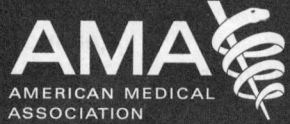

ICD-10-CM 2026
The Complete Official Codebook

AMA publications fund initiatives that drive improvements in patient health, practice innovation and medical education.

Publisher's Notice

The *ICD-10-CM: The Complete Official Codebook* is designed to be an accurate and authoritative source regarding coding and every reasonable effort has been made to ensure accuracy and completeness of the content. However, the American Medical Association (AMA) makes no guarantee, warranty, or representation that this publication is accurate, complete, or without errors. It is understood that the AMA is not rendering any legal or other professional services or advice in this publication and that the AMA bears no liability for any results or consequences that may arise from the use of this book.

Our Commitment to Accuracy

The AMA is committed to producing accurate and reliable materials. To report corrections, please call the AMA Unified Service Center at (800) 621-8335. To purchase additional copies, visit the AMA store at amastore.com. Refer to product number OP201426.

Acknowledgments

Marianne Randall, CPC, *Senior Product Manager*
Anita Schmidt, BS, RHIA, AHIMA-approved ICD-10-CM/PCS Trainer, *Subject Matter Expert*
Leanne Patterson, CPC, *Subject Matter Expert*
LaJuana Green, RHIA, CCS, *Subject Matter Expert*
Laura M. Anderson, RN, BSN, CCDS, *Subject Matter Expert*
Tara Rose, CPC, CPC-I, CPMA, RHIA, *Subject Matter Expert*
Stacy Perry, *Manager, Desktop Publishing*
Tracy Betzler, *Senior Desktop Publishing Specialist*
Hope M. Dunn, *Senior Desktop Publishing Specialist*
Katie Russell, *Senior Desktop Publishing Specialist*
Lynn Speirs, *Editor*

Copyright

Property of Optum360, LLC. Optum360, LLC and the Optum logo are trademarks of Optum, Inc. All other brand or product names are trademarks or registered trademarks of their respective owner.

© 2025 Optum360, LLC. All rights reserved.

Made in the USA
OP201426
BQ49:09/25

Leanne Patterson, CPC

Ms. Patterson has more than 20 years of experience in the healthcare profession. She has an extensive background in professional component coding, with proven expertise in assignment of E/M codes, general surgery coding, medical record documentation improvement, and HIPAA compliance. Her experience includes serving as Director of Compliance, conducting chart-to-claim audits, and physician education. She has been responsible for coding and denial management in large multi-specialty physician practices, and most recently has been part of a team developing content for products related to ICD-10-CM. Ms. Patterson is credentialed by and is a member of the AAPC.

Anita Schmidt, BS, RHIA, AHIMA-approved ICD-10-CM/PCS Trainer

Ms. Schmidt has expertise in ICD-10-CM/PCS, DRG, and CPT with more than 20 years' experience in coding in multiple settings, including inpatient, observation, and same-day surgery. Her experience includes analysis of medical record documentation, assignment of ICD-10-CM and PCS codes, and DRG validation. She has collaborated with clinical documentation specialists to identify documentation needs and potential areas for physician education. Most recently she has been developing content for resource and educational products related to ICD-10-CM, ICD-10-PCS, DRG, and CPT. Ms. Schmidt is an AHIMA-approved ICD-10-CM/PCS trainer and is an active member of the American Health Information Management Association (AHIMA) and the Minnesota Health Information Management Association (MHIMA).

Contents

How to Use ICD-10-CM: The Complete Official Codebook 2026 iii
Introduction iii
What's New for 2026 iii
Conversion Table iii
10 Steps to Correct Coding iii
Official ICD-10-CM Guidelines for Coding and Reporting iii
Indexes iii
    Index to Diseases and Injuries iii
    Neoplasm Table iii
    Table of Drugs and Chemicals iii
    External Causes Index iii
    Index Notations iv
Tabular List of Diseases v
    Code and Code Descriptions v
    Tabular Notations v
    Official Notations v
    Publisher Notations vi
    Icons vi
    Color Bars viii
Chapter-Level Notations viii
Appendixes viii
Illustrations viii

What's New for 2026 ix
Official Updates ix
Proprietary Updates x

Conversion Table of ICD-10-CM Codes xi

10 Steps to Correct Coding xiv

ICD-10-CM Official Guidelines for Coding and Reporting .... Coding Guidelines–1

ICD-10-CM Index to Diseases and Injuries 1

ICD-10-CM Neoplasm Table 342

ICD-10-CM Table of Drugs and Chemicals 361

ICD-10-CM Index to External Causes 411

ICD-10-CM Tabular List of Diseases and Injuries 449
Chapter 1.   Certain Infectious and Parasitic Diseases (A00–B99), U07.1, U09.9 449
Chapter 2.   Neoplasms (C00–D49) 475
Chapter 3.   Diseases of the Blood and Blood-forming Organs and Certain Disorders Involving the Immune Mechanism (D50–D89) 517
Chapter 4.   Endocrine, Nutritional, and Metabolic Diseases (E00–E89) 531
Chapter 5.   Mental, Behavioral, and Neurodevelopmental Disorders (F01–F99) 557
Chapter 6.   Diseases of the Nervous System (G00–G99) 589
Chapter 7.   Diseases of the Eye and Adnexa (H00–H59) 613
Chapter 8.   Diseases of the Ear and Mastoid Process (H60–H95) 649
Chapter 9.   Diseases of the Circulatory System (I00–I99) ... 661
Chapter 10. Diseases of the Respiratory System (J00–J99), U07.0 ... 707
Chapter 11. Diseases of the Digestive System (K00–K95) 725
Chapter 12. Diseases of the Skin and Subcutaneous Tissue (L00–L99) 751
Chapter 13. Diseases of the Musculoskeletal System and Connective Tissue (M00–M99) 775
Chapter 14. Diseases of Genitourinary System (N00–N99) ... 865
Chapter 15. Pregnancy, Childbirth, and the Puerperium (O00–O9A) 887
Chapter 16. Certain Conditions Originating in the Perinatal Period (P00–P96) 927
Chapter 17. Congenital Malformations, Deformations, and Chromosomal Abnormalities (Q00–QA0) 941
Chapter 18. Symptoms, Signs, and Abnormal Clinical and Laboratory Findings, Not Elsewhere Classified (R00–R99) 963
Chapter 19. Injury, Poisoning, and Certain Other Consequences of External Causes (S00–T88) 985
Chapter 20. External Causes of Morbidity (V00–Y99) 1189
Chapter 21. Factors Influencing Health Status and Contact with Health Services (Z00–Z99) 1255
Chapter 22. Codes for Special Purposes (U00–U85) 1295

Appendixes Appendixes–1
Appendix A: Valid 3-character ICD-10-CM Codes Appendixes–1
Appendix B: Pharmacology List 2026 .... Appendixes–3
Appendix C: Z Codes for Long-Term Drug Use with Associated Drugs Appendixes–21
Appendix D: Z Codes Only as Principal/First-Listed Diagnosis Appendixes–23
Appendix E: Centers for Medicare & Medicaid Services Hierarchical Condition Categories (CMS-HCC) Appendixes–25
Appendix F: Centers for Medicare & Medicaid Services Quality Payment Program Appendixes–29

Illustrations Illustrations–1
Chapter 3.   Diseases of the Blood and Blood-forming Organs and Certain Disorders Involving the Immune Mechanism (D50–D89) Illustrations–1
    Red Blood Cells Illustrations–1
    White Blood Cell Illustrations–1
    Platelet Illustrations–1
    Coagulation Illustrations–1
    Spleen Anatomical Location and External Structures Illustrations–2
    Spleen Interior Structures Illustrations–2
Chapter 4.   Endocrine, Nutritional, and Metabolic Diseases (E00–E89) Illustrations–3
    Endocrine System Illustrations–3
    Thyroid Illustrations–4
    Thyroid and Parathyroid Glands Illustrations–4
    Pancreas Illustrations–5
    Anatomy of the Adrenal Gland Illustrations–5
    Structure of an Ovary Illustrations–6
    Testis and Associated Structures Illustrations–6
    Thymus Illustrations–6
Chapter 6.   Diseases of the Nervous System (G00–G99) Illustrations–7
    Brain Illustrations–7
    Cranial Nerves Illustrations–7
    Peripheral Nervous System Illustrations–8
    Spinal Cord and Spinal Nerves Illustrations–9
    Nerve Cell Illustrations–9
    Trigeminal and Facial Nerve Branches Illustrations–9

Contents

Chapter 7. Diseases of the Eye and Adnexa (H00–H59) Illustrations-10
- Eye Illustrations-10
- Posterior Pole of Globe/Flow of Aqueous Humor Illustrations-10
- Lacrimal System Illustrations-10
- Eye Musculature Illustrations-10
- Eyelid Structures Illustrations-10

Chapter 8. Diseases of the Ear and Mastoid Process (H60–H95) Illustrations-11
- Ear Anatomy Illustrations-11

Chapter 9. Diseases of the Circulatory System (I00–I99) Illustrations-12
- Anatomy of the Heart Illustrations-12
- Heart Cross Section Illustrations-12
- Heart Valves Illustrations-12
- Heart Conduction System Illustrations-13
- Coronary Arteries Illustrations-13
- Arteries Illustrations-14
- Veins Illustrations-15
- Internal Carotid and Vertebral Arteries and Branches Illustrations-16
- External Carotid Artery and Branches Illustrations-16
- Branches of Abdominal Aorta Illustrations-16
- Portal Venous Circulation Illustrations-16
- Lymphatic System Illustrations-17
- Axillary Lymph Nodes Illustrations-18
- Lymphatic System of Head and Neck Illustrations-18
- Lymphatic Capillaries Illustrations-18
- Lymphatic Drainage Illustrations-18

Chapter 10. Diseases of the Respiratory System (J00–J99), U07.0 .... Illustrations-19
- Respiratory System Illustrations-19
- Upper Respiratory System Illustrations-19
- Nasal Cavity Illustrations-19
- Lower Respiratory System Illustrations-20
- Paranasal Sinuses Illustrations-20
- Alveoli Illustrations-20
- Lung Segments Illustrations-21

Chapter 11. Diseases of the Digestive System (K00–K95) Illustrations-22
- Digestive System Illustrations-22
- Omentum and Mesentery Illustrations-22
- Peritoneum and Retroperitoneum Illustrations-22

Chapter 12. Diseases of the Skin and Subcutaneous Tissue (L00–L99) Illustrations-23
- Nail Anatomy Illustrations-23
- Skin and Subcutaneous Tissue Illustrations-23

Chapter 13. Diseases of the Musculoskeletal System and Connective Tissue (M00–M99) Illustrations-24
- Bones and Joints Illustrations-24
- Shoulder Anterior View Illustrations-25
- Shoulder Posterior View Illustrations-25
- Elbow Anterior View Illustrations-25
- Elbow Posterior View Illustrations-25
- Hand Illustrations-25
- Hip Anterior View Illustrations-26
- Hip Posterior View Illustrations-26
- Knee Anterior View Illustrations-26
- Knee Posterior View Illustrations-26
- Foot Illustrations-26
- Muscles Illustrations-27

Chapter 14. Diseases of Genitourinary System (N00–N99) Illustrations-28
- Urinary System Illustrations-28
- Male Genitourinary System Illustrations-28
- Male Bladder Illustrations-28
- Female Genitourinary System Illustrations-29
- Female Bladder Illustrations-29
- Female Internal Genitalia Illustrations-29

Chapter 15. Pregnancy, Childbirth, and the Puerperium (O00–O9A) Illustrations-30
- Term Pregnancy – Single Gestation Illustrations-30
- Twin Gestation–Dichorionic–Diamniotic (DI-DI) Illustrations-30
- Twin Gestation–Monochorionic–Diamniotic (MO-DI) Illustrations-31
- Twin Gestation–Monochorionic–Monoamniotic (MO-MO) Illustrations-31

Chapter 19. Injury, Poisoning, and Certain Other Consequences of External Causes (S00–T88) Illustrations-32
- Types of Fractures Illustrations-32
- Salter-Harris Fracture Types Illustrations-32

How to Use ICD-10-CM: The Complete Official Codebook 2026

Introduction
ICD-10-CM: The Complete Official Codebook 2026 is your definitive coding resource, combining the work of the National Center for Health Statistics (NCHS), Centers for Medicare and Medicaid Services (CMS), American Hospital Association (AHA), and Publisher experts to provide the information you need for coding accuracy.

The International Classification of Diseases, 10th Revision, Clinical Modification (ICD-10-CM), is an adaptation of ICD-10, copyrighted by the World Health Organization (WHO). The development and maintenance of this clinical modification (CM) is the responsibility of the NCHS as authorized by WHO. Any new concepts added to ICD-10-CM are based on an established update process through the collaboration of WHO's Update and Revision Committee and the ICD-10-CM Coordination and Maintenance Committee.

In addition to the ICD-10-CM classification, other official government source information has been included in this manual. Depending on the source, updates to information may be annual or quarterly. This manual provides the most current information that was available at the time of publication. For updates to the source documents that may have occurred after this manual was published, please refer to the following:

- **NCHS, International Classification of Diseases, Tenth Revision, Clinical Modification (ICD-10-CM)**
  https://www.cms.gov/medicare/coding-billing/icd-10-codes
- **CMS Integrated Outpatient Code Editor (IOCE), version 26.2**
  https://www.cms.gov/Medicare/Coding/OutpatientCodeEdit/OCEQtrReleaseSpecs.html
- **CMS-HCC Risk Adjustment Model, version 28**
- **CMS ESRD-HCC Risk Adjustment Model, version 24**
- **CMS RxHCC Risk Adjustment Model, version 08**
  https://www.cms.gov/Medicare/Health-Plans/MedicareAdvtgSpecRateStats/Risk-Adjustors.html
- **HHS-HCC Commercial Risk Adjustment Model, version 07**
  https://www.cms.gov/CCIIO/Resources/Regulations-and-Guidance
- **CMS Quality Payment Program (QPP)**
  https://qpp.cms.gov/mips/explore-measures
- **AHA Coding Clinics**
  https://www.codingclinicadvisor.com/

The official NCHS ICD-10-CM classification includes three main sections: the guidelines, the indexes, and the tabular list, all of which make up the bulk of this coding manual. To complement the classification, Optum's coding experts have incorporated Medicare-related coding edits and proprietary features, such as supplementary notations, coding tools, and appendixes, into a comprehensive and easy-to-use reference. This publication is organized as follows:

What's New for 2026
This section provides a high-level overview of the code changes made for fiscal 2026. The list of codes provided identifies new, revised, and deleted codes. Asterisked codes identify prior midyear changes that were made to the classification, effective April 1, 2025. All changes are based on official addenda, provided by the NCHS.

Conversion Table
The conversion table was developed by NCHS to help facilitate data retrieval as new codes are added to the ICD-10-CM classification. This table provides a crosswalk from each fiscal 2026 new code to the equivalent code(s) assigned, prior to October 1, 2025, for that diagnosis or condition. Asterisked codes identify prior midyear additions, effective April 1, 2025. For the full conversion table, refer to the Conversion Table zip file at https://www.cms.gov/medicare/coding-billing/icd-10-codes.

10 Steps to Correct Coding
This step-by-step tutorial walks the coder through the process of finding the correct code — from locating the code in the official indexes to verifying the code in the tabular section — while following applicable conventions, guidelines, and instructional notes. Specific examples are provided with detailed explanations of each coding step along with advice for proper sequencing.

Official ICD-10-CM Guidelines for Coding and Reporting
This section provides the full official conventions and guidelines regulating the appropriate assignment and reporting of ICD-10-CM codes. These conventions and guidelines are published by the U.S. Department of Health and Human Services (DHHS) and approved by the cooperating parties (American Health Information Management Association [AHIMA], NCHS, Centers for Disease Control and Prevention [CDC], and the American Hospital Association [AHA]).

Indexes

Index to Diseases and Injuries
The Index to Diseases and Injuries is arranged in alphabetic order by terms specific to a disease, condition, illness, injury, eponym, or abbreviation as well as terms that describe circumstances other than a disease or injury that may require attention from a health care professional.

Neoplasm Table
The Neoplasm Table is arranged in alphabetic order by anatomical site. Codes are then listed in individual columns based upon the histological behavior (malignant, in situ, benign, uncertain, or unspecified) of the neoplasm.

Table of Drugs and Chemicals
The Table of Drugs and Chemicals is arranged in alphabetic order by the specific drug or chemical name. Codes are listed in individual columns based upon the associated intent (poisoning, adverse effect, or underdosing). Drugs with an asterisk identify substances added to the table by Optum subject matter experts.

External Causes Index
The External Causes Index is arranged in alphabetic order by main terms that describe the cause, the intent, the place of occurrence, the activity, and the status of the patient at the time the injury occurred or health condition arose.

Index Notations

With
The word "with" or "in" should be interpreted to mean "associated with" or "due to." The classification presumes a causal relationship between the two conditions linked by these terms in the index. These conditions should be coded as related even in the absence of provider documentation explicitly linking them unless the documentation clearly states the conditions are unrelated or when another guideline specifically requires a documented linkage between two conditions (e.g., the sepsis guideline for "acute organ dysfunction that is not clearly associated with the sepsis"). For conditions not specifically linked by these relational terms in the classification or when a guideline requires explicit documentation of a linkage between two conditions, provider documentation must link the conditions to code them as related.

The word "with" in the index is sequenced immediately following the main term, not in alphabetical order.

> **Dermatopolymyositis** M33.90
>   with
>   myopathy M33.92
>   respiratory involvement M33.91
>   specified organ involvement NEC M33.99
>   amyopathic M33.93

See
When the instruction "see" follows a term in the index, it indicates that another term must be referenced to locate the correct code.

> **Hematoperitoneum** — *see* Hemoperitoneum

See Also
The instructional note "see also" simply provides alternative terms the coder may reference that may be useful in determining the correct code but are not necessary to follow if the main term supplies the appropriate code.

> **Hematinuria** — *see also* Hemaglobinuria
>   malarial B50.8

Default Codes
In the index, the default code is the code listed next to the main term and represents the condition most commonly associated with that main term. This code may be assigned when documentation does not support reporting a more specific code. Alternatively, it may provide an unspecified code for the condition.

> **Hemiatrophy** R68.89
>   cerebellar G31.9
>   face, facial, progressive (Romberg) G51.8
>   tongue K14.8

Parentheses
Parentheses in the indexes enclose nonessential modifiers, supplementary words that may be present or absent in the statement of a disease without affecting the code.

> **Pseudomeningocele** (cerebral) (infective) (post-traumatic) G96.198
>   postprocedural (spinal) G97.82

Brackets
ICD-10-CM has a coding convention addressing code assignment for manifestations that occur as a result of an underlying condition. This convention requires the underlying condition to be sequenced first, followed by the code or codes for the associated manifestation. In the index, italicized codes in brackets identify manifestation codes.

> **Polyneuropathy** (peripheral) G62.9
>   alcoholic G62.1
>   amyloid (Portuguese) E85.1 *[G63]*
>   transthyretin-related (ATTR) familial E85.1 *[G63]*

Shaded Guides
Exclusive vertical shaded guides in the Index to Diseases and Injuries and External Causes Index help the user easily follow the indent levels for the subentries under a main term. Sequencing rules may apply depending on the level of indent for separate subentries.

> **Hemicrania**
>   congenital malformation Q00.0
>   continua G44.51
>   meaning migraine — *see also* Migraine G43.909
>   paroxysmal G44.039
>   chronic G44.049
>   intractable G44.041
>   not intractable G44.049
>   episodic G44.039
>   intractable G44.031
>   not intractable G44.039
>   intractable G44.031
>   not intractable G44.039

Following References
The Index to Diseases and Injuries includes "following" references to assist in locating out-of-sequence codes in the tabular list. Out-of-sequence codes contain an alphabetic character (letter) in the third- or fourth-character position. These codes are placed according to the classification rules — according to condition — not according to alphabetic or numeric sequencing rules.

> **Carcinoma** (malignant) — *see also* Neoplasm, by site, malignant
>   neuroendocrine — *see also* Tumor, neuroendocrine
>   high grade, any site C7A.1 (*following* C75)
>   poorly differentiated, any site C7A.1 (*following* C75)

Additional Character Required
The Index to Diseases and Injuries, Neoplasm Table, and External Causes Index provide an icon after certain codes to signify to the user that additional characters are required to make the code valid. The tabular list should be consulted for appropriate character selection.

> **Fall, falling** (accidental) W19 ☑
>   building W20.1 ☑

Tabular List of Diseases

ICD-10-CM codes and descriptions are arranged numerically within the tabular list of diseases with 19 separate chapters providing codes associated with a particular body system or nature of injury or disease. There is also a chapter providing codes for external causes of an injury or health conditions, a chapter for codes that address encounters with healthcare facilities for circumstances other than a disease or injury, and finally, a chapter for codes that capture special circumstances such as new diseases of uncertain etiology or emergency use codes..

Code and Code Descriptions

ICD-10-CM is an alphanumeric classification system that contains categories, subcategories, and valid codes. The first character is always a letter with any additional characters represented by either a letter or number. A three-character category without further subclassification is equivalent to a valid three-character code. Valid codes may be three, four, five, six, or seven characters in length, with each level of subdivision after a three-character category representing a subcategory. The final level of subdivision is a valid code.

Boldface

Boldface type is used for all codes and descriptions in the tabular list.

Italics

Italicized type is used to identify manifestation codes, those codes that should not be reported as first-listed diagnoses.

Deleted Text

~~Strikethrough~~ on a code and code description indicates a deletion from the classification for the current year.

Key Word

Green font is used throughout the Tabular List of Diseases to differentiate the key words that appear in similar code descriptions in a given category or subcategory. The key word convention is used only in those categories in which there are multiple codes with very similar descriptions with only a few words that differentiate them.

For example, refer to the list of codes below from category H55:

✓4th H55	**Nystagmus and other irregular eye movements**	
	✓5th H55.0 **Nystagmus**	
	H55.00	**Unspecified nystagmus**
	H55.01	**Congenital nystagmus**
	H55.02	**Latent nystagmus**
	H55.03	**Visual deprivation nystagmus**
	H55.04	**Dissociated nystagmus**
	H55.09	**Other forms of nystagmus**

The portion of the code description that appears in green font in the tabular list helps the coder quickly identify the key terms and the correct code. This convention is especially useful when the codes describe laterality, such as the following codes from subcategory H40.22:

✓6th H40.22	**Chronic angle-closure glaucoma**		
	Chronic primary angle closure glaucoma		
	✓7th H40.221	**Chronic angle-closure glaucoma, right eye**	Rx
	✓7th H40.222	**Chronic angle-closure glaucoma, left eye**	Rx
	✓7th H40.223	**Chronic angle-closure glaucoma, bilateral**	Rx
	✓7th H40.229	**Chronic angle-closure glaucoma, unspecified eye**	Rx

Tabular Notations

Official parenthetical notes as well as Optum's supplementary notations are provided at the chapter, code block, category, subcategory, and individual code level to help the user assign proper codes. The information in the notation can apply to one or more codes depending on where the citation is placed.

Official Notations

Includes Notes

The word **INCLUDES** appears immediately under certain categories to further define, clarify, or give examples of the content of a code category.

Inclusion Terms

Lists of inclusion terms are included under certain codes. These terms indicate some of the conditions for which that code number may be used. Inclusion terms may be synonyms with the code title, or, in the case of "other specified" codes, the terms may also provide a list of various conditions included within a classification code. The inclusion terms are not exhaustive. The index may provide additional terms that may also be assigned to a given code.

Excludes Notes

ICD-10-CM has two types of excludes notes. Each note has a different definition for use. However, they are similar in that they both indicate that codes excluded from each other are independent of each other.

Excludes 1

An **EXCLUDES 1** note is a "pure" excludes. It means "NOT CODED HERE!" An Excludes 1 note indicates mutually exclusive codes: two conditions that cannot be reported together. An Excludes1 note indicates that the code excluded should never be used at the same time as the code above the Excludes1 note. An Excludes1 is used when two conditions cannot occur together, such as a congenital form versus an acquired form of the same condition.

An exception to the Excludes 1 definition is when the two conditions are unrelated to each other. If it is not clear whether the two conditions involving an Excludes 1 note are related or not, query the provider. For example, code F45.8 Other somatoform disorders, has an Excludes 1 note for "sleep related teeth grinding (G47.63)" because "teeth grinding" is an inclusion term under F45.8. Only one of these two codes should be assigned for teeth grinding. However psychogenic dysmenorrhea is also an inclusion term under F45.8, and a patient could have both this condition and sleep-related teeth grinding. In this case, the two conditions are clearly unrelated to each other, so it would be appropriate to report F45.8 and G47.63 together.

Excludes 2

An **EXCLUDES 2** note means "NOT INCLUDED HERE." An Excludes 2 note indicates that although the excluded condition is not part of the condition it is excluded from, a patient may have both conditions at the same time. Therefore, when an Excludes 2 note appears under a code, it may be acceptable to use both the code and the excluded code together if supported by the medical documentation.

Note

The term "NOTE" appears as an icon and precedes the instructional information. These notes function as alerts to highlight coding instructions within the text.

Code First/Use additional code

These instructional notes provide sequencing instruction. They may appear independently of each other or to designate certain etiology/manifestation paired codes. These instructions signal the coder that an additional code should be reported to provide a more complete picture of that diagnosis.

In etiology/manifestation coding, ICD-10-CM requires the underlying condition to be sequenced first, followed by the manifestation. In these situations, codes with "In diseases classified elsewhere" in the code description are never permitted as a first-listed or principal diagnosis code and must be sequenced following the underlying condition code.

Code Also
A "code also" note alerts the coder that more than one code may be required to fully describe the condition. The sequencing depends on the circumstances of the encounter. Factors that may determine sequencing include severity and reason for the encounter.

Revised Text
The revised text ▶◀ "bow ties" alert the user to changes in official notations for the current year. Revised text may include the following:

- A change in a current parenthetical description
- A change in the code(s) associated with a current parenthetical note
- A change in how a current parenthetical note is classified (e.g., an Excludes 1 note that changed to an Excludes 2 note)
- Addition of a new parenthetical note(s) to a code

Deleted Text
~~Strikethrough~~ on official notations indicate a deletion from the classification for the current year.

Publisher Notations

AHA *Coding Clinic* Citations
Coding Clinics are official American Hospital Association (AHA) publications that provide coding advice specific to ICD-10-CM and ICD-10-PCS.

Coding Clinic citations included in this manual are current up to the second quarter of 2025.

These citations identify the year, quarter, and page number of one or more Coding Clinic publications that may have coding advice relevant to a particular code or group of codes. With the most current citation listed first, these notations are preceded by the symbol **AHA:** and appear in purple type.

> **I15.1** Hypertension secondary to other renal disorders   **Rx**
> **AHA:** 2016, 3Q, 22

Definitions
Definitions explain a specific term, condition, or disease process in layman's terms. These notations are preceded by the symbol **DEF:** and appear in purple type.

> ✓5th **M51.4** Schmorl's nodes
> **DEF:** Irregular bone defect in the margin of the vertebral body that causes herniation into the end plate of the vertebral body.

Coding Tips
The tips in the tabular list offer coding advice that is not readily available within the ICD-10-CM classification. It may relate official coding guidelines, indexing nuances, or advice from *AHA's Coding Clinic for ICD-10-CM/PCS*. These notations are preceded by the symbol **TIP:** and appear in brown type.

> ✓5th **M11.2** Other chondrocalcinosis
> Chondrocalcinosis NOS
> **AHA:** 2018,3Q,20
> **TIP:** Pseudogout is captured with codes in this subcategory.

Icons
Note: The following icons are placed to the left of the code.

Changes to ICD-10-CM codes since the last published edition of this manual are highlighted in two ways:

The following green icons identify new or revised codes effective April 1, 2025:

- ● **New Code — Midyear**
- ▲ **Revised Code — Midyear**

The following black icons identify new or revised codes effective October 1, 2025:

- ● **New Code**
- ▲ **Revised Code**
- ✓ **Additional Characters Required**
  - ✓4th This symbol indicates that the code requires a 4th character.
  - ✓5th This symbol indicates that the code requires a 5th character.
  - ✓6th This symbol indicates that the code requires a 6th character.
  - ✓7th This symbol indicates that the code requires a 7th character.

> ✓5th **H60.3** Other infective otitis externa
> ✓6th **H60.31** Diffuse otitis externa
>   **H60.311** Diffuse otitis externa, right ear
>   **H60.312** Diffuse otitis externa, left ear
>   **H60.313** Diffuse otitis externa, bilateral
>   **H60.319** Diffuse otitis externa, unspecified ear

✓x7th **Placeholder Alert**
This symbol indicates that the code requires a 7th character following the placeholder "X". Codes with fewer than six characters that require a 7th character must contain placeholder "X" to fill in the empty character(s).

> ✓x7th **T16.1** Foreign body in right ear

This manual provides the most current information that was available at the time of publication. Except where otherwise noted, the icons and/or color bars reflect edits provided in the Integrated Outpatient Code Editor (IOCE) quarterly files utilized under the outpatient prospective payment system (OPPS). Because the October 2025 quarterly files were not available at the time this book was printed, the edits in this manual are based on the July 2025 quarterly files.

The following is a list of IOCE edits specifically identified in this manual:

- Age
- Manifestation
- Unacceptable principal diagnosis

Note: The following icons are placed at the end of the code description.

Age Edits

🅽 Newborn Age: 0
These diagnoses are intended for newborns and neonates and the patient's age must be 0 years.

| N47.0 | Adherent prepuce, newborn | 🅽 |

🅿 Pediatric Age: 0-17
These diagnoses are intended for children and the patient's age must be between 0 and 17 years.

| L21.1 | Seborrheic infantile dermatitis | 🅿 |

Ⓜ Maternity Age: 9-64
These diagnoses are intended for childbearing patients between the age of 9 and 64 years.

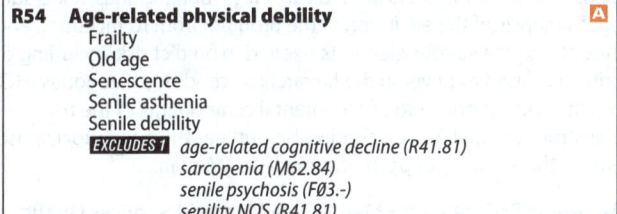

🅰 Adult Age: 15-124
These diagnoses are intended for patients between the age of 15 and 124 years.

R54	Age-related physical debility	🅰
	Frailty
	Old age
	Senescence
	Senile asthenia
	Senile debility
	EXCLUDES 1 age-related cognitive decline (R41.81)
	sarcopenia (M62.84)
	senile psychosis (F03.-)
	senility NOS (R41.81)

Sex Edits

Effective April 1, 2024, the Integrated Outpatient Code Editor (IOCE), a program used to process claims for outpatient providers, has deactivated the sex conflict edit. There will no longer be a female or male edit restriction for ICD-10-CM codes.

UPD Unacceptable Principal Diagnosis
This icon identifies codes that are not appropriate as a first-listed code for *outpatient* encounters. These codes describe circumstances that influence an individual's health status but are not a current illness or injury, or that are not specifically manifestations but may be due to an underlying cause.

| √7ᵗʰ T48.5X5 | Adverse effect of other anti-common-cold drugs | UPD |

HCC CMS-HCC Condition
This icon identifies codes that are considered a CMS-HCC (hierarchical condition category) diagnosis.

The HCC codes represented in this manual have been updated to reflect the 2026 Initial ICD-10-CM Mappings for CMS-HCC Model v28. Midyear final mappings were not available at the time this publication went to print; refer to the following CMS website for final mappings: https://www.cms.gov/Medicare/Health-Plans/MedicareAdvtgSpecRateStats/Risk-Adjustors.html.

| P12.2 | Epicranial subaponeurotic hemorrhage due to birth injury | HCC |
| | Subgaleal hemorrhage |

Rx Rx-HCC Condition
This icon identifies codes that are included in the Rx-HCC risk-adjustment model, which covers the Part D (prescription drug) benefit.

The Rx-HCC codes represented in this manual have been updated to reflect the 2026 Initial ICD-10-CM Mappings for CMS Rx-HCC Model v08. Midyear final mappings were not available at the time this publication went to print; refer to the following CMS website for final mappings: https://www.cms.gov/Medicare/Health-Plans/MedicareAdvtgSpecRateStats/Risk-Adjustors.html.

| Z21 | Asymptomatic human immunodeficiency virus [HIV] infection status | HCC Rx ESR COM |

ESR ESRD HCC Condition
This icon identifies codes that are included in the end-stage renal disease (ESRD) HCC risk-adjustment model.

The ESRD HCC codes represented in this manual have been updated to reflect the 2026 Initial ICD-10-CM Mappings for CMS ESRD HCC Model v24. Midyear final mappings were not available at the time this publication went to print; refer to the following CMS website for final mappings: https://www.cms.gov/Medicare/Health-Plans/MedicareAdvtgSpecRateStats/Risk-Adjustors.html.

| Z21 | Asymptomatic human immunodeficiency virus [HIV] infection status | HCC Rx ESR COM |

COM Commercial HCC Condition
This icon identifies codes that are included in the commercial HHS-HCC risk-adjustment model.

The commercial HCC codes represented in this manual are based on the commercial HCC Model v07. These mappings can be found at the following: https://www.cms.gov/CCIIO/Resources/Regulations-and-Guidance.

| Z21 | Asymptomatic human immunodeficiency virus [HIV] infection status | HCC Rx ESR COM |

Q QPP Condition
This icon identifies codes recognized as a quality measure for claims-based reporting under CMS's Merit-based Incentive Payment System (MIPS) Claims Single Source v6.0.

| K22.70 | Barrett's esophagus without dysplasia | Q |
| | Barrett's esophagus NOS |

PDx Z-code as First-Listed Diagnosis
Section IV of the official guidelines states that the term "first-listed diagnosis" is used instead of principal diagnosis in the outpatient setting and represents the diagnosis that is chiefly responsible for the services provided during the encounter. This icon identifies Z codes that, in general, may be reported only as a first-listed diagnosis. According to guideline I.C.21.c.16, these are the only Z codes that are specifically meant to be utilized as a first-listed diagnosis; all other Z codes may be either first-listed or secondary diagnoses, depending upon the circumstances of the encounter, coding instructions, and guidelines.

Note: The codes identified with this icon may be used as a secondary diagnosis if the patient has multiple encounters on the same day and those medical records are combined.

A comprehensive list of all Z codes primarily used as first-listed diagnoses appears in appendix D, at the back of this book.

| Z52.21 | Bone donor, autologous | PDx |

Color Bars

Manifestation Code
Codes defined as manifestation codes appear in italic type, with a blue color bar over the code description. A manifestation cannot be reported as a first-listed code; it is sequenced as a secondary diagnosis with the underlying disease code listed first.

G32.89	*Other specified degenerative disorders of nervous system in diseases classified elsewhere*
	Degenerative encephalopathy in diseases classified elsewhere

Unspecified Diagnosis
Codes that appear with a gray color bar over the alphanumeric code identify unspecified diagnoses. These codes should be used in limited circumstances, when neither the diagnostic statement nor the documentation provides enough information to assign a more specific diagnosis code. The abbreviation NOS, "not otherwise specified," in the tabular list may be interpreted as "unspecified."

G03.9	Meningitis, unspecified	COM
	Arachnoiditis (spinal) NOS	

Chapter-Level Notations

Chapter-specific Guidelines with Coding Examples
Each chapter begins with the Official Guidelines for Coding and Reporting specific to that chapter, where provided. Coding examples specific to outpatient care settings have been provided to illustrate the coding and/or sequencing guidance in these guidelines.

Muscle and Tendon Table
ICD-10-CM categorizes certain muscles and tendons in the upper and lower extremities by their action (e.g., extension or flexion) as well as their anatomical location. The Muscle/Tendon table is provided at the beginning of chapter 13 and chapter 19 to help users when code selection depends on the action of the muscle and/or tendon.

Note: This table is not all-inclusive, and proper code assignment should be based on the provider's documentation.

Appendixes

The additional resources described below have been included as appendixes for this book. These resources further instruct the professional coder on the appropriate application of the ICD-10-CM code set.

Appendix A: Valid 3-character ICD-10-CM Codes
The user may consult this table to confirm that no further specificity, such as the use of 4th, 5th, 6th, or 7th characters or placeholders (X), is necessary. All ICD-10-CM codes that are valid at the three-character level are listed.

Appendix B: Pharmacology List 2026
This reference is a comprehensive but not all-inclusive list of pharmacological agents used to treat acute and/or chronic conditions. Drugs are listed in alphabetical order by their brand and/or generic names along with their drug action and indications for which they may commonly be prescribed. Some drugs have also been mapped to their appropriate Z code for long-term drug use.

Appendix C: Z Codes for Long-Term Drug Use with Associated Drugs
This resource correlates Z codes that are used to identify current long-term drug use with a list of drugs that are typically categorized to that class of drug.

Note: These tables are not all-inclusive but list some of the more commonly used drugs.

Appendix D: Z Codes Only as Principal/First-Listed Diagnosis
This resource provides a comprehensive list of Z codes that are primarily used as first-listed diagnoses for outpatient encounters.

Appendix E: Centers for Medicare & Medicaid Services Hierarchical Condition Categories (CMS-HCC)
This resource provides the framework behind the Centers for Medicare and Medicaid Services' (CMS) Medicare Advantage (MA) program, a risk-adjustment model developed as a means of compensating health care plans with large numbers of Medicare Part C beneficiaries. It includes a brief synopsis of the evolution of the program from its inception and insight into the various elements needed to predict risk, including the principles used to develop the hierarchical condition categories (HCCs), which make up one of the fundamental components of the risk-adjustment model. This appendix also outlines the audit process used to ensure the accuracy of payments made to MA plans.

Appendix F: Centers for Medicare & Medicaid Services Quality Payment Program
This resource provides an overview of the Medicare Access and CHIP Reauthorization Act (MACRA), which replaced Medicare's sustainable growth rate (SGR) methodology with the Quality Payment Program (QPP). It summarizes the Merit-based Incentive Payment System (MIPS) track used by those who opt to participate in traditional Medicare and not an advanced alternative payment model (APM). This includes eligibility requirements and an overview of the four performance categories that combine to make up the MIPS.

Illustrations
This section includes illustrations of normal anatomy with ICD-10-CM-specific terminology.

What's New for 2026

Official Updates
A summary of changes to the official ICD-10-CM code set is provided below, identifying changes made for fiscal 2026, effective October 1, 2025, to September 30, 2026. Asterisked codes identify prior midyear changes that were made to the classification, effective April 1, 2025. All code changes were made by the agency charged with maintaining and updating the ICD-10-CM code set, the National Center for Health Statistics (NCHS), a section of the Centers for Disease Control and Prevention (CDC).

487 New Codes

B88.01	B88.09	C50.A0	C50.A1	C50.A2
D71.1	D71.8	D71.9	E11.A	E72.530
E72.538	E72.539	E72.540	E72.541	E72.548
E72.549	E78.010	E78.011	E78.019	E83.820
E83.821	E83.822	E83.823	E83.824	E83.825
E88.10	E88.11	E88.12	E88.13	E88.14
E88.19	G31.87	G35.A	G35.B0	G35.B1
G35.B2	G35.C0	G35.C1	G35.C2	G35.D
G71.036	H01.81	H01.82	H01.83	H01.84
H01.85	H01.86	H01.89	H01.8A	H01.8B
H05.831	H05.832	H05.833	H05.839	H40.841
H40.842	H40.843	H40.849	I27.840	I27.841
I27.848	I27.849	L02.217	L02.227	L03.31A
L03.32A	L98.431	L98.432	L98.433	L98.434
L98.435	L98.436	L98.438	L98.439	L98.441
L98.442	L98.443	L98.444	L98.445	L98.446
L98.448	L98.449	L98.451	L98.452	L98.453
L98.454	L98.455	L98.456	L98.458	L98.459
L98.461	L98.462	L98.463	L98.464	L98.465
L98.466	L98.468	L98.469	L98.471	L98.472
L98.473	L98.474	L98.475	L98.476	L98.478
L98.479	L98.A111	L98.A112	L98.A113	L98.A114
L98.A115	L98.A116	L98.A118	L98.A119	L98.A121
L98.A122	L98.A123	L98.A124	L98.A125	L98.A126
L98.A128	L98.A129	L98.A191	L98.A192	L98.A193
L98.A194	L98.A195	L98.A196	L98.A198	L98.A199
L98.A211	L98.A212	L98.A213	L98.A214	L98.A215
L98.A216	L98.A218	L98.A219	L98.A221	L98.A222
L98.A223	L98.A224	L98.A225	L98.A226	L98.A228
L98.A229	L98.A291	L98.A292	L98.A293	L98.A294
L98.A295	L98.A296	L98.A298	L98.A299	L98.A311
L98.A312	L98.A313	L98.A314	L98.A315	L98.A316
L98.A318	L98.A319	L98.A321	L98.A322	L98.A323
L98.A324	L98.A325	L98.A326	L98.A328	L98.A329
L98.A391	L98.A392	L98.A393	L98.A394	L98.A395
L98.A396	L98.A398	L98.A399	M05.A	N00.B1
N00.B2	N04.B1	N04.B2	N07.B	Q87.87
Q87.88	Q89.81	Q89.89	Q99.811	Q99.812
Q99.813	Q99.818	Q99.819	Q99.89	QA0.0101
QA0.0102	QA0.0109	QA0.011	QA0.012	QA0.0131
QA0.0139	QA0.0141	QA0.0142	QA0.0149	QA0.0151
QA0.0159	QA0.8	R10.20	R10.21	R10.22
R10.23	R10.24	R10.85	R10.8A1	R10.8A2
R10.8A3	R10.8A9	R10.A0	R10.A1	R10.A2
R10.A3	R11.16	R39.851	R39.852	R39.853
R39.859	R76.81	R76.89	S30.11XA	S30.11XD
S30.11XS	S30.12XA	S30.12XD	S30.12XS	S30.13XA
S30.13XD	S30.13XS	S30.81AA	S30.81AD	S30.81AS
S30.82AA	S30.82AD	S30.82AS	S30.84AA	S30.84AD
S30.84AS	S30.85AA	S30.85AD	S30.85AS	S30.86AA
S30.86AD	S30.86AS	S30.87AA	S30.87AD	S30.87AS
S30.9AXA	S30.9AXD	S30.9AXS	S31.106A	S31.106D
S31.106S	S31.107A	S31.107D	S31.107S	S31.10AA
S31.10AD	S31.10AS	S31.116A	S31.116D	S31.116S
S31.117A	S31.117D	S31.117S	S31.11AA	S31.11AD
S31.11AS	S31.126A	S31.126D	S31.126S	S31.127A
S31.127D	S31.127S	S31.12AA	S31.12AD	S31.12AS
S31.136A	S31.136D	S31.136S	S31.137A	S31.137D
S31.137S	S31.13AA	S31.13AD	S31.13AS	S31.146A
S31.146D	S31.146S	S31.147A	S31.147D	S31.147S
S31.14AA	S31.14AD	S31.14AS	S31.156A	S31.156D
S31.156S	S31.157A	S31.157D	S31.157S	S31.15AA
S31.15AD	S31.15AS	S31.606A	S31.606D	S31.606S
S31.607A	S31.607D	S31.607S	S31.60AA	S31.60AD
S31.60AS	S31.616A	S31.616D	S31.616S	S31.617A
S31.617D	S31.617S	S31.61AA	S31.61AD	S31.61AS
S31.626A	S31.626D	S31.626S	S31.627A	S31.627D
S31.627S	S31.62AA	S31.62AD	S31.62AS	S31.636A
S31.636D	S31.636S	S31.637A	S31.637D	S31.637S
S31.63AA	S31.63AD	S31.63AS	S31.646A	S31.646D
S31.646S	S31.647A	S31.647D	S31.647S	S31.64AA
S31.64AD	S31.64AS	S31.656A	S31.656D	S31.656S
S31.657A	S31.657D	S31.657S	S31.65AA	S31.65AD
S31.65AS	T36.AX1A	T36.AX1D	T36.AX1S	T36.AX2A
T36.AX2D	T36.AX2S	T36.AX3A	T36.AX3D	T36.AX3S
T36.AX4A	T36.AX4D	T36.AX4S	T36.AX5A	T36.AX5D
T36.AX5S	T36.AX6A	T36.AX6D	T36.AX6S	T65.841A
T65.841D	T65.841S	T65.842A	T65.842D	T65.842S
T65.843A	T65.843D	T65.843S	T65.844A	T65.844D
T65.844S	T75.830A	T75.830D	T75.830S	T75.838A
T75.838D	T75.838S	T78.070A	T78.070D	T78.070S
T78.071A	T78.071D	T78.071S	T78.079A	T78.079D
T78.079S	T78.080A	T78.080D	T78.080S	T78.081A
T78.081D	T78.081S	T78.089A	T78.089D	T78.089S
T78.110A	T78.110D	T78.110S	T78.111A	T78.111D
T78.111S	T78.119A	T78.119D	T78.119S	T78.120A
T78.120D	T78.120S	T78.121A	T78.121D	T78.121S
T78.129A	T78.129D	T78.129S	T78.19XA	T78.19XD
T78.19XS	W44.H9XA	W44.H9XD	W44.H9XS	W45.3XXA
W45.3XXD	W45.3XXS	Y36.A1XA	Y36.A1XD	Y36.A1XS
Y36.A2XA	Y36.A2XD	Y36.A2XS	Y37.A1XA	Y37.A1XD
Y37.A1XS	Y37.A2XA	Y37.A2XD	Y37.A2XS	Y93.L1
Y93.L9	Z15.05	Z15.060	Z15.068	Z15.07
Z15.3	Z40.81	Z40.82	Z40.89	Z59.861
Z59.868	Z59.869	Z77.31	Z77.39	Z80.44
Z84.11	Z84.19	Z84.A	Z85.4A	Z86.00A
Z91.0110	Z91.0111	Z91.0112	Z91.0120	Z91.0121
Z91.0122	Z91.B			

38 Revised Codes
Note: Each code is listed with its revised description only.

L02.212	Cutaneous abscess of back [any part, except buttock and flank]
L02.222	Furuncle of back [any part, except buttock and flank]
M21.159	Varus deformity, not elsewhere classified, unspecified hip
M24.076	Loose body in unspecified toe joint(s)
M61.129	Myositis ossificans progressiva, unspecified upper arm
P09.6	Abnormal findings on neonatal hearing screening
Q75.001	Craniosynostosis, unspecified type, unilateral
Q75.002	Craniosynostosis, unspecified type, bilateral
Q75.009	Craniosynostosis, unspecified
Q75.021	Coronal craniosynostosis, unilateral
Q75.022	Coronal craniosynostosis, bilateral
Q75.029	Coronal craniosynostosis, unspecified
S62.90XA	Unspecified fracture of unspecified hand, initial encounter for closed fracture
S62.90XB	Unspecified fracture of unspecified hand, initial encounter for open fracture
S62.90XD	Unspecified fracture of unspecified hand, subsequent encounter for fracture with routine healing
S62.90XG	Unspecified fracture of unspecified hand, subsequent encounter for fracture with delayed healing

What's New for 2026

S62.90XK	Unspecified fracture of unspecified hand, subsequent encounter for fracture with nonunion
S62.90XP	Unspecified fracture of unspecified hand, subsequent encounter for fracture with malunion
S62.90XS	Unspecified fracture of unspecified hand, sequela
S62.91XA	Unspecified fracture of right hand, initial encounter for closed fracture
S62.91XB	Unspecified fracture of right hand, initial encounter for open fracture
S62.91XD	Unspecified fracture of right hand, subsequent encounter for fracture with routine healing
S62.91XG	Unspecified fracture of right hand, subsequent encounter for fracture with delayed healing
S62.91XK	Unspecified fracture of right hand, subsequent encounter for fracture with nonunion
S62.91XP	Unspecified fracture of right hand, subsequent encounter for fracture with malunion
S62.91XS	Unspecified fracture of right hand, sequela
S62.92XA	Unspecified fracture of left hand, initial encounter for closed fracture
S62.92XB	Unspecified fracture of left hand, initial encounter for open fracture
S62.92XD	Unspecified fracture of left hand, subsequent encounter for fracture with routine healing
S62.92XG	Unspecified fracture of left hand, subsequent encounter for fracture with delayed healing
S62.92XK	Unspecified fracture of left hand, subsequent encounter for fracture with nonunion
S62.92XP	Unspecified fracture of left hand, subsequent encounter for fracture with malunion
S62.92XS	Unspecified fracture of left hand, sequela
S74.21XA	Injury of cutaneous sensory nerve at hip and thigh level, right leg, initial encounter
S74.21XD	Injury of cutaneous sensory nerve at hip and thigh level, right leg, subsequent encounter
S74.21XS	Injury of cutaneous sensory nerve at hip and thigh level, right leg, sequela
Y07.435	Stepbrother, perpetrator of maltreatment and neglect
Z83.718	Family history of other colon polyps

12 Deleted Codes

S30.1XXA	Contusion of abdominal wall, initial encounter
S30.1XXD	Contusion of abdominal wall, subsequent encounter
S30.1XXS	Contusion of abdominal wall, sequela
T78.07XA	Anaphylactic reaction due to milk and dairy products, initial encounter
T78.07XD	Anaphylactic reaction due to milk and dairy products, subsequent encounter
T78.07XS	Anaphylactic reaction due to milk and dairy products, sequela
T78.08XA	Anaphylactic reaction due to eggs, initial encounter
T78.08XD	Anaphylactic reaction due to eggs, subsequent encounter
T78.08XS	Anaphylactic reaction due to eggs, sequela
T78.1XXA	Other adverse food reactions, not elsewhere classified, initial encounter
T78.1XXD	Other adverse food reactions, not elsewhere classified, subsequent encounter
T78.1XXS	Other adverse food reactions, not elsewhere classified, sequela

Proprietary Updates

The following proprietary features have also been added:

- New definitions that describe, in lay terms, a specific condition or disease process
- New coding tips that provide coding advice beyond the code classification
- Updated *AHA Coding Clinic* references through second quarter 2025

Conversion Table of ICD-10-CM Codes

The FY 2026 (October 1, 2025-September 30, 2026) Conversion Table for new ICD-10-CM codes is provided to assist users in data retrieval. For each new code the table shows its previously assigned code equivalent. Asterisks identify new codes added to the classification April 1, 2025.

Code Assignment Beginning 10/1/2025	Previous Code(s) Assignment	Code Assignment Beginning 10/1/2025	Previous Code(s) Assignment	Code Assignment Beginning 10/1/2025	Previous Code(s) Assignment	Code Assignment Beginning 10/1/2025	Previous Code(s) Assignment	Code Assignment Beginning 10/1/2025	Previous Code(s) Assignment
B88.01	B88.0	G35.C1	G35	L98.443	L98.493	L98.A122	L98.492	L98.A311	L98.491
B88.09	B88.0	G35.C2	G35	L98.444	L98.494	L98.A123	L98.493	L98.A312	L98.492
C50.A0	C50.919, C50.929	G35.D	G35	L98.445	L98.495	L98.A124	L98.494	L98.A313	L98.493
		G71.036	G71.038	L98.446	L98.496	L98.A125	L98.495	L98.A314	L98.494
C50.A1	C50.911, C50.921	H01.81	H01.8	L98.448	L98.498	L98.A126	L98.496	L98.A315	L98.495
		H01.82	H01.8	L98.449	L98.499	L98.A128	L98.498	L98.A316	L98.496
C50.A2	C50.912, C50.922	H01.83	H01.8	L98.451	L98.491	L98.A129	L98.499	L98.A318	L98.498
D71.1	D71	H01.84	H01.8	L98.452	L98.492	L98.A191	L98.491	L98.A319	L98.499
D71.8	D71	H01.85	H01.8	L98.453	L98.493	L98.A192	L98.492	L98.A321	L98.491
D71.9	D71	H01.86	H01.8	L98.454	L98.494	L98.A193	L98.493	L98.A322	L98.492
E11.A	E11.9	H01.89	H01.8	L98.455	L98.495	L98.A194	L98.494	L98.A323	L98.493
E72.530	E72.53	H01.8A	H01.8	L98.456	L98.496	L98.A195	L98.495	L98.A324	L98.494
E72.538	E72.53	H01.8B	H01.8	L98.458	L98.498	L98.A196	L98.496	L98.A325	L98.495
E72.539	E72.53	H05.831	H05.83	L98.459	L98.499	L98.A198	L98.498	L98.A326	L98.496
E72.540	R82.992	H05.832	H05.83	L98.461	L98.491	L98.A199	L98.499	L98.A328	L98.498
E72.541	R82.992	H05.833	H05.83	L98.462	L98.492	L98.A211	L98.491	L98.A329	L98.499
E72.548	R82.992	H05.839	H05.83	L98.463	L98.493	L98.A212	L98.492	L98.A391	L98.491
E72.549	R82.992	H40.841	H40.84	L98.464	L98.494	L98.A213	L98.493	L98.A392	L98.492
E78.010	E78.01	H40.842	H40.84	L98.465	L98.495	L98.A214	L98.494	L98.A393	L98.493
E78.011	E78.01	H40.843	H40.84	L98.466	L98.496	L98.A215	L98.495	L98.A394	L98.494
E78.019	E78.01	H40.843	H40.84	L98.468	L98.498	L98.A216	L98.496	L98.A395	L98.495
E83.820	E83.89	I27.840	I27.89	L98.469	L98.499	L98.A218	L98.498	L98.A396	L98.496
E83.821	E83.89	I27.841	I27.89	L98.471	L98.491	L98.A219	L98.499	L98.A398	L98.498
E83.822	E83.89	I27.848	I27.89	L98.472	L98.492	L98.A221	L98.491	L98.A399	L98.499
E83.823	E83.89	I27.849	I27.89	L98.473	L98.493	L98.A222	L98.492	M05.A	M05.9
E83.824	E83.89	L02.217	L02.212	L98.474	L98.494	L98.A223	L98.493	N00.B1	N00.8
E83.825	E83.89	L02.227	L02.222	L98.475	L98.495	L98.A224	L98.494	N00.B2	N00.8
E88.10	E88.1	L03.31A	L03.312	L98.476	L98.496	L98.A225	L98.495	N04.B1	N04.8
E88.11	E88.1	L03.32A	L03.322	L98.478	L98.498	L98.A226	L98.496	N04.B2	N04.8
E88.12	E88.1	L98.431	L98.491	L98.479	L98.499	L98.A228	L98.498	N07.B	N07.8
E88.13	E88.1	L98.432	L98.492	L98.A111	L98.491	L98.A229	L98.499	Q87.87	Q87.89
E88.14	E88.1	L98.433	L98.493	L98.A112	L98.492	L98.A291	L98.491	Q87.88	Q87.89
E88.19	E88.1	L98.434	L98.494	L98.A113	L98.493	L98.A292	L98.492	Q89.81	Q89.8
G31.87	R48.2	L98.435	L98.495	L98.A114	L98.494	L98.A293	L98.493	Q89.89	Q89.8
G35.A	G35	L98.436	L98.496	L98.A115	L98.495	L98.A294	L98.494	Q99.811	Q99.8
G35.B0	G35	L98.438	L98.498	L98.A116	L98.496	L98.A295	L98.495	Q99.812	Q99.8
G35.B1	G35	L98.439	L98.499	L98.A118	L98.498	L98.A296	L98.496	Q99.813	Q99.8
G35.B2	G35	L98.441	L98.491	L98.A119	L98.499	L98.A298	L98.498	Q99.818	Q99.8
G35.C0	G35	L98.442	L98.492	L98.A121	L98.491	L98.A299	L98.499	Q99.819	Q99.8

Conversion Table of ICD-10-CM Codes

Code Assignment Beginning 10/1/2025	Previous Code(s) Assignment	Code Assignment Beginning 10/1/2025	Previous Code(s) Assignment	Code Assignment Beginning 10/1/2025	Previous Code(s) Assignment	Code Assignment Beginning 10/1/2025	Previous Code(s) Assignment	Code Assignment Beginning 10/1/2025	Previous Code(s) Assignment
Q99.89	Q99.8	S30.13XS	S30.1XXS	S31.127A	S31.129A	S31.616D	S31.619D	S31.65AS	S31.659S
QA0.0101	F89	S30.81AA	S30.811A	S31.127D	S31.129D	S31.616S	S31.619S	T36.AX1A	T36.8X1A
QA0.0102	F89	S30.81AD	S30.811D	S31.127S	S31.129S	S31.617A	S31.619A	T36.AX1D	T36.8X1D
QA0.0109	F89	S30.81AS	S30.811S	S31.12AA	S31.129A	S31.617D	S31.619D	T36.AX1S	T36.8X1S
QA0.011	F89	S30.82AA	S30.821A	S31.12AD	S31.129D	S31.617S	S31.619S	T36.AX2A	T36.8X2A
QA0.012	F89	S30.82AD	S30.821D	S31.12AS	S31.129S	S31.61AA	S31.619A	T36.AX2D	T36.8X2D
QA0.0131	F89	S30.82AS	S30.821S	S31.136A	S31.139A	S31.61AD	S31.619D	T36.AX2S	T36.8X2S
QA0.0139	F89	S30.84AA	S30.841A	S31.136D	S31.139D	S31.61AS	S31.619S	T36.AX3A	T36.8X3A
QA0.0141	F89	S30.84AD	S30.841D	S31.136S	S31.139S	S31.626A	S31.629A	T36.AX3D	T36.8X3D
QA0.0142	F89	S30.84AS	S30.841S	S31.137A	S31.139A	S31.626D	S31.629D	T36.AX3S	T36.8X3S
QA0.0149	F89	S30.85AA	S30.851A	S31.137D	S31.139D	S31.626S	S31.629S	T36.AX4A	T36.8X4A
QA0.0151	F89	S30.85AD	S30.851D	S31.137S	S31.139S	S31.627A	S31.629A	T36.AX4D	T36.8X4D
QA0.0159	F89	S30.85AS	S30.851S	S31.13AA	S31.139A	S31.627D	S31.629D	T36.AX4S	T36.8X4S
QA0.8	F89	S30.86AA	S30.861A	S31.13AD	S31.139D	S31.627S	S31.629S	T36.AX5A	T36.8X5A
R10.20	R10.2	S30.86AD	S30.861D	S31.13AS	S31.139S	S31.62AA	S31.629A	T36.AX5D	T36.8X5D
R10.21	R10.2	S30.86AS	S30.861S	S31.146A	S31.149A	S31.62AD	S31.629D	T36.AX5S	T36.8X5S
R10.22	R10.2	S30.87AA	S30.871A	S31.146D	S31.149D	S31.62AS	S31.629S	T36.AX6A	T36.8X6A
R10.23	R10.2	S30.87AD	S30.871D	S31.146S	S31.149S	S31.636A	S31.639A	T36.AX6D	T36.8X6D
R10.24	R10.2	S30.87AS	S30.871S	S31.147A	S31.149A	S31.636D	S31.639D	T36.AX6S	T36.8X6S
R10.85	R10.84	S30.9AXA	S30.92XA	S31.147D	S31.149D	S31.636S	S31.639S	T65.841A	T65.891A
R10.8A1	R10.84	S30.9AXD	S30.92XD	S31.147S	S31.149S	S31.637A	S31.639A	T65.841D	T65.891D
R10.8A2	R10.84	S30.9AXS	S30.92XS	S31.14AA	S31.149A	S31.637D	S31.639D	T65.841S	T65.891S
R10.8A3	R10.84	S31.106A	S31.109A	S31.14AD	S31.149D	S31.637S	S31.639S	T65.842A	T65.892A
R10.8A9	R10.84	S31.106D	S31.109D	S31.14AS	S31.149S	S31.63AA	S31.639A	T65.842D	T65.892D
R10.A0	R10.84	S31.106S	S31.109S	S31.156A	S31.159A	S31.63AD	S31.639D	T65.842S	T65.892S
R10.A1	R10.84	S31.107A	S31.109A	S31.156D	S31.159D	S31.63AS	S31.639S	T65.843A	T65.893A
R10.A2	R10.84	S31.107D	S31.109D	S31.156S	S31.159S	S31.646A	S31.649A	T65.843D	T65.893D
R10.A3	R10.84	S31.107S	S31.109S	S31.157A	S31.159A	S31.646D	S31.649D	T65.843S	T65.893S
R11.16	R11.10	S31.10AA	S31.109A	S31.157D	S31.159D	S31.646S	S31.649S	T65.844A	T65.894A
R39.851	R39.89	S31.10AD	S31.109D	S31.157S	S31.159S	S31.647A	S31.649A	T65.844D	T65.894D
R39.852	R39.89	S31.10AS	S31.109S	S31.15AA	S31.159A	S31.647D	S31.649D	T65.844S	T65.894S
R39.853	R39.89	S31.116A	S31.119A	S31.15AD	S31.159D	S31.647S	S31.649S	T75.830A	T75.89XA
R39.859	R39.89	S31.116D	S31.119D	S31.15AS	S31.159S	S31.64AA	S31.649A	T75.830D	T75.89XD
R76.81	R76.8	S31.116S	S31.119S	S31.606A	S31.609A	S31.64AD	S31.649D	T75.830S	T75.89XS
R76.89	R76.8	S31.117A	S31.119A	S31.606D	S31.609D	S31.64AS	S31.649S	T75.838A	T75.89XA
S30.11XA	S30.1XXA	S31.117D	S31.119D	S31.606S	S31.609S	S31.656A	S31.659A	T75.838D	T75.89XD
S30.11XD	S30.1XXD	S31.117S	S31.119S	S31.607A	S31.609A	S31.656D	S31.659D	T75.838S	T75.89XS
S30.11XS	S30.1XXS	S31.11AA	S31.119A	S31.607D	S31.609D	S31.656S	S31.659S	T78.070A	T78.07XA
S30.12XA	S30.1XXA	S31.11AD	S31.119D	S31.607S	S31.609S	S31.657A	S31.659A	T78.070D	T78.07XD
S30.12XD	S30.1XXD	S31.11AS	S31.119S	S31.60AA	S31.609A	S31.657D	S31.659D	T78.070S	T78.07XS
S30.12XS	S30.1XXS	S31.126A	S31.129A	S31.60AD	S31.609D	S31.657S	S31.659S	T78.071A	T78.07XA
S30.13XA	S30.1XXA	S31.126D	S31.129D	S31.60AS	S31.609S	S31.65AA	S31.659A	T78.071D	T78.07XD
S30.13XD	S30.1XXD	S31.126S	S31.129S	S31.616A	S31.619A	S31.65AD	S31.659D	T78.071S	T78.07XS

Code Assignment Beginning 10/1/2025	Previous Code(s) Assignment	Code Assignment Beginning 10/1/2025	Previous Code(s) Assignment	Code Assignment Beginning 10/1/2025	Previous Code(s) Assignment	Code Assignment Beginning 10/1/2025	Previous Code(s) Assignment	Code Assignment Beginning 10/1/2025	Previous Code(s) Assignment
T78.079A	T78.07XA	T78.119D	T78.1XXD	W44.H9XS	Codes in Categories T15-T19	Z15.05	Z15.09	Z91.0110	Z91.011
T78.079D	T78.07XD	T78.119S	T78.1XXS			Z15.060	Z15.09	Z91.0111	Z91.011
T78.079S	T78.07XS	T78.120A	T78.1XXA	W453XXA	W45.8XXA	Z15.068	Z15.09	Z91.0112	Z91.011
T78.080A	T78.08XA	T78.120D	T78.1XXD	W453XXD	W45.8XXD	Z15.07	Z15.09	Z91.0120	Z91.012
T78.080D	T78.08XD	T78.120S	T78.1XXS	W453XXS	W45.8XXS	Z15.3	Z15.89	Z91.0121	Z91.012
T78.080S	T78.08XS	T78.121A	T78.1XXA	Y36.A1XA	Y36.90XA	Z40.81	Z40.8	Z91.0122	Z91.012
T78.081A	T78.08XA	T78.121D	T78.1XXD	Y36.A1XD	Y36.90XD	Z40.82	Z40.8	Z91.B	Z91.89
T78.081D	T78.08XD	T78.121S	T78.1XXS	Y36.A1XS	Y36.90XS	Z40.89	Z40.8		
T78.081S	T78.08XS	T78.129A	T78.1XXA	Y36.A2XA	Y36.90XA	Z59.861	Z59.86		
T78.089A	T78.08XA	T78.129D	T78.1XXD	Y36.A2XD	Y36.90XD	Z59.868	Z59.86		
T78.089D	T78.08XD	T78.129S	T78.1XXS	Y36.A2XS	Y36.90XS	Z59.869	Z59.86		
T78.089S	T78.08XS	T78.19XA	T78.1XXA	Y37.A1XA	Y37.90XA	Z77.31	Z77.3		
T78.110A	T78.1XXA	T78.19XD	T78.1XXD	Y37.A1XD	Y37.90XD	Z77.39	Z77.3		
T78.110D	T78.1XXD	T78.19XS	T78.1XXS	Y37.A1XS	Y37.90XS	Z80.44	Z40.89		
T78.110S	T78.1XXS	W44.H9XA	Codes in Categories T15-T19	Y37.A2XA	Y37.90XA	Z84.11	Z84.1		
T78.111A	T78.1XXA			Y37.A2XD	Y37.90XD	Z84.19	Z84.1		
T78.111D	T78.1XXD	W44.H9XD	Codes in Categories T15-T19	Y37.A2XS	Y37.90XS	Z84.A	Z84.89		
T78.111S	T78.1XXS			Y93.L1	Y93.89	Z85.4A	Z85.44		
T78.119A	T78.1XXA			Y93.L9	Y93.89	Z86.00A	Z86.002		

10 Steps to Correct Coding

Follow the 10 steps below to correctly code encounters for health care services.

Step 1: Identify the reason for the visit or encounter (i.e., a sign, symptom, diagnosis and/or condition).

The medical record documentation should accurately reflect the patient's condition, using terminology that includes specific diagnoses and symptoms or clearly states the reasons for the encounter.

Choosing the main term that best describes the reason chiefly responsible for the service provided is the most important step in coding. If symptoms are present and documented but a definitive diagnosis has not yet been determined, code the symptoms. *For outpatient cases, do not code conditions that are referred to as "rule out," "suspected," "probable," or "questionable."* Diagnoses often are not established at the time of the initial encounter/visit and may require two or more visits to be established. Code only what is documented in the available outpatient records and only to the highest degree of certainty known at the time of the patient's visit. For inpatient medical records, uncertain diagnoses may be reported if documented at the time of discharge.

Step 2: After selecting the reason for the encounter, consult the alphabetic index.

The most critical rule is to begin code selection in the alphabetic index. Never turn first to the tabular list. The index provides cross-references, essential and nonessential modifiers, and other instructional notations that may not be found in the tabular list.

Step 3: Locate the main term entry.

The alphabetic index lists conditions, which may be expressed as nouns or eponyms, with critical use of adjectives. Some conditions known by several names have multiple main entries. Reasons for encounters may be located under general terms such as admission, encounter, and examination. Other general terms such as history, status (post), or presence (of) can be used to locate other factors influencing health.

Step 4: Scan subterm entries.

Scan the subterm entries, as appropriate, being sure to review continued lines and additional subterms that may appear in the next column or on the next page. Shaded vertical guidelines in the index indicate the indentation level for each subterm in relation to the main terms.

Step 5: Pay close attention to index instructions.

- Parentheses ( ) enclose nonessential modifiers, terms that are supplementary words or explanatory information that may or may not appear in the diagnostic statement and do not affect code selection.
- Brackets [ ] enclose manifestation codes that can be used only as secondary codes to the underlying condition code immediately preceding it. If used, manifestation codes must be reported with the appropriate etiology codes.
- Default codes are listed next to the main term and represent the condition most commonly associated with the main term or the unspecified code for the main term.
- "*See*" cross-references, identified by italicized type and "code by" cross-references indicate that another term *must be referenced* to locate the correct code.
- "*See also*" cross-references, identified by italicized type, provide alternative terms that may be useful to look up but *are not mandatory*.
- "Omit code" cross-references identify instances when a code is not applicable depending on the condition being coded.
- "With" subterms are listed out of alphabetic order and identify a presumed causal relationship between the two conditions they link.
- "Due to" subterms identify a relationship between the two conditions they link.
- "NEC," abbreviation for "not elsewhere classified," follows some main terms or subterms and indicates that there is no specific code for the condition even though the medical documentation may be very specific.
- "NOS," abbreviation for "not otherwise specified," follows some main terms or subterms and is the equivalent of unspecified; NOS signifies that the information in the medical record is insufficient for assigning a more specific code.
- *Following* references help coders locate alphanumeric codes that are out of sequence in the tabular section.
- Check-additional-character symbols flag codes that require additional characters to make the code valid; the characters available to complete the code should be verified in the tabular section.

Step 6: Choose a potential code and locate it in the tabular list.

To prevent coding errors, always use both the alphabetic index (to identify a code) and the tabular list (to verify a code), as the index does not include the important instructional notes found in the tabular list. An added benefit of using the tabular list, which groups like things together, is that while looking at one code in the list, a coder might see a more specific one that would have been missed had the coder relied solely on the alphabetic index. Additionally, many of the codes require a fourth, fifth, sixth, or seventh character to be valid, and many of these characters can be found only in the tabular list.

Step 7: Read all instructional material in the tabular section.

The coder must follow any Includes, Excludes 1 and Excludes 2 notes, and other instructional notes, such as "Code first" and "Use additional code," listed in the tabular list for the chapter, category, subcategory, and subclassification levels of code selection that direct the coder to use a different or additional code. Any codes in the tabular range A00.0–T88.9, Z00–Z99.8, and U00–U85 may be used to identify the diagnostic reason for the encounter. The tabular list encompasses many codes describing disease and injury classifications (e.g., infectious and parasitic diseases, neoplasms, symptoms, nervous and circulatory system, etc.).

Codes that describe symptoms and signs, as opposed to definitive diagnoses, should be reported when an established diagnosis has not been made (confirmed) by the physician. Chapter 18 of the ICD-10-CM code book, "Symptoms, Signs, and Abnormal Clinical and Laboratory Findings, Not Elsewhere Classified" (codes R00–R99), contains many, but not all, codes for symptoms.

ICD-10-CM classifies encounters with health care providers for circumstances other than a disease or injury in chapter 21, "Factors Influencing Health Status and Contact with Health Services" (codes Z00–Z99). Circumstances other than a disease or injury often are recorded as chiefly responsible for the encounter.

A code is invalid if it does not include the full number of characters (greatest level of specificity) required. Codes in ICD-10-CM can contain from three to seven alphanumeric characters. A three-character code is to be used only if the category is not further subdivided into four-, five-, six-, or seven-character codes. Placeholder character X is used as part of an alphanumeric code to allow for future expansion and as a placeholder for empty characters in a code that requires a seventh character but has no fourth, fifth, or sixth character. Note that certain categories require seventh characters that apply to all codes in that category. Always check the category level for applicable seventh characters for that category.

Step 8: Consult the official ICD-10-CM conventions and guidelines.

The *ICD-10-CM Official Guidelines for Coding and Reporting* govern the use of certain codes. These guidelines provide both general and chapter-specific coding guidance.

Step 9: Confirm and assign the code.
Having reviewed all relevant information concerning the possible code choices, assign the code that most completely describes the condition.

Repeat steps 1 through 9 for all additional documented conditions that meet the following criteria:

- They exist at the time of the visit *AND*
- They require or affect patient care, treatment, or management

Step 10: Sequence codes correctly.
Sequencing is the order in which the codes are listed on the claim. List first the ICD-10-CM code for the diagnosis, condition, problem, or other reason for the encounter/visit that is shown in the medical record to be chiefly responsible for the services provided. List additional codes that describe any coexisting conditions. Follow the official coding guidelines (see the guidelines, section II, "Selection of Principal Diagnosis"; section III, "Reporting Additional Diagnoses"; and section IV, "Diagnostic Coding and Reporting Guidelines for Outpatient Services") on proper sequencing of codes.

Coding Examples

Diagnosis: Anorexia

Step 1: The reason for the encounter was the condition, anorexia.

Step 2: Consult the alphabetic index.

Step 3: Locate the main term "Anorexia."

Step 4: Two possible subterms are available, "hysterical" and "nervosa." Neither is documented in this instance, however, so they cannot be used in code selection.

Step 5: The code listed next to the main term is called the default code selection. Because the two subentries (essential modifiers) do not apply in this instance, the default code (R63.0) should be used.

Step 6: Turn to code R63.0 in the tabular list and read all instructional notes.

Step 7: The Excludes 1 note at code R63.0 indicates that anorexia nervosa and loss of appetite determined to be of nonorganic origin should be reported with a code from chapter 5. The diagnostic statement does not describe the condition as anorexia nervosa, however, and does not indicate that the anorexia is of a nonorganic origin. There is no further division of the category past the fourth-character subcategory. Therefore, code R63.0 is at the highest level of specificity.

Step 8: Review of official guideline I.C.18 indicates that a symptom code is appropriate when a more definitive diagnosis is not documented.

Step 9: The default code, R63.0 Anorexia, is the correct code selection.

Repeat steps 1 through 9 for any concomitant diagnoses.

Step 10: Since anorexia is listed as the chief reason for the health care encounter, the first-listed, or principal, diagnosis is R63.0. Note that this is a chapter 18 symptom code but can be assigned for both inpatient and outpatient records since the provider did not establish a more definitive diagnosis, according to sections II.A and IV.D.

Diagnosis: Acute bronchitis

Step 1: The reason for the encounter was the condition, acute bronchitis.

Step 2: Consult the alphabetic index.

Step 3: Locate the main term "Bronchitis."

Step 4: There is a subterm for "acute or subacute." Additional subterms are not included in the diagnostic statement.

Step 5: Nonessential modifiers (with bronchospasm or obstruction) are terms that do not affect code assignment. Since no other subterms indented under "acute" apply here, the code listed next to this subentry—in this case J20.9—should be chosen.

Step 6: Turn to code J20.9 in the tabular list and read all instructional notes.

Step 7: The Includes note under category J20 lists alternative terms for acute bronchitis. Note that the list is not exhaustive but is only a representative selection of diagnoses that are included in the subcategory. The Excludes 1 note refers to category J40 for bronchitis and tracheobronchitis NOS. There are several conditions in the Excludes 2 notes that, if applicable, can be coded in addition to this code.

Note that the codes included in J20 represent acute bronchitis due to various infectious organisms that could be selected if identified in the documentation. In this case, the organism was not identified and there is no further division of the category past the fourth character subcategory. Therefore, code J20.9 is at the highest level of specificity.

Step 8: Review of official guideline I.C.10 provides no additional information affecting the code selected.

Step 9: Assign code J20.9 Acute bronchitis, unspecified.

Repeat steps 1 through 9 for any concomitant diagnoses.

Step 10: In the absence of additional diagnoses that may affect sequencing, code J20.9 should be sequenced as the first-listed, or principal, diagnosis.

Diagnosis: Cerebellar ataxia in myxedema

Step 1: The reason for the encounter was the condition, cerebellar ataxia.

Step 2: Consult the alphabetic index.

Step 3: Locate the main term "Ataxia."

Step 4: Available subterms include "cerebellar (hereditary)," with additional indented subterms for "in" and "myxedema," all essential modifiers that are included in the diagnostic statement. Two codes are provided, E03.9 and G13.2, the latter of which is in brackets.

Step 5: Note the nonessential modifier (in parentheses) after the subterm cerebellar includes the term "hereditary." Because it is in parentheses, this term is not required in the diagnostic statement for this subentry to apply. The brackets around G13.2 identify this code as a manifestation of the condition described by code E03.9 and indicate that the two must be reported together and sequencing rules apply.

Step 6: Locate codes E03.9 and G13.2 in the tabular list, and read all instructional notes.

Step 7: For code E03.9, there are no instructional notes in the tabular list at the category E03 or code level that indicate that this condition should be coded elsewhere in the classification or that additional codes are required. Without further information from the diagnostic statement, myxedema, not otherwise specified (NOS), is appropriately reported with code E03.9 Hypothyroidism, unspecified, according to the inclusion term at this code.

Code G13.2 in the tabular list has an instructional note to "Code first underlying disease," which includes conditions found in category E03.-. Based on this note, codes E03.9 and G13.2 are to be coded together, with G13.2 listed only as a secondary diagnosis. This correlates with what the alphabetic index indicated. As there is no further division of codes in category G13 beyond the fourth character, G13.2 is at the highest level of specificity.

Step 8: Although there are some general conventions, such as how to interpret brackets in the alphabetic index, no chapter-specific guidelines apply to this coding scenario.

Step 9: Assign codes E03.9 Hypothyroidism, unspecified, and G13.2 Systemic atrophy primarily affecting the central nervous system in myxedema.

Repeat steps 1 through 9 for any concomitant diagnoses.

Step 10: Based on the alphabetic index and tabular instructional notations, code E03.9 should be sequenced as the first-listed, or principal, diagnosis followed by G13.2 as a secondary diagnosis.

Diagnosis: Decubitus ulcer of right elbow with skin loss and necrosis of subcutaneous tissue

Step 1: The reason for the encounter was the condition, decubitus ulcer.

Step 2: Consult the alphabetic index.

Step 3: Locate the main term "Ulcer."

Step 4: For the subterm "decubitus," there is no code provided or additional subterms indented, but a cross-reference is listed.

Step 5: The italicized cross-reference instructs the coder to "*see* Ulcer, pressure, by site."

Repeat steps 3 through 5 for the cross-reference:

Step 3: Locate the main term "Ulcer."

Step 4: Review the subentries for the subterm "pressure." The next level of indent lists either the site of the ulcer or the specific stage of the ulcer (stage 1–4, unstageable, and unspecified stages). The diagnostic statement provides the site, right elbow, and the extent of tissue damage (skin loss and necrosis of subcutaneous tissue) but does not specifically state that the ulcer is stage 1, stage 2, etc. Nonessential modifiers (in parentheses) at each stage include a description of the typical extent of damage at each stage. For example, stage 1 describes "pre-ulcer skin changes limited to persistent focal edema." Based on the documentation in the record, the coder can correlate the documentation to the nonessential modifiers and choose the specific stage from the index. The coder can also go directly to the body site, choosing the stage of the ulcer after reviewing the code options and instructional notations in the tabular list.

The diagnostic statement indicates that the extent of the damage to the elbow includes skin loss and necrosis of subcutaneous tissue, coinciding with the nonessential modifier next to the subentry "stage 3." The body site of elbow (L89.0-) is listed as another level of indent with other body sites.

Step 5: Note that code L89.0 is followed by a dash and an additional-character-required icon, which indicate that more characters are needed to complete the code. From here, the tabular listing for L89.0- can be consulted.

Step 6: Locate code L89.0- in the tabular list and read all instructional notes.

Step 7: The tabular listing at category L89 has an Includes note for "decubitus ulcer," which confirms that category L89 is the appropriate category to represent what is documented in the diagnostic statement.

Several Excludes 2 notes are also listed at the category level. Excludes 2 notes represent conditions that can occur concomitantly with the decubitus ulcer and can be coded in addition to code L89, if supported by the documentation.

The subcategory codes under L89.0 indicate that the fifth character describes laterality. Locate the right elbow at subcategory L89.01. See that an additional sixth character to specify the stage of the ulcer is now needed to complete the code. The stage can be determined either by the specific documentation of the stage (e.g., stage 1, stage 2) or, in this case, a description that matches one of the inclusion terms that follow each stage code. For example, the diagnostic description in this case of "skin loss and necrosis of the subcutaneous tissue" matches the inclusion term under L89.013 Pressure ulcer of right elbow, stage 3. No additional characters are required because code L89.013 is at its highest level of specificity.

Step 8: The official guidelines contain quite a bit of information relating to pressure ulcers in chapter-specific guideline I.C.12 as well as information in general guideline I.B.14. These and any other pertinent guidelines should be reviewed to ensure appropriate code assignment.

Step 9: Assign code L89.013 Pressure ulcer of right elbow, stage 3.

Repeat steps 1 through 9 for any concomitant diagnoses.

Step 10: Since the decubitus ulcer is listed as the chief reason for the health care encounter, the first-listed, or principal, diagnosis is L89.013. However, according to the code first instructional note at the L89 category level, gangrene (I96) would be sequenced before the pressure ulcer if it were documented.

Diagnosis: Emergency department visit for bimalleolar fracture of the right ankle due to trauma

Step 1: The reason for the encounter was the condition, bimalleolar fracture.

Step 2: Consult the alphabetic index.

Step 3: Locate the main term "Fracture." Note that many main terms represent fractures: "Fracture, burst," "Fracture, chronic," "Fracture, insufficiency," "Fracture, nontraumatic NEC," "Fracture, pathological," and "Fracture, traumatic." Since the diagnostic statement specifically states that this fracture was the result of trauma, the main term "Fracture, traumatic" should be used.

Step 4: Subterms that should be referenced are "ankle" and "bimalleolar (displaced)," which lists code S82.84-.

Step 5: A nonessential modifier (in parentheses) next to the term bimalleolar for "displaced" indicates that S82.84- is the default category unless the fracture is specifically identified as "nondisplaced."

Note that code S82.84- is followed by a dash and an additional-character icon, both of which indicate that more characters are required. From here, the tabular list can be consulted.

Step 6: Locate code S82.84- in the tabular list and read all instructional notes.

Step 7: The instructional notes at category S82 indicate that fractures not specified as displaced or nondisplaced default to displaced and that fractures not designated as open or closed default to closed. Additional instructional notes can be found at the category level but none pertain to the current scenario.

Read through the subcategory codes under S82.84, and note that the sixth character specifies displaced or nondisplaced and laterality. Based on the index nonessential modifier (displaced) and the code note at category S82, code selection should identify a displaced fracture of the right side. A displaced bimalleolar fracture of the right lower leg is coded to S82.841.

To complete the code, a seventh character must be assigned to identify the type of encounter (initial, subsequent, or sequela) and whether the fracture is open or closed. Most of the codes in category S82 require a seventh character represented in the list at the category level. However, it is important to note that some subcategories have their own specific set of seventh characters. In this instance, subcategory S82.84- does not have a unique set of seventh characters and the list provided at the category level should be used. Without documentation of the fracture being open, the tabular notation indicates that the default is closed. Character A, representing "initial encounter for closed fracture," listed in the box at the category level is the most appropriate option.

Step 8: Assign code S82.841A Displaced bimalleolar fracture of right lower leg, initial encounter for closed fracture.

Step 9: Review chapter-specific guideline I.C.19. and any other official conventions or guidelines to ensure appropriate code assignment.

Repeat steps 1 through 9 for any concomitant diagnoses.

Step 10: Additional codes can be applied to relate the specific cause of the injury, the place of occurrence, the activity of the patient at the time of the injury, and the patient's status, when this information is available in the record. However, coding this information is voluntary and reporting requirements depend on state mandates and/or facility-specific reporting requirements. If assigned, the external cause codes should be reported as secondary diagnoses only with the injury (fracture) sequenced first. Most codes in chapter 20, "External Causes of Morbidity," require a seventh character to identify the type of encounter. The seventh character assigned to an external cause code should match the seventh character of the code assigned for the associated injury or condition for the encounter.

2026 ICD-10-CM Official Guidelines for Coding and Reporting

Narrative changes effective October 1, 2025 appear in **bold** text
Narrative changes effective April 1, 2025 appear in shaded text
Items underlined have been moved within the guidelines since the April 2025, FY 2025 version
Italics are used to indicate revisions to heading changes

The Centers for Medicare and Medicaid Services (CMS) and the National Center for Health Statistics (NCHS), two departments within the U.S. Federal Government's Department of Health and Human Services (DHHS) provide the following guidelines for coding and reporting using the International Classification of Diseases, 10th Revision, Clinical Modification (ICD-10-CM). These guidelines should be used as a companion document to the official version of the ICD-10-CM as published on the NCHS website. The ICD-10-CM is a morbidity classification published by the United States for classifying diagnoses and reason for visits in all health care settings. The ICD-10-CM is based on the ICD-10, the statistical classification of disease published by the World Health Organization (WHO).

These guidelines have been approved by the four organizations that make up the Cooperating Parties for the ICD-10-CM: the American Hospital Association (AHA), the American Health Information Management Association (AHIMA), CMS, and NCHS.

These guidelines are a set of rules that have been developed to accompany and complement the official conventions and instructions provided within the ICD-10-CM itself. The instructions and conventions of the classification take precedence over guidelines. These guidelines are based on the coding and sequencing instructions in the Tabular List and Alphabetic Index of ICD-10-CM, but provide additional instruction. Adherence to these guidelines when assigning ICD-10-CM diagnosis codes is required under the Health Insurance Portability and Accountability Act (HIPAA). The diagnosis codes (Tabular List and Alphabetic Index) have been adopted under HIPAA for all healthcare settings. A joint effort between the healthcare provider and the coder is essential to achieve complete and accurate documentation, code assignment, and reporting of diagnoses and procedures. These guidelines have been developed to assist both the healthcare provider and the coder in identifying those diagnoses that are to be reported. The importance of consistent, complete documentation in the medical record cannot be overemphasized. Without such documentation accurate coding cannot be achieved. The entire record should be reviewed to determine the specific reason for the encounter and the conditions treated.

The term encounter is used for all settings, including hospital admissions. In the context of these guidelines, the term provider is used throughout the guidelines to mean physician or any qualified health care practitioner who is legally accountable for establishing the patient's diagnosis. Only this set of guidelines, approved by the Cooperating Parties, is official.

The guidelines are organized into sections. Section I includes the structure and conventions of the classification and general guidelines that apply to the entire classification, and chapter-specific guidelines that correspond to the chapters as they are arranged in the classification. Section II includes guidelines for selection of principal diagnosis for non-outpatient settings. Section III includes guidelines for reporting additional diagnoses in non-outpatient settings. Section IV is for outpatient coding and reporting. It is necessary to review all sections of the guidelines to fully understand all of the rules and instructions needed to code properly.

Section I. Conventions, general coding guidelines and chapter specific guidelines 2
A. Conventions for the ICD-10-CM...2
  1. The Alphabetic Index and Tabular List 2
  2. Format and Structure:...2
  3. Use of codes for reporting purposes 3
  4. Placeholder character 3
  5. 7th Characters 3
  6. Abbreviations 3
     a. Alphabetic Index abbreviations 3
     b. Tabular List abbreviations 3
  7. Punctuation 3
  8. Use of "and" 3
  9. Other and Unspecified codes 3
     a. "Other" codes 3
     b. "Unspecified" codes 3
  10. Includes Notes...3
  11. Inclusion terms 3
  12. Excludes Notes 3
     a. Excludes1 3
     b. Excludes2 3
  13. Etiology/manifestation convention ("code first", "use additional code" and "in diseases classified elsewhere" notes) 3
  14. "And" 3
  15. "With" 3
  16. "See" and "See Also" 4
  17. "Code also" note 4
  18. Default codes 4
  19. Code assignment and Clinical Criteria 4
B. General Coding Guidelines 4
  1. Locating a code in the ICD-10-CM 4
  2. Level of Detail in Coding 4
  3. Code or codes from A00.0 through T88.9, Z00-Z99.8, U00-U85.................4
  4. Signs and symptoms 4
  5. Conditions that are an integral part of a disease process 4
  6. Conditions that are not an integral part of a disease process 4
  7. Multiple coding for a single condition 4
  8. Acute and Chronic Conditions 4
  9. Combination Code 4
  10. Sequela (Late Effects) 4
  11. Impending or Threatened Condition 4
  12. Reporting Same Diagnosis Code More than Once 4
  13. Laterality 4
  14. Documentation by Clinicians Other than the Patient's Provider..............5
  15. Syndromes..5
  16. Documentation of Complications of Care 5
  17. Borderline Diagnosis...5
  18. Use of Sign/Symptom/Unspecified Codes...5
  19. Coding for Healthcare Encounters in Hurricane Aftermath 5
     a. Use of External Cause of Morbidity Codes..5
     b. Sequencing of External Causes of Morbidity Codes..............................5
     c. Other External Causes of Morbidity Code Issues 5
     d. Use of Z codes 5
  20. Multiple Sites Coding..6
C. Chapter-Specific Coding Guidelines 6
  1. Chapter 1: Certain Infectious and Parasitic Diseases (A00-B99), U07.1, U09.9...6
     a. Human Immunodeficiency Virus (HIV) Infections..................................6
     b. Infectious agents as the cause of diseases classified to other chapters....6
     c. Infections resistant to antibiotics..6
     d. Sepsis, Severe Sepsis, and Septic Shock Infections resistant to antibiotics 6
     e. Methicillin Resistant Staphylococcus aureus (MRSA) Conditions 7
     f. Zika virus infections..8
     g. Coronavirus infections...8
  2. Chapter 2: Neoplasms (C00-D49) 9
     a. Admission/Encounter for treatment of primary site..............................9
     b. Admission/Encounter for treatment of secondary site 9
     c. Coding and sequencing of complications 9
     d. Primary malignancy previously excised 9
     e. Admissions/Encounters involving antineoplastic chemotherapy, immunotherapy and radiation therapy 9
     f. Admission/encounter to determine extent of malignancy..................10
     g. Symptoms, signs, and abnormal findings listed in Chapter 18 associated with neoplasms 10
     h. Admission/encounter for pain control/management 10
     i. Malignancy in two or more noncontiguous sites 10
     j. Disseminated malignant neoplasm, unspecified 10
     k. Malignant neoplasm without specification of site...............................10
     l. Sequencing of neoplasm codes 10
     m. Current malignancy versus personal history of malignancy.............10
     n. Leukemia, Multiple Myeloma, and Malignant Plasma Cell Neoplasms in remission versus personal history...10
     o. Aftercare following surgery for neoplasm 10
     p. Follow-up care for completed treatment of a malignancy..................10
     q. Prophylactic organ removal for prevention of malignancy 10
     r. Malignant neoplasm associated with transplanted organ 10
     s. Breast Implant Associated Anaplastic Large Cell Lymphoma 10
     t. Secondary malignant neoplasm of lymphoid tissue............................10
  3. Chapter 3: Disease of the blood and blood-forming organs and certain disorders involving the immune mechanism (D50-D89) 10
  4. Chapter 4: Endocrine, Nutritional, and Metabolic Diseases (E00-E89)....10
     a. Diabetes mellitus 10
     b. Obesity..11
  5. Chapter 5: Mental, Behavioral and Neurodevelopmental disorders (F01-F99) 11
     a. Pain disorders related to psychological factors....................................11
     b. Mental and behavioral disorders due to psychoactive substance use....11
     c. Factitious Disorder..12
     d. Dementia 12
  6. Chapter 6: Diseases of the Nervous System (G00-G99) 12
     a. Dominant/nondominant side..12
     b. Pain - Category G89 12
  7. Chapter 7: Diseases of the Eye and Adnexa (H00-H59) 13
     a. Glaucoma..13
     b. Blindness..13
  8. Chapter 8: Diseases of the Ear and Mastoid Process (H60-H95) 13
  9. Chapter 9: Diseases of the Circulatory System (I00-I99) 13
     a. Hypertension 13
     b. Atherosclerotic Coronary Artery Disease and Angina 14
     c. Intraoperative and Postprocedural Cerebrovascular Accident 14
     d. Sequelae of Cerebrovascular Disease 14
     e. Acute myocardial infarction (AMI) 14
  10. Chapter 10: Diseases of the Respiratory System (J00-J99), U07.0 14
     a. Chronic Obstructive Pulmonary Disease [COPD] and Asthma 14
     b. Acute Respiratory Failure 14
     c. Influenza due to certain identified influenza viruses 15
     d. Ventilator associated Pneumonia 15

e. Vaping-related disorders 15
11. Chapter 11: Diseases of the Digestive System (KØØ-K95) 15
12. Chapter 12: Diseases of the Skin and Subcutaneous Tissue (LØØ-L99) 15
a. Pressure ulcer stage codes 15
b. Non-Pressure Chronic Ulcers 15
13. Chapter 13: Diseases of the Musculoskeletal System and Connective Tissue (MØØ-M99) 15
a. Site and laterality 15
b. Acute traumatic versus chronic or recurrent musculoskeletal conditions 16
c. Coding of Pathologic Fractures 16
d. Osteoporosis 16
e. Multisystem Inflammatory Syndrome 16
14. Chapter 14: Diseases of Genitourinary System (NØØ-N99) 16
a. Chronic kidney disease 16
15. Chapter 15: Pregnancy, Childbirth, and the Puerperium (OØØ-O9A) 16
a. General Rules for Obstetric Cases 16
b. Selection of OB Principal or First-listed Diagnosis 16
c. Pre-existing conditions versus conditions due to the pregnancy 17
d. Pre-existing hypertension in pregnancy 17
e. Fetal Conditions Affecting the Management of the Mother 17
f. HIV Infection in Pregnancy, Childbirth and the Puerperium 17
g. Diabetes mellitus in pregnancy 17
h. Long term use of insulin and oral hypoglycemics 17
i. Gestational (pregnancy induced) diabetes 17
j. Sepsis and septic shock complicating abortion, pregnancy, childbirth and the puerperium 17
k. Puerperal sepsis 17
l. Alcohol, tobacco and drug use during pregnancy, childbirth and the puerperium 17
m. Poisoning, toxic effects, adverse effects and underdosing in a pregnant patient 17
n. Normal Delivery, Code O8Ø 17
o. The Peripartum and Postpartum Periods 18
p. Code O94, Sequelae of complication of pregnancy, childbirth, and the puerperium 18
q. Termination of Pregnancy and Spontaneous abortions 18
r. Abuse in a pregnant patient 18
s. COVID-19 infection in pregnancy, childbirth, and the puerperium 18
16. Chapter 16: Certain Conditions Originating in the Perinatal Period (PØØ-P96) 18
a. General Perinatal Rules 18
b. Observation and Evaluation of Newborns for Suspected Conditions not Found 18
c. Coding Additional Perinatal Diagnoses 18
d. Prematurity and Fetal Growth Retardation 19
e. Low birth weight and immaturity status 19
f. Bacterial Sepsis of Newborn 19
g. Stillbirth 19
h. COVID-19 Infection in Newborn 19
17. Chapter 17: Congenital malformations, deformations, and chromosomal abnormalities (QØØ-QA1) 19
18. Chapter 18: Symptoms, signs, and abnormal clinical and laboratory findings, not elsewhere classified (RØØ-R99) 19
a. Use of symptom codes 19
b. Use of a symptom code with a definitive diagnosis code 19
c. Combination codes that include symptoms 19
d. Repeated falls 19
e. Coma 19
f. Functional quadriplegia 19
g. SIRS due to Non-Infectious Process 19
h. Death NOS 19
i. NIHSS Stroke Scale 19
19. Chapter 19: Injury, poisoning, and certain other consequences of external causes (SØØ-T88) 20
a. Application of 7th Characters in Chapter 19 20
b. Coding of Injuries 20
c. Coding of Traumatic Fractures 20
d. Coding of Burns and Corrosions 20
e. Adverse Effects, Poisoning, Underdosing and Toxic Effects 21
f. Adult and child abuse, neglect and other maltreatment 21
g. Complications of care 21
20. Chapter 20: External Causes of Morbidity (VØØ-Y99) 22
a. General External Cause Coding Guidelines 22
b. Place of Occurrence Guideline 22
c. Activity Code 22
d. Place of Occurrence, Activity, and Status Codes Used with other External Cause Code 22
e. If the Reporting Format Limits the Number of External Cause Codes 22
f. Multiple External Cause Coding Guidelines 22
g. Child and Adult Abuse Guideline 23
h. Unknown or Undetermined Intent Guideline 23
i. Sequelae (Late Effects) of External Cause Guidelines 23
j. Terrorism Guidelines 23
k. External Cause Status 23
21. Chapter 21: Factors influencing health status and contact with health services (ZØØ-Z99) 23
a. Use of Z Codes in Any Healthcare Setting 23
b. Z Codes Indicate a Reason for an Encounter or Provide Additional Information about a Patient Encounter 23
c. Categories of Z Codes 23
22. Chapter 22: Codes for Special Purposes (UØØ-U85) 27
Section II. Selection of Principal Diagnosis 27
A. Codes for symptoms, signs, and ill-defined conditions 27
B. Two or more interrelated conditions, each potentially meeting the definition for principal diagnosis. 27
C. Two or more diagnoses that equally meet the definition for principal diagnosis 27
D. Two or more comparative or contrasting conditions 27
E. A symptom(s) followed by contrasting/comparative diagnoses 27
F. Original treatment plan not carried out 27
G. Complications of surgery and other medical care 27
H. Uncertain Diagnosis 27
I. Admission from Observation Unit 27
1. Admission Following Medical Observation 27
2. Admission Following Post-Operative Observation 27
J. Admission from Outpatient Surgery 27
K. Admissions/Encounters for Rehabilitation 27
Section III. Reporting Additional Diagnoses 28
A. Previous conditions 28
B. Abnormal findings 28
C. Uncertain Diagnosis 28
Section IV. Diagnostic Coding and Reporting Guidelines for Outpatient Services 28
A. Selection of first-listed condition 28
1. Outpatient Surgery 28
2. Observation Stay 28
B. Codes from AØØ.Ø through T88.9, ZØØ-Z99, UØØ-U85 28
C. Accurate reporting of ICD-10-CM diagnosis codes 28
D. Codes that describe symptoms and signs 28
E. Encounters for circumstances other than a disease or injury 28
F. Level of Detail in Coding 28
1. ICD-10-CM codes with 3, 4, 5, 6 or 7 characters 28
2. Use of full number of characters required for a code 28
3. Highest level of specificity 28
G. ICD-1Ø-CM code for the diagnosis, condition, problem, or other reason for encounter/visit 28
H. Uncertain diagnosis 29
I. Chronic diseases 29
J. Code all documented conditions that coexist 29
K. Patients receiving diagnostic services only 29
L. Patients receiving therapeutic services only 29
M. Patients receiving preoperative evaluations only 29
N. Ambulatory surgery 29
O. Routine outpatient prenatal visits 29
P. Encounters for general medical examinations with abnormal findings 29
Q. Encounters for routine health screenings 29
Appendix I. Present on Admission Reporting Guidelines 29

Section I. Conventions, general coding guidelines and chapter specific guidelines

The conventions, general guidelines and chapter-specific guidelines are applicable to all health care settings unless otherwise indicated. The conventions and instructions of the classification take precedence over guidelines.

A. Conventions for the ICD-10-CM

The conventions for the ICD-10-CM are the general rules for use of the classification independent of the guidelines. These conventions are incorporated within the Alphabetic Index and Tabular List of the ICD-10-CM as instructional notes.

1. The Alphabetic Index and Tabular List

The ICD-10-CM is divided into the Alphabetic Index, an alphabetical list of terms and their corresponding code, and the Tabular List, a structured list of codes divided into chapters based on body system or condition. The Alphabetic Index consists of the following parts: the Index of Diseases and Injury, the Index of External Causes of Injury, the Table of Neoplasms and the Table of Drugs and Chemicals.

See Section I.C.2. Neoplasms

See Section I.C.19. Adverse effects, poisoning, underdosing and toxic effects

2. Format and Structure:

The ICD-10-CM Tabular List contains categories, subcategories and codes. Characters for categories, subcategories and codes may be either a letter or a number. All categories are 3 characters. A three-character category that has no further subdivision is equivalent to a code. Subcategories are either 4 or 5 characters. Codes may be 3, 4, 5, 6 or 7 characters. That is, each level of subdivision after a category is a subcategory. The final level of subdivision is a code. Codes that have applicable 7th characters are still referred to as codes, not subcategories. A code that has an applicable 7th character is considered invalid without the 7th character.

The ICD-10-CM uses an indented format for ease in reference.

3. **Use of codes for reporting purposes**
   For reporting purposes only codes are permissible, not categories or subcategories, and any applicable 7th character is required.

4. **Placeholder character**
   The ICD-10-CM utilizes a placeholder character "X". The "X" is used as a placeholder at certain codes to allow for future expansion. An example of this is at the poisoning, adverse effect and underdosing codes, categories T36-T50. Where a placeholder exists, the X must be used in order for the code to be considered a valid code.

5. **7th Characters**
   Certain ICD-10-CM categories have applicable 7th characters. The applicable 7th character is required for all codes within the category, or as the notes in the Tabular List instruct. The 7th character must always be the 7th character in the data field. If a code that requires a 7th character is not 6 characters, a placeholder X must be used to fill in the empty characters.

6. **Abbreviations**
   a. **Alphabetic Index abbreviations**
      NEC "Not elsewhere classifiable"
      This abbreviation in the Alphabetic Index represents "other specified." When a specific code is not available for a condition, the Alphabetic Index directs the coder to the "other specified" code in the Tabular List.
      NOS "Not otherwise specified"
      This abbreviation is the equivalent of unspecified.
   b. **Tabular List abbreviations**
      NEC "Not elsewhere classifiable"
      This abbreviation in the Tabular List represents "other specified". When a specific code is not available for a condition, the Tabular List includes an NEC entry under a code to identify the code as the "other specified" code.
      NOS "Not otherwise specified"
      This abbreviation is the equivalent of unspecified.

7. **Punctuation**
   [ ] Brackets are used in the Tabular List to enclose synonyms, alternative wording or explanatory phrases. Brackets are used in the Alphabetic Index to identify manifestation codes.
   ( ) Parentheses are used in both the Alphabetic Index and Tabular List to enclose supplementary words that may be present or absent in the statement of a disease or procedure without affecting the code number to which it is assigned. The terms within the parentheses are referred to as nonessential modifiers. The nonessential modifiers in the Alphabetic Index to Diseases apply to subterms following a main term except when a nonessential modifier and a subentry are mutually exclusive, the subentry takes precedence. For example, in the ICD-10-CM Alphabetic Index under the main term Enteritis, "acute" is a nonessential modifier and "chronic" is a subentry. In this case, the nonessential modifier "acute" does not apply to the subentry "chronic".
   : Colons are used in the Tabular List after an incomplete term which needs one or more of the modifiers following the colon to make it assignable to a given category.
   , **Commas are used in the Alphabetic Index and have different meanings based on the context of the Index entry, including alternate verbiage, modifier (essential and nonessential), or alternative for "and/or."**

8. **Use of "and".**
   See Section I.A.14. Use of the term "And"

9. **Other and Unspecified codes**
   a. **"Other" codes**
      Codes titled "other" or "other specified" are for use when the information in the medical record provides detail for which a specific code does not exist. Alphabetic Index entries with NEC in the line designate "other" codes in the Tabular List. These Alphabetic Index entries represent specific disease entities for which no specific code exists, so the term is included within an "other" code.
   b. **"Unspecified" codes**
      Codes titled "unspecified" are for use when the information in the medical record is insufficient to assign a more specific code. For those categories for 7 which an unspecified code is not provided, the "other specified" code may represent both other and unspecified.
      See Section I.B.18. Use of Signs/Symptom/Unspecified Codes

10. **Includes Notes**
    This note appears immediately under a three-character code title to further define, or give examples of, the content of the category.

11. **Inclusion terms**
    List of terms is included under some codes. These terms are the conditions for which that code is to be used. The terms may be synonyms of the code title, or, in the case of "other specified" codes, the terms are a list of the various conditions assigned to that code. The inclusion terms are not necessarily exhaustive.

Additional terms found only in the Alphabetic Index may also be assigned to a code.

12. **Excludes Notes**
    The ICD-10-CM has two types of excludes notes. Each type of note has a different definition for use, but they are all similar in that they indicate that codes excluded from each other are independent of each other.

    a. **Excludes1**
       A type 1 Excludes note is a pure excludes note. It means "NOT CODED HERE!" An Excludes1 note indicates that the code excluded should never be used at the same time as the code above the Excludes1 note. An Excludes1 is used when two conditions cannot occur together, such as a congenital form versus an acquired form of the same condition.

       An exception to the Excludes1 definition is the circumstance when the two conditions are unrelated to each other. If it is not clear whether the two conditions involving an Excludes1 note are related or not, query the provider. For example, code F45.8, Other somatoform disorders, has an Excludes1 note for "sleep related teeth grinding (G47.63)," because "teeth grinding" is an inclusion term under F45.8. Only one of these two codes should be assigned for teeth grinding. However psychogenic dysmenorrhea is also an inclusion term under F45.8, and a patient could have both this condition and sleep related teeth grinding. In this case, the two conditions are clearly unrelated to each other, and so it would be appropriate to report F45.8 and G47.63 together.

    b. **Excludes2**
       A type 2 Excludes note represents "Not included here." An excludes2 note indicates that the condition excluded is not part of the condition represented by the code, but a patient may have both conditions at the same time. When an Excludes2 note appears under a code, it is acceptable to use both the code and the excluded code together, when appropriate.

13. **Etiology/manifestation convention ("code first", "use additional code" and "in diseases classified elsewhere" notes)**
    Certain conditions have both an underlying etiology and multiple body system manifestations due to the underlying etiology. For such conditions, the ICD-10-CM has a coding convention that requires the underlying condition be sequenced first, if applicable, followed by the manifestation. Wherever such a combination exists, there is a "use additional code" note at the etiology code, and a "code first" note at the manifestation code. These instructional notes indicate the proper sequencing order of the codes, etiology followed by manifestation.

    In most cases the manifestation codes will have in the code title, "in diseases classified elsewhere." Codes with this title are a component of the etiology/manifestation convention. The code title indicates that it is a manifestation code. "In diseases classified elsewhere" codes are never permitted to be used as first listed or principal diagnosis codes. They must be used in conjunction with an underlying condition code and they must be listed following the underlying condition. See category F02, Dementia in other diseases classified elsewhere, for an example of this convention.

    There are manifestation codes that do not have "in diseases classified elsewhere" in the title. For such codes, there is a "use additional code" note at the etiology code and a "code first" note at the manifestation code, and the rules for sequencing apply.

    In addition to the notes in the Tabular List, these conditions also have a specific Alphabetic Index entry structure. In the Alphabetic Index both conditions are listed together with the etiology code first followed by the manifestation codes in brackets. The code in brackets is always to be sequenced second.

    An example of the etiology/manifestation convention is dementia with Parkinson's disease. In the Alphabetic Index, a code from category G20 is listed first, followed by code F02.80 or F02.81- in brackets. A code from category G20- represents the underlying etiology, Parkinson's disease, and must be sequenced first, whereas codes F02.80 and F02.81- represent the manifestation of dementia in diseases classified elsewhere, with or without behavioral disturbance.

    "Code first" and "Use additional code" notes are also used as sequencing rules in the classification for certain codes that are not part of an etiology/ manifestation combination.
    See Section I.B.7. Multiple coding for a single condition.

14. **"And"**
    The word "and" should be interpreted to mean either "and" or "or" when it appears in a title.

    For example, cases of "tuberculosis of bones", "tuberculosis of joints" and "tuberculosis of bones and joints" are classified to subcategory A18.0, Tuberculosis of bones and joints.

15. **"With"**
    The word "with" or "in" should be interpreted to mean "associated with" or "due to" when it appears in a code title, the Alphabetic Index (either under a main term or subterm), or an instructional note in the Tabular List. The classification presumes a causal relationship between the two conditions linked by these terms in the Alphabetic Index or Tabular List. These conditions should be coded as related even in the absence of provider documentation explicitly linking them, unless the documentation clearly states the conditions are unrelated or when another guideline exists that specifically requires a documented linkage between two conditions (e.g., sepsis guideline for "acute organ dysfunction that is not clearly associated with the sepsis").

For conditions not specifically linked by these relational terms in the classification or when a guideline requires that a linkage between two conditions be explicitly documented, provider documentation must link the conditions in order to code them as related.

The word "with" in the Alphabetic Index is sequenced immediately following the main term or subterm, not in alphabetical order.

16. "See" and "See Also"
The "see" instruction following a main term in the Alphabetic Index indicates that another term should be referenced. It is necessary to go to the main term referenced with the "see" note to locate the correct code.

A "see also" instruction following a main term in the Alphabetic Index instructs that there is another main term that may also be referenced that may provide additional Alphabetic Index entries that may be useful. It is not necessary to follow the "see also" note when the original main term provides the necessary code.

17. "Code also" note
A "code also" note instructs that two codes may be required to fully describe a condition, but this note does not provide sequencing direction. The sequencing depends on the circumstances of the encounter.

18. Default codes
A code listed next to a main term in the ICD-10-CM Alphabetic Index is referred to as a default code. The default code represents that condition that is most commonly associated with the main term or is the unspecified code for the condition. If a condition is documented in a medical record (for example, appendicitis) without any additional information, such as acute or chronic, the default code should be assigned.

19. Code assignment and Clinical Criteria
The assignment of a diagnosis code is based on the provider's diagnostic statement that the condition exists. The provider's statement that the patient has a particular condition is sufficient. Code assignment is not based on clinical criteria used by the provider to establish the diagnosis. If there is conflicting medical record documentation, query the provider.

B. General Coding Guidelines

1. Locating a code in the ICD-10-CM
To select a code in the classification that corresponds to a diagnosis or reason for visit documented in a medical record, first locate the term in the Alphabetic Index, and then verify the code in the Tabular List. Read and be guided by instructional notations that appear in both the Alphabetic Index and the Tabular List.

It is essential to use both the Alphabetic Index and Tabular List when locating and assigning a code. The Alphabetic Index does not always provide the full code. Selection of the full code, including laterality and any applicable 7th character can only be done in the Tabular List. A dash (-) at the end of an Alphabetic Index entry indicates that additional characters are required. Even if a dash is not included at the Alphabetic Index entry, it is necessary to refer to the Tabular List to verify that no 7th character is required.

2. Level of Detail in Coding
Diagnosis codes are to be used and reported at their highest number of characters available and to the highest level of specificity documented in the medical record.

ICD-10-CM diagnosis codes are composed of codes with 3, 4, 5, 6 or 7 characters. Codes with three characters are included in ICD-10-CM as the heading of a category of codes that may be further subdivided by the use of fourth and/or fifth characters and/or sixth characters, which provide greater detail.

A three-character code is to be used only if it is not further subdivided. A code is invalid if it has not been coded to the full number of characters required for that code, including the 7th character, if applicable.

3. Code or codes from A00.0 through T88.9, Z00-Z99.8, U00-U85
The appropriate code or codes from A00.0 through T88.9, Z00-Z99.8, and U00-U85 must be used to identify diagnoses, symptoms, conditions, problems, complaints or other reason(s) for the encounter/visit.

4. Signs and symptoms
Codes that describe symptoms and signs, as opposed to diagnoses, are acceptable for reporting purposes when a related definitive diagnosis has not been established (confirmed) by the provider. Chapter 18 of ICD-10-CM, Symptoms, Signs, and Abnormal Clinical and Laboratory Findings, Not Elsewhere Classified (codes R00.0-R99) contains many, but not all, codes for symptoms.

See Section I.B.18. Use of Signs/Symptom/Unspecified Codes

5. Conditions that are an integral part of a disease process
Signs and symptoms that are associated routinely with a disease process should not be assigned as additional codes, unless otherwise instructed by the classification.

6. Conditions that are not an integral part of a disease process
Additional signs and symptoms that may not be associated routinely with a disease process should be coded when present.

7. Multiple coding for a single condition
In addition to the etiology/manifestation convention that requires two codes to fully describe a single condition that affects multiple body systems, there are other single conditions that also require more than one code. "Use additional code" notes are found in the Tabular List at codes that are not part of an etiology/manifestation pair where a secondary code is useful to fully describe a condition. The sequencing rule is the same as the etiology/manifestation pair, "use additional code" indicates that a secondary code should be added, if known.

For example, for bacterial infections that are not included in chapter 1, a secondary code from category B95, Streptococcus, Staphylococcus, and Enterococcus, as the cause of diseases classified elsewhere, or B96, Other bacterial agents as the cause of diseases classified elsewhere, may be required to identify the bacterial organism causing the infection. A "use additional code" note will normally be found at the infectious disease code, indicating a need for the organism code to be added as a secondary code.

"Code first" notes are also under certain codes that are not specifically manifestation codes but may be due to an underlying cause. When there is a "code first" note and an underlying condition is present, the underlying condition should be sequenced first, if known.

"Code, if applicable, any causal condition first" notes indicate that this code may be assigned as a principal diagnosis when the causal condition is unknown or not applicable. If a causal condition is known, then the code for that condition should be sequenced as the principal or first-listed diagnosis.

Multiple codes may be needed for sequela, complication codes and obstetric codes to more fully describe a condition. See the specific guidelines for these conditions for further instruction.

8. Acute and Chronic Conditions
If the same condition is described as both acute (subacute) and chronic, and separate subentries exist in the Alphabetic Index at the same indentation level, code both and sequence the acute (subacute) code first.

9. Combination Code
A combination code is a single code used to classify:

    Two diagnoses, or

    A diagnosis with an associated secondary process (manifestation)

    A diagnosis with an associated complication

Combination codes are identified by referring to subterm entries in the Alphabetic Index and by reading the inclusion and exclusion notes in the Tabular List.

Assign only the combination code when that code fully identifies the diagnostic conditions involved or when the Alphabetic Index so directs. Multiple coding should not be used when the classification provides a combination code that clearly identifies all of the elements documented in the diagnosis. When the combination code lacks necessary specificity in describing the manifestation or complication, an additional code should be used as a secondary code.

10. Sequela (Late Effects)
A sequela is the residual effect (condition produced) after the acute phase of an illness or injury has terminated. There is no time limit on when a sequela code can be used. The residual may be apparent early, such as in cerebral infarction, or it may occur months or years later, such as that due to a previous injury. Examples of sequela include: scar formation resulting from a burn, deviated septum due to a nasal fracture, and infertility due to tubal occlusion from old tuberculosis. Coding of sequela generally requires two codes sequenced in the following order: the condition or nature of the sequela is sequenced first. The sequela code is sequenced second.

An exception to the above guidelines are those instances where the code for the sequela is followed by a manifestation code identified in the Tabular List and title, or the sequela code has been expanded (at the fourth, fifth or sixth character levels) to include the manifestation(s). The code for the acute phase of an illness or injury that led to the sequela is never used with a code for the late effect.

See Section I.C.9. Sequelae of cerebrovascular disease

See Section I.C.15. Sequelae of complication of pregnancy, childbirth and the puerperium

See Section I.C.19. Application of 7th characters for Chapter 19

11. Impending or Threatened Condition
Code any condition described at the time of discharge as "impending" or "threatened" as follows:

    If it did occur, code as confirmed diagnosis.

    If it did not occur, reference the Alphabetic Index to determine if the condition has a subentry term for "impending" or "threatened" and also reference main term entries for "Impending" and for "Threatened."

    If the subterms are listed, assign the given code.

    If the subterms are not listed, code the existing underlying condition(s) and not the condition described as impending or threatened.

12. Reporting Same Diagnosis Code More than Once
Each unique ICD-10-CM diagnosis code may be reported only once for an encounter. This applies to bilateral conditions when there are no distinct codes identifying laterality or two different conditions classified to the same ICD-10-CM diagnosis code.

13. Laterality
Some ICD-10-CM codes indicate laterality, specifying whether the condition occurs on the left, right or is bilateral. If no bilateral code is provided and the condition is bilateral, assign separate codes for both the left and right side. If the side is not identified in the medical record, assign the code for the unspecified side.

When a patient has a bilateral condition and each side is treated during separate encounters, assign the "bilateral" code (as the condition still exists on both sides), including for the encounter to treat the first side. For the second encounter for treatment after one side has previously been treated and the condition no longer exists on that side, assign the appropriate unilateral code for the side where the condition still exists (e.g., cataract surgery performed on each eye in separate encounters). The bilateral code would not be assigned for the subsequent encounter, as the patient no longer has the condition in the previously-treated site. If the treatment on the first side did not completely resolve the condition, then the bilateral code would still be appropriate.

When laterality is not documented by the patient's provider, code assignment for the affected side may be based on medical record documentation from other clinicians. If there is conflicting medical record documentation regarding the affected side, the patient's provider should be queried for clarification. Codes for "unspecified" side should rarely be used, such as when the documentation in the record is insufficient to determine the affected side and it is not possible to obtain clarification.

14. Documentation by Clinicians Other than the Patient's Provider

Code assignment is based on the documentation by the patient's provider (i.e., physician or other qualified healthcare practitioner legally accountable for establishing the patient's diagnosis). There are a few exceptions when code assignment may be based on medical record documentation from clinicians who are not the patient's provider (i.e., physician or other qualified healthcare practitioner legally accountable for establishing the patient's diagnosis). In this context, "clinicians" other than the patient's provider refer to healthcare professionals permitted, based on regulatory or accreditation requirements or internal hospital policies, to document in a patient's official medical record.

These exceptions include codes for:
- Body Mass Index (BMI)
- Depth of non-pressure chronic ulcers
- Pressure ulcer stage
- Coma scale
- NIH stroke scale (NIHSS)
- Social determinants of health (SDOH) classified to Chapter 21
- Laterality
- Blood alcohol level
- Underimmunization status
- **Firearm injury intent**

This information is typically, or may be, documented by other clinicians involved in the care of the patient (e.g., a dietitian often documents the BMI, a nurse often documents the pressure ulcer stages, and an emergency medical technician often documents the coma scale). However, the associated diagnosis (such as overweight, obesity, acute stroke, pressure ulcer, or a condition classifiable to category F10, Alcohol related disorders) must be documented by the patient's provider. If there is conflicting medical record documentation, either from the same clinician or different clinicians, the patient's provider should be queried for clarification.

The BMI, coma scale, NIHSS, blood alcohol level codes, codes for social determinants of health and underimmunization status should only be reported as secondary diagnoses.

See Section I.C.21.c.17. for additional information regarding coding social determinants of health.

15. Syndromes

Follow the Alphabetic Index guidance when coding syndromes. In the absence of Alphabetic Index guidance, assign codes for the documented manifestations of the syndrome. Additional codes for manifestations that are not an integral part of the disease process may also be assigned when the condition does not have a unique code.

16. Documentation of Complications of Care

Code assignment is based on the provider's documentation of the relationship between the condition and the care or procedure, unless otherwise instructed by the classification. The guideline extends to any complications of care, regardless of the chapter the code is located in. It is important to note that not all conditions that occur during or following medical care or surgery are classified as complications. There must be a cause-and-effect relationship between the care provided and the condition, and the documentation must support that the condition is clinically significant. It is not necessary for the provider to explicitly document the term "complication." For example, if the condition alters the course of the surgery as documented in the operative report, then it would be appropriate to report a complication code. Query the provider for clarification if the documentation is not clear as to the relationship between the condition and the care or procedure.

17. Borderline Diagnosis

If the provider documents a "borderline" diagnosis at the time of discharge, the diagnosis is coded as confirmed, unless the classification provides a specific entry (e.g., borderline diabetes). If a borderline condition has a specific index entry in ICD-10-CM, it should be coded as such. Since borderline conditions are not uncertain diagnoses, no distinction is made between the care setting (inpatient versus outpatient). Whenever the documentation is unclear regarding a borderline condition, coders are encouraged to query for clarification.

18. Use of Sign/Symptom/Unspecified Codes

Sign/symptom and "unspecified" codes have acceptable, even necessary, uses. While specific diagnosis codes should be reported when they are supported by the available medical record documentation and clinical knowledge of the patient's health condition, there are instances when signs/symptoms or unspecified codes are the best choices for accurately reflecting the healthcare encounter. Each healthcare encounter should be coded to the level of certainty known for that encounter.

As stated in the introductory section of these official coding guidelines, a joint effort between the healthcare provider and the coder is essential to achieve complete and accurate documentation, code assignment, and reporting of diagnoses and procedures. The importance of consistent, complete documentation in the medical record cannot be overemphasized. Without such documentation accurate coding cannot be achieved. The entire record should be reviewed to determine the specific reason for the encounter and the conditions treated.

If a definitive diagnosis has not been established by the end of the encounter, it is appropriate to report codes for sign(s) and/or symptom(s) in lieu of a definitive diagnosis. When sufficient clinical information isn't known or available about a particular health condition to assign a more specific code, it is acceptable to report the appropriate "unspecified" code (e.g., a diagnosis of pneumonia has been determined, but not the specific type). Unspecified codes should be reported when they are the codes that most accurately reflect what is known about the patient's condition at the time of that particular encounter. It would be inappropriate to select a specific code that is not supported by the medical record documentation or conduct medically unnecessary diagnostic testing in order to determine a more specific code.

19. Coding for Healthcare Encounters in Hurricane Aftermath

a. Use of External Cause of Morbidity Codes

An external cause of morbidity code should be assigned to identify the cause of the injury(ies) incurred as a result of the hurricane. The use of external cause of morbidity codes is supplemental to the application of ICD-10-CM codes. External cause of morbidity codes are never to be recorded as a principal diagnosis (first-listed in non-inpatient settings). The appropriate injury code should be sequenced before any external cause codes. The external cause of morbidity codes capture how the injury or health condition happened (cause), the intent (unintentional or accidental; or intentional, such as suicide or assault), the place where the event occurred, the activity of the patient at the time of the event, and the person's status (e.g., civilian, military). They should not be assigned for encounters to treat hurricane victims' medical conditions when no injury, adverse effect or poisoning is involved. External cause of morbidity codes should be assigned for each encounter for care and treatment of the injury. External cause of morbidity codes may be assigned in all health care settings. For the purpose of capturing complete and accurate ICD-10-CM data in the aftermath of the hurricane, a healthcare setting should be considered as any location where medical care is provided by licensed healthcare professionals.

b. Sequencing of External Causes of Morbidity Codes

Codes for cataclysmic events, such as a hurricane, take priority over all other external cause codes except child and adult abuse and terrorism and should be sequenced before other external cause of injury codes. Assign as many external cause of morbidity codes as necessary to fully explain each cause. For example, if an injury occurs as a result of a building collapse during the hurricane, external cause codes for both the hurricane and the building collapse should be assigned, with the external causes code for hurricane being sequenced as the first external cause code. For injuries incurred as a direct result of the hurricane, assign the appropriate code(s) for the injuries, followed by the code X37.0-, Hurricane (with the appropriate 7th character), and any other applicable external cause of injury codes. Code X37.0- also should be assigned when an injury is incurred as a result of flooding caused by a levee breaking related to the hurricane. Code X38.-, Flood (with the appropriate 7th character), should be assigned when an injury is from flooding resulting directly from the storm. Code X36.0-, Collapse of dam or man-made structure, should not be assigned when the cause of the collapse is due to the hurricane. Use of code X36.0- is limited to collapses of man-made structures due to earth surface movements, not due to storm surges directly from a hurricane.

c. Other External Causes of Morbidity Code Issues

For injuries that are not a direct result of the hurricane, such as an evacuee that has incurred an injury as a result of a motor vehicle accident, assign the appropriate external cause of morbidity code(s) to describe the cause of the injury, but do not assign code X37.0-, Hurricane. If it is not clear whether the injury was a direct result of the hurricane, assume the injury is due to the hurricane and assign code X37.0-, Hurricane, as well as any other applicable external cause of morbidity codes. In addition to code X37.0-, Hurricane, other possible applicable external cause of morbidity codes include:

X30-, Exposure to excessive natural heat
X31-, Exposure to excessive natural cold
X38-, Flood

d. Use of Z codes

Z codes (other reasons for healthcare encounters) may be assigned as appropriate to further explain the reasons for presenting for healthcare services, including transfers between healthcare facilities, or provide additional information relevant to a patient encounter. The ICD-10-CM Official Guidelines for Coding and Reporting identify which codes maybe assigned as principal or first-listed diagnosis only, secondary diagnosis only, or principal/first-listed or secondary (depending on the circumstances). Possible applicable Z codes include:

Z59.0-, Homelessness
Z59.1, Inadequate housing
Z59.5, Extreme poverty
Z75.1, Person awaiting admission to adequate facility elsewhere

Z75.3, Unavailability and inaccessibility of health-care facilities
Z75.4, Unavailability and inaccessibility of other helping agencies
Z76.2, Encounter for health supervision and care of other healthy infant and child
Z99.12, Encounter for respirator [ventilator] dependence during power failure

The external cause of morbidity codes and the Z codes listed above are not an all-inclusive list. Other codes may be applicable to the encounter based upon the documentation. Assign as many codes as necessary to fully explain each healthcare encounter. Since patient history information may be very limited, use any available documentation to assign the appropriate external cause of morbidity and Z codes.

20. **Multiple Sites Coding**
The classification defines "multiple" as involving two or more sites. Follow chapter-specific guidelines for assigning codes for "multiple sites." In the absence of chapter-specific guidelines, assign codes describing specified sites individually when documented. When the specified site(s) are not documented, assign the appropriate code for "multiple sites."

C. Chapter-Specific Coding Guidelines

In addition to general coding guidelines, there are guidelines for specific diagnoses and/or conditions in the classification. Unless otherwise indicated, these guidelines apply to all health care settings. Please refer to Section II for guidelines on the selection of principal diagnosis.

1. **Chapter 1: Certain Infectious and Parasitic Diseases (A00-B99), U07.1, U09.9**
   a. **Human Immunodeficiency Virus (HIV) Infections**
      1) **Code only confirmed cases**
         Code only confirmed cases of HIV infection/illness. This is an exception to the hospital inpatient guideline Section II, H.
         In this context, "confirmation" does not require documentation of positive serology or culture for HIV; the provider's diagnostic statement that the patient is HIV positive or has an HIV-related illness is sufficient.
      2) **Selection and sequencing of HIV codes**
         (a) *HIV disease*
             If the term "AIDS" or "HIV disease" is documented or if the patient is treated for any HIV-related illness or is described as having any condition(s) resulting from the patient's HIV positive status; code B20, Human immunodeficiency virus [HIV], should be assigned.
         (b) **Patient admitted for HIV-related condition**
             If a patient is admitted for an HIV-related condition, the principal diagnosis should be B20, Human immunodeficiency virus [HIV] disease followed by additional diagnosis codes for all reported HIV-related conditions.
             An exception to this guideline is if the reason for admission is hemolytic-uremic syndrome associated with HIV disease. Assign code D59.31, Infection- associated hemolytic-uremic syndrome, followed by code B20, Human immunodeficiency virus [HIV] disease.
         (c) **Patient with HIV disease admitted for unrelated condition**
             If a patient with HIV disease is admitted for an unrelated condition (such as a traumatic injury), the code for the unrelated condition (e.g., the nature of injury code) should be the principal diagnosis. **Code B20 would be reported as a secondary diagnosis. Codes for other documented conditions should also be reported as secondary diagnoses.**
         (d) *Patient newly diagnosed with HIV disease*
             Whether the patient is newly diagnosed or has had previous admissions/encounters for HIV conditions is irrelevant to the sequencing decision.
         (e) **Asymptomatic human immunodeficiency virus**
             When "HIV positive," "HIV test positive," or similar terminology is documented, and there is no documentation of symptoms or HIV-related illness, code Z21, Asymptomatic human immunodeficiency virus [HIV] infection status, should be assigned.
         (f) *Inconclusive HIV serology*
             Patients with documentation of inconclusive HIV serology, may be assigned code R75, Inconclusive laboratory evidence of human immunodeficiency virus [HIV].
         (g) *Previously diagnosed HIV-related illness*
             Patients with documentation of a prior diagnosis of an HIV-related illness should be coded to B20. Once an HIV-related illness has developed, code B20 should always be assigned on every subsequent admission/encounter. Patients previously diagnosed with any HIV illness (B20) should never be assigned to R75, Inconclusive laboratory evidence of human immunodeficiency virus [HIV] or Z21, Asymptomatic human immunodeficiency virus [HIV] infection status.

      (h) **HIV Infection in Pregnancy, Childbirth and the Puerperium**
          When a patient presents during pregnancy, childbirth or the puerperium with documented symptomatic HIV disease or an HIV related illness, assign a code from subcategory O98.7, Human immunodeficiency [HIV] disease complicating pregnancy, childbirth and the puerperium, followed by code B20 and additional code(s) for any HIV-related illness(es). Codes from Chapter 15 always take sequencing priority.
          When a patient presents during pregnancy, childbirth or the puerperium with documented asymptomatic HIV infection status or is HIV-positive, assign a code from subcategory O98.7 followed by code Z21.
      (i) *Encounters for HIV testing*
          If a patient without signs or symptoms is tested for HIV, assign code Z11.4, Encounter for screening for human immunodeficiency virus [HIV]. Use additional codes for any associated high-risk behavior, if applicable.
          If a patient with signs or symptoms of HIV presents for HIV testing, code the signs and symptoms. An additional counseling code Z71.7, Human immunodeficiency virus [HIV] counseling, may be assigned if counseling is provided during the encounter for the test. Code Z11.4, Encounter for screening for human immunodeficiency virus [HIV], should not be assigned if HIV signs or symptoms are present.
          When a patient presents for follow up regarding their HIV test results and the test result is negative, assign code Z71.7, Human immunodeficiency virus [HIV] counseling.
          If the results are positive, see previous guidelines and assign codes as appropriate.
      (j) *HIV disease or HIV positive status managed by antiretroviral medication*
          If a patient with documented HIV disease, HIV-related illness or AIDS is currently managed on antiretroviral medications, assign code B20, Human immunodeficiency virus [HIV] disease.
          If a patient with documented HIV positive status is currently managed on antiretroviral medication, assign code Z21, Asymptomatic human immunodeficiency virus [HIV] infection status, in the absence of any additional documentation of HIV disease, HIV-related illness or AIDS.
          Code Z79.899, Other long term (current) drug therapy, may be assigned as an additional code to identify the long-term (current) use of antiretroviral medications.
      (k) **Encounter for HIV Prophylaxis Measures**
          When a patient is seen for administration of pre-exposure prophylaxis medication for HIV, assign code Z29.81, Encounter for HIV pre-exposure prophylaxis. Pre-exposure prophylaxis (PrEP) is intended to prevent infection in people who are at risk for getting HIV through sex or injection drug use. Any risk factors for HIV should also be coded.
   b. **Infectious agents as the cause of diseases classified to other chapters**
      Certain infections are classified in chapters other than Chapter 1 and no organism is identified as part of the infection code. In these instances, it is necessary to use an additional code from Chapter 1 to identify the organism. A code from category B95, Streptococcus, Staphylococcus, and Enterococcus as the cause of diseases classified to other chapters, B96, Other bacterial agents as the cause of diseases classified to other chapters, or B97, Viral agents as the cause of diseases classified to other chapters, is to be used as an additional code to identify the organism. An instructional note will be found at the infection code advising that an additional organism code is required.
   c. **Infections resistant to antibiotics**
      Many bacterial infections are resistant to current antibiotics. It is necessary to identify all infections documented as antibiotic resistant. Assign a code from category Z16, Resistance to antimicrobial drugs, following the infection code only if the infection code does not identify drug resistance.
   d. **Sepsis, Severe Sepsis, and Septic Shock Infections resistant to antibiotics**
      1) **Coding of Sepsis and Severe Sepsis**
         (a) **Sepsis**
             For a diagnosis of sepsis, assign the appropriate code for the underlying systemic infection. If the type of infection or causal organism is not further specified, assign code A41.9, Sepsis, unspecified organism.
             A code from subcategory R65.2, Severe sepsis, should not be assigned unless severe sepsis or an associated acute organ dysfunction is documented.
             (i) **Negative or inconclusive blood cultures and sepsis**
                 Negative or inconclusive blood cultures do not preclude a diagnosis of sepsis in patients with clinical evidence of the condition; however, the provider should be queried.

(ii) Urosepsis

The term urosepsis is a nonspecific term. It is not to be considered synonymous with sepsis. It has no default code in the Alphabetic Index. Should a provider use this term, he/she must be queried for clarification.

(iii) Sepsis with organ dysfunction

If a patient has sepsis and associated acute organ dysfunction or multiple organ dysfunction (MOD), follow the instructions for coding severe sepsis.

(iv) Acute organ dysfunction that is not clearly associated with the sepsis

If a patient has sepsis and an acute organ dysfunction, but the medical record documentation indicates that the acute organ dysfunction is related to a medical condition other than the sepsis, do not assign a code from subcategory R65.2, Severe sepsis. An acute organ dysfunction must be associated with the sepsis in order to assign the severe sepsis code. If the documentation is not clear as to whether an acute organ dysfunction is related to the sepsis or another medical condition, query the provider.

(b) Severe sepsis

The coding of severe sepsis requires a minimum of 2 codes: first a code for the underlying systemic infection, followed by a code from subcategory R65.2, Severe sepsis. If the causal organism is not documented, assign code A41.9, Sepsis, unspecified organism, for the infection. Additional code(s) for the associated acute organ dysfunction are also required.

Due to the complex nature of severe sepsis, some cases may require querying the provider prior to assignment of the codes.

2) Septic shock

Septic shock generally refers to circulatory failure associated with severe sepsis, and therefore, it represents a type of acute organ dysfunction.

For cases of septic shock, the code for the systemic infection should be sequenced first, followed by code R65.21, Severe sepsis with septic shock or code T81.12, Postprocedural septic shock.

Any additional codes for the other acute organ dysfunctions should also be assigned. As noted in the sequencing instructions in the Tabular List, the code for septic shock cannot be assigned as a principal diagnosis.

3) Sequencing of severe sepsis

If severe sepsis is present on admission, and meets the definition of principal diagnosis, the underlying systemic infection should be assigned as principal diagnosis followed by the appropriate code from subcategory R65.2 as required by the sequencing rules in the Tabular List. A code from subcategory R65.2 can never be assigned as a principal diagnosis.

When severe sepsis develops during an encounter (it was not present on admission), the underlying systemic infection and the appropriate code from subcategory R65.2 should be assigned as secondary diagnoses.

Severe sepsis may be present on admission, but the diagnosis may not be confirmed until sometime after admission. If the documentation is not clear whether severe sepsis was present on admission, the provider should be queried.

For infection-associated hemolytic-uremic syndrome with severe sepsis, see guideline I.C.1.d.9.

4) Sepsis or severe sepsis with a localized infection

If the reason for admission is sepsis or severe sepsis and a localized infection, such as pneumonia or cellulitis, a code(s) for the underlying systemic infection should be assigned first and the code for the localized infection should be assigned as a secondary diagnosis. If the patient has severe sepsis, a code from subcategory R65.2 should also be assigned as a secondary diagnosis. If the patient is admitted with a localized infection, such as pneumonia, and sepsis/severe sepsis doesn't develop until after admission, the localized infection should be assigned first, followed by the appropriate sepsis/severe sepsis codes.

For hemolytic-uremic syndrome associated with sepsis, see guideline I.C.1.d.9.

5) Sepsis due to a postprocedural infection

(a) Documentation of causal relationship

As with all postprocedural complications, code assignment is based on the provider's documentation of the relationship between the infection and the procedure.

(b) Sepsis due to a postprocedural infection

For sepsis following a postprocedural wound (surgical site) infection, a code from T81.41 to T81.43, Infection following a procedure, T81.49, Infection following a procedure, other surgical site, or a code from O86.00 to O86.03, Infection of obstetric surgical wound, or code O86.09, Infection of obstetric surgical wound, other surgical site, that identifies the site of the infection should be sequenced first, if known. Assign an additional code for sepsis following a procedure (T81.44) or sepsis following an obstetrical procedure (O86.04). Use an additional code to identify the infectious agent. If the patient has severe sepsis, the appropriate code from subcategory R65.2 should also be assigned with the additional code(s) for any acute organ dysfunction.

For infections following infusion, transfusion, therapeutic injection, or immunization, a code from subcategory T80.2, Infections following infusion, transfusion, and therapeutic injection, or code T88.0-, Infection following immunization, should be coded first, followed by the code for the specific infection. If the patient has severe sepsis, the appropriate code from subcategory R65.2 should also be assigned, with the additional codes(s) for any acute organ dysfunction.

(c) Postprocedural infection and postprocedural septic shock

If a postprocedural infection has resulted in postprocedural septic shock, assign the codes indicated above for sepsis due to a postprocedural infection, followed by code T81.12-, Postprocedural septic shock. Do not assign code R65.21, Severe sepsis with septic shock. Additional code(s) should be assigned for any acute organ dysfunction.

6) Sepsis and severe sepsis associated with a noninfectious process (condition)

In some cases, a noninfectious process (condition) such as trauma, may lead to an infection which can result in sepsis or severe sepsis. If sepsis or severe sepsis is documented as associated with a noninfectious condition, such as a burn or serious injury, and this condition meets the definition for principal diagnosis, the code for the noninfectious condition should be sequenced first, followed by the code for the resulting infection. If severe sepsis is present, a code from subcategory R65.2 should also be assigned with any associated organ dysfunction(s) codes. It is not necessary to assign a code from subcategory R65.1, Systemic inflammatory response syndrome (SIRS) of non-infectious origin, for these cases.

If the infection meets the definition of principal diagnosis, it should be sequenced before the non-infectious condition. When both the associated non-infectious condition and the infection meet the definition of principal diagnosis, either may be assigned as principal diagnosis.

Only one code from category R65, Symptoms and signs specifically associated with systemic inflammation and infection, should be assigned. Therefore, when a non-infectious condition leads to an infection resulting in severe sepsis, assign the appropriate code from subcategory R65.2, Severe sepsis. Do not additionally assign a code from subcategory R65.1, Systemic inflammatory response syndrome (SIRS) of non-infectious origin.

See Section I.C.18. SIRS due to non-infectious process

7) Sepsis and septic shock complicating abortion, pregnancy, childbirth, and the puerperium

See Section I.C.15. Sepsis and septic shock complicating abortion, pregnancy, childbirth and the puerperium

8) Newborn sepsis

See Section I.C.16. f. Bacterial sepsis of Newborn

9) Hemolytic-uremic syndrome associated with sepsis

If the reason for admission is hemolytic-uremic syndrome that is associated with sepsis, assign code D59.31, Infection-associated hemolytic-uremic syndrome, as the principal diagnosis. Codes for the underlying systemic infection and any other conditions (such as severe sepsis) should be assigned as secondary diagnoses.

e. Methicillin Resistant Staphylococcus aureus (MRSA) Conditions

1) Selection and sequencing of MRSA codes

(a) Combination codes for MRSA infection

When a patient is diagnosed with an infection that is due to methicillin resistant *Staphylococcus aureus* (MRSA), and that infection has a combination code that includes the causal organism (e.g., sepsis, pneumonia) assign the appropriate combination code for the condition (e.g., code A41.02, Sepsis due to Methicillin resistant Staphylococcus aureus or code J15.212, Pneumonia due to Methicillin resistant Staphylococcus aureus). Do not assign code B95.62, Methicillin resistant Staphylococcus aureus infection as the cause of diseases classified elsewhere, as an additional code, because the combination code includes the type of infection and the MRSA organism. Do not assign a code from subcategory Z16.11, Resistance to penicillins, as an additional diagnosis.

See Section C.1. for instructions on coding and sequencing of sepsis and severe sepsis

(b) Other codes for MRSA infection

When there is documentation of a current infection (e.g., wound infection, stitch abscess, urinary tract infection) due to MRSA, and that infection does not have a combination code that includes the causal organism, assign the appropriate code to identify the condition along with code B95.62, Methicillin resistant Staphylococcus aureus infection as the cause of diseases classified elsewhere for the MRSA infection. Do not assign a code from subcategory Z16.11, Resistance to penicillins.

(c) **Methicillin susceptible Staphylococcus aureus (MSSA) and MRSA colonization**

The condition or state of being colonized or carrying MSSA or MRSA is called colonization or carriage, while an individual person is described as being colonized or being a carrier.

Colonization means that MSSA or MSRA is present on or in the body without necessarily causing illness. A positive MRSA colonization test might be documented by the provider as "MRSA screen positive" or "MRSA nasal swab positive".

Assign code Z22.322, Carrier or suspected carrier of Methicillin resistant Staphylococcus aureus, for patients documented as having MRSA colonization. Assign code Z22.321, Carrier or suspected carrier of Methicillin susceptible Staphylococcus aureus, for patients documented as having MSSA colonization. Colonization is not necessarily indicative of a disease process or as the cause of a specific condition the patient may have unless documented as such by the provider.

(d) **MRSA colonization and infection**

If a patient is documented as having both MRSA colonization and infection during a hospital admission, code Z22.322, Carrier or suspected carrier of Methicillin resistant Staphylococcus aureus, and a code for the MRSA infection may both be assigned.

f. **Zika virus infections**

1) **Code only confirmed cases**

Code only a confirmed diagnosis of Zika virus (A92.5, Zika virus disease) as documented by the provider. This is an exception to the hospital inpatient guideline Section II, H. In this context, "confirmation" does not require documentation of the type of test performed; the provider's diagnostic statement that the condition is confirmed is sufficient. This code should be assigned regardless of the stated mode of transmission.

If the provider documents "suspected", "possible" or "probable" Zika, do not assign code A92.5. Assign a code(s) explaining the reason for encounter (such as fever, rash, or joint pain) or Z20.821, Contact with and (suspected) exposure to Zika virus.

g. **Coronavirus infections**

1) **COVID-19 infection (infection due to SARS-CoV-2)**

(a) **Code only confirmed cases**

Code only a confirmed diagnosis of the 2019 novel coronavirus disease (COVID-19) as documented by the provider. For a confirmed diagnosis, assign code U07.1, COVID-19. This is an exception to the hospital inpatient guideline Section II, H. In this context, "confirmation" does not require documentation of a positive test result for COVID-19; the provider's documentation that the individual has COVID-19 is sufficient.

If the provider documents "suspected," "possible," "probable," or "inconclusive" COVID-19, do not assign code U07.1. Instead, code the signs and symptoms reported. See guideline I.C.1.g.1.g.

(b) **Sequencing of codes**

When COVID-19 meets the definition of principal diagnosis, code U07.1, COVID-19, should be sequenced first, followed by the appropriate codes for associated manifestations, except when another guideline requires that certain codes be sequenced first, such as obstetrics, sepsis, or transplant complications.

For a COVID-19 infection that progresses to sepsis, see Section I.C.1.d. Sepsis, Severe Sepsis, and Septic Shock

See Section I.C.15.s. for COVID-19 infection in pregnancy, childbirth, and the puerperium

See Section I.C.16.h. for COVID-19 infection in newborn

For a COVID-19 infection in a lung transplant patient, see Section I.C.19.g.3.a. Transplant complications other than kidney.

(c) **Acute respiratory manifestations of COVID-19**

When the reason for the encounter/admission is a respiratory manifestation of COVID-19, assign code U07.1, COVID-19, as the principal/first-listed diagnosis and assign code(s) for the respiratory manifestation(s) as additional diagnoses.

The following conditions are examples of common respiratory manifestations of COVID-19.

(i) **Pneumonia**

For a patient with pneumonia confirmed as due to COVID-19, assign codes U07.1, COVID-19, and J12.82, Pneumonia due to coronavirus disease 2019.

(ii) **Acute bronchitis**

For a patient with acute bronchitis confirmed as due to COVID-19, assign codes U07.1, and J20.8, Acute bronchitis due to other specified organisms. Bronchitis not otherwise specified (NOS) due to COVID-19 should be coded using code U07.1 and J40, Bronchitis, not specified as acute or chronic.

(iii) **Lower respiratory infection**

If the COVID-19 is documented as being associated with a lower respiratory infection, not otherwise specified (NOS), or an acute respiratory infection, NOS, codes U07.1 and J22, Unspecified acute lower respiratory infection, should be assigned.

If the COVID-19 is documented as being associated with a respiratory infection, NOS, codes U07.1 and J98.8, Other specified respiratory disorders, should be assigned.

(iv) **Acute respiratory distress syndrome**

For acute respiratory distress syndrome (ARDS) due to COVID-19, assign codes U07.1, and J80, Acute respiratory distress syndrome.

(v) **Acute respiratory failure**

For acute respiratory failure due to COVID-19, assign code U07.1, and code J96.0-, Acute respiratory failure.

(d) **Non-respiratory manifestations of COVID-19**

When the reason for the encounter/admission is a non-respiratory manifestation (e.g., viral enteritis) of COVID-19, assign code U07.1, COVID-19, as the principal/first-listed diagnosis and assign code(s) for the manifestation(s) as additional diagnoses.

(e) **Exposure to COVID-19**

For asymptomatic individuals with actual or suspected exposure to COVID-19, assign code Z20.822, Contact with and (suspected) exposure to COVID-19.

For symptomatic individuals with actual or suspected exposure to COVID-19 and the infection has been ruled out, or test results are inconclusive or unknown, assign code Z20.822, Contact with and (suspected) exposure to COVID-19. See guideline I.C.21.c.1, Contact/Exposure, for additional guidance regarding the use of category Z20 codes.

If COVID-19 is confirmed, see guideline I.C.1.g.1.a.

(f) **Screening for COVID-19**

For screening for COVID-19, including preoperative testing, assign code Z11.52, Encounter for screening for COVID-19.

(g) **Signs and symptoms without definitive diagnosis of COVID-19**

For patients presenting with any signs/symptoms associated with COVID-19 (such as fever, etc.) but a definitive diagnosis has not been established, assign the appropriate code(s) for each of the presenting signs and symptoms such as:
- R05.1, Acute cough, or R05.9, Cough, unspecified
- R06.02 Shortness of breath
- R50.9 Fever, unspecified

If a patient with signs/symptoms associated with COVID-19 also has an actual or suspected contact with or exposure to COVID-19, assign Z20.822, Contact with and (suspected) exposure to COVID-19, as an additional code.

(h) **Asymptomatic individuals who test positive for COVID-19**

For asymptomatic individuals who test positive for COVID-19 and there is no provider documentation of a diagnosis of COVID-19, query the provider as to whether or not the individual has COVID-19. A false positive laboratory test is possible, and it is the provider's responsibility to confirm the diagnosis and document accordingly.

(i) **Personal history of COVID-19**

For patients with a history of COVID-19, assign code Z86.16, Personal history of COVID-19.

(j) **Follow-up visits after COVID-19 infection has resolved**

For individuals who previously had COVID-19, without residual symptom(s) or condition(s), and are being seen for follow-up evaluation, and COVID-19 test results are negative, assign codes Z09, Encounter for follow-up examination after completed treatment for conditions other than malignant neoplasm, and Z86.16, Personal history of COVID-19.

For follow-up visits for individuals with symptom(s) or condition(s) related to a previous COVID-19 infection, see guideline I.C.1.g.1.m.

See Section I.C.21.c.8, Factors influencing health states and contact with health services, Follow-up

(k) **Encounter for antibody testing**

For an encounter for antibody testing that is not being performed to confirm a current COVID-19 infection, nor is a follow-up test after resolution of COVID-19, assign Z01.84, Encounter for antibody response examination.

Follow the applicable guidelines above if the individual is being tested to confirm a current COVID-19 infection.

For follow-up testing after a COVID-19 infection, see guideline I.C.1.g.1.j.

(l) **Multisystem Inflammatory Syndrome**

For individuals with multisystem inflammatory syndrome (MIS) and COVID-19, assign code U07.1, COVID-19, as the principal/first-listed diagnosis and assign code M35.81, Multisystem inflammatory syndrome, as an additional diagnosis.

If an individual with a history of COVID-19 develops MIS, assign codes M35.81, Multisystem inflammatory syndrome, and U09.9, Post COVID-19 condition, unspecified.

If an individual with a known or suspected exposure to COVID-19, and no current COVID-19 infection or history of COVID-19, develops MIS, assign codes M35.81, Multisystem inflammatory syndrome, and Z20.822, Contact with and (suspected) exposure to COVID-19.

Additional codes should be assigned for any associated complications of MIS.

(m) **Post COVID-19 Condition**

For sequela of COVID-19, or associated symptoms or conditions that develop following a previous COVID-19 infection, assign a code(s) for the specific symptom(s) or condition(s) related to the previous COVID-19 infection, if known, and code U09.9, Post COVID-19 condition, unspecified.

Code U09.9 should not be assigned for manifestations of an active (current) COVID-19 infection.

If a patient has a condition(s) associated with a previous COVID-19 infection and develops a new active (current) COVID-19 infection, code U09.9 may be assigned in conjunction with code U07.1, COVID-19, to identify that the patient also has a condition(s) associated with a previous COVID-19 infection. Code(s) for the specific condition(s) associated with the previous COVID-19 infection and code(s) for manifestation(s) of the new active (current) COVID-19 infection should also be assigned.

(n) **Underimmunization for COVID-19 Status**

Code Z28.310, Unvaccinated for COVID-19, may be assigned when the patient has not received a COVID-19 vaccine of any type. Code Z28.311, Partially vaccinated for COVID-19, may be assigned when the patient has been partially vaccinated for COVID-19 as per the recommendations of the Centers for Disease Control and Prevention (CDC) in place at the time of the encounter. For information, visit the CDC's website https://www.cdc.gov/covidschedule.

See Section I.B.14. for underimmunization documentation by clinicians other than patient's provider.

2. **Chapter 2: Neoplasms (C00-D49)**
   General Guidelines

Chapter 2 of the ICD-10-CM contains the codes for most benign and all malignant neoplasms. Certain benign neoplasms, such as prostatic adenomas, may be found in the specific body system chapters. To properly code a neoplasm, it is necessary to determine from the record if the neoplasm is benign, in-situ, malignant, or of uncertain histologic behavior. If malignant, any secondary (metastatic) sites should also be determined.

Primary malignant neoplasms overlapping site boundaries

A primary malignant neoplasm that overlaps two or more contiguous (next to each other) sites should be classified to the subcategory/code .8 ('overlapping lesion'), unless the combination is specifically indexed elsewhere. For multiple neoplasms of the same site that are not contiguous such as tumors in different quadrants of the same breast, codes for each site should be assigned.

Malignant neoplasm of ectopic tissue

Malignant neoplasms of ectopic tissue are to be coded to the site of origin mentioned, e.g., ectopic pancreatic malignant neoplasms involving the stomach are coded to malignant neoplasm of pancreas, unspecified (C25.9).

The neoplasm table in the Alphabetic Index should be referenced first. However, if the histological term is documented, that term should be referenced first, rather than going immediately to the Neoplasm Table, in order to determine which column in the Neoplasm Table is appropriate. For example, if the documentation indicates "adenoma," refer to the term in the Alphabetic Index to review the entries under this term and the instructional note to "see also neoplasm, by site, benign." The table provides the proper code based on the type of neoplasm and the site. It is important to select the proper column in the table that corresponds to the type of neoplasm. The Tabular List should then be referenced to verify that the correct code has been selected from the table and that a more specific site code does not exist.

See Section I.C.21. Factors influencing health status and contact with health services, Status, for information regarding Z15.0, codes for genetic susceptibility to cancer.

a. **Admission/Encounter for treatment of primary site**

If the malignancy is chiefly responsible for occasioning the patient admission/encounter and treatment is directed at the primary site, designate the primary malignancy as the principal/first-listed diagnosis.

The only exception to this guideline is if the administration of chemotherapy, immunotherapy or external beam radiation therapy is chiefly responsible for occasioning the admission/encounter. In that case, assign the appropriate Z51.-- code as the first-listed or principal diagnosis, and the underlying diagnosis or problem for which the service is being performed as a secondary diagnosis.

b. **Admission/Encounter for treatment of secondary site**

When a patient is admitted because of a primary neoplasm with metastasis and treatment is directed toward the secondary site only, the secondary neoplasm is designated as the principal diagnosis even though the primary malignancy is still present.

c. **Coding and sequencing of complications**

Coding and sequencing of complications associated with the malignancies or with the therapy thereof are subject to the following guidelines:

1) **Anemia associated with malignancy**

When admission/encounter is for management of an anemia associated with the malignancy, and the treatment is only for anemia, the appropriate code for the malignancy is sequenced as the principal or first-listed diagnosis followed by the appropriate code for the anemia (such as code D63.0, Anemia in neoplastic disease).

2) **Anemia associated with chemotherapy, immunotherapy and radiation therapy**

When the admission/encounter is for management of an anemia associated with an adverse effect of the administration of chemotherapy or immunotherapy and the only treatment is for the anemia, the anemia code is sequenced first followed by the appropriate codes for the neoplasm and the adverse effect (T45.1X5-, Adverse effect of antineoplastic and immunosuppressive drugs).

When the admission/encounter is for management of an anemia associated with an adverse effect of radiotherapy, the anemia code should be sequenced first, followed by the appropriate neoplasm code and code Y84.2, Radiological procedure and radiotherapy as the cause of abnormal reaction of the patient, or of later complication, without mention of misadventure at the time of the procedure.

3) **Management of dehydration due to the malignancy**

When the admission/encounter is for management of dehydration due to the malignancy and only the dehydration is being treated (intravenous rehydration), the dehydration is sequenced first, followed by the code(s) for the malignancy.

4) **Treatment of a complication resulting from a surgical procedure**

When the admission/encounter is for treatment of a complication resulting from a surgical procedure, designate the complication as the principal or first-listed diagnosis if treatment is directed at resolving the complication.

d. **Primary malignancy previously excised**

When a primary malignancy has been previously excised or eradicated from its site and there is no further treatment directed to that site and there is no evidence of any existing primary malignancy at that site, a code from category Z85, Personal history of malignant neoplasm, should be used to indicate the former site of the malignancy. Any mention of extension, invasion, or metastasis to another site is coded as a secondary malignant neoplasm to that site. The secondary site may be the principal or first-listed diagnosis with the Z85 code used as a secondary code.

See section I.C.2.t. Secondary malignant neoplasm of lymphoid tissue.

e. *Admissions/Encounters involving antineoplastic chemotherapy, immunotherapy and radiation therapy*

1) **Episode of care involves surgical removal of neoplasm**

When an episode of care involves the surgical removal of a neoplasm, primary or secondary site, followed by adjunct chemotherapy or radiation treatment during the same episode of care, the code for the neoplasm should be assigned as principal or first-listed diagnosis.

2) *Patient admission/encounter chiefly for administration of antineoplastic chemotherapy, immunotherapy and radiation therapy*

If a patient admission/encounter is chiefly for the administration of chemotherapy, immunotherapy or external beam radiation therapy **for the treatment of a neoplasm,** assign code Z51.0, Encounter for antineoplastic radiation therapy, or Z51.11, Encounter for antineoplastic chemotherapy, or Z51.12, Encounter for antineoplastic immunotherapy as the first-listed or principal diagnosis. **If the reason for the encounter is more than one type of antineoplastic therapy, code Z51.0 and codes from subcategory Z51.1 may be assigned together, in which case one of these codes would be reported as a secondary diagnosis.**

The malignancy for which the therapy is being administered should be assigned as a secondary diagnosis.

If a patient admission/encounter is for the insertion or implantation of radioactive elements (e.g., brachytherapy) the appropriate code for the malignancy is sequenced as the principal or first-listed diagnosis. Code Z51.0 should not be assigned.

3) **Patient admitted for radiation therapy, chemotherapy or immunotherapy and develops complications**

When a patient is admitted for the purpose of external beam radiotherapy, immunotherapy or chemotherapy and develops complications such as uncontrolled nausea and vomiting or dehydration, the principal or first-listed diagnosis is Z51.0, Encounter for antineoplastic radiation therapy, or Z51.11, Encounter for antineoplastic chemotherapy, or Z51.12, Encounter for antineoplastic immunotherapy followed by any codes for the complications.

When a patient is admitted for the purpose of insertion or implantation of radioactive elements (e.g., brachytherapy) and develops complications such as uncontrolled nausea and vomiting or dehydration, the principal or first-listed diagnosis is the appropriate code for the malignancy followed by any codes for the complications.

f. **Admission/encounter to determine extent of malignancy**
When the reason for admission/encounter is to determine the extent of the malignancy, or for a procedure such as paracentesis or thoracentesis, the primary malignancy or appropriate metastatic site is designated as the principal or first-listed diagnosis, even though chemotherapy or radiotherapy is administered.

g. **Symptoms, signs, and abnormal findings listed in Chapter 18 associated with neoplasms**
Symptoms, signs, and ill-defined conditions listed in Chapter 18 characteristic of, or associated with, an existing primary or secondary site malignancy cannot be used to replace the malignancy as principal or first-listed diagnosis, regardless of the number of admissions or encounters for treatment and care of the neoplasm.
See section I.C.21. Factors influencing health status and contact with health services, Encounter for prophylactic organ removal.

h. **Admission/encounter for pain control/management**
See Section I.C.6. for information on coding admission/encounter for pain control/management.

i. **Malignancy in two or more noncontiguous sites**
A patient may have more than one malignant tumor in the same organ. These tumors may represent different primaries or metastatic disease, depending on the site. Should the documentation be unclear, the provider should be queried as to the status of each tumor so that the correct codes can be assigned.

j. **Disseminated malignant neoplasm, unspecified**
Code C80.0, Disseminated malignant neoplasm, unspecified, is for use only in those cases where the patient has advanced metastatic disease and no known primary or secondary sites are specified. It should not be used in place of assigning codes for the primary site and all known secondary sites.

k. **Malignant neoplasm without specification of site**
Code C80.1, Malignant (primary) neoplasm, unspecified, equates to Cancer, unspecified. This code should only be used when no determination can be made as to the primary site of a malignancy. This code should rarely be used in the inpatient setting.

l. **Sequencing of neoplasm codes**
1) **Encounter for treatment of primary malignancy**
If the reason for the encounter is for treatment of a primary malignancy, assign the malignancy as the principal/first-listed diagnosis. The primary site is to be sequenced first, followed by any metastatic sites.

2) **Encounter for treatment of secondary malignancy**
When an encounter is for a primary malignancy with metastasis and treatment is directed toward the metastatic (secondary) site(s) only, the metastatic site(s) is designated as the principal/first-listed diagnosis. The primary malignancy is coded as an additional code.

3) **Malignant neoplasm in a pregnant patient**
When a pregnant patient has a malignant neoplasm, a code from subcategory O9A.1-, Malignant neoplasm complicating pregnancy, childbirth, and the puerperium, should be sequenced first, followed by the appropriate code from Chapter 2 to indicate the type of neoplasm.

4) **Encounter for complication associated with a neoplasm**
When an encounter is for management of a complication associated with a neoplasm, such as dehydration, and the treatment is only for the complication, the complication is coded first, followed by the appropriate code(s) for the neoplasm.

The exception to this guideline is anemia. When the admission/encounter is for management of an anemia associated with the malignancy, and the treatment is only for anemia, the appropriate code for the malignancy is sequenced as the principal or first-listed diagnosis followed by code D63.0, Anemia in neoplastic disease.

5) **Complication from surgical procedure for treatment of a neoplasm**
When an encounter is for treatment of a complication resulting from a surgical procedure performed for the treatment of the neoplasm, designate the complication as the principal/first-listed diagnosis. See the guideline regarding the coding of a current malignancy versus personal history to determine if the code for the neoplasm should also be assigned.

6) **Pathologic fracture due to a neoplasm**
When an encounter is for a pathological fracture due to a neoplasm, and the focus of treatment is the fracture, a code from subcategory M84.5, Pathological fracture in neoplastic disease, should be sequenced first, followed by the code for the neoplasm.

If the focus of treatment is the neoplasm with an associated pathological fracture, the neoplasm code should be sequenced first, followed by a code from M84.5 for the pathological fracture.

m. **Current malignancy versus personal history of malignancy**
When a primary malignancy has been excised but further treatment, such as an additional surgery for the malignancy, radiation therapy or chemotherapy is directed to that site, the primary malignancy code should be used until treatment is completed.

When a primary malignancy has been previously excised or eradicated from its site, there is no further treatment (of the malignancy) directed to that site, and there is no evidence of any existing primary malignancy at that site, a code from category Z85, Personal history of malignant neoplasm, should be used to indicate the former site of the malignancy.

Codes from subcategories Z85.0 – Z85.85 should only be assigned for the former site of a primary malignancy, not the site of a secondary malignancy. Code Z85.89 may be assigned for the former site(s) of either a primary or secondary malignancy.

See Section I.C.21. Factors influencing health status and contact with health services, History (of)

n. **Leukemia, Multiple Myeloma, and Malignant Plasma Cell Neoplasms in remission versus personal history**
The categories for leukemia, and category C90, Multiple myeloma and malignant plasma cell neoplasms, have codes indicating whether or not the leukemia has achieved remission. There are also codes Z85.6, Personal history of leukemia, and Z85.79, Personal history of other malignant neoplasms of lymphoid, hematopoietic and related tissues. If the documentation is unclear as to whether the leukemia has achieved remission, the provider should be queried.

See Section I.C.21. Factors influencing health status and contact with health services, History (of)

o. **Aftercare following surgery for neoplasm**
See Section I.C.21. Factors influencing health status and contact with health services, Aftercare

p. **Follow-up care for completed treatment of a malignancy**
See Section I.C.21. Factors influencing health status and contact with health services, Follow-up

q. **Prophylactic organ removal for prevention of malignancy**
See Section I.C. 21, Factors influencing health status and contact with health services, Prophylactic organ removal

r. **Malignant neoplasm associated with transplanted organ**
A malignant neoplasm of a transplanted organ should be coded as a transplant complication. Assign first the appropriate code from category T86.-, Complications of transplanted organs and tissue, followed by code C80.2, Malignant neoplasm associated with transplanted organ. Use an additional code for the specific malignancy.

s. **Breast Implant Associated Anaplastic Large Cell Lymphoma**
Breast implant associated anaplastic large cell lymphoma (BIA-ALCL) is a type of lymphoma that can develop around breast implants. Assign code C84.7A, Anaplastic large cell lymphoma, ALK-negative, breast, for BIA-ALCL or C84.7B, Anaplastic large cell lymphoma, ALK-negative, in remission, for BIA-ALCL in remission. Do not assign a complication code from chapter 19.

t. **Secondary malignant neoplasm of lymphoid tissue**
When a malignant neoplasm of lymphoid tissue metastasizes beyond the lymph nodes, a code from categories C81-C85 with a final character identifying "extranodal and solid organ sites" should be assigned rather than a code for the secondary neoplasm of the affected solid organ. For example, for metastasis of diffuse large B-cell lymphoma to the lung, brain and left adrenal gland, assign code C83.398, Diffuse large B-cell lymphoma of other extranodal and solid organ sites.

3. **Chapter 3: Disease of the blood and blood-forming organs and certain disorders involving the immune mechanism (D50-D89)**
Reserved for future guideline expansion

4. **Chapter 4: Endocrine, Nutritional, and Metabolic Diseases (E00-E89)**
a. **Diabetes mellitus**
The diabetes mellitus codes are combination codes that include the type of diabetes mellitus, the body system affected, and the complications affecting that body system. As many codes within a particular category as are necessary to describe all of the complications of the disease may be used. They should be sequenced based on the reason for a particular encounter. Assign as many codes from categories E08 – E13 as needed to identify all of the associated conditions that the patient has.

1) **Type of diabetes**
The age of a patient is not the sole determining factor, though most type 1 diabetics develop the condition before reaching puberty. For this reason, type 1 diabetes mellitus is also referred to as juvenile diabetes.

(a) **Presymptomatic Type 1 Diabetes Mellitus**
Codes E10.A-, Type 1 diabetes mellitus, presymptomatic, are assigned for early-stage type 1 diabetes that predates the onset of symptoms.

(b) **Type 2 diabetes mellitus in remission**
Code E11.A, Type 2 diabetes mellitus without complications in remission, is assigned based on provider documentation that the diabetes mellitus is in remission. If the documentation is unclear as to whether the Type 2 diabetes mellitus has

achieved remission, the provider should be queried. For example, the term "resolved" is not synonymous with remission.

2) **Type of diabetes mellitus not documented**
If the type of diabetes mellitus is not documented in the medical record the default is E11.-, Type 2 diabetes mellitus.

3) **Diabetes mellitus and the use of insulin, oral hypoglycemics, and injectable non-insulin drugs**
If the documentation in a medical record does not indicate the type of diabetes but does indicate that the patient uses insulin, code E11-, Type 2 diabetes mellitus, should be assigned. Additional code(s) should be assigned from category Z79 to identify the long-term (current) use of insulin, oral hypoglycemic drugs, or injectable non-insulin antidiabetic, as follows:

If the patient is treated with both oral hypoglycemic drugs and insulin, both code Z79.4, Long term (current) use of insulin, and code Z79.84, Long term (current) use of oral hypoglycemic drugs, should be assigned.

If the patient is treated with both insulin and an injectable non-insulin antidiabetic drug, assign codes Z79.4, Long term (current) use of insulin, and Z79.85, Long-term (current) use of injectable non-insulin antidiabetic drugs.

If the patient is treated with both oral hypoglycemic drugs and an injectable non-insulin antidiabetic drug, assign codes Z79.84, Long term (current) use of oral hypoglycemic drugs, and Z79.85, Long-term (current) use of injectable non-insulin antidiabetic drugs.

Code Z79.4 should not be assigned if insulin is given temporarily to bring a type 2 patient's blood sugar under control during an encounter.

4) **Diabetes mellitus in pregnancy and gestational diabetes**
See Section I.C.15. Diabetes mellitus in pregnancy.
See Section I.C.15. Gestational (pregnancy induced) diabetes

5) **Complications due to insulin pump malfunction**
   (a) **Underdose of insulin due to insulin pump failure**
   An underdose of insulin due to an insulin pump failure should be assigned to a code from subcategory T85.6, Mechanical complication of other specified internal and external prosthetic devices, implants and grafts, that specifies the type of pump malfunction, as the principal or first-listed code, followed by code T38.3X6-, Underdosing of insulin and oral hypoglycemic [antidiabetic] drugs. Additional codes for the type of diabetes mellitus and any associated complications due to the underdosing should also be assigned.

   (b) **Overdose of insulin due to insulin pump failure**
   The principal or first-listed code for an encounter due to an insulin pump malfunction resulting in an overdose of insulin, should also be T85.6-, Mechanical complication of other specified internal and external prosthetic devices, implants and grafts, followed by code T38.3X1-, Poisoning by insulin and oral hypoglycemic [antidiabetic] drugs, accidental (unintentional).

6) **Secondary diabetes mellitus**
Codes under categories E08, Diabetes mellitus due to underlying condition, E09, Drug or chemical induced diabetes mellitus, and E13, Other specified diabetes mellitus, identify complications/manifestations associated with secondary diabetes mellitus. Secondary diabetes is always caused by another condition or event (e.g., cystic fibrosis, malignant neoplasm of pancreas, pancreatectomy, adverse effect of drug, or poisoning).

   (a) **Secondary diabetes mellitus and the use of insulin, oral hypoglycemic drugs, or injectable non-insulin drugs**
   For patients with secondary diabetes mellitus who routinely use insulin, oral hypoglycemic drugs, or injectable non-insulin drugs, additional code(s) from category Z79 should be assigned to identify the long-term (current) use of insulin, oral hypoglycemic drugs, or non-injectable non-insulin drugs as follows:

   If the patient is treated with both oral hypoglycemic drugs and insulin, both code Z79.4, Long term (current) use of insulin, and code Z79.84, Long term (current) use of oral hypoglycemic drugs, should be assigned.

   If the patient is treated with both insulin and an injectable non-insulin antidiabetic drug, assign codes Z79.4, Long-term (current) use of insulin, and Z79.85, Long-term (current) use of injectable non-insulin antidiabetic drugs.

   If the patient is treated with both oral hypoglycemic drugs and an injectable non-insulin antidiabetic drug, assign codes Z79.84, Long-term (current) use of oral hypoglycemic drugs, and Z79.85, Long-term (current) use of injectable non-insulin antidiabetic drugs.

   Code Z79.4 should not be assigned if insulin is given temporarily to bring a secondary diabetic patient's blood sugar under control during an encounter.

   (b) **Assigning and sequencing secondary diabetes codes and its causes**
   The sequencing of the secondary diabetes codes in relationship to codes for the cause of the diabetes is based on the Tabular List instructions for categories E08, E09 and E13.

   (i) **Secondary diabetes mellitus due to pancreatectomy**
   For postpancreatectomy diabetes mellitus (lack of insulin due to the surgical removal of all or part of the pancreas), assign code E89.1, Postprocedural hypoinsulinemia.
   Assign a code from category E13 as the principal or first-listed diagnosis and a code from subcategory Z90.41, Acquired absence of pancreas, as an additional code.

   (ii) **Secondary diabetes due to drugs**
   Secondary diabetes may be caused by an adverse effect of correctly administered medications, poisoning or sequela of poisoning.
   See section I.C.19.e. for coding of adverse effects and poisoning, and section I.C.20 for external cause code reporting.

b. **Obesity**
The obesity codes in category E66, Overweight and obesity, include codes related to the cause of obesity, such as drug-induced obesity (E66.1), and codes related to effects of obesity, such as code E66.2, Morbid (severe) obesity with alveolar hypoventilation. There are other codes related to obesity in other categories of the classification, such as E88.82, Obesity due to disruption of MC4R pathway; and codes in fifth character subcategory O99.21, Obesity complicating pregnancy, childbirth, and the puerperium.

1) **Obesity class**
The obesity class codes in subcategory E66.81, Obesity class, require a fifth character to convey the severity of obesity. The obesity class should be documented in the medical record by the provider for these codes to be assigned. The obesity class codes can be reported with other obesity codes in the classification found in Chapters 4 and 15 to fully describe the condition. However, if both class 3 obesity and morbid obesity are documented, only a code for class 3 obesity should be assigned as it is more specific.

5. **Chapter 5: Mental, Behavioral and Neurodevelopmental disorders (F01-F99)**

   a. **Pain disorders related to psychological factors**
   Assign code F45.41, for pain that is exclusively related to psychological disorders. As indicated by the Excludes 1 note under category G89, a code from category G89 should not be assigned with code F45.41.
   Code F45.42, Pain disorders with related psychological factors, should be used with a code from category G89, Pain, not elsewhere classified, if there is documentation of a psychological component for a patient with acute or chronic pain.
   See Section I.C.6. Pain

   b. **Mental and behavioral disorders due to psychoactive substance use**

   1) **In Remission**
   Selection of codes describing "in remission" for categories F10-F19, Mental and behavioral disorders due to psychoactive substance use (categories F10-F19 with -.11, -.21, -.91) requires the provider's clinical judgment and are assigned only on the basis of provider documentation (as defined in the Official Guidelines for Coding and Reporting), unless otherwise instructed by the classification.
   Mild substance use disorders in early or sustained remission are classified to the appropriate codes for substance abuse in remission, and moderate or severe substance use disorders in early or sustained remission are classified to the appropriate codes for substance dependence in remission.

   2) **Psychoactive Substance Use, Abuse and Dependence**
   When the provider documentation refers to use, abuse and dependence of the same substance (e.g. alcohol, opioid, cannabis, etc.), only one code should be assigned to identify the pattern of use based on the following hierarchy:
   - If both use and abuse are documented, assign only the code for abuse
   - If both abuse and dependence are documented, assign only the code for dependence
   - If use, abuse and dependence are all documented, assign only the code for dependence
   - If both use and dependence are documented, assign only the code for dependence.

   3) **Psychoactive Substance Use, Unspecified**
   As with all other unspecified diagnoses, the codes for unspecified psychoactive substance use (F10.9-, F11.9-, F12.9-, F13.9-, F14.9-, F15.9-, F16.9-, F18.9-, F19.9-) should only be assigned based on provider documentation and when they meet the definition of a reportable diagnosis (see Section III, Reporting Additional Diagnoses). These codes are to be used only when the psychoactive substance use is associated with a substance related disorder (chapter 5 disorders such as sexual dysfunction, sleep disorder, or a mental or behavioral disorder) or medical condition, and such a relationship is documented by the provider.

4) **Medical Conditions Due to Psychoactive Substance Use, Abuse and Dependence**

Medical conditions due to substance use, abuse, and dependence are not classified as substance-induced disorders. Assign the diagnosis code for the medical condition as directed by the Alphabetical Index along with the appropriate psychoactive substance use, abuse or dependence code. For example, for alcoholic pancreatitis due to alcohol dependence, assign the appropriate code from subcategory K85.2, Alcohol induced acute pancreatitis, and the appropriate code from subcategory F10.2, such as code F10.20, Alcohol dependence, uncomplicated. It would not be appropriate to assign code F10.288, Alcohol dependence with other alcohol-induced disorder.

5) **Blood Alcohol Level**

A code from category Y90, Evidence of alcohol involvement determined by blood alcohol level, may be assigned when this information is documented and the patient's provider has documented a condition classifiable to category F10, Alcohol related disorders. The blood alcohol level does not need to be documented by the patient's provider in order for it to be coded.

See Section I.B.14. for blood alcohol level documentation by clinicians other than patient's provider.

c. **Factitious Disorder**

Factitious disorder imposed on self or Munchausen's syndrome is a disorder in which a person falsely reports or causes his or her own physical or psychological signs or symptoms. For patients with documented factitious disorder on self or Munchausen's syndrome, assign the appropriate code from subcategory F68.1-, Factitious disorder imposed on self.

Munchausen's syndrome by proxy (MSBP) is a disorder in which a caregiver (perpetrator) falsely reports or causes an illness or injury in another person (victim) under his or her care, such as a child, an elderly adult, or a person who has a disability. The condition is also referred to as "factitious disorder imposed on another" or "factitious disorder by proxy." The perpetrator, not the victim, receives this diagnosis. Assign code F68.A, Factitious disorder imposed on another, to the perpetrator's record. For the victim of a patient suffering from MSBP, assign the appropriate code from categories T74, Adult and child abuse, neglect and other maltreatment, confirmed, or T76, Adult and child abuse, neglect and other maltreatment, suspected.

See Section I.C.19.f. Adult and child abuse, neglect and other maltreatment

d. **Dementia**

The ICD-10-CM classifies dementia (categories F01, F02, and F03) on the basis of the etiology and severity (unspecified, mild, moderate or severe). Selection of the appropriate severity level requires the provider's clinical judgment and codes should be assigned only on the basis of provider documentation (as defined in the *Official Guidelines for Coding and Reporting*), unless otherwise instructed by the classification. If the documentation does not provide information about the severity of the dementia, assign the appropriate code for unspecified severity.

If a patient is admitted to an inpatient acute care hospital or other inpatient facility setting with dementia at one severity level and it progresses to a higher severity level, assign one code for the highest severity level reported during the stay.

6. **Chapter 6: Diseases of the Nervous System (G00-G99)**

a. **Dominant/nondominant side**

Codes from category G81, Hemiplegia and hemiparesis, and subcategories G83.1, Monoplegia of lower limb, G83.2, Monoplegia of upper limb, and G83.3, Monoplegia, unspecified, identify whether the dominant or nondominant side is affected. Should the affected side be documented, but not specified as dominant or nondominant, and the classification system does not indicate a default, code selection is as follows:

- For ambidextrous patients, the default should be dominant.
- If the left side is affected, the default is non-dominant.
- If the right side is affected, the default is dominant.

b. **Pain - Category G89**

1) **General coding information**

Codes in category G89, Pain, not elsewhere classified, may be used in conjunction with codes from other categories and chapters to provide more detail about acute or chronic pain and neoplasm-related pain, unless otherwise indicated below.

If the pain is not specified as acute or chronic, post-thoracotomy, postprocedural, or neoplasm-related, do not assign codes from category G89.

A code from category G89 should not be assigned if the underlying (definitive) diagnosis is known, unless the reason for the encounter is pain control/ management and not management of the underlying condition.

When an admission or encounter is for a procedure aimed at treating the underlying condition (e.g., spinal fusion, kyphoplasty), a code for the underlying condition (e.g., vertebral fracture, spinal stenosis) should be assigned as the principal diagnosis. No code from category G89 should be assigned.

(a) **Category G89 Codes as Principal or First-Listed Diagnosis**

Category G89 codes are acceptable as principal diagnosis or the first-listed code:
- When pain control or pain management is the reason for the admission/encounter (e.g., a patient with displaced intervertebral disc, nerve impingement and severe back pain presents for injection of steroid into the spinal canal). The underlying cause of the pain should be reported as an additional diagnosis, if known.
- When a patient is admitted for the insertion of a neurostimulator for pain control, assign the appropriate pain code as the principal or first-listed diagnosis. When an admission or encounter is for a procedure aimed at treating the underlying condition and a neurostimulator is inserted for pain control during the same admission/encounter, a code for the underlying condition should be assigned as the principal diagnosis and the appropriate pain code should be assigned as a secondary diagnosis.

(b) **Use of Category G89 Codes in Conjunction with Site Specific Pain Codes**

(i) **Assigning Category G89 and Site-Specific Pain Codes**

Codes from category G89 may be used in conjunction with codes that identify the site of pain (including codes from chapter 18) if the category G89 code provides additional information. For example, if the code describes the site of the pain, but does not fully describe whether the pain is acute or chronic, then both codes should be assigned.

(ii) **Sequencing of Category G89 Codes with Site-Specific Pain Codes**

The sequencing of category G89 codes with site-specific pain codes (including chapter 18 codes), is dependent on the circumstances of the encounter/admission as follows:
- If the encounter is for pain control or pain management, assign the code from category G89 followed by the code identifying the specific site of pain (e.g., encounter for pain management for acute neck pain from trauma is assigned code G89.11, Acute pain due to trauma, followed by code M54.2, Cervicalgia, to identify the site of pain).
- If the encounter is for any other reason except pain control or pain management, and a related definitive diagnosis has not been established (confirmed) by the provider, assign the code for the specific site of pain first, followed by the appropriate code from category G89.

2) **Pain due to devices, implants and grafts**

See Section I.C.19. Pain due to medical devices

3) **Postoperative Pain**

The provider's documentation should be used to guide the coding of postoperative pain, as well as *Section III. Reporting Additional Diagnoses* and *Section IV. Diagnostic Coding and Reporting in the Outpatient Setting*.

The default for post-thoracotomy and other postoperative pain not specified as acute or chronic is the code for the acute form.

Routine or expected postoperative pain immediately after surgery should not be coded.

(a) **Postoperative pain not associated with specific postoperative complication**

Postoperative pain not associated with a specific postoperative complication is assigned to the appropriate postoperative pain code in category G89.

(b) **Postoperative pain associated with specific postoperative complication**

Postoperative pain associated with a specific postoperative complication (such as painful wire sutures) is assigned to the appropriate code(s) found in Chapter 19, Injury, poisoning, and certain other consequences of external causes. If appropriate, use additional code(s) from category G89 to identify acute or chronic pain (G89.18 or G89.28).

4) **Chronic pain**

Chronic pain is classified to subcategory G89.2. There is no time frame defining when pain becomes chronic pain. The provider's documentation should be used to guide use of these codes.

5) **Neoplasm Related Pain**

Code G89.3 is assigned to pain documented as being related, associated or due to cancer, primary or secondary malignancy, or tumor. This code is assigned regardless of whether the pain is acute or chronic.

This code may be assigned as the principal or first-listed code when the stated reason for the admission/encounter is documented as pain control/pain management. The underlying neoplasm should be reported as an additional diagnosis.

When the reason for the admission/encounter is management of the neoplasm and the pain associated with the neoplasm is also documented, code G89.3 may be assigned as an additional diagnosis. It is not necessary to assign an additional code for the site of the pain.

See Section I.C.2. for instructions on the sequencing of neoplasms for all other stated reasons for the admission/encounter (except for pain control/pain management).

6) **Chronic pain syndrome**
Central pain syndrome (G89.0) and chronic pain syndrome (G89.4) are different than the term "chronic pain," and therefore codes should only be used when the provider has specifically documented this condition.
See Section I.C.5. Pain disorders related to psychological factors

7. **Chapter 7: Diseases of the Eye and Adnexa (H00-H59)**
   a. **Glaucoma**
      1) **Assigning Glaucoma Codes**
         Assign as many codes from category H40, Glaucoma, as needed to identify the type of glaucoma, the affected eye, and the glaucoma stage.
      2) **Bilateral glaucoma with same type and stage**
         When a patient has bilateral glaucoma and both eyes are documented as being the same type and stage, and there is a code for bilateral glaucoma, report only the code for the type of glaucoma, bilateral, with the seventh character for the stage.

         When a patient has bilateral glaucoma and both eyes are documented as being the same type and stage, and the classification does not provide a code for bilateral glaucoma (i.e. subcategories H40.10, and H40.20) report only one code for the type of glaucoma with the appropriate seventh character for the stage.
      3) **Bilateral glaucoma stage with different types or stages**
         When a patient has bilateral glaucoma and each eye is documented as having a different type or stage, and the classification distinguishes laterality, assign the appropriate code for each eye rather than the code for bilateral glaucoma.

         When a patient has bilateral glaucoma and each eye is documented as having a different type, and the classification does not distinguish laterality (i.e., subcategories H40.10, and H40.20), assign one code for each type of glaucoma with the appropriate seventh character for the stage.

         When a patient has bilateral glaucoma and each eye is documented as having the same type, but different stage, and the classification does not distinguish laterality (i.e., subcategories H40.10 and H40.20), assign a code for the type of glaucoma for each eye with the seventh character for the specific glaucoma stage documented for each eye.
      4) **Patient admitted with glaucoma and stage evolves during the admission**
         If a patient is admitted with glaucoma and the stage progresses during the admission, assign the code for highest stage documented.
      5) **Indeterminate stage glaucoma**
         Assignment of the seventh character "4" for "indeterminate stage" should be based on the clinical documentation. The seventh character "4" is used for glaucomas whose stage cannot be clinically determined. This seventh character should not be confused with the seventh character "0", unspecified, which should be assigned when there is no documentation regarding the stage of the glaucoma.
   b. **Blindness**
      If "blindness" or "low vision" of both eyes is documented but the visual impairment category is not documented, assign code H54.3, Unqualified visual loss, both eyes. If "blindness" or "low vision" in one eye is documented but the visual impairment category is not documented, assign a code from H54.6-, Unqualified visual loss, one eye. If "blindness" or "visual loss" is documented without any information about whether one or both eyes are affected, assign code H54.7, Unspecified visual loss.

8. **Chapter 8: Diseases of the Ear and Mastoid Process (H60-H95)**
   Reserved for future guideline expansion

9. **Chapter 9: Diseases of the Circulatory System (I00-I99)**
   a. **Hypertension**
      The classification presumes a causal relationship between hypertension and heart involvement and between hypertension and kidney involvement, as the two conditions are linked by the term "with" in the Alphabetic Index. These conditions should be coded as related even in the absence of provider documentation explicitly linking them, unless the documentation clearly states the conditions are unrelated.

      For hypertension and conditions not specifically linked by relational terms such as "with," "associated with" or "due to" in the classification, provider documentation must link the conditions in order to code them as related.
      1) **Hypertension with Heart Disease**
         Hypertension with heart conditions classified to I50.-, Heart failure, I51.4, Myocarditis, unspecified, I51.89, Other ill-defined heart diseases, and I51.9, Heart disease, unspecified, is assigned to a code from category I11, Hypertensive heart disease. Use additional code(s) from category I50, Heart failure, or I51, Complications and ill-defined descriptions of heart disease, to identify the heart condition.

         Hypertension with heart conditions classified to I51.5, Myocardial degeneration, or I51.7, Cardiomegaly, is assigned to a code from category I11, Hypertensive heart disease. No additional code is assigned to identify the specific heart condition.

         The same heart conditions (I50.-, I51.4-I51.7, I51.89, I51.9) with hypertension are coded separately if the provider has documented they are unrelated to the hypertension. The applicable hypertension code I10, Essential (primary) hypertension, or a code from category I15, Secondary hypertension, should be assigned. Sequence according to the circumstances of the admission/encounter.
      2) **Hypertensive Chronic Kidney Disease**
         Assign codes from category I12, Hypertensive chronic kidney disease, when both hypertension and a condition classifiable to category N18, Chronic kidney disease (CKD), are present. CKD should not be coded as hypertensive if the provider indicates the CKD is not related to the hypertension.

         The appropriate code from category N18 should be used as a secondary code with a code from category I12 to identify the stage of chronic kidney disease.
         See Section I.C.14. Chronic kidney disease.
         If a patient has hypertensive chronic kidney disease and acute renal failure, the acute renal failure should also be coded. Sequence according to the circumstances of the admission/encounter.
      3) **Hypertensive Heart and Chronic Kidney Disease**
         The codes in category I13, Hypertensive heart and chronic kidney disease, are combination codes that include hypertension, heart disease and chronic kidney disease. Assign codes from combination category I13, Hypertensive heart and chronic kidney disease, when there is hypertension with both heart and chronic kidney disease. If heart failure is present, assign an additional code from category I50 to identify the type of heart failure.

         The appropriate code from category N18, Chronic kidney disease, should be used as a secondary code with a code from category I13 to identify the stage of chronic kidney disease.
         See Section I.C.14. Chronic kidney disease.

         The Includes note at I13 specifies that the conditions included at I11 and I12 are included together in I13. If a patient has hypertension, heart disease and chronic kidney disease, then a code from I13 should be used, not codes from I11 or I12.

         For patients with both acute renal failure and chronic kidney disease, the acute renal failure should also be coded. Sequence according to the circumstances of the admission/encounter.
      4) **Hypertensive Cerebrovascular Disease**
         For hypertensive cerebrovascular disease, first assign the appropriate code from categories I60-I69, followed by the appropriate hypertension code.
      5) **Hypertensive Retinopathy**
         Subcategory H35.0, Background retinopathy and retinal vascular changes, should be used along with a code from categories I10-I15, in the Hypertensive diseases section, to include the systemic hypertension. The sequencing is based on the reason for the encounter.
      6) **Hypertension, Secondary**
         Secondary hypertension is due to an underlying condition. Two codes are required: one to identify the underlying etiology and one from category I15 to identify the hypertension. Sequencing of codes is determined by the reason for admission/encounter.
      7) **Hypertension, Transient**
         Assign code R03.0, Elevated blood pressure reading without diagnosis of hypertension, unless patient has an established diagnosis of hypertension. Assign code O13.-, Gestational [pregnancy-induced] hypertension without significant proteinuria, or O14.-, Pre-eclampsia, for transient hypertension of pregnancy.
      8) **Hypertension, Controlled**
         This diagnostic statement usually refers to an existing state of hypertension under control by therapy. Assign the appropriate code from categories I10-I15, Hypertensive diseases.
      9) **Hypertension, Uncontrolled**
         Uncontrolled hypertension may refer to untreated hypertension or hypertension not responding to current therapeutic regimen. In either case, assign the appropriate code from categories I10-I15, Hypertensive diseases.
      10) **Hypertensive Crisis**
          Assign a code from category I16, Hypertensive crisis, for documented hypertensive urgency, hypertensive emergency or unspecified hypertensive crisis. Code also any identified hypertensive disease (I10-I15). The sequencing is based on the reason for the encounter.
      11) **Pulmonary Hypertension**
          Pulmonary hypertension is classified to category I27, Other pulmonary heart diseases. For secondary pulmonary hypertension (I27.1, I27.2-), code also any associated conditions or adverse effects of drugs or toxins.

The sequencing is based on the reason for the encounter, except for adverse effects of drugs (See Section I.C.19.e.).

12) **Hypertension, Resistant**
Resistant hypertension refers to blood pressure of a patient with hypertension that remains above goal in spite of the use of antihypertensive medications. Assign code I1A.0, Resistant hypertension, as an additional code when apparent treatment resistant hypertension, treatment resistant hypertension, or true resistant hypertension is documented by the provider. A code for the specific type of existing hypertension is sequenced first, if known.

b. **Atherosclerotic Coronary Artery Disease and Angina**
ICD-10-CM has combination codes for atherosclerotic heart disease with angina pectoris. The subcategories for these codes are I25.11, Atherosclerotic heart disease of native coronary artery with angina pectoris and I25.7, Atherosclerosis of coronary artery bypass graft(s) and coronary artery of transplanted heart with angina pectoris.

When using one of these combination codes it is not necessary to use an additional code for angina pectoris. A causal relationship can be assumed in a patient with both atherosclerosis and angina pectoris, unless the documentation indicates the angina is due to something other than the atherosclerosis.

If a patient with coronary artery disease is admitted due to an acute myocardial infarction (AMI), the AMI should be sequenced before the coronary artery disease.

See Section I.C.9. Acute myocardial infarction (AMI)

c. **Intraoperative and Postprocedural Cerebrovascular Accident**
Medical record documentation should clearly specify the cause- and-effect relationship between the medical intervention and the cerebrovascular accident in order to assign a code for intraoperative or postprocedural cerebrovascular accident.

Proper code assignment depends on whether it was an infarction or hemorrhage and whether it occurred intraoperatively or postoperatively. If it was a cerebral hemorrhage, code assignment depends on the type of procedure performed.

d. **Sequelae of Cerebrovascular Disease**
1) **Category I69, Sequelae of Cerebrovascular disease**
Category I69 is used to indicate conditions classifiable to categories I60-I67 as the causes of sequela (neurologic deficits), themselves classified elsewhere. These "late effects" include neurologic deficits that persist after initial onset of conditions classifiable to categories I60-I67. The neurologic deficits caused by cerebrovascular disease may be present from the onset or may arise at any time after the onset of the condition classifiable to categories I60-I67.

Codes from category I69, Sequelae of cerebrovascular disease, that specify hemiplegia, hemiparesis and monoplegia identify whether the dominant or nondominant side is affected. Should the affected side be documented, but not specified as dominant or nondominant, and the classification system does not indicate a default, code selection is as follows:
- For ambidextrous patients, the default should be dominant.
- If the left side is affected, the default is non-dominant.
- If the right side is affected, the default is dominant.

2) **Codes from category I69 with codes from I60-I67**
Codes from category I69 may be assigned on a health care record with codes from I60-I67, if the patient has a current cerebrovascular disease and deficits from an old cerebrovascular disease.

3) **Codes from category I69 and Personal history of transient ischemic attack (TIA) and cerebral infarction (Z86.73)**
Codes from category I69 should not be assigned if the patient does not have neurologic deficits.

See Section I.C.21.4. History (of) for use of personal history codes

e. **Acute myocardial infarction (AMI)**
1) **Type 1 ST elevation myocardial infarction (STEMI) and non-ST elevation myocardial infarction (NSTEMI)**
The ICD-10-CM codes for type 1 acute myocardial infarction (AMI) identify the site, such as anterolateral wall or true posterior wall. Subcategories I21.0-I21.2 and code I21.3 are used for type 1 ST elevation myocardial infarction (STEMI). Code I21.4, Non-ST elevation (NSTEMI) myocardial infarction, is used for type 1 non-ST elevation myocardial infarction (NSTEMI) and nontransmural MIs.

If a type 1 NSTEMI evolves to STEMI, assign the STEMI code. If a type 1 STEMI converts to NSTEMI due to thrombolytic therapy, it is still coded as STEMI.

For encounters occurring while the myocardial infarction is equal to, or less than, four weeks old, including transfers to another acute setting or a postacute setting, and the myocardial infarction meets the definition for "other diagnoses" (see Section III, Reporting Additional Diagnoses), codes from category I21 may continue to be reported. For encounters after the 4-week time frame and the patient is still receiving care related to the myocardial infarction, the appropriate aftercare code should be assigned, rather than a code from category I21. For old or healed myocardial infarctions not requiring further care, code I25.2, Old myocardial infarction, may be assigned.

2) **Acute myocardial infarction, unspecified**
Code I21.9, Acute myocardial infarction, unspecified, is the default for unspecified acute myocardial infarction or unspecified type. If only type 1 STEMI or transmural MI without the site is documented, assign code I21.3, ST elevation (STEMI) myocardial infarction of unspecified site.

3) **AMI documented as nontransmural or subendocardial but site provided**
If an AMI is documented as nontransmural or subendocardial, but the site is provided, it is still coded as a subendocardial AMI.

See Section I.C.21.3. for information on coding status post administration of tPA in a different facility within the last 24 hours.

4) **Subsequent acute myocardial infarction**
A code from category I22, Subsequent ST elevation (STEMI) and non-ST elevation (NSTEMI) myocardial infarction, is to be used when a patient who has suffered a type 1 or unspecified AMI has a new AMI within the 4 week time frame of the initial AMI. A code from category I22 must be used in conjunction with a code from category I21. The sequencing of the I22 and I21 codes depends on the circumstances of the encounter.

Do not assign code I22 for subsequent myocardial infarctions other than type 1 or unspecified. For subsequent type 2 AMI assign only code I21.A1. For subsequent type 4 or type 5 AMI, assign only code I21.A9.

If a subsequent myocardial infarction of one type occurs within 4 weeks of a myocardial infarction of a different type, assign the appropriate codes from category I21 to identify each type. Do not assign a code from I22. Codes from category I22 should only be assigned if both the initial and subsequent myocardial infarctions are type 1 or unspecified.

5) **Other Types of Myocardial Infarction**
The ICD-10-CM provides codes for different types of myocardial infarction. Type 1 myocardial infarctions are assigned to codes I21.0-I21.4.

Type 2 myocardial infarction (myocardial infarction due to demand ischemia or secondary to ischemic imbalance) is assigned to code I21.A1, Myocardial infarction type 2 with the underlying cause coded first, if applicable. Do not assign code I24.89, Other forms of acute ischemic heart disease, for the demand ischemia. If a type 2 AMI is described as NSTEMI or STEMI, only assign code I21.A1. Codes I21.01-I21.4 should only be assigned for type 1 AMIs.

Acute myocardial infarctions type 3, 4a, 4b, 4c and 5 are assigned to code I21.A9, Other myocardial infarction type.

The "Code also" and "Code first" notes should be followed related to complications, and for coding of postprocedural myocardial infarctions during or following cardiac surgery.

6) **Myocardial Infarction with Coronary Microvascular Dysfunction**
Coronary microvascular dysfunction (CMD) is a condition that impacts the microvasculature by restricting microvascular flow and increasing microvascular resistance. Code I21.B, Myocardial infarction with coronary microvascular dysfunction, is assigned for myocardial infarction with coronary microvascular disease, myocardial infarction with coronary microvascular dysfunction, and myocardial infarction with non-obstructive coronary arteries (MINOCA) with microvascular disease.

10. **Chapter 10: Diseases of the Respiratory System (J00-J99), U07.0**
a. **Chronic Obstructive Pulmonary Disease [COPD] and Asthma**
1) **Acute exacerbation of chronic obstructive bronchitis and asthma**
The codes in categories J44 and J45 distinguish between uncomplicated cases and those in acute exacerbation. An acute exacerbation is a worsening or a decompensation of a chronic condition. An acute exacerbation is not equivalent to an infection superimposed on a chronic condition, though an exacerbation may be triggered by an infection.

b. **Acute Respiratory Failure**
1) **Acute respiratory failure as principal diagnosis**
A code from subcategory J96.0, Acute respiratory failure, or subcategory J96.2, Acute and chronic respiratory failure, may be assigned as a principal diagnosis when it is the condition established after study to be chiefly responsible for occasioning the admission to the hospital, and the selection is supported by the Alphabetic Index and Tabular List. However, chapter-specific coding guidelines (such as obstetrics, poisoning, HIV, newborn) that provide sequencing direction take precedence.

2) **Acute respiratory failure as secondary diagnosis**
Respiratory failure may be listed as a secondary diagnosis if it occurs after admission, or if it is present on admission, but does not meet the definition of principal diagnosis.

3) **Sequencing of acute respiratory failure and another acute condition**
When a patient is admitted with respiratory failure and another acute condition, (e.g., myocardial infarction, cerebrovascular accident, aspiration pneumonia), the principal diagnosis will not be the same in every situation. This applies whether the other acute condition is a

respiratory or nonrespiratory condition. Selection of the principal diagnosis will be dependent on the circumstances of admission. If both the respiratory failure and the other acute condition are equally responsible for occasioning the admission to the hospital, and there are no chapter-specific sequencing rules, the guideline regarding two or more diagnoses that equally meet the definition for principal diagnosis (Section II, C.) may be applied in these situations.

If the documentation is not clear as to whether acute respiratory failure and another condition are equally responsible for occasioning the admission, query the provider for clarification.

c. **Influenza due to certain identified influenza viruses**
Code only confirmed cases of influenza due to certain identified influenza viruses (category J09), and due to other identified influenza virus (category J10). This is an exception to the hospital inpatient guideline Section II, H. (Uncertain Diagnosis).

In this context, "confirmation" does not require documentation of positive laboratory testing specific for avian or other novel influenza A or other identified influenza virus. However, coding should be based on the provider's diagnostic statement that the patient has avian influenza, or other novel influenza A, for category J09, or has another particular identified strain of influenza, such as H1N1 or H3N2, but not identified as novel or variant, for category J10.

If the provider records "suspected" or "possible" or "probable" avian influenza, or novel influenza, or other identified influenza, then the appropriate influenza code from category J11, Influenza due to unidentified influenza virus, should be assigned. A code from category J09, Influenza due to certain identified influenza viruses, should not be assigned nor should a code from category J10, Influenza due to other identified influenza virus.

d. **Ventilator associated Pneumonia**
   1) **Documentation of Ventilator associated Pneumonia**
   As with all procedural or postprocedural complications, code assignment is based on the provider's documentation of the relationship between the condition and the procedure.

   Code J95.851, Ventilator associated pneumonia, should be assigned only when the provider has documented ventilator associated pneumonia (VAP). An additional code to identify the organism (e.g., Pseudomonas aeruginosa, code B96.5) should also be assigned. Do not assign an additional code from categories J12-J18 to identify the type of pneumonia.

   Code J95.851 should not be assigned for cases where the patient has pneumonia and is on a mechanical ventilator and the provider has not specifically stated that the pneumonia is ventilator-associated pneumonia. If the documentation is unclear as to whether the patient has a pneumonia that is a complication attributable to the mechanical ventilator, query the provider.

   2) **Ventilator associated Pneumonia Develops after Admission**
   A patient may be admitted with one type of pneumonia (e.g., code J13, Pneumonia due to Streptococcus pneumonia) and subsequently develop VAP. In this instance, the principal diagnosis would be the appropriate code from categories J12-J18 for the pneumonia diagnosed at the time of admission. Code J95.851, Ventilator associated pneumonia, would be assigned as an additional diagnosis when the provider has also documented the presence of ventilator associated pneumonia.

e. **Vaping-related disorders**
For patients presenting with condition(s) related to vaping, assign code U07.0, Vaping-related disorder, as the principal diagnosis. For lung injury due to vaping, assign only code U07.0. Assign additional codes for other manifestations, such as acute respiratory failure (subcategory J96.0-) or pneumonitis (code J68.0).

Associated respiratory signs and symptoms due to vaping, such as cough, shortness of breath, etc., are not coded separately, when a definitive diagnosis has been established. However, it would be appropriate to code separately any gastrointestinal symptoms, such as diarrhea and abdominal pain.

See Section I.C.1.g.1.c.i. for Pneumonia confirmed as due to COVID-19

11. **Chapter 11: Diseases of the Digestive System (K00-K95)**
Reserved for future guideline expansion

12. **Chapter 12: Diseases of the Skin and Subcutaneous Tissue (L00-L99)**
    a. **Pressure ulcer stage codes**
       1) **Pressure ulcer stages**
       Codes in category L89, Pressure ulcer, identify the site and stage of the pressure ulcer.

       The ICD-10-CM classifies pressure ulcer stages based on severity, which is designated by stages 1-4, deep tissue pressure injury, unspecified stage, and unstageable.

       Assign as many codes from category L89 as needed to identify all the pressure ulcers the patient has, if applicable.

       See Section I.B.14. for pressure ulcer stage documentation by clinicians other than patient's provider.

       2) **Unstageable pressure ulcers**
       Assignment of the code for unstageable pressure ulcer (L89.--0) should be based on the clinical documentation. These codes are used for pressure ulcers whose stage cannot be clinically determined (e.g., the ulcer is covered by eschar or has been treated with a skin or muscle graft). This code should not be confused with the codes for unspecified stage (L89.--9). When there is no documentation regarding the stage of the pressure ulcer, assign the appropriate code for unspecified stage (L89.-- 9).

       If during an encounter, the stage of an unstageable pressure ulcer is revealed after debridement, assign only the code for the stage revealed following debridement.

       3) **Documented pressure ulcer stage**
       Assignment of the pressure ulcer stage code should be guided by clinical documentation of the stage or documentation of the terms found in the Alphabetic Index. For clinical terms describing the stage that are not found in the Alphabetic Index, and there is no documentation of the stage, the provider should be queried.

       4) **Patients admitted with pressure ulcers documented as healed**
       No code is assigned if the documentation states that the pressure ulcer is completely healed at the time of admission.

       5) **Pressure ulcers documented as healing**
       Pressure ulcers described as healing should be assigned the appropriate pressure ulcer stage code based on the documentation in the medical record. If the documentation does not provide information about the stage of the healing pressure ulcer, assign the appropriate code for unspecified stage.

       If the documentation is unclear as to whether the patient has a current (new) pressure ulcer or if the patient is being treated for a healing pressure ulcer, query the provider.

       For ulcers that were present on admission but healed at the time of discharge, assign the code for the site and stage of the pressure ulcer at the time of admission.

       6) **Patient admitted with pressure ulcer evolving into another stage during the admission**
       If a patient is admitted to an inpatient hospital with a pressure ulcer at one stage and it progresses to a higher stage, two separate codes should be assigned: one code for the site and stage of the ulcer on admission and a second code for the same ulcer site and the highest stage reported during the stay.

       7) **Pressure-induced deep tissue damage**
       For pressure-induced deep tissue damage or deep tissue pressure injury, assign only the appropriate code for pressure-induced deep tissue damage (L89.--6).

    b. **Non-Pressure Chronic Ulcers**
       1) **Patients admitted with non-pressure ulcers documented as healed**
       No code is assigned if the documentation states that the non-pressure ulcer is completely healed at the time of admission.

       2) **Non-pressure ulcers documented as healing**
       Non-pressure ulcers described as healing should be assigned the appropriate non-pressure ulcer code based on the documentation in the medical record. If the documentation does not provide information about the severity of the healing non-pressure ulcer, assign the appropriate code for unspecified severity.

       If the documentation is unclear as to whether the patient has a current (new) non-pressure ulcer or if the patient is being treated for a healing non-pressure ulcer, query the provider.

       For ulcers that were present on admission but healed at the time of discharge, assign the code for the site and severity of the non-pressure ulcer at the time of admission.

       3) **Patient admitted with non-pressure ulcer that progresses to another severity level during the admission**
       If a patient is admitted to an inpatient hospital with a non-pressure ulcer at one severity level and it progresses to a higher severity level, two separate codes should be assigned: one code for the site and severity level of the ulcer on admission and a second code for the same ulcer site and the highest severity level reported during the stay.

       See Section I.B.14. for pressure ulcer stage documentation by clinicians other than patient's provider

13. **Chapter 13: Diseases of the Musculoskeletal System and Connective Tissue (M00-M99)**
    a. **Site and laterality**
    Most of the codes within Chapter 13 have site and laterality designations. The site represents the bone, joint or the muscle involved.

       1) **Bone versus joint**
       For certain conditions, the bone may be affected at the upper or lower end, (e.g., avascular necrosis of bone, M87, Osteoporosis, M80, M81). Though the portion of the bone affected may be at the joint, the site designation will be the bone, not the joint.

2) **Multiple sites**
Codes describing specified sites are assigned individually by site when documented. When the specified site(s) are not documented, assign the appropriate code for "multiple sites."

b. **Acute traumatic versus chronic or recurrent musculoskeletal conditions**
Many musculoskeletal conditions are a result of previous injury or trauma to a site, or are recurrent conditions. Bone, joint or muscle conditions that are the result of a healed injury are usually found in chapter 13. Recurrent bone, joint or muscle conditions are also usually found in chapter 13. Any current, acute injury should be coded to the appropriate injury code from chapter 19. Chronic or recurrent conditions should generally be coded with a code from chapter 13. If it is difficult to determine from the documentation in the record which code is best to describe a condition, query the provider.

c. **Coding of Pathologic Fractures**
7th character A is for use as long as the patient is receiving active treatment for the fracture. While the patient may be seen by a new or different provider over the course of treatment for a pathological fracture, assignment of the 7th character is based on whether the patient is undergoing active treatment and not whether the provider is seeing the patient for the first time.

7th character D is to be used for encounters after the patient has completed active treatment for the fracture and is receiving routine care for the fracture during the healing or recovery phase. The other 7th characters, listed under each subcategory in the Tabular List, are to be used for subsequent encounters for treatment of problems associated with the healing, such as malunions, nonunions, and sequelae.

Care for complications of surgical treatment for fracture repairs during the healing or recovery phase should be coded with the appropriate complication codes.

See Section I.C.19. Coding of traumatic fractures.

d. **Osteoporosis**
Osteoporosis is a systemic condition, meaning that all bones of the musculoskeletal system are affected. Therefore, site is not a component of the codes under category M81, Osteoporosis without current pathological fracture. The site codes under category M80, Osteoporosis with current pathological fracture, identify the site of the fracture, not the osteoporosis.

1) **Osteoporosis without pathological fracture**
Category M81, Osteoporosis without current pathological fracture, is for use for patients with osteoporosis who do not currently have a pathologic fracture due to the osteoporosis, even if they have had a fracture in the past. For patients with a history of osteoporosis fractures, status code Z87.310, Personal history of (healed) osteoporosis fracture, should follow the code from M81.

2) **Osteoporosis with current pathological fracture**
Category M80, Osteoporosis with current pathological fracture, is for patients who have a current pathologic fracture at the time of an encounter. The codes under M80 identify the site of the fracture. A code from category M80, not a traumatic fracture code, should be used for any patient with known osteoporosis who suffers a fracture, even if the patient had a minor fall or trauma, if that fall or trauma would not usually break a normal, healthy bone.

e. **Multisystem Inflammatory Syndrome**
See Section I.C.1.g.1.l. for Multisystem Inflammatory Syndrome

14. **Chapter 14: Diseases of Genitourinary System (N00-N99)**
    a. **Chronic kidney disease**
       1) **Stages of chronic kidney disease (CKD)**
          The ICD-10-CM classifies CKD based on severity. The severity of CKD is designated by stages 1-5. Stage 2, code N18.2, equates to mild CKD; stage 3, codes N18.30-N18.32, equate to moderate CKD; and stage 4, code N18.4, equates to severe CKD. Code N18.6, End stage renal disease (ESRD), is assigned when the provider has documented end-stage renal disease (ESRD).

          If both a stage of CKD and ESRD are documented, assign code N18.6 only.

       2) **Chronic kidney disease and kidney transplant status**
          Patients who have undergone kidney transplant may still have some form of chronic kidney disease (CKD) because the kidney transplant may not fully restore kidney function. Therefore, the presence of CKD alone does not constitute a transplant complication. Assign the appropriate N18 code for the patient's stage of CKD and code Z94.0, Kidney transplant status. If a transplant complication such as failure or rejection or other transplant complication is documented, see section I.C.19.g for information on coding complications of a kidney transplant. If the documentation is unclear as to whether the patient has a complication of the transplant, query the provider.

       3) **Chronic kidney disease with other conditions**
          Patients with CKD may also suffer from other serious conditions, most commonly diabetes mellitus and hypertension. The sequencing of the CKD code in relationship to codes for other contributing conditions is based on the conventions in the Tabular List.

          See I.C.9. Hypertensive chronic kidney disease.
          See I.C.19. Chronic kidney disease and kidney transplant complications.

15. **Chapter 15: Pregnancy, Childbirth, and the Puerperium (O00-O9A)**
    a. **General Rules for Obstetric Cases**
       1) **Codes from chapter 15 and sequencing priority**
          Obstetric cases require codes from chapter 15, codes in the range O00-O9A, Pregnancy, Childbirth, and the Puerperium. Chapter 15 codes have sequencing priority over codes from other chapters. Additional codes from other chapters may be used in conjunction with chapter 15 codes to further specify conditions. Should the provider document that the pregnancy is incidental to the encounter, then code Z33.1, Pregnant state, incidental, should be used in place of any chapter 15 codes. It is the provider's responsibility to state that the condition being treated is not affecting the pregnancy.

       2) **Chapter 15 codes used only on the maternal record**
          Chapter 15 codes are to be used only on the maternal record, never on the record of the newborn.

       3) **Final character for trimester**
          The majority of codes in Chapter 15 have a final character indicating the trimester of pregnancy. The timeframes for the trimesters are indicated at the beginning of the chapter. If trimester is not a component of a code, it is because the condition always occurs in a specific trimester, or the concept of trimester of pregnancy is not applicable. Certain codes have characters for only certain trimesters because the condition does not occur in all trimesters, but it may occur in more than just one.

          Assignment of the final character for trimester should be based on the provider's documentation of the trimester (or number of weeks) for the current admission/encounter. This applies to the assignment of trimester for pre-existing conditions as well as those that develop during or are due to the pregnancy. The provider's documentation of the number of weeks may be used to assign the appropriate code identifying the trimester.

          Whenever delivery occurs during the current admission, and there is an "in childbirth" option for the obstetric complication being coded, the "in childbirth" code should be assigned. When the classification does not provide an obstetric code with an "in childbirth" option, it is appropriate to assign a code describing the current trimester.

       4) **Selection of trimester for inpatient admissions that encompass more than one trimester**
          In instances when a patient is admitted to a hospital for complications of pregnancy during one trimester and remains in the hospital into a subsequent trimester, the trimester character for the antepartum complication code should be assigned on the basis of the trimester when the complication developed, not the trimester of the discharge. If the condition developed prior to the current admission/encounter or represents a pre-existing condition, the trimester character for the trimester at the time of the admission/encounter should be assigned.

       5) **Unspecified trimester**
          Each category that includes codes for trimester has a code for "unspecified trimester." The "unspecified trimester" code should rarely be used, such as when the documentation in the record is insufficient to determine the trimester and it is not possible to obtain clarification.

       6) **7th character for fetus identification**
          Where applicable, a 7th character is to be assigned for certain categories (O31, O32, O33.3-O33.6, O35, O36, O40, O41, O60.1, O60.2, O64, and O69) to identify the fetus for which the complication code applies.

          Assign 7th character "0":
          - For single gestations
          - When the documentation in the record is insufficient to determine the fetus affected and it is not possible to obtain clarification.
          - When it is not possible to clinically determine which fetus is affected.

       7) **Completed weeks of gestation**
          In ICD-10-CM, "completed" weeks of gestation refers to full weeks. For example, if the provider documents gestation at 39 weeks and 6 days, the code for 39 weeks of gestation should be assigned, as the patient has not yet reached 40 completed weeks.

    b. **Selection of OB Principal or First-listed Diagnosis**
       1) **Routine outpatient prenatal visits**
          For routine outpatient prenatal visits when no complications are present, a code from category Z34, Encounter for supervision of normal pregnancy, should be used as the first-listed diagnosis. These codes should not be used in conjunction with chapter 15 codes.

       2) **Supervision of High-Risk Pregnancy**
          Codes from category O09, Supervision of high-risk pregnancy, are intended for use only during the prenatal period. For complications during the labor or delivery episode as a result of a high-risk pregnancy, assign the applicable complication codes from Chapter 15. If there are no complications during the labor or delivery episode, assign code O80, Encounter for full-term uncomplicated delivery.

          For routine prenatal outpatient visits for patients with high-risk pregnancies, a code from category O09, Supervision of high-risk pregnancy, should be used as the first-listed diagnosis. Secondary chapter 15 codes may be used in conjunction with these codes if appropriate.

3) **Episodes when no delivery occurs**
   In episodes when no delivery occurs, the principal diagnosis should correspond to the principal complication of the pregnancy which necessitated the encounter. Should more than one complication exist, all of which are treated or monitored, any of the complication codes may be sequenced first.

4) **When a delivery occurs**
   When an obstetric patient is admitted and delivers during that admission, the condition that prompted the admission should be sequenced as the principal diagnosis. If multiple conditions prompted the admission, sequence the one most related to the delivery as the principal diagnosis. A code for any complication of the delivery should be assigned as an additional diagnosis. In cases of cesarean delivery, if the patient was admitted with a condition that resulted in the performance of a cesarean procedure, that condition should be selected as the principal diagnosis. If the reason for the admission was unrelated to the condition resulting in the cesarean delivery, the condition related to the reason for the admission should be selected as the principal diagnosis.

5) **Outcome of delivery**
   A code from category Z37, Outcome of delivery, should be included on every maternal record when a delivery has occurred. These codes are not to be used on subsequent records or on the newborn record.

c. **Pre-existing conditions versus conditions due to the pregnancy**
Certain categories in Chapter 15 distinguish between conditions of the mother that existed prior to pregnancy (pre-existing) and those that are a direct result of pregnancy. When assigning codes from Chapter 15, it is important to assess if a condition was pre-existing prior to pregnancy or developed during or due to the pregnancy in order to assign the correct code.

Categories that do not distinguish between pre-existing and pregnancy-related conditions may be used for either. It is acceptable to use codes specifically for the puerperium with codes complicating pregnancy and childbirth if a condition arises postpartum during the delivery encounter.

d. **Pre-existing hypertension in pregnancy**
Category O10, Pre-existing hypertension complicating pregnancy, childbirth and the puerperium, includes codes for hypertensive heart and hypertensive chronic kidney disease. When assigning one of the O10 codes that includes hypertensive heart disease or hypertensive chronic kidney disease, it is necessary to add a secondary code from the appropriate hypertension category to specify the type of heart failure or chronic kidney disease.

See Section I.C.9. Hypertension.

e. **Fetal Conditions Affecting the Management of the Mother**
   1) **Codes from categories O35 and O36**
      Codes from categories O35, Maternal care for known or suspected fetal abnormality and damage, and O36, Maternal care for other fetal problems, are assigned only when the fetal condition is actually responsible for modifying the management of the mother, i.e., by requiring diagnostic studies, additional observation, special care, or termination of pregnancy. The fact that the fetal condition exists does not justify assigning a code from this series to the mother's record.

   2) **In utero surgery**
      In cases when surgery is performed on the fetus, a diagnosis code from category O35, Maternal care for known or suspected fetal abnormality and damage, should be assigned identifying the fetal condition. Assign the appropriate procedure code for the procedure performed.

      No code from Chapter 16, the perinatal codes, should be used on the mother's record to identify fetal conditions. Surgery performed in utero on a fetus is still to be coded as an obstetric encounter.

f. **HIV Infection in Pregnancy, Childbirth and the Puerperium**
During pregnancy, childbirth or the puerperium, a patient admitted because of an HIV-related illness should receive a principal diagnosis from subcategory O98.7-, Human immunodeficiency [HIV] disease complicating pregnancy, childbirth and the puerperium, followed by the code(s) for the HIV-related illness(es).

Patients with asymptomatic HIV infection status admitted during pregnancy, childbirth, or the puerperium should receive codes of O98.7- and Z21, Asymptomatic human immunodeficiency virus [HIV] infection status.

g. **Diabetes mellitus in pregnancy**
Diabetes mellitus is a significant complicating factor in pregnancy. Pregnant patients who are diabetic should be assigned a code from category O24, Diabetes mellitus in pregnancy, childbirth, and the puerperium, first, followed by the appropriate diabetes code(s) (E08-E13) from Chapter 4.

h. **Long term use of insulin and oral hypoglycemics**
See section I.C.4.a.3 for information on the long-term use of insulin and oral hypoglycemics.

i. **Gestational (pregnancy induced) diabetes**
Gestational (pregnancy induced) diabetes can occur during the second and third trimester of pregnancy in patients who were not diabetic prior to pregnancy. Gestational diabetes can cause complications in the pregnancy similar to those of pre-existing diabetes mellitus. It also puts the patient at greater risk of developing diabetes after the pregnancy.

Codes for gestational diabetes are in subcategory O24.4, Gestational diabetes mellitus. No other code from category O24, Diabetes mellitus in pregnancy, childbirth, and the puerperium, should be used with a code from O24.4.

The codes under subcategory O24.4 include diet controlled, insulin controlled, and controlled by oral hypoglycemic drugs. If a patient with gestational diabetes is treated with both diet and insulin, only the code for insulin-controlled is required. If a patient with gestational diabetes is treated with both diet and oral hypoglycemic medications, only the code for "controlled by oral hypoglycemic drugs" is required. Codes Z79.4, Long-term (current) use of insulin, Z79.84, Long-term (current) use of oral hypoglycemic drugs, and Z79.85, Long-term (current) use of injectable non-insulin antidiabetic drugs, should not be assigned with codes from subcategory O24.4.

An abnormal glucose tolerance in pregnancy is assigned a code from subcategory O99.81, Abnormal glucose complicating pregnancy, childbirth, and the puerperium.

j. **Sepsis and septic shock complicating abortion, pregnancy, childbirth and the puerperium**
When assigning a chapter 15 code for sepsis complicating abortion, pregnancy, childbirth, and the puerperium, a code for the specific type of infection should be assigned as an additional diagnosis. If severe sepsis is present, a code from subcategory R65.2, Severe sepsis, and code(s) for associated organ dysfunction(s) should also be assigned as additional diagnoses.

k. **Puerperal sepsis**
Code O85, Puerperal sepsis, should be assigned with a secondary code to identify the causal organism (e.g., for a bacterial infection, assign a code from category B95-B96, Bacterial infections in conditions classified elsewhere). A code from category A40, Streptococcal sepsis, or A41, Other sepsis, should not be used for puerperal sepsis. If applicable, use additional codes to identify severe sepsis (R65.2-) and any associated acute organ dysfunction.

Code O85 should not be assigned for sepsis following an obstetrical procedure (See Section I.C.1.d.5.b., Sepsis due to a postprocedural infection).

l. **Alcohol, tobacco and drug use during pregnancy, childbirth and the puerperium**
   1) **Alcohol use during pregnancy, childbirth and the puerperium**
      Codes under subcategory O99.31, Alcohol use complicating pregnancy, childbirth, and the puerperium, should be assigned for any pregnancy case when a patient uses alcohol during the pregnancy or postpartum. A secondary code from category F10, Alcohol related disorders, should also be assigned to identify manifestations of the alcohol use.

   2) **Tobacco use during pregnancy, childbirth and the puerperium**
      Codes under subcategory O99.33, Smoking (tobacco) complicating pregnancy, childbirth, and the puerperium, should be assigned for any pregnancy case when a patient uses any type of tobacco product during the pregnancy or postpartum.

      A secondary code from category F17, Nicotine dependence, should also be assigned to identify the type of nicotine dependence.

   3) **Drug use during pregnancy, childbirth and the puerperium**
      Codes under subcategory O99.32, Drug use complicating pregnancy, childbirth, and the puerperium, should be assigned for any pregnancy case when a patient uses drugs during the pregnancy or postpartum. This can involve illegal drugs, or inappropriate use or abuse of prescription drugs. Secondary code(s) from categories F11-F16 and F18-F19 should also be assigned to identify manifestations of the drug use.

m. **Poisoning, toxic effects, adverse effects and underdosing in a pregnant patient**
A code from subcategory O9A.2, Injury, poisoning and certain other consequences of external causes complicating pregnancy, childbirth, and the puerperium, should be sequenced first, followed by the appropriate injury, poisoning, toxic effect, adverse effect or underdosing code, and then the additional code(s) that specifies the condition caused by the poisoning, toxic effect, adverse effect or underdosing.

See Section I.C.19. Adverse effects, poisoning, underdosing and toxic effects.

n. **Normal Delivery, Code O80**
   1) **Encounter for full term uncomplicated delivery**
      Code O80 should be assigned when a patient is admitted for a full-term normal delivery and delivers a single, healthy infant without any complications antepartum, during the delivery, or postpartum during the delivery episode. Code O80 is always a principal diagnosis. It is not to be used if any other code from chapter 15 is needed to describe a current complication of the antenatal, delivery, or postnatal period. Additional codes from other chapters may be used with code O80 if they are not related to or are in any way complicating the pregnancy.

   2) **Uncomplicated delivery with resolved antepartum complication**
      Code O80 may be used if the patient had a complication at some point during the pregnancy, but the complication is not present at the time of the admission for delivery.

   3) **Outcome of delivery for O80**
      Z37.0, Single live birth, is the only outcome of delivery code appropriate for use with O80.

o. **The Peripartum and Postpartum Periods**
   1) **Peripartum and Postpartum periods**
      The postpartum period begins immediately after delivery and continues for six weeks following delivery. The peripartum period is defined as the last month of pregnancy to five months postpartum.
   2) **Peripartum and postpartum complication**
      A postpartum complication is any complication occurring within the six-week period.
   3) **Pregnancy-related complications after 6-week period**
      Chapter 15 codes may also be used to describe pregnancy-related complications after the peripartum or postpartum period if the provider documents that a condition is pregnancy related.
   4) **Admission for routine postpartum care following delivery outside hospital**
      When the mother delivers outside the hospital prior to admission and is admitted for routine postpartum care and no complications are noted, code Z39.0, Encounter for care and examination of mother immediately after delivery, should be assigned as the principal diagnosis.
   5) **Pregnancy associated cardiomyopathy**
      Pregnancy associated cardiomyopathy, code O90.3, is unique in that it may be diagnosed in the third trimester of pregnancy but may continue to progress months after delivery. For this reason, it is referred to as peripartum cardiomyopathy. Code O90.3 is only for use when the cardiomyopathy develops as a result of pregnancy in a patient who did not have pre-existing heart disease.

p. **Code O94, Sequelae of complication of pregnancy, childbirth, and the puerperium**
   1) **Code O94**
      Code O94, Sequelae of complication of pregnancy, childbirth, and the puerperium, is for use in those cases when an initial complication of a pregnancy develops a sequela or sequelae requiring care or treatment at a future date.
   2) **After the initial postpartum period**
      This code may be used at any time after the initial postpartum period.
   3) **Sequencing of Code O94**
      This code, like all sequela codes, is to be sequenced following the code describing the sequelae of the complication.

q. **Termination of Pregnancy and Spontaneous abortions**
   1) **Abortion with Liveborn Fetus**
      When an attempted termination of pregnancy results in a liveborn fetus, assign code Z33.2, Encounter for elective termination of pregnancy and a code from category Z37, Outcome of Delivery.
   2) **Retained Products of Conception following an abortion**
      Subsequent encounters for retained products of conception following a spontaneous abortion or elective termination of pregnancy, without complications are assigned O03.4, Incomplete spontaneous abortion without complication, or code O07.4, Failed attempted termination of pregnancy without complication. This advice is appropriate even when the patient was discharged previously with a discharge diagnosis of complete abortion. If the patient has a specific complication associated with the spontaneous abortion or elective termination of pregnancy in addition to retained products of conception, assign the appropriate complication code (e.g., O03.-, O04.-, O07.-) instead of code O03.4 or O07.4.
   3) **Complications leading to abortion**
      Codes from Chapter 15 may be used as additional codes to identify any documented complications of the pregnancy in conjunction with codes in categories in O04, O07 and O08.
   4) **Hemorrhage following elective abortion**
      For hemorrhage post elective abortion, assign code O04.6, Delayed or excessive hemorrhage following (induced) termination of pregnancy. Do not assign code O72.1, Other immediate postpartum hemorrhage, as this code should not be assigned for post abortion conditions.

r. **Abuse in a pregnant patient**
   For suspected or confirmed cases of abuse of a pregnant patient, a code(s) from subcategories O9A.3, Physical abuse complicating pregnancy, childbirth, and the puerperium, O9A.4, Sexual abuse complicating pregnancy, childbirth, and the puerperium, and O9A.5, Psychological abuse complicating pregnancy, childbirth, and the puerperium, should be sequenced first, followed by the appropriate codes (if applicable) to identify any associated current injury due to physical abuse, sexual abuse, and the perpetrator of abuse.
   See Section I.C.19. Adult and child abuse, neglect and other maltreatment.

s. **COVID-19 infection in pregnancy, childbirth, and the puerperium**
   During pregnancy, childbirth or the puerperium, when COVID-19 is the reason for admission/encounter , code O98.5-, Other viral diseases complicating pregnancy, childbirth and the puerperium, should be sequenced as the principal/first-listed diagnosis, and code U07.1, COVID-19, and the appropriate codes for associated manifestation(s) should be assigned as additional diagnoses. Codes from Chapter 15 always take sequencing priority.

If the reason for admission/encounter is unrelated to COVID-19 but the patient **has been diagnosed with** COVID-19 during the admission/encounter, the appropriate code for the reason for admission/encounter should be sequenced as the principal/first-listed diagnosis, and codes O98.5- and U07.1, as well as the appropriate codes for associated COVID-19 manifestations, should be assigned as additional diagnoses.

16. **Chapter 16: Certain Conditions Originating in the Perinatal Period (P00-P96)**
    For coding and reporting purposes the perinatal period is defined as before birth through the 28th day following birth. The following guidelines are provided for reporting purposes.

    a. **General Perinatal Rules**
       1) **Use of Chapter 16 Codes**
          Codes in this chapter are <u>never</u> for use on the maternal record. Codes from Chapter 15, the obstetric chapter, are never permitted on the newborn record. Chapter 16 codes may be used throughout the life of the patient if the condition is still present.
       2) **Principal Diagnosis for Birth Record**
          When coding the birth episode in a newborn record, assign a code from category Z38, Liveborn infants according to place of birth and type of delivery, as the principal diagnosis. A code from category Z38 is assigned only once, to a newborn at the time of birth. If a newborn is transferred to another institution, a code from category Z38 should not be used at the receiving hospital.
          A code from category Z38 is used only on the newborn record, not on the mother's record.
       3) **Use of Codes from other Chapters with Codes from Chapter 16**
          Codes from other chapters may be used with codes from chapter 16 if the codes from the other chapters provide more specific detail. Codes for signs and symptoms may be assigned when a definitive diagnosis has not been established. If the reason for the encounter is a perinatal condition, the code from chapter 16 should be sequenced first.
       4) **Use of Chapter 16 Codes after the Perinatal Period**
          Should a condition originate in the perinatal period, and continue throughout the life of the patient, the perinatal code should continue to be used regardless of the patient's age.
       5) **Birth process or community acquired conditions**
          If a newborn has a condition that may be either due to the birth process or community acquired and the documentation does not indicate which it is, the default is due to the birth process and the code from Chapter 16 should be used. If the condition is community-acquired, a code from Chapter 16 should not be assigned.
          For COVID-19 infection in a newborn, see guideline I.C.16.h.
       6) **Code all clinically significant conditions**
          All clinically significant conditions noted on routine newborn examination should be coded. A condition is clinically significant if it requires:
          - clinical evaluation; or
          - therapeutic treatment; or
          - diagnostic procedures; or
          - extended length of hospital stay; or
          - increased nursing care and/or monitoring; or
          - has implications for future health care needs
          Note: The perinatal guidelines listed above are the same as the general coding guidelines for "additional diagnoses," except for the final point regarding implications for future health care needs. Codes should be assigned for conditions that have been specified by the provider as having implications for future health care needs.

    b. **Observation and Evaluation of Newborns for Suspected Conditions not Found**
       1) **Use of Z05 codes**
          Assign a code from category Z05, Observation and evaluation of newborn for suspected diseases and conditions ruled out, to identify those instances when a healthy newborn is evaluated for a suspected condition/disease that is determined after study not to be present. Do not use a code from category Z05 when the patient is documented to have signs or symptoms of a suspected problem; in such cases code the sign or symptom.
       2) **Z05 on other than the birth record**
          A code from category Z05 may also be assigned as a principal or first-listed code for readmissions or encounters when the code from category Z38 code no longer applies. Codes from category Z05 are for use only for healthy newborns and infants for which no condition after study is found to be present.
       3) **Z05 on a birth record**
          A code from category Z05 is to be used as a secondary code after the code from category Z38, Liveborn infants according to place of birth and type of delivery.

    c. **Coding Additional Perinatal Diagnoses**
       1) **Assigning codes for conditions that require treatment**
          Assign codes for conditions that require treatment or further investigation, prolong the length of stay, or require resource utilization.

2) **Codes for conditions specified as having implications for future health care needs**
Assign codes for conditions that have been specified by the provider as having implications for future health care needs.
Note: This guideline should not be used for adult patients.

d. **Prematurity and Fetal Growth Retardation**
Providers utilize different criteria in determining prematurity. A code for prematurity should not be assigned unless it is documented. Assignment of codes in categories P05, Disorders of newborn related to slow fetal growth and fetal malnutrition, and P07, Disorders of newborn related to short gestation and low birth weight, not elsewhere classified, should be based on the recorded birth weight and estimated gestational age.

When both birth weight and gestational age are available, two codes from category P07 should be assigned, with the code for birth weight sequenced before the code for gestational age.

e. **Low birth weight and immaturity status**
Codes from category P07, Disorders of newborn related to short gestation and low birth weight, not elsewhere classified, are for use for a child or adult who was premature or had a low birth weight as a newborn and this is affecting the patient's current health status.

See Section I.C.21. Factors influencing health status and contact with health services, Status.

f. **Bacterial Sepsis of Newborn**
Category P36, Bacterial sepsis of newborn, includes congenital sepsis. If a perinate is documented as having sepsis without documentation of congenital or community acquired, the default is congenital and a code from category P36 should be assigned. If the P36 code includes the causal organism, an additional code from category B95, Streptococcus, Staphylococcus, and Enterococcus as the cause of diseases classified elsewhere, or B96, Other bacterial agents as the cause of diseases classified elsewhere, should not be assigned. If the P36 code does not include the causal organism, assign an additional code from category B96. If applicable, use additional codes to identify severe sepsis (R65.2-) and any associated acute organ dysfunction.

g. **Stillbirth**
Code P95, Stillbirth, is only for use in institutions that maintain separate records for stillbirths. No other code should be used with P95. Code P95 should not be used on the mother's record.

h. **COVID-19 Infection in Newborn**
For a newborn that tests positive for COVID-19, assign code U07.1, COVID-19, and the appropriate codes for associated manifestation(s) in neonates/newborns in the absence of documentation indicating a specific type of transmission. For a newborn that tests positive for COVID-19 and the provider documents the condition was contracted in utero or during the birth process, assign codes P35.8, Other congenital viral diseases, and U07.1, COVID-19. When coding the birth episode in a newborn record, the appropriate code from category Z38, Liveborn infants according to place of birth and type of delivery, should be assigned as the principal diagnosis.

17. *Chapter 17: Congenital malformations, deformations, and chromosomal abnormalities (Q00-QA1)*
Assign an appropriate code(s) from categories Q00-**QA1**, Congenital malformations, deformations, and chromosomal abnormalities when a malformation/deformation or chromosomal abnormality is documented. A malformation/deformation/or chromosomal abnormality may be the principal/first-listed diagnosis on a record or a secondary diagnosis.

When a malformation/deformation or chromosomal abnormality does not have a unique code assignment, assign additional code(s) for any manifestations that may be present.

When the code assignment specifically identifies the malformation/deformation or chromosomal abnormality, manifestations that are an inherent component of the anomaly should not be coded separately. Additional codes should be assigned for manifestations that are not an inherent component.

Codes from Chapter 17 may be used throughout the life of the patient. If a congenital malformation or deformity has been corrected, a personal history code should be used to identify the history of the malformation or deformity. Although present at birth, a malformation/deformation/or chromosomal abnormality may not be identified until later in life. Whenever the condition is diagnosed by the provider, it is appropriate to assign a code from codes Q00-**QA1**. For the birth admission, the appropriate code from category Z38, Liveborn infants, according to place of birth and type of delivery, should be sequenced as the principal diagnosis, followed by any congenital anomaly codes, Q00-**QA1**.

18. **Chapter 18: Symptoms, signs, and abnormal clinical and laboratory findings, not elsewhere classified (R00-R99)**
Chapter 18 includes symptoms, signs, abnormal results of clinical or other investigative procedures, and ill-defined conditions regarding which no diagnosis classifiable elsewhere is recorded. Signs and symptoms that point to a specific diagnosis have been assigned to a category in other chapters of the classification.

a. **Use of symptom codes**
Codes that describe symptoms and signs are acceptable for reporting purposes when a related definitive diagnosis has not been established (confirmed) by the provider.

b. **Use of a symptom code with a definitive diagnosis code**
Codes for signs and symptoms may be reported in addition to a related definitive diagnosis when the sign or symptom is not routinely associated with that diagnosis, such as the various signs and symptoms associated with complex syndromes. The definitive diagnosis code should be sequenced before the symptom code.

Signs or symptoms that are associated routinely with a disease process should not be assigned as additional codes, unless otherwise instructed by the classification.

c. **Combination codes that include symptoms**
ICD-10-CM contains a number of combination codes that identify both the definitive diagnosis and common symptoms of that diagnosis. When using one of these combination codes, an additional code should not be assigned for the symptom.

d. **Repeated falls**
Code R29.6, Repeated falls, is for use for encounters when a patient has recently fallen and the reason for the fall is being investigated.

Code Z91.81, History of falling, is for use when a patient has fallen in the past and is at risk for future falls. When appropriate, both codes R29.6 and Z91.81 may be assigned together.

e. **Coma**
Code R40.20, Unspecified coma, should be assigned when the underlying cause of the coma is not known, or the cause is a traumatic brain injury and the coma scale is not documented in the medical record.

Do not report codes for unspecified coma, individual or total Glasgow coma scale scores for a patient with a medically induced coma or a sedated patient.

1) **Coma Scale**
The coma scale codes (R40.21- to R40.24-) can be used in conjunction with traumatic brain injury codes. These codes cannot be used with code R40.2A, Nontraumatic coma due to underlying condition. They are primarily for use by trauma registries, but they may be used in any setting where this information is collected. The coma scale codes should be sequenced after the diagnosis code(s).

These codes, one from each subcategory, are needed to complete the scale. The 7th character indicates when the scale was recorded. The 7th character should match for all three codes.

At a minimum, report the initial score documented on presentation at your facility. This may be a score from the emergency medicine technician (EMT) or in the emergency department. If desired, a facility may choose to capture multiple coma scale scores.

Assign code R40.24-, Glasgow coma scale, total score, when only the total score is documented in the medical record and not the individual score(s).

If multiple coma scores are captured within the first 24 hours after hospital admission, assign only the code for the score at the time of admission. ICD-10-CM does not classify coma scores that are reported after admission but less than 24 hours later.

See Section I.B.14. for coma scale documentation by clinicians other than patient's provider

f. **Functional quadriplegia**
GUIDELINE HAS BEEN DELETED EFFECTIVE OCTOBER 1, 2017

g. **SIRS due to Non-Infectious Process**
The systemic inflammatory response syndrome (SIRS) can develop as a result of certain non-infectious disease processes, such as trauma, malignant neoplasm, or pancreatitis. When SIRS is documented with a noninfectious condition, and no subsequent infection is documented, the code for the underlying condition, such as an injury, should be assigned, followed by code R65.10, Systemic inflammatory response syndrome (SIRS) of non-infectious origin without acute organ dysfunction, or code R65.11, Systemic inflammatory response syndrome (SIRS) of non-infectious origin with acute organ dysfunction. If an associated acute organ dysfunction is documented, the appropriate code(s) for the specific type of organ dysfunction(s) should be assigned in addition to code R65.11. If acute organ dysfunction is documented, but it cannot be determined if the acute organ dysfunction is associated with SIRS or due to another condition (e.g., directly due to the trauma), the provider should be queried.

h. **Death NOS**
Code R99, Ill-defined and unknown cause of mortality, is only for use in the very limited circumstance when a patient who has already died is brought into an emergency department or other healthcare facility and is pronounced dead upon arrival. It does not represent the discharge disposition of death.

i. **NIHSS Stroke Scale**
The NIH stroke scale (NIHSS) codes (R29.7- -) can be used in conjunction with acute stroke codes (I60–I63) to identify the patient's neurological status and the severity of the stroke. The stroke scale codes should be sequenced after the acute stroke diagnosis code(s).

At a minimum, report the initial score documented. If desired, a facility may choose to capture multiple stroke scale scores.

See Section I.B.14. for NIHSS stroke scale documentation by clinicians other than patient's provider

19. Chapter 19: Injury, poisoning, and certain other consequences of external causes (S00-T88)

a. Application of 7th Characters in Chapter 19

Most categories in chapter 19 have a 7th character requirement for each applicable code. Most categories in this chapter have three 7th character values (with the exception of fractures): A, initial encounter, D, subsequent encounter and S, sequela. Categories for traumatic fractures have additional 7th character values. While the patient may be seen by a new or different provider over the course of treatment for an injury, assignment of the 7th character is based on whether the patient is undergoing active treatment and not whether the provider is seeing the patient for the first time.

For complication codes, active treatment refers to treatment for the condition described by the code, even though it may be related to an earlier precipitating problem. For example, code T84.50XA, Infection and inflammatory reaction due to unspecified internal joint prosthesis, initial encounter, is used when active treatment is provided for the infection, even though the condition relates to the prosthetic device, implant or graft that was placed at a previous encounter.

7th character "A", initial encounter is used for each encounter where the patient is receiving active treatment for the condition.

7th character "D" subsequent encounter is used for encounters after the patient has completed active treatment of the condition and is receiving routine care for the condition during the healing or recovery phase.

The aftercare Z codes should not be used for aftercare for conditions such as injuries or poisonings, where 7th characters are provided to identify subsequent care. For example, for aftercare of an injury, assign the acute injury code with the 7th character "D" (subsequent encounter).

7th character "S", sequela, is for use for complications or conditions that arise as a direct result of a condition, such as scar formation after a burn. The scars are sequelae of the burn. When using 7th character "S", it is necessary to use both the injury code that precipitated the sequela and the code for the sequela itself. The "S" is added only to the injury code, not the sequela code. The 7th character "S" identifies the injury responsible for the sequela. The specific type of sequela (e.g. scar) is sequenced first, followed by the injury code.

See Section I.B.10. Sequelae, (Late Effects)

b. Coding of Injuries

When coding injuries, assign separate codes for each injury unless a combination code is provided, in which case the combination code is assigned. Codes from category T07, Unspecified multiple injuries should not be assigned in the inpatient setting unless information for a more specific code is not available. Traumatic injury codes (S00-T14.9) are not to be used for normal, healing surgical wounds or to identify complications of surgical wounds.

The code for the most serious injury, as determined by the provider and the focus of treatment, is sequenced first.

1) **Superficial injuries**
   Superficial injuries such as abrasions or contusions are not coded when associated with more severe injuries of the same site.

2) **Primary injury with damage to nerves/blood vessels**
   When a primary injury results in minor damage to peripheral nerves or blood vessels, the primary injury is sequenced first with additional code(s) for injuries to nerves and spinal cord (such as category S04), and/or injury to blood vessels (such as category S15). When the primary injury is to the blood vessels or nerves, that injury should be sequenced first.

3) **Iatrogenic injuries**
   Injury codes from Chapter 19 should not be assigned for injuries that occur during, or as a result of, a medical intervention. Assign the appropriate complication code(s).

c. Coding of Traumatic Fractures

The principles of multiple coding of injuries should be followed in coding fractures. Fractures of specified sites are coded individually by site in accordance with both the provisions within categories S02, S12, S22, S32, S42, S49, S52, S59, S62, S72, S79, S82, S89 and S92 and the level of detail furnished by medical record content.

A fracture not indicated as open or closed should be coded to closed. A fracture not indicated whether displaced or not displaced should be coded to displaced.

More specific guidelines are as follows:

1) **Initial vs. subsequent encounter for fractures**
   Traumatic fractures are coded using the appropriate 7th character for initial encounter (A, B, C) for each encounter where the patient is receiving active treatment for the fracture. The appropriate 7th character for initial encounter should also be assigned for a patient who delayed seeking treatment for the fracture or nonunion.

   Fractures are coded using the appropriate 7th character for subsequent care for encounters after the patient has completed active treatment of the fracture and is receiving routine care for the fracture during the healing or recovery phase.

   Care for complications of surgical treatment for fracture repairs during the healing or recovery phase should be coded with the appropriate complication codes.

   Care of complications of fractures, such as malunion and nonunion, should be reported with the appropriate 7th character for subsequent care with nonunion (K, M, N,) or subsequent care with malunion (P, Q, R).

   Malunion/nonunion: The appropriate 7th character for initial encounter should also be assigned for a patient who delayed seeking treatment for the fracture or nonunion.

   The open fracture designations in the assignment of the 7th character for fractures of the forearm, femur and lower leg, including ankle are based on the Gustilo open fracture classification. When the Gustilo classification type is not specified for an open fracture, the 7th character for open fracture type I or II should be assigned (B, E, H, M, Q).

   A code from category M80, not a traumatic fracture code, should be used for any patient with known osteoporosis who suffers a fracture, even if the patient had a minor fall or trauma, if that fall or trauma would not usually break a normal, healthy bone.

   See Section I.C.13. Osteoporosis.

   The aftercare Z codes should not be used for aftercare for traumatic fractures. For aftercare of a traumatic fracture, assign the acute fracture code with the appropriate 7th character.

2) **Multiple fractures sequencing**
   Multiple fractures are sequenced in accordance with the severity of the fracture.

3) **Physeal fractures**
   For physeal fractures, assign only the code identifying the type of physeal fracture. Do not assign a separate code to identify the specific bone that is fractured.

d. Coding of Burns and Corrosions

The ICD-10-CM makes a distinction between burns and corrosions. The burn codes are for thermal burns, except sunburns, that come from a heat source, such as a fire or hot appliance. The burn codes are also for burns resulting from electricity and radiation. Corrosions are burns due to chemicals. The guidelines are the same for burns and corrosions.

Current burns (T20-T25) are classified by depth, extent and by agent (X code). Burns are classified by depth as first degree (erythema), second degree (blistering), and third degree (full-thickness involvement). Burns of the eye and internal organs (T26-T28) are classified by site, but not by degree.

1) **Sequencing of burn and related condition codes**
   Sequence first the code that reflects the highest degree of burn when more than one burn is present.

   a. When the reason for the admission or encounter is for treatment of external multiple burns, sequence first the code that reflects the burn of the highest degree.
   b. When a patient has both internal and external burns, the circumstances of admission govern the selection of the principal diagnosis or first-listed diagnosis.
   c. When a patient is admitted for burn injuries and other related conditions such as smoke inhalation and/or respiratory failure, the circumstances of admission govern the selection of the principal or first-listed diagnosis.

2) **Burns of the same anatomic site**
   Classify burns of the same anatomic site and on the same side but of different degrees to the subcategory identifying the highest degree recorded in the diagnosis (e.g., for second and third degree burns of right thigh, assign only code T24.311-).

3) **Non-healing burns**
   Non-healing burns are coded as acute burns.
   Necrosis of burned skin should be coded as a non-healed burn.

4) **Infected burn**
   For any documented infected burn site, use an additional code for the infection.

5) **Assign separate codes for each burn site**
   When coding burns, assign separate codes for each burn site. Category T30, Burn and corrosion, body region unspecified is extremely vague and should rarely be used.

   Codes for burns of "multiple sites" should only be assigned when the medical record documentation does not specify the individual sites.

6) **Burns and corrosions classified according to extent of body surface involved**
   Assign codes from category T31, Burns classified according to extent of body surface involved, or T32, Corrosions classified according to extent of body surface involved, for acute burns or corrosions when the site of the burn or corrosion is not specified or when there is a need for additional data. It is advisable to use category T31 as additional coding when needed to provide data for evaluating burn mortality, such as that needed by burn units. It is also advisable to use category T31 as an additional code for reporting purposes when there is mention of a third-degree burn involving 20 percent or more of the body surface.

Codes from categories T31 and T32 should not be used for sequelae of burns or corrosions.

Categories T31 and T32 are based on the classic "rule of nines" in estimating body surface involved: head and neck are assigned nine percent, each arm nine percent, each leg 18 percent, the anterior trunk 18 percent, posterior trunk 18 percent, and genitalia one percent. Providers may change these percentage assignments where necessary to accommodate infants and children who have proportionately larger heads than adults, and patients who have large buttocks, thighs, or abdomen that involve burns.

7) **Encounters for treatment of sequela of burns**
Encounters for the treatment of the late effects of burns or corrosions (i.e., scars or joint contractures) should be coded with a burn or corrosion code with the 7th character "S" for sequela.

8) **Sequelae with a late effect code and current burn**
When appropriate, both a code for a current burn or corrosion with 7th character "A" or "D" and a burn or corrosion code with 7th character "S" may be assigned on the same record (when both a current burn and sequelae of an old burn exist). Burns and corrosions do not heal at the same rate and a current healing wound may still exist with sequela of a healed burn or corrosion.

See Section I.B.10. Sequela (Late Effects)

9) **Use of an external cause code with burns and corrosions**
An external cause code should be used with burns and corrosions to identify the source and intent of the burn, as well as the place where it occurred.

e. **Adverse Effects, Poisoning, Underdosing and Toxic Effects**
Codes in categories T36-T65 are combination codes that include the substance that was taken as well as the intent. No additional external cause code is required for poisonings, toxic effects, adverse effects and underdosing codes.

1) **Do not code directly from the Table of Drugs**
Do not code directly from the Table of Drugs and Chemicals. Always refer back to the Tabular List.

2) **Use as many codes as necessary to describe**
Use as many codes as necessary to describe completely all drugs, medicinal or biological substances.

3) **If the same code would describe the causative agent**
If the same code would describe the causative agent for more than one adverse reaction, poisoning, toxic effect or underdosing, assign the code only once.

4) **If two or more drugs, medicinal or biological substances**
If two or more drugs, medicinal or biological substances are taken, code each individually unless a combination code is listed in the Table of Drugs and Chemicals.

If multiple unspecified drugs, medicinal or biological substances were taken, assign the appropriate code from subcategory T50.91, Poisoning by, adverse effect of and underdosing of multiple unspecified drugs, medicaments and biological substances.

5) **The occurrence of drug toxicity is classified in ICD-10-CM as follows:**

   (a) **Adverse Effect**
   When coding an adverse effect of a drug that has been correctly prescribed and properly administered, assign the appropriate code for the nature of the adverse effect followed by the appropriate code for the adverse effect of the drug (T36-T50). The code for the drug should have a 5th or 6th character "5" (for example T36.0X5-) Examples of the nature of an adverse effect are tachycardia, delirium, gastrointestinal hemorrhaging, vomiting, hypokalemia, hepatitis, renal failure, or respiratory failure.

   (b) **Poisoning**
   When coding a poisoning or reaction to the improper use of a medication (e.g., overdose, wrong substance given or taken in error, wrong route of administration), first assign the appropriate code from categories T36-T50. The poisoning codes have an associated intent as their 5th or 6th character (accidental, intentional self-harm, assault and undetermined). If the intent of the poisoning is unknown or unspecified, code the intent as accidental intent. The undetermined intent is only for use if the documentation in the record specifies that the intent cannot be determined. Use additional code(s) for all manifestations of poisonings.

   If there is also a diagnosis of abuse or dependence of the substance, the abuse or dependence is assigned as an additional code.

   Examples of poisoning include:
   (i) Error was made in drug prescription
   Errors made in drug prescription or in the administration of the drug by provider, nurse, patient, or other person.
   (ii) Overdose of a drug intentionally taken
   If an overdose of a drug was intentionally taken or administered and resulted in drug toxicity, it would be coded as a poisoning.
   (iii) Nonprescribed drug taken with correctly prescribed and properly administered drug
   If a nonprescribed drug or medicinal agent was taken in combination with a correctly prescribed and properly administered drug, any drug toxicity or other reaction resulting from the interaction of the two drugs would be classified as a poisoning.
   (iv) Interaction of drug(s) and alcohol
   When a reaction results from the interaction of a drug(s) and alcohol, this would be classified as poisoning.

   See Section I.C.4. if poisoning is the result of insulin pump malfunctions.

   For Sequela (Late Effects) see Section I.B.10.

   (c) **Underdosing**
   Underdosing refers to taking less of a medication than is prescribed by a provider or a manufacturer's instruction. Discontinuing the use of a prescribed medication on the patient's own initiative (not directed by the patient's provider) is also classified as an underdosing. For underdosing, assign the code from categories T36-T50 (fifth or sixth character "6"). Documentation of a change in the patient's condition is not required in order to assign an underdosing code. Documentation that the patient is taking less of a medication than is prescribed or discontinued the prescribed medication is sufficient for code assignment.

   Codes for underdosing should never be assigned as principal or first-listed codes. If a patient has a relapse or exacerbation of the medical condition for which the drug is prescribed because of the reduction in dose, then the medical condition itself should be coded.

   Noncompliance (Z91.12-, Z91.13-, Z91.14- and Z91.A4-) or complication of care (Y63.6-Y63.9) codes are to be used with an underdosing code to indicate intent, if known.

   (d) **Toxic Effects**
   When a harmful substance is ingested or comes in contact with a person, this is classified as a toxic effect. The toxic effect codes are in categories T51-T65. When coding a toxic effect, assign the toxic effect code first, followed by codes for all associated manifestations of the toxic effect.

   Toxic effect codes have an associated intent: accidental, intentional self-harm, assault and undetermined.

   For Sequela (Late Effects) see Section I.B.10. Sequela

f. **Adult and child abuse, neglect and other maltreatment**
Sequence first the appropriate code from categories T74, Adult and child abuse, neglect and other maltreatment, confirmed, or T76, Adult and child abuse, neglect and other maltreatment, suspected, for abuse, neglect and other maltreatment, followed by any accompanying mental health or injury code(s).

If the documentation in the medical record states abuse or neglect, it is coded as confirmed (T74.-). It is coded as suspected if it is documented as suspected (T76.-).

For cases of confirmed abuse or neglect an external cause code from the assault section (X92-Y09) should be added to identify the cause of any physical injuries. A perpetrator code (Y07) should be added when the perpetrator of the abuse is known. For suspected cases of abuse or neglect, do not report external cause or perpetrator code.

If a suspected case of abuse, neglect or mistreatment is ruled out during an encounter code Z04.71, Encounter for examination and observation following alleged physical adult abuse, ruled out, or code Z04.72, Encounter for examination and observation following alleged child physical abuse, ruled out, should be used, not a code from T76.

If a suspected case of alleged rape or sexual abuse is ruled out during an encounter code Z04.41, Encounter for examination and observation following alleged adult rape or code Z04.42, Encounter for examination and observation following alleged child rape, should be used, not a code from T76.

If a suspected case of forced sexual exploitation or forced labor exploitation is ruled out during an encounter, code Z04.81, Encounter for examination and observation of victim following forced sexual exploitation, or code Z04.82, Encounter for examination and observation of victim following forced labor exploitation, should be used, not a code from T76.

See Section I.C.15. Abuse in a pregnant patient.

g. **Complications of care**
1) **General guidelines for complications of care**
   (a) **Documentation of complications of care**
   See Section I.B.16. for information on documentation of complications of care.

2) **Pain due to medical devices**
Pain associated with devices, implants or grafts left in a surgical site (for example painful hip prosthesis) is assigned to the appropriate code(s) found in Chapter 19, Injury, poisoning, and certain other consequences of external causes. Specific codes for pain due to medical devices are found in the T code section of the ICD-10-CM. Use additional code(s) from category G89 to identify acute or chronic pain due to presence of the device, implant or graft (G89.18 or G89.28).

3) **Transplant complications**

(a) **Transplant complications other than kidney**
Codes under category T86, Complications of transplanted organs and tissues, are for use for both complications and rejection of transplanted organs. A transplant complication code is only assigned if the complication affects the function of the transplanted organ. Two codes are required to fully describe a transplant complication: the appropriate code from category T86 and a secondary code that identifies the complication.

Pre-existing conditions or conditions that develop after the transplant are not coded as complications unless they affect the function of the transplanted organs.

See I.C.21. for transplant organ removal status
See I.C.2. for malignant neoplasm associated with transplanted organ.
See I.C.1.d.4. for sequencing of sepsis due to infection in transplanted organ

(b) **Kidney transplant complications**
Patients who have undergone kidney transplant may still have some form of chronic kidney disease (CKD) because the kidney transplant may not fully restore kidney function. Code T86.1- should be assigned for documented complications of a kidney transplant, such as transplant failure or rejection or other transplant complication. Code T86.1- should not be assigned for post kidney transplant patients who have chronic kidney (CKD) unless a transplant complication such as transplant failure or rejection is documented. If the documentation is unclear as to whether the patient has a complication of the transplant, query the provider.

Conditions that affect the function of the transplanted kidney, other than CKD, should be assigned a code from subcategory T86.1, Complications of transplanted organ, Kidney, and a secondary code that identifies the complication.

For patients with CKD following a kidney transplant, but who do not have a complication such as failure or rejection, *see section I.C.14. Chronic kidney disease and kidney transplant status.*

See I.C.1.d.4. for sequencing of sepsis due to infection in transplanted organ

4) **Complication codes that include the external cause**
As with certain other T codes, some of the complications of care codes have the external cause included in the code. The code includes the nature of the complication as well as the type of procedure that caused the complication. No external cause code indicating the type of procedure is necessary for these codes.

5) **Complications of care codes within the body system chapters**
Intraoperative and postprocedural complication codes are found within the body system chapters with codes specific to the organs and structures of that body system. These codes should be sequenced first, followed by a code(s) for the specific complication, if applicable.

Complication codes from the body system chapters should be assigned for intraoperative and postprocedural complications (e.g., the appropriate complication code from chapter 9 would be assigned for a vascular intraoperative or postprocedural complication) unless the complication is specifically indexed to a T code in chapter 19.

20. **Chapter 20: External Causes of Morbidity (V00-Y99)**
The external causes of morbidity codes should never be sequenced as the first-listed or principal diagnosis.

External cause codes are intended to provide data for injury research and evaluation of injury prevention strategies. These codes capture how the injury or health condition happened (cause), the intent (unintentional or accidental; or intentional, such as suicide or assault), the place where the event occurred the activity of the patient at the time of the event, and the person's status (e.g., civilian, military).

There is no national requirement for mandatory ICD-10-CM external cause code reporting. Unless a provider is subject to a state-based external cause code reporting mandate or these codes are required by a particular payer, reporting of ICD-10-CM codes in Chapter 20, External Causes of Morbidity, is not required. In the absence of a mandatory reporting requirement, providers are encouraged to voluntarily report external cause codes, as they provide valuable data for injury research and evaluation of injury prevention strategies.

a. **General External Cause Coding Guidelines**

1) **Used with any code in the range of A00.0-T88.9, Z00-Z99**
An external cause code may be used with any code in the range of A00.0-T88.9, Z00-Z99, classification that represents a health condition due to an external cause. Though they are most applicable to injuries,
they are also valid for use with such things as infections or diseases due to an external source, and other health conditions, such as a heart attack that occurs during strenuous physical activity.

2) **External cause code used for length of treatment**
Assign the external cause code, with the appropriate 7th character (initial encounter, subsequent encounter or sequela) for each encounter for which the injury or condition is being treated.

Most categories in chapter 20 have a 7th character requirement for each applicable code. Most categories in this chapter have three 7th character values: A, initial encounter, D, subsequent encounter and S, sequela. While the patient may be seen by a new or different provider over the course of treatment for an injury or condition, assignment of the 7th character for external cause should match the 7th character of the code assigned for the associated injury or condition for the encounter.

3) **Use the full range of external cause codes**
Use the full range of external cause codes to completely describe the cause, the intent, the place of occurrence, and if applicable, the activity of the patient at the time of the event, and the patient's status, for all injuries, and other health conditions due to an external cause.

4) **Assign as many external cause codes as necessary**
Assign as many external cause codes as necessary to fully explain each cause. If only one external code can be recorded, assign the code most related to the principal diagnosis.

5) **The selection of the appropriate external cause code**
The selection of the appropriate external cause code is guided by the Alphabetic Index of External Causes and by Inclusion and Exclusion notes in the Tabular List.

6) **External cause code can never be a principal diagnosis**
An external cause code can never be a principal (first-listed) diagnosis.

7) **Combination external cause codes**
Certain of the external cause codes are combination codes that identify sequential events that result in an injury, such as a fall which results in striking against an object. The injury may be due to either event or both. The combination external cause code used should correspond to the sequence of events regardless of which caused the most serious injury.

8) **No external cause code needed in certain circumstances**
No external cause code from Chapter 20 is needed if the external cause and intent are included in a code from another chapter (e.g., T36.0X1-, Poisoning by penicillins, accidental (unintentional)).

b. **Place of Occurrence Guideline**
Codes from category Y92, Place of occurrence of the external cause, are secondary codes for use after other external cause codes to identify the location of the patient at the time of injury or other condition.

Generally, a place of occurrence code is assigned only once, at the initial encounter for treatment. However, in the rare instance that a new injury occurs during hospitalization, an additional place of occurrence code may be assigned. No 7th characters are used for Y92.

Do not use place of occurrence code Y92.9 if the place is not stated or is not applicable.

c. **Activity Code**
Assign a code from category Y93, Activity code, to describe the activity of the patient at the time the injury or other health condition occurred.

An activity code is used only once, at the initial encounter for treatment. Only one code from Y93 should be recorded on a medical record.

The activity codes are not applicable to poisonings, adverse effects, misadventures or sequela.

Do not assign Y93.9, Unspecified activity, if the activity is not stated.

A code from category Y93 is appropriate for use with external cause and intent codes if identifying the activity provides additional information about the event.

d. **Place of Occurrence, Activity, and Status Codes Used with other External Cause Code**
When applicable, place of occurrence, activity, and external cause status codes are sequenced after the main external cause code(s). Regardless of the number of external cause codes assigned, generally there should be only one place of occurrence code, one activity code, and one external cause status code assigned to an encounter. However, in the rare instance that a new injury occurs during hospitalization, an additional place of occurrence code may be assigned.

e. **If the Reporting Format Limits the Number of External Cause Codes**
If the reporting format limits the number of external cause codes that can be used in reporting clinical data, report the code for the cause/intent most related to the principal diagnosis. If the format permits capture of additional external cause codes, the cause/intent, including medical misadventures, of the additional events should be reported rather than the codes for place, activity, or external status.

f. **Multiple External Cause Coding Guidelines**
More than one external cause code is required to fully describe the external cause of an illness or injury. The assignment of external cause codes should be sequenced in the following priority:

If two or more events cause separate injuries, an external cause code should be assigned for each cause. The first-listed external cause code will be selected in the following order:

External codes for child and adult abuse take priority over all other external cause codes.

See Section I.C.19., Child and Adult abuse guidelines.

External cause codes for terrorism events take priority over all other external cause codes except child and adult abuse.

External cause codes for cataclysmic events take priority over all other external cause codes except child and adult abuse and terrorism.

External cause codes for transport accidents take priority over all other external cause codes except cataclysmic events, child and adult abuse and terrorism.

Activity and external cause status codes are assigned following all causal (intent) external cause codes.

The first-listed external cause code should correspond to the cause of the most serious diagnosis due to an assault, accident, or self-harm, following the order of hierarchy listed above.

g. **Child and Adult Abuse Guideline**
Adult and child abuse, neglect and maltreatment are classified as assault. Any of the assault codes may be used to indicate the external cause of any injury resulting from the confirmed abuse.

For confirmed cases of abuse, neglect and maltreatment, when the perpetrator is known, a code from Y07, Perpetrator of maltreatment and neglect, should accompany any other assault codes.

See Section I.C.19. Adult and child abuse, neglect and other maltreatment

h. **Unknown or Undetermined Intent Guideline**
If the intent (accident, self-harm, assault) of the cause of an injury or other condition is unknown or unspecified, code the intent as accidental intent. All transport accident categories assume accidental intent.

1) **Use of undetermined intent**
External cause codes for events of undetermined intent are only for use if the documentation in the record specifies that the intent cannot be determined.

i. **Sequelae (Late Effects) of External Cause Guidelines**
1) **Sequelae external cause codes**
Sequela are reported using the external cause code with the 7th character "S" for sequela. These codes should be used with any report of a late effect or sequela resulting from a previous injury.
See Section I.B.10. Sequela (Late Effects)

2) **Sequela external cause code with a related current injury**
A sequela external cause code should never be used with a related current nature of injury code.

3) **Use of sequela external cause codes for subsequent visits**
Use a late effect external cause code for subsequent visits when a late effect of the initial injury is being treated. Do not use a late effect external cause code for subsequent visits for follow-up care (e.g., to assess healing, to receive rehabilitative therapy) of the injury when no late effect of the injury has been documented.

j. **Terrorism Guidelines**
1) **Cause of injury identified by the Federal Government (FBI) as terrorism**
When the cause of an injury is identified by the Federal Government (FBI) as terrorism, the first-listed external cause code should be a code from category Y38, Terrorism. The definition of terrorism employed by the FBI is found at the inclusion note at the beginning of category Y38. Use additional code for place of occurrence (Y92.-). More than one Y38 code may be assigned if the injury is the result of more than one mechanism of terrorism.

2) **Cause of an injury is suspected to be the result of terrorism**
When the cause of an injury is suspected to be the result of terrorism a code from category Y38 should not be assigned. Suspected cases should be classified as assault.

3) **Code Y38.9, Terrorism, secondary effects**
Assign code Y38.9, Terrorism, secondary effects, for conditions occurring subsequent to the terrorist event. This code should not be assigned for conditions that are due to the initial terrorist act.

It is acceptable to assign code Y38.9 with another code from Y38 if there is an injury due to the initial terrorist event and an injury that is a subsequent result of the terrorist event.

k. **External Cause Status**
A code from category Y99, External cause status, should be assigned whenever any other external cause code is assigned for an encounter, including an Activity code, except for the events noted below. Assign a code from category Y99, External cause status, to indicate the work status of the person at the time the event occurred. The status code indicates whether the event occurred during military activity, whether a non-military person was at work, whether an individual including a student or volunteer was involved in a non-work activity at the time of the causal event.

A code from Y99, External cause status, should be assigned, when applicable, with other external cause codes, such as transport accidents and falls. The external cause status codes are not applicable to poisonings, adverse effects, misadventures or late effects.

Do not assign a code from category Y99 if no other external cause codes (cause, activity) are applicable for the encounter.

An external cause status code is used only once, at the initial encounter for treatment. Only one code from Y99 should be recorded on a medical record.

Do not assign code Y99.9, Unspecified external cause status, if the status is not stated.

21. **Chapter 21: Factors influencing health status and contact with health services (Z00-Z99)**
Note: The chapter specific guidelines provide additional information about the use of Z codes for specified encounters.

a. **Use of Z Codes in Any Healthcare Setting**
Z codes are for use in any healthcare setting. Z codes may be used as either a first-listed (principal diagnosis code in the inpatient setting) or secondary code, depending on the circumstances of the encounter. Certain Z codes may only be used as first-listed or principal diagnosis.

b. **Z Codes Indicate a Reason for an Encounter or Provide Additional Information about a Patient Encounter**
Z codes are not procedure codes. A corresponding procedure code must accompany a Z code to describe any procedure performed.

c. **Categories of Z Codes**
1) **Contact/Exposure**
Category Z20 indicates contact with, and suspected exposure to, communicable diseases. These codes are for patients who are suspected to have been exposed to a disease by close personal contact with an infected individual or are in an area where a disease is epidemic.

Category Z77, Other contact with and (suspected) exposures hazardous to health, indicates contact with and suspected exposures hazardous to health.

Contact/exposure codes may be used as a first-listed code to explain an encounter for testing, or, more commonly, as a secondary code to identify a potential risk.

2) **Inoculations and vaccinations**
Code Z23 is for encounters for inoculations and vaccinations. It indicates that a patient is being seen to receive a prophylactic inoculation against a disease. Procedure codes are required to identify the actual administration of the injection and the type(s) of immunizations given. Code Z23 may be used as a secondary code if the inoculation is given as a routine part of preventive health care, such as a well-baby visit.

3) **Status**
Status codes indicate that a patient is either a carrier of a disease or has the sequelae or residual of a past disease or condition. This includes such things as the presence of prosthetic or mechanical devices resulting from past treatment. A status code is informative, because the status may affect the course of treatment and its outcome. A status code is distinct from a history code. The history code indicates that the patient no longer has the condition.

A status code should not be used with a diagnosis code from one of the body system chapters, if the diagnosis code includes the information provided by the status code. For example, code Z94.1, Heart transplant status, should not be used with a code from subcategory T86.2, Complications of heart transplant. The status code does not provide additional information. The complication code indicates that the patient is a heart transplant patient.

For encounters for weaning from a mechanical ventilator, assign a code from subcategory J96.1, Chronic respiratory failure, followed by code Z99.11, Dependence on respirator [ventilator] status.

The status Z codes/categories are:

Z14   Genetic carrier
       Genetic carrier status indicates that a person carries a gene, associated with a particular disease, which may be passed to offspring who may develop that disease. The person does not have the disease and is not at risk of developing the disease.

Z15   Genetic susceptibility to disease
       Genetic susceptibility indicates that a person has a gene that increases the risk of that person developing the disease. Codes from category Z15 should **generally** not be used as principal or first-listed codes. If the patient has the condition to which he/she is susceptible, and that condition is the reason for the encounter, the code for the current condition should be sequenced first. If the patient is being seen for follow-up after completed treatment for this condition, and the condition no longer exists, a follow-up code should be sequenced first, followed by the appropriate personal history and genetic susceptibility codes. If the purpose of the encounter is genetic counseling associated with procreative management, code Z31.5, Encounter for genetic counseling, should be assigned as the first-listed code, followed by a code from category Z15.

	Additional codes should be assigned for any applicable family or personal history.
Z16	Resistance to antimicrobial drugs
	This **category** indicates that a patient has a condition that is resistant to antimicrobial drug treatment. Sequence the infection code first.
Z17	Estrogen, and other hormones and factors receptor status
Z18	Retained foreign body fragments
Z19	Hormone sensitivity malignancy status
Z21	Asymptomatic HIV infection status
	This code indicates that a patient has tested positive for HIV but has manifested no signs or symptoms of the disease.
Z22	Carrier of infectious disease
	Carrier status indicates that a person harbors the specific organisms of a disease without manifest symptoms and is capable of transmitting the infection.
Z28.3	Underimmunization status
	See Section I.B.14. for underimmunization documentation by clinicians other than the patient's provider.
Z33.1	Pregnant state, incidental
	This code is a secondary code only for use when the pregnancy is in no way complicating the reason for visit. Otherwise, a code from the obstetric chapter is required.
Z66	Do not resuscitate
	This code may be used when it is documented by the provider that a patient is on do not resuscitate status at any time during the stay.
Z67	Blood type
Z68	Body mass index (BMI)
	BMI codes should only be assigned when there is an associated, reportable diagnosis (such as obesity or anorexia) documented by the patient's provider.
	Do not assign BMI codes during pregnancy. When the documentation reflects fluctuating BMI values during the current encounter for an associated reportable condition, assign a code for the most severe value.
	See Section I.B.14. for BMI documentation by clinicians other than the patient's provider.
Z74.01	Bed confinement status
Z76.82	Awaiting organ transplant status
Z78	Other specified health status
	Code Z78.1, Physical restraint status, may be used when it is documented by the provider that a patient has been put in restraints during the current encounter. Please note that this code should not be reported when it is documented by the provider that a patient is temporarily restrained during a procedure.
Z79	Long-term (current) drug therapy
	Codes from this category indicate a patient's continuous use of a prescribed drug (including such things as aspirin therapy) for the long-term treatment of a condition or for prophylactic use. It is not for use for patients who have addictions to drugs. This subcategory is not for use of medications for detoxification or maintenance programs to prevent withdrawal symptoms (e.g., methadone maintenance for opiate dependence). Assign the appropriate code for the drug use, abuse, or dependence instead.
	Assign a code from Z79 if the patient is receiving a medication for an extended period as a prophylactic measure (such as for the prevention of deep vein thrombosis) or as treatment of a chronic condition (such as arthritis) or a disease requiring a lengthy course of treatment (such as cancer). Do not assign a code from category Z79 for medication being administered for a brief period of time to treat an acute illness or injury (such as a course of antibiotics to treat acute bronchitis).
Z88	Allergy status to drugs, medicaments and biological substances
	Except: Z88.9, Allergy status to unspecified drugs, medicaments and biological substances status
Z89	Acquired absence of limb
Z90	Acquired absence of organs, not elsewhere classified
Z91.0-	Allergy status, other than to drugs and biological substances
Z92.82	Status post administration of tPA (rtPA) in a different facility within the last 24 hours prior to admission to a current facility
	Assign code Z92.82, Status post administration of tPA (rtPA) in a different facility within the last 24 hours prior to admission to current facility, as a secondary diagnosis when a patient is received by transfer into a facility and documentation indicates they were administered tissue plasminogen activator (tPA) within the last 24 hours prior to admission to the current facility. This guideline applies even if the patient is still receiving the tPA at the time they are received into the current facility.
	The appropriate code for the condition for which the tPA was administered (such as cerebrovascular disease or myocardial infarction) should be assigned first.
	Code Z92.82 is only applicable to the receiving facility record and not to the transferring facility record.

Z93	Artificial opening status
Z94	Transplanted organ and tissue status
Z95	Presence of cardiac and vascular implants and grafts
Z96	Presence of other functional implants
Z97	Presence of other devices
Z98	Other postprocedural states
	Assign code Z98.85, Transplanted organ removal status, to indicate that a transplanted organ has been previously removed. This code should not be assigned for the encounter in which the transplanted organ is removed. The complication necessitating removal of the transplant organ should be assigned for that encounter.
	See section I.C.19. for information on the coding of organ transplant complications.
Z99	Dependence on enabling machines and devices, not elsewhere classified
	Note: Categories Z89-Z90 and Z93-Z99 are for use only if there are no complications or malfunctions of the organ or tissue replaced, the amputation site or the equipment on which the patient is dependent.

4) **History (of)**

There are two types of history Z codes, personal and family. Personal history codes explain a patient's past medical condition that no longer exists and is not receiving any treatment, but that has the potential for recurrence, and therefore may require continued monitoring.

Family history codes are for use when a patient has a family member(s) who has had a particular disease that causes the patient to be at higher risk of also contracting the disease.

Personal history codes may be used in conjunction with follow-up codes and family history codes may be used in conjunction with screening codes to explain the need for a test or procedure. History codes are also acceptable on any medical record regardless of the reason for visit. A history of an illness, even if no longer present, is important information that may alter the type of treatment ordered.

The reason for the encounter (for example, screening or counseling) should be sequenced first and the appropriate personal and/or family history code(s) should be assigned as additional diagnos(es).

The history Z code categories are:

Z80	Family history of primary malignant neoplasm
Z81	Family history of mental and behavioral disorders
Z82	Family history of certain disabilities and chronic diseases (leading to disablement)
Z83	Family history of other specific disorders
Z84	Family history of other conditions
Z85	Personal history of malignant neoplasm
Z86	Personal history of certain other diseases
Z87	Personal history of other diseases and conditions
Z91.4-	Personal history of psychological trauma, not elsewhere classified
Z91.5-	Personal history of self-harm
Z91.81	History of falling
Z91.82	Personal history of military deployment
Z91.85	Personal history of military service
Z92	Personal history of medical treatment
	Except: Z92.0, Personal history of contraception
	Except: Z92.82, Status post administration of tPA (rtPA) in a different facility within the last 24 hours prior to admission to a current facility

5) **Screening**

Screening is the testing for disease or disease precursors in seemingly well individuals so that early detection and treatment can be provided for those who test positive for the disease (e.g., screening mammogram).

The testing of a person to rule out or confirm a suspected diagnosis because the patient has some sign or symptom is a diagnostic examination, not a screening. In these cases, the sign or symptom is used to explain the reason for the test.

A screening code may be a first-listed code if the reason for the visit is specifically the screening exam. It may also be used as an additional code if the screening is done during an office visit for other health problems. A screening code is not necessary if the screening is inherent to a routine examination, such as a pap smear done during a routine pelvic examination.

Should a condition be discovered during the screening then the code for the condition may be assigned as an additional diagnosis.

The Z code indicates that a screening exam is planned. A procedure code is required to confirm that the screening was performed.

The screening Z codes/categories:

Z11	Encounter for screening for infectious and parasitic diseases
Z12	Encounter for screening for malignant neoplasms
Z13	Encounter for screening for other diseases and disorders Except: Z13.9, Encounter for screening, unspecified
Z36	Encounter for antenatal screening for mother

6) **Observation**
There are three observation Z code categories. They are for use in very limited circumstances when a person is being observed for a suspected condition that is ruled out. The observation codes are not for use if an injury or illness or any signs or symptoms related to the suspected condition are present. In such cases the diagnosis/symptom code is used with the corresponding external cause code.

The observation codes are primarily to be used as a principal/first-listed diagnosis. An observation code may be assigned as a secondary diagnosis code when the patient is being observed for a condition that is ruled out and is unrelated to the principal/first-listed diagnosis. Also, when the principal diagnosis is required to be a code from category Z38, Liveborn infants according to place of birth and type of delivery, then a code from category Z05, Encounter for observation and evaluation of newborn for suspected diseases and conditions ruled out, is sequenced after the Z38 code. Additional codes may be used in addition to the observation code, but only if they are unrelated to the suspected condition being observed.

Codes from subcategory Z03.7, Encounter for suspected maternal and fetal conditions ruled out, may either be used as a first-listed or as an additional code assignment depending on the case. They are for use in very limited circumstances on a maternal record when an encounter is for a suspected maternal or fetal condition that is ruled out during that encounter (for example, a maternal or fetal condition may be suspected due to an abnormal test result). These codes should not be used when the condition is confirmed. In those cases, the confirmed condition should be coded. In addition, these codes are not for use if an illness or any signs or symptoms related to the suspected condition or problem are present. In such cases the diagnosis/symptom code is used.

Additional codes may be used in addition to the code from subcategory Z03.7, but only if they are unrelated to the suspected condition being evaluated.

Codes from subcategory Z03.7 may not be used for encounters for antenatal screening of mother. *See Section I.C.21. Screening.*

For encounters for suspected fetal condition that are inconclusive following testing and evaluation, assign the appropriate code from category O35, O36, O40 or O41.

The observation Z code categories:

Z03   Encounter for medical observation for suspected diseases and conditions ruled out
Z04   Encounter for examination and observation for other reasons Except: Z04.9, Encounter for examination and observation for unspecified reason
Z05   Encounter for observation and evaluation of newborn for suspected diseases and conditions ruled out

7) **Aftercare**
Aftercare visit codes cover situations when the initial treatment of a disease has been performed and the patient requires continued care during the healing or recovery phase, or for the long-term consequences of the disease. The aftercare Z code should not be used if treatment is directed at a current, acute disease. The diagnosis code is to be used in these cases.

The aftercare Z codes should also not be used for aftercare for injuries. For aftercare of an injury, assign the acute injury code with the appropriate 7th character (for subsequent encounter).

The aftercare codes are generally first listed to explain the specific reason for the encounter. An aftercare code may be reported as an additional code when a specific type of aftercare is provided in addition to the reason for the encounter. An example of this would be the closure of a colostomy during an encounter for treatment of another condition.

Aftercare codes should be used in conjunction with other aftercare codes or diagnosis codes to provide better detail on the specifics of an aftercare encounter visit, unless otherwise directed by the classification. The sequencing of multiple aftercare codes depends on the circumstances of the encounter.

Certain aftercare Z code categories need a secondary diagnosis code to describe the resolving condition or sequelae. For others, the condition is included in the code title.

Additional Z code aftercare category terms include fitting and adjustment, and attention to artificial openings.

Status Z codes may be used with aftercare Z codes to indicate the nature of the aftercare. For example, code Z95.1, Presence of aortocoronary bypass graft, may be used with code Z48.812, Encounter for surgical aftercare following surgery on the circulatory system, to indicate the surgery for which the aftercare is being performed. A status code should not be used when the aftercare code indicates the type of status, such as using Z43.0, Encounter for attention to tracheostomy, with Z93.0, Tracheostomy status.

The aftercare codes are generally found in the following categories:

Z42   Encounter for plastic and reconstructive surgery following medical procedure or healed injury
Z43   Encounter for attention to artificial openings
Z44   Encounter for fitting and adjustment of external prosthetic device
Z45   Encounter for adjustment and management of implanted device
Z46   Encounter for fitting and adjustment of other devices
Z47   Orthopedic aftercare
Z48   Encounter for other postprocedural aftercare
Z49   Encounter for care involving renal dialysis
Z51   Encounter for other aftercare and medical care

8) **Follow-up**
The follow-up codes are used to explain continuing surveillance following completed treatment of a disease, condition, or injury. They imply that the condition has been fully treated and no longer exists. They should not be confused with aftercare codes, or injury codes with a 7th character for subsequent encounter, that explain ongoing care of a healing condition or its sequelae. Follow-up codes may be used in conjunction with history codes to provide the full picture of the healed condition and its treatment. The follow-up code is sequenced first, followed by the history code.

A follow-up code may be used to explain multiple visits. Should a condition be found to have recurred on the follow-up visit, then the diagnosis code for the condition should be assigned in place of the follow-up code.

The follow-up Z codes/categories:

Z08   Encounter for follow-up examination after completed treatment for malignant neoplasm
Z09   Encounter for follow-up examination after completed treatment for conditions other than malignant neoplasm

Codes Z08, Encounter for follow-up examination after completed treatment for malignant neoplasm, and Z09, Encounter for follow up examination after completed treatment for conditions other than malignant neoplasm, may be assigned following any type of completed treatment modality (including both medical and surgical treatments).

Z39   Encounter for maternal postpartum care and examination

9) **Donor**
Codes in category Z52, Donors of organs and tissues, are used for living individuals who are donating blood or other body tissue. These codes are for individuals donating for others, as well as for self-donations. They are not used to identify cadaveric donations.

10) **Counseling**
Counseling Z codes are used when a patient or family member receives assistance in the aftermath of an illness or injury, or when support is required in coping with family or social problems.

The counseling Z codes/categories:

Z30.0-   Encounter for general counseling and advice on contraception
Z31.5   Encounter for procreative genetic counseling
Z31.6-   Encounter for general counseling and advice on procreation
Z32.2   Encounter for childbirth instruction
Z32.3   Encounter for childcare instruction
Z69   Encounter for mental health services for victim and perpetrator of abuse
Z70   Counseling related to sexual attitude, behavior and orientation
Z71   Persons encountering health services for other counseling and medical advice, not elsewhere classified
Note: Code Z71.84, Encounter for health counseling related to travel, is to be used for health risk and safety counseling for future travel purposes.
Code Z71.85, Encounter for immunization safety counseling, is to be used for counseling of the patient or caregiver regarding the safety of a vaccine. This code should not be used for the provision of general information regarding risks and potential side effects during routine encounters for the administration of vaccines.
Code Z71.87, Encounter for pediatric-to-adult transition counseling, should be assigned when pediatric-to-adult transition counseling is the sole reason for the encounter or when this counseling is provided in addition to other services, such as treatment of a chronic condition. If both transition counseling and treatment of a medical condition are provided during the same encounter, the code(s) for the medical condition(s) treated and code Z71.87 should be assigned, with sequencing depending on the circumstances of the encounter.
Z76.81   Expectant mother prebirth pediatrician visit

11) **Encounters for Obstetrical and Reproductive Services**
See Section I.C.15. Pregnancy, Childbirth, and the Puerperium, for further instruction on the use of these codes.

Z codes for pregnancy are for use in those circumstances when none of the problems or complications included in the codes from the Obstetrics chapter exist (a routine prenatal visit or postpartum care). Codes in category Z34, Encounter for supervision of normal pregnancy, are always first listed and are not to be used with any other code from the OB chapter.

Codes in category Z3A, Weeks of gestation, may be assigned to provide additional information about the pregnancy. Category Z3A codes should not be assigned for pregnancies with abortive outcomes (categories O00-O08), elective termination of pregnancy (code Z33.2), nor for postpartum conditions, as category Z3A is not applicable to these conditions. The date of the admission should be used to determine weeks of gestation for inpatient admissions that encompass more than one gestational week.

The outcome of delivery, category Z37, should be included on all maternal delivery records. It is always a secondary code.

Codes in category Z37 should not be used on the newborn record.

Z codes for family planning (contraceptive) or procreative management and counseling should be included on an obstetric record either during the pregnancy or the postpartum stage, if applicable.

Z codes/categories for obstetrical and reproductive services:

Z30	Encounter for contraceptive management
Z31	Encounter for procreative management
Z32.2	Encounter for childbirth instruction
Z32.3	Encounter for childcare instruction
Z33	Pregnant state
Z34	Encounter for supervision of normal pregnancy
Z36	Encounter for antenatal screening of mother
Z3A	Weeks of gestation
Z37	Outcome of delivery
Z39	Encounter for maternal postpartum care and examination
Z76.81	Expectant mother prebirth pediatrician visit

12) Routine and Administrative Examinations

The Z codes allow for the description of encounters for routine examinations, such as, a general check-up, or, examinations for administrative purposes, such as, a pre-employment physical. The codes are not to be used if the examination is for diagnosis of a suspected condition or for treatment purposes. In such cases the diagnosis code is used. During a routine exam, should a diagnosis or condition be discovered, it should be coded as an additional code. Pre-existing and chronic conditions and history codes may also be included as additional codes as long as the examination is for administrative purposes and not focused on any particular condition.

Some of the codes for routine health examinations distinguish between "with" and "without" abnormal findings. Code assignment depends on the information that is known at the time the encounter is being coded. For example, if no abnormal findings were found during the examination, but the encounter is being coded before test results are back, it is acceptable to assign the code for "without abnormal findings." When assigning a code for "with abnormal findings," additional code(s) should be assigned to identify the specific abnormal finding(s).

Pre-operative examination and pre-procedural laboratory examination Z codes are for use only in those situations when a patient is being cleared for a procedure or surgery and no treatment is given.

The Z codes/categories for routine and administrative examinations:

Z00	Encounter for general examination without complaint, suspected or reported diagnosis
Z01	Encounter for other special examination without complaint, suspected or reported diagnosis
Z02	Encounter for administrative examination Except: Z02.9, Encounter for administrative examinations, unspecified
Z32.0-	Encounter for pregnancy test

13) Miscellaneous Z Codes

The miscellaneous Z codes capture a number of other health care encounters that do not fall into one of the other categories. Some of these codes identify the reason for the encounter; others are for use as additional codes that provide useful information on circumstances that may affect a patient's care and treatment.

Prophylactic Organ Removal
For encounters specifically for prophylactic removal of an organ (such as prophylactic removal of breasts due to a genetic susceptibility to cancer or a family history of cancer), the principal or first-listed code should be a code from subcategory Z40.0, Encounter for prophylactic surgery for risk factors related to malignant neoplasms, or subcategory Z40.8, Encounter for other prophylactic surgery. If applicable, assign additional code(s) to identify any associated risk factor (such as genetic susceptibility or family history).

If the patient has a malignancy of one site and is having prophylactic removal at another site to prevent either a new primary malignancy or metastatic disease, a code for the malignancy should also be assigned in addition to a code from subcategory Z40.0, Encounter for prophylactic surgery for risk factors related to malignant neoplasms. A Z40.0 code should not be assigned if the patient is having organ removal for treatment of a malignancy, such as the removal of the testes for the treatment of prostate cancer.

Miscellaneous Z codes/subcategories/categories:

Z28	Immunization not carried out Except: Z28.3-, Underimmunization status
Z29	Encounter for other prophylactic measures
Z40	Encounter for prophylactic surgery
Z41	Encounter for procedures for purposes other than remedying health state Except: Z41.9, Encounter for procedure for purposes other than remedying health state, unspecified
Z53	Persons encountering health services for specific procedures and treatment, not carried out
Z72	Problems related to lifestyle Note: These codes should be assigned only when the documentation specifies that the patient has an associated problem
Z73	Problems related to life management difficulty Note: These codes should be assigned only when the documentation specifies that the patient has an associated problem
Z74	Problems related to care provider dependency Except: Z74.01, Bed confinement status
Z75	Problems related to medical facilities and other health care
Z76.0	Encounter for issue of repeat prescription
Z76.3	Healthy person accompanying sick person
Z76.4	Other boarder to healthcare facility
Z76.5	Malingerer [conscious simulation]
Z91.1-	Patient's noncompliance with medical treatment and regimen
Z91.A-	Caregiver's noncompliance with patient's medical treatment and regimen
Z91.B	**Personal risk factor of exposure to diethylstilbestrol**
Z91.83	Wandering in diseases classified elsewhere
Z91.84-	Oral health risk factors
Z91.89	Other specified personal risk factors, not elsewhere classified

See Section I.B.14. for Z55-Z65 Persons with potential health hazards related to socioeconomic and psychosocial circumstances, documentation by clinicians other than the patient's provider

14) Nonspecific Z Codes

Certain Z codes are so non-specific, or potentially redundant with other codes in the classification, that there can be little justification for their use in the inpatient setting. Their use in the outpatient setting should be limited to those instances when there is no further documentation to permit more precise coding. Otherwise, any sign or symptom or any other reason for visit that is captured in another code should be used.

Nonspecific Z codes/categories:

Z02.9	Encounter for administrative examinations, unspecified
Z04.9	Encounter for examination and observation for unspecified reason
Z13.9	Encounter for screening, unspecified
Z41.9	Encounter for procedure for purposes other than remedying health state, unspecified
Z52.9	Donor of unspecified organ or tissue
Z86.59	Personal history of other mental and behavioral disorders
Z88.9	Allergy status to unspecified drugs, medicaments and biological substances status
Z92.0	Personal history of contraception

15) Z Codes That May Only be Principal/First-Listed Diagnosis

The following Z codes/**subcategories**/categories may only be reported as the principal/first-listed diagnosis, except when there are multiple encounters on the same day and the medical records for the encounters are combined:

Z00	Encounter for general examination without complaint, suspected or reported diagnosis Except: Z00.6
Z01	Encounter for other special examination without complaint, suspected or reported diagnosis
Z02	Encounter for administrative examination
Z04	Encounter for examination and observation for other reasons
Z33.2	Encounter for elective termination of pregnancy
Z31.81	Encounter for male factor infertility in female patient
Z31.83	Encounter for assisted reproductive fertility procedure cycle
Z31.84	Encounter for fertility preservation procedure
Z34	Encounter for supervision of normal pregnancy
Z39	Encounter for maternal postpartum care and examination
Z38	Liveborn infants according to place of birth and type of delivery
Z40	Encounter for prophylactic surgery
Z42	Encounter for plastic and reconstructive surgery following medical procedure or healed injury
Z51.0	Encounter for antineoplastic radiation therapy
Z51.1-	Encounter for antineoplastic chemotherapy and immunotherapy
Z52	Donors of organs and tissues Except: Z52.9, Donor of unspecified organ or tissue

Z76.1 Encounter for health supervision and care of foundling
Z76.2 Encounter for health supervision and care of other healthy infant and child
Z99.12 Encounter for respirator [ventilator] dependence during power failure

16) **Newborns and Infants**
See Section I.C.16. Newborn (Perinatal) Guidelines, for further instruction on the use of these codes.

Newborn Z codes/subcategories/categories:
Z76.1 Encounter for health supervision and care of foundling
Z00.1- Encounter for routine child health examination
Z38 Liveborn infants according to place of birth and type of delivery

17) **Social Determinants of Health**
Social determinants of health (SDOH) codes describing social problems, conditions, or risk factors that influence a patient's health should be assigned when this information is documented in the patient's medical record. Assign as many SDOH codes as are necessary to describe all of the social problems, conditions, or risk factors documented during the current episode of care. For example, a patient who lives alone may suffer an acute injury temporarily impacting their ability to perform routine activities of daily living. When documented as such, this would support assignment of code Z60.2, Problems related to living alone. However, merely living alone, without documentation of a risk or unmet need for assistance at home, would not support assignment of code Z60.2. Documentation by a clinician (or patient-reported information that is signed off by a clinician) that the patient expressed concerns with access and availability of food would support assignment of code Z59.41, Food insecurity. **Similarly, medical record documentation indicating the patient is experiencing homelessness would support assignment of a code from subcategory Z59.0-, Homelessness.**

For social determinants of health classified to chapter 21, such as information found in categories Z55-Z65, Persons with potential health hazards related to socioeconomic and psychosocial circumstances, code assignment may be based on medical record documentation from clinicians involved in the care of the patient who are not the patient's provider since this information represents social information, rather than medical diagnoses. For example, coding professionals may utilize documentation of social information from social workers, community health workers, case managers, or nurses, if their documentation is included in the official medical record.

Patient self-reported documentation may be used to assign codes for social determinants of health, as long as the patient self-reported information is signed-off by and incorporated into the medical record by either a clinician or provider.

Social determinants of health codes are located primarily in these Z code categories:

Z55 Problems related to education and literacy
Z56 Problems related to employment and unemployment
Z57 Occupational exposure to risk factors
Z58 Problems related to physical environment
Z59 Problems related to housing and economic circumstances
Z60 Problems related to social environment
Z62 Problems related to upbringing
Z63 Other problems related to primary support group, including family circumstances
Z64 Problems related to certain psychosocial circumstances
Z65 Problems related to other psychosocial circumstances

See Section I.B.14. Documentation by Clinicians Other than the Patient's Provider.

22. **Chapter 22: Codes for Special Purposes (U00-U85)**
U07.0 Vaping-related disorder (see Section I.C.10.e., Vaping-related disorders)
U07.1 COVID-19 (see Section I.C.1.g.1., COVID-19 infection)
U09.9 Post COVID-19 condition, unspecified (see Section I.C.1.g.1.m.)

Section II. Selection of Principal Diagnosis

The circumstances of inpatient admission always govern the selection of principal diagnosis. The principal diagnosis is defined in the Uniform Hospital Discharge Data Set (UHDDS) as "that condition established after study to be chiefly responsible for occasioning the admission of the patient to the hospital for care."

The UHDDS definitions are used by hospitals to report inpatient data elements in a standardized manner. These data elements and their definitions can be found in the July 31, 1985, Federal Register (Vol. 50, No, 147), pp. 31038-40.

Since that time, the application of the UHDDS definitions has been expanded to include all non-outpatient settings (acute care, short term, long term care and psychiatric hospitals; home health agencies; rehab facilities; nursing homes, etc.). The UHDDS definitions also apply to hospice services (all levels of care).

In determining principal diagnosis, coding conventions in the ICD-10-CM, the Tabular List and Alphabetic Index take precedence over these official coding guidelines. (See Section I.A., Conventions for the ICD-10-CM)

The importance of consistent, complete documentation in the medical record cannot be overemphasized. Without such documentation the application of all coding guidelines is a difficult, if not impossible, task.

A. **Codes for symptoms, signs, and ill-defined conditions**
Codes for symptoms, signs, and ill-defined conditions from Chapter 18 are not to be used as principal diagnosis when a related definitive diagnosis has been established.

B. **Two or more interrelated conditions, each potentially meeting the definition for principal diagnosis.**
When there are two or more interrelated conditions (such as diseases in the same ICD-10-CM chapter or manifestations characteristically associated with a certain disease) potentially meeting the definition of principal diagnosis, either condition may be sequenced first, unless the circumstances of the admission, the therapy provided, the Tabular List, or the Alphabetic Index indicate otherwise.

C. **Two or more diagnoses that equally meet the definition for principal diagnosis**
In the unusual instance when two or more diagnoses equally meet the criteria for principal diagnosis as determined by the circumstances of admission, diagnostic workup and/or therapy provided, and the Alphabetic Index, Tabular List, or another coding guidelines does not provide sequencing direction, any one of the diagnoses may be sequenced first.

D. **Two or more comparative or contrasting conditions**
In those rare instances when two or more contrasting or comparative diagnoses are documented as "either/or" (or similar terminology), they are coded as if the diagnoses were confirmed and the diagnoses are sequenced according to the circumstances of the admission. If no further determination can be made as to which diagnosis should be principal, either diagnosis may be sequenced first.

E. **A symptom(s) followed by contrasting/comparative diagnoses**
GUIDELINE HAS BEEN DELETED EFFECTIVE OCTOBER 1, 2014

F. **Original treatment plan not carried out**
Sequence as the principal diagnosis the condition, which after study occasioned the admission to the hospital, even though treatment may not have been carried out due to unforeseen circumstances.

G. **Complications of surgery and other medical care**
When the admission is for treatment of a complication resulting from surgery or other medical care, the complication code is sequenced as the principal diagnosis. If the complication is classified to the T80-T88 series and the code lacks the necessary specificity in describing the complication, an additional code for the specific complication should be assigned.

H. **Uncertain Diagnosis**
If the diagnosis documented at the time of discharge is qualified as "probable," "suspected," "likely," "questionable," "possible," or "still to be ruled out," "compatible with," "consistent with," or other similar terms indicating uncertainty, code the condition as if it existed or was established. The bases for these guidelines are the diagnostic workup, arrangements for further workup or observation, and initial therapeutic approach that correspond most closely with the established diagnosis.

Note: This guideline is applicable only to inpatient admissions to short-term, acute, long-term care and psychiatric hospitals.

I. **Admission from Observation Unit**
1. **Admission Following Medical Observation**
When a patient is admitted to an observation unit for a medical condition, which either worsens or does not improve, and is subsequently admitted as an inpatient of the same hospital for this same medical condition, the principal diagnosis would be the medical condition which led to the hospital admission.
2. **Admission Following Post-Operative Observation**
When a patient is admitted to an observation unit to monitor a condition (or complication) that develops following outpatient surgery, and then is subsequently admitted as an inpatient of the same hospital, hospitals should apply the Uniform Hospital Discharge Data Set (UHDDS) definition of principal diagnosis as "that condition established after study to be chiefly responsible for occasioning the admission of the patient to the hospital for care."

J. **Admission from Outpatient Surgery**
When a patient receives surgery in the hospital's outpatient surgery department and is subsequently admitted for continuing inpatient care at the same hospital, the following guidelines should be followed in selecting the principal diagnosis for the inpatient admission:
- If the reason for the inpatient admission is a complication, assign the complication as the principal diagnosis.
- If no complication, or other condition, is documented as the reason for the inpatient admission, assign the reason for the outpatient surgery as the principal diagnosis.
- If the reason for the inpatient admission is another condition unrelated to the surgery, assign the unrelated condition as the principal diagnosis.

K. **Admissions/Encounters for Rehabilitation**
When the purpose for the admission/encounter is rehabilitation, sequence first the code for the condition for which the service is being performed. For example, for an admission/encounter for rehabilitation for right-sided dominant hemiplegia following a cerebrovascular infarction, report code I69.351,

Hemiplegia and hemiparesis following cerebral infarction affecting right dominant side, as the first-listed or principal diagnosis.

If the condition for which the rehabilitation service is being provided is no longer present, report the appropriate aftercare code as the first-listed or principal diagnosis, unless the rehabilitation service is being provided following an injury. For rehabilitation services following active treatment of an injury, assign the injury code with the appropriate seventh character for subsequent encounter as the first-listed or principal diagnosis. For example, if a patient with severe degenerative osteoarthritis of the hip, underwent hip replacement and the current encounter/admission is for rehabilitation, report code Z47.1, Aftercare following joint replacement surgery, as the first-listed or principal diagnosis. If the patient requires rehabilitation post hip replacement for right intertrochanteric femur fracture, report code S72.141D, Displaced intertrochanteric fracture of right femur, subsequent encounter for closed fracture with routine healing, as the first-listed or principal diagnosis.

See Section I.C.21.c.7., Factors influencing health states and contact with health services, Aftercare.

See Section I.C.19.a., for additional information about the use of 7th characters for injury codes.

Section III. Reporting Additional Diagnoses

GENERAL RULES FOR OTHER (ADDITIONAL) DIAGNOSES
For reporting purposes, the definition for "other diagnoses" is interpreted as additional clinically significant conditions that affect patient care in terms of requiring:
- clinical evaluation; or
- therapeutic treatment; or
- diagnostic procedures; or
- extended length of hospital stay; or
- increased nursing care and/or monitoring.

The UHDDS item #11-b defines Other Diagnoses as "all conditions that coexist at the time of admission, that develop subsequently, or that affect the treatment received and/or the length of stay. Diagnoses that relate to an earlier episode which have no bearing on the current hospital stay are to be excluded." UHDDS definitions apply to inpatients in acute care, short-term, long term care and psychiatric hospital setting. The UHDDS definitions are used by acute care short-term hospitals to report inpatient data elements in a standardized manner. These data elements and their definitions can be found in the July 31, 1985, Federal Register (Vol. 50, No, 147), pp. 31038-40. Since that time, the application of the UHDDS definitions has been expanded to include all non-outpatient settings (acute care, short term, long term care and psychiatric hospitals; home health agencies; rehab facilities; nursing homes, etc.). The UHDDS definitions also apply to hospice services (all levels of care).

The following guidelines are to be applied in designating "other diagnoses" when neither the Alphabetic Index nor the Tabular List in ICD-10-CM provide direction. The listing of the diagnoses in the patient record is the responsibility of the provider.

A. Previous conditions

If the provider has included a diagnosis in the final diagnostic statement, such as the discharge summary or the face sheet, it should ordinarily be coded. Some providers include in the diagnostic statement resolved conditions or diagnoses and status-post procedures from previous admissions that have no bearing on the current stay. Such conditions are not to be reported and are coded only if required by hospital policy.

However, history codes (categories Z80-Z87) may be used as secondary codes if the historical condition or family history has an impact on current care or influences treatment.

B. Abnormal findings

Abnormal findings (laboratory, x-ray, pathologic, and other diagnostic results) are not coded and reported unless the provider indicates their clinical significance. If the findings are outside the normal range and the provider has ordered other tests to evaluate the condition or prescribed treatment, it is appropriate to ask the provider whether the abnormal finding should be added.

Please note: This differs from the coding practices in the outpatient setting for coding encounters for diagnostic tests that have been interpreted by a provider.

C. Uncertain Diagnosis

If the diagnosis documented at the time of discharge is qualified as "probable," "suspected," "likely," "questionable," "possible," or "still to be ruled out," "compatible with," "consistent with," or other similar terms indicating uncertainty, code the condition as if it existed or was established. The bases for these guidelines are the diagnostic workup, arrangements for further workup or observation, and initial therapeutic approach that correspond most closely with the established diagnosis.

Note: This guideline is applicable only to inpatient admissions to short-term, acute, long-term care and psychiatric hospitals.

Section IV. Diagnostic Coding and Reporting Guidelines for Outpatient Services

These coding guidelines for outpatient diagnoses have been approved for use by hospitals/ providers in coding and reporting hospital-based outpatient services and provider-based office visits. Guidelines in Section I, Conventions, general coding guidelines and chapter-specific guidelines, should also be applied for outpatient services and office visits.

Information about the use of certain abbreviations, punctuation, symbols, and other conventions used in the ICD-10-CM Tabular List (code numbers and titles), can be found in Section IA of these guidelines, under "Conventions Used in the Tabular List." Section I.B. contains general guidelines that apply to the entire classification. Section I.C. contains chapter-specific guidelines that correspond to the chapters as they are arranged in the classification. Information about the correct sequence to use in finding a code is also described in Section I.

The terms encounter and visit are often used interchangeably in describing outpatient service contacts and, therefore, appear together in these guidelines without distinguishing one from the other.

Though the conventions and general guidelines apply to all settings, coding guidelines for outpatient and provider reporting of diagnoses will vary in a number of instances from those for inpatient diagnoses, recognizing that:

The Uniform Hospital Discharge Data Set (UHDDS) definition of principal diagnosis does not apply to hospital-based outpatient services and provider-based office visits. Coding guidelines for inconclusive diagnoses (probable, suspected, rule out, etc.) were developed for inpatient reporting and do not apply to outpatients.

A. Selection of first-listed condition

In the outpatient setting, the term first-listed diagnosis is used in lieu of principal diagnosis.

In determining the first-listed diagnosis the coding conventions of ICD-10-CM, as well as the general and disease specific guidelines take precedence over the outpatient guidelines.

Diagnoses often are not established at the time of the initial encounter/visit. It may take two or more visits before the diagnosis is confirmed.

The most critical rule involves beginning the search for the correct code assignment through the Alphabetic Index. Never begin searching initially in the Tabular List as this will lead to coding errors.

1. **Outpatient Surgery**
   When a patient presents for outpatient surgery (same day surgery), code the reason for the surgery as the first-listed diagnosis (reason for the encounter), even if the surgery is not performed due to a contraindication.

2. **Observation Stay**
   When a patient is admitted for observation for a medical condition, assign a code for the medical condition as the first-listed diagnosis.

   When a patient presents for outpatient surgery and develops complications requiring admission to observation, code the reason for the surgery as the first reported diagnosis (reason for the encounter), followed by codes for the complications as secondary diagnoses.

B. Codes from A00.0 through T88.9, Z00-Z99, U00-U85

The appropriate code(s) from A00.0 through T88.9, Z00-Z99 and U00-U85 must be used to identify diagnoses, symptoms, conditions, problems, complaints, or other reason(s) for the encounter/visit.

C. Accurate reporting of ICD-10-CM diagnosis codes

For accurate reporting of ICD-10-CM diagnosis codes, the documentation should describe the patient's condition, using terminology which includes specific diagnoses as well as symptoms, problems, or reasons for the encounter. There are ICD-10-CM codes to describe all of these.

D. Codes that describe symptoms and signs

Codes that describe symptoms and signs, as opposed to diagnoses, are acceptable for reporting purposes when a diagnosis has not been established (confirmed) by the provider. Chapter 18 of ICD-10-CM, Symptoms, Signs, and Abnormal Clinical and Laboratory Findings Not Elsewhere Classified (codes R00-R99) contain many, but not all codes for symptoms.

E. Encounters for circumstances other than a disease or injury

ICD-10-CM provides codes to deal with encounters for circumstances other than a disease or injury. The Factors Influencing Health Status and Contact with Health Services codes (Z00-Z99) are provided to deal with occasions when circumstances other than a disease or injury are recorded as diagnosis or problems.

See Section I.C.21. Factors influencing health status and contact with health services.

F. Level of Detail in Coding

1. **ICD-10-CM codes with 3, 4, 5, 6 or 7 characters**
   ICD-10-CM is composed of codes with 3, 4, 5, 6 or 7 characters. Codes with three characters are included in ICD-10-CM as the heading of a category of codes that may be further subdivided by the use of fourth, fifth, sixth or seventh characters to provide greater specificity.

2. **Use of full number of characters required for a code**
   A three-character code is to be used only if it is not further subdivided. A code is invalid if it has not been coded to the full number of characters required for that code, including the 7th character, if applicable.

3. **Highest level of specificity**
   Code to the highest level of specificity when supported by the medical record documentation.

G. ICD-10-CM code for the diagnosis, condition, problem, or other reason for encounter/visit

List first the ICD-10-CM code for the diagnosis, condition, problem, or other reason for encounter/visit shown in the medical record to be chiefly responsible for the services provided. List additional codes that describe any coexisting conditions. In some cases, the first-listed diagnosis may be a symptom when a diagnosis has not been established (confirmed) by the provider.

H. Uncertain diagnosis
Do not code diagnoses documented as "probable," "suspected," "questionable," "rule out," "compatible with," "consistent with," or "working diagnosis" or other similar terms indicating uncertainty. Rather, code the condition(s) to the highest degree of certainty for that encounter/visit, such as symptoms, signs, abnormal test results, or other reason for the visit.

Please note: This differs from the coding practices used by short-term, acute care, long-term care and psychiatric hospitals.

I. Chronic diseases
Chronic diseases treated on an ongoing basis may be coded and reported as many times as the patient receives treatment and care for the condition(s).

J. Code all documented conditions that coexist
Code all documented conditions that coexist at the time of the encounter/visit and that require or affect patient care, treatment or management. Do not code conditions that were previously treated and no longer exist. However, history codes (categories Z80-Z87) may be used as secondary codes if the historical condition or family history has an impact on current care or influences treatment.

K. Patients receiving diagnostic services only
For patients receiving diagnostic services only during an encounter/visit, sequence first the diagnosis, condition, problem, or other reason for encounter/visit shown in the medical record to be chiefly responsible for the outpatient services provided during the encounter/visit. Codes for other diagnoses (e.g., chronic conditions) may be sequenced as additional diagnoses.

For encounters for routine laboratory/radiology testing in the absence of any signs, symptoms, or associated diagnosis, assign Z01.89, Encounter for other specified special examinations. If routine testing is performed during the same encounter as a test to evaluate a sign, symptom, or diagnosis, it is appropriate to assign both the Z code and the code describing the reason for the non-routine test.

For outpatient encounters for diagnostic tests that have been interpreted by a physician, and the final report is available at the time of coding, code any confirmed or definitive diagnosis(es) documented in the interpretation. Do not code related signs and symptoms as additional diagnoses.

Please note: This differs from the coding practice in the hospital inpatient setting regarding abnormal findings on test results.

L. Patients receiving therapeutic services only
For patients receiving therapeutic services only during an encounter/visit, sequence first the diagnosis, condition, problem, or other reason for encounter/visit shown in the medical record to be chiefly responsible for the outpatient services provided during the encounter/visit. Codes for other diagnoses (e.g., chronic conditions) may be sequenced as additional diagnoses.

The only exception to this rule is that when the primary reason for the admission/encounter is chemotherapy or radiation therapy, the appropriate Z code for the service is listed first, and the diagnosis or problem for which the service is being performed listed second.

M. Patients receiving preoperative evaluations only
For patients receiving preoperative evaluations only, sequence first a code from subcategory Z01.81, Encounter for pre-procedural examinations, to describe the pre-op consultations. Assign a code for the condition to describe the reason for the surgery as an additional diagnosis. Code also any findings related to the pre-op evaluation.

N. Ambulatory surgery
For ambulatory surgery, code the diagnosis for which the surgery was performed. If the postoperative diagnosis is known to be different from the preoperative diagnosis at the time the diagnosis is confirmed, select the postoperative diagnosis for coding, since it is the most definitive.

O. Routine outpatient prenatal visits
See Section I.C.15. Routine outpatient prenatal visits.

P. Encounters for general medical examinations with abnormal findings
The subcategories for encounters for general medical examinations, Z00.0- and encounter for routine child health examination, Z00.12-, provide codes for with and without abnormal findings. Should a general medical examination result in an abnormal finding, the code for general medical examination with abnormal finding should be assigned as the first-listed diagnosis. An examination with abnormal findings refers to a condition/diagnosis that is newly identified or a change in severity of a chronic condition (such as uncontrolled hypertension, or an acute exacerbation of chronic obstructive pulmonary disease) during a routine physical examination. A secondary code for the abnormal finding should also be coded.

Q. Encounters for routine health screenings
See Section I.C.21. Factors influencing health status and contact with health services, Screening

Appendix I. Present on Admission Reporting Guidelines

Introduction
These guidelines are to be used as a supplement to the *ICD-10-CM Official Guidelines for Coding and Reporting* to facilitate the assignment of the Present on Admission (POA) indicator for each diagnosis and external cause of injury code reported on claim forms (UB-04 and 837 Institutional).

These guidelines are not intended to replace any guidelines in the main body of the *ICD-10-CM Official Guidelines for Coding and Reporting*. The POA guidelines are not intended to provide guidance on when a condition should be coded, but rather, how to apply the POA indicator to the final set of diagnosis codes that have been assigned in accordance with Sections I, II, and III of the official coding guidelines. Subsequent to the assignment of the ICD-10-CM codes, the POA indicator should then be assigned to those conditions that have been coded.

As stated in the Introduction to the *ICD-10-CM Official Guidelines for Coding and Reporting*, a joint effort between the healthcare provider and the coder is essential to achieve complete and accurate documentation, code assignment, and reporting of diagnoses and procedures. The importance of consistent, complete documentation in the medical record cannot be overemphasized. Medical record documentation from any provider involved in the care and treatment of the patient may be used to support the determination of whether a condition was present on admission or not. In the context of the official coding guidelines, the term "provider" means a physician or any qualified healthcare practitioner who is legally accountable for establishing the patient's diagnosis.

These guidelines are not a substitute for the provider's clinical judgment as to the determination of whether a condition was/was not present on admission. The provider should be queried regarding issues related to the linking of signs/symptoms, timing of test results, and the timing of findings.

Please see the CDC website for the detailed list of ICD-10-CM codes that do not require the use of a POA indicator (https://www.cdc.gov/nchs/icd/icd-10-cm/files.html). The codes and categories on this exempt list are for circumstances regarding the healthcare encounter or factors influencing health status that do not represent a current disease or injury or that describe conditions that are always present on admission.

General Reporting Requirements
All claims involving inpatient admissions to general acute care hospitals or other facilities that are subject to a law or regulation mandating collection of present on admission information.

Present on admission is defined as present at the time the order for inpatient admission occurs -- conditions that develop during an outpatient encounter, including emergency department, observation, or outpatient surgery, are considered as present on admission.

POA indicator is assigned to principal and secondary diagnoses (as defined in Section II of the Official Guidelines for Coding and Reporting) and the external cause of injury codes.

Issues related to inconsistent, missing, conflicting or unclear documentation must still be resolved by the provider.

If a condition would not be coded and reported based on UHDDS definitions and current official coding guidelines, then the POA indicator would not be reported.

Reporting Options
    Y – Yes
    N – No
    U – Unknown
    W – Clinically undetermined
    Unreported/Not used – (Exempt from POA reporting)

Reporting Definitions
    Y = present at the time of inpatient admission
    N = not present at the time of inpatient admission
    U = documentation is insufficient to determine if condition is present on admission
    W = provider is unable to clinically determine whether condition was present on admission or not

Timeframe for POA Identification and Documentation
There is no required timeframe as to when a provider (per the definition of "provider" used in these guidelines) must identify or document a condition to be present on admission. In some clinical situations, it may not be possible for a provider to make a definitive diagnosis (or a condition may not be recognized or reported by the patient) for a period of time after admission. In some cases, it may be several days before the provider arrives at a definitive diagnosis. This does not mean that the condition was not present on admission. Determination of whether the condition was present on admission or not will be based on the applicable POA guideline as identified in this document, or on the provider's best clinical judgment.

If at the time of code assignment the documentation is unclear as to whether a condition was present on admission or not, it is appropriate to query the provider for clarification.

Assigning the POA Indicator
Condition is on the "Exempt from Reporting" list
    Leave the "present on admission" field blank if the condition is on the list of ICD-10-CM codes for which this field is not applicable. This is the only circumstance in which the field may be left blank.

POA Explicitly Documented
    Assign Y for any condition the provider explicitly documents as being present on admission.

    Assign N for any condition the provider explicitly documents as not present at the time of admission.

Conditions diagnosed prior to inpatient admission
Assign "Y" for conditions that were diagnosed prior to admission (example: hypertension, diabetes mellitus, asthma)

Conditions diagnosed during the admission but clearly present before admission
Assign "Y" for conditions diagnosed during the admission that were clearly present but not diagnosed until after admission occurred.

Diagnoses subsequently confirmed after admission are considered present on admission if at the time of admission they are documented as suspected, possible, rule out, differential diagnosis, or constitute an underlying cause of a symptom that is present at the time of admission.

Condition develops during outpatient encounter prior to inpatient admission
Assign Y for any condition that develops during an outpatient encounter prior to a written order for inpatient admission.

Documentation does not indicate whether condition was present on admission
Assign "U" when the medical record documentation is unclear as to whether the condition was present on admission. "U" should not be routinely assigned and used only in very limited circumstances. Coders are encouraged to query the providers when the documentation is unclear.

Documentation states that it cannot be determined whether the condition was or was not present on admission
Assign "W" when the medical record documentation indicates that it cannot be clinically determined whether or not the condition was present on admission.

Chronic condition with acute exacerbation during the admission
If a single code identifies both the chronic condition and the acute exacerbation, see POA guidelines pertaining to codes that contain multiple clinical concepts.

If a single code only identifies the chronic condition and not the acute exacerbation (e.g., acute exacerbation of chronic leukemia), assign "Y."

Conditions documented as possible, probable, suspected, or rule out at the time of discharge
If the final diagnosis contains a possible, probable, suspected, or rule out diagnosis, and this diagnosis was based on signs, symptoms or clinical findings suspected at the time of inpatient admission, assign "Y."

If the final diagnosis contains a possible, probable, suspected, or rule out diagnosis, and this diagnosis was based on signs, symptoms or clinical findings that were not present on admission, assign "N".

Conditions documented as impending or threatened at the time of discharge
If the final diagnosis contains an impending or threatened diagnosis, and this diagnosis is based on symptoms or clinical findings that were present on admission, assign "Y".

If the final diagnosis contains an impending or threatened diagnosis, and this diagnosis is based on symptoms or clinical findings that were not present on admission, assign "N".

Acute and Chronic Conditions
Assign "Y" for acute conditions that are present at time of admission and N for acute conditions that are not present at time of admission.

Assign "Y" for chronic conditions, even though the condition may not be diagnosed until after admission.

If a single code identifies both an acute and chronic condition, see the POA guidelines for codes that contain multiple clinical concepts.

Codes That Contain Multiple Clinical Concepts
Assign "N" if at least one of the clinical concepts included in the code was not present on admission (e.g., COPD with acute exacerbation and the exacerbation was not present on admission; gastric ulcer that does not start bleeding until after admission; asthma patient develops status asthmaticus after admission).

Assign "Y" if all of the clinical concepts included in the code were present on admission (e.g., duodenal ulcer that perforates prior to admission).

For infection codes that include the causal organism, assign "Y" if the infection (or signs of the infection) were present on admission, even though the culture results may not be known until after admission (e.g., patient is admitted with pneumonia and the provider documents Pseudomonas as the causal organism a few days later).

Same Diagnosis Code for Two or More Conditions
When the same ICD-10-CM diagnosis code applies to two or more conditions during the same encounter (e.g., two separate conditions classified to the same ICD-10-CM diagnosis code):

Assign "Y" if all conditions represented by the single ICD-10-CM code were present on admission (e.g., bilateral unspecified age-related cataracts).

Assign "N" if any of the conditions represented by the single ICD-10-CM code was not present on admission (e.g., traumatic secondary and recurrent hemorrhage and seroma is assigned to a single code T79.2, but only one of the conditions was present on admission).

Obstetrical conditions
Whether or not the patient delivers during the current hospitalization does not affect assignment of the POA indicator. The determining factor for POA assignment is whether the pregnancy complication or obstetrical condition described by the code was present at the time of admission or not.

If the pregnancy complication or obstetrical condition was present on admission (e.g., patient admitted in preterm labor), assign "Y".

If the pregnancy complication or obstetrical condition was not present on admission (e.g., 2nd degree laceration during delivery, postpartum hemorrhage that occurred during current hospitalization, fetal distress develops after admission), assign "N".

If the obstetrical code includes more than one diagnosis and any of the diagnoses identified by the code were not present on admission assign "N". (e.g., Category O11, Pre-existing hypertension with pre-eclampsia)

Perinatal conditions
Newborns are not considered to be admitted until after birth. Therefore, any condition present at birth or that developed in utero is considered present at admission and should be assigned "Y". This includes conditions that occur during delivery (e.g., injury during delivery, meconium aspiration, exposure to streptococcus B in the vaginal canal).

Congenital conditions and anomalies
Assign "Y" for congenital conditions and anomalies except for categories Q00-Q99, Congenital anomalies, which are on the exempt list. Congenital conditions are always considered present on admission.

External cause of injury codes
Assign "Y" for any external cause code representing an external cause of morbidity that occurred prior to inpatient admission (e.g., patient fell out of bed at home, patient fell out of bed in emergency room prior to admission)

Assign "N" for any external cause code representing an external cause of morbidity that occurred during inpatient hospitalization (e.g., patient fell out of hospital bed during hospital stay, patient experienced an adverse reaction to a medication administered after inpatient admission).

ICD-10-CM Index to Diseases and Injuries

A

Aarskog's syndrome Q87.19
Abandonment — *see* Maltreatment
Abasia (-astasia) (hysterical) F44.4
Abderhalden-Kaufmann-Lignac syndrome (cystinosis) E72.04
Abdomen, abdominal — *see also* condition
  acute R10.0
  angina K55.1
  muscle deficiency syndrome Q79.4
Abdominalgia — *see* Pain, abdominal
Abduction contracture, hip or other joint — *see* Contraction, joint
Aberrant (congenital) — *see also* Malposition, congenital
  adrenal gland Q89.1
  artery (peripheral) Q27.8
    basilar NEC Q28.1
    cerebral Q28.3
    coronary Q24.5
    digestive system Q27.8
    eye Q15.8
    lower limb Q27.8
    precerebral Q28.1
    pulmonary Q25.79
    renal Q27.2
    retina Q14.1
    specified site NEC Q27.8
    subclavian Q27.8
    upper limb Q27.8
    vertebral Q28.1
  breast Q83.8
  endocrine gland NEC Q89.2
  hepatic duct Q44.5
  pancreas Q45.3
  parathyroid gland Q89.2
  pituitary gland Q89.2
  sebaceous glands, mucous membrane, mouth, congenital Q38.6
  spleen Q89.09
  subclavian artery Q27.8
  thymus (gland) Q89.2
  thyroid gland Q89.2
  vein (peripheral) NEC Q27.8
    cerebral Q28.3
    digestive system Q27.8
    lower limb Q27.8
    precerebral Q28.1
    specified site NEC Q27.8
    upper limb Q27.8
Aberration
  distantial — *see* Disturbance, visual
  mental F99
Abetalipoproteinemia E78.6
Abiotrophy R68.89
Ablatio, ablation
  retinae — *see* Detachment, retina
Ablepharia, ablepharon Q10.3
Abnormal, abnormality, abnormalities — *see also* Anomaly
  acid-base balance (mixed) E87.4
  albumin R77.0
  alphafetoprotein R77.2
  alveolar ridge K08.9
  anatomical relationship Q89.9
  anti-CCP (cyclic citrullinated protein) R76.81
  anti-cyclic citrullinated protein antibody and rheumatoid factor R76.81
  apertures, congenital, diaphragm Q79.1
  atrial septal, specified NEC Q21.19
  auditory perception H93.29- ☑
    diplacusis — *see* Diplacusis
    hyperacusis — *see* Hyperacusis
    recruitment — *see* Recruitment, auditory
    threshold shift — *see* Shift, auditory threshold
  autosomes Q99.9
    fragile site Q95.5
  basal metabolic rate R94.8
  biosynthesis, testicular androgen E29.1
  bleeding time R79.1
  blood amino-acid level R79.83
  blood-gas level R79.81

Abnormal, abnormality, abnormalities — *continued*
  blood level (of)
    cobalt R79.0
    copper R79.0
    iron R79.0
    lithium R78.89
    magnesium R79.0
    mineral NEC R79.0
    zinc R79.0
  blood pressure
    elevated R03.0
    low reading (nonspecific) R03.1
  blood sugar R73.09
  bowel sounds R19.15
    absent R19.11
    hyperactive R19.12
  brain scan R94.02
  breathing R06.9
  caloric test R94.138
  cerebrospinal fluid R83.9
    cytology R83.6
    drug level R83.2
    enzyme level R83.0
    hormones R83.1
    immunology R83.4
    microbiology R83.5
    nonmedicinal level R83.3
    specified type NEC R83.8
  chemistry, blood R79.9
    C-reactive protein R79.82
    drugs — *see* Findings, abnormal, in blood
    gas level R79.81
    minerals R79.0
    pancytopenia D61.818
    PTT R79.1
    specified NEC R79.89
    toxins — *see* Findings, abnormal, in blood
  chest sounds (friction) (rales) R09.89
  chromosome, chromosomal Q99.9
    with more than three X chromosomes, female Q97.1
    analysis result R89.8
      bronchial washings R84.8
      cerebrospinal fluid R83.8
      cervix uteri NEC R87.89
      nasal secretions R84.8
      nipple discharge R89.8
      peritoneal fluid R85.89
      pleural fluid R84.8
      prostatic secretions R86.8
      saliva R85.89
      seminal fluid R86.8
      sputum R84.8
      synovial fluid R89.8
      throat scrapings R84.8
      vagina R87.89
      vulva R87.89
      wound secretions R89.8
    dicentric replacement Q93.2
    ring replacement Q93.2
    sex Q99.8- ☑
      female phenotype Q97.9
        specified NEC Q97.8
      male phenotype Q98.9
        specified NEC Q98.8
      structural male Q98.6
    specified NEC Q99.8- ☑
  clinical findings NEC R68.89
  coagulation D68.9
    newborn, transient P61.6
    profile R79.1
    time R79.1
  communication — *see* Fistula
  conjunctiva, vascular H11.41- ☑
  coronary artery Q24.5
  cortisol-binding globulin E27.8
  course, eustachian tube Q17.8
  creatinine clearance R94.4
  cytology
    anus R85.619
      atypical squamous cells cannot exclude high grade squamous intraepithelial lesion (ASC-H) R85.611

Abnormal, abnormality, abnormalities — *continued*
  cytology — *continued*
    anus — *continued*
      atypical squamous cells of undetermined significance (ASC-US) R85.610
      cytologic evidence of malignancy R85.614
      high grade squamous intraepithelial lesion (HGSIL) R85.613
      human papillomavirus (HPV) DNA test
        high risk positive R85.81
        low risk positive R85.82
      inadequate smear R85.615
      low grade squamous intraepithelial lesion (LGSIL) R85.612
      satisfactory anal smear but lacking transformation zone R85.616
      specified NEC R85.618
      unsatisfactory smear R85.615
    female genital organs — *see* Abnormal, Papanicolaou (smear)
  dark adaptation curve H53.61
  dentofacial NEC — *see* Anomaly, dentofacial
  development, developmental Q89.9
    central nervous system Q07.9
  diagnostic imaging
    abdomen, abdominal region NEC R93.5
    biliary tract R93.2
    bladder R93.41
    breast R92.8
    central nervous system NEC R90.89
    cerebrovascular NEC R90.89
    coronary circulation R93.1
    digestive tract NEC R93.3
    gastrointestinal (tract) R93.3
    genitourinary organs R93.89
    head R93.0
    heart R93.1
    intrathoracic organ NEC R93.89
    kidney R93.42- ☑
    limbs R93.6
    liver R93.2
    lung (field) R91.8
    musculoskeletal system NEC R93.7
    renal pelvis R93.41
    retroperitoneum R93.5
    site specified NEC R93.89
    skin and subcutaneous tissue R93.89
    skull R93.0
    testis R93.81- ☑
    ureter R93.41
    urinary organs specified NEC R93.49
  direction, teeth, fully erupted M26.30
  ear ossicles, acquired NEC H74.39- ☑
    ankylosis — *see* Ankylosis, ear ossicles
    discontinuity — *see* Discontinuity, ossicles, ear
    partial loss — *see* Loss, ossicles, ear (partial)
  Ebstein Q22.5
  echocardiogram R93.1
  echoencephalogram R90.81
  echogram — *see* Abnormal, diagnostic imaging
  electro-oculogram [EOG] R94.110
  electrocardiogram [ECG] [EKG] R94.31
  electroencephalogram [EEG] R94.01
  electrolyte — *see* Imbalance, electrolyte
  electromyogram [EMG] R94.131
  electrophysiological intracardiac studies R94.39
  electroretinogram [ERG] R94.111
  erythrocytes
    congenital, with perinatal jaundice D58.9
  feces (color) (contents) (mucus) R19.5
  finding — *see* Findings, abnormal, without diagnosis
  fluid
    amniotic — *see* Abnormal, specimen, specified
    cerebrospinal — *see* Abnormal, cerebrospinal fluid
    peritoneal — *see* Abnormal, specimen, digestive organs
    pleural — *see* Abnormal, specimen, respiratory organs
    synovial — *see* Abnormal, specimen, specified
    thorax (bronchial washings) (pleural fluid) — *see* Abnormal, specimen, respiratory organs
    vaginal — *see* Abnormal, specimen, female genital organs

☑ Additional Character Required — Refer to the Tabular List for Character Selection

Abnormal, abnormality, abnormalities — continued
  form
    teeth K00.2
    uterus — see Anomaly, uterus
  function studies
    auditory R94.120
    bladder R94.8
    brain R94.09
    cardiovascular R94.30
    ear R94.128
    endocrine NEC R94.7
    eye NEC R94.118
    kidney R94.4
    liver R94.5
    nervous system
      central NEC R94.09
      peripheral NEC R94.138
    pancreas R94.8
    placenta R94.8
    pulmonary R94.2
    special senses NEC R94.128
    spleen R94.8
    thyroid R94.6
    vestibular R94.121
  gait — see Gait
    hysterical F44.4
  gastrin secretion E16.4
  globulin R77.1
    cortisol-binding E27.8
    thyroid-binding E07.89
  glomerular, minor — see also N00-N07 with fourth character .0 N05.0
  glucagon secretion E16.3
  glucose tolerance (test) (non-fasting) R73.09
  gravitational (G) forces or states (effect of) T75.81- ☑
  hair (color) (shaft) L67.9
    specified NEC L67.8
  hard tissue formation in pulp (dental) K04.3
  head movement R25.0
  heart
    rate R00.9
      specified NEC R00.8
    shadow R93.1
    sounds NEC R01.2
  hemoglobin (disease) — see also Disease, hemoglobin D58.2
    trait — see Trait, hemoglobin, abnormal
  histology NEC R89.7
  immunological findings R89.4
    in serum R76.9
      specified NEC R76.89
  increase in appetite R63.2
  involuntary movement — see Abnormal, movement, involuntary
  jaw closure M26.51
  karyotype R89.8
  kidney function test R94.4
  knee jerk R29.2
  leukocyte (cell) (differential) NEC D72.9
  liver function test — see also Elevated, liver function, test R79.89
  loss of
    height R29.890
    weight R63.4
  mammogram NEC R92.8
    calcification (calculus) R92.1
    microcalcification R92.0
  Mantoux test R76.11
  movement (disorder) — see also Disorder, movement
    head R25.0
    involuntary R25.9
      fasciculation R25.3
      of head R25.0
      spasm R25.2
      specified type NEC R25.8
      tremor R25.1
  myoglobin (Aberdeen) (Annapolis) R89.7
  neonatal screening P09.9
    for
      congenital adrenal hyperplasia P09.2
      congenital endocrine disease P09.2
      congenital hematologic disorders P09.3
      critical congenital heart disease P09.5
      cystic fibrosis P09.4
      hemoglobinopathy P09.3
      hypothyroidism P09.2
      inborn errors of metabolism P09.1
      red cell membrane defects P09.3
      sickle cell P09.3

Abnormal, abnormality, abnormalities — continued
  neonatal screening — continued
    for — continued
      specified NEC P09.8
      hearing P09.6
  oculomotor study R94.113
  palmar creases Q82.8
  Papanicolaou (smear)
    anus R85.619
      atypical squamous cells cannot exclude high grade squamous intraepithelial lesion (ASC-H) R85.611
      atypical squamous cells of undetermined significance (ASC-US) R85.610
      cytologic evidence of malignancy R85.614
      high grade squamous intraepithelial lesion (HGSIL) R85.613
      human papillomavirus (HPV) DNA test
        high risk positive R85.81
        low risk positive R85.82
      inadequate smear R85.615
      low grade squamous intraepithelial lesion (LGSIL) R85.612
      satisfactory anal smear but lacking transformation zone R85.616
      specified NEC R85.618
      unsatisfactory smear R85.615
    bronchial washings R84.6
    cerebrospinal fluid R83.6
    cervix R87.629
      atypical squamous cells cannot exclude high grade squamous intraepithelial lesion (ASC-H) R87.611
      atypical squamous cells of undetermined significance (ASC-US) R87.610
      cytologic evidence of malignancy R87.614
      high grade squamous intraepithelial lesion (HGSIL) R87.613
      inadequate smear R87.615
      low grade squamous intraepithelial lesion (LGSIL) R87.612
      non-atypical endometrial cells R87.618
      satisfactory cervical smear but lacking transformation zone R87.616
      specified NEC R87.618
      thin preparation R87.619
      unsatisfactory smear R87.615
    nasal secretions R84.6
    nipple discharge R89.6
    peritoneal fluid R85.69
    pleural fluid R84.6
    prostatic secretions R86.6
    saliva R85.69
    seminal fluid R86.6
    sites NEC R89.6
    sputum R84.6
    synovial fluid R89.6
    throat scrapings R84.6
    vagina R87.629
      atypical squamous cells cannot exclude high grade squamous intraepithelial lesion (ASC-H) R87.621
      atypical squamous cells of undetermined significance (ASC-US) R87.620
      cytologic evidence of malignancy R87.624
      high grade squamous intraepithelial lesion (HGSIL) R87.623
      inadequate smear R87.625
      low grade squamous intraepithelial lesion (LGSIL) R87.622
      specified NEC R87.628
      thin preparation R87.629
      unsatisfactory smear R87.625
    vulva R87.69
    wound secretions R89.6
  partial thromboplastin time (PTT) R79.1
  pelvis (bony) — see Deformity, pelvis
  percussion, chest (tympany) R09.89
  periods (grossly) — see Menstruation
  phonocardiogram R94.39
  plantar reflex R29.2
  plasma
    protein R77.9
      specified NEC R77.8
    viscosity R70.1
  pleural (folds) Q34.0
  posture R29.3
  product of conception O02.9
    specified type NEC O02.89

Abnormal, abnormality, abnormalities — continued
  prothrombin time (PT) R79.1
  pulmonary
    artery, congenital Q25.79
    function, newborn P28.89
    test results R94.2
  pulsations in neck R00.2
  pupillary H21.56- ☑
    function (reaction) (reflex) — see Anomaly, pupil, function
  radiological examination — see Abnormal, diagnostic imaging
  red blood cell(s) (morphology) (volume) R71.8
  reflex — see Reflex
  renal function test R94.4
  response to nerve stimulation R94.130
  retinal correspondence H53.31
  retinal function study R94.111
  rheumatoid factor and anti-citrullinated protein antibody
    with rheumatoid arthritis M05.A
    without rheumatoid arthritis R76.81
  rhythm, heart — see also Arrhythmia
  saliva — see Abnormal, specimen, digestive organs
  scan
    kidney R94.4
    liver R93.2
    thyroid R94.6
  secretion
    gastrin E16.4
    glucagon E16.3
  semen, seminal fluid — see Abnormal, specimen, male genital organs
  serum level (of)
    acid phosphatase R74.8
    alkaline phosphatase R74.8
    amylase R74.8
    enzymes R74.9
      specified NEC R74.8
    lipase R74.8
    triacylglycerol lipase R74.8
  shape
    gravid uterus — see Anomaly, uterus
  sinus venosus Q21.16
  size, tooth, teeth K00.2
  spacing, tooth, teeth, fully erupted M26.30
  specimen
    digestive organs (peritoneal fluid) (saliva) R85.9
      cytology R85.69
      drug level R85.2
      enzyme level R85.0
      histology R85.7
      hormones R85.1
      immunology R85.4
      microbiology R85.5
      nonmedicinal level R85.3
      specified type NEC R85.89
    female genital organs (secretions) (smears) R87.9
      cytology R87.69
        cervix R87.619
          human papillomavirus (HPV) DNA test
            high risk positive R87.810
            low risk positive R87.820
          inadequate (unsatisfactory) smear R87.615
          non-atypical endometrial cells R87.618
          specified NEC R87.618
        vagina R87.629
          human papillomavirus (HPV) DNA test
            high risk positive R87.811
            low risk positive R87.821
          inadequate (unsatisfactory) smear R87.625
        vulva R87.69
      drug level R87.2
      enzyme level R87.0
      histological R87.7
      hormones R87.1
      immunology R87.4
      microbiology R87.5
      nonmedicinal level R87.3
      specified type NEC R87.89
    male genital organs (prostatic secretions) (semen) R86.9
      cytology R86.6
      drug level R86.2
      enzyme level R86.0
      histological R86.7
      hormones R86.1
      immunology R86.4
      microbiology R86.5
      nonmedicinal level R86.3

Abnormal, abnormality, abnormalities — continued
 specimen — continued
  male genital organs — continued
   specified type NEC R86.8
  nipple discharge — see Abnormal, specimen, specified
  respiratory organs (bronchial washings) (nasal secretions) (pleural fluid) (sputum) R84.9
   cytology R84.6
   drug level R84.2
   enzyme level R84.0
   histology R84.7
   hormones R84.1
   immunology R84.4
   microbiology R84.5
   nonmedicinal level R84.3
   specified type NEC R84.8
  specified organ, system and tissue NOS R89.9
   cytology R89.6
   drug level R89.2
   enzyme level R89.0
   histology R89.7
   hormones R89.1
   immunology R89.4
   microbiology R89.5
   nonmedicinal level R89.3
   specified type NEC R89.8
  synovial fluid — see Abnormal, specimen, specified
  thorax (bronchial washings) (pleural fluids) — see Abnormal, specimen, respiratory organs
  vagina (secretion) (smear) R87.629
  vulva (secretion) (smear) R87.69
  wound secretion — see Abnormal, specimen, specified
 spermatozoa — see Abnormal, specimen, male genital organs
 sputum (amount) (color) (odor) R09.3
 stool (color) (contents) (mucus) R19.5
  bloody K92.1
  guaiac positive R19.5
 synchondrosis Q78.8
 thermography — see also Abnormal, diagnostic imaging R93.89
 thyroid-binding globulin E07.89
 tooth, teeth (form) (size) K00.2
 toxicology (findings) R78.9
 transport protein E88.09
 tumor marker NEC R97.8
 ultrasound results — see Abnormal, diagnostic imaging
 umbilical cord complicating delivery O69.9- ☑
 urination NEC R39.198
 urine (constituents) R82.90
  bile R82.2
  cytological examination R82.89
  drugs R82.5
  fat R82.0
  glucose R81
  heavy metals R82.6
  hemoglobin R82.3
  histological examination R82.89
  ketones R82.4
  microbiological examination (culture) R82.79
  myoglobin R82.1
  positive culture R82.79
  protein — see Proteinuria
  specified substance NEC R82.998
   chromoabnormality NEC R82.91
  substances nonmedical R82.6
 uterine hemorrhage — see Hemorrhage, uterus
 vectorcardiogram R94.39
 visually evoked potential (VEP) R94.112
 white blood cells D72.9
  specified NEC D72.89
 X-ray examination — see Abnormal, diagnostic imaging
Abnormity (any organ or part) — see Anomaly
Abocclusion M26.29
 hemolytic disease (newborn) P55.1
 incompatibility reaction ABO — see Complication(s), transfusion, incompatibility reaction, ABO
Abolition, language R48.8
Aborter, habitual or recurrent — see Loss (of), pregnancy, recurrent
Abortion (complete) (spontaneous) O03.9
 with
  retained products of conception — see Abortion, incomplete
 attempted (elective) (failed) O07.4
  complicated by O07.30
   afibrinogenemia O07.1
   cardiac arrest O07.36

Abortion — continued
 attempted — continued
  complicated by — continued
   chemical damage of pelvic organ(s) O07.34
   circulatory collapse O07.31
   cystitis O07.38
   defibrination syndrome O07.1
   electrolyte imbalance O07.33
   embolism (air) (amniotic fluid) (blood clot) (fat) (pulmonary) (septic) (soap) O07.2
   endometritis O07.0
   genital tract and pelvic infection O07.0
   hemolysis O07.1
   hemorrhage (delayed) (excessive) O07.1
   infection
    genital tract or pelvic O07.0
    urinary tract O07.38
   intravascular coagulation O07.1
   laceration of pelvic organ(s) O07.34
   metabolic disorder O07.33
   oliguria O07.32
   oophoritis O07.0
   parametritis O07.0
   pelvic peritonitis O07.0
   perforation of pelvic organ(s) O07.34
   renal failure or shutdown O07.32
   salpingitis or salpingo-oophoritis O07.0
   sepsis O07.37
   shock O07.31
   specified condition NEC O07.39
   tubular necrosis (renal) O07.32
   uremia O07.32
   urinary tract infection O07.38
   venous complication NEC O07.35
    embolism (air) (amniotic fluid) (blood clot) (fat) (pulmonary) (septic) (soap) O07.2
 complicated (by) (following) O03.80
  afibrinogenemia O03.6
  cardiac arrest O03.86
  chemical damage of pelvic organ(s) O03.84
  circulatory collapse O03.81
  cystitis O03.88
  defibrination syndrome O03.6
  electrolyte imbalance O03.83
  embolism (air) (amniotic fluid) (blood clot) (fat) (pulmonary) (septic) (soap) O03.7
  endometritis O03.5
  genital tract and pelvic infection O03.5
  hemolysis O03.6
  hemorrhage (delayed) (excessive) O03.6
  infection
   genital tract or pelvic O03.5
   urinary tract O03.88
  intravascular coagulation O03.6
  laceration of pelvic organ(s) O03.84
  metabolic disorder O03.83
  oliguria O03.82
  oophoritis O03.5
  parametritis O03.5
  pelvic peritonitis O03.5
  perforation of pelvic organ(s) O03.84
  renal failure or shutdown O03.82
  salpingitis or salpingo-oophoritis O03.5
  sepsis O03.87
  shock O03.81
  specified condition NEC O03.89
  tubular necrosis (renal) O03.82
  uremia O03.82
  urinary tract infection O03.88
  venous complication NEC O03.85
   embolism (air) (amniotic fluid) (blood clot) (fat) (pulmonary) (septic) (soap) O03.7
 failed — see Abortion, attempted
 habitual or recurrent N96
  with current abortion — see categories O03-O04
  without current pregnancy N96
  care in current pregnancy O26.2- ☑
 incomplete (spontaneous) O03.4
  complicated (by) (following) O03.30
   afibrinogenemia O03.1
   cardiac arrest O03.36
   chemical damage of pelvic organ(s) O03.34
   circulatory collapse O03.31
   cystitis O03.38
   defibrination syndrome O03.1
   electrolyte imbalance O03.33
   embolism (air) (amniotic fluid) (blood clot) (fat) (pulmonary) (septic) (soap) O03.2
   endometritis O03.0

Abortion — continued
 incomplete — continued
  complicated — continued
   genital tract and pelvic infection O03.0
   hemolysis O03.1
   hemorrhage (delayed) (excessive) O03.1
   infection
    genital tract or pelvic O03.0
    urinary tract O03.38
   intravascular coagulation O03.1
   laceration of pelvic organ(s) O03.34
   metabolic disorder O03.33
   oliguria O03.32
   oophoritis O03.0
   parametritis O03.0
   pelvic peritonitis O03.0
   perforation of pelvic organ(s) O03.34
   renal failure or shutdown O03.32
   salpingitis or salpingo-oophoritis O03.0
   sepsis O03.37
   shock O03.31
   specified condition NEC O03.39
   tubular necrosis (renal) O03.32
   uremia O03.32
   urinary tract infection O03.38
   venous complication NEC O03.35
    embolism (air) (amniotic fluid) (blood clot) (fat) (pulmonary) (septic) (soap) O03.2
 induced (encounter for) Z33.2
  complicated by O04.80
   afibrinogenemia O04.6
   cardiac arrest O04.86
   chemical damage of pelvic organ(s) O04.84
   circulatory collapse O04.81
   cystitis O04.88
   defibrination syndrome O04.6
   electrolyte imbalance O04.83
   embolism (air) (amniotic fluid) (blood clot) (fat) (pulmonary) (septic) (soap) O04.7
   endometritis O04.5
   genital tract and pelvic infection O04.5
   hemolysis O04.6
   hemorrhage (delayed) (excessive) O04.6
   infection
    genital tract or pelvic O04.5
    urinary tract O04.88
   intravascular coagulation O04.6
   laceration of pelvic organ(s) O04.84
   metabolic disorder O04.83
   oliguria O04.82
   oophoritis O04.5
   parametritis O04.5
   pelvic peritonitis O04.5
   perforation of pelvic organ(s) O04.84
   renal failure or shutdown O04.82
   salpingitis or salpingo-oophoritis O04.5
   sepsis O04.87
   shock O04.81
   specified condition NEC O04.89
   tubular necrosis (renal) O04.82
   uremia O04.82
   urinary tract infection O04.88
   venous complication NEC O04.85
    embolism (air) (amniotic fluid) (blood clot) (fat) (pulmonary) (septic) (soap) O04.7
 inevitable O03.4
 missed O02.1
 spontaneous — see Abortion (complete) (spontaneous)
  threatened O20.0
 threatened (spontaneous) O20.0
 tubal O00.10-
  with intrauterine pregnancy O00.11- ☑
Abortus fever A23.1
Aboulomania F60.7
Abrami's disease D59.8
Abramov-Fiedler myocarditis (acute isolated myocarditis) I40.1
Abrasion T14.8- ☑
 abdomen, abdominal (wall) S30.811- ☑
 alveolar process S00.512- ☑
 ankle S90.51- ☑
 antecubital space — see Abrasion, elbow
 anus S30.817- ☑
 arm (upper) S40.81- ☑
 auditory canal — see Abrasion, ear
 auricle — see Abrasion, ear
 axilla — see Abrasion, arm
 back, lower S30.810- ☑

Abrasion — continued
- breast S20.11- ☑
- brow S00.81- ☑
- buttock S30.810- ☑
- calf — see Abrasion, leg
- canthus — see Abrasion, eyelid
- cheek S00.81- ☑
  - internal S00.512- ☑
- chest wall — see Abrasion, thorax
- chin S00.81- ☑
- clitoris S30.814- ☑
- cornea S05.0- ☑
- costal region — see Abrasion, thorax
- dental K03.1
- digit(s)
  - foot — see Abrasion, toe
  - hand — see Abrasion, finger
- ear S00.41- ☑
- elbow S50.31- ☑
- epididymis S30.813- ☑
- epigastric region S30.811- ☑
- epiglottis S10.11- ☑
- esophagus (thoracic) S27.818- ☑
  - cervical S10.11- ☑
- eyebrow — see Abrasion, eyelid
- eyelid S00.21- ☑
- face S00.81- ☑
- finger(s) S60.41- ☑
  - index S60.41- ☑
  - little S60.41- ☑
  - middle S60.41- ☑
  - ring S60.41- ☑
- flank S30.81A- ☑
- foot (except toe(s) alone) S90.81- ☑
  - toe — see Abrasion, toe
- forearm S50.81- ☑
  - elbow only — see Abrasion, elbow
- forehead S00.81- ☑
- genital organs, external
  - female S30.816- ☑
  - male S30.815- ☑
- groin S30.811- ☑
- gum S00.512- ☑
- hand S60.51- ☑
- head S00.91- ☑
  - ear — see Abrasion, ear
  - eyelid — see Abrasion, eyelid
  - lip S00.511- ☑
  - nose S00.31- ☑
  - oral cavity S00.512- ☑
  - scalp S00.01- ☑
  - specified site NEC S00.81- ☑
- heel — see Abrasion, foot
- hip S70.21- ☑
- inguinal region S30.811- ☑
- interscapular region S20.419- ☑
- jaw S00.81- ☑
- knee S80.21- ☑
- labium (majus) (minus) S30.814- ☑
- larynx S10.11- ☑
- leg (lower) S80.81- ☑
  - knee — see Abrasion, knee
  - upper — see Abrasion, thigh
- lip S00.511- ☑
- lower back S30.810- ☑
- lumbar region S30.810- ☑
- malar region S00.81- ☑
- mammary — see Abrasion, breast
- mastoid region S00.81- ☑
- mouth S00.512- ☑
- nail
  - finger — see Abrasion, finger
  - toe — see Abrasion, toe
- nape S10.81- ☑
- nasal S00.31- ☑
- neck S10.91- ☑
  - specified site NEC S10.81- ☑
  - throat S10.11- ☑
- nose S00.31- ☑
- occipital region S00.01- ☑
- oral cavity S00.512- ☑
- orbital region — see Abrasion, eyelid
- palate S00.512- ☑
- palm — see Abrasion, hand
- parietal region S00.01- ☑
- pelvis S30.810- ☑

Abrasion — continued
- penis S30.812- ☑
- perineum
  - female S30.814- ☑
  - male S30.815- ☑
- periocular area — see Abrasion, eyelid
- phalanges
  - finger — see Abrasion, finger
  - toe — see Abrasion, toe
- pharynx S10.11- ☑
- pinna — see Abrasion, ear
- popliteal space — see Abrasion, knee
- prepuce S30.812- ☑
- pubic region S30.810- ☑
- pudendum
  - female S30.816- ☑
  - male S30.815- ☑
- sacral region S30.810- ☑
- scalp S00.01- ☑
- scapular region — see Abrasion, shoulder
- scrotum S30.813- ☑
- shin — see Abrasion, leg
- shoulder S40.21- ☑
- skin NEC T14.8- ☑
- sternal region S20.319- ☑
- submaxillary region S00.81- ☑
- submental region S00.81- ☑
- subungual
  - finger(s) — see Abrasion, finger
  - toe(s) — see Abrasion, toe
- supraclavicular fossa S10.81- ☑
- supraorbital S00.81- ☑
- temple S00.81- ☑
- temporal region S00.81- ☑
- testis S30.813- ☑
- thigh S70.31- ☑
- thorax, thoracic (wall) S20.91- ☑
  - back S20.41- ☑
  - front S20.31- ☑
- throat S10.11- ☑
- thumb S60.31- ☑
- toe(s) (lesser) S90.416- ☑
  - great S90.41- ☑
- tongue S00.512- ☑
- tooth, teeth (dentifrice) (habitual) (hard tissues) (occupational) (ritual) (traditional) K03.1
- trachea S10.11- ☑
- tunica vaginalis S30.813- ☑
- tympanum, tympanic membrane — see Abrasion, ear
- uvula S00.512- ☑
- vagina S30.814- ☑
- vocal cords S10.11- ☑
- vulva S30.814- ☑
- wrist S60.81- ☑

Abrism — see Poisoning, food, noxious, plant

Abruptio placentae O45.9- ☑
- with
  - afibrinogenemia O45.01- ☑
  - coagulation defect O45.00- ☑
    - specified NEC O45.09- ☑
  - disseminated intravascular coagulation O45.02- ☑
  - hypofibrinogenemia O45.01- ☑
- specified NEC O45.8- ☑

Abruption, placenta — see Abruptio placentae

Abscess (connective tissue) (embolic) (fistulous) (infective) (metastatic) (multiple) (pernicious) (pyogenic) (septic) L02.91
- with
  - diverticular disease (intestine) K57.80
    - with bleeding K57.81
    - large intestine K57.20
      - with
        - bleeding K57.21
        - small intestine K57.40
          - with bleeding K57.41
    - small intestine K57.00
      - with
        - bleeding K57.01
        - large intestine K57.40
          - with bleeding K57.41
  - lymphangitis — code by site under Abscess
- abdomen, abdominal
  - cavity K65.1
  - wall L02.211
- abdominopelvic K65.1
- accessory sinus — see Sinusitis
- adrenal (capsule) (gland) E27.8

Abscess — continued
- alveolar K04.7
  - with sinus K04.6
- amebic A06.4
  - brain (and liver or lung abscess) A06.6
  - genitourinary tract A06.82
  - liver (without mention of brain or lung abscess) A06.4
  - lung (and liver) (without mention of brain abscess) A06.5
  - specified site NEC A06.89
  - spleen A06.89
- anerobic A48.0
- ankle — see Abscess, lower limb
- anorectal K61.2
- antecubital space — see Abscess, upper limb
- antrum (chronic) (Highmore) — see Sinusitis, maxillary
- anus K61.0
- apical (tooth) K04.7
  - with sinus (alveolar) K04.6
- appendix K35.33
- areola (acute) (chronic) (nonpuerperal) N61.1
  - puerperal, postpartum or gestational — see Infection, nipple
- arm (any part) — see Abscess, upper limb
- artery (wall) I77.89
- atheromatous I77.2
- auricle, ear — see Abscess, ear, external
- axilla (region) L02.41- ☑
  - lymph gland or node L04.2
- back (any part, except buttock and flank) L02.212
- Bartholin's gland N75.1
  - with
    - abortion — see Abortion, by type complicated by, sepsis
    - ectopic or molar pregnancy O08.0
  - following ectopic or molar pregnancy O08.0
- Bezold's — see Mastoiditis, acute
- bilharziasis B65.1
- bladder (wall) — see Cystitis, specified type NEC
- bone (subperiosteal) — see also Osteomyelitis, specified type NEC
  - accessory sinus (chronic) — see Sinusitis
  - chronic or old — see Osteomyelitis, chronic
  - jaw (lower) (upper) M27.2
  - mastoid — see Mastoiditis, acute, subperiosteal
  - petrous — see Petrositis
  - spinal (tuberculous) A18.01
    - nontuberculous — see Osteomyelitis, vertebra
- bowel K63.0
- brain (any part) (cystic) (otogenic) G06.0
  - amebic (with abscess of any other site) A06.6
  - gonococcal A54.82
  - pheomycotic (chromomycotic) B43.1
  - tuberculous A17.81
- breast (acute) (chronic) (nonpuerperal) N61.1
  - newborn P39.0
  - puerperal, postpartum, gestational — see Mastitis, obstetric, purulent
- broad ligament N73.2
  - acute N73.0
  - chronic N73.1
- Brodie's (localized) (chronic) M86.8X- ☑
- bronchi J98.09
- buccal cavity K12.2
- bulbourethral gland N34.0
- bursa M71.00
  - ankle M71.07- ☑
  - elbow M71.02- ☑
  - foot M71.07- ☑
  - hand M71.04- ☑
  - hip M71.05- ☑
  - knee M71.06- ☑
  - multiple sites M71.09
  - pharyngeal J39.1
  - shoulder M71.01- ☑
  - specified site NEC M71.08
  - wrist M71.03- ☑
- buttock L02.31
- canthus — see Blepharoconjunctivitis
- cartilage — see Disorder, cartilage, specified type NEC
- cecum K35.33
- cerebellum, cerebellar G06.0
  - sequelae G09
- cerebral (embolic) G06.0
  - sequelae G09
- cervical (meaning neck) L02.11
  - lymph gland or node L04.0
- cervix (stump) (uteri) — see Cervicitis

Abscess — *continued*
- cheek (external) L02.01
  - inner K12.2
- chest J86.9
  - with fistula J86.0
  - wall L02.213
- chin L02.01
- choroid — *see* Inflammation, chorioretinal
- circumtonsillar J36
- cold (lung) (tuberculous) — *see also* Tuberculosis, abscess, lung
  - articular — *see* Tuberculosis, joint
- colon (wall) K63.0
- colostomy K94.02
- conjunctiva — *see* Conjunctivitis, acute
- cornea H16.31- ☑
- corpus
  - cavernosum N48.21
  - luteum — *see* Oophoritis
- Cowper's gland N34.0
- cranium G06.0
- cul-de-sac (Douglas') (posterior) — *see* Peritonitis, pelvic, female
- cutaneous — *see* Abscess, by site
- dental K04.7
  - with sinus (alveolar) K04.6
- dentoalveolar K04.7
  - with sinus K04.6
- diaphragm, diaphragmatic K65.1
- Douglas' cul-de-sac or pouch — *see* Peritonitis, pelvic, female
- Dubois A50.59
- ear (middle) — *see also* Otitis, media, suppurative
  - acute — *see* Otitis, media, suppurative, acute
  - external H60.0- ☑
- entamebic — *see* Abscess, amebic
- enterostomy K94.12
- epididymis N45.4
- epidural G06.2
  - brain G06.0
  - spinal cord G06.1
- epiglottis J38.7
- epiploon, epiploic K65.1
- erysipelatous — *see* Erysipelas
- esophagus K20.80
- ethmoid (bone) (chronic) (sinus) J32.2
- external auditory canal — *see* Abscess, ear, external
- extradural G06.2
  - brain G06.0
    - sequelae G09
  - spinal cord G06.1
- extraperitoneal K68.19
- eye — *see* Endophthalmitis, purulent
- eyelid H00.03- ☑
- face (any part, except ear, eye and nose) L02.01
- fallopian tube — *see* Salpingitis
- fascia M72.8
- fauces J39.1
- fecal K63.0
- femoral (region) — *see* Abscess, lower limb
- filaria, filarial — *see* Infestation, filarial
- finger (any) — *see also* Abscess, hand
  - flank L02.217
  - nail — *see* Cellulitis, finger
- foot L02.61- ☑
- forehead L02.01
- frontal sinus (chronic) J32.1
- gallbladder K81.0
- genital organ or tract
  - female (external) N76.4
  - male N49.9
    - multiple sites N49.8
    - specified NEC N49.8
- gestational mammary O91.11- ☑
- gestational subareolar O91.11- ☑
- gingival
  - aggressive K05.20
    - generalized K05.229
      - moderate K05.222
      - severe K05.223
      - slight K05.221
    - localized K05.219
      - moderate K05.212
      - severe K05.213
      - slight K05.211
- gland, glandular (lymph) (acute) — *see* Lymphadenitis, acute
- gluteal (region) L02.31

Abscess — *continued*
- gonorrheal — *see* Gonococcus
- groin L02.214
- gum
  - aggressive K05.20
    - generalized K05.229
      - moderate K05.222
      - severe K05.223
      - slight K05.221
    - localized K05.219
      - moderate K05.212
      - severe K05.213
      - slight K05.211
- hand L02.51- ☑
- head NEC L02.811
  - face (any part, except ear, eye and nose) L02.01
- heart — *see* Carditis
- heel — *see* Abscess, foot
- helminthic — *see* Infestation, helminth
- hepatic (cholangitic) (hematogenic) (lymphogenic) (pylephlebitic) K75.0
  - amebic A06.4
- hip (region) — *see* Abscess, lower limb
- horseshoe K61.31
- ileocecal K35.33
- ileostomy (bud) K94.12
- iliac (region) L02.214
  - fossa K35.33
- infraclavicular (fossa) — *see* Abscess, upper limb
- inguinal (region) L02.214
  - lymph gland or node L04.1
- intersphincteric K61.4
- intestine, intestinal NEC K63.0
  - rectal K61.1
- intra-abdominal — *see also* Abscess, peritoneum K65.1
  - following procedure T81.43- ☑
    - obstetrical O86.03
  - postprocedural T81.43- ☑
  - retroperitoneal K68.11
- intracranial G06.0
- intramammary — *see* Abscess, breast
- intramuscular, following procedure T81.42- ☑
  - obstetrical O86.02
- intraorbital — *see* Abscess, orbit
- intraperitoneal K65.1
- intrasphincteric (anus) K61.4
- intraspinal G06.1
- intratonsillar J36
- ischiorectal (fossa) (specified NEC) K61.39
- jaw (bone) (lower) (upper) M27.2
- joint — *see* Arthritis, pyogenic or pyemic
  - spine (tuberculous) A18.01
    - nontuberculous — *see* Spondylopathy, infective
- kidney N15.1
  - with calculus N20.0
    - with hydronephrosis N13.6
  - puerperal (postpartum) O86.21
- knee — *see also* Abscess, lower limb
  - joint M00.9
- labium (majus) (minus) N76.4
- lacrimal
  - caruncle — *see* Inflammation, lacrimal, passages, acute
  - gland — *see* Dacryoadenitis
  - passages (duct) (sac) — *see* Inflammation, lacrimal, passages, acute
- lacunar N34.0
- larynx J38.7
- lateral (alveolar) K04.7
  - with sinus K04.6
- leg (any part) — *see* Abscess, lower limb
- lens H27.8
- lingual K14.0
  - tonsil J36
- lip K13.0
- Littre's gland N34.0
- liver (cholangitic) (hematogenic) (lymphogenic) (pylephlebitic) (pyogenic) K75.0
  - amebic (due to Entamoeba histolytica) (dysenteric) (tropical) A06.4
    - with
      - brain abscess (and liver or lung abscess) A06.6
      - lung abscess A06.5
- loin (region) L02.211
- lower limb L02.41- ☑
- lumbar (tuberculous) A18.01
  - nontuberculous L02.212
- lung (miliary) (putrid) J85.2

Abscess — *continued*
- lung — *continued*
  - with pneumonia J85.1
    - due to specified organism (*see* Pneumonia, in (due to))
  - amebic (with liver abscess) A06.5
    - with
      - brain abscess A06.6
      - pneumonia A06.5
- lymph, lymphatic, gland or node (acute) — *see also* Lymphadenitis, acute
- mesentery I88.0
- malar M27.2
- mammary gland — *see* Abscess, breast
- marginal, anus K61.0
- mastoid — *see* Mastoiditis, acute
- maxilla, maxillary M27.2
  - molar (tooth) K04.7
    - with sinus K04.6
  - premolar K04.7
  - sinus (chronic) J32.0
- mediastinum J85.3
- meibomian gland — *see* Hordeolum
- meninges G06.2
- mesentery, mesenteric K65.1
- mesosalpinx — *see* Salpingitis
- mons pubis L02.215
- mouth (floor) K12.2
- muscle — *see* Myositis, infective
- myocardium I40.0
- nabothian (follicle) — *see* Cervicitis
- nasal J32.9
- nasopharyngeal J39.1
- navel L02.216
  - newborn P38.9
    - with mild hemorrhage P38.1
    - without hemorrhage P38.9
- neck (region) L02.11
  - lymph gland or node L04.0
- nephritic — *see* Abscess, kidney
- nipple N61.1
  - associated with
    - lactation — *see* Pregnancy, complicated by
    - pregnancy — *see* Pregnancy, complicated by
- nose (external) (fossa) (septum) J34.0
  - sinus (chronic) — *see* Sinusitis
- omentum K65.1
- operative wound T81.49- ☑
- orbit, orbital — *see* Cellulitis, orbit
- otogenic G06.0
- ovary, ovarian (corpus luteum) — *see* Oophoritis
- oviduct — *see* Oophoritis
- palate (soft) K12.2
  - hard M27.2
- palmar (space) — *see* Abscess, hand
- pancreas (duct) — *see* Pancreatitis, acute
- parafrenal N48.21
- parametric, parametrium N73.2
  - acute N73.0
  - chronic N73.1
- paranephric N15.1
- parapancreatic — *see* Pancreatitis, acute
- parapharyngeal J39.0
- pararectal K61.1
- parasinus — *see* Sinusitis
- parauterine — *see also* Disease, pelvis, inflammatory N73.2
- paravaginal — *see* Vaginitis
- parietal region (scalp) L02.811
- parodontal — *see* Periodontitis, aggressive, localized
- parotid (duct) (gland) K11.3
  - region K12.2
- pectoral (region) L02.213
- pelvis, pelvic
  - female — *see* Disease, pelvis, inflammatory
  - male, peritoneal K65.1
- penis N48.21
  - gonococcal (accessory gland) (periurethral) A54.1
- perianal K61.0
- periapical K04.7
  - with sinus (alveolar) K04.6
- periappendicular K35.33
- pericardial I30.1
- pericecal K35.33
- pericemental — *see* Periodontitis, aggressive, localized
- pericholecystic — *see* Cholecystitis, acute
- pericoronal — *see* Periodontitis, aggressive, localized
- peridental — *see* Periodontitis, aggressive, localized
- perimetric — *see also* Disease, pelvis, inflammatory N73.2

Abscess — *continued*
- perinephric, perinephritic — *see* Abscess, kidney
- perineum, perineal (superficial) L02.215
  - urethra N34.0
- periodontal (parietal) — *see* Periodontitis, aggressive, localized
  - apical K04.7
- periosteum, periosteal — *see also* Osteomyelitis, specified type NEC
  - with osteomyelitis — *see also* Osteomyelitis, specified type NEC
    - acute — *see* Osteomyelitis, acute
    - chronic — *see* Osteomyelitis, chronic
- peripharyngeal J39.0
- peripleuritic J86.9
  - with fistula J86.0
- periprostatic N41.2
- perirectal K61.1
- perirenal (tissue) — *see* Abscess, kidney
- perisinuous (nose) — *see* Sinusitis
- peritoneum, peritoneal (perforated) (ruptured) K65.1
  - with appendicitis — *see also* Appendicitis K35.33
  - pelvic
    - female — *see* Peritonitis, pelvic, female
    - male K65.1
  - postoperative T81.43- ☑
  - puerperal, postpartum, childbirth O85
  - tuberculous A18.31
- peritonsillar J36
- perityphlic K35.33
- periureteral N28.89
- periurethral N34.0
  - gonococcal (accessory gland) (periurethral) A54.1
- periuterine — *see also* Disease, pelvis, inflammatory N73.2
- perivesical — *see* Cystitis, specified type NEC
- petrous bone — *see* Petrositis
- phagedenic NOS L02.91
  - chancroid A57
- pharynx, pharyngeal (lateral) J39.1
- pilonidal L05.01
- pituitary (gland) E23.6
- pleura J86.9
  - with fistula J86.0
- popliteal — *see* Abscess, lower limb
- postcecal K35.33
- postlaryngeal J38.7
- postnasal J34.0
- postoperative (any site) — *see also* Infection, postoperative wound T81.49- ☑
  - retroperitoneal K68.11
- postpharyngeal J39.0
- posttonsillar J36
- post-typhoid A01.09
- pouch of Douglas — *see* Peritonitis, pelvic, female
- premammary — *see* Abscess, breast
- prepatellar — *see* Abscess, lower limb
- presacral K68.19
- prostate N41.2
  - gonococcal (acute) (chronic) A54.22
- psoas muscle K68.12
- puerperal — *code by* site under Puerperal, abscess
- pulmonary — *see* Abscess, lung
- pulp, pulpal (dental) K04.01
  - irreversible K04.02
  - reversible K04.01
- rectovaginal septum K63.0
- rectovesical — *see* Cystitis, specified type NEC
- rectum K61.1
- renal — *see* Abscess, kidney
- retina — *see* Inflammation, chorioretinal
- retrobulbar — *see* Abscess, orbit
- retrocecal K65.1
- retrolaryngeal J38.7
- retromammary — *see* Abscess, breast
- retroperitoneal NEC K68.19
  - postprocedural K68.11
- retropharyngeal J39.0
- retrouterine — *see* Peritonitis, pelvic, female
- retrovesical — *see* Cystitis, specified type NEC
- root, tooth K04.7
  - with sinus (alveolar) K04.6
- round ligament — *see also* Disease, pelvis, inflammatory N73.2
- rupture (spontaneous) NOS L02.91
- sacrum (tuberculous) A18.01
  - nontuberculous M46.28
- salivary (duct) (gland) K11.3
- scalp (any part) L02.811

Abscess — *continued*
- scapular — *see* Osteomyelitis, specified type NEC
- sclera — *see* Scleritis
- scrofulous (tuberculous) A18.2
- scrotum N49.2
- seminal vesicle N49.0
- septal, dental K04.7
  - with sinus (alveolar) K04.6
- serous — *see* Periostitis
- shoulder (region) — *see* Abscess, upper limb
- sigmoid K63.0
- sinus (accessory) (chronic) (nasal) — *see also* Sinusitis
  - intracranial venous (any) G06.0
- Skene's duct or gland N34.0
- skin — *see* Abscess, by site
- specified site NEC L02.818
- spermatic cord N49.1
- sphenoidal (sinus) (chronic) J32.3
- spinal cord (any part) (staphylococcal) G06.1
  - tuberculous A17.81
- spine (column) (tuberculous) A18.01
  - epidural G06.1
  - nontuberculous — *see* Osteomyelitis, vertebra
- spleen D73.3
  - amebic A06.89
- stitch T81.41- ☑
  - following an obstetrical procedure O86.01
- sub-fascial, following an obstetrical procedure O86.02
- subarachnoid G06.2
  - brain G06.0
  - spinal cord G06.1
- subareolar — *see* Abscess, breast
- subcecal K35.33
- subcutaneous — *see also* Abscess, by site
  - following procedure T81.41- ☑
    - obstetrical O86.01
  - pheomycotic (chromomycotic) B43.2
- subdiaphragmatic K65.1
- subdural G06.2
  - brain G06.0
    - sequelae G09
  - spinal cord G06.1
- subgaleal L02.811
- subhepatic K65.1
- sublingual K12.2
  - gland K11.3
- submammary — *see* Abscess, breast
- submandibular (region) (space) (triangle) K12.2
  - gland K11.3
- submaxillary (region) L02.01
  - gland K11.3
- submental L02.01
  - gland K11.3
- subperiosteal — *see* Osteomyelitis, specified type NEC
- subphrenic K65.1
  - following an obstetrical procedure O86.03
  - postoperative T81.43- ☑
- suburethral N34.0
- sudoriparous L75.8
- supraclavicular (fossa) — *see* Abscess, upper limb
- supralevator K61.5
- suprapelvic, acute N73.0
- suprarenal (capsule) (gland) E27.8
- sweat gland L74.8
- tear duct — *see* Inflammation, lacrimal, passages, acute
- temple L02.01
- temporal region L02.01
- temporosphenoidal G06.0
- tendon (sheath) M65.00
  - ankle M65.07- ☑
  - foot M65.07- ☑
  - forearm M65.03- ☑
  - hand M65.04- ☑
  - lower leg M65.06- ☑
  - pelvic region M65.05- ☑
  - shoulder region M65.01- ☑
  - specified site NEC M65.08
  - thigh M65.05- ☑
  - upper arm M65.02- ☑
- testis N45.4
- thigh — *see* Abscess, lower limb
- thorax J86.9
  - with fistula J86.0
- throat J39.1
- thumb — *see also* Abscess, hand
  - nail — *see* Cellulitis, finger
- thymus (gland) E32.1
- thyroid (gland) E06.0

Abscess — *continued*
- toe (any) — *see also* Abscess, foot
  - nail — *see* Cellulitis, toe
- tongue (staphylococcal) K14.0
- tonsil(s) (lingual) J36
- tonsillopharyngeal J36
- tooth, teeth (root) K04.7
  - with sinus (alveolar) K04.6
  - supporting structures NEC — *see* Periodontitis, aggressive, localized
- trachea J39.8
- trunk L02.219
  - abdominal wall L02.211
  - back L02.212
  - chest wall L02.213
  - groin L02.214
  - perineum L02.215
  - umbilicus L02.216
- tubal — *see* Salpingitis
- tuberculous — *see* Tuberculosis, abscess
- tubo-ovarian — *see* Salpingo-oophoritis
- tunica vaginalis N49.1
- umbilicus L02.216
- upper
  - limb L02.41- ☑
  - respiratory J39.8
- urethral (gland) N34.0
- urinary N34.0
- uterus, uterine (wall) — *see also* Endometritis
  - ligament — *see also* Disease, pelvis, inflammatory N73.2
  - neck — *see* Cervicitis
- uvula K12.2
- vagina (wall) — *see* Vaginitis
- vaginorectal — *see* Vaginitis
- vas deferens N49.1
- vermiform appendix K35.33
- vertebra (column) (tuberculous) A18.01
  - nontuberculous — *see* Osteomyelitis, vertebra
- vesical — *see* Cystitis, specified type NEC
- vesico-uterine pouch — *see* Peritonitis, pelvic, female
- vitreous (humor) — *see* Endophthalmitis, purulent
- vocal cord J38.3
- von Bezold's — *see* Mastoiditis, acute
- vulva N76.4
- vulvovaginal gland N75.1
- web space — *see* Abscess, hand
- wound T81.49- ☑
- wrist — *see* Abscess, upper limb

Absence (of) (organ or part) (complete or partial)
- adrenal (gland) (congenital) Q89.1
  - acquired E89.6
- albumin in blood E88.09
- alimentary tract (congenital) Q45.8
  - upper Q40.8
- alveolar process (acquired) — *see* Anomaly, alveolar
- ankle (acquired) Z89.44- ☑
- anus (congenital) Q42.3
  - with fistula Q42.2
- aorta (congenital) Q25.41
- appendix, congenital Q42.8
- arm (acquired) Z89.20- ☑
  - above elbow Z89.22- ☑
    - congenital (with hand present) — *see* Agenesis, arm, with hand present
    - and hand — *see* Agenesis, forearm, and hand
  - below elbow Z89.21- ☑
    - congenital (with hand present) — *see* Agenesis, arm, with hand present
    - and hand — *see* Agenesis, forearm, and hand
  - congenital — *see* Defect, reduction, upper limb
  - shoulder (following explantation of shoulder joint prosthesis) (joint) (with or without presence of antibiotic-impregnated cement spacer) Z89.23- ☑
    - congenital (with hand present) — *see* Agenesis, arm, with hand present
- artery (congenital) (peripheral) Q27.8
  - brain Q28.3
  - coronary Q24.5
  - pulmonary Q25.79
  - specified NEC Q27.8
  - umbilical Q27.0
- atrial septum (congenital) Q21.19
- auditory canal (congenital) (external) Q16.1
- auricle (ear), congenital Q16.0
- bile, biliary duct, congenital Q44.5
- bladder (acquired) Z90.6

Absence — *continued*
  bladder — *continued*
    congenital Q64.5
  bowel sounds R19.11
  brain Q00.0
    part of Q04.3
  breast(s) (and nipple(s)) (acquired) Z90.1- ☑
    congenital Q83.8
  broad ligament Q50.6
  bronchus (congenital) Q32.4
  canaliculus lacrimalis, congenital Q10.4
  cerebellum (vermis) Q04.3
  cervix (acquired) (with uterus) Z90.710
    with remaining uterus Z90.712
    congenital Q51.5
  chin, congenital Q18.8
  cilia (congenital) Q10.3
    acquired — *see* Madarosis
  clitoris (congenital) Q52.6
  coccyx, congenital Q76.49
  cold sense R20.8
  congenital
    lumen — *see* Atresia
    organ or site NEC — *see* Agenesis
    septum — *see* Imperfect, closure
  corpus callosum Q04.0
  cricoid cartilage, congenital Q31.8
  diaphragm (with hernia), congenital Q79.1
  digestive organ(s) or tract, congenital Q45.8
    acquired NEC Z90.49
    upper Q40.8
  ductus arteriosus Q28.8
  duodenum (acquired) Z90.49
    congenital Q41.0
  ear, congenital Q16.9
    acquired H93.8- ☑
    auricle Q16.0
    external Q16.0
    inner Q16.5
    lobe, lobule Q17.8
    middle, except ossicles Q16.4
      ossicles Q16.3
    ossicles Q16.3
  ejaculatory duct (congenital) Q55.4
  endocrine gland (congenital) NEC Q89.2
    acquired E89.89
  epididymis (congenital) Q55.4
    acquired Z90.79
  epiglottis, congenital Q31.8
  esophagus (congenital) Q39.8
    acquired (partial) Z90.49
  eustachian tube (congenital) Q16.2
  extremity (acquired) Z89.9
    congenital Q73.0
    knee (following explantation of knee joint prosthesis) (joint) (with or without presence of antibiotic-impregnated cement spacer) Z89.52- ☑
    lower (above knee) Z89.619
      below knee Z89.51- ☑
    upper — *see* Absence, arm
  eye (acquired) Z90.01
    congenital Q11.1
    muscle (congenital) Q10.3
  eyeball (acquired) Z90.01
  eyelid (fold) (congenital) Q10.3
    acquired Z90.01
  face, specified part NEC Q18.8
  fallopian tube(s) (acquired) Z90.79
    congenital Q50.6
  family member (causing problem in home) NEC — *see also* Disruption, family Z63.32
  femur, congenital — *see* Defect, reduction, lower limb, longitudinal, femur
  fibrinogen (congenital) D68.2
    acquired D65
  finger(s) (acquired) Z89.02- ☑
    congenital — *see* Agenesis, hand
  foot (acquired) Z89.43- ☑
    congenital — *see* Agenesis, foot
  forearm (acquired) — *see* Absence, arm, below elbow
  gallbladder (acquired) Z90.49
    congenital Q44.0
  gamma globulin in blood D80.1
    hereditary D80.0
  genital organs
    acquired (female) (male) Z90.79
    female, congenital Q52.8
      external Q52.71

Absence — *continued*
  genital organs — *continued*
    female, congenital — *continued*
      internal NEC Q52.8
    male, congenital Q55.8
  genitourinary organs, congenital NEC
    female Q52.8
    male Q55.8
  globe (acquired) Z90.01
    congenital Q11.1
  glottis, congenital Q31.8
  hand and wrist (acquired) Z89.11- ☑
    congenital — *see* Agenesis, hand
  head, part (acquired) NEC Z90.09
  heat sense R20.8
  hip (following explantation of hip joint prosthesis) (joint) (with or without presence of antibiotic-impregnated cement spacer) Z89.62- ☑
  hymen (congenital) Q52.4
  ileum (acquired) Z90.49
    congenital Q41.2
  immunoglobulin, isolated NEC D80.3
    IgA D80.2
    IgG D80.3
    IgM D80.4
  incus (acquired) — *see* Loss, ossicles, ear
    congenital Q16.3
  inner ear, congenital Q16.5
  intestine (acquired) (small) Z90.49
    congenital Q41.9
      specified NEC Q41.8
    large Z90.49
      congenital Q42.9
        specified NEC Q42.8
  iris, congenital Q13.1
  jejunum (acquired) Z90.49
    congenital Q41.1
  joint
    acquired
      hip (following explantation of hip joint prosthesis) (with or without presence of antibiotic-impregnated cement spacer) Z89.62- ☑
      knee (following explantation of knee joint prosthesis) (with or without presence of antibiotic-impregnated cement spacer) Z89.52- ☑
      shoulder (following explantation of shoulder joint prosthesis) (with or without presence of antibiotic-impregnated cement spacer) Z89.23- ☑
    congenital NEC Q74.8
  kidney(s) (acquired) Z90.5
    congenital Q60.2
      bilateral Q60.1
      unilateral Q60.0
  knee (following explantation of knee joint prosthesis) (joint) (with or without presence of antibiotic-impregnated cement spacer) Z89.52- ☑
  labyrinth, membranous Q16.5
  larynx (congenital) Q31.8
    acquired Z90.02
  leg (acquired) (above knee) Z89.61- ☑
    below knee (acquired) Z89.51- ☑
    congenital — *see* Defect, reduction, lower limb
  lens (acquired) — *see also* Aphakia
    congenital Q12.3
    post cataract extraction Z98.4- ☑
  limb (acquired) — *see* Absence, extremity
  lip Q38.6
  liver (congenital) Q44.79
  lung (fissure) (lobe) (bilateral) (unilateral) (congenital) Q33.3
    acquired (any part) Z90.2
  menstruation — *see* Amenorrhea
  muscle (congenital) (pectoral) Q79.8
    ocular Q10.3
  neck, part Q18.8
  neutrophil — *see* Agranulocytosis
  nipple(s) (with breast(s)) (acquired) Z90.1- ☑
    congenital Q83.2
  nose (congenital) Q30.1
    acquired Z90.09
  organ
    of Corti, congenital Q16.5
    or site, congenital NEC Q89.89
      acquired NEC Z89.89
  osseous meatus (ear) Q16.4
  ovary (acquired)
    bilateral Z90.722

Absence — *continued*
  ovary — *continued*
    congenital
      bilateral Q50.02
      unilateral Q50.01
    unilateral Z90.721
  oviduct (acquired)
    bilateral Z90.722
    congenital Q50.6
    unilateral Z90.721
  pancreas (congenital) Q45.0
    acquired Z90.410
      complete Z90.410
      partial Z90.411
      total Z90.410
  parathyroid gland (acquired) E89.2
    congenital Q89.2
  patella, congenital Q74.1
  penis (congenital) Q55.5
    acquired Z90.79
  pericardium (congenital) Q24.8
  pituitary gland (congenital) Q89.2
    acquired E89.3
  prostate (acquired) Z90.79
    congenital Q55.4
  pulmonary valve Q22.0
  punctum lacrimale (congenital) Q10.4
  radius, congenital — *see* Defect, reduction, upper limb, longitudinal, radius
  rectum (congenital) Q42.1
    with fistula Q42.0
    acquired Z90.49
  respiratory organ NOS Q34.9
  rib (acquired) Z90.89
    congenital Q76.6
  sacrum, congenital Q76.49
  salivary gland(s), congenital Q38.4
  scrotum, congenital Q55.29
  seminal vesicles (congenital) Q55.4
    acquired Z90.79
  septum
    atrial (congenital) Q21.19
    between aorta and pulmonary artery Q21.4
    ventricular (congenital) Q20.4
  sex chromosome
    female phenotype Q97.8
    male phenotype Q98.8
  skull bone (congenital) Q75.8
    with
      anencephaly Q00.0
      encephalocele — *see* Encephalocele
      hydrocephalus Q03.9
        with spina bifida — *see* Spina bifida, by site, with hydrocephalus
      microcephaly Q02
  spermatic cord, congenital Q55.4
  spine, congenital Q76.49
  spleen (congenital) Q89.01
    acquired Z90.81
  sternum, congenital Q76.7
  stomach (acquired) (partial) Z90.3
    congenital Q40.2
  superior vena cava, congenital Q26.8
  teeth, tooth (congenital) K00.0
    acquired (complete) K08.109
      class I K08.101
      class II K08.102
      class III K08.103
      class IV K08.104
      due to
        caries K08.139
          class I K08.131
          class II K08.132
          class III K08.133
          class IV K08.134
        periodontal disease K08.129
          class I K08.121
          class II K08.122
          class III K08.123
          class IV K08.124
        specified NEC K08.199
          class I K08.191
          class II K08.192
          class III K08.193
          class IV K08.194
        trauma K08.119
          class I K08.111
          class II K08.112
          class III K08.113

☑ **Additional Character Required — Refer to the Tabular List for Character Selection**

Absence — continued
teeth, tooth — continued
acquired — continued
due to — continued
trauma — continued
class IV K08.114
partial K08.409
class I K08.401
class II K08.402
class III K08.403
class IV K08.404
due to
caries K08.439
class I K08.431
class II K08.432
class III K08.433
class IV K08.434
periodontal disease K08.429
class I K08.421
class II K08.422
class III K08.423
class IV K08.424
specified NEC K08.499
class I K08.491
class II K08.492
class III K08.493
class IV K08.494
trauma K08.419
class I K08.411
class II K08.412
class III K08.413
class IV K08.414
tendon (congenital) Q79.8
testis (congenital) Q55.0
  acquired Z90.79
thumb (acquired) Z89.01- ☑
  congenital — see Agenesis, hand
thymus gland Q89.2
thyroid (gland) (acquired) E89.0
  cartilage, congenital Q31.8
  congenital E03.1
toe(s) (acquired) Z89.42- ☑
  with foot — see Absence, foot and ankle
  congenital — see Agenesis, foot
  great Z89.41- ☑
tongue, congenital Q38.3
trachea (cartilage), congenital Q32.1
transverse aortic arch, congenital Q25.49
tricuspid valve Q22.4
umbilical artery, congenital Q27.0
upper arm and forearm with hand present, congenital — see Agenesis, arm, with hand present
ureter (congenital) Q62.4
  acquired Z90.6
urethra, congenital Q64.5
uterus (acquired) Z90.710
  with cervix Z90.710
  with remaining cervical stump Z90.711
  congenital Q51.0
uvula, congenital Q38.5
vagina, congenital Q52.0
vas deferens (congenital) Q55.4
  acquired Z90.79
vein (peripheral) congenital NEC Q27.8
  cerebral Q28.3
  digestive system Q27.8
  great Q26.8
  lower limb Q27.8
  portal Q26.5
  precerebral Q28.1
  specified site NEC Q27.8
  upper limb Q27.8
vena cava (inferior) (superior), congenital Q26.8
ventricular septum Q20.4
vertebra, congenital Q76.49
von Willebrand factor, complete (near) — see also Disease, von Willebrand D68.03
vulva, congenital Q52.71
wrist (acquired) Z89.12- ☑
Absorbent system disease I87.8
Absorption
  carbohydrate, disturbance K90.49
  chemical — see Table of Drugs and Chemicals
    through placenta (newborn) P04.9
      environmental substance P04.6
      nutritional substance P04.5
      obstetric anesthetic or analgesic drug P04.0
  drug NEC — see Table of Drugs and Chemicals

Absorption — continued
drug — see Table of Drugs and Chemicals — continued
  addictive
    through placenta (newborn) — see also Newborn, affected by, maternal, use of P04.40
      cocaine P04.41
      hallucinogens P04.42
      specified drug NEC P04.49
  medicinal
    through placenta (newborn) P04.19
    through placenta (newborn) P04.19
    obstetric anesthetic or analgesic drug P04.0
fat, disturbance K90.49
  pancreatic K90.3
noxious substance — see Table of Drugs and Chemicals
protein, disturbance K90.49
starch, disturbance K90.49
toxic substance — see Table of Drugs and Chemicals
uremic — see Uremia
Abstinence symptoms, syndrome
  alcohol F10.239
    with delirium F10.231
  cocaine F14.23
  neonatal P96.1
  nicotine — see Dependence, drug, nicotine, with, withdrawal
  opioid F11.93
    with dependence F11.23
  psychoactive NEC F19.939
    with
      delirium F19.931
      dependence F19.239
        with
          delirium F19.231
          perceptual disturbance F19.232
          uncomplicated F19.230
      perceptual disturbance F19.932
      uncomplicated F19.930
  sedative F13.939
    with
      delirium F13.931
      dependence F13.239
        with
          delirium F13.231
          perceptual disturbance F13.232
          uncomplicated F13.230
      perceptual disturbance F13.932
      uncomplicated F13.930
  stimulant NEC F15.93
    with dependence F15.23
Abulia R68.89
Abulomania F60.7
Abuse
  adult — see Maltreatment, adult
  as reason for
    couple seeking advice (including offender) Z63.0
  alcohol (non-dependent) F10.10
    with
      anxiety disorder F10.180
      intoxication F10.129
        with delirium F10.121
        uncomplicated F10.120
      mood disorder F10.14
      other specified disorder F10.188
      psychosis F10.159
        delusions F10.150
        hallucinations F10.151
      sexual dysfunction F10.181
      sleep disorder F10.182
      unspecified disorder F10.19
      withdrawal F10.139
        with
          perceptual disturbance F10.132
          delirium F10.131
          uncomplicated F10.130
      counseling and surveillance Z71.41
      in remission (early) (sustained) F10.11
  amphetamine (or related substance) — see also Abuse, drug, stimulant NEC
    stimulant NEC F15.10
      with
        anxiety disorder F15.180
        intoxication F15.129
          with
            delirium F15.121
            perceptual disturbance F15.122
        withdrawal F15.13
  analgesics (non-prescribed) (over the counter) F55.8

Abuse — continued
antacids F55.0
antidepressants — see Abuse, drug, psychoactive NEC
anxiolytic — see Abuse, drug, sedative
barbiturates — see Abuse, drug, sedative
caffeine — see Abuse, drug, stimulant NEC
cannabis, cannabinoids — see Abuse, drug, cannabis
child — see Maltreatment, child
cocaine — see Abuse, drug, cocaine
drug NEC (non-dependent) F19.10
  with sleep disorder F19.182
  amphetamine type — see Abuse, drug, stimulant NEC
  analgesics (non-prescribed) (over the counter) F55.8
  antacids F55.0
  antidepressants — see Abuse, drug, psychoactive NEC
  anxiolytics — see Abuse, drug, sedative
  barbiturates — see Abuse, drug, sedative
  caffeine — see Abuse, drug, stimulant NEC
  cannabis F12.10
    with
      anxiety disorder F12.180
      intoxication F12.129
        with
          delirium F12.121
          perceptual disturbance F12.122
          uncomplicated F12.120
      other specified disorder F12.188
      psychosis F12.159
        delusions F12.150
        hallucinations F12.151
      unspecified disorder F12.19
      withdrawal F12.13
    in remission (early) (sustained) F12.11
  cocaine F14.10
    with
      anxiety disorder F14.180
      intoxication F14.129
        with
          delirium F14.121
          perceptual disturbance F14.122
          uncomplicated F14.120
      mood disorder F14.14
      other specified disorder F14.188
      psychosis F14.159
        delusions F14.150
        hallucinations F14.151
      sexual dysfunction F14.181
      sleep disorder F14.182
      unspecified disorder F14.19
      withdrawal F14.13
    in remission (early) (sustained) F14.11
  counseling and surveillance Z71.51
  hallucinogen F16.10
    with
      anxiety disorder F16.180
      flashbacks F16.183
      intoxication F16.129
        with
          delirium F16.121
          perceptual disturbance F16.122
          uncomplicated F16.120
      mood disorder F16.14
      other specified disorder F16.188
      perception disorder, persisting F16.183
      psychosis F16.159
        delusions F16.150
        hallucinations F16.151
      unspecified disorder F16.19
    in remission (early) (sustained) F16.11
  hashish — see Abuse, drug, cannabis
  herbal or folk remedies F55.1
  hormones F55.3
  hypnotics — see Abuse, drug, sedative
  in remission (early) (sustained) F19.11
  inhalant F18.10
    with
      anxiety disorder F18.180
      dementia, persisting F18.17
      intoxication F18.129
        with delirium F18.121
        uncomplicated F18.120
      mood disorder F18.14
      other specified disorder F18.188
      psychosis F18.159
        delusions F18.150
        hallucinations F18.151
      unspecified disorder F18.19
    in remission (early) (sustained) F18.11
  laxatives F55.2

Abuse — continued
  drug — continued
    LSD — see Abuse, drug, hallucinogen
    marihuana — see Abuse, drug, cannabis
    morphine type (opioids) — see Abuse, drug, opioid
    opioid F11.10
      with
        intoxication F11.129
          with
            delirium F11.121
            perceptual disturbance F11.122
          uncomplicated F11.120
        mood disorder F11.14
        opioid-associated amnestic syndrome F11.188
        other specified disorder F11.188
        psychosis F11.159
          delusions F11.150
          hallucinations F11.151
        sexual dysfunction F11.181
        sleep disorder F11.182
        unspecified disorder F11.19
        withdrawal F11.13
      in remission (early) (sustained) F11.11
    PCP (phencyclidine) (or related substance) — see Abuse, drug, hallucinogen
    psychoactive NEC F19.10
      with
        amnestic disorder F19.16
        anxiety disorder F19.180
        dementia F19.17
        intoxication F19.129
          with
            delirium F19.121
            perceptual disturbance F19.122
          uncomplicated F19.120
        mood disorder F19.14
        other specified disorder F19.188
        psychosis F19.159
          delusions F19.150
          hallucinations F19.151
        sexual dysfunction F19.181
        sleep disorder F19.182
        unspecified disorder F19.19
        withdrawal F19.139
          with
            perceptual disturbance F19.132
          delirium F19.131
          uncomplicated F19.130
    sedative, hypnotic or anxiolytic F13.10
      with
        anxiety disorder F13.180
        intoxication F13.129
          with delirium F13.121
          uncomplicated F13.120
        mood disorder F13.14
        other specified disorder F13.188
        psychosis F13.159
          delusions F13.150
          hallucinations F13.151
        sexual dysfunction F13.181
        sleep disorder F13.182
        unspecified disorder F13.19
        withdrawal F13.139
          with
            perceptual disturbance F13.132
          delirium F13.131
          uncomplicated F13.130
      in remission (early) (sustained) F13.11
    solvent — see Abuse, drug, inhalant
    steroids F55.3
    stimulant NEC F15.10
      with
        anxiety disorder F15.180
        intoxication F15.129
          with
            delirium F15.121
            perceptual disturbance F15.122
          uncomplicated F15.120
        mood disorder F15.14
        other specified disorder F15.188
        psychosis F15.159
          delusions F15.150
          hallucinations F15.151
        sexual dysfunction F15.181
        sleep disorder F15.182
        unspecified disorder F15.19
        withdrawal F15.13
      in remission (early) (sustained) F15.11
    tranquilizers — see Abuse, drug, sedative

Abuse — continued
  drug — continued
    vitamins F55.4
  hallucinogens — see Abuse, drug, hallucinogen
  hashish — see Abuse, drug, cannabis
  herbal or folk remedies F55.1
  hormones F55.3
  hypnotic — see Abuse, drug, sedative
  inhalant — see Abuse, drug, inhalant
  laxatives F55.2
  LSD — see Abuse, drug, hallucinogen
  marihuana — see Abuse, drug, cannabis
  morphine type (opioids) — see Abuse, drug, opioid
  non-psychoactive substance NEC F55.8
    antacids F55.0
    folk remedies F55.1
    herbal remedies F55.1
    hormones F55.3
    laxatives F55.2
    steroids F55.3
    vitamins F55.4
  opioids — see Abuse, drug, opioid
  PCP (phencyclidine) (or related substance) — see Abuse, drug, hallucinogen
  physical (adult) (child) — see Maltreatment
  psychoactive substance — see Abuse, drug, psychoactive NEC
  psychological (adult) (child) — see Maltreatment
  sedative — see Abuse, drug, sedative
  sexual — see Maltreatment
  solvent — see Abuse, drug, inhalant
  steroids F55.3
  vitamins F55.4
Acalculia R48.8
  developmental F81.2
Acanthamebiasis (with) B60.10
  conjunctiva B60.12
  keratoconjunctivitis B60.13
  meningoencephalitis B60.11
  other specified B60.19
Acanthocephaliasis B83.8
Acanthocheilonemiasis B74.4
Acanthocytosis E78.6
Acantholysis L11.9
Acanthosis (acquired) (nigricans) L83
  benign Q82.8
  congenital Q82.8
  seborrheic L82.1
    inflamed L82.0
  tongue K14.3
Acapnia E87.3
Acarbia E87.29
Acardia, acardius Q89.89
Acardiacus amorphus Q89.89
Acardiotrophia I51.4
Acariasis B88.09
  scabies B86
Acarodermatitis (urticarioides) B88.09
Acarophobia F40.218
Acatalasemia, acatalasia E80.3
Acathisia (drug induced) G25.71
Accelerated atrioventricular conduction I45.6
Accentuation of personality traits (type A) Z73.1
Accessory (congenital)
  adrenal gland Q89.1
  anus Q43.4
  appendix Q43.4
  atrioventricular conduction I45.6
  auditory ossicles Q16.3
  auricle (ear) Q17.0
  biliary duct or passage Q44.5
  bladder Q64.79
  blood vessels NEC Q27.9
    coronary Q24.5
  bone NEC Q79.8
  breast tissue, axilla Q83.1
  carpal bones Q74.0
  cecum Q43.4
  chromosome(s) NEC (nonsex) Q92.9
    with complex rearrangements NEC Q92.5
      seen only at prometaphase Q92.8
    13 — see Trisomy, 13
    18 — see Trisomy, 18
    21 — see Trisomy, 21
    partial Q92.9
    sex
      female phenotype Q97.8
  coronary artery Q24.5
  cusp(s), heart valve NEC Q24.8

Accessory — continued
  cusp(s), heart valve — continued
    pulmonary Q22.3
  cystic duct Q44.5
  digit(s) Q69.9
  ear (auricle) (lobe) Q17.0
  endocrine gland NEC Q89.2
  eye muscle Q10.3
  eyelid Q10.3
  face bone(s) Q75.8
  fallopian tube (fimbria) (ostium) Q50.6
  finger(s) Q69.0
  foreskin N47.8
  frontonasal process Q75.8
  gallbladder Q44.1
  genital organ(s)
    female Q52.8
      external Q52.79
      internal NEC Q52.8
    male Q55.8
  genitourinary organs NEC Q89.89
    female Q52.8
    male Q55.8
  hallux Q69.2
  heart Q24.8
    valve NEC Q24.8
      pulmonary Q22.3
  hepatic ducts Q44.5
  hymen Q52.4
  intestine (large) (small) Q43.4
  kidney Q63.0
  lacrimal canal Q10.6
  leaflet, heart valve NEC Q24.8
  ligament, broad Q50.6
  liver Q44.79
    duct Q44.5
  lobule (ear) Q17.0
  lung (lobe) Q33.1
  muscle Q79.8
  navicular of carpus Q74.0
  nervous system, part NEC Q07.8
  nipple Q83.3
  nose Q30.8
  organ or site not listed — see Anomaly, by site
  ovary Q50.31
  oviduct Q50.6
  pancreas Q45.3
  parathyroid gland Q89.2
  parotid gland (and duct) Q38.4
  pituitary gland Q89.2
  preauricular appendage Q17.0
  prepuce N47.8
  renal arteries (multiple) Q27.2
  rib Q76.6
    cervical Q76.5
  roots (teeth) K00.2
  salivary gland Q38.4
  sesamoid bones Q74.8
    foot Q74.2
    hand Q74.0
  skin tags Q82.8
  spleen Q89.09
  sternum Q76.7
  submaxillary gland Q38.4
  tarsal bones Q74.2
  teeth, tooth K00.1
  tendon Q79.8
  thumb Q69.1
  thymus gland Q89.2
  thyroid gland Q89.2
  toes Q69.2
  tongue Q38.3
  tooth, teeth K00.1
  tragus Q17.0
  ureter Q62.5
  urethra Q64.79
  urinary organ or tract NEC Q64.8
  uterus Q51.28
  vagina Q52.10
  valve, heart NEC Q24.8
    pulmonary Q22.3
  vertebra Q76.49
  vocal cords Q31.8
  vulva Q52.79
Accident
  birth — see Birth, injury
  cardiac — see Infarct, myocardium
  cerebrovascular (ischemic) I63.9
    aborted I63.9

Accident — *continued*
  cerebrovascular — *continued*
    chronic (old) (remote) (imaging) (without sequelae) Z86.73
      with residual defects — *see* Sequelae, disease, cerebrovascular
    embolic I63.- ☑
    hemorrhagic — *see* Hemorrhage, intracranial, intracerebral
    old (without sequelae) Z86.73
      with sequelae (of) — *see* Sequelae, infarction, cerebral
    thrombotic I63.- ☑
  coronary — *see* Infarct, myocardium
  craniovascular I63.9
  vascular, brain I63.9
Accidental — *see* condition
Accommodation (disorder) — *see also* condition
  hysterical paralysis of F44.89
  insufficiency of H52.4
  paresis — *see* Paresis, of accommodation
  spasm — *see* Spasm, of accommodation
Accouchement — *see* Delivery
Accreta placenta O43.21- ☑
Accretio cordis (nonrheumatic) I31.0
Accretions, tooth, teeth K03.6
Acculturation difficulty Z60.3
Accumulation secretion, prostate N42.89
Acephalia, acephalism, acephalus, acephaly Q00.0
Acephalobrachia monster Q89.89
Acephalochirus monster Q89.89
Acephalogaster Q89.89
Acephalostomus monster Q89.89
Acephalothorax Q89.89
Acerophobia F40.298
Acetonemia R79.89
  in Type 1 diabetes E10.10
    with coma E10.11
Acetonuria R82.4
Achalasia (cardia) (esophagus) K22.0
  congenital Q39.5
  pylorus Q40.0
  sphincteral NEC K59.89
Ache(s) — *see* Pain
Acheilia Q38.6
Achillobursitis — *see* Tendinitis, Achilles
Achillodynia — *see* Tendinitis, Achilles
Achlorhydria, achlorhydric (neurogenic) K31.83
  anemia D50.8
  diarrhea K31.83
  psychogenic F45.8
  secondary to vagotomy K91.1
Achluophobia F40.228
Acholia K82.8
Acholuric jaundice (familial) (splenomegalic) — *see also* Spherocytosis
  acquired D59.8
Achondrogenesis Q77.0
Achondroplasia (osteosclerosis congenita) Q77.4
Achroma, cutis L80
Achromat (ism), achromatopsia (acquired) (congenital) H53.51
Achromia, congenital — *see* Albinism
Achromia parasitica B36.0
Achylia gastrica K31.89
  psychogenic F45.8
Acid
  burn — *see* Corrosion
  deficiency
    amide nicotinic E52
    ascorbic E54
    folic E53.8
    nicotinic E52
    pantothenic E53.8
  intoxication — *see also* Acidosis E87.29
  peptic disease K30
  phosphatase deficiency E83.39
  stomach K30
    psychogenic F45.8
Acidemia — *see also* Acidosis E87.20
  argininosuccinic E72.22
  isovaleric E71.110
  metabolic — *see also* Acidosis, metabolic
    newborn P19.9
      first noted before onset of labor P19.0
      first noted during labor P19.1
        noted at birth P19.2
  methylmalonic E71.120
  pipecolic E72.3

Acidemia — *continued*
  propionic E71.121
Acidity, gastric (high) K30
  psychogenic F45.8
Acidocytopenia — *see* Agranulocytosis
Acidocytosis D72.10
Acidopenia — *see* Agranulocytosis
Acidosis (lactic) E87.20
  in Type 1 diabetes E10.10
    with coma E10.11
  kidney, tubular N25.89
  lactic E87.20
    acute E87.21
    chronic E87.22
  metabolic NEC E87.20
    with respiratory acidosis E87.4
    acute E87.21
    chronic E87.22
    hyperchloremic, of newborn P74.421
    late, of newborn P74.0
  mixed metabolic and respiratory, newborn P84
  newborn P84
  renal (hyperchloremic) (tubular) N25.89
  respiratory E87.29
    acute J96.02
    chronic J96.12
    complicated by
      metabolic
        acidosis E87.4
        alkalosis E87.4
  specified NEC E87.29
Aciduria
  4-hydroxybutyric E72.81
  argininosuccinic E72.22
  gamma-hydroxybutyric E72.81
  glutaric (type I) E72.3
    type II E71.313
    type III E71.5- ☑
  orotic (congenital) (hereditary) (pyrimidine deficiency) E79.89
    anemia D53.0
Acladiosis (skin) B36.0
Aclasis, diaphyseal Q78.6
Acleistocardia Q21.19
Aclusion — *see* Anomaly, dentofacial, malocclusion
Acne L70.9
  artificialis L70.8
  atrophica L70.2
  cachecticorum (Hebra) L70.8
  conglobata L70.1
  cystic L70.0
  decalvans L66.2
  excoriee (des jeunes filles) L70.5
  frontalis L70.2
  indurata L70.0
  infantile L70.4
  keloid L73.0
  lupoid L70.2
  necrotic, necrotica (miliaris) L70.2
  neonatal L70.4
  nodular L70.0
  occupational L70.8
  picker's L70.5
  pustular L70.0
  rodens L70.2
  rosacea L71.9
  specified NEC L70.8
  tropica L70.3
  varioliformis L70.2
  vulgaris L70.0
Acnitis (primary) A18.4
Acosta's disease T70.29- ☑
Acoustic — *see* condition
Acousticophobia F40.298
ACPO (acute colonic pseudo-obstruction) K59.81
Acquired — *see also* condition
  immunodeficiency syndrome (AIDS) B20
Acrania Q00.0
Acroangiodermatitis I78.9
Acroasphyxia, chronic I73.89
Acrobystitis N47.7
Acrocephalopolysyndactyly Q87.0
Acrocephalosyndactyly Q87.0
Acrocephaly Q75.009
Acrochondrohyperplasia — *see* Syndrome, Marfan
Acrocyanosis I73.89
  newborn P28.2
    meaning transient blue hands and feet — *omit code*
Acrodermatitis L30.8

Acrodermatitis — *continued*
  atrophicans (chronica) L90.4
  continua (Hallopeau) L40.2
  enteropathica (hereditary) E83.2
  Hallopeau's L40.2
  infantile papular L44.4
  perstans L40.2
  pustulosa continua L40.2
  recalcitrant pustular L40.2
Acrodynia — *see* Poisoning, mercury
Acromegaly, acromegalia E22.0
Acromelalgia I73.81
Acromicria, acromikria Q79.8
Acronyx L60.0
Acropachy, thyroid — *see* Thyrotoxicosis
Acroparesthesia (simple) (vasomotor) I73.89
Acropathy, thyroid — *see* Thyrotoxicosis
Acrophobia F40.241
Acroposthitis N47.7
Acroscleriasis, acroscleroderma, acrosclerosis — *see* Sclerosis, systemic
Acrosphacelus I96
Acrospiroma, eccrine — *see* Neoplasm, skin, benign
Acrostealgia — *see* Osteochondropathy
Acrotrophodynia — *see* Immersion
ACTH ectopic syndrome E24.3
Actinic — *see* condition
Actinobacillosis, actinobacillus A28.8
  mallei A24.0
  muris A25.1
Actinomyces israelii (infection) — *see* Actinomycosis
Actinomycetoma (foot) B47.1
Actinomycosis, actinomycotic A42.9
  with pneumonia A42.0
  abdominal A42.1
  cervicofacial A42.2
  cutaneous A42.89
  gastrointestinal A42.1
  pulmonary A42.0
  sepsis A42.7
  specified site NEC A42.89
Actinoneuritis G62.82
Action, heart
  disorder I49.9
  irregular I49.9
    psychogenic F45.8
Activated protein C resistance D68.51
Activation
  mast cell (disorder) (syndrome) D89.40
    idiopathic D89.42
    monoclonal D89.41
    secondary D89.43
    specified type NEC D89.49
Active — *see* condition
Acute — *see also* condition
  abdomen R10.0
  gallbladder — *see* Cholecystitis, acute
Acyanotic heart disease (congenital) Q24.9
Acystia Q64.5
Adair-Dighton syndrome (brittle bones and blue sclera, deafness) Q78.0
Adamantinoblastoma — *see* Ameloblastoma
Adamantinoma — *see also* Cyst, calcifying odontogenic
  long bones C40.90
    lower limb C40.2- ☑
    upper limb C40.0- ☑
  malignant C41.1
    jaw (bone) (lower) C41.1
      upper C41.0
  tibial C40.2- ☑
Adamantoblastoma — *see* Ameloblastoma
Adams-Stokes (-Morgagni) **disease or syndrome** I45.9
Adaption reaction — *see* Disorder, adjustment
Addiction — *see also* Dependence F19.20
  alcohol, alcoholic (ethyl) (methyl) (wood) (without remission) F10.20
    with remission F10.21
  drug — *see* Dependence, drug
  ethyl alcohol (without remission) F10.20
    with remission F10.21
  heroin — *see* Dependence, drug, opioid
  methyl alcohol (without remission) F10.20
    with remission F10.21
  methylated spirit (without remission) F10.20
    with remission F10.21
  morphine (-like substances) — *see* Dependence, drug, opioid
  nicotine — *see* Dependence, drug, nicotine
  opium and opioids — *see* Dependence, drug, opioid

Addiction — continued
 tobacco — see Dependence, drug, nicotine
Addison-Biermer anemia (pernicious) D51.0
Addison-Schilder complex E71.528
Addisonian crisis E27.2
Addison's
 anemia (pernicious) D51.0
 disease (bronze) or syndrome E27.1
  tuberculous A18.7
 keloid L94.0
Additional — see also Accessory
 chromosome(s) — see also Trisomy Q99.8- ☑
  21 — see Trisomy, 21
  marker — see Extra, marker chromosomes
  sex — see Abnormal, chromosome, sex
Adduction contracture, hip or other joint — see Contraction, joint
Adenitis — see also Lymphadenitis
 acute, unspecified site L04.9
  axillary I88.9
   acute L04.2
   chronic or subacute I88.1
  Bartholin's gland N75.8
  bulbourethral gland — see Urethritis
  cervical I88.9
   acute L04.0
   chronic or subacute I88.1
  chancroid (Hemophilus ducreyi) A57
  chronic, unspecified site I88.1
  Cowper's gland — see Urethritis
  due to Pasteurella multocida (P. septica) A28.0
  epidemic, acute B27.09
  gangrenous L04.9
  gonorrheal NEC A54.89
  groin I88.9
   acute L04.1
   chronic or subacute I88.1
  infectious (acute) (epidemic) B27.09
  inguinal I88.9
   acute L04.1
   chronic or subacute I88.1
  lymph gland or node, except mesenteric I88.9
   acute — see Lymphadenitis, acute
   chronic or subacute I88.1
  mesenteric (acute) (chronic) (nonspecific) (subacute) I88.0
  parotid gland (suppurative) — see Sialoadenitis
  salivary gland (any) (suppurative) — see Sialoadenitis
  scrofulous (tuberculous) A18.2
  Skene's duct or gland — see Urethritis
  strumous, tuberculous A18.2
  subacute, unspecified site I88.1
  sublingual gland (suppurative) — see Sialoadenitis
  submandibular gland (suppurative) — see Sialoadenitis
  submaxillary gland (suppurative) — see Sialoadenitis
  tuberculous — see Tuberculosis, lymph gland
  urethral gland — see Urethritis
  Wharton's duct (suppurative) — see Sialoadenitis
Adenoacanthoma — see Neoplasm, malignant, by site
Adenoameloblastoma — see Cyst, calcifying odontogenic
Adenocarcinoid (tumor) — see Neoplasm, malignant, by site
Adenocarcinoma — see also Neoplasm, malignant, by site
 acidophil
  specified site — see Neoplasm, malignant, by site
  unspecified site C75.1
 adrenal cortical C74.0- ☑
 alveolar — see Neoplasm, lung, malignant
 apocrine
  breast — see Neoplasm, breast, malignant
  in situ
   breast D05.8- ☑
   specified site NEC — see Neoplasm, skin, in situ
   unspecified site D04.9
  specified site NEC — see Neoplasm, skin, malignant
  unspecified site C44.99
 basal cell
  specified site — see Neoplasm, skin, malignant
  unspecified site C08.9
 basophil
  specified site — see Neoplasm, malignant, by site
  unspecified site C75.1
 bile duct type C22.1
  liver C22.1
  specified site NEC — see Neoplasm, malignant, by site
  unspecified site C22.1
 bronchiolar — see Neoplasm, lung, malignant
 bronchioloalveolar — see Neoplasm, lung, malignant

Adenocarcinoma — continued
 ceruminous C44.29- ☑
 cervix, in situ — see also Carcinoma, cervix uteri, in situ D06.9
 chromophobe
  specified site — see Neoplasm, malignant, by site
  unspecified site C75.1
 diffuse type
  specified site — see Neoplasm, malignant, by site
  unspecified site C16.9
 duct
  infiltrating
   with Paget's disease — see Neoplasm, breast, malignant
   specified site — see Neoplasm, malignant, by site
   unspecified site (female) C50.91- ☑
    male C50.92- ☑
  specified site — see Neoplasm, malignant, by site
  unspecified site
   female C56.9
   male C61
 eosinophil
  specified site — see Neoplasm, malignant, by site
  unspecified site C75.1
 follicular
  with papillary C73
  moderately differentiated C73
  specified site — see Neoplasm, malignant, by site
  trabecular C73
  unspecified site C73
  well differentiated C73
 Hurthle cell C73
 in
  adenomatous
   polyposis coli C18.9
 infiltrating duct
  with Paget's disease — see Neoplasm, breast, malignant
  specified site — see Neoplasm, by site, malignant
  unspecified site (female) C50.91- ☑
   male C50.92- ☑
 inflammatory
  specified site — see Neoplasm, by site, malignant
  unspecified site (female) C50.91- ☑
   male C50.92- ☑
 intestinal type
  specified site — see Neoplasm, by site, malignant
  unspecified site C16.9
 intracystic papillary
 intraductal
  breast D05.1- ☑
  noninfiltrating
   breast D05.1- ☑
   papillary
    with invasion
     specified site — see Neoplasm, by site, malignant
     unspecified site (female) C50.91- ☑
      male C50.92- ☑
    breast D05.1- ☑
    specified site NEC — see Neoplasm, in situ, by site
    unspecified site D05.1- ☑
   specified site NEC — see Neoplasm, in situ, by site
   unspecified site D05.1- ☑
  papillary
   with invasion
    specified site — see Neoplasm, malignant, by site
    unspecified site (female) C50.91- ☑
     male C50.92- ☑
   breast D05.1- ☑
   specified site — see Neoplasm, in situ, by site
   unspecified site D05.1- ☑
  specified site NEC — see Neoplasm, in situ, by site
  unspecified site D05.1- ☑
 islet cell
  with exocrine, mixed
   specified site — see Neoplasm, malignant, by site
   unspecified site C25.9
  pancreas C25.4
  specified site NEC — see Neoplasm, malignant, by site
  unspecified site C25.4
 lobular
  in situ
   breast D05.0- ☑
   specified site NEC — see Neoplasm, in situ, by site

Adenocarcinoma — continued
 lobular — continued
  in situ — continued
   unspecified site D05.0- ☑
  specified site — see Neoplasm, malignant, by site
  unspecified site (female) C50.91- ☑
   male C50.92- ☑
 mucoid — see also Neoplasm, malignant, by site
  cell
   specified site — see Neoplasm, malignant, by site
   unspecified site C75.1
 nonencapsulated sclerosing C73
 papillary
  with follicular C73
  follicular variant C73
  intraductal (noninfiltrating)
   with invasion
    specified site — see Neoplasm, malignant, by site
    unspecified site (female) C50.91- ☑
     male C50.92- ☑
   breast D05.1- ☑
   specified site NEC — see Neoplasm, in situ, by site
   unspecified site D05.1- ☑
  serous
   specified site — see Neoplasm, malignant, by site
   unspecified site C56.9
 papillocystic
  specified site — see Neoplasm, malignant, by site
  unspecified site C56.9
 pseudomucinous
  specified site — see Neoplasm, malignant, by site
  unspecified site C56.9
 renal cell C64.- ☑
 sebaceous — see Neoplasm, skin, malignant
 serous — see also Neoplasm, malignant, by site
  papillary
   specified site — see Neoplasm, malignant, by site
   unspecified site C56.9
 sweat gland — see Neoplasm, skin, malignant
 water-clear cell C75.0
Adenocarcinoma-in-situ — see also Neoplasm, in situ, by site
 breast D05.9- ☑
Adenofibroma
 clear cell — see Neoplasm, benign, by site
 endometrioid D27.9
  borderline malignancy D39.10
  malignant C56.- ☑
 mucinous
  specified site — see Neoplasm, benign, by site
  unspecified site D27.9
 papillary
  specified site — see Neoplasm, benign, by site
  unspecified site D27.9
 prostate — see Enlargement, enlarged, prostate
 serous
  specified site — see Neoplasm, benign, by site
  unspecified site D27.9
 specified site — see Neoplasm, benign, by site
 unspecified site D27.9
Adenofibrosis
 breast — see Fibroadenosis, breast
 endometrioid N80.00
Adenoiditis (chronic) J35.02
 with tonsillitis J35.03
 acute J03.90
  recurrent J03.91
  specified organism NEC J03.80
   recurrent J03.81
  staphylococcal J03.80
   recurrent J03.81
  streptococcal J03.00
   recurrent J03.01
Adenoids — see condition
Adenolipoma — see Neoplasm, benign, by site
Adenolipomatosis, Launois-Bensaude E88.89
Adenolymphoma
 specified site — see Neoplasm, benign, by site
 unspecified site D11.9
Adenoma — see also Neoplasm, benign, by site
 acidophil
  specified site — see Neoplasm, benign, by site
  unspecified site D35.2
 acidophil-basophil, mixed
  specified site — see Neoplasm, benign, by site
  unspecified site D35.2
 adrenal (cortical) D35.00

☑ **Additional Character Required** — Refer to the Tabular List for Character Selection

Adenoma — *continued*
- adrenal — *continued*
  - clear cell D35.00
  - compact cell D35.00
  - glomerulosa cell D35.00
  - heavily pigmented variant D35.00
  - mixed cell D35.00
- alpha-cell
  - pancreas D13.7
  - specified site NEC — *see* Neoplasm, benign, by site
  - unspecified site D13.7
- alveolar D14.30
- apocrine
  - breast D24.- ☑
  - specified site NEC — *see* Neoplasm, skin, benign, by site
  - unspecified site D23.9
- basal cell D11.9
- basophil
  - specified site — *see* Neoplasm, benign, by site
  - unspecified site D35.2
- basophil-acidophil, mixed
  - specified site — *see* Neoplasm, benign, by site
  - unspecified site D35.2
- beta-cell
  - pancreas D13.7
  - specified site NEC — *see* Neoplasm, benign, by site
  - unspecified site D13.7
- bile duct D13.4
  - common D13.5
  - extrahepatic D13.5
  - intrahepatic D13.4
  - specified site NEC — *see* Neoplasm, benign, by site
  - unspecified site D13.4
- black D35.00
- bronchial D38.1
  - cylindroid type — *see* Neoplasm, lung, malignant
- ceruminous D23.2- ☑
- chief cell D35.1
- chromophobe
  - specified site — *see* Neoplasm, benign, by site
  - unspecified site D35.2
- colloid
  - specified site — *see* Neoplasm, benign, by site
  - unspecified site D34
- eccrine, papillary — *see* Neoplasm, skin, benign
- endocrine, multiple
  - single specified site — *see* Neoplasm, uncertain behavior, by site
  - two or more specified sites D44.- ☑
  - unspecified site D44.9
- endometrioid — *see also* Neoplasm, benign
  - borderline malignancy — *see* Neoplasm, uncertain behavior, by site
- eosinophil
  - specified site — *see* Neoplasm, benign, by site
  - unspecified site D35.2
- fetal
  - specified site — *see* Neoplasm, benign, by site
  - unspecified site D34
- follicular
  - specified site — *see* Neoplasm, benign, by site
  - unspecified site D34
- hepatocellular D13.4
- Hurthle cell D34
- islet cell
  - pancreas D13.7
  - specified site NEC — *see* Neoplasm, benign, by site
  - unspecified site D13.7
- liver cell D13.4
- macrofollicular
  - specified site — *see* Neoplasm, benign, by site
  - unspecified site D34
- malignant, malignum — *see* Neoplasm, malignant, by site
- microcystic
  - pancreas D13.6
  - specified site NEC — *see* Neoplasm, benign, by site
  - unspecified site D13.6
- microfollicular
  - specified site — *see* Neoplasm, benign, by site
  - unspecified site D34
- mucoid cell
  - specified site — *see* Neoplasm, benign, by site
  - unspecified site D35.2
- multiple endocrine
  - single specified site — *see* Neoplasm, uncertain behavior, by site
  - two or more specified sites D44.- ☑

Adenoma — *continued*
- multiple endocrine — *continued*
  - unspecified site D44.9
- nipple D24.- ☑
- papillary — *see also* Neoplasm, benign, by site
  - eccrine — *see* Neoplasm, skin, benign, by site
- Pick's tubular
  - specified site — *see* Neoplasm, benign, by site
  - unspecified site
    - female D27.9
    - male D29.20
- pleomorphic
  - carcinoma in — *see* Neoplasm, salivary gland, malignant
  - specified site — *see* Neoplasm, malignant, by site
  - unspecified site C08.9
- polypoid — *see also* Neoplasm, benign
  - adenocarcinoma in — *see* Neoplasm, malignant, by site
  - adenocarcinoma in situ — *see* Neoplasm, in situ, by site
- prostate — *see* Neoplasm, prostate, benign
- rete cell D29.20
- sebaceous — *see* Neoplasm, skin, benign
- Sertoli cell
  - specified site — *see* Neoplasm, benign, by site
  - unspecified site
    - female D27.9
    - male D29.20
- skin appendage — *see* Neoplasm, skin, benign
- sudoriferous gland — *see* Neoplasm, skin, benign
- sweat gland — *see* Neoplasm, skin, benign
- testicular
  - specified site — *see* Neoplasm, benign, by site
  - unspecified site
    - female D27.9
    - male D29.20
- tubular — *see also* Neoplasm, benign, by site
  - adenocarcinoma in — *see* Neoplasm, malignant, by site
  - adenocarcinoma in situ — *see* Neoplasm, in situ, by site
  - Pick's
    - specified site — *see* Neoplasm, benign, by site
    - unspecified site
      - female D27.9
      - male D29.20
- tubulovillous — *see also* Neoplasm, benign, by site
  - adenocarcinoma in — *see* Neoplasm, malignant, by site
  - adenocarcinoma in situ — *see* Neoplasm, in situ, by site
- villous — *see* Neoplasm, uncertain behavior, by site
  - adenocarcinoma in — *see* Neoplasm, malignant, by site
  - adenocarcinoma in situ — *see* Neoplasm, in situ, by site
- water-clear cell D35.1

Adenomatosis
- endocrine (multiple) E31.20
  - single specified site — *see* Neoplasm, uncertain behavior, by site
- erosive of nipple D24.- ☑
- pluriendocrine — *see* Adenomatosis, endocrine
- pulmonary D38.1
  - malignant — *see* Neoplasm, lung, malignant
- specified site — *see* Neoplasm, benign, by site
- unspecified site D12.6

Adenomatous
- goiter (nontoxic) E04.9
  - with hyperthyroidism — *see* Hyperthyroidism, with, goiter, nodular
  - toxic — *see* Hyperthyroidism, with, goiter, nodular

Adenomyoma — *see also* Neoplasm, benign, by site
- prostate — *see* Enlarged, prostate

Adenomyometritis N80.00

Adenomyosis (uterus) N80.03

Adenopathy (lymph gland) R59.9
- generalized R59.1
- inguinal R59.0
- localized R59.0
- mediastinal R59.0
- mesentery R59.0
- syphilitic (secondary) A51.49
- tracheobronchial R59.0
  - tuberculous A15.4
    - primary (progressive) A15.7
- tuberculous — *see also* Tuberculosis, lymph gland
  - tracheobronchial A15.4

Adenopathy — *continued*
- tuberculous — *see also* Tuberculosis, lymph gland — *continued*
  - tracheobronchial — *continued*
    - primary (progressive) A15.7

Adenosalpingitis — *see* Salpingitis

Adenosarcoma — *see* Neoplasm, malignant, by site

Adenosclerosis I88.8

Adenosis (sclerosing) breast — *see* Fibroadenosis, breast

Adenovirus, as cause of disease classified elsewhere B97.0

Adentia (complete) (partial) — *see* Absence, teeth

Adherent — *see also* Adhesions
- labia (minora) N90.89
- pericardium (nonrheumatic) I31.0
  - rheumatic I09.2
- placenta (with hemorrhage) O72.0
  - without hemorrhage O73.0
- prepuce, newborn N47.0
- scar (skin) L90.5
- tendon in scar L90.5

Adhesions, adhesive (postinfective) K66.0
- with intestinal obstruction K56.50
  - complete K56.52
  - incomplete K56.51
  - partial K56.51
- abdominal (wall) — *see* Adhesions, peritoneum
- appendix K38.8
- bile duct (common) (hepatic) K83.8
- bladder (sphincter) N32.89
- bowel — *see* Adhesions, peritoneum
- cardiac I31.0
  - rheumatic I09.2
- cecum — *see* Adhesions, peritoneum
- cervicovaginal N88.1
  - congenital Q52.8
  - postpartal O90.89
  - old N88.1
- cervix N88.1
- ciliary body NEC — *see* Adhesions, iris
- clitoris N90.89
- colon — *see* Adhesions, peritoneum
- common duct K83.8
- congenital — *see also* Anomaly, by site
  - fingers — *see* Syndactylism, complex, fingers
  - omental, anomalous Q43.3
  - peritoneal Q43.3
  - tongue (to gum or roof of mouth) Q38.3
- conjunctiva (acquired) H11.21- ☑
  - congenital Q15.8
- cystic duct K82.8
- diaphragm — *see* Adhesions, peritoneum
- due to foreign body — *see* Foreign body
- duodenum — *see* Adhesions, peritoneum
- ear
  - middle H74.1- ☑
- epididymis N50.89
- epidural — *see* Adhesions, meninges
- epiglottis J38.7
- eyelid H02.59
- female pelvis N73.6
- gallbladder K82.8
- globe H44.89
- heart I31.0
  - rheumatic I09.2
- ileocecal (coil) — *see* Adhesions, peritoneum
- ileum — *see* Adhesions, peritoneum
- intestine — *see also* Adhesions, peritoneum
  - with obstruction K56.50
    - complete K56.52
    - incomplete K56.51
    - partial K56.51
- intra-abdominal — *see* Adhesions, peritoneum
- iris H21.50- ☑
  - anterior H21.51- ☑
  - goniosynechiae H21.52- ☑
  - posterior H21.54- ☑
  - to corneal graft T85.898- ☑
- joint — *see* Ankylosis
  - knee M23.8X- ☑
  - temporomandibular M26.61- ☑
- labium (majus) (minus), congenital Q52.5
- liver — *see* Adhesions, peritoneum
- lung J98.4
- mediastinum J98.59
- meninges (cerebral) (spinal) G96.12
  - congenital Q07.8
  - tuberculous (cerebral) (spinal) A17.0

Adhesions, adhesive — *continued*
- mesenteric — *see* Adhesions, peritoneum
- nasal (septum) (to turbinates) J34.89
- ocular muscle — *see* Strabismus, mechanical
- omentum — *see* Adhesions, peritoneum
- ovary N73.6
  - congenital (to cecum, kidney or omentum) Q50.39
- paraovarian N73.6
- pelvic (peritoneal)
  - female N73.6
    - postprocedural N99.4
  - male — *see* Adhesions, peritoneum
  - postpartal (old) N73.6
  - tuberculous A18.17
- penis to scrotum (congenital) Q55.8
- periappendiceal — *see also* Adhesions, peritoneum
- pericardium (nonrheumatic) I31.0
  - focal I31.8
  - rheumatic I09.2
  - tuberculous A18.84
- pericholecystic K82.8
- perigastric — *see* Adhesions, peritoneum
- periovarian N73.6
- periprostatic N42.89
- perirectal — *see* Adhesions, peritoneum
- perirenal N28.89
- peritoneum, peritoneal (postinfective) K66.0
  - with obstruction (intestinal) K56.50
    - complete K56.52
    - incomplete K56.51
    - partial K56.51
  - congenital Q43.3
  - pelvic, female N73.6
    - postprocedural N99.4
  - postpartal, pelvic N73.6
  - postprocedural K66.0
  - to uterus N73.6
- peritubal N73.6
- periureteral N28.89
- periuterine N73.6
- perivesical N32.89
- perivesicular (seminal vesicle) N50.89
- pleura, pleuritic J94.8
  - tuberculous NEC A15.6
- pleuropericardial J94.8
- postoperative (gastrointestinal tract) K66.0
  - with obstruction — *see also* Obstruction, intestine, postoperative K91.30
  - due to foreign body accidentally left in wound — *see* Foreign body, accidentally left during a procedure
  - pelvic peritoneal N99.4
  - urethra — *see* Stricture, urethra, postprocedural
  - vagina N99.2
- postpartal, old (vulva or perineum) N90.89
- preputial, prepuce N47.5
- pulmonary J98.4
- pylorus — *see* Adhesions, peritoneum
- sciatic nerve — *see* Lesion, nerve, sciatic
- seminal vesicle N50.89
- shoulder (joint) — *see* Capsulitis, adhesive
- sigmoid flexure — *see* Adhesions, peritoneum
- spermatic cord (acquired) N50.89
  - congenital Q55.4
- spinal canal G96.12
- stomach — *see* Adhesions, peritoneum
- subscapular — *see* Capsulitis, adhesive
- temporomandibular M26.61- ☑
- tendinitis (*see also* Tenosynovitis, specified type NEC)
  - shoulder — *see* Capsulitis, adhesive
- testis N44.8
- tongue, congenital (to gum or roof of mouth) Q38.3
  - acquired K14.8
- trachea J39.8
- tubo-ovarian N73.6
- tunica vaginalis N44.8
- uterus N73.6
  - internal N85.6
  - to abdominal wall N73.6
- vagina (chronic) N89.5
  - postoperative N99.2
- vitreomacular H43.82- ☑
- vitreous H43.89
- vulva N90.89

Adiaspiromycosis B48.8
Adie (-Holmes) **pupil or syndrome** — *see* Anomaly, pupil, function, tonic pupil
Adiponecrosis neonatorum P83.88
Adiposis — *see also* Obesity

Adiposis — *continued*
- cerebralis E23.6
- dolorosa E88.2

Adiposity — *see also* Obesity
- heart — *see* Degeneration, myocardial
- localized E65

Adiposogenital dystrophy E23.6

Adjustment
- disorder — *see* Disorder, adjustment
- implanted device — *see* Encounter (for), adjustment (of)
- prosthesis, external — *see* Fitting
- reaction — *see* Disorder, adjustment

Administration of tPA (rtPA) in a different facility within the last 24 hours prior to admission to current facility Z92.82

Admission (for) — *see also* Encounter (for)
- adjustment (of)
  - artificial
    - arm Z44.00- ☑
      - complete Z44.01- ☑
      - partial Z44.02- ☑
    - eye Z44.2- ☑
    - leg Z44.10- ☑
      - complete Z44.11- ☑
      - partial Z44.12- ☑
  - brain neuropacemaker Z46.2
    - implanted Z45.42
  - breast
    - implant Z45.81- ☑
    - prosthesis (external) Z44.3- ☑
  - colostomy belt Z46.89
  - contact lenses Z46.0
  - cystostomy device Z46.6
  - dental prosthesis Z46.3
  - device NEC
    - abdominal Z46.89
    - implanted Z45.89
      - cardiac Z45.09
        - defibrillator (with synchronous cardiac pacemaker) Z45.02
        - pacemaker (cardiac resynchronization therapy (CRT-P)) Z45.018
          - pulse generator Z45.010
        - resynchronization therapy defibrillator (CRT-D) Z45.02
      - hearing device Z45.328
        - bone conduction Z45.320
        - cochlear Z45.321
      - infusion pump Z45.1
      - nervous system Z45.49
        - CSF drainage Z45.41
        - hearing device — *see* Admission, adjustment, device, implanted, hearing device
        - neuropacemaker Z45.42
        - visual substitution Z45.31
      - specified NEC Z45.89
      - vascular access Z45.2
    - visual substitution Z45.31
  - nervous system Z46.2
    - implanted — *see* Admission, adjustment, device, implanted, nervous system
  - orthodontic Z46.4
  - prosthetic Z44.9
    - arm — *see* Admission, adjustment, artificial, arm
    - breast Z44.3- ☑
    - dental Z46.3
    - eye Z44.2- ☑
    - leg — *see* Admission, adjustment, artificial, leg
    - specified type NEC Z44.8
  - substitution
    - auditory Z46.2
      - implanted — *see* Admission, adjustment, device, implanted, hearing device
    - nervous system Z46.2
      - implanted — *see* Admission, adjustment, device, implanted, nervous system
    - visual Z46.2
      - implanted Z45.31
  - urinary Z46.6
- hearing aid Z46.1
  - implanted — *see* Admission, adjustment, device, implanted, hearing device
- ileostomy device Z46.89
- intestinal appliance or device NEC Z46.89
- neuropacemaker (brain) (peripheral nerve) (spinal cord) Z46.2

Admission — *continued*
- adjustment — *continued*
  - neuropacemaker — *continued*
    - implanted Z45.42
  - orthodontic device Z46.4
  - orthopedic (brace) (cast) (device) (shoes) Z46.89
  - pacemaker (cardiac resynchronization therapy (CRT-P))
    - cardiac Z45.018
      - pulse generator Z45.010
    - nervous system Z46.2
      - implanted Z45.42
  - portacath (port-a-cath) Z45.2
  - prosthesis Z44.9
    - arm — *see* Admission, adjustment, artificial, arm
    - breast Z44.3- ☑
    - dental Z46.3
    - eye Z44.2- ☑
    - leg — *see* Admission, adjustment, artificial, leg
    - specified NEC Z44.8
  - spectacles Z46.0
- aftercare — *see also* Aftercare Z51.89
  - postpartum
    - immediately after delivery Z39.0
    - routine follow-up Z39.2
  - radiation therapy (antineoplastic) Z51.0
  - sepsis Z51.A
- attention to artificial opening (of) Z43.9
  - artificial vagina Z43.7
  - colostomy Z43.3
  - cystostomy Z43.5
  - enterostomy Z43.4
  - gastrostomy Z43.1
  - ileostomy Z43.2
  - jejunostomy Z43.4
  - nephrostomy Z43.6
  - specified site NEC Z43.8
    - intestinal tract Z43.4
    - urinary tract Z43.6
  - tracheostomy Z43.0
  - ureterostomy Z43.6
  - urethrostomy Z43.6
- breast augmentation or reduction Z41.1
- breast reconstruction following mastectomy Z42.1
- change of
  - dressing (nonsurgical) Z48.00
  - neuropacemaker device (brain) (peripheral nerve) (spinal cord) Z46.2
    - implanted Z45.42
  - surgical dressing Z48.01
- circumcision, ritual or routine (in absence of diagnosis) Z41.2
- clinical research investigation (control) (normal comparison) (participant) Z00.6
- contraceptive management Z30.9
- cosmetic surgery NEC Z41.1
- counseling — *see also* Counseling
  - dietary Z71.3
  - gestational carrier Z31.7
  - HIV Z71.7
  - human immunodeficiency virus Z71.7
  - nonattending third party Z71.0
  - procreative management NEC Z31.69
- delivery, full-term, uncomplicated O80
  - cesarean, without indication O82
- desensitization to allergens Z51.6
- dietary surveillance and counseling Z71.3
- ear piercing Z41.3
- examination at health care facility (adult) — *see also* Examination Z00.00
  - with abnormal findings Z00.01
  - clinical research investigation (control) (normal comparison) (participant) Z00.6
  - dental Z01.20
    - with abnormal findings Z01.21
  - donor (potential) Z00.5
  - ear Z01.10
    - with abnormal findings NEC Z01.118
  - eye Z01.00
    - with abnormal findings Z01.01
    - following failed vision screening Z01.020
      - with abnormal findings Z01.021
  - general, specified reason NEC Z00.8
  - hearing Z01.10
    - with abnormal findings NEC Z01.118
    - infant or child (over 28 days old) Z00.129
      - with abnormal findings Z00.121
  - postpartum checkup Z39.2
  - psychiatric (general) Z00.8

☑ Additional Character Required — Refer to the Tabular List for Character Selection

Admission — *continued*
- examination at health care facility — *see also* Examination — *continued*
  - psychiatric — *continued*
    - requested by authority Z04.6
  - vision Z01.00
    - with abnormal findings Z01.01
    - following failed vision screening Z01.020
      - with abnormal findings Z01.021
    - infant or child (over 28 days old) Z00.129
      - with abnormal findings Z00.121
- fitting (of)
  - artificial
    - arm — *see* Admission, adjustment, artificial, arm
    - eye Z44.2- ☑
    - leg — *see* Admission, adjustment, artificial, leg
  - brain neuropacemaker Z46.2
    - implanted Z45.42
  - breast prosthesis (external) Z44.3- ☑
  - colostomy belt Z46.89
  - contact lenses Z46.0
  - cystostomy device Z46.6
  - dental prosthesis Z46.3
  - dentures Z46.3
  - device NEC
    - abdominal Z46.89
    - nervous system Z46.2
      - implanted — *see* Admission, adjustment, device, implanted, nervous system
    - orthodontic Z46.4
    - prosthetic Z44.9
      - breast Z44.3- ☑
      - dental Z46.3
      - eye Z44.2- ☑
    - substitution
      - auditory Z46.2
        - implanted — *see* Admission, adjustment, device, implanted, hearing device
      - nervous system Z46.2
        - implanted — *see* Admission, adjustment, device, implanted, nervous system
      - visual Z46.2
        - implanted Z45.31
  - hearing aid Z46.1
  - ileostomy device Z46.89
  - intestinal appliance or device NEC Z46.89
  - neuropacemaker (brain) (peripheral nerve) (spinal cord) Z46.2
    - implanted Z45.42
  - orthodontic device Z46.4
  - orthopedic device (brace) (cast) (shoes) Z46.89
  - prosthesis Z44.9
    - arm — *see* Admission, adjustment, artificial, arm
    - breast Z44.3- ☑
    - dental Z46.3
    - eye Z44.2- ☑
    - leg — *see* Admission, adjustment, artificial, leg
    - specified type NEC Z44.8
  - spectacles Z46.0
- follow-up examination Z09
- intrauterine device management Z30.431
  - initial prescription Z30.014
- mental health evaluation Z00.8
  - requested by authority Z04.6
- observation — *see* Observation
- Papanicolaou smear, cervix Z12.4
  - for suspected malignant neoplasm Z12.4
- plastic and reconstructive surgery following medical procedure or healed injury NEC Z42.8
- plastic surgery, cosmetic NEC Z41.1
- postpartum observation
  - immediately after delivery Z39.0
  - routine follow-up Z39.2
- poststerilization (for restoration) Z31.0
  - aftercare Z31.42
- procreative management Z31.9
- prophylactic (measure) — *see also* Encounter, prophylactic measures
  - oophorectomy for persons without known genetic/familial risk factors Z40.81
  - organ removal Z40.00
    - breast Z40.01
    - fallopian tube(s) Z40.03
      - for persons without known genetic/familial risk factors Z40.82
    - ovary(s) Z40.02
      - for persons without known genetic/familial risk factors Z40.81

Admission — *continued*
- prophylactic — *see also* Encounter, prophylactic measures — *continued*
  - organ removal — *continued*
    - specified organ NEC Z40.09
    - testes Z40.09
  - salpingectomy for persons without known genetic/familial risk factors Z40.82
  - vaccination Z23
- psychiatric examination (general) Z00.8
  - requested by authority Z04.6
- radiation therapy (antineoplastic) Z51.0
- reconstructive surgery following medical procedure or healed injury NEC Z42.8
- removal of
  - cystostomy catheter Z43.5
  - drains Z48.03
  - dressing (nonsurgical) Z48.00
  - implantable subdermal contraceptive Z30.46
  - intrauterine contraceptive device Z30.432
  - neuropacemaker (brain) (peripheral nerve) (spinal cord) Z46.2
    - implanted Z45.42
  - staples Z48.02
  - surgical dressing Z48.01
  - sutures Z48.02
  - ureteral stent Z46.6
- respirator [ventilator] use during power failure Z99.12
- restoration of organ continuity (poststerilization) Z31.0
  - aftercare Z31.42
- sensitivity test — *see also* Test, skin
  - allergy NEC Z01.82
  - Mantoux Z11.1
- tuboplasty following previous sterilization Z31.0
  - aftercare Z31.42
- vasoplasty following previous sterilization Z31.0
  - aftercare Z31.42
- vision examination Z01.00
  - with abnormal findings Z01.01
  - following failed vision screening Z01.020
    - with abnormal findings Z01.021
  - infant or child (over 28 days old) Z00.129
    - with abnormal findings Z00.121
- waiting period for admission to other facility Z75.1

Adnexitis (suppurative) — *see* Salpingo-oophoritis
Adolescent X-linked adrenoleukodystrophy E71.521
Adrenal (gland) — *see* condition
Adrenalism, tuberculous A18.7
Adrenalitis, adrenitis E27.8
- autoimmune E27.1
- meningococcal, hemorrhagic A39.1

Adrenarche, premature E27.0
Adrenocortical syndrome — *see* Cushing's, syndrome
Adrenogenital syndrome E25.9
- acquired E25.8
- congenital E25.0
- salt loss E25.0

Adrenogenitalism, congenital E25.0
Adrenoleukodystrophy E71.529
- neonatal E71.511
- X-linked E71.529
  - Addison only phenotype E71.528
  - Addison-Schilder E71.528
  - adolescent E71.521
  - adrenomyeloneuropathy E71.522
  - childhood cerebral E71.520
  - other specified E71.528

Adrenomyeloneuropathy E71.522
Adventitious bursa — *see* Bursopathy, specified type NEC
Adverse effect — *see* Table of Drugs and Chemicals, categories T36-T50, with 6th character 5
Advice — *see* Counseling
Adynamia (episodica) (hereditary) (periodic) G72.3
Aeration lung imperfect, newborn — *see* Atelectasis
Aero-otitis media T70.0- ☑
Aerobullosis T70.3- ☑
Aerocele — *see* Embolism, air
Aerodermectasia
- subcutaneous (traumatic) T79.7- ☑

Aerodontalgia T70.29- ☑
Aeroembolism T70.3- ☑
Aerogenes capsulatus infection A48.0
Aerophagy, aerophagia (psychogenic) F45.8
Aerophobia F40.228
Aerosinusitis T70.1- ☑
Aerotitis T70.0- ☑
Affection — *see* Disease
Afibrinogenemia — *see also* Defect, coagulation D68.8

Afibrinogenemia — *continued*
- acquired D65
- congenital D68.2
- following ectopic or molar pregnancy O08.1
- in abortion — *see* Abortion, by type, complicated by, afibrinogenemia
- puerperal O72.3

African
- sleeping sickness B56.9
- tick fever A68.1
- trypanosomiasis B56.9
  - gambian B56.0
  - rhodesian B56.1

After-cataract — *see* Cataract, secondary
Aftercare — *see also* Care Z51.89
- following surgery (for) (on)
  - amputation Z47.81
  - attention to
    - drains Z48.03
    - dressings (nonsurgical) Z48.00
      - surgical Z48.01
    - sutures Z48.02
  - circulatory system Z48.812
  - delayed (planned) wound closure Z48.1
  - digestive system Z48.815
  - explantation of joint prosthesis (staged procedure)
    - hip Z47.32
    - knee Z47.33
    - shoulder Z47.31
  - genitourinary system Z48.816
  - joint replacement Z47.1
  - neoplasm Z48.3
  - nervous system Z48.811
  - oral cavity Z48.814
  - organ transplant
    - bone marrow Z48.290
    - heart Z48.21
    - heart-lung Z48.280
    - kidney Z48.22
    - liver Z48.23
    - lung Z48.24
    - multiple organs NEC Z48.288
    - specified NEC Z48.298
  - orthopedic NEC Z47.89
  - planned wound closure Z48.1
  - removal of internal fixation device Z47.2
  - respiratory system Z48.813
  - scoliosis Z47.82
  - sense organs Z48.810
  - skin and subcutaneous tissue Z48.817
  - specified body system
    - circulatory Z48.812
    - digestive Z48.815
    - genitourinary Z48.816
    - nervous Z48.811
    - oral cavity Z48.814
    - respiratory Z48.813
    - sense organs Z48.810
    - skin and subcutaneous tissue Z48.817
    - teeth Z48.814
  - specified NEC Z48.89
  - spinal Z47.89
  - teeth Z48.814
- fracture — *code to* fracture with seventh character D
- involving
  - removal of
    - drains Z48.03
    - dressings (nonsurgical) Z48.00
    - staples Z48.02
    - surgical dressings Z48.01
    - sutures Z48.02
  - neuropacemaker (brain) (peripheral nerve) (spinal cord) Z46.2
    - implanted Z45.42
  - orthopedic NEC Z47.89
- postprocedural — *see* Aftercare, following surgery

Agalactia (primary) O92.3
- elective, secondary or therapeutic O92.5

Agammaglobulinemia (acquired) (secondary) (nonfamilial) D80.1
- with
  - immunoglobulin-bearing B-lymphocytes D80.1
  - lymphopenia D81.9
- autosomal recessive (Swiss type) D80.0
- Bruton's X-linked D80.0
- common variable (CVAgamma) D80.1
- congenital sex-linked D80.0
- hereditary D80.0
- lymphopenic D81.9

Agammaglobulinemia — continued
　Swiss type (autosomal recessive) D80.0
　X-linked (with growth hormone deficiency) (Bruton) D80.0
Aganglionosis (bowel) (colon) Q43.1
Age (old) — see Senility
Agenesis
　adrenal (gland) Q89.1
　alimentary tract (complete) (partial) NEC Q45.8
　　upper Q40.8
　anus, anal (canal) Q42.3
　　with fistula Q42.2
　aorta Q25.41
　appendix Q42.8
　arm (complete) Q71.0- ☑
　　with hand present Q71.1- ☑
　artery (peripheral) Q27.9
　　brain Q28.3
　　coronary Q24.5
　　pulmonary Q25.79
　　specified NEC Q27.8
　　umbilical Q27.0
　auditory (canal) (external) Q16.1
　auricle (ear) Q16.0
　bile duct or passage Q44.5
　bladder Q64.5
　bone Q79.9
　brain Q00.0
　　part of Q04.3
　breast (with nipple present) Q83.8
　　with absent nipple Q83.0
　bronchus Q32.4
　canaliculus lacrimalis Q10.4
　carpus — see Agenesis, hand
　cartilage Q79.9
　cecum Q42.8
　cerebellum Q04.3
　cervix Q51.5
　chin Q18.8
　cilia Q10.3
　circulatory system, part NOS Q28.9
　clavicle Q74.0
　clitoris Q52.6
　coccyx Q76.49
　colon Q42.9
　　specified NEC Q42.8
　corpus callosum Q04.0
　cricoid cartilage Q31.8
　diaphragm (with hernia) Q79.1
　digestive organ(s) or tract (complete) (partial) NEC Q45.8
　　upper Q40.8
　ductus arteriosus Q28.8
　duodenum Q41.0
　ear Q16.9
　　auricle Q16.0
　　lobe Q17.8
　ejaculatory duct Q55.4
　endocrine (gland) NEC Q89.2
　epiglottis Q31.8
　esophagus Q39.8
　eustachian tube Q16.2
　eye Q11.1
　　adnexa Q15.8
　eyelid (fold) Q10.3
　face
　　bones NEC Q75.8
　　specified part NEC Q18.8
　fallopian tube Q50.6
　femur — see Defect, reduction, lower limb, longitudinal, femur
　fibula — see Defect, reduction, lower limb, longitudinal, fibula
　finger (complete) (partial) — see Agenesis, hand
　foot (and toes) (complete) (partial) Q72.3- ☑
　forearm (with hand present) — see Agenesis, arm, with hand present
　　and hand Q71.2- ☑
　gallbladder Q44.0
　gastric Q40.2
　genitalia, genital (organ(s))
　　female Q52.8
　　　external Q52.71
　　　internal NEC Q52.8
　　male Q55.8
　glottis Q31.8
　hair Q84.0
　hand (and fingers) (complete) (partial) Q71.3- ☑
　heart Q24.8

Agenesis — continued
　heart — continued
　　valve NEC Q24.8
　　　pulmonary Q22.0
　hepatic Q44.79
　humerus — see Defect, reduction, upper limb
　hymen Q52.4
　ileum Q41.2
　incus Q16.3
　intestine (small) Q41.9
　　large Q42.9
　　　specified NEC Q42.8
　iris (dilator fibers) Q13.1
　jaw M26.09
　jejunum Q41.1
　kidney(s) (partial) Q60.2
　　bilateral Q60.1
　　unilateral Q60.0
　labium (majus) (minus) Q52.71
　labyrinth, membranous Q16.5
　lacrimal apparatus Q10.4
　larynx Q31.8
　leg (complete) Q72.0- ☑
　　with foot present Q72.1- ☑
　　lower leg (with foot present) — see Agenesis, leg, with foot present
　　and foot Q72.2- ☑
　lens Q12.3
　limb (complete) Q73.0
　　lower — see Agenesis, leg
　　upper — see Agenesis, arm
　lip Q38.0
　liver Q44.79
　lung (fissure) (lobe) (bilateral) (unilateral) Q33.3
　mandible, maxilla M26.09
　metacarpus — see Agenesis, hand
　metatarsus — see Agenesis, foot
　muscle Q79.8
　　eyelid Q10.3
　　ocular Q15.8
　musculoskeletal system NEC Q79.8
　nail(s) Q84.3
　neck, part Q18.8
　nerve Q07.8
　nervous system, part NEC Q07.8
　nipple Q83.2
　nose Q30.1
　nuclear Q07.8
　organ
　　of Corti Q16.5
　　or site not listed — see Anomaly, by site
　osseous meatus (ear) Q16.1
　ovary
　　bilateral Q50.02
　　unilateral Q50.01
　oviduct Q50.6
　pancreas Q45.0
　parathyroid (gland) Q89.2
　parotid gland(s) Q38.4
　patella Q74.1
　pelvic girdle (complete) (partial) Q74.2
　penis Q55.5
　pericardium Q24.8
　pituitary (gland) Q89.2
　prostate Q55.4
　punctum lacrimale Q10.4
　radioulnar — see Defect, reduction, upper limb
　radius — see Defect, reduction, upper limb, longitudinal, radius
　rectum Q42.1
　　with fistula Q42.0
　renal Q60.2
　　bilateral Q60.1
　　unilateral Q60.0
　respiratory organ NEC Q34.8
　rib Q76.6
　roof of orbit Q75.8
　round ligament Q52.8
　sacrum Q76.49
　salivary gland Q38.4
　scapula Q74.0
　scrotum Q55.29
　seminal vesicles Q55.4
　septum
　　atrial Q21.19
　　between aorta and pulmonary artery Q21.4
　　ventricular Q20.4
　shoulder girdle (complete) (partial) Q74.0
　skull (bone) Q75.8

Agenesis — continued
　skull — continued
　　with
　　　anencephaly Q00.0
　　　encephalocele — see Encephalocele
　　　hydrocephalus Q03.9
　　　　with spina bifida — see Spina bifida, by site, with hydrocephalus
　　　microcephaly Q02
　spermatic cord Q55.4
　spinal cord Q06.0
　spine Q76.49
　spleen Q89.01
　sternum Q76.7
　stomach Q40.2
　submaxillary gland(s) (congenital) Q38.4
　tarsus — see Agenesis, foot
　tendon Q79.8
　testicle Q55.0
　thymus (gland) Q89.2
　thyroid (gland) E03.1
　　cartilage Q31.8
　tibia — see Defect, reduction, lower limb, longitudinal, tibia
　tibiofibular — see Defect, reduction, lower limb, specified type NEC
　toe (and foot) (complete) (partial) — see Agenesis, foot
　tongue Q38.3
　trachea (cartilage) Q32.1
　ulna — see Defect, reduction, upper limb, longitudinal, ulna
　upper limb — see Agenesis, arm
　ureter Q62.4
　urethra Q64.5
　urinary tract NEC Q64.8
　uterus Q51.0
　uvula Q38.5
　vagina Q52.0
　vas deferens Q55.4
　vein(s) (peripheral) Q27.9
　　brain Q28.3
　　great NEC Q26.8
　　portal Q26.5
　vena cava (inferior) (superior) Q26.8
　vermis of cerebellum Q04.3
　vertebra Q76.49
　vulva Q52.71
Ageusia R43.2
Agitated — see condition
Agitation R45.1
AGL (acquired generalized lipodystrophy) E88.12
Aglossia (congenital) Q38.3
Aglossia-adactylia syndrome Q87.0
Aglycogenosis E74.00
Agnosia (body image) (other senses) (tactile) R48.1
　developmental F88
　verbal R48.1
　　auditory R48.1
　　　developmental F80.2
　　developmental F80.2
　visual (object) R48.3
Agoraphobia F40.00
　with panic disorder F40.01
　without panic disorder F40.02
Agrammatism R48.8
Agranulocytopenia — see Agranulocytosis
Agranulocytosis (chronic) (cyclical) (genetic) (infantile) (periodic) (pernicious) — see also Neutropenia D70.9
　congenital D70.0
　cytoreductive cancer chemotherapy sequela D70.1
　drug-induced D70.2
　　due to cytoreductive cancer chemotherapy D70.1
　due to infection D70.3
　secondary D70.4
　　drug-induced D70.2
　　　due to cytoreductive cancer chemotherapy D70.1
Agraphia (absolute) R48.8
　with alexia R48.0
　developmental F81.81
Ague (dumb) — see Malaria
Agyria Q04.3
Ahumada-del Castillo syndrome E23.0
Aichomophobia F40.298
AIDS (related complex) B20
Ailment heart — see Disease, heart
Ailurophobia F40.218
AIN — see Neoplasia, intraepithelial, anal
Ainhum (disease) L94.6

AIPHI (acute idiopathic pulmonary hemorrhage in infants (over 28 days old)) R04.81
Air
    anterior mediastinum J98.2
    compressed, disease T70.3-
    conditioner lung or pneumonitis J67.7
    embolism (artery) (cerebral) (any site) T79.0-
        with ectopic or molar pregnancy O08.2
        due to implanted device NEC — see Complications, by site and type, specified NEC
        following
            abortion — see Abortion by type, complicated by, embolism
            ectopic or molar pregnancy O08.2
            infusion, therapeutic injection or transfusion T80.0-
        in pregnancy, childbirth or puerperium — see Embolism, obstetric
        traumatic T79.0-
    hunger, psychogenic F45.8
    rarefied, effects of — see Effect, adverse, high altitude
    sickness T75.3-
Airplane sickness T75.3-
Akathisia (drug-induced) (treatment-induced) G25.71
    neuroleptic induced (acute) G25.71
    tardive G25.71
Akinesia R29.898
Akinetic mutism R41.89
Akureyri's disease G93.39
Alactasia, congenital E73.0
Alagille (-Watson) syndrome Q44.71
Alastrim B03
Albers-Schonberg syndrome Q78.2
Albert's syndrome — see Tendinitis, Achilles
Albinism, albino E70.30
    with hematologic abnormality E70.339
        Chediak-Higashi syndrome E70.330
        Hermansky-Pudlak syndrome E70.331
        other specified E70.338
    I E70.320
    II E70.321
    ocular E70.319
        autosomal recessive E70.311
        other specified E70.318
        X-linked E70.310
    oculocutaneous E70.329
        other specified E70.328
        tyrosinase (ty) negative E70.320
        tyrosinase (ty) positive E70.321
    other specified E70.39
Albinismus E70.30
Albright (-McCune)(-Sternberg) **syndrome** Q78.1
Albuminous — see condition
Albuminuria, albuminuric (acute) (chronic) (subacute) — see also Proteinuria R80.9
    complicating pregnancy — see Proteinuria, gestational
        with
            gestational hypertension — see Pre-eclampsia
            pre-existing hypertension — see Hypertension, complicating pregnancy, pre-existing, with, pre-eclampsia
    gestational — see Proteinuria, gestational
        with
            gestational hypertension — see Pre-eclampsia
            pre-existing hypertension — see Hypertension, complicating pregnancy, pre-existing, with, pre-eclampsia
    orthostatic R80.2
    postural R80.2
    pre-eclamptic — see Pre-eclampsia
    scarlatinal A38.8
Albuminurophobia F40.298
Alcaptonuria E70.29
Alcohol, alcoholic, alcohol-induced
    addiction (without remission) F10.20
        with remission F10.21
    amnestic disorder, persisting F10.96
        with dependence F10.26
    anxiety disorder F10.980
    bipolar and related disorder F10.94
    brain syndrome, chronic F10.97
        with dependence F10.27
    cardiopathy I42.6
    counseling and surveillance Z71.41
        family member Z71.42
    delirium (acute) (tremens) (withdrawal) F10.921
        with intoxication F10.921

Alcohol, alcoholic, alcohol-induced — continued
    delirium — continued
        with intoxication — continued
            in
                abuse F10.121
                dependence F10.221
        abuse F10.131
            with intoxication F10.121
        dependence (acute) (tremens) (withdrawal) F10.231
            with intoxication F10.221
        use, unspecified F10.931
            with intoxication F10.921
    dementia F10.97
        with dependence F10.27
    depressive disorder F10.94
    deterioration F10.97
        with dependence F10.27
    hallucinosis (acute) F10.951
        in
            abuse F10.151
            dependence F10.251
    insanity F10.959
    intoxication (acute) (without dependence) F10.129
        with
            delirium F10.121
            dependence F10.229
                with delirium F10.221
                uncomplicated F10.220
            uncomplicated F10.120
    jealousy F10.988
    Korsakoff's, Korsakov's, Korsakow's F10.26
    liver K70.9
        acute — see Disease, liver, alcoholic, hepatitis
    major neurocognitive disorder, amnestic-confabulatory type F10.96
    major neurocognitive disorder, nonamnestic-confabulatory type F10.97
    mania (acute) (chronic) F10.959
    mild neurocognitive disorder F10.988
    paranoia, paranoid (type) psychosis F10.950
    pellagra E52
    poisoning, accidental (acute) NEC — see Table of Drugs and Chemicals, alcohol, poisoning
    psychosis — see Psychosis, alcoholic
    psychotic disorder F10.959
    sexual dysfunction F10.981
    sleep disorder F10.982
    withdrawal (without convulsions) F10.239
        with delirium F10.231
Alcoholism (chronic) (without remission) F10.20
    with
        psychosis — see Psychosis, alcoholic
        remission F10.21
    Korsakov's F10.96
        with dependence F10.26
Alder (-Reilly) **anomaly or syndrome** (leukocyte granulation) D72.0
Aldosteronism E26.9
    familial (type I) E26.02
    glucocorticoid-remediable E26.02
    primary (due to (bilateral) adrenal hyperplasia) E26.09
    primary NEC E26.09
    secondary E26.1
    specified NEC E26.89
Aldosteronoma D44.10
Aldrich (-Wiskott) **syndrome** (eczema-thrombocytopenia) D82.0
Alektorophobia F40.218
Aleppo boil B55.1
Aleukemic — see condition
Aleukia
    congenital D70.0
    hemorrhagica D61.9
        congenital D61.09
    splenica D73.1
Alexia R48.0
    developmental F81.0
    secondary to organic lesion R48.0
Algoneurodystrophy M89.00
    ankle M89.07-
    foot M89.07-
    forearm M89.03-
    hand M89.04-
    lower leg M89.06-
    multiple sites M89.09
    shoulder M89.01-
    specified site NEC M89.08
    thigh M89.05-

Algoneurodystrophy — continued
    upper arm M89.02-
Algophobia F40.298
Alienation, mental — see Psychosis
Alkalemia E87.3
Alkalosis E87.3
    metabolic E87.3
        with respiratory acidosis E87.4
        of newborn P74.41
    respiratory E87.3
Alkaptonuria E70.29
Allen-Masters syndrome N83.8
Allergy, allergic (reaction) (to) T78.40-
    air-borne substance NEC (rhinitis) J30.89
    alveolitis (extrinsic) J67.9
        due to
            Aspergillus clavatus J67.4
            Cryptostroma corticale J67.6
            organisms (fungal, thermophilic actinomycete) growing in ventilation (air conditioning) systems J67.7
            specified type NEC J67.8
    anaphylactic reaction or shock T78.2-
    angioneurotic edema T78.3-
    animal (dander) (epidermal) (hair) (rhinitis) J30.81
    bee sting (anaphylactic shock) T63.44-
    biological — see Allergy, drug
    colitis — see also Colitis, allergic K52.29
    dairy products T78.119-
        with
            reactivity to baked milk T78.111-
            tolerance to baked milk T78.110-
        anaphylactic reaction T78.079-
            with T78.079-
                reactivity to baked milk T78.071-
                tolerance to baked milk T78.070-
    dander (animal) (rhinitis) J30.81
    dandruff (rhinitis) J30.81
    dental restorative material (existing) K08.55
    dermatitis — see Dermatitis, contact, allergic
    diathesis — see History, allergy
    drug, medicament & biological (any) (external) (internal) T78.40-
        correct substance properly administered — see Table of Drugs and Chemicals, by drug, adverse effect
        wrong substance given or taken NEC (by accident) — see Table of Drugs and Chemicals, by drug, poisoning
    due to pollen J30.1
    dust (house) (stock) (rhinitis) J30.89
        with asthma — see Asthma, allergic extrinsic
    eczema — see Dermatitis, contact, allergic
    eggs T78.40-
        adverse reaction NEC T78.129-
            with
                reactivity to baked egg T78.121-
                tolerance to baked egg T78.120-
        anaphylactic reaction T78.089-
            with
                reactivity to baked egg T78.081-
                tolerance to baked egg T78.080-
    epidermal (animal) (rhinitis) J30.81
    feathers (rhinitis) J30.89
    food (any) (ingested) NEC T78.19-
        anaphylactic shock — see Shock, anaphylactic, due to food
        dermatitis — see Dermatitis, due to, food
        dietary counseling and surveillance Z71.3
        in contact with skin L23.6
        rhinitis J30.5
        status (without reaction) Z91.018
            beef Z91.014
            eggs Z91.0120
                with
                    reactivity to baked egg Z91.0122
                    tolerance to baked egg Z91.0121
            lamb Z91.014
            mammalian meats Z91.014
            milk products Z91.0110
                with
                    reactivity to baked milk Z91.0112
                    tolerance to baked milk Z91.0111
            peanuts Z91.010
            pork Z91.014
            red meats Z91.014
            seafood Z91.013
            specified NEC Z91.018

Allergy, allergic — *continued*
  gastrointestinal — *see also* specific type of allergic reaction
    meaning colitis — *see also* Colitis, allergic K52.29
    meaning gastroenteritis — *see also* Gastroenteritis, allergic K52.29
    meaning other adverse food reaction not elsewhere classified T78.19- ☑
  grain J30.1
  grass (hay fever) (pollen) J30.1
    asthma — *see* Asthma, allergic extrinsic
  hair (animal) (rhinitis) J30.81
  history (of) — *see* History, allergy
  horse serum — *see* Allergy, serum
  inhalant (rhinitis) J30.89
    pollen J30.1
  kapok (rhinitis) J30.89
  medicine — *see* Allergy, drug
  milk protein — *see also* Allergy, food Z91.0110
    with
      reactivity to baked milk Z91.0112
      tolerance to baked milk Z91.0111
    adverse reaction NEC T78.119- ☑
      with
        reactivity to baked milk T78.111- ☑
        tolerance to baked milk T78.110- ☑
      anaphylactic reaction T78.079- ☑
        with
          reactivity to baked milk T78.071- ☑
          tolerance to baked milk T78.070- ☑
      dermatitis L27.2
      enterocolitis syndrome K52.21
      enteropathy K52.22
      gastroenteritis K52.29
      gastroesophageal reflux — *see also* Reaction, adverse, food K21.9
        with esophagitis (without bleeding) K21.00
          with bleeding K21.01
      proctocolitis K52.29
  nasal, seasonal due to pollen J30.1
  pneumonia J82.89
  pollen (any) (hay fever) J30.1
    asthma — *see* Asthma, allergic extrinsic
  primrose J30.1
  primula J30.1
  proctocolitis K52.29
  purpura D69.0
  ragweed (hay fever) (pollen) J30.1
    asthma — *see* Asthma, allergic extrinsic
  rose (pollen) J30.1
  seasonal NEC J30.2
  Senecio jacobae (pollen) J30.1
  serum — *see also* Reaction, serum T80.69- ☑
    anaphylactic shock T80.59- ☑
  shock (anaphylactic) T78.2- ☑
    due to
      administration of blood and blood products T80.51- ☑
      adverse effect of correct medicinal substance properly administered T88.6- ☑
      immunization T80.52- ☑
      serum NEC T80.59- ☑
      vaccination T80.52- ☑
    specific NEC T78.49- ☑
  tree (any) (hay fever) (pollen) J30.1
    asthma — *see* Asthma, allergic extrinsic
  upper respiratory J30.9
  urticaria L50.0
  vaccine — *see* Allergy, serum
  wheat — *see* Allergy, food
Allescheriasis B48.2
Alligator skin disease Q80.9
Allocheiria, allochiria R20.8
Almeida's disease — *see* Paracoccidioidomycosis
Alopecia (hereditaria) (seborrheica) L65.9
  androgenic L64.9
    drug-induced L64.0
    specified NEC L64.8
  areata L63.9
    ophiasis L63.2
    specified NEC L63.8
    totalis L63.0
    universalis L63.1
  cicatricial L66.9
    central centrifugal L66.81
    specified NEC L66.89
  circumscripta L63.9
  congenital, congenitalis Q84.0

Alopecia — *continued*
  due to cytotoxic drugs NEC L65.8
  frontal fibrosing L66.12
  mucinosa L65.2
  postinfective NEC L65.8
  postpartum L65.0
  premature L64.8
  specific (syphilitic) A51.32
  specified NEC L65.8
  syphilitic (secondary) A51.32
  totalis (capitis) L63.0
  universalis (entire body) L63.1
  X-ray L58.1
Alpers' disease G31.81
Alpine sickness T70.29- ☑
Alport syndrome Q87.81
ALTE (apparent life threatening event) **in newborn and infant** R68.13
Alteration (of), **Altered**
  awareness
    transient R40.4
    unintended under general anesthesia, during procedure T88.53- ☑
  mental status R41.82
  pattern of family relationships affecting child Z62.898
  sensation
    following
      cerebrovascular disease I69.998
        cerebral infarction I69.398
        intracerebral hemorrhage I69.198
        nontraumatic intracranial hemorrhage NEC I69.298
        specified disease NEC I69.898
        subarachnoid hemorrhage I69.098
Alternating — *see* condition
Altitude, high (effects) — *see* Effect, adverse, high altitude
Aluminosis (of lung) J63.0
Alveolitis
  allergic (extrinsic) — *see* Pneumonitis, hypersensitivity
  due to
    Aspergillus clavatus J67.4
    Cryptostroma corticale J67.6
  fibrosing (cryptogenic) (idiopathic) J84.112
  jaw M27.3
  sicca dolorosa M27.3
Alveolus, alveolar — *see* condition
Alymphocytosis D72.810
  thymic (with immunodeficiency) D82.1
Alymphoplasia, thymic D82.1
Alzheimer's disease or sclerosis — *see* Disease, Alzheimer's
Amastia (with nipple present) Q83.8
  with absent nipple Q83.0
Amathophobia F40.228
Amaurosis (acquired) (congenital) — *see also* Blindness
  fugax G45.3
  hysterical F44.6
  Leber's congenital H35.50
  uremic — *see* Uremia
Amaurotic idiocy (infantile) (juvenile) (late) E75.4
Amaxophobia F40.248
Ambiguous genitalia Q56.4
Amblyopia (congenital) (ex anopsia) (partial) (suppression) H53.00- ☑
  anisometropic — *see* Amblyopia, refractive
  deprivation H53.01- ☑
  hysterical F44.6
  nocturnal — *see also* Blindness, night
    vitamin A deficiency E50.5
  refractive H53.02- ☑
  strabismic H53.03- ☑
  suspect H53.04- ☑
  tobacco H53.8
  toxic NEC H53.8
  uremic — *see* Uremia
Ameba, amebic (histolytica) — *see also* Amebiasis
  abscess (liver) A06.4
Amebiasis A06.9
  with abscess — *see* Abscess, amebic
  acute A06.0
  chronic (intestine) A06.1
    with abscess — *see* Abscess, amebic
  cutaneous A06.7
  cutis A06.7
  cystitis A06.81
  genitourinary tract NEC A06.82
  hepatic — *see* Abscess, liver, amebic
  intestine A06.0

Amebiasis — *continued*
  nondysenteric colitis A06.2
  skin A06.7
  specified site NEC A06.89
Ameboma (of intestine) A06.3
Amelia Q73.0
  lower limb — *see* Agenesis, leg
  upper limb — *see* Agenesis, arm
Ameloblastoma — *see also* Cyst, calcifying odontogenic
  long bones C40.9- ☑
    lower limb C40.2- ☑
    upper limb C40.0- ☑
  malignant C41.1
    jaw (bone) (lower) C41.1
      upper C41.0
  tibial C40.2- ☑
Amelogenesis imperfecta K00.5
  nonhereditaria (segmentalis) K00.4
Amenorrhea N91.2
  hyperhormonal E28.8
  primary N91.0
  secondary N91.1
Amentia — *see* Disability, intellectual
  Meynert's (nonalcoholic) F04
American
  leishmaniasis B55.2
  mountain tick fever A93.2
Ametropia — *see* Disorder, refraction
AMH (asymptomatic microscopic hematuria) R31.21
Amianthosis J61
Amimia R48.8
Amino-acid disorder E72.9
  anemia D53.0
Aminoacidopathy E72.9
Aminoaciduria E72.9
AMKD (APOL1-mediated kidney disease) (with glomerulonephritis) (with glomerulosclerosis) N07.B
Amnesia R41.3
  anterograde R41.1
  auditory R48.8
  dissociative F44.0
    with dissociative fugue F44.1
  hysterical F44.0
  postictal in epilepsy — *see* Epilepsy
  psychogenic F44.0
  retrograde R41.2
  transient global G45.4
Amnes(t)ic syndrome (post-traumatic) F04
  induced by
    alcohol F10.96
      with dependence F10.26
    psychoactive NEC F19.96
      with
        abuse F19.16
        dependence F19.26
    sedative F13.96
      with dependence F13.26
Amnion, amniotic — *see* condition
Amnionitis — *see* Pregnancy, complicated by
Amok F68.8
Amoral traits F60.89
Amphetamine (or other stimulant) **-induced**
  anxiety disorder F15.980
  bipolar and related disorder F15.94
  delirium F15.921
  depressive disorder F15.94
  obsessive-compulsive and related disorder F15.988
  psychotic disorder F15.959
  sexual dysfunction F15.981
  sleep disorder F15.982
  stimulant withdrawal F15.23
Ampulla
  lower esophagus K22.89
  phrenic K22.89
Amputation — *see also* Absence, by site, acquired
  neuroma (postoperative) (traumatic) — *see* Complications, amputation stump, neuroma
  stump (surgical)
    abnormal, painful, or with complication (late) — *see* Complications, amputation stump
    healed or old NOS Z89.9
  traumatic (complete) (partial)
    arm (upper) (complete) S48.91- ☑
      at
        elbow S58.01- ☑
          partial S58.02- ☑
        shoulder joint (complete) S48.01- ☑
          partial S48.02- ☑

Amputation — continued
  traumatic — continued
    arm — continued
      between
        elbow and wrist (complete) S58.11- ☑
          partial S58.12- ☑
        shoulder and elbow (complete) S48.11- ☑
          partial S48.12- ☑
      partial S48.92- ☑
    breast (complete) S28.21- ☑
      partial S28.22- ☑
    clitoris (complete) S38.211- ☑
      partial S38.212- ☑
    ear (complete) S08.11- ☑
      partial S08.12- ☑
    finger (complete) (metacarpophalangeal) S68.11- ☑
      index S68.11- ☑
      little S68.11- ☑
      middle S68.11- ☑
      partial S68.12- ☑
        index S68.12- ☑
        little S68.12- ☑
        middle S68.12- ☑
        ring S68.12- ☑
      ring S68.11- ☑
      thumb — see Amputation, traumatic, thumb
      transphalangeal (complete) S68.61- ☑
        index S68.61- ☑
        little S68.61- ☑
        middle S68.61- ☑
        partial S68.62- ☑
          index S68.62- ☑
          little S68.62- ☑
          middle S68.62- ☑
          ring S68.62- ☑
        ring S68.61- ☑
    foot (complete) S98.91- ☑
      at ankle level S98.01- ☑
        partial S98.02- ☑
      midfoot S98.31- ☑
        partial S98.32- ☑
      partial S98.92- ☑
    forearm (complete) S58.91- ☑
      at elbow level (complete) S58.01- ☑
        partial S58.02- ☑
      between elbow and wrist (complete) S58.11- ☑
        partial S58.12- ☑
      partial S58.92- ☑
    genital organ(s) (external)
      female (complete) S38.211- ☑
        partial S38.212- ☑
      male
        penis (complete) S38.221- ☑
          partial S38.222- ☑
        scrotum (complete) S38.231- ☑
          partial S38.232- ☑
        testes (complete) S38.231- ☑
          partial S38.232- ☑
    hand (complete) (wrist level) S68.41- ☑
      finger(s) alone — see Amputation, traumatic, finger
      partial S68.42- ☑
      thumb alone — see Amputation, traumatic, thumb
      transmetacarpal (complete) S68.71- ☑
        partial S68.72- ☑
    head
      ear — see Amputation, traumatic, ear
      nose (partial) S08.812- ☑
        complete S08.811- ☑
      part S08.89- ☑
        scalp S08.0- ☑
    hip (and thigh) (complete) S78.91- ☑
      at hip joint (complete) S78.01- ☑
        partial S78.02- ☑
      between hip and knee (complete) S78.11- ☑
        partial S78.12- ☑
      partial S78.92- ☑
    labium (majus) (minus) (complete) S38.21- ☑
      partial S38.21- ☑
    leg (lower) S88.91- ☑
      at knee level S88.01- ☑
        partial S88.02- ☑
      between knee and ankle S88.11- ☑
        partial S88.12- ☑
      partial S88.92- ☑

Amputation — continued
  traumatic — continued
    nose (partial) S08.812- ☑
      complete S08.811- ☑
    penis (complete) S38.221- ☑
      partial S38.222- ☑
    scrotum (complete) S38.231- ☑
      partial S38.232- ☑
    shoulder — see Amputation, traumatic, arm
      at shoulder joint — see Amputation, traumatic, arm, at shoulder joint
    testes (complete) S38.231- ☑
      partial S38.232- ☑
    thigh — see Amputation, traumatic, hip
    thorax, part of S28.1- ☑
      breast — see Amputation, traumatic, breast
    thumb (complete) (metacarpophalangeal) S68.01- ☑
      partial S68.02- ☑
      transphalangeal (complete) S68.51- ☑
        partial S68.52- ☑
    toe (lesser) S98.13- ☑
      great S98.11- ☑
        partial S98.12- ☑
      more than one S98.21- ☑
        partial S98.22- ☑
      partial S98.14- ☑
    vulva (complete) S38.211- ☑
      partial S38.212- ☑
Amputee (bilateral) (old) Z89.9
Amsterdam dwarfism Q87.19
Amusia R48.8
  developmental F80.89
Amyelencephalus, amyelencephaly Q00.0
Amyelia Q06.0
Amygdalitis — see Tonsillitis
Amygdalolith J35.8
Amyloid heart (disease) E85.4 [I43]
Amyloidosis (generalized) (primary) E85.9
  with lung involvement E85.4 [J99]
  familial E85.2
  genetic E85.2
  heart E85.4 [I43]
  hemodialysis-associated E85.3
  light chain (AL) E85.81
  liver E85.4 [K77]
  localized E85.4
  neuropathic heredofamilial E85.1
  non-neuropathic heredofamilial E85.0
  organ limited E85.4
  Portuguese E85.1
  pulmonary E85.4 [J99]
  secondary systemic E85.3
  senile systemic (SSA) E85.82
  skin (lichen) (macular) E85.4 [L99]
  specified NEC E85.89
  subglottic E85.4 [J99]
  wild-type transthyretin-related (ATTR) E85.82
Amylopectinosis (brancher enzyme deficiency) E74.03
Amylophagia — see Pica
Amyoplasia congenita Q79.8
Amyotonia M62.89
  congenita G70.2
Amyotrophia, amyotrophy, amyotrophic G71.8
  congenita Q79.8
  diabetic — see Diabetes, amyotrophy
  lateral sclerosis G12.21
  neuralgic G54.5
  spinal progressive G12.25
Anacidity, gastric K31.83
  psychogenic F45.8
Anaerosis of newborn P28.89
Analbuminemia E88.09
Analgesia — see Anesthesia
Analphalipoproteinemia E78.6
Anaphylactic
  purpura D69.0
  shock or reaction — see Shock, anaphylactic
Anaphylactoid shock or reaction — see Shock, anaphylactic
Anaphylactoid syndrome of pregnancy O88.01- ☑
Anaphylaxis — see Shock, anaphylactic
Anaplasia cervix — see also Dysplasia, cervix N87.9
Anaplasmosis [A. phagocytophilum] (transfusion transmitted) A79.82
  human A77.49
Anarthria R47.1
Anasarca R60.1
  cardiac — see Failure, heart, congestive

Anasarca — continued
  lung J18.2
  newborn P83.2
  nutritional E43
  pulmonary J18.2
  renal N04.9
Anastomosis
  aneurysmal — see Aneurysm
  arteriovenous ruptured brain I60.8
    intracerebral I61.8
    intraparenchymal I61.8
    intraventricular I61.5
    subarachnoid I60.8
  intestinal K63.89
    complicated NEC K91.89
      involving urinary tract N99.89
  retinal and choroidal vessels (congenital) Q14.8
Anatomical narrow angle H40.03- ☑
Ancylostoma, ancylostomiasis (braziliense) (caninum) (ceylanicum) (duodenale) B76.0
  Necator americanus B76.1
Andersen's disease (glycogen storage) E74.09
Anderson-Fabry disease E75.21
Andes disease T70.29- ☑
Andrews' disease (bacterid) L08.89
Androblastoma
  benign
    specified site — see Neoplasm, benign, by site
    unspecified site
      female D27.9
      male D29.20
  malignant
    specified site — see Neoplasm, malignant, by site
    unspecified site
      female C56.9
      male C62.90
  specified site — see Neoplasm, uncertain behavior, by site
  tubular
    with lipid storage
      specified site — see Neoplasm, benign, by site
      unspecified site
        female D27.9
        male D29.20
    specified site — see Neoplasm, benign, by site
    unspecified site
      female D27.9
      male D29.20
  unspecified site
    female D39.10
    male D40.10
Androgen insensitivity syndrome — see also Syndrome, androgen insensitivity E34.50
Androgen resistance syndrome — see also Syndrome, androgen insensitivity E34.50
Android pelvis Q74.2
  with disproportion (fetopelvic) O33.3- ☑
  causing obstructed labor O65.3
Androphobia F40.290
Anectasis, pulmonary (newborn) — see Atelectasis
Anemia (essential) (general) (hemoglobin deficiency) (infantile) (primary) (profound) D64.9
  with (due to) (in)
    disorder of
      anaerobic glycolysis D55.29
      pentose phosphate pathway D55.1
    koilonychia D50.9
  achlorhydric D50.8
  achrestic D53.1
  Addison (-Biermer) (pernicious) D51.0
  agranulocytic — see Agranulocytosis
  amino-acid-deficiency D53.0
  aplastic D61.9
    congenital D61.09
    drug-induced D61.1
    due to
      drugs D61.1
      external agents NEC D61.2
      infection D61.2
      radiation D61.2
    idiopathic D61.3
    red cell (pure) D60.9
      chronic D60.0
      congenital D61.01
      specified type NEC D60.8
      transient D60.1
    specified type NEC D61.89
    toxic D61.2

Anemia — continued
  aregenerative
    congenital D61.09
  asiderotic D50.9
  atypical (primary) D64.9
  Baghdad spring D55.0
  Balantidium coli A07.0
  Biermer's (pernicious) D51.0
  blood loss (chronic) D50.0
    acute D62
  bothriocephalus B70.0 [D63.8]
  brickmaker's B76.9 [D63.8]
  cerebral I67.89
  childhood D58.9
  chlorotic D50.8
  chronic
    blood loss D50.0
    hemolytic D58.9
      idiopathic D59.9
    simple D53.9
  chronica congenita aregenerativa D61.09
  combined system disease NEC D51.0 [G32.0]
    due to dietary vitamin B12 deficiency D51.3 [G32.0]
  complicating pregnancy, childbirth or puerperium — see Pregnancy, complicated by (management affected by), anemia
  congenital P61.4
    aplastic D61.09
    due to isoimmunization NOS P55.9
    dyserythropoietic, dyshematopoietic D64.4
    following fetal blood loss P61.3
    Heinz body D58.2
    hereditary hemolytic NOS D58.9
    pernicious D51.0
    spherocytic D58.0
  Cooley's (erythroblastic) D56.1
  cytogenic D51.0
  deficiency D53.9
    2, 3 diphosphoglycurate mutase D55.29
    2, 3 PG D55.29
    6-PGD D55.1
    6 phosphogluconate dehydrogenase D55.1
    amino-acid D53.0
    combined B12 and folate D53.1
    enzyme D55.9
      drug-induced (hemolytic) D59.2
      glucose-6-phosphate dehydrogenase (G6PD) D55.0
      glycolytic D55.29
      nucleotide metabolism D55.3
      related to hexose monophosphate (HMP) shunt pathway NEC D55.1
      specified type NEC D55.8
    erythrocytic glutathione D55.1
    folate D52.9
      dietary D52.0
      drug-induced D52.1
    folic acid D52.9
      dietary D52.0
      drug-induced D52.1
    G SH D55.1
    G6PD D55.0
    GGS-R D55.1
    glucose-6-phosphate dehydrogenase D55.0
    glutathione reductase D55.1
    glyceraldehyde phosphate dehydrogenase D55.29
    hexokinase D55.29
    iron D50.9
      secondary to blood loss (chronic) D50.0
    nutritional D53.9
      with
        poor iron absorption D50.8
        specified deficiency NEC D53.8
    phosphofructo-aldolase D55.29
    phosphoglycerate kinase D55.29
    PK D55.21
    protein D53.0
    pyruvate kinase D55.21
    transcobalamin II D51.2
    triose-phosphate isomerase D55.29
    vitamin B12 NOS D51.9
      dietary D51.3
      due to
        intrinsic factor deficiency D51.0
        selective vitamin B12 malabsorption with proteinuria D51.1
      pernicious D51.0
      specified type NEC D51.8
  Diamond-Blackfan (congenital hypoplastic) D61.01

Anemia — continued
  dibothriocephalus B70.0 [D63.8]
  dimorphic D53.1
  diphasic D53.1
  Diphyllobothrium (Dibothriocephalus) B70.0 [D63.8]
  due to (in) (with)
    antineoplastic chemotherapy D64.81
    blood loss (chronic) D50.0
      acute D62
    chemotherapy, antineoplastic D64.81
    chronic disease classified elsewhere NEC D63.8
    chronic kidney disease D63.1
    deficiency
      amino-acid D53.0
      copper D53.8
      folate (folic acid) D52.9
        dietary D52.0
        drug-induced D52.1
      molybdenum D53.8
      protein D53.0
      zinc D53.8
    dietary vitamin B12 deficiency D51.3
    disorder of
      glutathione metabolism D55.1
      nucleotide metabolism D55.3
    drug — see Anemia, by type — see also Table of Drugs and Chemicals
    end stage renal disease D63.1
    enzyme disorder D55.9
    fetal blood loss P61.3
    fish tapeworm (D. latum) infestation B70.0 [D63.8]
    hemorrhage (chronic) D50.0
      acute D62
    impaired absorption D50.9
    loss of blood (chronic) D50.0
      acute D62
    myxedema E03.9 [D63.8]
    Necator americanus B76.1 [D63.8]
    prematurity P61.2
    selective vitamin B12 malabsorption with proteinuria D51.1
    transcobalamin II deficiency D51.2
  Dyke-Young type (secondary) (symptomatic) D59.19
  dyserythropoietic (congenital) D64.4
  dyshematopoietic (congenital) D64.4
  Egyptian B76.9 [D63.8]
  elliptocytosis — see Elliptocytosis
  enzyme-deficiency, drug-induced D59.2
  epidemic — see also Ancylostomiasis B76.9 [D63.8]
  erythroblastic
    familial D56.1
    newborn — see also Disease, hemolytic P55.9
    of childhood D56.1
  erythrocytic glutathione deficiency D55.1
  erythropoietin-resistant anemia (EPO resistant anemia) D63.1
  Faber's (achlorhydric anemia) D50.9
  factitious (self-induced blood letting) D50.0
  familial erythroblastic D56.1
  Fanconi ('s) D61.03
  favism D55.0
  fish tapeworm (D. latum) infestation B70.0 [D63.8]
  folate (folic acid) deficiency D52.9
  glucose-6-phosphate dehydrogenase (G6PD) deficiency D55.0
  glutathione-reductase deficiency D55.1
  goat's milk D52.0
  granulocytic — see Agranulocytosis
  Heinz body, congenital D58.2
  hemolytic D58.9
    acquired D59.9
      with hemoglobinuria NEC D59.6
      autoimmune NEC D59.19
      infectious D59.4
      specified type NEC D59.8
      toxic D59.4
    acute D59.9
      due to enzyme deficiency specified type NEC D55.8
      Lederer's D59.19
    autoimmune D59.10
      cold D59.12
      drug-induced D59.0
      mixed D59.13
      warm D59.11
    chronic D58.9
      idiopathic D59.9
    cold type (primary) (secondary) (symptomatic) D59.12
    congenital (spherocytic) — see Spherocytosis

Anemia — continued
  hemolytic — continued
    due to
      cardiac conditions D59.4
      drugs (nonautoimmune) D59.2
        autoimmune D59.0
      enzyme disorder D55.9
        drug-induced D59.2
      presence of shunt or other internal prosthetic device D59.4
    familial D58.9
    hereditary D58.9
      due to enzyme disorder D55.9
        specified type NEC D55.8
      specified type NEC D58.8
    idiopathic (chronic) D59.9
    mechanical D59.4
    microangiopathic D59.4
    mixed type (primary) (secondary) (symptomatic) D59.13
    nonautoimmune D59.4
      drug-induced D59.2
    nonspherocytic
      congenital or hereditary NEC D55.8
        glucose-6-phosphate dehydrogenase deficiency D55.0
        pyruvate kinase deficiency D55.21
        type
          I D55.1
          II D55.29
      type
        I D55.1
        II D55.29
    primary
      autoimmune
        cold type D59.12
        mixed type D59.13
        warm type D59.11
    secondary D59.4
      autoimmune
        cold type D59.12
        mixed type D59.13
        warm type D59.11
    specified (hereditary) type NEC D58.8
    Stransky-Regala type — see also Hemoglobinopathy D58.8
    symptomatic D59.4
      autoimmune
        cold type D59.12
        mixed type D59.13
        warm type D59.11
    toxic D59.4
    warm type (primary) (secondary) (symptomatic) D59.11
  hemorrhagic (chronic) D50.0
    acute D62
  Herrick's D57.1
  hexokinase deficiency D55.29
  hookworm B76.9 [D63.8]
  hypochromic (idiopathic) (microcytic) (normoblastic) D50.9
    due to blood loss (chronic) D50.0
      acute D62
    familial sex-linked D64.0
    pyridoxine-responsive D64.3
    sideroblastic, sex-linked D64.0
  hypoplasia, red blood cells D61.9
    congenital or familial D61.01
  hypoplastic (idiopathic) D61.9
    congenital or familial (of childhood) D61.01
  hypoproliferative (refractive) D61.9
  idiopathic D64.9
    aplastic D61.3
    hemolytic, chronic D59.9
  in (due to) (with)
    chronic kidney disease D63.1
    end stage renal disease D63.1
    failure, kidney (renal) D63.1
    neoplastic disease — see also Neoplasm D63.0
  intertropical — see also Ancylostomiasis D63.8
  iron deficiency D50.9
    secondary to blood loss (chronic) D50.0
      acute D62
    specified type NEC D50.8
  Joseph-Diamond-Blackfan (congenital hypoplastic) D61.01
  Lederer's (hemolytic) D59.19
  leukoerythroblastic D61.82
  macrocytic D53.9

Anemia — continued
    macrocytic — continued
        nutritional D52.0
        tropical D52.8
    malarial — see also Malaria B54 [D63.8]
    malignant (progressive) D51.0
    malnutrition D53.9
    marsh — see also Malaria B54 [D63.8]
    Mediterranean (with other hemoglobinopathy) D56.9
    megaloblastic D53.1
        combined B12 and folate deficiency D53.1
        hereditary D51.1
        nutritional D52.0
        orotic aciduria D53.0
        refractory D53.1
        specified type NEC D53.1
    megalocytic D53.1
    microcytic (hypochromic) D50.9
        due to blood loss (chronic) D50.0
            acute D62
        familial D56.8
    microdrepanocytosis D57.40
    microelliptopoikilocytic (Rietti-Greppi- Micheli) D56.9
    miner's B76.9 [D63.8]
    myelodysplastic D46.9
    myelofibrosis D75.81
    myelogenous D64.89
    myelopathic D64.89
    myelophthisic D61.82
    myeloproliferative D47.Z9 (following D47.4)
    newborn P61.4
        due to
            ABO (antibodies, isoimmunization, maternal/fetal incompatibility) P55.1
            Rh (antibodies, isoimmunization, maternal/fetal incompatibility) P55.0
        following fetal blood loss P61.3
        posthemorrhagic (fetal) P61.3
    nonspherocytic hemolytic — see Anemia, hemolytic, nonspherocytic
    normocytic (infectional) D64.9
        due to blood loss (chronic) D50.0
            acute D62
        myelophthisic D61.82
    nutritional (deficiency) D53.9
        with
            poor iron absorption D50.8
            specified deficiency NEC D53.8
        megaloblastic D52.0
    of prematurity P61.2
    orotaciduric (congenital) (hereditary) D53.0
    osteosclerotic D64.89
    ovalocytosis (hereditary) — see Elliptocytosis
    paludal — see also Malaria B54 [D63.8]
    pernicious (congenital) (malignant) (progressive) D51.0
    pleochromic D64.89
        of sprue D52.8
    posthemorrhagic (chronic) D50.0
        acute D62
        newborn P61.3
    postoperative (postprocedural)
        due to (acute) blood loss D62
            chronic blood loss D50.0
        specified NEC D64.89
    postpartum O90.81
    pressure D64.89
    progressive D64.9
        malignant D51.0
        pernicious D51.0
    protein-deficiency D53.0
    pseudoleukemica infantum D64.89
    pure red cell D60.9
        congenital D61.01
    pyridoxine-responsive D64.3
    pyruvate kinase deficiency D55.21
    refractory D46.4
        with
            excess of blasts D46.20
                1 (RAEB 1) D46.21
                2 (RAEB 2) D46.22
                in transformation (RAEB T) — see Leukemia, acute myeloblastic
            hemochromatosis D46.1
            sideroblasts (ring) (RARS) D46.1
        megaloblastic D53.1
    sideroblastic D46.1
    sideropenic D50.9
    without ring sideroblasts, so stated D46.0
    without sideroblasts without excess of blasts D46.0

Anemia — continued
    Rietti-Greppi-Micheli D56.9
    scorbutic D53.2
    secondary to
        blood loss (chronic) D50.0
            acute D62
        hemorrhage (chronic) D50.0
            acute D62
    semiplastic D61.89
    sickle-cell — see Disease, sickle-cell
    sideroblastic D64.3
        hereditary D64.0
        hypochromic, sex-linked D64.0
        pyridoxine-responsive NEC D64.3
        refractory D46.1
        secondary (due to)
            disease D64.1
            drugs and toxins D64.2
        specified type NEC D64.3
    sideropenic (refractory) D50.9
        due to blood loss (chronic) D50.0
            acute D62
    simple chronic D53.9
    specified type NEC D64.89
    spherocytic (hereditary) — see Spherocytosis
    splenic D64.89
    splenomegalic D64.89
    stomatocytosis D58.8
    syphilitic (acquired) (late) A52.79 [D63.8]
    target cell D64.89
    thalassemia D56.9
    thrombocytopenic — see Thrombocytopenia
    toxic D61.2
    tropical B76.9 [D63.8]
        macrocytic D52.8
    tuberculous A18.89 [D63.8]
    vegan D51.3
    vitamin
        B6-responsive D64.3
        B12 deficiency (dietary) pernicious D51.0
    von Jaksch's D64.89
    Witts' (achlorhydric anemia) D50.8
Anemophobia F40.228
Anencephalus, anencephaly Q00.0
Anergasia — see Psychosis, organic
Anesthesia, anesthetic R20.0
    complication or reaction NEC — see also Complications, anesthesia T88.59- ☑
    due to
        correct substance properly administered — see Table of Drugs and Chemicals, by drug, adverse effect
        overdose or wrong substance given — see Table of Drugs and Chemicals, by drug, poisoning
    unintended awareness under general anesthesia during procedure T88.53- ☑
        personal history of Z92.84
    cornea H18.81- ☑
    dissociative F44.6
    functional (hysterical) F44.6
    hyperesthetic, thalamic G89.0
    hysterical F44.6
    local skin lesion R20.0
    sexual (psychogenic) F52.1
    shock (due to) T88.2- ☑
    skin R20.0
    testicular N50.9
Anetoderma (maculosum) (of) L90.8
    Jadassohn-Pellizzari L90.2
    Schweninger-Buzzi L90.1
Aneurin deficiency E51.9
Aneurysm (anastomotic) (artery) (cirsoid) (diffuse) (false) (fusiform) (multiple) (saccular) I72.9
    abdominal (aorta) I71.40
        infrarenal I71.43
            ruptured I71.33
        juxtarenal I71.42
            ruptured I71.32
        pararenal I71.41
            ruptured I71.31
        ruptured I71.30
        syphilitic A52.01
    aorta, aortic (nonsyphilitic) I71.9
        abdominal I71.40
            dissecting — see Dissection, aorta, abdominal
            ruptured I71.30
        arch I71.22
            ruptured I71.12
        arteriosclerotic I71.9

Aneurysm — continued
    aorta, aortic — continued
        arteriosclerotic — continued
            ruptured I71.8
        ascending I71.21
            ruptured I71.11
        congenital Q25.43
        descending I71.9
            abdominal I71.40
                ruptured I71.30
            ruptured I71.8
            thoracic I71.23
                ruptured I71.13
        dissecting — see Dissection, aorta
        root Q25.43
        ruptured I71.8
        sinus, congenital Q25.43
        syphilitic A52.01
        thoracic I71.20
            ruptured I71.10
        thoracoabdominal I71.60
            paravisceral I71.62
                ruptured I71.52
            ruptured I71.50
            supraceliac I71.61
                ruptured I71.51
        thorax, thoracic I71.20
            arch I71.22
                ruptured I71.12
            ascending I71.21
                ruptured I71.11
            descending I71.23
                ruptured I71.13
            ruptured I71.10
            arch I71.12
            ascending I71.11
            descending I71.13
        transverse I71.22
            ruptured I71.12
        valve (heart) — see also Endocarditis, aortic I35.8
    arteriosclerotic I72.9
        cerebral I67.1
            ruptured — see Hemorrhage, intracranial, subarachnoid
    arteriovenous (congenital) — see also Malformation, arteriovenous
        acquired I77.0
        brain I67.1
            ruptured — see Aneurysm, arteriovenous, brain, ruptured
        coronary I25.41
        pulmonary I28.0
        brain Q28.2
            ruptured I60.8
                intracerebral I61.8
                intraparenchymal I61.8
                intraventricular I61.5
                subarachnoid I60.8
        peripheral — see Malformation, arteriovenous, peripheral
        precerebral vessels Q28.0
        specified site NEC — see also Malformation, arteriovenous
            acquired I77.0
    basal — see Aneurysm, brain
    basilar (trunk) I72.5
    berry (congenital) (nonruptured) I67.1
        ruptured I60.7
    brain I67.1
        arteriosclerotic I67.1
            ruptured — see Hemorrhage, intracranial, subarachnoid
        arteriovenous (congenital) (nonruptured) Q28.2
            acquired I67.1
                ruptured — see Aneurysm, arteriovenous, brain, ruptured
            ruptured — see Aneurysm, arteriovenous, brain, ruptured
        berry (congenital) (nonruptured) I67.1
            ruptured — see also Hemorrhage, intracranial, subarachnoid I60.7
        congenital Q28.3
            ruptured I60.7
        meninges I67.1
            ruptured I60.8
        miliary (congenital) (nonruptured) I67.1
            ruptured — see also Hemorrhage, intracranial, subarachnoid I60.7
        mycotic I67.1

Aneurysm — continued
　brain — continued
　　mycotic — continued
　　　with endocarditis — see also Endocarditis
　　　ruptured — see Aneurysm, arteriovenous, brain, ruptured I60.8
　　　syphilitic (hemorrhage) A52.05
　　cardiac (false) — see also Aneurysm, heart I25.3
　　carotid artery (common) (external) I72.0
　　　internal (intracranial) I67.1
　　　　extracranial portion I72.0
　　　ruptured into brain I60.0- ☑
　　　syphilitic A52.09
　　　　intracranial A52.05
　　cavernous sinus I67.1
　　　arteriovenous (congenital) (nonruptured) Q28.3
　　　　ruptured I60.8
　　celiac I72.8
　　central nervous system, syphilitic A52.05
　　cerebral — see Aneurysm, brain
　　chest — see Aneurysm, thorax
　　circle of Willis I67.1
　　　congenital Q28.3
　　　　ruptured I60.6
　　　ruptured I60.6
　　common iliac artery I72.3
　　congenital (peripheral) Q27.8
　　　aorta (root) (sinus) Q25.43
　　　brain Q28.3
　　　　ruptured I60.7
　　　coronary Q24.5
　　　digestive system Q27.8
　　　lower limb Q27.8
　　　pulmonary Q25.79
　　　retina Q14.1
　　　specified site NEC Q27.8
　　　upper limb Q27.8
　　conjunctiva — see Abnormality, conjunctiva, vascular
　　conus arteriosus — see Aneurysm, heart
　　coronary (arteriosclerotic) (artery) I25.41
　　　arteriovenous, congenital Q24.5
　　　congenital Q24.5
　　　ruptured — see Infarct, myocardium
　　　syphilitic A52.06
　　　vein I25.89
　　cylindroid (aorta) I71.9
　　　ruptured I71.8
　　　syphilitic A52.01
　　ductus arteriosus Q25.0
　　endocardial, infective (any valve) I33.0
　　femoral (artery) (ruptured) I72.4
　　gastroduodenal I72.8
　　gastroepiploic I72.8
　　heart (wall) (chronic or with a stated duration of over 4 weeks) I25.3
　　　valve — see Endocarditis
　　hepatic I72.8
　　iliac (common) (artery) (ruptured) I72.3
　　infective I72.9
　　　endocardial (any valve) I33.0
　　innominate (nonsyphilitic) I72.8
　　　syphilitic A52.09
　　interauricular septum — see Aneurysm, heart
　　interventricular septum — see Aneurysm, heart
　　intrathoracic (nonsyphilitic) — see also Aneurysm, aorta, thorax I71.20
　　　ruptured — see also Aneurysm, aorta, thorax, ruptured I71.10
　　　syphilitic A52.01
　　lower limb I72.4
　　lung (pulmonary artery) I28.1
　　mediastinal (nonsyphilitic) I72.8
　　　syphilitic A52.09
　　miliary (congenital) I67.1
　　　ruptured — see Hemorrhage, intracerebral, subarachnoid, intracranial
　　mitral (heart) (valve) I34.89
　　mural — see Aneurysm, heart
　　mycotic I72.9
　　　endocardial (any valve) I33.0
　　　ruptured, brain — see Hemorrhage, intracerebral, subarachnoid
　　　myocardium — see Aneurysm, heart
　　neck I72.0
　　pancreaticoduodenal I72.8
　　patent ductus arteriosus Q25.0
　　peripheral NEC I72.8
　　　congenital Q27.8
　　　　digestive system Q27.8

Aneurysm — continued
　peripheral — continued
　　congenital — continued
　　　lower limb Q27.8
　　　specified site NEC Q27.8
　　　upper limb Q27.8
　popliteal (artery) (ruptured) I72.4
　precerebral
　　congenital (nonruptured) Q28.1
　　specified site, NEC I72.5
　pulmonary I28.1
　　arteriovenous Q25.72
　　　acquired I28.0
　　syphilitic A52.09
　　valve (heart) — see Endocarditis, pulmonary
　racemose (peripheral) I72.9
　　congenital — see Aneurysm, congenital
　radial I72.1
　Rasmussen NEC A15.0
　renal (artery) I72.2
　retina — see also Disorder, retina, microaneurysms
　　congenital Q14.1
　　diabetic — see E08-E13 with .3-
　sinus of Valsalva Q25.43
　specified NEC I72.8
　spinal (cord) I72.8
　　syphilitic (hemorrhage) A52.09
　splenic I72.8
　subclavian (artery) (ruptured) I72.8
　　syphilitic A52.09
　superior mesenteric I72.8
　syphilitic (aorta) A52.01
　　central nervous system A52.05
　　congenital (late) A50.54 [I79.0]
　　spine, spinal A52.09
　thoracoabdominal (aorta) I71.60
　　ruptured I71.50
　　syphilitic A52.01
　thorax, thoracic (aorta) (arch) (nonsyphilitic) — see Aneurysm, aorta, thorax
　　ruptured — see Aneurysm, aorta, thorax, ruptured
　　syphilitic A52.01
　traumatic (complication) (early), specified site — see Injury, blood vessel
　tricuspid (heart) (valve) I07.8
　ulnar I72.1
　upper limb (ruptured) I72.1
　valve, valvular — see Endocarditis
　venous — see also Varix I86.8
　　congenital Q27.8
　　　digestive system Q27.8
　　　lower limb Q27.8
　　　specified site NEC Q27.8
　　　upper limb Q27.8
　ventricle — see Aneurysm, heart
　vertebral artery I72.6
　visceral NEC I72.8
Angelman syndrome Q93.51
Anger R45.4
Angiectasis, angiectopia I99.8
Angiitis I77.6
　allergic granulomatous M30.1
　hypersensitivity M31.0
　necrotizing M31.9
　　specified NEC M31.8
　nervous system, granulomatous I67.7
Angina (attack) (cardiac) (chest) (heart) (pectoris) (syndrome) (vasomotor) I20.9
　with
　　atherosclerotic heart disease — see Arteriosclerosis, coronary (artery),
　　coronary microvascular disease I20.81
　　coronary microvascular dysfunction I20.81
　　documented spasm I20.1
　abdominal K55.1
　accelerated — see Angina, unstable
　agranulocytic — see Agranulocytosis
　angiospastic — see Angina, with documented spasm
　aphthous B08.5
　crescendo — see Angina, unstable
　croupous J05.0
　cruris I73.9
　de novo effort — see Angina, unstable
　diphtheritic, membranous A36.0
　equivalent I20.89
　exudative, chronic J37.0
　following acute myocardial infarction I23.7
　gangrenous diphtheritic A36.0
　intestinal K55.1

Angina — continued
　Ludovici K12.2
　Ludwig's K12.2
　malignant diphtheritic A36.0
　membranous J05.0
　　diphtheritic A36.0
　　Vincent's A69.1
　mesenteric K55.1
　monocytic — see Mononucleosis, infectious
　of effort — see Angina, specified NEC
　phlegmonous J36
　　diphtheritic A36.0
　post-infarctional I23.7
　pre-infarctional — see Angina, unstable
　Prinzmetal — see Angina, with documented spasm
　progressive — see Angina, unstable
　pseudomembranous A69.1
　pultaceous, diphtheritic A36.0
　refractory I20.2
　spasm-induced — see Angina, with documented spasm
　specified NEC I20.89
　stable I20.89
　stenocardia — see Angina, specified NEC
　stridulous, diphtheritic A36.2
　tonsil J36
　trachealis J05.0
　unstable I20.0
　variant — see Angina, with documented spasm
　Vincent's A69.1
　worsening effort — see Angina, unstable
Angioblastoma — see Neoplasm, connective tissue, uncertain behavior
Angiocholecystitis — see Cholecystitis, acute
Angiocholitis — see also Cholecystitis, acute K83.09
Angiodysgenesis spinalis G95.19
Angiodysplasia (cecum) (colon) K55.20
　with bleeding K55.21
　duodenum (and stomach) K31.819
　　with bleeding K31.811
　stomach (and duodenum) K31.819
　　with bleeding K31.811
Angioedema (allergic) (any site) (with urticaria) T78.3- ☑
　episodic, with eosinophilia D72.118
　hereditary D84.1
Angioendothelioma — see Neoplasm, uncertain behavior, by site
　benign D18.00
　　intra-abdominal D18.03
　　intracranial D18.02
　　skin D18.01
　　specified site NEC D18.09
　bone — see Neoplasm, bone, malignant
　Ewing's — see Neoplasm, bone, malignant
Angioendotheliomatosis C85.8- ☑
Angiofibroma — see also Neoplasm, benign, by site
　juvenile
　　specified site — see Neoplasm, benign, by site
　　unspecified site D10.6
Angiohemophilia (A) (B) — see Disease, von Willebrand
Angioid streaks (choroid) (macula) (retina) H35.33
Angiokeratoma — see Neoplasm, skin, benign
　corporis diffusum E75.21
Angioleiomyoma — see Neoplasm, connective tissue, benign
Angiolipoma — see also Lipoma
　infiltrating — see Lipoma
Angioma — see also Hemangioma, by site
　capillary I78.1
　hemorrhagicum hereditaria I78.0
　intra-abdominal D18.03
　intracranial D18.02
　malignant — see Neoplasm, connective tissue, malignant
　plexiform D18.00
　　intra-abdominal D18.03
　　intracranial D18.02
　　skin D18.01
　　specified site NEC D18.09
　senile I78.1
　serpiginosum L81.7
　skin D18.01
　specified site NEC D18.09
　spider I78.1
　stellate I78.1
　venous Q28.3
Angiomatosis Q82.8
　bacillary A79.89
　encephalotrigeminal Q85.89
　hemorrhagic familial I78.0
　hereditary familial I78.0

☑ Additional Character Required — Refer to the Tabular List for Character Selection

Angiomatosis — continued
  liver K76.4
Angiomyolipoma — see Lipoma
Angiomyoliposarcoma — see Neoplasm, connective tissue, malignant
Angiomyoma — see Neoplasm, connective tissue, benign
Angiomyosarcoma — see Neoplasm, connective tissue, malignant
Angiomyxoma — see Neoplasm, connective tissue, uncertain behavior
Angioneurosis F45.8
Angioneurotic edema (allergic) (any site) (with urticaria) T78.3- ☑
  hereditary D84.1
Angiopathia, angiopathy I99.9
  cerebral I67.9
    amyloid E85.4 [I68.0]
  diabetic (peripheral) — see Diabetes, angiopathy
  peripheral I73.9
    diabetic — see Diabetes, angiopathy
    specified type NEC I73.89
  retinae syphilitica A52.05
  retinalis (juvenilis)
    diabetic — see Diabetes, retinopathy
    proliferative — see Retinopathy, proliferative
Angiosarcoma — see also Neoplasm, connective tissue, malignant
  liver C22.3
Angiosclerosis — see Arteriosclerosis
Angiospasm (peripheral) (traumatic) (vessel) — see also Vasospasm I73.9
  brachial plexus G54.0
  cerebral G45.9
  cervical plexus G54.2
  nerve
    arm — see Mononeuropathy, upper limb
      axillary G54.0
      median — see Lesion, nerve, median
      ulnar — see Lesion, nerve, ulnar
    axillary G54.0
    leg — see Mononeuropathy, lower limb
    median — see Lesion, nerve, median
    plantar — see Lesion, nerve, plantar
    ulnar — see Lesion, nerve, ulnar
Angiospastic disease or edema I73.9
Angiostrongyliasis
  due to
    Parastrongylus
      cantonensis B83.2
      costaricensis B81.3
  intestinal B81.3
Anguillulosis — see Strongyloidiasis
Angulation
  cecum — see Obstruction, intestine
  coccyx (acquired) M43.8X8
    congenital NEC Q76.49
  femur (acquired) — see also Deformity, limb, specified type NEC, thigh
    congenital Q74.2
  intestine (large) (small) — see Obstruction, intestine
  sacrum (acquired) — see also subcategory M43.8- ☑
    congenital NEC Q76.49
  sigmoid (flexure) — see Obstruction, intestine
  spine — see Dorsopathy, deforming, specified NEC
  tibia (acquired) — see also Deformity, limb, specified type NEC, lower leg
    congenital Q74.2
  ureter N13.5
    with infection N13.6
  wrist (acquired) — see also Deformity, limb, specified type NEC, forearm
    congenital Q74.0
Angulus infectiosus (lips) K13.0
Anhedonia R45.84
  sexual F52.0
Anhidrosis L74.4
Anhydration E86.0
Anhydremia E86.0
Anidrosis L74.4
Aniridia (congenital) Q13.1
Anisakiasis (infection) (infestation) B81.0
Anisakis larvae infestation B81.0
Aniseikonia H52.32
Anisocoria (pupil) H57.02
  congenital Q13.2
Anisocytosis R71.8
Anisometropia (congenital) H52.31
Ankle — see condition

Ankyloblepharon (eyelid) (acquired) — see also Blepharophimosis
  filiforme (adnatum) (congenital) Q10.3
  total Q10.3
Ankyloglossia Q38.1
Ankylosis (fibrous) (osseous) (joint) M24.60
  ankle M24.67- ☑
  arthrodesis status Z98.1
  cricoarytenoid (cartilage) (joint) (larynx) J38.7
  dental K03.5
  ear ossicles H74.31- ☑
  elbow M24.62- ☑
  foot M24.67- ☑
  hand M24.64- ☑
  hip M24.65- ☑
  incostapedial joint (infectional) — see Ankylosis, ear ossicles
  jaw (temporomandibular) M26.61- ☑
  knee M24.66- ☑
  lumbosacral (joint) M43.27
  postoperative (status) Z98.1
  produced by surgical fusion, status Z98.1
  sacro-iliac (joint) M43.28
  shoulder M24.61- ☑
  specified site NEC M24.69
  spine (joint) — see also Fusion, spine
    spondylitic — see Spondylitis, ankylosing
  surgical Z98.1
  temporomandibular M26.61- ☑
  tooth, teeth (hard tissues) K03.5
  wrist M24.63- ☑
Ankylostoma — see Ancylostoma
Ankylostomiasis — see Ancylostomiasis
Ankylurethria — see Stricture, urethra
Annular — see also condition
  detachment, cervix N88.8
  organ or site, congenital NEC — see Distortion
  pancreas (congenital) Q45.1
Anoctaminopathy G71.035
Anodontia (complete) (partial) (vera) K00.0
  acquired K08.10- ☑
Anomaly, anomalous (congenital) (unspecified type) Q89.9
  abdominal wall NEC Q79.59
  acoustic nerve Q07.8
  adrenal (gland) Q89.1
  Alder (-Reilly) (leukocyte granulation) D72.0
  alimentary tract Q45.9
    upper Q40.9
  alveolar M26.70
    hyperplasia M26.79
      mandibular M26.72
      maxillary M26.71
    hypoplasia M26.79
      mandibular M26.74
      maxillary M26.73
    ridge (process) M26.79
    specified NEC M26.79
  ankle (joint) Q74.2
  anus Q43.9
  aorta (arch) NEC Q25.40
    coarctation (preductal) (postductal) Q25.1
  aortic cusp or valve Q23.9
  appendix Q43.8
  apple peel syndrome Q41.1
  aqueduct of Sylvius Q03.0
    with spina bifida — see Spina bifida, with hydrocephalus
  arm Q74.0
  arteriovenous NEC
    coronary Q24.5
    gastrointestinal Q27.33
      acquired — see Angiodysplasia
  artery (peripheral) Q27.9
    basilar NEC Q28.1
    cerebral Q28.3
    coronary Q24.5
    digestive system Q27.8
    eye Q15.8
    great Q25.9
      specified NEC Q25.8
    lower limb Q27.8
    peripheral Q27.9
      specified NEC Q27.8
    pulmonary NEC Q25.79
    renal Q27.2
    retina Q14.1
    specified site NEC Q27.8
    subclavian Q27.8

Anomaly, anomalous — continued
  artery — continued
    subclavian — continued
      origin Q25.48
    umbilical Q27.0
    upper limb Q27.8
    vertebral NEC Q28.1
  aryteno-epiglottic folds Q31.8
  atrial
    bands or folds Q20.8
    septa Q21.10
  atrioventricular
    excitation I45.6
    septum Q21.0
  auditory canal Q17.8
  auricle
    ear Q17.8
      causing impairment of hearing Q16.9
    heart Q20.8
  Axenfeld's Q15.0
  back Q89.9
  band
    atrial Q20.8
    heart Q24.8
    ventricular Q24.8
  Bartholin's duct Q38.4
  biliary duct or passage Q44.5
  bladder Q64.70
    absence Q64.5
    diverticulum Q64.6
    exstrophy Q64.10
      cloacal Q64.12
      extroversion Q64.19
      specified type NEC Q64.19
      supravesical fissure Q64.11
    neck obstruction Q64.31
    specified type NEC Q64.79
  bone Q79.9
    arm Q74.0
    face Q75.9
    leg Q74.2
    pelvic girdle Q74.2
    shoulder girdle Q74.0
    skull Q75.9
      with
        anencephaly Q00.0
        encephalocele — see Encephalocele
        hydrocephalus Q03.9
          with spina bifida — see Spina bifida, with hydrocephalus
        microcephaly Q02
  brain (multiple) Q04.9
    vessel Q28.3
  breast Q83.9
  broad ligament Q50.6
  bronchus Q32.4
  bulbus cordis Q21.9
  bursa Q79.9
  canal of Nuck Q52.4
  canthus Q10.3
  capillary Q27.9
  cardiac Q24.9
    chambers Q20.9
      specified NEC Q20.8
    septal closure Q21.9
      specified NEC Q21.8
    valve NEC Q24.8
      pulmonary Q22.3
  cardiovascular system Q28.8
  carpus Q74.0
  caruncle, lacrimal Q10.6
  cascade stomach Q40.2
  cauda equina Q06.3
  cecum Q43.9
  cerebral Q04.9
    vessels Q28.3
  cervix Q51.9
  Chediak-Higashi (-Steinbrinck) (congenital gigantism of peroxidase granules) E70.330
  cheek Q18.9
  chest wall Q67.8
    bones Q76.9
  chin Q18.9
  chordae tendineae Q24.8
  choroid Q14.3
    plexus Q07.8
  chromosomes, chromosomal Q99.9
    D (1) — see condition, chromosome 13
    E (3) — see condition, chromosome 18

Anomaly, anomalous — continued
- chromosomes, chromosomal — continued
  - G — see condition, chromosome 21
  - sex
    - female phenotype Q97.8
    - gonadal dysgenesis (pure) Q99.1
    - Klinefelter's Q98.4
    - male phenotype Q98.9
    - Turner's Q96.9
    - specified NEC Q99.8- ☑
- cilia Q10.3
- circulatory system Q28.9
- clavicle Q74.0
- clitoris Q52.6
- coccyx Q76.49
- colon Q43.9
- common duct Q44.5
- communication
  - coronary artery Q24.5
  - left ventricle with right atrium Q21.0
- concha (ear) Q17.3
- connection
  - portal vein Q26.5
  - pulmonary venous Q26.4
    - partial Q26.3
    - total Q26.2
  - renal artery with kidney Q27.2
- cornea (shape) Q13.4
- coronary artery or vein Q24.5
- cranium — see Anomaly, skull
- cricoid cartilage Q31.8
- cystic duct Q44.5
- dental
  - alveolar — see Anomaly, alveolar
  - arch relationship M26.20
    - specified NEC M26.29
- dentofacial M26.9
  - alveolar — see Anomaly, alveolar
  - dental arch relationship M26.20
    - specified NEC M26.29
  - functional M26.50
    - specified NEC M26.59
  - jaw-cranial base relationship M26.10
    - asymmetry M26.12
      - maxillary M26.11
    - specified type NEC M26.19
  - jaw size M26.00
    - macrogenia M26.05
    - mandibular
      - hyperplasia M26.03
      - hypoplasia M26.04
    - maxillary
      - hyperplasia M26.01
      - hypoplasia M26.02
    - microgenia M26.06
    - specified type NEC M26.09
  - malocclusion M26.4
    - dental arch relationship NEC M26.29
    - jaw-cranial base relationship — see Anomaly, dentofacial, jaw-cranial base relationship
    - jaw size — see Anomaly, dentofacial, jaw size
    - specified type NEC M26.89
  - temporomandibular joint M26.60- ☑
    - adhesions M26.61- ☑
    - ankylosis M26.61- ☑
    - arthralgia M26.62- ☑
    - articular disc M26.63- ☑
    - specified type NEC M26.69
  - tooth position, fully erupted M26.30
    - specified NEC M26.39
- dermatoglyphic Q82.8
- diaphragm (apertures) NEC Q79.1
- digestive organ(s) or tract Q45.9
  - lower Q43.9
  - upper Q40.9
- distance, interarch (excessive) (inadequate) M26.25
- distribution, coronary artery Q24.5
- ductus
  - arteriosus Q25.0
  - botalli Q25.0
- duodenum Q43.9
- dura (brain) Q04.9
  - spinal cord Q06.9
- ear (external) Q17.9
  - causing impairment of hearing Q16.9
  - inner Q16.5
  - middle (causing impairment of hearing) Q16.4
  - ossicles Q16.3

Anomaly, anomalous — continued
- Ebstein's (heart) (tricuspid valve) Q22.5
- ectodermal Q82.9
- Eisenmenger's (ventricular septal defect) Q21.8
- ejaculatory duct Q55.4
- elbow Q74.0
- endocrine gland NEC Q89.2
- epididymis Q55.4
- epiglottis Q31.8
- esophagus Q39.9
- eustachian tube Q17.8
- eye Q15.9
  - anterior segment Q13.9
    - specified NEC Q13.89
  - posterior segment Q14.9
    - specified NEC Q14.8
  - ptosis (eyelid) Q10.0
  - specified NEC Q15.8
- eyebrow Q18.8
- eyelid Q10.3
  - ptosis Q10.0
- face Q18.9
  - bone(s) Q75.9
- fallopian tube Q50.6
- fascia Q79.9
- femur NEC Q74.2
- fibula NEC Q74.2
- finger Q74.0
- fixation, intestine Q43.3
- flexion (joint) NOS Q74.9
  - hip or thigh Q65.89
- foot NEC Q74.2
  - varus (congenital) Q66.3- ☑
- foramen
  - Botalli Q21.12
  - ovale Q21.12
- forearm Q74.0
- forehead Q75.8
- form, teeth K00.2
- fovea centralis Q14.1
- frontal bone — see Anomaly, skull
- gallbladder (position) (shape) (size) Q44.1
- Gartner's duct Q52.4
- gastrointestinal tract Q45.9
- genitalia, genital organ(s) or system
  - female Q52.9
    - external Q52.70
    - internal NOS Q52.9
  - male Q55.9
    - hydrocele P83.5
    - specified NEC Q55.8
- genitourinary NEC
  - female Q52.9
  - male Q55.9
- Gerbode Q21.0
- glottis Q31.8
- granulation or granulocyte, genetic (constitutional) (leukocyte) D72.0
- gum Q38.6
- gyri Q07.9
- hair Q84.2
- hand Q74.0
- hard tissue formation in pulp K04.3
- head — see Anomaly, skull
- heart Q24.9
  - auricle Q20.8
  - bands or folds Q24.8
  - fibroelastosis cordis I42.4
  - obstructive NEC Q22.6
  - patent ductus arteriosus (Botalli) Q25.0
  - septum Q21.9
    - auricular Q21.19
    - interatrial Q21.19
    - interventricular Q21.0
      - with pulmonary stenosis or atresia, dextraposition of aorta and hypertrophy of right ventricle Q21.3
    - specified NEC Q21.8
    - ventricular Q21.0
      - with pulmonary stenosis or atresia, dextraposition of aorta and hypertrophy of right ventricle Q21.3
  - tetralogy of Fallot Q21.3
  - valve NEC Q24.8
    - aortic
      - bicuspid valve Q23.81
        - functional, with stenosis — see Stenosis, aortic (valve)
      - insufficiency Q23.1

Anomaly, anomalous — continued
- heart — continued
  - valve — continued
    - aortic — continued
      - stenosis Q23.0
        - subaortic Q24.4
    - mitral
      - insufficiency Q23.3
      - stenosis Q23.2
    - pulmonary Q22.3
      - atresia Q22.0
      - insufficiency Q22.2
      - stenosis Q22.1
        - infundibular Q24.3
        - subvalvular Q24.3
    - tricuspid
      - atresia Q22.4
      - stenosis Q22.4
  - ventricle Q20.8
- heel NEC Q74.2
- Hegglin's D72.0
- hemianencephaly Q00.0
- hemicephaly Q00.0
- hemicrania Q00.0
- hepatic duct Q44.5
- hip NEC Q74.2
- hourglass stomach Q40.2
- humerus Q74.0
- hydatid of Morgagni
  - female Q50.5
  - male (epididymal) Q55.4
  - testicular Q55.29
- hymen Q52.4
- hypersegmentation of neutrophils, hereditary D72.0
- hypophyseal Q89.2
- ileocecal (coil) (valve) Q43.9
- ileum Q43.9
- ilium NEC Q74.2
- integument Q84.9
  - specified NEC Q84.8
- interarch distance (excessive) (inadequate) M26.25
- intervertebral cartilage or disc Q76.49
- intestine (large) (small) Q43.9
  - with anomalous adhesions, fixation or malrotation Q43.3
- iris Q13.2
- ischium NEC Q74.2
- jaw — see Anomaly, dentofacial
  - alveolar — see Anomaly, alveolar
- jaw-cranial base relationship — see Anomaly, dentofacial, jaw-cranial base relationship
- jejunum Q43.8
- joint Q74.9
  - specified NEC Q74.8
- Jordan's D72.0
- kidney(s) (calyx) (pelvis) Q63.9
  - artery Q27.2
  - specified NEC Q63.8
- Klippel-Feil (brevicollis) Q76.1
- knee Q74.1
- labium (majus) (minus) Q52.70
- labyrinth, membranous Q16.5
- lacrimal apparatus or duct Q10.6
- larynx, laryngeal (muscle) Q31.9
  - web (bed) Q31.0
- lens Q12.9
- leukocytes, genetic D72.0
  - granulation (constitutional) D72.0
- lid (fold) Q10.3
- ligament Q79.9
  - broad Q50.6
  - round Q52.8
- limb Q74.9
  - lower NEC Q74.2
    - reduction deformity — see Defect, reduction, lower limb
  - upper Q74.0
- lip Q38.0
- liver Q44.70
  - duct Q44.5
- lower limb NEC Q74.2
- lumbosacral (joint) (region) Q76.49
  - kyphosis — see Kyphosis, congenital
  - lordosis — see Lordosis, congenital
- lung (fissure) (lobe) Q33.9
- mandible — see Anomaly, dentofacial
- maxilla — see Anomaly, dentofacial
- May (-Hegglin) D72.0
- meatus urinarius NEC Q64.79

Anomaly, anomalous — *continued*
- meningeal bands or folds Q07.9
  - constriction of Q07.8
  - spinal Q06.9
- meninges Q07.9
  - cerebral Q04.8
  - spinal Q06.9
- meningocele Q05.9
- mesentery Q45.9
- metacarpus Q74.0
- metatarsus NEC Q74.2
- middle ear Q16.4
  - ossicles Q16.3
- mitral (leaflets) (valve) Q23.9
  - cleft Q23.82
  - insufficiency Q23.3
  - specified NEC Q23.88
  - stenosis Q23.2
- mouth Q38.6
- Mullerian — *see also* Anomaly, by site
  - uterus NEC Q51.818
- multiple NEC Q89.7
- muscle Q79.9
  - eyelid Q10.3
- musculoskeletal system, except limbs Q79.9
- myocardium Q24.8
- nail Q84.6
- narrowness, eyelid Q10.3
- nasal sinus (wall) Q30.8
- neck (any part) Q18.9
- nerve Q07.9
  - acoustic Q07.8
  - optic Q07.8
- nervous system (central) Q07.9
- nipple Q83.9
- nose, nasal (bones) (cartilage) (septum) (sinus) Q30.9
  - specified NEC Q30.8
- ocular muscle Q15.8
- omphalomesenteric duct Q43.0
- opening, pulmonary veins Q26.4
- optic
  - disc Q14.2
  - nerve Q07.8
- opticociliary vessels Q13.2
- orbit (eye) Q10.7
- organ Q89.9
  - of Corti Q16.5
- origin
  - artery
    - innominate Q25.8
    - pulmonary Q25.79
    - renal Q27.2
    - subclavian Q25.48
- osseous meatus (ear) Q16.1
- ovary Q50.39
- oviduct Q50.6
- palate (hard) (soft) NEC Q38.5
- pancreas or pancreatic duct Q45.3
- papillary muscles Q24.8
- parathyroid gland Q89.2
- paraurethral ducts Q64.79
- parotid (gland) Q38.4
- patella Q74.1
- Pelger-Huet (hereditary hyposegmentation) D72.0
- pelvic girdle NEC Q74.2
- pelvis (bony) NEC Q74.2
  - rachitic E64.3
- penis (glans) Q55.69
- pericardium Q24.8
- peripheral vascular system Q27.9
- Peter's Q13.4
- pharynx Q38.8
- pigmentation L81.9
  - congenital Q82.8
- pituitary (gland) Q89.2
- pleural (folds) Q34.0
- portal vein Q26.5
  - connection Q26.5
- position, tooth, teeth, fully erupted M26.30
  - specified NEC M26.39
- precerebral vessel Q28.1
- prepuce Q55.69
- prostate Q55.4
- pulmonary Q33.9
  - artery NEC Q25.79
  - valve Q22.3
    - atresia Q22.0
    - insufficiency Q22.2
    - specified type NEC Q22.3

Anomaly, anomalous — *continued*
- pulmonary — *continued*
  - valve — *continued*
    - stenosis Q22.1
      - infundibular Q24.3
      - subvalvular Q24.3
  - venous connection Q26.4
    - partial Q26.3
    - total Q26.2
- pupil Q13.2
  - function H57.00
    - anisocoria H57.02
    - Argyll Robertson pupil H57.01
    - miosis H57.03
    - mydriasis H57.04
    - specified type NEC H57.09
    - tonic pupil H57.05- ☑
- pylorus Q40.3
- radius Q74.0
- rectum Q43.9
- reduction (extremity) (limb)
  - femur (longitudinal) — *see* Defect, reduction, lower limb, longitudinal, femur
  - fibula (longitudinal) — *see* Defect, reduction, lower limb, longitudinal, fibula
  - lower limb — *see* Defect, reduction, lower limb
  - radius (longitudinal) — *see* Defect, reduction, upper limb, longitudinal, radius
  - tibia (longitudinal) — *see* Defect, reduction, lower limb, longitudinal, tibia
  - ulna (longitudinal) — *see* Defect, reduction, upper limb, longitudinal, ulna
  - upper limb — *see* Defect, reduction, upper limb
- refraction — *see* Disorder, refraction
- renal Q63.9
  - artery Q27.2
  - pelvis Q63.9
    - specified NEC Q63.8
- respiratory system Q34.9
  - specified NEC Q34.8
- retina Q14.1
- rib Q76.6
  - cervical Q76.5
- Rieger Q13.81
- rotation — *see* Malrotation
  - hip or thigh Q65.89
- round ligament Q52.8
- sacroiliac (joint) NEC Q74.2
- sacrum NEC Q76.49
  - kyphosis — *see* Kyphosis, congenital
  - lordosis — *see* Lordosis, congenital
- saddle nose, syphilitic A50.57
- salivary duct or gland Q38.4
- scapula Q74.0
- scrotum — *see* Malformation, testis and scrotum
- sebaceous gland Q82.9
- seminal vesicles Q55.4
- sense organs NEC Q07.8
- sex chromosomes NEC — *see also* Anomaly, chromosomes
  - female phenotype Q97.8
  - male phenotype Q98.9
- shoulder (girdle) (joint) Q74.0
- sigmoid (flexure) Q43.9
- simian crease Q82.8
- sinus of Valsalva Q25.49
- skeleton generalized Q78.9
- skin (appendage) Q82.9
- skull Q75.9
  - with
    - anencephaly Q00.0
    - encephalocele — *see* Encephalocele
    - hydrocephalus Q03.9
      - with spina bifida — *see* Spina bifida, by site, with hydrocephalus
    - microcephaly Q02
- specified organ or site NEC Q89.89
- spermatic cord Q55.4
- spine, spinal NEC Q76.49
  - column NEC Q76.49
    - kyphosis — *see* Kyphosis, congenital
    - lordosis — *see* Lordosis, congenital
  - cord Q06.9
  - nerve root Q07.8
- spleen Q89.09
  - agenesis Q89.01
- stenonian duct Q38.4
- sternum NEC Q76.7
- stomach Q40.3

Anomaly, anomalous — *continued*
- submaxillary gland Q38.4
- tarsus NEC Q74.2
- tendon Q79.9
- testis — *see* Malformation, testis and scrotum
- thigh NEC Q74.2
- thorax (wall) Q67.8
  - bony Q76.9
- throat Q38.8
- thumb Q74.0
- thymus gland Q89.2
- thyroid (gland) Q89.2
  - cartilage Q31.8
- tibia NEC Q74.2
  - saber A50.56
- toe Q74.2
- tongue Q38.3
- tooth, teeth K00.9
  - eruption K00.6
  - position, fully erupted M26.30
  - spacing, fully erupted M26.30
- trachea (cartilage) Q32.1
- tragus Q17.9
- tricuspid (leaflet) (valve) Q22.9
  - atresia or stenosis Q22.4
  - Ebstein's Q22.5
- Uhl's (hypoplasia of myocardium, right ventricle) Q24.8
- ulna Q74.0
- umbilical artery Q27.0
- union
  - cricoid cartilage and thyroid cartilage Q31.8
  - thyroid cartilage and hyoid bone Q31.8
  - trachea with larynx Q31.8
- upper limb Q74.0
- urachus Q64.4
- ureter Q62.8
  - obstructive NEC Q62.39
    - cecoureterocele Q62.32
    - orthotopic ureterocele Q62.31
- urethra Q64.70
  - absence Q64.5
  - double Q64.74
  - fistula to rectum Q64.73
  - obstructive Q64.39
    - stricture Q64.32
  - prolapse Q64.71
  - specified type NEC Q64.79
- urinary tract Q64.9
- uterus Q51.9
  - with only one functioning horn Q51.4
- uvula Q38.5
- vagina Q52.4
- valleculae Q31.8
- valve (heart) NEC Q24.8
  - coronary sinus Q24.5
  - inferior vena cava Q24.8
  - pulmonary Q22.3
  - sinus coronario Q24.5
  - venae cavae inferioris Q24.8
- vas deferens Q55.4
- vascular Q27.9
  - brain Q28.3
  - ring Q25.45
- vein(s) (peripheral) Q27.9
  - brain Q28.3
  - cerebral Q28.3
  - coronary Q24.5
  - developmental Q28.3
  - great Q26.9
    - specified NEC Q26.8
- vena cava (inferior) (superior) Q26.9
- venous — *see* Anomaly, vein(s)
- venous return Q26.8
- ventricular
  - bands or folds Q24.8
  - septa Q21.0
- vertebra Q76.49
  - kyphosis — *see* Kyphosis, congenital
  - lordosis — *see* Lordosis, congenital
- vesicourethral orifice Q64.79
- vessel(s) Q27.9
  - optic papilla Q14.2
  - precerebral Q28.1
- vitelline duct Q43.0
- vitreous body or humor Q14.0
- vulva Q52.70
- wrist (joint) Q74.0

Anomia R48.8

Anonychia (congenital) Q84.3

Anonychia — *continued*
  acquired L60.8
Anophthalmos, anophthalmus (congenital) (globe) Q11.1
  acquired Z90.01
Anopia, anopsia H53.46- ☑
  quadrant H53.46- ☑
Anorchia, anorchism, anorchidism Q55.0
Anorexia R63.0
  hysterical F44.89
  nervosa F50.00
    atypical F50.9
    binge-eating type F50.2- ☑
      with purging F50.02- ☑
    restricting type F50.01- ☑
Anorgasmy, psychogenic (female) F52.31
  male F52.32
Anosmia R43.0
  hysterical F44.6
  postinfectional J39.8
Anosognosia R41.85
Anosteoplasia Q78.9
Anovulatory cycle N97.0
Anoxemia R09.02
  newborn P84
Anoxia (pathological) R09.02
  altitude T70.29- ☑
  cerebral G93.1
    complicating
      anesthesia (general) (local) or other sedation T88.59- ☑
        in labor and delivery O74.3
        in-pregnancy O29.21- ☑
        postpartum, puerperal O89.2
        delivery (cesarean) (instrumental) O75.4
      during a procedure G97.81
      newborn P84
      resulting from a procedure G97.82
    due to
      drowning T75.1- ☑
      high altitude T70.29- ☑
    heart — *see* Insufficiency, coronary
    intrauterine P84
    myocardial — *see* Insufficiency, coronary
    newborn P84
    spinal cord G95.11
    systemic (by suffocation) (low content in atmosphere) — *see* Asphyxia, traumatic
Anteflexion — *see* Anteversion
Antenatal
  care (normal pregnancy) Z34.90
  screening (encounter for) of mother — *see also* Encounter, antenatal screening Z36.9
Antepartum — *see* condition
Anterior — *see* condition
Antero-occlusion M26.220
Anteversion
  cervix — *see* Anteversion, uterus
  femur (neck), congenital Q65.89
  uterus, uterine (cervix) (postinfectional) (postpartal, old) N85.4
    congenital Q51.818
    in pregnancy or childbirth — *see* Pregnancy, complicated by
Anthophobia F40.228
Anthracosilicosis J60
Anthracosis (lung) (occupational) J60
  lingua K14.3
Anthrax A22.9
  with pneumonia A22.1
  cerebral A22.8
  colitis A22.2
  cutaneous A22.0
  gastrointestinal A22.2
  inhalation A22.1
  intestinal A22.2
  meningitis A22.8
  pulmonary A22.1
  respiratory A22.1
  sepsis A22.7
  specified manifestation NEC A22.8
Anthropoid pelvis Q74.2
  with disproportion (fetopelvic) O33.3
Anthropophobia F40.10
  generalized F40.11
Antibodies, maternal (blood group) — *see* Isoimmunization, affecting management of pregnancy
  anti-D — *see* Isoimmunization, affecting management of pregnancy, Rh

Antibodies, maternal — *continued*
  anti-D — *see* Isoimmunization, affecting management of pregnancy, Rh — *continued*
    newborn P55.0
Antibody
  anticardiolipin R76.0
    with
      hemorrhagic disorder D68.312
      hypercoagulable state D68.61
  antiphosphatidylglycerol R76.0
    with
      hemorrhagic disorder D68.312
      hypercoagulable state D68.61
  antiphosphatidylinositol R76.0
    with
      hemorrhagic disorder D68.312
      hypercoagulable state D68.61
  antiphosphatidylserine R76.0
    with
      hemorrhagic disorder D68.312
      hypercoagulable state D68.61
  antiphospholipid R76.0
    with
      hemorrhagic disorder D68.312
      hypercoagulable state D68.61
Anticardiolipin syndrome D68.61
Anticoagulant, circulating (intrinsic) — *see also* Disorder, hemorrhagic D68.318
  drug-induced (extrinsic) — *see also* Disorder, hemorrhagic D68.32
  iatrogenic D68.32
Antidiuretic hormone syndrome E22.2
Antimonial cholera — *see* Poisoning, antimony
Antiphospholipid
  antibody
    with hemorrhagic disorder D68.312
  syndrome D68.61
Antisocial personality F60.2
Antithrombinemia — *see* Circulating anticoagulants
Antithromboplastinemia D68.318
Antithromboplastinogenemia D68.318
Antitoxin complication or reaction — *see* Complications, vaccination
Antlophobia F40.228
Antritis J32.0
  maxilla J32.0
    acute J01.00
    recurrent J01.01
  stomach K29.50
    with bleeding K29.51
Antrum, antral — *see* condition
Anuria R34
  calculous (impacted) (recurrent) — *see also* Calculus, urinary N20.9
  following
    abortion — *see* Abortion by type complicated by, renal failure
    ectopic or molar pregnancy O08.4
  newborn P96.0
  postprocedural N99.0
  postrenal N13.8
  puerperal O90.49
  traumatic (following crushing) T79.5- ☑
Anus, anal — *see* condition
Anusitis K62.89
Anxiety F41.9
  depression F41.8
  episodic paroxysmal F41.0
  generalized F41.1
  hysteria F41.8
  neurosis F41.1
  panic type F41.0
  reaction F41.1
  separation, abnormal (of childhood) F93.0
  specified NEC F41.8
  state F41.1
Aorta, aortic — *see* condition
Aortectasia — *see* Ectasia, aorta
  with aneurysm — *see* Aneurysm, aorta
Aortitis (nonsyphilitic) (calcific) I77.6
  arteriosclerotic I70.0
  Doehle-Heller A52.02
  luetic A52.02
  rheumatic — *see* Endocarditis, acute, rheumatic
  specific (syphilitic) A52.02
  syphilitic A52.02
    congenital A50.54 *[I79.1]*
Apathetic thyroid storm — *see* Thyrotoxicosis
Apathy R45.3

Apeirophobia F40.228
Apepsia K30
  psychogenic F45.8
Aperistalsis, esophagus K22.0
Apertognathia M26.29
Apert's syndrome Q87.0
Aphagia R13.0
  psychogenic F50.9
Aphakia (acquired) (postoperative) H27.0- ☑
  congenital Q12.3
Aphasia (amnestic) (global) (nominal) (semantic) (syntactic) R47.01
  acquired, with epilepsy (Landau-Kleffner syndrome) — *see* Epilepsy, specified NEC
  auditory (developmental) F80.2
  developmental (receptive type) F80.2
    expressive type F80.1
    Wernicke's F80.2
  following
    cerebrovascular disease I69.920
      cerebral infarction I69.320
      intracerebral hemorrhage I69.120
      nontraumatic intracranial hemorrhage NEC I69.220
      specified disease NEC I69.820
      subarachnoid hemorrhage I69.020
    primary progressive — *see also* Dementia, in, diseases specified elsewhere G31.01 *[F02.80]*
      with behavioral disturbance — *see also* Dementia, in, diseases specified elsewhere G31.01 *[F02.81-]* ☑
    progressive isolated — *see also* Dementia, in, diseases specified elsewhere G31.01 *[F02.80]*
      with behavioral disturbance — *see also* Dementia, in, diseases specified elsewhere G31.01 *[F02.81-]* ☑
  sensory F80.2
  syphilis, tertiary A52.19
  Wernicke's (developmental) F80.2
Aphonia (organic) R49.1
  hysterical F44.4
  psychogenic F44.4
Aphthae, aphthous — *see also* condition
  Bednar's K12.0
  cachectic K14.0
  epizootic B08.8
  fever B08.8
  oral (recurrent) K12.0
  stomatitis (major) (minor) K12.0
  thrush B37.0
  ulcer (oral) (recurrent) K12.0
    genital organ(s) NEC
      female N76.6
      male N50.89
    larynx J38.7
Apical — *see* condition
Apiphobia F40.218
APL (acquired partial lipodystrophy) E88.11
Aplasia — *see also* Agenesis
  abdominal muscle syndrome Q79.4
  alveolar process (acquired) — *see* Anomaly, alveolar
    congenital Q38.6
  aorta (congenital) Q25.41
  axialis extracorticalis (congenita) E75.29
  bone marrow (myeloid) D61.9
    congenital D61.01
  brain Q00.0
    part of Q04.3
  bronchus Q32.4
  cementum K00.4
  cerebellum Q04.3
  cervix (congenital) Q51.5
  congenital pure red cell D61.01
  corpus callosum Q04.0
  cutis congenita Q84.8
  erythrocyte congenital D61.01
  extracortical axial E75.29
  eye Q11.1
  fovea centralis (congenital) Q14.1
  gallbladder, congenital Q44.0
  iris Q13.1
  labyrinth, membranous Q16.5
  limb (congenital) Q73.8
    lower — *see* Defect, reduction, lower limb
    upper — *see* Agenesis, arm
  lung, congenital (bilateral) (unilateral) Q33.3
  pancreas Q45.0
  parathyroid-thymic D82.1
  Pelizaeus-Merzbacher E75.27
  penis Q55.5

Aplasia — continued
prostate Q55.4
red cell (with thymoma) D60.9
- acquired D60.9
- due to drugs D60.9
- adult D60.9
- chronic D60.0
- congenital D61.01
- constitutional D61.01
- due to drugs D60.9
- hereditary D61.01
- of infants D61.01
- primary D61.01
- pure D61.01
  - due to drugs D60.9
- specified type NEC D60.8
- transient D60.1
round ligament Q52.8
skin Q84.8
spermatic cord Q55.4
spleen Q89.01
testicle Q55.0
thymic, with immunodeficiency D82.1
thyroid (congenital) (with myxedema) E03.1
uterus Q51.0
ventral horn cell Q06.1

Apnea, apneic (of) (spells) R06.81
newborn P28.40
- central P28.41
- mixed P28.43
- obstructive P28.42
- sleep
  - primary P28.30
    - central P28.31
    - mixed P28.33
    - obstructive P28.32
    - specified NEC P28.39
- specified NEC P28.49
prematurity P28.49
sleep G47.30
- central (primary) G47.31
  - idiopathic G47.31
  - in conditions classified elsewhere G47.37
- obstructive (adult) (pediatric) G47.33
  - hypopnea G47.33
- primary central G47.31
- specified NEC G47.39

Apneumatosis, newborn P28.0
Apocrine metaplasia (breast) — see Dysplasia, mammary, specified type NEC
Apophysitis (bone) — see also Osteochondropathy
- calcaneus M92.6- ☑
- juvenile M92.9

Apoplectiform convulsions (cerebral ischemia) I67.82
Apoplexy, apoplectic
adrenal A39.1
heart (auricle) (ventricle) — see Infarct, myocardium
heat T67.01- ☑
hemorrhagic (stroke) — see Hemorrhage, intracranial
meninges, hemorrhagic — see Hemorrhage, intracranial, subarachnoid
uremic N18.9 [I68.8]

Appearance
bizarre R46.1
specified NEC R46.89
very low level of personal hygiene R46.0

Appendage
epididymal (organ of Morgagni) Q55.4
intestine (epiploic) Q43.8
preauricular Q17.0
testicular (organ of Morgagni) Q55.29

Appendicitis (pneumococcal) (retrocecal) K37
with
- gangrene K35.891
  - with localized peritonitis K35.31
- perforation NOS K35.32
- peritoneal abscess K35.33
- peritonitis NEC K35.33
  - generalized K35.209
    - with
      - abscess K35.219
        - with perforation or rupture K35.211
        - following rupture or perforation of appendix NOS K35.211
        - without perforation or rupture K35.210
      - perforation or rupture K35.201
      - following rupture or perforation of appendix NOS K35.201

Appendicitis — continued
with — continued
- peritonitis — continued
  - generalized — continued
    - without rupture or perforation of appendix K35.200
  - localized K35.30
    - with
      - gangrene K35.31
      - perforation K35.32
        - and abscess K35.33
      - rupture (with localized peritonitis) K35.32
acute (catarrhal) (fulminating) (obstructive) (retrocecal) (suppurative) K35.80
- with
  - gangrene K35.891
  - peritoneal abscess K35.33
  - peritonitis NEC K35.33
    - generalized K35.209
      - with
        - abscess K35.219
          - with perforation or rupture K35.211
          - following rupture or perforation of appendix NOS K35.211
          - without perforation or rupture K35.210
        - perforation or rupture K35.201
        - following rupture or perforation of appendix NOS K35.201
        - without rupture or perforation of appendix K35.200
    - localized K35.30
      - with
        - gangrene K35.31
        - perforation K35.32
          - and abscess K35.33
  - specified NEC K35.890
    - with gangrene K35.891
      - with localized peritonitis K35.31
amebic A06.89
chronic (recurrent) K36
exacerbation — see Appendicitis, with, gangrene
gangrenous — see Appendicitis, acute
healed (obliterative) K36
interval K36
neurogenic K36
obstructive K36
recurrent K36
relapsing K36
ruptured NOS (with localized peritonitis) K35.32
subacute (adhesive) K36
subsiding K36
suppurative — see Appendicitis, acute
tuberculous A18.32

Appendicopathia oxyurica B80
Appendix, appendicular — see also condition
epididymis Q55.4
Morgagni
- female Q50.5
- male (epididymal) Q55.4
- testicular Q55.29
testis Q55.29

Appetite
depraved — see Pica
excessive R63.2
lack or loss — see also Anorexia R63.0
- nonorganic origin F50.89
- psychogenic F50.89
perverted (hysterical) — see Pica

Apple peel syndrome Q41.1
Apprehension state F41.1
Apprehensiveness, abnormal F41.9
Approximal wear K03.0
Apraxia (classic) (ideational) (ideokinetic) (ideomotor) (motor) (verbal) R48.2
following
- cerebrovascular disease I69.990
  - cerebral infarction I69.390
  - intracerebral hemorrhage I69.190
  - nontraumatic intracranial hemorrhage NEC I69.290
  - specified disease NEC I69.890
  - subarachnoid hemorrhage I69.090
oculomotor, congenital H51.8
primary progressive, of speech G31.87

Aptyalism K11.7
Apudoma — see Neoplasm, uncertain behavior, by site
Aqueous misdirection H40.83- ☑
Arabicum elephantiasis — see Infestation, filarial
Arachnitis — see Meningitis

Arachnodactyly — see Syndrome, Marfan
Arachnoiditis (acute) (adhesive) (basal) (brain) (cerebrospinal) — see Meningitis
Arachnophobia F40.210
Arboencephalitis, Australian A83.4
Arborization block (heart) I45.5
ARC (AIDS-related complex) B20
Arc-welder's lung J63.4
Arch
aortic Q25.49
bovine Q25.49
Arches — see condition
Arcuate uterus Q51.810
Arcuatus uterus Q51.810
Arcus (cornea) senilis — see Degeneration, cornea, senile
Areflexia R29.2
Areola — see condition
Argentaffinoma — see also Neoplasm, uncertain behavior, by site
malignant — see Neoplasm, malignant, by site
syndrome E34.09
Argininemia E72.21
Arginosuccinic aciduria E72.22
Argyll Robertson phenomenon, pupil or syndrome (syphilitic) A52.19
atypical H57.09
nonsyphilitic H57.09
Argyria, argyriasis
conjunctival H11.13- ☑
from drug or medicament — see Table of Drugs and Chemicals, by substance
Argyrosis, conjunctival H11.13- ☑
Arhinencephaly Q04.1
Ariboflavinosis E53.0
Arm — see condition
Arnold-Chiari disease, obstruction or syndrome (type II) Q07.00
with
- hydrocephalus Q07.02
  - with spina bifida Q07.03
- spina bifida Q07.01
  - with hydrocephalus Q07.03
type III — see Encephalocele
type IV Q04.8
Aromatic amino-acid metabolism disorder E70.9
specified NEC E70.89
Arousals, confusional G47.51
Arrest, arrested
cardiac I46.9
- complicating
  - abortion — see Abortion, by type, complicated by, cardiac arrest
  - anesthesia (general) (local) or other sedation — see Table of Drugs and Chemicals, by drug
    - in labor and delivery O74.2
    - in pregnancy O29.11- ☑
    - postpartum, puerperal O89.1
  - delivery (cesarean) (instrumental) O75.4
- due to
  - cardiac condition I46.2
  - specified condition NEC I46.8
- intraoperative I97.71- ☑
- newborn P29.81
- personal history, successfully resuscitated Z86.74
- postprocedural I97.12- ☑
  - obstetric procedure O75.4
cardiorespiratory — see Arrest, cardiac
circulatory — see Arrest, cardiac
deep transverse O64.0- ☑
development or growth
- bone — see Disorder, bone, development or growth
- child R62.50
- tracheal rings Q32.1
epiphyseal
- complete
  - femur M89.15- ☑
  - humerus M89.12- ☑
  - tibia M89.16- ☑
  - ulna M89.13- ☑
- forearm M89.13- ☑
  - specified NEC M89.13- ☑
  - ulna — see Arrest, epiphyseal, by type, ulna
- lower leg M89.16- ☑
  - specified NEC M89.168
  - tibia — see Arrest, epiphyseal, by type, tibia
- partial
  - femur M89.15- ☑
  - humerus M89.12- ☑

Arrest, arrested — *continued*
　epiphyseal — *continued*
　　partial — *continued*
　　　tibia M89.16- ☑
　　　ulna M89.13- ☑
　　　specified NEC M89.18
　granulopoiesis — *see* Agranulocytosis
　growth plate — *see* Arrest, epiphyseal
　heart — *see* Arrest, cardiac
　legal, anxiety concerning Z65.3
　physeal — *see* Arrest, epiphyseal
　respiratory R09.2
　　newborn P28.81
　sinus I45.5
　spermatogenesis (complete) — *see* Azoospermia
　　incomplete — *see* Oligospermia
　transverse (deep) O64.0- ☑
Arrhenoblastoma
　benign
　　specified site — *see* Neoplasm, benign, by site
　　unspecified site
　　　female D27.9
　　　male D29.20
　malignant
　　specified site — *see* Neoplasm, malignant, by site
　　unspecified site
　　　female C56.9
　　　male C62.90
　specified site — *see* Neoplasm, uncertain behavior, by site
　unspecified site
　　female D39.10
　　male D40.10
Arrhythmia (auricle) (cardiac) (juvenile) (nodal) (reflex) (supraventricular) (transitory) (ventricle) I49.9
　block I45.9
　extrasystolic I49.49
　newborn
　　bradycardia P29.12
　　　occurring before birth P03.819
　　　　before onset of labor P03.810
　　　　during labor P03.811
　　tachycardia P29.11
　psychogenic F45.8
　sinus I49.8
　specified NEC I49.8
　vagal R55
　ventricular re-entry I47.0
Arrillaga-Ayerza syndrome (pulmonary sclerosis with pulmonary hypertension) I27.0
Arsenical pigmentation L81.8
　from drug or medicament — *see* Table of Drugs and Chemicals
Arsenism — *see* Poisoning, arsenic
Arterial — *see* condition
Arteriofibrosis — *see* Arteriosclerosis
Arteriolar sclerosis — *see* Arteriosclerosis
Arteriolith — *see* Arteriosclerosis
Arteriolitis I77.6
　necrotizing, kidney I77.5
　renal — *see* Hypertension, kidney
Arteriolosclerosis — *see* Arteriosclerosis
Arterionephrosclerosis — *see* Hypertension, kidney
Arteriopathy I77.9
　cerebral autosomal dominant, with subcortical infarcts and leukoencephalopathy (CADASIL) I67.850
Arteriosclerosis, arteriosclerotic (diffuse) (obliterans) (of) (senile) (with calcification) I70.90
　with
　　chronic limb-threatening ischemia — *see* Arteriosclerosis, with critical limb ischemia
　　critical limb ischemia
　　　bypass graft I70.329
　　　　autologous vein graft I70.429
　　　　　leg I70.429
　　　　　　with
　　　　　　　gangrene (and intermittent claudication, rest pain, and ulcer) I70.469
　　　　　　　rest pain (and intermittent claudication) I70.429
　　　　　　bilateral I70.423
　　　　　　　with
　　　　　　　　gangrene (and intermittent claudication, rest pain, and ulcer) I70.463
　　　　　　　　rest pain (and intermittent claudication) I70.423
　　　　　　　left I70.422

Arteriosclerosis, arteriosclerotic — *continued*
　with — *continued*
　　critical limb ischemia — *continued*
　　　bypass graft — *continued*
　　　　autologous vein graft — *continued*
　　　　　leg — *continued*
　　　　　　left — *continued*
　　　　　　　with
　　　　　　　　gangrene (and intermittent claudication, rest pain, and ulcer) I70.462
　　　　　　　　rest pain (and intermittent claudication) I70.422
　　　　　　　　ulceration (and intermittent claudication and rest pain) I70.449
　　　　　　　　　ankle I70.443
　　　　　　　　　calf I70.442
　　　　　　　　　foot site NEC I70.445
　　　　　　　　　heel I70.444
　　　　　　　　　lower leg NEC I70.448
　　　　　　　　　mid foot I70.444
　　　　　　　　　thigh I70.441
　　　　　　right I70.421
　　　　　　　with
　　　　　　　　gangrene (and intermittent claudication, rest pain, and ulcer) I70.461
　　　　　　　　rest pain (and intermittent claudication) I70.421
　　　　　　　　ulceration (and intermittent claudication and rest pain) I70.439
　　　　　　　　　ankle I70.433
　　　　　　　　　calf I70.432
　　　　　　　　　foot site NEC I70.435
　　　　　　　　　heel I70.434
　　　　　　　　　lower leg NEC I70.438
　　　　　　　　　midfoot I70.434
　　　　　　　　　thigh I70.431
　　　　　leg I70.329
　　　　　　with
　　　　　　　gangrene (and intermittent claudication, rest pain, and ulcer) I70.369
　　　　　　　rest pain (and intermittent claudication) I70.329
　　　　　　bilateral I70.323
　　　　　　　with
　　　　　　　　gangrene (and intermittent claudication, rest pain, and ulcer) I70.363
　　　　　　　　rest pain (and intermittent claudication) I70.323
　　　　　　left I70.322
　　　　　　　with
　　　　　　　　gangrene (and intermittent claudication, rest pain, and ulcer) I70.362
　　　　　　　　rest pain (and intermittent claudication) I70.322
　　　　　　　　ulceration (and intermittent claudication and rest pain) I70.349
　　　　　　　　　ankle I70.343
　　　　　　　　　calf I70.342
　　　　　　　　　foot site NEC I70.345
　　　　　　　　　heel I70.344
　　　　　　　　　lower leg NEC I70.348
　　　　　　　　　midfoot I70.344
　　　　　　　　　thigh I70.341
　　　　　　right I70.321
　　　　　　　with
　　　　　　　　gangrene (and intermittent claudication, rest pain, and ulcer) I70.361
　　　　　　　　rest pain (and intermittent claudication) I70.321
　　　　　　　　ulceration (and intermittent claudication and rest pain) I70.339
　　　　　　　　　ankle I70.333
　　　　　　　　　calf I70.332
　　　　　　　　　foot site NEC I70.335
　　　　　　　　　heel I70.334
　　　　　　　　　lower leg NEC I70.338
　　　　　　　　　midfoot I70.334
　　　　　　　　　thigh I70.331
　　　　nonautologous biological graft I70.529
　　　　　leg I70.529

Arteriosclerosis, arteriosclerotic — *continued*
　with — *continued*
　　critical limb ischemia — *continued*
　　　bypass graft — *continued*
　　　　nonautologous biological graft — *continued*
　　　　　leg — *continued*
　　　　　　with
　　　　　　　gangrene (and intermittent claudication, rest pain, and ulcer) I70.569
　　　　　　　rest pain (and intermittent claudication) I70.529
　　　　　　bilateral I70.523
　　　　　　　with
　　　　　　　　gangrene (and intermittent claudication, rest pain, and ulcer) I70.563
　　　　　　　　rest pain (and intermittent claudication) I70.523
　　　　　　left I70.522
　　　　　　　with
　　　　　　　　gangrene (and intermittent claudication, rest pain, and ulcer) I70.562
　　　　　　　　rest pain (and intermittent claudication) I70.522
　　　　　　　　ulceration (and intermittent claudication and rest pain) I70.549
　　　　　　　　　ankle I70.543
　　　　　　　　　calf I70.542
　　　　　　　　　foot site NEC I70.545
　　　　　　　　　heel I70.544
　　　　　　　　　lower leg NEC I70.548
　　　　　　　　　midfoot I70.544
　　　　　　　　　thigh I70.541
　　　　　　right I70.521
　　　　　　　with
　　　　　　　　gangrene (and intermittent claudication, rest pain, and ulcer) I70.561
　　　　　　　　rest pain (and intermittent claudication) I70.521
　　　　　　　　ulceration (and intermittent claudication and rest pain) I70.539
　　　　　　　　　ankle I70.533
　　　　　　　　　calf I70.532
　　　　　　　　　foot site NEC I70.535
　　　　　　　　　heel I70.534
　　　　　　　　　lower leg NEC I70.538
　　　　　　　　　midfoot I70.534
　　　　　　　　　thigh I70.531
　　　　nonbiological graft I70.629
　　　　　leg I70.629
　　　　　　with
　　　　　　　gangrene (and intermittent claudication, rest pain, and ulcer) I70.669
　　　　　　　rest pain (and intermittent claudication) I70.629
　　　　　　bilateral I70.623
　　　　　　　with
　　　　　　　　gangrene (and intermittent claudication, rest pain, and ulcer) I70.663
　　　　　　　　rest pain (intermittent claudication) I70.623
　　　　　　left I70.622
　　　　　　　with
　　　　　　　　gangrene (and intermittent claudication, rest pain, and ulcer) I70.662
　　　　　　　　rest pain (and intermittent claudication) I70.622
　　　　　　　　ulceration (and intermittent claudication and rest pain) I70.649
　　　　　　　　　ankle I70.643
　　　　　　　　　calf I70.642
　　　　　　　　　foot site NEC I70.645
　　　　　　　　　heel I70.644
　　　　　　　　　lower leg NEC I70.648
　　　　　　　　　midfoot I70.644
　　　　　　　　　thigh I70.641
　　　　　　right I70.621

Arteriosclerosis, arteriosclerotic — *continued*
  with — *continued*
    critical limb ischemia — *continued*
      bypass graft — *continued*
        nonbiological graft — *continued*
          leg — *continued*
            right — *continued*
              with
                gangrene (and intermittent claudication, rest pain, and ulcer) I70.661
                rest pain (and intermittent claudication) I70.621
                ulceration (and intermittent claudication and rest pain) I70.639
                  ankle I70.633
                  calf I70.632
                  foot site NEC I70.635
                  heel I70.634
                  lower leg NEC I70.638
                  midfoot I70.634
                  thigh I70.631
        specified graft NEC I70.729
          leg I70.729
            with
              gangrene (and intermittent claudication, rest pain, and ulcer) I70.769
              rest pain (and intermittent claudication) I70.729
            bilateral I70.723
              with
                gangrene (and intermittent claudication, rest pain, and ulcer) I70.763
                rest pain (and intermittent claudication) I70.723
            left I70.722
              with
                gangrene (and intermittent claudication, rest pain, and ulcer) I70.762
                rest pain (and intermittent claudication) I70.722
                ulceration (and intermittent claudication and rest pain) I70.749
                  ankle I70.743
                  calf I70.742
                  foot site NEC I70.745
                  heel I70.744
                  lower leg NEC I70.748
                  midfoot I70.744
                  thigh I70.741
            right I70.721
              with
                gangrene (and intermittent claudication, rest pain, and ulcer) I70.761
                rest pain (and intermittent claudication) I70.721
                ulceration (and intermittent claudication and rest pain) I70.739
                  ankle I70.733
                  calf I70.732
                  foot site NEC I70.735
                  heel I70.734
                  lower leg NEC I70.738
                  midfoot I70.734
                  thigh I70.731
      leg I70.229
        with
          gangrene (and intermittent claudication, rest pain, and ulcer) I70.269
          rest pain (and intermittent claudication) I70.229
        bilateral I70.223
          with
            gangrene (and intermittent claudication, rest pain, and ulcer) I70.263
            rest pain (and intermittent claudication) I70.223
        left I70.222
          with
            gangrene (and intermittent claudication, rest pain, and ulcer) I70.262
            rest pain (and intermittent claudication) I70.222
            ulceration (and intermittent claudication and rest pain) I70.249
              ankle I70.243
              calf I70.242
              foot site NEC I70.245
              heel I70.244
              lower leg NEC I70.248
              midfoot I70.244
              thigh I70.241
        right I70.221
          with
            gangrene (and intermittent claudication, rest pain, and ulcer) I70.261
            rest pain (and intermittent claudication) I70.221
            ulceration (and intermittent claudication and rest pain) I70.239
              ankle I70.233
              calf I70.232
              foot site NEC I70.235
              heel I70.234
              lower leg NEC I70.238
              midfoot I70.234
              thigh I70.231
  aorta I70.0
  arteries of extremities — *see* Arteriosclerosis, extremities
    with
      chronic limb-threatening ischemia — *see* Arteriosclerosis, with critical limb ischemia
      critical limb ischemia — *see* Arteriosclerosis, with critical limb ischemia
  brain I67.2
    with infarction — *see* Occlusion, artery, brain or cerebral, with infarction
  bypass graft
    with
      chronic limb-threatening ischemia — *see* Arteriosclerosis, with critical limb ischemia
      critical limb ischemia — *see* Arteriosclerosis, with critical limb ischemia
    coronary — *see* Arteriosclerosis, coronary, bypass graft
    extremities — *see* Arteriosclerosis, extremities, bypass graft
  cardiac — *see* Disease, heart, ischemic, atherosclerotic
  cardiopathy — *see* Disease, heart, ischemic, atherosclerotic
  cardiorenal — *see* Hypertension, cardiorenal
  cardiovascular — *see* Disease, heart, ischemic, atherosclerotic
  carotid — *see also* Occlusion, artery, carotid I65.2- ☑
  central nervous system I67.2
    with infarction — *see* Occlusion, artery, cerebral or precerebral, with infarction
  cerebral I67.2
    with infarction — *see* Occlusion, artery, brain or cerebral, with infarction
  cerebrovascular I67.2
    with infarction — *see* Occlusion, artery, brain or cerebral, with infarction
  coronary (artery) I25.10
    due to
      calcified coronary lesion (severely) I25.84
      lipid rich plaque I25.83
    bypass graft I25.810
      with
        angina pectoris I25.709
          with documented spasm I25.701
          refractory I25.702
          specified type NEC I25.708
          unstable I25.700
        ischemic chest pain I25.709
      autologous artery I25.810
        with
          angina pectoris I25.729
            with documented spasm I25.721
            refractory I25.722
            specified type I25.728
            unstable I25.720
          ischemic chest pain I25.729
      autologous vein I25.810
        with
          angina pectoris I25.719
            with documented spasm I25.711
            refractory I25.712
            specified type I25.718
            unstable I25.710
          ischemic chest pain I25.719
      nonautologous biological I25.810
        with
          angina pectoris I25.739
            with documented spasm I25.731
            refractory I25.732
            specified type I25.738
            unstable I25.730
          ischemic chest pain I25.739
      specified type NEC I25.810
        with
          angina pectoris I25.799
            with documented spasm I25.791
            refractory I25.792
            specified type I25.798
            unstable I25.790
          ischemic chest pain I25.799
    native vessel
      with
        angina pectoris I25.119
          with documented spasm I25.111
          refractory I25.112
          specified type NEC I25.118
          unstable I25.110
        ischemic chest pain I25.119
    transplanted heart I25.811
      bypass graft I25.812
        with
          angina pectoris I25.769
            with documented spasm I25.761
            refractory I25.762
            specified type I25.768
            unstable I25.760
          ischemic chest pain I25.769
      native coronary artery I25.811
        with
          angina pectoris I25.759
            with documented spasm I25.751
            refractory I25.752
            specified type I25.758
            unstable I25.750
          ischemic chest pain I25.759
  extremities (native arteries) I70.209
    with
      chronic limb-threatening ischemia — *see* Arteriosclerosis, with critical limb ischemia
      critical limb ischemia — *see* Arteriosclerosis, with critical limb ischemia
    bypass graft I70.309
      with
        chronic limb-threatening ischemia — *see* Arteriosclerosis, with critical limb ischemia
        critical limb ischemia — *see* Arteriosclerosis, with critical limb ischemia
      autologous vein graft I70.409
        leg I70.409
          with
            gangrene (and intermittent claudication, rest pain and ulcer) I70.469
            intermittent claudication I70.419
            rest pain (and intermittent claudication) I70.429
        bilateral I70.403
          with
            gangrene (and intermittent claudication, rest pain and ulcer) I70.463
            intermittent claudication I70.463
            rest pain (and intermittent claudication) I70.423
          specified type NEC I70.493
        left I70.402
          with
            gangrene (and intermittent claudication, rest pain and ulcer) I70.462
            intermittent claudication I70.412
            rest pain (and intermittent claudication) I70.422

Arteriosclerosis, arteriosclerotic — *continued*
  extremities — *continued*
    bypass graft — *continued*
      autologous vein graft — *continued*
        leg — *continued*
          left — *continued*
            with — *continued*
              ulceration (and intermittent claudication and rest pain) I70.449
                ankle I70.443
                calf I70.442
                foot site NEC I70.445
                heel I70.444
                lower leg NEC I70.448
                midfoot I70.444
                thigh I70.441
            specified type NEC I70.492
          right I70.401
            with
              gangrene (and intermittent claudication, rest pain and ulcer) I70.461
              intermittent claudication I70.411
              rest pain (and intermittent claudication) I70.421
              ulceration (and intermittent claudication and rest pain) I70.439
                ankle I70.433
                calf I70.432
                foot site NEC I70.435
                heel I70.434
                lower leg NEC I70.438
                midfoot I70.434
                thigh I70.431
            specified type NEC I70.491
          specified type NEC I70.499
        specified NEC I70.408
          with
            gangrene (and intermittent claudication, rest pain and ulcer) I70.468
            intermittent claudication I70.418
            rest pain (and intermittent claudication) I70.428
            ulceration (and intermittent claudication and rest pain) I70.45
          specified type NEC I70.498
        leg I70.309
          with
            gangrene (and intermittent claudication, rest pain and ulcer) I70.369
            intermittent claudication I70.319
            rest pain (and intermittent claudication) I70.329
          bilateral I70.303
            with
              gangrene (and intermittent claudication, rest pain and ulcer) I70.363
              intermittent claudication I70.313
              rest pain (and intermittent claudication) I70.323
            specified type NEC I70.393
          left I70.302
            with
              gangrene (and intermittent claudication, rest pain and ulcer) I70.362
              intermittent claudication I70.312
              rest pain (and intermittent claudication) I70.322
              ulceration (and intermittent claudication and rest pain) I70.349
                ankle I70.343
                calf I70.342
                foot site NEC I70.345
                heel I70.344
                lower leg NEC I70.348
                midfoot I70.344
                thigh I70.341
            specified type NEC I70.392
          right I70.301
            with
              gangrene (and intermittent claudication, rest pain and ulcer) I70.361
              intermittent claudication I70.311
              rest pain (and intermittent claudication) I70.321
              ulceration (and intermittent claudication and rest pain) I70.339
                ankle I70.333
                calf I70.332

Arteriosclerosis, arteriosclerotic — *continued*
  extremities — *continued*
    bypass graft — *continued*
      leg — *continued*
        right — *continued*
          with — *continued*
            ulceration — *continued*
              foot site NEC I70.335
              heel I70.334
              lower leg NEC I70.338
              midfoot I70.334
              thigh I70.331
          specified type NEC I70.391
        specified type NEC I70.399
      nonautologous biological graft I70.509
        leg I70.509
          with
            gangrene (and intermittent claudication, rest pain and ulcer) I70.569
            intermittent claudication I70.519
            rest pain (and intermittent claudication) I70.529
          bilateral I70.503
            with
              gangrene (and intermittent claudication, rest pain and ulcer) I70.563
              intermittent claudication I70.513
              rest pain (and intermittent claudication) I70.523
            specified type NEC I70.593
          left I70.502
            with
              gangrene (and intermittent claudication, rest pain and ulcer) I70.562
              intermittent claudication I70.512
              rest pain (and intermittent claudication) I70.522
              ulceration (and intermittent claudication and rest pain) I70.549
                ankle I70.543
                calf I70.542
                foot site NEC I70.545
                heel I70.544
                lower leg NEC I70.548
                midfoot I70.544
                thigh I70.541
            specified type NEC I70.592
          right I70.501
            with
              gangrene (and intermittent claudication, rest pain and ulcer) I70.561
              intermittent claudication I70.511
              rest pain (and intermittent claudication) I70.521
              ulceration (and intermittent claudication and rest pain) I70.539
                ankle I70.533
                calf I70.532
                foot site NEC I70.535
                heel I70.534
                lower leg NEC I70.538
                midfoot I70.534
                thigh I70.531
            specified type NEC I70.591
          specified type NEC I70.599
        specified NEC I70.508
          with
            gangrene (and intermittent claudication, rest pain and ulcer) I70.568
            intermittent claudication I70.518
            rest pain (and intermittent claudication) I70.528
            ulceration (and intermittent claudication and rest pain) I70.55
          specified type NEC I70.598
      nonbiological graft I70.609
        leg I70.609
          with
            gangrene (and intermittent claudication, rest pain and ulcer) I70.669
            intermittent claudication I70.619
            rest pain (and intermittent claudication) I70.629
          bilateral I70.603

Arteriosclerosis, arteriosclerotic — *continued*
  extremities — *continued*
    bypass graft — *continued*
      nonbiological graft — *continued*
        leg — *continued*
          bilateral — *continued*
            with
              gangrene (and intermittent claudication, rest pain and ulcer) I70.663
              intermittent claudication I70.613
              rest pain (and intermittent claudication) I70.623
            specified type NEC I70.693
          left I70.602
            with
              gangrene (and intermittent claudication, rest pain and ulcer) I70.662
              intermittent claudication I70.612
              rest pain (and intermittent claudication) I70.622
              ulceration (and intermittent claudication and rest pain) I70.649
                ankle I70.643
                calf I70.642
                foot site NEC I70.645
                heel I70.644
                lower leg NEC I70.648
                midfoot I70.644
                thigh I70.641
            specified type NEC I70.692
          right I70.601
            with
              gangrene (and intermittent claudication, rest pain and ulcer) I70.661
              intermittent claudication I70.611
              rest pain (and intermittent claudication) I70.621
              ulceration (and intermittent claudication and rest pain) I70.639
                ankle I70.633
                calf I70.632
                foot site NEC I70.635
                heel I70.634
                lower leg NEC I70.638
                midfoot I70.634
                thigh I70.631
            specified type NEC I70.691
          specified type NEC I70.699
        specified NEC I70.608
          with
            gangrene (and intermittent claudication, rest pain and ulcer) I70.668
            intermittent claudication I70.618
            rest pain (and intermittent claudication) I70.628
            ulceration (and intermittent claudication and rest pain) I70.65
          specified type NEC I70.698
      specified graft NEC I70.709
        leg I70.709
          with
            gangrene (and intermittent claudication, rest pain and ulcer) I70.769
            intermittent claudication I70.719
            rest pain (and intermittent claudication) I70.729
          bilateral I70.703
            with
              gangrene (and intermittent claudication, rest pain and ulcer) I70.763
              intermittent claudication I70.713
              rest pain (and intermittent claudication) I70.723
            specified type NEC I70.793
          left I70.702
            with
              gangrene (and intermittent claudication, rest pain and ulcer) I70.762
              intermittent claudication I70.712
              rest pain (and intermittent claudication) I70.722
              ulceration (and intermittent claudication and rest pain) I70.749
                ankle I70.743

Arteriosclerosis, arteriosclerotic — continued
- extremities — continued
  - bypass graft — continued
    - specified graft — continued
      - leg — continued
        - left — continued
          - with — continued
            - ulceration — continued
              - calf I70.742
              - foot site NEC I70.745
              - heel I70.744
              - lower leg NEC I70.748
              - midfoot I70.744
              - thigh I70.741
            - specified type NEC I70.792
        - right I70.701
          - with
            - gangrene (and intermittent claudication, rest pain and ulcer) I70.761
            - intermittent claudication I70.711
            - rest pain (and intermittent claudication) I70.721
            - ulceration (and intermittent claudication and rest pain) I70.739
              - ankle I70.733
              - calf I70.732
              - foot site NEC I70.735
              - heel I70.734
              - lower leg NEC I70.738
              - midfoot I70.734
              - thigh I70.731
            - specified type NEC I70.791
          - specified type NEC I70.799
      - specified NEC I70.708
        - with
          - gangrene (and intermittent claudication, rest pain and ulcer) I70.768
          - intermittent claudication I70.718
          - rest pain (and intermittent claudication) I70.728
          - ulceration (and intermittent claudication and rest pain) I70.75
        - specified type NEC I70.798
    - specified NEC I70.308
      - with
        - gangrene (and intermittent claudication, rest pain and ulcer) I70.368
        - intermittent claudication I70.318
        - rest pain (and intermittent claudication) I70.328
        - ulceration (and intermittent claudication and rest pain) I70.35
      - specifiec type NEC I70.398
    - leg I70.209
      - with
        - gangrene (and intermittent claudication, rest pain and ulcer) I70.269
        - intermittent claudication I70.219
        - rest pain (and intermittent claudication) I70.229
      - bilateral I70.203
        - with
          - gangrene (and intermittent claudication, rest pain and ulcer) I70.263
          - intermittent claudication I70.213
          - rest pain (and intermittent claudication) I70.223
        - specified type NEC I70.293
      - left I70.202
        - with
          - gangrene (and intermittent claudication, rest pain and ulcer) I70.262
          - intermittent claudication I70.212
          - rest pain (and intermittent claudication) I70.222
          - ulceration (and intermittent claudication and rest pain) I70.249
            - ankle I70.243
            - calf I70.242
            - foot site NEC I70.245
            - heel I70.244
            - lower leg NEC I70.248
            - midfoot I70.244
            - thigh I70.241
          - specified type NEC I70.292
        - right I70.201
          - with
            - gangrene (and intermittent claudication, rest pain and ulcer) I70.261

Arteriosclerosis, arteriosclerotic — continued
- extremities — continued
  - leg — continued
    - right — continued
      - with — continued
        - intermittent claudication I70.211
        - rest pain (and intermittent claudication) I70.221
        - ulceration (and intermittent claudication and rest pain) I70.239
          - ankle I70.233
          - calf I70.232
          - foot site NEC I70.235
          - heel I70.234
          - lower leg NEC I70.238
          - midfoot I70.234
          - thigh I70.231
        - specified type NEC I70.291
    - specified site NEC I70.208
      - with
        - gangrene (and intermittent claudication, rest pain and ulcer) I70.268
        - intermittent claudication I70.218
        - rest pain (and intermittent claudication) I70.228
        - ulceration (and intermittent claudication and rest pain) I70.25
      - specified type NEC I70.298
  - generalized I70.91
  - heart (disease) — see Arteriosclerosis, coronary (artery)
  - kidney — see Hypertension, kidney
  - medial — see Arteriosclerosis, extremities
  - mesenteric (artery) K55.1
  - Monckeberg's — see Arteriosclerosis, extremities
  - myocarditis I51.4
  - peripheral (of extremities) — see Arteriosclerosis, extremities
  - pulmonary (idiopathic) I27.0
  - renal (arterioles) — see also Hypertension, kidney
    - artery I70.1
  - retina (vascular) I70.8 [H35.0-] ☑
  - specified artery NEC I70.8
  - spinal (cord) G95.19
  - vertebral (artery) I67.2
    - with infarction — see Occlusion, artery, vertebral, with infarction

Arteriospasm I73.9
Arteriovenous — see condition
Arteritis I77.6
- allergic M31.0
- aorta (nonsyphilitic) I77.6
  - syphilitic A52.02
- aortic arch M31.4
- brachiocephalic M31.4
- brain I67.7
  - syphilitic A52.04
- cerebral I67.7
  - in systemic lupus erythematosus M32.19
  - listerial A32.89
  - syphilitic A52.04
  - tuberculous A18.89
- coronary (artery) I25.89
  - rheumatic I01.8
    - chronic I09.89
  - syphilitic A52.06
- cranial (left) (right), giant cell M31.6
- deformans — see Arteriosclerosis
- giant cell NEC M31.6
  - with polymyalgia rheumatica M31.5
- necrosing or necrotizing M31.9
  - specified NEC M31.8
- nodosa M30.0
- obliterans — see Arteriosclerosis
- pulmonary I28.8
- rheumatic — see Fever, rheumatic
- senile — see Arteriosclerosis
- suppurative I77.2
- syphilitic (general) A52.09
  - brain A52.04
  - coronary A52.06
  - spinal A52.09
- temporal, giant cell M31.6
- young female aortic arch syndrome M31.4

Artery, arterial — see also condition
- abscess I77.89
- single umbilical Q27.0

Arthralgia (allergic) — see also Pain, joint
- in caisson disease T70.3- ☑
- temporomandibular M26.62- ☑

Arthritis, arthritic (acute) (chronic) (nonpyogenic) (subacute) M19.90
- allergic — see Arthritis, specified form NEC
- ankylosing (crippling) (spine) — see also Spondylitis, ankylosing
  - sites other than spine — see Arthritis, specified form NEC
- atrophic — see Osteoarthritis
  - spine — see Spondylitis, ankylosing
- back — see Spondylopathy, inflammatory
- blennorrhagic (gonococcal) A54.42
- Charcot's — see Arthropathy, neuropathic
  - diabetic — see Diabetes, arthropathy, neuropathic
  - syringomyelic G95.0
- chylous (filarial) — see also category M01 B74.9
- climacteric (any site) NEC — see Arthritis, specified form NEC
- crystal (-induced) — see Arthritis, in, crystals
- deformans — see Osteoarthritis
- degenerative — see Osteoarthritis
- due to or associated with
  - acromegaly E22.0
  - brucellosis — see Brucellosis
  - caisson disease T70.3- ☑
  - diabetes — see Diabetes, arthropathy
  - dracontiasis — see also category M01 B72
  - enteritis NEC
    - regional — see Enteritis, regional
  - erysipelas — see also category M01 A46
  - erythema
    - epidemic A25.1
    - nodosum L52
  - filariasis NOS B74.9
  - glanders A24.0
  - helminthiasis — see also category M01 B83.9
  - hemophilia D66 [M36.2]
  - Henoch- (Schonlein) purpura D69.0 [M36.4]
  - human parvovirus — see also category M01 B97.6
  - infectious disease NEC M01.- ☑
  - leprosy (see also category M01) — see also Leprosy A30.9
  - Lyme disease A69.23
  - mycobacteria — see also category M01 A31.8
  - parasitic disease NEC — see also category M01 B89
  - paratyphoid fever (see also category M01) — see also Fever, paratyphoid A01.4
  - rat bite fever — see also category M01 A25.1
  - regional enteritis — see Enteritis, regional
  - respiratory disorder NOS J98.9
  - serum sickness — see also Reaction, serum T80.69- ☑
  - syringomyelia G95.0
  - typhoid fever A01.04
- epidemic erythema A25.1
- facet joint — see also Spondylosis M47.819
- febrile — see Fever, rheumatic
- gonococcal A54.42
- gouty (acute) — see Gout
- in (due to)
  - acromegaly — see also subcategory M14.8- E22.0
  - amyloidosis — see also subcategory M14.8- E85.4
  - bacterial disease — see also subcategory M01 A49.9
  - Behcet's syndrome M35.2
  - caisson disease — see also subcategory M14.8- T70.3- ☑
  - coliform bacilli (Escherichia coli) — see Arthritis, in, pyogenic organism NEC
  - crystals M11.9
    - dicalcium phosphate — see Arthritis, in, crystals, specified type NEC
    - hydroxyapatite M11.0- ☑
    - pyrophosphate — see Arthritis, in, crystals, specified type NEC
    - specified type NEC M11.80
      - ankle M11.87- ☑
      - elbow M11.82- ☑
      - foot joint M11.87- ☑
      - hand joint M11.84- ☑
      - hip M11.85- ☑
      - knee M11.86- ☑
      - multiple sites M11.89
      - shoulder M11.81- ☑
      - vertebrae M11.88
      - wrist M11.83- ☑
  - dermatoarthritis, lipoid E78.81
  - dracontiasis (dracunculiasis) — see also category M01 B72
  - endocrine disorder NEC — see also subcategory M14.8- E34.9

Arthritis, arthritic — *continued*
- in — *continued*
  - enteritis, infectious NEC — *see also* category M01 A09
    - specified organism NEC — *see also* category M01 A08.8
  - erythema
    - multiforme — *see also* subcategory M14.8- L51.9
    - nodosum — *see also* subcategory M14.8- L52
  - gout — *see* Gout
  - helminthiasis NEC — *see also* category M01 B83.9
  - hemochromatosis — *see also* subcategory M14.8- E83.118
  - hemoglobinopathy NEC D58.2 *[M36.3]*
  - hemophilia NEC D66 *[M36.2]*
  - Hemophilus influenzae M00.8- ☑ *[B96.3]*
  - Henoch (-Schonlein) purpura D69.0 *[M36.4]*
  - hyperparathyroidism NEC — *see also* subcategory M14.8- E21.3
  - hypersensitivity reaction NEC T78.49- ☑ *[M36.4]*
  - hypogammaglobulinemia — *see also* subcategory M14.8- D80.1
  - hypothyroidism NEC — *see also* subcategory M14.8- E03.9
  - infection — *see* Arthritis, pyogenic or pyemic
    - spine — *see* Spondylopathy, infective
  - infectious disease NEC M01.- ☑
  - leprosy — *see also* category M01 A30.9
  - leukemia NEC C95.9- ☑ *[M36.1]*
  - lipoid dermatoarthritis E78.81
  - Lyme disease A69.23
  - Mediterranean fever, familial — *see also* subcategory M14.8- M04.1
  - Meningococcus A39.83
  - metabolic disorder NEC — *see also* subcategory M14.8- E88.9
  - multiple myelomatosis C90.0- ☑ *[M36.1]*
  - mumps B26.85
  - mycosis NEC — *see also* category M01 B49
  - myelomatosis (multiple) C90.0- ☑ *[M36.1]*
  - neurological disorder NEC G98.0
  - ochronosis — *see also* subcategory M14.8- E70.29
  - O'nyong-nyong — *see also* category M01 A92.1
  - parasitic disease NEC — *see also* category M01 B89
  - paratyphoid fever — *see also* category M01 A01.4
  - Pseudomonas — *see* Arthritis, pyogenic, bacterial NEC
  - psoriasis L40.50
  - pyogenic organism NEC — *see* Arthritis, pyogenic, bacterial NEC
  - Reiter's disease — *see* Reiter's disease
  - respiratory disorder NEC — *see also* subcategory M14.8- J98.9
  - reticulosis, malignant — *see also* subcategory M14.8- C86.0- ☑
  - rubella B06.82
  - Salmonella (arizonae) (cholerae-suis) (enteritidis) (typhimurium) A02.23
  - sarcoidosis D86.86
  - specified bacteria NEC — *see* Arthritis, pyogenic, bacterial NEC
  - sporotrichosis B42.82
  - syringomyelia G95.0
  - thalassemia NEC D56.9 *[M36.3]*
  - tuberculosis — *see* Tuberculosis, arthritis
  - typhoid fever A01.04
  - urethritis, Reiter's — *see* Reiter's disease
  - viral disease NEC — *see also* category M01 B34.9
- infectious or infective — *see also* Arthritis, pyogenic or pyemic
  - spine — *see* Spondylopathy, infective
- juvenile M08.90
  - with systemic onset — *see* Still's disease
  - ankle M08.97- ☑
  - elbow M08.92- ☑
  - foot joint M08.97- ☑
  - hand joint M08.94- ☑
  - hip M08.95- ☑
  - knee M08.96- ☑
  - multiple site M08.99
  - pauciarticular M08.40
    - ankle M08.47- ☑
    - elbow M08.42- ☑
    - foot joint M08.47- ☑
    - hand joint M08.44- ☑
    - hip M08.45- ☑
    - knee M08.46- ☑
    - shoulder M08.41- ☑
    - specified site NEC M08.4A

Arthritis, arthritic — *continued*
- juvenile — *continued*
  - pauciarticular — *continued*
    - vertebrae M08.48
    - wrist M08.43- ☑
  - psoriatic L40.54
  - rheumatoid — *see* Arthritis, rheumatoid, juvenile
  - shoulder M08.91- ☑
  - specified site NEC M08.9A
  - specified type NEC M08.80
    - ankle M08.87- ☑
    - elbow M08.82- ☑
    - foot joint M08.87- ☑
    - hand joint M08.84- ☑
    - hip M08.85- ☑
    - knee M08.86- ☑
    - multiple site M08.89
    - shoulder M08.81- ☑
    - specified joint NEC M08.88
    - vertebrae M08.88
    - wrist M08.83- ☑
  - wrist M08.93- ☑
- meaning osteoarthritis — *see* Osteoarthritis
- meningococcal A39.83
- menopausal (any site) NEC — *see* Arthritis, specified form NEC
- mutilans (psoriatic) L40.52
- mycotic NEC — *see also* category M01 B49
- neuropathic (Charcot) — *see* Arthropathy, neuropathic
  - diabetic — *see* Diabetes, arthropathy, neuropathic
  - nonsyphilitic NEC G98.0
  - syringomyelic G95.0
- ochronotic — *see also* subcategory M14.8- E70.29
- palindromic (any site) — *see* Rheumatism, palindromic
- pneumococcal M00.10
  - ankle M00.17- ☑
  - elbow M00.12- ☑
  - foot joint — *see* Arthritis, pneumococcal, ankle
  - hand joint M00.14- ☑
  - hip M00.15- ☑
  - knee M00.16- ☑
  - multiple site M00.19
  - shoulder M00.11- ☑
  - vertebra M00.18
  - wrist M00.13- ☑
- postdysenteric — *see* Arthropathy, postdysenteric
- postmeningococcal A39.84
- postrheumatic, chronic — *see* Arthropathy, postrheumatic, chronic
- primary progressive — *see also* Arthritis, specified form NEC
  - spine — *see* Spondylitis, ankylosing
- psoriatic L40.50
- purulent (any site except spine) — *see* Arthritis, pyogenic or pyemic
  - spine — *see* Spondylopathy, infective
- pyogenic or pyemic (any site except spine) M00.9
  - bacterial NEC M00.80
    - ankle M00.87- ☑
    - elbow M00.82- ☑
    - foot joint — *see* Arthritis, pyogenic, bacterial NEC, ankle
    - hand joint M00.84- ☑
    - hip M00.85- ☑
    - knee M00.86- ☑
    - multiple site M00.89
    - shoulder M00.81- ☑
    - vertebra M00.88
    - wrist M00.83- ☑
  - pneumococcal — *see* Arthritis, pneumococcal
  - spine — *see* Spondylopathy, infective
  - staphylococcal — *see* Arthritis, staphylococcal
  - streptococcal — *see* Arthritis, streptococcal NEC
    - pneumococcal — *see* Arthritis, pneumococcal
- reactive — *see* Reiter's disease
- rheumatic — *see also* Arthritis, rheumatoid
  - acute or subacute — *see* Fever, rheumatic
- rheumatoid M06.9
  - with
    - carditis — *see* Rheumatoid, carditis
    - endocarditis — *see* Rheumatoid, carditis
    - heart involvement NEC — *see* Rheumatoid, carditis
    - lung involvement — *see* Rheumatoid, lung
    - myocarditis — *see* Rheumatoid, carditis
    - myopathy — *see* Rheumatoid, myopathy
    - pericarditis — *see* Rheumatoid, carditis
    - polyneuropathy — *see* Rheumatoid, polyneuropathy

Arthritis, arthritic — *continued*
- rheumatoid — *continued*
  - with — *continued*
    - rheumatoid factor — *see* Arthritis, rheumatoid, seropositive
    - splenoadenomegaly and leukopenia — *see* Felty's syndrome
    - vasculitis — *see* Rheumatoid, vasculitis
    - visceral involvement NEC — *see* Rheumatoid, arthritis, with involvement of organs NEC
  - juvenile (with or without rheumatoid factor) M08.00
    - with systemic onset — *see* Still's disease
    - ankle M08.07- ☑
    - elbow M08.02- ☑
    - foot joint M08.07- ☑
    - hand joint M08.04- ☑
    - hip M08.05- ☑
    - knee M08.06- ☑
    - multiple site M08.09
    - shoulder M08.01- ☑
    - specified site NEC M08.0A
    - vertebra M08.08
    - wrist M08.03- ☑
  - seronegative M06.00
    - ankle M06.07- ☑
    - elbow M06.02- ☑
    - foot joint M06.07- ☑
    - hand joint M06.04- ☑
    - hip M06.05- ☑
    - knee M06.06- ☑
    - multiple site M06.09
    - shoulder M06.01- ☑
    - specified site NEC M06.0A
    - vertebra M06.08
    - wrist M06.03- ☑
  - seropositive M05.9
    - specified NEC M05.80
      - ankle M05.87- ☑
      - elbow M05.82- ☑
      - foot joint M05.87- ☑
      - hand joint M05.84- ☑
      - hip M05.85- ☑
      - knee M05.86- ☑
      - multiple sites M05.89
      - shoulder M05.81- ☑
      - specified site NEC M05.8A
      - vertebra — *see* Spondylitis, ankylosing
      - wrist M05.83- ☑
    - without organ involvement M05.70
      - ankle M05.77- ☑
      - elbow M05.72- ☑
      - foot joint M05.77- ☑
      - hand joint M05.74- ☑
      - hip M05.75- ☑
      - knee M05.76- ☑
      - multiple sites M05.79
      - shoulder M05.71- ☑
      - specified site NEC M05.7A
      - vertebra — *see* Spondylitis, ankylosing
      - wrist M05.73- ☑
  - specified type NEC M06.80
    - ankle M06.87- ☑
    - elbow M06.82- ☑
    - foot joint M06.87- ☑
    - hand joint M06.84- ☑
    - hip M06.85- ☑
    - knee M06.86- ☑
    - multiple site M06.89
    - shoulder M06.81- ☑
    - specified site NEC M06.8A
    - vertebra M06.88
    - wrist M06.83- ☑
  - spine — *see* Spondylitis, ankylosing
- rubella B06.82
- scorbutic — *see also* subcategory M14.8- E54
- senile or senescent — *see* Osteoarthritis
- septic (any site except spine) — *see* Arthritis, pyogenic or pyemic
  - spine — *see* Spondylopathy, infective
- serum (nontherapeutic) (therapeutic) — *see* Arthropathy, postimmunization
- specified form NEC M13.80
  - ankle M13.87- ☑
  - elbow M13.82- ☑
  - foot joint M13.87- ☑
  - hand joint M13.84- ☑
  - hip M13.85- ☑

Arthritis, arthritic — continued
- specified form — continued
  - knee M13.86- ☑
  - multiple site M13.89
  - shoulder M13.81- ☑
  - specified joint NEC M13.88
  - wrist M13.83- ☑
- spine — see also Spondylosis
  - infectious or infective NEC — see Spondylopathy, infective
  - Marie-Strumpell — see Spondylitis, ankylosing
  - pyogenic — see Spondylopathy, infective
  - rheumatoid — see Spondylitis, ankylosing
  - traumatic (old) — see Spondylopathy, traumatic
  - tuberculous A18.01
- staphylococcal M00.00
  - ankle M00.07- ☑
  - elbow M00.02- ☑
  - foot joint — see Arthritis, staphylococcal, ankle
  - hand joint M00.04- ☑
  - hip M00.05- ☑
  - knee M00.06- ☑
  - multiple site M00.09
  - shoulder M00.01- ☑
  - vertebra M00.08
  - wrist M00.03- ☑
- streptococcal NEC M00.20
  - ankle M00.27- ☑
  - elbow M00.22- ☑
  - foot joint — see Arthritis, streptococcal, ankle
  - hand joint M00.24- ☑
  - hip M00.25- ☑
  - knee M00.26- ☑
  - multiple site M00.29
  - shoulder M00.21- ☑
  - vertebra M00.28
  - wrist M00.23- ☑
- suppurative — see Arthritis, pyogenic or pyemic
- syphilitic (late) A52.16
  - congenital A50.55 [M12.80]
- syphilitica deformans (Charcot) A52.16
- temporomandibular joint M26.64- ☑
- toxic of menopause (any site) — see Arthritis, specified form NEC
- transient — see Arthropathy, specified form NEC
- traumatic (chronic) — see Arthropathy, traumatic
- tuberculous A18.02
  - spine A18.01
- uratic — see Gout
- urethritica (Reiter's) — see Reiter's disease
- vertebral — see Spondylopathy, inflammatory
- villous (any site) — see Arthropathy, specified form NEC

Arthrocele — see Effusion, joint
Arthrodesis status Z98.1
Arthrodynia — see also Pain, joint
Arthrodysplasia Q74.9
Arthrofibrosis, joint — see Ankylosis
Arthrogryposis (congenital) Q68.8
- multiplex congenita Q74.3
Arthrokatadysis M24.7
Arthropathy — see also Arthritis M12.9
- Charcot's — see Arthropathy, neuropathic
  - diabetic — see Diabetes, arthropathy, neuropathic
  - syringomyelic G95.0
- cricoarytenoid J38.7
- crystal (-induced) — see Arthritis, in, crystals
- diabetic NEC — see Diabetes, arthropathy
- distal interphalangeal, psoriatic L40.51
- enteropathic M07.60
  - ankle M07.67- ☑
  - elbow M07.62- ☑
  - foot joint M07.67- ☑
  - hand joint M07.64- ☑
  - hip M07.65- ☑
  - knee M07.66- ☑
  - multiple site M07.69
  - shoulder M07.61- ☑
  - vertebra M07.68
  - wrist M07.63- ☑
- facet joint — see also Spondylosis M47.819
- following intestinal bypass M02.00
  - ankle M02.07- ☑
  - elbow M02.02- ☑
  - foot joint M02.07- ☑
  - hand joint M02.04- ☑
  - hip M02.05- ☑
  - knee M02.06- ☑

Arthropathy — continued
- following intestinal bypass — continued
  - multiple site M02.09
  - shoulder M02.01- ☑
  - vertebra M02.08
  - wrist M02.03- ☑
- gouty — see also Gout
  - in (due to)
    - Lesch-Nyhan syndrome E79.1 [M14.8-] ☑
    - sickle-cell disorders D57.- ☑ [M14.8-] ☑
- hemophilic NEC D66 [M36.2]
  - in (due to)
    - hyperparathyroidism NEC E21.3 [M14.8-] ☑
    - metabolic disease NOS E88.9 [M14.8-] ☑
- in (due to)
  - acromegaly E22.0 [M14.8-] ☑
  - amyloidosis E85.4 [M14.8-] ☑
  - blood disorder NOS D75.9 [M36.3]
  - diabetes — see Diabetes, arthropathy
  - endocrine disease NOS E34.9 [M14.8-] ☑
  - erythema
    - multiforme L51.9 [M14.8-] ☑
    - nodosum L52 [M14.8-] ☑
  - hemochromatosis E83.118 [M14.8-] ☑
  - hemoglobinopathy NEC D58.2 [M36.3]
  - hemophilia NEC D66 [M36.2]
  - Henoch-Schonlein purpura D69.0 [M36.4]
  - hyperthyroidism E05.90 [M14.8-] ☑
  - hypothyroidism E03.9 [M14.8-] ☑
  - infective endocarditis I33.0 [M12.80]
  - leukemia NEC C95.9- ☑ [M36.1]
  - malignant histiocytosis C96.A [M36.1]
  - metabolic disease NOS E88.9 [M14.8-] ☑
  - multiple myeloma C90.0- ☑ [M36.1]
  - neoplastic disease NOS (see also Neoplasm) D49.9 [M36.1]
  - nutritional deficiency — see also subcategory M14.8- E63.9
  - psoriasis NOS L40.50
  - sarcoidosis D86.86
  - syphilis (late) A52.77
    - congenital A50.55 [M12.80]
  - thyrotoxicosis — see also subcategory M14.8- E05.90
  - ulcerative colitis NEC K51.90 [M07.6-] ☑
  - viral hepatitis (postinfectious) NEC B19.9 [M12.80]
  - Whipple's disease — see also subcategory M14.8- K90.81
- Jaccoud — see Arthropathy, postrheumatic, chronic
- juvenile — see Arthritis, juvenile
  - psoriatic L40.54
- mutilans (psoriatic) L40.52
- neuropathic (Charcot) M14.60
  - ankle M14.67- ☑
  - diabetic — see Diabetes, arthropathy, neuropathic
  - elbow M14.62- ☑
  - foot joint M14.67- ☑
  - hand joint M14.64- ☑
  - hip M14.65- ☑
  - knee M14.66- ☑
  - multiple site M14.69
  - nonsyphilitic NEC G98.0
  - shoulder M14.61- ☑
  - syringomyelic G95.0
  - vertebra M14.68
  - wrist M14.63- ☑
- osteopulmonary — see Osteoarthropathy, hypertrophic, specified NEC
- postdysenteric M02.10
  - ankle M02.17- ☑
  - elbow M02.12- ☑
  - foot joint M02.17- ☑
  - hand joint M02.14- ☑
  - hip M02.15- ☑
  - knee M02.16- ☑
  - multiple site M02.19
  - shoulder M02.11- ☑
  - vertebra M02.18
  - wrist M02.13- ☑
- postimmunization M02.20
  - ankle M02.27- ☑
  - elbow M02.22- ☑
  - foot joint M02.27- ☑
  - hand joint M02.24- ☑
  - hip M02.25- ☑
  - knee M02.26- ☑
  - multiple site M02.29
  - shoulder M02.21- ☑

Arthropathy — continued
- postimmunization — continued
  - vertebra M02.28
  - wrist M02.23- ☑
- postinfectious NEC B99.- ☑ [M12.80]
  - in (due to)
    - enteritis due to Yersinia enterocolitica A04.6 [M12.80]
    - syphilis A52.77
    - viral hepatitis NEC B19.9 [M12.80]
- postrheumatic, chronic (Jaccoud) M12.00
  - ankle M12.07- ☑
  - elbow M12.02- ☑
  - foot joint M12.07- ☑
  - hand joint M12.04- ☑
  - hip M12.05- ☑
  - knee M12.06- ☑
  - multiple site M12.09
  - shoulder M12.01- ☑
  - specified joint NEC M12.08
  - vertebrae M12.08
  - wrist M12.03- ☑
- psoriatic NEC L40.59
  - interphalangeal, distal L40.51
- reactive M02.9
  - in (due to)
    - infective endocarditis I33.0 [M02.9]
  - specified type NEC M02.80
    - ankle M02.87- ☑
    - elbow M02.82- ☑
    - foot joint M02.87- ☑
    - hand joint M02.84- ☑
    - hip M02.85- ☑
    - knee M02.86- ☑
    - multiple site M02.89
    - shoulder M02.81- ☑
    - vertebra M02.88
    - wrist M02.83- ☑
- specified form NEC M12.80
  - ankle M12.87- ☑
  - elbow M12.82- ☑
  - foot joint M12.87- ☑
  - hand joint M12.84- ☑
  - hip M12.85- ☑
  - knee M12.86- ☑
  - multiple site M12.89
  - shoulder M12.81- ☑
  - specified joint NEC M12.88
  - vertebrae M12.88
  - wrist M12.83- ☑
- syringomyelic G95.0
- tabes dorsalis A52.16
- tabetic A52.16
- temporomandibular joint M26.65- ☑
- transient — see Arthropathy, specified form NEC
- traumatic M12.50
  - ankle M12.57- ☑
  - elbow M12.52- ☑
  - foot joint M12.57- ☑
  - hand joint M12.54- ☑
  - hip M12.55- ☑
  - knee M12.56- ☑
  - multiple site M12.59
  - shoulder M12.51- ☑
  - specified joint NEC M12.58
  - vertebrae M12.58
  - wrist M12.53- ☑

Arthropyosis — see Arthritis, pyogenic or pyemic
Arthrosis (deformans) (degenerative) (localized) — see also Osteoarthritis M19.90
- spine — see Spondylosis
Arthus' phenomenon or reaction T78.41- ☑
- due to
  - drug — see Table of Drugs and Chemicals, by drug
Articular — see condition
Articulation, reverse (teeth) M26.24
Artificial
- insemination complication — see Complications, artificial, fertilization
- opening status (functioning) (without complication) Z93.9
  - anus (colostomy) Z93.3
  - colostomy Z93.3
  - cystostomy Z93.50
    - appendico-vesicostomy Z93.52
    - cutaneous Z93.51
    - specified NEC Z93.59

Artificial — continued
　　opening status — continued
　　　　enterostomy Z93.4
　　　　gastrostomy Z93.1
　　　　ileostomy (ileal pouch) (Kock pouch) Z93.2
　　　　intestinal tract NEC Z93.4
　　　　jejunostomy Z93.4
　　　　nephrostomy Z93.6
　　　　specified site NEC Z93.8
　　　　tracheostomy Z93.0
　　　　ureterostomy Z93.6
　　　　urethrostomy Z93.6
　　　　urinary tract NEC Z93.6
　　　　vagina Z93.8
　　　　vagina status Z93.8
Arytenoid — *see* condition
Asadollahi-Rauch syndrome Q87.85
Asbestosis (occupational) J61
ASC-H (atypical squamous cells cannot exclude high grade squamous intraepithelial lesion on cytologic smear)
　　anus R85.611
　　cervix R87.611
　　vagina R87.621
ASC-US (atypical squamous cells of undetermined significance on cytologic smear)
　　anus R85.610
　　cervix R87.610
　　vagina R87.620
Ascariasis B77.9
　　with
　　　　complications NEC B77.89
　　　　intestinal complications B77.0
　　　　pneumonia, pneumonitis B77.81
Ascaridosis, ascaridiasis — *see* Ascariasis
Ascaris (infection) (infestation) (lumbricoides) — *see* Ascariasis
Ascending — *see* condition
Aschoff's bodies — *see* Myocarditis, rheumatic
Ascites (abdominal) R18.8
　　cardiac — *see also* Failure, heart, right I50.810
　　chylous (nonfilarial) I89.8
　　　　filarial — *see* Infestation, filarial
　　due to
　　　　cirrhosis, alcoholic K70.31
　　　　hepatitis — *see also* Hepatitis
　　　　　　alcoholic K70.11
　　　　　　chronic active — *see also* Hepatitis, chronic active K73.2
　　　　　　　　with toxic liver disease K71.51
　　　　S. japonicum B65.2
　　heart — *see also* Failure, heart, right I50.810
　　malignant R18.0
　　pseudochylous R18.8
　　syphilitic A52.74
　　tuberculous A18.31
Aseptic — *see* condition
Asherman's syndrome N85.6
Asialia K11.7
Asiatic cholera — *see* Cholera
Asimultagnosia (simultanagnosia) R48.3
Askin's tumor — *see* Neoplasm, connective tissue, malignant
Asocial personality F60.2
Asomatognosia R41.4
Aspartylglucosaminuria E77.1
Asperger's disease or syndrome F84.5
Aspergilloma — *see* Aspergillosis
Aspergillosis (with pneumonia) B44.9
　　bronchopulmonary, allergic B44.81
　　disseminated B44.7
　　generalized B44.7
　　pulmonary NEC B44.1
　　　　allergic B44.81
　　　　invasive B44.0
　　specified NEC B44.89
　　tonsillar B44.2
Aspergillus (flavus) (fumigatus) (infection) (terreus) — *see* Aspergillosis
Aspermatogenesis — *see* Azoospermia
Aspermia (testis) — *see* Azoospermia
Asphyxia, asphyxiation (by) R09.01
　　antenatal P84
　　birth P84
　　bunny bag — *see* Asphyxia, due to, mechanical threat to breathing, trapped in bed clothes
　　crushing S28.0- ☑
　　drowning T75.1- ☑
　　gas, fumes, or vapor — *see* Table of Drugs and Chemicals
　　inhalation — *see* Inhalation

Asphyxia, asphyxiation — continued
　　intrauterine P84
　　local I73.00
　　　　with gangrene I73.01
　　mucus — *see also* Foreign body, respiratory tract, causing, asphyxiation
　　newborn P84
　　pathological R09.01
　　postnatal P84
　　　　mechanical — *see* Asphyxia, due to, mechanical threat to breathing
　　prenatal P84
　　reticularis R23.1
　　strangulation — *see* Asphyxia, due to, mechanical threat to breathing
　　submersion T75.1- ☑
　　traumatic T71.9- ☑
　　　　due to
　　　　　　crushed chest S28.0- ☑
　　　　　　foreign body (in) — *see* Foreign body, respiratory tract, causing asphyxia
　　　　　　low oxygen content of ambient air T71.20- ☑
　　　　　　　　due to
　　　　　　　　　　being trapped in
　　　　　　　　　　　　low oxygen environment T71.29- ☑
　　　　　　　　　　　　in car trunk T71.221- ☑
　　　　　　　　　　　　　　circumstances undetermined T71.224- ☑
　　　　　　　　　　　　　　done with intent to harm by
　　　　　　　　　　　　　　　　another person T71.223- ☑
　　　　　　　　　　　　　　　　self T71.222- ☑
　　　　　　　　　　　　in refrigerator T71.231- ☑
　　　　　　　　　　　　　　circumstances undetermined T71.234- ☑
　　　　　　　　　　　　　　done with intent to harm by
　　　　　　　　　　　　　　　　another person T71.233- ☑
　　　　　　　　　　　　　　　　self T71.232- ☑
　　　　　　　　　　cave-in T71.21- ☑
　　　　mechanical threat to breathing (accidental) T71.191- ☑
　　　　　　circumstances undetermined T71.194- ☑
　　　　　　done with intent to harm by
　　　　　　　　another person T71.193- ☑
　　　　　　　　self T71.192- ☑
　　　　　　hanging T71.161- ☑
　　　　　　　　circumstances undetermined T71.164- ☑
　　　　　　　　done with intent to harm by
　　　　　　　　　　another person T71.163- ☑
　　　　　　　　　　self T71.162- ☑
　　　　　　plastic bag T71.121- ☑
　　　　　　　　circumstances undetermined T71.124- ☑
　　　　　　　　done with intent to harm by
　　　　　　　　　　another person T71.123- ☑
　　　　　　　　　　self T71.122- ☑
　　　　　　smothering
　　　　　　　　in furniture T71.151- ☑
　　　　　　　　　　circumstances undetermined T71.154- ☑
　　　　　　　　　　done with intent to harm by
　　　　　　　　　　　　another person T71.153- ☑
　　　　　　　　　　　　self T71.152- ☑
　　　　　　　　under
　　　　　　　　　　another person's body T71.141- ☑
　　　　　　　　　　　　circumstances undetermined T71.144- ☑
　　　　　　　　　　　　done with intent to harm T71.143- ☑
　　　　　　　　　　pillow T71.111- ☑
　　　　　　　　　　　　circumstances undetermined T71.114- ☑
　　　　　　　　　　　　done with intent to harm by
　　　　　　　　　　　　　　another person T71.113- ☑
　　　　　　　　　　　　　　self T71.112- ☑
　　　　　　trapped in bed clothes T71.131- ☑
　　　　　　　　circumstances undetermined T71.134- ☑
　　　　　　　　done with intent to harm by
　　　　　　　　　　another person T71.133- ☑
　　　　　　　　　　self T71.132- ☑
　　vomiting, vomitus — *see* Foreign body, respiratory tract, causing asphyxia
Aspiration
　　amniotic (clear) fluid (newborn) P24.10
　　　　with
　　　　　　pneumonia (pneumonitis) P24.11
　　　　　　respiratory symptoms P24.11
　　blood
　　　　newborn (without respiratory symptoms) P24.20

Aspiration — continued
　　blood — continued
　　　　newborn — continued
　　　　　　with
　　　　　　　　pneumonia (pneumonitis) P24.21
　　　　　　　　respiratory symptoms P24.21
　　　　　　specified age NEC — *see* Foreign body, respiratory tract
　　bronchitis J69.0
　　food or foreign body — *see* Foreign body, by site
　　liquor (amnii) (newborn) P24.10
　　　　with
　　　　　　pneumonia (pneumonitis) P24.11
　　　　　　respiratory symptoms P24.11
　　meconium (newborn) (without respiratory symptoms) P24.00
　　　　with
　　　　　　pneumonitis (pneumonitis) P24.01
　　　　　　respiratory symptoms P24.01
　　milk (newborn) (without respiratory symptoms) P24.30
　　　　with
　　　　　　pneumonia (pneumonitis) P24.31
　　　　　　respiratory symptoms P24.31
　　　　specified age NEC — *see* Foreign body, respiratory tract
　　mucus — *see also* Foreign body, by site, causing asphyxia
　　　　newborn P24.10
　　　　　　with
　　　　　　　　pneumonia (pneumonitis) P24.11
　　　　　　　　respiratory symptoms P24.11
　　neonatal P24.9
　　　　specific NEC (without respiratory symptoms) P24.80
　　　　　　with
　　　　　　　　pneumonia (pneumonitis) P24.81
　　　　　　　　respiratory symptoms P24.81
　　newborn P24.9
　　　　specific NEC (without respiratory symptoms) P24.80
　　　　　　with
　　　　　　　　pneumonia (pneumonitis) P24.81
　　　　　　　　respiratory symptoms P24.81
　　pneumonia J69.0
　　pneumonitis J69.0
　　syndrome of newborn — *see* Aspiration, by substance, with pneumonia
　　vernix caseosa (newborn) P24.80
　　　　with
　　　　　　pneumonia (pneumonitis) P24.81
　　　　　　respiratory symptoms P24.81
　　vomitus — *see also* Foreign body, respiratory tract
　　　　newborn (without respiratory symptoms) P24.30
　　　　　　with
　　　　　　　　pneumonia (pneumonitis) P24.31
　　　　　　　　respiratory symptoms P24.31
Asplenia (congenital) Q89.01
　　functional D73.0
　　postsurgical Z90.81
Assam fever B55.0
Assault, sexual — *see* Maltreatment
Assmann's focus NEC A15.0
Astasia (-abasia) (hysterical) F44.4
Asteatosis cutis L85.3
Astereognosia, astereognosis R48.1
Asterixis R27.8
　　in liver disease K71.3
Asteroid hyalitis — *see* Deposit, crystalline
Asthenia, asthenic R53.1
　　cardiac — *see also* Failure, heart I50.9
　　　　psychogenic F45.8
　　cardiovascular — *see also* Failure, heart I50.9
　　　　psychogenic F45.8
　　heart — *see also* Failure, heart I50.9
　　　　psychogenic F45.8
　　hysterical F44.4
　　myocardial — *see also* Failure, heart I50.9
　　　　psychogenic F45.8
　　nervous F48.8
　　neurocirculatory F45.8
　　neurotic F48.8
　　psychogenic F48.8
　　psychoneurotic F48.8
　　psychophysiologic F48.8
　　reaction (psychophysiologic) F48.8
　　senile R54
Asthenopia — *see also* Discomfort, visual
　　hysterical F44.6
　　psychogenic F44.6
Asthenospermia — *see* Abnormal, specimen, male genital organs

☑ **Additional Character Required** — Refer to the Tabular List for Character Selection

Asthma, asthmatic (bronchial) (catarrh) (spasmodic) J45.909
- with
  - chronic obstructive bronchitis J44.89
    - with
      - acute lower respiratory infection J44.0
      - exacerbation (acute) J44.1
  - chronic obstructive pulmonary disease J44.89
    - with
      - acute lower respiratory infection J44.0
      - exacerbation (acute) J44.1
  - exacerbation (acute) J45.901
  - hay fever — see Asthma, allergic extrinsic
  - rhinitis, allergic — see Asthma, allergic extrinsic
  - status asthmaticus J45.902
- allergic extrinsic J45.909
  - with
    - exacerbation (acute) J45.901
    - status asthmaticus J45.902
- atopic — see Asthma, allergic extrinsic
- cardiac — see Failure, ventricular, left
- cardiobronchial I50.1
- childhood J45.909
  - with
    - exacerbation (acute) J45.901
    - status asthmaticus J45.902
- chronic obstructive J44.89
  - with
    - acute lower respiratory infection J44.0
    - exacerbation (acute) J44.1
- collier's J60
- cough variant J45.991
- detergent J69.8
- due to
  - detergent J69.8
  - inhalation of fumes J68.3
- eosinophilic J82.83
- extrinsic, allergic — see Asthma, allergic extrinsic
- grinder's J62.8
- hay — see Asthma, allergic extrinsic
- heart I50.1
- idiosyncratic — see Asthma, nonallergic
- intermittent (mild) J45.20
  - with
    - exacerbation (acute) J45.21
    - status asthmaticus J45.22
- intrinsic, nonallergic — see Asthma, nonallergic
- Kopp's E32.8
- late-onset J45.909
  - with
    - exacerbation (acute) J45.901
    - status asthmaticus J45.902
- mild intermittent J45.20
  - with
    - exacerbation (acute) J45.21
    - status asthmaticus J45.22
- mild persistent J45.30
  - with
    - exacerbation (acute) J45.31
    - status asthmaticus J45.32
- Millar's (laryngismus stridulus) J38.5
- miner's J60
- mixed J45.909
  - with
    - exacerbation (acute) J45.901
    - status asthmaticus J45.902
- moderate persistent J45.40
  - with
    - exacerbation (acute) J45.41
    - status asthmaticus J45.42
- nervous — see Asthma, nonallergic
- nonallergic (intrinsic) J45.909
  - with
    - exacerbation (acute) J45.901
    - status asthmaticus J45.902
- persistent
  - mild J45.30
    - with
      - exacerbation (acute) J45.31
      - status asthmaticus J45.32
  - moderate J45.40
    - with
      - exacerbation (acute) J45.41
      - status asthmaticus J45.42
  - severe J45.50
    - with
      - exacerbation (acute) J45.51
      - status asthmaticus J45.52
- platinum J45.998

Asthma, asthmatic — continued
- pneumoconiotic NEC J64
- potter's J62.8
- predominantly allergic J45.909
- psychogenic F54
- pulmonary eosinophilic J82.83
- red cedar J67.8
- Rostan's I50.1
- sandblaster's J62.8
- sequoiosis J67.8
- severe persistent J45.50
  - with
    - exacerbation (acute) J45.51
    - status asthmaticus J45.52
- specified NEC J45.998
- stonemason's J62.8
- thymic E32.8
- tuberculous — see Tuberculosis, pulmonary
- Wichmann's (laryngismus stridulus) J38.5
- wood J67.8

Astigmatism (compound) (congenital) H52.20- ☑
- irregular H52.21- ☑
- regular H52.22- ☑

Astraphobia F40.220

Astroblastoma
- specified site — see Neoplasm, malignant, by site
- unspecified site C71.9

Astrocytoma (cystic)
- anaplastic
  - specified site — see Neoplasm, malignant, by site
  - unspecified site C71.9
- fibrillary
  - specified site — see Neoplasm, malignant, by site
  - unspecified site C71.9
- fibrous
  - specified site — see Neoplasm, malignant, by site
  - unspecified site C71.9
- gemistocytic
  - specified site — see Neoplasm, malignant, by site
  - unspecified site C71.9
- juvenile
  - specified site — see Neoplasm, malignant, by site
  - unspecified site C71.9
- pilocytic
  - specified site — see Neoplasm, malignant, by site
  - unspecified site C71.9
- piloid
  - specified site — see Neoplasm, malignant, by site
  - unspecified site C71.9
- protoplasmic
  - specified site — see Neoplasm, malignant, by site
  - unspecified site C71.9
- specified site NEC — see Neoplasm, malignant, by site
- subependymal D43.2
  - giant cell
    - specified site — see Neoplasm, uncertain behavior, by site
    - unspecified site D43.2
  - specified site — see Neoplasm, uncertain behavior, by site
  - unspecified site D43.2
- unspecified site C71.9

Astroglioma
- specified site — see Neoplasm, malignant, by site
- unspecified site C71.9

Asymbolia R48.8

Asymmetry — see also Distortion
- between native and reconstructed breast N65.1
- face Q67.0
- jaw (lower) — see Anomaly, dentofacial, jaw-cranial base relationship, asymmetry

Asynergia, asynergy R27.8
- ventricular I51.89

Asystole (heart) — see Arrest, cardiac

At risk
- for
  - dental caries Z91.849
    - high Z91.843
    - low Z91.841
    - moderate Z91.842
  - falling Z91.81
  - feeling loneliness Z65.8
  - social isolation Z91.89

Ataxia, ataxy, ataxic R27.0
- acute R27.8
- autosomal recessive Friedreich G11.11
- brain (hereditary) G11.9
- cerebellar (hereditary) G11.9
  - with defective DNA repair G11.3

Ataxia, ataxy, ataxic — continued
- cerebellar — continued
  - alcoholic G31.2
  - early-onset G11.10
    - with
      - essential tremor G11.19
      - myoclonus [Hunt's ataxia] G11.19
      - retained tendon reflexes G11.19
    - in
      - alcoholism G31.2
      - myxedema E03.9 [G13.2]
      - neoplastic disease — see also Neoplasm D49.9 [G32.81]
      - specified disease NEC G32.81
  - late-onset (Marie's) G11.2
- cerebral (hereditary) G11.9
- congenital nonprogressive G11.0
- family, familial — see Ataxia, hereditary
- following
  - cerebrovascular disease I69.993
    - cerebral infarction I69.393
    - intracerebral hemorrhage I69.193
    - nontraumatic intracranial hemorrhage NEC I69.293
    - specified disease NEC I69.893
    - subarachnoid hemorrhage I69.093
- Friedreich's (heredofamilial) (cerebellar) (spinal) (with retained reflexes) G11.11
- gait R26.0
  - hysterical F44.4
- general R27.8
- gluten M35.9 [G32.81]
  - with celiac disease K90.0 [G32.81]
- hereditary G11.9
  - with neuropathy G60.2
  - cerebellar — see Ataxia, cerebellar
  - spastic G11.4
  - specified NEC G11.8
  - spinal (Friedreich's) G11.11
- heredofamilial — see Ataxia, hereditary
- Hunt's G11.19
- hysterical F44.4
- locomotor (progressive) (syphilitic) (partial) (spastic) A52.11
  - diabetic — see Diabetes, ataxia
- Marie's (cerebellar) (heredofamilial) (late-onset) G11.2
- nonorganic origin F44.4
- nonprogressive, congenital G11.0
- psychogenic F44.4
- Roussy-Levy G60.0
- Sanger-Brown's (hereditary) G11.2
- spastic hereditary G11.4
- spinal
  - hereditary (Friedreich's) G11.11
  - progressive (syphilitic) A52.11
- spinocerebellar, X-linked recessive G11.19
- telangiectasia (Louis-Bar) G11.3

Ataxia-telangiectasia (Louis-Bar) G11.3

Atelectasis (massive) (partial) (pressure) (pulmonary) J98.11
- newborn P28.10
  - due to resorption P28.11
  - partial P28.19
  - primary P28.0
  - secondary P28.19
- primary (newborn) P28.0
- tuberculous — see Tuberculosis, pulmonary

Atelocardia Q24.9

Atelomyelia Q06.1

Atheroembolism
- of
  - extremities
    - lower I75.02- ☑
    - upper I75.01- ☑
  - kidney I75.81
  - specified NEC I75.89

Atheroma, atheromatous — see also Arteriosclerosis I70.90
- aorta, aortic I70.0
  - valve — see also Endocarditis, aortic I35.8
- aorto-iliac I70.0
- artery — see Arteriosclerosis
- basilar (artery) I67.2
- carotid (artery) (common) (internal) I67.2
- cerebral (arteries) I67.2
- coronary (artery) I25.10
  - with angina pectoris — see Arteriosclerosis, coronary (artery),
- degeneration — see Arteriosclerosis
- heart, cardiac — see Disease, heart, ischemic, atherosclerotic
- mitral (valve) I34.89

Atheroma, atheromatous — continued
  myocardium, myocardial — see Disease, heart, ischemic, atherosclerotic
  pulmonary valve (heart) — see also Endocarditis, pulmonary I37.8
  tricuspid (heart) (valve) I36.8
  valve, valvular — see Endocarditis
  vertebral (artery) I67.2
Atheromatosis — see Arteriosclerosis
Atherosclerosis — see also Arteriosclerosis
  coronary
    artery I25.10
      with angina pectoris — see Arteriosclerosis, coronary (artery),
      due to
        calcified coronary lesion (severely) I25.84
        lipid rich plaque I25.83
    transplanted heart I25.811
      bypass graft I25.812
        with angina pectoris — see Arteriosclerosis, coronary (artery),
      native coronary artery I25.811
        with angina pectoris — see Arteriosclerosis, coronary (artery),
Athetosis (acquired) R25.8
  bilateral (congenital) G80.3
  congenital (bilateral) (double) G80.3
  double (congenital) G80.3
  unilateral R25.8
Athlete's
  foot B35.3
  heart I51.7
Athrepsia E41
Athyrea (acquired) — see also Hypothyroidism
  congenital E03.1
Atonia, atony, atonic
  bladder (sphincter) (neurogenic) N31.2
  capillary I78.8
  cecum K59.89
    psychogenic F45.8
  colon — see Atony, intestine
  congenital P94.2
  esophagus K22.89
  intestine K59.89
    psychogenic F45.8
  stomach K31.89
    neurotic or psychogenic F45.8
  uterus (during labor) O62.2
    with hemorrhage (postpartum) O72.1
    postpartum (with hemorrhage) O72.1
      without hemorrhage O75.89
Atopy — see History, allergy
Atransferrinemia, congenital E88.09
Atresia, atretic
  alimentary organ or tract NEC Q45.8
    upper Q40.8
  ani, anus, anal (canal) Q42.3
    with fistula Q42.2
  aorta (ring) Q25.29
  aortic (orifice) (valve) Q23.0
    arch Q25.21
    congenital with hypoplasia of ascending aorta and defective development of left ventricle (with mitral stenosis) Q23.4
    in hypoplastic left heart syndrome Q23.4
  aqueduct of Sylvius Q03.0
    with spina bifida — see Spina bifida, with hydrocephalus
  artery NEC Q27.8
    cerebral Q28.3
    coronary Q24.5
    digestive system Q27.8
    eye Q15.8
    lower limb Q27.8
    pulmonary Q25.5
    specified site NEC Q27.8
    umbilical Q27.0
    upper limb Q27.8
  auditory canal (external) Q16.1
  bile duct (common) (congenital) (hepatic) Q44.2
    acquired — see Obstruction, bile duct
  bladder (neck) Q64.39
    obstruction Q64.31
  bronchus Q32.4
  cecum Q42.8
  cervix (acquired) N88.2
    congenital Q51.828
    in pregnancy or childbirth — see Anomaly, cervix, in pregnancy or childbirth

Atresia, atretic — continued
  cervix — continued
    in pregnancy or childbirth — see Anomaly, cervix, in pregnancy or childbirth — continued
      causing obstructed labor O65.5
  choana Q30.0
  colon Q42.9
    specified NEC Q42.8
  common duct Q44.2
  cricoid cartilage Q31.8
  cystic duct Q44.2
    acquired K82.8
      with obstruction K82.0
  digestive organs NEC Q45.8
  duodenum Q41.0
  ear canal Q16.1
  ejaculatory duct Q55.4
  epiglottis Q31.8
  esophagus Q39.0
    with tracheoesophageal fistula Q39.1
  eustachian tube Q17.8
  fallopian tube (congenital) Q50.6
    acquired N97.1
  follicular cyst N83.0- ☑
  foramen of
    Luschka Q03.1
      with spina bifida — see Spina bifida, with hydrocephalus
    Magendie Q03.1
      with spina bifida — see Spina bifida, with hydrocephalus
  gallbladder Q44.1
  genital organ
    external
      female Q52.79
      male Q55.8
    internal
      female Q52.8
      male Q55.8
  glottis Q31.8
  gullet Q39.0
    with tracheoesophageal fistula Q39.1
  heart valve NEC Q24.8
    pulmonary Q22.0
    tricuspid Q22.4
  hymen Q52.3
    acquired (postinfective) N89.6
  ileum Q41.2
  intestine (small) Q41.9
    large Q42.9
      specified NEC Q42.8
  iris, filtration angle Q15.0
  jejunum Q41.1
  lacrimal apparatus Q10.4
  larynx Q31.8
  meatus urinarius Q64.33
  mitral valve Q23.2
    in hypoplastic left heart syndrome Q23.4
  nares (anterior) (posterior) Q30.0
  nasopharynx Q34.8
  nose, nostril Q30.0
    acquired J34.89
  organ or site NEC Q89.89
  osseous meatus (ear) Q16.1
  oviduct (congenital) Q50.6
    acquired N97.1
  parotid duct Q38.4
    acquired K11.8
  pulmonary (artery) Q25.5
    valve Q22.0
  pulmonic Q22.0
  pupil Q13.2
  rectum Q42.1
    with fistula Q42.0
  salivary duct Q38.4
    acquired K11.8
  sublingual duct Q38.4
    acquired K11.8
  submandibular duct Q38.4
    acquired K11.8
  submaxillary duct Q38.4
    acquired K11.8
  thyroid cartilage Q31.8
  trachea Q32.1
  tricuspid valve Q22.4
  ureter Q62.10
    pelvic junction Q62.11
    vesical orifice Q62.12
  ureteropelvic junction Q62.11

Atresia, atretic — continued
  ureterovesical orifice Q62.12
  urethra (valvular) Q64.39
    stricture Q64.32
  urinary tract NEC Q64.8
  uterus Q51.818
    acquired N85.8
  vagina (congenital) Q52.4
    acquired (postinfectional) (senile) N89.5
  vas deferens Q55.3
  vascular NEC Q27.8
    cerebral Q28.3
    digestive system Q27.8
    lower limb Q27.8
    specified site NEC Q27.8
    upper limb Q27.8
  vein NEC Q27.8
    digestive system Q27.8
    great Q26.8
    lower limb Q27.8
    portal Q26.5
    pulmonary Q26.4
      partial Q26.3
      total Q26.2
    specified site NEC Q27.8
    upper limb Q27.8
  vena cava (inferior) (superior) Q26.8
  vesicourethral orifice Q64.31
  vulva Q52.79
    acquired N90.5
Atrichia, atrichosis — see Alopecia
Atrophia — see also Atrophy
  cutis senilis L90.8
    due to radiation L57.8
  gyrata of choroid and retina H31.23
  senilis R54
    dermatological L90.8
      due to radiation (nonionizing) (solar) L57.8
  unguium L60.3
    congenita Q84.6
Atrophie blanche (en plaque) (de Milian) L95.0
Atrophoderma, atrophodermia (of) L90.9
  diffusum (idiopathic) L90.4
  maculatum L90.8
    et striatum L90.8
      due to syphilis A52.79
    syphilitic A51.39
  neuriticum L90.8
  Pasini and Pierini L90.3
  pigmentosum Q82.1
  reticulatum symmetricum faciei L66.4
  senile L90.8
    due to radiation (nonionizing) (solar) L57.8
  vermiculata (cheeks) L66.4
Atrophy, atrophic (of)
  adrenal (capsule) (gland) E27.49
    primary (autoimmune) E27.1
  alveolar process or ridge (edentulous) K08.20
  anal sphincter (disuse) N81.84
  appendix K38.8
  arteriosclerotic — see Arteriosclerosis
  bile duct (common) (hepatic) K83.8
  bladder N32.89
    neurogenic N31.8
  blanche (en plaque) (of Milian) L95.0
  bone (senile) NEC — see also Disorder, bone, specified type NEC
    due to
      tabes dorsalis (neurogenic) A52.11
  brain (cortex) (progressive) G31.9
    frontotemporal circumscribed — see also Dementia, in, diseases specified elsewhere G31.01 [F02.80]
      with behavioral disturbance — see also Dementia, in, diseases specified elsewhere G31.01 [F02.81-] ☑
    senile NEC G31.1
  breast N64.2
    obstetric — see Disorder, breast, specified type NEC
  buccal cavity K13.79
  cardiac — see Degeneration, myocardial
  cartilage (infectional) (joint) — see Disorder, cartilage, specified NEC
  cerebellar — see Atrophy, brain
  cerebral — see Atrophy, brain
  cervix (mucosa) (senile) (uteri) N88.8
    menopausal N95.8
  Charcot-Marie-Tooth G60.0
  choroid (central) (macular) (myopic) (retina) H31.10- ☑
    diffuse secondary H31.12- ☑

☑ **Additional Character Required** — Refer to the Tabular List for Character Selection

Atrophy, atrophic — *continued*
  choroid — *continued*
    gyrate H31.23
    senile H31.11- ☑
  ciliary body — *see* Atrophy, iris
  conjunctiva (senile) H11.89
  corpus cavernosum N48.89
  cortical — *see* Atrophy, brain
  cystic duct K82.8
  Dejerine-Thomas G23.8
  disuse NEC — *see* Atrophy, muscle
  Duchenne-Aran G12.21
  ear H93.8- ☑
  edentulous alveolar ridge K08.20
  endometrium (senile) N85.8
    cervix N88.8
  enteric K63.89
  epididymis N50.89
  eyeball — *see* Disorder, globe, degenerated condition, atrophy
  eyelid (senile) — *see* Disorder, eyelid, degenerative
  facial (skin) L90.9
  fallopian tube (senile) N83.32- ☑
    with ovary N83.33- ☑
  fascioscapulohumeral (Landouzy- Dejerine) G71.02
  fatty, thymus (gland) E32.8
  gallbladder K82.8
  gastric K29.40
    with bleeding K29.41
  gastrointestinal K63.89
  glandular I89.8
  globe H44.52- ☑
  gum — *see* Recession, gingival
  hair L67.8
  heart (brown) — *see* Degeneration, myocardial
  hemifacial Q67.4
    Romberg G51.8
  infantile E41
    paralysis, acute — *see* Poliomyelitis, paralytic
  intestine K63.89
  iris (essential) (progressive) H21.26- ☑
    specified NEC H21.29
  kidney (senile) (terminal) — *see also* Sclerosis, renal N26.1
    congenital or infantile Q60.5
      bilateral Q60.4
      unilateral Q60.3
    hydronephrotic — *see* Hydronephrosis
  lacrimal gland (primary) H04.14- ☑
    secondary H04.15- ☑
  Landouzy-Dejerine G71.02
  laryngitis, infective J37.0
  larynx J38.7
  Leber's optic (hereditary) H47.22
  lip K13.0
  liver (yellow) K72.90
    with coma K72.91
    acute, subacute K72.00
      with coma K72.01
    chronic K72.10
      with coma K72.11
  lung (senile) J98.4
  macular (dermatological) L90.8
    syphilitic, skin A51.39
      striated A52.79
  mandible (edentulous) K08.20
    minimal K08.21
    moderate K08.22
    severe K08.23
  maxilla K08.20
    minimal K08.24
    moderate K08.25
    severe K08.26
  muscle, muscular (diffuse) (general) (idiopathic) (primary) M62.50
    ankle M62.57- ☑
    back M62.5A9
      cervical M62.5A0
      lumbosacral M62.5A2
      thoracic M62.5A1
    Duchenne-Aran G12.21
    foot M62.57- ☑
    forearm M62.53- ☑
    hand M62.54- ☑
    infantile spinal G12.0
    lower leg M62.56- ☑
    multiple sites M62.59
    myelopathic — *see* Atrophy, muscle, spinal
    myotonic G71.11

Atrophy, atrophic — *continued*
  muscle, muscular — *continued*
    neuritic G58.9
    neuropathic (peroneal) (progressive) G60.0
    pelvic (disuse) N81.84
    peroneal G60.0
    progressive (bulbar) G12.21
      adult G12.1
      infantile (spinal) G12.0
      spinal G12.25
        adult G12.1
        infantile G12.0
    pseudohypertrophic G71.02
    shoulder region M62.51- ☑
    specified site NEC M62.58
    spinal G12.9
      adult form G12.1
      Aran-Duchenne G12.21
      childhood form, type II G12.1
      distal G12.1
      hereditary NEC G12.1
      infantile, type I (Werdnig-Hoffmann) G12.0
      juvenile form, type III (Kugelberg- Welander) G12.1
      progressive G12.25
      scapuloperoneal form G12.1
      specified NEC G12.8
    syphilitic A52.78
    thigh M62.55- ☑
    upper arm M62.52- ☑
  myocardium — *see* Degeneration, myocardial
  myometrium (senile) N85.8
    cervix N88.8
  myopathic NEC — *see* Atrophy, muscle
  myotonia G71.11
  nail L60.3
  nasopharynx J31.1
  nerve — *see also* Disorder, nerve
    abducens — *see* Strabismus, paralytic, sixth nerve
    accessory G52.8
    acoustic or auditory H93.3- ☑
    cranial G52.9
      eighth (auditory) H93.3- ☑
      eleventh (accessory) G52.8
      fifth (trigeminal) G50.8
      first (olfactory) G52.0
      fourth (trochlear) — *see* Strabismus, paralytic, fourth nerve
      second (optic) H47.20
      sixth (abducens) — *see* Strabismus, paralytic, sixth nerve
      tenth (pneumogastric) (vagus) G52.2
      third (oculomotor) — *see* Strabismus, paralytic, third nerve
      twelfth (hypoglossal) G52.3
    hypoglossal G52.3
    oculomotor — *see* Strabismus, paralytic, third nerve
    olfactory G52.0
    optic (papillomacular bundle)
      syphilitic (late) A52.15
        congenital A50.44
    pneumogastric G52.2
    trigeminal G50.8
    trochlear — *see* Strabismus, paralytic, fourth nerve
    vagus (pneumogastric) G52.2
  neurogenic, bone, tabetic A52.11
  nutritional E43
    with marasmus E41
  old age R54
  olivopontocerebellar G23.8
  optic (nerve) H47.20
    glaucomatous H47.23- ☑
    hereditary H47.22
    primary H47.21- ☑
    specified type NEC H47.29- ☑
    syphilitic (late) A52.15
      congenital A50.44
  orbit H05.31- ☑
  ovary (senile) N83.31- ☑
    with fallopian tube N83.33- ☑
  oviduct (senile) — *see* Atrophy, fallopian tube
  palsy, diffuse (progressive) G12.22
  pancreas (duct) (senile) K86.89
  parotid gland K11.0
  pelvic muscle N81.84
  penis N48.89
  pharynx J39.2
  pluriglandular E31.8
    autoimmune E31.0

Atrophy, atrophic — *continued*
  polyarthritis M15.9
  prostate N42.89
  pseudohypertrophic (muscle) G71.02
  renal — *see also* Sclerosis, renal N26.1
  retina, retinal (postinfectional) H35.89
  rhinitis J31.0
  salivary gland K11.0
  scar L90.5
  sclerosis, lobar (of brain) — *see also* Dementia, in, diseases specified elsewhere G31.09 *[F02.80]*
    with behavioral disturbance — *see also* Dementia, in, diseases specified elsewhere G31.09 *[F02.81-]* ☑
  scrotum N50.89
  seminal vesicle N50.89
  senile R54
    due to radiation (nonionizing) (solar) L57.8
  skin (patches) (spots) L90.9
    degenerative (senile) L90.8
    due to radiation (nonionizing) (solar) L57.8
    senile L90.8
  spermatic cord N50.89
  spinal (acute) (cord) G95.89
    muscular — *see* Atrophy, muscle, spinal
    paralysis G12.20
      acute — *see* Poliomyelitis, paralytic
      meaning progressive muscular atrophy G12.25
  spine (column) — *see* Spondylopathy, specified NEC
  spleen (senile) D73.0
  stomach K29.40
    with bleeding K29.41
  striate (skin) L90.6
    syphilitic A52.79
  subcutaneous L90.9
  sublingual gland K11.0
  submandibular gland K11.0
  submaxillary gland K11.0
  Sudeck's — *see* Algoneurodystrophy
  suprarenal (capsule) (gland) E27.49
    primary E27.1
  systemic affecting central nervous system in
    myxedema E03.9 *[G13.2]*
    neoplastic disease — *see also* Neoplasm D49.9 *[G13.1]*
    specified disease NEC G13.8
  tarso-orbital fascia, congenital Q10.3
  testis N50.0
  thenar, partial — *see* Syndrome, carpal tunnel
  thymus (fatty) E32.8
  thyroid (gland) (acquired) E03.4
    with cretinism E03.1
    congenital (with myxedema) E03.1
  tongue (senile) K14.8
    papillae K14.4
  trachea J39.8
  tunica vaginalis N50.89
  turbinate J34.89
  tympanic membrane (nonflaccid) H73.82- ☑
    flaccid H73.81- ☑
  upper respiratory tract J39.8
  uterus, uterine (senile) N85.8
    cervix N88.8
    due to radiation (intended effect) N85.8
      adverse effect or misadventure N99.89
  vagina (senile) N95.2
  vas deferens N50.89
  vascular I99.8
  vertebra (senile) — *see* Spondylopathy, specified NEC
  vulva (senile) N90.5
  Werdnig-Hoffmann G12.0
  yellow — *see* Failure, hepatic

Attack, attacks
  with alteration of consciousness (with automatisms) — *see* Epilepsy, localization-related, symptomatic, with complex partial seizures
  Adams-Stokes I45.9
  akinetic — *see* Epilepsy, generalized, specified NEC
  angina — *see* Angina
  atonic — *see* Epilepsy, generalized, specified NEC
  benign shuddering G25.83
  cataleptic — *see* Catalepsy
  coronary — *see* Infarct, myocardium
  cyanotic, newborn P28.2
  drop NEC R55
  epileptic — *see* Epilepsy
  heart — *see* Infarct, myocardium
  hysterical F44.9

Attack, attacks — continued
    jacksonian — see Epilepsy, localization-related, symptomatic, with simple partial seizures
    myocardium, myocardial — see Infarct, myocardium
    myoclonic — see Epilepsy, generalized, specified NEC
    panic F41.0
    psychomotor — see Epilepsy, localization-related, symptomatic, with complex partial seizures
    salaam — see Epilepsy, spasms
    schizophreniform, brief F23
    shuddering, benign G25.83
    Stokes-Adams I45.9
    syncope R55
    transient ischemic (TIA) G45.9
        specified NEC G45.8
    unconsciousness R55
        hysterical F44.89
    vasomotor R55
    vasovagal (paroxysmal) (idiopathic) R55
    without alteration of consciousness — see Epilepsy, localization-related, symptomatic, with simple partial seizures
Attention (to)
    artificial
        opening (of) Z43.9
            digestive tract NEC Z43.4
                colon Z43.3
                ilium Z43.2
                stomach Z43.1
            specified NEC Z43.8
            trachea Z43.0
            urinary tract NEC Z43.6
                cystostomy Z43.5
                nephrostomy Z43.6
                ureterostomy Z43.6
                urethrostomy Z43.6
            vagina Z43.7
        colostomy Z43.3
        cystostomy Z43.5
    deficit disorder or syndrome F98.8
        with hyperactivity — see Disorder, attention-deficit hyperactivity
    gastrostomy Z43.1
    ileostomy Z43.2
    jejunostomy Z43.4
    nephrostomy Z43.6
    surgical dressings Z48.01
    sutures Z48.02
    tracheostomy Z43.0
    ureterostomy Z43.6
    urethrostomy Z43.6
Attrition
    gum — see Recession, gingival
    tooth, teeth (excessive) (hard tissues) K03.0
Atypical, atypism — see also condition
    cells (on cytolgocial smear) (endocervical) (endometrial) (glandular)
        cervix R87.619
        vagina R87.629
    cervical N87.9
    endometrium N85.9
        hyperplasia N85.00
    parenting situation Z62.9
Auditory — see condition
Aujeszky's disease B33.8
Aurantiasis, cutis E67.1
Auricle, auricular — see also condition
    cervical Q18.2
Auriculotemporal syndrome G50.8
Austin Flint murmur (aortic insufficiency) I35.1
Australian
    Q fever A78
    X disease A83.4
Autism, autistic (childhood) (infantile) F84.0
    atypical F84.9
    spectrum disorder F84.0
Autoantibodies, multiple confirmed islet, with normoglycemia E10.A1
Autodigestion R68.89
Autoerythrocyte sensitization (syndrome) D69.2
Autographism L50.3
Autoimmune
    disease (systemic) M35.9
        inhibitors to clotting factors D68.311
    lymphoproliferative syndrome [ALPS] D89.82
    thyroiditis E06.3
Autoimmunity, confirmed islet, with dysglycemia E10.A2
Autointoxication R68.89
Automatism G93.89

Automatism — continued
    with temporal sclerosis G93.81
        epileptic — see Epilepsy, localization-related, symptomatic, with complex partial seizures
        paroxysmal, idiopathic — see Epilepsy, localization-related, symptomatic, with complex partial seizures
Autonomic, autonomous
    bladder (neurogenic) N31.2
    hysteria seizure F44.5
Autosensitivity, erythrocyte D69.2
Autosensitization, cutaneous L30.2
Autosome — see condition by chromosome involved
Autotopagnosia R48.1
Autotoxemia R68.89
Autumn — see condition
Avellis' syndrome G46.8
Aversion
    oral R63.39
        newborn P92.8
        nonorganic origin F98.2- ☑
    sexual F52.1
Aviator's
    disease or sickness — see Effect, adverse, high altitude
    ear T70.0- ☑
Avitaminosis (multiple) — see also Deficiency, vitamin E56.9
    B E53.9
        with
            beriberi E51.11
            pellagra E52
    B2 E53.0
    B6 E53.1
    B12 E53.8
    D E55.9
        with rickets E55.0
    G E53.0
    K E56.1
    nicotinic acid E52
AVNRT (atrioventricular nodal re-entrant tachycardia) I47.19
AVRT (atrioventricular nodal re-entrant tachycardia) I47.19
Avulsion (traumatic)
    blood vessel — see Injury, blood vessel
    bone — see Fracture, by site
    cartilage — see Dislocation, by site
        symphyseal (inner), complicating delivery O71.6
    external site other than limb — see Wound, open, by site
    eye S05.7- ☑
    head (intracranial)
        external site NEC S08.89- ☑
        scalp S08.0- ☑
    internal organ or site — see Injury, by site
    joint — see also Dislocation, by site
        capsule — see Sprain, by site
    kidney S37.06- ☑
    ligament — see Sprain, by site
    limb — see also Amputation, traumatic, by site
        skin and subcutaneous tissue — see Wound, open, by site
    muscle — see Injury, muscle
    nerve (root) — see Injury, nerve
    scalp S08.0- ☑
    skin and subcutaneous tissue — see Wound, open, by site
    spleen S36.032- ☑
    symphyseal cartilage (inner), complicating delivery O71.6
    tendon — see Injury, muscle
    tooth S03.2- ☑
Awareness of heart beat R00.2
Axenfeld's
    anomaly or syndrome Q15.0
    degeneration (calcareous) Q13.4
Axilla, axillary — see also condition
    breast Q83.1
Axonotmesis — see Injury, nerve
Ayerza's disease or syndrome (pulmonary artery sclerosis with pulmonary hypertension) I27.0
Azoospermia (organic) N46.01
    due to
        drug therapy N46.021
        efferent duct obstruction N46.023
        infection N46.022
        radiation N46.024
        specified cause NEC N46.029
        systemic disease N46.025
Azotemia R79.89
    meaning uremia N19
Aztec ear Q17.3
Azygos
    continuation inferior vena cava Q26.8

Azygos — continued
    lobe (lung) Q33.1

B

Baastrup's disease — see Kissing spine
Babesiosis B60.00
    due to
        Babesia
            divergens B60.03
            duncani B60.02
            KO-1 B60.09
            microti B60.01
            MO-1 B60.03
        species
            unspecified B60.00
            venatorum B60.09
        specified NEC B60.09
Babington's disease (familial hemorrhagic telangiectasia) I78.0
Babinski's syndrome A52.79
Baby
    crying constantly R68.11
    floppy (syndrome) P94.2
Bacillary — see condition
Bacilluria R82.71
Bacillus — see also Infection, bacillus
    abortus infection A23.1
    anthracis infection A22.9
    coli infection — see also Escherichia coli B96.20
    Flexner's A03.1
    mallei infection A24.0
    Shiga's A03.0
    suipestifer infection — see Infection, salmonella
Back — see condition
Backache (postural) M54.9
    sacroiliac M53.3
    specified NEC M54.89
Backflow — see Reflux
Backward reading (dyslexia) F81.0
Bacteremia R78.81
    with sepsis — see Sepsis
Bactericholia — see Cholecystitis, acute
Bacterid, bacteride (pustular) L40.3
Bacterium, bacteria, bacterial
    agent NEC, as cause of disease classified elsewhere B96.89
    in blood — see Bacteremia
    in urine — see Bacteriuria
Bacteriuria, bacteruria (asymptomatic) R82.71
Bacteroides
    fragilis, as cause of disease classified elsewhere B96.6
Bad
    heart — see Disease, heart
    trip
        due to drug abuse — see Abuse, drug, hallucinogen
        due to drug dependence — see Dependence, drug, hallucinogen
Baelz's disease (cheilitis glandularis apostematosa) K13.0
Baerensprung's disease (eczema marginatum) B35.6
Bagasse disease or pneumonitis J67.1
Bagassosis J67.1
Baker's cyst — see Cyst, Baker's
Bakwin-Krida syndrome (metaphyseal dysplasia) Q78.5
Balancing side interference M26.56
Balanitis (circinata) (erosiva) (gangrenosa) (phagedenic) (vulgaris) N48.1
    amebic A06.82
    candidal B37.42
    due to Haemophilus ducreyi A57
    gonococcal (acute) (chronic) A54.23
    xerotica obliterans N48.0
Balanoposthitis N47.6
    gonococcal (acute) (chronic) A54.23
    ulcerative (specific) A63.8
Balanorrhagia — see Balanitis
Balantidiasis, balantidiosis A07.0
Bald tongue K14.4
Baldness — see also Alopecia
    male-pattern — see Alopecia, androgenic
Balkan grippe A78
Balloon disease — see Effect, adverse, high altitude
Balo's disease (concentric sclerosis) G37.5
Bamberger-Marie disease — see Osteoarthropathy, hypertrophic, specified type NEC
Bancroft's filariasis B74.0
Band(s)
    adhesive — see Adhesions, peritoneum
    anomalous or congenital — see also Anomaly, by site

Band(s) — continued
  anomalous or congenital — see also Anomaly, by site — continued
    heart (atrial) (ventricular) Q24.8
    intestine Q43.3
    omentum Q43.3
  cervix N88.1
  constricting, congenital Q79.8
  gallbladder (congenital) Q44.1
  intestinal (adhesive) — see Adhesions, peritoneum
  obstructive
    intestine K56.50
      complete K56.52
      incomplete K56.51
      partial K56.51
    peritoneum K56.50
      complete K56.52
      incomplete K56.51
      partial K56.51
  periappendiceal, congenital Q43.3
  peritoneal (adhesive) — see Adhesions, peritoneum
  uterus N73.6
    internal N85.6
  vagina N89.5
Bandemia D72.825
Bandl's ring (contraction), complicating delivery O62.4
Bangkok hemorrhagic fever A91
Bang's disease (brucella abortus) A23.1
Bankruptcy (anxiety concerning) Z59.868
Bannister's disease T78.3- ☑
  hereditary D84.1
Banti's disease or syndrome (with cirrhosis) (with portal hypertension) K76.6
Bar, median, prostate — see Enlargement, enlarged, prostate
Barcoo disease or rot — see Ulcer, skin
Barlow's disease E54
Barodontalgia T70.29- ☑
Baron Munchausen syndrome — see Disorder, factitious
Barosinusitis T70.1- ☑
Barotitis T70.0- ☑
Barotrauma T70.29- ☑
  odontalgia T70.29- ☑
  otitic T70.0- ☑
  sinus T70.1- ☑
Barraquer (-Simons) **disease or syndrome** (progressive lipodystrophy) E88.11
Barre-Guillain disease or syndrome G61.0
Barre-Lieou syndrome (posterior cervical sympathetic) M53.0
Barrel chest M95.4
Barrett's
  disease — see Barrett's, esophagus
  esophagus K22.70
    with dysplasia K22.719
      high grade K22.711
      low grade K22.710
    without dysplasia K22.70
  syndrome — see Barrett's, esophagus
  ulcer K22.10
    with bleeding K22.11
    without bleeding K22.10
Barsony (-Polgar) (-Teschendorf) **syndrome** (corkscrew esophagus) K22.4
Barth syndrome E78.71
Bartholinitis (suppurating) N75.8
  gonococcal (acute) (chronic) (with abscess) A54.1
Bartonellosis A44.9
  cutaneous A44.1
  mucocutaneous A44.1
  specified NEC A44.8
  systemic A44.0
Barton's fracture S52.56- ☑
Bartter's syndrome E26.81
Basal — see condition
Basan's (hidrotic) ectodermal dysplasia Q82.4
Baseball finger — see Dislocation, finger
Basedow's disease (exophthalmic goiter) — see Hyperthyroidism, with, goiter
Basic — see condition
Basilar — see condition
Bason's (hidrotic) ectodermal dysplasia Q82.4
Basopenia — see Agranulocytosis
Basophilia D72.824
Basophilism (cortico-adrenal) (Cushing's) (pituitary) E24.0
Bassen-Kornzweig disease or syndrome E78.6
Bat ear Q17.5

Bateman's
  disease B08.1
  purpura (senile) D69.2
Bathing cramp T75.1- ☑
Bathophobia F40.248
Batten (-Mayou) **disease** E75.4
  retina E75.4 [H36.89]
Batten-Steinert syndrome G71.11
Battered — see Maltreatment
Battey Mycobacterium infection A31.0
Battle exhaustion F43.0
Battledore placenta O43.19- ☑
Baumgarten-Cruveilhier cirrhosis, disease or syndrome K74.69
Bauxite fibrosis (of lung) J63.1
Bayle's disease (general paresis) A52.17
Bazin's disease (primary) (tuberculous) A18.4
Beach ear — see Swimmer's, ear
Beaded hair (congenital) Q84.1
Beal conjunctivitis or syndrome B30.2
Beard's disease (neurasthenia) F48.8
Beat(s)
  atrial, premature I49.1
  ectopic I49.49
  elbow — see Bursitis, elbow
  escaped, heart I49.49
  hand — see Bursitis, hand
  knee — see Bursitis, knee
  premature I49.40
    atrial I49.1
    auricular I49.1
    supraventricular I49.1
Beau's
  disease or syndrome — see Degeneration, myocardial
  lines (transverse furrows on fingernails) L60.4
Bechterev's syndrome — see Spondylitis, ankylosing
Becker's
  cardiomyopathy I42.8
  disease
    idiopathic mural endomyocardial disease I42.3
    myotonia congenita, recessive form G71.12
  dystrophy G71.01
  pigmented hairy nevus D22.5
Beck's syndrome (anterior spinal artery occlusion) I65.8
Beckwith-Wiedemann syndrome Q87.3
Bed confinement status Z74.01
Bed-sharing, infant Z72.823
Bed sore — see Ulcer, pressure, by site
Bedbug bite(s) — see Bite(s), by site, superficial, insect
Bedclothes, asphyxiation or suffocation by — see Asphyxia, traumatic, due to, mechanical, trapped
Bednar's
  aphthae K12.0
  tumor — see Neoplasm, malignant, by site
Bedridden Z74.01
Bedsore — see Ulcer, pressure, by site
Bedwetting — see Enuresis
Bee sting (with allergic or anaphylactic shock) T63.44- ☑
Beer drinker's heart (disease) I42.6
Begbie's disease (exophthalmic goiter) — see Hyperthyroidism, with, goiter
Behavior
  antisocial
    adult Z72.811
    child or adolescent Z72.810
  disorder, disturbance — see Disorder, conduct
  disruptive — see Disorder, conduct
  drug seeking Z76.5
  inexplicable R46.2
  marked evasiveness R46.5
  obsessive-compulsive R46.81
  overactivity R46.3
  poor responsiveness R46.4
  self-damaging (life-style) Z72.89
  sleep-incompatible Z72.821
  slowness R46.4
  specified NEC R46.89
  strange (and inexplicable) R46.2
  suspiciousness R46.5
  type A pattern Z73.1
  undue concern or preoccupation with stressful events R46.6
  verbosity and circumstantial detail obscuring reason for contact R46.7
Behcet's disease or syndrome M35.2
Behr's disease — see Degeneration, macula
Beigel's disease or morbus (white piedra) B36.2
Bejel A65
Bekhterev's syndrome — see Spondylitis, ankylosing

Belching — see Eructation
Bell's
  mania F30.8
  palsy, paralysis G51.0
    infant or newborn P11.3
  spasm G51.3- ☑
Bence Jones albuminuria or proteinuria NEC R80.3
Bends T70.3- ☑
Benedikt's paralysis or syndrome G46.3
Benign — see also condition
  prostatic hyperplasia — see Hyperplasia, prostate
Bennett's fracture (displaced) S62.21- ☑
Benson's disease — see Deposit, crystalline
Bent
  back (hysterical) F44.4
  nose M95.0
    congenital Q67.4
Bereavement (uncomplicated) Z63.4
Bergeron's disease (hysterical chorea) F44.4
Berger's disease — see Nephropathy, IgA
Beriberi (dry) E51.11
  heart (disease) E51.12
  polyneuropathy E51.11
  wet E51.12
  involving circulatory system E51.11
Berlin's disease or edema (traumatic) S05.8X- ☑
Berlock (berloque) **dermatitis** L56.2
Bernard-Horner syndrome G90.2
Bernard-Soulier disease or thrombopathia D69.1
Bernhardt (-Roth) **disease** — see Mononeuropathy, lower limb, meralgia paresthetica
Bernheim's syndrome — see Failure, heart, right
Bertielliasis B71.8
Berylliosis (lung) J63.2
Besnier-Boeck (-Schaumann) **disease** — see Sarcoidosis
Besnier's
  lupus pernio D86.3
  prurigo L20.0
Bestiality F65.89
Best's disease H35.50
Beta-mercaptolactate-cysteine disulfiduria E72.09
Betalipoproteinemia, broad or floating E78.2
Betting and gambling Z72.6
  pathological (compulsive) F63.0
Bezoar T18.9- ☑
  intestine T18.3- ☑
  stomach T18.2- ☑
Bezold's abscess — see Mastoiditis, acute
BI-RADS — see Breast, Imaging Reporting and Data System
Bianchi's syndrome R48.8
Bicornate or bicornis uterus Q51.3
  in pregnancy or childbirth O34.00
    causing obstructed labor O65.5
Bicuspid aortic valve (at birth) (congenital) Q23.81
  functional, with stenosis — see Stenosis, aortic (valve)
Biedl-Bardet syndrome Q87.83
Bielschowsky (-Jansky) **disease** E75.4
Biermer's (pernicious) **anemia or disease** D51.0
Biett's disease L93.0
Bifid (congenital)
  apex, heart Q24.8
  clitoris Q52.6
  kidney Q63.8
  nose Q30.2
  patella Q74.1
  scrotum Q55.29
  toe NEC Q74.2
  tongue Q38.3
  ureter Q62.8
  uterus Q51.3
  uvula Q35.7
Biforis uterus (suprasimplex) Q51.3
Bifurcation (congenital)
  gallbladder Q44.1
  kidney pelvis Q63.8
  renal pelvis Q63.8
  rib Q76.6
  tongue, congenital Q38.3
  trachea Q32.1
  ureter Q62.8
  urethra Q64.74
  vertebra Q76.49
Big spleen syndrome D73.1
Bigeminal pulse R00.8
Bigorexia F45.22
Bilateral — see condition
Bile
  duct — see condition

Bile — continued
  pigments in urine R82.2
Bilharziasis — see also Schistosomiasis
  chyluria B65.0
  cutaneous B65.3
  galacturia B65.0
  hematochyluria B65.0
  intestinal B65.1
  lipemia B65.9
  lipuria B65.0
  oriental B65.2
  piarhemia B65.9
  pulmonary NOS B65.9 [J99]
    pneumonia B65.9 [J17]
  tropical hematuria B65.0
  vesical B65.0
Biliary — see condition
Bilirubin metabolism disorder E80.7
  specified NEC E80.6
Bilirubinemia, familial nonhemolytic E80.4
Bilirubinuria R82.2
Biliuria R82.2
Bilocular stomach K31.2
Binswanger's disease I67.3
Biparta, bipartite
  carpal scaphoid Q74.0
  patella Q74.1
  vagina Q52.10
Bird
  face Q75.8
  fancier's disease or lung J67.2
Birt-Hogg-Dube syndrome Q87.89
Birth
  complications in mother — see Delivery, complicated
  compression during NOS P15.9
  defect — see Anomaly
  immature (less than 37 completed weeks) — see Preterm, newborn
    extremely (less than 28 completed weeks) — see Immaturity, extreme
  inattention, at or after — see Maltreatment, child, neglect
  injury NOS P15.9
    basal ganglia P11.1
    brachial plexus NEC P14.3
    brain (compression) (pressure) P11.2
    central nervous system NOS P11.9
    cerebellum P11.1
    cerebral hemorrhage P10.1
    external genitalia P15.5
    eye P15.3
    face P15.4
    fracture
      bone P13.9
        specified NEC P13.8
      clavicle P13.4
      femur P13.2
      humerus P13.3
      long bone, except femur P13.3
      radius and ulna P13.3
      skull P13.0
      spine P11.5
      tibia and fibula P13.3
    intracranial P11.2
      laceration or hemorrhage P10.9
        specified NEC P10.8
    intraventricular hemorrhage P10.2
    laceration
      brain P10.1
      by scalpel P15.8
      peripheral nerve P14.9
    liver P15.0
    meninges
      brain P11.1
      spinal cord P11.5
    nerve
      brachial plexus P14.3
      cranial NEC (except facial) P11.4
      facial P11.3
      peripheral P14.9
      phrenic (paralysis) P14.2
    paralysis
      facial nerve P11.3
      spinal P11.5
    penis P15.5
    rupture
      spinal cord P11.5
    scalp P12.9
    scalpel wound P15.8
    scrotum P15.5

Birth — continued
  injury — continued
    skull NEC P13.1
      fracture P13.0
    specified type NEC P15.8
    spinal cord P11.5
    spine P11.5
    spleen P15.1
    sternomastoid (hematoma) P15.2
    subarachnoid hemorrhage P10.3
    subcutaneous fat necrosis P15.6
    subdural hemorrhage P10.0
    tentorial tear P10.4
    testes P15.5
    vulva P15.5
  lack of care, at or after — see Maltreatment, child, neglect
  neglect, at or after — see Maltreatment, child, neglect
  palsy or paralysis, newborn, NOS (birth injury) P14.9
  premature (infant) — see Preterm, newborn
  shock, newborn P96.89
  trauma — see Birth, injury
  weight
    low (2499 grams or less) — see Low, birthweight
      extremely (999 grams or less) — see Low, birthweight, extreme
    4000 grams to 4499 grams P08.1
    4500 grams or more P08.0
Birthmark Q82.5
Bisalbuminemia E88.09
Biskra's button B55.1
Bite(s) (animal) (human)
  abdomen, abdominal
    wall S31.159-
      with penetration into peritoneal cavity S31.659-
      epigastric region S31.152-
        with penetration into peritoneal cavity S31.652-
      left
        lower quadrant S31.154-
          with penetration into peritoneal cavity S31.654-
        upper quadrant S31.151-
          with penetration into peritoneal cavity S31.651-
      periumbilic region S31.155-
        with penetration into peritoneal cavity S31.655-
      right
        lower quadrant S31.153-
          with penetration into peritoneal cavity S31.653-
        upper quadrant S31.150-
          with penetration into peritoneal cavity S31.650-
      superficial NEC S30.871-
        insect S30.861-
  alveolar (process) — see Bite, oral cavity
  amphibian (venomous) — see Venom, bite, amphibian
  animal — see also Bite, by site
    venomous — see Venom
  ankle S91.05-
    superficial NEC S90.57-
      insect S90.56-
  antecubital space — see Bite, elbow
  anus S31.835-
    superficial NEC S30.877-
      insect S30.867-
  arm (upper) S41.15-
    lower — see Bite, forearm
    superficial NEC S40.87-
      insect S40.86-
  arthropod NEC — see Venom, bite, arthropod
  auditory canal (external) (meatus) — see Bite, ear
  auricle, ear — see Bite, ear
  axilla — see Bite, arm
  back — see also Bite, thorax, back
    lower S31.050-
      with penetration into retroperitoneal space S31.051-
      superficial NEC S30.870-
        insect S30.860-
  bedbug — see Bite(s), by site, superficial, insect
  breast S21.05-
    superficial NEC S20.17-
      insect S20.16-
  brow — see Bite, head, specified site NEC
  buttock S31.805-

Bite(s) — continued
  buttock — continued
    left S31.825-
    right S31.815-
    superficial NEC S30.870-
      insect S30.860-
  calf — see Bite, leg
  canaliculus lacrimalis — see Bite, eyelid
  canthus, eye — see Bite, eyelid
  centipede — see Toxicity, venom, arthropod, centipede
  cheek (external) S01.45-
    internal — see Bite, oral cavity
    superficial NEC S00.87-
      insect S00.86-
  chest wall — see Bite, thorax
  chigger B88.09
  chin — see Bite, head, specified site NEC
  clitoris — see Bite, vulva
  costal region — see Bite, thorax
  digit(s)
    hand — see Bite, finger
    toe — see Bite, toe
  ear (canal) (external) S01.35-
    superficial NEC S00.47-
      insect S00.46-
  elbow S51.05-
    superficial NEC S50.37-
      insect S50.36-
  epididymis — see Bite, testis
  epigastric region — see Bite, abdomen
  epiglottis — see Bite, neck, specified site NEC
  esophagus, cervical S11.25-
    superficial NEC S10.17-
      insect S10.16-
  eyebrow — see Bite, eyelid
  eyelid S01.15-
    superficial NEC S00.27-
      insect S00.26-
  face NEC — see Bite, head, specified site NEC
  finger(s) S61.259-
    with
      damage to nail S61.359-
    index S61.258-
      with
        damage to nail S61.358-
      left S61.251-
        with
          damage to nail S61.351-
      right S61.250-
        with
          damage to nail S61.350-
      superficial NEC S60.478-
        insect S60.46-
    little S61.25-
      with
        damage to nail S61.35-
      superficial NEC S60.47-
        insect S60.46-
    middle S61.25-
      with
        damage to nail S61.35-
      superficial NEC S60.47-
        insect S60.46-
    ring S61.25-
      with
        damage to nail S61.35-
      superficial NEC S60.47-
        insect S60.46-
    superficial NEC S60.479-
      insect S60.469-
    thumb — see Bite, thumb
  flank S31.15A-
    with penetration into peritoneal cavity S31.65A-
    left S31.157-
      with penetration into peritoneal cavity S31.657-
    right S31.156-
      with penetration into peritoneal cavity S31.656-
    superficial NEC S30.87A-
      insect S30.86A-
  flea — see Bite, by site, superficial, insect
  foot (except toe(s) alone) S91.35-
    superficial NEC S90.87-
      insect S90.86-
    toe — see Bite, toe
  forearm S51.85-
    elbow only — see Bite, elbow

Bite(s) — continued
    forearm — continued
        superficial NEC S50.87- ☑
            insect S50.86- ☑
    forehead — see Bite, head, specified site NEC
    genital organs, external
        female S31.552- ☑
            superficial NEC S30.876- ☑
                insect S30.866- ☑
            vagina and vulva — see Bite, vulva
        male S31.551- ☑
            penis — see Bite, penis
            scrotum — see Bite, scrotum
            superficial NEC S30.875- ☑
                insect S30.865- ☑
            testes — see Bite, testis
    groin — see Bite, abdomen, wall
    gum — see Bite, oral cavity
    hand S61.45- ☑
        finger — see Bite, finger
        superficial NEC S60.57- ☑
            insect S60.56- ☑
        thumb — see Bite, thumb
    head S01.95- ☑
        cheek — see Bite, cheek
        ear — see Bite, ear
        eyelid — see Bite, eyelid
        lip — see Bite, lip
        nose — see Bite, nose
        oral cavity — see Bite, oral cavity
        scalp — see Bite, scalp
        specified site NEC S01.85- ☑
            superficial NEC S00.87- ☑
                insect S00.86- ☑
            superficial NEC S00.97- ☑
                insect S00.96- ☑
        temporomandibular area — see Bite, cheek
    heel — see Bite, foot
    hip S71.05- ☑
        superficial NEC S70.27- ☑
            insect S70.26- ☑
    hymen S31.45- ☑
    hypochondrium — see Bite, abdomen, wall
    hypogastric region — see Bite, abdomen, wall
    inguinal region — see Bite, abdomen, wall
    insect — see Bite, by site, superficial, insect
    instep — see Bite, foot
    interscapular region — see Bite, thorax, back
    jaw — see Bite, head, specified site NEC
    knee S81.05- ☑
        superficial NEC S80.27- ☑
            insect S80.26- ☑
    labium (majus) (minus) — see Bite, vulva
    lacrimal duct — see Bite, eyelid
    larynx S11.015- ☑
        superficial NEC S10.17- ☑
            insect S10.16- ☑
    leg (lower) S81.85- ☑
        ankle — see Bite, ankle
        foot — see Bite, foot
        knee — see Bite, knee
        superficial NEC S80.87- ☑
            insect S80.86- ☑
        toe — see Bite, toe
        upper — see Bite, thigh
    lip S01.551- ☑
        superficial NEC S00.571- ☑
            insect S00.561- ☑
    lizard (venomous) — see Venom, bite, reptile
    loin — see Bite, abdomen, wall
    lower back — see Bite, back, lower
    lumbar region — see Bite, back, lower
    malar region — see Bite, head, specified site NEC
    mammary — see Bite, breast
    marine animals (venomous) — see Toxicity, venom, marine animal
    mastoid region — see Bite, head, specified site NEC
    mouth — see Bite, oral cavity
    nail
        finger — see Bite, finger
        toe — see Bite, toe
    nape — see Bite, neck, specified site NEC
    nasal (septum) (sinus) — see Bite, nose
    nasopharynx — see Bite, head, specified site NEC
    neck S11.95- ☑
        involving
            cervical esophagus — see Bite, esophagus, cervical

Bite(s) — continued
    neck — continued
        involving — continued
            larynx — see Bite, larynx
            pharynx — see Bite, pharynx
            thyroid gland S11.15- ☑
            trachea — see Bite, trachea
        specified site NEC S11.85- ☑
            superficial NEC S10.87- ☑
                insect S10.86- ☑
            superficial NEC S10.97- ☑
                insect S10.96- ☑
        throat S11.85- ☑
            superficial NEC S10.17- ☑
                insect S10.16- ☑
    nose (septum) (sinus) S01.25- ☑
        superficial NEC S00.37- ☑
            insect S00.36- ☑
    occipital region — see Bite, scalp
    oral cavity S01.552- ☑
        superficial NEC S00.572- ☑
            insect S00.562- ☑
    orbital region — see Bite, eyelid
    palate — see Bite, oral cavity
    palm — see Bite, hand
    parietal region — see Bite, scalp
    pelvis S31.050- ☑
        with penetration into retroperitoneal space S31.051- ☑
        superficial NEC S30.870- ☑
            insect S30.860- ☑
    penis S31.25- ☑
        superficial NEC S30.872- ☑
            insect S30.862- ☑
    perineum
        female — see Bite, vulva
        male — see Bite, pelvis
    periocular area (with or without lacrimal passages) — see Bite, eyelid
    phalanges
        finger — see Bite, finger
        toe — see Bite, toe
    pharynx S11.25- ☑
        superficial NEC S10.17- ☑
            insect S10.16- ☑
    pinna — see Bite, ear
    poisonous — see Venom
    popliteal space — see Bite, knee
    prepuce — see Bite, penis
    pubic region — see Bite, abdomen, wall
    rectovaginal septum — see Bite, vulva
    red bug B88.09
    reptile NEC — see also Venom, bite, reptile
        nonvenomous — see Bite, by site
        snake — see Venom, bite, snake
    sacral region — see Bite, back, lower
    sacroiliac region — see Bite, back, lower
    salivary gland — see Bite, oral cavity
    scalp S01.05- ☑
        superficial NEC S00.07- ☑
            insect S00.06- ☑
    scapular region — see Bite, shoulder
    scrotum S31.35- ☑
        superficial NEC S30.873- ☑
            insect S30.863- ☑
    sea-snake (venomous) — see Toxicity, venom, snake, sea snake
    shin — see Bite, leg
    shoulder S41.05- ☑
        superficial NEC S40.27- ☑
            insect S40.26- ☑
    snake — see also Venom, bite, snake
        nonvenomous — see Bite, by site
    spermatic cord — see Bite, testis
    spider (venomous) — see Toxicity, venom, spider
        nonvenomous — see Bite, by site, superficial, insect
    sternal region — see Bite, thorax, front
    submaxillary region — see Bite, head, specified site NEC
    submental region — see Bite, head, specified site NEC
    subungual
        finger(s) — see Bite, finger
        toe — see Bite, toe
    superficial — see Bite, by site, superficial
    supraclavicular fossa S11.85- ☑
    supraorbital — see Bite, head, specified site NEC
    temple, temporal region — see Bite, head, specified site NEC

Bite(s) — continued
    temporomandibular area — see Bite, cheek
    testis S31.35- ☑
        superficial NEC S30.873- ☑
            insect S30.863- ☑
    thigh S71.15- ☑
        superficial NEC S70.37- ☑
            insect S70.36- ☑
    thorax, thoracic (wall) S21.95- ☑
        back S21.25- ☑
            with penetration into thoracic cavity S21.45- ☑
        breast — see Bite, breast
        front S21.15- ☑
            with penetration into thoracic cavity S21.35- ☑
        superficial NEC S20.97- ☑
            back S20.47- ☑
            front S20.37- ☑
            insect S20.96- ☑
                back S20.46- ☑
                front S20.36- ☑
    throat — see Bite, neck, throat
    thumb S61.05- ☑
        with
            damage to nail S61.15- ☑
        superficial NEC S60.37- ☑
            insect S60.36- ☑
    thyroid S11.15- ☑
        superficial NEC S10.87- ☑
            insect S10.86- ☑
    toe(s) S91.15- ☑
        with
            damage to nail S91.25- ☑
        great S91.15- ☑
            with
                damage to nail S91.25- ☑
        lesser S91.15- ☑
            with
                damage to nail S91.25- ☑
        superficial NEC S90.47- ☑
            great S90.47- ☑
            insect S90.46- ☑
                great S90.46- ☑
    tongue S01.552- ☑
    trachea S11.025- ☑
        superficial NEC S10.17- ☑
            insect S10.16- ☑
    tunica vaginalis — see Bite, testis
    tympanum, tympanic membrane — see Bite, ear
    umbilical region S31.155- ☑
    uvula — see Bite, oral cavity
    vagina — see Bite, vulva
    venomous — see Venom
    vocal cords S11.035- ☑
        superficial NEC S10.17- ☑
            insect S10.16- ☑
    vulva S31.45- ☑
        superficial NEC S30.874- ☑
            insect S30.864- ☑
    wrist S61.55- ☑
        superficial NEC S60.87- ☑
            insect S60.86- ☑
Biting, cheek or lip K13.1
Biventricular failure (heart) I50.82
Bjorck (-Thorson) **syndrome** (malignant carcinoid) E34.09
Black
    death A20.9
    eye S00.1- ☑
    hairy tongue K14.3
    heel (foot) S90.3- ☑
    lung (disease) J60
    palm (hand) S60.22- ☑
Blackfan-Diamond anemia or syndrome (congenital hypoplastic anemia) D61.01
Blackhead L70.0
Blackout R55
Bladder — see condition
Blast (air) (hydraulic) (immersion) (underwater)
    blindness S05.8X- ☑
    injury
        abdomen or thorax — see Injury, by site
        ear (acoustic nerve trauma) — see Injury, nerve, acoustic, specified type NEC
        syndrome NEC T70.8- ☑
Blastoma — see Neoplasm, malignant, by site
    pulmonary — see Neoplasm, lung, malignant
Blastomycosis, blastomycotic B40.9

Blastomycosis, blastomycotic — continued
 Brazilian — see Paracoccidioidomycosis
 cutaneous B40.3
 disseminated B40.7
 European — see Cryptococcosis
 generalized B40.7
 keloidal B48.0
 North American B40.9
 primary pulmonary B40.0
 pulmonary B40.2
  acute B40.0
  chronic B40.1
 skin B40.3
 South American — see Paracoccidioidomycosis
 specified NEC B40.89
Bleb(s) R23.8
 emphysematous (lung) (solitary) J43.9
 endophthalmitis H59.43
 filtering (vitreous), after glaucoma surgery Z98.83
 inflamed (infected), postprocedural H59.40
  stage 1 H59.41
  stage 2 H59.42
  stage 3 H59.43
 lung (ruptured) J43.9
  congenital — see Atelectasis
  newborn P25.8
 subpleural (emphysematous) J43.9
Blebitis, postprocedural H59.40
 stage 1 H59.41
 stage 2 H59.42
 stage 3 H59.43
Bleeder (familial) (hereditary) — see Hemophilia
Bleeding — see also Hemorrhage
 anal K62.5
 anovulatory N97.0
 atonic, following delivery O72.1
 capillary I78.8
  puerperal O72.2
 contact (postcoital) N93.0
 due to uterine subinvolution N85.3
 ear — see Otorrhagia
 excessive, associated with menopausal onset N92.4
 familial — see Defect, coagulation
 following intercourse N93.0
 gastrointestinal K92.2
 hemorrhoids — see Hemorrhoids
 intermenstrual (regular) N92.3
  irregular N92.1
 intraoperative — see Complication, intraoperative, hemorrhage
 irregular N92.6
 menopausal N92.4
 newborn, intraventricular — see Newborn, affected by, hemorrhage, intraventricular
 nipple N64.59
 nose R04.0
 ovulation N92.3
 perimenopausal N92.4
 postclimacteric N95.0
 postcoital N93.0
 postmenopausal N95.0
 postoperative — see Complication, postprocedural, hemorrhage
 preclimacteric N92.4
 pre-pubertal vaginal N93.1
 puberty (excessive, with onset of menstrual periods) N92.2
 rectum, rectal K62.5
  newborn P54.2
 tendencies — see Defect, coagulation
 throat R04.1
 tooth socket (post-extraction) K91.840
 umbilical stump P51.9
 uterus, uterine NEC N93.9
  climacteric N92.4
  dysfunctional or functional N93.8
  menopausal N92.4
  preclimacteric or premenopausal N92.4
  unrelated to menstrual cycle N93.9
 vagina, vaginal (abnormal) N93.9
  dysfunctional or functional N93.8
  newborn P54.6
  pre-pubertal N93.1
 vicarious N94.89
Blennorrhagia, blennorrhagic — see Gonorrhea
Blennorrhea (acute) (chronic) — see also Gonorrhea
 inclusion (neonatal) (newborn) P39.1
 lower genitourinary tract (gonococcal) A54.00
 neonatorum (gonococcal ophthalmia) A54.31

Blepharelosis — see Entropion
Blepharitis (angularis) (ciliaris) (eyelid) (marginal) (nonulcerative) H01.009
 herpes zoster B02.39
 left H01.006
  lower H01.005
  upper H01.004
  upper and lower H01.00B
 right H01.003
  lower H01.002
  upper H01.001
  upper and lower H01.00A
 squamous H01.029
  left H01.026
   lower H01.025
   upper H01.024
   upper and lower H01.02B
  right H01.023
   lower H01.022
   upper H01.021
   upper and lower H01.02A
 ulcerative H01.019
  left H01.016
   lower H01.015
   upper H01.014
   upper and lower H01.01B
  right H01.013
   lower H01.012
   upper H01.011
   upper and lower H01.01A
Blepharochalasis H02.30
 congenital Q10.0
 left H02.36
  lower H02.35
  upper H02.34
 right H02.33
  lower H02.32
  upper H02.31
Blepharoclonus H02.59
Blepharoconjunctivitis H10.50- ☑
 angular H10.52- ☑
 contact H10.53- ☑
 ligneous H10.51- ☑
Blepharophimosis (eyelid) H02.529
 congenital Q10.3
 left H02.526
  lower H02.525
  upper H02.524
 right H02.523
  lower H02.522
  upper H02.521
Blepharoptosis H02.40- ☑
 congenital Q10.0
 mechanical H02.41- ☑
 myogenic H02.42- ☑
 neurogenic H02.43- ☑
 paralytic H02.43- ☑
Blepharopyorrhea, gonococcal A54.39
Blepharospasm G24.5
 drug induced G24.01
Blighted ovum O02.0
Blind — see also Blindness
 bronchus (congenital) Q32.4
 loop syndrome K90.2
  congenital Q43.8
 sac, fallopian tube (congenital) Q50.6
 spot, enlarged — see Defect, visual field, localized, scotoma, blind spot area
 tract or tube, congenital NEC — see Atresia, by site
Blindness (acquired) (congenital) (both eyes) H54.0X- ☑
 blast S05.8X- ☑
 color — see Deficiency, color vision
 concussion S05.8X- ☑
 cortical H47.619
  left brain H47.612
  right brain H47.611
 day H53.11
 due to injury (current episode) S05.9- ☑
  sequelae — code to injury with seventh character S
 eclipse (total) — see Retinopathy, solar
 emotional (hysterical) F44.6
 face H53.16
 hysterical F44.6
 legal (both eyes) (USA definition) H54.8
 mind R48.8
 night H53.60
  abnormal dark adaptation curve H53.61
  acquired H53.62

Blindness — continued
 night — continued
  congenital H53.63
  specified type NEC H53.69
  vitamin A deficiency E50.5
 one eye (other eye normal) H54.40
  left (normal vision on right) H54.42- ☑
   low vision on right H54.12- ☑
  low vision, other eye H54.10
  right (normal vision on left) H54.41- ☑
   low vision on left H54.11- ☑
 psychic R48.8
 river B73.01
 snow — see Photokeratitis
 sun, solar — see Retinopathy, solar
 transient — see Disturbance, vision, subjective, loss, transient
 traumatic (current episode) S05.9- ☑
 word (developmental) F81.0
  acquired R48.0
  secondary to organic lesion R48.0
Blister (nonthermal)
 abdominal wall S30.821- ☑
 alveolar process S00.522- ☑
 ankle S90.52- ☑
 antecubital space — see Blister, elbow
 anus S30.827- ☑
 arm (upper) S40.82- ☑
 auditory canal — see Blister, ear
 auricle — see Blister, ear
 axilla — see Blister, arm
 back, lower S30.820- ☑
 beetle dermatitis L24.89
 breast S20.12- ☑
 brow S00.82- ☑
 calf — see Blister, leg
 canthus — see Blister, eyelid
 cheek S00.82- ☑
  internal S00.522- ☑
 chest wall — see Blister, thorax
 chin S00.82- ☑
 costal region — see Blister, thorax
 digit(s)
  foot — see Blister, toe
  hand — see Blister, finger
 due to burn — see Burn, by site, second degree
 ear S00.42- ☑
 elbow S50.32- ☑
 epiglottis S10.12- ☑
 esophagus, cervical S10.12- ☑
 eyebrow — see Blister, eyelid
 eyelid S00.22- ☑
 face S00.82- ☑
 fever B00.1
 finger(s) S60.429- ☑
  index S60.42- ☑
  little S60.42- ☑
  middle S60.42- ☑
  ring S60.42- ☑
 flank S30.82A- ☑
 foot (except toe(s) alone) S90.82- ☑
  toe — see Blister, toe
 forearm S50.82- ☑
  elbow only — see Blister, elbow
 forehead S00.82- ☑
 fracture — omit code
 genital organ
  female S30.826- ☑
  male S30.825- ☑
 gum S00.522- ☑
 hand S60.52- ☑
 head S00.92- ☑
  ear — see Blister, ear
  eyelid — see Blister, eyelid
  lip S00.521- ☑
  nose S00.32- ☑
  oral cavity S00.522- ☑
  scalp S00.02- ☑
  specified site NEC S00.82- ☑
 heel — see Blister, foot
 hip S70.22- ☑
 interscapular region S20.429- ☑
 jaw S00.82- ☑
 knee S80.22- ☑
 larynx S10.12- ☑
 leg (lower) S80.82- ☑
  knee — see Blister, knee

☑ Additional Character Required — Refer to the Tabular List for Character Selection

Blister — continued
- leg — continued
  - upper — see Blister, thigh
- lip S00.521- ☑
- malar region S00.82- ☑
- mammary — see Blister, breast
- mastoid region S00.82- ☑
- mouth S00.522- ☑
- multiple, skin, nontraumatic R23.8
- nail
  - finger — see Blister, finger
  - toe — see Blister, toe
- nasal S00.32- ☑
- neck S10.92- ☑
  - specified site NEC S10.82- ☑
  - throat S10.12- ☑
- nose S00.32- ☑
- occipital region S00.02- ☑
- oral cavity S00.522- ☑
- orbital region — see Blister, eyelid
- palate S00.522- ☑
- palm — see Blister, hand
- parietal region S00.02- ☑
- pelvis S30.820- ☑
- penis S30.822- ☑
- periocular area — see Blister, eyelid
- phalanges
  - finger — see Blister, finger
  - toe — see Blister, toe
- pharynx S10.12- ☑
- pinna — see Blister, ear
- popliteal space — see Blister, knee
- scalp S00.02- ☑
- scapular region — see Blister, shoulder
- scrotum S30.823- ☑
- shin — see Blister, leg
- shoulder S40.22- ☑
- sternal region S20.329- ☑
- submaxillary region S00.82- ☑
- submental region S00.82- ☑
- subungual
  - finger(s) — see Blister, finger
  - toe(s) — see Blister, toe
- supraclavicular fossa S10.82- ☑
- supraorbital S00.82- ☑
- temple S00.82- ☑
- temporal region S00.82- ☑
- testis S30.823- ☑
- thermal — see Burn, by site, second degree
- thigh S70.32- ☑
- thorax, thoracic (wall) S20.92- ☑
  - back S20.42- ☑
  - front S20.32- ☑
- throat S10.12- ☑
- thumb S60.32- ☑
- toe(s) S90.42- ☑
  - great S90.42- ☑
- tongue S00.522- ☑
- trachea S10.12- ☑
- tympanum, tympanic membrane — see Blister, ear
- upper arm — see Blister, arm (upper)
- uvula S00.522- ☑
- vagina S30.824- ☑
- vocal cords S10.12- ☑
- vulva S30.824- ☑
- wrist S60.82- ☑

Bloating R14.0
Bloch-Sulzberger disease or syndrome Q82.3
Block, blocked
- alveolocapillary J84.10
- arborization (heart) I45.5
- arrhythmic I45.9
- atrioventricular (incomplete) (partial) I44.30
  - with atrioventricular dissociation I44.2
  - complete I44.2
    - congenital Q24.6
  - congenital Q24.6
  - first degree I44.0
  - second degree (types I and II) I44.1
  - specified NEC I44.39
  - third degree I44.2
  - types I and II I44.1
- auriculoventricular — see Block, atrioventricular
- bifascicular (cardiac) I45.3
- bundle-branch (complete) (false) (incomplete) I45.4
  - bilateral I45.2
  - left I44.7

Block, blocked — continued
- bundle-branch — continued
  - left — continued
    - with right bundle branch block I45.2
    - hemiblock I44.60
      - anterior I44.4
      - posterior I44.5
    - incomplete I44.7
      - with right bundle branch block I45.2
  - right I45.10
    - with
      - left bundle branch block I45.2
      - left fascicular block I45.2
    - specified NEC I45.19
  - Wilson's type I45.19
- cardiac I45.9
- conduction I45.9
  - complete I44.2
- fascicular (left) I44.60
  - anterior I44.4
  - posterior I44.5
  - right I45.0
  - specified NEC I44.69
- foramen Magendie (acquired) G91.1
  - congenital Q03.1
    - with spina bifida — see Spina bifida, by site, with hydrocephalus
- heart I45.9
  - bundle branch I45.4
    - bilateral I45.2
  - complete (atrioventricular) I44.2
  - congenital Q24.6
  - first degree (atrioventricular) I44.0
  - second degree (atrioventricular) I44.1
  - specified type NEC I45.5
  - third degree (atrioventricular) I44.2
- hepatic vein I82.0
- intraventricular (nonspecific) I45.4
  - bundle branch
    - bilateral I45.2
- kidney N28.9
  - postcystoscopic or postprocedural N99.0
- Mobitz (types I and II) I44.1
- myocardial — see Block, heart
- nodal I45.5
- organ or site, congenital NEC — see Atresia, by site
- portal (vein) I81
- second degree (types I and II) I44.1
- sinoatrial I45.5
- sinoauricular I45.5
- third degree I44.2
- trifascicular I45.3
- tubal N97.1
- vein NOS I82.90
- Wenckebach (types I and II) I44.1

Blockage — see Obstruction
Blocq's disease F44.4
Blood
- constituents, abnormal R78.9
- disease D75.9
- donor — see Donor, blood
- dyscrasia D75.9
  - with
    - abortion — see Abortion, by type, complicated by, hemorrhage
    - ectopic pregnancy O08.1
    - molar pregnancy O08.1
  - following ectopic or molar pregnancy O08.1
  - newborn P61.9
  - puerperal, postpartum O72.3
- flukes NEC — see Schistosomiasis
- in
  - feces K92.1
    - occult R19.5
  - urine — see Hematuria
- mole O02.0
- occult in feces R19.5
- pressure
  - decreased, due to shock following injury T79.4- ☑
  - examination only Z01.30
  - fluctuating I99.8
  - high — see Hypertension
    - borderline R03.0
    - incidental reading, without diagnosis of hypertension R03.0
  - low — see also Hypotension
    - incidental reading, without diagnosis of hypotension R03.1
- spitting — see Hemoptysis

Blood — continued
- staining cornea — see Pigmentation, cornea, stromal
- transfusion
  - reaction or complication — see Complications, transfusion
- type
  - A (Rh positive) Z67.10
    - Rh negative Z67.11
  - AB (Rh positive) Z67.30
    - Rh negative Z67.31
  - B (Rh positive) Z67.20
    - Rh negative Z67.21
  - O (Rh positive) Z67.40
    - Rh negative Z67.41
  - Rh (positive) Z67.90
    - negative Z67.91
- vessel rupture — see Hemorrhage
- vomiting — see Hematemesis

Blood-forming organs, disease D75.9
Bloodgood's disease — see Mastopathy, cystic
Bloom (-Machacek)(-Torre) **syndrome** Q82.8
Blount disease or osteochondrosis M92.51- ☑
Blue
- baby Q24.9
- diaper syndrome E72.09
- dome cyst (breast) — see Cyst, breast
- dot cataract Q12.0
- nevus D22.9
- sclera Q13.5
  - with fragility of bone and deafness Q78.0
- toe syndrome I75.02- ☑

Blueness — see Cyanosis
Blues, postpartal O90.6
- baby O90.6

Blurring, visual H53.8
Blushing (abnormal) (excessive) R23.2
BMI — see Body, mass index
Boarder, hospital NEC Z76.4
- accompanying sick person Z76.3
- healthy infant or child Z76.2
- foundling Z76.1

Bockhart's impetigo L01.02
Bodechtel-Guttman disease (subacute sclerosing panencephalitis) A81.1
Boder-Sedgwick syndrome (ataxia-telangiectasia) G11.3
Body, bodies
- Aschoff's — see Myocarditis, rheumatic
- asteroid, vitreous — see Deposit, crystalline
- cytoid (retina) — see Occlusion, artery, retina
- drusen (degenerative) (macula) (retinal) — see also Degeneration, macula, drusen
  - optic disc — see Drusen, optic disc
- foreign — see Foreign body
- loose
  - joint, except knee — see Loose, body, joint
  - knee M23.4- ☑
  - sheath, tendon — see Disorder, tendon, specified type NEC
- mass index (BMI)
  - adult
    - 19.9 or less Z68.1
    - 20.0-20.9 Z68.20
    - 21.0-21.9 Z68.21
    - 22.0-22.9 Z68.22
    - 23.0-23.9 Z68.23
    - 24.0-24.9 Z68.24
    - 25.0-25.9 Z68.25
    - 26.0-26.9 Z68.26
    - 27.0-27.9 Z68.27
    - 28.0-28.9 Z68.28
    - 29.0-29.9 Z68.29
    - 30.0-30.9 Z68.30
    - 31.0-31.9 Z68.31
    - 32.0-32.9 Z68.32
    - 33.0-33.9 Z68.33
    - 34.0-34.9 Z68.34
    - 35.0-35.9 Z68.35
    - 36.0-36.9 Z68.36
    - 37.0-37.9 Z68.37
    - 38.0-38.9 Z68.38
    - 39.0-39.9 Z68.39
    - 40.0-44.9 Z68.41
    - 45.0-49.9 Z68.42
    - 50.0-59.9 Z68.43
    - 60.0-69.9 Z68.44
    - 70 and over Z68.45
  - pediatric
    - 5th percentile to less than 85th percentile for age Z68.52

Body, bodies — continued
  mass index — continued
    pediatric — continued
      85th percentile to less than 95th percentile for age Z68.53
      95th percentile for age to less than 120% of the 95th percentile for age Z68.54
      120% of the 95th percentile for age to less than 140% of the 95th percentile for age Z68.55
      greater than or equal to 140% of the 95th percentile for age Z68.56
      less than fifth percentile for age Z68.51
  Mooser's A75.2
  rice — see also Loose, body, joint
    knee M23.4- ☑
  rocking F98.4
Boeck's
  disease or sarcoid — see Sarcoidosis
  lupoid (miliary) D86.3
Boerhaave's syndrome (spontaneous esophageal rupture) K22.3
Boggy
  cervix N88.8
  uterus N85.8
Boil — see also Furuncle, by site
  Aleppo B55.1
  Baghdad B55.1
  Delhi B55.1
  lacrimal
    gland — see Dacryoadenitis
    passages (duct) (sac) — see Inflammation, lacrimal, passages, acute
  Natal B55.1
  orbit, orbital — see Abscess, orbit
  tropical B55.1
Bold hives — see Urticaria
Bombé, iris — see Membrane, pupillary
Bone — see condition
Bonnevie-Ullrich syndrome — see also Turner's syndrome Q87.19
Bonnier's syndrome H81.8- ☑
Bonvale dam fever T73.3- ☑
Bony block of joint — see Ankylosis
BOOP (bronchiolitis obliterans organized pneumonia) J84.89
Borderline
  diabetes mellitus R73.03
  hypertension R03.0
  osteopenia M85.8- ☑
  pelvis, with obstruction during labor O65.1
  personality F60.3
Borna disease A83.9
Bornholm disease B33.0
Boston exanthem A88.0
Botalli, ductus (patent) (persistent) Q25.0
Bothriocephalus latus infestation B70.0
Botulism (foodborne intoxication) A05.1
  infant A48.51
  non-foodborne A48.52
  wound A48.52
Bouba — see Yaws
Bouchard's nodes (with arthropathy) M15.2
Bouffée délirante F23
Bouillaud's disease or syndrome (rheumatic heart disease) I01.9
Bourneville's disease Q85.1
Boutonniere deformity (finger) — see Deformity, finger, boutonniere
Bouveret (-Hoffmann) **syndrome** (paroxysmal tachycardia) I47.9
Bovine heart — see Hypertrophy, cardiac
Bowel — see condition
Bowen's
  dermatosis (precancerous) — see Neoplasm, skin, in situ
  disease — see Neoplasm, skin, in situ
  epithelioma — see Neoplasm, skin, in situ
  type
    epidermoid carcinoma-in-situ — see Neoplasm, skin, in situ
    intraepidermal squamous cell carcinoma — see Neoplasm, skin, in situ
Bowing
  femur — see also Deformity, limb, specified type NEC, thigh
    congenital Q68.3
  fibula — see also Deformity, limb, specified type NEC, lower leg
    congenital Q68.4
  forearm — see Deformity, limb, specified type NEC, forearm

Bowing — continued
  leg(s), long bones, congenital Q68.5
  radius — see Deformity, limb, specified type NEC, forearm
  tibia — see also Deformity, limb, specified type NEC, lower leg
    congenital Q68.4
Bowleg(s) (acquired) M21.16- ☑
  congenital Q68.5
  rachitic E64.3
Boyd's dysentery A03.2
Brachial — see condition
Brachycardia R00.1
Brachycephaly, non-deformational Q75.022
Bradley's disease A08.19
Bradyarrhythmia, cardiac I49.8
Bradycardia (sinoatrial) (sinus) (vagal) R00.1
  neonatal P29.12
  reflex G90.09
  tachycardia syndrome I49.5
Bradykinesia R25.8
Bradypnea R06.89
Bradytachycardia I49.5
Brailsford's disease or osteochondrosis — see Osteochondrosis, juvenile, radius
Brain
  death G93.82
  syndrome — see Syndrome, brain
Branched-chain amino-acid disorder E71.2
Branchial — see condition
  cartilage, congenital Q18.2
Branchiogenic remnant (in neck) Q18.0
Brandt's syndrome (acrodermatitis enteropathica) E83.2
Brash (water) R12
Bravais-jacksonian epilepsy — see Epilepsy, localization-related, symptomatic, with simple partial seizures
Braxton Hicks contractions — see False, labor
Brazilian leishmaniasis B55.2
BRBPR K62.5
Break, retina (without detachment) H33.30- ☑
  with retinal detachment — see Detachment, retina
  horseshoe tear H33.31- ☑
  multiple H33.33- ☑
  round hole H33.32- ☑
Breakdown
  device, graft or implant — see also Complications, by site and type, mechanical T85.618- ☑
    arterial graft NEC — see Complication, cardiovascular device, mechanical, vascular
    breast (implant) T85.41- ☑
    catheter NEC T85.618- ☑
      cystostomy T83.010- ☑
      dialysis (renal) T82.41- ☑
        intraperitoneal T85.611- ☑
      Hopkins T83.018- ☑
      ileostomy T83.018- ☑
      infusion NEC T82.514- ☑
        cranial T85.610- ☑
        epidural T85.610- ☑
        intrathecal T85.610- ☑
        spinal T85.610- ☑
        subarachnoid T85.610- ☑
        subdural T85.610- ☑
      nephrostomy T83.012- ☑
      urethral indwelling T83.011- ☑
      urinary NEC T83.018- ☑
      urostomy T83.018- ☑
    electronic (electrode) (pulse generator) (stimulator)
      bone T84.310- ☑
      cardiac T82.119- ☑
        electrode T82.110- ☑
        pulse generator T82.111- ☑
        specified type NEC T82.118- ☑
      nervous system — see Complication, prosthetic device, mechanical, electronic nervous system stimulator
      urinary — see Complication, genitourinary, device, urinary, mechanical
    fixation, internal (orthopedic) NEC — see Complication, fixation device, mechanical
    gastrointestinal — see Complications, prosthetic device, mechanical, gastrointestinal device
    genital NEC T83.418- ☑
      intrauterine contraceptive device T83.31- ☑
      penile prosthesis (cylinder) (implanted) (pump) (reservoir) T83.410- ☑
      testicular prosthesis T83.411- ☑

Breakdown — continued
  device, graft or implant — see also Complications, by site and type, mechanical — continued
    heart NEC — see Complication, cardiovascular device, mechanical
    intrathecal infusion pump T85.615- ☑
    joint prosthesis — see Complications, joint prosthesis, internal, mechanical, by site
    nervous system, specified device NEC T85.615- ☑
    ocular NEC — see Complications, prosthetic device, mechanical, ocular device
    orthopedic NEC — see Complication, orthopedic, device, mechanical
    specified NEC T85.618- ☑
    subcutaneous device pocket
      nervous system prosthetic device, implant, or graft T85.890- ☑
      other internal prosthetic device, implant, or graft T85.898- ☑
    sutures, permanent T85.612- ☑
      used in bone repair — see Complications, fixation device, internal (orthopedic), mechanical
    urinary NEC T83.118- ☑
      graft T83.21- ☑
      sphincter, implanted T83.111- ☑
      stent (ileal conduit) (nephroureteral) T83.113- ☑
      ureteral indwelling T83.112- ☑
    vascular NEC — see Complication, cardiovascular device, mechanical
    ventricular intracranial shunt T85.01- ☑
  nervous F48.8
  perineum O90.1
  respirator J95.850
    specified NEC J95.859
  ventilator J95.850
    specified NEC J95.859
Breast — see also condition
  buds E30.1
    in newborn P96.89
  dense R92.3-
  Imaging Reporting and Data System (BI-RADS) : A R92.31- ☑
  Imaging Reporting and Data System (BI-RADS) : B R92.32- ☑
  Imaging Reporting and Data System (BI-RADS) : C R92.33- ☑
  Imaging Reporting and Data System (BI-RADS) : D R92.34- ☑
  Imaging Reporting and Data System (BI-RADS) : 1 R92.31- ☑
  Imaging Reporting and Data System (BI-RADS) : 2 R92.32- ☑
  Imaging Reporting and Data System (BI-RADS) : 3 R92.33- ☑
  Imaging Reporting and Data System (BI-RADS) : 4 R92.34- ☑
  nodule — see also Lump, breast N63.0
Breath
  foul R19.6
  holder, child R06.89
  holding spell R06.89
  shortness R06.02
Breathing
  labored — see Hyperventilation
  mouth R06.5
    causing malocclusion M26.59
  periodic R06.3
    high altitude G47.32
Breathlessness R06.81
Breda's disease — see Yaws
Breech presentation (mother) O32.1- ☑
  causing obstructed labor O64.1- ☑
  footling O32.8- ☑
    causing obstructed labor O64.8- ☑
  incomplete O32.8- ☑
    causing obstructed labor O64.8- ☑
Breisky's disease N90.4
Brennemann's syndrome I88.0
Brenner
  tumor (benign) D27.9
    borderline malignancy D39.1- ☑
    malignant C56.- ☑
    proliferating D39.1- ☑
Bretonneau's disease or angina A36.0
Breus' mole O02.0
Brevicollis Q76.49
Brickmakers' anemia B76.9 [D63.8]

☑ Additional Character Required — Refer to the Tabular List for Character Selection

Bridge, myocardial Q24.5
Bright red blood per rectum (BRBPR) K62.5
Bright's disease — *see also* Nephritis
  arteriosclerotic — *see* Hypertension, kidney
Brill (-Zinsser) **disease** (recrudescent typhus) A75.1
Brill-Symmers' disease C82.90
Brion-Kayser disease — *see* Fever, paratyphoid
Briquet's disorder or syndrome F45.0
Brissaud's
  infantilism or dwarfism E23.0
  motor-verbal tic F95.2
Brittle
  bones disease Q78.0
  nails L60.3
    congenital Q84.6
Broad — *see also* condition
  beta disease E78.2
  ligament laceration syndrome N83.8
Broad- or floating-betalipoproteinemia E78.2
Brock's syndrome (atelectasis due to enlarged lymph nodes) J98.19
Brocq-Duhring disease (dermatitis herpetiformis) L13.0
Brodie's abscess or disease M86.8X- ☑
Broken
  arches — *see also* Deformity, limb, flat foot
  arm (meaning upper limb) — *see* Fracture, arm
  back — *see* Fracture, vertebra
  bone — *see* Fracture
  implant or internal device — *see* Complications, by site and type, mechanical
  leg (meaning lower limb) — *see* Fracture, leg
  nose S02.2- ☑
  tooth, teeth — *see* Fracture, tooth
Bromhidrosis, bromidrosis L75.0
Bromidism, bromism G92.8
  due to
    correct substance properly administered — *see* Table of Drugs and Chemicals, by drug, adverse effect
    overdose or wrong substance given or taken — *see* Table of Drugs and Chemicals, by drug, poisoning
  chronic (dependence) F13.20
Bromidrosiphobia F40.298
Bronchi, bronchial — *see* condition
Bronchiectasis (cylindrical) (diffuse) (fusiform) (localized) (saccular) J47.9
  with
    acute
      bronchitis J47.0
      lower respiratory infection J47.0
    exacerbation (acute) J47.1
  congenital Q33.4
  tuberculous NEC — *see* Tuberculosis, pulmonary
Bronchiolectasis — *see* Bronchiectasis
Bronchiolitis (acute) (infective) (subacute) J21.9
  with
    bronchospasm or obstruction J21.9
    influenza, flu or grippe — *see* Influenza, with, respiratory manifestations NEC
  chemical (chronic) J68.4
    acute J68.0
  chronic (fibrosing) J44.89
    obliterative J44.81
  due to
    external agent — *see* Bronchitis, acute, due to
    human metapneumovirus J21.1
    respiratory syncytial virus (RSV) J21.0
    specified organism NEC J21.8
  fibrosa obliterans J44.81
  influenzal — *see* Influenza, with, respiratory manifestations NEC
  obliterans — *see also* Bronchiolitis, obliterative J44.81
    with organizing pneumonia (BOOP) J84.89
    syndrome J44.81
  obliterative (chronic) (subacute) — *see also* Bronchiolitis, obliterans J44.81
    due to chemicals, gases, fumes or vapors (inhalation) — *see also* Disease, respiratory, chronic, due to chemicals, gases, fumes or vapors J42
    due to fumes or vapors — *see also* Disease, respiratory, chronic, due to chemicals, gases, fumes or vapors J44.81
  respiratory, interstitial lung disease J84.115
Bronchitis (diffuse) (fibrinous) (hypostatic) (infective) (membranous) J40
  with
    influenza, flu or grippe — *see* Influenza, with, respiratory manifestations NEC
    obstruction (airway) (lung) J44.89

Bronchitis — *continued*
  with — *continued*
    tracheitis (15 years of age and above) J40
      acute or subacute J20.9
      chronic J42
      under 15 years of age J20.9
  acute or subacute (with bronchospasm or obstruction) J20.9
    with
      bronchiectasis J47.0
      chronic obstructive pulmonary disease J44.0
    chemical (due to gases, fumes or vapors) J68.0
    due to
      fumes or vapors J68.0
      Haemophilus influenzae J20.1
      Mycoplasma pneumoniae J20.0
      radiation J70.0
      specified organism NEC J20.8
      Streptococcus J20.2
      virus
        coxsackie J20.3
        echovirus J20.7
        parainfluenzae J20.4
        respiratory syncytial (RSV) J20.5
        rhinovirus J20.6
      viral NEC J20.8
  allergic (acute) J45.909
    with
      exacerbation (acute) J45.901
      status asthmaticus J45.902
  arachidic T17.528- ☑
  aspiration (due to food and vomit) J69.0
  asthmatic J45.9-
    chronic J44.89
      with
        acute lower respiratory infection J44.0
        exacerbation (acute) J44.1
  capillary — *see* Pneumonia, broncho
  caseous (tuberculous) A15.5
  Castellani's A69.8
  catarrhal (15 years of age and above) J40
    acute — *see* Bronchitis, acute
    chronic J41.0
    under 15 years of age J20.9
  chemical (acute) (subacute) J68.0
    chronic — *see also* Disease, respiratory, chronic, due to chemicals, gases, fumes or vapors J42
    due to fumes or vapors — *see also* Disease, respiratory, chronic, due to chemicals, gases, fumes or vapors J42
    chronic J68.4
  chronic J42
    with
      airways obstruction J44.89
      tracheitis (chronic) J42
    asthmatic (obstructive) J44.89
    catarrhal J41.0
    chemical (due to fumes or vapors) — *see also* Disease, respiratory, chronic, due to chemicals, gases, fumes or vapors J42
    due to
      chemicals, gases, fumes or vapors (inhalation) — *see also* Disease, respiratory, chronic, due to chemicals, gases, fumes or vapors J42
      radiation J70.1
      tobacco smoking J41.0
    emphysematous J44.89
    mucopurulent J41.1
    non-obstructive J41.0
    obliterans — *see* Bronchiolitis, obliterans
    obstructive J44.89
    purulent J41.1
    simple J41.0
  croupous — *see* Bronchitis, acute
  due to gases, fumes or vapors (chemical) J68.0
  emphysematous (obstructive) J44.89
  exudative — *see* Bronchitis, acute
  fetid J41.1
  grippal — *see* Influenza, with, respiratory manifestations NEC
  in those under 15 years age — *see* Bronchitis, acute
    chronic — *see* Bronchitis, chronic
  influenzal — *see* Influenza, with, respiratory manifestations NEC
  mixed simple and mucopurulent J41.8
  moulder's J62.8
  mucopurulent (chronic) (recurrent) J41.1
    acute or subacute J20.9
    simple (mixed) J41.8

Bronchitis — *continued*
  obliterans (chronic) — *see* Bronchiolitis, obliterans
  obstructive (chronic) (diffuse) J44.89
  pituitous J41.1
  pneumococcal, acute or subacute J20.2
  pseudomembranous, acute or subacute — *see* Bronchitis, acute
  purulent (chronic) (recurrent) J41.1
    acute or subacute — *see* Bronchitis, acute
  putrid J41.1
  senile (chronic) J42
  simple and mucopurulent (mixed) J41.8
  smokers' J41.0
  spirochetal NEC A69.8
  subacute — *see* Bronchitis, acute
  suppurative (chronic) J41.1
    acute or subacute — *see* Bronchitis, acute
  tuberculous A15.5
  under 15 years of age — *see* Bronchitis, acute
    chronic — *see* Bronchitis, chronic
  viral NEC, acute or subacute — *see also* Bronchitis, acute J20.8
Bronchoalveolitis J18.0
Bronchoaspergillosis B44.1
Bronchocele meaning goiter E04.0
Broncholithiasis J98.09
  tuberculous NEC A15.5
Bronchomalacia J98.09
  congenital Q32.2
Bronchomycosis NOS B49 *[J99]*
  candidal B37.1
Bronchopleuropneumonia — *see* Pneumonia, broncho
Bronchopneumonia — *see* Pneumonia, broncho
Bronchopneumonitis — *see* Pneumonia, broncho
Bronchopulmonary — *see* condition
Bronchopulmonitis — *see* Pneumonia, broncho
Bronchorrhagia (see Hemoptysis)
Bronchorrhea J98.09
  acute J20.9
  chronic (infective) (purulent) J42
Bronchospasm (acute) J98.01
  with
    bronchiolitis, acute J21.9
    bronchitis, acute (conditions in J20) — *see* Bronchitis, acute
  due to external agent — *see* condition, respiratory, acute, due to
  exercise induced J45.990
Bronchospirochetosis A69.8
  Castellani A69.8
Bronchostenosis J98.09
Bronchus — *see* condition
Brontophobia F40.220
Bronze baby syndrome P83.88
Brooke's tumor — *see* Neoplasm, skin, benign
Brown enamel of teeth (hereditary) K00.5
Brown-Sequard disease, paralysis or syndrome G83.81
Brown's sheath syndrome H50.61- ☑
Bruce sepsis A23.0
Brucellosis (infection) A23.9
  abortus A23.1
  canis A23.3
  dermatitis A23.9
  melitensis A23.0
  mixed A23.8
  sepsis A23.9
    melitensis A23.0
    specified NEC A23.8
  suis A23.2
Bruck-de Lange disease Q87.19
Bruck's disease — *see* Deformity, limb
BRUE (brief resolved unexplained event) R68.13
Brugsch's syndrome Q82.8
Bruise (skin surface intact) — *see also* Contusion
  with
    open wound — *see* Wound, open
    internal organ — *see* Injury, by site
  newborn P54.5
    scalp, due to birth injury, newborn P12.3
    umbilical cord O69.5- ☑
Bruit (arterial) R09.89
  cardiac R01.1
Brush burn — *see* Abrasion, by site
Bruton's X-linked agammaglobulinemia D80.0
Bruxism
  psychogenic F45.8
  sleep related G47.63
Bubbly lung syndrome P27.0
Bubo I88.8

Bubo — *continued*
  blennorrhagic (gonococcal) A54.89
  chancroidal A57
  climatic A55
  due to Haemophilus ducreyi A57
  gonococcal A54.89
  indolent (nonspecific) I88.8
  inguinal (nonspecific) I88.8
    chancroidal A57
    climatic A55
    due to H. ducreyi A57
    infective I88.8
  scrofulous (tuberculous) A18.2
  soft chancre A57
  suppurating — *see* Lymphadenitis, acute
  syphilitic (primary) A51.0
    congenital A50.07
  tropical A55
  virulent (chancroidal) A57
Bubonic plague A20.0
Bubonocele — *see* Hernia, inguinal
Buccal — *see* condition
Buchanan's disease or osteochondrosis M91.0
Buchem's syndrome (hyperostosis corticalis) M85.2
Bucket-handle fracture or tear (semilunar cartilage) — *see* Tear, meniscus
Budd-Chiari syndrome (hepatic vein thrombosis) I82.0
Budgerigar fancier's disease or lung J67.2
Buds
  breast E30.1
    in newborn P96.89
Buerger's disease (thromboangiitis obliterans) I73.1
Bulbar — *see* condition
Bulbus cordis (left ventricle) (persistent) Q21.8
Bulimia (nervosa) F50.2- ☑
  atypical F50.9
  normal weight F50.9
Bulky
  stools R19.5
  uterus N85.2
Bulla (e) R23.8
  lung (emphysematous) (solitary) J43.9
    newborn P25.8
Bullet wound — *see also* Puncture
  fracture — *code as* Fracture, by site
  internal organ — *see* Injury, by site
Bundle
  branch block (complete) (false) (incomplete) — *see* Block, bundle-branch
  of His — *see* condition
Bunion M21.61- ☑
  tailor's M21.62- ☑
Bunionette M21.62- ☑
Buphthalmia, buphthalmos (congenital) Q15.0
Burdwan fever B55.0
Burger-Grutz disease or syndrome E78.3
Buried
  penis (congenital) Q55.64
    acquired N48.83
  roots K08.3
Burke's syndrome K86.89
Burkholderia
  cepacia A49.8
  mallei A24.0
  pseudomallei — *see* Melioidosis
Burkitt
  cell leukemia C91.0- ☑
  lymphoma (malignant) C83.7- ☑
    small noncleaved, diffuse C83.7- ☑
    spleen C83.77
    undifferentiated C83.7- ☑
  tumor C83.7- ☑
  type
    acute lymphoblastic leukemia C91.0- ☑
    undifferentiated C83.7- ☑
Burn (electricity) (flame) (hot gas, liquid or hot object) (radiation) (steam) (thermal) T30.0
  abdomen, abdominal (muscle) (wall) T21.02- ☑
    first degree T21.12- ☑
    second degree T21.22- ☑
    third degree T21.32- ☑
  above elbow T22.039- ☑
    first degree T22.139- ☑
    left T22.032- ☑
      first degree T22.132- ☑
      second degree T22.232- ☑
      third degree T22.332- ☑
    right T22.031- ☑

Burn — *continued*
  above elbow — *continued*
    right — *continued*
      first degree T22.131- ☑
      second degree T22.231- ☑
      third degree T22.331- ☑
    second degree T22.239- ☑
    third degree T22.339- ☑
  acid (caustic) (external) (internal) — *see* Corrosion, by site
  alimentary tract NEC T28.2- ☑
    esophagus T28.1- ☑
    mouth T28.0- ☑
    pharynx T28.0- ☑
  alkaline (caustic) (external) (internal) — *see* Corrosion, by site
  ankle T25.019- ☑
    first degree T25.119- ☑
    left T25.012- ☑
      first degree T25.112- ☑
      second degree T25.212- ☑
      third degree T25.312- ☑
    multiple with foot — *see* Burn, lower, limb, multiple, ankle and foot
    right T25.011- ☑
      first degree T25.111- ☑
      second degree T25.211- ☑
      third degree T25.311- ☑
    second degree T25.219- ☑
    third degree T25.319- ☑
  anus — *see* Burn, buttock
  arm (lower) (upper) — *see* Burn, upper, limb
  axilla T22.049- ☑
    first degree T22.149- ☑
    left T22.042- ☑
      first degree T22.142- ☑
      second degree T22.242- ☑
      third degree T22.342- ☑
    right T22.041- ☑
      first degree T22.141- ☑
      second degree T22.241- ☑
      third degree T22.341- ☑
    second degree T22.249- ☑
    third degree T22.349- ☑
  back (lower) T21.04- ☑
    first degree T21.14- ☑
    second degree T21.24- ☑
    third degree T21.34- ☑
    upper T21.03- ☑
      first degree T21.13- ☑
      second degree T21.23- ☑
      third degree T21.33- ☑
  blisters — *code as* Burn, second degree, by site
  breast(s) — *see* Burn, chest wall
  buttock(s) T21.05- ☑
    first degree T21.15- ☑
    second degree T21.25- ☑
    third degree T21.35- ☑
  calf T24.039- ☑
    first degree T24.139- ☑
    left T24.032- ☑
      first degree T24.132- ☑
      second degree T24.232- ☑
      third degree T24.332- ☑
    right T24.031- ☑
      first degree T24.131- ☑
      second degree T24.231- ☑
      third degree T24.331- ☑
    second degree T24.239- ☑
    third degree T24.339- ☑
  canthus (eye) — *see* Burn, eyelid
  caustic acid or alkaline — *see* Corrosion, by site
  cervix T28.3- ☑
  cheek T20.06- ☑
    first degree T20.16- ☑
    second degree T20.26- ☑
    third degree T20.36- ☑
  chemical (acids) (alkalines) (caustics) (external) (internal) — *see* Corrosion, by site
  chest wall T21.01- ☑
    first degree T21.11- ☑
    second degree T21.21- ☑
    third degree T21.31- ☑
  chin T20.03- ☑
    first degree T20.13- ☑

Burn — *continued*
  chin — *continued*
    second degree T20.23- ☑
    third degree T20.33- ☑
  colon T28.2- ☑
  conjunctiva (and cornea) — *see* Burn, cornea
  cornea (and conjunctiva) T26.1- ☑
    chemical — *see* Corrosion, cornea
  corrosion (external) (internal) — *see* Corrosion, by site
  deep necrosis of underlying tissue — *code as* Burn, third degree, by site
  dorsum of hand T23.069- ☑
    first degree T23.169- ☑
    left T23.062- ☑
      first degree T23.162- ☑
      second degree T23.262- ☑
      third degree T23.362- ☑
    right T23.061- ☑
      first degree T23.161- ☑
      second degree T23.261- ☑
      third degree T23.361- ☑
    second degree T23.269- ☑
    third degree T23.369- ☑
  due to ingested chemical agent — *see* Corrosion, by site
  ear (auricle) (external) (canal) T20.01- ☑
    first degree T20.11- ☑
    second degree T20.21- ☑
    third degree T20.31- ☑
  elbow T22.029- ☑
    first degree T22.129- ☑
    left T22.022- ☑
      first degree T22.122- ☑
      second degree T22.222- ☑
      third degree T22.322- ☑
    right T22.021- ☑
      first degree T22.121- ☑
      second degree T22.221- ☑
      third degree T22.321- ☑
    second degree T22.229- ☑
    third degree T22.329- ☑
  epidermal loss — *code as* Burn, second degree, by site
  erythema, erythematous — *code as* Burn, first degree, by site
  esophagus T28.1- ☑
  extent (percentage of body surface)
    less than 10 percent T31.0
    10-19 percent T31.10
      with 0-9 percent third degree burns T31.10
      with 10-19 percent third degree burns T31.11
    20-29 percent T31.20
      with 0-9 percent third degree burns T31.20
      with 10-19 percent third degree burns T31.21
      with 20-29 percent third degree burns T31.22
    30-39 percent T31.30
      with 0-9 percent third degree burns T31.30
      with 10-19 percent third degree burns T31.31
      with 20-29 percent third degree burns T31.32
      with 30-39 percent third degree burns T31.33
    40-49 percent T31.40
      with 0-9 percent third degree burns T31.40
      with 10-19 percent third degree burns T31.41
      with 20-29 percent third degree burns T31.42
      with 30-39 percent third degree burns T31.43
      with 40-49 percent third degree burns T31.44
    50-59 percent T31.50
      with 0-9 percent third degree burns T31.50
      with 10-19 percent third degree burns T31.51
      with 20-29 percent third degree burns T31.52
      with 30-39 percent third degree burns T31.53
      with 40-49 percent third degree burns T31.54
      with 50-59 percent third degree burns T31.55
    60-69 percent T31.60
      with 0-9 percent third degree burns T31.60
      with 10-19 percent third degree burns T31.61
      with 20-29 percent third degree burns T31.62
      with 30-39 percent third degree burns T31.63
      with 40-49 percent third degree burns T31.64
      with 50-59 percent third degree burns T31.65
      with 60-69 percent third degree burns T31.66
    70-79 percent T31.70
      with 0-9 percent third degree burns T31.70
      with 10-19 percent third degree burns T31.71
      with 20-29 percent third degree burns T31.72
      with 30-39 percent third degree burns T31.73
      with 40-49 percent third degree burns T31.74
      with 50-59 percent third degree burns T31.75
      with 60-69 percent third degree burns T31.76

Burn — *continued*
  extent — *continued*
    70-79 percent — *continued*
      with 70-79 percent third degree burns T31.77
    80-89 percent T31.80
      with 0-9 percent third degree burns T31.80
      with 10-19 percent third degree burns T31.81
      with 20-29 percent third degree burns T31.82
      with 30-39 percent third degree burns T31.83
      with 40-49 percent third degree burns T31.84
      with 50-59 percent third degree burns T31.85
      with 60-69 percent third degree burns T31.86
      with 70-79 percent third degree burns T31.87
      with 80-89 percent third degree burns T31.88
    90 percent or more T31.90
      with 0-9 percent third degree burns T31.90
      with 10-19 percent third degree burns T31.91
      with 20-29 percent third degree burns T31.92
      with 30-39 percent third degree burns T31.93
      with 40-49 percent third degree burns T31.94
      with 50-59 percent third degree burns T31.95
      with 60-69 percent third degree burns T31.96
      with 70-79 percent third degree burns T31.97
      with 80-89 percent third degree burns T31.98
      with 90 percent or more third degree burns T31.99
  extremity — *see* Burn, limb
  eye(s) and adnexa T26.4-
    with resulting rupture and destruction of eyeball T26.2-
    conjunctival sac — *see* Burn, cornea
    cornea — *see* Burn, cornea
    lid — *see* Burn, eyelid
    periocular area — *see* Burn, eyelid
    specified site NEC T26.3-
  eyeball — *see* Burn, eye
  eyelid(s) T26.0-
    chemical — *see* Corrosion, eyelid
  face — *see* Burn, head
  finger T23.029-
    first degree T23.129-
    left T23.022-
      first degree T23.122-
      second degree T23.222-
      third degree T23.322-
    multiple sites (without thumb) T23.039-
      with thumb T23.049-
        first degree T23.149-
        left T23.042-
          first degree T23.142-
          second degree T23.242-
          third degree T23.342-
        right T23.041-
          first degree T23.141-
          second degree T23.241-
          third degree T23.341-
      second degree T23.249-
      third degree T23.349-
    first degree T23.139-
    left T23.032-
      first degree T23.132-
      second degree T23.232-
      third degree T23.332-
    right T23.031-
      first degree T23.131-
      second degree T23.231-
      third degree T23.331-
    second degree T23.239-
    third degree T23.339-
    right T23.021-
      first degree T23.121-
      second degree T23.221-
      third degree T23.321-
    second degree T23.229-
    third degree T23.329-
  flank — *see* Burn, abdominal wall
  foot T25.029-
    first degree T25.129-
    left T25.022-
      first degree T25.122-
      second degree T25.222-
      third degree T25.322-
    multiple with ankle — *see* Burn, lower, limb, multiple, ankle and foot
    right T25.021-
      first degree T25.121-
      second degree T25.221-

Burn — *continued*
  foot — *continued*
    right — *continued*
      third degree T25.321-
    second degree T25.229-
    third degree T25.329-
  forearm T22.019-
    first degree T22.119-
    left T22.012-
      first degree T22.112-
      second degree T22.212-
      third degree T22.312-
    right T22.011-
      first degree T22.111-
      second degree T22.211-
      third degree T22.311-
    second degree T22.219-
    third degree T22.319-
  forehead T20.06-
    first degree T20.16-
    second degree T20.26-
    third degree T20.36-
  fourth degree — *code as* Burn, third degree, by site
  friction — *see* Burn, by site
  from swallowing caustic or corrosive substance NEC — *see* Corrosion, by site
  full thickness skin loss — *code as* Burn, third degree, by site
  gastrointestinal tract NEC T28.2-
    from swallowing caustic or corrosive substance T28.7-
  genital organs
    external
      female T21.07-
        first degree T21.17-
        second degree T21.27-
        third degree T21.37-
      male T21.06-
        first degree T21.16-
        second degree T21.26-
        third degree T21.36-
    internal T28.3-
      from caustic or corrosive substance T28.8-
  groin — *see* Burn, abdominal wall
  hand(s) T23.009-
    back — *see* Burn, dorsum of hand
    finger — *see* Burn, finger
    first degree T23.109-
    left T23.002-
      first degree T23.102-
      second degree T23.202-
      third degree T23.302-
    multiple sites with wrist T23.099-
      first degree T23.199-
      left T23.092-
        first degree T23.192-
        second degree T23.292-
        third degree T23.392-
      right T23.091-
        first degree T23.191-
        second degree T23.291-
        third degree T23.391-
      second degree T23.299-
      third degree T23.399-
    palm — *see* Burn, palm
    right T23.001-
      first degree T23.101-
      second degree T23.201-
      third degree T23.301-
    second degree T23.209-
    third degree T23.309-
    thumb — *see* Burn, thumb
  head (and face) (and neck) T20.00-
    cheek — *see* Burn, cheek
    chin — *see* Burn, chin
    ear — *see* Burn, ear
    eye(s) only — *see* Burn, eye
    first degree T20.10-
    forehead — *see* Burn, forehead
    lip — *see* Burn, lip
    multiple sites T20.09-
      first degree T20.19-
      second degree T20.29-
      third degree T20.39-
    neck — *see* Burn, neck
    nose — *see* Burn, nose

Burn — *continued*
  head — *continued*
    scalp — *see* Burn, scalp
    second degree T20.20-
    third degree T20.30-
  hip(s) — *see* Burn, thigh
  inhalation — *see* Burn, respiratory tract
    caustic or corrosive substance (fumes) — *see* Corrosion, respiratory tract
  internal organ(s) T28.40-
    alimentary tract T28.2-
      esophagus T28.1-
    eardrum T28.41-
    esophagus T28.1-
      from caustic or corrosive substance (swallowing) NEC — *see* Corrosion, by site
    genitourinary T28.3-
    mouth T28.0-
    pharynx T28.0-
    respiratory tract — *see* Burn, respiratory tract
    specified organ NEC T28.49-
  interscapular region — *see* Burn, back, upper
  intestine (large) (small) T28.2-
  knee T24.029-
    first degree T24.129-
    left T24.022-
      first degree T24.122-
      second degree T24.222-
      third degree T24.322-
    right T24.021-
      first degree T24.121-
      second degree T24.221-
      third degree T24.321-
    second degree T24.229-
    third degree T24.329-
  labium (majus) (minus) — *see* Burn, genital organs, external, female
  lacrimal apparatus, duct, gland or sac — *see* Burn, eye, specified site NEC
  larynx T27.0-
    with lung T27.1-
  leg(s) (lower) (upper) — *see* Burn, lower, limb
  lightning — *see* Burn, by site
  limb(s)
    lower (except ankle or foot alone) — *see* Burn, lower, limb
    upper — *see* Burn, upper limb
  lip(s) T20.02-
    first degree T20.12-
    second degree T20.22-
    third degree T20.32-
  lower
    back — *see* Burn, back
    limb T24.009-
      ankle — *see* Burn, ankle
      calf — *see* Burn, calf
      first degree T24.109-
      foot — *see* Burn, foot
      hip — *see* Burn, thigh
      knee — *see* Burn, knee
      left T24.002-
        first degree T24.102-
        second degree T24.202-
        third degree T24.302-
      multiple sites, except ankle and foot T24.099-
        ankle and foot T25.099-
          first degree T25.199-
          left T25.092-
            first degree T25.192-
            second degree T25.292-
            third degree T25.392-
          right T25.091-
            first degree T25.191-
            second degree T25.291-
            third degree T25.391-
          second degree T25.299-
          third degree T25.399-
        first degree T24.199-
        left T24.092-
          first degree T24.192-
          second degree T24.292-
          third degree T24.392-
        right T24.091-
          first degree T24.191-
          second degree T24.291-
          third degree T24.391-

Burn — *continued*
  lower — *continued*
    limb — *continued*
      multiple sites, except ankle and foot — *continued*
        second degree T24.299- ☑
        third degree T24.399- ☑
        right T24.001- ☑
          first degree T24.101- ☑
          second degree T24.201- ☑
          third degree T24.301- ☑
        second degree T24.209- ☑
        thigh — *see* Burn, thigh
        third degree T24.309- ☑
        toe — *see* Burn, toe
  lung (with larynx and trachea) T27.1- ☑
  mouth T28.0- ☑
  neck T20.07- ☑
    first degree T20.17- ☑
    second degree T20.27- ☑
    third degree T20.37- ☑
  nose (septum) T20.04- ☑
    first degree T20.14- ☑
    second degree T20.24- ☑
    third degree T20.34- ☑
  ocular adnexa — *see* Burn, eye
  orbit region — *see* Burn, eyelid
  palm T23.059- ☑
    first degree T23.159- ☑
    left T23.052- ☑
      first degree T23.152- ☑
      second degree T23.252- ☑
      third degree T23.352- ☑
    right T23.051- ☑
      first degree T23.151- ☑
      second degree T23.251- ☑
      third degree T23.351- ☑
    second degree T23.259- ☑
    third degree T23.359- ☑
  partial thickness — *code as* Burn, by site, second degree
  pelvis — *see* Burn, trunk
  penis — *see* Burn, genital organs, external, male
  perineum
    female — *see* Burn, genital organs, external, female
    male — *see* Burn, genital organs, external, male
  periocular area — *see* Burn, eyelid
  pharynx T28.0- ☑
  rectum T28.2- ☑
  respiratory tract T27.3- ☑
    larynx — *see* Burn, larynx
    specified part NEC T27.2- ☑
    trachea — *see* Burn, trachea
  sac, lacrimal — *see* Burn, eye, specified site NEC
  scalp T20.05- ☑
    first degree T20.15- ☑
    second degree T20.25- ☑
    third degree T20.35- ☑
  scapular region T22.069- ☑
    first degree T22.169- ☑
    left T22.062- ☑
      first degree T22.162- ☑
      second degree T22.262- ☑
      third degree T22.362- ☑
    right T22.061- ☑
      first degree T22.161- ☑
      second degree T22.261- ☑
      third degree T22.361- ☑
    second degree T22.269- ☑
    third degree T22.369- ☑
  sclera — *see* Burn, eye, specified site NEC
  scrotum — *see* Burn, genital organs, external, male
  shoulder T22.059- ☑
    first degree T22.159- ☑
    left T22.052- ☑
      first degree T22.152- ☑
      second degree T22.252- ☑
      third degree T22.352- ☑
    right T22.051- ☑
      first degree T22.151- ☑
      second degree T22.251- ☑
      third degree T22.351- ☑
    second degree T22.259- ☑
    third degree T22.359- ☑
  stomach T28.2- ☑
  temple — *see* Burn, head
  testis — *see* Burn, genital organs, external, male

Burn — *continued*
  thigh T24.019- ☑
    first degree T24.119- ☑
    left T24.012- ☑
      first degree T24.112- ☑
      second degree T24.212- ☑
      third degree T24.312- ☑
    right T24.011- ☑
      first degree T24.111- ☑
      second degree T24.211- ☑
      third degree T24.311- ☑
    second degree T24.219- ☑
    third degree T24.319- ☑
  thorax (external) — *see* Burn, trunk
  throat (meaning pharynx) T28.0- ☑
  thumb(s) T23.019- ☑
    first degree T23.119- ☑
    left T23.012- ☑
      first degree T23.112- ☑
      second degree T23.212- ☑
      third degree T23.312- ☑
    multiple sites with fingers T23.049- ☑
      first degree T23.149- ☑
      left T23.042- ☑
        first degree T23.142- ☑
        second degree T23.242- ☑
        third degree T23.342- ☑
      right T23.041- ☑
        first degree T23.141- ☑
        second degree T23.241- ☑
        third degree T23.341- ☑
      second degree T23.249- ☑
      third degree T23.349- ☑
    right T23.011- ☑
      first degree T23.111- ☑
      second degree T23.211- ☑
      third degree T23.311- ☑
    second degree T23.219- ☑
    third degree T23.319- ☑
  toe T25.039- ☑
    first degree T25.139- ☑
    left T25.032- ☑
      first degree T25.132- ☑
      second degree T25.232- ☑
      third degree T25.332- ☑
    right T25.031- ☑
      first degree T25.131- ☑
      second degree T25.231- ☑
      third degree T25.331- ☑
    second degree T25.239- ☑
    third degree T25.339- ☑
  tongue T28.0- ☑
  tonsil(s) T28.0- ☑
  trachea T27.0- ☑
    with lung T27.1- ☑
  trunk T21.00- ☑
    abdominal wall — *see* Burn, abdominal wall
    anus — *see* Burn, buttock
    axilla — *see* Burn, upper limb
    back — *see* Burn, back
    breast — *see* Burn, chest wall
    buttock — *see* Burn, buttock
    chest wall — *see* Burn, chest wall
    first degree T21.10- ☑
    flank — *see* Burn, abdominal wall
    genital
      female — *see* Burn, genital organs, external, female
      male — *see* Burn, genital organs, external, male
    groin — *see* Burn, abdominal wall
    interscapular region — *see* Burn, back, upper
    labia — *see* Burn, genital organs, external, female
    lower back — *see* Burn, back
    penis — *see* Burn, genital organs, external, male
    perineum
      female — *see* Burn, genital organs, external, female
      male — *see* Burn, genital organs, external, male
    scapula region — *see* Burn, scapular region
    scrotum — *see* Burn, genital organs, external, male
    second degree T21.20- ☑
    specified site NEC T21.09- ☑
      first degree T21.19- ☑
      second degree T21.29- ☑
      third degree T21.39- ☑
    testes — *see* Burn, genital organs, external, male

Burn — *continued*
  trunk — *continued*
    third degree T21.30- ☑
    upper back — *see* Burn, back, upper
    vulva — *see* Burn, genital organs, external, female
  unspecified site with extent of body surface involved specified
    less than 10 percent T31.0
    10-19 percent (0-9 percent third degree) T31.10
      with 10-19 percent third degree T31.11
    20-29 percent (0-9 percent third degree) T31.20
      with
        10-19 percent third degree T31.21
        20-29 percent third degree T31.22
    30-39 percent (0-9 percent third degree) T31.30
      with
        10-19 percent third degree T31.31
        20-29 percent third degree T31.32
        30-39 percent third degree T31.33
    40-49 percent (0-9 percent third degree) T31.40
      with
        10-19 percent third degree T31.41
        20-29 percent third degree T31.42
        30-39 percent third degree T31.43
        40-49 percent third degree T31.44
    50-59 percent (0-9 percent third degree) T31.50
      with
        10-19 percent third degree T31.51
        20-29 percent third degree T31.52
        30-39 percent third degree T31.53
        40-49 percent third degree T31.54
        50-59 percent third degree T31.55
    60-69 percent (0-9 percent third degree) T31.60
      with
        10-19 percent third degree T31.61
        20-29 percent third degree T31.62
        30-39 percent third degree T31.63
        40-49 percent third degree T31.64
        50-59 percent third degree T31.65
        60-69 percent third degree T31.66
    70-79 percent (0-9 percent third degree) T31.70
      with
        10-19 percent third degree T31.71
        20-29 percent third degree T31.72
        30-39 percent third degree T31.73
        40-49 percent third degree T31.74
        50-59 percent third degree T31.75
        60-69 percent third degree T31.76
        70-79 percent third degree T31.77
    80-89 percent (0-9 percent third degree) T31.80
      with
        10-19 percent third degree T31.81
        20-29 percent third degree T31.82
        30-39 percent third degree T31.83
        40-49 percent third degree T31.84
        50-59 percent third degree T31.85
        60-69 percent third degree T31.86
        70-79 percent third degree T31.87
        80-89 percent third degree T31.88
    90 percent or more (0-9 percent third degree) T31.90
      with
        10-19 percent third degree T31.91
        20-29 percent third degree T31.92
        30-39 percent third degree T31.93
        40-49 percent third degree T31.94
        50-59 percent third degree T31.95
        60-69 percent third degree T31.96
        70-79 percent third degree T31.97
        80-89 percent third degree T31.98
        90-99 percent third degree T31.99
  upper limb T22.00- ☑
    above elbow — *see* Burn, above elbow
    axilla — *see* Burn, axilla
    elbow — *see* Burn, elbow
    first degree T22.10- ☑
    forearm — *see* Burn, forearm
    hand — *see* Burn, hand
    interscapular region — *see* Burn, back, upper
    multiple sites T22.099- ☑
      first degree T22.199- ☑
      left T22.092- ☑
        first degree T22.192- ☑
        second degree T22.292- ☑
        third degree T22.392- ☑
      right T22.091- ☑
        first degree T22.191- ☑
        second degree T22.291- ☑
        third degree T22.391- ☑

☑ Additional Character Required — Refer to the Tabular List for Character Selection

Burn — continued
- upper limb — continued
  - multiple sites — continued
    - second degree T22.299- ☑
    - third degree T22.399- ☑
  - scapular region — see Burn, scapular region
  - second degree T22.20- ☑
  - shoulder — see Burn, shoulder
  - third degree T22.30- ☑
  - wrist — see Burn, wrist
- uterus T28.3- ☑
- vagina T28.3- ☑
- vulva — see Burn, genital organs, external, female
- wrist T23.079- ☑
  - first degree T23.179- ☑
  - left T23.072- ☑
    - first degree T23.172- ☑
    - second degree T23.272- ☑
    - third degree T23.372- ☑
  - multiple sites with hand T23.099- ☑
    - first degree T23.199- ☑
    - left T23.092- ☑
      - first degree T23.192- ☑
      - second degree T23.292- ☑
      - third degree T23.392- ☑
    - right T23.091- ☑
      - first degree T23.191- ☑
      - second degree T23.291- ☑
      - third degree T23.391- ☑
    - second degree T23.299- ☑
    - third degree T23.399- ☑
  - right T23.071- ☑
    - first degree T23.171- ☑
    - second degree T23.271- ☑
    - third degree T23.371- ☑
  - second degree T23.279- ☑
  - third degree T23.379- ☑

Burn-out (state) Z73.0
Burnett's syndrome E83.52
Burning
- feet syndrome E53.9
- sensation R20.8
- tongue K14.6

Burns' disease or osteochondrosis — see Osteochondrosis, juvenile, ulna
Bursa — see condition
Bursitis M71.9
- Achilles — see Tendinitis, Achilles
- adhesive — see Bursitis, specified NEC
- ankle — see Enthesopathy, ankle and tarsus
- calcaneal — see Enthesopathy, foot, specified type NEC
- collateral ligament, tibial — see Bursitis, tibial collateral
- due to use, overuse, pressure — see also Disorder, soft tissue, due to use, specified type NEC
  - specified NEC — see Disorder, soft tissue, due to use, specified NEC
- Duplay's M75.0- ☑
- elbow NEC M70.3- ☑
  - olecranon M70.2- ☑
- finger — see Disorder, soft tissue, due to use, specified type NEC, hand
- foot — see Enthesopathy, foot, specified type NEC
- gonococcal A54.49
- gouty — see Gout
- hand M70.1- ☑
- hip NEC M70.7- ☑
  - trochanteric M70.6- ☑
- infective NEC M71.10
  - abscess — see Abscess, bursa
  - ankle M71.17- ☑
  - elbow M71.12- ☑
  - foot M71.17- ☑
  - hand M71.14- ☑
  - hip M71.15- ☑
  - knee M71.16- ☑
  - multiple sites M71.19
  - shoulder M71.11- ☑
  - specified site NEC M71.18
  - wrist M71.13- ☑
- ischial — see Bursitis, hip
- knee NEC M70.5- ☑
  - prepatellar M70.4- ☑
- occupational NEC — see also Disorder, soft tissue, due to use
- olecranon — see Bursitis, elbow, olecranon
- pharyngeal J39.1
- popliteal — see Bursitis, knee

Bursitis — continued
- prepatellar M70.4- ☑
- radiohumeral M70.3- ☑
- rheumatoid M06.20
  - ankle M06.27- ☑
  - elbow M06.22- ☑
  - foot joint M06.27- ☑
  - hand joint M06.24- ☑
  - hip M06.25- ☑
  - knee M06.26- ☑
  - multiple site M06.29
  - shoulder M06.21- ☑
  - vertebra M06.28
  - wrist M06.23- ☑
- scapulohumeral — see Bursitis, shoulder
- semimembranous muscle (knee) — see Bursitis, knee
- shoulder M75.5- ☑
  - adhesive — see Capsulitis, adhesive
- specified NEC M71.50
  - ankle M71.57- ☑
  - due to use, overuse or pressure — see Disorder, soft tissue, due to, use
  - elbow M71.52- ☑
  - foot M71.57- ☑
  - hand M71.54- ☑
  - hip M71.55- ☑
  - knee M71.56- ☑
  - shoulder — see Bursitis, shoulder
  - specified site NEC M71.58
  - tibial collateral M76.4- ☑
  - wrist M71.53- ☑
- subacromial — see Bursitis, shoulder
- subcoracoid — see Bursitis, shoulder
- subdeltoid — see Bursitis, shoulder
- syphilitic A52.78
- Thornwaldt, Tornwaldt J39.2
- tibial collateral M76.4- ☑
- toe — see Enthesopathy, foot, specified type NEC
- trochanteric (area) — see Bursitis, hip, trochanteric
- wrist — see Bursitis, hand

Bursopathy M71.9
- specified type NEC M71.80
  - ankle M71.87- ☑
  - elbow M71.82- ☑
  - foot M71.87- ☑
  - hand M71.84- ☑
  - hip M71.85- ☑
  - knee M71.86- ☑
  - multiple sites M71.89
  - shoulder M71.81- ☑
  - specified site NEC M71.88
  - wrist M71.83- ☑

Burst stitches or sutures (complication of surgery) T81.31- ☑
- external operation wound T81.31- ☑
- internal operation wound — see also Dehiscence, closure T81.328- ☑
  - abdominal wall muscle or fascia T81.321- ☑
  - specified NEC T81.328- ☑

Buruli ulcer A31.1
Bury's disease L95.1
Buschke's
- disease — see Cryptococcosis by site
- scleredema — see Sclerosis, systemic

Busse-Buschke disease — see Cryptococcosis by site
Buttock — see condition
Button
- Biskra B55.1
- Delhi B55.1
- oriental B55.1

Buttonhole deformity (finger) — see Deformity, finger, boutonniere
Bwamba fever A92.8
Byssinosis J66.0
Bywaters' syndrome T79.5- ☑

C

Cachexia R64
- cancerous R64
- cardiac — see Disease, heart
- dehydration E86.0
- due to
  - malnutrition — see also Malnutrition, severe E88.A
  - underlying condition E88.A
- exophthalmic — see Hyperthyroidism
- heart — see Disease, heart

Cachexia — continued
- hypophyseal E23.0
- hypopituitary E23.0
- lead — see Poisoning, lead
- malignant R64
- marsh — see Malaria
- nervous F48.8
- old age R54
- paludal — see Malaria
- pituitary E23.0
- pulmonary R64
- renal N28.9
- saturnine — see Poisoning, lead
- senile R54
- Simmonds' E23.0
- splenica D73.0
- strumipriva E03.4
- tuberculous NEC — see Tuberculosis

CADASIL (cerebral autosomal dominant arteriopathy with subcortical infarcts and leukoencephalopathy) I67.850
Cafe, au lait spots L81.3
Caffeine-induced
- anxiety disorder F15.980
- sleep disorder F15.982

Caffey's syndrome Q78.8
Caisson disease T70.3- ☑
Cake kidney Q63.1
Caked breast (puerperal, postpartum) O92.79
Calabar swelling B74.3
Calcaneal spur — see Spur, bone, calcaneal
Calcaneo-apophysitis M92.6- ☑
Calcareous — see condition
Calcicosis J62.8
Calciferol (vitamin D) **deficiency** E55.9
- with rickets E55.0

Calcification
- adrenal (capsule) (gland) E27.49
  - tuberculous B90.8 [E35]
- aorta I70.0
- arterial
  - generalized, of infancy E83.820
    - with
      - ABCC6 deficiency E83.823
      - ENPP1 deficiency E83.821
      - unspecified genetic causality E83.820
- artery (annular) — see Arteriosclerosis
- auricle (ear) — see Disorder, pinna, specified type NEC
- basal ganglia G23.8
- bladder N32.89
  - due to Schistosoma hematobium B65.0
- brain (cortex) — see Calcification, cerebral
- bronchus J98.09
- bursa M71.40
  - ankle M71.47- ☑
  - elbow M71.42- ☑
  - foot M71.47- ☑
  - hand M71.44- ☑
  - hip M71.45- ☑
  - knee M71.46- ☑
  - multiple sites M71.49
  - shoulder M75.3- ☑
  - specified site NEC M71.48
  - wrist M71.43- ☑
- cardiac — see Degeneration, myocardial
- cerebral (cortex) G93.89
  - artery I67.2
- cervix (uteri) N88.8
- choroid plexus G93.89
- conjunctiva — see Concretion, conjunctiva
- corpora cavernosa (penis) N48.89
- cortex (brain) — see Calcification, cerebral
- dental pulp (nodular) K04.2
- dentinal papilla K00.4
- fallopian tube N83.8
- falx cerebri G96.198
- gallbladder K82.8
- general E83.59
- heart — see also Degeneration, myocardial
  - valve — see also Endocarditis
    - mitral — see Calcification, mitral
- idiopathic infantile arterial (IIAC) — see Calcification, arterial, generalized, of infancy
- intervertebral cartilage or disc (postinfective) — see Disorder, disc, specified NEC
- intracranial — see Calcification, cerebral
- joint — see Disorder, joint, specified type NEC
- kidney N28.89
  - tuberculous N29 [B90.1]

Calcification — continued
- larynx (senile) J38.7
- lens — see Cataract, specified NEC
- lung (active) (postinfectional) J98.4
  - tuberculous B90.9
- lymph gland or node (postinfectional) I89.8
  - tuberculous — see also Tuberculosis, lymph gland B90.8
- mammographic R92.1
- massive (paraplegic) — see Myositis, ossificans, in, quadriplegia
- medial — see Arteriosclerosis, extremities
- meninges (cerebral) (spinal) G96.198
- metastatic E83.59
- mitral (valve)
  - annular I34.81
    - nonrheumatic I34.81
    - rheumatic I05.8
  - annulus I34.81
    - nonrheumatic I34.81
    - rheumatic I05.8
- Monckeberg's — see Arteriosclerosis, extremities
- muscle M61.9
  - due to burns — see Myositis, ossificans, in, burns
  - paralytic — see Myositis, ossificans, in, quadriplegia
  - specified type NEC M61.40
    - ankle M61.47- ☑
    - foot M61.47- ☑
    - forearm M61.43- ☑
    - hand M61.44- ☑
    - lower leg M61.46- ☑
    - multiple sites M61.49
    - pelvic region M61.45- ☑
    - shoulder region M61.41- ☑
    - specified site NEC M61.48
    - thigh M61.45- ☑
    - upper arm M61.42- ☑
- myocardium, myocardial — see Degeneration, myocardial
- ovary N83.8
- pancreas K86.89
- penis N48.89
- periarticular — see Disorder, joint, specified type NEC
- pericardium — see also Pericarditis I31.1
- pineal gland E34.8
- pleura J94.8
  - postinfectional J94.8
  - tuberculous NEC B90.9
- pulpal (dental) (nodular) K04.2
- sclera H15.89
- spleen D73.89
- subcutaneous L94.2
- suprarenal (capsule) (gland) E27.49
- tendon (sheath) — see also Tenosynovitis, specified type NEC
  - with bursitis, synovitis or tenosynovitis — see Tendinitis, calcific
- trachea J39.8
- ureter N28.89
- uterus N85.8
- vitreous — see Deposit, crystalline

Calcified — see Calcification

Calcinosis (interstitial) (tumoral) (universalis) E83.59
- with Raynaud's phenomenon, esophageal dysfunction, sclerodactyly, telangiectasia (CREST syndrome) M34.1
- circumscripta (skin) L94.2
- cutis L94.2

Calciphylaxis — see also Calcification, by site E83.59

Calcium
- deposits — see Calcification, by site
- metabolism disorder E83.50
- salts or soaps in vitreous — see Deposit, crystalline

Calciuria R82.994

Calculi — see Calculus

Calculosis, intrahepatic — see Calculus, bile duct

Calculus, calculi, calculous
- ampulla of Vater — see Calculus, bile duct
- anuria (impacted) (recurrent) — see also Calculus, urinary N20.9
- appendix K38.1
- bile duct (common) (hepatic) K80.50
  - with
    - calculus of gallbladder — see Calculus, gallbladder and bile duct
    - cholangitis K80.30

Calculus, calculi, calculous — continued
- bile duct — continued
  - with — continued
    - cholangitis — continued
      - with
        - cholecystitis — see Calculus, bile duct, with cholecystitis
        - obstruction K80.31
      - acute K80.32
        - with
          - chronic cholangitis K80.36
            - with obstruction K80.37
          - obstruction K80.33
      - chronic K80.34
        - with
          - acute cholangitis K80.36
            - with obstruction K80.37
          - obstruction K80.35
    - cholecystitis (with cholangitis) K80.40
      - with obstruction K80.41
      - acute K80.42
        - with
          - chronic cholecystitis K80.46
            - with obstruction K80.47
          - obstruction K80.43
      - chronic K80.44
        - with
          - acute cholecystitis K80.46
            - with obstruction K80.47
          - obstruction K80.45
- biliary — see also Calculus, gallbladder
  - with bile duct involvement — see also Calculus, bile duct
  - specified NEC K80.80
    - with obstruction K80.81
- bilirubin, multiple — see Calculus, gallbladder
- bladder (encysted) (impacted) (urinary) (diverticulum) N21.0
- bronchus J98.09
- calyx (kidney) (renal) — see Calculus, kidney
- cholesterol (pure) (solitary) — see Calculus, gallbladder
- common duct (bile) — see Calculus, bile duct
- conjunctiva — see Concretion, conjunctiva
- cystic N21.0
  - duct — see Calculus, gallbladder
- dental (subgingival) (supragingival) K03.6
- diverticulum
  - bladder N21.0
  - kidney N20.0
- epididymis N50.89
- gallbladder K80.20
  - with
    - bile duct calculus — see Calculus, gallbladder and bile duct
    - cholecystitis K80.10
      - with obstruction K80.11
      - acute K80.00
        - with
          - chronic cholecystitis K80.12
            - with obstruction K80.13
          - obstruction K80.01
      - chronic K80.10
        - with
          - acute cholecystitis K80.12
            - with obstruction K80.13
          - obstruction K80.11
    - specified NEC K80.18
      - with obstruction K80.19
  - obstruction K80.21
- gallbladder and bile duct K80.70
  - with
    - cholecystitis K80.60
      - with obstruction K80.61
      - acute K80.62
        - with
          - chronic cholecystitis K80.66
            - with obstruction K80.67
          - obstruction K80.63
      - chronic K80.64
        - with
          - acute cholecystitis K80.66
            - with obstruction K80.67
          - obstruction K80.65
    - obstruction K80.71
- hepatic (duct) — see Calculus, bile duct
- ileal conduit N21.8
- intestinal (impaction) (obstruction) K56.49
- kidney (impacted) (multiple) (pelvis) (recurrent) (staghorn) N20.0

Calculus, calculi, calculous — continued
- kidney — continued
  - with calculus, ureter N20.2
    - with hydronephrosis N13.2
      - with infection N13.6
  - congenital Q63.8
    - with hydronephrosis N13.2
      - with infection N13.6
- lacrimal passages — see Dacryolith
- liver (impacted) — see Calculus, bile duct
- lung J98.4
- mammographic R92.1
- nephritic (impacted) (recurrent) — see Calculus, kidney
- nose J34.89
- pancreas (duct) K86.89
- parotid duct or gland K11.5
- pelvis, encysted — see Calculus, kidney
- prostate N42.0
- pulmonary J98.4
- pyelitis (impacted) (recurrent) N20.0
  - with hydronephrosis N13.6
- pyelonephritis (impacted) (recurrent) — see category N20.- ☑
  - with hydronephrosis N13.6
- renal (impacted) (recurrent) — see Calculus, kidney
- salivary (duct) (gland) K11.5
- seminal vesicle N50.89
- staghorn — see Calculus, kidney
- Stensen's duct K11.5
- stomach K31.89
- sublingual duct or gland K11.5
  - congenital Q38.4
- submandibular duct, gland or region K11.5
- submaxillary duct, gland or region K11.5
- suburethral N21.8
- tonsil J35.8
- tooth, teeth (subgingival) (supragingival) K03.6
- tunica vaginalis N50.89
- ureter (impacted) (recurrent) N20.1
  - with calculus, kidney N20.2
    - with hydronephrosis N13.2
      - with infection N13.6
  - with hydronephrosis N13.2
    - with infection N13.6
- ureteropelvic junction N20.1
- urethra (impacted) N21.1
- urinary (duct) (impacted) (passage) (tract) N20.9
  - with hydronephrosis N13.2
    - with infection N13.6
  - in (due to)
  - lower N21.9
    - specified NEC N21.8
- vagina N89.8
- vesical (impacted) N21.0
- Wharton's duct K11.5
- xanthine E79.82 [N22]

Calicectasis N28.89

Caliectasis N28.89

California
- disease B38.9
- encephalitis A83.5

Caligo cornea — see Opacity, cornea, central

Callositas, callosity (infected) L84

Callus (infected) L84
- bone — see Osteophyte
- excessive, following fracture — code as Sequelae of fracture

CALME (childhood asymmetric labium majus enlargement) N90.61

Calorie deficiency or malnutrition — see also Malnutrition E46

Calpainopathy (primary) G71.032
- autosomal dominant G71.031
- autosomal recessive G71.032

Calve-Perthes disease — see Legg-Calve-Perthes disease

Calve's disease — see Osteochondrosis, juvenile, spine

Calvities — see Alopecia, androgenic

Cameroon fever — see Malaria

Camptocormia (hysterical) F44.4

Camurati-Engelmann syndrome Q78.3

Canal — see also condition
- atrioventricular Q21.20
  - common Q21.23
  - incomplete Q21.21
  - intermediate Q21.22
  - partial Q21.21
  - transitional Q21.22

Canaliculitis (lacrimal) (acute) (subacute) H04.33- ☑
- Actinomyces A42.89

Canaliculitis

Canaliculitis — continued
- chronic H04.42- ☑

Canavan disease E75.28

Canceled procedure (surgical) Z53.9
- because of
  - contraindication Z53.09
    - smoking Z53.01
  - left against medical advice (AMA) Z53.29
  - patient's decision Z53.20
    - for reasons of belief or group pressure Z53.1
    - specified reason NEC Z53.29
  - specified reason NEC Z53.8

Cancer — see also Neoplasm, by site, malignant
- bile duct type liver C22.1
- blood — see Leukemia
- breast — see also Neoplasm, breast, malignant
  - C50.91- ☑
- hepatocellular C22.0
- lung — see also Neoplasm, lung, malignant C34.90
- ovarian — see also Neoplasm ovary, malignant C56.9
- unspecified site (primary) C80.1

Cancer (o) **phobia** F45.29

Cancerous — see Neoplasm, malignant, by site

Cancrum oris A69.0

Candidiasis, candidal B37.9
- balanitis B37.42
- bronchitis B37.1
- cheilitis B37.83
- congenital P37.5
- cystitis B37.41
- disseminated B37.7
- endocarditis B37.6
- enteritis B37.82
- esophagitis B37.81
- intertrigo B37.2
- lung B37.1
- meningitis B37.5
- mouth B37.0
- nails B37.2
- neonatal P37.5
- onychia B37.2
- oral B37.0
- osteomyelitis B37.89
- otitis externa B37.84
- paronychia B37.2
- perionyxis B37.2
- pneumonia B37.1
- proctitis B37.82
- pulmonary B37.1
- pyelonephritis B37.49
- sepsis B37.7
- skin B37.2
- specified site NEC B37.89
- stomatitis B37.0
- systemic B37.7
- urethritis B37.41
- urogenital site NEC B37.49
- vagina (acute) B37.31
  - chronic (recurrent) B37.32
- vulva (acute) B37.31
  - chronic (recurrent) B37.32
- vulvovaginitis (acute) B37.31
  - chronic (recurrent) B37.32

Candidid L30.2

Candidosis — see Candidiasis

Candiru infection or infestation B88.8

Canities (premature) L67.1
- congenital Q84.2

Canker (mouth) (sore) K12.0
- rash A38.9

Cannabinosis J66.2

Cannabis induced
- anxiety disorder F12.980
- psychotic disorder F12.959
- sleep disorder F12.988

Canton fever A75.9

Cantrell's syndrome Q87.89

Capillariasis (intestinal) B81.1
- hepatic B83.8

Capillary — see condition

Caplan's syndrome — see Rheumatoid, lung

Capsule — see condition

Capsulitis (joint) — see also Enthesopathy
- adhesive (shoulder) M75.0- ☑
- hepatic K65.8
- labyrinthine — see Otosclerosis, specified NEC
- thyroid E06.9

Caput
- crepitus Q75.8

Caput — continued
- medusae I86.8
- succedaneum P12.81

Car sickness T75.3- ☑

Carapata (disease) A68.0

Carate — see Pinta

Carbon lung J60

Carbuncle L02.93
- abdominal wall L02.231
- anus K61.0
- auditory canal, external — see Abscess, ear, external
- auricle ear — see Abscess, ear, external
- axilla L02.43- ☑
- back (any part) L02.232
- breast N61.1
- buttock L02.33
- cheek (external) L02.03
- chest wall L02.233
- chin L02.03
- corpus cavernosum N48.21
- ear (any part) (external) (middle) — see Abscess, ear, external
- external auditory canal — see Abscess, ear, external
- eyelid — see Abscess, eyelid
- face NEC L02.03
- femoral (region) — see Carbuncle, lower limb
- finger — see Carbuncle, hand
- flank L02.231
- foot L02.63- ☑
- forehead L02.03
- genital — see Abscess, genital
- gluteal (region) L02.33
- groin L02.234
- hand L02.53- ☑
- head NEC L02.831
- heel — see Carbuncle, foot
- hip — see Carbuncle, lower limb
- kidney — see Abscess, kidney
- knee — see Carbuncle, lower limb
- labium (majus) (minus) N76.4
- lacrimal
  - gland — see Dacryoadenitis
  - passages (duct) (sac) — see Inflammation, lacrimal, passages, acute
- leg — see Carbuncle, lower limb
- lower limb L02.43- ☑
- malignant A22.0
- navel L02.236
- neck L02.13
- nose (external) (septum) J34.0
- orbit, orbital — see Abscess, orbit
- palmar (space) — see Carbuncle, hand
- partes posteriores L02.33
- pectoral region L02.233
- penis N48.21
- perineum L02.235
- pinna — see Abscess, ear, external
- popliteal — see Carbuncle, lower limb
- scalp L02.831
- seminal vesicle N49.0
- shoulder — see Carbuncle, upper limb
- specified site NEC L02.838
- temple (region) L02.03
- thumb — see Carbuncle, hand
- toe — see Carbuncle, foot
- trunk L02.239
  - abdominal wall L02.231
  - back L02.232
  - chest wall L02.233
  - groin L02.234
  - perineum L02.235
  - umbilicus L02.236
- umbilicus L02.236
- upper limb L02.43- ☑
- urethra N34.0
- vulva N76.4

Carbunculus — see Carbuncle

Carcinoid (tumor) — see Tumor, carcinoid

Carcinoidosis E34.00
- heart E34.01

Carcinoma (malignant) — see also Neoplasm, by site, malignant
- acidophil
  - specified site — see Neoplasm, malignant, by site
  - unspecified site C75.1
- acidophil-basophil, mixed
  - specified site — see Neoplasm, malignant, by site
  - unspecified site C75.1

Carcinoma — continued
- adnexal (skin) — see Neoplasm, skin, malignant
- adrenal cortical C74.0- ☑
- alveolar — see Neoplasm, lung, malignant
  - cell — see Neoplasm, lung, malignant
- ameloblastic C41.1
  - upper jaw (bone) C41.0
- apocrine
  - breast — see Neoplasm, breast, malignant
  - specified site NEC — see Neoplasm, skin, malignant
  - unspecified site C44.99
- basal cell (pigmented) (also see Neoplasm, skin, malignant) C44.91
  - fibro-epithelial — see Neoplasm, skin, malignant
  - morphea — see Neoplasm, skin, malignant
  - multicentric — see Neoplasm, skin, malignant
- basal-squamous cell, mixed — see Neoplasm, skin, malignant
- basaloid
- basophil
  - specified site — see Neoplasm, malignant, by site
  - unspecified site C75.1
- basophil-acidophil, mixed
  - specified site — see Neoplasm, malignant, by site
  - unspecified site C75.1
- basosquamous — see Neoplasm, skin, malignant
- bile duct
  - with hepatocellular, mixed C22.0
  - liver C22.1
  - specified site NEC — see Neoplasm, malignant, by site
  - unspecified site C22.1
- branchial or branchiogenic C10.4
- bronchial or bronchogenic — see Neoplasm, lung, malignant
- bronchiolar — see Neoplasm, lung, malignant
- bronchioloalveolar — see Neoplasm, lung, malignant
- C cell
  - specified site — see Neoplasm, malignant, by site
  - unspecified site C73
- ceruminous C44.29- ☑
- cervix uteri
  - in situ D06.9
    - endocervix D06.0
    - exocervix D06.1
    - specified site NEC D06.7
- chorionic
  - specified site — see Neoplasm, malignant, by site
  - unspecified site
    - female C58
    - male C62.90
- chromophobe
  - specified site — see Neoplasm, malignant, by site
  - unspecified site C75.1
- cloacogenic
  - specified site — see Neoplasm, malignant, by site
  - unspecified site C21.2
- diffuse type
  - specified site — see Neoplasm, malignant, by site
  - unspecified site C16.9
- duct (cell)
  - with Paget's disease — see Neoplasm, breast, malignant
  - infiltrating
    - with lobular carcinoma (in situ)
      - specified site — see Neoplasm, malignant, by site
      - unspecified site (female) C50.91- ☑
        - male C50.92- ☑
    - specified site — see Neoplasm, malignant, by site
    - unspecified site (female) C50.91- ☑
      - male C50.92- ☑
- ductal
  - with lobular
    - specified site — see Neoplasm, malignant, by site
    - unspecified site (female) C50.91- ☑
      - male C50.92- ☑
- ductular, infiltrating
  - specified site — see Neoplasm, malignant, by site
  - unspecified site (female) C50.91- ☑
    - male C50.92- ☑
- embryonal
  - liver C22.7
- endometrioid
  - specified site — see Neoplasm, malignant, by site
  - unspecified site
    - female C56.9
    - male C61

Carcinoma — *continued*
  eosinophil
    specified site — *see* Neoplasm, malignant, by site
    unspecified site C75.1
  epidermoid — *see also* Neoplasm, skin, malignant
    in situ, Bowen's type — *see* Neoplasm, skin, in situ
  fibroepithelial, basal cell — *see* Neoplasm, skin, malignant
  follicular
    with papillary (mixed) C73
    moderately differentiated C73
    pure follicle C73
    specified site — *see* Neoplasm, malignant, by site
    trabecular C73
    unspecified site C73
    well differentiated C73
  generalized, with unspecified primary site C80.0
  glycogen-rich — *see* Neoplasm, breast, malignant
  granulosa cell C56.- ☑
  hepatic cell C22.0
  hepatocellular C22.0
    with bile duct, mixed C22.0
    fibrolamellar C22.0
  hepatocholangiolitic C22.0
  Hurthle cell C73
  in
    adenomatous
      polyposis coli C18.9
    pleomorphic adenoma — *see* Neoplasm, salivary gland or duct, malignant
    situ — *see* Carcinoma-in-situ
  infiltrating
    duct
      with lobular
        specified site — *see* Neoplasm, malignant, by site
        unspecified site (female) C50.91- ☑
          male C50.92- ☑
      with Paget's disease — *see* Neoplasm, breast, malignant
      specified site — *see* Neoplasm, malignant
      unspecified site (female) C50.91- ☑
        male C50.92- ☑
    ductular
      specified site — *see* Neoplasm, malignant
      unspecified site (female) C50.91- ☑
        male C50.92- ☑
    lobular
      specified site — *see* Neoplasm, malignant
      unspecified site (female) C50.91- ☑
        male C50.92- ☑
  inflammatory
    specified site — *see* Neoplasm, malignant
    unspecified site (female) C50.91- ☑
      male C50.92- ☑
  intestinal type
    specified site — *see* Neoplasm, malignant, by site
    unspecified site C16.9
  intracystic
    noninfiltrating — *see* Neoplasm, in situ, by site
  intraductal (noninfiltrating)
    with Paget's disease — *see* Neoplasm, breast, malignant
    breast D05.1- ☑
    papillary
      with invasion
        specified site — *see* Neoplasm, malignant, by site
        unspecified site (female) C50.91- ☑
          male C50.92- ☑
      breast D05.1- ☑
      specified site NEC — *see* Neoplasm, in situ, by site
      unspecified site (female) D05.1- ☑
    specified site NEC — *see* Neoplasm, in situ, by site
    unspecified site (female) D05.1- ☑
  intraepidermal — *see* Neoplasm, in situ
    squamous cell, Bowen's type — *see* Neoplasm, skin, in situ
  intraepithelial — *see* Neoplasm, in situ, by site
    squamous cell — *see* Neoplasm, in situ, by site
  intraosseous C41.1
    upper jaw (bone) C41.0
  islet cell
    with exocrine, mixed
      specified site — *see* Neoplasm, malignant, by site
      unspecified site C25.9
    pancreas C25.4

Carcinoma — *continued*
  islet cell — *continued*
    specified site NEC — *see* Neoplasm, malignant, by site
    unspecified site C25.4
  juvenile, breast — *see* Neoplasm, breast, malignant
  large cell
    small cell
      specified site — *see* Neoplasm, malignant, by site
      unspecified site C34.90
  Leydig cell (testis)
    specified site — *see* Neoplasm, malignant, by site
    unspecified site
      female C56.9
      male C62.90
  lipid-rich (female) C50.91- ☑
    male C50.92- ☑
  liver cell C22.0
  liver NEC C22.7
  lobular (infiltrating)
    with intraductal
      specified site — *see* Neoplasm, malignant, by site
      unspecified site (female) C50.91- ☑
        male C50.92- ☑
    noninfiltrating
      breast D05.0- ☑
      specified site NEC — *see* Neoplasm, in situ, by site
      unspecified site D05.0- ☑
    specified site — *see* Neoplasm, malignant, by site
    unspecified site (female) C50.91- ☑
      male C50.92- ☑
  medullary
    with
      amyloid stroma
        specified site — *see* Neoplasm, malignant, by site
        unspecified site C73
      lymphoid stroma
        specified site — *see* Neoplasm, malignant, by site
        unspecified site (female) C50.91- ☑
          male C50.92- ☑
  Merkel cell C4A.9 (*following* C43)
    anal margin C4A.51 (*following* C43)
    anal skin C4A.51 (*following* C43)
    canthus C4A.1- ☑ (*following* C43)
    ear and external auricular canal C4A.2- ☑ (*following* C43)
    external auricular canal C4A.2- ☑ (*following* C43)
    eyelid, including canthus C4A.1- ☑ (*following* C43)
    face C4A.30 (*following* C43)
      specified NEC C4A.39 (*following* C43)
    hip C4A.7- ☑ (*following* C43)
    lip C4A.0 (*following* C43)
    lower limb, including hip C4A.7- ☑ (*following* C43)
    neck C4A.4 (*following* C43)
    nodal presentation C7B.1 (*following* C75)
    nose C4A.31 (*following* C43)
    overlapping sites C4A.8 (*following* C43)
    perianal skin C4A.51 (*following* C43)
    scalp C4A.4 (*following* C43)
    secondary C7B.1 (*following* C75)
    shoulder C4A.6- ☑ (*following* C43)
    skin of breast C4A.52 (*following* C43)
    trunk NEC C4A.59 (*following* C43)
    upper limb, including shoulder C4A.6- ☑ (*following* C43)
    visceral metastatic C7B.1 (*following* C75)
  metastatic — *see* Neoplasm, secondary, by site
  metatypical — *see* Neoplasm, skin, malignant
  morphea, basal cell — *see* Neoplasm, skin, malignant
  mucoid
    cell
      specified site — *see* Neoplasm, malignant, by site
      unspecified site C75.1
  neuroendocrine — *see also* Tumor, neuroendocrine
    high grade, any site C7A.1 (*following* C75)
    poorly differentiated, any site C7A.1 (*following* C75)
  nonencapsulated sclerosing C73
  noninfiltrating
    intracystic — *see* Neoplasm, in situ, by site
    intraductal
      breast D05.1- ☑
      papillary
        breast D05.1- ☑
        specified site NEC — *see* Neoplasm, in situ, by site
        unspecified site D05.1- ☑

Carcinoma — *continued*
  noninfiltrating — *continued*
    intraductal — *continued*
      specified site — *see* Neoplasm, in situ, by site
      unspecified site D05.1- ☑
    lobular
      breast D05.0- ☑
      specified site NEC — *see* Neoplasm, in situ, by site
      unspecified site (female) D05.0- ☑
  oat cell
    specified site — *see* Neoplasm, malignant, by site
    unspecified site C34.90
  odontogenic C41.1
    upper jaw (bone) C41.0
  papillary
    with follicular (mixed) C73
    follicular variant C73
    intraductal (noninfiltrating)
      with invasion
        specified site — *see* Neoplasm, malignant, by site
        unspecified site (female) C50.91- ☑
          male C50.92- ☑
      breast D05.1- ☑
      specified site NEC — *see* Neoplasm, in situ, by site
      unspecified site D05.1- ☑
    serous
      specified site — *see* Neoplasm, malignant, by site
    surface
      specified site — *see* Neoplasm, malignant, by site
      unspecified site C56.9
    unspecified site C56.9
  papillocystic
    specified site — *see* Neoplasm, malignant, by site
    unspecified site C56.9
  parafollicular cell
    specified site — *see* Neoplasm, malignant, by site
    unspecified site C73
  pilomatrix — *see* Neoplasm, skin, malignant
  pseudomucinous
    specified site — *see* Neoplasm, malignant, by site
    unspecified site C56.9
  renal cell C64.- ☑
  Schmincke — *see* Neoplasm, nasopharynx, malignant
  Schneiderian
    specified site — *see* Neoplasm, malignant, by site
    unspecified site C30.0
  sebaceous — *see* Neoplasm, skin, malignant
  secondary — *see also* Neoplasm, secondary, by site
    Merkel cell C7B.1 (*following* C75)
  secretory, breast — *see* Neoplasm, breast, malignant
  serous
    papillary
      specified site — *see* Neoplasm, malignant, by site
      unspecified site C56.9
    surface, papillary
      specified site — *see* Neoplasm, malignant, by site
      unspecified site C56.9
  Sertoli cell
    specified site — *see* Neoplasm, malignant, by site
    unspecified site C62.90
      female C56.9
      male C62.90
  skin appendage — *see* Neoplasm, skin, malignant
  small cell
    fusiform cell
      specified site — *see* Neoplasm, malignant, by site
      unspecified site C34.90
    intermediate cell
      specified site — *see* Neoplasm, malignant, by site
      unspecified site C34.90
    large cell
      specified site — *see* Neoplasm, malignant, by site
      unspecified site C34.90
  solid
    with amyloid stroma
      specified site — *see* Neoplasm, malignant, by site
      unspecified site C73
    microinvasive
      specified site — *see* Neoplasm, malignant, by site
      unspecified site C53.9
  sweat gland — *see* Neoplasm, skin, malignant
  theca cell C56.- ☑
  thymic C37
  unspecified site (primary) C80.1
  water-clear cell C75.0
Carcinoma-in-situ — *see also* Neoplasm, in situ, by site

☑ **Additional Character Required** — Refer to the Tabular List for Character Selection

Carcinoma-in-situ — *continued*
- breast NOS D05.9- ☑
  - specified type NEC D05.8- ☑
- epidermoid — *see also* Neoplasm, in situ, by site
  - with questionable stromal invasion
    - cervix D06.9
    - specified site NEC — *see* Neoplasm, in situ, by site
    - unspecified site D06.9
- Bowen's type — *see* Neoplasm, skin, in situ
- intraductal
  - breast D05.1- ☑
  - specified site NEC — *see* Neoplasm, in situ, by site
  - unspecified site D05.1- ☑
- lobular
  - with
    - infiltrating duct
      - breast (female) C50.91- ☑
        - male C50.92- ☑
      - specified site NEC — *see* Neoplasm, malignant
      - unspecified site (female) C50.91- ☑
        - male C50.92- ☑
    - intraductal
      - breast D05.8- ☑
      - specified site NEC — *see* Neoplasm, in situ, by site
      - unspecified site (female) D05.8- ☑
  - breast D05.0- ☑
  - specified site NEC — *see* Neoplasm, in situ, by site
  - unspecified site D05.0- ☑
- squamous cell — *see also* Neoplasm, in situ, by site
  - with questionable stromal invasion
    - cervix D06.9
    - specified site NEC — *see* Neoplasm, in situ, by site
    - unspecified site D06.9

Carcinomaphobia F45.29
Carcinomatosis C80.0
- peritonei C78.6
- unspecified site (primary) (secondary) C80.0

Carcinosarcoma — *see* Neoplasm, malignant, by site
- embryonal — *see* Neoplasm, malignant, by site

Cardia, cardial — *see* condition
Cardiac — *see also* condition
- death, sudden — *see* Arrest, cardiac
- pacemaker
  - in situ Z95.0
    - management or adjustment Z45.018
- tamponade I31.4

Cardialgia — *see* Pain, precordial
Cardiectasis — *see* Hypertrophy, cardiac
Cardiochalasia K21.9
Cardiomalacia I51.5
Cardiomegalia glycogenica diffusa E74.02 [I43]
Cardiomegaly — *see also* Hypertrophy, cardiac
- congenital Q24.8
- glycogen E74.02 [I43]
- idiopathic I51.7

Cardiomyoliposis I51.5
Cardiomyopathy (familial) (idiopathic) I42.9
- alcoholic I42.6
- amyloid E85.4 [I43]
  - transthyretin-related (ATTR) familial E85.4 [I43]
- arteriosclerotic — *see* Disease, heart, ischemic, atherosclerotic
- beriberi E51.12
- cobalt-beer I42.6
- congenital I42.4
- congestive I42.0
- constrictive NOS I42.5
- dilated I42.0
- due to
  - alcohol I42.6
  - beriberi E51.12
  - cardiac glycogenosis E74.02 [I43]
  - drugs I42.7
  - external agents NEC I42.7
  - Friedreich's ataxia G11.11
  - myotonia atrophica G71.11 [I43]
  - progressive muscular dystrophy — *see also* Dystrophy, muscular, by type G71.09 [I43]
- glycogen storage E74.02 [I43]
- hypertensive — *see* Hypertension, heart
- hypertrophic (nonobstructive) I42.2
  - obstructive I42.1
    - congenital Q24.8
- in
  - Chagas' disease (chronic) B57.2
    - acute B57.0
  - sarcoidosis D86.85

Cardiomyopathy — *continued*
- ischemic I25.5
- metabolic E88.9 [I43]
  - thyrotoxic E05.90 [I43]
    - with thyroid storm E05.91 [I43]
- newborn I42.8
  - congenital I42.4
- non-ischemic — *see also* by cause I42.8
- nutritional E63.9 [I43]
  - beriberi E51.12
- obscure of Africa I42.8
- peripartum O90.3
- postpartum O90.3
- restrictive NEC I42.5
- rheumatic I09.0
- secondary I42.9
- specified NEC I42.8
- stress induced I51.81
- takotsubo I51.81
- thyrotoxic E05.90 [I43]
  - with thyroid storm E05.91 [I43]
- toxic NEC I42.7
- transthyretin-related (ATTR) familial amyloid E85.4
- tuberculous A18.84
- viral B33.24

Cardionephritis — *see* Hypertension, cardiorenal
Cardionephropathy — *see* Hypertension, cardiorenal
Cardionephrosis — *see* Hypertension, cardiorenal
Cardiopathia nigra I27.0
Cardiopathy — *see also* Disease, heart I51.9
- idiopathic I42.9
- mucopolysaccharidosis E76.3 [I52]

Cardiopericarditis — *see* Pericarditis
Cardiophobia F45.29
Cardiorenal — *see* condition
Cardiorrhexis — *see* Infarct, myocardium
Cardiosclerosis — *see* Disease, heart, ischemic, atherosclerotic
Cardiosis — *see* Disease, heart
Cardiospasm (esophagus) (reflex) (stomach) K22.0
- congenital Q39.5
  - with megaesophagus Q39.5

Cardiostenosis — *see* Disease, heart
Cardiosymphysis I31.0
Cardiovascular — *see* condition
Carditis (acute) (bacterial) (chronic) (subacute) I51.89
- meningococcal A39.50
- rheumatic — *see* Disease, heart, rheumatic
- rheumatoid — *see* Rheumatoid, carditis
- viral B33.20

Care (of) (for) (following)
- child (routine) Z76.2
- family member (handicapped) (sick)
  - creating problem for family Z63.6
  - provided away from home for holiday relief Z75.5
  - unavailable, due to
    - absence (person rendering care) (sufferer) Z74.2
    - inability (any reason) of person rendering care Z74.2
- foundling Z76.1
- holiday relief Z75.5
- improper — *see* Maltreatment
- lack of (at or after birth) (infant) — *see* Maltreatment, child, neglect
- lactating mother Z39.1
- palliative Z51.5
- postpartum
  - immediately after delivery Z39.0
  - routine follow-up Z39.2
- respite Z75.5
- unavailable, due to
  - absence of person rendering care Z74.2
  - inability (any reason) of person rendering care Z74.2
- well-baby Z76.2

Caries
- bone NEC A18.03
- dental (dentino enamel junction) (early childhood) (of dentine) (pre-eruptive) (recurrent) (to the pulp) K02.9
  - arrested (coronal) (root) K02.3
  - chewing surface
    - limited to enamel K02.51
    - penetrating into dentin K02.52
    - penetrating into pulp K02.53
  - coronal surface
    - chewing surface
      - limited to enamel K02.51
      - penetrating into dentin K02.52
      - penetrating into pulp K02.53

Caries — *continued*
- dental — *continued*
  - coronal surface — *continued*
    - pit and fissure surface
      - limited to enamel K02.51
      - penetrating into dentin K02.52
      - penetrating into pulp K02.53
    - smooth surface
      - limited to enamel K02.61
      - penetrating into dentin K02.62
      - penetrating into pulp K02.63
  - pit and fissure surface
    - limited to enamel K02.51
    - penetrating into dentin K02.52
    - penetrating into pulp K02.53
  - primary, cervical origin K02.52
  - root K02.7
  - smooth surface
    - limited to enamel K02.61
    - penetrating into dentin K02.62
    - penetrating into pulp K02.63
- external meatus — *see* Disorder, ear, external, specified type NEC
- hip (tuberculous) A18.02
- initial (tooth)
  - chewing surface K02.51
  - pit and fissure surface K02.51
  - smooth surface K02.61
- knee (tuberculous) A18.02
- labyrinth H83.8- ☑
- limb NEC (tuberculous) A18.03
- mastoid process (chronic) — *see* Mastoiditis, chronic
- tuberculous A18.03
- middle ear H74.8- ☑
- nose (tuberculous) A18.03
- orbit (tuberculous) A18.03
- ossicles, ear — *see* Abnormal, ear ossicles
- petrous bone — *see* Petrositis
- root (dental) (tooth) K02.7
- sacrum (tuberculous) A18.01
- spine, spinal (column) (tuberculous) A18.01
- syphilitic A52.77
  - congenital (early) A50.02 [M90.80]
- tooth, teeth — *see* Caries, dental
- tuberculous A18.03
- vertebra (column) (tuberculous) A18.01

Carious teeth — *see* Caries, dental
Carneous mole O02.0
Carnitine insufficiency E71.40
Carotenemia (dietary) E67.1
Carotenosis (cutis) (skin) E67.1
Carotid body or sinus syndrome G90.01
Carotidynia G90.01
Carpal tunnel syndrome — *see* Syndrome, carpal tunnel
Carpenter's syndrome Q87.0
Carpopedal spasm — *see* Tetany
Carr-Barr-Plunkett syndrome Q97.1
Carrier (suspected) of
- Acinetobacter baumannii Z22.349
  - carbapenem-resistant Z22.340
  - carbapenem-sensitive Z22.341
- amebiasis Z22.1
- bacterial disease NEC Z22.39
  - diphtheria Z22.2
  - intestinal infectious NEC Z22.1
    - typhoid Z22.0
  - meningococcal Z22.31
  - sexually transmitted Z22.4
  - specified NEC Z22.39
  - staphylococcal (Methicillin susceptible) Z22.321
    - Methicillin resistant Z22.322
  - streptococcal Z22.338
    - group B Z22.330
      - complicating pregnancy or delivery O99.82- ☑
  - typhoid Z22.0
- cholera Z22.1
- diphtheria Z22.2
- E. coli (Escherichia coli) Z22.35- ☑
- Enterobacterales Z22.359
  - carbapenem-resistant Z22.350
  - carbapenem-sensitive Z22.358
  - Enterobacterales, specified type NEC Z22.358
  - ESBL-producing Z22.358
  - extended-spectrum beta-lactamase producing Z22.358
- gastrointestinal pathogens NEC Z22.1
- genetic Z14.8
  - cystic fibrosis Z14.1
  - hemophilia A (asymptomatic) Z14.01

Carrier of — *continued*
  genetic — *continued*
    hemophilia A — *continued*
      symptomatic Z14.02
  gestational, pregnant Z33.1
  gonorrhea Z22.4
  HAA (hepatitis Australian-antigen) B18.8
  HB (c)(s)-AG B18.1
  hepatitis (viral) B18.9
    Australia-antigen (HAA) B18.8
    B surface antigen (HBsAg) B18.1
      with acute delta- (super)infection B17.0
    C B18.2
    specified NEC B18.8
  human T-cell lymphotropic virus type-1 (HTLV-1) infection Z22.6
  infectious organism Z22.9
    specified NEC Z22.8
  K. pneumoniae (Klebsiella pneumoniae) Z22.35- ☑
  meningococci Z22.31
  Salmonella typhosa Z22.0
  serum hepatitis — *see* Carrier, hepatitis
  staphylococci (Methicillin susceptible) Z22.321
    Methicillin resistant Z22.322
  streptococci Z22.338
    group B Z22.330
      complicating pregnancy or delivery O99.82- ☑
  syphilis Z22.4
  typhoid Z22.0
  venereal disease NEC Z22.4
Carrion's disease A44.0
Carter's relapsing fever (Asiatic) A68.1
Cartilage — *see* condition
Caruncle (inflamed)
  conjunctiva (acute) — *see* Conjunctivitis, acute
  labium (majus) (minus) N90.89
  lacrimal — *see* Inflammation, lacrimal, passages
  myrtiform N89.8
  urethral (benign) N36.2
Cascade stomach K31.2
Caseation lymphatic gland (tuberculous) A18.2
Cassidy (-Scholte) **syndrome** (malignant carcinoid) E34.09
Castellani's disease A69.8
Castration, traumatic, male S38.231- ☑
Casts in urine R82.998
Cat
  cry syndrome Q93.4
  ear Q17.3
  eye syndrome Q92.8
Cat-scratch — *see also* Abrasion
  disease or fever A28.1
Catabolism, senile R54
Catalepsy (hysterical) F44.2
  schizophrenic F20.2
Cataplexy (idiopathic) — *see* Narcolepsy
Cataract (cortical) (immature) (incipient) H26.9
  with
    neovascularization — *see* Cataract, complicated
  age-related — *see* Cataract, senile
  anterior
    and posterior axial embryonal Q12.0
    pyramidal Q12.0
  associated with
    galactosemia E74.21 *[H28]*
    myotonic disorders G71.19 *[H28]*
  blue Q12.0
  central Q12.0
  cerulean Q12.0
  complicated H26.20
    with
      neovascularization H26.21- ☑
      ocular disorder H26.22- ☑
      glaucomatous flecks H26.23- ☑
  congenital Q12.0
  coraliform Q12.0
  coronary Q12.0
  crystalline Q12.0
  diabetic — *see* Diabetes, cataract
  drug-induced H26.3- ☑
  due to
    ocular disorder — *see* Cataract, complicated
    radiation H26.8
  electric H26.8
  extraction status Z98.4- ☑
  glass-blower's H26.8
  heat ray H26.8
  heterochromic — *see* Cataract, complicated
  hypermature — *see* Cataract, senile, morgagnian type

Cataract — *continued*
  in (due to)
    chronic iridocyclitis — *see* Cataract, complicated
    diabetes — *see* Diabetes, cataract
    endocrine disease E34.9 *[H28]*
    eye disease — *see* Cataract, complicated
    hypoparathyroidism E20.9 *[H28]*
    malnutrition-dehydration E46 *[H28]*
    metabolic disease E88.9 *[H28]*
    myotonic disorders G71.19 *[H28]*
    nutritional disease E63.9 *[H28]*
  infantile — *see* Cataract, presenile
  irradiational — *see* Cataract, specified NEC
  juvenile — *see* Cataract, presenile
  malnutrition-dehydration E46 *[H28]*
  morgagnian — *see* Cataract, senile, morgagnian type
  myotonic G71.19 *[H28]*
  myxedema E03.9 *[H28]*
  nuclear
    embryonal Q12.0
    sclerosis — *see* Cataract, senile, nuclear
  presenile H26.00-
    combined forms H26.06- ☑
    cortical H26.01- ☑
    lamellar — *see* Cataract, presenile, cortical
    nuclear H26.03- ☑
    specified NEC H26.09
    subcapsular polar (anterior) H26.04- ☑
      posterior H26.05- ☑
    zonular — *see* Cataract, presenile, cortical
  secondary H26.40
    Soemmering's ring H26.41- ☑
    specified NEC H26.49- ☑
    to eye disease — *see* Cataract, complicated
  senile H25.9
    brunescens — *see* Cataract, senile, nuclear
    combined forms H25.81- ☑
    coronary — *see* Cataract, senile, incipient
    cortical H25.01- ☑
    hypermature — *see* Cataract, senile, morgagnian type
    incipient (mature) (total) H25.09- ☑
      cortical — *see* Cataract, senile, cortical
      subcapsular — *see* Cataract, senile, subcapsular
    morgagnian type (hypermature) H25.2- ☑
    nuclear (sclerosis) H25.1- ☑
    polar subcapsular (anterior) (posterior) — *see* Cataract, senile, incipient
    punctate — *see* Cataract, senile, incipient
    specified NEC H25.89
    subcapsular polar (anterior) H25.03- ☑
      posterior H25.04- ☑
  snowflake — *see* Diabetes, cataract
  specified NEC H26.8
  toxic — *see* Cataract, drug-induced
  traumatic H26.10- ☑
    localized H26.11- ☑
    partially resolved H26.12- ☑
    total H26.13- ☑
  zonular (perinuclear) Q12.0
Cataracta — *see also* Cataract
  brunescens — *see* Cataract, senile, nuclear
  centralis pulverulenta Q12.0
  cerulea Q12.0
  complicata — *see* Cataract, complicated
  congenita Q12.0
  coralliformis Q12.0
  coronaria Q12.0
  diabetic — *see* Diabetes, cataract
  membranacea
    accreta — *see* Cataract, secondary
    congenita Q12.0
  nigra — *see* Cataract, senile, nuclear
  sunflower — *see* Cataract, complicated
Catarrh, catarrhal (acute) (febrile) (infectious) (inflammation) — *see also* condition J00
  bronchial — *see* Bronchitis
  chest — *see* Bronchitis
  chronic J31.0
  due to congenital syphilis A50.03
  enteric — *see* Enteritis
  eustachian H68.009
  fauces — *see* Pharyngitis
  gastrointestinal — *see* Enteritis
  gingivitis K05.00
    nonplaque induced K05.01
    plaque induced K05.00
  hay — *see* Fever, hay
  intestinal — *see* Enteritis

Catarrh, catarrhal — *continued*
  larynx, chronic J37.0
  liver B15.9
    with hepatic coma B15.0
  lung — *see* Bronchitis
  middle ear, chronic — *see* Otitis, media, nonsuppurative, chronic, serous
  mouth K12.1
  nasal (chronic) — *see* Rhinitis
  nasobronchial J31.1
  nasopharyngeal (chronic) J31.1
    acute J00
  pulmonary — *see* Bronchitis
  spring (eye) (vernal) — *see* Conjunctivitis, acute, atopic
  summer (hay) — *see* Fever, hay
  throat J31.2
  tubotympanal — *see also* Otitis, media, nonsuppurative
    chronic — *see* Otitis, media, nonsuppurative, chronic, serous
Catatonia (schizophrenic) F20.2
Catatonic
  disorder due to known physiologic condition F06.1
  schizophrenia F20.2
  stupor R40.1
Cauda equina — *see* condition
Cauliflower ear M95.1- ☑
Causalgia (upper limb) G56.4- ☑
  lower limb G57.7- ☑
Cause
  external, general effects T75.89- ☑
Caustic burn — *see* Corrosion, by site
Cavare's disease (familial periodic paralysis) G72.3
Cave-in, injury
  crushing (severe) — *see* Crush
  suffocation — *see* Asphyxia, traumatic, due to low oxygen, due to cave-in
Cavernitis (penis) N48.29
Cavernositis N48.29
Cavernous — *see* condition
Cavitation of lung — *see also* Tuberculosis, pulmonary
  nontuberculous J98.4
Cavities, dental — *see* Caries, dental
Cavity
  lung — *see* Cavitation of lung
  optic papilla Q14.2
  pulmonary — *see* Cavitation of lung
Cavovarus foot, congenital Q66.1- ☑
Cavus foot (congenital) Q66.7- ☑
  acquired — *see* Deformity, limb, foot, specified NEC
Cazenave's disease L10.2
CCCA (central centrifugal cicatricial alopecia) L66.81
CDKL5 (Cyclin-Dependent Kinase-Like 5 Deficiency Disorder) G40.42
Cecitis K52.9
  with perforation, peritonitis, or rupture K65.8
Cecoureterocele Q62.32
Cecum — *see* condition
Celiac
  artery compression syndrome I77.4
  disease (with steatorrhea) K90.0
  infantilism K90.0
Cell(s), **cellular** — *see also* condition
  in urine R82.998
Cellulitis (diffuse) (phlegmonous) (septic) (suppurative) L03.90
  abdominal wall L03.311
  anaerobic A48.0
  ankle — *see* Cellulitis, lower limb
  anus K61.0
  arm — *see* Cellulitis, upper limb
  auricle (ear) — *see* Cellulitis, ear
  axilla L03.11- ☑
  back (any part) L03.312
  breast (acute) (nonpuerperal) (subacute) N61.0
    nipple N61.0
  broad ligament
    acute N73.0
  buttock L03.317
  cervical (meaning neck) L03.221
  cervix (uteri) — *see* Cervicitis
  cheek (external) L03.211
    internal K12.2
  chest wall L03.313
  chronic L03.90
  clostridial A48.0
  corpus cavernosum N48.22
  digit
    finger — *see* Cellulitis, finger

Cellulitis

Cellulitis — *continued*
- digit — *continued*
  - toe — *see* Cellulitis, toe
- Douglas' cul-de-sac or pouch
  - acute N73.0
- drainage site (following operation) T81.49- ☑
- ear (external) H60.1- ☑
- eosinophilic (granulomatous) L98.3
- erysipelatous — *see* Erysipelas
- external auditory canal — *see* Cellulitis, ear
- eyelid — *see* Abscess, eyelid
- face NEC L03.211
- finger (intrathecal) (periosteal) (subcutaneous) (subcuticular) L03.01- ☑
- flank L03.31A
- foot — *see* Cellulitis, lower limb
- gangrenous — *see* Gangrene
- genital organ NEC
  - female (external) N76.4
  - male N49.9
    - multiple sites N49.8
    - specified NEC N49.8
- gluteal (region) L03.317
- gonococcal A54.89
- groin L03.314
- hand — *see* Cellulitis, upper limb
- head NEC L03.811
  - face (any part, except ear, eye and nose) L03.211
- heel — *see* Cellulitis, lower limb
- hip — *see* Cellulitis, lower limb
- jaw (region) L03.211
- knee — *see* Cellulitis, lower limb
- labium (majus) (minus) — *see* Vulvitis
- lacrimal passages — *see* Inflammation, lacrimal, passages
- larynx J38.7
- leg — *see* Cellulitis, lower limb
- lip K13.0
- lower limb L03.11- ☑
  - toe — *see* Cellulitis, toe
- mouth (floor) K12.2
- multiple sites, so stated L03.90
- nasopharynx J39.1
- navel L03.316
  - newborn P38.9
    - with mild hemorrhage P38.1
    - without hemorrhage P38.9
- neck (region) L03.221
- nipple (acute) (nonpuerperal) (subacute) N61.0
- nose (septum) (external) J34.0
- orbit, orbital H05.01- ☑
- palate (soft) K12.2
- pectoral (region) L03.313
- pelvis, pelvic (chronic)
  - female — *see also* Disease, pelvis, inflammatory N73.2
    - acute N73.0
  - following ectopic or molar pregnancy O08.0
  - male K65.0
- penis N48.22
- perineal, perineum L03.315
- periorbital L03.213
- perirectal K61.1
- peritonsillar J36
- periurethral N34.0
- periuterine — *see also* Disease, pelvis, inflammatory N73.2
  - acute N73.0
- pharynx J39.1
- preseptal L03.213
- rectum K61.1
- retroperitoneal K68.9
- round ligament
  - acute N73.0
- scalp (any part) L03.811
- scrotum N49.2
- seminal vesicle N49.0
- shoulder — *see* Cellulitis, upper limb
- specified site NEC L03.818
- submandibular (region) (space) (triangle) K12.2
  - gland K11.3
- submaxillary (region) K12.2
  - gland K11.3
- thigh — *see* Cellulitis, lower limb
- thumb (intrathecal) (periosteal) (subcutaneous) (subcuticular) — *see* Cellulitis, finger
- toe (intrathecal) (periosteal) (subcutaneous) (subcuticular) L03.03- ☑
- tonsil J36
- trunk L03.319

Cellulitis — *continued*
- trunk — *continued*
  - abdominal wall L03.311
  - back (any part) L03.312
  - buttock L03.317
  - chest wall L03.313
  - groin L03.314
  - perineal, perineum L03.315
  - umbilicus L03.316
- tuberculous (primary) A18.4
- umbilicus L03.316
- upper limb L03.11- ☑
  - axilla — *see* Cellulitis, axilla
  - finger — *see* Cellulitis, finger
  - thumb — *see* Cellulitis, finger
- vaccinal T88.0- ☑
- vocal cord J38.3
- vulva — *see* Vulvitis
- wrist — *see* Cellulitis, upper limb

Cementoblastoma, benign — *see* Cyst, calcifying odontogenic
Cementoma — *see* Cyst, calcifying odontogenic
Cementoperiostitis — *see* Periodontitis
Cementosis K03.4
Central auditory processing disorder H93.25
Central pain syndrome G89.0
Cephalematocele, cephal(o)hematocele
- newborn P52.8
  - birth injury P10.8
- traumatic — *see* Hematoma, brain

Cephalematoma, cephalhematoma (calcified)
- newborn (birth injury) P12.0
- traumatic — *see* Hematoma, brain

Cephalgia, cephalalgia — *see also* Headache
- histamine G44.009
  - intractable G44.001
  - not intractable G44.009
- trigeminal autonomic (TAC) NEC G44.099
  - intractable G44.091
  - not intractable G44.099

Cephalic — *see* condition
Cephalitis — *see* Encephalitis
Cephalocele — *see* Encephalocele
Cephalomenia N94.89
Cephalopelvic — *see* condition
Cerclage (with cervical incompetence) in pregnancy — *see* Incompetence, cervix, in pregnancy
Cerebellitis — *see* Encephalitis
Cerebellum, cerebellar — *see* condition
Cerebral — *see* condition
Cerebritis — *see* Encephalitis
Cerebro-hepato-renal syndrome Q87.89
Cerebromalacia — *see* Softening, brain
- sequelae of cerebrovascular disease I69.398

Cerebroside lipidosis E75.22
Cerebrospasticity (congenital) G80.1
Cerebrospinal — *see* condition
Cerebrum — *see* condition
Ceroid-lipofuscinosis, neuronal E75.4
Cerumen (accumulation) (impacted) H61.2- ☑
Cervical — *see also* condition
- auricle Q18.2
- dysplasia in pregnancy — *see* Abnormal, cervix, in pregnancy or childbirth
- erosion in pregnancy — *see* Abnormal, cervix, in pregnancy or childbirth
- fibrosis in pregnancy — *see* Abnormal, cervix, in pregnancy or childbirth
- fusion syndrome Q76.1
- rib Q76.5
- shortening (complicating pregnancy) O26.87- ☑

Cervicalgia M54.2
Cervicitis (acute) (atrophic) (chronic) (nonvenereal) (senile) (subacute) (with ulceration) N72
- with
  - abortion — *see* Abortion, by type complicated by genital tract and pelvic infection
  - ectopic pregnancy O08.0
  - molar pregnancy O08.0
- chlamydial A56.09
- gonococcal A54.03
- herpesviral A60.03
- puerperal (postpartum) O86.11
- syphilitic A52.76
- trichomonal A59.09
- tuberculous A18.16

Cervicocolpitis (emphysematosa) — *see also* Cervicitis N72
Cervix — *see* condition

Cesarean delivery, previous, affecting management of pregnancy O34.219
- classical (vertical) scar O34.212
- isthmocele (non-pregnant state) N85.A
  - maternal care for O34.22
- low transverse scar O34.211
- mid-transverse T incision O34.218
- scar
  - defect (non-pregnant state) N85.A
    - maternal care for O34.22
  - specified type NEC O34.218

Cestan (-Chenais) **paralysis or syndrome** G46.3
Cestan-Raymond syndrome I65.8
Cestode infestation B71.9
- specified type NEC B71.8

Cestodiasis B71.9
CGL (congenital generalized lipodystrophy) E88.12
Chabert's disease A22.9
Chacaleh E53.8
Chafing L30.4
Chagas' (-Mazza) **disease** (chronic) B57.2
- with
  - cardiovascular involvement NEC B57.2
  - digestive system involvement B57.30
    - megacolon B57.32
    - megaesophagus B57.31
    - other specified B57.39
  - megacolon B57.32
  - megaesophagus B57.31
  - myocarditis B57.2
  - nervous system involvement B57.40
    - meningitis B57.41
    - meningoencephalitis B57.42
    - other specified B57.49
  - specified organ involvement NEC B57.5
- acute (with) B57.1
  - cardiovascular NEC B57.0
  - myocarditis B57.0

Chagres fever B50.9
Chairridden Z74.09
Chalasia (cardiac sphincter) K21.9
Chalazion H00.19
- left H00.16
  - lower H00.15
  - upper H00.14
- right H00.13
  - lower H00.12
  - upper H00.11

Chalcosis — *see also* Disorder, globe, degenerative, chalcosis
- cornea — *see* Deposit, cornea
- crystalline lens — *see* Cataract, complicated
- retina H35.89

Chalicosis (pulmonum) J62.8
Chancre (any genital site) (hard) (hunterian) (mixed) (primary) (seronegative) (seropositive) (syphilitic) A51.0
- congenital A50.07
- conjunctiva NEC A51.2
- ducreyi A57
- Ducrey's A57
- extragenital A51.2
- eyelid A51.2
- lip A51.2
- nipple A51.2
- Nisbet's A57
- of
  - carate A67.0
  - pinta A67.0
  - yaws A66.0
- palate, soft A51.2
- phagedenic A57
- simple A57
- soft A57
  - bubo A57
  - palate A51.2
- urethra A51.0
- yaws A66.0

Chancroid (anus) (genital) (penis) (perineum) (rectum) (urethra) (vulva) A57
Chandler's disease (osteochondritis dissecans, hip) — *see* Osteochondritis, dissecans, hip
Change(s) (in) (of) — *see also* Removal
- arteriosclerotic — *see* Arteriosclerosis
- bone — *see also* Disorder, bone
  - diabetic — *see* Diabetes, bone change
- bowel habit R19.4
- cardiorenal (vascular) — *see* Hypertension, cardiorenal
- cardiovascular — *see* Disease, cardiovascular
- circulatory I99.9

Change(s) (of) — *continued*
 cognitive (mild) (organic) R41.89
 color, tooth, teeth
  during formation K00.8
  posteruptive K03.7
 contraceptive device Z30.433
 corneal membrane H18.30
  Bowman's membrane fold or rupture H18.31- ☑
  Descemet's membrane
   fold H18.32- ☑
   rupture H18.33- ☑
 coronary — *see* Disease, heart, ischemic
 degenerative, spine or vertebra — *see* Spondylosis
 dental pulp, regressive K04.2
 dressing (nonsurgical) Z48.00
  surgical Z48.01
 heart — *see* Disease, heart
 hip joint — *see* Derangement, joint, hip
 hyperplastic larynx J38.7
 hypertrophic
  nasal sinus J34.89
  turbinate, nasal J34.3
  upper respiratory tract J39.8
 indwelling catheter Z46.6
 inflammatory — *see also* Inflammation
  sacroiliac M46.1
 job, anxiety concerning Z56.1
 joint — *see* Derangement, joint
 life — *see* Menopause
 mental status R41.82
 minimal (glomerular) — *see also* N00-N07 with fourth character .0 N05.0
 myocardium, myocardial — *see* Degeneration, myocardial
 of life — *see* Menopause
 pacemaker Z45.018
  pulse generator Z45.010
 personality (enduring) F68.8
  due to (secondary to)
   general medical condition F07.0
  secondary (nonspecific) F60.89
 regressive, dental pulp K04.2
 renal — *see* Disease, renal
 retina H35.9
  myopic — *see also* Myopia, degenerative H44.2- ☑
 sacroiliac joint M53.3
 senile — *see also* condition R54
 sensory R20.8
 skin R23.9
  acute, due to ultraviolet radiation L56.9
   specified NEC L56.8
  chronic, due to nonionizing radiation L57.9
   specified NEC L57.8
  cyanosis R23.0
  flushing R23.2
  pallor R23.1
  petechiae R23.3
  specified change NEC R23.8
  swelling — *see* Mass, localized
  texture R23.4
 trophic
  arm — *see* Mononeuropathy, upper limb
  leg — *see* Mononeuropathy, lower limb
 vascular I99.9
 vasomotor I73.9
 voice R49.9
  psychogenic F44.4
  specified NEC R49.8
Changing sleep-work schedule, affecting sleep G47.26
Changuinola fever A93.1
Chapping skin T69.8- ☑
Charcot-Marie-Tooth disease, paralysis or syndrome G60.0
Charcot's
 arthropathy — *see* Arthropathy, neuropathic
 cirrhosis K74.3
 disease (tabetic arthropathy) A52.16
 joint (disease) (tabetic) A52.16
  diabetic — *see* Diabetes, with, arthropathy
  syringomyelic G95.0
 syndrome (intermittent claudication) I73.9
CHARGE association Q89.89
Charley-horse (quadriceps) M62.831
 traumatic (quadriceps) S76.11- ☑
Charlouis' disease — *see* Yaws
Cheadle's disease E54
Check-up — *see* Examination

Checking (of)
 cardiac pacemaker (battery) (electrode(s)) Z45.018
  pulse generator Z45.010
 implantable subdermal contraceptive Z30.46
 intrauterine contraceptive device Z30.431
 wound Z48.0-
  due to injury — code to Injury, by site, using appropriate seventh character for subsequent encounter
  postoperative — *see* Aftercare
Chediak-Higashi (-Steinbrinck) **syndrome** (congenital gigantism of peroxidase granules) E70.330
Cheek — *see* condition
Cheese itch B88.09
Cheese-washer's lung J67.8
Cheese-worker's lung J67.8
Cheilitis (acute) (angular) (catarrhal) (chronic) (exfoliative) (gangrenous) (glandular) (infectional) (suppurative) (ulcerative) (vesicular) K13.0
 actinic (due to sun) L56.8
  other than from sun L59.8
 candidal B37.83
Cheilodynia K13.0
Cheiloschisis — *see* Cleft, lip
Cheilosis (angular) K13.0
 with pellagra E52
 due to
  vitamin B2 (riboflavin) deficiency E53.0
Cheiromegaly M79.89
Cheiropompholyx L30.1
Cheloid — *see* Keloid
Chemical burn — *see* Corrosion, by site
Chemodectoma — *see* Paraganglioma, nonchromaffin
Chemosis, conjunctiva — *see* Edema, conjunctiva
Chemotherapy (session) (for)
 cancer Z51.11
 neoplasm Z51.11
Cherubism M27.8
Chest — *see* condition
Cheyne-Stokes breathing (respiration) R06.3
Chiari's
 disease or syndrome (hepatic vein thrombosis) I82.0
 malformation
  type I G93.5
  type II — *see* Spina bifida
 net Q24.8
Chicago disease B40.9
Chickenpox — *see* Varicella
Chiclero ulcer or sore B55.1
Chigger (infestation) B88.09
Chignon (disease) B36.8
 newborn (from vacuum extraction) (birth injury) P12.1
Chilaiditi's syndrome (subphrenic displacement, colon) Q43.3
Chilblain(s) (lupus) T69.1- ☑
Child — *see also* Problem, child
 custody dispute Z65.3
Childbirth — *see* Delivery
Childhood
 cerebral X-linked adrenoleukodystrophy E71.520
 period of rapid growth Z00.2
Chill(s) R68.83
 with fever R50.9
 congestive in malarial regions B54
 without fever R68.83
Chilomastigiasis A07.8
Chimera 46,XX/46,XY Q99.0
Chin — *see* condition
Chinese dysentery A03.9
Chionophobia F40.228
Chitral fever A93.1
Chlamydia, chlamydial A74.9
 cervicitis A56.09
 conjunctivitis A74.0
 cystitis A56.01
 endometritis A56.11
 epididymitis A56.19
 female
  pelvic inflammatory disease A56.11
  pelviperitonitis A56.11
 orchitis A56.19
 peritonitis A74.81
 pharyngitis A56.4
 proctitis A56.3
 psittaci (infection) A70
 salpingitis A56.11
 sexually-transmitted infection NEC A56.8
 specified NEC A74.89
 urethritis A56.01

Chlamydia, chlamydial — *continued*
 vulvovaginitis A56.02
Chlamydiosis — *see* Chlamydia
Chloasma (skin) (idiopathic) (symptomatic) L81.1
 eyelid H02.71- ☑
  hyperthyroid E05.90 [H02.71-] ☑
   with thyroid storm E05.91 [H02.71-] ☑
  left H02.716
   lower H02.715
   upper H02.714
  right H02.713
   lower H02.712
   upper H02.711
Chloroma C92.3- ☑
Chlorosis D50.9
 Egyptian B76.9 [D63.8]
 miner's B76.9 [D63.8]
Chlorotic anemia D50.8
Chocolate cyst (ovary) N80.10- ☑
Choked
 disc or disk — *see* Papilledema
 on food, phlegm, or vomitus NOS — *see* Foreign body, by site
 while vomiting NOS — *see* Foreign body, by site
Chokes (resulting from bends) T70.3- ☑
Choking sensation R09.89
Cholangiectasis K83.8
Cholangiocarcinoma
 with hepatocellular carcinoma, combined C22.0
 liver C22.1
 specified site NEC — *see* Neoplasm, malignant, by site
 unspecified site C22.1
Cholangiohepatitis K83.8
 due to fluke infestation B66.1
Cholangiohepatoma C22.0
Cholangiolitis (acute) (chronic) (extrahepatic) (gangrenous) (intrahepatic) K83.09
 paratyphoidal — *see* Fever, paratyphoid
 typhoidal A01.09
Cholangioma D13.4
 malignant — *see* Cholangiocarcinoma
Cholangitis (ascending) (recurrent) (secondary) (stenosing) (suppurative) K83.09
 with calculus, bile duct — *see* Calculus, bile duct, with cholangitis
 chronic nonsuppurative destructive K74.3
 primary K83.09
  sclerosing K83.01
 sclerosing K83.09
Cholecystectasia K82.8
Cholecystitis K81.9
 with
  calculus, stones in
   bile duct (common) (hepatic) — *see* Calculus, bile duct, with cholecystitis
   cystic duct — *see* Calculus, gallbladder, with cholecystitis
   gallbladder — *see* Calculus, gallbladder, with cholecystitis
  choledocholithiasis — *see* Calculus, bile duct, with cholecystitis
  cholelithiasis — *see* Calculus, gallbladder, with cholecystitis
  gangrene of gallbladder K82.A1
  perforation of gallbladder K82.A2
 acute (emphysematous) (gangrenous) (suppurative) K81.0
  with
   calculus, stones in
    cystic duct — *see* Calculus, gallbladder, with cholecystitis, acute
    gallbladder — *see* Calculus, gallbladder, with cholecystitis, acute
   choledocholithiasis — *see* Calculus, bile duct, with cholecystitis, acute
   cholelithiasis — *see* Calculus, gallbladder, with cholecystitis, acute
   chronic cholecystitis K81.2
    with gallbladder calculus K80.12
     with obstruction K80.13
 chronic K81.1
  with acute cholecystitis K81.2
   with gallbladder calculus K80.12
    with obstruction K80.13
 emphysematous (acute) — *see* Cholecystitis, acute
 gangrenous — *see* Cholecystitis, acute
 paratyphoidal, current A01.4
 suppurative — *see* Cholecystitis, acute

Cholecystitis — continued
- typhoidal A01.09

Cholecystolithiasis — see Calculus, gallbladder
Choledochitis (suppurative) K83.09
Choledocholith — see Calculus, bile duct
Choledocholithiasis (common duct) (hepatic duct) — see Calculus, bile duct
- cystic — see Calculus, gallbladder
- typhoidal A01.09

Cholelithiasis (cystic duct) (gallbladder) (impacted) (multiple) — see Calculus, gallbladder
- bile duct (common) (hepatic) — see Calculus, bile duct
- hepatic duct — see Calculus, bile duct
- specified NEC K80.80
  - with obstruction K80.81

Cholemia — see also Jaundice
- familial (simple) (congenital) E80.4
- Gilbert's E80.4

Choleperitoneum, choleperitonitis K65.3
Cholera (Asiatic) (epidemic) (malignant) A00.9
- antimonial — see Poisoning, antimony
- classical A00.0
- due to Vibrio cholerae 01 A00.9
  - biovar cholerae A00.0
  - biovar eltor A00.1
  - el tor A00.1
- el tor A00.1

Cholerine — see Cholera
Cholestasis NEC K83.1
- with hepatocyte injury K71.0
- due to total parenteral nutrition (TPN) K76.89
- intrahepatic K76.89
- pure K71.0

Cholesteatoma (ear) (middle) (with reaction) H71.9- ☑
- attic H71.0- ☑
- external ear (canal) H60.4- ☑
- mastoid H71.2- ☑
- postmastoidectomy cavity (recurrent) — see Complications, postmastoidectomy, recurrent cholesteatoma
- recurrent (postmastoidectomy) — see Complications, postmastoidectomy, recurrent cholesteatoma
- tympanum H71.1- ☑

Cholesteatosis, diffuse H71.3- ☑
Cholesteremia E78.00
Cholesterin in vitreous — see Deposit, crystalline
Cholesterol
- deposit
  - retina H35.89
  - vitreous — see Deposit, crystalline
- elevated (high) E78.00
  - with elevated (high) triglycerides E78.2
  - screening for Z13.220
- imbibition of gallbladder K82.4

Cholesterolemia (essential) (pure) E78.00
- familial E78.019
  - heterozygous E78.011
  - homozygous E78.010
- hereditary E78.019

Cholesterolosis, cholesterosis (gallbladder) K82.4
- cerebrotendinous E75.5

Cholocolic fistula K82.3
Choluria R82.2
Chondritis M94.8X9
- auricle H61.03- ☑
- costal (Tietze's) M94.0
- external ear H61.03- ☑
- patella, posttraumatic — see Chondromalacia, patella
- pinna H61.03- ☑
- purulent M94.8X- ☑
- tuberculous NEC A18.02
  - intervertebral A18.01

Chondro-osteodysplasia (Morquio-Brailsford type) E76.219
Chondro-osteodystrophy E76.29
Chondro-osteoma — see Neoplasm, bone, benign
Chondroblastoma — see also Neoplasm, bone, benign
- malignant — see Neoplasm, bone, malignant

Chondrocalcinosis M11.20
- ankle M11.27- ☑
- elbow M11.22- ☑
- familial M11.10
  - ankle M11.17- ☑
  - elbow M11.12- ☑
  - foot joint M11.17- ☑
  - hand joint M11.14- ☑
  - hip M11.15- ☑
  - knee M11.16- ☑
  - multiple site M11.19

Chondrocalcinosis — continued
- familial — continued
  - shoulder M11.11- ☑
  - vertebrae M11.18
  - wrist M11.13- ☑
- foot joint M11.27- ☑
- hand joint M11.24- ☑
- hip M11.25- ☑
- knee M11.26- ☑
- multiple site M11.29
- shoulder M11.21- ☑
- specified type NEC M11.20
  - ankle M11.27- ☑
  - elbow M11.22- ☑
  - foot joint M11.27- ☑
  - hand joint M11.24- ☑
  - hip M11.25- ☑
  - knee M11.26- ☑
  - multiple site M11.29
  - shoulder M11.21- ☑
  - vertebrae M11.28
  - wrist M11.23- ☑
- vertebrae M11.28
- wrist M11.23- ☑

Chondrodermatitis nodularis helicis or anthelicis — see Perichondritis, ear
Chondrodysplasia Q78.9
- with hemangioma Q78.4
- calcificans congenita Q77.3
- fetalis Q77.4
- metaphyseal (Jansen's) (McKusick's) (Schmid's) Q78.8
- punctata Q77.3

Chondrodystrophy, chondrodystrophia (familial) (fetalis) (hypoplastic) Q78.9
- calcificans congenita Q77.3
- myotonic (congenital) G71.13
- punctata Q77.3

Chondroectodermal dysplasia Q77.6
Chondrogenesis imperfecta Q77.4
Chondrolysis M94.35-
Chondroma — see also Neoplasm, cartilage, benign
- juxtacortical — see Neoplasm, bone, benign
- periosteal — see Neoplasm, bone, benign

Chondromalacia (systemic) M94.20
- acromioclavicular joint M94.21- ☑
- ankle M94.27- ☑
- elbow M94.22- ☑
- foot joint M94.27- ☑
- glenohumeral joint M94.21- ☑
- hand joint M94.24- ☑
- hip M94.25- ☑
- knee M94.26- ☑
  - patella M22.4- ☑
- multiple sites M94.29
- patella M22.4- ☑
- rib M94.28
- sacroiliac joint M94.259
- shoulder M94.21- ☑
- sternoclavicular joint M94.21- ☑
- vertebral joint M94.28
- wrist M94.23- ☑

Chondromatosis — see also Neoplasm, cartilage, uncertain behavior
- internal Q78.4

Chondromyxosarcoma — see Neoplasm, cartilage, malignant
Chondropathia tuberosa M94.0
Chondrosarcoma — see also Neoplasm, cartilage, malignant
- juxtacortical — see Neoplasm, bone, malignant
- mesenchymal — see Neoplasm, connective tissue, malignant
- myxoid — see Neoplasm, cartilage, malignant

Chordee (nonvenereal) N48.89
- congenital Q54.4
- gonococcal A54.09

Chorditis (fibrinous) (nodosa) (tuberosa) J38.2
Chordoma — see Neoplasm, vertebral (column), malignant
Chorea (chronic) (gravis) (posthemiplegic) (senile) (spasmodic) G25.5
- with
  - heart involvement I02.0
    - active or acute (conditions in I01-) I02.0
    - rheumatic I02.9
      - with valvular disorder I02.0

Chorea — continued
- with — continued
  - rheumatic heart disease (chronic) (inactive) (quiescent) — code to rheumatic heart condition involved
- drug-induced G25.4
- habit F95.8
- hereditary G10
- Huntington's G10
- hysterical F44.4
- minor I02.9
  - with heart involvement I02.0
- progressive G25.5
  - hereditary G10
- rheumatic (chronic) I02.9
  - with heart involvement I02.0
- Sydenham's I02.9
  - with heart involvement — see Chorea, with rheumatic heart disease
- nonrheumatic G25.5

Choreoathetosis (paroxysmal) G25.5
Chorioadenoma (destruens) D39.2
Chorioamnionitis O41.12- ☑
Chorioangioma D26.7
Choriocarcinoma — see Neoplasm, malignant, by site
- combined with
  - embryonal carcinoma — see Neoplasm, malignant, by site
  - other germ cell elements — see Neoplasm, malignant, by site
  - teratoma — see Neoplasm, malignant, by site
- specified site — see Neoplasm, malignant, by site
- unspecified site
  - female C58
  - male C62.90

Chorioencephalitis (acute) (lymphocytic) (serous) A87.2
Chorioepithelioma — see Choriocarcinoma
Choriomeningitis (acute) (lymphocytic) (serous) A87.2
Chorionepithelioma — see Choriocarcinoma
Chorioretinitis — see also Inflammation, chorioretinal
- disseminated — see also Inflammation, chorioretinal, disseminated
  - in neurosyphilis A52.19
- Egyptian B76.9 [D63.8]
- focal — see also Inflammation, chorioretinal, focal
- histoplasmic B39.9 [H32]
- in (due to)
  - histoplasmosis B39.9 [H32]
  - syphilis (secondary) A51.43
    - late A52.71
  - toxoplasmosis (acquired) B58.01
    - congenital (active) P37.1 [H32]
  - tuberculosis A18.53
- juxtapapillary, juxtapapillaris — see Inflammation, chorioretinal, focal, juxtapapillary
- leprous A30.9 [H32]
- miner's B76.9 [D63.8]
- progressive myopia (degeneration) — see also Myopia, degenerative H44.2- ☑
- syphilitic (secondary) A51.43
  - congenital (early) A50.01 [H32]
  - late A50.32
  - late A52.71
- tuberculous A18.53

Chorioretinopathy, central serous H35.71- ☑
Choroid — see condition
Choroideremia H31.21
Choroiditis — see Chorioretinitis
Choroidopathy — see Disorder, choroid
Choroidoretinitis — see Chorioretinitis
Choroidoretinopathy, central serous — see Chorioretinopathy, central serous

Christian-Weber disease M35.6
Christmas disease D67
Chromaffinoma — see also Neoplasm, benign, by site
- malignant — see Neoplasm, malignant, by site

Chromatopsia — see Deficiency, color vision
Chromhidrosis, chromidrosis L75.1
Chromoblastomycosis — see Chromomycosis
Chromoconversion R82.91
Chromomycosis B43.9
- brain abscess B43.1
- cerebral B43.1
- cutaneous B43.0
- skin B43.0
- specified NEC B43.8
- subcutaneous abscess or cyst B43.2

Chromophytosis B36.0
Chromosome — see Anomaly, by chromosome involved

Chromosome — continued
  D (1) — see Anomaly, chromosome 13
  E (3) — see Anomaly, chromosome 18
  G — see Anomaly, chromosome 21
Chromotrichomycosis B36.8
Chronic — see condition
  fracture — see Fracture, pathological
Churg-Strauss syndrome M30.1
Chyle cyst, mesentery I89.8
Chylocele (nonfilarial) I89.8
  filarial — see also Infestation, filarial B74.9 [N51]
  tunica vaginalis N50.89
    filarial — see also Infestation, filarial B74.9 [N51]
Chylomicronemia (fasting) (with hyperprebetalipoproteinemia) E78.3
Chylopericardium I31.39
  acute I30.9
Chylothorax (nonfilarial) J94.0
  filarial — see also Infestation, filarial B74.9 [J91.8]
Chylous — see condition
Chyluria (nonfilarial) R82.0
  due to
    bilharziasis B65.0
    Brugia (malayi) B74.1
      timori B74.2
    schistosomiasis (bilharziasis) B65.0
    Wuchereria (bancrofti) B74.0
  filarial — see Infestation, filarial
Cicatricial (deformity) — see Cicatrix
Cicatrix (adherent) (contracted) (painful) (vicious) — see also Scar L90.5
  adenoid (and tonsil) J35.8
  alveolar process M26.79
  anus K62.89
  auricle — see Disorder, pinna, specified type NEC
  bile duct (common) (hepatic) K83.8
  bladder N32.89
  bone — see Disorder, bone, specified type NEC
  brain G93.89
  cervix (postoperative) (postpartal) N88.1
  common duct K83.8
  cornea H17.9
    tuberculous A18.59
  duodenum (bulb), obstructive K31.5
  esophagus K22.2
  eyelid — see Disorder, eyelid function
  hypopharynx J39.2
  lacrimal passages — see Obstruction, lacrimal
  larynx J38.7
  lung J98.4
  middle ear H74.8- ☑
  mouth K13.79
  muscle M62.89
    with contracture — see Contraction, muscle NEC
  nasopharynx J39.2
  palate (soft) K13.79
  penis N48.89
  pharynx J39.2
  prostate N42.89
  rectum K62.89
  retina — see Scar, chorioretinal
  semilunar cartilage — see Derangement, meniscus
  seminal vesicle N50.89
  skin L90.5
    infected L08.89
    postinfective L90.5
    tuberculous B90.8
  specified site NEC L90.5
  throat J39.2
  tongue K14.8
  tonsil (and adenoid) J35.8
  trachea J39.8
  tuberculous NEC B90.9
  urethra N36.8
  uterus N85.8
  vagina N89.8
    postoperative N99.2
  vocal cord J38.3
  wrist, constricting (annular) L90.5
CIDP (chronic inflammatory demyelinating polyneuropathy) G61.81
CIN — see Neoplasia, intraepithelial, cervix
CINCA (chronic infantile neurological, cutaneous and articular syndrome) M04.2
Cinchonism — see Deafness, ototoxic
  correct substance properly administered — see Table of Drugs and Chemicals, by drug, adverse effect
  overdose or wrong substance given or taken — see Table of Drugs and Chemicals, by drug, poisoning

Circle of Willis — see condition
Circular — see condition
Circulating anticoagulants — see also Disorder, hemorrhagic D68.318
  due to drugs — see also Disorder, hemorrhagic D68.32
  following childbirth O72.3
Circulation
  collateral, any site I99.8
  defective (lower extremity) I99.9
    congenital Q28.9
  embryonic Q28.9
  failure (peripheral) R57.9
    newborn P29.89
  fetal, persistent P29.38
  Fontan related I27.849
    with
      Fontan-associated condition, specified NEC I27.848
      Fontan-associated liver disease [FALD] I27.840
      Fontan-associated lymphatic dysfunction I27.841
  heart, incomplete Q28.9
Circulatory system — see condition
Circulus senilis (cornea) — see Degeneration, cornea, senile
Circumcision (in absence of medical indication) (ritual) (routine) Z41.2
Circumscribed — see condition
Circumvallate placenta O43.11- ☑
Cirrhosis, cirrhotic (hepatic) (liver) K74.60
  alcoholic K70.30
    with ascites K70.31
  atrophic — see Cirrhosis, liver
  Baumgarten-Cruveilhier K74.69
  biliary (cholangiolitic) (cholangitic) (hypertrophic) (obstructive) (pericholangiolitic) K74.5
    due to
      Clonorchiasis B66.1
      flukes B66.3
    primary K74.3
    secondary K74.4
  cardiac (of liver) K76.1
  Charcot's K74.3
  cholangiolitic, cholangitic, cholestatic (primary) K74.3
  congestive K76.1
  Cruveilhier-Baumgarten K74.69
  cryptogenic (liver) K74.69
  due to
    hepatolenticular degeneration E83.01
    Wilson's disease E83.01
    xanthomatosis E78.2
  fatty K76.0
    alcoholic K70.0
  Hanot's (hypertrophic) K74.3
  hepatic — see Cirrhosis, liver
  hypertrophic K74.3
  Indian childhood K74.69
  kidney — see Sclerosis, renal
  Laennec's K70.30
    with ascites K70.31
    alcoholic K70.30
      with ascites K70.31
    nonalcoholic K74.69
  liver K74.60
    alcoholic K70.30
      with ascites K70.31
    fatty K70.0
    congenital P78.81
    syphilitic A52.74
  lung (chronic) J84.10
  macronodular K74.69
    alcoholic K70.30
      with ascites K70.31
  micronodular K74.69
    alcoholic K70.30
      with ascites K70.31
  mixed type K74.69
  monolobular K74.3
  nephritis — see Sclerosis, renal
  nutritional K74.69
    alcoholic K70.30
      with ascites K70.31
  obstructive — see Cirrhosis, biliary
  ovarian N83.8
  pancreas (duct) K86.89
  pigmentary E83.110
  portal K74.69
    alcoholic K70.30
      with ascites K70.31
  postnecrotic K74.69
    alcoholic K70.30
      with ascites K70.31

Cirrhosis, cirrhotic — continued
  pulmonary J84.10
  renal — see Sclerosis, renal
  spleen D73.2
  stasis K76.1
  Todd's K74.3
  unilobar K74.3
  xanthomatous (biliary) K74.5
    due to xanthomatosis (familial) (metabolic) (primary) E78.2
Cistern, subarachnoid R93.0
Citrullinemia E72.23
Citrullinuria E72.23
Civatte's disease or poikiloderma L57.3
CLAD — see Dysfunction, chronic, lung allograft
Clam digger's itch B65.3
Clammy skin R23.1
Clap — see Gonorrhea
Clarke-Hadfield syndrome (pancreatic infantilism) K86.89
Clark's paralysis G80.9
Clastothrix L67.8
Claude Bernard-Horner syndrome G90.2
  traumatic — see Injury, nerve, cervical sympathetic
Claude's disease or syndrome G46.3
Claudicatio venosa intermittens I87.8
Claudication (intermittent) I73.9
  cerebral (artery) G45.9
  spinal cord (arteriosclerotic) G95.19
    syphilitic A52.09
  venous (axillary) I87.8
Claustrophobia F40.240
Clavus (infected) L84
Clawfoot (congenital) Q66.89
  acquired — see Deformity, limb, clawfoot
Clawhand (acquired) — see also Deformity, limb, clawhand
  congenital Q68.1
Clawtoe (congenital) Q66.89
  acquired — see Deformity, toe, specified NEC
Clay eating — see Pica
Cleansing of artificial opening — see Attention to, artificial, opening
Cleft (congenital) — see also Imperfect, closure
  alveolar process M26.79
  branchial (persistent) Q18.2
    cyst Q18.0
      fistula Q18.0
      sinus Q18.0
  cricoid cartilage, posterior Q31.8
  cyst Q18.0
    fistula Q18.0
    sinus Q18.0
  foot Q72.7- ☑
  hand Q71.6- ☑
  lip (unilateral) Q36.9
    with cleft palate Q37.9
      hard Q37.1
        with soft Q37.5
      soft Q37.3
        with hard Q37.5
    bilateral Q36.0
      with cleft palate Q37.8
        hard Q37.0
          with soft Q37.4
        soft Q37.2
          with hard Q37.4
    median Q36.1
  mitral valve leaflet (at birth) (congenital) Q23.82
  nose Q30.2
  palate Q35.9
    with cleft lip (unilateral) Q37.9
      bilateral Q37.8
    hard Q35.1
      with
        cleft lip (unilateral) Q37.1
          bilateral Q37.0
        soft Q35.5
          with cleft lip (unilateral) Q37.5
            bilateral Q37.4
    medial Q35.5
    soft Q35.3
      with
        cleft lip (unilateral) Q37.3
          bilateral Q37.2
        hard Q35.5
          with cleft lip (unilateral) Q37.5
            bilateral Q37.4
  penis Q55.69
  scrotum Q55.29
  thyroid cartilage Q31.8

☑ Additional Character Required — Refer to the Tabular List for Character Selection

Cleft — *continued*
  uvula Q35.7
Cleidocranial dysostosis Q74.0
Cleptomania F63.2
Clicking hip (newborn) R29.4
Climacteric (female) — *see also* Menopause
  arthritis (any site) NEC — *see* Arthritis, specified form NEC
  depression (single episode) F32.89
    recurrent episode F33.8
  male (symptoms) (syndrome) NEC N50.89
  melancholia (single episode) F32.89
    recurrent episode F33.8
  paranoid state F22
  polyarthritis NEC — *see* Arthritis, specified form NEC
  symptoms (female) N95.1
Clinical research investigation (clinical trial) (control subject) (normal comparison) (participant) Z00.6
Clitoris — *see* condition
Cloaca (persistent) Q43.7
Clonorchiasis, clonorchis infection (liver) B66.1
Clonus R25.8
Closed bite M26.29
Clostridium (C.) **perfringens, as cause of disease classified elsewhere** B96.7
Closure
  congenital, nose Q30.0
  cranial sutures, premature Q75.009
  defective or imperfect NEC — *see* Imperfect, closure
  fistula, delayed — *see* Fistula
  foramen ovale, imperfect Q21.12
  hymen N89.6
  interauricular septum, defective Q21.19
  interventricular septum, defective Q21.0
  lacrimal duct — *see also* Stenosis, lacrimal, duct
    congenital Q10.5
  nose (congenital) Q30.0
    acquired M95.0
  of artificial opening — *see* Attention to, artificial, opening
  vagina N89.5
  valve — *see* Endocarditis
  vulva N90.5
Clot (blood) — *see also* Embolism
  artery (obstruction) (occlusion) — *see* Embolism
  bladder N32.89
  brain (intradural or extradural) — *see* Occlusion, artery, cerebral
  circulation I74.9
  heart — *see also* Infarct, myocardium
    not resulting in infarction I51.3
  vein — *see* Thrombosis
Clouded state R40.1
  epileptic — *see* Epilepsy, specified NEC
  paroxysmal — *see* Epilepsy, specified NEC
Cloudy antrum, antra J32.0
Clouston's (hidrotic) **ectodermal dysplasia** Q82.4
Cloverleaf skull Q75.051
Clubbed nail pachydermoperiostosis M89.40 *[L62]*
Clubbing of finger(s) (nails) R68.3
Clubfinger R68.3
  congenital Q68.1
Clubfoot (congenital) Q66.89
  acquired — *see* Deformity, limb, clubfoot
  equinovarus Q66.0- ☑
  paralytic — *see* Deformity, limb, clubfoot
Clubhand (congenital) (radial) Q71.4- ☑
  acquired — *see* Deformity, limb, clubhand
Clubnail R68.3
  congenital Q84.6
Clump, kidney Q63.1
Clumsiness, clumsy child syndrome F82
Cluttering F80.81
Clutton's joints A50.51 *[M12.80]*
Coagulation, intravascular (diffuse) (disseminated) — *see also* Defibrination syndrome
  complicating abortion — *see* Abortion, by type, complicated by, intravascular coagulation
  COVID-19 associated — *see also* COVID-19 D65
  following ectopic or molar pregnancy O08.1
Coagulopathy — *see also* Defect, coagulation
  consumption D65
  intravascular D65
    newborn P60
Coalition
  calcaneo-scaphoid Q66.89
  tarsal Q66.89
Coalminer's
  elbow — *see* Bursitis, elbow, olecranon
  lung or pneumoconiosis J60

Coalworker's lung or pneumoconiosis J60
Coarctation
  aorta (preductal) (postductal) Q25.1
  pulmonary artery Q25.71
Coated tongue K14.3
Coats' disease (exudative retinopathy) — *see* Retinopathy, exudative
Cocaine-induced
  anxiety disorder F14.980
  bipolar and related disorder F14.94
  depressive disorder F14.94
  obsessive-compulsive and related disorder F14.988
  psychotic disorder F14.959
  sexual dysfunction F14.981
  sleep disorder F14.982
Cocainism — *see* Disorder, cocaine use
Coccidioidomycosis B38.9
  cutaneous B38.3
  disseminated B38.7
  generalized B38.7
  meninges B38.4
  prostate B38.81
  pulmonary B38.2
    acute B38.0
    chronic B38.1
  skin B38.3
  specified NEC B38.89
Coccidioidosis — *see* Coccidioidomycosis
Coccidiosis (intestinal) A07.3
Coccydynia, coccygodynia M53.3
Coccyx — *see* condition
Cochin-China diarrhea K90.1
Cockayne's syndrome Q87.19
Cocked up toe — *see* Deformity, toe, specified NEC
Cock's peculiar tumor L72.3
Codman's tumor — *see* Neoplasm, bone, benign
Coenurosis B71.8
Coffee-worker's lung J67.8
Cogan's syndrome H16.32- ☑
  oculomotor apraxia H51.8
Coitus, painful (female) N94.10
  male N53.12
  psychogenic F52.6
Cold J00
  with influenza, flu, or grippe — *see* Influenza, with, respiratory manifestations NEC
  agglutinin disease or hemoglobinuria (chronic) D59.12
  bronchial — *see* Bronchitis
  chest — *see* Bronchitis
  common (head) J00
  effects of T69.9- ☑
    specified effect NEC T69.8- ☑
  excessive, effects of T69.9- ☑
    specified effect NEC T69.8- ☑
  exhaustion from T69.8- ☑
  exposure to T69.9- ☑
    specified effect NEC T69.8- ☑
  head J00
  injury syndrome (newborn) P80.0
  on lung — *see* Bronchitis
  rose J30.1
  sensitivity, auto-immune D59.12
  symptoms J00
  virus J00
Coldsore B00.1
Colibacillosis A49.8
  as the cause of other disease — *see also* Escherichia coli B96.20
  generalized — *see also* Sepsis, Escherichia coli A41.51
Colic (bilious) (infantile) (intestinal) (recurrent) (spasmodic) R10.83
  abdomen R10.83
    psychogenic F45.8
  appendix, appendicular K38.8
  bile duct — *see* Calculus, bile duct
  biliary — *see* Calculus, bile duct
  common duct — *see* Calculus, bile duct
  cystic duct — *see* Calculus, gallbladder
  Devonshire NEC — *see* Poisoning, lead
  gallbladder — *see* Calculus, gallbladder
  gallstone — *see* Calculus, gallbladder
    gallbladder or cystic duct — *see* Calculus, gallbladder
  hepatic (duct) — *see* Calculus, bile duct
  hysterical F45.8
  kidney N23
  lead NEC — *see* Poisoning, lead
  mucous K58.9
    with diarrhea K58.0

Colic — *continued*
  mucous — *continued*
    psychogenic F54
  nephritic N23
  painter's NEC — *see* Poisoning, lead
  pancreas K86.89
  psychogenic F45.8
  renal N23
  saturnine NEC — *see* Poisoning, lead
  ureter N23
  urethral N36.8
    due to calculus N21.1
  uterus NEC N94.89
    menstrual — *see* Dysmenorrhea
  worm NOS B83.9
Colicystitis — *see* Cystitis
Colitis (acute) (catarrhal) (chronic) (noninfective) (hemorrhagic) — *see also* Enteritis K52.9
  allergic K52.29
    with
      food protein-induced enterocolitis syndrome K52.21
      proctocolitis K52.29
  amebic (acute) — *see also* Amebiasis A06.0
    nondysenteric A06.2
  anthrax A22.2
  bacillary — *see* Infection, Shigella
  balantidial A07.0
  Clostridioides difficile
    not specified as recurrent A04.72
    recurrent A04.71
  Clostridium difficile
    not specified as recurrent A04.72
    recurrent A04.71
  coccidial A07.3
  collagenous K52.831
  cystica superficialis K52.89
  dietary counseling and surveillance (for) Z71.3
  dietetic — *see also* Colitis, allergic K52.29
  drug-induced K52.1
  due to radiation K52.0
  eosinophilic K52.82
  food hypersensitivity — *see also* Colitis, allergic K52.29
  giardial A07.1
  granulomatous — *see* Enteritis, regional, large intestine
  indeterminate, so stated K52.3
  infectious — *see* Enteritis, infectious
  ischemic K55.9
    acute (subacute) — *see also* Ischemia, intestine, acute K55.039
    chronic K55.1
    due to mesenteric artery insufficiency K55.1
    fulminant (acute) — *see also* Ischemia, intestine, acute K55.039
  left sided K51.50
    with
      abscess K51.514
      complication K51.519
        specified NEC K51.518
      fistula K51.513
      obstruction K51.512
      rectal bleeding K51.511
  lymphocytic K52.832
  membranous
    psychogenic F54
  microscopic K52.839
    specified NEC K52.838
  mucous — *see* Syndrome, irritable, bowel
    psychogenic F54
  noninfective K52.9
    specified NEC K52.89
  polyposa — *see* Polyp, colon, inflammatory
  protozoal A07.9
  pseudomembranous
    not specified as recurrent A04.72
    recurrent A04.71
  pseudomucinous — *see* Syndrome, irritable, bowel
  regional — *see* Enteritis, regional, large intestine
    infectious A09
  segmental — *see* Enteritis, regional, large intestine
  septic — *see* Enteritis, infectious
  spastic K58.9
    with diarrhea K58.0
    psychogenic F54
  staphylococcal A04.8
    foodborne A05.0
  subacute ischemic — *see also* Ischemia, intestine, acute K55.039

Colitis — continued
- thromboulcerative — see also Ischemia, intestine, acute K55.039
- toxic NEC K52.1
  - due to
    - Clostridioides difficile
      - not specified as recurrent A04.72
      - recurrent A04.71
    - Clostridium difficile
      - not specified as recurrent A04.72
      - recurrent A04.71
- transmural — see Enteritis, regional, large intestine
- trichomonal A07.8
- tuberculous (ulcerative) A18.32
- ulcerative (chronic) K51.90
  - with
    - complication K51.919
      - abscess K51.914
      - fistula K51.913
      - obstruction K51.912
      - rectal bleeding K51.911
      - specified complication NEC K51.918
  - enterocolitis — see Enterocolitis, ulcerative
  - ileocolitis — see Ileocolitis, ulcerative
  - mucosal proctocolitis — see Proctocolitis, mucosal
  - proctitis — see Proctitis, ulcerative
  - pseudopolyposis — see Polyp, colon, inflammatory
  - psychogenic F54
  - rectosigmoiditis — see Rectosigmoiditis, ulcerative
  - specified type NEC K51.80
    - with
      - complication K51.819
        - abscess K51.814
        - fistula K51.813
        - obstruction K51.812
        - rectal bleeding K51.811
        - specified complication NEC K51.818

Collagenosis, collagen disease (nonvascular) (vascular) M35.9
- cardiovascular I42.8
- reactive perforating L87.1
- specified NEC M35.89

Collapse R55
- adrenal E27.2
- cardiorespiratory R57.0
- cardiovascular R57.0
  - newborn P29.89
- circulatory (peripheral) R57.9
  - during or after labor and delivery O75.1
  - following ectopic or molar pregnancy O08.3
  - newborn P29.89
- during or
  - after labor and delivery O75.1
  - resulting from a procedure, not elsewhere classified T81.10-
- external ear canal — see Stenosis, external ear canal
- general R55
- heart — see Disease, heart
- heat T67.1-
- hysterical F44.89
- labyrinth, membranous (congenital) Q16.5
- lung (massive) — see also Atelectasis J98.19
  - pressure due to anesthesia (general) (local) or other sedation T88.2- ☑
    - during labor and delivery O74.1
    - in pregnancy O29.02- ☑
    - postpartum, puerperal O89.09
- myocardial — see Disease, heart
- nasal valve J34.829
  - external J34.8210
    - dynamic J34.8212
    - static J34.8211
  - internal J34.8200
    - dynamic J34.8202
    - static J34.8201
- nervous F48.8
- neurocirculatory F45.8
- nose M95.0
  - lower sidewall or nostril, on inspiration J34.8212
  - upper, middle sidewall, on inspiration J34.8202
- postoperative T81.10- ☑
- pulmonary — see also Atelectasis J98.19
  - newborn — see Atelectasis
- trachea J39.8
- tracheobronchial J98.09
- valvular — see Endocarditis
- vascular (peripheral) R57.9
  - during or after labor and delivery O75.1

Collapse — continued
- vascular — continued
  - following ectopic or molar pregnancy O08.3
  - newborn P29.89
- vertebra M48.50- ☑
  - cervical region M48.52- ☑
  - cervicothoracic region M48.53- ☑
  - in (due to)
    - neoplasm (metastasis) M84.58- ☑
    - osteoporosis — see also Osteoporosis M80.88- ☑
      - cervical region M80.88- ☑
      - cervicothoracic region M80.88- ☑
      - lumbar region M80.88- ☑
      - lumbosacral region M80.88- ☑
      - multiple sites M80.88- ☑
      - occipito-atlanto-axial region M80.88- ☑
      - sacrococcygeal region M80.88- ☑
      - thoracic region M80.88- ☑
      - thoracolumbar region M80.88- ☑
  - specified disease NEC M48.50- ☑
    - cervical region M48.52- ☑
    - cervicothoracic region M48.53- ☑
    - lumbar region M48.56- ☑
    - lumbosacral region M48.57- ☑
    - occipito-atlanto-axial region M48.51- ☑
    - sacrococcygeal region M48.58- ☑
    - thoracic region M48.54- ☑
    - thoracolumbar region M48.55- ☑
  - lumbar region M48.56- ☑
  - lumbosacral region M48.57- ☑
  - occipito-atlanto-axial region M48.51- ☑
  - sacrococcygeal region M48.58- ☑
  - thoracic region M48.54- ☑
  - thoracolumbar region M48.55- ☑

Collateral — see also condition
- circulation (venous) I87.8
- dilation, veins I87.8

Colles' fracture S52.53- ☑

Collet (-Sicard) **syndrome** G52.7

Collier's asthma or lung J60

Collodion baby Q80.2

Colloid nodule (of thyroid) (cystic) E04.1

Coloboma (iris) Q13.0
- eyelid Q10.3
- fundus Q14.8
- lens Q12.2
- optic disc (congenital) Q14.2
  - acquired H47.31- ☑

Coloenteritis — see Enteritis

Colon — see condition

Colonization
- MRSA (Methicillin resistant Staphylococcus aureus) Z22.322
- MSSA (Methicillin susceptible Staphylococcus aureus) Z22.321
- status — see Carrier (suspected) of

Coloptosis K63.4

Color blindness — see Deficiency, color vision

Colostomy
- attention to Z43.3
- fitting or adjustment Z46.89
- malfunctioning K94.03
- status Z93.3

Colpitis (acute) — see Vaginitis

Colpocele N81.5

Colpocystitis — see Vaginitis

Colpospasm N94.2

Column, spinal, vertebral — see condition

Coma R40.20
- with
  - motor response (none) R40.231- ☑
    - abnormal extensor posturing to pain or noxious stimuli (< 2 years of age) R40.232- ☑
    - abnormal flexure posturing to pain or noxious stimuli (0-5 years of age) R40.233- ☑
    - extensor posturing to pain or noxious stimuli (2-5 years of age) R40.232- ☑
    - flexion/decorticate posturing (< 2 years of age) R40.233- ☑
    - localizes pain (2-5 years of age) R40.235- ☑
    - normal or spontaneous movement (< 2 years of age) R40.236- ☑
    - obeys commands (2-5 years of age) R40.236- ☑
    - score of
      - 1 R40.231- ☑
      - 2 R40.232- ☑
      - 3 R40.233- ☑

Coma — continued
- with — continued
  - motor response — continued
    - score of — continued
      - 4 R40.234- ☑
      - 5 R40.235- ☑
      - 6 R40.236- ☑
    - withdraws from pain or noxious stimuli (0-5 years of age) R40.234- ☑
    - withdraws to touch (< 2 years of age) R40.235- ☑
  - opening of eyes (never) R40.211- ☑
    - in response to
      - pain R40.212- ☑
      - sound R40.213- ☑
    - score of
      - 1 R40.211- ☑
      - 2 R40.212- ☑
      - 3 R40.213- ☑
      - 4 R40.214- ☑
    - spontaneous R40.214- ☑
  - verbal response (none) R40.221- ☑
    - confused conversation R40.224- ☑
    - cooing or babbling or crying appropriately (<2 years of age) R40.225- ☑
    - inappropriate crying or screaming (< 2 years of age) R40.223- ☑
    - inappropriate words R40.223- ☑
    - inappropriate words (2-5 years of age) R40.224- ☑
    - incomprehensible sounds (2-5 years of age) R40.222- ☑
    - incomprehensible words R40.222- ☑
    - irritable cries (< 2 years of age) R40.224- ☑
    - moans/grunts to pain; restless (< 2 years old) R40.222- ☑
    - oriented R40.225- ☑
    - score of
      - 1 R40.221- ☑
      - 2 R40.222- ☑
      - 3 R40.223- ☑
      - 4 R40.224- ☑
      - 5 R40.225- ☑
    - screaming (2-5 years of age) R40.223- ☑
    - uses appropriate words (2-5 years of age) R40.225- ☑
- eclamptic — see Eclampsia
- epileptic — see Epilepsy
- Glasgow, scale score — see Glasgow coma scale
- hepatic — see Failure, hepatic, by type, with coma
- hyperglycemic (diabetic) — see Diabetes, by type, with hyperosmolarity, with coma
- hyperosmolar (diabetic) — see Diabetes, by type, with hyperosmolarity, with coma
- hypoglycemic (diabetic) — see Diabetes, by type, with hypoglycemia, with coma
  - nondiabetic E15
- in diabetes — see Diabetes, coma
- insulin-induced — see Coma, hypoglycemic
- ketoacidotic (diabetic) — see Diabetes, by type, with ketoacidosis, with coma
- myxedematous E03.5
- newborn P91.5
- nontraumatic, due to underlying condition R40.2A
- persistent vegetative state R40.3
- secondary R40.2A
- specified NEC, without documented Glasgow coma scale score, or with partial Glasgow coma scale score reported R40.244- ☑

Comatose — see Coma

Combat fatigue F43.0

Combined — see condition

Comedo, comedones (giant) L70.0

Comedocarcinoma — see also Neoplasm, breast, malignant
- noninfiltrating
  - breast D05.8- ☑
  - specified site — see Neoplasm, in situ, by site
  - unspecified site D05.8- ☑

Comedomastitis — see Ectasia, mammary duct

Comminuted fracture — code as Fracture, closed

Common
- arterial trunk Q20.0
- atrioventricular canal Q21.23
- atrium Q21.19
- cold (head) J00
- truncus (arteriosus) Q20.0
- variable immunodeficiency — see Immunodeficiency, common variable
- ventricle Q20.4

Commotio, commotion (current)
- brain — *see* Injury, intracranial, concussion
- cerebri — *see* Injury, intracranial, concussion
- retinae S05.8X-
- spinal cord — *see* Injury, spinal cord, by region
- spinalis — *see* Injury, spinal cord, by region

Communication
- between
  - base of aorta and pulmonary artery Q21.4
  - left ventricle and right atrium Q20.5
  - pericardial sac and pleural sac Q34.8
  - pulmonary artery and pulmonary vein, congenital Q25.72
- congenital between uterus and digestive or urinary tract Q51.7

Compartment syndrome (deep) (posterior) (traumatic) T79.A0- ☑ (*following* T79.7)
- abdomen T79.A3- ☑ (*following* T79.7)
- lower extremity (hip, buttock, thigh, leg, foot, toes) T79.A2- ☑ (*following* T79.7)
- nontraumatic
  - abdomen M79.A3 (*following* M79.7)
  - lower extremity (hip, buttock, thigh, leg, foot, toes) M79.A2- ☑ (*following* M79.7)
  - specified site NEC M79.A9 (*following* M79.7)
  - upper extremity (shoulder, arm, forearm, wrist, hand, fingers) M79.A1- ☑ (*following* M79.7)
- specified site NEC T79.A9- ☑ (*following* T79.7)
- upper extremity (shoulder, arm, forearm, wrist, hand, fingers) T79.A1- ☑ (*following* T79.7)

Compensation
- failure — *see* Disease, heart
- neurosis, psychoneurosis — *see* Disorder, factitious

Complaint — *see also* Disease
- bowel, functional K59.9
  - psychogenic F45.8
- intestine, functional K59.9
  - psychogenic F45.8
- kidney — *see* Disease, renal
- miners' J60

Complete — *see* condition

Complex
- Addison-Schilder E71.528
- cardiorenal — *see* Hypertension, cardiorenal
- Costen's M26.69
- disseminated mycobacterium avium- intracellulare (DMAC) A31.2
- Eisenmenger's (ventricular septal defect) I27.83
- hypersexual F52.8
- jumped process, spine — *see* Dislocation, vertebra
- primary, tuberculous A15.7
- Schilder-Addison E71.528
- subluxation (vertebral) M99.19
  - abdomen M99.19
  - acromioclavicular M99.17
  - cervical region M99.11
  - cervicothoracic M99.11
  - costochondral M99.18
  - costovertebral M99.18
  - head region M99.10
  - hip M99.15
  - lower extremity M99.16
  - lumbar region M99.13
  - lumbosacral M99.13
  - occipitocervical M99.10
  - pelvic region M99.15
  - pubic M99.15
  - rib cage M99.18
  - sacral region M99.14
  - sacrococcygeal M99.14
  - sacroiliac M99.14
  - specified NEC M99.19
  - sternochondral M99.18
  - sternoclavicular M99.17
  - thoracic region M99.12
  - thoracolumbar M99.12
  - upper extremity M99.17
- Taussig-Bing (transposition, aorta and overriding pulmonary artery) Q20.1

Complication(s) (from) (of)
- accidental puncture or laceration during a procedure (of) — *see* Complications, intraoperative (intraprocedural), puncture or laceration
- amputation stump (surgical) (late) NEC T87.9
  - dehiscence T87.81
  - infection or inflammation T87.40
    - lower limb T87.4- ☑
    - upper limb T87.4- ☑

Complication(s) — *continued*
- amputation stump — *continued*
  - necrosis T87.50
    - lower limb T87.5- ☑
    - upper limb T87.5- ☑
  - neuroma T87.30
    - lower limb T87.3- ☑
    - upper limb T87.3- ☑
  - specified type NEC T87.89
- anastomosis (and bypass) — *see also* Complications, prosthetic device or implant
  - intestinal (internal) NEC K91.89
    - involving urinary tract N99.89
  - urinary tract (involving intestinal tract) N99.89
  - vascular — *see* Complications, cardiovascular device or implant
- anesthesia, anesthetic — *see also* Anesthesia, complication T88.59- ☑
  - brain, postpartum, puerperal O89.2
  - cardiac
    - in
      - labor and delivery O74.2
      - pregnancy O29.19- ☑
    - postpartum, puerperal O89.1
  - central nervous system
    - in
      - labor and delivery O74.3
      - pregnancy O29.29- ☑
    - postpartum, puerperal O89.2
  - difficult or failed intubation T88.4- ☑
    - in pregnancy O29.6- ☑
  - failed sedation (conscious) (moderate) during procedure T88.52- ☑
  - general, unintended awareness during procedure T88.53- ☑
  - hyperthermia, malignant T88.3- ☑
  - hypothermia T88.51- ☑
  - intubation failure T88.4- ☑
  - malignant hyperthermia T88.3- ☑
  - pulmonary
    - in
      - labor and delivery O74.1
      - pregnancy NEC O29.09- ☑
    - postpartum, puerperal O89.09
  - shock T88.2- ☑
  - spinal and epidural
    - in
      - labor and delivery NEC O74.6
        - headache O74.5
      - pregnancy NEC O29.5X- ☑
    - postpartum, puerperal NEC O89.5
      - headache O89.4
  - unintended awareness under general anesthesia during procedure T88.53- ☑
- anti-reflux device — *see* Complications, esophageal anti-reflux device
- aortic (bifurcation) graft — *see* Complications, graft, vascular
- aortocoronary (bypass) graft — *see* Complications, coronary artery (bypass) graft
- aortofemoral (bypass) graft — *see* Complications, extremity artery (bypass) graft
- arteriovenous
  - fistula, surgically created T82.9- ☑
    - embolism T82.818- ☑
    - fibrosis T82.828- ☑
    - hemorrhage T82.838- ☑
    - infection or inflammation T82.7- ☑
    - mechanical
      - breakdown T82.510- ☑
      - displacement T82.520- ☑
      - leakage T82.530- ☑
      - malposition T82.520- ☑
      - obstruction T82.590- ☑
      - perforation T82.590- ☑
      - protrusion T82.590- ☑
    - pain T82.848- ☑
    - specified type NEC T82.898- ☑
    - stenosis T82.858- ☑
    - thrombosis T82.868- ☑
  - shunt, surgically created T82.9- ☑
    - embolism T82.818- ☑
    - fibrosis T82.828- ☑
    - hemorrhage T82.838- ☑
    - infection or inflammation T82.7- ☑
    - mechanical
      - breakdown T82.511- ☑

Complication(s) — *continued*
- arteriovenous — *continued*
  - shunt, surgically created — *continued*
    - mechanical — *continued*
      - displacement T82.521- ☑
      - leakage T82.531- ☑
      - malposition T82.521- ☑
      - obstruction T82.591- ☑
      - perforation T82.591- ☑
      - protrusion T82.591- ☑
    - pain T82.848- ☑
    - specified type NEC T82.898- ☑
    - stenosis T82.858- ☑
    - thrombosis T82.868- ☑
- arthroplasty — *see* Complications, joint prosthesis
- artificial
  - fertilization or insemination N98.9
    - attempted introduction (of)
      - embryo in embryo transfer N98.3
      - ovum following in vitro fertilization N98.2
    - hyperstimulation of ovaries N98.1
    - infection N98.0
    - specified NEC N98.8
  - heart T82.9- ☑
    - embolism T82.817- ☑
    - fibrosis T82.827- ☑
    - hemorrhage T82.837- ☑
    - infection or inflammation T82.7- ☑
    - mechanical
      - breakdown T82.512- ☑
      - displacement T82.522- ☑
      - leakage T82.532- ☑
      - malposition T82.522- ☑
      - obstruction T82.592- ☑
      - perforation T82.592- ☑
      - protrusion T82.592- ☑
    - pain T82.847- ☑
    - specified type NEC T82.897- ☑
    - stenosis T82.857- ☑
    - thrombosis T82.867- ☑
  - opening
    - cecostomy — *see* Complications, colostomy
    - colostomy — *see* Complications, colostomy
    - cystostomy — *see* Complications, cystostomy
    - enterostomy — *see* Complications, enterostomy
    - gastrostomy — *see* Complications, gastrostomy
    - ileostomy — *see* Complications, enterostomy
    - jejunostomy — *see* Complications, enterostomy
    - nephrostomy — *see* Complications, stoma, urinary tract
    - tracheostomy — *see* Complications, tracheostomy
    - ureterostomy — *see* Complications, stoma, urinary tract
    - urethrostomy — *see* Complications, stoma, urinary tract
- balloon implant or device
  - gastrointestinal T85.9- ☑
    - embolism T85.818- ☑
    - fibrosis T85.828- ☑
    - hemorrhage T85.838- ☑
    - infection and inflammation T85.79- ☑
    - pain T85.848- ☑
    - specified type NEC T85.898- ☑
    - stenosis T85.858- ☑
    - thrombosis T85.868- ☑
  - vascular (counterpulsation) T82.9- ☑
    - embolism T82.818- ☑
    - fibrosis T82.828- ☑
    - hemorrhage T82.838- ☑
    - infection or inflammation T82.7- ☑
    - mechanical
      - breakdown T82.513- ☑
      - displacement T82.523- ☑
      - leakage T82.533- ☑
      - malposition T82.523- ☑
      - obstruction T82.593- ☑
      - perforation T82.593- ☑
      - protrusion T82.593- ☑
    - pain T82.848- ☑
    - specified type NEC T82.898- ☑
    - stenosis T82.858- ☑
    - thrombosis T82.868- ☑
- bariatric procedure
  - gastric band procedure K95.09
    - infection K95.01
  - specified procedure NEC K95.89

Complication(s) — *continued*
  bariatric procedure — *continued*
    specified procedure — *continued*
      infection K95.81
  bile duct implant (prosthetic) T85.9- ☑
    embolism T85.818- ☑
    fibrosis T85.828- ☑
    hemorrhage T85.838- ☑
    infection and inflammation T85.79- ☑
    mechanical
      breakdown T85.510- ☑
      displacement T85.520- ☑
      malfunction T85.510- ☑
      malposition T85.520- ☑
      obstruction T85.590- ☑
      perforation T85.590- ☑
      protrusion T85.590- ☑
      specified NEC T85.590- ☑
    pain T85.848- ☑
    specified type NEC T85.898- ☑
    stenosis T85.858- ☑
    thrombosis T85.868- ☑
  bladder device (auxiliary) — *see* Complications, genitourinary, device or implant, urinary system
  bleeding (postoperative) — *see* Complication, postoperative, hemorrhage
    intraoperative — *see* Complication, intraoperative, hemorrhage
  blood vessel graft — *see* Complications, graft, vascular
  bone
    device NEC T84.9- ☑
      embolism T84.81- ☑
      fibrosis T84.82- ☑
      hemorrhage T84.83- ☑
      infection or inflammation T84.7- ☑
      mechanical
        breakdown T84.318- ☑
        displacement T84.328- ☑
        malposition T84.328- ☑
        obstruction T84.398- ☑
        perforation T84.398- ☑
        protrusion T84.398- ☑
      pain T84.84- ☑
      specified type NEC T84.89- ☑
      stenosis T84.85- ☑
      thrombosis T84.86- ☑
    graft — *see* Complications, graft, bone
    growth stimulator (electrode) — *see* Complications, electronic stimulator device, bone
    marrow transplant — *see* Complications, transplant, bone, marrow
  brain neurostimulator (electrode) — *see* Complications, electronic stimulator device, brain
  breast implant (prosthetic) T85.9- ☑
    capsular contracture T85.44- ☑
    embolism T85.818- ☑
    fibrosis T85.828- ☑
    hemorrhage T85.838- ☑
    infection and inflammation T85.79- ☑
    mechanical
      breakdown T85.41- ☑
      displacement T85.42- ☑
      leakage T85.43- ☑
      malposition T85.42- ☑
      obstruction T85.49- ☑
      perforation T85.49- ☑
      protrusion T85.49- ☑
      specified NEC T85.49- ☑
    pain T85.848- ☑
    specified type NEC T85.898- ☑
    stenosis T85.858- ☑
    thrombosis T85.868- ☑
  bypass — *see also* Complications, prosthetic device or implant
    aortocoronary — *see* Complications, coronary artery (bypass) graft
    arterial — *see also* Complications, graft, vascular
      extremity — *see* Complications, extremity artery (bypass) graft
  cardiac — *see also* Disease, heart
    device, implant or graft T82.9- ☑
      embolism T82.817- ☑
      fibrosis T82.827- ☑
      hemorrhage T82.837- ☑
      infection or inflammation T82.7- ☑
        valve prosthesis T82.6- ☑

Complication(s) — *continued*
  cardiac — *see also* Disease, heart — *continued*
    device, implant or graft — *continued*
      mechanical
        breakdown T82.519- ☑
          specified device NEC T82.518- ☑
        displacement T82.529- ☑
          specified device NEC T82.528- ☑
        leakage T82.539- ☑
          specified device NEC T82.538- ☑
        malposition T82.529- ☑
          specified device NEC T82.528- ☑
        obstruction T82.599- ☑
          specified device NEC T82.598- ☑
        perforation T82.599- ☑
          specified device NEC T82.598- ☑
        protrusion T82.599- ☑
          specified device NEC T82.598- ☑
      pain T82.847- ☑
      specified type NEC T82.897- ☑
      stenosis T82.857- ☑
      thrombosis T82.867- ☑
  cardiovascular device, graft or implant T82.9- ☑
    aortic graft — *see* Complications, graft, vascular
    arteriovenous
      fistula, artificial — *see* Complication, arteriovenous, fistula, surgically created
      shunt — *see* Complication, arteriovenous, shunt, surgically created
    artificial heart — *see* Complication, artificial, heart
    balloon (counterpulsation) device — *see* Complication, balloon implant, vascular
    carotid artery graft — *see* Complications, graft, vascular
    coronary bypass graft — *see* Complication, coronary artery (bypass) graft
    dialysis catheter (vascular) — *see* Complication, catheter, dialysis
    electronic T82.9- ☑
      electrode T82.9- ☑
        embolism T82.817- ☑
        fibrosis T82.827- ☑
        hemorrhage T82.837- ☑
        infection T82.7- ☑
        mechanical
          breakdown T82.110- ☑
          displacement T82.120- ☑
          leakage T82.190- ☑
          obstruction T82.190- ☑
          perforation T82.190- ☑
          protrusion T82.190- ☑
          specified type NEC T82.190- ☑
        pain T82.847- ☑
        specified NEC T82.897- ☑
        stenosis T82.857- ☑
        thrombosis T82.867- ☑
      embolism T82.817- ☑
      fibrosis T82.827- ☑
      hemorrhage T82.837- ☑
      infection T82.7- ☑
      mechanical
        breakdown T82.119- ☑
        displacement T82.129- ☑
        leakage T82.199- ☑
        obstruction T82.199- ☑
        perforation T82.199- ☑
        protrusion T82.199- ☑
        specified type NEC T82.199- ☑
      pain T82.847- ☑
      pulse generator T82.9- ☑
        embolism T82.817- ☑
        fibrosis T82.827- ☑
        hemorrhage T82.837- ☑
        infection T82.7- ☑
        mechanical
          breakdown T82.111- ☑
          displacement T82.121- ☑
          leakage T82.191- ☑
          obstruction T82.191- ☑
          perforation T82.191- ☑
          protrusion T82.191- ☑
          specified type NEC T82.191- ☑
        pain T82.847- ☑
        specified NEC T82.897- ☑
        stenosis T82.857- ☑
        thrombosis T82.867- ☑

Complication(s) — *continued*
  cardiovascular device, graft or implant — *continued*
    electronic — *continued*
      specified condition NEC T82.897- ☑
      specified device NEC T82.9- ☑
        embolism T82.817- ☑
        fibrosis T82.827- ☑
        hemorrhage T82.837- ☑
        infection T82.7- ☑
        mechanical
          breakdown T82.118- ☑
          displacement T82.128- ☑
          leakage T82.198- ☑
          obstruction T82.198- ☑
          perforation T82.198- ☑
          protrusion T82.198- ☑
          specified type NEC T82.198- ☑
        pain T82.847- ☑
        specified NEC T82.897- ☑
        stenosis T82.857- ☑
        thrombosis T82.867- ☑
      stenosis T82.857- ☑
      thrombosis T82.867- ☑
    extremity artery graft — *see* Complication, extremity artery (bypass) graft
    femoral artery graft — *see* Complication, extremity artery (bypass) graft
    heart
      transplant — *see* Complication, transplant, heart
      valve — *see* Complication, prosthetic device, heart valve
        graft — *see* Complication, heart, valve, graft
    heart-lung transplant — *see* Complication, transplant, heart, with lung
    infection or inflammation T82.7- ☑
    umbrella device — *see* Complication, umbrella device, vascular
    vascular graft (or anastomosis) — *see* Complication, graft, vascular
  carotid artery (bypass) graft — *see* Complications, graft, vascular
  catheter (device) NEC — *see also* Complications, prosthetic device or implant
    cranial infusion
      infection and inflammation T85.735- ☑
      mechanical
        breakdown T85.610- ☑
        displacement T85.620- ☑
        leakage T85.630- ☑
        malfunction T85.690- ☑
        malposition T85.620- ☑
        obstruction T85.690- ☑
        perforation T85.690- ☑
        protrusion T85.690- ☑
        specified NEC T85.690- ☑
    cystostomy T83.9- ☑
      embolism T83.81- ☑
      fibrosis T83.82- ☑
      hemorrhage T83.83- ☑
      infection and inflammation T83.510- ☑
      mechanical
        breakdown T83.010- ☑
        displacement T83.020- ☑
        leakage T83.030- ☑
        malposition T83.020- ☑
        obstruction T83.090- ☑
        perforation T83.090- ☑
        protrusion T83.090- ☑
        specified NEC T83.090- ☑
      pain T83.84- ☑
      specified type NEC T83.89- ☑
      stenosis T83.85- ☑
      thrombosis T83.86- ☑
    dialysis (vascular) T82.9- ☑
      embolism T82.818- ☑
      fibrosis T82.828- ☑
      hemorrhage T82.838- ☑
      infection and inflammation T82.7- ☑
      intraperitoneal — *see* Complications, catheter, intraperitoneal dialysis
      mechanical
        breakdown T82.41- ☑
        displacement T82.42- ☑
        leakage T82.43- ☑
        malposition T82.42- ☑
        obstruction T82.49- ☑

☑ Additional Character Required — Refer to the Tabular List for Character Selection

Complication(s) — *continued*
  catheter — *see also* Complications, prosthetic device or implant — *continued*
    dialysis — *continued*
      mechanical — *continued*
        perforation T82.49- ☑
        protrusion T82.49- ☑
      pain T82.848- ☑
      specified type NEC T82.898- ☑
      stenosis T82.858- ☑
      thrombosis T82.868- ☑
    epidural infusion T85.9- ☑
      embolism T85.810- ☑
      fibrosis T85.820- ☑
      hemorrhage T85.830- ☑
      infection and inflammation T85.735- ☑
      mechanical
        breakdown T85.610- ☑
        displacement T85.620- ☑
        leakage T85.630- ☑
        malfunction T85.690- ☑
        malposition T85.620- ☑
        obstruction T85.690- ☑
        perforation T85.690- ☑
        protrusion T85.690- ☑
        specified NEC T85.690- ☑
      pain T85.840- ☑
      specified type NEC T85.890- ☑
      stenosis T85.850- ☑
      thrombosis T85.860- ☑
    intraperitoneal dialysis T85.9- ☑
      embolism T85.818- ☑
      fibrosis T85.828- ☑
      hemorrhage T85.838- ☑
      infection and inflammation T85.71- ☑
      mechanical
        breakdown T85.611- ☑
        displacement T85.621- ☑
        leakage T85.631- ☑
        malfunction T85.611- ☑
        malposition T85.621- ☑
        obstruction T85.691- ☑
        perforation T85.691- ☑
        protrusion T85.691- ☑
        specified NEC T85.691- ☑
      pain T85.848- ☑
      specified type NEC T85.898- ☑
      stenosis T85.858- ☑
      thrombosis T85.868- ☑
    intrathecal infusion
      infection and inflammation T85.735- ☑
      mechanical
        breakdown T85.610- ☑
        displacement T85.620- ☑
        leakage T85.630- ☑
        malfunction T85.690- ☑
        malposition T85.620- ☑
        obstruction T85.690- ☑
        perforation T85.690- ☑
        protrusion T85.690- ☑
        specified NEC T85.690- ☑
    intravenous infusion T82.9- ☑
      embolism T82.818- ☑
      fibrosis T82.828- ☑
      hemorrhage T82.838- ☑
      infection or inflammation T82.7- ☑
      mechanical
        breakdown T82.514- ☑
        displacement T82.524- ☑
        leakage T82.534- ☑
        malposition T82.524- ☑
        obstruction T82.594- ☑
        perforation T82.594- ☑
        protrusion T82.594- ☑
      pain T82.848- ☑
      specified type NEC T82.898- ☑
      stenosis T82.858- ☑
      thrombosis T82.868- ☑
    spinal infusion
      infection and inflammation T85.735- ☑
      mechanical
        breakdown T85.610- ☑
        displacement T85.620- ☑
        leakage T85.630- ☑
        malfunction T85.690- ☑

Complication(s) — *continued*
  catheter — *see also* Complications, prosthetic device or implant — *continued*
    spinal infusion — *continued*
      mechanical — *continued*
        malposition T85.620- ☑
        obstruction T85.690- ☑
        perforation T85.690- ☑
        protrusion T85.690- ☑
        specified NEC T85.690- ☑
    subarachnoid infusion
      infection and inflammation T85.735- ☑
      mechanical
        breakdown T85.610- ☑
        displacement T85.620- ☑
        leakage T85.630- ☑
        malfunction T85.690- ☑
        malposition T85.620- ☑
        obstruction T85.690- ☑
        perforation T85.690- ☑
        protrusion T85.690- ☑
        specified NEC T85.690- ☑
    subdural infusion T85.9- ☑
      embolism T85.810- ☑
      fibrosis T85.820- ☑
      hemorrhage T85.830- ☑
      infection and inflammation T85.735- ☑
      mechanical
        breakdown T85.610- ☑
        displacement T85.620- ☑
        leakage T85.630- ☑
        malfunction T85.690- ☑
        malposition T85.620- ☑
        obstruction T85.690- ☑
        perforation T85.690- ☑
        protrusion T85.690- ☑
        specified NEC T85.690- ☑
      pain T85.840- ☑
      specified type NEC T85.890- ☑
      stenosis T85.850- ☑
      thrombosis T85.860- ☑
    urethral T83.9-
      displacement T83.028- ☑
      embolism T83.81- ☑
      fibrosis T83.82- ☑
      hemorrhage T83.83- ☑
      indwelling
        breakdown T83.011- ☑
        displacement T83.021- ☑
        infection and inflammation T83.511- ☑
        leakage T83.031- ☑
        specified complication NEC T83.091- ☑
      infection and inflammation T83.511- ☑
      leakage T83.038- ☑
      malposition T83.028- ☑
      mechanical
        breakdown T83.011- ☑
      obstruction (mechanical) T83.091- ☑
      pain T83.84- ☑
      perforation T83.091- ☑
      protrusion T83.091- ☑
      specified type NEC T83.091- ☑
      stenosis T83.85- ☑
      thrombosis T83.86- ☑
    urinary NEC
      breakdown T83.018- ☑
      displacement T83.028- ☑
      infection and inflammation T83.518- ☑
      leakage T83.038- ☑
      specified complication NEC T83.098- ☑
  cecostomy (stoma) — *see* Complications, colostomy
  cesarean delivery wound NEC O90.89
    disruption O90.0
    hematoma O90.2
    infection (following delivery) O86.00
  chemotherapy (antineoplastic) NEC T88.7- ☑
  chimeric antigen receptor (CAR-T) cell therapy T80.82- ☑
  chin implant (prosthetic) — *see* Complication, prosthetic device or implant, specified NEC
  circulatory system I99.8
    intraoperative I97.88
    postprocedural I97.89
      following cardiac surgery — *see also* Infarct, myocardium, associated with revascularization procedure I97.190
        postcardiotomy syndrome I97.0

Complication(s) — *continued*
  circulatory system — *continued*
    postprocedural — *continued*
      hypertension I97.3
      lymphedema after mastectomy I97.2
      postcardiotomy syndrome I97.0
      specified NEC I97.89
  colostomy (stoma) K94.00
    hemorrhage K94.01
    infection K94.02
    malfunction K94.03
    mechanical K94.03
    specified complication NEC K94.09
  contraceptive device, intrauterine — *see* Complications, intrauterine, contraceptive device
  cord (umbilical) — *see* Complications, umbilical cord
  corneal graft — *see* Complications, graft, cornea
  coronary artery (bypass) graft T82.9- ☑
    atherosclerosis — *see* Arteriosclerosis, coronary (artery)
    embolism T82.817- ☑
    fibrosis T82.827- ☑
    hemorrhage T82.837- ☑
    infection and inflammation T82.7- ☑
    mechanical
      breakdown T82.211- ☑
      displacement T82.212- ☑
      leakage T82.213- ☑
      malfunction T82.212- ☑
      malposition T82.212- ☑
      obstruction T82.218- ☑
      perforation T82.218- ☑
      protrusion T82.218- ☑
      specified NEC T82.218- ☑
    pain T82.847- ☑
    specified type NEC T82.898- ☑
    stenosis T82.857- ☑
    thrombosis T82.867- ☑
  counterpulsation device (balloon), intra-aortic — *see* Complications, balloon implant, vascular
  cystostomy (stoma) N99.518
    catheter — *see* Complications, catheter, cystostomy
    hemorrhage N99.510
    infection N99.511
    malfunction N99.512
    specified type NEC N99.518
  delivery — *see also* Complications, obstetric O75.9
    procedure (instrumental) (manual) (surgical) O75.4
    specified NEC O75.89
  dialysis (peritoneal) (renal) — *see also* Complications, infusion
    catheter (vascular) — *see* Complication, catheter, dialysis
      peritoneal, intraperitoneal — *see* Complications, catheter, intraperitoneal
  dorsal column (spinal) neurostimulator — *see* Complications, electronic stimulator device, spinal cord
  drug NEC T88.7- ☑
  ear procedure — *see also* Disorder, ear
    intraoperative H95.88
      hematoma — *see* Complications, intraoperative, hemorrhage (hematoma) (of) ear
      hemorrhage — *see* Complications, intraoperative, hemorrhage (hematoma) (of), ear
      laceration — *see* Complications, intraoperative, puncture or laceration, ear
      specified NEC H95.88
    postoperative H95.89
      external ear canal stenosis H95.81- ☑
      hematoma — *see* Complications, postprocedural, hematoma (of), ear
      hemorrhage — *see* Complications, postprocedural, hemorrhage (of), ear
      postmastoidectomy — *see* Complications, post-mastoidectomy
      seroma — *see* Complications, postprocedural, seroma (of), mastoid process
      specified NEC H95.89
  ectopic pregnancy O08.9
    damage to pelvic organs O08.6
    embolism O08.2
    genital infection O08.0
    hemorrhage (delayed) (excessive) O08.1
    metabolic disorder O08.5
    renal failure O08.4
    shock O08.3
    specified type NEC O08.0
    venous complication NEC O08.7

☑ Additional Character Required — Refer to the Tabular List for Character Selection

Complication(s) — *continued*
  electronic stimulator device
    bladder (urinary) — *see* Complications, electronic stimulator device, urinary
    bone T84.9- ☑
      breakdown T84.310- ☑
      displacement T84.320- ☑
      embolism T84.81- ☑
      fibrosis T84.82- ☑
      hemorrhage T84.83- ☑
      infection or inflammation T84.7- ☑
      malfunction T84.310- ☑
      malposition T84.320- ☑
      mechanical NEC T84.390- ☑
      obstruction T84.390- ☑
      pain T84.84- ☑
      perforation T84.390- ☑
      protrusion T84.390- ☑
      specified type NEC T84.89- ☑
      stenosis T84.85- ☑
      thrombosis T84.86- ☑
    brain T85.9- ☑
      embolism T85.810- ☑
      fibrosis T85.820- ☑
      hemorrhage T85.830- ☑
      infection and inflammation T85.731- ☑
      mechanical
        breakdown T85.110- ☑
        displacement T85.120- ☑
        leakage T85.190- ☑
        malposition T85.120- ☑
        obstruction T85.190- ☑
        perforation T85.190- ☑
        protrusion T85.190- ☑
        specified NEC T85.190- ☑
      pain T85.840- ☑
      specified type NEC T85.890- ☑
      stenosis T85.850- ☑
      thrombosis T85.860- ☑
    cardiac (defibrillator) (pacemaker) — *see* Complications, cardiovascular device or implant, electronic
    generator (brain) (gastric) (peripheral) (sacral) (spinal)
      breakdown T85.113- ☑
      displacement T85.123- ☑
      leakage T85.193- ☑
      malposition T85.123- ☑
      obstruction T85.193- ☑
      perforation T85.193- ☑
      protrusion T85.193- ☑
      specified type NEC T85.193- ☑
    muscle T84.9- ☑
      breakdown T84.418- ☑
      displacement T84.428- ☑
      embolism T84.81- ☑
      fibrosis T84.82- ☑
      hemorrhage T84.83- ☑
      infection or inflammation T84.7- ☑
      mechanical NEC T84.498- ☑
      pain T84.84- ☑
      specified type NEC T84.89- ☑
      stenosis T84.85- ☑
      thrombosis T84.86- ☑
    nervous system T85.9- ☑
      brain — *see* Complications, electronic stimulator device, brain
      cranial nerve — *see* Complications, electronic stimulator device, peripheral nerve
      embolism T85.810- ☑
      fibrosis T85.820- ☑
      gastric nerve — *see* Complications, electronic stimulator device, peripheral nerve
      hemorrhage T85.830- ☑
      infection and inflammation T85.738- ☑
      mechanical
        breakdown T85.118- ☑
        displacement T85.128- ☑
        leakage T85.199- ☑
        malposition T85.128- ☑
        obstruction T85.199- ☑
        perforation T85.199- ☑
        protrusion T85.199- ☑
        specified NEC T85.199- ☑
      pain T85.840- ☑
      peripheral nerve — *see* Complications, electronic stimulator device, peripheral nerve

Complication(s) — *continued*
  electronic stimulator device — *continued*
    nervous system — *continued*
      sacral nerve — *see* Complications, electronic stimulator device, peripheral nerve
      specified type NEC T85.890- ☑
      spinal cord — *see* Complications, electronic stimulator device, spinal cord
      stenosis T85.850- ☑
      thrombosis T85.860- ☑
      vagal nerve — *see* Complications, electronic stimulator device, peripheral nerve
    peripheral nerve T85.9- ☑
      embolism T85.810- ☑
      fibrosis T85.820- ☑
      hemorrhage T85.830- ☑
      infection and inflammation T85.732- ☑
      mechanical
        breakdown T85.111- ☑
        displacement T85.121- ☑
        leakage T85.191- ☑
        malposition T85.121- ☑
        obstruction T85.191- ☑
        perforation T85.191- ☑
        protrusion T85.191- ☑
        specified NEC T85.191- ☑
      pain T85.840- ☑
      specified type NEC T85.890- ☑
      stenosis T85.850- ☑
      thrombosis T85.860- ☑
    spinal cord T85.9- ☑
      embolism T85.810- ☑
      fibrosis T85.820- ☑
      hemorrhage T85.830- ☑
      infection and inflammation T85.733- ☑
      mechanical
        breakdown T85.112- ☑
        displacement T85.122- ☑
        leakage T85.192- ☑
        malposition T85.122- ☑
        obstruction T85.192- ☑
        perforation T85.192- ☑
        protrusion T85.192- ☑
        specified NEC T85.192- ☑
      pain T85.840- ☑
      specified type NEC T85.890- ☑
      stenosis T85.850- ☑
      thrombosis T85.860- ☑
    urinary T83.9- ☑
      embolism T83.81- ☑
      fibrosis T83.82- ☑
      hemorrhage T83.83- ☑
      infection and inflammation T83.598- ☑
      mechanical
        breakdown T83.110- ☑
        displacement T83.120- ☑
        malposition T83.120- ☑
        perforation T83.190- ☑
        protrusion T83.190- ☑
        specified NEC T83.190- ☑
      pain T83.84- ☑
      specified type NEC T83.89- ☑
      stenosis T83.85- ☑
      thrombosis T83.86- ☑
  electroshock therapy T88.9- ☑
    specified NEC T88.8- ☑
  endocrine E34.9
    postprocedural
      adrenal hypofunction E89.6
      hypoinsulinemia E89.1
      hypoparathyroidism E89.2
      hypopituitarism E89.3
      hypothyroidism E89.0
      ovarian failure E89.40
        asymptomatic E89.40
        symptomatic E89.41
      specified NEC E89.89
      testicular hypofunction E89.5
  endodontic treatment NEC M27.59
  enterostomy (stoma) K94.10
    hemorrhage K94.11
    infection K94.12
    malfunction K94.13
    mechanical K94.13
    specified complication NEC K94.19
  episiotomy, disruption O90.1

Complication(s) — *continued*
  esophageal anti-reflux device T85.9- ☑
    embolism T85.818- ☑
    fibrosis T85.828- ☑
    hemorrhage T85.838- ☑
    infection and inflammation T85.79- ☑
    mechanical
      breakdown T85.511- ☑
      displacement T85.521- ☑
      malfunction T85.511- ☑
      malposition T85.521- ☑
      obstruction T85.591- ☑
      perforation T85.591- ☑
      protrusion T85.591- ☑
      specified NEC T85.591- ☑
    pain T85.848- ☑
    specified type NEC T85.898- ☑
    stenosis T85.858- ☑
    thrombosis T85.868- ☑
  esophagostomy K94.30
    hemorrhage K94.31
    infection K94.32
    malfunction K94.33
    mechanical K94.33
    specified complication NEC K94.39
  extracorporeal circulation T80.90- ☑
  extremity artery (bypass) graft T82.9- ☑
    arteriosclerosis — *see* Arteriosclerosis, extremities, bypass graft
    embolism T82.818- ☑
    fibrosis T82.828- ☑
    hemorrhage T82.838- ☑
    infection and inflammation T82.7- ☑
    mechanical
      breakdown T82.318- ☑
        femoral artery T82.312- ☑
      displacement T82.328- ☑
        femoral artery T82.322- ☑
      leakage T82.338- ☑
        femoral artery T82.332- ☑
      malposition T82.328- ☑
        femoral artery T82.322- ☑
      obstruction T82.398- ☑
        femoral artery T82.392- ☑
      perforation T82.398- ☑
        femoral artery T82.392- ☑
      protrusion T82.398- ☑
        femoral artery T82.392- ☑
    pain T82.848- ☑
    specified type NEC T82.898- ☑
    stenosis T82.858- ☑
    thrombosis T82.868- ☑
  eye H57.9
    corneal graft — *see* Complications, graft, cornea
    implant (prosthetic) T85.9- ☑
      embolism T85.818- ☑
      fibrosis T85.828- ☑
      hemorrhage T85.838- ☑
      infection and inflammation T85.79- ☑
      mechanical
        breakdown T85.318- ☑
        displacement T85.328- ☑
        leakage T85.398- ☑
        malposition T85.328- ☑
        obstruction T85.398- ☑
        perforation T85.398- ☑
        protrusion T85.398- ☑
        specified NEC T85.398- ☑
      pain T85.848- ☑
      specified type NEC T85.898- ☑
      stenosis T85.858- ☑
      thrombosis T85.868- ☑
    intraocular lens — *see* Complications, intraocular lens
    orbital prosthesis — *see* Complications, orbital prosthesis
  female genital N94.9
    device, implant or graft NEC — *see* Complications, genitourinary, device or implant, genital tract
  femoral artery (bypass) graft — *see* Complication, extremity artery (bypass) graft
  fixation device, internal (orthopedic) T84.9- ☑
    infection and inflammation T84.60- ☑
      arm T84.61- ☑
        humerus T84.61- ☑
        radius T84.61- ☑
        ulna T84.61- ☑

☑ Additional Character Required — Refer to the Tabular List for Character Selection

Complication(s) — *continued*
    fixation device, internal — *continued*
        infection and inflammation — *continued*
            leg T84.629- ☑
                femur T84.62- ☑
                fibula T84.62- ☑
                tibia T84.62- ☑
            specified site NEC T84.89- ☑
            spine T84.63- ☑
        mechanical
            breakdown
                limb T84.119- ☑
                    carpal T84.210- ☑
                    femur T84.11- ☑
                    fibula T84.11- ☑
                    humerus T84.11- ☑
                    metacarpal T84.210- ☑
                    metatarsal T84.213- ☑
                    phalanx
                        foot T84.213- ☑
                        hand T84.210- ☑
                    radius T84.11- ☑
                    tarsal T84.213- ☑
                    tibia T84.11- ☑
                    ulna T84.11- ☑
                specified bone NEC T84.218- ☑
                spine T84.216- ☑
            displacement
                limb T84.129- ☑
                    carpal T84.220- ☑
                    femur T84.12- ☑
                    fibula T84.12- ☑
                    humerus T84.12- ☑
                    metacarpal T84.220- ☑
                    metatarsal T84.223- ☑
                    phalanx
                        foot T84.223- ☑
                        hand T84.220- ☑
                    radius T84.12- ☑
                    tarsal T84.223- ☑
                    tibia T84.12- ☑
                    ulna T84.12- ☑
                specified bone NEC T84.228- ☑
                spine T84.226- ☑
            malposition — *see* Complications, fixation device, internal, mechanical, displacement
            obstruction — *see* Complications, fixation device, internal, mechanical, specified type NEC
            perforation — *see* Complications, fixation device, internal, mechanical, specified type NEC
            protrusion — *see* Complications, fixation device, internal, mechanical, specified type NEC
            specified type NEC
                limb T84.199- ☑
                    carpal T84.290- ☑
                    femur T84.19- ☑
                    fibula T84.19- ☑
                    humerus T84.19- ☑
                    metacarpal T84.290- ☑
                    metatarsal T84.293- ☑
                    phalanx
                        foot T84.293- ☑
                        hand T84.290- ☑
                    radius T84.19- ☑
                    tarsal T84.293- ☑
                    tibia T84.19- ☑
                    ulna T84.19- ☑
                specified bone NEC T84.298- ☑
                vertebra T84.296- ☑
        specified type NEC T84.89- ☑
            embolism T84.81- ☑
            fibrosis T84.82- ☑
            hemorrhage T84.83- ☑
            pain T84.84- ☑
            specified complication NEC T84.89- ☑
            stenosis T84.85- ☑
            thrombosis T84.86- ☑
    following
        acute myocardial infarction NEC I23.8
            aneurysm (false) (of cardiac wall) (of heart wall) (ruptured) I23.3
            angina I23.7
            atrial
                septal defect I23.1
                thrombosis I23.6
            cardiac wall rupture I23.3

Complication(s) — *continued*
    following — *continued*
        acute myocardial infarction — *continued*
            chordae tendinae rupture I23.4
            defect
                septal
                    atrial (heart) I23.1
                    ventricular (heart) I23.2
            hemopericardium I23.0
            papillary muscle rupture I23.5
            rupture
                cardiac wall I23.3
                    with hemopericardium I23.0
                chordae tendineae I23.4
                papillary muscle I23.5
            specified NEC I23.8
            thrombosis
                atrium I23.6
                auricular appendage I23.6
                ventricle (heart) I23.6
            ventricular
                septal defect I23.2
                thrombosis I23.6
        ectopic or molar pregnancy O08.9
            cardiac arrest O08.81
            sepsis O08.82
            specified type NEC O08.89
            urinary tract infection O08.83
        termination of pregnancy — *see* Abortion
    gastrointestinal K92.9
        bile duct prosthesis — *see* Complications, bile duct implant
        esophageal anti-reflux device — *see* Complications, esophageal anti-reflux device
        postoperative
            colostomy — *see* Complications, colostomy
            dumping syndrome K91.1
            enterostomy — *see* Complications, enterostomy
            gastrostomy — *see* Complications, gastrostomy
            malabsorption NEC K91.2
            obstruction — *see also* Obstruction, intestine, postoperative K91.30
            postcholecystectomy syndrome K91.5
            specified NEC K91.89
            vomiting after GI surgery K91.0
        prosthetic device or implant
            bile duct prosthesis — *see* Complications, bile duct implant
            esophageal anti-reflux device — *see* Complications, esophageal anti-reflux device
            specified type NEC
                embolism T85.818- ☑
                fibrosis T85.828- ☑
                hemorrhage T85.838- ☑
                mechanical
                    breakdown T85.518- ☑
                    displacement T85.528- ☑
                    malfunction T85.518- ☑
                    malposition T85.528- ☑
                    obstruction T85.598- ☑
                    perforation T85.598- ☑
                    protrusion T85.598- ☑
                    specified NEC T85.598- ☑
                pain T85.848- ☑
                specified complication NEC T85.898- ☑
                stenosis T85.858- ☑
                thrombosis T85.868- ☑
    gastrostomy (stoma) K94.20
        hemorrhage K94.21
        infection K94.22
        malfunction K94.23
        mechanical K94.23
        specified complication NEC K94.29
    genitourinary
        device or implant T83.9- ☑
            genital tract T83.9- ☑
                infection or inflammation T83.69- ☑
                intrauterine contraceptive device — *see* Complications, intrauterine, contraceptive device
                mechanical — *see* Complications, by device, mechanical
                mesh — *see* Complications, prosthetic device or implant, mesh
                penile prosthesis — *see* Complications, prosthetic device, penile
                specified type NEC T83.89- ☑
                    embolism T83.81- ☑

Complication(s) — *continued*
    genitourinary — *continued*
        device or implant — *continued*
            genital tract — *continued*
                specified type — *continued*
                    fibrosis T83.82- ☑
                    hemorrhage T83.83- ☑
                    pain T83.84- ☑
                    specified complication NEC T83.89- ☑
                    stenosis T83.85- ☑
                    thrombosis T83.86- ☑
                vaginal mesh — *see* Complications, prosthetic device or implant, mesh
            urinary system T83.9- ☑
                cystostomy catheter — *see* Complication, catheter, cystostomy
                electronic stimulator — *see* Complications, electronic stimulator device, urinary
                indwelling urethral catheter — *see* Complications, catheter, urethral, indwelling
                infection or inflammation T83.598- ☑
                    indwelling urethral catheter T83.511- ☑
                kidney transplant — *see* Complication, transplant, kidney
                organ graft — *see* Complication, graft, urinary organ
                specified type NEC T83.89- ☑
                    embolism T83.81- ☑
                    fibrosis T83.82- ☑
                    hemorrhage T83.83- ☑
                    mechanical T83.198- ☑
                        breakdown T83.118- ☑
                        displacement T83.128- ☑
                        malfunction T83.118- ☑
                        malposition T83.128- ☑
                        obstruction T83.198- ☑
                        perforation T83.198- ☑
                        protrusion T83.198- ☑
                        specified NEC T83.198- ☑
                sphincter implant — *see* Complications, implant, urinary sphincter
                sphincter, implanted T83.191- ☑
                stent (ileal conduit) (nephroureteral) T83.193- ☑
                    pain T83.84- ☑
                    specified complication NEC T83.89- ☑
                    stenosis T83.85- ☑
                    thrombosis T83.86- ☑
                    ureteral indwelling T83.192- ☑
        postprocedural
            pelvic peritoneal adhesions N99.4
            renal failure N99.0
            specified NEC N99.89
            stoma — *see* Complications, stoma, urinary tract
            urethral stricture — *see* Stricture, urethra, postprocedural
            vaginal
                adhesions N99.2
                vault prolapse N99.3
    graft (bypass) (patch) — *see also* Complications, prosthetic device or implant
        aorta — *see* Complications, graft, vascular
        arterial — *see* Complication, graft, vascular
        bone T86.839
            failure T86.831
            infection T86.832
            mechanical T84.318- ☑
                breakdown T84.318- ☑
                displacement T84.328- ☑
                protrusion T84.398- ☑
                specified type NEC T84.398- ☑
            rejection T86.830
            specified type NEC T86.838
        carotid artery — *see* Complications, graft, vascular
        cornea T86.849- ☑
            failure T86.841- ☑
            infection T86.842- ☑
            mechanical T85.398- ☑
                breakdown T85.318- ☑
                displacement T85.328- ☑
                protrusion T85.398- ☑
                specified type NEC T85.398- ☑
            rejection T86.840- ☑
            retroprosthetic membrane T85.398- ☑
            specified type NEC T86.848- ☑
        femoral artery (bypass) — *see* Complication, extremity artery (bypass) graft

Complication(s) — *continued*
  graft — *see also* Complications, prosthetic device or implant — *continued*
    genital organ or tract — *see* Complications, genitourinary, device or implant, genital tract
    muscle T84.9- ☑
      breakdown T84.410- ☑
      displacement T84.420- ☑
      embolism T84.81- ☑
      fibrosis T84.82- ☑
      hemorrhage T84.83- ☑
      infection and inflammation T84.7- ☑
      mechanical NEC T84.490- ☑
      pain T84.84- ☑
      specified type NEC T84.89- ☑
      stenosis T84.85- ☑
      thrombosis T84.86- ☑
    nerve — *see* Complication, prosthetic device or implant, specified NEC
    skin — *see* Complications, prosthetic device or implant, skin graft
    tendon T84.9- ☑
      breakdown T84.410- ☑
      displacement T84.420- ☑
      embolism T84.81- ☑
      fibrosis T84.82- ☑
      hemorrhage T84.83- ☑
      infection and inflammation T84.7- ☑
      mechanical NEC T84.490- ☑
      pain T84.84- ☑
      specified type NEC T84.89- ☑
      stenosis T84.85- ☑
      thrombosis T84.86- ☑
    urinary organ T83.9- ☑
      embolism T83.81- ☑
      fibrosis T83.82- ☑
      hemorrhage T83.83- ☑
      infection and inflammation T83.598- ☑
        indwelling urethral catheter T83.511- ☑
      mechanical
        breakdown T83.21- ☑
        displacement T83.22- ☑
        erosion T83.24- ☑
        exposure T83.25- ☑
        leakage T83.23- ☑
        malposition T83.22- ☑
        obstruction T83.29- ☑
        perforation T83.29- ☑
        protrusion T83.29- ☑
        specified NEC T83.29- ☑
      pain T83.84- ☑
      specified type NEC T83.89- ☑
      stenosis T83.85- ☑
      thrombosis T83.86- ☑
    vascular T82.9- ☑
      embolism T82.818- ☑
      femoral artery — *see* Complication, extremity artery (bypass) graft
      fibrosis T82.828- ☑
      hemorrhage T82.838- ☑
      mechanical
        breakdown T82.319- ☑
          aorta (bifurcation) T82.310- ☑
          carotid artery T82.311- ☑
          specified vessel NEC T82.318- ☑
        displacement T82.329- ☑
          aorta (bifurcation) T82.320- ☑
          carotid artery T82.321- ☑
          specified vessel NEC T82.328- ☑
        leakage T82.339- ☑
          aorta (bifurcation) T82.330- ☑
          carotid artery T82.331- ☑
          specified vessel NEC T82.338- ☑
        malposition T82.329- ☑
          aorta (bifurcation) T82.320- ☑
          carotid artery T82.321- ☑
          specified vessel NEC T82.328- ☑
        obstruction T82.399- ☑
          aorta (bifurcation) T82.390- ☑
          carotid artery T82.391- ☑
          specified vessel NEC T82.398- ☑
        perforation T82.399- ☑
          aorta (bifurcation) T82.390- ☑
          carotid artery T82.391- ☑
          specified vessel NEC T82.398- ☑

Complication(s) — *continued*
  graft — *see also* Complications, prosthetic device or implant — *continued*
    vascular — *continued*
      mechanical — *continued*
        protrusion T82.399- ☑
          aorta (bifurcation) T82.390- ☑
          carotid artery T82.391- ☑
          specified vessel NEC T82.398- ☑
      pain T82.848- ☑
      specified complication NEC T82.898- ☑
      stenosis T82.858- ☑
      thrombosis T82.868- ☑
  heart I51.9
    assist device
      infection and inflammation T82.7- ☑
      following acute myocardial infarction — *see* Complications, following, acute myocardial infarction
      postoperative — *see* Complications, circulatory system
      transplant — *see* Complication, transplant, heart and lung(s) — *see* Complications, transplant, heart, with lung
    valve
      graft (biological) T82.9- ☑
        embolism T82.817- ☑
        fibrosis T82.827- ☑
        hemorrhage T82.837- ☑
        infection and inflammation T82.7- ☑
        mechanical T82.228- ☑
          breakdown T82.221- ☑
          displacement T82.222- ☑
          leakage T82.223- ☑
          malposition T82.222- ☑
          obstruction T82.228- ☑
          perforation T82.228- ☑
          protrusion T82.228- ☑
        pain T82.847- ☑
        specified type NEC T82.897- ☑
        stenosis T82.857- ☑
        thrombosis T82.867- ☑
      prosthesis T82.9- ☑
        embolism T82.817- ☑
        fibrosis T82.827- ☑
        hemorrhage T82.837- ☑
        infection or inflammation T82.6- ☑
        mechanical T82.09- ☑
          breakdown T82.01- ☑
          displacement T82.02- ☑
          leakage T82.03- ☑
          malposition T82.02- ☑
          obstruction T82.09- ☑
          perforation T82.09- ☑
          protrusion T82.09- ☑
        pain T82.847- ☑
        specified type NEC T82.897- ☑
          mechanical T82.09- ☑
        stenosis T82.857- ☑
        thrombosis T82.867- ☑
  hematoma
    intraoperative — *see* Complication, intraoperative, hemorrhage
    postprocedural — *see* Complication, postprocedural, hematoma
  hemodialysis — *see* Complications, dialysis
  hemorrhage
    intraoperative — *see* Complication, intraoperative, hemorrhage
    postprocedural — *see* Complication, postprocedural, hemorrhage
  IEC (immune effector cellular) therapy T80.82- ☑
  ileostomy (stoma) — *see* Complications, enterostomy
  immune effector cellular (IEC) therapy T80.82- ☑
  immunization (procedure) — *see* Complications, vaccination
  implant — *see also* Complications, by site and type
    urinary sphincter T83.9- ☑
      embolism T83.81- ☑
      fibrosis T83.82- ☑
      hemorrhage T83.83- ☑
      infection and inflammation T83.591- ☑
      mechanical
        breakdown T83.111- ☑
        displacement T83.121- ☑
        leakage T83.191- ☑
        malposition T83.121- ☑

Complication(s) — *continued*
  implant — *see also* Complications, by site and type — *continued*
    urinary sphincter — *continued*
      mechanical — *continued*
        obstruction T83.191- ☑
        perforation T83.191- ☑
        protrusion T83.191- ☑
        specified NEC T83.191- ☑
      pain T83.84- ☑
      specified type NEC T83.89- ☑
      stenosis T83.85- ☑
      thrombosis T83.86- ☑
  infusion (procedure) T80.90- ☑
    air embolism T80.0- ☑
    blood — *see* Complications, transfusion
    catheter — *see* Complications, catheter
    infection T80.29- ☑
    pump — *see* Complications, cardiovascular, device or implant
    sepsis T80.29- ☑
    serum reaction — *see also* Reaction, serum T80.69- ☑
      anaphylactic shock — *see also* Shock, anaphylactic T80.59- ☑
    specified type NEC T80.89- ☑
  inhalation therapy NEC T81.81- ☑
  injection (procedure) T80.90- ☑
    drug reaction — *see* Reaction, drug
    infection T80.29- ☑
    sepsis T80.29- ☑
    serum (prophylactic) (therapeutic) — *see* Complications, vaccination
    specified type NEC T80.89- ☑
    vaccine (any) — *see* Complications, vaccination
  inoculation (any) — *see* Complications, vaccination
  insulin pump
    infection and inflammation T85.72- ☑
    mechanical
      breakdown T85.614- ☑
      displacement T85.624- ☑
      leakage T85.633- ☑
      malposition T85.624- ☑
      obstruction T85.694- ☑
      perforation T85.694- ☑
      protrusion T85.694- ☑
      specified NEC T85.694- ☑
  intestinal pouch NEC K91.858
  intraocular lens (prosthetic) T85.9- ☑
    embolism T85.818- ☑
    fibrosis T85.828- ☑
    hemorrhage T85.838- ☑
    infection and inflammation T85.79- ☑
    mechanical
      breakdown T85.21- ☑
      displacement T85.22- ☑
      malposition T85.22- ☑
      obstruction T85.29- ☑
      perforation T85.29- ☑
      protrusion T85.29- ☑
      specified NEC T85.29- ☑
    pain T85.848- ☑
    specified type NEC T85.898- ☑
    stenosis T85.858- ☑
    thrombosis T85.868- ☑
  intraoperative (intraprocedural)
    cardiac arrest — *see also* Infarct, myocardium, associated with revascularization procedure
      during cardiac surgery I97.710
      during other surgery I97.711
    cardiac functional disturbance NEC — *see also* Infarct, myocardium, associated with revascularization procedure
      during cardiac surgery I97.790
      during other surgery I97.791
    hemorrhage (hematoma) (of)
      circulatory system organ or structure
        during cardiac bypass I97.411
        during cardiac catheterization I97.410
        during other circulatory system procedure I97.418
        during other procedure I97.42
      digestive system organ
        during procedure on digestive system K91.61
        during procedure on other organ K91.62
      ear
        during procedure on ear and mastoid process H95.21

☑ Additional Character Required — Refer to the Tabular List for Character Selection

Complication(s) — *continued*
  intraoperative — *continued*
    hemorrhage — *continued*
      ear — *continued*
        during procedure on other organ H95.22
      endocrine system organ or structure
        during procedure on endocrine system organ or structure E36.01
        during procedure on other organ E36.02
      eye and adnexa
        during ophthalmic procedure H59.11- ☑
        during other procedure H59.12- ☑
      genitourinary organ or structure
        during procedure on genitourinary organ or structure N99.61
        during procedure on other organ N99.62
      mastoid process
        during procedure on ear and mastoid process H95.21
        during procedure on other organ H95.22
      musculoskeletal structure
        during musculoskeletal surgery M96.810
        during non-orthopedic surgery M96.811
        during orthopedic surgery M96.810
      nervous system
        during a nervous system procedure G97.31
        during other procedure G97.32
      respiratory system
        during other procedure J95.62
        during procedure on respiratory system organ or structure J95.61
      skin and subcutaneous tissue
        during a dermatologic procedure L76.01
        during a procedure on other organ L76.02
      spleen
        during a procedure on other organ D78.02
        during a procedure on the spleen D78.01
    puncture or laceration (accidental) (unintentional) (of)
      brain
        during a nervous system procedure G97.48
        during other procedure G97.49
      circulatory system organ or structure
        during circulatory system procedure I97.51
        during other procedure I97.52
      digestive system
        during procedure on digestive system K91.71
        during procedure on other organ K91.72
      ear
        during procedure on ear and mastoid process H95.31
        during procedure on other organ H95.32
      endocrine system organ or structure
        during procedure on endocrine system organ or structure E36.11
        during procedure on other organ E36.12
      eye and adnexa
        during ophthalmic procedure H59.21- ☑
        during other procedure H59.22- ☑
      genitourinary organ or structure
        during procedure on genitourinary organ or structure N99.71
        during procedure on other organ N99.72
      mastoid process
        during procedure on ear and mastoid process H95.31
        during procedure on other organ H95.32
      musculoskeletal structure
        during musculoskeletal surgery M96.820
        during non-orthopedic surgery M96.821
        during orthopedic surgery M96.820
      nervous system
        during a nervous system procedure G97.48
        during other procedure G97.49
      respiratory system
        during other procedure J95.72
        during procedure on respiratory system organ or structure J95.71
      skin and subcutaneous tissue
        during a dermatologic procedure L76.11
        during a procedure on other organ L76.12
      spleen
        during a procedure on other organ D78.12
        during a procedure on the spleen D78.11
    specified NEC
      circulatory system I97.88
      digestive system K91.81
      ear H95.88
      endocrine system E36.8

Complication(s) — *continued*
  intraoperative — *continued*
    specified — *continued*
      eye and adnexa H59.88
      genitourinary system N99.81
      mastoid process H95.88
      musculoskeletal structure M96.89
      nervous system G97.81
      respiratory system J95.88
      skin and subcutaneous tissue L76.81
      spleen D78.81
  intraperitoneal catheter (dialysis) (infusion) — *see* Complication(s), catheter, intraperitoneal dialysis
  intrathecal infusion pump
    infection and inflammation T85.738- ☑
    mechanical
      breakdown T85.615- ☑
      displacement T85.625- ☑
      leakage T85.635- ☑
      malfunction T85.695- ☑
      malposition T85.625- ☑
      obstruction T85.695- ☑
      perforation T85.695- ☑
      protrusion T85.695- ☑
      specified NEC T85.695- ☑
  intrauterine
    contraceptive device
      embolism T83.81- ☑
      fibrosis T83.82- ☑
      hemorrhage T83.83- ☑
      infection and inflammation T83.69- ☑
      mechanical
        breakdown T83.31- ☑
        displacement T83.32- ☑
        malposition T83.32- ☑
        obstruction T83.39- ☑
        perforation T83.39- ☑
        protrusion T83.39- ☑
        specified NEC T83.39- ☑
      pain T83.84- ☑
      specified type NEC T83.89- ☑
      stenosis T83.85- ☑
      thrombosis T83.86- ☑
    procedure (fetal), to newborn P96.5
  jejunostomy (stoma) — *see* Complications, enterostomy
  joint prosthesis, internal T84.9- ☑
    breakage (fracture) T84.01- ☑
    dislocation T84.02- ☑
    fracture T84.01- ☑
    infection or inflammation T84.50- ☑
      hip T84.5- ☑
      knee T84.5- ☑
      specified joint NEC T84.59- ☑
    instability T84.02- ☑
    malposition — *see* Complications, joint prosthesis, mechanical, displacement
    mechanical
      breakage, broken T84.01- ☑
      dislocation T84.02- ☑
      displacement T84.02- ☑
      fracture T84.01- ☑
      instability T84.02- ☑
      leakage — *see* Complications, joint prosthesis, mechanical, specified NEC
      loosening T84.039- ☑
        hip T84.03- ☑
        knee T84.03- ☑
        specified joint NEC T84.038- ☑
      obstruction — *see* Complications, joint prosthesis, mechanical, specified NEC
      osteolysis T84.059- ☑
        hip T84.05- ☑
        knee T84.05- ☑
      perforation — *see* Complications, joint prosthesis, mechanical, specified NEC
        osteolysis T84.059- ☑
        other specified joint T84.058- ☑
      periprosthetic osteolysis, by site T84.05- ☑
      protrusion — *see* Complications, joint prosthesis, mechanical, specified NEC
      specified complication NEC T84.099- ☑
        hip T84.09- ☑
        knee T84.09- ☑
        other specified joint T84.098- ☑
      subluxation T84.02- ☑
      wear of articular bearing surface T84.069- ☑

Complication(s) — *continued*
  joint prosthesis, internal — *continued*
    mechanical — *continued*
      wear of articular bearing surface — *continued*
        hip T84.06- ☑
        knee T84.06- ☑
        other specified joint T84.068- ☑
    specified joint NEC T84.89- ☑
      embolism T84.81- ☑
      fibrosis T84.82- ☑
      hemorrhage T84.83- ☑
      pain T84.84- ☑
      specified complication NEC T84.89- ☑
      stenosis T84.85- ☑
      thrombosis T84.86- ☑
    subluxation T84.02- ☑
  kidney transplant — *see* Complications, transplant, kidney
  labor O75.9
    specified NEC O75.89
  liver transplant (immune or nonimmune) — *see* Complications, transplant, liver
  lumbar puncture G97.1
    cerebrospinal fluid leak G97.0
    headache or reaction G97.1
  lung transplant — *see* Complications, transplant, lung
    and heart — *see* Complications, transplant, lung, with heart
  male genital N50.9
    device, implant or graft — *see* Complications, genitourinary, device or implant, genital tract
    postprocedural or postoperative — *see* Complications, genitourinary, postprocedural
    specified NEC N99.89
  mastoid (process) procedure
    intraoperative H95.88
      hematoma — *see* Complications, intraoperative, hemorrhage (hematoma) (of), mastoid process
      hemorrhage — *see* Complications, intraoperative, hemorrhage (hematoma) (of), mastoid process
      laceration — *see* Complications, intraoperative, puncture or laceration, mastoid process
      specified NEC H95.88
    postmastoidectomy — *see* Complications, postmastoidectomy
    postoperative H95.89
      external ear canal stenosis H95.81- ☑
      hematoma — *see* Complications, postprocedural, hematoma (of), mastoid process
      hemorrhage — *see* Complications, postprocedural, hemorrhage (of), mastoid process
      postmastoidectomy — *see* Complications, postmastoidectomy
      seroma — *see* Complications, postprocedural, seroma (of), mastoid process
      specified NEC H95.89
  mastoidectomy cavity — *see* Complications, postmastoidectomy
  mechanical — *see* Complications, by site and type, mechanical
  medical procedures — *see also* Complication(s), intraoperative T88.9- ☑
  metabolic E88.9
    postoperative E89.89
    specified NEC E89.89
  molar pregnancy NOS O08.9
    damage to pelvic organs O08.6
    embolism O08.2
    genital infection O08.0
    hemorrhage (delayed) (excessive) O08.1
    metabolic disorder O08.5
    renal failure O08.4
    shock O08.3
    specified type NEC O08.8
    venous complication NEC O08.7
  musculoskeletal system — *see also* Complication, intraoperative (intraprocedural), by site
    device, implant or graft NEC — *see* Complications, orthopedic, device or implant
    internal fixation (nail) (plate) (rod) — *see* Complications, fixation device, internal
    joint prosthesis — *see* Complications, joint prosthesis
    post radiation M96.89
      kyphosis M96.2
      scoliosis M96.5
      specified complication NEC M96.89

Complication(s) — *continued*
- musculoskeletal system — *see also* Complication, intraoperative, by site — *continued*
  - postoperative (postprocedural) M96.89
    - with osteoporosis — *see* Osteoporosis
    - fracture following insertion of device — *see* Fracture, following insertion of orthopedic implant, joint prosthesis or bone plate
    - joint instability after prosthesis removal M96.89
    - lordosis M96.4
    - postlaminectomy syndrome NEC M96.1
      - kyphosis M96.3
    - pseudarthrosis M96.0
    - specified complication NEC M96.89
- nephrostomy (stoma) — *see* Complications, stoma, urinary tract, external NEC
- nervous system G98.8
  - central G96.9
  - device, implant or graft — *see also* Complication, prosthetic device or implant, specified NEC
    - electronic stimulator (electrode(s)) — *see* Complications, electronic stimulator device
    - specified NEC
      - infection and inflammation T85.738- ☑
      - mechanical T85.695- ☑
        - breakdown T85.615- ☑
        - displacement T85.625- ☑
        - leakage T85.635- ☑
        - malfunction T85.695- ☑
        - malposition T85.625- ☑
        - obstruction T85.695- ☑
        - perforation T85.695- ☑
        - protrusion T85.695- ☑
        - specified NEC T85.695- ☑
    - ventricular shunt — *see* Complications, ventricular shunt
  - electronic stimulator (electrode(s)) — *see* Complications, electronic stimulator device
  - postprocedural G97.82
    - intracranial hypotension G97.2
    - specified NEC G97.82
    - spinal fluid leak G97.0
- newborn, due to intrauterine (fetal) procedure P96.5
- nonabsorbable (permanent) sutures — *see* Complication, sutures, permanent
- obstetric O75.9
  - procedure (instrumental) (manual) (surgical) specified NEC O75.4
  - specified NEC O75.89
  - surgical wound NEC O90.89
    - hematoma O90.2
    - infection O86.00
- ocular lens implant — *see* Complications, intraocular lens
- ophthalmologic
  - postprocedural bleb — *see* Blebitis
- orbital prosthesis T85.9- ☑
  - embolism T85.818- ☑
  - fibrosis T85.828- ☑
  - hemorrhage T85.838- ☑
  - infection and inflammation T85.79- ☑
  - mechanical
    - breakdown T85.31- ☑
    - displacement T85.32- ☑
    - malposition T85.32- ☑
    - obstruction T85.39- ☑
    - perforation T85.39- ☑
    - protrusion T85.39- ☑
    - specified NEC T85.39- ☑
  - pain T85.848- ☑
  - specified type NEC T85.898- ☑
  - stenosis T85.858- ☑
  - thrombosis T85.868- ☑
- organ or tissue transplant (partial) (total) — *see* Complications, transplant
- orthopedic — *see also* Disorder, soft tissue
  - device or implant T84.9- ☑
    - bone
      - device or implant — *see* Complication, bone, device NEC
      - graft — *see* Complication, graft, bone
      - breakdown T84.418- ☑
      - displacement T84.428- ☑
      - electronic bone stimulator — *see* Complications, electronic stimulator device, bone
      - embolism T84.81- ☑
      - fibrosis T84.82- ☑

Complication(s) — *continued*
- orthopedic — *see also* Disorder, soft tissue — *continued*
  - device or implant — *continued*
    - fixation device — *see* Complication, fixation device, internal
    - hemorrhage T84.83- ☑
    - infection or inflammation T84.7- ☑
    - joint prosthesis — *see* Complication, joint prosthesis, internal
    - malfunction T84.418- ☑
    - malposition T84.428- ☑
    - mechanical NEC T84.498- ☑
    - muscle graft — *see* Complications, graft, muscle
    - obstruction T84.498- ☑
    - pain T84.84- ☑
    - perforation T84.498- ☑
    - protrusion T84.498- ☑
    - specified complication NEC T84.89- ☑
    - stenosis T84.85- ☑
    - tendon graft — *see* Complications, graft, tendon
    - thrombosis T84.86- ☑
  - fracture (following insertion of device) — *see* Fracture, following insertion of orthopedic implant, joint prosthesis or bone plate
  - postprocedural M96.89
    - fracture — *see* Fracture, following insertion of orthopedic implant, joint prosthesis or bone plate
    - postlaminectomy syndrome NEC M96.1
      - kyphosis M96.3
      - lordosis M96.4
    - postradiation
      - kyphosis M96.2
      - scoliosis M96.5
    - pseudarthrosis post-fusion M96.0
    - specified type NEC M96.89
- pacemaker (cardiac) — *see* Complications, cardiovascular device or implant, electronic
- pancreas transplant — *see* Complications, transplant, pancreas
- penile prosthesis (implant) — *see* Complications, prosthetic device, penile
- perfusion NEC T80.90- ☑
- perineal repair (obstetrical) NEC O90.89
  - disruption O90.1
  - hematoma O90.2
  - infection (following delivery) O86.09
- phototherapy T88.9- ☑
  - specified NEC T88.8- ☑
- postmastoidectomy NEC H95.19- ☑
  - cyst, mucosal H95.13- ☑
  - granulation H95.12- ☑
  - inflammation, chronic H95.11- ☑
  - recurrent cholesteatoma H95.0- ☑
- postoperative — *see* Complications, postprocedural
  - circulatory — *see* Complications, circulatory system
  - ear — *see* Complications, ear
  - endocrine — *see* Complications, endocrine
  - eye — *see* Complications, eye
  - lumbar puncture G97.1
    - cerebrospinal fluid leak G97.0
  - nervous system (central) (peripheral) — *see* Complications, nervous system
  - respiratory system — *see* Complications, respiratory system
- postprocedural — *see also* Complications, surgical procedure
  - cardiac arrest — *see also* Infarct, myocardium, associated with revascularization procedure
    - following cardiac surgery I97.120
    - following other surgery I97.121
  - cardiac functional disturbance NEC — *see also* Infarct, myocardium, associated with revascularization procedure
    - following cardiac surgery I97.190
    - following other surgery I97.191
  - cardiac insufficiency
    - following cardiac surgery I97.110
    - following other surgery I97.111
  - chorioretinal scars following retinal surgery H59.81-
  - following cataract surgery
    - cataract (lens) fragments H59.02- ☑
    - cystoid macular edema H59.03- ☑
    - specified NEC H59.09- ☑
    - vitreous (touch) syndrome H59.01- ☑

Complication(s) — *continued*
- postprocedural — *see also* Complications, surgical procedure — *continued*
  - heart failure
    - following cardiac surgery I97.130
    - following other surgery I97.131
  - hematoma (of)
    - circulatory system organ or structure
      - following cardiac bypass I97.631
      - following cardiac catheterization I97.630
      - following other circulatory system procedure I97.638
      - following other procedure I97.621
    - digestive system
      - following procedure on digestive system K91.870
      - following procedure on other organ K91.871
    - ear
      - following other procedure H95.52
      - following procedure on ear and mastoid process H95.51
    - endocrine system
      - following endocrine system procedure E89.820
      - following other procedure E89.821
    - eye and adnexa
      - following ophthalmic procedure H59.33- ☑
      - following other procedure H59.34- ☑
    - genitourinary organ or structure
      - following procedure on genitourinary organ or structure N99.840
      - following procedure on other organ N99.841
    - mastoid process
      - following other procedure H95.52
      - following procedure on ear and mastoid process H95.51
    - musculoskeletal structure
      - following musculoskeletal surgery M96.840
      - following non-orthopedic surgery M96.841
      - following orthopedic surgery M96.840
    - nervous system
      - following nervous system procedure G97.61
      - following other procedure G97.62
    - respiratory system
      - following other procedure J95.861
      - following procedure on respiratory system organ or structure J95.860
    - skin and subcutaneous tissue
      - following dermatologic procedure L76.31
      - following procedure on other organ L76.32
    - spleen
      - following procedure on other organ D78.32
      - following procedure on the spleen D78.31
  - hemorrhage (of)
    - circulatory system organ or structure
      - following cardiac bypass I97.611
      - following cardiac catheterization I97.610
      - following other circulatory system procedure I97.618
      - following other procedure I97.620
    - digestive system
      - following procedure on digestive system K91.840
      - following procedure on other organ K91.841
    - ear
      - following other procedure H95.42
      - following procedure on ear and mastoid process H95.41
    - endocrine system
      - following endocrine system procedure E89.810
      - following other procedure E89.811
    - eye and adnexa
      - following ophthalmic procedure H59.31- ☑
      - following other procedure H59.32- ☑
    - genitourinary organ or structure
      - following procedure on genitourinary organ or structure N99.820
      - following procedure on other organ N99.821
    - mastoid process
      - following other procedure H95.42
      - following procedure on ear and mastoid process H95.41
    - musculoskeletal structure
      - following musculoskeletal surgery M96.830
      - following non-orthopedic surgery M96.831
      - following orthopedic surgery M96.830
    - nervous system
      - following nervous system procedure G97.51
      - following other procedure G97.52

☑ **Additional Character Required — Refer to the Tabular List for Character Selection**

Complication

Complication(s) — *continued*
- postprocedural — *see also* Complications, surgical procedure — *continued*
  - hemorrhage — *continued*
    - respiratory system
      - following a respiratory system procedure J95.830
      - following other procedure J95.831
    - skin and subcutaneous tissue
      - following a procedure on other organ L76.22
      - following dermatologic procedure L76.21
    - spleen
      - following procedure on other organ D78.22
      - following procedure on the spleen D78.21
  - seroma (of)
    - circulatory system organ or structure
      - following cardiac bypass I97.641
      - following cardiac catheterization I97.640
      - following other circulatory system procedure I97.648
      - following other procedure I97.622
    - digestive system
      - following procedure on digestive system K91.872
      - following procedure on other organ K91.873
    - ear
      - following other procedure H95.54
      - following procedure on ear and mastoid process H95.53
    - endocrine system
      - following endocrine system procedure E89.822
      - following other procedure E89.823
    - eye and adnexa
      - following ophthalmic procedure H59.35- ☑
      - following other procedure H59.36- ☑
    - genitourinary organ or structure
      - following procedure on genitourinary organ or structure N99.842
      - following procedure on other organ N99.843
    - mastoid process
      - following other procedure H95.54
      - following procedure on ear and mastoid process H95.53
    - musculoskeletal structure
      - following musculoskeletal surgery M96.842
      - following non-orthopedic surgery M96.843
      - following orthopedic surgery M96.842
    - nervous system
      - following nervous system procedure G97.63
      - following other procedure G97.64
    - respiratory system
      - following other procedure J95.863
      - following procedure on respiratory system organ or structure J95.862
    - skin and subcutaneous tissue
      - following dermatologic procedure L76.33
      - following procedure on other organ L76.34
    - spleen
      - following procedure on other organ D78.34
      - following procedure on the spleen D78.33
  - specified NEC
    - circulatory system I97.89
    - digestive K91.89
    - ear H95.89
    - endocrine E89.89
    - eye and adnexa H59.89
    - genitourinary N99.89
    - mastoid process H95.89
    - metabolic E89.89
    - musculoskeletal structure M96.89
    - nervous system G97.82
    - respiratory system J95.89
    - skin and subcutaneous tissue L76.82
    - spleen D78.89
- pregnancy NEC — *see* Pregnancy, complicated by
- prosthetic device or implant T85.9- ☑
  - bile duct — *see* Complications, bile duct implant
  - breast — *see* Complications, breast implant
  - bulking agent
    - ureteral
      - erosion T83.714- ☑
      - exposure T83.724- ☑
    - urethral
      - erosion T83.713- ☑
      - exposure T83.723- ☑
  - cardiac and vascular NEC — *see* Complications, cardiovascular device or implant
  - corneal transplant — *see* Complications, graft, cornea

Complication(s) — *continued*
- prosthetic device or implant — *continued*
  - electronic nervous system stimulator — *see* Complications, electronic stimulator device
  - epidural infusion catheter — *see* Complications, catheter, epidural
  - esophageal anti-reflux device — *see* Complications, esophageal anti-reflux device
  - genital organ or tract — *see* Complications, genitourinary, device or implant, genital tract
    - specified NEC T83.79- ☑
  - heart valve — *see* Complications, heart, valve, prosthesis
  - infection or inflammation T85.79- ☑
    - intestine transplant T86.852
    - liver transplant T86.43
    - lung transplant T86.812
    - pancreas transplant T86.892
    - skin graft T86.822
  - intraocular lens — *see* Complications, intraocular lens
  - intraperitoneal (dialysis) catheter — *see* Complication(s), catheter, intraperitoneal dialysis
  - joint — *see* Complications, joint prosthesis, internal
  - mechanical NEC T85.698- ☑
    - dialysis catheter (vascular) — *see also* Complication, catheter, dialysis, mechanical
      - peritoneal — *see* Complication(s), catheter, intraperitoneal dialysis
    - gastrointestinal device T85.598- ☑
    - ocular device T85.398- ☑
    - subdural (infusion) catheter T85.690- ☑
    - suture, permanent T85.692- ☑
      - that for bone repair — *see* Complications, fixation device, internal (orthopedic), mechanical
    - ventricular shunt
      - breakdown T85.01- ☑
      - displacement T85.02- ☑
      - leakage T85.03- ☑
      - malposition T85.02- ☑
      - obstruction T85.09- ☑
      - perforation T85.09- ☑
      - protrusion T85.09- ☑
      - specified NEC T85.09- ☑
  - mesh
    - erosion (to surrounding organ or tissue) T83.718- ☑
      - urethral (into pelvic floor muscles) T83.712- ☑
      - vaginal (into pelvic floor muscles) T83.711- ☑
    - exposure (into surrounding organ or tissue) T83.728- ☑
      - urethral (through urethral wall) T83.722- ☑
      - vaginal (into vagina) (through vaginal wall) T83.721- ☑
  - orbital — *see* Complications, orbital prosthesis
  - penile T83.9- ☑
    - embolism T83.81- ☑
    - fibrosis T83.82- ☑
    - hemorrhage T83.83- ☑
    - infection and inflammation T83.61- ☑
    - mechanical
      - breakdown T83.410- ☑
      - displacement T83.420- ☑
      - leakage T83.490- ☑
      - malposition T83.420- ☑
      - obstruction T83.490- ☑
      - perforation T83.490- ☑
      - protrusion T83.490- ☑
      - specified NEC T83.490- ☑
    - pain T83.84- ☑
    - specified type NEC T83.89- ☑
    - stenosis T83.85- ☑
    - thrombosis T83.86- ☑
  - prosthetic materials NEC
    - erosion (to surrounding organ or tissue) T83.718- ☑
    - exposure (into surrounding organ or tissue) T83.728- ☑
  - skin graft T86.829
    - artificial skin or decellularized allodermis
      - embolism T85.818- ☑
      - fibrosis T85.828- ☑
      - hemorrhage T85.838- ☑
      - infection and inflammation T85.79- ☑
      - mechanical
        - breakdown T85.613- ☑
        - displacement T85.623- ☑

Complication(s) — *continued*
- prosthetic device or implant — *continued*
  - skin graft — *continued*
    - artificial skin or decellularized allodermis — *continued*
      - mechanical — *continued*
        - malfunction T85.613- ☑
        - malposition T85.623- ☑
        - obstruction T85.693- ☑
        - perforation T85.693- ☑
        - protrusion T85.693- ☑
        - specified NEC T85.693- ☑
      - pain T85.848- ☑
      - specified type NEC T85.898- ☑
      - stenosis T85.858- ☑
      - thrombosis T85.868- ☑
    - failure T86.821
    - infection T86.822
    - rejection T86.820
    - specified NEC T86.828
  - sling
    - urethral (female) (male)
      - erosion T83.712- ☑
      - exposure T83.722- ☑
  - specified NEC T85.9- ☑
    - embolism T85.818- ☑
    - fibrosis T85.828- ☑
    - hemorrhage T85.838- ☑
    - infection and inflammation T85.79- ☑
    - mechanical
      - breakdown T85.618- ☑
      - displacement T85.628- ☑
      - leakage T85.638- ☑
      - malfunction T85.618- ☑
      - malposition T85.628- ☑
      - obstruction T85.698- ☑
      - perforation T85.698- ☑
      - protrusion T85.698- ☑
      - specified NEC T85.698- ☑
    - pain T85.848- ☑
    - specified type NEC T85.898- ☑
    - stenosis T85.858- ☑
    - thrombosis T85.868- ☑
  - subdural infusion catheter — *see* Complications, catheter, subdural
  - sutures — *see* Complications, sutures
  - urinary organ or tract NEC — *see* Complications, genitourinary, device or implant, urinary system
  - vascular — *see* Complications, cardiovascular device, graft or implant
  - ventricular shunt — *see* Complications, ventricular shunt (device)
- puerperium — *see* Puerperal
- puncture, spinal G97.1
  - cerebrospinal fluid leak G97.0
  - headache or reaction G97.1
- pyelogram N99.89
- radiation
  - kyphosis M96.2
  - scoliosis M96.5
- reattached
  - extremity (infection) (rejection)
    - lower T87.1X- ☑
    - upper T87.0X- ☑
  - specified body part NEC T87.2
- reconstructed breast
  - asymmetry between native and reconstructed breast N65.1
  - deformity N65.0
  - disproportion between native and reconstructed breast N65.1
  - excess tissue N65.0
  - misshappen N65.0
- reimplant NEC — *see also* Complications, prosthetic device or implant
  - limb (infection) (rejection) — *see* Complications, reattached, extremity
  - organ (partial) (total) — *see* Complications, transplant
  - prosthetic device NEC — *see* Complications, prosthetic device
- renal N28.9
  - allograft — *see* Complications, transplant, kidney
  - dialysis — *see* Complications, dialysis
- respirator
  - mechanical J95.850
    - specified NEC J95.859
- respiratory system J98.9

Complication(s) — *continued*
　respiratory system — *continued*
　　device, implant or graft — *see* Complication, prosthetic device or implant, specified NEC
　　lung transplant — *see* Complications, prosthetic device or implant, lung transplant
　　postoperative J95.89
　　　air leak J95.812
　　　Mendelson's syndrome (chemical pneumonitis) J95.4
　　　pneumothorax J95.811
　　　pulmonary insufficiency (acute) (after nonthoracic surgery) J95.2
　　　　chronic J95.3
　　　　following thoracic surgery J95.1
　　　respiratory failure (acute) J95.821
　　　　acute and chronic J95.822
　　　specified NEC J95.89
　　　subglottic stenosis J95.5
　　　tracheostomy complication — *see* Complications, tracheostomy
　　therapy T81.89- ☑
　sedation during labor and delivery O74.9
　　cardiac O74.2
　　central nervous system O74.3
　　pulmonary NEC O74.1
　shunt — *see also* Complications, prosthetic device or implant
　　arteriovenous — *see* Complications, arteriovenous, shunt
　　ventricular (communicating) — *see* Complications, ventricular shunt
　skin
　　graft T86.829
　　　failure T86.821
　　　infection T86.822
　　　rejection T86.820
　　　specified type NEC T86.828
　spinal
　　anesthesia — *see* Complications, anesthesia, spinal
　　catheter (epidural) (subdural) — *see* Complications, catheter
　　puncture or tap G97.1
　　　cerebrospinal fluid leak G97.0
　　　headache or reaction G97.1
　stent
　　bile duct — *see* Complications, bile duct prosthesis
　　ureteral indwelling
　　　breakdown T83.112- ☑
　　　displacement T83.122- ☑
　　　leakage T83.192- ☑
　　　malposition T83.122- ☑
　　　obstruction T83.192- ☑
　　　perforation T83.192- ☑
　　　protrusion T83.192- ☑
　　　specified NEC T83.192- ☑
　　urinary NEC (ileal conduit) (nephroureteral) T83.193- ☑
　　　embolism T83.81- ☑
　　　fibrosis T83.82- ☑
　　　hemorrhage T83.83- ☑
　　　infection and inflammation T83.593- ☑
　　　mechanical
　　　　breakdown T83.113- ☑
　　　　displacement T83.123- ☑
　　　　leakage T83.193- ☑
　　　　malposition T83.123- ☑
　　　　obstruction T83.193- ☑
　　　　perforation T83.193- ☑
　　　　protrusion T83.193- ☑
　　　　specified NEC T83.193- ☑
　　　pain T83.84- ☑
　　　specified type NEC T83.89- ☑
　　　stenosis T83.85- ☑
　　　thrombosis T83.86- ☑
　　vascular
　　　end stent stenosis — *see* Restenosis, stent
　　　in stent stenosis — *see* Restenosis, stent
　stoma
　　digestive tract
　　　colostomy — *see* Complications, colostomy
　　　enterostomy — *see* Complications, enterostomy
　　　esophagostomy — *see* Complications, esophagostomy
　　　gastrostomy — *see* Complications, gastrostomy
　　urinary tract N99.528
　　　continent N99.538
　　　　hemorrhage N99.530

Complication(s) — *continued*
　stoma — *continued*
　　urinary tract — *continued*
　　　continent — *continued*
　　　　herniation N99.533
　　　　infection N99.531
　　　　malfunction N99.532
　　　　specified type NEC N99.538
　　　　stenosis N99.534
　　　cystostomy — *see* Complications, cystostomy
　　　external NOS N99.528
　　　hemorrhage N99.520
　　　herniation N99.523
　　　incontinent N99.528
　　　　hemorrhage N99.520
　　　　herniation N99.523
　　　　infection N99.521
　　　　malfunction N99.522
　　　　specified type NEC N99.528
　　　　stenosis N99.524
　　　infection N99.521
　　　malfunction N99.522
　　　specified type NEC N99.528
　　　stenosis N99.524
　stomach banding — *see* Complication(s), bariatric procedure
　stomach stapling — *see* Complication(s), bariatric procedure
　surgical material, nonabsorbable — *see* Complication, suture, permanent
　surgical procedure (on) T81.9- ☑
　　amputation stump (late) — *see* Complications, amputation stump
　　cardiac — *see* Complications, circulatory system
　　cholesteatoma, recurrent — *see* Complications, postmastoidectomy, recurrent cholesteatoma
　　circulatory (early) — *see* Complications, circulatory system
　　digestive system — *see* Complications, gastrointestinal
　　dumping syndrome (postgastrectomy) K91.1
　　ear — *see* Complications, ear
　　elephantiasis or lymphedema I97.89
　　　postmastectomy I97.2
　　emphysema (surgical) T81.82- ☑
　　endocrine — *see* Complications, endocrine
　　eye — *see* Complications, eye
　　fistula (persistent postoperative) T81.83- ☑
　　foreign body inadvertently left in wound (sponge) (suture) (swab) — *see* Foreign body, accidentally left during a procedure
　　gastrointestinal — *see* Complications, gastrointestinal
　　genitourinary NEC N99.89
　　hematoma
　　　intraoperative — *see* Complication, intraoperative, hemorrhage
　　　postprocedural — *see* Complication, postprocedural, hematoma
　　hemorrhage
　　　intraoperative — *see* Complication, intraoperative, hemorrhage
　　　postprocedural — *see* Complication, postprocedural, hemorrhage
　　hepatic failure K91.82
　　hyperglycemia (postpancreatectomy) E89.1
　　hypoinsulinemia (postpancreatectomy) E89.1
　　hypoparathyroidism (postparathyroidectomy) E89.2
　　hypopituitarism (posthypophysectomy) E89.3
　　hypothyroidism (post-thyroidectomy) E89.0
　　intestinal obstruction — *see also* Obstruction, intestine, postoperative K91.30
　　intracranial hypotension following ventricular shunting (ventriculostomy) G97.2
　　lymphedema I97.89
　　　postmastectomy I97.2
　　malabsorption (postsurgical) NEC K91.2
　　　osteoporosis — *see* Osteoporosis, postsurgical malabsorption
　　mastoidectomy cavity NEC — *see* Complications, postmastoidectomy
　　metabolic E89.89
　　　specified NEC E89.89
　　musculoskeletal — *see* Complications, musculoskeletal system
　　nervous system (central) (peripheral) — *see* Complications, nervous system
　　ovarian failure E89.40
　　　asymptomatic E89.40
　　　symptomatic E89.41

Complication(s) — *continued*
　surgical procedure — *continued*
　　peripheral vascular — *see* Complications, surgical procedure, vascular
　　postcardiotomy syndrome I97.0
　　postcholecystectomy syndrome K91.5
　　postcommissurotomy syndrome I97.0
　　postgastrectomy dumping syndrome K91.1
　　postlaminectomy syndrome NEC M96.1
　　　kyphosis M96.3
　　postmastectomy lymphedema syndrome I97.2
　　postmastoidectomy cholesteatoma — *see* Complications, postmastoidectomy, recurrent cholesteatoma
　　postvagotomy syndrome K91.1
　　postvalvulotomy syndrome I97.0
　　pulmonary insufficiency (acute) J95.2
　　　chronic J95.3
　　　following thoracic surgery J95.1
　　reattached body part — *see* Complications, reattached
　　respiratory — *see* Complications, respiratory system
　　shock (hypovolemic) T81.19- ☑
　　spleen (postoperative) D78.89
　　　intraoperative D78.81
　　stitch abscess T81.41- ☑
　　subglottic stenosis (postsurgical) J95.5
　　testicular hypofunction E89.5
　　transplant — *see* Complications, organ or tissue transplant
　　urinary NEC N99.89
　　vaginal vault prolapse (posthysterectomy) N99.3
　　vascular (peripheral)
　　　artery T81.719- ☑
　　　　mesenteric T81.710- ☑
　　　　renal T81.711- ☑
　　　　specified NEC T81.718- ☑
　　　vein T81.72- ☑
　　wound infection T81.49- ☑
　suture, permanent (wire) NEC T85.9- ☑
　　with repair of bone — *see* Complications, fixation device, internal
　　embolism T85.818- ☑
　　fibrosis T85.828- ☑
　　hemorrhage T85.838- ☑
　　infection and inflammation T85.79- ☑
　　mechanical
　　　breakdown T85.612- ☑
　　　displacement T85.622- ☑
　　　malfunction T85.612- ☑
　　　malposition T85.622- ☑
　　　obstruction T85.692- ☑
　　　perforation T85.692- ☑
　　　protrusion T85.692- ☑
　　　specified NEC T85.692- ☑
　　pain T85.848- ☑
　　specified type NEC T85.898- ☑
　　stenosis T85.858- ☑
　　thrombosis T85.868- ☑
　tracheostomy J95.00
　　granuloma J95.09
　　hemorrhage J95.01
　　infection J95.02
　　malfunction J95.03
　　mechanical J95.03
　　obstruction J95.03
　　specified type NEC J95.09
　　tracheo-esophageal fistula J95.04
　transfusion (blood) (lymphocytes) (plasma) T80.92- ☑
　　air embolism T80.0- ☑
　　circulatory overload E87.71
　　febrile nonhemolytic transfusion reaction R50.84
　　hemochromatosis E83.111
　　hemolysis T80.89- ☑
　　hemolytic reaction (antigen unspecified) T80.919- ☑
　　incompatibility reaction (antigen unspecified) T80.919- ☑
　　　ABO T80.30- ☑
　　　　delayed serologic (DSTR) T80.39- ☑
　　　　hemolytic transfusion reaction (HTR) (unspecified time after transfusion) T80.319- ☑
　　　　　acute (AHTR) (less than 24 hours after transfusion) T80.310- ☑
　　　　　delayed (DHTR) (24 hours or more after transfusion) T80.311- ☑
　　　　specified NEC T80.39- ☑
　　　acute (antigen unspecified) T80.910- ☑

☑ **Additional Character Required — Refer to the Tabular List for Character Selection**

Complication(s) — *continued*
- transfusion — *continued*
  - incompatibility reaction — *continued*
    - delayed (antigen unspecified) T80.911- ☑
    - delayed serologic (DSTR) T80.89- ☑
    - non-ABO (minor antigens (Duffy) (K) (Kell) (Kidd) (Lewis) (M) (N) (P) (S)) T80.A0- ☑ (*following T80.4*)
      - delayed serologic (DSTR) T80.A9- ☑ (*following T80.4*)
      - hemolytic transfusion reaction (HTR) (unspecified time after transfusion) T80.A19- ☑ (*following T80.4*)
        - acute (AHTR) (less than 24 hours after transfusion) T80.A10- ☑ (*following T80.4*)
        - delayed (DHTR) (24 hours or more after transfusion) T80.A11- ☑ (*following T80.4*)
      - specified NEC T80.A9- ☑ (*following T80.4*)
    - Rh (antigens (C) (c) (D) (E) (e)) (factor) T80.40- ☑
      - delayed serologic (DSTR) T80.49- ☑
      - hemolytic transfusion reaction (HTR) (unspecified time after transfusion) T80.419- ☑
        - acute (AHTR) (less than 24 hours after transfusion) T80.410- ☑
        - delayed (DHTR) (24 hours or more after transfusion) T80.411- ☑
      - specified NEC T80.49- ☑
  - infection T80.29- ☑
    - acute T80.22- ☑
  - reaction NEC T80.89- ☑
  - sepsis T80.29- ☑
  - shock T80.89- ☑
- transplant T86.90
  - bone T86.839
    - failure T86.831
    - infection T86.832
    - rejection T86.830
    - specified type NEC T86.838
  - bone marrow T86.00
    - failure T86.02
    - infection T86.03
    - rejection T86.01
    - specified type NEC T86.09
  - cornea T86.849- ☑
    - failure T86.841- ☑
    - infection T86.842- ☑
    - rejection T86.840- ☑
    - specified type NEC T86.848- ☑
  - failure T86.92
  - heart T86.20
    - with lung T86.30
      - cardiac allograft vasculopathy T86.290
        - failure T86.32
        - infection T86.33
        - rejection T86.31
        - specified type NEC T86.39
    - failure T86.22
    - infection T86.23
    - rejection T86.21
    - specified type NEC T86.298
  - infection T86.93
  - intestine T86.859
    - failure T86.851
    - infection T86.852
    - rejection T86.850
    - specified type NEC T86.858
  - kidney T86.10
    - failure T86.12
    - infection T86.13
    - rejection T86.11
    - specified type NEC T86.19
  - liver T86.40
    - failure T86.42
    - infection T86.43
    - rejection T86.41
    - specified type NEC T86.49
  - lung T86.819
    - with heart T86.30
      - failure T86.32
      - infection T86.33
      - rejection T86.31
      - specified type NEC T86.39
    - failure T86.811
    - infection T86.812
    - rejection T86.810
    - specified type NEC T86.818

Complication(s) — *continued*
- transplant — *continued*
  - malignant neoplasm C80.2
  - pancreas T86.899
    - failure T86.891
    - infection T86.892
    - rejection T86.890
    - specified type NEC T86.898
  - peripheral blood stem cells T86.5
  - post-transplant lymphoproliferative disorder (PTLD) D47.Z1 (*following D47.4*)
  - rejection T86.91
  - skin T86.829
    - failure T86.821
    - infection T86.822
    - rejection T86.820
    - specified type NEC T86.828
  - specified
    - tissue T86.899
      - failure T86.891
      - infection T86.892
      - rejection T86.890
      - specified type NEC T86.898
    - type NEC T86.99
  - stem cell (from peripheral blood) (from umbilical cord) T86.5
  - umbilical cord stem cells T86.5
- trauma (early) T79.9- ☑
  - specified NEC T79.8- ☑
- ultrasound therapy NEC T88.9- ☑
- umbilical cord NEC
  - complicating delivery O69.9- ☑
    - specified NEC O69.89- ☑
- umbrella device, vascular T82.9- ☑
  - embolism T82.818- ☑
  - fibrosis T82.828- ☑
  - hemorrhage T82.838- ☑
  - infection or inflammation T82.7- ☑
  - mechanical
    - breakdown T82.515- ☑
    - displacement T82.525- ☑
    - leakage T82.535- ☑
    - malposition T82.525- ☑
    - obstruction T82.595- ☑
    - perforation T82.595- ☑
    - protrusion T82.595- ☑
  - pain T82.848- ☑
  - specified type NEC T82.898- ☑
  - stenosis T82.858- ☑
  - thrombosis T82.868- ☑
- urethral catheter — *see* Complications, catheter, urethral, indwelling
- vaccination T88.1- ☑
  - anaphylaxis NEC T80.52- ☑
  - arthropathy — *see* Arthropathy, postimmunization
  - cellulitis T88.0- ☑
  - encephalitis or encephalomyelitis G04.02
  - infection (general) (local) NEC T88.0- ☑
  - meningitis G03.8
  - myelitis G04.02
  - protein sickness T80.62- ☑
  - rash T88.1- ☑
  - reaction (allergic) T88.1- ☑
    - serum T80.62- ☑
  - sepsis T88.0- ☑
  - serum intoxication, sickness, rash, or other serum reaction NEC T80.62- ☑
    - anaphylactic shock T80.52- ☑
  - shock (allergic) (anaphylactic) T80.52- ☑
  - vaccinia (generalized) (localized) T88.1- ☑
- vas deferens device or implant — *see* Complications, genitourinary, device or implant, genital tract
- vascular I99.9
  - device or implant T82.9- ☑
    - embolism T82.818- ☑
    - fibrosis T82.828- ☑
    - hemorrhage T82.838- ☑
    - infection or inflammation T82.7- ☑
    - mechanical
      - breakdown T82.519- ☑
        - specified device NEC T82.518- ☑
      - displacement T82.529- ☑
        - specified device NEC T82.528- ☑
      - leakage T82.539- ☑
        - specified device NEC T82.538- ☑
      - malposition T82.529- ☑
        - specified device NEC T82.528- ☑

Complication(s) — *continued*
- vascular — *continued*
  - device or implant — *continued*
    - mechanical — *continued*
      - obstruction T82.599- ☑
        - specified device NEC T82.598- ☑
      - perforation T82.599- ☑
        - specified device NEC T82.598- ☑
      - protrusion T82.599- ☑
        - specified device NEC T82.598- ☑
    - pain T82.848- ☑
    - specified type NEC T82.898- ☑
    - stenosis T82.858- ☑
    - thrombosis T82.868- ☑
  - dialysis catheter — *see* Complication, catheter, dialysis
  - following infusion, therapeutic injection or transfusion T80.1- ☑
  - graft T82.9- ☑
    - embolism T82.818- ☑
    - fibrosis T82.828- ☑
    - hemorrhage T82.838- ☑
    - mechanical
      - breakdown T82.319- ☑
        - aorta (bifurcation) T82.310- ☑
        - carotid artery T82.311- ☑
        - specified vessel NEC T82.318- ☑
      - displacement T82.329- ☑
        - aorta (bifurcation) T82.320- ☑
        - carotid artery T82.321- ☑
        - specified vessel NEC T82.328- ☑
      - leakage T82.339- ☑
        - aorta (bifurcation) T82.330- ☑
        - carotid artery T82.331- ☑
        - femoral artery T82.332- ☑
        - specified vessel NEC T82.338- ☑
      - malposition T82.329- ☑
        - aorta (bifurcation) T82.320- ☑
        - carotid artery T82.321- ☑
        - specified vessel NEC T82.328- ☑
      - obstruction T82.399- ☑
        - aorta (bifurcation) T82.390- ☑
        - carotid artery T82.391- ☑
        - specified vessel NEC T82.398- ☑
      - perforation T82.399- ☑
        - aorta (bifurcation) T82.390- ☑
        - carotid artery T82.391- ☑
        - specified vessel NEC T82.398- ☑
      - protrusion T82.399- ☑
        - aorta (bifurcation) T82.390- ☑
        - carotid artery T82.391- ☑
        - specified vessel NEC T82.398- ☑
    - pain T82.848- ☑
    - specified complication NEC T82.898- ☑
    - stenosis T82.858- ☑
    - thrombosis T82.868- ☑
  - postoperative — *see* Complications, postoperative, circulatory
  - vena cava device (filter) (sieve) (umbrella) — *see* Complications, umbrella device, vascular
- ventilation therapy NEC T81.81- ☑
- ventilator
  - mechanical J95.850
  - specified NEC J95.859
- ventricular (communicating) shunt (device) T85.9- ☑
  - embolism T85.810- ☑
  - fibrosis T85.820- ☑
  - hemorrhage T85.830- ☑
  - infection and inflammation T85.730- ☑
  - mechanical
    - breakdown T85.01- ☑
    - displacement T85.02- ☑
    - leakage T85.03- ☑
    - malposition T85.02- ☑
    - obstruction T85.09- ☑
    - perforation T85.09- ☑
    - protrusion T85.09- ☑
    - specified NEC T85.09- ☑
  - pain T85.840- ☑
  - specified type NEC T85.890- ☑
  - stenosis T85.850- ☑
  - thrombosis T85.860- ☑
- wire suture, permanent (implanted) — *see* Complications, suture, permanent

Compressed air disease T70.3- ☑

Compression
  with injury — code by Nature of injury
  artery I77.1
    celiac, syndrome I77.4
  brachial plexus G54.0
  brain (stem) G93.5
    due to
      contusion (diffuse) — see also Injury, intracranial, diffuse S06.A0- ☑
        with herniation S06.A1- ☑
        focal — see also Injury, intracranial, focal S06.A0- ☑
          with herniation S06.A1- ☑
      injury NEC — see also Injury, intracranial, diffuse S06.A0- ☑
    nontraumatic G93.5
    traumatic — see also Injury, intracranial, diffuse S06.A0- ☑
      with herniation S06.A1- ☑
  bronchus J98.09
  cauda equina G83.4
  celiac (artery) (axis) I77.4
  cerebral — see Compression, brain
  cervical plexus G54.2
  cord
    spinal — see Compression, spinal
    umbilical — see Compression, umbilical cord
  cranial nerve G52.9
    eighth H93.3- ☑
    eleventh G52.8
    fifth G50.8
    first G52.0
    fourth — see Strabismus, paralytic, fourth nerve
    ninth G52.1
    second — see Disorder, nerve, optic
    seventh G51.8
    sixth — see Strabismus, paralytic, sixth nerve
    tenth G52.2
    third — see Strabismus, paralytic, third nerve
    twelfth G52.3
  diver's squeeze T70.3- ☑
  during birth (newborn) P15.9
  esophagus K22.2
  eustachian tube — see Obstruction, eustachian tube, cartilagenous
  facies Q67.1
  fracture
    nontraumatic NOS — see Collapse, vertebra
    pathological — see Fracture, pathological
    traumatic — see Fracture, traumatic
  heart — see Disease, heart
  intestine — see Obstruction, intestine
  laryngeal nerve, recurrent G52.2
    with paralysis of vocal cords and larynx J38.00
      bilateral J38.02
      unilateral J38.01
  lumbosacral plexus G54.1
  lung J98.4
  lymphatic vessel I89.0
  medulla — see Compression, brain
  nerve — see also Disorder, nerve G58.9
    arm NEC — see Mononeuropathy, upper limb
    axillary G54.0
    cranial — see Compression, cranial nerve
    leg NEC — see Mononeuropathy, lower limb
    median (in carpal tunnel) — see Syndrome, carpal tunnel
    optic — see Disorder, nerve, optic
    plantar — see Lesion, nerve, plantar
    posterior tibial (in tarsal tunnel) — see Syndrome, tarsal tunnel
    root or plexus NOS (in) G54.9
      intervertebral disc disorder NEC — see Disorder, disc, with, radiculopathy
        with myelopathy — see Disorder, disc, with, myelopathy
      neoplastic disease — see also Neoplasm D49.9 [G55]
      spondylosis — see Spondylosis, with radiculopathy
    sciatic (acute) — see Lesion, nerve, sciatic
    sympathetic G90.89
    traumatic — see Injury, nerve
    ulnar — see Lesion, nerve, ulnar
    upper extremity NEC — see Mononeuropathy, upper limb
  spinal (cord) G95.20
    by displacement of intervertebral disc NEC — see also Disorder, disc, with, myelopathy

Compression — continued
  spinal — continued
    nerve root NOS G54.9
      due to displacement of intervertebral disc NEC — see Disorder, disc, with, radiculopathy
        with myelopathy — see Disorder, disc, with, myelopathy
      specified NEC G95.29
      spondylogenic (cervical) (lumbar, lumbosacral) (thoracic) — see Spondylosis, with myelopathy NEC
      anterior — see Syndrome, anterior, spinal artery, compression
      traumatic — see Injury, spinal cord, by region
    subcostal nerve (syndrome) — see Mononeuropathy, upper limb, specified NEC
    sympathetic nerve NEC G90.89
    syndrome T79.5- ☑
    trachea J39.8
    ulnar nerve (by scar tissue) — see Lesion, nerve, ulnar
  umbilical cord
    complicating delivery O69.2- ☑
      cord around neck O69.1- ☑
      prolapse O69.0- ☑
      specified NEC O69.2- ☑
  ureter N13.5
  vein I87.1
  vena cava (inferior) (superior) I87.1
Compulsion, compulsive
  gambling F63.0
  neurosis F42.8
  personality F60.5
  states F42.8
  swearing F42.8
    in Gilles de la Tourette's syndrome F95.2
  tics and spasms F95.9
Concato's disease (pericardial polyserositis) A19.9
  nontubercular I31.1
  pleural — see Pleurisy, with effusion
Concavity chest wall M95.4
Concealed penis Q55.64
Concern (normal) **about sick person in family** Z63.6
Concrescence (teeth) K00.2
Concretio cordis I31.1
  rheumatic I09.2
Concretion — see also Calculus
  appendicular K38.1
  canaliculus — see Dacryolith
  clitoris N90.89
  conjunctiva H11.12- ☑
  eyelid — see Disorder, eyelid, specified type NEC
  lacrimal passages — see Dacryolith
  prepuce (male) N47.8
  salivary gland (any) K11.5
  seminal vesicle N50.89
  tonsil J35.8
Concussion (brain) (cerebral) (current) S06.0X9- ☑
  with
    loss of consciousness
      30 minutes or less S06.0X1- ☑
      brief S06.0X1- ☑
      status unknown S06.0XA- ☑
      unspecified duration S06.0X9- ☑
    no loss of consciousness S06.0X0- ☑
  blast (air) (hydraulic) (immersion) (underwater)
    abdomen or thorax — see Injury, blast, by site
    ear with acoustic nerve injury — see Injury, nerve, acoustic, specified type NEC
  cauda equina S34.3- ☑
  conus medullaris S34.02- ☑
  ocular S05.8X- ☑
  spinal (cord)
    cervical S14.0- ☑
    lumbar S34.01- ☑
    sacral S34.02- ☑
    thoracic S24.0- ☑
  syndrome F07.81
  without loss of consciousness S06.0X0- ☑
Condition — see also Disease
  Fontan-associated, specified NEC I27.848
  post COVID-19 U09.9
Conditions arising in the perinatal period — see Newborn, affected by
Conduct disorder — see Disorder, conduct
Condyloma A63.0
  acuminatum A63.0
  gonorrheal A54.09
  latum A51.31
  syphilitic A51.31

Condyloma — continued
  syphilitic — continued
    congenital A50.07
  venereal, syphilitic A51.31
Conflagration — see also Burn
  asphyxia (by inhalation of gases, fumes or vapors) — see also Table of Drugs and Chemicals T59.9- ☑
Conflict (with) — see also Discord
  family Z63.8
  grandparent-child Z62.831
  group home staff-child Z62.833
  kinship-care child Z62.831
  marital Z63.0
    involving divorce or estrangement Z63.5
  non-parental relative-child Z62.831
  non-parental relative legal guardian-child Z62.831
  non-relative guardian-child Z62.832
  other relative-child Z62.831
  parent-child Z62.820
    parent-adopted child Z62.821
    parent-biological child Z62.820
    parent-foster child Z62.822
    parent-step child Z62.823
  social role NEC Z73.5
Confluent — see condition
Confusion, confused R41.0
  epileptic F05
  mental state (psychogenic) F44.89
  psychogenic F44.89
  reactive (from emotional stress, psychological trauma) F44.89
Confusional arousals G47.51
Congelation T69.9- ☑
Congenital — see also condition
  aortic septum Q25.49
  intrinsic factor deficiency D51.0
  malformation — see Anomaly
Congestion, congestive
  bladder N32.89
  bowel K63.89
  brain G93.89
  breast N64.59
  bronchial J98.09
  catarrhal J31.0
  chest R09.89
  chill, malarial — see Malaria
  circulatory NEC I99.8
  duodenum K31.89
  eye — see Hyperemia, conjunctiva
  facial, due to birth injury P15.4
  general R68.89
  glottis J37.0
  heart — see Failure, heart, congestive
  hepatic K76.1
  hypostatic (lung) — see Edema, lung
  intestine K63.89
  kidney N28.89
  labyrinth H83.8- ☑
  larynx J37.0
  liver K76.1
  lung R09.89
    active or acute — see Pneumonia
  malaria, malarial — see Malaria
  nasal R09.81
  nose R09.81
  orbit, orbital — see also Exophthalmos
    inflammatory (chronic) — see Inflammation, orbit
  ovary N83.8
  pancreas K86.89
  pelvic, female N94.89
  pleural J94.8
  prostate (active) N42.1
  pulmonary — see Congestion, lung
  renal N28.89
  retina H35.81
  seminal vesicle N50.1
  spinal cord G95.19
  spleen (chronic) D73.2
  stomach K31.89
  trachea — see Tracheitis
  urethra N36.8
  uterus N85.8
    with subinvolution N85.3
  venous (passive) I87.8
  viscera R68.89
Congestive — see Congestion
Conical
  cervix (hypertrophic elongation) N88.4
  cornea — see Keratoconus

Conical — *continued*
  teeth K00.2
Conjoined twins Q89.4
Conjugal maladjustment Z63.0
  involving divorce or estrangement Z63.5
Conjunctiva — *see* condition
Conjunctivitis (staphylococcal) (streptococcal) NOS H10.9
  Acanthamoeba B60.12
  acute H10.3- ☑
    atopic H10.1- ☑
    chemical — *see also* Corrosion, cornea H10.21- ☑
    mucopurulent H10.02- ☑
      follicular H10.01- ☑
      pseudomembranous H10.22- ☑
    serous except viral H10.23- ☑
      viral — *see* Conjunctivitis, viral
    toxic H10.21- ☑
  adenoviral (acute) (follicular) B30.1
  allergic (acute) — *see* Conjunctivitis, acute, atopic
    chronic H10.45
      vernal H10.44
  anaphylactic — *see* Conjunctivitis, acute, atopic
  Apollo B30.3
  atopic (acute) — *see* Conjunctivitis, acute, atopic
  Beal's B30.2
  blennorrhagic (gonococcal) (neonatorum) A54.31
  chemical (acute) — *see also* Corrosion, cornea H10.21- ☑
  chlamydial A74.0
    due to trachoma A71.1
    neonatal P39.1
  chronic (nodosa) (petrificans) (phlyctenular) H10.40- ☑
    allergic H10.45
      vernal H10.44
    follicular H10.43- ☑
    giant papillary H10.41- ☑
    simple H10.42- ☑
    vernal H10.44
  coxsackievirus 24 B30.3
  diphtheritic A36.86
  due to
    dust — *see* Conjunctivitis, acute, atopic
    filariasis B74.9
    mucocutaneous leishmaniasis B55.2
  enterovirus type 70 (hemorrhagic) B30.3
  epidemic (viral) B30.9
    hemorrhagic B30.3
  gonococcal (neonatorum) A54.31
  granular (trachomatous) A71.1
    sequelae (late effect) B94.0
  hemorrhagic (acute) (epidemic) B30.3
  herpes zoster B02.31
  in (due to)
    Acanthamoeba B60.12
    adenovirus (acute) (follicular) B30.1
    Chlamydia A74.0
    coxsackievirus 24 B30.3
    diphtheria A36.86
    enterovirus type 70 (hemorrhagic) B30.3
    filariasis B74.9
    gonococci A54.31
    herpes (simplex) virus B00.53
      zoster B02.31
    infectious disease NEC B99.- ☑
    meningococci A39.89
    mucocutaneous leishmaniasis B55.2
    rosacea H10.82- ☑
    syphilis (late) A52.71
    zoster B02.31
  inclusion A74.0
  infantile P39.1
    gonococcal A54.31
  Koch-Weeks' — *see* Conjunctivitis, acute, mucopurulent
  light — *see* Conjunctivitis, acute, atopic
  ligneous — *see* Blepharoconjunctivitis, ligneous
  meningococcal A39.89
  mucopurulent — *see* Conjunctivitis, acute, mucopurulent
  neonatal P39.1
    gonococcal A54.31
  Newcastle B30.8
  of Beal B30.2
  parasitic
    filariasis B74.9
    mucocutaneous leishmaniasis B55.2
  Parinaud's H10.89
  petrificans H10.89
  rosacea H10.82- ☑
  specified NEC H10.89
  swimming-pool B30.1

Conjunctivitis — *continued*
  trachomatous A71.1
    acute A71.0
    sequelae (late effect) B94.0
  traumatic NEC H10.89
  tuberculous A18.59
  tularemic A21.1
  tularensis A21.1
  viral B30.9
    due to
      adenovirus B30.1
      enterovirus B30.3
    specified NEC B30.8
Conjunctivochalasis H11.82- ☑
Connective tissue — *see* condition
Conn's syndrome E26.01
Conradi (-Hunermann) **disease** Q77.3
Consanguinity Z84.3
  counseling Z71.89
Conscious simulation (of illness) Z76.5
Consecutive — *see* condition
Consolidation lung (base) — *see* Pneumonia, lobar
Constipation (atonic) (neurogenic) (simple) (spastic) K59.00
  chronic K59.09
    idiopathic K59.04
  drug-induced K59.03
  functional K59.04
  outlet dysfunction K59.02
  psychogenic F45.8
  slow transit K59.01
  specified NEC K59.09
Constitutional — *see also* condition
  substandard F60.7
Constitutionally substandard F60.7
Constriction — *see also* Stricture
  auditory canal — *see* Stenosis, external ear canal
  bronchial J98.09
  duodenum K31.5
  esophagus K22.2
  external
    abdomen, abdominal (wall) S30.841- ☑
    alveolar process S00.542- ☑
    ankle S90.54- ☑
    antecubital space — *see* Constriction, external, forearm
    arm (upper) S40.84- ☑
    auricle — *see* Constriction, external, ear
    axilla — *see* Constriction, external, arm
    back, lower S30.840- ☑
    breast S20.14- ☑
    brow S00.84- ☑
    buttock S30.840- ☑
    calf — *see* Constriction, external, leg
    canthus — *see* Constriction, external, eyelid
    cheek S00.84- ☑
      internal S00.542- ☑
    chest wall — *see* Constriction, external, thorax
    chin S00.84- ☑
    clitoris S30.844- ☑
    costal region — *see* Constriction, external, thorax
    digit(s)
      foot — *see* Constriction, external, toe
      hand — *see* Constriction, external, finger
    ear S00.44- ☑
    elbow S50.34- ☑
    epididymis S30.843- ☑
    epigastric region S30.841- ☑
    esophagus, cervical S10.14- ☑
    eyebrow — *see* Constriction, external, eyelid
    eyelid S00.24- ☑
    face S00.84- ☑
    finger(s) S60.44- ☑
      index S60.44- ☑
      little S60.44- ☑
      middle S60.44- ☑
      ring S60.44- ☑
    flank S30.84A- ☑
    foot (except toe(s) alone) S90.84- ☑
      toe — *see* Constriction, external, toe
    forearm S50.84- ☑
      elbow only — *see* Constriction, external, elbow
    forehead S00.84- ☑
    genital organs, external
      female S30.846- ☑
      male S30.845- ☑
    groin S30.841- ☑
    gum S00.542- ☑

Constriction — *continued*
  external — *continued*
    hand S60.54- ☑
    head S00.94- ☑
      ear — *see* Constriction, external, ear
      eyelid — *see* Constriction, external, eyelid
      lip S00.541- ☑
      nose S00.34- ☑
      oral cavity S00.542- ☑
      scalp S00.04- ☑
      specified site NEC S00.84- ☑
    heel — *see* Constriction, external, foot
    hip S70.24- ☑
    inguinal region S30.841- ☑
    interscapular region S20.449- ☑
    jaw S00.84- ☑
    knee S80.24- ☑
    labium (majus) (minus) S30.844- ☑
    larynx S10.14- ☑
    leg (lower) S80.84- ☑
      knee — *see* Constriction, external, knee
      upper — *see* Constriction, external, thigh
    lip S00.541- ☑
    lower back S30.840- ☑
    lumbar region S30.840- ☑
    malar region S00.84- ☑
    mammary — *see* Constriction, external, breast
    mastoid region S00.84- ☑
    mouth S00.542- ☑
    nail
      finger — *see* Constriction, external, finger
      toe — *see* Constriction, external, toe
    nasal S00.34- ☑
    neck S10.94- ☑
      specified site NEC S10.84- ☑
      throat S10.14- ☑
    nose S00.34- ☑
    occipital region S00.04- ☑
    oral cavity S00.542- ☑
    orbital region — *see* Constriction, external, eyelid
    palate S00.542- ☑
    palm — *see* Constriction, external, hand
    parietal region S00.04- ☑
    pelvis S30.840- ☑
    penis S30.842- ☑
    perineum
      female S30.844- ☑
      male S30.840- ☑
    periocular area — *see* Constriction, external, eyelid
    phalanges
      finger — *see* Constriction, external, finger
      toe — *see* Constriction, external, toe
    pharynx S10.14- ☑
    pinna — *see* Constriction, external, ear
    popliteal space — *see* Constriction, external, knee
    prepuce S30.842- ☑
    pubic region S30.840- ☑
    pudendum
      female S30.846- ☑
      male S30.845- ☑
    sacral region S30.840- ☑
    scalp S00.04- ☑
    scapular region — *see* Constriction, external, shoulder
    scrotum S30.843- ☑
    shin — *see* Constriction, external, leg
    shoulder S40.24- ☑
    sternal region S20.349- ☑
    submaxillary region S00.84- ☑
    submental region S00.84- ☑
    subungual
      finger(s) — *see* Constriction, external, finger
      toe(s) — *see* Constriction, external, toe
    supraclavicular fossa S10.84- ☑
    supraorbital S00.84- ☑
    temple S00.84- ☑
    temporal region S00.84- ☑
    testis S30.843- ☑
    thigh S70.34- ☑
    thorax, thoracic (wall) S20.94- ☑
      back S20.44- ☑
      front S20.34- ☑
    throat S10.14- ☑
    thumb S60.34- ☑
    toe(s) (lesser) S90.44- ☑
      great S90.44- ☑
    tongue S00.542- ☑

Constriction — *continued*
　external — *continued*
　　　trachea S10.14- ☑
　　　tunica vaginalis S30.843- ☑
　　　uvula S00.542- ☑
　　　vagina S30.844- ☑
　　　vulva S30.844- ☑
　　　wrist S60.84- ☑
　gallbladder — *see* Obstruction, gallbladder
　intestine — *see* Obstruction, intestine
　larynx J38.6
　　congenital Q31.8
　　　specified NEC Q31.8
　　　subglottic Q31.1
　organ or site, congenital NEC — *see* Atresia, by site
　prepuce (acquired) (congenital) N47.1
　pylorus (adult hypertrophic) K31.1
　　congenital or infantile Q40.0
　　newborn Q40.0
　ring dystocia (uterus) O62.4
　spastic — *see also* Spasm
　　ureter N13.5
　ureter N13.5
　　with infection N13.6
　urethra — *see* Stricture, urethra
　visual field (peripheral) (functional) — *see* Defect, visual field
Constrictive — *see* condition
Consultation
　medical — *see* Counseling, medical
　religious Z71.81
　specified reason NEC Z71.89
　spiritual Z71.81
　without complaint or sickness Z71.9
　　feared complaint unfounded Z71.1
　　specified reason NEC Z71.89
Consumption — *see* Tuberculosis
Contact (with) — *see also* Exposure (to)
　acariasis Z20.7
　AIDS virus Z20.6
　air pollution Z77.110
　algae and algae toxins Z77.121
　algae bloom Z77.121
　anthrax Z20.810
　aromatic amines Z77.020
　aromatic (hazardous) compounds NEC Z77.028
　aromatic dyes NOS Z77.028
　arsenic Z77.010
　asbestos Z77.090
　bacterial disease NEC Z20.818
　benzene Z77.021
　blue-green algae bloom Z77.121
　body fluids (potentially hazardous) Z77.21
　brown tide Z77.121
　chemicals (chiefly nonmedicinal) (hazardous) NEC Z77.098
　cholera Z20.09
　chromium compounds Z77.018
　communicable disease Z20.9
　　bacterial NEC Z20.818
　　specified NEC Z20.89
　　viral NEC Z20.828
　　Zika virus Z20.821
　coronavirus (disease) (novel) 2019 Z20.822
　COVID-19 Z20.822
　cyanobacteria bloom Z77.121
　dyes Z77.098
　Escherichia coli (E. coli) Z20.01
　fiberglass — *see* Table of Drugs and Chemicals, fiberglass
　German measles Z20.4
　gonorrhea Z20.2
　hazardous metals NEC Z77.018
　hazardous substances NEC Z77.29
　hazards in the physical environment NEC Z77.128
　hazards to health NEC Z77.9
　HIV Z20.6
　HTLV-III/LAV Z20.6
　human immunodeficiency virus (HIV) Z20.6
　infection Z20.9
　　specified NEC Z20.89
　infestation (parasitic) NEC Z20.7
　intestinal infectious disease NEC Z20.09
　　Escherichia coli (E. coli) Z20.01
　lead Z77.011
　meningococcus Z20.811
　mold (toxic) Z77.120
　nickel dust Z77.018
　noise Z77.122

Contact — *continued*
　parasitic disease Z20.7
　pediculosis Z20.7
　pfiesteria piscicida Z77.121
　poliomyelitis Z20.89
　pollution
　　air Z77.110
　　environmental NEC Z77.118
　　soil Z77.112
　　water Z77.111
　polycyclic aromatic hydrocarbons Z77.028
　positive maternal group B streptococcus P00.82
　rabies Z20.3
　radiation, naturally occurring NEC Z77.123
　radon Z77.123
　red tide (Florida) Z77.121
　rubella Z20.4
　SARS-CoV-2 Z20.822
　sexually-transmitted disease Z20.2
　smallpox (laboratory) Z20.89
　syphilis Z20.2
　tuberculosis Z20.1
　uranium Z77.012
　varicella Z20.820
　venereal disease Z20.2
　viral disease NEC Z20.828
　viral hepatitis Z20.5
　war theater (Gulf) (Persian Gulf) Z77.31
　　specified Z77.39
　water pollution Z77.111
　Zika virus Z20.821
Contamination, food — *see* Intoxication, foodborne
Contraception, contraceptive
　advice Z30.09
　counseling Z30.09
　device (intrauterine) (in situ) Z97.5
　　causing menorrhagia T83.83- ☑
　　checking Z30.431
　　complications — *see* Complications, intrauterine, contraceptive device
　　in place Z97.5
　　initial prescription Z30.014
　　reinsertion Z30.433
　　removal Z30.432
　　replacement Z30.433
　emergency (postcoital) Z30.012
　initial prescription Z30.019
　　barrier Z30.018
　　diaphragm Z30.018
　　injectable Z30.013
　　intrauterine device Z30.014
　　pills Z30.011
　　postcoital (emergency) Z30.012
　　specified type NEC Z30.018
　　subdermal implantable Z30.017
　　transdermal patch hormonal Z30.016
　　vaginal ring hormonal Z30.015
　maintenance Z30.40
　　barrier Z30.49
　　diaphragm Z30.49
　　examination Z30.8
　　injectable Z30.42
　　intrauterine device Z30.431
　　pills Z30.41
　　specified type NEC Z30.49
　　subdermal implantable Z30.46
　　transdermal patch hormonal Z30.45
　　vaginal ring hormonal Z30.44
　management Z30.9
　　specified NEC Z30.8
　postcoital (emergency) Z30.012
　prescription Z30.019
　　repeat Z30.40
　sterilization Z30.2
　surveillance (drug) — *see* Contraception, maintenance
Contraction(s), contracture, contracted
　Achilles tendon — *see also* Short, tendon, Achilles
　　congenital Q66.89
　amputation stump (surgical) (flexion) (late) (next proximal joint) T87.89
　anus K59.89
　bile duct (common) (hepatic) K83.8
　bladder N32.89
　　neck or sphincter N32.0
　bowel, cecum, colon or intestine, any part — *see* Obstruction, intestine
　Braxton Hicks — *see* False, labor
　breast implant, capsular T85.44- ☑
　bronchial J98.09

Contraction(s), contracture, contracted — *continued*
　burn (old) — *see* Cicatrix
　cervix — *see* Stricture, cervix
　cicatricial — *see* Cicatrix
　conjunctiva, trachomatous, active A71.1
　　sequelae (late effect) B94.0
　Dupuytren's M72.0
　eyelid — *see* Disorder, eyelid function
　fascia (lata) (postural) M72.8
　　Dupuytren's M72.0
　　palmar M72.0
　　plantar M72.2
　finger NEC — *see also* Deformity, finger
　　congenital Q68.1
　　joint — *see* Contraction, joint, hand
　flaccid — *see* Contraction, paralytic
　gallbladder K82.0
　heart valve — *see* Endocarditis
　hip — *see* Contraction, joint, hip
　hourglass
　　bladder N32.89
　　　congenital Q64.79
　　gallbladder K82.0
　　　congenital Q44.1
　　stomach K31.89
　　　congenital Q40.2
　　　psychogenic F45.8
　　uterus (complicating delivery) O62.4
　hysterical F44.4
　internal os — *see* Stricture, cervix
　joint (abduction) (acquired) (adduction) (flexion) (rotation) M24.50
　　ankle M24.57- ☑
　　congenital NEC Q68.8
　　　hip Q65.89
　　elbow M24.52- ☑
　　foot joint M24.57- ☑
　　hand joint M24.54- ☑
　　hip M24.55- ☑
　　　congenital Q65.89
　　hysterical F44.4
　　knee M24.56- ☑
　　shoulder M24.51- ☑
　　specified site NEC M24.59
　　wrist M24.53- ☑
　kidney (granular) (secondary) N26.9
　　congenital Q63.8
　　hydronephritic — *see* Hydronephrosis
　　Page N26.2
　　pyelonephritic — *see* Pyelitis, chronic
　　tuberculous A18.11
　ligament — *see also* Disorder, ligament
　　congenital Q79.8
　muscle (postinfective) (postural) NEC M62.40
　　with contracture of joint — *see* Contraction, joint
　　ankle M62.47- ☑
　　congenital Q79.8
　　　sternocleidomastoid Q68.0
　　extraocular — *see* Strabismus
　　eye (extrinsic) — *see* Strabismus
　　foot M62.47- ☑
　　forearm M62.43- ☑
　　hand M62.44- ☑
　　hysterical F44.4
　　ischemic (Volkmann's) T79.6- ☑
　　lower leg M62.46- ☑
　　multiple sites M62.49
　　pelvic region M62.45- ☑
　　posttraumatic — *see* Strabismus, paralytic
　　psychogenic F45.8
　　　conversion reaction F44.4
　　shoulder region M62.41- ☑
　　specified site NEC M62.48
　　thigh M62.45- ☑
　　upper arm M62.42- ☑
　neck — *see* Torticollis
　ocular muscle — *see* Strabismus
　organ or site, congenital NEC — *see* Atresia, by site
　outlet (pelvis) — *see* Contraction, pelvis
　palmar fascia M72.0
　paralytic
　　joint — *see* Contraction, joint
　　muscle — *see also* Contraction, muscle NEC
　　ocular — *see* Strabismus, paralytic
　pelvis (acquired) (general) M95.5
　　with disproportion (fetopelvic) O33.1
　　　causing obstructed labor O65.1
　　　inlet O33.2

☑ **Additional Character Required** — Refer to the Tabular List for Character Selection

Contraction(s), contracture, contracted — *continued*
- pelvis — *continued*
  - with disproportion — *continued*
    - mid-cavity O33.3- ☑
    - outlet O33.3- ☑
- plantar fascia M72.2
- premature
  - atrium I49.1
  - auriculoventricular I49.49
  - heart I49.49
  - junctional I49.2
  - supraventricular I49.1
  - ventricular I49.3
- prostate N42.89
- pylorus NEC — *see also* Pylorospasm
  - psychogenic F45.8
- rectum, rectal (sphincter) K59.89
- ring (Bandl's) (complicating delivery) O62.4
- scar — *see* Cicatrix
- spine — *see* Dorsopathy, deforming
- sternocleidomastoid (muscle), congenital Q68.0
- stomach K31.89
  - hourglass K31.89
    - congenital Q40.2
    - psychogenic F45.8
  - psychogenic F45.8
- tendon (sheath) M62.40
  - with contracture of joint — *see* Contraction, joint
  - Achilles — *see* Short, tendon, Achilles
  - ankle M62.47- ☑
    - Achilles — *see* Short, tendon, Achilles
  - foot M62.47- ☑
  - forearm M62.43- ☑
  - hand M62.44- ☑
  - lower leg M62.46- ☑
  - multiple sites M62.49
  - neck M62.48
  - pelvic region M62.45- ☑
  - shoulder region M62.41- ☑
  - specified site NEC M62.48
  - thigh M62.45- ☑
  - thorax M62.48
  - trunk M62.48
  - upper arm M62.42- ☑
- toe — *see* Deformity, toe, specified NEC
- ureterovesical orifice (postinfectional) N13.5
  - with infection N13.6
- urethra — *see also* Stricture, urethra
  - orifice N32.0
- uterus N85.8
  - abnormal NEC O62.9
  - clonic (complicating delivery) O62.4
  - dyscoordinate (complicating delivery) O62.4
  - hourglass (complicating delivery) O62.4
  - hypertonic O62.4
  - hypotonic NEC O62.2
  - inadequate
    - primary O62.0
    - secondary O62.1
  - incoordinate (complicating delivery) O62.4
  - poor O62.2
  - tetanic (complicating delivery) O62.4
- vagina (outlet) N89.5
- vesical N32.89
  - neck or urethral orifice N32.0
- visual field — *see* Defect, visual field, generalized
- Volkmann's (ischemic) T79.6- ☑

Contusion (skin surface intact) T14.8- ☑
- abdomen, abdominal (muscle) (wall) S30.11- ☑
- adnexa, eye NEC S05.8X- ☑
- adrenal gland S37.812- ☑
- alveolar process S00.532- ☑
- ankle S90.0- ☑
- antecubital space — *see* Contusion, forearm
- anus S30.3- ☑
- arm (upper) S40.02- ☑
  - lower (with elbow) — *see* Contusion, forearm
- auditory canal — *see* Contusion, ear
- auricle — *see* Contusion, ear
- axilla — *see* Contusion, arm, upper
- back — *see also* Contusion, thorax, back
  - lower S30.0- ☑
- bile duct S36.13- ☑
- bladder S37.22- ☑
- bone NEC T14.8- ☑
- brain (diffuse) — *see* Injury, intracranial, diffuse
  - focal — *see* Injury, intracranial, focal
- brainstem S06.38- ☑

Contusion — *continued*
- breast S20.0- ☑
- broad ligament S37.892- ☑
- brow S00.83- ☑
- buttock S30.0- ☑
- canthus, eye S00.1- ☑
- cauda equina S34.3- ☑
- cerebellar, traumatic S06.37- ☑
- cerebral S06.33- ☑
  - left side S06.32- ☑
  - right side S06.31- ☑
- cheek S00.83- ☑
  - internal S00.532- ☑
- chest (wall) — *see* Contusion, thorax
- chin S00.83- ☑
- clitoris S30.23- ☑
- colon — *see* Injury, intestine, large, contusion
- common bile duct S36.13- ☑
- conjunctiva S05.1- ☑
  - with foreign body (in conjunctival sac) — *see* Foreign body, conjunctival sac
- conus medullaris (spine) S34.139- ☑
- cornea — *see* Contusion, eyeball
  - with foreign body — *see* Foreign body, cornea
- corpus cavernosum S30.21- ☑
- cortex (brain) (cerebral) — *see* Injury, intracranial, diffuse
  - focal — *see* Injury, intracranial, focal
- costal region — *see* Contusion, thorax
- cystic duct S36.13- ☑
- diaphragm S27.802- ☑
- duodenum S36.420- ☑
- ear S00.43- ☑
- elbow S50.0- ☑
  - with forearm — *see* Contusion, forearm
- epididymis S30.22- ☑
- epigastric region S30.11- ☑
- epiglottis S10.0- ☑
- esophagus (thoracic) S27.812- ☑
  - cervical S10.0- ☑
- eyeball S05.1- ☑
- eyebrow S00.1- ☑
- eyelid (and periocular area) S00.1- ☑
- face NEC S00.83- ☑
- fallopian tube S37.529- ☑
  - bilateral S37.522- ☑
  - unilateral S37.521- ☑
- femoral triangle S30.11- ☑
- finger(s) S60.00- ☑
  - with damage to nail (matrix) S60.10- ☑
  - index S60.02- ☑
    - with damage to nail S60.12- ☑
  - little S60.05- ☑
    - with damage to nail S60.15- ☑
  - middle S60.03- ☑
    - with damage to nail S60.13- ☑
  - ring S60.04- ☑
    - with damage to nail S60.14- ☑
  - thumb — *see* Contusion, thumb
- flank (latus) region S30.13- ☑
- foot (except toe(s) alone) S90.3- ☑
  - toe — *see* Contusion, toe
- forearm S50.1- ☑
  - elbow only — *see* Contusion, elbow
- forehead S00.83- ☑
- gallbladder S36.122- ☑
- genital organs, external
  - female S30.202- ☑
  - male S30.201- ☑
- globe (eye) — *see* Contusion, eyeball
- groin S30.12- ☑
- gum S00.532- ☑
- hand S60.22- ☑
  - finger(s) — *see* Contusion, finger
  - wrist — *see* Contusion, wrist
- head S00.93- ☑
  - ear — *see* Contusion, ear
  - eyelid — *see* Contusion, eyelid
  - lip S00.531- ☑
  - nose S00.33- ☑
  - oral cavity S00.532- ☑
  - scalp S00.03- ☑
  - specified part NEC S00.83- ☑
- heart — *see also* Injury, heart S26.91- ☑
- heel — *see* Contusion, foot
- hepatic duct S36.13- ☑
- hip S70.0- ☑

Contusion — *continued*
- ileum S36.428- ☑
- iliac region S30.12- ☑
- inguinal region S30.12- ☑
- interscapular region S20.229- ☑
- intra-abdominal organ S36.92- ☑
  - colon — *see* Injury, intestine, large, contusion
  - liver S36.112- ☑
  - pancreas — *see* Contusion, pancreas
  - rectum S36.62- ☑
  - small intestine — *see* Injury, intestine, small, contusion
  - specified organ NEC S36.892- ☑
  - spleen — *see* Contusion, spleen
  - stomach S36.32- ☑
- iris (eye) — *see* Contusion, eyeball
- jaw S00.83- ☑
- jejunum S36.428- ☑
- kidney S37.01- ☑
  - major (greater than 2 cm) S37.02- ☑
  - minor (less than 2 cm) S37.01- ☑
- knee S80.0- ☑
- labium (majus) (minus) S30.23- ☑
- lacrimal apparatus, gland or sac S05.8X- ☑
- larynx S10.0- ☑
- leg (lower) S80.1- ☑
  - knee — *see* Contusion, knee
- lens — *see* Contusion, eyeball
- lip S00.531- ☑
- liver S36.112- ☑
- lower back S30.0- ☑
- lumbar region S30.0- ☑
- lung S27.329- ☑
  - bilateral S27.322- ☑
  - unilateral S27.321- ☑
- malar region S00.83- ☑
- mastoid region S00.83- ☑
- membrane, brain — *see* Injury, intracranial, diffuse
  - focal — *see* Injury, intracranial, focal
- mesentery S36.892- ☑
- mesosalpinx S37.892- ☑
- mouth S00.532- ☑
- muscle — *see* Contusion, by site
- nail
  - finger — *see* Contusion, finger, with damage to nail
  - toe — *see* Contusion, toe, with damage to nail
- nasal S00.33- ☑
- neck S10.93- ☑
  - specified site NEC S10.83- ☑
  - throat S10.0- ☑
- nerve — *see* Injury, nerve
- newborn P54.5
- nose S00.33- ☑
- occipital
  - lobe (brain) — *see* Injury, intracranial, diffuse
    - focal — *see* Injury, intracranial, focal
  - region (scalp) S00.03- ☑
- orbit (region) (tissues) S05.1- ☑
- ovary S37.429- ☑
  - bilateral S37.422- ☑
  - unilateral S37.421- ☑
- palate S00.532- ☑
- pancreas S36.229- ☑
  - body S36.221- ☑
  - head S36.220- ☑
  - tail S36.222- ☑
- parietal
  - lobe (brain) — *see* Injury, intracranial, diffuse
    - focal — *see* Injury, intracranial, focal
  - region (scalp) S00.03- ☑
- pelvic organ S37.92- ☑
  - adrenal gland S37.812- ☑
  - bladder S37.22- ☑
  - fallopian tube — *see* Contusion, fallopian tube
  - kidney — *see* Contusion, kidney
  - ovary — *see* Contusion, ovary
  - prostate S37.822- ☑
  - specified organ NEC S37.892- ☑
  - ureter S37.12- ☑
  - urethra S37.32- ☑
  - uterus S37.62- ☑
- pelvis S30.0- ☑
- penis S30.21- ☑
- perineum
  - female S30.23- ☑
  - male S30.0- ☑

☑ **Additional Character Required — Refer to the Tabular List for Character Selection**

Contusion — *continued*
- periocular area S00.1- ☑
- peritoneum S36.81- ☑
- periurethral tissue — *see* Contusion, urethra
- pharynx S10.0- ☑
- pinna — *see* Contusion, ear
- popliteal space — *see* Contusion, knee
- prepuce S30.21- ☑
- prostate S37.822- ☑
- pubic region S30.11- ☑
- pudendum
  - female S30.202- ☑
  - male S30.201- ☑
- quadriceps femoris — *see* Contusion, thigh
- rectum S36.62- ☑
- retroperitoneum S36.892- ☑
- round ligament S37.892- ☑
- sacral region S30.0- ☑
- scalp S00.03- ☑
  - due to birth injury P12.3
- scapular region — *see* Contusion, shoulder
- sclera — *see* Contusion, eyeball
- scrotum S30.22- ☑
- seminal vesicle S37.892- ☑
- shoulder S40.01- ☑
- skin NEC T14.8- ☑
- small intestine — *see* Injury, intestine, small, contusion
- spermatic cord S30.22- ☑
- spinal cord — *see* Injury, spinal cord, by region
  - cauda equina S34.3- ☑
  - conus medullaris S34.139- ☑
- spleen S36.029- ☑
  - major S36.021- ☑
  - minor S36.020- ☑
- sternal region S20.219- ☑
- stomach S36.32- ☑
- subconjunctival S05.1- ☑
- subcutaneous NEC T14.8- ☑
- submaxillary region S00.83- ☑
- submental region S00.83- ☑
- subperiosteal NEC T14.8- ☑
- subungual
  - finger — *see* Contusion, finger, with damage to nail
  - toe — *see* Contusion, toe, with damage to nail
- supraclavicular fossa S10.83- ☑
- supraorbital S00.83- ☑
- suprarenal gland S37.812- ☑
- temple (region) S00.83- ☑
- temporal
  - lobe (brain) — *see* Injury, intracranial, diffuse
  - focal — *see* Injury, intracranial, focal
  - region S00.83- ☑
- testis S30.22- ☑
- thigh S70.1- ☑
- thorax (wall) S20.20- ☑
  - back S20.22- ☑
  - front S20.21- ☑
- throat S10.0- ☑
- thumb S60.01- ☑
  - with damage to nail S60.11- ☑
- toe(s) (lesser) S90.12- ☑
  - with damage to nail S90.22- ☑
  - great S90.11- ☑
    - with damage to nail S90.21- ☑
- tongue S00.532- ☑
- trachea (cervical) S10.0- ☑
  - thoracic S27.52- ☑
- tunica vaginalis S30.22- ☑
- tympanum, tympanic membrane — *see* Contusion, ear
- ureter S37.12- ☑
- urethra S37.32- ☑
- urinary organ NEC S37.892- ☑
- uterus S37.62- ☑
- uvula S00.532- ☑
- vagina S30.23- ☑
- vas deferens S37.892- ☑
- vesical S37.22- ☑
- vocal cord(s) S10.0- ☑
- vulva S30.23- ☑
- wrist S60.21- ☑

Conus (congenital) (any type) Q14.8
- cornea — *see* Keratoconus
- medullaris syndrome G95.81

Conversion hysteria, neurosis or reaction F44.9
Converter, tuberculosis (test reaction) R76.11
Conviction (legal), anxiety concerning Z65.0

Conviction (legal), **anxiety concerning** — *continued*
- with imprisonment Z65.1

Convulsions (idiopathic) — *see also* Seizure(s) R56.9
- apoplectiform (cerebral ischemia) I67.82
- dissociative F44.5
- epileptic — *see* Epilepsy
- epileptiform, epileptoid — *see* Epilepsy
- ether (anesthetic) — *see* Table of Drugs and Chemicals, by drug
- febrile R56.00
  - with status epilepticus G40.901
    - complex R56.01
      - with status epilepticus G40.901
    - simple R56.00
- hysterical F44.5
- infantile P90
  - epilepsy — *see* Epilepsy
- jacksonian — *see* Epilepsy, localization-related, symptomatic, with simple partial seizures
- myoclonic G25.3
- newborn P90
- obstetrical (nephritic) (uremic) — *see* Eclampsia
- paretic A52.17
- post traumatic R56.1
- psychomotor — *see* Epilepsy, localization-related, symptomatic, with complex partial seizures
- recurrent R56.9
- reflex R25.8
- scarlatinal A38.8
- tetanus, tetanic — *see* Tetanus
- thymic E32.8

Convulsive — *see also* Convulsions
Cooley's anemia D56.1
Coolie itch B76.9
Cooper's
- disease — *see* Mastopathy, cystic
- hernia — *see* Hernia, abdomen, specified site NEC

Copra itch B88.09
Coprophagy F50.89
Coprophobia F40.298
Coproporphyria, hereditary E80.29
Cor
- biloculare Q20.8
- bovis, bovinum — *see* Hypertrophy, cardiac
- pulmonale I27.81
  - acute I26.09
    - without pulmonary embolism I27.81
  - chronic I27.81
    - with chronic pulmonary embolism I27.82
- triatriatum, triatrium Q24.2
- triloculare Q20.8
  - biatrium Q20.4
  - biventriculare Q21.19

Corbus' disease (gangrenous balanitis) N48.1
Cord — *see also* condition
- around neck
  - complicating delivery O69.81- ☑
    - with compression O69.1- ☑
- bladder G95.89
  - tabetic A52.19

Cordis ectopia Q24.8
Corditis (spermatic) N49.1
Corectopia Q13.2
Cori's disease (glycogen storage) E74.03
Corkhandler's disease or lung J67.3
Corkscrew esophagus K22.4
Corkworker's disease or lung J67.3
Corn (infected) L84
Cornea — *see also* condition
- donor Z52.5
- plana Q13.4

Cornelia de Lange syndrome Q87.19
Cornu cutaneum L85.8
Cornual gestation or pregnancy O00.80
- with intrauterine pregnancy O00.81

Coronary (artery) — *see* condition
Coronavirus (infection)
- 2019 — *see also* COVID-19 U07.1
- as cause of diseases classified elsewhere B97.29
- coronavirus-19 — *see also* COVID-19 U07.1
- COVID-19 — *see also* COVID-19 U07.1
- SARS-associated B97.21

Corpora — *see also* condition
- amylacea, prostate N42.89
- cavernosa — *see* condition

Corpulence — *see* Obesity
Corpus — *see* condition
Corrected transposition Q20.5

Corrosion (injury) (acid) (caustic) (chemical) (lime) (external) (internal) T30.4
- abdomen, abdominal (muscle) (wall) T21.42- ☑
  - first degree T21.52- ☑
  - second degree T21.62- ☑
  - third degree T21.72- ☑
- above elbow T22.439- ☑
  - first degree T22.539- ☑
  - left T22.432- ☑
    - first degree T22.532- ☑
    - second degree T22.632- ☑
    - third degree T22.732- ☑
  - right T22.431- ☑
    - first degree T22.531- ☑
    - second degree T22.631- ☑
    - third degree T22.731- ☑
  - second degree T22.639- ☑
  - third degree T22.739- ☑
- alimentary tract NEC T28.7- ☑
- ankle T25.419- ☑
  - first degree T25.519- ☑
  - left T25.412- ☑
    - first degree T25.512- ☑
    - second degree T25.612- ☑
    - third degree T25.712- ☑
  - multiple with foot — *see* Corrosion, lower, limb, multiple, ankle and foot
  - right T25.411- ☑
    - first degree T25.511- ☑
    - second degree T25.611- ☑
    - third degree T25.711- ☑
  - second degree T25.619- ☑
  - third degree T25.719- ☑
- anus — *see* Corrosion, buttock
- arm(s) (meaning upper limb(s)) — *see* Corrosion, upper limb
- axilla T22.449- ☑
  - first degree T22.549- ☑
  - left T22.442- ☑
    - first degree T22.542- ☑
    - second degree T22.642- ☑
    - third degree T22.742- ☑
  - right T22.441- ☑
    - first degree T22.541- ☑
    - second degree T22.641- ☑
    - third degree T22.741- ☑
  - second degree T22.649- ☑
  - third degree T22.749- ☑
- back (lower) T21.44- ☑
  - first degree T21.54- ☑
  - second degree T21.64- ☑
  - third degree T21.74- ☑
  - upper T21.43- ☑
    - first degree T21.53- ☑
    - second degree T21.63- ☑
    - third degree T21.73- ☑
- blisters — *code as* Corrosion, second degree, by site
- breast(s) — *see* Corrosion, chest wall
- buttock(s) T21.45- ☑
  - first degree T21.55- ☑
  - second degree T21.65- ☑
  - third degree T21.75- ☑
- calf T24.439- ☑
  - first degree T24.539- ☑
  - left T24.432- ☑
    - first degree T24.532- ☑
    - second degree T24.632- ☑
    - third degree T24.732- ☑
  - right T24.431- ☑
    - first degree T24.531- ☑
    - second degree T24.631- ☑
    - third degree T24.731- ☑
  - second degree T24.639- ☑
  - third degree T24.739- ☑
- canthus (eye) — *see* Corrosion, eyelid
- cervix T28.8- ☑
- cheek T20.46- ☑
  - first degree T20.56- ☑
  - second degree T20.66- ☑
  - third degree T20.76- ☑
- chest wall T21.41- ☑
  - first degree T21.51- ☑
  - second degree T21.61- ☑
  - third degree T21.71- ☑
- chin T20.43- ☑

Corrosion — *continued*
- chin — *continued*
  - first degree T20.53- ☑
  - second degree T20.63- ☑
  - third degree T20.73- ☑
- colon T28.7- ☑
- conjunctiva (and cornea) — *see* Corrosion, cornea
- cornea (and conjunctiva) T26.6- ☑
- deep necrosis of underlying tissue — *code as* Corrosion, third degree, by site
- dorsum of hand T23.469- ☑
  - first degree T23.569- ☑
  - left T23.462- ☑
    - first degree T23.562- ☑
    - second degree T23.662- ☑
    - third degree T23.762- ☑
  - right T23.461- ☑
    - first degree T23.561- ☑
    - second degree T23.661- ☑
    - third degree T23.761- ☑
  - second degree T23.669- ☑
  - third degree T23.769- ☑
- ear (auricle) (external) (canal) T20.41- ☑
  - drum T28.91- ☑
  - first degree T20.51- ☑
  - second degree T20.61- ☑
  - third degree T20.71- ☑
- elbow T22.429- ☑
  - first degree T22.529- ☑
  - left T22.422- ☑
    - first degree T22.522- ☑
    - second degree T22.622- ☑
    - third degree T22.722- ☑
  - right T22.421- ☑
    - first degree T22.521- ☑
    - second degree T22.621- ☑
    - third degree T22.721- ☑
  - second degree T22.629- ☑
  - third degree T22.729- ☑
- entire body — *see* Corrosion, multiple body regions
- epidermal loss — *code as* Corrosion, second degree, by site
- epiglottis T27.4- ☑
- erythema, erythematous — *code as* Corrosion, first degree, by site
- esophagus T28.6- ☑
- extent (percentage of body surface)
  - less than 10 percent T32.0
  - 10-19 percent (0-9 percent third degree) T32.10
    - with 10-19 percent third degree T32.11
  - 20-29 percent (0-9 percent third degree) T32.20
    - with
      - 10-19 percent third degree T32.21
      - 20-29 percent third degree T32.22
  - 30-39 percent (0-9 percent third degree) T32.30
    - with
      - 10-19 percent third degree T32.31
      - 20-29 percent third degree T32.32
      - 30-39 percent third degree T32.33
  - 40-49 percent (0-9 percent third degree) T32.40
    - with
      - 10-19 percent third degree T32.41
      - 20-29 percent third degree T32.42
      - 30-39 percent third degree T32.43
      - 40-49 percent third degree T32.44
  - 50-59 percent (0-9 percent third degree) T32.50
    - with
      - 10-19 percent third degree T32.51
      - 20-29 percent third degree T32.52
      - 30-39 percent third degree T32.53
      - 40-49 percent third degree T32.54
      - 50-59 percent third degree T32.55
  - 60-69 percent (0-9 percent third degree) T32.60
    - with
      - 10-19 percent third degree T32.61
      - 20-29 percent third degree T32.62
      - 30-39 percent third degree T32.63
      - 40-49 percent third degree T32.64
      - 50-59 percent third degree T32.65
      - 60-69 percent third degree T32.66
  - 70-79 percent (0-9 percent third degree) T32.70
    - with
      - 10-19 percent third degree T32.71
      - 20-29 percent third degree T32.72
      - 30-39 percent third degree T32.73
      - 40-49 percent third degree T32.74
      - 50-59 percent third degree T32.75

Corrosion — *continued*
- extent — *continued*
  - 70-79 percent — *continued*
    - with — *continued*
      - 60-69 percent third degree T32.76
      - 70-79 percent third degree T32.77
  - 80-89 percent (0-9 percent third degree) T32.80
    - with
      - 10-19 percent third degree T32.81
      - 20-29 percent third degree T32.82
      - 30-39 percent third degree T32.83
      - 40-49 percent third degree T32.84
      - 50-59 percent third degree T32.85
      - 60-69 percent third degree T32.86
      - 70-79 percent third degree T32.87
      - 80-89 percent third degree T32.88
  - 90 percent or more (0-9 percent third degree) T32.90
    - with
      - 10-19 percent third degree T32.91
      - 20-29 percent third degree T32.92
      - 30-39 percent third degree T32.93
      - 40-49 percent third degree T32.94
      - 50-59 percent third degree T32.95
      - 60-69 percent third degree T32.96
      - 70-79 percent third degree T32.97
      - 80-89 percent third degree T32.98
      - 90-99 percent third degree T32.99
- extremity — *see* Corrosion, limb
- eye(s) and adnexa T26.9- ☑
  - with resulting rupture and destruction of eyeball T26.7- ☑
  - conjunctival sac — *see* Corrosion, cornea
  - cornea — *see* Corrosion, cornea
  - lid — *see* Corrosion, eyelid
  - periocular area — *see* Corrosion eyelid
  - specified site NEC T26.8- ☑
- eyeball — *see* Corrosion, eye
- eyelid(s) T26.5- ☑
- face — *see* Corrosion, head
- finger T23.429- ☑
  - first degree T23.529- ☑
  - left T23.422- ☑
    - first degree T23.522- ☑
    - second degree T23.622- ☑
    - third degree T23.722- ☑
  - multiple sites (without thumb) T23.439- ☑
    - with thumb T23.449- ☑
      - first degree T23.549- ☑
      - left T23.442- ☑
        - first degree T23.542- ☑
        - second degree T23.642- ☑
        - third degree T23.742- ☑
      - right T23.441- ☑
        - first degree T23.541- ☑
        - second degree T23.641- ☑
        - third degree T23.741- ☑
      - second degree T23.649- ☑
      - third degree T23.749- ☑
    - first degree T23.539- ☑
    - left T23.432- ☑
      - first degree T23.532- ☑
      - second degree T23.632- ☑
      - third degree T23.732- ☑
    - right T23.431- ☑
      - first degree T23.531- ☑
      - second degree T23.631- ☑
      - third degree T23.731- ☑
    - second degree T23.639- ☑
    - third degree T23.739- ☑
  - right T23.421- ☑
    - first degree T23.521- ☑
    - second degree T23.621- ☑
    - third degree T23.721- ☑
  - second degree T23.629- ☑
  - third degree T23.729- ☑
- flank — *see* Corrosion, abdomen
- foot T25.429- ☑
  - first degree T25.529- ☑
  - left T25.422- ☑
    - first degree T25.522- ☑
    - second degree T25.622- ☑
    - third degree T25.722- ☑
  - multiple with ankle — *see* Corrosion, lower, limb, multiple, ankle and foot
  - right T25.421- ☑
    - first degree T25.521- ☑

Corrosion — *continued*
- foot — *continued*
  - right — *continued*
    - second degree T25.621- ☑
    - third degree T25.721- ☑
  - second degree T25.629- ☑
  - third degree T25.729- ☑
- forearm T22.419- ☑
  - first degree T22.519- ☑
  - left T22.412- ☑
    - first degree T22.512- ☑
    - second degree T22.612- ☑
    - third degree T22.712- ☑
  - right T22.411- ☑
    - first degree T22.511- ☑
    - second degree T22.611- ☑
    - third degree T22.711- ☑
  - second degree T22.619- ☑
  - third degree T22.719- ☑
- forehead T20.46- ☑
  - first degree T20.56- ☑
  - second degree T20.66- ☑
  - third degree T20.76- ☑
- fourth degree — *code as* Corrosion, third degree, by site
- full thickness skin loss — *code as* Corrosion, third degree, by site
- gastrointestinal tract NEC T28.7- ☑
- genital organs
  - external
    - female T21.47- ☑
      - first degree T21.57- ☑
      - second degree T21.67- ☑
      - third degree T21.77- ☑
    - male T21.46- ☑
      - first degree T21.56- ☑
      - second degree T21.66- ☑
      - third degree T21.76- ☑
  - internal T28.8- ☑
- groin — *see* Corrosion, abdominal wall
- hand(s) T23.409- ☑
  - back — *see* Corrosion, dorsum of hand
  - finger — *see* Corrosion, finger
  - first degree T23.509- ☑
  - left T23.402- ☑
    - first degree T23.502- ☑
    - second degree T23.602- ☑
    - third degree T23.702- ☑
  - multiple sites with wrist T23.499- ☑
    - first degree T23.599- ☑
    - left T23.492- ☑
      - first degree T23.592- ☑
      - second degree T23.692- ☑
      - third degree T23.792- ☑
    - right T23.491- ☑
      - first degree T23.591- ☑
      - second degree T23.691- ☑
      - third degree T23.791- ☑
    - second degree T23.699- ☑
    - third degree T23.799- ☑
  - palm — *see* Corrosion, palm
  - right T23.401- ☑
    - first degree T23.501- ☑
    - second degree T23.601- ☑
    - third degree T23.701- ☑
  - second degree T23.609- ☑
  - third degree T23.709- ☑
  - thumb — *see* Corrosion, thumb
- head (and face) (and neck) T20.40- ☑
  - cheek — *see* Corrosion, cheek
  - chin — *see* Corrosion, chin
  - ear — *see* Corrosion, ear
  - eye(s) only — *see* Corrosion, eye
  - first degree T20.50- ☑
  - forehead — *see* Corrosion, forehead
  - lip — *see* Corrosion, lip
  - multiple sites T20.49- ☑
    - first degree T20.59- ☑
    - second degree T20.69- ☑
    - third degree T20.79- ☑
  - neck — *see* Corrosion, neck
  - nose — *see* Corrosion, nose
  - scalp — *see* Corrosion, scalp
  - second degree T20.60- ☑
  - third degree T20.70- ☑
- hip(s) — *see* Corrosion, lower, limb
- inhalation — *see* Corrosion, respiratory tract

Corrosion — *continued*
- internal organ(s) — *see also* Corrosion, by site T28.90- ☑
  - alimentary tract T28.7- ☑
    - esophagus T28.6- ☑
  - esophagus T28.6- ☑
  - genitourinary T28.8- ☑
  - mouth T28.5- ☑
  - pharynx T28.5- ☑
  - specified organ NEC T28.99- ☑
- interscapular region — *see* Corrosion, back, upper
- intestine (large) (small) T28.7- ☑
- knee T24.429- ☑
  - first degree T24.529- ☑
  - left T24.422- ☑
    - first degree T24.522- ☑
    - second degree T24.622- ☑
    - third degree T24.722- ☑
  - right T24.421- ☑
    - first degree T24.521- ☑
    - second degree T24.621- ☑
    - third degree T24.721- ☑
  - second degree T24.629- ☑
  - third degree T24.729- ☑
- labium (majus) (minus) — *see* Corrosion, genital organs, external, female
- lacrimal apparatus, duct, gland or sac — *see* Corrosion, eye, specified site NEC
- larynx T27.4- ☑
  - with lung T27.5- ☑
- leg(s) (meaning lower limb(s)) — *see* Corrosion, lower limb
- limb(s)
  - lower — *see* Corrosion, lower, limb
  - upper — *see* Corrosion, upper limb
- lip(s) T20.42- ☑
  - first degree T20.52- ☑
  - second degree T20.62- ☑
  - third degree T20.72- ☑
- lower
  - back — *see* Corrosion, back
  - limb T24.409- ☑
    - ankle — *see* Corrosion, ankle
    - calf — *see* Corrosion, calf
    - first degree T24.509- ☑
    - foot — *see* Corrosion, foot
    - knee — *see* Corrosion, knee
    - left T24.402- ☑
      - first degree T24.502- ☑
      - second degree T24.602- ☑
      - third degree T24.702- ☑
    - multiple sites, except ankle and foot T24.499- ☑
      - ankle and foot T25.499- ☑
        - first degree T25.599- ☑
        - left T25.492- ☑
          - first degree T25.592- ☑
          - second degree T25.692- ☑
          - third degree T25.792- ☑
        - right T25.491- ☑
          - first degree T25.591- ☑
          - second degree T25.691- ☑
          - third degree T25.791- ☑
        - second degree T25.699- ☑
        - third degree T25.799- ☑
      - first degree T24.599- ☑
      - left T24.492- ☑
        - first degree T24.592- ☑
        - second degree T24.692- ☑
        - third degree T24.792- ☑
      - right T24.491- ☑
        - first degree T24.591- ☑
        - second degree T24.691- ☑
        - third degree T24.791- ☑
      - second degree T24.699- ☑
      - third degree T24.799- ☑
    - right T24.401- ☑
      - first degree T24.501- ☑
      - second degree T24.601- ☑
      - third degree T24.701- ☑
    - second degree T24.609- ☑
    - thigh — *see* Corrosion, thigh
    - third degree T24.709- ☑
- lung (with larynx and trachea) T27.5- ☑
- mouth T28.5- ☑
- neck T20.47- ☑
  - first degree T20.57- ☑
  - second degree T20.67- ☑

Corrosion — *continued*
- neck — *continued*
  - third degree T20.77- ☑
- nose (septum) T20.44- ☑
  - first degree T20.54- ☑
  - second degree T20.64- ☑
  - third degree T20.74- ☑
- ocular adnexa — *see* Corrosion, eye
- orbit region — *see* Corrosion, eyelid
- palm T23.459- ☑
  - first degree T23.559- ☑
  - left T23.452- ☑
    - first degree T23.552- ☑
    - second degree T23.652- ☑
    - third degree T23.752- ☑
  - right T23.451- ☑
    - first degree T23.551- ☑
    - second degree T23.651- ☑
    - third degree T23.751- ☑
  - second degree T23.659- ☑
  - third degree T23.759- ☑
- partial thickness — *code as* Corrosion, unspecified degree, by site
- pelvis — *see* Corrosion, trunk
- penis — *see* Corrosion, genital organs, external, male
- perineum
  - female — *see* Corrosion, genital organs, external, female
  - male — *see* Corrosion, genital organs, external, male
- periocular area — *see* Corrosion, eyelid
- pharynx T28.5- ☑
- rectum T28.7- ☑
- respiratory tract T27.7- ☑
  - larynx — *see* Corrosion, larynx
  - specified part NEC T27.6- ☑
  - trachea — *see* Corrosion, larynx
- sac, lacrimal — *see* Corrosion, eye, specified site NEC
- scalp T20.45- ☑
  - first degree T20.55- ☑
  - second degree T20.65- ☑
  - third degree T20.75- ☑
- scapular region T22.469- ☑
  - first degree T22.569- ☑
  - left T22.462- ☑
    - first degree T22.562- ☑
    - second degree T22.662- ☑
    - third degree T22.762- ☑
  - right T22.461- ☑
    - first degree T22.561- ☑
    - second degree T22.661- ☑
    - third degree T22.761- ☑
  - second degree T22.669- ☑
  - third degree T22.769- ☑
- sclera — *see* Corrosion, eye, specified site NEC
- scrotum — *see* Corrosion, genital organs, external, male
- shoulder T22.459- ☑
  - first degree T22.559- ☑
  - left T22.452- ☑
    - first degree T22.552- ☑
    - second degree T22.652- ☑
    - third degree T22.752- ☑
  - right T22.451- ☑
    - first degree T22.551- ☑
    - second degree T22.651- ☑
    - third degree T22.751- ☑
  - second degree T22.659- ☑
  - third degree T22.759- ☑
- stomach T28.7- ☑
- temple — *see* Corrosion, head
- testis — *see* Corrosion, genital organs, external, male
- thigh T24.419- ☑
  - first degree T24.519- ☑
  - left T24.412- ☑
    - first degree T24.512- ☑
    - second degree T24.612- ☑
    - third degree T24.712- ☑
  - right T24.411- ☑
    - first degree T24.511- ☑
    - second degree T24.611- ☑
    - third degree T24.711- ☑
  - second degree T24.619- ☑
  - third degree T24.719- ☑
- thorax (external) — *see* Corrosion, trunk
- throat (meaning pharynx) T28.5- ☑
- thumb(s) T23.419- ☑
  - first degree T23.519- ☑

Corrosion — *continued*
- thumb(s) — *continued*
  - left T23.412- ☑
    - first degree T23.512- ☑
    - second degree T23.612- ☑
    - third degree T23.712- ☑
  - multiple sites with fingers T23.449- ☑
    - first degree T23.549- ☑
    - left T23.442- ☑
      - first degree T23.542- ☑
      - second degree T23.642- ☑
      - third degree T23.742- ☑
    - right T23.441- ☑
      - first degree T23.541- ☑
      - second degree T23.641- ☑
      - third degree T23.741- ☑
    - second degree T23.649- ☑
    - third degree T23.749- ☑
  - right T23.411- ☑
    - first degree T23.511- ☑
    - second degree T23.611- ☑
    - third degree T23.711- ☑
  - second degree T23.619- ☑
  - third degree T23.719- ☑
- toe T25.439- ☑
  - first degree T25.539- ☑
  - left T25.432- ☑
    - first degree T25.532- ☑
    - second degree T25.632- ☑
    - third degree T25.732- ☑
  - right T25.431- ☑
    - first degree T25.531- ☑
    - second degree T25.631- ☑
    - third degree T25.731- ☑
  - second degree T25.639- ☑
  - third degree T25.739- ☑
- tongue T28.5- ☑
- tonsil(s) T28.5- ☑
- total body — *see* Corrosion, multiple body regions
- trachea T27.4- ☑
  - with lung T27.5- ☑
- trunk T21.40- ☑
  - abdominal wall — *see* Corrosion, abdominal wall
  - anus — *see* Corrosion, buttock
  - axilla — *see* Corrosion, upper limb
  - back — *see* Corrosion, back
  - breast — *see* Corrosion, chest wall
  - buttock — *see* Corrosion, buttock
  - chest wall — *see* Corrosion, chest wall
  - first degree T21.50- ☑
  - flank — *see* Corrosion, abdominal wall
  - genital
    - female — *see* Corrosion, genital organs, external, female
    - male — *see* Corrosion, genital organs, external, male
  - groin — *see* Corrosion, abdominal wall
  - interscapular region — *see* Corrosion, back, upper
  - labia — *see* Corrosion, genital organs, external, female
  - lower back — *see* Corrosion, back
  - penis — *see* Corrosion, genital organs, external, male
  - perineum
    - female — *see* Corrosion, genital organs, external, female
    - male — *see* Corrosion, genital organs, external, male
  - scapular region — *see* Corrosion, upper limb
  - scrotum — *see* Corrosion, genital organs, external, male
  - second degree T21.60- ☑
  - shoulder — *see* Corrosion, upper limb
  - specified site NEC T21.49- ☑
    - first degree T21.59- ☑
    - second degree T21.69- ☑
    - third degree T21.79- ☑
  - testes — *see* Corrosion, genital organs, external, male
  - third degree T21.70- ☑
  - upper back — *see* Corrosion, back, upper
  - vagina T28.8- ☑
  - vulva — *see* Corrosion, genital organs, external, female
- unspecified site with extent of body surface involved specified
  - less than 10 percent T32.0
  - 10-19 percent (0-9 percent third degree) T32.10
    - with 10-19 percent third degree T32.11
  - 20-29 percent (0-9 percent third degree) T32.20

☑ Additional Character Required — Refer to the Tabular List for Character Selection

Corrosion — continued
  unspecified site with extent of body surface involved specified — continued
    20-29 percent — continued
      with
        10-19 percent third degree T32.21
        20-29 percent third degree T32.22
    30-39 percent (0-9 percent third degree) T32.30
      with
        10-19 percent third degree T32.31
        20-29 percent third degree T32.32
        30-39 percent third degree T32.33
    40-49 percent (0-9 percent third degree) T32.40
      with
        10-19 percent third degree T32.41
        20-29 percent third degree T32.42
        30-39 percent third degree T32.43
        40-49 percent third degree T32.44
    50-59 percent (0-9 percent third degree) T32.50
      with
        10-19 percent third degree T32.51
        20-29 percent third degree T32.52
        30-39 percent third degree T32.53
        40-49 percent third degree T32.54
        50-59 percent third degree T32.55
    60-69 percent (0-9 percent third degree) T32.60
      with
        10-19 percent third degree T32.61
        20-29 percent third degree T32.62
        30-39 percent third degree T32.63
        40-49 percent third degree T32.64
        50-59 percent third degree T32.65
        60-69 percent third degree T32.66
    70-79 percent (0-9 percent third degree) T32.70
      with
        10-19 percent third degree T32.71
        20-29 percent third degree T32.72
        30-39 percent third degree T32.73
        40-49 percent third degree T32.74
        50-59 percent third degree T32.75
        60-69 percent third degree T32.76
        70-79 percent third degree T32.77
    80-89 percent (0-9 percent third degree) T32.80
      with
        10-19 percent third degree T32.81
        20-29 percent third degree T32.82
        30-39 percent third degree T32.83
        40-49 percent third degree T32.84
        50-59 percent third degree T32.85
        60-69 percent third degree T32.86
        70-79 percent third degree T32.87
        80-89 percent third degree T32.88
    90 percent or more (0-9 percent third degree) T32.90
      with
        10-19 percent third degree T32.91
        20-29 percent third degree T32.92
        30-39 percent third degree T32.93
        40-49 percent third degree T32.94
        50-59 percent third degree T32.95
        60-69 percent third degree T32.96
        70-79 percent third degree T32.97
        80-89 percent third degree T32.98
        90-99 percent third degree T32.99
  upper limb (axilla) (scapular region) T22.40- ☑
    above elbow — see Corrosion, above elbow
    axilla — see Corrosion, axilla
    elbow — see Corrosion, elbow
    first degree T22.50- ☑
    forearm — see Corrosion, forearm
    hand — see Corrosion, hand
    interscapular region — see Corrosion, back, upper
    multiple sites T22.499- ☑
      first degree T22.599- ☑
      left T22.492- ☑
        first degree T22.592- ☑
        second degree T22.692- ☑
        third degree T22.792- ☑
      right T22.491- ☑
        first degree T22.591- ☑
        second degree T22.691- ☑
        third degree T22.791- ☑
      second degree T22.699- ☑
      third degree T22.799- ☑
    scapular region — see Corrosion, scapular region
    second degree T22.60- ☑
    shoulder — see Corrosion, shoulder
    third degree T22.70- ☑
    wrist — see Corrosion, hand

Corrosion — continued
  uterus T28.8- ☑
  vagina T28.8- ☑
  vulva — see Corrosion, genital organs, external, female
  wrist T23.479-
    first degree T23.579- ☑
    left T23.472-
      first degree T23.572- ☑
      second degree T23.672- ☑
      third degree T23.772- ☑
    multiple sites with hand T23.499- ☑
      first degree T23.599- ☑
      left T23.492-
        first degree T23.592- ☑
        second degree T23.692- ☑
        third degree T23.792- ☑
      right T23.491-
        first degree T23.591- ☑
        second degree T23.691- ☑
        third degree T23.791- ☑
      second degree T23.699- ☑
      third degree T23.799- ☑
    right T23.471-
      first degree T23.571- ☑
      second degree T23.671- ☑
      third degree T23.771- ☑
    second degree T23.679- ☑
    third degree T23.779- ☑
Corrosive burn — see Corrosion
Corsican fever — see Malaria
Cortical — see condition
Cortico-adrenal — see condition
Coryza (acute) J00
  with grippe or influenza — see Influenza, with, respiratory manifestations NEC
  syphilitic
    congenital (chronic) A50.05
Co-sleeping, child-caregiver Z72.823
Costen's syndrome or complex M26.69
Costiveness — see Constipation
Costochondritis M94.0
Cot death R99
Cotard's syndrome F22
Cotia virus B08.8
Cotton wool spots (retinal) H35.81
Cotugno disease — see Sciatica
Cough (affected) (epidemic) (nervous) R05.9
  with hemorrhage — see Hemoptysis
  acute R05.1
  bronchial R05.8
    with grippe or influenza — see Influenza, with, respiratory manifestations NEC
  chronic R05.3
  functional F45.8
  hysterical F45.8
  laryngeal, spasmodic R05.8
  paroxysmal, due to Bordetella pertussis (without pneumonia) A37.00
    with pneumonia A37.01
  persistent R05.3
  psychogenic F45.8
  refractory R05.3
  smokers' J41.0
  specified NEC R05.8
  subacute R05.2
  syncope R05.4
  tea taster's B49
  unexplained R05.3
Counseling (for) Z71.9
  abuse NEC
    perpetrator Z69.82
    victim Z69.81
  alcohol abuser Z71.41
    family Z71.42
  child abuse
    nonparental
      perpetrator Z69.021
      victim Z69.020
    parental
      perpetrator Z69.011
      victim Z69.010
  consanguinity Z71.89
  contraceptive Z30.09
  dietary Z71.3
  drug abuser Z71.51
    family member Z71.52
  exercise Z71.82
  family Z71.89

Counseling — continued
  fertility preservation (prior to cancer therapy) (prior to removal of gonads) Z31.62
  for non-attending third party Z71.0
    related to sexual behavior or orientation Z70.2
  genetic
    nonprocreative Z71.83
    procreative NEC Z31.5
  gestational carrier Z31.7
  health (advice) (education) (instruction) — see Counseling, medical
    risk for travel (international) Z71.84
  human immunodeficiency virus (HIV) Z71.7
  immunization safety Z71.85
  impotence Z70.1
  insulin pump use Z46.81
  medical (for) Z71.9
    boarding school resident Z59.3
    consanguinity Z71.89
    feared complaint and no disease found Z71.1
    human immunodeficiency virus (HIV) Z71.7
    institutional resident Z59.3
    on behalf of another Z71.0
      related to sexual behavior or orientation Z70.2
    person living alone — see also Consultation, specified reason NEC Z60.2
    specified reason NEC Z71.89
  natural family planning
    procreative Z31.61
    to avoid pregnancy Z30.02
  pediatric-to-adult transition Z71.87
  perpetrator (of)
    abuse NEC Z69.82
    child abuse
      non-parental Z69.021
      parental Z69.011
    rape NEC Z69.82
    spousal abuse Z69.12
  procreative NEC Z31.69
    fertility preservation (prior to cancer therapy) (prior to removal of gonads) Z31.62
    using natural family planning Z31.61
  promiscuity Z70.1
  rape victim Z69.81
  religious Z71.81
  safety for travel (international) Z71.84
  sex, sexual (related to) Z70.9
    attitude(s) Z70.0
    behavior or orientation Z70.1
    combined concerns Z70.3
    non-responsiveness Z70.1
    on behalf of third party Z70.2
    specified reason NEC Z70.8
  socioeconomic factors Z71.88
  specified reason NEC Z71.89
  spiritual Z71.81
  spousal abuse (perpetrator) Z69.12
    victim Z69.11
  substance abuse Z71.89
    alcohol Z71.41
    drug Z71.51
    tobacco Z71.6
  tobacco use Z71.6
  travel (international) Z71.84
  use (of)
    insulin pump Z46.81
  vaccine product safety Z71.85
  victim (of)
    abuse Z69.81
    child abuse
      by parent Z69.010
      non-parental Z69.020
    rape NEC Z69.81
Coupled rhythm R00.8
Couvelaire syndrome or uterus (complicating delivery) O45.8X- ☑
COVID-19 U07.1
  condition post U09.9
  contact (with) Z20.822
  exposure (to) Z20.822
  history of (personal) Z86.16
  long (haul) U09.9
  partially vaccinated (for) Z28.311
  pneumonia J12.82
  screening Z11.52
  sequelae (post acute) U09.9
  unvaccinated (for) Z28.310
Cowperitis — see Urethritis
Cowper's gland — see condition

Cowpox B08.010
  due to vaccination T88.1- ☑
Coxa
  magna M91.4- ☑
  plana M91.2- ☑
  valga (acquired) — *see also* Deformity, limb, specified type NEC, thigh
    congenital Q65.81
    sequelae (late effect) of rickets E64.3
  vara (acquired) — *see also* Deformity, limb, specified type NEC, thigh
    congenital Q65.82
    sequelae (late effect) of rickets E64.3
Coxalgia, coxalgic (nontuberculous) — *see also* Pain, joint, hip
  tuberculous A18.02
Coxitis — *see* Monoarthritis, hip
Coxsackie (virus) (infection) B34.1
  as cause of disease classified elsewhere B97.11
  carditis B33.20
  central nervous system NEC A88.8
  endocarditis B33.21
  enteritis A08.39
  meningitis (aseptic) A87.0
  myocarditis B33.22
  pericarditis B33.23
  pharyngitis B08.5
  pleurodynia B33.0
  specific disease NEC B33.8
Crabs, meaning pubic lice B85.3
Crack baby P04.41
Cracked nipple N64.0
  associated with
    lactation O92.13
    pregnancy O92.11- ☑
    puerperium O92.12
Cracked tooth K03.81
Cradle cap L21.0
Craft neurosis F48.8
Cramp(s) R25.2
  abdominal — *see* Pain, abdominal
  bathing T75.1- ☑
  colic R10.83
    psychogenic F45.8
  due to immersion T75.1- ☑
  fireman T67.2- ☑
  heat T67.2- ☑
  immersion T75.1- ☑
  intestinal — *see* Pain, abdominal
    psychogenic F45.8
  leg, sleep related G47.62
  limb (lower) (upper) NEC R25.2
    sleep related G47.62
  linotypist's F48.8
    organic G25.89
  muscle (limb) (general) R25.2
    due to immersion T75.1- ☑
    psychogenic F45.8
  occupational (hand) F48.8
    organic G25.89
  salt-depletion E87.1
  sleep related, leg G47.62
  stoker's T67.2- ☑
  swimmer's T75.1- ☑
  telegrapher's F48.8
    organic G25.89
  typist's F48.8
    organic G25.89
  uterus N94.89
    menstrual — *see* Dysmenorrhea
  writer's F48.8
    organic G25.89
Cranial — *see* condition
Craniocleidodysostosis Q74.0
Craniofenestria (skull) Q75.8
Craniolacunia (skull) Q75.8
Craniopagus Q89.4
Craniopathy, metabolic M85.2
Craniopharyngeal — *see* condition
Craniopharyngioma D44.4
Craniorachischisis (totalis) Q00.1
Cranioschisis Q75.8
Craniostenosis Q75.009
Craniosynostosis Q75.009
  bilateral Q75.002
  coronal Q75.029
    bilateral Q75.022
    unilateral Q75.021

Craniosynostosis — *continued*
  lambdoid Q75.049
    bilateral Q75.042
    unilateral Q75.041
  metopic Q75.03
  multi-suture, specified NEC Q75.058
  sagittal Q75.01
  single-suture, specified NEC Q75.08
  unilateral Q75.001
Craniotabes (cause unknown) M83.8
  neonatal P96.3
  rachitic E64.3
  syphilitic A50.56
Cranium — *see* condition
Craw-craw — *see* Onchocerciasis
Creaking joint — *see* Derangement, joint, specified type NEC
Creeping
  eruption B76.9
  palsy or paralysis G12.22
Crenated tongue K14.8
Creotoxism A05.9
Crepitus
  caput Q75.8
  joint — *see* Derangement, joint, specified type NEC
Crescent or conus choroid, congenital Q14.3
CREST syndrome M34.1
Cretin, cretinism (congenital) (endemic) (nongoitrous) (sporadic) E00.9
  pelvis
    with disproportion (fetopelvic) O33.0
      causing obstructed labor O65.0
  type
    hypothyroid E00.1
    mixed E00.2
    myxedematous E00.1
    neurological E00.0
Creutzfeldt-Jakob disease or syndrome (with dementia) A81.00
  familial A81.09
  iatrogenic A81.09
  specified NEC A81.09
  sporadic A81.09
  variant (vCJD) A81.01
Cri-du-chat syndrome Q93.4
Crib death R99
Cribriform hymen Q52.3
Crigler-Najjar disease or syndrome E80.5
Crime, victim of Z65.4
Crimean hemorrhagic fever A98.0
Criminalism F60.2
Crisis
  abdomen R10.0
  acute reaction F43.0
  addisonian E27.2
  adrenal (cortical) E27.2
  celiac K90.0
  Dietl's N13.8
  emotional — *see also* Disorder, adjustment
    acute reaction to stress F43.0
    specific to childhood and adolescence F93.8
  glaucomatocyclitic — *see* Glaucoma, secondary, inflammation
  heart — *see* Failure, heart
  nitritoid I95.2
    correct substance properly administered — *see* Table of Drugs and Chemicals, by drug, adverse effect
    overdose or wrong substance given or taken — *see* Table of Drugs and Chemicals, by drug, poisoning
  oculogyric H51.8
    psychogenic F45.8
  Pel's (tabetic) A52.11
  psychosexual identity F64.2
  renal N28.0
  sickle-cell — *see also* Disease, sickle-cell, by type, with crisis D57.00
    with
      acute chest syndrome D57.01
      cerebral vascular involvement D57.03
      complication specified NEC D57.09
      pain (vaso-occlusive) D57.00
      splenic sequestration D57.02
  state (acute reaction) F43.0
  tabetic A52.11
  thyroid — *see* Thyrotoxicosis with thyroid storm
  thyrotoxic — *see* Thyrotoxicosis with thyroid storm
Crocq's disease (acrocyanosis) I73.89
Crohn's disease — *see* Enteritis, regional

Crooked septum, nasal J34.2
Cross-eye — *see* Strabismus, convergent concomitant
Cross syndrome E70.328
Crossbite (anterior) (posterior) M26.24
Croup, croupous (catarrhal) (infectious) (inflammatory) (nondiphtheritic) J05.0
  bronchial J20.9
  diphtheritic A36.2
  false J38.5
  spasmodic J38.5
    diphtheritic A36.2
  stridulous J38.5
    diphtheritic A36.2
Crouzon's disease Q75.1
Crowding, tooth, teeth, fully erupted M26.31
CRST syndrome M34.1
Cruchet's disease A85.8
Cruelty in children — *see also* Disorder, conduct
Crural ulcer — *see* Ulcer, lower limb
Crush, crushed, crushing T14.8- ☑
  abdomen S38.1- ☑
  ankle S97.0- ☑
  arm (upper) (and shoulder) S47.- ☑
  axilla — *see* Crush, arm
  back, lower S38.1- ☑
  buttock S38.1- ☑
  cheek S07.0- ☑
  chest S28.0- ☑
  cranium S07.1- ☑
  ear S07.0- ☑
  elbow S57.0- ☑
  extremity
    lower
      ankle — *see* Crush, ankle
      below knee — *see* Crush, leg
      foot — *see* Crush, foot
      hip — *see* Crush, hip
      knee — *see* Crush, knee
      thigh — *see* Crush, thigh
      toe — *see* Crush, toe
    upper
      below elbow S67.9- ☑
      elbow — *see* Crush, elbow
      finger — *see* Crush, finger
      forearm — *see* Crush, forearm
      hand — *see* Crush, hand
      thumb — *see* Crush, thumb
      upper arm — *see* Crush, arm
      wrist — *see* Crush, wrist
  face S07.0- ☑
  finger(s) S67.1- ☑
    with hand (and wrist) — *see* Crush, hand, specified site NEC
    index S67.19- ☑
    little S67.19- ☑
    middle S67.19- ☑
    ring S67.19- ☑
    thumb — *see* Crush, thumb
  foot S97.8- ☑
    toe — *see* Crush, toe
  forearm S57.8- ☑
  genitalia, external
    female S38.002- ☑
      vagina S38.03- ☑
      vulva S38.03- ☑
    male S38.001- ☑
      penis S38.01- ☑
      scrotum S38.02- ☑
      testis S38.02- ☑
  hand (except fingers alone) S67.2- ☑
    with wrist S67.4- ☑
  head S07.9- ☑
    specified NEC S07.8- ☑
  heel — *see* Crush, foot
  hip S77.0- ☑
    with thigh S77.2- ☑
  internal organ (abdomen, chest, or pelvis) NEC T14.8- ☑
  knee S87.0- ☑
  labium (majus) (minus) S38.03- ☑
  larynx S17.0- ☑
  leg (lower) S87.8- ☑
    knee — *see* Crush, knee
  lip S07.0- ☑
  lower
    back S38.1- ☑
    leg — *see* Crush, leg
  neck S17.9- ☑

☑ Additional Character Required — Refer to the Tabular List for Character Selection

Crush, crushed, crushing — continued
- nerve — see Injury, nerve
- nose S07.0- ☑
- pelvis S38.1- ☑
- penis S38.01- ☑
- scalp S07.8- ☑
- scapular region — see Crush, arm
- scrotum S38.02- ☑
- severe, unspecified site T14.8- ☑
- shoulder (and upper arm) — see Crush, arm
- skull S07.1- ☑
- syndrome (complication of trauma) T79.5- ☑
- testis S38.02- ☑
- thigh S77.1- ☑
  - with hip S77.2- ☑
- throat S17.8- ☑
- thumb S67.0- ☑
  - with hand (and wrist) — see Crush, hand, specified site NEC
- toe(s) S97.10- ☑
  - great S97.11- ☑
  - lesser S97.12- ☑
- trachea S17.0- ☑
- vagina S38.03- ☑
- vulva S38.03- ☑
- wrist S67.3- ☑
  - with hand S67.4- ☑

Crusta lactea L21.0
Crusts R23.4
Crutch paralysis — see Injury, brachial plexus
Cruveilhier-Baumgarten cirrhosis, disease or syndrome K74.69
Cruveilhier's atrophy or disease G12.8
Crying (constant) (continuous) (excessive)
- child, adolescent, or adult R45.83
- infant (baby) (newborn) R68.11

Cryofibrinogenemia D89.2
Cryoglobulinemia (essential) (idiopathic) (mixed) (primary) (purpura) (secondary) (vasculitis) D89.1
- with lung involvement D89.1 [J99]

Cryptitis (anal) (rectal) K62.89
Cryptococcosis, cryptococcus (infection) (neoformans) B45.9
- bone B45.3
- cerebral B45.1
- cutaneous B45.2
- disseminated B45.7
- generalized B45.7
- meningitis B45.1
- meningocerebralis B45.1
- osseous B45.3
- pulmonary B45.0
- skin B45.2
- specified NEC B45.8

Cryptopapillitis (anus) K62.89
Cryptophthalmos Q11.2
- syndrome Q87.0

Cryptorchid, cryptorchism, cryptorchidism Q53.9
- bilateral Q53.20
  - abdominal Q53.211
  - perineal Q53.22
- unilateral Q53.10
  - abdominal Q53.111
  - perineal Q53.12

Cryptosporidiosis A07.2
- hepatobiliary B88.8
- respiratory B88.8

Cryptostromosis J67.6
Crystalluria R82.998
Cubitus
- congenital Q68.8
- valgus (acquired) M21.02- ☑
  - congenital Q68.8
  - sequelae (late effect) of rickets E64.3
- varus (acquired) M21.12- ☑
  - congenital Q68.8
  - sequelae (late effect) of rickets E64.3

Cultural deprivation or shock Z60.3
Curling esophagus K22.4
Curling's ulcer — see Ulcer, peptic, acute
Curschmann (-Batten) (-Steinert) **disease or syndrome** G71.11
Curse, Ondine's — see Apnea, sleep
Curvature
- organ or site, congenital NEC — see Distortion
- penis (lateral) Q55.61
- Pott's (spinal) A18.01
- radius, idiopathic, progressive (congenital) Q74.0

Curvature — continued
- spine (acquired) (angular) (idiopathic) (incorrect) (postural) — see Dorsopathy, deforming
  - congenital Q67.5
  - due to or associated with
    - Charcot-Marie-Tooth disease — see also subcategory M49.8 G60.0
    - osteitis
      - deformans M88.88
      - fibrosa cystica — see also subcategory M49.8 E21.0
    - tuberculosis (Pott's curvature) A18.01
  - sequelae (late effect) of rickets E64.3
  - tuberculous A18.01

Cushingoid due to steroid therapy E24.2
- correct substance properly administered — see Table of Drugs and Chemicals, by drug, adverse effect
- overdose or wrong substance given or taken — see Table of Drugs and Chemicals, by drug, poisoning

Cushing's
- syndrome or disease E24.9
  - drug-induced E24.2
  - iatrogenic E24.2
  - pituitary-dependent E24.0
  - specified NEC E24.8
- ulcer — see Ulcer, peptic, acute

Cusp, Carabelli — omit code
Cut (external) — see also Laceration
- muscle — see Injury, muscle

Cutaneous — see also condition
- hemorrhage R23.3
- larva migrans B76.9

Cutis — see also condition
- hyperelastica Q82.8
  - acquired L57.4
- laxa (hyperelastica) — see Dermatolysis
- marmorata R23.8
- osteosis L94.2
- pendula — see Dermatolysis
- rhomboidalis nuchae L57.2
- verticis gyrata Q82.8
  - acquired L91.8

Cyanosis R23.0
- due to
  - patent foramen botalli Q21.12
  - persistent foramen ovale Q21.12
- enterogenous D74.8
- paroxysmal digital — see Raynaud's disease
  - with gangrene I73.01
- retina, retinal H35.89

Cyanotic heart disease I24.9
- congenital Q24.9

Cycle
- anovulatory N97.0
- menstrual, irregular N92.6

Cyclencephaly Q04.9
Cyclical vomiting, in migraine — see also Vomiting, cyclical G43.A0 (following G43.7)
- psychogenic F50.89

Cyclitis — see also Iridocyclitis H20.9
- chronic — see Iridocyclitis, chronic
- Fuchs' heterochromic H20.81- ☑
- granulomatous — see Iridocyclitis, chronic
- lens-induced — see Iridocyclitis, lens-induced
- posterior H30.2- ☑

Cycloid personality F34.0
Cyclophoria H50.54
Cyclopia, cyclops Q87.0
Cyclopism Q87.0
Cyclosporiasis A07.4
Cyclothymia F34.0
Cyclothymic personality F34.0
Cyclotropia H50.41- ☑
Cylindroma — see also Neoplasm, malignant, by site
- eccrine dermal — see Neoplasm, skin, benign
- skin — see Neoplasm, skin, benign

Cylindruria R82.998
Cynanche
- diphtheritic A36.2
- tonsillaris J36

Cynophobia F40.218
Cynorexia R63.2
Cyphosis — see Kyphosis
Cyprus fever — see Brucellosis
Cyst (colloid) (mucous) (simple) (retention)
- adenoid (infected) J35.8
- adrenal gland E27.8
  - congenital Q89.1
- air, lung J98.4

Cyst — continued
- allantoic Q64.4
- alveolar process (jaw bone) M27.40
- amnion, amniotic O41.8X-
- aneurysmal M27.49
- anterior
  - chamber (eye) — see Cyst, iris
  - nasopalatine K09.1
- antrum J34.1
- anus K62.89
- apical (tooth) (periodontal) K04.8
- appendix K38.8
- arachnoid, brain (acquired) G93.0
  - congenital Q04.6
- arytenoid J38.7
- Baker's M71.2- ☑
  - ruptured M66.0
  - tuberculous A18.02
- Bartholin's gland N75.0
- bile duct (common) (hepatic) K83.5
- bladder (multiple) (trigone) N32.89
- blue dome (breast) — see Cyst, breast
- bone (local) NEC M85.60
  - aneurysmal M85.50
    - ankle M85.57- ☑
    - foot M85.57- ☑
    - forearm M85.53- ☑
    - hand M85.54- ☑
    - jaw M27.49
    - lower leg M85.56- ☑
    - multiple site M85.59
    - neck M85.58
    - rib M85.58
    - shoulder M85.51- ☑
    - skull M85.58
    - specified site NEC M85.58
    - thigh M85.55- ☑
    - toe M85.57- ☑
    - upper arm M85.52- ☑
    - vertebra M85.58
  - solitary M85.40
    - ankle M85.47- ☑
    - fibula M85.46- ☑
    - foot M85.47- ☑
    - hand M85.44- ☑
    - humerus M85.42- ☑
    - jaw M27.49
    - neck M85.48
    - pelvis M85.45- ☑
    - radius M85.43- ☑
    - rib M85.48
    - shoulder M85.41- ☑
    - skull M85.48
    - specified site NEC M85.48
    - tibia M85.46- ☑
    - toe M85.47- ☑
    - ulna M85.43- ☑
    - vertebra M85.48
  - specified type NEC M85.60
    - ankle M85.67- ☑
    - foot M85.67- ☑
    - forearm M85.63- ☑
    - hand M85.64- ☑
    - jaw M27.40
      - developmental (nonodontogenic) K09.1
      - odontogenic K09.0
      - latent M27.0
    - lower leg M85.66- ☑
    - multiple site M85.69
    - neck M85.68
    - rib M85.68
    - shoulder M85.61- ☑
    - skull M85.68
    - specified site NEC M85.68
    - thigh M85.65- ☑
    - toe M85.67- ☑
    - upper arm M85.62- ☑
    - vertebra M85.68
- brain (acquired) G93.0
  - congenital Q04.6
  - hydatid B67.99 [G94]
  - third ventricle (colloid), congenital Q04.6
- branchial (cleft) Q18.0
- branchiogenic Q18.0
- breast (benign) (blue dome) (pedunculated) (solitary) N60.0- ☑

Cyst — continued
 breast — continued
  involution — see Dysplasia, mammary, specified type NEC
  sebaceous — see Dysplasia, mammary, specified type NEC
 broad ligament (benign) N83.8
 bronchogenic (mediastinal) (sequestration) J98.4
  congenital Q33.0
 buccal K09.8
 bulbourethral gland N36.8
 bursa, bursal NEC M71.30
  with rupture — see Rupture, synovium
  ankle M71.37-
  elbow M71.32- ☑
  foot M71.37-
  hand M71.34- ☑
  hip M71.35- ☑
  multiple sites M71.39
  pharyngeal J39.2
  popliteal space — see Cyst, Baker's
  shoulder M71.31- ☑
  specified site NEC M71.38
  wrist M71.33- ☑
 calcifying odontogenic D16.5
  upper jaw (bone) (maxilla) D16.4
 canal of Nuck (female) N94.89
  congenital Q52.4
 canthus — see Cyst, conjunctiva
 carcinomatous — see Neoplasm, malignant, by site
 cauda equina G95.89
 cavum septi pellucidi — see Cyst, brain
 celomic (pericardium) Q24.8
 cerebellopontine (angle) — see Cyst, brain
 cerebellum — see Cyst, brain
 cerebral — see Cyst, brain
 cervical lateral Q18.0
 cervix NEC N88.8
  embryonic Q51.6
  nabothian N88.8
 chiasmal optic NEC — see Disorder, optic, chiasm
 chocolate (ovary) N80.10- ☑
 choledochus, congenital Q44.4
 chorion O41.8X- ☑
 choroid plexus G93.0
  congenital Q04.6
 ciliary body — see Cyst, iris
 clitoris N90.7
 colon K63.89
 common (bile) duct K83.5
 congenital NEC Q89.89
  adrenal gland Q89.1
  epiglottis Q31.8
  esophagus Q39.8
  fallopian tube Q50.4
  kidney Q61.00
   more than one (multiple) Q61.02
    specified as polycystic Q61.3
     adult type Q61.2
     infantile type NEC Q61.19
      collecting duct dilation Q61.11
   solitary Q61.01
  larynx Q31.8
  liver Q44.6
  lung Q33.0
  mediastinum Q34.1
  ovary Q50.1
  oviduct Q50.4
  periurethral (tissue) Q64.79
  prepuce Q55.69
  salivary gland (any) Q38.4
  sublingual Q38.6
  submaxillary gland Q38.6
  thymus (gland) Q89.2
  tongue Q38.3
  ureterovesical orifice Q62.8
  vulva Q52.79
 conjunctiva H11.44- ☑
 cornea H18.89- ☑
 corpora quadrigemina G93.0
 corpus
  albicans N83.29- ☑
  luteum (hemorrhagic) (ruptured) N83.1- ☑
 Cowper's gland (benign) (infected) N36.8
 cranial meninges G93.0
 craniobuccal pouch E23.6
 craniopharyngeal pouch E23.6
 cystic duct K82.8

Cyst — continued
 Cysticercus — see Cysticercosis
 Dandy-Walker Q03.1
  with spina bifida — see Spina bifida
 dental (root) K04.8
  developmental K09.0
  eruption K09.0
  primordial K09.0
 dentigerous (mandible) (maxilla) K09.0
 dermoid — see Neoplasm, benign, by site
  with malignant transformation C56.- ☑
  implantation
   external area or site (skin) NEC L72.0
   iris — see Cyst, iris, implantation
   vagina N89.8
   vulva N90.7
  mouth K09.8
  oral soft tissue K09.8
  sacrococcygeal — see Cyst, pilonidal
 developmental K09.1
  odontogenic K09.0
  oral region (nonodontogenic) K09.1
  ovary, ovarian Q50.1
 dura (cerebral) G93.0
  spinal G96.198
 ear (external) Q18.1
 echinococcal — see Echinococcus
 embryonic
  cervix uteri Q51.6
  fallopian tube Q50.4
  vagina Q52.4
 endometrium, endometrial (uterus) N85.8
  ectopic — see Endometriosis
 enterogenous Q43.8
 epidermal, epidermoid (inclusion) (see also Cyst, skin) L72.0
  mouth K09.8
  oral soft tissue K09.8
 epididymis N50.3
 epiglottis J38.7
 epiphysis cerebri E34.8
 epithelial (inclusion) L72.0
 epoophoron Q50.5
 eruption K09.0
 esophagus K22.89
 ethmoid sinus J34.1
 external female genital organs NEC N90.7
 eye NEC H57.89
  congenital Q15.8
 eyelid (sebaceous) H02.829
  infected — see Hordeolum
  left H02.826
   lower H02.825
   upper H02.824
  right H02.823
   lower H02.822
   upper H02.821
 fallopian tube N83.8
  congenital Q50.4
 fimbrial (twisted) Q50.4
 fissural (oral region) K09.1
 follicle (graafian) (hemorrhagic) N83.0- ☑
  nabothian N88.8
 follicular (atretic) (hemorrhagic) (ovarian) N83.0- ☑
  dentigerous K09.0
  odontogenic K09.0
  skin L72.9
   specified NEC L72.8
 frontal sinus J34.1
 gallbladder K82.8
 ganglion — see Ganglion
 Gartner's duct Q52.4
 gingiva K09.0
 gland of Moll — see Cyst, eyelid
 globulomaxillary K09.1
 graafian follicle (hemorrhagic) N83.0- ☑
 granulosal lutein (hemorrhagic) N83.1- ☑
 hemangiomatous D18.00
  intra-abdominal D18.03
  intracranial D18.02
  skin D18.01
  specified site NEC D18.09
 hemorrhagic M27.49
 hydatid — see also Echinococcus B67.90
  brain B67.99 [G94]
  liver — see also Cyst, liver, hydatid B67.8
  lung NEC B67.99 [J99]

Cyst — continued
 hydatid — see also Echinococcus — continued
  Morgagni
   female Q50.5
   male (epididymal) Q55.4
    testicular Q55.29
  specified site NEC B67.99
 hymen N89.8
  embryonic Q52.4
 hypopharynx J39.2
 hypophysis, hypophyseal (duct) (recurrent) E23.6
  cerebri E23.6
 implantation (dermoid)
  external area or site (skin) NEC L72.0
  iris — see Cyst, iris, implantation
  vagina N89.8
  vulva N90.7
 incisive canal K09.1
 inclusion (epidermal) (epithelial) (epidermoid) (squamous) L72.0
  not of skin — code under Cyst, by site
 intestine (large) (small) K63.89
 intracranial — see Cyst, brain
 intraligamentous — see also Disorder, ligament
  knee — see Derangement, knee
 intrasellar E23.6
 iris H21.309
  exudative H21.31- ☑
  idiopathic H21.30- ☑
  implantation H21.32- ☑
  parasitic H21.33- ☑
  pars plana (primary) H21.34- ☑
   exudative H21.35- ☑
 jaw (bone) M27.40
  aneurysmal M27.49
  developmental (odontogenic) K09.0
  fissural K09.1
  hemorrhagic M27.49
  traumatic M27.49
 joint NEC — see Disorder, joint, specified type NEC
 kidney N28.1
  acquired N28.1
  calyceal — see Hydronephrosis
  congenital Q61.00
   more than one (multiple) Q61.02
    specified as polycystic Q61.3
     adult type (autosomal dominant) Q61.2
     infantile type (autosomal recessive) NEC Q61.19
      collecting duct dilation Q61.11
  pyelogenic — see Hydronephrosis
  simple N28.1
  solitary (single) N28.1
   acquired N28.1
   congenital Q61.01
 labium (majus) (minus) N90.7
  sebaceous N90.7
 lacrimal — see also Disorder, lacrimal system, specified NEC
  gland H04.13- ☑
  passages or sac — see Disorder, lacrimal system, specified NEC
 larynx J38.7
 lateral periodontal K09.0
 lens H27.8
  congenital Q12.8
 lip (gland) K13.0
 liver (idiopathic) (simple) K76.89
  congenital Q44.6
  hydatid B67.8
   granulosus B67.0
   multilocularis B67.5
 lung J98.4
  congenital Q33.0
  giant bullous J43.9
 lutein N83.1- ☑
 lymphangiomatous D18.1
 lymphoepithelial, oral soft tissue K09.8
 macula — see Degeneration, macula, hole
 malignant — see Neoplasm, malignant, by site
 mammary gland — see Cyst, breast
 mandible M27.40
  dentigerous K09.0
  radicular K04.8
 maxilla M27.40
  dentigerous K09.0
  radicular K04.8
 medial, face and neck Q18.8

Cyst — *continued*
 median
  anterior maxillary K09.1
  palatal K09.1
 mediastinum, congenital Q34.1
 meibomian (gland) — *see* Chalazion
  infected — *see* Hordeolum
 membrane, brain G93.0
 meninges (cerebral) G93.0
  spinal G96.198
 meniscus, knee — *see* Derangement, knee, meniscus, cystic
 mesentery, mesenteric K66.8
  chyle I89.8
 mesonephric duct
  female Q50.5
  male Q55.4
 milk N64.89
 Morgagni (hydatid)
  female Q50.5
  male (epididymal) Q55.4
   testicular Q55.29
 mouth K09.8
 Mullerian duct Q50.4
  appendix testis Q55.29
  cervix Q51.6
  fallopian tube Q50.4
  female Q50.4
  male Q55.29
  prostatic utricle Q55.4
  vagina (embryonal) Q52.4
 multilocular (ovary) D39.10
  benign — *see* Neoplasm, benign, by site
 myometrium N85.8
 nabothian (follicle) (ruptured) N88.8
 nasoalveolar K09.1
 nasolabial K09.1
 nasopalatine (anterior) (duct) K09.1
 nasopharynx J39.2
 neoplastic — *see* Neoplasm, uncertain behavior, by site
  benign — *see* Neoplasm, benign, by site
 nerve root
  cervical G96.191
  lumbar G96.191
  sacral G96.191
  thoracic G96.191
 nervous system NEC G96.89
 neuroenteric (congenital) Q06.8
 nipple — *see* Cyst, breast
 nose (turbinates) J34.1
  sinus J34.1
 odontogenic, developmental K09.0
 omentum (lesser) K66.8
  congenital Q45.8
 ora serrata — *see* Cyst, retina, ora serrata
 oral
  region K09.9
   developmental (nonodontogenic) K09.1
   specified NEC K09.8
  soft tissue K09.9
   specified NEC K09.8
 orbit H05.81- ☑
 ovary, ovarian (twisted) N83.20- ☑
  adherent N83.20- ☑
  chocolate N80.10- ☑
  corpus
   albicans N83.29- ☑
   luteum (hemorrhagic) N83.1- ☑
  dermoid D27.9
  developmental Q50.1
  due to failure of involution NEC N83.20- ☑
  endometrial N80.10- ☑
  follicular (graafian) (hemorrhagic) N83.0- ☑
  hemorrhagic N83.20- ☑
  in pregnancy or childbirth O34.8- ☑
   with obstructed labor O65.5
  multilocular D39.10
  pseudomucinous D27.9
  retention N83.29- ☑
  serous N83.20- ☑
  specified NEC N83.29- ☑
  theca lutein (hemorrhagic) N83.1- ☑
  tuberculous A18.18
 oviduct N83.8
 palate (median) (fissural) K09.1
 palatine papilla (jaw) K09.1
 pancreas, pancreatic (hemorrhagic) (true) K86.2
  congenital Q45.2

Cyst — *continued*
 pancreas, pancreatic — *continued*
  false K86.3
 paralabral
  hip M24.85- ☑
  shoulder S43.43- ☑
 paramesonephric duct Q50.4
  female Q50.4
  male Q55.29
 paranephric N28.1
 paraphysis, cerebri, congenital Q04.6
 parasitic B89
 parathyroid (gland) E21.4
 paratubal N83.8
 paraurethral duct N36.8
 paroophoron Q50.5
 parotid gland K11.6
 parovarian Q50.5
 pelvis, female N94.89
  in pregnancy or childbirth O34.8- ☑
   causing obstructed labor O65.5
 penis (sebaceous) N48.89
 periapical K04.8
 pericardial (congenital) Q24.8
  acquired (secondary) I31.8
 pericoronal K09.0
 perineural G96.191
 periodontal K04.8
  lateral K09.0
 peripelvic (lymphatic) N28.1
 peritoneum K66.8
  chylous I89.8
 periventricular, acquired, newborn P91.1
 pharynx (wall) J39.2
 pilar L72.11
 pilonidal (infected) (rectum) L05.91
  with abscess L05.01
  malignant C44.59- ☑
 pituitary (duct) (gland) E23.6
 placenta O43.19- ☑
 pleura J94.8
 popliteal — *see* Cyst, Baker's
 porencephalic Q04.6
  acquired G93.0
 postanal (infected) — *see* Cyst, pilonidal
 postmastoidectomy cavity (mucosal) — *see* Complications, postmastoidectomy, cyst
 preauricular Q18.1
 prepuce N47.4
  congenital Q55.69
 primordial (jaw) K09.0
 prostate N42.83
 pseudomucinous (ovary) D27.9
 pupillary, miotic H21.27- ☑
 radicular (residual) K04.8
 radiculodental K04.8
 ranular K11.8
 Rathke's pouch E23.6
 rectum (epithelium) (mucous) K62.89
 renal — *see* Cyst, kidney
 residual (radicular) K04.8
 retention (ovary) N83.29- ☑
  salivary gland K11.6
 retina H33.19- ☑
  ora serrata H33.11- ☑
  parasitic H33.12- ☑
 retroperitoneal K68.9
 sacrococcygeal (dermoid) — *see* Cyst, pilonidal
 salivary gland or duct (mucous extravasation or retention) K11.6
 Sampson's N80.10- ☑
 sclera H15.89
 scrotum L72.9
  sebaceous L72.3
 sebaceous (duct) (gland) L72.3
  breast — *see* Dysplasia, mammary, specified type NEC
  eyelid — *see* Cyst, eyelid
  genital organ NEC
   female N94.89
   male N50.89
  scrotum L72.3
 semilunar cartilage (knee) (multiple) — *see* Derangement, knee, meniscus, cystic
 seminal vesicle N50.89
 serous (ovary) N83.20- ☑
 sinus (accessory) (nasal) J34.1
 Skene's gland N36.8
 skin L72.9

Cyst — *continued*
 skin — *continued*
  breast — *see* Dysplasia, mammary, specified type NEC
  epidermal, epidermoid L72.0
  epithelial L72.0
  eyelid — *see* Cyst, eyelid
  genital organ NEC
   female N90.7
   male N50.89
  inclusion L72.0
  scrotum L72.9
  sebaceous L72.3
  sweat gland or duct L74.8
 solitary
  bone — *see* Cyst, bone, solitary
  jaw M27.40
  kidney N28.1
 spermatic cord N50.89
 sphenoid sinus J34.1
 spinal meninges G96.198
 spleen NEC D73.4
  congenital Q89.09
  hydatid — *see also* Echinococcus B67.99 [D77]
 Stafne's M27.0
 subarachnoid intrasellar R93.0
 subcutaneous, pheomycotic (chromomycotic) B43.2
 subdural (cerebral) G93.0
  spinal cord G96.198
 sublingual gland K11.6
 submandibular gland K11.6
 submaxillary gland K11.6
 suburethral N36.8
 suprarenal gland E27.8
 suprasellar — *see* Cyst, brain
 sweat gland or duct L74.8
 synovial — *see also* Cyst, bursa
  ruptured — *see* Rupture, synovium
 Tarlov G96.191
 tarsal — *see* Chalazion
 tendon (sheath) — *see* Disorder, tendon, specified type NEC
 testis N44.2
  tunica albuginea N44.1
 theca lutein (ovary) N83.1- ☑
 Thornwaldt's J39.2
 thymus (gland) E32.8
 thyroglossal duct (infected) (persistent) Q89.2
 thyroid (gland) E04.1
 thyrolingual duct (infected) (persistent) Q89.2
 tongue K14.8
 tonsil J35.8
 tooth — *see* Cyst, dental
 Tornwaldt's J39.2
 trichilemmal (proliferating) L72.12
 trichodermal L72.12
 tubal (fallopian) N83.8
  inflammatory — *see* Salpingitis, chronic
 tubo-ovarian N83.8
  inflammatory N70.13
 tunica
  albuginea testis N44.1
  vaginalis N50.89
 turbinate (nose) J34.1
 Tyson's gland N48.89
 urachus, congenital Q64.4
 ureter N28.89
 ureterovesical orifice N28.89
 urethra, urethral (gland) N36.8
 uterine ligament N83.8
 uterus (body) (corpus) (recurrent) N85.8
  embryonic Q51.818
   cervix Q51.6
 vagina, vaginal (implantation) (inclusion) (squamous cell) (wall) N89.8
  embryonic Q52.4
 vallecula, vallecular (epiglottis) J38.7
 vesical (orifice) N32.89
 vitreous body H43.89
 vulva (implantation) (inclusion) N90.7
  congenital Q52.79
  sebaceous gland N90.7
 vulvovaginal gland N90.7
 wolffian
  female Q50.5
  male Q55.4
Cystadenocarcinoma — *see* Neoplasm, malignant, by site
 bile duct C22.1
 endometrioid — *see* Neoplasm, malignant, by site
  specified site — *see* Neoplasm, malignant, by site

Cystadenocarcinoma — *continued*
  endometrioid — *see* Neoplasm, malignant, by site — *continued*
    unspecified site
      female C56.9
      male C61
  mucinous
    papillary
      specified site — *see* Neoplasm, malignant, by site
      unspecified site C56.9
    specified site — *see* Neoplasm, malignant, by site
    unspecified site C56.9
  papillary
    mucinous
      specified site — *see* Neoplasm, malignant, by site
      unspecified site C56.9
    pseudomucinous
      specified site — *see* Neoplasm, malignant, by site
      unspecified site C56.9
    serous
      specified site — *see* Neoplasm, malignant, by site
      unspecified site C56.9
    specified site — *see* Neoplasm, malignant, by site
    unspecified site C56.9
  pseudomucinous
    papillary
      specified site — *see* Neoplasm, malignant, by site
      unspecified site C56.9
    specified site — *see* Neoplasm, malignant, by site
    unspecified site C56.9
  serous
    papillary
      specified site — *see* Neoplasm, malignant, by site
      unspecified site C56.9
    specified site — *see* Neoplasm, malignant, by site
    unspecified site C56.9

Cystadenofibroma
  clear cell — *see* Neoplasm, benign, by site
  endometrioid D27.9
    borderline malignancy D39.1- ☑
    malignant C56.- ☑
  mucinous
    specified site — *see* Neoplasm, benign, by site
    unspecified site D27.9
  serous
    specified site — *see* Neoplasm, benign, by site
    unspecified site D27.9
  specified site — *see* Neoplasm, benign, by site
  unspecified site D27.9

Cystadenoma — *see also* Neoplasm, benign, by site
  bile duct D13.4
  endometrioid — *see* Neoplasm, benign, by site
    borderline malignancy — *see* Neoplasm, uncertain behavior, by site
    malignant — *see* Neoplasm, malignant, by site
  mucinous
    borderline malignancy
      ovary C56.- ☑
      specified site NEC — *see* Neoplasm, uncertain behavior, by site
      unspecified site C56.9
    papillary
      borderline malignancy
        ovary C56.- ☑
        specified site NEC — *see* Neoplasm, uncertain behavior, by site
        unspecified site C56.9
      specified site — *see* Neoplasm, benign, by site
      unspecified site D27.9
    specified site — *see* Neoplasm, benign, by site
    unspecified site D27.9
  papillary
    borderline malignancy
      ovary C56.- ☑
      specified site NEC — *see* Neoplasm, uncertain behavior, by site
      unspecified site C56.9
    lymphomatosum
      specified site — *see* Neoplasm, benign, by site
      unspecified site D11.9
    mucinous
      borderline malignancy
        ovary C56.- ☑
        specified site NEC — *see* Neoplasm, uncertain behavior, by site
        unspecified site C56.9
      specified site — *see* Neoplasm, benign, by site
      unspecified site D27.9

Cystadenoma — *continued*
  papillary — *continued*
    pseudomucinous
      borderline malignancy
        ovary C56.- ☑
        specified site NEC — *see* Neoplasm, uncertain behavior, by site
        unspecified site C56.9
      specified site — *see* Neoplasm, benign, by site
      unspecified site D27.9
    serous
      borderline malignancy
        ovary C56.- ☑
        specified site NEC — *see* Neoplasm, uncertain behavior, by site
        unspecified site C56.9
      specified site — *see* Neoplasm, benign, by site
      unspecified site D27.9
    specified site — *see* Neoplasm, benign, by site
    unspecified site D27.9
  pseudomucinous
    borderline malignancy
      ovary C56.- ☑
      specified site NEC — *see* Neoplasm, uncertain behavior, by site
      unspecified site C56.9
    papillary
      borderline malignancy
        ovary C56.- ☑
        specified site NEC — *see* Neoplasm, uncertain behavior, by site
        unspecified site C56.9
      specified site — *see* Neoplasm, benign, by site
      unspecified site D27.9
    specified site — *see* Neoplasm, benign, by site
    unspecified site D27.9
  serous
    borderline malignancy
      ovary C56.- ☑
      specified site NEC — *see* Neoplasm, uncertain behavior, by site
      unspecified site C56.9
    papillary
      borderline malignancy
        ovary C56.- ☑
        specified site NEC — *see* Neoplasm, uncertain behavior, by site
        unspecified site C56.9
      specified site — *see* Neoplasm, benign, by site
      unspecified site D27.9
    specified site — *see* Neoplasm, benign, by site
    unspecified site D27.9

Cystathionine synthase deficiency E72.11
Cystathioninemia E72.19
Cystathioninuria E72.19
Cystic — *see also* condition
  breast (chronic) — *see* Mastopathy, cystic
  corpora lutea (hemorrhagic) N83.1- ☑
  duct — *see* condition
  eyeball (congenital) Q11.0
  fibrosis — *see* Fibrosis, cystic
  kidney (congenital) Q61.9
    adult type Q61.2
    infantile type NEC Q61.19
      collecting duct dilatation Q61.11
    medullary Q61.5
  liver, congenital Q44.6
  lung disease J98.4
    congenital Q33.0
  mastitis, chronic — *see* Mastopathy, cystic
  medullary, kidney Q61.5
  meniscus — *see* Derangement, knee, meniscus, cystic
  ovary N83.20- ☑
Cysticercosis, cysticerciasis B69.9
  with
    epileptiform fits B69.0
    myositis B69.81
  brain B69.0
  central nervous system B69.0
  cerebral B69.0
  ocular B69.1
  specified NEC B69.89
Cysticercus cellulose infestation — *see* Cysticercosis
Cystinosis (malignant) E72.04
Cystinuria E72.01
Cystitis (exudative) (hemorrhagic) (septic) (suppurative) N30.90

Cystitis — *continued*
  with
    fibrosis — *see* Cystitis, chronic, interstitial
    hematuria N30.91
    leukoplakia — *see* Cystitis, chronic, interstitial
    malakoplakia — *see* Cystitis, chronic, interstitial
    metaplasia — *see* Cystitis, chronic, interstitial
    prostatitis N41.3
  acute N30.00
    with hematuria N30.01
    of trigone N30.30
      with hematuria N30.31
  allergic — *see* Cystitis, specified type NEC
  amebic A06.81
  bilharzial B65.9 *[N33]*
  blennorrhagic (gonococcal) A54.01
  bullous — *see* Cystitis, specified type NEC
  calculous N21.0
  chlamydial A56.01
  chronic N30.20
    with hematuria N30.21
    interstitial N30.10
      with hematuria N30.11
    of trigone N30.30
      with hematuria N30.31
    specified NEC N30.20
      with hematuria N30.21
  cystic (a) — *see* Cystitis, specified type NEC
  diphtheritic A36.85
  echinococcal
    granulosus B67.39
    multilocularis B67.69
  emphysematous — *see* Cystitis, specified type NEC
  encysted — *see* Cystitis, specified type NEC
  eosinophilic — *see* Cystitis, specified type NEC
  follicular — *see* Cystitis, of trigone
  gangrenous — *see* Cystitis, specified type NEC
  glandularis — *see* Cystitis, specified type NEC
  gonococcal A54.01
  incrusted — *see* Cystitis, specified type NEC
  interstitial (chronic) — *see* Cystitis, chronic, interstitial
  irradiation N30.40
    with hematuria N30.41
  irritation — *see* Cystitis, specified type NEC
  malignant — *see* Cystitis, specified type NEC
  of trigone N30.30
    with hematuria N30.31
  panmural — *see* Cystitis, chronic, interstitial
  polyposa — *see* Cystitis, specified type NEC
  prostatic N41.3
  puerperal (postpartum) O86.22
  radiation — *see* Cystitis, irradiation
  specified type NEC N30.80
    with hematuria N30.81
  subacute — *see* Cystitis, chronic
  submucous — *see* Cystitis, chronic, interstitial
  syphilitic (late) A52.76
  trichomonal A59.03
  tuberculous A18.12
  ulcerative — *see* Cystitis, chronic, interstitial
Cystocele (-urethrocele)
  female N81.10
    with prolapse of uterus — *see* Prolapse, uterus
    lateral N81.12
    midline N81.11
    paravaginal N81.12
  in pregnancy or childbirth O34.8- ☑
    causing obstructed labor O65.5
  male N32.89
Cystolithiasis N21.0
Cystoma — *see also* Neoplasm, benign, by site
  endometrial, ovary N80.10- ☑
  mucinous
    specified site — *see* Neoplasm, benign, by site
    unspecified site D27.9
  serous
    specified site — *see* Neoplasm, benign, by site
    unspecified site D27.9
  simple (ovary) N83.29- ☑
Cystoplegia N31.2
Cystoptosis N32.89
Cystopyelitis — *see* Pyelonephritis
Cystorrhagia N32.89
Cystosarcoma phyllodes D48.6- ☑
  benign D24.- ☑
  malignant — *see* Neoplasm, breast, malignant
Cystostomy
  attention to Z43.5

Cystostomy — *continued*
  complication — *see* Complications, cystostomy
  status Z93.50
    appendico-vesicostomy Z93.52
    cutaneous Z93.51
    specified NEC Z93.59
Cystourethritis — *see* Urethritis
Cystourethrocele — *see also* Cystocele
  female N81.10

Cystourethrocele — *continued*
  female — *continued*
    with uterine prolapse — *see* Prolapse, uterus
    lateral N81.12
    midline N81.11
    paravaginal N81.12
  male N32.89
Cytomegalic inclusion disease
  congenital P35.1

Cytomegalovirus infection B25.9
Cytomycosis (reticuloendothelial) B39.4
Cytopenia D75.9
  refractory
    with multilineage dysplasia D46.A (*following* D46.2)
    and ring sideroblasts (RCMD RS) D46.B (*following* D46.2)
Czerny's disease (periodic hydrarthrosis of the knee) — *see* Effusion, joint, knee

D

d-glycericacidemia E72.59
Da Costa's syndrome F45.8
Daae (-Finsen) **disease** (epidemic pleurodynia) B33.0
Dabney's grip B33.0
Dacryoadenitis, dacryadenitis H04.00- ☑
  acute H04.01- ☑
  chronic H04.02- ☑
Dacryocystitis H04.30- ☑
  acute H04.32- ☑
  chronic H04.41- ☑
  neonatal P39.1
  phlegmonous H04.31- ☑
  syphilitic A52.71
    congenital (early) A50.01
  trachomatous, active A71.1
    sequelae (late effect) B94.0
Dacryocystoblennorrhea — see Inflammation, lacrimal, passages, chronic
Dacryocystocele — see Disorder, lacrimal system, changes
Dacryolith, dacryolithiasis H04.51- ☑
Dacryoma — see Disorder, lacrimal system, changes
Dacryopericystitis — see Dacryocystitis
Dacryops H04.11- ☑
Dacryostenosis — see also Stenosis, lacrimal
  congenital Q10.5
Dactylitis
  bone — see Osteomyelitis
  sickle-cell D57.04
    Beta plus D57.454
    Beta zero D57.434
    Hb C D57.214
    Hb SD D57.814
    Hb SE D57.814
    Hb SS D57.04
    specified NEC D57.814
    thalassemia D57.414
  skin L08.9
  syphilitic A52.77
  tuberculous A18.03
Dactylolysis spontanea (ainhum) L94.6
Dactylosymphysis Q70.9
  fingers — see Syndactylism, complex, fingers
  toes — see Syndactylism, complex, toes
Damage
  arteriosclerotic — see Arteriosclerosis
  brain (nontraumatic) G93.9
    anoxic, hypoxic G93.1
      resulting from a procedure G97.82
      child NEC G80.9
      due to birth injury P11.2
  cardiorenal (vascular) — see Hypertension, cardiorenal
  cerebral NEC — see Damage, brain
  coccyx, complicating delivery O71.6
  coronary — see Disease, heart, ischemic
  deep tissue, pressure-induced — see also L89 with final character .6
  eye, birth injury P15.3
  liver (nontraumatic) K76.9
    alcoholic K70.9
    due to drugs — see Disease, liver, toxic
    toxic — see Disease, liver, toxic
  lung
    dabbing (related) U07.0
    electronic cigarette (related) U07.0
    vaping (associated) (device) (product) (use) U07.0
  medication T88.7- ☑
  organ
    dabbing (related) U07.0
    electronic cigarette (related) U07.0
    vaping (associated) (device) (product) (use) U07.0
  pelvic
    joint or ligament, during delivery O71.6
    organ NEC
      during delivery O71.5
      following ectopic or molar pregnancy O08.6
  renal — see Disease, renal
  subendocardium, subendocardial — see Degeneration, myocardial
  vascular I99.9
Dana-Putnam syndrome (subacute combined sclerosis with pernicious anemia) — see Degeneration, combined
Danbolt (-Cross) **syndrome** (acrodermatitis enteropathica) E83.2
Dandruff L21.0

Dandy-Walker syndrome Q03.1
  with spina bifida — see Spina bifida
Danlos' syndrome — see also Syndrome, Ehlers-Danlos Q79.60
Darier (-White) **disease** (congenital) Q82.8
  meaning erythema annulare centrifugum L53.1
Darier-Roussy sarcoid D86.3
Darling's disease or histoplasmosis B39.4
Darwin's tubercle Q17.8
Dawson's (inclusion body) **encephalitis** A81.1
De Beurmann (-Gougerot) **disease** B42.1
De la Tourette's syndrome F95.2
De Lange's syndrome Q87.19
De Morgan's spots (senile angiomas) I78.1
De Quervain's
  disease (tendon sheath) M65.4
  syndrome E34.51
  thyroiditis (subacute granulomatous thyroiditis) E06.1
De Toni-Fanconi (-Debre) **syndrome** E72.09
  with cystinosis E72.04
Dead
  fetus, retained (mother) O36.4- ☑
    early pregnancy O02.1
  labyrinth H83.2- ☑
  ovum, retained O02.0
Deaf nonspeaking NEC H91.3
Deafmutism (acquired) (congenital) NEC H91.3
  hysterical F44.6
  syphilitic, congenital — see also subcategory H94.8 A50.09
Deafness (acquired) (complete) (hereditary) (partial) H91.9-
  with blue sclera and fragility of bone Q78.0
  auditory fatigue — see Deafness, specified type NEC
  aviation T70.0- ☑
    nerve injury — see Injury, nerve, acoustic, specified type NEC
  boilermaker's H83.3- ☑
  central — see Deafness, sensorineural
  conductive H90.2
    and sensorineural
      mixed H90.8
        bilateral H90.6
      bilateral H90.0
      unilateral H90.1- ☑
        with restricted hearing on the contralateral side H90.A- ☑
  congenital H90.5
    with blue sclera and fragility of bone Q78.0
  due to toxic agents — see Deafness, ototoxic
  emotional (hysterical) F44.6
  functional (hysterical) F44.6
  high frequency H91.9- ☑
  hysterical F44.6
  low frequency H91.9- ☑
  mental R48.8
  mixed conductive and sensorineural H90.8
    bilateral H90.6
    unilateral H90.7- ☑
  nerve — see Deafness, sensorineural
  neural — see Deafness, sensorineural
  noise-induced — see also subcategory H83.3- ☑
    nerve injury — see Injury, nerve, acoustic, specified type NEC
  nonspeaking H91.3
  ototoxic H91.0- ☑
  perceptive — see Deafness, sensorineural
  psychogenic (hysterical) F44.6
  sensorineural H90.5
    and conductive
      bilateral H90.6
      mixed H90.8
        bilateral H90.6
      bilateral H90.3
      unilateral H90.4- ☑
        with restricted hearing on the contralateral side H90.A- ☑
  sensory — see Deafness, sensorineural
  specified type NEC H91.8- ☑
  sudden (idiopathic) H91.2- ☑
  syphilitic A52.15
  transient ischemic H93.01- ☑
  traumatic — see Injury, nerve, acoustic, specified type NEC
  word (developmental) H93.25
Death (cause unknown) (of) (unexplained) (unspecified cause) R99
  brain G93.82

Death — continued
  cardiac (sudden) (with successful resuscitation) — see Arrest, cardiac
    family history of Z82.41
    personal history of Z86.74
  family member (assumed) Z63.4
Debility (chronic) (general) (nervous) R53.81
  congenital or neonatal NOS P96.9
  nervous R53.81
  old age R54
  senile R54
Debove's disease (splenomegaly) R16.1
Debt, burdensome Z59.868
Decalcification
  bone — see Osteoporosis
  teeth K03.89
Decapsulation, kidney N28.89
Decay
  dental — see Caries, dental
  senile R54
  tooth, teeth — see Caries, dental
Deciduitis (acute)
  following ectopic or molar pregnancy O08.0
Decline (general) — see Debility
  cognitive, age-associated R41.81
Decompensation
  cardiac (acute) (chronic) — see Disease, heart
  cardiovascular — see Disease, cardiovascular
  heart — see Disease, heart
  hepatic — see Failure, hepatic
  myocardial (acute) (chronic) — see Disease, heart
  respiratory J98.8
Decompression sickness T70.3- ☑
Decrease (d)
  absolute neutrophile count — see Neutropenia
  blood
    glucose E16.2
      level 1 E16.A1
      level 2 E16.A2
      level 3 E16.A3
    platelets — see Thrombocytopenia
    pressure R03.1
      due to shock following
        injury T79.4- ☑
        operation T81.19- ☑
  estrogen E28.39
    postablative E89.40
      asymptomatic E89.40
      symptomatic E89.41
  fragility of erythrocytes D58.8
  function
    lipase (pancreatic) K90.3
    ovary in hypopituitarism E23.0
    parenchyma of pancreas K86.89
    pituitary (gland) (anterior) (lobe) E23.0
      posterior (lobe) E23.0
  functional activity R68.89
  glucose E16.2
  hematocrit R71.0
  hemoglobin R71.0
  leukocytes D72.819
    specified NEC D72.818
  libido R68.82
  lymphocytes D72.810
  platelets D69.6
  respiration, due to shock following injury T79.4- ☑
  sexual desire R68.82
  tear secretion NEC — see Syndrome, dry eye
  tolerance
    fat K90.49
    glucose R73.09
    pancreatic K90.3
    salt and water E87.8
  vision NEC H54.7
  white blood cell count D72.819
    specified NEC D72.818
Decubitus (ulcer) — see Ulcer, pressure, by site
  cervix N86
Deepening acetabulum — see Derangement, joint, specified type NEC, hip
Defect, defective Q89.9
  3-beta-hydroxysteroid dehydrogenase E25.0
  11-hydroxylase E25.0
  21-hydroxylase E25.0
  abdominal wall, congenital Q79.59
  antibody immunodeficiency D80.9
  aorticopulmonary septum Q21.4
  atrial septal Q21.10
    coronary sinus Q21.13

Defect, defective — continued
  atrial septal — continued
    following acute myocardial infarction (current complication) I23.1
    ostium primum type (type I) Q21.20
      with
        common atrioventricular valves and moderate or larger inlet VSD Q21.23
        separate atrioventricular valves Q21.21
          and small or restrictive inlet VSD Q21.22
    ostium secundum type (patent persistent) (type II) Q21.11
    sinus venosus Q21.16
      inferior Q21.15
      superior Q21.14
    specified NEC Q21.19
    vena cava type
      inferior Q21.15
      superior Q21.14
  atrioventricular
    canal Q21.20
    septal
      common Q21.23
      complete Q21.23
      incomplete Q21.21
      intermediate Q21.22
      partial Q21.21
      transitional Q21.22
      unspecified as to partial or complete Q21.20
    septum Q21.20
  auricular septal Q21.10
  bilirubin excretion NEC E80.6
  biosynthesis, androgen (testicular) E29.1
  bulbar septum Q21.0
  catalase E80.3
  cell membrane receptor complex (CR3) D71.8
  circulation I99.9
    congenital Q28.9
    newborn Q28.9
  coagulation (factor) — see also Deficiency, factor D68.9
    with
      COVID-19 associated coagulopathy D68.8
      ectopic pregnancy O08.1
      molar pregnancy O08.1
    acquired D68.4
    antepartum with hemorrhage — see Hemorrhage, antepartum, with coagulation defect
    due to
      liver disease D68.4
      vitamin K deficiency D68.4
    hereditary NEC D68.2
    intrapartum O67.0
    newborn, transient P61.6
    postpartum O99.13
      with hemorrhage O72.3
    specified type NEC D68.8
  complement system D84.1
  conduction (heart) I45.9
    bone — see Deafness, conductive
  congenital, organ or site not listed — see Anomaly, by site
  coronary sinus Q21.13
  cushion, endocardial Q21.20
    common Q21.23
    incomplete Q21.21
    intermediate Q21.22
    transitional Q21.22
  degradation, glycoprotein E77.1
  dental bridge, crown, fillings — see Defect, dental restoration
  dental restoration K08.50
    specified NEC K08.59
  dentin (hereditary) K00.5
  Descemet's membrane, congenital Q13.89
  developmental — see also Anomaly
    cauda equina Q06.3
  diaphragm
    with elevation, eventration or hernia — see Hernia, diaphragm
    congenital Q79.1
      with hernia Q79.0
      gross (with hernia) Q79.0
  ectodermal, congenital Q82.9
  Eisenmenger's Q21.8
  enzyme
    catalase E80.3
    peroxidase E80.3
  esophagus, congenital Q39.9
  extensor retinaculum M62.89

Defect, defective — continued
  fibrin polymerization D68.2
  filling
    bladder R93.41
    kidney R93.42-
    renal pelvis R93.41
    stomach R93.3
    ureter R93.41
    urinary organs, specified NEC R93.49
  GABA (gamma aminobutyric acid) metabolic E72.81
  Gerbode Q21.0
  glucose transport, blood-brain barrier E74.810
  glycoprotein degradation E77.1
  Hageman (factor) D68.2
  hearing — see Deafness
  high grade F70
  home, technical, preventing adequate care Z59.19
  interatrial septal Q21.19
  interauricular septal Q21.19
  interventricular septal Q21.0
    with dextroposition of aorta, pulmonary stenosis and hypertrophy of right ventricle Q21.3
    in tetralogy of Fallot Q21.3
  intervertebral annular fibrosis — see also Disease, intervertebral disc, by site M51.9
    lumbar M51.A0
      large M51.A2
      small M51.A1
    lumbosacral M51.A3
      large M51.A5
      small M51.A4
  learning (specific) — see Disorder, learning
  lymphocyte function antigen-1 (LFA-1) D84.0
  lysosomal enzyme, post-translational modification E77.0
  major osseous M89.70
    ankle M89.77- ☑
    carpus M89.74- ☑
    clavicle M89.71- ☑
    femur M89.75- ☑
    fibula M89.76- ☑
    fingers M89.74- ☑
    foot M89.77- ☑
    forearm M89.73- ☑
    hand M89.74- ☑
    humerus M89.72- ☑
    lower leg M89.76- ☑
    metacarpus M89.74- ☑
    metatarsus M89.77- ☑
    multiple sites M89.79
    pelvic region M89.75- ☑
    pelvis M89.75- ☑
    radius M89.73- ☑
    scapula M89.71- ☑
    shoulder region M89.71- ☑
    specified NEC M89.78
    tarsus M89.77- ☑
    thigh M89.75- ☑
    tibia M89.76- ☑
    toes M89.77- ☑
    ulna M89.73- ☑
  mental — see Disability, intellectual
  modification, lysosomal enzymes, post-translational E77.0
  obstructive, congenital
    renal pelvis Q62.39
    ureter Q62.39
      atresia — see Atresia, ureter
      cecoureterocele Q62.32
      megaureter Q62.2
      orthotopic ureterocele Q62.31
  osseous, major M89.70
    ankle M89.77- ☑
    carpus M89.74- ☑
    clavicle M89.71- ☑
    femur M89.75- ☑
    fibula M89.76- ☑
    fingers M89.74- ☑
    foot M89.77- ☑
    forearm M89.73- ☑
    hand M89.74- ☑
    humerus M89.72- ☑
    lower leg M89.76- ☑
    metacarpus M89.74- ☑
    metatarsus M89.77- ☑
    multiple sites M89.9
    pelvic region M89.75- ☑
    pelvis M89.75- ☑
    radius M89.73- ☑

Defect, defective — continued
  osseous, major — continued
    scapula M89.71- ☑
    shoulder region M89.71- ☑
    specified NEC M89.78
    tarsus M89.77- ☑
    thigh M89.75- ☑
    tibia M89.76- ☑
    toes M89.77- ☑
    ulna M89.73- ☑
  osteochondral NEC — see also Deformity M95.8
  ostium
    primum Q21.20
    secundum Q21.11
  peroxidase E80.3
  placental blood supply — see Insufficiency, placental
  platelets, qualitative D69.1
    constitutional — see Disease, von Willebrand
  postural NEC, spine — see Dorsopathy, deforming
  qualitative, of von Willebrand factor
    with
      decreased platelet adhesion and selective deficiency of high-molecular-weight multimers — see also Disease, von Willebrand D68.020
      defective platelet adhesion with a normal size distribution of von Willebrand factor multimers — see also Disease, von Willebrand D68.022
      defective von Willebrand factor to factor VIII binding — see also Disease, von Willebrand D68.023
      high-molecular-weight von Willebrand factor loss — see also Disease, von Willebrand D68.021
      hyper-adhesive forms — see also Disease, von Willebrand D68.021
      increased affinity for platelet glycoprotein Ib — see also Disease, von Willebrand D68.021
      markedly decreased affinity for factor VIII — see also Disease, von Willebrand D68.023
      in von Willebrand factor function, with no further subtyping — see also Disease, von Willebrand D68.029
  reduction
    limb Q73.8
      lower Q72.9- ☑
        absence — see Agenesis, leg
          foot — see Agenesis, foot
        longitudinal
          femur Q72.4- ☑
          fibula Q72.6- ☑
          tibia Q72.5- ☑
        specified type NEC Q72.89- ☑
        split foot Q72.7- ☑
      specified type NEC Q73.8
      upper Q71.9- ☑
        absence — see Agenesis, arm
          forearm — see Agenesis, forearm
          hand — see Agenesis, hand
        lobster-claw hand Q71.6- ☑
        longitudinal
          radius Q71.4- ☑
          ulna Q71.5- ☑
        specified type NEC Q71.89- ☑
  renal pelvis Q63.8
    obstructive Q62.39
  respiratory system, congenital Q34.9
  restoration, dental K08.50
    specified NEC K08.59
  retinal nerve bundle fibers H35.89
  septal (heart) NOS Q21.9
    acquired (atrial) (auricular) (ventricular) (old) I51.0
    atrial — see also Defect, atrial septal Q21.10
      concurrent with acute myocardial infarction — see Infarct, myocardium
      following acute myocardial infarction (current complication) I23.1
    ventricular — see also Defect, ventricular septal Q21.0
  sinus venosus — see also Defect, atrial septal, sinus venosus Q21.16
  speech — see Disorder, speech
    developmental F80.9
    specified NEC R47.89
  Taussig-Bing (aortic transposition and overriding pulmonary artery) Q20.1
  teeth, wedge K03.1
  vascular (local) I99.9
    congenital Q27.9
  ventricular septal Q21.0

Defect, defective — *continued*
 ventricular septal — *continued*
  concurrent with acute myocardial infarction — *see* Infarct, myocardium
  following acute myocardial infarction (current complication) I23.2
  in tetralogy of Fallot Q21.3
 vision NEC H54.7
 visual field H53.40
  bilateral
   heteronymous H53.47
   homonymous H53.46- ☑
  generalized contraction H53.48- ☑
  localized
   arcuate H53.43- ☑
   scotoma (central area) H53.41- ☑
    blind spot area H53.42- ☑
   sector H53.43- ☑
   specified type NEC H53.45- ☑
 voice R49.9
  specified NEC R49.8
 wedge, tooth, teeth (abrasion) K03.1
Deferentitis N49.1
 gonorrheal (acute) (chronic) A54.23
Defibrination (syndrome) D65
 antepartum — *see* Hemorrhage, antepartum, with coagulation defect, disseminated intravascular coagulation
 following ectopic or molar pregnancy O08.1
 intrapartum O67.0
 newborn P60
 postpartum O72.3
Deficiency, deficient
 3-beta hydroxysteroid dehydrogenase E25.0
 5-alpha reductase (with male pseudohermaphroditism) E29.1
 11-hydroxylase E25.0
 21-hydroxylase E25.0
 ABCC6
  causing generalized arterial calcification of infancy E83.823
  pseudoxanthoma elasticum E83.824
 AADC (aromatic L-amino acid decarboxylase) E70.81
 abdominal muscle syndrome Q79.4
 AC globulin (congenital) (hereditary) D68.2
  acquired D68.4
 accelerator globulin (Ac G) (blood) D68.2
 acid phosphatase E83.39
 acid sphingomyelinase (ASMD) E75.249
  type
   A E75.240
   A/B E75.244
   B E75.241
 activating factor (blood) D68.2
 ADA2 (adenosine deaminase 2) D81.32
 adenosine deaminase (ADA) D81.30
  with severe combined immunodeficiency (SCID) D81.31
  partial (type 1) D81.39
  specified NEC D81.39
  type 1 (without SCID) (without severe combined immunodeficiency) D81.39
  type 2 D81.32
 aldolase (hereditary) E74.19
 alpha-1-antitrypsin E88.01
 amino-acids E72.9
 anemia — *see* Anemia
 aneurin E51.9
 anti-hemophilic
  factor (A) D66
   B D67
   C D68.1
  globulin (AHG) NEC D66
 antibody with
  hyperimmunoglobulinemia D80.6
  near-normal immunoglobins D80.6
 antidiuretic hormone E23.2
 antithrombin (antithrombin III) D68.59
 aromatic L-amino acid decarboxylase (AADC) E70.81
 ascorbic acid E54
 attention (disorder) (syndrome) F98.8
  with hyperactivity — *see* Disorder, attention-deficit hyperactivity
 autoprothrombin
  I D68.2
  II D67
  C D68.2
 beta-glucuronidase E76.29

Deficiency, deficient — *continued*
 biotin E53.8
 biotin-dependent carboxylase D81.819
 biotinidase D81.810
 brancher enzyme (amylopectinosis) E74.03
 C1 esterase inhibitor (C1-INH) D84.1
 calciferol E55.9
  with
   adult osteomalacia M83.8
   rickets — *see* Rickets
 calcium (dietary) E58
 calorie, severe E43
  with marasmus E41
   and kwashiorkor E42
 cardiac — *see* Insufficiency, myocardial
 carnitine E71.40
  due to
   hemodialysis E71.43
   inborn errors of metabolism E71.42
   Valproic acid therapy E71.43
  iatrogenic E71.43
  muscle palmityltransferase E71.314
  primary E71.41
  secondary E71.448
 carotene E50.9
 CD73 deficiency causing arterial calcification E83.825
 central nervous system G96.89
 ceruloplasmin (Wilson) E83.01
 choline E53.8
 Christmas factor D67
 chromium E61.4
 chronic neurovisceral acid sphingomyelinase E75.244
 chronic visceral acid sphingomyelinase E75.241
 clotting (blood) — *see also* Deficiency, coagulation factor D68.9
 clotting factor NEC (hereditary) — *see also* Deficiency, factor D68.2
 coagulation NOS D68.9
  with
   ectopic pregnancy O08.1
   molar pregnancy O08.1
  acquired (any) D68.4
  antepartum hemorrhage — *see* Hemorrhage, antepartum, with coagulation defect
  clotting factor NEC — *see also* Deficiency, factor D68.2
  due to
   hyperprothrombinemia D68.4
   liver disease D68.4
   vitamin K deficiency D68.4
  newborn, transient P61.6
  postpartum O72.3
  specified NEC D68.8
 cognitive F09
 color vision H53.50
  achromatopsia H53.51
  acquired H53.52
  deuteranomaly H53.53
  protanomaly H53.54
  specified type NEC H53.59
  tritanomaly H53.55
 combined glucocorticoid and mineralocorticoid E27.49
 contact factor D68.2
 copper (nutritional) E61.0
 corticoadrenal E27.40
  primary E27.1
 craniofacial axis Q75.009
 cyanocobalamin E53.8
 debrancher enzyme (limit dextrinosis) E74.03
 dehydrogenase
  long chain/very long chain acyl CoA E71.310
  medium chain acyl CoA E71.311
  short chain acyl CoA E71.312
 diet E63.9
 dihydropyrimidine dehydrogenase (DPD) E88.89
 disaccharidase E73.9
 edema — *see* Malnutrition, severe
 endocrine E34.9
 energy-supply — *see* Malnutrition
 ENPP1
  causing
   autosomal recessive hypophosphatemic rickets type 2 E83.822
   generalized arterial calcification of infancy E83.821
 enzymes, circulating NEC E88.09
 ergosterol E55.9
  with
   adult osteomalacia M83.8
   rickets — *see* Rickets
 essential fatty acid (EFA) E63.0

Deficiency, deficient — *continued*
 eye movements
  saccadic H55.81
  smooth pursuit H55.82
 factor — *see also* Deficiency, coagulation
  Hageman D68.2
  I (congenital) (hereditary) D68.2
  II (congenital) (hereditary) D68.2
  IX (congenital) (functional) (hereditary) (with functional defect) D67
  multiple (congenital) D68.8
   acquired D68.4
  V (congenital) (hereditary) D68.2
  VII (congenital) (hereditary) D68.2
  VIII (congenital) (functional) (hereditary) (with functional defect) D66
   with vascular defect — *see* Disease, von Willebrand
  X (congenital) (hereditary) D68.2
  XI (congenital) (hereditary) D68.1
  XII (congenital) (hereditary) D68.2
  XIII (congenital) (hereditary) D68.2
 femoral, proximal focal (congenital) — *see* Defect, reduction, lower limb, longitudinal, femur
 fibrin-stabilizing factor (congenital) (hereditary) D68.2
  acquired D68.4
 fibrinase D68.2
 fibrinogen (congenital) (hereditary) D68.2
  acquired D65
 folate E53.8
 folic acid E53.8
 foreskin N47.3
 fructokinase E74.11
 fructose-1-phosphate aldolase E74.19
 fructose 1,6-diphosphatase E74.19
 GABA-T (gamma aminobutyric acid transaminase) E72.81
 GABA (gamma aminobutyric acid) transaminase E72.81
 GABA transporter 1 QA0.0131
 galactokinase E74.29
 galactose-1-phosphate uridyl transferase E74.29
 gammaglobulin in blood D80.1
  hereditary D80.0
 glass factor D68.2
 glucocorticoid E27.49
  mineralocorticoid E27.49
 glucose-6-phosphatase E74.01
 glucose-6-phosphate dehydrogenase
  anemia D55.0
  without anemia D75.A
 glucose transporter protein type 1 E74.810
 glucuronyl transferase E80.5
 Glut1 E74.810
 glycogen synthetase E74.09
 gonadotropin (isolated) E23.0
 growth hormone (idiopathic) (isolated) E23.0
 Hageman factor D68.2
 hemoglobin D64.9
 hepatophosphorylase E74.09
 homogentisate 1,2-dioxygenase E70.29
 hormone
  anterior pituitary (partial) NEC E23.0
   growth E23.0
  growth (isolated) E23.0
  pituitary E23.0
  testicular E29.1
 hypoxanthine- (guanine)-phosphoribosyltransferase (HG- PRT) (total H-PRT) E79.1
 immunity D84.9
  cell-mediated D84.89
   with thrombocytopenia and eczema D82.0
  combined D81.9
  humoral D80.9
  IgA (secretory) D80.2
  IgG D80.3
  IgM D80.4
 immuno — *see* Immunodeficiency
 immunoglobulin, selective
  A (IgA) D80.2
  G (IgG) (subclasses) D80.3
  M (IgM) D80.4
 infantile neurovisceral acid sphingomyelinase E75.240
 inositol (B complex) E53.8
 intrinsic
  factor (congenital) D51.0
  sphincter N36.42
   with urethral hypermobility N36.43
 iodine E61.8
  congenital syndrome — *see* Syndrome, iodine-deficiency, congenital
 iron E61.1

Deficiency, deficient — continued
- iron — continued
  - anemia D50.9
- kalium E87.6
- kappa-light chain D80.8
- labile factor (congenital) (hereditary) D68.2
  - acquired D68.4
- lacrimal fluid (acquired) — see also Syndrome, dry eye
  - congenital Q10.6
- lactase
  - congenital E73.0
  - secondary E73.1
- Laki-Lorand factor D68.2
- LCAD (long chain acyl CoA dehydrogenase deficiency) E71.310
- lecithin cholesterol acyltransferase E78.6
- leukocyte adhesion (LAD-I) (LAD-II) (LAD-III) D71.1
  - type I D71.1
  - type II D71.1
  - type III D71.1
- lipocaic K86.89
- lipoprotein (familial) (high density) E78.6
- liver phosphorylase E74.09
- lysosomal alpha-1, 4 glucosidase E74.02
- lysosome-associated membrane protein 2 [LAMP2] E74.05
- magnesium E61.2
- major histocompatibility complex
  - class I D81.6
  - class II D81.7
- manganese E61.3
- MCAD (medium chain acyl CoA dehydrogenase deficiency) E71.311
- menadione (vitamin K) E56.1
  - newborn P53
- mental (familial) (hereditary) — see Disability, intellectual
- methylenetetrahydrofolate reductase (MTHFR) E72.12
- mevalonate kinase M04.1
- mineral NEC E61.8
- mineralocorticoid E27.49
  - with glucocorticoid E27.49
- molybdenum (nutritional) E61.5
- moral F60.2
- multiple nutrient elements E61.7
- multiple sulfatase (MSD) E75.26
- muscle
  - carnitine (palmityltransferase) E71.314
  - phosphofructokinase E74.09
- myoadenylate deaminase E79.2
- myocardial — see Insufficiency, myocardial
- myophosphorylase E74.04
- NADH diaphorase or reductase (congenital) D74.0
- NADH-methemoglobin reductase (congenital) D74.0
- natrium E87.1
- niacin (amide) (-tryptophan) E52
- nicotinamide E52
- nicotinic acid E52
- number of teeth — see Anodontia
- nutrient element E61.9
  - multiple E61.7
  - specified NEC E61.8
- nutrition, nutritional — see also Nutrition deficient E63.9
  - sequelae — see Sequelae, nutritional deficiency
  - specified NEC E63.8
- of interleukin 1 receptor antagonist [DIRA] M04.8
- ornithine transcarbamylase E72.4
- ovarian E28.39
- oxygen — see Anoxia
- pantothenic acid E53.8
- parathyroid (gland) E20.9
- perineum (female) N81.89
- phenylalanine hydroxylase E70.1
- phosphoenolpyruvate carboxykinase E74.4
- phosphofructokinase E74.19
- phosphomannomutase E74.818
- phosphomannose isomerase E74.818
- phosphomannosyl mutase E74.818
- phosphorylase kinase, liver E74.09
- pituitary hormone (isolated) E23.0
- plasma thromboplastin
  - antecedent (PTA) D68.1
  - component (PTC) D67
- plasminogen (type 1) (type 2) E88.02
- platelet NEC D69.1
  - constitutional — see Disease, von Willebrand
- polyglandular E31.8
  - autoimmune E31.0
- potassium (K) E87.6
- prepuce N47.3

Deficiency, deficient — continued
- proaccelerin (congenital) (hereditary) D68.2
  - acquired D68.4
- proconvertin factor (congenital) (hereditary) D68.2
  - acquired D68.4
- protein — see also Malnutrition E46
  - anemia D53.0
  - C D68.59
  - S D68.59
- prothrombin (congenital) (hereditary) D68.2
  - acquired D68.4
- Prower factor D68.2
- pseudocholinesterase E88.09
- PTA (plasma thromboplastin antecedent) D68.1
- PTC (plasma thromboplastin component) D67
- purine nucleoside phosphorylase (PNP) D81.5
- pyracin (alpha) (beta) E53.1
- pyridoxal E53.1
- pyridoxamine E53.1
- pyridoxine (derivatives) E53.1
- pyruvate
  - carboxylase E74.4
  - dehydrogenase E74.4
- riboflavin (vitamin B2) E53.0
- salt E87.1
- SCAD (short chain acyl CoA dehydrogenase deficiency) E71.312
- secretion
  - ovary E28.39
  - salivary gland (any) K11.7
  - urine R34
- selenium (dietary) E59
- serum antitrypsin, familial E88.01
- short stature homeobox gene (SHOX)
  - with
    - dyschondrosteosis Q78.8
    - short stature (idiopathic) E34.328
    - Turner's syndrome Q96.9
- sodium (Na) E87.1
- SPCA (factor VII) D68.2
- sphincter, intrinsic N36.42
  - with urethral hypermobility N36.43
- stable factor (congenital) (hereditary) D68.2
  - acquired D68.4
- Stuart-Prower (factor X) D68.2
- succinic semialdehyde dehydrogenase E72.81
- sucrase E74.39
- sulfatase E75.26
- sulfite oxidase E72.19
- thiamin, thiaminic (chloride) E51.9
  - beriberi (dry) E51.11
  - wet E51.12
- thrombokinase D68.2
  - newborn P53
- thyroid (gland) — see Hypothyroidism
- tocopherol E56.0
- tooth bud K00.0
- transcobalamine II (anemia) D51.2
- vanadium E61.6
- vascular I99.9
- vasopressin E23.2
- vertical ridge K06.8
- viosterol — see Deficiency, calciferol
- vitamin (multiple) NOS E56.9
  - A E50.9
    - with
      - Bitot's spot (corneal) E50.1
      - follicular keratosis E50.8
      - keratomalacia E50.4
      - manifestations NEC E50.8
      - night blindness E50.5
      - scar of cornea, xerophthalmic E50.6
      - xeroderma E50.8
      - xerophthalmia E50.7
      - xerosis
        - conjunctival E50.0
        - and Bitot's spot E50.1
        - cornea E50.2
        - and ulceration E50.3
    - sequelae E64.1
  - B (complex) NOS E53.9
    - with
      - beriberi (dry) E51.11
      - wet E51.12
      - pellagra E52
  - B1 NOS E51.9
    - beriberi (dry) E51.11
      - with circulatory system manifestations E51.11
      - wet E51.12

Deficiency, deficient — continued
- vitamin — continued
  - B12 E53.8
  - B2 (riboflavin) E53.0
  - B6 E53.1
  - C E54
    - sequelae E64.2
  - D E55.9
    - with
      - adult osteomalacia M83.8
      - rickets — see Rickets
    - 25-hydroxylase E83.32
  - E E56.0
  - folic acid E53.8
  - G E53.0
  - group B E53.9
    - specified NEC E53.8
  - H (biotin) E53.8
  - K E56.1
    - of newborn P53
  - nicotinic E52
  - P E56.8
  - PP (pellagra-preventing) E52
  - specified NEC E56.8
  - thiamin E51.9
    - beriberi — see Beriberi
- VLCAD (very long chain acyl CoA dehydrogenase deficiency) E71.310
- von Willebrand factor
  - partial quantitative — see also Disease, von Willebrand D68.01
  - total quantitative — see also Disease, von Willebrand D68.03
- zinc, dietary E60

Deficit — see also Deficiency
- attention and concentration R41.840
  - disorder — see Attention, deficit
  - following
    - cerebral infarction I69.310
    - cerebrovascular disease I69.910
      - specified disease NEC I69.810
    - nontraumatic
      - intracerebral hemorrhage I69.110
      - specified intracranial hemorrhage NEC I69.210
      - subarachnoid hemorrhage I69.010
- cognitive
  - communication R41.841
  - emotional
    - following
      - cerebral infarction I69.315
      - cerebrovascular disease I69.915
        - specified disease NEC I69.815
      - nontraumatic
        - intracerebral hemorrhage I69.115
        - specified intracranial hemorrhage NEC I69.215
        - subarachnoid hemorrhage I69.015
  - following
    - cerebral infarction I69.319
    - cerebrovascular disease I69.919
      - specified disease NEC I69.819
    - nontraumatic
      - intracerebral hemorrhage I69.119
      - specified intracranial hemorrhage NEC I69.219
      - subarachnoid hemorrhage I69.019
  - social
    - following
      - cerebral infarction I69.315
      - cerebrovascular disease I69.915
        - specified disease NEC I69.815
      - nontraumatic
        - intracerebral hemorrhage I69.115
        - specified intracranial hemorrhage NEC I69.215
        - subarachnoid hemorrhage I69.015
- cognitive NEC R41.89
  - following
    - cerebral infarction I69.318
    - cerebrovascular disease I69.918
      - specified disease NEC I69.818
    - nontraumatic
      - intracerebral hemorrhage I69.118
      - specified intracranial hemorrhage NEC I69.218
      - subarachnoid hemorrhage I69.018
- concentration R41.840
- executive function R41.844
  - following
    - cerebral infarction I69.314
    - cerebrovascular disease I69.914

Deficit — *continued*
    executive function — *continued*
        following — *continued*
            cerebrovascular disease — *continued*
                specified disease NEC I69.814
                nontraumatic
                    intracerebral hemorrhage I69.114
                    specified intracranial hemorrhage NEC I69.214
                    subarachnoid hemorrhage I69.014
        frontal lobe R41.844
            following
                cerebral infarction I69.314
                cerebrovascular disease I69.914
                    specified disease NEC I69.814
                nontraumatic
                    intracerebral hemorrhage I69.114
                    specified intracranial hemorrhage NEC I69.214
                    subarachnoid hemorrhage I69.014
        memory
            following
                cerebral infarction I69.311
                cerebrovascular disease I69.911
                    specified disease NEC I69.811
                nontraumatic
                    intracerebral hemorrhage I69.111
                    specified intracranial hemorrhage NEC I69.211
                    subarachnoid hemorrhage I69.011
    neurologic NEC R29.818
        ischemic
            reversible (RIND) I63.9
                prolonged (PRIND) I63.9
    oxygen R09.02
    prolonged reversible ischemic neurologic (PRIND) I63.9
    psychomotor R41.843
        following
            cerebral infarction I69.313
            cerebrovascular disease I69.913
                specified disease NEC I69.813
            nontraumatic
                intracerebral hemorrhage I69.113
                specified intracranial hemorrhage NEC I69.213
                subarachnoid hemorrhage I69.013
    visuospatial R41.842
        following
            cerebral infarction I69.312
            cerebrovascular disease I69.912
                specified disease NEC I69.812
            nontraumatic
                intracerebral hemorrhage I69.112
                specified intracranial hemorrhage NEC I69.212
                subarachnoid hemorrhage I69.012
Deflection
    radius — *see* Deformity, limb, specified type NEC, forearm
    septum (acquired) (nasal) (nose) J34.2
    spine — *see* Curvature, spine
    turbinate (nose) J34.2
Defluvium
    capillorum — *see* Alopecia
    ciliorum — *see* Madarosis
    unguium L60.8
Deformity Q89.9
    abdomen, congenital Q89.9
    abdominal wall
        acquired M95.8
        congenital Q79.59
    acquired (unspecified site) M95.9
    adrenal gland Q89.1
    alimentary tract, congenital Q45.9
        upper Q40.9
    ankle (joint) (acquired) — *see also* Deformity, limb, lower leg
        abduction — *see* Contraction, joint, ankle
        congenital Q68.8
        contraction — *see* Contraction, joint, ankle
        specified type NEC — *see* Deformity, limb, foot, specified NEC
    anus (acquired) K62.89
        congenital Q43.9
    aorta (arch) (congenital) Q25.40
        acquired I77.89
    aortic
        arch, acquired I77.89
        cusp or valve (congenital) Q23.88
            acquired — *see also* Endocarditis, aortic I35.8
    arm (acquired) (upper) — *see also* Deformity, limb, upper arm
        congenital Q68.8
        forearm — *see* Deformity, limb, forearm
    artery (congenital) (peripheral) NOS Q27.9

Deformity — *continued*
    artery — *continued*
        acquired I77.89
        coronary (acquired) I25.9
            congenital Q24.5
        umbilical Q27.0
    atrial septal — *see also* Defect, atrial septal Q21.10
    auditory canal (external) (congenital) — *see also* Malformation, ear, external
        acquired — *see* Disorder, ear, external, specified type NEC
    auricle
        ear (congenital) — *see also* Malformation, ear, external
            acquired — *see* Disorder, pinna, deformity
    back — *see* Dorsopathy, deforming
    bile duct (common) (congenital) (hepatic) Q44.5
        acquired K83.8
    biliary duct or passage (congenital) Q44.5
        acquired K83.8
    bladder (neck) (trigone) (sphincter) (acquired) N32.89
        congenital Q64.79
    bone (acquired) NOS M95.9
        congenital Q79.9
        turbinate M95.0
    brain (congenital) Q04.9
        acquired G93.89
        reduction Q04.3
    breast (acquired) N64.89
        congenital Q83.9
        reconstructed N65.0
    bronchus (congenital) Q32.4
        acquired NEC J98.09
    bursa, congenital Q79.9
    canaliculi (lacrimalis) (acquired) — *see also* Disorder, lacrimal system, changes
        congenital Q10.6
    canthus, acquired — *see* Disorder, eyelid, specified type NEC
    capillary (acquired) I78.8
    cardiovascular system, congenital Q28.9
    caruncle, lacrimal (acquired) — *see also* Disorder, lacrimal system, changes
        congenital Q10.6
    cascade, stomach K31.2
    cecum (congenital) Q43.9
        acquired K63.89
    cerebral, acquired G93.89
        congenital Q04.9
    cervix (uterus) (acquired) NEC N88.8
        congenital Q51.9
    cheek (acquired) M95.2
        congenital Q18.9
    chest (acquired) (wall) M95.4
        congenital Q67.8
        sequelae (late effect) of rickets E64.3
    chin (acquired) M95.2
        congenital Q18.9
    choroid (congenital) Q14.3
        acquired H31.8
        plexus Q07.8
            acquired G96.198
    cicatricial — *see* Cicatrix
    cilia, acquired — *see* Disorder, eyelid, specified type NEC
    clavicle (acquired) M95.8
        congenital Q68.8
    clitoris (congenital) Q52.6
        acquired N90.89
    clubfoot — *see* Clubfoot
    coccyx (acquired) — *see* subcategory M43.8- ☑
    colon (congenital) Q43.9
        acquired K63.89
    concha (ear), congenital — *see also* Malformation, ear, external
        acquired — *see* Disorder, pinna, deformity
    cornea (acquired) H18.70
        congenital Q13.4
        descemetocele — *see* Descemetocele
        ectasia — *see* Ectasia, cornea
        specified NEC H18.79- ☑
        staphyloma — *see* Staphyloma, cornea
    coronary artery (acquired) I25.9
        congenital Q24.5
    cranium (acquired) — *see* Deformity, skull
    cricoid cartilage (congenital) Q31.8
        acquired J38.7
    cystic duct (congenital) Q44.5
        acquired K82.8
    Dandy-Walker Q03.1
        with spina bifida — *see* Spina bifida

Deformity — *continued*
    diaphragm (congenital) Q79.1
        acquired J98.6
    digestive organ NOS Q45.9
    ductus arteriosus Q25.0
    duodenal bulb K31.89
    duodenum (congenital) Q43.9
        acquired K31.89
    dura — *see* Deformity, meninges
    ear (acquired) — *see also* Disorder, pinna, deformity
        congenital (external) Q17.9
            internal Q16.5
            middle Q16.4
                ossicles Q16.3
            ossicles Q16.3
    ectodermal (congenital) NEC Q84.9
    ejaculatory duct (congenital) Q55.4
        acquired N50.89
    elbow (joint) (acquired) — *see also* Deformity, limb, upper arm
        congenital Q68.8
        contraction — *see* Contraction, joint, elbow
    endocrine gland NEC Q89.2
    epididymis (congenital) Q55.4
        acquired N50.89
    epiglottis (congenital) Q31.8
        acquired J38.7
    esophagus (congenital) Q39.9
        acquired K22.89
    eustachian tube (congenital) NEC Q17.8
    eye, congenital Q15.9
    eyebrow (congenital) Q18.8
    eyelid (acquired) — *see also* Disorder, eyelid, specified type NEC
        congenital Q10.3
    face (acquired) M95.2
        congenital Q18.9
    fallopian tube, acquired N83.8
    femur (acquired) — *see* Deformity, limb, specified type NEC, thigh
    fetal
        with fetopelvic disproportion O33.7- ☑
        causing obstructed labor O66.3
    finger (acquired) M20.00- ☑
        boutonniere M20.02- ☑
        congenital Q68.1
        flexion contracture — *see* Contraction, joint, hand
        mallet finger M20.01- ☑
        specified NEC M20.09- ☑
        swan-neck M20.03- ☑
    flexion (joint) (acquired) — *see also* Deformity, limb, flexion M21.20
        congenital NOS Q74.9
        hip Q65.89
    foot (acquired) — *see also* Deformity, limb, lower leg
        cavovarus (congenital) Q66.1- ☑
        congenital NOS Q66.9- ☑
            specified type NEC Q66.89
        specified type NEC — *see* Deformity, limb, foot, specified NEC
        valgus (congenital) Q66.6
            acquired — *see* Deformity, valgus, ankle
        varus (congenital) NEC Q66.3- ☑
            acquired — *see* Deformity, varus, ankle
    forearm (acquired) — *see also* Deformity, limb, forearm
        congenital Q68.8
    forehead (acquired) M95.2
        congenital Q75.8
    frontal bone (acquired) M95.2
        congenital Q75.8
    gallbladder (congenital) Q44.1
        acquired K82.8
    gastrointestinal tract (congenital) NOS Q45.9
        acquired K63.89
    genitalia, genital organ(s) or system NEC
        female (congenital) Q52.9
            acquired N94.89
            external Q52.70
        male (congenital) Q55.9
            acquired N50.89
    globe (eye) (congenital) Q15.8
        acquired H44.89
    gum, acquired NEC K06.8
    hand (acquired) — *see* Deformity, limb, hand
        congenital Q68.1
    head (acquired) M95.2
        congenital Q75.8
    heart (congenital) Q24.9

☑ **Additional Character Required** — Refer to the Tabular List for Character Selection

Deformity

Deformity — continued
- heart — continued
  - septum Q21.9
    - auricular — see also Defect, atrial septal Q21.10
    - ventricular Q21.0
  - valve (congenital) NEC Q24.8
    - acquired — see Endocarditis
- heel (acquired) — see Deformity, foot
- hepatic duct (congenital) Q44.5
  - acquired K83.8
- hip (joint) (acquired) (see also Deformity, limb, thigh)
  - congenital Q65.9
  - due to (previous) juvenile osteochondrosis — see Coxa, plana
  - flexion — see Contraction, joint, hip
- hourglass — see Contraction, hourglass
- humerus (acquired) M21.82- ☑
  - congenital Q74.0
- hypophyseal (congenital) Q89.2
- ileocecal (coil) (valve) (acquired) K63.89
  - congenital Q43.9
- ileum (congenital) Q43.9
  - acquired K63.89
- ilium (acquired) M95.5
  - congenital Q74.2
- integument (congenital) Q84.9
- intervertebral cartilage or disc (acquired) — see Disorder, disc, specified NEC
- intestine (large) (small) (congenital) NOS Q43.9
  - acquired K63.89
- intrinsic minus or plus (hand) — see Deformity, limb, specified type NEC, forearm
- iris (acquired) H21.89
  - congenital Q13.2
- ischium (acquired) M95.5
  - congenital Q74.2
- jaw (acquired) (congenital) M26.9
- joint (acquired) NEC M21.90
  - congenital Q68.8
  - elbow M21.92- ☑
  - hand M21.94- ☑
  - hip M21.95- ☑
  - knee M21.96- ☑
  - shoulder M21.92- ☑
  - wrist M21.93- ☑
- kidney(s) (calyx) (pelvis) (congenital) Q63.9
  - acquired N28.89
  - artery (congenital) Q27.2
    - acquired I77.89
- Klippel-Feil (brevicollis) Q76.1
- knee (acquired) NEC — see also Deformity, limb, lower leg
  - congenital Q68.2
- labium (majus) (minus) (congenital) Q52.79
  - acquired N90.89
- lacrimal passages or duct (congenital) NEC Q10.6
  - acquired — see Disorder, lacrimal system, changes
- larynx (muscle) (congenital) Q31.8
  - acquired J38.7
  - web (glottic) Q31.0
- leg (upper) (acquired) NEC — see also Deformity, limb, thigh
  - congenital Q68.8
  - lower leg — see Deformity, limb, lower leg
- lens (acquired) H27.8
  - congenital Q12.9
- lid (fold) (acquired) — see also Disorder, eyelid, specified type NEC
  - congenital Q10.3
- ligament (acquired) — see Disorder, ligament
  - congenital Q79.9
- limb (acquired) M21.90
  - clawfoot M21.53- ☑
  - clawhand M21.51- ☑
    - congenital Q68.1
  - clubfoot M21.54- ☑
  - clubhand M21.52- ☑
  - congenital, except reduction deformity Q74.9
  - flat foot M21.4- ☑
  - flexion M21.20
    - ankle M21.27- ☑
    - elbow M21.22- ☑
    - finger M21.24- ☑
    - hip M21.25- ☑
    - knee M21.26- ☑
    - shoulder M21.21- ☑
    - toe M21.27- ☑
    - wrist M21.23- ☑

Deformity — continued
- limb — continued
  - foot
    - claw — see Deformity, limb, clawfoot
    - club — see Deformity, limb, clubfoot
    - drop M21.37- ☑
    - flat — see Deformity, limb, flat foot
    - specified NEC M21.6X- ☑
  - forearm M21.93- ☑
  - hand M21.94- ☑
  - lower leg M21.96- ☑
  - specified type NEC M21.80
    - forearm M21.83- ☑
    - lower leg M21.86- ☑
    - thigh M21.85- ☑
    - upper arm M21.82- ☑
  - thigh M21.95- ☑
  - unequal length M21.70
    - short site is
      - femur M21.75- ☑
      - fibula M21.76- ☑
      - humerus M21.72- ☑
      - radius M21.73- ☑
      - tibia M21.76- ☑
      - ulna M21.73- ☑
  - upper arm M21.92- ☑
  - valgus — see Deformity, valgus
  - varus — see Deformity, varus
  - wrist drop M21.33- ☑
- lip (acquired) NEC K13.0
  - congenital Q38.0
- liver (congenital) Q44.70
  - acquired K76.89
- lumbosacral (congenital) (joint) (region) Q76.49
  - acquired — see subcategory M43.8- ☑
  - kyphosis — see Kyphosis, congenital
  - lordosis — see Lordosis, congenital
- lung (congenital) Q33.9
  - acquired J98.4
- lymphatic system, congenital Q89.9
- Madelung's (radius) Q74.0
- mandible (acquired) (congenital) M26.9
- maxilla (acquired) (congenital) M26.9
- meninges or membrane (congenital) Q07.9
  - cerebral Q04.8
    - acquired G96.198
  - spinal cord (congenital) Q06.- ☑
    - acquired G96.198
- metacarpus (acquired) — see Deformity, limb, forearm
  - congenital Q74.0
- metatarsus (acquired) — see Deformity, foot
  - congenital Q66.9- ☑
- middle ear (congenital) Q16.4
  - ossicles Q16.3
- mitral (leaflets) (valve) I05.8
  - parachute Q23.2
  - stenosis, congenital Q23.2
- mouth (acquired) K13.79
  - congenital Q38.6
- multiple, congenital NEC Q89.7
- muscle (acquired) M62.89
  - congenital Q79.9
    - sternocleidomastoid Q68.0
- musculoskeletal system (acquired) M95.9
  - congenital Q79.9
  - specified NEC M95.8
- nail (acquired) L60.8
  - congenital Q84.6
- nasal — see Deformity, nose
- neck (acquired) M95.3
  - congenital Q18.9
    - sternocleidomastoid Q68.0
- nervous system (congenital) Q07.9
- nipple (congenital) Q83.9
  - acquired N64.89
- nose (acquired) (cartilage) M95.0
  - bone (turbinate) M95.0
  - congenital Q30.9
    - bent or squashed Q67.4
  - saddle M95.0
    - syphilitic A50.57
  - septum (acquired) J34.2
    - congenital Q30.8
  - sinus (wall) (congenital) Q30.8
    - acquired M95.0
  - syphilitic (congenital) A50.57
    - late A52.73
- ocular muscle (congenital) Q10.3

Deformity — continued
- ocular muscle — continued
  - acquired — see Strabismus, mechanical
- opticociliary vessels (congenital) Q13.2
- orbit (eye) (acquired) H05.30
  - atrophy — see Atrophy, orbit
  - congenital Q10.7
  - due to
    - bone disease NEC H05.32- ☑
    - trauma or surgery H05.33- ☑
  - enlargement — see Enlargement, orbit
  - exostosis — see Exostosis, orbit
- organ of Corti (congenital) Q16.5
- ovary (congenital) Q50.39
  - acquired N83.8
- oviduct, acquired N83.8
- palate (congenital) Q38.5
  - acquired M27.8
  - cleft (congenital) — see Cleft, palate
- pancreas (congenital) Q45.3
  - acquired K86.89
- parathyroid (gland) Q89.2
- parotid (gland) (congenital) Q38.4
  - acquired K11.8
- patella (acquired) — see Disorder, patella, specified NEC
- pelvis, pelvic (acquired) (bony) M95.5
  - with disproportion (fetopelvic) O33.0
    - causing obstructed labor O65.0
  - congenital Q74.2
  - rachitic sequelae (late effect) E64.3
- penis (glans) (congenital) Q55.69
  - acquired N48.89
- pericardium (congenital) Q24.8
  - acquired — see Pericarditis
- pharynx (congenital) Q38.8
  - acquired J39.2
- pinna, acquired — see also Disorder, pinna, deformity
  - congenital Q17.9
- pituitary (congenital) Q89.2
- posture — see Dorsopathy, deforming
- prepuce (congenital) Q55.69
  - acquired N47.8
- prostate (congenital) Q55.4
  - acquired N42.89
- pupil (congenital) Q13.2
  - acquired — see Abnormality, pupillary
- pylorus (congenital) Q40.3
  - acquired K31.89
- rachitic (acquired), old or healed E64.3
- radius (acquired) — see also Deformity, limb, forearm
  - congenital Q68.8
- rectum (congenital) Q43.9
  - acquired K62.89
- reduction (extremity) (limb), congenital — see also condition and site Q73.8
  - brain Q04.3
  - lower — see Defect, reduction, lower limb
  - upper — see Defect, reduction, upper limb
- renal — see Deformity, kidney
- respiratory system (congenital) Q34.9
- rib (acquired) M95.4
  - congenital Q76.6
  - cervical Q76.5
- rotation (joint) (acquired) — see Deformity, limb, specified site NEC
  - congenital Q74.9
  - hip — see Deformity, limb, specified type NEC, thigh
    - congenital Q65.89
- sacroiliac joint (congenital) — see subcategory Q74.2
  - acquired — see subcategory M43.8- ☑
- sacrum (acquired) — see subcategory M43.8- ☑
- saddle
  - back — see Lordosis
  - nose M95.0
    - syphilitic A50.57
- salivary gland or duct (congenital) Q38.4
  - acquired K11.8
- scapula (acquired) M95.8
  - congenital Q68.8
- scrotum (congenital) — see also Malformation, testis and scrotum
  - acquired N50.89
- seminal vesicles (congenital) Q55.4
  - acquired N50.89
- septum, nasal (acquired) J34.2
- shoulder (joint) (acquired) — see Deformity, limb, upper arm
  - congenital Q74.0
  - contraction — see Contraction, joint, shoulder

☑ Additional Character Required — Refer to the Tabular List for Character Selection

Deformity — continued
  sigmoid (flexure) (congenital) Q43.9
    acquired K63.89
  skin (congenital) Q82.9
  skull (acquired) M95.2
    congenital Q75.8
      with
        anencephaly Q00.0
        encephalocele — see Encephalocele
        hydrocephalus Q03.9
          with spina bifida — see Spina bifida, by site, with hydrocephalus
        microcephaly Q02
  soft parts, organs or tissues (of pelvis)
    in pregnancy or childbirth NEC O34.8-
      causing obstructed labor O65.5
  spermatic cord (congenital) Q55.4
    acquired N50.89
    torsion — see Torsion, spermatic cord
  spinal — see Dorsopathy, deforming
    column (acquired) — see Dorsopathy, deforming
      congenital Q67.5
    cord (congenital) Q06.9
      acquired G95.89
    nerve root (congenital) Q07.9
  spine (acquired) — see also Dorsopathy, deforming
    congenital Q67.5
    rachitic E64.3
    specified NEC — see Dorsopathy, deforming, specified NEC
  spleen
    acquired D73.89
    congenital Q89.09
  Sprengel's (congenital) Q74.0
  sternocleidomastoid (muscle), congenital Q68.0
  sternum (acquired) M95.4
    congenital NEC Q76.7
  stomach (congenital) Q40.3
    acquired K31.89
  submandibular gland (congenital) Q38.4
  submaxillary gland (congenital) Q38.4
    acquired K11.8
  talipes — see Talipes
  testis (congenital) — see also Malformation, testis and scrotum
    acquired N44.8
    torsion — see Torsion, testis
  thigh (acquired) — see also Deformity, limb, thigh
    congenital NEC Q68.8
  thorax (acquired) (wall) M95.4
    congenital Q67.8
    sequelae of rickets E64.3
  thumb (acquired) — see also Deformity, finger
    congenital NEC Q68.1
  thymus (tissue) (congenital) Q89.2
  thyroid (gland) (congenital) Q89.2
    cartilage Q31.8
      acquired J38.7
  tibia (acquired) — see also Deformity, limb, specified type NEC, lower leg
    congenital NEC Q68.8
    saber (syphilitic) A50.56
  toe (acquired) M20.6- ☑
    congenital Q66.9- ☑
    hallux rigidus M20.2- ☑
    hallux valgus M20.1- ☑
    hallux varus M20.3- ☑
    hammer toe M20.4- ☑
    specified NEC M20.5X- ☑
  tongue (congenital) Q38.3
    acquired K14.8
  tooth, teeth K00.2
  trachea (rings) (congenital) Q32.1
    acquired J39.8
  transverse aortic arch (congenital) Q25.49
  tricuspid (leaflets) (valve) I07.8
    atresia or stenosis Q22.4
    Ebstein's Q22.5
  trunk (acquired) M95.8
    congenital Q89.9
  ulna (acquired) — see also Deformity, limb, forearm
    congenital NEC Q68.8
  urachus, congenital Q64.4
  ureter (opening) (congenital) Q62.8
    acquired N28.89
  urethra (congenital) Q64.79
    acquired N36.8
  urinary tract (congenital) Q64.9

Deformity — continued
  urinary tract — continued
    urachus Q64.4
  uterus (congenital) Q51.9
    acquired N85.8
  uvula (congenital) Q38.5
  vagina (acquired) N89.8
    congenital Q52.4
  valgus NEC M21.00
    ankle M21.07- ☑
    elbow M21.02- ☑
    hip M21.05- ☑
    knee M21.06- ☑
  valve, valvular (congenital) (heart) Q24.8
    acquired — see Endocarditis
  varus NEC M21.10
    ankle M21.17- ☑
    elbow M21.12- ☑
    hip M21.15- ☑
    knee M21.16- ☑
    tibia — see Osteochondrosis, juvenile, tibia
  vas deferens (congenital) Q55.4
    acquired N50.89
  vein (congenital) Q27.9
    great Q26.9
  vertebra — see Dorsopathy, deforming
  vertical talus (congenital) Q66.80
    left foot Q66.82
    right foot Q66.81
  vesicourethral orifice (acquired) N32.89
    congenital NEC Q64.79
  vessels of optic papilla (congenital) Q14.2
  visual field (contraction) — see Defect, visual field
  vitreous body, acquired H43.89
  vulva (congenital) Q52.79
    acquired N90.89
  wrist (joint) (acquired) — see also Deformity, limb, forearm
    congenital Q68.8
    contraction — see Contraction, joint, wrist
Degeneration, degenerative
  adrenal (capsule) (fatty) (gland) (hyaline) (infectional) E27.8
  amyloid — see also Amyloidosis E85.9
  anterior cornua, spinal cord G12.29
  anterior labral S43.49- ☑
  aorta, aortic I70.0
    fatty I77.89
  aortic valve (heart) — see Endocarditis, aortic
  arteriovascular — see Arteriosclerosis
  artery, arterial (atheromatous) (calcareous) — see also Arteriosclerosis
    cerebral, amyloid E85.4 [I68.0]
    medial — see Arteriosclerosis, extremities
  articular cartilage NEC — see Derangement, joint, articular cartilage, by site
  atheromatous — see Arteriosclerosis
  basal nuclei or ganglia G23.9
    specified NEC G23.8
  bone NEC — see Disorder, bone, specified type NEC
  brachial plexus G54.0
  brain (cortical) (progressive) G31.9
    alcoholic G31.2
    arteriosclerotic I67.2
    childhood G31.9
      specified NEC G31.89
    cystic G31.89
      congenital Q04.6
    in
      alcoholism G31.2
      beriberi E51.2
      cerebrovascular disease I67.9
      congenital hydrocephalus Q03.9
        with spina bifida — see Spina bifida
      Fabry-Anderson disease E75.21
      Gaucher's disease E75.22
      Hunter's syndrome E76.1
      lipidosis
        cerebral E75.4
        generalized E75.6
      mucopolysaccharidosis — see Mucopolysaccharidosis
      myxedema E03.9 [G32.89]
      neoplastic disease — see also Neoplasm D49.9 [G32.89]
      Niemann-Pick disease E75.249 [G32.89]
      sphingolipidosis E75.3 [G32.89]
      vitamin B12 deficiency E53.8 [G32.89]

Degeneration, degenerative — continued
  brain — continued
    senile NEC G31.1
  breast N64.89
  Bruch's membrane — see Degeneration, choroid
  capillaries (fatty) I78.8
    amyloid E85.89 [I79.8]
  cardiac — see also Degeneration, myocardial
    valve, valvular — see Endocarditis
  cardiorenal — see Hypertension, cardiorenal
  cardiovascular — see also Disease, cardiovascular
    renal — see Hypertension, cardiorenal
  cerebellar NOS G31.9
    alcoholic G31.2
    primary (hereditary) (sporadic) G11.9
  cerebral — see Degeneration, brain
  cerebrovascular I67.9
    due to hypertension I67.4
  cervical plexus G54.2
  cervix N88.8
    due to radiation (intended effect) N88.8
      adverse effect or misadventure N99.89
  chamber angle H21.21- ☑
  changes, spine or vertebra — see Spondylosis
  chorioretinal — see also Degeneration, choroid
    hereditary H31.20
  choroid (colloid) (drusen) H31.10- ☑
    atrophy — see Atrophy, choroidal
    hereditary — see Dystrophy, choroidal, hereditary
  ciliary body H21.22- ☑
  cochlear — see subcategory H83.8- ☑
  combined (spinal cord) (subacute) E53.8 [G32.0]
    with anemia (pernicious) D51.0 [G32.0]
      due to dietary vitamin B12 deficiency D51.3 [G32.0]
    in (due to)
      vitamin B12 deficiency E53.8 [G32.0]
        anemia D51.9 [G32.0]
  conjunctiva H11.10
    concretions — see Concretion, conjunctiva
    deposits — see Deposit, conjunctiva
    pigmentations — see Pigmentation, conjunctiva
    pinguecula — see Pinguecula
    xerosis — see Xerosis, conjunctiva
  cornea H18.40
    calcerous H18.43
      band keratopathy H18.42- ☑
    familial, hereditary — see Dystrophy, cornea
    hyaline (of old scars) H18.49
    keratomalacia — see Keratomalacia
    nodular H18.45- ☑
    peripheral H18.46- ☑
    senile H18.41- ☑
    specified type NEC H18.49
  cortical (cerebellar) (parenchymatous) G31.89
    alcoholic G31.2
    diffuse, due to arteriopathy I67.2
  corticobasal G31.85
  cutis L98.8
    amyloid E85.4 [L99]
  dental pulp K04.2
  disc disease — see Degeneration, intervertebral disc, by site
  dorsolateral (spinal cord) — see Degeneration, combined
  extrapyramidal G25.9
  eye, macular — see also Degeneration, macula
    congenital or hereditary — see Dystrophy, retina
  facet joints — see Spondylosis
  fatty
    liver NEC K76.0
      alcoholic K70.0
  grey matter (brain) (Alpers') G31.81
  heart — see also Degeneration, myocardial
    amyloid E85.4 [I43]
    atheromatous — see Disease, heart, ischemic, atherosclerotic
    ischemic — see Disease, heart, ischemic
  hepatolenticular (Wilson's) E83.01
  hepatorenal K76.7
  hyaline (diffuse) (generalized)
    localized — see Degeneration, by site
  infrapatellar fat pad M79.4
  intervertebral disc
    with
      myelopathy — see Disorder, disc, with, myelopathy
      radiculitis or radiculopathy — see Disorder, disc, with, radiculopathy
    cervical, cervicothoracic — see Disorder, disc, cervical, degeneration

Degeneration, degenerative — continued
- intervertebral disc — continued
  - cervical, cervicothoracic — see Disorder, disc, cervical, degeneration — continued
    - with
      - myelopathy — see Disorder, disc, cervical, with myelopathy
      - neuritis, radiculitis or radiculopathy — see Disorder, disc, cervical, with neuritis
  - lumbar region M51.36- ☑
    - with
      - myelopathy M51.06
      - neuritis, radiculitis, radiculopathy or sciatica M51.16
  - lumbosacral region M51.37- ☑
    - with
      - neuritis, radiculitis, radiculopathy or sciatica M51.17
  - sacrococcygeal region M53.3
  - thoracic region M51.34
    - with
      - myelopathy M51.04
      - neuritis, radiculitis, radiculopathy M51.14
  - thoracolumbar region M51.35
    - with
      - myelopathy M51.05
      - neuritis, radiculitis, radiculopathy M51.15
- intestine, amyloid E85.4
- iris (pigmentary) H21.23- ☑
- ischemic — see Ischemia
- joint disease — see Osteoarthritis
- kidney N28.89
  - amyloid E85.4 [N29]
  - cystic, congenital Q61.9
  - fatty N28.89
  - polycystic Q61.3
    - adult type (autosomal dominant) Q61.2
    - infantile type (autosomal recessive) NEC Q61.19
      - collecting duct dilatation Q61.11
  - Kuhnt-Junius — see also Degeneration, macula H35.32- ☑
- lens — see Cataract
- lenticular (familial) (progressive) (Wilson's) (with cirrhosis of liver) E83.01
- liver (diffuse) NEC K76.89
  - amyloid E85.4 [K77]
  - cystic K76.89
    - congenital Q44.6
  - fatty NEC K76.0
    - alcoholic K70.0
  - hypertrophic K76.89
  - parenchymatous, acute or subacute K72.00
    - with coma K72.01
  - pigmentary K76.89
  - toxic (acute) K71.9
- lung J98.4
- lymph gland I89.8
  - hyaline I89.8
- macula, macular (acquired) (age-related) (senile) H35.30
  - angioid streaks H35.33
  - atrophic age-related H35.31- ☑
  - congenital or hereditary — see Dystrophy, retina
  - cystoid H35.35- ☑
  - drusen H35.36- ☑
  - dry age-related H35.31- ☑
  - exudative H35.32- ☑
  - hole H35.34- ☑
  - nonexudative H35.31- ☑
  - puckering H35.37- ☑
  - toxic H35.38- ☑
  - wet age-related H35.32- ☑
- membranous labyrinth, congenital (causing impairment of hearing) Q16.5
- meniscus — see Derangement, meniscus
- mitral — see Insufficiency, mitral
- Monckeberg's — see Arteriosclerosis, extremities
- motor centers, senile G31.1
- multi-system G90.3
- mural — see Degeneration, myocardial
- muscle (fatty) (fibrous) (hyaline) (progressive) M62.89
  - heart — see Degeneration, myocardial
- myelin, central nervous system G37.9
- myocardial, myocardium (fatty) (hyaline) (senile) I51.5
  - with rheumatic fever (conditions in I00) I09.0
    - active, acute or subacute I01.2
      - with chorea I02.0
    - inactive or quiescent (with chorea) I09.0
  - hypertensive — see Hypertension, heart

Degeneration, degenerative — continued
- myocardial, myocardium — continued
  - rheumatic — see Degeneration, myocardial, with rheumatic fever
  - syphilitic A52.06
- nasal sinus (mucosa) J32.9
  - frontal J32.1
  - maxillary J32.0
- nerve — see Disorder, nerve
- nervous system G31.9
  - alcoholic G31.2
  - amyloid E85.4 [G99.8]
  - autonomic G90.9
  - fatty G31.89
  - specified NEC G31.89
- nipple N64.89
- olivopontocerebellar (hereditary) (familial) G23.8
- osseous labyrinth — see subcategory H83.8- ☑
- ovary N83.8
  - cystic N83.20- ☑
  - microcystic N83.20- ☑
- pallidal pigmentary (progressive) G23.0
- pancreas K86.89
  - tuberculous A18.83
- penis N48.89
- pigmentary (diffuse) (general)
  - localized — see Degeneration, by site
  - pallidal (progressive) G23.0
- pineal gland E34.8
- pituitary (gland) E23.6
- popliteal fat pad M79.4
- posterolateral (spinal cord) — see Degeneration, combined
- pulmonary valve (heart) I37.8
- pulp (tooth) K04.2
- pupillary margin H21.24- ☑
- renal — see Degeneration, kidney
- retina H35.9
  - hereditary (cerebroretinal) (congenital) (juvenile) (macula) (peripheral) (pigmentary) — see Dystrophy, retina
  - Kuhnt-Junius — see also Degeneration, macula H35.32- ☑
  - macula (cystic) (exudative) (hole) (nonexudative) (pseudohole) (senile) (toxic) — see Degeneration, macula
  - peripheral H35.40
    - lattice H35.41- ☑
    - microcystoid H35.42- ☑
    - paving stone H35.43- ☑
    - secondary
      - pigmentary H35.45- ☑
      - vitreoretinal H35.46- ☑
    - senile reticular H35.44- ☑
  - pigmentary (primary) — see also Dystrophy, retina
    - secondary — see Degeneration, retina, peripheral, secondary
  - posterior pole — see Degeneration, macula
- saccule, congenital (causing impairment of hearing) Q16.5
- senile R54
  - brain G31.1
  - cardiac, heart or myocardium — see Degeneration, myocardial
  - motor centers G31.1
  - vascular — see Arteriosclerosis
- sinus (cystic) — see also Sinusitis
  - polypoid J33.1
- skin L98.8
  - amyloid E85.4 [L99]
  - colloid L98.8
- spinal (cord) G31.89
  - amyloid E85.4 [G32.89]
  - combined (subacute) — see Degeneration, combined
  - dorsolateral — see Degeneration, combined
  - familial NEC G31.89
  - fatty G31.89
  - funicular — see Degeneration, combined
  - posterolateral — see Degeneration, combined
  - subacute combined — see Degeneration, combined
  - tuberculous A17.81
- spleen D73.0
  - amyloid E85.4 [D77]
- stomach K31.89
- striatonigral G23.2
- suprarenal (capsule) (gland) E27.8
- synovial membrane (pulpy) — see Disorder, synovium, specified type NEC

Degeneration, degenerative — continued
- tapetoretinal — see Dystrophy, retina
- thymus (gland) E32.8
  - fatty E32.8
- thyroid (gland) E07.89
- tricuspid (heart) (valve) I07.9
- tuberculous NEC — see Tuberculosis
- turbinate J34.89
- uterus (cystic) N85.8
- vascular (senile) — see Arteriosclerosis
  - hypertensive — see Hypertension
- vitreoretinal, secondary — see Degeneration, retina, peripheral, secondary, vitreoretinal
- vitreous (body) H43.81- ☑
- Wallerian — see Disorder, nerve
- Wilson's hepatolenticular E83.01

Deglutition
- paralysis R13.0
  - hysterical F44.4
- pneumonia J69.0

Degos' disease I77.89

Dehiscence (of)
- amputation stump T87.81
- cesarean wound O90.0
- closure of
  - abdominal wall muscle or fascia T81.321- ☑
  - cornea T81.31- ☑
  - craniotomy T81.328- ☑
  - fascia (muscular) (superficial) T81.328- ☑
  - gastrointestinal tract anastomosis, repair, or closure T81.320- ☑
  - internal organ or tissue T81.328- ☑
  - laceration (external) (internal) T81.33- ☑
  - ligament T81.328- ☑
  - mucosa T81.31- ☑
  - muscle or muscle flap T81.328- ☑
  - ribs or rib cage T81.328- ☑
  - skin and subcutaneous tissue (full-thickness) (superficial) T81.31- ☑
  - skull T81.328- ☑
  - sternum (sternotomy) T81.328- ☑
  - tendon T81.328- ☑
  - traumatic laceration (external) (internal) T81.33- ☑
- episiotomy O90.1
- operation wound NEC T81.31- ☑
  - deep T81.329- ☑
  - external operation wound (superficial) T81.31- ☑
  - internal operation wound (deep) T81.329- ☑
    - abdominal wall muscle or fascia T81.321- ☑
    - specified NEC T81.328- ☑
- perineal wound (postpartum) O90.1
- traumatic injury wound repair T81.33- ☑
- wound T81.30- ☑
  - traumatic repair T81.33- ☑

Dehydration E86.0
- newborn P74.1

Dejerine-Roussy syndrome G89.0

Dejerine-Sottas disease or neuropathy (hypertrophic) G60.0

Dejerine-Thomas atrophy G23.8

Delay, delayed
- any plane in pelvis
  - complicating delivery O66.9
- birth or delivery NOS O63.9
- closure, ductus arteriosus (Botalli) P29.38
- coagulation — see Defect, coagulation
- conduction (cardiac) (ventricular) I45.9
- delivery, second twin, triplet, etc O63.2
- development R62.50
  - global F88
  - intellectual (specific) F81.9
  - language F80.9
    - due to hearing loss F80.4
  - learning F81.9
  - milestone R62.0
  - pervasive F84.9
  - physiological R62.50
    - specified stage NEC R62.0
  - reading F81.0
  - sexual E30.0
  - speech F80.9
    - due to hearing loss F80.4
  - spelling F81.81
- ejaculation F52.32
- gastric emptying K30
- menarche E30.0
- menstruation (cause unknown) N91.0
- milestone R62.0

Delay, delayed — *continued*
  passage of meconium (newborn) P76.0
  primary respiration P28.9
  puberty (constitutional) E30.0
  separation of umbilical cord P96.82
  sexual maturation, female E30.0
  sleep phase syndrome G47.21
  union, fracture — *see* Fracture, by site
  vaccination Z28.9
Deletion(s)
  autosome Q93.9
    identified by fluorescence in situ hybridization (FISH) Q93.89
    identified by in situ hybridization (ISH) Q93.89
  chromosome
    with complex rearrangements NEC Q93.7
    part of NEC Q93.59
    seen only at prometaphase Q93.89
    short arm
      4 Q93.3
      5p Q93.4
      22q11.2 Q93.81
    specified NEC Q93.89
  long arm chromosome 18 or 21 Q93.89
    with complex rearrangements NEC Q93.7
  microdeletions NEC Q93.88
Delhi boil or button B55.1
Delinquency (juvenile) (neurotic) F91.8
  group Z72.810
Delinquent immunization status Z28.39
  COVID-19 Z28.31- ☑
Delirium, delirious (acute or subacute) (not alcohol- or drug-induced) R41.0
  with
    dementia — *see also* Dementia F05
  alcoholic (acute) (tremens) (withdrawal) F10.921
    with intoxication F10.921
      in
        abuse F10.121
        dependence F10.221
  due to (secondary to)
    alcohol
      intoxication F10.921
        in
          abuse F10.121
          dependence F10.221
      withdrawal F10.231
    amphetamine intoxication F15.921
      in
        abuse F15.121
        dependence F15.221
    anxiolytic
      intoxication F13.921
        in
          abuse F13.121
          dependence F13.221
      withdrawal F13.231
    cannabis intoxication (acute) F12.921
      in
        abuse F12.121
        dependence F12.221
    cocaine intoxication (acute) F14.921
      in
        abuse F14.121
        dependence F14.221
    general medical condition F05
    hallucinogen intoxication F16.921
      in
        abuse F16.121
        dependence F16.221
    hypnotic
      intoxication F13.921
        in
          abuse F13.121
          dependence F13.221
      withdrawal F13.231
    inhalant intoxication (acute) F18.921
      in
        abuse F18.121
        dependence F18.221
    multiple etiologies F05
    opioid intoxication (acute) F11.921
      in
        abuse F11.121
        dependence F11.221
    other (or unknown) substance F19.921
    phencyclidine intoxication (acute) F16.921
      in
        abuse F16.121

Delirium, delirious — *continued*
  due to — *continued*
    phencyclidine intoxication — *continued*
      in — *continued*
        dependence F16.221
    psychoactive substance NEC intoxication (acute) F19.921
      in
        abuse F19.121
        dependence F19.221
    sedative
      intoxication F13.921
        in
          abuse F13.121
          dependence F13.221
      withdrawal F13.231
    unknown etiology R41.0
  exhaustion F43.0
  hysterical F44.89
  postprocedural (postoperative) F05
  puerperal F05
  thyroid — *see* Thyrotoxicosis with thyroid storm
  traumatic — *see* Injury, intracranial
  tremens (alcohol-induced) F10.231
    sedative-induced F13.231
Delivery (childbirth) (labor)
  arrested active phase O62.1
  cesarean (for)
    abnormal
      pelvis (bony) (deformity) (major) NEC with disproportion (fetopelvic) O33.0
        with obstructed labor O65.0
      presentation or position O32.9- ☑
    abruptio placentae — *see also* Abruptio placentae O45.9- ☑
    acromion presentation O32.2- ☑
    atony, uterus O62.2
    breech presentation O32.1- ☑
      incomplete O32.8- ☑
    brow presentation O32.3- ☑
    cephalopelvic disproportion O33.9
    cerclage O34.3- ☑
    chin presentation O32.3- ☑
    cicatrix of cervix O34.4- ☑
    contracted pelvis (general)
      inlet O33.2
      outlet O33.3- ☑
    cord presentation or prolapse O69.0- ☑
    cystocele O34.8- ☑
    deformity (acquired) (congenital)
      pelvic organs or tissues NEC O34.8- ☑
      pelvis (bony) NEC O33.0
    disproportion NOS O33.9
    eclampsia — *see* Eclampsia
    face presentation O32.3- ☑
    failed
      forceps O66.5
      induction of labor O61.9
        instrumental O61.1
        mechanical O61.1
        medical O61.0
        specified NEC O61.8
        surgical O61.1
      trial of labor NOS O66.40
        following previous cesarean delivery O66.41
      vacuum extraction O66.5
      ventouse O66.5
    fetal-maternal hemorrhage O43.01- ☑
    hemorrhage (intrapartum) O67.9
      with coagulation defect O67.0
      specified cause NEC O67.8
    high head at term O32.4- ☑
    hydrocephalic fetus O33.6- ☑
    incarceration of uterus O34.51- ☑
    incoordinate uterine action O62.4
    increased size, fetus O33.5- ☑
    inertia, uterus O62.2
      primary O62.0
      secondary O62.1
    isthmocele O34.22
    lateroversion, uterus O34.59- ☑
    mal lie O32.9- ☑
    malposition
      fetus O32.9- ☑
      pelvic organs or tissues NEC O34.8- ☑
      uterus NEC O34.59- ☑
    malpresentation NOS O32.9- ☑
    oblique presentation O32.2- ☑

Delivery — *continued*
  cesarean — *continued*
    occurring after 37 completed weeks of gestation but before 39 completed weeks gestation due to (spontaneous) onset of labor O75.82
    oversize fetus O33.5- ☑
    pelvic tumor NEC O34.8- ☑
    placenta previa O44.0- ☑
      complete O44.0- ☑
        with hemorrhage O44.1- ☑
    placental insufficiency O36.51- ☑
    planned, occurring after 37 completed weeks of gestation but before 39 completed weeks gestation due to (spontaneous) onset of labor O75.82
    polyp, cervix O34.4- ☑
      causing obstructed labor O65.5
    poor dilatation, cervix O62.0
    pre-eclampsia O14.94
      mild O14.04
      moderate O14.04
      severe O14.14
        with hemolysis, elevated liver enzymes and low platelet count (HELLP) O14.24
    previous
      cesarean delivery O34.219
        classical (vertical) scar O34.212
        isthmocele O34.22
        low transverse scar O34.211
        mid-transverse T incision O34.218
        scar
          defect (isthmocele) O34.22
          specified type NEC O34.218
      surgery (to)
        cervix O34.4- ☑
        gynecological NEC O34.8- ☑
        rectum O34.7- ☑
        uterus O34.29
        vagina O34.6- ☑
    prolapse
      arm or hand O32.2- ☑
      uterus O34.52- ☑
    prolonged labor NOS O63.9
    rectocele O34.8- ☑
    retroversion
      uterus O34.53- ☑
    rigid
      cervix O34.4- ☑
      pelvic floor O34.8- ☑
      perineum O34.7- ☑
      vagina O34.6- ☑
      vulva O34.7- ☑
    sacculation, pregnant uterus O34.59- ☑
    scar(s)
      cervix O34.4- ☑
      cesarean delivery O34.219
        classical (vertical) O34.212
        isthmocele O34.22
        low transverse O34.211
        mid-transverse T incision O34.218
        scar
          defect (isthmocele) O34.22
          specified type NEC O34.218
      defect (isthmocele) O34.22
      transmural uterine O34.29
      uterus O34.29
    Shirodkar suture in situ O34.3- ☑
    shoulder presentation O32.2- ☑
    stenosis or stricture, cervix O34.4- ☑
    streptococcus group B (GBS) carrier state O99.824
    transmural uterine scar O34.29
    transverse presentation or lie O32.2- ☑
    tumor, pelvic organs or tissues NEC O34.8- ☑
      cervix O34.4- ☑
    umbilical cord presentation or prolapse O69.0- ☑
    without indication O82
  completely normal case O80
  complicated O75.9
    by
      abnormal, abnormality (of)
        forces of labor O62.9
          specified type NEC O62.8
        glucose O99.814
        uterine contractions NOS O62.9
      abruptio placentae — *see also* Abruptio placentae O45.9- ☑
      abuse
        physical O9A.32 (*following* O99)

Delivery — continued
  complicated — continued
    by — continued
      abuse — continued
        psychological O9A.52 (following O99)
        sexual O9A.42 (following O99)
      adherent placenta O72.0
        without hemorrhage O73.0
      alcohol use O99.314
      anemia (pre-existing) O99.02
      anesthetic death O74.8
      annular detachment of cervix O71.3
      atony, uterus O62.2
      attempted vacuum extraction and forceps O66.5
      Bandl's ring O62.4
      bariatric surgery status O99.844
      biliary tract disorder O26.62
      bleeding — see Delivery, complicated by, hemorrhage
      blood disorder NEC O99.12
      cervical dystocia (hypotonic) O62.2
        primary O62.0
        secondary O62.1
      circulatory system disorder O99.42
      compression of cord (umbilical) NEC O69.2- ☑
      condition NEC O99.892
      contraction, contracted ring O62.4
      cord (umbilical)
        around neck
          with compression O69.1- ☑
          without compression O69.81- ☑
        bruising O69.5- ☑
        complication O69.9- ☑
          specified NEC O69.89- ☑
        compression NEC O69.2- ☑
        entanglement O69.2- ☑
          without compression O69.82- ☑
        hematoma O69.5- ☑
        presentation O69.0- ☑
        prolapse O69.0- ☑
        short O69.3- ☑
        thrombosis (vessels) O69.5- ☑
        vascular lesion O69.5- ☑
      Couvelaire uterus O45.8X- ☑
      damage to (injury to) NEC
        perineum O71.82
        periurethral tissue O71.82
        vulva O71.82
      delay following rupture of membranes (spontaneous) — see Pregnancy, complicated by, premature rupture of membranes
      depressed fetal heart tones O76
      diabetes O24.92
        gestational O24.429
          diet controlled O24.420
          insulin controlled O24.424
          oral drug controlled (antidiabetic) (hypoglycemic) O24.425
        pre-existing O24.32
          specified NEC O24.82
          type 1 O24.02
          type 2 O24.12
      diastasis recti (abdominis) O71.89
      dilatation
        bladder O66.8
        cervix incomplete, poor or slow O62.0
      disease NEC O99.892
      disruptio uteri — see Delivery, complicated by, rupture, uterus
      drug use O99.324
      dysfunction, uterus NOS O62.9
        hypertonic O62.4
        hypotonic O62.2
          primary O62.0
          secondary O62.1
        incoordinate O62.4
      eclampsia O15.1
      embolism (pulmonary) — see Embolism, obstetric
      endocrine, nutritional or metabolic disease NEC O99.284
      failed
        attempted vaginal birth after previous cesarean delivery O66.41
        induction of labor O61.9
          instrumental O61.1
          mechanical O61.1
          medical O61.0
          specified NEC O61.8

Delivery — continued
  complicated — continued
    by — continued
      failed — continued
        induction of labor — continued
          surgical O61.1
        trial of labor O66.40
      female genital mutilation O65.5
      fetal
        abnormal acid-base balance O68
        acidemia O68
        acidosis O68
        alkalosis O68
        death, early O02.1
        deformity O66.3
        heart rate or rhythm (abnormal) (non-reassuring) O76
        hypoxia O77.8
        stress O77.9
          due to drug administration O77.1
          electrocardiographic evidence of O77.8
          specified NEC O77.8
          ultrasound evidence of O77.8
      fever during labor O75.2
      gastric banding status O99.844
      gastric bypass status O99.844
      gastrointestinal disease NEC O99.62
      gestational
        diabetes O24.429
          diet controlled O24.420
          insulin (and diet) controlled O24.424
          oral drug controlled (antidiabetic) (hypoglycemic) O24.425
        edema O12.04
          with proteinuria O12.24
        proteinuria O12.14
      gonorrhea O98.22
      hematoma O71.7
        ischial spine O71.7
        pelvic O71.7
        vagina O71.7
        vulva or perineum O71.7
      hemorrhage (uterine) O67.9
        associated with
          afibrinogenemia O67.0
          coagulation defect O67.0
          hyperfibrinolysis O67.0
          hypofibrinogenemia O67.0
        due to
          low implantation of placenta O44.5- ☑
          low-lying placenta O44.5- ☑
          placenta previa O44.1- ☑
            marginal O44.3- ☑
            partial O44.3- ☑
          premature separation of placenta (normally implanted) — see also Abruptio placentae O45.9- ☑
          retained placenta O72.0
          uterine leiomyoma O67.8
        placenta NEC O67.8
        postpartum NEC (atonic) (immediate) O72.1
          with retained or trapped placenta O72.0
          delayed O72.2
          secondary O72.2
          third stage O72.0
      hourglass contraction, uterus O62.4
      hypertension, hypertensive (pre-existing) — see Hypertension, complicated by, childbirth (labor)
      hypotension O26.5- ☑
      incomplete dilatation (cervix) O62.0
      incoordinate uterus contractions O62.4
      inertia, uterus O62.2
        during latent phase of labor O62.0
        primary O62.0
        secondary O62.1
      infection (maternal) O98.92
        carrier state NEC O99.834
        gonorrhea O98.22
        human immunodeficiency virus (HIV) O98.72
        sexually transmitted NEC O98.32
        specified NEC O98.82
        syphilis O98.12
        tuberculosis O98.02
        viral hepatitis O98.42
        viral NEC O98.52
      injury (to mother) — see also Delivery, complicated, by, damage to O71.9

Delivery — continued
  complicated — continued
    by — continued
      injury — see also Delivery, complicated, by, damage to — continued
        nonobstetric O9A.22 (following O99)
          caused by abuse — see Delivery, complicated by, abuse
      intrauterine fetal death, early O02.1
      inversion, uterus O71.2
      laceration (perineal) O70.9
        anus (sphincter) O70.4
          with third degree laceration — see also Delivery, complicated, by, laceration, perineum, third degree O70.20
            with mucosa O70.3
          without third degree laceration O70.2- ☑
        bladder (urinary) O71.5
        bowel O71.5
        cervix (uteri) O71.3
        fourchette O70.0
        hymen O70.0
        labia O70.0
        pelvic
          floor O70.1
          organ NEC O71.5
        perineum, perineal O70.9
          first degree O70.0
          fourth degree O70.3
          muscles O70.1
          second degree O70.1
          skin O70.0
          slight O70.0
          third degree O70.20
            with
              both external anal sphincter (EAS) and internal anal sphincter (IAS) torn (IIIc) O70.23
              less than 50% of external anal sphincter (EAS) thickness torn (IIIa) O70.21
              more than 50% external anal sphincter (EAS) thickness torn (IIIb) O70.22
            IIIa O70.21
            IIIb O70.22
            IIIc O70.23
        peritoneum (pelvic) O71.5
        rectovaginal (septum) (without perineal laceration) O71.4
          with perineum — see also Delivery, complicated, by, laceration, perineum, third degree O70.20
          with anal or rectal mucosa O70.3
        specified NEC O71.89
        sphincter ani — see Delivery, complicated, by, laceration, anus (sphincter)
        urethra O71.5
        uterus O71.81
          before labor O71.81
        vagina, vaginal (deep) (high) (without perineal laceration) O71.4
          with perineum O70.0
          muscles, with perineum O70.1
        vulva O70.0
      liver disorder O26.62
      malignancy O9A.12 (following O99)
      malnutrition O25.2
      malposition, malpresentation
        uterus or cervix O65.5
        placenta O44.0- ☑
          with hemorrhage O44.1- ☑
        without obstruction — see also Delivery, complicated by, obstruction O32.9- ☑
          breech O32.1- ☑
          compound O32.6- ☑
          face (brow) (chin) O32.3- ☑
          footling O32.8- ☑
          high head O32.4- ☑
          oblique O32.2- ☑
          specified NEC O32.8- ☑
          transverse O32.2- ☑
          unstable lie O32.0- ☑
      meconium in amniotic fluid O77.0
      mental disorder NEC O99.344
      metrorrhexis — see Delivery, complicated by, rupture, uterus
      nervous system disorder O99.354

Delivery — continued
  complicated — continued
    by — continued
      obesity (pre-existing) O99.214
      obesity surgery status O99.844
      obstetric trauma O71.9
        specified NEC O71.89
      obstructed labor
        due to
          breech (complete) (frank) presentation O64.1- ☑
            incomplete O64.8- ☑
          brow presentation O64.3- ☑
          buttock presentation O64.1- ☑
          chin presentation O64.2- ☑
          compound presentation O64.5- ☑
          contracted pelvis O65.1
          deep transverse arrest O64.0- ☑
          deformed pelvis O65.0
          dystocia (fetal) O66.9
            due to
              conjoined twins O66.3
              fetal
                abnormality NEC O66.3
                ascites O66.3
                hydrops O66.3
                meningomyelocele O66.3
                sacral teratoma O66.3
                tumor O66.3
              hydrocephalic fetus O66.3
              shoulder O66.0
          face presentation O64.2- ☑
          fetopelvic disproportion O65.4
          footling presentation O64.8- ☑
          impacted shoulders O66.0
          incomplete rotation of fetal head O64.0- ☑
          large fetus O66.2
          locked twins O66.1
          malposition O64.9- ☑
            specified NEC O64.8- ☑
          malpresentation O64.9- ☑
            specified NEC O64.8- ☑
          multiple fetuses NEC O66.6
          pelvic
            abnormality (maternal) O65.9
              organ O65.5
              specified NEC O65.8
            contraction
              inlet O65.2
              mid-cavity O65.3
              outlet O65.3
          persistent (position)
            occipitoiliac O64.0- ☑
            occipitoposterior O64.0- ☑
            occipitosacral O64.0- ☑
            occipitotransverse O64.0- ☑
          prolapsed arm O64.4- ☑
          shoulder presentation O64.4- ☑
          specified NEC O66.8
      pathological retraction ring, uterus O62.4
      penetration, pregnant uterus by instrument O71.1
      perforation — see Delivery, complicated by, laceration
      placenta, placental
        ablatio — see also Abruptio placentae O45.9- ☑
        abnormality O43.9- ☑
          specified NEC O43.89- ☑
        abruptio — see also Abruptio placentae O45.9- ☑
        accreta O43.21- ☑
        adherent (with hemorrhage) O72.0
          without hemorrhage O73.0
        detachment (premature) — see also Abruptio placentae O45.9- ☑
        disorder O43.9- ☑
          specified NEC O43.89- ☑
        hemorrhage NEC O67.8
        increta O43.22- ☑
        low (implantation) (lying) O44.4- ☑
          with hemorrhage O44.5- ☑
        malformation O43.10- ☑
        malposition O44.0- ☑
          without hemorrhage O44.1- ☑
        percreta O43.23- ☑
        previa (central) (complete) (lateral) (total) O44.0- ☑

Delivery — continued
  complicated — continued
    by — continued
      placenta, placental — continued
        previa — continued
          with hemorrhage O44.1- ☑
          marginal O44.2- ☑
            with hemorrhage O44.3- ☑
          partial O44.2- ☑
            with hemorrhage O44.3- ☑
        retained (with hemorrhage) O72.0
          without hemorrhage O73.0
        separation (premature) O45.9- ☑
          specified NEC O45.8X- ☑
        vicious insertion O44.1- ☑
      precipitate labor O62.3
      premature rupture, membranes — see also Pregnancy, complicated by, premature rupture of membranes O42.90
      prolapse
        arm or hand O32.2- ☑
        cord (umbilical) O69.0- ☑
        foot or leg O32.8- ☑
        uterus O34.52- ☑
      prolonged labor O63.9
        first stage O63.0
        second stage O63.1
      protozoal disease (maternal) O98.62
      respiratory disease NEC O99.52
      retained membranes or portions of placenta O72.2
        without hemorrhage O73.1
      retarded birth O63.9
      retention of secundines (with hemorrhage) O72.0
        without hemorrhage O73.0
        partial O72.2
          without hemorrhage O73.1
      rupture
        bladder (urinary) O71.5
        cervix O71.3
        pelvic organ NEC O71.5
        urethra O71.5
        uterus (during or after labor) O71.1
          before labor O71.0- ☑
      separation, pubic bone (symphysis pubis) O71.6
      shock O75.1
      shoulder presentation O64.4- ☑
      skin disorder NEC O99.72
      spasm, cervix O62.4
      stenosis or stricture, cervix O65.5
      streptococcus group B (GBS) carrier state O99.824
      subluxation of symphysis (pubis) O26.72
      syphilis (maternal) O98.12
      tear — see Delivery, complicated by, laceration
      tetanic uterus O62.4
      trauma (obstetrical) — see also Delivery, complicated, by, damage to O71.9
        non-obstetric O9A.22 (following O99)
        periurethral O71.82
        specified NEC O71.89
      tuberculosis (maternal) O98.02
      tumor, pelvic organs or tissues NEC O65.5
      umbilical cord around neck
        with compression O69.1- ☑
        without compression O69.81- ☑
      uterine inertia O62.2
        during latent phase of labor O62.0
        primary O62.0
        secondary O62.1
      vasa previa O69.4- ☑
      velamentous insertion of cord O43.12- ☑
    specified complication NEC O75.89
  delayed NOS O63.9
    following rupture of membranes
      artificial O75.5
    second twin, triplet, etc. O63.2
  forceps, low following failed vacuum extraction O66.5
  missed (at or near term) O36.4- ☑
  normal O80
  obstructed — see Delivery, complicated by, obstructed labor
  precipitate O62.3
  preterm — see also Pregnancy, complicated by, preterm labor O60.10- ☑
  spontaneous O80
  term pregnancy NOS O80
  uncomplicated O80
  vaginal, following previous cesarean delivery O34.219
    classical (vertical) scar O34.212

Delivery — continued
  vaginal, following previous cesarean delivery — continued
    low transverse scar O34.211
    mid-transverse T incision O34.218
    scar
      defect (isthmocele) O34.22
      specified type NEC O34.218
Delusions (paranoid) — see Disorder, delusional
Dementia (degenerative (primary)) (persisting) (unspecified severity) (without behavioral disturbance, psychotic disturbance, mood disturbance, and anxiety) F03.90
  with
    aberrant motor behavior (exit-seeking) (pacing) (restlessness) (rocking) F03.911
    acute confusional state F05
    agitation F03.911
    anxiety F03.94
    behavioral disturbances (sexual disinhibition) (sleep disturbance) (social disinhibition) F03.918
      specified NEC F03.918
    Lewy bodies — see also Dementia, in, diseases specified elsewhere G31.83 [F02.80]
      with behavioral disturbance — see also Dementia, in, diseases specified elsewhere G31.83 [F02.81-] ☑
    mood disturbance (anhedonia) (apathy) (depression) F03.93
    Parkinsonism — see also Dementia, in, diseases specified elsewhere G20.C [F02.80]
      with behavioral disturbance — see also Dementia, in, diseases specified elsewhere G20.C [F02.81-] ☑
    Parkinson's disease — see also Dementia, in, diseases specified elsewhere G20.A1 [F02.80]
      with behavioral disturbance — see also Dementia, in, diseases specified elsewhere G20.A1 [F02.81-] ☑
    psychotic disturbance (delusional state) (hallucinations) (paranoia) (suspiciousness) F03.92
    verbal or physical behaviors (anger) (aggression) (combativeness) (profanity) (shouting) (threatening) (violence) F03.911
  alcoholic F10.97
    with dependence F10.27
  Alzheimer's type — see Disease, Alzheimer's
  arteriosclerotic — see Dementia, vascular
  atypical, Alzheimer's type — see Disease, Alzheimer's, specified NEC
  congenital — see Disability, intellectual
  frontal (lobe) — see also Dementia, in, diseases specified elsewhere G31.09 [F02.80]
    with behavioral disturbance — see also Dementia, in, diseases specified elsewhere G31.09 [F02.81-] ☑
  frontotemporal G31.09 [F02.80]
    with behavioral disturbance G31.09 [F02.81-] ☑
    specified NEC — see also Dementia, in, diseases specified elsewhere G31.09 [F02.80]
      with behavioral disturbance — see also Dementia, in, diseases specified elsewhere G31.09 [F02.81-] ☑
  in (due to)
    alcohol F10.97
      with dependence F10.27
    Alzheimer's disease — see Disease, Alzheimer's
    arteriosclerotic brain disease — see Dementia, vascular
    cerebral lipidoses — see also Dementia, in, diseases specified elsewhere E75.- ☑ [F02.80]
      with behavioral disturbance — see also Dementia, in, diseases specified elsewhere E75.- ☑ [F02.81-] ☑
    Creutzfeldt-Jakob disease — see also Creutzfeldt-Jakob disease or syndrome (with dementia) A81.00
    diseases specified elsewhere (unspecified severity) (without behavioral disturbance, psychotic disturbance, mood disturbance, and anxiety) F02.80
      with
        aberrant motor behavior (exit-seeking) (pacing) (restlessness) (rocking) F02.811
        agitation F02.811
        anxiety F02.84
        behavioral disturbances (sexual disinhibition) (sleep disturbance) (social disinhibition) F02.818

☑ **Additional Character Required** — Refer to the Tabular List for Character Selection

Dementia — *continued*
- in — *continued*
  - diseases specified elsewhere — *continued*
    - with — *continued*
      - behavioral disturbances — *continued*
        - specified NEC F02.818
      - mood disturbance (anhedonia) (apathy) (depression) F02.83
      - psychotic disturbance (delusional state) (hallucinations) (paranoia) (suspiciousness) F02.82
      - verbal or physical behaviors (anger) (aggression) (combativeness) (profanity) (shouting) (threatening) (violence) F02.811
    - mild F02.A0
      - with
        - aberrant motor behavior (exit-seeking) (pacing) (restlessness) (rocking) F02.A11
        - agitation F02.A11
        - anxiety F02.A4
        - behavioral disturbances (sexual disinhibition) (sleep disturbance) (social disinhibition) F02.A18
          - specified NEC F02.A18
        - mood disturbance (anhedonia) (apathy) (depression) F02.A3
        - psychotic disturbance (delusional state) (hallucinations) (paranoia) (suspiciousness) F02.A2
        - verbal or physical behaviors (anger) (aggression) (combativeness) (profanity) (shouting) (threatening) (violence) F02.A11
    - moderate F02.B0
      - with
        - aberrant motor behavior (exit-seeking) (pacing) (restlessness) (rocking) F02.B11
        - agitation F02.B11
        - anxiety F02.B4
        - behavioral disturbances (sexual disinhibition) (sleep disturbance) (social disinhibition) F02.B18
          - specified NEC F02.B18
        - mood disturbance (anhedonia) (apathy) (depression) F02.B3
        - psychotic disturbance (delusional state) (hallucinations) (paranoia) (suspiciousness) F02.B2
        - verbal or physical behaviors (anger) (aggression) (combativeness) (profanity) (shouting) (threatening) (violence) F02.B11
    - severe F02.C0
      - with
        - aberrant motor behavior (exit-seeking) (pacing) (restlessness) (rocking) F02.C11
        - agitation F02.C11
        - anxiety F02.C4
        - behavioral disturbances (sexual disinhibition) (sleep disturbance) (social disinhibition) F02.C18
          - specified NEC F02.C18
        - mood disturbance (anhedonia) (apathy) (depression) F02.C3
        - psychotic disturbance (delusional state) (hallucinations) (paranoia) (suspiciousness) F02.C2
        - verbal or physical behaviors (anger) (aggression) (combativeness) (profanity) (shouting) (threatening) (violence) F02.C11
    - epilepsy — *see also* Dementia, in, diseases specified elsewhere G40.- ☑ *[F02.80]*
      - with behavioral disturbance — *see also* Dementia, in, diseases specified elsewhere G40.- ☑ *[F02.81-]* ☑
    - hepatolenticular degeneration — *see also* Dementia, in, diseases specified elsewhere E83.01 *[F02.80]*
      - with behavioral disturbance — *see also* Dementia, in, diseases specified elsewhere E83.01 *[F02.81-]* ☑
    - human immunodeficiency virus (HIV) disease — *see also* Dementia, in, diseases specified elsewhere B20 *[F02.80]*

Dementia — *continued*
- in — *continued*
  - human immunodeficiency virus disease — *see also* Dementia, in, diseases specified elsewhere — *continued*
    - with behavioral disturbance — *see also* Dementia, in, diseases specified elsewhere B20 *[F02.81-]* ☑
  - Huntington's disease or chorea — *see also* Dementia, in, diseases specified elsewhere G10 *[F02.80]*
    - with behavioral disturbance — *see also* Dementia, in, diseases specified elsewhere G10 *[F02.81-]* ☑
  - hypercalcemia — *see also* Dementia, in, diseases specified elsewhere E83.52 *[F02.80]*
    - with behavioral disturbance — *see also* Dementia, in, diseases specified elsewhere E83.52 *[F02.81-]* ☑
  - hypothyroidism, acquired — *see also* Dementia, in, diseases specified elsewhere E03.9 *[F02.80]*
    - with behavioral disturbance — *see also* Dementia, in, diseases specified elsewhere E03.9 *[F02.81-]* ☑
    - due to iodine deficiency — *see also* Dementia, in, diseases specified elsewhere E01.8 *[F02.80]*
      - with behavioral disturbance — *see also* Dementia, in, diseases specified elsewhere E01.8 *[F02.81-]* ☑
  - inhalants F18.97
    - with dependence F18.27
  - multiple
    - etiologies F03.- ☑
    - sclerosis — *see also* Dementia, in, diseases specified elsewhere G35.D *[F02.80]*
      - with behavioral disturbance — *see also* Dementia, in, diseases specified elsewhere G35.D *[F02.81-]* ☑
  - neurosyphilis — *see also* Dementia, in, diseases specified elsewhere A52.17 *[F02.80]*
    - with behavioral disturbance — *see also* Dementia, in, diseases specified elsewhere A52.17 *[F02.81-]* ☑
    - juvenile — *see also* Dementia, in, diseases specified elsewhere A50.49 *[F02.80]*
      - with behavioral disturbance — *see also* Dementia, in, diseases specified elsewhere A50.49 *[F02.81-]* ☑
  - niacin deficiency — *see also* Dementia, in, diseases specified elsewhere E52 *[F02.80]*
    - with behavioral disturbance — *see also* Dementia, in, diseases specified elsewhere E52 *[F02.81-]* ☑
  - paralysis agitans — *see also* Dementia, in, diseases specified elsewhere G20.C *[F02.80]*
    - with behavioral disturbance — *see also* Dementia, in, diseases specified elsewhere G20.C *[F02.81-]* ☑
  - Parkinson's disease — *see also* Dementia, in, diseases specified elsewhere G20.A1 *[F02.80]*
  - pellagra — *see also* Dementia, in, diseases specified elsewhere E52 *[F02.80]*
    - with behavioral disturbance — *see also* Dementia, in, diseases specified elsewhere E52 *[F02.81-]* ☑
  - Pick's — *see also* Dementia, in, diseases specified elsewhere G31.01 *[F02.80]*
    - with behavioral disturbance — *see also* Dementia, in, diseases specified elsewhere G31.01 *[F02.81-]* ☑
  - polyarteritis nodosa — *see also* Dementia, in, diseases specified elsewhere M30.0 *[F02.80]*
    - with behavioral disturbance — *see also* Dementia, in, diseases specified elsewhere M30.0 *[F02.81-]* ☑
  - psychoactive drug F19.97
    - with dependence F19.27
    - inhalants F18.97
      - with dependence F18.27
    - sedatives, hypnotics or anxiolytics F13.97
      - with dependence F13.27
  - sedatives, hypnotics or anxiolytics F13.97
    - with dependence F13.27
  - systemic lupus erythematosus — *see also* Dementia, in, diseases specified elsewhere M32.- ☑ *[F02.80]*
    - with behavioral disturbance — *see also* Dementia, in, diseases specified elsewhere M32.- ☑ *[F02.81-]* ☑

Dementia — *continued*
- in — *continued*
  - trypanosomiasis
    - African — *see also* Dementia, in, diseases specified elsewhere B56.9 *[F02.80]*
      - with behavioral disturbance — *see also* Dementia, in, diseases specified elsewhere B56.9 *[F02.81-]* ☑
  - unknown etiology F03.- ☑
  - vitamin B12 deficiency — *see also* Dementia, in, diseases specified elsewhere E53.8 *[F02.80]*
    - with behavioral disturbance — *see also* Dementia, in, diseases specified elsewhere E53.8 *[F02.81-]* ☑
  - volatile solvents F18.97
    - with dependence F18.27
- infantile, infantilis F84.3
- Lewy body — *see also* Dementia, in, diseases specified elsewhere G31.83 *[F02.80]*
  - with behavioral disturbance — *see also* Dementia, in, diseases specified elsewhere G31.83 *[F02.81-]* ☑
- mild F03.A0
  - with
    - aberrant motor behavior (exit-seeking) (pacing) (restlessness) (rocking) F03.A11
    - agitation F03.A11
    - anxiety F03.A4
    - behavioral disturbances (sexual disinhibition) (sleep disturbance) (social disinhibition) F03.A18
      - specified NEC F03.A18
    - mood disturbance (anhedonia) (apathy) (depression) F03.A3
    - psychotic disturbance (delusional state) (hallucinations) (paranoia) (suspiciousness) F03.A2
    - verbal or physical behaviors (anger) (aggression) (combativeness) (profanity) (shouting) (threatening) (violence) F03.A11
- moderate F03.B0
  - with
    - aberrant motor behavior (exit-seeking) (pacing) (restlessness) (rocking) F03.B11
    - agitation F03.B11
    - anxiety F03.B4
    - behavioral disturbances (sexual disinhibition) (sleep disturbance) (social disinhibition) F03.B18
      - specified NEC F03.B18
    - mood disturbance (anhedonia) (apathy) (depression) F03.B3
    - psychotic disturbance (delusional state) (hallucinations) (paranoia) (suspiciousness) F03.B2
    - verbal or physical behaviors (anger) (aggression) (combativeness) (profanity) (shouting) (threatening) (violence) F03.B11
- multi-infarct — *see* Dementia, vascular
- old age (senile) F03.- ☑
  - Alzheimer's type — *see* Disease, Alzheimer's, late onset
- paralytica, paralytic (syphilitic) — *see also* Dementia, in, diseases specified elsewhere A52.17 *[F02.80]*
  - with behavioral disturbance — *see also* Dementia, in, diseases specified elsewhere A52.17 *[F02.81-]* ☑
  - juvenilis A50.45
- paretic A52.17
- praecox — *see* Schizophrenia
- presenile F03.- ☑
  - Alzheimer's type — *see* Disease, Alzheimer's, early onset
- primary degenerative F03.- ☑
- progressive, syphilitic A52.17
- senile F03.- ☑
  - Alzheimer's type — *see* Disease, Alzheimer's, late onset
  - depressed or paranoid type F03.- ☑
- severe F03.C0
  - with
    - aberrant motor behavior (exit-seeking) (pacing) (restlessness) (rocking) F03.C11
    - agitation F03.C11
    - anxiety F03.C4
    - behavioral disturbances (sexual disinhibition) (sleep disturbance) (social disinhibition) F03.C18
      - specified NEC F03.C18

Dementia — continued
  severe — continued
    with — continued
      mood disturbance (anhedonia) (apathy) (depression) F03.C3
      psychotic disturbance (delusional state) (hallucinations) (paranoia) (suspiciousness) F03.C2
      verbal or physical behaviors (anger) (aggression) (combativeness) (profanity) (shouting) (threatening) (violence) F03.C11
  vascular (acute onset) (mixed) (multi-infarct) (subcortical) (unspecified severity) (without behavioral disturbance, psychotic disturbance, mood disturbance, and anxiety) F01.50
    with
      aberrant motor behavior (exit-seeking) (pacing) (restlessness) (rocking) F01.511
      agitation F01.511
      anxiety F01.54
      behavioral disturbances (sleep disturbance) (sexual disinhibition) (social disinhibition) F01.518
        specified NEC F01.518
      mood disturbance (anhedonia) (apathy) (depression) F01.53
      psychotic disturbance (delusional state) (hallucinations) (paranoia) (suspiciousness) F01.52
      verbal or physical behaviors (anger) (aggression) (combativeness) (profanity) (shouting) (threatening) (violence) F01.511
    mild F01.A0
      with
        aberrant motor behavior (exit-seeking) (pacing) (restlessness) (rocking) F01.A11
        agitation F01.A11
        anxiety F01.A4
        behavioral disturbances (sleep disturbance) (sexual disinhibition) (social disinhibition) F01.A18
          specified NEC F01.A18
        mood disturbance (anhedonia) (apathy) (depression) F01.A3
        psychotic disturbance (delusional state) (hallucinations) (paranoia) (suspiciousness) F01.A2
        verbal or physical behaviors (anger) (aggression) (combativeness) (profanity) (shouting) (threatening) (violence) F01.A11
    moderate F01.B0
      with
        aberrant motor behavior (exit-seeking) (pacing) (restlessness) (rocking) F01.B11
        agitation F01.B11
        anxiety F01.B4
        behavioral disturbances (sleep disturbance) (sexual disinhibition) (social disinhibition) F01.B18
          specified NEC F01.B18
        mood disturbance (anhedonia) (apathy) (depression) F01.B3
        psychotic disturbance (delusional state) (hallucinations) (paranoia) (suspiciousness) F01.B2
        verbal or physical behaviors (anger) (aggression) (combativeness) (profanity) (shouting) (threatening) (violence) F01.B11
    severe F01.C0
      with
        aberrant motor behavior (exit-seeking) (pacing) (restlessness) (rocking) F01.C11
        agitation F01.C11
        anxiety F01.C4
        behavioral disturbances (sleep disturbance) (sexual disinhibition) (social disinhibition) F01.C18
          specified NEC F01.C18
        mood disturbance (anhedonia) (apathy) (depression) F01.C3
        psychotic disturbance (delusional state) (hallucinations) (paranoia) (suspiciousness) F01.C2
        verbal or physical behaviors (anger) (aggression) (combativeness) (profanity) (shouting) (threatening) (violence) F01.C11

Demineralization, bone — see Osteoporosis
Demodex folliculorum (infestation) B88.01
Demophobia F40.248
Demoralization R45.3
Demyelination, demyelinization
  central nervous system G37.9
    specified NEC G37.89
  corpus callosum (central) G37.1
  disseminated, acute G36.9
    specified NEC G36.8
  global G35.D
  in optic neuritis G36.0
Dengue (classical) (fever) A90
  hemorrhagic A91
  sandfly A93.1
Dennie-Marfan syphilitic syndrome A50.45
Dens evaginatus, in dente or invaginatus K00.2
Dense breasts — see also Density, breast R92.30
Density
  breast R92.30
    low R92.30
    mammographic
      extreme R92.34- ☑
      fatty tissue R92.31- ☑
      fibroglandular R92.32- ☑
      heterogeneous R92.33- ☑
  increased, bone (disseminated) (generalized) (spotted) — see Disorder, bone, density and structure, specified type NEC
  lung (nodular) J98.4
Dental — see also condition
  examination Z01.20
    with abnormal findings Z01.21
  restoration
    aesthetically inadequate or displeasing K08.56
    defective K08.50
      specified NEC K08.59
    failure of marginal integrity K08.51
    failure of periodontal anatomical integrity K08.54
Dentia praecox K00.6
Denticles (pulp) K04.2
Dentigerous cyst K09.0
Dentin
  irregular (in pulp) K04.3
  opalescent K00.5
  secondary (in pulp) K04.3
  sensitive K03.89
Dentinogenesis imperfecta K00.5
Dentinoma — see Cyst, calcifying odontogenic
Dentition (syndrome) K00.7
  delayed K00.6
  difficult K00.7
  precocious K00.6
  premature K00.6
  retarded K00.6
Dependence (on) (syndrome) F19.20
  with remission F19.21
  alcohol (ethyl) (methyl) (without remission) F10.20
    with
      amnestic disorder, persisting F10.26
      anxiety disorder F10.280
      dementia, persisting F10.27
      intoxication F10.229
        with delirium F10.221
        uncomplicated F10.220
      mood disorder F10.24
      psychotic disorder F10.259
        with
          delusions F10.250
          hallucinations F10.251
      remission F10.21
      sexual dysfunction F10.281
      sleep disorder F10.282
      specified disorder NEC F10.288
      withdrawal F10.239
        with
          delirium F10.231
          perceptual disturbance F10.232
          uncomplicated F10.230
    counseling and surveillance Z71.41
    in remission F10.21
  amobarbital — see Dependence, drug, sedative
  amphetamine(s) (type) — see Dependence, drug, stimulant NEC
  amytal (sodium) — see Dependence, drug, sedative
  analgesic NEC F55.8
  anesthetic (agent) (gas) (general) (local) NEC — see Dependence, drug, psychoactive NEC
  anxiolytic NEC — see Dependence, drug, sedative
  barbital(s) — see Dependence, drug, sedative
  barbiturate(s) (compounds) (drugs classifiable to T42) — see Dependence, drug, sedative

Dependence — continued
  benzedrine — see Dependence, drug, stimulant NEC
  bhang — see Dependence, drug, cannabis
  bromide(s) NEC — see Dependence, drug, sedative
  caffeine — see Dependence, drug, stimulant NEC
  cannabis (sativa) (indica) (resin) (derivatives) (type) — see Dependence, drug, cannabis
  chloral (betaine) (hydrate) — see Dependence, drug, sedative
  chlordiazepoxide — see Dependence, drug, sedative
  coca (leaf) (derivatives) — see Dependence, drug, cocaine
  cocaine — see Dependence, drug, cocaine
  codeine — see Dependence, drug, opioid
  combinations of drugs F19.20
  D-lysergic acid diethylamide — see Dependence, drug, hallucinogen
  dagga — see Dependence, drug, cannabis
  demerol — see Dependence, drug, opioid
  dexamphetamine — see Dependence, drug, stimulant NEC
  dexedrine — see Dependence, drug, stimulant NEC
  dextro-nor-pseudo-ephedrine — see Dependence, drug, stimulant NEC
  dextromethorphan — see Dependence, drug, opioid
  dextromoramide — see Dependence, drug, opioid
  dextrorphan — see Dependence, drug, opioid
  diazepam — see Dependence, drug, sedative
  dilaudid — see Dependence, drug, opioid
  drug NEC F19.20
    with sleep disorder F19.282
    cannabis F12.20
      with
        anxiety disorder F12.280
        intoxication F12.229
          with
            delirium F12.221
            perceptual disturbance F12.222
          uncomplicated F12.220
        other specified disorder F12.288
        psychosis F12.259
          delusions F12.250
          hallucinations F12.251
        unspecified disorder F12.29
        withdrawal F12.23
      in remission F12.21
    cocaine F14.20
      with
        anxiety disorder F14.280
        intoxication F14.229
          with
            delirium F14.221
            perceptual disturbance F14.222
          uncomplicated F14.220
        mood disorder F14.24
        other specified disorder F14.288
        psychosis F14.259
          delusions F14.250
          hallucinations F14.251
        sexual dysfunction F14.281
        sleep disorder F14.282
        unspecified disorder F14.29
        withdrawal F14.23
      in remission F14.21
    withdrawal symptoms in newborn P96.1
  counseling and surveillance Z71.51
  hallucinogen F16.20
    with
      anxiety disorder F16.280
      flashbacks F16.283
      intoxication F16.229
        with delirium F16.221
        uncomplicated F16.220
      mood disorder F16.24
      other specified disorder F16.288
      perception disorder, persisting F16.283
      psychosis F16.259
        delusions F16.250
        hallucinations F16.251
      unspecified disorder F16.29
    in remission F16.21
  in remission F19.21
  inhalant F18.20
    with
      anxiety disorder F18.280
      dementia, persisting F18.27
      intoxication F18.229
        with delirium F18.221
        uncomplicated F18.220
      mood disorder F18.24

Dependence — *continued*
 drug — *continued*
  inhalant — *continued*
   with — *continued*
    other specified disorder F18.288
    psychosis F18.259
     delusions F18.250
     hallucinations F18.251
    unspecified disorder F18.29
   in remission F18.21
  nicotine F17.200
   with disorder F17.209
    in remission F17.201
    specified disorder NEC F17.208
    withdrawal F17.203
   chewing tobacco F17.220
    with disorder F17.229
     in remission F17.221
     specified disorder NEC F17.228
     withdrawal F17.223
   cigarettes F17.210
    with disorder F17.219
     in remission F17.211
     specified disorder NEC F17.218
     withdrawal F17.213
   specified product NEC F17.290
    with disorder F17.299
     remission F17.291
     specified disorder NEC F17.298
     withdrawal F17.293
  opioid F11.20
   with
    intoxication F11.229
     with
      delirium F11.221
      perceptual disturbance F11.222
     uncomplicated F11.220
    mood disorder F11.24
    opioid-associated amnestic syndrome F11.288
    other specified disorder F11.288
    psychosis F11.259
     delusions F11.250
     hallucinations F11.251
    sexual dysfunction F11.281
    sleep disorder F11.282
    unspecified disorder F11.29
    withdrawal F11.23
   in remission F11.21
  psychoactive NEC F19.20
   with
    amnestic disorder F19.26
    anxiety disorder F19.280
    dementia F19.27
    intoxication F19.229
     with
      delirium F19.221
      perceptual disturbance F19.222
     uncomplicated F19.220
    mood disorder F19.24
    other specified disorder F19.288
    psychosis F19.259
     delusions F19.250
     hallucinations F19.251
    sexual dysfunction F19.281
    sleep disorder F19.282
    unspecified disorder F19.29
    withdrawal F19.239
     with
      delirium F19.231
      perceptual disturbance F19.232
     uncomplicated F19.230
   in remission F19.21
  sedative, hypnotic or anxiolytic F13.20
   with
    amnestic disorder F13.26
    anxiety disorder F13.280
    dementia, persisting F13.27
    intoxication F13.229
     with delirium F13.221
     uncomplicated F13.220
    mood disorder F13.24
    other specified disorder F13.288
    psychosis F13.259
     delusions F13.250
     hallucinations F13.251
    sexual dysfunction F13.281
    sleep disorder F13.282
    unspecified disorder F13.29
    withdrawal F13.239

Dependence — *continued*
 drug — *continued*
  sedative, hypnotic or anxiolytic — *continued*
   with — *continued*
    withdrawal — *continued*
     with
      delirium F13.231
      perceptual disturbance F13.232
     uncomplicated F13.230
   in remission F13.21
  stimulant NEC F15.20
   with
    anxiety disorder F15.280
    intoxication F15.229
     with
      delirium F15.221
      perceptual disturbance F15.222
     uncomplicated F15.220
    mood disorder F15.24
    other specified disorder F15.288
    psychosis F15.259
     delusions F15.250
     hallucinations F15.251
    sexual dysfunction F15.281
    sleep disorder F15.282
    unspecified disorder F15.29
    withdrawal F15.23
   in remission F15.21
 ethyl
  alcohol (without remission) F10.20
   with remission F10.21
  bromide — *see* Dependence, drug, sedative
 carbamate F19.20
 chloride F19.20
  morphine — *see* Dependence, drug, opioid
 ganja — *see* Dependence, drug, cannabis
 glue (airplane) (sniffing) — *see* Dependence, drug, inhalant
 glutethimide — *see* Dependence, drug, sedative
 hallucinogenics — *see* Dependence, drug, hallucinogen
 hashish — *see* Dependence, drug, cannabis
 hemp — *see* Dependence, drug, cannabis
 heroin (salt) (any) — *see* Dependence, drug, opioid
 hypnotic NEC — *see* Dependence, drug, sedative
 Indian hemp — *see* Dependence, drug, cannabis
 inhalants — *see* Dependence, drug, inhalant
 khat — *see* Dependence, drug, stimulant NEC
 laudanum — *see* Dependence, drug, opioid
 LSD (-25) (derivatives) — *see* Dependence, drug, hallucinogen
 luminal — *see* Dependence, drug, sedative
 lysergic acid — *see* Dependence, drug, hallucinogen
 maconha — *see* Dependence, drug, cannabis
 marihuana — *see* Dependence, drug, cannabis
 meprobamate — *see* Dependence, drug, sedative
 mescaline — *see* Dependence, drug, hallucinogen
 methadone — *see* Dependence, drug, opioid
 methamphetamine(s) — *see* Dependence, drug, stimulant NEC
 methaqualone — *see* Dependence, drug, sedative
 methyl
  alcohol (without remission) F10.20
   with remission F10.21
  bromide — *see* Dependence, drug, sedative
  morphine — *see* Dependence, drug, opioid
  phenidate — *see* Dependence, drug, stimulant NEC
  sulfonal — *see* Dependence, drug, sedative
 morphine (sulfate) (sulfite) (type) — *see* Dependence, drug, opioid
 narcotic (drug) NEC — *see* Dependence, drug, opioid
 nembutal — *see* Dependence, drug, sedative
 neraval — *see* Dependence, drug, sedative
 neravan — *see* Dependence, drug, sedative
 neurobarb — *see* Dependence, drug, sedative
 nicotine — *see* Dependence, drug, nicotine
 nitrous oxide F19.20
 nonbarbiturate sedatives and tranquilizers with similar effect — *see* Dependence, drug, sedative
on
 artificial heart (fully implantable) (mechanical) Z95.812
 aspirator Z99.0
 care provider (because of) Z74.9
  impaired mobility Z74.09
  need for
   assistance with personal care Z74.1
   continuous supervision Z74.3
   no other household member able to render care Z74.2

Dependence — *continued*
on — *continued*
 care provider — *continued*
  specified reason NEC Z74.8
 machine Z99.89
  enabling NEC Z99.89
  specified type NEC Z99.89
 renal dialysis (hemodialysis) (peritoneal) Z99.2
 respirator Z99.11
 ventilator Z99.11
 wheelchair Z99.3
opiate — *see* Dependence, drug, opioid
opioids — *see* Dependence, drug, opioid
opium (alkaloids) (derivatives) (tincture) — *see* Dependence, drug, opioid
oxygen (long-term) (supplemental) Z99.81
paraldehyde — *see* Dependence, drug, sedative
paregoric — *see* Dependence, drug, opioid
PCP (phencyclidine) (or related substance) — *see* Dependence, drug, hallucinogen
pentobarbital — *see* Dependence, drug, sedative
pentobarbitone (sodium) — *see* Dependence, drug, sedative
pentothal — *see* Dependence, drug, sedative
peyote — *see* Dependence, drug, hallucinogen
phencyclidine (PCP) (or related substance) — *see* Dependence, drug, hallucinogen
phenmetrazine — *see* Dependence, drug, stimulant NEC
phenobarbital — *see* Dependence, drug, sedative
polysubstance F19.20
psilocibin, psilocin, psilocyn, psilocyline — *see* Dependence, drug, hallucinogen
psychostimulant NEC — *see* Dependence, drug, stimulant NEC
secobarbital — *see* Dependence, drug, sedative
seconal — *see* Dependence, drug, sedative
sedative NEC — *see* Dependence, drug, sedative
specified drug NEC — *see* Dependence, drug
stimulant NEC — *see* Dependence, drug, stimulant NEC
substance NEC — *see* Dependence, drug
supplemental oxygen Z99.81
tobacco — *see* Dependence, drug, nicotine
 counseling and surveillance Z71.6
tranquilizer NEC — *see* Dependence, drug, sedative
vitamin B6 E53.1
volatile solvents — *see* Dependence, drug, inhalant
Dependency
 care-provider Z74.9
 passive F60.7
 reactions (persistent) F60.7
Depersonalization (in neurotic state) (neurotic) (syndrome) F48.1
Depletion
 extracellular fluid E86.9
 plasma E86.1
 potassium E87.6
  nephropathy N25.89
 salt or sodium E87.1
  causing heat exhaustion or prostration T67.4- ☑
  nephropathy N28.9
 volume NOS E86.9
Deployment (current) (military) status Z56.82
 in theater or in support of military war, peacekeeping and humanitarian operations Z56.82
 personal history of Z91.82
  military war, peacekeeping and humanitarian deployment (current or past conflict) Z91.82
 returned from Z91.82
Depolarization, premature I49.40
 atrial I49.1
 junctional I49.2
 specified NEC I49.49
 ventricular I49.3
Deposit
 bone in Boeck's sarcoid D86.89
 calcareous, calcium — *see* Calcification
 cholesterol
  retina H35.89
  vitreous (body) (humor) — *see* Deposit, crystalline
 conjunctiva H11.11- ☑
 cornea H18.00- ☑
  argentous H18.02- ☑
  due to metabolic disorder H18.03- ☑
  Kayser-Fleischer ring H18.04- ☑
  pigmentation — *see* Pigmentation, cornea
 crystalline, vitreous (body) (humor) H43.2- ☑
 hemosiderin in old scars of cornea — *see* Pigmentation, cornea, stromal

Deposit — *continued*
- metallic in lens — *see* Cataract, specified NEC
- skin R23.8
- tooth, teeth (betel) (black) (green) (materia alba) (orange) (tobacco) K03.6
- urate, kidney — *see* Calculus, kidney

Depraved appetite — *see* Pica

Depressed
- HDL cholesterol E78.6

Depression (acute) (mental) F32.A
- agitated (single episode) F32.2
- anaclitic — *see* Disorder, adjustment
- anxiety F41.8
  - persistent F34.1
- arches — *see also* Deformity, limb, flat foot
- atypical (single episode) F32.89
  - recurrent episode F33.8
- basal metabolic rate R94.8
- bone marrow D75.89
- central nervous system G96.9
- cerebral R29.818
  - newborn P91.4
- cerebrovascular I67.9
- chest wall M95.4
- climacteric (single episode) F32.89
  - recurrent episode F33.8
- endogenous (without psychotic symptoms) F33.2
  - with psychotic symptoms F33.3
- functional activity R68.89
- hysterical F44.89
- involutional (single episode) F32.89
  - recurrent episode F33.8
- major F32.9
  - with psychotic symptoms F32.3
  - recurrent — *see* Disorder, depressive, recurrent
- manic-depressive — *see* Disorder, depressive, recurrent
- masked (single episode) F32.89
- medullary G93.89
- menopausal (single episode) F32.89
  - recurrent episode F33.8
- metatarsus — *see* Depression, arches
- monopolar F33.9
- nervous F34.1
- neurotic F34.1
- nose M95.0
- postnatal (NOS) F53.0
- postpartum (NOS) F53.0
- post-psychotic of schizophrenia F32.89
- post-schizophrenic F32.89
- psychogenic (reactive) (single episode) F32.9
- psychoneurotic F34.1
- psychotic (single episode) F32.3
  - recurrent F33.3
- reactive (psychogenic) (single episode) F32.9
  - psychotic (single episode) F32.3
- recurrent — *see* Disorder, depressive, recurrent
- respiratory center G93.89
- seasonal — *see* Disorder, depressive, recurrent
- senile F03.- ☑
- severe, single episode F32.2
- situational F43.21
- skull Q67.4
- specified NEC (single episode) F32.89
- sternum M95.4
- visual field — *see* Defect, visual field
- vital (recurrent) (without psychotic symptoms) F33.2
  - with psychotic symptoms F33.3
  - single episode F32.2

Deprivation
- cultural Z60.3
- effects NOS T73.9- ☑
  - specified NEC T73.8- ☑
- emotional NEC Z65.8
  - affecting infant or child — *see* Maltreatment, child, psychological
- food T73.0- ☑
- material due to limited financial resources, specified NEC Z59.87
- protein — *see* Malnutrition
- sleep Z72.820
- social Z60.4
  - affecting infant or child — *see* Maltreatment, child, psychological
- specified NEC T73.8- ☑
- vitamins — *see* Deficiency, vitamin
- water T73.1- ☑

Derangement
- ankle (internal) — *see* Derangement, joint, articular cartilage, ankle
- cartilage (articular) NEC — *see* Derangement, joint, articular cartilage, by site
  - recurrent — *see* Dislocation, recurrent
- cruciate ligament, anterior, current injury — *see* Sprain, knee, cruciate, anterior
- elbow (internal) — *see* Derangement, joint, articular cartilage, elbow
- hip (joint) (internal) (old) — *see* Derangement, joint, articular cartilage, hip
- joint (internal) M24.9
  - ankylosis — *see* Ankylosis
  - articular cartilage M24.10
    - ankle M24.17- ☑
    - elbow M24.12- ☑
    - foot M24.17- ☑
    - hand M24.14- ☑
    - hip M24.15- ☑
    - knee NEC M23.9- ☑
    - loose body — *see* Loose, body
    - shoulder M24.11- ☑
    - specified site NEC M24.19
    - wrist M24.13- ☑
  - contracture — *see* Contraction, joint
  - current injury — *see also* Dislocation
    - knee, meniscus or cartilage — *see* Tear, meniscus
  - dislocation
    - pathological — *see* Dislocation, pathological
    - recurrent — *see* Dislocation, recurrent
  - knee — *see* Derangement, knee
  - ligament — *see* Disorder, ligament
  - loose body — *see* Loose, body
  - recurrent — *see* Dislocation, recurrent
  - specified type NEC M24.80
    - ankle M24.87- ☑
    - elbow M24.82- ☑
    - foot joint M24.87- ☑
    - hand joint M24.84- ☑
    - hip M24.85- ☑
    - shoulder M24.81- ☑
    - specified site NEC M24.89
    - wrist M24.83- ☑
  - temporomandibular M26.69
- knee (recurrent) M23.9- ☑
  - ligament disruption, spontaneous M23.60- ☑
    - anterior cruciate M23.61- ☑
    - capsular M23.67- ☑
    - instability, chronic M23.5- ☑
    - lateral collateral M23.64- ☑
    - medial collateral M23.63- ☑
    - posterior cruciate M23.62- ☑
  - loose body M23.4- ☑
  - meniscus M23.30- ☑
    - cystic M23.0- ☑
      - lateral M23.002
        - anterior horn M23.04- ☑
        - posterior horn M23.05- ☑
        - specified NEC M23.06- ☑
      - medial M23.005
        - anterior horn M23.01- ☑
        - posterior horn M23.02- ☑
        - specified NEC M23.03- ☑
    - degenerate — *see* Derangement, knee, meniscus, specified NEC
    - detached — *see* Derangement, knee, meniscus, specified NEC
    - due to old tear or injury M23.20- ☑
      - lateral M23.20- ☑
        - anterior horn M23.24- ☑
        - posterior horn M23.25- ☑
        - specified NEC M23.26- ☑
      - medial M23.20- ☑
        - anterior horn M23.21- ☑
        - posterior horn M23.22- ☑
        - specified NEC M23.23- ☑
    - retained — *see* Derangement, knee, meniscus, specified NEC
    - specified NEC M23.30- ☑
      - lateral M23.30- ☑
        - anterior horn M23.34- ☑
        - posterior horn M23.35- ☑
        - specified NEC M23.36- ☑
      - medial M23.30- ☑
        - anterior horn M23.31- ☑

Derangement — *continued*
- knee — *continued*
  - meniscus — *continued*
    - specified — *continued*
      - medial — *continued*
        - posterior horn M23.32- ☑
        - specified NEC M23.33- ☑
    - old M23.8X- ☑
  - specified NEC — *see* subcategory M23.8- ☑
- low back NEC — *see* Dorsopathy, specified NEC
- meniscus — *see* Derangement, knee, meniscus
- mental — *see* Psychosis
- patella, specified NEC — *see* Disorder, patella, derangement NEC
- semilunar cartilage (knee) — *see* Derangement, knee, meniscus, specified NEC
- shoulder (internal) — *see* Derangement, joint, shoulder

Dercum's disease E88.2
Derealization (neurotic) F48.1
Dermal — *see* condition
Dermaphytid — *see* Dermatophytosis
Dermatitis (eczematous) L30.9
- ab igne L59.0
- acarine B88.09
- actinic (due to sun) L57.8
  - other than from sun L59.8
- allergic — *see* Dermatitis, contact, allergic
- ambustionis, due to burn or scald — *see* Burn
- amebic A06.7
- ammonia L22
- arsenical (ingested) L27.8
- artefacta L98.1
  - psychogenic F54
- atopic L20.9
  - psychogenic F54
  - specified NEC L20.89
- autoimmune progesterone L30.8
- berlock, berloque L56.2
- blastomycotic B40.3
- blister beetle L24.89
- bullous, bullosa L13.9
  - mucosynechial, atrophic L12.1
  - seasonal L30.8
  - specified NEC L13.8
- calorica L59.0
  - due to burn or scald — *see* Burn
- caterpillar L24.89
- cercarial B65.3
- combustionis L59.0
  - due to burn or scald — *see* Burn
- congelationis T69.1- ☑
- contact (occupational) L25.9
  - allergic L23.9
    - due to
      - adhesives L23.1
      - cement L23.5
      - chemical products NEC L23.5
      - chromium L23.0
      - cosmetics L23.2
      - dander (cat) (dog) L23.81
      - drugs in contact with skin L23.3
      - dyes L23.4
      - food in contact with skin L23.6
      - hair (cat) (dog) L23.81
      - insecticide L23.5
      - metals L23.0
      - nickel L23.0
      - plants, non-food L23.7
      - plastic L23.5
      - rubber L23.5
      - specified agent NEC L23.89
  - due to
    - cement L25.3
    - chemical products NEC L25.3
    - cosmetics L25.0
    - dander (cat) (dog) L23.81
    - drugs in contact with skin L25.1
    - dyes L25.2
    - food in contact with skin L25.4
    - hair (cat) (dog) L23.81
    - plants, non-food L25.5
    - specified agent NEC L25.8
  - irritant L24.9
    - due to
      - body fluids L24.A0
        - feces L24.A2
        - incontinence (dual) (fecal) (urinary) L24.A2
        - saliva L24.A1

Dermatitis — *continued*
  contact — *continued*
    irritant — *continued*
      due to — *continued*
        body fluids — *continued*
          specified NEC L24.A9
          urine L24.A2
          wound exudate L24.A9
        cement L24.5
        chemical products NEC L24.5
        cosmetics L24.3
        detergents L24.0
        drugs in contact with skin L24.4
        exudate L24.A9
        food in contact with skin L24.6
        friction L24.A0
        oils and greases L24.1
        plants, non-food L24.7
        solvents L24.2
        specified agent NEC L24.89
      related to
        colostomy L24.B3
        endotracheal tube L24.A9
        enterocutaneous fistula L24.B3
        gastrostomy L24.B1
        ileostomy L24.B3
        jejunostomy L24.B1
        saliva or spit fistula L24.B1
        stoma or fistula L24.B0
          digestive L24.B1
          fecal or urinary L24.B3
          respiratory L24.B2
        tracheostomy L24.B2
contusiformis L52
desquamative L30.8
diabetic — *see* E08-E13 with .620
diaper L22
diphtheritica A36.3
dry skin L85.3
due to
  acetone (contact) (irritant) L24.2
  acids (contact) (irritant) L24.5
  adhesive(s) (allergic) (contact) (plaster) L23.1
    irritant L24.5
  alcohol (irritant) (skin contact) (substances in category T51) L24.2
    taken internally L27.8
  alkalis (contact) (irritant) L24.5
  arsenic (ingested) L27.8
  carbon disulfide (contact) (irritant) L24.2
  caustics (contact) (irritant) L24.5
  cement (contact) L25.3
  cereal (ingested) L27.2
  chemical(s) NEC L25.3
    taken internally L27.8
  chlorocompounds L24.2
  chromium (contact) (irritant) L24.81
  coffee (ingested) L27.2
  cold weather L30.8
  cosmetics (contact) L25.0
    allergic L23.2
    irritant L24.3
  cyclohexanes L24.2
  dander (cat) (dog) L23.81
  Demodex species B88.01
  Dermanyssus gallinae B88.09
  detergents (contact) (irritant) L24.0
  dichromate L24.81
  drugs and medicaments (generalized) (internal use) L27.0
    external — *see* Dermatitis, due to, drugs, in contact with skin
    in contact with skin L25.1
      allergic L23.3
      irritant L24.4
    localized skin eruption L27.1
    specified substance — *see* Table of Drugs and Chemicals
  dyes (contact) L25.2
    allergic L23.4
    irritant L24.89
  epidermophytosis — *see* Dermatophytosis
  esters L24.2
  external irritant NEC L24.9
  exudate (wound fluids) L24.A9
  fish (ingested) L27.2
  flour (ingested) L27.2
  food (ingested) L27.2
    in contact with skin L25.4

Dermatitis — *continued*
  due to — *continued*
    fruit (ingested) L27.2
    furs (allergic) (contact) L23.81
    glues — *see* Dermatitis, due to, adhesives
    glycols L24.2
    greases NEC (contact) (irritant) L24.1
    hair (cat) (dog) L23.81
    hot
      objects and materials — *see* Burn
      weather or places L59.0
    hydrocarbons L24.2
    infrared rays L59.8
    ingestion, ingested substance L27.9
      chemical NEC L27.8
      drugs and medicaments — *see* Dermatitis, due to, drugs
      food L27.2
      specified NEC L27.8
    insecticide in contact with skin L24.5
    internal agent L27.9
      drugs and medicaments (generalized) — *see* Dermatitis, due to, drugs
      food L27.2
    irradiation — *see* Dermatitis, due to, radioactive substance
    ketones L24.2
    lacquer tree (allergic) (contact) L23.7
    light (sun) NEC L57.8
      acute L56.8
      other L59.8
    Liponyssoides sanguineus B88.09
    low temperature L30.8
    meat (ingested) L27.2
    metals, metal salts (contact) (irritant) L24.81
    milk (ingested) L27.2
    nickel (contact) (irritant) L24.81
    nylon (contact) (irritant) L24.5
    oils NEC (contact) (irritant) L24.1
    paint solvent (contact) (irritant) L24.2
    petroleum products (contact) (irritant) (substances in T52.0) L24.2
    plants NEC (contact) L25.5
      allergic L23.7
      irritant L24.7
    plasters (adhesive) (any) (allergic) (contact) L23.1
      irritant L24.5
    plastic (contact) L25.3
    preservatives (contact) — *see* Dermatitis, due to, chemical, in contact with skin
    primrose (allergic) (contact) L23.7
    primula (allergic) (contact) L23.7
    radiation L59.8
      nonionizing (chronic exposure) L57.8
      sun NEC L57.8
        acute L56.8
    radioactive substance L58.9
      acute L58.0
      chronic L58.1
    radium L58.9
      acute L58.0
      chronic L58.1
    ragweed (allergic) (contact) L23.7
    Rhus (allergic) (contact) (diversiloba) (radicans) (toxicodendron) (venenata) (verniciflua) L23.7
    rubber (contact) L24.5
    Senecio jacobaea (allergic) (contact) L23.7
    solvents (contact) (irritant) (substances in category T52) L24.2
    specified agent NEC (contact) L25.8
      allergic L23.89
      irritant L24.89
    sunshine NEC L57.8
      acute L56.8
    tetrachlorethylene (contact) (irritant) L24.2
    toluene (contact) (irritant) L24.2
    turpentine (contact) (irritant) L24.2
    ultraviolet rays (sun NEC) (chronic exposure) L57.8
      acute L56.8
    vaccine or vaccination L27.0
      specified substance — *see* Table of Drugs and Chemicals
    varicose veins — *see* Varix, leg, with, inflammation
    X-rays L58.9
      acute L58.0
      chronic L58.1
dyshydrotic L30.1
dysmenorrheica N94.6
escharotica — *see* Burn

Dermatitis — *continued*
exfoliative, exfoliativa (generalized) L26
  neonatorum L00
eyelid — *see also* Dermatosis, eyelid H01.9
  allergic H01.119
    left H01.116
      lower H01.115
      upper H01.114
    right H01.113
      lower H01.112
      upper H01.111
  contact — *see* Dermatitis, eyelid, allergic
  due to
    Demodex species B88.01
    herpes (zoster) B02.39
      simplex B00.59
  eczematous H01.139
    left H01.136
      lower H01.135
      upper H01.134
    right H01.133
      lower H01.132
      upper H01.131
  specified NEC H01.8- ☑
facta, factitia, factitial L98.1
  psychogenic F54
flexural NEC L20.82
friction L30.4
fungus B36.9
  specified type NEC B36.8
gangrenosa, gangrenous infantum L08.0
harvest mite B88.09
heat L59.0
herpesviral, vesicular (ear) (lip) B00.1
herpetiformis (bullous) (erythematous) (pustular) (vesicular) L13.0
  juvenile L12.2
  senile L12.0
hiemalis L30.8
hypostatic, hypostatica — *see* Varix, leg, with, inflammation
infectious eczematoid L30.3
infective L30.3
irritant — *see* Dermatitis, contact, irritant
Jacquet's (diaper dermatitis) L22
Leptus B88.09
lichenified NEC L28.0
medicamentosa (generalized) (internal use) — *see* Dermatitis, due to drugs
mite B88.09
multiformis L13.0
  juvenile L12.2
napkin L22
neurotica L13.0
nummular L30.0
papillaris capillitii L73.0
pellagrous E52
perioral L71.0
photocontact L56.2
polymorpha dolorosa L13.0
pruriginosa L13.0
pruritic NEC L30.8
psychogenic F54
purulent L08.0
pustular
  contagious B08.02
  subcorneal L13.1
pyococcal L08.0
pyogenica L08.0
repens L40.2
Ritter's (exfoliativa) L00
Schamberg's L81.7
schistosome B65.3
seasonal bullous L30.8
seborrheic L21.9
  infantile L21.1
  specified NEC L21.8
sensitization NOS L23.9
septic L08.0
solare L57.8
specified NEC L30.8
stasis I87.2
  with
    varicose ulcer — *see* Varix, leg, with ulcer, with inflammation
    varicose veins — *see* Varix, leg, with, inflammation
  due to postthrombotic syndrome — *see* Syndrome, postthrombotic
suppurative L08.0

Dermatitis — continued
    traumatic NEC L30.4
    trophoneurotica L13.0
    ultraviolet (sun) (chronic exposure) L57.8
        acute L56.8
    varicose — see Varix, leg, with, inflammation
    vegetans L10.1
    verrucosa B43.0
    vesicular, herpesviral B00.1
Dermatoarthritis, lipoid E78.81
Dermatochalasis, eyelid H02.839
    left H02.836
        lower H02.835
        upper H02.834
    right H02.833
        lower H02.832
        upper H02.831
Dermatofibroma (lenticulare) — see Neoplasm, skin, benign
    protuberans — see Neoplasm, skin, uncertain behavior
Dermatofibrosarcoma (pigmented) (protuberans) — see Neoplasm, skin, malignant
Dermatographia L50.3
Dermatolysis (exfoliativa) (congenital) Q82.8
    acquired L57.4
    eyelids — see Blepharochalasis
    palpebrarum — see Blepharochalasis
    senile L57.4
Dermatomegaly NEC Q82.8
Dermatomucosomyositis — see also Dermatomyositis M33.10
    with
        myopathy M33.12
        respiratory involvement M33.11
        specified organ involvement NEC M33.19
Dermatomycosis B36.9
    furfuracea B36.0
    specified type NEC B36.8
Dermatomyositis (acute) (chronic) — see also Dermatopolymyositis
    adult — see also Dermatomyositis, specified NEC M33.10
    in (due to) neoplastic disease — see also Neoplasm D49.9 [M36.0]
    juvenile M33.00
        with
            myopathy M33.02
            respiratory involvement M33.01
            specified organ involvement NEC M33.09
        amyopathic M33.03
        without myopathy M33.03
    specified NEC M33.10
        with
            myopathy M33.12
            respiratory involvement M33.11
            specified organ involvement NEC M33.19
        amyopathic M33.13
        without myopathy M33.13
Dermatoneuritis of children — see Poisoning, mercury
Dermatophilosis A48.8
Dermatophytid L30.2
Dermatophytide — see Dermatophytosis
Dermatophytosis (epidermophyton) (infection) (Microsporum) (tinea) (Trichophyton) B35.9
    beard B35.0
    body B35.4
    capitis B35.0
    corporis B35.4
    deep-seated B35.8
    disseminated B35.8
    foot B35.3
    granulomatous B35.8
    groin B35.6
    hand B35.2
    nail B35.1
    perianal (area) B35.6
    scalp B35.0
    specified NEC B35.8
Dermatopolymyositis M33.90
    with
        myopathy M33.92
        respiratory involvement M33.91
        specified organ involvement NEC M33.99
    amyopathic M33.93
    in neoplastic disease — see also Neoplasm D49.9 [M36.0]
    juvenile M33.00
        with
            myopathy M33.02
            respiratory involvement M33.01
            specified organ involvement NEC M33.09

Dermatopolymyositis — continued
    juvenile — continued
        amyopathic M33.03
        without myopathy M33.03
    specified NEC M33.10
        amyopathic M33.13
        myopathy M33.12
        respiratory involvement M33.11
        specified organ involvement NEC M33.19
        without myopathy M33.13
    without myopathy M33.93
Dermatopolyneuritis — see Poisoning, mercury
Dermatorrhexis — see also Syndrome, Ehlers-Danlos Q79.60
    acquired L57.4
Dermatosclerosis — see also Scleroderma
    localized L94.0
Dermatosis L98.9
    Andrews' L08.89
    Bowen's — see Neoplasm, skin, in situ
    bullous L13.9
        specified NEC L13.8
    exfoliativa L26
    eyelid (noninfectious) — see also Dermatitis, eyelid H01.9
        discoid lupus erythematosus — see Lupus, erythematosus, eyelid
        xeroderma — see Xeroderma, acquired, eyelid
    factitial L98.1
    febrile neutrophilic L98.2
    gonococcal A54.89
    herpetiformis L13.0
        juvenile L12.2
    linear IgA L13.8
    menstrual NEC L98.8
    neutrophilic, febrile L98.2
    occupational — see Dermatitis, contact
    papulosa nigra L82.1
    pigmentary L81.9
        progressive L81.7
        Schamberg's L81.7
    psychogenic F54
    purpuric, pigmented L81.7
    pustular, subcorneal L13.1
    transient acantholytic L11.1
Dermographia, dermographism L50.3
Dermoid (cyst) — see also Neoplasm, benign, by site
    with malignant transformation C56.- ☑
    due to radiation (nonionizing) L57.8
Dermopathy
    infiltrative with thyrotoxicosis — see Thyrotoxicosis
    nephrogenic fibrosing L90.8
Dermophytosis — see Dermatophytosis
DES
    child (daughter) (son) Z91.B
    grandchild (granddaughter) (grandson) Z84.A
    second generation Z91.B
    third generation Z84.A
Descemetocele H18.73- ☑
Descemet's membrane — see condition
Descending — see condition
Descensus uteri — see Prolapse, uterus
Desert
    rheumatism B38.0
    sore — see Ulcer, skin
Desertion (newborn) — see Maltreatment
Desmoid (extra-abdominal) (tumor)
    abdominal wall D48.113
    back D48.117
    buttock D48.116
    chest wall D48.111
    extremity
        lower D48.116
        upper D48.115
    head and neck D48.110
    intraabdominal D48.114
    intrathoracic D48.112
    pelvic cavity D48.114
    pelvic girdle D48.116
    peritoneal D48.114
    retroperitoneal D48.114
    shoulder girdle D48.115
    site unspecified D48.119
    specified site NEC D48.118
Despondency F32.A
Desquamation, skin R23.4
Destruction, destructive — see also Damage
    articular facet — see also Derangement, joint, specified type NEC
        knee M23.8X- ☑

Destruction, destructive — continued
    articular facet — see also Derangement, joint, specified type — continued
        vertebra — see Spondylosis
    bone — see also Disorder, bone, specified type NEC
        syphilitic A52.77
    joint — see also Derangement, joint, specified type NEC
        sacroiliac M53.3
    rectal sphincter K62.89
    septum (nasal) J34.89
    tuberculous NEC — see Tuberculosis
    tympanum, tympanic membrane (nontraumatic) — see Disorder, tympanic membrane, specified NEC
    vertebral disc — see Degeneration, intervertebral disc
Destructiveness — see also Disorder, conduct
    adjustment reaction — see Disorder, adjustment
Desultory labor O62.2
Detachment
    cartilage — see Sprain
    cervix, annular N88.8
        complicating delivery O71.3
    choroid (old) (postinfectional) (simple) (spontaneous) H31.40- ☑
        hemorrhagic H31.41- ☑
        serous H31.42- ☑
    ligament — see Sprain
    meniscus (knee) — see also Derangement, knee, meniscus, specified NEC
        current injury — see Tear, meniscus
        due to old tear or injury — see Derangement, knee, meniscus, due to old tear
    retina (without retinal break) (serous) H33.2- ☑
        with retinal:
            break H33.00- ☑
                giant H33.03- ☑
                multiple H33.02- ☑
                single H33.01- ☑
            dialysis H33.04- ☑
        pigment epithelium — see Degeneration, retina, separation of layers, pigment epithelium detachment
        rhegmatogenous — see Detachment, retina, with retinal, break
        specified NEC H33.8
        total H33.05- ☑
        traction H33.4- ☑
    vitreous (body) H43.81- ☑
Detergent asthma J69.8
Deterioration
    epileptic F06.8
    general physical R53.81
    heart, cardiac — see Degeneration, myocardial
    mental — see Psychosis
    myocardial, myocardium — see Degeneration, myocardial
    senile (simple) R54
Deuteranomaly (anomalous trichromat) H53.53
Deuteranopia (complete) (incomplete) H53.53
Development
    abnormal, bone Q79.9
    arrested R62.50
        bone — see Arrest, development or growth, bone
        child R62.50
        due to malnutrition E45
    defective, congenital — see also Anomaly, by site
        cauda equina Q06.3
        left ventricle Q24.8
            in hypoplastic left heart syndrome Q23.4
        valve Q24.8
            pulmonary Q22.3
    delayed — see also Delay, development R62.50
        arithmetical skills F81.2
        language (skills) (expressive) F80.1
        learning skill F81.9
        mixed skills F88
        motor coordination F82
        reading F81.0
        specified learning skill NEC F81.89
        speech F80.9
        spelling F81.81
        written expression F81.81
    imperfect, congenital — see also Anomaly, by site
        heart Q24.9
        lungs Q33.6
    incomplete
        bronchial tree Q32.4
        organ or site not listed — see Hypoplasia, by site
        respiratory system Q34.9

Development — *continued*
  sexual, precocious NEC E30.1
  tardy, mental — *see also* Disability, intellectual F79
Developmental — *see* condition
  testing, infant or child — *see* Examination, child
Devergie's disease (pityriasis rubra pilaris) L44.0
Deviation (in)
  conjugate palsy (eye) (spastic) H51.0
  esophagus (acquired) K22.89
  eye, skew H51.8
  midline (jaw) (teeth) (dental arch) M26.29
    specified site NEC — *see* Malposition
  nasal septum J34.2
    congenital Q67.4
  opening and closing of the mandible M26.53
  organ or site, congenital NEC — *see* Malposition, congenital
  septum (nasal) (acquired) J34.2
    congenital Q67.4
  sexual F65.9
    bestiality F65.89
    erotomania F52.8
    exhibitionism F65.2
    fetishism, fetishistic F65.0
      transvestism F65.1
    frotteurism F65.81
    masochism F65.51
    multiple F65.89
    necrophilia F65.89
    nymphomania F52.8
    pederosis F65.4
    pedophilia F65.4
    sadism, sadomasochism F65.52
    satyriasis F52.8
    specified type NEC F65.89
    transvestism F64.1
    voyeurism F65.3
  teeth, midline M26.29
  trachea J39.8
  ureter, congenital Q62.61
Device
  cerebral ventricle (communicating) in situ Z98.2
  contraceptive — *see* Contraceptive, device
  drainage, cerebrospinal fluid, in situ Z98.2
Devic's disease G36.0
Devil's
  grip B33.0
  pinches (purpura simplex) D69.2
Devitalized tooth K04.99
Devonshire colic — *see* Poisoning, lead
Dextraposition, aorta Q20.3
  in tetralogy of Fallot Q21.3
Dextrinosis, limit (debrancher enzyme deficiency) E74.03
Dextrocardia (true) Q24.0
  with
    complete transposition of viscera Q89.3
    situs inversus Q89.3
Dextrotransposition, aorta Q20.3
Dhat syndrome F48.8
Dhobi itch B35.6
Di George's syndrome D82.1
Di Guglielmo's disease C94.0- ☑
Diabetes, diabetic (mellitus) (sugar) E11.9
  with
    amyotrophy E11.44
    arthropathy NEC E11.618
    autonomic (poly)neuropathy E11.43
    cataract E11.36
    Charcot's joints E11.610
    chronic kidney disease E11.22
    circulatory complication NEC E11.59
    coma due to
      hyperosmolarity E11.01
      hypoglycemia E11.641
      ketoacidosis E11.11
    complication E11.8
      specified NEC E11.69
    dermatitis E11.620
    foot ulcer E11.621
    gangrene E11.52
    gastroparalysis E11.43
    gastroparesis E11.43
    glomerulonephrosis, intracapillary E11.21
    glomerulosclerosis, intercapillary E11.21
    hyperglycemia E11.65
    hyperosmolarity E11.00
      with coma E11.01
    hypoglycemia E11.649
      with coma E11.641

Diabetes, diabetic — *continued*
  with — *continued*
    ketoacidosis E11.10
      with coma E11.11
    kidney complications NEC E11.29
    Kimmelstiel-Wilson disease E11.21
    loss of protective sensation (LOPS) — *see* Diabetes, by type, with neuropathy
    mononeuropathy E11.41
    myasthenia E11.44
    necrobiosis lipoidica E11.620
    nephropathy E11.21
    neuralgia E11.42
    neurologic complication NEC E11.49
    neuropathic arthropathy E11.610
    neuropathy E11.40
    ophthalmic complication NEC E11.39
    oral complication NEC E11.638
    osteomyelitis E11.69
    periodontal disease E11.630
    peripheral angiopathy E11.51
      with gangrene E11.52
    polyneuropathy E11.42
    renal complication NEC E11.29
    renal tubular degeneration E11.29
    retinopathy E11.319
      with macular edema E11.311
        resolved following treatment E11.37- ☑
      nonproliferative E11.329- ☑
        with macular edema E11.321- ☑
        mild E11.329- ☑
          with macular edema E11.321- ☑
        moderate E11.339- ☑
          with macular edema E11.331- ☑
        severe E11.349- ☑
          with macular edema E11.341- ☑
      proliferative E11.359- ☑
        with
          combined traction retinal detachment and rhegmatogenous retinal detachment E11.354- ☑
          macular edema E11.351- ☑
          stable proliferative diabetic retinopathy E11.355- ☑
          traction retinal detachment involving the macula E11.352- ☑
          traction retinal detachment not involving the macula E11.353- ☑
    skin complication NEC E11.628
    skin ulcer NEC E11.622
  brittle — *see* Diabetes, type 1
  bronzed E83.110
  complicating pregnancy — *see* Pregnancy, complicated by, diabetes
  dietary counseling and surveillance Z71.3
  due to
    autoimmune process — *see* Diabetes, type 1
    immune mediated pancreatic islet beta-cell destruction — *see* Diabetes, type 1
    pancreatectomy — *see* Diabetes, specified type NEC
  due to drug or chemical E09.9
    with
      amyotrophy E09.44
      arthropathy NEC E09.618
      autonomic (poly)neuropathy E09.43
      cataract E09.36
      Charcot's joints E09.610
      chronic kidney disease E09.22
      circulatory complication NEC E09.59
      complication E09.8
        specified NEC E09.69
      dermatitis E09.620
      foot ulcer E09.621
      gangrene E09.52
      gastroparalysis E09.43
      gastroparesis E09.43
      glomerulonephrosis, intracapillary E09.21
      glomerulosclerosis, intercapillary E09.21
      hyperglycemia E09.65
      hyperosmolarity E09.00
        with coma E09.01
      hypoglycemia E09.649
        with coma E09.641
      ketoacidosis E09.10
        with coma E09.11
      kidney complications NEC E09.29
      Kimmelstiel-Wilson disease E09.21
      mononeuropathy E09.41

Diabetes, diabetic — *continued*
  due to drug or chemical — *continued*
    with — *continued*
      myasthenia E09.44
      necrobiosis lipoidica E09.620
      nephropathy E09.21
      neuralgia E09.42
      neurologic complication NEC E09.49
      neuropathic arthropathy E09.610
      neuropathy E09.40
      ophthalmic complication NEC E09.39
      oral complication NEC E09.638
      periodontal disease E09.630
      peripheral angiopathy E09.51
        with gangrene E09.52
      polyneuropathy E09.42
      renal complication NEC E09.29
      renal tubular degeneration E09.29
      retinal, hemorrhage E09.39
      retinopathy E09.319
        with macular edema E09.311
          resolved following treatment E09.37- ☑
        nonproliferative E09.329- ☑
          with macular edema E09.321- ☑
          mild E09.329- ☑
            with macular edema E09.321- ☑
          moderate E09.339- ☑
            with macular edema E09.331- ☑
          severe E09.349- ☑
            with macular edema E09.341- ☑
        proliferative E09.359- ☑
          with
            combined traction retinal detachment and rhegmatogenous retinal detachment E09.354- ☑
            macular edema E09.351- ☑
            stable proliferative diabetic retinopathy E09.355- ☑
            traction retinal detachment involving the macula E09.352- ☑
            traction retinal detachment not involving the macula E09.353- ☑
      skin complication NEC E09.628
      skin ulcer NEC E09.622
  due to underlying condition E08.9
    with
      amyotrophy E08.44
      arthropathy NEC E08.618
      autonomic (poly)neuropathy E08.43
      cataract E08.36
      Charcot's joints E08.610
      chronic kidney disease E08.22
      circulatory complication NEC E08.59
      complication E08.8
        specified NEC E08.69
      dermatitis E08.620
      foot ulcer E08.621
      gangrene E08.52
      gastroparalysis E08.43
      gastroparesis E08.43
      glomerulonephrosis, intracapillary E08.21
      glomerulosclerosis, intercapillary E08.21
      hyperglycemia E08.65
      hyperosmolarity E08.00
        with coma E08.01
      hypoglycemia E08.649
        with coma E08.641
      ketoacidosis E08.10
        with coma E08.11
      kidney complications NEC E08.29
      Kimmelstiel-Wilson disease E08.21
      mononeuropathy E08.41
      myasthenia E08.44
      necrobiosis lipoidica E08.620
      nephropathy E08.21
      neuralgia E08.42
      neurologic complication NEC E08.49
      neuropathic arthropathy E08.610
      neuropathy E08.40
      ophthalmic complication NEC E08.39
      oral complication NEC E08.638
      periodontal disease E08.630
      peripheral angiopathy E08.51
        with gangrene E08.52
      polyneuropathy E08.42
      renal complication NEC E08.29
      renal tubular degeneration E08.29
      retinal, hemorrhage E08.39

Diabetes, diabetic — *continued*
　due to underlying condition — *continued*
　　with — *continued*
　　　retinopathy E08.319
　　　　with macular edema E08.311
　　　　resolved following treatment E08.37- ☑
　　　　nonproliferative E08.329- ☑
　　　　　with macular edema E08.321- ☑
　　　　　mild E08.329- ☑
　　　　　　with macular edema E08.321- ☑
　　　　　moderate E08.339- ☑
　　　　　　with macular edema E08.331- ☑
　　　　　severe E08.349- ☑
　　　　　　with macular edema E08.341- ☑
　　　　proliferative E08.359- ☑
　　　　　with
　　　　　　combined traction retinal detachment and rhegmatogenous retinal detachment E08.354- ☑
　　　　　　macular edema E08.351- ☑
　　　　　　stable proliferative diabetic retinopathy E08.355- ☑
　　　　　　traction retinal detachment involving the macula E08.352- ☑
　　　　　　traction retinal detachment not involving the macula E08.353- ☑
　　　skin complication NEC E08.628
　　　skin ulcer NEC E08.622
　gestational (in pregnancy) O24.419
　　affecting newborn P70.0
　　diet controlled O24.410
　　in childbirth O24.429
　　　diet controlled O24.420
　　　insulin (and diet) controlled O24.424
　　　oral drug controlled (antidiabetic) (hypoglycemic) O24.425
　　insulin (and diet) controlled O24.414
　　oral drug controlled (antidiabetic) (hypoglycemic) O24.415
　　puerperal O24.439
　　　diet controlled O24.430
　　　insulin (and diet) controlled O24.434
　　　oral drug controlled (antidiabetic) (hypoglycemic) O24.435
　hepatogenous E13.9
　idiopathic — *see* Diabetes, type 1
　inadequately controlled — *see* Diabetes, by type, with hyperglycemia
　insipidus E23.2
　　nephrogenic N25.1
　　pituitary E23.2
　　vasopressin resistant N25.1
　insulin dependent — *code to* type of diabetes
　juvenile-onset — *see* Diabetes, type 1
　ketosis-prone — *see* Diabetes, type 1
　latent R73.03
　neonatal (transient) P70.2
　non-insulin dependent — *code to* type of diabetes
　out of control — *see* Diabetes, by type, with hyperglycemia
　phosphate E83.39
　poorly controlled — *see* Diabetes, by type, with hyperglycemia
　postpancreatectomy — *see* Diabetes, specified type NEC
　postprocedural — *see* Diabetes, specified type NEC
　retina, hemorrhage E13.39
　secondary diabetes mellitus NEC — *see* Diabetes, specified type NEC
　specified type NEC E13.9
　　with
　　　amyotrophy E13.44
　　　arthropathy NEC E13.618
　　　autonomic (poly)neuropathy E13.43
　　　cataract E13.36
　　　Charcot's joints E13.610
　　　chronic kidney disease E13.22
　　　circulatory complication NEC E13.59
　　　complication E13.8
　　　　specified NEC E13.69
　　　dermatitis E13.620
　　　foot ulcer E13.621
　　　gangrene E13.52
　　　gastroparalysis E13.43
　　　gastroparesis E13.43
　　　glomerulonephrosis, intracapillary E13.21
　　　glomerulosclerosis, intercapillary E13.21
　　　hyperglycemia E13.65
　　　hyperosmolarity E13.00

Diabetes, diabetic — *continued*
　specified type — *continued*
　　with — *continued*
　　　hyperosmolarity — *continued*
　　　　with coma E13.01
　　　hypoglycemia E13.649
　　　　with coma E13.641
　　　ketoacidosis E13.10
　　　　with coma E13.11
　　　kidney complications NEC E13.29
　　　Kimmelstiel-Wilson disease E13.21
　　　mononeuropathy E13.41
　　　myasthenia E13.44
　　　necrobiosis lipoidica E13.620
　　　nephropathy E13.21
　　　neuralgia E13.42
　　　neurologic complication NEC E13.49
　　　neuropathic arthropathy E13.610
　　　neuropathy E13.40
　　　ophthalmic complication NEC E13.39
　　　oral complication NEC E13.638
　　　periodontal disease E13.630
　　　peripheral angiopathy E13.51
　　　　with gangrene E13.52
　　　polyneuropathy E13.42
　　　renal complication NEC E13.29
　　　renal tubular degeneration E13.29
　　　retinal, hemorrhage E13.39
　　　retinopathy E13.319
　　　　with macular edema E13.311
　　　　resolved following treatment E13.37- ☑
　　　　nonproliferative E13.329- ☑
　　　　　with macular edema E13.321- ☑
　　　　　mild E13.329- ☑
　　　　　　with macular edema E13.321- ☑
　　　　　moderate E13.339- ☑
　　　　　　with macular edema E13.331- ☑
　　　　　severe E13.349- ☑
　　　　　　with macular edema E13.341- ☑
　　　　proliferative E13.359- ☑
　　　　　with
　　　　　　combined traction retinal detachment and rhegmatogenous retinal detachment E13.354- ☑
　　　　　　macular edema E13.351- ☑
　　　　　　stable proliferative diabetic retinopathy E13.355- ☑
　　　　　　traction retinal detachment involving the macula E13.352- ☑
　　　　　　traction retinal detachment not involving the macula E13.353- ☑
　　　skin complication NEC E13.628
　　　skin ulcer NEC E13.622
　steroid-induced — *see* Diabetes, due to, drug or chemical
　type 1 E10.9
　　with
　　　amyotrophy E10.44
　　　arthropathy NEC E10.618
　　　autonomic (poly)neuropathy E10.43
　　　cataract E10.36
　　　Charcot's joints E10.610
　　　chronic kidney disease E10.22
　　　circulatory complication NEC E10.59
　　　coma due to
　　　　hypoglycemia E10.641
　　　　ketoacidosis E10.11
　　　complication E10.8
　　　　specified NEC E10.69
　　　dermatitis E10.620
　　　foot ulcer E10.621
　　　gangrene E10.52
　　　gastroparalysis E10.43
　　　gastroparesis E10.43
　　　glomerulonephrosis, intracapillary E10.21
　　　glomerulosclerosis, intercapillary E10.21
　　　hyperglycemia E10.65
　　　hypoglycemia E10.649
　　　　with coma E10.641
　　　ketoacidosis E10.10
　　　　with coma E10.11
　　　kidney complications NEC E10.29
　　　Kimmelstiel-Wilson disease E10.21
　　　mononeuropathy E10.41
　　　myasthenia E10.44
　　　necrobiosis lipoidica E10.620
　　　nephropathy E10.21
　　　neuralgia E10.42
　　　neurologic complication NEC E10.49

Diabetes, diabetic — *continued*
　type 1 — *continued*
　　with — *continued*
　　　neuropathic arthropathy E10.610
　　　neuropathy E10.40
　　　ophthalmic complication NEC E10.39
　　　oral complication NEC E10.638
　　　osteomyelitis E10.69
　　　periodontal disease E10.630
　　　peripheral angiopathy E10.51
　　　　with gangrene E10.52
　　　polyneuropathy E10.42
　　　renal complication NEC E10.29
　　　renal tubular degeneration E10.29
　　　retinal, hemorrhage E10.39
　　　retinopathy E10.319
　　　　with macular edema E10.311
　　　　resolved following treatment E10.37- ☑
　　　　nonproliferative E10.329- ☑
　　　　　with macular edema E10.321- ☑
　　　　　mild E10.329- ☑
　　　　　　with macular edema E10.321- ☑
　　　　　moderate E10.339- ☑
　　　　　　with macular edema E10.331- ☑
　　　　　severe E10.349- ☑
　　　　　　with macular edema E10.341- ☑
　　　　proliferative E10.359- ☑
　　　　　with
　　　　　　combined traction retinal detachment and rhegmatogenous retinal detachment E10.354- ☑
　　　　　　macular edema E10.351- ☑
　　　　　　stable proliferative diabetic retinopathy E10.355- ☑
　　　　　　traction retinal detachment involving the macula E10.352- ☑
　　　　　　traction retinal detachment not involving the macula E10.353- ☑
　　　skin complication NEC E10.628
　　　skin ulcer NEC E10.622
　　early-stage E10.A- ☑
　　presymptomatic E10.A0
　　　Stage 1 E10.A1
　　　Stage 2 E10.A2
　type 2 E11.9
　　with
　　　amyotrophy E11.44
　　　arthropathy NEC E11.618
　　　autonomic (poly)neuropathy E11.43
　　　cataract E11.36
　　　Charcot's joints E11.610
　　　chronic kidney disease E11.22
　　　circulatory complication NEC E11.59
　　　coma due to
　　　　hyperosmolarity E11.01
　　　　hypoglycemia E11.641
　　　　ketoacidosis E11.1- ☑
　　　complication E11.8
　　　　specified NEC E11.69
　　　dermatitis E11.620
　　　foot ulcer E11.621
　　　gangrene E11.52
　　　gastroparalysis E11.43
　　　gastroparesis E11.43
　　　glomerulonephrosis, intracapillary E11.21
　　　glomerulosclerosis, intercapillary E11.21
　　　hyperglycemia E11.65
　　　hyperosmolarity E11.00
　　　　with coma E11.01
　　　hypoglycemia E11.649
　　　　with coma E11.641
　　　ketoacidosis E11.10
　　　　with coma E11.11
　　　kidney complications NEC E11.29
　　　Kimmelstiel-Wilson disease E11.21
　　　mononeuropathy E11.41
　　　myasthenia E11.44
　　　necrobiosis lipoidica E11.620
　　　nephropathy E11.21
　　　neuralgia E11.42
　　　neurologic complication NEC E11.49
　　　neuropathic arthropathy E11.610
　　　neuropathy E11.40
　　　ophthalmic complication NEC E11.39
　　　oral complication NEC E11.638
　　　osteomyelitis E11.69
　　　periodontal disease E11.630
　　　peripheral angiopathy E11.51

Diabetes, diabetic — *continued*
  type 2 — *continued*
    with — *continued*
      peripheral angiopathy — *continued*
        with gangrene E11.52
      polyneuropathy E11.42
      renal complication NEC E11.29
      renal tubular degeneration E11.29
      retinal, hemorrhage E11.39
      retinopathy E11.319
        with macular edema E11.311
        resolved following treatment E11.37- ☑
        nonproliferative E11.329- ☑
          with macular edema E11.321- ☑
          mild E11.329- ☑
            with macular edema E11.321- ☑
          moderate E11.339- ☑
            with macular edema E11.331- ☑
          severe E11.349- ☑
            with macular edema E11.341- ☑
        proliferative E11.359- ☑
          with
            combined traction retinal detachment and rhegmatogenous retinal detachment E11.354- ☑
            macular edema E11.351- ☑
            stable proliferative diabetic retinopathy E11.355- ☑
            traction retinal detachment involving the macula E11.352- ☑
            traction retinal detachment not involving the macula E11.353- ☑
      skin complication NEC E11.628
      skin ulcer NEC E11.622
    without complications in remission E11.A
    uncontrolled
      meaning
        hyperglycemia — *see* Diabetes, by type, with, hyperglycemia
        hypoglycemia — *see* Diabetes, by type, with, hypoglycemia
    without complications in remission E11.A
Diacyclothrombopathia D69.1
Diagnosis deferred R69
Dialysis (intermittent) (treatment)
  noncompliance (with) Z91.158
    due to financial hardship Z91.151
  renal (hemodialysis) (peritoneal), status Z99.2
  retina, retinal — *see* Detachment, retina, with retinal, dialysis
Diamond-Blackfan anemia (congenital hypoplastic) D61.01
Diamond-Gardener syndrome (autoerythrocyte sensitization) D69.2
Diaper rash L22
Diaphoresis (excessive) R61
Diaphragm — *see* condition
Diaphragmalgia R07.1
Diaphragmatitis, diaphragmitis J98.6
Diaphysial aclasis Q78.6
Diaphysitis — *see* Osteomyelitis, specified type NEC
Diarrhea, diarrheal (disease) (infantile) (inflammatory) R19.7
  achlorhydric K31.83
  allergic K52.29
    due to
      colitis — *see* Colitis, allergic
      enteritis — *see* Enteritis, allergic
  amebic — *see also* Amebiasis A06.0
    with abscess — *see* Abscess, amebic
    acute A06.0
    chronic A06.1
    nondysenteric A06.2
  bacillary — *see* Dysentery, bacillary
  balantidial A07.0
  cachectic NEC K52.89
  Chilomastix A07.8
  choleriformis A00.1
  chronic (noninfectious) K52.9
  coccidial A07.3
  Cochin-China K90.1
    strongyloidiasis B78.0
  Dientamoeba A07.8
  dietetic — *see also* Diarrhea, allergic K52.29
  drug-induced K52.1
  due to
    bacteria A04.9
      specified NEC A04.8
    Campylobacter A04.5

Diarrhea, diarrheal — *continued*
  due to — *continued*
    Capillaria philippinensis B81.1
    Clostridium difficile
      not specified as recurrent A04.72
      recurrent A04.71
    Clostridium perfringens (C) (F) A04.8
    Cryptosporidium A07.2
    drugs K52.1
    Escherichia coli A04.4
      enteroaggregative A04.4
      enterohemorrhagic A04.3
      enteroinvasive A04.2
      enteropathogenic A04.0
      enterotoxigenic A04.1
      specified NEC A04.4
    food hypersensitivity — *see also* Diarrhea, allergic K52.29
    Necator americanus B76.1
    S. japonicum B65.2
    specified organism NEC A08.8
      bacterial A04.8
      viral A08.39
    Staphylococcus A04.8
    Trichuris trichiuria B79
    virus — *see* Enteritis, viral
    Yersinia enterocolitica A04.6
  dysenteric A09
  endemic A09
  epidemic A09
  flagellate A07.9
  Flexner's (ulcerative) A03.1
  functional K59.1
    following gastrointestinal surgery K91.89
    psychogenic F45.8
  Giardia lamblia A07.1
  giardial A07.1
  hill K90.1
  infectious A09
  malarial — *see* Malaria
  mite B88.09
  mycotic NEC B49
  neonatal (noninfectious) P78.3
  nervous F45.8
  neurogenic K59.1
  noninfectious K52.9
  postgastrectomy K91.1
  postvagotomy K91.1
  protozoal A07.9
    specified NEC A07.8
  psychogenic F45.8
  specified
    bacterium NEC A04.8
    virus NEC A08.39
  strongyloidiasis B78.0
  toxic K52.1
  trichomonal A07.8
  tropical K90.1
  tuberculous A18.32
  viral — *see* Enteritis, viral
Diastasis
  cranial bones M84.88
    congenital NEC Q75.8
  joint (traumatic) — *see* Dislocation
  muscle M62.00
    ankle M62.07- ☑
    congenital Q79.8
    foot M62.07- ☑
    forearm M62.03- ☑
    hand M62.04- ☑
    lower leg M62.06- ☑
    pelvic region M62.05- ☑
    shoulder region M62.01- ☑
    specified site NEC M62.08
    thigh M62.05- ☑
    upper arm M62.02- ☑
  recti (abdomen)
    complicating delivery O71.89
    congenital Q79.59
Diastema, tooth, teeth, fully erupted M26.32
Diastematomyelia Q06.2
Diataxia, cerebral G80.4
Diathesis
  allergic — *see* History, allergy
  bleeding (familial) D69.9
  cystine (familial) E72.00
  gouty — *see* Gout
  hemorrhagic (familial) D69.9

Diathesis — *continued*
  hemorrhagic — *continued*
    newborn NEC P53
  spasmophilic R29.0
Diaz's disease or osteochondrosis (juvenile) (talus) — *see* Osteochondrosis, juvenile, tarsus
Dibothriocephalus, dibothriocephaliasis (latus) (infection) (infestation) B70.0
  larval B70.1
Dicephalus, dicephaly Q89.4
Dichotomy, teeth K00.2
Dichromat, dichromatopsia (congenital) — *see* Deficiency, color vision
Dichuchwa A65
Dicroceliasis B66.2
Didelphia, didelphys — *see* Double uterus
Didymytis N45.1
  with orchitis N45.3
Dietary
  inadequacy or deficiency E63.9
  surveillance and counseling Z71.3
Dietl's crisis N13.8
Dieulafoy lesion (hemorrhagic)
  duodenum K31.82
  esophagus K22.89
  intestine (colon) K63.81
  stomach K31.82
Difficult, difficulty (in)
  acculturation Z60.3
  feeding R63.30
    elderly R63.39
    infant NOS R63.39
    newborn P92.9
      breast P92.5
      specified NEC P92.8
    nonorganic (infant or child) F98.29
    specified NEC R63.39
  intubation, in anesthesia T88.4- ☑
  mechanical, gastroduodenal stoma K91.89
    causing obstruction — *see also* Obstruction, intestine, postoperative K91.30
  micturition
    need to immediately re-void R39.191
    position dependent R39.192
    specified NEC R39.198
  reading (developmental) F81.0
    secondary to emotional disorders F93.9
  spelling (specific) F81.81
    with reading disorder F81.89
    due to inadequate teaching Z55.8
  swallowing — *see* Dysphagia
  understanding
    health related information Z55.6
    medication instructions Z55.6
  walking R26.2
  work
    conditions NEC Z56.5
    schedule Z56.3
Diffuse — *see* condition
Digestive — *see* condition
Dihydropyrimidine dehydrogenase disease (DPD) E88.89
Diktyoma — *see* Neoplasm, malignant, by site
Dilaceration, tooth K00.4
Dilatation
  anus K59.89
  venule — *see* Hemorrhoids
  aorta (focal) (general) — *see* Ectasia, aorta
    with aneuysm — *see* Aneurysm, aorta
    congenital Q25.44
  artery — *see* Aneurysm
  bladder (sphincter) N32.89
    congenital Q64.79
  blood vessel I99.8
  bronchial J47.9
    with
      exacerbation (acute) J47.1
      lower respiratory infection J47.0
  calyx N28.89
    due to obstruction — *see* Hydronephrosis
  capillaries I78.8
  cardiac (acute) (chronic) — *see also* Hypertrophy, cardiac
    congenital Q24.8
      valve NEC Q24.8
        pulmonary Q22.3
    valve — *see* Endocarditis
  cavum septi pellucidi Q06.8
  cervix (uteri) — *see also* Incompetency, cervix
    incomplete, poor, slow complicating delivery O62.0
  colon K59.39

Dilatation — continued
 colon — continued
  congenital Q43.1
  psychogenic F45.8
  toxic K59.31
 common duct (acquired) K83.8
  congenital Q44.5
 cystic duct (acquired) K82.8
  congenital Q44.5
 duct, mammary — see Ectasia, mammary duct
 duodenum K59.89
 esophagus K22.89
  congenital Q39.5
  due to achalasia K22.0
 eustachian tube, congenital Q17.8
 gallbladder K82.8
 gastric — see Dilatation, stomach
 heart (acute) (chronic) — see also Hypertrophy, cardiac
  congenital Q24.8
  valve — see Endocarditis
 ileum K59.89
  psychogenic F45.8
 jejunum K59.89
  psychogenic F45.8
 kidney (calyx) (collecting structures) (cystic) (parenchyma) (pelvis) (idiopathic) N28.89
  due to obstruction — see Hydronephrosis
 lacrimal passages or duct — see Disorder, lacrimal system, changes
 lymphatic vessel I89.0
 mammary duct — see Ectasia, mammary duct
 Meckel's diverticulum (congenital) Q43.0
  malignant — see Table of Neoplasms, small intestine, malignant
 myocardium (acute) (chronic) — see Hypertrophy, cardiac
 organ or site, congenital NEC — see Distortion
 pancreatic duct K86.89
 pericardium — see Pericarditis
 pharynx J39.2
 prostate N42.89
 pulmonary
  artery (idiopathic) I28.8
  valve, congenital Q22.3
 pupil H57.04
 rectum K59.39
 saccule, congenital Q16.5
 salivary gland (duct) K11.8
 sphincter ani K62.89
 stomach K31.89
  acute K31.0
  psychogenic F45.8
 submaxillary duct K11.8
 trachea, congenital Q32.1
 ureter (idiopathic) N28.82
  congenital Q62.2
  due to obstruction N13.4
 urethra (acquired) N36.8
 vasomotor I73.9
 vein I86.8
 ventricular, ventricle (acute) (chronic) — see also Hypertrophy, cardiac
  cerebral, congenital Q04.8
 venule NEC I86.8
 vesical orifice N32.89
Dilated, dilation — see Dilatation
Diminished, diminution
 hearing (acuity) — see Deafness
 sense or sensation (cold) (heat) (tactile) (vibratory) R20.8
 vision NEC H54.7
 vital capacity R94.2
Diminuta taenia B71.0
Dimitri-Sturge-Weber disease Q85.89
Dimple
 congenital sacral Q82.6
 parasacral Q82.6
 pilonidal or postanal — see Cyst, pilonidal
Dioctophyme renalis (infection) (infestation) B83.8
Dipetalonemiasis B74.4
Diphallus Q55.69
Diphtheria, diphtheritic (gangrenous) (hemorrhagic) A36.9
 carrier (suspected) Z22.2
 cutaneous A36.3
 faucial A36.0
 infection of wound A36.3
 laryngeal A36.2
 myocarditis A36.81
 nasal, anterior A36.89
 nasopharyngeal A36.1
 neurological complication A36.89

Diphtheria, diphtheritic — continued
 pharyngeal A36.0
 specified site NEC A36.89
 tonsillar A36.0
Diphyllobothriasis (intestine) B70.0
 larval B70.1
Diplacusis H93.22- ☑
Diplegia (upper limbs) G83.0
 congenital (cerebral) G80.8
 facial G51.0
 lower limbs G82.20
 spastic G80.1
Diplococcus, diplococcal — see condition
Diplopia H53.2
Dipsomania F10.20
 with
  psychosis — see Psychosis, alcoholic
  remission F10.21
Dipylidiasis B71.1
DIRA (deficiency of interleukin 1 receptor antagonist) M04.8
Direction, teeth, abnormal, fully erupted M26.30
Dirofilariasis B74.8
Dirt-eating child F98.3
Disability, disabilities
 heart — see Disease, heart
 intellectual F79
  with
   autistic features F84.9
   pathogenic CHAMP1 (genetic) (variant) F78.A9
   pathogenic HNRNPH2 (genetic) (variant) F78.A9
   pathogenic SATB2 (genetic) (variant) F78.A9
   pathogenic SETBP1 (genetic) (variant) F78.A9
   pathogenic STXBP1 (genetic) (variant) F78.A9
   pathogenic SYNGAP1 (genetic) (variant) F78.A1
  autosomal dominant F78.A9
  autosomal recessive F78.A9
  genetic related F78.A9
   with
    pathogenic CHAMP1 (variant) F78.A9
    pathogenic HNRNPH2 (variant) F78.A9
    pathogenic SATB2 (variant) F78.A9
    pathogenic SETBP1 (variant) F78.A9
    pathogenic STXBP1 (variant) F78.A9
    pathogenic SYNGAP1 (variant) F78.A1
   specified NEC F78.A9
   SYNGAP1-related F78.A1
  in
   autosomal dominant mental retardation F78.A9
   autosomal recessive mental retardation F78.A9
   SATB2-associated syndrome F78.A9
   SETBP1 disorder F78.A9
   STXBP1 encephalopathy with epilepsy — see also Encephalopathy; and — see also Epilepsy
   X-linked mental retardation (syndromic) (Bain type) F78.A9
  mild (I.Q. 50-69) F70
  moderate (I.Q. 35-49) F71
  profound (I.Q. under 20) F73
  severe (I.Q. 20-34) F72
  specified level NEC F78.A9
  SYNGAP1-related F78.A1
  X-linked (syndromic) (Bain type) F78.A9
 knowledge acquisition F81.9
 learning F81.9
 limiting activities Z73.6
 spelling, specific F81.81
Disappearance of family member Z63.4
Disarticulation — see Amputation
 meaning traumatic amputation — see Amputation, traumatic
Discharge (from)
 abnormal finding in — see Abnormal, specimen
 breast (female) (male) N64.52
 diencephalic autonomic idiopathic — see Epilepsy, specified NEC
 ear — see also Otorrhea
  blood — see Otorrhagia
 excessive urine R35.89
 nipple N64.52
 penile R36.9
 postnasal R09.82
 prison, anxiety concerning Z65.2
 urethral R36.9
  without blood R36.0
  hematospermia R36.1
 vaginal N89.8
Discitis, diskitis M46.40
 cervical region M46.42
 cervicothoracic region M46.43

Discitis, diskitis — continued
 lumbar region M46.46
 lumbosacral region M46.47
 multiple sites M46.49
 occipito-atlanto-axial region M46.41
 pyogenic — see Infection, intervertebral disc, pyogenic
 sacrococcygeal region M46.48
 thoracic region M46.44
 thoracolumbar region M46.45
Discoid
 meniscus (congenital) Q68.6
 semilunar cartilage (congenital) — see Derangement, knee, meniscus, specified NEC
Discoloration
 nails L60.8
 teeth (posteruptive) K03.7
  during formation K00.8
Discomfort
 chest R07.89
 visual H53.14- ☑
Discontinuity, ossicles, ear H74.2- ☑
Discord (with)
 boss Z56.4
 classmates Z55.4
 counselor Z64.4
 employer Z56.4
 family Z63.8
 fellow employees Z56.4
 in-laws Z63.1
 landlord Z59.2
 lodgers Z59.2
 neighbors Z59.2
 probation officer Z64.4
 social worker Z64.4
 teachers Z55.4
 workmates Z56.4
Discordant connection
 atrioventricular (congenital) Q20.5
 ventriculoarterial Q20.3
Discrepancy
 centric occlusion maximum intercuspation M26.55
 leg length (acquired) — see Deformity, limb, unequal length
  congenital — see Defect, reduction, lower limb
 uterine size date O26.84- ☑
Discrimination
 ethnic Z60.5
 political Z60.5
 racial Z60.5
 religious Z60.5
 sex Z60.5
Disease, diseased — see also Syndrome
 absorbent system I87.8
 acid-peptic K30
 Acosta's T70.29- ☑
 Adams-Stokes (-Morgagni) (syncope with heart block) I45.9
 Addison's anemia (pernicious) D51.0
 adenoids (and tonsils) J35.9
 adrenal (capsule) (cortex) (gland) (medullary) E27.9
  hyperfunction E27.0
  specified NEC E27.8
 ainhum L94.6
 airway
  obstructive, chronic J44.9
   due to
    cotton dust J66.0
    specific organic dusts NEC J66.8
   reactive — see Asthma
 akamushi (scrub typhus) A75.3
 Albers-Schonberg (marble bones) Q78.2
 Albert's — see Tendinitis, Achilles
 Alexander G31.86
 alimentary canal K63.9
 alligator-skin Q80.9
  acquired L85.0
 alpha heavy chain C88.3- ☑
 alpine T70.29- ☑
 altitude T70.20- ☑
 alveolar ridge
  edentulous K06.9
   specified NEC K06.8
 alveoli, teeth K08.9
 Alzheimer's — see also Dementia, in, diseases specified elsewhere G30.9 [F02.80]
  with behavioral disturbance — see also Dementia, in, diseases specified elsewhere G30.9 [F02.81-]

☑ Additional Character Required — Refer to the Tabular List for Character Selection

Disease, diseased — continued
  Alzheimer's — see also Dementia, in, diseases specified elsewhere — continued
    early onset — see also Dementia, in, diseases specified elsewhere G30.0 [F02.80]
      with behavioral disturbance — see also Dementia, in, diseases specified elsewhere G30.0 [F02.81-] ☑
    late onset — see also Dementia, in, diseases specified elsewhere G30.1 [F02.80]
      with behavioral disturbance — see also Dementia, in, diseases specified elsewhere G30.1 [F02.81-] ☑
    specified NEC — see also Dementia, in, diseases specified elsewhere G30.8 [F02.80]
      with behavioral disturbance — see also Dementia, in, diseases specified elsewhere G30.8 [F02.81-] ☑
  amyloid — see Amyloidosis
  Andersen's (glycogenosis IV) E74.09
  Andes T70.29- ☑
  Andrews' (bacterid) L08.89
  angiospastic I73.9
    cerebral G45.9
    vein I87.8
  anterior
    chamber H21.9
    horn cell G12.29
  antiglomerular basement membrane (anti- GBM) antibody M31.0
    tubulo-interstitial nephritis N12
  Antopol E74.05
  antral — see Sinusitis, maxillary
  anus K62.9
    specified NEC K62.89
  aorta (nonsyphilitic) I77.9
    syphilitic NEC A52.02
  aortic (heart) (valve) I35.9
    rheumatic I06.9
  Apollo B30.3
  aponeuroses — see Enthesopathy
  appendix K38.9
    specified NEC K38.8
  aqueous (chamber) H21.9
  Arnold-Chiari — see Arnold-Chiari disease
  arterial — see also Disease, artery I77.9
    occlusive — see also Occlusion, by site
      due to stricture or stenosis I77.1
    peripheral I73.9
  arteriocardiorenal — see Hypertension, cardiorenal
  arteriolar (generalized) (obliterative) I77.9
  arteriorenal — see Hypertension, kidney
  arteriosclerotic — see also Arteriosclerosis
    cardiovascular — see Disease, heart, ischemic, atherosclerotic
    coronary (artery) — see Disease, heart, ischemic, atherosclerotic
    heart — see Disease, heart, ischemic, atherosclerotic
  artery — see also Disease, arterial I77.9
    cerebral I67.9
    coronary I25.10
      with angina pectoris — see Arteriosclerosis, coronary (artery)
    peripheral I73.9
  arthropod-borne NOS (viral) A94
    specified type NEC A93.8
  atticoantral, chronic H66.20
    left H66.22
      with right H66.23
    right H66.21
      with left H66.23
  auditory canal — see Disorder, ear, external
  auricle, ear NEC — see Disorder, pinna
  Australian X A83.4
  autoimmune (systemic) NOS M35.9
    hemolytic D59.10
      cold type (primary) (secondary) (symptomatic) D59.12
      drug-induced D59.0
      mixed type (primary) (secondary) (symptomatic) D59.13
      warm type (primary) (secondary) (symptomatic) D59.11
    thyroid E06.3
  autoinflammatory M04.9
    NOD2-associated M04.8
    specified type NEC M04.8
  aviator's — see Effect, adverse, high altitude

Disease, diseased — continued
  Ayerza's (pulmonary artery sclerosis with pulmonary hypertension) I27.0
  Babington's (familial hemorrhagic telangiectasia) I78.0
  bacterial A49.9
    specified NEC A48.8
    zoonotic A28.9
      specified type NEC A28.8
  Baelz's (cheilitis glandularis apostematosa) K13.0
  bagasse J67.1
  balloon — see Effect, adverse, high altitude
  Bang's (brucella abortus) A23.1
  Bannister's T78.3- ☑
  barometer makers' — see Poisoning, mercury
  Barraquer (-Simons') (progressive lipodystrophy) E88.11
  Barrett's — see Barrett's, esophagus
  Bartholin's gland N75.9
  basal ganglia G25.9
    degenerative G23.9
      specified NEC G23.8
    specified NEC G25.89
  Basedow's (exophthalmic goiter) — see Hyperthyroidism, with, goiter (diffuse)
  Bateman's B08.1
  Batten-Steinert G71.11
  Battey A31.0
  Beard's (neurasthenia) F48.8
  Becker
    idiopathic mural endomyocardial I42.3
    myotonia congenita G71.12
  Begbie's (exophthalmic goiter) — see Hyperthyroidism, with, goiter (diffuse)
  behavioral, organic F07.9
  Beigel's (white piedra) B36.2
  Benson's — see Deposit, crystalline
  Bernard-Soulier (thrombopathy) D69.1
  Bernhardt (-Roth) — see Mononeuropathy, lower limb, meralgia paresthetica
  Biermer's (pernicious anemia) D51.0
  bile duct (common) (hepatic) K83.9
    with calculus, stones — see Calculus, bile duct
    specified NEC K83.8
  biliary (tract) K83.9
    specified NEC K83.8
  Billroth's — see Spina bifida
  bird fancier's J67.2
  black lung J60
  bladder N32.9
    in (due to)
      schistosomiasis (bilharziasis) B65.0 [N33]
    specified NEC N32.89
  bleeder's D66
  blood D75.9
    forming organs D75.9
    vessel I99.9
  Bloodgood's — see Mastopathy, cystic
  Blount M92.51- ☑
  Bodechtel-Guttmann (subacute sclerosing panencephalitis) A81.1
  bone — see also Disorder, bone
    aluminum M83.4
    fibrocystic NEC
      jaw M27.49
  bone-marrow D75.9
  Borna A83.9
  Bornholm (epidemic pleurodynia) B33.0
  Bouchard's (myopathic dilatation of the stomach) K31.8
  Bouillaud's (rheumatic heart disease) I01.9
  Bourneville (-Brissaud) (tuberous sclerosis) Q85.1
  Bouveret (-Hoffmann) (paroxysmal tachycardia) I47.9
  bowel K63.9
    functional K59.9
      psychogenic F45.8
  brain — see also Dementia, in, diseases specified elsewhere G93.9
    arterial, artery I67.9
    arteriosclerotic I67.2
    congenital Q04.9
    degenerative — see Degeneration, brain
    inflammatory — see Encephalitis
    organic G93.9
      arteriosclerotic I67.2
    parasitic NEC B71.9 [G94]
    senile NEC G31.1
    specified NEC G93.89
  breast — see also Disorder, breast N64.9
    cystic (chronic) — see Mastopathy, cystic
    fibrocystic — see Mastopathy, cystic

Disease, diseased — continued
  breast — see also Disorder, breast — continued
    Paget's
      female, unspecified side C50.91- ☑
      male, unspecified side C50.92- ☑
    specified NEC N64.89
  Breda's — see Yaws
  Bretonneau's (diphtheritic malignant angina) A36.0
  Bright's — see Nephritis
    arteriosclerotic — see Hypertension, kidney
  Brill-Zinsser (recrudescent typhus) A75.1
  Brill's (recrudescent typhus) A75.1
  Brion-Kayser — see Fever, paratyphoid
  broad
    beta E78.2
    ligament (noninflammatory) N83.9
      inflammatory — see Disease, pelvis, inflammatory
      specified NEC N83.8
  Brocq-Duhring (dermatitis herpetiformis) L13.0
  Brocq's
    meaning
      dermatitis herpetiformis L13.0
      prurigo L28.2
  bronchopulmonary J98.4
  bronchus NEC J98.09
  bronze Addison's E27.1
    tuberculous A18.7
  budgerigar fancier's J67.2
  Buerger's (thromboangiitis obliterans) I73.1
  bullous L13.9
    chronic of childhood L12.2
    specified NEC L13.8
  Burger-Grutz (essential familial hyperlipemia) E78.3
  bursa — see Bursopathy
  caisson T70.3- ☑
  California — see Coccidioidomycosis
  Canavan E75.28
  capillaries I78.9
    specified NEC I78.8
  Carapata A68.0
  carcinoid E34.00
    heart E34.01
    specified NEC E34.09
  cardiac — see Disease, heart
  cardiopulmonary, chronic I27.9
  cardiorenal (hepatic) (hypertensive) (vascular) — see Hypertension, cardiorenal
  cardiovascular (atherosclerotic) I25.10
    with angina pectoris — see Arteriosclerosis, coronary (artery)
    congenital Q28.9
    hypertensive — see Hypertension, heart
    newborn P29.9
      specified NEC P29.89
    renal (hypertensive) — see Hypertension, cardiorenal
    syphilitic (asymptomatic) A52.00
  cartilage — see Disorder, cartilage
  Castellani's A69.8
  Castleman (unicentric) (multicentric) D47.Z2
    HHV-8-associated — see also Herpesvirus, human, 8 D47.Z2
  cat-scratch A28.1
  Cavare's (familial periodic paralysis) G72.3
  cecum K63.9
  celiac (adult) (infantile) (with steatorrhea) K90.0
  cellular tissue L98.9
  central core G71.29
  cerebellar, cerebellum — see Disease, brain
  cerebral — see also Disease, brain
    degenerative — see Degeneration, brain
  cerebrospinal G96.9
  cerebrovascular I67.9
    acute I67.89
      embolic I63.4- ☑
      thrombotic I63.3- ☑
    arteriosclerotic I67.2
    hereditary NEC I67.858
    specified NEC I67.89
  cervix (uteri) (noninflammatory) N88.9
    inflammatory — see Cervicitis
    specified NEC N88.8
  Chabert's A22.9
  Chandler's (osteochondritis dissecans, hip) — see Osteochondritis, dissecans, hip
  Charlouis — see Yaws
  Chediak-Steinbrinck (-Higashi) (congenital gigantism of peroxidase granules) E70.330
  chest J98.9

Disease, diseased — continued
 Chiari's (hepatic vein thrombosis) I82.0
 Chicago B40.9
 Chignon B36.8
 chigo, chigoe B88.1
 childhood granulomatous D71.8
 Chinese liver fluke B66.1
 chlamydial A74.9
  specified NEC A74.89
 cholecystic K82.9
 choroid H31.9
  specified NEC H31.8
 Christmas D67
 chronic bullous of childhood L12.2
 chylomicron retention E78.3
 ciliary body H21.9
  specified NEC H21.89
 circulatory (system) NEC I99.8
  newborn P29.9
  syphilitic A52.00
   congenital A50.54
 coagulation factor deficiency (congenital) — see Defect, coagulation
 coccidioidal — see Coccidioidomycosis
 cold
  agglutinin or hemoglobinuria D59.12
   paroxysmal D59.6
  hemagglutinin (chronic) D59.12
 collagen NOS (nonvascular) (vascular) M35.9
  specified NEC M35.89
 colon K63.9
  functional K59.9
   congenital Q43.2
  ischemic — see also Ischemia, intestine, acute K55.039
 colonic inflammatory bowel, unclassified (IBDU) K52.3
 combined system — see Degeneration, combined
 compressed air T70.3- ☑
 Concato's (pericardial polyserositis) A19.9
  nontubercular I31.1
  pleural — see Pleurisy, with effusion
 conjunctiva H11.9
  chlamydial A74.0
  specified NEC H11.89
  viral B30.9
   specified NEC B30.8
 connective tissue, systemic (diffuse) M35.9
  in (due to)
   hypogammaglobulinemia D80.1 [M36.8]
   ochronosis E70.29 [M36.8]
  specified NEC M35.89
 Conor and Bruch's (boutonneuse fever) A77.1
 Cooper's — see Mastopathy, cystic
 Cori's (glycogenosis III) E74.03
 corkhandler's or corkworker's J67.3
 cornea H18.9
  specified NEC H18.89- ☑
 coronary (artery) — see Disease, heart, ischemic, atherosclerotic
  congenital Q24.5
  microvascular
   with
    angina pectoris I20.81
    myocardial infarction I21.B
     acute I24.81
     chronic I25.85
  ostial, syphilitic (aortic) (mitral) (pulmonary) A52.03
 corpus cavernosum N48.9
  specified NEC N48.89
 Cotugno — see Sciatica
 COVID-19 U07.1
 coxsackie (virus) NEC B34.1
 cranial nerve NOS G52.9
 Creutzfeldt-Jakob — see Creutzfeldt-Jakob disease or syndrome
 Crocq's (acrocyanosis) I73.89
 Crohn's — see Enteritis, regional
 Curschmann G71.11
 cystic
  breast (chronic) — see Mastopathy, cystic
  kidney, congenital Q61.9
  liver, congenital Q44.6
  lung J98.4
   congenital Q33.0
 cytomegalic inclusion (generalized) B25.9
  with pneumonia B25.0
  congenital P35.1
 cytomegaloviral B25.9
  specified NEC B25.8

Disease, diseased — continued
 Czerny's (periodic hydrarthrosis of the knee) — see Effusion, joint, knee
 Daae (-Finsen) (epidemic pleurodynia) B33.0
 Danon E74.05
 Darling's — see Histoplasmosis capsulati
 de Quervain's (tendon sheath) M65.4
  thyroid (subacute granulomatous thyroiditis) E06.1
 Debove's (splenomegaly) R16.1
 deer fly — see Tularemia
 Degos' I77.89
 demyelinating, demyelinizing (nervous system) G37.9
  multiple sclerosis G35.D
  specified NEC G37.89
 dense deposit — see also N00-N07 with fourth character .6 N05.6
 deposition, hydroxyapatite — see Disease, hydroxyapatite deposition
 Devergie's (pityriasis rubra pilaris) L44.0
 Devic's G36.0
 diaphorase deficiency D74.0
 diaphragm J98.6
 diarrheal, infectious NEC A09
 digestive system K92.9
  specified NEC K92.89
 disc, degenerative — see Degeneration, intervertebral disc
 discogenic — see also Displacement, intervertebral disc NEC
  with myelopathy — see Disorder, disc, with, myelopathy
 diverticular — see Diverticula
 Dubois (thymus) A50.59 [E35]
 Duchenne-Griesinger G71.01
 Duchenne's
  muscular dystrophy G71.01
  pseudohypertrophy, muscles G71.01
 ductless glands E34.9
 duodenum K31.9
  specified NEC K31.89
 Dupre's (meningism) R29.1
 Dupuytren's (muscle contracture) M72.0
 Durand-Nicholas-Favre (climatic bubo) A55
 Duroziez's (congenital mitral stenosis) Q23.2
 ear — see Disorder, ear
 Eberth's — see Fever, typhoid
 Ebola (virus) A98.4
 Ebstein's heart Q22.5
 Echinococcus — see Echinococcus
 echovirus NEC B34.1
 Eddowes' (brittle bones and blue sclera) Q78.0
 edentulous (alveolar) ridge K06.9
  specified NEC K06.8
 Edsall's T67.2- ☑
 Eichstedt's (pityriasis versicolor) B36.0
 Eisenmenger's (irreversible) I27.83
 Ellis-van Creveld (chondroectodermal dysplasia) Q77.6
 end stage renal (ESRD) N18.6
  due to hypertension I12.0
 endocrine glands or system NEC E34.9
 endomyocardial (eosinophilic) I42.3
 English (rickets) E55.0
 enteroviral, enterovirus NEC B34.1
  central nervous system NEC A88.8
 epidemic B99.9
  specified NEC B99.8
 epididymis N50.9
 Erb (-Landouzy) G71.02
 Erdheim-Chester (ECD) E88.89
 esophagus K22.9
  functional K22.4
  psychogenic F45.8
  specified NEC K22.89
 Eulenburg's (congenital paramyotonia) G71.19
 eustachian tube — see Disorder, eustachian tube
 external
  auditory canal — see Disorder, ear, external
  ear — see Disorder, ear, external
 extrapyramidal G25.9
  specified NEC G25.89
 eye H57.9
  anterior chamber H21.9
  inflammatory NEC H57.89
  muscle (external) — see Strabismus
  specified NEC H57.89
  syphilitic — see Oculopathy, syphilitic
  thyroid H05.83- ☑
 eyeball H44.9

Disease, diseased — continued
 eyeball — continued
  specified NEC H44.89
 eyelid — see Disorder, eyelid
  specified NEC — see Disorder, eyelid, specified type NEC
 eyeworm of Africa B74.3
 facial nerve (seventh) G51.9
  newborn (birth injury) P11.3
 Fahr (of brain) G23.8
 Fahr Volhard (of kidney) I12.- ☑
 fallopian tube (noninflammatory) N83.9
  inflammatory — see Salpingo-oophoritis
  specified NEC N83.8
 familial periodic paralysis G72.3
 Fanconi ('s) D61.03
 fascia NEC — see also Disorder, muscle
  inflammatory — see Myositis
  specified NEC M62.89
 Fauchard's (periodontitis) — see Periodontitis
 Favre-Durand-Nicolas (climatic bubo) A55
 Fede's K14.0
 Feer's — see Poisoning, mercury
 female pelvic inflammatory — see also Disease, pelvis, inflammatory N73.9
  syphilitic (secondary) A51.42
  tuberculous A18.17
 Fernels' (aortic aneurysm) I71.9
 fibrocaseous of lung — see Tuberculosis, pulmonary
 fibrocystic — see Fibrocystic disease
 Fiedler's (leptospiral jaundice) A27.0
 fifth B08.3
 file-cutter's — see Poisoning, lead
 fish-skin Q80.9
  acquired L85.0
 Flajani (-Basedow) (exophthalmic goiter) — see Hyperthyroidism, with, goiter (diffuse)
 flax-dresser's J66.1
 fluke — see Infestation, fluke
 foot and mouth B08.8
 foot process N04.9
 Forbes' (glycogenosis III) E74.03
 Fordyce-Fox (apocrine miliaria) L75.2
 Fordyce's (ectopic sebaceous glands) (mouth) Q38.6
 Forestier's (rhizomelic pseudopolyarthritis) M35.3
  meaning ankylosing hyperostosis — see Hyperostosis, ankylosing
 Fothergill's
  neuralgia — see Neuralgia, trigeminal
  scarlatina anginosa A38.9
 Fournier (gangrene) N49.3
  female N76.82
  vagina and vulva N76.82
 fourth B08.8
 Fox (-Fordyce) (apocrine miliaria) L75.2
 Francis' — see Tularemia
 Franklin C88.2- ☑
 Frei's (climatic bubo) A55
 Friedreich's
  combined systemic or ataxia G11.11
  myoclonia G25.3
 frontal sinus — see Sinusitis, frontal
 fungus NEC B49
 Gaisbock's (polycythemia hypertonica) D75.1
 gallbladder K82.9
  calculus — see Calculus, gallbladder
  cholecystitis — see Cholecystitis
  cholesterolosis K82.4
  fistula — see Fistula, gallbladder
  hydrops K82.1
  obstruction — see Obstruction, gallbladder
  perforation K82.2
  specified NEC K82.89
 gamma heavy chain C88.2- ☑
 Gamna's (siderotic splenomegaly) D73.2
 Gamstorp's (adynamia episodica hereditaria) G72.3
 Gandy-Nanta (siderotic splenomegaly) D73.2
 ganister J62.8
 gastric — see Disease, stomach
 gastroesophageal reflux (GERD) K21.9
  with esophagitis (without bleeding) K21.00
   with bleeding K21.01
 gastrointestinal (tract) K92.9
  amyloid E85.4
  functional K59.9
   psychogenic F45.8
  specified NEC K92.89
 Gee (-Herter) (-Heubner) (-Thaysen) (nontropical sprue) K90.0

☑ Additional Character Required — Refer to the Tabular List for Character Selection

Disease, diseased — continued
  genital organs
    female N94.9
    male N50.9
  Gerhardt's (erythromelalgia) I73.81
  Gibert's (pityriasis rosea) L42
  Gierke's (glycogenosis I) E74.01
  Gilles de la Tourette's (motor-verbal tic) F95.2
  gingiva K06.9
    plaque induced K05.00
    specified NEC K06.8
  gland (lymph) I89.9
  Glanzmann's (hereditary hemorrhagic thrombasthenia) D69.1
  glass-blower's (cataract) — see Cataract, specified NEC
    salivary gland hypertrophy K11.1
  Glisson's — see Rickets
  globe H44.9
    specified NEC H44.89
  glomerular — see also Glomerulonephritis
    with edema — see Nephrosis
    acute — see Nephritis, acute
    chronic — see Nephritis, chronic
    minimal change N05.0
    rapidly progressive N01.9
  glycogen storage E74.00
    Andersen's E74.09
    Cori's E74.03
    Forbes' E74.03
    generalized E74.00
    glucose-6-phosphatase deficiency E74.01
    heart E74.02 [I43]
    hepatorenal E74.09
    Hers' E74.09
    liver and kidney E74.09
    lysosomal E74.02
      with acid maltase deficiency E74.02
      without acid maltase deficiency E74.05
    McArdle's E74.04
    muscle phosphofructokinase E74.09
    myocardium E74.02 [I43]
    Pompe's E74.02
    Tauri's E74.09
    type 0 E74.09
    type I E74.01
    type II E74.02
    type IIB E74.05
    type III E74.03
    type IV E74.09
    type V E74.04
    type VI-XI E74.09
    Von Gierke's E74.01
  Goldstein's (familial hemorrhagic telangiectasia) I78.0
  gonococcal NOS A54.9
  graft-versus-host (GVH) D89.813
    acute D89.810
    acute on chronic D89.812
    chronic D89.811
  grainhandler's J67.8
  granulomatous (childhood) (chronic) D71.8
  Graves' (exophthalmic goiter) — see Hyperthyroidism, with, goiter (diffuse)
  Griesinger's — see Ancylostomiasis
  Grisel's M43.6
  Gruby's (tinea tonsurans) B35.0
  Guillain-Barre G61.0
  Guinon's (motor-verbal tic) F95.2
  gum K06.9
  gynecological N94.9
  H (Hartnup's) E72.02
  Haff — see Poisoning, mercury
  Hageman (congenital factor XII deficiency) D68.2
  hair (color) (shaft) L67.9
    follicles L73.9
      specified NEC L73.8
  Hamman's (spontaneous mediastinal emphysema) J98.2
  hand, foot and mouth B08.4
  Hansen's — see Leprosy
  Hantavirus, with pulmonary manifestations B33.4
    with renal manifestations A98.5
  Harada's H30.81-
  Hartnup (pellagra-cerebellar ataxia-renal aminoaciduria) E72.02
  Hart's (pellagra-cerebellar ataxia-renal aminoaciduria) E72.02
  Hashimoto's (struma lymphomatosa) E06.3
  Hb — see Disease, hemoglobin
  heart (organic) I51.9

Disease, diseased — continued
  heart — continued
    with
      pulmonary edema (acute) — see also Failure, ventricular, left I50.1
      rheumatic fever (conditions in I00)
        active I01.9
          with chorea I02.0
          specified NEC I01.8
        inactive or quiescent (with chorea) I09.9
          specified NEC I09.89
    amyloid E85.4 [I43]
    aortic (valve) I35.9
    arteriosclerotic or sclerotic (senile) — see Disease, heart, ischemic, atherosclerotic
    artery, arterial — see Disease, heart, ischemic, atherosclerotic
    beer drinkers' I42.6
    beriberi (wet) E51.12
    black I27.0
    congenital Q24.9
      cyanotic Q24.9
      specified NEC Q24.8
    coronary — see Disease, heart, ischemic
    cryptogenic I51.9
    fibroid — see Myocarditis
    functional I51.89
      psychogenic F45.8
    glycogen storage E74.02 [I43]
    gonococcal A54.83
    hypertensive — see Hypertension, heart
    hyperthyroid — see also Hyperthyroidism E05.90 [I43]
      with thyroid storm E05.91 [I43]
    ischemic (chronic or with a stated duration of over 4 weeks) I25.9
      atherosclerotic (of) I25.10
        with angina pectoris — see Arteriosclerosis, coronary (artery)
        coronary artery bypass graft — see Arteriosclerosis, coronary (artery),
      cardiomyopathy I25.5
      diagnosed on ECG or other special investigation, but currently presenting no symptoms I25.6
      silent I25.6
      specified form NEC
        acute I24.89
        chronic I25.89
    kyphoscoliotic I27.1
    meningococcal A39.50
      endocarditis A39.51
      myocarditis A39.52
      pericarditis A39.53
    mitral I05.9
      specified NEC I05.8
    muscular — see Degeneration, myocardial
    psychogenic (functional) F45.8
    pulmonary (chronic) I27.9
      in schistosomiasis B65.9 [I52]
      specified NEC I27.89
    rheumatic (chronic) (inactive) (old) (quiescent) (with chorea) I09.9
      active or acute I01.9
        with chorea (acute) (rheumatic) (Sydenham's) I02.0
      specified NEC I09.89
    senile — see Myocarditis
    syphilitic A52.06
      aortic A52.03
        aneurysm A52.01
      congenital A50.54 [I52]
    thyrotoxic — see also Thyrotoxicosis E05.90 [I43]
      with thyroid storm E05.91 [I43]
    valve, valvular (obstructive) (regurgitant) — see also Endocarditis
      congenital NEC Q24.8
      pulmonary Q22.3
    vascular — see Disease, cardiovascular
  Heartland A93.8
  heavy chain NEC C88.2-
    alpha C88.3-
    gamma C88.2-
    mu C88.2-
  Hebra's
    pityriasis
      maculata et circinata L42
      rubra pilaris L44.0
    prurigo L28.2
  hematopoietic organs D75.9

Disease, diseased — continued
  hemoglobin or Hb
    abnormal (mixed) NEC D58.2
      with thalassemia D56.9
    AS genotype D57.3
    Bart's D56.0
    C (Hb-C) D58.2
      with other abnormal hemoglobin NEC D58.2
      elliptocytosis D58.1
      Hb-S D57.2-
      sickle-cell D57.2-
      thalassemia D56.8
    Constant Spring D58.2
    D (Hb-D) D58.2
    E (Hb-E) D58.2
    E-beta thalassemia D56.5
    elliptocytosis D58.1
    H (Hb-H) (thalassemia) D56.0
      with other abnormal hemoglobin NEC D56.9
      Constant Spring D56.0
    I thalassemia D56.9
    M D74.0
    S or SS D57.1
      with
        acute chest syndrome D57.01
        cerebral vascular involvement D57.03
        crisis (painful) D57.00
          with
            dactylitis D57.04
            specified complication D57.09
        pain (vaso-occlusive) D57.00
        splenic sequestration D57.02
    beta plus D57.44
      with
        acute chest syndrome D57.451
        cerebral vascular involvement D57.453
        crisis D57.459
          with
            dactylitis D57.454
            specified complication D57.458
        pain (vaso-occlusive) D57.459
        splenic sequestration D57.452
      without crisis D57.44
    beta zero D57.42
      with
        acute chest syndrome D57.431
        cerebral vascular involvement D57.433
        crisis D57.439
          with
            dactylitis D57.434
            specified complication D57.438
        pain (vaso-occlusive) D57.439
        splenic sequestration D57.432
      without crisis D57.42
    SC D57.2-
    SD D57.8-
    SE D57.8-
    spherocytosis D58.0
    unstable, hemolytic D58.2
  hemolytic (newborn) P55.9
    autoimmune D59.10
      cold type (primary) (secondary) (symptomatic) D59.12
      mixed type (primary) (secondary) (symptomatic) D59.13
      warm type (primary) (secondary) (symptomatic) D59.11
    drug-induced D59.0
    due to or with
      incompatibility
        ABO (blood group) P55.1
        blood (group) (Duffy) (K) (Kell) (Kidd) (Lewis) (M) (S) NEC P55.8
        Rh (blood group) (factor) P55.0
      Rh negative mother P55.0
    specified type NEC P55.8
    unstable hemoglobin D58.2
  hemorrhagic D69.9
    newborn P53
  Henoch (-Schonlein) (purpura nervosa) D69.0
  hepatic — see Disease, liver
  hepatolenticular E83.01
  heredodegenerative NEC
    spinal cord G95.89
  herpesviral, disseminated B00.7
  Hers' (glycogenosis VI) E74.09
  Herter (-Gee) (-Heubner) (nontropical sprue) K90.0
  Heubner-Herter (nontropical sprue) K90.0

Disease, diseased — continued
- high fetal gene or hemoglobin thalassemia D56.9
- Hildenbrand's — see Typhus
- hip (joint) M25.9
  - congenital Q65.89
  - suppurative M00.9
  - tuberculous A18.02
- His (-Werner) (trench fever) A79.0
- Hodgson's — see also Aneurysm, aorta, thorax I71.20
  - ruptured — see also Aneurysm, aorta, thorax, ruptured I71.10
- Holla — see Spherocytosis
- hookworm B76.9
  - specified NEC B76.8
- host-versus-graft D89.813
  - acute D89.810
  - acute on chronic D89.812
  - chronic D89.811
- human immunodeficiency virus (HIV) B20
- Huntington's G10
  - with dementia — see also Dementia, in, diseases specified elsewhere G10 [F02.80]
- Hunt's (herpetic geniculate ganglionitis) (neuralgia) B02.21
  - dyssynergia cerebellaris myoclonica G11.19
- Hutchinson's (cheiropompholyx) — see Hutchinson's disease
- hyaline (diffuse) (generalized)
  - membrane (lung) (newborn) P22.0
    - adult J80
- hydatid — see Echinococcus
- hydroxyapatite deposition M11.00
  - ankle M11.07- ☑
  - elbow M11.02- ☑
  - foot joint M11.07- ☑
  - hand joint M11.04- ☑
  - hip M11.05- ☑
  - knee M11.06- ☑
  - multiple site M11.09
  - shoulder M11.01- ☑
  - vertebra M11.08
  - wrist M11.03- ☑
- hyperkinetic — see Hyperkinesia
- hypertensive — see Hypertension
- hypophysis E23.7
- I-cell E77.0
- Iceland G93.39
- IgG4-related D89.84
- immune D89.9
- immunoglobulin G4-related D89.84
- immunoproliferative (malignant) C88.9- ☑
  - small intestinal C88.3- ☑
  - specified NEC C88.8- ☑
- inclusion B25.9
  - salivary gland B25.9
- infectious, infective B99.9
  - congenital P37.9
    - specified NEC P37.8
    - viral P35.9
      - specified type NEC P35.8
  - specified NEC B99.8
- inflammatory
  - penis N48.29
    - abscess N48.21
    - cellulitis N48.22
  - prepuce N47.7
    - balanoposthitis N47.6
  - tubo-ovarian — see Salpingo-oophoritis
- intervertebral disc — see also Disorder, disc
  - with myelopathy — see Disorder, disc, with, myelopathy
  - cervical, cervicothoracic — see Disorder, disc, cervical
    - with
      - myelopathy — see Disorder, disc, cervical, with myelopathy
      - neuritis, radiculitis or radiculopathy — see Disorder, disc, cervical, with neuritis
      - specified NEC — see Disorder, disc, cervical, specified type NEC
  - lumbar (with)
    - myelopathy M51.06
    - neuritis, radiculitis, radiculopathy or sciatica M51.16
    - specified NEC M51.86
  - lumbosacral (with)
    - neuritis, radiculitis, radiculopathy or sciatica M51.17
    - specified NEC M51.87

Disease, diseased — continued
- intervertebral disc — see also Disorder, disc — continued
  - specified NEC — see Disorder, disc, specified NEC
  - thoracic (with)
    - myelopathy M51.04
    - neuritis, radiculitis or radiculopathy M51.14
    - specified NEC M51.84
  - thoracolumbar (with)
    - myelopathy M51.05
    - neuritis, radiculitis or radiculopathy M51.15
    - specified NEC M51.85
- intestine K63.9
  - functional K59.9
    - psychogenic F45.8
    - specified NEC K59.89
  - organic K63.9
  - protozoal A07.9
  - specified NEC K63.89
- iris H21.9
  - specified NEC H21.89
- iron metabolism or storage E83.10
- island (scrub typhus) A75.3
- itai-itai — see Poisoning, cadmium
- Jakob-Creutzfeldt — see Creutzfeldt-Jakob disease or syndrome
- jaw M27.9
  - fibrocystic M27.49
  - specified NEC M27.8
- jigger B88.1
- joint M25.9
  - see also Disorder, joint
  - Charcot's — see Arthropathy, neuropathic (Charcot)
  - degenerative — see Osteoarthritis
    - multiple M15.9
    - spine — see Spondylosis
  - facet joint — see also Spondylosis M47.819
  - hypertrophic — see Osteoarthritis
  - sacroiliac M53.3
  - specified NEC — see Disorder, joint, specified type NEC
  - spine NEC — see Dorsopathy
  - suppurative — see Arthritis, pyogenic or pyemic
- Jourdain's (acute gingivitis) K05.00
  - nonplaque induced K05.01
  - plaque induced K05.00
- Kaschin-Beck (endemic polyarthritis) M12.10
  - ankle M12.17- ☑
  - elbow M12.12- ☑
  - foot joint M12.17- ☑
  - hand joint M12.14- ☑
  - hip M12.15- ☑
  - knee M12.16- ☑
  - multiple site M12.19
  - shoulder M12.11- ☑
  - vertebra M12.18
  - wrist M12.13- ☑
- Katayama B65.2
- Kedani (scrub typhus) A75.3
- Keshan E59
- kidney (functional) (pelvis) N28.9
  - chronic N18.9
    - hypertensive — see Hypertension, kidney
    - stage 1 N18.1
    - stage 2 (mild) N18.2
    - stage 3 (moderate) N18.30
    - stage 3a N18.31
    - stage 3b N18.32
    - stage 4 (severe) N18.4
    - stage 5 N18.5
  - complicating pregnancy — see Pregnancy, complicated by, renal disease
  - cystic (congenital) Q61.9
  - fibrocystic (congenital) Q61.8
  - hypertensive — see Hypertension, kidney
  - in (due to)
    - schistosomiasis (bilharziasis) B65.9 [N29]
  - multicystic Q61.4
  - polycystic Q61.3
    - adult type Q61.2
    - childhood type NEC Q61.19
      - collecting duct dilatation Q61.11
- Kimmelstiel (-Wilson) (intercapillary polycystic (congenital) glomerulosclerosis) — see E08-E13 with .21
- Kinnier Wilson's (hepatolenticular degeneration) E83.01
- kissing — see Mononucleosis, infectious
- Klebs' — see also Glomerulonephritis N05.- ☑
- Klippel-Feil (brevicollis) Q76.1

Disease, diseased — continued
- Kohler-Pellegrini-Stieda (calcification, knee joint) — see Bursitis, tibial collateral
- Kok Q89.89
- Konig's (osteochondritis dissecans) — see Osteochondritis, dissecans
- Korsakoff's (nonalcoholic) F04
  - alcoholic F10.96
    - with dependence F10.26
- Kostmann's (infantile genetic agranulocytosis) D70.0
- kuru A81.81
- Kyasanur Forest A98.2
- labyrinth, ear — see Disorder, ear, inner
- lacrimal system — see Disorder, lacrimal system
- Lafora body — see also Epilepsy, progressive, Lafora G40.C09
- Lancereaux-Mathieu (leptospiral jaundice) A27.0
- Landry's G61.0
- Larrey-Weil (leptospiral jaundice) A27.0
- larynx J38.7
- legionnaires' A48.1
  - nonpneumonic A48.2
- Lenegre's I44.2
- lens H27.9
  - specified NEC H27.8
- Lev's (acquired complete heart block) I44.2
- Lewy body (dementia) — see also Dementia, in, diseases specified elsewhere G31.83 [F02.80]
  - with behavioral disturbance — see also Dementia, in, diseases specified elsewhere G31.83 [F02.81-] ☑
- Lichtheim's (subacute combined sclerosis with pernicious anemia) D51.0
- Lightwood's (renal tubular acidosis) N25.89
- Lignac's (cystinosis) E72.04
- lip K13.0
- lipid-storage E75.6
  - specified NEC E75.5
- Lipschutz's N76.6
- liver (chronic) (organic) K76.9
  - alcoholic (chronic) K70.9
    - acute — see Disease, liver, alcoholic, hepatitis
    - cirrhosis K70.30
      - with ascites K70.31
    - failure K70.40
      - with coma K70.41
    - fatty liver K70.0
    - fibrosis K70.2
    - hepatitis K70.10
      - with ascites K70.11
    - sclerosis K70.2
  - cystic, congenital Q44.6
  - drug-induced (idiosyncratic) (toxic) (predictable) (unpredictable) — see Disease, liver, toxic
  - end stage K72.1- ☑
    - due to hepatitis — see Hepatitis
    - with coma K72.11
  - fatty, nonalcoholic (NAFLD) K76.0
    - alcoholic K70.0
  - fibrocystic (congenital) Q44.6
  - fluke
    - Chinese B66.1
    - oriental B66.1
    - sheep B66.3
  - Fontan-associated (FALD) I27.840
  - gestational alloimmune (GALD) P78.84
  - glycogen storage E74.09 [K77]
  - in (due to)
    - schistosomiasis (bilharziasis) B65.9 [K77]
  - inflammatory K75.9
    - alcoholic K70.1- ☑
    - specified NEC K75.89
  - metabolic dysfunction-associated steatotic (MASLD) K76.0
  - polycystic (congenital) Q44.6
  - toxic K71.9
    - with
      - cholestasis K71.0
      - cirrhosis (liver) K71.7
      - fibrosis (liver) K71.7
      - focal nodular hyperplasia K71.8
      - hepatic granuloma K71.8
      - hepatic necrosis K71.10
        - with coma K71.11
      - hepatitis NEC K71.6
        - acute K71.2
        - chronic
          - active K71.50
            - with ascites K71.51

☑ Additional Character Required — Refer to the Tabular List for Character Selection

Disease, diseased — continued
- liver — continued
  - toxic — continued
    - with — continued
      - hepatitis — continued
        - chronic — continued
          - lobular K71.4
          - persistent K71.3
          - lupoid K71.50
            - with ascites K71.51
        - peliosis hepatis K71.8
        - veno-occlusive disease (VOD) of liver K71.8
    - veno-occlusive K76.5
- Lobo's (keloid blastomycosis) B48.0
- Lobstein's (brittle bones and blue sclera) Q78.0
- Ludwig's (submaxillary cellulitis) K12.2
- lumbosacral region M53.87
- lung J98.4
  - black J60
  - congenital Q33.9
  - cystic J98.4
    - congenital Q33.0
  - dabbing (related) U07.0
  - electronic cigarette (related) U07.0
  - fibroid (chronic) — see Fibrosis, lung
  - fluke B66.4
    - oriental B66.4
  - in
    - amyloidosis E85.4 [J99]
    - sarcoidosis D86.0
    - Sjogren's syndrome M35.02
    - systemic
      - lupus erythematosus M32.13
      - sclerosis M34.81
  - interstitial J84.9
    - with progressive fibrotic phenotype, in diseases classified elsewhere J84.170
    - drug-induced — see Disorder, lung, interstitial, drug-induced
    - of childhood, specified NEC J84.848
      - drug-induced — see Disorder, lung, interstitial, drug-induced
    - respiratory bronchiolitis J84.115
    - specified NEC J84.89
  - obstructive (chronic) J44.9
    - with
      - acute
        - bronchitis J44.0
        - exacerbation NEC J44.1
        - lower respiratory infection J44.0
      - alveolitis, allergic J67.9
      - asthma J44.89
      - bronchiectasis J47.9
        - with
          - exacerbation (acute) J47.1
          - lower respiratory infection J47.0
      - bronchitis J44.89
        - with
          - exacerbation (acute) J44.1
          - lower respiratory infection J44.0
      - emphysema J43.9
      - hypersensitivity pneumonitis J67.9
    - decompensated J44.1
      - with
        - exacerbation (acute) J44.1
  - polycystic J98.4
    - congenital Q33.0
  - rheumatoid (diffuse) (interstitial) — see Rheumatoid, lung
  - vaping (associated) (device) (product) (use) U07.0
- Lutembacher's (atrial septal defect with mitral stenosis) Q21.19
- Lyme A69.20
- lymphatic (gland) (system) (channel) (vessel) I89.9
- lymphoproliferative D47.9
  - specified NEC D47.Z9 (following D47.4)
  - T-gamma D47.Z9 (following D47.4)
  - X-linked D82.3
- Magitot's M27.2
- malarial — see Malaria
- malignant — see also Neoplasm, malignant, by site
- Manson's B65.1
- maple bark J67.6
- maple-syrup-urine E71.0
- Marburg (virus) A98.3
- Marion's (bladder neck obstruction) N32.0
- Marsh's (exophthalmic goiter) — see Hyperthyroidism, with, goiter (diffuse)
- mastoid (process) — see Disorder, ear, middle

Disease, diseased — continued
- Mathieu's (leptospiral jaundice) A27.0
- Maxcy's A75.2
- McArdle (-Schmid-Pearson) (glycogenosis V) E74.04
- mediastinum J98.59
- medullary center (idiopathic) (respiratory) G93.89
- Meige's (chronic hereditary edema) Q82.0
- meningococcal — see Infection, meningococcal
- mental F99
  - organic F09
- mesenchymal M35.9
- mesenteric embolic — see also Ischemia, intestine, acute K55.039
- metabolic, metabolism E88.9
  - bilirubin E80.7
- metal-polisher's J62.8
- metastatic — see also Neoplasm, secondary, by site C79.9
- microvascular - code to condition
- microvillus
  - atrophy Q43.8
  - inclusion (MVD) Q43.8
- middle ear — see Disorder, ear, middle
- Mikulicz' (dryness of mouth, absent or decreased lacrimation) K11.8
- Milroy's (chronic hereditary edema) Q82.0
- Minamata — see Poisoning, mercury
- minicore G71.29
- Minor's G95.19
- Minot-von Willebrand-Jurgens (angiohemophilia) — see Disease, von Willebrand
- Minot's (hemorrhagic disease, newborn) P53
- Mitchell's (erythromelalgia) I73.81
- mitral (valve) I05.9
  - nonrheumatic I34.9
- mixed connective tissue M35.1
- MOG antibody G37.81
- moldy hay J67.0
- Monge's T70.29- ☑
- Morgagni-Adams-Stokes (syncope with heart block) I45.9
- Morgagni's (syndrome) (hyperostosis frontalis interna) M85.2
- Morton's (with metatarsalgia) — see Lesion, nerve, plantar
- Morvan's G60.8
- motor neuron (bulbar) (mixed type) (spinal) G12.20
  - amyotrophic lateral sclerosis G12.21
  - familial G12.24
  - progressive bulbar palsy G12.22
  - specified NEC G12.29
- moyamoya I67.5
- mu heavy chain disease C88.2- ☑
- multicore G71.29
- multiminicore G71.29
- muscle — see also Disorder, muscle
  - inflammatory — see Myositis
  - ocular (external) — see Strabismus
- musculoskeletal system, soft tissue — see also Disorder, soft tissue
  - specified NEC — see Disorder, soft tissue, specified type NEC
- mushroom workers' J67.5
- mycotic B49
- myelin oligodendrocyte glycoprotein antibody G37.81
- myelodysplastic — see also Syndrome, myelodysplastic C94.6
- myelodysplastic/myeloproliferative neoplasm, unclassifiable C94.6
- myeloproliferative D47.1
  - chronic D47.1
  - not classified C94.6
  - specified NEC C94.6
  - unclassifiable C94.6
- myocardium, myocardial — see also Degeneration, myocardial I51.5
  - primary (idiopathic) I42.9
- myoneural G70.9
- Naegeli's D69.1
- nails L60.9
  - specified NEC L60.8
- Nairobi (sheep virus) A93.8
- nasal J34.9
- nemaline body G71.21
- nerve — see Disorder, nerve
- nervous system G98.8
  - autonomic G90.9
  - central G96.9
    - specified NEC G96.89
  - congenital Q07.9
  - parasympathetic G90.9

Disease, diseased — continued
- nervous system — continued
  - specified NEC G98.8
  - sympathetic G90.9
  - vegetative G90.9
- neuromuscular system G70.9
- Newcastle B30.8
- Nicolas (-Durand)-Favre (climatic bubo) A55
- nipple N64.9
  - Paget's C50.01- ☑
    - female C50.01- ☑
    - male C50.02- ☑
- Nishimoto (-Takeuchi) I67.5
- nonarthropod-borne NOS (viral) B34.9
  - enterovirus NEC B34.1
- nonautoimmune hemolytic D59.4
  - drug-induced D59.2
- Nonne-Milroy-Meige (chronic hereditary edema) Q82.0
- nose J34.9
- nucleus pulposus — see Disorder, disc
- nutritional E63.9
- oast-house-urine E72.19
- ocular
  - herpesviral B00.50
  - zoster B02.30
- obliterative vascular I77.1
- Ohara's — see Tularemia
- Opitz's (congestive splenomegaly) D73.2
- Oppenheim-Urbach (necrobiosis lipoidica diabeticorum) — see E08-E13 with .620
- optic nerve NEC — see Disorder, nerve, optic
- orbit — see Disorder, orbit
- organ
  - dabbing (related) U07.0
  - electronic cigarette (related) U07.0
  - vaping (associated) (device) (product) (use) U07.0
- Oriental liver fluke B66.1
- Oriental lung fluke B66.4
- Ormond's N13.5
- Oropouche virus A93.0
- Osler-Rendu (familial hemorrhagic telangiectasia) I78.0
- osteofibrocystic E21.0
- Otto's M24.7
- outer ear — see Disorder, ear, external
- ovary (noninflammatory) N83.9
  - cystic N83.20- ☑
  - inflammatory — see Salpingo-oophoritis
  - polycystic E28.2
  - specified NEC N83.8
- Owren's (congenital) — see Defect, coagulation
- p110d-activating mutation causing senescent T cells, lymphadenopathy, and immunodeficiency [PASLI] D81.82
- pancreas K86.9
  - cystic K86.2
  - fibrocystic E84.9
  - specified NEC K86.89
- panvalvular I08.9
  - specified NEC I08.8
- parametrium (noninflammatory) N83.9
- parasitic B89
  - cerebral NEC B71.9 [G94]
  - intestinal NOS B82.9
  - mouth B37.0
  - skin NOS B88.9
  - specified type — see Infestation
  - tongue B37.0
- parathyroid (gland) E21.5
  - specified NEC E21.4
- Parkinson's G20.A1
  - with dyskinesia
    - with
      - fluctuations G20.B2
      - OFF episodes G20.B2
    - without mention of
      - fluctuations G20.B1
      - OFF episodes G20.B1
  - without dyskinesia
    - with
      - fluctuations G20.A2
      - OFF episodes G20.A2
    - without mention of
      - fluctuations G20.A1
      - OFF episodes G20.A1
- parodontal K05.6
- Parrot's (syphilitic osteochondritis) A50.02
- Parry's (exophthalmic goiter) — see Hyperthyroidism, with, goiter (diffuse)

Disease, diseased — continued
  Parson's (exophthalmic goiter) — see Hyperthyroidism, with, goiter (diffuse)
  Paxton's (white piedra) B36.2
  pearl-worker's — see Osteomyelitis, specified type NEC
  Pellegrini-Stieda (calcification, knee joint) — see Bursitis, tibial collateral
  pelvis, pelvic
    female NOS N94.9
      specified NEC N94.89
    gonococcal (acute) (chronic) A54.24
    inflammatory (female) N73.9
      acute N73.0
      chlamydial A56.11
      chronic N73.1
      specified NEC N73.8
      syphilitic (secondary) A51.42
        late A52.76
      tuberculous A18.17
    organ, female N94.9
    peritoneum, female NEC N94.89
  penis N48.9
    inflammatory N48.29
      abscess N48.21
      cellulitis N48.22
    specified NEC N48.89
  periapical tissues NOS K04.90
  periodontal K05.6
    specified NEC K05.5
  periosteum — see Disorder, bone, specified type NEC
  peripheral
    arterial I73.9
    autonomic nervous system G90.9
    nerves — see Polyneuropathy
    vascular NOS I73.9
      in diabetes mellitus — see Diabetes, by type, with peripheral angiopathy
  peritoneum K66.9
    pelvic, female NEC N94.89
    specified NEC K66.8
  persistent mucosal (middle ear) H66.20
    left H66.22
      with right H66.23
    right H66.21
      with left H66.23
  Petit's — see Hernia, abdomen, specified site NEC
  pharynx J39.2
    specified NEC J39.2
  Phocas' — see Mastopathy, cystic
  photochromogenic (acid-fast bacilli) (pulmonary) A31.0
    nonpulmonary A31.9
  Pick's — see also Dementia, in, diseases specified elsewhere G31.01 [F02.80]
    with behavioral disturbance — see also Dementia, in, diseases specified elsewhere G31.01 [F02.81-] ☑
    brain G31.01 [F02.80]
      with behavioral disturbance — see also Dementia, in, diseases specified elsewhere G31.01 [F02.81-] ☑
    of pericardium (pericardial pseudocirrhosis of liver) I31.1
  pigeon fancier's J67.2
  pineal gland E34.8
  pink — see Poisoning, mercury
  Pinkus' (lichen nitidus) L44.1
  pinworm B80
  Piry virus A93.8
  pituitary (gland) E23.7
  pituitary-snuff-taker's J67.8
  pleura (cavity) J94.9
    specified NEC J94.8
  pneumatic drill (hammer) T75.21- ☑
  Pollitzer's (hidradenitis suppurativa) L73.2
  polycystic
    kidney or renal Q61.3
      adult type Q61.2
      childhood type NEC Q61.19
        collecting duct dilatation Q61.11
    liver or hepatic Q44.6
    lung or pulmonary J98.4
      congenital Q33.0
    ovary, ovaries E28.2
    spleen Q89.09
  polyethylene T84.05- ☑
  Pompe's (glycogenosis II) E74.02
  Posadas-Wernicke B38.9
  Potain's (pulmonary edema) — see Edema, lung
  prepuce N47.8

Disease, diseased — continued
  prepuce — continued
    inflammatory N47.7
      balanoposthitis N47.6
  Pringle's (tuberous sclerosis) Q85.1
  prion, central nervous system A81.9
    specified NEC A81.89
  prostate N42.9
    specified NEC N42.89
  protozoal B64
    acanthamebiasis — see Acanthamebiasis
    African trypanosomiasis — see African trypanosomiasis
    babesiosis — see also Babesiosis B60.00
    Chagas disease — see Chagas disease
    intestine, intestinal A07.9
    leishmaniasis — see Leishmaniasis
    malaria — see Malaria
    naegleriasis B60.2
    pneumocystosis B59
    specified organism NEC B60.8
    toxoplasmosis — see Toxoplasmosis
  pseudo-Hurler's E77.0
  psychiatric F99
  psychotic — see Psychosis
  Puente's (simple glandular cheilitis) K13.0
  puerperal — see also Puerperal O90.89
  pulmonary — see also Disease, lung
    artery I28.9
    chronic obstructive J44.9
      with
        acute bronchitis J44.0
        exacerbation (acute) J44.1
        lower respiratory infection (acute) J44.0
      decompensated J44.1
        with
          exacerbation (acute) J44.1
    heart I27.9
      specified NEC I27.89
    hypertensive (vascular) — see also Hypertension, pulmonary I27.20
      NEC I27.2- ☑
      primary (idiopathic) I27.0
    valve I37.9
      rheumatic I09.89
  pulp (dental) NOS K04.90
  pulseless M31.4
  Putnam's (subacute combined sclerosis with pernicious anemia) D51.0
  Pyle (-Cohn) (metaphyseal dysplasia) Q78.5
  ragpicker's or ragsorter's A22.1
  Raynaud's — see Raynaud's disease
  reactive airway — see Asthma
  Reclus' (cystic) — see Mastopathy, cystic
  rectum K62.9
    specified NEC K62.89
  Refsum's (heredopathia atactica polyneuritiformis) G60.1
  renal (functional) (pelvis) — see also Disease, kidney N28.9
    with
      edema — see Nephrosis
      glomerular lesion — see Glomerulonephritis
        with edema — see Nephrosis
      interstitial nephritis N12
    acute N28.9
    chronic — see also Disease, kidney, chronic N18.9
    cystic, congenital Q61.9
    diabetic — see E08-E13 with .22
    end-stage (failure) N18.6
      due to hypertension I12.0
    fibrocystic (congenital) Q61.8
    hypertensive — see Hypertension, kidney
    lupus M32.14
    phosphate-losing (tubular) N25.0
    polycystic (congenital) Q61.3
      adult type Q61.2
      childhood type NEC Q61.19
        collecting duct dilatation Q61.11
    rapidly progressive N01.9
    subacute N01.9
  Rendu-Osler-Weber (familial hemorrhagic telangiectasia) I78.0
  renovascular (arteriosclerotic) — see Hypertension, kidney
  respiratory (tract) J98.9
    acute or subacute NOS J06.9
      due to
        chemicals, gases, fumes or vapors (inhalation) J68.3

Disease, diseased — continued
  respiratory — continued
    acute or subacute — continued
      due to — continued
        external agent J70.9
          specified NEC J70.8
        radiation J70.0
        smoke inhalation J70.5
      noninfectious J39.8
    chronic NOS J98.9
      due to
        chemicals, gases, fumes or vapors J68.4
        external agent J70.9
          specified NEC J70.8
        radiation J70.1
      newborn P27.9
        specified NEC P27.8
    due to
      chemicals, gases, fumes or vapors J68.9
        acute or subacute NEC J68.3
        chronic J68.4
      external agent J70.9
        specified NEC J70.8
    newborn P28.9
      specified type NEC P28.89
    upper J39.9
      acute or subacute J06.9
      noninfectious NEC J39.8
      specified NEC J39.8
      streptococcal J06.9
  retina, retinal H35.9
    Batten's or Batten-Mayou E75.4 [H36.89]
    specified NEC H35.89
  rheumatoid — see Arthritis, rheumatoid
  rickettsial NOS A79.9
    specified type NEC A79.89
  Riga (-Fede) (cachectic aphthae) K14.0
  Riggs' (compound periodontitis) — see Periodontitis
  Ritter's L00
  Rivalta's (cervicofacial actinomycosis) A42.2
  Robles' (onchocerciasis) B73.01
  rod body G71.21
  Roger's (congenital interventricular septal defect) Q21.0
  Rosenthal's (factor XI deficiency) D68.1
  Ross River B33.1
  Rossbach's (hyperchlorhydria) K31.89
    psychogenic F45.8
  Rotes Querol — see Hyperostosis, ankylosing
  Roth (-Bernhardt) — see Mononeuropathy, lower limb, meralgia paresthetica
  Runeberg's (progressive pernicious anemia) D51.0
  sacroiliac NEC M53.3
  salivary gland or duct K11.9
    inclusion B25.9
    specified NEC K11.8
    virus B25.9
  sandworm B76.9
  Schimmelbusch's — see Mastopathy, cystic
  Schmorl's — see Schmorl's disease or nodes
  Schonlein (-Henoch) (purpura rheumatica) D69.0
  Schottmuller's — see Fever, paratyphoid
  Schultz's (agranulocytosis) — see Agranulocytosis
  Schwalbe-Ziehen-Oppenheim G24.1
  Schwartz-Jampel G71.13
  sclera H15.9
    specified NEC H15.89
  scrofulous (tuberculous) A18.2
  scrotum N50.9
  sebaceous glands L73.9
  semilunar cartilage, cystic — see also Derangement, knee, meniscus, cystic
  seminal vesicle N50.9
  serum NEC — see also Reaction, serum T80.69- ☑
  sexually transmitted A64
    anogenital
      herpesviral infection — see Herpes, anogenital
      warts A63.0
    chancroid A57
    chlamydial infection — see Chlamydia
    gonorrhea — see Gonorrhea
    granuloma inguinale A58
    specified organism NEC A63.8
    syphilis — see Syphilis
    trichomoniasis — see Trichomoniasis
  Sezary C84.1- ☑
  shimamushi (scrub typhus) A75.3
  shipyard B30.0
  sickle-cell D57.1

☑ Additional Character Required — Refer to the Tabular List for Character Selection

Disease, diseased — continued
  sickle-cell — continued
    with
      acute chest syndrome D57.01
      cerebral vascular involvement D57.03
      crisis (painful) D57.00
        with
          complication specified NEC D57.09
            dactylitis D57.04
      dactylitis D57.04
      pain (vaso-occlusive) D57.00
      priapism D57.09
      splenic sequestration D57.02
    elliptocytosis D57.8- ☑
    Hb-C D57.20
      with
        acute chest syndrome D57.211
        cerebral vascular involvement D57.213
        crisis D57.219
          with
            dactylitis D57.214
            specified complication NEC D57.218
        dactylitis D57.214
        pain (vaso-occlusive) D57.219
        priapism D57.218
        splenic sequestration D57.212
      without crisis D57.20
    Hb-SD D57.80
      with
        acute chest syndrome D57.811
        cerebral vascular involvement D57.813
        crisis D57.819
          with
            complication specified NEC D57.818
              dactylitis D57.814
        dactylitis D57.814
        pain (vaso-occlusive) D57.819
        priapism D57.818
        splenic sequestration D57.812
      without crisis D57.80
    Hb-SE D57.80
      with
        acute chest syndrome D57.811
        cerebral vascular involvement D57.813
        crisis D57.819
          with
            complication specified NEC D57.818
              dactylitis D57.814
        dactylitis D57.814
        pain (vaso-occlusive) D57.819
        priapism D57.818
        splenic sequestration D57.812
      without crisis D57.80
    specified NEC D57.80
      with
        acute chest syndrome D57.811
        cerebral vascular involvement D57.813
        crisis D57.819
          with
            complication specified NEC D57.818
              dactylitis D57.814
        dactylitis D57.814
        pain (vaso-occlusive) D57.819
        priapism D57.818
        splenic sequestration D57.812
      without crisis D57.80
    spherocytosis D57.80
      with
        acute chest syndrome D57.811
        cerebral vascular involvement D57.813
        crisis D57.819
          with complication specified NEC D57.818
        pain (vaso-occlusive) D57.819
        priapism D57.818
        splenic sequestration D57.812
      without crisis D57.80
    thalassemia D57.40
      with
        acute chest syndrome D57.411
          with dactylitis D57.414
          with specified complication NEC D57.418
        cerebral vascular involvement D57.413
        crisis (painful) D57.419
          with specified complication NEC D57.418
        dactylitis D57.414
        pain (vaso-occlusive) D57.419
        priapism D57.418
        splenic sequestration D57.412
      beta plus D57.44

Disease, diseased — continued
  sickle-cell — continued
    thalassemia — continued
      beta plus — continued
        with
          acute chest syndrome D57.451
            with dactylitis D57.454
          cerebral vascular involvement D57.453
          crisis D57.459
            with specified complication NEC D57.458
          dactylitis D57.454
          pain (vaso-occlusive) D57.459
          priapism D57.458
          splenic sequestration D57.452
        without crisis D57.44
      beta zero D57.42
        with
          acute chest syndrome D57.431
            with dactylitis D57.434
          cerebral vascular involvement D57.433
          crisis D57.439
            with specified complication NEC D57.438
          dactylitis D57.434
          pain (vaso-occlusive) D57.439
          priapism D57.438
          splenic sequestration D57.432
        without crisis D57.42
  silo-filler's J68.8
    bronchitis J68.0
    pneumonitis J68.0
    pulmonary edema J68.1
  simian B B00.4
  Simons' (progressive lipodystrophy) E88.11
  sin nombre virus B33.4
  sinus — see Sinusitis
  Sirkari's B55.0
  sixth B08.20
    due to human herpesvirus 6 B08.21
    due to human herpesvirus 7 B08.22
  skin L98.9
    due to metabolic disorder NEC E88.9 [L99]
    specified NEC L98.8
  slim (HIV) B20
  small vessel I73.9
  Sneddon-Wilkinson (subcorneal pustular dermatosis) L13.1
  South African creeping B88.09
  spinal (cord) G95.9
    congenital Q06.9
    specified NEC G95.89
  spine — see also Spondylopathy
    joint — see Dorsopathy
    tuberculous A18.01
  spinocerebellar (hereditary) G11.9
    specified NEC G11.8
  spleen D73.9
    amyloid E85.4 [D77]
    organic D73.9
    polycystic Q89.09
    postinfectional D73.89
  sponge-diver's — see Toxicity, venom, marine animal, sea anemone
  Startle Q89.89
  Steinert's G71.11
  Sticker's (erythema infectiosum) B08.3
  Stieda's (calcification, knee joint) — see Bursitis, tibial collateral
  Stokes' (exophthalmic goiter) — see Hyperthyroidism, with, goiter (diffuse)
  Stokes-Adams (syncope with heart block) I45.9
  stomach K31.9
    functional, psychogenic F45.8
    specified NEC K31.89
  stonemason's J62.8
  storage
    glycogen — see Disease, glycogen storage
    mucopolysaccharide — see Mucopolysaccharidosis
  striatopallidal system NEC G25.89
  Stuart-Prower (congenital factor X deficiency) D68.2
  Stuart's (congenital factor X deficiency) D68.2
  subcutaneous tissue — see Disease, skin
  supporting structures of teeth K08.9
    specified NEC K08.89
  suprarenal (capsule) (gland) E27.9
    hyperfunction E27.0
    specified NEC E27.8
  sweat glands L74.9

Disease, diseased — continued
  sweat glands — continued
    specified NEC L74.8
  Sweeley-Klionsky E75.21
  Swift (-Feer) — see Poisoning, mercury
  swimming-pool granuloma A31.1
  Sylvest's (epidemic pleurodynia) B33.0
  sympathetic nervous system G90.9
  synovium — see Disorder, synovium
  syphilitic — see Syphilis
  systemic tissue mast cell D47.02
  tanapox (virus) B08.71
  Tangier E78.6
  Tarral-Besnier (pityriasis rubra pilaris) L44.0
  Tauri's E74.09
  tear duct — see Disorder, lacrimal system
  tendon, tendinous — see also Disorder, tendon
    nodular — see Trigger finger
  terminal vessel I73.9
  testis N50.9
  thalassemia Hb-S — see Disease, sickle-cell, thalassemia
  Thaysen-Gee (nontropical sprue) K90.0
  Thomsen G71.12
  throat J39.2
    septic J02.0
  thromboembolic — see Embolism
  thymus (gland) E32.9
    specified NEC E32.8
  thyroid (gland) E07.9
    heart — see also Hyperthyroidism E05.90 [I43]
      with thyroid storm E05.91 [I43]
    specified NEC E07.89
  Tietze's M94.0
  tongue K14.9
    specified NEC K14.8
  tonsils, tonsillar (and adenoids) J35.9
  tooth, teeth K08.9
    hard tissues K03.9
      specified NEC K03.89
    pulp NEC K04.99
    specified NEC K08.89
  Tourette's F95.2
  trachea NEC J39.8
  tricuspid I07.9
    nonrheumatic I36.9
  triglyceride-storage E75.5
  trophoblastic — see Mole, hydatidiform
  tsutsugamushi A75.3
  tube (fallopian) (noninflammatory) N83.9
    inflammatory — see Salpingitis
    specified NEC N83.8
  tuberculous NEC — see Tuberculosis
  tubo-ovarian (noninflammatory) N83.9
    inflammatory — see Salpingo-oophoritis
    specified NEC N83.8
  tubotympanic, chronic — see Otitis, media, suppurative, chronic, tubotympanic
  tubulo-interstitial N15.9
    specified NEC N15.8
  tympanum — see Disorder, tympanic membrane
  Uhl's Q24.8
  Underwood's (sclerema neonatorum) P83.0
  Unverricht (-Lundborg) — see Epilepsy, generalized, idiopathic
  Urbach-Oppenheim (necrobiosis lipoidica diabeticorum) — see E08-E13 with .620
  ureter N28.9
    in (due to)
      schistosomiasis (bilharziasis) B65.0 [N29]
  urethra N36.9
    specified NEC N36.8
  urinary (tract) N39.9
    bladder N32.9
      specified NEC N32.89
    specified NEC N39.8
  uterus (noninflammatory) N85.9
    infective — see Endometritis
    inflammatory — see Endometritis
    specified NEC N85.8
  uveal tract (anterior) H21.9
    posterior H31.9
  vagabond's B85.1
  vagina, vaginal (noninflammatory) N89.9
    inflammatory NEC N76.89
    specified NEC N89.8
  valve, valvular I38
    multiple I08.9
      specified NEC I08.8
  van Creveld-von Gierke (glycogenosis I) E74.01

☑ Additional Character Required — Refer to the Tabular List for Character Selection

Disease, diseased — *continued*
vas deferens N50.9
vascular I99.9
  arteriosclerotic — *see* Arteriosclerosis
  ciliary body NEC — *see* Disorder, iris, vascular
  hypertensive — *see* Hypertension
  iris NEC — *see* Disorder, iris, vascular
  obliterative I77.1
    peripheral I73.9
  occlusive I99.8
  peripheral (occlusive) I73.9
    in diabetes mellitus — *see* E08-E13 with .51
vasomotor I73.9
vasospastic I73.9
vein I87.9
venereal — *see also* Disease, sexually transmitted A64
  chlamydial NEC A56.8
    anus A56.3
    genitourinary NOS A56.2
    pharynx A56.4
    rectum A56.3
  fifth A55
  sixth A55
  specified nature or type NEC A63.8
vertebra, vertebral — *see also* Spondylopathy
  disc — *see* Disorder, disc
vibration — *see* Vibration, adverse effects
viral, virus — *see also* Disease, by type of virus B34.9
  arbovirus NOS A94
  arthropod-borne NOS A94
  congenital P35.9
    specified NEC P35.8
  Hanta (with renal manifestations) (Dobrava) (Puumala) (Seoul) A98.5
    with pulmonary manifestations (Andes) (Bayou) (Bermejo) (Black Creek Canal) (Choclo) (Juquitiba) (Laguna negra) (Lechiguanas) (New York) (Oran) (Sin nombre) B33.4
  Hantaan (Korean hemorrhagic fever) A98.5
  human immunodeficiency (HIV) B20
  Kunjin A83.4
  nonarthropod-borne NOS B34.9
  Powassan A84.81
  Rocio (encephalitis) A83.6
  Sin nombre (Hantavirus) (cardio)-pulmonary syndrome) B33.4
  Tahyna B33.8
  vesicular stomatitis A93.8
vitreous H43.9
  specified NEC H43.89
vocal cord J38.3
Volkmann's, acquired T79.6- ☑
von Eulenburg's (congenital paramyotonia) G71.19
von Gierke's (glycogenosis I) E74.01
von Graefe's — *see* Strabismus, paralytic, ophthalmoplegia, progressive
von Willebrand (-Jurgens) (angiohemophilia) D68.00
  acquired D68.04
  platelet-type D68.09
  pseudo D68.09
  specified NEC D68.09
  type 1 D68.01
  type 1C D68.01
  type 2 D68.029
    type 2A D68.020
    type 2B D68.021
    type 2M D68.022
    type 2N D68.023
  type 3 D68.03
Vrolik's (osteogenesis imperfecta) Q78.0
vulva (noninflammatory) N90.9
  inflammatory NEC N76.89
  specified NEC N90.89
Wallgren's (obstruction of splenic vein with collateral circulation) I87.8
Wassilieff's (leptospiral jaundice) A27.0
wasting NEC E88.A
  due to
    malnutrition E43
      with marasmus E41
    underlying condition E88.A
      with marasmus E41
Waterhouse-Friderichsen A39.1
Wegner's (syphilitic osteochondritis) A50.02
Weil's (leptospiral jaundice of lung) A27.0
Weir Mitchell's (erythromelalgia) I73.81
Werdnig-Hoffmann G12.0
Wermer's E31.21
Werner-His (trench fever) A79.0

Disease, diseased — *continued*
Werner-Schultz (neutropenic splenomegaly) D73.81
Wernicke-Posadas B38.9
whipworm B79
white blood cells D72.9
  specified NEC D72.89
white matter R90.82
white-spot, meaning lichen sclerosus et atrophicus L90.0
  penis N48.0
  vulva N90.4
Wilkie's K55.1
Wilkinson-Sneddon (subcorneal pustular dermatosis) L13.1
Willis' — *see* Diabetes
Wilson's (hepatolenticular degeneration) E83.01
woolsorter's A22.1
yaba monkey tumor B08.72
yaba pox (virus) B08.72
Zika virus A92.5
  congenital P35.4
zoonotic, bacterial A28.9
  specified type NEC A28.8
Disfigurement (due to scar) L90.5
Disgerminoma — *see* Dysgerminoma
DISH (diffuse idiopathic skeletal hyperostosis) — *see* Hyperostosis, ankylosing
Disinsertion, retina — *see* Detachment, retina
Dislocatable hip, congenital Q65.6
Dislocation (articular)
  with fracture — *see* Fracture
  acromioclavicular (joint) S43.10- ☑
    with displacement
      100%-200% S43.12- ☑
      more than 200% S43.13- ☑
    inferior S43.14- ☑
    posterior S43.15- ☑
  ankle S93.0- ☑
  astragalus — *see* Dislocation, ankle
  atlantoaxial S13.121- ☑
  atlantooccipital S13.111- ☑
  atloidooccipital S13.111- ☑
  breast bone S23.29- ☑
  capsule, joint — *code by* site under Dislocation
  carpal (bone) — *see* Dislocation, wrist
  carpometacarpal (joint) NEC S63.05- ☑
    thumb S63.04- ☑
  cartilage (joint) — *code by* site under Dislocation
  cervical spine (vertebra) — *see* Dislocation, vertebra, cervical
  chronic — *see* Dislocation, recurrent
  clavicle — *see* Dislocation, acromioclavicular joint
  coccyx S33.2- ☑
  congenital NEC Q68.8
  coracoid — *see* Dislocation, shoulder
  costal cartilage S23.29- ☑
  costochondral S23.29- ☑
  cricoarytenoid articulation S13.29- ☑
  cricothyroid articulation S13.29- ☑
  dorsal vertebra — *see* Dislocation, vertebra, thoracic
  ear ossicle — *see* Discontinuity, ossicles, ear
  elbow S53.10- ☑
    congenital Q68.8
    pathological — *see* Dislocation, pathological NEC, elbow
    radial head alone — *see* Dislocation, radial head
    recurrent — *see* Dislocation, recurrent, elbow
    traumatic S53.10- ☑
      anterior S53.11- ☑
      lateral S53.14- ☑
      medial S53.13- ☑
      posterior S53.12- ☑
      specified type NEC S53.19- ☑
  eye, nontraumatic — *see* Luxation, globe
  eyeball, nontraumatic — *see* Luxation, globe
  femur
    distal end — *see* Dislocation, knee
    proximal end — *see* Dislocation, hip
  fibula
    distal end — *see* Dislocation, ankle
    proximal end — *see* Dislocation, knee
  finger S63.25- ☑
    index S63.25- ☑
    interphalangeal S63.27- ☑
      distal S63.29- ☑
        index S63.29- ☑
        little S63.29- ☑
        middle S63.29- ☑

Dislocation — *continued*
finger — *continued*
  interphalangeal — *continued*
    distal — *continued*
      ring S63.29- ☑
      index S63.27- ☑
      little S63.27- ☑
      middle S63.27- ☑
      proximal S63.28- ☑
        index S63.28- ☑
        little S63.28- ☑
        middle S63.28- ☑
        ring S63.28- ☑
      ring S63.27- ☑
    little S63.25- ☑
    metacarpophalangeal S63.26- ☑
      index S63.26- ☑
      little S63.26- ☑
      middle S63.26- ☑
      ring S63.26- ☑
    middle S63.25- ☑
    recurrent — *see* Dislocation, recurrent, finger
    ring S63.25- ☑
    thumb — *see* Dislocation, thumb
  foot S93.30- ☑
    recurrent — *see* Dislocation, recurrent, foot
    specified site NEC S93.33- ☑
    tarsal joint S93.31- ☑
    tarsometatarsal joint S93.32- ☑
    toe — *see* Dislocation, toe
  fracture — *see* Fracture
  glenohumeral (joint) — *see* Dislocation, shoulder
  glenoid — *see* Dislocation, shoulder
  habitual — *see* Dislocation, recurrent
  hip S73.00- ☑
    anterior S73.03- ☑
      obturator S73.02- ☑
    central S73.04- ☑
    congenital (total) Q65.2
      bilateral Q65.1
      partial Q65.5
        bilateral Q65.4
        unilateral Q65.3- ☑
      unilateral Q65.0- ☑
    developmental M24.85- ☑
    pathological — *see* Dislocation, pathological NEC, hip
    posterior S73.01- ☑
    recurrent — *see* Dislocation, recurrent, hip
  humerus, proximal end — *see* Dislocation, shoulder
  incomplete — *see* Subluxation, by site
  incus — *see* Discontinuity, ossicles, ear
  infracoracoid — *see* Dislocation, shoulder
  innominate (pubic junction) (sacral junction) S33.39- ☑
    acetabulum — *see* Dislocation, hip
  interphalangeal (joint(s))
    finger S63.279- ☑
      distal S63.29- ☑
        index S63.29- ☑
        little S63.29- ☑
        middle S63.29- ☑
        ring S63.29- ☑
      index S63.27- ☑
      little S63.27- ☑
      middle S63.27- ☑
      proximal S63.28- ☑
        index S63.28- ☑
        little S63.28- ☑
        middle S63.28- ☑
        ring S63.28- ☑
      ring S63.27- ☑
    foot or toe — *see* Dislocation, toe
    thumb S63.12- ☑
  jaw (cartilage) (meniscus) S03.0- ☑
  joint prosthesis — *see* Complications, joint prosthesis, mechanical, displacement, by site
  knee S83.106- ☑
    cap — *see* Dislocation, patella
    congenital Q68.2
    old M23.8X- ☑
    patella — *see* Dislocation, patella
    pathological — *see* Dislocation, pathological NEC, knee
    proximal tibia
      anteriorly S83.11- ☑
      laterally S83.14- ☑
      medially S83.13- ☑

☑ **Additional Character Required** — Refer to the Tabular List for Character Selection

Dislocation — *continued*
  knee — *continued*
    proximal tibia — *continued*
      posteriorly S83.12- ☑
    recurrent — *see also* Derangement, knee, specified NEC
    specified type NEC S83.19- ☑
  lacrimal gland H04.16-
  lens (complete) H27.10
    anterior H27.12- ☑
    congenital Q12.1
    ocular implant — *see* Complications, intraocular lens
    partial H27.11- ☑
    posterior H27.13- ☑
    traumatic S05.8X- ☑
  ligament — *code by* site under Dislocation
  lumbar (vertebra) — *see* Dislocation, vertebra, lumbar
  lumbosacral (vertebra) — *see also* Dislocation, vertebra, lumbar
    congenital Q76.49
  mandible S03.0- ☑
  meniscus (knee) — *see* Tear, meniscus
    other sites - code by site under Dislocation
  metacarpal (bone)
    distal end — *see* Dislocation, finger
    proximal end S63.06- ☑
  metacarpophalangeal (joint)
    finger S63.26- ☑
      index S63.26- ☑
      little S63.26- ☑
      middle S63.26- ☑
      ring S63.26- ☑
    thumb S63.11- ☑
  metatarsal (bone) — *see* Dislocation, foot
  metatarsophalangeal (joint(s)) — *see* Dislocation, toe
  midcarpal (joint) S63.03- ☑
  midtarsal (joint) — *see* Dislocation, foot
  neck S13.20- ☑
    specified site NEC S13.29- ☑
    vertebra — *see* Dislocation, vertebra, cervical
  nose (septal cartilage) S03.1- ☑
  occipitoatloid S13.111- ☑
  old — *see* Derangement, joint, specified type NEC
  ossicles, ear — *see* Discontinuity, ossicles, ear
  partial — *see* Subluxation, by site
  patella S83.006- ☑
    congenital Q74.1
    lateral S83.01- ☑
    recurrent (nontraumatic) M22.0- ☑
      incomplete M22.1- ☑
    specified type NEC S83.09- ☑
  pathological NEC M24.30
    ankle M24.37- ☑
    elbow M24.32- ☑
    foot joint M24.37- ☑
    hand joint M24.34- ☑
    hip M24.35- ☑
    knee M24.36- ☑
    lumbosacral joint — *see* subcategory M53.2- ☑
    pelvic region — *see* Dislocation, pathological, hip
    sacroiliac — *see* subcategory M53.2- ☑
    shoulder M24.31- ☑
    specified site NEC M24.39
    wrist M24.33- ☑
  pelvis NEC S33.30- ☑
    specified NEC S33.39- ☑
  phalanx
    finger or hand — *see* Dislocation, finger
    foot or toe — *see* Dislocation, toe
  prosthesis, internal — *see* Complications, prosthetic device, by site, mechanical
  radial head S53.006- ☑
    anterior S53.01- ☑
    posterior S53.02- ☑
    specified type NEC S53.09- ☑
  radiocarpal (joint) S63.02- ☑
  radiohumeral (joint) — *see* Dislocation, radial head
  radioulnar (joint)
    distal S63.01- ☑
    proximal — *see* Dislocation, elbow
  radius
    distal end — *see* Dislocation, wrist
    proximal end — *see* Dislocation, radial head
  recurrent M24.40
    ankle M24.47- ☑
    elbow M24.42- ☑
    finger M24.44- ☑

Dislocation — *continued*
  recurrent — *continued*
    foot joint M24.47- ☑
    hand joint M24.44- ☑
    hip M24.45- ☑
    knee M24.46- ☑
      patella — *see* Dislocation, patella, recurrent
    patella — *see* Dislocation, patella, recurrent
    sacroiliac — *see* subcategory M53.2- ☑
    shoulder M24.41- ☑
    specified site NEC M24.49
    toe M24.47- ☑
    vertebra — *see also* subcategory M43.5- ☑
      atlantoaxial M43.4
        with myelopathy M43.3
    wrist M24.43- ☑
  rib (cartilage) S23.29- ☑
  sacrococcygeal S33.2- ☑
  sacroiliac (joint) (ligament) S33.2- ☑
    congenital Q74.2
    recurrent — *see* subcategory M53.2- ☑
  sacrum S33.2- ☑
  scaphoid (bone) (hand) (wrist) — *see* Dislocation, wrist
    foot — *see* Dislocation, foot
  scapula — *see* Dislocation, shoulder, girdle, scapula
  semilunar cartilage, knee — *see* Tear, meniscus
  septal cartilage (nose) S03.1- ☑
  septum (nasal) (old) J34.2
  sesamoid bone — *code by* site under Dislocation
  shoulder (blade) (ligament) (joint) (traumatic) S43.006- ☑
    acromioclavicular — *see* Dislocation, acromioclavicular
    chronic — *see* Dislocation, recurrent, shoulder
    congenital Q68.8
    girdle S43.30- ☑
      scapula S43.31- ☑
      specified site NEC S43.39- ☑
    humerus S43.00- ☑
      anterior S43.01- ☑
      inferior S43.03- ☑
      posterior S43.02- ☑
    pathological — *see* Dislocation, pathological NEC, shoulder
    recurrent — *see* Dislocation, recurrent, shoulder
    specified type NEC S43.08- ☑
  spine
    cervical — *see* Dislocation, vertebra, cervical
    congenital Q76.49
    due to birth trauma P11.5
    lumbar — *see* Dislocation, vertebra, lumbar
    thoracic — *see* Dislocation, vertebra, thoracic
  spontaneous — *see* Dislocation, pathological
  sternoclavicular (joint) S43.206- ☑
    anterior S43.21- ☑
    posterior S43.22- ☑
  sternum S23.29- ☑
  subglenoid — *see* Dislocation, shoulder
  symphysis pubis S33.4- ☑
  talus — *see* Dislocation, ankle
  tarsal (bone(s)) (joint(s)) — *see* Dislocation, foot
  tarsometatarsal (joint(s)) — *see* Dislocation, foot
  temporomandibular (joint) S03.0- ☑
  thigh, proximal end — *see* Dislocation, hip
  thorax S23.20- ☑
    specified site NEC S23.29- ☑
    vertebra — *see* Dislocation, vertebra
  thumb S63.10- ☑
    interphalangeal joint — *see* Dislocation, interphalangeal (joint), thumb
    metacarpophalangeal joint — *see* Dislocation, metacarpophalangeal (joint), thumb
  thyroid cartilage S13.29- ☑
  tibia
    distal end — *see* Dislocation, ankle
    proximal end — *see* Dislocation, knee
  tibiofibular (joint)
    distal — *see* Dislocation, ankle
    superior — *see* Dislocation, knee
  toe(s) S93.106- ☑
    great S93.10- ☑
      interphalangeal joint S93.11- ☑
      metatarsophalangeal joint S93.12- ☑
    interphalangeal joint S93.119- ☑
    lesser S93.106- ☑
      interphalangeal joint S93.11- ☑
      metatarsophalangeal joint S93.12- ☑

Dislocation — *continued*
  toe(s) — *continued*
    metatarsophalangeal joint S93.12- ☑
    tooth S03.2- ☑
    trachea S23.29- ☑
  ulna
    distal end S63.07- ☑
    proximal end — *see* Dislocation, elbow
  ulnohumeral (joint) — *see* Dislocation, elbow
  vertebra (articular process) (body) (traumatic)
    cervical S13.101- ☑
      atlantoaxial joint S13.121- ☑
      atlantooccipital joint S13.111- ☑
      atloidooccipital joint S13.111- ☑
      joint between
        C0 and C1 S13.111- ☑
        C1 and C2 S13.121- ☑
        C2 and C3 S13.131- ☑
        C3 and C4 S13.141- ☑
        C4 and C5 S13.151- ☑
        C5 and C6 S13.161- ☑
        C6 and C7 S13.171- ☑
        C7 and T1 S13.181- ☑
      occipitoatloid joint S13.111- ☑
    congenital Q76.49
    lumbar S33.101- ☑
      joint between
        L1 and L2 S33.111- ☑
        L2 and L3 S33.121- ☑
        L3 and L4 S33.131- ☑
        L4 and L5 S33.141- ☑
    nontraumatic — *see* Displacement, intervertebral disc
    partial — *see* Subluxation, by site
    recurrent NEC — *see* subcategory M43.5- ☑
    thoracic S23.101- ☑
      joint between
        T1 and T2 S23.111- ☑
        T2 and T3 S23.121- ☑
        T3 and T4 S23.123- ☑
        T4 and T5 S23.131- ☑
        T5 and T6 S23.133- ☑
        T6 and T7 S23.141- ☑
        T7 and T8 S23.143- ☑
        T8 and T9 S23.151- ☑
        T9 and T10 S23.153- ☑
        T10 and T11 S23.161- ☑
        T11 and T12 S23.163- ☑
        T12 and L1 S23.171- ☑
  wrist (carpal bone) S63.006- ☑
    carpometacarpal joint — *see* Dislocation, carpometacarpal (joint)
    distal radioulnar joint — *see* Dislocation, radioulnar (joint), distal
    metacarpal bone, proximal — *see* Dislocation, metacarpal (bone), proximal end
    midcarpal — *see* Dislocation, midcarpal (joint)
    radiocarpal joint — *see* Dislocation, radiocarpal (joint)
    recurrent — *see* Dislocation, recurrent, wrist
    specified site NEC S63.09- ☑
    ulna — *see* Dislocation, ulna, distal end
  xiphoid cartilage S23.29- ☑
Disorder (of) — *see also* Disease
  acantholytic L11.9
    specified NEC L11.8
  acute
    psychotic — *see* Psychosis, acute
    stress F43.0
  adjustment (grief) F43.20
    with
      anxiety F43.22
        with depressed mood F43.23
      conduct disturbance F43.24
        with emotional disturbance F43.25
      depressed mood F43.21
        with anxiety F43.23
      other specified symptom F43.29
  adrenal (capsule) (gland) (medullary) E27.9
    specified NEC E27.8
  adrenogenital — *see also* Adrenogenital syndrome E25.9
    drug-induced E25.8
    iatrogenic E25.8
    idiopathic E25.8
  adult personality (and behavior) F69
    specified NEC F68.8
  affective (mood) — *see* Disorder, mood
  aggressive, unsocialized F91.1
  alcohol-related F10.99

Disorder — continued
  alcohol-related — continued
    with
      amnestic disorder, persisting F10.96
      anxiety disorder F10.980
      dementia, persisting F10.97
      intoxication F10.929
        with delirium F10.921
        uncomplicated F10.920
      mood disorder F10.94
      other specified F10.988
      psychotic disorder F10.959
        with
          delusions F10.950
          hallucinations F10.951
      sexual dysfunction F10.981
      sleep disorder F10.982
  alcohol use
    mild F10.10
      with
        alcohol-induced
          anxiety disorder F10.180
          bipolar and related disorder F10.14
          depressive disorder F10.14
          psychotic disorder F10.159
          sexual dysfunction F10.181
          sleep disorder F10.182
        alcohol intoxication F10.129
          delirium F10.121
      in remission (early) (sustained) F10.11
    moderate or severe F10.20
      with
        alcohol-induced
          anxiety disorder F10.280
          bipolar and related disorder F10.24
          depressive disorder F10.24
          major neurocognitive disorder, amnestic-confabulatory type F10.26
          major neurocognitive disorder, nonamnestic-confabulatory type F10.27
          mild neurocognitive disorder F10.288
          psychotic disorder F10.259
          sexual dysfunction F10.281
          sleep disorder F10.282
        alcohol intoxication F10.229
          delirium F10.221
      in remission (early) (sustained) F10.21
  allergic — see Allergy
  alveolar NEC J84.09
  amino-acid
    cystathioninuria E72.19
    cystinosis E72.04
    cystinuria E72.01
    glycinuria E72.09
    homocystinuria E72.11
    metabolism — see Disturbance, metabolism, amino-acid
    specified NEC E72.89
    neonatal, transitory P74.8
    renal transport NEC E72.09
    transport NEC E72.09
  amnesic, amnestic
    alcohol-induced F10.96
      with dependence F10.26
    due to (secondary to) general medical condition F04
    psychoactive NEC-induced F19.96
      with
        abuse F19.16
        dependence F19.26
    sedative, hypnotic or anxiolytic-induced F13.96
      with dependence F13.26
  amphetamine-type substance use
    mild F15.10
      in remission (early) (sustained) F15.11
    moderate F15.20
      in remission (early) (sustained) F15.21
    severe F15.20
      in remission (early) (sustained) F15.21
  amphetamine (or other stimulant) use
    mild
      with
        amphetamine, cocaine, or other stimulant intoxication
          with perceptual disturbances F15.122
          without perceptual disturbances F15.129
        amphetamine (or other stimulant) -induced
          anxiety disorder F15.180
          bipolar and related disorder F15.14
          depressive disorder F15.14

Disorder — continued
  amphetamine use — continued
    mild — continued
      with — continued
        amphetamine -induced — continued
          obsessive-compulsive and related disorder F15.188
          psychotic disorder F15.159
          sexual dysfunction F15.181
        intoxication delirium F15.121
    moderate or severe
      with
        amphetamine, cocaine, or other stimulant intoxication
          with perceptual disturbances F15.222
          without perceptual disturbances F15.229
        amphetamine (or other stimulant) -induced
          anxiety disorder F15.280
          bipolar and related disorder F15.24
          depressive disorder F15.24
          obsessive-compulsive and related disorder F15.288
          psychotic disorder F15.259
          sexual dysfunction F15.281
        intoxication delirium F15.221
  anaerobic glycolysis with anemia D55.29
  anxiety F41.9
    due to (secondary to)
      alcohol F10.980
        in
          abuse F10.180
          dependence F10.280
      amphetamine F15.980
        in
          abuse F15.180
          dependence F15.280
      anxiolytic F13.980
        in
          abuse F13.180
          dependence F13.280
      caffeine F15.980
        in
          abuse F15.180
          dependence F15.280
      cannabis F12.980
        in
          abuse F12.180
          dependence F12.280
      cocaine F14.980
        in
          abuse F14.180
          dependence F14.180
      general medical condition F06.4
      hallucinogen F16.980
        in
          abuse F16.180
          dependence F16.280
      hypnotic F13.980
        in
          abuse F13.180
          dependence F13.280
      inhalant F18.980
        in
          abuse F18.180
          dependence F18.280
      phencyclidine F16.980
        in
          abuse F16.180
          dependence F16.280
      psychoactive substance NEC F19.980
        in
          abuse F19.180
          dependence F19.280
      sedative F13.980
        in
          abuse F13.180
          dependence F13.280
      volatile solvents F18.980
        in
          abuse F18.180
          dependence F18.280
    generalized F41.1
    illness F45.21
    mixed
      with depression (mild) F41.8
      specified NEC F41.3
    organic F06.4
    phobic F40.9
      of childhood F40.8

Disorder — continued
  anxiety — continued
    specified NEC F41.8
  aortic valve — see Endocarditis, aortic
  aromatic amino-acid metabolism E70.9
    specified NEC E70.89
  arteriole NEC I77.89
  artery NEC I77.89
  articulation — see Disorder, joint
  attachment (childhood)
    disinhibited F94.2
    reactive F94.1
  attention-deficit hyperactivity (adolescent) (adult) (child) F90.9
    combined
      presentation F90.2
      type F90.2
    hyperactive
      impulsive presentation F90.1
      type F90.1
    inattentive
      presentation F90.0
      type F90.0
    specified type NEC F90.8
  attention-deficit without hyperactivity (adolescent) (adult) (child) F98.8
  auditory processing (central) H93.25
  autism spectrum F84.0
  autistic F84.0
  autoimmune D89.89
  autonomic nervous system G90.9
    specified NEC G90.89
  avoidant
    child or adolescent F40.10
    restrictive food intake F50.82
  balance
    acid-base E87.8
      mixed E87.4
    electrolyte E87.8
    fluid NEC E87.8
  behavioral (disruptive) — see Disorder, conduct
  bereavement, persistent complex F43.81
  beta-amino-acid metabolism E72.89
  bile acid and cholesterol metabolism E78.70
    Barth syndrome E78.71
    other specified E78.79
    Smith-Lemli-Opitz syndrome E78.72
  bilirubin excretion E80.6
  binge eating F50.81- ☑
  binocular
    movement H51.9
      convergence
        excess H51.12
        insufficiency H51.11
      internuclear ophthalmoplegia — see Ophthalmoplegia, internuclear
      palsy of conjugate gaze H51.0
      specified type NEC H51.8
    vision NEC — see Disorder, vision, binocular
  bipolar (I) (seasonal) (type I) F31.9
    and related due to a known physiological condition
      with
        manic features F06.33
        manic- or hypomanic-like episodes F06.33
        mixed features F06.34
    current (or most recent) episode
      depressed F31.9
        with psychotic features F31.5
        without psychotic features F31.30
          mild F31.31
          moderate F31.32
          severe (without psychotic features) F31.4
            with psychotic features F31.5
      hypomanic F31.0
      manic F31.9
        with psychotic features F31.2
        without psychotic features F31.10
          mild F31.11
          moderate F31.12
          severe (without psychotic features) F31.13
            with psychotic features F31.2
      mixed F31.60
        mild F31.61
        moderate F31.62
        severe (without psychotic features) F31.63
          with psychotic features F31.64
      severe depression (without psychotic features) F31.4
        with psychotic features F31.5

☑ Additional Character Required — Refer to the Tabular List for Character Selection

Disorder — continued
- bipolar — continued
  - II (type 2) F31.81
  - in remission (currently) F31.70
    - in full remission
      - most recent episode
        - depressed F31.76
        - hypomanic F31.72
        - manic F31.74
        - mixed F31.78
    - in partial remission
      - most recent episode
        - depressed F31.75
        - hypomanic F31.71
        - manic F31.73
        - mixed F31.77
  - organic F06.30
  - single manic episode F30.9
    - mild F30.11
    - moderate F30.12
    - severe (without psychotic symptoms) F30.13
      - with psychotic symptoms F30.2
    - specified NEC F31.89
- bladder N32.9
  - functional NEC N31.9
  - in schistosomiasis B65.0 [N33]
  - specified NEC N32.89
- bleeding D68.9
- blood D75.9
  - in congenital early syphilis A50.09 [D77]
- body dysmorphic F45.22
- bone M89.9
  - continuity M84.9
    - specified type NEC M84.80
      - ankle M84.87- ☑
      - fibula M84.86- ☑
      - foot M84.87- ☑
      - hand M84.84- ☑
      - humerus M84.82- ☑
      - neck M84.88
      - pelvis M84.859
      - radius M84.83- ☑
      - rib M84.88
      - shoulder M84.81- ☑
      - skull M84.88
      - thigh M84.85- ☑
      - tibia M84.86- ☑
      - ulna M84.83- ☑
      - vertebra M84.88
  - density and structure M85.9
    - cyst — see also Cyst, bone, specified type NEC
      - aneurysmal — see Cyst, bone, aneurysmal
      - solitary — see Cyst, bone, solitary
    - diffuse idiopathic skeletal hyperostosis — see Hyperostosis, ankylosing
    - fibrous dysplasia (monostotic) — see Dysplasia, fibrous, bone
    - fluorosis — see Fluorosis, skeletal
    - hyperostosis of skull M85.2
    - osteitis condensans — see Osteitis, condensans
    - specified type NEC M85.8- ☑
      - ankle M85.87-
      - foot M85.87- ☑
      - forearm M85.83- ☑
      - hand M85.84- ☑
      - lower leg M85.86- ☑
      - multiple sites M85.89
      - neck M85.88
      - rib M85.88
      - shoulder M85.81- ☑
      - skull M85.88
      - thigh M85.85- ☑
      - upper arm M85.82- ☑
      - vertebra M85.88
  - development and growth NEC M89.20
    - carpus M89.24- ☑
    - clavicle M89.21- ☑
    - femur M89.25- ☑
    - fibula M89.26- ☑
    - finger M89.24- ☑
    - humerus M89.22- ☑
    - ilium M89.28
    - ischium M89.28
    - metacarpus M89.24- ☑
    - metatarsus M89.27- ☑
    - multiple sites M89.29
    - neck M89.28

Disorder — continued
- bone — continued
  - development and growth — continued
    - radius M89.23- ☑
    - rib M89.28
    - scapula M89.21- ☑
    - skull M89.28
    - tarsus M89.27- ☑
    - tibia M89.26- ☑
    - toe M89.27- ☑
    - ulna M89.23- ☑
    - vertebra M89.28
  - specified type NEC M89.8X- ☑
- brachial plexus G54.0
- branched-chain amino-acid metabolism E71.2
  - specified NEC E71.19
- breast N64.9
  - agalactia — see Agalactia
  - associated with
    - lactation O92.70
      - specified NEC O92.79
    - pregnancy O92.20
      - specified NEC O92.29
    - puerperium O92.20
      - specified NEC O92.29
  - cracked nipple — see Cracked nipple
  - galactorrhea — see Galactorrhea
  - hypogalactia O92.4
  - lactation disorder NEC O92.79
  - mastitis — see Mastitis
  - nipple infection — see Infection, nipple
  - retracted nipple — see Retraction, nipple
  - specified type NEC N64.89
- Briquet's F45.0
- bullous, in diseases classified elsewhere L14
- caffeine use
  - mild
    - with
      - caffeine-induced
        - anxiety disorder F15.180
        - sleep disorder F15.182
  - moderate or severe
    - with
      - caffeine-induced
        - anxiety disorder F15.280
        - sleep disorder F15.282
- cannabis use
  - mild F12.10
    - with
      - cannabis-induced
        - anxiety disorder F12.180
        - psychotic disorder F12.159
        - sleep disorder F12.188
      - cannabis intoxication delirium F12.121
        - with perceptual disturbances F12.122
        - without perceptual disturbances F12.129
    - in remission (early) (sustained) F12.11
  - moderate or severe F12.20
    - with
      - cannabis-induced
        - anxiety disorder F12.280
        - psychotic disorder F12.259
        - sleep disorder F12.288
      - cannabis intoxication
        - with perceptual disturbances F12.222
        - without perceptual disturbances F12.229
        - delirium F12.221
    - in remission (early) (sustained) F12.21
- carbohydrate
  - absorption, intestinal NEC E74.39
  - metabolism (congenital) E74.9
    - specified NEC E74.89
- cardiac, functional I51.89
- carnitine metabolism E71.40
- cartilage M94.9
  - articular NEC — see Derangement, joint, articular cartilage
  - chondrocalcinosis — see Chondrocalcinosis
  - specified type NEC M94.8X- ☑
    - articular — see Derangement, joint, articular cartilage
    - multiple sites M94.8X0
- catatonia (due to known physiological condition) (with another mental disorder) F06.1
- catatonic NOS F06.1
  - due to (secondary to) known physiological condition F06.1
  - organic NOS F06.1

Disorder — continued
- central auditory processing H93.25
- cervical
  - region NEC M53.82
  - root (nerve) NEC G54.2
- character NOS F60.9
- childhood disintegrative NEC F84.3
- cholesterol and bile acid metabolism E78.70
  - Barth syndrome E78.71
  - other specified E78.79
  - Smith-Lemli-Opitz syndrome E78.72
- choroid H31.9
  - atrophy — see Atrophy, choroid
  - degeneration — see Degeneration, choroid
  - detachment — see Detachment, choroid
  - dystrophy — see Dystrophy, choroid
  - hemorrhage — see Hemorrhage, choroid
  - rupture — see Rupture, choroid
  - scar — see Scar, chorioretinal
  - solar retinopathy — see Retinopathy, solar
  - specified type NEC H31.8
- ciliary body — see Disorder, iris
  - degeneration — see Degeneration, ciliary body
- citrate metabolism NEC E74.829
- citrate transporter, SLC13A5 E74.820
- coagulation (factor) — see also Defect, coagulation D68.9
  - newborn, transient P61.6
- cocaine use
  - mild F14.10
    - with
      - amphetamine, cocaine, or other stimulant intoxication
        - with perceptual disturbances F14.122
        - without perceptual disturbances F14.129
      - cocaine-induced
        - anxiety disorder F14.180
        - bipolar and related disorder F14.14
        - depressive disorder F14.14
        - obsessive-compulsive and related disorder F14.188
        - psychotic disorder F14.159
        - sexual dysfunction F14.181
        - sleep disorder F14.182
      - cocaine intoxication delirium F14.121
    - in remission (early) (sustained) F14.11
  - moderate or severe F14.20
    - with
      - amphetamine, cocaine, or other stimulant intoxication
        - with perceptual disturbances F14.222
        - without perceptual disturbances F14.229
      - cocaine-induced
        - anxiety disorder F14.280
        - bipolar and related disorder F14.24
        - depressive disorder F14.24
        - obsessive-compulsive and related disorder F14.288
        - psychotic disorder F14.259
        - sexual dysfunction F14.281
        - sleep disorder F14.282
      - cocaine intoxication delirium F14.221
    - in remission (early) (sustained) F14.21
- coccyx NEC M53.3
- cognitive F09
  - due to (secondary to) general medical condition F09
  - persisting R41.89
    - due to
      - alcohol F10.97
        - with dependence F10.27
      - anxiolytics F13.97
        - with dependence F13.27
      - hypnotics F13.97
        - with dependence F13.27
      - sedatives F13.97
        - with dependence F13.27
      - specified substance NEC F19.97
        - with
          - abuse F19.17
          - dependence F19.27
- communication F80.9
  - social pragmatic F80.82
- conduct (childhood) F91.9
  - adjustment reaction — see Disorder, adjustment
  - adolescent onset type F91.2
  - childhood onset type F91.1
  - compulsive F63.9
  - confined to family context F91.0
  - depressive F91.8
  - group type F91.2

Disorder — *continued*
- conduct — *continued*
  - hyperkinetic — *see* Disorder, attention-deficit hyperactivity
  - oppositional defiance F91.3
  - socialized F91.2
  - solitary aggressive type F91.1
  - specified NEC F91.8
  - unsocialized (aggressive) F91.1
- conduction, heart I45.9
- congenital glycosylation (CDG) E74.89
- conjunctiva H11.9
  - infection — *see* Conjunctivitis
- connective tissue, localized L94.9
  - specified NEC L94.8
- conversion (functional neurological symptom disorder)
  - with
    - abnormal movement F44.4
    - anesthesia or sensory loss F44.6
    - attacks or seizures F44.5
    - mixed symptoms F44.7
    - special sensory symptoms F44.6
    - speech symptoms F44.4
    - swallowing symptoms F44.4
    - weakness or paralysis F44.4
- convulsive (secondary) — *see* Convulsions
- cornea H18.9
  - deformity — *see* Deformity, cornea
  - degeneration — *see* Degeneration, cornea
  - deposits — *see* Deposit, cornea
  - due to contact lens H18.82- ☑
    - specified as edema — *see* Edema, cornea
  - edema — *see* Edema, cornea
  - keratitis — *see* Keratitis
  - keratoconjunctivitis — *see* Keratoconjunctivitis
  - membrane change — *see* Change, corneal membrane
  - neovascularization — *see* Neovascularization, cornea
  - scar — *see* Opacity, cornea
  - specified type NEC H18.89- ☑
  - ulcer — *see* Ulcer, cornea
- corpus cavernosum N48.9
- cranial nerve — *see* Disorder, nerve, cranial
- Cyclin-Dependent Kinase-Like 5 Deficiency (CDKL5) G40.42
- cyclothymic F34.0
- defiant oppositional F91.3
- delusional (persistent) (systematized) F22
  - induced F24
- depersonalization F48.1
- depressive F32.A
  - due to known physiological condition
    - with
      - depressive features F06.31
      - major depressive-like episode F06.32
      - mixed features F06.34
  - major F32.9
    - with psychotic symptoms F32.3
    - in remission (full) F32.5
      - partial F32.4
    - recurrent F33.9
      - with psychotic features F33.3
    - single episode F32.9
      - mild F32.0
      - moderate F32.1
      - severe (without psychotic symptoms) F32.2
        - with psychotic symptoms F32.3
  - organic F06.31
  - persistent F34.1
  - recurrent F33.9
    - current episode
      - mild F33.0
      - moderate F33.1
      - severe (without psychotic symptoms) F33.2
        - with psychotic symptoms F33.3
    - in remission F33.40
      - full F33.42
      - partial F33.41
    - specified NEC F33.8
  - single episode — *see* Episode, depressive
  - specified NEC F32.89
- developmental F89
  - arithmetical skills F81.2
  - coordination (motor) F82
  - expressive writing F81.81
  - language F80.9
    - expressive F80.1
    - mixed receptive and expressive F80.2
    - receptive type F80.2
    - specified NEC F80.89

Disorder — *continued*
- developmental — *continued*
  - learning F81.9
    - arithmetical F81.2
    - reading F81.0
  - mixed F88
  - motor coordination or function F82
  - pervasive F84.9
    - specified NEC F84.8
  - phonological F80.0
  - reading F81.0
  - scholastic skills — *see also* Disorder, learning
    - mixed F81.89
  - specified NEC F88
  - speech F80.9
    - articulation F80.0
    - specified NEC F80.89
  - written expression F81.81
- diaphragm J98.6
- digestive (system) K92.9
  - newborn P78.9
    - specified NEC P78.89
  - postprocedural — *see* Complication, gastrointestinal
  - psychogenic F45.8
- disc (intervertebral) M51.9
  - with
    - myelopathy
      - cervical region M50.00
      - cervicothoracic region M50.03
      - high cervical region M50.01
      - lumbar region M51.06
      - mid-cervical region M50.020
      - sacrococcygeal region M53.3
      - thoracic region M51.04
      - thoracolumbar region M51.05
    - radiculopathy
      - cervical region M50.10
      - cervicothoracic region M50.13
      - high cervical region M50.11
      - lumbar region M51.16
      - lumbosacral region M51.17
      - mid-cervical region M50.120
      - sacrococcygeal region M53.3
      - thoracic region M51.14
      - thoracolumbar region M51.15
  - cervical M50.90
    - with
      - myelopathy M50.00
        - C2-C3 M50.01
        - C3-C4 M50.01
        - C4-C5 M50.021
        - C5-C6 M50.022
        - C6-C7 M50.023
        - C7-T1 M50.03
        - cervicothoracic region M50.03
        - high cervical region M50.01
        - mid-cervical region M50.020
      - neuritis, radiculitis or radiculopathy M50.10
        - C2-C3 M50.11
        - C3-C4 M50.11
        - C4-C5 M50.121
        - C5-C6 M50.122
        - C6-C7 M50.123
        - C7-T1 M50.13
        - cervicothoracic region M50.13
        - high cervical region M50.11
        - mid-cervical region M50.120
    - C2-C3 M50.91
    - C3-C4 M50.91
    - C4-C5 M50.921
    - C5-C6 M50.922
    - C6-C7 M50.923
    - C7-T1 M50.93
    - cervicothoracic region M50.93
    - degeneration M50.30
      - C2-C3 M50.31
      - C3-C4 M50.31
      - C4-C5 M50.321
      - C5-C6 M50.322
      - C6-C7 M50.323
      - C7-T1 M50.33
      - cervicothoracic region M50.33
      - high cervical region M50.31
      - mid-cervical region M50.320
    - displacement M50.20
      - C2-C3 M50.21
      - C3-C4 M50.21
      - C4-C5 M50.221
      - C5-C6 M50.222

Disorder — *continued*
- disc — *continued*
  - cervical — *continued*
    - displacement — *continued*
      - C6-C7 M50.223
      - C7-T1 M50.23
      - cervicothoracic region M50.23
      - high cervical region M50.21
      - mid-cervical region M50.220
    - high cervical region M50.91
    - mid-cervical region M50.920
    - specified type NEC M50.80
      - C2-C3 M50.81
      - C3-C4 M50.81
      - C4-C5 M50.821
      - C5-C6 M50.822
      - C6-C7 M50.823
      - C7-T1 M50.83
      - cervicothoracic region M50.83
      - high cervical region M50.81
      - mid-cervical region M50.820
  - specified NEC
    - lumbar region M51.86
    - lumbosacral region M51.87
    - sacrococcygeal region M53.3
    - thoracic region M51.84
    - thoracolumbar region M51.85
- disinhibited attachment (childhood) F94.2
- disintegrative, childhood NEC F84.3
- disruptive F91.9
  - mood dysregulation F34.81
  - specified NEC F91.8
- disruptive behavior — *see* Disorder, conduct
- dissocial personality F60.2
- dissociative F44.9
  - affecting
    - motor function F44.4
      - and sensation F44.7
    - sensation F44.6
      - and motor function F44.7
  - brief reactive F43.0
  - due to (secondary to) general medical condition F06.8
  - mixed F44.7
  - organic F06.8
  - other specified NEC F44.89
- double heterozygous sickling — *see* Disease, sickle-cell
- dream anxiety F51.5
- drug induced hemorrhagic D68.32
- drug related F19.99
  - abuse — *see* Abuse, drug
  - dependence — *see* Dependence, drug
- dysmorphic body F45.22
- dysthymic F34.1
- ear H93.9- ☑
  - bleeding — *see* Otorrhagia
  - deafness — *see* Deafness
  - degenerative H93.09- ☑
  - discharge — *see* Otorrhea
  - external H61.9- ☑
    - auditory canal stenosis — *see* Stenosis, external ear canal
    - exostosis — *see* Exostosis, external ear canal
    - impacted cerumen — *see* Impaction, cerumen
    - otitis — *see* Otitis, externa
    - perichondritis — *see* Perichondritis, ear
    - pinna — *see* Disorder, pinna
    - specified type NEC H61.89- ☑
  - inner H83.9- ☑
    - vestibular dysfunction — *see* Disorder, vestibular function
  - middle H74.9- ☑
    - adhesive H74.1- ☑
    - ossicle — *see* Abnormal, ear ossicles
    - polyp — *see* Polyp, ear (middle)
    - specified NEC, in diseases classified elsewhere H75.8- ☑
  - postprocedural — *see* Complications, ear, procedure
  - specified NEC, in diseases classified elsewhere H94.8- ☑
- eating (adult) (psychogenic) F50.9
  - anorexia — *see* Anorexia
  - binge F50.81- ☑
  - bulimia F50.2- ☑
  - child F98.29
    - pica (in remission) F98.3
    - rumination disorder (in remission) F98.21
  - pica F50.89
    - adult (in remission) F50.83

Disorder — continued
- eating — continued
  - pica — continued
    - childhood (in remission) F98.3
  - rumination — see also Rumination R11.10
    - adult (in remission) F50.84
    - infancy or childhood (in remission) F98.21
  - specified NEC F50.89
- electrolyte (balance) NEC E87.8
  - with
    - abortion — see Abortion by type complicated by specified condition NEC
    - ectopic pregnancy O08.5
    - molar pregnancy O08.5
  - acidosis (lactic) (metabolic) E87.20
    - acute E87.21
    - chronic E87.22
    - respiratory E87.29
    - specified NEC E87.29
  - alkalosis (metabolic) (respiratory) E87.3
- elimination, transepidermal L87.9
  - specified NEC L87.8
- emotional (persistent) F34.9
  - of childhood F93.9
  - specified NEC F93.8
- endocrine E34.9
  - postprocedural E89.89
  - specified NEC E89.89
- erectile (male) (organic) — see also Dysfunction, sexual, male, erectile N52.9
  - nonorganic F52.21
- erythematous — see Erythema
- esophagus K22.9
  - functional K22.4
  - psychogenic F45.8
- eustachian tube H69.9- ☑
  - infection — see Salpingitis, eustachian
  - obstruction — see Obstruction, eustachian tube
  - patulous — see Patulous, eustachian tube
  - specified NEC H69.8- ☑
- exhibitionistic F65.2
- extrapyramidal G25.9
  - in deseases classified elsewhere — see category G26
  - specified type NEC G25.89
- eye H57.9
  - postprocedural — see Complication, postprocedural, eye
- eyelid H02.9
  - cyst — see Cyst, eyelid
  - degenerative H02.70
    - chloasma — see Chloasma, eyelid
    - madarosis — see Madarosis
    - specified type NEC H02.79
    - vitiligo — see Vitiligo, eyelid
    - xanthelasma — see Xanthelasma
  - dermatochalasis — see Dermatochalasis
  - edema — see Edema, eyelid
  - elephantiasis — see Elephantiasis, eyelid
  - foreign body, retained — see Foreign body, retained, eyelid
  - function H02.59
    - abnormal innervation syndrome — see Syndrome, abnormal innervation
    - blepharochalasis — see Blepharochalasis
    - blepharoclonus — see Blepharoclonus
    - blepharophimosis — see Blepharophimosis
    - blepharoptosis — see Blepharoptosis
    - lagophthalmos — see Lagophthalmos
    - lid retraction — see Retraction, lid
  - hypertrichosis — see Hypertrichosis, eyelid
  - specified type NEC H02.89
  - vascular H02.879
    - left H02.876
      - lower H02.875
      - upper H02.874
    - right H02.873
      - lower H02.872
      - upper H02.871
- factitious
  - by proxy F68.A
  - imposed on another F68.A
  - imposed on self F68.10
    - with predominantly
      - psychological symptoms F68.11
        - with physical symptoms F68.13
      - physical symptoms F68.12
        - with psychological symptoms F68.13
- factor, coagulation — see Defect, coagulation

Disorder — continued
- fatty acid
  - metabolism E71.30
    - specified NEC E71.39
  - oxidation
    - LCAD E71.310
    - MCAD E71.311
    - SCAD E71.312
    - specified deficiency NEC E71.318
- feeding (infant or child) — see also Disorder, eating R63.30
  - or eating disorder F50.9
  - pediatric
    - acute R63.31
    - chronic R63.32
  - specified NEC F50.9
- feigned (with obvious motivation) Z76.5
  - without obvious motivation — see Disorder, factitious
- female
  - hypoactive sexual desire F52.0
  - orgasmic F52.31
  - sexual interest/arousal F52.22
- fetishistic F65.0
- fibroblastic M72.9
  - specified NEC M72.8
- fluency
  - adult onset F98.5
  - childhood onset F80.81
  - following
    - cerebral infarction I69.323
    - cerebrovascular disease I69.923
      - specified disease NEC I69.823
    - intracerebral hemorrhage I69.123
    - nontraumatic intracranial hemorrhage NEC I69.223
    - subarachnoid hemorrhage I69.023
  - in conditions classified elsewhere R47.82
- fluid balance E87.8
- follicular (skin) L73.9
  - specified NEC L73.8
- FOXG1-related Q A0.0151
- frotteuristic F65.81
- fructose metabolism E74.10
  - essential fructosuria E74.11
  - fructokinase deficiency E74.11
  - fructose-1, 6-diphosphatase deficiency E74.19
  - hereditary fructose intolerance E74.12
  - other specified E74.19
- functional polymorphonuclear neutrophils D71.9
  - specified NEC D71.8
- gallbladder, biliary tract and pancreas in diseases classified elsewhere K87
- gambling F63.0
- gamma aminobutyric acid (GABA) metabolism E72.81
- gamma-glutamyl cycle E72.89
- gastric (functional) K31.9
  - motility K30
  - psychogenic F45.8
  - secretion K30
- gastrointestinal (functional) NOS K92.9
  - newborn P78.9
  - psychogenic F45.8
- gender-identity or -role F64.9
  - childhood F64.2
  - effect on relationship F66
  - of adolescence or adulthood F64.0
    - nontranssexual F64.8
  - specified NEC F64.8
  - uncertainty F66
- gender incongruence F64.9
  - in adolescents and adults F64.0
  - of childhood F64.2
- genito-pelvic pain penetration F52.6
- genitourinary system
  - female N94.9
  - male N50.9
  - psychogenic F45.8
- globe H44.9
  - degenerated condition H44.50
    - absolute glaucoma H44.51- ☑
    - atrophy H44.52- ☑
    - leucocoria H44.53- ☑
  - degenerative H44.30
    - chalcosis H44.31- ☑
    - myopia — see also Myopia, degenerative H44.2- ☑
    - siderosis H44.32- ☑
    - specified type NEC H44.39- ☑
  - endophthalmitis — see Endophthalmitis

Disorder — continued
- globe — continued
  - foreign body, retained — see Foreign body, intraocular, old, retained
  - hemophthalmos — see Hemophthalmos
  - hypotony H44.40
    - due to
      - ocular fistula H44.42- ☑
      - specified disorder NEC H44.43- ☑
    - flat anterior chamber H44.41- ☑
    - primary H44.44- ☑
  - luxation — see Luxation, globe
  - specified type NEC H44.89
- glomerular (in) N05.9
  - amyloidosis E85.4 [N08]
  - cryoglobulinemia D89.1 [N08]
  - disseminated intravascular coagulation D65 [N08]
  - Fabry's disease E75.21 [N08]
  - familial lecithin cholesterol acyltransferase deficiency E78.6 [N08]
  - Goodpasture's syndrome M31.0
  - hemolytic-uremic syndrome — see Syndrome, hemolytic-uremic
  - Henoch (-Schonlein) purpura D69.0 [N08]
  - malariae malaria B52.0
  - microscopic polyangiitis M31.7 [N08]
  - multiple myeloma C90.0- ☑ [N08]
  - mumps B26.83
  - schistosomiasis B65.9 [N08]
  - sepsis NEC A41.- ☑ [N08]
    - streptococcal A40.- ☑ [N08]
  - sickle-cell disorders D57.- ☑ [N08]
  - strongyloidiasis B78.9 [N08]
  - subacute bacterial endocarditis I33.0 [N08]
  - syphilis A52.75
  - systemic lupus erythematosus M32.14
  - thrombotic thrombocytopenic purpura M31.19 [N08]
  - Waldenstrom macroglobulinemia C88.0- ☑ [N08]
  - Wegener's granulomatosis M31.31
- gluconeogenesis E74.4
- glucosaminoglycan metabolism — see Disorder, metabolism, glucosaminoglycan
- glucose transport E74.819
  - specified NEC E74.818
- glycine metabolism E72.50
  - d-glycericacidemia E72.59
  - hyperhydroxyprolinemia E72.59
  - hyperoxaluria R82.992
    - dietary E72.540
    - enteric E72.541
    - primary E72.539
      - specified type NEC E72.538
      - type 1 E72.530
      - type 2 E72.538
      - type 3 E72.538
    - secondary E72.549
      - specified type NEC E72.548
  - hyperprolinemia E72.59
  - non-ketotic hyperglycinemia E72.51
  - oxalosis E72.53- ☑
  - oxaluria E72.53- ☑
  - sarcosinemia E72.59
  - trimethylaminuria E72.52
- glycoprotein metabolism E77.9
  - specified NEC E77.8
- grief
  - complicated F43.81
  - prolonged F43.81
- habit (and impulse) F63.9
  - involving sexual behavior NEC F65.9
  - specified NEC F63.89
- hallucinogen use
  - mild F16.10
    - with
      - hallucinogen-induced
        - anxiety disorder F16.180
        - bipolar and related disorder F16.14
        - depressive disorder F16.14
        - psychotic disorder F16.159
      - hallucinogen intoxication delirium F16.121
      - other hallucinogen intoxication F16.129
    - in remission (early) (sustained) F16.11
  - moderate or severe F16.20
    - with
      - hallucinogen-induced
        - anxiety disorder F16.280
        - bipolar and related disorder F16.24
        - depressive disorder F16.24

Disorder — *continued*
- hallucinogen use — *continued*
  - moderate or severe — *continued*
    - with — *continued*
      - hallucinogen-induced — *continued*
        - psychotic disorder F16.259
      - hallucinogen intoxication delirium F16.221
      - other hallucinogen intoxication F16.229
    - in remission (early) (sustained) F16.21
- heart action I49.9
- hematological D75.9
  - newborn (transient) P61.9
    - specified NEC P61.8
- hematopoietic organs D75.9
- hemorrhagic NEC D69.9
  - drug-induced D68.32
  - due to
    - extrinsic circulating anticoagulants D68.32
    - increase in
      - anti-IIa D68.32
      - anti-Xa D68.32
    - intrinsic
      - circulating anticoagulants D68.318
      - increase in
        - anti-VIIIa D68.318
        - anti-IXa D68.318
        - anti-XIa D68.318
        - antithrombin D68.318
    - following childbirth O72.3
- hemostasis — *see* Defect, coagulation
- histidine metabolism E70.40
  - histidinemia E70.41
  - other specified E70.49
- hoarding F42.3
- hyperkinetic — *see* Disorder, attention-deficit hyperactivity
- hyperleucine-isoleucinemia E71.19
- hypervalinemia E71.19
- hypoactive sexual desire F52.0
- hypochondriacal F45.20
  - body dysmorphic F45.22
  - neurosis F45.21
  - other specified F45.29
- identity
  - dissociative F44.81
  - illness anxiety F45.21
  - of childhood F93.8
- immune mechanism (immunity) D89.9
  - specified type NEC D89.89
- impaired renal tubular function N25.9
  - specified NEC N25.89
- impulse (control) F63.9
- inflammatory
  - pelvic, in diseases classified elsewhere — *see* category N74
  - penis N48.29
    - abscess N48.21
    - cellulitis N48.22
- inhalant use
  - mild F18.10
    - with
      - inhalant-induced
        - anxiety disorder F18.180
        - depressive disorder F18.14
        - major neurocognitive disorder F18.17
        - mild neurocognitive disorder F18.188
        - psychotic disorder F18.159
      - inhalant intoxication F18.129
      - inhalant intoxication delirium F18.121
    - in remission (early) (sustained) F18.11
  - moderate or severe F18.20
    - with
      - inhalant-induced
        - anxiety disorder F18.280
        - depressive disorder F18.24
        - major neurocognitive disorder F18.27
        - mild neurocognitive disorder F18.288
        - psychotic disorder F18.259
      - inhalant intoxication F18.229
      - inhalant intoxication delirium F18.221
    - in remission (early) (sustained) F18.21
- integument, newborn P83.9
  - specified NEC P83.88
- intermittent explosive F63.81
- internal secretion pancreas — *see* Increased, secretion, pancreas, endocrine
- intestine, intestinal
  - carbohydrate absorption NEC E74.39
    - postoperative K91.2

Disorder — *continued*
- intestine, intestinal — *continued*
  - functional NEC K59.9
    - postoperative K91.89
  - psychogenic F45.8
  - vascular K55.9
    - chronic K55.1
    - specified NEC K55.8
- intraoperative (intraprocedural) — *see* Complications, intraoperative
- involuntary emotional expression (IEED) F07.89
- iris H21.9
  - adhesions — *see* Adhesions, iris
  - atrophy — *see* Atrophy, iris
  - chamber angle recession — *see* Recession, chamber angle
  - cyst — *see* Cyst, iris
  - degeneration — *see* Degeneration, iris
  - in diseases classified elsewhere H22
  - iridodialysis — *see* Iridodialysis
  - iridoschisis — *see* Iridoschisis
  - miotic pupillary cyst — *see* Cyst, pupillary
  - pupillary
    - abnormality — *see* Abnormality, pupillary
    - membrane — *see* Membrane, pupillary
  - specified type NEC H21.89
  - vascular NEC H21.1X- ☑
- iron metabolism E83.10
  - specified NEC E83.19
- isovaleric acidemia E71.110
- jaw, developmental M27.0
  - temporomandibular — *see also* Anomaly, dentofacial, temporomandibular joint M26.60- ☑
- joint M25.9
  - derangement — *see* Derangement, joint
  - effusion — *see* Effusion, joint
  - fistula — *see* Fistula, joint
  - hemarthrosis — *see* Hemarthrosis
  - instability — *see* Instability, joint
  - osteophyte — *see* Osteophyte
  - pain — *see* Pain, joint
  - psychogenic F45.8
  - specified type NEC M25.80
    - ankle M25.87- ☑
    - elbow M25.82- ☑
    - foot joint M25.87- ☑
    - hand joint M25.84- ☑
    - hip M25.85- ☑
    - knee M25.86- ☑
    - shoulder M25.81- ☑
    - wrist M25.83- ☑
  - stiffness — *see* Stiffness, joint
- ketone metabolism E71.32
- kidney N28.9
  - functional (tubular) N25.9
  - in
    - schistosomiasis B65.9 *[N29]*
  - tubular function N25.9
    - specified NEC N25.89
- lacrimal system H04.9
  - changes H04.69
    - fistula — *see* Fistula, lacrimal
  - gland H04.19
    - atrophy — *see* Atrophy, lacrimal gland
    - cyst — *see* Cyst, lacrimal, gland
    - dacryops — *see* Dacryops
    - dislocation — *see* Dislocation, lacrimal gland
    - dry eye syndrome — *see* Syndrome, dry eye
    - infection — *see* Dacryoadenitis
    - granuloma — *see* Granuloma, lacrimal
    - inflammation — *see* Inflammation, lacrimal
    - obstruction — *see* Obstruction, lacrimal
  - specified NEC H04.89
- lactation NEC O92.79
- language (developmental) F80.9
  - expressive F80.1
  - mixed receptive and expressive F80.2
  - receptive F80.2
- late luteal phase dysphoric N94.89
- learning (specific) F81.9
  - acalculia R48.8
  - alexia R48.0
  - mathematics F81.2
  - reading F81.0
  - specified
    - with impairment in
      - mathematics F81.2
      - reading F81.0

Disorder — *continued*
- learning — *continued*
  - specified — *continued*
    - with impairment in — *continued*
      - written expression F81.81
    - specified NEC F81.89
    - spelling F81.81
    - written expression F81.81
- lens H27.9
  - aphakia — *see* Aphakia
  - cataract — *see* Cataract
  - dislocation — *see* Dislocation, lens
  - specified type NEC H27.8
- ligament M24.20
  - ankle M24.27- ☑
  - attachment, spine — *see* Enthesopathy, spinal
  - elbow M24.22- ☑
  - foot joint M24.27- ☑
  - hand joint M24.24- ☑
  - hip M24.25- ☑
  - knee — *see* Derangement, knee, specified NEC
  - shoulder M24.21- ☑
  - specified site NEC M24.29
  - vertebra M24.28
  - wrist M24.23- ☑
- ligamentous attachments — *see also* Enthesopathy
  - spine — *see* Enthesopathy, spinal
- lipid
  - metabolism, congenital E78.9
  - storage E75.6
    - specified NEC E75.5
- lipoprotein
  - deficiency (familial) E78.6
  - metabolism E78.9
    - specified NEC E78.89
- liver K76.9
  - malarial B54 *[K77]*
- low back — *see also* Dorsopathy, specified NEC
- lumbosacral
  - plexus G54.1
  - root (nerve) NEC G54.4
- lung, interstitial, drug-induced J70.4
  - acute J70.2
  - chronic J70.3
  - dabbing (related) U07.0
  - e-cigarette (related) U07.0
  - electronic cigarette (related) U07.0
  - vaping (associated) (device) (product) (related) (use) U07.0
- lymphoproliferative, post-transplant (PTLD) D47.Z1 (*following* D47.4)
- lysine and hydroxylysine metabolism E72.3
- major neurocognitive — *see also* Dementia, in (due to) F03.- ☑
- male
  - erectile (organic) — *see also* Dysfunction, sexual, male, erectile N52.9
    - nonorganic F52.21
  - hypoactive sexual desire F52.0
  - orgasmic F52.32
- manic F30.9
  - organic F06.33
- mast cell activation — *see* Activation, mast cell
- mastoid — *see also* Disorder, ear, middle
  - postprocedural — *see* Complications, ear, procedure
- meninges, specified type NEC G96.198
- meniscus — *see* Derangement, knee, meniscus
- menopausal N95.9
  - specified NEC N95.8
- menstrual N92.6
  - psychogenic F45.8
  - specified NEC N92.5
- mental (or behavioral) (nonpsychotic) F99
  - due to (secondary to)
    - amphetamine
      - due to drug abuse — *see* Abuse, drug, stimulant
      - due to drug dependence — *see* Dependence, drug, stimulant
    - brain disease, damage and dysfunction F09
    - caffeine use
      - due to drug abuse — *see* Abuse, drug, stimulant
      - due to drug dependence — *see* Dependence, drug, stimulant
    - cannabis use
      - due to drug abuse — *see* Abuse, drug, cannabis

Disorder — continued
- mental — continued
  - due to — continued
    - cannabis use — continued
      - due to drug dependence — see Dependence, drug, cannabis
    - general medical condition F09
    - sedative or hypnotic use
      - due to drug abuse — see Abuse, drug, sedative
      - due to drug dependence — see Dependence, drug, sedative
    - tobacco (nicotine) use — see Dependence, drug, nicotine
  - following organic brain damage F07.9
    - frontal lobe syndrome F07.0
    - personality change F07.0
    - postconcussional syndrome F07.81
    - specified NEC F07.89
  - infancy, childhood or adolescence F98.9
  - neurotic — see Neurosis
  - organic or symptomatic F09
  - presenile, psychotic F03.- ☑
  - problem NEC
  - psychoneurotic — see Neurosis
  - psychotic — see Psychosis
  - puerperal F53.0
  - senile, psychotic NEC F03.- ☑
- metabolic, amino acid, transitory, newborn P74.8
- metabolism NOS E88.9
  - amino-acid E72.9
    - aromatic E70.9
      - albinism — see Albinism
      - histidine E70.40
        - histidinemia E70.41
        - other specified E70.49
      - hyperphenylalaninemia E70.1
        - classical phenylketonuria E70.0
      - other specified E70.89
      - tryptophan E70.5
      - tyrosine E70.20
        - hypertyrosinemia E70.21
        - other specified E70.29
    - branched chain E71.2
      - 3-methylglutaconic aciduria E71.111
      - hyperleucine-isoleucinemia E71.19
      - hypervalinemia E71.19
      - isovaleric acidemia E71.110
      - maple syrup urine disease E71.0
      - methylmalonic acidemia E71.120
      - organic aciduria NEC E71.118
      - other specified E71.19
      - propionate NEC E71.128
      - propionic acidemia E71.121
    - glycine E72.50
      - d-glycericacidemia E72.59
      - hyperhydroxyprolinemia E72.59
      - hyperoxaluria R82.992
        - primary E72.53- ☑
      - hyperprolinemia E72.59
      - non-ketotic hyperglycinemia E72.51
      - other specified E72.59
      - sarcosinemia E72.59
      - trimethylaminuria E72.52
    - hydroxylysine E72.3
    - lysine E72.3
    - ornithine E72.4
    - other specified E72.89
      - beta-amino acid E72.89
      - gamma-glutamyl cycle E72.89
    - straight-chain E72.89
    - sulfur-bearing E72.10
      - homocystinuria E72.11
      - methylenetetrahydrofolate reductase deficiency E72.12
      - other specified E72.19
  - bile acid and cholesterol metabolism E78.70
  - bilirubin E80.7
    - specified NEC E80.6
  - calcium E83.50
    - hypercalcemia E83.52
    - hypocalcemia E83.51
    - other specified E83.59
  - carbohydrate E74.9
    - specified NEC E74.89
  - cholesterol and bile acid metabolism E78.70
  - citrate NEC E74.829
  - congenital E88.9
  - copper E83.00
    - specified type NEC E83.09

Disorder — continued
- metabolism — continued
  - copper — continued
    - Wilson's disease E83.01
  - cystinuria E72.01
  - fructose E74.10
  - galactose E74.20
  - glucosaminoglycan E76.9
    - mucopolysaccharidosis — see Mucopolysaccharidosis
    - specified NEC E76.8
  - glutamine E72.89
  - glycine E72.50
  - glycogen storage (hepatorenal) E74.09
  - glycoprotein E77.9
    - specified NEC E77.8
  - glycosaminoglycan E76.9
    - specified NEC E76.8
  - in labor and delivery O75.89
  - iron E83.10
  - isoleucine E71.19
  - leucine E71.19
  - lipoid E78.9
  - lipoprotein E78.9
    - specified NEC E78.89
  - magnesium E83.40
    - hypermagnesemia E83.41
    - hypomagnesemia E83.42
    - other specified E83.49
  - mineral E83.9
    - specified NEC E83.89
  - mitochondrial E88.40
    - aminoacyl-tRNA synthetase E88.43
    - ARS2-related E88.43
    - MELAS syndrome E88.41
    - MERRF syndrome (myoclonic epilepsy associated with ragged-red fibers) E88.42
    - other specified E88.49
    - tRNA synthetases E88.43
  - ornithine E72.4
  - phosphatases E83.30
  - phosphorus E83.30
    - acid phosphatase deficiency E83.39
    - hypophosphatasia E83.39
    - hypophosphatemia E83.39
      - familial E83.31
    - other specified E83.39
    - pseudovitamin D deficiency E83.32
  - plasma protein NEC E88.09
  - porphyrin — see Porphyria
  - postprocedural E89.89
    - specified NEC E89.89
  - purine E79.9
    - specified NEC E79.89
  - pyrimidine E79.9
    - specified NEC E79.89
  - pyruvate E74.4
  - serine E72.89
  - sodium E87.8
  - specified NEC E88.89
  - threonine E72.89
  - valine E71.19
  - zinc E83.2
- methylmalonic acidemia E71.120
- micturition NEC — see also Difficulty, micturition R39.198
  - feeling of incomplete emptying R39.14
  - hesitancy R39.11
  - poor stream R39.12
  - psychogenic F45.8
  - split stream R39.13
  - straining R39.16
  - urgency R39.15
- mild neurocognitive G31.84
  - due to known physiological condition (without behavioral disturbance) F06.70
  - with behavioral disturbance F06.71
- mitochondrial metabolism E88.40
- mitral (valve) — see Endocarditis, mitral
- mixed
  - anxiety and depressive F41.8
  - of scholastic skills (developmental) F81.89
  - receptive expressive language F80.2
- mood F39
  - bipolar — see Disorder, bipolar
  - depressive — see Disorder, depressive
  - due to (secondary to)
    - alcohol F10.94
    - amphetamine F15.94

Disorder — continued
- mood — continued
  - due to — continued
    - amphetamine — continued
      - in
        - abuse F15.14
        - dependence F15.24
    - anxiolytic F13.94
      - in
        - abuse F13.14
        - dependence F13.24
    - cocaine F14.94
      - in
        - abuse F14.14
        - dependence F14.24
    - general medical condition F06.30
    - hallucinogen F16.94
      - in
        - abuse F16.14
        - dependence F16.24
    - hypnotic F13.94
      - in
        - abuse F13.14
        - dependence F13.24
    - inhalant F18.94
      - in
        - abuse F18.14
        - dependence F18.24
    - opioid F11.94
      - in
        - abuse F11.14
        - dependence F11.24
    - phencyclidine (PCP) F16.94
      - in
        - abuse F16.14
        - dependence F16.24
    - physiological condition F06.30
      - with
        - depressive features F06.31
        - major depressive-like episode F06.32
        - manic features F06.33
        - mixed features F06.34
    - psychoactive substance NEC F19.94
      - in
        - abuse F19.14
        - dependence F19.24
    - sedative F13.94
      - in
        - abuse F13.14
        - dependence F13.24
    - volatile solvents F18.94
      - in
        - abuse F18.14
        - dependence F18.24
  - manic episode F30.9
    - with psychotic symptoms F30.2
    - in remission (full) F30.4
      - partial F30.3
    - specified type NEC F30.8
    - without psychotic symptoms F30.10
      - mild F30.11
      - moderate F30.12
      - severe F30.13
  - organic F06.30
    - right hemisphere F07.89
  - persistent F34.9
    - cyclothymia F34.0
    - dysthymia F34.1
    - specified type NEC F34.89
  - recurrent F39
  - right hemisphere organic F07.89
- movement G25.9
  - drug-induced G25.70
    - akathisia G25.71
    - specified NEC G25.79
  - hysterical F44.4
  - in diseases classified elsewhere — see category G26
  - periodic limb G47.61
    - sleep related G47.61
  - sleep related NEC G47.69
  - specified NEC G25.89
  - stereotyped F98.4
  - treatment-induced G25.9
- multiple personality F44.81
- muscle M62.9
  - attachment, spine — see Enthesopathy, spinal
  - in trichinellosis — see Trichinellosis, with muscle disorder
  - psychogenic F45.8

Disorder — *continued*
- muscle — *continued*
    - specified type NEC M62.89
    - tone, newborn P94.9
        - specified NEC P94.8
- muscular
    - attachments — *see also* Enthesopathy
        - spine — *see* Enthesopathy, spinal
    - urethra N36.44
- musculoskeletal system, soft tissue — *see* Disorder, soft tissue
    - postprocedural M96.89
    - psychogenic F45.8
- myoneural G70.9
    - due to lead G70.1
    - specified NEC G70.89
    - toxic G70.1
- myotonic NEC G71.19
- nail, in diseases classified elsewhere L62
- neck region NEC — *see* Dorsopathy, specified NEC
- neonatal onset multisystemic inflammatory (NOMID) M04.2
- nerve G58.9
    - abducent NEC — *see* Strabismus, paralytic, sixth nerve
    - accessory G52.8
    - acoustic — *see* subcategory H93.3- ☑
    - auditory — *see* subcategory H93.3- ☑
    - auriculotemporal G50.8
    - axillary G54.0
    - cerebral — *see* Disorder, nerve, cranial
    - cranial G52.9
        - eighth — *see* subcategory H93.3- ☑
        - eleventh G52.8
        - fifth G50.9
        - first G52.0
        - fourth NEC — *see* Strabismus, paralytic, fourth nerve
        - multiple G52.7
        - ninth G52.1
        - second NEC — *see* Disorder, nerve, optic
        - seventh NEC G51.8
        - sixth NEC — *see* Strabismus, paralytic, sixth nerve
        - specified NEC G52.8
        - tenth G52.2
        - third NEC — *see* Strabismus, paralytic, third nerve
        - twelfth G52.3
    - entrapment — *see* Neuropathy, entrapment
    - facial G51.9
        - specified NEC G51.8
    - femoral — *see* Lesion, nerve, femoral
    - glossopharyngeal NEC G52.1
    - hypoglossal G52.3
    - intercostal G58.0
    - lateral
        - cutaneous of thigh — *see* Mononeuropathy, lower limb, meralgia paresthetica
        - popliteal — *see* Lesion, nerve, popliteal
    - lower limb — *see* Mononeuropathy, lower limb
    - medial popliteal — *see* Lesion, nerve, popliteal, medial
    - median NEC — *see* Lesion, nerve, median
    - multiple G58.7
    - oculomotor NEC — *see* Strabismus, paralytic, third nerve
    - olfactory G52.0
    - optic NEC H47.09- ☑
        - hemorrhage into sheath — *see* Hemorrhage, optic nerve
        - ischemic H47.01- ☑
    - peroneal — *see* Lesion, nerve, popliteal
    - phrenic G58.8
    - plantar — *see* Lesion, nerve, plantar
    - pneumogastric G52.2
    - posterior tibial — *see* Syndrome, tarsal tunnel
    - radial — *see* Lesion, nerve, radial
    - recurrent laryngeal G52.2
    - root G54.9
        - cervical G54.2
        - lumbosacral G54.1
        - specified NEC G54.8
        - thoracic G54.3
    - sciatic NEC — *see* Lesion, nerve, sciatic
    - specified NEC G58.8
        - lower limb — *see* Mononeuropathy, lower limb, specified NEC
        - upper limb — *see* Mononeuropathy, upper limb, specified NEC
    - sympathetic G90.9
    - tibial — *see* Lesion, nerve, popliteal, medial

Disorder — *continued*
- nerve — *continued*
    - trigeminal G50.9
        - specified NEC G50.8
    - trochlear NEC — *see* Strabismus, paralytic, fourth nerve
    - ulnar — *see* Lesion, nerve, ulnar
    - upper limb — *see* Mononeuropathy, upper limb
    - vagus G52.2
- nervous system G98.8
    - autonomic (peripheral) G90.9
        - specified NEC G90.89
    - central G96.9
        - specified NEC G96.89
    - parasympathetic G90.9
    - specified NEC G98.8
    - sympathetic G90.9
    - vegetative G90.9
- neurocognitive R41.9
    - with Lewy bodies — *see also* Dementia, in, diseases specified elsewhere G31.83 [F02.-] ☑
    - frontotemporal, specified NEC — *see also* Dementia, in, diseases specified elsewhere G31.09 [F02.-] ☑
    - major — *see also* Dementia F03.- ☑
        - due to vascular disease — *see* Dementia, vascular
            - mild — *see* Dementia, vascular, mild
            - moderate — *see* Dementia, vascular, moderate
            - severe — *see* Dementia, vascular, severe
        - in (due to) (other diseases classified elsewhere) — *see also* Dementia, in (due to) F02.80
            - with
                - aggressive behavior — *see also* Dementia, in (due to) F02.81- ☑
                - combative behavior — *see also* Dementia, in (due to) F02.81- ☑
                - violent behavior — *see also* Dementia, in (due to) F02.81- ☑
    - mild (of uncertain or unknown etiology) — *see also* Disorder, mild neurocognitive G31.84
- neurodevelopmental F89
    - CACNA1A-related QA0.0102
    - DLG4-related synaptopathy QA0.0142
    - FOXG1-related QA0.0151
    - GRIA1-related QA0.011
    - GRIA2-related QA0.011
    - GRIA3-related QA0.011
    - GRIA4-related QA0.011
    - GRIK2-related QA0.011
    - GRIN1-related QA0.011
    - GRIN2A-related QA0.011
    - GRIN2B-related QA0.011
    - GRIN2D-related QA0.011
    - other
        - glutamate receptor, ionotropic, related QA0.011
        - ion channel gene related QA0.0109
        - receptor gene related QA0.012
        - related to other genes associated with transcription and gene expression QA0.0159
        - synapse related gene QA0.0149
        - transporter or solute carrier gene related QA0.0139
    - SCN2A-related QA0.0101
    - SLC6A1-related QA0.0131
    - specified NEC F88
        - related to pathogenic variants in specific genes NEC QA0.8
    - STXBP1-related QA0.0141
    - syntaxin-binding protein 1-related QA0.0141
- neurohypophysis NEC E23.3
- neurological NEC R29.818
    - TUBB4A-related G23.3
- neuromuscular G70.9
    - hereditary NEC G71.9
    - specified NEC G70.89
    - toxic G70.1
- neurotic F48.9
    - specified NEC F48.8
- neutrophil, polymorphonuclear D71.9
    - specified NEC D71.8
- nicotine use — *see* Dependence, drug, nicotine
- nightmare F51.5
- non-rapid eye movement sleep arousal
    - sleep terror type F51.4
    - sleepwalking type F51.3
- nose J34.9
    - specified NEC J34.89
- obsessive-compulsive F42.9

Disorder — *continued*
- obsessive-compulsive — *continued*
    - and related disorder due to a known physiological condition F06.8
- odontogenesis NOS K00.9
- opioid use
    - with
        - opioid-induced psychotic disorder F11.959
            - with
                - delusions F11.950
                - hallucinations F11.951
        - due to drug dependence — *see* Dependence, drug, opioid
    - mild F11.10
        - with
            - opioid-induced
                - anxiety disorder F11.188
                - depressive disorder F11.14
                - sexual dysfunction F11.181
            - opioid intoxication
                - with perceptual disturbances F11.122
                - delirium F11.121
                - without perceptual disturbances F11.129
        - in remission (early) (sustained) F11.11
    - moderate or severe F11.20
        - with
            - opioid-induced
                - anxiety disorder F11.288
                - depressive disorder F11.24
                - sexual dysfunction F11.281
            - opioid intoxication
                - with perceptual disturbances F11.222
                - delirium F11.221
                - without perceptual disturbances F11.229
        - in remission (early) (sustained) F11.21
- oppositional defiant F91.3
- optic
    - chiasm H47.49
        - due to
            - inflammatory disorder H47.41
            - neoplasm H47.42
            - vascular disorder H47.43
    - disc H47.39- ☑
        - coloboma — *see* Coloboma, optic disc
        - drusen — *see* Drusen, optic disc
        - pseudopapilledema — *see* Pseudopapilledema
    - radiations — *see* Disorder, visual, pathway
    - tracts — *see* Disorder, visual, pathway
- orbit H05.9
    - cyst — *see* Cyst, orbit
    - deformity — *see* Deformity, orbit
    - edema — *see* Edema, orbit
    - enophthalmos — *see* Enophthalmos
    - exophthalmos — *see* Exophthalmos
    - hemorrhage — *see* Hemorrhage, orbit
    - inflammation — *see* Inflammation, orbit
    - myopathy — *see* Myopathy, extraocular muscles
    - retained foreign body — *see* Foreign body, orbit, old
    - specified type NEC H05.89
- organic
    - anxiety F06.4
    - catatonic NOS F06.1
    - delusional F06.2
    - dissociative F06.8
    - emotionally labile (asthenic) F06.8
    - mood (affective) F06.30
    - schizophrenia-like F06.2
- orgasmic (female) F52.31
    - male F52.32
- ornithine metabolism E72.4
- overanxious F41.1
    - of childhood F93.8
- pain
    - with related psychological factors F45.42
    - exclusively related to psychological factors F45.41
    - genito-pelvic penetration disorder F52.6
- pancreatic internal secretion E16.9
    - specified NEC E16.8
- panic F41.0
    - with agoraphobia F40.01
- papulosquamous L44.9
    - in diseases classified elsewhere L45
    - specified NEC L44.8
- paranoid F22
    - induced F24
    - shared F24
- paraphilic F65.9
    - specified NEC F65.89
- parathyroid (gland) E21.5

Disorder — continued
- parathyroid — continued
  - specified NEC E21.4
- parietoalveolar NEC J84.09
- paroxysmal, mixed R56.9
- patella M22.9- ☑
  - chondromalacia — see Chondromalacia, patella
  - derangement NEC M22.3X- ☑
  - recurrent
    - dislocation — see Dislocation, patella, recurrent
    - subluxation — see Dislocation, patella, recurrent, incomplete
  - specified NEC M22.8X- ☑
- patellofemoral M22.2X- ☑
- pedophilic F65.4
- pentose phosphate pathway with anemia D55.1
- perception, due to hallucinogens F16.983
  - in
    - abuse F16.183
    - dependence F16.283
- peripheral nervous system NEC G64
- peroxisomal E71.50
  - biogenesis
    - neonatal adrenoleukodystrophy E71.511
    - specified disorder NEC E71.518
    - Zellweger syndrome E71.510
  - rhizomelic chondrodysplasia punctata E71.540
  - specified form NEC E71.548
    - group 1 E71.518
    - group 2 E71.53
    - group 3 E71.542
  - X-linked adrenoleukodystrophy E71.529
    - adolescent E71.521
    - adrenomyeloneuropathy E71.522
    - childhood E71.520
    - specified form NEC E71.528
  - Zellweger-like syndrome E71.541
- persistent
  - (somatoform) pain F45.41
  - affective (mood) F34.9
- personality — see also Personality F60.9
  - affective F34.0
  - aggressive F60.3
  - amoral F60.2
  - anankastic F60.5
  - antisocial F60.2
  - anxious F60.6
  - asocial F60.2
  - asthenic F60.7
  - avoidant F60.6
  - borderline F60.3
  - change (secondary) due to general medical condition F07.0
  - compulsive F60.5
  - cyclothymic F34.0
  - dependent (passive) F60.7
  - depressive F34.1
  - dissocial F60.2
  - emotional instability F60.3
  - expansive paranoid F60.0
  - explosive F60.3
  - following organic brain damage F07.9
  - histrionic F60.4
  - hyperthymic F34.0
  - hypothymic F34.1
  - hysterical F60.4
  - immature F60.89
  - inadequate F60.7
  - labile F60.3
  - mixed (nonspecific) F60.89
  - moral deficiency F60.2
  - narcissistic F60.81
  - negativistic F60.89
  - obsessional F60.5
  - obsessive (-compulsive) F60.5
  - organic F07.9
  - overconscientious F60.5
  - paranoid F60.0
  - passive (-dependent) F60.7
  - passive-aggressive F60.89
  - pathological NEC F60.9
  - pseudosocial F60.2
  - psychopathic F60.2
  - schizoid F60.1
  - schizotypal F21
  - self-defeating F60.7
  - specified NEC F60.89
  - type A F60.5
  - unstable (emotional) F60.3

Disorder — continued
- pervasive, developmental F84.9
- phencyclidine use
  - mild F16.10
    - with
      - phencyclidine-induced
        - anxiety disorder F16.180
        - bipolar and related disorder F16.14
        - depressive disorder F16.14
        - psychotic disorder F16.159
      - phencyclidine intoxication F16.129
      - phencyclidine intoxication delirium F16.121
    - in remission (early) (sustained) F16.11
  - moderate or severe F16.20
    - with
      - phencyclidine-induced
        - anxiety disorder F16.280
        - bipolar and related disorder F16.14
        - depressive disorder F16.24
        - psychotic disorder F16.259
      - phencyclidine intoxication F16.229
      - phencyclidine intoxication delirium F16.221
    - in remission (early) (sustained) F16.21
- phobic anxiety, childhood F40.8
- phosphate-losing tubular N25.0
- pigmentation L81.9
  - choroid, congenital Q14.3
  - diminished melanin formation L81.6
  - iron L81.8
  - specified NEC L81.8
- pinna (noninfective) H61.10- ☑
  - deformity, acquired H61.11- ☑
  - hematoma H61.12- ☑
  - perichondritis — see Perichondritis, ear
  - specified type NEC H61.19- ☑
- pituitary gland E23.7
  - iatrogenic (postprocedural) E89.3
  - specified NEC E23.6
- platelet-activating anti-PF4, specified NEC D75.84
- platelets D69.1
- plexus G54.9
  - specified NEC G54.8
- polymorphonuclear neutrophils D71.9
  - specified NEC D71.8
- porphyrin metabolism — see Porphyria
- postconcussional F07.81
- posthallucinogen perception F16.983
  - in
    - abuse F16.183
    - dependence F16.283
- postmenopausal N95.9
  - specified NEC N95.8
- postprocedural (postoperative) — see Complications, postprocedural
- post-transplant lymphoproliferative D47.Z1 (following D47.4)
- post-traumatic stress (PTSD) F43.10
  - acute F43.11
  - chronic F43.12
- premenstrual dysphoric (PMDD) F32.81
- prepuce N47.8
- propionic acidemia E71.121
- prostate N42.9
  - specified NEC N42.89
- psychogenic NOS — see also condition F45.9
  - anxiety F41.8
  - appetite F50.9
  - asthenic F48.8
  - cardiovascular (system) F45.8
  - compulsive F42.8
  - cutaneous F54
  - depressive F32.9
  - digestive (system) F45.8
  - dysmenorrheic F45.8
  - dyspneic F45.8
  - endocrine (system) F54
  - eye NEC F45.8
  - feeding — see Disorder, eating
  - functional NEC F45.8
  - gastric F45.8
  - gastrointestinal (system) F45.8
  - genitourinary (system) F45.8
  - heart (function) (rhythm) F45.8
  - hyperventilatory F45.8
  - hypochondriacal — see Disorder, hypochondriacal
  - intestinal F45.8
  - joint F45.8
  - learning F81.9
  - limb F45.8

Disorder — continued
- psychogenic — see also condition — continued
  - lymphatic (system) F45.8
  - menstrual F45.8
  - micturition F45.8
  - monoplegic NEC F44.4
  - motor F44.4
  - muscle F45.8
  - musculoskeletal F45.8
  - neurocirculatory F45.8
  - obsessive F42.8
  - occupational F48.8
  - organ or part of body NEC F45.8
  - paralytic NEC F44.4
  - phobic F40.9
  - physical NEC F45.8
  - rectal F45.8
  - respiratory (system) F45.8
  - rheumatic F45.8
  - sexual (function) F52.9
  - skin (allergic) (eczematous) F54
  - sleep F51.9
  - specified part of body NEC F45.8
  - stomach F45.8
- psychological F99
  - associated with
    - disease classified elsewhere F54
    - sexual
      - development F66
      - relationship F66
    - uncertainty about gender identity F64.9
- psychomotor NEC F44.4
  - hysterical F44.4
- psychoneurotic — see also Neurosis
  - mixed NEC F48.8
- psychophysiologic — see Disorder, somatoform
- psychosexual F65.9
  - development F66
  - identity of childhood F64.2
- psychosomatic NOS — see Disorder, somatoform
  - multiple F45.0
  - undifferentiated F45.1
- psychotic — see Psychosis
  - transient (acute) F23
- puberty E30.9
  - specified NEC E30.8
- pulmonary (valve) — see Endocarditis, pulmonary
- purine metabolism E79.9
- pyrimidine metabolism E79.9
- pyruvate metabolism E74.4
- reactive attachment (childhood) F94.1
- reading R48.0
  - developmental (specific) F81.0
- receptive language F80.2
- receptor, hormonal, peripheral — see also Syndrome, androgen insensitivity E34.50
- recurrent brief depressive F33.8
- reflex R29.2
- refraction H52.7
  - aniseikonia H52.32
  - anisometropia H52.31
  - astigmatism — see Astigmatism
  - hypermetropia — see Hypermetropia
  - myopia — see Myopia
  - presbyopia H52.4
  - specified NEC H52.6
- relationship F68.8
  - due to sexual orientation F66
- REM sleep behavior G47.52
- renal function, impaired (tubular) N25.9
- resonance R49.9
  - specified NEC R49.8
- respiratory function, impaired — see also Failure, respiration
  - postprocedural — see Complication, postoperative, respiratory system
  - psychogenic F45.8
- retina H35.9
  - angioid streaks H35.33
  - changes in vascular appearance H35.01- ☑
  - degeneration — see Degeneration, retina
  - dystrophy (hereditary) — see Dystrophy, retina
  - edema H35.81
  - hemorrhage — see Hemorrhage, retina
  - ischemia H35.82
  - macular degeneration — see Degeneration, macula
  - microaneurysms H35.04- ☑
  - microvascular abnormality NEC H35.09
  - neovascularization — see Neovascularization, retina

Disorder — continued
  retina — continued
    retinopathy — see Retinopathy
    separation of layers H35.70
      central serous chorioretinopathy H35.71- ☑
      pigment epithelium detachment (serous) H35.72- ☑
        hemorrhagic H35.73- ☑
    specified type NEC H35.89
    telangiectasis — see Telangiectasis, retina
    vasculitis — see Vasculitis, retina
  retroperitoneal K68.9
  right hemisphere organic affective F07.89
  rumination (infant or child) (in remission) F98.21
    adult (in remission) F50.84
  sacrum, sacrococcygeal NEC M53.3
  schizoaffective F25.9
    bipolar type F25.0
    depressive type F25.1
    manic type F25.0
    mixed type F25.0
    specified NEC F25.8
  schizoid of childhood F84.5
  schizophrenia spectrum and other psychotic disorder F29
    specified NEC F28
  schizophreniform F20.81
    brief F23
  schizotypal (personality) F21
  seasonal affective, recurrent episodes F33.- ☑
  secretion, thyrocalcitonin E07.0
  sedative, hypnotic, or anxiolytic use
    mild F13.10
      with
        sedative, hypnotic, or anxiolytic-induced
          anxiety disorder F13.180
          bipolar and related disorder F13.14
          depressive disorder F13.14
          psychotic disorder F13.159
          sexual dysfunction F13.181
        sedative, hypnotic, or anxiolytic intoxication F13.129
        sedative, hypnotic, or anxiolytic intoxication delirium F13.121
      in remission (early) (sustained) F13.11
    moderate or severe F13.20
      with
        sedative, hypnotic, or anxiolytic-induced
          anxiety disorder F13.280
          bipolar and related disorder F13.24
          depressive disorder F13.24
          major neurocognitive disorder F13.27
          mild neurocognitive disorder F13.288
          psychotic disorder F13.259
          sexual dysfunction F13.281
        sedative, hypnotic, or anxiolytic intoxication F13.229
        sedative, hypnotic, or anxiolytic intoxication delirium F13.221
      in remission (early) (sustained) F13.21
  seizure — see also Epilepsy G40.909
    intractable G40.919
      with status epilepticus G40.911
  semantic pragmatic F80.89
    with autism F84.0
  sense of smell R43.1
    psychogenic F45.8
  separation anxiety, of childhood F93.0
  sexual
    aversion F52.1
    function, psychogenic F52.9
    interest/arousal, female F52.22
    masochism F65.51
    maturation F66
    nonorganic F52.9
    preference — see also Deviation, sexual F65.9
      fetishistic transvestism F65.1
    relationship F66
    sadism F65.52
  shyness, of childhood and adolescence F40.10
  sibling rivalry F93.8
  sickle-cell (sickling) (homozygous) — see Disease, sickle-cell
    heterozygous D57.3
    specified type NEC D57.8- ☑
    trait D57.3
  sinus (nasal) J34.9
    specified NEC J34.89

Disorder — continued
  skin L98.9
    atrophic L90.9
      specified NEC L90.8
    granulomatous L92.9
      specified NEC L92.8
    hypertrophic L91.9
      specified NEC L91.8
    infiltrative L98.6
    newborn P83.9
      specified NEC P83.88
    picking F42.4
    psychogenic (allergic) (eczematous) F54
  SLC13A5 Citrate Transporter Disorder E74.820
  sleep G47.9
    breathing-related — see Apnea, sleep
    circadian rhythm G47.20
      advance sleep phase type G47.22
      delayed sleep phase type G47.21
      due to
        alcohol
          abuse F10.182
          dependence F10.282
          use F10.982
        amphetamines
          abuse F15.182
          dependence F15.282
          use F15.982
        caffeine
          abuse F15.182
          dependence F15.282
          use F15.982
        cocaine
          abuse F14.182
          dependence F14.282
          use F14.982
        drug NEC
          abuse F19.182
          dependence F19.282
          use F19.982
        opioid
          abuse F11.182
          dependence F11.282
          use F11.982
        psychoactive substance NEC
          abuse F19.182
          dependence F19.282
          use F19.982
        sedative, hypnotic, or anxiolytic
          abuse F13.182
          dependence F13.282
          use F13.982
        stimulant NEC
          abuse F15.182
          dependence F15.282
          use F15.982
      free running type G47.24
      in conditions classified elsewhere G47.27
      irregular sleep wake type G47.23
      jet lag type G47.25
      non-24-hour sleep-wake type G47.24
      shift work type G47.26
      specified NEC G47.29
    due to
      alcohol
        abuse F10.182
        dependence F10.282
        use F10.982
      amphetamine
        abuse F15.182
        dependence F15.282
        use F15.982
      anxiolytic
        abuse F13.182
        dependence F13.282
        use F13.982
      caffeine
        abuse F15.182
        dependence F15.282
        use F15.982
      cocaine
        abuse F14.182
        dependence F14.282
        use F14.982
      drug NEC
        abuse F19.182
        dependence F19.282
        use F19.982

Disorder — continued
  sleep — continued
    due to — continued
      hypnotic
        abuse F13.182
        dependence F13.282
        use F13.982
      opioid
        abuse F11.182
        dependence F11.282
        use F11.982
      psychoactive substance NEC
        abuse F19.182
        dependence F19.282
        use F19.982
      sedative
        abuse F13.182
        dependence F13.282
        use F13.982
      stimulant NEC
        abuse F15.182
        dependence F15.282
        use F15.982
    emotional F51.9
    excessive somnolence — see Hypersomnia
    hypersomnia type — see Hypersomnia
    initiating or maintaining — see Insomnia
    nightmares F51.5
    nonorganic F51.9
      specified NEC F51.8
    parasomnia type G47.50
    specified NEC G47.8
    terrors F51.4
    walking F51.3
  sleep-wake pattern or schedule — see also Disorder, sleep, circadian rhythm G47.9
    specified NEC G47.8
  social
    anxiety (of childhood) F40.10
      generalized F40.11
    functioning in childhood F94.9
      specified NEC F94.8
    pragmatic F80.82
  soft tissue M79.9
    ankle M79.9
    due to use, overuse and pressure M70.90
      ankle M70.97- ☑
      bursitis — see Bursitis
      foot M70.97- ☑
      forearm M70.93- ☑
      hand M70.94- ☑
      lower leg M70.96- ☑
      multiple sites M70.99
      pelvic region M70.95- ☑
      shoulder region M70.91- ☑
      specified site NEC M70.98
      specified type NEC M70.80
        ankle M70.87- ☑
        foot M70.87- ☑
        forearm M70.83- ☑
        hand M70.84- ☑
        lower leg M70.86- ☑
        multiple sites M70.89
        pelvic region M70.85- ☑
        shoulder region M70.81- ☑
        specified site NEC M70.88
        thigh M70.85- ☑
        upper arm M70.82- ☑
      thigh M70.95- ☑
      upper arm M70.92- ☑
    foot M79.9
    forearm M79.9
    hand M79.9
    lower leg M79.9
    multiple sites M79.9
    occupational — see Disorder, soft tissue, due to use, overuse and pressure
    pelvic region M79.9
    shoulder region M79.9
    specified type NEC M79.89
    thigh M79.9
    upper arm M79.9
  somatic symptom F45.1
  somatization F45.0
  somatoform F45.9
    pain (persistent) F45.41
    somatization (multiple) (long-lasting) F45.0
    specified NEC F45.8

Disorder — continued
  somatoform — continued
    undifferentiated F45.1
  somnolence, excessive — see Hypersomnia
  specific
    arithmetical F81.2
    developmental, of motor F82
    reading F81.0
    speech and language F80.9
    spelling F81.81
    written expression F81.81
  speech R47.9
    articulation (functional) (specific) F80.0
    developmental F80.9
    specified NEC R47.89
  speech-sound F80.0
  spelling (specific) F81.81
  spine — see also Dorsopathy
    ligamentous or muscular attachments, peripheral — see Enthesopathy, spinal
    specified NEC — see Dorsopathy, specified NEC
  stereotyped, habit or movement F98.4
  stimulant use (other) (unspecified)
    mild F15.10
      in remission (early) (sustained) F15.11
    moderate or severe F15.20
      in remission (early) (sustained) F15.21
  stomach (functional) — see Disorder, gastric
  stress F43.9
    acute F43.0
    post-traumatic F43.10
      acute F43.11
      chronic F43.12
  substance use (other) (unknown)
    mild F19.10
      with substance-induced
        anxiety disorder F19.180
        bipolar and related disorder F19.14
        depressive disorder F19.14
        major neurocognitive disorder F19.17
        mild neurocognitive disorder F19.188
        obsessive-compulsive and related disorder F19.188
        sexual dysfunction F19.181
      substance intoxication F19.129
      substance intoxication delirium F19.121
    moderate or severe F19.20
      with substance-induced
        anxiety disorder F19.280
        bipolar and related disorder F19.24
        depressive disorder F19.24
        major neurocognitive disorder F19.27
        mild neurocognitive disorder F19.288
        obsessive-compulsive and related disorder F19.288
        sexual dysfunction F19.281
      in remission (early) (sustained) F19.21
      substance intoxication F19.229
      substance intoxication delirium F19.221
  sulfur-bearing amino-acid metabolism E72.10
  sweat gland (eccrine) L74.9
    apocrine L75.9
      specified NEC L75.8
    specified NEC L74.8
  synovium M67.90
    acromioclavicular M67.91- ☑
    ankle M67.97- ☑
    elbow M67.92- ☑
    foot M67.97- ☑
    forearm M67.93- ☑
    hand M67.94- ☑
    hip M67.95- ☑
    knee M67.96- ☑
    multiple sites M67.99
    rupture — see Rupture, synovium
    shoulder M67.91- ☑
    specified type NEC M67.80
      acromioclavicular M67.81- ☑
      ankle M67.87- ☑
      elbow M67.82- ☑
      foot M67.87- ☑
      hand M67.84- ☑
      hip M67.85- ☑
      knee M67.86- ☑
      multiple sites M67.89
      wrist M67.83- ☑
    synovitis — see Synovitis
    upper arm M67.92- ☑

Disorder — continued
  synovium — continued
    wrist M67.93- ☑
  temperature regulation, newborn P81.9
    specified NEC P81.8
  temporomandibular joint M26.60- ☑
  tendon M67.90
    acromioclavicular M67.91- ☑
    ankle M67.97- ☑
    contracture — see Contracture, tendon
    elbow M67.92- ☑
    foot M67.97- ☑
    forearm M67.93- ☑
    hand M67.94- ☑
    hip M67.95- ☑
    knee M67.96- ☑
    multiple sites M67.99
    rupture — see Rupture, tendon
    shoulder M67.91- ☑
    specified type NEC M67.80
      acromioclavicular M67.81- ☑
      ankle M67.87- ☑
      elbow M67.82- ☑
      foot M67.87- ☑
      hand M67.84- ☑
      hip M67.85- ☑
      knee M67.86- ☑
      multiple sites M67.89
      trunk M67.88
      wrist M67.83- ☑
    synovitis — see Synovitis
    tendinitis — see Tendinitis
    tenosynovitis — see Tenosynovitis
    trunk M67.98
    upper arm M67.92- ☑
    wrist M67.93- ☑
  thoracic root (nerve) NEC G54.3
  thyrocalcitonin hypersecretion E07.0
  thyroid (gland) E07.9
    function NEC, neonatal, transitory P72.2
    iodine-deficiency related E01.8
    specified NEC E07.89
  tic — see Tic
  tobacco use
    chewing tobacco (mild) (moderate) (severe)
      in remission (early) (sustained) F17.221
    cigarettes (mild) (moderate) (severe)
      in remission (early) (sustained) F17.211
    mild F17.200
      in remission (early) (sustained) F17.201
    moderate F17.200
      in remission (early) (sustained) F17.201
    severe F17.200
      in remission (early) (sustained) F17.201
    specified product NEC (mild) (moderate) (severe)
      in remission (early) (sustained) F17.291
  tooth K08.9
    development K00.9
      specified NEC K00.8
    eruption K00.6
  Tourette's F95.2
  trance and possession F44.89
  transvestic F65.1
  trauma and stressor-related NOS F43.9
    other specified F43.89
    unspecified F43.9
  tricuspid (valve) — see Endocarditis, tricuspid
  tryptophan metabolism E70.5
  tubular, phosphate-losing N25.0
  tubulo-interstitial (in)
    brucellosis A23.9 [N16]
    cystinosis E72.04
    diphtheria A36.84
    glycogen storage disease E74.00 [N16]
    leukemia NEC C95.9- ☑ [N16]
    lymphoma NEC C85.9- ☑ [N16]
    mixed cryoglobulinemia D89.1 [N16]
    multiple myeloma C90.0- ☑ [N16]
    Salmonella infection A02.25
    sarcoidosis D86.84
    sepsis A41.9 [N16]
      streptococcal A40.9 [N16]
    systemic lupus erythematosus M32.15
    toxoplasmosis B58.83
    transplant rejection T86.91 [N16]
    Wilson's disease E83.01 [N16]
  tubulo-renal function, impaired N25.9
    specified NEC N25.89

Disorder — continued
  tympanic membrane H73.9- ☑
    atrophy — see Atrophy, tympanic membrane
    infection — see Myringitis
    perforation — see Perforation, tympanum
    specified NEC H73.89- ☑
  unsocialized aggressive F91.1
  urea cycle metabolism E72.20
    argininemia E72.21
    argininosuccinic aciduria E72.22
    citrullinemia E72.23
    ornithine transcarbamylase deficiency E72.4
    other specified E72.29
  ureter (in) N28.9
    schistosomiasis B65.0 [N29]
    tuberculosis A18.11
  urethra N36.9
    specified NEC N36.8
  urinary system N39.9
    specified NEC N39.8
  valve, heart
    aortic — see Endocarditis, aortic
    mitral — see Endocarditis, mitral
    pulmonary — see Endocarditis, pulmonary
    rheumatic
      aortic — see Endocarditis, aortic, rheumatic
      mitral — see Endocarditis, mitral
      pulmonary — see Endocarditis, pulmonary, rheumatic
      tricuspid — see Endocarditis, tricuspid
    tricuspid — see Endocarditis, tricuspid
  vestibular function H81.9- ☑
    specified NEC — see subcategory H81.8- ☑
    in diseases classified elsewhere H82.- ☑
    vertigo — see Vertigo
  vision, binocular H53.30
    abnormal retinal correspondence H53.31
    diplopia H53.2
    fusion with defective stereopsis H53.32
    simultaneous perception H53.33
    suppression H53.34
  visual
    cortex
      blindness H47.619
        left brain H47.612
        right brain H47.611
      due to
        inflammatory disorder H47.629
          left brain H47.622
          right brain H47.621
        neoplasm H47.639
          left brain H47.632
          right brain H47.631
        vascular disorder H47.649
          left brain H47.642
          right brain H47.641
    pathway H47.9
      due to
        inflammatory disorder H47.51- ☑
        neoplasm H47.52- ☑
        vascular disorder H47.53- ☑
      optic chiasm — see Disorder, optic, chiasm
  vitreous body H43.9
    crystalline deposits — see Deposit, crystalline
    degeneration — see Degeneration, vitreous
    hemorrhage — see Hemorrhage, vitreous
    opacities — see Opacity, vitreous
    prolapse — see Prolapse, vitreous
    specified type NEC H43.89
  voice R49.9
    specified type NEC R49.8
  volatile solvent use
    due to drug abuse — see Abuse, drug, inhalant
    due to drug dependence — see Dependence, drug, inhalant
  voyeuristic F65.3
  white blood cells D72.9
    specified NEC D72.89
  withdrawing, child or adolescent F40.10
Disorientation R41.0
Displacement, displaced
  acquired traumatic of bone, cartilage, joint, tendon NEC — see Dislocation
  adrenal gland (congenital) Q89.1
  appendix, retrocecal (congenital) Q43.8
  auricle (congenital) Q17.4
  bladder (acquired) N32.89
    congenital Q64.19

Displacement, displaced — *continued*
- brachial plexus (congenital) Q07.8
- brain stem, caudal (congenital) Q04.8
- canaliculus (lacrimalis), congenital Q10.6
- cardia through esophageal hiatus (congenital) Q40.1
- cerebellum, caudal (congenital) Q04.8
- cervix — *see* Malposition, uterus
- colon (congenital) Q43.3
- device, implant or graft — *see also* Complications, by site and type, mechanical T85.628- ☑
  - arterial graft NEC — *see* Complication, cardiovascular device, mechanical, vascular
  - breast (implant) T85.42- ☑
  - catheter NEC T85.628- ☑
    - dialysis (renal) T82.42- ☑
      - intraperitoneal T85.621- ☑
    - infusion NEC T82.524- ☑
      - spinal (epidural) (subdural) T85.620- ☑
    - urinary
      - cystostomy T83.020- ☑
      - Hopkins T83.028- ☑
      - ileostomy T83.028- ☑
      - indwelling T83.021- ☑
      - nephrostomy T83.022- ☑
      - specified NEC T83.028- ☑
      - urostomy T83.028- ☑
  - electronic (electrode) (pulse generator) (stimulator) — *see* Complication, electronic stimulator
  - fixation, internal (orthopedic) NEC — *see* Complication, fixation device, mechanical
  - gastrointestinal — *see* Complications, prosthetic device, mechanical, gastrointestinal device
  - genital NEC T83.428- ☑
    - intrauterine contraceptive device (string) T83.32- ☑
    - penile prosthesis (cylinder) (implanted) (pump) (reservoir) T83.420- ☑
    - testicular prosthesis T83.421- ☑
  - heart NEC — *see* Complication, cardiovascular device, mechanical
  - joint prosthesis — *see* Complications, joint prosthesis, mechanical
  - ocular — *see* Complications, prosthetic device, mechanical, ocular device
  - orthopedic NEC — *see* Complication, orthopedic, device or graft, mechanical
  - specified NEC T85.628- ☑
  - urinary NEC T83.128- ☑
    - graft T83.22- ☑
    - sphincter, implanted T83.121- ☑
    - stent (ileal conduit) (nephroureteral) T83.123- ☑
    - ureteral indwelling T83.122- ☑
  - vascular NEC — *see* Complication, cardiovascular device, mechanical
  - ventricular intracranial shunt T85.02- ☑
- electronic stimulator
  - bone T84.320- ☑
  - cardiac — *see* Complications, cardiac device, electronic
  - nervous system — *see* Complication, prosthetic device, mechanical, electronic nervous system stimulator
  - urinary — *see* Complications, electronic stimulator, urinary
- esophageal mucosa into cardia of stomach, congenital Q39.8
- esophagus (acquired) K22.89
  - congenital Q39.8
- eyeball (acquired) (lateral) (old) — *see* Displacement, globe
  - congenital Q15.8
  - current — *see* Avulsion, eye
- fallopian tube (acquired) N83.4- ☑
  - congenital Q50.6
  - opening (congenital) Q50.6
- gallbladder (congenital) Q44.1
- gastric mucosa (congenital) Q40.2
- globe (acquired) (old) (lateral) H05.21- ☑
  - current — *see* Avulsion, eye
- heart (congenital) Q24.8
  - acquired I51.89
- hymen (upward) (congenital) Q52.4
- intervertebral disc NEC
  - with myelopathy — *see* Disorder, disc, with, myelopathy
  - cervical, cervicothoracic (with) M50.20

Displacement, displaced — *continued*
- intervertebral disc — *continued*
  - cervical, cervicothoracic — *continued*
    - myelopathy — *see* Disorder, disc, cervical, with myelopathy
    - neuritis, radiculitis or radiculopathy — *see* Disorder, disc, cervical, with neuritis
  - due to trauma — *see* Dislocation, vertebra
  - lumbar region M51.26
    - with
      - myelopathy M51.06
      - neuritis, radiculitis, radiculopathy or sciatica M51.16
  - lumbosacral region M51.27
    - with
      - neuritis, radiculitis, radiculopathy or sciatica M51.17
  - sacrococcygeal region M53.3
  - thoracic region M51.24
    - with
      - myelopathy M51.04
      - neuritis, radiculitis, radiculopathy M51.14
  - thoracolumbar region M51.25
    - with
      - myelopathy M51.05
      - neuritis, radiculitis, radiculopathy M51.15
- intrauterine device (string) T83.32- ☑
- kidney (acquired) N28.83
  - congenital Q63.2
- lachrymal, lacrimal apparatus or duct (congenital) Q10.6
- lens, congenital Q12.1
- macula (congenital) Q14.1
- Meckel's diverticulum Q43.0
  - malignant — *see* Table of Neoplasms, small intestine, malignant
- nail (congenital) Q84.6
  - acquired L60.8
- opening of Wharton's duct in mouth Q38.4
- organ or site, congenital NEC — *see* Malposition, congenital
- ovary (acquired) N83.4- ☑
  - congenital Q50.39
  - free in peritoneal cavity (congenital) Q50.39
  - into hernial sac N83.4- ☑
- oviduct (acquired) N83.4- ☑
  - congenital Q50.6
- parathyroid (gland) E21.4
- parotid gland (congenital) Q38.4
- punctum lacrimale (congenital) Q10.6
- sacro-iliac (joint) (congenital) Q74.2
  - current injury S33.2- ☑
  - old — *see* subcategory M53.2- ☑
- salivary gland (any) (congenital) Q38.4
- spleen (congenital) Q89.09
- stomach, congenital Q40.2
- sublingual duct Q38.4
- tongue (downward) (congenital) Q38.3
- tooth, teeth, fully erupted M26.30
  - horizontal M26.33
  - vertical M26.34
- trachea (congenital) Q32.1
- ureter or ureteric opening or orifice (congenital) Q62.62
- uterine opening of oviducts or fallopian tubes Q50.6
- uterus, uterine — *see* Malposition, uterus
- ventricular septum Q21.0
  - with rudimentary ventricle Q20.4

Disproportion
- between native and reconstructed breast N65.1
- fiber-type G71.20
  - congenital G71.29

Disruptio uteri — *see* Rupture, uterus

Disruption (of)
- ciliary body NEC H21.89
- closure of
  - abdominal wall muscle or fascia T81.321- ☑
  - cornea T81.31- ☑
  - craniotomy T81.328- ☑
  - fascia (muscular) (superficial) T81.328- ☑
  - gastrointestinal tract anastomosis, repair, or closure T81.320- ☑
  - internal organ or tissue T81.328- ☑
  - laceration (external) (internal) T81.33- ☑
  - ligament T81.328- ☑
  - mucosa T81.31- ☑
  - muscle or muscle flap T81.328- ☑
  - ribs or rib cage T81.328- ☑
  - skin and subcutaneous tissue (full-thickness) (superficial) T81.31- ☑

Disruption — *continued*
- closure of — *continued*
  - skull T81.328- ☑
  - sternum (sternotomy) T81.328- ☑
  - tendon T81.328- ☑
  - traumatic laceration (external) (internal) T81.33- ☑
- family Z63.8
  - due to
    - absence of family member due to military deployment Z63.31
    - absence of family member NEC Z63.32
    - alcoholism and drug addiction in family Z63.72
    - bereavement Z63.4
    - death (assumed) or disappearance of family member Z63.4
    - divorce or separation Z63.5
    - drug addiction in family Z63.72
    - return of family member from military deployment (current or past conflict) Z63.71
    - stressful life events NEC Z63.79
- iris NEC H21.89
- ligament(s) — *see also* Sprain
  - knee
    - current injury — *see* Dislocation, knee
    - old (chronic) — *see* Derangement, knee, instability
    - spontaneous NEC — *see* Derangement, knee, disruption ligament
- ossicular chain — *see* Discontinuity, ossicles, ear
- pelvic ring (stable) S32.810- ☑
  - unstable S32.811- ☑
- traumatic injury wound repair T81.33- ☑
- wound T81.30- ☑
  - episiotomy O90.1
  - operation T81.31- ☑
    - cesarean O90.0
    - deep T81.329- ☑
    - external operation wound (superficial) T81.31- ☑
    - internal operation wound (deep) T81.329- ☑
      - abdominal wall muscle or fascia T81.321- ☑
      - specified NEC T81.328- ☑
  - perineal (obstetric) O90.1
  - traumatic injury repair T81.33- ☑

Dissatisfaction with
- employment Z56.9
- school environment Z55.4

Dissecting — *see* condition

Dissection
- aorta I71.00
  - abdominal I71.02
  - thoracic I71.019
    - aortic arch I71.011
    - ascending aorta I71.010
    - descending thoracic aorta I71.012
  - thoracoabdominal I71.03
- artery I77.70
  - basilar (trunk) I77.75
  - carotid I77.71
  - cerebral (nonruptured) I67.0
    - ruptured — *see* Hemorrhage, intracranial, subarachnoid
  - coronary I25.42
  - extremity
    - lower I77.77
    - upper I77.76
  - iliac I77.72
  - precerebral
    - congenital (nonruptured) Q28.1
    - specified site NEC I77.75
  - renal I77.73
  - specified NEC I77.79
  - vertebral I77.74
- precerebral artery, congenital (nonruptured) Q28.1
- traumatic — *see* Wound, open, by site
- vascular I99.8
- wound — *see* Wound, open

Disseminated — *see* condition

Dissociation
- auriculoventricular or atrioventricular (AV) (any degree) (isorhythmic) I45.89
  - with heart block I44.2
- interference I45.89

Dissociative reaction, state F44.9

Dissolution, vertebra — *see* Osteoporosis

Distension, distention
- abdomen R14.0
- bladder N32.89
- cecum K63.89
- colon K63.89

Distension, distention — *continued*
- gallbladder K82.8
- intestine K63.89
- kidney N28.89
- liver K76.89
- seminal vesicle N50.89
- stomach K31.89
  - acute K31.0
  - psychogenic F45.8
- ureter — *see* Dilatation, ureter
- uterus N85.8

Disto-occlusion (Division I) (Division II) M26.212
Distoma hepaticum infestation B66.3
Distomiasis B66.9
- bile passages B66.3
- hemic B65.9
- hepatic B66.3
  - due to Clonorchis sinensis B66.1
- intestinal B66.5
- liver B66.3
  - due to Clonorchis sinensis B66.1
- lung B66.4
- pulmonary B66.4

Distomolar (fourth molar) K00.1
Distortion(s) (congenital)
- adrenal (gland) Q89.1
- arm NEC Q68.8
- bile duct or passage Q44.5
- bladder Q64.79
- brain Q04.9
- cervix (uteri) Q51.9
- chest (wall) Q67.8
  - bones Q76.8
- clavicle Q74.0
- clitoris Q52.6
- coccyx Q76.49
- common duct Q44.5
- coronary Q24.5
- cystic duct Q44.5
- ear (auricle) (external) Q17.3
  - inner Q16.5
  - middle Q16.4
    - ossicles Q16.3
- endocrine NEC Q89.2
- eustachian tube Q17.8
- eye (adnexa) Q15.8
- face bone(s) NEC Q75.8
- fallopian tube Q50.6
- femur NEC Q68.8
- fibula NEC Q68.8
- finger(s) Q68.1
- foot Q66.9- ☑
- genitalia, genital organ(s)
  - female Q52.8
    - external Q52.79
    - internal NEC Q52.8
- gyri Q04.8
- hand bone(s) Q68.1
- heart (auricle) (ventricle) Q24.8
  - valve (cusp) Q24.8
- hepatic duct Q44.5
- humerus NEC Q68.8
- hymen Q52.4
- intrafamilial communications Z63.8
- jaw NEC M26.89
- labium (majus) (minus) Q52.79
- leg NEC Q68.8
- lens Q12.8
- liver Q44.79
- lumbar spine Q76.49
  - with disproportion O33.8
    - causing obstructed labor O65.0
- lumbosacral (joint) (region) Q76.49
  - kyphosis — *see* Kyphosis, congenital
  - lordosis — *see* Lordosis, congenital
- nerve Q07.8
- nose Q30.8
- organ
  - of Corti Q16.5
  - or site not listed — *see* Anomaly, by site
- ossicles, ear Q16.3
- oviduct Q50.6
- pancreas Q45.2
- parathyroid (gland) Q89.2
- pituitary (gland) Q89.2
- radius NEC Q68.8
- sacroiliac joint Q74.2
- sacrum Q76.49
- scapula Q74.0

Distortion(s) — *continued*
- shoulder girdle Q74.0
- skull bone(s) NEC Q75.8
  - with
    - anencephalus Q00.0
    - encephalocele — *see* Encephalocele
    - hydrocephalus Q03.9
      - with spina bifida — *see* Spina bifida, with hydrocephalus
    - microcephaly Q02
- spinal cord Q06.8
- spine Q76.49
  - kyphosis — *see* Kyphosis, congenital
  - lordosis — *see* Lordosis, congenital
- spleen Q89.09
- sternum NEC Q76.7
- thorax (wall) Q67.8
  - bony Q76.8
- thymus (gland) Q89.2
- thyroid (gland) Q89.2
- tibia NEC Q68.8
- toe(s) Q66.9- ☑
- tongue Q38.3
- trachea (cartilage) Q32.1
- ulna NEC Q68.8
- ureter Q62.8
- urethra Q64.79
  - causing obstruction Q64.39
- uterus Q51.9
- vagina Q52.4
- vertebra Q76.49
  - kyphosis — *see* Kyphosis, congenital
  - lordosis — *see* Lordosis, congenital
- visual — *see also* Disturbance, vision
  - shape and size H53.15
- vulva Q52.79
- wrist (bones) (joint) Q68.8

Distress
- abdomen — *see* Pain, abdominal
- acute respiratory R06.03
  - syndrome (adult) (child) J80
- epigastric R10.13
- fetal P84
  - complicating pregnancy — *see* Stress, fetal
- gastrointestinal (functional) K30
  - psychogenic F45.8
- intestinal (functional) NOS K59.9
  - psychogenic F45.8
- maternal, during labor and delivery O75.0
- relationship, with spouse or intimate partner Z63.0
- respiratory (adult) (child) R06.03
  - newborn P22.9
    - specified NEC P22.8
  - orthopnea R06.01
  - psychogenic F45.8
  - shortness of breath R06.02
  - specified type NEC R06.09

Distribution vessel, atypical Q27.9
- coronary artery Q24.5
- precerebral Q28.1

Districhiasis L68.8
Disturbance(s) — *see also* Disease
- absorption K90.9
  - calcium E58
  - carbohydrate K90.49
  - fat K90.49
    - pancreatic K90.3
  - protein K90.49
  - starch K90.49
  - vitamin — *see* Deficiency, vitamin
- acid-base equilibrium E87.8
  - mixed E87.4
- activity and attention (with hyperkinesis) — *see* Disorder, attention-deficit hyperactivity
- amino acid transport E72.00
- assimilation, food K90.9
- auditory nerve, except deafness — *see* subcategory H93.3- ☑
- behavior — *see* Disorder, conduct
- blood clotting (mechanism) — *see also* Defect, coagulation D68.9
- cerebral
  - nerve — *see* Disorder, nerve, cranial
  - status, newborn P91.9
    - specified NEC P91.88
- circulatory I99.9
- conduct — *see also* Disorder, conduct F91.9
  - adjustment reaction — *see* Disorder, adjustment
  - compulsive F63.9

Disturbance(s) — *continued*
- conduct — *see also* Disorder, conduct — *continued*
  - disruptive F91.9
  - hyperkinetic — *see* Disorder, attention-deficit hyperactivity
  - socialized F91.2
  - specified NEC F91.8
  - unsocialized F91.1
- coordination R27.8
- cranial nerve — *see* Disorder, nerve, cranial
- deep sensibility — *see* Disturbance, sensation
- digestive K30
  - psychogenic F45.8
- electrolyte — *see also* Imbalance, electrolyte
  - newborn, transitory P74.49
    - hyperammonemia P74.6
    - hyperchloremia P74.421
    - hyperchloremic metabolic acidosis P74.421
    - hypochloremia P74.422
    - potassium balance
      - hyperkalemia P74.31
      - hypokalemia P74.32
    - sodium balance
      - hypernatremia P74.21
      - hyponatremia P74.22
    - specified type NEC P74.49
- emotions specific to childhood and adolescence F93.9
  - with
    - anxiety and fearfulness NEC F93.8
    - elective mutism F94.0
    - oppositional disorder F91.3
    - sensitivity (withdrawal) F40.10
    - shyness F40.10
    - social withdrawal F40.10
  - involving relationship problems F93.8
  - mixed F93.8
  - specified NEC F93.8
- endocrine (gland) E34.9
  - neonatal, transitory P72.9
    - specified NEC P72.8
- equilibrium R42
- fructose metabolism E74.10
- gait — *see* Gait
  - hysterical F44.4
  - psychogenic F44.4
- gastrointestinal (functional) K30
  - psychogenic F45.8
- habit, child F98.9
- hearing, except deafness and tinnitus — *see* Abnormal, auditory perception
- heart, functional (conditions in I44-I50)
  - due to presence of (cardiac) prosthesis I97.19- ☑
  - postoperative I97.89
    - cardiac surgery — *see also* Infarct, myocardium, associated with revascularization procedure I97.190
    - other surgery I97.191
- hormones E34.9
- innervation uterus (parasympathetic) (sympathetic) N85.8
- keratinization NEC
  - gingiva K05.10
    - nonplaque induced K05.11
    - plaque induced K05.10
  - lip K13.0
  - oral (mucosa) (soft tissue) K13.29
  - tongue K13.29
- learning (specific) — *see* Disorder, learning
- memory — *see* Amnesia
  - mild, following organic brain damage F06.8
- mental F99
  - associated with diseases classified elsewhere F54
- metabolism E88.9
  - with
    - abortion — *see* Abortion, by type with other specified complication
    - ectopic pregnancy O08.5
    - molar pregnancy O08.5
  - amino-acid E72.9
    - aromatic E70.9
    - branched-chain E71.2
    - straight-chain E72.89
    - sulfur-bearing E72.10
  - ammonia E72.20
  - arginine E72.21
  - arginosuccinic acid E72.22
  - carbohydrate E74.9
  - cholesterol E78.9
  - citrulline E72.23

Disturbance(s) — continued
- metabolism — continued
  - cystathionine E72.19
  - general E88.9
  - glutamine E72.89
  - histidine E70.40
  - homocystine E72.19
  - hydroxylysine E72.3
  - in labor or delivery O75.89
  - iron E83.10
  - lipoid E78.9
  - lysine E72.3
  - methionine E72.19
  - neonatal, transitory P74.9
    - calcium and magnesium P71.9
      - specified type NEC P71.8
    - carbohydrate metabolism P70.9
      - specified type NEC P70.8
    - specified NEC P74.8
  - ornithine E72.4
  - phosphate E83.39
  - sodium NEC E87.8
  - threonine E72.89
  - tryptophan E70.5
  - tyrosine E70.20
  - urea cycle E72.20
- motor R29.2
- nervous, functional R45.0
- neuromuscular mechanism (eye), due to syphilis A52.15
- nutritional E63.9
  - nail L60.3
- ocular motion H51.9
  - psychogenic F45.8
- oculogyric H51.8
  - psychogenic F45.8
- oculomotor H51.9
  - psychogenic F45.8
- olfactory nerve R43.1
- optic nerve NEC — see Disorder, nerve, optic
- oral epithelium, including tongue NEC K13.29
- perceptual due to
  - alcohol withdrawal F10.232
  - amphetamine intoxication F15.922
    - in
      - abuse F15.122
      - dependence F15.222
  - anxiolytic withdrawal F13.232
  - cannabis intoxication (acute) F12.922
    - in
      - abuse F12.122
      - dependence F12.222
  - cocaine intoxication (acute) F14.922
    - in
      - abuse F14.122
      - dependence F14.222
  - hypnotic withdrawal F13.232
  - opioid intoxication (acute) F11.922
    - in
      - abuse F11.122
      - dependence F11.222
  - phencyclidine intoxication (acute) F16.122
  - sedative withdrawal F13.232
- personality (pattern) (trait) — see also Disorder, personality F60.9
  - following organic brain damage F07.9
- polyglandular E31.9
  - specified NEC E31.8
- potassium balance, newborn
  - hyperkalemia P74.31
  - hypokalemia P74.32
- psychogenic F45.9
- psychomotor F44.4
- psychophysical visual H53.16
- pupillary — see Anomaly, pupil, function
- reflex R29.2
- rhythm, heart I49.9
- salivary secretion K11.7
- sensation (cold) (heat) (localization) (tactile discrimination) (texture) (vibratory) NEC R20.9
  - hysterical F44.6
  - skin R20.9
    - anesthesia R20.0
    - hyperesthesia R20.3
    - hypoesthesia R20.1
    - paresthesia R20.2
    - specified type NEC R20.8
  - smell R43.9
    - and taste (mixed) R43.8
    - anosmia R43.0

Disturbance(s) — continued
- sensation — continued
  - smell — continued
    - parosmia R43.1
    - specified NEC R43.8
  - taste R43.9
    - and smell (mixed) R43.8
    - parageusia R43.2
    - specified NEC R43.8
- sensory — see Disturbance, sensation
- situational (transient) — see also Disorder, adjustment
  - acute F43.0
- sleep G47.9
  - nonorganic origin F51.9
- smell — see Disturbance, sensation, smell
- sociopathic F60.2
- sodium balance, newborn
  - hypernatremia P74.21
  - hyponatremia P74.22
- speech R47.9
  - developmental F80.9
  - specified NEC R47.89
- stomach (functional) K31.9
- sympathetic (nerve) G90.9
- taste — see Disturbance, sensation, taste
- temperature
  - regulation, newborn P81.9
    - specified NEC P81.8
  - sense R20.8
    - hysterical F44.6
- tooth
  - eruption K00.6
  - formation K00.4
  - structure, hereditary NEC K00.5
- touch — see Disturbance, sensation
- vascular I99.9
  - arteriosclerotic — see Arteriosclerosis
- vasomotor I73.9
- vasospastic I73.9
- vision, visual H53.9
  - following
    - cerebral infarction I69.398
    - cerebrovascular disease I69.998
      - specified NEC I69.898
    - intracerebral hemorrhage I69.198
    - nontraumatic intracranial hemorrhage NEC I69.298
    - specified disease NEC I69.898
    - subarachnoid hemorrhage I69.098
  - psychophysical H53.16
  - specified NEC H53.8
  - subjective H53.10
    - day blindness H53.11
    - discomfort H53.14- ☑
    - distortions of shape and size H53.15
    - loss
      - sudden H53.13- ☑
      - transient H53.12- ☑
    - specified type NEC H53.19
- voice R49.9
  - psychogenic F44.4
  - specified NEC R49.8
- **Diuresis** R35.89
- **Diver's palsy, paralysis or squeeze** T70.3- ☑
- **Diverticulitis** (acute) K57.92
  - bladder — see Cystitis
  - ileum — see Diverticulitis, intestine, small
  - intestine K57.92
    - with
      - abscess, perforation K57.80
        - with bleeding K57.81
      - bleeding K57.93
    - congenital Q43.8
    - large K57.32
      - with
        - abscess, perforation K57.20
          - with bleeding K57.21
        - bleeding K57.33
        - small intestine K57.52
          - with
            - abscess, perforation K57.40
              - with bleeding K57.41
            - bleeding K57.53
    - small K57.12
      - with
        - abscess, perforation K57.00
          - with bleeding K57.01
        - bleeding K57.13
        - large intestine K57.52

Diverticulitis — continued
- intestine — continued
  - small — continued
    - with — continued
      - large intestine — continued
        - with
          - abscess, perforation K57.40
            - with bleeding K57.41
          - bleeding K57.53
- **Diverticulosis** K57.90
  - with bleeding K57.91
  - large intestine K57.30
    - with
      - bleeding K57.31
      - small intestine K57.50
        - with bleeding K57.51
  - small intestine K57.10
    - with
      - bleeding K57.11
      - large intestine K57.50
        - with bleeding K57.51
- **Diverticulum, diverticula** (multiple) K57.90
  - appendix (noninflammatory) K38.2
  - bladder (sphincter) N32.3
    - congenital Q64.6
  - bronchus (congenital) Q32.4
    - acquired J98.09
  - calyx, calyceal (kidney) N28.89
  - cardia (stomach) K31.4
  - cecum — see Diverticulosis, intestine, large
    - congenital Q43.8
  - colon — see Diverticulosis, intestine, large
    - congenital Q43.8
  - duodenum — see Diverticulosis, intestine, small
    - congenital Q43.8
  - epiphrenic (esophagus) K22.5
  - esophagus (congenital) Q39.6
    - acquired (epiphrenic) (pulsion) (traction) K22.5
  - eustachian tube — see Disorder, eustachian tube, specified NEC
  - fallopian tube N83.8
  - gastric K31.4
  - heart (congenital) Q24.8
  - ileum — see Diverticulosis, intestine, small
  - jejunum — see Diverticulosis, intestine, small
  - kidney (pelvis) (calyces) N28.89
    - with calculus — see Calculus, kidney
  - Meckel's (displaced) (hypertrophic) Q43.0
    - malignant — see Table of Neoplasms, small intestine, malignant
  - midthoracic K22.5
  - organ or site, congenital NEC — see Distortion
  - pericardium (congenital) (cyst) Q24.8
    - acquired I31.8
  - pharyngoesophageal (congenital) Q39.6
    - acquired K22.5
  - pharynx (congenital) Q38.7
  - rectosigmoid — see Diverticulosis, intestine, large
    - congenital Q43.8
  - rectum — see Diverticulosis, intestine, large
  - Rokitansky's K22.5
  - seminal vesicle N50.89
  - sigmoid — see Diverticulosis, intestine, large
    - congenital Q43.8
  - stomach (acquired) K31.4
    - congenital Q40.2
  - trachea (acquired) J39.8
  - ureter (acquired) N28.89
    - congenital Q62.8
  - ureterovesical orifice N28.89
  - urethra (acquired) N36.1
    - congenital Q64.79
  - ventricle, left (congenital) Q24.8
  - vesical N32.3
    - congenital Q64.6
  - Zenker's (esophagus) K22.5
- **Division**
  - cervix uteri (acquired) N88.8
  - glans penis Q55.69
  - labia minora (congenital) Q52.79
  - ligament (partial or complete) (current) — see also Sprain
    - with open wound — see Wound, open
  - muscle (partial or complete) (current) — see also Injury, muscle
    - with open wound — see Wound, open
  - nerve (traumatic) — see Injury, nerve
  - spinal cord — see Injury, spinal cord, by region
  - vein I87.8
- **Divorce, causing family disruption** Z63.5

☑ Additional Character Required — Refer to the Tabular List for Character Selection

Dix-Hallpike neurolabyrinthitis — see Neuronitis, vestibular
Dizziness R42
  hysterical F44.89
  psychogenic F45.8
DMAC (disseminated mycobacterium avium-intracellulare complex) A31.2
DNR (do not resuscitate) Z66
Doan-Wiseman syndrome (primary splenic neutropenia) — see Agranulocytosis
Doehle-Heller aortitis A52.02
Dog bite — see Bite
Dohle body panmyelopathic syndrome D72.0
Dolichocephaly Q67.2
  non-deformational Q75.01
Dolichocolon Q43.8
Dolichostenomelia — see Syndrome, Marfan
Donohue's syndrome E34.8
Donor (organ or tissue) Z52.9
  blood (whole) Z52.000
    autologous Z52.010
    specified component (lymphocytes) (platelets) NEC Z52.008
      autologous Z52.018
      specified donor NEC Z52.098
    specified donor NEC Z52.090
    stem cells Z52.001
      autologous Z52.011
      specified donor NEC Z52.091
  bone Z52.20
    autologous Z52.21
    marrow Z52.3
    specified type NEC Z52.29
  cornea Z52.5
  egg (Oocyte) Z52.819
    age 35 and over Z52.812
      anonymous recipient Z52.812
      designated recipient Z52.813
    under age 35 Z52.810
      anonymous recipient Z52.810
      designated recipient Z52.811
  kidney Z52.4
  liver Z52.6
  lung Z52.89
  lymphocyte — see Donor, blood, specified components NEC
  Oocyte — see Donor, egg
  platelets Z52.008
  potential, examination of Z00.5
  semen Z52.89
  skin Z52.10
    autologous Z52.11
    specified type NEC Z52.19
  specified organ or tissue NEC Z52.89
  sperm Z52.89
Donovanosis A58
Dorsalgia M54.9
  psychogenic F45.41
  specified NEC M54.89
Dorsopathy M53.9
  deforming M43.9
    specified NEC — see subcategory M43.8-
  specified NEC M53.80
    cervical region M53.82
    cervicothoracic region M53.83
    lumbar region M53.86
    lumbosacral region M53.87
    occipito-atlanto-axial region M53.81
    sacrococcygeal region M53.88
    thoracic region M53.84
    thoracolumbar region M53.85
Double
  albumin E88.09
  aortic arch Q25.45
  auditory canal Q17.8
  auricle (heart) Q20.8
  bladder Q64.79
  cervix Q51.820
    with doubling of uterus (and vagina) Q51.10
      with obstruction Q51.11
  inlet ventricle Q20.4
  kidney with double pelvis (renal) Q63.0
  meatus urinarius Q64.75
  monster Q89.4
  outlet
    left ventricle Q20.2
    right ventricle Q20.1
  pelvis (renal) with double ureter Q62.5
  tongue Q38.3

Double — continued
  ureter (one or both sides) Q62.5
    with double pelvis (renal) Q62.5
  urethra Q64.74
  urinary meatus Q64.75
  uterus Q51.28
    with
      doubling of cervix (and vagina) Q51.10
        with obstruction Q51.11
      complete Q51.21
    in pregnancy or childbirth O34.0-
      causing obstructed labor O65.5
    partial Q51.22
    specified NEC Q51.28
    vagina Q52.10
      with doubling of uterus (and cervix) Q51.10
        with obstruction Q51.11
    vision H53.2
    vulva Q52.79
Doubled up Z59.01
Douglas' pouch, cul-de-sac — see condition
Down syndrome Q90.9
  meiotic nondisjunction Q90.0
  mitotic nondisjunction Q90.1
  mosaicism Q90.1
  translocation Q90.2
DPD (dihydropyrimidine dehydrogenase deficiency) E88.89
Dracontiasis B72
Dracunculiasis, dracunculosis B72
Dream state, hysterical F44.89
Drepanocytic anemia — see Disease, sickle-cell
Dresbach's syndrome (elliptocytosis) D58.1
Dreschlera (hawaiiensis) (infection) B43.8
Dressler's syndrome I24.1
Drift, ulnar — see Deformity, limb, specified type NEC, forearm
Drinking (alcohol)
  excessive, to excess NEC (without dependence) F10.10
  habitual (continual) (without remission) F10.20
    with remission F10.21
Drip, postnasal (chronic) R09.82
  due to
    allergic rhinitis — see Rhinitis, allergic
    common cold J00
    gastroesophageal reflux — see Reflux, gastroesophageal
    nasopharyngitis — see Nasopharyngitis
    other known condition — code to condition
    sinusitis — see Sinusitis
Droop
  facial R29.810
    cerebrovascular disease I69.992
      cerebral infarction I69.392
      intracerebral hemorrhage I69.192
      nontraumatic intracranial hemorrhage NEC I69.292
      specified disease NEC I69.892
      subarachnoid hemorrhage I69.092
Drop (in)
  attack NEC R55
  finger — see Deformity, finger
  foot — see Deformity, limb, foot, drop
  hematocrit (precipitous) R71.0
  hemoglobin R71.0
  toe — see Deformity, toe, specified NEC
  wrist — see Deformity, limb, wrist drop
Dropped heart beats I45.9
Dropsy, dropsical — see also Hydrops
  abdomen R18.8
  brain — see Hydrocephalus
  cardiac, heart — see Failure, heart, congestive
  gangrenous — see Gangrene
  heart — see Failure, heart, congestive
  kidney — see Nephrosis
  lung — see Edema, lung
  newborn due to isoimmunization P56.0
  pericardium — see Pericarditis
Drowned, drowning (near) T75.1-
Drowsiness R40.0
Drug
  abuse counseling and surveillance Z71.51
  addiction — see Dependence
  dependence — see Dependence
  habit — see Dependence
  harmful use — see Abuse, drug
  induced fever R50.2
  overdose — see Table of Drugs and Chemicals, by drug, poisoning
  poisoning — see Table of Drugs and Chemicals, by drug, poisoning

Drug — continued
  resistant organism infection — see also Resistant, organism, to, drug Z16.30
  therapy
    long term (current) (prophylactic) — see Therapy, drug long-term (current) (prophylactic)
    short term — omit code
  wrong substance given or taken in error — see Table of Drugs and Chemicals, by drug, poisoning
Drunkenness (without dependence) F10.129
  acute in alcoholism F10.229
  chronic (without remission) F10.20
    with remission F10.21
  pathological (without dependence) F10.129
    with dependence F10.229
  sleep F51.9
Drusen
  macula (degenerative) (retina) — see Degeneration, macula, drusen
  optic disc H47.32-
Dry, dryness — see also condition
  larynx J38.7
  mouth R68.2
    due to dehydration E86.0
  nose J34.89
  socket (teeth) M27.3
  throat J39.2
DSAP L56.5
Duane's syndrome H50.81-
Dubin-Johnson disease or syndrome E80.6
Dubois' disease (thymus gland) A50.59 [E35]
Dubowitz' syndrome Q87.19
Duchenne-Aran muscular atrophy G12.21
Duchenne-Griesinger disease G71.01
Duchenne's
  disease or syndrome
    motor neuron disease G12.22
    muscular dystrophy G71.01
    locomotor ataxia (syphilitic) A52.11
  paralysis
    birth injury P14.0
    due to or associated with
      motor neuron disease G12.22
      muscular dystrophy G71.01
Ducreyi chancre A57
Ducrey's chancre A57
Duct, ductus — see condition
Duffy phenotype — see Phenotype, Duffy
Duhring's disease (dermatitis herpetiformis) L13.0
Dullness, cardiac (decreased) (increased) R01.2
Dumb ague — see Malaria
Dumbness — see Aphasia
Dumdum fever B55.0
Dumping syndrome (postgastrectomy) K91.1
Duodenitis (nonspecific) (peptic) K29.80
  with bleeding K29.81
  erosive — see Ulcer, duodenum
Duodenocholangitis — see Cholangitis
Duodenum, duodenal — see condition
Duplay's bursitis or periarthritis M75.0-
Duplication, duplex — see also Accessory
  alimentary tract Q45.8
  anus Q43.4
  appendix (and cecum) Q43.4
  biliary duct (any) Q44.5
  bladder Q64.79
  cecum (and appendix) Q43.4
  cervix Q51.820
  chromosome NEC — see also Trisomy
    with complex rearrangements NEC Q92.5
    seen only at prometaphase Q92.8
  cystic duct Q44.5
  digestive organs Q45.8
  esophagus Q39.8
  frontonasal process Q75.8
  intestine (large) (small) Q43.4
  kidney Q63.0
  liver Q44.79
  pancreas Q45.3
  penis Q55.69
  respiratory organs NEC Q34.8
  salivary duct Q38.4
  spinal cord (incomplete) Q06.2
  stomach Q40.2
Dupre's disease (meningism) R29.1
Dupuytren's contraction or disease M72.0
Durand-Nicolas-Favre disease A55
Durotomy (inadvertent) (incidental) G97.41
Duroziez's disease (congenital mitral stenosis) Q23.2

Dutton's relapsing fever (West African) A68.1
Dwarfism — see also Short, stature E34.328
  achondroplastic Q77.4
  congenital — see also Short, stature E34.328
  constitutional E34.31
  hypochondroplastic Q77.4
  hypophyseal E23.0
  infantile — see also Short, stature E34.328
  Laron-type — see also Short, stature E34.321
  Lorain (-Levi) type E23.0
  metatropic Q77.8
  nephrotic-glycosuric (with hypophosphatemic rickets) E72.09
  nutritional E45
  pancreatic K86.89
  pituitary E23.0
  renal N25.0
  thanatophoric Q77.1
Dyke-Young anemia (secondary) (symptomatic) D59.19
Dysacusis — see Abnormal, auditory perception
Dysadrenocortism E27.9
  hyperfunction E27.0
Dysarthria R47.1
  following
    cerebral infarction I69.322
    cerebrovascular disease I69.922
      specified disease NEC I69.822
    intracerebral hemorrhage I69.122
    nontraumatic intracranial hemorrhage NEC I69.222
    subarachnoid hemorrhage I69.022
Dysautonomia (familial) G90.1
Dysbarism T70.3- ☑
Dysbasia R26.2
  angiosclerotica intermittens I73.9
  hysterical F44.4
  lordotica (progressiva) G24.1
  nonorganic origin F44.4
  psychogenic F44.4
Dysbetalipoproteinemia (familial) E78.2
Dyscalculia R48.8
  developmental F81.2
Dyschezia K59.00
Dyschondroplasia (with hemangiomata) Q78.4
Dyschromia (skin) L81.9
Dyscollagenosis M35.9
Dyscranio-pygo-phalangy Q87.0
Dyscrasia
  blood (with) D75.9
    antepartum hemorrhage — see Hemorrhage, antepartum, with coagulation defect
    intrapartum hemorrhage O67.0
    newborn P61.9
      specified type NEC P61.8
    puerperal, postpartum O72.3
  polyglandular, pluriglandular E31.9
Dysendocrinism E34.9
Dysentery, dysenteric (catarrhal) (diarrhea) (epidemic) (hemorrhagic) (infectious) (sporadic) (tropical) A09
  abscess, liver A06.4
  amebic — see also Amebiasis A06.0
    with abscess — see Abscess, amebic
    acute A06.0
    chronic A06.1
  arthritis — see also category M01 A09
    bacillary (see also category M01) A03.9
  bacillary A03.9
    arthritis — see also category M01 A03.9
    Boyd A03.2
    Flexner A03.1
    Schmitz (-Stutzer) A03.0
    Shiga (-Kruse) A03.0
    Shigella A03.9
      boydii A03.2
      dysenteriae A03.0
      flexneri A03.1
      group A A03.0
      group B A03.1
      group C A03.2
      group D A03.3
      sonnei A03.3
      specified type NEC A03.8
    Sonne A03.3
    specified type NEC A03.8
  balantidial A07.0
  Balantidium coli A07.0
  Boyd's A03.2
  candidal B37.82
  Chilomastix A07.8
  Chinese A03.9

Dysentery, dysenteric — continued
  coccidial A07.3
  Dientamoeba (fragilis) A07.8
  Embadomonas A07.8
  Entamoeba, entamebic — see Dysentery, amebic
  Flexner-Boyd A03.2
  Flexner's A03.1
  Giardia lamblia A07.1
  Hiss-Russell A03.1
  Lamblia A07.1
  leishmanial B55.0
  malarial — see Malaria
  metazoal B82.0
  monilial B37.82
  protozoal A07.9
  Salmonella A02.0
  schistosomal B65.1
  Schmitz (-Stutzer) A03.0
  Shiga (-Kruse) A03.0
  Shigella NOS — see Dysentery, bacillary
  Sonne A03.3
  strongyloidiasis B78.0
  trichomonal A07.8
  viral — see also Enteritis, viral A08.4
Dysequilibrium R42
Dysesthesia R20.8
  hysterical F44.6
Dysferlinopathy G71.033
Dysfibrinogenemia (congenital) D68.2
Dysfunction
  adrenal E27.9
    hyperfunction E27.0
  autonomic
    due to alcohol G31.2
    somatoform F45.8
  bladder N31.9
    neurogenic NOS — see Dysfunction, bladder, neuromuscular
    neuromuscular NOS N31.9
      atonic (motor) (sensory) N31.2
      autonomous N31.2
      flaccid N31.2
      nonreflex N31.2
      reflex N31.1
      specified NEC N31.8
      uninhibited N31.0
  bleeding, uterus N93.8
  cerebral G93.89
  chronic
    coronary microvascular I25.85
    lung allograft J4A.9
      mixed J4A.0
      specified NEC J4A.8
  colon K59.9
    psychogenic F45.8
  colostomy K94.03
  coronary microvascular I25.85
    with
      angina pectoris I20.81
      myocardial infarction I21.B
    acute I24.81
    chronic I25.85
  cystic duct K82.8
  cystostomy (stoma) — see Complications, cystostomy
  ejaculatory N53.19
    anejaculatory orgasm N53.13
    painful N53.12
    premature F52.4
    retarded N53.11
  endocrine NOS E34.9
  endometrium N85.8
  enterostomy K94.13
  erectile — see Dysfunction, sexual, male, erectile
  feeding, pediatric
    acute R63.31
    chronic R63.32
  gallbladder K82.8
  gastrostomy (stoma) K94.23
  gland, glandular NOS E34.9
    meibomian, of eyelid — see Dysfunction, meibomian gland
  heart I51.89
  hemoglobin D75.89
  hepatic K76.89
  hypophysis E23.7
  hypothalamic NEC E23.3
  ileostomy (stoma) K94.13
  jejunostomy (stoma) K94.13
  kidney — see Disease, renal

Dysfunction — continued
  labyrinthine — see subcategory H83.2- ☑
  left ventricular, following sudden emotional stress I51.81
  liver K76.89
  lymphatic
    Fontan-associated I27.841
  male — see Dysfunction, sexual, male
  meibomian gland, of eyelid H02.889
    left H02.886
      lower H02.885
      upper H02.884
      upper and lower eyelids H02.88B
    right H02.883
      lower H02.882
      upper H02.881
      upper and lower eyelids H02.88A
  multifidus muscles, lumbar region M62.85
  orgasmic (female) F52.31
    male F52.32
  ovary E28.9
    specified NEC E28.8
  papillary muscle I51.89
  parathyroid E21.4
  physiological NEC R68.89
    psychogenic F59
  pineal gland E34.8
  pituitary (gland) E23.3
  platelets D69.1
  polyglandular E31.9
    specified NEC E31.8
  psychophysiologic F59
  psychosexual F52.9
    with
      dyspareunia F52.6
      premature ejaculation F52.4
      vaginismus F52.5
  pylorus K31.9
  rectum K59.9
    psychogenic F45.8
  reflex (sympathetic) — see Syndrome, pain, complex regional I
  segmental — see Dysfunction, somatic
  senile R54
  sexual (due to) R37
    alcohol F10.981
    amphetamine F15.981
      in
        abuse F15.181
        dependence F15.281
    anxiolytic F13.981
      in
        abuse F13.181
        dependence F13.281
    cocaine F14.981
      in
        abuse F14.181
        dependence F14.281
    excessive sexual drive F52.8
    failure of genital response (male) F52.21
      female F52.22
    female N94.9
      aversion F52.1
      dyspareunia N94.10
        psychogenic F52.6
      frigidity F52.22
      nymphomania F52.8
      orgasmic F52.31
      psychogenic F52.9
        aversion F52.1
        dyspareunia F52.6
        frigidity F52.22
        nymphomania F52.8
        orgasmic F52.31
        vaginismus F52.5
      vaginismus N94.2
        psychogenic F52.5
    hypnotic F13.981
      in
        abuse F13.181
        dependence F13.281
    inhibited orgasm (female) F52.31
      male F52.32
    lack
      of sexual enjoyment F52.1
      or loss of sexual desire F52.0
    male N53.9
      anejaculatory orgasm N53.13
      ejaculatory N53.19
        painful N53.12

Dysfunction — continued
　sexual — continued
　　male — continued
　　　ejaculatory — continued
　　　　　premature F52.4
　　　　　retarded N53.11
　　　erectile N52.9
　　　　drug induced N52.2
　　　　due to
　　　　　disease classified elsewhere N52.1
　　　　　drug N52.2
　　　　postoperative (postprocedural) N52.39
　　　　　following
　　　　　　cryotherapy N52.37
　　　　　　interstitial seed therapy N52.36
　　　　　　prostate ablative therapy N52.37
　　　　　　prostatectomy N52.34
　　　　　　　radical N52.31
　　　　　　radiation therapy N52.35
　　　　　　radical cystectomy N52.32
　　　　　　ultrasound ablative therapy N52.37
　　　　　　urethral surgery N52.33
　　　　psychogenic F52.21
　　　　specified cause NEC N52.8
　　　　vasculogenic
　　　　　arterial insufficiency N52.01
　　　　　　with corporo-venous occlusive N52.03
　　　　　corporo-venous occlusive N52.02
　　　　　　with arterial insufficiency N52.03
　　　impotence — see Dysfunction, sexual, male, erectile
　　　psychogenic F52.9
　　　　aversion F52.1
　　　　erectile F52.21
　　　　orgasmic F52.32
　　　　premature ejaculation F52.4
　　　　satyriasis F52.8
　　　　specified type NEC F52.8
　　　specified type NEC N53.8
　　nonorganic F52.9
　　　specified NEC F52.8
　　opioid F11.981
　　　in
　　　　abuse F11.181
　　　　dependence F11.281
　　orgasmic dysfunction (female) F52.31
　　　male F52.32
　　premature ejaculation F52.4
　　psychoactive substances NEC F19.981
　　　in
　　　　abuse F19.181
　　　　dependence F19.281
　　psychogenic F52.9
　　sedative F13.981
　　　in
　　　　abuse F13.181
　　　　dependence F13.281
　　sexual aversion F52.1
　　vaginismus (nonorganic) (psychogenic) F52.5
　sinoatrial node I49.5
　somatic M99.09
　　abdomen M99.09
　　acromioclavicular M99.07
　　cervical region M99.01
　　cervicothoracic M99.01
　　costochondral M99.08
　　costovertebral M99.08
　　head region M99.00
　　hip M99.05
　　lower extremity M99.06
　　lumbar region M99.03
　　lumbosacral M99.03
　　occipitocervical M99.00
　　pelvic region M99.05
　　pubic M99.05
　　rib cage M99.08
　　sacral region M99.04
　　sacrococcygeal M99.04
　　sacroiliac M99.04
　　specified NEC M99.09
　　sternochondral M99.08
　　sternoclavicular M99.07
　　thoracic region M99.02
　　thoracolumbar M99.02
　　upper extremity M99.07
　somatoform autonomic F45.8
　stomach K31.89
　　psychogenic F45.8
　suprarenal E27.9

Dysfunction — continued
　suprarenal — continued
　　hyperfunction E27.0
　symbolic R48.9
　　specified type NEC R48.8
　temporomandibular (joint) M26.69
　　joint-pain syndrome M26.62- ☑
　testicular (endocrine) E29.9
　　specified NEC E29.8
　thymus E32.9
　thyroid E07.9
　ureterostomy (stoma) — see Complications, stoma, urinary tract
　urethrostomy (stoma) — see Complications, stoma, urinary tract
　uterus, complicating delivery O62.9
　　hypertonic O62.4
　　hypotonic O62.2
　　　primary O62.0
　　　secondary O62.1
　ventricular I51.9
　　with congestive heart failure — see also Failure, heart I50.9
　　left, reversible, following sudden emotional stress I51.81
Dysgenesis
　gonadal (due to chromosomal anomaly) Q96.9
　　pure Q99.1
　renal Q60.5
　　bilateral Q60.4
　　unilateral Q60.3
　reticular D72.0
　tidal platelet D69.3
Dysgerminoma
　specified site — see Neoplasm, malignant, by site
　unspecified site
　　female C56.9
　　male C62.90
Dysgeusia R43.2
Dysgraphia R27.8
Dyshidrosis, dysidrosis L30.1
Dyskaryotic cervical smear R87.619
Dyskeratosis L85.8
　cervix — see Dysplasia, cervix
　congenital Q82.8
　uterus NEC N85.8
Dyskinesia G24.9
　biliary (cystic duct or gallbladder) K82.8
　drug induced
　　orofacial G24.01
　esophagus K22.4
　hysterical F44.4
　intestinal K59.89
　nonorganic origin F44.4
　orofacial (idiopathic) G24.4
　　drug induced G24.01
　psychogenic F44.4
　subacute, drug induced G24.01
　tardive G24.01
　　neuroleptic induced G24.01
　trachea J39.8
　tracheobronchial J98.09
Dyslalia (developmental) F80.0
Dyslexia R48.0
　developmental F81.0
Dyslipidemia E78.5
　depressed HDL cholesterol E78.6
　elevated fasting triglycerides E78.1
Dysmaturity — see also Light for dates
　pulmonary (newborn) (Wilson-Mikity) P27.0
Dysmenorrhea (essential) (exfoliative) N94.6
　congestive (syndrome) N94.6
　primary N94.4
　psychogenic F45.8
　secondary N94.5
Dysmetabolic syndrome X E88.810
Dysmetria R27.8
Dysmorphia
　muscle F45.22
Dysmorphism (due to)
　alcohol Q86.0
　exogenous cause NEC Q86.8
　hydantoin Q86.1
　warfarin Q86.2
Dysmorphophobia (nondelusional) F45.22
　delusional F22
Dysnomia R47.01
Dysorexia R63.0
　psychogenic F50.89

Dysostosis
　cleidocranial, cleidocranialis Q74.0
　craniofacial Q75.1
　Fairbank's (idiopathic familial generalized osteophytosis) Q78.9
　mandibulofacial (incomplete) Q75.4
　multiplex E76.01
　oculomandibular Q75.5
Dyspareunia (female) N94.10
　deep N94.12
　male N53.12
　nonorganic F52.6
　psychogenic F52.6
　secondary N94.19
　specified NEC N94.19
　superficial (introital) N94.11
Dyspepsia R10.13
　atonic K30
　functional (allergic) (congenital) (gastrointestinal) (occupational) (reflex) K30
　intestinal K59.89
　nervous F45.8
　neurotic F45.8
　psychogenic F45.8
Dysphagia R13.10
　cervical R13.19
　following
　　cerebral infarction I69.391
　　cerebrovascular disease I69.991
　　　specified NEC I69.891
　　intracerebral hemorrhage I69.191
　　nontraumatic intracranial hemorrhage NEC I69.291
　　specified disease NEC I69.891
　　subarachnoid hemorrhage I69.091
　functional (hysterical) F45.8
　hysterical F45.8
　nervous (hysterical) F45.8
　neurogenic R13.19
　oral phase R13.11
　oropharyngeal phase R13.12
　pharyngeal phase R13.13
　pharyngoesophageal phase R13.14
　psychogenic F45.8
　sideropenic D50.1
　spastica K22.4
　specified NEC R13.19
Dysphagocytosis, congenital D71.8
Dysphasia R47.02
　developmental
　　expressive type F80.1
　　receptive type F80.2
　following
　　cerebrovascular disease I69.921
　　　cerebral infarction I69.321
　　intracerebral hemorrhage I69.121
　　nontraumatic intracranial hemorrhage NEC I69.221
　　specified disease NEC I69.821
　　subarachnoid hemorrhage I69.021
Dysphonia R49.0
　functional F44.4
　hysterical F44.4
　psychogenic F44.4
　spastica J38.3
Dysphoria
　gender F64.9
　　in
　　　adolescence and adulthood F64.0
　　　children F64.2
　　specified NEC F64.8
　postpartal O90.6
Dyspituitarism E23.3
Dysplasia — see also Anomaly
　acetabular, congenital Q65.89
　alveolar capillary, with vein misalignment J84.843
　anus (histologically confirmed) (mild) (moderate) K62.82
　　severe D01.3
　arrhythmogenic right ventricular I42.8
　arterial, fibromuscular I77.3
　asphyxiating thoracic (congenital) Q77.2
　brain Q07.9
　bronchopulmonary, perinatal P27.1
　cervix (uteri) N87.9
　　mild N87.0
　　moderate N87.1
　　severe D06.9
　chondroectodermal Q77.6
　colon D12.6
　craniometaphyseal Q78.8
　dentinal K00.5

Dysplasia — continued
  diaphyseal, progressive Q78.3
  dystrophic Q77.5
  ectodermal (anhidrotic) (congenital) (hereditary) Q82.4
    hydrotic Q82.8
  epithelial, uterine cervix — see Dysplasia, cervix
  eye (congenital) Q11.2
  fibrous
    bone NEC (monostotic) M85.00
      ankle M85.07- ☑
      foot M85.07- ☑
      forearm M85.03- ☑
      hand M85.04- ☑
      lower leg M85.06- ☑
      multiple site M85.09
      neck M85.08
      rib M85.08
      shoulder M85.01- ☑
      skull M85.08
      specified site NEC M85.08
      thigh M85.05- ☑
      toe M85.07- ☑
      upper arm M85.02- ☑
      vertebra M85.08
    diaphyseal, progressive Q78.3
    jaw M27.8
    polyostotic Q78.1
  florid osseous — see also Cyst, calcifying odontogenic
  high grade, focal D12.6
  hip, congenital Q65.89
  joint, congenital Q74.8
  kidney Q61.4
    multicystic Q61.4
  leg Q74.2
  lung, congenital (not associated with short gestation) Q33.6
  mammary (gland) (benign) N60.9- ☑
    cyst (solitary) — see Cyst, breast
    cystic — see Mastopathy, cystic
    duct ectasia — see Ectasia, mammary duct
    fibroadenosis — see Fibroadenosis, breast
    fibrosclerosis — see Fibrosclerosis, breast
    specified type NEC N60.8- ☑
  metaphyseal Q78.5
  muscle Q79.8
  oculodentodigital Q87.0
  periapical (cemental) (cemento-osseous) — see Cyst, calcifying odontogenic
  periosteum — see Disorder, bone, specified type NEC
  polyostotic fibrous Q78.1
  prostate — see also Neoplasia, intraepithelial, prostate N42.30
    severe D07.5
    specified NEC N42.39
  renal Q61.4
    multicystic Q61.4
  retinal, congenital Q14.1
  right ventricular, arrhythmogenic I42.8
  septo-optic Q04.4
  skin L98.8
  spinal cord Q06.1
  spondyloepiphyseal Q77.7
  thymic, with immunodeficiency D82.1
  vagina N89.3
    mild N89.0
    moderate N89.1
    severe NEC D07.2
  vulva N90.3
    mild N90.0
    moderate N90.1
    severe NEC D07.1
Dysplasminogenemia E88.02
Dyspnea (nocturnal) (paroxysmal) R06.00
  asthmatic (bronchial) J45.909
    with
      bronchitis J45.909
        with
          exacerbation (acute) J45.901
          status asthmaticus J45.902
      chronic J44.89
    exacerbation (acute) J45.901
    status asthmaticus J45.902
  cardiac — see Failure, ventricular, left
  functional F45.8
  hyperventilation R06.4
  hysterical F45.8
  newborn P28.89
  orthopnea R06.01

Dyspnea — continued
  psychogenic F45.8
  shortness of breath R06.02
  specified type NEC R06.09
  transfusion-associated [TAD] J95.87
Dyspraxia R27.8
  developmental (syndrome) F82
Dysproteinemia E88.09
Dysreflexia, autonomic G90.4
Dysrhythmia
  cardiac I49.9
    newborn
      bradycardia P29.12
      occurring before birth P03.819
        before onset of labor P03.810
        during labor P03.811
      tachycardia P29.11
    postoperative I97.89
  cerebral or cortical — see Epilepsy
Dyssomnia — see Disorder, sleep
Dyssynergia
  biliary K83.8
  bladder sphincter N36.44
  cerebellaris myoclonica (Hunt's ataxia) G11.19
Dysthymia F34.1
Dysthyroidism E07.9
Dystocia O66.9
  affecting newborn P03.1
  cervical (hypotonic) O62.2
    affecting newborn P03.6
    primary O62.0
    secondary O62.1
  contraction ring O62.4
  fetal O66.9
    abnormality NEC O66.3
    conjoined twins O66.3
    oversize O66.2
  maternal O66.9
  positional O64.9- ☑
  shoulder (girdle) O66.0
    causing obstructed labor O66.0
  uterine NEC O62.4
Dystonia G24.9
  cervical G24.3
  deformans progressiva G24.1
  drug induced NEC G24.09
    acute G24.02
    specified NEC G24.09
  familial G24.1
  idiopathic G24.1
    familial G24.1
    nonfamilial G24.2
    orofacial G24.4
  lenticularis G24.8
  musculorum deformans G24.1
  neuroleptic induced (acute) G24.02
  orofacial (idiopathic) G24.4
  oromandibular G24.4
    due to drug G24.01
  specified NEC G24.8
  torsion (familial) (idiopathic) G24.1
    acquired G24.8
    genetic G24.1
    symptomatic (nonfamilial) G24.2
Dystonic movements R25.8
Dystrophy, dystrophia
  adiposogenital E23.6
  autosomal recessive, childhood type, muscular dystrophy resembling Duchenne or Becker G71.01
  Becker's type G71.01
  cervical sympathetic G90.2
  choroid (hereditary) H31.20
    central areolar H31.22
    choroideremia H31.21
    gyrate atrophy H31.23
    specified type NEC H31.29
  cornea (hereditary) H18.50- ☑
    endothelial H18.51- ☑
    epithelial H18.52- ☑
    granular H18.53- ☑
    lattice H18.54- ☑
    macular H18.55- ☑
    specified type NEC H18.59- ☑
  Duchenne's type G71.01
  due to malnutrition E45
  Erb's G71.02
  Fuchs' H18.51- ☑
  Gower's muscular G71.01

Dystrophy, dystrophia — continued
  hair L67.8
  infantile neuraxonal G31.89
  Landouzy-Dejerine G71.02
  Leyden-Mobius — see also Dystrophy, muscular, limb-girdle, by type G71.039
    meaning Limb girdle muscular dystrophy NOS G71.039
    meaning Limb girdle muscular dystrophy, other specified type — see by type
    meaning Limb girdle muscular dystrophy, specified type NEC G71.038
    meaning Limb girdle muscular dystrophy type 2A (autosomal recessive) G71.032
  muscular G71.00
    autosomal recessive, childhood type, muscular dystrophy resembling Duchenne or Becker G71.01
    benign (Becker type) G71.01
      scapuloperoneal with early contractures [Emery-Dreifuss] G71.09
    congenital (hereditary) (progressive) (with specific morphological abnormalities of the muscle fiber) G71.09
      myotonic G71.11
    distal G71.09
    Duchenne type G71.01
    Emery-Dreifuss G71.09
    Erb type G71.02
    facioscapulohumeral G71.02
    Gower's G71.01
    hereditary (progressive) — see also Dystrophy, muscular, by type G71.09
    Landouzy-Dejerine type G71.02
    limb-girdle G71.039
      alpha-sarcoglycan-relate G71.0341
      anoctamin-5-related autosomal recessive (R12) G71.035
      autosomal recessive NEC G71.038
      beta-sarcoglycan-related G71.0342
      calpain-3-related G71.032
        autosomal dominant G71.031
        autosomal recessive G71.032
      collagen VI related
        autosomal dominant G71.031
        autosomal recessive G71.038
      D1 (autosomal dominant) G71.031
      D2 (autosomal dominant) G71.031
      D3 (autosomal dominant) G71.031
      D4 (autosomal dominant) G71.031
      D5 (autosomal dominant) G71.031
      delta-sarcoglycan-related G71.0349
      due to
        alpha sarcoglycan dysfunction G71.0341
        anoctamin-5 dysfunction G71.035
        beta sarcoglycan dysfunction G71.0342
        fukutin related protein dysfunction G71.036
        sarcoglycan dysfunction, specified NEC G71.0349
      FKRP-related autosomal recessive G71.038
      gamma-sarcoglycan-related G71.0349
      R1 (autosomal recessive) G71.032
      R2 (autosomal recessive) G71.033
      R3 (autosomal recessive) G71.0341
      R4 (autosomal recessive) G71.0342
      R5 (autosomal recessive) G71.0349
      R6 (autosomal recessive) G71.0349
      R7 (autosomal recessive) G71.038
      R8 (autosomal recessive) G71.038
      R9 (autosomal recessive) G71.036
      R10 (autosomal recessive) G71.038
      R11 (autosomal recessive) G71.038
      R12 (autosomal recessive) G71.035
      R13 (autosomal recessive) G71.038
      R14 (autosomal recessive) G71.038
      R15 (autosomal recessive) G71.038
      R16 (autosomal recessive) G71.038
      R17 (autosomal recessive) G71.038
      R18 (autosomal recessive) G71.038
      R19 (autosomal recessive) G71.038
      R20 (autosomal recessive) G71.038
      R21 (autosomal recessive) G71.038
      R22 (autosomal recessive) G71.038
      R23 (autosomal recessive) G71.038
      R24 (autosomal recessive) G71.038
      type 1 (autosomal dominant) G71.031
      type 1A (autosomal dominant) G71.031
      type 1B (autosomal dominant) G71.031
      type 1C (autosomal dominant) G71.031
      type 1E (autosomal dominant) G71.031

☑ **Additional Character Required — Refer to the Tabular List for Character Selection**

Dystrophy, dystrophia — continued
- muscular — continued
  - limb-girdle — continued
    - type 1H (autosomal dominant) G71.031
    - type 1I (autosomal dominant) G71.031
    - type 2 (autosomal recessive) G71.038
      - specified NEC G71.038
    - type 2A (autosomal recessive) G71.032
    - type 2B (autosomal recessive) G71.033
    - type 2C (autosomal recessive) G71.0349
    - type 2D (autosomal recessive) G71.0341
    - type 2E (autosomal recessive) G71.0342
    - type 2F (autosomal recessive) G71.0349
    - type 2G (autosomal recessive) G71.038
    - type 2H (autosomal recessive) G71.038
    - type 2I (autosomal recessive) G71.036
    - type 2J (autosomal recessive) G71.038
    - type 2K (autosomal recessive) G71.038
    - type 2L (autosomal recessive) G71.035
    - type 2M (autosomal recessive) G71.038
    - type 2N (autosomal recessive) G71.038
    - type 2O (autosomal recessive) G71.038
    - type 2P (autosomal recessive) G71.038
    - type 2Q (autosomal recessive) G71.038
    - type 2S (autosomal recessive) G71.038
    - type 2T (autosomal recessive) G71.038
    - type 2U (autosomal recessive) G71.038
  - myotonic G71.11
  - progressive (hereditary) — see also Dystrophy, muscular, by type G71.09
    - Charcot-Marie (-Tooth) type G60.0
  - pseudohypertrophic (infantile) G71.01
  - scapulohumeral G71.02
  - scapuloperoneal G71.02
  - severe (Duchenne type) G71.01
  - specified type NEC G71.09
- myocardium, myocardial — see Degeneration, myocardial
- nail L60.3
  - congenital Q84.6
- nutritional E45
- ocular G71.09
- oculocerebrorenal E72.03
- oculopharyngeal G71.09
- ovarian N83.8
- polyglandular E31.8
- reflex (neuromuscular) (sympathetic) — see Syndrome, pain, complex regional I
- retinal (hereditary) H35.50
  - in
    - lipid storage disorders E75.6 [H36.89]
    - systemic lipidoses E75.6 [H36.89]
  - involving
    - pigment epithelium H35.54
    - sensory area H35.53
  - pigmentary H35.52
  - vitreoretinal H35.51
- Salzmann's nodular — see Degeneration, cornea, nodular
- scapuloperoneal G71.09
- skin NEC L98.8
- sympathetic (reflex) — see Syndrome, pain, complex regional I
  - cervical G90.2
- tapetoretinal H35.54
- thoracic, asphyxiating Q77.2
- unguium L60.3
  - congenital Q84.6
- vitreoretinal H35.51
- vulva N90.4
- yellow (liver) — see Failure, hepatic

Dysuria R30.0
- psychogenic F45.8

E

Eales' disease H35.06- ☑
Ear — see also condition
- piercing Z41.3
- tropical NEC B36.9 [H62.4-] ☑
  - in
    - aspergillosis B44.89
    - candidiasis B37.84
    - moniliasis B37.84
- wax (impacted) H61.20
  - left H61.22
    - with right H61.23
  - right H61.21
    - with left H61.23

Earache — see subcategory H92.0- ☑
Early satiety R68.81
Eaton-Lambert syndrome — see Syndrome, Lambert-Eaton
Eberth's disease (typhoid fever) A01.00
Ebola virus disease A98.4
Ebstein's anomaly or syndrome (heart) Q22.5
Eccentro-osteochondrodysplasia E76.29
Ecchondroma — see Neoplasm, bone, benign
Ecchondrosis D48.0
Ecchymosis R58
- conjunctiva — see Hemorrhage, conjunctiva
- eye (traumatic) — see Contusion, eyeball
- eyelid (traumatic) — see Contusion, eyelid
- newborn P54.5
- spontaneous R23.3
- traumatic — see Contusion

Echinococciasis — see Echinococcus
Echinococcosis — see Echinococcus
Echinococcus (infection) B67.90
- granulosus B67.4
  - bone B67.2
  - liver B67.0
  - lung B67.1
  - multiple sites B67.32
  - specified site NEC B67.39
  - thyroid B67.31
- liver NOS B67.8
  - granulosus B67.0
  - multilocularis B67.5
- lung NEC B67.99
  - granulosus B67.1
  - multilocularis B67.69
- multilocularis B67.7
  - liver B67.5
  - multiple sites B67.61
  - specified site NEC B67.69
- specified site NEC B67.99
  - granulosus B67.39
  - multilocularis B67.69
- thyroid NEC B67.99
  - granulosus B67.31
  - multilocularis B67.69 [E35]

Echinorhynchiasis B83.8
Echinostomiasis B66.8
Echolalia R48.8
Echovirus, as cause of disease classified elsewhere B97.12
Eclampsia, eclamptic (coma) (convulsions) (delirium) (with hypertension) NEC O15.9
- complicating
  - labor and delivery O15.1
  - postpartum O15.2
  - pregnancy O15.0- ☑
  - puerperium O15.2

Economic circumstances affecting care Z59.9
Economo's disease A85.8
Ectasia, ectasis
- annuloaortic I35.8
- aorta I77.819
  - with aneurysm — see Aneurysm, aorta
  - abdominal I77.811
  - thoracic I77.810
  - thoracoabdominal I77.812
- breast — see Ectasia, mammary duct
- capillary I78.8
- cornea H18.71- ☑
- gastric antral vascular (GAVE) K31.819
  - with hemorrhage K31.811
  - without hemorrhage K31.819
- mammary duct N60.4- ☑
- salivary gland (duct) K11.8
- sclera — see Sclerectasia

Ecthyma L08.0
- contagiosum B08.02
- gangrenosum L08.0
- infectiosum B08.02

Ectocardia Q24.8
Ectodermal dysplasia (anhidrotic) Q82.4
Ectodermosis erosiva pluriorificialis L51.1
Ectopic, ectopia (congenital)
- abdominal viscera Q45.8
  - due to defect in anterior abdominal wall Q79.59
- ACTH syndrome E24.3
- adrenal gland Q89.1
- anus Q43.5
- atrial beats I49.1
- beats I49.49
  - atrial I49.1

Ectopic, ectopia — continued
- beats — continued
  - ventricular I49.3
- bladder Q64.10
- bone and cartilage in lung Q33.5
- brain Q04.8
- breast tissue Q83.8
- cardiac Q24.8
- cerebral Q04.8
- cordis Q24.8
- endometrium — see Endometriosis
- gastric mucosa Q40.2
- gestation — see Pregnancy, by site
- heart Q24.8
- hormone secretion NEC E34.2
- kidney (crossed) (pelvis) Q63.2
- lens, lentis Q12.1
- mole — see Pregnancy, by site
- organ or site NEC — see Malposition, congenital
- pancreas Q45.3
- pregnancy — see Pregnancy, ectopic
- pupil — see Abnormality, pupillary
- renal Q63.2
- sebaceous glands of mouth Q38.6
- spleen Q89.09
- testis Q53.00
  - bilateral Q53.02
  - unilateral Q53.01
- thyroid Q89.2
- tissue in lung Q33.5
- ureter Q62.63
- ventricular beats I49.3
- vesicae Q64.10

Ectromelia Q73.8
- lower limb — see Defect, reduction, limb, lower, specified type NEC
- upper limb — see Defect, reduction, limb, upper, specified type NEC

Ectropion H02.109
- cervix N86
  - with cervicitis N72
- congenital Q10.1
- eyelid H02.109
  - cicatricial H02.119
    - left H02.116
      - lower H02.115
      - upper H02.114
    - right H02.113
      - lower H02.112
      - upper H02.111
  - congenital Q10.1
  - left H02.106
    - lower H02.105
    - upper H02.104
  - mechanical H02.129
    - left H02.126
      - lower H02.125
      - upper H02.124
    - right H02.123
      - lower H02.122
      - upper H02.121
  - paralytic H02.159
    - left H02.156
      - lower H02.155
      - upper H02.154
    - right H02.153
      - lower H02.152
      - upper H02.151
  - right H02.103
    - lower H02.102
    - upper H02.101
  - senile H02.139
    - left H02.136
      - lower H02.135
      - upper H02.134
    - right H02.133
      - lower H02.132
      - upper H02.131
  - spastic H02.149
    - left H02.146
      - lower H02.145
      - upper H02.144
    - right H02.143
      - lower H02.142
      - upper H02.141
- iris H21.89
- lip (acquired) K13.0
  - congenital Q38.0
- urethra N36.8

Ectropion — *continued*
  uvea H21.89
Eczema (acute) (chronic) (erythematous) (fissum) (rubrum) (squamous) — *see also* Dermatitis L30.9
  contact — *see* Dermatitis, contact
  dyshydrotic L30.1
  external ear — *see* Otitis, externa, acute, eczematoid
  flexural L20.82
  herpeticum B00.0
  hypertrophicum L28.0
  hypostatic — *see* Varix, leg, with, inflammation
  impetiginous L01.1
  infantile (due to any substance) L20.83
    intertriginous L21.1
    seborrheic L21.1
  intertriginous NEC L30.4
    infantile L21.1
  intrinsic (allergic) L20.84
  lichenified NEC L28.0
  marginatum (hebrae) B35.6
  pustular L30.3
  stasis I87.2
    with varicose veins — *see* Varix, leg, with, inflammation
  vaccination, vaccinatum T88.1- ☑
  varicose — *see* Varix, leg, with, inflammation
Eczematid L30.2
Eddowes (-Spurway) **syndrome** Q78.0
Edema, edematous (infectious) (pitting) (toxic) R60.9
  with nephritis — *see* Nephrosis
  allergic T78.3- ☑
  amputation stump (surgical) (sequelae (late effect)) T87.89
  angioneurotic (allergic) (any site) (with urticaria) T78.3- ☑
    hereditary D84.1
  angiospastic I73.9
  Berlin's (traumatic) S05.8X- ☑
  brain (cytotoxic) (vasogenic) G93.6
    due to birth injury P11.0
    newborn (anoxia or hypoxia) P52.4
      birth injury P11.0
    traumatic — *see* Injury, intracranial, cerebral edema
  cardiac — *see* Failure, heart, congestive
  cardiovascular — *see* Failure, heart, congestive
  cerebral — *see* Edema, brain
  cerebrospinal — *see* Edema, brain
  cervix (uteri) (acute) N88.8
    puerperal, postpartum O90.89
  chronic hereditary Q82.0
  circumscribed, acute T78.3- ☑
    hereditary D84.1
  conjunctiva H11.42- ☑
  cornea H18.2- ☑
    idiopathic H18.22- ☑
    secondary H18.23- ☑
      due to contact lens H18.21- ☑
  due to
    lymphatic obstruction I89.0
    salt retention E87.0
  epiglottis — *see* Edema, glottis
  essential, acute T78.3- ☑
    hereditary D84.1
  extremities, lower — *see* Edema, legs
  eyelid NEC H02.849
    left H02.846
      lower H02.845
      upper H02.844
    right H02.843
      lower H02.842
      upper H02.841
  familial, hereditary Q82.0
  famine — *see* Malnutrition, severe
  generalized R60.1
  glottis, glottic, glottidis (obstructive) (passive) J38.4
    allergic T78.3- ☑
    hereditary D84.1
  heart — *see* Failure, heart, congestive
  heat T67.7- ☑
  hereditary Q82.0
  inanition — *see* Malnutrition, severe
  intracranial G93.6
  iris H21.89
  joint — *see* Effusion, joint
  larynx — *see* Edema, glottis
  legs R60.0
    due to venous obstruction I87.1
    hereditary Q82.0

Edema, edematous — *continued*
  localized R60.0
    due to venous obstruction I87.1
  lower limbs — *see* Edema, legs
  lung J81.1
    with heart condition or failure — *see* Failure, ventricular, left
    newborn P29.0
    acute J81.0
    chemical (acute) J68.1
      chronic J68.1
    chronic J81.1
      due to
        chemicals, gases, fumes or vapors (inhalation) J68.1
        external agent J70.9
          specified NEC J70.8
        radiation J70.1
    due to
      chemicals, fumes or vapors (inhalation) J68.1
      external agent J70.9
        specified NEC J70.8
      high altitude T70.29- ☑
      near drowning T75.1- ☑
      radiation J70.0
    meaning failure, left ventricle I50.1
  lymphatic I89.0
    due to mastectomy I97.2
  macula H35.81
    cystoid, following cataract surgery — *see* Complications, postprocedural, following cataract surgery
    diabetic — *see* Diabetes, by type, with, retinopathy, with macular edema
  malignant — *see* Gangrene, gas
  Milroy's Q82.0
  nasopharynx J39.2
  newborn P83.30
    hydrops fetalis — *see* Hydrops, fetalis
    specified NEC P83.39
  nutritional — *see also* Malnutrition, severe
    with dyspigmentation, skin and hair E40
  optic disc or nerve — *see* Papilledema
  orbit H05.22- ☑
  pancreas K86.89
  papilla, optic — *see* Papilledema
  penis N48.89
  periodic T78.3- ☑
    hereditary D84.1
  pharynx J39.2
  pulmonary — *see* Edema, lung
  Quincke's T78.3- ☑
    hereditary D84.1
  renal — *see* Nephrosis
  retina H35.81
    diabetic — *see* Diabetes, by type, with, retinopathy, with macular edema
  salt E87.0
  scrotum N50.89
  seminal vesicle N50.89
  spermatic cord N50.89
  spinal (cord) (vascular) (nontraumatic) G95.19
  starvation — *see* Malnutrition, severe
  stasis — *see* Hypertension, venous, (chronic)
  subglottic — *see* Edema, glottis
  supraglottic — *see* Edema, glottis
  testis N44.8
  tunica vaginalis N50.89
  vas deferens N50.89
  vulva (acute) N90.89
Edentulism — *see* Absence, teeth, acquired
Edsall's disease T67.2- ☑
Educational handicap Z55.9
  less than a high school diploma Z55.5
  no general equivalence degree (GED) Z55.5
  specified NEC Z55.8
Edward's syndrome — *see* Trisomy, 18
Effect(s) (of) (from) — *see* Effect, adverse NEC
Effect, adverse
  abnormal gravitational (G) forces or states T75.81- ☑
  abuse — *see* Maltreatment
  air pressure T70.9- ☑
    specified NEC T70.8- ☑
  altitude (high) — *see* Effect, adverse, high altitude
  anesthesia — *see also* Anesthesia T88.59- ☑
    in labor and delivery O74.9
    local, toxic
      in labor and delivery O74.4

Effect, adverse — *continued*
  anesthesia — *see also* Anesthesia — *continued*
    local, toxic — *continued*
      in pregnancy NEC O29.3- ☑
      postpartum, puerperal O89.3
    postpartum, puerperal O89.9
    specified NEC T88.59- ☑
      in labor and delivery O74.8
      postpartum, puerperal O89.8
    spinal and epidural T88.59- ☑
      headache T88.59- ☑
        in labor and delivery O74.5
        postpartum, puerperal O89.4
      specified NEC
        in labor and delivery O74.6
        postpartum, puerperal O89.5
  antitoxin — *see* Complications, vaccination
  atmospheric pressure T70.9- ☑
    due to explosion T70.8- ☑
    high T70.3- ☑
    low — *see* Effect, adverse, high altitude
    specified effect NEC T70.8- ☑
  biological, correct substance properly administered — *see* Effect, adverse, drug
  blood (derivatives) (serum) (transfusion) — *see* Complications, transfusion
  chemical substance — *see* Table of Drugs and Chemicals
  cold (temperature) (weather) T69.9- ☑
    chilblains T69.1- ☑
    frostbite — *see* Frostbite
    specified effect NEC T69.8- ☑
  drugs and medicaments T88.7- ☑
    specified drug — *see* Table of Drugs and Chemicals, by drug, adverse effect
    specified effect — *code to* condition
  electric current, electricity (shock) T75.4- ☑
    burn — *see* Burn
  exertion (excessive) T73.3- ☑
  exposure — *see* Exposure
  external cause NEC T75.89- ☑
  foodstuffs T78.19- ☑
    allergic reaction — *see* Allergy, food
      causing anaphylaxis — *see* Shock, anaphylactic, due to food
    noxious — *see* Poisoning, food, noxious
  gases, fumes, or vapors T59.9- ☑
    specified agent — *see* Table of Drugs and Chemicals
  glue (airplane) sniffing
    due to drug abuse — *see* Abuse, drug, inhalant
    due to drug dependence — *see* Dependence, drug, inhalant
  heat — *see* Heat
  high altitude NEC T70.29- ☑
    anoxia T70.29- ☑
    on
      ears T70.0- ☑
      sinuses T70.1- ☑
    polycythemia D75.1
  high pressure fluids T70.4- ☑
  hot weather — *see* Heat
  hunger T73.0- ☑
  immersion, foot — *see* Immersion
  immunization — *see* Complications, vaccination
  immunological agents — *see* Complications, vaccination
  infrared (radiation) (rays) NOS T66.- ☑
    dermatitis or eczema L59.8
  infusion — *see* Complications, infusion
  lack of care of infants — *see* Maltreatment, child
  lightning — *see* Lightning
  medical care T88.9- ☑
    specified NEC T88.8- ☑
  medicinal substance, correct, properly administered — *see* Effect, adverse, drug
  motion T75.3- ☑
  noise, on inner ear — *see* subcategory H83.3- ☑
  overheated places — *see* Heat
  psychosocial, of work environment Z56.5
  radiation (diagnostic) (infrared) (natural source) (therapeutic) (ultraviolet) (X-ray) NOS T66.- ☑
    dermatitis or eczema — *see* Dermatitis, due to, radiation
    fibrosis of lung J70.1
    pneumonitis J70.0
    pulmonary manifestations
      acute J70.0
      chronic J70.1
  skin L59.9

Effect, adverse — *continued*
  radioactive substance NOS
    dermatitis or eczema — *see* Radiodermatitis
  reduced temperature T69.9- ☑
    immersion foot or hand — *see* Immersion
    specified effect NEC T69.8- ☑
  serum NEC — *see also* Reaction, serum T80.69- ☑
  specified NEC T78.8- ☑
    external cause NEC T75.89- ☑
  strangulation — *see* Asphyxia, traumatic
  submersion T75.1- ☑
  thirst T73.1- ☑
  toxic — *see* Toxicity
  transfusion — *see* Complications, transfusion
  ultraviolet (radiation) (rays) NOS T66.- ☑
    burn — *see* Burn
    dermatitis or eczema — *see* Dermatitis, due to, ultraviolet rays
      acute L56.8
  vaccine (any) — *see* Complications, vaccination
  vibration — *see* Vibration, adverse effects
  war theater, specified NEC T75.838- ☑
  water pressure NEC T70.9- ☑
    specified NEC T70.8- ☑
  weightlessness T75.82- ☑
  whole blood — *see* Complications, transfusion
  work environment Z56.5
Effects, late — *see* Sequelae
Effluvium
  anagen L65.1
  telogen L65.0
Effort syndrome (psychogenic) F45.8
Effusion
  amniotic fluid — *see* Pregnancy, complicated by, premature rupture of membranes
  brain (serous) G93.6
  bronchial — *see* Bronchitis
  cerebral G93.6
  cerebrospinal — *see also* Meningitis
    vessel G93.6
  chest — *see* Effusion, pleura
  chylous, chyliform (pleura) J94.0
  intracranial G93.6
  joint M25.40
    ankle M25.47- ☑
    elbow M25.42- ☑
    foot joint M25.47- ☑
    hand joint M25.44- ☑
    hip M25.45- ☑
    knee M25.46- ☑
    shoulder M25.41- ☑
    specified joint NEC M25.48
    wrist M25.43- ☑
  malignant pleural J91.0
  meninges — *see* Meningitis
  pericardium, pericardial (noninflammatory) I31.39
    acute — *see* Pericarditis, acute
    malignant, in disease classified elsewhere I31.31
    specified type, NEC I31.39
  peritoneal (chronic) R18.8
  pleura, pleurisy, pleuritic, pleuropericardial J90
    chylous, chyliform J94.0
    due to systemic lupus erythematosis M32.13
    in conditions classified elsewhere J91.8
    influenzal — *see* Influenza, with, respiratory manifestations NEC
    malignant J91.0
    newborn P28.89
    tuberculous NEC A15.6
      primary (progressive) A15.7
  spinal — *see* Meningitis
  thorax, thoracic — *see* Effusion, pleura
Egg shell nails L60.3
  congenital Q84.6
EGPA (eosinophilic granulomatosis with polyangiitis) M30.1
Egyptian splenomegaly B65.1
Ehlers-Danlos syndrome — *see also* Syndrome, Ehlers-Danlos Q79.60
Ehrlichiosis A77.40
  due to
    E. chaffeensis A77.41
    E. ewingii A77.49
    E. muris euclairensis A77.49
    E. sennetsu A79.81
    specified organism NEC A77.49
Eichstedt's disease B36.0
Eisenmenger's
  complex or syndrome I27.83

Eisenmenger's — *continued*
  defect Q21.8
Ejaculation
  delayed F52.32
  painful N53.12
  premature F52.4
  retarded N53.11
  retrograde N53.14
  semen, painful N53.12
    psychogenic F52.6
Ekbom's syndrome (restless legs) G25.81
Ekman's syndrome (brittle bones and blue sclera) Q78.0
Elastic skin Q82.8
  acquired L57.4
Elastofibroma — *see* Neoplasm, connective tissue, benign
Elastoma (juvenile) Q82.8
  Miescher's L87.2
Elastomyofibrosis I42.4
Elastosis
  actinic, solar L57.8
  atrophicans (senile) L57.4
  perforans serpiginosa L87.2
  senilis L57.4
Elbow — *see* condition
Electric current, electricity, effects (concussion) (fatal) (nonfatal) (shock) T75.4- ☑
  burn — *see* Burn
Electric feet syndrome E53.8
Electrocution T75.4- ☑
  from electroshock gun (taser) T75.4- ☑
Electrolyte imbalance E87.8
  with
    abortion — *see* Abortion by type, complicated by, electrolyte imbalance
    ectopic pregnancy O08.5
    molar pregnancy O08.5
Elephantiasis (nonfilarial) I89.0
  arabicum — *see* Infestation, filarial
  bancroftian B74.0
  congenital (any site) (hereditary) Q82.0
  due to
    Brugia (malayi) B74.1
      timori B74.2
    mastectomy I97.2
    Wuchereria (bancrofti) B74.0
  eyelid H02.859
    left H02.856
      lower H02.855
      upper H02.854
    right H02.853
      lower H02.852
      upper H02.851
  filarial, filariensis — *see* Infestation, filarial
  glandular I89.0
  graecorum A30.9
  lymphangiectatic I89.0
  lymphatic vessel I89.0
    due to mastectomy I97.2
  scrotum (nonfilarial) I89.0
  streptococcal I89.0
  surgical I97.89
    postmastectomy I97.2
  telangiectodes I89.0
  vulva (nonfilarial) N90.89
Elevated, elevation
  alanine transaminase (ALT) R74.01
  ALT (alanine transaminase) R74.01
  antibody titer R76.0
  aspartate transaminase (AST) R74.01
  AST (aspartate transaminase) R74.01
  basal metabolic rate R94.8
  blood pressure — *see also* Hypertension
    reading (incidental) (isolated) (nonspecific), no diagnosis of hypertension R03.0
  blood sugar R73.9
  body temperature (of unknown origin) R50.9
  C-reactive protein (CRP) R79.82
  cancer antigen 125 [CA 125] R97.1
  carcinoembryonic antigen [CEA] R97.0
  cholesterol E78.00
    with high triglycerides E78.2
  conjugate, eye H51.0
  diaphragm, congenital Q79.1
  erythrocyte sedimentation rate R70.0
  fasting glucose R73.01
  fasting triglycerides E78.1
  finding on laboratory examination — *see* Findings, abnormal, inconclusive, without diagnosis, by type of exam

Elevated, elevation — *continued*
  GFR (glomerular filtration rate) — *see* Findings, abnormal, inconclusive, without diagnosis, by type of exam
  glucose tolerance (oral) R73.02
  immunoglobulin level R76.89
  indoleacetic acid R82.5
  lactic acid dehydrogenase (LDH) level R74.02
  leukocytes D72.829
  lipoprotein a (Lp(a)) level E78.41
  liver function
    study R94.5
    test R79.89
      alkaline phosphatase R74.8
      aminotransferase R74.01
      bilirubin R17
      hepatic enzyme R74.8
      lactate dehydrogenase R74.02
  Lp(a) (lipoprotein(a)) E78.41
  lymphocytes D72.820
  prostate specific antigen [PSA] R97.20
  Rh titer — *see* Complication(s), transfusion, incompatibility reaction, Rh (factor)
  scapula, congenital Q74.0
  sedimentation rate R70.0
  SGOT R74.01
  SGPT R74.01
  transaminase level R74.01
  triglycerides E78.1
    with high cholesterol E78.2
  troponin R79.89
  tumor associated antigens [TAA] NEC R97.8
  tumor specific antigens [TSA] NEC R97.8
  urine level of
    17-ketosteroids R82.5
    catecholamine R82.5
    indoleacetic acid R82.5
    steroids R82.5
    vanillylmandelic acid (VMA) R82.5
  venous pressure I87.8
  white blood cell count D72.829
    specified NEC D72.828
Elliptocytosis (congenital) (hereditary) D58.1
  Hb C (disease) D58.1
  hemoglobin disease D58.1
  sickle-cell (disease) D57.8- ☑
  trait D57.3
Ellis-van Creveld syndrome (chondroectodermal dysplasia) Q77.6
Ellison-Zollinger syndrome E16.4
Elongated, elongation (congenital) — *see also* Distortion
  bone Q79.9
  cervix (uteri) Q51.828
    acquired N88.4
    hypertrophic N88.4
  colon Q43.8
  common bile duct Q44.5
  cystic duct Q44.5
  frenulum, penis Q55.69
  labia minora (acquired) N90.69
  ligamentum patellae Q74.1
  petiolus (epiglottidis) Q31.8
  tooth, teeth K00.2
  uvula Q38.6
Eltor cholera A00.1
Emaciation R64
  due to malnutrition E43
Embadomoniasis A07.8
Embedded tooth, teeth K01.0
  root only K08.3
Embolic — *see* condition
Embolism (multiple) (paradoxical) I74.9
  air (any site) (traumatic) T79.0- ☑
    following
      abortion — *see* Abortion by type complicated by embolism
      ectopic pregnancy O08.2
      infusion, therapeutic injection or transfusion T80.0- ☑
      molar pregnancy O08.2
      procedure NEC
        artery T81.719- ☑
          mesenteric T81.710- ☑
          renal T81.711- ☑
          specified NEC T81.718- ☑
        vein T81.72- ☑
    in pregnancy, childbirth or puerperium — *see* Embolism, obstetric

Embolism — continued
- amniotic fluid (pulmonary) — see also Embolism, obstetric
  - following
    - abortion — see Abortion by type complicated by embolism
    - ectopic pregnancy O08.2
    - molar pregnancy O08.2
- aorta, aortic I74.10
  - abdominal I74.09
    - saddle I74.01
  - bifurcation I74.09
  - saddle I74.01
  - thoracic I74.11
- artery I74.9
  - auditory, internal I65.8
  - basilar — see Occlusion, artery, basilar
  - carotid (common) (internal) — see Occlusion, artery, carotid
  - cerebellar (anterior inferior) (posterior inferior) (superior) I66.3
  - cerebral — see Occlusion, artery, cerebral
  - choroidal (anterior) I65.8
  - communicating posterior I65.8
  - coronary — see also Infarct, myocardium
    - not resulting in infarction I24.0
  - extremity I74.4
    - lower I74.3
    - upper I74.2
  - hypophyseal I65.8
  - iliac I74.5
  - limb I74.4
    - lower I74.3
    - upper I74.2
  - mesenteric (with gangrene) — see also Ischemia, intestine, acute K55.059
  - ophthalmic — see Occlusion, artery, retina
  - peripheral I74.4
  - pontine I65.8
  - precerebral — see Occlusion, artery, precerebral
  - pulmonary — see Embolism, pulmonary
  - renal N28.0
  - retinal — see Occlusion, artery, retina
  - septic I76
  - specified NEC I74.8
  - vertebral — see Occlusion, artery, vertebral
- basilar (artery) I65.1
- blood clot
  - following
    - abortion — see Abortion by type complicated by embolism
    - ectopic or molar pregnancy O08.2
  - in pregnancy, childbirth or puerperium — see Embolism, obstetric
- brain — see also Occlusion, artery, cerebral
  - following
    - abortion — see Abortion by type complicated by embolism
    - ectopic or molar pregnancy O08.2
    - puerperal, postpartum, childbirth — see Embolism, obstetric
- capillary I78.8
- cardiac — see also Infarct, myocardium
  - not resulting in infarction I51.3
- carotid (artery) (common) (internal) — see Occlusion, artery, carotid
- cavernous sinus (venous) — see Embolism, intracranial, venous sinus
- cement
  - pulmonary artery I26.95
    - with acute cor pulmonale I26.03
- cerebral — see Occlusion, artery, cerebral
- cholesterol — see Atheroembolism
- coronary (artery or vein) (systemic) — see Occlusion, coronary
- due to device, implant or graft — see also Complications, by site and type, specified NEC
  - arterial graft NEC T82.818- ☑
  - breast (implant) T85.818- ☑
  - catheter NEC T85.818- ☑
    - dialysis (renal) T82.818- ☑
      - intraperitoneal T85.818- ☑
    - infusion NEC T82.818- ☑
      - spinal (epidural) (subdural) T85.810- ☑
    - urinary (indwelling) T83.81- ☑
  - electronic (electrode) (pulse generator) (stimulator)
    - bone T84.81- ☑
    - cardiac T82.817- ☑

Embolism — continued
- due to device, implant or graft — see also Complications, by site and type, specified — continued
  - electronic — continued
    - nervous system (brain) (peripheral nerve) (spinal) T85.810- ☑
    - urinary T83.81- ☑
  - fixation, internal (orthopedic) NEC T84.81- ☑
  - gastrointestinal (bile duct) (esophagus) T85.818- ☑
  - genital NEC T83.81- ☑
  - heart (graft) (valve) T82.817- ☑
  - joint prosthesis T84.81- ☑
  - ocular (corneal graft) (orbital implant) T85.818- ☑
  - orthopedic (bone graft) NEC T86.838
  - specified NEC T85.818- ☑
  - urinary (graft) NEC T83.81- ☑
  - vascular NEC T82.818- ☑
  - ventricular intracranial shunt T85.810- ☑
- extremities
  - lower — see Embolism, vein, lower extremity
    - arterial I74.3
  - upper I74.2
- eye H34.9
- fat (cerebral) (pulmonary) (systemic) T79.1- ☑
  - complicating delivery — see Embolism, obstetric
  - following
    - abortion — see Abortion by type complicated by embolism
    - ectopic or molar pregnancy O08.2
  - pulmonary artery I26.96
    - with acute cor pulmonale I26.04
- following
  - abortion — see Abortion by type complicated by embolism
  - ectopic or molar pregnancy O08.2
  - infusion, therapeutic injection or transfusion
    - air T80.0- ☑
- heart (fatty) — see also Infarct, myocardium
  - not resulting in infarction I51.3
- hepatic (vein) I82.0
- in pregnancy, childbirth or puerperium — see Embolism, obstetric
- intestine (artery) (vein) (with gangrene) — see also Ischemia, intestine, acute K55.039
- intracranial — see also Occlusion, artery, cerebral
  - venous sinus (any) G08
    - nonpyogenic I67.6
- intraspinal venous sinuses or veins G08
  - nonpyogenic G95.19
- kidney (artery) N28.0
- lateral sinus (venous) — see Embolism, intracranial, venous sinus
- leg — see Embolism, vein, lower extremity
  - arterial I74.3
- longitudinal sinus (venous) — see Embolism, intracranial, venous sinus
- lung (massive) — see Embolism, pulmonary
- meninges I66.8
- mesenteric (artery) (vein) (with gangrene) — see also Ischemia, intestine, acute K55.059
- obstetric (in) (pulmonary)
  - childbirth O88.22
    - air O88.02
    - amniotic fluid O88.12
    - blood clot O88.22
    - fat O88.82
    - pyemic O88.32
    - septic O88.32
    - specified type NEC O88.82
  - pregnancy O88.21- ☑
    - air O88.01- ☑
    - amniotic fluid O88.11- ☑
    - blood clot O88.21- ☑
    - fat O88.81- ☑
    - pyemic O88.31- ☑
    - septic O88.31- ☑
    - specified type NEC O88.81- ☑
  - puerperal O88.23
    - air O88.03
    - amniotic fluid O88.13
    - blood clot O88.23
    - fat O88.83
    - pyemic O88.33
    - septic O88.33
    - specified type NEC O88.83
- ophthalmic — see Occlusion, artery, retina
- penis N48.81
- peripheral artery NOS I74.4

Embolism — continued
- pituitary E23.6
- popliteal (artery) I74.3
- portal (vein) I81
- postoperative, postprocedural
  - artery T81.719- ☑
    - mesenteric T81.710- ☑
    - renal T81.711- ☑
    - specified NEC T81.718- ☑
  - vein T81.72- ☑
- precerebral artery — see Occlusion, artery, precerebral
- puerperal — see Embolism, obstetric
- pulmonary (acute) (artery) (vein) I26.99
  - with acute cor pulmonale I26.09
  - cement I26.95
    - with acute cor pulmonale I26.03
  - chronic I27.82
  - fat I26.96
    - with acute cor pulmonale I26.04
  - following
    - abortion — see Abortion by type complicated by embolism
    - ectopic or molar pregnancy O08.2
  - healed or old Z86.711
  - in pregnancy, childbirth or puerperium — see Embolism, obstetric
  - multiple subsegmental without acute cor pulmonale I26.94
  - personal history of Z86.711
  - saddle I26.92
    - with acute cor pulmonale I26.02
  - septic I26.90
    - with acute cor pulmonale I26.01
  - single subsegmental without acute cor pulmonale I26.93
  - subsegmental NOS I26.93
- pyemic (multiple) I76
  - following
    - abortion — see Abortion by type complicated by embolism
    - ectopic or molar pregnancy O08.2
  - Hemophilus influenzae A41.3
  - pneumococcal A40.3
    - with pneumonia J13
  - puerperal, postpartum, childbirth (any organism) — see Embolism, obstetric
  - specified organism NEC A41.89
  - staphylococcal A41.2
  - streptococcal A40.9
- renal (artery) N28.0
  - vein I82.3
- retina, retinal — see Occlusion, artery, retina
- saddle
  - abdominal aorta I74.01
  - pulmonary artery I26.92
    - with acute cor pulmonale I26.02
- septic (arterial) I76
  - complicating abortion — see Abortion, by type, complicated by, embolism
- sinus — see Embolism, intracranial, venous sinus
- soap complicating abortion — see Abortion, by type, complicated by, embolism
- spinal cord G95.19
  - pyogenic origin G06.1
- spleen, splenic (artery) I74.8
- thrombotic
  - specified NEC I26.99
    - with acute cor pulmonale I26.09
- upper extremity I74.2
- vein (acute) I82.90
  - antecubital I82.61- ☑
    - chronic I82.71- ☑
  - axillary I82.A1- ☑ (following I82.7)
    - chronic I82.A2- ☑ (following I82.7)
  - basilic I82.61- ☑
    - chronic I82.71- ☑
  - brachial I82.62- ☑
    - chronic I82.72- ☑
  - brachiocephalic (innominate) I82.290
    - chronic I82.291
  - calf, muscle I82.46- ☑
    - chronic I82.56- ☑
  - cephalic I82.61- ☑
    - chronic I82.71- ☑
  - chronic I82.91
  - deep (DVT) I82.40- ☑
    - calf I82.4Z- ☑
      - chronic I82.5Z- ☑

☑ Additional Character Required — Refer to the Tabular List for Character Selection

Embolism — continued
  vein — continued
    deep — continued
      lower leg I82.4Z- ☑
        chronic I82.5Z- ☑
      thigh I82.4Y- ☑
        chronic I82.5Y- ☑
      upper leg I82.4Y- ☑
        chronic I82.5Y- ☑
    femoral I82.41- ☑
      chronic I82.51- ☑
    gastrocnemial I82.46- ☑
      chronic I82.56- ☑
    iliac (iliofemoral) I82.42- ☑
      chronic I82.52- ☑
    innominate I82.290
      chronic I82.291
    internal jugular I82.C1- ☑ (*following* I82.7)
      chronic I82.C2- ☑ (*following* I82.7)
    lower extremity
      deep I82.40- ☑
        chronic I82.50- ☑
        specified NEC I82.49- ☑
          chronic NEC I82.59- ☑
      distal
        deep I82.4Z- ☑
      proximal
        deep I82.4Y- ☑
          chronic I82.5Y- ☑
      superficial I82.81- ☑
    peroneal I82.45- ☑
      chronic I82.55- ☑
    popliteal I82.43- ☑
      chronic I82.53- ☑
    radial I82.62- ☑
      chronic I82.72- ☑
    renal I82.3
    saphenous (greater) (lesser) I82.81- ☑
    soleal I82.46- ☑
      chronic I82.56- ☑
    specified NEC I82.890
      chronic NEC I82.891
    subclavian I82.B1- ☑ (*following* I82.7)
      chronic I82.B2- ☑ (*following* I82.7)
    thoracic NEC I82.290
      chronic I82.291
    tibial I82.44- ☑
      chronic I82.54- ☑
    ulnar I82.62- ☑
      chronic I82.72- ☑
    upper extremity I82.60- ☑
      chronic I82.70- ☑
      deep I82.62- ☑
        chronic I82.72- ☑
      superficial I82.61- ☑
        chronic I82.71- ☑
  vena cava
    inferior (acute) I82.220
      chronic I82.221
    superior (acute) I82.210
      chronic I82.211
  venous sinus G08
  vessels of brain — *see* Occlusion, artery, cerebral

Embolus — *see* Embolism

Embryoma — *see also* Neoplasm, uncertain behavior, by site
  benign — *see* Neoplasm, benign, by site
  kidney C64.- ☑
  liver C22.0
  malignant — *see also* Neoplasm, malignant, by site
    kidney C64.- ☑
    liver C22.0
    testis C62.9- ☑
      descended (scrotal) C62.1- ☑
      undescended C62.0- ☑
  testis C62.9- ☑
    descended (scrotal) C62.1- ☑
    undescended C62.0- ☑

Embryonic
  circulation Q28.9
  heart Q28.9
  vas deferens Q55.4

Embryopathia NOS Q89.9
Embryotoxon Q13.4
Emesis — *see* Vomiting
Emotional lability R45.86
Emotionality, pathological F60.3
Emotogenic disease — *see* Disorder, psychogenic
Emphysema (atrophic) (bullous) (chronic) (interlobular) (lung) (obstructive) (pulmonary) (senile) (vesicular) J43.9
  cellular tissue (traumatic) T79.7- ☑
    surgical T81.82- ☑
  centrilobular J43.2
  compensatory J98.3
  congenital (interstitial) P25.0
  conjunctiva H11.89
  connective tissue (traumatic) T79.7- ☑
    surgical T81.82- ☑
  due to chemicals, gases, fumes or vapors — *see also* Disease, respiratory, chronic, due to chemicals, gases, fumes or vapors J43.- ☑
  eyelid(s) — *see* Disorder, eyelid, specified type NEC
    surgical T81.82- ☑
    traumatic T79.7- ☑
  interstitial J98.2
    congenital P25.0
    perinatal period P25.0
  laminated tissue T79.7- ☑
    surgical T81.82- ☑
  mediastinal J98.2
    newborn P25.2
  orbit, orbital — *see* Disorder, orbit, specified type NEC
  panacinar J43.1
  panlobular J43.1
  specified NEC J43.8
  subcutaneous (traumatic) T79.7- ☑
    nontraumatic J98.2
    postprocedural T81.82- ☑
    surgical T81.82- ☑
  surgical T81.82- ☑
  thymus (gland) (congenital) E32.8
  traumatic (subcutaneous) T79.7- ☑
  unilateral J43.0

Empty nest syndrome Z60.0
Empyema (acute) (chest) (double) (pleura) (supradiaphragmatic) (thorax) J86.9
  with fistula J86.0
  accessory sinus (chronic) — *see* Sinusitis
  antrum (chronic) — *see* Sinusitis, maxillary
  brain (any part) — *see* Abscess, brain
  ethmoidal (chronic) (sinus) — *see* Sinusitis, ethmoidal
  extradural — *see* Abscess, extradural
  frontal (chronic) (sinus) — *see* Sinusitis, frontal
  gallbladder K81.0
  mastoid (process) (acute) — *see* Mastoiditis, acute
  maxilla, maxillary M27.2
    sinus (chronic) — *see* Sinusitis, maxillary
  nasal sinus (chronic) — *see* Sinusitis
  sinus (accessory) (chronic) (nasal) — *see* Sinusitis
  sphenoidal (sinus) (chronic) — *see* Sinusitis, sphenoidal
  subarachnoid — *see* Abscess, extradural
  subdural — *see* Abscess, subdural
  tuberculous A15.6
  ureter — *see* Ureteritis
  ventricular — *see* Abscess, brain

En coup de sabre lesion L94.1
Enamel pearls K00.2
Enameloma K00.2
Enanthema, viral B09
Encephalitis (chronic) (hemorrhagic) (idiopathic) (nonepidemic) (spurious) (subacute) G04.90
  acute — *see also* Encephalitis, viral A86
    disseminated G04.00
      infectious G04.01
      noninfectious G04.81
      postimmunization (postvaccination) G04.02
      postinfectious G04.01
    inclusion body A85.8
    necrotizing hemorrhagic G04.30
      postimmunization G04.32
      postinfectious G04.31
      specified NEC G04.39
  arboviral, arbovirus NEC A85.2
  arthropod-borne NEC (viral) A85.2
  Australian A83.4
  California (virus) A83.5
  Central European (tick-borne) A84.1
  Czechoslovakian A84.1
  Dawson's (inclusion body) A81.1
  diffuse sclerosing A81.1
  disseminated, acute G04.00
  due to
    cat scratch disease A28.1

Encephalitis — continued
  due to — continued
    human immunodeficiency virus (HIV) disease B20 *[G05.3]*
    malaria — *see* Malaria
    rickettsiosis — *see* Rickettsiosis
    smallpox inoculation G04.02
    typhus — *see* Typhus
  Eastern equine A83.2
  endemic (viral) A86
  epidemic NEC (viral) A86
  equine (acute) (infectious) (viral) A83.9
    Eastern A83.2
    Venezuelan A92.2
    Western A83.1
  Far Eastern (tick-borne) A84.0
  following vaccination or other immunization procedure G04.02
  herpes zoster B02.0
  herpesviral B00.4
    due to herpesvirus 6 B10.01
    due to herpesvirus 7 B10.09
    specified NEC B10.09
  Ilheus (virus) A83.8
  in (due to)
    actinomycosis A42.82
    adenovirus A85.1
    African trypanosomiasis B56.9 *[G05.3]*
    Chagas' disease (chronic) B57.42
    cytomegalovirus B25.8
    enterovirus A85.0
    herpes (simplex) virus B00.4
      due to herpesvirus 6 B10.01
      due to herpesvirus 7 B10.09
      specified NEC B10.09
    infectious disease NEC B99.- ☑ *[G05.3]*
    influenza — *see* Influenza, with, encephalopathy
    listeriosis A32.12
    measles B05.0
    mumps B26.2
    naegleriasis B60.2
    parasitic disease NEC B89 *[G05.3]*
    poliovirus A80.9 *[G05.3]*
    rubella B06.01
    syphilis
      congenital A50.42
      late A52.14
    systemic lupus erythematosus M32.19 *[G05.3]*
    toxoplasmosis (acquired) B58.2
      congenital P37.1
    tuberculosis A17.82
    zoster B02.0
  inclusion body A81.1
  infectious (acute) (virus) NEC A86
  Japanese (B type) A83.0
  La Crosse A83.5
  lead — *see* Poisoning, lead
  lethargica (acute) (infectious) A85.8
  louping ill A84.89
  lupus erythematosus, systemic M32.19 *[G05.3]*
  lymphatica A87.2
  Mengo A85.8
  meningococcal A39.81
  Murray Valley A83.4
  otitic NEC H66.40 *[G05.3]*
  parasitic NOS B71.9
  periaxial G37.0
  periaxialis (concentrica) (diffuse) G37.5
  postchickenpox B01.11
  postexanthematous NEC B09
  postimmunization G04.02
  postinfectious NEC G04.01
  postmeasles B05.0
  postvaccinal G04.02
  postvaricella B01.11
  postviral NEC A86
  Powassan A84.81
  Rasmussen G04.81
  Rio Bravo A85.8
  Russian
    autumnal A83.0
    spring-summer (taiga) A84.0
  saturnine — *see* Poisoning, lead
  specified NEC G04.81
  St. Louis A83.3
  subacute sclerosing A81.1
  summer A83.0
  suppurative G04.81
  tick-borne A84.9

Encephalitis — continued
  Torula, torular (cryptococcal) B45.1
  toxic NEC G92.8
  trichinosis B75 *[G05.3]*
  type
    B A83.0
    C A83.3
  van Bogaert's A81.1
  Venezuelan equine A92.2
  Vienna A85.8
  viral, virus A86
    arthropod-borne NEC A85.2
      mosquito-borne A83.9
        Australian X disease A83.4
        California virus A83.5
        Eastern equine A83.2
        Japanese (B type) A83.0
        Murray Valley A83.4
        specified NEC A83.8
        St. Louis A83.3
        type B A83.0
        type C A83.3
        Western equine A83.1
      tick-borne A84.9
        biundulant A84.1
        central European A84.1
        Czechoslovakian A84.1
        diphasic meningoencephalitis A84.1
        Far Eastern A84.0
        Russian spring-summer (taiga) A84.0
        specified NEC A84.89
    specified type NEC A85.8
    tick-borne, specified NEC A84.89
    Western equine A83.1
Encephalocele Q01.9
  frontal Q01.0
  nasofrontal Q01.1
  occipital Q01.2
  specified NEC Q01.8
Encephalocystocele — *see* Encephalocele
Encephaloduroarteriomyosynangiosis (EDAMS) I67.5
Encephalomalacia (brain) (cerebellar) (cerebral) — *see* Softening, brain
Encephalomeningitis — *see* Meningoencephalitis
Encephalomeningocele — *see* Encephalocele
Encephalomeningomyelitis — *see* Meningoencephalitis
Encephalomyelitis — *see also* Encephalitis G04.90
  acute disseminated G04.00
    infectious G04.01
    noninfectious G04.81
    postimmunization G04.02
    postinfectious G04.01
  acute necrotizing hemorrhagic G04.30
    postimmunization G04.32
    postinfectious G04.31
    specified NEC G04.39
  equine A83.9
    Eastern A83.2
    Venezuelan A92.2
    Western A83.1
  in diseases classified elsewhere G05.3
  myalgic G93.32
    chronic fatigue syndrome [ME/CFS] G93.32
  postchickenpox B01.11
  postinfectious NEC G04.01
  postmeasles B05.0
  postvaccinal G04.02
  postvaricella B01.11
  rubella B06.01
  specified NEC G04.81
  Venezuelan equine A92.2
Encephalomyelocele — *see* Encephalocele
Encephalomyelomeningitis — *see* Meningoencephalitis
Encephalomyelopathy G96.9
Encephalomyeloradiculitis (acute) G61.0
Encephalomyeloradiculoneuritis (acute) (Guillain-Barre) G61.0
Encephalomyeloradiculopathy G96.9
Encephalopathia hyperbilirubinemica, newborn P57.9
  due to isoimmunization (conditions in P55) P57.0
Encephalopathy (acute) G93.40
  acute necrotizing hemorrhagic G04.30
    postimmunization G04.32
    postinfectious G04.31
    specified NEC G04.39
  alcoholic G31.2
  anoxic — *see* Damage, brain, anoxic
  arteriosclerotic I67.2
  centrolobar progressive (Schilder) G37.0

Encephalopathy — continued
  congenital Q07.9
  degenerative, in specified disease NEC G32.89
  demyelinating callosal G37.1
  developmental and epileptic G93.45
  due to
    drugs — *see also* Table of Drugs and Chemicals G92.8
  early infantile epileptic G93.45
  FOXG1-related QA0.0151
  hepatic (without coma) K76.82
  hyperbilirubinemic, newborn P57.9
    due to isoimmunization (conditions in P55) P57.0
  hypertensive I67.4
  hypoglycemic E16.2
  hypoxic — *see* Damage, brain, anoxic
  hypoxic ischemic P91.60
    mild P91.61
    moderate P91.62
    severe P91.63
  in (due to) (with)
    birth injury P11.1
    hyperinsulinism E16.1 *[G94]*
    influenza — *see* Influenza, with, encephalopathy
    lack of vitamin — *see also* Deficiency, vitamin E56.9 *[G32.89]*
    neoplastic disease — *see also* Neoplasm D49.9 *[G13.1]*
    serum — *see also* Reaction, serum T80.69- ☑
    syphilis A52.17
    trauma (postconcussional) F07.81
      current injury — *see* Injury, intracranial
    vaccination G04.02
  lead — *see* Poisoning, lead
  metabolic G93.41
    drug induced G92.8
    toxic G92.8
  myoclonic, early, symptomatic — *see* Epilepsy, generalized, specified NEC
  necrotizing, subacute (Leigh) G31.82
  neonatal P91.819
    in diseases classified elsewhere P91.811
  pellagrous E52 *[G32.89]*
  portal-systemic K76.82
  postcontusional F07.81
    current injury — *see* Injury, intracranial, diffuse
  posthypoglycemic (coma) E16.1 *[G94]*
  postradiation G93.89
  saturnine — *see* Poisoning, lead
  septic G93.41
  specified NEC G93.49
  spongiform, subacute (viral) A81.09
  toxic G92.9
    metabolic G92.8
  traumatic (postconcussional) F07.81
    current injury — *see* Injury, intracranial
  vitamin B deficiency NEC E53.9 *[G32.89]*
    vitamin B1 E51.2
  Wernicke's E51.2
Encephalorrhagia — *see* Hemorrhage, intracranial, intracerebral
Encephalosis, posttraumatic F07.81
Enchondroma — *see also* Neoplasm, bone, benign
Enchondromatosis (cartilaginous) (multiple) Q78.4
Encopresis R15.9
  functional F98.1
  nonorganic origin F98.1
  psychogenic F98.1
Encounter (with health service) (for) Z76.89
  adjustment and management (of)
    breast implant Z45.81- ☑
    implanted device NEC Z45.89
    myringotomy device (stent) (tube) Z45.82
    neurostimulator (brain) (gastric) (peripheral nerve) (sacral nerve) (spinal cord) (vagus nerve) Z45.42
  administrative purpose only Z02.9
    examination for
      adoption Z02.82
      armed forces Z02.3
      child welfare Z02.84
      disability determination Z02.71
      driving license Z02.4
      employment Z02.1
      insurance Z02.6
      medical certificate NEC Z02.79
      paternity testing Z02.81
      residential institution admission Z02.2
      school admission Z02.0
      sports Z02.5
    specified reason NEC Z02.89
  aftercare — *see* Aftercare

Encounter — continued
  antenatal screening Z36.9
    cervical length Z36.86
    chromosomal anomalies Z36.0
    congenital cardiac abnormalities Z36.83
    elevated maternal serum alphafetoprotein Z36.1
    fetal growth retardation Z36.4
    fetal lung maturity Z36.84
    fetal macrosomia Z36.88
    hydrops fetalis Z36.81
    intrauterine growth restriction (IUGR) /small-for-dates Z36.4
    isoimmunization Z36.5
    large-for-dates Z36.88
    malformations Z36.3
    non-visualized anatomy on a previous scan Z36.2
    nuchal translucency Z36.82
    raised alphafetoprotein level Z36.1
    risk of pre-term labor Z36.86
    specified follow-up NEC Z36.2
    specified genetic defects NEC Z36.8A
    specified type NEC Z36.89
    Streptococcus B Z36.85
    suspected anomaly Z36.3
    uncertain dates Z36.87
  assisted reproductive fertility procedure cycle Z31.83
  blood typing Z01.83
    Rh typing Z01.83
  breast augmentation or reduction Z41.1
  breast implant exchange (different material) (different size) Z45.81- ☑
  breast reconstruction following mastectomy Z42.1
  check-up — *see* Examination
  chemotherapy for neoplasm Z51.11
  child welfare screening exam Z02.84
  colonoscopy, screening Z12.11
  counseling — *see* Counseling
  delivery, full-term, uncomplicated O80
    cesarean, without indication O82
  desensitization to allergens Z51.6
  ear piercing Z41.3
  examination — *see* Examination
  expectant parent(s) (adoptive) pre-birth pediatrician visit Z76.81
  fertility preservation procedure (prior to cancer therapy) (prior to removal of gonads) Z31.84
  fitting (of) — *see* Fitting (and adjustment) (of)
  genetic
    counseling
      nonprocreative Z71.83
      procreative Z31.5
    testing — *see* Test, genetic
  hearing conservation and treatment Z01.12
  HIV
    pre-exposure prophylaxis Z29.81
    PrEP Z29.81
  immunotherapy for neoplasm Z51.12
  in vitro fertilization cycle Z31.83
  instruction (in)
    child care (postpartal) (prenatal) Z32.3
    childbirth Z32.2
    natural family planning
      procreative Z31.61
      to avoid pregnancy Z30.02
  insulin pump titration Z46.81
  joint prosthesis insertion following prior explantation of joint prosthesis (staged procedure)
    hip Z47.32
    knee Z47.33
    shoulder Z47.31
  laboratory (as part of a general medical examination) Z00.00
    with abnormal findings Z00.01
  mental health services (for)
    abuse NEC
      perpetrator Z69.82
      victim Z69.81
    child abuse
      nonparental
        perpetrator Z69.021
        victim Z69.020
      parental
        perpetrator Z69.011
        victim Z69.010
    child neglect
      nonparental
        perpetrator Z69.021
        victim Z69.020

☑ **Additional Character Required** — Refer to the Tabular List for Character Selection

Encounter — continued
- mental health services — continued
  - child neglect — continued
    - parental
      - perpetrator Z69.011
      - victim Z69.010
  - child psychological abuse
    - nonparental
      - perpetrator Z69.021
      - victim Z69.020
    - parental
      - perpetrator Z69.011
      - victim Z69.010
  - child sexual abuse
    - nonparental
      - perpetrator Z69.021
      - victim Z69.020
    - parental
      - perpetrator Z69.011
      - victim Z69.010
  - non-spousal adult abuse
    - perpetrator Z69.82
    - victim Z69.81
  - spousal or partner
    - abuse
      - perpetrator Z69.12
      - victim Z69.11
    - neglect
      - perpetrator Z69.12
      - victim Z69.11
    - psychological abuse
      - perpetrator Z69.12
      - victim Z69.11
    - violence
      - perpetrator (physical) (sexual) Z69.12
      - victim (physical) Z69.11
        - sexual Z69.81
- observation (for) (ruled out)
  - alarm, without findings
    - apnea Z03.83
    - bradycardia Z03.83
    - oximeter Z03.83
  - condition suspected related to home physiologic monitoring device Z03.83
    - newborn Z05.81
      - apnea alarm Z05.81
      - bradycardia alarm Z05.81
      - malfunction of home cardiorespiratory monitor Z05.81
      - non-specific findings home physiologic monitoring device Z05.81
      - pulse oximeter alarm without findings Z05.81
  - exposure to (suspected)
    - anthrax Z03.810
    - biological agent NEC Z03.818
  - malfunction of home cardiorespiratory monitor Z03.83
  - non-specific findings home physiologic monitoring device Z03.83
- palliative care Z51.5
- pediatrician visit, by expectant parent(s) (adoptive) Z76.81
- placental sample (taken vaginally) — see also Encounter, antenatal screening Z36.9
- plastic and reconstructive surgery following medical procedure or healed injury NEC Z42.8
- postoperative — see Aftercare
- pregnancy
  - supervision of — see Pregnancy, supervision of
  - test Z32.00
    - result negative Z32.02
    - result positive Z32.01
- procreative management and counseling for gestational carrier Z31.7
- prophylactic measures Z29.9
  - antivenin Z29.12
  - fluoride administration Z29.3
  - HIV pre-exposure Z29.81
  - immunotherapy for respiratory syncytial virus (RSV) Z29.11
  - rabies immune globin Z29.14
  - Rho (D) immune globulin Z29.13
  - specified NEC Z29.89
- radiation therapy (antineoplastic) Z51.0
- radiological (as part of a general medical examination) Z00.00
  - with abnormal findings Z00.01
- reconstructive surgery following medical procedure or healed injury NEC Z42.8
- removal (of) — see also Removal

Encounter — continued
- removal — see also Removal — continued
  - artificial
    - arm Z44.00- ☑
      - complete Z44.01- ☑
      - partial Z44.02- ☑
    - eye Z44.2- ☑
    - leg Z44.10- ☑
      - complete Z44.11- ☑
      - partial Z44.12- ☑
  - breast implant Z45.81- ☑
    - tissue expander (with or without synchronous insertion of permanent implant) Z45.81- ☑
  - device Z46.9
    - specified NEC Z46.89
  - external
    - fixation device — code to fracture with seventh character D
    - prosthesis, prosthetic device Z44.9
      - breast Z44.3- ☑
      - specified NEC Z44.8
  - implanted device NEC Z45.89
  - insulin pump Z46.81
  - internal fixation device Z47.2
  - myringotomy device (stent) (tube) Z45.82
  - nervous system device NEC Z46.2
    - brain neuropacemaker Z46.2
    - visual substitution device Z46.2
      - implanted Z45.31
  - non-vascular catheter Z46.82
  - orthodontic device Z46.4
  - stent
    - ureteral Z46.6
  - urinary device Z46.6
- repeat cervical smear to confirm findings of recent normal smear following initial abnormal smear Z01.42
- respirator [ventilator] use during power failure Z99.12
- Rh typing Z01.83
- screening — see Screening
- specified NEC Z76.89
- sterilization Z30.2
- suspected condition, ruled out
  - amniotic cavity and membrane Z03.71
  - cervical shortening Z03.75
  - fetal anomaly Z03.73
  - fetal growth Z03.74
  - maternal and fetal conditions NEC Z03.79
  - oligohydramnios Z03.71
  - placental problem Z03.72
  - polyhydramnios Z03.71
- suspected exposure (to), ruled out
  - anthrax Z03.810
  - biological agents NEC Z03.818
- termination of pregnancy, elective Z33.2
- testing — see Test
- therapeutic drug level monitoring Z51.81
- titration, insulin pump Z46.81
- to determine fetal viability of pregnancy O36.80- ☑
- training
  - insulin pump Z46.81
- X-ray of chest (as part of a general medical examination) Z00.00
  - with abnormal findings Z00.01

Encystment — see Cyst
Endarteritis (bacterial, subacute) (infective) I77.6
- brain I67.7
- cerebral or cerebrospinal I67.7
- deformans — see Arteriosclerosis
- embolic — see Embolism
- obliterans — see also Arteriosclerosis
  - pulmonary I28.8
- pulmonary I28.8
- retina — see Vasculitis, retina
- senile — see Arteriosclerosis
- syphilitic A52.09
  - brain or cerebral A52.04
  - congenital A50.54 [I79.8]
- tuberculous A18.89

Endemic — see condition
Endocarditis (chronic) (marantic) (nonbacterial) (thrombotic) (valvular) I38
- with rheumatic fever (conditions in I00)
  - active — see Endocarditis, acute, rheumatic
  - inactive or quiescent (with chorea) I09.1
- acute or subacute I33.9
  - infective I33.0
  - rheumatic (aortic) (mitral) (pulmonary) (tricuspid) I01.1

Endocarditis — continued
- acute or subacute — continued
  - rheumatic — continued
    - with chorea (acute) (rheumatic) (Sydenham's) I02.0
- aortic (heart) (nonrheumatic) (valve) I35.8
  - with
    - mitral disease I08.0
      - with tricuspid (valve) disease I08.3
        - active or acute I01.1
          - with chorea (acute) (rheumatic) (Sydenham's) I02.0
      - rheumatic fever (conditions in I00)
        - active — see Endocarditis, acute, rheumatic
        - inactive or quiescent (with chorea) I06.9
    - tricuspid (valve) disease I08.2
      - with mitral (valve) disease I08.3
  - acute or subacute I33.9
  - arteriosclerotic I35.8
  - rheumatic I06.9
    - with mitral disease I08.0
      - with tricuspid (valve) disease I08.3
        - active or acute I01.1
          - with chorea (acute) (rheumatic) (Sydenham's) I02.0
    - active or acute I01.1
      - with chorea (acute) (rheumatic) (Sydenham's) I02.0
    - specified NEC I06.8
  - specified cause NEC I35.8
  - syphilitic A52.03
- arteriosclerotic I38
- atypical verrucous (Libman-Sacks) M32.11
- bacterial (acute) (any valve) (subacute) I33.0
- candidal B37.6
- congenital Q24.8
- constrictive I33.0
- Coxiella burnetii A78 [I39]
- Coxsackie B33.21
- due to
  - prosthetic cardiac valve T82.6- ☑
  - Q fever A78 [I39]
  - Serratia marcescens I33.0
  - typhoid (fever) A01.02
- gonococcal A54.83
- infectious or infective (acute) (any valve) (subacute) I33.0
- lenta (acute) (any valve) (subacute) I33.0
- Libman-Sacks M32.11
- listerial A32.82
- Loffler's I42.3
- malignant (acute) (any valve) (subacute) I33.0
- meningococcal A39.51
- mitral (chronic) (double) (fibroid) (heart) (inactive) (valve) (with chorea) I05.9
  - with
    - aortic (valve) disease I08.0
      - with tricuspid (valve) disease I08.3
        - active or acute I01.1
          - with chorea (acute) (rheumatic) (Sydenham's) I02.0
    - rheumatic fever (conditions in I00)
      - active — see Endocarditis, acute, rheumatic
      - inactive or quiescent (with chorea) I05.9
    - tricuspid (valve) disease I08.1
      - with aortic (valve) disease I08.3
  - active or acute I01.1
    - with chorea (acute) (rheumatic) (Sydenham's) I02.0
    - bacterial I33.0
  - arteriosclerotic I34.89
  - nonrheumatic I34.89
    - acute or subacute I33.9
  - specified NEC I05.8
- monilial B37.6
- multiple valves I08.9
  - specified disorders I08.8
- mycotic (acute) (any valve) (subacute) I33.0
- pneumococcal (acute) (any valve) (subacute) I33.0
- pulmonary (chronic) (heart) (valve) I37.8
  - with rheumatic fever (conditions in I00)
    - active — see Endocarditis, acute, rheumatic
    - inactive or quiescent (with chorea) I09.89
      - with aortic, mitral or tricuspid disease I08.8
  - acute or subacute I33.9
    - rheumatic I01.1
      - with chorea (acute) (rheumatic) (Sydenham's) I02.0
  - arteriosclerotic I37.8
  - congenital Q22.2
  - rheumatic (chronic) (inactive) (with chorea) I09.89
    - active or acute I01.1

Endocarditis — *continued*
  pulmonary — *continued*
    rheumatic — *continued*
      active or acute — *continued*
        with chorea (acute) (rheumatic) (Sydenham's) I02.0
      syphilitic A52.03
  purulent (acute) (any valve) (subacute) I33.0
  Q fever A78 [I39]
  rheumatic (chronic) (inactive) (with chorea) I09.1
    active or acute (aortic) (mitral) (pulmonary) (tricuspid) I01.1
      with chorea (acute) (rheumatic) (Sydenham's) I02.0
  rheumatoid — *see* Rheumatoid, carditis
  septic (acute) (any valve) (subacute) I33.0
  streptococcal (acute) (any valve) (subacute) I33.0
  subacute — *see* Endocarditis, acute
  suppurative (acute) (any valve) (subacute) I33.0
  syphilitic A52.03
  toxic I33.9
  tricuspid (chronic) (heart) (inactive) (rheumatic) (valve) (with chorea) I07.9
    with
      aortic (valve) disease I08.2
        mitral (valve) disease I08.3
      mitral (valve) disease I08.1
        aortic (valve) disease I08.3
      rheumatic fever (conditions in I00)
        active — *see* Endocarditis, acute, rheumatic
        inactive or quiescent (with chorea) I07.8
    active or acute I01.1
      with chorea (acute) (rheumatic) (Sydenham's) I02.0
    arteriosclerotic I36.8
    nonrheumatic I36.8
      acute or subacute I33.9
    specified cause, except rheumatic I36.8
  tuberculous — *see* Tuberculosis, endocarditis
  typhoid A01.02
  ulcerative (acute) (any valve) (subacute) I33.0
  vegetative (acute) (any valve) (subacute) I33.0
  verrucous (atypical) (nonbacterial) (nonrheumatic) M32.11
Endocardium, endocardial — *see also* condition
  cushion defect Q21.20
Endocervicitis — *see also* Cervicitis
  due to intrauterine (contraceptive) device T83.69- ☑
  hyperplastic N72
Endocrine — *see* condition
Endocrinopathy, pluriglandular E31.9
Endodontic
  overfill M27.52
  underfill M27.53
Endodontitis K04.01
  irreversible K04.02
  reversible K04.01
Endomastoiditis — *see* Mastoiditis
Endometrioma N80.12- ☑
Endometriosis N80.9
  abdomen, abdominal N80.C0
    specified site, NEC N80.C9
    wall N80.C19
      fascia and muscular layers N80.C11
      subcutaneous tissue N80.C10
      unspecified depth N80.C19
  appendix N80.549
    deep N80.542
    superficial N80.541
  bladder (unspecified depth) N80.A0
    deep N80.A2
    superficial N80.A1
  bowel N80.50
  broad ligament N80.3C- ☑
  cardiothoracic space N80.B6
  cecum N80.539
    deep N80.532
    superficial N80.531
  cervix N80.0- ☑
  colon N80.559
    descending N80.559
      deep N80.552
      superficial N80.551
    sigmoid N80.529
      deep N80.522
      superficial N80.521
    transverse N80.559
      deep N80.552
      superficial N80.551
  cul-de-sac (Douglas')
    anterior (unspecified depth) N80.319

Endometriosis — *continued*
  cul-de-sac — *continued*
    anterior — *continued*
      deep N80.312
      superficial N80.311
    posterior (unspecified depth) N80.329
      deep N80.322
      superficial N80.321
  deep
    involving muscular wall of fallopian tube N80.22- ☑
    retrocervical N80.02
  diaphragm N80.B39
    deep N80.B32
    superficial N80.B31
    unspecified depth N80.B39
  exocervix N80.01
  extra-pelvic abdominal peritoneum N80.C4
  fallopian tube (unspecified depth) N80.20- ☑
    deep N80.22- ☑
    superficial N80.21- ☑
  female genital organ NEC N80.8
  gallbladder N80.8
  in scar of skin N80.6
  inguinal canal N80.C3
  internal N80.02
  intestine N80.50
    small N80.569
      deep (multifocal) N80.562
      superficial N80.561
  lung N80.B2
  mediastinal space N80.B5
  myometrium N80.03
  nerve
    femoral N80.D6
    obturator N80.D3
    pelvic N80.D0
      splanchnic N80.D1
    pudendal N80.D5
    retroperitoneum, NEC N80.D9
    sacral splanchnic N80.D1
    sciatic N80.D4
    specified, NEC N80.D9
  ovary (unspecified depth) N80.10- ☑
    deep N80.12- ☑
    superficial N80.11- ☑
  parametrium N80.399
  pelvic
    brim N80.38- ☑
      deep N80.37- ☑
      superficial N80.36- ☑
    peritoneum N80.30
      specified sites, NEC N80.399
        deep N80.392
        superficial N80.391
    sidewall N80.35- ☑
      deep N80.34- ☑
      superficial N80.33- ☑
  pericardial space N80.B4
  peritoneal (pelvic) N80.30
  pleura N80.B1
  rectovaginal septum N80.40
    with involvement of vagina N80.42
    without involvement of vagina N80.41
  rectum N80.519
    deep (multifocal) N80.512
    superficial N80.511
  retroperitoneum N80.30
  round ligament N80.3C9
  sacral nerve roots N80.D2
  skin (scar) N80.6
  specified site NEC N80.8
  stromal D39.0
  thorax N80.B- ☑
  umbilicus N80.C2
  ureter N80.A69
    deep N80.A5- ☑
    extrinsic N80.A4- ☑
    intrinsic N80.A5- ☑
    superficial N80.A4- ☑
    unspecified depth N80.A6- ☑
  uterosacral ligament(s) N80.3C- ☑
    deep N80.3B- ☑
    superficial N80.3A- ☑
  uterus N80.00
    deep N80.02
    internal N80.02
    superficial N80.01
  vagina N80.42

Endometriosis — *continued*
  vulva N80.8
Endometritis (decidual) (nonspecific) (purulent) (senile) (atrophic) (suppurative) N71.9
  with ectopic pregnancy O08.0
  acute N71.0
  blennorrhagic (gonococcal) (acute) (chronic) A54.24
  cervix, cervical (with erosion or ectropion) — *see also* Cervicitis
    hyperplastic N72
  chlamydial A56.11
  chronic N71.1
  following
    abortion — *see* Abortion by type complicated by genital infection
    ectopic or molar pregnancy O08.0
  gonococcal, gonorrheal (acute) (chronic) A54.24
  hyperplastic — *see also* Hyperplasia, endometrial N85.00
    cervix N72
  puerperal, postpartum, childbirth O86.12
  subacute N71.0
  tuberculous A18.17
Endometrium — *see* condition
Endomyocardiopathy, South African I42.3
Endomyocarditis — *see* Endocarditis
Endomyofibrosis I42.3
Endomyometritis — *see* Endometritis
Endopericarditis — *see* Endocarditis
Endoperineuritis — *see* Disorder, nerve
Endophlebitis — *see* Phlebitis
Endophthalmia — *see* Endophthalmitis, purulent
Endophthalmitis (acute) (infective) (metastatic) (subacute) H44.009
  bleb associated — *see also* Bleb, inflamed (infected), postprocedural H59.4- ☑
  gonorrheal A54.39
  in (due to)
    cysticercosis B69.1
    onchocerciasis B73.01
    toxocariasis B83.0
  panuveitis — *see* Panuveitis
  parasitic H44.12- ☑
  purulent H44.00- ☑
    panophthalmitis — *see* Panophthalmitis
    vitreous abscess H44.02- ☑
  specified NEC H44.19
  sympathetic — *see* Uveitis, sympathetic
Endosalpingioma D28.2
Endosalpingiosis N94.89
Endosteitis — *see* Osteomyelitis
Endothelioma, bone — *see* Neoplasm, bone, malignant
Endotheliosis (hemorrhagic infectional) D69.8
Endotoxemia — code to condition
Endotrachelitis — *see* Cervicitis
Engelmann (-Camurati) **syndrome** Q78.3
English disease — *see* Rickets
Engman's disease L30.3
Engorgement
  breast N64.59
    newborn P83.4
    puerperal, postpartum O92.79
  lung (passive) — *see* Edema, lung
  pulmonary (passive) — *see* Edema, lung
  stomach K31.89
  venous, retina — *see* Occlusion, retina, vein, engorgement
Enlargement, enlarged — *see also* Hypertrophy
  adenoids J35.2
    with tonsils J35.3
  alveolar ridge K08.89
    congenital — *see* Anomaly, alveolar
  apertures of diaphragm (congenital) Q79.1
  gingival K06.1
  heart, cardiac — *see* Hypertrophy, cardiac
  labium majus, childhood asymmetric (CALME) N90.61
  lacrimal gland, chronic H04.03- ☑
  liver — *see* Hypertrophy, liver
  lymph gland or node R59.9
    generalized R59.1
    localized R59.0
  orbit H05.34- ☑
  organ or site, congenital NEC — *see* Anomaly, by site
  parathyroid (gland) E21.0
  pituitary fossa R93.0
  prostate N40.9
    with lower urinary tract symptoms (LUTS) N40.1
      nodular N40.3
    nodular N40.2

Enlargement, enlarged — continued
- prostate — continued
  - nodular — continued
    - with lower urinary tract symptoms (LUTS) N40.3
    - without lower urinary tract symptoms (LUTS) N40.0
      - nodular N40.2
- sella turcica R93.0
- spleen — see Splenomegaly
- thymus (gland) (congenital) E32.0
- thyroid (gland) — see Goiter
- tongue K14.8
- tonsils J35.1
  - with adenoids J35.3
- uterus N85.2
- vestibular aqueduct Q16.5

Enophthalmos H05.40- ☑
- due to
  - orbital tissue atrophy H05.41- ☑
  - trauma or surgery H05.42- ☑

Enostosis M27.8

Entamebic, entamebiasis — see Amebiasis

Entanglement
- umbilical cord(s) O69.82- ☑
  - with compression O69.2- ☑
  - around neck
    - with compression O69.1- ☑
    - without compression O69.81- ☑
  - of twins in monoamniotic sac O69.2- ☑
  - other, with compression O69.2- ☑
  - other, without compression O69.82- ☑
    - without compression O69.82- ☑

Enteralgia — see Pain, abdominal

Enteric — see condition

Enteritis (acute) (diarrheal) (hemorrhagic) (noninfective) K52.9
- adenovirus A08.2
- aertrycke infection A02.0
- allergic K52.29
  - with
    - eosinophilic gastritis or gastroenteritis K52.81
    - food protein-induced enterocolitis syndrome K52.21
    - food protein-induced enteropathy K52.22
      - FPIES K52.21
- amebic (acute) A06.0
  - with abscess — see Abscess, amebic
  - chronic A06.1
    - with abscess — see Abscess, amebic
    - nondysenteric A06.2
  - nondysenteric A06.2
- astrovirus A08.32
- bacillary NOS A03.9
- bacterial A04.9
  - specified NEC A04.8
- calicivirus A08.31
- candidal B37.82
- Chilomastix A07.8
- choleriformis A00.1
- chronic (noninfectious) K52.9
  - ulcerative — see Colitis, ulcerative
- cicatrizing (chronic) — see Enteritis, regional, small intestine
- Clostridioides difficile
  - not specified as recurrent A04.72
  - recurrent A04.71
- Clostridium
  - botulinum (food poisoning) A05.1
  - difficile
    - not specified as recurrent A04.72
    - recurrent A04.71
- coccidial A07.3
- coxsackie virus A08.39
- dietetic — see also Enteritis, allergic K52.29
- drug-induced K52.1
  - due to
    - astrovirus A08.32
    - calicivirus A08.31
    - coxsackie virus A08.39
    - drugs K52.1
    - echovirus A08.39
    - enterovirus NEC A08.39
    - food hypersensitivity — see also Enteritis, allergic K52.29
    - infectious organism (bacterial) (viral) — see Enteritis, infectious
    - torovirus A08.39
    - Yersinia enterocolitica A04.6
  - echovirus A08.39

Enteritis — continued
- eltor A00.1
- enterovirus NEC A08.39
- eosinophilic K52.81
- epidemic (infectious) A09
- fulminant — see also Ischemia, intestine, acute K55.019
- gangrenous — see Enteritis, infectious
- giardial A07.1
- infectious NOS A09
  - due to
    - adenovirus A08.2
    - Aerobacter aerogenes A04.8
    - Arizona (bacillus) A02.0
    - bacteria NOS A04.9
      - specified NEC A04.8
    - Campylobacter A04.5
    - Clostridioides difficile
      - not specified as recurrent A04.72
      - recurrent A04.71
    - Clostridium difficile
      - not specified as recurrent A04.72
      - recurrent A04.71
    - Clostridium perfringens A04.8
    - Enterobacter aerogenes A04.8
    - enterovirus A08.39
    - Escherichia coli A04.4
      - enteroaggregative A04.4
      - enterohemorrhagic A04.3
      - enteroinvasive A04.2
      - enteropathogenic A04.0
      - enterotoxigenic A04.1
      - specified NEC A04.4
    - specified
      - bacteria NEC A04.8
      - virus NEC A08.39
    - Staphylococcus A04.8
    - virus NEC A08.4
      - specified type NEC A08.39
    - Yersinia enterocolitica A04.6
  - specified organism NEC A08.8
- influenzal — see Influenza, with, digestive manifestations
- ischemic K55.9
  - acute — see also Ischemia, intestine, acute K55.019
  - chronic K55.1
- microsporidial A07.8
- mucomembranous, myxomembranous — see Syndrome, irritable bowel
- mucous — see Syndrome, irritable bowel
- necroticans A05.2
- necrotizing of newborn — see Enterocolitis, necrotizing, in newborn
- neurogenic — see Syndrome, irritable bowel
- newborn necrotizing — see Enterocolitis, necrotizing, in newborn
- noninfectious K52.9
- norovirus A08.11
- parasitic NEC B82.9
- paratyphoid (fever) — see Fever, paratyphoid
- protozoal A07.9
  - specified NEC A07.8
- radiation K52.0
- regional (of) K50.90
  - with
    - complication K50.919
      - abscess K50.914
      - fistula K50.913
      - intestinal obstruction K50.912
      - rectal bleeding K50.911
      - specified complication NEC K50.918
  - colon — see Enteritis, regional, large intestine
  - duodenum — see Enteritis, regional, small intestine
  - ileum — see Enteritis, regional, small intestine
  - jejunum — see Enteritis, regional, small intestine
  - large bowel — see Enteritis, regional, large intestine
  - large intestine (colon) (rectum) K50.10
    - with
      - complication K50.119
        - abscess K50.114
        - fistula K50.113
        - intestinal obstruction K50.112
        - rectal bleeding K50.111
        - small intestine (duodenum) (ileum) (jejunum) involvement K50.80
          - with
            - complication K50.819
              - abscess K50.814
              - fistula K50.813
              - intestinal obstruction K50.812
              - rectal bleeding K50.811

Enteritis — continued
- regional — continued
  - large intestine — continued
    - with — continued
      - complication — continued
        - small intestine involvement — continued
          - with — continued
            - complication — continued
              - specified complication NEC K50.818
        - specified complication NEC K50.118
  - rectum — see Enteritis, regional, large intestine
  - small intestine (duodenum) (ileum) (jejunum) K50.00
    - with
      - complication K50.019
        - abscess K50.014
        - fistula K50.013
        - intestinal obstruction K50.012
        - large intestine (colon) (rectum) involvement K50.80
          - with
            - complication K50.819
              - abscess K50.814
              - fistula K50.813
              - intestinal obstruction K50.812
              - rectal bleeding K50.811
              - specified complication NEC K50.818
        - rectal bleeding K50.011
        - specified complication NEC K50.018
- rotaviral A08.0
- Salmonella, salmonellosis (arizonae) (cholerae-suis) (enteritidis) (typhimurium) A02.0
- segmental — see Enteritis, regional
- septic A09
- Shigella — see Infection, Shigella
- small round structured NEC A08.19
- spasmodic, spastic — see Syndrome, irritable bowel
- staphylococcal A04.8
  - due to food A05.0
- torovirus A08.39
- toxic NEC K52.1
  - due to
    - Clostridioides difficile
      - not specified as recurrent A04.72
      - recurrent A04.71
    - Clostridium difficile
      - not specified as recurrent A04.72
      - recurrent A04.71
- trichomonal A07.8
- tuberculous A18.32
- typhosa A01.00
- ulcerative (chronic) — see Colitis, ulcerative
- viral A08.4
  - adenovirus A08.2
  - enterovirus A08.39
  - Rotavirus A08.0
  - small round structured NEC A08.19
  - specified NEC A08.39
  - virus specified NEC A08.39

Enterobiasis B80

Enterobius vermicularis (infection) (infestation) B80

Enterocele — see also Hernia, abdomen
- pelvic, pelvis (acquired) (congenital) N81.5
- vagina, vaginal (acquired) (congenital) NEC N81.5

Enterocolitis — see also Enteritis K52.9
- due to
  - Clostridioides difficile
    - not specified as recurrent A04.72
    - recurrent A04.71
  - Clostridium difficile
    - not specified as recurrent A04.72
    - recurrent A04.71
- fulminant ischemic — see also Ischemia, intestine, acute K55.059
- granulomatous — see Enteritis, regional
- hemorrhagic (acute) — see also Ischemia, intestine, acute K55.059
- chronic K55.1
- infectious NEC A09
- ischemic K55.9
- necrotizing K55.30
  - with
    - perforation K55.33
    - pneumatosis K55.32
      - and perforation K55.33

Enterocolitis — *continued*
  necrotizing — *continued*
   due to
    Clostridioides difficile
     not specified as recurrent A04.72
     recurrent A04.71
    Clostridium difficile
     not specified as recurrent A04.72
     recurrent A04.71
   in non-newborn K55.30
    stage 1 (without pneumatosis, without perforation) K55.31
    stage 2 (with pneumatosis, without perforation) K55.32
    stage 3 (with pneumatosis, with perforation) K55.33
   in newborn P77.9
    stage 1 (without pneumatosis, without perforation) P77.1
    stage 2 (with pneumatosis, without perforation) P77.2
    stage 3 (with pneumatosis, with perforation) P77.3
   without pneumatosis or perforation K55.31
  noninfectious K52.9
   newborn — *see* Enterocolitis, necrotizing, in newborn
  pseudomembranous (newborn)
   not specified as recurrent A04.72
   recurrent A04.71
  radiation K52.0
   newborn — *see* Enterocolitis, necrotizing, in newborn
  ulcerative (chronic) — *see* Pancolitis, ulcerative (chronic)
Enterogastritis — *see* Enteritis
Enteropathy K63.9
  celiac-gluten-sensitive K90.0
   non-celiac K90.41
  food protein-induced K52.22
  hemorrhagic, terminal — *see also* Ischemia, intestine, acute K55.059
  protein-losing K90.49
Enteroperitonitis — *see* Peritonitis
Enteroptosis K63.4
Enterorrhagia K92.2
Enterospasm — *see also* Syndrome, irritable, bowel
  psychogenic F45.8
Enterostenosis — *see also* Obstruction, intestine, specified NEC K56.699
Enterostomy
  complication — *see* Complication, enterostomy
  status Z93.4
Enterovirus, as cause of disease classified elsewhere B97.10
  coxsackievirus B97.11
  echovirus B97.12
  other specified B97.19
Enthesopathy (peripheral) M77.9
  Achilles tendinitis — *see* Tendinitis, Achilles
  ankle and tarsus M77.5- ☑
   specified type NEC — *see* Enthesopathy, foot, specified type NEC
  anterior tibial syndrome M76.81- ☑
  calcaneal spur — *see* Spur, bone, calcaneal
  elbow region M77.8
   lateral epicondylitis — *see* Epicondylitis, lateral
   medial epicondylitis — *see* Epicondylitis, medial
  foot NEC M77.8
   metatarsalgia — *see* Metatarsalgia
   specified type NEC M77.5- ☑
  forearm M77.8
  gluteal tendinitis — *see* Tendinitis, gluteal
  hand M77.8
  hip — *see* Enthesopathy, lower limb, specified type NEC
  iliac crest spur — *see* Spur, bone, iliac crest
  iliotibial band syndrome — *see* Syndrome, iliotibial band
  knee — *see* Enthesopathy, lower limb, lower leg, specified type NEC
  lateral epicondylitis — *see* Epicondylitis, lateral
  lower limb (excluding foot) M76.9
   Achilles tendinitis — *see* Tendinitis, Achilles
   ankle and tarsus M77.5- ☑
    specified type NEC — *see* Enthesopathy, foot, specified type NEC
   anterior tibial syndrome M76.81- ☑
   gluteal tendinitis — *see* Tendinitis, gluteal
   iliac crest spur — *see* Spur, bone, iliac crest
   iliotibial band syndrome — *see* Syndrome, iliotibial band
   patellar tendinitis — *see* Tendinitis, patellar

Enthesopathy — *continued*
 lower limb — *continued*
  pelvic region — *see* Enthesopathy, lower limb, specified type NEC
  peroneal tendinitis — *see* Tendinitis, peroneal
  posterior tibial syndrome M76.82- ☑
  psoas tendinitis — *see* Tendinitis, psoas
  specified type NEC M76.89- ☑
  tibial collateral bursitis — *see* Bursitis, tibial collateral
 medial epicondylitis — *see* Epicondylitis, medial
 metatarsalgia — *see* Metatarsalgia
 multiple sites M77.8
 patellar tendinitis — *see* Tendinitis, patellar
 pelvis M77.8
 periarthritis of wrist — *see* Periarthritis, wrist
 peroneal tendinitis — *see* Tendinitis, peroneal
 posterior tibial syndrome M76.82- ☑
 psoas tendinitis — *see* Tendinitis, psoas
 shoulder region — *see* Lesion, shoulder
 specified type NEC M77.8
 spinal M46.00
  cervical region M46.02
  cervicothoracic region M46.03
  lumbar region M46.06
  lumbosacral region M46.07
  multiple sites M46.09
  occipito-atlanto-axial region M46.01
  sacrococcygeal region M46.08
  thoracic region M46.04
  thoracolumbar region M46.05
 tibial collateral bursitis — *see* Bursitis, tibial collateral
 upper arm M77.8
 wrist and carpus NEC M77.8
  calcaneal spur — *see* Spur, bone, calcaneal
  periarthritis of wrist — *see* Periarthritis, wrist
Entomophobia F40.218
Entomophthoromycosis B46.8
Entrance, air into vein — *see* Embolism, air
Entrapment
 muscle
  eye
   extraocular H50.68- ☑
   oblique
    inferior H50.62- ☑
    superior H50.66- ☑
   rectus
    inferior H50.63- ☑
    lateral H50.64- ☑
    medial H50.65- ☑
    superior H50.67- ☑
 nerve — *see* Neuropathy, entrapment
Entropion (eyelid) (paralytic) H02.009
 cicatricial H02.019
  left H02.016
   lower H02.015
   upper H02.014
  right H02.013
   lower H02.012
   upper H02.011
 congenital Q10.2
 left H02.006
  lower H02.005
  upper H02.004
 mechanical H02.029
  left H02.026
   lower H02.025
   upper H02.024
  right H02.023
   lower H02.022
   upper H02.021
 right H02.003
  lower H02.002
  upper H02.001
 senile H02.039
  left H02.036
   lower H02.035
   upper H02.034
  right H02.033
   lower H02.032
   upper H02.031
 spastic H02.049
  left H02.046
   lower H02.045
   upper H02.044
  right H02.043
   lower H02.042
   upper H02.041
Enucleated eye (traumatic, current) S05.7- ☑

Enuresis R32
 functional F98.0
 habit disturbance F98.0
 nocturnal N39.44
  psychogenic F98.0
 nonorganic origin F98.0
 psychogenic F98.0
Eosinopenia — *see* Agranulocytosis
Eosinophilia (allergic) (idiopathic) (secondary) D72.10
 with
  angiolymphoid hyperplasia (ALHE) D18.01
 familial D72.19
 hereditary D72.19
 in disease classified elsewhere D72.18
 infiltrative — *see* Eosinophilia, pulmonary
 Loffler's J82.89
 peritoneal — *see* Peritonitis, eosinophilic
 pulmonary NEC J82.89
  acute J82.82
  asthmatic J82.83
  chronic J82.81
 specified NEC D72.19
 tropical (pulmonary) J82.89
Eosinophilia-myalgia syndrome M35.89
Ependymitis (acute) (cerebral) (chronic) (granular) — *see* Encephalomyelitis
Ependymoblastoma
 specified site — *see* Neoplasm, malignant, by site
 unspecified site C71.9
Ependymoma (epithelial) (malignant)
 anaplastic
  specified site — *see* Neoplasm, malignant, by site
  unspecified site C71.9
 benign
  specified site — *see* Neoplasm, benign, by site
  unspecified site D33.2
 myxopapillary D43.2
  specified site — *see* Neoplasm, uncertain behavior, by site
  unspecified site D43.2
 papillary D43.2
  specified site — *see* Neoplasm, uncertain behavior, by site
  unspecified site D43.2
 specified site — *see* Neoplasm, malignant, by site
 unspecified site C71.9
Ependymopathy G93.89
Ephelis, ephelides L81.2
Epiblepharon (congenital) Q10.3
Epicanthus, epicanthic fold (eyelid) (congenital) Q10.3
Epicondylitis (elbow)
 lateral M77.1- ☑
 medial M77.0- ☑
Epicystitis — *see* Cystitis
Epidemic — *see* condition
Epidermidalization, cervix — *see* Dysplasia, cervix
Epidermis, epidermal — *see* condition
Epidermodysplasia verruciformis B07.8
Epidermolysis
 bullosa (congenital) Q81.9
  acquired L12.30
   drug-induced L12.31
   specified cause NEC L12.35
  dystrophica Q81.2
  letalis Q81.1
  simplex Q81.0
  specified NEC Q81.8
 necroticans combustiformis L51.2
  due to drug — *see* Table of Drugs and Chemicals, by drug
Epidermophytid — *see* Dermatophytosis
Epidermophytosis (infected) — *see* Dermatophytosis
Epididymis — *see* condition
Epididymitis (acute) (nonvenereal) (recurrent) (residual) N45.1
 with orchitis N45.3
 blennorrhagic (gonococcal) A54.23
 caseous (tuberculous) A18.15
 chlamydial A56.19
 filarial — *see also* Infestation, filarial B74.9 [N51]
 gonococcal A54.23
 syphilitic A52.76
 tuberculous A18.15
Epididymo-orchitis — *see also* Epididymitis N45.3
Epidural — *see* condition
Epigastrium, epigastric — *see* condition
Epigastrocele — *see* Hernia, ventral
Epiglottis — *see* condition
Epiglottitis, epiglottiditis (acute) J05.10

Epiglottitis, epiglottiditis — continued
  with obstruction J05.11
  chronic J37.0
Epignathus Q89.4
Epilepsia partialis continua — see also Kozhevnikof's epilepsy G40.1- ☑
Epilepsy, epileptic, epilepsia (attack) (cerebral) (convulsion) (fit) (seizure) G40.909

> Note: the following terms are to be considered equivalent to intractable: pharmacoresistant (pharmacologically resistant), treatment resistant, refractory (medically) and poorly controlled

  with
    complex partial seizures — see Epilepsy, localization-related, symptomatic, with complex partial seizures
    grand mal seizures on awakening — see Epilepsy, generalized, specified NEC
    myoclonic absences — see Epilepsy, generalized, specified NEC
    myoclonic-astatic seizures — see Epilepsy, generalized, specified NEC
    simple partial seizures — see Epilepsy, localization-related, symptomatic, with simple partial seizures
  akinetic — see Epilepsy, generalized, specified NEC
  benign childhood with centrotemporal EEG spikes — see Epilepsy, localization-related, idiopathic
  benign myoclonic in infancy G40.80- ☑
  Bravais-jacksonian — see Epilepsy, localization-related, symptomatic, with simple partial seizures
  childhood
    with occipital EEG paroxysms — see Epilepsy, localization-related, idiopathic
    absence G40.A09 (following G40.3)
      intractable G40.A19 (following G40.3)
        with status epilepticus G40.A11 (following G40.3)
        without status epilepticus G40.A19 (following G40.3)
      not intractable G40.A09 (following G40.3)
        with status epilepticus G40.A01 (following G40.3)
        without status epilepticus G40.A09 (following G40.3)
  climacteric — see Epilepsy, specified NEC
  cysticercosis B69.0
  deterioration (mental) F06.8
  due to syphilis A52.19
  focal — see Epilepsy, localization-related, symptomatic, with simple partial seizures
  generalized
    idiopathic G40.309
      intractable G40.319
        with status epilepticus G40.311
        without status epilepticus G40.319
      not intractable G40.309
        with status epilepticus G40.301
        without status epilepticus G40.309
    specified NEC G40.409
      intractable G40.419
        with status epilepticus G40.411
        without status epilepticus G40.419
      not intractable G40.409
        with status epilepticus G40.401
        without status epilepticus G40.409
  impulsive petit mal — see Epilepsy, juvenile myoclonic
  intractable G40.919
    with status epilepticus G40.911
    without status epilepticus G40.919
  juvenile absence G40.A09 (following G40.3)
    intractable G40.A19 (following G40.3)
      with status epilepticus G40.A11 (following G40.3)
      without status epilepticus G40.A19 (following G40.3)
    not intractable G40.A09 (following G40.3)
      with status epilepticus G40.A01 (following G40.3)
      without status epilepticus G40.A09 (following G40.3)
  juvenile myoclonic G40.B09 (following G40.3)
    intractable G40.B19 (following G40.3)
      with status epilepticus G40.B11 (following G40.3)
      without status epilepticus G40.B19 (following G40.3)
    not intractable G40.B09 (following G40.3)
      with status epilepticus G40.B01 (following G40.3)
      without status epilepticus G40.B09 (following G40.3)

Epilepsy, epileptic, epilepsia — continued
  KCNQ2-related G40.842
    intractable G40.844
      with status epilepticus G40.843
      without status epilepticus G40.844
    not intractable G40.842
      with status epilepticus G40.841
      without status epilepticus G40.842
  Lafora progressive myoclonus — see also Epilepsy, myoclonus, progressive, Lafora G40.C09
  localization-related (focal) (partial)
    idiopathic G40.009
      with seizures of localized onset G40.009
        intractable G40.019
          with status epilepticus G40.011
          without status epilepticus G40.019
        not intractable G40.009
          with status epilepticus G40.001
          without status epilepticus G40.009
    symptomatic
      with complex partial seizures G40.209
        intractable G40.219
          with status epilepticus G40.211
          without status epilepticus G40.219
        not intractable G40.209
          with status epilepticus G40.201
          without status epilepticus G40.209
      with simple partial seizures G40.109
        intractable G40.119
          with status epilepticus G40.111
          without status epilepticus G40.119
        not intractable G40.109
          with status epilepticus G40.101
          without status epilepticus G40.109
  myoclonus, myoclonic — see also Epilepsy, generalized, specified NEC
    progressive — see also Epilepsy, generalized, idiopathic
      Lafora G40.C09
        intractable G40.C19
          with status epilepticus G40.C11
          without status epilepticus G40.C19
        not intractable G40.C09
          with status epilepticus G40.C01
          without status epilepticus G40.C09
      type 1 — see Epilepsy, generalized, idiopathic
      type 2 — see Epilepsy, myoclonus, progressive, Lafora
    severe, in infancy (SMEI) G40.83- ☑
  not intractable G40.909
    with status epilepticus G40.901
    without status epilepticus G40.909
  on awakening — see Epilepsy, generalized, specified NEC
  parasitic NOS B71.9 [G94]
  partial — see Epilepsy, localization-related, symptomatic, with simple partial seizures
  partialis continua — see also Kozhevnikof's epilepsy G40.1- ☑
  peripheral — see Epilepsy, specified NEC
  polymorphic, in infancy (PMEI) G40.83- ☑
  procursiva — see Epilepsy, localization-related, symptomatic, with simple partial seizures
  progressive (familial) myoclonic — see Epilepsy, myoclonus, progressive
    Lafora — see also Epilepsy, myoclonus, progressive, Lafora G40.C09
  reflex — see Epilepsy, specified NEC
  related to
    alcohol G40.509
      not intractable G40.509
        with status epilepticus G40.501
        without status epilepticus G40.509
    drugs G40.509
      not intractable G40.509
        with status epilepticus G40.501
        without status epilepticus G40.509
    external causes G40.509
      not intractable G40.509
        with status epilepticus G40.501
        without status epilepticus G40.509
    hormonal changes G40.509
      not intractable G40.509
        with status epilepticus G40.501
        without status epilepticus G40.509
    sleep deprivation G40.509
      not intractable G40.509
        with status epilepticus G40.501
        without status epilepticus G40.509
    stress G40.509

Epilepsy, epileptic, epilepsia — continued
  related to — continued
    stress — continued
      not intractable G40.509
        with status epilepticus G40.501
        without status epilepticus G40.509
  somatomotor — see Epilepsy, localization-related, symptomatic, with simple partial seizures
  somatosensory — see Epilepsy, localization-related, symptomatic, with simple partial seizures
  spasms G40.822
    intractable G40.824
      with status epilepticus G40.823
      without status epilepticus G40.824
    not intractable G40.822
      with status epilepticus G40.821
      without status epilepticus G40.822
  specified NEC G40.802
    intractable G40.804
      with status epilepticus G40.803
      without status epilepticus G40.804
    not intractable G40.802
      with status epilepticus G40.801
      without status epilepticus G40.802
  syndromes
    generalized
      idiopathic G40.309
        intractable G40.319
          with status epilepticus G40.311
          without status epilepticus G40.319
        not intractable G40.309
          with status epilepticus G40.301
          without status epilepticus G40.309
      specified NEC G40.409
        intractable G40.419
          with status epilepticus G40.411
          without status epilepticus G40.419
        not intractable G40.409
          with status epilepticus G40.401
          without status epilepticus G40.409
    localization-related (focal) (partial)
      idiopathic G40.009
        with seizures of localized onset G40.009
          intractable G40.019
            with status epilepticus G40.011
            without status epilepticus G40.019
          not intractable G40.009
            with status epilepticus G40.001
            without status epilepticus G40.009
      symptomatic
        with complex partial seizures G40.209
          intractable G40.219
            with status epilepticus G40.211
            without status epilepticus G40.219
          not intractable G40.209
            with status epilepticus G40.201
            without status epilepticus G40.209
        with simple partial seizures G40.109
          intractable G40.119
            with status epilepticus G40.111
            without status epilepticus G40.119
          not intractable G40.109
            with status epilepticus G40.101
            without status epilepticus G40.109
    specified NEC G40.802
      intractable G40.804
        with status epilepticus G40.803
        without status epilepticus G40.804
      not intractable G40.802
        with status epilepticus G40.801
        without status epilepticus G40.802
  tonic (-clonic) — see Epilepsy, generalized, specified NEC
  twilight F05
  uncinate (gyrus) — see Epilepsy, localization-related, symptomatic, with complex partial seizures
  Unverricht (-Lundborg) (familial myoclonic) — see Epilepsy, generalized, idiopathic
  visceral — see Epilepsy, specified NEC
  visual — see Epilepsy, specified NEC
Epiloia Q85.1
Epimenorrhea N92.0
Epipharyngitis — see Nasopharyngitis
Epiphora H04.20- ☑
  due to
    excess lacrimation H04.21- ☑
    insufficient drainage H04.22- ☑
Epiphyseal arrest — see Arrest, epiphyseal
Epiphyseolysis, epiphysiolysis — see Osteochondropathy
Epiphysitis — see also Osteochondropathy

Epiphysitis — *continued*
  juvenile M92.9
  syphilitic (congenital) A50.02
Epiplocele — *see* Hernia, abdomen
Epiploitis — *see* Peritonitis
Epiplosarcomphalocele — *see* Hernia, umbilicus
Episcleritis (suppurative) H15.10- ☑
  in (due to)
    syphilis A52.71
    tuberculosis A18.51
  nodular H15.12- ☑
  periodica fugax H15.11- ☑
    angioneurotic — *see* Edema, angioneurotic
    syphilitic (late) A52.71
    tuberculous A18.51
Episode
  affective, mixed F39
  depersonalization (in neurotic state) F48.1
  depressive F32.A
    major F32.9
      mild F32.0
      moderate F32.1
      severe (without psychotic symptoms) F32.2
        with psychotic symptoms F32.3
      recurrent F33.9
        brief F33.8
      specified NEC F32.89
  hypomanic F30.8
  manic F30.9
    with
      psychotic symptoms F30.2
      remission (full) F30.4
        partial F30.3
    other specified F30.8
    recurrent F31.89
    without psychotic symptoms F30.10
      mild F30.11
      moderate F30.12
      severe (without psychotic symptoms) F30.13
        with psychotic symptoms F30.2
  psychotic F23
    organic F06.8
  schizophrenic (acute) NEC, brief F23
Epispadias (female) (male) Q64.0
Episplenitis D73.89
Epistaxis (multiple) R04.0
  hereditary I78.0
  vicarious menstruation N94.89
Epithelioma (malignant) — *see also* Neoplasm, malignant, by site
  adenoides cysticum — *see* Neoplasm, skin, benign
  basal cell — *see* Neoplasm, skin, malignant
  benign — *see* Neoplasm, benign, by site
  Bowen's — *see* Neoplasm, skin, in situ
  calcifying, of Malherbe — *see* Neoplasm, skin, benign
  external site — *see* Neoplasm, skin, malignant
  intraepidermal, Jadassohn — *see* Neoplasm, skin, benign
  squamous cell — *see* Neoplasm, malignant, by site
Epitheliomatosis pigmented Q82.1
Epitheliopathy, multifocal placoid pigment H30.14- ☑
Epithelium, epithelial — *see* condition
Epituberculosis (with atelectasis) (allergic) A15.7
Eponychia Q84.6
Epstein's
  nephrosis or syndrome — *see* Nephrosis
  pearl K09.8
Epulis (gingiva) (fibrous) (giant cell) K06.8
Equinia A24.0
Equinovarus (congenital) (talipes) Q66.0- ☑
  acquired — *see* Deformity, limb, clubfoot
Equivalent
  convulsive (abdominal) — *see* Epilepsy, specified NEC
  epileptic (psychic) — *see* Epilepsy, localization-related, symptomatic, with complex partial seizures
Erb-Goldflam disease or syndrome G70.00
  with exacerbation (acute) G70.01
  in crisis G70.01
Erb (-Duchenne) **paralysis** (birth injury) (newborn) P14.0
Erb's
  disease G71.02
  palsy, paralysis (brachial) (birth) (newborn) P14.0
    spinal (spastic) syphilitic A52.17
  pseudohypertrophic muscular dystrophy G71.02
Erdheim's syndrome (acromegalic macrospondylitis) E22.0
Erection, painful (persistent) — *see* Priapism
Ergosterol deficiency (vitamin D) E55.9
  with
    adult osteomalacia M83.8

Ergosterol deficiency — *continued*
  with — *continued*
    rickets — *see* Rickets
Ergotism — *see also* Poisoning, food, noxious, plant
  from ergot used as drug (migraine therapy) — *see* Table of Drugs and Chemicals
Erosio interdigitalis blastomycetica B37.2
Erosion
  artery I77.2
    without rupture I77.89
  bone — *see* Disorder, bone, density and structure, specified NEC
  bronchus J98.09
  cameron — *see* Ulcer, stomach
  cartilage (joint) — *see* Disorder, cartilage, specified type NEC
  cervix (uteri) (acquired) (chronic) (congenital) N86
    with cervicitis N72
  cornea (nontraumatic) — *see* Ulcer, cornea
    recurrent H18.83- ☑
    traumatic — *see* Abrasion, cornea
  dental (idiopathic) (occupational) (due to diet, drugs or vomiting) K03.2
  duodenum, postpyloric — *see* Ulcer, duodenum
  esophagus K22.10
    with bleeding K22.11
  gastric — *see* Ulcer, stomach
  gastrojejunal — *see* Ulcer, gastrojejunal
  implanted mesh — *see* Complications, prosthetic device or implant, mesh
  intestine K63.3
  lymphatic vessel I89.8
  pylorus, pyloric (ulcer) — *see* Ulcer, stomach
  spine, aneurysmal A52.09
  stomach — *see* Ulcer, stomach
  subcutaneous device pocket
    nervous system prosthetic device, implant, or graft T85.890- ☑
    other internal prosthetic device, implant, or graft T85.898- ☑
  teeth (idiopathic) (occupational) (due to diet, drugs or vomiting) K03.2
  urethra N36.8
  uterus N85.8
Erotomania F52.8
Error
  metabolism, inborn — *see* Disorder, metabolism
  refractive — *see* Disorder, refraction
Eructation R14.2
  nervous or psychogenic F45.8
Eruption
  creeping B76.9
  drug (generalized) (taken internally) L27.0
    fixed L27.1
    in contact with skin — *see* Dermatitis, due to drugs
    localized L27.1
  Hutchinson, summer L56.4
  Kaposi's varicelliform B00.0
  napkin L22
  polymorphous light (sun) L56.4
  recalcitrant pustular L13.8
  ringed R23.8
  skin (nonspecific) R21
    creeping (meaning hookworm) B76.9
    due to inoculation/vaccination (generalized) — *see also* Dermatitis, due to, vaccine L27.0
      localized L27.1
    erysipeloid A26.0
    feigned L98.1
    Kaposi's varicelliform B00.0
    lichenoid L28.0
    meaning dermatitis — *see* Dermatitis
    toxic NEC L53.0
  tooth, teeth, abnormal (incomplete) (late) (premature) (sequence) K00.6
  vesicular R23.8
Erysipelas (gangrenous) (infantile) (newborn) (phlegmonous) (suppurative) A46
  external ear A46 [H62.4-] ☑
  puerperal, postpartum O86.89
Erysipeloid A26.9
  cutaneous (Rosenbach's) A26.0
  disseminated A26.8
  sepsis A26.7
  specified NEC A26.8
Erythema, erythematous (infectional) (inflammation) L53.9
  ab igne L59.0
  annulare (centrifugum) (rheumaticum) L53.1
  arthriticum epidemicum A25.1

Erythema, erythematous — *continued*
  brucellum — *see* Brucellosis
  chronic figurate NEC L53.3
  chronicum migrans (Borrelia burgdorferi) A69.20
  diaper L22
  due to
    chemical NEC L53.0
      in contact with skin L24.5
    drug (internal use) — *see* Dermatitis, due to, drugs
  elevatum diutinum L95.1
  endemic E52
  epidemic, arthritic A25.1
  figuratum perstans L53.3
  gluteal L22
  heat — *code by site under* Burn, first degree
  ichthyosiforme congenitum bullous Q80.3
  in diseases classified elsewhere L54
  induratum (nontuberculous) L52
    tuberculous A18.4
  infectiosum B08.3
  intertrigo L30.4
  iris L51.9
  marginatum L53.2
    in (due to) acute rheumatic fever I00
  medicamentosum — *see* Dermatitis, due to, drugs
  migrans A26.0
    chronicum A69.20
    tongue K14.1
  multiforme (major) (minor) L51.9
    bullous, bullosum L51.1
    conjunctiva L51.1
    nonbullous L51.0
    pemphigoides L12.0
    specified NEC L51.8
  napkin L22
  neonatorum P83.88
    toxic P83.1
  nodosum L52
    tuberculous A18.4
  palmar L53.8
  pernio T69.1- ☑
  rash, newborn P83.88
  scarlatiniform (recurrent) (exfoliative) L53.8
  solare L55.0
  specified NEC L53.8
  toxic, toxicum NEC L53.0
    newborn P83.1
  tuberculous (primary) A18.4
Erythematous, erythematosus — *see* condition
Erythermalgia (primary) I73.81
Erythralgia I73.81
Erythrasma L08.1
Erythredema (polyneuropathy) — *see* Poisoning, mercury
Erythremia (acute) C94.0- ☑
  chronic D45
  secondary D75.1
Erythroblastopenia — *see also* Aplasia, red cell D60.9
  congenital D61.01
Erythroblastophthisis D61.09
Erythroblastosis (fetalis) (newborn) P55.9
  due to
    ABO (antibodies) (incompatibility) (isoimmunization) P55.1
    Rh (antibodies) (incompatibility) (isoimmunization) P55.0
Erythrocyanosis (crurum) I73.89
Erythrocythemia — *see* Erythremia
Erythrocytosis (megalosplenic) (secondary) D75.1
  familial D75.0
  oval, hereditary — *see* Elliptocytosis
  secondary D75.1
  stress D75.1
Erythroderma (secondary) — *see also* Erythema L53.9
  bullous ichthyosiform, congenital Q80.3
  desquamativum L21.1
  ichthyosiform, congenital (bullous) Q80.3
  neonatorum P83.88
  psoriaticum L40.8
Erythrodysesthesia, palmar plantar (PPE) L27.1
Erythrogenesis imperfecta D61.09
Erythroleukemia C94.0- ☑
Erythromelalgia I73.81
Erythrophagocytosis D75.89
Erythrophobia F40.298
Erythroplakia, oral epithelium, and tongue K13.29
Erythroplasia (Queyrat) D07.4
  specified site — *see* Neoplasm, skin, in situ
  unspecified site D07.4

☑ **Additional Character Required** — Refer to the Tabular List for Character Selection

Escherichia coli (E. coli), **as cause of disease classified elsewhere** B96.20
- non-O157 Shiga toxin-producing (with known O group) B96.22
- non-Shiga toxin-producing B96.29
- O157 B96.21
- O157 with confirmation of Shiga toxin when H antigen is unknown, or is not H7 B96.21
- O157:H- (nonmotile) with confirmation of Shiga toxin B96.21
- O157:H7 with or without confirmation of Shiga toxin-production B96.21
- specified NEC B96.22
- Shiga toxin-producing (with unspecified O group) (STEC) B96.23
- specified NEC B96.29

Esophagismus K22.4
Esophagitis (acute) (alkaline) (chemical) (chronic) (infectional) (necrotic) (peptic) (postoperative) (without bleeding) K20.90
- with bleeding K20.91
- candidal B37.81
- due to gastrointestinal reflux disease (without bleeding) K21.00
  - with bleeding K21.01
- eosinophilic K20.0
- reflux K21.00
  - with bleeding K21.01
- specified NEC (without bleeding) K20.80
  - with bleeding K20.81
- tuberculous A18.83
- ulcerative K22.10
  - with bleeding K22.11

Esophagocele K22.5
Esophagomalacia K22.89
Esophagospasm K22.4
Esophagostenosis K22.2
Esophagostomiasis B81.8
Esophagotracheal — see condition
Esophagus — see condition
Esophoria H50.51
- convergence, excess H51.12
- divergence, insufficiency H51.8

Esotropia — see Strabismus, convergent concomitant
Espundia B55.2
Essential — see condition
Esthesioneuroblastoma C30.0
Esthesioneurocytoma C30.0
Esthesioneuroepithelioma C30.0
Esthiomene A55
Estivo-autumnal malaria (fever) B50.9
Estrangement (marital) Z63.5
- parent-child NEC Z62.890

Estriasis — see Myiasis
Ethanolism — see Alcoholism
Etherism — see Dependence, drug, inhalant
Ethmoid, ethmoidal — see condition
Ethmoiditis (chronic) (nonpurulent) (purulent) — see also Sinusitis, ethmoidal
- influenzal — see Influenza, with, respiratory manifestations NEC
- Woakes' J33.1

Ethylism — see Alcoholism
Eulenburg's disease (congenital paramyotonia) G71.19
Eumycetoma B47.0
Eunuchoidism E29.1
- hypogonadotropic E23.0

European blastomycosis — see Cryptococcosis
Eustachian — see condition
EVALI (e-cigarette, or vaping, product use associated lung injury) U07.0
Evaluation (for) (of)
- development state
  - adolescent Z00.3
  - period of
    - delayed growth in childhood Z00.70
      - with abnormal findings Z00.71
    - rapid growth in childhood Z00.2
  - puberty Z00.3
- growth and developmental state (period of rapid growth) Z00.2
  - delayed growth Z00.70
    - with abnormal findings Z00.71
- mental health (status) Z00.8
  - requested by authority Z04.6
- period of
  - delayed growth in childhood Z00.70
    - with abnormal findings Z00.71
  - rapid growth in childhood Z00.2

Evaluation — continued
- suspected condition — see Observation

Evans syndrome D69.41
Event
- apparent life threatening in newborn and infant (ALTE) R68.13
- brief resolved unexplained event (BRUE) R68.13

Eventration — see also Hernia, ventral
- colon into chest — see Hernia, diaphragm
- diaphragm (congenital) Q79.1

Eversion
- bladder N32.89
- cervix (uteri) N86
  - with cervicitis N72
- foot NEC — see also Deformity, valgus, ankle
  - congenital Q66.6
- punctum lacrimale (postinfectional) (senile) H04.52- ☑
- ureter (meatus) N28.89
- urethra (meatus) N36.8
- uterus N81.4

Evidence
- cytologic
  - of malignancy on anal smear R85.614
  - of malignancy on cervical smear R87.614
  - of malignancy on vaginal smear R87.624

Evisceration
- birth injury P15.8
- traumatic NEC
  - eye — see Enucleated eye

Evulsion — see Avulsion
Ewing's sarcoma or tumor — see Neoplasm, bone, malignant

Examination (for) (following) (general) (of) (routine) Z00.00
- with abnormal findings Z00.01
- abuse, physical (alleged), ruled out
  - adult Z04.71
  - child Z04.72
- adolescent (development state) Z00.3
- alleged rape or sexual assault (victim), ruled out
  - adult Z04.41
  - child Z04.42
- allergy Z01.82
- annual (adult) (periodic) (physical) Z00.00
  - with abnormal findings Z00.01
  - gynecological Z01.419
    - with abnormal findings Z01.411
- antibody response Z01.84
- blood — see Examination, laboratory
- blood pressure Z01.30
  - with abnormal findings Z01.31
- cancer staging — see Neoplasm, malignant, by site
- cervical Papanicolaou smear Z12.4
  - as part of routine gynecological examination Z01.419
    - with abnormal findings Z01.411
- child (over 28 days old) Z00.129
  - with abnormal findings Z00.121
  - under 28 days old — see Newborn, examination
- clinical research control or normal comparison (control) (participant) Z00.6
- contraceptive (drug) maintenance (routine) Z30.8
  - device (intrauterine) Z30.431
- dental Z01.20
  - with abnormal findings Z01.21
- developmental — see Examination, child
- donor (potential) Z00.5
- ear Z01.10
  - with abnormal findings NEC Z01.118
- eye Z01.00
  - with abnormal findings Z01.01
  - following failed vision screening Z01.020
    - with abnormal findings Z01.021
- follow-up (routine) (following) Z09
  - chemotherapy NEC Z09
    - malignant neoplasm Z08
  - fracture Z09
  - malignant neoplasm Z08
  - postpartum Z39.2
  - psychotherapy Z09
  - radiotherapy NEC Z09
    - malignant neoplasm Z08
  - surgery NEC Z09
    - malignant neoplasm Z08
- following
  - accident NEC Z04.3
    - transport Z04.1
    - work Z04.2
  - assault, alleged, ruled out
    - adult Z04.71
    - child Z04.72

Examination — continued
- following — continued
  - motor vehicle accident Z04.1
  - treatment (for) Z09
    - combined NEC Z09
      - fracture Z09
      - malignant neoplasm Z08
    - malignant neoplasm Z08
    - mental disorder Z09
    - specified condition NEC Z09
- forced sexual exploitation Z04.81
- forced labor exploitation Z04.82
- gynecological Z01.419
  - with abnormal findings Z01.411
  - for contraceptive maintenance Z30.8
- health — see Examination, medical
- hearing Z01.10
  - with abnormal findings NEC Z01.118
  - following failed hearing screening Z01.110
  - infant or child (over 28 days old) Z00.129
    - with abnormal findings Z00.121
- immunity status testing Z01.84
- laboratory (as part of a general medical examination) Z00.00
  - with abnormal findings Z00.01
  - preprocedural Z01.812
- lactating mother Z39.1
- medical (adult) (for) (of) Z00.00
  - with abnormal findings Z00.01
  - administrative purpose only Z02.9
    - specified NEC Z02.89
  - admission to
    - armed forces Z02.3
    - old age home Z02.2
    - prison Z02.89
    - residential institution Z02.2
    - school Z02.0
      - following illness or medical treatment Z02.0
    - summer camp Z02.89
  - adoption Z02.82
  - blood alcohol or drug level Z02.83
  - camp (summer) Z02.89
  - clinical research, normal subject (control) (participant) Z00.6
  - control subject in clinical research (normal comparison) (participant) Z00.6
  - donor (potential) Z00.5
  - driving license Z02.4
  - general (adult) Z00.00
    - with abnormal findings Z00.01
  - immigration Z02.89
  - insurance purposes Z02.6
  - marriage Z02.89
  - medicolegal reasons NEC Z04.89
  - naturalization Z02.89
  - participation in sport Z02.5
  - paternity testing Z02.81
  - population survey Z00.8
  - pre-employment Z02.1
  - pre-operative — see Examination, pre-procedural
  - pre-procedural
    - cardiovascular Z01.810
    - respiratory Z01.811
    - specified NEC Z01.818
  - preschool children
    - for admission to school Z02.0
  - prisoners
    - for entrance into prison Z02.89
  - recruitment for armed forces Z02.3
  - specified NEC Z00.8
  - sport competition Z02.5
- medicolegal reason NEC Z04.89
- following
  - forced sexual exploitation Z04.81
  - forced labor exploitation Z04.82
- newborn — see Newborn, examination
- pelvic (annual) (periodic) Z01.419
  - with abnormal findings Z01.411
- period of rapid growth in childhood Z00.2
- periodic (adult) (annual) (routine) Z00.00
  - with abnormal findings Z00.01
- physical (adult) — see also Examination, medical Z00.00
  - sports Z02.5
- postpartum
  - immediately after delivery Z39.0
  - routine follow-up Z39.2
- pre-chemotherapy (antineoplastic) Z01.818
- prenatal (normal pregnancy) — see also Pregnancy, normal Z34.9- ☑

Examination — *continued*
  pre-procedural (pre-operative)
    cardiovascular Z01.810
    laboratory Z01.812
    respiratory Z01.811
    specified NEC Z01.818
  prior to chemotherapy (antineoplastic) Z01.818
  psychiatric NEC Z00.8
    follow-up not needing further care Z09
    requested by authority Z04.6
  radiological (as part of a general medical examination) Z00.00
    with abnormal findings Z00.01
  repeat cervical smear to confirm findings of recent normal smear following initial abnormal smear Z01.42
  skin (hypersensitivity) Z01.82
  special — *see also* Examination, by type Z01.89
    specified type NEC Z01.89
  specified type or reason NEC Z04.89
  teeth Z01.20
    with abnormal findings Z01.21
  urine — *see* Examination, laboratory
  vision Z01.00
    with abnormal findings Z01.01
    following failed vision screening Z01.020
      with abnormal findings Z01.021
    infant or child (over 28 days old) Z00.129
      with abnormal findings Z00.121
Exanthem, exanthema — *see also* Rash
  with enteroviral vesicular stomatitis B08.4
  Boston A88.0
  epidemic with meningitis A88.0 [G02]
  subitum B08.20
    due to human herpesvirus 6 B08.21
    due to human herpesvirus 7 B08.22
  viral, virus B09
    specified type NEC B08.8
Excess, excessive, excessively
  alcohol level in blood R78.0
  androgen (ovarian) E28.1
  attrition, tooth, teeth K03.0
  carotene, carotin (dietary) E67.1
  cold, effects of T69.9- ☑
    specified effect NEC T69.8- ☑
  convergence H51.12
  crying
    in child, adolescent, or adult R45.83
    in infant R68.11
  development, breast N62
  divergence H51.8
  drinking (alcohol) NEC (without dependence) F10.10
    habitual (continual) (without remission) F10.20
  eating R63.2
  estrogen E28.0
  fat — *see also* Obesity
    in heart — *see* Degeneration, myocardial
    localized E65
  foreskin N47.8
  gas R14.0
  glucagon E16.3
  heat — *see* Heat
  intermaxillary vertical dimension of fully erupted teeth M26.37
  interocclusal distance of fully erupted teeth M26.37
  kalium E87.5
  large
    colon K59.39
      congenital Q43.8
    infant P08.0
    organ or site, congenital NEC — *see* Anomaly, by site
  long
    organ or site, congenital NEC — *see* Anomaly, by site
  menstruation (with regular cycle) N92.0
    with irregular cycle N92.1
  napping Z72.821
  natrium E87.0
  number of teeth K00.1
  nutrient (dietary) NEC R63.2
  potassium (K) E87.5
  salivation K11.7
  secretion — *see also* Hypersecretion
    milk O92.6
    sputum R09.3
    sweat R61
  sexual drive F52.8
  short
    organ or site, congenital NEC — *see* Anomaly, by site
    umbilical cord in labor or delivery O69.3- ☑
  skin L98.7

Excess, excessive, excessively — *continued*
  skin — *continued*
    and subcutaneous tissue L98.7
    eyelid (acquired) — *see* Blepharochalasis
      congenital Q10.3
  sodium (Na) E87.0
  spacing of fully erupted teeth M26.32
  sputum R09.3
  sweating R61
  thirst R63.1
    due to deprivation of water T73.1- ☑
  transportation time Z59.82
  tuberosity of jaw M26.07
  vitamin
    A (dietary) E67.0
      administered as drug (prolonged intake) — *see* Table of Drugs and Chemicals, vitamins, adverse effect
      overdose or wrong substance given or taken — *see* Table of Drugs and Chemicals, vitamins, poisoning
    D (dietary) E67.3
      administered as drug (prolonged intake) — *see* Table of Drugs and Chemicals, vitamins, adverse effect
      overdose or wrong substance given or taken — *see* Table of Drugs and Chemicals, vitamins, poisoning
  weight
    gain R63.5
    loss R63.4
Excitability, abnormal, under minor stress (personality disorder) F60.3
Excitation
  anomalous atrioventricular I45.6
  psychogenic F30.8
  reactive (from emotional stress, psychological trauma) F30.8
Excitement
  hypomanic F30.8
  manic F30.9
  mental, reactive (from emotional stress, psychological trauma) F30.8
  state, reactive (from emotional stress, psychological trauma) F30.8
Excoriation (traumatic) — *see also* Abrasion
  neurotic L98.1
  skin picking disorder F42.4
Exfoliation
  due to erythematous conditions according to extent of body surface involved L49.0
    10-19 percent of body surface L49.1
    20-29 percent of body surface L49.2
    30-39 percent of body surface L49.3
    40-49 percent of body surface L49.4
    50-59 percent of body surface L49.5
    60-69 percent of body surface L49.6
    70-79 percent of body surface L49.7
    80-89 percent of body surface L49.8
    90-99 percent of body surface L49.9
    less than 10 percent of body surface L49.0
  teeth, due to systemic causes K08.0
Exfoliative — *see* condition
Exhaustion, exhaustive (physical NEC) R53.83
  battle F43.0
  cardiac — *see* Failure, heart
  delirium F43.0
  due to
    cold T69.8- ☑
    excessive exertion T73.3- ☑
    exposure T73.2- ☑
    neurasthenia F48.8
  heart — *see* Failure, heart
  heat — *see also* Heat, exhaustion T67.5- ☑
    due to
      salt depletion T67.4- ☑
      water depletion T67.3- ☑
  maternal, complicating delivery O75.81
  mental F48.8
  myocardium, myocardial — *see* Failure, heart
  nervous F48.8
  old age R54
  psychogenic F48.8
  psychosis F43.0
  senile R54
  vital NEC Z73.0
Exhibitionism F65.2
Exocervicitis — *see* Cervicitis

Exomphalos Q79.2
  meaning hernia — *see* Hernia, umbilical
Exophoria H50.52
  convergence, insufficiency H51.11
  divergence, excess H51.8
Exophthalmos H05.2- ☑
  congenital Q15.8
  constant NEC H05.24- ☑
  displacement, globe — *see* Displacement, globe
  due to thyrotoxicosis (hyperthyroidism) — *see* Hyperthyroidism, with, goiter (diffuse)
  dysthyroid — *see* Hyperthyroidism, with, goiter (diffuse)
  goiter — *see* Hyperthyroidism, with, goiter (diffuse)
  intermittent NEC H05.25- ☑
  malignant — *see* Hyperthyroidism, with, goiter (diffuse)
  orbital
    edema — *see* Edema, orbit
    hemorrhage — *see* Hemorrhage, orbit
  pulsating NEC H05.26- ☑
  thyrotoxic, thyrotropic — *see* Hyperthyroidism, with, goiter (diffuse)
Exostosis — *see also* Disorder, bone
  cartilaginous — *see* Neoplasm, bone, benign
  congenital (multiple) Q78.6
  external ear canal H61.81- ☑
  gonococcal A54.49
  jaw (bone) M27.8
  multiple, congenital Q78.6
  orbit H05.35- ☑
  osteocartilaginous — *see* Neoplasm, bone, benign
  syphilitic A52.77
Exotropia — *see* Strabismus, divergent concomitant
Explanation of
  investigation finding Z71.2
  medication Z71.89
Exploitation
  labor
    confirmed
      adult forced T74.61- ☑
      child forced T74.62- ☑
    suspected
      adult forced T76.61- ☑
      child forced T76.62- ☑
  sexual
    confirmed
      adult forced T74.51- ☑
      child T74.52- ☑
    suspected
      adult forced T76.51- ☑
      child T76.52- ☑
Exposure (to) — *see also* Contact, with T75.89- ☑
  acariasis Z20.7
  Agent Orange Z77.39
  AIDS virus Z20.6
  air pollution Z77.110
  algae and algae toxins Z77.121
  algae bloom Z77.121
  anthrax Z20.810
  aromatic amines Z77.020
  aromatic (hazardous) compounds NEC Z77.028
  aromatic dyes NOS Z77.028
  arsenic Z77.010
  asbestos Z77.090
  bacterial disease NEC Z20.818
  benzene Z77.021
  blue-green algae bloom Z77.121
  body fluids (potentially hazardous) Z77.21
  brown tide Z77.121
  chemicals (chiefly nonmedicinal) (hazardous) NEC Z77.098
  cholera Z20.09
  chromium compounds Z77.018
  cold, effects of T69.9- ☑
    specified effect NEC T69.8- ☑
  communicable disease Z20.9
    bacterial NEC Z20.818
    specified NEC Z20.89
    viral NEC Z20.828
    Zika virus Z20.821
  coronavirus (disease) (novel) 2019 Z20.822
  COVID-19 Z20.822
  cyanobacteria bloom Z77.121
  disaster Z65.5
  discrimination Z60.5
  dyes Z77.098
  effects of T73.9- ☑
  environmental tobacco smoke (acute) (chronic) Z77.22
  Escherichia coli (E. coli) Z20.01

Exposure — *continued*
- exhaustion due to T73.2- ☑
- fiberglass — *see* Table of Drugs and Chemicals, fiberglass
- German measles Z20.4
- gonorrhea Z20.2
- hazardous metals NEC Z77.018
- hazardous substances NEC Z77.29
- hazards in the physical environment NEC Z77.128
- hazards to health NEC Z77.9
- human immunodeficiency virus (HIV) Z20.6
- human T-lymphotropic virus type-1 (HTLV-1) Z20.89
- implanted
  - mesh — *see* Complications, prosthetic device or implant, mesh
  - prosthetic materials NEC — *see* Complications, prosthetic materials NEC
- infestation (parasitic) NEC Z20.7
- intestinal infectious disease NEC Z20.09
  - Escherichia coli (E. coli) Z20.01
- lead Z77.011
- meningococcus Z20.811
- mold (toxic) Z77.120
- nickel dust Z77.018
- noise Z77.122
- occupational
  - air contaminants NEC Z57.39
  - dust Z57.2
  - environmental tobacco smoke Z57.31
  - extreme temperature Z57.6
  - noise Z57.0
  - radiation Z57.1
  - risk factors Z57.9
    - specified NEC Z57.8
  - toxic agents (gases) (liquids) (solids) (vapors) in agriculture Z57.4
  - toxic agents (gases) (liquids) (solids) (vapors) in industry NEC Z57.5
  - vibration Z57.7
- parasitic disease NEC Z20.7
- pediculosis Z20.7
- persecution Z60.5
- pfiesteria piscicida Z77.121
- poliomyelitis Z20.89
- pollution
  - air Z77.110
  - environmental NEC Z77.118
  - soil Z77.112
  - water Z77.111
- polycyclic aromatic hydrocarbons Z77.028
- prenatal (drugs) (toxic chemicals) — *see* Newborn, affected by, noxious substances transmitted via placenta or breast milk
- rabies Z20.3
- radiation, naturally occurring NEC Z77.123
- radon Z77.123
- red tide (Florida) Z77.121
- risk factor, personal, to diethylstilbestrol (DES) (in utero) Z91.B
- rubella Z20.4
- SARS-CoV-2 Z20.822
- second hand tobacco smoke (acute) (chronic) Z77.22
  - in the perinatal period P96.81
- sexually-transmitted disease Z20.2
- smallpox (laboratory) Z20.89
- syphilis Z20.2
- terrorism Z65.4
- torture Z65.4
- tuberculosis Z20.1
- uranium Z77.012
- varicella Z20.820
- venereal disease Z20.2
- viral disease NEC Z20.828
- war Z65.5
- water pollution Z77.111
- Zika virus Z20.821

Exsanguination — *see* Hemorrhage

Exstrophy
- abdominal contents Q45.8
- bladder Q64.10
  - cloacal Q64.12
  - specified type NEC Q64.19
  - supravesical fissure Q64.11

Extensive — *see* condition

Extra — *see also* Accessory
- marker chromosomes (normal individual) Q92.61
  - in abnormal individual Q92.62
- rib Q76.6
  - cervical Q76.5

Extrasystoles (supraventricular) I49.49

Extrasystoles — *continued*
- atrial I49.1
- auricular I49.1
- junctional I49.2
- ventricular I49.3

Extrauterine gestation or pregnancy — *see* Pregnancy, by site

Extravasation
- blood R58
- chyle into mesentery I89.8
- pelvicalyceal N13.8
- pyelosinus N13.8
- urine (from ureter) R39.0
- vesicant agent
  - antineoplastic chemotherapy T80.810- ☑
  - other agent NEC T80.818- ☑

Extremity — *see* condition, limb

Extrophy — *see* Exstrophy

Extroversion
- bladder Q64.19
- uterus N81.4
  - complicating delivery O71.2
  - postpartal (old) N81.4

Extruded tooth (teeth) M26.34

Extrusion
- breast implant (prosthetic) T85.42- ☑
- eye implant (globe) (ball) T85.328- ☑
- intervertebral disc — *see* Displacement, intervertebral disc
- ocular lens implant (prosthetic) — *see* Complications, intraocular lens
- vitreous — *see* Prolapse, vitreous

Exudate
- causing irritant dermatitis L24.A9
- pleural — *see* Effusion, pleura
- retina H35.89
- wound fluids causing irritant dermatitis L24.A9

Exudative — *see* condition

Eye, eyeball, eyelid — *see* condition

Eyestrain — *see* Disturbance, vision, subjective

Eyeworm disease of Africa B74.3

F

Faber's syndrome (achlorhydric anemia) D50.9
Fabry (-Anderson) disease E75.21
Facet syndrome M47.89- ☑
Faciocephalalgia, autonomic — *see also* Neuropathy, peripheral, autonomic G90.09
Factor(s)
- psychic, associated with diseases classified elsewhere F54
- psychological
  - affecting physical conditions F54
  - or behavioral
    - affecting general medical condition F54
    - associated with disorders or diseases classified elsewhere F54

Fahr disease (of brain) G23.8
Fahr Volhard disease (of kidney) I12.- ☑
Failure, failed
- abortion — *see* Abortion, attempted
- aortic (valve) I35.8
  - rheumatic I06.8
- attempted abortion — *see* Abortion, attempted
- biventricular I50.82
  - due to left heart failure I50.814
- bone marrow — *see* Anemia, aplastic
- cardiac — *see* Failure, heart
- cardiorenal (chronic) — *see also* Failure, renal, and Failure, heart I50.9
  - hypertensive I13.2
- cardiorespiratory — *see also* Failure, heart R09.2
- cardiovascular (chronic) — *see* Failure, heart
- cerebrovascular I67.9
- cervical dilatation in labor O62.0
- circulation, circulatory (peripheral) R57.9
  - newborn P29.89
- compensation — *see* Disease, heart
- compliance with medical treatment or regimen — *see* Noncompliance
- congestive — *see* Failure, heart, congestive
- dental implant (endosseous) M27.69
  - due to
    - failure of dental prosthesis M27.63
    - lack of attached gingiva M27.62
    - occlusal trauma (poor prosthetic design) M27.62
    - parafunctional habits M27.62

Failure, failed — *continued*
- dental implant — *continued*
  - due to — *continued*
    - periodontal infection (peri-implantitis) M27.62
    - poor oral hygiene M27.62
  - osseointegration M27.61
    - due to
      - complications of systemic disease M27.61
      - poor bone quality M27.61
    - iatrogenic M27.61
  - post-osseointegration
    - biological M27.62
    - due to complications of systemic disease M27.62
    - iatrogenic M27.62
    - mechanical M27.63
  - pre-integration M27.61
  - pre-osseointegration M27.61
  - specified NEC M27.69
- descent of head (at term) of pregnancy (mother) O32.4- ☑
- endosseous dental implant — *see* Failure, dental implant
- engagement of head (term of pregnancy) (mother) O32.4- ☑
- erection (penile) — *see also* Dysfunction, sexual, male, erectile N52.9
  - nonorganic F52.21
- examination(s), anxiety concerning Z55.2
- expansion terminal respiratory units (newborn) (primary) P28.0
- forceps NOS (with subsequent cesarean delivery) O66.5
- gain weight (child over 28 days old) R62.51
  - adult R62.7
  - newborn P92.6
- genital response (male) F52.21
  - female F52.22
- heart (acute) (senile) (sudden) I50.9
  - with
    - acute pulmonary edema — *see* Failure, ventricular, left
    - decompensation I50.9
      - with
        - normal ejection fraction I50.33
        - preserved ejection fraction I50.33
        - reduced ejection fraction I50.23
          - with diastolic dysfunction I50.43
    - combined systolic and diastolic I50.43
    - diastolic I50.33
      - right I50.813
    - systolic I50.23
  - dilatation — *see* Disease, heart
  - hypertension — *see* Hypertension, heart
  - normal ejection fraction — *see* Failure, heart, diastolic
  - preserved ejection fraction — *see* Failure, heart, diastolic
  - reduced ejection fraction — *see* Failure, heart, systolic
  - arteriosclerotic I70.90
  - biventricular I50.82
    - due to left heart failure I50.814
  - combined left-right sided I50.82
    - due to left heart failure I50.814
  - compensated — *see also* Failure, heart, by type as diastolic or systolic, chronic I50.9
  - complicating
    - anesthesia (general) (local) or other sedation
      - in labor and delivery O74.2
      - in pregnancy O29.12- ☑
      - postpartum, puerperal O89.1
    - delivery (cesarean) (instrumental) O75.4
  - congestive I50.9
    - with rheumatic fever (conditions in I00)
      - active I01.8
      - inactive or quiescent (with chorea) I09.81
    - newborn P29.0
    - rheumatic (chronic) (inactive) (with chorea) I09.81
      - active or acute I01.8
        - with chorea I02.0
  - decompensated — *see also* Failure, heart, by type as diastolic or systolic, acute and chronic I50.9
  - degenerative — *see* Degeneration, myocardial
  - diastolic (congestive) (left ventricular) I50.30
    - acute (congestive) I50.31
      - and (on) chronic (congestive) I50.33
    - chronic (congestive) I50.32
      - and (on) acute (congestive) I50.33
    - combined with systolic (congestive) I50.40
      - acute (congestive) I50.41
        - and (on) chronic (congestive) I50.43

Failure, failed — continued
  heart — continued
    diastolic — continued
      combined with systolic — continued
        chronic (congestive) I50.42
          and (on) acute (congestive) I50.43
      due to presence of cardiac prosthesis I97.13- ☑
      end stage — see also Failure, heart, by type as diastolic or systolic, chronic I50.84
      following cardiac surgery I97.130
      following other surgery I97.131
      high output NOS I50.83
      hypertensive — see Hypertension, heart
      left (ventricular) — see also Failure, heart, ventricular, left
        combined diastolic and systolic — see Failure, heart, diastolic, combined with systolic
        diastolic — see Failure, heart, diastolic
        systolic — see Failure, heart, systolic
      low output (syndrome) NOS I50.9
      newborn P29.0
      organic — see Disease, heart
      peripartum O90.3
      postprocedural I97.13- ☑
      rheumatic (chronic) (inactive) I09.9
      right (isolated) (ventricular) I50.810
        acute I50.811
          and (on) chronic I50.813
        chronic I50.812
          and acute I50.813
        secondary to left heart failure I50.814
      specified NEC I50.89

    Note: heart failure stages A, B, C, and D are based on the American College of Cardiology and American Heart Association stages of heart failure, which complement and should not be confused with the New York Heart Association Classification of Heart Failure, into Class I, Class II, Class III, and Class IV

      stage A Z91.89
      stage B — see also Failure, heart, by type as diastolic or systolic, if known I50.9
      stage C — see also Failure, heart, by type as diastolic or systolic, if known I50.9
      stage D — see also Failure, heart, by type as diastolic or systolic, chronic I50.84
      systolic (congestive) (left ventricular) I50.20
        acute (congestive) I50.21
          and (on) chronic (congestive) I50.23
        chronic (congestive) I50.22
          and (on) acute (congestive) I50.23
        combined with diastolic (congestive) I50.40
          acute (congestive) I50.41
            and (on) chronic (congestive) I50.43
          chronic (congestive) I50.42
            and (on) acute (congestive) I50.43
      thyrotoxic — see also Thyrotoxicosis E05.90 [I43]
        with
          high output — see also Thyrotoxicosis I50.83
          thyroid storm E05.91 [I43]
            high output — see also Thyrotoxicosis I50.83
      valvular — see Endocarditis
  hepatic K72.90
    with coma K72.91
    acute or subacute K72.00
      with coma K72.01
      due to drugs K71.10
        with coma K71.11
    alcoholic (acute) (chronic) (subacute) K70.40
      with coma K70.41
    chronic K72.10
      with coma K72.11
      due to drugs (acute) (subacute) (chronic) K71.10
        with coma K71.11
    due to drugs (acute) (subacute) (chronic) K71.10
      with coma K71.11
    end stage K72.10
      with coma K72.11
    postprocedural K91.82
  hepatorenal K76.7
  induction (of labor) O61.9
    abortion — see Abortion, attempted
    by
      oxytocic drugs O61.0
      prostaglandins O61.0
    instrumental O61.1
    mechanical O61.1
    medical O61.0
    specified NEC O61.8

Failure, failed — continued
  induction — continued
    surgical O61.1
  intestinal K90.83
  intubation during anesthesia T88.4- ☑
    in pregnancy O29.6- ☑
    labor and delivery O74.7
    postpartum, puerperal O89.6
  involution, thymus (gland) E32.0
  kidney — see also Disease, kidney, chronic N19
    acute — see also Failure, renal, acute N17.9
  lactation (complete) O92.3
    partial O92.4
  Leydig's cell, adult E29.1
  liver — see Failure, hepatic
  menstruation at puberty N91.0
  mitral I05.8
  myocardial, myocardium — see also Failure, heart I50.9
    chronic — see also Failure, heart, congestive I50.9
    congestive — see also Failure, heart, congestive I50.9
  newborn screening — see Abnormal, neonatal screening
    neonatal congenital heart disease P09.5
  orgasm (female) (psychogenic) F52.31
    male F52.32
  ovarian (primary) E28.39
    iatrogenic E89.40
      asymptomatic E89.40
      symptomatic E89.41
    postprocedural (postablative) (postirradiation) (postsurgical) E89.40
      asymptomatic E89.40
      symptomatic E89.41
  ovulation causing infertility N97.0
  polyglandular, autoimmune E31.0
  prosthetic joint implant — see Complications, joint prosthesis, mechanical, breakdown, by site
  renal N19
    with
      tubular necrosis (acute) N17.0
    acute N17.9
      with
        cortical necrosis N17.1
        medullary necrosis N17.2
        tubular necrosis N17.0
      specified NEC N17.8
    chronic N18.9
      hypertensive — see Hypertension, kidney
    congenital P96.0
    end stage (chronic) N18.6
      due to hypertension I12.0
    following
      abortion — see Abortion by type complicated by specified condition NEC
      crushing T79.5- ☑
      ectopic or molar pregnancy O08.4
      labor and delivery (acute) O90.49
    hypertensive — see Hypertension, kidney
    postprocedural N99.0
  respiration, respiratory J96.90
    with
      hypercapnia J96.92
      hypercarbia J96.92
      hypoxia J96.91
    acute J96.00
      with
        hypercapnia J96.02
        hypercarbia J96.02
        hypoxia J96.01
      center G93.89
    acute and (on) chronic J96.20
      with
        hypercapnia J96.22
        hypercarbia J96.22
        hypoxia J96.21
    chronic J96.10
      with
        hypercapnia J96.12
        hypercarbia J96.12
        hypoxia J96.11
    newborn P28.5
    postprocedural (acute) J95.821
      acute and chronic J95.822
  rotation
    cecum Q43.3
    colon Q43.3
    intestine Q43.3
    kidney Q63.2
  sedation (conscious) (moderate) during procedure T88.52- ☑

Failure, failed — continued
  sedation during procedure — continued
    history of Z92.83
  segmentation — see also Fusion
    fingers — see Syndactylism, complex, fingers
    vertebra Q76.49
      with scoliosis Q76.3
  seminiferous tubule, adult E29.1
  senile (general) R54
  sexual arousal (male) F52.21
    female F52.22
  testicular endocrine function E29.1
  to thrive (child over 28 days old) R62.51
    adult R62.7
    newborn P92.6
  transplant T86.92
    bone T86.831
      marrow T86.02
    cornea T86.841- ☑
    heart T86.22
      with lung(s) T86.32
    intestine T86.851
    kidney T86.12
    liver T86.42
    lung(s) T86.811
      with heart T86.32
    pancreas T86.891
    skin (allograft) (autograft) T86.821
    specified organ or tissue NEC T86.891
    stem cell (peripheral blood) (umbilical cord) T86.5
    trial of labor (with subsequent cesarean delivery) O66.40
      following previous cesarean delivery O66.41
  tubal ligation N99.89
  urinary — see Disease, kidney, chronic
  vacuum extraction NOS (with subsequent cesarean delivery) O66.5
  vasectomy N99.89
  ventouse NOS (with subsequent cesarean delivery) O66.5
  ventricular — see also Failure, heart I50.9
    left — see also Failure, heart, left I50.1
      with rheumatic fever (conditions in I00)
        active I01.8
          with chorea I02.0
        inactive or quiescent (with chorea) I09.81
      rheumatic (chronic) (inactive) (with chorea) I09.81
        active or acute I01.8
          with chorea I02.0
    right — see Failure, heart, right
  vital centers, newborn P91.88
Fainting (fit) R55
Fallen arches — see Deformity, limb, flat foot
Falling, falls (repeated) R29.6
  any organ or part — see Prolapse
Fallopian
  insufflation Z31.41
  tube — see condition
Fallot's
  pentalogy Q21.8
  tetrad or tetralogy Q21.3
  triad or trilogy Q22.3
False — see also condition
  croup J38.5
  joint — see Nonunion, fracture
  labor (pains) O47.9
    at or after 37 completed weeks of gestation O47.1
    before 37 completed weeks of gestation O47.0- ☑
  passage, urethra (prostatic) N36.5
  pregnancy F45.8
Faltering growth R62.51
Family, familial — see also condition
  disruption Z63.8
    involving divorce or separation Z63.5
  Li-Fraumeni (syndrome) Z15.01
  planning advice Z30.09
  problem Z63.9
    specified NEC Z63.8
  retinoblastoma C69.2- ☑
Famine (effects of) T73.0- ☑
  edema — see Malnutrition, severe
Fanconi ('s) anemia D61.03
Fanconi hypoplastic anemia D61.03
Fanconi panmyelopathy D61.03
Fanconi (-de Toni)(-Debre) syndrome E72.09
  with cystinosis E72.04
Farber's disease or syndrome E75.29
Farcy A24.0
Farmer's
  lung J67.0
  skin L57.8

Farsightedness — see Hypermetropia
Fascia — see condition
Fasciculation R25.3
Fasciitis M72.9
- diffuse (eosinophilic) M35.4
- infective M72.8
  - necrotizing M72.6
- necrotizing M72.6
- nodular M72.4
- perirenal (with ureteral obstruction) N13.5
  - with infection N13.6
- plantar M72.2
- specified NEC M72.8
- traumatic (old) M72.8
  - current — code by site under Sprain

Fascioliasis B66.3
Fasciolopsis, fasciolopsiasis (intestinal) B66.5
Fascioscapulohumeral myopathy G71.02
Fast pulse R00.0
Fat
- embolism — see Embolism, fat
- excessive — see also Obesity
  - in heart — see Degeneration, myocardial
- in stool R19.5
- localized (pad) E65
  - heart — see Degeneration, myocardial
  - knee M79.4
  - retropatellar M79.4
- necrosis
  - breast N64.1
  - mesentery K65.4
  - omentum K65.4
- pad E65
  - knee M79.4

Fatigue R53.83
- auditory deafness — see Deafness
- chronic R53.82
- combat F43.0
- general R53.83
  - psychogenic F48.8
- heat (transient) T67.6- ☑
- muscle M62.89
- myocardium — see Failure, heart
- neoplasm-related R53.0
- nervous, neurosis F48.8
- operational F48.8
- psychogenic (general) F48.8
- senile R54
- voice R49.8

Fatness — see Obesity
Fatty — see also condition
- apron E65
- degeneration — see Degeneration, fatty
- heart (enlarged) — see Degeneration, myocardial
- liver NEC K76.0
  - alcoholic K70.0
  - nonalcoholic K76.0
- necrosis — see Degeneration, fatty

Fauces — see condition
Fauchard's disease (periodontitis) — see Periodontitis
Faucitis J02.9
Favism (anemia) D55.0
Favus — see Dermatophytosis
Fazio-Londe disease or syndrome G12.1
Fear complex or reaction F40.9
Fear of — see Phobia
Feared complaint unfounded Z71.1
Febris, febrile — see also Fever
- flava — see also Fever, yellow A95.9
- melitensis A23.0
- pestis — see Plague
- recurrens — see Fever, relapsing
- rubra A38.9

Fecal
- incontinence R15.9
- smearing R15.1
- soiling R15.1
- urgency R15.2

Fecalith (impaction) K56.41
- appendix K38.1
- congenital P76.8

Fede's disease K14.0
Feeble-minded F70
Feeble rapid pulse due to shock following injury T79.4- ☑
Feeding
- difficulties R63.30
- problem (elderly) (infant) R63.39
  - newborn P92.9

Feeding — continued
- problem — continued
  - newborn — continued
    - specified NEC P92.8
  - nonorganic (adult) — see Disorder, eating

Feeling (of)
- foreign body in throat R09.A2

Feer's disease — see Poisoning, mercury
Feet — see condition
Feigned illness Z76.5
Feil-Klippel syndrome (brevicollis) Q76.1
Feinmesser's (hidrotic) **ectodermal dysplasia** Q82.4
Felinophobia F40.218
Felon — see also Cellulitis, digit
- with lymphangitis — see Lymphangitis, acute, digit

Felty's syndrome M05.00
- ankle M05.07- ☑
- elbow M05.02- ☑
- foot joint M05.07- ☑
- hand joint M05.04- ☑
- hip M05.05- ☑
- knee M05.06- ☑
- multiple site M05.09
- shoulder M05.01- ☑
- vertebra — see Spondylitis, ankylosing
- wrist M05.03- ☑

Female genital cutting status — see Female genital mutilation status (FGM)
Female genital mutilation status (FGM) N90.810
- specified NEC N90.818
- type I (clitorectomy status) N90.811
- type II (clitorectomy with excision of labia minora status) N90.812
- type III (infibulation status) N90.813
- type IV N90.818

Femur, femoral — see condition
Fenestration, fenestrated — see also Imperfect, closure
- aortico-pulmonary Q21.4
- atrial septum Q21.11
- cusps, heart valve NEC Q24.8
  - pulmonary Q22.3
- pulmonic cusps Q22.3

Fernell's disease (aortic aneurysm) I71.9
Fertile eunuch syndrome E23.0
Fetid
- breath R19.6
- sweat L75.0

Fetishism F65.0
- transvestic F65.1

Fetus, fetal — see also condition
- alcohol syndrome (dysmorphic) Q86.0
- compressus O31.0- ☑
- hydantoin syndrome Q86.1
- lung tissue P28.0
- papyraceous O31.0- ☑

Fever (inanition) (of unknown origin) (persistent) (with chills) (with rigor) R50.9
- abortus A23.1
- Aden (dengue) A90
- African tick bite A77.8
- African tick-borne A68.1
- American
  - mountain (tick) A93.2
  - spotted A77.0
- aphthous B08.8
- arbovirus, arboviral A94
  - hemorrhagic A94
  - specified NEC A93.8
- Argentinian hemorrhagic A96.0
- Assam B55.0
- Australian Q A78
- Bangkok hemorrhagic A91
- Barmah forest A92.8
- Bartonella A44.0
- bilious, hemoglobinuric B50.8
- blackwater B50.8
- blister B00.1
- Bolivian hemorrhagic A96.1
- Bonvale dam T73.3- ☑
- boutonneuse A77.1
- brain — see Encephalitis
- Brazilian purpuric A48.4
- breakbone A90
- Bullis A77.0
- Bunyamwera A92.8
- Burdwan B55.0
- Bwamba A92.8
- Cameroon — see Malaria

Fever — continued
- Canton A75.9
- cat-scratch A28.1
- catarrhal (acute) J00
  - chronic J31.0
- Central Asian hemorrhagic A98.0
- cerebral — see Encephalitis
- cerebrospinal meningococcal A39.0
- Chagres B50.9
- Chandipura A92.8
- Changuinola A93.1
- Charcot's (biliary) (hepatic) (intermittent) — see Calculus, bile duct
- Chikungunya (viral) (hemorrhagic) A92.0
- Chitral A93.1
- Colombo — see Fever, paratyphoid
- Colorado tick (virus) A93.2
- congestive (remittent) — see Malaria
- Congo virus A98.0
- continued malarial B50.9
- Corsican — see Malaria
- Crimean-Congo hemorrhagic A98.0
- Cyprus — see Brucellosis
- dandy A90
- deer fly — see Tularemia
- dengue (virus) A90
  - hemorrhagic A91
  - sandfly A93.1
- desert B38.0
- drug induced R50.2
- due to
  - conditions classified elsewhere R50.81
  - heat T67.01- ☑
- enteric A01.00
- enteroviral exanthematous (Boston exanthem) A88.0
- ephemeral (of unknown origin) R50.9
- epidemic hemorrhagic A98.5
- erysipelatous — see Erysipelas
- estivo-autumnal (malarial) B50.9
- famine A75.0
- five day A79.0
- following delivery O86.4
- Fort Bragg A27.89
- gastroenteric A01.00
- gastromalarial — see Malaria
- Gibraltar — see Brucellosis
- glandular — see Mononucleosis, infectious
- Guama (viral) A92.8
- Haverhill A25.1
- hay (allergic) J30.1
  - with asthma (bronchial) J45.909
    - with
      - exacerbation (acute) J45.901
      - status asthmaticus J45.902
    - due to
      - allergen other than pollen J30.89
      - pollen, any plant or tree J30.1
- heat (effects) T67.01- ☑
- hematuric, bilious B50.8
- hemoglobinuric (malarial) (bilious) B50.8
- hemorrhagic (arthropod-borne) NOS A94
  - with renal syndrome A98.5
  - arenaviral A96.9
    - specified NEC A96.8
  - Argentinian A96.0
  - Bangkok A91
  - Bolivian A96.1
  - Central Asian A98.0
  - Chikungunya A92.0
  - Crimean-Congo A98.0
  - dengue (virus) A91
  - epidemic A98.5
  - Junin (virus) A96.0
  - Korean A98.5
  - Kyasanur forest A98.2
  - Machupo (virus) A96.1
  - mite-borne A93.8
  - mosquito-borne A92.8
  - Omsk A98.1
  - Philippine A91
  - Russian A98.5
  - Singapore A91
  - Southeast Asia A91
  - Thailand A91
  - tick-borne NEC A93.8
  - viral A99
    - specified NEC A98.8
- hepatic — see Cholecystitis
- herpetic — see Herpes

Fever — *continued*
  icterohemorrhagic A27.0
  Indiana A93.8
  infective B99.9
    specified NEC B99.8
  intermittent (bilious) — *see also* Malaria
    of unknown origin R50.9
      pernicious B50.9
  iodide R50.2
  Japanese river A75.3
  jungle — *see also* Malaria
    yellow A95.0
  Junin (virus) hemorrhagic A96.0
  Katayama B65.2
  kedani A75.3
  Kenya (tick) A77.1
  Kew Garden A79.1
  Korean hemorrhagic A98.5
  Lassa A96.2
  Lone Star A77.0
  Machupo (virus) hemorrhagic A96.1
  malaria, malarial — *see* Malaria
  Malta A23.9
  Marseilles A77.1
  marsh — *see* Malaria
  Mayaro (viral) A92.8
  Mediterranean — *see also* Brucellosis A23.9
    familial M04.1
    tick A77.1
  meningeal — *see* Meningitis
  Meuse A79.0
  Mexican A75.2
  mianeh A68.1
  miasmatic — *see* Malaria
  mosquito-borne (viral) A92.9
    hemorrhagic A92.8
  mountain — *see also* Brucellosis
    meaning Rocky Mountain spotted fever A77.0
    tick (American) (Colorado) (viral) A93.2
  Mucambo (viral) A92.8
  mud A27.9
  Neapolitan — *see* Brucellosis
  neutropenic D70.9
  newborn P81.9
    environmental P81.0
  Nine-Mile A78
  non-exanthematous tick A93.2
  North Asian tick-borne A77.2
  Omsk hemorrhagic A98.1
  O'nyong-nyong (viral) A92.1
  Oropouche (viral) A93.0
  Oroya A44.0
  pacific coast tick A77.8
  paludal — *see* Malaria
  Panama (malarial) B50.9
  Pappataci A93.1
  paratyphoid A01.4
    A A01.1
    B A01.2
    C A01.3
  parrot A70
  periodic (Mediterranean) M04.1
  persistent (of unknown origin) R50.9
  petechial A39.0
  pharyngoconjunctival B30.2
  Philippine hemorrhagic A91
  phlebotomus A93.1
  Piry (virus) A93.8
  Pixuna (viral) A92.8
  Plasmodium ovale B53.0
  polioviral (nonparalytic) A80.4
  Pontiac A48.2
  postimmunization R50.83
  postoperative R50.82
    due to infection T81.40- ☑
  posttransfusion R50.84
  postvaccination R50.83
  presenting with conditions classified elsewhere R50.81
  pretibial A27.89
  puerperal O86.4
  Q A78
  quadrilateral A78
  quartan (malaria) B52.9
  Queensland (coastal) (tick) A77.3
  quintan A79.0
  rabbit — *see* Tularemia
  rat-bite A25.9
    due to
      Spirillum A25.0

Fever — *continued*
  rat-bite — *continued*
    due to — *continued*
      Streptobacillus moniliformis A25.1
  recurrent — *see* Fever, relapsing
  relapsing (Borrelia) A68.9
    Carter's (Asiatic) A68.1
    Dutton's (West African) A68.1
    Koch's A68.9
    louse-borne A68.0
    Novy's
      louse-borne A68.0
      tick-borne A68.1
    Obermeyer's (European) A68.0
    tick-borne A68.1
  remittent (bilious) (congestive) (gastric) — *see* Malaria
  rheumatic (active) (acute) (chronic) (subacute) I00
    with central nervous system involvement I02.9
    active with heart involvement — *see* category I01.- ☑
    inactive or quiescent with
      cardiac hypertrophy I09.89
      carditis I09.9
      endocarditis I09.1
        aortic (valve) I06.9
          with mitral (valve) disease I08.0
        mitral (valve) I05.9
          with aortic (valve) disease I08.0
        pulmonary (valve) I09.89
        tricuspid (valve) I07.8
      heart disease NEC I09.89
      heart failure (congestive) (conditions in category I50.) I09.81
      left ventricular failure (conditions in I50.1-I50.4-) I09.81
      myocarditis, myocardial degeneration (conditions in I51.4) I09.0
      pancarditis I09.9
      pericarditis I09.2
  Rift Valley (viral) A92.4
  Rocky Mountain spotted A77.0
  rose J30.1
  Ross River B33.1
  Russian hemorrhagic A98.5
  San Joaquin (Valley) B38.0
  sandfly A93.1
  Sao Paulo A77.0
  scarlet A38.9
  seven day (leptospirosis) (autumnal) (Japanese) A27.89
    dengue A90
  shin-bone A79.0
  Singapore hemorrhagic A91
  solar A90
  Songo A98.5
  sore B00.1
  South African tick-bite A68.1
  Southeast Asia hemorrhagic A91
  spinal — *see* Meningitis
  spirillary A25.0
  splenic — *see* Anthrax
  spotted A77.9
    American A77.0
    Brazilian A77.0
    cerebrospinal meningitis A39.0
    Colombian A77.0
    due to Rickettsia
      africae (African tick bite fever) A77.8
      australis A77.3
      conorii A77.1
      parkeri A77.8
      rickettsii A77.0
      sibirica A77.2
      specified type NEC A77.8
    Ehrlichiosis A77.40
      due to
        E. chaffeensis A77.41
        specified organism NEC A77.49
    Rocky Mountain A77.0
  steroid R50.2
  streptobacillary A25.1
  subtertian B50.9
  Sumatran mite A75.3
  sun A90
  swamp A27.9
  swine A02.8
  sylvatic, yellow A95.0
  Tahyna B33.8
  tertian — *see* Malaria, tertian
  Thailand hemorrhagic A91
  thermic T67.01- ☑

Fever — *continued*
  three-day A93.1
  tick
    American mountain A93.2
    Colorado A93.2
    Kemerovo A93.8
    Mediterranean A77.1
    mountain A93.2
    nonexanthematous A93.2
    Quaranfil A93.8
  tick-bite NEC A93.8
  tick-borne (hemorrhagic) NEC A93.8
  trench A79.0
  tsutsugamushi A75.3
  typhogastric A01.00
  typhoid (abortive) (hemorrhagic) (intermittent) (malignant) A01.00
    complicated by
      arthritis A01.04
      heart involvement A01.02
      meningitis A01.01
      osteomyelitis A01.05
      pneumonia A01.03
      specified NEC A01.09
  typhomalarial — *see* Malaria
  typhus — *see* Typhus (fever)
  undulant — *see* Brucellosis
  unknown origin R50.9
  uveoparotid D86.89
  valley B38.0
  Venezuelan equine A92.2
  vesicular stomatitis A93.8
  viral hemorrhagic — *see* Fever, hemorrhagic, by type of virus
  Volhynian A79.0
  Wesselsbron (viral) A92.8
  West
    African B50.8
    Nile (viral) A92.30
      with
        complications NEC A92.39
        cranial nerve disorders A92.32
        encephalitis A92.31
        encephalomyelitis A92.31
        neurologic manifestation NEC A92.32
        optic neuritis A92.32
        polyradiculitis A92.32
  Whitmore's — *see* Melioidosis
  Wolhynian A79.0
  worm B83.9
  yellow A95.9
    jungle A95.0
    sylvatic A95.0
    urban A95.1
  Zika virus A92.5
FFA (frontal fibrosing alopecia) L66.12
Fibrillation
  atrial or auricular (established) I48.91
    chronic I48.20
      persistent I48.19
    paroxysmal I48.0
    permanent I48.21
    persistent (chronic) (NOS) (other) I48.19
      longstanding I48.11
  cardiac I49.8
  heart I49.8
  muscular M62.89
  ventricular I49.01
Fibrin
  ball or bodies, pleural (sac) J94.1
  chamber, anterior (eye) (gelatinous exudate) — *see* Iridocyclitis, acute
Fibrinogenolysis — *see* Fibrinolysis
Fibrinogenopenia D68.8
  acquired D65
  congenital D68.2
Fibrinolysis (hemorrhagic) (acquired) D65
  antepartum hemorrhage — *see* Hemorrhage, antepartum, with coagulation defect
  following
    abortion — *see* Abortion by type complicated by hemorrhage
    ectopic or molar pregnancy O08.1
  intrapartum O67.0
  newborn, transient P60
  postpartum O72.3
Fibrinopenia (hereditary) D68.2
  acquired D68.4
Fibrinopurulent — *see* condition

Fibrinous — see condition
Fibro-odontoma, ameloblastic — see Cyst, calcifying odontogenic
Fibro-osteoma — see Neoplasm, bone, benign
Fibroadenoma
 cellular intracanalicular D24.- ☑
  giant D24.- ☑
 intracanalicular
  cellular D24.- ☑
   giant D24.- ☑
  specified site — see Neoplasm, benign, by site
  unspecified site D24.- ☑
 juvenile D24.- ☑
 pericanalicular
  specified site — see Neoplasm, benign, by site
  unspecified site D24.- ☑
 phyllodes D24.- ☑
 prostate D29.1
 specified site NEC — see Neoplasm, benign, by site
 unspecified site D24.- ☑
Fibroadenosis, breast (chronic) (cystic) (diffuse) (periodic) (segmental) N60.2- ☑
Fibroangioma — see also Neoplasm, benign, by site
 juvenile
  specified site — see Neoplasm, benign, by site
  unspecified site D10.6
Fibrochondrosarcoma — see Neoplasm, cartilage, malignant
Fibrocystic
 disease — see also Fibrosis, cystic
  breast — see Mastopathy, cystic
  jaw M27.49
  kidney (congenital) Q61.8
  liver Q44.6
  pancreas E84.9
 kidney (congenital) Q61.8
Fibrodysplasia ossificans progressiva — see Myositis, ossificans, progressiva
Fibroelastosis (cordis) (endocardial) (endomyocardial) I42.4
Fibroid (tumor) — see also Neoplasm, connective tissue, benign
 disease, lung (chronic) — see Fibrosis, lung
 heart (disease) — see Myocarditis
 in pregnancy or childbirth O34.1- ☑
  causing obstructed labor O65.5
 induration, lung (chronic) — see Fibrosis, lung
 lung — see Fibrosis, lung
 pneumonia (chronic) — see Fibrosis, lung
 uterus — see also Leiomyoma, uterus D25.9
Fibrolipoma — see Lipoma
Fibroliposarcoma — see Neoplasm, connective tissue, malignant
Fibroma — see also Neoplasm, connective tissue, benign
 ameloblastic — see Cyst, calcifying odontogenic
 bone (nonossifying) — see Disorder, bone, specified type NEC
  ossifying — see Neoplasm, bone, benign
 cementifying — see Neoplasm, bone, benign
 chondromyxoid — see Neoplasm, bone, benign
 desmoplastic — see Neoplasm, connective tissue, uncertain behavior
 durum — see Neoplasm, connective tissue, benign
 fascial — see Neoplasm, connective tissue, benign
 invasive — see Neoplasm, connective tissue, uncertain behavior
 molle — see Lipoma
 myxoid — see Neoplasm, connective tissue, benign
 nasopharynx, nasopharyngeal (juvenile) D10.6
 nonosteogenic (nonossifying) — see Dysplasia, fibrous
 odontogenic (central) — see Cyst, calcifying odontogenic
 ossifying — see Neoplasm, bone, benign
 periosteal — see Neoplasm, bone, benign
 soft — see Lipoma
Fibromatosis M72.9
 abdominal — see Neoplasm, connective tissue, uncertain behavior
 aggressive D48.11- ☑
 congenital generalized — see Neoplasm, connective tissue, uncertain behavior
 Dupuytren's M72.0
 gingival K06.1
 palmar (fascial) M72.0
 plantar (fascial) M72.2
 pseudosarcomatous (proliferative) (subcutaneous) M72.4
 retroperitoneal D48.3
 specified NEC M72.8
Fibromyalgia M79.7

Fibromyoma — see also Neoplasm, connective tissue, benign
 uterus (corpus) — see also Leiomyoma, uterus
  in pregnancy or childbirth — see Fibroid, in pregnancy or childbirth
   causing obstructed labor O65.5
Fibromyositis M79.7
Fibromyxolipoma D17.9
Fibromyxoma — see Neoplasm, connective tissue, benign
Fibromyxosarcoma — see Neoplasm, connective tissue, malignant
Fibroplasia, retrolental H35.17- ☑
Fibropurulent — see condition
Fibrosarcoma — see also Neoplasm, connective tissue, malignant
 ameloblastic C41.1
  upper jaw (bone) C41.0
 congenital — see Neoplasm, connective tissue, malignant
 fascial — see Neoplasm, connective tissue, malignant
 infantile — see Neoplasm, connective tissue, malignant
 odontogenic C41.1
  upper jaw (bone) C41.0
 periosteal — see Neoplasm, bone, malignant
Fibrosclerosis
 breast N60.3- ☑
 multifocal M35.5
 penis (corpora cavernosa) N48.6
Fibrosis, fibrotic
 adrenal (gland) E27.8
 amnion O41.8X- ☑
 anal papillae K62.89
 arteriocapillary — see Arteriosclerosis
 bladder N32.89
  interstitial — see Cystitis, chronic, interstitial
  localized submucosal — see Cystitis, chronic, interstitial
  panmural — see Cystitis, chronic, interstitial
 breast — see Fibrosclerosis, breast
 capillary — see also Arteriosclerosis I70.90
  lung (chronic) — see Fibrosis, lung
 cardiac — see Myocarditis
 cervix N88.8
 chorion O41.8X- ☑
 corpus cavernosum (sclerosing) N48.6
 cystic (of pancreas) E84.9
  with
   distal intestinal obstruction syndrome E84.19
   fecal impaction E84.19
   intestinal manifestations NEC E84.19
   pulmonary manifestations E84.0
   specified manifestations NEC E84.8
 due to device, implant or graft — see also Complications, by site and type, specified NEC T85.828- ☑
  arterial graft NEC T82.828- ☑
  breast (implant) T85.828- ☑
  catheter NEC T85.828- ☑
   dialysis (renal) T82.828- ☑
    intraperitoneal T85.828- ☑
   infusion NEC T82.828- ☑
    spinal (epidural) (subdural) T85.820- ☑
   urinary (indwelling) T83.82- ☑
  electronic (electrode) (pulse generator) (stimulator)
   bone T84.82- ☑
   cardiac T82.827- ☑
   nervous system (brain) (peripheral nerve) (spinal) T85.820- ☑
   urinary T83.82- ☑
  fixation, internal (orthopedic) NEC T84.82- ☑
  gastrointestinal (bile duct) (esophagus) T85.828- ☑
  genital NEC T83.82- ☑
  heart NEC T82.827- ☑
  joint prosthesis T84.82- ☑
  ocular (corneal graft) (orbital implant) NEC T85.828- ☑
  orthopedic NEC T84.82- ☑
  specified NEC T85.828- ☑
  urinary NEC T83.82- ☑
  vascular NEC T82.828- ☑
  ventricular intracranial shunt T85.820- ☑
 ejaculatory duct N50.89
 endocardium — see Endocarditis
 endomyocardial (tropical) I42.3
 epididymis N50.89
 eye muscle — see Strabismus, mechanical
 heart — see Myocarditis
 hepatic — see Fibrosis, liver
 hepatolienal (portal hypertension) K76.6

Fibrosis, fibrotic — continued
 hepatosplenic (portal hypertension) K76.6
 infrapatellar fat pad M79.4
 intrascrotal N50.89
 kidney N26.9
 liver K74.00
  with sclerosis K74.2
  advanced K74.02
  alcoholic K70.2
  early K74.01
  stage
   F1 or F2 K74.01
   F3 K74.02
 lung (atrophic) (chronic) (confluent) (massive) (perialveolar) (peribronchial) J84.10
  with
   anthracosilicosis J60
   anthracosis J60
   asbestosis J61
   bagassosis J67.1
   bauxite J63.1
   berylliosis J63.2
   byssinosis J66.0
   calcicosis J62.8
   chalicosis J62.8
   dust reticulation J64
   farmer's lung J67.0
   ganister disease J62.8
   graphite J63.3
   pneumoconiosis NOS J64
   siderosis J63.4
   silicosis J62.8
  capillary J84.10
  congenital P27.8
  diffuse (idiopathic) J84.10
   chemicals, gases, fumes or vapors (inhalation) — see also Disease, respiratory, chronic, due to chemicals, gases, fumes or vapors J84.10
   interstitial J84.10
    acute J84.114
   talc J62.0
  following radiation J70.1
  idiopathic J84.112
  postinflammatory J84.10
  silicotic J62.8
  tuberculous — see Tuberculosis, pulmonary
 lymphatic gland I89.8
 median bar — see Hyperplasia, prostate
 mediastinum (idiopathic) J98.59
 meninges G96.198
 myocardium, myocardial — see Myocarditis
 ovary N83.8
 oviduct N83.8
 pancreas K86.89
 penis NEC N48.6
 pericardium I31.0
 perineum, in pregnancy or childbirth O34.7- ☑
  causing obstructed labor O65.5
 pleura J94.1
 popliteal fat pad M79.4
 prostate (chronic) — see Hyperplasia, prostate
 pulmonary — see also Fibrosis, lung J84.10
  congenital P27.8
  idiopathic J84.112
 rectal sphincter K62.89
 retroperitoneal K68.2
  with infection N13.6
  idiopathic (with ureteral obstruction) N13.5
 sclerosing mesenteric (idiopathic) K65.4
 scrotum N50.89
 seminal vesicle N50.89
 senile R54
 skin L90.5
 spermatic cord N50.89
 spleen D73.89
  in schistosomiasis (bilharziasis) B65.9 [D77]
 subepidermal nodular — see Neoplasm, skin, benign
 submucous (oral) (tongue) K13.5
 testis N44.8
  chronic, due to syphilis A52.76
 thymus (gland) E32.8
 tongue, submucous K13.5
 tunica vaginalis N50.89
 uterus (non-neoplastic) N85.8
 vagina N89.8
 valve, heart — see Endocarditis
 vas deferens N50.89
 vein I87.8
Fibrositis (periarticular) M79.7

Fibrositis — continued
  nodular, chronic (Jaccoud's) (rheumatoid) — see Arthropathy, postrheumatic, chronic
Fibrothorax J94.1
Fibrotic — see Fibrosis
Fibrous — see condition
Fibroxanthoma — see also Neoplasm, connective tissue, benign
  atypical — see Neoplasm, connective tissue, uncertain behavior
  malignant — see Neoplasm, connective tissue, malignant
Fibroxanthosarcoma — see Neoplasm, connective tissue, malignant
Fiedler's
  disease (icterohemorrhagic leptospirosis) A27.0
  myocarditis (acute) I40.1
Fifth disease B08.3
  venereal A55
Filaria, filarial, filariasis — see Infestation, filarial
Filatov's disease — see Mononucleosis, infectious
File-cutter's disease — see Poisoning, lead
Filling defect
  biliary tract R93.2
  bladder R93.41
  duodenum R93.3
  gallbladder R93.2
  gastrointestinal tract R93.3
  intestine R93.3
  kidney R93.42- ☑
  stomach R93.3
  ureter R93.41
  urinary organs, specified NEC R93.49
Fimbrial cyst Q50.4
Financial problem affecting care NOS Z59.9
  bankruptcy Z59.868
  foreclosure on loan Z59.89
    home loan Z59.81- ☑
  insecurity Z59.869
    paying for utilities (electricity) (heat) (oil) (water bill) Z59.861
  strain Z59.868
Findings, abnormal, inconclusive, without diagnosis — see also Abnormal
  17-ketosteroids, elevated R82.5
  acetonuria R82.4
  alcohol in blood R78.0
  anisocytosis R71.8
  antenatal screening of mother O28.9
    biochemical O28.1
    chromosomal O28.5
    cytological O28.2
    genetic O28.5
    hematological O28.0
    radiological O28.4
    specified NEC O28.8
    ultrasonic O28.3
  antibody titer, elevated R76.0
  anticardiolipin antibody R76.0
  antiphosphatidylglycerol antibody R76.0
  antiphosphatidylinositol antibody R76.0
  antiphosphatidylserine antibody R76.0
  antiphospholipid antibody R76.0
  bacteriuria R82.71
  bicarbonate E87.8
  bile in urine R82.2
  blood sugar R73.09
    high R73.9
    low (transient) E16.2
  body fluid or substance, specified NEC R88.8
  casts, urine R82.998
  catecholamines R82.5
  cells, urine R82.998
  chloride E87.8
  cholesterol E78.9
    high E78.00
      with high triglycerides E78.2
  chyluria R82.0
  cloudy
    dialysis effluent R88.0
    urine R82.90
  creatinine clearance R94.4
  crystals, urine R82.998
  culture
    blood R78.81
    positive — see Positive, culture
  echocardiogram R93.1
  electrolyte level, urinary R82.998
  function study NEC R94.8
    bladder R94.8

Findings, abnormal, inconclusive, without diagnosis — continued
  function study — continued
    endocrine NEC R94.7
      thyroid R94.6
    kidney R94.4
    liver R94.5
    pancreas R94.8
    placenta R94.8
    pulmonary R94.2
    spleen R94.8
  gallbladder, nonvisualization R93.2
  glucose (tolerance test) (non-fasting) R73.09
  glycosuria R81
  heart
    shadow R93.1
    sounds R01.2
  hematinuria R82.3
  hematocrit drop (precipitous) R71.0
  hemoglobinuria R82.3
  human papillomavirus (HPV) DNA test positive
    cervix
      high risk R87.810
      low risk R87.820
    vagina
      high risk R87.811
      low risk R87.821
  in blood (of substance not normally found in blood) R78.9
    addictive drug NEC R78.4
    alcohol (excessive level) R78.0
    cocaine R78.2
    hallucinogen R78.3
    heavy metals (abnormal level) R78.79
    lead R78.71
    lithium (abnormal level) R78.89
    opiate drug R78.1
    psychotropic drug R78.5
    specified substance NEC R78.89
    steroid agent R78.6
  indoleacetic acid, elevated R82.5
  ketonuria R82.4
  lactic acid dehydrogenase (LDH) R74.02
  liver function test — see also Elevated, liver function, test R79.89
  mammogram NEC R92.8
    calcification (calculus) R92.1
    inconclusive result R92.2
    microcalcification R92.0
  mediastinal shift R93.89
  melanin, urine R82.998
  myoglobinuria R82.1
  neonatal screening — see Abnormal, neonatal screening
  newborn screens, state mandated — see Abnormal, neonatal screening
  nonvisualization of gallbladder R93.2
  odor of urine NOS R82.90
  Papanicolaou cervix R87.619
    non-atypical endometrial cells R87.618
  pneumoencephalogram R93.0
  poikilocytosis R71.8
  potassium (deficiency) E87.6
    excess E87.5
  PPD R76.11
  radiologic (X-ray) R93.89
    abdomen R93.5
    biliary tract R93.2
    breast R92.8
    gastrointestinal tract R93.3
    genitourinary organs R93.89
    head R93.0
    inconclusive due to excess body fat of patient R93.9
    intrathoracic organs NEC R93.1
    musculoskeletal
      limbs R93.6
      other than limb R93.7
    placenta R93.89
    retroperitoneum R93.5
    skin R93.89
    skull R93.0
    subcutaneous tissue R93.89
    testis R93.81- ☑
  red blood cell (count) (morphology) (sickling) (volume) R71.8
  scan NEC R94.8
    bladder R94.8
    bone R94.8
    kidney R94.4
    liver R93.2
    lung R94.2

Findings, abnormal, inconclusive, without diagnosis — continued
  scan — continued
    pancreas R94.8
    placental R94.8
    spleen R94.8
    thyroid R94.6
  sedimentation rate, elevated R70.0
  SGOT R74.01
  SGPT R74.01
  sodium (deficiency) E87.1
    excess E87.0
  specified body fluid NEC R88.8
  stress test R94.39
  testis R93.81- ☑
  thyroid (function) (metabolic rate) (scan) (uptake) R94.6
  transaminase (level) R74.01
  triglycerides E78.9
    high E78.1
      with high cholesterol E78.2
  tuberculin skin test (without active tuberculosis) R76.11
  urine R82.90
    acetone R82.4
    bacteria R82.71
    bile R82.2
    casts or cells R82.998
    chyle R82.0
    culture positive R82.79
    glucose R81
    hemoglobin R82.3
    ketone R82.4
    sugar R81
  vanillylmandelic acid (VMA), elevated R82.5
  vectorcardiogram (VCG) R94.39
  ventriculogram R93.0
  white blood cell (count) (differential) (morphology) D72.9
  xerography R92.8
Finger — see condition
Fire, Saint Anthony's — see Erysipelas
Fire-setting
  pathological (compulsive) F63.1
Fish hook stomach K31.89
Fishmeal-worker's lung J67.8
Fissure, fissured
  anus, anal K60.2
    acute K60.0
    chronic K60.1
    congenital Q43.8
  ear, lobule, congenital Q17.8
  epiglottis (congenital) Q31.8
  larynx J38.7
    congenital Q31.8
  lip K13.0
    congenital — see Cleft, lip
  nipple N64.0
    associated with
      lactation O92.13
      pregnancy O92.11- ☑
      puerperium O92.12
  nose Q30.2
  palate (congenital) — see Cleft, palate
  skin R23.4
  spine (congenital) — see also Spina bifida
    with hydrocephalus — see Spina bifida, by site, with hydrocephalus
  tongue (acquired) K14.5
    congenital Q38.3
Fistula (cutaneous) L98.8
  abdomen (wall) K63.2
    bladder N32.2
    intestine NEC K63.2
    ureter N28.89
    uterus N82.5
  abdominorectal K63.2
  abdominosigmoidal K63.2
  abdominothoracic J86.0
  abdominouterine N82.5
    congenital Q51.7
  abdominovesical N32.2
  accessory sinuses — see Sinusitis
  actinomycotic — see Actinomycosis
  alveolar antrum — see Sinusitis, maxillary
  alveolar process K04.6
  anorectal (infectional) K60.50
    complex K60.529
      chronic K60.522
      initial K60.521
      new K60.521
      occurring following complete healing K60.523

Fistula — *continued*
- anorectal — *continued*
  - complex — *continued*
    - persistent K60.522
    - recurrent K60.523
  - extrasphincteric K60.52- ☑
  - high intersphincteric K60.52- ☑
  - low intersphincteric K60.51- ☑
  - simple K60.519
    - chronic K60.512
    - initial K60.511
    - new K60.511
    - occurring following complete healing K60.513
    - persistent K60.512
    - recurrent K60.513
  - superficial K60.51- ☑
  - suprasphincteric K60.52- ☑
  - transsphincteric K60.52- ☑
- antrobuccal — *see* Sinusitis, maxillary
- antrum — *see* Sinusitis, maxillary
- anus, anal (recurrent) (infectional) K60.30
  - complex K60.329
    - chronic K60.322
    - initial K60.321
    - new K60.321
    - occurring following complete healing K60.323
    - persistent K60.322
    - recurrent K60.323
  - congenital Q43.6
    - with absence, atresia and stenosis Q42.2
  - extrasphincteric K60.32- ☑
  - high intersphincteric K60.32- ☑
  - low intersphincteric K60.31- ☑
  - simple K60.319
    - chronic K60.312
    - initial K60.311
    - new K60.311
    - occurring following complete healing K60.313
    - persistent K60.312
    - recurrent K60.313
  - superficial K60.31- ☑
  - suprasphincteric K60.32- ☑
  - transsphincteric K60.32- ☑
  - tuberculous A18.32
- aorta-duodenal I77.2
- appendix, appendicular K38.3
- arteriovenous (acquired) (nonruptured) I77.0
  - brain I67.1
    - congenital Q28.2
      - ruptured — *see* Fistula, arteriovenous, brain, ruptured
    - ruptured I60.8
      - intracerebral I61.8
      - intraparenchymal I61.8
      - intraventricular I61.5
      - subarachnoid I60.8
  - cerebral — *see* Fistula, arteriovenous, brain
  - congenital (peripheral) — *see also* Malformation, arteriovenous
    - brain Q28.2
      - ruptured — *see* Fistula, arteriovenous, brain, ruptured
    - coronary Q24.5
    - pulmonary Q25.72
  - coronary I25.41
    - congenital Q24.5
  - pulmonary I28.0
    - congenital Q25.72
  - surgically created (for dialysis) Z99.2
    - complication — *see* Complication, arteriovenous, fistula, surgically created
  - traumatic — *see* Injury, blood vessel
- artery I77.2
- aural (mastoid) — *see* Mastoiditis, chronic
- auricle — *see also* Disorder, pinna, specified type NEC
  - congenital Q18.1
- Bartholin's gland N82.8
- bile duct (common) (hepatic) K83.3
  - with calculus, stones — *see also* Calculus, bile duct K83.3
- biliary (tract) — *see* Fistula, bile duct
- bladder (sphincter) NEC — *see also* Fistula, vesico- N32.2
  - into seminal vesicle N32.2
- bone — *see also* Disorder, bone, specified type NEC
  - with osteomyelitis, chronic — *see* Osteomyelitis, chronic, with draining sinus
- brain G93.89

Fistula — *continued*
- brain — *continued*
  - arteriovenous (acquired) — *see also* Fistula, arteriovenous, brain I67.1
    - congenital Q28.2
- branchial (cleft) Q18.0
- branchiogenous Q18.0
- breast N61.0
  - puerperal, postpartum or gestational, due to mastitis (purulent) — *see* Mastitis, obstetric, purulent
- bronchial J86.0
- bronchocutaneous, bronchomediastinal, bronchopleural, bronchopleuromediastinal (infective) J86.0
  - tuberculous NEC A15.5
- bronchoesophageal J86.0
  - congenital Q39.2
    - with atresia of esophagus Q39.1
- bronchovisceral J86.0
- buccal cavity (infective) K12.2
- cecosigmoidal K63.2
- cecum K63.2
- cerebrospinal (fluid) G96.08
- cervical, lateral Q18.1
- cervicoaural Q18.1
- cervicosigmoidal N82.4
- cervicovesical N82.1
- cervix N82.8
- chest (wall) J86.0
- cholecystenteric — *see* Fistula, gallbladder
- cholecystocolic — *see* Fistula, gallbladder
- cholecystocolonic — *see* Fistula, gallbladder
- cholecystoduodenal — *see* Fistula, gallbladder
- cholecystogastric — *see* Fistula, gallbladder
- cholecystointestinal — *see* Fistula, gallbladder
- choledochoduodenal — *see* Fistula, bile duct
- cholocolic K82.3
- coccyx — *see* Sinus, pilonidal
- colon K63.2
- colostomy K94.09
- colovesical N32.1
- common duct — *see* Fistula, bile duct
- congenital, site not listed — *see* Anomaly, by site
- coronary, arteriovenous I25.41
  - congenital Q24.5
- costal region J86.0
- cul-de-sac, Douglas' N82.8
- cystic duct — *see also* Fistula, gallbladder
  - congenital Q44.5
- dental K04.6
- diaphragm J86.0
- duodenum K31.6
- ear (external) (canal) — *see* Disorder, ear, external, specified type NEC
- enterocolic K63.2
- enterocutaneous K63.2
- enterouterine N82.4
  - congenital Q51.7
- enterovaginal N82.4
  - congenital Q52.2
  - large intestine N82.3
  - small intestine N82.2
- enterovesical N32.1
- epididymis N50.89
  - tuberculous A18.15
- esophagobronchial J86.0
  - congenital Q39.2
    - with atresia of esophagus Q39.1
- esophagocutaneous K22.89
- esophagopleural-cutaneous J86.0
- esophagotracheal J86.0
  - congenital Q39.2
    - with atresia of esophagus Q39.1
- esophagus K22.89
  - congenital Q39.2
    - with atresia of esophagus Q39.1
- ethmoid — *see* Sinusitis, ethmoidal
- eyeball (cornea) (sclera) — *see* Disorder, globe, hypotony
- eyelid H01.8- ☑
- fallopian tube, external N82.5
- fecal K63.2
  - congenital Q43.6
- from periapical abscess K04.6
- frontal sinus — *see* Sinusitis, frontal
- gallbladder K82.3
  - with calculus, cholelithiasis, stones — *see* Calculus, gallbladder
- gastric K31.6
- gastrocolic K31.6
  - congenital Q40.2

Fistula — *continued*
- gastrocolic — *continued*
  - tuberculous A18.32
- gastroenterocolic K31.6
- gastroesophageal K31.6
- gastrojejunal K31.6
- gastrojejunocolic K31.6
- genital tract (female) N82.9
  - specified NEC N82.8
  - to intestine NEC N82.4
  - to skin N82.5
- hepatic artery-portal vein, congenital Q26.6
- hepatopleural J86.0
- hepatopulmonary J86.0
- ileorectal or ileosigmoidal K63.2
- ileovaginal N82.2
- ileovesical N32.1
- ileum K63.2
- in ano K60.30
  - tuberculous A18.32
- inner ear (labyrinth) — *see* subcategory H83.1- ☑
- intestine NEC K63.2
- intestinocolonic (abdominal) K63.2
- intestinoureteral N28.89
- intestinouterine N82.4
- intestinovaginal N82.4
  - large intestine N82.3
  - small intestine N82.2
- intestinovesical N32.1
- ischiorectal (fossa) K61.39
- jejunum K63.2
- joint M25.10
  - ankle M25.17- ☑
  - elbow M25.12- ☑
  - foot joint M25.17- ☑
  - hand joint M25.14- ☑
  - hip M25.15- ☑
  - knee M25.16- ☑
  - shoulder M25.11- ☑
  - specified joint NEC M25.18
  - tuberculous — *see* Tuberculosis, joint
  - vertebrae M25.18
  - wrist M25.13- ☑
- kidney N28.89
- labium (majus) (minus) N82.8
- labyrinth — *see* subcategory H83.1- ☑
- lacrimal (gland) (sac) H04.61- ☑
- lacrimonasal duct — *see* Fistula, lacrimal
- laryngotracheal, congenital Q34.8
- larynx J38.7
- lip K13.0
  - congenital Q38.0
- lumbar, tuberculous A18.01
- lung J86.0
- lymphatic I89.8
- mammary (gland) N61.0
- mastoid (process) (region) — *see* Mastoiditis, chronic
- maxillary J32.0
- medial, face and neck Q18.8
- mediastinal J86.0
- mediastinobronchial J86.0
- mediastinocutaneous J86.0
- middle ear — *see* subcategory H74.8- ☑
- mouth K12.2
- nasal J34.89
  - sinus — *see* Sinusitis
- nasopharynx J39.2
- nipple N64.0
- nose J34.89
- oral (cutaneous) K12.2
  - maxillary J32.0
  - nasal (with cleft palate) — *see* Cleft, palate
- orbit, orbital — *see* Disorder, orbit, specified type NEC
- oroantral J32.0
- oviduct, external N82.5
- palate (hard) M27.8
- pancreatic K86.89
- pancreaticoduodenal K86.89
- parotid (gland) K11.4
  - region K12.2
- penis N48.89
- perianal K60.30
- pericardium (pleura) (sac) — *see* Pericarditis
- pericecal K63.2
- perineorectal K60.40
- perineosigmoidal K63.2
- perineum, perineal (with urethral involvement) NEC N36.0

Fistula — *continued*
  perineum, perineal — *continued*
    tuberculous A18.13
    ureter N28.89
  perirectal K60.40
    tuberculous A18.32
  peritoneum K65.9
  pharyngoesophageal J39.2
  pharynx J39.2
    branchial cleft (congenital) Q18.0
  pilonidal (infected) (rectum) — *see* Sinus, pilonidal
  pleura, pleural, pleurocutaneous, pleuroperitoneal J86.0
    tuberculous NEC A15.6
  pleuropericardial I31.8
  portal vein-hepatic artery, congenital Q26.6
  postauricular H70.81- ☑
  postoperative, persistent T81.83- ☑
    specified site — *see* Fistula, by site
  preauricular (congenital) Q18.1
  prostate N42.89
  pulmonary J86.0
    arteriovenous I28.0
      congenital Q25.72
    tuberculous — *see* Tuberculosis, pulmonary
  pulmonoperitoneal J86.0
  rectal (infectional) K60.40
    complex K60.429
      chronic K60.422
      initial K60.421
      new K60.421
      occurring following complete healing K60.423
      persistent K60.422
      recurrent K60.423
    extrasphincteric K60.42- ☑
    high intersphincteric K60.42- ☑
    low intersphincteric K60.41- ☑
    simple K60.419
      chronic K60.412
      initial K60.411
      new K60.411
      occurring following complete healing K60.413
      persistent K60.412
      recurrent K60.413
    superficial K60.41- ☑
    suprasphincteric K60.42- ☑
    transsphincteric K60.42- ☑
  rectolabial N82.4
  rectosigmoid (intercommunicating) K63.2
  rectoureteral N28.89
  rectourethral N36.0
    congenital Q64.73
  rectouterine N82.4
    congenital Q51.7
  rectovaginal N82.3
    congenital Q52.2
    tuberculous A18.18
  rectovesical N32.1
    congenital Q64.79
  rectovesicovaginal N82.3
  rectovulval N82.4
    congenital Q52.79
  rectum (to skin) K60.40
    congenital Q43.6
      with absence, atresia and stenosis Q42.0
    tuberculous A18.32
  renal N28.89
  retroauricular — *see* Fistula, postauricular
  salivary duct or gland (any) K11.4
    congenital Q38.4
  scrotum (urinary) N50.89
    tuberculous A18.15
  semicircular canals — *see* subcategory H83.1- ☑
  sigmoid K63.2
    to bladder N32.1
  sinus — *see* Sinusitis
  skin L98.8
    to genital tract (female) N82.5
  splenocolic D73.89
  stercoral K63.2
  stomach K31.6
  sublingual gland K11.4
  submandibular gland K11.4
  submaxillary (gland) K11.4
    region K12.2
  thoracic J86.0
    duct I89.8
  thoracoabdominal J86.0
  thoracogastric J86.0

Fistula — *continued*
  thoracointestinal J86.0
  thorax J86.0
  thyroglossal duct Q89.2
  thyroid E07.89
  trachea, congenital (external) (internal) Q32.1
  tracheoesophageal J86.0
    congenital Q39.2
      with atresia of esophagus Q39.1
    following tracheostomy J95.04
  traumatic arteriovenous — *see* Injury, blood vessel, by site
  tuberculous — *code by* site under Tuberculosis
  typhoid A01.09
  umbilicourinary Q64.8
  urachus, congenital Q64.4
  ureter (persistent) N28.89
  ureteroabdominal N28.89
  ureterorectal N28.89
  ureterosigmoido-abdominal N28.89
  ureterovaginal N82.1
  ureterovesical N32.2
  urethra N36.0
    congenital Q64.79
    tuberculous A18.13
  urethroperineal N36.0
  urethroperineovesical N32.2
  urethrorectal N36.0
    congenital Q64.73
  urethroscrotal N50.89
  urethrovaginal N82.1
  urethrovesical N32.2
  urinary (tract) (persistent) (recurrent) N36.0
  uteroabdominal N82.5
    congenital Q51.7
  uteroenteric, uterointestinal N82.4
    congenital Q51.7
  uterorectal N82.4
    congenital Q51.7
  uteroureteric N82.1
  uterourethral Q51.7
  uterovaginal N82.8
  uterovesical N82.1
    congenital Q51.7
  uterus N82.8
  vagina (postpartal) (wall) N82.8
  vaginocutaneous (postpartal) N82.5
  vaginointestinal NEC N82.4
    large intestine N82.3
    small intestine N82.2
  vaginoperineal N82.5
  vasocutaneous, congenital Q55.7
  vesical NEC N32.2
  vesicoabdominal N32.2
  vesicocervicovaginal N82.1
  vesicocolic N32.1
  vesicocutaneous N32.2
  vesicoenteric N32.1
  vesicointestinal N32.1
  vesicometrorectal N82.4
  vesicoperineal N32.2
  vesicorectal N32.1
    congenital Q64.79
  vesicosigmoidal N32.1
  vesicosigmoidovaginal N82.3
  vesicoureteral N32.2
  vesicoureterovaginal N82.1
  vesicourethral N32.2
  vesicourethrorectal N32.1
  vesicouterine N82.1
    congenital Q51.7
  vesicovaginal N82.0
  vulvorectal N82.4
    congenital Q52.79
Fit R56.9
  epileptic — *see* Epilepsy
  fainting R55
  hysterical F44.5
  newborn P90
Fitting (and adjustment) (of)
  artificial
    arm — *see* Admission, adjustment, artificial, arm
    breast Z44.3- ☑
    eye Z44.2- ☑
    leg — *see* Admission, adjustment, artificial, leg
  automatic implantable cardiac defibrillator (with synchronous cardiac pacemaker) Z45.02
  brain neuropacemaker Z46.2
    implanted Z45.42

Fitting — *continued*
  cardiac defibrillator — *see* Fitting (and adjustment) (of), automatic implantable cardiac defibrillator
  catheter, non-vascular Z46.82
  colostomy belt Z46.89
  contact lenses Z46.0
  CRT-D (resynchronization therapy defibrillator) Z45.02
  CRT-P (cardiac resynchronization therapy pacemaker) Z45.018
    pulse generator Z45.010
  cystostomy device Z46.6
  defibrillator, cardiac — *see* Fitting (and adjustment) (of), automatic implantable cardiac defibrillator
  dentures Z46.3
  device NOS Z46.9
    abdominal Z46.89
    gastrointestinal NEC Z46.59
    implanted NEC Z45.89
    nervous system Z46.2
      implanted — *see* Admission, adjustment, device, implanted, nervous system
    orthodontic Z46.4
    orthoptic Z46.0
    orthotic Z46.89
    prosthetic (external) Z44.9
      breast Z44.3- ☑
      dental Z46.3
      eye Z44.2- ☑
      specified NEC Z44.8
    specified NEC Z46.89
    substitution
      auditory Z46.2
        implanted — *see* Admission, adjustment, device, implanted, hearing device
      nervous system Z46.2
        implanted — *see* Admission, adjustment, device, implanted, nervous system
      visual Z46.2
        implanted Z45.31
    urinary Z46.6
  gastric lap band Z46.51
  gastrointestinal appliance NEC Z46.59
  glasses (reading) Z46.0
  hearing aid Z46.1
  ileostomy device Z46.89
  insulin pump Z46.81
  intestinal appliance NEC Z46.89
  myringotomy device (stent) (tube) Z45.82
  neuropacemaker Z46.2
    implanted Z45.42
  non-vascular catheter Z46.82
  orthodontic device Z46.4
  orthopedic device (brace) (cast) (corset) (shoes) Z46.89
  pacemaker (cardiac) (cardiac resynchronization therapy (CRT-P)) Z45.018
    nervous system (brain) (peripheral nerve) (spinal cord) Z46.2
      implanted Z45.42
    pulse generator Z45.010
  portacath (port-a-cath) Z45.2
  prosthesis (external) Z44.9
    arm — *see* Admission, adjustment, artificial, arm
    breast Z44.3- ☑
    dental Z46.3
    eye Z44.2- ☑
    leg — *see* Admission, adjustment, artificial, leg
    specified NEC Z44.8
  spectacles Z46.0
  wheelchair Z46.89
Fitzhugh-Curtis syndrome
  due to
    Chlamydia trachomatis A74.81
    Neisseria gonorrhea (gonococcal peritonitis) A54.85
Fitz's syndrome (acute hemorrhagic pancreatitis) — *see also* Pancreatitis, acute K85.80
Fixation
  joint — *see* Ankylosis
  larynx J38.7
  stapes — *see* Ankylosis, ear ossicles
    deafness — *see* Deafness, conductive
  uterus (acquired) — *see* Malposition, uterus
  vocal cord J38.3
Flabby ridge K06.8
Flaccid — *see also* condition
  palate, congenital Q38.5
Flail
  chest S22.5- ☑

Flail — *continued*
  chest — *continued*
    associated with chest compression and cardiopulmonary resuscitation M96.A4
    newborn (birth injury) P13.8
  joint (paralytic) M25.20
    ankle M25.27- ☑
    elbow M25.22- ☑
    foot joint M25.27- ☑
    hand joint M25.24- ☑
    hip M25.25- ☑
    knee M25.26- ☑
    shoulder M25.21- ☑
    specified joint NEC M25.28
    wrist M25.23- ☑
Flajani's disease — *see* Hyperthyroidism, with, goiter (diffuse)
Flap, liver K71.3
Flashbacks (residual to hallucinogen use) F16.283
Flat
  affect R45.89
  chamber (eye) — *see* Disorder, globe, hypotony, flat anterior chamber
  chest, congenital Q67.8
  foot (acquired) (fixed type) (painful) (postural) — *see also* Deformity, limb, flat foot
    congenital (rigid) (spastic) (everted)) Q66.5- ☑
    rachitic sequelae (late effect) E64.3
  organ or site, congenital NEC — *see* Anomaly, by site
  pelvis M95.5
    with disproportion (fetopelvic) O33.0
      causing obstructed labor O65.0
    congenital Q74.2
Flatau-Schilder disease G37.0
Flatback syndrome M40.30
  lumbar region M40.36
  lumbosacral region M40.37
  thoracolumbar region M40.35
Flattening
  head, femur M89.8X5
  hip — *see* Coxa, plana
  lip (congenital) Q18.8
  nose (congenital) Q67.4
    acquired M95.0
Flatulence R14.3
  psychogenic F45.8
Flatus R14.3
  vaginalis N89.8
Flax-dresser's disease J66.1
Flea bite — *see* Injury, bite, by site, superficial, insect
Flecks, glaucomatous (subcapsular) — *see* Cataract, complicated
Fleischer (-Kayser) **ring** (cornea) H18.04- ☑
Fleshy mole O02.0
Flexibilitas cerea — *see* Catalepsy
Flexion
  amputation stump (surgical) T87.89
  cervix — *see* Malposition, uterus
  contracture, joint — *see* Contraction, joint
  deformity, joint — *see also* Deformity, limb, flexion M21.20
    hip, congenital Q65.89
  uterus — *see also* Malposition, uterus
    lateral — *see* Lateroversion, uterus
Flexner-Boyd dysentery A03.2
Flexner's dysentery A03.1
Flexure — *see* Flexion
Flint murmur (aortic insufficiency) I35.1
Floater, vitreous — *see* Opacity, vitreous
Floating
  cartilage (joint) — *see also* Loose, body, joint
    knee — *see* Derangement, knee, loose body
  gallbladder, congenital Q44.1
  kidney N28.89
    congenital Q63.8
  spleen D73.89
Flooding N92.0
Floor — *see* condition
Floppy
  baby syndrome (nonspecific) P94.2
  iris syndrome (intraoperative) (IFIS) H21.81
  nonrheumatic mitral valve syndrome I34.1
Flu — *see also* Influenza
  avian — *see also* Influenza, due to, identified novel influenza A virus J09.X2
  bird — *see also* Influenza, due to, identified novel influenza A virus J09.X2
  intestinal NEC A08.4

Flu — *continued*
  swine (viruses that normally cause infections in pigs) — *see also* Influenza, due to, identified novel influenza A virus J09.X2
Fluctuating blood pressure I99.8
Fluid
  abdomen R18.8
  chest J94.8
  heart — *see* Failure, heart, congestive
  joint — *see* Effusion, joint
  loss (acute) E86.9
  lung — *see* Edema, lung
  overload E87.70
    specified NEC E87.79
  peritoneal cavity R18.8
  pleural cavity J94.8
  retention R60.9
Flukes NEC — *see also* Infestation, fluke
  blood NEC — *see* Schistosomiasis
  liver B66.3
Fluor (vaginalis) N89.8
  trichomonal or due to Trichomonas (vaginalis) A59.00
Fluorosis
  dental K00.3
  skeletal M85.10
    ankle M85.17- ☑
    foot M85.17- ☑
    forearm M85.13- ☑
    hand M85.14- ☑
    lower leg M85.16- ☑
    multiple site M85.19
    neck M85.18
    rib M85.18
    shoulder M85.11- ☑
    skull M85.18
    specified site NEC M85.18
    thigh M85.15- ☑
    toe M85.17- ☑
    upper arm M85.12- ☑
    vertebra M85.18
Flush syndrome E34.09
Flushing R23.2
  menopausal N95.1
Flutter
  atrial or auricular I48.92
    atypical I48.4
    type I I48.3
    type II I48.4
    typical I48.3
  heart I49.8
    atrial or auricular I48.92
      atypical I48.4
      type I I48.3
      type II I48.4
      typical I48.3
    ventricular I49.02
  ventricular I49.02
FNHTR (febrile nonhemolytic transfusion reaction) R50.84
Fochier's abscess — *code by* site under Abscess
Focus, Assmann's — *see* Tuberculosis, pulmonary
Fogo selvagem L10.3
Foix-Alajouanine syndrome G95.19
Fold, folds (anomalous) — *see also* Anomaly, by site
  Descemet's membrane — *see* Change, corneal membrane, Descemet's, fold
  epicanthic Q10.3
  heart Q24.8
Folie a deux F24
Follicle
  cervix (nabothian) (ruptured) N88.8
  graafian, ruptured, with hemorrhage N83.0- ☑
  nabothian N88.8
Follicular — *see* condition
Folliculitis (superficial) L73.9
  abscedens et suffodiens L66.3
  cyst N83.0- ☑
  decalvans L66.2
  deep — *see* Furuncle, by site
  gonococcal (acute) (chronic) A54.01
  keloid, keloidalis L73.0
  pustular L01.02
  ulerythematosa reticulata L66.4
Folliculome lipidique
  specified site — *see* Neoplasm, benign, by site
  unspecified site
    female D27.9
    male D29.20
Følling's disease E70.0

Follow-up — *see* Examination, follow-up
Fong's syndrome (hereditary osteo-onychodysplasia) Q87.2
Food
  allergy L27.2
  asphyxia (from aspiration or inhalation) — *see* Foreign body, by site
  choked on — *see* Foreign body, by site
  deprivation T73.0- ☑
    specified kind of food NEC E63.8
  insecurity Z59.41
  intoxication — *see* Poisoning, food
  lack of T73.0- ☑
  poisoning — *see* Poisoning, food
  rejection NEC — *see* Disorder, eating
  strangulation or suffocation — *see* Foreign body, by site
  toxemia — *see* Poisoning, food
Foot — *see* condition
Foramen ovale (nonclosure) (patent) (persistent) Q21.12
Forbes' glycogen storage disease E74.03
Fordyce-Fox disease L75.2
Fordyce's disease (mouth) Q38.6
Forearm — *see* condition
Foreclosure on loan Z59.89
Foreign body
  with
    laceration — *see* Laceration, by site, with foreign body
    puncture wound — *see* Puncture, by site, with foreign body
  accidentally left following a procedure T81.509- ☑
  aspiration T81.506- ☑
    resulting in
      adhesions T81.516- ☑
      obstruction T81.526- ☑
      perforation T81.536- ☑
      specified complication NEC T81.596- ☑
  cardiac catheterization T81.505- ☑
    resulting in
      acute reaction T81.60- ☑
        aseptic peritonitis T81.61- ☑
        specified NEC T81.69- ☑
      adhesions T81.515- ☑
      obstruction T81.525- ☑
      perforation T81.535- ☑
      specified complication NEC T81.595- ☑
  causing
    acute reaction T81.60- ☑
      aseptic peritonitis T81.61- ☑
      specified complication NEC T81.69- ☑
    adhesions T81.519- ☑
    aseptic peritonitis T81.61- ☑
    obstruction T81.529- ☑
    perforation T81.539- ☑
    specified complication NEC T81.599- ☑
  endoscopy T81.504- ☑
    resulting in
      adhesions T81.514- ☑
      obstruction T81.524- ☑
      perforation T81.534- ☑
      specified complication NEC T81.594- ☑
  immunization T81.503- ☑
    resulting in
      adhesions T81.513- ☑
      obstruction T81.523- ☑
      perforation T81.533- ☑
      specified complication NEC T81.593- ☑
  infusion T81.501- ☑
    resulting in
      adhesions T81.511- ☑
      obstruction T81.521- ☑
      perforation T81.531- ☑
      specified complication NEC T81.591- ☑
  injection T81.503- ☑
    resulting in
      adhesions T81.513- ☑
      obstruction T81.523- ☑
      perforation T81.533- ☑
      specified complication NEC T81.593- ☑
  kidney dialysis T81.502- ☑
    resulting in
      adhesions T81.512- ☑
      obstruction T81.522- ☑
      perforation T81.532- ☑
      specified complication NEC T81.592- ☑
  packing removal T81.507- ☑
    resulting in
      acute reaction T81.60- ☑

Foreign body — continued
  accidentally left following a procedure — continued
    packing removal — continued
      resulting in — continued
        acute reaction — continued
          aseptic peritonitis T81.61- ☑
          specified NEC T81.69- ☑
        adhesions T81.517- ☑
        obstruction T81.527- ☑
        perforation T81.537- ☑
        specified complication NEC T81.597- ☑
      puncture T81.506- ☑
        resulting in
          adhesions T81.516- ☑
          obstruction T81.526- ☑
          perforation T81.536- ☑
          specified complication NEC T81.596- ☑
      specified procedure NEC T81.508- ☑
        resulting in
          acute reaction T81.60- ☑
            aseptic peritonitis T81.61- ☑
            specified NEC T81.69- ☑
          adhesions T81.518- ☑
          obstruction T81.528- ☑
          perforation T81.538- ☑
          specified complication NEC T81.598- ☑
      surgical operation T81.500- ☑
        resulting in
          acute reaction T81.60- ☑
            aseptic peritonitis T81.61- ☑
            specified NEC T81.69- ☑
          adhesions T81.510- ☑
          obstruction T81.520- ☑
          perforation T81.530- ☑
          specified complication NEC T81.590- ☑
      transfusion T81.501- ☑
        resulting in
          adhesions T81.511- ☑
          obstruction T81.521- ☑
          perforation T81.531- ☑
          specified complication NEC T81.591- ☑
  alimentary tract T18.9- ☑
    anus T18.5- ☑
    colon T18.4- ☑
    esophagus — see Foreign body, esophagus
    mouth T18.0- ☑
    multiple sites T18.8- ☑
    rectosigmoid (junction) T18.5- ☑
    rectum T18.5- ☑
    small intestine T18.3- ☑
    specified site NEC T18.8- ☑
    stomach T18.2- ☑
  anterior chamber (eye) S05.5- ☑
  auditory canal — see Foreign body, entering through orifice, ear
  bronchus T17.508- ☑
    causing
      asphyxiation T17.500- ☑
        food (bone) (seed) T17.520- ☑
        gastric contents (vomitus) T17.510- ☑
        specified type NEC T17.590- ☑
      injury NEC T17.508- ☑
        food (bone) (seed) T17.528- ☑
        gastric contents (vomitus) T17.518- ☑
        specified type NEC T17.598- ☑
  canthus — see Foreign body, conjunctival sac
  ciliary body (eye) S05.5- ☑
  conjunctival sac T15.1- ☑
  cornea T15.0- ☑
  entering through orifice
    accessory sinus T17.0- ☑
    alimentary canal T18.9- ☑
      multiple parts T18.8- ☑
      specified part NEC T18.8- ☑
    alveolar process T18.0- ☑
    antrum (Highmore's) T17.0- ☑
    anus T18.5- ☑
    appendix T18.4- ☑
    auditory canal — see Foreign body, entering through orifice, ear
    auricle — see Foreign body, entering through orifice, ear
    bladder T19.1- ☑
    bronchioles — see Foreign body, respiratory tract, specified site NEC
    bronchus (main) — see Foreign body, bronchus

Foreign body — continued
  entering through orifice — continued
    buccal cavity T18.0- ☑
    canthus (inner) — see Foreign body, conjunctival sac
    cecum T18.4- ☑
    cervix (canal) (uteri) T19.3- ☑
    colon T18.4- ☑
    conjunctival sac — see Foreign body, conjunctival sac
    cornea — see Foreign body, cornea
    digestive organ or tract NOS T18.9- ☑
      multiple parts T18.8- ☑
      specified part NEC T18.8- ☑
    duodenum T18.3- ☑
    ear (external) T16.- ☑
    esophagus — see Foreign body, esophagus
    eye (external) NOS T15.9- ☑
      conjunctival sac — see Foreign body, conjunctival sac
      cornea — see Foreign body, cornea
      specified part NEC T15.8- ☑
    eyeball — see also Foreign body, entering through orifice, eye, specified part NEC
      with penetrating wound — see Puncture, eyeball
    eyelid — see also Foreign body, conjunctival sac
      with
        laceration — see Laceration, eyelid, with foreign body
        puncture — see Puncture, eyelid, with foreign body
        superficial injury — see Foreign body, superficial, eyelid
    gastrointestinal tract T18.9- ☑
      multiple parts T18.8- ☑
      specified part NEC T18.8- ☑
    genitourinary tract T19.9- ☑
      multiple parts T19.8- ☑
      specified part NEC T19.8- ☑
    globe — see Foreign body, entering through orifice, eyeball
    gum T18.0- ☑
    Highmore's antrum T17.0- ☑
    hypopharynx — see Foreign body, pharynx
    ileum T18.3- ☑
    intestine (small) T18.3- ☑
      large T18.4- ☑
    lacrimal apparatus (punctum) — see Foreign body, entering through orifice, eye, specified part NEC
    large intestine T18.4- ☑
    larynx — see Foreign body, larynx
    lung — see Foreign body, respiratory tract, specified site NEC
    maxillary sinus T17.0- ☑
    mouth T18.0- ☑
    nasal sinus T17.0- ☑
    nasopharynx — see Foreign body, pharynx
    nose (passage) T17.1- ☑
    nostril T17.1- ☑
    oral cavity T18.0- ☑
    palate T18.0- ☑
    penis T19.4- ☑
    pharynx — see Foreign body, pharynx
    piriform sinus — see Foreign body, pharynx
    rectosigmoid (junction) T18.5- ☑
    rectum T18.5- ☑
    respiratory tract — see Foreign body, respiratory tract
    sinus (accessory) (frontal) (maxillary) (nasal) T17.0- ☑
      piriform — see Foreign body, pharynx
    small intestine T18.3- ☑
    stomach T18.2- ☑
    suffocation by — see Foreign body, by site
    tear ducts or glands — see Foreign body, entering through orifice, eye, specified part NEC
    throat — see Foreign body, pharynx
    tongue T18.0- ☑
    tonsil, tonsillar (fossa) — see Foreign body, pharynx
    trachea — see Foreign body, trachea
    ureter T19.8- ☑
    urethra T19.0- ☑
    uterus (any part) T19.3- ☑
    vagina T19.2- ☑
    vulva T19.2- ☑
  esophagus T18.108- ☑
    causing
      injury NEC T18.108- ☑
        food (bone) (seed) T18.128- ☑
        gastric contents (vomitus) T18.118- ☑

Foreign body — continued
  esophagus — continued
    causing — continued
      injury — continued
        specified type NEC T18.198- ☑
      tracheal compression T18.100- ☑
        food (bone) (seed) T18.120- ☑
        gastric contents (vomitus) T18.110- ☑
        specified type NEC T18.190- ☑
  feeling of, in throat R09.89
  fragment — see Retained, foreign body fragments (type of)
  genitourinary tract T19.9- ☑
    bladder T19.1- ☑
    multiple parts T19.8- ☑
    penis T19.4- ☑
    specified site NEC T19.8- ☑
    urethra T19.0- ☑
    uterus T19.3- ☑
      IUD Z97.5
    vagina T19.2- ☑
      contraceptive device Z97.5
    vulva T19.2- ☑
  granuloma (old) (soft tissue) — see also Granuloma, foreign body
    skin L92.3
  in
    laceration — see Laceration, by site, with foreign body
    puncture wound — see Puncture, by site, with foreign body
    soft tissue (residual) M79.5
  inadvertently left in operation wound — see Foreign body, accidentally left during a procedure
  ingestion, ingested NOS T18.9- ☑
  inhalation or inspiration — see Foreign body, by site
  internal organ, not entering through a natural orifice — code as specific injury with foreign body
  intraocular S05.5- ☑
    old, retained (nonmagnetic) H44.70- ☑
      anterior chamber H44.71- ☑
      ciliary body H44.72- ☑
      iris H44.72- ☑
      lens H44.73- ☑
      magnetic H44.60- ☑
        anterior chamber H44.61- ☑
        ciliary body H44.62- ☑
        iris H44.62- ☑
        lens H44.63- ☑
        posterior wall H44.64- ☑
        specified site NEC H44.69- ☑
        vitreous body H44.65- ☑
      posterior wall H44.74- ☑
      specified site NEC H44.79- ☑
      vitreous body H44.75- ☑
  iris — see Foreign body, intraocular
  lacrimal punctum — see Foreign body, entering through orifice, eye, specified part NEC
  larynx T17.308- ☑
    causing
      asphyxiation T17.300- ☑
        food (bone) (seed) T17.320- ☑
        gastric contents (vomitus) T17.310- ☑
        specified type NEC T17.390- ☑
      injury NEC T17.308- ☑
        food (bone) (seed) T17.328- ☑
        gastric contents (vomitus) T17.318- ☑
        specified type NEC T17.398- ☑
  lens — see Foreign body, intraocular
  ocular muscle S05.4- ☑
    old, retained — see Foreign body, orbit, old
  old or residual
    soft tissue (residual) M79.5
  operation wound, left accidentally — see Foreign body, accidentally left during a procedure
  orbit S05.4- ☑
    old, retained H05.5- ☑
  pharynx T17.208- ☑
    causing
      asphyxiation T17.200- ☑
        food (bone) (seed) T17.220- ☑
        gastric contents (vomitus) T17.210- ☑
        specified type NEC T17.290- ☑
      injury NEC T17.208- ☑
        food (bone) (seed) T17.228- ☑
        gastric contents (vomitus) T17.218- ☑
        specified type NEC T17.298- ☑

☑ Additional Character Required — Refer to the Tabular List for Character Selection

Foreign body — *continued*
respiratory tract T17.908- ☑
  bronchioles — *see* Foreign body, respiratory tract, specified site NEC
  bronchus — *see* Foreign body, bronchus
  causing
    asphyxiation T17.900- ☑
      food (bone) (seed) T17.920- ☑
      gastric contents (vomitus) T17.910- ☑
      specified type NEC T17.990- ☑
    injury NEC T17.908- ☑
      food (bone) (seed) T17.928- ☑
      gastric contents (vomitus) T17.918- ☑
      specified type NEC T17.998- ☑
  larynx — *see* Foreign body, larynx
  lung — *see* Foreign body, respiratory tract, specified site NEC
  multiple parts — *see* Foreign body, respiratory tract, specified site NEC
  nasal sinus T17.0- ☑
  nasopharynx — *see* Foreign body, pharynx
  nose T17.1- ☑
  nostril T17.1- ☑
  pharynx — *see* Foreign body, pharynx
  specified site NEC T17.808- ☑
    causing
      asphyxiation T17.800- ☑
        food (bone) (seed) T17.820- ☑
        gastric contents (vomitus) T17.810- ☑
        specified type NEC T17.890- ☑
      injury NEC T17.808- ☑
        food (bone) (seed) T17.828- ☑
        gastric contents (vomitus) T17.818- ☑
        specified type NEC T17.898- ☑
  throat — *see* Foreign body, pharynx
  trachea — *see* Foreign body, trachea
retained (old) (nonmagnetic) (in)
  anterior chamber (eye) — *see* Foreign body, intraocular, old, retained, anterior chamber
    magnetic — *see* Foreign body, intraocular, old, retained, magnetic, anterior chamber
  ciliary body — *see* Foreign body, intraocular, old, retained, ciliary body
    magnetic — *see* Foreign body, intraocular, old, retained, magnetic, ciliary body
  eyelid H02.819
    left H02.816
      lower H02.815
      upper H02.814
    right H02.813
      lower H02.812
      upper H02.811
  fragments — *see* Retained, foreign body fragments (type of)
  globe — *see* Foreign body, intraocular, old, retained
    magnetic — *see* Foreign body, intraocular, old, retained, magnetic
  intraocular — *see* Foreign body, intraocular, old, retained
    magnetic — *see* Foreign body, intraocular, old, retained, magnetic
  iris — *see* Foreign body, intraocular, old, retained, iris
    magnetic — *see* Foreign body, intraocular, old, retained, magnetic, iris
  lens — *see* Foreign body, intraocular, old, retained, lens
    magnetic — *see* Foreign body, intraocular, old, retained, magnetic, lens
  muscle — *see* Foreign body, retained, soft tissue
  orbit — *see* Foreign body, orbit, old
  posterior wall of globe — *see* Foreign body, intraocular, old, retained, posterior wall
    magnetic — *see* Foreign body, intraocular, old, retained, magnetic, posterior wall
  retrobulbar — *see* Foreign body, orbit, old, retrobulbar
  soft tissue M79.5
  vitreous — *see* Foreign body, intraocular, old, retained, vitreous body
    magnetic — *see* Foreign body, intraocular, old, retained, magnetic, vitreous body
  retina S05.5- ☑
sensation — *see* Sensation, foreign body
superficial, without open wound
  abdomen, abdominal (wall) S30.851- ☑
  alveolar process S00.552- ☑
  ankle S90.55- ☑

Foreign body — *continued*
superficial, without open wound — *continued*
  antecubital space — *see* Foreign body, superficial, forearm
  anus S30.857- ☑
  arm (upper) S40.85- ☑
    auditory canal — *see* Foreign body, superficial, ear
    auricle — *see* Foreign body, superficial, ear
    axilla — *see* Foreign body, superficial, arm
  back, lower S30.850- ☑
  breast S20.15- ☑
  brow S00.85- ☑
  buttock S30.850- ☑
  calf — *see* Foreign body, superficial, leg
  canthus — *see* Foreign body, superficial, eyelid
  cheek S00.85- ☑
    internal S00.552- ☑
  chest wall — *see* Foreign body, superficial, thorax
  chin S00.85- ☑
  clitoris S30.854- ☑
  costal region — *see* Foreign body, superficial, thorax
  digit(s)
    foot — *see* Foreign body, superficial, toe
    hand — *see* Foreign body, superficial, finger
  ear S00.45- ☑
  elbow S50.35- ☑
  epididymis S30.853- ☑
  epigastric region S30.851- ☑
  epiglottis S10.15- ☑
  esophagus, cervical S10.15- ☑
  eyebrow — *see* Foreign body, superficial, eyelid
  eyelid S00.25- ☑
  face S00.85- ☑
  finger(s) S60.459- ☑
    index S60.45- ☑
    little S60.45- ☑
    middle S60.45- ☑
    ring S60.45- ☑
  flank S30.85A- ☑
  foot (except toe(s) alone) S90.85- ☑
    toe — *see* Foreign body, superficial, toe
  forearm S50.85- ☑
    elbow only — *see* Foreign body, superficial, elbow
  forehead S00.85- ☑
  genital organs, external
    female S30.856- ☑
    male S30.855- ☑
  groin S30.851- ☑
  gum S00.552- ☑
  hand S60.55- ☑
  head S00.95- ☑
    ear — *see* Foreign body, superficial, ear
    eyelid — *see* Foreign body, superficial, eyelid
    lip S00.551- ☑
    nose S00.35- ☑
    oral cavity S00.552- ☑
    scalp S00.05- ☑
    specified site NEC S00.85- ☑
  heel — *see* Foreign body, superficial, foot
  hip S70.25- ☑
  inguinal region S30.851- ☑
  interscapular region S20.459- ☑
  jaw S00.85- ☑
  knee S80.25- ☑
  labium (majus) (minus) S30.854- ☑
  larynx S10.15- ☑
  leg (lower) S80.85- ☑
    knee — *see* Foreign body, superficial, knee
    upper — *see* Foreign body, superficial, thigh
  lip S00.551- ☑
  lower back S30.850- ☑
  lumbar region S30.850- ☑
  malar region S00.85- ☑
  mammary — *see* Foreign body, superficial, breast
  mastoid region S00.85- ☑
  mouth S00.552- ☑
  nail
    finger — *see* Foreign body, superficial, finger
    toe — *see* Foreign body, superficial, toe
  nape S10.85- ☑
  nasal S00.35- ☑
  neck S10.95- ☑
    specified site NEC S10.85- ☑
    throat S10.15- ☑
  nose S00.35- ☑
  occipital region S00.05- ☑

Foreign body — *continued*
superficial, without open wound — *continued*
  oral cavity S00.552- ☑
  orbital region — *see* Foreign body, superficial, eyelid
  palate S00.552- ☑
  palm — *see* Foreign body, superficial, hand
  parietal region S00.05- ☑
  pelvis S30.850- ☑
  penis S30.852- ☑
  perineum
    female S30.854- ☑
    male S30.850- ☑
  periocular area — *see* Foreign body, superficial, eyelid
  phalanges
    finger — *see* Foreign body, superficial, finger
    toe — *see* Foreign body, superficial, toe
  pharynx S10.15- ☑
  pinna — *see* Foreign body, superficial, ear
  popliteal space — *see* Foreign body, superficial, knee
  prepuce S30.852- ☑
  pubic region S30.850- ☑
  pudendum
    female S30.856- ☑
    male S30.855- ☑
  sacral region S30.850- ☑
  scalp S00.05- ☑
  scapular region — *see* Foreign body, superficial, shoulder
  scrotum S30.853- ☑
  shin — *see* Foreign body, superficial, leg
  shoulder S40.25- ☑
  sternal region S20.359- ☑
  submaxillary region S00.85- ☑
  submental region S00.85- ☑
  subungual
    finger(s) — *see* Foreign body, superficial, finger
    toe(s) — *see* Foreign body, superficial, toe
  supraclavicular fossa S10.85- ☑
  supraorbital S00.85- ☑
  temple S00.85- ☑
  temporal region S00.85- ☑
  testis S30.853- ☑
  thigh S70.35- ☑
  thorax, thoracic (wall) S20.95- ☑
    back S20.45- ☑
    front S20.35- ☑
  throat S10.15- ☑
  thumb S60.35- ☑
  toe(s) (lesser) S90.456- ☑
    great S90.45- ☑
  tongue S00.552- ☑
  trachea S10.15- ☑
  tunica vaginalis S30.853- ☑
  tympanum, tympanic membrane — *see* Foreign body, superficial, ear
  uvula S00.552- ☑
  vagina S30.854- ☑
  vocal cords S10.15- ☑
  vulva S30.854- ☑
  wrist S60.85- ☑
swallowed T18.9- ☑
trachea T17.408- ☑
  causing
    asphyxiation T17.400- ☑
      food (bone) (seed) T17.420- ☑
      gastric contents (vomitus) T17.410- ☑
      specified type NEC T17.490- ☑
    injury NEC T17.408- ☑
      food (bone) (seed) T17.428- ☑
      gastric contents (vomitus) T17.418- ☑
      specified type NEC T17.498- ☑
type of fragment — *see* Retained, foreign body fragments (type of)
vitreous (humor) S05.5- ☑

Forestier's disease (rhizomelic pseudopolyarthritis) M35.3
  meaning ankylosing hyperostosis — *see* Hyperostosis, ankylosing

Formation
  hyalin in cornea — *see* Degeneration, cornea
  sequestrum in bone (due to infection) — *see* Osteomyelitis, chronic
  valve
    colon, congenital Q43.8
    ureter (congenital) Q62.39

Formication R20.2
Fort Bragg fever A27.89

Fossa — see also condition
 pyriform — see condition
Foster-Kennedy syndrome H47.14- ☑
Fothergill's
 disease (trigeminal neuralgia) — see also Neuralgia, trigeminal
  scarlatina anginosa A38.9
Foul breath R19.6
Foundling Z76.1
Fournier disease or gangrene N49.3
 female N76.82
 vagina and vulva N76.82
Fourth
 cranial nerve — see condition
 molar K00.1
Foville's (peduncular) **disease or syndrome** G46.3
Fox (-Fordyce) disease (apocrine miliaria) L75.2
FPIES (food protein-induced enterocolitis syndrome) K52.21
Fracture, burst — see Fracture, traumatic, by site
Fracture, chronic — see Fracture, pathological, by site
Fracture, insufficiency — see Fracture, pathological, by site
Fracture, nontraumatic, NEC
 atypical
  femur M84.750-
   complete
    oblique M84.759- ☑
     left side M84.758- ☑
     right side M84.757- ☑
    transverse M84.756- ☑
     left side M84.755- ☑
     right side M84.754- ☑
   incomplete M84.753- ☑
    left side M84.752- ☑
    right side M84.751- ☑
Fracture, pathological (pathologic) — see also Fracture, traumatic M84.40- ☑
 ankle M84.47- ☑
 carpus M84.44- ☑
 clavicle M84.41- ☑
 compression (not due to trauma) — see also Collapse, vertebra M48.50- ☑
 dental implant M27.63
 dental restorative material K08.539
  with loss of material K08.531
  without loss of material K08.530
 due to
  neoplastic disease NEC — see also Neoplasm M84.50- ☑
   ankle M84.57- ☑
   carpus M84.54- ☑
   clavicle M84.51- ☑
   femur M84.55- ☑
   fibula M84.56- ☑
   finger M84.54- ☑
   hip M84.559- ☑
   humerus M84.52- ☑
   ilium M84.550- ☑
   ischium M84.550- ☑
   metacarpus M84.54- ☑
   metatarsus M84.57- ☑
   neck M84.58- ☑
   pelvis M84.550- ☑
   radius M84.53- ☑
   rib M84.58- ☑
   scapula M84.51- ☑
   skull M84.58- ☑
   specified site NEC M84.58- ☑
   tarsus M84.57- ☑
   tibia M84.56- ☑
   toe M84.57- ☑
   ulna M84.53- ☑
   vertebra M84.58- ☑
  osteoporosis M80.00- ☑
   disuse — see Osteoporosis, specified type NEC, with pathological fracture
   drug-induced — see Osteoporosis, drug induced, with pathological fracture
   idiopathic — see Osteoporosis, specified type NEC, with pathological fracture
   postmenopausal — see Osteoporosis, postmenopausal, with pathological fracture
   postoophorectomy — see Osteoporosis, postoophorectomy, with pathological fracture

Fracture, pathological — continued
 due to — continued
  osteoporosis — continued
   postsurgical malabsorption — see Osteoporosis, specified type NEC, with pathological fracture
   specified cause NEC — see Osteoporosis, specified type NEC, with pathological fracture
  specified disease NEC M84.60- ☑
   ankle M84.67- ☑
   carpus M84.64- ☑
   clavicle M84.61- ☑
   femur M84.65- ☑
   fibula M84.66- ☑
   finger M84.64- ☑
   hip M84.65- ☑
   humerus M84.62- ☑
   ilium M84.650- ☑
   ischium M84.650- ☑
   metacarpus M84.64- ☑
   metatarsus M84.67- ☑
   neck M84.68- ☑
   radius M84.63- ☑
   rib M84.68- ☑
   scapula M84.61- ☑
   skull M84.68- ☑
   tarsus M84.67- ☑
   tibia M84.66- ☑
   toe M84.67- ☑
   ulna M84.63- ☑
   vertebra M84.68- ☑
 femur M84.45- ☑
 fibula M84.46- ☑
 finger M84.44- ☑
 hip M84.459- ☑
 humerus M84.42- ☑
 ilium M84.454- ☑
 ischium M84.454- ☑
 joint prosthesis — see Complications, joint prosthesis, mechanical, breakdown, by site
  periprosthetic — see Fracture, pathological, periprosthetic
 metacarpus M84.44- ☑
 metatarsus M84.47- ☑
 neck M84.48- ☑
 pelvis M84.454- ☑
 periprosthetic M97.9- ☑
  ankle M97.2- ☑
  elbow M97.4- ☑
  finger M97.8- ☑
  hip M97.0- ☑
  knee M97.1- ☑
  other specified joint M97.8- ☑
  shoulder M97.3- ☑
  spinal joint M97.8- ☑
  toe joint M97.8- ☑
  wrist joint M97.8- ☑
 radius M84.43- ☑
 restorative material (dental) K08.539
  with loss of material K08.531
  without loss of material K08.530
 rib M84.48- ☑
 scapula M84.41- ☑
 skull M84.48- ☑
 tarsus M84.47- ☑
 tibia M84.46- ☑
 toe M84.47- ☑
 ulna M84.43- ☑
 vertebra M84.48- ☑
Fracture, traumatic (abduction) (adduction) (separation) — see also Fracture, pathological T14.8- ☑
 acetabulum S32.40- ☑
  column
   anterior (displaced) (iliopubic) S32.43- ☑
    nondisplaced S32.436- ☑
   posterior (displaced) (ilioischial) S32.443- ☑
    nondisplaced S32.44- ☑
  dome (displaced) S32.48- ☑
   nondisplaced S32.48- ☑
  specified NEC S32.49- ☑
  transverse (displaced) S32.45- ☑
   with associated posterior wall fracture (displaced) S32.46- ☑
    nondisplaced S32.46- ☑
   nondisplaced S32.45- ☑

Fracture, traumatic — continued
 acetabulum — continued
  wall
   anterior (displaced) S32.41- ☑
    nondisplaced S32.41- ☑
   medial (displaced) S32.47- ☑
    nondisplaced S32.47- ☑
   posterior (displaced) S32.42- ☑
    with associated transverse fracture (displaced) S32.46- ☑
     nondisplaced S32.46- ☑
    nondisplaced S32.42- ☑
 acromion — see Fracture, scapula, acromial process
 ankle S82.899- ☑
  bimalleolar (displaced) S82.84- ☑
   nondisplaced S82.84- ☑
  lateral malleolus only (displaced) S82.6- ☑
   nondisplaced S82.6- ☑
  medial malleolus (displaced) S82.5- ☑
   associated with Maisonneuve's fracture — see Fracture, Maisonneuve's
   nondisplaced S82.5- ☑
  talus — see Fracture, tarsal, talus
  trimalleolar (displaced) S82.85- ☑
   nondisplaced S82.85- ☑
 arm (upper) — see also Fracture, humerus, shaft
  humerus — see Fracture, humerus
  radius — see Fracture, radius
  ulna — see Fracture, ulna
 associated with chest compression and cardiopulmonary resuscitation M96.A9
 astragalus — see Fracture, tarsal, talus
 atlas — see Fracture, neck, cervical vertebra, first
 axis — see Fracture, neck, cervical vertebra, second
 back — see Fracture, vertebra
 Barton's — see Barton's fracture
 base of skull — see Fracture, skull, base
 basicervical (basal) (femoral) S72.04- ☑
 Bennett's — see Bennett's fracture
 bimalleolar — see Fracture, ankle, bimalleolar
 blow-out S02.3- ☑
 bone NEC T14.8- ☑
  birth injury P13.9
  following insertion of orthopedic implant, joint prosthesis or bone plate — see Fracture, following insertion of orthopedic implant, joint prosthesis or bone plate
  in (due to) neoplastic disease NEC — see Fracture, pathological, due to, neoplastic disease
  pathological (cause unknown) — see Fracture, pathological
 breast bone — see Fracture, sternum
 bucket handle (semilunar cartilage) — see Tear, meniscus
 buckle — see Fracture, by site, torus
 burst — see Fracture, traumatic, by site
 calcaneus — see Fracture, tarsal, calcaneus
 carpal bone(s) S62.10- ☑
  capitate (displaced) S62.13- ☑
   nondisplaced S62.13- ☑
  cuneiform — see Fracture, carpal bone, triquetrum
  hamate (body) (displaced) S62.143- ☑
   hook process (displaced) S62.15- ☑
    nondisplaced S62.15- ☑
   nondisplaced S62.14- ☑
  larger multangular — see Fracture, carpal bones, trapezium
  lunate (displaced) S62.12- ☑
   nondisplaced S62.12- ☑
  navicular S62.00- ☑
   distal pole (displaced) S62.01- ☑
    nondisplaced S62.01- ☑
   middle third (displaced) S62.02- ☑
    nondisplaced S62.02- ☑
   proximal third (displaced) S62.03- ☑
    nondisplaced S62.03- ☑
   volar tuberosity — see Fracture, carpal bones, navicular, distal pole
  os magnum — see Fracture, carpal bones, capitate
  pisiform (displaced) S62.16- ☑
   nondisplaced S62.16- ☑
  semilunar — see Fracture, carpal bones, lunate
  smaller multangular — see Fracture, carpal bones, trapezoid
  trapezium (displaced) S62.17- ☑
   nondisplaced S62.17- ☑
  trapezoid (displaced) S62.18- ☑
   nondisplaced S62.18- ☑

Fracture, traumatic — *continued*
- carpal bone(s) — *continued*
  - triquetrum (displaced) S62.11- ☑
    - nondisplaced S62.11- ☑
  - unciform — *see* Fracture, carpal bones, hamate
- cervical — *see* Fracture, vertebra, cervical
- clavicle S42.00- ☑
  - acromial end (displaced) S42.03- ☑
    - nondisplaced S42.03- ☑
  - birth injury P13.4
  - lateral end — *see* Fracture, clavicle, acromial end
  - shaft (displaced) S42.02- ☑
    - nondisplaced S42.02- ☑
  - sternal end (anterior) (displaced) S42.01- ☑
    - nondisplaced S42.01- ☑
    - posterior S42.01- ☑
- coccyx S32.2- ☑
- collapsed — *see* Collapse, vertebra
- collar bone — *see* Fracture, clavicle
- Colles' — *see* Colles' fracture
- coronoid process — *see* Fracture, ulna, upper end, coronoid process
- corpus cavernosum penis S39.840- ☑
- costochondral cartilage S23.41- ☑
- costochondral, costosternal junction — *see* Fracture, rib
- cranium — *see* Fracture, skull
- cricoid cartilage S12.8- ☑
- cuboid (ankle) — *see* Fracture, tarsal, cuboid
- cuneiform
  - foot — *see* Fracture, tarsal, cuneiform
  - wrist — *see* Fracture, carpal, triquetrum
- delayed union — *see* Delay, union, fracture
- dental restorative material K08.539
  - with loss of material K08.531
  - without loss of material K08.530
- due to
  - birth injury — *see* Birth, injury, fracture
  - osteoporosis — *see* Osteoporosis, with fracture
- Dupuytren's — *see* Fracture, ankle, lateral malleolus
- elbow S42.40- ☑
- ethmoid (bone) (sinus) — *see* Fracture, skull, base
- face bone S02.92- ☑
- fatigue — *see also* Fracture, stress
  - vertebra M48.40- ☑
    - cervical region M48.42- ☑
    - cervicothoracic region M48.43- ☑
    - lumbar region M48.46- ☑
    - lumbosacral region M48.47- ☑
    - occipito-atlanto-axial region M48.41- ☑
    - sacrococcygeal region M48.48- ☑
    - thoracic region M48.44- ☑
    - thoracolumbar region M48.45- ☑
- femur, femoral S72.9- ☑
  - basicervical (basal) S72.04- ☑
  - birth injury P13.2
  - capital epiphyseal S79.01- ☑
  - condyles, epicondyles — *see* Fracture, femur, lower end
  - distal end — *see* Fracture, femur, lower end
  - epiphysis
    - head — *see* Fracture, femur, upper end, epiphysis
    - lower — *see* Fracture, femur, lower end, epiphysis
    - upper — *see* Fracture, femur, upper end, epiphysis
  - following insertion of implant, prosthesis or plate M96.66- ☑
  - head — *see* Fracture, femur, upper end, head
  - intertrochanteric — *see* Fracture, femur, trochanteric
  - intratrochanteric — *see* Fracture, femur, trochanteric
  - lower end S72.40- ☑
    - condyle (displaced) S72.41- ☑
      - lateral (displaced) S72.42- ☑
        - nondisplaced S72.42- ☑
      - medial (displaced) S72.43- ☑
        - nondisplaced S72.43- ☑
      - nondisplaced S72.41- ☑
    - epiphysis (displaced) S72.44- ☑
      - nondisplaced S72.44- ☑
    - physeal S79.10- ☑
      - Salter-Harris
        - Type I S79.11- ☑
        - Type II S79.12- ☑
        - Type III S79.13- ☑
        - Type IV S79.14- ☑
        - specified NEC S79.19- ☑
    - specified NEC S72.49- ☑
    - supracondylar (displaced) S72.45- ☑

Fracture, traumatic — *continued*
- femur, femoral — *continued*
  - lower end — *continued*
    - supracondylar — *continued*
      - with intracondylar extension (displaced) S72.46- ☑
        - nondisplaced S72.46- ☑
      - nondisplaced S72.45- ☑
    - torus S72.47- ☑
  - neck — *see* Fracture, femur, upper end, neck
  - pertrochanteric — *see* Fracture, femur, trochanteric
  - shaft (lower third) (middle third) (upper third) S72.30- ☑
    - comminuted (displaced) S72.35- ☑
      - nondisplaced S72.35- ☑
    - oblique (displaced) S72.33- ☑
      - nondisplaced S72.33- ☑
    - segmental (displaced) S72.36- ☑
      - nondisplaced S72.36- ☑
    - specified NEC S72.39- ☑
    - spiral (displaced) S72.34- ☑
      - nondisplaced S72.34- ☑
    - transverse (displaced) S72.32- ☑
      - nondisplaced S72.32- ☑
  - specified site NEC — *see* subcategory S72.8- ☑
  - subcapital (displaced) S72.01- ☑
  - subtrochanteric (region) (section) (displaced) S72.2- ☑
    - nondisplaced S72.2- ☑
  - transcervical — *see* Fracture, femur, midcervical
  - transtrochanteric — *see* Fracture, femur, trochanteric
  - trochanteric S72.10- ☑
    - apophyseal (displaced) S72.13- ☑
      - nondisplaced S72.13- ☑
    - greater trochanter (displaced) S72.11- ☑
      - nondisplaced S72.11- ☑
    - intertrochanteric (displaced) S72.14- ☑
      - nondisplaced S72.14- ☑
    - lesser trochanter (displaced) S72.12- ☑
      - nondisplaced S72.12- ☑
  - upper end S72.00- ☑
    - apophyseal (displaced) S72.13- ☑
      - nondisplaced S72.13- ☑
    - cervicotrochanteric — *see* Fracture, femur, upper end, neck, base
    - epiphysis (displaced) S72.02- ☑
      - nondisplaced S72.02- ☑
    - head S72.05- ☑
      - articular (displaced) S72.06- ☑
        - nondisplaced S72.06- ☑
      - specified NEC S72.09- ☑
    - intertrochanteric (displaced) S72.14- ☑
      - nondisplaced S72.14- ☑
    - intracapsular S72.01- ☑
    - midcervical (displaced) S72.03- ☑
      - nondisplaced S72.03- ☑
    - neck S72.00- ☑
      - base (displaced) S72.04- ☑
        - nondisplaced S72.04- ☑
      - specified NEC S72.09- ☑
    - pertrochanteric — *see* Fracture, femur, upper end, trochanteric
    - physeal S79.00- ☑
      - Salter-Harris type I S79.01- ☑
      - specified NEC S79.09- ☑
    - subcapital (displaced) S72.01- ☑
    - subtrochanteric (displaced) S72.2- ☑
      - nondisplaced S72.2- ☑
    - transcervical — *see* Fracture, femur, upper end, midcervical
    - trochanteric S72.10- ☑
      - greater (displaced) S72.11- ☑
        - nondisplaced S72.11- ☑
      - lesser (displaced) S72.12- ☑
        - nondisplaced S72.12- ☑
- fibula (shaft) (styloid) S82.40- ☑
  - comminuted (displaced) S82.45- ☑
    - nondisplaced S82.45- ☑
  - following insertion of implant, prosthesis or plate M96.67- ☑
  - involving ankle or malleolus — *see* Fracture, fibula, lateral malleolus
  - lateral malleolus (displaced) S82.6- ☑
    - nondisplaced S82.6- ☑
  - lower end
    - physeal S89.30- ☑

Fracture, traumatic — *continued*
- fibula — *continued*
  - lower end — *continued*
    - physeal — *continued*
      - Salter-Harris
        - Type I S89.31- ☑
        - Type II S89.32- ☑
        - specified NEC S89.39- ☑
      - specified NEC S82.83- ☑
    - torus S82.82- ☑
  - oblique (displaced) S82.43- ☑
    - nondisplaced S82.43- ☑
  - segmental (displaced) S82.46- ☑
    - nondisplaced S82.46- ☑
  - specified NEC S82.49- ☑
  - spiral (displaced) S82.44- ☑
    - nondisplaced S82.44- ☑
  - transverse (displaced) S82.42- ☑
    - nondisplaced S82.42- ☑
  - upper end
    - physeal S89.20- ☑
      - Salter-Harris
        - Type I S89.21- ☑
        - Type II S89.22- ☑
      - specified NEC S89.29- ☑
    - specified NEC S82.83- ☑
    - torus S82.81- ☑
- finger (except thumb) S62.60- ☑
  - distal phalanx (displaced) S62.63- ☑
    - nondisplaced S62.66- ☑
  - index S62.60- ☑
    - distal phalanx (displaced) S62.63- ☑
      - nondisplaced S62.66- ☑
    - middle phalanx (displaced) S62.62- ☑
      - nondisplaced S62.65- ☑
    - proximal phalanx (displaced) S62.61- ☑
      - nondisplaced S62.64- ☑
  - little S62.60- ☑
    - distal phalanx (displaced) S62.63- ☑
      - nondisplaced S62.66- ☑
    - middle phalanx (displaced) S62.62- ☑
      - nondisplaced S62.65- ☑
    - proximal phalanx (displaced) S62.61- ☑
      - nondisplaced S62.64- ☑
  - middle S62.60- ☑
    - distal phalanx (displaced) S62.63- ☑
      - nondisplaced S62.66- ☑
    - middle phalanx (displaced) S62.62- ☑
      - nondisplaced S62.65- ☑
    - proximal phalanx (displaced) S62.61- ☑
      - nondisplaced S62.64- ☑
  - ring S62.60- ☑
    - distal phalanx (displaced) S62.63- ☑
      - nondisplaced S62.66- ☑
    - middle phalanx (displaced) S62.62- ☑
      - nondisplaced S62.65- ☑
    - proximal phalanx (displaced) S62.61- ☑
      - nondisplaced S62.64- ☑
  - thumb — *see* Fracture, thumb
- following insertion (intraoperative) (postoperative) of orthopedic implant, joint prosthesis or bone plate M96.69
  - femur M96.66- ☑
  - fibula M96.67- ☑
  - humerus M96.62- ☑
  - pelvis M96.65
  - radius M96.63- ☑
  - specified bone NEC M96.69
  - tibia M96.67- ☑
  - ulna M96.63- ☑
- foot S92.90- ☑
  - astragalus — *see* Fracture, tarsal, talus
  - calcaneus — *see* Fracture, tarsal, calcaneus
  - cuboid — *see* Fracture, tarsal, cuboid
  - cuneiform — *see* Fracture, tarsal, cuneiform
  - metatarsal — *see* Fracture, metatarsal
  - navicular — *see* Fracture, tarsal, navicular
  - sesamoid S92.81- ☑
  - specified NEC S92.81- ☑
  - talus — *see* Fracture, tarsal, talus
  - tarsal — *see* Fracture, tarsal
  - toe — *see* Fracture, toe

☑ **Additional Character Required** — Refer to the Tabular List for Character Selection

Fracture, traumatic — continued
- forearm S52.9- ☑
  - radius — see Fracture, radius
  - ulna — see Fracture, ulna
- fossa (anterior) (middle) (posterior) S02.19- ☑
- fragility — see Fracture, pathological, due to osteoporosis
- frontal (bone) (skull) S02.0- ☑
  - sinus S02.19- ☑
- glenoid (cavity) (scapula) — see Fracture, scapula, glenoid cavity
- greenstick — see Fracture, by site
- hallux — see Fracture, toe, great
- hand S62.9- ☑
  - carpal — see Fracture, carpal bone
  - finger (except thumb) — see Fracture, finger
  - metacarpal — see Fracture, metacarpal
  - navicular (scaphoid) (hand) — see Fracture, carpal bone, navicular
  - thumb — see Fracture, thumb
- healed or old
  - with complications — code by Nature of the complication
- heel bone — see Fracture, tarsal, calcaneus
- Hill-Sachs S42.29- ☑
- hip — see Fracture, femur, neck
- humerus S42.30- ☑
  - anatomical neck — see Fracture, humerus, upper end
  - articular process — see Fracture, humerus, lower end
  - capitellum — see Fracture, humerus, lower end, condyle, lateral
  - distal end — see Fracture, humerus, lower end
  - epiphysis
    - lower — see Fracture, humerus, lower end, physeal
    - upper — see Fracture, humerus, upper end, physeal
  - external condyle — see Fracture, humerus, lower end, condyle, lateral
  - following insertion of implant, prosthesis or plate M96.62-
  - great tuberosity — see Fracture, humerus, upper end, greater tuberosity
  - intercondylar — see Fracture, humerus, lower end
  - internal epicondyle — see Fracture, humerus, lower end, epicondyle, medial
  - lesser tuberosity — see Fracture, humerus, upper end, lesser tuberosity
  - lower end S42.40- ☑
    - condyle
      - lateral (displaced) S42.45- ☑
        - nondisplaced S42.45- ☑
      - medial (displaced) S42.46- ☑
        - nondisplaced S42.46- ☑
    - epicondyle
      - lateral (displaced) S42.43- ☑
        - nondisplaced S42.43- ☑
      - medial (displaced) S42.44- ☑
        - incarcerated S42.44- ☑
        - nondisplaced S42.44- ☑
    - physeal S49.10- ☑
      - Salter-Harris
        - Type I S49.11- ☑
        - Type II S49.12- ☑
        - Type III S49.13- ☑
        - Type IV S49.14- ☑
      - specified NEC S49.19- ☑
    - specified NEC (displaced) S42.49- ☑
      - nondisplaced S42.49- ☑
    - supracondylar (simple) (displaced) S42.41- ☑
      - with intercondylar fracture — see Fracture, humerus, lower end
      - comminuted (displaced) S42.42- ☑
        - nondisplaced S42.42- ☑
      - nondisplaced S42.41- ☑
    - torus S42.48- ☑
    - transcondylar (displaced) S42.47- ☑
      - nondisplaced S42.47- ☑
  - proximal end — see Fracture, humerus, upper end
  - shaft S42.30- ☑
    - comminuted (displaced) S42.35- ☑
      - nondisplaced S42.35- ☑
    - greenstick S42.31- ☑
    - oblique (displaced) S42.33- ☑
      - nondisplaced S42.33- ☑
    - segmental (displaced) S42.36- ☑
      - nondisplaced S42.36- ☑
    - specified NEC S42.39- ☑
    - spiral (displaced) S42.34- ☑

Fracture, traumatic — continued
- humerus — continued
  - shaft — continued
    - spiral — continued
      - nondisplaced S42.34- ☑
    - transverse (displaced) S42.32- ☑
      - nondisplaced S42.32- ☑
  - supracondylar — see Fracture, humerus, lower end
  - surgical neck — see Fracture, humerus, upper end, surgical neck
  - trochlea — see Fracture, humerus, lower end, condyle, medial
  - tuberosity — see Fracture, humerus, upper end
  - upper end S42.20- ☑
    - anatomical neck — see Fracture, humerus, upper end, specified NEC
    - articular head — see Fracture, humerus, upper end, specified NEC
    - epiphysis — see Fracture, humerus, upper end, physeal
    - greater tuberosity (displaced) S42.25- ☑
      - nondisplaced S42.25- ☑
    - lesser tuberosity (displaced) S42.26- ☑
      - nondisplaced S42.26- ☑
    - physeal S49.00- ☑
      - Salter-Harris
        - Type I S49.01- ☑
        - Type II S49.02- ☑
        - Type III S49.03- ☑
        - Type IV S49.04- ☑
      - specified NEC S49.09- ☑
    - specified NEC (displaced) S42.29- ☑
      - nondisplaced S42.29- ☑
    - surgical neck (displaced) S42.21- ☑
      - four-part S42.24- ☑
      - nondisplaced S42.21- ☑
      - three-part S42.23- ☑
      - two-part (displaced) S42.22- ☑
        - nondisplaced S42.22- ☑
    - torus S42.27- ☑
    - transepiphyseal — see Fracture, humerus, upper end, physeal
- hyoid bone S12.8- ☑
- ilium S32.30- ☑
  - with disruption of pelvic ring — see Disruption, pelvic ring
  - avulsion (displaced) S32.31- ☑
    - nondisplaced S32.31- ☑
  - specified NEC S32.39- ☑
- impaction, impacted — code as Fracture, by site
- innominate bone — see Fracture, ilium
- instep — see Fracture, foot
- ischium S32.60- ☑
  - with disruption of pelvic ring — see Disruption, pelvic ring
  - avulsion (displaced) S32.61- ☑
    - nondisplaced S32.61- ☑
  - specified NEC S32.69- ☑
- jaw (bone) (lower) — see Fracture, mandible
  - upper — see Fracture, maxilla
- joint prosthesis — see Complications, joint prosthesis, mechanical, breakdown, by site
  - periprosthetic — see Fracture, traumatic, periprosthetic
- knee cap — see Fracture, patella
- larynx S12.8- ☑
- late effects — see Sequelae, fracture
- leg (lower) S82.9- ☑
  - ankle — see Fracture, ankle
  - femur — see Fracture, femur
  - fibula — see Fracture, fibula
  - malleolus — see Fracture, ankle
  - patella — see Fracture, patella
  - specified site NEC S82.89- ☑
  - tibia — see Fracture, tibia
- lumbar spine — see Fracture, vertebra, lumbar
- lumbosacral spine S32.9- ☑
- Maisonneuve's (displaced) S82.86- ☑
  - nondisplaced S82.86- ☑
- malar bone — see also Fracture, maxilla S02.400- ☑
  - left side S02.40B- ☑
  - right side S02.40A- ☑
- malleolus — see Fracture, ankle
- malunion — see Fracture, by site
- mandible (lower jaw (bone)) S02.609- ☑
  - alveolus S02.67- ☑
  - angle (of jaw) S02.65- ☑

Fracture, traumatic — continued
- mandible — continued
  - body, unspecified S02.600- ☑
    - left side S02.602- ☑
    - right side S02.601- ☑
  - condylar process S02.61- ☑
  - coronoid process S02.63- ☑
  - ramus, unspecified S02.64- ☑
  - specified site S02.69- ☑
  - subcondylar process S02.62- ☑
  - symphysis S02.66- ☑
- manubrium (sterni) S22.21- ☑
  - dissociation from sternum S22.23- ☑
- march — see Fracture, traumatic, stress, by site
- maxilla, maxillary (bone) (sinus) (superior) (upper jaw) S02.401- ☑
  - alveolus S02.42- ☑
  - inferior — see Fracture, mandible
  - LeFort I S02.411- ☑
  - LeFort II S02.412- ☑
  - LeFort III S02.413- ☑
  - left side S02.40D- ☑
  - right side S02.40C- ☑
- metacarpal S62.309- ☑
  - base (displaced) S62.319- ☑
    - nondisplaced S62.349- ☑
  - fifth S62.30- ☑
    - base (displaced) S62.31- ☑
      - nondisplaced S62.34- ☑
    - neck (displaced) S62.33- ☑
      - nondisplaced S62.36- ☑
    - shaft (displaced) S62.32- ☑
      - nondisplaced S62.35- ☑
    - specified NEC S62.398- ☑
  - first S62.20- ☑
    - base NEC (displaced) S62.23- ☑
      - nondisplaced S62.23- ☑
    - Bennett's — see Bennett's fracture
    - neck (displaced) S62.25- ☑
      - nondisplaced S62.25- ☑
    - shaft (displaced) S62.24- ☑
      - nondisplaced S62.24- ☑
    - specified NEC S62.29- ☑
  - fourth S62.30- ☑
    - base (displaced) S62.31- ☑
      - nondisplaced S62.34- ☑
    - neck (displaced) S62.33- ☑
      - nondisplaced S62.36- ☑
    - shaft (displaced) S62.32- ☑
      - nondisplaced S62.35- ☑
    - specified NEC S62.39- ☑
  - neck (displaced) S62.33- ☑
    - nondisplaced S62.36- ☑
  - Rolando's — see Rolando's fracture
  - second S62.30- ☑
    - base (displaced) S62.31- ☑
      - nondisplaced S62.34- ☑
    - neck (displaced) S62.33- ☑
      - nondisplaced S62.36- ☑
    - shaft (displaced) S62.32- ☑
      - nondisplaced S62.35- ☑
    - specified NEC S62.39- ☑
  - shaft (displaced) S62.32- ☑
    - nondisplaced S62.35- ☑
  - specified NEC S62.399- ☑
  - third S62.30- ☑
    - base (displaced) S62.31- ☑
      - nondisplaced S62.34- ☑
    - neck (displaced) S62.33- ☑
      - nondisplaced S62.36- ☑
    - shaft (displaced) S62.32- ☑
      - nondisplaced S62.35- ☑
    - specified NEC S62.39- ☑
- metaphyseal — see Fracture, traumatic, by site, shaft
- metastatic — see Fracture, pathological, due to, neoplastic disease — see also Neoplasm
- metatarsal bone S92.30- ☑
  - fifth (displaced) S92.35- ☑
    - nondisplaced S92.35- ☑
  - first (displaced) S92.31- ☑
    - nondisplaced S92.31- ☑
  - fourth (displaced) S92.34- ☑
    - nondisplaced S92.34- ☑
  - physeal S99.10- ☑

☑ Additional Character Required — Refer to the Tabular List for Character Selection

Fracture, traumatic — *continued*
   metatarsal bone — *continued*
      physeal — *continued*
         Salter-Harris
            Type I S99.11- ☑
            Type II S99.12- ☑
            Type III S99.13- ☑
            Type IV S99.14- ☑
         specified NEC S99.19- ☑
      second (displaced) S92.32- ☑
         nondisplaced S92.32- ☑
      third (displaced) S92.33- ☑
         nondisplaced S92.33- ☑
   Monteggia's — *see* Monteggia's fracture
   multiple
      hand (and wrist) NEC — *see* Fracture, by site
      ribs — *see* Fracture, rib, multiple
   nasal (bone(s)) S02.2- ☑
   navicular (scaphoid) (foot) — *see also* Fracture, tarsal, navicular
      hand — *see* Fracture, carpal, navicular
   neck S12.9- ☑
      cervical vertebra S12.9- ☑
         fifth (displaced) S12.400- ☑
            nondisplaced S12.401- ☑
            specified type NEC (displaced) S12.490- ☑
               nondisplaced S12.491- ☑
         first (displaced) S12.000- ☑
            burst (stable) S12.01- ☑
               unstable S12.02- ☑
            lateral mass (displaced) S12.040- ☑
               nondisplaced S12.041- ☑
            nondisplaced S12.001- ☑
            posterior arch (displaced) S12.030- ☑
               nondisplaced S12.031- ☑
            specified type NEC (displaced) S12.090- ☑
               nondisplaced S12.091- ☑
         fourth (displaced) S12.300- ☑
            nondisplaced S12.301- ☑
            specified type NEC (displaced) S12.390- ☑
               nondisplaced S12.391- ☑
         second (displaced) S12.100- ☑
            dens (anterior) (displaced) (type II) S12.110- ☑
               nondisplaced S12.112- ☑
               posterior S12.111- ☑
            specified type NEC (displaced) S12.120- ☑
               nondisplaced S12.121- ☑
            nondisplaced S12.101- ☑
            specified type NEC (displaced) S12.190- ☑
               nondisplaced S12.191- ☑
         seventh (displaced) S12.600- ☑
            nondisplaced S12.601- ☑
            specified type NEC (displaced) S12.690- ☑
               nondisplaced S12.691- ☑
         sixth (displaced) S12.500- ☑
            nondisplaced S12.501- ☑
            specified type NEC (displaced) S12.590- ☑
               nondisplaced S12.591- ☑
         third (displaced) S12.200- ☑
            nondisplaced S12.201- ☑
            specified type NEC (displaced) S12.290- ☑
               nondisplaced S12.291- ☑
      hyoid bone S12.8- ☑
      larynx S12.8- ☑
      specified site NEC S12.8- ☑
      thyroid cartilage S12.8- ☑
      trachea S12.8- ☑
   neoplastic NEC — *see* Fracture, pathological, due to, neoplastic disease
   neural arch — *see* Fracture, vertebra
   newborn — *see* Birth, injury, fracture
   nontraumatic — *see* Fracture, pathological
   nonunion — *see* Nonunion, fracture
   nose, nasal (bone) (septum) S02.2- ☑
   occiput — *see* Fracture, skull, base, occiput
   odontoid process — *see* Fracture, neck, cervical vertebra, second
   olecranon (process) (ulna) — *see* Fracture, ulna, upper end, olecranon process
   orbit, orbital (bone) (region) S02.85- ☑
      floor (blow-out) S02.3- ☑
      roof S02.12- ☑
      wall S02.85- ☑
         lateral S02.84- ☑
         medial S02.83- ☑

Fracture, traumatic — *continued*
   os
      calcis — *see* Fracture, tarsal, calcaneus
      magnum — *see* Fracture, carpal, capitate
      pubis — *see* Fracture, pubis
   palate S02.8- ☑
   parietal bone (skull) S02.0- ☑
   patella S82.00- ☑
      comminuted (displaced) S82.04- ☑
         nondisplaced S82.04- ☑
      longitudinal (displaced) S82.02- ☑
         nondisplaced S82.02- ☑
      osteochondral (displaced) S82.01- ☑
         nondisplaced S82.01- ☑
      specified NEC S82.09- ☑
      transverse (displaced) S82.03- ☑
         nondisplaced S82.03- ☑
   pedicle (of vertebral arch) — *see* Fracture, vertebra
   pelvis, pelvic (bone) S32.9- ☑
      acetabulum — *see* Fracture, acetabulum
      circle — *see* Disruption, pelvic ring
      following insertion of implant, prosthesis or plate M96.65
      ilium — *see* Fracture, ilium
      ischium — *see* Fracture, ischium
      multiple
         with disruption of pelvic ring (circle) — *see* Disruption, pelvic ring
         without disruption of pelvic ring (circle) S32.82- ☑
      pubis — *see* Fracture, pubis
      sacrum — *see* Fracture, sacrum
      specified site NEC S32.89- ☑
   periprosthetic, around internal prosthetic joint M97.9- ☑
      ankle M97.2- ☑
      elbow M97.4- ☑
      finger M97.8- ☑
      hip M97.0- ☑
      knee M97.1- ☑
      shoulder M97.3- ☑
      specified joint NEC M97.8- ☑
      spine M97.8- ☑
      toe M97.8- ☑
      wrist M97.8- ☑
   phalanx
      foot — *see* Fracture, toe
      hand — *see* Fracture, finger
   pisiform — *see* Fracture, carpal, pisiform
   pond — *see* Fracture, skull
   prosthetic device, internal — *see* Complications, prosthetic device, by site, mechanical
   pubis S32.50- ☑
      with disruption of pelvic ring — *see* Disruption, pelvic ring
      specified site NEC S32.59- ☑
      superior rim S32.51- ☑
   radius S52.9- ☑
      distal end — *see* Fracture, radius, lower end
      following insertion of implant, prosthesis or plate M96.63- ☑
      head — *see* Fracture, radius, upper end, head
      lower end S52.50- ☑
         Barton's — *see* Barton's fracture
         Colles' — *see* Colles' fracture
         extraarticular NEC S52.55- ☑
         intraarticular NEC S52.57- ☑
         physeal S59.20- ☑
            Salter-Harris
               Type I S59.21- ☑
               Type II S59.22- ☑
               Type III S59.23- ☑
               Type IV S59.24- ☑
            specified NEC S59.29- ☑
         Smith's — *see* Smith's fracture
         specified NEC S52.59- ☑
         styloid process (displaced) S52.51- ☑
            nondisplaced S52.51- ☑
         torus S52.52- ☑
      neck — *see* Fracture, radius, upper end
      proximal end — *see* Fracture, radius, upper end
      shaft S52.30- ☑
         bent bone S52.38- ☑
         comminuted (displaced) S52.35- ☑
            nondisplaced S52.35- ☑
         Galeazzi's — *see* Galeazzi's fracture
         greenstick S52.31- ☑
         oblique (displaced) S52.33- ☑

Fracture, traumatic — *continued*
   radius — *continued*
      shaft — *continued*
         oblique — *continued*
            nondisplaced S52.33- ☑
         segmental (displaced) S52.36- ☑
            nondisplaced S52.36- ☑
         specified NEC S52.39- ☑
         spiral (displaced) S52.34- ☑
            nondisplaced S52.34- ☑
         transverse (displaced) S52.32- ☑
            nondisplaced S52.32- ☑
      upper end S52.10- ☑
         head (displaced) S52.12- ☑
            nondisplaced S52.12- ☑
         neck (displaced) S52.13- ☑
            nondisplaced S52.13- ☑
         physeal S59.10- ☑
            Salter-Harris
               Type I S59.11- ☑
               Type II S59.12- ☑
               Type III S59.13- ☑
               Type IV S59.14- ☑
            specified NEC S59.19- ☑
         specified NEC S52.18- ☑
         torus S52.11- ☑
   ramus
      inferior or superior, pubis — *see* Fracture, pubis
      mandible — *see* Fracture, mandible
   restorative material (dental) K08.539
      with loss of material K08.531
      without loss of material K08.530
   rib S22.3- ☑
      with flail chest — *see* Flail, chest
      associated with chest compression and cardiopulmonary resuscitation M96.A2
      multiple S22.4- ☑
         with flail chest — *see* Flail, chest
         associated with chest compression and cardiopulmonary resuscitation M96.A3
   root, tooth — *see* Fracture, tooth
   sacrum S32.10- ☑
      specified NEC S32.19- ☑
      Type
         1 S32.14- ☑
         2 S32.15- ☑
         3 S32.16- ☑
         4 S32.17- ☑
      Zone
         I S32.119- ☑
            displaced (minimally) S32.111- ☑
               severely S32.112- ☑
            nondisplaced S32.110- ☑
         II S32.129- ☑
            displaced (minimally) S32.121- ☑
               severely S32.122- ☑
            nondisplaced S32.120- ☑
         III S32.139- ☑
            displaced (minimally) S32.131- ☑
               severely S32.132- ☑
            nondisplaced S32.130- ☑
   scaphoid (hand) — *see also* Fracture, carpal, navicular
      foot — *see* Fracture, tarsal, navicular
   scapula S42.10- ☑
      acromial process (displaced) S42.12- ☑
         nondisplaced S42.12- ☑
      body (displaced) S42.11- ☑
         nondisplaced S42.11- ☑
      coracoid process (displaced) S42.13- ☑
         nondisplaced S42.13- ☑
      glenoid cavity (displaced) S42.14- ☑
         nondisplaced S42.14- ☑
      neck (displaced) S42.15- ☑
         nondisplaced S42.15- ☑
      specified NEC S42.19- ☑
   semilunar bone, wrist — *see* Fracture, carpal, lunate
   sequelae — *see* Sequelae, fracture
   sesamoid bone
      foot S92.81- ☑
      hand — *see* Fracture, carpal
      other — *see* Fracture, traumatic, by site
   shepherd's — *see* Fracture, tarsal, talus
   shoulder (girdle) S42.9- ☑
      blade — *see* Fracture, scapula
   sinus (ethmoid) (frontal) S02.19- ☑
   skull S02.91- ☑

Fracture, traumatic — continued
- skull — continued
  - base S02.10- ☑
    - occiput S02.119- ☑
      - condyle S02.113- ☑
        - specified NEC S02.118- ☑
          - left side S02.11H- ☑
          - right side S02.11G- ☑
        - type I S02.110- ☑
          - left side S02.11B- ☑
          - right side S02.11A- ☑
        - type II S02.111- ☑
          - left side S02.11D- ☑
          - right side S02.11C- ☑
        - type III S02.112- ☑
          - left side S02.11F- ☑
          - right side S02.11E- ☑
      - specified NEC S02.19- ☑
    - birth injury P13.0
    - frontal bone S02.0- ☑
    - parietal bone S02.0- ☑
    - specified site NEC S02.8- ☑
    - temporal bone S02.19- ☑
    - vault S02.0- ☑
- Smith's — see Smith's fracture
- sphenoid (bone) (sinus) S02.19- ☑
- spine — see Fracture, vertebra
- spinous process — see Fracture, vertebra
- spontaneous (cause unknown) — see Fracture, pathological
- stave (of thumb) — see Fracture, metacarpal, first
- sternum S22.20- ☑
  - with flail chest — see Flail, chest
  - associated with chest compression and cardiopulmonary resuscitation M96.A1
  - body S22.22- ☑
  - manubrium S22.21- ☑
  - xiphoid (process) S22.24- ☑
    - associated with chest compression and cardiopulmonary resuscitation M96.A1
- stress M84.30- ☑
  - ankle M84.37- ☑
  - carpus M84.34- ☑
  - clavicle M84.31- ☑
  - femoral neck M84.359- ☑
  - femur M84.35- ☑
  - fibula M84.36- ☑
  - finger M84.34- ☑
  - hip M84.35- ☑
  - humerus M84.32- ☑
  - ilium M84.350- ☑
  - ischium M84.350- ☑
  - metacarpus M84.34- ☑
  - metatarsus M84.37- ☑
  - neck — see Fracture, fatigue, vertebra
  - pelvis M84.350- ☑
  - radius M84.33- ☑
  - rib M84.38- ☑
  - scapula M84.31- ☑
  - skull M84.38- ☑
  - tarsus M84.37- ☑
  - tibia M84.36- ☑
  - toe M84.37- ☑
  - ulna M84.33- ☑
  - vertebra — see Fracture, fatigue, vertebra
- supracondylar, elbow — see Fracture, humerus, lower end, supracondylar
- symphysis pubis — see Fracture, pubis
- talus (ankle bone) — see Fracture, tarsal, talus
- tarsal bone(s) S92.20- ☑
  - astragalus — see Fracture, tarsal, talus
  - calcaneus S92.00- ☑
    - anterior process (displaced) S92.02- ☑
      - nondisplaced S92.02- ☑
    - body (displaced) S92.01- ☑
      - nondisplaced S92.01- ☑
    - extraarticular NEC (displaced) S92.05- ☑
      - nondisplaced S92.05- ☑
    - intraarticular (displaced) S92.06- ☑
      - nondisplaced S92.06- ☑
    - physeal S99.00- ☑
      - Salter-Harris
        - Type I S99.01- ☑
        - Type II S99.02- ☑
        - Type III S99.03- ☑
        - Type IV S99.04- ☑

Fracture, traumatic — continued
- tarsal bone(s) — continued
  - calcaneus — continued
    - physeal — continued
      - specified NEC S99.09- ☑
    - tuberosity (displaced) S92.04- ☑
      - avulsion (displaced) S92.03- ☑
        - nondisplaced S92.03- ☑
      - nondisplaced S92.04- ☑
  - cuboid (displaced) S92.21- ☑
    - nondisplaced S92.21- ☑
  - cuneiform
    - intermediate (displaced) S92.23- ☑
      - nondisplaced S92.23- ☑
    - lateral (displaced) S92.22- ☑
      - nondisplaced S92.22- ☑
    - medial (displaced) S92.24- ☑
      - nondisplaced S92.24- ☑
  - navicular (displaced) S92.25- ☑
    - nondisplaced S92.25- ☑
  - scaphoid — see Fracture, tarsal, navicular
  - talus S92.10- ☑
    - avulsion (displaced) S92.15- ☑
      - nondisplaced S92.15- ☑
    - body (displaced) S92.12- ☑
      - nondisplaced S92.12- ☑
    - dome (displaced) S92.14- ☑
      - nondisplaced S92.14- ☑
    - head (displaced) S92.12- ☑
      - nondisplaced S92.12- ☑
    - lateral process (displaced) S92.14- ☑
      - nondisplaced S92.14- ☑
    - neck (displaced) S92.11- ☑
      - nondisplaced S92.11- ☑
    - posterior process (displaced) S92.13- ☑
      - nondisplaced S92.13- ☑
    - specified NEC S92.19- ☑
- temporal bone (styloid) S02.19- ☑
- thorax (bony) S22.9- ☑
  - with flail chest — see Flail, chest
  - rib S22.3- ☑
    - multiple S22.4- ☑
      - with flail chest — see Flail, chest
  - sternum S22.20- ☑
    - body S22.22- ☑
    - manubrium S22.21- ☑
    - xiphoid process S22.24- ☑
      - associated with chest compression and cardiopulmonary resuscitation M96.A1
  - vertebra (displaced) S22.009- ☑
    - burst (stable) S22.001- ☑
      - unstable S22.002- ☑
    - eighth S22.069- ☑
      - burst (stable) S22.061- ☑
        - unstable S22.062- ☑
      - specified type NEC S22.068- ☑
      - wedge compression S22.060- ☑
    - eleventh S22.089- ☑
      - burst (stable) S22.081- ☑
        - unstable S22.082- ☑
      - specified type NEC S22.088- ☑
      - wedge compression S22.080- ☑
    - fifth S22.059- ☑
      - burst (stable) S22.051- ☑
        - unstable S22.052- ☑
      - specified type NEC S22.058- ☑
      - wedge compression S22.050- ☑
    - first S22.019- ☑
      - burst (stable) S22.011- ☑
        - unstable S22.012- ☑
      - specified type NEC S22.018- ☑
      - wedge compression S22.010- ☑
    - fourth S22.049- ☑
      - burst (stable) S22.041- ☑
        - unstable S22.042- ☑
      - specified type NEC S22.048- ☑
      - wedge compression S22.040- ☑
    - ninth S22.079- ☑
      - burst (stable) S22.071- ☑
        - unstable S22.072- ☑
      - specified type NEC S22.078- ☑
      - wedge compression S22.070- ☑
    - nondisplaced S22.001- ☑
    - second S22.029- ☑
      - burst (stable) S22.021- ☑

Fracture, traumatic — continued
- thorax — continued
  - vertebra — continued
    - second — continued
      - burst — continued
        - unstable S22.022- ☑
      - specified type NEC S22.028- ☑
      - wedge compression S22.020- ☑
    - seventh S22.069- ☑
      - burst (stable) S22.061- ☑
        - unstable S22.062- ☑
      - specified type NEC S22.068- ☑
      - wedge compression S22.060- ☑
    - sixth S22.059- ☑
      - burst (stable) S22.051- ☑
        - unstable S22.052- ☑
      - specified type NEC S22.058- ☑
      - wedge compression S22.050- ☑
    - specified type NEC S22.008- ☑
    - tenth S22.079- ☑
      - burst (stable) S22.071- ☑
        - unstable S22.072- ☑
      - specified type NEC S22.078- ☑
      - wedge compression S22.070- ☑
    - third S22.039- ☑
      - burst (stable) S22.031- ☑
        - unstable S22.032- ☑
      - specified type NEC S22.038- ☑
      - wedge compression S22.030- ☑
    - twelfth S22.089- ☑
      - burst (stable) S22.081- ☑
        - unstable S22.082- ☑
      - specified type NEC S22.088- ☑
      - wedge compression S22.080- ☑
    - wedge compression S22.000- ☑
- thumb S62.50- ☑
  - distal phalanx (displaced) S62.52- ☑
    - nondisplaced S62.52- ☑
  - proximal phalanx (displaced) S62.51- ☑
    - nondisplaced S62.51- ☑
- thyroid cartilage S12.8- ☑
- tibia (shaft) S82.20- ☑
  - comminuted (displaced) S82.25- ☑
    - nondisplaced S82.25- ☑
  - condyles — see Fracture, tibia, upper end
  - distal end — see Fracture, tibia, lower end
  - epiphysis
    - lower — see Fracture, tibia, lower end
    - upper — see Fracture, tibia, upper end
  - following insertion of implant, prosthesis or plate M96.67- ☑
  - head (involving knee joint) — see Fracture, tibia, upper end
  - intercondyloid eminence — see Fracture, tibia, upper end
  - involving ankle or malleolus — see Fracture, ankle, medial malleolus
  - lower end S82.30- ☑
    - physeal S89.10- ☑
      - Salter-Harris
        - Type I S89.11- ☑
        - Type II S89.12- ☑
        - Type III S89.13- ☑
        - Type IV S89.14- ☑
      - specified NEC S89.19- ☑
    - pilon (displaced) S82.87- ☑
      - nondisplaced S82.87- ☑
    - specified NEC S82.39- ☑
    - torus S82.31- ☑
  - malleolus — see Fracture, ankle, medial malleolus
  - oblique (displaced) S82.23- ☑
    - nondisplaced S82.23- ☑
  - pilon — see Fracture, tibia, lower end, pilon
  - proximal end — see Fracture, tibia, upper end
  - segmental (displaced) S82.26- ☑
    - nondisplaced S82.26- ☑
  - specified NEC S82.29- ☑
  - spine — see Fracture, tibia, upper end, spine
  - spiral (displaced) S82.24- ☑
    - nondisplaced S82.24- ☑
  - transverse (displaced) S82.22- ☑
    - nondisplaced S82.22- ☑
  - tuberosity — see Fracture, tibia, upper end, tuberosity
  - upper end S82.10- ☑
    - bicondylar (displaced) S82.14- ☑
      - nondisplaced S82.14- ☑

Fracture, traumatic — continued
  tibia — continued
    upper end — continued
      lateral condyle (displaced) S82.12- ☑
        nondisplaced S82.12- ☑
      medial condyle (displaced) S82.13- ☑
        nondisplaced S82.13- ☑
      physeal S89.00- ☑
        Salter-Harris
          Type I S89.01- ☑
          Type II S89.02- ☑
          Type III S89.03- ☑
          Type IV S89.04- ☑
        specified NEC S89.09- ☑
      plateau — see Fracture, tibia, upper end, bicondylar
      specified NEC S82.19- ☑
      spine (displaced) S82.11- ☑
        nondisplaced S82.11- ☑
      torus S82.16- ☑
      tuberosity (displaced) S82.15- ☑
        nondisplaced S82.15- ☑
  toe S92.91- ☑
    great (displaced) S92.40- ☑
      distal phalanx (displaced) S92.42- ☑
        nondisplaced S92.42- ☑
      nondisplaced S92.40- ☑
      proximal phalanx (displaced) S92.41- ☑
        nondisplaced S92.41- ☑
      specified NEC S92.49- ☑
    lesser (displaced) S92.50- ☑
      distal phalanx (displaced) S92.53- ☑
        nondisplaced S92.53- ☑
      middle phalanx (displaced) S92.52- ☑
        nondisplaced S92.52- ☑
      nondisplaced S92.50- ☑
      proximal phalanx (displaced) S92.51- ☑
        nondisplaced S92.51- ☑
      specified NEC S92.59- ☑
    physeal
      phalanx S99.20- ☑
        Salter-Harris
          Type I S99.21- ☑
          Type II S99.22- ☑
          Type III S99.23- ☑
          Type IV S99.24- ☑
        specified NEC S99.29- ☑
  tooth (root) S02.5- ☑
  trachea (cartilage) S12.8- ☑
  transverse process — see Fracture, vertebra
  trapezium or trapezoid bone — see Fracture, carpal
  trimalleolar — see Fracture, ankle, trimalleolar
  triquetrum (cuneiform of carpus) — see Fracture, carpal, triquetrum
  trochanter — see Fracture, femur, trochanteric
  tuberosity (external) — see Fracture, traumatic, by site
  ulna (shaft) S52.20- ☑
    bent bone S52.28- ☑
    coronoid process — see Fracture, ulna, upper end, coronoid process
    distal end — see Fracture, ulna, lower end
    following insertion of implant, prosthesis or plate M96.63- ☑
    head S52.60- ☑
    lower end S52.60- ☑
      physeal S59.00- ☑
        Salter-Harris
          Type I S59.01- ☑
          Type II S59.02- ☑
          Type III S59.03- ☑
          Type IV S59.04- ☑
        specified NEC S59.09- ☑
      specified NEC S52.69- ☑
      styloid process (displaced) S52.61- ☑
        nondisplaced S52.61- ☑
      torus S52.62- ☑
    proximal end — see Fracture, ulna, upper end
    shaft S52.20- ☑
      comminuted (displaced) S52.25- ☑
        nondisplaced S52.25- ☑
      greenstick S52.21- ☑
      Monteggia's — see Monteggia's fracture
      oblique (displaced) S52.23- ☑
        nondisplaced S52.23- ☑
      segmental (displaced) S52.26- ☑
        nondisplaced S52.26- ☑

Fracture, traumatic — continued
  ulna — continued
    shaft — continued
      specified NEC S52.29- ☑
      spiral (displaced) S52.24- ☑
        nondisplaced S52.24- ☑
      transverse (displaced) S52.22- ☑
        nondisplaced S52.22- ☑
    upper end S52.00- ☑
      coronoid process (displaced) S52.04- ☑
        nondisplaced S52.04- ☑
      olecranon process (displaced) S52.02- ☑
        with intraarticular extension S52.03- ☑
        nondisplaced S52.02- ☑
          with intraarticular extension S52.03- ☑
      specified NEC S52.09- ☑
      torus S52.01- ☑
  unciform — see Fracture, carpal, hamate
  vault of skull S02.0- ☑
  vertebra, vertebral (arch) (body) (column) (neural arch) (pedicle) (spinous process) (transverse process)
    atlas — see Fracture, neck, cervical vertebra, first
    axis — see Fracture, neck, cervical vertebra, second
    cervical (teardrop) S12.9- ☑
      axis — see Fracture, neck, cervical vertebra, second
      first (atlas) — see Fracture, neck, cervical vertebra, first
      second (axis) — see Fracture, neck, cervical vertebra, second
    chronic M84.48- ☑
    coccyx S32.2- ☑
    dorsal — see Fracture, thorax, vertebra
    lumbar S32.009- ☑
      burst (stable) S32.001- ☑
        unstable S32.002- ☑
      fifth S32.059- ☑
        burst (stable) S32.051- ☑
          unstable S32.052- ☑
        specified type NEC S32.058- ☑
        wedge compression S32.050- ☑
      first S32.019- ☑
        burst (stable) S32.011- ☑
          unstable S32.012- ☑
        specified type NEC S32.018- ☑
        wedge compression S32.010- ☑
      fourth S32.049- ☑
        burst (stable) S32.041- ☑
          unstable S32.042- ☑
        specified type NEC S32.048- ☑
        wedge compression S32.040- ☑
      second S32.029- ☑
        burst (stable) S32.021- ☑
          unstable S32.022- ☑
        specified type NEC S32.028- ☑
        wedge compression S32.020- ☑
      specified type NEC S32.008- ☑
      third S32.039- ☑
        burst (stable) S32.031- ☑
          unstable S32.032- ☑
        specified type NEC S32.038- ☑
        wedge compression S32.030- ☑
      wedge compression S32.000- ☑
    metastatic — see Collapse, vertebra, in, specified disease NEC — see also Neoplasm
    newborn (birth injury) P11.5
    sacrum S32.10- ☑
      specified NEC S32.19- ☑
      Type
        1 S32.14- ☑
        2 S32.15- ☑
        3 S32.16- ☑
        4 S32.17- ☑
      Zone
        I S32.119- ☑
          displaced (minimally) S32.111- ☑
          severely S32.112- ☑
          nondisplaced S32.110- ☑
        II S32.129- ☑
          displaced (minimally) S32.121- ☑
          severely S32.122- ☑
          nondisplaced S32.120- ☑
        III S32.139- ☑
          displaced (minimally) S32.131- ☑
          severely S32.132- ☑
          nondisplaced S32.130- ☑
    thoracic — see Fracture, thorax, vertebra

Fracture, traumatic — continued
  vertex S02.0- ☑
  vomer (bone) S02.2- ☑
  wrist S62.10- ☑
    carpal — see Fracture, carpal bone
    navicular (scaphoid) (hand) — see Fracture, carpal, navicular
  xiphisternum, xiphoid (process) S22.24- ☑
    associated with chest compression and cardiopulmonary resuscitation M96.A1
  zygoma S02.402- ☑
    left side S02.40F- ☑
    right side S02.40E- ☑
Fragile, fragility
  autosomal site Q95.5
  bone, congenital (with blue sclera) Q78.0
  capillary (hereditary) D69.8
  hair L67.8
  nails L60.3
  non-sex chromosome site Q95.5
  X chromosome Q99.2
Fragilitas
  crinium L67.8
  ossium (with blue sclerae) (hereditary) Q78.0
  unguium L60.3
    congenital Q84.6
Fragments, cataract (lens), **following cataract surgery** H59.02- ☑
  retained foreign body — see Retained, foreign body fragments (type of)
Frailty (frail) R54
  mental R41.81
Frambesia, frambesial (tropica) — see also Yaws
  initial lesion or ulcer A66.0
  primary A66.0
Frambeside
  gummatous A66.4
  of early yaws A66.2
Frambesioma A66.1
Franceschetti-Klein (-Wildervanck) **disease or syndrome** Q75.4
Francis' disease — see Tularemia
Franklin disease C88.2- ☑
Frank's essential thrombocytopenia D69.3
Fraser's syndrome Q87.0
Freckle(s) L81.2
  malignant melanoma in — see Melanoma
  melanotic (Hutchinson's) — see Melanoma, in situ
  retinal D49.81
Frederickson's hyperlipoproteinemia, type
  I and V E78.3
  IIA E78.00
  IIB and III E78.2
  IV E78.1
Freeman Sheldon syndrome Q87.0
Freezing — see also Effect, adverse, cold T69.9- ☑
Freiberg's disease (infraction of metatarsal head or osteochondrosis) — see Osteochondrosis, juvenile, metatarsus
Frei's disease A55
Fremitus, friction, cardiac R01.2
Frenum, frenulum
  external os Q51.828
  tongue (shortening) (congenital) Q38.1
Frequency micturition (nocturnal) R35.0
  psychogenic F45.8
Frey's syndrome
  auriculotemporal G50.8
  hyperhidrosis L74.52
Friction
  burn — see Burn, by site
  fremitus, cardiac R01.2
  precordial R01.2
  sounds, chest R09.89
Friderichsen-Waterhouse syndrome or disease A39.1
Friedlander's B (bacillus) **NEC** — see also condition A49.8
Friedreich's
  ataxia G11.11
  combined systemic disease G11.11
  facial hemihypertrophy Q67.4
  sclerosis (cerebellum) (spinal cord) G11.11
Frigidity F52.22
Frohlich's syndrome E23.6
Frontal — see also condition
  lobe syndrome F07.0
Frostbite (superficial) T33.90- ☑

Frostbite — *continued*
  with
    partial thickness skin loss — *see* Frostbite (superficial), by site
    tissue necrosis T34.90- ☑
  abdominal wall T33.3- ☑
    with tissue necrosis T34.3- ☑
  ankle T33.81- ☑
    with tissue necrosis T34.81- ☑
  arm T33.4- ☑
    with tissue necrosis T34.4- ☑
    finger(s) — *see* Frostbite, finger
    hand — *see* Frostbite, hand
    wrist — *see* Frostbite, wrist
  ear T33.01- ☑
    with tissue necrosis T34.01- ☑
  face T33.09- ☑
    with tissue necrosis T34.09- ☑
  finger T33.53- ☑
    with tissue necrosis T34.53- ☑
  foot T33.82- ☑
    with tissue necrosis T34.82- ☑
  hand T33.52- ☑
    with tissue necrosis T34.52- ☑
  head T33.09- ☑
    with tissue necrosis T34.09- ☑
    ear — *see* Frostbite, ear
    nose — *see* Frostbite, nose
  hip (and thigh) T33.6- ☑
    with tissue necrosis T34.6- ☑
  knee T33.7- ☑
    with tissue necrosis T34.7- ☑
  leg T33.99- ☑
    with tissue necrosis — *see also* Frostbite, by specific site on leg, if specified T34.99- ☑
    ankle — *see* Frostbite, ankle
    foot — *see* Frostbite, foot
    knee — *see* Frostbite, knee
    lower T33.7- ☑
      with tissue necrosis T34.7- ☑
    thigh — *see* Frostbite, hip
    toe — *see* Frostbite, toe
  limb
    lower T33.99- ☑
      with tissue necrosis T34.99- ☑
    upper — *see* Frostbite, arm
  neck T33.1- ☑
    with tissue necrosis T34.1- ☑
  nose T33.02- ☑
    with tissue necrosis T34.02- ☑
  pelvis T33.3- ☑
    with tissue necrosis T34.3- ☑
  specified site NEC T33.99- ☑
    with tissue necrosis T34.99- ☑
  thigh — *see* Frostbite, hip
  thorax T33.2- ☑
    with tissue necrosis T34.2- ☑
  toes T33.83- ☑
    with tissue necrosis T34.83- ☑
  trunk T33.99- ☑
    with tissue necrosis T34.99- ☑
  wrist T33.51- ☑
    with tissue necrosis T34.51- ☑
Frotteurism F65.81
Frozen — *see also* Effect, adverse, cold T69.9- ☑
  pelvis (female) N94.89
    male K66.8
  shoulder — *see* Capsulitis, adhesive
Fructokinase deficiency E74.11
Fructose 1,6 diphosphatase deficiency E74.19
Fructosemia (benign) (essential) E74.12
Fructosuria (benign) (essential) E74.11
Fuchs'
  black spot (myopic) — *see also* Myopia, degenerative H44.2-
  dystrophy (corneal endothelium) H18.51- ☑
  heterochromic cyclitis — *see* Cyclitis, Fuchs' heterochromic
Fucosidosis E77.1
Fugue R68.89
  dissociative F44.1
  hysterical (dissociative) F44.1
  postictal in epilepsy — *see* Epilepsy
  reaction to exceptional stress (transient) F43.0
Fulminant, fulminating — *see* condition

Functional — *see also* condition
  bleeding (uterus) N93.8
Functioning, intellectual, borderline R41.83
Fundus — *see* condition
Fungemia NOS B49
  candida B37.7
Fungus, fungous
  cerebral G93.89
  disease NOS B49
  infection — *see* Infection, fungus
Funiculitis (acute) (chronic) (endemic) N49.1
  gonococcal (acute) (chronic) A54.23
  tuberculous A18.15
Funnel
  breast (acquired) M95.4
    congenital Q67.6
    sequelae (late effect) of rickets E64.3
  chest (acquired) M95.4
    congenital Q67.6
    sequelae (late effect) of rickets E64.3
  pelvis (acquired) M95.5
    with disproportion (fetopelvic) O33.3- ☑
      causing obstructed labor O65.3
    congenital Q74.2
FUO (fever of unknown origin) R50.9
Furfur L21.0
  microsporon B36.0
Furloughed Z56.89
Furrier's lung J67.8
Furrowed K14.5
  nail(s) (transverse) L60.4
    congenital Q84.6
  tongue K14.5
    congenital Q38.3
Furuncle L02.92
  abdominal wall L02.221
  ankle — *see* Furuncle, lower limb
  antecubital space — *see* Furuncle, upper limb
  anus K61.0
  arm — *see* Furuncle, upper limb
  auditory canal, external — *see* Abscess, ear, external
  auricle (ear) — *see* Abscess, ear, external
  axilla (region) L02.42- ☑
  back (any part except buttock and flank) L02.222
  breast N61.1
  buttock L02.32
  cheek (external) L02.02
  chest wall L02.223
  chin L02.02
  corpus cavernosum N48.21
  ear, external — *see* Abscess, ear, external
  external auditory canal — *see* Abscess, ear, external
  eyelid — *see* Abscess, eyelid
  face L02.02
  femoral (region) — *see* Furuncle, lower limb
  finger — *see* Furuncle, hand
  flank L02.227
  foot L02.62- ☑
  forehead L02.02
  gluteal (region) L02.32
  groin L02.224
  hand L02.52- ☑
  head L02.821
    face L02.02
  hip — *see* Furuncle, lower limb
  kidney — *see* Abscess, kidney
  knee — *see* Furuncle, lower limb
  labium (majus) (minus) N76.4
  lacrimal
    gland — *see* Dacryoadenitis
    passages (duct) (sac) — *see* Inflammation, lacrimal, passages, acute
  leg (any part) — *see* Furuncle, lower limb
  lower limb L02.42- ☑
  malignant A22.0
  mouth K12.2
  navel L02.226
  neck L02.12
  nose J34.0
  orbit, orbital — *see* Abscess, orbit
  palmar (space) — *see* Furuncle, hand
  partes posteriores L02.32
  pectoral region L02.223
  penis N48.21
  perineum L02.225
  pinna — *see* Abscess, ear, external
  popliteal — *see* Furuncle, lower limb

Furuncle — *continued*
  prepatellar — *see* Furuncle, lower limb
  scalp L02.821
  seminal vesicle N49.0
  shoulder — *see* Furuncle, upper limb
  specified site NEC L02.828
  submandibular K12.2
  temple (region) L02.02
  thumb — *see* Furuncle, hand
  toe — *see* Furuncle, foot
  trunk L02.229
    abdominal wall L02.221
    back L02.222
    chest wall L02.223
    groin L02.224
    perineum L02.225
    umbilicus L02.226
  umbilicus L02.226
  upper limb L02.42- ☑
  vulva N76.4
Furunculosis — *see* Furuncle
Fused — *see* Fusion, fused
Fusion, fused (congenital)
  astragaloscaphoid Q74.2
  atria Q21.19
  auditory canal Q16.1
  auricles, heart Q21.19
  binocular with defective stereopsis H53.32
  bone Q79.8
  cervical spine M43.22
  choanal Q30.0
  commissure, mitral valve Q23.2
  cusps, heart valve NEC Q24.8
    mitral Q23.2
    pulmonary Q22.1
    tricuspid Q22.4
  ear ossicles Q16.3
  fingers Q70.0- ☑
  hymen Q52.3
  joint (acquired) — *see also* Ankylosis
    congenital Q74.8
  kidneys (incomplete) Q63.1
  labium (majus) (minus) Q52.5
  larynx and trachea Q34.8
  limb, congenital Q74.8
    lower Q74.2
    upper Q74.0
  lobes, lung Q33.8
  lumbosacral (acquired) M43.27
    arthrodesis status Z98.1
    congenital Q76.49
    postprocedural status Z98.1
  nares, nose, nasal, nostril(s) Q30.0
  organ or site not listed — *see* Anomaly, by site
  ossicles Q79.9
    auditory Q16.3
  pulmonic cusps Q22.1
  ribs Q76.6
  sacroiliac (joint) (acquired) M43.28
    arthrodesis status Z98.1
    congenital Q74.2
    postprocedural status Z98.1
  spine (acquired) NEC M43.20
    arthrodesis status Z98.1
    cervical region M43.22
    cervicothoracic region M43.23
    congenital Q76.49
    lumbar M43.26
    lumbosacral region M43.27
    occipito-atlanto-axial region M43.21
    postoperative status Z98.1
    sacrococcygeal region M43.28
    thoracic region M43.24
    thoracolumbar region M43.25
  sublingual duct with submaxillary duct at opening in mouth Q38.4
  testes Q55.1
  toes Q70.2- ☑
  tooth, teeth K00.2
  trachea and esophagus Q39.8
  twins Q89.4
  vagina Q52.4
  ventricles, heart Q21.0
  vertebra (arch) — *see* Fusion, spine
  vulva Q52.5
Fusospirillosis (mouth) (tongue) (tonsil) A69.1
Fussy baby R68.12

G

Gain in weight (abnormal) (excessive) — see also Weight, gain
Gaisbock's disease (polycythemia hypertonica) D75.1
Gait abnormality R26.9
- ataxic R26.0
- falling R29.6
- hysterical (ataxic) (staggering) F44.4
- paralytic R26.1
- spastic R26.1
- specified type NEC R26.89
- staggering R26.0
- unsteadiness R26.81
- walking difficulty NEC R26.2

Galactocele (breast) N64.89
- puerperal, postpartum O92.79

Galactokinase deficiency E74.29
Galactophoritis N61.0
- gestational, puerperal, postpartum O91.2- ☑

Galactorrhea O92.6
- not associated with childbirth N64.3

Galactosemia (classic) (congenital) E74.21
Galactosuria E74.29
Galacturia R82.0
- schistosomiasis (bilharziasis) B65.0

GALD (gestational alloimmune liver disease) P78.84
Galeazzi's fracture S52.37- ☑
Galen's vein — see condition
Galeophobia F40.218
Gall duct — see condition
Gallbladder — see also condition
- acute K81.0

Gallop rhythm R00.8
Gallstone (colic) (cystic duct) (gallbladder) (impacted) (multiple) — see also Calculus, gallbladder
- with
  - cholecystitis — see Calculus, gallbladder, with cholecystitis
- bile duct (common) (hepatic) — see Calculus, bile duct
- causing intestinal obstruction K56.3
- specified NEC K80.80
  - with obstruction K80.81

Gambling Z72.6
- pathological (compulsive) F63.0

Gammopathy (of undetermined significance [MGUS]) D47.2
- associated with lymphoplasmacytic dyscrasia D47.2
- monoclonal D47.2
- polyclonal D89.0

Gamna's disease (siderotic splenomegaly) D73.1
Gamophobia F40.298
Gampsodactylia (congenital) Q66.7- ☑
Gamstorp's disease (adynamia episodica hereditaria) G72.3
Gandy-Nanta disease (siderotic splenomegaly) D73.1
Gang
- membership offenses Z72.810

Gangliocytoma D36.10
Ganglioglioma — see Neoplasm, uncertain behavior, by site
Ganglion (compound) (diffuse) (joint) (tendon (sheath)) M67.40
- ankle M67.47- ☑
- foot M67.47- ☑
- forearm M67.43- ☑
- hand M67.44- ☑
- lower leg M67.46- ☑
- multiple sites M67.49
- of yaws (early) (late) A66.6
- pelvic region M67.45- ☑
- periosteal — see Periostitis
- shoulder region M67.41- ☑
- specified site NEC M67.48
- thigh region M67.45- ☑
- tuberculous A18.09
- upper arm M67.42- ☑
- wrist M67.43- ☑

Ganglioneuroblastoma — see Neoplasm, nerve, malignant
Ganglioneuroma D36.10
- malignant — see Neoplasm, nerve, malignant

Ganglioneuromatosis D36.10
Ganglionitis
- fifth nerve — see Neuralgia, trigeminal
- gasserian (postherpetic) (postzoster) B02.21
- geniculate G51.1
  - newborn (birth injury) P11.3
  - postherpetic, postzoster B02.21
- herpes zoster B02.21

Ganglionitis — continued
- postherpetic geniculate B02.21

Gangliosidosis E75.10
- GM1 E75.19
- GM2 E75.00
  - other specified E75.09
  - Sandhoff disease E75.01
  - Tay-Sachs disease E75.02
- GM3 E75.19
- mucolipidosis IV E75.11

Gangosa A66.5
Gangrene, gangrenous (connective tissue) (dropsical) (dry) (moist) (skin) (ulcer) — see also Necrosis I96
- with diabetes (mellitus) — see Diabetes, with, gangrene
- abdomen (wall) I96
- alveolar M27.3
- appendix K35.80
  - with
    - peritonitis, localized — see also Appendicitis K35.31
- arteriosclerotic (general) (senile) — see Arteriosclerosis, extremities, with, gangrene
- auricle I96
- Bacillus welchii A48.0
- bladder (infectious) — see Cystitis, specified type NEC
- bowel, cecum, or colon — see Gangrene, intestine
- Clostridium perfringens or welchii A48.0
- cornea H18.89- ☑
- corpora cavernosa N48.29
  - noninfective N48.89
- cutaneous, spreading I96
- decubital — see Ulcer, pressure, by site
- diabetic (any site) — see Diabetes, with, gangrene
- emphysematous — see Gangrene, gas
- epidemic — see Poisoning, food, noxious, plant
- epididymis (infectional) N45.1
- erysipelas — see Erysipelas
- extremity (lower) (upper) I96
- Fournier N49.3
  - female N76.82
  - vagina and vulva N76.82
- fusospirochetal A69.0
- gallbladder — see Cholecystitis, acute
- gas (bacillus) A48.0
  - following
    - abortion — see Abortion by type complicated by infection
    - ectopic or molar pregnancy O08.0
- glossitis K14.0
- hernia — see Hernia, by site, with gangrene
- intestine, intestinal (hemorrhagic) (massive) — see also Infarct, intestine K55.069
  - with
    - mesenteric embolism — see also Infarct, intestine K55.069
    - obstruction — see Obstruction, intestine
- laryngitis J04.0
- limb (lower) (upper) I96
- lung J85.0
  - spirochetal A69.8
- lymphangitis I89.1
- Meleney's (synergistic) — see Ulcer, skin
- mesentery — see also Infarct, intestine K55.069
  - with
    - embolism — see also Infarct, intestine K55.069
    - intestinal obstruction — see Obstruction, intestine
- mouth A69.0
- ovary — see Oophoritis
- pancreas — see Pancreatitis, acute
- penis N48.29
  - noninfective N48.89
- perineum I96
- pharynx — see also Pharyngitis
  - Vincent's A69.1
- presenile I73.1
- progressive synergistic — see Ulcer, skin
- pulmonary J85.0
- pulpal (dental) K04.1
- quinsy J36
- Raynaud's (symmetric gangrene) I73.01
- retropharyngeal J39.2
- scrotum N49.3
  - noninfective N50.89
- senile (atherosclerotic) — see Arteriosclerosis, extremities, with, gangrene
- spermatic cord N49.1
  - noninfective N50.89
- spine I96
- spirochetal NEC A69.8

Gangrene, gangrenous — continued
- spreading cutaneous I96
- stomatitis A69.0
- symmetrical I73.01
- testis (infectional) N45.2
  - noninfective N44.8
- throat — see also Pharyngitis
  - diphtheritic A36.0
  - Vincent's A69.1
- thyroid (gland) E07.89
- tooth (pulp) K04.1
- tuberculous NEC — see Tuberculosis
- tunica vaginalis N49.1
  - noninfective N50.89
- umbilicus I96
- uterus — see Endometritis
- uvulitis K12.2
- vas deferens N49.1
  - noninfective N50.89
- vulva N76.82

Ganister disease J62.8
Ganser's syndrome (hysterical) F44.89
Gardner-Diamond syndrome (autoerythrocyte sensitization) D69.2
Gargoylism E76.01
Garre's disease, osteitis (sclerosing), osteomyelitis — see Osteomyelitis, specified type NEC
Garrod's pad, knuckle M72.1
Gartner's duct
- cyst Q52.4
- persistent Q50.6

Gas R14.3
- asphyxiation, inhalation, poisoning, suffocation NEC — see Table of Drugs and Chemicals
- excessive R14.0
- gangrene A48.0
- following
  - abortion — see Abortion by type complicated by infection
  - ectopic or molar pregnancy O08.0
- on stomach R14.0
- pains R14.1

Gastralgia — see also Pain, abdominal
Gastrectasis K31.0
- psychogenic F45.8

Gastric — see condition
Gastrinoma
- malignant
  - pancreas C25.4
  - specified site NEC — see Neoplasm, malignant, by site
  - unspecified site C25.4
- specified site — see Neoplasm, uncertain behavior
- unspecified site D37.9

Gastritis (simple) K29.70
- with bleeding K29.71
- acute (erosive) K29.00
  - with bleeding K29.01
- alcoholic K29.20
  - with bleeding K29.21
- allergic K29.60
  - with bleeding K29.61
- atrophic (chronic) K29.40
  - with bleeding K29.41
- chronic (antral) (fundal) K29.50
  - with bleeding K29.51
  - atrophic K29.40
    - with bleeding K29.41
  - superficial K29.30
    - with bleeding K29.31
- dietary counseling and surveillance Z71.3
- due to diet deficiency E63.9
- eosinophilic K52.81
- giant hypertrophic K29.60
  - with bleeding K29.61
- granulomatous K29.60
  - with bleeding K29.61
- hypertrophic (mucosa) K29.60
  - with bleeding K29.61
- nervous F54
- spastic K29.60
  - with bleeding K29.61
- specified NEC K29.60
  - with bleeding K29.61
- superficial chronic K29.30
  - with bleeding K29.31
- tuberculous A18.83
- viral NEC A08.4

Gastrocarcinoma — see Neoplasm, malignant, stomach

Gastrocolic — see condition
Gastrodisciasis, gastrodiscoidiasis B66.8
Gastroduodenitis K29.90
- with bleeding K29.91
- virus, viral A08.4
  - specified type NEC A08.39
Gastrodynia — see Pain, abdominal
Gastroenteritis (acute) (chronic) (noninfectious) — see also Enteritis K52.9
- allergic K52.29
  - with
    - eosinophilic gastritis or gastroenteritis K52.81
    - food protein-induced enterocolitis syndrome K52.21
    - food protein-induced enteropathy K52.22
- dietetic — see also Gastroenteritis, allergic K52.29
- drug-induced K52.1
- due to
  - Cryptosporidium A07.2
  - drugs K52.1
  - food poisoning — see Intoxication, foodborne
  - radiation K52.0
- eosinophilic K52.81
- epidemic (infectious) A09
- food hypersensitivity — see also Gastroenteritis, allergic K52.29
- infectious — see Enteritis, infectious
- influenzal — see Influenza, with gastroenteritis
- noninfectious K52.9
  - specified NEC K52.89
- rotaviral A08.0
- Salmonella A02.0
- toxic K52.1
- viral NEC A08.4
  - acute infectious A08.39
    - type Norwalk A08.11
  - infantile (acute) A08.39
  - Norwalk agent A08.11
  - rotaviral A08.0
  - severe of infants A08.39
  - specified type NEC A08.39
Gastroenteropathy — see also Gastroenteritis K52.9
- acute, due to Norovirus A08.11
- acute, due to Norwalk agent A08.11
- infectious A09
Gastroenteroptosis K63.4
Gastroesophageal laceration- hemorrhage syndrome K22.6
Gastrointestinal — see condition
Gastrojejunal — see condition
Gastrojejunitis — see also Enteritis K52.9
Gastrojejunocolic — see condition
Gastroliths K31.89
Gastromalacia K31.89
Gastroparalysis K31.84
- diabetic — see Diabetes, gastroparalysis
Gastroparesis K31.84
- diabetic — see Diabetes, by type, with gastroparesis
Gastropathy K31.9
- congestive portal — see also Hypertension, portal K31.89
- erythematous K29.70
- exudative K90.89
- portal hypertensive — see also Hypertension, portal K31.89
- specified NEC K31.89
Gastroptosis K31.89
Gastrorrhagia K92.2
- psychogenic F45.8
Gastroschisis (congenital) Q79.3
Gastrospasm (neurogenic) (reflex) K31.89
- neurotic F45.8
- psychogenic F45.8
Gastrostaxis — see Gastritis, with bleeding
Gastrostenosis K31.89
Gastrostomy
- attention to Z43.1
- status Z93.1
Gastrosuccorrhea (continuous) (intermittent) K31.89
- neurotic F45.8
- psychogenic F45.8
Gatophobia F40.218
Gaucher's disease or splenomegaly (adult) (infantile) E75.22
Gee (-Herter)(-Thaysen) **disease** (nontropical sprue) K90.0
Gelineau's syndrome G47.419
- with cataplexy G47.411
Gemination, tooth, teeth K00.2
Gemistocytoma
- specified site — see Neoplasm, malignant, by site

Gemistocytoma — continued
- unspecified site C71.9
General, generalized — see condition
Genetic
- carrier (status)
  - cystic fibrosis Z14.1
  - hemophilia A (asymptomatic) Z14.01
    - symptomatic Z14.02
  - specified NEC Z14.8
- susceptibility to disease NEC Z15.89
  - epilepsy Z15.1
  - kidney disease Z15.3
  - malignant neoplasm Z15.09
    - biliary tract Z15.068
    - breast Z15.01
    - colorectal Z15.060
    - digestive system NEC Z15.068
    - endometrium Z15.04
    - fallopian tube(s) Z15.05
    - gastric Z15.068
    - ovary Z15.02
    - pancreas Z15.068
    - prostate Z15.03
    - small bowel Z15.068
    - specified NEC Z15.09
    - urinary tract Z15.07
  - multiple endocrine neoplasia Z15.81
  - neurodevelopmental disorders Z15.1
  - obesity Z15.2
Genital — see condition
Genito-anorectal syndrome A55
Genitourinary system — see condition
Genu
- congenital Q74.1
- extrorsum (acquired) — see also Deformity, varus, knee
  - congenital Q74.1
  - sequelae (late effect) of rickets E64.3
- introrsum (acquired) — see also Deformity, valgus, knee
  - congenital Q74.1
  - sequelae (late effect) of rickets E64.3
- rachitic (old) E64.3
- recurvatum (acquired) — see also Deformity, limb, specified type NEC, lower leg
  - congenital Q68.2
  - sequelae (late effect) of rickets E64.3
- valgum (acquired) (knock-knee) M21.06- ☑
  - congenital Q74.1
  - sequelae (late effect) of rickets E64.3
- varum (acquired) (bowleg) M21.16- ☑
  - congenital Q74.1
  - sequelae (late effect) of rickets E64.3
Geographic tongue K14.1
Geophagia — see Pica
Geotrichosis B48.3
- stomatitis B48.3
Gephyrophobia F40.242
Gerbode defect Q21.0
GERD (gastroesophageal reflux disease) — see also Disease, gastroesophageal reflux K21.9
Gerhardt's
- disease (erythromelalgia) I73.81
- syndrome (vocal cord paralysis) J38.00
  - bilateral J38.02
  - unilateral J38.01
German measles — see also Rubella
- exposure to Z20.4
Germinoblastoma (diffuse) C85.9- ☑
- follicular C82.9- ☑
Germinoma — see Neoplasm, malignant, by site
Gerontoxon — see Degeneration, cornea, senile
Gerstmann-Straussler-Scheinker syndrome (GSS) A81.82
Gerstmann's syndrome R48.8
- developmental F81.2
Gestation (period) — see also Pregnancy
- ectopic — see Pregnancy, by site
- multiple O30.9- ☑
  - greater than quadruplets — see Pregnancy, multiple (gestation), specified NEC
  - specified NEC — see Pregnancy, multiple (gestation), specified NEC
Gestational
- mammary abscess O91.11- ☑
- purulent mastitis O91.11- ☑
- subareolar abscess O91.11- ☑
Ghon tubercle, primary infection A15.7
Ghost
- teeth K00.4
- vessels (cornea) H16.41- ☑

Ghoul hand A66.3
Gianotti-Crosti disease L44.4
Giant
- cell
  - epulis K06.8
  - peripheral granuloma K06.8
- esophagus, congenital Q39.5
- kidney, congenital Q63.3
- urticaria T78.3- ☑
  - hereditary D84.1
Giardiasis A07.1
Gibert's disease or pityriasis L42
Giddiness R42
- hysterical F44.89
- psychogenic F45.8
Gierke's disease (glycogenosis I) E74.01
Gigantism (cerebral) (hypophyseal) (pituitary) E22.0
- constitutional E34.4
Gilbert's disease or syndrome E80.4
Gilchrist's disease B40.9
Gilford-Hutchinson disease E34.8
Gilles de la Tourette's disease or syndrome (motor-verbal tic) F95.2
Gingivitis K05.10
- acute (catarrhal) K05.00
  - necrotizing A69.1
  - nonplaque induced K05.01
  - plaque induced K05.00
- chronic (desquamative) (hyperplastic) (simple marginal) (pregnancy associated) (ulcerative) K05.10
  - nonplaque induced K05.11
  - plaque induced K05.10
- expulsiva — see Periodontitis
- necrotizing ulcerative (acute) A69.1
- pellagrous E52
  - acute necrotizing A69.1
- Vincent's A69.1
Gingivoglossitis K14.0
Gingivopericementitis — see Periodontitis
Gingivosis — see Gingivitis, chronic
Gingivostomatitis K05.10
- herpesviral B00.2
- necrotizing ulcerative (acute) A69.1
Gland, glandular — see condition
Glanders A24.0
Glanzmann (-Naegeli) **disease or thrombasthenia** D69.1
Glasgow coma scale
- total score
  - 3-8 R40.243- ☑
  - 9-12 R40.242- ☑
  - 13-15 R40.241- ☑
Glass-blower's disease (cataract) — see Cataract, specified NEC
Glaucoma H40.9
- with
  - increased episcleral venous pressure H40.81- ☑
  - pseudoexfoliation of lens — see Glaucoma, open angle, primary, capsular
- absolute H44.51- ☑
- angle-closure (primary) H40.20- ☑
  - acute (attack) (crisis) H40.21- ☑
  - chronic H40.22- ☑
  - intermittent H40.23- ☑
  - residual stage H40.24- ☑
  - secondary, neovascular H40.84- ☑
- borderline H40.00- ☑
- capsular (with pseudoexfoliation of lens) — see Glaucoma, open angle, primary, capsular
- childhood Q15.0
- closed angle — see Glaucoma, angle-closure
- congenital Q15.0
- corticosteroid-induced — see Glaucoma, secondary, drugs
- hypersecretion H40.82- ☑
- in (due to)
  - amyloidosis E85.4 [H42]
  - aniridia Q13.1 [H42]
  - concussion of globe — see Glaucoma, secondary, trauma
  - dislocation of lens — see Glaucoma, secondary
  - disorder of lens NEC — see Glaucoma, secondary
  - drugs — see Glaucoma, secondary, drugs
  - endocrine disease NOS E34.9 [H42]
  - eye
    - inflammation — see Glaucoma, secondary, inflammation
    - trauma — see Glaucoma, secondary, trauma
  - hypermature cataract — see Glaucoma, secondary

Glaucoma — continued
- in — continued
  - iridocyclitis — see Glaucoma, secondary, inflammation
  - lens disorder — see Glaucoma, secondary
  - Lowe's syndrome E72.03 [H42]
  - metabolic disease NOS E88.9 [H42]
  - ocular disorders NEC — see Glaucoma, secondary
  - onchocerciasis B73.02
  - pupillary block — see Glaucoma, secondary
  - retinal vein occlusion — see Glaucoma, secondary
  - Rieger anomaly Q13.81 [H42]
  - rubeosis of iris — see Glaucoma, secondary
  - tumor of globe — see Glaucoma, secondary
- infantile Q15.0
- low tension — see Glaucoma, open angle, primary, low-tension
- malignant H40.83- ☑
- narrow angle — see Glaucoma, angle-closure
- neovascular secondary angle closure H40.84- ☑
- newborn Q15.0
- noncongestive (chronic) — see Glaucoma, open angle
- nonobstructive — see Glaucoma, open angle
- obstructive — see also Glaucoma, angle-closure
  - due to lens changes — see Glaucoma, secondary
- open angle H40.10- ☑
  - primary H40.11- ☑
    - capsular (with pseudoexfoliation of lens) H40.14- ☑
    - low-tension H40.12- ☑
    - pigmentary H40.13- ☑
    - residual stage H40.15- ☑
- phacolytic — see Glaucoma, secondary
- pigmentary — see Glaucoma, open angle, primary, pigmentary
- postinfectious — see Glaucoma, secondary, inflammation
- secondary (to) H40.5- ☑
  - drugs H40.6- ☑
  - inflammation H40.4- ☑
  - trauma H40.3- ☑
- simple (chronic) H40.11- ☑
- simplex H40.11- ☑
- specified type NEC H40.89
- suspect H40.00- ☑
- syphilitic A52.71
- traumatic — see also Glaucoma, secondary, trauma
  - newborn (birth injury) P15.3
- tuberculous A18.59

Glaucomatous flecks (subcapsular) — see Cataract, complicated

Glazed tongue K14.4

Gleet (gonococcal) A54.01

Glenard's disease K63.4

Glioblastoma (multiforme)
- with sarcomatous component
  - specified site — see Neoplasm, malignant, by site
  - unspecified site C71.9
- giant cell
  - specified site — see Neoplasm, malignant, by site
  - unspecified site C71.9
- specified site — see Neoplasm, malignant, by site
- unspecified site C71.9

Glioma (malignant)
- astrocytic
  - specified site — see Neoplasm, malignant, by site
  - unspecified site C71.9
- mixed
  - specified site — see Neoplasm, malignant, by site
  - unspecified site C71.9
- nose Q30.8
- specified site NEC — see Neoplasm, malignant, by site
- subependymal D43.2
  - specified site — see Neoplasm, uncertain behavior, by site
  - unspecified site D43.2
- unspecified site C71.9

Gliomatosis cerebri C71.0

Glioneuroma — see Neoplasm, uncertain behavior, by site

Gliosarcoma
- specified site — see Neoplasm, malignant, by site
- unspecified site C71.9

Gliosis (cerebral) G93.89
- spinal G95.89

Glisson's disease — see Rickets

Globinuria R82.3

Globus (hystericus) F45.8

Glomangioma D18.00
- intra-abdominal D18.03
- intracranial D18.02

Glomangioma — continued
- skin D18.01
- specified site NEC D18.09

Glomangiomyoma D18.00
- intra-abdominal D18.03
- intracranial D18.02
- skin D18.01
- specified site NEC D18.09

Glomangiosarcoma — see Neoplasm, connective tissue, malignant

Glomerular
- disease in syphilis A52.75
- nephritis — see Glomerulonephritis

Glomerulitis — see Glomerulonephritis

Glomerulonephritis — see also Nephritis N05.9
- with
  - C3
    - glomerulonephritis N05.A
    - glomerulopathy N05.A
      - with dense deposit disease N05.6
  - edema — see Nephrosis
  - minimal change N05.0
  - minor glomerular abnormality N05.0
- acute N00.9
- chronic N03.9
- crescentic (diffuse) NEC — see also N00-N07 with fourth character .7 N05.7
- dense deposit — see also N00-N07 with fourth character .6 N05.6
- diffuse
  - crescentic — see also N00-N07 with fourth character .7 N05.7
  - endocapillary proliferative — see also N00-N07 with fourth character .4 N05.4
  - membranous — see also N00-N07 with fourth character .2 N05.2
  - mesangial proliferative — see also N00-N07 with fourth character .3 N05.3
  - mesangiocapillary — see also N00-N07 with fourth character .5 N05.5
  - sclerosing N18.9
- endocapillary proliferative (diffuse) NEC — see also N00-N07 with fourth character .4 N05.4
- extracapillary NEC — see also N00-N07 with fourth character .7 N05.7
- focal (and segmental) — see also N00-N07 with fourth character .1 N05.1
- hypocomplementemic — see Glomerulonephritis, membranoproliferative
- IgA — see Nephropathy, IgA
- immune complex (circulating) NEC N05.8
- in (due to)
  - amyloidosis E85.4 [N08]
  - bilharziasis B65.9 [N08]
  - cryoglobulinemia D89.1 [N08]
  - defibrination syndrome D65 [N08]
  - diabetes mellitus — see Diabetes, glomerulosclerosis
  - disseminated intravascular coagulation D65 [N08]
  - Fabry (-Anderson) disease E75.21 [N08]
  - Goodpasture's syndrome M31.0
  - hemolytic-uremic syndrome — see Syndrome, hemolytic-uremic
  - Henoch (-Schonlein) purpura D69.0 [N08]
  - lecithin cholesterol acyltransferase deficiency E78.6 [N08]
  - microscopic polyangiitis M31.7 [N08]
  - multiple myeloma C90.0- ☑ [N08]
  - Plasmodium malariae B52.0
  - schistosomiasis B65.9 [N08]
  - sepsis A41.9 [N08]
    - streptococcal A40.- ☑ [N08]
  - sickle-cell disorders D57.- ☑ [N08]
  - strongyloidiasis B78.9 [N08]
  - subacute bacterial endocarditis I33.0 [N08]
  - syphilis (late) congenital A50.59 [N08]
  - systemic lupus erythematosus M32.14
  - thrombotic thrombocytopenic purpura M31.19 [N08]
  - typhoid fever A01.09
  - Waldenstrom macroglobulinemia C88.0- ☑ [N08]
  - Wegener's granulomatosis M31.31
- latent or quiescent N03.9
- lobular, lobulonodular — see Glomerulonephritis, membranoproliferative
- membranoproliferative (diffuse)(type 1 or 3) — see also N00-N07 with fourth character .5 N05.5
  - dense deposit (type 2) NEC — see also N00-N07 with fourth character .6 N05.6
- membranous (diffuse) NEC — see also N00-N07 with fourth character .2 N05.2

Glomerulonephritis — continued
- mesangial
  - IgA/IgG — see Nephropathy, IgA
  - proliferative (diffuse) NEC — see also N00-N07 with fourth character .3 N05.3
- mesangiocapillary (diffuse) NEC — see also N00-N07 with fourth character .5 N05.5
- necrotic, necrotizing NEC — see also N00-N07 with fourth character .8 N05.8
- nodular — see Glomerulonephritis, membranoproliferative
- poststreptococcal NEC N05.9
  - acute N00.9
  - chronic N03.9
  - rapidly progressive N01.9
- proliferative NEC — see also N00-N07 with fourth character .8 N05.8
  - diffuse (lupus) M32.14
- rapidly progressive N01.9
- sclerosing, diffuse N18.9
- specified pathology NEC — see also N00-N07 with fourth character .8 N05.8
- subacute N01.9

Glomerulopathy — see Glomerulonephritis

Glomerulosclerosis — see also Sclerosis, renal
- intercapillary (nodular) (with diabetes) — see Diabetes, glomerulosclerosis
- intracapillary — see Diabetes, glomerulosclerosis

Glossagra K14.6

Glossalgia K14.6

Glossitis (chronic superficial) (gangrenous) (Moeller's) K14.0
- areata exfoliativa K14.1
- atrophic K14.4
- benign migratory K14.1
- cortical superficial, sclerotic K14.0
- Hunter's D51.0
- interstitial, sclerous K14.0
- median rhomboid K14.2
- pellagrous E52
- superficial, chronic K14.0

Glossocele K14.8

Glossodynia K14.6
- exfoliativa K14.4

Glossoncus K14.8

Glossopathy K14.9

Glossophytia K14.3

Glossoplegia K14.8

Glossoptosis K14.8

Glossopyrosis K14.6

Glossotrichia K14.3

Glossy skin L90.8

Glottis — see condition

Glottitis — see also Laryngitis J04.0

Glucagonoma
- pancreas
  - benign D13.7
  - malignant C25.4
  - uncertain behavior D37.8
- specified site NEC
  - benign — see Neoplasm, benign, by site
  - malignant — see Neoplasm, malignant, by site
  - uncertain behavior — see Neoplasm, uncertain behavior, by site
- unspecified site
  - benign D13.7
  - malignant C25.4
  - uncertain behavior D37.8

Glucoglycinuria E72.51

Glucose-galactose malabsorption E74.39

Glue
- ear — see Otitis, media, nonsuppurative, chronic, mucoid
- sniffing (airplane) — see Abuse, drug, inhalant
- dependence — see Dependence, drug, inhalant

GLUT1 deficiency syndrome 1, infantile onset E74.810

GLUT1 deficiency syndrome 2, childhood onset E74.810

Glutaric aciduria E72.3

Glycinemia E72.51

Glycinuria (renal) (with ketosis) E72.09

Glycogen
- infiltration — see Disease, glycogen storage
- storage disease — see Disease, glycogen storage

Glycogenosis (diffuse) (generalized) — see also Disease, glycogen storage
- cardiac E74.02 [I43]
- diabetic, secondary — see Diabetes, glycogenosis, secondary
- pulmonary interstitial J84.842

Glycopenia E16.2

Glycosuria R81

Glycosuria — continued
  renal E74.818
Gnathostoma spinigerum (infection) (infestation), **gnathostomiasis** (wandering swelling) B83.1
Goiter (plunging) (substernal) E04.9
  with
    hyperthyroidism (recurrent) — see Hyperthyroidism, with, goiter
    thyrotoxicosis — see Hyperthyroidism, with, goiter
  adenomatous — see Goiter, nodular
  cancerous C73
  congenital (nontoxic) E03.0
    diffuse E03.0
    parenchymatous E03.0
    transitory, with normal functioning P72.0
  cystic E04.2
    due to iodine-deficiency E01.1
  due to
    enzyme defect in synthesis of thyroid hormone E07.1
    iodine-deficiency (endemic) E01.2
  dyshormonogenetic (familial) E07.1
  endemic (iodine-deficiency) E01.2
    diffuse E01.0
    multinodular E01.1
  exophthalmic — see Hyperthyroidism, with, goiter
  iodine-deficiency (endemic) E01.2
    diffuse E01.0
    multinodular E01.1
    nodular E01.1
  lingual Q89.2
  lymphadenoid E06.3
  malignant C73
  multinodular (cystic) (nontoxic) E04.2
    toxic or with hyperthyroidism E05.20
      with thyroid storm E05.21
  neonatal NEC P72.0
  nodular (nontoxic) (due to) E04.9
    with
      hyperthyroidism E05.20
        with thyroid storm E05.21
      thyrotoxicosis E05.20
        with thyroid storm E05.21
    endemic E01.1
    iodine-deficiency E01.1
    sporadic E04.9
    toxic E05.20
      with thyroid storm E05.21
  nontoxic E04.9
    diffuse (colloid) E04.0
    multinodular E04.2
    simple E04.0
    specified NEC E04.8
    uninodular E04.1
  simple E04.0
  toxic — see Hyperthyroidism, with, goiter
  uninodular (nontoxic) E04.1
    toxic or with hyperthyroidism E05.10
      with thyroid storm E05.11
Goiter-deafness syndrome E07.1
Goldberg-Maxwell syndrome E34.51
Goldberg syndrome Q89.89
Goldblatt's hypertension or kidney I70.1
Goldenhar (-Gorlin) syndrome Q87.0
Goldflam-Erb disease or syndrome G70.00
  with exacerbation (acute) G70.01
  in crisis G70.01
Goldscheider's disease Q81.8
Goldstein's disease (familial hemorrhagic telangiectasia) I78.0
Golfer's elbow — see Epicondylitis, medial
Gonadoblastoma
  specified site — see Neoplasm, uncertain behavior, by site
  unspecified site
    female D39.10
    male D40.10
Gonecystitis — see Vesiculitis
Gongylonemiasis B83.8
Goniosynechiae — see Adhesions, iris, goniosynechiae
Gonococcemia A54.86
Gonococcus, gonococcal (disease) (infection) — see also condition A54.9
  anus A54.6
  bursa, bursitis A54.49
  conjunctiva, conjunctivitis (neonatorum) A54.31
  endocardium A54.83
  eye A54.30
    conjunctivitis A54.31
    iridocyclitis A54.32

Gonococcus, gonococcal — continued
  eye — continued
    keratitis A54.33
    newborn A54.31
    other specified A54.39
  fallopian tubes (acute) (chronic) A54.24
  genitourinary (organ) (system) (tract) (acute)
    lower A54.00
      with abscess (accessory gland) (periurethral) A54.1
    upper — see also condition A54.29
  heart A54.83
  iridocyclitis A54.32
  joint A54.42
  lymphatic (gland) (node) A54.89
  meninges, meningitis A54.81
  musculoskeletal A54.40
    arthritis A54.42
    osteomyelitis A54.43
    other specified A54.49
    spondylopathy A54.41
  pelviperitonitis A54.24
  pelvis (acute) (chronic) A54.24
  pharynx A54.5
  proctitis A54.6
  pyosalpinx (acute) (chronic) A54.24
  rectum A54.6
  skin A54.89
  specified site NEC A54.89
  tendon sheath A54.49
  throat A54.5
  urethra (acute) (chronic) A54.01
    with abscess (accessory gland) (periurethral) A54.1
  vulva (acute) (chronic) A54.02
Gonocytoma
  specified site — see Neoplasm, uncertain behavior, by site
  unspecified site
    female D39.10
    male D40.10
Gonorrhea (acute) (chronic) A54.9
  Bartholin's gland (acute) (chronic) (purulent) A54.02
    with abscess (accessory gland) (periurethral) A54.1
  bladder A54.01
  cervix A54.03
  conjunctiva, conjunctivitis (neonatorum) A54.31
  contact Z20.2
  Cowper's gland (with abscess) A54.1
  exposure to Z20.2
  fallopian tube (acute) (chronic) A54.24
  kidney (acute) (chronic) A54.21
  lower genitourinary tract A54.00
    with abscess (accessory gland) (periurethral) A54.1
  ovary (acute) (chronic) A54.24
  pelvis (acute) (chronic) A54.24
    female pelvic inflammatory disease A54.24
  penis A54.09
  prostate (acute) (chronic) A54.22
  seminal vesicle (acute) (chronic) A54.23
  specified site not listed — see also Gonococcus A54.89
  spermatic cord (acute) (chronic) A54.23
  urethra A54.01
    with abscess (accessory gland) (periurethral) A54.1
  vagina A54.02
  vas deferens (acute) (chronic) A54.23
  vulva A54.02
Goodall's disease A08.19
Goodpasture's syndrome M31.0
Gopalan's syndrome (burning feet) E53.0
Gorlin-Chaudry-Moss syndrome Q87.0
Gottron's papules L94.4
Gougerot-Blum syndrome (pigmented purpuric lichenoid dermatitis) L81.7
Gougerot-Carteaud disease or syndrome (confluent reticulate papillomatosis) L83
Gougerot's syndrome (trisymptomatic) L81.7
Gouley's syndrome (constrictive pericarditis) I31.1
Goundou A66.6
Gout, chronic — see also Gout, gouty M1A.9- ☑ (following M08)
  drug-induced M1A.20- ☑ (following M08)
    ankle M1A.27- ☑ (following M08)
    elbow M1A.22- ☑ (following M08)
    foot joint M1A.27- ☑ (following M08)
    hand joint M1A.24- ☑ (following M08)
    hip M1A.25- ☑ (following M08)
    knee M1A.26- ☑ (following M08)
    multiple site M1A.29- ☑ (following M08)
    shoulder M1A.21- ☑ (following M08)

Gout, chronic — continued
  drug-induced — continued
    vertebrae M1A.28- ☑ (following M08)
    wrist M1A.23- ☑ (following M08)
  idiopathic M1A.00- ☑ (following M08)
    ankle M1A.07- ☑ (following M08)
    elbow M1A.02- ☑ (following M08)
    foot joint M1A.07- ☑ (following M08)
    hand joint M1A.04- ☑ (following M08)
    hip M1A.05- ☑ (following M08)
    knee M1A.06- ☑ (following M08)
    multiple site M1A.09- ☑ (following M08)
    shoulder M1A.01- ☑ (following M08)
    vertebrae M1A.08- ☑ (following M08)
    wrist M1A.03- ☑ (following M08)
  in (due to) renal impairment M1A.30- ☑ (following M08)
    ankle M1A.37- ☑ (following M08)
    elbow M1A.32- ☑ (following M08)
    foot joint M1A.37- ☑ (following M08)
    hand joint M1A.34- ☑ (following M08)
    hip M1A.35- ☑ (following M08)
    knee M1A.36- ☑ (following M08)
    multiple site M1A.39- ☑ (following M08)
    shoulder M1A.31- ☑ (following M08)
    vertebrae M1A.38- ☑ (following M08)
    wrist M1A.33- ☑ (following M08)
  lead-induced M1A.10- ☑ (following M08)
    ankle M1A.17- ☑ (following M08)
    elbow M1A.12- ☑ (following M08)
    foot joint M1A.17- ☑ (following M08)
    hand joint M1A.14- ☑ (following M08)
    hip M1A.15- ☑ (following M08)
    knee M1A.16- ☑ (following M08)
    multiple site M1A.19- ☑ (following M08)
    shoulder M1A.11- ☑ (following M08)
    vertebrae M1A.18- ☑ (following M08)
    wrist M1A.13- ☑ (following M08)
  primary — see Gout, chronic, idiopathic
  saturnine — see Gout, chronic, lead-induced
  secondary NEC M1A.40- ☑ (following M08)
    ankle M1A.47- ☑ (following M08)
    elbow M1A.42- ☑ (following M08)
    foot joint M1A.47- ☑ (following M08)
    hand joint M1A.44- ☑ (following M08)
    hip M1A.45- ☑ (following M08)
    knee M1A.46- ☑ (following M08)
    multiple site M1A.49- ☑ (following M08)
    shoulder M1A.41- ☑ (following M08)
    vertebrae M1A.48- ☑ (following M08)
    wrist M1A.43- ☑ (following M08)
  syphilitic — see also subcategory M14.8- A52.77
  tophi M1A.9- ☑ (following M08)
Gout, gouty (acute) (attack) (flare) — see also Gout, chronic M10.9
  drug-induced M10.20
    ankle M10.27- ☑
    elbow M10.22- ☑
    foot joint M10.27- ☑
    hand joint M10.24- ☑
    hip M10.25- ☑
    knee M10.26- ☑
    multiple site M10.29
    shoulder M10.21- ☑
    vertebrae M10.28
    wrist M10.23- ☑
  idiopathic M10.00
    ankle M10.07- ☑
    elbow M10.02- ☑
    foot joint M10.07- ☑
    hand joint M10.04- ☑
    hip M10.05- ☑
    knee M10.06- ☑
    multiple site M10.09
    shoulder M10.01- ☑
    vertebrae M10.08
    wrist M10.03- ☑
  in (due to) renal impairment M10.30
    ankle M10.37- ☑
    elbow M10.32- ☑
    foot joint M10.37- ☑
    hand joint M10.34- ☑
    hip M10.35- ☑
    knee M10.36- ☑
    multiple site M10.39
    shoulder M10.31- ☑

Gout, gouty — continued
- in renal impairment — continued
  - vertebrae M10.38
  - wrist M10.33- ☑
- lead-induced M10.10
  - ankle M10.17- ☑
  - elbow M10.12- ☑
  - foot joint M10.17- ☑
  - hand joint M10.14- ☑
  - hip M10.15- ☑
  - knee M10.16- ☑
  - multiple site M10.19
  - shoulder M10.11- ☑
  - vertebrae M10.18
  - wrist M10.13- ☑
- primary — see Gout, idiopathic
- saturnine — see Gout, lead-induced
- secondary NEC M10.40
  - ankle M10.47- ☑
  - elbow M10.42- ☑
  - foot joint M10.47- ☑
  - hand joint M10.44- ☑
  - hip M10.45- ☑
  - knee M10.46- ☑
  - multiple site M10.49
  - shoulder M10.41- ☑
  - vertebrae M10.48
  - wrist M10.43- ☑
- syphilitic — see also subcategory M14.8- A52.77
- tophi — see Gout, chronic

Gower's
- muscular dystrophy G71.01
- syndrome (vasovagal attack) R55

Gradenigo's syndrome — see Otitis, media, suppurative, acute

Graefe's disease — see Strabismus, paralytic, ophthalmoplegia, progressive

Graft-versus-host disease D89.813
- acute D89.810
- acute on chronic D89.812
- chronic D89.811

Grain mite (itch) B88.09
Grainhandler's disease or lung J67.8
Grand mal — see Epilepsy, generalized, specified NEC
Grand multipara status only (not pregnant) Z64.1
- pregnant — see Pregnancy, complicated by, grand multiparity

Granite worker's lung J62.8
Granular — see also condition
- inflammation, pharynx J31.2
- kidney (contracting) — see Sclerosis, renal
- liver K74.69

Granulation tissue (abnormal) (excessive) L92.9
- postmastoidectomy cavity — see Complications, postmastoidectomy, granulation

Granulocytopenia (primary) (malignant) — see Agranulocytosis

Granuloma L92.9
- abdomen K66.8
  - from residual foreign body L92.3
  - pyogenicum L98.0
- actinic L57.5
- annulare (perforating) L92.0
- apical K04.5
- aural — see Otitis, externa, specified NEC
- beryllium (skin) L92.3
- bone
  - eosinophilic C96.6
  - from residual foreign body — see Osteomyelitis, specified type NEC
  - lung C96.6
- brain (any site) G06.0
  - schistosomiasis B65.9 [G07]
- canaliculus lacrimalis — see Granuloma, lacrimal
- candidal (cutaneous) B37.2
- cerebral (any site) G06.0
- coccidioidal (primary) (progressive) B38.7
  - lung B38.1
  - meninges B38.4
- colon K63.89
- conjunctiva H11.22- ☑
- dental K04.5
- ear, middle — see Cholesteatoma
- eosinophilic C96.6
  - bone C96.6
  - lung C96.6
  - oral mucosa K13.4
  - skin L92.2

Granuloma — continued
- eyelid H01.8- ☑
- facial (e) L92.2
- foreign body (in soft tissue) NEC M60.20
  - ankle M60.27- ☑
  - foot M60.27- ☑
  - forearm M60.23- ☑
  - hand M60.24- ☑
  - in operation wound — see Foreign body, accidentally left during a procedure
  - lower leg M60.26- ☑
  - pelvic region M60.25- ☑
  - shoulder region M60.21- ☑
  - skin L92.3
  - specified site NEC M60.28
  - subcutaneous tissue L92.3
  - thigh M60.25- ☑
  - upper arm M60.22- ☑
- gangraenescens M31.2
- genito-inguinale A58
- giant cell (central) (reparative) (jaw) M27.1
  - gingiva (peripheral) K06.8
- gland (lymph) I88.8
- hepatic NEC K75.3
  - in (due to)
    - berylliosis J63.2 [K77]
    - sarcoidosis D86.89
- Hodgkin C81.9- ☑
- ileum K63.89
- infectious B99.9
  - specified NEC B99.8
- inguinale (Donovan) (venereal) A58
- intestine NEC K63.89
- intracranial (any site) G06.0
- intraspinal (any part) G06.1
- iridocyclitis — see Iridocyclitis, chronic
- jaw (bone) (central) M27.1
  - reparative giant cell M27.1
- kidney — see also Infection, kidney N15.8
- lacrimal H04.81- ☑
- larynx J38.7
- lethal midline (faciale(e)) M31.2
- liver NEC — see Granuloma, hepatic
- lung (infectious) — see also Fibrosis, lung
  - coccidioidal B38.1
  - eosinophilic C96.6
- Majocchi's B35.8
- malignant (facial(e)) M31.2
- mandible (central) M27.1
- midline (lethal) M31.2
- monilial (cutaneous) B37.2
- nasal sinus — see Sinusitis
- operation wound T81.89- ☑
  - foreign body — see Foreign body, accidentally left during a procedure
  - stitch T81.89- ☑
  - talc — see Foreign body, accidentally left during a procedure
- oral mucosa K13.4
- orbit, orbital H05.11- ☑
- paracoccidioidal B41.8
- penis, venereal A58
- periapical K04.5
- peritoneum K66.8
  - due to ova of helminths NOS — see also Helminthiasis B83.9 [K67]
- postmastoidectomy cavity — see Complications, postmastoidectomy, recurrent cholesteatoma
- prostate N42.89
- pudendi (ulcerating) A58
- pulp, internal (tooth) K03.3
- pyogenic, pyogenicum (of) (skin) L98.0
  - gingiva K06.8
  - maxillary alveolar ridge K04.5
  - oral mucosa K13.4
- rectum K62.89
- reticulohistiocytic D76.3
- rubrum nasi L74.8
- Schistosoma — see Schistosomiasis
- septic (skin) L98.0
- silica (skin) L92.3
- sinus (accessory) (infective) (nasal) — see Sinusitis
- skin L92.9
  - from residual foreign body L92.3
  - pyogenicum L98.0
- spine
  - syphilitic (epidural) A52.19
  - tuberculous A18.01

Granuloma — continued
- stitch (postoperative) T81.89- ☑
- suppurative (skin) L98.0
- swimming pool A31.1
- talc — see also Granuloma, foreign body
  - in operation wound — see Foreign body, accidentally left during a procedure
- telangiectaticum (skin) L98.0
- tracheostomy J95.09
- trichophyticum B35.8
- tropicum A66.4
- umbilical P83.81
- umbilicus P83.81
- urethra N36.8
- uveitis — see Iridocyclitis, chronic
- vagina A58
- venereum A58
- vocal cord J38.3

Granulomatosis L92.9
- with polyangiitis M31.3- ☑
- eosinophilic, with polyangiitis [EGPA] M30.1
- lymphoid C83.8- ☑
- miliary (listerial) A32.89
- necrotizing, respiratory M31.30
- progressive septic D71.8
- specified NEC L92.8
- Wegener's M31.30
  - with renal involvement M31.31

Granulomatous tissue (abnormal) (excessive) L92.9
Granulosis rubra nasi L74.8
Graphite fibrosis (of lung) J63.3
Graphospasm F48.8
- organic G25.89

Grating scapula M89.8X1
Gravel (urinary) — see Calculus, urinary
Graves' disease — see Hyperthyroidism, with, goiter
Gravis — see condition
Grawitz tumor C64.- ☑
Gray syndrome (newborn) P93.0
Grayness, hair (premature) L67.1
- congenital Q84.2

Green sickness D50.8
Greenfield's disease
- meaning
  - concentric sclerosis (encephalitis periaxialis concentrica) G37.5
  - metachromatic leukodystrophy E75.25

Greenstick fracture — code as Fracture, by site
Grey syndrome (newborn) P93.0
Grief F43.21
- complicated F43.81
- prolonged F43.81
- reaction — see also Disorder, adjustment F43.20

Griesinger's disease B76.0
Grinder's lung or pneumoconiosis J62.8
Grinding, teeth
- psychogenic F45.8
- sleep related G47.63

Grip
- Dabney's B33.0
- devil's B33.0

Grippe, grippal — see also Influenza
- Balkan A78
- summer, of Italy A93.1

Grisel's disease M43.6
Groin — see condition
Grooved tongue K14.5
Ground itch B76.9
Grover's disease or syndrome L11.1
Growing pains, children R29.898
Growth (fungoid) (neoplastic) (new) — see also Neoplasm
- adenoid (vegetative) J35.8
- benign — see Neoplasm, benign, by site
- malignant — see Neoplasm, malignant, by site
- rapid, childhood Z00.2
- secondary — see Neoplasm, secondary, by site

Gruby's disease B35.0
Guardianship by non-parental relative Z62.23
Gubler-Millard paralysis or syndrome G46.3
Guerin-Stern syndrome Q74.3
Guidance, insufficient anterior (occlusal) M26.54
Guillain-Barre disease or syndrome G61.0
- sequelae G65.0

Guinea worms (infection) (infestation) B72
Guinon's disease (motor-verbal tic) F95.2
Gull's disease E03.4
Gum — see condition
Gumboil K04.7
- with sinus K04.6

Gumma (syphilitic) A52.79
- artery A52.09
  - cerebral A52.04
- bone A52.77
  - of yaws (late) A66.6
- brain A52.19
- cauda equina A52.19
- central nervous system A52.3
- ciliary body A52.71
- congenital A50.59
- eyelid A52.71
- heart A52.06
- intracranial A52.19
- iris A52.71
- kidney A52.75
- larynx A52.73
- leptomeninges A52.19
- liver A52.74
- meninges A52.19
- myocardium A52.06
- nasopharynx A52.73
- neurosyphilitic A52.3
- nose A52.73
- orbit A52.71
- palate (soft) A52.79
- penis A52.76
- pericardium A52.06
- pharynx A52.73
- pituitary A52.79
- scrofulous (tuberculous) A18.4
- skin A52.79
- specified site NEC A52.79
- spinal cord A52.19
- tongue A52.79
- tonsil A52.73
- trachea A52.73
- tuberculous A18.4
- ulcerative due to yaws A66.4
- ureter A52.75
- yaws A66.4
  - bone A66.6

Gunn's syndrome Q07.8
Gunshot wound — *see also* Puncture, open
- fracture — *code as* Fracture, by site
- internal organs — *see* Injury, by site

Gynandrism Q56.0
Gynandroblastoma
- specified site — *see* Neoplasm, uncertain behavior, by site
- unspecified site
  - female D39.10
  - male D40.10

Gynecological examination (periodic) (routine) Z01.419
- with abnormal findings Z01.411

Gynecomastia N62
Gynephobia F40.291
Gyrate scalp Q82.8

H

H-ABC (hypomyelination with atrophy of the basal ganglia and cerebellum) G23.3
H (Hartnup's) **disease** E72.02
Haas' disease or osteochondrosis (juvenile) (head of humerus) — *see* Osteochondrosis, juvenile, humerus
Habit, habituation
- bad sleep Z72.821
- chorea F95.8
- disturbance, child F98.9
- drug — *see* Dependence, drug
- irregular sleep Z72.821
- laxative F55.2
- spasm — *see* Tic
- tic — *see* Tic

Haemophilus (H.) **influenzae, as cause of disease classified elsewhere** B96.3
Haff disease — *see* Poisoning, mercury
HAFOUS (Hao-Fountain syndrome) Q87.87
Hageman's factor defect, deficiency or disease D68.2
Haglund's disease or osteochondrosis (juvenile) (os tibiale externum) — *see* Osteochondrosis, juvenile, tarsus
Hailey-Hailey disease Q82.8
Hair — *see also* condition
- plucking F63.3
  - in stereotyped movement disorder F98.4
- tourniquet syndrome — *see also* Constriction, external, by site
  - finger S60.44- ☑

Hair — *continued*
- tourniquet syndrome — *see also* Constriction, external, by site — *continued*
  - penis S30.842- ☑
  - thumb S60.34- ☑
  - toe S90.44- ☑

Hair-pulling, pathological (compulsive) F63.3
Hairball in stomach T18.2- ☑
Hairy black tongue K14.3
Half vertebra Q76.49
Halitosis R19.6
Hallerman-Streiff syndrome Q87.0
Hallervorden-Spatz disease G23.0
Hallopeau's acrodermatitis or disease L40.2
Hallucination R44.3
- auditory R44.0
- gustatory R44.2
- olfactory R44.2
- specified NEC R44.2
- tactile R44.2
- visual R44.1

Hallucinosis (chronic) F28
- alcoholic (acute) F10.951
  - in
    - abuse F10.151
    - dependence F10.251
- drug-induced F19.951
  - cannabis F12.951
  - cocaine F14.951
  - hallucinogen F16.151
    - in
      - abuse F19.151
        - cannabis F12.151
        - cocaine F14.151
        - hallucinogen F16.151
        - inhalant F18.151
        - opioid F11.151
        - sedative, anxiolytic or hypnotic F13.151
        - stimulant NEC F15.151
      - dependence F19.251
        - cannabis F12.251
        - cocaine F14.251
        - hallucinogen F16.251
        - inhalant F18.251
        - opioid F11.251
        - sedative, anxiolytic or hypnotic F13.251
        - stimulant NEC F15.251
  - inhalant F18.951
  - opioid F11.951
  - sedative, anxiolytic or hypnotic F13.951
  - stimulant NEC F15.951
- organic F06.0

Hallux
- deformity (acquired) NEC M20.5X- ☑
- limitus M20.5X- ☑
- malleus (acquired) NEC M20.3- ☑
- rigidus (acquired) M20.2- ☑
  - congenital Q74.2
  - sequelae (late effect) of rickets E64.3
- valgus (acquired) M20.1- ☑
  - congenital Q66.6
- varus (acquired) M20.3- ☑
  - congenital Q66.3- ☑

Halo, visual H53.19
Hamartoma, hamartoblastoma Q85.9
- epithelial (gingival), odontogenic, central or peripheral — *see* Cyst, calcifying odontogenic

Hamartosis Q85.9
Hamman-Rich syndrome J84.114
Hammer toe (acquired) NEC — *see also* Deformity, toe, hammer toe
- congenital Q66.89
- sequelae (late effect) of rickets E64.3

Hand — *see* condition
Hand-foot syndrome L27.1
Hand-Schuller-Christian disease or syndrome C96.5
Handicap, handicapped
- educational Z55.9
  - specified NEC Z55.8

Hanging (asphyxia) (strangulation) (suffocation) — *see* Asphyxia, traumatic, due to mechanical threat
Hangnail — *see also* Cellulitis, digit
- with lymphangitis — *see* Lymphangitis, acute, digit

Hangover (alcohol) F10.129
Hanhart's syndrome Q87.0
Hanot-Chauffard (-Troisier) **syndrome** E83.19
Hanot's cirrhosis or disease K74.3
Hansen's disease — *see* Leprosy

Hantaan virus disease (Korean hemorrhagic fever) A98.5
Hantavirus disease (with renal manifestations) (Dobrava) (Puumala) (Seoul) A98.5
- with pulmonary manifestations (Andes) (Bayou) (Bermejo) (Black Creek Canal) (Choclo) (Juquitiba) (Laguna negra) (Lechiguanas) (New York) (Oran) (Sin nombre) B33.4

Happy puppet syndrome Q93.51
Harada's disease or syndrome H30.81- ☑
Hardening
- artery — *see* Arteriosclerosis
- brain G93.89

Hardship, material, due to limited financial resources, specified NEC Z59.87
Harelip (complete) (incomplete) — *see* Cleft, lip
Harlequin (newborn) Q80.4
Harley's disease D59.6
Harmful use (of)
- alcohol F10.10
- anxiolytics — *see* Abuse, drug, sedative
- cannabinoids — *see* Abuse, drug, cannabis
- cocaine — *see* Abuse, drug, cocaine
- drug — *see* Abuse, drug
- hallucinogens — *see* Abuse, drug, hallucinogen
- hypnotics — *see* Abuse, drug, sedative
- opioids — *see* Abuse, drug, opioid
- PCP (phencyclidine) — *see* Abuse, drug, hallucinogen
- sedatives — *see* Abuse, drug, sedative
- stimulants NEC — *see* Abuse, drug, stimulant

Harris' lines — *see* Arrest, epiphyseal
Hartnup's disease E72.02
Harvester's lung J67.0
Harvesting ovum for in vitro fertilization Z31.83
Hashimoto's disease or thyroiditis E06.3
Hashitoxicosis (transient) E06.3
Hassal-Henle bodies or warts (cornea) H18.49
Haut mal — *see* Epilepsy, generalized, specified NEC
Haverhill fever A25.1
Hay fever — *see also* Fever, hay J30.1
Hayem-Widal syndrome D59.8
Haygarth's nodes M15.8
Haymaker's lung J67.0
Hb (abnormal)
- Bart's disease D56.0
- disease — *see* Disease, hemoglobin
- trait — *see* Trait

Head — *see* condition
Headache R51.9
- with
  - orthostatic component NEC R51.0
  - positional component NEC R51.0
- allergic NEC G44.89
- associated with sexual activity G44.82
- cervicogenic G44.86
- chronic daily R51.9
- cluster G44.009
  - chronic G44.029
    - intractable G44.021
    - not intractable G44.029
  - episodic G44.019
    - intractable G44.011
    - not intractable G44.019
  - intractable G44.001
  - not intractable G44.009
- cough (primary) G44.83
- daily chronic R51.9
- drug-induced NEC G44.40
  - intractable G44.41
  - not intractable G44.40
- exertional (primary) G44.84
- histamine G44.009
  - intractable G44.001
  - not intractable G44.009
- hypnic G44.81
- lumbar puncture G97.1
- medication overuse G44.40
  - intractable G44.41
  - not intractable G44.40
- menstrual — *see* Migraine, menstrual
- migraine (type) — *see also* Migraine G43.909
- nasal septum R51.9
- neuralgiform, short lasting unilateral, with conjunctival injection and tearing (SUNCT) G44.059
  - intractable G44.051
  - not intractable G44.059
- new daily persistent (NDPH) G44.52
- orgasmic G44.82
- periodic syndromes in adults and children G43.C0 (*following* G43.7)

Headache — *continued*
  periodic syndromes in adults and children — *continued*
    with refractory migraine G43.C1 (*following* G43.7)
    intractable G43.C1 (*following* G43.7)
    not intractable G43.C0 (*following* G43.7)
    without refractory migraine G43.C0 (*following* G43.7)
  postspinal puncture G97.1
  post-traumatic G44.309
    acute G44.319
      intractable G44.311
      not intractable G44.319
    chronic G44.329
      intractable G44.321
      not intractable G44.329
    intractable G44.301
    not intractable G44.309
  pre-menstrual — *see* Migraine, menstrual
  preorgasmic G44.82
  primary
    cough G44.83
    exertional G44.84
    stabbing G44.85
    thunderclap G44.53
  rebound G44.40
    intractable G44.41
    not intractable G44.40
  short lasting unilateral neuralgiform, with conjunctival injection and tearing (SUNCT) G44.059
    intractable G44.051
    not intractable G44.059
  specified syndrome NEC G44.89
  spinal and epidural anesthesia - induced T88.59- ☑
    in labor and delivery O74.5
    in pregnancy O29.4- ☑
      postpartum, puerperal O89.4
  spinal fluid loss (from puncture) G97.1
  stabbing (primary) G44.85
  tension (-type) G44.209
    chronic G44.229
      intractable G44.221
      not intractable G44.229
    episodic G44.219
      intractable G44.211
      not intractable G44.219
    intractable G44.201
    not intractable G44.209
  thunderclap (primary) G44.53
  vascular NEC G44.1
Healthy
  infant
    accompanying sick mother Z76.3
    receiving care Z76.2
  person accompanying sick person Z76.3
Hearing examination Z01.10
  with abnormal findings NEC Z01.118
  following failed hearing screening Z01.110
  for hearing conservation and treatment Z01.12
  infant or child (over 28 days old) Z00.129
    with abnormal findings Z00.121
Heart — *see* condition
  carcinoid — *see* Syndrome, carcinoid, heart
Heart beat
  abnormality R00.9
    specified NEC R00.8
  awareness R00.2
  rapid R00.0
  slow R00.1
Heartburn R12
  psychogenic F45.8
Heartland virus disease A93.8
Heat (effects) T67.9- ☑
  apoplexy T67.01- ☑
  burn — *see also* Burn L55.9
  collapse T67.1- ☑
  cramps T67.2- ☑
  dermatitis or eczema L59.0
  edema T67.7- ☑
  erythema — *code by site under* Burn, first degree
  excessive T67.9- ☑
    specified effect NEC T67.8- ☑
  exhaustion T67.5- ☑
    anhydrotic T67.3- ☑
    due to
      salt (and water) depletion T67.4- ☑
      water depletion T67.3- ☑
        with salt depletion T67.4- ☑
  fatigue (transient) T67.6- ☑

Heat — *continued*
  fever T67.01- ☑
  hyperpyrexia T67.01- ☑
  prickly L74.0
  prostration — *see* Heat, exhaustion
  pyrexia T67.01- ☑
  rash L74.0
  specified effect NEC T67.8- ☑
  stroke T67.01- ☑
    exertional T67.02- ☑
    specified NEC T67.09- ☑
  sunburn — *see* Sunburn
  syncope T67.1- ☑
Heavy-for-dates NEC (infant) (4000g to 4499g) P08.1
  exceptionally (4500g or more) P08.0
Hebephrenia, hebephrenic (schizophrenia) F20.1
Heberden's disease or nodes (with arthropathy) M15.1
Hebra's
  pityriasis L26
  prurigo L28.2
Heel — *see* condition
Heerfordt's disease D86.89
HeFH (heterozygous familial hypercholesterolemia) E78.011
Hegglin's anomaly or syndrome D72.0
Heilmeyer-Schoner disease D45
Heine-Medin disease A80.9
Heinz body anemia, congenital D58.2
Heliophobia F40.228
Heller's disease or syndrome F84.3
HELLP syndrome (hemolysis, elevated liver enzymes and low platelet count) O14.2- ☑
  complicating
    childbirth O14.24
    puerperium O14.25
Helminthiasis — *see also* Infestation, helminth
  Ancylostoma B76.0
  intestinal B82.0
    mixed types (types classifiable to more than one of the titles B65.0-B81.3 and B81.8) B81.4
      specified type NEC B81.8
  mixed types (intestinal) (types classifiable to more than one of the titles B65.0-B81.3 and B81.8) B81.4
  Necator (americanus) B76.1
  specified type NEC B83.8
Heloma L84
Hemangioblastoma — *see* Neoplasm, connective tissue, uncertain behavior
  malignant — *see* Neoplasm, connective tissue, malignant
Hemangioendothelioma — *see also* Neoplasm, uncertain behavior, by site
  benign D18.00
    intra-abdominal D18.03
    intracranial D18.02
    skin D18.01
    specified site NEC D18.09
  bone (diffuse) — *see* Neoplasm, bone, malignant
  epithelioid — *see also* Neoplasm, uncertain behavior, by site
    malignant — *see* Neoplasm, malignant, by site
  malignant — *see* Neoplasm, connective tissue, malignant
Hemangiofibroma — *see* Neoplasm, benign, by site
Hemangiolipoma — *see* Lipoma
Hemangioma D18.00
  arteriovenous D18.00
    intra-abdominal D18.03
    intracranial D18.02
    skin D18.01
    specified site NEC D18.09
  capillary I78.1
    intra-abdominal D18.03
    intracranial D18.02
    skin D18.01
    specified site NEC D18.09
  cavernous D18.00
    intra-abdominal D18.03
    intracranial D18.02
    skin D18.01
    specified site NEC D18.09
  epithelioid D18.00
    intra-abdominal D18.03
    intracranial D18.02
    skin D18.01
    specified site NEC D18.09
  histiocytoid D18.00
    intra-abdominal D18.03
    intracranial D18.02
    skin D18.01
    specified site NEC D18.09

Hemangioma — *continued*
  infantile D18.00
    intra-abdominal D18.03
    intracranial D18.02
    skin D18.01
    specified site NEC D18.09
  intra-abdominal D18.03
  intracranial D18.02
  intramuscular D18.00
    intra-abdominal D18.03
    intracranial D18.02
    skin D18.01
    specified site NEC D18.09
  intrathoracic structures D18.09
  juvenile D18.00
  malignant — *see* Neoplasm, connective tissue, malignant
  plexiform D18.00
    intra-abdominal D18.03
    intracranial D18.02
    skin D18.01
    specified site NEC D18.09
  racemose D18.00
    intra-abdominal D18.03
    intracranial D18.02
    skin D18.01
    specified site NEC D18.09
  sclerosing — *see* Neoplasm, skin, benign
  simplex D18.00
    intra-abdominal D18.03
    intracranial D18.02
    skin D18.01
    specified site NEC D18.09
  skin D18.01
  specified site NEC D18.09
  venous D18.00
    intra-abdominal D18.03
    intracranial D18.02
    skin D18.01
    specified site NEC D18.09
  verrucous keratotic D18.00
    intra-abdominal D18.03
    intracranial D18.02
    skin D18.01
    specified site NEC D18.09
Hemangiomatosis (systemic) I78.8
  involving single site — *see* Hemangioma
Hemangiopericytoma — *see also* Neoplasm, connective tissue, uncertain behavior
  benign — *see* Neoplasm, connective tissue, benign
  malignant — *see* Neoplasm, connective tissue, malignant
Hemangiosarcoma — *see* Neoplasm, connective tissue, malignant
Hemarthrosis (nontraumatic) M25.00
  ankle M25.07- ☑
  elbow M25.02- ☑
  foot joint M25.07- ☑
  hand joint M25.04- ☑
  hip M25.05- ☑
  in hemophilic arthropathy — *see* Arthropathy, hemophilic
  knee M25.06- ☑
  shoulder M25.01- ☑
  specified joint NEC M25.08
  traumatic — *see* Sprain, by site
  vertebrae M25.08
  wrist M25.03- ☑
Hematemesis K92.0
  with ulcer — *code by site under* Ulcer, with hemorrhage K27.4
  newborn, neonatal P54.0
    due to swallowed maternal blood P78.2
Hematidrosis L74.8
Hematinuria — *see also* Hemoglobinuria
  malarial B50.8
Hematobilia K83.8
Hematocele
  female NEC N94.89
    with ectopic pregnancy O00.90
      with intrauterine pregnancy O00.91
    ovary N83.8
  male N50.1
Hematochezia — *see also* Melena K92.1
Hematochyluria — *see also* Infestation, filarial
  schistosomiasis (bilharziasis) B65.0
Hematocolpos (with hematometra or hematosalpinx) N89.7
Hematocornea — *see* Pigmentation, cornea, stromal
Hematogenous — *see* condition

Hematoma (traumatic) (skin surface intact) — *see also* Contusion
- with
  - injury of internal organs — *see* Injury, by site
  - open wound — *see* Wound, open
- amputation stump (surgical) (late) T87.89
- aorta, dissecting I71.00
  - abdominal I71.02
  - thoracic — *see also* Dissection, aorta, thoracic I71.019
  - thoracoabdominal I71.03
- aortic intramural — *see* Dissection, aorta
- arterial (complicating trauma) — *see* Injury, blood vessel, by site
- auricle — *see* Contusion, ear
  - nontraumatic — *see* Disorder, pinna, hematoma
- birth injury NEC P15.8
- brain (traumatic)
  - with
    - cerebral laceration or contusion (diffuse) — *see* Injury, intracranial, diffuse
      - focal — *see* Injury, intracranial, focal
  - cerebellar, traumatic S06.37- ☑
  - intracerebral, traumatic — *see* Injury, intracranial, intracerebral hemorrhage
  - newborn NEC P52.4
    - birth injury P10.1
  - nontraumatic — *see* Hemorrhage, intracranial
  - subarachnoid, arachnoid, traumatic — *see* Injury, intracranial, subarachnoid hemorrhage
  - subdural, traumatic — *see* Injury, intracranial, subdural hemorrhage
- breast (nontraumatic) N64.89
- broad ligament (nontraumatic) N83.7
  - traumatic S37.892- ☑
- cerebellar, traumatic S06.37- ☑
- cerebral — *see* Hematoma, brain
- cerebrum S06.36- ☑
  - left S06.35- ☑
  - right S06.34- ☑
- cesarean delivery wound O90.2
- complicating delivery (perineal) (pelvic) (vagina) (vulva) O71.7
- corpus cavernosum (nontraumatic) N48.89
- epididymis (nontraumatic) N50.1
- epidural (traumatic) — *see* Injury, intracranial, epidural hemorrhage
  - spinal — *see* Injury, spinal cord, by region
- episiotomy O90.2
- face, birth injury P15.4
- genital organ NEC (nontraumatic)
  - female (nonobstetric) N94.89
    - traumatic S30.202- ☑
  - male N50.1
    - traumatic S30.201- ☑
- internal organs — *see* Injury, by site
- intracerebral, traumatic — *see* Injury, intracranial, intracerebral hemorrhage
- intraoperative — *see* Complications, intraoperative, hemorrhage
- labia (nontraumatic) (nonobstetric) N90.89
- liver (subcapsular) (nontraumatic) K76.89
  - birth injury P15.0
- mediastinum — *see* Injury, intrathoracic
- mesosalpinx (nontraumatic) N83.7
  - traumatic S37.898- ☑
- muscle — code by site under Contusion
- nontraumatic
  - muscle M79.81
  - soft tissue M79.81
- obstetrical surgical wound O90.2
- orbit, orbital (nontraumatic) — *see also* Hemorrhage, orbit
  - traumatic — *see* Contusion, orbit
- pelvis (female) (nontraumatic) (nonobstetric) N94.89
  - obstetric O71.7
  - traumatic — *see* Injury, by site
- penis (nontraumatic) N48.89
  - birth injury P15.5
- perianal (nontraumatic) K64.5
- perineal S30.23-
  - complicating delivery O71.7
- perirenal — *see* Injury, kidney
- peritoneal K66.1
- pinna — *see* Contusion, ear
  - nontraumatic — *see* Disorder, pinna, hematoma
- placenta O43.89- ☑
- postoperative (postprocedural) — *see* Complication, postprocedural, hematoma

Hematoma — *continued*
- retroperitoneal (nontraumatic) K68.3
  - traumatic S36.892- ☑
- scrotum, superficial S30.22- ☑
  - birth injury P15.5
- seminal vesicle (nontraumatic) N50.1
  - traumatic S37.892- ☑
- spermatic cord (traumatic) S37.892- ☑
  - nontraumatic N50.1
- spinal (cord) (meninges) — *see also* Injury, spinal cord, by region
  - newborn (birth injury) P11.5
- spleen D73.5
  - intraoperative — *see* Complications, intraoperative, hemorrhage, spleen
  - postprocedural (postoperative) — *see* Complications, postprocedural, hemorrhage, spleen
- sternocleidomastoid, birth injury P15.2
- sternomastoid, birth injury P15.2
- subarachnoid (traumatic) — *see* Injury, intracranial, subarachnoid hemorrhage
  - newborn (nontraumatic) P52.5
    - due to birth injury P10.3
  - nontraumatic — *see* Hemorrhage, intracranial, subarachnoid
- subdural (traumatic) — *see* Injury, intracranial, subdural hemorrhage
  - newborn (localized) P52.8
    - birth injury P10.0
  - nontraumatic — *see* Hemorrhage, intracranial, subdural
- superficial, newborn P54.5
- testis (nontraumatic) N50.1
  - birth injury P15.5
- tunica vaginalis (nontraumatic) N50.1
- umbilical cord, complicating delivery O69.5- ☑
- uterine ligament (broad) (nontraumatic) N83.7
  - traumatic S37.892- ☑
- vagina (ruptured) (nontraumatic) N89.8
  - complicating delivery O71.7
- vas deferens (nontraumatic) N50.1
  - traumatic S37.892- ☑
- vitreous — *see* Hemorrhage, vitreous
- vulva (nontraumatic) (nonobstetric) N90.89
  - complicating delivery O71.7
  - newborn (birth injury) P15.5

Hematometra N85.7
- with hematocolpos N89.7

Hematomyelia (central) G95.19
- newborn (birth injury) P11.5
- traumatic T14.8- ☑

Hematomyelitis G04.90
Hematoperitoneum — *see* Hemoperitoneum
Hematophobia F40.230
Hematopneumothorax (see Hemothorax)
Hematopoiesis, cyclic D70.4
Hematoporphyria — *see* Porphyria
Hematorachis, hematorrhachis G95.19
- newborn (birth injury) P11.5

Hematosalpinx N83.6
- with
  - hematocolpos N89.7
  - hematometra N85.7
    - with hematocolpos N89.7
- infectional — *see* Salpingitis

Hematospermia R36.1
Hematothorax (see Hemothorax)
Hematuria R31.9
- benign (familial) (of childhood) — *see also* Hematuria, idiopathic
  - essential microscopic R31.1
- due to sulphonamide, sulfonamide — *see* Table of Drugs and Chemicals, by drug
- endemic — *see also* Schistosomiasis B65.0
- gross R31.0
- idiopathic N02.9
  - with glomerular lesion
    - C3
      - glomerulonephritis N02.A
      - glomerulopathy N02.A
        - with dense deposit disease N02.6
    - crescentic (diffuse) glomerulonephritis N02.7
    - dense deposit disease N02.6
    - endocapillary proliferative glomerulonephritis N02.4
    - focal and segmental hyalinosis or sclerosis N02.1
    - membranoproliferative (diffuse) N02.5
    - membranous (diffuse) N02.2

Hematuria — *continued*
- idiopathic — *continued*
  - with glomerular lesion — *continued*
    - mesangial proliferative (diffuse) N02.3
    - mesangiocapillary (diffuse) N02.5
    - minor abnormality N02.0
    - proliferative NEC N02.8
    - specified pathology NEC N02.8
- intermittent — *see* Hematuria, idiopathic
- malarial B50.8
- microscopic NEC (with symptoms) R31.29
  - asymptomatic R31.21
  - benign essential R31.1
- paroxysmal — *see also* Hematuria, idiopathic
  - nocturnal D59.5
- persistent — *see* Hematuria, idiopathic
- recurrent — *see* Hematuria, idiopathic
- tropical — *see also* Schistosomiasis B65.0
- tuberculous A18.13

Hemeralopia (day blindness) H53.11
- vitamin A deficiency E50.5

Hemi-akinesia R41.4
Hemi-inattention R41.4
Hemianalgesia R20.0
Hemianencephaly Q00.0
Hemianesthesia R20.0
Hemianopia, hemianopsia (heteronymous) H53.47
- homonymous H53.46- ☑
- syphilitic A52.71

Hemiathetosis R25.8
Hemiatrophy R68.89
- cerebellar G31.9
- face, facial, progressive (Romberg) G51.8
- tongue K14.8

Hemiballism (us) G25.5
Hemicardia Q24.8
Hemicephalus, hemicephaly Q00.0
Hemichorea G25.5
Hemicolitis, left — *see* Colitis, left sided
Hemicrania
- congenital malformation Q00.0
- continua G44.51
- meaning migraine — *see also* Migraine G43.909
- paroxysmal G44.039
  - chronic G44.049
    - intractable G44.041
    - not intractable G44.049
  - episodic G44.039
    - intractable G44.031
    - not intractable G44.039
  - intractable G44.031
  - not intractable G44.039

Hemidystrophy — *see* Hemiatrophy
Hemiectromelia Q73.8
Hemihypalgesia R20.8
Hemihypesthesia R20.1
Hemimegalencephaly Q04.5
Hemimelia Q73.8
- lower limb — *see* Defect, reduction, lower limb, specified type NEC
- upper limb — *see* Defect, reduction, upper limb, specified type NEC

Hemiparalysis — *see* Hemiplegia
Hemiparesis — *see* Hemiplegia
Hemiparesthesia R20.2
Hemiparkinsonism G20.C
Hemiplegia G81.9- ☑
- alternans facialis G83.89
- ascending NEC G81.90
  - spinal G95.89
- congenital (cerebral) G80.8
  - spastic G80.2
- embolic (current episode) I63.4- ☑
- flaccid G81.0- ☑
- following
  - cerebrovascular disease I69.959
    - cerebral infarction I69.35- ☑
    - intracerebral hemorrhage I69.15- ☑
    - nontraumatic intracranial hemorrhage NEC I69.25- ☑
    - specified disease NEC I69.85- ☑
    - stroke NOS I69.35- ☑
    - subarachnoid hemorrhage I69.05- ☑
- hysterical F44.4
- newborn NEC P91.88
  - birth injury P11.9
- spastic G81.1- ☑
  - congenital G80.2

Hemiplegia — *continued*
    thrombotic (current episode) I63.3- ☑
Hemisection, spinal cord — *see* Injury, spinal cord, by region
Hemispasm (facial) R25.2
Hemisporosis B48.8
Hemitremor R25.1
Hemivertebra Q76.49
    failure of segmentation with scoliosis Q76.3
    fusion with scoliosis Q76.3
Hemochromatosis E83.119
    with refractory anemia D46.1
    due to repeated red blood cell transfusion E83.111
    hereditary (primary) E83.110
    neonatal P78.84
    primary E83.110
    specified NEC E83.118
Hemoglobin — *see also* condition
    abnormal (disease) — *see* Disease, hemoglobin
    AS genotype D57.3
    Constant Spring D58.2
    E-beta thalassemia D56.5
    fetal, hereditary persistence (HPFH) D56.4
    H Constant Spring D56.0
    low NOS D64.9
    S (Hb S), heterozygous D57.3
Hemoglobinemia D59.9
    due to blood transfusion T80.89- ☑
    paroxysmal D59.6
        nocturnal D59.5
Hemoglobinopathy (mixed) D58.2
    with thalassemia D56.8
    sickle-cell D57.1
        with thalassemia D57.40
            with
                acute chest syndrome D57.411
                cerebral vascular involvement D57.413
                crisis (painful) D57.419
                      with
                          dactylitis D57.414
                          specified complication NEC D57.418
                pain (vaso-occlusive) D57.419
                splenic sequestration D57.412
        without crisis D57.40
Hemoglobinuria R82.3
    with anemia, hemolytic, acquired (chronic) NEC D59.6
    cold (paroxysmal) (with Raynaud's syndrome) D59.6
        agglutinin D59.12
    due to exertion or hemolysis NEC D59.6
    intermittent D59.6
    malarial B50.8
    march D59.6
    nocturnal (paroxysmal) D59.5
    paroxysmal (cold) D59.6
        nocturnal D59.5
Hemolymphangioma D18.1
Hemolysis
    intravascular
        with
            abortion — *see* Abortion, by type, complicated by, hemorrhage
            ectopic or molar pregnancy O08.1
            hemorrhage
                antepartum — *see* Hemorrhage, antepartum, with coagulation defect
                intrapartum — *see also* Hemorrhage, complicating, delivery O67.0
            postpartum O72.3
    neonatal (excessive) P58.9
        specified NEC P58.8
Hemolytic — *see* condition
Hemopericardium I31.2
    following acute myocardial infarction (current complication) I23.0
    newborn P54.8
    traumatic — *see* Injury, heart, with hemopericardium
Hemoperitoneum K66.1
    infectional K65.9
    traumatic S36.899- ☑
        with open wound — *see* Wound, open, abdominal, wall, by site if known, with penetration into peritoneal cavity
Hemophilia (classical) (familial) (hereditary) D66
    A D66
    acquired D68.311
    autoimmune D68.311
    B D67
    C D68.1
    calcipriva — *see also* Defect, coagulation D68.4

Hemophilia — *continued*
    nonfamilial — *see also* Defect, coagulation D68.4
    secondary D68.311
    vascular — *see* Disease, von Willebrand
Hemophthalmos H44.81- ☑
Hemopneumothorax — *see also* Hemothorax
    traumatic S27.2- ☑
Hemoptysis R04.2
    newborn P26.9
    tuberculous — *see* Tuberculosis, pulmonary
Hemorrhage, hemorrhagic (concealed) R58
    abdomen R58
    accidental antepartum — *see* Hemorrhage, antepartum
    acute idiopathic pulmonary, in infants R04.81
    adenoid J35.8
    adrenal (capsule) (gland) E27.49
        medulla E27.8
        newborn P54.4
    after delivery — *see* Hemorrhage, postpartum
    alveolar
        lung, newborn P26.8
        process K08.89
    alveolus K08.89
    amputation stump (surgical) T87.89
    anemia (chronic) D50.0
        acute D62
    antepartum (with) O46.90
        with coagulation defect O46.00- ☑
            afibrinogenemia O46.01- ☑
            disseminated intravascular coagulation O46.02- ☑
            hypofibrinogenemia O46.01- ☑
            specified defect NEC O46.09- ☑
        before 20 weeks gestation O20.9
            specified type NEC O20.8
            threatened abortion O20.0
        due to
            abruptio placenta — *see also* Abruptio placentae O45.9- ☑
            leiomyoma, uterus — *see* Hemorrhage, antepartum, specified cause NEC
            placenta previa O44.1- ☑
        specified cause NEC — *see* subcategory O46.8X- ☑
    anus (sphincter) K62.5
    apoplexy (stroke) — *see* Hemorrhage, intracranial, intracerebral
    arachnoid — *see* Hemorrhage, intracranial, subarachnoid
    artery R58
        brain — *see* Hemorrhage, intracranial, intracerebral
    basilar (ganglion) I61.0
    bladder N32.89
    bowel K92.2
        newborn P54.3
    brain (miliary) (nontraumatic) — *see* Hemorrhage, intracranial, intracerebral
        due to
            birth injury P10.1
            syphilis A52.05
        epidural or extradural (traumatic) — *see* Injury, intracranial, epidural hemorrhage
        newborn P52.4
            birth injury P10.1
        subarachnoid — *see* Hemorrhage, intracranial, subarachnoid
        subdural — *see* Hemorrhage, intracranial, subdural
    brainstem (nontraumatic) I61.3
        traumatic S06.38- ☑
    breast N64.59
    bronchial tube — *see* Hemorrhage, lung
    bronchopulmonary — *see* Hemorrhage, lung
    bronchus — *see* Hemorrhage, lung
    bulbar I61.5
    capillary I78.8
        primary D69.8
    cecum K92.2
    cerebellar, cerebellum (nontraumatic) I61.4
        newborn P52.6
        traumatic S06.37- ☑
    cerebral, cerebrum — *see also* Hemorrhage, intracranial, intracerebral
        lobe I61.1
        newborn (anoxic) P52.4
            birth injury P10.1
    cerebromeningeal I61.8
    cerebrospinal — *see* Hemorrhage, intracranial, intracerebral
    cervix (uteri) (stump) NEC N88.8
    chamber, anterior (eye) — *see* Hyphema
    childbirth — *see* Hemorrhage, complicating, delivery

Hemorrhage, hemorrhagic — *continued*
    choroid H31.30- ☑
        expulsive H31.31- ☑
    ciliary body — *see* Hyphema
    cochlea — *see* subcategory H83.8- ☑
    colon K92.2
    complicating
        abortion — *see* Abortion, by type, complicated by, hemorrhage
        delivery O67.9
            associated with coagulation defect (afibrinogenemia) (DIC) (hyperfibrinolysis) O67.0
            specified cause NEC O67.8
        surgical procedure — *see* Hemorrhage, intraoperative
    conjunctiva H11.3- ☑
        newborn P54.8
    cord, newborn (stump) P51.9
    corpus luteum (ruptured) cyst N83.1- ☑
    cortical (brain) I61.1
    cranial — *see* Hemorrhage, intracranial
    cutaneous R23.3
        due to autosensitivity, erythrocyte D69.2
        newborn P54.5
    delayed
        following ectopic or molar pregnancy O08.1
        postpartum O72.2
    diathesis (familial) D69.9
    disease D69.9
        newborn P53
        specified type NEC D69.8
    due to or associated with
        afibrinogenemia or other coagulation defect (conditions in categories D65- D69)
            antepartum — *see* Hemorrhage, antepartum, with coagulation defect
            intrapartum O67.0
    dental implant M27.61
    device, implant or graft — *see also* Complications, by site and type, specified NEC T85.838- ☑
        arterial graft NEC T82.838- ☑
        breast T85.838- ☑
        catheter NEC T85.838- ☑
            dialysis (renal) T82.838- ☑
                intraperitoneal T85.838- ☑
            infusion NEC T82.838- ☑
                spinal (epidural) (subdural) T85.830- ☑
            urinary (indwelling) T83.83- ☑
        electronic (electrode) (pulse generator) (stimulator)
            bone T84.83- ☑
            cardiac T82.837- ☑
            nervous system (brain) (peripheral nerve) (spinal) T85.830- ☑
            urinary T83.83- ☑
        fixation, internal (orthopedic) NEC T84.83- ☑
        gastrointestinal (bile duct) (esophagus) T85.838- ☑
        genital NEC T83.83- ☑
        heart NEC T82.837- ☑
        joint prosthesis T84.83- ☑
        ocular (corneal graft) (orbital implant) NEC T85.838- ☑
        orthopedic NEC T84.83- ☑
            bone graft T86.838
        specified NEC T85.838- ☑
        urinary NEC T83.83- ☑
        vascular NEC T82.838- ☑
        ventricular intracranial shunt T85.830- ☑
    duodenum, duodenal K92.2
        ulcer — *see* Ulcer, duodenum, with hemorrhage
    dura mater — *see* Hemorrhage, intracranial, subdural
    endotracheal — *see* Hemorrhage, lung
    epicranial subaponeurotic (massive), birth injury P12.2
    epidural (traumatic) — *see also* Injury, intracranial, epidural hemorrhage
        nontraumatic I62.1
    esophagus K22.89
        varix I85.01
            secondary I85.11
    excessive, following ectopic gestation (subsequent episode) O08.1
    extradural (traumatic) — *see* Injury, intracranial, epidural hemorrhage
        birth injury P10.8
        newborn (anoxic) (nontraumatic) P52.8
        nontraumatic I62.1
    eye NEC H57.89

Hemorrhage, hemorrhagic — *continued*
- eye — *continued*
  - fundus — *see* Hemorrhage, retina
  - lid — *see* Disorder, eyelid, specified type NEC
- fallopian tube N83.6
- fibrinogenolysis — *see* Fibrinolysis
- fibrinolytic (acquired) — *see* Fibrinolysis
- from
  - ear (nontraumatic) — *see* Otorrhagia
  - tracheostomy stoma J95.01
- fundus, eye — *see* Hemorrhage, retina
- funis — *see* Hemorrhage, umbilicus, cord
- gastric — *see* Hemorrhage, stomach
- gastroenteric K92.2
  - newborn P54.3
- gastrointestinal (tract) K92.2
  - newborn P54.3
- genital organ, male N50.1
- genitourinary (tract) NOS R31.9
- gingiva K06.8
- globe (eye) — *see* Hemophthalmos
- graafian follicle cyst (ruptured) N83.0- ☑
- gum K06.8
- heart I51.89
- hypopharyngeal (throat) R04.1
- intermenstrual (regular) N92.3
  - irregular N92.1
- internal (organs) NEC R58
  - capsule I61.0
  - ear — *see* subcategory H83.8- ☑
  - newborn P54.8
- intestine K92.2
  - newborn P54.3
- intra-abdominal R58
- intra-alveolar (lung), newborn P26.8
- intracerebral (nontraumatic) — *see* Hemorrhage, intracranial, intracerebral
- intracranial (nontraumatic) I62.9
  - birth injury P10.9
  - epidural, nontraumatic I62.1
  - extradural, nontraumatic I62.1
  - intracerebral (nontraumatic) (in) I61.9
    - brain stem I61.3
    - cerebellum I61.4
    - hemisphere I61.2
      - cortical (superficial) I61.1
      - subcortical (deep) I61.0
    - intraoperative
      - during a nervous system procedure G97.31
      - during other procedure G97.32
    - intraventricular I61.5
    - multiple localized I61.6
    - newborn P52.4
      - birth injury P10.1
    - postprocedural
      - following a nervous system procedure G97.51
      - following other procedure G97.52
    - specified NEC I61.8
    - superficial I61.1
    - traumatic — *see* Injury, intracranial, intracerebral hemorrhage, traumatic
  - newborn P52.9
    - specified NEC P52.8
  - subarachnoid (nontraumatic) (from) I60.9
    - intracranial (cerebral) artery I60.7
      - anterior communicating I60.2
      - basilar I60.4
      - carotid siphon and bifurcation I60.0- ☑
      - communicating I60.7
        - anterior I60.2
        - posterior I60.3- ☑
      - middle cerebral I60.1- ☑
      - posterior communicating I60.3- ☑
      - specified artery NEC I60.6
      - vertebral I60.5- ☑
    - newborn P52.5
      - birth injury P10.3
    - specified NEC I60.8
    - traumatic S06.6X- ☑
  - subdural (nontraumatic) I62.00
    - acute I62.01
    - birth injury P10.0
    - chronic I62.03
    - newborn (anoxic) (hypoxic) P52.8
      - birth injury P10.0
    - spinal G95.19
    - subacute I62.02

Hemorrhage, hemorrhagic — *continued*
- intracranial — *continued*
  - subdural — *continued*
    - traumatic — *see* Injury, intracranial, subdural hemorrhage
  - traumatic — *see* Injury, intracranial, focal brain injury
- intramedullary NEC G95.19
- intraocular — *see* Hemophthalmos
- intraoperative, intraprocedural — *see* Complication, hemorrhage (hematoma), intraoperative (intraprocedural), by site
- intrapartum — *see* Hemorrhage, complicating, delivery
- intrapelvic
  - female N94.89
  - male K66.1
- intraperitoneal K66.1
- intrapontine I61.3
- intraprocedural — *see* Complication, hemorrhage (hematoma), intraoperative (intraprocedural), by site
- intrauterine N85.7
  - complicating delivery — *see also* Hemorrhage, complicating, delivery O67.9
  - postpartum — *see* Hemorrhage, postpartum
- intraventricular I61.5
  - newborn (nontraumatic) — *see also* Newborn, affected by, hemorrhage P52.3
    - due to birth injury P10.2
    - grade
      - 1 P52.0
      - 2 P52.1
      - 3 P52.21
      - 4 P52.22
- intravesical N32.89
- iris (postinfectional) (postinflammatory) (toxic) — *see* Hyphema
- joint (nontraumatic) — *see* Hemarthrosis
- kidney N28.89
- knee (joint) (nontraumatic) — *see* Hemarthrosis, knee
- labyrinth — *see* subcategory H83.8- ☑
- lenticular striate artery I61.0
- ligature, vessel — *see* Hemorrhage, postoperative
- liver K76.89
- lung R04.89
  - newborn P26.9
    - massive P26.1
    - specified NEC P26.8
  - tuberculous — *see* Tuberculosis, pulmonary
- massive umbilical, newborn P51.0
- mediastinum — *see* Hemorrhage, lung
- medulla I61.3
- membrane (brain) I60.8
  - spinal cord — *see* Hemorrhage, spinal cord
- meninges, meningeal (brain) (middle) I60.8
  - spinal cord — *see* Hemorrhage, spinal cord
- mesentery K66.1
- metritis — *see* Endometritis
- mouth K13.79
- mucous membrane NEC R58
  - newborn P54.8
- muscle M62.89
- nail (subungual) L60.8
- nasal turbinate R04.0
  - newborn P54.8
- navel, newborn P51.9
- newborn P54.9
  - specified NEC P54.8
- nipple N64.59
- nose R04.0
  - newborn P54.8
- omentum K66.1
- optic nerve (sheath) H47.02- ☑
- orbit, orbital H05.23- ☑
- ovary NEC N83.8
- oviduct N83.6
- pancreas K86.89
- parathyroid (gland) (spontaneous) E21.4
- parturition — *see* Hemorrhage, complicating, delivery
- penis N48.89
- pericardium, pericarditis I31.2
- peritoneum, peritoneal K66.1
- peritonsillar tissue J35.8
  - due to infection J36
- petechial R23.3
  - due to autosensitivity, erythrocyte D69.2
- pituitary (gland) E23.6
- pleura — *see* Hemorrhage, lung
- polioencephalitis, superior E51.2
- polymyositis — *see* Polymyositis

Hemorrhage, hemorrhagic — *continued*
- pons, pontine I61.3
- posterior fossa (nontraumatic) I61.8
  - newborn P52.6
- postmenopausal N95.0
- postnasal R04.0
- postoperative — *see* Complications, postprocedural, hemorrhage, by site
- postpartum NEC (following delivery of placenta) O72.1
  - delayed or secondary O72.2
  - retained placenta O72.0
  - third stage O72.0
- pregnancy — *see* Hemorrhage, antepartum
- preretinal — *see* Hemorrhage, retina
- prostate N42.1
- puerperal — *see* Hemorrhage, postpartum
  - delayed or secondary O72.2
- pulmonary R04.89
  - newborn P26.9
    - massive P26.1
    - specified NEC P26.8
  - tuberculous — *see* Tuberculosis, pulmonary
- purpura (primary) D69.3
- rectum (sphincter) K62.5
  - newborn P54.2
- recurring, following initial hemorrhage at time of injury T79.2- ☑
- renal N28.89
- respiratory passage or tract R04.9
  - specified NEC R04.89
- retina, retinal (vessels) H35.6- ☑
  - diabetic — *see* Microaneurysm, retinal, diabetic
- retroperitoneal K68.3
- scalp R58
- scrotum N50.1
- secondary (nontraumatic) R58
  - following initial hemorrhage at time of injury T79.2- ☑
- seminal vesicle N50.1
- skin R23.3
  - newborn P54.5
- slipped umbilical ligature P51.8
- spermatic cord N50.1
- spinal (cord) G95.19
  - newborn (birth injury) P11.5
- spleen D73.5
  - intraoperative — *see* Complications, intraoperative, hemorrhage, spleen
  - postprocedural — *see* Complications, postprocedural, hemorrhage, spleen
- stomach K92.2
  - newborn P54.3
  - ulcer — *see* Ulcer, stomach, with hemorrhage
- subarachnoid (nontraumatic) — *see* Hemorrhage, intracranial, subarachnoid
- subconjunctival — *see also* Hemorrhage, conjunctiva
  - birth injury P15.3
- subcortical (brain) I61.0
- subcutaneous R23.3
- subdiaphragmatic R58
- subdural (acute) (nontraumatic) — *see* Hemorrhage, intracranial, subdural
- subependymal
  - newborn P52.0
    - with intraventricular extension P52.1
      - and intracerebral extension P52.22
- subgaleal P12.2
- subhyaloid — *see* Hemorrhage, retina
- subperiosteal — *see* Disorder, bone, specified type NEC
- subretinal — *see* Hemorrhage, retina
- subtentorial — *see* Hemorrhage, intracranial, subdural
- subungual L60.8
- suprarenal (capsule) (gland) E27.49
  - newborn P54.4
- tentorium (traumatic) NEC — *see* Hemorrhage, brain
  - newborn (birth injury) P10.4
- testis N50.1
- third stage (postpartum) O72.0
- thorax — *see* Hemorrhage, lung
- throat R04.1
- thymus (gland) E32.8
- thyroid (cyst) (gland) E07.89
- tongue K14.8
- tonsil J35.8
- trachea — *see* Hemorrhage, lung
- tracheobronchial R04.89
  - newborn P26.0
- traumatic — *code to* specific injury
  - cerebellar — *see* Hemorrhage, brain

Hemorrhage, hemorrhagic — continued
- traumatic — *code to* specific injury — *continued*
  - intracranial — *see* Hemorrhage, brain
  - recurring or secondary (following initial hemorrhage at time of injury) T79.2- ☑
- tuberculous NEC — *see also* Tuberculosis, pulmonary A15.0
- tunica vaginalis N50.1
- ulcer — *code by* site under Ulcer, with hemorrhage K27.4
- umbilicus, umbilical
  - cord
    - after birth, newborn P51.9
    - complicating delivery O69.5- ☑
  - newborn P51.9
    - massive P51.0
    - slipped ligature P51.8
    - stump P51.9
- urethra (idiopathic) N36.8
- uterus, uterine (abnormal) N93.9
  - climacteric N92.4
  - complicating delivery — *see* Hemorrhage, complicating, delivery
  - dysfunctional or functional N93.8
  - intermenstrual (regular) N92.3
    - irregular N92.1
  - postmenopausal N95.0
  - postpartum — *see* Hemorrhage, postpartum
  - preclimacteric or premenopausal N92.4
  - prepubertal N93.8
  - pubertal N92.2
- vagina (abnormal) N93.9
  - newborn P54.6
- vas deferens N50.1
- vasa previa O69.4- ☑
- ventricular I61.5
- vesical N32.89
- viscera NEC R58
  - newborn P54.8
- vitreous (humor) (intraocular) H43.1- ☑
- vulva N90.89

Hemorrhoids (bleeding) (without mention of degree) K64.9
- 1st degree (grade/stage I) (without prolapse outside of anal canal) K64.0
- 2nd degree (grade/stage II) (that prolapse with straining but retract spontaneously) K64.1
- 3rd degree (grade/stage III) (that prolapse with straining and require manual replacement back inside anal canal) K64.2
- 4th degree (grade/stage IV) (with prolapsed tissue that cannot be manually replaced) K64.3
- complicating
  - pregnancy O22.4- ☑
  - puerperium O87.2
- external K64.4
  - with
    - thrombosis K64.5
- internal (without mention of degree) K64.8
- prolapsed K64.8
- skin tags
  - anus K64.4
  - residual K64.4
- specified NEC K64.8
- strangulated — *see also* Hemorrhoids, by degree K64.8
- thrombosed — *see also* Hemorrhoids, by degree K64.5
- ulcerated — *see also* Hemorrhoids, by degree K64.8

Hemosalpinx N83.6
- with
  - hematocolpos N89.7
  - hematometra N85.7
    - with hematocolpos N89.7

Hemosiderosis (dietary) E83.19
- pulmonary, idiopathic E83.1- ☑ *[J84.03]*
- transfusion T80.89- ☑

Hemothorax (bacterial) (nontuberculous) J94.2
- newborn P54.8
- traumatic S27.1- ☑
  - with pneumothorax S27.2- ☑
- tuberculous NEC A15.6

Henoch (-Schonlein) **disease or syndrome** (purpura) D69.0
Henpue, henpuye A66.6
Hepar lobatum (syphilitic) A52.74
Hepatalgia K76.89
Hepatitis K75.9
- A — *see* Hepatitis, viral, type, A
- acute B17.9
  - with coma K72.01
  - with hepatic failure — *see* Failure, hepatic
  - alcoholic — *see* Hepatitis, alcoholic

Hepatitis — continued
- acute — *continued*
  - infectious B17.9
  - non-viral K72.0- ☑
  - viral — *see also*, Hepatitis, viral B17.9
- alcoholic (acute) (chronic) K70.10
  - with ascites K70.11
- amebic — *see* Abscess, liver, amebic
- anicteric, (viral) — *see* Hepatitis, viral
- antigen-associated (HAA) — *see* Hepatitis, B
- Australia-antigen (positive) — *see* Hepatitis, B
- autoimmune K75.4
- B B19.10
  - with B19.11
    - delta (agent) — *see* Hepatitis, D
    - hepatic coma B19.11
  - acute B16.9
    - with
      - delta-agent (coinfection) (without hepatic coma) B16.1
        - with hepatic coma B16.0
      - hepatic coma (without delta-agent coinfection) B16.2
  - chronic B18.1
    - with delta-agent B18.0
- bacterial NEC K75.89
- C (viral) B19.20
  - with hepatic coma B19.21
  - acute B17.10
    - with hepatic coma B17.11
  - chronic B18.2
- catarrhal (acute) B15.9
  - with hepatic coma B15.0
- cholangiolitic K75.89
- cholestatic K75.89
- chronic K73.9
  - active NEC K73.2
    - toxic — *see* Disease, liver, toxic, with, hepatitis, chronic, active
  - lobular NEC K73.1
  - persistent NEC K73.0
  - specified NEC K73.8
  - toxic — *see* Disease, liver, toxic, with, hepatitis, chronic
  - viral — *see* Hepatitis, viral, chronic
- cytomegaloviral B25.1
- D B16.1
  - acute B16.1
    - with hepatic coma B16.0
    - in hepatitis B carrier B17.0
  - chronic B18.0
- delta (agent) — *see* Hepatitis, D
- due to ethanol (acute) (chronic) — *see* Hepatitis, alcoholic
- epidemic B15.9
  - with hepatic coma B15.0
- fulminant NEC (viral) — *see* Hepatitis, viral
- granulomatous NEC K75.3
- herpesviral B00.81
- history of
  - B Z86.19
  - C Z86.19
- homologous serum — *see* Hepatitis, viral, type B
- in (due to)
  - mumps B26.81
  - toxoplasmosis (acquired) B58.1
    - congenital (active) P37.1 *[K77]*
- infectious, infective B15.9
  - acute (subacute) B17.9
  - chronic B18.9
- inoculation — *see* Hepatitis, viral, type B
- interstitial (chronic) K74.69
- ischemia, ischemic K72.00
- lupoid NEC K75.4
- malignant NEC (with hepatic failure) K72.90
  - with coma K72.91
- neonatal (idiopathic) (toxic) P59.29
- neonatal giant cell P59.29
- newborn P59.29
- non-viral K72.0- ☑
- postimmunization — *see* Hepatitis, viral, type B
- post-transfusion — *see* Hepatitis, viral, type B
- reactive, nonspecific K75.2
- serum — *see* Hepatitis, viral, type B
- shock K72.00
- specified type NEC
  - with hepatic failure — *see* Failure, hepatic
- syphilitic (late) A52.74
  - congenital (early) A50.08 *[K77]*
    - late A50.59 *[K77]*

Hepatitis — continued
- syphilitic — *continued*
  - secondary A51.45
- toxic — *see also* Disease, liver, toxic K71.6
- tuberculous A18.83
- viral, virus B19.9
  - with hepatic coma B19.0
  - acute B17.9
  - chronic B18.9
    - specified NEC B18.8
    - type
      - B B18.1
        - with delta-agent B18.0
      - C B18.2
      - D B18.0
  - congenital P35.3
  - coxsackie B33.8 *[K77]*
  - cytomegalic inclusion B25.1
  - in remission, any type — *code to* Hepatitis, chronic, by type
  - non-A, non-B B17.8
  - specified type NEC (with or without coma) B17.8
  - type
    - A B15.9
      - with hepatic coma B15.0
    - B B19.10
      - with hepatic coma B19.11
      - acute B16.9
        - with
          - delta-agent (coinfection) (without hepatic coma) B16.1
            - with hepatic coma B16.0
          - hepatic coma (without delta-agent coinfection) B16.2
      - chronic B18.1
        - with delta-agent B18.0
    - C B19.20
      - with hepatic coma B19.21
      - acute B17.10
        - with hepatic coma B17.11
      - chronic B18.2
    - D B16.1
      - acute B16.1
        - with hepatic coma B16.0
        - in hepatitis B carrier B17.0
      - chronic B18.0
    - delta (agent) — *see* Hepatitis, viral, type, D
    - E B17.2
  - non-A, non-B B17.8

Hepatization lung (acute) — *see* Pneumonia, lobar
Hepatoblastoma C22.2
Hepatocarcinoma C22.0
Hepatocholangiocarcinoma C22.0
Hepatocholangioma, benign D13.4
Hepatocholangitis K75.89
Hepatolenticular degeneration E83.01
Hepatoma (malignant) C22.0
- benign D13.4
- embryonal C22.0

Hepatomegaly — *see also* Hypertrophy, liver
- with splenomegaly R16.2
- congenital Q44.79
- in mononucleosis
  - gammaherpesviral B27.09
  - infectious specified NEC B27.89

Hepatoptosis K76.89
Hepatorenal syndrome following labor and delivery O90.41
Hepatosis K76.89
Hepatosplenomegaly R16.2
- hyperlipemic (Burger-Grutz type) E78.3 *[K77]*
Hereditary — *see* condition
Hereditary alpha tryptasemia (syndrome) D89.44
Heredodegeneration, macular — *see* Dystrophy, retina
Heredopathia atactica polyneuritiformis G60.1
Heredosyphilis — *see* Syphilis, congenital
Herlitz' syndrome Q81.1
Hermansky-Pudlak syndrome E70.331
Hermaphrodite, hermaphroditism (true) Q56.0
- 46,XX/46,XY Q99.0
- 46,XX with streak gonads Q99.1
- 46,XY with streak gonads Q99.1
- chimera 46,XX/46,XY Q99.0

Hernia, hernial (acquired) (recurrent) K46.9
- with
  - gangrene — *see* Hernia, by site, with, gangrene
  - incarceration — *see* Hernia, by site, with, obstruction
  - irreducible — *see* Hernia, by site, with, obstruction
  - obstruction — *see* Hernia, by site, with, obstruction

Hernia, hernial — *continued*
 with — *continued*
  strangulation — *see* Hernia, by site, with, obstruction
 abdomen, abdominal K46.9
  with
   gangrene (and obstruction) K46.1
   obstruction K46.0
  femoral — *see* Hernia, femoral
  incisional — *see* Hernia, incisional
  inguinal — *see* Hernia, inguinal
  specified site NEC K45.8
   with
    gangrene (and obstruction) K45.1
    obstruction K45.0
  umbilical — *see* Hernia, umbilical
  wall — *see* Hernia, ventral
 appendix — *see* Hernia, abdomen
 bladder (mucosa) (sphincter)
  congenital (female) (male) Q79.51
  female — *see* Cystocele
  male N32.89
 brain, congenital — *see* Encephalocele
 cartilage, vertebra — *see* Displacement, intervertebral disc
 cerebral, congenital — *see also* Encephalocele
  endaural Q01.8
 ciliary body (traumatic) S05.2- ☑
 colon — *see* Hernia, abdomen
 Cooper's — *see* Hernia, abdomen, specified site NEC
 crural — *see* Hernia, femoral
 diaphragm, diaphragmatic K44.9
  with
   gangrene (and obstruction) K44.1
   obstruction K44.0
  congenital Q79.0
 direct (inguinal) — *see* Hernia, inguinal
 diverticulum, intestine — *see* Hernia, abdomen
 double (inguinal) — *see* Hernia, inguinal, bilateral
 due to adhesions (with obstruction) K56.50
 epigastric — *see also* Hernia, ventral K43.9
 esophageal hiatus — *see* Hernia, hiatal
 external (inguinal) — *see* Hernia, inguinal
 fallopian tube N83.4- ☑
 fascia M62.89
 femoral K41.90
  with
   gangrene (and obstruction) K41.40
    not specified as recurrent K41.40
    recurrent K41.41
   obstruction K41.30
    not specified as recurrent K41.30
    recurrent K41.31
   not specified as recurrent K41.90
   recurrent K41.91
  bilateral K41.20
   with
    gangrene (and obstruction) K41.10
     not specified as recurrent K41.10
     recurrent K41.11
    obstruction K41.00
     not specified as recurrent K41.00
     recurrent K41.01
    not specified as recurrent K41.20
    recurrent K41.21
  unilateral K41.90
   with
    gangrene (and obstruction) K41.40
     not specified as recurrent K41.40
     recurrent K41.41
    obstruction K41.30
     not specified as recurrent K41.30
     recurrent K41.31
    not specified as recurrent K41.90
    recurrent K41.91
 foramen magnum G93.5
  congenital Q01.8
 funicular (umbilical) — *see also* Hernia, umbilicus
  spermatic (cord) — *see* Hernia, inguinal
 gastrointestinal tract — *see* Hernia, abdomen
 Hesselbach's — *see* Hernia, femoral, specified site NEC
 hiatal (esophageal) (sliding) K44.9
  with
   gangrene (and obstruction) K44.1
   obstruction K44.0
  congenital Q40.1
 hypogastric — *see* Hernia, ventral
 incarcerated — *see also* Hernia, by site, with obstruction
  with gangrene — *see* Hernia, by site, with gangrene
 incisional K43.2

Hernia, hernial — *continued*
 incisional — *continued*
  with
   gangrene (and obstruction) K43.1
   obstruction K43.0
 indirect (inguinal) — *see* Hernia, inguinal
 inguinal (direct) (external) (funicular) (indirect) (internal) (oblique) (scrotal) (sliding) K40.90
  with
   gangrene (and obstruction) K40.40
    not specified as recurrent K40.40
    recurrent K40.41
   obstruction K40.30
    not specified as recurrent K40.30
    recurrent K40.31
   not specified as recurrent K40.90
   recurrent K40.91
  bilateral K40.20
   with
    gangrene (and obstruction) K40.10
     not specified as recurrent K40.10
     recurrent K40.11
    obstruction K40.00
     not specified as recurrent K40.00
     recurrent K40.01
    not specified as recurrent K40.20
    recurrent K40.21
  unilateral K40.90
   with
    gangrene (and obstruction) K40.40
     not specified as recurrent K40.40
     recurrent K40.41
    obstruction K40.30
     not specified as recurrent K40.30
     recurrent K40.31
    not specified as recurrent K40.90
    recurrent K40.91
 internal — *see also* Hernia, abdomen
  inguinal — *see* Hernia, inguinal
 interstitial — *see* Hernia, abdomen
 intervertebral cartilage or disc — *see* Displacement, intervertebral disc
 intestine, intestinal — *see* Hernia, by site
 intra-abdominal — *see* Hernia, abdomen
 iris (traumatic) S05.2- ☑
 irreducible — *see also* Hernia, by site, with obstruction
  with gangrene — *see* Hernia, by site, with gangrene
 ischiatic — *see* Hernia, abdomen, specified site NEC
 ischiorectal — *see* Hernia, abdomen, specified site NEC
 lens (traumatic) S05.2- ☑
 linea (alba) (semilunaris) — *see* Hernia, ventral
 Littre's — *see* Hernia, abdomen
 lumbar — *see* Hernia, abdomen, specified site NEC
 lung (subcutaneous) J98.4
 mediastinum J98.59
 mesenteric (internal) — *see* Hernia, abdomen
 midline — *see* Hernia, ventral
 muscle (sheath) M62.89
 nucleus pulposus — *see* Displacement, intervertebral disc
 oblique (inguinal) — *see* Hernia, inguinal
 obstructive — *see also* Hernia, by site, with obstruction
  with gangrene — *see* Hernia, by site, with gangrene
 obturator — *see* Hernia, abdomen, specified site NEC
 omental — *see* Hernia, abdomen
 ovary N83.4- ☑
 oviduct N83.4- ☑
 paraesophageal — *see also* Hernia, diaphragm
  congenital Q40.1
 parastomal K43.5
  with
   gangrene (and obstruction) K43.4
   obstruction K43.3
 paraumbilical — *see* Hernia, umbilicus
 perineal — *see* Hernia, abdomen, specified site NEC
 Petit's — *see* Hernia, abdomen, specified site NEC
 postoperative — *see* Hernia, incisional
 pregnant uterus — *see* Abnormal, uterus in pregnancy or childbirth
 prevesical N32.89
 properitoneal — *see* Hernia, abdomen, specified site NEC
 pudendal — *see* Hernia, abdomen, specified site NEC
 rectovaginal N81.6
 retroperitoneal — *see* Hernia, abdomen, specified site NEC
 Richter's — *see* Hernia, abdomen, with obstruction
 Rieux's, Riex's — *see* Hernia, abdomen, specified site NEC

Hernia, hernial — *continued*
 sac condition (adhesion) (dropsy) (inflammation) (laceration) (suppuration) — *code by site under* Hernia
 sciatic — *see* Hernia, abdomen, specified site NEC
 scrotum, scrotal — *see* Hernia, inguinal
 sliding (inguinal) — *see also* Hernia, inguinal
  hiatus — *see* Hernia, hiatal
 spigelian — *see* Hernia, ventral
 spinal — *see* Spina bifida
 strangulated — *see also* Hernia, by site, with obstruction
  with gangrene — *see* Hernia, by site, with gangrene
 subxiphoid — *see* Hernia, ventral
 supra-umbilicus — *see* Hernia, ventral
 tendon — *see* Disorder, tendon, specified type NEC
 Treitz's (fossa) — *see* Hernia, abdomen, specified site NEC
 tunica vaginalis Q55.29
 umbilicus, umbilical K42.9
  with
   gangrene (and obstruction) K42.1
   obstruction K42.0
 ureter N28.89
 urethra, congenital Q64.79
 urinary meatus, congenital Q64.79
 uterus N81.4
  pregnant — *see* Abnormal, uterus in pregnancy or childbirth
 vaginal (anterior) (wall) — *see* Cystocele
 Velpeau's — *see* Hernia, femoral
 ventral K43.9
  with
   gangrene (and obstruction) K43.7
   obstruction K43.6
  incisional K43.2
   with
    gangrene (and obstruction) K43.1
    obstruction K43.0
   recurrent — *see* Hernia, incisional
  specified NEC K43.9
   with
    gangrene (and obstruction) K43.7
    obstruction K43.6
 vesical
  congenital (female) (male) Q79.51
  female — *see* Cystocele
  male N32.89
 vitreous (into wound) S05.2- ☑
  into anterior chamber — *see* Prolapse, vitreous
Herniation — *see also* Hernia
 brain (stem) G93.5
  nontraumatic G93.5
  traumatic S06.A1- ☑
   cerebellar S06.A1- ☑
   subfalcine (cingulate) S06.A1- ☑
   tonsillar S06.A1- ☑
   transtentorial (central) (upward cerebellar) S06.A1- ☑
   uncal S06.A1- ☑
 cerebral G93.5
  nontraumatic G93.5
  traumatic S06.A1- ☑
 mediastinum J98.59
 nucleus pulposus — *see* Displacement, intervertebral disc
Herpangina B08.5
Herpes, herpesvirus, herpetic B00.9
 anogenital A60.9
  perianal skin A60.1
  rectum A60.1
  urogenital tract A60.00
   cervix A60.03
   male genital organ NEC A60.02
   penis A60.01
   specified site NEC A60.09
   vagina A60.04
   vulva A60.04
 blepharitis (zoster) B02.39
  simplex B00.59
 circinatus B35.4
  bullosus L12.0
 conjunctivitis (simplex) B00.53
  zoster B02.31
 cornea B02.33
 encephalitis B00.4
  due to herpesvirus 6 B10.01
  due to herpesvirus 7 B10.09
  specified NEC B10.09
 eye (zoster) B02.30

☑ Additional Character Required — Refer to the Tabular List for Character Selection

Herpes, herpesvirus, herpetic — continued
- eye — continued
  - simplex B00.50
- eyelid (zoster) B02.39
  - simplex B00.59
- facialis B00.1
- febrilis B00.1
- geniculate ganglionitis B02.21
- genital, genitalis A60.00
  - female A60.09
  - male A60.02
- gestational, gestationis O26.4- ☑
- gingivostomatitis B00.2
- human B00.9
  - 1 — see Herpes, simplex
  - 2 — see Herpes, simplex
  - 3 — see Varicella
  - 4 — see Mononucleosis, Epstein-Barr (virus)
  - 5 — see Disease, cytomegalic inclusion (generalized)
  - 6
    - encephalitis B10.01
    - specified NEC B10.81
  - 7
    - encephalitis B10.09
    - specified NEC B10.82
  - 8 B10.89
- infection NEC B10.89
  - Kaposi's sarcoma associated B10.89
- iridocyclitis (simplex) B00.51
  - zoster B02.32
- iris (vesicular erythema multiforme) L51.9
- iritis (simplex) B00.51
- Kaposi's sarcoma associated B10.89
- keratitis (simplex) (dendritic) (disciform) (interstitial) B00.52
  - zoster (interstitial) B02.33
- keratoconjunctivitis (simplex) B00.52
  - zoster B02.33
- labialis B00.1
- lip B00.1
- meningitis (simplex) B00.3
  - zoster B02.1
- ophthalmicus (zoster) NEC B02.30
  - simplex B00.50
- penis A60.01
- perianal skin A60.1
- pharyngitis, pharyngotonsillitis B00.2
- rectum A60.1
- scrotum A60.02
- sepsis B00.7
- simplex B00.9
  - complicated NEC B00.89
  - congenital P35.2
  - conjunctivitis B00.53
  - external ear B00.1
  - eyelid B00.59
  - hepatitis B00.81
  - keratitis (interstitial) B00.52
  - myelitis B00.82
  - specified complication NEC B00.89
  - visceral B00.89
- stomatitis B00.2
- tonsurans B35.0
- visceral B00.89
- vulva A60.04
- whitlow B00.89
- zoster — see also condition B02.9
  - auricularis B02.21
  - complicated NEC B02.8
  - conjunctivitis B02.31
  - disseminated B02.7
  - encephalitis B02.0
  - eye (lid) B02.39
  - geniculate ganglionitis B02.21
  - keratitis (interstitial) B02.33
  - meningitis B02.1
  - myelitis B02.24
  - neuritis, neuralgia B02.29
  - ophthalmicus NEC B02.30
  - oticus B02.21
  - polyneuropathy B02.23
  - specified complication NEC B02.8
  - trigeminal neuralgia B02.22

Herpesvirus (human) — see Herpes
Herpetophobia F40.218
Herrick's anemia — see Disease, sickle-cell
Hers' disease E74.09
Herter-Gee syndrome K90.0
Herxheimer's reaction R68.89

Hesitancy
- of micturition R39.11
- urinary R39.11

Hesselbach's hernia — see Hernia, femoral, specified site NEC
Heterochromia (congenital) Q13.2
- cataract — see Cataract, complicated
- cyclitis (Fuchs) — see Cyclitis, Fuchs' heterochromic
- hair L67.1
- iritis — see Cyclitis, Fuchs' heterochromic
- retained metallic foreign body (nonmagnetic) — see Foreign body, intraocular, old, retained
  - magnetic — see Foreign body, intraocular, old, retained, magnetic
- uveitis — see Cyclitis, Fuchs' heterochromic

Heterophoria — see Strabismus, heterophoria
Heterophyes, heterophyiasis (small intestine) B66.8
Heterotopia, heterotopic — see also Malposition, congenital
- cerebralis Q04.8

Heterotropia — see Strabismus
Heubner-Herter disease K90.0
Hexadactylism Q69.9
HGSIL (cytology finding) (high grade squamous intraepithelial lesion on cytologic smear) (Pap smear finding)
- anus R85.613
- cervix R87.613
  - biopsy (histology) finding — see Neoplasia, intraepithelial, cervix, grade II or grade III
- vagina R87.623
  - biopsy (histology) finding — see Neoplasia, intraepithelial, cervix, grade II or grade III

Hibernoma — see Lipoma
Hiccup, hiccough R06.6
- epidemic B33.0
- psychogenic F45.8

Hidden penis (congenital) Q55.64
- acquired N48.83

Hidradenitis (axillaris) (suppurative) L73.2
Hidradenoma (nodular) — see also Neoplasm, skin, benign
- clear cell — see Neoplasm, skin, benign
- papillary — see Neoplasm, skin, benign

Hidrocystoma — see Neoplasm, skin, benign
High
- altitude effects T70.20- ☑
  - anoxia T70.29- ☑
  - on
    - ears T70.0- ☑
    - sinuses T70.1- ☑
  - polycythemia D75.1
- arch
  - foot Q66.7- ☑
  - palate, congenital Q38.5
- arterial tension — see Hypertension
- basal metabolic rate R94.8
- blood pressure — see also Hypertension
  - borderline R03.0
  - reading (incidental) (isolated) (nonspecific), without diagnosis of hypertension R03.0
- cholesterol E78.00
  - with high triglycerides E78.2
- diaphragm (congenital) Q79.1
- expressed emotional level within family Z63.8
- head at term O32.4- ☑
- palate, congenital Q38.5
- risk
  - infant NEC Z76.2
  - sexual behavior (heterosexual) Z72.51
    - bisexual Z72.53
    - homosexual Z72.52
- scrotal testis, testes
  - bilateral Q53.23
  - unilateral Q53.13
- temperature (of unknown origin) R50.9
- thoracic rib Q76.6
- triglycerides E78.1
  - with high cholesterol E78.2

Hildenbrand's disease A75.0
Hilum — see condition
Hip — see condition
Hippel's disease Q85.83
Hippophobia F40.218
Hippus H57.09
Hirschsprung's disease or megacolon Q43.1
Hirsutism, hirsuties L68.0
Hirudiniasis
- external B88.3
- internal B83.4

His-Werner disease A79.0
Hiss-Russell dysentery A03.1
Histidinemia, histidinuria E70.41
Histiocytoma — see also Neoplasm, skin, benign
- fibrous — see also Neoplasm, skin, benign
  - atypical — see Neoplasm, connective tissue, uncertain behavior
  - malignant — see Neoplasm, connective tissue, malignant

Histiocytosis D76.3
- acute differentiated progressive C96.0
- Langerhans' cell NEC C96.6
  - multifocal X
    - multisystemic (disseminated) C96.0
    - unisystemic C96.5
  - pulmonary, adult (adult PLCH) J84.82
  - unifocal (X) C96.6
- lipid, lipoid D76.3
  - essential E75.29
- malignant C96.A (following C96.6)
- mononuclear phagocytes NEC D76.1
  - Langerhans' cells C96.6
- non-Langerhans cell D76.3
- polyostotic sclerosing D76.3
- sinus, with massive lymphadenopathy D76.3
- syndrome NEC D76.3
- X NEC C96.6
  - acute (progressive) C96.0
  - chronic C96.6
  - multifocal C96.5
  - multisystemic C96.0
  - unifocal C96.6

Histoplasmosis B39.9
- with pneumonia NEC B39.2
- African B39.5
- American — see Histoplasmosis, capsulati
- capsulati B39.4
  - disseminated B39.3
  - generalized B39.3
  - pulmonary B39.2
    - acute B39.0
    - chronic B39.1
- Darling's B39.4
- duboisii B39.5
- lung NEC B39.2

History
- family (of) — see also History, personal (of)
  - adenomatous polyposis Z83.72
  - alcohol abuse Z81.1
  - allergy NEC Z84.89
  - anemia Z83.2
  - arthritis Z82.61
  - asthma Z82.5
  - blindness Z82.1
  - cardiac death (sudden) Z82.41
  - carrier of genetic disease Z84.81
  - chromosomal anomaly Z82.79
  - chronic
    - disabling disease NEC Z82.8
    - lower respiratory disease Z82.5
  - colonic polyps Z83.719
    - adenomatous and serrated Z83.710
    - hyperplastic Z83.711
    - inflammatory Z83.718
    - specified, NEC Z83.718
    - tubular adenoma Z83.710
    - tubulovillous adenoma Z83.710
    - villous adenoma Z83.710
  - congenital malformations and deformations Z82.79
    - polycystic kidney Z82.71
  - consanguinity Z84.3
  - deafness Z82.2
  - diabetes mellitus Z83.3
  - disability NEC Z82.8
  - disease or disorder (of)
    - allergic NEC Z84.89
    - behavioral NEC Z81.8
    - blood and blood-forming organs Z83.2
    - cardiovascular NEC Z82.49
    - chronic disabling NEC Z82.8
    - digestive Z83.79
    - ear NEC Z83.52
    - elevated lipoprotein (a) (Lp(a)) Z83.430
    - endocrine NEC Z83.49
    - eye NEC Z83.518
      - glaucoma Z83.511
    - familial hypercholesterolemia Z83.42
    - genitourinary NEC Z84.2
    - glaucoma Z83.511

History — continued
  family — see also History, personal — continued
    disease or disorder — continued
      hematological Z83.2
      immune mechanism Z83.2
      infectious NEC Z83.1
      ischemic heart Z82.49
      kidney Z84.19
        APOL1-mediated (AMKD) Z84.11
      lipoprotein metabolism Z83.438
      mental NEC Z81.8
      metabolic Z83.49
      musculoskeletal NEC Z82.69
      neurological NEC Z82.0
      nutritional Z83.49
      parasitic NEC Z83.1
      psychiatric NEC Z81.8
      respiratory NEC Z83.6
      skin and subcutaneous tissue NEC Z84.0
      specified NEC Z84.89
    drug abuse NEC Z81.3
    elevated lipoprotein (a) (Lp(a)) Z83.430
    epilepsy Z82.0
    exposure to diethylstilbestrol (DES) Z84.A
    familial hypercholesterolemia Z83.42
    genetic disease carrier Z84.81
    glaucoma Z83.511
    hearing loss Z82.2
    human immunodeficiency virus (HIV) infection Z83.0
    Huntington's chorea Z82.0
    hyperlipidemia, familial combined Z83.438
    intellectual disability Z81.0
    leukemia Z80.6
    lipidemia NEC Z83.438
    malignant neoplasm (of) NOS Z80.9
      bladder Z80.52
      breast Z80.3
      bronchus Z80.1
      digestive organ Z80.0
      fallopian tube(s) Z80.44
      gastrointestinal tract Z80.0
      genital organ Z80.49
        fallopian tube(s) Z80.44
        ovary Z80.41
        prostate Z80.42
        specified organ NEC Z80.49
        testis Z80.43
      hematopoietic NEC Z80.7
      intrathoracic organ NEC Z80.2
      kidney Z80.51
      lung Z80.1
      lymphatic NEC Z80.7
      ovary Z80.41
      prostate Z80.42
      respiratory organ NEC Z80.2
      specified site NEC Z80.8
      testis Z80.43
      trachea Z80.1
      urinary organ or tract Z80.59
        bladder Z80.52
        kidney Z80.51
    mental
      disorder NEC Z81.8
    multiple endocrine neoplasia (MEN) syndrome Z83.41
    osteoporosis Z82.62
    polycystic kidney Z82.71
    polyposis, adenomatous Z83.72
    polyps (colon) — see also History, family, colonic
      polyps Z83.719
    psychiatric disorder Z81.8
    psychoactive substance abuse NEC Z81.3
    respiratory condition NEC Z83.6
      asthma and other lower respiratory conditions
        Z82.5
    self-harmful behavior Z81.8
    SIDS (sudden infant death syndrome) Z84.82
    skin condition Z84.0
    specified condition NEC Z84.89
    stroke (cerebrovascular) Z82.3
    substance abuse NEC Z81.4
      alcohol Z81.1
      drug NEC Z81.3
        psychoactive NEC Z81.3
      tobacco Z81.2
    sudden
      cardiac death Z82.41
      infant death syndrome (SIDS) Z84.82
    tobacco abuse Z81.2
    violence, violent behavior Z81.8

History — continued
  family — see also History, personal — continued
    visual loss Z82.1
  personal (of) — see also History, family (of)
    abuse
      adult Z91.419
        financial Z91.413
        forced labor or sexual exploitation Z91.42
        intimate partner Z91.414
        physical and sexual Z91.410
        psychological Z91.411
      childhood Z62.819
        financial Z62.814
        forced labor or sexual exploitation in childhood
          Z62.813
        intimate partner Z62.815
        physical Z62.810
        psychological Z62.811
        sexual Z62.810
      in adolescence — see History, personal, abuse,
        childhood
    alcohol dependence F10.21
    allergy (to) Z88.9
      analgesic agent NEC Z88.6
      anesthetic Z88.4
      anti-infective agent NEC Z88.3
      antibiotic agent NEC Z88.1
      contrast media Z91.041
      drugs, medicaments and biological substances
        Z88.9
        specified NEC Z88.8
      food Z91.018
        additives Z91.02
        beef Z91.014
        eggs Z91.0120
          with
            reactivity to baked egg Z91.0122
            tolerance to baked egg Z91.0121
        lamb Z91.014
        mammalian meats Z91.014
        milk products Z91.0110
          with
            reactivity to baked milk Z91.0112
            tolerance to baked milk Z91.0111
        peanuts Z91.010
        pork Z91.014
        red meats Z91.014
        seafood Z91.013
        specified food NEC Z91.018
      insect Z91.038
        bee Z91.030
      latex Z91.040
      medicinal agents Z88.9
        specified NEC Z88.8
      narcotic agent NEC Z88.5
      nonmedicinal agents Z91.048
      penicillin Z88.0
      serum Z88.7
      specified NEC Z91.09
      sulfonamides Z88.2
      vaccine Z88.7
    anaphylactic shock Z87.892
    anaphylaxis Z87.892
    behavioral disorders Z86.59
    benign carcinoid tumor Z86.012
    benign neoplasm Z86.018
      brain Z86.011
      carcinoid Z86.012
      colonic polyps — see History, personal, neoplasm,
        benign, colon polyp
    brain injury (traumatic) Z87.820
    breast implant removal Z98.86
    calculi, renal Z87.442
    cancer — see History, personal (of), malignant neo-
      plasm (of)
    CAR-T (Chimeric Antigen Receptor T-cell) therapy
      Z92.850
    cardiac arrest (death), successfully resuscitated Z86.74
    cellular therapy Z92.859
      specified NEC Z92.858
    cerebral infarction without residual deficit Z86.73
    certain (corrected) conditions arising in the perinatal
      period, specified NEC Z87.68
    cervical dysplasia Z87.410
    chemotherapy for neoplastic condition Z92.21
    childhood abuse — see History, personal (of), abuse
    Chimeric Antigen Receptor T-cell (CAR-T) therapy
      Z92.850
    cleft lip (corrected) Z87.730

History — continued
  personal — see also History, family — continued
    cleft palate (corrected) Z87.730
    cloaca, persistent Z87.732
    cloacal malformations Z87.732
    collapsed vertebra (healed) Z87.311
      due to osteoporosis Z87.310
    combat and operational stress reaction Z86.51
    congenital malformation (corrected) Z87.798
      circulatory system (corrected) Z87.74
      diaphragmatic hernia Z87.760
      digestive system (corrected) NEC Z87.738
      ear (corrected) Z87.721
      eye (corrected) Z87.720
      face and neck (corrected) Z87.790
      gastroschisis Z87.761
      genitourinary system (corrected) NEC Z87.718
      heart (corrected) Z87.74
      integument (corrected) Z87.768
      limb(s) (corrected) Z87.768
      malformations
        abdominal wall Z87.763
        diaphragm NEC Z87.760
        integument Z87.768
        limbs Z87.768
        musculoskeletal system Z87.768
        prune belly Z87.762
      musculoskeletal system (corrected) Z87.768
      neck (corrected) Z87.790
      nervous system (corrected) NEC Z87.728
      respiratory system (corrected) Z87.75
      sense organs (corrected) NEC Z87.728
      specified NEC Z87.798
    contraception Z92.0
    coronavirus (disease) (novel) 2019 Z86.16
    COVID-19 Z86.16
    deployment (military) Z91.82
    diabetic foot ulcer Z86.31
    disease or disorder (of) Z87.898
      anaphylaxis Z87.892
      blood and blood-forming organs Z86.2
      circulatory system Z86.79
        specified condition NEC Z86.79
      connective tissue Z87.39
      digestive system Z87.19
        colonic polyp — see History, personal, neo-
          plasm, benign, colon polyp
        peptic ulcer disease Z87.11
        specified condition NEC Z87.19
      ear Z86.69
      endocrine Z86.39
        diabetic foot ulcer Z86.31
        gestational diabetes Z86.32
        specified type NEC Z86.39
      eye Z86.69
      genital (track) system NEC
        female Z87.42
        male Z87.438
      hematological Z86.2
      Hodgkin Z85.71
      immune mechanism Z86.2
      infectious Z86.19
        coronavirus (disease) (novel) 2019 Z86.16
        COVID-19 Z86.16
        malaria Z86.13
        Methicillin resistant Staphylococcus aureus
          (MRSA) Z86.14
        poliomyelitis Z86.12
        SARS-CoV-2 Z86.16
        specified NEC Z86.19
        tuberculosis Z86.11
      mental NEC Z86.59
      metabolic Z86.39
        diabetic foot ulcer Z86.31
        gestational diabetes Z86.32
        specified type NEC Z86.39
      musculoskeletal NEC Z87.39
      nervous system Z86.69
      nutritional Z86.39
      parasitic Z86.19
      respiratory system NEC Z87.09
      sense organs Z86.69
      skin Z87.2
      specified site or type NEC Z87.898
      subcutaneous tissue Z87.2
      trophoblastic Z87.59
      urinary system NEC Z87.448
    drug dependence — see Dependence, drug, by type,
      in remission

History — continued
  personal — see also History, family — continued
    drug therapy
      antineoplastic chemotherapy Z92.21
      estrogen Z92.23
      ICI (immune checkpoint inhibitor) drug therapy Z92.26
      immunosuppression Z92.25
      inhaled steroids Z92.240
      monoclonal drug Z92.22
      specified NEC Z92.29
      steroid Z92.241
      systemic steroids Z92.241
    dysplasia
      cervical (mild) (moderate) Z87.410
        severe (grade III) Z86.001
      prostatic Z87.430
      vaginal (mild) (moderate) Z87.411
        severe (grade III) Z86.002
      vulvar (mild) (moderate) Z87.412
        severe (grade III) Z86.002
    embolism (venous) Z86.718
      pulmonary Z86.711
    encephalitis Z86.61
    estrogen therapy Z92.23
    extracorporeal membrane oxygenation (ECMO) Z92.81
    failed conscious sedation Z92.83
    failed moderate sedation Z92.83
    fall, falling Z91.81
    forced labor or sexual exploitation Z91.42
      in childhood Z62.813
    fracture (healed)
      fatigue Z87.312
      fragility Z87.310
      osteoporosis Z87.310
      pathological NEC Z87.311
      stress Z87.312
      traumatic Z87.81
    gene therapy Z92.86
    gestational diabetes Z86.32
    hepatitis
      B Z86.19
      C Z86.19
    Hodgkin disease Z85.71
    hyperthermia, malignant Z88.4
    hypospadias (corrected) Z87.710
    hysterectomy Z90.710
    ICI (immune checkpoint inhibitor) drug therapy Z92.26
    immune checkpoint inhibitor (ICI) therapy Z92.26
    immunosuppression therapy Z92.25
    in situ neoplasm
      breast Z86.000
      cervix uteri Z86.001
      digestive organs, specified NEC Z86.004
      esophagus Z86.003
      fallopian tube(s) Z86.00A
      genital organs, specified NEC Z86.002
      melanoma Z86.006
      middle ear Z86.005
      oral cavity Z86.003
      respiratory system Z86.005
      skin Z86.007
      specified NEC Z86.008
      stomach Z86.003
    in utero procedure during pregnancy Z98.870
    in utero procedure while a fetus Z98.871
    infection NEC Z86.19
      central nervous system Z86.61
      coronavirus (disease) (novel) 2019 Z86.16
      COVID-19 Z86.16
      latent tuberculosis Z86.15
      Methicillin resistant Staphylococcus aureus (MRSA) Z86.14
      SARS-CoV-2 Z86.16
      urinary (recurrent) (tract) Z87.440
    injury NEC Z87.828
    irradiation Z92.3
    kidney stones Z87.442
    latent tuberculosis infection Z86.15
    leukemia Z85.6
    lymphoma (non-Hodgkin) Z85.72
    malignant melanoma (skin) Z85.820
    malignant neoplasm (of) Z85.9
      accessory sinuses Z85.22
      anus NEC Z85.048
        carcinoid Z85.040
      bladder Z85.51
      bone Z85.830

History — continued
  personal — see also History, family — continued
    malignant neoplasm — continued
      brain Z85.841
      breast Z85.3
      bronchus NEC Z85.118
        carcinoid Z85.110
      carcinoid — see History, personal (of), malignant neoplasm, by site, carcinoid
      cervix Z85.41
      colon NEC Z85.038
        carcinoid Z85.030
      digestive organ Z85.00
        specified NEC Z85.09
      endocrine gland NEC Z85.858
      epididymis Z85.48
      esophagus Z85.01
      eye Z85.840
      fallopian tube(s) Z85.4A
      gastrointestinal tract — see History, malignant neoplasm, digestive organ
      genital organ
        female Z85.40
          specified NEC Z85.44
        male Z85.45
          specified NEC Z85.49
      hematopoietic NEC Z85.79
      intrathoracic organ Z85.20
      kidney NEC Z85.528
        carcinoid Z85.520
      large intestine NEC Z85.038
        carcinoid Z85.030
      larynx Z85.21
      liver Z85.05
      lung NEC Z85.118
        carcinoid Z85.110
      mediastinum Z85.29
      Merkel cell Z85.821
      middle ear Z85.22
      nasal cavities Z85.22
      nervous system NEC Z85.848
      oral cavity Z85.819
        specified site NEC Z85.818
      ovary Z85.43
      pancreas Z85.07
      pelvis Z85.53
      pharynx Z85.819
        specified site NEC Z85.818
      pleura Z85.29
      prostate Z85.46
      rectosigmoid junction NEC Z85.048
        carcinoid Z85.040
      rectum NEC Z85.048
        carcinoid Z85.040
      respiratory organ Z85.20
      sinuses, accessory Z85.22
      skin NEC Z85.828
        melanoma Z85.820
        Merkel cell Z85.821
      small intestine NEC Z85.068
        carcinoid Z85.060
      soft tissue Z85.831
      specified site NEC Z85.89
      stomach NEC Z85.028
        carcinoid Z85.020
      testis Z85.47
      thymus NEC Z85.238
        carcinoid Z85.230
      thyroid Z85.850
      tongue Z85.810
      trachea Z85.12
      urinary organ or tract Z85.50
        specified NEC Z85.59
      uterus Z85.42
    maltreatment Z91.89
    medical treatment NEC Z92.89
    melanoma Z85.820
      in situ Z86.006
      malignant (skin) Z85.820
    meningitis Z86.61
    mental disorder Z86.59
    Merkel cell carcinoma (skin) Z85.821
    Methicillin resistant Staphylococcus aureus (MRSA) Z86.14
    military deployment Z91.82
    military service Z91.85
    military war, peacekeeping and humanitarian deployment (current or past conflict) Z91.82
    myocardial infarction (old) I25.2

History — continued
  personal — see also History, family — continued
    necrotizing enterocolitis of newborn (corrected) Z87.61
    neglect (in)
      adult Z91.412
      childhood Z62.812
    neoplasia
      anal intraepithelial, III [AIN III] Z86.004
      high-grade prostatic intraepithelial, III [HGPIN III] Z86.002
      vaginal intraepithelial, III [VAIN III] Z86.002
      vulvar intraepithelial, III [VIN III] Z86.002
    neoplasm
      benign Z86.018
        brain Z86.011
        colon polyp Z86.0100
          adenomatous (sessile) Z86.0101
          hyperplastic Z86.0102
          serrated (sessile) Z86.0101
          specified NEC Z86.0109
          traditional serrated adenoma Z86.0101
          tubular adenoma Z86.0101
          tubulovillous adenoma Z86.0101
          villous adenoma Z86.0101
      in situ
        breast Z86.000
        cervix uteri Z86.001
        digestive organs, specified NEC Z86.004
        esophagus Z86.003
        genital organs, specified NEC Z86.002
        melanoma Z86.006
        middle ear Z86.005
        oral cavity Z86.003
        respiratory system Z86.005
        skin Z86.007
        specified NEC Z86.008
        stomach Z86.003
      malignant — see History of, malignant neoplasm
      uncertain behavior Z86.03
    nephrotic syndrome Z87.441
    nicotine dependence Z87.891
    noncompliance with medical treatment or regimen — see Noncompliance
    nutritional deficiency Z86.39
    obstetric complications Z87.59
      childbirth Z87.59
      pregnancy Z87.59
      pre-term labor Z87.51
      puerperium Z87.59
    osteoporosis fractures Z87.310
    parasuicide (attempt) Z91.51
    physical trauma NEC Z87.828
      self-harm or suicide attempt Z91.51
    pneumonia (recurrent) Z87.01
    poisoning NEC Z91.89
      self-harm or suicide attempt Z91.51
    poor personal hygiene Z91.89
    preterm labor Z87.51
    procedure during pregnancy Z98.870
    procedure while a fetus Z98.871
    prolonged reversible ischemic neurologic deficit (PRIND) Z86.73
    prostatic dysplasia Z87.430
    psychological
      abuse
        adult Z91.411
        child Z62.811
      trauma, specified NEC Z91.49
    radiation therapy Z92.3
    removal
      implant
        breast Z98.86
    renal calculi Z87.442
    respiratory condition NEC Z87.09
    retained foreign body fully removed Z87.821
    risk factors NEC Z91.89
    SARS-CoV-2 infection Z86.16
    self-harm
      nonsuicidal Z91.52
      suicidal Z91.51
    self-inflicted injury without suicidal intent Z91.52
    self-injury
      nonsuicidal Z91.52
    self-mutilation Z91.52
    self-poisoning attempt Z91.51
    sex reassignment Z87.890
    sleep-wake cycle problem Z72.821
    specified NEC Z87.898

History — continued
  personal — see also History, family — continued
    steroid therapy (systemic) Z92.241
      inhaled Z92.240
    stroke without residual deficits Z86.73
    substance abuse NEC F10-F19
    sudden cardiac arrest Z86.74
    sudden cardiac death successfully resuscitated Z86.74
    suicidal behavior Z91.51
    suicide attempt Z91.51
    surgery NEC Z98.890
      with uterine scar Z98.891
      sex reassignment Z87.890
      transplant — see Transplant
    thrombophlebitis Z86.72
    thrombosis (venous) Z86.718
      pulmonary Z86.711
    tobacco dependence Z87.891
    tracheoesophageal
      atresia Z87.731
      fistula Z87.731
    transient ischemic attack (TIA) without residual deficits Z86.73
    trauma (physical) NEC Z87.828
      psychological NEC Z91.49
      self-harm Z91.51
    traumatic brain injury Z87.820
    tuberculosis, latent infection Z86.15
    unhealthy sleep-wake cycle Z72.821
    unintended awareness under general anesthesia Z92.84
    urinary calculi Z87.442
    urinary (recurrent) (tract) infection(s) Z87.440
    uterine scar from previous surgery Z98.891
    vaginal dysplasia Z87.411
    venous thrombosis or embolism Z86.718
      pulmonary Z86.711
    vulvar dysplasia Z87.412
HIV — see also Human, immunodeficiency virus B20
  laboratory evidence (nonconclusive) R75
  nonconclusive test (in infants) R75
  positive, seropositive Z21
Hives (bold) — see Urticaria
Hoarseness R49.0
Hobo Z59.00
Hodgkin disease — see Lymphoma, Hodgkin
Hodgson's — see also Aneurysm, aorta, thorax I71.20
  ruptured — see also Aneurysm, aorta, thorax, ruptured I71.10
Hoffa-Kastert disease E88.89
Hoffa's disease E88.89
Hoffmann-Bouveret syndrome I47.9
Hoffmann's syndrome E03.9 [G73.7]
HoFH (homozygous familial hypercholesterolemia) E78.010
Hole (round)
  macula H35.34- ☑
  retina (without detachment) — see Break, retina, round hole
    with detachment — see Detachment, retina, with retinal, break
Holiday relief care Z75.5
Hollenhorst's plaque — see Occlusion, artery, retina
Hollow foot (congenital) Q66.7- ☑
  acquired — see Deformity, limb, foot, specified NEC
Holoprosencephaly Q04.2
Holt-Oram syndrome Q87.2
Homelessness Z59.00
  sheltered Z59.01
  unsheltered Z59.02
Homesickness — see Disorder, adjustment
Homocysteinemia R79.83
Homocystinemia R79.83
Homocystinuria E72.11
Homogentisate 1,2-dioxygenase deficiency E70.29
Homologous serum hepatitis (prophylactic) (therapeutic) — see Hepatitis, viral, type B
Honeycomb lung J98.4
  congenital Q33.0
Hooded
  clitoris Q52.6
  penis Q55.69
Hookworm (disease) (infection) (infestation) B76.9
  with anemia B76.9 [D63.8]
  specified NEC B76.8
Hordeolum (eyelid) (externum) (recurrent) H00.019
  internum H00.029
    left H00.026
      lower H00.025
      upper H00.024

Hordeolum — continued
  internum — continued
    right H00.023
      lower H00.022
      upper H00.021
    left H00.016
      lower H00.015
      upper H00.014
    right H00.013
      lower H00.012
      upper H00.011
Horn
  cutaneous L85.8
  nail L60.2
    congenital Q84.6
Horner (-Claude Bernard) **syndrome** G90.2
  traumatic — see Injury, nerve, cervical sympathetic
Horseshoe kidney (congenital) Q63.1
Horton's headache or neuralgia G44.099
  intractable G44.091
  not intractable G44.099
Hospital hopper syndrome — see Disorder, factitious
Hospitalism in children — see Disorder, adjustment
Hostility R45.5
  towards child Z62.3
Hot flashes
  menopausal N95.1
Hourglass (contracture) — see also Contraction, hourglass
  stomach K31.89
    congenital Q40.2
    stricture K31.2
Household, housing circumstance affecting care Z59.9
  specified NEC Z59.89
Housemaid's knee — see Bursitis, prepatellar
HSCT-TMA (hematopoietic stem cell transplantation-associated thrombotic microangiopathy) M31.11
Hudson (-Stahli) **line** (cornea) — see Pigmentation, cornea, anterior
Human
  bite (open wound) — see also Bite
    intact skin surface — see Bite, superficial
  herpesvirus — see Herpes
  immunodeficiency virus (HIV) disease (infection) B20
    asymptomatic status Z21
    contact Z20.6
    counseling Z71.7
    dementia — see also Dementia, in, diseases specified elsewhere B20 [F02.80]
      with behavioral disturbance — see also Dementia, in, diseases specified elsewhere B20 [F02.81-] ☑
    exposure to Z20.6
    laboratory evidence R75
    type-2 (HIV 2) as cause of disease classified elsewhere B97.35
  papillomavirus (HPV)
    DNA test positive
      high risk
        cervix R87.810
        vagina R87.811
      low risk
        cervix R87.820
        vagina R87.821
    screening for Z11.51
  T-cell lymphotropic virus
    type-1 (HTLV-I) infection B33.3
      as cause of disease classified elsewhere B97.33
      carrier Z22.6
    type-2 (HTLV-II) as cause of disease classified elsewhere B97.34
Humidifier lung or pneumonitis J67.7
Humiliation (experience) **in childhood** Z62.898
Humpback (acquired) — see Kyphosis
Hunchback (acquired) — see Kyphosis
Hunger T73.0- ☑
  air, psychogenic F45.8
Hungry bone syndrome E83.81
Hunner's ulcer — see Cystitis, chronic, interstitial
Hunter's
  glossitis D51.0
  syndrome E76.1
Huntington's disease or chorea G10
  with dementia — see also Dementia, in, diseases specified elsewhere G10 [F02.80]
    with behavioral disturbance — see also Dementia, in, diseases specified elsewhere G10 [F02.81-] ☑
Hunt's
  disease or syndrome (herpetic geniculate ganglionitis) B02.21

Hunt's — continued
  disease or syndrome — continued
    dyssynergia cerebellaris myoclonica G11.19
    neuralgia B02.21
Hurler (-Scheie) **disease or syndrome** E76.02
Hurst's disease G36.1
Hurthle cell
  adenocarcinoma C73
  adenoma D34
  carcinoma C73
  tumor D34
Hutchinson-Boeck disease or syndrome — see Sarcoidosis
Hutchinson-Gilford disease or syndrome E34.8
Hutchinson's
  disease, meaning
    angioma serpiginosum L81.7
    pompholyx (cheiropompholyx) L30.1
    prurigo estivalis L56.4
    summer eruption or summer prurigo L56.4
  melanotic freckle — see Melanoma, in situ
    malignant melanoma in — see Melanoma
  teeth or incisors (congenital syphilis) A50.52
  triad (congenital syphilis) A50.53
Hyalin plaque, sclera, senile H15.89
Hyaline membrane (disease) (lung) (pulmonary) (newborn) P22.0
Hyalinosis
  cutis (et mucosae) E78.89
  focal and segmental (glomerular) — see also N00-N07 with fourth character .1 N05.1
Hyalitis, hyalosis, asteroid — see also Deposit, crystalline
  syphilitic (late) A52.71
Hydatid
  cyst or tumor — see Echinococcus
  mole — see Hydatidiform mole
  Morgagni
    female Q50.5
    male (epididymal) Q55.4
    testicular Q55.29
Hydatidiform mole (benign) (complicating pregnancy) (delivered) (undelivered) O01.9
  classical O01.0
  complete O01.0
  incomplete O01.1
  invasive D39.2
  malignant D39.2
  partial O01.1
Hydatidosis — see Echinococcus
Hydradenitis (axillaris) (suppurative) L73.2
Hydradenoma — see Hidradenoma
Hydramnios O40.- ☑
Hydrancephaly, hydranencephaly Q04.3
  with spina bifida — see Spina bifida, with hydrocephalus
Hydrargyrism NEC — see Poisoning, mercury
Hydrarthrosis — see also Effusion, joint
  gonococcal A54.42
  intermittent M12.40
    ankle M12.47- ☑
    elbow M12.42- ☑
    foot joint M12.47- ☑
    hand joint M12.44- ☑
    hip M12.45- ☑
    knee M12.46- ☑
    multiple site M12.49
    shoulder M12.41- ☑
    specified joint NEC M12.48
    wrist M12.43- ☑
  of yaws (early) (late) — see also subcategory M14.8- A66.6
  syphilitic (late) A52.77
    congenital A50.55 [M12.80]
Hydremia D64.89
Hydrencephalocele (congenital) — see Encephalocele
Hydrencephalomeningocele (congenital) — see Encephalocele
Hydroa R23.8
  aestivale L56.4
  vacciniforme L56.4
Hydroadenitis (axillaris) (suppurative) L73.2
Hydrocalycosis — see Hydronephrosis
Hydrocele (spermatic cord) (testis) (tunica vaginalis) N43.3
  canal of Nuck N94.89
  communicating N43.2
    congenital P83.5
  congenital P83.5
  encysted N43.0
  female NEC N94.89
  infected N43.1
  newborn P83.5

Hydrocele — *continued*
- round ligament N94.89
- specified NEC N43.2
- spinalis — *see* Spina bifida
- vulva N90.89

Hydrocephalus (acquired) (external) (internal) (malignant) (recurrent) G91.9
- aqueduct Sylvius stricture Q03.0
- causing disproportion O33.6- ☑
  - with obstructed labor O66.3
- communicating G91.0
- congenital (external) (internal) Q03.9
  - with spina bifida Q05.4
    - cervical Q05.0
    - dorsal Q05.1
    - lumbar Q05.2
    - lumbosacral Q05.2
    - sacral Q05.3
    - thoracic Q05.1
    - thoracolumbar Q05.1
  - specified NEC Q03.8
- due to toxoplasmosis (congenital) P37.1
- foramen Magendie block (acquired) G91.1
  - congenital — *see also* Hydrocephalus, congenital Q03.1
- in (due to)
  - infectious disease NEC B89 [G91.4]
  - neoplastic disease NEC — *see also* Neoplasm G91.4
  - parasitic disease B89 [G91.4]
- newborn Q03.9
  - with spina bifida — *see* Spina bifida, with hydrocephalus
- noncommunicating G91.1
- normal pressure G91.2
  - secondary G91.0
- obstructive G91.1
- otitic G93.2
- post-traumatic NEC G91.3
- secondary G91.4
  - post-traumatic G91.3
- specified NEC G91.8
- syphilitic, congenital A50.49

Hydrocolpos (congenital) N89.8
Hydrocystoma — *see* Neoplasm, skin, benign
Hydroencephalocele (congenital) — *see* Encephalocele
Hydroencephalomeningocele (congenital) — *see* Encephalocele
Hydrohematopneumothorax — *see* Hemothorax
Hydromeningitis — *see* Meningitis
Hydromeningocele (spinal) — *see also* Spina bifida
- cranial — *see* Encephalocele

Hydrometra N85.8
Hydrometrocolpos N89.8
Hydromicrocephaly Q02
Hydromphalos (since birth) Q45.8
Hydromyelia Q06.4
Hydromyelocele — *see* Spina bifida
Hydronephrosis (atrophic) (early) (functionless) (intermittent) (primary) (secondary) NEC N13.30
- with
  - infection N13.6
  - obstruction (by) (of)
    - renal calculus N13.2
      - with infection N13.6
    - ureteral NEC N13.1
      - with infection N13.6
        - calculus N13.2
          - with infection N13.6
    - ureteropelvic junction (congenital) Q62.11
      - acquired N13.0
        - with infection N13.6
    - ureteral stricture NEC N13.1
      - with infection N13.6
- congenital Q62.0
  - due to acquired occlusion of ureteropelvic junction N13.0
- specified type NEC N13.39
- tuberculous A18.11

Hydropericarditis — *see* Pericarditis
Hydropericardium — *see* Pericarditis
Hydroperitoneum R18.8
Hydrophobia — *see* Rabies
Hydrophthalmos Q15.0
Hydropneumohemothorax — *see* Hemothorax
Hydropneumopericarditis — *see* Pericarditis
Hydropneumopericardium — *see* Pericarditis
Hydropneumothorax J94.8
- traumatic — *see* Injury, intrathoracic, lung
- tuberculous NEC A15.6

Hydrops R60.9
- abdominis R18.8
- articulorum intermittens — *see* Hydrarthrosis, intermittent
- cardiac — *see* Failure, heart, congestive
- causing obstructed labor (mother) O66.3
- endolymphatic H81.0- ☑
- fetal — *see* Pregnancy, complicated by, hydrops, fetalis
- fetalis P83.2
  - due to
    - ABO isoimmunization P56.0
    - alpha thalassemia D56.0
    - hemolytic disease P56.90
      - specified NEC P56.99
    - isoimmunization (ABO) (Rh) P56.0
    - other specified nonhemolytic disease NEC P83.2
    - Rh incompatibility P56.0
  - during pregnancy — *see* Pregnancy, complicated by, hydrops, fetalis
- gallbladder K82.1
- joint — *see* Effusion, joint
- labyrinth H81.0- ☑
- newborn (idiopathic) P83.2
  - due to
    - ABO isoimmunization P56.0
    - alpha thalassemia D56.0
    - hemolytic disease P56.90
      - specified NEC P56.99
    - isoimmunization (ABO) (Rh) P56.0
    - Rh incompatibility P56.0
- nutritional — *see* Malnutrition, severe
- pericardium — *see* Pericarditis
- pleura — *see* Hydrothorax
- spermatic cord — *see* Hydrocele

Hydropyonephrosis N13.6
Hydrorachis Q06.4
Hydrorrhea (nasal) J34.89
- pregnancy — *see* Rupture, membranes, premature

Hydrosadenitis (axillaris) (suppurativa) L73.2
Hydrosalpinx (fallopian tube) (follicularis) N70.11
Hydrothorax (double) (pleura) J94.8
- chylous (nonfilarial) I89.8
  - filarial — *see also* Infestation, filarial B74.9 [J91.8]
- traumatic — *see* Injury, intrathoracic
- tuberculous NEC (non primary) A15.6

Hydroureter — *see also* Hydronephrosis N13.4
- with infection N13.6
- congenital Q62.39

Hydroureteronephrosis — *see* Hydronephrosis
Hydrourethra N36.8
Hydroxykynureninuria E70.89
Hydroxylysinemia E72.3
Hydroxyprolinemia E72.59
Hygiene, sleep
- abuse Z72.821
- inadequate Z72.821
- poor Z72.821

Hygroma (congenital) (cystic) D18.1
- praepatellare, prepatellar — *see* Bursitis, prepatellar
- subdural — *see* Leak, cerebrospinal fluid

Hymen — *see* condition
Hymenolepis, hymenolepiasis (diminuta) (infection) (infestation) (nana) B71.0
Hypalgesia R20.8
Hyper-reflexia R29.2
Hyperacidity (gastric) K31.89
- psychogenic F45.8

Hyperactive, hyperactivity F90.9
- basal cell, uterine cervix — *see* Dysplasia, cervix
- bowel sounds R19.12
- cervix epithelial (basal) — *see* Dysplasia, cervix
- child F90.9
  - attention deficit — *see* Disorder, attention-deficit hyperactivity
- detrusor muscle N32.81
- gastrointestinal K31.89
  - psychogenic F45.8
- nasal mucous membrane J34.3
- stomach K31.89
- thyroid (gland) — *see* Hyperthyroidism

Hyperacusis H93.23- ☑
Hyperadrenalism E27.5
Hyperadrenocorticism E24.9
- congenital E25.0
- iatrogenic E24.2
  - correct substance properly administered — *see* Table of Drugs and Chemicals, by drug, adverse effect

Hyperadrenocorticism — *continued*
- iatrogenic — *continued*
  - overdose or wrong substance given or taken — *see* Table of Drugs and Chemicals, by drug, poisoning
- not associated with Cushing's syndrome E27.0
- pituitary-dependent E24.0

Hyperaldosteronism E26.9
- familial (type I) E26.02
- glucocorticoid-remediable E26.02
- primary (due to (bilateral) adrenal hyperplasia) E26.09
- primary NEC E26.09
- secondary E26.1
- specified NEC E26.89

Hyperalgesia R20.8
Hyperalimentation R63.2
- carotene, carotin E67.1
- specified NEC E67.8
- vitamin
  - A E67.0
  - D E67.3

Hyperaminoaciduria
- arginine E72.21
- cystine E72.01
- lysine E72.3
- ornithine E72.4

Hyperammonemia (congenital) E72.20
Hyperazotemia — *see* Uremia
Hyperbetalipoproteinemia (familial) E78.00
- with prebetalipoproteinemia E78.2

Hyperbicarbonatemia P74.41
Hyperbilirubinemia
- constitutional E80.6
- familial conjugated E80.6
- neonatal (transient) — *see* Jaundice, newborn

Hypercalcemia, hypocalciuric, familial E83.52
Hypercalciuria, idiopathic R82.994
Hypercapnia R06.89
- newborn P84

Hypercarotenemia (dietary) E67.1
Hypercementosis K03.4
Hyperchloremia E87.8
Hyperchlorhydria K31.89
- neurotic F45.8
- psychogenic F45.8

Hypercholesterinemia — *see* Hypercholesterolemia
Hypercholesterolemia (essential) (primary) (pure) E78.00
- with hyperglyceridemia, endogenous E78.2
- dietary counseling and surveillance Z71.3
- familial E78.019
  - heterozygous [HeFH] E78.011
  - homozygous [HoFH] E78.010
- hereditary E78.019

Hyperchylia gastrica, psychogenic F45.8
Hyperchylomicronemia (familial) (primary) E78.3
- with hyperbetalipoproteinemia E78.3

Hypercoagulable (state) D68.59
- activated protein C resistance D68.51
- antithrombin (III) deficiency D68.59
- factor V Leiden mutation D68.51
- primary NEC D68.59
- protein C deficiency D68.59
- protein S deficiency D68.59
- prothrombin gene mutation D68.52
- secondary D68.69
- specified NEC D68.69

Hypercoagulation (state) D68.59
Hypercorticalism, pituitary-dependent E24.0
Hypercorticosolism — *see* Cushing's, syndrome
Hypercorticosteronism E24.2
- correct substance properly administered — *see* Table of Drugs and Chemicals, by drug, adverse effect
- overdose or wrong substance given or taken — *see* Table of Drugs and Chemicals, by drug, poisoning

Hypercortisonism E24.2
- correct substance properly administered — *see* Table of Drugs and Chemicals, by drug, adverse effect
- overdose or wrong substance given or taken — *see* Table of Drugs and Chemicals, by drug, poisoning

Hyperekplexia Q89.89
Hyperelectrolytemia E87.8
Hyperemesis R11.10
- with nausea R11.2
- gravidarum (mild) O21.0
  - with
    - carbohydrate depletion O21.1
    - dehydration O21.1
    - electrolyte imbalance O21.1
    - metabolic disturbance O21.1

Hyperemesis — continued
  gravidarum — continued
    severe (with metabolic disturbance) O21.1
  projectile R11.12
  psychogenic F45.8
Hyperemia (acute) (passive) R68.89
  anal mucosa K62.89
  bladder N32.89
  cerebral I67.89
  conjunctiva H11.43- ☑
  ear internal, acute — see subcategory H83.0- ☑
  enteric K59.89
  eye — see Hyperemia, conjunctiva
  eyelid (active) (passive) — see Disorder, eyelid, specified type NEC
  intestine K59.89
  iris — see Disorder, iris, vascular
  kidney N28.89
  labyrinth — see subcategory H83.0- ☑
  liver (active) K76.89
  lung (passive) — see Edema, lung
  pulmonary (passive) — see Edema, lung
  renal N28.89
  retina H35.89
  stomach K31.89
Hyperesthesia (body surface) R20.3
  larynx (reflex) J38.7
    hysterical F44.89
  pharynx (reflex) J39.2
    hysterical F44.89
Hyperestrogenism (drug-induced) (iatrogenic) E28.0
Hyperexplexia Q89.89
Hyperfibrinolysis — see Fibrinolysis
Hyperfructosemia E74.19
Hyperfunction
  adrenal cortex, not associated with Cushing's syndrome E27.0
    medulla E27.5
      adrenomedullary E27.5
    virilism E25.9
      congenital E25.0
  ovarian E28.8
  pancreas K86.89
  parathyroid (gland) E21.3
  pituitary (gland) (anterior) E22.9
    specified NEC E22.8
  polyglandular E31.1
  testicular E29.0
Hypergammaglobulinemia D89.2
  polyclonal D89.0
  Waldenstrom D89.0
Hypergastrinemia E16.4
Hyperglobulinemia R77.1
Hyperglycemia, hyperglycemic (transient) R73.9
  coma — see Diabetes, by type, with coma
  postpancreatectomy E89.1
Hyperglyceridemia (endogenous) (essential) (familial) (hereditary) (pure) E78.1
  mixed E78.3
Hyperglycinemia (non-ketotic) E72.51
Hypergonadism
  ovarian E28.8
  testicular (primary) (infantile) E29.0
Hyperheparinemia D68.32
Hyperhidrosis, hyperidrosis R61
  focal
    primary L74.519
      axilla L74.510
      face L74.511
      palms L74.512
      soles L74.513
    secondary L74.52
  generalized R61
  localized
    primary L74.519
      axilla L74.510
      face L74.511
      palms L74.512
      soles L74.513
    secondary L74.52
  psychogenic F45.8
  secondary R61
    focal L74.52
Hyperhistidinemia E70.41
Hyperhomocysteinemia E72.11
Hyperhydroxyprolinemia E72.59
Hyperinsulinism (functional) E16.1
  with
    coma (hypoglycemic) E15

Hyperinsulinism — continued
  with — continued
    encephalopathy E16.1 [G94]
  ectopic E16.1
  therapeutic misadventure (from administration of insulin) — see subcategory T38.3- ☑
Hyperkalemia E87.5
Hyperkeratosis — see also Keratosis L85.9
  cervix N88.0
  due to yaws (early) (late) (palmar or plantar) A66.3
  follicularis Q82.8
    penetrans (in cutem) L87.0
  palmoplantaris climacterica L85.1
  pinta A67.1
  senile (with pruritus) L57.0
  universalis congenita Q80.8
  vocal cord J38.3
  vulva N90.4
Hyperkinesia, hyperkinetic (disease) (reaction) (syndrome) (childhood) (adolescence) — see also Disorder, attention-deficit hyperactivity
  heart I51.89
Hyperleucine-isoleucinemia E71.19
Hyperlipemia, hyperlipidemia E78.5
  combined E78.2
  familial E78.49
  group
    A E78.00
    B E78.1
    C E78.2
    D E78.3
  mixed E78.2
  specified NEC E78.49
Hyperlipidosis E75.6
  hereditary NEC E75.5
Hyperlipoproteinemia E78.5
  Fredrickson's type
    I E78.3
    IIa E78.00
    IIb E78.2
    III E78.2
    IV E78.1
    V E78.3
  low-density-lipoprotein-type (LDL) E78.00
  very-low-density-lipoprotein-type (VLDL) E78.1
Hyperlucent lung, unilateral J43.0
Hyperlysinemia E72.3
Hypermagnesemia E83.41
  neonatal P71.8
Hypermenorrhea N92.0
Hypermethioninemia E72.19
Hypermetropia (congenital) H52.0- ☑
Hypermobility, hypermotility
  cecum — see Syndrome, irritable bowel
  coccyx — see subcategory M53.2- ☑
  colon — see Syndrome, irritable bowel
    psychogenic F45.8
  ileum K58.9
  intestine — see also Syndrome, irritable bowel K58.9
    psychogenic F45.8
  meniscus (knee) — see Derangement, knee, meniscus
  scapula — see Instability, joint, shoulder
  stomach K31.89
    psychogenic F45.8
  syndrome M35.7
  urethra N36.41
    with intrinsic sphincter deficiency N36.43
Hypernasality R49.21
Hypernatremia E87.0
Hypernephroma C64.- ☑
Hyperopia — see Hypermetropia
Hyperorexia nervosa F50.2- ☑
Hyperornithinemia E72.4
Hyperosmia R43.1
Hyperosmolality — see also Diabetes, by type, with hyperosmolarity E87.0
Hyperostosis (monomelic) — see also Disorder, bone, density and structure, specified NEC
  ankylosing (spine) M48.10
    cervical region M48.12
    cervicothoracic region M48.13
    lumbar region M48.16
    lumbosacral region M48.17
    multiple sites M48.19
    occipito-atlanto-axial region M48.11
    sacrococcygeal region M48.18
    thoracic region M48.14
    thoracolumbar region M48.15

Hyperostosis — continued
  cortical (skull) M85.2
    infantile M89.8X- ☑
  frontal, internal of skull M85.2
  interna frontalis M85.2
  skeletal, diffuse idiopathic — see Hyperostosis, ankylosing
  skull M85.2
    congenital Q75.8
  vertebral, ankylosing — see Hyperostosis, ankylosing
Hyperovarism E28.8
Hyperoxaluria R82.992
  primary E72.53- ☑
Hyperparathyroidism E21.3
  primary E21.0
  secondary (renal) N25.81
    non-renal E21.1
  specified NEC E21.2
  tertiary E21.2
Hyperpathia R20.8
Hyperperistalsis R19.2
  psychogenic F45.8
Hyperpermeability, capillary I78.8
Hyperphagia R63.2
Hyperphenylalaninemia NEC E70.1
Hyperphoria (alternating) H50.53
Hyperphosphatemia E83.39
Hyperpiesis, hyperpiesia — see Hypertension
Hyperpigmentation — see also Pigmentation
  melanin NEC L81.4
  postinflammatory L81.0
Hyperpinealism E34.8
Hyperpituitarism E22.9
Hyperplasia, hyperplastic
  adenoids J35.2
  adrenal (capsule) (cortex) (gland) E27.8
    with
      sexual precocity (male) E25.9
        congenital E25.0
      virilism, adrenal E25.9
        congenital E25.0
      virilization (female) E25.9
        congenital E25.0
    congenital E25.0
    salt-losing E25.0
  adrenomedullary E27.5
  angiolymphoid, eosinophilia (ALHE) D18.01
  appendix (lymphoid) K38.8
  artery, fibromuscular I77.3
  bone — see also Hypertrophy, bone
    marrow D75.89
  breast — see also Hypertrophy, breast
    atypical, atypia N60.9- ☑
      ductal N60.9- ☑
      lobular N60.9- ☑
  C-cell, thyroid E07.0
  cementation (tooth) (teeth) K03.4
  cervical gland R59.0
  cervix (uteri) (basal cell) (endometrium) (polypoid) — see also Dysplasia, cervix
    congenital Q51.828
  clitoris, congenital Q52.6
  denture K06.2
  endocervicitis N72
  endometrium, endometrial (adenomatous) (cystic) (glandular) (glandular-cystic) (polypoid) N85.00
    with atypia N85.02
    benign N85.01
    cervix — see Dysplasia, cervix
    complex (without atypia) N85.01
    simple (without atypia) N85.01
  epithelial L85.9
    focal, oral, including tongue K13.29
    nipple N62
    skin L85.9
    tongue K13.29
    vaginal wall N89.3
  erythroid D75.89
  fibromuscular of artery (carotid) (renal) I77.3
  genital
    female NEC N94.89
    male N50.89
  gingiva K06.1
  glandularis cystica uteri (interstitialis) — see also Hyperplasia, endometrial N85.00
  gum K06.1
  hymen, congenital Q52.4
  irritative, edentulous (alveolar) K06.2

☑ Additional Character Required — Refer to the Tabular List for Character Selection

Hyperplasia, hyperplastic — continued
- jaw M26.09
  - alveolar M26.79
    - lower M26.03
      - alveolar M26.72
    - upper M26.01
      - alveolar M26.71
- kidney (congenital) Q63.3
- labia N90.69
  - epithelial N90.3
- liver (congenital) Q44.79
  - nodular, focal K76.89
- lymph gland or node R59.9
- mandible, mandibular M26.03
  - alveolar M26.72
  - unilateral condylar M27.8
- maxilla, maxillary M26.01
  - alveolar M26.71
- myometrium, myometrial N85.2
- neuroendocrine cell, of infancy J84.841
- nose
  - lymphoid J34.89
  - polypoid J33.9
- oral mucosa (irritative) K13.6
- organ or site, congenital NEC — see Anomaly, by site
- ovary N83.8
- palate, papillary (irritative) K13.6
- pancreatic islet cells E16.9
  - alpha E16.8
    - with excess
      - gastrin E16.4
      - glucagon E16.3
  - beta E16.1
- parathyroid (gland) E21.0
- pharynx (lymphoid) J39.2
- prostate (adenofibromatous) N40.0
  - with lower urinary tract symptoms (LUTS) N40.1
    - nodular N40.3
  - nodular N40.2
    - with lower urinary tract symptoms (LUTS) N40.3
    - without lower urinary tract symptoms (LUTS) N40.0
      - nodular N40.2
- renal artery I77.89
- reticulo-endothelial (cell) D75.89
- salivary gland (any) K11.1
- Schimmelbusch's — see Mastopathy, cystic
- suprarenal capsule (gland) E27.8
- thymus (gland) (persistent) E32.0
- thyroid (gland) — see Goiter
- tonsils (faucial) (infective) (lingual) (lymphoid) J35.1
  - with adenoids J35.3
- unilateral condylar M27.8
- uterus, uterine N85.2
  - endometrium (glandular) — see also Hyperplasia, endometrial N85.00
- vulva N90.69
  - epithelial N90.3

Hyperpnea — see Hyperventilation
Hyperpotassemia E87.5
Hyperprebetalipoproteinemia (familial) E78.1
Hyperprolactinemia E22.1
Hyperprolinemia (type I) (type II) E72.59
Hyperproteinemia E88.09
Hyperprothrombinemia, causing coagulation factor deficiency D68.4
Hyperpyrexia R50.9
- heat (effects) T67.01- ☑
- malignant, due to anesthetic T88.3- ☑
- rheumatic — see Fever, rheumatic
- unknown origin R50.9

Hypersalivation K11.7
Hypersecretion
- ACTH (not associated with Cushing's syndrome) E27.0
  - pituitary E24.0
- adrenaline E27.5
- adrenomedullary E27.5
- androgen (testicular) E29.0
  - ovarian (drug-induced) (iatrogenic) E28.1
- calcitonin E07.0
- catecholamine E27.5
- corticoadrenal E24.9
- cortisol E24.9
- epinephrine E27.5
- estrogen E28.0
- gastric K31.89
  - psychogenic F45.8
- gastrin E16.4
- glucagon E16.3

Hypersecretion — continued
- hormone(s)
  - ACTH (not associated with Cushing's syndrome) E27.0
    - pituitary E24.0
  - antidiuretic E22.2
  - growth E22.0
  - intestinal NEC E34.1
  - ovarian androgen E28.1
  - pituitary E22.9
  - testicular E29.0
  - thyroid stimulating E05.80
    - with thyroid storm E05.81
- insulin — see Hyperinsulinism
- lacrimal glands — see Epiphora
- medulloadrenal E27.5
- milk O92.6
- ovarian androgens E28.1
- salivary gland (any) K11.7
- thyrocalcitonin E07.0
- upper respiratory J39.8

Hypersegmentation, leukocytic, hereditary D72.0
Hypersensitive, hypersensitiveness, hypersensitivity — see also Allergy
- carotid sinus G90.01
- colon — see Irritable, colon
- drug T88.7- ☑
- gastrointestinal K52.29
  - immediate K52.29
  - psychogenic F45.8
- labyrinth — see subcategory H83.2- ☑
- pain R20.8
- pneumonitis — see Pneumonitis, allergic
- reaction T78.40- ☑
- upper respiratory tract NEC J39.3

Hypersomnia (organic) G47.10
- due to
  - alcohol
    - abuse F10.182
    - dependence F10.282
    - use F10.982
  - amphetamines
    - abuse F15.182
    - dependence F15.282
    - use F15.982
  - caffeine
    - abuse F15.182
    - dependence F15.282
    - use F15.982
  - cocaine
    - abuse F14.182
    - dependence F14.282
    - use F14.982
  - drug NEC
    - abuse F19.182
    - dependence F19.282
    - use F19.982
  - medical condition G47.14
  - mental disorder F51.13
  - opioid
    - abuse F11.182
    - dependence F11.282
    - use F11.982
  - psychoactive substance NEC
    - abuse F19.182
    - dependence F19.282
    - use F19.982
  - sedative, hypnotic, or anxiolytic
    - abuse F13.182
    - dependence F13.282
    - use F13.982
  - stimulant NEC
    - abuse F15.182
    - dependence F15.282
    - use F15.982
- idiopathic G47.11
  - with long sleep time G47.11
  - without long sleep time G47.12
- menstrual related G47.13
- nonorganic origin F51.11
  - specified NEC F51.19
- not due to a substance or known physiological condition F51.11
  - specified NEC F51.19
- primary F51.11
- recurrent G47.13
- specified NEC G47.19

Hypersplenia, hypersplenism D73.1
Hyperstimulation, ovaries (associated with induced ovulation) N98.1

Hypersusceptibility — see Allergy
Hypertelorism (ocular) (orbital) Q75.2
Hypertension, hypertensive (accelerated) (benign) (essential) (idiopathic) (malignant) (systemic) I10
- with
  - heart failure (congestive) I11.0
  - heart involvement (conditions in I50.- or I51.4-I51.7, I51.89, I51.9, due to hypertension) — see Hypertension, heart
  - kidney involvement — see Hypertension, kidney
- benign, intracranial G93.2
- borderline R03.0
- cardiorenal (disease) I13.10
  - with heart failure I13.0
    - with stage 1 through stage 4 chronic kidney disease I13.0
    - with stage 5 or end stage renal disease I13.2
  - without heart failure I13.10
    - with stage 1 through stage 4 chronic kidney disease I13.10
    - with stage 5 or end stage renal disease I13.11
- cardiovascular
  - disease (arteriosclerotic) (sclerotic) — see Hypertension, heart
  - renal (disease) — see Hypertension, cardiorenal
- chronic venous — see Hypertension, venous (chronic)
- complicating
  - childbirth (labor) O16.4
  - pre-existing O10.92
    - with
      - heart disease O10.12
        - with renal disease O10.32
      - pre-eclampsia O11.4
      - renal disease O10.22
        - with heart disease O10.32
      - essential O10.02
      - secondary O10.42
  - pregnancy O16.- ☑ — see also Pre-eclampsia O14.9- ☑
    - with edema — see Pre-eclampsia O14.9- ☑
    - gestational (pregnancy induced) (without proteinuria) O13.- ☑
      - with proteinuria O14.9- ☑
        - mild pre-eclampsia O14.0- ☑
        - moderate pre-eclampsia O14.0- ☑
        - severe pre-eclampsia O14.1- ☑
          - with hemolysis, elevated liver enzymes and low platelet count (HELLP) O14.2- ☑
    - pre-existing O10.91- ☑
      - with
        - heart disease O10.11- ☑
          - with renal disease O10.31- ☑
        - pre-eclampsia — see category O11
        - renal disease O10.21- ☑
          - with heart disease O10.31- ☑
        - essential O10.01- ☑
        - secondary O10.41- ☑
    - transient O13.- ☑
  - puerperium, pre-existing O16.5
    - pre-existing
      - with
        - heart disease O10.13
          - with renal disease O10.33
        - pre-eclampsia O11.5
        - renal disease O10.23
          - with heart disease O10.33
        - essential O10.03
    - pregnancy-induced O13.9
    - secondary O10.43
- crisis I16.9
- due to
  - endocrine disorders I15.2
  - pheochromocytoma — see also Pheochromocytoma, by type I15.2
  - renal disorders NEC I15.1
    - arterial I15.0
  - renovascular disorders I15.0
  - specified disease NEC I15.8
- emergency I16.1
- encephalopathy I67.4
- gestational (without significant proteinuria) (pregnancy-induced) (transient) O13.- ☑
  - with significant proteinuria — see Pre-eclampsia
  - complicating
    - delivery O13.4
    - puerperium O13.5
- Goldblatt's I70.1

Hypertension, hypertensive — *continued*
- heart (disease) (conditions in I51.4-I51.9 due to hypertension) I11.9
  - with
    - heart failure (congestive) I11.0
    - kidney disease (chronic) — *see* Hypertension, cardiorenal
- intracranial, benign G93.2
- kidney I12.9
  - with
    - heart disease — *see* Hypertension, cardiorenal
    - stage 1 through stage 4 chronic kidney disease I12.9
    - stage 5 chronic kidney disease (CKD) or end stage renal disease (ESRD) I12.0
- lesser circulation I27.0
- maternal O16.- ☑
- newborn P29.2
  - pulmonary (persistent) P29.30
- ocular H40.05- ☑
- pancreatic duct — *code to* underlying condition
  - with chronic pancreatitis K86.1
- portal (due to chronic liver disease) (idiopathic) K76.6
  - gastropathy K31.89
  - in (due to) schistosomiasis (bilharziasis) B65.9 *[K77]*
- postoperative I97.3
- psychogenic F45.8
- pulmonary I27.20
  - with
    - cor pulmonale (chronic) I27.29
      - acute I26.09
    - right heart ventricular strain/failure I27.29
      - acute I26.09
    - right to left shunt related to congenital heart disease I27.83
    - unclear multifactorial mechanisms I27.29
  - arterial (associated) (drug-induced) (toxin-induced) I27.21
  - chronic thromboembolic I27.24
  - due to
    - hematologic disorders I27.29
    - kyphoscoliotic heart disease I27.1
    - left heart disease I27.22
    - lung diseases and hypoxia I27.23
    - metabolic disorders I27.29
    - specified systemic disorders I27.29
  - group 1 (associated) (drug-induced) (toxin-induced) I27.21
  - group 2 I27.22
  - group 3 I27.23
  - group 4 I27.24
  - group 5 I27.29
  - of newborn (persistent) P29.30
  - primary (idiopathic) I27.0
  - secondary
    - arterial I27.21
    - specified NEC I27.29
- renal — *see* Hypertension, kidney
- renovascular I15.0
- resistant (apparent treatment) (treatment) (true) I1A.0
- secondary NEC I15.9
  - due to
    - endocrine disorders I15.2
    - pheochromocytoma — *see also* Pheochromocytoma, by type I15.2
    - renal disorders NEC I15.1
      - arterial I15.0
    - renovascular disorders I15.0
  - specified NEC I15.8
- transient R03.0
  - of pregnancy O13.- ☑
- urgency I16.0
- venous (chronic)
  - due to
    - deep vein thrombosis — *see* Syndrome, postthrombotic
  - idiopathic I87.309
    - with
      - inflammation I87.32- ☑
        - with ulcer I87.33- ☑
      - specified complication NEC I87.39- ☑
      - ulcer I87.31- ☑
        - with inflammation I87.33- ☑
    - asymptomatic I87.30- ☑

Hypertensive urgency — *see* Hypertension
Hyperthecosis ovary E28.8
Hyperthermia (of unknown origin) — *see also* Hyperpyrexia
- malignant, due to anesthesia T88.3- ☑

Hyperthermia — *continued*
- newborn P81.9
  - environmental P81.0
Hyperthyroid (recurrent) — *see* Hyperthyroidism
Hyperthyroidism (latent) (pre-adult) (recurrent) E05.90
- with
  - goiter (diffuse) E05.00
    - with thyroid storm E05.01
  - nodular (multinodular) E05.20
    - with thyroid storm E05.21
    - uninodular E05.10
      - with thyroid storm E05.11
  - storm E05.91
- due to ectopic thyroid tissue E05.30
  - with thyroid storm E05.31
- neonatal, transitory P72.1
- specified NEC E05.80
  - with thyroid storm E05.81
Hypertony, hypertonia, hypertonicity
- bladder N31.8
- congenital P94.1
- stomach K31.89
  - psychogenic F45.8
- uterus, uterine (contractions) (complicating delivery) O62.4
Hypertrichosis L68.9
- congenital Q84.2
- eyelid H02.869
  - left H02.866
    - lower H02.865
    - upper H02.864
  - right H02.863
    - lower H02.862
    - upper H02.861
- lanuginosa Q84.2
  - acquired L68.1
- localized L68.2
- specified NEC L68.8
Hypertriglyceridemia, essential E78.1
Hypertrophy, hypertrophic
- adenofibromatous, prostate — *see* Enlargement, enlarged, prostate
- adenoids (infective) J35.2
  - with tonsils J35.3
- adrenal cortex E27.8
- alveolar process or ridge — *see* Anomaly, alveolar
- anal papillae K62.89
- artery I77.89
  - congenital NEC Q27.8
    - digestive system Q27.8
    - lower limb Q27.8
    - specified site NEC Q27.8
    - upper limb Q27.8
- auricular — *see* Hypertrophy, cardiac
- Bartholin's gland N75.8
- bile duct (common) (hepatic) K83.8
- bladder (sphincter) (trigone) N32.89
- bone M89.30
  - carpus M89.34- ☑
  - clavicle M89.31- ☑
  - femur M89.35- ☑
  - fibula M89.36- ☑
  - finger M89.34- ☑
  - humerus M89.32- ☑
  - ilium M89.38
  - ischium M89.38
  - metacarpus M89.34- ☑
  - metatarsus M89.37- ☑
  - multiple sites M89.39
  - neck M89.38
  - pubic ramus [pubis] M89.38
  - radius M89.33- ☑
  - rib M89.38
  - scapula M89.31- ☑
  - skull M89.38
  - tarsus M89.37- ☑
  - tibia M89.36- ☑
  - toe M89.37- ☑
  - ulna M89.33- ☑
  - vertebra M89.38
- brain G93.89
- breast N62
  - cystic — *see* Mastopathy, cystic
  - newborn P83.4
  - pubertal, massive N62
  - puerperal, postpartum — *see* Disorder, breast, specified type NEC
  - senile (parenchymatous) N62

Hypertrophy, hypertrophic — *continued*
- cardiac (chronic) (idiopathic) I51.7
  - with rheumatic fever (conditions in I00)
    - active I01.8
    - inactive or quiescent (with chorea) I09.89
  - congenital NEC Q24.8
  - fatty — *see* Degeneration, myocardial
  - hypertensive — *see* Hypertension, heart
  - rheumatic (with chorea) I09.89
    - active or acute I01.8
      - with chorea I02.0
  - valve — *see* Endocarditis
- cartilage — *see* Disorder, cartilage, specified type NEC
- cecum — *see* Megacolon
- cervix (uteri) N88.8
  - congenital Q51.828
  - elongation N88.4
- clitoris (cirrhotic) N90.89
  - congenital Q52.6
- colon — *see also* Megacolon
  - congenital Q43.2
- conjunctiva, lymphoid H11.89
- corpora cavernosa N48.89
- cystic duct K82.8
- duodenum K31.89
- endometrium (glandular) — *see also* Hyperplasia, endometrial N85.00
  - cervix N88.8
- epididymis N50.89
- esophageal hiatus (congenital) Q79.1
  - with hernia — *see* Hernia, hiatal
- eyelid — *see* Disorder, eyelid, specified type NEC
- facet joint — *see also* Spondylosis M47.819
- fat pad E65
  - knee (infrapatellar) (popliteal) (prepatellar) (retropatellar) M79.4
- foot (congenital) Q74.2
- frenulum, frenum (tongue) K14.8
  - lip K13.0
- gallbladder K82.8
- gastric mucosa K29.60
  - with bleeding K29.61
- gland, glandular R59.9
  - generalized R59.1
  - localized R59.0
- gum (mucous membrane) K06.1
- heart (idiopathic) — *see also* Hypertrophy, cardiac
  - valve — *see also* Endocarditis I38
- hemifacial Q67.4
- hepatic — *see* Hypertrophy, liver
- hiatus (esophageal) Q79.1
- hilus gland R59.0
- hymen, congenital Q52.4
- ileum K63.89
- intestine NEC K63.89
- jejunum K63.89
- kidney (compensatory) N28.81
  - congenital Q63.3
- labium (majus) (minus) N90.60
- ligament — *see* Disorder, ligament
- lingual tonsil (infective) J35.1
  - with adenoids J35.3
- lip K13.0
  - congenital Q18.6
- liver R16.0
  - acute K76.89
  - cirrhotic — *see* Cirrhosis, liver
  - congenital Q44.79
  - fatty — *see* Fatty, liver
- lymph, lymphatic gland R59.9
  - generalized R59.1
  - localized R59.0
  - tuberculous — *see* Tuberculosis, lymph gland
- mammary gland — *see* Hypertrophy, breast
- Meckel's diverticulum (congenital) Q43.0
  - malignant — *see* Table of Neoplasms, small intestine, malignant
- median bar — *see* Hyperplasia, prostate
- meibomian gland — *see* Chalazion
- meniscus, knee, congenital Q74.1
- metatarsal head — *see* Hypertrophy, bone, metatarsus
- metatarsus — *see* Hypertrophy, bone, metatarsus
- mucous membrane
  - alveolar ridge K06.2
  - gum K06.1
  - nose (turbinate) J34.3
- muscle M62.89
- muscular coat, artery I77.89
- myocardium — *see also* Hypertrophy, cardiac

☑ **Additional Character Required** — Refer to the Tabular List for Character Selection

Hypertrophy, hypertrophic — continued
- myocardium — see also Hypertrophy, cardiac — continued
  - idiopathic I42.2
- myometrium N85.2
- nail L60.2
  - congenital Q84.5
- nasal J34.89
  - alae J34.89
  - bone J34.89
  - cartilage J34.89
  - mucous membrane (septum) J34.3
  - sinus J34.89
  - turbinate J34.3
- nasopharynx, lymphoid (infectional) (tissue) (wall) J35.2
- nipple N62
- organ or site, congenital NEC — see Anomaly, by site
- ovary N83.8
- palate (hard) M27.8
  - soft K13.79
- pancreas, congenital Q45.3
- parathyroid (gland) E21.0
- parotid gland K11.1
- penis N48.89
- pharyngeal tonsil J35.2
- pharynx J39.2
  - lymphoid (infectional) (tissue) (wall) J35.2
- pituitary (anterior) (fossa) (gland) E23.6
- prepuce (congenital) N47.8
  - female N90.89
- prostate — see Enlargement, enlarged, prostate
  - congenital Q55.4
- pseudomuscular — see also Dystrophy, muscular, by type, if applicable G71.09
- pylorus (adult) (muscle) (sphincter) K31.1
  - congenital or infantile Q40.0
- rectal, rectum (sphincter) K62.89
- rhinitis (turbinate) J31.0
- salivary gland (any) K11.1
  - congenital Q38.4
- scaphoid (tarsal) — see Hypertrophy, bone, tarsus
- scar L91.0
- scrotum N50.89
- seminal vesicle N50.89
- sigmoid — see Megacolon
- skin L91.9
  - specified NEC L91.8
- spermatic cord N50.89
- spleen — see Splenomegaly
- spondylitis — see Spondylosis
- stomach K31.89
- sublingual gland K11.1
- submandibular gland K11.1
- suprarenal cortex (gland) E27.8
- synovial NEC M67.20
  - acromioclavicular M67.21- ☑
  - ankle M67.27- ☑
  - elbow M67.22- ☑
  - foot M67.27- ☑
  - hand M67.24- ☑
  - hip M67.25- ☑
  - knee M67.26- ☑
  - multiple sites M67.29
  - specified site NEC M67.28
  - wrist M67.23- ☑
- tendon — see Disorder, tendon, specified type NEC
- testis N44.8
  - congenital Q55.29
- thymic, thymus (gland) (congenital) E32.0
- thyroid (gland) — see Goiter
- toe (congenital) Q74.2
  - acquired — see also Deformity, toe, specified NEC
- tongue K14.8
  - congenital Q38.2
  - papillae (foliate) K14.3
- tonsils (faucial) (infective) (lingual) (lymphoid) J35.1
  - with adenoids J35.3
- tunica vaginalis N50.89
- ureter N28.89
- urethra N36.8
- uterus N85.2
  - neck (with elongation) N88.4
  - puerperal O90.89
- uvula K13.79
- vagina N89.8
- vas deferens N50.89
- vein I87.8

Hypertrophy, hypertrophic — continued
- ventricle, ventricular (heart) — see also Hypertrophy, cardiac
  - congenital Q24.8
  - in tetralogy of Fallot Q21.3
- verumontanum N36.8
- vocal cord J38.3
- vulva N90.60
  - stasis (nonfilarial) N90.69

Hypertropia H50.2- ☑
Hypertyrosinemia E70.21
Hyperuricemia (asymptomatic) E79.0
Hyperuricosuria R82.993
Hypervalinemia E71.19
Hyperventilation (tetany) R06.4
- hysterical F45.8
- psychogenic F45.8
- syndrome F45.8

Hypervitaminosis (dietary) NEC E67.8
- A E67.0
  - administered as drug (prolonged intake) — see Table of Drugs and Chemicals, vitamins, adverse effect
  - overdose or wrong substance given or taken — see Table of Drugs and Chemicals, vitamins, poisoning
- B6 E67.2
- D E67.3
  - administered as drug (prolonged intake) — see Table of Drugs and Chemicals, vitamins, adverse effect
  - overdose or wrong substance given or taken — see Table of Drugs and Chemicals, vitamins, poisoning
- K E67.8
  - administered as drug (prolonged intake) — see Table of Drugs and Chemicals, vitamins, adverse effect
  - overdose or wrong substance given or taken — see Table of Drugs and Chemicals, vitamins, poisoning

Hypervolemia E87.70
- specified NEC E87.79

Hypesthesia R20.1
- cornea — see Anesthesia, cornea

Hyphema H21.0- ☑
- traumatic S05.1- ☑

Hypo-osmolality E87.1
Hypo-ovarianism, hypo-ovarism E28.39
Hypoacidity, gastric K31.89
- psychogenic F45.8

Hypoadrenalism, hypoadrenia E27.40
- primary E27.1
- tuberculous A18.7

Hypoadrenocorticism E27.40
- pituitary E23.0
- primary E27.1

Hypoalbuminemia E88.09
Hypoaldosteronism E27.40
Hypoalphalipoproteinemia E78.6
Hypobarism T70.29- ☑
Hypobaropathy T70.29- ☑
Hypobetalipoproteinemia (familial) E78.6
Hypocalcemia E83.51
- autosomal dominant E20.810
  - type 1 (ADH1) E20.810
  - type 2 (ADH2) E20.810
- dietary E58
- neonatal P71.1
  - due to cow's milk P71.0
- phosphate-loading (newborn) P71.1

Hypochloremia E87.8
Hypochlorhydria K31.89
- neurotic F45.8
- psychogenic F45.8

Hypochondria, hypochondriac, hypochondriasis (reaction) F45.21
- sleep F51.03

Hypochondrogenesis Q77.0
Hypochondroplasia Q77.4
Hypochromasia, blood cells D50.8
Hypocitraturia R82.991
Hypodontia — see Anodontia
Hypoeosinophilia D72.89
Hypoesthesia R20.1
Hypofibrinogenemia D68.8
- acquired D65
- congenital (hereditary) D68.2

Hypofunction
- adrenocortical E27.40
  - drug-induced E27.3
  - postprocedural E89.6
  - primary E27.1
- adrenomedullary, postprocedural E89.6
- cerebral R29.818
- corticoadrenal NEC E27.40
- intestinal K59.89
- labyrinth — see subcategory H83.2- ☑
- ovary E28.39
- pituitary (gland) (anterior) E23.0
- testicular E29.1
  - postprocedural (postsurgical) (postirradiation) (iatrogenic) E89.5

Hypogalactia O92.4
Hypogammaglobulinemia — see also Agammaglobulinemia D80.1
- hereditary D80.0
- nonfamilial D80.1
- transient, of infancy D80.7

Hypogenitalism (congenital) — see Hypogonadism
Hypoglossia Q38.3
Hypoglycemia (spontaneous) E16.2
- coma E15
  - diabetic — see Diabetes, by type, with hypoglycemia, with coma
- diabetic — see Diabetes, hypoglycemia
- dietary counseling and surveillance Z71.3
- drug-induced E16.0
  - with coma (nondiabetic) E15
- due to insulin E16.0
  - with coma (nondiabetic) E15
  - therapeutic misadventure — see subcategory T38.3- ☑
- functional, nonhyperinsulinemic E16.1
- iatrogenic E16.0
  - with coma (nondiabetic) E15
- in infant of diabetic mother P70.1
  - gestational diabetes P70.0
- infantile E16.1
- leucine-induced E71.19
- level
  - 1 E16.A1
  - 2 E16.A2
  - 3 E16.A3
- neonatal (transitory) P70.4
  - iatrogenic P70.3
- reactive (not drug-induced) E16.1
- transitory neonatal P70.4

Hypogonadism
- female E28.39
- hypogonadotropic E23.0
- male E29.1
- ovarian (primary) E28.39
- pituitary E23.0
- testicular (primary) E29.1

Hypohidrosis, hypoidrosis L74.4
Hypoinsulinemia, postprocedural E89.1
Hypokalemia E87.6
Hypoleukocytosis — see Agranulocytosis
Hypolipoproteinemia (alpha) (beta) E78.6
Hypomagnesemia E83.42
- neonatal P71.2

Hypomania, hypomanic reaction F30.8
Hypomenorrhea — see Oligomenorrhea
Hypometabolism R63.8
Hypomotility
- gastrointestinal (tract) K31.89
  - psychogenic F45.8
- intestine K59.89
  - psychogenic F45.8
- stomach K31.89
  - psychogenic F45.8

Hypomyelination - hypogonadotropic hypogonadism - hypodontia G11.5
Hypomyelination with atrophy of the basal ganglia and cerebellum (H-ABC) G23.3
Hyponasality R49.22
Hyponatremia E87.1
Hypoparathyroidism E20.9
- autoimmune E20.812
- due to impaired parathyroid hormone secretion, unspecified E20.819
- familial E20.89
  - isolated E20.818
- idiopathic E20.0
- neonatal, transitory P71.4
- postprocedural E89.2

Hypoparathyroidism — continued
- secondary, in diseases classified elsewhere E20.811
- specified NEC E20.89
  - due to impaired parathyroid hormone secretion E20.818

Hypoperfusion (in)
- newborn P96.89

Hypopharyngitis — see Laryngopharyngitis

Hypophoria H50.53

Hypophosphatemia, hypophosphatasia (acquired) (congenital) (renal) E83.39
- familial E83.31

Hypophyseal, hypophysis — see also condition
- dwarfism E23.0
- gigantism E22.0

Hypopiesis — see Hypotension

Hypopinealism E34.8

Hypopituitarism (juvenile) E23.0
- drug-induced E23.1
- due to
  - hypophysectomy E89.3
  - radiotherapy E89.3
- iatrogenic NEC E23.1
- postirradiation E89.3
- postpartum O99.285
- postprocedural E89.3

Hypoplasia, hypoplastic
- adrenal (gland), congenital Q89.1
- alimentary tract, congenital Q45.8
  - upper Q40.8
- anus, anal (canal) Q42.3
  - with fistula Q42.2
- aorta, aortic Q25.42
  - ascending, in hypoplastic left heart syndrome Q23.4
  - valve Q23.1
    - in hypoplastic left heart syndrome Q23.4
- areola, congenital Q83.8
- arm (congenital) — see Defect, reduction, upper limb
- artery (peripheral) Q27.8
  - brain (congenital) Q28.3
  - coronary Q24.5
  - digestive system Q27.8
  - lower limb Q27.8
  - pulmonary Q25.79
    - functional, unilateral J43.0
  - retinal (congenital) Q14.1
  - specified site NEC Q27.8
  - umbilical Q27.0
  - upper limb Q27.8
- auditory canal Q17.8
  - causing impairment of hearing Q16.9
- biliary duct or passage Q44.5
- bone NOS Q79.9
  - face Q75.8
  - marrow D61.9
    - megakaryocytic D69.49
  - skull — see Hypoplasia, skull
- brain Q02
  - gyri Q04.3
  - part of Q04.3
- breast (areola) N64.82
- bronchus Q32.4
- cardiac Q24.8
- carpus — see Defect, reduction, upper limb, specified type NEC
- cartilage hair Q78.8
- cecum Q42.8
- cementum K00.4
- cephalic Q02
- cerebellum Q04.3
- cervix (uteri), congenital Q51.821
- clavicle (congenital) Q74.0
- coccyx Q76.49
- colon Q42.9
  - specified NEC Q42.8
- corpus callosum Q04.0
- cricoid cartilage Q31.2
- digestive organ(s) or tract NEC Q45.8
  - upper (congenital) Q40.8
- ear (auricle) (lobe) Q17.2
  - middle Q16.4
- enamel of teeth (neonatal) (postnatal) (prenatal) K00.4
- endocrine (gland) NEC Q89.2
- endometrium N85.8
- epididymis (congenital) Q55.4
- epiglottis Q31.2
- erythroid, congenital D61.01
- esophagus (congenital) Q39.8
- eustachian tube Q17.8

Hypoplasia, hypoplastic — continued
- eye Q11.2
- eyelid (congenital) Q10.3
- face Q18.8
  - bone(s) Q75.8
- femur (congenital) — see Defect, reduction, lower limb, specified type NEC
- fibula (congenital) — see Defect, reduction, lower limb, specified type NEC
- finger (congenital) — see Defect, reduction, upper limb, specified type NEC
- focal dermal Q82.8
- foot — see Defect, reduction, lower limb, specified type NEC
- gallbladder Q44.0
- genitalia, genital organ(s)
  - female, congenital Q52.8
    - external Q52.79
    - internal NEC Q52.8
  - in adiposogenital dystrophy E23.6
- glottis Q31.2
- hair Q84.2
- hand (congenital) — see Defect, reduction, upper limb, specified type NEC
- heart Q24.8
- humerus (congenital) — see Defect, reduction, upper limb, specified type NEC
- intestine (small) Q41.9
  - large Q42.9
    - specified NEC Q42.8
- jaw M26.09
  - alveolar M26.79
  - lower M26.04
    - alveolar M26.74
  - upper M26.02
    - alveolar M26.73
- kidney(s) Q60.5
  - bilateral Q60.4
  - unilateral Q60.3
- labium (majus) (minus), congenital Q52.79
- larynx Q31.2
- left heart syndrome Q23.4
- leg (congenital) — see Defect, reduction, lower limb
- limb Q73.8
  - lower (congenital) — see Defect, reduction, lower limb
  - upper (congenital) — see Defect, reduction, upper limb
- liver Q44.79
- lung (lobe) (not associated with short gestation) Q33.6
  - associated with immaturity, low birth weight, prematurity, or short gestation P28.0
- mammary (areola), congenital Q83.8
- mandible, mandibular M26.04
  - alveolar M26.74
  - unilateral condylar M27.8
- maxillary M26.02
  - alveolar M26.73
- medullary D61.9
- megakaryocytic D69.49
- metacarpus — see Defect, reduction, upper limb, specified type NEC
- metatarsus — see Defect, reduction, lower limb, specified type NEC
- muscle Q79.8
- nail(s) Q84.6
- nose, nasal Q30.1
- optic nerve H47.03- ☑
- osseous meatus (ear) Q17.8
- ovary, congenital Q50.39
- pancreas Q45.0
- parathyroid (gland) Q89.2
- parotid gland Q38.4
- patella Q74.1
- pelvis, pelvic girdle Q74.2
- penis (congenital) Q55.62
- peripheral vascular system Q27.8
  - digestive system Q27.8
  - lower limb Q27.8
  - specified site NEC Q27.8
  - upper limb Q27.8
- pituitary (gland) (congenital) Q89.2
- pulmonary (not associated with short gestation) Q33.6
  - artery, functional J43.0
  - associated with short gestation P28.0
- radioulnar — see Defect, reduction, upper limb, specified type NEC
- radius — see Defect, reduction, upper limb
- rectum Q42.1

Hypoplasia, hypoplastic — continued
- rectum — continued
  - with fistula Q42.0
- respiratory system NEC Q34.8
- rib Q76.6
- right heart syndrome Q22.6
- sacrum Q76.49
- scapula Q74.0
- scrotum Q55.1
- shoulder girdle Q74.0
- skin Q82.8
- skull (bone) Q75.8
  - with
    - anencephaly Q00.0
    - encephalocele — see Encephalocele
    - hydrocephalus Q03.9
      - with spina bifida — see Spina bifida, by site, with hydrocephalus
    - microcephaly Q02
- spinal (cord) (ventral horn cell) Q06.1
- spine Q76.49
- sternum Q76.7
- tarsus — see Defect, reduction, lower limb, specified type NEC
- testis Q55.1
- thymic, with immunodeficiency D82.1
- thymus (gland) Q89.2
  - with immunodeficiency D82.1
- thyroid (gland) E03.1
  - cartilage Q31.2
- tibiofibular (congenital) — see Defect, reduction, lower limb, specified type NEC
- toe — see Defect, reduction, lower limb, specified type NEC
- tongue Q38.3
- Turner's K00.4
- ulna (congenital) — see Defect, reduction, upper limb
- umbilical artery Q27.0
- unilateral condylar M27.8
- ureter Q62.8
- uterus, congenital Q51.811
- vagina Q52.4
- vascular NEC peripheral Q27.8
  - brain Q28.3
  - digestive system Q27.8
  - lower limb Q27.8
  - specified site NEC Q27.8
  - upper limb Q27.8
- vein(s) (peripheral) Q27.8
  - brain Q28.3
  - digestive system Q27.8
  - great Q26.8
  - lower limb Q27.8
  - specified site NEC Q27.8
  - upper limb Q27.8
- vena cava (inferior) (superior) Q26.8
- vertebra Q76.49
- vulva, congenital Q52.79
- zonule (ciliary) Q12.8

Hypoplasminogenemia E88.02

Hypopnea, obstructive sleep apnea G47.33

Hypopotassemia E87.6

Hypoproconvertinemia, congenital (hereditary) D68.2

Hypoproteinemia E77.8

Hypoprothrombinemia (congenital) (hereditary) (idiopathic) D68.2
- acquired D68.4
- newborn, transient P61.6

Hypoptyalism K11.7

Hypopyon (eye) (anterior chamber) — see Iridocyclitis, acute, hypopyon

Hypopyrexia R68.0

Hyporeflexia R29.2

Hyposecretion
- ACTH E23.0
- antidiuretic hormone E23.2
- ovary E28.39
- salivary gland (any) K11.7
- vasopressin E23.2

Hyposegmentation, leukocytic, hereditary D72.0

Hyposiderinemia D50.9

Hypospadias Q54.9
- balanic Q54.0
- coronal Q54.0
- glandular Q54.0
- penile Q54.1
- penoscrotal Q54.2
- perineal Q54.3
- specified NEC Q54.8

☑ **Additional Character Required** — Refer to the Tabular List for Character Selection

Hypospermatogenesis — see Oligospermia
Hyposplenism D73.0
Hypostasis pulmonary, passive — see Edema, lung
Hypostatic — see condition
Hyposthenuria N28.89
Hypotension (arterial) (constitutional) I95.9
- chronic I95.89
- due to (of) hemodialysis I95.3
- drug-induced I95.2
- iatrogenic I95.89
- idiopathic (permanent) I95.0
- intra-dialytic I95.3
- intracranial G96.810
  - following
    - lumbar cerebrospinal fluid shunting G97.83
    - specified procedure NEC G97.84
    - ventricular shunting (ventriculostomy) G97.2
  - specified NEC G96.819
  - spontaneous G96.811
- maternal, syndrome (following labor and delivery) O26.5-
- neurogenic, orthostatic G90.3
- orthostatic (chronic) I95.1
  - due to drugs I95.2
  - neurogenic G90.3
- postoperative I95.81
- postural I95.1
- specified NEC I95.89

Hypothermia (accidental) T68.- ☑
- due to anesthesia, anesthetic T88.51- ☑
- low environmental temperature T68.- ☑
- neonatal P80.9
  - environmental (mild) NEC P80.8
  - mild P80.8
  - severe (chronic) (cold injury syndrome) P80.0
  - specified NEC P80.8
- not associated with low environmental temperature R68.0

Hypothyroidism (acquired) E03.9
- autoimmune — see Thyroiditis, autoimmune
- congenital (without goiter) E03.1
  - with goiter (diffuse) E03.0
- due to
  - exogenous substance NEC E03.2
  - iodine-deficiency, acquired E01.8
    - subclinical E02
  - irradiation therapy E89.0
  - medicament NEC E03.2
  - P-aminosalicylic acid (PAS) E03.2
  - phenylbutazone E03.2
  - resorcinol E03.2
  - sulfonamide E03.2
  - surgery E89.0
  - thiourea group drugs E03.2
- iatrogenic NEC E03.2
- iodine-deficiency (acquired) E01.8
  - congenital — see Syndrome, iodine- deficiency, congenital
  - subclinical E02
- neonatal, transitory P72.2
- postinfectious E03.3
- postirradiation E89.0
- postprocedural E89.0
- postsurgical E89.0
- specified NEC E03.8
- subclinical, iodine-deficiency related E02

Hypotonia, hypotonicity, hypotony
- bladder N31.2
- congenital (benign) P94.2
- eye — see Disorder, globe, hypotony

Hypotrichosis — see Alopecia
Hypotropia H50.2- ☑
Hypoventilation R06.89
- congenital central alveolar G47.35
- sleep related
  - idiopathic nonobstructive alveolar G47.34
  - in conditions classified elsewhere G47.36

Hypovitaminosis — see Deficiency, vitamin
Hypovolemia E86.1
- surgical shock T81.19- ☑
- traumatic (shock) T79.4- ☑

Hypoxemia R09.02
- newborn P84
- sleep related, in conditions classified elsewhere G47.36

Hypoxia — see also Anoxia R09.02
- cerebral, during a procedure NEC G97.81
  - postprocedural NEC G97.82
- intrauterine P84

Hypoxia — continued
- myocardial — see Insufficiency, coronary
- newborn P84
- sleep-related G47.34

Hypsarrhythmia — see Epilepsy, generalized, specified NEC
Hysteralgia, pregnant uterus O26.89- ☑
Hysteria, hysterical (conversion) (dissociative state) F44.9
- anxiety F41.8
- convulsions F44.5
- psychosis, acute F44.9

Hysteroepilepsy F44.5

IBDU (colonic inflammatory bowel dissease unclassified) K52.3
ICANS (immune effector cell-associated neurotoxicity syndrome) — see Syndrome, immune effector cell-associated neurotoxicity
Ichthyoparasitism due to Vandellia cirrhosa B88.8
Ichthyosis (congenital) Q80.9
- acquired L85.0
- fetalis Q80.4
- hystrix Q80.8
- lamellar Q80.2
- lingual K13.29
- palmaris and plantaris Q82.8
- simplex Q80.0
- vera Q80.8
- vulgaris Q80.0
- X-linked Q80.1

Ichthyotoxism — see Poisoning, fish
- bacterial — see Intoxication, foodborne

Icteroanemia, hemolytic (acquired) D59.9
- congenital — see Spherocytosis

Icterus — see also Jaundice
- conjunctiva R17
- gravis, newborn P55.0
- hematogenous (acquired) D59.9
- hemolytic (acquired) D59.9
  - congenital — see Spherocytosis
- hemorrhagic (acute) (leptospiral) (spirochetal) A27.0
  - newborn P53
- infectious B15.9
  - with hepatic coma B15.0
  - leptospiral A27.0
  - spirochetal A27.0
- neonatorum — see Jaundice, newborn
- newborn P59.9
- spirochetal A27.0

Ictus solaris, solis T67.01- ☑
Id reaction (due to bacteria) L30.2
Ideation
- homicidal R45.850
- suicidal R45.851

Identity disorder (child) F64.9
- gender role F64.2
- psychosexual F64.2

Idioglossia F80.0
Idiopathic — see condition
Idiot, idiocy (congenital) F73
- amaurotic (Bielschowsky(-Jansky)) (family) (infantile (late)) (juvenile (late)) (Vogt-Spielmeyer) E75.4
- microcephalic Q02

IgE asthma J45.909
IIAC (idiopathic infantile arterial calcification) — see Calcification, arterial, generalized, of infancy
Ileitis (chronic) (noninfectious) — see also Enteritis K52.9
- backwash — see Pancolitis, ulcerative (chronic)
- infectious A09
- regional (ulcerative) — see Enteritis, regional, small intestine
- segmental — see Enteritis, regional
- terminal (ulcerative) — see Enteritis, regional, small intestine

Ileocolitis — see also Enteritis K52.9
- infectious A09
- regional — see Enteritis, regional
- ulcerative K51.0- ☑

Ileostomy
- attention to Z43.2
- malfunctioning K94.13
- status (ileal pouch) (Kock pouch) Z93.2
  - with complication — see Complications, enterostomy

Ileotyphus — see Typhoid
Ileum — see condition
Ileus (bowel) (colon) (inhibitory) (intestine) K56.7

Ileus — continued
- adynamic K56.0
- due to gallstone (in intestine) K56.3
- duodenal (chronic) K31.5
- gallstone K56.3
- mechanical NEC — see also Obstruction, intestine, specified NEC K56.699
- meconium P76.0
  - in cystic fibrosis E84.11
  - meaning meconium plug (without cystic fibrosis) P76.0
- myxedema K59.89
- neurogenic K56.0
  - Hirschsprung's disease or megacolon Q43.1
- newborn
  - due to meconium P76.0
    - in cystic fibrosis E84.11
    - meaning meconium plug (without cystic fibrosis) P76.0
  - transitory P76.1
- obstructive — see also Obstruction, intestine, specified NEC K56.699
- paralytic K56.0
- postoperative K91.89

Iliac — see condition
Iliotibial band syndrome M76.3- ☑
Illiteracy Z55.0
- health Z55.6

Illness — see also Disease R69
- Gulf war T75.830- ☑
- manic-depressive — see Disorder, bipolar

Imbalance R26.89
- autonomic G90.89
- constituents of food intake E63.1
- electrolyte E87.8
  - with
    - abortion — see Abortion by type, complicated by, electrolyte imbalance
    - molar pregnancy O08.5
  - due to hyperemesis gravidarum O21.1
  - following ectopic or molar pregnancy O08.5
  - neonatal, transitory NEC P74.49
    - potassium
      - hyperkalemia P74.31
      - hypokalemia P74.32
    - sodium
      - hypernatremia P74.21
      - hyponatremia P74.22
- endocrine E34.9
- eye muscle NOS H50.9
- hormone E34.9
- hysterical F44.4
- labyrinth — see subcategory H83.2- ☑
- posture R29.3
- protein-energy — see Malnutrition
- sympathetic G90.89

Imbecile, imbecility (I.Q. 35-49) F71
Imbedding, intrauterine device T83.39- ☑
Imbibition, cholesterol (gallbladder) K82.4
Imbrication, teeth,, fully erupted M26.30
Imerslund (-Gräsbeck) **syndrome** D51.1
Immature — see also Immaturity
- birth (less than 37 completed weeks) — see Preterm, newborn
- extremely (less than 28 completed weeks) — see Immaturity, extreme
- personality F60.89

Immaturity (less than 37 completed weeks) — see also Preterm, newborn
- extreme of newborn (less than 28 completed weeks of gestation) (less than 196 completed days of gestation) (unspecified weeks of gestation) P07.20
- gestational age
  - 23 completed weeks (23 weeks, 0 days through 23 weeks, 6 days) P07.22
  - 24 completed weeks (24 weeks, 0 days through 24 weeks, 6 days) P07.23
  - 25 completed weeks (25 weeks, 0 days through 25 weeks, 6 days) P07.24
  - 26 completed weeks (26 weeks, 0 days through 26 weeks, 6 days) P07.25
  - 27 completed weeks (27 weeks, 0 days through 27 weeks, 6 days) P07.26
  - less than 23 completed weeks P07.21
- fetus or infant light-for-dates — see Light-for-dates
- lung, newborn P28.0
- organ or site NEC — see Hypoplasia
- pulmonary, newborn P28.0
- reaction F60.89

Immaturity — continued
  sexual (female) (male), after puberty E30.0
Immersion T75.1- ☑
  foot T69.02- ☑
  hand T69.01- ☑
Immobile, immobility
  complete, due to severe physical disability or frailty R53.2
  intestine K59.89
  syndrome (paraplegic) M62.3
Immune reconstitution (inflammatory) syndrome [IRIS] D89.3
Immunization — *see also* Vaccination
  ABO — *see* Incompatibility, ABO
    in newborn P55.1
  appropriate for age
    child (over 28 days old) Z00.129
      with abnormal findings Z00.121
  complication — *see* Complications, vaccination
  encounter for Z23
  not done (not carried out) — *see also* Underimmunization status Z28.9
    because (of)
      acute illness of patient Z28.01
      allergy to vaccine (or component) Z28.04
      caregiver refusal Z28.82
      chronic illness of patient Z28.02
      contraindication NEC Z28.09
      delay in delivery of vaccine Z28.83
      group pressure Z28.1
      guardian refusal Z28.82
      immune compromised state of patient Z28.03
      lack of availability of vaccine Z28.83
      manufacturer delay of vaccine Z28.83
      parent refusal Z28.82
      patient had disease being vaccinated against Z28.81
      patient refusal Z28.21
      patient's belief Z28.1
      religious beliefs of patient Z28.1
      specified reason NEC Z28.89
        of patient Z28.29
      unavailability of vaccine Z28.83
      unspecified patient reason Z28.20
  partial — *see also* Underimmunization status
    for COVID-19 Z28.311
  Rh factor
    affecting management of pregnancy NEC O36.09- ☑
      anti-D antibody O36.01- ☑
    from transfusion — *see* Complication(s), transfusion, incompatibility reaction, Rh (factor)
Immunocompromised NOS D84.9
Immunocytoma C83.0- ☑
Immunodeficiency D84.9
  with
    adenosine-deaminase deficiency — *see also* Deficiency, adenosine deaminase D81.30
    antibody defects D80.9
      specified type NEC D80.8
    hyperimmunoglobulinemia D80.6
    increased immunoglobulin M (IgM) D80.5
    major defect D82.9
      specified type NEC D82.8
    partial albinism D82.8
    short-limbed stature D82.2
    thrombocytopenia and eczema D82.0
  antibody with
    hyperimmunoglobulinemia D80.6
    near-normal immunoglobulins D80.6
  autosomal recessive, Swiss type D80.0
  combined D81.9
    biotin-dependent carboxylase D81.819
      biotinidase D81.810
      holocarboxylase synthetase D81.818
      specified type NEC D81.818
    severe (SCID) D81.9
      with
        low or normal B-cell numbers D81.2
        low T- and B-cell numbers D81.1
        reticular dysgenesis D81.0
    specified type NEC D81.89
  common variable D83.9
    with
      abnormalities of B-cell numbers and function D83.0
      autoantibodies to B- or T-cells D83.2
      immunoregulatory T-cell disorders D83.1
    specified type NEC D83.8

Immunodeficiency — continued
  due to
    conditions classified elsewhere D84.81
    drugs D84.821
    external causes D84.822
    medication (current or past) D84.821
  following hereditary defective response to Epstein-Barr virus (EBV) D82.3
  selective, immunoglobulin
    A (IgA) D80.2
    G (IgG) (subclasses) D80.3
    M (IgM) D80.4
  severe combined (SCID) D81.9
    due to adenosine deaminase deficiency D81.31
  specified type NEC D84.89
  X-linked, with increased IgM D80.5
Immunodeficient NOS D84.9
Immunosuppressed NOS D84.9
Immunotherapy (encounter for)
  antineoplastic Z51.12
Impaction, impacted
  bowel, colon, rectum — *see also* Impaction, fecal K56.49
    by gallstone K56.3
  calculus — *see* Calculus
  cerumen (ear) (external) H61.2- ☑
  cuspid — *see* Impaction, tooth
  dental (same or adjacent tooth) K01.1
  fecal, feces K56.41
  fracture — *see* Fracture, by site
  gallbladder — *see* Calculus, gallbladder
  gallstone(s) — *see* Calculus, gallbladder
    bile duct (common) (hepatic) — *see* Calculus, bile duct
    cystic duct — *see* Calculus, gallbladder
    in intestine, with obstruction (any part) K56.3
  intestine (calculous) NEC — *see also* Impaction, fecal K56.49
    gallstone, with ileus K56.3
  intrauterine device (IUD) T83.39- ☑
  molar — *see* Impaction, tooth
  shoulder, causing obstructed labor O66.0
  tooth, teeth K01.1
  turbinate J34.89
Impaired, impairment (function)
  auditory discrimination — *see* Abnormal, auditory perception
  cognitive, mild, of uncertain or unknown etiology G31.84
  dual sensory Z73.82
  fasting glucose R73.01
  glucose tolerance (oral) R73.02
  hearing — *see* Deafness
  heart — *see* Disease, heart
  kidney N28.9
    disorder resulting from N25.9
      specified NEC N25.89
  liver K72.90
    with coma K72.91
  mastication K08.89
  mild cognitive G31.84
    of uncertain or unknown etiology G31.84
  mild neurocognitive
    due to known physiological condition (without behavioral disturbance) F06.70
      with behavioral disturbance F06.71
  mobility
    ear ossicles — *see* Ankylosis, ear ossicles
    requiring care provider Z74.09
  myocardium, myocardial — *see* Insufficiency, myocardial
  rectal sphincter R19.8
  renal (acute) (chronic) N28.9
    disorder resulting from N25.9
      specified NEC N25.89
  vision NEC H54.7
    both eyes H54.3
Impediment, speech — *see also* Disorder, speech R47.9
  psychogenic (childhood) F98.8
  slurring R47.81
  specified NEC R47.89
Impending
  coronary syndrome I20.0
  delirium tremens F10.239
  myocardial infarction I20.0
Imperception auditory (acquired) — *see also* Deafness
  congenital H93.25
Imperfect
  aeration, lung (newborn) NEC — *see* Atelectasis
  closure (congenital)
    alimentary tract NEC Q45.8
      lower Q43.8

Imperfect — continued
  closure — continued
    alimentary tract — continued
      upper Q40.8
    atrioventricular ostium Q21.20
    atrium (secundum) Q21.11
    branchial cleft NOS Q18.2
      cyst Q18.0
      fistula Q18.0
      sinus Q18.0
    choroid Q14.3
    cricoid cartilage Q31.8
    cusps, heart valve NEC Q24.8
      pulmonary Q22.3
    ductus
      arteriosus Q25.0
      Botalli Q25.0
    ear drum (causing impairment of hearing) Q16.4
    esophagus with communication to bronchus or trachea Q39.1
    eyelid Q10.3
    foramen
      botalli Q21.12
      ovale Q21.12
    genitalia, genital organ(s) or system
      female Q52.8
        external Q52.79
        internal NEC Q52.8
      male Q55.8
    glottis Q31.8
    interatrial ostium or septum Q21.19
    interauricular ostium or septum Q21.19
    interventricular ostium or septum Q21.0
    larynx Q31.8
    lip — *see* Cleft, lip
    nasal septum Q30.3
    nose Q30.2
    omphalomesenteric duct Q43.0
    optic nerve entry Q14.2
    organ or site not listed — *see* Anomaly, by site
    ostium
      interatrial Q21.19
      interauricular Q21.19
      interventricular Q21.0
    palate — *see* Cleft, palate
    preauricular sinus Q18.1
    retina Q14.1
    roof of orbit Q75.8
    sclera Q13.5
    septum
      aorticopulmonary Q21.4
      atrial (secundum) Q21.19
      between aorta and pulmonary artery Q21.4
      heart Q21.9
      interatrial (secundum) Q21.19
      interauricular (secundum) Q21.19
      interventricular Q21.0
        in tetralogy of Fallot Q21.3
      nasal Q30.3
      ventricular Q21.0
        with pulmonary stenosis or atresia, dextraposition of aorta, and hypertrophy of right ventricle Q21.3
        in tetralogy of Fallot Q21.3
    skull Q75.009
      with
        anencephaly Q00.0
        encephalocele — *see* Encephalocele
        hydrocephalus Q03.9
          with spina bifida — *see* Spina bifida, by site, with hydrocephalus
        microcephaly Q02
    spine (with meningocele) — *see* Spina bifida
    trachea Q32.1
    tympanic membrane (causing impairment of hearing) Q16.4
    uterus Q51.818
    vitelline duct Q43.0
  erection — *see* Dysfunction, sexual, male, erectile
  fusion — *see* Imperfect, closure
  inflation, lung (newborn) — *see* Atelectasis
  posture R29.3
  rotation, intestine Q43.3
  septum, ventricular Q21.0
Imperfectly descended testis — *see* Cryptorchid
Imperforate (congenital) — *see also* Atresia
  anus Q42.3
    with fistula Q42.2
  cervix (uteri) Q51.828

Imperforate — continued
- esophagus Q39.0
  - with tracheoesophageal fistula Q39.1
- hymen Q52.3
- jejunum Q41.1
- pharynx Q38.8
- rectum Q42.1
  - with fistula Q42.0
- urethra Q64.39
- vagina Q52.4

Impervious (congenital) — see also Atresia
- anus Q42.3
  - with fistula Q42.2
- bile duct Q44.2
- esophagus Q39.0
  - with tracheoesophageal fistula Q39.1
- intestine (small) Q41.9
  - large Q42.9
    - specified NEC Q42.8
- rectum Q42.1
  - with fistula Q42.0
- ureter — see Atresia, ureter
- urethra Q64.39

Impetiginization of dermatoses L01.1
Impetigo (any organism) (any site) (circinate) (contagiosa) (simplex) (vulgaris) L01.00
- Bockhart's L01.02
- bullous, bullosa L01.03
- external ear L01.00 [H62.4-] ☑
- follicularis L01.02
- furfuracea L30.5
- herpetiformis L40.1
  - nonobstetrical L40.1
- neonatorum L01.03
- nonbullous L01.01
- specified type NEC L01.09
- ulcerative L01.09

Impingement (on teeth)
- joint — see Disorder, joint, specified type NEC
- soft tissue
  - anterior M26.81
  - posterior M26.82

Implant, endometrial N80.9
Implantation
- anomalous — see Anomaly, by site
  - ureter Q62.63
- cyst
  - external area or site (skin) NEC L72.0
  - iris — see Cyst, iris, implantation
  - vagina N89.8
  - vulva N90.7
- dermoid (cyst) — see Implantation, cyst

Impotence (sexual) N52.9
- counseling Z70.1
- organic origin — see also Dysfunction, sexual, male, erectile N52.9
- psychogenic F52.21

Impression, basilar Q75.8
Imprisonment, anxiety concerning Z65.1
Improper care (child) (newborn) — see Maltreatment
Improperly tied umbilical cord (causing hemorrhage) P51.8
Impulsiveness (impulsive) R45.87
Inability to
- comply with dietary regimen Z91.118
- pay for utilities Z59.861
- swallow — see Aphagia

Inaccessible, inaccessibility
- health care NEC Z75.3
  - due to
    - waiting period Z75.2
      - for admission to facility elsewhere Z75.1
  - other helping agencies Z75.4
- transportation Z59.82

Inactive — see condition
Inadequate, inadequacy
- aesthetics of dental restoration K08.56
- biologic, constitutional, functional, or social F60.7
- development
  - child R62.50
  - genitalia
    - after puberty NEC E30.0
    - congenital
      - female Q52.8
        - external Q52.79
        - internal Q52.8
      - male Q55.8
  - lungs Q33.6
    - associated with short gestation P28.0

Inadequate, inadequacy — continued
- development — continued
  - organ or site not listed — see Anomaly, by site
- diet (causing nutritional deficiency) E63.9
- drinking-water supply Z58.6
- eating habits Z72.4
- environment, household Z59.11
- family support Z63.8
- food (supply) NEC Z59.48
  - hunger effects T73.0- ☑
- functional F60.7
- household care, due to
  - family member
    - handicapped or ill Z74.2
    - on vacation Z75.5
    - temporarily away from home Z74.2
  - technical defects in home Z59.19
  - temporary absence from home of person rendering care Z74.2
- housing Z59.10
  - environmental temperature Z59.11
  - heating Z59.11
  - space Z59.19
  - specified NEC Z59.19
  - utilities Z59.12
- income (financial) Z59.6
- intrafamilial communication Z63.8
- material resources due to limited financial resources, specified NEC Z59.87
- mental — see Disability, intellectual
- parental supervision or control of child Z62.0
- personality F60.7
- pulmonary
  - function R06.89
    - newborn P28.5
  - ventilation, newborn P28.5
- sample of cytologic smear
  - anus R85.615
  - cervix R87.615
  - vagina R87.625
- social F60.7
  - insurance Z59.71
  - skills NEC Z73.4
  - social support Z60.8
- supervision of child by parent Z62.0
- teaching affecting education Z55.8
- transportation Z59.82
- welfare support Z59.72

Inanition R64
- with edema — see Malnutrition, severe
- due to
  - deprivation of food T73.0- ☑
  - malnutrition — see Malnutrition
- fever R50.9

Inappropriate
- change in quantitative human chorionic gonadotropin (hCG) in early pregnancy O02.81
- diet or eating habits Z72.4
- level of quantitative human chorionic gonadotropin (hCG) for gestational age in early pregnancy O02.81
- secretion
  - antidiuretic hormone (ADH) (excessive) E22.2
    - deficiency E23.2
  - pituitary (posterior) E22.2
- sinus tachycardia, so stated (IST) I47.11

Inattention at or after birth — see Neglect
Incarceration, incarcerated
- enterocele K46.0
  - gangrenous K46.1
- epiplocele K46.0
  - gangrenous K46.1
- exomphalos K42.0
  - gangrenous K42.1
- hernia — see also Hernia, by site, with obstruction
  - with gangrene — see Hernia, by site, with gangrene
- iris, in wound — see Injury, eye, laceration, with prolapse
- lens, in wound — see Injury, eye, laceration, with prolapse
- omphalocele K42.0
- prison, anxiety concerning Z65.1
- rupture — see Hernia, by site
- sarcoepiplocele K46.0
  - gangrenous K46.1
- sarcoepiplomphalocele K42.0
  - with gangrene K42.1
- uterus N85.8
  - gravid O34.51- ☑
    - causing obstructed labor O65.5

Incised wound
- external — see Laceration
- internal organs — see Injury, by site

Incision, incisional
- hernia K43.2
  - with
    - gangrene (and obstruction) K43.1
    - obstruction K43.0
  - surgical, complication — see Complications, surgical procedure
  - traumatic
    - external — see Laceration
    - internal organs — see Injury, by site

Inclusion
- azurophilic leukocytic D72.0
- blennorrhea (neonatal) (newborn) P39.1
- gallbladder in liver (congenital) Q44.1

Incompatibility
- ABO
  - affecting management of pregnancy O36.11- ☑
    - anti-A sensitization O36.11- ☑
    - anti-B sensitization O36.19- ☑
    - specified NEC O36.19- ☑
  - infusion or transfusion reaction — see Complication(s), transfusion, incompatibility reaction, ABO
  - newborn P55.1
- blood (group) (Duffy) (K) (Kell) (Kidd) (Lewis) (M) (S) NEC
  - affecting management of pregnancy O36.11- ☑
    - anti-A sensitization O36.11- ☑
    - anti-B sensitization O36.19- ☑
  - infusion or transfusion reaction T80.89- ☑
  - newborn P55.8
- divorce or estrangement Z63.5
- Rh (blood group) (factor) Z31.82
  - affecting management of pregnancy NEC O36.09- ☑
    - anti-D antibody O36.01- ☑
  - infusion or transfusion reaction — see Complication(s), transfusion, incompatibility reaction, Rh (factor)
  - newborn P55.0
- rhesus — see Incompatibility, Rh

Incompetency, incompetent, incompetence
- annular
  - aortic (valve) — see Insufficiency, aortic
  - mitral (valve) I34.0
  - pulmonary valve (heart) I37.1
- aortic (valve) — see Insufficiency, aortic
- cardiac valve — see Endocarditis
- cervix, cervical (os) N88.3
  - in pregnancy O34.3- ☑
- chronotropic I45.89
  - with
    - autonomic dysfunction G90.89
    - ischemic heart disease I25.89
    - left ventricular dysfunction I51.89
    - sinus node dysfunction I49.8
- esophagogastric (junction) (sphincter) K22.0
- mitral (valve) — see Insufficiency, mitral
- pelvic fundus N81.89
- pubocervical tissue N81.82
- pulmonary valve (heart) I37.1
  - congenital Q22.3
- rectovaginal tissue N81.83
- tricuspid (annular) (valve) — see Insufficiency, tricuspid
- valvular — see Endocarditis
  - congenital Q24.8
- vein, venous (saphenous) (varicose) — see Varix, leg

Incomplete — see also condition
- atrioventricular
  - canal Q21.21
  - septal defect Q21.21
- bladder, emptying R33.9
- defecation R15.0
- endocardial cushion defect Q21.21
- expansion lungs (newborn) NEC — see Atelectasis
- rotation, intestine Q43.3

Inconclusive
- diagnostic imaging due to excess body fat of patient R93.9
- findings on diagnostic imaging of breast NEC R92.8
- mammogram R92.2

Incontinence R32
- anal sphincter R15.9
- coital N39.491
- feces R15.9
  - nonorganic origin F98.1
- insensible (urinary) N39.42

Incontinence — continued
- overflow N39.490
- postural (urinary) N39.492
- psychogenic F45.8
- rectal R15.9
- reflex N39.498
- stress (female) (male) N39.3
  - and urge N39.46
- urethral sphincter R32
- urge N39.41
  - and stress (female) (male) N39.46
- urine (urinary) R32
  - continuous N39.45
  - due to cognitive impairment, or severe physical disability or immobility R39.81
  - functional R39.81
  - insensible N39.42
  - mixed (stress and urge) N39.46
  - nocturnal N39.44
  - nonorganic origin F98.0
  - overflow N39.490
  - post dribbling N39.43
  - postural N39.492
  - reflex N39.498
  - specified NEC N39.498
  - stress (female) (male) N39.3
    - and urge N39.46
  - total N39.498
  - unaware N39.42
  - urge N39.41
    - and stress (female) (male) N39.46

Incontinentia pigmenti Q82.3
Incoordinate, incoordination
- esophageal-pharyngeal (newborn) — see Dysphagia
- muscular R27.8
- uterus (action) (contractions) (complicating delivery) O62.4

Increase, increased
- abnormal, in development R63.8
- androgens (ovarian) E28.1
- anticoagulants (antithrombin) (anti-VIIIa) (anti-IXa) (anti-Xa) (anti-XIa) — see Circulating anticoagulants
- cold sense R20.8
- estrogen E28.0
- function
  - adrenal
    - cortex — see Cushing's, syndrome
    - medulla E27.5
  - pituitary (gland) (anterior) (lobe) E22.9
    - posterior E22.2
- heat sense R20.8
- intracranial pressure (benign) G93.2
- permeability, capillaries I78.8
- pressure, intracranial G93.2
- secretion
  - gastrin E16.4
  - glucagon E16.3
  - pancreas, endocrine E16.9
    - growth hormone-releasing hormone E16.8
    - pancreatic polypeptide E16.8
    - somatostatin E16.8
    - vasoactive-intestinal polypeptide E16.8
- sphericity, lens Q12.4
- splenic activity D73.1
- venous pressure I87.8
  - portal K76.6

Increta placenta O43.22- ☑
Incrustation, cornea, foreign body (lead)(zinc) — see Foreign body, cornea
Incyclophoria H50.54
Incyclotropia — see Cyclotropia
Indeterminate sex Q56.4
India rubber skin Q82.8
Indigestion (acid) (bilious) (functional) K30
- catarrhal K31.89
- due to decomposed food NOS A05.9
- nervous F45.8
- psychogenic F45.8

Indirect — see condition
Induratio penis plastica N48.6
Induration, indurated
- brain G93.89
- breast (fibrous) N64.51
  - puerperal, postpartum O92.29
- broad ligament N83.8
- chancre
  - anus A51.1
  - congenital A50.07
  - extragenital NEC A51.2

Induration, indurated — continued
- corpora cavernosa (penis) (plastic) N48.6
- liver (chronic) K76.89
- lung (black) (chronic) (fibroid) — see also Fibrosis, lung J84.10
  - essential brown J84.03
- penile (plastic) N48.6
- phlebitic — see Phlebitis
- skin R23.4

Inebriety (without dependence) — see Alcohol, intoxication
Inefficiency, kidney N28.9
Inelasticity, skin R23.4
Inequality, leg (length) (acquired) — see also Deformity, limb, unequal length
- congenital — see Defect, reduction, lower limb
- lower leg — see Deformity, limb, unequal length

Inertia
- bladder (neurogenic) N31.2
- stomach K31.89
  - psychogenic F45.8
- uterus, uterine during labor O62.2
  - during latent phase of labor O62.0
  - primary O62.0
  - secondary O62.1
- vesical (neurogenic) N31.2

Infancy, infantile, infantilism — see also condition
- celiac K90.0
- genitalia, genitals (after puberty) E30.0
- Herter's (nontropical sprue) K90.0
- intestinal K90.0
- Lorain E23.0
- pancreatic K86.89
- pelvis M95.5
  - with disproportion (fetopelvic) O33.1
    - causing obstructed labor O65.1
- pituitary E23.0
- renal N25.0
- uterus — see Infantile, genitalia

Infant(s) — see also Infancy
- excessive crying R68.11
- irritable child R68.12
- lack of care — see Neglect
- liveborn (singleton) Z38.2
  - born in hospital Z38.00
    - by cesarean Z38.01
  - born outside hospital Z38.1
  - multiple NEC Z38.8
    - born in hospital Z38.68
      - by cesarean Z38.69
    - born outside hospital Z38.7
  - quadruplet Z38.8
    - born in hospital Z38.63
      - by cesarean Z38.64
    - born outside hospital Z38.7
  - quintuplet Z38.8
    - born in hospital Z38.65
      - by cesarean Z38.66
    - born outside hospital Z38.7
  - triplet Z38.8
    - born in hospital Z38.61
      - by cesarean Z38.62
    - born outside hospital Z38.7
  - twin Z38.5
    - born in hospital Z38.30
      - by cesarean Z38.31
    - born outside hospital Z38.4
- of diabetic mother (syndrome of) P70.1
  - gestational diabetes P70.0

Infantile — see also condition
- genitalia, genitals E30.0
- os, uterine E30.0
- penis E30.0
- testis E29.1
- uterus E30.0

Infantilism — see Infancy
Infarct, infarction
- adrenal (capsule) (gland) E27.49
- appendices epiploicae — see also Infarct, intestine K55.069
- bowel — see also Infarct, intestine K55.069
- brain (stem) — see Infarct, cerebral
- breast N64.89
- brewer's (kidney) N28.0
- cardiac — see Infarct, myocardium
- cerebellar — see Infarct, cerebral
- cerebral (acute) — see also Occlusion, artery cerebral or precerebral, with infarction I63.9
  - aborted I63.9

Infarct, infarction — continued
- cerebral — see also Occlusion, artery cerebral or precerebral, with infarction — continued
  - chronic (imaging) (old) (remote) (without sequelae) Z86.73
    - with residual defects — see Sequelae, disease, cerebrovascular
  - cortical I63.9
  - due to
    - cerebral venous thrombosis, nonpyogenic I63.6
    - embolism
      - cerebral arteries I63.4- ☑
      - precerebral arteries I63.1- ☑
    - occlusion NEC
      - cerebral arteries I63.5- ☑
      - precerebral arteries I63.2- ☑
      - small artery I63.81
    - stenosis NEC
      - cerebral arteries I63.5- ☑
      - precerebral arteries I63.2- ☑
      - small artery I63.81
    - thrombosis
      - cerebral artery I63.3- ☑
      - precerebral artery I63.0- ☑
  - intraoperative
    - during cardiac surgery I97.810
    - during other surgery I97.811
  - neonatal P91.82- ☑
  - perinatal (arterial ischemic) P91.82- ☑
  - postprocedural
    - following cardiac surgery I97.820
    - following other surgery I97.821
  - specified NEC I63.89
- colon (acute) (agnogenic) (embolic) (hemorrhagic) (nonocclusive) (nonthrombotic) (occlusive) (segmental) (thrombotic) (with gangrene) — see also Infarct, intestine K55.049
- coronary artery — see Infarct, myocardium
- embolic — see Embolism
- fallopian tube N83.8
- gallbladder K82.8
- heart — see Infarct, myocardium
- hepatic K76.3
- hypophysis (anterior lobe) E23.6
- impending (myocardium) I20.0
- intestine (acute) (agnogenic) (embolic) (hemorrhagic) (nonocclusive) (nonthrombotic) (occlusive) (thrombotic) (with gangrene) K55.069
  - diffuse K55.062
  - focal K55.061
  - large K55.049
    - diffuse K55.042
    - focal K55.041
  - small K55.029
    - diffuse K55.022
    - focal K55.021
- kidney N28.0
- lacunar I63.81
- liver K76.3
- lung (embolic) (thrombotic) — see Embolism, pulmonary
- lymph node I89.8
- mesentery, mesenteric (embolic) (thrombotic) (with gangrene) — see also Infarct, intestine K55.069
- muscle (ischemic) M62.20
  - ankle M62.27- ☑
  - foot M62.27- ☑
  - forearm M62.23- ☑
  - hand M62.24- ☑
  - lower leg M62.26- ☑
  - pelvic region M62.25- ☑
  - shoulder region M62.21- ☑
  - specified site NEC M62.28
  - thigh M62.25- ☑
  - upper arm M62.22- ☑
- myocardium, myocardial (acute) (with stated duration of 4 weeks or less) I21.9
  - with
    - coronary microvascular disease I21.B
    - coronary microvascular dysfunction I21.B
    - nonobstructive coronary arteries [MINOCA] with microvascular disease I21.B
  - associated with revascularization procedure I21.A9
  - diagnosed on ECG, but presenting no symptoms I25.2
  - due to
    - demand ischemia I21.A1
    - ischemic imbalance I21.A1
  - healed or old I25.2

☑ Additional Character Required — Refer to the Tabular List for Character Selection

Infarct, infarction — continued
- myocardium, myocardial — continued
  - intraoperative — see also Infarct, myocardium, associated with revascularization procedure
    - during cardiac surgery I97.790
    - during other surgery I97.791
  - non-Q wave I21.4
  - non-ST elevation (NSTEMI) I21.4
    - subsequent I22.2
  - nontransmural I21.4
  - past (diagnosed on ECG or other investigation, but currently presenting no symptoms) I25.2
  - postprocedural — see also Infarct, myocardium, associated with revascularization procedure
    - following cardiac surgery — see also Infarct, myocardium, type 4 or type 5 I97.190
    - following other surgery I97.191
  - Q wave — see also Infarct, myocardium, ST elevation, by site I21.3
  - secondary to
    - demand ischemia I21.A1
    - ischemic imbalance I21.A1
  - ST elevation (STEMI) I21.3
    - anterior (anteroapical) (anterolateral) (anteroseptal) (Q wave) (wall) I21.09
      - subsequent I22.0
    - inferior (diaphragmatic) (inferolateral) (inferoposterior) (wall) NEC I21.19
      - subsequent I22.1
    - inferoposterior transmural (Q wave) I21.11
    - involving
      - coronary artery of anterior wall NEC I21.09
      - coronary artery of inferior wall NEC I21.19
      - diagonal coronary artery I21.02
      - left anterior descending coronary artery I21.02
      - left circumflex coronary artery I21.21
      - left main coronary artery I21.01
      - oblique marginal coronary artery I21.21
      - right coronary artery I21.11
    - lateral (apical-lateral) (basal-lateral) (high) I21.29
      - subsequent I22.8
    - posterior (posterobasal) (posterolateral) (posteroseptal) (true) I21.29
      - subsequent I22.8
    - septal I21.29
      - subsequent I22.8
    - specified NEC I21.29
      - subsequent I22.8
  - subsequent I22.9
    - subsequent (recurrent) (reinfarction) I22.9
      - anterior (anteroapical) (anterolateral) (anteroseptal) (wall) I22.0
      - diaphragmatic (wall) I22.1
      - inferior (diaphragmatic) (inferolateral) (inferoposterior) (wall) I22.1
      - lateral (apical-lateral) (basal-lateral) (high) I22.8
      - non-ST elevation (NSTEMI) I22.2
      - posterior (posterobasal) (posterolateral) (posteroseptal) (true) I22.8
      - septal I22.8
      - specified NEC I22.8
      - ST elevation I22.9
        - anterior (anteroapical) (anterolateral) (anteroseptal) (wall) I22.0
        - inferior (diaphragmatic) (inferolateral) (inferoposterior) (wall) I22.1
        - specified NEC I22.8
      - subendocardial I22.2
      - transmural I22.9
        - anterior (anteroapical) (anterolateral) (anteroseptal) (wall) I22.0
        - diaphragmatic (wall) I22.1
        - inferior (diaphragmatic) (inferolateral) (inferoposterior) (wall) I22.1
        - lateral (apical-lateral) (basal-lateral) (high) I22.8
        - posterior (posterobasal) (posterolateral) (posteroseptal) (true) I22.8
        - specified NEC I22.8
      - type 1 — see also Infarction, myocardial, subsequent, by site, or by ST elevation or non-ST elevation I22.9
        - type 2 I21.A1
        - type 3 I21.A9
        - type 4 I21.A9
        - type 5 I21.A9
  - syphilitic A52.06
  - transmural — see also, Infarct, myocardium, ST elevation, by site I21.3

Infarct, infarction — continued
- myocardium, myocardial — continued
  - transmural — see also, Infarct, myocardium, ST elevation, by site — continued
    - anterior (anteroapical) (anterolateral) (anteroseptal) (Q wave) (wall) NEC I21.09
    - inferior (diaphragmatic) (inferolateral) (inferoposterior) (Q wave) (wall) NEC I21.19
    - inferoposterior (Q wave) (wall) I21.11
    - lateral (apical-lateral) (basal-lateral) (high) NEC I21.29
    - posterior (posterobasal) (posterolateral) (posteroseptal) (true) NEC I21.29
    - septal NEC I21.29
    - specified NEC I21.29
  - type 1 — see also Infarction, myocardial, by site, or by ST elevation or non-ST elevation I21.9
  - type 2 I21.A1
  - type 3 I21.A9
  - type 4 (a) (b) (c) I21.A9
  - type 5 I21.A9
- nontransmural I21.4
- omentum — see also Infarct, intestine K55.069
- ovary N83.8
- pancreas K86.89
- papillary muscle — see Infarct, myocardium
- parathyroid gland E21.4
- pituitary (gland) E23.6
- placenta O43.81- ☑
- prostate N42.89
- pulmonary (artery) (vein) (hemorrhagic) — see Embolism, pulmonary
- renal (embolic) (thrombotic) N28.0
- retina, retinal (artery) — see Occlusion, artery, retina
- spinal (cord) (acute) (embolic) (nonembolic) G95.11
- spleen D73.5
  - embolic or thrombotic I74.8
- subendocardial (acute) (nontransmural) I21.4
- suprarenal (capsule) (gland) E27.49
- testis N50.1
- thrombotic — see also Thrombosis
  - artery, arterial — see Embolism
- thyroid (gland) E07.89
- ventricle (heart) — see Infarct, myocardium

Infecting — see condition

Infection, infected, infective (opportunistic) B99.9
- with
  - drug resistant organism — see Resistance (to), drug — see also specific organism
  - lymphangitis — see Lymphangitis
  - organ dysfunction (acute) R65.20
    - with septic shock R65.21
- abscess (skin) — code by site under Abscess
- Absidia — see Mucormycosis
- Acanthamoeba — see Acanthamebiasis
- Acanthocheilonema (perstans) (streptocerca) B74.4
- accessory sinus (chronic) — see Sinusitis
- achorion — see Dermatophytosis
- Acinetobacter baumannii, as cause of disease classified elsewhere B96.83
- Acremonium falciforme B47.0
- acromioclavicular M00.9
- Actinobacillus (actinomycetem-comitans) A28.8
  - mallei A24.0
  - muris A25.1
- Actinomadura B47.1
- Actinomyces (israelii) — see also Actinomycosis A42.9
- Actinomycetales — see Actinomycosis
- actinomycotic NOS — see Actinomycosis
- adenoid (and tonsil) J03.90
  - chronic J35.02
- adenovirus NEC
  - as cause of disease classified elsewhere B97.0
  - unspecified nature or site B34.0
- aerogenes capsulatus A48.0
- aertrycke — see Infection, salmonella
- alimentary canal NOS — see Enteritis, infectious
- Allescheria boydii B48.2
- Alternaria B48.8
- alveolus, alveolar (process) K04.7
- Ameba, amebic (histolytica) — see Amebiasis
- amniotic fluid, sac or cavity O41.10- ☑
  - chorioamnionitis O41.12- ☑
  - placentitis O41.14- ☑
- amputation stump (surgical) — see Complication, amputation stump, infection
- Ancylostoma (duodenalis) B76.0
- Anisakiasis, Anisakis larvae B81.0
- anthrax — see Anthrax

Infection, infected, infective — continued
- antrum (chronic) — see Sinusitis, maxillary
- anus, anal (papillae) (sphincter) K62.89
- arbovirus (arbor virus) A94
  - specified type NEC A93.8
- artificial insemination N98.0
- Ascaris lumbricoides — see Ascariasis
- Ascomycetes B47.0
- Aspergillus (flavus) (fumigatus) (terreus) — see Aspergillosis
- atypical
  - acid-fast (bacilli) — see Mycobacterium, atypical
  - mycobacteria — see Mycobacterium, atypical
  - virus A81.9
    - specified type NEC A81.89
- auditory meatus (external) — see Otitis, externa, infective
- auricle (ear) — see Otitis, externa, infective
- axillary gland (lymph) L04.2
- Bacillus A49.9
  - abortus A23.1
  - anthracis — see Anthrax
  - ducreyi (any location) A57
  - Flexner's A03.1
  - Friedlander's NEC A49.8
  - gas (gangrene) A48.0
  - mallei A24.0
  - melitensis A23.0
  - paratyphoid, paratyphosus A01.4
    - A A01.1
    - B A01.2
    - C A01.3
  - Shiga (-Kruse) A03.0
  - suipestifer — see Infection, salmonella
  - swimming pool A31.1
  - typhosa A01.00
  - welchii — see Gangrene, gas
- bacterial NOS A49.9
  - as cause of disease classified elsewhere B96.89
    - Acinetobacter baumannii B96.83
    - Bacteroides fragilis [B. fragilis] B96.6
    - Clostridium perfringens [C. perfringens] B96.7
    - Cronobacter (sakazakii) A49.8
    - Enterobacter sakazakii B96.89
    - Enterococcus B95.2
    - Escherichia coli [E. coli] — see also Escherichia coli B96.20
    - Helicobacter pylori [H.pylori] B96.81
    - Hemophilus influenzae [H. influenzae] B96.3
    - Klebsiella pneumoniae [K. pneumoniae] B96.1
    - Mycoplasma pneumoniae [M. pneumoniae] B96.0
    - Proteus (mirabilis) (morganii) B96.4
    - Pseudomonas (aeruginosa) (mallei) (pseudomallei) B96.5
    - Staphylococcus B95.8
      - aureus (methicillin susceptible) (MSSA) B95.61
        - methicillin resistant (MRSA) B95.62
      - specified NEC B95.7
    - Streptococcus B95.5
      - group A B95.0
      - group B B95.1
      - pneumoniae B95.3
      - specified NEC B95.4
    - Vibrio vulnificus B96.82
  - specified NEC A48.8
- Bacterium
  - paratyphosum A01.4
    - A A01.1
    - B A01.2
    - C A01.3
  - typhosum A01.00
- Bacteroides NEC A49.8
  - fragilis, as cause of disease classified elsewhere B96.6
- Balantidium coli A07.0
- Bartholin's gland N75.8
- Basidiobolus B46.8
- bile duct (common) (hepatic) — see Cholangitis
- bladder — see Cystitis
- Blastomyces, blastomycotic — see also Blastomycosis
  - brasiliensis — see Paracoccidioidomycosis
  - dermatitidis — see Blastomycosis
  - European — see Cryptococcosis
  - Loboi B48.0
  - North American B40.9
  - South American — see Paracoccidioidomycosis
- bleb, postprocedure — see Blebitis
- bone — see Osteomyelitis
- Bordetella — see Whooping cough
- Borrelia bergdorfi A69.20
- brain — see also Encephalitis G04.90

Infection, infected, infective — *continued*
- brain — *see also* Encephalitis — *continued*
  - membranes — *see* Meningitis
  - septic G06.0
    - meninges — *see* Meningitis, bacterial
- branchial cyst Q18.0
- breast — *see* Mastitis
- bronchus — *see* Bronchitis
- Brucella A23.9
  - abortus A23.1
  - canis A23.3
  - melitensis A23.0
  - mixed A23.8
  - specified NEC A23.8
  - suis A23.2
- Brugia (malayi) B74.1
  - timori B74.2
- bursa — *see* Bursitis, infective
- buttocks (skin) L08.9
- Campylobacter, intestinal A04.5
  - as cause of disease classified elsewhere B96.81
- Candida (albicans) (tropicalis) — *see* Candidiasis
- candiru B88.8
- Capillaria (intestinal) B81.1
  - hepatica B83.8
  - philippinensis B81.1
- cartilage — *see* Disorder, cartilage, specified type NEC
- cat liver fluke B66.0
- catheter-related bloodstream (CRBSI) T80.211- ☑
- cellulitis — *code by* site under Cellulitis
- central line-associated T80.219- ☑
  - bloodstream (CLABSI) T80.211- ☑
  - specified NEC T80.218- ☑
- Cephalosporium falciforme B47.0
- cerebrospinal — *see* Meningitis
- cervical gland (lymph) L04.0
- cervix — *see* Cervicitis
- cesarean delivery wound (puerperal) O86.00
- cestodes — *see* Infestation, cestodes
- chest J22
- Chilomastix (intestinal) A07.8
- Chlamydia, chlamydial A74.9
  - anus A56.3
  - genitourinary tract A56.2
    - lower A56.00
    - specified NEC A56.19
  - lymphogranuloma A55
  - pharynx A56.4
  - psittaci A70
  - rectum A56.3
  - sexually transmitted NEC A56.8
- cholera — *see* Cholera
- Cladosporium
  - bantianum (brain abscess) B43.1
  - carrionii B43.0
  - castellanii B36.1
  - trichoides (brain abscess) B43.1
  - werneckii B36.1
- Clonorchis (sinensis) (liver) B66.1
- Clostridioides
  - difficile
    - as cause of disease classified elsewhere B96.89
    - foodborne (disease)
      - not specified as recurrent A04.72
      - recurrent A04.71
    - gas gangrene A48.0
    - necrotizing enterocolitis
      - not specified as recurrent A04.72
      - recurrent A04.71
    - sepsis A41.4
- Clostridium NEC
  - bifermentans A48.0
  - botulinum (food poisoning) A05.1
    - infant A48.51
    - wound A48.52
  - difficile
    - as cause of disease classified elsewhere B96.89
    - foodborne (disease)
      - not specified as recurrent A04.72
      - recurrent A04.71
    - gas gangrene A48.0
    - necrotizing enterocolitis
      - not specified as recurrent A04.72
      - recurrent A04.71
    - sepsis A41.4
  - gas-forming NEC A48.0
  - histolyticum A48.0
  - novyi, causing gas gangrene A48.0
  - oedematiens A48.0

Infection, infected, infective — *continued*
- Clostridium — *continued*
  - perfringens
    - as cause of disease classified elsewhere B96.7
    - due to food A05.2
    - foodborne (disease) A05.2
    - gas gangrene A48.0
    - sepsis A41.4
  - septicum, causing gas gangrene A48.0
  - sordellii, causing gas gangrene A48.0
  - welchii
    - as cause of disease classified elsewhere B96.7
    - foodborne (disease) A05.2
    - gas gangrene A48.0
    - necrotizing enteritis A05.2
    - sepsis A41.4
- Coccidioides (immitis) — *see* Coccidioidomycosis
- colon — *see* Enteritis, infectious
- colostomy K94.02
- common duct — *see* Cholangitis
- congenital P39.9
  - Candida (albicans) P37.5
  - cytomegalovirus P35.1
  - hepatitis, viral P35.3
  - herpes simplex P35.2
  - infectious or parasitic disease P37.9
    - specified NEC P37.8
  - listeriosis (disseminated) P37.2
  - malaria NEC P37.4
    - falciparum P37.3
  - Plasmodium falciparum P37.3
  - poliomyelitis P35.8
  - rubella P35.0
  - skin P39.4
  - toxoplasmosis (acute) (subacute) (chronic) P37.1
  - tuberculosis P37.0
  - urinary (tract) P39.3
  - vaccinia P35.8
  - virus P35.9
    - specified type NEC P35.8
- Conidiobolus B46.8
- coronavirus-2019 U07.1
- coronavirus NEC B34.2
  - as cause of disease classified elsewhere B97.29
  - severe acute respiratory syndrome (SARS associated) B97.21
- corpus luteum — *see* Salpingo-oophoritis
- Corynebacterium diphtheriae — *see* Diphtheria
- cotia virus B08.8
- COVID-19 — *see also* COVID-19 U07.1
- Coxiella burnetii A78
- coxsackie — *see* Coxsackie
- Cronobacter (sakazakii) A49.8
  - as cause of disease classified elsewhere B96.89
  - generalized A41.59
- Cryptococcus neoformans — *see* Cryptococcosis
- Cryptosporidium A07.2
- Cunninghamella — *see* Mucormycosis
- cyst — *see* Cyst
- cystic duct — *see also* Cholecystitis K81.9
- Cysticercus cellulosae — *see* Cysticercosis
- cytomegalovirus, cytomegaloviral B25.9
  - congenital P35.1
  - maternal, maternal care for (suspected) damage to fetus O35.3- ☑
  - mononucleosis B27.10
    - with
      - complication NEC B27.19
      - meningitis B27.12
      - polyneuropathy B27.11
- delta-agent (acute), in hepatitis B carrier B17.0
- dental (pulpal origin) K04.7
- Deuteromycetes B47.0
- Dicrocoelium dendriticum B66.2
- diphtherial — *see* Diphtheria
- Diphyllobothrium (adult) (latum) (pacificum) B70.0
  - larval B70.1
- Diplogonoporus (grandis) B71.8
- Dipylidium caninum B67.4
- Dirofilaria B74.8
- Dracunculus medinensis B72
- Drechslera (hawaiiensis) B43.8
- ducreyi Haemophilus (any location) A57
- due to or resulting from
  - artificial insemination N98.0
  - Babesia
    - divergens (-like) strain B60.03
    - duncani (-type) species B60.02

Infection, infected, infective — *continued*
- due to or resulting from — *continued*
  - Babesia — *continued*
    - microti B60.01
    - species
      - specified NEC B60.09
  - central venous catheter T80.219- ☑
    - bloodstream T80.211- ☑
    - exit or insertion site T80.212- ☑
    - localized T80.212- ☑
    - port or reservoir T80.212- ☑
    - specified NEC T80.218- ☑
    - tunnel T80.212- ☑
  - device, implant or graft — *see also* Complications, by site and type, infection or inflammation T85.79- ☑
    - arterial graft NEC T82.7- ☑
    - breast (implant) T85.79- ☑
    - catheter NEC T85.79- ☑
      - dialysis (renal) T82.7- ☑
        - central line T80.211- ☑
        - intraperitoneal T85.71- ☑
      - infusion NEC T82.7- ☑
        - cranial T85.735- ☑
        - intrathecal T85.735- ☑
        - spinal (epidural) (subdural) T85.735- ☑
        - subarachnoid T85.735- ☑
      - urinary T83.518- ☑
        - cystostomy T83.510- ☑
        - Hopkins T83.518- ☑
        - ileostomy T83.518- ☑
        - nephrostomy T83.512- ☑
        - specified NEC T83.518- ☑
        - urethral indwelling T83.511- ☑
        - urostomy T83.518- ☑
    - electronic (electrode) (pulse generator) (stimulator)
      - bone T84.7- ☑
      - cardiac T82.7- ☑
      - nervous system T85.738- ☑
        - brain T85.731- ☑
        - cranial nerve T85.732- ☑
        - gastric nerve T85.732- ☑
        - generator pocket T85.734- ☑
        - neurostimulator generator T85.734- ☑
        - peripheral nerve T85.732- ☑
        - sacral nerve T85.732- ☑
        - spinal cord T85.733- ☑
        - vagal nerve T85.732- ☑
      - urinary (indwelling) T83.51- ☑
    - fixation, internal (orthopedic) NEC — *see* Complication, fixation device, infection
    - gastrointestinal (bile duct) (esophagus) T85.79- ☑
      - neurostimulator electrode (lead) T85.732- ☑
    - genital NEC T83.69- ☑
    - heart NEC T82.7- ☑
      - valve (prosthesis) T82.6- ☑
        - graft T82.7- ☑
    - joint prosthesis — *see* Complication, joint prosthesis, infection
    - ocular (corneal graft) (orbital implant) NEC T85.79- ☑
    - orthopedic NEC T84.7- ☑
    - penile (cylinder) (pump) (reservoir) T83.61- ☑
    - specified NEC T85.79- ☑
    - testicular T83.62- ☑
    - urinary NEC T83.598- ☑
      - ileal conduit stent T83.593- ☑
      - implanted neurostimulation T83.590- ☑
      - implanted sphincter T83.591- ☑
      - indwelling ureteral stent T83.592- ☑
      - nephroureteral stent T83.593- ☑
      - specified stent NEC T83.593- ☑
    - vascular NEC T82.7- ☑
    - ventricular intracranial (communicating) shunt T85.730- ☑
  - Hickman catheter T80.219- ☑
    - bloodstream T80.211- ☑
    - localized T80.212- ☑
    - specified NEC T80.218- ☑
  - immunization or vaccination T88.0- ☑
  - infusion, injection or transfusion NEC T80.29- ☑
  - injury NEC — *code by* site under Wound, open
  - peripherally inserted central catheter (PICC) T80.219- ☑
    - bloodstream T80.211- ☑

☑ Additional Character Required — Refer to the Tabular List for Character Selection

Infection, infected, infective — continued
- due to or resulting from — continued
  - peripherally inserted central catheter — continued
    - localized T80.212- ☑
    - specified NEC T80.218- ☑
  - portacath (port-a-cath) T80.219- ☑
    - bloodstream T80.211- ☑
    - localized T80.212- ☑
    - specified NEC T80.218- ☑
  - protozoa of the order Piroplasmida NEC B60.09
  - pulmonary artery catheter — see Infection, due to or resulting from, central venous catheter
  - surgery T81.40-
  - Swan Ganz catheter — see Infection, due to or resulting from, central venous catheter
  - triple lumen catheter T80.219- ☑
    - bloodstream T80.211- ☑
    - localized T80.212- ☑
    - specified NEC T80.218- ☑
  - umbilical venous catheter T80.219- ☑
    - bloodstream T80.211- ☑
    - localized T80.212- ☑
    - specified NEC T80.218- ☑
- during labor NEC O75.3
- ear (middle) — see also Otitis media
  - external — see Otitis, externa, infective
  - inner — see subcategory H83.0- ☑
- Eberthella typhosa A01.00
- Echinococcus — see Echinococcus
- echovirus
  - as cause of disease classified elsewhere B97.12
  - unspecified nature or site B34.1
- endocardium I33.0
- endocervix — see Cervicitis
- Entamoeba — see Amebiasis
- enteric — see Enteritis, infectious
- Enterobacter sakazakii B96.89
- Enterobius vermicularis B80
- enterostomy K94.12
- enterovirus B34.1
  - as cause of disease classified elsewhere B97.10
    - coxsackievirus B97.11
    - echovirus B97.12
    - specified NEC B97.19
- Entomophthora B46.8
- Epidermophyton — see Dermatophytosis
- epididymis — see Epididymitis
- episiotomy (puerperal) O86.09
- Erysipelothrix (insidiosa) (rhusiopathiae) — see Erysipeloid
- erythema infectiosum B08.3
- Escherichia (E.) coli NEC A49.8
  - as cause of disease classified elsewhere — see also Escherichia coli B96.20
  - congenital P39.8
    - sepsis P36.4
  - generalized A41.51
  - intestinal — see Enteritis, infectious, due to, Escherichia coli
- ethmoidal (chronic) (sinus) — see Sinusitis, ethmoidal
- eustachian tube (ear) — see Salpingitis, eustachian
- external auditory canal (meatus) NEC — see Otitis, externa, infective
- eye (purulent) — see Endophthalmitis, purulent
- eyelid — see Inflammation, eyelid
- fallopian tube — see Salpingo-oophoritis
- Fasciola (gigantica) (hepatica) (indica) B66.3
- Fasciolopsis (buski) B66.5
- filarial — see Infestation, filarial
- finger (skin) L08.9
  - nail L03.01- ☑
    - fungus B35.1
- fish tapeworm B70.0
  - larval B70.1
- flagellate, intestinal A07.9
- fluke — see Infestation, fluke
- focal
  - teeth (pulpal origin) K04.7
  - tonsils J35.01
- Fonsecaea (compactum) (pedrosoi) B43.0
- food — see Intoxication, foodborne
- foot (skin) L08.9
  - dermatophytic fungus B35.3
- Francisella tularensis — see Tularemia
- frontal (sinus) (chronic) — see Sinusitis, frontal
- fungus NOS B49
  - beard B35.0

Infection, infected, infective — continued
- fungus — continued
  - dermatophytic — see Dermatophytosis
  - foot B35.3
  - groin B35.6
  - hand B35.2
  - nail B35.1
  - pathogenic to compromised host only B48.8
  - perianal (area) B35.6
  - scalp B35.0
  - skin B36.9
    - foot B35.3
    - hand B35.2
    - toenails B35.1
- Fusarium B48.8
- gallbladder — see Cholecystitis
- gas bacillus — see Gangrene, gas
- gastrointestinal — see Enteritis, infectious
- generalized NEC — see Sepsis
- generator pocket, implanted electronic neurostimulator T85.734- ☑
- genital organ or tract
  - female — see Disease, pelvis, inflammatory
  - male N49.9
    - multiple sites N49.8
    - specified NEC N49.8
- Ghon tubercle, primary A15.7
- Giardia lamblia A07.1
- gingiva (chronic) K05.10
  - acute K05.00
    - nonplaque induced K05.01
    - plaque induced K05.00
  - nonplaque induced K05.11
  - plaque induced K05.10
- glanders A24.0
- glenosporopsis B48.0
- Gnathostoma (spinigerum) B83.1
- Gongylonema B83.8
- gonococcal — see Gonococcus
- gram-negative bacilli NOS A49.9
- guinea worm B72
- gum (chronic) K05.10
  - acute K05.00
    - nonplaque induced K05.01
    - plaque induced K05.00
  - nonplaque induced K05.11
  - plaque induced K05.10
- Haemophilus — see Infection, Hemophilus
- heart — see Carditis
- Helicobacter pylori A04.8
  - as cause of disease classified elsewhere B96.81
- helminths B83.9
  - intestinal B82.0
    - mixed (types classifiable to more than one of the titles B65.0-B81.3 and B81.8) B81.4
    - specified type NEC B81.8
  - specified type NEC B83.8
- Hemophilus
  - aegyptius, systemic A48.4
  - ducreyi (any location) A57
  - generalized A41.3
  - influenzae NEC A49.2
    - as cause of disease classified elsewhere B96.3
- herpes (simplex) — see also Herpes
  - congenital P35.2
  - disseminated B00.7
  - zoster B02.9
- herpesvirus, herpesviral — see Herpes
- Heterophyes (heterophyes) B66.8
- hip (joint) NEC M00.9
  - due to internal joint prosthesis
    - left T84.52- ☑
    - right T84.51- ☑
  - skin NEC L08.9
- Histoplasma — see Histoplasmosis
  - American B39.4
  - capsulatum B39.4
- hookworm B76.9
- human
  - papilloma virus A63.0
  - T-cell lymphotropic virus type-1 (HTLV-1) B33.3
- hydrocele N43.0
- Hymenolepis B71.0
- hypopharynx — see Pharyngitis
- inguinal (lymph) glands L04.1
  - due to soft chancre A57
- intervertebral disc, pyogenic M46.30
  - cervical region M46.32
  - cervicothoracic region M46.33

Infection, infected, infective — continued
- intervertebral disc, pyogenic — continued
  - lumbar region M46.36
  - lumbosacral region M46.37
  - multiple sites M46.39
  - occipito-atlanto-axial region M46.31
  - sacrococcygeal region M46.38
  - thoracic region M46.34
  - thoracolumbar region M46.35
- intestine, intestinal — see Enteritis, infectious
  - specified NEC A08.8
- intra-amniotic affecting newborn NEC P39.2
- intrauterine inflammation O41.12- ☑
- Isospora belli or hominis A07.3
- Japanese B encephalitis A83.0
- jaw (bone) (lower) (upper) M27.2
- joint NEC M00.9
  - due to internal joint prosthesis T84.50- ☑
- kidney (cortex) (hematogenous) N15.9
  - with calculus N20.0
    - with hydronephrosis N13.6
  - following ectopic gestation O08.83
  - pelvis and ureter (cystic) N28.85
  - puerperal (postpartum) O86.21
  - specified NEC N15.8
- Klebsiella (K.) pneumoniae NEC A49.8
  - as cause of disease classified elsewhere B96.1
- knee (joint) NEC M00.9
  - joint M00.9
  - due to internal joint prosthesis
    - left T84.54- ☑
    - right T84.53- ☑
  - skin L08.9
- Koch's — see Tuberculosis
- labia (majora) (minora) (acute) — see Vulvitis
- lacrimal
  - gland — see Dacryoadenitis
  - passages (duct) (sac) — see Inflammation, lacrimal, passages
- lancet fluke B66.2
- larynx NEC J37.0
- leg (skin) NOS L08.9
- Legionella pneumophila A48.1
  - nonpneumonic A48.2
- Leishmania — see also Leishmaniasis
  - aethiopica B55.1
  - braziliensis B55.2
  - chagasi B55.0
  - donovani B55.0
  - infantum B55.0
  - major B55.1
  - mexicana B55.1
  - tropica B55.1
- lentivirus, as cause of disease classified elsewhere B97.31
- Leptosphaeria senegalensis B47.0
- Leptospira interrogans A27.9
  - autumnalis A27.89
  - canicola A27.89
  - hebdomadis A27.89
  - icterohaemorrhagiae A27.0
  - pomona A27.89
  - specified type NEC A27.89
- leptospirochetal NEC — see Leptospirosis
- Listeria monocytogenes — see also Listeriosis
  - congenital P37.2
- Loa loa B74.3
  - with conjunctival infestation B74.3
  - eyelid B74.3
- Loboa loboi B48.0
- local, skin (staphylococcal) (streptococcal) L08.9
  - abscess — code by site under Abscess
  - cellulitis — code by site under Cellulitis
  - specified NEC L08.89
  - ulcer — see Ulcer, skin
- Loefflerella mallei A24.0
- lung — see also Pneumonia J18.9
  - atypical Mycobacterium A31.0
  - spirochetal A69.8
  - tuberculous — see Tuberculosis, pulmonary
  - virus — see Pneumonia, viral
- lymph gland — see also Lymphadenitis, acute
  - mesenteric I88.0
- lymphoid tissue, base of tongue or posterior pharynx, NEC (chronic) J35.03
- Madurella (grisea) (mycetomii) B47.0
- major
  - following ectopic or molar pregnancy O08.0
  - puerperal, postpartum, childbirth O85
- Malassezia furfur B36.0

Infection, infected, infective — *continued*
  Malleomyces
    mallei A24.0
    pseudomallei (whitmori) — *see* Melioidosis
  mammary gland N61.0
  Mansonella (ozzardi) (perstans) (streptocerca) B74.4
  mastoid — *see* Mastoiditis
  maxilla, maxillary M27.2
    sinus (chronic) — *see* Sinusitis, maxillary
  mediastinum J98.51
  Medina (worm) B72
  meibomian cyst or gland — *see* Hordeolum
  meninges — *see* Meningitis, bacterial
  meningococcal — *see also* condition A39.9
    adrenals A39.1
    brain A39.81
    cerebrospinal A39.0
    conjunctiva A39.89
    endocardium A39.51
    heart A39.50
      endocardium A39.51
      myocardium A39.52
      pericardium A39.53
    joint A39.83
    meninges A39.0
    meningococcemia A39.4
      acute A39.2
      chronic A39.3
    myocardium A39.52
    pericardium A39.53
    retrobulbar neuritis A39.82
    specified site NEC A39.89
  mesenteric lymph nodes or glands NEC I88.0
  Metagonimus B66.8
  metatarsophalangeal M00.9
  methicillin
    resistant Staphylococcus aureus (MRSA) A49.02
    susceptible Staphylococcus aureus (MSSA) A49.01
  Microsporum, microsporic — *see* Dermatophytosis
  mixed flora (bacterial) NEC A49.8
  Monilia — *see* Candidiasis
  Monosporium apiospermum B48.2
  mouth, parasitic B37.0
  Mucor — *see* Mucormycosis
  muscle NEC — *see* Myositis, infective
  mycelium NOS B49
  mycetoma B47.9
    actinomycotic NEC B47.1
    mycotic NEC B47.0
  Mycobacterium, mycobacterial — *see* Mycobacterium
  Mycoplasma NEC A49.3
    pneumoniae, as cause of disease classified elsewhere B96.0
  mycotic NOS B49
    pathogenic to compromised host only B48.8
    skin NOS B36.9
  myocardium NEC I40.0
  nail (chronic)
    with lymphangitis — *see* Lymphangitis, acute, digit
    finger L03.01- ☑
      fungus B35.1
    ingrowing L60.0
    toe L03.03- ☑
      fungus B35.1
  nasal sinus (chronic) — *see* Sinusitis
  nasopharynx — *see* Nasopharyngitis
  navel L08.82
  Necator americanus B76.1
  Neisseria — *see* Gonococcus
  Neotestudina rosatii B47.0
  newborn P39.9
    intra-amniotic NEC P39.2
    skin P39.4
    specified type NEC P39.8
  nipple N61.0
    associated with
      lactation O91.03
      pregnancy O91.01- ☑
      puerperium O91.02
  Nocardia — *see* Nocardiosis
  obstetrical surgical wound (puerperal) O86.00
    incisional site
      deep O86.02
      superficial O86.01
    organ and space site O86.03
    surgical site specified NEC O86.09
  Oesophagostomum (apiostomum) B81.8
  Oestrus ovis — *see* Myiasis
  Oidium albicans B37.9

Infection, infected, infective — *continued*
  Onchocerca (volvulus) — *see* Onchocerciasis
  oncovirus, as cause of disease classified elsewhere B97.32
  operation wound T81.49- ☑
  Opisthorchis (felineus) (viverrini) B66.0
  orbit, orbital — *see* Inflammation, orbit
  orthopoxvirus NEC B08.09
  ovary — *see* Salpingo-oophoritis
  Oxyuris vermicularis B80
  pancreas (acute) — *see* Pancreatitis, acute
    abscess — *see* Pancreatitis, acute
    specified NEC — *see also* Pancreatitis, acute K85.80
  papillomavirus, as cause of disease classified elsewhere B97.7
  papovavirus NEC B34.4
  Paracoccidioides brasiliensis — *see* Paracoccidioidomycosis
  Paragonimus (westermani) B66.4
  parainfluenza virus B34.8
  parameningococcus NOS A39.9
  parapoxvirus B08.60
    specified NEC B08.69
  parasitic B89
  Parastrongylus
    cantonensis B83.2
    costaricensis B81.3
  paratyphoid A01.4
    Type A A01.1
    Type B A01.2
    Type C A01.3
  paraurethral ducts N34.2
  parotid gland — *see* Sialoadenitis
  parvovirus NEC B34.3
    as cause of disease classified elsewhere B97.6
  Pasteurella NEC A28.9
    multocida A28.0
    pestis — *see* Plague
    pseudotuberculosis A28.0
    septica (cat bite) (dog bite) A28.0
    tularensis — *see* Tularemia
  pelvic, female — *see* Disease, pelvis, inflammatory
  Penicillium (marneffei) B48.4
  penis (glans) (retention) NEC N48.29
  periapical K04.5
  peridental, periodontal K05.20
    generalized — *see* Periodontitis, aggressive, generalized
    localized — *see* Periodontitis, aggressive, localized
  perinatal period P39.9
    specified type NEC P39.8
  perineal repair (puerperal) O86.09
  periorbital — *see* Inflammation, orbit
  perirectal K62.89
  perirenal — *see* Infection, kidney
  peritoneal — *see* Peritonitis
  periureteral N28.89
  Petriellidium boydii B48.2
  pharynx — *see also* Pharyngitis
    coxsackievirus B08.5
    posterior, lymphoid (chronic) J35.03
  Phialophora
    gougerotii (subcutaneous abscess or cyst) B43.2
    jeanselmei (subcutaneous abscess or cyst) B43.2
    verrucosa (skin) B43.0
  Piedraia hortae B36.3
  pinta A67.9
    intermediate A67.1
    late A67.2
    mixed A67.3
    primary A67.0
  pinworm B80
  pityrosporum furfur B36.0
  pleuro-pneumonia-like organism (PPLO) NEC A49.3
    as cause of disease classified elsewhere B96.0
  pneumococcus, pneumococcal NEC A49.1
    as cause of disease classified elsewhere B95.3
    generalized (purulent) A40.3
      with pneumonia J13
  Pneumocystis carinii (pneumonia) B59
  Pneumocystis jirovecii (pneumonia) B59
  port or reservoir T80.212- ☑
  postoperative T81.40- ☑
  postoperative wound T81.49- ☑
    surgical site
      deep incisional T81.42- ☑
      organ and space T81.43- ☑
      specified NEC T81.49- ☑
      superficial incisional T81.41- ☑

Infection, infected, infective — *continued*
  postprocedural T81.40- ☑
  postvaccinal T88.0- ☑
  prepuce NEC N47.7
    with penile inflammation N47.6
  prion — *see* Disease, prion, central nervous system
  prostate (capsule) — *see* Prostatitis
  Proteus (mirabilis) (morganii) (vulgaris) NEC A49.8
    as cause of disease classified elsewhere B96.4
  protozoal NEC B64
    intestinal A07.9
      specified NEC A07.8
    specified NEC B60.8
  Pseudoallescheria boydii B48.2
  Pseudomonas NEC A49.8
    as cause of disease classified elsewhere B96.5
    generalized A41.52
    mallei A24.0
    pneumonia J15.1
    pseudomallei — *see* Melioidosis
  puerperal O86.4
    genitourinary tract NEC O86.89
    major or generalized O85
    minor O86.4
    specified NEC O86.89
  pulmonary — *see* Infection, lung
  purulent — *see* Abscess
  Pyrenochaeta romeroi B47.0
  Q fever A78
  rectum (sphincter) K62.89
  renal — *see also* Infection, kidney
    pelvis and ureter (cystic) N28.85
  reovirus, as cause of disease classified elsewhere B97.5
  respiratory (tract) NEC J98.8
    acute J22
    chronic J98.8
    influenzal (upper) (acute) — *see* Influenza, with, respiratory manifestations NEC
    lower (acute) J22
      chronic — *see* Bronchitis, chronic
    rhinovirus J00
    syncytial virus (RSV) — *see* Infection, virus, respiratory syncytial (RSV)
    upper (acute) NOS J06.9
      chronic J39.8
      streptococcal J06.9
      viral NOS J06.9
        due to respiratory syncytial virus (RSV) J06.9 [B97.4]
  resulting from
    presence of internal prosthesis, implant, graft — *see* Complications, by site and type, infection
  retortamoniasis A07.8
  retroperitoneal NEC K68.9
  retrovirus B33.3
    as cause of disease classified elsewhere B97.30
    human
      immunodeficiency, type 2 (HIV 2) B97.35
      T-cell lymphotropic
        type I (HTLV-I) B97.33
        type II (HTLV-II) B97.34
    lentivirus B97.31
    oncovirus B97.32
    specified NEC B97.39
  Rhinosporidium (seeberi) B48.1
  rhinovirus
    as cause of disease classified elsewhere B97.89
    unspecified nature or site B34.8
  Rhizopus — *see* Mucormycosis
  rickettsial NOS A79.9
  roundworm (large) NEC B82.0
    Ascariasis — *see also* Ascariasis B77.9
  rubella — *see* Rubella
  Saccharomyces — *see* Candidiasis
  salivary duct or gland (any) — *see* Sialoadenitis
  Salmonella (aertrycke) (arizonae) (cholerae-suis) (enteritidis) (gallinarum) (suipestifer) (typhimurium) A02.9
    with
      (gastro)enteritis A02.0
      sepsis A02.1
      specified manifestation NEC A02.8
    due to food (poisoning) A02.9
    hirschfeldii A01.3
    localized A02.20
      arthritis A02.23
      meningitis A02.21
      osteomyelitis A02.24
      pneumonia A02.22

Infection, infected, infective — continued
  Salmonella — continued
    localized — continued
      pyelonephritis A02.25
      specified NEC A02.29
    paratyphi A01.4
      A A01.1
      B A01.2
      C A01.3
    schottmuelleri A01.2
    typhi, typhosa — see Typhoid
  Sarcocystis A07.8
  SARS-CoV-2 — see Infection, COVID-19
  scabies B86
  Schistosoma — see Infestation, Schistosoma
  scrotum (acute) NEC N49.2
  seminal vesicle — see Vesiculitis
  septic
    localized, skin — see Abscess
  Serratia NEC A49.8
    as cause of disease classified elsewhere B96.89
    generalized A41.53
  sheep liver fluke B66.3
  Shigella A03.9
    boydii A03.2
    dysenteriae A03.0
    flexneri A03.1
    group
      A A03.0
      B A03.1
      C A03.2
      D A03.3
    Schmitz (-Stutzer) A03.0
    schmitzii A03.0
    shigae A03.0
    sonnei A03.3
    specified NEC A03.8
  shoulder (joint) NEC M00.9
    due to internal joint prosthesis T84.59- ☑
  skin NEC L08.9
  sinus (accessory) (chronic) (nasal) — see also Sinusitis
    pilonidal — see Sinus, pilonidal
    skin NEC L08.89
  Skene's duct or gland — see Urethritis
  skin (local) (staphylococcal) (streptococcal) L08.9
    abscess — code by site under Abscess
    cellulitis — code by site under Cellulitis
    due to fungus B36.9
      specified type NEC B36.8
    mycotic B36.9
      specified type NEC B36.8
    newborn P39.4
    ulcer — see Ulcer, skin
  slow virus A81.9
    specified NEC A81.89
  Sparganum (mansoni) (proliferum) (baxteri) B70.1
  specific — see also Syphilis
    to perinatal period — see Infection, congenital
  specified NEC B99.8
  spermatic cord NEC N49.1
  sphenoidal (sinus) — see Sinusitis, sphenoidal
  spinal cord NOS — see also Myelitis G04.91
    abscess G06.1
    meninges — see Meningitis
    streptococcal G04.89
  Spirillum A25.0
  spirochetal NOS A69.9
    lung A69.8
    specified NEC A69.8
  Spirometra larvae B70.1
  spleen D73.89
  Sporotrichum, Sporothrix (schenckii) — see Sporotrichosis
  staphylococcal, unspecified site
    as cause of disease classified elsewhere B95.8
      aureus (methicillin susceptible) (MSSA) B95.61
        methicillin resistant (MRSA) B95.62
      specified NEC B95.7
    aureus (methicillin susceptible) (MSSA) A49.01
      methicillin resistant (MRSA) A49.02
    food poisoning A05.0
    generalized (purulent) A41.2
    pneumonia — see Pneumonia, staphylococcal
  Stellantchasmus falcatus B66.8
  streptobacillus moniliformis A25.1
  streptococcal NEC A49.1
    as cause of disease classified elsewhere B95.5
    B genitourinary complicating
      childbirth O98.82

Infection, infected, infective — continued
  streptococcal — continued
    B genitourinary complicating — continued
      pregnancy O98.81- ☑
      puerperium O98.83
    congenital
      sepsis P36.10
        group B P36.0
        specified NEC P36.19
    generalized (purulent) A40.9
  Streptomyces B47.1
  Strongyloides (stercoralis) — see Strongyloidiasis
  stump (amputation) (surgical) — see Complication, amputation stump, infection
  subcutaneous tissue, local L08.9
  suipestifer — see Infection, salmonella
  swimming pool bacillus A31.1
  Taenia — see Infestation, Taenia
  Taeniarhynchus saginatus B68.1
  tapeworm — see Infestation, tapeworm
  tendon (sheath) — see Tenosynovitis, infective NEC
  Ternidens diminutus B81.8
  testis — see Orchitis
  threadworm B80
  throat — see Pharyngitis
  thyroglossal duct K14.8
  toe (skin) L08.9
    cellulitis L03.03- ☑
      fungus B35.1
    nail L03.03- ☑
      fungus B35.1
  tongue NEC K14.0
    parasitic B37.0
  tonsil (and adenoid) (faucial) (lingual) (pharyngeal) — see Tonsillitis
  tooth, teeth K04.7
    periapical K04.7
    peridental, periodontal K05.20
      generalized — see Periodontitis, aggressive, generalized
      localized — see Periodontitis, aggressive, localized
    pulp K04.01
      irreversible K04.02
      reversible K04.01
    socket M27.3
  TORCH — see Infection, congenital
    without active infection P00.2
  Torula histolytica — see Cryptococcosis
  Toxocara (canis) (cati) (felis) B83.0
  Toxoplasma gondii — see Toxoplasma
  trachea, chronic J42
  trematode NEC — see Infestation, fluke
  trench fever A79.0
  Treponema pallidum — see Syphilis
  Trichinella (spiralis) B75
  Trichomonas A59.9
    cervix A59.09
    intestine A07.8
    prostate A59.02
    specified site NEC A59.8
    urethra A59.03
    urogenitalis A59.00
    vagina A59.01
    vulva A59.01
  Trichophyton, trichophytic — see Dermatophytosis
  Trichosporon (beigelii) cutaneum B36.2
  Trichostrongylus B81.2
  Trichuris (trichiura) B79
  Trombicula (irritans) B88.09
  Trypanosoma
    brucei
      gambiense B56.0
      rhodesiense B56.1
    cruzi — see Chagas' disease
  tubal — see Salpingo-oophoritis
  tuberculous
    latent (LTBI) Z22.7
    NEC — see Tuberculosis
  tubo-ovarian — see Salpingo-oophoritis
  tunica vaginalis N49.1
  tunnel T80.212- ☑
  tympanic membrane NEC — see Myringitis
  typhoid (abortive) (ambulant) (bacillus) — see Typhoid
  typhus A75.9
    flea-borne A75.2
    mite-borne A75.3
    recrudescent A75.1
    tick-borne A77.9
      African A77.1

Infection, infected, infective — continued
  typhus — continued
    tick-borne — continued
      North Asian A77.2
  umbilicus L08.82
  ureter — see Ureteritis
  urethra — see Urethritis
  urinary (tract) N39.0
    bladder — see Cystitis
    complicating
      pregnancy O23.4- ☑
        specified type NEC O23.3- ☑
    kidney — see Infection, kidney
    newborn P39.3
    puerperal (postpartum) O86.20
    tuberculous A18.13
    urethra — see Urethritis
  uterus, uterine — see Endometritis
  vaccination T88.0- ☑
  vaccinia not from vaccination B08.011
  vagina (acute) — see Vaginitis
  varicella B01.9
  varicose veins — see Varix
  vas deferens NEC N49.1
  vesical — see Cystitis
  Vibrio
    cholerae A00.0
      El Tor A00.1
    parahaemolyticus (food poisoning) A05.3
    vulnificus
      as cause of disease classified elsewhere B96.82
      foodborne intoxication A05.5
  Vincent's (gum) (mouth) (tonsil) A69.1
  virus, viral NOS B34.9
    adenovirus
      as cause of disease classified elsewhere B97.0
      unspecified nature or site B34.0
    arborvirus, arbovirus arthropod-borne A94
    as cause of disease classified elsewhere B97.89
      adenovirus B97.0
      coronavirus B97.29
        SARS-associated B97.21
      coxsackievirus B97.11
      echovirus B97.12
      enterovirus B97.10
        coxsackievirus B97.11
        echovirus B97.12
        specified NEC B97.19
      human
        immunodeficiency, type 2 (HIV 2) B97.35
        metapneumovirus B97.81
        T-cell lymphotropic,
          type I (HTLV-I) B97.33
          type II (HTLV-II) B97.34
      papillomavirus B97.7
      parvovirus B97.6
      reovirus B97.5
      respiratory syncytial (RSV) — see Infection, virus, respiratory syncytial (RSV)
      retrovirus B97.30
        human
          immunodeficiency, type 2 (HIV 2) B97.35
          T-cell lymphotropic,
            type I (HTLV-I) B97.33
            type II (HTLV-II) B97.34
        lentivirus B97.31
        oncovirus B97.32
        specified NEC B97.39
      specified NEC B97.89
    central nervous system A89
      atypical A81.9
        specified NEC A81.89
      enterovirus NEC A88.8
        meningitis A87.0
      slow virus A81.9
        specified NEC A81.89
      specified NEC A88.8
    chest J98.8
    cotia B08.8
    COVID-19 U07.1
    coxsackie — see also Infection, coxsackie B34.1
      as cause of disease classified elsewhere B97.11
    ECHO
      as cause of disease classified elsewhere B97.12
      unspecified nature or site B34.1
    encephalitis, tick-borne A84.9
    enterovirus, as cause of disease classified elsewhere B97.10
      coxsackievirus B97.11

Infection, infected, infective — *continued*
　virus, viral — *continued*
　　enterovirus, as cause of disease classified elsewhere
　　　— *continued*
　　　echovirus B97.12
　　　specified NEC B97.19
　　exanthem NOS B09
　　human metapneumovirus as cause of disease classified elsewhere B97.81
　　human papilloma as cause of disease classified elsewhere B97.7
　　intestine — *see* Enteritis, viral
　　respiratory syncytial (RSV)
　　　as cause of disease classified elsewhere B97.4
　　　bronchiolitis J21.0
　　　bronchitis J20.5
　　　bronchopneumonia J12.1
　　　otitis media H65.- ☑ *[B97.4]*
　　　pneumonia J12.1
　　　upper respiratory infection J06.9 *[B97.4]*
　　rhinovirus
　　　as cause of disease classified elsewhere B97.89
　　　unspecified nature or site B34.8
　　slow A81.9
　　　specified NEC A81.89
　　specified type NEC B33.8
　　　as cause of disease classified elsewhere B97.89
　　　unspecified nature or site B34.8
　　unspecified nature or site B34.9
　　West Nile — *see* Virus, West Nile
　　vulva (acute) — *see* Vulvitis
　West Nile — *see* Virus, West Nile
　whipworm B79
　worms B83.9
　　specified type NEC B83.8
　Wuchereria (bancrofti) B74.0
　　malayi B74.1
　yatapoxvirus B08.70
　　specified NEC B08.79
　yeast — *see also* Candidiasis B37.9
　yellow fever — *see* Fever, yellow
　Yersinia
　　enterocolitica (intestinal) A04.6
　　pestis — *see* Plague
　　pseudotuberculosis A28.2
　Zeis' gland — *see* Hordeolum
　Zika virus A92.5
　　congenital P35.4
　zoonotic bacterial NOS A28.9
　Zopfia senegalensis B47.0
Infective, infectious — *see* condition
Infertility
　female N97.9
　　age-related N97.8
　　associated with
　　　anovulation N97.0
　　　cervical (mucus) disease or anomaly N88.3
　　　congenital anomaly
　　　　cervix N88.3
　　　　fallopian tube N97.1
　　　　uterus N97.2
　　　　vagina N97.8
　　　dysmucorrhea N88.3
　　　fallopian tube disease or anomaly N97.1
　　　pituitary-hypothalamic origin E23.0
　　　specified origin NEC N97.8
　　　Stein-Leventhal syndrome E28.2
　　　uterine disease or anomaly N97.2
　　　vaginal disease or anomaly N97.8
　　due to
　　　cervical anomaly N88.3
　　　fallopian tube anomaly N97.1
　　　ovarian failure E28.39
　　　Stein-Leventhal syndrome E28.2
　　　uterine anomaly N97.2
　　　vaginal anomaly N97.8
　　nonimplantation N97.2
　　origin
　　　cervical N88.3
　　　tubal (block) (occlusion) (stenosis) N97.1
　　　uterine N97.2
　　　vaginal N97.8
　male N46.9
　　azoospermia N46.01
　　　extratesticular cause N46.029
　　　　drug therapy N46.021
　　　　efferent duct obstruction N46.023
　　　　infection N46.022
　　　　radiation N46.024

Infertility — *continued*
　male — *continued*
　　azoospermia — *continued*
　　　extratesticular cause — *continued*
　　　　specified cause NEC N46.029
　　　　systemic disease N46.025
　　oligospermia N46.11
　　　extratesticular cause N46.129
　　　　drug therapy N46.121
　　　　efferent duct obstruction N46.123
　　　　infection N46.122
　　　　radiation N46.124
　　　　specified cause NEC N46.129
　　　　systemic disease N46.125
　　specified type NEC N46.8
Infestation B88.9
　Acanthocheilonema (perstans) (streptocerca) B74.4
　Acariasis B88.09
　　demodex folliculorum B88.01
　　sarcoptes scabiei B86
　　trombiculae B88.09
　Agamofilaria streptocerca B74.4
　Ancylostoma, ankylostoma (braziliense) (caninum) (ceylanicum) (duodenale) B76.0
　　americanum B76.1
　　new world B76.1
　Anisakis larvae, anisakiasis B81.0
　arthropod NEC B88.2
　Ascaris lumbricoides — *see* Ascariasis
　Balantidium coli A07.0
　beef tapeworm B68.1
　Bothriocephalus (latus) B70.0
　　larval B70.1
　broad tapeworm B70.0
　　larval B70.1
　Brugia (malayi) B74.1
　　timori B74.2
　candiru B88.8
　Capillaria
　　hepatica B83.8
　　philippinensis B81.1
　cat liver fluke B66.0
　cestodes B71.9
　　diphyllobothrium — *see* Infestation, diphyllobothrium
　　dipylidiasis B71.1
　　hymenolepiasis B71.0
　　specified type NEC B71.8
　chigger B88.09
　chigo, chigoe B88.1
　Clonorchis (sinensis) (liver) B66.1
　coccidial A07.3
　crab-lice B85.3
　Cysticercus cellulosae — *see* Cysticercosis
　Demodex (brevis) (folliculorum) B88.01
　Dermanyssus gallinae B88.09
　Dermatobia (hominis) — *see* Myiasis
　Dibothriocephalus (latus) B70.0
　　larval B70.1
　Dicrocoelium dendriticum B66.2
　Diphyllobothrium (adult) (latum) (intestinal) (pacificum) B70.0
　　larval B70.1
　Diplogonoporus (grandis) B71.8
　Dipylidium caninum B67.4
　Distoma hepaticum B66.3
　dog tapeworm B67.4
　Dracunculus medinensis B72
　dragon worm B72
　dwarf tapeworm B71.0
　Echinococcus — *see* Echinococcus
　Echinostomum ilocanum B66.8
　Entamoeba (histolytica) — *see* Infection, Ameba
　Enterobius vermicularis B80
　eyelid
　　in (due to)
　　　leishmaniasis B55.1
　　　loiasis B74.3
　　　onchocerciasis B73.09
　　　phthiriasis B85.3
　　parasitic NOS B89
　eyeworm B74.3
　Fasciola (gigantica) (hepatica) (indica) B66.3
　Fasciolopsis (buski) (intestine) B66.5
　filarial B74.9
　　bancroftian B74.0
　　conjunctiva B74.9
　　due to
　　　Acanthocheilonema (perstans) (streptocerca) B74.4
　　　Brugia (malayi) B74.1

Infestation — *continued*
　filarial — *continued*
　　due to — *continued*
　　　Brugia — *continued*
　　　　timori B74.2
　　　Dracunculus medinensis B72
　　　guinea worm B72
　　　loa loa B74.3
　　　Mansonella (ozzardi) (perstans) (streptocerca) B74.4
　　　Onchocerca volvulus B73.00
　　　　eye B73.00
　　　　eyelid B73.09
　　　Wuchereria (bancrofti) B74.0
　　Malayan B74.1
　　ozzardi B74.4
　　specified type NEC B74.8
　fish tapeworm B70.0
　　larval B70.1
　fluke B66.9
　　blood NOS — *see* Schistosomiasis
　　cat liver B66.0
　　intestinal B66.5
　　lancet B66.2
　　liver (sheep) B66.3
　　　cat B66.0
　　　Chinese B66.1
　　　due to clonorchiasis B66.1
　　　oriental B66.1
　　lung (oriental) B66.4
　　sheep liver B66.3
　　specified type NEC B66.8
　fly larvae — *see* Myiasis
　Gasterophilus (intestinalis) — *see* Myiasis
　Gastrodiscoides hominis B66.8
　Giardia lamblia A07.1
　Gnathostoma (spinigerum) B83.1
　Gongylonema B83.8
　guinea worm B72
　helminth B83.9
　　angiostrongyliasis B83.2
　　　intestinal B81.3
　　gnathostomiasis B83.1
　　hirudiniasis, internal B83.4
　　intestinal B82.0
　　　angiostrongyliasis B81.3
　　　anisakiasis B81.0
　　　ascariasis — *see* Ascariasis
　　　capillariasis B81.1
　　　cysticercosis — *see* Cysticercosis
　　　diphyllobothriasis — *see* Infestation, diphyllobothriasis
　　　dracunculiasis B72
　　　echinococcus — *see* Echinococcosis
　　　enterobiasis B80
　　　filariasis — *see* Infestation, filarial
　　　fluke — *see* Infestation, fluke
　　　hookworm — *see* Infestation, hookworm
　　　mixed (types classifiable to more than one of the titles B65.0-B81.3 and B81.8) B81.4
　　　onchocerciasis — *see* Onchocerciasis
　　　schistosomiasis — *see* Infestation, schistosoma
　　　specified
　　　　cestode NEC — *see* Infestation, cestode
　　　　type NEC B81.8
　　　strongyloidiasis — *see* Strongyloidiasis
　　　taenia — *see* Infestation, taenia
　　　trichinellosis B75
　　　trichostrongyliasis B81.2
　　　trichuriasis B79
　　specified type NEC B83.8
　　syngamiasis B83.3
　　visceral larva migrans B83.0
　Heterophyes (heterophyes) B66.8
　hookworm B76.9
　　ancylostomiasis B76.0
　　necatoriasis B76.1
　　specified type NEC B76.8
　Hymenolepis (diminuta) (nana) B71.0
　intestinal NEC B82.9
　leeches (aquatic) (land) — *see* Hirudiniasis
　Leishmania — *see* Leishmaniasis
　lice, louse — *see* Infestation, Pediculus
　Linguatula B88.8
　Liponyssoides sanguineus B88.09
　Loa loa B74.3
　　conjunctival B74.3
　　eyelid B74.3
　louse — *see* Infestation, Pediculus

Infestation — continued
- maggots — see Myiasis
- Mansonella (ozzardi) (perstans) (streptocerca) B74.4
- Medina (worm) B72
- Metagonimus (yokogawai) B66.8
- microfilaria streptocerca — see Onchocerciasis
  - eye B73.00
  - eyelid B73.09
- mites B88.9
  - Demodex B88.01
  - scabic B86
- Monilia (albicans) — see Candidiasis
- mouth B37.0
- Necator americanus B76.1
- nematode NEC (intestinal) B82.0
  - Ancylostoma B76.0
  - conjunctiva NEC B83.9
  - Enterobius vermicularis B80
  - Gnathostoma spinigerum B83.1
  - physaloptera B80
  - specified NEC B81.8
  - trichostrongylus B81.2
  - trichuris (trichuria) B79
- Oesophagostomum (apiostomum) B81.8
- Oestrus ovis — see also Myiasis B87.9
- Onchocerca (volvulus) — see Onchocerciasis
- Opisthorchis (felineus) (viverrini) B66.0
- orbit, parasitic NOS B89
- Oxyuris vermicularis B80
- Paragonimus (westermani) B66.4
- parasite, parasitic B89
  - eyelid B89
  - intestinal NOS B82.9
  - mouth B37.0
  - skin B88.9
  - tongue B37.0
- Parastrongylus
  - cantonensis B83.2
  - costaricensis B81.3
- Pediculus B85.2
  - body B85.1
  - capitis (humanus) (any site) B85.0
  - corporis (humanus) (any site) B85.1
  - head B85.0
  - mixed (classifiable to more than one of the titles B85.0 - B85.3) B85.4
  - pubis (any site) B85.3
- Pentastoma B88.8
- pest Z59.19
- Phthirus (pubis) (any site) B85.3
  - with any infestation classifiable to B85.0 - B85.2 B85.4
- pinworm B80
- pork tapeworm (adult) B68.0
- protozoal NEC B64
  - intestinal A07.9
    - specified NEC A07.8
  - specified NEC B60.8
- pubic, louse B85.3
- rat tapeworm B71.0
- red bug B88.09
- roundworm (large) NEC B82.0
  - Ascariasis — see also Ascariasis B77.9
- sandflea B88.1
- Sarcoptes scabiei B86
- scabies B86
- Schistosoma B65.9
  - bovis B65.8
  - cercariae B65.3
  - haematobium B65.0
  - intercalatum B65.8
  - japonicum B65.2
  - mansoni B65.1
  - mattheei B65.8
  - mekongi B65.8
  - specified type NEC B65.8
  - spindale B65.8
- screw worms — see Myiasis
- skin NOS B88.9
- Sparganum (mansoni) (proliferum) (baxteri) B70.1
  - larval B70.1
- specified type NEC B88.8
- Spirometra larvae B70.1
- Stellantchasmus falcatus B66.8
- Strongyloides stercoralis — see Strongyloidiasis
- Taenia B68.9
  - diminuta B71.0
  - echinococcus — see Echinococcus
  - mediocanellata B68.1
  - nana B71.0

Infestation — continued
- Taenia — continued
  - saginata B68.1
  - solium (intestinal form) B68.0
    - larval form — see Cysticercosis
- Taeniarhynchus saginatus B68.1
- tapeworm B71.9
  - beef B68.1
  - broad B70.0
    - larval B70.1
  - dog B67.4
  - dwarf B71.0
  - fish B70.0
    - larval B70.1
  - pork B68.0
  - rat B71.0
- Ternidens diminutus B81.8
- Tetranychus molestissimus B88.09
- threadworm B80
- tongue B37.0
- Toxocara (canis) (cati) (felis) B83.0
- trematode(s) NEC — see Infestation, fluke
- Trichinella (spiralis) B75
- Trichocephalus B79
- Trichomonas — see Trichomoniasis
- Trichostrongylus B81.2
- Trichuris (trichiura) B79
- Trombicula (irritans) B88.09
- Tunga penetrans B88.1
- Uncinaria americana B76.1
- Vandellia cirrhosa B88.8
- whipworm B79
- worms B83.9
  - intestinal B82.0
- Wuchereria (bancrofti) B74.0

Infiltrate, infiltration
- amyloid (generalized) (localized) — see Amyloidosis
- calcareous NEC R89.7
  - localized — see Degeneration, by site
- calcium salt R89.7
- cardiac
  - fatty — see Degeneration, myocardial
  - glycogenic E74.02 [I43]
- corneal — see Edema, cornea
- eyelid — see Inflammation, eyelid
- glycogen, glycogenic — see Disease, glycogen storage
- heart, cardiac
  - fatty — see Degeneration, myocardial
  - glycogenic E74.02 [I43]
- inflammatory in vitreous H43.89
- kidney N28.89
- leukemic — see Leukemia
- liver K76.89
  - fatty — see Fatty, liver NEC
  - glycogen — see also Disease, glycogen storage E74.03 [K77]
- lung R91.8
  - eosinophilic — see Eosinophilia, pulmonary
- lymphatic — see also Leukemia, lymphatic C91.9-
  - gland I88.9
- muscle, fatty M62.89
- myocardium, myocardial
  - fatty — see Degeneration, myocardial
  - glycogenic E74.02 [I43]
- on chest x-ray R91.8
- pulmonary R91.8
  - with eosinophilia — see Eosinophilia, pulmonary
- skin (lymphocytic) L98.6
- thymus (gland) (fatty) E32.8
- urine R39.0
- vesicant agent
  - antineoplastic chemotherapy T80.810- ☑
  - other agent NEC T80.818- ☑
- vitreous body H43.89

Infirmity R68.89
- senile R54

Inflammation, inflamed, inflammatory (with exudation)
- abducent (nerve) — see Strabismus, paralytic, sixth nerve
- accessory sinus (chronic) — see Sinusitis
- adrenal (gland) E27.8
- alveoli, teeth M27.3
  - scorbutic E54
- anal canal, anus K62.89
- antrum (chronic) — see Sinusitis, maxillary
- appendix — see Appendicitis
- arachnoid — see Meningitis
- areola N61.0
  - puerperal, postpartum or gestational — see Infection, nipple

Inflammation, inflamed, inflammatory — continued
- areolar tissue NOS L08.9
- artery — see Arteritis
- auditory meatus (external) — see Otitis, externa
- Bartholin's gland N75.8
- bile duct (common) (hepatic) or passage — see Cholangitis
- bladder — see Cystitis
- bone — see Osteomyelitis
- brain — see also Encephalitis
  - membrane — see Meningitis
- breast N61.0
  - cancer — see Table of Neoplasms
  - neoplasm — see Table of Neoplasms
  - puerperal, postpartum, gestational — see Mastitis, obstetric
- broad ligament — see Disease, pelvis, inflammatory
- bronchi — see Bronchitis
- catarrhal J00
- cecum — see Appendicitis
- cerebral — see also Encephalitis
  - membrane — see Meningitis
- cerebrospinal
  - meningococcal A39.0
- cervix (uteri) — see Cervicitis
- chest J98.8
- chorioretinal H30.9- ☑
  - cyclitis — see Cyclitis
  - disseminated H30.10- ☑
    - generalized H30.13- ☑
    - peripheral H30.12- ☑
    - posterior pole H30.11- ☑
  - epitheliopathy — see Epitheliopathy
  - focal H30.00- ☑
    - juxtapapillary H30.01- ☑
    - macular H30.04- ☑
    - paramacular — see Inflammation, chorioretinal, focal, macular
    - peripheral H30.03- ☑
    - posterior pole H30.02- ☑
  - specified type NEC H30.89- ☑
- choroid — see Inflammation, chorioretinal
- chronic, postmastoidectomy cavity — see Complications, postmastoidectomy, inflammation
- colon — see Enteritis
- connective tissue (diffuse) NEC — see Disorder, soft tissue, specified type NEC
- cornea — see Keratitis
- corpora cavernosa N48.29
- cranial nerve — see Disorder, nerve, cranial
- Douglas' cul-de-sac or pouch (chronic) N73.0
- due to device, implant or graft — see also Complications, by site and type, infection or inflammation
  - arterial graft T82.7- ☑
  - breast (implant) T85.79- ☑
  - catheter T85.79- ☑
    - dialysis (renal) T82.7- ☑
      - intraperitoneal T85.71- ☑
    - infusion T82.7- ☑
      - cranial T85.735- ☑
      - intrathecal T85.735- ☑
      - spinal (epidural) (subdural) T85.735- ☑
      - subarachnoid T85.735- ☑
    - urinary T83.518- ☑
      - cystostomy T83.510- ☑
      - Hopkins T83.518- ☑
      - ileostomy T83.518- ☑
      - nephrostomy T83.512- ☑
      - specified NEC T83.518- ☑
      - urethral indwelling T83.511- ☑
      - urostomy T83.518- ☑
  - electronic (electrode) (pulse generator) (stimulator)
    - bone T84.7- ☑
    - cardiac T82.7- ☑
    - nervous system T85.738- ☑
      - brain T85.731- ☑
      - cranial nerve T85.732- ☑
      - gastric nerve T85.732- ☑
      - neurostimulator generator T85.734- ☑
      - peripheral nerve T85.732- ☑
      - sacral nerve T85.732- ☑
      - spinal cord T85.733- ☑
      - vagal nerve T85.732- ☑
    - urinary T83.590- ☑
  - fixation, internal (orthopedic) NEC — see Complication, fixation device, infection
  - gastrointestinal (bile duct) (esophagus) T85.79- ☑

Inflammation, inflamed, inflammatory — *continued*
  due to device, implant or graft — *see also* Complications, by site and type, infection or inflammation — *continued*
    gastrointestinal — *continued*
      neurostimulator electrode (lead) T85.732- ☑
      genital NEC T83.69- ☑
      heart NEC T82.7- ☑
        valve (prosthesis) T82.6- ☑
          graft T82.7- ☑
      joint prosthesis — *see* Complication, joint prosthesis, infection
      ocular (corneal graft) (orbital implant) NEC T85.79- ☑
      orthopedic NEC T84.7- ☑
      penile (cylinder) (pump) (reservoir) T83.61- ☑
      specified NEC T85.79- ☑
      testicular T83.62- ☑
      urinary NEC T83.598- ☑
        ileal conduit stent T83.593- ☑
        implanted neurostimulation T83.590- ☑
        implanted sphincter T83.591- ☑
        indwelling ureteral stent T83.592- ☑
        nephroureteral stent T83.593- ☑
        specified stent NEC T83.593- ☑
      vascular NEC T82.7- ☑
      ventricular intracranial (communicating) shunt T85.730- ☑
  duodenum K29.80
    with bleeding K29.81
  dura mater — *see* Meningitis
  ear (middle) — *see also* Otitis, media
    external — *see* Otitis, externa
    inner — *see* subcategory H83.0- ☑
  epididymis — *see* Epididymitis
  esophagus — *see* Esophagitis
  ethmoidal (sinus) (chronic) — *see* Sinusitis, ethmoidal
  eustachian tube (catarrhal) — *see* Salpingitis, eustachian
  eyelid H01.9
    abscess — *see* Abscess, eyelid
    blepharitis — *see* Blepharitis
    chalazion — *see* Chalazion
    dermatosis (noninfectious) — *see* Dermatosis, eyelid
    hordeolum — *see* Hordeolum
    specified NEC H01.8- ☑
  fallopian tube — *see* Salpingo-oophoritis
  fascia — *see* Myositis
  follicular, pharynx J31.2
  frontal (sinus) (chronic) — *see* Sinusitis, frontal
  gallbladder — *see* Cholecystitis
  gastric — *see* Gastritis
  gastrointestinal — *see* Enteritis
  genital organ (internal) (diffuse)
    female — *see* Disease, pelvis, inflammatory
    male N49.9
      multiple sites N49.8
      specified NEC N49.8
  gland (lymph) — *see* Lymphadenitis
  glottis — *see* Laryngitis
  granular, pharynx J31.2
  gum K05.10
    nonplaque induced K05.11
    plaque induced K05.10
  heart — *see* Carditis
  hepatic duct — *see* Cholangitis
  ileoanal (internal) pouch K91.850
  ileum — *see also* Enteritis
    regional or terminal — *see* Enteritis, regional
  intestinal pouch K91.850
  intestine (any part) — *see* Enteritis
  jaw (acute) (bone) (chronic) (lower) (suppurative) (upper) M27.2
  joint NEC — *see* Arthritis
    sacroiliac M46.1
  kidney — *see* Nephritis
  knee (joint) M13.169
    tuberculous A18.02
  labium (majus) (minus) — *see* Vulvitis
  lacrimal
    gland — *see* Dacryoadenitis
    passages (duct) (sac) — *see also* Dacryocystitis
      canaliculitis — *see* Canaliculitis, lacrimal
  larynx — *see* Laryngitis
  leg NOS L08.9
  lip K13.0
  liver (capsule) — *see also* Hepatitis
    chronic K73.9
    suppurative K75.0
  lung (acute) — *see also* Pneumonia

Inflammation, inflamed, inflammatory — *continued*
  lung — *see also* Pneumonia — *continued*
    chronic J98.4
  lymph gland or node — *see* Lymphadenitis
  lymphatic vessel — *see* Lymphangitis
  maxilla, maxillary M27.2
    sinus (chronic) — *see* Sinusitis, maxillary
  membranes of brain or spinal cord — *see* Meningitis
  meninges — *see* Meningitis
  mouth K12.1
  muscle — *see* Myositis
  myocardium — *see* Myocarditis
  nasal sinus (chronic) — *see* Sinusitis
  nasopharynx — *see* Nasopharyngitis
  navel L08.82
  nerve NEC — *see* Neuritis
  nipple N61.0
    puerperal, postpartum or gestational — *see* Infection, nipple
  nose — *see* Rhinitis
  oculomotor (nerve) — *see* Strabismus, paralytic, third nerve
  optic nerve — *see* Neuritis, optic
  orbit (chronic) H05.10
    acute H05.00
      abscess — *see* Abscess, orbit
      cellulitis — *see* Cellulitis, orbit
      osteomyelitis — *see* Osteomyelitis, orbit
      periostitis — *see* Periostitis, orbital
      tenonitis — *see* Tenonitis, eye
      granuloma — *see* Granuloma, orbit
      myositis — *see* Myositis, orbital
  ovary — *see* Salpingo-oophoritis
  oviduct — *see* Salpingo-oophoritis
  pancreas (acute) — *see* Pancreatitis
  parametrium N73.0
  parotid region L08.9
  pelvis, female — *see* Disease, pelvis, inflammatory
  penis (corpora cavernosa) N48.29
  perianal K62.89
  pericardium — *see* Pericarditis
  perineum (female) (male) L08.9
  perirectal K62.89
  peritoneum — *see* Peritonitis
  periuterine — *see* Disease, pelvis, inflammatory
  perivesical — *see* Cystitis
  petrous bone (acute) (chronic) — *see* Petrositis
  pharynx (acute) — *see* Pharyngitis
  pia mater — *see* Meningitis
  pleura — *see* Pleurisy
  polyp, colon — *see also* Polyp, colon, inflammatory K51.40
  prostate — *see also* Prostatitis
    specified type NEC N41.8
  rectosigmoid — *see* Rectosigmoiditis
  rectum — *see also* Proctitis K62.89
  respiratory, upper — *see also* Infection, respiratory, upper J06.9
    acute, due to radiation J70.0
    chronic, due to external agent — *see* condition, respiratory, chronic, due to
    due to
      chemicals, gases, fumes or vapors (inhalation) J68.2
      radiation J70.1
  retina — *see* Chorioretinitis
  retrocecal — *see* Appendicitis
  retroperitoneal — *see* Peritonitis
  salivary duct or gland (any) (suppurative) — *see* Sialoadenitis
  scorbutic, alveoli, teeth E54
  scrotum N49.2
  seminal vesicle — *see* Vesiculitis
  sigmoid — *see* Enteritis
  sinus — *see* Sinusitis
  Skene's duct or gland — *see* Urethritis
  skin L08.9
  spermatic cord N49.1
  sphenoidal (sinus) — *see* Sinusitis, sphenoidal
  spinal
    cord — *see* Encephalitis
    membrane — *see* Meningitis
    nerve — *see* Disorder, nerve
  spine — *see* Spondylopathy, inflammatory
  spleen (capsule) D73.89
  stomach — *see* Gastritis
  subcutaneous tissue L08.9
  suprarenal (gland) E27.8
  synovial — *see* Tenosynovitis

Inflammation, inflamed, inflammatory — *continued*
  tendon (sheath) NEC — *see* Tenosynovitis
  testis — *see* Orchitis
  throat (acute) — *see* Pharyngitis
  thymus (gland) E32.8
  thyroid (gland) — *see* Thyroiditis
  tongue K14.0
  tonsil — *see* Tonsillitis
  trachea — *see* Tracheitis
  trochlear (nerve) — *see* Strabismus, paralytic, fourth nerve
  tubal — *see* Salpingo-oophoritis
  tuberculous NEC — *see* Tuberculosis
  tubo-ovarian — *see* Salpingo-oophoritis
  tunica vaginalis N49.1
  tympanic membrane — *see* Tympanitis
  umbilicus, umbilical L08.82
  uterine ligament — *see* Disease, pelvis, inflammatory
  uterus (catarrhal) — *see* Endometritis
  uveal tract (anterior) NOS — *see also* Iridocyclitis
    posterior — *see* Chorioretinitis
  vagina — *see* Vaginitis
  vas deferens N49.1
  vein — *see also* Phlebitis
    intracranial or intraspinal (septic) G08
    thrombotic I80.9
      leg — *see* Phlebitis, leg
    lower extremity — *see* Phlebitis, leg
  vocal cord J38.3
  vulva — *see* Vulvitis
  Wharton's duct (suppurative) — *see* Sialoadenitis
Inflation, lung, imperfect (newborn) — *see* Atelectasis
Influenza (bronchial) (epidemic) (respiratory (upper)) (unidentified influenza virus) J11.1
  with
    digestive manifestations J11.2
    encephalopathy J11.81
    enteritis J11.2
    gastroenteritis J11.2
    gastrointestinal manifestations J11.2
    laryngitis J11.1
    myocarditis J11.82
    otitis media J11.83
    pharyngitis J11.1
    pneumonia J11.00
      specified type J11.08
    respiratory manifestations NEC J11.1
    specified manifestation NEC J11.89
  A (non-novel) J10.- ☑
  A/H5N1 — *see also* Influenza, due to, identified novel influenza A virus J09.X2
  avian — *see also* Influenza, due to, identified novel influenza A virus J09.X2
  B J10.- ☑
  bird — *see also* Influenza, due to, identified novel influenza A virus J09.X2
  C J10.- ☑
  due to
    avian — *see also* Influenza, due to, identified novel influenza A virus J09.X2
    identified influenza virus NEC J10.1
      with
        digestive manifestations J10.2
        encephalopathy J10.81
        enteritis J10.2
        gastroenteritis J10.2
        gastrointestinal manifestations J10.2
        laryngitis J10.1
        myocarditis J10.82
        otitis media J10.83
        pharyngitis J10.1
        pneumonia (unspecified type) J10.00
          with same identified influenza virus J10.01
          specified type NEC J10.08
        respiratory manifestations NEC J10.1
        specified manifestation NEC J10.89
    identified novel influenza A virus J09.X2
      with
        digestive manifestations J09.X3
        encephalopathy J09.X9
        enteritis J09.X3
        gastroenteritis J09.X3
        gastrointestinal manifestations J09.X3
        laryngitis J09.X2
        myocarditis J09.X9
        otitis media J09.X9
        pharyngitis J09.X2
        pneumonia J09.X1
        respiratory manifestations NEC J09.X2

☑ **Additional Character Required** — Refer to the Tabular List for Character Selection

Influenza — *continued*
  due to — *continued*
    identified novel influenza A virus — *continued*
      with — *continued*
        specified manifestation NEC J09.X9
        upper respiratory symptoms J09.X2
  novel (2009) H1N1 influenza — *see also* Influenza, due to, identified influenza virus NEC J10.1
  novel influenza A/H1N1 — *see also* Influenza, due to, identified influenza virus NEC J10.1
  of other animal origin, not bird or swine — *see also* Influenza, due to, identified novel influenza A virus J09.X2
  swine (viruses that normally cause infections in pigs) — *see also* Influenza, due to, identified novel influenza A virus J09.X2

Influenza-like disease — *see* Influenza
Influenzal — *see* Influenza
Infraction, Freiberg's (metatarsal head) — *see* Osteochondrosis, juvenile, metatarsus
Infraeruption of tooth (teeth) M26.34
Infusion complication, misadventure, or reaction — *see* Complications, infusion
Ingestion
  chemical — *see* Table of Drugs and Chemicals, by substance, poisoning
  drug or medicament
    correct substance properly administered — *see* Table of Drugs and Chemicals, by drug, adverse effect
    overdose or wrong substance given or taken — *see* Table of Drugs and Chemicals, by drug, poisoning
  foreign body — *see* Foreign body, alimentary tract
  multiple drug — *see* Table of Drugs and Chemicals, multiple
  tularemia A21.3

Ingrowing
  hair (beard) L73.1
  nail (finger) (toe) L60.0

Inguinal — *see also* condition
  testicle Q53.9
    bilateral Q53.212
    unilateral Q53.112

Inhalant-induced
  anxiety disorder F18.980
  depressive disorder F18.94
  major neurocognitive disorder F18.97
  mild neurocognitive disorder F18.988
  psychotic disorder F18.959

Inhalation
  anthrax A22.1
  flame T27.3-
  food or foreign body — *see* Foreign body, by site
  gases, fumes, or vapors T59.9- ☑
    specified agent NEC — *see* Table of Drugs and Chemicals, by substance T59.89- ☑
  liquid or vomitus — *see* Asphyxia
  meconium (newborn) P24.00
    with
      with respiratory symptoms P24.01
      pneumonia (pneumonitis) P24.01
  mucus — *see* Asphyxia, mucus
  oil or gasoline (causing suffocation) — *see* Foreign body, by site
  smoke T59.81- ☑
    with respiratory conditions J70.5
      due to chemicals, gases, fumes and vapors J68.9
  steam — *see also* Burn, respiratory tract T59.9- ☑
  stomach contents or secretions — *see* Foreign body, by site
    due to anesthesia (general) (local) or other sedation T88.59- ☑
      in labor and delivery O74.0
      in pregnancy O29.01- ☑
      postpartum, puerperal O89.01

Inhibition, orgasm
  female F52.31
  male F52.32

Inhibitor, systemic lupus erythematosus (presence of) D68.62
Iniencephalus, iniencephaly Q00.2
Injection, traumatic jet (air) (industrial) (water) (paint or dye) T70.4-
Injury — *see also* specified injury type T14.90- ☑
  abdomen, abdominal S39.91- ☑
    blood vessel — *see* Injury, blood vessel, abdomen
    cavity — *see* Injury, intra-abdominal
    contusion S30.11- ☑

Injury — *continued*
  abdomen, abdominal — *continued*
    internal — *see* Injury, intra-abdominal
    intra-abdominal organ — *see* Injury, intra-abdominal
    nerve — *see* Injury, nerve, abdomen
    open — *see* Wound, open, abdomen
    specified NEC S39.81- ☑
    superficial — *see* Injury, superficial, abdomen
  Achilles tendon S86.00- ☑
    laceration S86.02- ☑
    specified type NEC S86.09- ☑
    strain S86.01- ☑
  acoustic, resulting in deafness — *see* Injury, nerve, acoustic
  adrenal (gland) S37.819- ☑
    contusion S37.812- ☑
    laceration S37.813- ☑
    specified type NEC S37.818- ☑
  alveolar (process) S09.93- ☑
  ankle S99.91- ☑
    contusion — *see* Contusion, ankle
    dislocation — *see* Dislocation, ankle
    fracture — *see* Fracture, ankle
    nerve — *see* Injury, nerve, ankle
    open — *see* Wound, open, ankle
    specified type NEC S99.81- ☑
    sprain — *see* Sprain, ankle
    superficial — *see* Injury, superficial, ankle
  anterior chamber, eye — *see* Injury, eye, specified site NEC
  anus — *see* Injury, abdomen
  aorta (thoracic) S25.00- ☑
    abdominal S35.00- ☑
      laceration (minor) (superficial) S35.01- ☑
        major S35.02- ☑
      specified type NEC S35.09- ☑
    laceration (minor) (superficial) S25.01- ☑
      major S25.02- ☑
    specified type NEC S25.09- ☑
  arm (upper) S49.9- ☑
    blood vessel — *see* Injury, blood vessel, arm
    contusion — *see* Contusion, arm, upper
    fracture — *see* Fracture, humerus
    lower — *see* Injury, forearm
    muscle — *see* Injury, muscle, shoulder
    nerve — *see* Injury, nerve, arm
    open — *see* Wound, open, arm
    specified type NEC S49.8- ☑
    superficial — *see* Injury, superficial, arm
  artery (complicating trauma) — *see also* Injury, blood vessel, by site
    cerebral or meningeal — *see* Injury, intracranial
  auditory canal (external) (meatus) S09.91- ☑
  auricle, auris, ear S09.91- ☑
  axilla — *see* Injury, shoulder
  back — *see* Injury, back, lower
  bile duct S36.13- ☑
  birth — *see also* Birth, injury P15.9
  bladder (sphincter) S37.20- ☑
    at delivery O71.5
    contusion S37.22- ☑
    laceration S37.23- ☑
    obstetrical trauma O71.5
    specified type NEC S37.29- ☑
  blast (air) (hydraulic) (immersion) (underwater) NEC T14.8- ☑
    acoustic nerve trauma — *see* Injury, nerve, acoustic
    bladder — *see* Injury, bladder
    brain — *see* Concussion
      primary, specified NEC S06.8A- ☑
    colon — *see* Injury, intestine, large
    ear (primary) S09.31- ☑
      secondary S09.39- ☑
    generalized T70.8- ☑
    lung — *see* Injury, intrathoracic, lung
    multiple body organs T70.8- ☑
    peritoneum S36.81- ☑
    rectum S36.61- ☑
    retroperitoneum S36.898- ☑
    small intestine S36.419- ☑
      duodenum S36.410- ☑
      specified site NEC S36.418- ☑
    specified
      intra-abdominal organ NEC S36.898- ☑
      pelvic organ NEC S37.899- ☑
  blood vessel NEC T14.8- ☑
    abdomen S35.9- ☑

Injury — *continued*
  blood vessel — *continued*
    abdomen — *continued*
      aorta — *see* Injury, aorta, abdominal
      celiac artery — *see* Injury, blood vessel, celiac artery
      iliac vessel — *see* Injury, blood vessel, iliac
      laceration S35.91- ☑
      mesenteric vessel — *see* Injury, mesenteric
      portal vein — *see* Injury, blood vessel, portal vein
      renal vessel — *see* Injury, blood vessel, renal
      specified vessel NEC S35.8X- ☑
      splenic vessel — *see* Injury, blood vessel, splenic
      vena cava — *see* Injury, vena cava, inferior
    ankle — *see* Injury, blood vessel, foot
    aorta (abdominal) (thoracic) — *see* Injury, aorta
    arm (upper) NEC S45.90- ☑
      forearm — *see* Injury, blood vessel, forearm
      laceration S45.91- ☑
      specified
        site NEC S45.80- ☑
          laceration S45.81- ☑
          specified type NEC S45.89- ☑
        type NEC S45.99- ☑
      superficial vein S45.30- ☑
        laceration S45.31- ☑
        specified type NEC S45.39- ☑
    axillary
      artery S45.00- ☑
        laceration S45.01- ☑
        specified type NEC S45.09- ☑
      vein S45.20- ☑
        laceration S45.21- ☑
        specified type NEC S45.29- ☑
    azygos vein — *see* Injury, blood vessel, thoracic, specified site NEC
    brachial
      artery S45.10- ☑
        laceration S45.11- ☑
        specified type NEC S45.19- ☑
      vein S45.20- ☑
        laceration S45.219- ☑
        specified type NEC S45.29- ☑
    carotid artery (common) (external) (internal, extracranial) S15.00- ☑
      internal, intracranial S06.8- ☑
      laceration (minor) (superficial) S15.01- ☑
        major S15.02- ☑
      specified type NEC S15.09- ☑
    celiac artery S35.219- ☑
      branch S35.299- ☑
        laceration (minor) (superficial) S35.291- ☑
          major S35.292- ☑
        specified NEC S35.298- ☑
      laceration (minor) (superficial) S35.211- ☑
        major S35.212- ☑
      specified type NEC S35.218- ☑
    cerebral — *see* Injury, intracranial
    deep plantar — *see* Injury, blood vessel, plantar artery
    digital (hand) — *see* Injury, blood vessel, finger
    dorsal
      artery (foot) S95.00- ☑
        laceration S95.01- ☑
        specified type NEC S95.09- ☑
      vein (foot) S95.20- ☑
        laceration S95.21- ☑
        specified type NEC S95.29- ☑
    due to accidental laceration during procedure — *see* Laceration, accidental complicating surgery
    extremity — *see* Injury, blood vessel, limb
    femoral
      artery (common) (superficial) S75.00- ☑
        laceration (minor) (superficial) S75.01- ☑
          major S75.02- ☑
        specified type NEC S75.09- ☑
      vein (hip level) (thigh level) S75.10- ☑
        laceration (minor) (superficial) S75.11- ☑
          major S75.12- ☑
        specified type NEC S75.19- ☑
    finger S65.50- ☑
      index S65.50- ☑
        laceration S65.51- ☑
        specified type NEC S65.59- ☑
      laceration S65.51- ☑
      little S65.50- ☑
        laceration S65.51- ☑

Injury — continued
  blood vessel — continued
    finger — continued
      little — continued
        specified type NEC S65.59- ☑
      middle S65.50- ☑
        laceration S65.51- ☑
        specified type NEC S65.59- ☑
      specified type NEC S65.59- ☑
      thumb — see Injury, blood vessel, thumb
    foot S95.90- ☑
      dorsal
        artery — see Injury, blood vessel, dorsal, artery
        vein — see Injury, blood vessel, dorsal, vein
      laceration S95.91- ☑
      plantar artery — see Injury, blood vessel, plantar artery
      specified
        site NEC S95.80- ☑
          laceration S95.81- ☑
          specified type NEC S95.89- ☑
        specified type NEC S95.99- ☑
    forearm S55.90- ☑
      laceration S55.91- ☑
      radial artery — see Injury, blood vessel, radial artery
      specified
        site NEC S55.80- ☑
          laceration S55.81- ☑
          specified type NEC S55.89- ☑
        type NEC S55.99- ☑
      ulnar artery — see Injury, blood vessel, ulnar artery
      vein S55.20- ☑
        laceration S55.21- ☑
        specified type NEC S55.29- ☑
    gastric
      artery — see Injury, mesenteric, artery, branch
      vein — see Injury, blood vessel, abdomen
    gastroduodenal artery — see Injury, mesenteric, artery, branch
    greater saphenous vein (lower leg level) S85.30- ☑
      hip (and thigh) level S75.20- ☑
        laceration (minor) (superficial) S75.21- ☑
          major S75.22- ☑
        specified type NEC S75.29- ☑
      laceration S85.31- ☑
      specified type NEC S85.39- ☑
    hand (level) S65.90- ☑
      finger — see Injury, blood vessel, finger
      laceration S65.91- ☑
      palmar arch — see Injury, blood vessel, palmar arch
      radial artery — see Injury, blood vessel, radial artery, hand
      specified
        site NEC S65.80- ☑
          laceration S65.81- ☑
          specified type NEC S65.89- ☑
        type NEC S65.99- ☑
      thumb — see Injury, blood vessel, thumb
      ulnar artery — see Injury, blood vessel, ulnar artery, hand
    head S09.0- ☑
      intracranial — see Injury, intracranial
      multiple S09.0- ☑
    hepatic
      artery — see Injury, mesenteric, artery
      vein — see Injury, vena cava, inferior
    hip S75.90- ☑
      femoral artery — see Injury, blood vessel, femoral, artery
      femoral vein — see Injury, blood vessel, femoral, vein
      greater saphenous vein — see Injury, blood vessel, greater saphenous, hip level
      laceration S75.91- ☑
      specified
        site NEC S75.80- ☑
          laceration S75.81- ☑
          specified type NEC S75.89- ☑
        type NEC S75.99- ☑
      hypogastric (artery) (vein) — see Injury, blood vessel, iliac
    iliac S35.5- ☑
      artery S35.51- ☑
      specified vessel NEC S35.5- ☑
      uterine vessel — see Injury, blood vessel, uterine
  blood vessel — continued
    iliac — continued
      vein S35.51- ☑
    innominate — see Injury, blood vessel, thoracic, innominate
    intercostal (artery) (vein) — see Injury, blood vessel, thoracic, intercostal
    jugular vein (external) S15.20- ☑
      internal S15.30- ☑
        laceration (minor) (superficial) S15.31- ☑
          major S15.32- ☑
        specified type NEC S15.39- ☑
      laceration (minor) (superficial) S15.21- ☑
        major S15.22- ☑
      specified type NEC S15.29- ☑
    leg (level) (lower) S85.90- ☑
      greater saphenous — see Injury, blood vessel, greater saphenous
      laceration S85.91- ☑
      lesser saphenous — see Injury, blood vessel, lesser saphenous
      peroneal artery — see Injury, blood vessel, peroneal artery
      popliteal
        artery — see Injury, blood vessel, popliteal, artery
        vein — see Injury, blood vessel, popliteal, vein
      specified
        site NEC S85.80- ☑
          laceration S85.81- ☑
          specified type NEC S85.89- ☑
        type NEC S85.99- ☑
      thigh — see Injury, blood vessel, hip
      tibial artery — see Injury, blood vessel, tibial artery
    lesser saphenous vein (lower leg level) S85.40- ☑
      laceration S85.41- ☑
      specified type NEC S85.49- ☑
    limb
      lower — see Injury, blood vessel, leg
      upper — see Injury, blood vessel, arm
    lower back — see Injury, blood vessel, abdomen
    specified NEC — see Injury, blood vessel, abdomen, specified, site NEC
    mammary (artery) (vein) — see Injury, blood vessel, thoracic, specified site NEC
    mesenteric (inferior) (superior)
      artery — see Injury, mesenteric, artery
      vein — see Injury, blood vessel, mesenteric, vein
    neck S15.9- ☑
      specified site NEC S15.8- ☑
    ovarian (artery) (vein) — see subcategory S35.8- ☑
    palmar arch (superficial) S65.20- ☑
      deep S65.30- ☑
        laceration S65.31- ☑
        specified type NEC S65.39- ☑
      laceration S65.21- ☑
      specified type NEC S65.29- ☑
    pelvis — see Injury, blood vessel, abdomen
    specified NEC — see Injury, blood vessel, abdomen, specified, site NEC
    peroneal artery S85.20- ☑
      laceration S85.21- ☑
      specified type NEC S85.29- ☑
    plantar artery (deep) (foot) S95.10- ☑
      laceration S95.11- ☑
      specified type NEC S95.19- ☑
    popliteal
      artery S85.00- ☑
        laceration S85.01- ☑
        specified type NEC S85.09- ☑
      vein S85.50- ☑
        laceration S85.51- ☑
        specified type NEC S85.59- ☑
    portal vein S35.319- ☑
      laceration S35.311- ☑
      specified type NEC S35.318- ☑
    precerebral — see Injury, blood vessel, neck
    pulmonary (artery) (vein) — see Injury, blood vessel, thoracic, pulmonary
    radial artery (forearm level) S55.10- ☑
      hand and wrist (level) S65.10- ☑
        laceration S65.11- ☑
        specified type NEC S65.19- ☑
      laceration S55.11- ☑
      specified type NEC S55.19- ☑
  blood vessel — continued
    renal
      artery S35.40- ☑
        laceration S35.41- ☑
        specified NEC S35.49- ☑
      vein S35.40- ☑
        laceration S35.41- ☑
        specified NEC S35.49- ☑
    saphenous vein (greater) (lower leg level) — see Injury, blood vessel, greater saphenous
      hip and thigh level — see Injury, blood vessel, greater saphenous, hip level
      lesser — see Injury, blood vessel, lesser saphenous
    shoulder
      specified NEC — see Injury, blood vessel, arm, specified site NEC
      superficial vein — see Injury, blood vessel, arm, superficial vein
    specified NEC T14.8- ☑
    splenic
      artery — see Injury, blood vessel, celiac artery, branch
      vein S35.329- ☑
        laceration S35.321- ☑
        specified NEC S35.328- ☑
    subclavian — see Injury, blood vessel, thoracic, innominate
    thigh — see Injury, blood vessel, hip
    thoracic S25.90- ☑
      aorta S25.00- ☑
        laceration (minor) (superficial) S25.01- ☑
          major S25.02- ☑
        specified type NEC S25.09- ☑
      azygos vein — see Injury, blood vessel, thoracic, specified, site NEC
      innominate
        artery S25.10- ☑
          laceration (minor) (superficial) S25.11- ☑
            major S25.12- ☑
          specified type NEC S25.19- ☑
        vein S25.30- ☑
          laceration (minor) (superficial) S25.31- ☑
            major S25.32- ☑
          specified type NEC S25.39- ☑
      intercostal S25.50- ☑
        laceration S25.51- ☑
        specified type NEC S25.59- ☑
      laceration S25.91- ☑
      mammary vessel — see Injury, blood vessel, thoracic, specified, site NEC
      pulmonary S25.40- ☑
        laceration (minor) (superficial) S25.41- ☑
          major S25.42- ☑
        specified type NEC S25.49- ☑
      specified
        site NEC S25.80- ☑
          laceration S25.81- ☑
          specified type NEC S25.89- ☑
        type NEC S25.99- ☑
      subclavian — see Injury, blood vessel, thoracic, innominate
      vena cava (superior) S25.20- ☑
        laceration (minor) (superficial) S25.21- ☑
          major S25.22- ☑
        specified type NEC S25.29- ☑
    thumb S65.40- ☑
      laceration S65.41- ☑
      specified type NEC S65.49- ☑
    tibial artery S85.10- ☑
      anterior S85.13- ☑
        laceration S85.14- ☑
        specified injury NEC S85.15- ☑
      laceration S85.11- ☑
      posterior S85.16- ☑
        laceration S85.17- ☑
        specified injury NEC S85.18- ☑
      specified injury NEC S85.12- ☑
    ulnar artery (forearm level) S55.00- ☑
      hand and wrist (level) S65.00- ☑
        laceration S65.01- ☑
        specified type NEC S65.09- ☑
      laceration S55.01- ☑
      specified type NEC S55.09- ☑
    upper arm (level) — see Injury, blood vessel, arm

Injury

Injury — *continued*
- blood vessel — *continued*
  - upper arm — *see* Injury, blood vessel, arm — *continued*
    - superficial vein — *see* Injury, blood vessel, arm, superficial vein
  - uterine S35.5- ☑
    - artery S35.53- ☑
    - vein S35.53- ☑
  - vena cava — *see* Injury, vena cava
  - vertebral artery S15.10- ☑
    - laceration (minor) (superficial) S15.11- ☑
      - major S15.12- ☑
    - specified type NEC S15.19- ☑
  - wrist (level) — *see* Injury, blood vessel, hand
- brachial plexus S14.3- ☑
  - newborn P14.3
- brain (traumatic) S06.9- ☑
  - diffuse (axonal) S06.2X- ☑
  - focal S06.30- ☑
- brainstem S06.38- ☑
- breast NOS S29.9- ☑
- broad ligament — *see* Injury, pelvic organ, specified site NEC
- bronchus, bronchi — *see* Injury, intrathoracic, bronchus
- brow S09.90- ☑
- buttock S39.92- ☑
- canthus, eye S05.90- ☑
- cardiac plexus — *see* Injury, nerve, thorax, sympathetic
- cauda equina S34.3- ☑
- cavernous sinus — *see* Injury, intracranial
- cecum — *see* Injury, colon
- celiac ganglion or plexus — *see* Injury, nerve, lumbosacral, sympathetic
- cerebellum — *see* Injury, intracranial
- cerebral — *see* Injury, intracranial
- cervix (uteri) — *see* Injury, uterus
- cheek (wall) S09.93- ☑
- chest — *see* Injury, thorax
- childbirth (newborn) — *see also* Birth, injury
  - maternal NEC O71.9
- chin S09.93- ☑
- choroid (eye) — *see* Injury, eye, specified site NEC
- clitoris S39.94- ☑
- coccyx — *see also* Injury, back, lower
  - complicating delivery O71.6
- colon — *see* Injury, intestine, large
- common bile duct — *see* Injury, liver
- conjunctiva (superficial) — *see* Injury, eye, conjunctiva
- conus medullaris — *see* Injury, spinal, sacral
- cord
  - spermatic (pelvic region) S37.898- ☑
    - scrotal region S39.848- ☑
  - spinal — *see* Injury, spinal cord, by region
- cornea — *see* Injury, eye, specified site NEC
  - abrasion — *see* Injury, eye, cornea, abrasion
- cortex (cerebral) — *see also* Injury, intracranial
  - visual — *see* Injury, nerve, optic
- costal region NEC S29.9- ☑
- costochondral NEC S29.9- ☑
- cranial
  - cavity — *see* Injury, intracranial
  - nerve — *see* Injury, nerve, cranial
- crushing — *see* Crush
- cutaneous sensory nerve
- cystic duct — *see* Injury, liver
- deep tissue — *see* Contusion, by site
  - meaning pressure ulcer — *see* Ulcer, pressure L89 with final character .6
- delivery (newborn) P15.9
  - maternal NEC O71.9
- Descemet's membrane — *see* Injury, eyeball, penetrating
- diaphragm — *see* Injury, intrathoracic, diaphragm
- duodenum — *see* Injury, intestine, small, duodenum
- ear (auricle) (external) (canal) S09.91- ☑
  - abrasion — *see* Abrasion, ear
  - bite — *see* Bite, ear
  - blister — *see* Blister, ear
  - bruise — *see* Contusion, ear
  - contusion — *see* Contusion, ear
  - external constriction — *see* Constriction, external, ear
  - hematoma — *see* Hematoma, ear
  - inner — *see* Injury, ear, middle
  - laceration — *see* Laceration, ear
  - middle S09.30- ☑
    - blast — *see* Injury, blast, ear
    - specified NEC S09.39- ☑

Injury — *continued*
- ear — *continued*
  - puncture — *see* Puncture, ear
  - superficial — *see* Injury, superficial, ear
- eighth cranial nerve (acoustic or auditory) — *see* Injury, nerve, acoustic
- elbow S59.90- ☑
  - contusion — *see* Contusion, elbow
  - dislocation — *see* Dislocation, elbow
  - fracture — *see* Fracture, ulna, upper end
  - open — *see* Wound, open, elbow
  - specified NEC S59.80- ☑
  - sprain — *see* Sprain, elbow
  - superficial — *see* Injury, superficial, elbow
- eleventh cranial nerve (accessory) — *see* Injury, nerve, accessory
- epididymis S39.94- ☑
- epigastric region S39.91- ☑
- epiglottis NEC S19.89- ☑
- esophageal plexus — *see* Injury, nerve, thorax, sympathetic
- esophagus (thoracic part) — *see also* Injury, intrathoracic, esophagus
  - cervical NEC S19.85- ☑
- eustachian tube S09.30- ☑
- eye S05.9- ☑
  - avulsion S05.7- ☑
  - ball — *see* Injury, eyeball
  - conjunctiva S05.0- ☑
  - cornea
    - abrasion S05.0- ☑
    - laceration S05.3- ☑
      - with prolapse S05.2- ☑
  - lacrimal apparatus S05.8X- ☑
  - orbit penetration S05.4- ☑
  - specified site NEC S05.8X- ☑
- eyeball S05.8X- ☑
  - contusion S05.1- ☑
  - penetrating S05.6- ☑
    - with
      - foreign body S05.5- ☑
      - prolapse or loss of intraocular tissue S05.2- ☑
      - without prolapse or loss of intraocular tissue S05.3- ☑
  - specified type NEC S05.8- ☑
- eyebrow S09.93- ☑
- eyelid S09.93- ☑
  - abrasion — *see* Abrasion, eyelid
  - contusion — *see* Contusion, eyelid
  - open — *see* Wound, open, eyelid
- face S09.93- ☑
- fallopian tube S37.509- ☑
  - bilateral S37.502- ☑
    - blast injury S37.512- ☑
    - contusion S37.522- ☑
    - laceration S37.532- ☑
    - specified type NEC S37.592- ☑
  - blast injury (primary) S37.519- ☑
    - bilateral S37.512- ☑
    - secondary — *see* Injury, fallopian tube, specified type NEC
    - unilateral S37.511- ☑
  - contusion S37.529- ☑
    - bilateral S37.522- ☑
    - unilateral S37.521- ☑
  - laceration S37.539- ☑
    - bilateral S37.532- ☑
    - unilateral S37.531- ☑
  - specified type NEC S37.599- ☑
    - bilateral S37.592- ☑
    - unilateral S37.591- ☑
  - unilateral S37.501- ☑
    - blast injury S37.511- ☑
    - contusion S37.521- ☑
    - laceration S37.531- ☑
    - specified type NEC S37.591- ☑
- fascia — *see* Injury, muscle
- fifth cranial nerve (trigeminal) — *see* Injury, nerve, trigeminal
- finger (nail) S69.9- ☑
  - blood vessel — *see* Injury, blood vessel, finger
  - contusion — *see* Contusion, finger
  - dislocation — *see* Dislocation, finger
  - fracture — *see* Fracture, finger
  - muscle — *see* Injury, muscle, finger
  - nerve — *see* Injury, nerve, digital, finger

Injury — *continued*
- finger — *continued*
  - open — *see* Wound, open, finger
  - specified NEC S69.8- ☑
  - sprain — *see* Sprain, finger
  - superficial — *see* Injury, superficial, finger
- first cranial nerve (olfactory) — *see* Injury, nerve, olfactory
- flank — *see* Injury, abdomen
- foot S99.92- ☑
  - blood vessel — *see* Injury, blood vessel, foot
  - contusion — *see* Contusion, foot
  - dislocation — *see* Dislocation, foot
  - fracture — *see* Fracture, foot
  - muscle — *see* Injury, muscle, foot
  - open — *see* Wound, open, foot
  - specified type NEC S99.82- ☑
  - sprain — *see* Sprain, foot
  - superficial — *see* Injury, superficial, foot
- forceps NOS P15.9
- forearm S59.91- ☑
  - blood vessel — *see* Injury, blood vessel, forearm
  - contusion — *see* Contusion, forearm
  - fracture — *see* Fracture, forearm
  - muscle — *see* Injury, muscle, forearm
  - nerve — *see* Injury, nerve, forearm
  - open — *see* Wound, open, forearm
  - specified NEC S59.81- ☑
  - superficial — *see* Injury, superficial, forearm
- forehead S09.90- ☑
- fourth cranial nerve (trochlear) — *see* Injury, nerve, trochlear
- gallbladder S36.129- ☑
  - contusion S36.122- ☑
  - laceration S36.123- ☑
  - specified NEC S36.128- ☑
- ganglion
  - celiac, coeliac — *see* Injury, nerve, lumbosacral, sympathetic
  - gasserian — *see* Injury, nerve, trigeminal
  - stellate — *see* Injury, nerve, thorax, sympathetic
  - thoracic sympathetic — *see* Injury, nerve, thorax, sympathetic
- gasserian ganglion — *see* Injury, nerve, trigeminal
- gastric artery — *see* Injury, blood vessel, celiac artery, branch
- gastroduodenal artery — *see* Injury, blood vessel, celiac artery, branch
- gastrointestinal tract — *see* Injury, intra-abdominal
  - with open wound into abdominal cavity — *see* Wound, open, with penetration into peritoneal cavity
  - colon — *see* Injury, intestine, large
  - rectum — *see* Injury, intestine, large, rectum
    - with open wound into abdominal cavity S36.61- ☑
  - small intestine — *see* Injury, intestine, small
  - specified site NEC — *see* Injury, intra-abdominal, specified, site NEC
  - stomach — *see* Injury, stomach
- genital organ(s)
  - external S39.94- ☑
    - specified NEC S39.848- ☑
  - internal S37.90- ☑
    - fallopian tube — *see* Injury, fallopian tube
    - ovary — *see* Injury, ovary
    - prostate — *see* Injury, prostate
    - seminal vesicle — *see* Injury, pelvis, organ, specified site NEC
    - uterus — *see* Injury, uterus
    - vas deferens — *see* Injury, pelvis, organ, specified site NEC
  - obstetrical trauma O71.9
- gland
  - lacrimal laceration — *see* Injury, eye, specified site NEC
  - salivary S09.93- ☑
  - thyroid NEC S19.84- ☑
- globe (eye) S05.90- ☑
  - specified NEC S05.8X- ☑
- groin — *see* Injury, abdomen
- gum S09.90- ☑
- hand S69.9- ☑
  - blood vessel — *see* Injury, blood vessel, hand
  - contusion — *see* Contusion, hand
  - fracture — *see* Fracture, hand
  - muscle — *see* Injury, muscle, hand
  - nerve — *see* Injury, nerve, hand
  - open — *see* Wound, open, hand
  - specified NEC S69.8- ☑

☑ **Additional Character Required — Refer to the Tabular List for Character Selection**

Injury — *continued*
  hand — *continued*
    sprain — *see* Sprain, hand
    superficial — *see* Injury, superficial, hand
  head S09.90- ☑
    with loss of consciousness S06.9- ☑
    specified NEC S09.8- ☑
  heart (traumatic) S26.90- ☑
    with hemopericardium S26.00- ☑
      contusion S26.01- ☑
      laceration (mild) S26.020- ☑
        major S26.022- ☑
        moderate S26.021- ☑
      specified type NEC S26.09- ☑
    contusion S26.91- ☑
    laceration S26.92- ☑
    non-traumatic (acute) (chronic) (non-ischemic) I5A
    specified type NEC S26.99- ☑
    without hemopericardium S26.10- ☑
      contusion S26.11- ☑
      laceration S26.12- ☑
      specified type NEC S26.19- ☑
  heel — *see* Injury, foot
  hepatic
    artery — *see* Injury, blood vessel, celiac artery, branch
    duct — *see* Injury, liver
    vein — *see* Injury, vena cava, inferior
  hip S79.91- ☑
    blood vessel — *see* Injury, blood vessel, hip
    contusion — *see* Contusion, hip
    dislocation — *see* Dislocation, hip
    fracture — *see* Fracture, femur, neck
    muscle — *see* Injury, muscle, hip
    nerve — *see* Injury, nerve, hip
    open — *see* Wound, open, hip
    specified NEC S79.81- ☑
    sprain — *see* Sprain, hip
    superficial — *see* Injury, superficial, hip
  hymen S39.94- ☑
  hypogastric
    blood vessel — *see* Injury, blood vessel, iliac
    plexus — *see* Injury, nerve, lumbosacral, sympathetic
  ileum — *see* Injury, intestine, small
  iliac region S39.91- ☑
  instrumental (during surgery) — *see* Laceration, accidental complicating surgery
  birth injury — *see* Birth, injury
  nonsurgical — *see* Injury, by site
  obstetrical O71.9
    bladder O71.5
    cervix O71.3
    high vaginal O71.4
    perineal NOS O70.9
    urethra O71.5
    uterus O71.5
      with rupture or perforation O71.1
  internal T14.8- ☑
    aorta — *see* Injury, aorta
    bladder (sphincter) — *see* Injury, bladder
      with
        ectopic or molar pregnancy O08.6
        following ectopic or molar pregnancy O08.6
        obstetrical trauma O71.5
    bronchus, bronchi — *see* Injury, intrathoracic, bronchus
    cecum — *see* Injury, intestine, large
    cervix (uteri) — *see also* Injury, uterus
      with ectopic or molar pregnancy O08.6
      following ectopic or molar pregnancy O08.6
      obstetrical trauma O71.3
    chest — *see* Injury, intrathoracic
    gastrointestinal tract — *see* Injury, intra-abdominal
    heart — *see* Injury, heart
    intestine NEC — *see* Injury, intestine
    intrauterine — *see* Injury, uterus
    mesentery — *see* Injury, intra-abdominal, specified, site NEC
    pelvis, pelvic (organ) S37.90- ☑
      following ectopic or molar pregnancy (subsequent episode) O08.6
      obstetrical trauma NEC O71.5
        rupture or perforation O71.1
      specified NEC S39.83- ☑
    rectum — *see* Injury, intestine, large, rectum
    stomach — *see* Injury, stomach
    ureter — *see* Injury, ureter
    urethra (sphincter) following ectopic or molar pregnancy O08.6

Injury — *continued*
  internal — *continued*
    uterus — *see* Injury, uterus
  interscapular area — *see* Injury, thorax
  intestine
    large S36.509- ☑
      ascending (right) S36.500- ☑
        blast injury (primary) S36.510- ☑
          secondary S36.590- ☑
        contusion S36.520- ☑
        laceration S36.530- ☑
        specified type NEC S36.590- ☑
      blast injury (primary) S36.519- ☑
        ascending (right) S36.510- ☑
        descending (left) S36.512- ☑
        rectum S36.61- ☑
        sigmoid S36.513- ☑
        specified site NEC S36.518- ☑
        transverse S36.511- ☑
      contusion S36.529- ☑
        ascending (right) S36.520- ☑
        descending (left) S36.522- ☑
        rectum S36.62- ☑
        sigmoid S36.523- ☑
        specified site NEC S36.528- ☑
        transverse S36.521- ☑
      descending (left) S36.502- ☑
        blast injury (primary) S36.512- ☑
          secondary S36.592- ☑
        contusion S36.522- ☑
        laceration S36.532- ☑
        specified type NEC S36.592- ☑
      laceration S36.539- ☑
        ascending (right) S36.530- ☑
        descending (left) S36.532- ☑
        rectum S36.63- ☑
        sigmoid S36.533- ☑
        specified site NEC S36.538- ☑
        transverse S36.531- ☑
      rectum S36.60- ☑
        blast injury (primary) S36.61- ☑
          secondary S36.69- ☑
        contusion S36.62- ☑
        laceration S36.63- ☑
        specified type NEC S36.69- ☑
      sigmoid S36.503- ☑
        blast injury (primary) S36.513- ☑
          secondary S36.593- ☑
        contusion S36.523- ☑
        laceration S36.533- ☑
        specified type NEC S36.593- ☑
      specified
        site NEC S36.508- ☑
          blast injury (primary) S36.518- ☑
            secondary S36.598- ☑
          contusion S36.528- ☑
          laceration S36.538- ☑
          specified type NEC S36.598- ☑
        type NEC S36.599- ☑
          ascending (right) S36.590- ☑
          descending (left) S36.592- ☑
          rectum S36.69- ☑
          sigmoid S36.593- ☑
          specified site NEC S36.598- ☑
          transverse S36.591- ☑
      transverse S36.501- ☑
        blast injury (primary) S36.511- ☑
          secondary S36.591- ☑
        contusion S36.521- ☑
        laceration S36.531- ☑
        specified type NEC S36.591- ☑
    small S36.409- ☑
      blast injury (primary) S36.419- ☑
        duodenum S36.410- ☑
        secondary S36.499- ☑
          duodenum S36.490- ☑
          specified site NEC S36.498- ☑
        specified site NEC S36.418- ☑
      contusion S36.429- ☑
        duodenum S36.420- ☑
        specified site NEC S36.428- ☑
      duodenum S36.400- ☑
        blast injury (primary) S36.410- ☑
          secondary S36.490- ☑
        contusion S36.420- ☑

Injury — *continued*
  intestine — *continued*
    small — *continued*
      duodenum — *continued*
        laceration S36.430- ☑
        specified NEC S36.490- ☑
      laceration S36.439- ☑
        duodenum S36.430- ☑
        specified site NEC S36.438- ☑
      specified
        site NEC S36.408- ☑
        type NEC S36.499- ☑
          duodenum S36.490- ☑
          specified site NEC S36.498- ☑
  intra-abdominal S36.90- ☑
    adrenal gland — *see* Injury, adrenal gland
    bladder — *see* Injury, bladder
    colon — *see* Injury, intestine, large
    contusion S36.92- ☑
    fallopian tube — *see* Injury, fallopian tube
    gallbladder — *see* Injury, gallbladder
    intestine — *see* Injury, intestine
    kidney — *see* Injury, kidney
    laceration S36.93- ☑
    liver — *see* Injury, liver
    ovary — *see* Injury, ovary
    pancreas — *see* Injury, pancreas
    pelvic NOS S37.90- ☑
    peritoneum — *see* Injury, intra-abdominal, specified, site NEC
    prostate — *see* Injury, prostate
    rectum — *see* Injury, intestine, large, rectum
    retroperitoneum — *see* Injury, intra-abdominal, specified, site NEC
    seminal vesicle — *see* Injury, pelvis, organ, specified site NEC
    small intestine — *see* Injury, intestine, small
    specified
      pelvic S37.90- ☑
        specified
          site NEC S37.899- ☑
            specified type NEC S37.898- ☑
          type NEC S37.99- ☑
      site NEC S36.899- ☑
        contusion S36.892- ☑
        laceration S36.893- ☑
        specified type NEC S36.898- ☑
      type NEC S36.99- ☑
    spleen — *see* Injury, spleen
    stomach — *see* Injury, stomach
    ureter — *see* Injury, ureter
    urethra — *see* Injury, urethra
    uterus — *see* Injury, uterus
    vas deferens — *see* Injury, pelvis, organ, specified site NEC
  intracranial (traumatic) — *see also* if applicable, Compression, brain, traumatic S06.9- ☑
    cerebellar — *see also* Injury, intracranial, focal brain injury
    cerebral edema, traumatic S06.1X- ☑
      diffuse S06.1X- ☑
      focal S06.1X- ☑
      hemorrhage, traumatic — *see* Injury, intracranial, intracerebral hemorrhage, traumatic
    diffuse (axonal) S06.2X- ☑
    epidural hemorrhage (traumatic) S06.4X- ☑
    focal brain injury S06.30- ☑
      contusion — *see* Contusion, cerebral
      laceration — *see* Laceration, cerebral
      intracerebral hemorrhage, traumatic S06.36- ☑
        left side S06.35- ☑
        right side S06.34- ☑
      specified NEC S06.89- ☑
    subarachnoid hemorrhage, traumatic S06.6X- ☑
    subdural hemorrhage, traumatic S06.5X- ☑
  intraocular — *see* Injury, eyeball, penetrating
  intrathoracic S27.9- ☑
    bronchus S27.409- ☑
      bilateral S27.402- ☑
      blast injury (primary) S27.419- ☑
        bilateral S27.412- ☑
        secondary — *see* Injury, intrathoracic, bronchus, specified type NEC
        unilateral S27.411- ☑
      contusion S27.429- ☑
        bilateral S27.422- ☑
        unilateral S27.421- ☑

Injury

Injury — continued
- intrathoracic — continued
  - bronchus — continued
    - laceration S27.439- ☑
      - bilateral S27.432- ☑
      - unilateral S27.431- ☑
    - specified type NEC S27.499- ☑
      - bilateral S27.492- ☑
      - unilateral S27.491- ☑
    - unilateral S27.401- ☑
  - diaphragm S27.809- ☑
    - contusion S27.802- ☑
    - laceration S27.803- ☑
    - specified type NEC S27.808- ☑
  - esophagus (thoracic) S27.819- ☑
    - contusion S27.812- ☑
    - laceration S27.813- ☑
    - specified type NEC S27.818- ☑
  - heart — see Injury, heart
  - hemopneumothorax S27.2- ☑
  - hemothorax S27.1- ☑
  - lung S27.309- ☑
    - aspiration J69.0
    - bilateral S27.302- ☑
    - blast injury (primary) S27.319- ☑
      - bilateral S27.312- ☑
      - secondary — see Injury, intrathoracic, lung, specified type NEC
      - unilateral S27.311- ☑
    - contusion S27.329- ☑
      - bilateral S27.322- ☑
      - unilateral S27.321- ☑
    - laceration S27.339- ☑
      - bilateral S27.332- ☑
      - unilateral S27.331- ☑
    - specified type NEC S27.399- ☑
      - bilateral S27.392- ☑
      - unilateral S27.391- ☑
    - unilateral S27.301- ☑
  - pleura S27.60- ☑
    - laceration S27.63- ☑
    - specified type NEC S27.69- ☑
  - pneumothorax S27.0- ☑
  - specified organ NEC S27.899- ☑
    - contusion S27.892- ☑
    - laceration S27.893- ☑
    - specified type NEC S27.898- ☑
  - thoracic duct — see Injury, intrathoracic, specified organ NEC
  - thymus gland — see Injury, intrathoracic, specified organ NEC
  - trachea, thoracic S27.50- ☑
    - blast (primary) S27.51- ☑
    - contusion S27.52- ☑
    - laceration S27.53- ☑
    - specified type NEC S27.59- ☑
- iris — see Injury, eye, specified site NEC
  - penetrating — see Injury, eyeball, penetrating
- jaw S09.93- ☑
- jejunum — see Injury, intestine, small
- joint NOS T14.8- ☑
  - old or residual — see Disorder, joint, specified type NEC
- kidney S37.00- ☑
  - acute (nontraumatic) N17.9
  - contusion — see Contusion, kidney
  - laceration — see Laceration, kidney
  - specified NEC S37.09- ☑
- knee S89.9- ☑
  - contusion — see Contusion, knee
  - dislocation — see Dislocation, knee
  - meniscus (lateral) (medial) — see Sprain, knee, specified site NEC
    - old injury or tear — see Derangement, knee, meniscus, due to old injury
  - open — see Wound, open, knee
  - specified NEC S89.8- ☑
  - sprain — see Sprain, knee
  - superficial — see Injury, superficial, knee
- labium (majus) (minus) S39.94- ☑
- labyrinth, ear S09.30- ☑
- lacrimal apparatus, duct, gland, or sac — see Injury, eye, specified site NEC
- larynx NEC S19.81- ☑
- leg (lower) S89.9- ☑
  - blood vessel — see Injury, blood vessel, leg

Injury — continued
- leg — continued
  - contusion — see Contusion, leg
  - fracture — see Fracture, leg
  - muscle — see Injury, muscle, leg
  - nerve — see Injury, nerve, leg
  - open — see Wound, open, leg
  - specified NEC S89.8- ☑
  - superficial — see Injury, superficial, leg
- lens, eye — see Injury, eye, specified site NEC
  - penetrating — see Injury, eyeball, penetrating
- limb NEC T14.8- ☑
- lip S09.93- ☑
- liver S36.119- ☑
  - contusion S36.112- ☑
  - laceration S36.113- ☑
    - major (stellate) S36.116- ☑
    - minor S36.114- ☑
    - moderate S36.115- ☑
  - specified NEC S36.118- ☑
- lower back S39.92- ☑
  - specified NEC S39.82- ☑
- lumbar, lumbosacral (region) S39.92- ☑
  - plexus — see Injury, lumbosacral plexus
- lumbosacral plexus S34.4- ☑
- lung — see also Injury, intrathoracic, lung
  - aspiration J69.0
  - dabbing (related) U07.0
  - electronic cigarette (related) U07.0
  - EVALI [e-cigarette, or vaping, product use associated] U07.0
  - transfusion-related (TRALI) J95.84
  - vaping (associated) (device) (product) (use) U07.0
- lymphatic thoracic duct — see Injury, intrathoracic, specified organ NEC
- malar region S09.93- ☑
- mastoid region S09.90- ☑
- maxilla S09.93- ☑
- mediastinum — see Injury, intrathoracic, specified organ NEC
- membrane, brain — see Injury, intracranial
- meningeal artery — see Injury, intracranial, subdural hemorrhage
- meninges (cerebral) — see Injury, intracranial
- mesenteric
  - artery
    - branch S35.299- ☑
      - laceration (minor) (superficial) S35.291- ☑
      - major S35.292- ☑
      - specified NEC S35.298- ☑
    - inferior S35.239- ☑
      - laceration (minor) (superficial) S35.231- ☑
      - major S35.232- ☑
      - specified NEC S35.238- ☑
    - superior S35.229- ☑
      - laceration (minor) (superficial) S35.221- ☑
      - major S35.222- ☑
      - specified NEC S35.228- ☑
  - plexus (inferior) (superior) — see Injury, nerve, lumbosacral, sympathetic
  - vein
    - inferior S35.349- ☑
      - laceration S35.341- ☑
      - specified NEC S35.348- ☑
    - superior S35.339- ☑
      - laceration S35.331- ☑
      - specified NEC S35.338- ☑
- mesentery — see Injury, intra-abdominal, specified site NEC
- mesosalpinx — see Injury, pelvic organ, specified site NEC
- middle ear S09.30- ☑
- midthoracic region NOS S29.9- ☑
- mouth S09.93- ☑
- multiple NOS T07.- ☑
- muscle (and fascia) (and tendon)
  - abdomen S39.001- ☑
    - laceration S39.021- ☑
    - specified type NEC S39.091- ☑
    - strain S39.011- ☑
  - abductor
    - thumb, forearm level — see Injury, muscle, thumb, abductor
  - adductor
    - thigh S76.20- ☑
      - laceration S76.22- ☑
      - specified type NEC S76.29- ☑

Injury — continued
- muscle — continued
  - adductor — continued
    - thigh — continued
      - strain S76.21- ☑
    - ankle — see Injury, muscle, foot
    - anterior muscle group, at leg level (lower) S86.20- ☑
      - laceration S86.22- ☑
      - specified type NEC S86.29- ☑
      - strain S86.21- ☑
    - arm (upper) — see Injury, muscle, shoulder
    - biceps (parts NEC) S46.20- ☑
      - laceration S46.22- ☑
      - long head S46.10- ☑
        - laceration S46.12- ☑
        - specified type NEC S46.19- ☑
        - strain S46.11- ☑
      - specified type NEC S46.29- ☑
      - strain S46.21- ☑
    - extensor
      - finger(s) (other than thumb) — see Injury, muscle, finger by site, extensor
      - forearm level, specified NEC — see Injury, muscle, forearm, extensor
      - thumb — see Injury, muscle, thumb, extensor
      - toe (large) (ankle level) (foot level) — see Injury, muscle, toe, extensor
    - finger
      - extensor (forearm level) S56.40- ☑
        - hand level S66.309- ☑
          - laceration S66.329- ☑
          - specified type NEC S66.399- ☑
          - strain S66.319- ☑
        - laceration S56.429- ☑
        - specified type NEC S56.499- ☑
        - strain S56.419- ☑
      - flexor (forearm level) S56.10- ☑
        - hand level S66.109- ☑
          - laceration S66.129- ☑
          - specified type NEC S66.199- ☑
          - strain S66.119- ☑
        - laceration S56.129- ☑
        - specified type NEC S56.199- ☑
        - strain S56.119- ☑
      - index
        - extensor (forearm level)
          - hand level S66.308- ☑
            - laceration S66.32- ☑
            - specified type NEC S66.39- ☑
            - strain S66.31- ☑
          - specified type NEC S56.492- ☑
        - flexor (forearm level)
          - hand level S66.108- ☑
            - laceration S66.12- ☑
            - specified type NEC S66.19- ☑
            - strain S66.11- ☑
          - specified type NEC S56.19- ☑
          - strain S56.11- ☑
        - intrinsic S66.50- ☑
          - laceration S66.52- ☑
          - specified type NEC S66.59- ☑
          - strain S66.51- ☑
      - intrinsic S66.509- ☑
        - laceration S66.529- ☑
        - specified type NEC S66.599- ☑
        - strain S66.519- ☑
      - little
        - extensor (forearm level)
          - hand level S66.30- ☑
            - laceration S66.32- ☑
            - specified type NEC S66.39- ☑
            - strain S66.31- ☑
          - laceration S56.42- ☑
          - specified type NEC S56.49- ☑
          - strain S56.41- ☑
        - flexor (forearm level)
          - hand level S66.10- ☑
            - laceration S66.12- ☑
            - specified type NEC S66.19- ☑
            - strain S66.11- ☑
          - laceration S56.12- ☑
          - specified type NEC S56.19- ☑
          - strain S56.11- ☑
        - intrinsic S66.50- ☑
          - laceration S66.52- ☑
          - specified type NEC S66.59- ☑

Injury — continued
  muscle — continued
    finger — continued
      little — continued
        intrinsic — continued
          strain S66.51- ☑
      middle
        extensor (forearm level)
          hand level S66.30- ☑
            laceration S66.32- ☑
            specified type NEC S66.39- ☑
            strain S66.31- ☑
          laceration S56.42- ☑
          specified type NEC S56.49- ☑
          strain S56.41- ☑
        flexor (forearm level)
          hand level S66.10- ☑
            laceration S66.12- ☑
            specified type NEC S66.19- ☑
            strain S66.11- ☑
          laceration S56.12- ☑
          specified type NEC S56.19- ☑
          strain S56.11- ☑
        intrinsic S66.50- ☑
          laceration S66.52- ☑
          specified type NEC S66.59- ☑
          strain S66.51- ☑
      ring
        extensor (forearm level)
          hand level S66.30- ☑
            laceration S66.32- ☑
            specified type NEC S66.39- ☑
            strain S66.31- ☑
          laceration S56.42- ☑
          specified type NEC S56.49- ☑
          strain S56.41- ☑
        flexor (forearm level)
          hand level S66.10- ☑
            laceration S66.12- ☑
            specified type NEC S66.19- ☑
            strain S66.11- ☑
          laceration S56.12- ☑
          specified type NEC S56.19- ☑
          strain S56.11- ☑
        intrinsic S66.50- ☑
          laceration S66.52- ☑
          specified type NEC S66.59- ☑
          strain S66.51- ☑
    flexor
      finger(s) (other than thumb) — see Injury, muscle, finger
      forearm level, specified NEC — see Injury, muscle, forearm, flexor
      thumb — see Injury, muscle, thumb, flexor
      toe (long) (ankle level) (foot level) — see Injury, muscle, toe, flexor
    foot S96.90- ☑
      intrinsic S96.20- ☑
        laceration S96.22- ☑
        specified type NEC S96.29- ☑
        strain S96.21- ☑
      laceration S96.92- ☑
      long extensor, toe — see Injury, muscle, toe, extensor
      long flexor, toe — see Injury, muscle, toe, flexor
      specified
        site NEC S96.80- ☑
          laceration S96.82- ☑
          specified type NEC S96.89- ☑
          strain S96.81- ☑
        type S96.99- ☑
      strain S96.91- ☑
    forearm (level) S56.90- ☑
      extensor S56.50- ☑
        laceration S56.52- ☑
        specified type NEC S56.59- ☑
        strain S56.51- ☑
      flexor S56.20- ☑
        laceration S56.22- ☑
        specified type NEC S56.29- ☑
        strain S56.21- ☑
      laceration S56.92- ☑
      specified S56.99- ☑
        site NEC S56.80- ☑
          laceration S56.82- ☑
          strain S56.81- ☑

Injury — continued
  muscle — continued
    forearm — continued
      specified — continued
        site — continued
          type NEC S56.89- ☑
      strain S56.91- ☑
    hand (level) S66.90- ☑
      laceration S66.92- ☑
      specified
        site NEC S66.80- ☑
          laceration S66.82- ☑
          specified type NEC S66.89- ☑
          strain S66.81- ☑
        type NEC S66.99- ☑
      strain S66.91- ☑
    head S09.10- ☑
      laceration S09.12- ☑
      specified type NEC S09.19- ☑
      strain S09.11- ☑
    hip NEC S76.00- ☑
      laceration S76.02- ☑
      specified type NEC S76.09- ☑
      strain S76.01- ☑
    intrinsic
      ankle and foot level — see Injury, muscle, foot, intrinsic
      finger (other than thumb) — see Injury, muscle, finger by site, intrinsic
      foot (level) — see Injury, muscle, foot, intrinsic
      thumb — see Injury, muscle, thumb, intrinsic
    leg (level) (lower) S86.90- ☑
      Achilles tendon — see Injury, Achilles tendon
      anterior muscle group — see Injury, muscle, anterior muscle group
      laceration S86.92- ☑
      peroneal muscle group — see Injury, muscle, peroneal muscle group
      posterior muscle group — see Injury, muscle, posterior muscle group, leg level
      specified
        site NEC S86.80- ☑
          laceration S86.82- ☑
          specified type NEC S86.89- ☑
          strain S86.81- ☑
        type NEC S86.99- ☑
      strain S86.91- ☑
    long
      extensor toe, at ankle and foot level — see Injury, muscle, toe, extensor
      flexor, toe, at ankle and foot level — see Injury, muscle, toe, flexor
      head, biceps — see Injury, muscle, biceps, long head
    lower back S39.002- ☑
      laceration S39.022- ☑
      specified type NEC S39.092- ☑
      strain S39.012- ☑
    neck (level) S16.9- ☑
      laceration S16.2- ☑
      specified type NEC S16.8- ☑
      strain S16.1- ☑
    pelvis S39.003- ☑
      laceration S39.023- ☑
      specified type NEC S39.093- ☑
      strain S39.013- ☑
    peroneal muscle group, at leg level (lower) S86.30- ☑
      laceration S86.32- ☑
      specified type NEC S86.39- ☑
      strain S86.31- ☑
    posterior muscle (group)
      leg level (lower) S86.10- ☑
        laceration S86.12- ☑
        specified type NEC S86.19- ☑
        strain S86.11- ☑
      thigh level S76.30- ☑
        laceration S76.32- ☑
        specified type NEC S76.39- ☑
        strain S76.31- ☑
    quadriceps (thigh) S76.10- ☑
      laceration S76.12- ☑
      specified type NEC S76.19- ☑
      strain S76.11- ☑
    shoulder S46.90- ☑
      laceration S46.92- ☑
      rotator cuff — see Injury, rotator cuff

Injury — continued
  muscle — continued
    shoulder — continued
      specified site NEC S46.80- ☑
        laceration S46.82- ☑
        specified type NEC S46.89- ☑
        strain S46.81- ☑
      specified type NEC S46.99- ☑
      strain S46.91- ☑
    thigh NEC (level) S76.90- ☑
      adductor — see Injury, muscle, adductor, thigh
      laceration S76.92- ☑
      posterior muscle (group) — see Injury, muscle, posterior muscle, thigh level
      quadriceps — see Injury, muscle, quadriceps
      specified
        site NEC S76.80- ☑
          laceration S76.82- ☑
          specified type NEC S76.89- ☑
          strain S76.81- ☑
        type NEC S76.99- ☑
      strain S76.91- ☑
    thorax (level) S29.009- ☑
      back wall S29.002- ☑
      front wall S29.001- ☑
      laceration S29.029- ☑
        back wall S29.022- ☑
        front wall S29.021- ☑
      specified type NEC S29.099- ☑
        back wall S29.092- ☑
        front wall S29.091- ☑
      strain S29.019- ☑
        back wall S29.012- ☑
        front wall S29.011- ☑
    thumb
      abductor (forearm level) S56.30- ☑
        laceration S56.32- ☑
        specified type NEC S56.39- ☑
        strain S56.31- ☑
      extensor (forearm level) S56.30- ☑
        hand level S66.20- ☑
          laceration S66.22- ☑
          specified type NEC S66.29- ☑
          strain S66.21- ☑
        laceration S56.32- ☑
        specified type NEC S56.39- ☑
        strain S56.31- ☑
      flexor (forearm level) S56.00- ☑
        hand level S66.00- ☑
          laceration S66.02- ☑
          specified type NEC S66.09- ☑
          strain S66.01- ☑
        laceration S56.02- ☑
        specified type NEC S56.09- ☑
        strain S56.01- ☑
        wrist level — see Injury, muscle, thumb, flexor, hand level
      intrinsic S66.40- ☑
        laceration S66.42- ☑
        specified type NEC S66.49- ☑
        strain S66.41- ☑
    toe — see also Injury, muscle, foot
      extensor, long S96.10- ☑
        laceration S96.12- ☑
        specified type NEC S96.19- ☑
        strain S96.11- ☑
      flexor, long S96.00- ☑
        laceration S96.02- ☑
        specified type NEC S96.09- ☑
        strain S96.01- ☑
    triceps S46.30- ☑
      laceration S46.32- ☑
      specified type NEC S46.39- ☑
      strain S46.31- ☑
    wrist (and hand) level — see Injury, muscle, hand
  musculocutaneous nerve — see Injury, nerve, musculocutaneous
  myocardial (acute) (chronic) (non-ischemic) (non-traumatic) I5A
    traumatic — see Injury, heart
  myocardium — see also Injury, heart
    non-traumatic — see Injury, myocardial
  nape — see Injury, neck
  nasal (septum) (sinus) S09.92- ☑
  nasopharynx S09.92- ☑
  neck S19.9- ☑

☑ Additional Character Required — Refer to the Tabular List for Character Selection

Injury — continued
- neck — continued
  - specified NEC S19.80- ☑
    - specified site NEC S19.89- ☑
- nerve NEC T14.8- ☑
  - abdomen S34.9- ☑
    - peripheral S34.6- ☑
    - specified site NEC S34.8- ☑
  - abducens S04.4- ☑
    - contusion S04.4- ☑
    - laceration S04.4- ☑
    - specified type NEC S04.4- ☑
  - abducent — see Injury, nerve, abducens
  - accessory S04.7- ☑
    - contusion S04.7- ☑
    - laceration S04.7- ☑
    - specified type NEC S04.7- ☑
  - acoustic S04.6- ☑
    - contusion S04.6- ☑
    - laceration S04.6- ☑
    - specified type NEC S04.6- ☑
  - ankle S94.9- ☑
    - cutaneous sensory S94.3- ☑
    - specified site NEC — see subcategory S94.8- ☑
  - anterior crural, femoral — see Injury, nerve, femoral
  - arm (upper) S44.9- ☑
    - axillary — see Injury, nerve, axillary
    - cutaneous — see Injury, nerve, cutaneous, arm
    - median — see Injury, nerve, median, upper arm
    - musculocutaneous — see Injury, nerve, musculocutaneous
    - radial — see Injury, nerve, radial, upper arm
    - specified site NEC — see subcategory S44.8- ☑
    - ulnar — see Injury, nerve, ulnar, arm
  - auditory — see Injury, nerve, acoustic
  - axillary S44.3- ☑
  - brachial plexus — see Injury, brachial plexus
  - cervical sympathetic S14.5- ☑
  - cranial S04.9- ☑
    - contusion S04.9- ☑
    - eighth (acoustic or auditory) — see Injury, nerve, acoustic
    - eleventh (accessory) — see Injury, nerve, accessory
    - fifth (trigeminal) — see Injury, nerve, trigeminal
    - first (olfactory) — see Injury, nerve, olfactory
    - fourth (trochlear) — see Injury, nerve, trochlear
    - laceration S04.9- ☑
    - ninth (glossopharyngeal) — see Injury, nerve, glossopharyngeal
    - second (optic) — see Injury, nerve, optic
    - seventh (facial) — see Injury, nerve, facial
    - sixth (abducent) — see Injury, nerve, abducens
    - specified
      - nerve NEC S04.89- ☑
        - contusion S04.89- ☑
        - laceration S04.89- ☑
        - specified type NEC S04.89- ☑
      - type NEC S04.9- ☑
    - tenth (pneumogastric or vagus) — see Injury, nerve, vagus
    - third (oculomotor) — see Injury, nerve, oculomotor
    - twelfth (hypoglossal) — see Injury, nerve, hypoglossal
  - cutaneous sensory
    - ankle (level) S94.3- ☑
    - arm (upper) (level) S44.5- ☑
    - foot (level) — see Injury, nerve, cutaneous sensory, ankle
    - forearm (level) S54.3- ☑
    - hip (level) S74.2- ☑
    - leg (lower level) S84.2- ☑
    - shoulder (level) — see Injury, nerve, cutaneous sensory, arm
    - thigh (level) — see Injury, nerve, cutaneous sensory, hip
  - deep peroneal — see Injury, nerve, peroneal, foot
  - digital
    - finger S64.4- ☑
      - index S64.49- ☑
      - little S64.49- ☑
      - middle S64.49- ☑
      - ring S64.49- ☑
    - thumb S64.3- ☑
    - toe — see Injury, nerve, ankle, specified site NEC
  - eighth cranial (acoustic or auditory) — see Injury, nerve, acoustic

Injury — continued
- nerve — continued
  - eleventh cranial (accessory) — see Injury, nerve, accessory
  - facial S04.5- ☑
    - contusion S04.5- ☑
    - laceration S04.5- ☑
    - newborn P11.3
    - specified type NEC S04.5- ☑
  - femoral (hip level) (thigh level) S74.1- ☑
  - fifth cranial (trigeminal) — see Injury, nerve, trigeminal
  - finger (digital) — see Injury, nerve, digital, finger
  - first cranial (olfactory) — see Injury, nerve, olfactory
  - foot S94.9- ☑
    - cutaneous sensory S94.3- ☑
    - deep peroneal S94.2- ☑
    - lateral plantar S94.0- ☑
    - medial plantar S94.1- ☑
    - specified site NEC — see subcategory S94.8- ☑
  - forearm (level) S54.9- ☑
    - cutaneous sensory — see Injury, nerve, cutaneous sensory, forearm
    - median — see Injury, nerve, median
    - radial — see Injury, nerve, radial
    - specified site NEC — see subcategory S54.8- ☑
    - ulnar — see Injury, nerve, ulnar
  - fourth cranial (trochlear) — see Injury, nerve, trochlear
  - glossopharyngeal S04.89- ☑
    - specified type NEC S04.89- ☑
  - hand S64.9- ☑
    - median — see Injury, nerve, median, hand
    - radial — see Injury, nerve, radial, hand
    - specified NEC — see subcategory S64.8- ☑
    - ulnar — see Injury, nerve, ulnar, hand
  - hip (level) S74.9- ☑
    - cutaneous sensory — see Injury, nerve, cutaneous sensory, hip
    - femoral — see Injury, nerve, femoral
    - sciatic — see Injury, nerve, sciatic
    - specified site NEC — see subcategory S74.8- ☑
  - hypoglossal S04.89- ☑
    - specified type NEC S04.89- ☑
  - lateral plantar S94.0- ☑
  - leg (lower) S84.9- ☑
    - cutaneous sensory — see Injury, nerve, cutaneous sensory, leg
    - peroneal — see Injury, nerve, peroneal
    - specified site NEC — see subcategory S84.8- ☑
    - tibial — see Injury, nerve, tibial
    - upper — see Injury, nerve, thigh
  - lower
    - back — see Injury, nerve, abdomen, specified site NEC
      - peripheral — see Injury, nerve, abdomen, peripheral
    - limb — see Injury, nerve, leg
  - lumbar plexus — see Injury, nerve, lumbosacral, sympathetic
  - lumbar spinal — see Injury, spinal, lumbar
    - peripheral S34.6- ☑
    - root S34.21- ☑
    - sympathetic S34.5- ☑
  - lumbosacral
    - plexus — see Injury, nerve, lumbosacral, sympathetic
    - sympathetic S34.5- ☑
  - medial plantar S94.1- ☑
  - median (forearm level) S54.1- ☑
    - hand (level) S64.1- ☑
    - upper arm (level) S44.1- ☑
    - wrist (level) — see Injury, nerve, median, hand
  - musculocutaneous S44.4- ☑
  - musculospiral (upper arm level) — see Injury, nerve, radial, upper arm
  - neck S14.9- ☑
    - peripheral S14.4- ☑
    - specified site NEC S14.8- ☑
    - sympathetic S14.5- ☑
  - ninth cranial (glossopharyngeal) — see Injury, nerve, glossopharyngeal
  - oculomotor S04.1- ☑
    - contusion S04.1- ☑
    - laceration S04.1- ☑
    - specified type NEC S04.1- ☑
  - olfactory S04.81- ☑
    - specified type NEC S04.81- ☑

Injury — continued
- nerve — continued
  - optic S04.01- ☑
    - contusion S04.01- ☑
    - laceration S04.01- ☑
    - specified type NEC S04.01- ☑
  - pelvic girdle — see Injury, nerve, hip
  - pelvis — see Injury, nerve, abdomen, specified site NEC
    - peripheral — see Injury, nerve, abdomen, peripheral
  - peripheral NEC T14.8- ☑
    - abdomen — see Injury, nerve, abdomen, peripheral
    - lower back — see Injury, nerve, abdomen, peripheral
    - neck — see Injury, nerve, neck, peripheral
    - pelvis — see Injury, nerve, abdomen, peripheral
    - specified NEC T14.8- ☑
  - peroneal (lower leg level) S84.1- ☑
    - foot S94.2- ☑
  - plexus
    - brachial — see Injury, brachial plexus
    - celiac, coeliac — see Injury, nerve, lumbosacral, sympathetic
    - mesenteric, inferior — see Injury, nerve, lumbosacral, sympathetic
    - sacral — see Injury, lumbosacral plexus
    - spinal
      - brachial — see Injury, brachial plexus
      - lumbosacral — see Injury, lumbosacral plexus
  - pneumogastric — see Injury, nerve, vagus
  - radial (forearm level) S54.2- ☑
    - hand (level) S64.2- ☑
    - upper arm (level) S44.2- ☑
    - wrist (level) — see Injury, nerve, radial, hand
  - root — see Injury, nerve, spinal, root
  - sacral plexus — see Injury, lumbosacral plexus
  - sacral spinal — see Injury, spinal, sacral
    - peripheral S34.6- ☑
    - root S34.22- ☑
    - sympathetic S34.5- ☑
  - sciatic (hip level) (thigh level) S74.0- ☑
  - second cranial (optic) — see Injury, nerve, optic
  - seventh cranial (facial) — see Injury, nerve, facial
  - shoulder — see Injury, nerve, arm
  - sixth cranial (abducent) — see Injury, nerve, abducens
  - spinal
    - plexus — see Injury, nerve, plexus, spinal
    - root
      - cervical S14.2- ☑
      - dorsal S24.2- ☑
      - lumbar S34.21- ☑
      - sacral S34.22- ☑
      - thoracic — see Injury, nerve, spinal, root, dorsal
  - splanchnic — see Injury, nerve, lumbosacral, sympathetic
  - sympathetic NEC — see Injury, nerve, lumbosacral, sympathetic
    - cervical — see Injury, nerve, cervical sympathetic
  - tenth cranial (pneumogastric or vagus) — see Injury, nerve, vagus
  - thigh (level) — see Injury, nerve, hip
    - cutaneous sensory — see Injury, nerve, cutaneous sensory, hip
    - femoral — see Injury, nerve, femoral
    - sciatic — see Injury, nerve, sciatic
    - specified NEC — see Injury, nerve, hip
  - third cranial (oculomotor) — see Injury, nerve, oculomotor
  - thorax S24.9- ☑
    - peripheral S24.3- ☑
    - specified site NEC S24.8- ☑
    - sympathetic S24.4- ☑
  - thumb, digital — see Injury, nerve, digital, thumb
  - tibial (lower leg level) (posterior) S84.0- ☑
  - toe — see Injury, nerve, ankle
  - trigeminal S04.3- ☑
    - contusion S04.3- ☑
    - laceration S04.3- ☑
    - specified type NEC S04.3- ☑
  - trochlear S04.2- ☑
    - contusion S04.2- ☑
    - laceration S04.2- ☑
    - specified type NEC S04.2- ☑
  - twelfth cranial (hypoglossal) — see Injury, nerve, hypoglossal

Injury — *continued*
  nerve — *continued*
    ulnar (forearm level) S54.0- ☑
      arm (upper) (level) S44.0- ☑
      hand (level) S64.0- ☑
      wrist (level) — *see* Injury, nerve, ulnar, hand
    vagus S04.89- ☑
      specified type NEC S04.89- ☑
      wrist (level) — *see* Injury, nerve, hand
    ninth cranial nerve (glossopharyngeal) — *see* Injury, nerve, glossopharyngeal
  nose (septum) S09.92- ☑
  obstetrical O71.9
    specified NEC O71.89
  occipital (region) (scalp) S09.90- ☑
    lobe — *see* Injury, intracranial
  optic chiasm S04.02- ☑
  optic radiation S04.03- ☑
  optic tract and pathways S04.03- ☑
  orbit, orbital (region) — *see* Injury, eye
    penetrating (with foreign body) — *see* Injury, eye, orbit, penetrating
    specified NEC — *see* Injury, eye, specified site NEC
  ovary, ovarian S37.409- ☑
    bilateral S37.402- ☑
      contusion S37.422- ☑
      laceration S37.432- ☑
      specified type NEC S37.492- ☑
    blood vessel — *see* Injury, blood vessel, ovarian
    contusion S37.429- ☑
      bilateral S37.422- ☑
      unilateral S37.421- ☑
    laceration S37.439- ☑
      bilateral S37.432- ☑
      unilateral S37.431- ☑
    specified type NEC S37.499- ☑
      bilateral S37.492- ☑
      unilateral S37.491- ☑
    unilateral S37.401- ☑
      contusion S37.421- ☑
      laceration S37.431- ☑
      specified type NEC S37.491- ☑
  palate (hard) (soft) S09.93- ☑
  pancreas S36.209- ☑
    body S36.201- ☑
      contusion S36.221- ☑
      laceration S36.231- ☑
        major S36.261- ☑
        minor S36.241- ☑
        moderate S36.251- ☑
      specified type NEC S36.291- ☑
    contusion S36.229- ☑
    head S36.200- ☑
      contusion S36.220- ☑
      laceration S36.230- ☑
        major S36.260- ☑
        minor S36.240- ☑
        moderate S36.250- ☑
      specified type NEC S36.290- ☑
    laceration S36.239- ☑
      major S36.269- ☑
      minor S36.249- ☑
      moderate S36.259- ☑
    specified type NEC S36.299- ☑
    tail S36.202- ☑
      contusion S36.222- ☑
      laceration S36.232- ☑
        major S36.262- ☑
        minor S36.242- ☑
        moderate S36.252- ☑
      specified type NEC S36.292- ☑
  parietal (region) (scalp) S09.90- ☑
    lobe — *see* Injury, intracranial
  patellar ligament (tendon) S76.10- ☑
    laceration S76.12- ☑
    specified NEC S76.19- ☑
    strain S76.11- ☑
  pelvis, pelvic (floor) S39.93- ☑
    complicating delivery O70.1
    joint or ligament, complicating delivery O71.6
    organ S37.90- ☑
      with ectopic or molar pregnancy O08.6
      complication of abortion — *see* Abortion
      contusion S37.92- ☑
      following ectopic or molar pregnancy O08.6
      laceration S37.93- ☑

Injury — *continued*
  pelvis, pelvic — *continued*
    organ — *continued*
      obstetrical trauma NEC O71.5
      specified
        site NEC S37.899- ☑
          contusion S37.892- ☑
          laceration S37.893- ☑
          specified type NEC S37.898- ☑
        type NEC S37.99- ☑
      specified NEC S39.83- ☑
  penis S39.94- ☑
  perineum S39.94- ☑
  peritoneum S36.81- ☑
    laceration S36.893- ☑
  periurethral tissue — *see* Injury, urethra
    complicating delivery O71.82
  phalanges
    foot — *see* Injury, foot
    hand — *see* Injury, hand
  pharynx NEC S19.85- ☑
  pleura — *see* Injury, intrathoracic, pleura
  plexus
    brachial — *see* Injury, brachial plexus
    cardiac — *see* Injury, nerve, thorax, sympathetic
    celiac, coeliac — *see* Injury, nerve, lumbosacral, sympathetic
    esophageal — *see* Injury, nerve, thorax, sympathetic
    hypogastric — *see* Injury, nerve, lumbosacral, sympathetic
    lumbar, lumbosacral — *see* Injury, lumbosacral plexus
    mesenteric — *see* Injury, nerve, lumbosacral, sympathetic
    pulmonary — *see* Injury, nerve, thorax, sympathetic
  postcardiac surgery (syndrome) I97.0
  prepuce S39.94- ☑
  pressure
    injury — *see* Ulcer, pressure, by site
  prostate S37.829- ☑
    contusion S37.822- ☑
    laceration S37.823- ☑
    specified type NEC S37.828- ☑
  pubic region S39.94- ☑
  pudendum S39.94- ☑
  pulmonary plexus — *see* Injury, nerve, thorax, sympathetic
  rectovaginal septum NEC S39.83- ☑
  rectum — *see* Injury, intestine, large, rectum
  retina — *see* Injury, eye, specified site NEC
    penetrating — *see* Injury, eyeball, penetrating
  retroperitoneal — *see* Injury, intra-abdominal, specified site NEC
  rotator cuff (muscle(s)) (tendon(s)) S46.00- ☑
    laceration S46.02- ☑
    specified type NEC S46.09- ☑
    strain S46.01- ☑
  round ligament — *see* Injury, pelvic organ, specified site NEC
  sacral plexus — *see* Injury, lumbosacral plexus
  salivary duct or gland S09.93- ☑
  scalp S09.90- ☑
    newborn (birth injury) P12.9
      due to monitoring (electrode) (sampling incision) P12.4
      specified NEC P12.89
        caput succedaneum P12.81
  scapular region — *see* Injury, shoulder
  sclera — *see* Injury, eye, specified site NEC
    penetrating — *see* Injury, eyeball, penetrating
  scrotum S39.94- ☑
  second cranial nerve (optic) — *see* Injury, nerve, optic
  self-inflicted, without suicidal intent R45.88
  seminal vesicle — *see* Injury, pelvic organ, specified site NEC
  seventh cranial nerve (facial) — *see* Injury, nerve, facial
  shoulder S49.9- ☑
    blood vessel — *see* Injury, blood vessel, arm
    contusion — *see* Contusion, shoulder
    dislocation — *see* Dislocation, shoulder
    fracture — *see* Fracture, shoulder
    muscle — *see* Injury, muscle, shoulder
    nerve — *see* Injury, nerve, shoulder
    open — *see* Wound, open, shoulder
    specified type NEC S49.8- ☑
    sprain — *see* Sprain, shoulder girdle
    superficial — *see* Injury, superficial, shoulder

Injury — *continued*
  sinus
    cavernous — *see* Injury, intracranial
    nasal S09.92- ☑
  sixth cranial nerve (abducent) — *see* Injury, nerve, abducens
  skeleton, birth injury P13.9
    specified part NEC P13.8
  skin NEC T14.8- ☑
    surface intact — *see* Injury, superficial
  skull NEC S09.90- ☑
  specified NEC T14.8- ☑
  spermatic cord (pelvic region) S37.898- ☑
    scrotal region S39.848- ☑
  spinal (cord)
    cervical (neck) S14.109- ☑
      anterior cord syndrome S14.139- ☑
        C1 level S14.131- ☑
        C2 level S14.132- ☑
        C3 level S14.133- ☑
        C4 level S14.134- ☑
        C5 level S14.135- ☑
        C6 level S14.136- ☑
        C7 level S14.137- ☑
        C8 level S14.138- ☑
      Brown-Sequard syndrome S14.149- ☑
        C1 level S14.141- ☑
        C2 level S14.142- ☑
        C3 level S14.143- ☑
        C4 level S14.144- ☑
        C5 level S14.145- ☑
        C6 level S14.146- ☑
        C7 level S14.147- ☑
        C8 level S14.148- ☑
      C1 level S14.101- ☑
      C2 level S14.102- ☑
      C3 level S14.103- ☑
      C4 level S14.104- ☑
      C5 level S14.105- ☑
      C6 level S14.106- ☑
      C7 level S14.107- ☑
      C8 level S14.108- ☑
      central cord syndrome S14.129- ☑
        C1 level S14.121- ☑
        C2 level S14.122- ☑
        C3 level S14.123- ☑
        C4 level S14.124- ☑
        C5 level S14.125- ☑
        C6 level S14.126- ☑
        C7 level S14.127- ☑
        C8 level S14.128- ☑
      complete lesion S14.119- ☑
        C1 level S14.111- ☑
        C2 level S14.112- ☑
        C3 level S14.113- ☑
        C4 level S14.114- ☑
        C5 level S14.115- ☑
        C6 level S14.116- ☑
        C7 level S14.117- ☑
        C8 level S14.118- ☑
      concussion S14.0- ☑
      edema S14.0- ☑
      incomplete lesion specified NEC S14.159- ☑
        C1 level S14.151- ☑
        C2 level S14.152- ☑
        C3 level S14.153- ☑
        C4 level S14.154- ☑
        C5 level S14.155- ☑
        C6 level S14.156- ☑
        C7 level S14.157- ☑
        C8 level S14.158- ☑
      posterior cord syndrome S14.159- ☑
        C1 level S14.151- ☑
        C2 level S14.152- ☑
        C3 level S14.153- ☑
        C4 level S14.154- ☑
        C5 level S14.155- ☑
        C6 level S14.156- ☑
        C7 level S14.157- ☑
        C8 level S14.158- ☑
    dorsal — *see* Injury, spinal, thoracic
    lumbar S34.109- ☑
      complete lesion S34.119- ☑
        L1 level S34.111- ☑
        L2 level S34.112- ☑

☑ **Additional Character Required** — Refer to the Tabular List for Character Selection

Injury — *continued*
  spinal — *continued*
    lumbar — *continued*
      complete lesion — *continued*
        L3 level S34.113- ☑
        L4 level S34.114- ☑
        L5 level S34.115- ☑
      concussion S34.01- ☑
      edema S34.01- ☑
      incomplete lesion S34.129- ☑
        L1 level S34.121- ☑
        L2 level S34.122- ☑
        L3 level S34.123- ☑
        L4 level S34.124- ☑
        L5 level S34.125- ☑
      L1 level S34.101- ☑
      L2 level S34.102- ☑
      L3 level S34.103- ☑
      L4 level S34.104- ☑
      L5 level S34.105- ☑
    nerve root NEC
      cervical — *see* Injury, nerve, spinal, root, cervical
      dorsal — *see* Injury, nerve, spinal, root, dorsal
      lumbar S34.21- ☑
      sacral S34.22- ☑
      thoracic — *see* Injury, nerve, spinal, root, dorsal
    plexus
      brachial — *see* Injury, brachial plexus
      lumbosacral — *see* Injury, lumbosacral plexus
    sacral S34.139- ☑
      complete lesion S34.131- ☑
      incomplete lesion S34.132- ☑
    thoracic S24.109- ☑
      anterior cord syndrome S24.139- ☑
        T1 level S24.131- ☑
        T2-T6 level S24.132- ☑
        T7-T10 level S24.133- ☑
        T11-T12 level S24.134- ☑
      Brown-Sequard syndrome S24.149- ☑
        T1 level S24.141- ☑
        T2-T6 level S24.142- ☑
        T7-T10 level S24.143- ☑
        T11-T12 level S24.144- ☑
      complete lesion S24.119- ☑
        T1 level S24.111- ☑
        T2-T6 level S24.112- ☑
        T7-T10 level S24.113- ☑
        T11-T12 level S24.114- ☑
      concussion S24.0- ☑
      edema S24.0- ☑
      incomplete lesion specified NEC S24.159- ☑
        T1 level S24.151- ☑
        T2-T6 level S24.152- ☑
        T7-T10 level S24.153- ☑
        T11-T12 level S24.154- ☑
      posterior cord syndrome S24.159- ☑
        T1 level S24.151- ☑
        T2-T6 level S24.152- ☑
        T7-T10 level S24.153- ☑
        T11-T12 level S24.154- ☑
      T1 level S24.101- ☑
      T2-T6 level S24.102- ☑
      T7-T10 level S24.103- ☑
      T11-T12 level S24.104- ☑
  splanchnic nerve — *see* Injury, nerve, lumbosacral, sympathetic
  spleen S36.00- ☑
    contusion S36.029- ☑
      major S36.021- ☑
      minor S36.020- ☑
    laceration S36.039- ☑
      major (massive) (stellate) S36.032- ☑
      moderate S36.031- ☑
      superficial (capsular) (minor) S36.030- ☑
    specified type NEC S36.09- ☑
  splenic artery — *see* Injury, blood vessel, celiac artery, branch
  stellate ganglion — *see* Injury, nerve, thorax, sympathetic
  sternal region S29.9- ☑
  stomach S36.30- ☑
    contusion S36.32- ☑
    laceration S36.33- ☑
    specified type NEC S36.39- ☑
  subconjunctival — *see* Injury, eye, conjunctiva
  subcutaneous NEC T14.8- ☑

Injury — *continued*
  submaxillary region S09.93- ☑
  submental region S09.93- ☑
  subungual
    fingers — *see* Injury, hand
    toes — *see* Injury, foot
  superficial NEC T14.8- ☑
    abdomen, abdominal (wall) S30.92- ☑
      abrasion S30.811- ☑
      bite S30.871- ☑
        insect S30.861- ☑
      contusion S30.11- ☑
      external constriction S30.841- ☑
      foreign body S30.851- ☑
    abrasion — *see* Abrasion, by site
    adnexa, eye NEC — *see* Injury, eye, specified site NEC
    alveolar process — *see* Injury, superficial, oral cavity
    ankle S90.91- ☑
      abrasion — *see* Abrasion, ankle
      bite — *see* Bite, ankle
      blister — *see* Blister, ankle
      contusion — *see* Contusion, ankle
      external constriction — *see* Constriction, external, ankle
      foreign body — *see* Foreign body, superficial, ankle
    anus S30.98- ☑
    arm (upper) S40.92- ☑
      abrasion — *see* Abrasion, arm
      bite — *see* Bite, superficial, arm
      blister — *see* Blister, arm (upper)
      contusion — *see* Contusion, arm
      external constriction — *see* Constriction, external, arm
      foreign body — *see* Foreign body, superficial, arm
    auditory canal (external) (meatus) — *see* Injury, superficial, ear
    auricle — *see* Injury, superficial, ear
    axilla — *see* Injury, superficial, arm
    back — *see also* Injury, superficial, thorax, back
      lower S30.91- ☑
        abrasion S30.810- ☑
        contusion S30.0- ☑
        external constriction S30.840- ☑
        superficial
          bite NEC S30.870- ☑
            insect S30.860- ☑
          foreign body S30.850- ☑
    bite NEC — *see* Bite, superficial NEC, by site
    blister — *see* Blister, by site
    breast S20.10- ☑
      abrasion — *see* Abrasion, breast
      bite — *see* Bite, superficial, breast
      contusion — *see* Contusion, breast
      external constriction — *see* Constriction, external, breast
      foreign body — *see* Foreign body, superficial, breast
    brow — *see* Injury, superficial, head, specified NEC
    buttock S30.91- ☑
    calf — *see* Injury, superficial, leg
    canthus, eye — *see* Injury, superficial, periocular area
    cheek (external) — *see* Injury, superficial, head, specified NEC
      internal — *see* Injury, superficial, oral cavity
    chest wall — *see* Injury, superficial, thorax
    chin — *see* Injury, superficial, head NEC
    clitoris S30.95- ☑
    conjunctiva — *see* Injury, eye, conjunctiva
      with foreign body (in conjunctival sac) — *see* Foreign body, conjunctival sac
    contusion — *see* Contusion, by site
    costal region — *see* Injury, superficial, thorax
    digit(s)
      hand — *see* Injury, superficial, finger
    ear (auricle) (canal) (external) S00.40- ☑
      abrasion — *see* Abrasion, ear
      bite — *see* Bite, superficial, ear
      contusion — *see* Contusion, ear
      external constriction — *see* Constriction, external, ear
      foreign body — *see* Foreign body, superficial, ear
    elbow S50.90- ☑
      abrasion — *see* Abrasion, elbow
      bite — *see* Bite, superficial, elbow
      blister — *see* Blister, elbow
      contusion — *see* Contusion, elbow
      external constriction — *see* Constriction, external, elbow

Injury — *continued*
  superficial — *continued*
    elbow — *continued*
      foreign body — *see* Foreign body, superficial, elbow
    epididymis S30.94- ☑
    epigastric region S30.92- ☑
    epiglottis — *see* Injury, superficial, throat
    esophagus
      cervical — *see* Injury, superficial, throat
    external constriction — *see* Constriction, external, by site
    extremity NEC T14.8- ☑
    eyeball NEC — *see* Injury, eye, specified site NEC
    eyebrow — *see* Injury, superficial, periocular area
    eyelid S00.20- ☑
      abrasion — *see* Abrasion, eyelid
      bite — *see* Bite, superficial, eyelid
      contusion — *see* Contusion, eyelid
      external constriction — *see* Constriction, external, eyelid
      foreign body — *see* Foreign body, superficial, eyelid
    face NEC — *see* Injury, superficial, head, specified NEC
    finger(s) S60.949- ☑
      abrasion — *see* Abrasion, finger
      bite — *see* Bite, superficial, finger
      blister — *see* Blister, finger
      contusion — *see* Contusion, finger
      external constriction — *see* Constriction, external, finger
      foreign body — *see* Foreign body, superficial, finger
      index S60.94- ☑
      insect bite — *see* Bite, by site, superficial, insect
      little S60.94- ☑
      middle S60.94- ☑
      ring S60.94- ☑
    flank S30.9A- ☑
    foot S90.92- ☑
      abrasion — *see* Abrasion, foot
      bite — *see* Bite, foot
      blister — *see* Blister, foot
      contusion — *see* Contusion, foot
      external constriction — *see* Constriction, external, foot
      foreign body — *see* Foreign body, superficial, foot
    forearm S50.91- ☑
      abrasion — *see* Abrasion, forearm
      bite — *see* Bite, forearm, superficial
      blister — *see* Blister, forearm
      contusion — *see* Contusion, forearm
      elbow only — *see* Injury, superficial, elbow
      external constriction — *see* Constriction, external, forearm
      foreign body — *see* Foreign body, superficial, forearm
    forehead — *see* Injury, superficial, head NEC
    foreign body — *see* Foreign body, superficial
    genital organs, external
      female S30.97- ☑
      male S30.96- ☑
    globe (eye) — *see* Injury, eye, specified site NEC
    groin S30.92- ☑
    gum — *see* Injury, superficial, oral cavity
    hand S60.92- ☑
      abrasion — *see* Abrasion, hand
      bite — *see* Bite, superficial, hand
      contusion — *see* Contusion, hand
      external constriction — *see* Constriction, external, hand
      foreign body — *see* Foreign body, superficial, hand
    head S00.90- ☑
      ear — *see* Injury, superficial, ear
      eyelid — *see* Injury, superficial, eyelid
      nose S00.30- ☑
      oral cavity S00.502- ☑
      scalp S00.00- ☑
      specified site NEC S00.80- ☑
    heel — *see* Injury, superficial, foot
    hip S70.91- ☑
      abrasion — *see* Abrasion, hip
      bite — *see* Bite, superficial, hip
      blister — *see* Blister, hip
      contusion — *see* Contusion, hip
      external constriction — *see* Constriction, external, hip
      foreign body — *see* Foreign body, superficial, hip

Injury — *continued*
  superficial — *continued*
    iliac region — *see* Injury, superficial, abdomen
    inguinal region — *see* Injury, superficial, abdomen
    insect bite — *see* Bite, by site, superficial, insect
    interscapular region — *see* Injury, superficial, thorax, back
    jaw — *see* Injury, superficial, head, specified NEC
    knee S80.91- ☑
      abrasion — *see* Abrasion, knee
      bite — *see* Bite, superficial, knee
      blister — *see* Blister, knee
      contusion — *see* Contusion, knee
      external constriction — *see* Constriction, external, knee
      foreign body — *see* Foreign body, superficial, knee
    labium (majus) (minus) S30.95- ☑
    lacrimal (apparatus) (gland) (sac) — *see* Injury, eye, specified site NEC
    larynx — *see* Injury, superficial, throat
    leg (lower) S80.92- ☑
      abrasion — *see* Abrasion, leg
      bite — *see* Bite, superficial, leg
      contusion — *see* Contusion, leg
      external constriction — *see* Constriction, external, leg
      foreign body — *see* Foreign body, superficial, leg
      knee — *see* Injury, superficial, knee
    limb NEC T14.8- ☑
    lip S00.501- ☑
    lower back S30.91- ☑
    lumbar region S30.91- ☑
    malar region — *see* Injury, superficial, head, specified NEC
    mammary — *see* Injury, superficial, breast
    mastoid region — *see* Injury, superficial, head, specified NEC
    mouth — *see* Injury, superficial, oral cavity
    muscle NEC T14.8- ☑
    nail NEC T14.8- ☑
      finger — *see* Injury, superficial, finger
      toe — *see* Injury, superficial, toe
    nasal (septum) — *see* Injury, superficial, nose
    neck S10.90- ☑
      specified site NEC S10.80- ☑
    nose (septum) S00.30- ☑
    occipital region — *see* Injury, superficial, scalp
    oral cavity S00.502- ☑
    orbital region — *see* Injury, superficial, periocular area
    palate — *see* Injury, superficial, oral cavity
    palm — *see* Injury, superficial, hand
    parietal region — *see* Injury, superficial, scalp
    pelvis S30.91- ☑
      girdle — *see* Injury, superficial, hip
    penis S30.93- ☑
    perineum
      female S30.95- ☑
      male S30.91- ☑
    periocular area S00.20- ☑
      abrasion — *see* Abrasion, eyelid
      bite — *see* Bite, superficial, eyelid
      contusion — *see* Contusion, eyelid
      external constriction — *see* Constriction, external, eyelid
      foreign body — *see* Foreign body, superficial, eyelid
    phalanges
      finger — *see* Injury, superficial, finger
      toe — *see* Injury, superficial, toe
    pharynx — *see* Injury, superficial, throat
    pinna — *see* Injury, superficial, ear
    popliteal space — *see* Injury, superficial, knee
    prepuce S30.93- ☑
    pubic region S30.91- ☑
    pudendum
      female S30.97- ☑
      male S30.96- ☑
    sacral region S30.91- ☑
    scalp S00.00- ☑
    scapular region — *see* Injury, superficial, shoulder
    sclera — *see* Injury, eye, specified site NEC
    scrotum S30.94- ☑
    shin — *see* Injury, superficial, leg
    shoulder S40.91- ☑
      abrasion — *see* Abrasion, shoulder
      bite — *see* Bite, superficial, shoulder
      blister — *see* Blister, shoulder
      contusion — *see* Contusion, shoulder

Injury — *continued*
  superficial — *continued*
    shoulder — *continued*
      external constriction — *see* Constriction, external, shoulder
      foreign body — *see* Foreign body, superficial, shoulder
    skin NEC T14.8- ☑
    sternal region — *see* Injury, superficial, thorax, front
    subconjunctival — *see* Injury, eye, specified site NEC
    subcutaneous NEC T14.8- ☑
    submaxillary region — *see* Injury, superficial, head, specified NEC
    submental region — *see* Injury, superficial, head, specified NEC
    subungual
      finger(s) — *see* Injury, superficial, finger
      toe(s) — *see* Injury, superficial, toe
    supraclavicular fossa — *see* Injury, superficial, neck
    supraorbital — *see* Injury, superficial, head, specified NEC
    temple — *see* Injury, superficial, head, specified NEC
    temporal region — *see* Injury, superficial, head, specified NEC
    testis S30.94- ☑
    thigh S70.92- ☑
      abrasion — *see* Abrasion, thigh
      bite — *see* Bite, superficial, thigh
      blister — *see* Blister, thigh
      contusion — *see* Contusion, thigh
      external constriction — *see* Constriction, external, thigh
      foreign body — *see* Foreign body, superficial, thigh
    thorax, thoracic (wall) S20.90- ☑
      abrasion — *see* Abrasion, thorax
      back S20.40- ☑
      bite — *see* Bite, thorax, superficial
      blister — *see* Blister, thorax
      contusion — *see* Contusion, thorax
      external constriction — *see* Constriction, external, thorax
      foreign body — *see* Foreign body, superficial, thorax
      front S20.30- ☑
    throat S10.10- ☑
      abrasion S10.11- ☑
      bite S10.17- ☑
        insect S10.16- ☑
      blister S10.12- ☑
      contusion S10.0- ☑
      external constriction S10.14- ☑
      foreign body S10.15- ☑
    thumb S60.93- ☑
      abrasion — *see* Abrasion, thumb
      bite — *see* Bite, superficial, thumb
      blister — *see* Blister, thumb
      contusion — *see* Contusion, thumb
      external constriction — *see* Constriction, external, thumb
      foreign body — *see* Foreign body, superficial, thumb
      insect bite — *see* Bite, by site, superficial, insect
      specified type NEC S60.39- ☑
    toe(s) S90.93- ☑
      abrasion — *see* Abrasion, toe
      bite — *see* Bite, toe
      blister — *see* Blister, toe
      contusion — *see* Contusion, toe
      external constriction — *see* Constriction, external, toe
      foreign body — *see* Foreign body, superficial, toe
      great S90.93- ☑
    tongue — *see* Injury, superficial, oral cavity
    tooth, teeth — *see* Injury, superficial, oral cavity
    trachea S10.10- ☑
    tunica vaginalis S30.94- ☑
    tympanum, tympanic membrane — *see* Injury, superficial, ear
    uvula — *see* Injury, superficial, oral cavity
    vagina S30.95- ☑
    vocal cords — *see* Injury, superficial, throat
    vulva S30.95- ☑
    wrist S60.91- ☑
  supraclavicular region — *see* Injury, neck
  supraorbital S09.93- ☑
  suprarenal gland (multiple) — *see* Injury, adrenal
  surgical complication (external or internal site) — *see* Laceration, accidental complicating surgery

Injury — *continued*
  temple S09.90- ☑
  temporal region S09.90- ☑
  tendon — *see also* Injury, muscle, by site
    abdomen — *see* Injury, muscle, abdomen
    Achilles — *see* Injury, Achilles tendon
    lower back — *see* Injury, muscle, lower back
    pelvic organs — *see* Injury, muscle, pelvis
  tenth cranial nerve (pneumogastric or vagus) — *see* Injury, nerve, vagus
  testis S39.94- ☑
  thalamic, thalamus — *see also* Injury, intracranial, focal brain injury
    hemorrhage, traumatic — *see* Injury, intracranial, intracerebral hemorrhage, traumatic
  thigh S79.92- ☑
    blood vessel — *see* Injury, blood vessel, hip
    contusion — *see* Contusion, thigh
    fracture — *see* Fracture, femur
    muscle — *see* Injury, muscle, thigh
    nerve — *see* Injury, nerve, thigh
    open — *see* Wound, open, thigh
    specified NEC S79.82- ☑
    superficial — *see* Injury, superficial, thigh
  third cranial nerve (oculomotor) — *see* Injury, nerve, oculomotor
  thorax, thoracic S29.9- ☑
    blood vessel — *see* Injury, blood vessel, thorax
    cavity — *see* Injury, intrathoracic
    dislocation — *see* Dislocation, thorax
    external (wall) S29.9- ☑
      contusion — *see* Contusion, thorax
      nerve — *see* Injury, nerve, thorax
      open — *see* Wound, open, thorax
      specified NEC S29.8- ☑
      sprain — *see* Sprain, thorax
      superficial — *see* Injury, superficial, thorax
    fracture — *see* Fracture, thorax
    internal — *see* Injury, intrathoracic
    intrathoracic organ — *see* Injury, intrathoracic
    sympathetic ganglion — *see* Injury, nerve, thorax, sympathetic
  throat — *see also* Injury, neck S19.9- ☑
  thumb S69.9- ☑
    blood vessel — *see* Injury, blood vessel, thumb
    contusion — *see* Contusion, thumb
    dislocation — *see* Dislocation, thumb
    fracture — *see* Fracture, thumb
    muscle — *see* Injury, muscle, thumb
    nerve — *see* Injury, nerve, digital, thumb
    open — *see* Wound, open, thumb
    specified NEC S69.8- ☑
    sprain — *see* Sprain, thumb
    superficial — *see* Injury, superficial, thumb
  thymus (gland) — *see* Injury, intrathoracic, specified organ NEC
  thyroid (gland) NEC S19.84- ☑
  toe S99.92- ☑
    contusion — *see* Contusion, toe
    dislocation — *see* Dislocation, toe
    fracture — *see* Fracture, toe
    muscle — *see* Injury, muscle, toe
    open — *see* Wound, open, toe
    specified type NEC S99.82- ☑
    sprain — *see* Sprain, toe
    superficial — *see* Injury, superficial, toe
  tongue S09.93- ☑
  tonsil S09.93- ☑
  tooth S09.93- ☑
  trachea (cervical) NEC S19.82- ☑
    thoracic — *see* Injury, intrathoracic, trachea, thoracic
  transfusion-related acute lung (TRALI) J95.84
  tunica vaginalis S39.94- ☑
  twelfth cranial nerve (hypoglossal) — *see* Injury, nerve, hypoglossal
  ureter S37.10- ☑
    contusion S37.12- ☑
    laceration S37.13- ☑
    specified type NEC S37.19- ☑
  urethra (sphincter) S37.30- ☑
    at delivery O71.5
    contusion S37.32- ☑
    laceration S37.33- ☑
    specified type NEC S37.39- ☑
  urinary organ S37.90- ☑
    contusion S37.92- ☑
    laceration S37.93- ☑

☑ **Additional Character Required — Refer to the Tabular List for Character Selection**

Injury — *continued*
  urinary organ — *continued*
    specified
      site NEC S37.899- ☑
        contusion S37.892- ☑
        laceration S37.893- ☑
        specified type NEC S37.898- ☑
      type NEC S37.99- ☑
  uterus, uterine S37.60- ☑
    with ectopic or molar pregnancy O08.6
    blood vessel — *see* Injury, blood vessel, iliac
    contusion S37.62- ☑
    laceration S37.63- ☑
      cervix at delivery O71.3
    rupture associated with obstetrics — *see* Rupture, uterus
    specified type NEC S37.69- ☑
  uvula S09.93- ☑
  vagina S39.93- ☑
    abrasion S30.814- ☑
    bite S31.45- ☑
      insect S30.864- ☑
      superficial NEC S30.874- ☑
    contusion S30.23- ☑
    crush S38.03- ☑
    during delivery — *see* Laceration, vagina, during delivery
    external constriction S30.844- ☑
    insect bite S30.864- ☑
    laceration S31.41- ☑
      with foreign body S31.42- ☑
    open wound S31.40- ☑
    puncture S31.43- ☑
      with foreign body S31.44- ☑
    superficial S30.95- ☑
      foreign body S30.854- ☑
  vas deferens — *see* Injury, pelvic organ, specified site NEC
  vascular NEC T14.8- ☑
  vein — *see* Injury, blood vessel
  vena cava (superior) S25.20- ☑
    inferior S35.10- ☑
      laceration (minor) (superficial) S35.11- ☑
        major S35.12- ☑
      specified type NEC S35.19- ☑
    laceration (minor) (superficial) S25.21- ☑
      major S25.22- ☑
    specified type NEC S25.29- ☑
  vesical (sphincter) — *see* Injury, bladder
  visual cortex S04.04- ☑
  vitreous (humor) S05.90- ☑
    specified NEC S05.8X- ☑
  vocal cord NEC S19.83- ☑
  vulva S39.94- ☑
    abrasion S30.814- ☑
    bite S31.45- ☑
      insect S30.864- ☑
      superficial NEC S30.874- ☑
    contusion S30.23- ☑
    crush S38.03- ☑
    during delivery — *see* Laceration, perineum, female, during delivery
    external constriction S30.844- ☑
    insect bite S30.864- ☑
    laceration S31.41- ☑
      with foreign body S31.42- ☑
    open wound S31.40- ☑
    puncture S31.43- ☑
      with foreign body S31.44- ☑
    superficial S30.95- ☑
      foreign body S30.854- ☑
  whiplash (cervical spine) S13.4- ☑
  wrist S69.9- ☑
    blood vessel — *see* Injury, blood vessel, hand
    contusion — *see* Contusion, wrist
    dislocation — *see* Dislocation, wrist
    fracture — *see* Fracture, wrist
    muscle — *see* Injury, muscle, hand
    nerve — *see* Injury, nerve, hand
    open — *see* Wound, open, wrist
    specified NEC S69.8- ☑
    sprain — *see* Sprain, wrist
    superficial — *see* Injury, superficial, wrist
Inoculation — *see also* Vaccination
  complication or reaction — *see* Complications, vaccination

Insanity, insane — *see also* Psychosis
  adolescent — *see* Schizophrenia
  confusional F28
    acute or subacute F05
  delusional F22
  senile F03.- ☑
Insect
  bite — *see* Bite, by site, superficial, insect
  venomous, poisoning NEC (by) — *see* Venom, arthropod
Insecurity
  financial Z59.869
  food Z59.41
  transportation Z59.82
Insensitivity
  adrenocorticotropin hormone (ACTH) E27.49
  androgen E34.50
    complete E34.51
    partial E34.52
Insertion
  cord (umbilical) lateral or velamentous O43.12- ☑
  intrauterine contraceptive device (encounter for) — *see* Intrauterine contraceptive device
Insolation (sunstroke) T67.01- ☑
Insomnia (organic) G47.00
  adjustment F51.02
  adjustment disorder F51.02
  behavioral, of childhood Z73.819
    combined type Z73.812
    limit setting type Z73.811
    sleep-onset association type Z73.810
  childhood Z73.819
  chronic F51.04
    somatized tension F51.04
  conditioned F51.04
  due to
    alcohol
      abuse F10.182
      dependence F10.282
      use F10.982
    amphetamines
      abuse F15.182
      dependence F15.282
      use F15.982
    anxiety disorder F51.05
    caffeine
      abuse F15.182
      dependence F15.282
      use F15.982
    cocaine
      abuse F14.182
      dependence F14.282
      use F14.982
    depression F51.05
    drug NEC
      abuse F19.182
      dependence F19.282
      use F19.982
    medical condition G47.01
    mental disorder NEC F51.05
    opioid
      abuse F11.182
      dependence F11.282
      use F11.982
    psychoactive substance NEC
      abuse F19.182
      dependence F19.182
      use F19.982
    sedative, hypnotic, or anxiolytic
      abuse F13.182
      dependence F13.282
      use F13.982
    stimulant NEC
      abuse F15.182
      dependence F15.282
      use F15.982
  fatal familial (FFI) A81.83
  idiopathic F51.01
  learned F51.3
  nonorganic origin F51.01
  not due to a substance or known physiological condition F51.01
    specified NEC F51.09
  paradoxical F51.03
  primary F51.01
  psychiatric F51.05
  psychophysiologic F51.04
  related to psychopathology F51.05
  short-term F51.02
  specified NEC G47.09

Insomnia — *continued*
  stress-related F51.02
  transient F51.02
  without objective findings F51.02
Inspiration
  food or foreign body — *see* Foreign body, by site
  mucus — *see* Asphyxia, mucus
Inspissated bile syndrome (newborn) P59.1
Instability
  emotional (excessive) F60.3
  housing
    housed Z59.819
      with risk of homelessness Z59.811
      homelessness in past 12 months Z59.812
  joint (post-traumatic) M25.30
    ankle M25.37- ☑
    due to old ligament injury — *see* Disorder, ligament
    elbow M25.32- ☑
    flail — *see* Flail, joint
    foot M25.37- ☑
    hand M25.34- ☑
    hip M25.35- ☑
    knee M25.36- ☑
    lumbosacral — *see* subcategory M53.2- ☑
    prosthesis — *see* Complications, joint prosthesis, mechanical, displacement, by site
    sacroiliac — *see* subcategory M53.2- ☑
    secondary to
      old ligament injury — *see* Disorder, ligament
      removal of joint prosthesis M96.89
    shoulder (region) M25.31- ☑
    specified site NEC M25.39
    spine — *see* subcategory M53.2- ☑
    wrist M25.33- ☑
  knee (chronic) M23.5- ☑
  lumbosacral — *see* subcategory M53.2- ☑
  nervous F48.8
  personality (emotional) F60.3
  spine — *see* Instability, joint, spine
  vasomotor R55
Institutional syndrome (childhood) F94.2
Institutionalization, affecting child Z62.22
  disinhibited attachment F94.2
Insufficiency, insufficient
  accommodation, old age H52.4
  adrenal (gland) E27.40
    primary E27.1
  adrenocortical E27.40
    drug-induced E27.3
    iatrogenic E27.3
    primary E27.1
  anatomic crown height K08.89
  anterior (occlusal) guidance M26.54
  anus K62.89
  aortic (valve) I35.1
    with
      mitral (valve) disease I08.0
        with tricuspid (valve) disease I08.3
      stenosis I35.2
      tricuspid (valve) disease I08.2
        with mitral (valve) disease I08.3
    congenital Q23.1
    rheumatic I06.1
      with
        mitral (valve) disease I08.0
          with tricuspid (valve) disease I08.3
        stenosis I06.2
          with mitral (valve) disease I08.0
            with tricuspid (valve) disease I08.3
        tricuspid (valve) disease I08.2
          with mitral (valve) disease I08.3
    specified cause NEC I35.1
    syphilitic A52.03
  arterial I77.1
    basilar G45.0
    carotid (hemispheric) G45.1
    cerebral I67.81
    coronary (acute or subacute) I24.89
    mesenteric K55.1
    peripheral I73.9
    precerebral (multiple) (bilateral) G45.2
    vertebral G45.0
  arteriovenous I99.8
  biliary K83.8
  cardiac — *see also* Insufficiency, myocardial
    due to presence of (cardiac) prosthesis I97.11- ☑
      postprocedural I97.11- ☑
  cardiorenal, hypertensive I13.2

Insufficiency, insufficient — *continued*
  cardiovascular — *see* Disease, cardiovascular
  cerebrovascular (acute) I67.81
    with transient focal neurological signs and symptoms G45.8
  circulatory NEC I99.8
    newborn P29.89
  clinical crown length K08.89
  convergence H51.11
  coronary (acute or subacute) I24.89
    chronic or with a stated duration of over 4 weeks I25.89
  corticoadrenal E27.40
    primary E27.1
  dietary E63.9
  divergence H51.8
  food T73.0- ☑
  gastroesophageal K22.89
  gonadal
    ovary E28.39
    testis E29.1
  health insurance coverage Z59.71
  heart — *see also* Insufficiency, myocardial
    newborn P29.0
    valve — *see* Endocarditis
  hepatic — *see* Failure, hepatic
  idiopathic autonomic G90.09
  interocclusal distance of fully erupted teeth (ridge) M26.36
  kidney N28.9
    acute N28.9
    chronic N18.9
  lacrimal (secretion) H04.12- ☑
    passages — *see* Stenosis, lacrimal
  liver — *see* Failure, hepatic
  lung — *see* Insufficiency, pulmonary
  mental (congenital) — *see* Disability, intellectual
  mesenteric K55.1
  mitral (valve) I34.0
    with
      aortic valve disease I08.0
        with tricuspid (valve) disease I08.3
      obstruction or stenosis I05.2
        with aortic valve disease I08.0
      tricuspid (valve) disease I08.1
        with aortic (valve) disease I08.3
    congenital Q23.3
    rheumatic I05.1
      with
        aortic valve disease I08.0
          with tricuspid (valve) disease I08.3
        obstruction or stenosis I05.2
          with aortic valve disease I08.0
            with tricuspid (valve) disease I08.3
        tricuspid (valve) disease I08.1
          with aortic (valve) disease I08.3
      active or acute I01.1
        with chorea, rheumatic (Sydenham's) I02.0
    specified cause, except rheumatic I34.0
  muscle — *see also* Disease, muscle
    heart — *see* Insufficiency, myocardial
    ocular NEC H50.9
  myocardial, myocardium (with arteriosclerosis) — *see also* Failure, heart I50.9
    with
      rheumatic fever (conditions in I00) I09.0
        active, acute or subacute I01.2
          with chorea I02.0
        inactive or quiescent (with chorea) I09.0
    congenital Q24.8
    hypertensive — *see* Hypertension, heart
    newborn P29.0
    rheumatic I09.0
      active, acute, or subacute I01.2
    syphilitic A52.06
  nourishment — *see also* Nutrition deficient T73.0- ☑
  pancreatic K86.89
    exocrine K86.81
  parathyroid (gland) E20.9
  peripheral vascular (arterial) I73.9
  pituitary E23.0
  placental (mother) O36.51- ☑
  platelets D69.6
  prenatal care affecting management of pregnancy O09.3- ☑
  progressive pluriglandular E31.0
  pulmonary J98.4
    acute, following surgery (nonthoracic) J95.2

Insufficiency, insufficient — *continued*
  pulmonary — *continued*
    acute, following surgery — *continued*
      thoracic J95.1
    chronic, following surgery J95.3
    following
      shock J98.4
      trauma J98.4
    newborn P28.89
    valve I37.1
      with stenosis I37.2
      congenital Q22.2
      rheumatic I09.89
        with aortic, mitral or tricuspid (valve) disease I08.8
  pyloric K31.89
  renal (acute) N28.9
    chronic N18.9
  respiratory R06.89
    newborn P28.5
  rotation — *see* Malrotation
  sleep syndrome F51.12
  social insurance Z59.71
  suprarenal E27.40
    primary E27.1
  tarso-orbital fascia, congenital Q10.3
  testis E29.1
  thyroid (gland) (acquired) E03.9
    congenital E03.1
  tricuspid (valve) (rheumatic) I07.1
    with
      aortic (valve) disease I08.2
        with mitral (valve) disease I08.3
      mitral (valve) disease I08.1
        with aortic (valve) disease I08.3
      obstruction or stenosis I07.2
        with aortic (valve) disease I08.2
          with mitral (valve) disease I08.3
    congenital Q22.8
    nonrheumatic I36.1
      with stenosis I36.2
  urethral sphincter R32
  valve, valvular (heart) I38
    aortic — *see* Insufficiency, aortic (valve)
    congenital Q24.8
    mitral — *see* Insufficiency, mitral (valve)
    pulmonary — *see* Insufficiency, pulmonary, valve
    tricuspid — *see* Insufficiency, tricuspid (valve)
  vascular I99.8
    intestine K55.9
      acute — *see also* Ischemia, intestine, acute K55.059
    mesenteric K55.1
    peripheral I73.9
    renal — *see* Hypertension, kidney
  velopharyngeal
    acquired K13.79
    congenital Q38.8
  venous (chronic) (peripheral) I87.2
  ventricular — *see* Insufficiency, myocardial
  welfare support Z59.72
Insufflation, fallopian Z31.41
Insular — *see* condition
Insulinoma
  pancreas
    benign D13.7
    malignant C25.4
    uncertain behavior D37.8
  specified site
    benign — *see* Neoplasm, by site, benign
    malignant — *see* Neoplasm, by site, malignant
    uncertain behavior — *see* Neoplasm, by site, uncertain behavior
  unspecified site
    benign D13.7
    malignant C25.4
    uncertain behavior D37.8
Insuloma — *see* Insulinoma
Interference
  balancing side M26.56
  non-working side M26.56
Intermenstrual — *see* condition
Intermittent — *see* condition
Internal — *see* condition
Interrogation
  cardiac defibrillator (automatic) (implantable) Z45.02
  cardiac pacemaker Z45.018
  cardiac (event) (loop) recorder Z45.09
  infusion pump (implanted) (intrathecal) Z45.1
  neurostimulator Z46.2

Interruption
  aortic arch Q25.21
  bundle of His I44.30
  phase-shift, sleep cycle — *see* Disorder, sleep, circadian rhythm
  sleep phase-shift, or 24 hour sleep-wake cycle — *see* Disorder, sleep, circadian rhythm
Interstitial — *see* condition
Intertrigo L30.4
  labialis K13.0
Intervertebral disc — *see* condition
Intestine, intestinal — *see* condition
Intolerance
  carbohydrate K90.49
  disaccharide, hereditary E73.0
  fat NEC K90.49
    pancreatic K90.3
  food K90.49
    dietary counseling and surveillance Z71.3
  fructose E74.10
    hereditary E74.12
  glucose (-galactose) E74.39
  gluten K90.41
  lactose E73.9
    specified NEC E73.8
  lysine E72.3
  milk NEC K90.49
    lactose E73.9
  orthostatic, chronic G90.A
  protein K90.49
  starch NEC K90.49
  sucrose (-isomaltose) E74.31
Intoxicated NEC (without dependence) — *see* Alcohol, intoxication
Intoxication
  acid — *see also* Acidosis E87.29
  alcoholic (acute) (without dependence) — *see* Alcohol, intoxication
  alimentary canal K52.1
  amphetamine (without dependence) — *see also* Abuse, drug, stimulant, with intoxication
    with dependence — *see* Dependence, drug, stimulant, with intoxication
    stimulant NEC F15.10
      with
        anxiety disorder F15.180
        intoxication F15.129
          with
            delirium F15.121
            perceptual disturbance F15.122
  anxiolytic (acute) (without dependence) — *see* Abuse, drug, sedative, with intoxication
    with dependence — *see* Dependence, drug, sedative, with intoxication
  caffeine F15.929
    with dependence — *see* Dependence, drug, stimulant, with intoxication
  cannabinoids (acute) (without dependence) — *see* Use, cannabis, with intoxication
    with
      abuse — *see* Abuse, drug, cannabis, with intoxication
      dependence — *see* Dependence, drug, cannabis, with intoxication
  chemical — *see* Table of Drugs and Chemicals
    via placenta or breast milk — *see* - Absorption, chemical, through placenta
  cocaine (acute) (without dependence) — *see* Abuse, drug, cocaine, with intoxication
    with dependence — *see* Dependence, drug, cocaine, with intoxication
  drug
    acute (without dependence) — *see* Abuse, drug, by type with intoxication
      with dependence — *see* Dependence, drug, by type with intoxication
    addictive
      via placenta or breast milk — *see* Absorption, drug, addictive, through placenta
      newborn P93.8
        gray baby syndrome P93.0
      overdose or wrong substance given or taken — *see* Table of Drugs and Chemicals, by drug, poisoning
  enteric K52.1
  foodborne A05.9
    bacterial A05.9
    classical (Clostridium botulinum) A05.1

Intoxication — continued
  foodborne — continued
    due to
      Bacillus cereus A05.4
      bacterium A05.9
        specified NEC A05.8
      Clostridium
        botulinum A05.1
        perfringens A05.2
        welchii A05.2
      Salmonella A02.9
        with
          (gastro)enteritis A02.0
          localized infection(s) A02.20
            arthritis A02.23
            meningitis A02.21
            osteomyelitis A02.24
            pneumonia A02.22
            pyelonephritis A02.25
            specified NEC A02.29
          sepsis A02.1
          specified manifestation NEC A02.8
      Staphylococcus A05.0
      Vibrio
        parahaemolyticus A05.3
        vulnificus A05.5
    enterotoxin, staphylococcal A05.0
    noxious — see Poisoning, food, noxious
  gastrointestinal K52.1
  hallucinogenic (without dependence) — see Abuse, drug, hallucinogen, with intoxication
    with dependence — see Dependence, drug, hallucinogen, with intoxication
  hepatocerebral K76.82
  hypnotic (acute) (without dependence) — see Abuse, drug, sedative, with intoxication
    with dependence — see Dependence, drug, sedative, with intoxication
  inhalant (acute) (without dependence) — see Abuse, drug, inhalant, with intoxication
    with dependence — see Dependence, drug, inhalant, with intoxication
  meaning
    inebriation — see category F10.- ☑
    poisoning — see Table of Drugs and Chemicals
  methyl alcohol (acute) (without dependence) — see Alcohol, intoxication
  opioid (acute) (without dependence) — see Abuse, drug, opioid, with intoxication
    with dependence — see Dependence, drug, opioid, with intoxication
  pathologic NEC (without dependence) — see Alcohol, intoxication
  phencyclidine (acute) (without dependence) — see Abuse, drug, hallucinogen, with intoxication
    with dependence — see Dependence, drug, hallucinogen, with intoxication
  potassium (K) E87.5
  psychoactive substance NEC (without dependence) — see Abuse, drug, psychoactive NEC, with intoxication
    with dependence — see Dependence, drug, psychoactive NEC, with intoxication
  sedative (acute) (without dependence) — see Abuse, drug, sedative, with intoxication
    with dependence — see Dependence, drug, sedative, with intoxication
  serum — see also Reaction, serum T80.69- ☑
  uremic — see Uremia
  volatile solvents (acute) (without dependence) — see Abuse, drug, inhalant, with intoxication
    with dependence — see Dependence, drug, inhalant, with intoxication
  water E87.79
Intraabdominal testis, testes
  bilateral Q53.211
  unilateral Q53.111
Intracranial — see condition
Intrahepatic gallbladder Q44.1
Intraligamentous — see condition
Intrathoracic — see also condition
  kidney Q63.2
Intrauterine contraceptive device
  checking Z30.431
  in situ Z97.5
  insertion Z30.430
    immediately following removal Z30.433
  management Z30.431
  reinsertion Z30.433

Intrauterine contraceptive device — continued
  removal Z30.432
  replacement Z30.433
  retention in pregnancy O26.3- ☑
Intraventricular — see condition
Intrinsic deformity — see Deformity
Intubation, difficult or failed T88.4- ☑
Intumescence, lens (eye) (cataract) — see Cataract
Intussusception (bowel) (colon) (enteric) (ileocecal) (ileocolic) (intestine) (rectum) K56.1
  appendix K38.8
  congenital Q43.8
  ureter (with obstruction) N13.5
Invagination (bowel, colon, intestine or rectum) K56.1
Inversion
  albumin-globulin (A-G) ratio E88.09
  bladder N32.89
  cecum — see Intussusception
  cervix N88.8
  chromosome in normal individual Q95.1
  circadian rhythm — see Disorder, sleep, circadian rhythm
  nipple N64.59
    congenital Q83.8
    gestational — see Retraction, nipple
    puerperal, postpartum — see Retraction, nipple
  nyctohemeral rhythm — see Disorder, sleep, circadian rhythm
  optic papilla Q14.2
  organ or site, congenital NEC — see Anomaly, by site
  sleep rhythm — see Disorder, sleep, circadian rhythm
  testis (congenital) Q55.29
  uterus (chronic) (postinfectional) (postpartal, old) N85.5
    postpartum O71.2
  vagina (posthysterectomy) N99.3
  ventricular Q20.5
Investigation — see also Examination Z04.9
  clinical research subject (control) (normal comparison) (participant) Z00.6
Involuntary movement, abnormal R25.9
Involution, involutional — see also condition
  breast, cystic — see Dysplasia, mammary, specified type NEC
  depression (single episode) F32.89
    recurrent episode F33.9
  melancholia (single episode) F32.89
    recurrent episode F33.8
  ovary, senile — see Atrophy, ovary
  thymus failure E32.8
I.Q.
  20-34 F72
  35-49 F71
  50-69 F70
  under 20 F73
IRDS (type I) P22.0
  type II P22.1
Irideremia Q13.1
Iridis rubeosis — see Disorder, iris, vascular
Iridochoroiditis (panuveitis) — see Panuveitis
Iridocyclitis H20.9
  acute H20.0- ☑
    hypopyon H20.05- ☑
    primary H20.01- ☑
    recurrent H20.02- ☑
    secondary (noninfectious) H20.04- ☑
      infectious H20.03- ☑
  chronic H20.1- ☑
  due to allergy — see Iridocyclitis, acute, secondary
  endogenous — see Iridocyclitis, acute, primary
  Fuchs' — see Cyclitis, Fuchs' heterochromic
  gonococcal A54.32
  granulomatous — see Iridocyclitis, chronic
  herpes, herpetic (simplex) B00.51
    zoster B02.32
  hypopyon — see Iridocyclitis, acute, hypopyon
  in (due to)
    ankylosing spondylitis M45.9
    gonococcal infection A54.32
    herpes (simplex) virus B00.51
      zoster B02.32
    infectious disease NOS B99.- ☑
    parasitic disease NOS B89 [H22]
    sarcoidosis D86.83
    syphilis A51.43
    tuberculosis A18.54
    zoster B02.32
  lens-induced H20.2- ☑
  nongranulomatous — see Iridocyclitis, acute
  recurrent — see Iridocyclitis, acute, recurrent

Iridocyclitis — continued
  rheumatic — see Iridocyclitis, chronic
  subacute — see Iridocyclitis, acute
  sympathetic — see Uveitis, sympathetic
  syphilitic (secondary) A51.43
  tuberculous (chronic) A18.54
  Vogt-Koyanagi H20.82- ☑
Iridocyclochoroiditis (panuveitis) — see Panuveitis
Iridodialysis H21.53- ☑
Iridodonesis H21.89
Iridoplegia (complete) (partial) (reflex) H57.09
Iridoschisis H21.25- ☑
Iris — see also condition
  bombé — see Membrane, pupillary
Iritis — see also Iridocyclitis
  chronic — see Iridocyclitis, chronic
  diabetic — see E08-E13 with .39
  due to
    herpes simplex B00.51
    leprosy A30.9 [H22]
  gonococcal A54.32
  gouty — see also Gout, by type M10.9 [H22]
  granulomatous — see Iridocyclitis, chronic
  lens induced — see Iridocyclitis, lens-induced
  papulosa (syphilitic) A52.71
  rheumatic — see Iridocyclitis, chronic
  syphilitic (secondary) A51.43
    congenital (early) A50.01
    late A52.71
  tuberculous A18.54
Iron — see condition
Iron-miner's lung J63.4
Irradiated enamel (tooth, teeth) K03.89
Irradiation effects, adverse T66.- ☑
Irreducible, irreducibility — see condition
Irregular, irregularity
  action, heart I49.9
  alveolar process K08.89
  bleeding N92.6
  breathing R06.89
  contour of cornea (acquired) — see Deformity, cornea
    congenital Q13.4
  contour, reconstructed breast N65.0
  dentin (in pulp) K04.3
  eye movements H55.89
    deficient
      saccadic H55.81
      smooth H55.82
    nystagmus — see Nystagmus
  labor O62.2
  menstruation (cause unknown) N92.6
  periods N92.6
  prostate N42.9
  pupil — see Abnormality, pupillary
  reconstructed breast N65.0
  respiratory R06.89
  septum (nasal) J34.2
  shape, organ or site, congenital NEC — see Distortion
  sleep-wake pattern (rhythm) G47.23
Irritable, irritability R45.4
  bladder N32.89
  bowel (syndrome) K58.9
    with
      constipation K58.1
      diarrhea K58.0
    mixed K58.2
    psychogenic F45.8
    specified NEC K58.8
  bronchial — see Bronchitis
  cerebral, in newborn P91.3
  colon — see also Irritable, bowel K58.9
    with diarrhea K58.0
    psychogenic F45.8
  duodenum K59.89
  heart (psychogenic) F45.8
  hip — see Derangement, joint, specified type NEC, hip
  ileum K59.89
  infant R68.12
  jejunum K59.89
  rectum K59.89
  stomach K31.89
    psychogenic F45.8
  sympathetic G90.89
  urethra N36.8
  without diarrhea K58.9
Irritation
  anus K62.89
  axillary nerve G54.0
  bladder N32.89

Irritation — *continued*
 brachial plexus G54.0
 bronchial — *see* Bronchitis
 cervical plexus G54.2
 cervix — *see* Cervicitis
 choroid, sympathetic — *see* Endophthalmitis
 cranial nerve — *see* Disorder, nerve, cranial
 gastric K31.89
  psychogenic F45.8
 globe, sympathetic — *see* Uveitis, sympathetic
 labyrinth — *see* subcategory H83.2- ☑
 lumbosacral plexus G54.1
 meninges (traumatic) — *see* Injury, intracranial
  nontraumatic — *see* Meningismus
 nerve — *see* Disorder, nerve
 nervous R45.0
 penis N48.89
 perineum NEC L29.3
 peripheral autonomic nervous system G90.89
 peritoneum — *see* Peritonitis
 pharynx J39.2
 plantar nerve — *see* Lesion, nerve, plantar
 spinal (cord) (traumatic) — *see also* Injury, spinal cord, by region
  nerve G58.9
   root NEC — *see* Radiculopathy
  nontraumatic — *see* Myelopathy
 stomach K31.89
  psychogenic F45.8
 sympathetic nerve NEC G90.89
 ulnar nerve — *see* Lesion, nerve, ulnar
 vagina N89.8
Ischemia, ischemic I99.8
 bowel (transient)
  acute — *see also* Ischemia, intestine, acute K55.059
  chronic K55.1
  due to mesenteric artery insufficiency K55.1
 brain — *see* Ischemia, cerebral
 cardiac — *see* Disease, heart, ischemic
 cardiomyopathy I25.5
 cerebral (chronic) (generalized) I67.82
  arteriosclerotic I67.2
  intermittent G45.9
  newborn P91.0
  recurrent focal G45.8
  transient G45.9
 colon chronic (due to mesenteric artery insufficiency) K55.1
 coronary — *see* Disease, heart, ischemic
 demand (coronary) — *see also* Angina I24.89
  with myocardial infarction I21.A1
  resulting in myocardial infarction I21.A1
 heart (chronic or with a stated duration of over 4 weeks) I25.9
  acute or with a stated duration of 4 weeks or less I24.9
  subacute I24.9
 infarction, muscle — *see* Infarct, muscle
 intestine (large) (small) (transient) K55.9
  acute K55.059
   diffuse K55.052
   focal K55.051
   large K55.039
    diffuse K55.032
    focal K55.031
   small K55.019
    diffuse K55.012
    focal K55.011
  chronic K55.1
  due to mesenteric artery insufficiency K55.1
 kidney N28.0
 limb, critical — *see* Arteriosclerosis, with critical limb ischemia
 limb-threatening, chronic — *see* Arteriosclerosis, with critical limb ischemia
 mesenteric, acute — *see also* Ischemia, intestine, acute K55.059
 muscle, traumatic T79.6- ☑
 myocardium, myocardial (chronic or with a stated duration of over 4 weeks) I25.9
  acute, without myocardial infarction I51.3
  silent (asymptomatic) I25.6
  transient of newborn P29.4
 renal N28.0
 retina, retinal — *see* Occlusion, artery, retina
 small bowel
  acute K55.019
   diffuse K55.012
   focal K55.011
  chronic K55.1

Ischemia, ischemic — *continued*
 small bowel — *continued*
  due to mesenteric artery insufficiency K55.1
 spinal cord G95.11
 subendocardial — *see* Insufficiency, coronary
 supply (coronary) — *see also* Angina I25.9
  due to vasospasm I20.1
Ischial spine — *see* condition
Ischialgia — *see* Sciatica
Ischiopagus Q89.4
Ischium, ischial — *see* condition
Ischuria R34
Iselin's disease or osteochondrosis — *see* Osteochondrosis, juvenile, metatarsus
Islands of
 parotid tissue in
  lymph nodes Q38.6
  neck structures Q38.6
 submaxillary glands in
  fascia Q38.6
  lymph nodes Q38.6
  neck muscles Q38.6
Islet cell tumor, pancreas D13.7
Isoimmunization NEC — *see also* Incompatibility
 affecting management of pregnancy (ABO) (with hydrops fetalis) O36.11- ☑
  anti-A sensitization O36.11- ☑
  anti-B sensitization O36.19- ☑
  anti-C sensitization O36.09- ☑
  anti-c sensitization O36.09- ☑
  anti-E sensitization O36.09- ☑
  anti-e sensitization O36.09- ☑
  Rh NEC O36.09- ☑
   anti-D antibody O36.01- ☑
  specified NEC O36.19- ☑
 newborn P55.9
  with
   hydrops fetalis P56.0
   kernicterus P57.0
  ABO (blood groups) P55.1
  Rhesus (Rh) factor P55.0
  specified type NEC P55.8
Isolation, isolated
 dwelling Z59.89
 family Z63.79
 social Z60.4
Isoleucinosis E71.19
Isomerism atrial appendages (with asplenia or polysplenia) Q20.6
Isosporiasis, isosporosis A07.3
Isovaleric acidemia E71.110
Issue of
 medical certificate Z02.79
  for disability determination Z02.71
 repeat prescription (appliance) (glasses) (medicinal substance, medicament, medicine) Z76.0
  contraception — *see* Contraception
IST (inappropriate sinus tachycardia, so stated) I47.11
Itch, itching — *see also* Pruritus
 baker's L23.6
 barber's B35.0
 bricklayer's L24.5
 cheese B88.09
 clam digger's B65.3
 coolie B76.9
 copra B88.09
 dew B76.9
 dhobi B35.6
 filarial — *see* Infestation, filarial
 grain B88.09
 grocer's B88.09
 ground B76.9
 harvest B88.09
 jock B35.6
 Malabar B35.5
  beard B35.0
  foot B35.3
  scalp B35.0
 meaning scabies B86
 Norwegian B86
 perianal L29.3
 poultrymen's B88.09
 sarcoptic B86
 scabies B86
 scrub B88.09
 straw B88.09
 swimmer's B65.3
 water B76.9

Itch, itching — *continued*
 winter L29.89
Ivemark's syndrome (asplenia with congenital heart disease) Q89.01
Ivory bones Q78.2
Ixodiasis NEC B88.8

J

Jaccoud's syndrome — *see* Arthropathy, postrheumatic, chronic
Jackson's
 membrane Q43.3
 paralysis or syndrome G83.89
 veil Q43.3
Jacquet's dermatitis (diaper dermatitis) L22
Jadassohn-Pellizari's disease or anetoderma L90.2
Jadassohn's
 blue nevus — *see* Nevus
 intraepidermal epithelioma — *see* Neoplasm, skin, benign
Jaffe-Lichtenstein (-Uehlinger) **syndrome** — *see* Dysplasia, fibrous, bone NEC
Jakob-Creutzfeldt disease or syndrome — *see* Creutzfeldt-Jakob disease or syndrome
Jaksch-Luzet disease D64.89
Jamaican
 neuropathy G92.8
 paraplegic tropical ataxic-spastic syndrome G92.8
Janet's disease F48.8
Janiceps Q89.4
Jansky-Bielschowsky amaurotic idiocy E75.4
Japanese
 B-type encephalitis A83.0
 river fever A75.3
Jaundice (yellow) R17
 acholuric (familial) (splenomegalic) — *see also* Spherocytosis
  acquired D59.8
 breast-milk (inhibitor) P59.3
 catarrhal (acute) B15.9
  with hepatic coma B15.0
 cholestatic (benign) R17
 due to or associated with
  delayed conjugation P59.8
   associated with (due to) preterm delivery P59.0
  preterm delivery P59.0
 epidemic (catarrhal) B15.9
  with hepatic coma B15.0
  leptospiral A27.0
  spirochetal A27.0
 familial nonhemolytic (congenital) (Gilbert) E80.4
  Crigler-Najjar E80.5
 febrile (acute) B15.9
  with hepatic coma B15.0
  leptospiral A27.0
  spirochetal A27.0
 hematogenous D59.9
 hemolytic (acquired) D59.9
  congenital — *see* Spherocytosis
 hemorrhagic (acute) (leptospiral) (spirochetal) A27.0
 infectious (acute) (subacute) B15.9
  with hepatic coma B15.0
  leptospiral A27.0
  spirochetal A27.0
 leptospiral (hemorrhagic) A27.0
 malignant (without coma) K72.90
  with coma K72.91
 neonatal — *see* Jaundice, newborn
 newborn P59.9
  due to or associated with
   ABO
    antibodies P55.1
    incompatibility, maternal/fetal P55.1
    isoimmunization P55.1
   absence or deficiency of enzyme system for bilirubin conjugation (congenital) P59.8
   bleeding P58.1
   breast milk inhibitors to conjugation P59.3
    associated with preterm delivery P59.0
   bruising P58.0
   Crigler-Najjar syndrome E80.5
   delayed conjugation P59.8
    associated with preterm delivery P59.0
   drugs or toxins
    given to newborn P58.42
    transmitted from mother P58.41
   excessive hemolysis P58.9

Jaundice — continued
  newborn — continued
    due to or associated with — continued
      excessive hemolysis — continued
        due to
          bleeding P58.1
          bruising P58.0
          drugs or toxins
            given to newborn P58.42
            transmitted from mother P58.41
          infection P58.2
          polycythemia P58.3
          swallowed maternal blood P58.5
        specified type NEC P58.8
    galactosemia E74.21
    Gilbert syndrome E80.4
    hemolytic disease P55.9
      ABO isoimmunization P55.1
      Rh isoimmunization P55.0
      specified NEC P55.8
    hepatocellular damage P59.20
      specified NEC P59.29
    hereditary hemolytic anemia P58.8
    hypothyroidism, congenital E03.1
    incompatibility, maternal/fetal NOS P55.9
    infection P58.2
    inspissated bile syndrome P59.1
    isoimmunization NOS P55.9
    mucoviscidosis E84.9
    polycythemia P58.3
    preterm delivery P59.0
    Rh
      antibodies P55.0
      incompatibility, maternal/fetal P55.0
      isoimmunization P55.0
    specified cause NEC P59.8
    swallowed maternal blood P58.5
    spherocytosis (congenital) D58.0
  nonhemolytic congenital familial (Gilbert) E80.4
  nuclear, newborn — see also Kernicterus of newborn P57.9
  obstructive — see also Obstruction, bile duct K83.1
  post-immunization — see Hepatitis, viral, type, B
  post-transfusion — see Hepatitis, viral, type, B
  regurgitation — see also Obstruction, bile duct K83.1
  serum (homologous) (prophylactic) (therapeutic) — see Hepatitis, viral, type, B
  spirochetal (hemorrhagic) A27.0
  symptomatic R17
    newborn P59.9
Jaw — see condition
Jaw-winking phenomenon or syndrome Q07.8
Jealousy
  alcoholic F10.988
  childhood F93.8
  sibling F93.8
Jejunitis — see Enteritis
Jejunostomy status Z93.4
Jejunum, jejunal — see condition
Jensen's disease — see Inflammation, chorioretinal, focal, juxtapapillary
Jerks, myoclonic G25.3
Jervell-Lange-Nielsen syndrome I45.81
Jeune's disease Q77.2
Jigger disease B88.1
Job's syndrome (chronic granulomatous disease) D71.8
Joint — see also condition
  mice — see Loose, body, joint
    knee M23.4- ☑
Jordan's anomaly or syndrome D72.0
Joseph-Diamond-Blackfan anemia (congenital hypoplastic) D61.01
Jungle yellow fever A95.0
Jüngling's disease — see Sarcoidosis
Juvenile — see condition

K

Kahler's disease C90.0- ☑
Kakke E51.11
Kala-azar B55.0
Kallmann's syndrome E23.0
Kanner's syndrome (autism) — see Psychosis, childhood
Kaposi's
  dermatosis (xeroderma pigmentosum) Q82.1
  lichen ruber L44.0
    acuminatus L44.0

Kaposi's — continued
  sarcoma
    colon C46.4
    connective tissue C46.1
    gastrointestinal organ C46.4
    lung C46.5- ☑
    lymph node (multiple) C46.3
    palate (hard) (soft) C46.2
    rectum C46.4
    skin (multiple sites) C46.0
    specified site NEC C46.7
    stomach C46.4
    unspecified site C46.9
  varicelliform eruption B00.0
    vaccinia T88.1- ☑
Kartagener's syndrome or triad (sinusitis, bronchiectasis, situs inversus) Q89.3
Karyotype
  with abnormality except iso (Xq) Q96.2
  45,X Q96.0
  46,X
    iso (Xq) Q96.1
  46,XX Q98.3
    with streak gonads Q50.32
    hermaphrodite (true) Q99.1
    male Q98.3
  46,XY
    with streak gonads Q56.1
    female Q97.3
    hermaphrodite (true) Q99.1
  47,XXX Q97.0
  47,XXY Q98.0
  47,XYY Q98.5
Kaschin-Beck disease — see Disease, Kaschin-Beck
Katayama's disease or fever B65.2
Kawasaki's syndrome M30.3
Kayser-Fleischer ring (cornea) (pseudosclerosis) H18.04- ☑
Kaznelson's syndrome (congenital hypoplastic anemia) D61.01
Kearns-Sayre syndrome H49.81- ☑
Kedani fever A75.3
Kelis L91.0
Kelly (-Patterson) **syndrome** (sideropenic dysphagia) D50.1
Keloid, cheloid L91.0
  acne L73.0
  Addison's L94.0
  cornea — see Opacity, cornea
  Hawkin's L91.0
  scar L91.0
Keloma L91.0
Kenya fever A77.1
Keratectasia — see also Ectasia, cornea
  congenital Q13.4
Keratinization of alveolar ridge mucosa
  excessive K13.23
  minimal K13.22
Keratinized residual ridge mucosa
  excessive K13.23
  minimal K13.22
Keratitis (nodular) (nonulcerative) (simple) (zonular) H16.9
  with ulceration (central) (marginal) (perforated) (ring) — see Ulcer, cornea
  actinic — see Photokeratitis
  arborescens (herpes simplex) B00.52
  areolar H16.11- ☑
  bullosa H16.8
  deep H16.309
    specified type NEC H16.399
  dendritic (a) (herpes simplex) B00.52
  disciform (is) (herpes simplex) B00.52
    varicella B01.81
  filamentary H16.12- ☑
  gonococcal (congenital or prenatal) A54.33
  herpes, herpetic (simplex) B00.52
    zoster B02.33
  in (due to)
    acanthamebiasis B60.13
    adenovirus B30.0
    exanthema — see also Exanthem B09
    herpes (simplex) virus B00.52
    measles B05.81
    syphilis A50.31
    tuberculosis A18.52
    zoster B02.33
  interstitial (nonsyphilitic) H16.30- ☑
    diffuse H16.32- ☑
    herpes, herpetic (simplex) B00.52
      zoster B02.33

Keratitis — continued
  interstitial — continued
    sclerosing H16.33- ☑
    specified type NEC H16.39- ☑
    syphilitic (congenital) (late) A50.31
    tuberculous A18.52
  macular H16.11- ☑
  nummular H16.11- ☑
  oyster shuckers' H16.8
  parenchymatous — see Keratitis, interstitial
  petrificans H16.8
  postmeasles B05.81
  punctata
    leprosa A30.9 [H16.14-] ☑
    syphilitic (profunda) A50.31
  punctate H16.14- ☑
  purulent H16.8
  rosacea L71.8
  sclerosing H16.33- ☑
  specified type NEC H16.8
  stellate H16.11- ☑
  striate H16.11- ☑
  superficial H16.10- ☑
    with conjunctivitis — see Keratoconjunctivitis
    due to light — see Photokeratitis
  suppurative H16.8
  syphilitic (congenital) (prenatal) A50.31
  trachomatous A71.1
    sequelae B94.0
  tuberculous A18.52
  vesicular H16.8
  xerotic — see also Keratomalacia H16.8
    vitamin A deficiency E50.4
Kerato-uveitis — see Iridocyclitis
Keratoacanthoma L85.8
Keratocele — see Descemetocele
Keratoconjunctivitis H16.20- ☑
  Acanthamoeba B60.13
  adenoviral B30.0
  epidemic B30.0
  exposure H16.21- ☑
  herpes, herpetic (simplex) B00.52
    zoster B02.33
  in exanthema — see also Exanthem B09
  infectious B30.0
  lagophthalmic — see Keratoconjunctivitis, specified type NEC
  neurotrophic H16.23- ☑
  phlyctenular H16.25- ☑
  postmeasles B05.81
  shipyard B30.0
  sicca (Sjogren's) M35.0- ☑
    not Sjogren's H16.22- ☑
  specified type NEC H16.29- ☑
  tuberculous (phlyctenular) A18.52
  vernal H16.26- ☑
Keratoconus H18.60- ☑
  congenital Q13.4
  stable H18.61- ☑
  unstable H18.62- ☑
Keratocyst (dental) (odontogenic) — see Cyst, calcifying odontogenic
Keratoderma, keratodermia (congenital) (palmaris et plantaris) (symmetrical) Q82.8
  acquired L85.1
    in diseases classified elsewhere L86
  climactericum L85.1
  gonococcal A54.89
  gonorrheal A54.89
  punctata L85.2
  Reiter's — see Reiter's disease
Keratodermatocele — see Descemetocele
Keratoglobus H18.79- ☑
  congenital Q15.8
    with glaucoma Q15.0
Keratohemia — see Pigmentation, cornea, stromal
Keratoiritis — see also Iridocyclitis
  syphilitic A50.39
  tuberculous A18.54
Keratoma L57.0
  palmaris and plantaris hereditarium Q82.8
  senile L57.0
Keratomalacia H18.44- ☑
  vitamin A deficiency E50.4
Keratomegaly Q13.4
Keratomycosis B49
  nigrans, nigricans (palmaris) B36.1
Keratopathy H18.9

Keratopathy — *continued*
 band H18.42- ☑
 bullous H18.1- ☑
 bullous (aphakic), following cataract surgery H59.01- ☑
Keratoscleritis, tuberculous A18.52
Keratosis L57.0
 actinic L57.0
 arsenical L85.8
 congenital, specified NEC Q80.8
 female genital NEC N94.89
 follicularis Q82.8
  acquired L11.0
  congenita Q82.8
  et parafollicularis in cutem penetrans L87.0
  spinulosa (decalvans) Q82.8
  vitamin A deficiency E50.8
 gonococcal A54.89
 lichenoid L82.0
 male genital (external) N50.89
 nigricans L83
 obturans, external ear (canal) — *see* Cholesteatoma, external ear
 palmaris et plantaris (inherited) (symmetrical) Q82.8
  acquired L85.1
 penile N48.89
 pharynx J39.2
 pilaris, acquired L85.8
 punctata (palmaris et plantaris) L85.2
 scrotal N50.89
 seborrheic L82.1
  inflamed L82.0
 senile L57.0
 solar L57.0
 tonsillaris J35.8
 vagina N89.4
 vegetans Q82.8
 vitamin A deficiency E50.8
 vocal cord J38.3
Keraunoparalysis T75.09- ☑
Kerion (celsi) B35.0
Kernicterus of newborn (not due to isoimmunization) P57.9
 due to isoimmunization (conditions in P55.0-P55.9) P57.0
 specified type NEC P57.8
Keshan disease E59
Ketoacidosis E87.29
 diabetic — *see* Diabetes, by type, with ketoacidosis
Ketonuria R82.4
Ketosis NEC E88.89
 diabetic — *see* Diabetes, by type, with ketoacidosis
Kew Garden fever A79.1
Kidney — *see* condition
Kienbock's disease — *see also* Osteochondrosis, juvenile, hand, carpal lunate
 adult M93.1
Kimmelstiel (-Wilson) **disease** — *see* Diabetes, Kimmelstiel (-Wilson) disease
Kink, kinking
 artery I77.1
 hair (acquired) L67.8
 ileum or intestine — *see* Obstruction, intestine
 Lane's — *see* Obstruction, intestine
 organ or site, congenital NEC — *see* Anomaly, by site
 ureter (pelvic junction) N13.5
  with
   hydronephrosis N13.1
    with infection N13.6
   pyelonephritis (chronic) N11.1
  congenital Q62.39
 vein(s) I87.8
  caval I87.1
  peripheral I87.1
Kinnier Wilson's disease (hepatolenticular degeneration) E83.01
Kissing spine M48.20
 cervical region M48.22
 cervicothoracic region M48.23
 lumbar region M48.26
 lumbosacral region M48.27
 occipito-atlanto-axial region M48.21
 thoracic region M48.24
 thoracolumbar region M48.25
Klatskin's tumor C22.1
Klauder's disease A26.8
Klebs' disease — *see also* Glomerulonephritis N05.-
Klebsiella (K.) **pneumoniae, as cause of disease classified elsewhere** B96.1
Kleeblattschaedel skull Q75.051

Klein (e)-**Levin syndrome** G47.13
Kleptomania F63.2
Klinefelter's syndrome Q98.4
 karyotype 47,XXY Q98.0
 male with more than two X chromosomes Q98.1
Klippel-Feil deficiency, disease, or syndrome (brevicollis) Q76.1
Klippel-Trenaunay (-Weber) **syndrome** Q87.2
Klippel's disease I67.2
Klumpke (-Dejerine) **palsy, paralysis** (birth) (newborn) P14.1
Knee — *see* condition
Knock knee (acquired) M21.06- ☑
 congenital Q74.1
Knot(s)
 intestinal, syndrome (volvulus) K56.2
 surfer S89.8- ☑
 umbilical cord (true) O69.2- ☑
Knotting (of)
 hair L67.8
 intestine K56.2
Knuckle pad (Garrod's) M72.1
Koch-Weeks' conjunctivitis — *see* Conjunctivitis, acute, mucopurulent
Koch's
 infection — *see* Tuberculosis
 relapsing fever A68.9
Koebner's syndrome Q81.8
Koenig's disease (osteochondritis dissecans) — *see* Osteochondritis, dissecans
Kohler-Pellegrini-Stieda disease or syndrome (calcification, knee joint) — *see* Bursitis, tibial collateral
Kohler's disease
 patellar — *see* Osteochondrosis, juvenile, patella
 tarsal navicular — *see* Osteochondrosis, juvenile, tarsus
Koilonychia L60.3
 congenital Q84.6
Kojevnikov's, epilepsy — *see* Kozhevnikof's epilepsy
Koplik's spots B05.9
Kopp's asthma E32.8
Korsakoff's (Wernicke) **disease, psychosis or syndrome** (alcoholic) F10.96
 with dependence F10.26
 drug-induced
  due to drug abuse — *see* Abuse, drug, by type, with amnestic disorder
  due to drug dependence — *see* Dependence, drug, by type, with amnestic disorder
 nonalcoholic F04
Korsakov's disease, psychosis or syndrome — *see* Korsakoff's disease
Korsakow's disease, psychosis or syndrome — *see* Korsakoff's disease
Kostmann's disease or syndrome (infantile genetic agranulocytosis) — *see* Agranulocytosis
Kozhevnikof's epilepsy G40.109
 intractable G40.119
  with status epilepticus G40.111
  without status epilepticus G40.119
 not intractable G40.109
  with status epilepticus G40.101
  without status epilepticus G40.109
Krabbe's
 disease E75.23
 syndrome, congenital muscle hypoplasia Q79.8
Kraepelin-Morel disease — *see* Schizophrenia
Kraft-Weber-Dimitri disease Q85.89
Kraurosis
 ani K62.89
 penis N48.0
 vagina N89.8
 vulva N90.4
Kreotoxism A05.9
Krukenberg's
 spindle — *see* Pigmentation, cornea, posterior
 tumor C79.6-
Kufs' disease E75.4
Kugelberg-Welander disease G12.1
Kuhnt-Junius degeneration — *see also* Degeneration, macula H35.32- ☑
Kummell's disease or spondylitis — *see* Spondylopathy, traumatic
Kupffer cell sarcoma C22.3
Kuru A81.81
Kussmaul's
 disease M30.0
 respiration E87.29

Kussmaul's — *continued*
 respiration — *continued*
  in diabetic acidosis — *see* Diabetes, by type, with ketoacidosis
Kwashiorkor E40
 marasmic, marasmus type E42
Kyasanur Forest disease A98.2
Kyphoscoliosis, kyphoscoliotic (acquired) — *see also* Scoliosis M41.9
 congenital Q67.5
 heart (disease) I27.1
 sequelae of rickets E64.3
 tuberculous A18.01
Kyphosis, kyphotic (acquired) M40.209
 cervical region M40.202
 cervicothoracic region M40.203
 congenital Q76.419
  cervical region Q76.412
  cervicothoracic region Q76.413
  occipito-atlanto-axial region Q76.411
  thoracic region Q76.414
  thoracolumbar region Q76.415
 Morquio-Brailsford type (spinal) — *see also* subcategory M49.8 E76.219
 postlaminectomy M96.3
 postradiation therapy M96.2
 postural (adolescent) M40.00
  cervicothoracic region M40.03
  thoracic region M40.04
  thoracolumbar region M40.05
 secondary NEC M40.10
  cervical region M40.12
  cervicothoracic region M40.13
  thoracic region M40.14
  thoracolumbar region M40.15
 sequelae of rickets E64.3
 specified type NEC M40.299
  cervical region M40.292
  cervicothoracic region M40.293
  thoracic region M40.294
  thoracolumbar region M40.295
 syphilitic, congenital A50.56
 thoracic region M40.204
 thoracolumbar region M40.205
 tuberculous A18.01
Kyrle disease L87.0

L

L-shaped kidney Q63.8
Labia, labium — *see* condition
Labile
 blood pressure R09.89
 vasomotor system I73.9
Labioglossal paralysis G12.29
Labium leporinum — *see* Cleft, lip
Labor — *see* Delivery
Labored breathing — *see* Hyperventilation
Labyrinthitis (circumscribed) (destructive) (diffuse) (inner ear) (latent) (purulent) (suppurative) — *see also* subcategory H83.0- ☑
 syphilitic A52.79
Laceration
 with abortion — *see* Abortion, by type, complicated by laceration of pelvic organs
 abdomen, abdominal
  wall S31.119- ☑
   with
    foreign body S31.129- ☑
    penetration into peritoneal cavity S31.619- ☑
     with foreign body S31.629- ☑
   epigastric region S31.112- ☑
    with
     foreign body S31.122- ☑
     penetration into peritoneal cavity S31.612- ☑
      with foreign body S31.622- ☑
   left
    lower quadrant S31.114- ☑
     with
      foreign body S31.124- ☑
      penetration into peritoneal cavity S31.614- ☑
       with foreign body S31.624- ☑
    upper quadrant S31.111- ☑
     with
      foreign body S31.121- ☑

Laceration — continued
  abdomen, abdominal — continued
    wall — continued
      left — continued
        upper quadrant — continued
          with — continued
            penetration into peritoneal cavity S31.611- ☑
              with foreign body S31.621- ☑
        periumbilic region S31.115- ☑
          with
            foreign body S31.125- ☑
            penetration into peritoneal cavity S31.615- ☑
              with foreign body S31.625- ☑
        right
          lower quadrant S31.113- ☑
            with
              foreign body S31.123- ☑
              penetration into peritoneal cavity S31.613- ☑
                with foreign body S31.623- ☑
          upper quadrant S31.110- ☑
            with
              foreign body S31.120- ☑
              penetration into peritoneal cavity S31.610- ☑
                with foreign body S31.620- ☑
  accidental, complicating surgery — see Complications, surgical, accidental puncture or laceration
  Achilles tendon S86.02- ☑
  adrenal gland S37.813- ☑
  alveolar (process) — see Laceration, oral cavity
  ankle S91.01- ☑
    with
      foreign body S91.02- ☑
  antecubital space — see Laceration, elbow
  anus (sphincter) S31.831- ☑
    with
      ectopic or molar pregnancy O08.6
      foreign body S31.832- ☑
    complicating delivery — see Delivery, complicated, by, laceration, anus (sphincter)
    following ectopic or molar pregnancy O08.6
    nontraumatic, nonpuerperal — see Fissure, anus
  arm (upper) S41.11- ☑
    with foreign body S41.12- ☑
    lower — see Laceration, forearm
  auditory canal (external) (meatus) — see Laceration, ear
  auricle, ear — see Laceration, ear
  axilla — see Laceration, arm
  back — see also Laceration, thorax, back
    lower S31.010- ☑
      with
        foreign body S31.020- ☑
        with penetration into retroperitoneal space S31.021- ☑
        penetration into retroperitoneal space S31.011- ☑
  bile duct S36.13- ☑
  bladder S37.23- ☑
    with ectopic or molar pregnancy O08.6
    following ectopic or molar pregnancy O08.6
    obstetrical trauma O71.5
  blood vessel — see Injury, blood vessel
  bowel — see also Laceration, intestine
    with ectopic or molar pregnancy O08.6
    complicating abortion — see Abortion, by type, complicated by, specified condition NEC
    following ectopic or molar pregnancy O08.6
    obstetrical trauma O71.5
  brain (any part) (cortex) (diffuse) (membrane) — see also Injury, intracranial, diffuse
    during birth P10.8
      with hemorrhage P10.1
    focal — see Injury, intracranial, focal brain injury
  brainstem S06.38- ☑
  breast S21.01- ☑
    with foreign body S21.02- ☑
  broad ligament S37.893- ☑
    with ectopic or molar pregnancy O08.6
    following ectopic or molar pregnancy O08.6
    laceration syndrome N83.8
    obstetrical trauma O71.6
    syndrome (laceration) N83.8
  buttock S31.801- ☑
    with foreign body S31.802- ☑

Laceration — continued
  buttock — continued
    left S31.821- ☑
      with foreign body S31.822- ☑
    right S31.811- ☑
      with foreign body S31.812- ☑
  calf — see Laceration, leg
  canaliculus lacrimalis — see Laceration, eyelid
  canthus, eye — see Laceration, eyelid
  capsule, joint — see Sprain
  causing eversion of cervix uteri (old) N86
  central (perineal), complicating delivery O70.9
  cerebellum, traumatic S06.37- ☑
  cerebral S06.33- ☑
    during birth P10.8
      with hemorrhage P10.1
    left side S06.32- ☑
    right side S06.31- ☑
  cervix (uteri)
    with ectopic or molar pregnancy O08.6
    following ectopic or molar pregnancy O08.6
    nonpuerperal, nontraumatic N88.1
    obstetrical trauma (current) O71.3
    old (postpartal) N88.1
    traumatic S37.63- ☑
  cheek (external) S01.41- ☑
    with foreign body S01.42- ☑
    internal — see Laceration, oral cavity
  chest wall — see Laceration, thorax
  chin — see Laceration, head, specified site NEC
  chordae tendinae NEC I51.1
    concurrent with acute myocardial infarction — see Infarct, myocardium
    following acute myocardial infarction (current complication) I23.4
  clitoris — see Laceration, vulva
  colon — see Laceration, intestine, large, colon
  common bile duct S36.13- ☑
  cortex (cerebral) — see Injury, intracranial, diffuse
  costal region — see Laceration, thorax
  cystic duct S36.13- ☑
  diaphragm S27.803- ☑
  digit(s)
    foot — see Laceration, toe
    hand — see Laceration, finger
  duodenum S36.430- ☑
  ear (canal) (external) S01.31- ☑
    with foreign body S01.32- ☑
    drum S09.2- ☑
  elbow S51.01- ☑
    with
      foreign body S51.02- ☑
  epididymis — see Laceration, testis
  epigastric region — see Laceration, abdomen, wall, epigastric region
  esophagus K22.89
    traumatic
      cervical S11.21- ☑
        with foreign body S11.22- ☑
      thoracic S27.813- ☑
  eye (ball) S05.3- ☑
    with prolapse or loss of intraocular tissue S05.2- ☑
    penetrating S05.6- ☑
  eyebrow — see Laceration, eyelid
  eyelid S01.11- ☑
    with foreign body S01.12- ☑
  face NEC — see Laceration, head, specified site NEC
  fallopian tube S37.539- ☑
    bilateral S37.532- ☑
    unilateral S37.531- ☑
  finger(s) S61.219- ☑
    with
      damage to nail S61.319- ☑
        with
          foreign body S61.329- ☑
      foreign body S61.229- ☑
    index S61.218- ☑
      with
        damage to nail S61.318- ☑
          with
            foreign body S61.328- ☑
        foreign body S61.228- ☑
      left S61.211- ☑
        with
          damage to nail S61.311- ☑
            with
              foreign body S61.321- ☑

Laceration — continued
  finger(s) — continued
    index — continued
      left — continued
        with — continued
          foreign body S61.221- ☑
      right S61.210- ☑
        with
          damage to nail S61.310- ☑
            with
              foreign body S61.320- ☑
          foreign body S61.220- ☑
    little S61.218- ☑
      with
        damage to nail S61.318- ☑
          with
            foreign body S61.328- ☑
        foreign body S61.228- ☑
      left S61.217- ☑
        with
          damage to nail S61.317- ☑
            with
              foreign body S61.327- ☑
          foreign body S61.227- ☑
      right S61.216- ☑
        with
          damage to nail S61.316- ☑
            with
              foreign body S61.326- ☑
          foreign body S61.226- ☑
    middle S61.218- ☑
      with
        damage to nail S61.318- ☑
          with
            foreign body S61.328- ☑
        foreign body S61.228- ☑
      left S61.213- ☑
        with
          damage to nail S61.313- ☑
            with
              foreign body S61.323- ☑
          foreign body S61.223- ☑
      right S61.212- ☑
        with
          damage to nail S61.312- ☑
            with
              foreign body S61.322- ☑
          foreign body S61.222- ☑
    ring S61.218- ☑
      with
        damage to nail S61.318- ☑
          with
            foreign body S61.328- ☑
        foreign body S61.228- ☑
      left S61.215- ☑
        with
          damage to nail S61.315- ☑
            with
              foreign body S61.325- ☑
          foreign body S61.225- ☑
      right S61.214- ☑
        with
          damage to nail S61.314- ☑
            with
              foreign body S61.324- ☑
          foreign body S61.224- ☑
  flank S31.11A- ☑
    with
      foreign body S31.12A- ☑
      penetration into peritoneal cavity S31.61A- ☑
        with foreign body S31.62A- ☑
    left S31.117- ☑
      with
        foreign body S31.127- ☑
        penetration into peritoneal cavity S31.617- ☑
          with foreign body S31.627- ☑
    right S31.116- ☑
      with
        foreign body S31.126- ☑
        penetration into peritoneal cavity S31.616- ☑
          with foreign body S31.626- ☑
  foot (except toe(s) alone) S91.319- ☑
    with foreign body S91.329- ☑
    left S91.312- ☑
      with foreign body S91.322- ☑
    right S91.311- ☑

☑ ADDITIONAL CHARACTER REQUIRED — Refer to the Tabular List for Character Selection

Laceration — *continued*
- foot(s alone) — *continued*
  - right — *continued*
    - with foreign body S91.321- ☑
    - toe — *see* Laceration, toe
- forearm S51.819- ☑
  - with
    - foreign body S51.829- ☑
  - elbow only — *see* Laceration, elbow
  - left S51.812- ☑
    - with
      - foreign body S51.822- ☑
  - right S51.811- ☑
    - with
      - foreign body S51.821- ☑
- forehead S01.81- ☑
  - with foreign body S01.82- ☑
- fourchette O70.0
  - with ectopic or molar pregnancy O08.6
  - complicating delivery O70.0
  - following ectopic or molar pregnancy O08.6
- gallbladder S36.123- ☑
- genital organs, external
  - female S31.512- ☑
    - with foreign body S31.522- ☑
    - vagina — *see* Laceration, vagina
    - vulva — *see* Laceration, vulva
  - male S31.511- ☑
    - with foreign body S31.521- ☑
    - penis — *see* Laceration, penis
    - scrotum — *see* Laceration, scrotum
    - testis — *see* Laceration, testis
- groin — *see* Laceration, abdomen, wall
- gum — *see* Laceration, oral cavity
- hand S61.419- ☑
  - with
    - foreign body S61.429- ☑
  - finger — *see* Laceration, finger
  - left S61.412- ☑
    - with
      - foreign body S61.422- ☑
  - right S61.411- ☑
    - with
      - foreign body S61.421- ☑
  - thumb — *see* Laceration, thumb
- head S01.91- ☑
  - with foreign body S01.92- ☑
  - cheek — *see* Laceration, cheek
  - ear — *see* Laceration, ear
  - eyelid — *see* Laceration, eyelid
  - lip — *see* Laceration, lip
  - nose — *see* Laceration, nose
  - oral cavity — *see* Laceration, oral cavity
  - scalp S01.01- ☑
    - with foreign body S01.02- ☑
  - specified site NEC S01.81- ☑
    - with foreign body S01.82- ☑
  - temporomandibular area — *see* Laceration, cheek
- heart — *see* Injury, heart, laceration
- heel — *see* Laceration, foot
- hepatic duct S36.13- ☑
- hip S71.019- ☑
  - with foreign body S71.029- ☑
  - left S71.012- ☑
    - with foreign body S71.022- ☑
  - right S71.011- ☑
    - with foreign body S71.021- ☑
- hymen — *see* Laceration, vagina
- hypochondrium — *see* Laceration, abdomen, wall
- hypogastric region — *see* Laceration, abdomen, wall
- ileum S36.438- ☑
- inguinal region — *see* Laceration, abdomen, wall
- instep — *see* Laceration, foot
- internal organ — *see* Injury, by site
- interscapular region — *see* Laceration, thorax, back
- intestine
  - large
    - colon S36.539- ☑
      - ascending S36.530- ☑
      - descending S36.532- ☑
      - sigmoid S36.533- ☑
      - specified site NEC S36.538- ☑
      - rectum S36.63- ☑
      - transverse S36.531- ☑
  - small S36.439- ☑
    - duodenum S36.430- ☑
    - specified site NEC S36.438- ☑

Laceration — *continued*
- intra-abdominal organ S36.93- ☑
  - intestine — *see* Laceration, intestine
  - liver — *see* Laceration, liver
  - pancreas — *see* Laceration, pancreas
  - peritoneum S36.81- ☑
  - specified site NEC S36.893- ☑
  - spleen — *see* Laceration, spleen
  - stomach — *see* Laceration, stomach
- intracranial NEC — *see also* Injury, intracranial, diffuse
  - birth injury P10.9
- jaw — *see* Laceration, head, specified site NEC
- jejunum S36.438- ☑
- joint capsule — *see* Sprain, by site
- kidney S37.03- ☑
  - major (greater than 3 cm) (massive) (stellate) S37.06- ☑
  - minor (less than 1 cm) S37.04- ☑
  - moderate (1 to 3 cm) S37.05- ☑
    - multiple S37.06- ☑
- knee S81.01- ☑
  - with foreign body S81.02- ☑
- labium (majus) (minus) — *see* Laceration, vulva
- lacrimal duct — *see* Laceration, eyelid
- large intestine — *see* Laceration, intestine, large
- larynx S11.011- ☑
  - with foreign body S11.012- ☑
- leg (lower) S81.819- ☑
  - with foreign body S81.829- ☑
  - foot — *see* Laceration, foot
  - knee — *see* Laceration, knee
  - left S81.812- ☑
    - with foreign body S81.822- ☑
  - right S81.811- ☑
    - with foreign body S81.821- ☑
  - upper — *see* Laceration, thigh
- ligament — *see* Sprain
- lip S01.511- ☑
  - with foreign body S01.521- ☑
- liver S36.113- ☑
  - major (stellate) S36.116- ☑
  - minor S36.114- ☑
  - moderate S36.115- ☑
- loin — *see* Laceration, abdomen, wall
- lower back — *see* Laceration, back, lower
- lumbar region — *see* Laceration, back, lower
- lung S27.339- ☑
  - bilateral S27.332- ☑
  - unilateral S27.331- ☑
- malar region — *see* Laceration, head, specified site NEC
- mammary — *see* Laceration, breast
- mastoid region — *see* Laceration, head, specified site NEC
- meninges — *see* Injury, intracranial, diffuse
- meniscus — *see* Tear, meniscus
- mesentery S36.893- ☑
- mesosalpinx S37.893- ☑
- mouth — *see* Laceration, oral cavity
- muscle — *see* Injury, muscle, by site, laceration
- nail
  - finger — *see* Laceration, finger, with damage to nail
  - toe — *see* Laceration, toe, with damage to nail
- nasal (septum) (sinus) — *see* Laceration, nose
- nasopharynx — *see* Laceration, head, specified site NEC
- neck S11.91- ☑
  - with foreign body S11.92- ☑
  - involving
    - cervical esophagus S11.21- ☑
      - with foreign body S11.22- ☑
    - larynx — *see* Laceration, larynx
    - pharynx — *see* Laceration, pharynx
    - thyroid gland — *see* Laceration, thyroid gland
    - trachea — *see* Laceration, trachea
  - specified site NEC S11.81- ☑
    - with foreign body S11.82- ☑
- nerve — *see* Injury, nerve
- nose (septum) (sinus) S01.21- ☑
  - with foreign body S01.22- ☑
- ocular NOS S05.3- ☑
  - adnexa NOS S01.11- ☑
- oral cavity S01.512- ☑
  - with foreign body S01.522- ☑
- orbit (eye) — *see* Wound, open, ocular, orbit
- ovary S37.439- ☑
  - bilateral S37.432- ☑
  - unilateral S37.431- ☑
- palate — *see* Laceration, oral cavity

Laceration — *continued*
- palm — *see* Laceration, hand
- pancreas S36.239- ☑
- pelvic S31.010- ☑
  - with
    - foreign body S31.020- ☑
      - penetration into retroperitoneal cavity S31.021- ☑
    - penetration into retroperitoneal cavity S31.011- ☑
  - floor — *see also* Laceration, back, lower
    - with ectopic or molar pregnancy O08.6
    - complicating delivery O70.1
    - following ectopic or molar pregnancy O08.6
    - old (postpartal) N81.89
  - organ S37.93- ☑
- penis S31.21- ☑
  - with foreign body S31.22- ☑
- perineum
  - female S31.41- ☑
    - with
      - ectopic or molar pregnancy O08.6
      - foreign body S31.42- ☑
    - during delivery O70.9
      - first degree O70.0
      - fourth degree O70.3
      - second degree O70.1
      - third degree — *see also* Delivery, complicated, by, laceration, perineum, third degree O70.20
    - old (postpartal) N81.89
    - postpartal N81.89
    - secondary (postpartal) O90.1
  - male S31.119- ☑
    - with foreign body S31.129- ☑
- periocular area (with or without lacrimal passages) — *see* Laceration, eyelid
- peritoneum S36.81- ☑
- periumbilic region — *see* Laceration, abdomen, wall, periumbilic
- periurethral tissue — *see* Laceration, urethra
- phalanges
  - finger — *see* Laceration, finger
  - toe — *see* Laceration, toe
- pharynx S11.21- ☑
  - with foreign body S11.22- ☑
- pinna — *see* Laceration, ear
- popliteal space — *see* Laceration, knee
- prepuce — *see* Laceration, penis
- prostate S37.823- ☑
- pubic region S31.119- ☑
  - with foreign body S31.129- ☑
- pudendum — *see* Laceration, genital organs, external
- rectovaginal septum — *see* Laceration, vagina
- rectum S36.63- ☑
- retroperitoneum S36.893- ☑
- round ligament S37.893- ☑
- sacral region — *see* Laceration, back, lower
- sacroiliac region — *see* Laceration, back, lower
- salivary gland — *see* Laceration, oral cavity
- scalp S01.01- ☑
  - with foreign body S01.02- ☑
- scapular region — *see* Laceration, shoulder
- scrotum S31.31- ☑
  - with foreign body S31.32- ☑
- seminal vesicle S37.893- ☑
- shin — *see* Laceration, leg
- shoulder S41.019- ☑
  - with foreign body S41.029- ☑
  - left S41.012- ☑
    - with foreign body S41.022- ☑
  - right S41.011- ☑
    - with foreign body S41.021- ☑
- small intestine — *see* Laceration, intestine, small
- spermatic cord — *see* Laceration, testis
- spinal cord (meninges) — *see also* Injury, spinal cord, by region
  - due to injury at birth P11.5
  - newborn (birth injury) P11.5
- spleen S36.039- ☑
  - major (massive) (stellate) S36.032- ☑
  - moderate S36.031- ☑
  - superficial (minor) S36.030- ☑
- sternal region — *see* Laceration, thorax, front
- stomach S36.33- ☑
- submaxillary region — *see* Laceration, head, specified site NEC

☑ Additional Character Required — Refer to the Tabular List for Character Selection

Laceration — continued
- submental region — see Laceration, head, specified site NEC
- subungual
  - finger(s) — see Laceration, finger, with damage to nail
  - toe(s) — see Laceration, toe, with damage to nail
- suprarenal gland — see Laceration, adrenal gland
- temple, temporal region — see Laceration, head, specified site NEC
- temporomandibular area — see Laceration, cheek
- tendon — see Injury, muscle, by site, laceration
  - Achilles S86.02-
- tentorium cerebelli — see Injury, intracranial, diffuse
- testis S31.31-
  - with foreign body S31.32-
- thigh S71.11-
  - with foreign body S71.12-
- thorax, thoracic (wall) S21.91-
  - with foreign body S21.92-
  - back S21.22-
    - with penetration into thoracic cavity S21.42-
  - front S21.12-
    - with penetration into thoracic cavity S21.32-
  - back S21.21-
    - with
      - foreign body S21.22-
        - with penetration into thoracic cavity S21.42-
      - penetration into thoracic cavity S21.41-
  - breast — see Laceration, breast
  - front S21.11-
    - with
      - foreign body S21.12-
        - with penetration into thoracic cavity S21.32-
      - penetration into thoracic cavity S21.31-
- thumb S61.019-
  - with
    - damage to nail S61.119-
      - with
        - foreign body S61.129-
    - foreign body S61.029-
  - left S61.012-
    - with
      - damage to nail S61.112-
        - with
          - foreign body S61.122-
      - foreign body S61.022-
  - right S61.011-
    - with
      - damage to nail S61.111-
        - with
          - foreign body S61.121-
      - foreign body S61.021-
- thyroid gland S11.11-
  - with foreign body S11.12-
- toe(s) S91.119-
  - with
    - damage to nail S91.219-
      - with
        - foreign body S91.229-
    - foreign body S91.129-
  - great S91.113-
    - with
      - damage to nail S91.213-
        - with
          - foreign body S91.223-
      - foreign body S91.123-
    - left S91.112-
      - with
        - damage to nail S91.212-
          - with
            - foreign body S91.222-
        - foreign body S91.122-
    - right S91.111-
      - with
        - damage to nail S91.211-
          - with
            - foreign body S91.221-
        - foreign body S91.121-
  - lesser S91.116-
    - with
      - damage to nail S91.216-
        - with
          - foreign body S91.226-

Laceration — continued
- toe(s) — continued
  - lesser — continued
    - with — continued
      - foreign body S91.126-
    - left S91.115-
      - with
        - damage to nail S91.215-
          - with
            - foreign body S91.225-
        - foreign body S91.125-
    - right S91.114-
      - with
        - damage to nail S91.214-
          - with
            - foreign body S91.224-
        - foreign body S91.124-
- tongue — see Laceration, oral cavity
- trachea S11.021-
  - with foreign body S11.022-
- tunica vaginalis — see Laceration, testis
- tympanum, tympanic membrane — see Laceration, ear, drum
- umbilical region S31.115-
  - with foreign body S31.125-
- ureter S37.13-
- urethra S37.33-
  - with or following ectopic or molar pregnancy O08.6
  - obstetrical trauma O71.5
- urinary organ NEC S37.893-
- uterus S37.63-
  - with ectopic or molar pregnancy O08.6
  - following ectopic or molar pregnancy O08.6
  - nonpuerperal, nontraumatic N85.8
  - obstetrical trauma NEC O71.81
  - old (postpartal) N85.8
- uvula — see Laceration, oral cavity
- vagina S31.41-
  - with
    - ectopic or molar pregnancy O08.6
    - foreign body S31.42-
  - during delivery O71.4
    - with perineal laceration — see Laceration, perineum, female, during delivery
  - following ectopic or molar pregnancy O08.6
  - nonpuerperal, nontraumatic N89.8
  - old (postpartal) N89.8
- vas deferens S37.893-
- vesical — see Laceration, bladder
- vocal cords S11.031-
  - with foreign body S11.032-
- vulva S31.41-
  - with
    - ectopic or molar pregnancy O08.6
    - foreign body S31.42-
  - complicating delivery O70.0
  - following ectopic or molar pregnancy O08.6
  - nonpuerperal, nontraumatic N90.89
  - old (postpartal) N90.89
- wrist S61.519-
  - with
    - foreign body S61.529-
  - left S61.512-
    - with
      - foreign body S61.522-
  - right S61.511-
    - with
      - foreign body S61.521-

Lack of
- achievement in school Z55.3
- adequate
  - food Z59.48
  - intermaxillary vertical dimension of fully erupted teeth M26.36
  - sleep Z72.820
- air conditioning Z59.11
- appetite (see Anorexia) R63.0
- awareness R41.9
- basic services in physical environment Z58.81
- care
  - in home Z74.2
  - of infant (at or after birth) T76.02-
    - confirmed T74.02-
- cognitive functions R41.9
- coordination R27.9
  - ataxia R27.0
  - specified type NEC R27.8

Lack of — continued
- development (physiological) R62.50
  - failure to thrive (child over 28 days old) R62.51
    - adult R62.7
    - newborn P92.6
  - short stature R62.52
  - specified type NEC R62.59
- electricity services Z59.12
- emotional support Z60.8
- energy R53.83
- financial resources Z59.6
- food Z59.48
- gas services Z59.12
- growth R62.52
- heating Z59.11
- housing (permanent) (temporary) Z59.00
  - adequate Z59.10
- learning experiences in childhood Z62.898
- leisure time (affecting life-style) Z73.2
- material resources due to limited financial resources, specified NEC Z59.87
- memory — see also Amnesia
  - mild, following organic brain damage F06.8
- oil services Z59.12
- ovulation N97.0
- parental supervision or control of child Z62.0
- person able to render necessary care Z74.2
- physical exercise Z72.3
- play experience in childhood Z62.898
- posterior occlusal support M26.57
- relaxation (affecting life-style) Z73.2
- safe drinking water Z58.6
- sexual
  - desire F52.0
  - enjoyment F52.1
- shelter Z59.02
- sleep (adequate) Z72.820
- supervision of child by parent Z62.0
- support, posterior occlusal M26.57
- transportation Z59.82
- water T73.1-
  - safe drinking Z58.6
  - services Z59.12

Lacrimal — see condition
Lacrimation, abnormal — see Epiphora
Lacrimonasal duct — see condition
Lactate, elevated — see Acidosis, lactic
Lactation, lactating (breast) (puerperal, postpartum)
- associated
  - cracked nipple O92.13
  - retracted nipple O92.03
- defective O92.4
- disorder NEC O92.79
- excessive O92.6
- failed (complete) O92.3
  - partial O92.4
- mastitis NEC — see Mastitis, obstetric
- mother (care and/or examination) Z39.1
- nonpuerperal N64.3

Lacticemia, excessive — see also Acidosis E87.20
Lacunar skull Q75.8
LAD (leukocyte adhesion deficiency) (LAD-I) (LAD-II) (LAD-III) D71.1
Laennec's cirrhosis K70.30
- with ascites K70.31
- nonalcoholic K74.69

Lafora disease — see also Epilepsy, progressive, Lafora G40.C09
Lag, lid (nervous) — see Retraction, lid
Lagophthalmos (eyelid) (nervous) H02.209
- bilateral, upper and lower eyelids H02.20C
- cicatricial H02.219
  - bilateral, upper and lower eyelids H02.21C
  - left H02.216
    - lower H02.215
    - upper H02.214
    - upper and lower eyelids H02.21B
  - right H02.213
    - lower H02.212
    - upper H02.211
    - upper and lower eyelids H02.21A
- keratoconjunctivitis — see Keratoconjunctivitis
- left H02.206
  - lower H02.205
  - upper H02.204
  - upper and lower eyelids H02.20B
- mechanical H02.229
  - bilateral, upper and lower eyelids H02.22C
  - left H02.226

Lagophthalmos — *continued*
  mechanical — *continued*
    left — *continued*
      lower H02.225
      upper H02.224
      upper and lower eyelids H02.22B
    right H02.223
      lower H02.222
      upper H02.221
      upper and lower eyelids H02.22A
  paralytic H02.239
    bilateral, upper and lower eyelids H02.23C
    left H02.236
      lower H02.235
      upper H02.234
      upper and lower eyelids H02.23B
    right H02.233
      lower H02.232
      upper H02.231
      upper and lower eyelids H02.23A
  right H02.203
    lower H02.202
    upper H02.201
    upper and lower eyelids H02.20A
Laki-Lorand factor deficiency — *see* Defect, coagulation, specified type NEC
Lalling F80.0
Lambert-Eaton syndrome — *see* Syndrome, Lambert-Eaton
Lambliasis, lambliosis A07.1
Landau-Kleffner syndrome — *see* Epilepsy, specified NEC
Landouzy-Dejerine dystrophy or facioscapulohumeral atrophy G71.02
Landouzy's disease (icterohemorrhagic leptospirosis) A27.0
Landry-Guillain-Barre, syndrome or paralysis G61.0
Landry's disease or paralysis G61.0
Lane's
  band Q43.3
  kink — *see* Obstruction, intestine
  syndrome K90.2
Langdon Down syndrome — *see* Trisomy, 21
Lapsed immunization schedule status Z28.39
Large
  baby (regardless of gestational age) (4000g to 4499g) P08.1
  ear, congenital Q17.1
  physiological cup Q14.2
  stature R68.89
Large-for-dates NEC (infant) (4000g to 4499g) P08.1
  affecting management of pregnancy O36.6- ☑
  exceptionally (4500g or more) P08.0
Larsen-Johansson disease or osteochondrosis — *see* Osteochondrosis, juvenile, patella
Larsen's syndrome (flattened facies and multiple congenital dislocations) Q74.8
Larva migrans
  cutaneous B76.9
    Ancylostoma B76.0
  visceral B83.0
Laryngeal — *see* condition
Laryngismus (stridulus) J38.5
  congenital P28.89
  diphtheritic A36.2
Laryngitis (acute) (edematous) (fibrinous) (infective) (infiltrative) (malignant) (membranous) (phlegmonous) (pneumococcal) (pseudomembranous) (septic) (subglottic) (suppurative) (ulcerative) J04.0
  with
    influenza, flu, or grippe — *see* Influenza, with, laryngitis
    tracheitis (acute) — *see* Laryngotracheitis
  atrophic J37.0
  catarrhal J37.0
  chronic J37.0
    with tracheitis (chronic) J37.1
  diphtheritic A36.2
  due to external agent — *see* Inflammation, respiratory, upper, due to
  H. influenzae J04.0
  Hemophilus influenzae J04.0
  hypertrophic J37.0
  influenzal — *see* Influenza, with, respiratory manifestations NEC
  obstructive J05.0
  sicca J37.0
  spasmodic J05.0
    acute J04.0
  streptococcal J04.0
  stridulous J05.0

Laryngitis — *continued*
  syphilitic (late) A52.73
    congenital A50.59 *[J99]*
    early A50.03 *[J99]*
  tuberculous A15.5
  Vincent's A69.1
Laryngocele (congenital) (ventricular) Q31.3
Laryngofissure J38.7
  congenital Q31.8
Laryngomalacia (congenital) Q31.5
Laryngopharyngitis (acute) J06.0
  chronic J37.0
  due to external agent — *see* Inflammation, respiratory, upper, due to
Laryngoplegia J38.00
  bilateral J38.02
  unilateral J38.01
Laryngoptosis J38.7
Laryngospasm J38.5
Laryngostenosis J38.6
Laryngotracheitis (acute) (Infectional) (infective) (viral) J04.2
  atrophic J37.1
  catarrhal J37.1
  chronic J37.1
  diphtheritic A36.2
  due to external agent — *see* Inflammation, respiratory, upper, due to
  Hemophilus influenzae J04.2
  hypertrophic J37.1
  influenzal — *see* Influenza, with, respiratory manifestations NEC
  pachydermic J38.7
  sicca J37.1
  spasmodic J38.5
    acute J05.0
  streptococcal J04.2
  stridulous J38.5
  syphilitic (late) A52.73
    congenital A50.59 *[J99]*
    early A50.03 *[J99]*
  tuberculous A15.5
  Vincent's A69.1
Laryngotracheobronchitis — *see* Bronchitis
Larynx, laryngeal — *see* condition
Lassa fever A96.2
Lassitude — *see* Weakness
Late
  talker R62.0
  walker R62.0
Late effect(s) — *see* Sequelae
Latent — *see* condition
Laterocession — *see* Lateroversion
Lateroflexion — *see* Lateroversion
Lateroversion
  cervix — *see* Lateroversion, uterus
  uterus, uterine (cervix) (postinfectional) (postpartal, old) N85.4
    congenital Q51.818
    in pregnancy or childbirth O34.59- ☑
Lathyrism — *see* Poisoning, food, noxious, plant
Launois-Bensaude adenolipomatosis E88.89
Launois' syndrome (pituitary gigantism) E22.0
Laurence-Moon syndrome Q87.84
Lax, laxity — *see also* Relaxation
  ligament (ous) — *see also* Disorder, ligament
    familial M35.7
    knee — *see* Derangement, knee
  skin (acquired) L57.4
    congenital Q82.8
Laxative habit F55.2
Lazy leukocyte syndrome D70.8
LBSL (leukoencephalopathy with brainstem - spinal cord involvement - lactate elevation) E88.43
Lead miner's lung J63.6
Leak, leakage
  air NEC J93.82
    postprocedural J95.812
  amniotic fluid — *see* Rupture, membranes, premature
  blood (microscopic), fetal, into maternal circulation affecting management of pregnancy — *see* Pregnancy, complicated by
  cerebrospinal fluid G96.00
    cranial
      postoperative G96.08
      specified NEC G96.08
      spontaneous G96.01
      traumatic G96.08
      from spinal (lumbar) puncture G97.0

Leak, leakage — *continued*
  cerebrospinal fluid — *continued*
    spinal
      postoperative G96.09
      post-traumatic G96.09
      specified NEC G96.09
      spontaneous G96.02
    spontaneous
      from
        skull base G96.01
        spine G96.02
  CSF — *see* Leak, cerebrospinal fluid
  device, implant or graft — *see also* Complications, by site and type, mechanical
    arterial graft NEC — *see* Complication, vascular, graft, mechanical, leakage T82.838- ☑
    breast (implant) T85.43- ☑
    catheter NEC T85.638- ☑
      dialysis (renal) T82.43- ☑
        intraperitoneal T85.631- ☑
      infusion NEC T82.534- ☑
        spinal (epidural) (subdural) T85.630- ☑
      urinary T83.038- ☑
        cystostomy T83.030- ☑
        Hopkins T83.038- ☑
        ileostomy T83.038- ☑
        indwelling T83.031- ☑
        nephrostomy T83.032- ☑
        specified T83.038- ☑
        urostomy T83.038- ☑
    gastrointestinal — *see* Complications, prosthetic device, mechanical, gastrointestinal device
    genital NEC T83.498- ☑
      penile prosthesis (cylinder) (implanted) (pump) (reservoir) T83.490- ☑
      testicular prosthesis T83.491- ☑
    heart NEC — *see* Complication, cardiovascular device, mechanical
    joint prosthesis — *see* Complications, joint prosthesis, mechanical, specified NEC, by site
    ocular NEC — *see* Complications, prosthetic device, mechanical, ocular device
    orthopedic NEC — *see* Complication, orthopedic, device, mechanical
    persistent air J93.82
    specified NEC T85.638- ☑
    urinary NEC — *see also* Complication, genitourinary, device, urinary, mechanical
      graft T83.23- ☑
    vascular NEC — *see* Complication, cardiovascular device, mechanical
    ventricular intracranial shunt T85.03- ☑
  urine — *see* Incontinence
Leaky heart — *see* Endocarditis
Learning defect (specific) F81.9
Leather bottle stomach C16.9
Leber's
  congenital amaurosis H35.50
  optic atrophy (hereditary) H47.22
Lederer's anemia D59.19
Leeches (external) — *see* Hirudiniasis
Leg — *see* condition
Legg (-Calve)-Perthes disease, syndrome or osteochondrosis M91.1- ☑
Legionellosis A48.1
  nonpneumonic A48.2
Legionnaires'
  disease A48.1
    nonpneumonic A48.2
  pneumonia A48.1
Leigh's disease G31.82
Leiner's disease L21.1
Leiofibromyoma — *see* Leiomyoma
Leiomyoblastoma — *see* Neoplasm, connective tissue, benign
Leiomyofibroma — *see also* Neoplasm, connective tissue, benign
  uterus (cervix) (corpus) D25.9
Leiomyoma — *see also* Neoplasm, connective tissue, benign
  bizarre — *see* Neoplasm, connective tissue, benign
  cellular — *see* Neoplasm, connective tissue, benign
  epithelioid — *see* Neoplasm, connective tissue, benign
  uterus (cervix) (corpus) D25.9
    intramural D25.1
    submucous D25.0
    subserosal D25.2
  vascular — *see* Neoplasm, connective tissue, benign

☑ **Additional Character Required** — Refer to the Tabular List for Character Selection

Leiomyoma, leiomyomatosis (intravascular) — see Neoplasm, connective tissue, uncertain behavior
Leiomyosarcoma — see also Neoplasm, connective tissue, malignant
　epithelioid — see Neoplasm, connective tissue, malignant
　myxoid — see Neoplasm, connective tissue, malignant
Leishmaniasis B55.9
　American (mucocutaneous) B55.2
　　cutaneous B55.1
　Asian Desert B55.1
　Brazilian B55.2
　cutaneous (any type) B55.1
　dermal — see also Leishmaniasis, cutaneous
　　post-kala-azar B55.0
　eyelid B55.1
　infantile B55.0
　Mediterranean B55.0
　mucocutaneous (American) (New World) B55.2
　naso-oral B55.2
　nasopharyngeal B55.2
　old world B55.1
　tegumentaria diffusa B55.1
　visceral B55.0
Leishmanoid, dermal — see also Leishmaniasis, cutaneous
　post-kala-azar B55.0
Lenegre's disease I44.2
Lengthening, leg — see Deformity, limb, unequal length
Lennert's lymphoma — see Lymphoma, Lennert's
Lennox-Gastaut syndrome G40.812
　intractable G40.814
　　with status epilepticus G40.813
　　without status epilepticus G40.814
　not intractable G40.812
　　with status epilepticus G40.811
　　without status epilepticus G40.812
Lens — see condition
Lenticonus (anterior) (posterior) (congenital) Q12.8
Lenticular degeneration, progressive E83.01
Lentiglobus (posterior) (congenital) Q12.8
Lentigo (congenital) L81.4
　maligna — see also Melanoma, in situ
　　melanoma — see Melanoma
Lentivirus, as cause of disease classified elsewhere B97.31
Leontiasis
　ossium M85.2
　syphilitic (late) A52.78
　　congenital A50.59
Lepothrix A48.8
Lepra — see Leprosy
Leprechaunism E34.8
Leprosy A30.- ☑
　with muscle disorder A30.9 [M63.80]
　　ankle A30.9 [M63.87-] ☑
　　foot A30.9 [M63.87-] ☑
　　forearm A30.9 [M63.83-] ☑
　　hand A30.9 [M63.84-] ☑
　　lower leg A30.9 [M63.86-] ☑
　　multiple sites A30.9 [M63.89]
　　pelvic region A30.9 [M63.85-] ☑
　　shoulder region A30.9 [M63.81-] ☑
　　specified site NEC A30.9 [M63.88]
　　thigh A30.9 [M63.85-] ☑
　　upper arm A30.9 [M63.82-] ☑
　anesthetic A30.9
　BB A30.3
　BL A30.4
　borderline (infiltrated) (neuritic) A30.3
　　lepromatous A30.4
　　tuberculoid A30.2
　BT A30.2
　dimorphous (infiltrated) (neuritic) A30.3
　I A30.0
　indeterminate (macular) (neuritic) A30.0
　lepromatous (diffuse) (infiltrated) (macular) (neuritic) (nodular) A30.5
　LL A30.5
　macular (early) (neuritic) (simple) A30.9
　maculoanesthetic A30.9
　mixed A30.3
　neural A30.9
　nodular A30.5
　primary neuritic A30.3
　specified type NEC A30.8
　TT A30.1
　tuberculoid (major) (minor) A30.1
Leptocytosis, hereditary D56.9

Leptomeningitis (chronic) (circumscribed) (hemorrhagic) (nonsuppurative) — see Meningitis
Leptomeningopathy G96.198
Leptospiral — see condition
Leptospirochetal — see condition
Leptospirosis A27.9
　canicola A27.89
　due to Leptospira interrogans serovar icterohaemorrhagiae A27.0
　icterohemorrhagica A27.0
　pomona A27.89
　Weil's disease A27.0
Leptus dermatitis B88.09
Leri-Weill syndrome Q77.8
Leriche's syndrome (aortic bifurcation occlusion) I74.09
Leri's pleonosteosis Q78.8
Lermoyez' syndrome — see Vertigo, peripheral NEC
Lesch-Nyhan syndrome E79.1
Leser-Trélat disease L82.1
　inflamed L82.0
Lesion(s) (nontraumatic)
　abducens nerve — see Strabismus, paralytic, sixth nerve
　alveolar process K08.9
　angiocentric immunoproliferative D47.Z9 (following D47.4)
　anorectal K62.9
　aortic (valve) I35.9
　auditory nerve — see subcategory H93.3- ☑
　basal ganglion G25.9
　bile duct — see Disease, bile duct
　biomechanical M99.9
　　specified type NEC M99.89
　　　abdomen M99.89
　　　acromioclavicular M99.87
　　　cervical region M99.81
　　　cervicothoracic M99.81
　　　costochondral M99.88
　　　costovertebral M99.88
　　　head region M99.80
　　　hip M99.85
　　　lower extremity M99.86
　　　lumbar region M99.83
　　　lumbosacral M99.83
　　　occipitocervical M99.80
　　　pelvic region M99.85
　　　pubic M99.85
　　　rib cage M99.88
　　　sacral region M99.84
　　　sacrococcygeal M99.84
　　　sacroiliac M99.84
　　　specified NEC M99.89
　　　sternochondral M99.88
　　　sternoclavicular M99.87
　　　thoracic region M99.82
　　　thoracolumbar M99.82
　　　upper extremity M99.87
　bladder N32.9
　bone — see Disorder, bone
　brachial plexus G54.0
　brain G93.9
　　congenital Q04.9
　　vascular I67.9
　　　degenerative I67.9
　　　hypertensive I67.4
　buccal cavity K13.79
　calcified — see Calcification
　cameron — see Ulcer, stomach
　canthus — see Disorder, eyelid
　carate — see Pinta, lesions
　cardia K31.9
　cardiac — see also Disease, heart I51.9
　　congenital Q24.9
　　valvular — see Endocarditis
　cauda equina G83.4
　cecum K63.9
　cerebral — see Lesion, brain
　cerebrovascular I67.9
　　degenerative I67.9
　　hypertensive I67.4
　cervical (nerve) root NEC G54.2
　chiasmal — see Disorder, optic, chiasm
　chorda tympani G51.8
　coin, lung R91.1
　colon K63.9
　combined periodontic - endodontic K05.5
　congenital — see Anomaly, by site
　conjunctiva H11.9
　conus medullaris — see Injury, conus medullaris
　coronary artery — see Ischemia, heart

Lesion(s) — continued
　cranial nerve G52.9
　　eighth — see Disorder, ear
　　eleventh G52.9
　　fifth G50.9
　　first G52.0
　　fourth — see Strabismus, paralytic, fourth nerve
　　seventh G51.9
　　sixth — see Strabismus, paralytic, sixth nerve
　　tenth G52.2
　　twelfth G52.3
　cystic — see Cyst
　degenerative — see Degeneration
　duodenum K31.9
　edentulous (alveolar) ridge, associated with trauma, due to traumatic occlusion K06.2
　en coup de sabre L94.1
　eyelid — see Disorder, eyelid
　gasserian ganglion G50.8
　gastric K31.9
　gastroduodenal K31.9
　gastrointestinal K63.9
　gingiva, associated with trauma K06.2
　glomerular
　　focal and segmental — see also N00-N07 with fourth character .1 N05.1
　　minimal change — see also N00-N07 with fourth character .0 N05.0
　heart (organic) — see Disease, heart
　hyperchromic, due to pinta (carate) A67.1
　hyperkeratotic — see Hyperkeratosis
　hypothalamic E23.7
　ileocecal K63.9
　ileum K63.9
　iliohypogastric nerve G57.8- ☑
　inflammatory — see Inflammation
　intestine K63.9
　intracerebral — see Lesion, brain
　intrachiasmal (optic) — see Disorder, optic, chiasm
　intracranial, space-occupying R90.0
　joint — see Disorder, joint
　　sacroiliac (old) M53.3
　keratotic — see Keratosis
　kidney — see Disease, renal
　laryngeal nerve (recurrent) G52.2
　lip K13.0
　liver K76.9
　lumbosacral
　　plexus G54.1
　　root (nerve) NEC G54.4
　lung (coin) R91.1
　maxillary sinus J32.0
　mitral I05.9
　Morel-Lavallée — see Hematoma, by site
　motor cortex NEC G93.89
　mouth K13.79
　nerve G58.9
　　femoral G57.2- ☑
　　median G56.1- ☑
　　　carpal tunnel syndrome — see Syndrome, carpal tunnel
　　plantar G57.6- ☑
　　popliteal (lateral) G57.3- ☑
　　　medial G57.4- ☑
　　radial G56.3- ☑
　　sciatic G57.0- ☑
　　spinal — see Injury, nerve, spinal
　　ulnar G56.2- ☑
　nervous system, congenital Q07.9
　nonallopathic — see Lesion, biomechanical
　nose (internal) J34.89
　obstructive — see Obstruction
　obturator nerve G57.8- ☑
　oral mucosa K13.70
　organ or site NEC — see Disease, by site
　osteolytic — see Osteolysis
　peptic K27.9
　periodontal, due to traumatic occlusion K05.5
　pharynx J39.2
　pigment, pigmented (skin) L81.9
　pinta — see Pinta, lesions
　polypoid — see Polyp
　prechiasmal (optic) — see Disorder, optic, chiasm
　primary — see also Syphilis, primary A51.0
　　carate A67.0
　　pinta A67.0
　　yaws A66.0
　pulmonary J98.4

Lesion(s) — continued
  pulmonary — continued
    valve I37.9
  pylorus K31.9
  rectosigmoid K63.9
  retina, retinal H35.9
  sacroiliac (joint) (old) M53.3
  salivary gland K11.9
    benign lymphoepithelial K11.8
  saphenous nerve G57.8- ☑
  sciatic nerve G57.0- ☑
  secondary — see Syphilis, secondary
  shoulder (region) M75.9- ☑
    specified NEC M75.8- ☑
  sigmoid K63.9
  sinus (accessory) (nasal) J34.89
  skin L98.9
    suppurative L08.0
  SLAP S43.43- ☑
  spinal cord G95.9
    congenital Q06.9
  spleen D73.89
  stomach K31.9
  superior glenoid labrum S43.43- ☑
  syphilitic — see Syphilis
  tertiary — see Syphilis, tertiary
  thoracic root (nerve) NEC G54.3
  tonsillar fossa J35.9
  tooth, teeth K08.9
    white spot
      chewing surface K02.51
      pit and fissure surface K02.51
      smooth surface K02.61
  traumatic — see specific type of injury by site
  tricuspid (valve) I07.9
    nonrheumatic I36.9
  trigeminal nerve G50.9
  ulcerated or ulcerative — see Ulcer, skin
  uterus N85.9
  vagina N89.8
  vagus nerve G52.2
  valvular — see Endocarditis
  vascular I99.9
    affecting central nervous system I67.9
    following trauma NEC T14.8- ☑
    umbilical cord, complicating delivery O69.5- ☑
  vulva N90.89
  warty — see Verruca
  white spot (tooth)
    chewing surface K02.51
    pit and fissure surface K02.51
    smooth surface K02.61
Less than a high school diploma Z55.5
Lethargic — see condition
Lethargy R53.83
Letterer-Siwe's disease C96.0
Leukemia, leukemic C95.9- ☑
  acute basophilic C94.8- ☑
  acute bilineal C95.0- ☑
  acute erythroid C94.0- ☑
  acute lymphoblastic C91.0- ☑
  acute megakaryoblastic C94.2- ☑
  acute megakaryocytic C94.2- ☑
  acute mixed lineage C95.0- ☑
  acute monoblastic (monoblastic/monocytic) C93.0- ☑
  acute monocytic (monoblastic/monocytic) C93.0- ☑
  acute myeloblastic (minimal differentiation) (with maturation) C92.0- ☑
  acute myeloid, NOS C92.0- ☑
    with
      11q23-abnormality C92.6- ☑
      dysplasia of remaining hematopoesis and/or myelodysplastic disease in its history C92.A- ☑ (following C92.6)
      multilineage dysplasia C92.A- ☑ (following C92.6)
      variation of MLL-gene C92.6- ☑
    M6 (a)(b) C94.0- ☑
    M7 C94.2- ☑
  acute myelomonocytic C92.5- ☑
  acute promyelocytic C92.4- ☑
  adult T-cell (HTLV-1-associated) (acute variant) (chronic variant) (lymphomatoid variant) (smouldering variant) C91.5- ☑
  aggressive NK-cell C94.8- ☑
  AML (1/ETO) (M0) (M1) (M2) (without a FAB classification) C92.0- ☑
  AML M3 C92.4- ☑

Leukemia, leukemic — continued
  AML M4 (Eo with inv(16) or t(16;16)) C92.5- ☑
  AML M5 C93.0- ☑
  AML M5a C93.0- ☑
  AML M5b C93.0- ☑
  AML Me with t (15;17) and variants C92.4- ☑
  atypical chronic myeloid, BCR/ABL-negative C92.2- ☑
  biphenotypic acute C95.0- ☑
  blast cell C95.0- ☑
  Burkitt-type, mature B-cell C91.A- ☑ (following C91.6)
  chronic eosinophilic — see also Syndrome, hypereosinophilic, myeloid C94.8- ☑
  chronic lymphocytic, of B-cell type C91.1- ☑
  chronic monocytic C93.1- ☑
  chronic myelogenous (Philadelphia chromosome (Ph1) positive) (t(9;22)) (q34;q11) (with crisis of blast cells) C92.1- ☑
  chronic myeloid, BCR/ABL-positive C92.1- ☑
    atypical, BCR/ABL-negative C92.2- ☑
  chronic myelomonocytic C93.1- ☑
  chronic neutrophilic D47.1
  CMML (-1) (-2) (with eosinophilia) C93.1- ☑
  granulocytic — see also Category C92 C92.9- ☑
  hairy cell C91.4- ☑
  juvenile myelomonocytic C93.3- ☑
  lymphoid C91.9- ☑
    specified NEC C91.Z- ☑ (following C91.6)
  mast cell C94.3- ☑
  mature B-cell, Burkitt-type C91.A- ☑ (following C91.6)
  monocytic (subacute) C93.9- ☑
    specified NEC C93.Z- ☑ (following C93.3)
  myelogenous — see also Category C92 C92.9- ☑
  myeloid C92.9- ☑
    specified NEC C92.Z- ☑ (following C92.6)
  plasma cell C90.1- ☑
  plasmacytic C90.1- ☑
  prolymphocytic
    of B-cell type C91.3- ☑
    of T-cell type C91.6- ☑
  specified NEC C94.8- ☑
  stem cell, of unclear lineage C95.0- ☑
  subacute lymphocytic C91.9- ☑
  T-cell large granular lymphocytic C91.Z- ☑ (following C91.6)
  unspecified cell type C95.9- ☑
    acute C95.0- ☑
    chronic C95.1- ☑
Leukemoid reaction — see also Reaction, leukemoid D72.823
Leukoaraiosis (hypertensive) I67.81
Leukoariosis — see Leukoaraiosis
Leukocoria — see Disorder, globe, degenerated condition, leucocoria
Leukocytopenia D72.819
Leukocytosis D72.829
  eosinophilic D72.19
Leukoderma, leukodermia NEC L81.5
  syphilitic A51.39
    late A52.79
Leukodystrophy G31.80
  with vanishing white matter disease G11.6
  LMNB1-related autosomal dominant G90.B
  metachromatic E75.25
  pol III-related G11.5
Leukoedema, oral epithelium K13.29
Leukoencephalitis G04.81
  acute (subacute) hemorrhagic G36.1
    postimmunization or postvaccinal G04.02
  postinfectious G04.01
  subacute sclerosing A81.1
  van Bogaert's (sclerosing) A81.1
Leukoencephalopathy — see also Encephalopathy G93.49
  with
    brainstem - spinal cord involvement - lactate elevation E88.43
    calcifications and cysts G93.43
    thalamus - brainstem involvement - high lactate E88.43
  adult-onset, with axonal spheroids (and pigmented glia) G93.44
  Binswanger's I67.3
  heroin vapor G92.8
  megalencephalic, with subcortical cysts G93.42
  metachromatic E75.25
  multifocal (progressive) A81.2
  postimmunization and postvaccinal G04.02
  progressive multifocal A81.2

Leukoencephalopathy — continued
  reversible, posterior G93.6
  van Bogaert's (sclerosing) A81.1
  vascular, progressive I67.3
Leukoerythroblastosis D75.9
Leukokeratosis — see also Leukoplakia
  mouth K13.21
  nicotina palati K13.24
  oral mucosa K13.21
  tongue K13.21
  vocal cord J38.3
Leukokraurosis vulva(e) N90.4
Leukoma (cornea) — see also Opacity, cornea
  adherent H17.0- ☑
  interfering with central vision — see Opacity, cornea, central
Leukomalacia, cerebral, newborn P91.2
  periventricular P91.2
Leukomelanopathy, hereditary D72.0
Leukonychia (punctata) (striata) L60.8
  congenital Q84.4
Leukopathia unguium L60.8
  congenital Q84.4
Leukopenia D72.819
  basophilic D72.818
  chemotherapy (cancer) induced D70.1
  congenital D70.0
  cyclic D70.0
  drug induced NEC D70.2
    due to cytoreductive cancer chemotherapy D70.1
  eosinophilic D72.818
  familial D70.0
  infantile genetic D70.0
  malignant D70.9
  periodic D70.0
  transitory neonatal P61.5
Leukopenic — see condition
Leukoplakia
  anus K62.89
  bladder (postinfectional) N32.89
  buccal K13.21
  cervix (uteri) N88.0
  esophagus K22.89
  gingiva K13.21
  hairy (oral mucosa) (tongue) K13.3
  kidney (pelvis) N28.89
  larynx J38.7
  lip K13.21
  mouth K13.21
  oral epithelium, including tongue (mucosa) K13.21
  palate K13.21
  pelvis (kidney) N28.89
  penis (infectional) N48.0
  rectum K62.89
  syphilitic (late) A52.79
  tongue K13.21
  ureter (postinfectional) N28.89
  urethra (postinfectional) N36.8
  uterus N85.8
  vagina N89.4
  vocal cord J38.3
  vulva N90.4
Leukorrhea N89.8
  due to Trichomonas (vaginalis) A59.00
  trichomonal A59.00
Leukosarcoma C85.9- ☑
Levocardia (isolated) Q24.1
  with situs inversus Q89.3
Levotransposition Q20.5
Lev's disease or syndrome (acquired complete heart block) I44.2
Levulosuria — see Fructosuria
Levurid L30.2
Lewy body (ies) (disease) G31.83
Leyden-Mobius dystrophy — see Dystrophy, Leyden-Mobius
Leydig cell
  carcinoma
    specified site — see Neoplasm, malignant, by site
    unspecified site
      female C56.9
      male C62.9- ☑
  tumor
    benign
      specified site — see Neoplasm, benign, by site
      unspecified site
        female D27.- ☑
        male D29.2- ☑

☑ Additional Character Required — Refer to the Tabular List for Character Selection

Leydig cell — *continued*
- tumor — *continued*
  - malignant
    - specified site — *see* Neoplasm, malignant, by site
    - unspecified site
      - female C56.- ☑
      - male C62.9- ☑
  - specified site — *see* Neoplasm, uncertain behavior, by site
  - unspecified site
    - female D39.1- ☑
    - male D40.1- ☑

Leydig-Sertoli cell tumor
- specified site — *see* Neoplasm, benign, by site
- unspecified site
  - female D27.- ☑
  - male D29.2- ☑

LGMD — *see* Dystrophy, muscular, limb-girdle
LGSIL (Low grade squamous intraepithelial lesion on cytologic smear of)
- anus R85.612
- cervix R87.612
- vagina R87.622

Liar, pathologic F60.2
Libido
- decreased R68.82

Libman-Sacks disease M32.11
Lice (infestation) B85.2
- body (Pediculus corporis) B85.1
- crab B85.3
- head (Pediculus capitis) B85.0
- mixed (classifiable to more than one of the titles B85.0-B85.3) B85.4
- pubic (Phthirus pubis) B85.3

Lichen L28.0
- albus L90.0
  - penis N48.0
  - vulva N90.4
- amyloidosis E85.4 [L99]
- atrophicus L90.0
  - penis N48.0
  - vulva N90.4
- congenital Q82.8
- myxedematosus L98.5
- nitidus L44.1
- pilaris Q82.8
  - acquired L85.8
- planopilaris L66.10
  - classic L66.11
  - follicular L66.11
  - specified NEC L66.19
- planus (chronicus) L43.9
  - annularis L43.8
  - bullous L43.1
  - follicular L66.11
  - hypertrophic L43.0
  - moniliformis L44.3
  - of Wilson L43.9
  - specified NEC L43.8
  - subacute (active) L43.3
  - tropicus L43.3
- ruber
  - acuminatus L44.0
  - moniliformis L44.3
  - planus L43.9
- sclerosus (et atrophicus) L90.0
  - penis N48.0
  - vulva N90.4
- scrofulosus (primary) (tuberculous) A18.4
- simplex (chronicus) (circumscriptus) L28.0
- striatus L44.2
- urticatus L28.2

Lichenification L28.0
Lichenoid keratosis — *see* Keratosis, lichenoid
Lichenoides tuberculosis (primary) A18.4
Lichtheim's disease or syndrome D51.0
Lien migrans D73.89
Ligament — *see* condition
Light
- for gestational age — *see* Light for dates
- headedness R42

Light-for-dates (infant) P05.00
- with weight of
  - 499 grams or less P05.01
  - 500-749 grams P05.02
  - 750-999 grams P05.03
  - 1000-1249 grams P05.04
  - 1250-1499 grams P05.05

Light-for-dates — *continued*
- with weight of — *continued*
  - 1500-1749 grams P05.06
  - 1750-1999 grams P05.07
  - 2000-2499 grams P05.08
  - 2500 grams and over P05.09
- affecting management of pregnancy O36.59- ☑
- and small-for-dates — *see* Small for dates
- specified NEC P05.09

Lightning (effects) (stroke) (struck by) T75.00- ☑
- burn — *see* Burn
- foot E53.8
- shock T75.01- ☑
- specified effect NEC T75.09- ☑

Lightwood-Albright syndrome N25.89
Lightwood's disease or syndrome (renal tubular acidosis) N25.89
Lignac (-de Toni) (-Fanconi) (-Debre) **disease or syndrome** E72.09
- with cystinosis E72.04

Ligneous thyroiditis E06.5
Likoff's syndrome I20.89
Limb — *see* condition
Limbic epilepsy personality syndrome F07.0
Limitation, limited
- activities due to disability Z73.6
- cardiac reserve — *see* Disease, heart
- eye muscle duction, traumatic — *see* Strabismus, mechanical
- mandibular range of motion M26.52

Lindau (-von Hippel) **disease** Q85.83
Line(s)
- Beau's L60.4
- Harris' — *see* Arrest, epiphyseal
- Hudson's (cornea) — *see* Pigmentation, cornea, anterior
- Stahli's (cornea) — *see* Pigmentation, cornea, anterior

Linea corneae senilis — *see* Change, cornea, senile
Lingua
- geographica K14.1
- nigra (villosa) K14.3
- plicata K14.5
- tylosis K13.29

Lingual — *see* condition
Linguatulosis B88.8
Linitis (gastric) **plastica** C16.9
Lip — *see* condition
Lipedema — *see* Edema
Lipemia — *see also* Hyperlipidemia
- retina, retinalis E78.3

Lipidosis E75.6
- cerebral (infantile) (juvenile) (late) E75.4
- cerebroretinal E75.4
- cerebroside E75.22
- cholesterol (cerebral) E75.5
- glycolipid E75.21
- hepatosplenomegalic E78.3
- sphingomyelin — *see* Niemann-Pick disease or syndrome
- sulfatide E75.29

Lipoadenoma — *see* Neoplasm, benign, by site
Lipoblastoma — *see* Lipoma
Lipoblastomatosis — *see* Lipoma
Lipochondrodystrophy E76.01
Lipochrome histiocytosis (familial) D71.8
Lipodermatosclerosis — *see also* Insufficiency, venous M79.3
- with
  - varicose veins — *see* Varix, leg, with, inflammation
  - ulcerated — *see* Varix, leg, with, ulcer, with inflammation by site
- ulcerated — *see* Ulcer, by site

Lipodystrophia progressiva E88.11
Lipodystrophy E88.10
- generalized (acquired) (congenital) E88.12
- HIV-associated E88.14
- injection E88.13
- insulin E88.13
- intestinal K90.81
- localized E88.13
  - mesenteric K65.4
- partial (acquired) (familial) E88.11
- progressive E88.11
- specified type NEC E88.19

Lipofibroma — *see* Lipoma
Lipofuscinosis, neuronal (with ceroidosis) E75.4
Lipogranuloma, sclerosing L92.8
Lipogranulomatosis E78.89
Lipoid — *see also* condition
- histiocytosis D76.3
  - essential E75.29

Lipoid — *continued*
- nephrosis N04.9
- proteinosis of Urbach E78.89

Lipoidemia — *see* Hyperlipidemia
Lipoidosis — *see* Lipidosis
Lipoma D17.9
- fetal D17.9
  - fat cell D17.9
- infiltrating D17.9
- intramuscular D17.9
- pleomorphic D17.9
- site classification
  - arms (skin) (subcutaneous) D17.2- ☑
  - connective tissue D17.30
    - intra-abdominal D17.5
    - intrathoracic D17.4
    - peritoneum D17.79
    - retroperitoneum D17.79
    - specified site NEC D17.39
    - spermatic cord D17.6
  - face (skin) (subcutaneous) D17.0
  - genitourinary organ NEC D17.72
  - head (skin) (subcutaneous) D17.0
  - intra-abdominal D17.5
  - intrathoracic D17.4
  - kidney D17.71
  - legs (skin) (subcutaneous) D17.2- ☑
  - neck (skin) (subcutaneous) D17.0
  - peritoneum D17.79
  - retroperitoneum D17.79
  - skin D17.30
    - specified site NEC D17.39
  - spermatic cord D17.6
  - subcutaneous D17.30
    - specified site NEC D17.39
  - trunk (skin) (subcutaneous) D17.1
  - unspecified D17.9
- spindle cell D17.9

Lipomatosis E88.2
- dolorosa (Dercum) E88.2
- fetal — *see* Lipoma
- Launois-Bensaude E88.89

Lipomyoma — *see* Lipoma
Lipomyxoma — *see* Lipoma
Lipomyxosarcoma — *see* Neoplasm, connective tissue, malignant
Lipoprotein metabolism disorder E78.9
Lipoproteinemia E78.5
- broad-beta E78.2
- floating-beta E78.2
- hyper-pre-beta E78.1

Liposarcoma — *see also* Neoplasm, connective tissue, malignant
- dedifferentiated — *see* Neoplasm, connective tissue, malignant
- differentiated type — *see* Neoplasm, connective tissue, malignant
- embryonal — *see* Neoplasm, connective tissue, malignant
- mixed type — *see* Neoplasm, connective tissue, malignant
- myxoid — *see* Neoplasm, connective tissue, malignant
- pleomorphic — *see* Neoplasm, connective tissue, malignant
- round cell — *see* Neoplasm, connective tissue, malignant
- well differentiated type — *see* Neoplasm, connective tissue, malignant

Liposynovitis prepatellaris E88.89
Lipping, cervix N86
Lipschütz disease or ulcer N76.6
Lipuria R82.0
- schistosomiasis (bilharziasis) B65.0

Lisping F80.0
Lissauer's paralysis A52.17
Lissencephalia, lissencephaly Q04.3
Listeriosis, listerellosis A32.9
- congenital (disseminated) P37.2
- cutaneous A32.0
- neonatal, newborn (disseminated) P37.2
- oculoglandular A32.81
- specified NEC A32.89

Lithemia E79.0
Lithiasis — *see* Calculus
Lithosis J62.8
Lithuria R82.998
Litigation, anxiety concerning Z65.3
Little leaguer's elbow — *see* Epicondylitis, medial
Little's disease G80.9

Littre's
　gland — see condition
　hernia — see Hernia, abdomen
Littritis — see Urethritis
Livedo (annularis) (racemosa) (reticularis) R23.1
Liver — see condition
Lives in a homeless encampment Z59.02
Living alone (problems with) Z60.2
　with handicapped person Z74.2
Living in a shelter (motel) (scattered site housing) (temporary or transitional living situation) Z59.01
Lloyd's syndrome — see Adenomatosis, endocrine
Loa loa (loiasis) B74.3
Lobar — see condition
Lobomycosis B48.0
Lobo's disease B48.0
Lobotomy syndrome F07.0
Lobstein (-Ekman) **disease or syndrome** Q78.0
Lobster-claw hand Q71.6- ☑
Lobulation (congenital) — see also Anomaly, by site
　kidney, Q63.1
　liver, abnormal Q44.79
　spleen Q89.09
Lobule, lobular — see condition
Local, localized — see condition
Locked-in state G83.5
Locked twins causing obstructed labor O66.1
Locking
　joint — see Derangement, joint, specified type NEC
　knee — see Derangement, knee
Lockjaw — see Tetanus
Loffler's
　endocarditis I42.3
　eosinophilia J82.89
　pneumonia J82.89
　syndrome (eosinophilic pneumonitis) J82.89
Loiasis (with conjunctival infestation) (eyelid) B74.3
Lone Star fever A77.0
Loneliness R45.89
Long
　COVID (-19) — see also COVID-19 U09.9
　labor O63.9
　　first stage O63.0
　　second stage O63.1
　QT syndrome I45.81
Long-term (current) (prophylactic) **drug therapy** (use of)
　5-fluorouracil Z79.631
　6-mercaptopurine Z79.631
　adalimumab Z79.620
　agents affecting estrogen receptors and estrogen levels NEC Z79.818
　alkylating agent Z79.630
　anastrozole (Arimidex) Z79.811
　anti-inflammatory, non-steroidal (NSAID) Z79.1
　antibiotics Z79.2
　　short-term use — omit code
　anticoagulants Z79.01
　antidiabetic drugs, injectable, non-insulin Z79.85
　antimetabolite agent Z79.631
　antiplatelet Z79.02
　antithrombotics Z79.02
　antitumor antibiotic Z79.632
　apremilast Z79.61
　aromatase inhibitors Z79.811
　aspirin Z79.82
　azathioprine Z79.624
　birth control pill or patch Z79.3
　bisphosphonates Z79.83
　bleomycin Z79.632
　calcineurin inhibitor Z79.621
　chlorambucil Z79.630
　cisplatin Z79.630
　contraceptive, oral Z79.3
　cyclophosphamide Z79.630
　cyclosporine Z79.621
　cytarabine Z79.631
　doxorubicin Z79.632
　drug, specified NEC Z79.899
　estrogen receptor downregulators Z79.818
　etanercept Z79.620
　etoposide Z79.634
　Evista Z79.810
　exemestane (Aromasin) Z79.811
　Fareston Z79.810
　fulvestrant (Faslodex) Z79.818
　gonadotropin-releasing hormone (GnRH) agonist Z79.818
　goserelin acetate (Zoladex) Z79.818
　hormone replacement Z79.890
　hydroxyurea Z79.64

Long-term (current) (prophylactic) **drug therapy** — continued
　immunomodulators, unspecified Z79.60
　　specified NEC Z79.69
　immunomodulatory imide drug Z79.61
　immunosuppressants, unspecified Z79.60
　　specified NEC Z79.69
　immunosuppressive biologic Z79.620
　infliximab Z79.620
　inhibitors of nucleotide synthesis Z79.624
　insulin Z79.4
　irinotecan Z79.634
　Janus kinase inhibitor Z79.622
　lenalidomide Z79.61
　letrozole (Femara) Z79.811
　leuprolide acetate (leuprorelin) (Lupron) Z79.818
　mammalian target of rapamycin (mTOR) inhibitor Z79.623
　megestrol acetate (Megace) Z79.818
　methadone for pain management Z79.891
　mitomycin C Z79.632
　mitotic inhibitor Z79.633
　monoclonal antibodies Z79.620
　mycophenolate Z79.624
　myelosuppressive agent Z79.64
　Nolvadex Z79.810
　non-insulin antidiabetic drug, injectable Z79.85
　non-steroidal anti-inflammatories (NSAID) Z79.1
　opiate analgesic Z79.891
　oral
　　antidiabetic Z79.84
　　contraceptive Z79.3
　　hypoglycemic Z79.84
　paclitaxel Z79.633
　plant alkaloids Z79.633
　pomalidomide Z79.61
　purine synthesis (IMDH) inhibitors Z79.624
　raloxifene (Evista) Z79.810
　selective estrogen receptor modulators (SERMs) Z79.810
　sirolimus Z79.623
　steroids
　　inhaled Z79.51
　　systemic Z79.52
　tacrolimus Z79.621
　tamoxifen (Nolvadex) Z79.810
　tofacitinib Z79.622
　topoisomerase inhibitor Z79.634
　topotecan Z79.634
　toremifene (Fareston) Z79.810
　vinblastine Z79.633
　vincristine Z79.633
Longitudinal stripes or grooves, nails L60.8
　congenital Q84.6
Loop
　intestine — see Volvulus
　vascular on papilla (optic) Q14.2
Loose — see also condition
　body
　　joint M24.00
　　　ankle M24.07- ☑
　　　elbow M24.02- ☑
　　　hand M24.04- ☑
　　　hip M24.05- ☑
　　　knee M23.4-
　　　shoulder (region) M24.01- ☑
　　　specified site NEC M24.08
　　　temporomandibular M24.08
　　　toe M24.07- ☑
　　　vertebra M24.08
　　　wrist M24.03- ☑
　　knee M23.4- ☑
　　sheath, tendon — see Disorder, tendon, specified type NEC
　cartilage — see Loose, body, joint
　skin and subcutaneous tissue (following bariatric surgery weight loss) (following dietary weight loss) L98.7
　tooth, teeth K08.89
Loosening
　aseptic
　　joint prosthesis — see Complications, joint prosthesis, mechanical, loosening, by site
　epiphysis — see Osteochondropathy
　mechanical
　　joint prosthesis — see Complications, joint prosthesis, mechanical, loosening, by site
Looser-Milkman (-Debray) **syndrome** M83.8
Lop ear (deformity) Q17.3
Lorain (-Levi) **short stature syndrome** E23.0

Lordosis M40.50
　acquired — see Lordosis, specified type NEC
　congenital Q76.429
　　lumbar region Q76.426
　　lumbosacral region Q76.427
　　sacral region Q76.428
　　sacrococcygeal region Q76.428
　　thoracolumbar region Q76.425
　lumbar region M40.56
　lumbosacral region M40.57
　postsurgical M96.4
　postural — see Lordosis, specified type NEC
　rachitic (late effect) (sequelae) E64.3
　sequelae of rickets E64.3
　specified type NEC M40.40
　　lumbar region M40.46
　　lumbosacral region M40.47
　　thoracolumbar region M40.45
　thoracolumbar region M40.55
　tuberculous A18.01
Loss (of)
　appetite — see also Anorexia R63.0
　　hysterical F50.89
　　nonorganic origin F50.89
　　psychogenic F50.89
　blood —see Hemorrhage
　bone —see Loss, substance of, bone
　consciousness, transient R55
　　traumatic — see Injury, intracranial
　control, sphincter, rectum R15.9
　　nonorganic origin F98.1
　elasticity, skin R23.4
　family (member) in childhood Z62.898
　fluid (acute) E86.9
　function of labyrinth — see subcategory H83.2- ☑
　hair, nonscarring — see Alopecia
　hearing — see also Deafness
　　central NOS H90.5
　　conductive H90.2
　　　bilateral H90.0
　　　unilateral
　　　　with
　　　　　restricted hearing on the contralateral side H90.A1- ☑
　　　　　unrestricted hearing on the contralateral side H90.1- ☑
　　mixed conductive and sensorineural hearing loss H90.8
　　　bilateral H90.6
　　　unilateral
　　　　with
　　　　　restricted hearing on the contralateral side H90.A3- ☑
　　　　　unrestricted hearing on the contralateral side H90.7- ☑
　　neural NOS H90.5
　　perceptive NOS H90.5
　　sensorineural NOS H90.5
　　　bilateral H90.3
　　　unilateral
　　　　with
　　　　　restricted hearing on the contralateral side H90.A2- ☑
　　　　　unrestricted hearing on the contralateral side H90.4- ☑
　　sensory NOS H90.5
　height R29.890
　limb or member, traumatic, current — see Amputation, traumatic
　love relationship in childhood Z62.898
　memory — see also Amnesia
　　mild, following organic brain damage F06.8
　mind — see Psychosis
　occlusal vertical dimension of fully erupted teeth M26.37
　organ or part — see Absence, by site, acquired
　ossicles, ear (partial) H74.32- ☑
　parent in childhood Z63.4
　pregnancy, recurrent N96
　　care in current pregnancy O26.2- ☑
　　without current pregnancy N96
　recurrent pregnancy — see Loss, pregnancy, recurrent
　self-esteem, in childhood Z62.898
　sense of
　　smell — see Disturbance, sensation, smell
　　taste — see Disturbance, sensation, taste
　　touch R20.8
　sensory R44.9
　　dissociative F44.6

Loss — *continued*
- sexual desire F52.0
- sight (acquired) (complete) (congenital) — *see* Blindness
- substance of
  - bone — *see* Disorder, bone, density and structure, specified NEC
    - horizontal alveolar K06.3
  - cartilage — *see* Disorder, cartilage, specified type NEC
    - auricle (ear) — *see* Disorder, pinna, specified type NEC
  - vitreous (humor) H15.89
- tooth, teeth — *see* Absence, teeth, acquired
- vision, visual H54.7
  - both eyes H54.3
  - one eye H54.60
    - left (normal vision on right) H54.62
    - right (normal vision on left) H54.61
  - specified as blindness — *see* Blindness
  - subjective
    - sudden H53.13- ☑
    - transient H53.12- ☑
- vitreous — *see* Prolapse, vitreous
- voice — *see* Aphonia
- weight (abnormal) (cause unknown) R63.4

Louis-Bar syndrome (ataxia-telangiectasia) G11.3
Louping ill (encephalitis) A84.89
Louse, lousiness — *see* Lice
Low
- achiever, school Z55.3
- back syndrome M54.50
- basal metabolic rate R94.8
- birthweight (2499 grams or less) P07.10
  - with weight of
    - 1000-1249 grams P07.14
    - 1250-1499 grams P07.15
    - 1500-1749 grams P07.16
    - 1750-1999 grams P07.17
    - 2000-2499 grams P07.18
  - extreme (999 grams or less) P07.00
    - with weight of
      - 499 grams or less P07.01
      - 500-749 grams P07.02
      - 750-999 grams P07.03
  - for gestational age — *see* Light for dates
- blood pressure — *see also* Hypotension
  - reading (incidental) (isolated) (nonspecific) R03.1
- cardiac reserve — *see* Disease, heart
- function — *see also* Hypofunction
  - kidney N28.9
- hematocrit D64.9
- hemoglobin D64.9
- income Z59.6
- level of literacy Z55.0
- lying
  - kidney N28.89
- organ or site, congenital — *see* Malposition, congenital
- output syndrome (cardiac) — *see* Failure, heart
- platelets (blood) — *see* Thrombocytopenia
- reserve, kidney N28.89
- salt syndrome E87.1
- self esteem R45.81
- set ears Q17.4
- vision H54.2X- ☑
  - one eye (other eye normal) H54.50
    - left (normal vision on right)
      - category 1 H54.52A1
      - category 2 H54.52A2
    - other eye blind — *see* Blindness
    - right (normal vision on left)
      - category 1 H54.511A
      - category 2 H54.512A
- von Willebrand factor R79.1

Low-density-lipoprotein-type (LDL) **hyperlipoproteinemia** E78.00
Lowe's syndrome E72.03
Lown-Ganong-Levine syndrome I45.6
LSD reaction (acute) (without dependence) F16.90
- with dependence F16.20

LTBI (latent tuberculosis infection) Z22.7
LTBL (leukoencephalopathy with thalamus - brainstem involvement - high lactate) E88.43
Ludwig's angina or disease K12.2
Lues (venerea), **luetic** — *see* Syphilis
Luetscher's syndrome (dehydration) E86.0
Lumbago, lumbalgia M54.50
- with sciatica M54.4- ☑
  - due to intervertebral disc disorder M51.17
- due to displacement, intervertebral disc M51.27

Lumbago, lumbalgia — *continued*
- due to displacement, intervertebral disc — *continued*
  - with sciatica M51.17

Lumbar — *see* condition
Lumbarization, vertebra, congenital Q76.49
Lumbermen's itch B88.09
Lump — *see also* Mass
- breast N63.0
  - axillary tail
    - left N63.32
    - right N63.31
  - left
    - lower inner quadrant N63.24
    - lower outer quadrant N63.23
    - overlapping quadrants N63.25
    - unspecified quadrant N63.20
    - upper inner quadrant N63.22
    - upper outer quadrant N63.21
  - right
    - lower inner quadrant N63.14
    - lower outer quadrant N63.13
    - overlapping quadrants N63.15
    - unspecified quadrant N63.10
    - upper inner quadrant N63.12
    - upper outer quadrant N63.11
  - subareolar
    - left N63.42
    - right N63.41

Lunacy — *see* Psychosis
Lung — *see* condition
Lupoid (miliary) **of Boeck** D86.3
Lupus
- anticoagulant D68.62
  - with
    - hemorrhagic disorder D68.312
    - hypercoagulable state D68.62
  - finding without diagnosis R76.0
- discoid (local) L93.0
- erythematosus (discoid) (local) L93.0
  - disseminated — *see* Lupus, erythematosus, systemic
  - eyelid H01.129
    - left H01.126
      - lower H01.125
      - upper H01.124
    - right H01.123
      - lower H01.122
      - upper H01.121
  - profundus L93.2
  - specified NEC L93.2
  - subacute cutaneous L93.1
  - systemic M32.9
    - with organ or system involvement M32.10
      - endocarditis M32.11
      - lung M32.13
      - pericarditis M32.12
      - renal (glomerular) M32.14
        - tubulo-interstitial M32.15
      - specified organ or system NEC M32.19
    - drug-induced M32.0
    - inhibitor (presence of) D68.62
      - with
        - hemorrhagic disorder D68.312
        - hypercoagulable state D68.62
      - finding without diagnosis R76.0
    - specified NEC M32.8
- exedens A18.4
- hydralazine M32.0
  - correct substance properly administered — *see* Table of Drugs and Chemicals, by drug, adverse effect
  - overdose or wrong substance given or taken — *see* Table of Drugs and Chemicals, by drug, poisoning
- nephritis (chronic) M32.14
- nontuberculous, not disseminated L93.0
- panniculitis L93.2
- pernio (Besnier) D86.3
- systemic — *see* Lupus, erythematosus, systemic
- tuberculous A18.4
  - eyelid A18.4
- vulgaris A18.4
  - eyelid A18.4

Luteinoma D27.- ☑
Lutembacher's disease or syndrome (atrial septal defect with mitral stenosis) Q21.19
Luteoma D27.- ☑
Lutz (-Splendore-de Almeida) **disease** — *see* Paracoccidioidomycosis
Luxation — *see also* Dislocation

Luxation — *continued*
- eyeball (nontraumatic) — *see* Luxation, globe
  - birth injury P15.3
- globe, nontraumatic H44.82- ☑
- lacrimal gland — *see* Dislocation, lacrimal gland
- lens (old) (partial) (spontaneous)
  - congenital Q12.1
  - syphilitic A50.39

Lycanthropy F22
Lyell's syndrome L51.2
- due to drug L51.2
  - correct substance properly administered — *see* Table of Drugs and Chemicals, by drug, adverse effect
  - overdose or wrong substance given or taken — *see* Table of Drugs and Chemicals, by drug, poisoning

Lyme disease A69.20
Lymph
- gland or node — *see* condition
- scrotum — *see* Infestation, filarial

Lymphadenitis I88.9
- with ectopic or molar pregnancy O08.0
- acute L04.9
  - axilla L04.2
  - face L04.0
  - flank L03.32A
  - head L04.0
  - hip L04.3
  - limb
    - lower L04.3
    - upper L04.2
  - neck L04.0
  - shoulder L04.2
  - specified site NEC L04.8
  - trunk L04.1
- anthracosis (occupational) J60
- any site, except mesenteric I88.9
  - chronic I88.1
  - subacute I88.1
- breast
  - gestational — *see* Mastitis, obstetric
  - puerperal, postpartum (nonpurulent) O91.22
- chancroidal (congenital) A57
- chronic I88.1
  - mesenteric I88.0
- due to
  - Brugia (malayi) B74.1
    - timori B74.2
  - chlamydial lymphogranuloma A55
  - diphtheria (toxin) A36.89
  - lymphogranuloma venereum A55
  - Wuchereria bancrofti B74.0
- following ectopic or molar pregnancy O08.0
- gonorrheal A54.89
- infective — *see* Lymphadenitis, acute
- mesenteric (acute) (chronic) (nonspecific) (subacute) I88.0
  - due to Salmonella typhi A01.09
  - tuberculous A18.39
- mycobacterial A31.8
- purulent — *see* Lymphadenitis, acute
- pyogenic — *see* Lymphadenitis, acute
- regional, nonbacterial I88.8
- septic — *see* Lymphadenitis, acute
- subacute, unspecified site I88.1
- suppurative — *see* Lymphadenitis, acute
- syphilitic (early) (secondary) A51.49
  - late A52.79
- tuberculous — *see* Tuberculosis, lymph gland
- venereal (chlamydial) A55

Lymphadenoid goiter E06.3
Lymphadenopathy (generalized) R59.1
- angioimmunoblastic, with dysproteinemia (AILD) C86.5- ☑
- due to toxoplasmosis (acquired) B58.89
  - congenital (acute) (subacute) (chronic) P37.1
- localized R59.0
- syphilitic (early) (secondary) A51.49

Lymphadenosis R59.1
Lymphangiectasis I89.0
- conjunctiva H11.89
- postinfectional I89.0
- scrotum I89.0

Lymphangiectatic elephantiasis, nonfilarial I89.0
Lymphangioendothelioma D18.1
- malignant — *see* Neoplasm, connective tissue, malignant

Lymphangioleiomyomatosis J84.81
Lymphangioma D18.1
- capillary D18.1

Lymphangioma — continued
  cavernous D18.1
  cystic D18.1
  malignant — see Neoplasm, connective tissue, malignant
Lymphangiomyoma D18.1
Lymphangiomyomatosis J84.81
Lymphangiosarcoma — see Neoplasm, connective tissue, malignant
Lymphangitis I89.1
  with
    abscess — code by site under Abscess
    cellulitis — code by site under Cellulitis
    ectopic or molar pregnancy O08.0
  acute L03.91
    abdominal wall L03.321
    ankle — see Lymphangitis, acute, lower limb
    arm — see Lymphangitis, acute, upper limb
    auricle (ear) — see Lymphangitis, acute, ear
    axilla L03.12- ☑
    back (any part) L03.322
    buttock L03.327
    cervical (meaning neck) L03.222
    cheek (external) L03.212
    chest wall L03.323
    digit
      finger — see Lymphangitis, acute, finger
      toe — see Lymphangitis, acute, toe
    ear (external) H60.1- ☑
    external auditory canal — see Lymphangitis, acute, ear
    eyelid — see Abscess, eyelid
    face NEC L03.212
    finger (intrathecal) (periosteal) (subcutaneous) (subcuticular) L03.02- ☑
    flank L03.32A
    foot — see Lymphangitis, acute, lower limb
    gluteal (region) L03.327
    groin L03.324
    hand — see Lymphangitis, acute, upper limb
    head NEC L03.891
      face (any part, except ear, eye and nose) L03.212
    heel — see Lymphangitis, acute, lower limb
    hip — see Lymphangitis, acute, lower limb
    jaw (region) L03.212
    knee — see Lymphangitis, acute, lower limb
    leg — see Lymphangitis, acute, lower limb
    lower limb L03.12- ☑
      toe — see Lymphangitis, acute, toe
    navel L03.326
    neck (region) L03.222
    orbit, orbital — see Cellulitis, orbit
    pectoral (region) L03.323
    perineal, perineum L03.325
    scalp (any part) L03.891
    shoulder — see Lymphangitis, acute, upper limb
    specified site NEC L03.898
    thigh — see Lymphangitis, acute, lower limb
    thumb (intrathecal) (periosteal) (subcutaneous) (subcuticular) — see Lymphangitis, acute, finger
    toe (intrathecal) (periosteal) (subcutaneous) (subcuticular) L03.04- ☑
    trunk L03.329
      abdominal wall L03.321
      back (any part) L03.322
      buttock L03.327
      chest wall L03.323
      groin L03.324
      perineal, perineum L03.325
      umbilicus L03.326
    umbilicus L03.326
    upper limb L03.12- ☑
      axilla — see Lymphangitis, acute, axilla
      finger — see Lymphangitis, acute, finger
      thumb — see Lymphangitis, acute, finger
    wrist — see Lymphangitis, acute, upper limb
  breast
    gestational — see Mastitis, obstetric
  chancroidal A57
  chronic (any site) I89.1
  due to
    Brugia (malayi) B74.1
      timori B74.2
    Wuchereria bancrofti B74.0
  following ectopic or molar pregnancy O08.89
  penis
    acute N48.29
    gonococcal (acute) (chronic) A54.09

Lymphangitis — continued
  puerperal, postpartum, childbirth O86.89
  strumous, tuberculous A18.2
  subacute (any site) I89.1
  tuberculous — see Tuberculosis, lymph gland
Lymphatic (vessel) — see condition
Lymphatism E32.8
Lymphectasia I89.0
Lymphedema (acquired) — see also Elephantiasis
  congenital Q82.0
  hereditary (chronic) (idiopathic) Q82.0
  postmastectomy I97.2
  praecox I89.0
  secondary I89.0
  surgical NEC I97.89
    postmastectomy (syndrome) I97.2
Lymphoblastic — see condition
Lymphoblastoma (diffuse) — see Lymphoma, lymphoblastic (diffuse)
  giant follicular — see Lymphoma, lymphoblastic (diffuse)
  macrofollicular — see Lymphoma, lymphoblastic (diffuse)
Lymphocele I89.8
Lymphocytic
  chorioencephalitis (acute) (serous) A87.2
  choriomeningitis (acute) (serous) A87.2
  meningoencephalitis A87.2
Lymphocytoma, benign cutis L98.8
Lymphocytopenia D72.810
Lymphocytosis (symptomatic) D72.820
  infectious (acute) B33.8
Lymphoepithelioma — see Neoplasm, malignant, by site
Lymphogranuloma (malignant) — see also Lymphoma, Hodgkin
  chlamydial A55
  inguinale A55
  venereum (any site) (chlamydial) (with stricture of rectum) A55
Lymphogranulomatosis (malignant) — see also Lymphoma, Hodgkin
  benign (Boeck's sarcoid) (Schaumann's) D86.1
Lymphohistiocytosis, hemophagocytic (familial) D76.1
Lymphoid — see condition
Lymphoma (of) (malignant) C85.90
  adult T-cell (HTLV-1-associated) (acute variant) (chronic variant) (lymphomatoid variant) (smouldering variant) C91.5-
  anaplastic large cell
    ALK-negative C84.7- ☑
    ALK-positive C84.6- ☑
    breast implant associated (BIA-ALCL) C84.7A
    CD30-positive C84.6- ☑
    primary cutaneous C86.6- ☑
  angioimmunoblastic T-cell C86.5- ☑
  B-cell C85.1- ☑
  B-precursor C83.5- ☑
  BALT C88.4- ☑
  blastic NK-cell C86.4- ☑
  blastic plasmacytoid dendritic cell neoplasm (BPDCN) C86.4- ☑
  brain, primary — see Lymphoma, primary central nervous system
  bronchial-associated lymphoid tissue [BALT-lymphoma] C88.4- ☑
  Burkitt (atypical) C83.7- ☑
  Burkitt-like C83.7- ☑
  central nervous system, primary — see Lymphoma, primary central nervous system
  centrocytic C83.1- ☑
  cutaneous follicle center C82.6- ☑
  cutaneous T-cell C84.A- ☑ (following C84.7)
  diffuse follicle center C82.5- ☑
  diffuse large cell C83.3- ☑
    anaplastic C83.3- ☑
    B-cell C83.3- ☑
    CD30-positive C83.3- ☑
    centroblastic C83.3- ☑
    extranodal and solid organ sites NEC C83.398
    immunoblastic C83.3- ☑
    plasmablastic C83.3- ☑
    primary central nervous system (brain) (meninges) (PCNSL) (spinal cord) C83.390
    subtype not specified C83.3- ☑
    T-cell rich C83.3- ☑
  enteropathy-type (associated) (intestinal) T-cell C86.2- ☑
  extranodal marginal zone B-cell lymphoma of mucosa-associated lymphoid tissue [MALT-lymphoma] C88.4- ☑

Lymphoma — continued
  extranodal NK/T-cell, nasal type C86.0- ☑
  follicular C82.9- ☑
    grade
      I C82.0- ☑
      II C82.1- ☑
      III C82.2- ☑
      IIIa C82.3- ☑
      IIIb C82.4- ☑
    specified NEC C82.8- ☑
  hepatosplenic T-cell (alpha-beta) (gamma-delta) C86.1- ☑
  histiocytic C85.9- ☑
    true C96.A (following C96.6)
  Hodgkin C81.9- ☑
    lymphocyte depleted (classical) C81.3- ☑
    lymphocyte-rich (classical) C81.4- ☑
    mixed cellularity (classical) C81.2- ☑
    nodular
      lymphocyte predominant C81.0- ☑
      sclerosis (classical) C81.1- ☑
    nodular sclerosis (classical) C81.1- ☑
    specified NEC (classical) C81.7- ☑
  intravascular large B-cell C83.8- ☑
  Lennert's C84.4- ☑
  lymphoblastic (diffuse) C83.5- ☑
  lymphoblastic B-cell C83.5- ☑
  lymphoblastic T-cell C83.5- ☑
  lymphoepithelioid C84.4- ☑
  lymphoplasmacytic C83.0- ☑
    with IgM-production C88.0- ☑
  MALT C88.4- ☑
  mantle cell C83.1- ☑
  mature T-cell NEC C84.4- ☑
  mature T/NK-cell C84.9- ☑
    specified NEC C84.Z- ☑ (following C84.7)
  mediastinal (thymic) large B-cell C85.2- ☑
  Mediterranean C88.3- ☑
  meninges, primary — see Lymphoma, primary central nervous system
  mucosa-associated lymphoid tissue [MALT-lymphoma] C88.4- ☑
  NK/T cell C84.9- ☑
  nodal marginal zone C83.0- ☑
  non-follicular (diffuse) C83.9- ☑
    specified NEC C83.8- ☑
  non-Hodgkin — see also Lymphoma, by type C85.9- ☑
    specified NEC C85.8- ☑
  non-leukemic variant of B-CLL C83.0- ☑
  peripheral T-cell NEC C84.4- ☑
  primary central nervous system (brain) (meninges) (PCNSL) (spinal cord) C83.390
    Burkitt C83.79
    diffuse large B-cell C83.390
    lymphoblastic C83.59
    peripheral T-cell C84.49
  primary cutaneous
    anaplastic large cell C86.6- ☑
    CD30-positive large T-cell C86.6- ☑
  primary effusion B-cell C83.8- ☑
  SALT C88.4- ☑
  skin-associated lymphoid tissue [SALT-lymphoma] C88.4- ☑
  small cell B-cell C83.0- ☑
  spinal cord, primary — see Lymphoma, primary central nervous system
  splenic marginal zone C83.0- ☑
  subcutaneous panniculitis-like T-cell C86.3- ☑
  T-precursor C83.5- ☑
  true histiocytic C96.A (following C96.6)
Lymphomatosis — see Lymphoma
Lymphopathia venereum, veneris A55
Lymphopenia D72.810
Lymphoplasmacytic leukemia — see Leukemia, chronic lymphocytic, B-cell type
Lymphoproliferation, X-linked disease D82.3
Lymphoreticulosis, benign (of inoculation) A28.1
Lymphorrhea I89.8
Lymphosarcoma (diffuse) — see also Lymphoma C85.9- ☑
Lymphostasis I89.8
Lypemania — see Melancholia
Lysine and hydroxylysine metabolism disorder E72.3
Lyssa — see Rabies

M

Macacus ear Q17.3
Maceration, wet feet, tropical (syndrome) T69.02- ☑
MacLeod's syndrome J43.0
Macrocephalia, macrocephaly Q75.3
Macrocheilia, macrochilia (congenital) Q18.6
Macrocolon — see also Megacolon Q43.1
Macrocornea Q15.8
  with glaucoma Q15.0
Macrocytic — see condition
Macrocytosis D75.89
Macrodactylia, macrodactylism (fingers) (thumbs) Q74.0
  toes Q74.2
Macrodontia K00.2
Macrogenia M26.05
Macrogenitosomia (adrenal) (male) (praecox) E25.9
  congenital E25.0
Macroglobulinemia (idiopathic) (primary) C88.0- ☑
  monoclonal (essential) D47.2
  Waldenstrom C88.0- ☑
Macroglossia (congenital) Q38.2
  acquired K14.8
Macrognathia, macrognathism (congenital) (mandibular) (maxillary) M26.09
Macrogyria (congenital) Q04.8
Macrohydrocephalus — see Hydrocephalus
Macromastia — see Hypertrophy, breast
Macrophthalmos Q11.3
  in congenital glaucoma Q15.0
Macropsia H53.15
Macrosigmoid K59.39
  congenital Q43.2
Macrospondylitis, acromegalic E22.0
Macrostomia (congenital) Q18.4
Macrotia (external ear) (congenital) Q17.1
Macula
  cornea, corneal — see Opacity, cornea
  degeneration (atrophic) (exudative) (senile) — see also Degeneration, macula
  hereditary — see Dystrophy, retina
Maculae ceruleae B85.1
Maculopathy, toxic — see Degeneration, macula, toxic
Madarosis (eyelid) H02.729
  left H02.726
    lower H02.725
    upper H02.724
  right H02.723
    lower H02.722
    upper H02.721
Madelung's
  deformity (radius) Q74.0
  disease
    radial deformity Q74.0
    symmetrical lipomas, neck E88.89
Madness — see Psychosis
Madura
  foot B47.9
    actinomycotic B47.1
    mycotic B47.0
Maduromycosis B47.0
Maffucci's syndrome Q78.4
Magnesium metabolism disorder — see Disorder, metabolism, magnesium
Main en griffe (acquired) — see also Deformity, limb, clawhand
  congenital Q68.1
Maintenance (encounter for)
  antineoplastic chemotherapy Z51.11
  antineoplastic radiation therapy Z51.0
  methadone F11.20
Majocchi's
  disease L81.7
  granuloma B35.8
Major — see condition
Mal de los pintos — see Pinta
Mal de mer T75.3- ☑
Malabar itch (any site) B35.5
Malabsorption K90.9
  calcium K90.89
  carbohydrate K90.49
  disaccharide E73.9
  fat K90.49
  galactose E74.20
  glucose (-galactose) E74.39
  intestinal K90.9
    specified NEC K90.89

Malabsorption — continued
  isomaltose E74.31
  lactose E73.9
  methionine E72.19
  monosaccharide E74.39
  postgastrectomy K91.2
  postsurgical K91.2
  protein K90.49
  starch K90.49
  sucrose E74.39
  syndrome K90.9
    postsurgical K91.2
Malacia, bone (adult) M83.9
  juvenile — see Rickets
Malacoplakia
  bladder N32.89
  pelvis (kidney) N28.89
  ureter N28.89
  urethra N36.8
Malacosteon, juvenile — see Rickets
Maladaptation — see Maladjustment
Maladie de Roger Q21.0
Maladjustment
  conjugal Z63.0
    involving divorce or estrangement Z63.5
  educational Z55.4
  family Z63.9
  marital Z63.0
    involving divorce or estrangement Z63.5
  occupational NEC Z56.89
  simple, adult — see Disorder, adjustment
  situational — see Disorder, adjustment
  social Z60.9
    due to
      acculturation difficulty Z60.3
      discrimination and persecution (perceived) Z60.5
      exclusion and isolation Z60.4
      life-cycle (phase of life) transition Z60.0
      rejection Z60.4
      specified reason NEC Z60.8
Malaise R53.81
Malakoplakia — see Malacoplakia
Malaria, malarial (fever) B54
  with
    blackwater fever B50.8
      hemoglobinuric (bilious) B50.8
    hemoglobinuria B50.8
  accidentally induced (therapeutically) — code by type under Malaria
  algid B50.9
  cerebral B50.0 [G94]
  clinically diagnosed (without parasitological confirmation) B54
  congenital NEC P37.4
    falciparum P37.3
  congestion, congestive B54
  continued (fever) B50.9
  estivo-autumnal B50.9
  falciparum B50.9
    with complications NEC B50.8
      cerebral B50.0 [G94]
      severe B50.8
  hemorrhagic B54
  malariae B52.9
    with
      complications NEC B52.8
      glomerular disorder B52.0
  malignant (tertian) — see Malaria, falciparum
  mixed infections — code to first listed type in B50-B53
  ovale B53.0
  parasitologically confirmed NEC B53.8
  pernicious, acute — see Malaria, falciparum
  Plasmodium (P.)
    falciparum NEC — see Malaria, falciparum
    malariae NEC B52.9
      with Plasmodium
        falciparum (and or vivax) — see Malaria, falciparum
        vivax — see also Malaria, vivax
          and falciparum — see Malaria, falciparum
    ovale B53.0
      with Plasmodium malariae — see also Malaria, malariae
      and vivax — see also Malaria, vivax
        and falciparum — see Malaria, falciparum
    simian B53.1
      with Plasmodium malariae — see also Malaria, malariae
      and vivax — see also Malaria, vivax

Malaria, malarial — continued
  Plasmodium — continued
    simian — continued
      with Plasmodium malariae — see also Malaria, malariae — continued
        and vivax — see also Malaria, vivax — continued
          and falciparum — see Malaria, falciparum
    vivax NEC B51.9
      with Plasmodium falciparum — see Malaria, falciparum
  quartan — see Malaria, malariae
  quotidian — see Malaria, falciparum
  recurrent B54
  remittent B54
  specified type NEC (parasitologically confirmed) B53.8
  spleen B54
  subtertian (fever) — see Malaria, falciparum
  tertian (benign) — see also Malaria, vivax
    malignant B50.9
  tropical B50.9
  typhoid B54
  vivax B51.9
    with
      complications NEC B51.8
      ruptured spleen B51.0
Malassez's disease (cystic) N50.89
Malassimilation K90.9
Maldescent, testis Q53.9
  bilateral Q53.20
    abdominal Q53.211
    perineal Q53.22
  unilateral Q53.10
    abdominal Q53.111
    perineal Q53.12
Maldevelopment — see also Anomaly
  brain Q07.9
  colon Q43.9
  hip Q74.2
    congenital dislocation Q65.2
      bilateral Q65.1
      unilateral Q65.0- ☑
  mastoid process Q75.8
  middle ear Q16.4
    except ossicles Q16.4
    ossicles Q16.3
  ossicles Q16.3
  spine Q76.49
  toe Q74.2
Male type pelvis Q74.2
  with disproportion (fetopelvic) O33.3- ☑
    causing obstructed labor O65.3
Malformation (congenital) — see also Anomaly
  adrenal gland Q89.1
  affecting multiple systems with skeletal changes NEC Q87.5
  alimentary tract Q45.9
    specified type NEC Q45.8
    upper Q40.9
      specified type NEC Q40.8
  aorta Q25.40
    absence Q25.41
    aneurysm, congenital Q25.43
    aplasia Q25.41
    atresia Q25.29
      aortic arch Q25.21
    coarctation (preductal) (postductal) Q25.1
    dilatation, congenital Q25.44
    hypoplasia Q25.42
    patent ductus arteriosus Q25.0
    specified type NEC Q25.49
    stenosis Q25.1
      supravalvular Q25.3
  aortic valve Q23.9
    specified NEC Q23.88
  arteriovenous, aneurysmatic (congenital) Q27.30
    brain Q28.2
      ruptured I60.8
        intracerebral I61.8
        intraparenchymal I61.8
        intraventricular I61.5
        subarachnoid I60.8
    cerebral — see also Malformation, arteriovenous, brain Q28.2
    peripheral Q27.30
      digestive system — see Angiodysplasia
      congenital Q27.33
      lower limb Q27.32
      other specified site Q27.39

Malformation — *continued*
　arteriovenous, aneurysmatic — *continued*
　　peripheral — *continued*
　　　renal vessel Q27.34
　　　upper limb Q27.31
　　precerebral vessels (nonruptured) Q28.0
　auricle
　　ear (congenital) Q17.3
　　　acquired H61.119
　　　　left H61.112
　　　　　with right H61.113
　　　　right H61.111
　　　　　with left H61.113
　bile duct Q44.5
　bladder Q64.79
　　aplasia Q64.5
　　diverticulum Q64.6
　　exstrophy — *see* Exstrophy, bladder
　　neck obstruction Q64.31
　bone Q79.9
　　face Q75.9
　　　specified type NEC Q75.8
　　skull Q75.9
　　　specified type NEC Q75.8
　brain (multiple) Q04.9
　　arteriovenous Q28.2
　　specified type NEC Q04.8
　branchial cleft Q18.2
　breast Q83.9
　　specified type NEC Q83.8
　broad ligament Q50.6
　bronchus Q32.4
　bursa Q79.9
　cardiac
　　chambers Q20.9
　　　specified type NEC Q20.8
　　septum Q21.9
　　　specified type NEC Q21.8
　cerebral Q04.9
　　vessels Q28.3
　cervix uteri Q51.9
　　specified type NEC Q51.828
　Chiari
　　Type I G93.5
　　Type II Q07.01
　choroid (congenital) Q14.3
　　plexus Q07.8
　circulatory system Q28.9
　cochlea Q16.5
　cornea Q13.4
　coronary vessels Q24.5
　corpus callosum (congenital) Q04.0
　diaphragm Q79.1
　digestive system NEC, specified type NEC Q45.8
　dura Q07.9
　　brain Q04.9
　　spinal Q06.9
　ear Q17.9
　　causing impairment of hearing Q16.9
　　external Q17.9
　　　accessory auricle Q17.0
　　　causing impairment of hearing Q16.9
　　　　absence of
　　　　　auditory canal Q16.1
　　　　　auricle Q16.0
　　　macrotia Q17.1
　　　microtia Q17.2
　　　misplacement Q17.4
　　　misshapen NEC Q17.3
　　　prominence Q17.5
　　　specified type NEC Q17.8
　　inner Q16.5
　　middle Q16.4
　　　absence of eustachian tube Q16.2
　　　ossicles (fusion) Q16.3
　　ossicles Q16.3
　　specified type NEC Q17.8
　epididymis Q55.4
　esophagus Q39.9
　　specified type NEC Q39.8
　eye Q15.9
　　lid Q10.3
　　specified NEC Q15.8
　fallopian tube Q50.6
　genital organ — *see* Anomaly, genitalia
　great
　　artery Q25.9
　　　aorta — *see* Malformation, aorta

Malformation — *continued*
　great — *continued*
　　artery — *continued*
　　　pulmonary artery — *see* Malformation, pulmonary, artery
　　　specified type NEC Q25.8
　　vein Q26.9
　　　anomalous
　　　　portal venous connection Q26.5
　　　　pulmonary venous connection Q26.4
　　　　　partial Q26.3
　　　　　total Q26.2
　　　persistent left superior vena cava Q26.1
　　　portal vein-hepatic artery fistula Q26.6
　　　specified type NEC Q26.8
　　　vena cava stenosis, congenital Q26.0
　gum Q38.6
　hair Q84.2
　heart Q24.9
　　specified type NEC Q24.8
　integument Q84.9
　　specified type NEC Q84.8
　internal ear Q16.5
　intestine Q43.9
　　specified type NEC Q43.8
　iris Q13.2
　joint Q74.9
　　ankle Q74.2
　　lumbosacral Q76.49
　　sacroiliac Q74.2
　　specified type NEC Q74.8
　kidney Q63.9
　　accessory Q63.0
　　giant Q63.3
　　horseshoe Q63.1
　　hydronephrosis Q62.0
　　malposition Q63.2
　　specified type NEC Q63.8
　lacrimal apparatus Q10.6
　lingual Q38.3
　lip Q38.0
　liver Q44.70
　lung Q33.9
　meninges or membrane (congenital) Q07.9
　　cerebral Q04.8
　　spinal (cord) Q06.9
　middle ear Q16.4
　　ossicles Q16.3
　mitral valve Q23.9
　　specified NEC Q23.88
　Mondini's (congenital) (malformation, cochlea) Q16.5
　mouth (congenital) Q38.6
　multiple types NEC Q89.7
　musculoskeletal system Q79.9
　myocardium Q24.8
　nail Q84.6
　nervous system (central) Q07.9
　nose Q30.9
　　specified type NEC Q30.8
　optic disc Q14.2
　orbit Q10.7
　ovary Q50.39
　palate Q38.5
　parathyroid gland Q89.2
　pelvic organs or tissues NEC
　　in pregnancy or childbirth O34.8- ☑
　　　causing obstructed labor O65.5
　penis Q55.69
　　aplasia Q55.5
　　curvature (lateral) Q55.61
　　hypoplasia Q55.62
　pericardium Q24.8
　peripheral vascular system Q27.9
　　specified type NEC Q27.8
　pharynx Q38.8
　precerebral vessels Q28.1
　prostate Q55.4
　pulmonary
　　arteriovenous Q25.72
　　artery Q25.9
　　　atresia Q25.5
　　　specified type NEC Q25.79
　　　stenosis Q25.6
　　valve Q22.3
　renal artery Q27.2
　respiratory system Q34.9
　retina Q14.1
　scrotum — *see* Malformation, testis and scrotum
　seminal vesicles Q55.4

Malformation — *continued*
　sense organs NEC Q07.9
　skin Q82.9
　specified NEC Q89.89
　spinal
　　cord Q06.9
　　nerve root Q07.8
　spine Q76.49
　　kyphosis — *see* Kyphosis, congenital
　　lordosis — *see* Lordosis, congenital
　spleen Q89.09
　stomach Q40.3
　　specified type NEC Q40.2
　teeth, tooth K00.9
　tendon Q79.9
　testis and scrotum Q55.20
　　aplasia Q55.0
　　hypoplasia Q55.1
　　polyorchism Q55.21
　　retractile testis Q55.22
　　scrotal transposition Q55.23
　　specified NEC Q55.29
　thorax, bony Q76.9
　throat Q38.8
　thyroid gland Q89.2
　tongue (congenital) Q38.3
　　hypertrophy Q38.2
　　tie Q38.1
　trachea Q32.1
　tricuspid valve Q22.9
　　specified type NEC Q22.8
　umbilical cord NEC (complicating delivery) O69.89- ☑
　umbilicus Q89.9
　ureter Q62.8
　　agenesis Q62.4
　　duplication Q62.5
　　malposition — *see* Malposition, congenital, ureter
　　obstructive defect — *see* Defect, obstructive, ureter
　　vesico-uretero-renal reflux Q62.7
　urethra Q64.79
　　aplasia Q64.5
　　duplication Q64.74
　　posterior valves Q64.2
　　prolapse Q64.71
　　stricture Q64.32
　urinary system Q64.9
　uterus Q51.9
　　specified type NEC Q51.818
　vagina Q52.4
　vas deferens Q55.4
　　atresia Q55.3
　vascular system, peripheral Q27.9
　venous — *see* Anomaly, vein(s)
　vulva Q52.70
Malfunction — *see also* Dysfunction
　cardiac electronic device T82.119- ☑
　　electrode T82.110- ☑
　　pulse generator T82.111- ☑
　　specified type NEC T82.118- ☑
　catheter device NEC T85.618- ☑
　　cystostomy T83.010- ☑
　　dialysis (renal) (vascular) T82.41- ☑
　　　intraperitoneal T85.611- ☑
　　infusion NEC T82.514- ☑
　　　cranial — *see also* Complication(s), catheter, cranial infusion, mechanical T85.690- ☑
　　　epidural — *see also* Complication(s), catheter, cranial infusion, mechanical T85.690- ☑
　　　intrathecal — *see also* Complication(s), catheter, cranial infusion, mechanical T85.690- ☑
　　　spinal — *see also* Complication(s), catheter, cranial infusion, mechanical T85.690- ☑
　　　subarachnoid — *see also* Complication(s), catheter, cranial infusion, mechanical T85.690- ☑
　　　subdural — *see also* Complication(s), catheter, cranial infusion, mechanical T85.690- ☑
　　　urinary — *see also* Breakdown, device, catheter T83.018- ☑
　colostomy K94.03
　　valve K94.03
　cystostomy (stoma) N99.512
　　catheter T83.010- ☑
　enteric stoma K94.13
　enterostomy K94.13
　esophagostomy K94.33
　gastroenteric K31.89
　gastrostomy K94.23
　ileostomy K94.13

Malfunction — continued
- ileostomy — continued
  - valve K94.13
- intrathecal infusion pump T85.615- ☑
- jejunostomy K94.13
- nervous system device, implant or graft, specified NEC T85.615- ☑
- pacemaker — see Malfunction, cardiac electronic device
- prosthetic device, internal — see Complications, prosthetic device, by site, mechanical
- tracheostomy J95.03
- urinary device NEC — see Complication, genitourinary, device, urinary, mechanical
- valve
  - colostomy K94.03
  - heart T82.09- ☑
  - ileostomy K94.13
- vascular graft or shunt NEC — see Complication, cardiovascular device, mechanical, vascular
- ventricular (communicating shunt) T85.01- ☑

Malherbe's tumor — see Neoplasm, skin, benign
Malibu disease L98.8
Malignancy — see also Neoplasm, malignant, by site
- unspecified site (primary) C80.1

Malignant — see condition
Malingerer, malingering Z76.5
Mallet finger (acquired) — see Deformity, finger, mallet finger
- congenital Q74.0
- sequelae of rickets E64.3

Malleus A24.0
Mallory-Weiss syndrome K22.6
Mallory's bodies R89.7
Malnutrition E46
- degree
  - first E44.1
  - mild (protein) E44.1
  - moderate (protein) E44.0
  - second E44.0
  - severe (protein-energy) E43
    - with
      - kwashiorkor E40
      - marasmus E41
      - intermediate form E42
        - with
          - kwashiorkor E42
  - third E43
- following gastrointestinal surgery K91.2
- intrauterine
  - light-for-dates — see Light for dates
  - small-for-dates — see Small for dates
- lack of care, or neglect (child) (infant) T76.02- ☑
  - confirmed T74.02- ☑
- malignant E40
- protein E46
  - calorie E46
    - mild E44.1
    - moderate E44.0
    - severe E43
      - with
        - kwashiorkor E40
        - marasmus E41
        - intermediate form E42
          - with
            - kwashiorkor (and marasmus) E42
  - energy E46
    - mild E44.1
    - moderate E44.0
    - severe E43
      - with
        - kwashiorkor E40
        - marasmus E41
        - intermediate form E42
          - with
            - kwashiorkor (and marasmus) E42
  - severe (protein-energy) E43
    - with
      - kwashiorkor E40
        - with marasmus E42
      - intermediate form E42
        - with
          - kwashiorkor (and marasmus) E42
          - marasmus E41

Malocclusion (teeth) M26.4
- Angle's M26.219
  - class I M26.211
  - class II M26.212
  - class III M26.213

Malocclusion — continued
- due to
  - abnormal swallowing M26.59
  - mouth breathing M26.59
  - tongue, lip or finger habits M26.59
- temporomandibular (joint) M26.69

Malposition
- cervix — see Malposition, uterus
- congenital
  - adrenal (gland) Q89.1
  - alimentary tract Q45.8
    - lower Q43.8
    - upper Q40.8
  - aorta Q25.49
  - appendix Q43.8
  - arterial trunk Q20.0
  - artery (peripheral) Q27.8
    - coronary Q24.5
    - digestive system Q27.8
    - lower limb Q27.8
    - pulmonary Q25.79
    - specified site NEC Q27.8
    - upper limb Q27.8
  - auditory canal Q17.8
    - causing impairment of hearing Q16.9
  - auricle (ear) Q17.4
    - causing impairment of hearing Q16.9
    - cervical Q18.2
  - biliary duct or passage Q44.5
  - bladder (mucosa) — see Exstrophy, bladder
  - brachial plexus Q07.8
  - brain tissue Q04.8
  - breast Q83.8
  - bronchus Q32.4
  - cecum Q43.8
  - clavicle Q74.0
  - colon Q43.8
  - digestive organ or tract NEC Q45.8
    - lower Q43.8
    - upper Q40.8
  - ear (auricle) (external) Q17.4
    - ossicles Q16.3
  - endocrine (gland) NEC Q89.2
  - epiglottis Q31.8
  - eustachian tube Q17.8
  - eye Q15.8
  - facial features Q18.8
  - fallopian tube Q50.6
  - finger(s) Q68.1
    - supernumerary Q69.0
  - foot Q66.9- ☑
  - gallbladder Q44.1
  - gastrointestinal tract Q45.8
  - genitalia, genital organ(s) or tract
    - female Q52.8
      - external Q52.79
      - internal NEC Q52.8
    - male Q55.8
  - glottis Q31.8
  - hand Q68.1
  - heart Q24.8
    - dextrocardia Q24.0
      - with complete transposition of viscera Q89.3
  - hepatic duct Q44.5
  - hip (joint) Q65.89
  - intestine (large) (small) Q43.8
    - with anomalous adhesions, fixation or malrotation Q43.3
  - joint NEC Q68.8
  - kidney Q63.2
  - larynx Q31.8
  - limb Q68.8
    - lower Q68.8
    - upper Q68.8
  - liver Q44.79
  - lung (lobe) Q33.8
  - nail(s) Q84.6
  - nerve Q07.8
  - nervous system NEC Q07.8
  - nose, nasal (septum) Q30.8
  - organ or site not listed — see Anomaly, by site
  - ovary Q50.39
  - pancreas Q45.3
  - parathyroid (gland) Q89.2
  - patella Q74.1
  - peripheral vascular system Q27.8
  - pituitary (gland) Q89.2
  - respiratory organ or system NEC Q34.8
  - rib (cage) Q76.6

Malposition — continued
- congenital — continued
  - rib — continued
    - supernumerary in cervical region Q76.5
  - scapula Q74.0
  - shoulder Q74.0
  - spinal cord Q06.8
  - spleen Q89.09
  - sternum NEC Q76.7
  - stomach Q40.2
  - symphysis pubis Q74.2
  - thymus (gland) Q89.2
  - thyroid (gland) (tissue) Q89.2
    - cartilage Q31.8
  - toe(s) Q66.9- ☑
    - supernumerary Q69.2
  - tongue Q38.3
  - trachea Q32.1
  - ureter Q62.60
    - deviation Q62.61
    - displacement Q62.62
    - ectopia Q62.63
    - specified type NEC Q62.69
  - uterus Q51.818
  - vein(s) (peripheral) Q27.8
    - great Q26.8
  - vena cava (inferior) (superior) Q26.8
- device, implant or graft — see also Complications, by site and type, mechanical T85.628- ☑
  - arterial graft NEC — see Complication, cardiovascular device, mechanical, vascular
  - breast (implant) T85.42- ☑
  - catheter NEC T85.628- ☑
    - cystostomy T83.020- ☑
    - dialysis (renal) T82.42- ☑
      - intraperitoneal T85.621- ☑
    - infusion NEC T82.524- ☑
      - spinal (epidural) (subdural) T85.620- ☑
    - urinary — see also Displacement, device, catheter, urinary T83.028- ☑
  - electronic (electrode) (pulse generator) (stimulator)
    - bone T84.320- ☑
    - cardiac T82.129- ☑
      - electrode T82.120- ☑
      - pulse generator T82.121- ☑
      - specified type NEC T82.128- ☑
    - nervous system — see Complication, prosthetic device, mechanical, electronic nervous system stimulator
    - urinary — see Complication, genitourinary, device, urinary, mechanical
  - fixation, internal (orthopedic) NEC — see Complication, fixation device, mechanical
  - gastrointestinal — see Complications, prosthetic device, mechanical, gastrointestinal device
  - genital NEC T83.428- ☑
    - intrauterine contraceptive device (string) T83.32- ☑
    - penile prosthesis (cylinder) (implanted) (pump) (reservoir) T83.420- ☑
    - testicular prosthesis T83.421- ☑
  - heart NEC — see Complication, cardiovascular device, mechanical
  - joint prosthesis — see Complication, joint prosthesis, mechanical
  - ocular NEC — see Complications, prosthetic device, mechanical, ocular device
  - orthopedic NEC — see Complication, orthopedic, device, mechanical
  - specified NEC T85.628- ☑
  - urinary NEC — see also Complication, genitourinary device, urinary, mechanical
    - graft T83.22- ☑
  - vascular NEC — see Complication, cardiovascular device, mechanical
  - ventricular intracranial shunt T85.02- ☑
- fetus — see Pregnancy, complicated by (management affected by), presentation, fetal
- gallbladder K82.8
- gastrointestinal tract, congenital Q45.8
- heart, congenital NEC Q24.8
- joint prosthesis — see Complications, joint prosthesis, mechanical, displacement, by site
- stomach K31.89
  - congenital Q40.2
- tooth, teeth, fully erupted M26.30
- uterus (acute) (acquired) (adherent) (asymptomatic) (postinfectional) (postpartal, old) N85.4

Malposition — continued
  uterus — continued
    anteflexion or anteversion N85.4
      congenital Q51.818
    flexion N85.4
      lateral — see Lateroversion, uterus
    inversion N85.5
    lateral (flexion) (version) — see Lateroversion, uterus
    in pregnancy or childbirth — see subcategory O34.5-
    retroflexion or retroversion — see Retroversion, uterus
Malposture R29.3
Malrotation
  cecum Q43.3
  colon Q43.3
  intestine Q43.3
  kidney Q63.2
Malta fever — see Brucellosis
Maltreatment
  adult
    abandonment
      confirmed T74.01- ☑
      suspected T76.01- ☑
    bullying
      confirmed T74.31- ☑
      suspected T76.31- ☑
    confirmed T74.91- ☑
    financial
      confirmed T74.A1- ☑
      suspected T76.A1- ☑
    history of Z91.419
    intimidation (through social media)
      confirmed T74.31- ☑
      suspected T76.31- ☑
    neglect
      confirmed T74.01- ☑
      suspected T76.01- ☑
    physical abuse
      confirmed T74.11- ☑
      suspected T76.11- ☑
    psychological abuse
      confirmed T74.31- ☑
      history of Z91.411
      suspected T76.31- ☑
    sexual abuse
      confirmed T74.21- ☑
      suspected T76.21- ☑
    suspected T76.91- ☑
    threatened abuse (harm) (physical violence) (sexual abuse)
      confirmed T74.31- ☑
      suspected T76.31- ☑
  child
    abandonment
      confirmed T74.02- ☑
      suspected T76.02- ☑
    bullying
      confirmed T74.32- ☑
      suspected T76.32- ☑
    confirmed T74.92- ☑
    financial
      confirmed T74.A2- ☑
      suspected T76.A2- ☑
    history of — see History, personal (of), abuse
    intimidation (through social media)
      confirmed T74.32- ☑
      suspected T76.32- ☑
    neglect
      confirmed T74.02- ☑
      history of — see History, personal (of), abuse
      suspected T76.02- ☑
    physical abuse
      confirmed T74.12- ☑
      history of — see History, personal (of), abuse
      suspected T76.12- ☑
    psychological abuse
      confirmed T74.32- ☑
      history of — see History, personal (of), abuse
      suspected T76.32- ☑
    sexual abuse
      confirmed T74.22- ☑
      history of — see History, personal (of), abuse
      suspected T76.22- ☑
    suspected T76.92- ☑
    threatened abuse (harm) (physical violence) (sexual abuse)
      confirmed T74.32- ☑

Maltreatment — continued
  child — continued
    threatened abuse — continued
      suspected T76.32- ☑
    personal history of Z91.89
Maltworker's lung J67.4
Malunion, fracture — see Fracture, by site
Mammillitis N61.0
  puerperal, postpartum O91.02
Mammitis — see Mastitis
Mammogram (examination) Z12.39
  routine Z12.31
Mammoplasia N62
Management (of)
  bone conduction hearing device (implanted) Z45.320
  cardiac pacemaker NEC Z45.018
  cerebrospinal fluid drainage device Z45.41
  cochlear device (implanted) Z45.321
  contraceptive Z30.9
    specified NEC Z30.8
  implanted device Z45.9
    specified NEC Z45.89
  infusion pump Z45.1
  procreative Z31.9
    male factor infertility in female Z31.81
    specified NEC Z31.89
  prosthesis (external) — see also Fitting Z44.9
    implanted Z45.9
      specified NEC Z45.89
  renal dialysis catheter Z49.01
  vascular access device Z45.2
Mangled — see specified injury by site
Mania (monopolar) — see also Disorder, mood, manic episode
  with psychotic symptoms F30.2
  without psychotic symptoms F30.10
    mild F30.11
    moderate F30.12
    severe F30.13
  Bell's F30.8
  chronic (recurrent) F31.89
  hysterical F44.89
  puerperal F30.8
  recurrent F31.89
Manic depression F31.9
Manic-depressive insanity, psychosis, or syndrome — see Disorder, bipolar
Mannosidosis E77.1
Mansonelliasis, mansonellosis B74.4
Manson's
  disease B65.1
  schistosomiasis B65.1
Manual — see condition
Maple-bark-stripper's lung (disease) J67.6
Maple-syrup-urine disease E71.0
Marable's syndrome (celiac artery compression) I77.4
Marasmus E41
  due to malnutrition E41
  intestinal E41
  nutritional E41
  senile R54
  tuberculous NEC — see Tuberculosis
Marble
  bones Q78.2
  skin R23.8
Marburg virus disease A98.3
March
  fracture — see Fracture, traumatic, stress, by site
  hemoglobinuria D59.6
Marchesani (-Weill) **syndrome** Q87.0
Marchiafava-Micheli syndrome D59.5
Marchiafava (-Bignami) **syndrome or disease** G37.1
Marcus Gunn's syndrome Q07.8
Marfan syndrome — see Syndrome, Marfan
Marie-Bamberger disease — see Osteoarthropathy, hypertrophic, specified NEC
Marie-Charcot-Tooth neuropathic muscular atrophy G60.0
Marie-Strumpell arthritis, disease or spondylitis — see Spondylitis, ankylosing
Marie's
  cerebellar ataxia (late-onset) G11.2
  disease or syndrome (acromegaly) E22.0
Marion's disease (bladder neck obstruction) N32.0
Marital conflict Z63.0
Mark
  port wine Q82.5
  raspberry Q82.5
  strawberry Q82.5

Mark — continued
  stretch L90.6
  tattoo L81.8
Marker heterochromatin — see Extra, marker chromosomes
Maroteaux-Lamy syndrome (mild) (severe) E76.29
Marrow (bone)
  arrest D61.9
  poor function D75.89
Marseilles fever A77.1
Marsh fever — see Malaria
Marshall's (hidrotic) **ectodermal dysplasia** Q82.4
Marsh's disease (exophthalmic goiter) E05.00
  with storm E05.01
Masculinization (female) **with adrenal hyperplasia** E25.9
  congenital E25.0
Masculinovoblastoma D27.- ☑
Masochism (sexual) F65.51
Mason's lung J62.8
Mass
  abdominal R19.00
    epigastric R19.06
    generalized R19.07
    left lower quadrant R19.04
    left upper quadrant R19.02
    periumbilic R19.05
    right lower quadrant R19.03
    right upper quadrant R19.01
    specified site NEC R19.09
  breast — see also Lump, breast N63.0
  chest R22.2
  cystic — see Cyst
  ear H93.8- ☑
  head R22.0
  intra-abdominal (diffuse) (generalized) — see Mass, abdominal
  kidney N28.89
  liver R16.0
  localized (skin) R22.9
    chest R22.2
    head R22.0
    limb
      lower R22.4- ☑
      upper R22.3- ☑
    neck R22.1
    trunk R22.2
  lung R91.8
  malignant — see Neoplasm, malignant, by site
  neck R22.1
  pelvic (diffuse) (generalized) — see Mass, abdominal
  specified organ NEC — see Disease, by site
  splenic R16.1
  substernal thyroid — see Goiter
  superficial (localized) R22.9
  umbilical (diffuse) (generalized) R19.09
Massive — see condition
Mast cell
  disease, systemic tissue D47.02
  leukemia C94.3- ☑
  neoplasm
    malignant C96.20
      specified type NEC C96.29
    of uncertain behavior NEC D47.09
  sarcoma C96.22
  tumor D47.09
Mastalgia N64.4
Masters-Allen syndrome N83.8
Mastitis (acute) (diffuse) (nonpuerperal) (subacute) N61.0
  with abscess N61.1
  chronic (cystic) — see Mastopathy, cystic
  cystic (Schimmelbusch's type) — see Mastopathy, cystic
  fibrocystic — see Mastopathy, cystic
  granulomatous N61.2- ☑
  infective N61.0
    newborn P39.0
  interstitial, gestational or puerperal — see Mastitis, obstetric
  neonatal (noninfective) P83.4
    infective P39.0
  obstetric (interstitial) (nonpurulent)
    associated with
      lactation O91.23
      pregnancy O91.21- ☑
      puerperium O91.22
    purulent
      associated with
        lactation O91.13
        pregnancy O91.11- ☑

Mastitis

Mastitis — continued
- obstetric — continued
  - purulent — continued
    - associated with — continued
      - puerperium O91.12
  - periductal — see Ectasia, mammary duct
  - phlegmonous — see Mastopathy, cystic
  - plasma cell — see Ectasia, mammary duct
  - without abscess N61.0
- **Mastocytoma** (extracutaneous) D47.09
  - malignant C96.29
  - solitary D47.01
- **Mastocytosis** D47.09
  - aggressive systemic C96.21
  - cutaneous (diffuse) (maculopapular) D47.01
    - congenital Q82.2
    - of neonatal onset Q82.2
    - of newborn onset Q82.2
  - indolent systemic D47.02
  - isolated bone marrow D47.02
  - malignant C96.29
  - systemic (indolent) (smoldering)
    - with an associated hematological non-mast cell lineage disease (SM-AHNMD) D47.02
- **Mastodynia** N64.4
- **Mastoid** — see condition
- **Mastoidalgia** — see subcategory H92.0- ☑
- **Mastoiditis** (coalescent) (hemorrhagic) (suppurative) H70.9- ☑
  - acute, subacute H70.00- ☑
    - complicated NEC H70.09- ☑
    - subperiosteal H70.01- ☑
  - chronic (necrotic) (recurrent) H70.1- ☑
  - in (due to)
    - infectious disease NEC B99.- ☑ [H75.0-] ☑
    - parasitic disease NEC B89 [H75.0-] ☑
    - tuberculosis A18.03
  - petrositis — see Petrositis
  - postauricular fistula — see Fistula, postauricular
  - specified NEC H70.89- ☑
  - tuberculous A18.03
- **Mastopathy, mastopathia** N64.9
  - chronica cystica — see Mastopathy, cystic
  - cystic (chronic) (diffuse) N60.1- ☑
    - with epithelial proliferation N60.3- ☑
  - diffuse cystic — see Mastopathy, cystic
  - estrogenic, oestrogenica, oestrogenic N64.89
  - ovarian origin N64.89
- **Mastoplasia, mastoplastia** N62
- **Masturbation** (excessive) F98.8
- **Maternal care** (for) — see Pregnancy (complicated by) (management affected by)
- **Matheiu's disease** (leptospiral jaundice) A27.0
- **Mauclaire's disease or osteochondrosis** — see Osteochondrosis, juvenile, hand, metacarpal
- **Maxcy's disease** A75.2
- **Maxilla, maxillary** — see condition
- **May** (-Hegglin) **anomaly or syndrome** D72.0
- **McArdle** (-Schmid)(-Pearson) **disease** (glycogen storage) E74.04
- **McCune-Albright syndrome** Q78.1
- **McQuarrie's syndrome** (idiopathic familial hypoglycemia) E16.2
- **ME/CFS** (myalgic encephalomyelitis/chronic fatigue syndrome) G93.32
- **Meadow's syndrome** Q86.1
- **Measles** (black) (hemorrhagic) (suppressed) B05.9
  - with
    - complications NEC B05.89
    - encephalitis B05.0
    - intestinal complications B05.4
    - keratitis (keratoconjunctivitis) B05.81
    - meningitis B05.1
    - otitis media B05.3
    - pneumonia B05.2
  - French — see Rubella
  - German — see Rubella
  - Liberty — see Rubella
- **Meat-wrappers' asthma** J68.9
- **Meatitis, urethral** — see Urethritis
- **Meatus, meatal** — see condition
- **Meckel-Gruber syndrome** Q61.9
- **Meckel's diverticulitis, diverticulum** (displaced) (hypertrophic) Q43.0
  - malignant — see Table of Neoplasms, small intestine, malignant
- **Meconium**
  - ileus, newborn P76.0

Meconium — continued
- ileus, newborn — continued
  - in cystic fibrosis E84.11
  - meaning meconium plug (without cystic fibrosis) P76.0
- obstruction, newborn P76.0
  - due to fecaliths P76.0
  - in mucoviscidosis E84.11
- peritonitis P78.0
- plug syndrome (newborn) NEC P76.0
- **MED13L** (mediator complex subunit 13L) **syndrome** Q87.85
- **Median** — see also condition
  - arcuate ligament syndrome I77.4
  - bar (prostate) (vesical orifice) — see Hyperplasia, prostate
  - rhomboid glossitis K14.2
- **Mediastinal shift** R93.89
- **Mediastinitis** (acute) (chronic) J98.51
  - syphilitic A52.73
  - tuberculous A15.8
- **Mediastinopericarditis** — see also Pericarditis
  - acute I30.9
  - adhesive I31.0
  - chronic I31.8
    - rheumatic I09.2
- **Mediastinum, mediastinal** — see condition
- **Mediator complex subunit 13L** (MED13L) **syndrome** Q87.85
- **Medicine poisoning** — see Table of Drugs and Chemicals, by drug, poisoning
- **Mediterranean**
  - fever — see Brucellosis
    - familial M04.1
    - tick A77.1
  - kala-azar B55.0
  - leishmaniasis B55.0
  - tick fever A77.1
- **Medulla** — see condition
- **Medullary cystic kidney** Q61.5
- **Medullated fibers**
  - optic (nerve) Q14.8
  - retina Q14.1
- **Medulloblastoma**
  - desmoplastic C71.6
  - specified site — see Neoplasm, malignant, by site
  - unspecified site C71.6
- **Medulloepithelioma** — see also Neoplasm, malignant, by site
  - teratoid — see Neoplasm, malignant, by site
- **Medullomyoblastoma**
  - specified site — see Neoplasm, malignant, by site
  - unspecified site C71.6
- **Meekeren-Ehlers-Danlos syndrome** — see also Syndrome, Ehlers-Danlos Q79.69
- **Megacolon** (acquired) (functional) (not Hirschsprung's disease) (in) K59.39
  - Chagas' disease B57.32
  - congenital, congenitum (aganglionic) Q43.1
  - Hirschsprung's (disease) Q43.1
  - toxic NEC K59.31
    - due to
      - Clostridioides difficile
        - not specified as recurrent A04.72
        - recurrent A04.71
      - Clostridium difficile
        - not specified as recurrent A04.72
        - recurrent A04.71
- **Megaesophagus** (functional) K22.0
  - congenital Q39.5
  - in (due to) Chagas' disease B57.31
- **Megalencephaly** Q04.5
- **Megalerythema** (epidemic) B08.3
- **Megaloappendix** Q43.8
- **Megalocephalus, megalocephaly** NEC Q75.3
- **Megalocornea** Q15.8
  - with glaucoma Q15.0
- **Megalocytic anemia** D53.1
- **Megalodactylia** (fingers) (thumbs) (congenital) Q74.0
  - toes Q74.2
- **Megaloduodenum** Q43.8
- **Megaloesophagus** (functional) K22.0
  - congenital Q39.5
- **Megalogastria** (acquired) K31.89
  - congenital Q40.2
- **Megalophthalmos** Q11.3
- **Megalopsia** H53.15
- **Megalosplenia** — see Splenomegaly
- **Megaloureter** N28.82
  - congenital Q62.2
- **Megarectum** K62.89

Megasigmoid K59.39
- congenital Q43.2
- **Megaureter** N28.82
  - congenital Q62.2
- **Megavitamin-B6 syndrome** E67.2
- **Megrim** — see Migraine
- **Meibomian**
  - cyst, infected — see Hordeolum
  - gland — see condition
  - sty, stye — see Hordeolum
- **Meibomitis** — see Hordeolum
- **Meige-Milroy disease** (chronic hereditary edema) Q82.0
- **Meige's syndrome** Q82.0
- **Melalgia, nutritional** E53.8
- **Melancholia** F32.A
  - climacteric (single episode) F32.89
    - recurrent episode F33.8
  - hypochondriac F45.29
  - intermittent (single episode) F32.89
    - recurrent episode F33.8
  - involutional (single episode) F32.89
    - recurrent episode F33.8
  - menopausal (single episode) F32.89
    - recurrent episode F33.8
  - puerperal F32.89
  - reactive (emotional stress or trauma) F32.3
  - recurrent F33.9
  - senile F03.- ☑
  - stuporous (single episode) F32.89
    - recurrent episode F33.8
- **Melanemia** R79.89
- **Melanoameloblastoma** — see Neoplasm, bone, benign
- **Melanoblastoma** — see Melanoma
- **Melanocarcinoma** — see Melanoma
- **Melanocytoma, eyeball** D31.9- ☑
- **Melanocytosis, neurocutaneous** Q82.8
- **Melanoderma, melanodermia** L81.4
- **Melanodontia, infantile** K03.89
- **Melanodontoclasia** K03.89
- **Melanoepithelioma** — see Melanoma
- **Melanoma** (malignant) C43.9
  - acral lentiginous, malignant — see Melanoma, skin, by site
  - amelanotic — see Melanoma, skin, by site
  - balloon cell — see Melanoma, skin, by site
  - benign — see Nevus
  - desmoplastic, malignant — see Melanoma, skin, by site
  - epithelioid cell — see Melanoma, skin, by site
    - with spindle cell, mixed — see Melanoma, skin, by site
  - in
    - giant pigmented nevus — see Melanoma, skin, by site
    - Hutchinson's melanotic freckle — see Melanoma, skin, by site
    - junctional nevus — see Melanoma, skin, by site
    - precancerous melanosis — see Melanoma, skin, by site
  - in situ D03.9
    - abdominal wall D03.59
    - ala nasi D03.39
    - ankle D03.7- ☑
    - anus, anal (margin) (skin) D03.51
    - arm D03.6- ☑
    - auditory canal D03.2- ☑
    - auricle (ear) D03.2- ☑
    - auricular canal (external) D03.2- ☑
    - axilla, axillary fold D03.59
    - back D03.59
    - breast D03.52
    - brow D03.39
    - buttock D03.59
    - canthus (eye) D03.1- ☑
    - cheek (external) D03.39
    - chest wall D03.59
    - chin D03.39
    - choroid D03.8
    - conjunctiva D03.8
    - ear (external) D03.2- ☑
    - external meatus (ear) D03.2- ☑
    - eye D03.8
    - eyebrow D03.39
    - eyelid (lower) (upper) D03.1- ☑
    - face D03.30
      - specified NEC D03.39
    - female genital organ (external) NEC D03.8
    - finger D03.6- ☑
    - flank D03.59

Melanoma — *continued*
　in situ — *continued*
　　foot D03.7- ☑
　　forearm D03.6- ☑
　　forehead D03.39
　　foreskin D03.8
　　gluteal region D03.59
　　groin D03.59
　　hand D03.6- ☑
　　heel D03.7- ☑
　　helix D03.2- ☑
　　hip D03.7- ☑
　　interscapular region D03.59
　　iris D03.8
　　jaw D03.39
　　knee D03.7- ☑
　　labium (majus) (minus) D03.8
　　lacrimal gland D03.8
　　leg D03.7- ☑
　　lip (lower) (upper) D03.0
　　lower limb NEC D03.7- ☑
　　male genital organ (external) NEC D03.8
　　nail D03.9
　　　finger D03.6- ☑
　　　toe D03.7- ☑
　　neck D03.4
　　nose (external) D03.39
　　orbit D03.8
　　penis D03.8
　　perianal skin D03.51
　　perineum D03.51
　　pinna D03.2- ☑
　　popliteal fossa or space D03.7- ☑
　　prepuce D03.8
　　pudendum D03.8
　　retina D03.8
　　retrobulbar D03.8
　　scalp D03.4
　　scrotum D03.8
　　shoulder D03.6- ☑
　　specified site NEC D03.8
　　submammary fold D03.52
　　temple D03.39
　　thigh D03.7- ☑
　　toe D03.7- ☑
　　trunk NEC D03.59
　　umbilicus D03.59
　　upper limb NEC D03.6- ☑
　　vulva D03.8
　juvenile — *see* Nevus
　malignant, of soft parts except skin — *see* Neoplasm, connective tissue, malignant
　metastatic
　　breast C79.81
　　genital organ C79.82
　　specified site NEC C79.89
　neurotropic, malignant — *see* Melanoma, skin, by site
　nodular — *see* Melanoma, skin, by site
　regressing, malignant — *see* Melanoma, skin, by site
　skin C43.9
　　abdominal wall C43.59
　　ala nasi C43.31
　　ankle C43.7- ☑
　　anus, anal (skin) C43.51
　　arm C43.6- ☑
　　auditory canal (external) C43.2- ☑
　　auricle (ear) C43.2- ☑
　　auricular canal (external) C43.2- ☑
　　axilla, axillary fold C43.59
　　back C43.59
　　breast (female) (male) C43.52
　　brow C43.39
　　buttock C43.59
　　canthus (eye) C43.1- ☑
　　cheek (external) C43.39
　　chest wall C43.59
　　chin C43.39
　　ear (external) C43.2- ☑
　　elbow C43.6- ☑
　　external meatus (ear) C43.2- ☑
　　eyebrow C43.39
　　eyelid (lower) (upper) C43.1- ☑
　　face C43.30
　　　specified NEC C43.39
　　female genital organ (external) NEC C51.9
　　finger C43.6- ☑
　　flank C43.59

Melanoma — *continued*
　skin — *continued*
　　foot C43.7- ☑
　　forearm C43.6- ☑
　　forehead C43.39
　　foreskin C60.0
　　glabella C43.39
　　gluteal region C43.59
　　groin C43.59
　　hand C43.6- ☑
　　heel C43.7- ☑
　　helix C43.2- ☑
　　hip C43.7- ☑
　　interscapular region C43.59
　　jaw (external) C43.39
　　knee C43.7- ☑
　　labium C51.9
　　　majus C51.0
　　　minus C51.1
　　leg C43.7- ☑
　　lip (lower) (upper) C43.0
　　lower limb NEC C43.7- ☑
　　male genital organ (external) NEC C63.9
　　nail
　　　finger C43.6- ☑
　　　toe C43.7- ☑
　　nasolabial groove C43.39
　　nates C43.59
　　neck C43.4
　　nose (external) C43.31
　　overlapping site C43.8
　　palpebra C43.1- ☑
　　penis C60.9
　　perianal skin C43.51
　　perineum C43.51
　　pinna C43.2- ☑
　　popliteal fossa or space C43.7- ☑
　　prepuce C60.0
　　pudendum C51.9
　　scalp C43.4
　　scrotum C63.2
　　shoulder C43.6- ☑
　　skin NEC C43.9
　　submammary fold C43.52
　　temple C43.39
　　thigh C43.7- ☑
　　toe C43.7- ☑
　　trunk NEC C43.59
　　umbilicus C43.59
　　upper limb NEC C43.6- ☑
　　vulva C51.9
　　　overlapping sites C51.8
　spindle cell
　　with epithelioid, mixed — *see* Melanoma, skin, by site
　　type A C69.4- ☑
　　type B C69.4- ☑
　superficial spreading — *see* Melanoma, skin, by site
Melanosarcoma — *see also* Melanoma
　epithelioid cell — *see* Melanoma
Melanosis L81.4
　addisonian E27.1
　　tuberculous A18.7
　adrenal E27.1
　colon K63.89
　conjunctiva — *see* Pigmentation, conjunctiva
　　congenital Q13.89
　cornea (presenile) (senile) — *see also* Pigmentation, cornea
　　congenital Q13.4
　eye NEC H57.89
　　congenital Q15.8
　lenticularis progressiva Q82.1
　liver K76.89
　precancerous — *see also* Melanoma, in situ
　　malignant melanoma in — *see* Melanoma
　Riehl's L81.4
　sclera H15.89
　　congenital Q13.89
　suprarenal E27.1
　tar L81.4
　toxic L81.4
Melanuria R82.998
MELAS syndrome E88.41
Melasma L81.1
　adrenal (gland) E27.1
　suprarenal (gland) E27.1
Melena K92.1

Melena — *continued*
　with ulcer — *code by* site under Ulcer, with hemorrhage K27.4
　due to swallowed maternal blood P78.2
　newborn, neonatal P54.1
　　due to swallowed maternal blood P78.2
Meleney's
　gangrene (cutaneous) — *see* Ulcer, skin
　ulcer (chronic undermining) — *see* Ulcer, skin
Melioidosis A24.9
　acute A24.1
　chronic A24.2
　fulminating A24.1
　pneumonia A24.1
　pulmonary (chronic) A24.2
　　acute A24.1
　　subacute A24.2
　sepsis A24.1
　specified NEC A24.3
　subacute A24.2
Melitensis, febris A23.0
Melkersson (-Rosenthal) **syndrome** G51.2
Mellitus, diabetes — *see* Diabetes
Melorheostosis (bone) — *see* Disorder, bone, density and structure, specified NEC
Meloschisis Q18.4
Melotia Q17.4
Membrana
　capsularis lentis posterior Q13.89
　epipapillaris Q14.2
Membranacea placenta O43.19- ☑
Membranaceous uterus N85.8
Membrane(s), membranous — *see also* condition
　cyclitic — *see* Membrane, pupillary
　folds, congenital — *see* Web
　Jackson's Q43.3
　over face of newborn P28.9
　premature rupture — *see* Rupture, membranes, premature
　pupillary H21.4- ☑
　　persistent Q13.89
　retained (with hemorrhage) (complicating delivery) O72.2
　　without hemorrhage O73.1
　secondary cataract — *see* Cataract, secondary
　unruptured (causing asphyxia) — *see* Asphyxia, newborn
　vitreous — *see* Opacity, vitreous, membranes and strands
Membranitis — *see* Chorioamnionitis
Memory disturbance, lack or loss — *see also* Amnesia
　mild, following organic brain damage F06.8
Menadione deficiency E56.1
Menarche
　delayed E30.0
　precocious E30.1
Mendacity, pathologic F60.2
Mendelson's syndrome (due to anesthesia) J95.4
　in labor and delivery O74.0
　in pregnancy O29.01- ☑
　obstetric O74.0
　postpartum, puerperal O89.01
Menetrier's disease or syndrome K29.60
　with bleeding K29.61
Meniere's disease, syndrome or vertigo H81.0- ☑
Meninges, meningeal — *see* condition
Meningioma — *see also* Neoplasm, meninges, benign
　angioblastic — *see* Neoplasm, meninges, benign
　angiomatous — *see* Neoplasm, meninges, benign
　atypical — *see* Neoplasm, meninges, uncertain behavior
　endotheliomatous — *see* Neoplasm, meninges, benign
　fibroblastic — *see* Neoplasm, meninges, benign
　fibrous — *see* Neoplasm, meninges, benign
　hemangioblastic — *see* Neoplasm, meninges, benign
　hemangiopericytic — *see* Neoplasm, meninges, benign
　malignant — *see* Neoplasm, meninges, malignant
　meningiothelial — *see* Neoplasm, meninges, benign
　meningotheliomatous — *see* Neoplasm, meninges, benign
　mixed — *see* Neoplasm, meninges, benign
　multiple — *see* Neoplasm, meninges, uncertain behavior
　papillary — *see* Neoplasm, meninges, uncertain behavior
　psammomatous — *see* Neoplasm, meninges, benign
　syncytial — *see* Neoplasm, meninges, benign
　transitional — *see* Neoplasm, meninges, benign
Meningiomatosis (diffuse) — *see* Neoplasm, meninges, uncertain behavior
Meningism — *see* Meningismus
Meningismus (infectional) (pneumococcal) R29.1
　due to serum or vaccine R29.1
　influenzal — *see* Influenza, with, manifestations NEC

Meningitis (basal) (basic) (brain) (cerebral) (cervical) (congestive) (diffuse) (hemorrhagic) (infantile) (membranous) (metastatic) (nonspecific) (pontine) (progressive) (simple) (spinal) (subacute) (sympathetic) (toxic) G03.9
- abacterial G03.0
- actinomycotic A42.81
- adenoviral A87.1
- arbovirus A87.8
- aseptic (acute) G03.0
- bacterial G00.9
  - Escherichia coli (E. coli) G00.8
  - Friedlander (bacillus) G00.8
  - gram-negative G00.9
  - H. influenzae G00.0
  - Klebsiella G00.8
  - pneumococcal G00.1
  - specified organism NEC G00.8
  - staphylococcal G00.3
  - streptococcal (acute) G00.2
- benign recurrent (Mollaret) G03.2
- candidal B37.5
- caseous (tuberculous) A17.0
- cerebrospinal A39.0
- chronic NEC G03.1
- clear cerebrospinal fluid NEC G03.0
- coxsackievirus A87.0
- cryptococcal B45.1
- diplococcal (gram positive) A39.0
- echovirus A87.0
- enteroviral A87.0
- eosinophilic B83.2
- epidemic NEC A39.0
- Escherichia coli (E. coli) G00.8
- fibrinopurulent G00.9
  - specified organism NEC G00.8
- Friedlander (bacillus) G00.8
- gonococcal A54.81
- gram-negative cocci G00.9
- gram-positive cocci G00.9
- H. influenzae G00.0
- Haemophilus (influenzae) G00.0
- in (due to)
  - adenovirus A87.1
  - African trypanosomiasis B56.9 [G02]
  - anthrax A22.8
  - bacterial disease NEC A48.8 [G01]
  - Chagas' disease (chronic) B57.41
  - chickenpox B01.0
  - coccidioidomycosis B38.4
  - Diplococcus pneumoniae G00.1
  - enterovirus A87.0
  - herpes (simplex) virus B00.3
    - zoster B02.1
  - infectious mononucleosis B27.92
  - leptospirosis A27.81
  - Listeria monocytogenes A32.11
  - Lyme disease A69.21
  - measles B05.1
  - mumps (virus) B26.1
  - neurosyphilis (late) A52.13
  - parasitic disease NEC B89 [G02]
  - poliovirus A80.9 [G02]
  - preventive immunization, inoculation or vaccination G03.8
  - rubella B06.02
  - Salmonella infection A02.21
  - specified cause NEC G03.8
  - Streptococcal pneumoniae G00.1
  - typhoid fever A01.01
  - varicella B01.0
  - viral disease NEC A87.8
  - whooping cough A37.90
  - zoster B02.1
- infectious G00.9
- influenzal (H. influenzae) G00.0
- Klebsiella G00.8
- leptospiral (aseptic) A27.81
- lymphocytic (acute) (benign) (serous) A87.2
- meningococcal A39.0
- Mima polymorpha G00.8
- Mollaret (benign recurrent) G03.2
- monilial B37.5
- mycotic NEC B49 [G02]
- Neisseria A39.0
- nonbacterial G03.0
- nonpyogenic NEC G03.0
- ossificans G96.198
- pneumococcal streptococcus pneumoniae G00.1

Meningitis — continued
- poliovirus A80.9 [G02]
- postmeasles B05.1
- purulent G00.9
  - specified organism NEC G00.8
- pyogenic G00.9
  - specified organism NEC G00.8
- Salmonella (arizonae) (Cholerae-Suis) (enteritidis) (typhimurium) A02.21
- septic G00.9
  - specified organism NEC G00.8
- serosa circumscripta NEC G03.0
- serous NEC G93.2
- specified organism NEC G00.8
- sporotrichosis B42.81
- staphylococcal G00.3
- sterile G03.0
- Streptococcal (acute) G00.2
  - pneumoniae G00.1
- suppurative G00.9
  - specified organism NEC G00.8
- syphilitic (late) (tertiary) A52.13
  - acute A51.41
  - congenital A50.41
  - secondary A51.41
- Torula histolytica (cryptococcal) B45.1
- traumatic (complication of injury) T79.8- ☑
- tuberculous A17.0
- typhoid A01.01
- viral NEC A87.9
- Yersinia pestis A20.3

Meningocele (spinal) — see also Spina bifida
- with hydrocephalus — see Spina bifida, by site, with hydrocephalus
- acquired (traumatic) G96.198
- cerebral — see Encephalocele

Meningocerebritis — see Meningoencephalitis

Meningococcemia A39.4
- acute A39.2
- chronic A39.3

Meningococcus, meningococcal — see also condition A39.9
- adrenalitis, hemorrhagic A39.1
- carrier (suspected) of Z22.31
- meningitis (cerebrospinal) A39.0

Meningoencephalitis — see also Encephalitis G04.90
- acute NEC — see also Encephalitis, viral A86
- bacterial NEC G04.2
- California A83.5
- diphasic A84.1
- eosinophilic B83.2
- epidemic A39.81
- herpesviral, herpetic B00.4
  - due to herpesvirus 6 B10.01
  - due to herpesvirus 7 B10.09
  - specified NEC B10.09
- in (due to)
  - blastomycosis NEC B40.81
  - diseases classified elsewhere G05.3
  - free-living amebae B60.2
  - H. influenzae G00.0
  - Hemophilus influenzae (H. influenzae) G00.0
  - herpes B00.4
    - due to herpesvirus 6 B10.01
    - due to herpesvirus 7 B10.09
    - specified NEC B10.09
  - Lyme disease A69.22
  - mercury — see subcategory T56.1- ☑
  - mumps B26.2
  - Naegleria (amebae) (organisms) (fowleri) B60.2
  - Parastrongylus cantonensis B83.2
  - toxoplasmosis (acquired) B58.2
    - congenital P37.1
- infectious (acute) (viral) A86
- influenzal (H. influenzae) G00.0
- Listeria monocytogenes A32.12
- lymphocytic (serous) A87.2
- mumps B26.2
- parasitic NEC B89 [G05.3]
- pneumococcal G00.1
- primary amebic B60.2
- specific (syphilitic) A52.14
- specified organism NEC G04.81
- staphylococcal G04.2
- streptococcal G04.2
- syphilitic A52.14
- toxic NEC G92.8
  - due to mercury — see subcategory T56.1- ☑
- tuberculous A17.82

Meningoencephalitis — continued
- virus NEC A86

Meningoencephalocele — see also Encephalocele
- syphilitic A52.19
- congenital A50.49

Meningoencephalomyelitis — see also Meningoencephalitis
- acute NEC (viral) A86
  - disseminated G04.00
    - postimmunization or postvaccination G04.02
    - postinfectious G04.01
- due to
  - actinomycosis A42.82
  - Torula B45.1
  - Toxoplasma or toxoplasmosis (acquired) B58.2
    - congenital P37.1
- postimmunization or postvaccination G04.02

Meningoencephalomyelopathy G96.9

Meningoencephalopathy G96.9

Meningomyelitis — see also Meningoencephalitis
- bacterial NEC G04.2
- blastomycotic NEC B40.81
- cryptococcal B45.1
- in diseases classified elsewhere G05.4
- meningococcal A39.81
- syphilitic A52.14
- tuberculous A17.82

Meningomyelocele — see also Spina bifida
- syphilitic A52.19

Meningomyeloneuritis — see Meningoencephalitis

Meningoradiculitis — see Meningitis

Meningovascular — see condition

Menkes' disease or syndrome E83.09
- meaning maple-syrup-urine disease E71.0

Menometrorrhagia N92.1

Menopause, menopausal (asymptomatic) (state) Z78.0
- arthritis (any site) NEC — see Arthritis, specified form NEC
- bleeding N92.4
- depression (single episode) F32.89
  - agitated (single episode) F32.2
    - recurrent episode F33.9
  - psychotic (single episode) F32.89
    - recurrent episode F33.9
  - recurrent episode F33.8
- melancholia (single episode) F32.89
  - recurrent episode F33.8
- paranoid state F22
- postirradiation (postprocedural)
  - asymptomatic E89.40
  - symptomatic E89.41
- premature E28.319
  - asymptomatic E28.319
    - postirradiation E89.40
    - postsurgical E89.40
  - symptomatic E28.310
    - postirradiation E89.41
    - postsurgical E89.41
- psychosis NEC F28
- symptomatic N95.1
- toxic polyarthritis NEC — see Arthritis, specified form NEC

Menorrhagia (primary) N92.0
- climacteric N92.4
  - menopausal N92.4
- menopausal N92.4
- perimenopausal N92.4
- postclimacteric N95.0
- postmenopausal N95.0
- preclimacteric or premenopausal N92.4
- pubertal (menses retained) N92.2

Menostaxis N92.0

Menses, retention N94.89

Menstrual — see Menstruation

Menstruation
- absent — see Amenorrhea
- anovulatory N97.0
- cycle, irregular N92.6
- delayed N91.0
- disorder N93.9
  - psychogenic F45.8
- during pregnancy O20.8
- excessive (with regular cycle) N92.0
  - with irregular cycle N92.1
  - at puberty N92.2
- frequent N92.0
- infrequent — see Oligomenorrhea
- irregular N92.6
  - specified NEC N92.5

Menstruation — continued
  latent N92.5
  membranous N92.5
  painful — see also Dysmenorrhea N94.6
    primary N94.4
    psychogenic F45.8
    secondary N94.5
  passage of clots N92.0
  precocious E30.1
  protracted N92.5
  rare — see Oligomenorrhea
  retained N94.89
  retrograde N92.5
  scanty — see Oligomenorrhea
  suppression N94.89
  vicarious (nasal) N94.89
Mental — see also condition
  deficiency — see Disability, intellectual
  deterioration — see Psychosis
  disorder — see Disorder, mental
  exhaustion F48.8
  insufficiency (congenital) — see Disability, intellectual
  observation without need for further medical care Z03.89
  retardation — see Disability, intellectual
  subnormality — see Disability, intellectuall
  upset — see Disorder, mental
Meralgia paresthetica G57.1- ☑
Mercurial — see condition
Mercurialism — see subcategory T56.1- ☑
Merkel cell tumor — see Carcinoma, Merkel cell
Merocele — see Hernia, femoral
Meromelia
  lower limb — see Defect, reduction, lower limb
    intercalary
      femur — see Defect, reduction, lower limb, specified type NEC
      tibiofibular (complete) (incomplete) — see Defect, reduction, lower limb
  upper limb — see Defect, reduction, upper limb
    intercalary, humeral, radioulnar — see Agenesis, arm, with hand present
MERRF syndrome (myoclonic epilepsy associated with ragged-red fiber) E88.42
Merzbacher-Pelizaeus disease E75.27
Mesaortitis — see Aortitis
Mesarteritis — see Arteritis
Mesencephalitis — see Encephalitis
Mesenchymoma — see also Neoplasm, connective tissue, uncertain behavior
  benign — see Neoplasm, connective tissue, benign
  malignant — see Neoplasm, connective tissue, malignant
Mesenteritis
  retractile K65.4
  sclerosing K65.4
Mesentery, mesenteric — see condition
Mesio-occlusion M26.213
Mesiodens, mesiodentes K00.1
Mesocolon — see condition
Mesonephroma (malignant) — see Neoplasm, malignant, by site
  benign — see Neoplasm, benign, by site
Mesophlebitis — see Phlebitis
Mesostromal dysgenesia Q13.89
Mesothelioma (malignant) C45.9
  benign
    mesentery D19.1
    mesocolon D19.1
    omentum D19.1
    peritoneum D19.1
    pleura D19.0
    specified site NEC D19.7
    unspecified site D19.9
  biphasic C45.9
    benign
      mesentery D19.1
      mesocolon D19.1
      omentum D19.1
      peritoneum D19.1
      pleura D19.0
      specified site NEC D19.7
      unspecified site D19.9
  cystic D48.4
  epithelioid C45.9
    benign
      mesentery D19.1
      mesocolon D19.1
      omentum D19.1
      peritoneum D19.1
      pleura D19.0

Mesothelioma — continued
  epithelioid — continued
    benign — continued
      specified site NEC D19.7
      unspecified site D19.9
  fibrous C45.9
    benign
      mesentery D19.1
      mesocolon D19.1
      omentum D19.1
      peritoneum D19.1
      pleura D19.0
      specified site NEC D19.7
      unspecified site D19.9
  site classification
    liver C45.7
    lung C45.7
    mediastinum C45.7
    mesentery C45.1
    mesocolon C45.1
    omentum C45.1
    pericardium C45.2
    peritoneum C45.1
    pleura C45.0
      parietal C45.0
    retroperitoneum C45.7
    specified site NEC C45.7
    unspecified C45.9
Metabolic syndrome E88.810
Metagonimiasis B66.8
Metagonimus infestation (intestine) B66.8
Metal
  pigmentation L81.8
  polisher's disease J62.8
Metamorphopsia H53.15
Metaplasia
  apocrine (breast) — see Dysplasia, mammary, specified type NEC
  cervix (squamous) — see Dysplasia, cervix
  endometrium (squamous) (uterus) N85.8
  esophagus K22.7- ☑
  gastric intestinal K31.A0
    with dysplasia K31.A29
      high grade K31.A22
      low grade K31.A21
    indefinite for dysplasia K31.A0
    without dysplasia K31.A19
    involving
      antrum K31.A11
      body (corpus) K31.A12
      cardia K31.A14
      fundus K31.A13
      multiple sites K31.A15
  kidney (pelvis) (squamous) N28.89
  myelogenous D73.1
  myeloid (agnogenic) (megakaryocytic) D73.1
  spleen D73.1
  squamous cell, bladder N32.89
Metastasis, metastatic
  abscess — see Abscess
  calcification E83.59
  cancer
    from specified site — see Neoplasm, malignant, by site
    to specified site — see Neoplasm, secondary, by site
  deposits (in) — see Neoplasm, secondary, by site
  disease — see also Neoplasm, secondary, by site C79.9
  spread (to) — see Neoplasm, secondary, by site
Metastrongyliasis B83.8
Metatarsalgia M77.4- ☑
  anterior G57.6- ☑
  Morton's G57.6- ☑
Metatarsus, metatarsal — see also condition
  adductus, congenital Q66.22- ☑
  valgus (abductus), congenital Q66.6
  varus (congenital) Q66.22- ☑
    primus Q66.21- ☑
Methadone use — see Use, opioid
Methemoglobinemia D74.9
  acquired (with sulfhemoglobinemia) D74.8
  congenital D74.0
  enzymatic (congenital) D74.0
  Hb M disease D74.0
  hereditary D74.0
  toxic D74.8
Methemoglobinuria — see Hemoglobinuria
Methioninemia E72.19
Methylmalonic acidemia E71.120

Metritis (catarrhal) (hemorrhagic) (septic) (suppurative) — see also Endometritis
  cervical — see Cervicitis
Metropathia hemorrhagica N93.8
Metroperitonitis — see Peritonitis, pelvic, female
Metrorrhagia N92.1
  climacteric N92.4
  menopausal N92.4
  perimenopausal N92.4
  postpartum NEC (atonic) (following delivery of placenta) O72.1
    delayed or secondary O72.2
  preclimacteric or premenopausal N92.4
  psychogenic F45.8
Metrorrhexis — see Rupture, uterus
Metrosalpingitis N70.91
Metrostaxis N93.8
Metrovaginitis — see Endometritis
Meyer-Schwickerath and Weyers syndrome Q87.0
Meynert's amentia (nonalcoholic) F04
  alcoholic F10.96
    with dependence F10.26
Mibelli's disease (porokeratosis) Q82.8
Mice, joint — see Loose, body, joint
  knee M23.4- ☑
Micrencephalon, micrencephaly Q02
Microalbuminuria R80.9
Microaneurysm, retinal — see also Disorder, retina, microaneurysms
  diabetic — see E08-E13 with .31
Microangiopathy (peripheral) I73.9
  thrombotic M31.10
    hematopoietic stem cell transplantation-associated [HSCT-TMA] M31.11
Microcalcifications, breast R92.0
Microcephalus, microcephalic, microcephaly Q02
  due to toxoplasmosis (congenital) P37.1
Microcheilia Q18.7
Microcolon (congenital) Q43.8
Microcornea (congenital) Q13.4
Microcytic — see condition
Microdeletions NEC Q93.88
Microdontia K00.2
Microdrepanocytosis D57.40
  with
    acute chest syndrome D57.411
    cerebral vascular involvement D57.413
    crisis (painful) D57.419
      with specified complication NEC D57.418
    pain (vaso-occlusive) D57.419
    splenic sequestration D57.412
Microembolism
  atherothrombotic — see Atheroembolism
  retinal — see Occlusion, artery, retina
Microencephalon Q02
Microfilaria streptocerca infestation — see Onchocerciasis
Microgastria (congenital) Q40.2
Microgenia M26.06
Microgenitalia, congenital
  female Q52.8
  male Q55.8
Microglioma — see Lymphoma, non-Hodgkin, specified NEC
Microglossia (congenital) Q38.3
Micrognathia, micrognathism (congenital) (mandibular) (maxillary) M26.09
Microgyria (congenital) Q04.3
Microinfarct of heart — see Insufficiency, coronary
Microlentia (congenital) Q12.8
Microlithiasis, alveolar, pulmonary J84.02
Micromastia N64.82
Micromyelia (congenital) Q06.8
Micropenis Q55.62
Microphakia (congenital) Q12.8
Microphthalmos, microphthalmia (congenital) Q11.2
  due to toxoplasmosis P37.1
Micropsia H53.15
Microscopic polyangiitis (polyarteritis) M31.7
Microsporidiosis B60.8
  intestinal A07.8
Microsporon furfur infestation B36.0
Microsporosis — see also Dermatophytosis
  nigra B36.1
Microstomia (congenital) Q18.5
Microtia (congenital) (external ear) Q17.2
Microtropia H50.40
Microvillus inclusion disease (MVD) (MVID) Q43.8

Micturition
- disorder NEC — *see also* Difficulty, micturition R39.198
  - psychogenic F45.8
- frequency R35.0
  - psychogenic F45.8
- hesitancy R39.11
- incomplete emptying R39.14
- nocturnal R35.1
- painful R30.9
  - dysuria R30.0
  - psychogenic F45.8
  - tenesmus R30.1
- poor stream R39.12
- position dependent R39.192
- split stream R39.13
- straining R39.16
- urgency R39.15

Mid plane — *see* condition

Middle
- ear — *see* condition
- lobe (right) syndrome J98.19

Miescher's elastoma L87.2
Mietens' syndrome Q87.2
Migraine (idiopathic) G43.909
- with refractory migraine G43.919
  - with status migrainosus G43.911
  - without status migrainosus G43.919
- with aura (acute-onset) (prolonged) (typical) (without headache) G43.109
  - with refractory migraine G43.119
    - with status migrainosus G43.111
    - without status migrainosus G43.119
  - chronic G43.E09
    - with refractory migraine G43.E19
      - with status migrainosus G43.E11
      - without status migrainosus G43.E19
    - intractable
      - with status migrainosus G43.E11
      - without status migrainosus G43.E19
    - not intractable
      - with status migrainosus G43.E01
      - without status migrainosus G43.E09
    - without refractory migraine G43.E09
      - with status migrainosus G43.E01
      - without status migrainosus G43.E09
  - intractable G43.119
    - with status migrainosus G43.111
    - without status migrainosus G43.119
  - not intractable G43.109
    - with status migrainosus G43.101
    - without status migrainosus G43.109
  - persistent G43.509
    - with cerebral infarction G43.609
      - with refractory migraine G43.619
        - with status migrainosus G43.611
        - without status migrainosus G43.619
      - intractable G43.619
        - with status migrainosus G43.611
        - without status migrainosus G43.619
      - not intractable G43.609
        - with status migrainosus G43.601
        - without status migrainosus G43.609
      - without refractory migraine G43.609
        - with status migrainosus G43.601
        - without status migrainosus G43.609
    - without cerebral infarction G43.509
      - with refractory migraine G43.519
        - with status migrainosus G43.511
        - without status migrainosus G43.519
      - intractable G43.519
        - with status migrainosus G43.511
        - without status migrainosus G43.519
      - not intractable G43.509
        - with status migrainosus G43.501
        - without status migrainosus G43.509
      - without refractory migraine G43.509
        - with status migrainosus G43.501
        - without status migrainosus G43.509
  - without mention of refractory migraine G43.109
    - with status migrainosus G43.101
    - without status migrainosus G43.109
  - abdominal G43.D0 (*following* G43.7)
    - with refractory migraine G43.D1 (*following* G43.7)
    - intractable G43.D1 (*following* G43.7)
    - not intractable G43.D0 (*following* G43.7)
    - without refractory migraine G43.D0 (*following* G43.7)
  - basilar — *see* Migraine, with aura
  - classical — *see* Migraine, with aura
  - common — *see* Migraine, without aura

Migraine — *continued*
- complicated G43.109
- equivalents — *see* Migraine, with aura
- familiar — *see* Migraine, hemiplegic
- hemiplegic G43.409
  - with refractory migraine G43.419
    - with status migrainosus G43.411
    - without status migrainosus G43.419
  - intractable G43.419
    - with status migrainosus G43.411
    - without status migrainosus G43.419
  - not intractable G43.409
    - with status migrainosus G43.401
    - without status migrainosus G43.409
  - without refractory migraine G43.409
    - with status migrainosus G43.401
    - without status migrainosus G43.409
- intractable G43.919
  - with status migrainosus G43.911
  - without status migrainosus G43.919
- menstrual G43.829
  - with refractory migraine G43.839
    - with status migrainosus G43.831
    - without status migrainosus G43.839
  - intractable G43.839
    - with status migrainosus G43.831
    - without status migrainosus G43.839
  - not intractable G43.829
    - with status migrainosus G43.821
    - without status migrainosus G43.829
  - without refractory migraine G43.829
    - with status migrainosus G43.821
    - without status migrainosus G43.829
- menstrually related — *see* Migraine, menstrual
- not intractable G43.909
  - with status migrainosus G43.901
  - without status migrainosus G43.909
- ophthalmoplegic G43.B0 (*following* G43.7)
  - with refractory migraine G43.B1 (*following* G43.7)
  - intractable G43.B1 (*following* G43.7)
  - not intractable G43.B0 (*following* G43.7)
  - without refractory migraine G43.B0 (*following* G43.7)
- persistent aura (with, without) cerebral infarction — *see* Migraine, with aura, persistent
- preceded or accompanied by transient focal neurological phenomena — *see* Migraine, with aura
- pre-menstrual — *see* Migraine, menstrual
- pure menstrual — *see* Migraine, menstrual
- retinal — *see* Migraine, with aura
- specified NEC G43.809
  - intractable G43.819
    - with status migrainosus G43.811
    - without status migrainosus G43.819
  - not intractable G43.809
    - with status migrainosus G43.801
    - without status migrainosus G43.809
- sporadic — *see* Migraine, hemiplegic
- transformed — *see* Migraine, without aura, chronic
- triggered seizures — *see* Migraine, with aura
- without aura G43.009
  - with refractory migraine G43.019
    - with status migrainosus G43.011
    - without status migrainosus G43.019
  - chronic G43.709
    - with refractory migraine G43.719
      - with status migrainosus G43.711
      - without status migrainosus G43.719
    - intractable
      - with status migrainosus G43.711
      - without status migrainosus G43.719
    - not intractable
      - with status migrainosus G43.701
      - without status migrainosus G43.709
    - without refractory migraine G43.709
      - with status migrainosus G43.701
      - without status migrainosus G43.709
  - intractable
    - with status migrainosus G43.011
    - without status migrainosus G43.019
  - not intractable
    - with status migrainosus G43.001
    - without status migrainosus G43.009
  - without mention of refractory migraine G43.009
    - with status migrainosus G43.001
    - without status migrainosus G43.009
  - without refractory migraine G43.909
    - with status migrainosus G43.901
    - without status migrainosus G43.909

Migrant, social Z59.00

Migration, anxiety concerning Z60.3
Migratory, migrating — *see also* condition
- person Z59.00
- testis Q55.29

Mikity-Wilson disease or syndrome P27.0
Mikulicz' disease or syndrome K11.8
Miliaria L74.3
- alba L74.1
- apocrine L75.2
- crystallina L74.1
- profunda L74.2
- rubra L74.0
- tropicalis L74.2

Miliary — *see* condition
Milium L72.0
- colloid L57.8

Milk
- crust L21.0
- excessive secretion O92.6
- poisoning — *see* Poisoning, food, noxious
- retention O92.79
- sickness — *see* Poisoning, food, noxious
- spots I31.0

Milk-alkali disease or syndrome E83.52
Milk-leg (deep vessels) (nonpuerperal) — *see* Embolism, vein, lower extremity
- complicating pregnancy O22.3- ☑
- puerperal, postpartum, childbirth O87.1

Milkman's disease or syndrome M83.8
Milky urine — *see* Chyluria
Millard-Gubler (-Foville) **paralysis or syndrome** G46.3
Millar's asthma J38.5
Miller Fisher syndrome G61.0
Mills' disease — *see* Hemiplegia
Millstone maker's pneumoconiosis J62.8
Milroy's disease (chronic hereditary edema) Q82.0
Minamata disease T56.1- ☑
Miners' asthma or lung J60
Minkowski-Chauffard syndrome — *see* Spherocytosis
Minor — *see* condition
Minor's disease (hematomyelia) G95.19
Minot-von Willebrand-Jurgens disease or syndrome (angiohemophilia) — *see* Disease, von Willebrand
Minot's disease (hemorrhagic disease), newborn P53
Minus (and plus) **hand** (intrinsic) — *see* Deformity, limb, specified type NEC, forearm
Miosis (pupil) H57.03
Mirizzi's syndrome (hepatic duct stenosis) K83.1
Mirror writing F81.0
MIS-A M35.81
MIS-C M35.81
Misadventure (of) (prophylactic) (therapeutic) — *see also* Complications T88.9- ☑
- administration of insulin (by accident) — *see* subcategory T38.3- ☑
- infusion — *see* Complications, infusion
- local applications (of fomentations, plasters, etc.) T88.9- ☑
  - burn or scald — *see* Burn
  - specified NEC T88.8- ☑
- medical care (early) (late) T88.9- ☑
  - adverse effect of drugs or chemicals — *see* Table of Drugs and Chemicals
  - burn or scald — *see* Burn
  - specified NEC T88.8- ☑
- specified NEC T88.8- ☑
- surgical procedure (early) (late) — *see* Complications, surgical procedure
- transfusion — *see* Complications, transfusion
- vaccination or other immunological procedure — *see* Complications, vaccination

Miscarriage O03.9
Misdirection, aqueous H40.83- ☑
Misperception, sleep state F51.02
Misplaced, misplacement
- ear Q17.4
- kidney (acquired) N28.89
  - congenital Q63.2
- organ or site, congenital NEC — *see* Malposition, congenital

Missed
- abortion O02.1
- delivery O36.4- ☑

Missing — *see also* Absence
- string of intrauterine contraceptive device T83.32- ☑

Misuse of drugs F19.99
Mitchell's disease (erythromelalgia) I73.81
Mite(s) (infestation) B88.9

Mite(s) — continued
 diarrhea B88.09
 grain (itch) B88.09
 hair follicle (itch) B88.09
 in sputum B88.09
Mitral — see condition
Mittelschmerz N94.0
Mixed — see condition
MMN (multifocal motor neuropathy) G61.82
MNGIE (Mitochondrial Neurogastrointestinal Encephalopathy) **syndrome** E88.49
Mobile, mobility
 cecum Q43.3
 excessive — see Hypermobility
 gallbladder, congenital Q44.1
 kidney N28.89
 organ or site, congenital NEC — see Malposition, congenital
Mobitz heart block (atrioventricular) I44.1
Moebius, Möbius
 disease (ophthalmoplegic migraine) — see Migraine, ophthalmoplegic
 syndrome Q87.0
  congenital oculofacial paralysis (with other anomalies) Q87.0
  ophthalmoplegic migraine — see Migraine, ophthalmoplegic
Moeller's glossitis K14.0
MOGAD (myelin oligodendrocyte glycoprotein antibody disease) G37.81
Mohr's syndrome (Types I and II) Q87.0
Mola destruens D39.2
Molar pregnancy O02.0
Molarization of premolars K00.2
Molding, head (during birth) — omit code
Mole (pigmented) — see also Nevus
 blood O02.0
 Breus' O02.0
 cancerous — see Melanoma
 carneous O02.0
 destructive D39.2
 fleshy O02.0
 hydatid, hydatidiform (benign) (complicating pregnancy) (delivered) (undelivered) O01.9
  classical O01.0
  complete O01.0
  incomplete O01.1
  invasive D39.2
  malignant D39.2
  partial O01.1
 intrauterine O02.0
 invasive (hydatidiform) D39.2
 malignant
  meaning
   malignant hydatidiform mole D39.2
   melanoma — see Melanoma
 nonhydatidiform O02.0
 nonpigmented — see Nevus
 pregnancy NEC O02.0
 skin — see Nevus
 tubal O00.10- ☑
  with intrauterine pregnancy O00.11- ☑
 vesicular — see Mole, hydatidiform
Molimen, molimina (menstrual) N94.3
Molluscum contagiosum (epitheliale) B08.1
Monckeberg's arteriosclerosis, disease, or sclerosis — see Arteriosclerosis, extremities
Mondini's malformation (cochlea) Q16.5
Mondor's disease I80.8
Monge's disease T70.29- ☑
Monilethrix (congenital) Q84.1
Moniliasis — see also Candidiasis B37.9
 neonatal P37.5
Monitoring (encounter for)
 therapeutic drug level Z51.81
Monkey malaria B53.1
Monkeypox B04
Monoarthritis M13.10
 ankle M13.17- ☑
 elbow M13.12- ☑
 foot joint M13.17- ☑
 hand joint M13.14- ☑
 hip M13.15- ☑
 knee M13.16- ☑
 shoulder M13.11- ☑
 wrist M13.13- ☑
Monoblastic — see condition

Monochromat (ism), monochromatopsia (acquired) (congenital) H53.51
Monocytic — see condition
Monocytopenia D72.818
Monocytosis (symptomatic) D72.821
Monomania — see Psychosis
Mononeuritis G58.9
 cranial nerve — see Disorder, nerve, cranial
 femoral nerve G57.2- ☑
 lateral
  cutaneous nerve of thigh G57.1- ☑
  popliteal nerve G57.3- ☑
 lower limb G57.9- ☑
  specified nerve NEC G57.8- ☑
 medial popliteal nerve G57.4- ☑
 median nerve G56.1- ☑
 multiplex G58.7
 plantar nerve G57.6- ☑
 posterior tibial nerve G57.5- ☑
 radial nerve G56.3- ☑
 sciatic nerve G57.0- ☑
 specified NEC G58.8
 tibial nerve G57.4- ☑
 ulnar nerve G56.2- ☑
 upper limb G56.9- ☑
  specified nerve NEC G56.8- ☑
 vestibular — see subcategory H93.3- ☑
Mononeuropathy G58.9
 carpal tunnel syndrome — see Syndrome, carpal tunnel
 diabetic NEC — see E08-E13 with .41
 femoral nerve — see Lesion, nerve, femoral
 ilioinguinal nerve G57.8- ☑
 in diseases classified elsewhere — see category G59
 intercostal G58.0
 lower limb G57.9- ☑
  causalgia — see Causalgia, lower limb
  femoral nerve — see Lesion, nerve, femoral
  meralgia paresthetica G57.1- ☑
  plantar nerve — see Lesion, nerve, plantar
  popliteal nerve — see Lesion, nerve, popliteal
  sciatic nerve — see Lesion, nerve, sciatic
  specified NEC G57.8- ☑
  tarsal tunnel syndrome — see Syndrome, tarsal tunnel
 median nerve — see Lesion, nerve, median
 multiplex G58.7
 obturator nerve G57.8- ☑
 popliteal nerve — see Lesion, nerve, popliteal
 radial nerve — see Lesion, nerve, radial
 saphenous nerve G57.8- ☑
 specified NEC G58.8
 tarsal tunnel syndrome — see Syndrome, tarsal tunnel
 tuberculous A17.83
 ulnar nerve — see Lesion, nerve, ulnar
 upper limb G56.9- ☑
  carpal tunnel syndrome — see Syndrome, carpal tunnel
  causalgia — see Causalgia
  median nerve — see Lesion, nerve, median
  radial nerve — see Lesion, nerve, radial
  specified site NEC G56.8- ☑
  ulnar nerve — see Lesion, nerve, ulnar
Mononucleosis, infectious B27.90
 with
  complication NEC B27.99
  meningitis B27.92
  polyneuropathy B27.91
 cytomegaloviral B27.10
  with
   complication NEC B27.19
   meningitis B27.12
   polyneuropathy B27.11
 Epstein-Barr (virus) B27.00
  with
   complication NEC B27.09
   meningitis B27.02
   polyneuropathy B27.01
 gammaherpesviral B27.00
  with
   complication NEC B27.09
   meningitis B27.02
   polyneuropathy B27.01
 specified NEC B27.80
  with
   complication NEC B27.89
   meningitis B27.82
   polyneuropathy B27.81
Monoparesis — see Monoplegia
Monoplegia G83.3- ☑

Monoplegia — continued
 congenital (cerebral) G80.8
  spastic G80.1
 embolic (current episode) I63.4- ☑
 following
  cerebrovascular disease
   cerebral infarction
    lower limb I69.34- ☑
    upper limb I69.33- ☑
   intracerebral hemorrhage
    lower limb I69.14- ☑
    upper limb I69.13- ☑
   lower limb I69.94- ☑
   nontraumatic intracranial hemorrhage NEC
    lower limb I69.24- ☑
    upper limb I69.23- ☑
   specified disease NEC
    lower limb I69.84- ☑
    upper limb I69.83- ☑
   stroke NOS
    lower limb I69.34- ☑
    upper limb I69.33- ☑
   subarachnoid hemorrhage
    lower limb I69.04- ☑
    upper limb I69.03- ☑
   upper limb I69.93- ☑
 hysterical (transient) F44.4
 lower limb G83.1- ☑
 psychogenic (conversion reaction) F44.4
 thrombotic (current episode) I63.3- ☑
 transient R29.818
 upper limb G83.2- ☑
Monorchism, monorchidism Q55.0
Monosomy — see also Deletion, chromosome Q93.9
 specified NEC Q93.89
 whole chromosome
  meiotic nondisjunction Q93.0
  mitotic nondisjunction Q93.1
  mosaicism Q93.1
 X Q96.9
Monster, monstrosity (single) Q89.7
 acephalic Q00.0
 twin Q89.4
Monteggia's fracture (-dislocation) S52.27- ☑
Mooren's ulcer (cornea) — see Ulcer, cornea, Mooren's
Moore's syndrome — see Epilepsy, specified NEC
Mooser-Neill reaction A75.2
Mooser's bodies A75.2
Morbidity not stated or unknown R69
Morbilli — see Measles
Morbus — see also Disease
 angelicus, anglorum E55.0
 Beigel B36.2
 caducus — see Epilepsy
 celiacus K90.0
 comitialis — see Epilepsy
 cordis — see also Disease, heart I51.9
  valvulorum — see Endocarditis
 coxae senilis M16.9
  tuberculous A18.02
 hemorrhagicus neonatorum P53
 maculosus neonatorum P54.5
Morel-Kraepelin disease — see Schizophrenia
Morel-Moore syndrome M85.2
Morel (-Stewart)(-Morgagni) **syndrome** M85.2
Morgagni-Stewart-Morel syndrome M85.2
Morgagni-Stokes-Adams syndrome I45.9
Morgagni-Turner (-Albright) **syndrome** Q96.9
Morgagni's
 cyst, organ, hydatid, or appendage
  female Q50.5
  male (epididymal) Q55.4
   testicular Q55.29
 syndrome M85.2
Moria F07.0
Moron (I.Q. 50-69) F70
Morphea L94.0
Morphinism (without remission) F11.20
 with remission F11.21
Morphinomania (without remission) F11.20
 with remission F11.21
Morquio (-Ullrich)(-Brailsford) **disease or syndrome** — see Mucopolysaccharidosis
Mortification (dry) (moist) — see Gangrene
Morton's metatarsalgia (neuralgia) (neuroma) (syndrome) G57.6- ☑
Morvan's disease or syndrome G60.8

Mosaicism, mosaic (autosomal) (chromosomal)
- 45,X/46,XX Q96.3
- 45,X/other cell lines NEC with abnormal sex chromosome Q96.4
- sex chromosome
  - female Q97.8
  - lines with various numbers of X chromosomes Q97.2
  - male Q98.7
- XY Q96.3

Moschowitz' disease M31.19
Mother yaw A66.0
Motion sickness (from travel, any vehicle) (from roundabouts or swings) T75.3- ☑
Mottled, mottling, teeth (enamel) (endemic) (nonendemic) K00.3
Mounier-Kuhn syndrome Q32.4
- with bronchiectasis J47.9
  - exacerbation (acute) J47.1
  - lower respiratory infection J47.0
- acquired J98.09
  - with bronchiectasis J47.9
    - with
      - exacerbation (acute) J47.1
      - lower respiratory infection J47.0

Mountain
- sickness T70.29- ☑
  - with polycythemia, acquired (acute) D75.1
- tick fever A93.2

Mouse, joint — see Loose, body, joint
- knee M23.4- ☑

Mouth — see condition
Movable
- coccyx — see subcategory M53.2- ☑
- kidney N28.89
  - congenital Q63.8
- spleen D73.89

Movements, dystonic R25.8
Moyamoya disease I67.5
Mpox B04
MRSA (Methicillin resistant Staphylococcus aureus)
- infection A49.02
  - as the cause of diseases classified elsewhere B95.62
- sepsis A41.02

MSD (multiple sulfatase deficiency) E75.26
MSSA (Methicillin susceptible Staphylococcus aureus)
- infection A49.01
  - as the cause of diseases classified elsewhere B95.61
- sepsis A41.01

Mucha-Habermann disease L41.0
Mucinosis (cutaneous) (focal) (papular) (skin) L98.5
- oral K13.79

Mucocele
- appendix K38.8
- buccal cavity K13.79
- gallbladder K82.1
- lacrimal sac, chronic H04.43- ☑
- nasal sinus J34.1
- nose J34.1
- salivary gland (any) K11.6
- sinus (accessory) (nasal) J34.1
- turbinate (bone) (middle) (nasal) J34.1
- uterus N85.8

Mucolipidosis
- I E77.1
- II, III E77.0
- IV E75.11

Mucopolysaccharidosis E76.3
- beta-gluduronidase deficiency E76.29
- cardiopathy E76.3 [I52]
- Hunter's syndrome E76.1
- Hurler-Scheie syndrome E76.02
- Hurler's syndrome E76.01
- Maroteaux-Lamy syndrome E76.29
- Morquio syndrome E76.219
  - A E76.210
  - B E76.211
  - classic E76.210
- Sanfilippo syndrome E76.22
- Scheie's syndrome E76.03
- specified NEC E76.29
- type
  - I
    - Hurler-Scheie syndrome E76.02
    - Hurler's syndrome E76.01
    - Scheie's syndrome E76.03
  - II E76.1
  - III E76.22
  - IV E76.219

Mucopolysaccharidosis — continued
- type — continued
  - IVA E76.210
  - IVB E76.211
  - VI E76.29
  - VII E76.29

Mucormycosis B46.5
- cutaneous B46.3
- disseminated B46.4
- gastrointestinal B46.2
- generalized B46.4
- pulmonary B46.0
- rhinocerebral B46.1
- skin B46.3
- subcutaneous B46.3

Mucositis (ulcerative) K12.30
- due to drugs NEC K12.32
- gastrointestinal K92.81
- mouth (oral) (oropharyngeal) K12.30
  - due to antineoplastic therapy K12.31
  - due to drugs NEC K12.32
  - due to radiation K12.33
  - specified NEC K12.39
  - viral K12.39
- nasal J34.81
- oral cavity — see Mucositis, mouth
- oral soft tissues — see Mucositis, mouth
- vagina and vulva N76.81

Mucositis necroticans agranulocytica — see Agranulocytosis
Mucous — see also condition
- patches (syphilitic) A51.39
  - congenital A50.07

Mucoviscidosis E84.9
- with meconium obstruction E84.11

Mucus
- asphyxia or suffocation — see Asphyxia, mucus
- in stool R19.5
- plug — see Asphyxia, mucus

Muguet B37.0
Mulberry molars (congenital syphilis) A50.52
Mullerian mixed tumor
- specified site — see Neoplasm, malignant, by site
- unspecified site C54.9

Multicystic kidney (development) Q61.4
Multiparity (grand) Z64.1
- affecting management of pregnancy, labor and delivery (supervision only) O09.4- ☑
- requiring contraceptive management — see Contraception

Multipartita placenta O43.19- ☑
Multiple, multiplex — see also condition
- digits (congenital) Q69.9
- endocrine neoplasia — see Neoplasia, endocrine, multiple (MEN)
- personality F44.81

Multisystem inflammatory syndrome (in adult) (in children) M35.81
Mumps B26.9
- arthritis B26.85
- complication NEC B26.89
- encephalitis B26.2
- hepatitis B26.81
- meningitis (aseptic) B26.1
- meningoencephalitis B26.2
- myocarditis B26.82
- oophoritis B26.89
- orchitis B26.0
- pancreatitis B26.3
- polyneuropathy B26.84

Mumu — see also Infestation, filarial B74.9 [N51]
Munchhausen's syndrome — see Disorder, factitious
Munchmeyer's syndrome — see Myositis, ossificans, progressiva
Mural — see condition
Murmur (cardiac) (heart) (organic) R01.1
- abdominal R19.15
- aortic (valve) — see Endocarditis, aortic
- benign R01.0
- diastolic — see Endocarditis
- Flint I35.1
- functional R01.0
- Graham Steell I37.1
- innocent R01.0
- mitral (valve) — see Insufficiency, mitral
- nonorganic R01.0
- presystolic, mitral — see Insufficiency, mitral
- pulmonic (valve) I37.8
- systolic R01.1

Murmur — continued
- tricuspid (valve) I07.9
- valvular — see Endocarditis

Murri's disease (intermittent hemoglobinuria) D59.6
Muscle, muscular — see also condition
- carnitine (palmityltransferase) deficiency E71.314

Musculoneuralgia — see Neuralgia
Mushroom-workers' (pickers') **disease or lung** J67.5
Mushrooming hip — see Derangement, joint, specified NEC, hip

Mutation(s)
- factor V Leiden D68.51
- prothrombin gene D68.52
- surfactant, of lung J84.83

Mutism — see also Aphasia
- deaf (acquired) (congenital) NEC H91.3
- elective (adjustment reaction) (childhood) F94.0
- hysterical F44.4
- selective (childhood) F94.0

MVD (microvillus inclusion disease) Q43.8
MVID (microvillus inclusion disease) Q43.8
Myalgia M79.10
- auxiliary muscles, head and neck M79.12
- epidemic (cervical) B33.0
- mastication muscle M79.11
- site specified NEC M79.18
- traumatic NEC T14.8- ☑

Myasthenia G70.9
- congenital G70.2
- cordis — see Failure, heart
- developmental G70.2
- gravis G70.00
  - with exacerbation (acute) G70.01
  - in crisis G70.01
  - neonatal, transient P94.0
  - pseudoparalytica G70.00
    - with exacerbation (acute) G70.01
    - in crisis G70.01
- stomach, psychogenic F45.8
- syndrome
  - in
    - diabetes mellitus — see E08-E13 with .44
    - neoplastic disease — see also Neoplasm D49.9 [G73.3]
    - pernicious anemia D51.0 [G73.3]
    - thyrotoxicosis E05.90 [G73.3]
      - with thyroid storm E05.91 [G73.3]

Myasthenic M62.81
Mycelium infection B49
Mycetismus — see Poisoning, food, noxious, mushroom
Mycetoma B47.9
- actinomycotic B47.1
- bone (mycotic) B47.9 [M90.80]
- eumycotic B47.0
- foot B47.9
  - actinomycotic B47.1
  - mycotic B47.0
- madurae NEC B47.9
  - mycotic B47.0
- maduromycotic B47.0
- mycotic B47.0
- nocardial B47.1

Mycobacteriosis — see Mycobacterium
Mycobacterium, mycobacterial (infection) A31.9
- anonymous A31.9
- atypical A31.9
  - cutaneous A31.1
  - pulmonary A31.0
    - tuberculous — see Tuberculosis, pulmonary
  - specified site NEC A31.8
- avium (intracellulare complex) A31.0
- balnei A31.1
- Battey A31.0
- chelonei A31.8
- cutaneous A31.1
- extrapulmonary systemic A31.8
- fortuitum A31.8
- intracellulare (Battey bacillus) A31.0
- kakaferifu A31.8
- kansasii (yellow bacillus) A31.0
- kasongo A31.8
- leprae — see also Leprosy A30.9
- luciflavum A31.1
- marinum (M. balnei) A31.1
- nonspecific — see Mycobacterium, atypical
- pulmonary (atypical) A31.0
  - tuberculous — see Tuberculosis, pulmonary
- scrofulaceum A31.8
- simiae A31.8

Mycobacterium, mycobacterial — *continued*
  systemic, extrapulmonary A31.8
  szulgai A31.8
  terrae A31.8
  triviale A31.8
  tuberculosis (human, bovine) — *see* Tuberculosis
  ulcerans A31.1
  xenopi A31.8
Mycoplasma (M.) pneumoniae, as cause of disease classified elsewhere B96.0
Mycosis, mycotic B49
  cutaneous NEC B36.9
  ear B36.9
    in
      aspergillosis B44.89
      candidiasis B37.84
      moniliasis B37.84
  fungoides (extranodal) (solid organ) C84.0- ☑
  mouth B37.0
  nails B35.1
  opportunistic B48.8
  skin NEC B36.9
  specified NEC B48.8
  stomatitis B37.0
  vagina, vaginitis (candidal) (acute) B37.31
    chronic (recurrent) B37.32
Mydriasis (pupil) H57.04
Myelatelia Q06.1
Myelinolysis, pontine, central G37.2
Myelitis (acute) (ascending) (childhood) (chronic) (descending) (diffuse) (disseminated) (idiopathic) (pressure) (progressive) (spinal cord) (subacute) — *see also* Encephalitis G04.91
  flaccid G04.82
  herpes simplex B00.82
  herpes zoster B02.24
  in diseases classified elsewhere G05.4
  necrotizing, subacute G37.4
  optic neuritis in G36.0
  postchickenpox B01.12
  postherpetic B02.24
  postimmunization G04.02
  postinfectious NEC G04.89
  postvaccinal G04.02
  specified NEC G04.89
  syphilitic (transverse) A52.14
  toxic G92.9
  transverse (in demyelinating diseases of central nervous system) G37.3
  tuberculous A17.82
  varicella B01.12
Myelo-osteo-musculodysplasia hereditaria Q79.8
Myeloblastic — *see* condition
Myeloblastoma
  granular cell — *see also* Neoplasm, connective tissue, malignant — *see* Neoplasm, connective tissue, malignant
    tongue D10.1
Myelocele — *see* Spina bifida
Myelocystocele — *see* Spina bifida
Myelocytic — *see* condition
Myelodysplasia D46.9
  specified NEC D46.Z (*following* D46.4)
  spinal cord (congenital) Q06.1
Myelodysplastic syndrome — *see also* Syndrome, myelodysplastic D46.9
  with
    5q deletion D46.C (*following* D46.2)
    isolated del (5q) chromosomal abnormality D46.C (*following* D46.2)
    pancytopenia, acquired — *see* Syndrome, myelodysplastic, pancytopenia
  specified NEC D46.Z (*following* D46.4)
Myeloencephalitis — *see* Encephalitis
Myelofibrosis D75.81
  with myeloid metaplasia D47.4
  acute C94.4- ☑
  idiopathic (chronic) D47.4
  primary D47.1
  secondary D75.81
    in myeloproliferative disease D47.4
Myelogenous — *see* condition
Myeloid — *see* condition
Myelokathexis D70.9
Myeloleukodystrophy E75.29
Myelolipoma — *see* Lipoma
Myeloma (multiple) C90.0- ☑
  monostotic C90.3- ☑

Myeloma — *continued*
  monostotic — *continued*
    plasma cell C90.0- ☑
  plasma cell C90.0- ☑
  solitary — *see also* Plasmacytoma, solitary C90.3- ☑
Myelomalacia G95.89
Myelomatosis C90.0- ☑
Myelomeningitis — *see* Meningoencephalitis
Myelomeningocele (spinal cord) — *see* Spina bifida
Myelopathic
  anemia D64.89
  muscle atrophy — *see* Atrophy, muscle, spinal
  pain syndrome G89.0
Myelopathy (spinal cord) G95.9
  drug-induced G95.89
  in (due to)
    degeneration or displacement, intervertebral disc NEC — *see* Disorder, disc, with, myelopathy
    disease classified elsewhere G99.2
    infection — *see* Encephalitis
    intervertebral disc disorder — *see also* Disorder, disc, with, myelopathy
    mercury — *see* subcategory T56.1- ☑
    neoplastic disease — *see also* Neoplasm D49.9 [G99.2]
    pernicious anemia D51.0 [G99.2]
    spondylosis — *see* Spondylosis, with myelopathy NEC
  necrotic (subacute) (vascular) G95.19
  radiation-induced G95.89
  spondylogenic NEC — *see* Spondylosis, with myelopathy NEC
  toxic G95.89
  transverse, acute G37.3
  vascular G95.19
  vitamin B12 E53.8 [G32.0]
Myelophthisis D61.82
Myeloradiculitis G04.91
Myeloradiculodysplasia (spinal) Q06.1
Myelosarcoma C92.3- ☑
Myelosclerosis D75.89
  with myeloid metaplasia D47.4
  disseminated, of nervous system G35.D
  megakaryocytic D47.4
    with myeloid metaplasia D47.4
Myelosis
  acute C92.0- ☑
  aleukemic C92.9- ☑
  chronic D47.1
  erythremic (acute) C94.0- ☑
  megakaryocytic C94.2- ☑
  nonleukemic D72.828
  subacute C92.9- ☑
Myiasis (cavernous) B87.9
  aural B87.4
  creeping B87.0
  cutaneous B87.0
  dermal B87.0
  ear (external) (middle) B87.4
  eye B87.2
  genitourinary B87.81
  intestinal B87.82
  laryngeal B87.3
  nasopharyngeal B87.3
  ocular B87.2
  orbit B87.2
  skin B87.0
  specified site NEC B87.89
  traumatic B87.1
  wound B87.1
Myoadenoma, prostate — *see* Hyperplasia, prostate
Myoblastoma
  granular cell — *see also* Neoplasm, connective tissue, benign
    malignant — *see* Neoplasm, connective tissue, malignant
  tongue D10.1
Myocardial — *see* condition
Myocardiopathy (congestive) (constrictive) (familial) (hypertrophic nonobstructive) (idiopathic) (infiltrative) (obstructive) (primary) (restrictive) (sporadic) — *see also* Cardiomyopathy I42.9
  alcoholic I42.6
  cobalt-beer I42.6
  glycogen storage E74.02 [I43]
  hypertrophic obstructive I42.1
  in (due to)
    beriberi E51.12
    cardiac glycogenosis E74.02 [I43]
    Friedreich's ataxia G11.11 [I43]

Myocardiopathy — *continued*
  in — *continued*
    myotonia atrophica G71.11 [I43]
    progressive muscular dystrophy — *see also* Dystrophy, muscular, by type G71.09 [I43]
  obscure (African) I42.8
  secondary I42.9
  thyrotoxic E05.90 [I43]
    with storm E05.91 [I43]
  toxic NEC I42.7
Myocarditis (with arteriosclerosis) (chronic) (fibroid) (interstitial) (old) (progressive) (senile) I51.4
  with
    rheumatic fever (conditions in I00) I09.0
      active — *see* Myocarditis, acute, rheumatic
      inactive or quiescent (with chorea) I09.0
  active I40.9
    rheumatic I01.2
      with chorea (acute) (rheumatic) (Sydenham's) I02.0
  acute or subacute (interstitial) I40.9
    due to
      streptococcus (beta-hemolytic) I01.2
    idiopathic I40.1
    rheumatic I01.2
      with chorea (acute) (rheumatic) (Sydenham's) I02.0
    specified NEC I40.8
  aseptic of newborn B33.22
  bacterial (acute) I40.0
  Coxsackie (virus) B33.22
  diphtheritic A36.81
  eosinophilic I40.1
  epidemic of newborn (Coxsackie) B33.22
  Fiedler's (acute) (isolated) I40.1
  giant cell (acute) (subacute) I40.1
  gonococcal A54.83
  granulomatous (idiopathic) (isolated) (nonspecific) I40.1
  hypertensive — *see* Hypertension, heart
  idiopathic (granulomatous) I40.1
  in (due to)
    diphtheria A36.81
    epidemic louse-borne typhus A75.0 [I41]
    Lyme disease A69.29
    sarcoidosis D86.85
    scarlet fever A38.1
    toxoplasmosis (acquired) B58.81
    typhoid A01.02
    typhus NEC A75.9 [I41]
  infective I40.0
  influenzal — *see* Influenza, with, myocarditis
  isolated (acute) I40.1
  meningococcal A39.52
  mumps B26.82
  nonrheumatic, active I40.9
  parenchymatous I40.9
  pneumococcal I40.0
  rheumatic (chronic) (inactive) (with chorea) I09.0
    active or acute I01.2
      with chorea (acute) (rheumatic) (Sydenham's) I02.0
  rheumatoid — *see* Rheumatoid, carditis
  septic I40.0
  staphylococcal I40.0
  suppurative I40.0
  syphilitic (chronic) A52.06
  toxic I40.8
    rheumatic — *see* Myocarditis, acute, rheumatic
  tuberculous A18.84
  typhoid A01.02
  valvular — *see* Endocarditis
  virus, viral B33.22
    of newborn (Coxsackie) B33.22
Myocardium, myocardial — *see* condition
Myocardosis — *see* Cardiomyopathy
Myoclonus, myoclonic, myoclonia (familial) (essential) (multifocal) (simplex) G25.3
  drug-induced G25.3
  epilepsy — *see also* Epilepsy, generalized, specified NEC G40.4- ☑
    familial (progressive) — *see* Epilepsy, myoclonus
    Lafora — *see* Epilepsy, myoclonus, progressive, Lafora
  epileptica — *see also* Epilepsy, myoclonus G40.409
    with status epilepticus G40.401
  facial G51.3- ☑
  familial progressive G25.3
    epilepsy — *see* Epilepsy, myoclonus, progressive
  Friedreich's G25.3
  jerks G25.3
  massive G25.3
  palatal G25.3
  pharyngeal G25.3

Myocytolysis I51.5
Myodiastasis — see Diastasis, muscle
Myoendocarditis — see Endocarditis
Myoepithelioma — see Neoplasm, benign, by site
Myofasciitis (acute) — see Myositis
Myofibroma — see also Neoplasm, connective tissue, benign
   uterus (cervix) (corpus) — see Leiomyoma
Myofibromatosis D48.19
   infantile Q89.89
Myofibrosis M62.89
   heart — see Myocarditis
   scapulohumeral — see Lesion, shoulder, specified NEC
Myofibrositis M79.7
   scapulohumeral — see Lesion, shoulder, specified NEC
Myoglobulinuria, myoglobinuria (primary) R82.1
Myokymia, facial G51.4
Myolipoma — see Lipoma
Myoma — see also Neoplasm, connective tissue, benign
   malignant — see Neoplasm, connective tissue, malignant
   prostate D29.1
   uterus (cervix) (corpus) — see Leiomyoma
Myomalacia M62.89
Myometritis — see Endometritis
Myometrium — see condition
Myonecrosis, clostridial A48.0
Myopathy G72.9
   acute
      necrotizing G72.81
      quadriplegic G72.81
   alcoholic G72.1
   benign congenital G71.20
   central core G71.29
   centronuclear G71.228
      autosomal (dominant) (recessive) G71.228
      other specified NEC G71.228
   congenital (benign) G71.20
   critical illness G72.81
   distal G71.09
   drug-induced G72.0
   endocrine NEC E34.9 [G73.7]
   extraocular muscles H05.82-
   facioscapulohumeral G71.02
   hereditary G71.9
      specified NEC G71.8
   hyaline body G71.29
   immune NEC G72.49
   in (due to)
      Addison's disease E27.1 [G73.7]
      alcohol G72.1
      amyloidosis E85.0 [G73.7]
      cretinism E00.9 [G73.7]
      Cushing's syndrome E24.9 [G73.7]
      drugs G72.0
      endocrine disease NEC E34.9 [G73.7]
      giant cell arteritis M31.6 [G73.7]
      glycogen storage disease E74.00 [G73.7]
      hyperadrenocorticism E24.9 [G73.7]
      hyperparathyroidism NEC E21.3 [G73.7]
      hypoparathyroidism E20.9 [G73.7]
      hypopituitarism E23.0 [G73.7]
      hypothyroidism E03.9 [G73.7]
      infectious disease NEC B99.- ☑ [G73.7]
      lipid storage disease E75.6 [G73.7]
      metabolic disease NEC E88.9 [G73.7]
      myxedema E03.9 [G73.7]
      parasitic disease NEC B89 [G73.7]
      polyarteritis nodosa M30.0 [G73.7]
      rheumatoid arthritis — see Rheumatoid, myopathy
      sarcoidosis D86.87
      scleroderma M34.82
      sicca syndrome M35.03
      Sjogren's syndrome M35.03
      systemic lupus erythematosus M32.19
      thyrotoxicosis (hyperthyroidism) E05.90 [G73.7]
         with thyroid storm E05.91 [G73.7]
      toxic agent NEC G72.2
   inflammatory NEC G72.49
   intensive care (ICU) G72.81
   limb-girdle — see Dystrophy, muscular, limb-girdle
   mitochondrial NEC G71.3
   Miyoshi, type 3 G71.035
   myosin storage G71.29
   myotubular (centronuclear) G71.220
      X-linked G71.220
   mytonic, proximal (PROMM) G71.11
   nemaline G71.21
   ocular G71.09
   oculopharyngeal G71.09

Myopathy — continued
   of critical illness G72.81
   primary G71.9
      specified NEC G71.8
   progressive NEC G72.89
   proximal myotonic (PROMM) G71.11
   rod (body) G71.21
   scapulohumeral G71.02
   specified NEC G72.89
   toxic G72.2
Myopericarditis — see also Pericarditis
   chronic rheumatic I09.2
Myopia (axial) (congenital) H52.1-
   degenerative (malignant) H44.20
      with
         choroidal neovascularization H44.2A- ☑
         foveoschisis H44.2D- ☑
         macular hole H44.2B- ☑
         retinal detachment H44.2C- ☑
         specified maculopathy NEC H44.2E- ☑
      bilateral H44.23
      left eye H44.22
      right eye H44.21
   malignant — see also Myopia, degenerative H44.2- ☑
   pernicious — see also Myopia, degenerative H44.2- ☑
   progressive high (degenerative) — see also Myopia, degenerative H44.2- ☑
Myosarcoma — see Neoplasm, connective tissue, malignant
Myosis (pupil) H57.03
   stromal (endolymphatic) D39.0
Myositis M60.9
   clostridial A48.0
   due to posture — see Myositis, specified type NEC
   epidemic B33.0
   fibrosa or fibrous (chronic), Volkmann's T79.6- ☑
   foreign body granuloma — see Granuloma, foreign body
   in (due to)
      bilharziasis B65.9 [M63.8-] ☑
      cysticercosis B69.81
      leprosy A30.9 [M63.8-] ☑
      mycosis B49 [M63.8-] ☑
      sarcoidosis D86.87
      schistosomiasis B65.9 [M63.8-] ☑
      syphilis
         late A52.78
         secondary A51.49
      toxoplasmosis (acquired) B58.82
      trichinellosis B75 [M63.8-] ☑
      tuberculosis A18.09
   inclusion body [IBM] G72.41
   infective M60.009
      arm M60.002
         left M60.001
         right M60.000
      leg M60.005
         left M60.004
         right M60.003
      lower limb M60.005
         ankle M60.07- ☑
         foot M60.07- ☑
         lower leg M60.06- ☑
         thigh M60.05- ☑
         toe M60.07- ☑
      multiple sites M60.09
      specified site NEC M60.08
      upper limb M60.002
         finger M60.04- ☑
         forearm M60.03- ☑
         hand M60.04- ☑
         shoulder region M60.01- ☑
         upper arm M60.02- ☑
   interstitial M60.10
      ankle M60.17- ☑
      foot M60.17- ☑
      forearm M60.13- ☑
      hand M60.14- ☑
      lower leg M60.16- ☑
      multiple sites M60.19
      shoulder region M60.11- ☑
      specified site NEC M60.18
      thigh M60.15- ☑
      upper arm M60.12- ☑
   mycotic B49 [M63.8-] ☑
   orbital, chronic H05.12- ☑
   ossificans or ossifying (circumscripta) — see also Ossification, muscle, specified NEC

Myositis — continued
   ossificans or ossifying — see also Ossification, muscle, specified — continued
      in (due to)
         burns M61.30
            ankle M61.37- ☑
            foot M61.37- ☑
            forearm M61.33- ☑
            hand M61.34- ☑
            lower leg M61.36- ☑
            multiple sites M61.39
            pelvic region M61.35- ☑
            shoulder region M61.31- ☑
            specified site NEC M61.38
            thigh M61.35- ☑
            upper arm M61.32- ☑
      quadriplegia or paraplegia M61.20
         ankle M61.27- ☑
         foot M61.27- ☑
         forearm M61.23- ☑
         hand M61.24- ☑
         lower leg M61.26- ☑
         multiple sites M61.29
         pelvic region M61.25- ☑
         shoulder region M61.21- ☑
         specified site NEC M61.28
         thigh M61.25- ☑
         upper arm M61.22- ☑
      progressiva M61.10
         ankle M61.17- ☑
         finger M61.14- ☑
         foot M61.17- ☑
         forearm M61.13- ☑
         hand M61.14- ☑
         lower leg M61.16- ☑
         multiple sites M61.19
         pelvic region M61.15- ☑
         shoulder region M61.11- ☑
         specified site NEC M61.18
         thigh M61.15- ☑
         toe M61.17- ☑
         upper arm M61.12- ☑
      traumatica M61.00
         ankle M61.07- ☑
         foot M61.07- ☑
         forearm M61.03- ☑
         hand M61.04- ☑
         lower leg M61.06- ☑
         multiple sites M61.09
         pelvic region M61.05- ☑
         shoulder region M61.01- ☑
         specified site NEC M61.08
         thigh M61.05- ☑
         upper arm M61.02- ☑
   purulent — see Myositis, infective
   specified type NEC M60.80
      ankle M60.87- ☑
      foot M60.87- ☑
      forearm M60.83- ☑
      hand M60.84- ☑
      lower leg M60.86- ☑
      multiple sites M60.89
      pelvic region M60.85- ☑
      shoulder region M60.81- ☑
      specified site NEC M60.88
      thigh M60.85- ☑
      upper arm M60.82- ☑
   suppurative — see Myositis, infective
   traumatic (old) — see Myositis, specified type NEC
Myospasia impulsiva F95.2
Myotonia (acquisita) (intermittens) M62.89
   atrophica G71.11
   chondrodystrophic G71.13
   congenita (acetazolamide responsive) (dominant) (recessive) G71.12
   drug-induced G71.14
   dystrophica G71.11
   fluctuans G71.19
   levior G71.12
   permanens G71.19
   symptomatic G71.19
Myotonic pupil — see Anomaly, pupil, function, tonic pupil
Myriapodiasis B88.2
Myringitis H73.2- ☑
   with otitis media — see Otitis, media
   acute H73.00- ☑

Myringitis — continued
  acute — continued
    bullous H73.01- ☑
    specified NEC H73.09- ☑
  bullous — see Myringitis, acute, bullous
  chronic H73.1- ☑
Mysophobia F40.228
Mytilotoxism — see Poisoning, fish
Myxadenitis labialis K13.0
Myxedema (adult) (idiocy) (infantile) (juvenile) — see also Hypothyroidism E03.9

Myxedema — continued
  circumscribed E05.90
    with storm E05.91
  coma E03.5
  congenital E00.1
  cutis L98.5
  localized (pretibial) E05.90
    with storm E05.91
  papular L98.5
Myxochondrosarcoma — see Neoplasm, cartilage, malignant
Myxofibroma — see Neoplasm, connective tissue, benign

Myxofibroma — continued
  odontogenic — see Cyst, calcifying odontogenic
Myxofibrosarcoma — see Neoplasm, connective tissue, malignant
Myxolipoma D17.9
Myxoliposarcoma — see Neoplasm, connective tissue, malignant
Myxoma — see also Neoplasm, connective tissue, benign
  nerve sheath — see Neoplasm, nerve, benign
  odontogenic — see Cyst, calcifying odontogenic
Myxosarcoma — see Neoplasm, connective tissue, malignant

N

Naegeli's
  disease Q82.8
  leukemia, monocytic C93.1- ☑
Naegleriasis (with meningoencephalitis) B60.2
Naffziger's syndrome G54.0
Naga sore — see Ulcer, skin
Nägele's pelvis M95.5
  with disproportion (fetopelvic) O33.0
    causing obstructed labor O65.0
Nail — see also condition
  biting F98.8
  patella syndrome Q87.2
Nanism, nanosomia — see Dwarfism
Nanophyetiasis B66.8
Nanukayami A27.89
Napkin rash L22
Narcolepsy G47.419
  with cataplexy G47.411
  in conditions classified elsewhere G47.429
    with cataplexy G47.421
Narcosis R06.89
Narcotism — see Dependence
NARP (Neuropathy, Ataxia and Retinitis pigmentosa) syndrome E88.49
Narrow
  anterior chamber angle H40.03- ☑
  gingival width (of periodontal soft tissue) K05.5
  pelvis — see Contraction, pelvis
Narrowing — see also Stenosis
  artery I77.1
    auditory, internal I65.8
    basilar — see Occlusion, artery, basilar
    carotid — see Occlusion, artery, carotid
    cerebellar — see Occlusion, artery, cerebellar
    cerebral — see Occlusion artery, cerebral
    choroidal — see Occlusion, artery, precerebral, specified NEC
    communicating posterior — see Occlusion, artery, precerebral, specified NEC
    coronary — see also Disease, heart, ischemic, atherosclerotic
      congenital Q24.5
        syphilitic A50.54 [I52]
      due to syphilis NEC A52.06
    hypophyseal — see Occlusion, artery, precerebral, specified NEC
    pontine — see Occlusion, artery, precerebral, specified NEC
    precerebral — see Occlusion, artery, precerebral
    vertebral — see Occlusion, artery, vertebral
  auditory canal (external) — see Stenosis, external ear canal
  caudal septum, fixed, lower lateral cartilage, alar rim and nasal sill J34.8211
  eustachian tube — see Obstruction, eustachian tube
  eyelid — see Disorder, eyelid function
  larynx J38.6
  mesenteric artery — see also Ischemia, intestine, acute K55.059
  nasal septum, head of the inferior turbinate and the upper lateral cartilage J34.8201
  palate M26.89
  palpebral fissure — see Disorder, eyelid function
  ureter N13.5
    with infection N13.6
  urethra — see Stricture, urethra
Narrowness, abnormal, eyelid Q10.3
Nasal — see condition
Nasolachrymal, nasolacrimal — see condition
Nasopharyngeal — see also condition
  pituitary gland Q89.2
  torticollis M43.6
Nasopharyngitis (acute) (infective) (streptococcal) (subacute) J00
  chronic (suppurative) (ulcerative) J31.1
Nasopharynx, nasopharyngeal — see condition
Natal tooth, teeth K00.6
Nausea (without vomiting) R11.0
  with vomiting R11.2
  gravidarum — see Hyperemesis, gravidarum
  marina T75.3- ☑
  navalis T75.3- ☑
Navel — see condition
Neapolitan fever — see Brucellosis
Near drowning T75.1- ☑

Near-syncope R55
Nearsightedness — see Myopia
Nebula, cornea — see Opacity, cornea
Necator americanus infestation B76.1
Necatoriasis B76.1
Neck — see condition
Necrobiosis R68.89
  lipoidica NEC L92.1
    with diabetes — see E08-E13 with .620
Necrolysis, toxic epidermal L51.2
  due to drug
    correct substance properly administered — see Table of Drugs and Chemicals, by drug, adverse effect
    overdose or wrong substance given or taken — see Table of Drugs and Chemicals, by drug, poisoning
Necrophilia F65.89
Necrosis, necrotic (ischemic) — see also Gangrene
  adrenal (capsule) (gland) E27.49
  amputation stump (surgical) (late) T87.50
    arm T87.5- ☑
    leg T87.5- ☑
  antrum J32.0
  aorta (hyaline) — see also Aneurysm, aorta
    cystic medial — see Dissection, aorta
  artery I77.5
  bladder (aseptic) (sphincter) N32.89
  bone — see also Osteonecrosis M87.9
    aseptic or avascular — see Osteonecrosis
    idiopathic M87.00
    ethmoid J32.2
    jaw M27.2
    tuberculous — see Tuberculosis, bone
  brain I67.89
  breast (aseptic) (fat) (segmental) N64.1
  bronchus J98.09
  central nervous system NEC I67.89
  cerebellar I67.89
  cerebral I67.89
  colon — see also Infarct, intestine K55.049
  cornea H18.89- ☑
  cortical (acute) (renal) N17.1
  cystic medial (aorta) — see Dissection, aorta
  dental pulp K04.1
  esophagus K22.89
  ethmoid (bone) J32.2
  eyelid — see Disorder, eyelid, degenerative
  fat, fatty (generalized) — see also Disorder, soft tissue, specified type NEC)
    abdominal wall K65.4
    breast (aseptic) (segmental) N64.1
    localized — see Degeneration, by site, fatty
    mesentery K65.4
    omentum K65.4
    pancreas K86.89
    peritoneum K65.4
    skin (subcutaneous), newborn P83.0
    subcutaneous, due to birth injury P15.6
  gallbladder — see Cholecystitis, acute
  heart — see Infarct, myocardium
  hip, aseptic or avascular — see Osteonecrosis, by type, femur
  intestine (acute) (hemorrhagic) (massive) — see also Infarct, intestine K55.069
  jaw M27.2
  kidney (bilateral) N28.0
    acute N17.9
    cortical (acute) (bilateral) N17.1
      with ectopic or molar pregnancy O08.4
    medullary (bilateral) (in acute renal failure) (papillary) N17.2
    papillary (bilateral) (in acute renal failure) N17.2
    tubular N17.0
      with ectopic or molar pregnancy O08.4
      complicating
        abortion — see Abortion, by type, complicated by, tubular necrosis
        ectopic or molar pregnancy O08.4
      pregnancy — see Pregnancy, complicated by, diseases of, specified type or system NEC
      following ectopic or molar pregnancy O08.4
      traumatic T79.5- ☑
  larynx J38.7
  liver (with hepatic failure) (cell) — see Failure, hepatic
    hemorrhagic, central K76.2
  lung J85.0
  lymphatic gland — see Lymphadenitis, acute
  mammary gland (fat) (segmental) N64.1
  mastoid (chronic) — see Mastoiditis, chronic

Necrosis, necrotic — continued
  medullary (acute) (renal) N17.2
  mesentery — see also Infarct, intestine K55.069
    fat K65.4
  mitral valve — see Insufficiency, mitral
  myocardium, myocardial — see Infarct, myocardium
  nose J34.0
  omentum (with mesenteric infarction) — see also Infarct, intestine K55.069
    fat K65.4
  orbit, orbital — see Osteomyelitis, orbit
  ossicles, ear — see Abnormal, ear ossicles
  ovary N70.92
  pancreas (aseptic) (duct) (fat) K86.89
    acute (infective) — see Pancreatitis, acute
    infective — see Pancreatitis, acute
  papillary (acute) (renal) N17.2
  perineum N90.89
  peritoneum (with mesenteric infarction) — see also Infarct, intestine K55.069
    fat K65.4
  pharynx J02.9
    in granulocytopenia — see Neutropenia
    Vincent's A69.1
  phosphorus — see subcategory T54.2- ☑
  pituitary (gland) E23.0
    postpartum O99.285
    Sheehan O99.285
  pressure — see Ulcer, pressure, by site
  pulmonary J85.0
  pulp (dental) K04.1
  radiation — see Necrosis, by site
  radium — see Necrosis, by site
  renal — see Necrosis, kidney
  sclera H15.89
  scrotum N50.89
  skin or subcutaneous tissue NEC I96
  spine, spinal (column) — see also Osteonecrosis, by type, vertebra
    cord G95.19
  spleen D73.5
  stomach K31.89
  stomatitis (ulcerative) A69.0
  subcutaneous fat, newborn P83.88
  subendocardial (acute) I21.4
    chronic I25.89
  suprarenal (capsule) (gland) E27.49
  testis N50.89
  thymus (gland) E32.8
  tonsil J35.8
  trachea J39.8
  tuberculous NEC — see Tuberculosis
  tubular (acute) (anoxic) (renal) (toxic) N17.0
    postprocedural N99.0
  vagina N89.8
  vertebra — see also Osteonecrosis, by type, vertebra
    tuberculous A18.01
  vulva N90.89
  X-ray — see Necrosis, by site
Necrospermia — see Infertility, male
Need (for)
  care provider because (of)
    assistance with personal care Z74.1
    continuous supervision required Z74.3
    impaired mobility Z74.09
    no other household member able to render care Z74.2
    specified reason NEC Z74.8
  immunization — see Vaccination
  vaccination — see Vaccination
Neglect
  adult
    confirmed T74.01- ☑
    history of Z91.412
    suspected T76.01- ☑
  child (childhood)
    confirmed T74.02- ☑
    history of Z62.812
    suspected T76.02- ☑
  emotional, in childhood Z62.898
  hemispatial R41.4
  left-sided R41.4
  sensory R41.4
  visuospatial R41.4
Neisserian infection NEC — see Gonococcus
Nelaton's syndrome G60.8
Nelson's syndrome E24.1
Nematodiasis (intestinal) B82.0
  Ancylostoma B76.0

Neonatal — *see also* Newborn
  acne L70.4
  bradycardia P29.12
  screening, abnormal findings on — *see* Abnormal, neonatal screening
  tachycardia P29.11
  tooth, teeth K00.6
Neonatorum — *see* condition
Neoplasia
  endocrine, multiple (MEN) E31.20
    type I E31.21
    type IIA E31.22
    type IIB E31.23
  intraepithelial (histologically confirmed)
    anal (AIN) (histologically confirmed) K62.82
      grade I K62.82
      grade II K62.82
      severe D01.3
    cervical glandular (histologically confirmed) D06.9
    cervix (uteri) (CIN) (histologically confirmed) N87.9
      glandular D06.9
      grade I N87.0
      grade II N87.1
      grade III (severe dysplasia) — *see also* Carcinoma, cervix uteri, in situ D06.9
    prostate (histologically confirmed) (PIN) N42.31
      grade I N42.31
      grade II N42.31
      grade III (severe dysplasia) D07.5
    vagina (histologically confirmed) (VAIN) N89.3
      grade I N89.0
      grade II N89.1
      grade III (severe dysplasia) D07.2
    vulva (histologically confirmed) (VIN) N90.3
      grade I N90.0
      grade II N90.1
      grade III (severe dysplasia) D07.1
Neoplasm, neoplastic — *see also* Table of Neoplasms
  lipomatous, benign — *see* Lipoma
  malignant mast cell C96.20
    specified type NEC C96.29
  mast cell, of uncertain behavior NEC D47.09
  myelodysplastic/myeloproliferative, unclassifiable C94.6
Neovascularization
  ciliary body — *see* Disorder, iris, vascular
  cornea H16.40- ☑
    deep H16.44- ☑
    ghost vessels — *see* Ghost, vessels
    localized H16.43- ☑
    pannus — *see* Pannus
  iris — *see* Disorder, iris, vascular
  retina H35.05- ☑
Nephralgia N23
Nephritis, nephritic (albuminuric) (azotemic) (congenital) (disseminated) (epithelial) (familial) (focal) (granulomatous) (hemorrhagic) (infantile) (nonsuppurative, excretory) (uremic) N05.9
  with
    C3
      glomerulonephritis N05.A
      glomerulopathy N05.A
        with dense deposit disease N05.6
      dense deposit disease N05.6
      diffuse
        crescentic glomerulonephritis N05.7
        endocapillary proliferative glomerulonephritis N05.4
        membranous glomerulonephritis N05.2
        mesangial proliferative glomerulonephritis N05.3
        mesangiocapillary glomerulonephritis N05.5
      edema — *see* Nephrosis
      focal and segmental glomerular lesions N05.1
      foot process disease N04.9
      glomerular lesion
        diffuse sclerosing N05.8
          hypocomplementemic — *see* Nephritis, membranoproliferative
        idiopathic immune membranoproliferative glomerulonephritis (IC-MPGN) N04.B1
        IgA — *see* Nephropathy, IgA
        lobular, lobulonodular — *see* Nephritis, membranoproliferative
        nodular — *see* Nephritis, membranoproliferative
        secondary immune complex membranoproliferative glomerulonephritis (IC-MPGN) N04.B2
      lesion of
        glomerulonephritis, proliferative N05.8
        renal necrosis N05.9
      minor glomerular abnormality N05.0

Nephritis, nephritic — *continued*
  with — *continued*
    specified morphological changes NEC N05.8
  acute N00.9
    with
      C3
        glomerulonephritis N00.A
        glomerulopathy N00.A
          with dense deposit disease N00.6
        dense deposit disease N00.6
        diffuse
          crescentic glomerulonephritis N00.7
          endocapillary proliferative glomerulonephritis N00.4
          membranous glomerulonephritis N00.2
          mesangial proliferative glomerulonephritis N00.3
          mesangiocapillary glomerulonephritis N00.5
        focal and segmental glomerular lesions N00.1
        idiopathic immune membranoproliferative glomerulonephritis (IC-MPGN) N00.B1
        minor glomerular abnormality N00.0
        secondary immune complex membranoproliferative glomerulonephritis (IC-MPGN) N00.B2
        specified morphological changes NEC N00.8
  amyloid E85.4 [N08]
  antiglomerular basement membrane (anti-GBM) antibody NEC
    in Goodpasture's syndrome M31.0
  antitubular basement membrane (tubulo-interstitial) NEC N12
    toxic — *see* Nephropathy, toxic
  arteriolar — *see* Hypertension, kidney
  arteriosclerotic — *see* Hypertension, kidney
  ascending — *see* Nephritis, tubulo-interstitial
  atrophic N03.9
  Balkan (endemic) N15.0
  calculous, calculus — *see* Calculus, kidney
  cardiac — *see* Hypertension, kidney
  cardiovascular — *see* Hypertension, kidney
  chronic N03.9
    with
      C3
        glomerulonephritis N03.A
        glomerulopathy N03.A
          with dense deposit disease N03.6
        dense deposit disease N03.6
        diffuse
          crescentic glomerulonephritis N03.7
          endocapillary proliferative glomerulonephritis N03.4
          membranous glomerulonephritis N03.2
          mesangial proliferative glomerulonephritis N03.3
          mesangiocapillary glomerulonephritis N03.5
        focal and segmental glomerular lesions N03.1
        minor glomerular abnormality N03.0
        specified morphological changes NEC N03.8
    arteriosclerotic — *see* Hypertension, kidney
  cirrhotic N26.9
  complicating pregnancy O26.83- ☑
  croupous N00.9
  degenerative — *see* Nephrosis
  diffuse sclerosing N05.8
  due to
    diabetes mellitus — *see* E08-E13 with .21
    subacute bacterial endocarditis I33.0
    systemic lupus erythematosus (chronic) M32.14
    typhoid fever A01.09
  gonococcal (acute) (chronic) A54.21
  hypocomplementemic — *see* Nephritis, membranoproliferative
  IgA — *see* Nephropathy, IgA
  immune complex (circulating) NEC N05.8
  infective — *see* Nephritis, tubulo-interstitial
  interstitial — *see* Nephritis, tubulo-interstitial
  lead N14.3
  membranoproliferative (diffuse) (type 1 or 3) — *see also* N00-N07 with fourth character .5 N05.5
    type 2 — *see also* N00-N07 with fourth character .6 N05.6
  minimal change N05.0
  necrotic, necrotizing NEC — *see also* N00-N07 with fourth character .8 N05.8
  nephrotic — *see* Nephrosis
  nodular — *see* Nephritis, membranoproliferative
  polycystic Q61.3
    adult type Q61.2

Nephritis, nephritic — *continued*
  polycystic — *continued*
    autosomal
      dominant Q61.2
      recessive NEC Q61.19
    childhood type NEC Q61.19
    infantile type NEC Q61.19
  poststreptococcal N05.9
    acute N00.9
    chronic N03.9
    rapidly progressive N01.9
  proliferative NEC — *see also* N00-N07 with fourth character .8 N05.8
  purulent — *see* Nephritis, tubulo-interstitial
  rapidly progressive N01.9
    with
      C3
        glomerulonephritis N01.A
        glomerulopathy N01.A
          with dense deposit disease N01.6
        dense deposit disease N01.6
        diffuse
          crescentic glomerulonephritis N01.7
          endocapillary proliferative glomerulonephritis N01.4
          membranous glomerulonephritis N01.2
          mesangial proliferative glomerulonephritis N01.3
          mesangiocapillary glomerulonephritis N01.5
        focal and segmental glomerular lesions N01.1
        minor glomerular abnormality N01.0
        specified morphological changes NEC N01.8
  salt losing or wasting NEC N28.89
  saturnine N14.3
  sclerosing, diffuse N05.8
  septic — *see* Nephritis, tubulo-interstitial
  specified pathology NEC — *see also* N00-N07 with fourth character .8 N05.8
  subacute N01.9
  suppurative — *see* Nephritis, tubulo-interstitial
  syphilitic (late) A52.75
    congenital A50.59 [N08]
    early (secondary) A51.44
  toxic — *see* Nephropathy, toxic
  tubal, tubular — *see* Nephritis, tubulo-interstitial
  tuberculous A18.11
  tubulo-interstitial (in) N12
    acute (infectious) N10
    chronic (infectious) N11.9
      nonobstructive N11.8
        reflux-associated N11.0
      obstructive N11.1
      specified NEC N11.8
    due to
      brucellosis A23.9 [N16]
      cryoglobulinemia D89.1 [N16]
      glycogen storage disease E74.00 [N16]
      Sjogren's syndrome M35.04
  vascular — *see* Hypertension, kidney
  war N00.9
Nephroblastoma (epithelial) (mesenchymal) C64.- ☑
Nephrocalcinosis E83.59 [N29]
Nephrocystitis, pustular — *see* Nephritis, tubulo-interstitial
Nephrolithiasis (congenital) (pelvis) (recurrent) — *see also* Calculus, kidney
Nephroma C64.- ☑
  mesoblastic D41.0- ☑
Nephronephritis — *see* Nephrosis
Nephronophthisis Q61.5
Nephropathia epidemica A98.5
Nephropathy — *see also* Nephritis N28.9
  with
    edema — *see* Nephrosis
    glomerular lesion — *see* Glomerulonephritis
  amyloid, hereditary E85.0
  analgesic N14.0
    with medullary necrosis, acute N17.2
  Balkan (endemic) N15.0
  chemical — *see* Nephropathy, toxic
  contrast-induced N14.11
  contrast medium, radiography N14.11
  diabetic — *see* E08-E13 with .21
  drug-induced N14.2
    contrast-induced N14.11
    specified NEC N14.19
  focal and segmental hyalinosis or sclerosis N02.1
  heavy metal-induced N14.3
  hereditary NEC N07.9

Nephropathy — *continued*
- hereditary — *continued*
  - with
    - APOL1-mediated kidney disease (AMKD) N07.B
    - C3
      - glomerulonephritis N07.A
      - glomerulopathy N07.A
        - with dense deposit disease N07.6
    - dense deposit disease N07.6
    - diffuse
      - crescentic glomerulonephritis N07.7
      - endocapillary proliferative glomerulonephritis N07.4
      - membranous glomerulonephritis N07.2
      - mesangial proliferative glomerulonephritis N07.3
      - mesangiocapillary glomerulonephritis N07.5
    - focal and segmental glomerular lesions N07.1
    - minor glomerular abnormality N07.0
    - specified morphological changes NEC N07.8
- hypercalcemic N25.89
- hypertensive — *see* Hypertension, kidney
- hypokalemic (vacuolar) N25.89
- IgA N02.B- ☑
  - with
    - focal and segmental hyalinosis or sclerosis N02.B2
    - glomerular lesion N02.B1
      - focal and segmental N02.B2
    - glomerulonephritis
      - membranoproliferative (diffuse) N02.B3
      - membranous (diffuse) N02.B4
      - mesangial proliferative (diffuse) N02.B5
      - mesangiocapillary (diffuse) N02.B6
    - proliferative NEC N02.B9
    - specified pathology NEC N02.B9
- lead N14.3
- membranoproliferative (diffuse) N02.5
- membranous (diffuse) N06.20
  - with
    - nephrotic syndrome N04.20
      - primary N04.21
      - secondary N04.22
    - idiopathic, with nephrotic syndrome N04.21
    - primary N06.21
      - with nephrotic syndrome N04.21
    - secondary N06.22
      - with nephrotic syndrome N04.22
- mesangial (IgA/IgG) — *see* Nephropathy, IgA
  - proliferative (diffuse) N02.3
- mesangiocapillary (diffuse) N02.5
- obstructive N13.8
- phenacetin N17.2
- phosphate-losing N25.0
- potassium depletion N25.89
- pregnancy-related O26.83- ☑
- proliferative NEC — *see also* N00-N07 with fourth character .8 N05.8
- protein-losing N25.89
- saturnine N14.3
- sickle-cell D57.- ☑ [N08]
- toxic NEC N14.4
  - due to
    - drugs N14.2
      - analgesic N14.0
      - specified NEC N14.19
    - heavy metals N14.3
- vasomotor N17.0
- water-losing N25.89

Nephroptosis N28.83
Nephropyosis — *see* Abscess, kidney
Nephrorrhagia N28.89
Nephrosclerosis (arteriolar) (arteriosclerotic) (chronic) (hyaline) — *see also* Hypertension, kidney
- hyperplastic — *see* Hypertension, kidney
- senile N26.9

Nephrosis, nephrotic (Epstein's) (syndrome) (congenital) N04.9
- with
  - foot process disease N04.9
  - glomerular lesion N04.1
  - hypocomplementemic N04.5
- acute N04.9
- anoxic — *see* Nephrosis, tubular
- chemical — *see* Nephrosis, tubular
- cholemic K76.7
- diabetic — *see* E08-E13 with .21
- Finnish type (congenital) Q89.89
- hemoglobin N10
- hemoglobinuric — *see* Nephrosis, tubular

Nephrosis, nephrotic — *continued*
- in
  - amyloidosis E85.4 [N08]
  - diabetes mellitus — *see* E08-E13 with .21
  - epidemic hemorrhagic fever A98.5
  - malaria (malariae) B52.0
- ischemic — *see* Nephrosis, tubular
- lipoid N04.9
- lower nephron — *see* Nephrosis, tubular
- malarial (malariae) B52.0
- minimal change N04.0
- myoglobin N10
- necrotizing — *see* Nephrosis, tubular
- osmotic (sucrose) N25.89
- radiation N04.9
- syphilitic (late) A52.75
- toxic — *see* Nephrosis, tubular
- tubular (acute) N17.0
  - postprocedural N99.0
  - radiation N04.9

Nephrosonephritis, hemorrhagic (endemic) A98.5
Nephrostomy
- attention to Z43.6
- status Z93.6

Nerve — *see also* condition
- injury — *see* Injury, nerve, by body site

Nerves R45.0
Nervous — *see also* condition R45.0
- heart F45.8
- stomach F45.8
- tension R45.0

Nervousness R45.0
Nesidioblastoma
- pancreas D13.7
- specified site NEC — *see* Neoplasm, benign, by site
- unspecified site D13.7

Nettleship's syndrome — *see* Urticaria pigmentosa
Neumann's disease or syndrome L10.1
Neuralgia, neuralgic (acute) M79.2
- accessory (nerve) G52.8
- acoustic (nerve) — *see* subcategory H93.3- ☑
- auditory (nerve) — *see* subcategory H93.3- ☑
- ciliary G44.009
  - intractable G44.001
  - not intractable G44.009
- cranial
  - nerve — *see also* Disorder, nerve, cranial
    - fifth or trigeminal — *see* Neuralgia, trigeminal
  - postherpetic, postzoster B02.29
- ear — *see* subcategory H92.0- ☑
- facialis vera G51.1
- Fothergill's — *see* Neuralgia, trigeminal
- glossopharyngeal (nerve) G52.1
- Horton's G44.099
  - intractable G44.091
  - not intractable G44.099
- Hunt's B02.21
- hypoglossal (nerve) G52.3
- infraorbital — *see* Neuralgia, trigeminal
- malarial — *see* Malaria
- migrainous G44.009
  - intractable G44.001
  - not intractable G44.009
- Morton's G57.6- ☑
- nerve, cranial — *see* Disorder, nerve, cranial
- nose G52.0
- occipital M54.81
- olfactory G52.0
- penis N48.9
- perineum R10.20
  - bilateral R10.23
  - left R10.22
  - right R10.21
- postherpetic NEC B02.29
  - trigeminal B02.22
- pubic region R10.20
  - bilateral R10.23
  - left R10.22
  - right R10.21
- scrotum R10.20
- Sluder's G44.89
- specified nerve NEC G58.8
- spermatic cord R10.20
- sphenopalatine (ganglion) G90.09
- trifacial — *see* Neuralgia, trigeminal
- trigeminal G50.0
  - postherpetic, postzoster B02.22
- vagus (nerve) G52.2
- writer's F48.8

Neuralgia, neuralgic — *continued*
- writer's — *continued*
  - organic G25.89

Neurapraxia — *see* Injury, nerve
Neurasthenia F48.8
- cardiac F45.8
- gastric F45.8
- heart F45.8

Neurilemmoma — *see also* Neoplasm, nerve, benign
- acoustic (nerve) D33.3
- malignant — *see also* Neoplasm, nerve, malignant
  - acoustic (nerve) C72.4- ☑

Neurilemmosarcoma — *see* Neoplasm, nerve, malignant
Neurinoma — *see* Neoplasm, nerve, benign
Neurinomatosis — *see* Neoplasm, nerve, uncertain behavior

Neuritis (rheumatoid) M79.2
- abducens (nerve) — *see* Strabismus, paralytic, sixth nerve
- accessory (nerve) G52.8
- acoustic (nerve) — *see also* subcategory H93.3- ☑
  - in (due to)
    - infectious disease NEC B99.- ☑ [H94.0-] ☑
    - parasitic disease NEC B89 [H94.0-] ☑
  - syphilitic A52.15
- alcoholic G62.1
  - with psychosis — *see* Psychosis, alcoholic
- amyloid, any site E85.4 [G63]
- auditory (nerve) — *see* subcategory H93.3- ☑
- brachial — *see* Radiculopathy
  - due to displacement, intervertebral disc — *see* Disorder, disc, cervical, with neuritis
- cranial nerve
  - due to Lyme disease A69.22
  - eighth or acoustic or auditory — *see* subcategory H93.3- ☑
  - eleventh or accessory G52.8
  - fifth or trigeminal G50.- ☑
  - first or olfactory G52.0
  - fourth or trochlear — *see* Strabismus, paralytic, fourth nerve
  - second or optic — *see* Neuritis, optic
  - seventh or facial G51.8
    - newborn (birth injury) P11.3
  - sixth or abducent — *see* Strabismus, paralytic, sixth nerve
  - tenth or vagus G52.2
  - third or oculomotor — *see* Strabismus, paralytic, third nerve
  - twelfth or hypoglossal G52.3
- Dejerine-Sottas G60.0
- diabetic (mononeuropathy) — *see* E08-E13 with .41
  - polyneuropathy — *see* E08-E13 with .42
- due to
  - beriberi E51.11
  - displacement, prolapse or rupture, intervertebral disc — *see* Disorder, disc, with, radiculopathy
  - herniation, nucleus pulposus M51.9 [G55]
- endemic E51.11
- facial G51.8
  - newborn (birth injury) P11.3
- general — *see* Polyneuropathy
- geniculate ganglion G51.1
  - due to herpes (zoster) B02.21
- gouty — *see also* Gout, by type M10.9 [G63]
- hypoglossal (nerve) G52.3
- ilioinguinal (nerve) G57.9- ☑
- infectious (multiple) NEC G61.0
- interstitial hypertrophic progressive G60.0
- lumbar M54.16
- lumbosacral M54.17
- multiple — *see also* Polyneuropathy
  - endemic E51.11
  - infective, acute G61.0
- multiplex endemica E51.11
- nerve root — *see* Radiculopathy
- oculomotor (nerve) — *see* Strabismus, paralytic, third nerve
- olfactory nerve G52.0
- optic (nerve) (hereditary) (sympathetic) H46.9
  - with demyelination G36.0
  - in myelitis G36.0
  - nutritional H46.2
  - papillitis — *see* Papillitis, optic
  - retrobulbar H46.1- ☑
  - specified type NEC H46.8
  - toxic H46.3
- peripheral (nerve) G62.9
  - multiple — *see* Polyneuropathy

Neuritis — continued
  peripheral — continued
    single — see Mononeuritis
  pneumogastric (nerve) G52.2
  postherpetic, postzoster B02.29
  progressive hypertrophic interstitial G60.0
  retrobulbar — see also Neuritis, optic, retrobulbar
    in (due to)
      late syphilis A52.15
      meningococcal infection A39.82
    meningococcal A39.82
    syphilitic A52.15
  sciatic (nerve) — see also Sciatica
    due to displacement of intervertebral disc — see Disorder, disc, with, radiculopathy
  serum — see also Reaction, serum T80.69- ☑
  shoulder-girdle G54.5
  specified nerve NEC G58.8
  spinal (nerve) root — see Radiculopathy
  syphilitic A52.15
  thenar (median) G56.1- ☑
  thoracic M54.14
  toxic NEC G62.2
  trochlear (nerve) — see Strabismus, paralytic, fourth nerve
  vagus (nerve) G52.2
Neuroastrocytoma — see Neoplasm, uncertain behavior, by site
Neuroavitaminosis E56.9 [G99.8]
Neuroblastoma
  olfactory C30.0
  specified site — see Neoplasm, malignant, by site
  unspecified site C74.90
Neurochorioretinitis — see Chorioretinitis
Neurocirculatory asthenia F45.8
Neurocysticercosis B69.0
Neurocytoma — see Neoplasm, benign, by site
Neurodermatitis (circumscribed) (circumscripta) (local) L28.0
  atopic L20.81
  diffuse (Brocq) L20.81
  disseminated L20.81
Neuroencephalomyelopathy, optic G36.0
Neuroepithelioma — see also Neoplasm, malignant, by site
  olfactory C30.0
Neurofibroma — see also Neoplasm, nerve, benign
  melanotic — see Neoplasm, nerve, benign
  multiple — see Neurofibromatosis
  plexiform — see Neoplasm, nerve, benign
Neurofibromatosis (multiple) (nonmalignant) Q85.00
  acoustic Q85.02
  malignant — see Neoplasm, nerve, malignant
  specified NEC Q85.09
  type 1 (von Recklinghausen) Q85.01
  type 2 Q85.02
Neurofibrosarcoma — see Neoplasm, nerve, malignant
Neurogenic — see also condition
  bladder — see also Dysfunction, bladder, neuromuscular N31.9
    cauda equina syndrome G83.4
  bowel NEC K59.2
  heart F45.8
Neuroglioma — see Neoplasm, uncertain behavior, by site
Neurolabyrinthitis (of Dix and Hallpike) — see Neuronitis, vestibular
Neurolathyrism — see Poisoning, food, noxious, plant
Neuroleprosy A30.9
Neuroma — see also Neoplasm, nerve, benign
  acoustic (nerve) D33.3
  amputation (stump) (traumatic) (surgical complication) (late) T87.3- ☑
    arm T87.3- ☑
    leg T87.3- ☑
  digital (toe) G57.6- ☑
  interdigital G58.8
    lower limb (toe) G57.8- ☑
    upper limb G56.8- ☑
  intermetatarsal G57.8- ☑
  Morton's G57.6- ☑
  nonneoplastic
    arm G56.9- ☑
    leg G57.9- ☑
    lower extremity G57.9- ☑
    upper extremity G56.9- ☑
  optic (nerve) D33.3
  plantar G57.6- ☑
  plexiform — see Neoplasm, nerve, benign

Neuroma — continued
  surgical (nonneoplastic)
    arm G56.9- ☑
    leg G57.9- ☑
    lower extremity G57.9- ☑
    upper extremity G56.9- ☑
Neuromyalgia — see Neuralgia
Neuromyasthenia (epidemic) (postinfectious) G93.39
Neuromyelitis G36.9
  ascending G61.0
  optica G36.0
Neuromyopathy G70.9
  paraneoplastic — see also, Neoplasm, by site, if known D49.9 [G13.0]
Neuromyotonia (Isaacs) G71.19
Neuronevus — see Nevus
Neuronitis G58.9
  ascending (acute) G57.2- ☑
  vestibular H81.2- ☑
Neuroparalytic — see condition
Neuropathy, neuropathic G62.9
  acute motor G62.81
  alcoholic G62.1
    with psychosis — see Psychosis, alcoholic
  arm G56.9- ☑
  autonomic, peripheral — see Neuropathy, peripheral, autonomic
  axillary G56.9- ☑
  bladder N31.9
    atonic (motor) (sensory) N31.2
    autonomous N31.2
    flaccid N31.2
    nonreflex N31.2
    reflex N31.1
    uninhibited N31.0
  brachial plexus G54.0
  cervical plexus G54.2
  chronic
    progressive segmentally demyelinating G62.89
    relapsing demyelinating G62.89
  Dejerine-Sottas G60.0
  diabetic — see E08-E13 with .40
    mononeuropathy — see E08-E13 with .41
    polyneuropathy — see E08-E13 with .42
  entrapment G58.9
    iliohypogastric nerve G57.8- ☑
    ilioinguinal nerve G57.8- ☑
    lateral cutaneous nerve of thigh G57.1- ☑
    median nerve G56.0- ☑
    obturator nerve G57.8- ☑
    peroneal nerve G57.3- ☑
    posterior tibial nerve G57.5- ☑
    saphenous nerve G57.8- ☑
    ulnar nerve G56.2- ☑
  facial nerve G51.9
  hereditary G60.9
    motor and sensory (types I-IV) G60.0
    sensory G60.8
    specified NEC G60.8
  hypertrophic G60.0
    Charcot-Marie-Tooth G60.0
    Dejerine-Sottas G60.0
    interstitial progressive G60.0
    of infancy G60.0
    Refsum G60.1
  idiopathic G60.9
    progressive G60.3
    specified NEC G60.8
  in association with hereditary ataxia G60.2
  intercostal G58.0
  ischemic — see Disorder, nerve
  Jamaica (ginger) G62.2
  leg NEC G57.9- ☑
  lower extremity G57.9- ☑
  lumbar plexus G54.1
  median nerve G56.1- ☑
  motor and sensory — see also Polyneuropathy
    hereditary (types I-IV) G60.0
  multifocal motor (MMN) G61.82
  multiple (acute) (chronic) — see Polyneuropathy
  optic (nerve) — see also Neuritis, optic
    ischemic H47.01- ☑
  paraneoplastic (sensorial) (Denny Brown) — see also, Neoplasm, by site, if known D49.9 [G13.0]
  peripheral (nerve) — see also Polyneuropathy G62.9
    autonomic G90.9
      idiopathic G90.09

Neuropathy, neuropathic — continued
  peripheral — see also Polyneuropathy — continued
    autonomic — continued
      in (due to)
        amyloidosis E85.4 [G99.0]
        diabetes mellitus — see E08-E13 with .43
        endocrine disease NEC E34.9 [G99.0]
        gout M10.00 [G99.0]
        hyperthyroidism E05.90 [G99.0]
          with thyroid storm E05.91 [G99.0]
        metabolic disease NEC E88.9 [G99.0]
      idiopathic G60.9
      progressive G60.3
    in (due to)
      antitetanus serum G62.0
      arsenic G62.2
      drugs NEC G62.0
      lead G62.2
      organophosphate compounds G62.2
      toxic agent NEC G62.2
  plantar nerves G57.6- ☑
  progressive
    hypertrophic interstitial G60.0
    inflammatory G62.81
  radicular NEC — see Radiculopathy
  sacral plexus G54.1
  sciatic G57.0- ☑
  serum G61.1
  toxic NEC G62.2
  trigeminal sensory G50.8
  ulnar nerve G56.2- ☑
  uremic N18.9 [G63]
  vitamin B12 E53.8 [G63]
    with anemia (pernicious) D51.0 [G63]
    due to dietary deficiency D51.3 [G63]
Neurophthisis — see also Disorder, nerve
  peripheral, diabetic — see E08-E13 with .42
Neuroretinitis — see Chorioretinitis
Neuroretinopathy, hereditary optic H47.22
Neurosarcoma — see Neoplasm, nerve, malignant
Neurosclerosis — see Disorder, nerve
Neurosis, neurotic F48.9
  anankastic F42.8
  anxiety (state) F41.1
    panic type F41.0
  asthenic F48.8
  bladder F45.8
  cardiac (reflex) F45.8
  cardiovascular F45.8
  character F60.9
  colon F45.8
  compensation F68.10
  compulsive, compulsion F42.8
  conversion F44.9
  craft F48.8
  cutaneous F45.8
  depersonalization F48.1
  depressive (reaction) (type) F34.1
  environmental F48.8
  excoriation L98.1
  fatigue F48.8
  functional — see Disorder, somatoform
  gastric F45.8
  gastrointestinal F45.8
  heart F45.8
  hypochondriacal F45.21
  hysterical F44.9
  incoordination F45.8
    larynx F45.8
    vocal cord F45.8
  intestine F45.8
  larynx (sensory) F45.8
    hysterical F44.4
  mixed NEC F48.8
  musculoskeletal F45.8
  obsessional F42.8
  obsessive-compulsive F42.8
  occupational F48.8
  ocular NEC F45.8
  organ — see Disorder, somatoform
  pharynx F45.8
  phobic F40.9
  posttraumatic (situational) F43.10
    acute F43.11
    chronic F43.12
  psychasthenic (type) F48.8
  railroad F48.8
  rectum F45.8
  respiratory F45.8

Neurosis, neurotic — continued
- rumination F45.8
- sexual F65.9
- situational F48.8
- social F40.10
  - generalized F40.11
- specified type NEC F48.8
- state F48.9
  - with depersonalization episode F48.1
- stomach F45.8
- traumatic F43.10
  - acute F43.11
  - chronic F43.12
- vasomotor F45.8
- visceral F45.8
- war F48.8

Neurospongioblastosis diffusa Q85.1

Neurosyphilis (arrested) (early) (gumma) (late) (latent) (recurrent) (relapse) A52.3
- with ataxia (cerebellar) (locomotor) (spastic) (spinal) A52.19
- aneurysm (cerebral) A52.05
- arachnoid (adhesive) A52.13
- arteritis (any artery) (cerebral) A52.04
- asymptomatic A52.2
- congenital A50.40
- dura (mater) A52.13
- general paresis A52.17
- hemorrhagic A52.05
- juvenile (asymptomatic) (meningeal) A50.40
- leptomeninges (aseptic) A52.13
- meningeal, meninges (adhesive) A52.13
- meningitis A52.13
- meningovascular (diffuse) A52.13
- optic atrophy A52.15
- parenchymatous (degenerative) A52.19
- paresis, paretic A52.17
  - juvenile A50.45
- remission in (sustained) A52.3
- serological (without symptoms) A52.2
- specified nature or site NEC A52.19
- tabes, tabetic (dorsalis) A52.11
  - juvenile A50.45
- taboparesis (taboparetic) A52.17
  - juvenile A50.45
- thrombosis (cerebral) A52.05
- vascular (cerebral) NEC A52.05

Neurothekeoma — see Neoplasm, nerve, benign

Neurotic — see Neurosis

Neurotoxemia — see Toxemia

Neuroclusion M26.211

Neutropenia, neutropenic (chronic) (genetic) (idiopathic) (immune) (infantile) (malignant) (pernicious) (splenic) D70.9
- benign ethnic — see Phenotype, Duffy, null
- congenital (primary) D70.0
- cyclic D70.4
- cytoreductive cancer chemotherapy sequela D70.1
- drug-induced D70.2
  - due to cytoreductive cancer chemotherapy D70.1
- due to infection D70.3
- fever D70.9
- neonatal, transitory (isoimmune) (maternal transfer) P61.5
- periodic D70.4
- secondary (cyclic) (periodic) (splenic) D70.4
  - drug-induced D70.2
    - due to cytoreductive cancer chemotherapy D70.1
- specified NEC D70.8
- toxic D70.8

Neutrophilia, hereditary giant D72.0

Nevocarcinoma — see Melanoma

Nevus D22.9
- achromic — see Neoplasm, skin, benign
- amelanotic — see Neoplasm, skin, benign
- angiomatous D18.00
  - intra-abdominal D18.03
  - intracranial D18.02
  - skin D18.01
  - specified site NEC D18.09
- araneus I78.1
- balloon cell — see Neoplasm, skin, benign
- bathing trunk D48.5
- blue — see Neoplasm, skin, benign
  - cellular — see Neoplasm, skin, benign
  - giant — see Neoplasm, skin, benign
  - Jadassohn's — see Neoplasm, skin, benign
- malignant — see Melanoma
- capillary D18.00

Nevus — continued
- capillary — continued
  - intra-abdominal D18.03
  - intracranial D18.02
  - skin D18.01
  - specified site NEC D18.09
- cavernous D18.00
  - intra-abdominal D18.03
  - intracranial D18.02
  - skin D18.01
  - specified site NEC D18.09
- cellular — see Neoplasm, skin, benign
  - blue — see Neoplasm, skin, benign
- choroid D31.3- ☑
- comedonicus Q82.5
- conjunctiva D31.0- ☑
- dermal — see Neoplasm, skin, benign
  - with epidermal nevus — see Neoplasm, skin, benign
- dysplastic — see Neoplasm, skin, benign
- eye D31.9- ☑
- flammeus Q82.5
- hemangiomatous D18.00
  - intra-abdominal D18.03
  - intracranial D18.02
  - skin D18.01
  - specified site NEC D18.09
- iris D31.4- ☑
- lacrimal gland D31.5- ☑
- lymphatic D18.1
- magnocellular
  - specified site — see Neoplasm, benign, by site
  - unspecified site D31.40
- malignant — see Melanoma
- meaning hemangioma D18.00
  - intra-abdominal D18.03
  - intracranial D18.02
  - skin D18.01
  - specified site NEC D18.09
- mouth (mucosa) D10.30
  - specified site NEC D10.39
  - white sponge Q38.6
- multiplex Q85.1
- non-neoplastic I78.1
- oral mucosa D10.30
  - specified site NEC D10.39
  - white sponge Q38.6
- orbit D31.6- ☑
- pigmented
  - giant — see also Neoplasm, skin, uncertain behavior D48.5
    - malignant melanoma in — see Melanoma
- portwine Q82.5
- retina D31.2- ☑
- retrobulbar D31.6- ☑
- sanguineous Q82.5
- senile I78.1
- skin D22.9
  - abdominal wall D22.5
  - ala nasi D22.39
  - ankle D22.7- ☑
  - anus, anal D22.5
  - arm D22.6- ☑
  - auditory canal (external) D22.2- ☑
  - auricle (ear) D22.2- ☑
  - auricular canal (external) D22.2- ☑
  - axilla, axillary fold D22.5
  - back D22.5
  - breast D22.5
  - brow D22.39
  - buttock D22.5
  - canthus (eye) D22.1- ☑
  - cheek (external) D22.39
  - chest wall D22.5
  - chin D22.39
  - ear (external) D22.2- ☑
  - external meatus (ear) D22.2- ☑
  - eyebrow D22.39
  - eyelid (lower) (upper) D22.1- ☑
  - face D22.30
    - specified NEC D22.39
  - female genital organ (external) NEC D28.0
  - finger D22.6- ☑
  - flank D22.5
  - foot D22.7- ☑
  - forearm D22.6- ☑
  - forehead D22.39
  - foreskin D29.0

Nevus — continued
- skin — continued
  - genital organ (external) NEC
    - female D28.0
    - male D29.9
  - gluteal region D22.5
  - groin D22.5
  - hand D22.6- ☑
  - heel D22.7- ☑
  - helix D22.2- ☑
  - hip D22.7- ☑
  - interscapular region D22.5
  - jaw D22.39
  - knee D22.7- ☑
  - labium (majus) (minus) D28.0
  - leg D22.7- ☑
  - lip (lower) (upper) D22.0
  - lower limb D22.7- ☑
  - male genital organ (external) D29.9
  - nail D22.9
    - finger D22.6- ☑
    - toe D22.7- ☑
  - nasolabial groove D22.39
  - nates D22.5
  - neck D22.4
  - nose (external) D22.39
  - palpebra D22.1- ☑
  - penis D29.0
  - perianal skin D22.5
  - perineum D22.5
  - pinna D22.2- ☑
  - popliteal fossa or space D22.7- ☑
  - prepuce D29.0
  - pudendum D28.0
  - scalp D22.4
  - scrotum D29.4
  - shoulder D22.6- ☑
  - submammary fold D22.5
  - temple D22.39
  - thigh D22.7- ☑
  - toe D22.7- ☑
  - trunk NEC D22.5
  - umbilicus D22.5
  - upper limb D22.6- ☑
  - vulva D28.0
- specified site NEC — see Neoplasm, by site, benign
- spider I78.1
- stellar I78.1
- strawberry Q82.5
- Sutton's benign D22.9
- unius lateris Q82.5
- Unna's Q82.5
- vascular Q82.5
- verrucous Q82.5

Newborn (infant) (liveborn) (singleton) Z38.2
- abstinence syndrome P96.1
- acne L70.4
- affected by
  - abnormalities of membranes P02.9
    - specified NEC P02.8
  - abruptio placenta P02.1
  - amino-acid metabolic disorder, transitory P74.8
  - amniocentesis (while in utero) P00.6
  - amnionitis P02.78
  - apparent life threatening event (ALTE) R68.13
  - bleeding (into)
    - cerebral cortex P52.22
    - germinal matrix P52.0
    - ventricles P52.1
  - breech delivery P03.0
  - cardiac arrest P29.81
  - cardiomyopathy I42.8
    - congenital I42.4
  - cerebral ischemia P91.0
  - Cesarean delivery P03.4
  - chemotherapy agents P04.11
  - chorioamnionitis P02.78
  - cocaine (crack) P04.41
  - complications of labor and delivery P03.9
    - specified NEC P03.89
  - compression of umbilical cord NEC P02.5
  - contracted pelvis P03.1
  - cyanosis P28.2
  - delivery P03.9
    - Cesarean P03.4
    - forceps P03.2
    - vacuum extractor P03.3
  - drugs of addiction P04.40

Newborn — *continued*
affected by — *continued*
  drugs of addiction — *continued*
    cocaine P04.41
    hallucinogens P04.42
    specified drug NEC P04.49
  entanglement (knot) in umbilical cord P02.5
  environmental chemicals P04.6
  fetal (intrauterine)
    growth retardation P05.9
    inflammatory response syndrome (FIRS) P02.70
    malnutrition not light or small for gestational age P05.2
  FIRS (fetal inflammatory response syndrome) P02.70
  forceps delivery P03.2
  heart rate abnormalities
    bradycardia P29.12
    intrauterine P03.819
      before onset of labor P03.810
      during labor P03.811
    tachycardia P29.11
  hemorrhage (antepartum) P02.1
    cerebellar (nontraumatic) P52.6
    intracerebral (nontraumatic) P52.4
    intracranial (nontraumatic) P52.9
      specified NEC P52.8
    intraventricular (nontraumatic) P52.3
      grade 1 P52.0
      grade 2 P52.1
      grade 3 P52.21
      grade 4 P52.22
    posterior fossa (nontraumatic) P52.6
    subarachnoid (nontraumatic) P52.5
    subependymal P52.0
      with intracerebral extension P52.22
      with intraventricular extension P52.1
        with enlargement of ventricles P52.21
      without intraventricular extension P52.0
  hypoxic ischemic encephalopathy [HIE] P91.60
    mild P91.61
    moderate P91.62
    severe P91.63
  induction of labor P03.89
  intestinal perforation P78.0
  intrauterine (fetal) blood loss P50.9
    due to (from)
      cut end of co-twin cord P50.5
      hemorrhage into
        co-twin P50.3
          maternal circulation P50.4
      placenta P50.2
      ruptured cord blood P50.1
      vasa previa P50.0
    specified NEC P50.8
  intrauterine (fetal) hemorrhage P50.9
  intrauterine (in utero) procedure P96.5
  malpresentation (malposition) NEC P03.1
  maternal (complication of) (use of)
    alcohol P04.3
    amphetamines P04.16
    analgesia (maternal) P04.0
    anesthesia (maternal) P04.0
    anticonvulsants P04.13
    antidepressants P04.15
    antineoplastic chemotherapy P04.11
    anxiolytics P04.1A
    blood loss P02.1
    cannabis P04.81
    circulatory disease P00.3
    condition P00.9
      specified NEC P00.89
    cytotoxic drugs P04.12
    delivery P03.9
      Cesarean P03.4
      forceps P03.2
      vacuum extractor P03.3
    diabetes mellitus (pre-existing) P70.1
    disorder P00.9
      specified NEC P00.89
    drugs (addictive) (illegal) NEC P04.49
    ectopic pregnancy P01.4
    gestational diabetes P70.0
    group B streptococcus (GBS) colonization (positive) P00.82
    hemorrhage P02.1
    hypertensive disorder P00.0
    incompetent cervix P01.0
    infectious disease P00.2
    injury P00.5

Newborn — *continued*
affected by — *continued*
  maternal — *continued*
    labor and delivery P03.9
    malpresentation before labor P01.7
    maternal death P01.6
    medical procedure P00.7
    medication P04.19
      specified type NEC P04.18
    multiple pregnancy P01.5
    nutritional disorder P00.4
    oligohydramnios P01.2
    opiates P04.14
      administered for procedures during pregnancy or labor and delivery P04.0
    parasitic disease P00.2
    periodontal disease P00.81
    placenta previa P02.0
    polyhydramnios P01.3
    precipitate delivery P03.5
    pregnancy P01.9
      specified P01.8
    premature rupture of membranes P01.1
    renal disease P00.1
    respiratory disease P00.3
    sedative-hypnotics P04.17
    surgical procedure P00.6
    tranquilizers administered for procedures during pregnancy or labor and delivery P04.0
    urinary tract disease P00.1
    uterine contraction (abnormal) P03.6
  meconium peritonitis P78.0
  medication (legal) (maternal use) (prescribed) P04.19
  membrane abnormalities P02.9
    specified NEC P02.8
  membranitis P02.78
  methamphetamine(s) P04.49
  mixed metabolic and respiratory acidosis P84
  neonatal abstinence syndrome P96.1
  noxious substances transmitted via placenta or breast milk P04.9
    cannabis P04.81
    specified NEC P04.89
  nutritional supplements P04.5
  placenta previa P02.0
  placental
    abnormality (functional) (morphological) P02.20
      specified NEC P02.29
    dysfunction P02.29
    infarction P02.29
    insufficiency P02.29
    separation NEC P02.1
    transfusion syndromes P02.3
  placentitis P02.78
  precipitate delivery P03.5
  prolapsed cord P02.4
  respiratory arrest P28.81
  slow intrauterine growth P05.9
  tobacco P04.2
  twin to twin transplacental transfusion P02.3
  umbilical cord (tightly) around neck P02.5
  umbilical cord condition P02.60
    short cord P02.69
    specified NEC P02.69
  uterine contractions (abnormal) P03.6
  vasa previa P02.69
    from intrauterine blood loss P50.0
apnea — *see also* Apnea, newborn P28.40
  obstructive P28.42
  primary — *see also* Apnea, newborn, sleep, primary P28.30
  sleep (central) (obstructive) (primary) — *see also* Apnea, newborn, sleep, primary P28.30
born in hospital Z38.00
  by cesarean Z38.01
born outside hospital Z38.1
breast buds P96.89
breast engorgement P83.4
check-up — *see* Newborn, examination
convulsion P90
dehydration P74.1
examination
  8 to 28 days old Z00.111
  under 8 days old Z00.110
fever P81.9
  environmentally-induced P81.0
hyperbilirubinemia P59.9
  of prematurity P59.0
hypernatremia P74.21

Newborn — *continued*
hyponatremia P74.22
infection P39.9
  candidal P37.5
  specified NEC P39.8
  urinary tract P39.3
jaundice P59.9
  due to
    breast milk inhibitor P59.3
    hepatocellular damage P59.20
      specified NEC P59.29
    preterm delivery P59.0
  of prematurity P59.0
  specified NEC P59.8
late metabolic acidosis P74.0
mastitis P39.0
  infective P39.0
  noninfective P83.4
multiple born NEC Z38.8
  born in hospital Z38.68
    by cesarean Z38.69
  born outside hospital Z38.7
omphalitis P38.9
  with mild hemorrhage P38.1
  without hemorrhage P38.9
post-term P08.21
prolonged gestation (over 42 completed weeks) P08.22
quadruplet Z38.8
  born in hospital Z38.63
    by cesarean Z38.64
  born outside hospital Z38.7
quintuplet Z38.8
  born in hospital Z38.65
    by cesarean Z38.66
  born outside hospital Z38.7
seizure P90
sepsis (congenital) P36.9
  due to
    anaerobes NEC P36.5
    Escherichia coli P36.4
    Staphylococcus P36.30
      aureus P36.2
      specified NEC P36.39
    Streptococcus P36.10
      group B P36.0
      specified NEC P36.19
  specified NEC P36.8
triplet Z38.8
  born in hospital Z38.61
    by cesarean Z38.62
  born outside hospital Z38.7
twin Z38.5
  born in hospital Z38.30
    by cesarean Z38.31
  born outside hospital Z38.4
vomiting P92.09
  bilious P92.01
weight check Z00.111
Newcastle conjunctivitis or disease B30.8
Nezelof's syndrome (pure alymphocytosis) D81.4
Niacin (amide) **deficiency** E52
Nicolas (-Durand)-**Favre disease** A55
Nicotine — *see* Tobacco
Nicotinic acid deficiency E52
Niemann-Pick disease or syndrome E75.249
  specified NEC E75.248
  type
    A E75.240
    A/B E75.244
    B E75.241
    C E75.242
    D E75.243
Night
  blindness — *see* Blindness, night
  sweats R61
  terrors (child) F51.4
Nightmares (REM sleep type) F51.5
NIHSS (National Institutes of Health Stroke Scale) **score** R29.7- ☑
Nipple — *see* condition
Nisbet's chancre A57
Nishimoto (-Takeuchi) **disease** I67.5
Nitritoid crisis or reaction — *see* Crisis, nitritoid
Nitrosohemoglobinemia D74.8
Njovera A65
No
  general equivalence degree (GED) Z55.5
  health insurance coverage Z59.71
Nocardiosis, nocardiasis A43.9

Nocardiosis, nocardiasis — *continued*
- cutaneous A43.1
- lung A43.0
- pneumonia A43.0
- pulmonary A43.0
- specified site NEC A43.8

Nocturia R35.1
- psychogenic F45.8

Nocturnal — *see* condition

Nodal rhythm I49.8

Node(s) — *see also* Nodule
- Bouchard's (with arthropathy) M15.2
- Haygarth's M15.8
- Heberden's (with arthropathy) M15.1
- larynx J38.7
- lymph — *see* condition
- milker's B08.03
- Osler's I33.0
- Schmorl's — *see* Schmorl's disease
- singer's J38.2
- teacher's J38.2
- tuberculous — *see* Tuberculosis, lymph gland
- vocal cord J38.2

Nodule(s), **nodular**
- actinomycotic — *see* Actinomycosis
- breast NEC — *see also* Lump, breast N63.0
- colloid (cystic), thyroid E04.1
- cutaneous — *see* Swelling, localized
- endometrial (stromal) D26.1
- Haygarth's M15.8
- inflammatory — *see* Inflammation
- juxta-articular
  - syphilitic A52.77
  - yaws A66.7
- larynx J38.7
- lung, solitary (subsegmental branch of the bronchial tree) R91.1
  - multiple R91.8
- milker's B08.03
- prostate N40.2
  - with lower urinary tract symptoms (LUTS) N40.3
  - without lower urinary tract symptoms (LUTS) N40.2
- pulmonary, solitary (subsegmental branch of the bronchial tree) R91.1
- retrocardiac R09.89
- rheumatoid M06.30
  - ankle M06.37- ☑
  - elbow M06.32- ☑
  - foot joint M06.37- ☑
  - hand joint M06.34- ☑
  - hip M06.35- ☑
  - knee M06.36- ☑
  - multiple site M06.39
  - shoulder M06.31- ☑
  - vertebra M06.38
  - wrist M06.33- ☑
- scrotum (inflammatory) N49.2
- singer's J38.2
- solitary, lung (subsegmental branch of the bronchial tree) R91.1
  - multiple R91.8
- subcutaneous — *see* Swelling, localized
- teacher's J38.2
- thyroid (cold) (gland) (nontoxic) E04.1
  - with thyrotoxicosis E05.20
    - with thyroid storm E05.21
  - toxic or with hyperthyroidism E05.20
    - with thyroid storm E05.21
- vocal cord J38.2

Noma (gangrenous) (hospital) (infective) A69.0
- auricle I96
- mouth A69.0
- pudendi N76.89
- vulvae N76.89

Nomad, nomadism Z59.00

NOMID (neonatal onset multisystemic inflammatory disorder) M04.2

Non-accidental trauma — *see* Abuse, physical

Non-Hodgkin lymphoma NEC — *see* Lymphoma, non-Hodgkin

Non-ketotic hyperglycinemia E72.51

Non-palpable testicle(s)
- bilateral R39.84
- unilateral R39.83

Non-working side interference M26.56

Nonadherence to medical treatment, specified NEC Z91.199

Nonadherence to medical treatment, specified — *continued*
- due to
  - financial hardship Z91.190
  - specified reason NEC Z91.198

Nonautoimmune hemolytic anemia D59.4
- drug-induced D59.2

Nonclosure — *see also* Imperfect, closure
- ductus arteriosus (Botallo's) Q25.0
- foramen
  - botalli Q21.12
  - ovale Q21.12

Noncompliance Z91.199
- with
  - dialysis Z91.158
    - due to financial hardship Z91.151
  - dietary regimen Z91.119
    - due to
      - financial hardship Z91.110
      - specified reason NEC Z91.118
  - medical treatment, specified NEC Z91.199
    - due to
      - financial hardship Z91.190
      - specified reason NEC Z91.198
  - medication regimen NEC Z91.148
    - due to financial hardship Z91.141
    - underdosing — *see also* Table of Drugs and Chemicals, categories T36-T50, with final character 6 Z91.148
      - intentional NEC Z91.128
        - by caregiver
          - due to
            - financial hardship Z91.A20
            - specified reason NEC Z91.A28
          - due to financial hardship of patient Z91.120
      - unintentional NEC Z91.138
        - by caregiver Z91.A3
        - due to patient's age related debility Z91.130
  - renal dialysis Z91.158
    - due to financial hardship Z91.151
- caregiver
  - with patient's
    - dietary regimen
      - due to
        - financial hardship Z91.A10
        - specified reason NEC Z91.A18
    - medical treatment and regimen
      - due to financial hardship Z91.A91
      - specified reason NEC Z91.A98
    - medication regimen
      - due to financial hardship Z91.A41
      - specified reason NEC Z91.A48
    - renal dialysis
      - due to financial hardship Z91.A51
      - specified reason NEC Z91.A58

Nondescent (congenital) — *see also* Malposition, congenital
- cecum Q43.3
- colon Q43.3
- testicle Q53.9
  - bilateral Q53.20
    - abdominal Q53.211
    - perineal Q53.22
  - unilateral Q53.10
    - abdominal Q53.111
    - perineal Q53.12

Nondevelopment
- brain Q02
  - part of Q04.3
- heart Q24.8
- organ or site, congenital NEC — *see* Hypoplasia

Nonengagement
- head NEC O32.4- ☑
- in labor, causing obstructed labor O64.8- ☑

Nonexanthematous tick fever A93.2

Nonexpansion, lung (newborn) P28.0

Nonfunctioning
- cystic duct — *see also* Disease, gallbladder K82.8
- gallbladder — *see also* Disease, gallbladder K82.8
- kidney N28.9
- labyrinth — *see* subcategory H83.2- ☑

Nonimplantation, ovum N97.2

Noninsufflation, fallopian tube N97.1

Nonne-Milroy syndrome Q82.0

Nonovulation N97.0

Nonpatent fallopian tube N97.1

Nonpneumatization, lung NEC P28.0

Nonrotation — *see* Malrotation

Nonsecretion, urine — *see* Anuria

Nonunion
- fracture — *see* Fracture, by site
- joint, following fusion or arthrodesis M96.0
- organ or site, congenital NEC — *see* Imperfect, closure
- symphysis pubis, congenital Q74.2

Nonvisualization, gallbladder R93.2

Nonvital, nonvitalized tooth K04.99

Noonan's syndrome Q87.19

Normocytic anemia (infectional) due to blood loss (chronic) D50.0
- acute D62

Norrie's disease (congenital) Q15.8

North American blastomycosis B40.9

Norwegian itch B86

Nose, nasal — *see* condition

Nose-picking F98.8

Nosebleed R04.0

Nosomania F45.21

Nosophobia F45.22

Nostalgia F43.20

Notch of iris Q13.2

Notching nose, congenital (tip) Q30.2

Nothnagel's
- syndrome — *see* Strabismus, paralytic, third nerve
- vasomotor acroparesthesia I73.89

Novy's relapsing fever A68.9
- louse-borne A68.0
- tick-borne A68.1

Noxious
- foodstuffs, poisoning by — *see* Poisoning, food, noxious, plant
- substances transmitted through placenta or breast milk P04.9

Nucleus pulposus — *see* condition

Numbness R20.0

Nuns' knee — *see* Bursitis, prepatellar

Nursemaid's elbow S53.03- ☑

Nutcracker esophagus K22.4

Nutmeg liver K76.1

Nutrient element deficiency E61.9
- specified NEC E61.8

Nutrition deficient or insufficient — *see also* Malnutrition E63.9
- due to
  - insufficient food T73.0- ☑
  - lack of
    - care (child) T76.02- ☑
      - adult T76.01- ☑
    - food T73.0- ☑
  - specific element deficiency — *see* Nutrient element deficiency, or by element
- sequelae — *see* Sequelae, nutritional deficiency
- specified NEC E63.8

Nutritional stunting E45

Nyctalopia (night blindness) — *see* Blindness, night

Nycturia R35.1
- psychogenic F45.8

Nymphomania F52.8

Nystagmus H55.00
- benign paroxysmal — *see* Vertigo, benign paroxysmal
- central positional H81.4
- congenital H55.01
- dissociated H55.04
- latent H55.02
- miners' H55.09
- positional
  - benign paroxysmal H81.4
  - central H81.4
- specified form NEC H55.09
- visual deprivation H55.03

O

Obermeyer's relapsing fever (European) A68.0

Obesity E66.9
- with alveolar hypoventilation E66.2
- adrenal E27.8
- class
  - 1 E66.811
  - 2 E66.812
  - 3 E66.813
- complicating
  - childbirth O99.214
  - pregnancy O99.21- ☑
  - puerperium O99.215
- constitutional E66.89
- dietary counseling and surveillance Z71.3

Obesity — continued
　drug-induced E66.1
　due to
　　disruption of MC4R pathway E88.82
　　drug E66.1
　　excess calories E66.09
　　　morbid E66.01
　　　severe E66.01
　　gene mutation
　　　leptin (LEP) E88.82
　　　leptin receptor (LEPR) E88.82
　　　melanocortin 4 Receptor (MC4R) E88.82
　　　nuclear receptor coactivator 1 (NCOA1) E88.82
　　　proopiomelanocortin (POMC) E88.82
　　　proprotein convertase subtilisin/kexin type 1 (PC-SK1) E88.82
　　　src homology 2B adaptor signaling protein (SH2B1) E88.82
　endocrine E66.89
　endogenous E66.89
　exogenous E66.09
　familial E66.89
　glandular E66.89
　hypothyroid — see Hypothyroidism
　hypoventilation syndrome (OHS) E66.2
　morbid E66.01
　　with
　　　alveolar hypoventilation E66.2
　　　obesity hypoventilation syndrome (OHS) E66.2
　　due to excess calories E66.01
　nutritional E66.09
　pituitary E23.6
　severe E66.01
　specified type NEC E66.89
Oblique — see condition
Obliteration
　appendix (lumen) K38.8
　artery I77.1
　bile duct (noncalculous) K83.1
　common duct (noncalculous) K83.1
　cystic duct — see Obstruction, gallbladder
　disease, arteriolar I77.1
　endometrium N85.8
　eye, anterior chamber — see Disorder, globe, hypotony
　fallopian tube N97.1
　lymphatic vessel I89.0
　　due to mastectomy I97.2
　organ or site, congenital NEC — see Atresia, by site
　ureter N13.5
　　with infection N13.6
　urethra — see Stricture, urethra
　vein I87.8
　vestibule (oral) K08.89
Observation (following) (for) (without need for further medical care) Z04.9
　accident NEC Z04.3
　　at work Z04.2
　　transport Z04.1
　adverse effect of drug Z03.6
　alleged rape or sexual assault (victim), ruled out
　　adult Z04.41
　　child Z04.42
　criminal assault Z04.89
　development state
　　adolescent Z00.3
　　period of rapid growth in childhood Z00.2
　　puberty Z00.3
　disease, specified NEC Z03.89
　following work accident Z04.2
　forced sexual exploitation Z04.81
　forced labor exploitation Z04.82
　growth and development state — see Observation, development state
　injuries (accidental) NEC — see also Observation, accident
　newborn (for)
　　suspected condition, related to exposure from the mother or birth process — see Newborn, affected by, maternal
　　　ruled out Z05.9
　　　　cardiac Z05.0
　　　　connective tissue Z05.73
　　　　gastrointestinal Z05.5
　　　　genetic Z05.41
　　　　genitourinary Z05.6
　　　　immunologic Z05.43
　　　　infectious Z05.1
　　　　metabolic Z05.42
　　　　musculoskeletal Z05.72
　　　　neurological Z05.2

Observation — continued
　newborn — continued
　　suspected condition, related to exposure from the mother or birth process — see Newborn, affected by, maternal — continued
　　　ruled out — continued
　　　　respiratory Z05.3
　　　　skin and subcutaneous tissue Z05.71
　　　　specified condition NEC Z05.89
　postpartum
　　immediately after delivery Z39.0
　　routine follow-up Z39.2
　pregnancy (normal) (without complication) Z34.9- ☑
　　high risk O09.9- ☑
　suicide attempt, alleged NEC Z03.89
　　self-poisoning Z03.6
　suspected, ruled out — see also Suspected condition, ruled out
　　abuse, physical
　　　adult Z04.71
　　　child Z04.72
　　accident at work Z04.2
　　adult battering victim Z04.71
　　child battering victim Z04.72
　　condition NEC Z03.89
　　　newborn — see also Observation, newborn (for), suspected condition, ruled out Z05.9
　　drug poisoning or adverse effect Z03.6
　　exposure (to)
　　　anthrax Z03.810
　　　biological agent NEC Z03.818
　　foreign body
　　　aspirated (inhaled) Z03.822
　　　ingested Z03.821
　　　inserted (injected), in (eye) (orifice) (skin) Z03.823
　　inflicted injury NEC Z04.89
　　suicide attempt, alleged Z03.89
　　　self-poisoning Z03.6
　　toxic effects from ingested substance (drug) (poison) Z03.6
　toxic effects from ingested substance (drug) (poison) Z03.6
Obsession, obsessional state F42.8
　mixed thoughts and acts F42.2
Obsessive-compulsive neurosis or reaction F42.8
Obstetric embolism, septic — see Embolism, obstetric, septic
Obstetrical trauma (complicating delivery) O71.9
　with or following ectopic or molar pregnancy O08.6
　specified type NEC O71.89
Obstipation — see Constipation
Obstruction, obstructed, obstructive
　airway J98.8
　　with
　　　allergic alveolitis J67.9
　　　asthma J45.909
　　　　with
　　　　　exacerbation (acute) J45.901
　　　　　status asthmaticus J45.902
　　　bronchiectasis J47.9
　　　　with
　　　　　exacerbation (acute) J47.1
　　　　　lower respiratory infection J47.0
　　　bronchitis (chronic) J44.89
　　　emphysema J43.9
　　chronic J44.9
　　　with
　　　　allergic alveolitis — see Pneumonitis, hypersensitivity
　　　　bronchiectasis J47.9
　　　　　with
　　　　　　exacerbation (acute) J47.1
　　　　　　lower respiratory infection J47.0
　　due to
　　　foreign body — see Foreign body, by site, causing asphyxia
　　　inhalation of fumes or vapors J68.9
　　　laryngospasm J38.5
　ampulla of Vater K83.1
　aortic (heart) (valve) — see Stenosis, aortic
　aortoiliac I74.09
　aqueduct of Sylvius G91.1
　　congenital Q03.0
　　　with spina bifida — see Spina bifida, by site, with hydrocephalus
　Arnold-Chiari — see Arnold-Chiari disease
　artery — see also Atherosclerosis, artery I70.9- ☑
　　basilar (complete) (partial) — see Occlusion, artery, basilar

Obstruction, obstructed, obstructive — continued
　artery — see also Atherosclerosis, artery — continued
　　carotid (complete) (partial) — see Occlusion, artery, carotid
　　cerebellar — see Occlusion, artery, cerebellar
　　cerebral (anterior) (middle) (posterior) — see Occlusion, artery, cerebral
　　precerebral — see Occlusion, artery, precerebral
　　renal N28.0
　　retinal NEC — see Occlusion, artery, retina
　　stent — see Restenosis, stent
　　vertebral (complete) (partial) — see Occlusion, artery, vertebral
　band (intestinal) — see also Obstruction, intestine, specified NEC K56.699
　bile duct or passage (common) (hepatic) (noncalculous) K83.1
　　with calculus K80.51
　　congenital (causing jaundice) Q44.3
　biliary (duct) (tract) K83.1
　　gallbladder K82.0
　bladder-neck (acquired) N32.0
　　congenital Q64.31
　　due to hyperplasia (hypertrophy) of prostate — see Hyperplasia, prostate
　bowel — see Obstruction, intestine
　bronchus J98.09
　canal, ear — see Stenosis, external ear canal
　cardia K22.2
　caval veins (inferior) (superior) I87.1
　cecum — see Obstruction, intestine
　circulatory I99.8
　colon — see Obstruction, intestine
　common duct (noncalculous) K83.1
　coronary (artery) — see Occlusion, coronary
　cystic duct — see also Obstruction, gallbladder
　　with calculus K80.21
　device, implant or graft — see also Complications, by site and type, mechanical T85.698- ☑
　　arterial graft NEC — see Complication, cardiovascular device, mechanical, vascular
　　catheter NEC T85.628- ☑
　　　cystostomy T83.090- ☑
　　　dialysis (renal) T82.49- ☑
　　　　intraperitoneal T85.691- ☑
　　　Hopkins T83.098- ☑
　　　ileostomy T83.098- ☑
　　　infusion NEC T82.594- ☑
　　　　spinal (epidural) (subdural) T85.690- ☑
　　　nephrostomy T83.092- ☑
　　　urethral indwelling T83.091- ☑
　　　urinary T83.098- ☑
　　　urostomy T83.098- ☑
　　due to infection T85.79- ☑
　　gastrointestinal — see Complications, prosthetic device, mechanical, gastrointestinal device
　　genital NEC T83.498- ☑
　　　intrauterine contraceptive device T83.39- ☑
　　　penile prosthesis (cylinder) (implanted) (pump) (reservoir) T83.490- ☑
　　　testicular prosthesis T83.491- ☑
　　heart NEC — see Complication, cardiovascular device, mechanical
　　joint prosthesis — see Complications, joint prosthesis, mechanical, specified NEC, by site
　　orthopedic NEC — see Complication, orthopedic, device, mechanical
　　specified NEC T85.628- ☑
　　urinary NEC — see also Complication, genitourinary, device, urinary, mechanical
　　　graft T83.29- ☑
　　vascular NEC — see Complication, cardiovascular device, mechanical
　　ventricular intracranial shunt T85.09- ☑
　due to foreign body accidentally left in operative wound T81.529- ☑
　duodenum K31.5
　ejaculatory duct N50.89
　esophagus K22.2
　eustachian tube (complete) (partial) H68.10- ☑
　　cartilagenous (extrinsic) H68.13- ☑
　　　intrinsic H68.12- ☑
　　osseous H68.11- ☑
　fallopian tube (bilateral) N97.1
　fecal K56.41
　　with hernia — see Hernia, by site, with obstruction
　foramen of Monro (congenital) Q03.8

Obstruction, obstructed, obstructive — continued
- foramen of Monro — continued
  - with spina bifida — see Spina bifida, by site, with hydrocephalus
- foreign body — see Foreign body
- gallbladder K82.0
  - with calculus, stones K80.21
  - congenital Q44.1
- gastric outlet K31.1
- gastrointestinal — see Obstruction, intestine
- hepatic K76.89
  - duct (noncalculous) K83.1
- ileum — see Obstruction, intestine
- iliofemoral (artery) I74.5
- intestine K56.609
  - with
    - adhesions (intestinal) (peritoneal) K56.50
      - complete K56.52
      - incomplete K56.51
      - partial K56.51
  - adynamic K56.0
  - by gallstone K56.3
  - complete K56.601
  - congenital (small) Q41.9
    - large Q42.9
      - specified part NEC Q42.8
  - incomplete K56.600
  - neurogenic K56.0
    - Hirschsprung's disease or megacolon Q43.1
  - newborn P76.9
    - due to
      - fecaliths P76.8
      - inspissated milk P76.2
      - meconium (plug) P76.0
        - in mucoviscidosis E84.11
    - specified NEC P76.8
  - partial K56.600
  - postoperative K91.30
    - complete K91.32
    - incomplete K91.31
    - partial K91.31
  - reflex K56.0
  - specified NEC K56.699
    - complete K56.691
    - incomplete K56.690
    - partial K56.690
  - volvulus K56.2
- intracardiac ball valve prosthesis T82.09- ☑
- jejunum — see Obstruction, intestine
- joint prosthesis — see Complications, joint prosthesis, mechanical, specified NEC, by site
- kidney (calices) — see also Hydronephrosis N28.89
- labor — see Delivery
- lacrimal (passages) (duct)
  - by
    - dacryolith — see Dacryolith
    - stenosis — see Stenosis, lacrimal
  - congenital Q10.5
  - neonatal H04.53- ☑
- lacrimonasal duct — see Obstruction, lacrimal
- lacteal, with steatorrhea K90.2
- laryngitis — see Laryngitis
- larynx NEC J38.6
  - congenital Q31.8
- lung J98.4
  - disease, chronic J44.9
- lymphatic I89.0
- meconium (plug)
  - newborn P76.0
    - due to fecaliths P76.0
  - in mucoviscidosis E84.11
- mitral — see Stenosis, mitral
- nasal J34.89
- nasolacrimal duct — see also Obstruction, lacrimal
  - congenital Q10.5
- nasopharynx J39.2
- nose J34.89
- organ or site, congenital NEC — see Atresia, by site
- pancreatic duct K86.89
- parotid duct or gland K11.8
- pelviureteral junction N13.5
  - with hydronephrosis N13.0
  - congenital Q62.39
- pharynx J39.2
- portal (circulation) (vein) I81
- prostate — see also Hyperplasia, prostate
  - valve (urinary) N32.0
- pulmonary valve (heart) I37.0
- pyelonephritis (chronic) N11.1

Obstruction, obstructed, obstructive — continued
- pylorus
  - adult K31.1
  - congenital or infantile Q40.0
- rectosigmoid — see Obstruction, intestine
- rectum K62.4
- renal — see also Hydronephrosis N28.89
  - outflow N13.8
  - pelvis, congenital Q62.39
- respiratory J98.8
  - chronic J44.9
- retinal (vessels) H34.9
- salivary duct (any) K11.8
  - with calculus K11.5
- sigmoid — see Obstruction, intestine
- sinus (accessory) (nasal) J34.89
- Stensen's duct K11.8
- stomach NEC K31.89
  - acute K31.0
  - congenital Q40.2
  - due to pylorospasm K31.3
- submandibular duct K11.8
- submaxillary gland K11.8
  - with calculus K11.5
- thoracic duct I89.0
- thrombotic — see Thrombosis
- trachea J39.8
- tracheostomy airway J95.03
- tricuspid (valve) — see Stenosis, tricuspid
- upper respiratory, congenital Q34.8
- ureter (functional) (pelvic junction) NEC N13.5
  - with
    - hydronephrosis N13.1
      - with infection N13.6
    - congenital Q62.39
    - pyelonephritis (chronic) N11.1
  - congenital Q62.39
  - due to calculus — see Calculus, ureter
- urethra NEC N36.8
  - congenital Q64.39
- urinary (moderate) N13.9
  - due to hyperplasia (hypertrophy) of prostate — see Hyperplasia, prostate
  - organ or tract (lower) N13.9
  - prostatic valve N32.0
  - specified NEC N13.8
- uropathy N13.9
- uterus N85.8
- vagina N89.5
- valvular — see Endocarditis
- vein, venous I87.1
  - caval (inferior) (superior) I87.1
  - thrombotic — see Thrombosis
- vena cava (inferior) (superior) I87.1
- vesical NEC N32.0
- vesicourethral orifice N32.0
  - congenital Q64.31
- vessel NEC I99.8
  - stent — see Restenosis, stent
- **Obturator** — see condition
- **Occlusal wear, teeth** K03.0
- **Occlusio pupillae** — see Membrane, pupillary
- **Occlusion, occluded**
  - anus K62.4
    - congenital Q42.3
      - with fistula Q42.2
  - aortoiliac (chronic) I74.09
  - aqueduct of Sylvius G91.1
    - congenital Q03.0
      - with spina bifida — see Spina bifida, by site, with hydrocephalus
  - artery — see also Atherosclerosis, artery I70.9- ☑
    - auditory, internal I65.8
    - basilar I65.1
      - with
        - infarction I63.22
          - due to
            - embolism I63.12
            - thrombosis I63.02
      - brain or cerebral I66.9
        - with infarction (due to) I63.5- ☑
          - embolism I63.4- ☑
          - thrombosis I63.3- ☑
      - carotid I65.2- ☑
        - with
          - infarction I63.23- ☑
            - due to
              - embolism I63.13- ☑

Occlusion, occluded — continued
- artery — see also Atherosclerosis, artery — continued
  - carotid — continued
    - with — continued
      - infarction — continued
        - due to — continued
          - thrombosis I63.03- ☑
  - cerebellar (anterior inferior) (posterior inferior) (superior) I66.3
    - with infarction I63.54- ☑
      - due to
        - embolism I63.44- ☑
        - thrombosis I63.34- ☑
  - cerebral I66.9
    - with infarction I63.50
      - due to
        - embolism I63.40
          - specified NEC I63.49
        - thrombosis I63.30
          - specified NEC I63.39
  - anterior I66.1- ☑
    - with infarction I63.52- ☑
      - due to
        - embolism I63.42- ☑
        - thrombosis I63.32- ☑
  - middle I66.0- ☑
    - with infarction I63.51- ☑
      - due to
        - embolism I63.41- ☑
        - thrombosis I63.31- ☑
  - posterior I66.2- ☑
    - with infarction I63.53- ☑
      - due to
        - embolism I63.43- ☑
        - thrombosis I63.33- ☑
  - specified NEC I66.8
    - with infarction I63.59
      - due to
        - embolism I63.4- ☑
        - thrombosis I63.3- ☑
  - choroidal (anterior) — see Occlusion, artery, precerebral, specified NEC
  - communicating posterior — see Occlusion, artery, precerebral, specified NEC
  - complete
    - coronary I25.82
    - extremities I70.92
  - coronary (acute) (thrombotic) (without myocardial infarction) I24.0
    - with myocardial infarction — see Infarction, myocardium
    - chronic total I25.82
    - complete I25.82
    - healed or old I25.2
    - total (chronic) I25.82
  - hypophyseal — see Occlusion, artery, precerebral, specified NEC
  - iliac I74.5
  - lower extremities due to stenosis or stricture I77.1
  - mesenteric (embolic) (thrombotic) — see also Infarct, intestine K55.069
  - perforating — see Occlusion, artery, cerebral, specified NEC
  - peripheral I77.9
    - thrombotic or embolic I74.4
  - pontine — see Occlusion, artery, precerebral, specified NEC
  - precerebral I65.9
    - with infarction I63.20
      - specified NEC I63.29
      - due to
        - embolism I63.10
          - specified NEC I63.19
        - thrombosis I63.00
          - specified NEC I63.09
    - basilar — see Occlusion, artery, basilar
    - carotid — see Occlusion, artery, carotid
    - puerperal O88.23
    - specified NEC I65.8
      - with infarction I63.29
        - due to
          - embolism I63.19
          - thrombosis I63.09
    - vertebral — see Occlusion, artery, vertebral
  - renal N28.0
  - retinal
    - branch H34.23- ☑
    - central H34.1- ☑

Occlusion, occluded — continued
   artery — see also Atherosclerosis, artery — continued
      retinal — continued
         partial H34.21- ☑
         transient H34.0- ☑
      spinal — see Occlusion, artery, precerebral, vertebral
      total (chronic)
         coronary I25.82
         extremities I70.92
      vertebral I65.0- ☑
         with
            infarction I63.21- ☑
               due to
                   embolism I63.11- ☑
                   thrombosis I63.01- ☑
   basilar artery — see Occlusion, artery, basilar
   bile duct (common) (hepatic) (noncalculous) K83.1
   bowel — see Obstruction, intestine
   carotid (artery) (common) (internal) — see Occlusion, artery, carotid
   centric (of teeth) M26.59
      maximum intercuspation discrepancy M26.55
   cerebellar (artery) — see Occlusion, artery, cerebellar
   cerebral (artery) — see Occlusion, artery, cerebral
   cerebrovascular — see also Occlusion, artery, cerebral
      with infarction I63.5- ☑
   cervical canal — see Stricture, cervix
   cervix (uteri) — see Stricture, cervix
   choanal Q30.0
   choroidal (artery) — see Occlusion, artery, precerebral, specified NEC
   colon — see Obstruction, intestine
   communicating posterior artery — see Occlusion, artery, precerebral, specified NEC
   coronary (artery) (vein) (thrombotic) — see also Infarct, myocardium
      chronic total I25.82
      healed or old I25.2
      not resulting in infarction I24.0
      total (chronic) I25.82
   cystic duct — see Obstruction, gallbladder
   embolic — see Embolism
   fallopian tube N97.1
      congenital Q50.6
   gallbladder — see also Obstruction, gallbladder
      congenital (causing jaundice) Q44.1
   gingiva, traumatic K06.2
   hymen N89.6
      congenital Q52.3
   hypophyseal (artery) — see Occlusion, artery, precerebral, specified NEC
   iliac artery I74.5
   intestine — see Obstruction, intestine
   lacrimal passages — see Obstruction, lacrimal
   lung J98.4
   lymph or lymphatic channel I89.0
   mammary duct N64.89
   mesenteric artery (embolic) (thrombotic) — see also Infarct, intestine K55.069
   nose J34.89
      congenital Q30.0
   organ or site, congenital NEC — see Atresia, by site
   oviduct N97.1
      congenital Q50.6
   peripheral arteries
      due to stricture or stenosis I77.1
      upper extremity I74.2
   pontine (artery) — see Occlusion, artery, precerebral, specified NEC
   posterior lingual, of mandibular teeth M26.29
   precerebral artery — see Occlusion, artery, precerebral
   punctum lacrimale — see Obstruction, lacrimal
   pupil — see Membrane, pupillary
   pylorus, adult — see also Stricture, pylorus K31.1
   renal artery N28.0
   retina, retinal
      artery — see Occlusion, artery, retinal
      vein (central) H34.81- ☑
         engorgement H34.82- ☑
         tributary H34.83- ☑
      vessels H34.9
   spinal artery — see Occlusion, artery, precerebral, vertebral
   teeth (mandibular) (posterior lingual) M26.29
   thoracic duct I89.0
   thrombotic — see Thrombosis, artery
   traumatic
      edentulous (alveolar) ridge K06.2

Occlusion, occluded — continued
   traumatic — continued
      gingiva K06.2
      periodontal K05.5
   tubal N97.1
   ureter (complete) (partial) N13.5
      congenital Q62.10
   ureteropelvic junction N13.5
      congenital Q62.11
   ureterovesical orifice N13.5
      congenital Q62.12
   urethra — see Stricture, urethra
   uterus N85.8
   vagina N89.5
   vascular NEC I99.8
   vein — see Thrombosis
      retinal — see Occlusion, retinal, vein
   vena cava (inferior) (superior) — see Embolism, vena cava
   ventricle (brain) NEC G91.1
   vertebral (artery) — see Occlusion, artery, vertebral
   vessel (blood) I99.8
   vulva N90.5
Occult
   blood in feces (stools) R19.5
Occupational
   problems NEC Z56.89
Ochlophobia — see Agoraphobia
Ochronosis (endogenous) E70.29
Ocular muscle — see condition
Oculogyric crisis or disturbance H51.8
   psychogenic F45.8
Oculomotor syndrome H51.9
Oculopathy
   syphilitic NEC A52.71
      congenital
         early A50.01
         late A50.30
      early (secondary) A51.43
      late A52.71
Oddi's sphincter spasm K83.4
Odontalgia K08.89
Odontoameloblastoma — see Cyst, calcifying odontogenic
Odontoclasia K03.89
Odontodysplasia, regional K00.4
Odontogenesis imperfecta K00.5
Odontoma (ameloblastic) (complex) (compound) (fibroameloblastic) — see Cyst, calcifying odontogenic
Odontomyelitis (closed) (open) K04.01
   irreversible K04.02
   reversible K04.01
Odontorrhagia K08.89
Odontosarcoma, ameloblastic C41.1
   upper jaw (bone) C41.0
Oestriasis — see Myiasis
Oguchi's disease H53.63
Ohara's disease — see Tularemia
OHS (obesity hypoventilation syndrome) E66.2
Oidiomycosis — see Candidiasis
Oidium albicans infection — see Candidiasis
Old age (without mention of debility) R54
   dementia F03.- ☑
Old (previous) **myocardial infarction** I25.2
Olfactory — see condition
Oligemia — see Anemia
Oligoastrocytoma
   specified site — see Neoplasm, malignant, by site
   unspecified site C71.9
Oligocythemia D64.9
Oligodendroblastoma
   specified site — see Neoplasm, malignant
   unspecified site C71.9
Oligodendroglioma
   anaplastic type
      specified site — see Neoplasm, malignant, by site
      unspecified site C71.9
   specified site — see Neoplasm, malignant, by site
   unspecified site C71.9
Oligodontia — see Anodontia
Oligoencephalon Q02
Oligohidrosis L74.4
Oligohydramnios O41.0- ☑
Oligohydrosis L74.4
Oligomenorrhea N91.5
   primary N91.3
   secondary N91.4
Oligophrenia — see also Disability, intellectual
   phenylpyruvic E70.0
Oligospermia N46.11

Oligospermia — continued
   due to
      drug therapy N46.121
      efferent duct obstruction N46.123
      infection N46.122
      radiation N46.124
      specified cause NEC N46.129
      systemic disease N46.125
Oligotrichia — see Alopecia
Oliguria R34
   with, complicating or following ectopic or molar pregnancy O08.4
   postprocedural N99.0
   puerperal O90.49
Ollier's disease Q78.4
Omentitis — see Peritonitis
Omentocele — see Hernia, abdomen, specified site NEC
Omentum, omental — see condition
Omphalitis (congenital) (newborn) P38.9
   with mild hemorrhage P38.1
   without hemorrhage P38.9
   not of newborn L08.82
   tetanus A33
Omphalocele Q79.2
Omphalomesenteric duct, persistent Q43.0
Omphalorrhagia, newborn P51.9
Omsk hemorrhagic fever A98.1
Onanism (excessive) F98.8
Onchocerciasis, onchocercosis B73.1
   with
      eye disease B73.00
         endophthalmitis B73.01
         eyelid B73.09
         glaucoma B73.02
         specified NEC B73.09
      eye NEC B73.00
      eyelid B73.09
Oncocytoma — see Neoplasm, benign, by site
Oncovirus, as cause of disease classified elsewhere B97.32
Ondine's curse — see Apnea, sleep
Oneirophrenia F23
Onychauxis L60.2
   congenital Q84.5
Onychia — see also Cellulitis, digit
   with lymphangitis — see Lymphangitis, acute, digit
   candidal B37.2
   dermatophytic B35.1
Onychitis — see also Cellulitis, digit
   with lymphangitis — see Lymphangitis, acute, digit
Onycho-osteodysplasia Q87.2
Onychocryptosis L60.0
Onychodystrophy L60.3
   congenital Q84.6
Onychogryphosis, onychogryposis L60.2
Onycholysis L60.1
Onychomadesis L60.8
Onychomalacia L60.3
Onychomycosis (finger) (toe) B35.1
Onychophagia F98.8
Onychophosis L60.8
Onychoptosis L60.8
Onychorrhexis L60.3
   congenital Q84.6
Onychoschizia L60.3
Onyxis (finger) (toe) L60.0
Onyxitis — see also Cellulitis, digit
   with lymphangitis — see Lymphangitis, acute, digit
Oophoritis (cystic) (infectional) (interstitial) N70.92
   with salpingitis N70.93
   acute N70.02
      with salpingitis N70.03
   chronic N70.12
      with salpingitis N70.13
   complicating abortion — see Abortion, by type, complicated by, oophoritis
Oophorocele N83.4- ☑
Opacity, opacities
   cornea H17.- ☑
      central H17.1- ☑
      congenital Q13.3
      degenerative — see Degeneration, cornea
      hereditary — see Dystrophy, cornea
      inflammatory — see Keratitis
      minor H17.81- ☑
      peripheral H17.82- ☑
      sequelae of trachoma (healed) B94.0
      specified NEC H17.89

Opacity, opacities — continued
- enamel (teeth) (fluoride) (nonfluoride) K00.3
- lens — see Cataract
- snowball — see Deposit, crystalline
- vitreous (humor) NEC H43.39- ☑
  - congenital Q14.0
  - membranes and strands H43.31- ☑

Opalescent dentin (hereditary) K00.5

Open, opening
- abnormal, organ or site, congenital — see Imperfect, closure
- angle with
  - borderline
    - findings
      - high risk H40.02- ☑
      - low risk H40.01- ☑
  - intraocular pressure H40.00- ☑
- cupping of discs H40.01- ☑
- glaucoma (primary) — see Glaucoma, open angle
- bite
  - anterior M26.220
  - posterior M26.221
- false — see Imperfect, closure
- margin on tooth restoration K08.51
- restoration margins of tooth K08.51
- wound — see Wound, open

Operational fatigue F48.8
Operative — see condition
Operculitis — see Periodontitis
Operculum — see Break, retina
Ophiasis L63.2
Ophthalmia — see also Conjunctivitis H10.9
- actinic rays — see Photokeratitis
- allergic (acute) — see Conjunctivitis, acute, atopic
- blennorrhagic (gonococcal) (neonatorum) A54.31
- diphtheritic A36.86
- Egyptian A71.1
- electrica — see Photokeratitis
- gonococcal (neonatorum) A54.31
- metastatic — see Endophthalmitis, purulent
- migraine — see Migraine, ophthalmoplegic
- neonatorum, newborn P39.1
  - gonococcal A54.31
- nodosa H16.24- ☑
- purulent — see Conjunctivitis, acute, mucopurulent
- spring — see Conjunctivitis, acute, atopic
- sympathetic — see Uveitis, sympathetic

Ophthalmitis — see Ophthalmia
Ophthalmocele (congenital) Q15.8
Ophthalmoneuromyelitis G36.0
Ophthalmopathy, Graves' H05.83- ☑
Ophthalmoplegia — see also Strabismus, paralytic
- anterior internuclear — see Ophthalmoplegia, internuclear
- ataxia-areflexia G61.0
- diabetic — see E08-E13 with .39
- exophthalmic E05.00
  - with thyroid storm E05.01
- external H49.88- ☑
  - progressive H49.4- ☑
    - with pigmentary retinopathy — see Kearns-Sayre syndrome
  - total H49.3- ☑
- internal (complete) (total) H52.51- ☑
- internuclear H51.2- ☑
- migraine — see Migraine, ophthalmoplegic
- Parinaud's H49.88- ☑
- progressive external — see Ophthalmoplegia, external, progressive
- supranuclear, progressive G23.1
- total (external) — see Ophthalmoplegia, external, total

Opioid(s)
- abuse — see Abuse, drug, opioids
- dependence — see Dependence, drug, opioids
- induced, without use disorder
  - anxiety disorder F11.988
  - delirium F11.921
  - depressive disorder F11.94
  - sexual dysfunction F11.981
  - sleep disorder F11.982

Opisthognathism M26.09
Opisthorchiasis (felineus) (viverrini) B66.0
Opitz' disease D73.2
Opiumism — see Dependence, drug, opioid
Oppenheim-Urbach disease (necrobiosis lipoidica diabeticorum) — see E08-E13 with .620
Oppenheim's disease G70.2
Opportunistic salpingectomy Z40.82

Optic nerve — see condition
Orbit — see condition
Orbitopathy (Graves') (thyroid) H05.83- ☑
Orchioblastoma C62.9- ☑
Orchitis (gangrenous) (nonspecific) (septic) (suppurative) N45.2
- blennorrhagic (gonococcal) (acute) (chronic) A54.23
- chlamydial A56.19
- filarial — see also Infestation, filarial B74.9 [N51]
- gonococcal (acute) (chronic) A54.23
- mumps B26.0
- syphilitic A52.76
- tuberculous A18.15

Orf (virus disease) B08.02
Organic — see also condition
- brain syndrome F09
- heart — see Disease, heart
- mental disorder F09
- psychosis F09

Orgasm
- anejaculatory N53.13

Oriental
- bilharziasis B65.2
- schistosomiasis B65.2

Orifice — see condition
Origin of both great vessels from right ventricle Q20.1
Ormond's disease (with ureteral obstruction) N13.5
- with infection N13.6

Ornithine metabolism disorder E72.4
Ornithinemia (Type I) (Type II) E72.4
Ornithosis A70
Orotaciduria, oroticaciduria (congenital) (hereditary) (pyrimidine deficiency) E79.89
- anemia D53.0

Orthodontics
- adjustment Z46.4
- fitting Z46.4

Orthopnea R06.01
Orthopoxvirus B08.09
Os, uterus — see condition
Osgood-Schlatter disease or osteochondrosis M92.52- ☑
Osler (-Weber)-**Rendu disease** I78.0
Osler's nodes I33.0
Osmidrosis L75.0
Osseous — see condition
Ossification
- artery — see Arteriosclerosis
- auricle (ear) — see Disorder, pinna, specified type NEC
- bronchial J98.09
- cardiac — see Degeneration, myocardial
- cartilage (senile) — see Disorder, cartilage, specified type NEC
- coronary (artery) — see Disease, heart, ischemic, atherosclerotic
- diaphragm J98.6
- ear, middle — see Otosclerosis
- falx cerebri G96.198
- fontanel, premature Q75.009
- heart — see also Degeneration, myocardial
  - valve — see Endocarditis
- larynx J38.7
- ligament — see Disorder, tendon, specified type NEC
  - posterior longitudinal — see Spondylopathy, specified NEC
- meninges (cerebral) (spinal) G96.198
- multiple, eccentric centers — see Disorder, bone, development or growth
- muscle — see also Calcification, muscle
  - due to burns — see Myositis, ossificans, in, burns
  - paralytic — see Myositis, ossificans, in, quadriplegia
  - progressive — see Myositis, ossificans, progressiva
  - specified NEC M61.50
    - ankle M61.57- ☑
    - foot M61.57- ☑
    - forearm M61.53- ☑
    - hand M61.54- ☑
    - lower leg M61.56- ☑
    - multiple sites M61.59
    - pelvic region M61.55- ☑
    - shoulder region M61.51- ☑
    - specified site NEC M61.58
    - thigh M61.55- ☑
    - upper arm M61.52- ☑
  - traumatic — see Myositis, ossificans, traumatica
- myocardium, myocardial — see Degeneration, myocardial
- penis N48.89
- periarticular — see Disorder, joint, specified type NEC

Ossification — continued
- pinna — see Disorder, pinna, specified type NEC
- rider's bone — see Ossification, muscle, specified NEC
- sclera H15.89
- subperiosteal, post-traumatic M89.8X- ☑
- tendon — see Disorder, tendon, specified type NEC
- trachea J39.8
- tympanic membrane — see Disorder, tympanic membrane, specified NEC
- vitreous (humor) — see Deposit, crystalline

Osteitis — see also Osteomyelitis
- alveolar M27.3
- condensans M85.30
  - ankle M85.37- ☑
  - foot M85.37- ☑
  - forearm M85.33- ☑
  - hand M85.34- ☑
  - lower leg M85.36- ☑
  - multiple site M85.39
  - neck M85.38
  - rib M85.38
  - shoulder M85.31- ☑
  - skull M85.38
  - specified site NEC M85.38
  - thigh M85.35- ☑
  - toe M85.37- ☑
  - upper arm M85.32- ☑
  - vertebra M85.38
- deformans — see also Paget's disease, bone M88.9
  - in (due to)
    - malignant neoplasm of bone — see also Neoplasm, malignant, by site C41.9 [M90.60]
    - neoplastic disease — see also Neoplasm, by type and site D49.9 [M90.60]
      - carpus D49.2 [M90.64-] ☑
      - clavicle D49.2 [M90.61-] ☑
      - femur D49.2 [M90.65-] ☑
      - fibula D49.2 [M90.66-] ☑
      - finger D49.2 [M90.64-] ☑
      - humerus D49.2 [M90.62-] ☑
      - ilium D49.2 [M90.68]
      - ischium D49.2 [M90.68]
      - metacarpus D49.2 [M90.64-] ☑
      - metatarsus D49.2 [M90.67-] ☑
      - multiple sites D49.89 [M90.69]
      - neck D49.2 [M90.68]
      - pubic ramus [pubis] D49.2 [M90.68]
      - radius D49.2 [M90.63-] ☑
      - rib D49.2 [M90.68]
      - scapula D49.2 [M90.61-] ☑
      - skull D49.2 [M90.68]
      - tarsus D49.2 [M90.67-] ☑
      - tibia D49.2 [M90.66-] ☑
      - toe D49.2 [M90.67-] ☑
      - ulna D49.2 [M90.63-] ☑
      - vertebra D49.2 [M90.68]
  - skull M88.0
  - specified NEC — see Paget's disease, bone, by site
  - vertebra M88.1
- due to yaws A66.6
- fibrosa NEC — see Cyst, bone, by site
  - circumscripta — see Dysplasia, fibrous, bone NEC
  - cystica (generalisata) E21.0
  - disseminata Q78.1
  - osteoplastica E21.0
- fragilitans Q78.0
- Garr's (sclerosing) — see Osteomyelitis, specified type NEC
- jaw (acute) (chronic) (lower) (suppurative) (upper) M27.2
- parathyroid E21.0
- petrous bone (acute) (chronic) — see Petrositis
- sclerotic, nonsuppurative — see Osteomyelitis, specified type NEC
- tuberculosa A18.09
  - cystica D86.89
  - multiplex cystoides D86.89

Osteo-onycho-arthro-dysplasia Q87.2
Osteo-onychodysplasia, hereditary Q87.2
Osteoarthritis M19.90
- ankle M19.07- ☑
  - post-traumatic M19.17- ☑
  - primary M19.07- ☑
  - secondary M19.27- ☑
- elbow M19.02- ☑
  - post-traumatic M19.12- ☑
  - primary M19.02- ☑
  - secondary M19.22- ☑

Osteoarthritis — continued
  foot joint M19.07- ☑
    post-traumatic M19.17- ☑
    primary M19.07- ☑
    secondary M19.27- ☑
  generalized (multiple joints) M15.9
    erosive M15.4
    primary M15.0
    specified NEC M15.8
  hand joint M19.04- ☑
    first carpometacarpal joint M18.9
      post-traumatic — see Osteoarthritis, post-traumatic NEC, hand joint, first carpometacarpal joint
      primary — see Osteoarthritis, primary, hand joint, first carpometacarpal joint
      secondary — see Osteoarthritis, secondary, hand joint, first carpometacarpal joint
    post-traumatic M19.14- ☑
    primary M19.04- ☑
    secondary M19.24- ☑
  hip M16.9
    bilateral M16.0
      due to hip dysplasia M16.2
      post-traumatic M16.4
      secondary M16.6
    due to hip dysplasia (unilateral) M16.3- ☑
      bilateral M16.2
    post-traumatic — see Osteoarthritis, post-traumatic, hip
    primary M16.1- ☑
    secondary — see Osteoarthritis, secondary, hip
    unilateral M16.1- ☑
      due to hip dysplasia M16.3- ☑
      post-traumatic M16.5- ☑
      primary M16.1- ☑
      secondary NEC M16.7
  interphalangeal
    distal (Heberden) M15.1
    proximal (Bouchard) M15.2
  knee M17.9
    bilateral M17.0
      post-traumatic M17.2
      secondary M17.4
    post-traumatic — see Osteoarthritis, post-traumatic, knee
    primary M17.1- ☑
      bilateral M17.0
    secondary — see Osteoarthritis, secondary, knee
    unilateral M17.1- ☑
      post-traumatic M17.3- ☑
      primary M17.1- ☑
      secondary NEC M17.5
  post-traumatic NEC M19.92
    ankle M19.17- ☑
    elbow M19.12- ☑
    foot joint M19.17- ☑
    hand joint M19.14- ☑
      first carpometacarpal joint M18.3- ☑
        bilateral M18.2
    hip M16.5- ☑
      bilateral M16.4
    knee M17.3- ☑
      bilateral M17.2
    shoulder M19.11- ☑
    specified site NEC M19.19
    wrist M19.13- ☑
  primary M19.91
    ankle M19.07- ☑
    elbow M19.02- ☑
    foot joint M19.07- ☑
    hand joint M19.04- ☑
      first carpometacarpal joint M18.1- ☑
        bilateral M18.0
    hip M16.1- ☑
      bilateral M16.0
    knee M17.1- ☑
      bilateral M17.0
    multiple sites M15.9
    shoulder M19.01- ☑
    specified site NEC M19.09
    spine — see Spondylosis
    wrist M19.03- ☑
  secondary M19.93
    ankle M19.27- ☑
    elbow M19.22- ☑
    foot joint M19.27- ☑

Osteoarthritis — continued
  secondary — continued
    hand joint M19.24- ☑
      first carpometacarpal joint M18.5- ☑
        bilateral M18.4
    hip M16.7
      bilateral M16.6
    knee M17.5
      bilateral M17.4
    multiple M15.3
    shoulder M19.21- ☑
    specified site NEC M19.29
    spine — see Spondylosis
    wrist M19.23- ☑
  shoulder M19.01- ☑
    post-traumatic M19.11- ☑
    primary M19.01- ☑
    secondary M19.21- ☑
  specified site NEC M19.09
  spine — see Spondylosis
  wrist M19.03- ☑
    first carpometacarpal joint — see Osteoarthritis, hand joint, first carpometacarpal joint
    post-traumatic M19.13- ☑
    primary M19.03- ☑
    secondary M19.23- ☑
Osteoarthropathy (hypertrophic) M19.90
  ankle — see Osteoarthritis, primary, ankle
  elbow — see Osteoarthritis, primary, elbow
  foot joint — see Osteoarthritis, primary, foot
  hand joint — see Osteoarthritis, primary, hand joint
  knee joint — see Osteoarthritis, primary, knee
  multiple site — see Osteoarthritis, primary, multiple joint
  pulmonary — see also Osteoarthropathy, specified type NEC
    hypertrophic — see Osteoarthropathy, hypertrophic, specified type NEC
  secondary — see Osteoarthropathy, specified type NEC
  secondary hypertrophic — see Osteoarthropathy, specified type NEC
  shoulder — see Osteoarthritis, primary, shoulder
  specified joint NEC — see Osteoarthritis, primary, specified joint NEC
  specified type NEC M89.40
    carpus M89.44- ☑
    clavicle M89.41- ☑
    femur M89.45- ☑
    fibula M89.46- ☑
    finger M89.44- ☑
    humerus M89.42- ☑
    ilium M89.48
    ischium M89.48
    metacarpus M89.44- ☑
    metatarsus M89.47- ☑
    multiple sites M89.49
    neck M89.48
    pubic ramus [pubis] M89.48
    radius M89.43- ☑
    rib M89.48
    scapula M89.41- ☑
    skull M89.48
    tarsus M89.47- ☑
    tibia M89.46- ☑
    toe M89.47- ☑
    ulna M89.43- ☑
    vertebra M89.48
  spine — see Spondylosis
  wrist — see Osteoarthritis, primary, wrist
Osteoarthrosis (degenerative) (hypertrophic) (joint) — see also Osteoarthritis
  deformans alkaptonurica E70.29 [M36.8]
  erosive M15.4
  generalized M15.9
    primary M15.0
  polyarticular M15.9
  spine — see Spondylosis
Osteoblastoma — see Neoplasm, bone, benign
  aggressive — see Neoplasm, bone, uncertain behavior
Osteochondritis — see also Osteochondropathy, by site
  Brailsford's — see Osteochondrosis, juvenile, radius
  dissecans M93.20
    ankle M93.27- ☑
    elbow M93.22- ☑
    foot M93.27- ☑
    hand M93.24- ☑
    hip M93.25- ☑
    knee M93.26- ☑

Osteochondritis — continued
  dissecans — continued
    multiple sites M93.29
    shoulder joint M93.21- ☑
    specified site NEC M93.28
    wrist M93.23- ☑
  juvenile M92.9
    patellar — see Osteochondrosis, juvenile, patella
  syphilitic (congenital) (early) A50.02 [M90.80]
    ankle A50.02 [M90.87-] ☑
    elbow A50.02 [M90.82-] ☑
    foot A50.02 [M90.87-] ☑
    forearm A50.02 [M90.83-] ☑
    hand A50.02 [M90.84-] ☑
    hip A50.02 [M90.85-] ☑
    knee A50.02 [M90.86-] ☑
    multiple sites A50.02 [M90.89]
    shoulder joint A50.02 [M90.81-] ☑
    specified site NEC A50.02 [M90.88]
Osteochondroarthrosis deformans endemica — see Disease, Kaschin-Beck
Osteochondrodysplasia Q78.9
  with defects of growth of tubular bones and spine Q77.9
    specified NEC Q77.8
  specified NEC Q78.8
Osteochondrodystrophy E78.9
Osteochondrolysis — see Osteochondritis, dissecans
Osteochondroma — see Neoplasm, bone, benign
Osteochondromatosis D16.9
  syndrome Q78.4
Osteochondromyxosarcoma — see Neoplasm, bone, malignant
Osteochondropathy M93.90
  ankle M93.97- ☑
  elbow M93.92- ☑
  foot M93.97- ☑
  hand M93.94- ☑
  hip M93.95- ☑
  Kienbock's disease of adults M93.1
  knee M93.96- ☑
  multiple joints M93.99
  osteochondritis dissecans — see Osteochondritis, dissecans
  osteochondrosis — see Osteochondrosis
  shoulder region M93.91- ☑
  slipped upper femoral epiphysis — see Slipped, epiphysis, upper femoral
  specified joint NEC M93.98
  specified type NEC M93.80
    ankle M93.87- ☑
    elbow M93.82- ☑
    foot M93.87- ☑
    hand M93.84- ☑
    hip M93.85- ☑
    knee M93.86- ☑
    multiple joints M93.89
    shoulder region M93.81- ☑
    specified joint NEC M93.88
    wrist M93.83- ☑
  syphilitic, congenital
    early A50.02 [M90.80]
    late A50.56 [M90.80]
  wrist M93.93- ☑
Osteochondrosarcoma — see Neoplasm, bone, malignant
Osteochondrosis — see also Osteochondropathy, by site
  acetabulum (juvenile) M91.0
  adult — see Osteochondropathy, specified type NEC, by site
  astragalus (juvenile) — see Osteochondrosis, juvenile, tarsus
  Blount M92.51- ☑
  Buchanan's M91.0
  Burns' — see Osteochondrosis, juvenile, ulna
  calcaneus (juvenile) — see Osteochondrosis, juvenile, tarsus
  capitular epiphysis (femur) (juvenile) — see Legg-Calve-Perthes disease
  carpal (juvenile) (lunate) (scaphoid) — see Osteochondrosis, juvenile, hand, carpal lunate
    adult M93.1
  coxae juvenilis — see Legg-Calve-Perthes disease
  deformans juvenilis, coxae — see Legg-Calve-Perthes disease
  Diaz's — see Osteochondrosis, juvenile, tarsus
  dissecans (knee) (shoulder) — see Osteochondritis, dissecans

☑ Additional Character Required — Refer to the Tabular List for Character Selection

Osteochondrosis — *continued*
- femoral capital epiphysis (juvenile) — *see* Legg-Calve-Perthes disease
- femur (head), juvenile — *see* Legg-Calve-Perthes disease
- fibula (juvenile) — *see* Osteochondrosis, juvenile, fibula
- foot NEC (juvenile) M92.8
- Freiberg's — *see* Osteochondrosis, juvenile, metatarsus
- Haas' (juvenile) — *see* Osteochondrosis, juvenile, humerus
- Haglund's — *see* Osteochondrosis, juvenile, tarsus
- hip (juvenile) — *see* Legg-Calve-Perthes disease
- humerus (capitulum) (head) (juvenile) — *see* Osteochondrosis, juvenile, humerus
- ilium, iliac crest (juvenile) M91.0
- ischiopubic synchondrosis M91.0
- Iselin's — *see* Osteochondrosis, juvenile, metatarsus
- juvenile, juvenilis M92.9
  - after congenital dislocation of hip reduction — *see* Osteochondrosis, juvenile, hip, specified NEC
  - arm — *see* Osteochondrosis, juvenile, upper limb NEC
  - capitular epiphysis (femur) — *see* Legg-Calve-Perthes disease
  - clavicle, sternal epiphysis — *see* Osteochondrosis, juvenile, upper limb NEC
  - coxae — *see* Legg-Calve-Perthes disease
  - deformans M92.9
  - fibula M92.50- ☑
  - foot NEC M92.8
  - hand M92.20- ☑
    - carpal lunate M92.21- ☑
    - metacarpal head M92.22- ☑
    - specified site NEC M92.29- ☑
  - head of femur — *see* Legg-Calve-Perthes disease
  - hip and pelvis M91.9- ☑
    - coxa plana — *see* Coxa, plana
    - femoral head — *see* Legg-Calve-Perthes disease
    - pelvis M91.0
    - pseudocoxalgia — *see* Pseudocoxalgia
    - specified NEC M91.8- ☑
  - humerus M92.0- ☑
  - limb
    - lower NEC M92.8
    - upper NEC — *see* Osteochondrosis, juvenile, upper limb NEC
  - medial cuneiform bone — *see* Osteochondrosis, juvenile, tarsus
  - metatarsus M92.7- ☑
  - patella M92.4- ☑
  - radius M92.1- ☑
  - specified
    - site NEC M92.8
    - type NEC M92.8
      - tibia and fibula M92.59- ☑
  - spine M42.00
    - cervical region M42.02
    - cervicothoracic region M42.03
    - lumbar region M42.06
    - lumbosacral region M42.07
    - multiple sites M42.09
    - occipito-atlanto-axial region M42.01
    - sacrococcygeal region M42.08
    - thoracic region M42.04
    - thoracolumbar region M42.05
  - tarsus M92.6- ☑
  - tibia M92.50- ☑
    - proximal M92.51- ☑
    - tubercle M92.52- ☑
  - ulna M92.1- ☑
  - upper limb NEC M92.3- ☑
  - vertebra (body) (epiphyseal plates) (Calve's) (Scheuermann's) — *see* Osteochondrosis, juvenile, spine
- Kienbock's — *see* Osteochondrosis, juvenile, hand, carpal lunate
  - adult M93.1
- Kohler's
  - patellar — *see* Osteochondrosis, juvenile, patella
  - tarsal navicular — *see* Osteochondrosis, juvenile, tarsus
- Legg-Perthes (-Calve) (-Waldenstrom) — *see* Legg-Calve-Perthes disease
- limb
  - lower NEC (juvenile) M92.8
    - tibia and fibula M92.59- ☑
  - upper NEC (juvenile) — *see* Osteochondrosis, juvenile, upper limb NEC
- lunate bone (carpal) (juvenile) — *see also* Osteochondrosis, juvenile, hand, carpal lunate

Osteochondrosis — *continued*
- lunate bone — *see also* Osteochondrosis, juvenile, hand, carpal lunate — *continued*
  - adult M93.1
- Mauclaire's — *see* Osteochondrosis, juvenile, hand, metacarpal
- metacarpal (head) (juvenile) — *see* Osteochondrosis, juvenile, hand, metacarpal
- metatarsus (fifth) (head) (juvenile) (second) — *see* Osteochondrosis, juvenile, metatarsus
- navicular (juvenile) — *see* Osteochondrosis, juvenile, tarsus
- os
  - calcis (juvenile) — *see* Osteochondrosis, juvenile, tarsus
  - tibiale externum (juvenile) — *see* Osteochondrosis, juvenile, tarsus
- Osgood-Schlatter M92.52- ☑
- Panner's — *see* Osteochondrosis, juvenile, humerus
- patellar center (juvenile) (primary) (secondary) — *see* Osteochondrosis, juvenile, patella
- pelvis (juvenile) M91.0
- Pierson's M91.0
- radius (head) (juvenile) — *see* Osteochondrosis, juvenile, radius
- Scheuermann's — *see* Osteochondrosis, juvenile, spine
- Sever's — *see* Osteochondrosis, juvenile, tarsus
- Sinding-Larsen — *see* Osteochondrosis, juvenile, patella
- spine M42.9
  - adult M42.10
    - cervical region M42.12
    - cervicothoracic region M42.13
    - lumbar region M42.16
    - lumbosacral region M42.17
    - multiple sites M42.19
    - occipito-atlanto-axial region M42.11
    - sacrococcygeal region M42.18
    - thoracic region M42.14
    - thoracolumbar region M42.15
  - juvenile — *see* Osteochondrosis, juvenile, spine
- symphysis pubis (juvenile) M91.0
- syphilitic (congenital) A50.02
- talus (juvenile) — *see* Osteochondrosis, juvenile, tarsus
- tarsus (navicular) (juvenile) — *see* Osteochondrosis, juvenile, tarsus
- tibia (proximal) (tubercle) (juvenile) — *see* Osteochondrosis, juvenile, tibia
- tuberculous — *see* Tuberculosis, bone
- ulna (lower) (juvenile) — *see* Osteochondrosis, juvenile, ulna
- van Neck's M91.0
- vertebral — *see* Osteochondrosis, spine

Osteoclastoma D48.0
- malignant — *see* Neoplasm, bone, malignant

Osteodynia — *see* Disorder, bone, specified type NEC

Osteodystrophy Q78.9
- azotemic N25.0
- congenital Q78.9
- parathyroid, secondary E21.1
- renal N25.0

Osteofibroma — *see* Neoplasm, bone, benign
Osteofibrosarcoma — *see* Neoplasm, bone, malignant
Osteogenesis imperfecta Q78.0
Osteogenic — *see* condition
Osteolysis M89.50
- carpus M89.54- ☑
- clavicle M89.51- ☑
- femur M89.55- ☑
- fibula M89.56- ☑
- finger M89.54- ☑
- humerus M89.52- ☑
- ilium M89.58
- ischium M89.58
- joint prosthesis (periprosthetic) — *see* Complications, joint prosthesis, mechanical, periprosthetic, osteolysis, by site
- metacarpus M89.54- ☑
- metatarsus M89.57- ☑
- multiple sites M89.59
- neck M89.58
- periprosthetic — *see* Complications, joint prosthesis, mechanical, periprosthetic, osteolysis, by site
- pubic ramus [pubis] M89.58
- radius M89.53- ☑
- rib M89.58
- scapula M89.51- ☑
- skull M89.58
- tarsus M89.57- ☑

Osteolysis — *continued*
- tibia M89.56- ☑
- toe M89.57- ☑
- ulna M89.53- ☑
- vertebra M89.58

Osteoma — *see also* Neoplasm, bone, benign
- osteoid — *see also* Neoplasm, bone, benign
  - giant — *see* Neoplasm, bone, benign

Osteomalacia M83.9
- adult M83.9
  - drug-induced NEC M83.5
  - due to
    - malabsorption (postsurgical) M83.2
    - malnutrition M83.3
  - specified NEC M83.8
- aluminium-induced M83.4
- infantile — *see* Rickets
- juvenile — *see* Rickets
- oncogenic E83.89
- pelvis M83.8
- puerperal M83.0
- senile M83.1
- vitamin-D-resistant in adults E83.31 [M90.8-] ☑
  - carpus E83.31 [M90.84-] ☑
  - clavicle E83.31 [M90.81-] ☑
  - femur E83.31 [M90.85-] ☑
  - fibula E83.31 [M90.86-] ☑
  - finger E83.31 [M90.84-] ☑
  - humerus E83.31 [M90.82-] ☑
  - ilium E83.31 [M90.88]
  - ischium E83.31 [M90.88]
  - metacarpus E83.31 [M90.84-] ☑
  - metatarsus E83.31 [M90.87-] ☑
  - multiple sites E83.31 [M90.89]
  - neck E83.31 [M90.88]
  - pubic ramus [pubis] E83.31 [M90.88]
  - radius E83.31 [M90.83-] ☑
  - rib E83.31 [M90.88]
  - scapula E83.31 [M90.819]
  - skull E83.31 [M90.88]
  - tarsus E83.31 [M90.87-] ☑
  - tibia E83.31 [M90.869]
  - toe E83.31 [M90.879]
  - ulna E83.31 [M90.839]
  - vertebra E83.31 [M90.88]

Osteomyelitis (general) (infective) (localized) (neonatal) (purulent) (septic) (staphylococcal) (streptococcal) (suppurative) (with periostitis) M86.9
- acute M86.10
  - carpus M86.14- ☑
  - clavicle M86.11- ☑
  - femur M86.15- ☑
  - fibula M86.16- ☑
  - finger M86.14- ☑
  - hematogenous M86.00
    - carpus M86.04- ☑
    - clavicle M86.01- ☑
    - femur M86.05- ☑
    - fibula M86.06- ☑
    - finger M86.04- ☑
    - humerus M86.02- ☑
    - ilium M86.08
    - ischium M86.08
    - mandible M27.2
    - metacarpus M86.04- ☑
    - metatarsus M86.07- ☑
    - multiple sites M86.09
    - neck M86.08
    - orbit H05.02- ☑
    - petrous bone — *see* Petrositis
    - radius M86.03- ☑
    - rib M86.08
    - scapula M86.01- ☑
    - skull M86.08
    - tarsus M86.07- ☑
    - tibia M86.06- ☑
    - toe M86.07- ☑
    - ulna M86.03- ☑
    - vertebra — *see* Osteomyelitis, vertebra
  - humerus M86.12- ☑
  - ilium M86.18
  - ischium M86.18
  - mandible M27.2
  - metacarpus M86.14- ☑
  - metatarsus M86.17- ☑
  - multiple sites M86.19
  - neck M86.18

Osteomyelitis — continued
- acute — continued
  - orbit H05.02- ☑
  - petrous bone — see Petrositis
  - radius M86.13- ☑
  - rib M86.18
  - scapula M86.11- ☑
  - skull M86.18
  - tarsus M86.17- ☑
  - tibia M86.16- ☑
  - toe M86.17- ☑
  - ulna M86.13- ☑
  - vertebra — see Osteomyelitis, vertebra
- chronic (or old) M86.60
  - with draining sinus M86.40
    - carpus M86.44- ☑
    - clavicle M86.41- ☑
    - femur M86.45- ☑
    - fibula M86.46- ☑
    - finger M86.44- ☑
    - humerus M86.42- ☑
    - ilium M86.48
    - ischium M86.48
    - mandible M27.2
    - metacarpus M86.44- ☑
    - metatarsus M86.47- ☑
    - multiple sites M86.49
    - neck M86.48
    - orbit H05.02- ☑
    - petrous bone — see Petrositis
    - pubic ramus [pubis] M86.48
    - radius M86.43- ☑
    - rib M86.48
    - scapula M86.41- ☑
    - skull M86.48
    - tarsus M86.47- ☑
    - tibia M86.46- ☑
    - toe M86.47- ☑
    - ulna M86.43- ☑
    - vertebra — see Osteomyelitis, vertebra
  - carpus M86.64- ☑
  - clavicle M86.61- ☑
  - femur M86.65- ☑
  - fibula M86.66- ☑
  - finger M86.64- ☑
  - hematogenous NEC M86.50
    - carpus M86.54- ☑
    - clavicle M86.51- ☑
    - femur M86.55- ☑
    - fibula M86.56- ☑
    - finger M86.54- ☑
    - humerus M86.52- ☑
    - ilium M86.58
    - ischium M86.58
    - mandible M27.2
    - metacarpus M86.54- ☑
    - metatarsus M86.57- ☑
    - multifocal M86.30
      - carpus M86.34- ☑
      - clavicle M86.31- ☑
      - femur M86.35- ☑
      - fibula M86.36- ☑
      - finger M86.34- ☑
      - humerus M86.32- ☑
      - ilium M86.38
      - ischium M86.38
      - metacarpus M86.34- ☑
      - metatarsus M86.37- ☑
      - multiple sites M86.39
      - neck M86.38
      - pubic ramus [pubis] M86.38
      - radius M86.33- ☑
      - rib M86.38
      - scapula M86.31- ☑
      - skull M86.38
      - tarsus M86.37- ☑
      - tibia M86.36- ☑
      - toe M86.37- ☑
      - ulna M86.33- ☑
      - vertebra — see Osteomyelitis, vertebra
    - multiple sites M86.59
    - neck M86.58
    - orbit H05.02- ☑
    - petrous bone — see Petrositis
    - pubic ramus [pubis] M86.58
    - radius M86.53- ☑

Osteomyelitis — continued
- chronic — continued
  - hematogenous — continued
    - rib M86.58
    - scapula M86.51- ☑
    - skull M86.58
    - tarsus M86.57- ☑
    - tibia M86.56- ☑
    - toe M86.57- ☑
    - ulna M86.53- ☑
    - vertebra — see Osteomyelitis, vertebra
  - humerus M86.62- ☑
  - ilium M86.659
  - ischium M86.659
  - mandible M27.2
  - metacarpus M86.64- ☑
  - metatarsus M86.67- ☑
  - multifocal — see Osteomyelitis, chronic, hematogenous, multifocal
  - multiple sites M86.69
  - neck M86.68
  - orbit H05.02- ☑
  - petrous bone — see Petrositis
  - radius M86.63- ☑
  - rib M86.68
  - scapula M86.61- ☑
  - skull M86.68
  - tarsus M86.67- ☑
  - tibia M86.66- ☑
  - toe M86.67- ☑
  - ulna M86.63- ☑
  - vertebra — see Osteomyelitis, vertebra
- echinococcal B67.2
- Garré's — see Osteomyelitis, specified type NEC
- in diabetes mellitus — see E08-E13 with .69
- jaw (acute) (chronic) (lower) (neonatal) (suppurative) (upper) M27.2
- nonsuppurating — see Osteomyelitis, specified type NEC
- orbit H05.02- ☑
- petrous bone — see Petrositis
- Salmonella (arizonae) (cholerae-suis) (enteritidis) (typhimurium) A02.24
- sclerosing, nonsuppurative — see Osteomyelitis, specified type NEC
- specified type NEC — see also subcategory M86.8X- ☑
  - mandible M27.2
  - orbit H05.02- ☑
  - petrous bone — see Petrositis
  - vertebra — see Osteomyelitis, vertebra
- subacute M86.20
  - carpus M86.24- ☑
  - clavicle M86.21- ☑
  - femur M86.25- ☑
  - fibula M86.26- ☑
  - finger M86.24- ☑
  - humerus M86.22- ☑
  - mandible M27.2
  - metacarpus M86.24- ☑
  - metatarsus M86.27- ☑
  - multiple sites M86.29
  - neck M86.28
  - orbit H05.02- ☑
  - petrous bone — see Petrositis
  - radius M86.23- ☑
  - rib M86.28
  - scapula M86.21- ☑
  - skull M86.28
  - tarsus M86.27- ☑
  - tibia M86.26- ☑
  - toe M86.27- ☑
  - ulna M86.23- ☑
  - vertebra — see Osteomyelitis, vertebra
- syphilitic A52.77
  - congenital (early) A50.02 [M90.80]
- tuberculous — see Tuberculosis, bone
- typhoid A01.05
- vertebra M46.20
  - cervical region M46.22
  - cervicothoracic region M46.23
  - lumbar region M46.26
  - lumbosacral region M46.27
  - occipito-atlanto-axial region M46.21
  - sacrococcygeal region M46.28
  - thoracic region M46.24
  - thoracolumbar region M46.25

Osteomyelofibrosis D47.4
Osteomyelosclerosis D75.89

Osteonecrosis M87.9
- due to
  - drugs — see Osteonecrosis, secondary, due to, drugs
  - trauma — see Osteonecrosis, secondary, due to, trauma
- idiopathic aseptic M87.00
  - ankle M87.07- ☑
  - carpus M87.03- ☑
  - clavicle M87.01- ☑
  - femur M87.05- ☑
  - fibula M87.06- ☑
  - finger M87.04- ☑
  - humerus M87.02- ☑
  - ilium M87.050
  - ischium M87.050
  - metacarpus M87.04- ☑
  - metatarsus M87.07- ☑
  - multiple sites M87.09
  - neck M87.08
  - pelvis M87.050
  - pubic ramus [pubis] M87.050
  - radius M87.03- ☑
  - rib M87.08
  - scapula M87.01- ☑
  - skull M87.08
  - tarsus M87.07- ☑
  - tibia M87.06- ☑
  - toe M87.07- ☑
  - ulna M87.03- ☑
  - vertebra M87.08
- secondary NEC M87.30
  - carpus M87.33- ☑
  - clavicle M87.31- ☑
  - due to
    - drugs M87.10
      - carpus M87.13- ☑
      - clavicle M87.11- ☑
      - femur M87.15- ☑
      - fibula M87.16- ☑
      - finger M87.14- ☑
      - humerus M87.12- ☑
      - ilium M87.150
      - ischium M87.150
      - jaw M87.180
      - metacarpus M87.14- ☑
      - metatarsus M87.17- ☑
      - multiple sites M87.19
      - neck M87.188
      - pubic ramus [pubis] M87.150
      - radius M87.13- ☑
      - rib M87.188
      - scapula M87.11- ☑
      - skull M87.188
      - tarsus M87.17- ☑
      - tibia M87.16- ☑
      - toe M87.17- ☑
      - ulna M87.13- ☑
      - vertebra M87.188
    - hemoglobinopathy NEC D58.2 [M90.50]
      - carpus D58.2 [M90.54-] ☑
      - clavicle D58.2 [M90.51-] ☑
      - femur D58.2 [M90.55-] ☑
      - fibula D58.2 [M90.56-] ☑
      - finger D58.2 [M90.54-] ☑
      - humerus D58.2 [M90.52-] ☑
      - ilium D58.2 [M90.58]
      - ischium D58.2 [M90.58]
      - metacarpus D58.2 [M90.54-] ☑
      - metatarsus D58.2 [M90.57-] ☑
      - multiple sites D58.2 [M90.59]
      - neck D58.2 [M90.58]
      - pubic ramus [pubis] D58.2 [M90.58]
      - radius D58.2 [M90.53-] ☑
      - rib D58.2 [M90.58]
      - scapula D58.2 [M90.51-] ☑
      - skull D58.2 [M90.58]
      - specified NEC D58.2 [M90.58]
      - tarsus D58.2 [M90.57-] ☑
      - tibia D58.2 [M90.56-] ☑
      - toe D58.2 [M90.57-] ☑
      - ulna D58.2 [M90.53-] ☑
      - vertebra D58.2 [M90.58]
    - trauma (previous) M87.20
      - carpus M87.23- ☑
      - clavicle M87.21- ☑
      - femur M87.25- ☑

☑ Additional Character Required — Refer to the Tabular List for Character Selection

Osteonecrosis — continued
  secondary — continued
    due to — continued
      trauma — continued
        fibula M87.26- ☑
        finger M87.24- ☑
        humerus M87.22- ☑
        ilium M87.250
        ischium M87.250
        metacarpus M87.24- ☑
        metatarsus M87.27- ☑
        multiple sites M87.29
        neck M87.28
        pubic ramus [pubis] M87.250
        radius M87.23- ☑
        rib M87.28
        scapula M87.21- ☑
        skull M87.28
        tarsus M87.27- ☑
        tibia M87.26- ☑
        toe M87.27- ☑
        ulna M87.23- ☑
        vertebra M87.28
    femur M87.35- ☑
    fibula M87.36- ☑
    finger M87.34- ☑
    humerus M87.32- ☑
    ilium M87.350
    in
      caisson disease T70.3- ☑ [M90.50]
        carpus T70.3- ☑ [M90.54-]
        clavicle T70.3- ☑ [M90.51-] ☑
        femur T70.3- ☑ [M90.55-] ☑
        fibula T70.3- ☑ [M90.56-] ☑
        finger T70.3- ☑ [M90.54-] ☑
        humerus T70.3- ☑ [M90.52-] ☑
        ilium T70.3- ☑ [M90.58]
        ischium T70.3- ☑ [M90.58]
        metacarpus T70.3- ☑ [M90.54-] ☑
        metatarsus T70.3- ☑ [M90.57-] ☑
        multiple sites T70.3- ☑ [M90.59]
        neck T70.3- ☑ [M90.58]
        pubic ramus [pubis] T70.3- ☑ [M90.58]
        radius T70.3- ☑ [M90.53-] ☑
        rib T70.3- ☑ [M90.58]
        scapula T70.3- ☑ [M90.51-] ☑
        skull T70.3- ☑ [M90.58]
        tarsus T70.3- ☑ [M90.57-] ☑
        tibia T70.3- ☑ [M90.56-] ☑
        toe T70.3- ☑ [M90.57-] ☑
        ulna T70.3- ☑ [M90.53-] ☑
        vertebra T70.3- ☑ [M90.58]
    ischium M87.350
    metacarpus M87.34- ☑
    metatarsus M87.37- ☑
    multiple site M87.39
    neck M87.38
    pubic ramus [pubis] M87.350
    radius M87.33- ☑
    rib M87.38
    scapula M87.319
    skull M87.38
    tarsus M87.379
    tibia M87.366
    toe M87.379
    ulna M87.33- ☑
    vertebra M87.38
  specified type NEC M87.80
    carpus M87.83- ☑
    clavicle M87.81- ☑
    femur M87.85- ☑
    fibula M87.86- ☑
    finger M87.84- ☑
    humerus M87.82- ☑
    ilium M87.850
    ischium M87.850
    metacarpus M87.84- ☑
    metatarsus M87.87- ☑
    multiple sites M87.89
    neck M87.88
    pubic ramus [pubis] M87.850
    radius M87.83- ☑
    rib M87.88
    scapula M87.81- ☑
    skull M87.88
    tarsus M87.87- ☑

Osteonecrosis — continued
  specified type — continued
    tibia M87.86- ☑
    toe M87.87- ☑
    ulna M87.83- ☑
    vertebra M87.88
Osteopathia condensans disseminata Q78.8
Osteopathy — see also Osteomyelitis, Osteonecrosis, Osteoporosis
  after poliomyelitis M89.60
    carpus M89.64- ☑
    clavicle M89.61- ☑
    femur M89.65- ☑
    fibula M89.66- ☑
    finger M89.64- ☑
    humerus M89.62- ☑
    ilium M89.68
    ischium M89.68
    metacarpus M89.64- ☑
    metatarsus M89.67- ☑
    multiple sites M89.69
    neck M89.68
    pubic ramus [pubis] M89.68
    radius M89.63- ☑
    rib M89.68
    scapula M89.61- ☑
    skull M89.68
    tarsus M89.67- ☑
    tibia M89.66- ☑
    toe M89.67- ☑
    ulna M89.63- ☑
    vertebra M89.68
  in (due to)
    renal osteodystrophy N25.0
    specified diseases classified elsewhere — see subcategory M90.8- ☑
Osteopenia M85.8- ☑
  borderline M85.8- ☑
Osteoperiostitis — see Osteomyelitis, specified type NEC
Osteopetrosis (familial) Q78.2
Osteophyte M25.70
  ankle M25.77- ☑
  elbow M25.72- ☑
  foot joint M25.77- ☑
  hand joint M25.74- ☑
  hip M25.75- ☑
  knee M25.76- ☑
  shoulder M25.71- ☑
  spine M25.78
  vertebrae M25.78
  wrist M25.73- ☑
Osteopoikilosis Q78.8
Osteoporosis (female) (male) M81.0
  with current pathological fracture M80.00- ☑
  age-related M81.0
    with current pathologic fracture M80.00- ☑
      carpus M80.04- ☑
      clavicle M80.01- ☑
      femur M80.05- ☑
      fibula M80.06- ☑
      finger M80.04- ☑
      hip M80.05- ☑
      humerus M80.02- ☑
      ilium M80.0B- ☑
      ischium M80.0B- ☑
      metacarpus M80.04- ☑
      metatarsus M80.07- ☑
      pelvis M80.0B- ☑
      pubic ramus [pubis] M80.0B- ☑
      radius M80.03- ☑
      rib(s) M80.0A- ☑
      scapula M80.01- ☑
      site specified NEC M80.0A- ☑
      tarsus M80.07- ☑
      tibia M80.06- ☑
      toe M80.07- ☑
      ulna M80.03- ☑
      vertebra M80.08- ☑
  disuse M81.8
    with current pathological fracture M80.80- ☑
      carpus M80.84- ☑
      clavicle M80.81- ☑
      femur M80.85- ☑
      fibula M80.86- ☑
      finger M80.84- ☑
      hip M80.85- ☑

Osteoporosis — continued
  disuse — continued
    with current pathological fracture — continued
      humerus M80.82- ☑
      ilium M80.8B- ☑
      ischium M80.8B- ☑
      metacarpus M80.84- ☑
      metatarsus M80.87- ☑
      pelvis M80.8B- ☑
      pubic ramus [pubis] M80.8B- ☑
      radius M80.83- ☑
      scapula M80.81- ☑
      site specified NEC M80.8A- ☑
      tarsus M80.87- ☑
      tibia M80.86- ☑
      toe M80.87- ☑
      ulna M80.83- ☑
      vertebra M80.88- ☑
  drug-induced — see Osteoporosis, specified type NEC
  idiopathic — see Osteoporosis, specified type NEC
  involutional — see Osteoporosis, age-related
  Lequesne M81.6
  localized M81.6
  postmenopausal M81.0
    with pathological fracture M80.00- ☑
      carpus M80.04- ☑
      clavicle M80.01- ☑
      femur M80.05- ☑
      fibula M80.06- ☑
      finger M80.04- ☑
      hip M80.05- ☑
      humerus M80.02- ☑
      ilium M80.0A- ☑
      ischium M80.0A- ☑
      metacarpus M80.04- ☑
      metatarsus M80.07- ☑
      pelvis M80.0B- ☑
      pubic ramus [pubis] M80.8B- ☑
      radius M80.03- ☑
      scapula M80.01- ☑
      site specified NEC M80.0A- ☑
      tarsus M80.07- ☑
      tibia M80.06- ☑
      toe M80.07- ☑
      ulna M80.03- ☑
      vertebra M80.08- ☑
  postoophorectomy — see Osteoporosis, specified type NEC
  postsurgical malabsorption — see Osteoporosis, specified type NEC
  post-traumatic — see Osteoporosis, specified type NEC
  senile — see Osteoporosis, age-related
  specified type NEC M81.8
    with pathological fracture M80.80- ☑
      carpus M80.84- ☑
      clavicle M80.81- ☑
      femur M80.85- ☑
      fibula M80.86- ☑
      finger M80.84- ☑
      hip M80.85- ☑
      humerus M80.82- ☑
      ilium M80.8B- ☑
      ischium M80.8B- ☑
      metacarpus M80.84- ☑
      metatarsus M80.87- ☑
      pelvis M80.8B- ☑
      pubic ramus [pubis] M80.8B- ☑
      radius M80.83- ☑
      scapula M80.81- ☑
      site specified NEC M80.8A- ☑
      tarsus M80.87- ☑
      tibia M80.86- ☑
      toe M80.87- ☑
      ulna M80.83- ☑
      vertebra M80.88- ☑
Osteopsathyrosis (idiopathica) Q78.0
Osteoradionecrosis, jaw (acute) (chronic) (lower) (suppurative) (upper) M27.2
Osteosarcoma (any form) — see Neoplasm, bone, malignant
Osteosclerosis Q78.2
  acquired M85.8- ☑
  congenita Q77.4
  fragilitas (generalisata) Q78.2
  myelofibrosis D75.81
Osteosclerotic anemia D64.89

☑ Additional Character Required — Refer to the Tabular List for Character Selection

Osteosis
 cutis L94.2
 renal fibrocystic N25.0
Österreicher-Turner syndrome Q87.2
Ostium
 atrioventriculare commune Q21.23
 primum (arteriosum) (defect) (persistent) Q21.20
 secundum (arteriosum) (defect) (patent) (persistent) Q21.11
Ostrum-Furst syndrome Q75.8
Otalgia H92.0- ☑
Otitis (acute) H66.90
 with effusion — *see also* Otitis, media, nonsuppurative
  purulent — *see* Otitis, media, suppurative
 adhesive — *see* subcategory H74.1- ☑
 chronic — *see also* Otitis, media, chronic
  with effusion — *see also* Otitis, media, nonsuppurative, chronic
 externa H60.9- ☑
  abscess — *see* Abscess, ear, external
  acute (noninfective) H60.50- ☑
   actinic H60.51- ☑
   chemical H60.52- ☑
   contact H60.53- ☑
   eczematoid H60.54- ☑
   infective — *see* Otitis, externa, infective
   reactive H60.55- ☑
   specified NEC H60.59- ☑
  cellulitis — *see* Cellulitis, ear
  chronic H60.6- ☑
  diffuse — *see* Otitis, externa, infective, diffuse
  hemorrhagic — *see* Otitis, externa, infective, hemorrhagic
  in (due to)
   aspergillosis B44.89
   candidiasis B37.84
   erysipelas A46 *[H62.4-]* ☑
   herpes (simplex) virus infection B00.1
    zoster B02.8
   impetigo L01.00 *[H62.4-]* ☑
   infectious disease NEC B99.- *[H62.4-]* ☑
   mycosis NEC B36.9 *[H62.4-]* ☑
   parasitic disease NEC B89 *[H62.4-]* ☑
   viral disease NEC B34.9 *[H62.4-]* ☑
   zoster B02.8
  infective NEC H60.39- ☑
   abscess — *see* Abscess, ear, external
   cellulitis — *see* Cellulitis, ear
   diffuse H60.31- ☑
   hemorrhagic H60.32- ☑
   swimmer's ear — *see* Swimmer's, ear
  malignant H60.2- ☑
  mycotic NEC B36.9 *[H62.4-]* ☑
   in
    aspergillosis B44.89
    candidiasis B37.84
    moniliasis B37.84
  necrotizing — *see* Otitis, externa, malignant
  Pseudomonas aeruginosa — *see* Otitis, externa, malignant
  reactive — *see* Otitis, externa, acute, reactive
  specified NEC — *see* subcategory H60.8- ☑
  tropical NEC B36.9 *[H62.4-]* ☑
   in
    aspergillosis B44.89
    candidiasis B37.84
    moniliasis B37.84
 insidiosa — *see* Otosclerosis
 interna H83.0- ☑
 media (hemorrhagic) (staphylococcal) (streptococcal) H66.9- ☑
  with effusion (nonpurulent) — *see* Otitis, media, nonsuppurative
  acute, subacute H66.90
   allergic — *see* Otitis, media, nonsuppurative, acute, allergic
   exudative — *see* Otitis, media, suppurative, acute
   mucoid — *see* Otitis, media, suppurative, acute
   necrotizing — *see also* Otitis, media, suppurative, acute
    in
     measles B05.3
     scarlet fever A38.0
   nonsuppurative NEC — *see* Otitis, media, nonsuppurative, acute
   purulent — *see* Otitis, media, suppurative, acute
   sanguinous — *see* Otitis, media, nonsuppurative, acute

Otitis — *continued*
 media — *continued*
  acute, subacute — *continued*
   secretory — *see* Otitis, media, nonsuppurative, acute, serous
   seromucinous — *see* Otitis, media, nonsuppurative, acute
   serous — *see* Otitis, media, nonsuppurative, acute, serous
   suppurative — *see* Otitis, media, suppurative, acute
  allergic — *see* Otitis, media, nonsuppurative
  catarrhal — *see* Otitis, media, nonsuppurative
  chronic H66.90
   with effusion (nonpurulent) — *see* Otitis, media, nonsuppurative, chronic
   allergic — *see* Otitis, media, nonsuppurative, chronic, allergic
   benign suppurative — *see* Otitis, media, suppurative, chronic, tubotympanic
   catarrhal — *see* Otitis, media, nonsuppurative, chronic, serous
   exudative — *see* Otitis, media, nonsuppurative, chronic
   mucinous — *see* Otitis, media, nonsuppurative, chronic, mucoid
   mucoid — *see* Otitis, media, nonsuppurative, chronic, mucoid
   nonsuppurative NEC — *see* Otitis, media, nonsuppurative, chronic
   purulent — *see* Otitis, media, suppurative, chronic
   secretory — *see* Otitis, media, nonsuppurative, chronic, mucoid
   seromucinous — *see* Otitis, media, nonsuppurative, chronic
   serous — *see* Otitis, media, nonsuppurative, chronic, serous
   suppurative — *see* Otitis, media, suppurative, chronic
   transudative — *see* Otitis, media, nonsuppurative, chronic, mucoid
  exudative — *see* Otitis, media, suppurative
  in (due to) (with)
   influenza — *see* Influenza, with, otitis media
   measles B05.3
   scarlet fever A38.0
   tuberculosis A18.6
   viral disease NEC B34.- *[H67.-]* ☑
  mucoid — *see* Otitis, media, nonsuppurative
  nonsuppurative H65.9- ☑
   acute or subacute NEC H65.19- ☑
    allergic H65.11- ☑
     recurrent H65.11- ☑
    recurrent H65.19- ☑
    secretory — *see* Otitis, media, nonsuppurative, serous
    serous H65.0- ☑
     recurrent H65.0- ☑
   chronic H65.49- ☑
    allergic H65.41- ☑
    mucoid H65.3- ☑
    serous H65.2- ☑
  postmeasles B05.3
  purulent — *see* Otitis, media, suppurative
  secretory — *see* Otitis, media, nonsuppurative
  seromucinous — *see* Otitis, media, nonsuppurative
  serous — *see* Otitis, media, nonsuppurative
  suppurative H66.4- ☑
   acute H66.00- ☑
    with rupture of ear drum H66.01- ☑
    recurrent H66.00- ☑
     with rupture of ear drum H66.01- ☑
   chronic — *see also* subcategory H66.3- ☑
    atticoantral H66.2- ☑
    benign — *see* Otitis, media, suppurative, chronic, tubotympanic
    tubotympanic H66.1- ☑
   transudative — *see* Otitis, media, nonsuppurative
   tuberculous A18.6
Otocephaly Q18.2
Otolith syndrome — *see* subcategory H81.8- ☑
Otomycosis (diffuse) NEC B36.9 *[H62.4-]* ☑
 in
  aspergillosis B44.89
  candidiasis B37.84
  moniliasis B37.84
Otoporosis — *see* Otosclerosis
Otorrhagia (nontraumatic) H92.2- ☑

Otorrhagia — *continued*
 traumatic — *code by* Type of injury
Otorrhea H92.1- ☑
 cerebrospinal (fluid) G96.01
  postoperative G96.08
  specified NEC G96.08
  spontaneous G96.01
  traumatic G96.08
Otosclerosis (general) H80.9- ☑
 cochlear (endosteal) H80.2- ☑
 involving
  otic capsule — *see* Otosclerosis, cochlear
  oval window
   nonobliterative H80.0- ☑
   obliterative H80.1- ☑
  round window — *see* Otosclerosis, cochlear
 nonobliterative — *see* Otosclerosis, involving, oval window, nonobliterative
 obliterative — *see* Otosclerosis, involving, oval window, obliterative
 specified NEC H80.8- ☑
Otospongiosis — *see* Otosclerosis
Otto's disease or pelvis M24.7
Outcome of delivery Z37.9
 multiple births Z37.9
  all liveborn Z37.50
   quadruplets Z37.52
   quintuplets Z37.53
   sextuplets Z37.54
   specified number NEC Z37.59
   triplets Z37.51
  all stillborn Z37.7
  some liveborn Z37.60
   quadruplets Z37.62
   quintuplets Z37.63
   sextuplets Z37.64
   specified number NEC Z37.69
   triplets Z37.61
 single NEC Z37.9
  liveborn Z37.0
  stillborn Z37.1
 twins NEC Z37.9
  both liveborn Z37.2
  both stillborn Z37.4
  one liveborn, one stillborn Z37.3
Outlet — *see* condition
Ovalocytosis (congenital) (hereditary) — *see* Elliptocytosis
Ovarian — *see* Condition
Ovariocele N83.4- ☑
Ovaritis (cystic) — *see* Oophoritis
Ovary, ovarian — *see also* condition
 resistant syndrome E28.39
 vein syndrome N13.8
Overactive — *see also* Hyperfunction
 adrenal cortex NEC E27.0
 bladder N32.81
 hypothalamus E23.3
 thyroid — *see* Hyperthyroidism
Overactivity R46.3
 child — *see* Disorder, attention-deficit hyperactivity
Overbite (deep) (excessive) (horizontal) (vertical) M26.29
Overbreathing — *see* Hyperventilation
Overconscientious personality F60.5
Overdevelopment — *see* Hypertrophy
Overdistension — *see* Distension
Overdose, overdosage (drug) — *see* Table of Drugs and Chemicals, by drug, poisoning
Overeating R63.2
 nonorganic origin F50.89
 psychogenic F50.89
Overexertion (effects) (exhaustion) T73.3- ☑
Overexposure (effects) T73.9- ☑
 exhaustion T73.2- ☑
Overfeeding — *see* Overeating
 newborn P92.4
Overfill, endodontic M27.52
Overgrowth
 bacterial
  small intestinal K63.8219
   hydrogen-subtype K63.8211
   hydrogen sulfide-subtype K63.8212
 bone — *see* Hypertrophy, bone
 fungal
  small intestinal K63.822
 intestinal methanogen K63.829
Overhanging of dental restorative material (unrepairable) K08.52
Overheated (places) (effects) — *see* Heat

Overjet (excessive horizontal) M26.23
Overlaid, overlying (suffocation) — see Asphyxia, traumatic, due to mechanical threat
Overlap, excessive horizontal (teeth) M26.23
Overlapping toe (acquired) — see also Deformity, toe, specified NEC
  congenital (fifth toe) Q66.89
Overload
  circulatory, due to transfusion (blood) (blood components) (TACO) E87.71
  fluid E87.70
    due to transfusion (blood) (blood components) E87.71
    specified NEC E87.79
  iron, due to repeated red blood cell transfusions E83.111
  potassium (K) E87.5
  sodium (Na) E87.0
Overnutrition — see Hyperalimentation
Overproduction — see also Hypersecretion
  ACTH E27.0
  catecholamine E27.5
  growth hormone E22.0
Overprotection, child by parent Z62.1
Overriding
  aorta Q25.49
  finger (acquired) — see Deformity, finger
    congenital Q68.1
  toe (acquired) — see also Deformity, toe, specified NEC
    congenital Q66.89
Overstrained R53.83
  heart — see Hypertrophy, cardiac
Overuse, muscle NEC M70.8- ☑
Overweight E66.3
Overworked R53.83
Oviduct — see condition
Ovotestis Q56.0
Ovulation (cycle)
  failure or lack of N97.0
  pain N94.0
Ovum — see condition
Owren's disease or syndrome (parahemophilia) D68.2
Ox heart — see Hypertrophy, cardiac
Oxalosis E72.53- ☑
Oxaluria E72.53- ☑
Oxycephaly, oxycephalic Q75.009
  syphilitic, congenital A50.02
Oxyuriasis B80
Oxyuris vermicularis (infestation) B80
Ozena J31.0

P

Pachyderma, pachydermia L85.9
  larynx (verrucosa) J38.7
Pachydermatocele (congenital) Q82.8
Pachydermoperiostosis — see also Osteoarthropathy, hypertrophic, specified type NEC
  clubbed nail M89.40 [L62]
Pachygyria Q04.3
Pachymeningitis (adhesive) (basal) (brain) (cervical) (chronic) (circumscribed) (external) (fibrous) (hemorrhagic) (hypertrophic) (internal) (purulent) (spinal) (suppurative) — see Meningitis
Pachyonychia (congenital) Q84.5
Pacinian tumor — see Neoplasm, skin, benign
Pad, knuckle or Garrod's M72.1
Paget-Schroetter syndrome I82.890
Paget's disease
  with infiltrating duct carcinoma — see Neoplasm, breast, malignant
  bone M88.9
    carpus M88.84- ☑
    clavicle M88.81- ☑
    femur M88.85- ☑
    fibula M88.86- ☑
    finger M88.84- ☑
    humerus M88.82- ☑
    ilium M88.88
    in neoplastic disease — see Osteitis, deformans, in neoplastic disease
    ischium M88.88
    metacarpus M88.84- ☑
    metatarsus M88.87- ☑
    multiple sites M88.89
    neck M88.88
    pubic ramus [pubis] M88.88
    radius M88.83- ☑
    rib M88.88
    scapula M88.81- ☑

Paget's disease — continued
  bone — continued
    skull M88.0
    specified NEC M88.88
    tarsus M88.87- ☑
    tibia M88.86- ☑
    toe M88.87- ☑
    ulna M88.83- ☑
    vertebra M88.1
  breast (female) C50.01- ☑
    male C50.02- ☑
  extramammary — see also Neoplasm, skin, malignant
    anus C21.0
    margin C44.590
    skin C44.590
  intraductal carcinoma — see Neoplasm, breast, malignant
  malignant — see Neoplasm, skin, malignant
    breast (female) C50.01- ☑
      male C50.02- ☑
    unspecified site (female) C50.01- ☑
      male C50.02- ☑
  mammary — see Paget's disease, breast
  nipple — see Paget's disease, breast
  osteitis deformans — see Paget's disease, bone
Pain(s) — see also Painful R52
  abdominal R10.9
    colic R10.83
    generalized R10.84
      with acute abdomen R10.0
    lower R10.30
      left quadrant R10.32
      pelvic or perineal R10.20
        bilateral R10.23
        left R10.22
        right R10.21
      periumbilical R10.33
      right quadrant R10.31
    multiple sites R10.85
    rebound — see Tenderness, abdominal, rebound
    severe with abdominal rigidity R10.0
    tenderness — see Tenderness, abdominal
    upper R10.10
      epigastric R10.13
      left quadrant R10.12
      right quadrant R10.11
  acute R52
    due to trauma G89.11
    neoplasm related G89.3
    postprocedural NEC G89.18
    post-thoracotomy G89.12
    specified by site — code to Pain, by site
  adnexa (uteri) R10.20
  anginoid — see Pain, precordial
  anus K62.89
  arm — see Pain, limb, upper
  axillary (axilla) M79.62- ☑
  back (postural) M54.9
  bladder R39.89
    associated with micturition — see Micturition, painful
    chronic R39.82
  bone — see Disorder, bone, specified type NEC
  breast N64.4
  broad ligament R10.20
  cancer associated (acute) (chronic) G89.3
  cecum — see Pain, abdominal
  cervicobrachial M53.1
  chest (central) R07.9
    anterior wall R07.89
    atypical R07.89
    ischemic I20.9
    musculoskeletal R07.89
    non-cardiac R07.89
    on breathing R07.1
    pleurodynia R07.81
    precordial R07.2
    wall (anterior) R07.89
  chronic G89.29
    associated with significant psychosocial dysfunction G89.4
    due to trauma G89.21
    neoplasm related G89.3
    postoperative NEC G89.28
    postprocedural NEC G89.28
    post-thoracotomy G89.22
    specified NEC G89.29
  coccyx M53.3
  colon — see Pain, abdominal

Pain(s) — continued
  coronary — see Angina
  costochondral R07.1
  diaphragm R07.1
  due to cancer G89.3
  due to device, implant or graft — see also Complications, by site and type, specified NEC T85.848- ☑
    arterial graft NEC T82.848- ☑
    breast (implant) T85.848- ☑
    catheter NEC T85.848- ☑
      dialysis (renal) T82.848- ☑
        intraperitoneal T85.848- ☑
      infusion NEC T82.848- ☑
        spinal (epidural) (subdural) T85.840- ☑
      urinary (indwelling) T83.84- ☑
    electronic (electrode) (pulse generator) (stimulator)
      bone T85.840- ☑
      cardiac T82.847- ☑
      nervous system (brain) (peripheral nerve) (spinal) T85.84- ☑
      urinary T83.84- ☑
    fixation, internal (orthopedic) NEC T84.84- ☑
    gastrointestinal (bile duct) (esophagus) T85.848- ☑
    genital NEC T83.84- ☑
    heart NEC T82.847- ☑
    infusion NEC T85.848- ☑
    joint prosthesis T84.84- ☑
    ocular (corneal graft) (orbital implant) NEC T85.848- ☑
    orthopedic NEC T84.84- ☑
    specified NEC T85.848- ☑
    urinary NEC T83.84- ☑
    vascular NEC T82.848- ☑
    ventricular intracranial shunt T85.840- ☑
  due to malignancy (primary) (secondary) G89.3
  ear — see subcategory H92.0- ☑
  epigastric, epigastrium R10.13
  eye — see Pain, ocular
  face, facial R51.9
    atypical G50.1
  female genital organs NEC N94.89
  finger — see Pain, limb, upper
  flank R10.A0
    bilateral R10.A3
    left R10.A2
    right R10.A1
  foot — see Pain, limb, lower
  gallbladder K82.9
  gas (intestinal) R14.1
  gastric — see Pain, abdominal
  generalized NOS R52
  genital organ
    female N94.89
    male N50.89
  groin — see Pain, abdominal, lower
  hand — see Pain, limb, upper
  head — see Headache
  heart — see Pain, precordial
  infra-orbital — see Neuralgia, trigeminal
  intercostal R07.82
  intermenstrual N94.0
  jaw R68.84
  joint M25.50
    ankle M25.57- ☑
    elbow M25.52- ☑
    finger M25.54- ☑
    foot M25.57- ☑
    hand M25.54- ☑
    hip M25.55- ☑
    knee M25.56- ☑
    shoulder M25.51- ☑
    specified site NEC M25.59
    toe M25.57- ☑
    wrist M25.53- ☑
  kidney N23
  laryngeal R07.0
  leg — see Pain, limb, lower
  limb M79.609
    lower M79.60- ☑
      foot M79.67- ☑
      lower leg M79.66- ☑
      thigh M79.65- ☑
      toe M79.67- ☑
    upper M79.60- ☑
      axilla M79.62- ☑
      finger M79.64- ☑
      forearm M79.63- ☑

Pain(s) — continued
- limb — continued
  - upper — continued
    - hand M79.64- ☑
    - upper arm M79.62- ☑
- loin M54.50
- low back M54.50
  - specified NEC M54.59
  - vertebral end plate M54.51
  - vertebrogenic M54.51
- lumbar region M54.50
  - vertebral end plate M54.51
  - vertebrogenic M54.51
- mandibular R68.84
- mastoid — see subcategory H92.0- ☑
- maxilla R68.84
- menstrual — see also Dysmenorrhea N94.6
- metacarpophalangeal (joint) — see Pain, joint, hand
- metatarsophalangeal (joint) — see Pain, joint, foot
- mouth K13.79
- muscle — see Myalgia
- musculoskeletal — see also Pain, by site M79.18
- myofascial M79.18
- nasal J34.89
- nasopharynx J39.2
- neck NEC M54.2
- nerve NEC — see Neuralgia
- neuromuscular — see Neuralgia
- nose J34.89
- ocular H57.1- ☑
- ophthalmic — see Pain, ocular
- orbital region — see Pain, ocular
- ovary N94.89
- over heart — see Pain, precordial
- ovulation N94.0
- pelvic (female) R10.20
  - bilateral R10.23
  - left R10.22
  - right R10.21
- penis N48.89
- pericardial — see Pain, precordial
- perineal, perineum R10.20
  - bilateral R10.23
  - left R10.22
  - right R10.21
- pharynx J39.2
- pleura, pleural, pleuritic R07.81
- postoperative NOS G89.18
- postprocedural NOS G89.18
- post-thoracotomy G89.12
- precordial (region) R07.2
- premenstrual N94.3
- psychogenic (persistent) (any site) F45.41
- radicular (spinal) — see Radiculopathy
- rectum K62.89
- respiration R07.1
- retrosternal R07.2
- rheumatoid, muscular — see Myalgia
- rib R07.89
- root (spinal) — see Radiculopathy
- round ligament (stretch) R10.20
- sacroiliac M53.3
- sciatic — see Sciatica
- scrotum N50.82
- seminal vesicle N50.89
- shoulder M25.51- ☑
- spermatic cord N50.89
- spinal root — see Radiculopathy
- spine M54.9
  - cervical M54.2
  - low back M54.50
    - with sciatica M54.4- ☑
  - thoracic M54.6
- stomach — see Pain, abdominal
- substernal R07.2
- suprapubic R10.24
- temporomandibular (joint) M26.62- ☑
- testis N50.81- ☑
- thoracic spine M54.6
  - with radicular and visceral pain M54.14
- throat R07.0
- tibia — see Pain, limb, lower
- toe — see Pain, limb, lower
- tongue K14.6
- tooth K08.89
- trigeminal — see Neuralgia, trigeminal
- tumor associated G89.3
- ureter N23

Pain(s) — continued
- urinary (organ) (system) N23
- uterus NEC N94.89
- vagina R10.20
- vertebral end plate — see Pain, vertebrogenic
- vertebrogenic M54.89
  - low back M54.51
  - lumbar M54.51
  - syndrome M54.89
- vesical R39.89
  - associated with micturition — see Micturition, painful
- vulva R10.20

Painful — see also Pain
- coitus
  - female N94.10
  - male N53.12
  - psychogenic F52.6
- ejaculation (semen) N53.12
  - psychogenic F52.6
- erection — see Priapism
- feet syndrome E53.8
- joint replacement (hip) (knee) T84.84- ☑
- menstruation — see Dysmenorrhea
  - psychogenic F45.8
- micturition — see Micturition, painful
- respiration R07.1
- scar NEC L90.5
- wire sutures T81.89- ☑

Painter's colic — see subcategory T56.0- ☑
Palate — see condition
Palatoplegia K13.79
Palatoschisis — see Cleft, palate
Palilalia R48.8
Palliative care Z51.5
Pallor R23.1
- optic disc, temporal — see Atrophy, optic

Palmar — see also condition
- fascia — see condition

Palpable
- cecum K63.89
- kidney N28.89
- ovary N83.8
- prostate N42.9
- spleen — see Splenomegaly

Palpitations (heart) R00.2
- psychogenic F45.8

Palsy — see also Paralysis G83.9
- atrophic diffuse (progressive) G12.22
- Bell's — see also Palsy, facial
  - newborn P11.3
- brachial plexus NEC G54.0
  - newborn (birth injury) P14.3
- brain — see Palsy, cerebral
- bulbar (progressive) (chronic) G12.22
  - of childhood (Fazio-Londe) G12.1
  - pseudo NEC G12.29
  - supranuclear (progressive) G23.1
- cerebral (congenital) G80.9
  - ataxic G80.4
  - athetoid G80.3
  - choreathetoid G80.3
  - diplegic G80.8
    - spastic G80.1
  - dyskinetic G80.3
    - athetoid G80.3
    - choreathetoid G80.3
    - distonic G80.3
  - dystonic G80.3
  - hemiplegic G80.8
    - spastic G80.2
  - mixed G80.8
  - monoplegic G80.8
    - spastic G80.1
  - paraplegic G80.8
    - spastic G80.1
  - quadriplegic G80.8
    - spastic G80.0
  - spastic G80.1
    - diplegic G80.1
    - hemiplegic G80.2
    - monoplegic G80.1
    - quadriplegic G80.0
    - specified NEC G80.1
    - tetrapelgic G80.0
  - specified NEC G80.8
  - syphilitic A52.12
    - congenital A50.49
  - tetraplegic G80.8
    - spastic G80.0

Palsy — continued
- cranial nerve — see also Disorder, nerve, cranial
  - multiple G52.7
  - in
    - infectious disease B99.- ☑ [G53]
    - neoplastic disease — see also Neoplasm D49.9 [G53]
    - parasitic disease B89 [G53]
    - sarcoidosis D86.82
- creeping G12.22
- diver's T70.3- ☑
- Erb's P14.0
- facial G51.0
  - newborn (birth injury) P11.3
- glossopharyngeal G52.1
- Klumpke (-Dejerine) P14.1
- lead — see subcategory T56.0- ☑
- median nerve (tardy) G56.1- ☑
- nerve G58.9
  - specified NEC G58.8
- peroneal nerve (acute) (tardy) G57.3- ☑
- progressive supranuclear G23.1
- pseudobulbar NEC G12.29
- radial nerve (acute) G56.3- ☑
- seventh nerve — see also Palsy, facial
  - newborn P11.3
- shaking — see Parkinsonism
- spastic (cerebral) (spinal) G80.1
- ulnar nerve (tardy) G56.2- ☑
- wasting G12.29

Paludism — see Malaria
Panangiitis M30.0
Panaris, panaritium — see also Cellulitis, digit
- with lymphangitis — see Lymphangitis, acute, digit

Panarteritis nodosa M30.0
- brain or cerebral I67.7

Pancake heart R93.1
- with cor pulmonale (chronic) I27.81

Pancarditis (acute) (chronic) I51.89
- rheumatic I09.89
  - active or acute I01.8

Pancoast's syndrome or tumor C34.1- ☑
Pancolitis — see also Colitis
- ulcerative (chronic) K51.00
  - with
    - abscess K51.014
    - complication K51.019
    - fistula K51.013
    - obstruction K51.012
    - rectal bleeding K51.011
    - specified complication NEC K51.018

Pancreas, pancreatic — see condition
Pancreatitis (annular) (apoplectic) (calcareous) (edematous) (hemorrhagic) (malignant) (subacute) (suppurative) K85.90
- with necrosis (uninfected) K85.91
  - infected K85.92
- acute (without necrosis or infection) K85.90
  - with necrosis (uninfected) K85.91
    - infected K85.92
  - alcohol induced (without necrosis or infection) K85.20
    - with necrosis (uninfected) K85.21
      - infected K85.22
  - biliary (without necrosis or infection) K85.10
    - with necrosis (uninfected) K85.11
      - infected K85.12
  - drug induced (without necrosis or infection) K85.30
    - with necrosis (uninfected) K85.31
      - infected K85.32
  - gallstone (without necrosis or infection) K85.10
    - with necrosis (uninfected) K85.11
      - infected K85.12
  - idiopathic (without necrosis or infection) K85.00
    - with necrosis (uninfected) K85.01
      - infected K85.02
  - specified NEC (without necrosis or infection) K85.80
    - with necrosis (uninfected) K85.81
      - infected K85.82
- chronic (infectious) K86.1
  - alcohol-induced K86.0
  - recurrent K86.1
  - relapsing K86.1
- cystic (chronic) K86.1
- cytomegaloviral B25.2
- fibrous (chronic) K86.1
- gallstone (without necrosis or infection) K85.10
  - with necrosis (uninfected) K85.11
    - infected K85.12

Pancreatitis — *continued*
   gangrenous — *see* Pancreatitis, acute
   interstitial (chronic) K86.1
     acute — *see also* Pancreatitis, acute K85.80
   mumps B26.3
   recurrent
     acute — *see* Pancreatitis, acute by type
     chronic K86.1
   relapsing, chronic K86.1
   syphilitic A52.74
Pancreatoblastoma — *see* Neoplasm, pancreas, malignant
Pancreolithiasis K86.89
Pancytolysis D75.89
Pancytopenia (acquired) D61.818
   with
     malformations D61.09
     myelodysplastic syndrome — *see* Syndrome, myelodysplastic, pancytopenia (acquired)
   antineoplastic chemotherapy induced D61.810
   congenital D61.09
   drug-induced NEC D61.811
   Fanconi D61.03
PANDAS (pediatric autoimmune neuropsychiatric disorders associated with streptococcal infections syndrome) D89.89
Panencephalitis, subacute, sclerosing A81.1
Panhematopenia D61.9
   congenital D61.09
   constitutional D61.09
   splenic, primary D73.1
Panhemocytopenia D61.9
   congenital D61.09
   constitutional D61.09
Panhypogonadism E29.1
Panhypopituitarism E23.0
   prepubertal E23.0
Panic (attack) (state) F41.0
   reaction to exceptional stress (transient) F43.0
Panmyelopathy, familial, constitutional D61.09
Panmyelophthisis D61.82
   congenital D61.09
Panmyelosis (acute) (with myelofibrosis) C94.4- ☑
Panner's disease — *see* Osteochondrosis, juvenile, humerus
Panneuritis endemica E51.11
Panniculitis (nodular) (nonsuppurative) M79.3
   back M54.00
     cervical region M54.02
     cervicothoracic region M54.03
     lumbar region M54.06
     lumbosacral region M54.07
     multiple sites M54.09
     occipito-atlanto-axial region M54.01
     sacrococcygeal region M54.08
     thoracic region M54.04
     thoracolumbar region M54.05
   lupus L93.2
   mesenteric K65.4
   neck M54.02
     cervicothoracic region M54.03
     occipito-atlanto-axial region M54.01
   relapsing M35.6
Panniculus adiposus (abdominal) E65
Pannus (allergic) (cornea) (degenerativus) (keratic) H16.42- ☑
   abdominal (symptomatic) E65
   trachomatosus, trachomatous (active) A71.1
Panophthalmitis H44.01- ☑
Pansinusitis (chronic) (hyperplastic) (nonpurulent) (purulent) J32.4
   acute J01.40
     recurrent J01.41
   tuberculous A15.8
Pansynostosis Q75.052
Panuveitis (sympathetic) H44.11- ☑
Panvalvular disease I08.9
   specified NEC I08.8
PAPA (pyogenic arthritis, pyoderma gangrenosum, and acne syndrome) M04.8
Papanicolaou smear, cervix Z12.4
   as part of routine gynecological examination Z01.419
     with abnormal findings Z01.411
   for suspected neoplasm Z12.4
   nonspecific abnormal finding R87.619
   routine Z01.419
     with abnormal findings Z01.411
Papilledema (choked disc) H47.10
   associated with
     decreased ocular pressure H47.12
     increased intracranial pressure H47.11

Papilledema — *continued*
   associated with — *continued*
     retinal disorder H47.13
     Foster-Kennedy syndrome H47.14- ☑
Papillitis H46.00
   anus K62.89
   chronic lingual K14.4
   necrotizing, kidney N17.2
   optic H46.0- ☑
   rectum K62.89
   renal, necrotizing N17.2
   tongue K14.0
Papilloma — *see also* Neoplasm, benign, by site
   acuminatum (female) (male) (anogenital) A63.0
   basal cell L82.1
     inflamed L82.0
   benign pinta (primary) A67.0
   bladder (urinary) (transitional cell) D41.4
   choroid plexus (lateral ventricle) (third ventricle) D33.0
     anaplastic C71.5
     fourth ventricle D33.1
     malignant C71.5
   renal pelvis (transitional cell) D41.1- ☑
     benign D30.1- ☑
   Schneiderian
     specified site — *see* Neoplasm, benign, by site
     unspecified site D14.0
   serous surface
     borderline malignancy
       specified site — *see* Neoplasm, uncertain behavior, by site
       unspecified site D39.10
     specified site — *see* Neoplasm, benign, by site
     unspecified site D27.9
   transitional (cell)
     bladder (urinary) D41.4
     inverted type — *see* Neoplasm, uncertain behavior, by site
     renal pelvis D41.1- ☑
     ureter D41.2- ☑
   ureter (transitional cell) D41.2- ☑
     benign D30.2- ☑
   urothelial — *see* Neoplasm, uncertain behavior, by site
   villous — *see* Neoplasm, uncertain behavior, by site
     adenocarcinoma in — *see* Neoplasm, malignant, by site
     in situ — *see* Neoplasm, in situ
   yaws, plantar or palmar A66.1
Papillomata, multiple, of yaws A66.1
Papillomatosis — *see also* Neoplasm, benign, by site
   confluent and reticulated L83
   cystic, breast — *see* Mastopathy, cystic
   ductal, breast — *see* Mastopathy, cystic
   intraductal (diffuse) — *see* Neoplasm, benign, by site
   subareolar duct D24.- ☑
Papillomavirus, as cause of disease classified elsewhere B97.7
Papillon-Léage and Psaume syndrome Q87.0
Papule(s) R23.8
   carate (primary) A67.0
   fibrous, of nose D22.39
   Gottron's L94.4
   pinta (primary) A67.0
Papulosis
   lymphomatoid C86.6- ☑
   malignant I77.89
Papyraceous fetus O31.0- ☑
Para-albuminemia E88.09
Paracephalus Q89.7
Parachute mitral valve Q23.2
Paracoccidioidomycosis B41.9
   disseminated B41.7
   generalized B41.7
   mucocutaneous-lymphangitic B41.8
   pulmonary B41.0
   specified NEC B41.8
   visceral B41.8
Paradentosis K05.4
Paraffinoma T88.8- ☑
Paraganglioma D44.7
   adrenal D35.0- ☑
     malignant C74.1- ☑
   aortic body D44.7
     malignant C75.5
   carotid body D44.6
     malignant C75.4
   chromaffin — *see also* Neoplasm, benign, by site
     malignant — *see* Neoplasm, malignant, by site

Paraganglioma — *continued*
   extra-adrenal D44.7
     malignant C75.5
       specified site — *see* Neoplasm, malignant, by site
       unspecified site C75.5
     specified site — *see* Neoplasm, uncertain behavior, by site
     unspecified site D44.7
   gangliocytic D13.2
     specified site — *see* Neoplasm, benign, by site
     unspecified site D13.2
   glomus jugulare D44.7
     malignant C75.5
   jugular D44.7
   malignant C75.5
     specified site — *see* Neoplasm, malignant, by site
     unspecified site C75.5
   nonchromaffin D44.7
     malignant C75.5
       specified site — *see* Neoplasm, malignant, by site
       unspecified site C75.5
     specified site — *see* Neoplasm, uncertain behavior, by site
     unspecified site D44.7
   parasympathetic D44.7
     specified site — *see* Neoplasm, uncertain behavior, by site
     unspecified site D44.7
   specified site — *see* Neoplasm, uncertain behavior, by site
   sympathetic D44.7
     specified site — *see* Neoplasm, uncertain behavior, by site
     unspecified site D44.7
   unspecified site D44.7
Parageusia R43.2
   psychogenic F45.8
Paragonimiasis B66.4
Paragranuloma, Hodgkin — *see* Lymphoma, Hodgkin, specified NEC
Parahemophilia — *see also* Defect, coagulation D68.2
Parakeratosis R23.4
   variegata L41.0
Paralysis, paralytic (complete) (incomplete) G83.9
   with
     syphilis A52.17
   abducens, abducent (nerve) — *see* Strabismus, paralytic, sixth nerve
   abductor, lower extremity G57.9- ☑
   accessory nerve G52.8
   accommodation — *see also* Paresis, of accommodation
     hysterical F44.89
   acoustic nerve (except Deafness) H93.3- ☑
   agitans — *see also* Parkinsonism G20.C
     arteriosclerotic G21.4
   alternating (oculomotor) G83.89
   amyotrophic G12.21
   ankle G57.9- ☑
   anus (sphincter) K62.89
   arm — *see* Monoplegia, upper limb
   ascending (spinal), acute G61.0
   association G12.29
   asthenic bulbar G70.00
     with exacerbation (acute) G70.01
     in crisis G70.01
   ataxic (hereditary) G11.9
     general (syphilitic) A52.17
   atrophic G58.9
     infantile, acute — *see* Poliomyelitis, paralytic
     progressive G12.22
     spinal (acute) — *see* Poliomyelitis, paralytic
   axillary G54.0
   Babinski-Nageotte's G83.89
   Bell's G51.0
     newborn P11.3
   Benedikt's G46.3
   birth injury P14.9
     spinal cord P11.5
   bladder (neurogenic) (sphincter) N31.2
   bowel, colon or intestine K56.0
   brachial plexus G54.0
     birth injury P14.3
     newborn (birth injury) P14.3
   brain G83.9
     diplegia G83.0
     triplegia G83.89
   bronchial J98.09
   Brown-Sequard G83.81
   bulbar (chronic) (progressive) G12.22

Paralysis, paralytic — continued
- bulbar — continued
  - infantile — see Poliomyelitis, paralytic
  - poliomyelitic — see Poliomyelitis, paralytic
  - pseudo G12.29
- bulbospinal G70.00
  - with exacerbation (acute) G70.01
  - in crisis G70.01
- cardiac — see also Failure, heart I50.9
- cerebrocerebellar, diplegic G80.1
- cervical
  - plexus G54.2
  - sympathetic G90.09
- Céstan-Chenais G46.3
- Charcot-Marie-Tooth type G60.0
- Clark's G80.9
- colon K56.0
- compressed air T70.3- ☑
- compression
  - arm G56.9- ☑
  - leg G57.9- ☑
  - lower extremity G57.9- ☑
  - upper extremity G56.9- ☑
- congenital (cerebral) — see Palsy, cerebral
- conjugate movement (gaze) (of eye) H51.0
  - cortical (nuclear) (supranuclear) H51.0
- cordis — see Failure, heart
- cranial or cerebral nerve G52.9
- creeping G12.22
- crossed leg G83.89
- crutch — see Injury, brachial plexus
- deglutition R13.0
  - hysterical F44.4
- dementia A52.17
- descending (spinal) NEC G12.29
- diaphragm (flaccid) J98.6
  - due to accidental dissection of phrenic nerve during procedure — see Puncture, accidental complicating surgery
- digestive organs NEC K59.89
- diplegic — see Diplegia
- divergence (nuclear) H51.8
- diver's T70.3- ☑
- Duchenne's
  - birth injury P14.0
  - due to or associated with
    - motor neuron disease G12.22
    - muscular dystrophy G71.01
  - due to intracranial or spinal birth injury — see Palsy, cerebral
- embolic (current episode) I63.4- ☑
- Erb (-Duchenne) (birth) (newborn) P14.0
- Erb's syphilitic spastic spinal A52.17
- esophagus K22.89
- eye muscle (extrinsic) H49.9
  - intrinsic — see also Paresis, of accommodation
- facial (nerve) G51.0
  - birth injury P11.3
  - congenital P11.3
  - following operation NEC — see Puncture, accidental complicating surgery
  - newborn (birth injury) P11.3
- familial (recurrent) (periodic) G72.3
  - spastic G11.4
- fauces J39.2
- finger G56.9- ☑
- gait R26.1
- gastric nerve (nondiabetic) G52.2
- gaze, conjugate H51.0
- general (progressive) (syphilitic) A52.17
  - juvenile A50.45
- glottis J38.00
  - bilateral J38.02
  - unilateral J38.01
- gluteal G54.1
- Gubler (-Millard) G46.3
- hand — see Monoplegia, upper limb
- heart — see Arrest, cardiac
- hemiplegic — see Hemiplegia
- hyperkalemic periodic (familial) G72.3
- hypoglossal (nerve) G52.3
- hypokalemic periodic G72.3
- hysterical F44.4
- ileus K56.0
- infantile — see also Poliomyelitis, paralytic A80.30
  - bulbar — see Poliomyelitis, paralytic
  - cerebral — see Palsy, cerebral
  - spastic — see Palsy, cerebral, spastic

Paralysis, paralytic — continued
- infective — see Poliomyelitis, paralytic
- inferior nuclear G83.9
- internuclear — see Ophthalmoplegia, internuclear
- intestine K56.0
- iris H57.09
  - due to diphtheria (toxin) A36.89
- ischemic, Volkmann's (complicating trauma) T79.6- ☑
- Jackson's G83.89
- jake — see Poisoning, food, noxious, plant
- Jamaica ginger (jake) G62.2
- juvenile general A50.45
- Klumpke (-Dejerine) (birth) (newborn) P14.1
- labioglossal (laryngeal) (pharyngeal) G12.29
- Landry's G61.0
- laryngeal nerve (recurrent) (superior) (unilateral) J38.00
  - bilateral J38.02
  - unilateral J38.01
- larynx J38.00
  - bilateral J38.02
  - due to diphtheria (toxin) A36.2
  - unilateral J38.01
- lateral G12.23
- lead T56.0- ☑
- left side — see Hemiplegia
- leg G83.1- ☑
  - both — see Paraplegia
  - crossed G83.89
  - hysterical F44.4
  - psychogenic F44.4
  - transient or transitory R29.818
    - traumatic NEC — see Injury, nerve, leg
- levator palpebrae superioris — see Blepharoptosis, paralytic
- limb — see Monoplegia
- lip K13.0
- Lissauer's A52.17
- lower limb — see Monoplegia, lower limb
  - both — see Paraplegia
- lung J98.4
- median nerve G56.1- ☑
- medullary (tegmental) G83.89
- mesencephalic NEC G83.89
  - tegmental G83.89
- middle alternating G83.89
- Millard-Gubler-Foville G46.3
- monoplegic — see Monoplegia
- motor G83.9
- muscle, muscular NEC G72.89
  - due to nerve lesion G58.9
  - eye (extrinsic) H49.9
    - intrinsic — see Paresis, of accommodation
    - oblique — see Strabismus, paralytic, fourth nerve
  - iris sphincter H21.9
  - ischemic (Volkmann's) (complicating trauma) T79.6- ☑
  - progressive G12.21
  - progressive, spinal G12.25
  - pseudohypertrophic G71.02
  - spinal progressive G12.25
- musculocutaneous nerve G56.9- ☑
- musculospiral G56.9- ☑
- nerve — see also Disorder, nerve
  - abducent — see Strabismus, paralytic, sixth nerve
  - accessory G52.8
  - auditory (except Deafness) H93.3- ☑
  - birth injury P14.9
  - cranial or cerebral G52.9
  - facial
    - birth injury P11.3
    - congenital P11.3
    - newborn (birth injury) P11.3
  - fourth or trochlear — see Strabismus, paralytic, fourth nerve
  - newborn (birth injury) P14.9
  - oculomotor — see Strabismus, paralytic, third nerve
  - phrenic (birth injury) P14.2
  - radial G56.3- ☑
  - seventh or facial G51.0
    - newborn (birth injury) P11.3
  - sixth or abducent — see Strabismus, paralytic, sixth nerve
  - syphilitic A52.15
  - third or oculomotor — see Strabismus, paralytic, third nerve
  - trigeminal G50.9
  - trochlear — see Strabismus, paralytic, fourth nerve
- ulnar G56.2- ☑

Paralysis, paralytic — continued
- normokalemic periodic G72.3
- ocular H49.9
  - alternating G83.89
- oculofacial, congenital (Moebius) Q87.0
- oculomotor (external bilateral) (nerve) — see Strabismus, paralytic, third nerve
- palate (soft) K13.79
- paratrigeminal G50.9
- periodic (familial) (hyperkalemic) (hypokalemic) (myotonic) (normokalemic) (potassium sensitive) (secondary) G72.3
- peripheral autonomic nervous system — see Neuropathy, peripheral, autonomic
- peroneal (nerve) G57.3- ☑
- pharynx J39.2
- phrenic nerve G56.8- ☑
- plantar nerve(s) G57.6- ☑
- pneumogastric nerve G52.2
- poliomyelitis (current) — see Poliomyelitis, paralytic
- popliteal nerve G57.3- ☑
- postepileptic transitory G83.84
- progressive (atrophic) (bulbar) (spinal) G12.22
  - general A52.17
  - infantile acute — see Poliomyelitis, paralytic
  - supranuclear G23.1
- pseudobulbar G12.29
- pseudohypertrophic (muscle) — see also Dystrophy, muscular, by type, if applicable G71.09
- psychogenic F44.4
- quadriceps G57.9- ☑
- quadriplegic — see Tetraplegia
- radial nerve G56.3- ☑
- rectus muscle (eye) H49.9
- recurrent isolated sleep G47.53
- respiratory (muscle) (system) (tract) R06.81
  - center NEC G93.89
  - congenital P28.89
  - newborn P28.89
- right side — see Hemiplegia
- saturnine T56.0- ☑
- sciatic nerve G57.0- ☑
- senile G83.9
- shaking — see Parkinsonism
- shoulder G56.9- ☑
- sleep, recurrent isolated G47.53
- spastic G83.9
  - cerebral — see Palsy, cerebral, spastic
  - congenital (cerebral) — see Palsy, cerebral, spastic
  - familial G11.4
  - hereditary G11.4
  - quadriplegic G80.0
  - syphilitic (spinal) A52.17
- sphincter, bladder — see Paralysis, bladder
- spinal (cord) G83.9
  - accessory nerve G52.8
  - acute — see Poliomyelitis, paralytic
  - ascending acute G61.0
  - atrophic (acute) — see also Poliomyelitis, paralytic
    - spastic, syphilitic A52.17
  - congenital NEC — see Palsy, cerebral
  - hereditary G95.89
  - infantile — see Poliomyelitis, paralytic
  - progressive G12.21
    - muscle G12.25
  - sequelae NEC G83.89
- sternomastoid G52.8
- stomach K31.84
  - diabetic — see Diabetes, by type, with gastroparesis
  - nerve G52.2
    - diabetic — see Diabetes, by type, with gastroparesis
- stroke — see Infarct, brain
- subscapularis G56.8- ☑
- supranuclear (progressive) G23.1
- sympathetic G90.89
  - cervical G90.09
  - nervous system — see Neuropathy, peripheral, autonomic
- syndrome G83.9
  - specified NEC G83.89
- syphilitic spastic spinal (Erb's) A52.17
- thigh G57.9- ☑
- throat J39.2
  - diphtheritic A36.0
  - muscle J39.2
- thrombotic (current episode) I63.3- ☑
- thumb G56.9- ☑

☑ Additional Character Required — Refer to the Tabular List for Character Selection

Paralysis, paralytic — continued
- tick — see Toxicity, venom, arthropod, specified NEC
- Todd's (postepileptic transitory paralysis) G83.84
- toe G57.6- ☑
- tongue K14.8
- transient R29.5
  - arm or leg NEC R29.818
  - traumatic NEC — see Injury, nerve
- trapezius G52.8
- traumatic, transient NEC — see Injury, nerve
- trembling — see Parkinsonism
- triceps brachii G56.9- ☑
- trigeminal nerve G50.9
- trochlear (nerve) — see Strabismus, paralytic, fourth nerve
- ulnar nerve G56.2- ☑
- upper limb — see Monoplegia, upper limb
- uremic N18.9 [G99.8]
- uveoparotitic D86.89
- uvula K13.79
  - postdiphtheritic A36.0
- vagus nerve G52.2
- vasomotor NEC G90.89
- velum palati K13.79
- vesical — see Paralysis, bladder
- vestibular nerve (except Vertigo) H93.3- ☑
- vocal cords J38.00
  - bilateral J38.02
  - unilateral J38.01
- Volkmann's (complicating trauma) T79.6- ☑
- wasting G12.29
- Weber's G46.3
- wrist G56.9- ☑

Paramedial urethrovesical orifice Q64.79
Paramenia N92.6
Parametritis — see also Disease, pelvis, inflammatory N73.2
- acute N73.0
- complicating abortion — see Abortion, by type, complicated by, parametritis

Parametrium, parametric — see condition
Paramnesia — see Amnesia
Paramolar K00.1
Paramyloidosis E85.89
Paramyoclonus multiplex G25.3
Paramyotonia (congenita) G71.19
Parangi — see Yaws
Paranoia (querulans) F22
- senile F03.- ☑

Paranoid
- dementia (senile) F03.- ☑
  - praecox — see Schizophrenia
- personality F60.0
- psychosis (climacteric) (involutional) (menopausal) F22
  - psychogenic (acute) F23
  - senile F03.- ☑
- reaction (acute) F23
  - chronic F22
- schizophrenia F20.0
- state (climacteric) (involutional) (menopausal) (simple) F22
  - senile F03.- ☑
- tendencies F60.0
- traits F60.0
- trends F60.0
- type, psychopathic personality F60.0

Paraparesis — see Paraplegia
Paraphasia R47.02
Paraphilia F65.9
Paraphimosis (congenital) N47.2
- chancroidal A57

Paraphrenia, paraphrenic (late) F22
- schizophrenia F20.0

Paraplegia (lower) G82.20
- ataxic — see Degeneration, combined, spinal cord
- complete G82.21
- congenital (cerebral) G80.8
  - spastic G80.1
- familial spastic G11.4
- functional (hysterical) F44.4
- hereditary, spastic G11.4
- hysterical F44.4
- incomplete G82.22
- Pott's A18.01
- psychogenic F44.4
- spastic
  - Erb's spinal, syphilitic A52.17
  - hereditary G11.4
  - tropical G04.1

Paraplegia — continued
- syphilitic (spastic) A52.17
- traumatic
  - current injury — code to injury with seventh character A
  - sequela of previous injury — code to injury with seventh character S
- tropical spastic G04.1

Parapoxvirus B08.60
- specified NEC B08.69

Paraproteinemia D89.2
- benign (familial) D89.2
- monoclonal D47.2
- secondary to malignant disease D47.2

Parapsoriasis L41.9
- en plaques L41.4
- guttata L41.1
- large plaque L41.4
- retiform, retiformis L41.5
- small plaque L41.3
- specified NEC L41.8
- varioliformis (acuta) L41.0

Parasitic — see also condition
- disease NEC B89
- stomatitis B37.0
- sycosis (beard) (scalp) B35.0
- twin Q89.4

Parasitism B89
- intestinal B82.9
- skin B88.9
- specified — see Infestation

Parasitophobia F40.218
Parasomnia G47.50
- due to
  - alcohol
    - abuse F10.182
    - dependence F10.282
    - use F10.982
  - amphetamines
    - abuse F15.182
    - dependence F15.282
    - use F15.982
  - caffeine
    - abuse F15.182
    - dependence F15.282
    - use F15.982
  - cocaine
    - abuse F14.182
    - dependence F14.282
    - use F14.982
  - drug NEC
    - abuse F19.182
    - dependence F19.282
    - use F19.982
  - opioid
    - abuse F11.182
    - dependence F11.282
    - use F11.982
  - psychoactive substance NEC
    - abuse F19.182
    - dependence F19.282
    - use F19.982
  - sedative, hypnotic, or anxiolytic
    - abuse F13.182
    - dependence F13.282
    - use F13.982
  - stimulant NEC
    - abuse F15.182
    - dependence F15.282
    - use F15.982
- in conditions classified elsewhere G47.54
- nonorganic origin F51.8
- organic G47.50
- specified NEC G47.59

Paraspadias Q54.9
Paraspasmus facialis G51.8
Parasuicide (attempt)
- history of (personal) Z91.51
  - in family Z81.8

Parathyroid gland — see condition
Parathyroid tetany E20.9
Paratrachoma A74.0
Paratyphilitis — see Appendicitis
Paratyphoid (fever) — see Fever, paratyphoid
Paratyphus — see Fever, paratyphoid
Paraurethral duct Q64.79
Paraurethritis — see also Urethritis
- gonococcal (acute) (chronic) (with abscess) A54.1

Paravaccinia NEC B08.04

Paravaginitis — see Vaginitis
Parencephalitis — see also Encephalitis
- sequelae G09

Parent-child conflict — see Conflict, parent-child
- estrangement NEC Z62.890

Paresis — see also Paralysis
- accommodation — see Paresis, of accommodation
- Bernhardt's G57.1- ☑
- bladder (sphincter) — see also Paralysis, bladder
  - tabetic A52.17
- bowel, colon or intestine K56.0
- extrinsic muscle, eye H49.9
- general (progressive) (syphilitic) A52.17
  - juvenile A50.45
- heart — see Failure, heart
- insane (syphilitic) A52.17
- juvenile (general) A50.45
- of accommodation H52.52- ☑
- peripheral progressive (idiopathic) G60.3
- pseudohypertrophic — see also Dystrophy, muscular, by type, if applicable G71.09
- senile G83.9
- syphilitic (general) A52.17
  - congenital A50.45
- vesical NEC N31.2

Paresthesia — see also Disturbance, sensation, skin R20.2
- Bernhardt G57.1- ☑

Paretic — see condition
Parinaud's
- conjunctivitis H10.89
- oculoglandular syndrome H10.89
- ophthalmoplegia H49.88- ☑

Parkinsonism (idiopathic) (primary) G20.C
- with neurogenic orthostatic hypotension (symptomatic) G90.3
- arteriosclerotic G21.4
- dementia — see also Dementia, in, diseases specified elsewhere G20.C [F02.80]
  - with behavioral disturbance — see also Dementia, in, diseases specified elsewhere G20.C [F02.81-] ☑
- due to
  - drugs NEC G21.19
  - neuroleptic G21.11
- medication-induced NEC G21.19
- neuroleptic induced G21.11
- postencephalitic G21.3
- secondary G21.9
  - due to
    - arteriosclerosis G21.4
    - drugs NEC G21.19
      - neuroleptic G21.11
    - encephalitis G21.3
    - external agents NEC G21.2
    - syphilis A52.19
  - specified NEC G21.8
- syphilitic A52.19
- treatment-induced NEC G21.19
- vascular G21.4

Parkinson's disease, syndrome or tremor — see Parkinsonism

Parodontitis — see Periodontitis
Parodontosis K05.4
Paronychia — see also Cellulitis, digit
- with lymphangitis — see Lymphangitis, acute, digit
- candidal (chronic) B37.2
- tuberculous (primary) A18.4

Parorexia (psychogenic) F50.89
Parosmia R43.1
- psychogenic F45.8

Parotid gland — see condition
Parotitis, parotiditis (allergic) (nonspecific toxic) (purulent) (septic) (suppurative) — see also Sialoadenitis
- epidemic — see Mumps
- infectious — see Mumps
- postoperative K91.89
- surgical K91.89

Parrot fever A70
Parrot's disease (early congenital syphilitic pseudoparalysis) A50.02
Parry-Romberg syndrome G51.8
Parry's disease or syndrome E05.00
- with thyroid storm E05.01

Pars planitis — see Cyclitis
Parsonage (-Aldren)-Turner syndrome G54.5
Parson's disease (exophthalmic goiter) E05.00
- with thyroid storm E05.01

Particolored infant Q82.8
Parturition — see Delivery

Parulis K04.7
- with sinus K04.6

Parvovirus, as cause of disease classified elsewhere B97.6

Pasini and Pierini's atrophoderma L90.3

Passage
- false, urethra N36.5
- meconium (newborn) during delivery P03.82
- of sounds or bougies — see Attention to, artificial, opening

Passive — see condition
- smoking Z77.22

Past due on rent or mortgage Z59.81- ☑

Pasteurella septica A28.0

Pasteurellosis — see Infection, Pasteurella

PAT (paroxysmal atrial tachycardia) I47.19

Patau's syndrome — see Trisomy, 13

Patches
- mucous (syphilitic) A51.39
  - congenital A50.07
- smokers' (mouth) K13.24

Patellar — see condition

Patent — see also Imperfect, closure
- canal of Nuck Q52.4
- cervix N88.3
- ductus arteriosus or Botallo's Q25.0
- foramen
  - botalli Q21.12
  - ovale Q21.12
- interauricular septum Q21.19
- interventricular septum Q21.0
- omphalomesenteric duct Q43.0
- os (uteri) — see Patent, cervix
- ostium secundum (type II) Q21.11
- urachus Q64.4
- vitelline duct Q43.0

Paterson (-Brown) (-Kelly) **syndrome or web** D50.1

Pathologic, pathological — see also condition
- asphyxia R09.01
- fire-setting F63.1
- gambling F63.0
- ovum O02.0
- resorption, tooth K03.3
- stealing F63.2

Pathology (of) — see Disease
- periradicular, associated with previous endodontic treatment NEC M27.59

Pattern, sleep-wake, irregular G47.23

Patulous — see also Imperfect, closure (congenital)
- alimentary tract Q45.8
  - lower Q43.8
  - upper Q40.8
- eustachian tube H69.0- ☑

Pause, sinoatrial I49.5

Paxton's disease B36.2

Pearl(s)
- enamel K00.2
- Epstein's K09.8

Pearl-worker's disease — see Osteomyelitis, specified type NEC

Pectenosis K62.4

Pectoral — see condition

Pectus
- carinatum (congenital) Q67.7
  - acquired M95.4
  - rachitic sequelae (late effect) E64.3
- excavatum (congenital) Q67.6
  - acquired M95.4
  - rachitic sequelae (late effect) E64.3
- recurvatum (congenital) Q67.6

Pedatrophia E41

Pederosis F65.4

Pediatric inflammatory multisystem syndrome M35.81

Pediculosis (infestation) B85.2
- capitis (head-louse) (any site) B85.0
- corporis (body-louse) (any site) B85.1
- eyelid B85.0
- mixed (classifiable to more than one of the titles B85.0-B85.3) B85.4
- pubis (pubic louse) (any site) B85.3
- vestimenti B85.1
- vulvae B85.3

Pediculus (infestation) — see Pediculosis

Pedophilia F65.4

Peg-shaped teeth K00.2

Pelade — see Alopecia, areata

Pelger-Huet anomaly or syndrome D72.0

Peliosis (rheumatica) D69.0
- hepatis K76.4

Peliosis — continued
- hepatis — continued
  - with toxic liver disease K71.8

Pelizaeus-Merzbacher disease E75.27

Pellagra (alcoholic) E52
- with
  - polyneuropathy E52 [G63]

Pellagra-cerebellar-ataxia-renal aminoaciduria syndrome E72.02

Pellegrini (-Stieda) **disease or syndrome** — see Bursitis, tibial collateral

Pellizzi's syndrome E34.8

Pel's crisis A52.11

Pelvic — see also condition
- examination (periodic) (routine) Z01.419
  - with abnormal findings Z01.411
- kidney, congenital Q63.2

Pelviolithiasis — see Calculus, kidney

Pelviperitonitis — see also Peritonitis, pelvic
- gonococcal A54.24
- puerperal O85

Pelvis — see condition or type

Pemphigoid L12.9
- benign, mucous membrane L12.1
- bullous L12.0
- cicatricial L12.1
- juvenile L12.2
- ocular L12.1
- specified NEC L12.8

Pemphigus L10.9
- benign familial (chronic) Q82.8
- Brazilian L10.3
- circinatus L13.0
- conjunctiva L12.1
- drug-induced L10.5
- erythematosus L10.4
- foliaceus L10.2
- gangrenous — see Gangrene
- neonatorum L01.03
- ocular L12.1
- paraneoplastic L10.81
- specified NEC L10.89
- syphilitic (congenital) A50.06
- vegetans L10.1
- vulgaris L10.0
- wildfire L10.3

Pendred's syndrome E07.1

Pendulous
- abdomen, in pregnancy — see Pregnancy, complicated by, abnormal, pelvic organs or tissues NEC
- breast N64.89

Penetrating wound — see also Puncture
- with internal injury — see Injury, by site
- eyeball — see Puncture, eyeball
- orbit (with or without foreign body) — see Puncture, orbit
- uterus by instrument with or following ectopic or molar pregnancy O08.6

Penicillosis B48.4

Penis — see condition

Penitis N48.29

Pentalogy of Fallot Q21.8

Pentasomy X syndrome Q97.1

Pentosuria (essential) E74.89

Percreta placenta - O43.23- ☑

Peregrinating patient — see Disorder, factitious

Perforation, perforated (nontraumatic) (of)
- accidental during procedure (blood vessel) (nerve) (organ) — see Complication, accidental puncture or laceration
- antrum — see Sinusitis, maxillary
- appendix K35.32
  - with localized peritonitis K35.32
- atrial septum, multiple Q21.19
- attic, ear — see Perforation, tympanum, attic
- bile duct (common) (hepatic) K83.2
  - cystic K82.2
- bladder (urinary)
  - with or following ectopic or molar pregnancy O08.6
  - obstetrical trauma O71.5
  - traumatic S37.29- ☑
    - at delivery O71.5
- bowel K63.1
  - with or following ectopic or molar pregnancy O08.6
  - newborn P78.0
  - obstetrical trauma O71.5
  - traumatic — see Laceration, intestine
- broad ligament N83.8
  - with or following ectopic or molar pregnancy O08.6

Perforation, perforated — continued
- broad ligament — continued
  - obstetrical trauma O71.6
- by
  - device, implant or graft — see also Complications, by site and type, mechanical T85.628- ☑
    - arterial graft NEC — see Complication, cardiovascular device, mechanical, vascular
    - breast (implant) T85.49- ☑
    - catheter NEC T85.698- ☑
      - cystostomy T83.090- ☑
      - dialysis (renal) T82.49- ☑
        - intraperitoneal T85.691- ☑
      - infusion NEC T82.594- ☑
        - spinal (epidural) (subdural) T85.690- ☑
      - urinary — see also Complications, catheter, urinary T83.098- ☑
    - electronic (electrode) (pulse generator) (stimulator)
      - bone T84.390- ☑
      - cardiac T82.199- ☑
        - electrode T82.190- ☑
        - pulse generator T82.191- ☑
        - specified type NEC T82.198- ☑
      - nervous system — see Complication, prosthetic device, mechanical, electronic nervous system stimulator
      - urinary — see Complication, genitourinary, device, urinary, mechanical
    - fixation, internal (orthopedic) NEC — see Complication, fixation device, mechanical
    - gastrointestinal — see Complications, prosthetic device, mechanical, gastrointestinal device
    - genital NEC T83.498- ☑
      - intrauterine contraceptive device T83.39- ☑
      - penile prosthesis T83.490- ☑
    - heart NEC — see Complication, cardiovascular device, mechanical
    - joint prosthesis — see Complications, joint prosthesis, mechanical, specified NEC, by site
    - ocular NEC — see Complications, prosthetic device, mechanical, ocular device
    - orthopedic NEC — see Complication, orthopedic, device, mechanical
    - specified NEC T85.628- ☑
    - urinary NEC — see also Complication, genitourinary, device, urinary, mechanical
      - graft T83.29- ☑
    - vascular NEC — see Complication, cardiovascular device, mechanical
    - ventricular intracranial shunt T85.09- ☑
  - foreign body left accidentally in operative wound T81.539- ☑
  - instrument (any) during a procedure, accidental — see Puncture, accidental complicating surgery
- cecum K35.32
  - with localized peritonitis K35.32
- cervix (uteri) N88.8
  - with or following ectopic or molar pregnancy O08.6
  - obstetrical trauma O71.3
- colon K63.1
  - newborn P78.0
  - obstetrical trauma O71.5
  - traumatic — see Laceration, intestine, large
- common duct (bile) K83.2
- cornea (due to ulceration) — see Ulcer, cornea, perforated
- cystic duct K82.2
- diverticulum (intestine) K57.80
  - with bleeding K57.81
  - large intestine K57.20
    - with
      - bleeding K57.21
      - small intestine K57.40
        - with bleeding K57.41
  - small intestine K57.00
    - with
      - bleeding K57.01
      - large intestine K57.40
        - with bleeding K57.41
- ear drum — see Perforation, tympanum
- esophagus K22.3
- ethmoidal sinus — see Sinusitis, ethmoidal
- frontal sinus — see Sinusitis, frontal
- gallbladder K82.2
- heart valve — see Endocarditis
- ileum K63.1
  - newborn P78.0

Perforation, perforated — continued
  ileum — continued
    obstetrical trauma O71.5
    traumatic — see Laceration, intestine, small
  instrumental, surgical (accidental) (blood vessel) (nerve) (organ) — see Puncture, accidental complicating surgery
  intestine NEC K63.1
    with ectopic or molar pregnancy O08.6
    newborn P78.0
    obstetrical trauma O71.5
    traumatic — see Laceration, intestine
    ulcerative NEC K63.1
      newborn P78.0
  jejunum, jejunal K63.1
    obstetrical trauma O71.5
    traumatic — see Laceration, intestine, small
    ulcer — see Ulcer, gastrojejunal, with perforation
  joint prosthesis — see Complications, joint prosthesis, mechanical, specified NEC, by site
  mastoid (antrum) (cell) — see Disorder, mastoid, specified NEC
  maxillary sinus — see Sinusitis, maxillary
  membrana tympani — see Perforation, tympanum
  nasal
    septum J34.89
      congenital Q30.3
      syphilitic A52.73
    sinus J34.89
      congenital Q30.8
      due to sinusitis — see Sinusitis
  palate — see also Cleft, palate Q35.9
    syphilitic A52.79
  palatine vault — see also Cleft, palate, hard Q35.1
    syphilitic A52.79
    congenital A50.59
  pars flaccida (ear drum) — see Perforation, tympanum, attic
  pelvic
    floor S31.030- ☑
      with
        ectopic or molar pregnancy O08.6
        penetration into retroperitoneal space S31.031- ☑
        retained foreign body S31.040- ☑
          with penetration into retroperitoneal space S31.041- ☑
    following ectopic or molar pregnancy O08.6
    obstetrical trauma O70.1
    organ S37.99- ☑
      adrenal gland S37.818- ☑
      bladder — see Perforation, bladder
      fallopian tube S37.599- ☑
        bilateral S37.592- ☑
        unilateral S37.591- ☑
      kidney S37.09- ☑
      obstetrical trauma O71.5
      ovary S37.499- ☑
        bilateral S37.492- ☑
        unilateral S37.491- ☑
      prostate S37.828- ☑
      specified organ NEC S37.898- ☑
      ureter — see Perforation, ureter
      urethra — see Perforation, urethra
      uterus — see Perforation, uterus
  perineum — see Laceration, perineum
  pharynx J39.2
  rectum K63.1
    newborn P78.0
    obstetrical trauma O71.5
    traumatic S36.63- ☑
  root canal space due to endodontic treatment M27.51
  sigmoid K63.1
    newborn P78.0
    obstetrical trauma O71.5
    traumatic S36.533- ☑
  sinus (accessory) (chronic) (nasal) J34.89
  sphenoidal sinus — see Sinusitis, sphenoidal
  surgical (accidental) (by instrument) (blood vessel) (nerve) (organ) — see Puncture, accidental complicating surgery
  traumatic
    external — see Puncture
    eye — see Puncture, eyeball
    internal organ — see Injury, by site
  tympanum, tympanic (membrane) (persistent posttraumatic) (postinflammatory) H72.9- ☑
    attic H72.1- ☑

Perforation, perforated — continued
  tympanum, tympanic — continued
    attic — continued
      multiple — see Perforation, tympanum, multiple
      total — see Perforation, tympanum, total
    central H72.0- ☑
      multiple — see Perforation, tympanum, multiple
      total — see Perforation, tympanum, total
    marginal NEC — see subcategory H72.2- ☑
    multiple H72.81- ☑
    pars flaccida — see Perforation, tympanum, attic
    total H72.82- ☑
    traumatic, current episode S09.2- ☑
  typhoid, gastrointestinal — see Typhoid
  ulcer — see Ulcer, by site, with perforation
  ureter N28.89
    traumatic S37.19- ☑
  urethra N36.8
    with ectopic or molar pregnancy O08.6
    following ectopic or molar pregnancy O08.6
    obstetrical trauma O71.5
    traumatic S37.39- ☑
      at delivery O71.5
  uterus
    with ectopic or molar pregnancy O08.6
    by intrauterine contraceptive device T83.39- ☑
    following ectopic or molar pregnancy O08.6
    obstetrical trauma O71.1
    traumatic S37.69- ☑
      obstetric O71.1
  uvula K13.79
    syphilitic A52.79
  vagina O71.4
    obstetrical trauma O71.4
    other trauma — see Puncture, vagina
Periadenitis mucosa necrotica recurrens K12.0
Periappendicitis (acute) — see Appendicitis
Periarteritis nodosa (disseminated) (infectious) (necrotizing) M30.0
Periarthritis (joint) — see also Enthesopathy
  Duplay's M75.0- ☑
  gonococcal A54.42
  humeroscapularis — see Capsulitis, adhesive
  scapulohumeral — see Capsulitis, adhesive
  shoulder — see Capsulitis, adhesive
  wrist M77.2- ☑
Periarthrosis (angioneural) — see Enthesopathy
Pericapsulitis, adhesive (shoulder) — see Capsulitis, adhesive
Pericarditis (with decompensation) (with effusion) I31.9
  with rheumatic fever (conditions in I00)
    active — see Pericarditis, rheumatic
    inactive or quiescent I09.2
  acute (hemorrhagic) (nonrheumatic) (Sicca) I30.9
    with chorea (acute) (rheumatic) (Sydenham's) I02.0
    benign I30.8
    nonspecific I30.8
    rheumatic I01.0
      with chorea (acute) (Sydenham's) I02.0
  adhesive or adherent (chronic) (external) (internal) I31.0
    acute — see Pericarditis, acute
    rheumatic I09.2
  bacterial (acute) (subacute) (with serous or seropurulent effusion) I30.1
  calcareous I31.1
  cholesterol (chronic) I31.8
    acute I30.9
  chronic (nonrheumatic) I31.9
    rheumatic I09.2
  constrictive (chronic) I31.1
  coxsackie B33.23
  fibrinocaseous (tuberculous) A18.84
  fibrinopurulent I30.1
  fibrinous I30.8
  fibrous I31.0
  gonococcal A54.83
  idiopathic I30.0
  in systemic lupus erythematosus M32.12
  infective I30.1
  meningococcal A39.53
  neoplastic (chronic) I31.8
    acute I30.9
  obliterans, obliterating I31.0
  plastic I31.0
  pneumococcal I30.1
  postinfarction I24.1
  purulent I30.1

Pericarditis — continued
  rheumatic (active) (acute) (with effusion) (with pneumonia) I01.0
    with chorea (acute) (rheumatic) (Sydenham's) I02.0
    chronic or inactive (with chorea) I09.2
  rheumatoid — see Rheumatoid, carditis
  septic I30.1
  serofibrinous I30.8
  staphylococcal I30.1
  streptococcal I30.1
  suppurative I30.1
  syphilitic A52.06
  tuberculous A18.84
  uremic N18.9 [I32]
  viral I30.1
Pericardium, pericardial — see condition
Pericellulitis — see Cellulitis
Pericementitis (chronic) (suppurative) — see also Periodontitis
  acute K05.20
    generalized — see Periodontitis, aggressive, generalized
    localized — see Periodontitis, aggressive, localized
Perichondritis
  auricle — see Perichondritis, ear
  bronchus J98.09
  ear (external) H61.00- ☑
    acute H61.01- ☑
    chronic H61.02- ☑
  external auditory canal — see Perichondritis, ear
  larynx J38.7
    syphilitic A52.73
    typhoid A01.09
  nose J34.89
  pinna — see Perichondritis, ear
  trachea J39.8
Periclasia K05.4
Pericoronitis — see Periodontitis
Pericystitis N30.90
  with hematuria N30.91
Peridiverticulitis (intestine) K57.92
  cecum — see Diverticulitis, intestine, large
  colon — see Diverticulitis, intestine, large
  duodenum — see Diverticulitis, intestine, small
  intestine — see Diverticulitis, intestine
  jejunum — see Diverticulitis, intestine, small
  rectosigmoid — see Diverticulitis, intestine, large
  rectum — see Diverticulitis, intestine, large
  sigmoid — see Diverticulitis, intestine, large
Periendocarditis — see Endocarditis
Periepididymitis N45.1
Perifolliculitis L01.02
  abscedens, caput, scalp L66.3
  capitis, abscedens (et suffodiens) L66.3
  superficial pustular L01.02
Perihepatitis K65.8
Perilabyrinthitis (acute) — see subcategory H83.0- ☑
Perimeningitis — see Meningitis
Perimetritis — see Endometritis
Perimetrosalpingitis — see Salpingo-oophoritis
Perineocele N81.81
Perinephric, perinephritic — see condition
Perinephritis — see also Infection, kidney
  purulent — see Abscess, kidney
Perineum, perineal — see condition
Perineuritis NEC — see Neuralgia
Periodic — see condition
Periodontitis (chronic) (complex) (compound) (local) (simplex) K05.30
  acute K05.20
    generalized K05.229
      moderate K05.222
      severe K05.223
      slight K05.221
    localized K05.219
      moderate K05.212
      severe K05.213
      slight K05.211
  aggressive K05.20
    generalized K05.229
      moderate K05.222
      severe K05.223
      slight K05.221
    localized K05.219
      moderate K05.212
      severe K05.213
      slight K05.211
  apical K04.5
    acute (pulpal origin) K04.4

Periodontitis — continued
  generalized K05.329
    moderate K05.322
    severe K05.323
    slight K05.321
  localized K05.319
    moderate K05.312
    severe K05.313
    slight K05.311
Periodontoclasia K05.4
Periodontosis (juvenile) K05.4
Periods — see also Menstruation
  heavy N92.0
  irregular N92.6
  shortened intervals (irregular) N92.1
Perionychia — see also Cellulitis, digit
  with lymphangitis — see Lymphangitis, acute, digit
Perioophoritis — see Salpingo-oophoritis
Periorchitis N45.2
Periosteum, periosteal — see condition
Periostitis (albuminosa) (circumscribed) (diffuse) (infective) (monomelic) — see also Osteomyelitis
  alveolar M27.3
  alveolodental M27.3
  dental M27.3
  gonorrheal A54.43
  jaw (lower) (upper) M27.2
  orbit H05.03- ☑
  syphilitic A52.77
    congenital (early) A50.02 [M90.80]
    secondary A51.46
  tuberculous — see Tuberculosis, bone
  yaws (hypertrophic) (early) (late) A66.6 [M90.80]
Periostosis (hyperplastic) — see also Disorder, bone, specified type NEC
  with osteomyelitis — see Osteomyelitis, specified type NEC
Peripartum
  cardiomyopathy O90.3
Periphlebitis — see Phlebitis
Periproctitis K62.89
Periprostatitis — see Prostatitis
Perirectal — see condition
Perirenal — see condition
Perisalpingitis — see Salpingo-oophoritis
Perisplenitis (infectional) D73.89
Peristalsis, visible or reversed R19.2
Peritendinitis — see Enthesopathy
Peritoneum, peritoneal — see condition
Peritonitis (adhesive) (bacterial) (fibrinous) (hemorrhagic) (idiopathic) (localized) (perforative) (primary) (with adhesions) (with effusion) K65.9
  with or following
    abscess K65.1
    appendicitis
      with perforation or rupture K35.32
        generalized — see also Appendicitis K35.209
        localized — see also Appendicitis K35.30
    diverticular disease (intestine) K57.80
      with bleeding K57.81
    ectopic or molar pregnancy O08.0
    large intestine K57.20
      with
        bleeding K57.21
        small intestine K57.40
          with bleeding K57.41
    small intestine K57.00
      with
        bleeding K57.01
        large intestine K57.40
          with bleeding K57.41
  acute (generalized) K65.0
  aseptic T81.61- ☑
  bile, biliary K65.3
  chemical T81.61- ☑
  chlamydial A74.81
  chronic proliferative K65.8
  complicating abortion — see Abortion, by type, complicated by, pelvic peritonitis
  congenital P78.1
  diaphragmatic K65.0
  diffuse K65.0
  diphtheritic A36.89
  disseminated K65.0
  due to
    bile K65.3
    foreign
      body or object accidentally left during a procedure (instrument) (sponge) (swab) T81.599- ☑

Peritonitis — continued
  due to — continued
    foreign — continued
      substance accidentally left during a procedure (chemical) (powder) (talc) T81.61- ☑
    talc T81.61- ☑
    urine K65.8
  eosinophilic K65.8
    acute K65.0
  fibrocaseous (tuberculous) A18.31
  fibropurulent K65.0
  following ectopic or molar pregnancy O08.0
  general (ized) K65.0
  gonococcal A54.85
  meconium (newborn) P78.0
  neonatal P78.1
    meconium P78.0
  pancreatic K65.0
  paroxysmal, familial E85.0
    benign E85.0
  pelvic
    female N73.5
      acute N73.3
      chronic N73.4
        with adhesions N73.6
    male K65.0
  periodic, familial E85.0
  proliferative, chronic K65.8
  puerperal, postpartum, childbirth O85
  purulent K65.0
  septic K65.0
  specified NEC K65.8
  spontaneous bacterial K65.2
  subdiaphragmatic K65.0
  subphrenic K65.0
  suppurative K65.0
  syphilitic A52.74
    congenital (early) A50.08 [K67]
  talc T81.61- ☑
  tuberculous A18.31
  urine K65.8
Peritonsillar — see condition
Peritonsillitis J36
Perityphlitis — see also Cecitis K37
Periureteritis N28.89
Periurethral — see condition
Periurethritis (gangrenous) — see Urethritis
Periuterine — see condition
Perivaginitis — see Vaginitis
Perivasculitis, retinal H35.06- ☑
Perivasitis (chronic) N49.1
Perivesiculitis (seminal) — see Vesiculitis
Perlèche NEC K13.0
  due to
    candidiasis B37.83
    moniliasis B37.83
    riboflavin deficiency E53.0
    vitamin B2 (riboflavin) deficiency E53.0
Pernicious — see condition
Pernio, perniosis T69.1- ☑
Perpetrator (of abuse) — see Index to External Causes of Injury, Perpetrator
Persecution
  delusion F22
  social Z60.5
Perseveration (tonic) R48.8
Persistence, persistent (congenital)
  anal membrane Q42.3
    with fistula Q42.2
  arteria stapedia Q16.3
  atrioventricular canal Q21.20
  branchial cleft NOS Q18.2
    cyst Q18.0
    fistula Q18.0
    sinus Q18.0
  bulbus cordis in left ventricle Q21.8
  canal of Cloquet Q14.0
  capsule (opaque) Q12.8
  cilioretinal artery or vein Q14.8
  cloaca Q43.7
  communication — see Fistula, congenital
  convolutions
    aortic arch Q25.46
    fallopian tube Q50.6
    oviduct Q50.6
    uterine tube Q50.6
  double aortic arch Q25.45
  ductus arteriosus (Botalli) Q25.0

Persistence, persistent — continued
  fetal
    circulation P29.38
    form of cervix (uteri) Q51.828
    hemoglobin, hereditary (HPFH) D56.4
  foramen
    Botalli Q21.12
    ovale Q21.12
  Gartner's duct Q52.4
  hemoglobin, fetal (hereditary) (HPFH) D56.4
  hyaloid
    artery (generally incomplete) Q14.0
    system Q14.8
  hymen, in pregnancy or childbirth — see Pregnancy, complicated by, abnormal, vulva
  lanugo Q84.2
  left
    posterior cardinal vein Q26.8
    root with right arch of aorta Q25.49
    superior vena cava Q26.1
  Meckel's diverticulum Q43.0
    malignant — see Table of Neoplasms, small intestine, malignant
  mucosal disease (middle ear) — see Otitis, media, suppurative, chronic, tubotympanic
  nail(s), anomalous Q84.6
  omphalomesenteric duct Q43.0
  organ or site not listed — see Anomaly, by site
  ostium
    atrioventriculare commune Q21.23
    primum Q21.20
    secundum Q21.11
  ovarian rests in fallopian tube Q50.6
  pancreatic tissue in intestinal tract Q43.8
  primary (deciduous)
    teeth K00.6
    vitreous hyperplasia Q14.0
  pupillary membrane Q13.89
  rhesus (Rh) titer — see Complication(s), transfusion, incompatibility reaction, Rh (factor)
  right aortic arch Q25.47
  sinus
    urogenitalis
      female Q52.8
      male Q55.8
    venosus with imperfect incorporation in right auricle Q26.8
  thymus (gland) (hyperplasia) E32.0
  thyroglossal duct Q89.2
  thyrolingual duct Q89.2
  truncus arteriosus or communis Q20.0
  tunica vasculosa lentis Q12.2
  umbilical sinus Q64.4
  urachus Q64.4
  vitelline duct Q43.0
Person (with)
  admitted for clinical research, as a control subject (normal comparison) (participant) Z00.6
  awaiting admission to adequate facility elsewhere Z75.1
  concern (normal) about sick person in family Z63.6
  consulting on behalf of another Z71.0
  feigning illness Z76.5
  living (in)
    alone Z60.2
    boarding school Z59.3
    residential institution Z59.3
    without
      adequate housing Z59.10
        air conditioning Z59.11
        environmental temperature Z59.11
          heating Z59.11
          space Z59.19
        housing (permanent) (temporary) Z59.00
      person able to render necessary care Z74.2
      shelter Z59.02
  on waiting list Z75.1
  sick or handicapped in family Z63.6
Personality (disorder) F60.9
  accentuation of traits (type A pattern) Z73.1
  affective F34.0
  aggressive F60.3
  amoral F60.2
  anacastic, anankastic F60.5
  antisocial F60.2
  anxious F60.6
  asocial F60.2
  asthenic F60.7
  avoidant F60.6
  borderline F60.3

Personality — *continued*
  change due to organic condition (enduring) F07.0
  compulsive F60.5
  cycloid F34.0
  cyclothymic F34.0
  dependent F60.7
  depressive F34.1
  dissocial F60.2
  dual F44.81
  eccentric F60.89
  emotionally unstable F60.3
  expansive paranoid F60.0
  explosive F60.3
  fanatic F60.0
  haltlose type F60.89
  histrionic F60.4
  hyperthymic F34.0
  hypothymic F34.1
  hysterical F60.4
  immature F60.89
  inadequate F60.7
  labile (emotional) F60.3
  mixed (nonspecific) F60.89
  morally defective F60.2
  multiple F44.81
  narcissistic F60.81
  obsessional F60.5
  obsessive (-compulsive) F60.5
  organic F07.0
  overconscientious F60.5
  paranoid F60.0
  passive (-dependent) F60.7
  passive-aggressive F60.89
  pathologic F60.9
  pattern defect or disturbance F60.9
  pseudopsychopathic (organic) F07.0
  pseudoretarded (organic) F07.0
  psychoinfantile F60.4
  psychoneurotic NEC F60.89
  psychopathic F60.2
  querulant F60.0
  sadistic F60.89
  schizoid F60.1
  self-defeating F60.89
  sensitive paranoid F60.0
  sociopathic (amoral) (antisocial) (asocial) (dissocial) F60.2
  specified NEC F60.89
  type A Z73.1
  unstable (emotional) F60.3
Perthes' disease — *see* Legg-Calve-Perthes disease
Pertussis — *see also* Whooping cough A37.90
Perversion, perverted
  appetite F50.89
    psychogenic F50.89
  function
    pituitary gland E23.2
      posterior lobe E22.2
  sense of smell and taste R43.8
    psychogenic F45.8
  sexual — *see* Deviation, sexual
Pervious, congenital — *see also* Imperfect, closure
  ductus arteriosus Q25.0
Pes (congenital) — *see also* Talipes
  acquired — *see also* Deformity, limb, foot, specified NEC
    planus — *see* Deformity, limb, flat foot
  adductus Q66.89
  cavus Q66.7- ☑
  deformity NEC, acquired — *see* Deformity, limb, foot, specified NEC
  planus (acquired) (any degree) — *see also* Deformity, limb, flat foot
    rachitic sequelae (late effect) E64.3
  valgus Q66.6
Pest, pestis — *see* Plague
Petechia, petechiae R23.3
  newborn P54.5
Petechial typhus A75.9
Peter's anomaly Q13.4
Petit mal seizure — *see* Epilepsy, childhood, absence
Petit's hernia — *see* Hernia, abdomen, specified site NEC
Petrellidosis B48.2
Petrositis H70.20- ☑
  acute H70.21- ☑
  chronic H70.22- ☑
Peutz-Jeghers disease or syndrome Q85.89
Peyronie's disease N48.6
PFAPA (periodic fever, aphthous stomatitis, pharyngitis, and adenopathy syndrome) M04.8
Pfeiffer's disease — *see* Mononucleosis, infectious

Phagedena (dry) (moist) (sloughing) — *see also* Gangrene
  geometric L88
  penis N48.29
  tropical — *see* Ulcer, skin
  vulva N76.6
Phagedenic — *see* condition
Phakoma H35.89
Phakomatosis — *see also* specific eponymous syndromes Q85.9
  Bourneville's Q85.1
  specified NEC Q85.89
Phantom limb syndrome (without pain) G54.7
  with pain G54.6
Pharyngeal pouch syndrome D82.1
Pharyngitis (acute) (catarrhal) (gangrenous) (infective) (malignant) (membranous) (phlegmonous) (pseudomembranous) (simple) (subacute) (suppurative) (ulcerative) (viral) J02.9
  with influenza, flu, or grippe — *see* Influenza, with, pharyngitis
  aphthous B08.5
  atrophic J31.2
  chlamydial A56.4
  chronic (atrophic) (granular) (hypertrophic) J31.2
  coxsackievirus B08.5
  diphtheritic A36.0
  enteroviral vesicular B08.5
  follicular (chronic) J31.2
  fusospirochetal A69.1
  gonococcal A54.5
  granular (chronic) J31.2
  herpesviral B00.2
  hypertrophic J31.2
  infectional, chronic J31.2
  influenzal — *see* Influenza, with, respiratory manifestations NEC
  lymphonodular, acute (enteroviral) B08.8
  pneumococcal J02.8
  purulent J02.9
  putrid J02.9
  septic J02.0
  sicca J31.2
  specified organism NEC J02.8
  staphylococcal J02.8
  streptococcal J02.0
  syphilitic, congenital (early) A50.03
  tuberculous A15.8
  vesicular, enteroviral B08.5
  viral NEC J02.8
Pharyngoconjunctivitis, viral B30.2
Pharyngolaryngitis (acute) J06.0
  chronic J37.0
Pharyngoplegia J39.2
Pharyngotonsillitis, herpesviral B00.2
Pharyngotracheitis, chronic J42
Pharynx, pharyngeal — *see* condition
Phelan-McDermid syndrome Q93.52
Phencyclidine-induced
  anxiety disorder F16.980
  bipolar and related disorder F16.94
  depressive disorder F16.94
  psychotic disorder F16.959
Phenomenon
  Arthus' — *see* Arthus' phenomenon
  jaw-winking Q07.8
  lupus erythematosus (LE) cell M32.9
  Raynaud's (secondary) I73.00
    with gangrene I73.01
  vasomotor R55
  vasospastic I73.9
  vasovagal R55
  Wenckebach's I44.1
Phenotype
  Duffy
    a positive Z67.A2
    a and b positive Z67.A4
    b positive Z67.A3
    Fy (a+b-) Z67.A2
    Fy (a-b-) Z67.A1
    Fy (a-b+) Z67.A3
    Fy (a+b+) Z67.A4
    null Z67.A1
Phenylketonuria E70.1
  classical E70.0
  maternal E70.1
Pheochromoblastoma
  specified site — *see* Neoplasm, malignant, by site
  unspecified site C74.10

Pheochromocytoma
  malignant
    specified site — *see* Neoplasm, malignant, by site
    unspecified site C74.10
  specified site — *see* Neoplasm, benign, by site
  unspecified site D35.00
Pheohyphomycosis — *see* Chromomycosis
Pheomycosis — *see* Chromomycosis
Phimosis (congenital) (due to infection) N47.1
  chancroidal A57
Phlebectasia — *see also* Varix
  congenital Q27.4
Phlebitis (infective) (pyemic) (septic) (suppurative) I80.9
  antepartum — *see* Thrombophlebitis, antepartum
  blue — *see* Phlebitis, leg, deep
  breast, superficial I80.8
  calf muscular vein (NOS) I80.25- ☑
  cavernous (venous) sinus — *see* Phlebitis, intracranial (venous) sinus
  cerebral (venous) sinus — *see* Phlebitis, intracranial (venous) sinus
  chest wall, superficial I80.8
  cranial (venous) sinus — *see* Phlebitis, intracranial (venous) sinus
  deep (vessels) — *see* Phlebitis, leg, deep
  due to implanted device — *see* Complications, by site and type, specified NEC
  during or resulting from a procedure T81.72- ☑
  femoral vein (superficial) I80.1- ☑
  femoropopliteal vein I80.0- ☑
  gastrocnemial vein I80.25- ☑
  gestational — *see* Phlebopathy, gestational
  hepatic veins I80.8
  iliac vein (common) (external) (internal) I80.21- ☑
  iliofemoral — *see* Phlebitis, femoral vein
  intracranial (venous) sinus (any) G08
    nonpyogenic I67.6
  intraspinal venous sinuses and veins G08
    nonpyogenic G95.19
  lateral (venous) sinus — *see* Phlebitis, intracranial (venous) sinus
  leg I80.3
    antepartum — *see* Thrombophlebitis, antepartum
    deep (vessels) NEC I80.20- ☑
      iliac I80.21- ☑
      popliteal vein I80.22- ☑
      specified vessel NEC I80.29- ☑
      tibial vein (anterior) (posterior) I80.23- ☑
    femoral vein (superficial) I80.1- ☑
    superficial (vessels) I80.0- ☑
  longitudinal sinus — *see* Phlebitis, intracranial (venous) sinus
  lower limb — *see* Phlebitis, leg
  migrans, migrating (superficial) I82.1
  pelvic
    with ectopic or molar pregnancy O08.0
    following ectopic or molar pregnancy O08.0
    puerperal, postpartum O87.1
  peroneal vein I80.24- ☑
  popliteal vein — *see* Phlebitis, leg, deep, popliteal
  portal (vein) K75.1
  postoperative T81.72- ☑
  pregnancy — *see* Thrombophlebitis, antepartum
  puerperal, postpartum, childbirth O87.0
    deep O87.1
    pelvic O87.1
    superficial O87.0
  retina — *see* Vasculitis, retina
  saphenous (accessory) (great) (long) (small) — *see* Phlebitis, leg, superficial
  sinus (meninges) — *see* Phlebitis, intracranial (venous) sinus
  soleal vein I80.25- ☑
  specified site NEC I80.8
  syphilitic A52.09
  tibial vein — *see* Phlebitis, leg, deep, tibial
  ulcerative I80.9
    leg — *see* Phlebitis, leg
  umbilicus I80.8
  uterus (septic) — *see* Endometritis
  varicose (leg) (lower limb) — *see* Varix, leg, with, inflammation
Phlebofibrosis I87.8
Phleboliths I87.8
Phlebopathy,
  gestational O22.9- ☑
  puerperal O87.9
Phlebosclerosis I87.8

Phlebothrombosis — *see also* Thrombosis
- antepartum — *see* Thrombophlebitis, antepartum
- pregnancy — *see* Thrombophlebitis, antepartum
- puerperal — *see* Thrombophlebitis, puerperal

Phlebotomus fever A93.1

Phlegmasia
- alba dolens O87.1
  - nonpuerperal — *see* Phlebitis, femoral vein
- cerulea dolens — *see* Phlebitis, leg, deep

Phlegmon — *see* Abscess

Phlegmonous — *see* condition

Phlyctenulosis (allergic) (keratoconjunctivitis) (nontuberculous) — *see also* Keratoconjunctivitis
- cornea — *see* Keratoconjunctivitis
- tuberculous A18.52

Phobia, phobic F40.9
- animal F40.218
  - spiders F40.210
- examination F40.298
- reaction F40.9
- simple F40.298
- social F40.10
  - generalized F40.11
- specific (isolated) F40.298
  - animal F40.218
    - spiders F40.210
  - blood F40.230
  - injection F40.231
  - injury F40.233
  - men F40.290
  - natural environment F40.228
    - thunderstorms F40.220
  - situational F40.248
    - bridges F40.242
    - closed in spaces F40.240
    - flying F40.243
    - heights F40.241
  - specified focus NEC F40.298
  - transfusion F40.231
  - women F40.291
- specified NEC F40.8
  - medical care NEC F40.232
- state F40.9

Phocas' disease — *see* Mastopathy, cystic

Phocomelia Q73.1
- lower limb — *see* Agenesis, leg, with foot present
- upper limb — *see* Agenesis, arm, with hand present

Phoria H50.50

Phosphate-losing tubular disorder N25.0

Phosphatemia E83.39

Phosphaturia E83.39

Photodermatitis (sun) L56.8
- chronic L57.8
- due to drug L56.8
- light other than sun L59.8

Photokeratitis H16.13- ☑

Photophobia H53.14- ☑

Photophthalmia — *see* Photokeratitis

Photopsia H53.19

Photoretinitis — *see* Retinopathy, solar

Photosensitivity, photosensitization (sun) skin L56.8
- light other than sun L59.8

Phrenitis — *see* Encephalitis

Phrynoderma (vitamin A deficiency) E50.8

Phthiriasis (pubis) B85.3
- with any infestation classifiable to B85.0-B85.2 B85.4

Phthirus infestation — *see* Phthiriasis

Phthisis — *see also* Tuberculosis
- bulbi (infectional) — *see* Disorder, globe, degenerated condition, atrophy
- eyeball (due to infection) — *see* Disorder, globe, degenerated condition, atrophy

PHTS Q85.81

Phycomycosis — *see* Zygomycosis

Physalopteriasis B81.8

Physical restraint status Z78.1

Phytobezoar T18.9- ☑
- intestine T18.3- ☑
- stomach T18.2- ☑

Pian — *see* Yaws

Pianoma A66.1

Pica F50.89
- in adults (in remission) F50.83
- infant or child (in remission) F98.3

Pick-Niemann disease — *see* Niemann-Pick disease or syndrome

Picking, nose F98.8

Pick's
- cerebral atrophy — *see also* Dementia, in, diseases specified elsewhere G31.01 [F02.80]
  - with behavioral disturbance — *see also* Dementia, in, diseases specified elsewhere G31.01 [F02.81-] ☑
- disease or syndrome (brain) — *see also* Dementia, in, diseases specified elsewhere G31.01 [F02.80]
  - with behavioral disturbance — *see also* Dementia, in, diseases specified elsewhere G31.01 [F02.81-] ☑
- brain — *see also* Dementia, in, diseases specified elsewhere G31.01 [F02.80]
  - with behavioral disturbance — *see also* Dementia, in, diseases specified elsewhere G31.01 [F02.81-] ☑
- pericardium (pericardial pseudocirrhosis of liver) I31.1
- syndrome
  - brain — *see also* Dementia, in, diseases specified elsewhere G31.01 [F02.80]
    - with behavioral disturbance — *see also* Dementia, in, diseases specified elsewhere G31.01 [F02.81-] ☑
  - of heart (pericardial pseudocirrhosis of liver) I31.1

Pickwickian syndrome E66.2

Piebaldism E70.39

Piedra (beard) (scalp) B36.8
- black B36.3
- white B36.2

Pierre Robin deformity or syndrome Q87.0

Pierson's disease or osteochondrosis M91.0

Pig-bel A05.2

Pigeon
- breast or chest (acquired) M95.4
  - congenital Q67.7
  - rachitic sequelae (late effect) E64.3
- breeder's disease or lung J67.2
- fancier's disease or lung J67.2
- toe — *see* Deformity, toe, specified NEC

Pigmentation (abnormal) (anomaly) L81.9
- conjunctiva H11.13- ☑
- cornea (anterior) H18.01- ☑
  - posterior H18.05- ☑
  - stromal H18.06- ☑
- diminished melanin formation NEC L81.6
- iron L81.8
- lids, congenital Q82.8
- limbus corneae — *see* Pigmentation, cornea
- metals L81.8
- optic papilla, congenital Q14.2
- retina, congenital (grouped) (nevoid) Q14.1
- scrotum, congenital Q82.8
- tattoo L81.8

Piles — *see also* Hemorrhoids K64.9

Pili
- annulati or torti (congenital) Q84.1
- incarnati L73.1

Pill roller hand (intrinsic) — *see* Parkinsonism

Pilomatrixoma — *see* Neoplasm, skin, benign
- malignant — *see* Neoplasm, skin, malignant

Pilonidal — *see* condition

Pimple R23.8

PIMS M35.81

PIN — *see* Neoplasia, intraepithelial, prostate

Pinched nerve — *see* Neuropathy, entrapment

Pindborg tumor — *see* Cyst, calcifying odontogenic

Pineal body or gland — *see* condition

Pinealoblastoma C75.3

Pinealoma D44.5
- malignant C75.3

Pineoblastoma C75.3

Pineocytoma D44.5

Pinguecula H11.15- ☑

Pingueculitis H10.81- ☑

Pinhole meatus — *see also* Stricture, urethra N35.919

Pink
- disease — *see* subcategory T56.1- ☑
- eye — *see* Conjunctivitis, acute, mucopurulent

Pinkus' disease (lichen nitidus) L44.1

Pinpoint
- meatus — *see* Stricture, urethra
- os (uteri) — *see* Stricture, cervix

Pins and needles R20.2

Pinta A67.9
- cardiovascular lesions A67.2
- chancre (primary) A67.0
- erythematous plaques A67.1
- hyperchromic lesions A67.1

Pinta — *continued*
- hyperkeratosis A67.1
- lesions A67.9
  - cardiovascular A67.2
  - hyperchromic A67.1
  - intermediate A67.1
  - late A67.2
  - mixed A67.3
  - primary A67.0
  - skin (achromic) (cicatricial) (dyschromic) A67.2
    - hyperchromic A67.1
    - mixed (achromic and hyperchromic) A67.3
- papule (primary) A67.0
- skin lesions (achromic) (cicatricial) (dyschromic) A67.2
  - hyperchromic A67.1
  - mixed (achromic and hyperchromic) A67.3
- vitiligo A67.2

Pintids A67.1

Pinworm (disease) (infection) (infestation) B80

Piroplasmosis — *see also* Babesiosis B60.00
- specified NEC B60.09

Pistol wound — *see* Gunshot wound

Pitchers' elbow — *see* Derangement, joint, specified type NEC, elbow

Pithecoid pelvis Q74.2
- with disproportion (fetopelvic) O33.0
  - causing obstructed labor O65.0

Pithiatism F48.8

Pitted — *see* Pitting

Pitting — *see also* Edema R60.9
- lip R60.0
- nail L60.8
- teeth K00.4

Pituitary gland — *see* condition

Pituitary-snuff-taker's disease J67.8

Pityriasis (capitis) L21.0
- alba L30.5
- circinata (et maculata) L42
- furfuracea L21.0
- Hebra's L26
- lichenoides L41.0
  - chronica L41.1
  - et varioliformis (acuta) L41.0
- maculata (et circinata) L30.5
- nigra B36.1
- pilaris, Hebra's L44.0
- rosea L42
- rotunda L44.8
- rubra (Hebra) pilaris L44.0
- simplex L30.5
- specified type NEC L30.5
- streptogenes L30.5
- versicolor (scrotal) B36.0

Placenta, placental — *see* Pregnancy, complicated by (care of) (management affected by), specified condition

Placentitis O41.14- ☑

Plagiocephaly Q67.3
- non-deformational
  - anterior Q75.021
  - posterior Q75.04- ☑

Plague A20.9
- abortive A20.8
- ambulatory A20.8
- asymptomatic A20.8
- bubonic A20.0
- cellulocutaneous A20.1
- cutaneobubonic A20.1
- lymphatic gland A20.0
- meningitis A20.3
- pharyngeal A20.8
- pneumonic (primary) (secondary) A20.2
- pulmonary, pulmonic A20.2
- septicemic A20.7
- tonsillar A20.8
  - septicemic A20.7

Planning, family
- contraception Z30.9
- procreation Z31.69

Plaque(s)
- artery, arterial — *see* Arteriosclerosis
- calcareous — *see* Calcification
- coronary, lipid rich I25.83
- epicardial I31.8
- erythematous, of pinta A67.1
- Hollenhorst's — *see* Occlusion, artery, retina
- lipid rich, coronary I25.83
- pleural (without asbestos) J92.9
  - with asbestos J92.0
- tongue K13.29

Plasmacytoma C90.3- ☑
  extramedullary C90.2- ☑
  medullary C90.0- ☑
  solitary C90.3- ☑
Plasmacytopenia D72.818
Plasmacytosis D72.822
Plaster ulcer — see Ulcer, pressure, by site
Plateau iris syndrome (post-iridectomy) (postprocedural) (without glaucoma) H21.82
  with glaucoma H40.22- ☑
Platybasia Q75.8
Platyonychia (congenital) Q84.6
  acquired L60.8
Platypelloid pelvis M95.5
  with disproportion (fetopelvic) O33.0
    causing obstructed labor O65.0
  congenital Q74.2
Platyspondylisis Q76.49
Plaut (-Vincent) **disease** — see also Vincent's A69.1
Plethora R23.2
  newborn P61.1
Pleura, pleural — see condition
Pleuralgia R07.81
Pleurisy (acute) (adhesive) (chronic) (costal) (diaphragmatic) (double) (dry) (fibrinous) (fibrous) (interlobar) (latent) (plastic) (primary) (residual) (sicca) (sterile) (subacute) (unresolved) R09.1
  with
    adherent pleura J86.0
    effusion J90
      chylous, chyliform J94.0
      tuberculous (non primary) A15.6
        primary (progressive) A15.7
    tuberculosis — see Pleurisy, tuberculous (non primary)
  encysted — see Pleurisy, with effusion
  exudative — see Pleurisy, with effusion
  fibrinopurulent, fibropurulent — see Pyothorax
  hemorrhagic — see Hemothorax
  pneumococcal J90
  purulent — see Pyothorax
  septic — see Pyothorax
  serofibrinous — see Pleurisy, with effusion
  seropurulent — see Pyothorax
  serous — see Pleurisy, with effusion
  staphylococcal J86.9
  streptococcal J90
  suppurative — see Pyothorax
  traumatic (post) (current) — see Injury, intrathoracic, pleura
  tuberculous (with effusion) (non primary) A15.6
    primary (progressive) A15.7
Pleuritis sicca — see Pleurisy
Pleuro-pneumonia-like-organism (PPLO), as cause of disease classified elsewhere B96.0
Pleurobronchopneumonia — see Pneumonia, broncho-
Pleurodynia R07.81
  epidemic B33.0
  viral B33.0
Pleuropericarditis — see also Pericarditis
  acute I30.9
Pleuropneumonia (acute) (bilateral) (double) (septic) — see also Pneumonia J18.8
  chronic — see Fibrosis, lung
Pleurorrhea — see Pleurisy, with effusion
Plexitis, brachial G54.0
Plica
  polonica B85.0
  syndrome, knee M67.5- ☑
  tonsil J35.8
Plicated tongue K14.5
Plug
  bronchus NEC J98.09
  meconium (newborn) NEC syndrome P76.0
  mucus — see Asphyxia, mucus
Plumbism — see subcategory T56.0- ☑
Plummer-Vinson syndrome D50.1
Plummer's disease E05.20
  with thyroid storm E05.21
Pluricarential syndrome of infancy E40
Plus (and minus) **hand** (intrinsic) — see Deformity, limb, specified type NEC, forearm
PMEI (polymorphic epilepsy in infancy) G40.83- ☑
Pneumathemia — see Air, embolism
Pneumatic hammer (drill) syndrome T75.21- ☑
Pneumatocele (lung) J98.4
  intracranial G93.89
  tension J98.8

Pneumatosis
  cystoides intestinalis K63.89
  intestinalis K63.89
  peritonei K66.8
Pneumaturia R39.89
Pneumoblastoma — see Neoplasm, lung, malignant
Pneumocephalus G93.89
Pneumococcemia A40.3
Pneumococcus, pneumococcal — see condition
Pneumoconiosis (due to) (inhalation of) J64
  with tuberculosis (any type in A15) J65
  aluminum J63.0
  asbestos J61
  bagasse, bagassosis J67.1
  bauxite J63.1
  beryllium J63.2
  coal miners' (simple) J60
  coalworkers' (simple) J60
  collier's J60
  cotton dust J66.0
  diatomite (diatomaceous earth) J62.8
  dust
    inorganic NEC J63.6
    lime J62.8
    marble J62.8
    organic NEC J66.8
  fumes or vapors (from silo) J68.9
  graphite J63.3
  grinder's J62.8
  kaolin J62.8
  mica J62.8
  millstone maker's J62.8
  mineral fibers NEC J61
  miner's J60
  moldy hay J67.0
  potter's J62.8
  rheumatoid — see Rheumatoid, lung
  sandblaster's J62.8
  silica, silicate NEC J62.8
    with carbon J60
  stonemason's J62.8
  talc (dust) J62.0
Pneumocystis carinii pneumonia B59
Pneumocystis jirovecii (pneumonia) B59
Pneumocystosis (with pneumonia) B59
Pneumohemopericardium I31.2
Pneumohemothorax J94.2
  traumatic S27.2- ☑
Pneumohydropericardium — see Pericarditis
Pneumohydrothorax — see Hydrothorax
Pneumomediastinum J98.2
  congenital or perinatal P25.2
Pneumomycosis B49 [J99]
Pneumonia (acute) (double) (migratory) (purulent) (septic) (unresolved) J18.9
  with
    influenza — see Influenza, with, pneumonia
    lung abscess J85.1
      due to specified organism — see Pneumonia, in (due to)
  2019 (novel) coronavirus J12.82
  adenoviral J12.0
  adynamic J18.2
  alba A50.04
  allergic — see also Pneumonitis, hypersensitivity J82.89
  alveolar — see Pneumonia, lobar
  anaerobes J15.8
  anthrax A22.1
  apex, apical — see Pneumonia, lobar
  Ascaris B77.81
  aspiration J69.0
    due to
      aspiration of microorganisms
        bacterial J15.9
        viral J12.9
      food (regurgitated) J69.0
      gastric secretions J69.0
      milk (regurgitated) J69.0
      oils, essences J69.1
      solids, liquids NEC J69.8
      vomitus J69.0
    newborn P24.81
      amniotic fluid (clear) P24.11
      blood P24.21
      food (regurgitated) P24.31
      liquor (amnii) P24.11
      meconium P24.01
      milk P24.31
      mucus P24.11

Pneumonia — continued
  aspiration — continued
    newborn — continued
      specified NEC P24.81
      stomach contents P24.31
    postprocedural J95.4
  atypical NEC J18.9
  bacillus J15.9
    specified NEC J15.8
  bacterial J15.9
    specified NEC J15.8
  Bacteroides (fragilis) (oralis) (melaninogenicus) J15.8
  basal, basic, basilar — see Pneumonia, by type
  bronchiolitis obliterans organized (BOOP) J84.89
  broncho-, bronchial (confluent) (croupous) (diffuse) (disseminated) (hemorrhagic) (involving lobes) (lobar) (terminal) J18.0
    allergic — see also Pneumonitis, hypersensitivity J82.89
    aspiration — see Pneumonia, aspiration
    bacterial J15.9
      specified NEC J15.8
    chronic — see Fibrosis, lung
    diplococcal J13
    Eaton's agent J15.7
    Escherichia coli (E. coli) J15.5
    Friedlander's bacillus J15.0
    Hemophilus influenzae J14
    hypostatic J18.2
    inhalation — see also Pneumonia, aspiration
      due to fumes or vapors (chemical) J68.0
      of oils or essences J69.1
    Klebsiella (pneumoniae) J15.0
    lipid, lipoid J69.1
      endogenous J84.89
    Mycoplasma (pneumoniae) J15.7
    pleuro-pneumonia-like-organisms (PPLO) J15.7
    pneumococcal J13
    Proteus J15.69
    Pseudomonas J15.1
    Serratia marcescens J15.69
    specified organism NEC J16.8
    staphylococcal — see Pneumonia, staphylococcal
    streptococcal NEC J15.4
      group B J15.3
      pneumoniae J13
    viral, virus — see Pneumonia, viral
  Butyrivibrio (fibriosolvens) J15.8
  Candida B37.1
  caseous — see Tuberculosis, pulmonary
  catarrhal — see Pneumonia, broncho
  chlamydial J16.0
    congenital P23.1
  cholesterol J84.89
  cirrhotic (chronic) — see Fibrosis, lung
  Clostridium (haemolyticum) (novyi) J15.8
  confluent — see Pneumonia, broncho
  congenital (infective) P23.9
    due to
      bacterium NEC P23.6
      Chlamydia P23.1
      Escherichia coli P23.4
      Haemophilus influenzae P23.6
      infective organism NEC P23.8
      Klebsiella pneumoniae P23.6
      Mycoplasma P23.6
      Pseudomonas P23.5
      Staphylococcus P23.2
      Streptococcus (except group B) P23.6
        group B P23.3
      viral agent P23.0
    specified NEC P23.8
  coronavirus (novel) (disease) 2019 J12.82
  COVID-19 J12.82
  croupous — see Pneumonia, lobar
  cryptogenic organizing J84.116
  cytomegalic inclusion B25.0
  cytomegaloviral B25.0
  deglutition — see Pneumonia, aspiration
  desquamative interstitial J84.117
  diffuse — see Pneumonia, broncho
  diplococcal, diplococcus (broncho-) (lobar) J13
  disseminated (focal) — see Pneumonia, broncho
  Eaton's agent J15.7
  embolic, embolism — see Embolism, pulmonary
  Enterobacter J15.69
  eosinophilic J82.81
    acute J82.82
    chronic J82.81

Pneumonia — *continued*
- Escherichia coli (E. coli) J15.5
- Eubacterium J15.8
- fibrinous — *see* Pneumonia, lobar
- fibroid, fibrous (chronic) — *see* Fibrosis, lung
- Friedlander's bacillus J15.0
- Fusobacterium (nucleatum) J15.8
- gangrenous J85.0
- giant cell (measles) B05.2
- gonococcal A54.84
- gram-negative bacteria NEC J15.69
  - anaerobic J15.8
- Hemophilus influenzae (broncho) (lobar) J14
- human metapneumovirus J12.3
- hypostatic (broncho) (lobar) J18.2
- in (due to)
  - Acinetobacter baumannii J15.61
  - actinomycosis A42.0
  - adenovirus J12.0
  - anthrax A22.1
  - ascariasis B77.81
  - aspergillosis B44.9
  - Bacillus anthracis A22.1
  - Bacterium anitratum J15.69
  - candidiasis B37.1
  - chickenpox B01.2
  - Chlamydia J16.0
    - neonatal P23.1
  - coccidioidomycosis B38.2
    - acute B38.0
    - chronic B38.1
  - cytomegalovirus disease B25.0
  - Diplococcus (pneumoniae) J13
  - Eaton's agent J15.7
  - Enterobacter J15.69
  - Escherichia coli (E. coli) J15.5
  - Friedlander's bacillus J15.0
  - fumes and vapors (chemical) (inhalation) J68.0
  - gonorrhea A54.84
  - Hemophilus influenzae (H. influenzae) J14
  - Herellea J15.69
  - histoplasmosis B39.2
    - acute B39.0
    - chronic B39.1
  - human metapneumovirus J12.3
  - Klebsiella (pneumoniae) J15.0
  - measles B05.2
  - Mycoplasma (pneumoniae) J15.7
  - nocardiosis, nocardiasis A43.0
  - ornithosis A70
  - parainfluenza virus J12.2
  - pleuro-pneumonia-like-organism (PPLO) J15.7
  - pneumococcus J13
  - pneumocystosis (Pneumocystis carinii) (Pneumocystis jirovecii) B59
  - Proteus J15.69
  - Pseudomonas NEC J15.1
    - pseudomallei A24.1
  - psittacosis A70
  - Q fever A78
  - respiratory syncytial virus (RSV) J12.1
  - rheumatic fever I00 *[J17]*
  - rubella B06.81
  - Salmonella (infection) A02.22
    - typhi A01.03
  - schistosomiasis B65.9 *[J17]*
  - Serratia marcescens J15.69
  - specified
    - bacterium NEC J15.8
    - organism NEC J16.8
  - spirochetal NEC A69.8
  - Staphylococcus J15.20
    - aureus (methicillin susceptible) (MSSA) J15.211
      - methicillin resistant (MRSA) J15.212
    - specified NEC J15.29
  - Streptococcus J15.4
    - group B J15.3
    - pneumoniae J13
    - specified NEC J15.4
  - toxoplasmosis B58.3
  - tularemia A21.2
  - typhoid (fever) A01.03
  - varicella B01.2
  - virus — *see* Pneumonia, viral
  - whooping cough A37.91
    - due to
      - Bordetella parapertussis A37.11
      - Bordetella pertussis A37.01
      - specified NEC A37.81

Pneumonia — *continued*
- in — *continued*
  - Yersinia pestis A20.2
- inhalation of food or vomit — *see* Pneumonia, aspiration
- interstitial J84.9
  - chronic J84.111
  - desquamative J84.117
  - due to
    - collagen vascular disease J84.178
    - known underlying cause J84.178
  - idiopathic NOS J84.111
  - in disease classified elsewhere J84.178
  - lymphocytic (due to collagen vascular disease) (in diseases classified elsewhere) J84.178
  - lymphoid J84.2
  - non-specific J84.89
    - due to
      - collagen vascular disease J84.178
      - known underlying cause J84.178
    - idiopathic J84.113
    - in diseases classified elsewhere J84.178
  - plasma cell B59
  - pseudomonas J15.1
  - usual J84.112
    - due to collagen vascular disease J84.178
    - idiopathic J84.112
    - in diseases classified elsewhere J84.178
- Klebsiella (pneumoniae) J15.0
- lipid, lipoid (exogenous) J69.1
  - endogenous J84.89
- lobar (disseminated) (double) (interstitial) J18.1
  - bacterial J15.9
    - specified NEC J15.8
  - chronic — *see* Fibrosis, lung
  - Escherichia coli (E. coli) J15.5
  - Friedlander's bacillus J15.0
  - Hemophilus influenzae J14
  - hypostatic J18.2
  - Klebsiella (pneumoniae) J15.0
  - pneumococcal J13
  - Proteus J15.69
  - Pseudomonas J15.1
  - specified organism NEC J16.8
  - staphylococcal — *see* Pneumonia, staphylococcal
  - streptococcal NEC J15.4
  - Streptococcus pneumoniae J13
  - viral, virus — *see* Pneumonia, viral
- lobular — *see* Pneumonia, broncho
- Loffler's J82.89
- lymphoid interstitial J84.2
- massive — *see* Pneumonia, lobar
- meconium P24.01
- MRSA (methicillin resistant Staphylococcus aureus) J15.212
- MSSA (methicillin susceptible Staphylococcus aureus) J15.211
- multilobar — *see* Pneumonia, by type
- Mycoplasma (pneumoniae) J15.7
- necrotic J85.0
- neonatal P23.9
  - aspiration — *see* Aspiration, by substance, with pneumonia
- nitrogen dioxide J68.0
- organizing J84.89
  - due to
    - collagen vascular disease J84.178
    - known underlying cause J84.178
  - in diseases classified elsewhere J84.178
- orthostatic J18.2
- parainfluenza virus J12.2
- parenchymatous — *see* Fibrosis, lung
- passive J18.2
- patchy — *see* Pneumonia, broncho
- Peptococcus J15.8
- Peptostreptococcus J15.8
- plasma cell (of infants) B59
- pleuro-pneumonia-like organism (PPLO) J15.7
- pleurolobar — *see* Pneumonia, lobar
- pneumococcal (broncho) (lobar) J13
- Pneumocystis (carinii) (jirovecii) B59
- postinfectional NEC B99.- ☑ *[J17]*
- postmeasles B05.2
- Proteus J15.69
- Pseudomonas J15.1
- psittacosis A70
- radiation J70.0
- respiratory syncytial virus (RSV) J12.1
- resulting from a procedure J95.89
- rheumatic I00 *[J17]*

Pneumonia — *continued*
- Salmonella (arizonae) (cholerae-suis) (enteritidis) (typhimurium) A02.22
  - typhi A01.03
  - typhoid fever A01.03
- SARS-associated coronavirus J12.81
- SARS-CoV-2 J12.82
- segmented, segmental — *see* Pneumonia, broncho-
- Serratia marcescens J15.69
- specified NEC J18.8
  - bacterium NEC J15.8
  - organism NEC J16.8
  - virus NEC J12.89
- spirochetal NEC A69.8
- staphylococcal (broncho) (lobar) J15.20
  - aureus (methicillin susceptible) (MSSA) J15.211
    - methicillin resistant (MRSA) J15.212
  - specified NEC J15.29
- static, stasis J18.2
- streptococcal NEC (broncho) (lobar) J15.4
  - group
    - A J15.4
    - B J15.3
  - specified NEC J15.4
- Streptococcus pneumoniae J13
- syphilitic, congenital (early) A50.04
- traumatic (complication) (early) (secondary) T79.8- ☑
- tuberculous (any) — *see* Tuberculosis, pulmonary
- tularemic A21.2
- varicella B01.2
- Veillonella J15.8
- ventilator associated J95.851
- viral, virus (broncho) (interstitial) (lobar) J12.9
  - adenoviral J12.0
  - congenital P23.0
  - human metapneumovirus J12.3
  - parainfluenza J12.2
  - respiratory syncytial (RSV) J12.1
  - SARS-associated coronavirus J12.81
  - specified NEC J12.89
- white (congenital) A50.04

Pneumonic — *see* condition

Pneumonitis (acute) (primary) — *see also* Pneumonia J98.4
- air-conditioner J67.7
- allergic (due to) J67.9
  - organic dust NEC J67.8
  - red cedar dust J67.8
  - sequoiosis J67.8
  - wood dust J67.8
- aspiration J69.0
  - due to
    - anesthesia J95.4
      - during
        - labor and delivery O74.0
        - pregnancy O29.01- ☑
        - puerperium O89.01
    - fumes or gases J68.0
    - obstetric O74.0
- chemical (due to gases, fumes or vapors) (inhalation) J68.0
  - due to anesthesia J95.4
- cholesterol J84.89
- chronic — *see* Fibrosis, lung
- congenital rubella P35.0
- crack (cocaine) J68.0
- due to
  - beryllium J68.0
  - cadmium J68.0
  - crack (cocaine) J68.0
  - detergent J69.8
  - fluorocarbon-polymer J68.0
  - food, vomit (aspiration) J69.0
  - fumes or vapors J68.0
  - gases, fumes or vapors (inhalation) J68.0
  - inhalation
    - blood J69.8
    - essences J69.1
    - food (regurgitated), milk, vomit J69.0
    - oils, essences J69.1
    - saliva J69.0
    - solids, liquids NEC J69.8
  - manganese J68.0
  - nitrogen dioxide J68.0
  - oils, essences J69.1
  - solids, liquids NEC J69.8
  - toxoplasmosis (acquired) B58.3
    - congenital P37.1
  - vanadium J68.0
  - ventilator J95.851

Pneumonitis — continued
　eosinophilic J82.81
　　acute J82.82
　　chronic J82.81
　hypersensitivity J67.9
　　air conditioner lung J67.7
　　bagassosis J67.1
　　bird fancier's lung J67.2
　　farmer's lung J67.0
　　maltworker's lung J67.4
　　maple bark-stripper's lung J67.6
　　mushroom worker's lung J67.5
　　specified organic dust NEC J67.8
　　suberosis J67.3
　interstitial (chronic) J84.89
　　acute J84.114
　　lymphoid J84.2
　　non-specific J84.89
　　　idiopathic J84.113
　lymphoid, interstitial J84.2
　meconium P24.01
　noninfectious J98.4
　postanesthetic J95.4
　　correct substance properly administered — see Table of Drugs and Chemicals, by drug, adverse effect
　　in labor and delivery O74.0
　　in pregnancy O29.01- ☑
　　obstetric O74.0
　　overdose or wrong substance given or taken (by accident) — see Table of Drugs and Chemicals, by drug, poisoning
　postpartum, puerperal O89.01
　postoperative J95.4
　　obstetric O74.0
　radiation J70.0
　rubella, congenital P35.0
　specified NEC J98.4
　ventilation (air-conditioning) J67.7
　ventilator associated J95.851
　wood-dust J67.8
Pneumonoconiosis — see Pneumoconiosis
Pneumoparotid K11.8
Pneumopathy NEC J98.4
　alveolar J84.09
　due to organic dust NEC J66.8
　parietoalveolar J84.09
Pneumopericarditis — see also Pericarditis
　acute I30.9
Pneumopericardium — see also Pericarditis
　congenital P25.3
　newborn P25.3
　traumatic (post) — see Injury, heart
Pneumophagia (psychogenic) F45.8
Pneumopleurisy, pneumopleuritis — see also Pneumonia J18.8
Pneumopyopericardium I30.1
Pneumopyothorax — see Pyopneumothorax
　with fistula J86.0
Pneumorrhagia — see also Hemorrhage, lung
　tuberculous — see Tuberculosis, pulmonary
Pneumothorax NOS J93.9
　acute J93.83
　chronic J93.81
　congenital P25.1
　perinatal period P25.1
　postprocedural J95.811
　specified NEC J93.83
　spontaneous NOS J93.83
　　newborn P25.1
　　primary J93.11
　　secondary J93.12
　　tension J93.0
　tense valvular, infectional J93.0
　tension (spontaneous) J93.0
　traumatic S27.0- ☑
　　with hemothorax S27.2- ☑
　tuberculous — see Tuberculosis, pulmonary
Podagra — see also Gout M10.9
Podencephalus Q01.9
Poikilocytosis R71.8
Poikiloderma L81.6
　Civatte's L57.3
　congenital Q82.8
　vasculare atrophicans L94.5
Poikilodermatomyositis M33.10
　with
　　myopathy M33.12
　　respiratory involvement M33.11
　　specified organ involvement NEC M33.19

Poikilodermatomyositis — continued
　amyopathic M33.13
　without myopathy M33.13
Pointed ear (congenital) Q17.3
Poison ivy, oak, sumac or other plant dermatitis (allergic) (contact) L23.7
Poisoning (acute) — see also Table of Drugs and Chemicals
　algae and toxins T65.82- ☑
　Bacillus B (aertrycke) (cholerae (suis)) (paratyphosus) (suipestifer) A02.9
　　botulinus A05.1
　bacterial toxins A05.9
　berries, noxious — see Poisoning, food, noxious, berries
　botulism A05.1
　ciguatera fish T61.0- ☑
　Clostridium botulinum A05.1
　death-cap (Amanita phalloides) (Amanita verna) — see Poisoning, food, noxious, mushrooms
　drug — see Table of Drugs and Chemicals, by drug, poisoning
　epidemic, fish (noxious) — see Poisoning, seafood
　　bacterial A05.9
　fava bean D55.0
　fish (noxious) T61.9- ☑
　　bacterial — see Intoxication, foodborne, by agent
　　ciguatera fish — see Poisoning, ciguatera fish
　　scombroid fish — see Poisoning, scombroid fish
　　specified type NEC T61.77- ☑
　food NEC A05.9
　　bacterial — see Intoxication, foodborne, by agent
　　due to
　　　Bacillus (aertrycke) (choleraesuis) (paratyphosus) (suipestifer) A02.9
　　　　botulinus A05.1
　　　Clostridium (perfringens) (Welchii) A05.2
　　　salmonella (aertrycke) (choleraesuis) (enteritidis) (gallinarum) (paratyphi) (suipestifer) A02.9
　　　　with
　　　　　gastroenteritis A02.0
　　　　　sepsis A02.1
　　　staphylococcus A05.0
　　　Vibrio
　　　　parahaemolyticus A05.3
　　　　vulnificus A05.5
　　noxious or naturally toxic T62.9- ☑
　　　berries — see subcategory T62.1- ☑
　　　fish — see Poisoning, seafood
　　　mushrooms — see subcategory T62.0X- ☑
　　　plants NEC — see subcategory T62.2X- ☑
　　　seafood — see Poisoning, seafood
　　　specified NEC — see subcategory T62.8X- ☑
　ichthyotoxism — see Poisoning, seafood
　kreotoxism, food A05.9
　latex T65.81- ☑
　lead T56.0- ☑
　mushroom — see Poisoning, food, noxious, mushroom
　mussels — see also Poisoning, shellfish
　　bacterial — see Intoxication, foodborne, by agent
　nicotine (tobacco) T65.2- ☑
　noxious foodstuffs — see Poisoning, food, noxious
　plants, noxious — see Poisoning, food, noxious, plants NEC
　ptomaine — see Poisoning, food
　radiation J70.0
　Salmonella (arizonae) (cholerae-suis) (enteritidis) (typhimurium) A02.9
　scombroid fish T61.1- ☑
　seafood (noxious) T61.9- ☑
　　bacterial — see Intoxication, foodborne, by agent
　　fish — see Poisoning, fish
　　shellfish — see Poisoning, shellfish
　　specified NEC — see subcategory T61.8X- ☑
　shellfish (amnesic) (azaspiracid) (diarrheic) (neurotoxic) (noxious) (paralytic) T61.78- ☑
　　bacterial — see Intoxication, foodborne, by agent
　　ciguatera mollusk — see Poisoning, ciguatera fish
　specified substance NEC T65.891- ☑
　Staphylococcus, food A05.0
　tobacco (nicotine) T65.2- ☑
　water E87.79
Poker spine — see Spondylitis, ankylosing
Poland syndrome Q79.8
Polioencephalitis (acute) (bulbar) A80.9
　inferior G12.22
　influenzal — see Influenza, with, encephalopathy
　superior hemorrhagic (acute) (Wernicke's) E51.2
　Wernicke's E51.2
Polioencephalomyelitis (acute) (anterior) A80.9

Polioencephalomyelitis — continued
　with beriberi E51.2
Polioencephalopathy, superior hemorrhagic E51.2
　with
　　beriberi E51.11
　　pellagra E52
Poliomeningoencephalitis — see Meningoencephalitis
Poliomyelitis (acute) (anterior) (epidemic) A80.9
　with paralysis (bulbar) — see Poliomyelitis, paralytic
　abortive A80.4
　ascending (progressive) — see Poliomyelitis, paralytic
　bulbar (paralytic) — see Poliomyelitis, paralytic
　congenital P35.8
　nonepidemic A80.9
　nonparalytic A80.4
　paralytic A80.30
　　specified NEC A80.39
　　vaccine-associated A80.0
　　wild virus
　　　imported A80.1
　　　indigenous A80.2
　spinal, acute A80.9
Poliosis (eyebrow) (eyelashes) L67.1
　circumscripta, acquired L67.1
Pollakiuria R35.0
　psychogenic F45.8
Pollinosis J30.1
Pollitzer's disease L73.2
Polyadenitis — see also Lymphadenitis
　malignant A20.0
Polyalgia M79.89
Polyangiitis M30.0
　microscopic M31.7
　overlap syndrome M30.8
Polyarteritis
　microscopic M31.7
　nodosa M30.0
　　with lung involvement M30.1
　　juvenile M30.2
　　related condition NEC M30.8
Polyarthralgia — see Pain, joint
Polyarthritis, polyarthropathy — see also Arthritis M13.0
　due to or associated with other specified conditions — see Arthritis
　epidemic (Australian) (with exanthema) B33.1
　infective — see Arthritis, pyogenic or pyemic
　inflammatory M06.4
　juvenile (chronic) (seronegative) M08.3
　migratory M13.8- ☑
　rheumatic, acute — see Fever, rheumatic
Polyarthrosis M15.9
　post-traumatic M15.3
　primary M15.0
　specified NEC M15.8
Polycarential syndrome of infancy E40
Polychondritis (atrophic) (chronic) — see also Disorder, cartilage, specified type NEC
　relapsing M94.1
Polycoria Q13.2
Polycystic (disease)
　degeneration, kidney Q61.3
　　autosomal dominant (adult type) Q61.2
　　autosomal recessive (infantile type) NEC Q61.19
　kidney Q61.3
　　autosomal
　　　dominant Q61.2
　　　recessive NEC Q61.19
　　autosomal dominant (adult type) Q61.2
　　autosomal recessive (childhood type) NEC Q61.19
　　infantile type NEC Q61.19
　liver Q44.6
　lung J98.4
　　congenital Q33.0
　ovary, ovaries E28.2
　spleen Q89.09
Polycythemia (secondary) D75.1
　acquired D75.1
　benign (familial) D75.0
　due to
　　donor twin P61.1
　　erythropoietin D75.1
　　fall in plasma volume D75.1
　　high altitude D75.1
　　maternal-fetal transfusion P61.1
　　stress D75.1
　emotional D75.1
　erythropoietin D75.1
　familial (benign) D75.0
　Gaisböck's (hypertonica) D75.1

Polycythemia — *continued*
- high altitude D75.1
- hypertonica D75.1
- hypoxemic D75.1
- neonatorum P61.1
- nephrogenous D75.1
- relative D75.1
- secondary D75.1
- spurious D75.1
- stress D75.1
- vera D45

Polycytosis cryptogenica D75.1

Polydactylism, polydactyly Q69.9
- fingers Q69.0
- thumb Q69.1
- toes Q69.2

Polydipsia R63.1

Polydystrophy, pseudo-Hurler E77.0

Polyembryoma — *see* Neoplasm, malignant, by site

Polyglandular
- deficiency E31.0
- dyscrasia E31.9
- dysfunction E31.9
- syndrome E31.8

Polyhydramnios O40.- ☑

Polymastia Q83.1

Polymenorrhea N92.0

Polymyalgia M35.3
- arteritica, giant cell M31.5
- rheumatica M35.3
  - with giant cell arteritis M31.5

Polymyositis (acute) (chronic) (hemorrhagic) M33.20
- with
  - myopathy M33.22
  - respiratory involvement M33.21
  - skin involvement — *see* Dermatopolymyositis
  - specified organ involvement NEC M33.29
- ossificans (generalisata) (progressiva) — *see* Myositis, ossificans, progressiva

Polyneuritis, polyneuritic — *see also* Polyneuropathy
- acute (post-)infective G61.0
- alcoholic G62.1
- cranialis G52.7
- demyelinating, chronic inflammatory (CIDP) G61.81
- diabetic — *see* Diabetes, polyneuropathy
- diphtheritic A36.83
- due to lack of vitamin NEC E56.9 *[G63]*
- endemic E51.11
- erythredema — *see* subcategory T56.1- ☑
- febrile, acute G61.0
- hereditary ataxic G60.1
- idiopathic, acute G61.0
- infective (acute) G61.0
- inflammatory, chronic demyelinating (CIDP) G61.81
- nutritional E63.9 *[G63]*
- postinfective (acute) G61.0
- specified NEC G62.89

Polyneuropathy (peripheral) G62.9
- alcoholic G62.1
- amyloid (Portuguese) E85.1 *[G63]*
  - transthyretin-related (ATTR) familial E85.1 *[G63]*
- arsenical G62.2
- critical illness G62.81
- demyelinating, chronic inflammatory (CIDP) G61.81
- diabetic — *see* Diabetes, polyneuropathy
- drug-induced G62.0
- hereditary G60.9
  - specified NEC G60.8
- idiopathic G60.9
  - progressive G60.3
- in (due to)
  - alcohol G62.1
    - sequelae G65.2
  - amyloidosis, familial (Portuguese) E85.1 *[G63]*
  - antitetanus serum G61.1
  - arsenic G62.2
    - sequelae G65.2
  - avitaminosis NEC E56.9 *[G63]*
  - beriberi E51.11
  - collagen vascular disease NEC M35.9 *[G63]*
  - deficiency (of)
    - B (-complex) vitamins E53.9 *[G63]*
      - vitamin B6 E53.1 *[G63]*
  - diabetes — *see* Diabetes, polyneuropathy
  - diphtheria A36.83
  - drug or medicament G62.0
    - correct substance properly administered — *see* Table of Drugs and Chemicals, by drug, adverse effect

Polyneuropathy — *continued*
- in — *continued*
  - drug or medicament — *continued*
    - overdose or wrong substance given or taken — *see* Table of Drugs and Chemicals, by drug, poisoning
  - endocrine disease NEC E34.9 *[G63]*
  - herpes zoster B02.23
  - hypoglycemia E16.2 *[G63]*
  - infectious
    - disease NEC B99.- ☑ *[G63]*
    - mononucleosis B27.91
  - lack of vitamin NEC E56.9 *[G63]*
  - lead G62.2
    - sequelae G65.2
  - leprosy A30.9 *[G63]*
  - Lyme disease A69.22
  - metabolic disease NEC E88.9 *[G63]*
  - microscopic polyangiitis M31.7 *[G63]*
  - mumps B26.84
  - neoplastic disease — *see also* Neoplasm D49.9 *[G63]*
  - nutritional deficiency NEC E63.9 *[G63]*
  - organophosphate compounds G62.2
    - sequelae G65.2
  - parasitic disease NEC B89 *[G63]*
  - pellagra E52 *[G63]*
  - polyarteritis nodosa M30.0
  - porphyria E80.20 *[G63]*
  - radiation G62.82
  - rheumatoid arthritis — *see* Rheumatoid, polyneuropathy
  - sarcoidosis D86.89
  - serum G61.1
  - syphilis (late) A52.15
    - congenital A50.43
  - systemic
    - connective tissue disorder M35.9 *[G63]*
    - lupus erythematosus M32.19
  - toxic agent NEC G62.2
    - sequelae G65.2
  - transthyretin-related (ATTR) familial amyloid E85.1
  - triorthocresyl phosphate G62.2
    - sequelae G65.2
  - tuberculosis A17.89
  - uremia N18.9 *[G63]*
  - vitamin B12 deficiency E53.8 *[G63]*
    - with anemia (pernicious) D51.0 *[G63]*
      - due to dietary deficiency D51.3 *[G63]*
  - zoster B02.23
- inflammatory G61.9
  - chronic demyelinating (CIDP) G61.81
  - sequelae G65.1
  - specified NEC G61.89
- lead G62.2
  - sequelae G65.2
- nutritional NEC E63.9 *[G63]*
- postherpetic (zoster) B02.23
- progressive G60.3
- radiation-induced G62.82
- sensory (hereditary) (idiopathic) G60.8
- specified NEC G62.89
- syphilitic (late) A52.15
  - congenital A50.43

Polyopia H53.8

Polyorchism, polyorchidism Q55.21

Polyosteoarthritis — *see also* Osteoarthritis, generalized M15.9
- post-traumatic M15.3
- specified NEC M15.8

Polyostotic fibrous dysplasia Q78.1

Polyotia Q17.0

Polyp, polypus
- accessory sinus J33.8
- adenocarcinoma in — *see* Neoplasm, malignant, by site
- adenocarcinoma in situ in — *see* Neoplasm, in situ, by site
- adenoid tissue J33.0
- adenomatous — *see also* Neoplasm, benign, by site
  - adenocarcinoma in — *see* Neoplasm, malignant, by site
  - adenocarcinoma in situ in — *see* Neoplasm, in situ, by site
  - carcinoma in — *see* Neoplasm, malignant, by site
  - carcinoma in situ in — *see* Neoplasm, in situ, by site
  - multiple — *see* Neoplasm, benign
    - adenocarcinoma in — *see* Neoplasm, malignant, by site
    - adenocarcinoma in situ in — *see* Neoplasm, in situ, by site

Polyp, polypus — *continued*
- antrum J33.8
- anus, anal (canal) K62.0
- Bartholin's gland N84.3
- bladder D41.4
- carcinoma in — *see* Neoplasm, malignant, by site
- carcinoma in situ in — *see* Neoplasm, in situ, by site
- cecum D12.0
- cervix (uteri) N84.1
  - in pregnancy or childbirth — *see* Pregnancy, complicated by, abnormal, cervix
  - mucous N84.1
  - nonneoplastic N84.1
- choanal J33.0
- cholesterol K82.4
- clitoris N84.3
- colon K63.5
  - adenomatous D12.6
    - ascending D12.2
    - cecum D12.0
    - descending D12.4
    - sigmoid D12.5
    - transverse D12.3
  - ascending K63.5
  - cecum K63.5
  - descending K63.5
  - hyperplastic, (any site) K63.5
  - inflammatory K51.40
    - with
      - abscess K51.414
      - complication K51.419
        - specified NEC K51.418
      - fistula K51.413
      - intestinal obstruction K51.412
      - rectal bleeding K51.411
  - sigmoid K63.5
  - transverse K63.5
- corpus uteri N84.0
- dental K04.01
  - irreversible K04.02
  - reversible K04.01
- duodenum K31.7
- ear (middle) H74.4- ☑
- endometrium N84.0
- esophageal K22.81
- esophagogastric junction K22.82
- ethmoidal (sinus) J33.8
- fallopian tube N84.8
- female genital tract N84.9
  - specified NEC N84.8
- frontal (sinus) J33.8
- gallbladder K82.4
- gingiva, gum K06.8
- labia, labium (majus) (minus) N84.3
- larynx (mucous) J38.1
  - adenomatous D14.1
- malignant — *see* Neoplasm, malignant, by site
- maxillary (sinus) J33.8
- middle ear — *see* Polyp, ear (middle)
- myometrium N84.0
- nares
  - anterior J33.9
  - posterior J33.0
- nasal (mucous) J33.9
  - cavity J33.0
  - septum J33.0
- nasopharyngeal J33.0
- nose (mucous) J33.9
- oviduct N84.8
- pharynx J39.2
- placenta O90.89
- prostate — *see* Enlargement, enlarged, prostate
- pudenda, pudendum N84.3
- pulpal (dental) K04.01
  - irreversible K04.02
  - reversible K04.01
- rectum (nonadenomatous) K62.1
  - adenomatous — *see* Polyp, adenomatous
- septum (nasal) J33.0
- sinus (accessory) (ethmoidal) (frontal) (maxillary) (sphenoidal) J33.8
- sphenoidal (sinus) J33.8
- stomach K31.7
  - adenomatous D13.1
- tube, fallopian N84.8
- turbinate, mucous membrane J33.8
- umbilical, newborn P83.6
- ureter N28.89
- urethra N36.2

☑ Additional Character Required — Refer to the Tabular List for Character Selection

Polyp, polypus — continued
  uterus (body) (corpus) (mucous) N84.0
    cervix N84.1
      in pregnancy or childbirth — see Pregnancy, complicated by, tumor, uterus
  vagina N84.2
  vocal cord (mucous) J38.1
  vulva N84.3
Polyphagia R63.2
Polyploidy Q92.7
Polypoid — see condition
Polyposis — see also Polyp
  adenomatous D13.91
  coli D12.6
    adenocarcinoma in C18.9
    adenocarcinoma in situ in — see Neoplasm, in situ, by site
    carcinoma in C18.9
  colon D12.6
  familial D12.6
    adenocarcinoma in situ in — see Neoplasm, in situ, by site
    adenomatous D13.91
  intestinal D12.6
  malignant lymphomatous C83.1- ☑
  multiple, adenomatous — see also Neoplasm, benign D36.9
Polyradiculitis — see Polyneuropathy
Polyradiculoneuropathy (acute) (postinfective) (segmentally demyelinating) G61.0
Polyserositis
  due to pericarditis I31.1
  pericardial I31.1
  periodic, familial E85.0
  tuberculous A19.9
    acute A19.1
    chronic A19.8
Polysplenia syndrome Q89.09
Polysyndactyly — see also Syndactylism, syndactyly Q70.4
Polytrichia L68.3
Polyunguia Q84.6
Polyuria R35.89
  nocturnal R35.81
  psychogenic F45.8
  specified NEC R35.89
Pompe's disease (glycogen storage) E74.02
Pompholyx L30.1
Poncet's disease (tuberculous rheumatism) A18.09
Pond fracture — see Fracture, skull
Ponos B55.0
Pons, pontine — see condition
Poor
  aesthetic of existing restoration of tooth K08.56
  contractions, labor O62.2
  gingival margin to tooth restoration K08.51
  housing weatherization Z59.19
  personal hygiene R46.0
  prenatal care, affecting management of pregnancy — see Pregnancy, complicated by, insufficient, prenatal care
  sucking reflex (newborn) R29.2
  urinary stream R39.12
  vision NEC H54.7
Poradenitis, nostras inguinalis or venerea A55
Porencephaly (congenital) (developmental) (true) Q04.6
  acquired G93.0
  nondevelopmental G93.0
  traumatic (post) F07.89
Porocephaliasis B88.8
Porokeratosis Q82.8
Poroma, eccrine — see Neoplasm, skin, benign
Porphyria (South African) E80.20
  acquired E80.20
  acute intermittent (hepatic) (Swedish) E80.21
  cutanea tarda (hereditary) (symptomatic) E80.1
  due to drugs E80.20
    correct substance properly administered — see Table of Drugs and Chemicals, by drug, adverse effect
    overdose or wrong substance given or taken — see Table of Drugs and Chemicals, by drug, poisoning
  erythropoietic (congenital) (hereditary) E80.0
  hepatocutaneous type E80.1
  secondary E80.20
  toxic NEC E80.20
  variegata E80.20
Porphyrinuria — see Porphyria
Porphyruria — see Porphyria

Port wine nevus, mark, or stain Q82.5
Portal — see condition
Posadas-Wernicke disease B38.9
Positive
  culture (nonspecific)
    blood R78.81
    bronchial washings R84.5
    cerebrospinal fluid R83.5
    cervix uteri R87.5
    nasal secretions R84.5
    nipple discharge R89.5
    nose R84.5
      staphylococcus (Methicillin susceptible) Z22.321
        Methicillin resistant Z22.322
    peritoneal fluid R85.5
    pleural fluid R84.5
    prostatic secretions R86.5
    saliva R85.5
    seminal fluid R86.5
    sputum R84.5
    synovial fluid R89.5
    throat scrapings R84.5
    urine R82.79
    vagina R87.5
    vulva R87.5
    wound secretions R89.5
  PPD (skin test) R76.11
  serology for syphilis A53.0
    false R76.89
    with signs or symptoms — code as Syphilis, by site and stage
  skin test, tuberculin (without active tuberculosis) R76.11
  test, human immunodeficiency virus (HIV) R75
  VDRL A53.0
    with signs or symptoms — code by site and stage under Syphilis A53.9
  Wassermann reaction A53.0
Post COVID-19 condition, unspecified U09.9
Postcardiotomy syndrome I97.0
Postcaval ureter Q62.62
Postcholecystectomy syndrome K91.5
Postclimacteric bleeding N95.0
Postcommissurotomy syndrome I97.0
Postconcussional syndrome F07.81
Postcontusional syndrome F07.81
Postcricoid region — see condition
Post-dates (40-42 weeks) (pregnancy) (mother) O48.0
  more than 42 weeks gestation O48.1
Postencephalitic syndrome F07.89
Posterior — see condition
Posterolateral sclerosis (spinal cord) — see Degeneration, combined
Postexanthematous — see condition
Postfebrile — see condition
Postgastrectomy dumping syndrome K91.1
Posthemiplegic chorea — see Monoplegia
Posthemorrhagic anemia (chronic) D50.0
  acute D62
  newborn P61.3
Postherpetic neuralgia (zoster) B02.29
  trigeminal B02.22
Posthitis N47.7
Postimmunization complication or reaction — see Complications, vaccination
Postinfectious — see condition
Postlaminectomy syndrome NEC M96.1
Postleukotomy syndrome F07.0
Postmastectomy lymphedema (syndrome) I97.2
Postmaturity, postmature (over 42 weeks)
  maternal (over 42 weeks gestation) O48.1
  newborn P08.22
Postmeasles complication NEC — see also condition B05.89
Postmenopausal
  endometrium (atrophic) N95.8
    suppurative — see also Endometritis N71.9
  osteoporosis — see Osteoporosis, postmenopausal
Postnasal drip R09.82
  due to
    allergic rhinitis — see Rhinitis, allergic
    common cold J00
    gastroesophageal reflux — see Reflux, gastroesophageal
    nasopharyngitis — see Nasopharyngitis
    other known condition — code to condition
    sinusitis — see Sinusitis
Postnatal — see condition
Postoperative (postprocedural) — see also Complication, postoperative

Postoperative — continued
  pneumothorax, therapeutic Z98.3
  state NEC Z98.890
  visit — see Aftercare
  wound check — see Aftercare
Postpancreatectomy hyperglycemia E89.1
Postpartum — see Puerperal
Postphlebitic syndrome — see Syndrome, postthrombotic
Postpolio (myelitic) **syndrome** G14
Postpoliomyelitic — see also condition
  osteopathy — see Osteopathy, after poliomyelitis
Postprocedural — see also Postoperative
  hypoinsulinemia E89.1
Postschizophrenic depression F32.89
Postsurgery status — see also Status (post)
  pneumothorax, therapeutic Z98.3
Post-term (40-42 weeks) (pregnancy) (mother) O48.0
  infant P08.21
  more than 42 weeks gestation (mother) O48.1
Post-traumatic brain syndrome, nonpsychotic F07.81
Post-typhoid abscess A01.09
Postures, hysterical F44.2
Postvaccinal reaction or complication — see Complications, vaccination
Postvalvulotomy syndrome I97.0
Potain's
  disease (pulmonary edema) — see Edema, lung
  syndrome (gastrectasis with dyspepsia) K31.0
POTS (postural orthostatic tachycardia syndrome) G90.A
Potter's
  asthma J62.8
  facies Q60.6
  lung J62.8
  syndrome (with renal agenesis) Q60.6
Pott's
  curvature (spinal) A18.01
  disease or paraplegia A18.01
  spinal curvature A18.01
  tumor, puffy — see Osteomyelitis, specified type NEC
Pouch
  bronchus Q32.4
  Douglas' — see condition
  esophagus, esophageal, congenital Q39.6
    acquired K22.5
  gastric K31.4
  Hartmann's K82.8
  pharynx, pharyngeal (congenital) Q38.7
Pouchitis K91.850
Poultrymen's itch B88.09
Poverty NEC Z59.6
  extreme Z59.5
Poxvirus NEC B08.8
Prader-Willi-like syndrome Q87.19
Prader-Willi syndrome Q87.11
Preauricular appendage or tag Q17.0
Prebetalipoproteinemia (acquired) (essential) (familial) (hereditary) (primary) (secondary) E78.1
  with chylomicronemia E78.3
Precipitate labor or delivery O62.3
Preclimacteric bleeding (menorrhagia) N92.4
Precocious
  adrenarche E30.1
  menarche E30.1
  menstruation E30.1
  pubarche E30.1
  puberty E30.1
    central E22.8
  sexual development NEC E30.1
  thelarche E30.8
Precocity, sexual (constitutional) (cryptogenic) (female) (idiopathic) (male) E30.1
  with adrenal hyperplasia E25.9
    congenital E25.0
Precordial pain R07.2
Predeciduous teeth K00.2
Prediabetes, prediabetic R73.03
  complicating
    pregnancy — see Pregnancy, complicated by, diseases of, specified type or system NEC
    puerperium O99.893
Predislocation status of hip at birth Q65.6
Pre-eclampsia O14.9- ☑
  with pre-existing hypertension — see Hypertension, complicating pregnancy, pre-existing, with, pre-eclampsia
  complicating
    childbirth O14.94
    puerperium O14.95
  mild O14.0- ☑

Pre-eclampsia — *continued*
  mild — *continued*
    complicating
      childbirth O14.04
      puerperium O14.05
  moderate O14.0- ☑
    complicating
      childbirth O14.04
      puerperium O14.05
  severe O14.1- ☑
    with hemolysis, elevated liver enzymes and low platelet count (HELLP) O14.2- ☑
      complicating
        childbirth O14.24
        puerperium O14.25
    complicating
      childbirth O14.14
      puerperium O14.15
Pre-eruptive color change, teeth, tooth K00.8
Pre-excitation atrioventricular conduction I45.6
Preglaucoma H40.00- ☑
Pregnancy (single) (uterine) — *see also* Delivery and Puerperal Z33.1

> Note: The Tabular must be reviewed for assignment of appropriate seventh character for multiple gestation codes in Chapter 15

> Note: The Tabular must be reviewed for assignment of the appropriate character indicating the trimester of the pregnancy

  abdominal (ectopic) O00.00
    with intrauterine pregnancy O00.01
    with viable fetus O36.7- ☑
  ampullar O00.10- ☑
    with intrauterine pregnancy O00.11- ☑
  biochemical O02.81
  broad ligament O00.80
    with intrauterine pregnancy O00.81
  cervical O00.80
    with intrauterine pregnancy O00.81
  chemical O02.81
  complicated by (care of) (management affected by)
    abnormal, abnormality
      cervix O34.4- ☑
        causing obstructed labor O65.5
      cord (umbilical) O69.9- ☑
      fetal heart rate or rhythm O36.83- ☑
      findings on antenatal screening of mother O28.9
        biochemical O28.1
        chromosomal O28.5
        cytological O28.2
        genetic O28.5
        hematological O28.0
        radiological O28.4
        specified NEC O28.8
        ultrasonic O28.3
      glucose (tolerance) NEC O99.810
      pelvic organs O34.9- ☑
        specified NEC O34.8- ☑
          causing obstructed labor O65.5
      pelvis (bony) (major) NEC O33.0
      perineum O34.7- ☑
      position
        placenta O44.0- ☑
          with hemorrhage O44.1- ☑
        uterus O34.59- ☑
      uterus O34.59- ☑
        causing obstructed labor O65.5
        congenital O34.0- ☑
      vagina O34.6- ☑
        causing obstructed labor O65.5
      vulva O34.7- ☑
        causing obstructed labor O65.5
    abruptio placentae — *see* Abruptio placentae
    abscess or cellulitis
      bladder O23.1- ☑
      breast O91.11- ☑
      genital organ or tract O23.9- ☑
    abuse
      physical O9A.31- ☑ (*following* O99)
      psychological O9A.51- ☑ (*following* O99)
      sexual O9A.41- ☑ (*following* O99)
    adverse effect anesthesia O29.9- ☑
      aspiration pneumonitis O29.01- ☑
      cardiac arrest O29.11- ☑
      cardiac complication NEC O29.19- ☑

Pregnancy — *continued*
  complicated by — *continued*
    adverse effect anesthesia — *continued*
      cardiac failure O29.12- ☑
      central nervous system complication NEC O29.29- ☑
      cerebral anoxia O29.21- ☑
      failed or difficult intubation O29.6- ☑
      inhalation of stomach contents or secretions NOS O29.01- ☑
      local, toxic reaction O29.3X- ☑
      Mendelson's syndrome O29.01- ☑
      pressure collapse of lung O29.02- ☑
      pulmonary complications NEC O29.09- ☑
      specified NEC O29.8X- ☑
      spinal and epidural type NEC O29.5X- ☑
        induced headache O29.4- ☑
    albuminuria — *see also* Proteinuria, gestational O12.1- ☑
    alcohol use O99.31- ☑
    amnionitis O41.12- ☑
    anaphylactoid syndrome of pregnancy O88.01- ☑
    anemia (conditions in D50-D64) (pre-existing) O99.01- ☑
      complicating childbirth O99.02
      complicating the puerperium O99.03
    antepartum hemorrhage O46.9- ☑
      with coagulation defect — *see* Hemorrhage, antepartum, with coagulation defect
      specified NEC O46.8X- ☑
    appendicitis O99.61- ☑
    atrophy (yellow) (acute) liver (subacute) O26.61- ☑
    bariatric surgery status O99.84- ☑
    bicornis or bicornuate uterus O34.0- ☑
    biliary tract problems O26.61- ☑
    breech presentation O32.1- ☑
    cardiovascular diseases (conditions in I00-I09, I20-I52, I70-I99) O99.41- ☑
    cerebrovascular disorders (conditions in I60-I69) O99.41- ☑
    cervical shortening O26.87- ☑
    cervicitis O23.51- ☑
    cesarean scar defect (isthmocele) O34.22
    chloasma (gravidarum) O26.89- ☑
    cholecystitis O99.61- ☑
    cholestasis (intrahepatic) O26.64- ☑
    chorioamnionitis O41.12- ☑
    circulatory system disorder (conditions in I00-I09, I20-I99, O99.41-)
    compound presentation O32.6- ☑
    conjoined twins O30.02- ☑
    connective system disorders (conditions in M00-M99) O99.891
    contracted pelvis (general) O33.1
      inlet O33.2
      outlet O33.3- ☑
    convulsions (eclamptic) (uremic) — *see also* Eclampsia O15.9
    cracked nipple O92.11- ☑
    cystitis O23.1- ☑
    cystocele O34.8- ☑
    death of fetus (near term) O36.4- ☑
      early pregnancy O02.1
      of one fetus or more in multiple gestation O31.2- ☑
    deciduitis O41.14- ☑
    decreased fetal movement O36.81- ☑
    dental problems O99.61- ☑
    diabetes (mellitus) O24.91- ☑
      gestational (pregnancy induced) — *see* Diabetes, gestational
      pre-existing O24.31- ☑
        specified NEC O24.81- ☑
        type 1 O24.01- ☑
        type 2 O24.11- ☑
    digestive system disorders (conditions in K00-K93) O99.61- ☑
    diseases of — *see* Pregnancy, complicated by, specified body system disease
      biliary tract O26.61- ☑
      blood NEC (conditions in D65-D77) O99.11- ☑
      liver O26.61- ☑
      specified NEC O99.891
    disorders of — *see* Pregnancy, complicated by, specified body system disorder
      amniotic fluid and membranes O41.9- ☑

Pregnancy — *continued*
  complicated by — *continued*
    disorders of — *see* Pregnancy, complicated by, specified body system disorder — *continued*
      amniotic fluid and membranes — *continued*
        specified NEC O41.8X- ☑
      biliary tract O26.61- ☑
      ear and mastoid process (conditions in H60-H95) O99.891
      eye and adnexa (conditions in H00-H59) O99.891
      liver O26.61- ☑
      skin (conditions in L00-L99) O99.71- ☑
      specified NEC O99.891
    displacement, uterus NEC O34.59- ☑
      causing obstructed labor O65.5
    disproportion (due to) O33.9
      fetal (ascites) (hydrops) (meningomyelocele) (sacral teratoma) (tumor) deformities NEC O33.7- ☑
      generally contracted pelvis O33.1
      hydrocephalic fetus O33.6- ☑
      inlet contraction of pelvis O33.2
      mixed maternal and fetal origin O33.4- ☑
      specified NEC O33.8
    double uterus O34.0- ☑
      causing obstructed labor O65.5
    drug use (conditions in F11-F19) O99.32- ☑
    eclampsia, eclamptic (coma) (convulsions) (delirium) (nephritis) (uremia) — *see also* Eclampsia O15.- ☑
    ectopic pregnancy — *see* Pregnancy, ectopic
    edema O12.0- ☑
      with
        gestational hypertension, mild — *see also* Pre-eclampsia O14.0- ☑
        proteinuria O12.2- ☑
    effusion, amniotic fluid — *see* Pregnancy, complicated by, premature rupture of membranes
    elderly
      multigravida O09.52- ☑
      primigravida O09.51- ☑
    embolism — *see also* Embolism, obstetric, pregnancy O88.- ☑
    endocrine diseases NEC O99.28- ☑
    endometritis O86.12
    excessive weight gain O26.0- ☑
    exhaustion O26.81- ☑
      during labor and delivery O75.81
    face presentation O32.3- ☑
    failed induction of labor O61.9
      instrumental O61.1
      mechanical O61.1
      medical O61.0
      specified NEC O61.8
      surgical O61.1
    failed or difficult intubation for anesthesia O29.6- ☑
    false labor (pains) O47.9
      at or after 37 completed weeks of pregnancy O47.1
      before 37 completed weeks of pregnancy O47.0- ☑
    fatigue O26.81- ☑
      during labor and delivery O75.81
    fatty metamorphosis of liver O26.61- ☑
    female genital mutilation O34.8- ☑ [N90.81-]
    fetal (maternal care for)
      abnormality or damage O35.9- ☑
        acid-base balance O68
        specified type NEC O35.8- ☑
      acidemia O68
      acidosis O68
      agenesis of corpus callosum O35.01- ☑
      alkalosis O68
      anemia and thrombocytopenia O36.82- ☑
      anencephaly O35.02- ☑
      bradycardia O36.83- ☑
      cardiac anomalies O35.B- ☑
      central nervous system malformation or damage O35.00- ☑
        specified type NEC O35.09- ☑
      choroid plexus cysts O35.03- ☑
      chromosomal abnormality (conditions in Q90-Q99) O35.10- ☑
        sex chromosome O35.15- ☑
        specified NEC O35.19- ☑
        Trisomy 13 O35.11- ☑
        Trisomy 18 O35.12- ☑
        Trisomy 21 O35.13- ☑

Pregnancy — continued
- complicated by — continued
  - fetal — continued
    - chromosomal abnormality — continued
      - Turner Syndrome O35.14- ☑
    - conjoined twins O30.02- ☑
    - damage from
      - amniocentesis O35.7- ☑
      - biopsy procedures O35.7- ☑
      - drug addiction O35.5- ☑
      - hematological investigation O35.7- ☑
      - intrauterine contraceptive device O35.7- ☑
      - maternal
        - alcohol addiction O35.4- ☑
        - cytomegalovirus infection O35.3- ☑
        - disease NEC O35.8- ☑
        - drug addiction O35.5- ☑
        - listeriosis O35.8- ☑
        - rubella O35.3- ☑
        - toxoplasmosis O35.8- ☑
        - viral infection O35.3- ☑
      - medical procedure NEC O35.7- ☑
      - radiation O35.6- ☑
    - death (near term) O36.4- ☑
      - early pregnancy O02.1
    - decreased movement O36.81- ☑
    - depressed heart rate tones O36.83- ☑
    - disproportion due to deformity (fetal) O33.7- ☑
    - encephalocele O35.04- ☑
    - excessive growth (large for dates) O36.6- ☑
    - facial anomalies O35.A- ☑
    - gastrointestinal anomalies O35.D- ☑
    - genitourinary anomalies O35.E- ☑
    - growth retardation O36.59- ☑
      - light for dates O36.59- ☑
      - small for dates O36.59- ☑
    - heart rate irregularity (abnormal variability) (bradycardia) (decelerations) (tachycardia) O36.83- ☑
    - hereditary disease O35.2- ☑
    - holoprosencephaly O35.05- ☑
    - hydrocephalus O35.06- ☑
    - hydrocephaly O35.06- ☑
    - intrauterine death O36.4- ☑
    - microcephaly O35.07- ☑
    - musculoskeletal anomalies
      - lower extremities O35.H- ☑
      - trunk O35.F- ☑
      - upper extremities O35.G- ☑
    - non-reassuring heart rate or rhythm O36.83- ☑
    - poor growth O36.59- ☑
      - light for dates O36.59- ☑
      - small for dates O36.59- ☑
    - problem O36.9- ☑
      - specified NEC O36.89- ☑
    - pulmonary anomalies O35.C- ☑
    - reduction (elective) O31.3- ☑
    - selective termination O31.3- ☑
    - spina bifida O35.08- ☑
    - thrombocytopenia O36.82- ☑
  - fibroid (tumor) (uterus) O34.1- ☑
  - fissure of nipple O92.11- ☑
  - gallstones O99.61- ☑
  - gastric banding status O99.84- ☑
  - gastric bypass status O99.84- ☑
  - genital herpes (asymptomatic) (history of) (inactive) O98.3- ☑
  - genital tract infection O23.9- ☑
  - glomerular diseases (conditions in N00-N07) O26.83- ☑
    - with hypertension, pre-existing — see Hypertension, complicating, pregnancy, pre-existing, with, renal disease
  - gonorrhea O98.21- ☑
  - grand multiparity O09.4- ☑
  - habitual aborter — see Pregnancy, complicated by, recurrent pregnancy loss
  - HELLP syndrome (hemolysis, elevated liver enzymes and low platelet count) O14.2- ☑
  - hemorrhage
    - antepartum — see Hemorrhage, antepartum
    - before 20 completed weeks gestation O20.9
      - specified NEC O20.8
      - due to premature separation, placenta — see also Abruptio placentae O45.9- ☑
      - early O20.9

Pregnancy — continued
- complicated by — continued
  - hemorrhage — continued
    - early — continued
      - specified NEC O20.8
      - threatened abortion O20.0
  - hemorrhoids O22.4- ☑
  - hepatitis (viral) O98.41- ☑
  - herniation of uterus O34.59- ☑
  - high
    - head at term O32.4- ☑
    - risk — see Supervision (of) (for), high-risk
  - history of in utero procedure during previous pregnancy O09.82- ☑
  - HIV O98.71- ☑
  - human immunodeficiency virus (HIV) disease O98.71- ☑
  - hydatidiform mole — see also Mole, hydatidiform O01.9
  - hydramnios O40.- ☑
  - hydrocephalic fetus (disproportion) O33.6- ☑
  - hydrops
    - amnii O40.- ☑
    - fetalis O36.2- ☑
      - associated with isoimmunization — see also Pregnancy, complicated by, isoimmunization O36.11- ☑
  - hydrorrhea O42.90
  - hyperemesis (gravidarum) (mild) — see also Hyperemesis, gravidarum O21.0
  - hypertension — see Hypertension, complicating pregnancy
  - hypertensive
    - heart and renal disease, pre-existing — see Hypertension, complicating, pregnancy, pre-existing, with, heart disease, with renal disease
    - heart disease, pre-existing — see Hypertension, complicating, pregnancy, pre-existing, with, heart disease
    - renal disease, pre-existing — see Hypertension, complicating, pregnancy, pre-existing, with, renal disease
  - hypotension O26.5- ☑
  - immune disorders NEC (conditions in D80-D89) O99.11- ☑
  - incarceration, uterus O34.51- ☑
  - incompetent cervix O34.3- ☑
  - inconclusive fetal viability O36.80- ☑
  - infection(s) O98.91- ☑
    - amniotic fluid or sac O41.10- ☑
    - bladder O23.1- ☑
    - carrier state NEC O99.830
      - streptococcus B O99.820
    - genital organ or tract O23.9- ☑
      - specified NEC O23.59- ☑
    - genitourinary tract O23.9- ☑
    - gonorrhea O98.21- ☑
    - hepatitis (viral) O98.41- ☑
    - HIV O98.71- ☑
    - human immunodeficiency virus (HIV) O98.71- ☑
    - intrauterine O41.12- ☑
    - kidney O23.0- ☑
    - nipple O91.01- ☑
    - parasitic disease O98.91- ☑
      - specified NEC O98.81- ☑
    - protozoal disease O98.61- ☑
    - sexually transmitted NEC O98.31- ☑
    - specified type NEC O98.81- ☑
    - syphilis O98.11- ☑
    - tuberculosis O98.01- ☑
    - urethra O23.2- ☑
    - urinary (tract) O23.4- ☑
      - specified NEC O23.3- ☑
    - viral disease O98.51- ☑
  - inflammation
    - intrauterine O41.12- ☑
  - injury or poisoning (conditions in S00-T88) O9A.21- ☑ (following O99)
    - due to abuse
      - physical O9A.31- ☑ (following O99)
      - psychological O9A.51- ☑ (following O99)
      - sexual O9A.41- ☑ (following O99)
  - insufficient
    - prenatal care O09.3- ☑
    - weight gain O26.1- ☑
  - insulin resistance O26.89- ☑

Pregnancy — continued
- complicated by — continued
  - intrauterine fetal death (near term) O36.4- ☑
    - early pregnancy O02.1
    - multiple gestation (one fetus or more) O31.2- ☑
  - isoimmunization O36.11- ☑
    - anti-A sensitization O36.11- ☑
    - anti-B sensitization O36.19- ☑
    - Rh O36.09- ☑
      - anti-D antibody O36.01- ☑
    - specified NEC O36.19- ☑
  - laceration of uterus NEC O71.81
  - malformation
    - central nervous system O35.00- ☑
      - specified type NEC O35.09- ☑
    - placenta, placental (vessel) O43.10- ☑
      - specified NEC O43.19- ☑
    - uterus (congenital) O34.0- ☑
  - malnutrition (conditions in E40-E46) O25.1- ☑
  - maternal hypotension syndrome O26.5- ☑
  - mental disorders (conditions in F01-F09, F20-F52 and F54-F99) O99.34- ☑
    - alcohol use O99.31- ☑
    - drug use O99.32- ☑
    - smoking O99.33- ☑
  - mentum presentation O32.3- ☑
  - metabolic disorders O99.28- ☑
  - missed
    - abortion O02.1
    - delivery O36.4- ☑
  - multiple gestations O30.9- ☑
    - conjoined twins O30.02- ☑
    - quadruplet — see Pregnancy, quadruplet
    - specified complication NEC O31.8X- ☑
    - specified number of multiples NEC — see Pregnancy, multiple (gestation), specified NEC
    - triplet — see Pregnancy, triplet
    - twin — see Pregnancy, twin
  - musculoskeletal condition (conditions is M00-M99) O99.891
  - necrosis, liver (conditions in K72) O26.61- ☑
  - neoplasm
    - benign
      - cervix O34.4- ☑
      - corpus uteri O34.1- ☑
      - uterus O34.1- ☑
    - malignant O9A.11- ☑ (following O99)
  - nephropathy NEC O26.83- ☑
  - nervous system condition (conditions in G00-G99) O99.35- ☑
  - nutritional diseases NEC O99.28- ☑
  - obesity (pre-existing) O99.21- ☑
  - obesity surgery status O99.84- ☑
  - oblique lie or presentation O32.2- ☑
  - older mother — see Pregnancy, complicated by, elderly
  - oligohydramnios O41.0- ☑
    - with premature rupture of membranes — see also Pregnancy, complicated by, premature rupture of membranes O42.- ☑
  - onset (spontaneous) of labor after 37 completed weeks of gestation but before 39 completed weeks gestation, with delivery by (planned) cesarean section O75.82
  - oophoritis O23.52- ☑
  - overdose, drug — see also Table of Drugs and Chemicals, by drug, poisoning O9A.21- ☑ (following O99)
  - oversize fetus O33.5- ☑
  - papyraceous fetus O31.0- ☑
  - pelvic inflammatory disease O99.891
  - periodontal disease O99.61- ☑
  - peripheral neuritis O26.82- ☑
  - peritoneal (pelvic) adhesions O99.891
  - phlebitis O22.9- ☑
  - phlebopathy O22.9- ☑
  - phlebothrombosis (superficial) O22.2- ☑
    - deep O22.3- ☑
  - placenta accreta O43.21- ☑
  - placenta increta O43.22- ☑
  - placenta percreta O43.23- ☑
  - placenta previa O44.0- ☑
    - complete O44.0- ☑
      - with hemorrhage O44.1- ☑
    - marginal O44.2- ☑
      - with hemorrhage O44.3- ☑

Pregnancy — *continued*
- complicated by — *continued*
  - placenta previa — *continued*
    - partial O44.2-
      - with hemorrhage O44.3- ☑
  - placental disorder O43.9-
    - specified NEC O43.89- ☑
  - placental dysfunction O43.89- ☑
  - placental infarction O43.81- ☑
  - placental insufficiency O36.51- ☑
  - placental transfusion syndromes
    - fetomaternal O43.01- ☑
    - fetus to fetus O43.02- ☑
    - maternofetal O43.01- ☑
  - placentitis O41.14- ☑
  - pneumonia O99.51- ☑
  - poisoning — *see also* Table of Drugs and Chemicals O9A.21- ☑ (*following* O99)
  - polyhydramnios O40.- ☑
  - polymorphic eruption of pregnancy O26.86
  - poor obstetric history NEC O09.29- ☑
  - postmaturity (post-term) (40 to 42 weeks) O48.0
    - more than 42 completed weeks gestation (prolonged) O48.1
  - pre-eclampsia O14.9- ☑
    - mild O14.0- ☑
    - moderate O14.0- ☑
    - severe O14.1- ☑
      - with hemolysis, elevated liver enzymes and low platelet count (HELLP) O14.2- ☑
  - premature labor — *see* Pregnancy, complicated by, preterm labor
  - premature rupture of membranes O42.90
    - with onset of labor
      - within 24 hours O42.00
        - at or after 37 weeks gestation, onset of labor within 24 hours of rupture O42.02
        - pre-term (before 37 completed weeks of gestation) O42.01- ☑
      - after 24 hours O42.10
        - at or after 37 weeks gestation, onset of labor more than 24 hours following rupture O42.12
        - pre-term (before 37 completed weeks of gestation) O42.11- ☑
      - at or after 37 weeks gestation, unspecified as to length of time between rupture and onset of labor O42.92
      - full-term, unspecified as to length of time between rupture and onset of labor O42.92
      - pre-term (before 37 completed weeks of gestation) O42.91- ☑
  - premature separation of placenta — *see also* Abruptio placentae O45.9- ☑
  - presentation, fetal — *see* Delivery, complicated by, malposition
  - preterm delivery O60.10- ☑
  - preterm labor
    - with delivery O60.10- ☑
      - preterm O60.10- ☑
      - term O60.20- ☑
    - second trimester
      - with term delivery O60.22- ☑
      - without delivery O60.02
      - with preterm delivery
        - second trimester O60.12- ☑
        - third trimester O60.13- ☑
    - third trimester
      - with term delivery O60.23- ☑
      - without delivery O60.03
      - with third trimester preterm delivery O60.14- ☑
    - without delivery O60.00
      - second trimester O60.02
      - third trimester O60.03
  - previous history of — *see* Pregnancy, supervision of, high-risk
  - prolapse, uterus O34.52- ☑
  - proteinuria (gestational) — *see also* Proteinuria, gestational O12.1- ☑
    - with edema O12.2- ☑
  - pruritic urticarial papules and plaques of pregnancy (PUPPP) O26.86
  - pruritus (neurogenic) O26.89- ☑
  - psychosis or psychoneurosis (puerperal) F53.1
  - ptyalism O26.89- ☑

Pregnancy — *continued*
- complicated by — *continued*
  - PUPPP (pruritic urticarial papules and plaques of pregnancy) O26.86
  - pyelitis O23.0-
  - recurrent pregnancy loss O26.2- ☑
  - renal disease or failure NEC O26.83- ☑
    - with secondary hypertension, pre-existing — *see* Hypertension, complicating, pregnancy, pre-existing, secondary
    - hypertensive, pre-existing — *see* Hypertension, complicating, pregnancy, pre-existing, with, renal disease
  - respiratory condition (conditions in J00-J99) O99.51- ☑
  - retained, retention
    - dead ovum O02.0
    - intrauterine contraceptive device O26.3- ☑
  - retroversion, uterus O34.53- ☑
  - Rh immunization, incompatibility or sensitization NEC O36.09- ☑
    - anti-D antibody O36.01- ☑
  - rupture
    - amnion (premature) — *see also* Pregnancy, complicated by, premature rupture of membranes O42.- ☑
    - membranes (premature) — *see also* Pregnancy, complicated by, premature rupture of membranes O42.- ☑
    - uterus (during labor) O71.1
      - before onset of labor O71.0- ☑
  - salivation (excessive) O26.89- ☑
  - salpingitis O23.52- ☑
  - salpingo-oophoritis O23.52- ☑
  - sepsis (conditions in A40, A41) O98.81- ☑
  - size date discrepancy (uterine) O26.84- ☑
  - skin condition (conditions in L00-L99) O99.71- ☑
  - smoking (tobacco) O99.33- ☑
  - social problem O09.7- ☑
  - specified condition NEC O26.89- ☑
  - spotting O26.85- ☑
  - streptococcus group B (GBS) carrier state O99.820
  - subluxation of symphysis (pubis) O26.71- ☑
  - syphilis (conditions in A50-A53) O98.11- ☑
  - threatened
    - abortion O20.0
    - labor O47.9
      - at or after 37 completed weeks of gestation O47.1
      - before 37 completed weeks of gestation O47.0- ☑
  - thrombophlebitis (superficial) O22.2- ☑
  - thrombosis O22.9- ☑
    - cerebral venous O22.5- ☑
    - cerebrovenous sinus O22.5- ☑
    - deep O22.3- ☑
  - tobacco use disorder (smoking) O99.33- ☑
  - torsion of uterus O34.59- ☑
  - toxemia O14.9- ☑
  - transverse lie or presentation O32.2- ☑
  - tuberculosis (conditions in A15-A19) O98.01- ☑
  - tumor (benign)
    - cervix O34.4- ☑
    - malignant O9A.11- ☑ (*following* O99)
    - uterus O34.1- ☑
  - unstable lie O32.0- ☑
  - upper respiratory infection O99.51- ☑
  - urethritis O23.2- ☑
  - uterine size date discrepancy O26.84- ☑
  - vaginitis or vulvitis O23.59- ☑
  - varicose veins (lower extremities) O22.0- ☑
    - genitals O22.1- ☑
    - legs O22.0- ☑
    - perineal O22.1- ☑
    - vaginal or vulval O22.1- ☑
  - venereal disease NEC (conditions in A63.8) O98.31- ☑
  - venous disorders O22.9- ☑
    - specified NEC O22.8X- ☑
  - very young mother — *see* Pregnancy, complicated by, young mother
  - viral diseases (conditions in A80-B09, B25-B34) O98.51- ☑
  - vomiting O21.9
    - due to diseases classified elsewhere O21.8
    - hyperemesis gravidarum (mild) — *see also* Hyperemesis, gravidarum O21.0

Pregnancy — *continued*
- complicated by — *continued*
  - vomiting — *continued*
    - late (occurring after 20 weeks of gestation) O21.2
  - young mother
    - multigravida O09.62- ☑
    - primigravida O09.61- ☑
  - complicated NOS O26.9- ☑
- concealed O09.3- ☑
- continuing following
  - elective fetal reduction of one or more fetus O31.3- ☑
  - intrauterine death of one or more fetus O31.2- ☑
  - spontaneous abortion of one or more fetus O31.1- ☑
- cornual O00.80
  - with intrauterine pregnancy O00.81
- ectopic (ruptured) O00.90
  - with intrauterine pregnancy O00.91
  - abdominal O00.00
    - with
      - intrauterine pregnancy O00.01
      - viable fetus O36.7- ☑
  - cervical O00.80
    - with intrauterine pregnancy O00.81
  - complicated (by) O08.9
    - afibrinogenemia O08.1
    - cardiac arrest O08.81
    - chemical damage of pelvic organ(s) O08.6
    - circulatory collapse O08.3
    - defibrination syndrome O08.1
    - electrolyte imbalance O08.5
    - embolism (amniotic fluid) (blood clot) (pulmonary) (septic) O08.2
    - endometritis O08.0
    - genital tract and pelvic infection O08.0
    - hemorrhage (delayed) (excessive) O08.1
    - infection
      - genital tract or pelvic O08.0
      - kidney O08.83
      - urinary tract O08.83
    - intravascular coagulation O08.1
    - laceration of pelvic organ(s) O08.6
    - metabolic disorder O08.5
    - oliguria O08.4
    - oophoritis O08.0
    - parametritis O08.0
    - pelvic peritonitis O08.0
    - perforation of pelvic organ(s) O08.6
    - renal failure or shutdown O08.4
    - salpingitis or salpingo-oophoritis O08.0
    - sepsis O08.82
    - shock O08.83
      - septic O08.82
    - specified condition NEC O08.89
    - tubular necrosis (renal) O08.4
    - uremia O08.4
    - urinary infection O08.83
    - venous complication NEC O08.7
      - embolism O08.2
  - cornual O00.80
    - with intrauterine pregnancy O00.81
  - intraligamentous O00.80
    - with intrauterine pregnancy O00.81
  - mural O00.80
    - with intrauterine pregnancy O00.81
  - ovarian O00.20- ☑
    - with intrauterine pregnancy O00.21- ☑
  - specified site NEC O00.80
    - with intrauterine pregnancy O00.81
  - tubal (ruptured) O00.10- ☑
    - with intrauterine pregnancy O00.11- ☑
- examination (normal) Z34.9- ☑
  - first Z34.0- ☑
  - high-risk — *see* Pregnancy, supervision of, high-risk
  - specified Z34.8- ☑
- extrauterine — *see* Pregnancy, ectopic
- fallopian O00.10- ☑
  - with intrauterine pregnancy O00.11- ☑
- false F45.8
- gestational carrier Z33.3
- heptachorionic, hepta-amniotic (septuplets) O30.83- ☑
- hexachorionic, hexa-amniotic (sextuplets) O30.83- ☑
- hidden O09.3- ☑
- high-risk — *see* Pregnancy, supervision of, high-risk
- incidental finding Z33.1
- interstitial O00.80
  - with intrauterine pregnancy O00.81
- intraligamentous O00.80
  - with intrauterine pregnancy O00.81

☑ **Additional Character Required** — Refer to the Tabular List for Character Selection

Pregnancy

Pregnancy — *continued*
- intramural O00.80
  - with intrauterine pregnancy O00.81
- intraperitoneal O00.00
  - with intrauterine pregnancy O00.01
- isthmian O00.10- ☑
  - with intrauterine pregnancy O00.11- ☑
- mesometric (mural) O00.80
  - with intrauterine pregnancy O00.81
- molar NEC O02.0
- complicated (by) O08.9
  - afibrinogenemia O08.1
  - cardiac arrest O08.81
  - chemical damage of pelvic organ(s) O08.6
  - circulatory collapse O08.3
  - defibrination syndrome O08.1
  - electrolyte imbalance O08.5
  - embolism (amniotic fluid) (blood clot) (pulmonary) (septic) O08.2
  - endometritis O08.0
  - genital tract and pelvic infection O08.0
  - hemorrhage (delayed) (excessive) O08.1
  - infection
    - genital tract or pelvic O08.0
    - kidney O08.83
    - urinary tract O08.83
  - intravascular coagulation O08.1
  - laceration of pelvic organ(s) O08.6
  - metabolic disorder O08.5
  - oliguria O08.4
  - oophoritis O08.0
  - parametritis O08.0
  - pelvic peritonitis O08.0
  - perforation of pelvic organ(s) O08.6
  - renal failure or shutdown O08.4
  - salpingitis or salpingo-oophoritis O08.0
  - sepsis O08.82
  - shock O08.3
    - septic O08.82
  - specified condition NEC O08.89
  - tubular necrosis (renal) O08.4
  - uremia O08.4
  - urinary infection O08.83
  - venous complication NEC O08.7
    - embolism O08.2
- hydatidiform — *see also* Mole, hydatidiform O01.9
- multiple (gestation) O30.9- ☑
  - greater than quadruplets — *see* Pregnancy, multiple (gestation), specified NEC
  - specified NEC O30.80- ☑
    - with
      - two or more monoamniotic fetuses O30.82- ☑
      - two or more monochorionic fetuses O30.81- ☑
      - number of chorions and amnions are both equal to the number of fetuses O30.83- ☑
      - two or more monoamniotic fetuses O30.82- ☑
      - two or more monochorionic fetuses O30.81- ☑
      - unable to determine number of placenta and number of amniotic sacs O30.89- ☑
      - unspecified number of placenta and unspecified number of amniotic sacs O30.80- ☑
- mural O00.80
  - with intrauterine pregnancy O00.81
- normal (supervision of) Z34.9- ☑
  - first Z34.0- ☑
  - high-risk — *see* Pregnancy, supervision of, high-risk
  - specified Z34.8- ☑
- ovarian O00.20- ☑
  - with intrauterine pregnancy O00.21- ☑
- pentachorionic, penta-amniotic (quintuplets) O30.83- ☑
- postmature (40 to 42 weeks) O48.0
  - more than 42 weeks gestation O48.1
- post-term (40 to 42 weeks) O48.0
- prenatal care only Z34.9- ☑
  - first Z34.0- ☑
  - high-risk — *see* Pregnancy, supervision of, high-risk
  - specified Z34.8- ☑
- prolonged (more than 42 weeks gestation) O48.1
- quadruplet O30.20- ☑
  - with
    - two or more monoamniotic fetuses O30.22- ☑
    - two or more monochorionic fetuses O30.21- ☑
    - quadrachorionic/quadra-amniotic O30.23- ☑
    - two or more monoamniotic fetuses O30.22- ☑
    - two or more monochorionic fetuses O30.21- ☑
    - unable to determine number of placenta and number of amniotic sacs O30.29- ☑

Pregnancy — *continued*
- quadruplet — *continued*
  - unspecified number of placenta and unspecified number of amniotic sacs O30.20- ☑
- quintuplet — *see* Pregnancy, multiple (gestation), specified NEC
- sextuplet — *see* Pregnancy, multiple (gestation), specified NEC
- supervision of
  - concealed pregnancy O09.3- ☑
  - elderly mother
    - multigravida O09.52- ☑
    - primigravida O09.51- ☑
  - hidden pregnancy O09.3- ☑
  - high-risk O09.9- ☑
    - due to (history of)
      - ectopic pregnancy O09.1- ☑
      - elderly — *see* Pregnancy, supervision, elderly mother
      - grand multiparity O09.4- ☑
      - in utero procedure during previous pregnancy O09.82- ☑
      - in vitro fertilization O09.81- ☑
      - infertility O09.0- ☑
      - insufficient prenatal care O09.3- ☑
      - molar pregnancy O09.A- ☑
      - multiple previous pregnancies O09.4- ☑
      - older mother — *see* Pregnancy, supervision of, elderly mother
      - poor reproductive or obstetric history NEC O09.29- ☑
      - pre-term labor O09.21- ☑
      - previous
        - neonatal death O09.29- ☑
        - social problems O09.7- ☑
      - specified NEC O09.89- ☑
      - very young mother — *see* Pregnancy, supervision, young mother
    - resulting from in vitro fertilization O09.81- ☑
  - normal Z34.9-
    - first Z34.0- ☑
    - specified NEC Z34.8- ☑
  - young mother
    - multigravida O09.62- ☑
    - primigravida O09.61- ☑
- triplet O30.10- ☑
  - with
    - two or more monoamniotic fetuses O30.12- ☑
    - two or more monochorionic fetuses O30.11- ☑
    - trichorionic/triamniotic O30.13- ☑
    - two or more monoamniotic fetuses O30.12- ☑
    - two or more monochorionic fetuses O30.11- ☑
    - unable to determine number of placenta and number of amniotic sacs O30.19- ☑
    - unspecified number of placenta and unspecified number of amniotic sacs O30.10- ☑
- tubal (with abortion) (with rupture) O00.10- ☑
  - with intrauterine pregnancy O00.11- ☑
- twin O30.00- ☑
  - conjoined O30.02- ☑
  - dichorionic/diamniotic (two placenta, two amniotic sacs) O30.04- ☑
  - monochorionic/diamniotic (one placenta, two amniotic sacs) O30.03- ☑
  - monochorionic/monoamniotic (one placenta, one amniotic sac) O30.01- ☑
  - unable to determine number of placenta and number of amniotic sacs O30.09- ☑
  - unspecified number of placenta and unspecified number of amniotic sacs O30.00- ☑
- unwanted Z64.0
- weeks of gestation
  - 8 weeks Z3A.08 (*following* Z36)
  - 9 weeks Z3A.09 (*following* Z36)
  - 10 weeks Z3A.10 (*following* Z36)
  - 11 weeks Z3A.11 (*following* Z36)
  - 12 weeks Z3A.12 (*following* Z36)
  - 13 weeks Z3A.13 (*following* Z36)
  - 14 weeks Z3A.14 (*following* Z36)
  - 15 weeks Z3A.15 (*following* Z36)
  - 16 weeks Z3A.16 (*following* Z36)
  - 17 weeks Z3A.17 (*following* Z36)
  - 18 weeks Z3A.18 (*following* Z36)
  - 19 weeks Z3A.19 (*following* Z36)
  - 20 weeks Z3A.20 (*following* Z36)
  - 21 weeks Z3A.21 (*following* Z36)
  - 22 weeks Z3A.22 (*following* Z36)

Pregnancy — *continued*
- weeks of gestation — *continued*
  - 23 weeks Z3A.23 (*following* Z36)
  - 24 weeks Z3A.24 (*following* Z36)
  - 25 weeks Z3A.25 (*following* Z36)
  - 26 weeks Z3A.26 (*following* Z36)
  - 27 weeks Z3A.27 (*following* Z36)
  - 28 weeks Z3A.28 (*following* Z36)
  - 29 weeks Z3A.29 (*following* Z36)
  - 30 weeks Z3A.30 (*following* Z36)
  - 31 weeks Z3A.31 (*following* Z36)
  - 32 weeks Z3A.32 (*following* Z36)
  - 33 weeks Z3A.33 (*following* Z36)
  - 34 weeks Z3A.34 (*following* Z36)
  - 35 weeks Z3A.35 (*following* Z36)
  - 36 weeks Z3A.36 (*following* Z36)
  - 37 weeks Z3A.37 (*following* Z36)
  - 38 weeks Z3A.38 (*following* Z36)
  - 39 weeks Z3A.39 (*following* Z36)
  - 40 weeks Z3A.40 (*following* Z36)
  - 41 weeks Z3A.41 (*following* Z36)
  - 42 weeks Z3A.42 (*following* Z36)
  - greater than 42 weeks Z3A.49 (*following* Z36)
  - less than 8 weeks Z3A.01 (*following* Z36)
  - not specified Z3A.00 (*following* Z36)

Preiser's disease — *see* Osteonecrosis, secondary, due to, trauma, metacarpus
Pre-kwashiorkor — *see* Malnutrition, severe
Preleukemia (syndrome) D46.9
Preluxation, hip, congenital Q65.6
Premature — *see also* condition
- adrenarche E27.0
- aging E34.8
- beats I49.40
  - atrial I49.1
  - auricular I49.1
  - supraventricular I49.1
- birth NEC — *see* Preterm, newborn
- closure, foramen ovale Q21.8
- contraction
  - atrial I49.1
  - atrioventricular I49.2
  - auricular I49.1
  - auriculoventricular I49.49
  - heart (extrasystole) I49.49
  - junctional I49.2
  - ventricular I49.3
- delivery — *see also* Pregnancy, complicated by, preterm labor O60.10- ☑
- ejaculation F52.4
- infant NEC — *see* Preterm, newborn
  - light-for-dates — *see* Light for dates
- labor — *see* Pregnancy, complicated by, preterm labor
- lungs P28.0
- menopause E28.319
  - asymptomatic E28.319
  - symptomatic E28.310
- newborn
  - extreme (less than 28 completed weeks) — *see* Immaturity, extreme
  - less than 37 completed weeks — *see* Preterm, newborn
- puberty E30.1
- rupture membranes or amnion — *see* Pregnancy, complicated by, premature rupture of membranes
- senility E34.8
- thelarche E30.8
- ventricular systole I49.3

Prematurity NEC (less than 37 completed weeks) — *see* Preterm, newborn
- extreme (less than 28 completed weeks) — *see* Immaturity, extreme

Premenstrual
- dysphoric disorder (PMDD) F32.81
- tension (syndrome) N94.3

Premolarization, cuspids K00.2
Prenatal
- care, normal pregnancy — *see* Pregnancy, normal
- screening of mother — *see also* Encounter, antenatal screening Z36.9
- teeth K00.6

Preparatory care for subsequent treatment NEC
- for dialysis Z49.01
  - peritoneal Z49.02

Prepartum — *see* condition
Preponderance, left or right ventricular I51.7
Prepuce — *see* condition
PRES (posterior reversible encephalopathy syndrome) I67.83
Presbycardia R54

Presbycusis, presbyacusia H91.1- ☑
Presbyesophagus K22.89
Presbyophrenia F03.- ☑
Presbyopia H52.4
Prescription of contraceptives (initial) Z30.019
  barrier Z30.018
  diaphragm Z30.018
  emergency (postcoital) Z30.012
  implantable subdermal Z30.017
  injectable Z30.013
  intrauterine contraceptive device Z30.014
  pills Z30.011
  postcoital (emergency) Z30.012
  repeat Z30.40
    barrier Z30.49
    diaphragm Z30.49
    implantable subdermal Z30.46
    injectable Z30.42
    pills Z30.41
    specified type NEC Z30.49
    transdermal patch hormonal Z30.45
    vaginal ring hormonal Z30.44
  specified type NEC Z30.018
    transdermal patch hormonal Z30.016
    vaginal ring hormonal Z30.015
Presence (of)
  ankle-joint implant (functional) (prosthesis) Z96.66-
  aortocoronary (bypass) graft Z95.1
  arterial-venous shunt (dialysis) Z99.2
  artificial
    eye (globe) Z97.0
    heart (fully implantable) (mechanical) Z95.812
      valve Z95.2
    larynx Z96.3
    lens (intraocular) Z96.1
    limb (complete) (partial) Z97.1- ☑
      arm Z97.1- ☑
        bilateral Z97.15
      leg Z97.1- ☑
        bilateral Z97.16
  audiological implant (functional) Z96.29
  bladder implant (functional) Z96.0
  bone
    conduction hearing device Z96.29
    implant (functional) NEC Z96.7
    joint (prosthesis) — see Presence, joint implant
  cardiac
    defibrillator (functional) (with synchronous cardiac pacemaker) Z95.810
    implant or graft Z95.9
      specified type NEC Z95.818
    pacemaker Z95.0
    resynchronization therapy
      defibrillator Z95.810
      pacemaker Z95.0
  cardioverter-defibrillator (ICD) Z95.810
  cerebrospinal fluid drainage device Z98.2
  cochlear implant (functional) Z96.21
  contact lens (es) Z97.3
  coronary artery graft or prosthesis Z95.5
  CRT-D (cardiac resynchronization therapy defibrillator) Z95.810
  CRT-P (cardiac resynchronization therapy pacemaker) Z95.0
  CSF shunt Z98.2
  dental prosthesis device Z97.2
  dentures Z97.2
  device (external) NEC Z97.8
    cardiac NEC Z95.818
    heart assist Z95.811
    implanted (functional) Z96.9
      specified NEC Z96.89
    prosthetic Z97.8
  ear implant Z96.20
    cochlear implant Z96.21
    myringotomy tube Z96.22
    specified type NEC Z96.29
  elbow-joint implant (functional) (prosthesis) Z96.62- ☑
  endocrine implant (functional) NEC Z96.49
  eustachian tube stent or device (functional) Z96.29
  external hearing-aid or device Z97.4
  finger-joint implant (functional) (prosthesis) Z96.69- ☑
  functional implant Z96.9
    specified NEC Z96.89
  graft
    cardiac NEC Z95.818
    vascular NEC Z95.828
  hearing-aid or device (external) Z97.4

Presence — continued
  hearing-aid or device — continued
    implant (bone) (cochlear) (functional) Z96.21
  heart assist device Z95.811
  heart valve implant (functional) Z95.2
    prosthetic Z95.2
    specified type NEC Z95.4
    xenogenic Z95.3
  hip-joint implant (functional) (prosthesis) Z96.64- ☑
  ICD (cardioverter-defibrillator) Z95.810
  implanted device (artificial) (functional) (prosthetic) Z96.9
    automatic cardiac defibrillator (with synchronous cardiac pacemaker) Z95.810
    cardiac pacemaker Z95.0
    cochlear Z96.21
    dental Z96.5
    heart Z95.812
    heart valve Z95.2
      prosthetic Z95.2
      specified NEC Z95.4
      xenogenic Z95.3
    insulin pump Z96.41
    intraocular lens Z96.1
    joint Z96.60
      ankle Z96.66- ☑
      elbow Z96.62- ☑
      finger Z96.69- ☑
      hip Z96.64- ☑
      knee Z96.65- ☑
      shoulder Z96.61- ☑
      specified NEC Z96.698
      wrist Z96.63- ☑
    larynx Z96.3
    myringotomy tube Z96.22
    otological Z96.20
      cochlear Z96.21
      eustachian stent Z96.29
      myringotomy Z96.22
      specified NEC Z96.29
      stapes Z96.29
    skin Z96.81
    skull plate Z96.7
    specified NEC Z96.89
    urogenital Z96.0
  insulin pump (functional) Z96.41
  intestinal bypass or anastomosis Z98.0
  intraocular lens (functional) Z96.1
  intrauterine contraceptive device (IUD) Z97.5
  intravascular implant (functional) (prosthetic) NEC Z95.9
    coronary artery Z95.5
    defibrillator (with synchronous cardiac pacemaker) Z95.810
    peripheral vessel (with angioplasty) Z95.820
  joint implant (prosthetic) (any) Z96.60
    ankle — see Presence, ankle joint implant
    elbow — see Presence, elbow joint implant
    finger — see Presence, finger joint implant
    hip — see Presence, hip joint implant
    knee — see Presence, knee joint implant
    shoulder — see Presence, shoulder joint implant
    specified joint NEC Z96.698
    wrist — see Presence, wrist joint implant
  knee-joint implant (functional) (prosthesis) Z96.65- ☑
  laryngeal implant (functional) Z96.3
  mandibular implant (dental) Z96.5
  myringotomy tube(s) Z96.22
  neurostimulator (brain) (gastric) (peripheral nerve) (sacral nerve) (spinal cord) (vagus nerve) Z96.82
  orthopedic-joint implant (prosthetic) (any) — see Presence, joint implant
  otological implant (functional) Z96.29
  shoulder-joint implant (functional) (prosthesis) Z96.61- ☑
  skull-plate implant Z96.7
  spectacles Z97.3
  stapes implant (functional) Z96.29
  systemic lupus erythematosus [SLE] inhibitor D68.62
  tendon implant (functional) (graft) Z96.7
  tooth root(s) implant Z96.5
  ureteral stent Z96.0
  urethral stent Z96.0
  urogenital implant (functional) Z96.0
  vascular implant or device Z95.9
    access port device Z95.828
    specified type NEC Z95.828
  wrist-joint implant (functional) (prosthesis) Z96.63- ☑
Presenile — see also condition
  dementia F03.- ☑

Presenile — continued
  premature aging E34.8
Presentation, fetal — see Delivery, complicated by, malposition
Prespondylolisthesis (congenital) Q76.2
Pressure
  area, skin — see Ulcer, pressure, by site
  brachial plexus G54.0
  brain G93.5
    injury at birth NEC P11.1
  cerebral — see Pressure, brain
  chest R07.89
  cone, tentorial G93.5
  hyposystolic — see also Hypotension
    incidental reading, without diagnosis of hypotension R03.1
  increased
    intracranial benign G93.2
      injury at birth P11.0
    intraocular H40.05- ☑
  injury — see Ulcer, pressure, by site
  lumbosacral plexus G54.1
  mediastinum J98.59
  necrosis (chronic) — see Ulcer, pressure, by site
  parental, inappropriate (excessive) Z62.6
  sore (chronic) — see Ulcer, pressure, by site
  spinal cord G95.20
  ulcer (chronic) — see Ulcer, pressure, by site
  venous, increased I87.8
Pre-syncope R55
Preterm
  delivery — see also Pregnancy, complicated by, preterm labor O60.10- ☑
  labor — see Pregnancy, complicated by, preterm labor
  newborn (infant) P07.30
    gestational age
      28 completed weeks (28 weeks, 0 days through 28 weeks, 6 days) P07.31
      29 completed weeks (29 weeks, 0 days through 29 weeks, 6 days) P07.32
      30 completed weeks (30 weeks, 0 days through 30 weeks, 6 days) P07.33
      31 completed weeks (31 weeks, 0 days through 31 weeks, 6 days) P07.34
      32 completed weeks (32 weeks, 0 days through 32 weeks, 6 days) P07.35
      33 completed weeks (33 weeks, 0 days through 33 weeks, 6 days) P07.36
      34 completed weeks (34 weeks, 0 days through 34 weeks, 6 days) P07.37
      35 completed weeks (35 weeks, 0 days through 35 weeks, 6 days) P07.38
      36 completed weeks (36 weeks, 0 days through 36 weeks, 6 days) P07.39
Previa
  placenta (total) (without hemorrhage) O44.0- ☑
    with hemorrhage O44.1- ☑
    complete O44.0- ☑
      with hemorrhage O44.1- ☑
    low — see also Delivery, complicated, by, placenta, low O44.4- ☑
      with hemorrhage O44.5- ☑
    marginal O44.2- ☑
      with hemorrhage O44.3- ☑
    partial O44.2- ☑
      with hemorrhage O44.3- ☑
  vasa O69.4- ☑
Priapism N48.30
  due to
    disease classified elsewhere N48.32
    drug N48.33
    sickle-cell disease — see Disease, sickle-cell, by type, with priapism
    specified cause NEC N48.39
    trauma N48.31
Prickling sensation (skin) R20.2
Prickly heat L74.0
Primary — see condition
Primigravida
  elderly, affecting management of pregnancy, labor and delivery (supervision only) — see Pregnancy, complicated by, elderly, primigravida
  older, affecting management of pregnancy, labor and delivery (supervision only) — see Pregnancy, complicated by, elderly, primigravida
  very young, affecting management of pregnancy, labor and delivery (supervision only) — see Pregnancy, complicated by, young mother, primigravida

Primipara
- elderly, affecting management of pregnancy, labor and delivery (supervision only) — see Pregnancy, complicated by, elderly, primigravida
- older, affecting management of pregnancy, labor and delivery (supervision only) — see Pregnancy, complicated by, elderly, primigravida
- very young, affecting management of pregnancy, labor and delivery (supervision only) — see Pregnancy, complicated by, young mother, primigravida

Primus varus Q66.21- ☑
PRIND (Prolonged reversible ischemic neurologic deficit) I63.9
Pringle's disease (tuberous sclerosis) Q85.1
Prinzmetal angina I20.1
Prizefighter ear — see Cauliflower ear
Problem (with) (related to)
- academic Z55.8
- acculturation Z60.3
- adjustment (to)
  - change of job Z56.1
  - life-cycle transition Z60.0
  - pension Z60.0
  - retirement Z60.0
- adopted child Z62.821
- alcoholism in family Z63.72
- atypical parenting situation Z62.9
- bankruptcy Z59.89
- behavioral (adult) F69
  - drug seeking Z76.5
- birth of sibling affecting child Z62.898
- care (of)
  - provider dependency Z74.9
  - specified NEC Z74.8
  - sick or handicapped person in family or household Z63.6
- child
  - abuse (affecting the child) — see Maltreatment, child
  - custody or support proceedings Z65.3
  - in
    - care of non-parental family member Z62.23
    - custody of
      - grandparent Z62.23
      - non-parental relative Z62.23
      - non-relative guardian Z62.24
    - foster care Z62.21
    - kinship care Z62.23
    - welfare
      - custody Z62.21
      - guardianship Z62.21
  - leaving living situation without permission Z62.892
  - living in
    - group home Z62.22
    - orphanage Z62.22
- child-rearing Z62.9
  - specified NEC Z62.898
- communication (developmental) F80.9
- completing medical forms Z55.6
- conflict or discord (with)
  - boss Z56.4
  - classmates Z55.4
  - counselor Z64.4
  - employer Z56.4
  - family Z63.9
    - specified NEC Z63.8
  - probation officer Z64.4
  - social worker Z64.4
  - teachers Z55.4
  - workmates Z56.4
- conviction in legal proceedings Z65.0
  - with imprisonment Z65.1
- counselor Z64.4
- creditors Z59.89
- digestive K92.9
- drug addict in family Z63.72
- ear — see Disorder, ear
- economic Z59.9
  - affecting care Z59.9
  - specified NEC Z59.89
  - strain Z59.868
- education Z55.9
  - specified NEC Z55.8
- employment Z56.9
  - change of job Z56.1
  - discord Z56.4
  - environment Z56.5
  - sexual harassment Z56.81
  - specified NEC Z56.89
  - stress NEC Z56.6

Problem — continued
- employment — continued
  - stressful schedule Z56.3
  - threat of job loss Z56.2
  - unemployment Z56.0
- enuresis, child F98.0
- eye H57.9
- failed examinations (school) Z55.2
- falling Z91.81
- family — see also Disruption, family Z63.9
  - specified NEC Z63.8
- feeding (elderly) (infant) NOS R63.39
  - newborn P92.9
    - breast P92.5
    - overfeeding P92.4
    - slow P92.2
    - specified NEC P92.8
    - underfeeding P92.3
  - nonorganic F50.89
- finance Z59.9
  - specified NEC Z59.89
- foreclosure on loan Z59.89
- foster child Z62.822
- frightening experience(s) in childhood Z62.898
- genital NEC
  - female N94.9
  - male N50.9
- health care Z75.9
  - specified NEC Z75.8
- health literacy Z55.6
- hearing — see Deafness
- homelessness Z59.00
- housing Z59.9
  - inadequate Z59.10
  - isolated Z59.89
  - specified NEC Z59.89
- identity (of childhood) F93.8
- illegitimate pregnancy (unwanted) Z64.0
- illiteracy Z55.0
- impaired mobility Z74.09
- imprisonment or incarceration Z65.1
- in-law Z63.1
- inadequate teaching affecting education Z55.8
- inappropriate (excessive) parental pressure Z62.6
- influencing health status NEC Z78.9
- institutionalization, affecting child Z62.22
- intrafamilial communication Z63.8
- jealousy, child F93.8
- landlord Z59.2
- language (developmental) F80.9
- learning (developmental) F81.9
- legal Z65.3
  - conviction without imprisonment Z65.0
  - imprisonment Z65.1
  - release from prison Z65.2
- life-management Z73.9
  - specified NEC Z73.89
- life-style Z72.9
  - gambling Z72.6
  - high-risk sexual behavior (heterosexual) Z72.51
    - bisexual Z72.53
    - homosexual Z72.52
  - inappropriate eating habits Z72.4
  - self-damaging behavior NEC Z72.89
  - specified NEC Z72.89
  - tobacco use Z72.0
- literacy Z55.9
  - low level Z55.0
  - specified NEC Z55.8
- living alone Z60.2
- lodgers Z59.2
- loss of love relationship in childhood Z62.898
- marital Z63.0
  - involving
    - divorce Z63.5
    - estrangement Z63.5
    - gender identity F66
- mastication K08.89
- medical
  - care, within family Z63.6
  - facilities Z75.9
    - specified NEC Z75.8
- mental F48.9
- money Z59.868
- multiparity Z64.1
- negative life events in childhood Z62.9
  - altered pattern of family relationships Z62.898
  - frightening experience Z62.898

Problem — continued
- negative life events in childhood — continued
  - loss of
    - love relationship Z62.898
    - self-esteem Z62.898
  - physical abuse (alleged) — see Maltreatment, child
  - removal from home Z62.29
  - specified event NEC Z62.898
- neighbor Z59.2
- neurological NEC R29.818
- new step-parent affecting child Z62.898
- none (feared complaint unfounded) Z71.1
- occupational NEC Z56.89
- parent-child — see Conflict, parent-child
- personal hygiene Z91.89
- personality F69
- phase-of-life transition, adjustment Z60.0
- presence of sick or disabled person in family or household Z63.79
  - needing care Z63.6
- primary support group (family) Z63.9
  - specified NEC Z63.8
- probation officer Z64.4
- psychiatric F99
- psychosexual (development) F66
- psychosocial Z65.9
  - religious or spiritual Z65.8
  - specified NEC Z65.8
- related to physical environment, specified NEC Z58.89
- relationship Z63.9
  - childhood F93.8
- release from prison Z65.2
  - religious or spiritual Z65.8
- removal from home affecting child Z62.29
- seeking and accepting known hazardous and harmful
  - behavioral or psychological interventions Z65.8
  - chemical, nutritional or physical interventions Z65.8
- sexual function (nonorganic) F52.9
- sight H54.7
- sleep disorder, child F51.9
- smell — see Disturbance, sensation, smell
- social
  - environment Z60.9
    - specified NEC Z60.8
  - exclusion and rejection Z60.4
  - worker Z64.4
- speech R47.9
  - developmental F80.9
  - specified NEC R47.89
- swallowing — see Dysphagia
- taste — see Disturbance, sensation, taste
- tic, child F95.0
- underachievement in school Z55.3
- unemployment Z56.0
  - threatened Z56.2
- unwanted pregnancy Z64.0
- upbringing Z62.9
  - specified NEC Z62.898
- urinary N39.9
- voice production R47.89
- work schedule (stressful) Z56.3

Procedure (surgical)
- converted
  - arthroscopic to open Z53.33
  - laparoscopic to open Z53.31
  - specified procedure NEC to open Z53.39
  - thoracoscopic to open Z53.32
- for purpose other than remedying health state Z41.9
  - specified NEC Z41.8
- not done Z53.9
  - because of
    - administrative reasons Z53.8
    - contraindication Z53.09
      - smoking Z53.01
    - patient's decision Z53.20
      - for reasons of belief or group pressure Z53.1
      - left against medical advice (AMA) Z53.29
      - left without being seen Z53.21
      - specified reason NEC Z53.29
    - specified reason NEC Z53.8

Procidentia (uteri) N81.3
Proctalgia K62.89
- fugax K59.4
- spasmodic K59.4

Proctitis K62.89
- amebic (acute) A06.0
- chlamydial A56.3
- gonococcal A54.6
- granulomatous — see Enteritis, regional, large intestine

Proctitis — continued
- herpetic A60.1
- radiation K62.7
- tuberculous A18.32
- ulcerative (chronic) K51.20
  - with
    - complication K51.219
      - abscess K51.214
      - fistula K51.213
      - obstruction K51.212
      - rectal bleeding K51.211
      - specified NEC K51.218

Proctocele
- female (without uterine prolapse) N81.6
  - with uterine prolapse N81.2
    - complete N81.3
- male K62.3

Proctocolitis
- allergic K52.29
- food-induced eosinophilic K52.29
- food protein-induced K52.29
- milk protein-induced K52.29
- mucosal — see Rectosigmoiditis, ulcerative

Proctoptosis K62.3
Proctorrhagia K62.5
Proctosigmoiditis K63.89
- ulcerative (chronic) — see Rectosigmoiditis, ulcerative

Proctospasm K59.4
- psychogenic F45.8

Profichet's disease — see Disorder, soft tissue, specified type NEC
Progeria E34.8
Prognathism (mandibular) (maxillary) M26.19
Progonoma (melanotic) — see Neoplasm, benign, by site
Progressive — see condition
Prolactinoma
- specified site — see Neoplasm, benign, by site
- unspecified site D35.2

Prolapse, prolapsed
- anus, anal (canal) (sphincter) K62.2
- arm or hand O32.2- ☑
  - causing obstructed labor O64.4- ☑
- bladder (mucosa) (sphincter) (acquired)
  - congenital Q79.4
  - female — see Cystocele
  - male N32.89
- breast implant (prosthetic) T85.49- ☑
- cecostomy K94.09
- cecum K63.4
- cervix, cervical (hypertrophied) N81.2
  - anterior lip, obstructing labor O65.5
  - postpartal, old N81.2
  - stump N81.85
- ciliary body (traumatic) — see Laceration, eye(ball), with prolapse or loss of interocular tissue
- colon (pedunculated) K63.4
- colostomy K94.09
- disc (intervertebral) — see Displacement, intervertebral disc
- eye implant (orbital) T85.398- ☑
  - lens (ocular) — see Complications, intraocular lens
- fallopian tube N83.4- ☑
- gastric (mucosa) K31.89
- genital, female N81.9
  - specified NEC N81.89
- globe, nontraumatic — see Luxation, globe
- ileostomy bud K94.19
- intervertebral disc — see Displacement, intervertebral disc
- intestine (small) K63.4
- iris (traumatic) — see Laceration, eye(ball), with prolapse or loss of interocular tissue
  - nontraumatic H21.89
- kidney N28.83
  - congenital Q63.2
- laryngeal muscles or ventricle J38.7
- liver K76.89
- meatus urinarius N36.8
- mitral (valve) I34.1
- ocular lens implant — see Complications, intraocular lens
- organ or site, congenital NEC — see Malposition, congenital
- ovary N83.4- ☑
- pelvic floor, female N81.89
- perineum, female N81.89
- rectum (mucosa) (sphincter) K62.3

Prolapse, prolapsed — continued
- rectum — continued
  - due to trichuris trichuria B79
- spleen D73.89
- stomach K31.89
- umbilical cord
  - complicating delivery O69.0- ☑
- urachus, congenital Q64.4
- ureter N28.89
  - with obstruction N13.5
    - with infection N13.6
- ureterovesical orifice N28.89
- urethra (acquired) (infected) (mucosa) N36.8
  - congenital Q64.71
- urinary meatus N36.8
  - congenital Q64.72
- uterovaginal N81.4
  - complete N81.3
  - incomplete N81.2
- uterus (with prolapse of vagina) N81.4
  - complete N81.3
  - congenital Q51.818
  - first degree N81.2
  - in pregnancy or childbirth — see Pregnancy, complicated by, abnormal, uterus
  - incomplete N81.2
  - postpartal (old) N81.4
  - second degree N81.2
  - third degree N81.3
- uveal (traumatic) — see Laceration, eye(ball), with prolapse or loss of interocular tissue
- vagina (anterior) (wall) — see Cystocele
  - with prolapse of uterus N81.4
    - complete N81.3
    - incomplete N81.2
  - posterior wall N81.6
  - posthysterectomy N99.3
- vitreous (humor) H43.0- ☑
  - in wound — see Laceration, eye(ball), with prolapse or loss of interocular tissue
- womb — see Prolapse, uterus

Prolapsus, female N81.9
- specified NEC N81.89

Proliferation(s)
- primary cutaneous CD30-positive large T-cell C86.6- ☑
- prostate, atypical small acinar N42.32

Proliferative — see condition
Prolonged, prolongation (of)
- bleeding (time) (idiopathic) R79.1
- coagulation (time) R79.1
- gestation (over 42 completed weeks)
  - mother O48.1
  - newborn P08.22
- interval I44.0
- labor O63.9
  - first stage O63.0
  - second stage O63.1
- partial thromboplastin time (PTT) R79.1
- pregnancy (more than 42 weeks gestation) O48.1
- prothrombin time R79.1
- QT interval R94.31
- uterine contractions in labor O62.4

Prominence, prominent
- auricle (congenital) (ear) Q17.5
- ischial spine or sacral promontory with disproportion (fetopelvic) O33.0
  - causing obstructed labor O65.0
- nose (congenital) acquired M95.0

Promiscuity — see High, risk, sexual behavior
Pronation
- ankle — see Deformity, limb, foot, specified NEC
- foot — see also Deformity, limb, foot, specified NEC
  - congenital Q74.2

Prophylactic
- administration of
  - antibiotics, long-term Z79.2
    - short-term use — omit code
  - drug — see also Long-term (current) drug therapy (use of) Z79.899
  - medication Z79.899
- organ removal (for neoplasia management) Z40.00
  - breast Z40.01
  - fallopian tube(s) Z40.03
    - with ovary(s) Z40.02
  - ovary(s) Z40.02
  - specified site NEC Z40.09
- surgery Z40.9
  - for risk factors related to malignant neoplasm — see Prophylactic, organ removal

Prophylactic — continued
- surgery — continued
  - specified NEC Z40.89
- vaccination Z23

Propionic acidemia E71.121
Proptosis (ocular) — see also Exophthalmos
- thyroid — see Hyperthyroidism, with goiter

Prosecution, anxiety concerning Z65.3
Prosopagnosia R48.3
Prostadynia N42.81
Prostate, prostatic — see condition
Prostatism — see Hyperplasia, prostate
Prostatitis (congestive) (suppurative) (with cystitis) N41.9
- acute N41.0
- cavitary N41.8
- chronic N41.1
- diverticular N41.8
- due to Trichomonas (vaginalis) A59.02
- fibrous N41.1
- gonococcal (acute) (chronic) A54.22
- granulomatous N41.4
- hypertrophic N41.1
- subacute N41.1
- trichomonal A59.02
- tuberculous A18.14

Prostatocystitis N41.3
Prostatorrhea N42.89
Prostatosis N42.82
Prostration R53.83
- heat — see also Heat, exhaustion
  - anhydrotic T67.3- ☑
  - due to
    - salt (and water) depletion T67.4- ☑
    - water depletion T67.3- ☑
- nervous F48.8
- senile R54

Protanomaly (anomalous trichromat) H53.54
Protanopia (complete) (incomplete) H53.54
Protection (against) (from) — see Prophylactic
Protein
- deficiency NEC — see Malnutrition
- malnutrition — see Malnutrition
- sickness — see also Reaction, serum T80.69- ☑

Proteinemia R77.9
Proteinosis
- alveolar (pulmonary) J84.01
- lipid or lipoid (of Urbach) E78.89

Proteinuria R80.9
- Bence Jones R80.3
- complicating pregnancy — see Proteinuria, gestational
- gestational
  - complicating
    - childbirth O12.14
    - pregnancy O12.1- ☑
      - with edema O12.2- ☑
    - puerperium O12.15
- idiopathic R80.0
- isolated R80.0
  - with glomerular lesion N06.9
    - C3
      - glomerulonephritis N06.A
      - glomerulopathy N06.A
        - with dense deposit disease N06.6
    - dense deposit disease N06.6
    - diffuse
      - crescentic glomerulonephritis N06.7
      - endocapillary proliferative glomerulonephritis N06.4
      - mesangiocapillary glomerulonephritis N06.5
    - focal and segmental hyalinosis or sclerosis N06.1
    - membranous (diffuse) — see also Nephropathy, membranous N06.20
      - with diffuse membranous glomerulonephritis N06.29
    - mesangial proliferative (diffuse) N06.3
    - minimal change N06.0
    - specified pathology NEC N06.8
- orthostatic R80.2
  - with glomerular lesion — see Proteinuria, isolated, with glomerular lesion
- persistent R80.1
  - with glomerular lesion — see Proteinuria, isolated, with glomerular lesion
- postural R80.2
  - with glomerular lesion — see Proteinuria, isolated, with glomerular lesion
- pre-eclamptic — see Pre-eclampsia
- puerperal O12.15

☑ **Additional Character Required — Refer to the Tabular List for Character Selection**

Proteinuria — continued
  specified type NEC R80.8
Proteolysis, pathologic D65
Proteus (mirabilis) (morganii), **as cause of disease classified elsewhere** B96.4
Prothrombin gene mutation D68.52
Protoporphyria, erythropoietic E80.0
Protozoal — see also condition
  disease B64
    specified NEC B60.8
Protrusion, protrusio
  acetabuli M24.7
  acetabulum (into pelvis) M24.7
  device, implant or graft — see also Complications, by site and type, mechanical T85.698- ☑
    arterial graft NEC — see Complication, cardiovascular device, mechanical, vascular
    breast (implant) T85.49- ☑
    catheter NEC T85.698- ☑
      cystostomy T83.090- ☑
      dialysis (renal) T82.49- ☑
        intraperitoneal T85.691- ☑
      infusion NEC T82.594- ☑
        spinal (epidural) (subdural) T85.690- ☑
      urinary — see also Complications, catheter, urinary T83.098- ☑
    electronic (electrode) (pulse generator) (stimulator)
      bone T84.390- ☑
      nervous system — see Complication, prosthetic device, mechanical, electronic nervous system stimulator
    fixation, internal (orthopedic) NEC — see Complication, fixation device, mechanical
    gastrointestinal — see Complications, prosthetic device, mechanical, gastrointestinal device
    genital NEC T83.498- ☑
      intrauterine contraceptive device T83.39- ☑
      penile prosthesis (cylinder) (implanted) (pump) (reservoir) T83.490- ☑
      testicular prosthesis T83.491- ☑
    heart NEC — see Complication, cardiovascular device, mechanical
    joint prosthesis — see Complications, joint prosthesis, mechanical, specified NEC, by site
    ocular NEC — see Complications, prosthetic device, mechanical, ocular device
    orthopedic NEC — see Complication, orthopedic, device, mechanical
    specified NEC T85.628- ☑
    urinary NEC — see also Complication, genitourinary, device, urinary, mechanical
      graft T83.29- ☑
    vascular NEC — see Complication, cardiovascular device, mechanical
    ventricular intracranial shunt T85.09- ☑
  intervertebral disc — see Displacement, intervertebral disc
  joint prosthesis — see Complications, joint prosthesis, mechanical, specified NEC, by site
  nucleus pulposus — see Displacement, intervertebral disc
Prune belly (syndrome) Q79.4
Prurigo (ferox) (gravis) (Hebrae) (Hebra's) (mitis) (simplex) L28.2
  Besnier's L20.0
  estivalis L56.4
  nodularis L28.1
  psychogenic F45.8
Pruritus, pruritic (essential) L29.9
  ani, anus L29.0
    psychogenic F45.8
  anogenital L29.3
    psychogenic F45.8
  cholestatic L29.81
  due to onchocerca volvulus B73.1
  gravidarum — see Pregnancy, complicated by, specified pregnancy-related condition NEC
  hiemalis L29.89
  neurogenic (any site) F45.8
  perianal L29.0
  psychogenic (any site) F45.8
  scroti, scrotum L29.1
    psychogenic F45.8
  senile, senilis L29.89
  specified NEC L29.89
    psychogenic F45.8
  Trichomonas A59.9
  vulva, vulvae L29.2

Pruritus, pruritic — continued
  vulva, vulvae — continued
    psychogenic F45.8
Psearthrosis, pseudoarthrosis (bone) — see Nonunion, fracture
  clavicle, congenital Q74.0
  joint, following fusion or arthrodesis M96.0
Pseudo-Cushing's syndrome, alcohol-induced E24.4
Pseudo-Hurler's polydystrophy E77.0
Pseudo-obstruction intestine (acute) (chronic) (idiopathic) (intermittent secondary) (primary) K59.89
  colonic K59.81
Pseudoaneurysm — see Aneurysm
Pseudoangina (pectoris) — see Angina
Pseudoangioma I81
Pseudoarteriosus Q28.8
Pseudoarthrosis — see Pseudarthrosis
Pseudobulbar affect (PBA) F48.2
Pseudochromhidrosis L67.8
Pseudocirrhosis, liver, pericardial I31.1
Pseudocowpox B08.03
Pseudocoxalgia M91.3- ☑
Pseudocroup J38.5
Pseudocyesis F45.8
Pseudocyst
  lung J98.4
  pancreas K86.3
  retina — see Cyst, retina
Pseudoelephantiasis neuroarthritica Q82.0
Pseudoexfoliation, capsule (lens) — see Cataract, specified NEC
Pseudofolliculitis barbae L73.1
Pseudoglioma H44.89
Pseudohemophilia (Bernuth's) (hereditary) (type B) — see Disease, von Willebrand
  Type A D69.8
  vascular D69.8
Pseudohermaphroditism Q56.3
  adrenal E25.8
  female — see also Disorder, adrenogenital Q56.2
    with adrenocortical disorder E25.8
    without adrenocortical disorder Q56.2
    adrenal (congenital) E25.0
  male — see also Disorder, adrenogenital Q56.1
    with
      5-alpha-reductase deficiency E29.1
      adrenocortical disorder E25.8
      androgen resistance E34.51
      cleft scrotum Q56.1
      feminizing testis E34.51
    without gonadal disorder Q56.1
      adrenal E25.8
Pseudohydrocephalus G93.2
Pseudohypertrophic muscular dystrophy (Erb's) G71.02
Pseudohypertrophy, muscle — see also Dystrophy, muscular, by type, if applicable G71.09
Pseudohypoparathyroidism E20.1
Pseudoinsomnia F51.03
Pseudoleukemia, infantile D64.89
Pseudomembranous — see condition
Pseudomeningocele (cerebral) (infective) (post-traumatic) G96.198
  postprocedural (spinal) G97.82
Pseudomenses (newborn) P54.6
Pseudomenstruation (newborn) P54.6
Pseudomonas
  aeruginosa, as cause of disease classified elsewhere B96.5
  mallei infection A24.0
    as cause of disease classified elsewhere B96.5
  pseudomallei, as cause of disease classified elsewhere B96.5
Pseudomyotonia G71.19
Pseudomyxoma peritonei C78.6
Pseudoneuritis, optic (nerve) (disc) (papilla), **congenital** Q14.2
Pseudopapilledema H47.33- ☑
  congenital Q14.2
Pseudoparalysis
  arm or leg R29.818
  atonic, congenital P94.2
Pseudopelade L66.0
Pseudophakia Z96.1
Pseudopolyarthritis, rhizomelic M35.3
Pseudopolycythemia D75.1
Pseudopseudohypoparathyroidism E20.1
Pseudopterygium H11.81- ☑
Pseudoptosis (eyelid) — see Blepharochalasis
Pseudopuberty, precocious
  female heterosexual E25.8

Pseudopuberty, precocious — continued
  male isosexual E25.8
Pseudorickets (renal) N25.0
Pseudorubella B08.20
Pseudosclerma, newborn P83.88
Pseudosclerosis (brain)
  Jakob's — see Creutzfeldt-Jakob disease or syndrome of Westphal (Strumpell) E83.01
  spastic — see Creutzfeldt-Jakob disease or syndrome
Pseudotetanus — see Convulsions
Pseudotetany R29.0
  hysterical F44.5
Pseudotruncus arteriosus Q25.49
Pseudotuberculosis A28.2
  enterocolitis A04.8
  pasteurella (infection) A28.0
Pseudotumor G93.2
  cerebri G93.2
  orbital H05.11- ☑
Pseudoxanthoma elasticum Q82.8
Psilosis (sprue) (tropical) K90.1
  nontropical K90.0
Psittacosis A70
Psoitis M60.88
Psoriasis L40.9
  arthropathic L40.50
    arthritis mutilans L40.52
    distal interphalangeal L40.51
    juvenile L40.54
    other specified L40.59
    spondylitis L40.53
  buccal K13.29
  flexural L40.8
  guttate L40.4
  mouth K13.29
  nummular L40.0
  plaque L40.0
  psychogenic F54
  pustular (generalized) L40.1
    palmaris et plantaris L40.3
  specified NEC L40.8
  vulgaris L40.0
Psychasthenia F48.8
Psychiatric disorder or problem F99
Psychogenic — see also condition
  factors associated with physical conditions F54
Psychological and behavioral factors affecting medical condition F59
Psychoneurosis, psychoneurotic — see also Neurosis
  anxiety (state) F41.1
  depersonalization F48.1
  hypochondriacal F45.21
  hysteria F44.9
  neurasthenic F48.8
  personality NEC F60.89
Psychopathy, psychopathic
  affectionless F94.2
  autistic F84.5
  constitution, post-traumatic F07.81
  personality — see Disorder, personality
  sexual — see Deviation, sexual
  state F60.2
Psychosexual identity disorder of childhood F64.2
Psychosis, psychotic F29
  acute (transient) F23
    hysterical F44.9
  affective — see Disorder, mood
  alcoholic F10.959
    with
      abuse F10.159
      anxiety disorder F10.980
        with
          abuse F10.180
          dependence F10.280
      delirium tremens F10.231
      delusions F10.950
        with
          abuse F10.150
          dependence F10.250
      dementia F10.97
        with dependence F10.27
      dependence F10.259
      hallucinosis F10.951
        with
          abuse F10.151
          dependence F10.251
      mood disorder F10.94
        with
          abuse F10.14

Psychosis, psychotic — continued
  alcoholic — continued
    with — continued
      mood disorder — continued
        with — continued
          dependence F10.24
        paranoia F10.950
          with
            abuse F10.150
            dependence F10.250
        persisting amnesia F10.96
          with dependence F10.26
      amnestic confabulatory F10.96
        with dependence F10.26
      delirium tremens F10.231
      Korsakoff's, Korsakov's, Korsakow's F10.26
      paranoid type F10.950
        with
          abuse F10.150
          dependence F10.250
  anergastic — see Psychosis, organic
  arteriosclerotic (simple type) (uncomplicated) — see also Dementia, vascular F01.50
    with behavioral disturbance — see Dementia, vascular
  childhood F84.0
    atypical F84.8
  climacteric — see Psychosis, involutional
  confusional F29
    acute or subacute F05
    reactive F23
  cycloid F23
  depressive — see Disorder, depressive
  disintegrative (childhood) F84.3
  drug-induced — see F11-F19 with .X59
    paranoid and hallucinatory states — see F11-F19 with .X50 or .X51
  due to or associated with
    addiction, drug — see F11-F19 with .X59
    dependence
      alcohol F10.259
      drug — see F11-F19 with .X59
    epilepsy F06.8
    Huntington's chorea F06.8
    ischemia, cerebrovascular (generalized) F06.8
    multiple sclerosis F06.8
    physical disease F06.8
    presenile dementia F03.- ☑
    senile dementia F03.- ☑
    vascular disease (arteriosclerotic) (cerebral) — see also Dementia, vascular F01.50
      with behavioral disturbance — see Dementia, vascular
  epileptic F06.8
  episode F23
    due to or associated with physical condition F06.8
  exhaustive F43.0
  hallucinatory, chronic F28
  hypomanic F30.8
  hysterical (acute) F44.9
  induced F24
  infantile F84.0
    atypical F84.8
  infective (acute) (subacute) F05
  involutional F28
    depressive — see Disorder, depressive
    melancholic — see Disorder, depressive
    paranoid (state) F22
  Korsakoff's, Korsakov's, Korsakow's (nonalcoholic) F04
    alcoholic F10.96
      in dependence F10.26
    induced by other psychoactive substance — see categories F11-F19 with .X5X
  mania, manic (single episode) F30.2
    recurrent type F31.89
  manic-depressive — see Disorder, bipolar
  menopausal — see Psychosis, involutional
  mixed schizophrenic and affective F25.8
  multi-infarct (cerebrovascular) — see also Dementia, vascular F01.50
    with behavioral disturbance — see Dementia, vascular
  nonorganic F29
    specified NEC F28
  organic F09
    due to or associated with
      arteriosclerosis (cerebral) — see Psychosis, arteriosclerotic
      cerebrovascular disease, arteriosclerotic — see Psychosis, arteriosclerotic
      childbirth — see Psychosis, puerperal

Psychosis, psychotic — continued
  organic — continued
    due to or associated with — continued
      Creutzfeldt-Jakob disease or syndrome — see Creutzfeldt-Jakob disease or syndrome
      dependence, alcohol F10.259
      disease
        alcoholic liver F10.259
        brain, arteriosclerotic — see Psychosis, arteriosclerotic
        cerebrovascular — see also Dementia, vascular F01.50
          with behavioral disturbance — see Dementia, vascular
        Creutzfeldt-Jakob — see Creutzfeldt-Jakob disease or syndrome
        endocrine or metabolic F06.8
          acute or subacute F05
        liver, alcoholic F10.259
      epilepsy transient (acute) F05
      infection
        brain (intracranial) F06.8
          acute or subacute F05
      intoxication
        alcoholic (acute) F10.259
        drug F11-F19 with .x59
      ischemia, cerebrovascular (generalized) — see Psychosis, arteriosclerotic
      puerperium — see Psychosis, puerperal
      trauma, brain (birth) (from electric current) (surgical) F06.8
        acute or subacute F05
    infective F06.8
      acute or subacute F05
    post-traumatic F06.8
      acute or subacute F05
  paranoiac F22
  paranoid (climacteric) (involutional) (menopausal) F22
    psychogenic (acute) F23
    schizophrenic F20.0
    senile F03.- ☑
  postpartum (NOS) F53.1
  presbyophrenic (type) F03.- ☑
  presenile F03.- ☑
  psychogenic (paranoid) F23
    depressive F32.3
  puerperal (NOS) F53.1
    specified type — see Psychosis, by type
  reactive (brief) (transient) (emotional stress) (psychological trauma) F23
    depressive F32.3
      recurrent F33.3
    excitative type F30.8
  schizoaffective F25.9
    depressive type F25.1
    manic type F25.0
  schizophrenia-like, in epilepsy F06.2
  schizophrenia, schizophrenic — see Schizophrenia
  schizophreniform F20.81
    affective type F25.9
    brief F23
    confusional type F23
    mixed type F25.0
  senile NEC F03.- ☑
    depressed or paranoid type F03.- ☑
    simple deterioration F03.- ☑
    specified type — code to condition
  shared F24
  situational (reactive) F23
  symbiotic (childhood) F84.3
  symptomatic F09
Psychosomatic — see Disorder, psychosomatic
Psychosyndrome, organic F07.9
Psychotic episode due to or associated with physical condition F06.8
Pterygium (eye) H11.00- ☑
  amyloid H11.01- ☑
  central H11.02- ☑
  colli Q18.3
  double H11.03- ☑
  peripheral
    progressive H11.05- ☑
    stationary H11.04- ☑
  recurrent H11.06- ☑
Ptilosis (eyelid) — see Madarosis
Ptomaine (poisoning) — see Poisoning, food
Ptosis — see also Blepharoptosis
  adiposa (false) — see Blepharoptosis

Ptosis — continued
  breast N64.81
  brow H57.81- ☑
  cecum K63.4
  colon K63.4
  congenital (eyelid) Q10.0
    specified site NEC — see Anomaly, by site
  eyebrow H57.81- ☑
  eyelid — see Blepharoptosis
    congenital Q10.0
  gastric K31.89
  intestine K63.4
  kidney N28.83
  liver K76.89
  renal N28.83
  splanchnic K63.4
  spleen D73.89
  stomach K31.89
  viscera K63.4
PTP D69.51
Ptyalism (periodic) K11.7
  hysterical F45.8
  pregnancy — see Pregnancy, complicated by, specified pregnancy-related condition NEC
  psychogenic F45.8
Ptyalolithiasis K11.5
Pubarche, precocious E30.1
Pubertas praecox E30.1
Puberty (development state) Z00.3
  bleeding (excessive) N92.2
  delayed E30.0
  precocious (constitutional) (cryptogenic) (idiopathic) E30.1
    central E22.8
    due to
      ovarian hyperfunction E28.1
        estrogen E28.0
      testicular hyperfunction E29.0
  premature E30.1
    due to
      adrenal cortical hyperfunction E25.8
      pineal tumor E34.8
      pituitary (anterior) hyperfunction E22.8
Puckering, macula — see Degeneration, macula, puckering
Pudenda, pudendum — see condition
Puente's disease (simple glandular cheilitis) K13.0
Puerperal, puerperium (complicated by, complications)
  abnormal glucose (tolerance test) O99.815
  abscess
    areola O91.02
      associated with lactation O91.03
    Bartholin's gland O86.19
    breast O91.12
      associated with lactation O91.13
    cervix (uteri) O86.11
    genital organ NEC O86.19
    kidney O86.21
    mammary O91.12
      associated with lactation O91.13
    nipple O91.02
      associated with lactation O91.03
    peritoneum O85
    subareolar O91.12
      associated with lactation O91.13
    urinary tract — see Puerperal, infection, urinary
    uterus O86.12
    vagina (wall) O86.13
    vaginorectal O86.13
    vulvovaginal gland O86.13
  adnexitis O86.19
  afibrinogenemia, or other coagulation defect O72.3
  albuminuria (acute) (subacute) — see Proteinuria, gestational
  alcohol use O99.315
  anemia O90.81
    pre-existing (pre-pregnancy) O99.03
  anesthetic death O89.8
  apoplexy O99.43
  bariatric surgery status O99.845
  blood disorder NEC O99.13
  blood dyscrasia O72.3
  cardiomyopathy O90.3
  cerebrovascular disorder (conditions in I60-I69) O99.43
  cervicitis O86.11
  circulatory system disorder O99.43
  coagulopathy (any) O99.13
    with hemorrhage O72.3
  complications O90.9
    specified NEC O90.89

Puerperal, puerperium — continued
- convulsions — see Eclampsia
- cystitis O86.22
- cystopyelitis O86.29
- delirium NEC F05
- diabetes O24.93
  - gestational — see Puerperal, gestational diabetes
  - pre-existing O24.33
    - specified NEC O24.83
    - type 1 O24.03
    - type 2 O24.13
- digestive system disorder O99.63
- disease O90.9
  - breast NEC O92.29
  - cerebrovascular (acute) O99.43
  - nonobstetric NEC O99.893
  - tubo-ovarian O86.19
  - Valsuani's O99.03
- disorder O90.9
  - biliary tract O26.63
  - lactation O92.70
  - liver O26.63
  - nonobstetric NEC O99.893
- disruption
  - cesarean wound O90.0
  - episiotomy wound O90.1
  - perineal laceration wound O90.1
- drug use O99.325
- eclampsia (with pre-existing hypertension) O15.2
- embolism (pulmonary) (blood clot) — see Embolism, obstetric, puerperal
- endocrine, nutritional or metabolic disease NEC O99.285
- endophlebitis — see Puerperal, phlebitis
- endotrachelitis O86.11
- failure
  - lactation (complete) O92.3
    - partial O92.4
  - renal, acute O90.49
- fever (of unknown origin) O86.4
  - septic O85
- fissure, nipple O92.12
  - associated with lactation O92.13
- fistula
  - breast (due to mastitis) O91.12
    - associated with lactation O91.13
  - nipple O91.02
    - associated with lactation O91.03
- galactophoritis O91.22
  - associated with lactation O91.23
- galactorrhea O92.6
- gastric banding status O99.845
- gastric bypass status O99.845
- gastrointestinal disease NEC O99.63
- gestational
  - diabetes O24.439
    - diet controlled O24.430
    - insulin (and diet) controlled O24.434
    - oral drug controlled (antidiabetic) (hypoglycemic) O24.435
  - edema O12.05
    - with proteinuria O12.25
  - proteinuria O12.15
- gonorrhea O98.23
- hematoma, subdural O99.43
- hemiplegia, cerebral O99.355
  - due to cerebrovascular disorder O99.43
- hemorrhage O72.1
  - brain O99.43
  - bulbar O99.43
  - cerebellar O99.43
  - cerebral O99.43
  - cortical O99.43
  - delayed or secondary O72.2
  - extradural O99.43
  - internal capsule O99.43
  - intracranial O99.43
  - intrapontine O99.43
  - meningeal O99.43
  - pontine O99.43
  - retained placenta O72.0
  - subarachnoid O99.43
  - subcortical O99.43
  - subdural O99.43
  - third stage O72.0
  - uterine, delayed O72.2
  - ventricular O99.43
- hemorrhoids O87.2
- hepatorenal syndrome O90.41

Puerperal, puerperium — continued
- hypertension — see Hypertension, complicating, puerperium
- hypertrophy, breast O92.29
- induration breast (fibrous) O92.29
- infection O86.4
  - cervix O86.11
  - generalized O85
  - genital tract NEC O86.19
    - obstetric surgical wound O86.09
  - kidney (bacillus coli) O86.21
  - maternal O98.93
    - carrier state NEC O99.835
    - gonorrhea O98.23
    - human immunodeficiency virus (HIV) O98.73
    - protozoal O98.63
    - sexually transmitted NEC O98.33
    - specified NEC O98.83
    - streptococcus group B (GBS) carrier state O99.825
    - syphilis O98.13
    - tuberculosis O98.03
    - viral hepatitis O98.43
    - viral NEC O98.53
  - nipple O91.02
    - associated with lactation O91.03
  - peritoneum O85
  - renal O86.21
  - specified NEC O86.89
  - urinary (asymptomatic) (tract) NEC O86.20
    - bladder O86.22
    - kidney O86.21
    - specified site NEC O86.29
    - urethra O86.22
  - vagina O86.13
  - vein — see Puerperal, phlebitis
- ischemia, cerebral O99.43
- lymphangitis O86.89
  - breast O91.22
    - associated with lactation O91.23
- malignancy O9A.13 (following O99)
- malnutrition O25.3
- mammillitis O91.02
  - associated with lactation O91.03
- mammitis O91.22
  - associated with lactation O91.23
- mania F30.8
- mastitis O91.22
  - associated with lactation O91.23
  - purulent O91.12
    - associated with lactation O91.13
- melancholia — see Disorder, depressive
- mental disorder NEC O99.345
- metroperitonitis O85
- metrorrhagia — see Hemorrhage, postpartum
- metrosalpingitis O86.19
- metrovaginitis O86.13
- milk leg O87.1
- monoplegia, cerebral O99.43
- mood disturbance O90.6
- necrosis, liver (acute) (subacute) (conditions in subcategory K72.0) O26.63
  - with renal failure O90.49
- nervous system disorder O99.355
- neuritis O90.89
- obesity (pre-existing prior to pregnancy) O99.215
- obesity surgery status O99.845
- occlusion, precerebral artery O99.43
- paralysis
  - bladder (sphincter) O90.89
  - cerebral O99.43
- paralytic stroke O99.43
- parametritis O85
- paravaginitis O86.13
- pelviperitonitis O85
- perimetritis O86.12
- perimetrosalpingitis O86.19
- perinephritis O86.21
- periphlebitis — see Puerperal phlebitis
- peritoneal infection O85
- peritonitis (pelvic) O85
- perivaginitis O86.13
- phlebitis O87.0
  - deep O87.1
  - pelvic O87.1
  - superficial O87.0
- phlebothrombosis, deep O87.1
- phlegmasia alba dolens O87.1
- placental polyp O90.89

Puerperal, puerperium — continued
- pneumonia, embolic — see Embolism, obstetric, puerperal
- pre-eclampsia — see Pre-eclampsia
- psychosis (NOS) F53.1
- pyelitis O86.21
- pyelocystitis O86.29
- pyelonephritis O86.21
- pyelonephrosis O86.21
- pyemia O85
- pyocystitis O86.29
- pyohemia O85
- pyometra O86.12
- pyonephritis O86.21
- pyosalpingitis O86.19
- pyrexia (of unknown origin) O86.4
- renal
  - disease NEC O90.89
  - failure O90.49
- respiratory disease NEC O99.53
- retention
  - decidua — see Retention, decidua
  - placenta O72.0
  - secundines — see Retention, secundines
- retracted nipple O92.02
- salpingo-ovaritis O86.19
- salpingoperitonitis O85
- secondary perineal tear O90.1
- sepsis (pelvic) O85
- septic thrombophlebitis O86.81
- skin disorder NEC O99.73
- specified condition NEC O99.893
- stroke O99.43
- subinvolution (uterus) O90.89
- subluxation of symphysis (pubis) O26.73
- suppuration — see Puerperal, abscess
- tetanus A34
- thelitis O91.02
  - associated with lactation O91.03
- thrombocytopenia O72.3
- thrombophlebitis (superficial) O87.0
  - deep O87.1
  - pelvic O87.1
  - septic O86.81
- thrombosis (venous) — see Thrombosis, puerperal
- thyroiditis O90.5
- toxemia (eclamptic) (pre-eclamptic) (with convulsions) O15.2
- trauma, non-obstetric O9A.23 (following O99)
  - caused by abuse (physical) (suspected) O9A.33 (following O99)
    - confirmed O9A.33 (following O99)
    - psychological (suspected) O9A.53 (following O99)
      - confirmed O9A.53 (following O99)
    - sexual (suspected) O9A.43 (following O99)
      - confirmed O9A.43 (following O99)
- uremia (due to renal failure) O90.49
- urethritis O86.22
- vaginitis O86.13
- varicose veins (legs) O87.4
  - vulva or perineum O87.8
- venous O87.9
- vulvitis O86.19
- vulvovaginitis O86.13
- white leg O87.1

Puerperium — see Puerperal
Pulmolithiasis J98.4
Pulmonary — see condition
Pulpitis (acute) (anachoretic) (chronic) (hyperplastic) (putrescent) (suppurative) (ulcerative) K04.01
- irreversible K04.02
- reversible K04.01

Pulpless tooth K04.99
Pulse
- alternating R00.8
- bigeminal R00.8
- fast R00.0
- feeble, rapid due to shock following injury T79.4- ☑
- rapid R00.0
- weak R09.89

Pulsus alternans or trigeminus R00.8
Punch drunk F07.81
Punctum lacrimale occlusion — see Obstruction, lacrimal
Puncture
- abdomen, abdominal
  - wall S31.139- ☑
    - with
      - foreign body S31.149- ☑
      - penetration into peritoneal cavity S31.639- ☑

Puncture — *continued*
  abdomen, abdominal — *continued*
    wall — *continued*
      with — *continued*
        penetration into peritoneal cavity — *continued*
          with foreign body S31.649- ☑
      epigastric region S31.132- ☑
        with
          foreign body S31.142- ☑
          penetration into peritoneal cavity S31.632- ☑
            with foreign body S31.642- ☑
      left
        lower quadrant S31.134- ☑
          with
            foreign body S31.144- ☑
            penetration into peritoneal cavity S31.634- ☑
              with foreign body S31.644- ☑
        upper quadrant S31.131- ☑
          with
            foreign body S31.141- ☑
            penetration into peritoneal cavity S31.631- ☑
              with foreign body S31.641- ☑
      periumbilic region S31.135- ☑
        with
          foreign body S31.145- ☑
          penetration into peritoneal cavity S31.635- ☑
            with foreign body S31.645- ☑
      right
        lower quadrant S31.133- ☑
          with
            foreign body S31.143- ☑
            penetration into peritoneal cavity S31.633- ☑
              with foreign body S31.643- ☑
        upper quadrant S31.130- ☑
          with
            foreign body S31.140- ☑
            penetration into peritoneal cavity S31.630- ☑
              with foreign body S31.640- ☑
  accidental, complicating surgery — *see* Complication, accidental puncture or laceration
  alveolar (process) — *see* Puncture, oral cavity
  ankle S91.039- ☑
    with
      foreign body S91.049- ☑
    left S91.032- ☑
      with
        foreign body S91.042- ☑
    right S91.031- ☑
      with
        foreign body S91.041- ☑
  anus S31.833- ☑
    with foreign body S31.834- ☑
  arm (upper) S41.139- ☑
    with foreign body S41.149- ☑
    left S41.132- ☑
      with foreign body S41.142- ☑
    lower — *see* Puncture, forearm
    right S41.131- ☑
      with foreign body S41.141- ☑
  auditory canal (external) (meatus) — *see* Puncture, ear
  auricle, ear — *see* Puncture, ear
  axilla — *see* Puncture, arm
  back — *see also* Puncture, thorax, back
    lower S31.030- ☑
      with
        foreign body S31.040- ☑
          with penetration into retroperitoneal space S31.041- ☑
        penetration into retroperitoneal space S31.031- ☑
  bladder (traumatic) S37.29- ☑
    nontraumatic N32.89
  breast S21.039- ☑
    with foreign body S21.049- ☑
    left S21.032- ☑
      with foreign body S21.042- ☑
    right S21.031- ☑
      with foreign body S21.041- ☑
  buttock S31.803- ☑

Puncture — *continued*
  buttock — *continued*
    with foreign body S31.804- ☑
    left S31.823- ☑
      with foreign body S31.824- ☑
    right S31.813- ☑
      with foreign body S31.814- ☑
  by
    device, implant or graft — *see* Complications, by site and type, mechanical
    foreign body left accidentally in operative wound T81.539- ☑
    instrument (any) during a procedure, accidental — *see* Puncture, accidental complicating surgery
  calf — *see* Puncture, leg
  canaliculus lacrimalis — *see* Puncture, eyelid
  canthus, eye — *see* Puncture, eyelid
  cervical esophagus S11.23- ☑
    with foreign body S11.24- ☑
  cheek (external) S01.439- ☑
    with foreign body S01.449- ☑
    internal — *see* Puncture, oral cavity
    left S01.432- ☑
      with foreign body S01.442- ☑
    right S01.431- ☑
      with foreign body S01.441- ☑
  chest wall — *see* Puncture, thorax
  chin — *see* Puncture, head, specified site NEC
  clitoris — *see* Puncture, vulva
  costal region — *see* Puncture, thorax
  digit(s)
    foot — *see* Puncture, toe
    hand — *see* Puncture, finger
  ear (canal) (external) S01.339- ☑
    with foreign body S01.349- ☑
    drum S09.2- ☑
    left S01.332- ☑
      with foreign body S01.342- ☑
    right S01.331- ☑
      with foreign body S01.341- ☑
  elbow S51.039- ☑
    with
      foreign body S51.049- ☑
    left S51.032- ☑
      with
        foreign body S51.042- ☑
    right S51.031- ☑
      with
        foreign body S51.041- ☑
  epididymis — *see* Puncture, testis
  epigastric region — *see* Puncture, abdomen, wall, epigastric
  epiglottis S11.83- ☑
    with foreign body S11.84- ☑
  esophagus
    cervical S11.23- ☑
      with foreign body S11.24- ☑
    thoracic S27.818- ☑
  eyeball S05.6- ☑
    with foreign body S05.5- ☑
  eyebrow — *see* Puncture, eyelid
  eyelid S01.13- ☑
    with foreign body S01.14- ☑
    left S01.132- ☑
      with foreign body S01.142- ☑
    right S01.131- ☑
      with foreign body S01.141- ☑
  face NEC — *see* Puncture, head, specified site NEC
  finger(s) S61.239- ☑
    with
      damage to nail S61.339- ☑
        with
          foreign body S61.349- ☑
      foreign body S61.249- ☑
    index S61.238- ☑
      with
        damage to nail S61.338- ☑
          with
            foreign body S61.348- ☑
        foreign body S61.248- ☑
      left S61.231- ☑
        with
          damage to nail S61.331- ☑
            with
              foreign body S61.341- ☑
          foreign body S61.241- ☑

Puncture — *continued*
  finger(s) — *continued*
    index — *continued*
      right S61.230- ☑
        with
          damage to nail S61.330- ☑
            with
              foreign body S61.340- ☑
          foreign body S61.240- ☑
    little S61.238- ☑
      with
        damage to nail S61.338- ☑
          with
            foreign body S61.348- ☑
        foreign body S61.248- ☑
      left S61.237- ☑
        with
          damage to nail S61.337- ☑
            with
              foreign body S61.347- ☑
          foreign body S61.247- ☑
      right S61.236- ☑
        with
          damage to nail S61.336- ☑
            with
              foreign body S61.346- ☑
          foreign body S61.246- ☑
    middle S61.238- ☑
      with
        damage to nail S61.338- ☑
          with
            foreign body S61.348- ☑
        foreign body S61.248- ☑
      left S61.233- ☑
        with
          damage to nail S61.333- ☑
            with
              foreign body S61.343- ☑
          foreign body S61.243- ☑
      right S61.232- ☑
        with
          damage to nail S61.332- ☑
            with
              foreign body S61.342- ☑
          foreign body S61.242- ☑
    ring S61.238- ☑
      with
        damage to nail S61.338- ☑
          with
            foreign body S61.348- ☑
        foreign body S61.248- ☑
      left S61.235- ☑
        with
          damage to nail S61.335- ☑
            with
              foreign body S61.345- ☑
          foreign body S61.245- ☑
      right S61.234- ☑
        with
          damage to nail S61.334- ☑
            with
              foreign body S61.344- ☑
          foreign body S61.244- ☑
  flank S31.13A- ☑
    with
      foreign body S31.14A- ☑
      penetration into peritoneal cavity S31.63A- ☑
        with foreign body S31.64A- ☑
    left S31.137- ☑
      with
        foreign body S31.147- ☑
        penetration into peritoneal cavity S31.637- ☑
          with foreign body S31.647- ☑
    right S31.136- ☑
      with
        foreign body S31.146- ☑
        penetration into peritoneal cavity S31.636- ☑
          with foreign body S31.646- ☑
  foot (except toe(s) alone) S91.339- ☑
    with foreign body S91.349- ☑
    left S91.332- ☑
      with foreign body S91.342- ☑
    right S91.331- ☑
      with foreign body S91.341- ☑
    toe — *see* Puncture, toe
  forearm S51.839- ☑

Puncture — *continued*
   forearm — *continued*
     with
       foreign body S51.849- ☑
     elbow only — *see* Puncture, elbow
     left S51.832- ☑
      with
       foreign body S51.842- ☑
     right S51.831- ☑
      with
       foreign body S51.841- ☑
   forehead — *see* Puncture, head, specified site NEC
   genital organs, external
     female S31.532- ☑
      with foreign body S31.542- ☑
      vagina — *see* Puncture, vagina
      vulva — *see* Puncture, vulva
     male S31.531- ☑
      with foreign body S31.541- ☑
      penis — *see* Puncture, penis
      scrotum — *see* Puncture, scrotum
      testis — *see* Puncture, testis
   groin — *see* Puncture, abdomen, wall
   gum — *see* Puncture, oral cavity
   hand S61.439- ☑
     with
      foreign body S61.449- ☑
     finger — *see* Puncture, finger
     left S61.432- ☑
      with
       foreign body S61.442- ☑
     right S61.431- ☑
      with
       foreign body S61.441- ☑
     thumb — *see* Puncture, thumb
   head S01.93- ☑
     with foreign body S01.94- ☑
     cheek — *see* Puncture, cheek
     ear — *see* Puncture, ear
     eyelid — *see* Puncture, eyelid
     lip — *see* Puncture, oral cavity
     nose — *see* Puncture, nose
     oral cavity — *see* Puncture, oral cavity
     scalp S01.03- ☑
      with foreign body S01.04- ☑
     specified site NEC S01.83- ☑
      with foreign body S01.84- ☑
     temporomandibular area — *see* Puncture, cheek
   heart S26.99- ☑
     with hemopericardium S26.09- ☑
     without hemopericardium S26.19- ☑
   heel — *see* Puncture, foot
   hip S71.039- ☑
     with foreign body S71.049- ☑
     left S71.032- ☑
      with foreign body S71.042- ☑
     right S71.031- ☑
      with foreign body S71.041- ☑
   hymen — *see* Puncture, vagina
   hypochondrium — *see* Puncture, abdomen, wall
   hypogastric region — *see* Puncture, abdomen, wall
   inguinal region — *see* Puncture, abdomen, wall
   instep — *see* Puncture, foot
   internal organs — *see* Injury, by site
   interscapular region — *see* Puncture, thorax, back
   intestine
     large
      colon S36.599- ☑
       ascending S36.590- ☑
       descending S36.592- ☑
       sigmoid S36.593- ☑
       specified site NEC S36.598- ☑
       transverse S36.591- ☑
      rectum S36.69- ☑
     small S36.499- ☑
      duodenum S36.490- ☑
      specified site NEC S36.498- ☑
   intra-abdominal organ S36.99- ☑
     gallbladder S36.128- ☑
     intestine — *see* Puncture, intestine
     liver S36.118- ☑
     pancreas — *see* Puncture, pancreas
     peritoneum S36.81- ☑
     specified site NEC S36.898- ☑
     spleen S36.09- ☑
     stomach S36.39- ☑
   jaw — *see* Puncture, head, specified site NEC

Puncture — *continued*
   knee S81.039- ☑
     with foreign body S81.049- ☑
     left S81.032- ☑
      with foreign body S81.042- ☑
     right S81.031- ☑
      with foreign body S81.041- ☑
   labium (majus) (minus) — *see* Puncture, vulva
   lacrimal duct — *see* Puncture, eyelid
   larynx S11.013- ☑
     with foreign body S11.014- ☑
   leg (lower) S81.839- ☑
     with foreign body S81.849- ☑
     foot — *see* Puncture, foot
     knee — *see* Puncture, knee
     left S81.832- ☑
      with foreign body S81.842- ☑
     right S81.831- ☑
      with foreign body S81.841- ☑
     upper — *see* Puncture, thigh
   lip S01.531- ☑
     with foreign body S01.541- ☑
   loin — *see* Puncture, abdomen, wall
   lower back — *see* Puncture, back, lower
   lumbar region — *see* Puncture, back, lower
   malar region — *see* Puncture, head, specified site NEC
   mammary — *see* Puncture, breast
   mastoid region — *see* Puncture, head, specified site NEC
   mouth — *see* Puncture, oral cavity
   nail
     finger — *see* Puncture, finger, with damage to nail
     toe — *see* Puncture, toe, with damage to nail
   nasal (septum) (sinus) — *see* Puncture, nose
   nasopharynx — *see* Puncture, head, specified site NEC
   neck S11.93- ☑
     with foreign body S11.94- ☑
     involving
      cervical esophagus — *see* Puncture, cervical esophagus
      larynx — *see* Puncture, larynx
      pharynx — *see* Puncture, pharynx
      thyroid gland — *see* Puncture, thyroid gland
      trachea — *see* Puncture, trachea
     specified site NEC S11.83- ☑
      with foreign body S11.84- ☑
   nose (septum) (sinus) S01.23- ☑
     with foreign body S01.24- ☑
   ocular — *see* Puncture, eyeball
   oral cavity S01.532- ☑
     with foreign body S01.542- ☑
   orbit S05.4- ☑
   palate — *see* Puncture, oral cavity
   palm — *see* Puncture, hand
   pancreas S36.299- ☑
     body S36.291- ☑
     head S36.290- ☑
     tail S36.292- ☑
   pelvis — *see* Puncture, back, lower
   penis S31.23- ☑
     with foreign body S31.24- ☑
   perineum
     female S31.43- ☑
      with foreign body S31.44- ☑
     male S31.139- ☑
      with foreign body S31.149- ☑
   periocular area (with or without lacrimal passages) — *see* Puncture, eyelid
   phalanges
     finger — *see* Puncture, finger
     toe — *see* Puncture, toe
   pharynx S11.23- ☑
     with foreign body S11.24- ☑
   pinna — *see* Puncture, ear
   popliteal space — *see* Puncture, knee
   prepuce — *see* Puncture, penis
   pubic region S31.139- ☑
     with foreign body S31.149- ☑
   pudendum — *see* Puncture, genital organs, external
   rectovaginal septum — *see* Puncture, vagina
   sacral region — *see* Puncture, back, lower
   sacroiliac region — *see* Puncture, back, lower
   salivary gland — *see* Puncture, oral cavity
   scalp S01.03- ☑
     with foreign body S01.04- ☑
   scapular region — *see* Puncture, shoulder
   scrotum S31.33- ☑
     with foreign body S31.34- ☑

Puncture — *continued*
   shin — *see* Puncture, leg
   shoulder S41.039- ☑
     with foreign body S41.049- ☑
     left S41.032- ☑
      with foreign body S41.042- ☑
     right S41.031- ☑
      with foreign body S41.041- ☑
   spermatic cord — *see* Puncture, testis
   sternal region — *see* Puncture, thorax, front
   submaxillary region — *see* Puncture, head, specified site NEC
   submental region — *see* Puncture, head, specified site NEC
   subungual
     finger(s) — *see* Puncture, finger, with damage to nail
     toe — *see* Puncture, toe, with damage to nail
   supraclavicular fossa — *see* Puncture, neck, specified site NEC
   temple, temporal region — *see* Puncture, head, specified site NEC
   temporomandibular area — *see* Puncture, cheek
   testis S31.33- ☑
     with foreign body S31.34- ☑
   thigh S71.139- ☑
     with foreign body S71.149- ☑
     left S71.132- ☑
      with foreign body S71.142- ☑
     right S71.131- ☑
      with foreign body S71.141- ☑
   thorax, thoracic (wall) S21.93- ☑
     with foreign body S21.94- ☑
     back S21.23- ☑
      with
       foreign body S21.24- ☑
        with penetration S21.44- ☑
       penetration S21.43- ☑
     breast — *see* Puncture, breast
     front S21.13- ☑
      with
       foreign body S21.14- ☑
        with penetration S21.34- ☑
       penetration S21.33- ☑
   throat — *see* Puncture, neck
   thumb S61.039- ☑
     with
      damage to nail S61.139- ☑
       with
        foreign body S61.149- ☑
      foreign body S61.049- ☑
     left S61.032- ☑
      with
       damage to nail S61.132- ☑
        with
         foreign body S61.142- ☑
       foreign body S61.042- ☑
     right S61.031- ☑
      with
       damage to nail S61.131- ☑
        with
         foreign body S61.141- ☑
       foreign body S61.041- ☑
   thyroid gland S11.13- ☑
     with foreign body S11.14- ☑
   toe(s) S91.139- ☑
     with
      damage to nail S91.239- ☑
       with
        foreign body S91.249- ☑
      foreign body S91.149- ☑
     great S91.133- ☑
      with
       damage to nail S91.233- ☑
        with
         foreign body S91.243- ☑
       foreign body S91.143- ☑
     left S91.132- ☑
      with
       damage to nail S91.232- ☑
        with
         foreign body S91.242- ☑
       foreign body S91.142- ☑
     right S91.131- ☑
      with
       damage to nail S91.231- ☑

Puncture — continued
　toe(s) — continued
　　great — continued
　　　right — continued
　　　　with — continued
　　　　　damage to nail — continued
　　　　　　with
　　　　　　　foreign body S91.241- ☑
　　　　　foreign body S91.141- ☑
　　lesser S91.136- ☑
　　　with
　　　　damage to nail S91.236- ☑
　　　　　with
　　　　　　foreign body S91.246- ☑
　　　　foreign body S91.146- ☑
　　left S91.135- ☑
　　　with
　　　　damage to nail S91.235- ☑
　　　　　with
　　　　　　foreign body S91.245- ☑
　　　　foreign body S91.145- ☑
　　right S91.134- ☑
　　　with
　　　　damage to nail S91.234- ☑
　　　　　with
　　　　　　foreign body S91.244- ☑
　　　　foreign body S91.144- ☑
　tongue — see Puncture, oral cavity
　trachea S11.023- ☑
　　with foreign body S11.024- ☑
　tunica vaginalis — see Puncture, testis
　tympanum, tympanic membrane S09.2- ☑
　umbilical region S31.135- ☑
　　with foreign body S31.145- ☑
　uvula — see Puncture, oral cavity
　vagina S31.43- ☑
　　with foreign body S31.44- ☑
　vocal cords S11.033- ☑
　　with foreign body S11.034- ☑
　vulva S31.43- ☑
　　with foreign body S31.44- ☑
　wrist S61.539- ☑
　　with
　　　foreign body S61.549- ☑
　　left S61.532- ☑
　　　with
　　　　foreign body S61.542- ☑
　　right S61.531- ☑
　　　with
　　　　foreign body S61.541- ☑
PUO (pyrexia of unknown origin) R50.9
Pupillary membrane (persistent) Q13.89
Pupillotonia — see Anomaly, pupil, function, tonic pupil
Purpura D69.2
　abdominal D69.0
　allergic D69.0
　anaphylactoid D69.0
　annularis telangiectodes L81.7
　arthritic D69.0
　autoerythrocyte sensitization D69.2
　autoimmune D69.0
　bacterial D69.0
　Bateman's (senile) D69.2
　capillary fragility (hereditary) (idiopathic) D69.8
　cryoglobulinemic D89.1
　Devil's pinches D69.2
　fibrinolytic — see Fibrinolysis
　fulminans, fulminous D65
　gangrenous D65
　hemorrhagic, hemorrhagica D69.3
　　not due to thrombocytopenia D69.0
　Henoch (-Schonlein) (allergic) D69.0
　hypergammaglobulinemic (benign) (Waldenstrom) D89.0
　idiopathic (thrombocytopenic) D69.3
　　nonthrombocytopenic D69.0
　immune thrombocytopenic D69.3
　infectious D69.0
　malignant D69.0
　neonatorum P54.5
　nervosa D69.0
　newborn P54.5
　nonthrombocytopenic D69.2
　　hemorrhagic D69.0
　　idiopathic D69.0
　nonthrombopenic D69.2
　peliosis rheumatica D69.0

Purpura — continued
　posttransfusion (post-transfusion) (from (fresh) whole
　　blood or blood products) D69.51
　primary D69.49
　red cell membrane sensitivity D69.2
　rheumatica D69.0
　Schonlein (-Henoch) (allergic) D69.0
　scorbutic E54 [D77]
　senile D69.2
　simplex D69.2
　symptomatica D69.0
　telangiectasia annularis L81.7
　thrombocytopenic D69.49
　　congenital D69.42
　　hemorrhagic D69.3
　　hereditary D69.42
　　idiopathic D69.3
　　immune D69.3
　　neonatal, transitory P61.0
　　thrombotic M31.19
　thrombohemolytic — see Fibrinolysis
　thrombolytic — see Fibrinolysis
　thrombopenic D69.49
　thrombotic, thrombocytopenic M31.19
　toxic D69.0
　vascular D69.0
　visceral symptoms D69.0
Purpuric spots R23.3
Purulent — see condition
Pus
　in
　　stool R19.5
　　urine N39.0
　tube (rupture) — see Salpingo-oophoritis
Pustular rash L08.0
Pustule (nonmalignant) L08.9
　malignant A22.0
Pustulosis palmaris et plantaris L40.3
Putnam (-Dana) **disease or syndrome** — see Degeneration,
　combined
Putrescent pulp (dental) K04.1
Pyarthritis, pyarthrosis — see Arthritis, pyogenic or pyemic
　tuberculous — see Tuberculosis, joint
Pyelectasis — see Hydronephrosis
Pyelitis (congenital) (uremic) — see also Pyelonephritis
　with
　　calculus — see category N20.-
　　　with hydronephrosis N13.6
　　contracted kidney N11.9
　acute N10
　chronic N11.9
　　with calculus — see category N20.- ☑
　　　with hydronephrosis N13.6
　cystica N28.84
　puerperal (postpartum) O86.21
　tuberculous A18.11
Pyelocystitis — see Pyelonephritis
Pyelonephritis — see also Nephritis, tubulo-interstitial
　with
　　calculus — see category N20.- ☑
　　　with hydronephrosis N13.6
　　contracted kidney N11.9
　acute N10
　calculous — see category N20.- ☑
　　with hydronephrosis N13.6
　chronic N11.9
　　with calculus — see category N20.- ☑
　　　with hydronephrosis N13.6
　　associated with ureteral obstruction or stricture N11.1
　　nonobstructive N11.8
　　　with reflux (vesicoureteral) N11.0
　　obstructive N11.1
　　specified NEC N11.8
　in (due to)
　　brucellosis A23.9 [N16]
　　cryoglobulinemia (mixed) D89.1 [N16]
　　cystinosis E72.04
　　diphtheria A36.84
　　glycogen storage disease E74.09 [N16]
　　leukemia NEC C95.9- ☑ [N16]
　　lymphoma NEC C85.90 [N16]
　　multiple myeloma C90.0- ☑ [N16]
　　obstruction N11.1
　　Salmonella infection A02.25
　　sarcoidosis D86.84
　　sepsis A41.9 [N16]
　　Sjogren's disease M35.04
　　toxoplasmosis B58.83

Pyelonephritis — continued
　in — continued
　　transplant rejection T86.91 [N16]
　　Wilson's disease E83.01 [N16]
　nonobstructive N12
　　with reflux (vesicoureteral) N11.0
　　chronic N11.8
　syphilitic A52.75
Pyelonephrosis (obstructive) N11.1
　chronic N11.9
Pyelophlebitis I80.8
Pyeloureteritis cystica N28.85
Pyemia, pyemic (fever) (infection) (purulent) — see also
　　Sepsis
　joint — see Arthritis, pyogenic or pyemic
　liver K75.1
　pneumococcal A40.3
　portal K75.1
　postvaccinal T88.0- ☑
　puerperal, postpartum, childbirth O85
　specified organism NEC A41.89
　tuberculous — see Tuberculosis, miliary
Pygopagus Q89.4
Pyknoepilepsy (idiopathic) — see Pyknolepsy
Pyknolepsy G40.A09 (following G40.3)
　intractable G40.A19 (following G40.3)
　　with status epilepticus G40.A11 (following G40.3)
　　without status epilepticus G40.A19 (following G40.3)
　not intractable G40.A09 (following G40.3)
　　with status epilepticus G40.A01 (following G40.3)
　　without status epilepticus G40.A09 (following G40.3)
Pylephlebitis K75.1
Pyle's syndrome Q78.5
Pylethrombophlebitis K75.1
Pylethrombosis K75.1
Pyloritis K29.90
　with bleeding K29.91
Pylorospasm (reflex) **NEC** K31.3
　congenital or infantile Q40.0
　neurotic F45.8
　newborn Q40.0
　psychogenic F45.8
Pylorus, pyloric — see condition
Pyo-oophoritis — see Salpingo-oophoritis
Pyo-ovarium — see Salpingo-oophoritis
Pyoarthrosis — see Arthritis, pyogenic or pyemic
Pyocele
　mastoid — see Mastoiditis, acute
　sinus (accessory) — see Sinusitis
　turbinate (bone) J32.9
　urethra — see also Urethritis N34.0
Pyocolpos — see Vaginitis
Pyocystitis N30.80
　with hematuria N30.81
Pyoderma, pyodermia L08.0
　gangrenosum L88
　newborn P39.4
　phagedenic L88
　vegetans L08.81
Pyodermatitis L08.0
　vegetans L08.81
Pyogenic — see condition
Pyohydronephrosis N13.6
Pyometra, pyomentrium, pyometritis — see Endometritis
Pyomyositis (tropical) — see Myositis, infective
Pyonephritis N12
Pyonephrosis N13.6
　tuberculous A18.11
Pyopericarditis, pyopericardium I30.1
Pyophlebitis — see Phlebitis
Pyopneumopericardium I30.1
Pyopneumothorax (infective) J86.9
　with fistula J86.0
　tuberculous NEC A15.6
Pyosalpinx, pyosalpingitis — see also Salpingo-oophoritis
Pyothorax J86.9
　with fistula J86.0
　tuberculous NEC A15.6
Pyoureter N28.89
　tuberculous A18.11
Pyramidopallidonigral syndrome G20.C
Pyrexia (of unknown origin) R50.9
　atmospheric T67.01- ☑
　during labor NEC O75.2
　heat T67.01- ☑
　newborn P81.9
　　environmentally-induced P81.0
　persistent R50.9
　puerperal O86.4

Pyroglobulinemia NEC E88.09
Pyromania F63.1
Pyrosis R12
Pyuria (bacterial) (sterile) R82.81

Q

Q fever A78
  with pneumonia A78
Quadricuspid aortic valve Q23.88
Quadrilateral fever A78
Quadriparesis — *see* Quadriplegia
  meaning muscle weakness M62.81
Quadriplegia G82.50
  complete
    C1-C4 level G82.51
    C5-C7 level G82.53
  congenital (cerebral) (spinal) G80.8
    spastic G80.0
  embolic (current episode) I63.4- ☑
  functional R53.2
  incomplete
    C1-C4 level G82.52
    C5-C7 level G82.54
  thrombotic (current episode) I63.3- ☑
  traumatic — *code to* injury with seventh character S
    current episode — *see* Injury, spinal (cord), cervical
Quadruplet, pregnancy — *see* Pregnancy, quadruplet
Quarrelsomeness F60.3
Queensland fever A77.3
Quervain's disease M65.4
  thyroid E06.1
Queyrat's erythroplasia D07.4
  penis D07.4
  specified site — *see* Neoplasm, skin, in situ
  unspecified site D07.4
Quincke's disease or edema T78.3- ☑
  hereditary D84.1
Quinsy (gangrenous) J36
Quintan fever A79.0
Quintuplet, pregnancy — *see* Pregnancy, quintuplet

R

Rabbit fever — *see* Tularemia
Rabies A82.9
  contact Z20.3
  exposure to Z20.3
  inoculation reaction — *see* Complications, vaccination
  sylvatic A82.0
  urban A82.1
Rachischisis — *see* Spina bifida
Rachitic — *see also* condition
  deformities of spine (late effect) (sequelae) E64.3
  pelvis (late effect) (sequelae) E64.3
    with disproportion (fetopelvic) O33.0
      causing obstructed labor O65.0
Rachitis, rachitism (acute) (tarda) — *see also* Rickets
  renalis N25.0
  sequelae E64.3
Radial nerve — *see* condition
Radiation
  burn — *see* Burn
  effects NOS T66.- ☑
  sickness NOS T66.- ☑
  therapy, encounter for Z51.0
Radiculitis (pressure) (vertebrogenic) — *see* Radiculopathy
Radiculomyelitis — *see also* Encephalitis
  toxic, due to
    Clostridium tetani A35
    Corynebacterium diphtheriae A36.82
Radiculopathy M54.10
  cervical region M54.12
  cervicothoracic region M54.13
  due to
    disc disorder
      C3 M50.11
      C4 M50.11
      C5 M50.121
      C6 M50.122
      C7 M50.123
    displacement of intervertebral disc — *see* Disorder, disc, with, radiculopathy
  leg M54.1- ☑
  lumbar region M54.16
  lumbosacral region M54.17
  occipito-atlanto-axial region M54.11
  postherpetic B02.29

Radiculopathy — *continued*
  sacrococcygeal region M54.18
  syphilitic A52.11
  thoracic region (with visceral pain) M54.14
  thoracolumbar region M54.15
Radiodermal burns (acute, chronic, or occupational) — *see* Burn
Radiodermatitis L58.9
  acute L58.0
  chronic L58.1
Radiotherapy session Z51.0
RAEB (refractory anemia with excess blasts) D46.2- ☑
Rage, meaning rabies — *see* Rabies
Ragpicker's disease A22.1
Ragsorter's disease A22.1
Raillietiniasis B71.8
Railroad neurosis F48.8
Railway spine F48.8
Raised — *see also* Elevated
  antibody titer R76.0
Rake teeth, tooth M26.39
Rales R09.89
Ramifying renal pelvis Q63.8
Ramsay-Hunt disease or syndrome — *see also* Hunt's, disease B02.21
  meaning dyssynergia cerebellaris myoclonica G11.19
Ranula K11.6
  congenital Q38.4
Rape
  adult
    confirmed T74.21- ☑
    suspected T76.21- ☑
  alleged, observation or examination, ruled out
    adult Z04.41
    child Z04.42
  child
    confirmed T74.22- ☑
    suspected T76.22- ☑
Rapid
  feeble pulse, due to shock, following injury T79.4- ☑
  heart (beat) R00.0
    psychogenic F45.8
  second stage (delivery) O62.3
  time-zone change syndrome G47.25
Rarefaction, bone — *see* Disorder, bone, density and structure, specified NEC
Rash (toxic) R21
  canker A38.9
  diaper L22
  drug (internal use) L27.0
    contact — *see also* Dermatitis, due to, drugs, external L25.1
  following immunization T88.1- ☑
  food — *see* Dermatitis, due to, food
  heat L74.0
  napkin (psoriasiform) L22
  nettle — *see* Urticaria
  pustular L08.0
  rose R21
    epidemic B06.9
  scarlet A38.9
  serum — *see also* Reaction, serum T80.69- ☑
  wandering tongue K14.1
Rasmussen aneurysm — *see* Tuberculosis, pulmonary
Rasmussen encephalitis G04.81
Rat-bite fever A25.9
  due to Streptobacillus moniliformis A25.1
  spirochetal (morsus muris) A25.0
Rathke's pouch tumor D44.3
Raymond (-Cestan) **syndrome** I65.8
Raynaud's disease, phenomenon or syndrome (secondary) I73.00
  with gangrene (symmetric) I73.01
RDS (newborn) (type I) P22.0
  type II P22.1
Reaction — *see also* Disorder
  adaptation — *see* Disorder, adjustment
  adjustment (anxiety) (conduct disorder) (depressiveness) (distress) — *see* Disorder, adjustment
  with
    mutism, elective (child) (adolescent) F94.0
  adverse
    food (any) (ingested) NEC T78.19- ☑
      anaphylactic — *see* Shock, anaphylactic, due to food
  affective — *see* Disorder, mood
  allergic — *see* Allergy
  anaphylactic — *see* Shock, anaphylactic

Reaction — *continued*
  anaphylactoid — *see* Shock, anaphylactic
  anesthesia — *see* Anesthesia, complication
  antitoxin (prophylactic) (therapeutic) — *see* Complications, vaccination
  anxiety F41.1
  Arthus — *see* Arthus' phenomenon
  asthenic F48.8
  combat and operational stress F43.0
  compulsive F42.8
  conversion F44.9
  crisis, acute F43.0
  deoxyribonuclease (DNA) (DNase) hypersensitivity D69.2
  depressive (single episode) F32.9
    affective (single episode) F31.4
      recurrent episode F33.9
    neurotic F34.1
    psychoneurotic F34.1
    psychotic F32.3
    recurrent — *see* Disorder, depressive, recurrent
  dissociative F44.9
  drug NEC T88.7- ☑
    addictive — *see* Dependence, drug
      transmitted via placenta or breast milk — *see* Absorption, drug, addictive, through placenta
    allergic — *see* Allergy, drug
    lichenoid L43.2
    newborn P93.8
      gray baby syndrome P93.0
    overdose or poisoning (by accident) — *see* Table of Drugs and Chemicals, by drug, poisoning
    photoallergic L56.1
    phototoxic L56.0
    withdrawal — *see* Dependence, by drug, with, withdrawal
      infant of dependent mother P96.1
      newborn P96.1
    wrong substance given or taken (by accident) — *see* Table of Drugs and Chemicals, by drug, poisoning
  fear F40.9
    child (abnormal) F93.8
  febrile nonhemolytic transfusion (FNHTR) R50.84
  fluid loss, cerebrospinal G97.1
  foreign
    body NEC — *see* Granuloma, foreign body
      in operative wound (inadvertently left) — *see* Foreign body, accidentally left during a procedure
    substance accidentally left during a procedure (chemical) (powder) (talc) T81.60- ☑
      aseptic peritonitis T81.61- ☑
      body or object (instrument) (sponge) (swab) — *see* Foreign body, accidentally left during a procedure
      specified reaction NEC T81.69- ☑
  grief — *see* Disorder, adjustment
  Herxheimer's R68.89
  hyperkinetic — *see* Hyperkinesia
  hypochondriacal F45.20
  hypoglycemic, due to insulin E16.0
    with coma (diabetic) — *see* Diabetes, coma
      nondiabetic E15
    therapeutic misadventure — *see* subcategory T38.3- ☑
  hypomanic F30.8
  hysterical F44.9
  immunization — *see* Complications, vaccination
  incompatibility
    ABO blood group (infusion) (transfusion) — *see* Complication(s), transfusion, incompatibility reaction, ABO
    delayed serologic T80.39- ☑
    minor blood group (Duffy) (E) (K) (Kell) (Kidd) (Lewis) (M) (N) (P) (S) T80.89- ☑
    Rh (factor) (infusion) (transfusion) — *see* Complication(s), transfusion, incompatibility reaction, Rh (factor)
  inflammatory — *see* Infection
  infusion — *see* Complications, infusion
  inoculation (immune serum) — *see* Complications, vaccination
  insulin T38.3- ☑
  involutional psychotic — *see* Disorder, depressive
  leukemoid D72.823
    basophilic D72.823
    lymphocytic D72.823
    monocytic D72.823

Reaction — *continued*
  leukemoid — *continued*
   myelocytic D72.823
   neutrophilic D72.823
  LSD (acute)
   due to drug abuse — *see* Abuse, drug, hallucinogen
   due to drug dependence — *see* Dependence, drug, hallucinogen
  lumbar puncture G97.1
  manic-depressive — *see* Disorder, bipolar
  neurasthenic F48.8
  neurogenic — *see* Neurosis
  neurotic F48.9
  neurotic-depressive F34.1
  nitritoid — *see* Crisis, nitritoid
  nonspecific
   to
    cell mediated immunity measurement of gamma interferon antigen response without active tuberculosis R76.12
    QuantiFERON-TB test (QFT) without active tuberculosis R76.12
    tuberculin test — *see also* Reaction, tuberculin skin test R76.11
  obsessive-compulsive F42.8
  organic, acute or subacute — *see* Delirium
  paranoid (acute) F23
   chronic F22
   senile F03.- ☑
  passive dependency F60.7
  phobic F40.9
  post-traumatic stress, uncomplicated Z73.3
  psychogenic F99
  psychoneurotic — *see also* Neurosis
   compulsive F42.8
   depersonalization F48.1
   depressive F34.1
   hypochondriacal F45.20
   neurasthenic F48.8
   obsessive F42.8
  psychophysiologic — *see* Disorder, somatoform
  psychosomatic — *see* Disorder, somatoform
  psychotic — *see* Psychosis
  scarlet fever toxin — *see* Complications, vaccination
  schizophrenic F23
   acute (brief) (undifferentiated) F23
   latent F21
   undifferentiated (acute) (brief) F23
  serological for syphilis — *see* Serology for syphilis
  serum T80.69- ☑
   anaphylactic (immediate) — *see also* Shock, anaphylactic T80.59- ☑
   specified reaction NEC
    due to
     administration of blood and blood products T80.61- ☑
     immunization T80.62- ☑
     serum specified NEC T80.69- ☑
     vaccination T80.62- ☑
  situational — *see* Disorder, adjustment
  somatization — *see* Disorder, somatoform
  spinal puncture G97.1
   dural G97.1
  stress (severe) F43.9
   acute (agitation) ("daze") (disorientation) (disturbance of consciousness) (flight reaction) (fugue) F43.0
   specified NEC F43.89
  surgical procedure — *see* Complications, surgical procedure
  tetanus antitoxin — *see* Complications, vaccination
  toxic, to local anesthesia T88.59- ☑
   in labor and delivery O74.4
   in pregnancy O29.3X- ☑
   postpartum, puerperal O89.3
  toxin-antitoxin — *see* Complications, vaccination
  transfusion (blood) (bone marrow) (lymphocytes) (allergic) — *see* Complications, transfusion
  tuberculin skin test, abnormal R76.11
  vaccination (any) — *see* Complications, vaccination
  withdrawing, child or adolescent F93.8
Reactive airway disease — *see* Asthma
Reactive depression — *see* Reaction, depressive
Rearrangement
  chromosomal
   balanced (in) Q95.9
    abnormal individual (autosomal) Q95.2
     non-sex (autosomal) chromosomes Q95.2
     sex/non-sex chromosomes Q95.3

Rearrangement — *continued*
  chromosomal — *continued*
   balanced — *continued*
    specified NEC Q95.8
Recalcitrant patient — *see* Noncompliance
Recanalization, thrombus — *see* Thrombosis
Recession, receding
  chamber angle (eye) H21.55- ☑
  chin M26.09
  gingival (postinfective) (postoperative)
   generalized K06.020
    minimal K06.021
    moderate K06.022
    severe K06.023
   localized K06.010
    minimal K06.011
    moderate K06.012
    severe K06.013
Recklinghausen disease Q85.01
  bones E21.0
Reclus' disease (cystic) — *see* Mastopathy, cystic
Recrudescence
  deficit
   cerebral infarction — *see* Sequelae, infarction, cerebral
   stroke — *see* Sequelae, infarction, cerebral
  sequelae
   cerebral infarction — *see* Sequelae, infarction, cerebral
   stroke — *see* Sequelae, infarction, cerebral
Recrudescent typhus (fever) A75.1
Recruitment, auditory H93.21- ☑
Rectalgia K62.89
Rectitis K62.89
Rectocele
  female (without uterine prolapse) N81.6
   with uterine prolapse N81.4
    complete N81.3
    incomplete N81.2
  in pregnancy — *see* Pregnancy, complicated by, abnormal, pelvic organs or tissues NEC
  male K62.3
Rectosigmoid junction — *see* condition
Rectosigmoiditis K63.89
  ulcerative (chronic) K51.30
   with
    complication K51.319
     abscess K51.314
     fistula K51.313
     obstruction K51.312
     rectal bleeding K51.311
     specified NEC K51.318
Rectourethral — *see* condition
Rectovaginal — *see* condition
Rectovesical — *see* condition
Rectum, rectal — *see* condition
Recurrent — *see* condition
  pregnancy loss — *see* Loss (of), pregnancy, recurrent
Red bugs B88.09
Red-cedar lung or pneumonitis J67.8
Red tide — *see also* Table of Drugs and Chemicals T65.82- ☑
Reduced
  mobility Z74.09
  ventilatory or vital capacity R94.2
Redundant, redundancy
  anus (congenital) Q43.8
  clitoris N90.89
  colon (congenital) Q43.8
  foreskin (congenital) N47.8
  intestine (congenital) Q43.8
  labia N90.69
  organ or site, congenital NEC — *see* Accessory
  panniculus (abdominal) E65
  prepuce (congenital) N47.8
  pylorus K31.89
  rectum (congenital) Q43.8
  scrotum N50.89
  sigmoid (congenital) Q43.8
  skin L98.7
   and subcutaneous tissue L98.7
   of face L57.4
    eyelids — *see* Blepharochalasis
  stomach K31.89
Reduplication — *see* Duplication
Reflex R29.2
  hyperactive gag J39.2
  pupillary, abnormal — *see* Anomaly, pupil, function
  vasoconstriction I73.9
  vasovagal R55
Reflux K21.9

Reflux — *continued*
  acid K21.9
  esophageal K21.9
   with esophagitis (without bleeding) K21.00
    with bleeding K21.01
   newborn P78.83
  gastroesophageal K21.9
   with esophagitis (without bleeding) K21.00
    with bleeding K21.01
  mitral — *see* Insufficiency, mitral
  ureteral — *see* Reflux, vesicoureteral
  vesicoureteral (with scarring) N13.70
   with
    nephropathy N13.729
     with hydroureter N13.739
      bilateral N13.732
      unilateral N13.731
     bilateral N13.722
     unilateral N13.721
     without hydroureter N13.729
      bilateral N13.722
      unilateral N13.721
    pyelonephritis (chronic) N11.0
   congenital Q62.7
   without nephropathy N13.71
Reforming, artificial openings — *see* Attention to, artificial, opening
Refractive error — *see* Disorder, refraction
Refsum's disease or syndrome G60.1
Refusal of
  food, psychogenic F50.89
  treatment (because of) Z53.20
   left against medical advice (AMA) Z53.29
   left without being seen Z53.21
   patient's decision NEC Z53.29
   reasons of belief or group pressure Z53.1
Regional — *see* condition
Regurgitation R11.10
  aortic (valve) — *see* Insufficiency, aortic
  food — *see also* Vomiting
   with reswallowing — *see* Rumination
   newborn P92.1
  gastric contents — *see* Vomiting
  heart — *see* Endocarditis
  mitral (valve) — *see* Insufficiency, mitral
   congenital Q23.3
  myocardial — *see* Endocarditis
  pulmonary (valve) (heart) I37.1
   congenital Q22.2
   syphilitic A52.03
  tricuspid — *see* Insufficiency, tricuspid
  valve, valvular — *see* Endocarditis
   congenital Q24.8
  vesicoureteral — *see* Reflux, vesicoureteral
Reichmann's disease or syndrome K31.89
Reifenstein syndrome E34.52
Reinsertion
  implantable subdermal contraceptive Z30.46
  intrauterine contraceptive device Z30.433
Reiter's disease, syndrome, or urethritis M02.30
  ankle M02.37- ☑
  elbow M02.32- ☑
  foot joint M02.37- ☑
  hand joint M02.34- ☑
  hip M02.35- ☑
  knee M02.36- ☑
  multiple site M02.39
  shoulder M02.31- ☑
  vertebra M02.38
  wrist M02.33- ☑
Rejection
  food, psychogenic F50.89
  transplant T86.91
   bone T86.830
    marrow T86.01
   cornea T86.840- ☑
   heart T86.21
    with lung(s) T86.31
   intestine T86.850
   kidney T86.11
   liver T86.41
   lung(s) T86.810
    with heart T86.31
   organ (immune or nonimmune cause) T86.91
   pancreas T86.890
   skin (allograft) (autograft) T86.820
   specified NEC T86.890
   stem cell (peripheral blood) (umbilical cord) T86.5

Relapsing fever A68.9
- Carter's (Asiatic) A68.1
- Dutton's (West African) A68.1
- Koch's A68.9
- louse-borne (epidemic) A68.0
- Novy's (American) A68.1
- Obermeyer's (European) A68.0
- Spirillum A68.9
- tick-borne (endemic) A68.1

Relationship
- occlusal
  - open anterior M26.220
  - open posterior M26.221

Relaxation
- anus (sphincter) K62.89
  - psychogenic F45.8
- arch (foot) — see also Deformity, limb, flat foot
- back ligaments — see Instability, joint, spine
- bladder (sphincter) N31.2
- cardioesophageal K21.9
- cervix — see Incompetency, cervix
- diaphragm J98.6
- joint (capsule) (ligament) (paralytic) — see Flail, joint
  - congenital NEC Q74.8
- lumbosacral (joint) — see subcategory M53.2- ☑
- pelvic floor N81.89
- perineum N81.89
- posture R29.3
- rectum (sphincter) K62.89
- sacroiliac (joint) — see subcategory M53.2- ☑
- scrotum N50.89
- urethra (sphincter) N36.44
- vesical N31.2

Release from prison, anxiety concerning Z65.2

Remains
- canal of Cloquet Q14.0
- capsule (opaque) Q14.8

Remittent fever (malarial) B54

Remnant
- canal of Cloquet Q14.0
- capsule (opaque) Q14.8
- cervix, cervical stump (acquired) (postoperative) N88.8
- cystic duct, postcholecystectomy K91.5
- fingernail L60.8
  - congenital Q84.6
- meniscus, knee — see Derangement, knee, meniscus, specified NEC
- thyroglossal duct Q89.2
- tonsil J35.8
  - infected (chronic) J35.01
- urachus Q64.4

Removal (from) (of)
- artificial
  - arm Z44.00- ☑
    - complete Z44.01- ☑
    - partial Z44.02- ☑
  - eye Z44.2- ☑
  - leg Z44.10- ☑
    - complete Z44.11- ☑
    - partial Z44.12- ☑
- breast implant Z45.81- ☑
- cardiac pulse generator (battery) (end-of-life) Z45.010
- catheter (urinary) (indwelling) Z46.6
  - from artificial opening — see Attention to, artificial, opening
  - non-vascular Z46.82
  - vascular NEC Z45.2
- device Z46.9
  - contraceptive Z30.432
    - implantable subdermal Z30.46
  - implanted NEC Z45.89
  - specified NEC Z46.89
- drains Z48.03
- dressing (nonsurgical) Z48.00
  - surgical Z48.01
- external
  - fixation device — code to fracture with seventh character D
  - prosthesis, prosthetic device Z44.9
    - breast Z44.3- ☑
    - specified NEC Z44.8
- home in childhood (to foster home or institution) Z62.29
- ileostomy Z43.2
- insulin pump Z46.81
- myringotomy device (stent) (tube) Z45.82
- nervous system device NEC Z46.2
  - brain neuropacemaker Z46.2
  - visual substitution device Z46.2

Removal — continued
- nervous system device — continued
  - visual substitution device — continued
    - implanted Z45.31
  - non-vascular catheter Z46.82
- organ, prophylactic (for neoplasia management) — see Prophylactic, organ removal
- orthodontic device Z46.4
- staples Z48.02
- stent
  - ureteral Z46.6
- suture Z48.02
- urinary device Z46.6
- vascular access device or catheter Z45.2

Ren
- arcuatus Q63.1
- mobile, mobilis N28.89
  - congenital Q63.8
- unguliformis Q63.1

Renal — see condition

Rendu-Osler-Weber disease or syndrome I78.0

Reninoma D41.0- ☑

Renon-Delille syndrome E23.3

Reovirus, as cause of disease classified elsewhere B97.5

Repeated falls NEC R29.6

Replaced chromosome by dicentric ring Q93.2

Replacement by artificial or mechanical device or prosthesis of
- bladder Z96.0
- blood vessel NEC Z95.828
- bone NEC Z96.7
- cochlea Z96.21
- coronary artery Z95.5
- eustachian tube Z96.29
- eye globe Z97.0
- heart Z95.812
  - valve Z95.2
    - prosthetic Z95.2
    - specified NEC Z95.4
    - xenogenic Z95.3
- intestine Z96.89
- joint Z96.60
  - hip — see Presence, hip joint implant
  - knee — see Presence, knee joint implant
  - specified site NEC Z96.698
- larynx Z96.3
- lens Z96.1
- limb(s) — see Presence, artificial, limb
- mandible NEC (for tooth root implant(s)) Z96.5
- organ NEC Z96.89
- peripheral vessel NEC Z95.828
- stapes Z96.29
- teeth Z97.2
- tendon Z96.7
- tissue NEC Z96.89
- tooth root(s) Z96.5
- vessel NEC Z95.828
  - coronary (artery) Z95.5

Request for expert evidence Z04.89

Reserve, decreased or low
- cardiac — see Disease, heart
- kidney N28.89

Residing
- in place not meant for human habitation (abandoned building) (car) (park) (sidewalk) Z59.02
- on the street Z59.02

Residual — see also condition
- ovary syndrome N99.83
- state, schizophrenic F20.5
- urine R39.198

Resistance, resistant (to)
- activated protein C D68.51
- insulin E88.819
  - complicating pregnancy O26.89- ☑
  - specified type NEC E88.818
- organism(s)
  - to
    - drug Z16.30
      - aminoglycosides Z16.29
      - amoxicillin Z16.11
      - ampicillin Z16.11
      - antibiotic(s) Z16.20
        - multiple Z16.24
        - specified NEC Z16.29
      - antifungal Z16.32
      - antimicrobial (single) Z16.30
        - multiple Z16.35
        - specified NEC Z16.39
      - antimycobacterial (single) Z16.341

Resistance, resistant — continued
- organism(s) — continued
  - to — continued
    - drug — continued
      - antimycobacterial — continued
        - multiple Z16.342
      - antiparasitic Z16.31
      - antiviral Z16.33
      - beta lactam antibiotics Z16.10
        - specified NEC Z16.19
      - carbapenem Z16.13
      - cephalosporins Z16.19
      - extended beta lactamase (ESBL) Z16.12
      - fluoroquinolones Z16.23
      - macrolides Z16.29
      - methicillin — see MRSA
      - multiple drugs (MDRO)
        - antibiotics Z16.24
        - antimicrobial Z16.35
        - antimycobacterials Z16.342
      - penicillins Z16.11
      - quinine (and related compounds) Z16.31
      - quinolones Z16.23
      - sulfonamides Z16.29
      - tetracyclines Z16.29
      - tuberculostatics (single) Z16.341
        - multiple Z16.342
      - vancomycin Z16.21
        - related antibiotics Z16.22
- thyroid hormone E07.89

Resorption
- dental (roots) K03.3
  - alveoli M26.79
- teeth (external) (internal) (pathological) (roots) K03.3

Respiration
- Cheyne-Stokes R06.3
- decreased due to shock, following injury T79.4- ☑
- disorder of, psychogenic F45.8
- insufficient, or poor R06.89
  - newborn P28.5
- painful R07.1
- sighing, psychogenic F45.8

Respiratory — see also condition
- distress syndrome (newborn) (type I) P22.0
  - type II P22.1
- syncytial virus, as cause of disease classified elsewhere — see also Virus, respiratory syncytial (RSV) B97.4

Respite care Z75.5

Response (drug)
- photoallergic L56.1
- phototoxic L56.0

Restenosis
- stent
  - vascular
    - end stent
      - adjacent to stent — see Arteriosclerosis
      - within the stent
        - coronary T82.855- ☑
        - peripheral T82.856- ☑
    - in stent
      - coronary vessel T82.855- ☑
      - peripheral vessel T82.856- ☑

Restless legs (syndrome) G25.81

Restlessness R45.1

Restoration (of)
- dental
  - aesthetically inadequate or displeasing K08.56
  - defective K08.50
    - specified NEC K08.59
  - failure of marginal integrity K08.51
  - failure of periodontal anatomical integrity K08.54
- organ continuity from previous sterilization (tuboplasty) (vasoplasty) Z31.0
  - aftercare Z31.42
- tooth (existing)
  - contours biologically incompatible with oral health K08.54
  - open margins K08.51
  - overhanging K08.52
  - poor aesthetic K08.56
  - poor gingival margins K08.51
  - unsatisfactory, of tooth K08.50
    - specified NEC K08.59

Restorative material (dental)
- allergy to K08.55
- fractured K08.539
  - with loss of material K08.531
  - without loss of material K08.530

Restorative material — continued
  unrepairable overhanging of K08.52
Restriction
  growth
    fetal O36.59- ☑
  of housing space Z59.19
Rests, ovarian, in fallopian tube Q50.6
Restzustand (schizophrenic) F20.5
Retained — see also Retention
  cholelithiasis following cholecystectomy K91.86
  foreign body fragments (type of) Z18.9
    acrylics Z18.2
    animal quill(s) or spines Z18.31
    cement Z18.83
    concrete Z18.83
    crystalline Z18.83
    depleted isotope Z18.09
    depleted uranium Z18.01
    diethylhexyl phthalates Z18.2
    glass Z18.81
    isocyanate Z18.2
    magnetic metal Z18.11
    metal Z18.10
    nonmagnectic metal Z18.12
    nontherapeutic radioactive Z18.09
    organic NEC Z18.39
    plastic Z18.2
    quill(s) (animal) Z18.31
    radioactive (nontherapeutic) NEC Z18.09
    specified NEC Z18.89
    spine(s) (animal) Z18.31
    stone Z18.83
    tooth (teeth) Z18.32
    wood Z18.33
  fragments (type of) Z18.9
    acrylics Z18.2
    animal quill(s) or spines Z18.31
    cement Z18.83
    concrete Z18.83
    crystalline Z18.83
    depleted isotope Z18.09
    depleted uranium Z18.01
    diethylhexyl phthalates Z18.2
    glass Z18.81
    isocyanate Z18.2
    magnetic metal Z18.11
    metal Z18.10
    nonmagnectic metal Z18.12
    nontherapeutic radioactive Z18.09
    organic NEC Z18.39
    plastic Z18.2
    quill(s) (animal) Z18.31
    radioactive (nontherapeutic) NEC Z18.09
    specified NEC Z18.89
    spine(s) (animal) Z18.31
    stone Z18.83
    tooth (teeth) Z18.32
    wood Z18.33
  gallstones, following cholecystectomy K91.86
Retardation
  development, developmental, specific — see Disorder, developmental
  endochondral bone growth — see Disorder, bone, development or growth
  growth R62.50
    due to malnutrition E45
  mental — see Disability, intellectual
  motor function, specific F82
  physical (child) R62.52
    due to malnutrition E45
  reading (specific) F81.0
  spelling (specific) (without reading disorder) F81.81
Retching — see Vomiting
Retention — see also Retained
  bladder — see Retention, urine
  carbon dioxide E87.29
  cholelithiasis following cholecystectomy K91.86
  cyst — see Cyst
  dead
    fetus (at or near term) (mother) O36.4- ☑
      early fetal death O02.1
    ovum O02.0
  decidua (fragments) (following delivery) (with hemorrhage) O72.2
    without hemorrhage O73.1
  deciduous tooth K00.6
  dental root K08.3
  fecal — see Constipation

Retention — continued
  fetus
    dead O36.4- ☑
      early O02.1
  fluid R60.9
  foreign body — see also Foreign body, retained
    current trauma — code as Foreign body, by site or type
  gallstones, following cholecystectomy K91.86
  gastric K31.89
  intrauterine contraceptive device, in pregnancy — see Pregnancy, complicated by, retention, intrauterine device
  membranes (complicating delivery) (with hemorrhage) O72.2
    with abortion — see Abortion, by type
    without hemorrhage O73.1
  meniscus — see Derangement, meniscus
  menses N94.89
  milk (puerperal, postpartum) O92.79
  nitrogen, extrarenal R39.2
  ovary syndrome N99.83
  placenta (total) (with hemorrhage) O72.0
    without hemorrhage O73.0
    portions or fragments (with hemorrhage) O72.2
      without hemorrhage O73.1
  products of conception
    early pregnancy (dead fetus) O02.1
    following
      delivery (with hemorrhage) O72.2
        without hemorrhage O73.1
  secundines (following delivery) (with hemorrhage) O72.0
    without hemorrhage O73.0
  complicating puerperium (delayed hemorrhage) O72.2
  partial O72.2
    without hemorrhage O73.1
  smegma, clitoris N90.89
  urine R33.9
    due to hyperplasia (hypertrophy) of prostate — see Hyperplasia, prostate
    drug-induced R33.0
    organic R33.8
      drug-induced R33.0
    psychogenic F45.8
    specified NEC R33.8
  water (in tissues) — see Edema
Reticulation, dust — see Pneumoconiosis
Reticulocytosis R70.1
Reticuloendotheliosis
  acute infantile C96.0
  leukemic C91.4- ☑
  nonlipid C96.0
Reticulohistiocytoma (giant-cell) D76.3
Reticuloid, actinic L57.1
Reticulosis (skin)
  acute of infancy C96.0
  hemophagocytic, familial D76.1
  histiocytic medullary C96.A (following C96.6)
  lipomelanotic I89.8
  malignant (midline) C86.0- ☑
  polymorphic C86.0- ☑
  Sezary — see Sezary disease
Retina, retinal — see also condition
  dark area D49.81
Retinitis — see also Inflammation, chorioretinal
  albuminurica N18.9 [H32]
  diabetic — see Diabetes, retinitis
  disciformis — see Degeneration, macula
  focal — see Inflammation, chorioretinal, focal
  gravidarum — see Pregnancy, complicated by, specified pregnancy-related condition NEC
  juxtapapillaris — see Inflammation, chorioretinal, focal, juxtapapillary
  luetic — see Retinitis, syphilitic
  pigmentosa H35.52
  proliferans — see Disorder, globe, degenerative, specified type NEC
  proliferating — see Disorder, globe, degenerative, specified type NEC
  renal N18.9 [H32]
  syphilitic (early) (secondary) A51.43
    central, recurrent A52.71
    congenital (early) A50.01 [H32]
    late A52.71
  tuberculous A18.53
Retinoblastoma C69.2- ☑
  differentiated C69.2- ☑

Retinoblastoma — continued
  undifferentiated C69.2- ☑
Retinochoroiditis — see also Inflammation, chorioretinal
  disseminated — see Inflammation, chorioretinal, disseminated
    syphilitic A52.71
  focal — see Inflammation, chorioretinal
  juxtapapillaris — see Inflammation, chorioretinal, focal, juxtapapillary
Retinopathy (background) H35.00
  arteriosclerotic I70.8 [H35.0-] ☑
  atherosclerotic I70.8 [H35.0-] ☑
  central serous — see Chorioretinopathy, central serous
  Coats H35.02- ☑
  diabetic — see Diabetes, retinopathy
  exudative H35.02- ☑
  hypertensive H35.03- ☑
  in (due to)
    diabetes — see Diabetes, retinopathy
    sickle-cell disorders
      nonproliferative D57.- ☑ [H36.81-] ☑
      proliferative D57.- ☑ [H36.82-] ☑
  of prematurity H35.10- ☑
    stage 0 H35.11- ☑
    stage 1 H35.12- ☑
    stage 2 H35.13- ☑
    stage 3 H35.14- ☑
    stage 4 H35.15- ☑
    stage 5 H35.16- ☑
  pigmentary, congenital — see Dystrophy, retina
  proliferative NEC H35.2- ☑
    diabetic — see Diabetes, retinopathy, proliferative
    sickle-cell D57.- ☑ [H36.82-] ☑
  thalassemia H35.2- ☑
  solar H31.02- ☑
Retinoschisis H33.10- ☑
  congenital Q14.1
  specified type NEC H33.19- ☑
Retortamoniasis A07.8
Retractile testis Q55.22
Retraction
  cervix — see Retroversion, uterus
  drum (membrane) — see Disorder, tympanic membrane, specified NEC
  finger — see Deformity, finger
  lid H02.539
    left H02.536
      lower H02.535
      upper H02.534
    right H02.533
      lower H02.532
      upper H02.531
  lung J98.4
  mediastinum J98.59
  nipple N64.53
    associated with
      lactation O92.03
      pregnancy O92.01- ☑
      puerperium O92.02
    congenital Q83.8
  palmar fascia M72.0
  pleura — see Pleurisy
  ring, uterus (Bandl's) (pathological) O62.4
  sternum (congenital) Q76.7
    acquired M95.4
  uterus — see Retroversion, uterus
  valve (heart) — see Endocarditis
Retrobulbar — see condition
Retrocecal — see condition
Retrocession — see Retroversion
Retrodisplacement — see Retroversion
Retroflection, retroflexion — see Retroversion
Retrognathia, retrognathism (mandibular) (maxillary) M26.19
Retrograde menstruation N92.5
Retroperineal — see condition
Retroperitoneal — see condition
Retroperitonitis K68.9
Retropharyngeal — see condition
Retroplacental — see condition
Retroposition — see Retroversion
Retroprosthetic membrane T85.398- ☑
Retrosternal thyroid (congenital) Q89.2
Retroversion, retroverted
  cervix — see Retroversion, uterus
  female NEC — see Retroversion, uterus
  iris H21.89
  testis (congenital) Q55.29

Retroversion, retroverted — continued
- uterus (acquired) (acute) (any degree) (asymptomatic) (cervix) (postinfectional) (postpartal, old) N85.4
  - congenital Q51.818
  - in pregnancy O34.53- ☑
Retrovirus, as cause of disease classified elsewhere B97.30
- human
  - immunodeficiency, type 2 (HIV 2) B97.35
  - T-cell lymphotropic
    - type I (HTLV-I) B97.33
    - type II (HTLV-II) B97.34
- lentivirus B97.31
- oncovirus B97.32
- specified NEC B97.39
Retrusion, premaxilla (developmental) M26.09
Rett's disease or syndrome F84.2
Reverse peristalsis R19.2
Reye's syndrome G93.7
Rh (factor)
- hemolytic disease (newborn) P55.0
- incompatibility, immunization or sensitization
  - affecting management of pregnancy NEC O36.09- ☑
    - anti-D antibody O36.01- ☑
  - newborn P55.0
  - transfusion reaction — see Complication(s), transfusion, incompatibility reaction, Rh (factor)
- negative mother affecting newborn P55.0
- titer elevated — see Complication(s), transfusion, incompatibility reaction, Rh (factor)
- transfusion reaction — see Complication(s), transfusion, incompatibility reaction, Rh (factor)
Rhabdomyolysis (idiopathic) NEC M62.82
- traumatic T79.6- ☑
Rhabdomyoma — see also Neoplasm, connective tissue, benign
- adult — see Neoplasm, connective tissue, benign
- fetal — see Neoplasm, connective tissue, benign
- glycogenic — see Neoplasm, connective tissue, benign
Rhabdomyosarcoma (any type) — see Neoplasm, connective tissue, malignant
Rhabdosarcoma — see Rhabdomyosarcoma
Rhesus (factor) **incompatibility** — see Rh, incompatibility
Rheumatic (acute) (subacute)
- adherent pericardium I09.2
- chronic I09.89
- coronary arteritis I01.8
- degeneration, myocardium I09.0
- fever (acute) — see Fever, rheumatic
- heart — see Disease, heart, rheumatic
- myocardial degeneration — see Degeneration, myocardium
- myocarditis (chronic) (inactive) (with chorea) I09.0
  - active or acute I01.2
    - with chorea (acute) (rheumatic) (Sydenham's) I02.0
- pancarditis, acute I01.8
  - with chorea (acute) (rheumatic) Sydenham's) I02.0
- pericarditis (active) (acute) (with effusion) (with pneumonia) I01.0
  - with chorea (acute) (rheumatic) (Sydenham's) I02.0
  - chronic or inactive I09.2
- pneumonia I00 [J17]
- torticollis M43.6
- typhoid fever A01.09
Rheumatism (articular) (neuralgic) (nonarticular) M79.0
- gout — see Arthritis, rheumatoid
- intercostal, meaning Tietze's disease M94.0
- palindromic (any site) M12.30
  - ankle M12.37- ☑
  - elbow M12.32- ☑
  - foot joint M12.37- ☑
  - hand joint M12.34- ☑
  - hip M12.35- ☑
  - knee M12.36- ☑
  - multiple site M12.39
  - shoulder M12.31- ☑
  - specified joint NEC M12.38
  - vertebrae M12.38
  - wrist M12.33- ☑
- sciatic M54.4- ☑
Rheumatoid — see also condition
- arthritis — see also Arthritis, rheumatoid
  - with involvement of organs NEC M05.60
    - ankle M05.67- ☑
    - elbow M05.62- ☑
    - foot joint M05.67- ☑
    - hand joint M05.64- ☑
    - hip M05.65- ☑

Rheumatoid — continued
- arthritis — see also Arthritis, rheumatoid — continued
  - with involvement of organs — continued
    - knee M05.66- ☑
    - multiple site M05.69
    - shoulder M05.61- ☑
    - vertebra — see Spondylitis, ankylosing
    - wrist M05.63- ☑
  - seronegative — see Arthritis, rheumatoid, seronegative
  - seropositive — see Arthritis, rheumatoid, seropositive
- carditis M05.30
  - ankle M05.37- ☑
  - elbow M05.32- ☑
  - foot joint M05.37- ☑
  - hand joint M05.34- ☑
  - hip M05.35- ☑
  - knee M05.36- ☑
  - multiple site M05.39
  - shoulder M05.31- ☑
  - vertebra — see Spondylitis, ankylosing
  - wrist M05.33- ☑
- endocarditis — see Rheumatoid, carditis
- lung (disease) M05.10
  - ankle M05.17- ☑
  - elbow M05.12- ☑
  - foot joint M05.17- ☑
  - hand joint M05.14- ☑
  - hip M05.15- ☑
  - knee M05.16- ☑
  - multiple site M05.19
  - shoulder M05.11- ☑
  - vertebra — see Spondylitis, ankylosing
  - wrist M05.13- ☑
- myocarditis — see Rheumatoid, carditis
- myopathy M05.40
  - ankle M05.47- ☑
  - elbow M05.42- ☑
  - foot joint M05.47- ☑
  - hand joint M05.44- ☑
  - hip M05.45- ☑
  - knee M05.46- ☑
  - multiple site M05.49
  - shoulder M05.41- ☑
  - vertebra — see Spondylitis, ankylosing
  - wrist M05.43- ☑
- pericarditis — see Rheumatoid, carditis
- polyarthritis — see Arthritis, rheumatoid
- polyneuropathy M05.50
  - ankle M05.57- ☑
  - elbow M05.52- ☑
  - foot joint M05.57- ☑
  - hand joint M05.54- ☑
  - hip M05.55- ☑
  - knee M05.56- ☑
  - multiple site M05.59
  - shoulder M05.51- ☑
  - vertebra — see Spondylitis, ankylosing
  - wrist M05.53- ☑
- vasculitis M05.20
  - ankle M05.27- ☑
  - elbow M05.22- ☑
  - foot joint M05.27- ☑
  - hand joint M05.24- ☑
  - hip M05.25- ☑
  - knee M05.26- ☑
  - multiple site M05.29
  - shoulder M05.21- ☑
  - vertebra — see Spondylitis, ankylosing
  - wrist M05.23- ☑
Rhinitis (atrophic) (catarrhal) (chronic) (croupous) (fibrinous) (granulomatous) (hyperplastic) (hypertrophic) (membranous) (obstructive) (purulent) (suppurative) (ulcerative) J31.0
- with
  - sore throat — see Nasopharyngitis
- acute J00
- allergic J30.9
  - with asthma J45.909
    - with
      - exacerbation (acute) J45.901
      - status asthmaticus J45.902
  - due to
    - food J30.5
    - pollen J30.1
  - nonseasonal J30.89

Rhinitis — continued
- allergic — continued
  - perennial J30.89
  - seasonal NEC J30.2
  - specified NEC J30.89
- infective J00
- pneumococcal J00
- syphilitic A52.73
  - congenital A50.05 [J99]
- tuberculous A15.8
- vasomotor J30.0
Rhinoantritis (chronic) — see Sinusitis, maxillary
Rhinodacryolith — see Dacryolith
Rhinolith (nasal sinus) J34.89
Rhinomegaly J34.89
Rhinopharyngitis (acute) (subacute) — see also Nasopharyngitis
- chronic J31.1
- destructive ulcerating A66.5
- mutilans A66.5
Rhinophyma L71.1
Rhinorrhea J34.89
- cerebrospinal (fluid) G96.01
  - postoperative G96.08
  - specified NEC G96.08
  - spontaneous G96.01
  - traumatic G96.08
- paroxysmal — see Rhinitis, allergic
- spasmodic — see Rhinitis, allergic
Rhinosalpingitis — see Salpingitis, eustachian
Rhinoscleroma A48.8
Rhinosinusitis — see Sinusitis
Rhinosporidiosis B48.1
Rhinovirus infection NEC B34.8
Rhizomelic chondrodysplasia punctata E71.540
Rhythm
- atrioventricular nodal I49.8
- disorder I49.9
  - coronary sinus I49.8
  - ectopic I49.8
  - nodal I49.8
- escape I49.9
- heart, abnormal I49.9
- idioventricular I44.2
- nodal I49.8
- sleep, inversion G47.2- ☑
  - nonorganic origin — see Disorder, sleep, circadian rhythm, psychogenic
Rhytidosis facialis L98.8
Rib — see also condition
- cervical Q76.5
Riboflavin deficiency E53.0
Rice bodies — see also Loose, body, joint
- knee M23.4- ☑
Richter syndrome — see Leukemia, chronic lymphocytic, B-cell type
Richter's hernia — see Hernia, abdomen, with obstruction
Ricinism — see Poisoning, food, noxious, plant
Rickets (active) (acute) (adolescent) (chest wall) (congenital) (current) (infantile) (intestinal) E55.0
- adult — see Osteomalacia
- celiac K90.0
- hypophosphatemic with nephrotic-glycosuric dwarfism E72.09
- inactive E64.3
- kidney N25.0
- renal N25.0
- sequelae, any E64.3
- vitamin-D-resistant E83.31 [M90.80]
Rickettsia 364D/R. philipii (Pacific Coast tick fever) A77.8
Rickettsial disease A79.9
- specified type NEC A79.89
Rickettsialpox (Rickettsia akari) A79.1
Rickettsiosis A79.9
- due to
  - Ehrlichia sennetsu A79.81
  - Neorickettsia sennetsu A79.81
  - Rickettsia akari (rickettsialpox) A79.1
- specified type NEC A79.89
- tick-borne A77.9
- vesicular A79.1
Rider's bone — see Ossification, muscle, specified NEC
Ridge, alveolus — see also condition
- flabby K06.8
Ridged ear, congenital Q17.3
Riedel's
- lobe, liver Q44.79
- struma, thyroiditis or disease E06.5
Rieger anomaly or syndrome Q13.81

Riehl's melanosis L81.4
Rietti-Greppi-Micheli anemia D56.9
Rieux's hernia — see Hernia, abdomen, specified site NEC
Riga (-Fede) **disease** K14.0
Riggs' disease — see Periodontitis
Right aortic arch Q25.47
Right middle lobe syndrome J98.11
Rigid, rigidity — see also condition
　abdominal R19.30
　　with severe abdominal pain R10.0
　　epigastric R19.36
　　generalized R19.37
　　left lower quadrant R19.34
　　left upper quadrant R19.32
　　periumbilic R19.35
　　right lower quadrant R19.33
　　right upper quadrant R19.31
　articular, multiple, congenital Q68.8
　cervix (uteri) in pregnancy — see Pregnancy, complicated by, abnormal, cervix
　hymen (acquired) (congenital) N89.6
　nuchal R29.1
　pelvic floor in pregnancy — see Pregnancy, complicated by, abnormal, pelvic organs or tissues NEC
　perineum or vulva in pregnancy — see Pregnancy, complicated by, abnormal, vulva
　spine — see Dorsopathy, specified NEC
　vagina in pregnancy — see Pregnancy, complicated by, abnormal, vagina
Rigors R68.89
　with fever R50.9
Riley-Day syndrome G90.1
RIND (reversible ischemic neurologic deficit) I63.9
Ring(s)
　aorta (vascular) Q25.45
　Bandl's O62.4
　contraction, complicating delivery O62.4
　esophageal, lower (muscular) K22.2
　Fleischer's (cornea) H18.04- ☑
　hymenal, tight (acquired) (congenital) N89.6
　Kayser-Fleischer (cornea) H18.04- ☑
　retraction, uterus, pathological O62.4
　Schatzki's (esophagus) (lower) K22.2
　　congenital Q39.3
　Soemmerring's — see Cataract, secondary
　vascular (congenital) Q25.8
　　aorta Q25.45
Ringed hair (congenital) Q84.1
Ringworm B35.9
　beard B35.0
　black dot B35.0
　body B35.4
　Burmese B35.5
　corporeal B35.4
　foot B35.3
　groin B35.6
　hand B35.2
　honeycomb B35.0
　nails B35.1
　perianal (area) B35.6
　scalp B35.0
　specified NEC B35.8
　Tokelau B35.5
Rise, venous pressure I87.8
Rising, PSA following treatment for malignant neoplasm of prostate R97.21
Risk
　for
　　dental caries Z91.849
　　　high Z91.843
　　　low Z91.841
　　　moderate Z91.842
　　homelessness, imminent Z59.811
　　suffocation (smothering) under another while sleeping Z72.823
　suicidal
　　meaning personal history of attempted suicide Z91.51
　　meaning suicidal ideation — see Ideation, suicidal
Ritter's disease L00
Rivalry, sibling Z62.891
Rivalta's disease A42.2
River blindness B73.01
Robert's pelvis Q74.2
　with disproportion (fetopelvic) O33.0
　　causing obstructed labor O65.0
Robin (-Pierre) **syndrome** Q87.0
Robinow-Silverman-Smith syndrome Q87.19
Robinson's (hidrotic) **ectodermal dysplasia or syndrome** Q82.4

Robles' disease B73.01
Rocky Mountain (spotted) **fever** A77.0
Roetheln — see Rubella
Roger's disease Q21.0
Rokitansky-Aschoff sinuses (gallbladder) K82.8
Rolando's fracture (displaced) S62.22- ☑
　nondisplaced S62.22- ☑
Romano-Ward (prolonged QT interval) **syndrome** I45.81
Romberg's disease or syndrome G51.8
Roof, mouth — see condition
Rosacea L71.9
　acne L71.9
　keratitis L71.8
　specified NEC L71.8
Rosary, rachitic E55.0
Rose
　cold J30.1
　fever J30.1
　rash R21
　　epidemic B06.9
Rosenbach's erysipeloid A26.0
Rosenthal's disease or syndrome D68.1
Roseola B09
　infantum B08.20
　　due to human herpesvirus 6 B08.21
　　due to human herpesvirus 7 B08.22
Ross River disease or fever B33.1
Rossbach's disease K31.89
　psychogenic F45.8
Rostan's asthma (cardiac) — see Failure, ventricular, left
Rotation
　anomalous, incomplete or insufficient, intestine Q43.3
　cecum (congenital) Q43.3
　colon (congenital) Q43.3
　spine, incomplete or insufficient — see Dorsopathy, deforming, specified NEC
　tooth, teeth, fully erupted M26.35
　vertebra, incomplete or insufficient — see Dorsopathy, deforming, specified NEC
Rotes Querol disease or syndrome — see Hyperostosis, ankylosing
Roth (-Bernhardt) **disease or syndrome** — see Meralgia paraesthetica
Rothmund (-Thomson) **syndrome** Q82.8
Rotor's disease or syndrome E80.6
Round
　back (with wedging of vertebrae) — see Kyphosis
　sequelae (late effect) of rickets E64.3
　worms (large) (infestation) NEC B82.0
　　Ascariasis — see also Ascariasis B77.9
Roussy-Levy syndrome G60.0
Rubella (German measles) B06.9
　complication NEC B06.09
　　neurological B06.00
　congenital P35.0
　contact Z20.4
　exposure to Z20.4
　maternal
　　care for (suspected) damage to fetus O35.3- ☑
　　manifest rubella in infant P35.0
　　suspected damage to fetus affecting management of pregnancy O35.3- ☑
　specified complications NEC B06.89
Rubeola (meaning measles) — see Measles
　meaning rubella — see Rubella
Rubeosis, iris — see Disorder, iris, vascular
Rubinstein-Taybi syndrome Q87.2
Rudimentary (congenital) — see also Agenesis
　arm — see Defect, reduction, upper limb
　bone Q79.9
　cervix uteri Q51.828
　eye Q11.2
　lobule of ear Q17.3
　patella Q74.1
　respiratory organs in thoracopagus Q89.4
　tracheal bronchus Q32.4
　uterus Q51.818
　　in male Q56.1
　vagina Q52.0
Ruled out condition — see Observation, suspected
Rumination R11.10
　with nausea R11.2
　disorder of infancy or childhood (in remission) F98.21
　in adults (in remission) F50.84
　neurotic F42.8
　newborn P92.1
　obsessional F42.8
　psychogenic F42.8
Runaway [from current living environment] Z62.892

Runeberg's disease D51.0
Running out of money Z59.868
Runny nose R09.89
Rupia (syphilitic) A51.39
　congenital A50.06
　tertiary A52.79
Rupture, ruptured
　abscess (spontaneous) — code by site under Abscess
　aneurysm — see Aneurysm
　anus (sphincter) — see Laceration, anus
　aorta, aortic I71.8
　　abdominal I71.30
　　　infrarenal I71.33
　　　juxtarenal I71.32
　　　pararenal I71.31
　　arch I71.12
　　ascending I71.11
　　descending I71.8
　　　abdominal I71.30
　　　thoracic I71.13
　　syphilitic A52.01
　　thoracoabdominal I71.50
　　　paravisceral I71.52
　　　supraceliac I71.51
　　thorax, thoracic I71.10
　　transverse I71.12
　　traumatic — see Injury, aorta, laceration, major
　　valve or cusp — see also Endocarditis, aortic I35.8
　appendix (with peritonitis) — see also Appendicitis K35.32
　　with localized peritonitis — see also Appendicitis K35.32
　arteriovenous fistula, brain — see Fistula, arteriovenous, brain, ruptured
　artery I77.2
　　brain — see Hemorrhage, intracranial, intracerebral
　　coronary — see Infarct, myocardium
　　heart — see Infarct, myocardium
　　pulmonary I28.8
　　traumatic (complication) — see Injury, blood vessel
　bile duct (common) (hepatic) K83.2
　　cystic K82.2
　bladder (sphincter) (nontraumatic) (spontaneous) N32.89
　　following ectopic or molar pregnancy O08.6
　　obstetrical trauma O71.5
　　traumatic S37.29- ☑
　blood vessel — see also Hemorrhage
　　brain — see Hemorrhage, intracranial, intracerebral
　　heart — see Infarct, myocardium
　　traumatic (complication) — see Injury, blood vessel, laceration, major, by site
　bone — see Fracture
　bowel (nontraumatic) K63.1
　brain
　　aneurysm (congenital) — see also Hemorrhage, intracranial, subarachnoid
　　　syphilitic A52.05
　　hemorrhagic — see Hemorrhage, intracranial, intracerebral
　capillaries I78.8
　cardiac (auricle) (ventricle) (wall) I23.3
　　with hemopericardium I23.0
　　infectional I40.9
　　traumatic — see Injury, heart
　cartilage (articular) (current) — see also Sprain
　　knee S83.3- ☑
　　semilunar — see Tear, meniscus
　cecum (with peritonitis) K65.0
　　with peritoneal abscess K35.33
　　traumatic S36.598- ☑
　celiac artery, traumatic — see Injury, blood vessel, celiac artery, laceration, major
　cerebral aneurysm (congenital) (see Hemorrhage, intracranial, subarachnoid)
　cervix (uteri)
　　with ectopic or molar pregnancy O08.6
　　following ectopic or molar pregnancy O08.6
　　obstetrical trauma O71.3
　　traumatic S37.69- ☑
　chordae tendineae NEC I51.1
　　concurrent with acute myocardial infarction — see Infarct, myocardium
　　following acute myocardial infarction (current complication) I23.4
　choroid (direct) (indirect) (traumatic) H31.32- ☑
　circle of Willis I60.6
　colon (nontraumatic) K63.1
　　traumatic — see Injury, intestine, large

☑ Additional Character Required — Refer to the Tabular List for Character Selection

Rupture, ruptured — continued
- cornea (traumatic) — see Injury, eye, laceration
- coronary (artery) (thrombotic) — see Infarct, myocardium
- corpus luteum (infected) (ovary) N83.1- ☑
- cyst — see Cyst
- cystic duct K82.2
- Descemet's membrane — see Change, corneal membrane, Descemet's, rupture
  - traumatic — see Injury, eye, laceration
- diaphragm, traumatic — see Injury, intrathoracic, diaphragm
- disc — see Rupture, intervertebral disc
- diverticulum (intestine) K57.80
  - with bleeding K57.81
  - bladder N32.3
  - large intestine K57.20
    - with
      - bleeding K57.21
        - small intestine K57.40
          - with bleeding K57.41
  - small intestine K57.00
    - with
      - bleeding K57.01
        - large intestine K57.40
          - with bleeding K57.41
- duodenal stump K31.89
- ear drum (nontraumatic) — see also Perforation, tympanum
  - traumatic S09.2- ☑
    - due to blast injury — see Injury, blast, ear
- esophagus K22.3
- eye (without prolapse or loss of intraocular tissue) — see Injury, eye, laceration
- fallopian tube NEC (nonobstetric) (nontraumatic) N83.8
  - due to pregnancy O00.10- ☑
    - with intrauterine pregnancy O00.11- ☑
- fontanel P13.1
- gallbladder K82.2
  - traumatic S36.128- ☑
- gastric — see also Rupture, stomach
  - vessel K92.2
- globe (eye) (traumatic) — see Injury, eye, laceration
  - nontraumatic — see also Disorder, globe H44.89
- graafian follicle (hematoma) N83.0- ☑
- heart — see Rupture, cardiac
- hymen (nontraumatic) (nonintentional) N89.8
- internal organ, traumatic — see Injury, by site
- intervertebral disc — see Displacement, intervertebral disc
  - traumatic — see Rupture, traumatic, intervertebral disc
- intestine NEC (nontraumatic) K63.1
  - traumatic — see Injury, intestine
- iris — see also Abnormality, pupillary
  - traumatic — see Injury, eye, laceration
- joint capsule, traumatic — see Sprain
- kidney (traumatic) S37.06- ☑
  - birth injury P15.8
  - nontraumatic N28.89
- lacrimal duct (traumatic) — see Injury, eye, specified site NEC
- lens (cataract) (traumatic) — see Cataract, traumatic
- ligament, traumatic — see Rupture, traumatic, ligament, by site
- liver S36.116- ☑
  - birth injury P15.0
- lymphatic vessel I89.8
- marginal sinus (placental) (with hemorrhage) — see Hemorrhage, antepartum, specified cause NEC
- membrana tympani (nontraumatic) — see Perforation, tympanum
- membranes (spontaneous)
  - artificial
    - delayed delivery following O75.5
  - delayed delivery following — see Pregnancy, complicated by, premature rupture of membranes
- meningeal artery I60.8
- meniscus (knee) — see also Tear, meniscus
  - old — see Derangement, meniscus
  - site other than knee — code as Sprain
- mesenteric artery, traumatic — see Injury, mesenteric, artery, laceration, major
- mesentery (nontraumatic) K66.8
  - traumatic — see Injury, intra-abdominal, specified, site NEC
- mitral (valve) I34.89
- muscle (traumatic) — see also Strain
  - diastasis — see Diastasis, muscle

Rupture, ruptured — continued
- muscle — see also Strain — continued
  - nontraumatic M62.10
    - ankle M62.17- ☑
    - foot M62.17- ☑
    - forearm M62.13- ☑
    - hand M62.14- ☑
    - lower leg M62.16- ☑
    - pelvic region M62.15- ☑
    - shoulder region M62.11- ☑
    - specified site NEC M62.18
    - thigh M62.15- ☑
    - upper arm M62.12- ☑
  - traumatic — see Strain, by site
- musculotendinous junction NEC, nontraumatic — see Rupture, tendon, spontaneous
- mycotic aneurysm causing cerebral hemorrhage — see Hemorrhage, intracranial, subarachnoid
- myocardium, myocardial — see Rupture, cardiac
  - traumatic — see Injury, heart
- nontraumatic, meaning hernia — see Hernia
- obstructed — see Hernia, by site, obstructed
- operation wound — see Disruption, wound, operation
- ovary, ovarian N83.8
  - corpus luteum cyst N83.1- ☑
  - follicle (graafian) N83.0- ☑
- oviduct (nonobstetric) (nontraumatic) N83.8
  - due to pregnancy O00.10- ☑
    - with intrauterine pregnancy O00.11- ☑
- pancreas (nontraumatic) K86.89
  - traumatic S36.299- ☑
- papillary muscle NEC I51.2
  - following acute myocardial infarction (current complication) I23.5
- pelvic
  - floor, complicating delivery O70.1
  - organ NEC, obstetrical trauma O71.5
- perineum (nonobstetric) (nontraumatic) N90.89
  - complicating delivery — see Delivery, complicated, by, laceration, anus (sphincter)
- postoperative wound — see Disruption, wound, operation
- prostate (traumatic) S37.828- ☑
- pulmonary
  - artery I28.8
  - valve (heart) I37.8
  - vein I28.8
  - vessel I28.8
- pus tube — see Salpingitis
- pyosalpinx — see Salpingitis
- rectum (nontraumatic) K63.1
  - traumatic S36.69- ☑
- retina, retinal (traumatic) (without detachment) — see also Break, retina
  - with detachment — see Detachment, retina, with retinal, break
- rotator cuff (nontraumatic) M75.10- ☑
  - complete M75.12- ☑
  - incomplete M75.11- ☑
- sclera — see Injury, eye, laceration
- sigmoid (nontraumatic) K63.1
  - traumatic S36.593- ☑
- spinal cord — see also Injury, spinal cord, by region
  - due to injury at birth P11.5
  - newborn (birth injury) P11.5
- spleen (traumatic) S36.09- ☑
  - birth injury P15.1
  - congenital (birth injury) P15.1
  - due to P. vivax malaria B51.0
  - nontraumatic D73.5
  - spontaneous D73.5
- splenic vein R58
  - traumatic — see Injury, blood vessel, splenic vein
- stomach (nontraumatic) (spontaneous) K31.89
  - traumatic S36.39- ☑
- supraspinatus (complete) (incomplete) (nontraumatic) — see Tear, rotator cuff
- symphysis pubis
  - obstetric O71.6
  - traumatic S33.4- ☑
- synovium (cyst) M66.10
  - ankle M66.17- ☑
  - elbow M66.12- ☑
  - finger M66.14- ☑
  - foot M66.17- ☑
  - forearm M66.13- ☑
  - hand M66.14- ☑

Rupture, ruptured — continued
- synovium — continued
  - pelvic region M66.15- ☑
  - shoulder region M66.11- ☑
  - specified site NEC M66.18
  - thigh M66.15- ☑
  - toe M66.17- ☑
  - upper arm M66.12- ☑
  - wrist M66.13- ☑
- tendon (traumatic) — see Strain
  - nontraumatic (spontaneous) M66.9
    - ankle M66.87- ☑
    - extensor M66.20
      - ankle M66.27- ☑
      - foot M66.27- ☑
      - forearm M66.23- ☑
      - hand M66.24- ☑
      - lower leg M66.26- ☑
      - multiple sites M66.29
      - pelvic region M66.25- ☑
      - shoulder region M66.21- ☑
      - specified site NEC M66.28
      - thigh M66.25- ☑
      - upper arm M66.22- ☑
    - flexor M66.30
      - ankle M66.37- ☑
      - foot M66.37- ☑
      - forearm M66.33- ☑
      - hand M66.34- ☑
      - lower leg M66.36- ☑
      - multiple sites M66.39
      - pelvic region M66.35- ☑
      - shoulder region M66.31- ☑
      - specified site NEC M66.38
      - thigh M66.35- ☑
      - upper arm M66.32- ☑
    - foot M66.87- ☑
    - forearm M66.83- ☑
    - hand M66.84- ☑
    - lower leg M66.86- ☑
    - multiple sites M66.89
    - pelvic region M66.85- ☑
    - shoulder region M66.81- ☑
    - specified
      - site NEC M66.88
      - tendon M66.80
    - thigh M66.85- ☑
    - upper arm M66.82- ☑
- thoracic duct I89.8
- tonsil J35.8
- traumatic
  - aorta — see Injury, aorta, laceration, major
  - diaphragm — see Injury, intrathoracic, diaphragm
  - external site — see Wound, open, by site
  - eye — see Injury, eye, laceration
  - internal organ — see Injury, by site
  - intervertebral disc
    - cervical S13.0- ☑
    - lumbar S33.0- ☑
    - thoracic S23.0- ☑
  - kidney S37.06- ☑
  - ligament — see also Sprain
    - ankle — see Sprain, ankle
    - carpus — see Rupture, traumatic, ligament, wrist
    - collateral (hand) — see Rupture, traumatic, ligament, finger, collateral
    - finger (metacarpophalangeal) (interphalangeal) S63.40- ☑
      - collateral S63.41- ☑
        - index S63.41- ☑
        - little S63.41- ☑
        - middle S63.41- ☑
        - ring S63.41- ☑
      - index S63.40- ☑
      - little S63.40- ☑
      - middle S63.40- ☑
      - palmar S63.42- ☑
        - index S63.42- ☑
        - little S63.42- ☑
        - middle S63.42- ☑
        - ring S63.42- ☑
      - ring S63.40- ☑
      - specified site NEC S63.499- ☑
        - index S63.49- ☑
        - little S63.49- ☑
        - middle S63.49- ☑

Rupture, ruptured — *continued*
  traumatic — *continued*
    ligament — *see also* Sprain — *continued*
      finger — *continued*
        specified site — *continued*
          ring S63.49- ☑
          volar plate S63.43- ☑
            index S63.43- ☑
            little S63.43- ☑
            middle S63.43- ☑
            ring S63.43- ☑
      foot — *see* Sprain, foot
      radial collateral S53.2- ☑
      radiocarpal — *see* Rupture, traumatic, ligament, wrist, radiocarpal
      ulnar collateral S53.3- ☑
      ulnocarpal — *see* Rupture, traumatic, ligament, wrist, ulnocarpal
      wrist S63.30- ☑
        collateral S63.31- ☑
        radiocarpal S63.32- ☑
        specified site NEC S63.39- ☑
        ulnocarpal (palmar) S63.33- ☑
    liver S36.116- ☑
    membrana tympani — *see* Rupture, ear drum, traumatic
    muscle or tendon — *see* Strain
    myocardium — *see* Injury, heart
    pancreas S36.299- ☑
    rectum S36.69- ☑
    sigmoid S36.593- ☑
    spleen S36.09- ☑
    stomach S36.39- ☑
    symphysis pubis S33.4- ☑
    tympanum, tympanic (membrane) — *see* Rupture, ear drum, traumatic
    ureter S37.19- ☑
    uterus S37.69- ☑
    vagina — *see* Injury, vagina
    vena cava — *see* Injury, vena cava, laceration, major
  tricuspid (heart) (valve) I07.8
  tube, tubal (nonobstetric) (nontraumatic) N83.8
    abscess — *see* Salpingitis
    due to pregnancy O00.10- ☑
      with intrauterine pregnancy O00.11- ☑
  tympanum, tympanic (membrane) (nontraumatic) — *see also* Perforation, tympanic membrane H72.9- ☑
    traumatic — *see* Rupture, ear drum, traumatic
  umbilical cord, complicating delivery O69.89- ☑
  ureter (traumatic) S37.19- ☑
    nontraumatic N28.89
  urethra (nontraumatic) N36.8
    with ectopic or molar pregnancy O08.6
    following ectopic or molar pregnancy O08.6
    obstetrical trauma O71.5
    traumatic S37.39- ☑
  uterosacral ligament (nonobstetric) (nontraumatic) N83.8
  uterus (traumatic) S37.69- ☑
    before labor O71.0- ☑
    during or after labor O71.1
    nonpuerperal, nontraumatic N85.8
    pregnant (during labor) O71.1
      before labor O71.0- ☑
  vagina — *see* Injury, vagina
  valve, valvular (heart) — *see* Endocarditis
  varicose vein — *see* Varix
  varix — *see* Varix
  vena cava R58
    traumatic — *see* Injury, vena cava, laceration, major
  vesical (urinary) N32.89
  vessel (blood) R58
    pulmonary I28.8
    traumatic — *see* Injury, blood vessel
  viscus R19.8
  vulva complicating delivery O70.0
Russell-Silver syndrome Q87.19
Russian spring-summer type encephalitis A84.0
Rust's disease (tuberculous cervical spondylitis) A18.01
Ruvalcaba-Myhre-Smith syndrome E71.440
Rytand-Lipsitch syndrome I44.2

S

Saber, sabre shin or tibia (syphilitic) A50.56 [M90.86-] ☑
Sac lacrimal — *see* condition
Saccharomyces infection B37.9
Saccharopinuria E72.3
Saccular — *see* condition
Sacculation
  aorta (nonsyphilitic) — *see* Aneurysm, aorta
  bladder N32.3
  intralaryngeal (congenital) (ventricular) Q31.3
  larynx (congenital) (ventricular) Q31.3
  organ or site, congenital — *see* Distortion
  pregnant uterus — *see* Pregnancy, complicated by, abnormal, uterus
  ureter N28.89
  urethra N36.1
  vesical N32.3
Sachs' amaurotic familial idiocy or disease E75.02
Sachs-Tay disease E75.02
Sacks-Libman disease M32.11
Sacralgia M53.3
Sacralization Q76.49
Sacrodynia M53.3
Sacroiliac joint — *see* condition
Sacroiliitis NEC M46.1
Sacrum — *see* condition
Saddle
  back — *see* Lordosis
  embolus
    abdominal aorta I74.01
    pulmonary artery I26.92
      with acute cor pulmonale I26.02
  injury — *code to* condition
  nose M95.0
    due to syphilis A50.57
Sadism (sexual) F65.52
Sadness, postpartal O90.6
Sadomasochism F65.50
Saemisch's ulcer (cornea) — *see* Ulcer, cornea, central
Sagging
  skin and subcutaneous tissue (following bariatric surgery weight loss) (following dietary weight loss) L98.7
Sahib disease B55.0
Sailors' skin L57.8
Saint
  Anthony's fire — *see* Erysipelas
  triad — *see* Hernia, diaphragm
  Vitus' dance — *see* Chorea, Sydenham's
Salaam
  attack(s) — *see* Epilepsy, spasms
  tic R25.8
Salicylism
  abuse F55.8
  overdose or wrong substance given — *see* Table of Drugs and Chemicals, by drug, poisoning
Salivary duct or gland — *see* condition
Salivation, excessive K11.7
Salmonella — *see* Infection, Salmonella
Salmonellosis A02.0
Salpingitis (catarrhal) (fallopian tube) (nodular) (pseudofollicular) (purulent) (septic) N70.91
  with oophoritis N70.93
  acute N70.01
    with oophoritis N70.03
  chlamydial A56.11
  chronic N70.11
    with oophoritis N70.13
  complicating abortion — *see* Abortion, by type, complicated by, salpingitis
  ear — *see* Salpingitis, eustachian
  eustachian (tube) H68.00- ☑
    acute H68.01- ☑
    chronic H68.02- ☑
  follicularis N70.11
    with oophoritis N70.13
  gonococcal (acute) (chronic) A54.24
  interstitial, chronic N70.11
    with oophoritis N70.13
  isthmica nodosa N70.11
    with oophoritis N70.13
  specific (gonococcal) (acute) (chronic) A54.24
  tuberculous (acute) (chronic) A18.17
  venereal (gonococcal) (acute) (chronic) A54.24
Salpingo-oophoritis (catarrhal) (purulent) (ruptured) (septic) (suppurative) N70.93
  acute N70.03
    with ectopic or molar pregnancy O08.0
    following ectopic or molar pregnancy O08.0
    gonococcal A54.24
  chronic N70.13
  following ectopic or molar pregnancy O08.0
  gonococcal (acute) (chronic) A54.24
  puerperal O86.19
Salpingo-oophoritis — *continued*
  specific (gonococcal) (acute) (chronic) A54.24
  subacute N70.03
  tuberculous (acute) (chronic) A18.17
  venereal (gonococcal) (acute) (chronic) A54.24
Salpingo-ovaritis — *see* Salpingo-oophoritis
Salpingocele N83.4- ☑
Salpingoperitonitis — *see* Salpingo-oophoritis
Salzmann's nodular dystrophy — *see* Degeneration, cornea, nodular
Sampson's cyst or tumor N80.10- ☑
San Joaquin (Valley) **fever** B38.0
Sandblaster's asthma, lung or pneumoconiosis J62.8
Sander's disease (paranoia) F22
Sandfly fever A93.1
Sandhoff's disease E75.01
Sanfilippo (Type B) (Type C) (Type D) **syndrome** E76.22
Sanger-Brown ataxia G11.2
Sao Paulo fever or typhus A77.0
Saponification, mesenteric K65.8
Sarcocele (benign)
  syphilitic A52.76
    congenital A50.59
Sarcocystosis A07.8
Sarcoepiplocele — *see* Hernia
Sarcoepiplomphalocele Q79.2
Sarcoglycanopathy G71.0340
  alpha G71.0341
  beta G71.0342
  delta G71.0349
  gamma G71.0349
Sarcoid — *see also* Sarcoidosis
  arthropathy D86.86
  Boeck's D86.9
  Darier-Roussy D86.3
  iridocyclitis D86.83
  meningitis D86.81
  myocarditis D86.85
  myositis D86.87
  pyelonephritis D86.84
  Spiegler-Fendt L08.89
Sarcoidosis D86.9
  with
    cranial nerve palsies D86.82
    hepatic granuloma D86.89
    polyarthritis D86.86
    tubulo-interstitial nephropathy D86.84
  combined sites NEC D86.89
  lung D86.0
    and lymph nodes D86.2
  lymph nodes D86.1
    and lung D86.2
  meninges D86.81
  skin D86.3
  specified type NEC D86.89
Sarcoma (of) — *see also* Neoplasm, connective tissue, malignant
  alveolar soft part — *see* Neoplasm, connective tissue, malignant
  ameloblastic C41.1
    upper jaw (bone) C41.0
  botryoid — *see* Neoplasm, connective tissue, malignant
  botryoides — *see* Neoplasm, connective tissue, malignant
  cerebellar C71.6
    circumscribed (arachnoidal) C71.6
  circumscribed (arachnoidal) cerebellar C71.6
  clear cell — *see also* Neoplasm, connective tissue, malignant
    kidney C64.- ☑
  dendritic cells (accessory cells) C96.4
  embryonal — *see* Neoplasm, connective tissue, malignant
  endometrial (stromal) C54.1
    isthmus C54.0
  epithelioid (cell) — *see* Neoplasm, connective tissue, malignant
  Ewing's — *see* Neoplasm, bone, malignant
  follicular dendritic cell C96.4
  germinoblastic (diffuse) — *see* Lymphoma, diffuse large cell
  follicular — *see* Lymphoma, follicular, specified NEC
  giant cell (except of bone) — *see also* Neoplasm, connective tissue, malignant
    bone — *see* Neoplasm, bone, malignant
  glomoid — *see* Neoplasm, connective tissue, malignant
  granulocytic C92.3- ☑
  hemangioendothelial — *see* Neoplasm, connective tissue, malignant
  hemorrhagic, multiple — *see* Sarcoma, Kaposi's

Sarcoma — continued
- histiocytic C96.A (following C96.6)
- Hodgkin — see Lymphoma, Hodgkin
- immunoblastic (diffuse) — see Lymphoma, diffuse large cell
- interdigitating dendritic cell C96.4
- Kaposi's
  - colon C46.4
  - connective tissue C46.1
  - gastrointestinal organ C46.4
  - lung C46.5- ☑
  - lymph node(s) C46.3
  - palate (hard) (soft) C46.2
  - rectum C46.4
  - skin C46.0
  - specified site NEC C46.7
  - stomach C46.4
  - unspecified site C46.9
- Kupffer cell C22.3
- Langerhans cell C96.4
- leptomeningeal — see Neoplasm, meninges, malignant
- liver NEC C22.4
- lymphangioendothelial — see Neoplasm, connective tissue, malignant
- lymphoblastic — see Lymphoma, lymphoblastic (diffuse)
- lymphocytic — see Lymphoma, small cell B-cell
- mast cell C96.22
- melanotic — see Melanoma
- meningeal — see Neoplasm, meninges, malignant
- meningothelial — see Neoplasm, meninges, malignant
- mesenchymal — see also Neoplasm, connective tissue, malignant
  - mixed — see Neoplasm, connective tissue, malignant
- mesothelial — see Mesothelioma
- monstrocellular
  - specified site — see Neoplasm, malignant, by site
  - unspecified site C71.9
- myeloid C92.3- ☑
- neurogenic — see Neoplasm, nerve, malignant
- odontogenic C41.1
  - upper jaw (bone) C41.0
- osteoblastic — see Neoplasm, bone, malignant
- osteogenic — see also Neoplasm, bone, malignant
  - juxtacortical — see Neoplasm, bone, malignant
  - periosteal — see Neoplasm, bone, malignant
- periosteal — see also Neoplasm, bone, malignant
  - osteogenic — see Neoplasm, bone, malignant
- pleomorphic cell — see Neoplasm, connective tissue, malignant
- reticulum cell (diffuse) — see Lymphoma, diffuse large cell
  - nodular — see Lymphoma, follicular
  - pleomorphic cell type — see Lymphoma, diffuse large cell
- rhabdoid — see Neoplasm, malignant, by site
- round cell — see Neoplasm, connective tissue, malignant
- small cell — see Neoplasm, connective tissue, malignant
- soft tissue — see Neoplasm, connective tissue, malignant
- spindle cell — see Neoplasm, connective tissue, malignant
- stromal (endometrial) C54.1
  - isthmus C54.0
- synovial — see also Neoplasm, connective tissue, malignant
  - biphasic — see Neoplasm, connective tissue, malignant
  - epithelioid cell — see Neoplasm, connective tissue, malignant
  - spindle cell — see Neoplasm, connective tissue, malignant

Sarcomatosis
- meningeal — see Neoplasm, meninges, malignant
- specified site NEC — see Neoplasm, connective tissue, malignant
- unspecified site C80.1

Sarcopenia (age-related) M62.84
Sarcosinemia E72.59
Sarcosporidiosis (intestinal) A07.8
SARS-CoV-2 — see also COVID-19
- sequelae (post acute) U09.9

Satiety, early R68.81
Saturnine — see condition
Saturnism
- overdose or wrong substance given or taken — see Table of Drugs and Chemicals, by drug, poisoning

Satyriasis F52.8
Sauriasis — see Ichthyosis
SBE (subacute bacterial endocarditis) I33.0
Scabies (any site) B86

Scabs R23.4
Scaglietti-Dagnini syndrome E22.0
Scald — see Burn
Scalenus anticus (anterior) **syndrome** G54.0
Scales R23.4
Scaling, skin R23.4
Scalp — see condition
Scapegoating affecting child Z62.3
Scaphocephaly, non-deformational Q75.01
Scapulalgia M89.8X1
Scapulohumeral myopathy G71.02
Scar, scarring — see also Cicatrix L90.5
- adherent L90.5
- atrophic L90.5
- cervix
  - in pregnancy or childbirth — see Pregnancy, complicated by, abnormal cervix
- cheloid L91.0
- chorioretinal H31.00- ☑
  - posterior pole macula H31.01- ☑
  - postsurgical H59.81- ☑
  - solar retinopathy H31.02- ☑
  - specified type NEC H31.09- ☑
- choroid — see Scar, chorioretinal
- conjunctiva H11.24- ☑
- cornea H17.9
  - xerophthalmic — see also Opacity, cornea
    - vitamin A deficiency E50.6
- defect (isthmocele) O34.22
- duodenum, obstructive K31.5
- hypertrophic L91.0
- keloid L91.0
- labia N90.89
- lung (base) J98.4
- macula — see Scar, chorioretinal, posterior pole
- muscle M62.89
- myocardium, myocardial I25.2
- painful L90.5
- posterior pole (eye) — see Scar, chorioretinal, posterior pole
- retina — see Scar, chorioretinal
- trachea J39.8
- transmural uterine, in pregnancy O34.29
- uterus N85.8
  - in pregnancy O34.29
- vagina N89.8
  - postoperative N99.2
- vulva N90.89

Scarabiasis B88.2
Scarlatina (anginosa) (maligna) A38.9
- myocarditis (acute) A38.1
- old — see Myocarditis
- otitis media A38.0
- ulcerosa A38.8

Scarlet fever (albuminuria) (angina) A38.9
Schamberg's disease (progressive pigmentary dermatosis) L81.7
Schatzki's ring (acquired) (esophagus) (lower) K22.2
- congenital Q39.3

Schaufenster krankheit I20.89
Schaumann's
- benign lymphogranulomatosis D86.1
- disease or syndrome — see Sarcoidosis

Scheie's syndrome E76.03
Schenck's disease B42.1
Scheuermann's disease or osteochondrosis — see Osteochondrosis, juvenile, spine
Schilder (-Flatau) **disease** G37.0
Schilling-type monocytic leukemia C93.0- ☑
Schimmelbusch's disease, cystic mastitis, or hyperplasia — see Mastopathy, cystic
Schistosoma infestation — see Infestation, Schistosoma
Schistosomiasis B65.9
- with muscle disorder B65.9 [M63.80]
  - ankle B65.9 [M63.87-] ☑
  - foot B65.9 [M63.87-] ☑
  - forearm B65.9 [M63.83-] ☑
  - hand B65.9 [M63.84-] ☑
  - lower leg B65.9 [M63.86-] ☑
  - multiple sites B65.9 [M63.89]
  - pelvic region B65.9 [M63.85-] ☑
  - shoulder region B65.9 [M63.81-] ☑
  - specified site NEC B65.9 [M63.88]
  - thigh B65.9 [M63.85-] ☑
  - upper arm B65.9 [M63.82-] ☑
- Asiatic B65.2
- bladder B65.0
- chestermani B65.8

Schistosomiasis — continued
- colon B65.1
- cutaneous B65.3
- due to
  - S. haematobium B65.0
  - S. japonicum B65.2
  - S. mansoni B65.1
  - S. mattheii B65.8
- Eastern B65.2
- genitourinary tract B65.0
- intestinal B65.1
- lung NEC B65.9 [J99]
  - pneumonia B65.9 [J17]
- Manson's (intestinal) B65.1
- oriental B65.2
- pulmonary NEC B65.9 [J99]
  - pneumonia B65.9
- Schistosoma
  - haematobium B65.0
  - japonicum B65.2
  - mansoni B65.1
- specified type NEC B65.8
- urinary B65.0
- vesical B65.0

Schizencephaly Q04.6
Schizoaffective psychosis F25.9
Schizodontia K00.2
Schizoid personality F60.1
Schizophrenia, schizophrenic F20.9
- acute (brief) (undifferentiated) F23
- atypical (form) F20.3
- borderline F21
- catalepsy F20.2
- catatonic (type) (excited) (withdrawn) F20.2
- cenesthopathic, cenesthesiopathic F20.89
- childhood type F20.9
- chronic undifferentiated F20.9
- cyclic F25.0
- disorganized (type) F20.1
- flexibilitas cerea F20.2
- hebephrenic (type) F20.1
- incipient F21
- latent F21
- negative type F20.5
- paranoid (type) F20.0
- paraphrenic F20.0
- post-psychotic depression F32.89
- prepsychotic F21
- prodromal F21
- pseudoneurotic F21
- pseudopsychopathic F21
- reaction F23
- residual (state) (type) F20.5
- restzustand F20.5
- schizoaffective (type) — see Psychosis, schizoaffective
- simple (type) F20.89
- simplex F20.89
- specified type NEC F20.89
- spectrum and other psychotic disorder F29
  - specified NEC F28
- stupor F20.2
- syndrome of childhood F84.5
- undifferentiated (type) F20.3
  - chronic F20.9

Schizothymia (persistent) F60.1
Schlatter-Osgood disease or osteochondrosis M92.52- ☑
Schlatter's tibia — see Osteochondrosis, juvenile, tibia
Schmidt's syndrome (polyglandular, autoimmune) E31.0
Schmincke's carcinoma or tumor — see Neoplasm, nasopharynx, malignant
Schmitz (-Stutzer) **dysentery** A03.0
Schmorl's disease or nodes
- lumbar region M51.46
- lumbosacral region M51.47
- sacrococcygeal region M53.3
- thoracic region M51.44
- thoracolumbar region M51.45

Schneiderian
- papilloma — see Neoplasm, nasopharynx, benign
  - specified site — see Neoplasm, benign, by site
  - unspecified site D14.0
- specified site — see Neoplasm, malignant, by site
  - unspecified site C30.0

Scholte's syndrome (malignant carcinoid) E34.09
Scholz (-Bielschowsky-Henneberg) **disease or syndrome** E75.25
Schonlein (-Henoch) **disease or purpura** (primary) (rheumatic) D69.0
Schottmuller's disease A01.4

Schroeder's syndrome (endocrine hypertensive) E27.0
Schuller-Christian disease or syndrome C96.5
Schultze's type acroparesthesia, simple I73.89
Schultz's disease or syndrome — *see* Agranulocytosis
Schwalbe-Ziehen-Oppenheim disease G24.1
Schwannoma — *see also* Neoplasm, nerve, benign
 malignant — *see also* Neoplasm, nerve, malignant
  with rhabdomyoblastic differentiation — *see* Neoplasm, nerve, malignant
 melanocytic — *see* Neoplasm, nerve, benign
 pigmented — *see* Neoplasm, nerve, benign
Schwannomatosis Q85.03
Schwartz-Bartter syndrome E22.2
Schwartz (-Jampel) **syndrome** G71.13
Schweninger-Buzzi anetoderma L90.1
Sciatic — *see* condition
Sciatica (infective) M54.3- ☑
 with lumbago M54.4- ☑
  due to intervertebral disc disorder — *see* Disorder, disc, with, radiculopathy
 due to displacement of intervertebral disc (with lumbago) — *see* Disorder, disc, with, radiculopathy
 wallet M54.3- ☑
Scimitar syndrome Q26.8
Sclera — *see* condition
Sclerectasia H15.84- ☑
Scleredema
 adultorum — *see* Sclerosis, systemic
 Buschke's — *see* Sclerosis, systemic
 newborn P83.0
Sclerema (adiposum) (edematosum) (neonatorum) (newborn) P83.0
 adultorum — *see* Sclerosis, systemic
Scleriasis — *see* Scleroderma
Scleritis H15.00- ☑
 with corneal involvement H15.04- ☑
 anterior H15.01- ☑
 brawny H15.02- ☑
 in (due to) zoster B02.34
 posterior H15.03- ☑
 specified type NEC H15.09- ☑
 syphilitic A52.71
 tuberculous (nodular) A18.51
Sclerochoroiditis H31.8
Scleroconjunctivitis — *see* Scleritis
Sclerocystic ovary syndrome E28.2
Sclerodactyly, sclerodactylia L94.3
Scleroderma, sclerodermia (acrosclerotic) (diffuse) (generalized) (progressive) (pulmonary) — *see also* Sclerosis, systemic M34.9
 circumscribed L94.0
 linear L94.1
 localized L94.0
 newborn P83.88
 systemic M34.9
Sclerokeratitis H16.8
 tuberculous A18.52
Scleroma nasi A48.8
Scleromalacia (perforans) H15.05- ☑
Scleromyxedema L98.5
Sclerose en plaques G35.D
Sclerosis, sclerotic
 adrenal (gland) E27.8
 Alzheimer's — *see* Disease, Alzheimer's
 amyotrophic (lateral) G12.21
 aorta, aortic I70.0
  valve — *see* Endocarditis, aortic
 artery, arterial, arteriolar, arteriovascular — *see* Arteriosclerosis
 ascending multiple G35.D
 brain (generalized) (lobular) G37.9
  artery, arterial I67.2
  diffuse G37.0
  disseminated G35.D
  insular G35.D
  Krabbe's E75.23
  miliary G35.D
  multiple G35.D
  presenile (Alzheimer's) — *see* Disease, Alzheimer's, early onset
  senile (arteriosclerotic) I67.2
  stem, multiple G35.D
  tuberous Q85.1
 bulbar, multiple G35.D
 bundle of His I44.39
 cardiac — *see* Disease, heart, ischemic, atherosclerotic
 cardiorenal — *see* Hypertension, cardiorenal
 cardiovascular — *see also* Disease, cardiovascular

Sclerosis, sclerotic — *continued*
 cardiovascular — *see also* Disease, cardiovascular — *continued*
  renal — *see* Hypertension, cardiorenal
 cerebellar — *see* Sclerosis, brain
 cerebral — *see* Sclerosis, brain
 cerebrospinal (disseminated) (multiple) G35.D
 cerebrovascular I67.2
 choroid — *see* Degeneration, choroid
 combined (spinal cord) — *see also* Degeneration, combined
  multiple G35.D
 concentric (Balo) G37.5
 cornea — *see* Opacity, cornea
 coronary (artery) I25.10
  with angina pectoris — *see* Arteriosclerosis, coronary (artery),
 corpus cavernosum
  female N90.89
  male N48.6
 diffuse (brain) (spinal cord) G37.0
 disseminated G35.D
 dorsal G35.D
 dorsolateral (spinal cord) — *see* Degeneration, combined
 endometrium N85.5
 extrapyramidal G25.9
 eye, nuclear (senile) — *see* Cataract, senile, nuclear
 focal and segmental (glomerular) — *see also* N00-N07
  with fourth character .1 N05.1
 Friedreich's (spinal cord) G11.11
 funicular (spermatic cord) N50.89
 general (vascular) — *see* Arteriosclerosis
 gland (lymphatic) I89.8
 hepatic K74.1
  alcoholic K70.2
 hereditary
  cerebellar G11.9
  spinal (Friedreich's ataxia) G11.11
 hippocampal G93.81
 insular G35.D
 kidney — *see* Sclerosis, renal
 larynx J38.7
 lateral (amyotrophic) (descending) (spinal) G12.21
  primary G12.23
 lens, senile nuclear — *see* Cataract, senile, nuclear
 liver K74.1
  with fibrosis K74.2
   alcoholic K70.2
  alcoholic K70.2
  cardiac K76.1
 lung — *see* Fibrosis, lung
 mastoid — *see* Mastoiditis, chronic
 mesial temporal G93.81
 mitral I05.8
 Monckeberg's (medial) — *see* Arteriosclerosis, extremities
 multiple (brain stem) (cerebral) (disseminated) (generalized) (spinal cord) G35.D
  progressive
   primary G35.B0
    with
     evidence of inflammatory disease activity G35.B1
     active G35.B1
     non-active G35.B2
    without evidence of inflammatory disease activity G35.B2
   secondary G35.C0
    with
     evidence of inflammatory disease activity G35.C1
     active G35.C1
     non-active G35.C2
    without evidence of inflammatory disease activity G35.C2
  relapsing-remitting G35.A
 myocardium, myocardial — *see* Disease, heart, ischemic, atherosclerotic
 nuclear (senile), eye — *see* Cataract, senile, nuclear
 ovary N83.8
 pancreas K86.89
 penis N48.6
 peripheral arteries — *see* Arteriosclerosis, extremities
 plaques G35.D
 pluriglandular E31.8
 polyglandular E31.8
 posterolateral (spinal cord) — *see* Degeneration, combined
 presenile (Alzheimer's) — *see* Disease, Alzheimer's, early onset

Sclerosis, sclerotic — *continued*
 primary, lateral G12.23
 progressive, systemic M34.0
 pulmonary — *see* Fibrosis, lung
  artery I27.0
  valve (heart) — *see* Endocarditis, pulmonary
 renal N26.9
  with
   cystine storage disease E72.09
   hypertensive heart disease (conditions in I11) — *see* Hypertension, cardiorenal
  arteriolar (hyaline) (hyperplastic) — *see* Hypertension, kidney
 retina (senile) (vascular) H35.00
 senile (vascular) — *see* Arteriosclerosis
 spinal (cord) (progressive) G95.89
  ascending G61.0
  combined — *see also* Degeneration, combined
   multiple G35.D
   syphilitic A52.11
  disseminated G35.D
  dorsolateral — *see* Degeneration, combined
  hereditary (Friedreich's) (mixed form) G11.11
  lateral (amyotrophic) G12.21
   progressive G12.23
  multiple G35.D
  posterior (syphilitic) A52.11
 stomach K31.89
 subendocardial, congenital I42.4
 systemic M34.9
  with
   lung involvement M34.81
   myopathy M34.82
   polyneuropathy M34.83
  drug-induced M34.2
  due to chemicals NEC M34.2
  progressive M34.0
  specified NEC M34.89
 temporal (mesial) G93.81
 tricuspid (heart) (valve) I07.8
 tuberous (brain) Q85.1
 tympanic membrane — *see* Disorder, tympanic membrane, specified NEC
 valve, valvular (heart) — *see* Endocarditis
 vascular — *see* Arteriosclerosis
 vein I87.8
Scoliosis (acquired) (postural) M41.9
 adolescent (idiopathic) — *see* Scoliosis, idiopathic, adolescent
 congenital Q67.5
  due to bony malformation Q76.3
  failure of segmentation (hemivertebra) Q76.3
  hemivertebra fusion Q76.3
  postural Q67.5
 degenerative M41.5- ☑
 idiopathic M41.20
  adolescent M41.129
   cervical region M41.122
   cervicothoracic region M41.123
   lumbar region M41.126
   lumbosacral region M41.127
   thoracic region M41.124
   thoracolumbar region M41.125
  cervical region M41.22
  cervicothoracic region M41.23
  infantile M41.00
   cervical region M41.02
   cervicothoracic region M41.03
   lumbar region M41.06
   lumbosacral region M41.07
   sacrococcygeal region M41.08
   thoracic region M41.04
   thoracolumbar region M41.05
  juvenile M41.119
   cervical region M41.112
   cervicothoracic region M41.113
   lumbar region M41.116
   lumbosacral region M41.117
   thoracic region M41.114
   thoracolumbar region M41.115
  lumbar region M41.26
  lumbosacral region M41.27
  thoracic region M41.24
  thoracolumbar region M41.25
 infantile — *see* Scoliosis, idiopathic, infantile
 neuromuscular M41.40
  cervical region M41.42
  cervicothoracic region M41.43
  lumbar region M41.46

☑ Additional Character Required — Refer to the Tabular List for Character Selection

Scoliosis — continued

Scoliosis — continued
- neuromuscular — continued
  - lumbosacral region M41.47
  - occipito-atlanto-axial region M41.41
  - thoracic region M41.44
  - thoracolumbar region M41.45
- paralytic — see Scoliosis, neuromuscular
- postprocedural M96.89
- postradiation therapy M96.5
- rachitic (late effect or sequelae) E64.3 [M49.80]
  - cervical region E64.3 [M49.82]
  - cervicothoracic region E64.3 [M49.83]
  - lumbar region E64.3 [M49.86]
  - lumbosacral region E64.3 [M49.87]
  - multiple sites E64.3 [M49.89]
  - occipito-atlanto-axial region E64.3 [M49.81]
  - sacrococcygeal region E64.3 [M49.88]
  - thoracic region E64.3 [M49.84]
  - thoracolumbar region E64.3 [M49.85]
- sciatic M54.4- ☑
- secondary (to) NEC M41.50
  - cerebral palsy, Friedreich's ataxia, poliomyelitis, neuromuscular disorders — see Scoliosis, neuromuscular
  - cervical region M41.52
  - cervicothoracic region M41.53
  - lumbar region M41.56
  - lumbosacral region M41.57
  - thoracic region M41.54
  - thoracolumbar region M41.55
- specified form NEC M41.80
  - cervical region M41.82
  - cervicothoracic region M41.83
  - lumbar region M41.86
  - lumbosacral region M41.87
  - thoracic region M41.84
  - thoracolumbar region M41.85
- thoracogenic M41.30
  - thoracic region M41.34
  - thoracolumbar region M41.35
- tuberculous A18.01

Scoliotic pelvis
- with disproportion (fetopelvic) O33.0
  - causing obstructed labor O65.0

Scorbutus, scorbutic — see also Scurvy
- anemia D53.2

Score, NIHSS (National Institutes of Health Stroke Scale) R29.7- ☑

Scotoma (arcuate) (Bjerrum) (central) (ring) — see also Defect, visual field, localized, scotoma
- scintillating H53.12- ☑

Scratch — see Abrasion

Scratchy throat R09.89

Screening (for) Z13.9
- alcoholism Z13.39
- anemia Z13.0
- anomaly, congenital Z13.89
- antenatal, of mother — see also Encounter, antenatal screening Z36.9
- arterial hypertension Z13.6
- arthropod-borne viral disease NEC Z11.59
- autism Z13.41
- bacteriuria, asymptomatic Z13.89
- behavioral disorder Z13.30
  - specified NEC Z13.39
- brain injury, traumatic Z13.850
- bronchitis, chronic Z13.83
- brucellosis Z11.2
- cardiovascular disorder Z13.6
- cataract Z13.5
- chlamydial diseases Z11.8
- cholera Z11.0
- chromosomal abnormalities (nonprocreative) NEC Z13.79
- colonoscopy Z12.11
- congenital
  - dislocation of hip Z13.89
  - eye disorder Z13.5
  - malformation or deformation Z13.89
- contamination NEC Z13.88
- coronavirus (disease) (novel) 2019 Z11.52
- COVID-19 Z11.52
- cystic fibrosis Z13.228
- dengue fever Z11.59
- dental disorder Z13.84
- depression (adult) (adolescent) (child) Z13.31
  - maternal Z13.32
  - perinatal Z13.32
- developmental
  - delays Z13.40

Screening — continued
- developmental — continued
  - delays — continued
    - global (milestones) Z13.42
    - specified NEC Z13.49
  - handicap Z13.42
  - in early childhood Z13.42
- diabetes mellitus Z13.1
- diphtheria Z11.2
- disability, intellectual Z13.39
- disease or disorder Z13.9
  - bacterial NEC Z11.2
    - intestinal infectious Z11.0
    - respiratory tuberculosis Z11.1
  - behavioral Z13.30
    - specified NEC Z13.39
  - blood or blood-forming organ Z13.0
  - cardiovascular Z13.6
  - Chagas' Z11.6
  - chlamydial Z11.8
  - coronavirus (novel) 2019 Z11.52
  - COVID-19 Z11.52
  - dental Z13.89
  - developmental delays Z13.40
    - global (milestones) Z13.42
    - specified NEC Z13.49
  - digestive tract NEC Z13.818
    - lower GI Z13.811
    - upper GI Z13.810
  - ear Z13.5
  - endocrine Z13.29
  - eye Z13.5
  - genitourinary Z13.89
  - heart Z13.6
  - human immunodeficiency virus (HIV) infection Z11.4
  - immunity Z13.0
  - infection
    - intestinal Z11.0
      - specified NEC Z11.6
  - infectious Z11.9
  - mental health and behavioral Z13.30
    - specified NEC Z13.39
  - metabolic Z13.228
  - neurological Z13.89
  - nutritional Z13.21
    - metabolic Z13.228
      - lipoid disorders Z13.220
  - protozoal Z11.6
    - intestinal Z11.0
  - respiratory Z13.83
  - rheumatic Z13.828
  - rickettsial Z11.8
  - sexually-transmitted NEC Z11.3
    - human immunodeficiency virus (HIV) Z11.4
  - sickle-cell (trait) Z13.0
  - skin Z13.89
  - specified NEC Z13.89
  - spirochetal Z11.8
  - thyroid Z13.29
  - vascular Z13.6
  - venereal Z11.3
  - viral NEC Z11.59
    - coronavirus (novel) 2019 Z11.52
    - COVID-19 Z11.52
    - human immunodeficiency virus (HIV) Z11.4
    - intestinal Z11.0
    - SARS-CoV-2 Z11.52
- elevated titer Z13.89
- emphysema Z13.83
- encephalitis, viral (mosquito- or tick-borne) Z11.59
- exposure to contaminants (toxic) Z13.88
- fever
  - dengue Z11.59
  - hemorrhagic Z11.59
  - yellow Z11.59
- filariasis Z11.6
- galactosemia Z13.228
- gastrointestinal condition Z13.818
- genetic (nonprocreative) - for procreative management — see Testing, genetic, for procreative management
  - disease carrier status (nonprocreative) Z13.71
  - specified NEC (nonprocreative) Z13.79
- genitourinary condition Z13.89
- glaucoma Z13.5
- gonorrhea Z11.3
- gout Z13.89
- helminthiasis (intestinal) Z11.6
- hematopoietic malignancy Z12.89

Screening — continued
- hemoglobinopathies NEC Z13.0
- hemorrhagic fever Z11.59
- Hodgkin disease Z12.89
- human immunodeficiency virus (HIV) Z11.4
- human papillomavirus Z11.51
- hypertension Z13.6
- immunity disorders Z13.0
- infant or child (over 28 days old) Z00.129
  - with abnormal findings Z00.121
- infection
  - mycotic Z11.8
  - parasitic Z11.8
- ingestion of radioactive substance Z13.88
- intellectual disability Z13.39
- intestinal
  - helminthiasis Z11.6
  - infectious disease Z11.0
- leishmaniasis Z11.6
- leprosy Z11.2
- leptospirosis Z11.8
- leukemia Z12.89
- lymphoma Z12.89
- malaria Z11.6
- malnutrition Z13.29
  - metabolic Z13.228
  - nutritional Z13.21
- measles Z11.59
- mental health disorder Z13.30
  - specified NEC Z13.39
- metabolic errors, inborn Z13.228
- multiphasic Z13.89
- musculoskeletal disorder Z13.828
  - osteoporosis Z13.820
- mycoses Z11.8
- myocardial infarction (acute) Z13.6
- neoplasm (malignant) (of) Z12.9
  - bladder Z12.6
  - blood Z12.89
  - breast Z12.39
    - routine mammogram Z12.31
  - cervix Z12.4
  - colon Z12.11
  - genitourinary organs NEC Z12.79
    - bladder Z12.6
    - cervix Z12.4
    - ovary Z12.73
    - prostate Z12.5
    - testis Z12.71
    - vagina Z12.72
  - hematopoietic system Z12.89
  - intestinal tract Z12.10
    - colon Z12.11
    - rectum Z12.12
    - small intestine Z12.13
  - lung Z12.2
  - lymph (glands) Z12.89
  - nervous system Z12.82
  - oral cavity Z12.81
  - prostate Z12.5
  - rectum Z12.12
  - respiratory organs Z12.2
  - skin Z12.83
  - small intestine Z12.13
  - specified site NEC Z12.89
  - stomach Z12.0
- nephropathy Z13.89
- nervous system disorders NEC Z13.858
- neurological condition Z13.89
- osteoporosis Z13.820
- parasitic infestation Z11.9
  - specified NEC Z11.8
- phenylketonuria Z13.228
- plague Z11.2
- poisoning (chemical) (heavy metal) Z13.88
- poliomyelitis Z11.59
- postnatal, chromosomal abnormalities Z13.89
- prenatal, of mother — see also Encounter, antenatal screening Z36.9
- protozoal disease Z11.6
  - intestinal Z11.0
- pulmonary tuberculosis Z11.1
- radiation exposure Z13.88
- respiratory condition Z13.83
- respiratory tuberculosis Z11.1
- rheumatoid arthritis Z13.828
- rubella Z11.59
- SARS-CoV-2 Z11.52
- schistosomiasis Z11.6

Screening — *continued*
  sexually-transmitted disease NEC Z11.3
    human immunodeficiency virus (HIV) Z11.4
  sickle-cell disease or trait Z13.0
  skin condition Z13.89
  sleeping sickness Z11.6
  special Z13.9
    specified NEC Z13.89
  syphilis Z11.3
  tetanus Z11.2
  trachoma Z11.8
  traumatic brain injury Z13.850
  trypanosomiasis Z11.6
  tuberculosis, respiratory Z11.1
    active Z11.1
    latent Z11.7
  venereal disease Z11.3
  viral encephalitis (mosquito- or tick-borne) Z11.59
  whooping cough Z11.2
  worms, intestinal Z11.6
  yaws Z11.8
  yellow fever Z11.59
Scrofula, scrofulosis (tuberculosis of cervical lymph glands) A18.2
Scrofulide (primary) (tuberculous) A18.4
Scrofuloderma, scrofulodermia (any site) (primary) A18.4
Scrofulosus lichen (primary) (tuberculous) A18.4
Scrofulous — *see* condition
Scrotal tongue K14.5
Scrotum — *see* condition
Scurvy, scorbutic E54
  anemia D53.2
  gum E54
  infantile E54
  rickets E55.0 *[M90.80]*
Sealpox B08.62
Seasickness T75.3- ☑
Seatworm (infection) (infestation) B80
Sebaceous — *see also* condition
  cyst — *see* Cyst, sebaceous
Seborrhea, seborrheic L21.9
  capillitii R23.8
  capitis L21.0
  dermatitis L21.9
    infantile L21.1
  eczema L21.9
    infantile L21.1
  sicca L21.0
Seckel's syndrome Q87.19
Seclusion, pupil — *see* Membrane, pupillary
Second hand tobacco smoke exposure (acute) (chronic) Z77.22
  in the perinatal period P96.81
Secondary
  dentin (in pulp) K04.3
  neoplasm, secondaries — *see* Table of Neoplasms, secondary
Secretion
  antidiuretic hormone, inappropriate E22.2
  catecholamine, by pheochromocytoma — *see also* Pheochromocytoma, by type E27.5
  hormone
    antidiuretic, inappropriate (syndrome) E22.2
    by
      carcinoid tumor — *see also* Tumor, carcinoid E34.09
      pheochromocytoma — *see also* Pheochromocytoma, by type E27.5
    ectopic NEC E34.2
  urinary
    excessive R35.89
    suppression R34
Section
  nerve, traumatic — *see* Injury, nerve
Sedative, hypnotic, or anxiolytic-induced
  anxiety disorder F13.980
  bipolar and related disorder F13.94
  delirium F13.921
  depressive disorder F13.94
  major neurocognitive disorder F13.97
  mild neurocognitive disorder F13.988
  psychotic disorder F13.959
  sexual dysfunction F13.981
  sleep disorder F13.982
Segmentation, incomplete (congenital) — *see also* Fusion
  bone NEC Q78.8
  lumbosacral (joint) (vertebra) Q76.49
SEID (systemic exertion intolerance disease) G93.32

Seitelberger's syndrome (infantile neuraxonal dystrophy) G31.89
Seizure(s) — *see also* Convulsions R56.9
  absence G40.A- ☑ (*following* G40.3)
  akinetic — *see* Epilepsy, generalized, specified NEC
  atonic — *see* Epilepsy, generalized, specified NEC
  autonomic (hysterical) F44.5
  convulsive — *see* Convulsions
  cortical (focal) (motor) — *see* Epilepsy, localization-related, symptomatic, with simple partial seizures
  disorder — *see also* Epilepsy G40.909
  due to stroke — *see* Sequelae (of), disease, cerebrovascular, by type, specified NEC
  epileptic — *see* Epilepsy
  febrile (simple) R56.00
    with status epilepticus G40.901
    complex (atypical) (complicated) R56.01
      with status epilepticus G40.901
  grand mal G40.409
    intractable G40.419
      with status epilepticus G40.411
      without status epilepticus G40.419
    not intractable G40.409
      with status epilepticus G40.401
      without status epilepticus G40.409
  heart — *see* Disease, heart
  hysterical F44.5
  intractable G40.919
    with status epilepticus G40.911
  Jacksonian (focal) (motor type) (sensory type) — *see* Epilepsy, localization-related, symptomatic, with simple partial seizures
  newborn P90
  nonspecific epileptic
    atonic — *see* Epilepsy, generalized, specified NEC
    clonic — *see* Epilepsy, generalized, specified NEC
    myoclonic — *see* Epilepsy, generalized, specified NEC
    tonic — *see* Epilepsy, generalized, specified NEC
    tonic-clonic — *see* Epilepsy, generalized, specified NEC
  partial, developing into secondarily generalized seizures
    complex — *see* Epilepsy, localization-related, symptomatic, with complex partial seizures
    simple — *see* Epilepsy, localization-related, symptomatic, with simple partial seizures
  petit mal G40.A- ☑ (*following* G40.3)
    intractable G40.A1- ☑ (*following* G40.3)
      with status epilepticus G40.A11 (*following* G40.3)
      without status epilepticus G40.A19 (*following* G40.3)
    not intractable G40.A0- ☑ (*following* G40.3)
      with status epilepticus G40.A01 (*following* G40.3)
      without status epilepticus G40.A09 (*following* G40.3)
  post traumatic R56.1
  recurrent G40.909
  specified NEC G40.89
  uncinate — *see* Epilepsy, localization-related, symptomatic, with complex partial seizures
Selenium deficiency, dietary E59
Self-damaging behavior (life-style) Z72.89
Self-harm (attempted)
  history (personal)
    in family Z81.8
    nonsuicidal Z91.52
    suicidal Z91.51
  nonsuicidal R45.88
Self-injury, nonsuicidal R45.88
  personal history Z91.52
Self-mutilation (attempted)
  history (personal)
    in family Z81.8
    nonsuicidal Z91.52
    suicidal Z91.51
  nonsuicidal R45.88
Self-poisoning
  history (personal) Z91.51
    in family Z81.8
  observation following (alleged) attempt Z03.6
Semicoma R40.1
Seminal vesiculitis N49.0
Seminoma C62.9- ☑
  specified site — *see* Neoplasm, malignant, by site
Senear-Usher disease or syndrome L10.4
Senectus R54
Senescence (without mention of psychosis) R54
Senile, senility — *see also* condition R41.81

Senile, senility — *continued*
  with
    acute confusional state F05
    mental changes NOS F03.- ☑
    psychosis NEC — *see* Psychosis, senile
  asthenia R54
  cervix (atrophic) N88.8
  debility R54
  endometrium (atrophic) N85.8
  fallopian tube (atrophic) — *see* Atrophy, fallopian tube
  heart (failure) R54
  ovary (atrophic) — *see* Atrophy, ovary
  premature E34.8
  vagina, vaginitis (atrophic) N95.2
  wart L82.1
Sensation
  burning (skin) R20.8
    tongue K14.6
  foreign body R09.A0
    eye H57.8A- ☑
    globus R09.A2
    nose R09.A1
    specified site NEC R09.A9
    throat R09.A2
  loss of R20.8
  prickling (skin) R20.2
  tingling (skin) R20.2
Sense loss
  smell — *see* Disturbance, sensation, smell
  taste — *see* Disturbance, sensation, taste
  touch R20.8
Sensibility disturbance (cortical) (deep) (vibratory) R20.9
Sensitive, sensitivity — *see also* Allergy
  carotid sinus G90.01
  child (excessive) F93.8
  cold, autoimmune D59.12
  dentin K03.89
  gluten (non-celiac) K90.41
  latex Z91.040
  methemoglobin D74.8
  tuberculin, without clinical or radiological symptoms R76.11
  visual
    glare H53.71
    impaired contrast H53.72
Sensitiver Beziehungswahn F22
Sensitization, auto-erythrocytic D69.2
Separation
  anxiety, abnormal (of childhood) F93.0
  apophysis, traumatic — *code as* Fracture, by site
  choroid — *see* Detachment, choroid
  epiphysis, epiphyseal
    nontraumatic — *see also* Osteochondropathy, specified type NEC
    upper femoral — *see* Slipped, epiphysis, upper femoral
    traumatic — *code as* Fracture, by site
  fracture — *see* Fracture
  infundibulum cardiac from right ventricle by a partition Q24.3
  joint (traumatic) (current) — *code by* site under Dislocation
  muscle (nontraumatic) — *see* Diastasis, muscle
  pubic bone, obstetrical trauma O71.6
  retina, retinal — *see* Detachment, retina
  symphysis pubis, obstetrical trauma O71.6
  tracheal ring, incomplete, congenital Q32.1
Sepsis (generalized) (unspecified organism) A41.9
  with
    ectopic or molar pregnancy O08.82
    organ dysfunction (acute) (multiple) R65.20
      with septic shock R65.21
  Acinetobacter baumannii A41.54
  actinomycotic A42.7
  adrenal hemorrhage syndrome (meningococcal) A39.1
  anaerobic A41.4
  Bacillus anthracis A22.7
  Brucella — *see also* Brucellosis A23.9
  candidal B37.7
  Cronobacter A41.59
  cryptogenic A41.9
  due to device, implant or graft T85.79- ☑
    arterial graft NEC T82.7- ☑
    breast (implant) T85.79- ☑
    catheter NEC T85.79- ☑
      dialysis (renal) T82.7- ☑
        intraperitoneal T85.71- ☑
      infusion NEC T82.7- ☑

☑ **Additional Character Required** — Refer to the Tabular List for Character Selection

Sepsis

Sepsis — *continued*
  due to device, implant or graft — *continued*
    catheter — *continued*
      infusion — *continued*
        spinal (cranial) (epidural) (intrathecal) (spinal) (subarachnoid) (subdural) T85.735- ☑
      urethral indwelling T83.511- ☑
      urinary T83.518- ☑
    electronic (electrode) (pulse generator) (stimulator)
      bone T84.7- ☑
      cardiac T82.7- ☑
      nervous system T85.738- ☑
        brain T85.731- ☑
        neurostimulator generator T85.734- ☑
        peripheral nerve T85.732- ☑
        spinal cord T85.733- ☑
      urinary T83.590- ☑
    fixation, internal (orthopedic) — *see* Complication, fixation device, infection
    gastrointestinal (bile duct) (esophagus) T85.79- ☑
      neurostimulator electrode (lead) T85.732- ☑
    genital T83.69- ☑
    heart NEC T82.7- ☑
      valve (prosthesis) T82.6- ☑
        graft T82.7- ☑
    joint prosthesis — *see* Complication, joint prosthesis, infection
    ocular (corneal graft) (orbital implant) T85.79- ☑
    orthopedic NEC T84.7- ☑
      fixation device, internal — *see* Complication, fixation device, infection
    specified NEC T85.79- ☑
    vascular T82.7- ☑
    ventricular intracranial (communicating) shunt T85.730- ☑
  during labor O75.3
  Enterococcus A41.81
  Erysipelothrix (rhusiopathiae) (erysipeloid) A26.7
  Escherichia coli (E. coli) A41.51
  extraintestinal yersiniosis A28.2
  following
    abortion (subsequent episode) O08.0
      current episode — *see* Abortion
    ectopic or molar pregnancy O08.82
    immunization T88.0- ☑
    infusion, therapeutic injection or transfusion NEC T80.29- ☑
    obstetrical procedure O86.04
  gangrenous A41.9
  gonococcal A54.86
  Gram-negative (organism) A41.50
    anaerobic A41.4
  Haemophilus influenzae A41.3
  herpesviral B00.7
  intra-abdominal K65.1
  intraocular — *see* Endophthalmitis, purulent
  Listeria monocytogenes A32.7
  localized — *code to* specific localized infection
    in operation wound T81.49- ☑
    skin — *see* Abscess
  malleus A24.0
  melioidosis A24.1
  meningeal — *see* Meningitis
  meningococcal A39.4
    acute A39.2
    chronic A39.3
  MRSA (Methicillin resistant Staphylococcus aureus) A41.02
  MSSA (Methicillin susceptible Staphylococcus aureus) A41.01
  newborn P36.9
    due to
      anaerobes NEC P36.5
      Escherichia coli P36.4
      Staphylococcus P36.30
        aureus P36.2
        specified NEC P36.39
      Streptococcus P36.10
        group B P36.0
        specified NEC P36.19
      specified NEC P36.8
  other gram-negative A41.59
  Pasteurella multocida A28.0
  pelvic, puerperal, postpartum, childbirth O85
  pneumococcal A40.3
  postprocedural T81.44- ☑
  Pseudomonas (pseudomonas aeruginosa) A41.52
  puerperal, postpartum, childbirth (pelvic) O85

Sepsis — *continued*
  Salmonella (arizonae) (cholerae-suis) (enteritidis) (typhimurium) A02.1
  Serratia A41.53
  severe R65.20
    with septic shock R65.21
  Shigella — *see also* Dysentery, bacillary A03.9
  skin, localized — *see* Abscess
  specified organism NEC A41.89
  Staphylococcus, staphylococcal A41.2
    aureus (methicillin susceptible) (MSSA) A41.01
      methicillin resistant (MRSA) A41.02
    coagulase-negative A41.1
    specified NEC A41.1
  Streptococcus, streptococcal A40.9
    agalactiae A40.1
    group
      A A40.0
      B A40.1
      D A41.81
    neonatal P36.10
      group B P36.0
      specified NEC P36.19
    pneumoniae A40.3
    pyogenes A40.0
    specified NEC A40.8
  tracheostomy stoma J95.02
  tularemic A21.7
  umbilical, umbilical cord (newborn) — *see* Sepsis, newborn
  Yersinia pestis A20.7
Septate — *see* Septum
Septic — *see* condition
  arm — *see* Cellulitis, upper limb
    with lymphangitis — *see* Lymphangitis, acute, upper limb
  embolus — *see* Embolism
  finger — *see* Cellulitis, digit
    with lymphangitis — *see* Lymphangitis, acute, digit
  foot — *see* Cellulitis, lower limb
    with lymphangitis — *see* Lymphangitis, acute, lower limb
  gallbladder (acute) K81.0
  hand — *see* Cellulitis, upper limb
    with lymphangitis — *see* Lymphangitis, acute, upper limb
  joint — *see* Arthritis, pyogenic or pyemic
  leg — *see* Cellulitis, lower limb
    with lymphangitis — *see* Lymphangitis, acute, lower limb
  nail — *see also* Cellulitis, digit
    with lymphangitis — *see* Lymphangitis, acute, digit
  sore — *see also* Abscess
    throat J02.0
      streptococcal J02.0
  spleen (acute) D73.89
  teeth, tooth (pulpal origin) K04.4
  throat — *see* Pharyngitis
  thrombus — *see* Thrombosis
  toe — *see* Cellulitis, digit
    with lymphangitis — *see* Lymphangitis, acute, digit
  tonsils, chronic J35.01
    with adenoiditis J35.03
  uterus — *see* Endometritis
Septicemia A41.9
  meaning sepsis — *see* Sepsis
Septum, septate (congenital) — *see also* Anomaly, by site
  anal Q42.3
    with fistula Q42.2
  aqueduct of Sylvius Q03.0
    with spina bifida — *see* Spina bifida, by site, with hydrocephalus
  uterus Q51.28
    complete Q51.21
    partial Q51.22
    specified NEC Q51.28
  vagina Q52.10
    in pregnancy — *see* Pregnancy, complicated by, abnormal vagina
      causing obstructed labor O65.5
    longitudinal Q52.129
      microperforate
        left side Q52.124
        right side Q52.123
      nonobstruction Q52.120
      obstructing Q52.129
        left side Q52.122
        right side Q52.121
    transverse Q52.11

Sequelae (of) — *see also* condition
  abscess, intracranial or intraspinal (conditions in G06) G09
  amputation — *code to* injury with seventh character S
  burn and corrosion — *code to* injury with seventh character S
  calcium deficiency E64.8
  cerebrovascular disease — *see* Sequelae, disease, cerebrovascular
  childbirth O94
  contusion — *code to* injury with seventh character S
  corrosion — *see* Sequelae, burn and corrosion
  COVID-19 (post acute) U09.9
  crushing injury — *code to* injury with seventh character S
  disease
    cerebrovascular I69.90
      alteration of sensation I69.998
      aphasia I69.920
      apraxia I69.990
      ataxia I69.993
      cognitive deficits I69.91- ☑
      disturbance of vision I69.998
      dysarthria I69.922
      dysphagia I69.991
      dysphasia I69.921
      facial droop I69.992
      facial weakness I69.992
      fluency disorder I69.923
      hemiplegia I69.95- ☑
      hemorrhage
        intracerebral — *see* Sequelae, hemorrhage, intracerebral
        intracranial, nontraumatic NEC — *see* Sequelae, hemorrhage, intracranial, nontraumatic
        subarachnoid — *see* Sequelae, hemorrhage, subarachnoid
      language deficit I69.928
      monoplegia
        lower limb I69.94- ☑
        upper limb I69.93- ☑
      paralytic syndrome I69.96- ☑
      specified effect NEC I69.998
      specified type NEC I69.80
        alteration of sensation I69.898
        aphasia I69.820
        apraxia I69.890
        ataxia I69.893
        cognitive deficits I69.81- ☑
        disturbance of vision I69.898
        dysarthria I69.822
        dysphagia I69.891
        dysphasia I69.821
        facial droop I69.892
        facial weakness I69.892
        fluency disorder I69.823
        hemiplegia I69.85- ☑
        language deficit I69.828
        monoplegia
          lower limb I69.84- ☑
          upper limb I69.83- ☑
        paralytic syndrome I69.86- ☑
        specified effect NEC I69.898
      speech deficit I69.928
      speech deficit I69.828
      stroke NOS — *see* Sequelae, stroke NOS
  dislocation — *code to* injury with seventh character S
  encephalitis or encephalomyelitis (conditions in G04) G09
    in infectious disease NEC B94.8
    viral B94.1
  external cause — *code to* injury with seventh character S
  foreign body entering natural orifice — *code to* injury with seventh character S
  fracture — *code to* injury with seventh character S
  frostbite — *code to* injury with seventh character S
  Hansen's disease B92
  hemorrhage
    intracerebral I69.10
      alteration of sensation I69.198
      aphasia I69.120
      apraxia I69.190
      ataxia I69.193
      cognitive deficits I69.11- ☑
      disturbance of vision I69.198
      dysarthria I69.122
      dysphagia I69.191

Sequelae — *continued*
  hemorrhage — *continued*
    intracerebral — *continued*
      dysphasia I69.121
      facial droop I69.192
      facial weakness I69.192
      fluency disorder I69.123
      hemiplegia I69.15- ☑
      language deficit NEC I69.128
      monoplegia
        lower limb I69.14- ☑
        upper limb I69.13- ☑
      paralytic syndrome I69.16- ☑
      specified effect NEC I69.198
      speech deficit NEC I69.128
    intracranial, nontraumatic NEC I69.20
      alteration of sensation I69.298
      aphasia I69.220
      apraxia I69.290
      ataxia I69.293
      cognitive deficits I69.21- ☑
      disturbance of vision I69.298
      dysarthria I69.222
      dysphagia I69.291
      dysphasia I69.221
      facial droop I69.292
      facial weakness I69.292
      fluency disorder I69.223
      hemiplegia I69.25- ☑
      language deficit NEC I69.228
      monoplegia
        lower limb I69.24- ☑
        upper limb I69.23- ☑
      paralytic syndrome I69.26- ☑
      specified effect NEC I69.298
      speech deficit NEC I69.228
    subarachnoid I69.00
      alteration of sensation I69.098
      aphasia I69.020
      apraxia I69.090
      ataxia I69.093
      cognitive deficits — *see* subcategory I69.01- ☑
      disturbance of vision I69.098
      dysarthria I69.022
      dysphagia I69.091
      dysphasia I69.021
      facial droop I69.092
      facial weakness I69.092
      fluency disorder I69.023
      hemiplegia I69.05- ☑
      language deficit NEC I69.028
      monoplegia
        lower limb I69.04- ☑
        upper limb I69.03- ☑
      paralytic syndrome I69.06- ☑
      specified effect NEC I69.098
      speech deficit NEC I69.028
  hepatitis, viral B94.2
  hyperalimentation E68
  infarction
    cerebral I69.30
      alteration of sensation I69.398
      aphasia I69.320
      apraxia I69.390
      ataxia I69.393
      cognitive deficits I69.31- ☑
      disturbance of vision I69.398
      dysarthria I69.322
      dysphagia I69.391
      dysphasia I69.321
      facial droop I69.392
      facial weakness I69.392
      fluency disorder I69.323
      hemiplegia I69.35- ☑
      language deficit NEC I69.328
      monoplegia
        lower limb I69.34- ☑
        upper limb I69.33- ☑
      paralytic syndrome I69.36- ☑
      specified effect NEC I69.398
      speech deficit NEC I69.328
  infection, pyogenic, intracranial or intraspinal G09
  infectious disease B94.9
    specified NEC B94.8
  injury — *code to* injury with seventh character S
  leprosy B92
  meningitis
    bacterial (conditions in G00) G09

Sequelae — *continued*
  meningitis — *continued*
    other or unspecified cause (conditions in G03) G09
  muscle (and tendon) injury — *code to* injury with seventh character S
  myelitis — *see* Sequelae, encephalitis
  niacin deficiency E64.8
  nutritional deficiency E64.9
    specified NEC E64.8
  obstetrical condition O94
  parasitic disease B94.9
  phlebitis or thrombophlebitis of intracranial or intraspinal venous sinuses and veins (conditions in G08) G09
  poisoning — *code to* poisoning with seventh character S
    nonmedicinal substance — *see* Sequelae, toxic effect, nonmedicinal substance
  poliomyelitis (acute) B91
  pregnancy O94
  protein-energy malnutrition E64.0
  puerperium O94
  rickets E64.3
  SARS-CoV-2 (post acute) U09.9
  selenium deficiency E64.8
  sprain and strain — *code to* injury with seventh character S
  stroke NOS I69.30
    alteration in sensation I69.398
    aphasia I69.320
    apraxia I69.390
    ataxia I69.393
    cognitive deficits I69.31- ☑
    disturbance of vision I69.398
    dysarthria I69.322
    dysphagia I69.391
    dysphasia I69.321
    facial droop I69.392
    facial weakness I69.392
    hemiplegia I69.35- ☑
    language deficit NEC I69.328
    monoplegia
      lower limb I69.34- ☑
      upper limb I69.33- ☑
    paralytic syndrome I69.36- ☑
    specified effect NEC I69.398
    speech deficit NEC I69.328
  tendon and muscle injury — *code to* injury with seventh character S
  thiamine deficiency E64.8
  trachoma B94.0
  tuberculosis B90.9
    bones and joints B90.2
    central nervous system B90.0
    genitourinary B90.1
    pulmonary (respiratory) B90.9
    specified organs NEC B90.8
  viral
    encephalitis B94.1
    hepatitis B94.2
  vitamin deficiency NEC E64.8
    A E64.1
    B E64.8
    C E64.2
  wound, open — *code to* injury with seventh character S
Sequestration — *see also* Sequestrum
  disc — *see* Displacement, intervertebral disc
  lung, congenital Q33.2
Sequestrum
  bone — *see* Osteomyelitis, chronic
  dental M27.2
  jaw bone M27.2
  orbit — *see* Osteomyelitis, orbit
  sinus (accessory) (nasal) — *see* Sinusitis
Sequoiosis lung or pneumonitis J67.8
Serology for syphilis
  doubtful
    with signs or symptoms — *code by* site and stage under Syphilis
    follow-up of latent syphilis — *see* Syphilis, latent
  negative, with signs or symptoms — *code by* site and stage under Syphilis
  positive A53.0
    with signs or symptoms — *code by* site and stage under Syphilis
  reactivated A53.0
Seroma — *see also* Hematoma
  postprocedural — *see* Complication, postprocedural, seroma

Seroma — *continued*
  traumatic, secondary and recurrent T79.2- ☑
Seropurulent — *see* condition
Serositis, multiple K65.8
  pericardial I31.1
  peritoneal K65.8
Serous — *see* condition
Sertoli cell
  adenoma
    specified site — *see* Neoplasm, benign, by site
    unspecified site
      female D27.9
      male D29.20
  carcinoma
    specified site — *see* Neoplasm, malignant, by site
    unspecified site (male) C62.9- ☑
      female C56.9
  tumor
    with lipid storage
      specified site — *see* Neoplasm, benign, by site
      unspecified site
        female D27.9
        male D29.20
    specified site — *see* Neoplasm, benign, by site
    unspecified site
      female D27.9
      male D29.20
Sertoli-Leydig cell tumor — *see* Neoplasm, benign, by site
  specified site — *see* Neoplasm, benign, by site
  unspecified site
    female D27.9
    male D29.20
Serum
  allergy, allergic reaction — *see also* Reaction, serum T80.69- ☑
    shock — *see also* Shock, anaphylactic T80.59- ☑
  arthritis — *see also* Reaction, serum T80.69- ☑
  complication or reaction NEC — *see also* Reaction, serum T80.69- ☑
  disease NEC — *see also* Reaction, serum T80.69- ☑
  hepatitis — *see also* Hepatitis, viral, type B
    carrier (suspected) of B18.1
  intoxication — *see also* Reaction, serum T80.69- ☑
  neuritis — *see also* Reaction, serum T80.69- ☑
  neuropathy G61.1
  poisoning NEC — *see also* Reaction, serum T80.69- ☑
  rash NEC — *see also* Reaction, serum T80.69- ☑
  reaction NEC — *see also* Reaction, serum T80.69- ☑
  sickness NEC — *see also* Reaction, serum T80.69- ☑
  urticaria — *see also* Reaction, serum T80.69- ☑
Sesamoiditis M25.8- ☑
Severe sepsis R65.20
  with septic shock R65.21
Sever's disease or osteochondrosis — *see* Osteochondrosis, juvenile, tarsus
Sex
  chromosome mosaics Q97.8
    lines with various numbers of X chromosomes Q97.2
  education Z70.8
  reassignment surgery status Z87.890
Sextuplet pregnancy — *see* Pregnancy, sextuplet
Sexual
  function, disorder of (psychogenic) F52.9
  immaturity (female) (male) E30.0
  impotence (psychogenic) organic origin NEC — *see* Dysfunction, sexual, male
  precocity (constitutional) (cryptogenic) (female) (idiopathic) (male) E30.1
Sexuality, pathologic — *see* Deviation, sexual
Sezary disease C84.1- ☑
Shadow, lung R91.8
Shaking palsy or paralysis — *see* Parkinsonism
Shallowness, acetabulum — *see* Derangement, joint, specified type NEC, hip
Shaver's disease J63.1
Sheath (tendon) — *see* condition
Sheathing, retinal vessels H35.01- ☑
Shedding
  nail L60.8
  premature, primary (deciduous) teeth K00.6
Sheehan's disease or syndrome E23.0
Shelf, rectal K62.89
Shell teeth K00.5
Shellshock (current) F43.0
  lasting state — *see* Disorder, post-traumatic stress
Shield kidney Q63.1
Shift
  auditory threshold (temporary) H93.24- ☑

Shift — continued
    mediastinal R93.89
Shifting sleep-work schedule (affecting sleep) G47.26
Shiga (-Kruse) **dysentery** A03.0
Shiga's bacillus A03.0
Shigella (dysentery) — see Dysentery, bacillary
Shigellosis A03.9
    Group A A03.0
    Group B A03.1
    Group C A03.2
    Group D A03.3
Shin splints S86.89- ☑
Shingles — see Herpes, zoster
Shipyard disease or eye B30.0
Shirodkar suture, in pregnancy — see Pregnancy, complicated by, incompetent cervix
Shock R57.9
    with ectopic or molar pregnancy O08.3
    adrenal (cortical) (Addisonian) E27.2
    adverse food reaction (anaphylactic) — see Shock, anaphylactic, due to food
    allergic — see Shock, anaphylactic
    anaphylactic T78.2- ☑
        chemical — see Table of Drugs and Chemicals
        due to drug or medicinal substance
            correct substance properly administered T88.6- ☑
            overdose or wrong substance given or taken (by accident) — see Table of Drugs and Chemicals, by drug, poisoning
        due to food (nonpoisonous) T78.00- ☑
            additives T78.06- ☑
            dairy products T78.079- ☑
                with
                    reactivity to baked milk T78.071- ☑
                    tolerance to baked milk T78.070- ☑
            eggs T78.089- ☑
                with
                    reactivity to baked egg T78.081- ☑
                    tolerance to baked egg T78.080- ☑
            fish T78.03- ☑
                shellfish T78.02- ☑
            fruit T78.04- ☑
            milk T78.079- ☑
                with
                    reactivity to baked milk T78.071- ☑
                    tolerance to baked milk T78.070- ☑
            nuts T78.05- ☑
                multiple types T78.05- ☑
                peanuts T78.01- ☑
            peanuts T78.01- ☑
            seeds T78.05- ☑
            specified type NEC T78.09- ☑
            vegetable T78.04- ☑
        following sting(s) — see Venom
        immunization T80.52- ☑
        serum T80.59- ☑
            blood and blood products T80.51- ☑
            immunization T80.52- ☑
            specified NEC T80.59- ☑
            vaccination T80.52- ☑
    anaphylactoid — see Shock, anaphylactic
    anesthetic
        correct substance properly administered T88.2- ☑
        overdose or wrong substance given or taken — see Table of Drugs and Chemicals, by drug, poisoning
            specified anesthetic — see Table of Drugs and Chemicals, by drug, poisoning
    cardiogenic R57.0
    chemical substance — see Table of Drugs and Chemicals
    complicating ectopic or molar pregnancy O08.3
    culture — see Disorder, adjustment
    drug
        due to correct substance properly administered T88.6- ☑
        overdose or wrong substance given or taken (by accident) — see Table of Drugs and Chemicals, by drug, poisoning
    during or after labor and delivery O75.1
    electric T75.4- ☑
        (taser) T75.4- ☑
    endotoxic R65.21
        postprocedural (resulting from a procedure, not elsewhere classified) T81.12- ☑
        following
            ectopic or molar pregnancy O08.3
            injury (immediate) (delayed) T79.4- ☑

Shock — continued
    following — continued
        labor and delivery O75.1
    food (anaphylactic) — see Shock, anaphylactic, due to food
    from electroshock gun (taser) T75.4- ☑
    gram-negative R65.21
        postprocedural (resulting from a procedure, not elsewhere classified) T81.12- ☑
    hematologic R57.8
    hemorrhagic R57.8
        surgery (intraoperative) (postoperative) T81.19- ☑
        trauma T79.4- ☑
    hypovolemic R57.1
        surgical T81.19- ☑
        traumatic T79.4- ☑
    insulin E15
        therapeutic misadventure — see subcategory T38.3- ☑
    kidney N17.0
        traumatic (following crushing) T79.5- ☑
    lightning T75.01- ☑
    liver K72.00
    lung J80
    obstetric O75.1
        with ectopic or molar pregnancy O08.3
        following ectopic or molar pregnancy O08.3
    pleural (surgical) T81.19- ☑
        due to trauma T79.4- ☑
    postprocedural (postoperative) T81.10- ☑
        with ectopic or molar pregnancy O08.3
        cardiogenic T81.11- ☑
        endotoxic T81.12- ☑
        following ectopic or molar pregnancy O08.3
        gram-negative T81.12- ☑
        hypovolemic T81.19- ☑
        septic T81.12- ☑
        specified type NEC T81.19- ☑
    psychic F43.0
    septic (due to severe sepsis) R65.21
    specified NEC R57.8
    surgical T81.10- ☑
    taser gun (taser) T75.4- ☑
    therapeutic misadventure NEC T81.10- ☑
    thyroxin
        overdose or wrong substance given or taken — see Table of Drugs and Chemicals, by drug, poisoning
    toxic, syndrome A48.3
    transfusion — see Complications, transfusion
    traumatic (immediate) (delayed) T79.4- ☑
Shoemaker's chest M95.4
Short, shortening, shortness
    arm (acquired) — see also Deformity, limb, unequal length
        congenital Q71.81- ☑
        forearm — see Deformity, limb, unequal length
    bowel syndrome — see Syndrome, short bowel
    breath R06.02
    cervical (complicating pregnancy) O26.87- ☑
        non-gravid uterus N88.3
    common bile duct, congenital Q44.5
    cord (umbilical), complicating delivery O69.3- ☑
    cystic duct, congenital Q44.5
    esophagus (congenital) Q39.8
    femur (acquired) — see Deformity, limb, unequal length, femur
        congenital — see Defect, reduction, lower limb, longitudinal, femur
    frenum, frenulum, linguae (congenital) Q38.1
    hip (acquired) — see also Deformity, limb, unequal length
        congenital Q65.89
    leg (acquired) — see also Deformity, limb, unequal length
        congenital Q72.81- ☑
        lower leg — see also Deformity, limb, unequal length
    limbed stature, with immunodeficiency D82.2
    lower limb (acquired) — see also Deformity, limb, unequal length
        congenital Q72.81- ☑
    organ or site, congenital NEC — see Distortion
    palate, congenital Q38.5
    radius (acquired) — see also Deformity, limb, unequal length
        congenital — see Defect, reduction, upper limb, longitudinal, radius
    rib syndrome Q77.2
    stature (child) (hereditary) (idiopathic) NEC R62.52

Short, shortening, shortness — continued
    stature — continued
        constitutional E34.31
        due to
            endocrine disorder E34.30
                specified type NEC, due to endocrine dosorder E34.39
            genetic causes E34.329
                ACAN gene variant E34.328
                acid-labile subunit gene (IGFALS) defect E34.321
                aggrecan deficiency E34.328
                genetic syndrome with resistance to insulin-like growth factor-1 E34.322
                growth hormone gene 1 (GH1) defect with growth hormone neutralizing antibodies E34.321
                growth hormone insensitivity syndrome (GHIS) E34.321
                insulin-like growth factor 1 gene (IGF1) defect E34.321
                insulin-like growth factor-1 receptor (IGF-1R) defect E34.322
                insulin-like growth factor-1 (IGF-1) resistance E34.322
                NPR-2 gene variant E34.328
                post-insulin-like growth factor-1 receptor signaling defect E34.322
                primary insulin-like growth factor-1 (IGF-1) deficiency E34.321
                severe primary insulin-like growth factor-1 deficiency (SPIGFD) E34.321
                signal transducer and activator of transcription 5B gene (STAT5b) defect E34.321
                specified genetic cause NEC E34.328
            Laron-type E34.321
    tendon — see also Contraction, tendon
        with contracture of joint — see Contraction, joint
        Achilles (acquired) M67.0- ☑
            congenital Q66.89
        congenital Q79.8
    thigh (acquired) — see also Deformity, limb, unequal length, femur
        congenital — see Defect, reduction, lower limb, longitudinal, femur
    tibialis anterior (tendon) — see Contraction, tendon
    umbilical cord
        complicating delivery O69.3- ☑
    upper limb, congenital — see Defect, reduction, upper limb, specified type NEC
    urethra N36.8
    uvula, congenital Q38.5
    vagina (congenital) Q52.4
Shortsightedness — see Myopia
Shoshin (acute fulminating beriberi) E51.11
Shoulder — see condition
Shovel-shaped incisors K00.2
Shower, thromboembolic — see Embolism
Shunt
    arterial-venous (dialysis) Z99.2
    arteriovenous, pulmonary (acquired) I28.0
        congenital Q25.72
    cerebral ventricle (communicating) in situ Z98.2
    surgical, prosthetic, with complications — see Complications, cardiovascular, device or implant
Shutdown, renal N28.9
Shy-Drager syndrome G90.3
Sialadenitis, sialadenosis (any gland) (chronic) (periodic) (suppurative) — see Sialoadenitis
Sialectasia K11.8
Sialidosis E77.1
Sialitis, silitis (any gland) (chronic) (suppurative) — see Sialoadenitis
Sialoadenitis (any gland) (periodic) (suppurative) K11.20
    acute K11.21
        recurrent K11.22
    chronic K11.23
Sialoadenopathy K11.9
Sialoangitis — see Sialoadenitis
Sialodochitis (fibrinosa) — see Sialoadenitis
Sialodocholithiasis K11.5
Sialolithiasis K11.5
Sialometaplasia, necrotizing K11.8
Sialorrhea — see also Ptyalism
    periodic — see Sialoadenitis
Sialosis K11.7
Siamese twin Q89.4
Sibling rivalry Z62.891
Sicard's syndrome G52.7

Sicca syndrome — see Syndrome, Sjogren
Sick R69
  or handicapped person in family Z63.79
    needing care at home Z63.6
  sinus (syndrome) I49.5
Sick-euthyroid syndrome E07.81
Sickle-cell
  anemia — see Disease, sickle-cell
  beta plus — see Disease, sickle-cell, thalassemia, beta plus
  beta zero — see Disease, sickle-cell, thalassemia, beta zero
  trait D57.3
Sicklemia — see also Disease, sickle-cell
  trait D57.3
Sickness
  air (travel) T75.3- ☑
  airplane T75.3- ☑
  alpine T70.29- ☑
  altitude T70.20- ☑
  Andes T70.29- ☑
  aviator's T70.29- ☑
  balloon T70.29- ☑
  car T75.3- ☑
  compressed air T70.3- ☑
  decompression T70.3- ☑
  green D50.8
  milk — see Poisoning, food, noxious
  motion T75.3- ☑
  mountain T70.29- ☑
    acute D75.1
  protein — see also Reaction, serum T80.69- ☑
  radiation T66.- ☑
  roundabout (motion) T75.3- ☑
  sea T75.3- ☑
  serum NEC — see also Reaction, serum T80.69- ☑
  sleeping (African) B56.9
    by Trypanosoma B56.9
      brucei
        gambiense B56.0
        rhodesiense B56.1
    East African B56.1
    Gambian B56.0
    Rhodesian B56.1
    West African B56.0
  swing (motion) T75.3- ☑
  train (railway) (travel) T75.3- ☑
  travel (any vehicle) T75.3- ☑
Sideropenia — see Anemia, iron deficiency
Siderosilicosis J62.8
Siderosis (lung) J63.4
  brain G93.89
  eye (globe) — see Disorder, globe, degenerative, siderosis
Siemens' syndrome (ectodermal dysplasia) Q82.8
Sighing R06.89
  psychogenic F45.8
Sigmoid — see also condition
  flexure — see condition
  kidney Q63.1
Sigmoiditis — see also Enteritis K52.9
  infectious A09
  noninfectious K52.9
Silfverskold's syndrome Q78.9
Silicosiderosis J62.8
Silicosis, silicotic (simple) (complicated) J62.8
  with tuberculosis J65
Silicotuberculosis J65
Silo-fillers' disease J68.8
  bronchitis J68.0
  pneumonitis J68.1
  pulmonary edema J68.1
Silver's syndrome Q87.19
Simian malaria B53.1
Simmonds' cachexia or disease E23.0
Simons' disease or syndrome (progressive lipodystrophy) E88.11
Simple, simplex — see condition
Simulation, conscious (of illness) Z76.5
Simultanagnosia (asimultagnosia) R48.3
Sin Nombre virus disease (Hantavirus) (cardio)-pulmonary syndrome B33.4
Sinding-Larsen disease or osteochondrosis — see Osteochondrosis, juvenile, patella
Singapore hemorrhagic fever A91
Singer's node or nodule J38.2
Single
  atrium Q21.20

Single — continued
  coronary artery Q24.5
  umbilical artery Q27.0
  ventricle Q20.4
Singultus R06.6
  epidemicus B33.0
Sinus — see also Fistula
  abdominal K63.89
  arrest I45.5
  arrhythmia I49.8
  bradycardia R00.1
  branchial cleft (internal) (external) Q18.0
  coccygeal — see Sinus, pilonidal
  dental K04.6
  dermal (congenital) Q06.8
    with abscess Q06.8
    coccygeal, pilonidal — see Sinus, coccygeal
  infected, skin NEC L08.89
  marginal, ruptured or bleeding — see Hemorrhage, antepartum, specified cause NEC
  medial, face and neck Q18.8
  pause I45.5
  pericranii Q01.9
  pilonidal (infected) (rectum) L05.92
    with abscess L05.02
  preauricular Q18.1
  rectovaginal N82.3
  Rokitansky-Aschoff (gallbladder) K82.8
  sacrococcygeal (dermoid) (infected) — see Sinus, pilonidal
  tachycardia R00.0
    paroxysmal I47.19
  tarsi syndrome M25.57- ☑
  testis N50.89
  tract (postinfective) — see Fistula
  urachus Q64.4
Sinusitis (accessory) (chronic) (hyperplastic) (nasal) (nonpurulent) (purulent) J32.9
  acute J01.90
    ethmoidal J01.20
      recurrent J01.21
    frontal J01.10
      recurrent J01.11
    involving more than one sinus, other than pansinusitis J01.80
      recurrent J01.81
    maxillary J01.00
      recurrent J01.01
    pansinusitis J01.40
      recurrent J01.41
    recurrent J01.91
    specified NEC J01.80
      recurrent J01.81
    sphenoidal J01.30
      recurrent J01.31
  allergic — see Rhinitis, allergic
  due to high altitude T70.1- ☑
  ethmoidal J32.2
    acute J01.20
      recurrent J01.21
  frontal J32.1
    acute J01.10
      recurrent J01.11
  influenzal — see Influenza, with, respiratory manifestations NEC
  involving more than one sinus but not pansinusitis J32.8
    acute J01.80
      recurrent J01.81
  maxillary J32.0
    acute J01.00
      recurrent J01.01
  sphenoidal J32.3
    acute J01.30
      recurrent J01.31
  tuberculous, any sinus A15.8
Sinusitis-bronchiectasis-situs inversus (syndrome) (triad) Q89.3
Sipple's syndrome E31.22
Sirenomelia (syndrome) Q87.2
Siriasis T67.01- ☑
Sirkari's disease B55.0
Siti A65
Situation, psychiatric F99
Situational
  disturbance (transient) — see Disorder, adjustment
    acute F43.0
  maladjustment — see Disorder, adjustment
  reaction — see Disorder, adjustment
    acute F43.0

Situs inversus or transversus (abdominalis) (thoracis) Q89.3
Sixth disease B08.20
  due to human herpesvirus 6 B08.21
  due to human herpesvirus 7 B08.22
Sjogren-Larsson syndrome Q87.19
Sjogren's syndrome or disease — see Syndrome, Sjogren
Skeletal — see condition
Skene's gland — see condition
Skenitis — see Urethritis
Skerljevo A65
Skevas-Zerfus disease — see Toxicity, venom, marine animal, sea anemone
Skin — see also condition
  clammy R23.1
  donor — see Donor, skin
  dry L85.3
  hidebound M35.9
Slate-dressers' or slate-miners' lung J62.8
Sleep
  apnea — see Apnea, sleep
  deprivation Z72.820
  disorder or disturbance G47.9
    child F51.9
    nonorganic origin F51.9
    specified NEC G47.8
  disturbance G47.9
    nonorganic origin F51.9
  drunkenness F51.9
  rhythm inversion G47.2- ☑
  terrors F51.4
  walking F51.3
    hysterical F44.89
Sleep hygiene
  abuse Z72.821
  inadequate Z72.821
  poor Z72.821
Sleep-wake schedule disorder G47.20
Sleeping sickness — see Sickness, sleeping
Sleeplessness — see Insomnia
  menopausal N95.1
Slim disease (in HIV infection) B20
Slipped, slipping
  epiphysis (traumatic) — see also Osteochondropathy, specified type NEC
    capital femoral (traumatic) [SCFE]
      acute (on chronic) S79.01- ☑
      nontraumatic M93.00- ☑
    current traumatic — code as Fracture, by site
    upper femoral (nontraumatic) [SUFE] M93.00- ☑
      acute M93.01- ☑
        on chronic M93.03- ☑
      chronic M93.02- ☑
  intervertebral disc — see Displacement, intervertebral disc
  ligature, umbilical P51.8
  patella — see Disorder, patella, derangement NEC
  rib M89.8X8
  sacroiliac joint — see subcategory M53.2- ☑
  tendon — see Disorder, tendon
  ulnar nerve, nontraumatic — see Lesion, nerve, ulnar
  vertebra NEC — see Spondylolisthesis
Slocumb's syndrome E27.0
Sloughing (multiple) (phagedena) (skin) — see also Gangrene
  abscess — see Abscess
  appendix K38.8
  fascia — see Disorder, soft tissue, specified type NEC
  scrotum N50.89
  tendon — see Disorder, tendon
  transplanted organ — see Rejection, transplant
  ulcer — see Ulcer, skin
Slow
  feeding, newborn P92.2
  flow syndrome, coronary I20.89
  heart (beat) R00.1
Slowing, urinary stream R39.198
Sluder's neuralgia (syndrome) G44.89
Slurred, slurring speech R47.81
Small (ness)
  for gestational age — see Small for dates
  introitus, vagina N89.6
  kidney (unknown cause) N27.9
    bilateral N27.1
    unilateral N27.0
  ovary (congenital) Q50.39
  pelvis
    with disproportion (fetopelvic) O33.1

☑ Additional Character Required — Refer to the Tabular List for Character Selection

Small — continued
- pelvis — continued
  - with disproportion — continued
    - causing obstructed labor O65.1
  - uterus N85.8
  - white kidney N03.9

Small-and-light-for-dates — see Small for dates

Small-for-dates (infant) P05.10
- with weight of
  - 499 grams or less P05.11
  - 500-749 grams P05.12
  - 750-999 grams P05.13
  - 1000-1249 grams P05.14
  - 1250-1499 grams P05.15
  - 1500-1749 grams P05.16
  - 1750-1999 grams P05.17
  - 2000-2499 grams P05.18
  - 2500 grams and over P05.19
- specified NEC P05.19

Smallpox B03

Smearing, fecal R15.1

SMEI (severe myoclonic epilepsy in infancy) G40.83- ☑

Smith-Lemli-Opitz syndrome E78.72

Smith's fracture S52.54- ☑

Smoker — see Dependence, drug, nicotine

Smoker's
- bronchitis J41.0
- cough J41.0
- palate K13.24
- throat J31.2
- tongue K13.24

Smoking
- passive Z77.22

Smothering spells R06.81

Snaggle teeth, tooth M26.39

Snapping
- finger — see Trigger finger
- hip — see Derangement, joint, specified type NEC, hip
  - involving the iliotibial band M76.3- ☑
- knee — see Derangement, knee
  - involving the iliotibial band M76.3- ☑

Sneddon-Wilkinson disease or syndrome (sub-corneal pustular dermatosis) L13.1

Sneezing (intractable) R06.7

Sniffing
- cocaine
  - abuse — see Abuse, drug, cocaine
  - dependence — see Dependence, drug, cocaine
- gasoline
  - abuse — see Abuse, drug, inhalant
  - dependence — see Dependence, drug, inhalant
- glue (airplane)
  - abuse — see Abuse, drug, inhalant
  - drug dependence — see Dependence, drug, inhalant

Sniffles
- newborn P28.89

Snoring R06.83

Snow blindness — see Photokeratitis

Snuffles (non-syphilitic) R06.5
- newborn P28.89
- syphilitic (infant) A50.05 [J99]

Social
- exclusion Z60.4
  - due to discrimination or persecution (perceived) Z60.5
- migrant Z59.00
  - acculturation difficulty Z60.3
- rejection Z60.4
  - due to discrimination or persecution Z60.5
- role conflict NEC Z73.5
- skills inadequacy NEC Z73.4
- transplantation Z60.3

Sodoku A25.0

Soemmerring's ring — see Cataract, secondary

Soft — see also condition
- nails L60.3

Softening
- bone — see Osteomalacia
- brain (necrotic) (progressive) G93.89
  - congenital Q04.8
  - embolic I63.4- ☑
  - hemorrhagic — see Hemorrhage, intracranial, intracerebral
  - occlusive I63.5- ☑
  - thrombotic I63.3- ☑
- cartilage M94.2- ☑
  - patella M22.4- ☑
- cerebellar — see Softening, brain
- cerebral — see Softening, brain

Softening — continued
- cerebrospinal — see Softening, brain
- myocardial, heart — see Degeneration, myocardial
- spinal cord G95.89
- stomach K31.89

Soldier's
- heart F45.8
- patches I31.0

Solitary
- cyst, kidney N28.1
- kidney, congenital Q60.0

Solvent abuse — see Abuse, drug, inhalant
- dependence — see Dependence, drug, inhalant

Somatization reaction, somatic reaction — see Disorder, somatoform

Somnambulism F51.3
- hysterical F44.89

Somnolence R40.0
- nonorganic origin F51.11

Sonne dysentery A03.3

Soor B37.0

Sore
- bed — see Ulcer, pressure, by site
- chiclero B55.1
- Delhi B55.1
- desert — see Ulcer, skin
- eye H57.1- ☑
- Lahore B55.1
- mouth K13.79
  - canker K12.0
- muscle M79.10
- Naga — see Ulcer, skin
- of skin — see Ulcer, skin
- oriental B55.1
- pressure — see Ulcer, pressure, by site
- skin L98.9
- soft A57
- throat (acute) — see also Pharyngitis
  - with influenza, flu, or grippe — see Influenza, with, respiratory manifestations NEC
  - chronic J31.2
  - coxsackie (virus) B08.5
  - diphtheritic A36.0
  - herpesviral B00.2
  - influenzal — see Influenza, with, respiratory manifestations NEC
  - septic J02.0
  - streptococcal (ulcerative) J02.0
  - viral NEC J02.8
    - coxsackie B08.5
- tropical — see Ulcer, skin
- veldt — see Ulcer, skin

Soto's syndrome (cerebral gigantism) Q87.3

South African cardiomyopathy syndrome I42.8

Southeast Asian hemorrhagic fever A91

Spacing
- abnormal, tooth, teeth, fully erupted M26.30
- excessive, tooth, fully erupted M26.32

Spade-like hand (congenital) Q68.1

Spading nail L60.8
- congenital Q84.6

Spanish collar N47.1

Sparganosis B70.1

Spasm(s), spastic, spasticity — see also condition R25.2
- accommodation — see Spasm, of accommodation
- ampulla of Vater K83.4
- anus, ani (sphincter) (reflex) K59.4
  - psychogenic F45.8
- artery I73.9
  - cerebral G45.9
- Bell's G51.3- ☑
- bladder (sphincter, external or internal) N32.89
  - psychogenic F45.8
- bronchus, bronchiole J98.01
- cardia K22.0
- cardiac I20.1
- carpopedal — see Tetany
- cerebral (arteries) (vascular) G45.9
- cervix, complicating delivery O62.4
- ciliary body (of accommodation) — see Spasm, of accommodation
- colon — see also Irritable, bowel K58.9
  - with diarrhea K58.0
  - psychogenic F45.8
- common duct K83.4
- compulsive — see Tic
- conjugate H51.8
- coronary (artery) I20.1
- diaphragm (reflex) R06.6

Spasm(s), spastic, spasticity — continued
- diaphragm — continued
  - epidemic B33.0
  - psychogenic F45.8
- duodenum K59.89
- epidemic diaphragmatic (transient) B33.0
- esophagus (diffuse) K22.4
  - psychogenic F45.8
- facial G51.3- ☑
- fallopian tube N83.8
- gastrointestinal (tract) K31.89
  - psychogenic F45.8
- glottis J38.5
  - hysterical F44.4
  - psychogenic F45.8
    - conversion reaction F44.4
  - reflex through recurrent laryngeal nerve J38.5
- habit — see Tic
- heart I20.1
- hemifacial (clonic) G51.3- ☑
- hourglass — see Contraction, hourglass
- hysterical F44.4
- infantile — see Epilepsy, spasms
- inferior oblique, eye H51.8
- intestinal — see also Syndrome, irritable bowel K58.9
  - psychogenic F45.8
- larynx, laryngeal J38.5
  - hysterical F44.4
  - psychogenic F45.8
    - conversion reaction F44.4
- levator palpebrae superioris — see Disorder, eyelid function
- muscle NEC M62.838
  - back M62.830
- nerve, trigeminal G50.0
- nervous F45.8
- nodding F98.4
- occupational F48.8
- oculogyric H51.8
  - psychogenic F45.8
- of accommodation H52.53- ☑
- ophthalmic artery — see Occlusion, artery, retina
- perineal, female N94.89
- peroneo-extensor — see also Deformity, limb, flat foot
- pharynx (reflex) J39.2
  - hysterical F45.8
  - psychogenic F45.8
- psychogenic F45.8
- pylorus NEC K31.3
  - adult hypertrophic K31.89
  - congenital or infantile Q40.0
  - psychogenic F45.8
- rectum (sphincter) K59.4
  - psychogenic F45.8
- retinal (artery) — see Occlusion, artery, retina
- sigmoid — see also Syndrome, irritable bowel K58.9
  - psychogenic F45.8
- sphincter of Oddi K83.4
- stomach K31.89
  - neurotic F45.8
- throat J39.2
  - hysterical F45.8
  - psychogenic F45.8
- tic F95.9
  - chronic F95.1
  - transient of childhood F95.0
- tongue K14.8
- torsion (progressive) G24.1
- trigeminal nerve — see Neuralgia, trigeminal
- ureter N13.5
- urethra (sphincter) N35.919
- uterus N85.8
  - complicating labor O62.4
- vagina N94.2
  - psychogenic F52.5
- vascular I73.9
- vasomotor I73.9
- vein NEC I87.8
- viscera — see Pain, abdominal

Spasmodic — see condition

Spasmophilia — see Tetany

Spasmus nutans F98.4

Spastic, spasticity — see also Spasm
- child (cerebral) (congenital) (paralysis) G80.1

Speaker's throat R49.8

Specific, specified — see condition

Speech
- defect, disorder, disturbance, impediment — see Disorder, speech R47.9

Speech — continued
    defect, disorder, disturbance, impediment — see Disorder, speech — continued
        psychogenic, in childhood and adolescence F98.8
        slurring R47.81
        specified NEC R47.89
Spells, transient oxygen desaturation of newborn —
    see also Apnea, newborn P28.40
    during sleep — see also Apnea, newborn, sleep, primary P28.30
Spencer's disease A08.19
Spens' syndrome (syncope with heart block) I45.9
Sperm counts (fertility testing) Z31.41
    postvasectomy Z30.8
    reversal Z31.42
Spermatic cord — see condition
Spermatocele N43.40
    congenital Q55.4
    multiple N43.42
    single N43.41
Spermatocystitis N49.0
Spermatocytoma C62.9-
    specified site — see Neoplasm, malignant, by site
Spermatorrhea N50.89
Sphacelus — see Gangrene
Sphenoidal — see condition
Sphenoiditis (chronic) — see Sinusitis, sphenoidal
Sphenopalatine ganglion neuralgia G90.09
Sphericity, increased, lens (congenital) Q12.4
Spherocytosis (congenital) (familial) (hereditary) D58.0
    hemoglobin disease D58.0
    sickle-cell (disease) D57.8-
Spherophakia Q12.4
Sphincter — see condition
Sphincteritis, sphincter of Oddi — see Cholangitis
Sphingolipidosis E75.3
    specified NEC E75.29
Sphingomyelinosis E75.3
Spicule tooth K00.2
Spider
    bite — see Toxicity, venom, spider
        nonvenomous — see Bite, by site, superficial, insect
    fingers — see Syndrome, Marfan
    nevus I78.1
    toes — see Syndrome, Marfan
    vascular I78.1
Spiegler-Fendt
    benign lymphocytoma L98.8
    sarcoid L08.89
Spielmeyer-Vogt disease E75.4
Spina bifida (aperta) Q05.9
    with hydrocephalus NEC Q05.4
    cervical Q05.5
        with hydrocephalus Q05.0
    dorsal Q05.6
        with hydrocephalus Q05.1
    lumbar Q05.7
        with hydrocephalus Q05.2
    lumbosacral Q05.7
        with hydrocephalus Q05.2
    occulta Q76.0
    sacral Q05.8
        with hydrocephalus Q05.3
    thoracic Q05.6
        with hydrocephalus Q05.1
    thoracolumbar Q05.6
        with hydrocephalus Q05.1
Spindle, Krukenberg's — see Pigmentation, cornea, posterior
Spine, spinal — see condition
Spiradenoma (eccrine) — see Neoplasm, skin, benign
Spirillosis A25.0
Spirillum
    minus A25.0
    obermeieri infection A68.0
Spirochetal — see condition
Spirochetosis A69.9
    arthritic, arthritica A69.9
    bronchopulmonary A69.8
    icterohemorrhagic A27.0
    lung A69.8
Spirometrosis B70.1
Spitting blood — see Hemoptysis
Splanchnoptosis K63.4
Spleen, splenic — see condition
Splenectasis — see Splenomegaly
Splenitis (interstitial) (malignant) (nonspecific) D73.89
    malarial — see also Malaria B54 [D77]
    tuberculous A18.85

Splenocele D73.89
Splenomegaly, splenomegalia (Bengal) (cryptogenic) (idiopathic) (tropical) R16.1
    with hepatomegaly R16.2
    cirrhotic D73.2
    congenital Q89.09
    congestive, chronic D73.2
    Egyptian B65.1
    Gaucher's E75.22
    malarial — see also Malaria B54 [D77]
    neutropenic D73.81
    Niemann-Pick — see Niemann-Pick disease or syndrome
    siderotic D73.2
    syphilitic A52.79
        congenital (early) A50.08 [D77]
Splenopathy D73.9
Splenoptosis D73.89
Splenosis D73.89
Splinter — see Foreign body, superficial, by site
Split, splitting
    foot Q72.7-
    hand Q71.6-
    heart sounds R01.2
    lip, congenital — see Cleft, lip
    nails L60.3
    urinary stream R39.13
Spondylarthrosis — see Spondylosis
Spondylitis (chronic) — see also Spondylopathy, inflammatory
    ankylopoietica — see Spondylitis, ankylosing
    ankylosing (chronic) M45.9
        with lung involvement M45.9 [J99]
        cervical region M45.2
        cervicothoracic region M45.3
        juvenile M08.1
        lumbar region M45.6
        lumbosacral region M45.7
        multiple sites M45.0
        occipito-atlanto-axial region M45.1
        sacrococcygeal region M45.8
        thoracic region M45.4
        thoracolumbar region M45.5
    atrophic (ligamentous) — see Spondylitis, ankylosing
    deformans (chronic) — see Spondylosis
    gonococcal A54.41
    gouty — see also Gout, by type, vertebrae M10.08
    in (due to)
        brucellosis A23.9 [M49.80]
            cervical region A23.9 [M49.82]
            cervicothoracic region A23.9 [M49.83]
            lumbar region A23.9 [M49.86]
            lumbosacral region A23.9 [M49.87]
            multiple sites A23.9 [M49.89]
            occipito-atlanto-axial region A23.9 [M49.81]
            sacrococcygeal region A23.9 [M49.88]
            thoracic region A23.9 [M49.84]
            thoracolumbar region A23.9 [M49.85]
        enterobacteria — see also subcategory M49.8 A04.9
        tuberculosis A18.01
    infectious NEC — see Spondylopathy, infective
    juvenile ankylosing (chronic) M08.1
    Kummell's — see Spondylopathy, traumatic
    Marie-Strumpell — see Spondylitis, ankylosing
    muscularis — see Spondylopathy, specified NEC
    psoriatic L40.53
    rheumatoid — see Spondylitis, ankylosing
    rhizomelica — see Spondylitis, ankylosing
    sacroiliac NEC M46.1
    senescent, senile — see Spondylosis
    traumatic (chronic) or post-traumatic — see Spondylopathy, traumatic
    tuberculous A18.01
    typhosa A01.05
Spondyloarthritis
    axial — see also Spondylitis, ankylosing
        non-radiographic M45.A0
            cervical M45.A2
            cervicothoracic M45.A3
            lumbar M45.A6
            lumbosacral M45.A7
            multiple sites M45.AB
            occipito-atlanto-axial region M45.A1
            sacral and sacrococcygeal M45.A8
            thoracic M45.A4
            thoracolumbar M45.A5
Spondylolisthesis (acquired) (degenerative) M43.10
    with disproportion (fetopelvic) O33.0
        causing obstructed labor O65.0
    cervical region M43.12

Spondylolisthesis — continued
    cervicothoracic region M43.13
    congenital Q76.2
    lumbar region M43.16
    lumbosacral region M43.17
    multiple sites M43.19
    occipito-atlanto-axial region M43.11
    sacrococcygeal region M43.18
    thoracic region M43.14
    thoracolumbar region M43.15
    traumatic (old) M43.10
        acute
            fifth cervical (displaced) S12.430-
                nondisplaced S12.431-
                specified type NEC (displaced) S12.450-
                    nondisplaced S12.451-
                type III S12.44-
            fourth cervical (displaced) S12.330-
                nondisplaced S12.331-
                specified type NEC (displaced) S12.350-
                    nondisplaced S12.351-
                type III S12.34-
            second cervical (displaced) S12.130-
                nondisplaced S12.131-
                specified type NEC (displaced) S12.150-
                    nondisplaced S12.151-
                type III S12.14-
            seventh cervical (displaced) S12.630-
                nondisplaced S12.631-
                specified type NEC (displaced) S12.650-
                    nondisplaced S12.651-
                type III S12.64-
            sixth cervical (displaced) S12.530-
                nondisplaced S12.531-
                specified type NEC (displaced) S12.550-
                    nondisplaced S12.551-
                type III S12.54-
            third cervical (displaced) S12.230-
                nondisplaced S12.231-
                specified type NEC (displaced) S12.250-
                    nondisplaced S12.251-
                type III S12.24-
Spondylolysis (acquired) M43.00
    cervical region M43.02
    cervicothoracic region M43.03
    congenital Q76.2
    lumbar region M43.06
    lumbosacral region M43.07
        with disproportion (fetopelvic) O33.0
            causing obstructed labor O65.8
    multiple sites M43.09
    occipito-atlanto-axial region M43.01
    sacrococcygeal region M43.08
    thoracic region M43.04
    thoracolumbar region M43.05
Spondylopathy M48.9
    infective NEC M46.50
        cervical region M46.52
        cervicothoracic region M46.53
        lumbar region M46.56
        lumbosacral region M46.57
        multiple sites M46.59
        occipito-atlanto-axial region M46.51
        sacrococcygeal region M46.58
        thoracic region M46.54
        thoracolumbar region M46.55
    inflammatory M46.90
        cervical region M46.92
        cervicothoracic region M46.93
        lumbar region M46.96
        lumbosacral region M46.97
        multiple sites M46.99
        occipito-atlanto-axial region M46.91
        sacrococcygeal region M46.98
        specified type NEC M46.80
            cervical region M46.82
            cervicothoracic region M46.83
            lumbar region M46.86
            lumbosacral region M46.87
            multiple sites M46.89
            occipito-atlanto-axial region M46.81
            sacrococcygeal region M46.88
            thoracic region M46.84
            thoracolumbar region M46.85
        thoracic region M46.94
        thoracolumbar region M46.95

Spondylopathy — continued
- neuropathic, in
  - syringomyelia and syringobulbia G95.0
  - tabes dorsalis A52.11
- specified NEC — see subcategory M48.8- ☑
- traumatic M48.30
  - cervical region M48.32
  - cervicothoracic region M48.33
  - lumbar region M48.36
  - lumbosacral region M48.37
  - occipito-atlanto-axial region M48.31
  - sacrococcygeal region M48.38
  - thoracic region M48.34
  - thoracolumbar region M48.35

Spondylosis M47.9
- with
  - disproportion (fetopelvic) O33.0
    - causing obstructed labor O65.0
- myelopathy NEC M47.10
  - cervical region M47.12
  - cervicothoracic region M47.13
  - lumbar region M47.16
  - occipito-atlanto-axial region M47.11
  - thoracic region M47.14
  - thoracolumbar region M47.15
- radiculopathy M47.20
  - cervical region M47.22
  - cervicothoracic region M47.23
  - lumbar region M47.26
  - lumbosacral region M47.27
  - occipito-atlanto-axial region M47.21
  - sacrococcygeal region M47.28
  - thoracic region M47.24
  - thoracolumbar region M47.25
- specified NEC M47.899
  - cervical region M47.892
  - cervicothoracic region M47.893
  - facet joint M47.819
  - lumbar region M47.896
  - lumbosacral region M47.897
  - occipito-atlanto-axial region M47.891
  - sacrococcygeal region M47.898
  - thoracic region M47.894
  - thoracolumbar region M47.895
- traumatic — see Spondylopathy, traumatic
- without myelopathy or radiculopathy M47.819
  - cervical region M47.812
  - cervicothoracic region M47.813
  - lumbar region M47.816
  - lumbosacral region M47.817
  - occipito-atlanto-axial region M47.811
  - sacrococcygeal region M47.818
  - thoracic region M47.814
  - thoracolumbar region M47.815

Sponge
- inadvertently left in operation wound — see Foreign body, accidentally left during a procedure
- kidney (medullary) Q61.5

Sponge-diver's disease — see Toxicity, venom, marine animal, sea anemone

Spongioblastoma (any type) — see Neoplasm, malignant, by site
- specified site — see Neoplasm, malignant, by site
- unspecified site C71.9

Spongioneuroblastoma — see Neoplasm, malignant, by site

Spontaneous — see also condition
- fracture (cause unknown) — see Fracture, pathological

Spoon nail L60.3
- congenital Q84.6

Sporadic — see condition

Sporothrix schenckii infection — see Sporotrichosis

Sporotrichosis B42.9
- arthritis B42.82
- disseminated B42.7
- generalized B42.7
- lymphocutaneous (fixed) (progressive) B42.1
- pulmonary B42.0
- specified NEC B42.89

Spots, spotting (in) (of)
- Bitot's — see also Pigmentation, conjunctiva
  - in the young child E50.1
  - vitamin A deficiency E50.1
- cafe, au lait L81.3
- Cayenne pepper I78.1
- cotton wool, retina — see Occlusion, artery, retina
- de Morgan's (senile angiomas) I78.1
- Fuchs' black (myopic) — see also Myopia, degenerative H44.2- ☑

Spots, spotting — continued
- intermenstrual (regular) N92.0
  - irregular N92.1
- Koplik's B05.9
- liver L81.4
- pregnancy O26.85- ☑
- purpuric R23.3
- ruby I78.1

Spotted fever — see Fever, spotted A77.9

Sprain (joint) (ligament)
- acromioclavicular joint or ligament S43.5- ☑
- ankle S93.40- ☑
  - calcaneofibular ligament S93.41- ☑
  - deltoid ligament S93.42- ☑
  - internal collateral ligament — see Sprain, ankle, specified ligament NEC
  - specified ligament NEC S93.49- ☑
  - talofibular ligament — see Sprain, ankle, specified ligament NEC
  - tibiofibular ligament S93.43- ☑
- anterior longitudinal, cervical S13.4- ☑
- atlas, atlanto-axial, atlanto-occipital S13.4- ☑
- breast bone — see Sprain, sternum
- calcaneofibular — see Sprain, ankle
- carpal — see Sprain, wrist
- carpometacarpal — see Sprain, hand, specified site NEC
- cartilage
  - costal S23.41- ☑
  - semilunar (knee) — see Sprain, knee, specified site NEC
    - with current tear — see Tear, meniscus
  - thyroid region S13.5- ☑
  - xiphoid — see Sprain, sternum
- cervical, cervicodorsal, cervicothoracic S13.4- ☑
- chondrosternal S23.421- ☑
- coracoclavicular S43.8- ☑
- coracohumeral S43.41- ☑
- coronary, knee — see Sprain, knee, specified site NEC
- costal cartilage S23.41- ☑
- cricoarytenoid articulation or ligament S13.5- ☑
- cricothyroid articulation S13.5- ☑
- cruciate, knee — see Sprain, knee, cruciate
- deltoid, ankle — see Sprain, ankle
- dorsal (spine) S23.3- ☑
- elbow S53.40- ☑
  - radial collateral ligament S53.43- ☑
  - radiohumeral S53.41- ☑
  - rupture
    - radial collateral ligament — see Rupture, traumatic, ligament, radial collateral
    - ulnar collateral ligament — see Rupture, traumatic, ligament, ulnar collateral
  - specified type NEC S53.49- ☑
  - ulnar collateral ligament S53.44- ☑
  - ulnohumeral S53.42- ☑
- femur, head — see Sprain, hip
- fibular collateral, knee — see Sprain, knee, collateral
- fibulocalcaneal — see Sprain, ankle
- finger(s) S63.61- ☑
  - index S63.61- ☑
  - interphalangeal (joint) S63.63- ☑
    - index S63.63- ☑
    - little S63.63- ☑
    - middle S63.63- ☑
    - ring S63.63- ☑
  - little S63.61- ☑
  - metacarpophalangeal (joint) S63.65- ☑
  - middle S63.61- ☑
  - ring S63.61- ☑
  - specified site NEC S63.69- ☑
    - index S63.69- ☑
    - little S63.69- ☑
    - middle S63.69- ☑
    - ring S63.69- ☑
- foot S93.60- ☑
  - specified ligament NEC S93.69- ☑
  - tarsal ligament S93.61- ☑
  - tarsometatarsal ligament S93.62- ☑
  - toe — see Sprain, toe
- hand S63.9- ☑
  - finger — see Sprain, finger
  - specified site NEC — see subcategory S63.8- ☑
  - thumb — see Sprain, thumb
- head S03.9- ☑
- hip S73.10- ☑
  - iliofemoral ligament S73.11- ☑

Sprain — continued
- hip — continued
  - ischiocapsular (ligament) S73.12- ☑
  - specified NEC S73.19- ☑
- iliofemoral — see Sprain, hip
- innominate
  - acetabulum — see Sprain, hip
  - sacral junction S33.6- ☑
- internal
  - collateral, ankle — see Sprain, ankle
  - semilunar cartilage — see Sprain, knee, specified site NEC
- interphalangeal
  - finger — see Sprain, finger, interphalangeal (joint)
  - toe — see Sprain, toe, interphalangeal joint
- ischiocapsular — see Sprain, hip
- ischiofemoral — see Sprain, hip
- jaw (articular disc) (cartilage) (meniscus) S03.4- ☑
  - old M26.69
- knee S83.9- ☑
  - collateral ligament S83.40- ☑
    - lateral (fibular) S83.42- ☑
    - medial (tibial) S83.41- ☑
  - cruciate ligament S83.50- ☑
    - anterior S83.51- ☑
    - posterior S83.52- ☑
  - lateral (fibular) collateral ligament S83.42- ☑
  - medial (tibial) collateral ligament S83.41- ☑
  - patellar ligament S76.11- ☑
  - specified site NEC S83.8X- ☑
  - superior tibiofibular joint (ligament) S83.6- ☑
- lateral collateral, knee — see Sprain, knee, collateral
- lumbar (spine) S33.5- ☑
- lumbosacral S33.9- ☑
- mandible (articular disc) S03.4- ☑
  - old M26.69
- medial collateral, knee — see Sprain, knee, collateral
- meniscus
  - jaw S03.4- ☑
    - old M26.69
  - knee — see Sprain, knee, specified site NEC
    - with current tear — see Tear, meniscus
      - old — see Derangement, knee, meniscus, due to old tear
  - mandible S03.4- ☑
    - old M26.69
- metacarpal (distal) (proximal) — see Sprain, hand, specified site NEC
- metacarpophalangeal — see Sprain, finger, metacarpophalangeal (joint)
- metatarsophalangeal — see Sprain, toe, metatarsophalangeal joint
- midcarpal — see Sprain, hand, specified site NEC
- midtarsal — see Sprain, foot, specified site NEC
- neck S13.9- ☑
  - anterior longitudinal cervical ligament S13.4- ☑
  - atlanto-axial joint S13.4- ☑
  - atlanto-occipital joint S13.4- ☑
  - cervical spine S13.4- ☑
  - cricoarytenoid ligament S13.5- ☑
  - cricothyroid ligament S13.5- ☑
  - specified site NEC S13.8- ☑
  - thyroid region (cartilage) S13.5- ☑
- nose S03.8- ☑
- orbicular, hip — see Sprain, hip
- patella — see Sprain, knee, specified site NEC
- patellar ligament S76.11- ☑
- pelvis NEC S33.8- ☑
- phalanx
  - finger — see Sprain, finger
  - toe — see Sprain, toe
- pubofemoral — see Sprain, hip
- radiocarpal — see Sprain, wrist
- radiohumeral — see Sprain, elbow
- radius, collateral — see Rupture, traumatic, ligament, radial collateral
- rib (cage) S23.41- ☑
- rotator cuff (capsule) S43.42- ☑
- sacroiliac (region)
  - chronic or old — see subcategory M53.2- ☑
  - joint S33.6- ☑
- scaphoid (hand) — see Sprain, hand, specified site NEC
- scapula (r) — see Sprain, shoulder girdle, specified site NEC
- semilunar cartilage (knee) — see Sprain, knee, specified site NEC
  - with current tear — see Tear, meniscus

Sprain — continued
  semilunar cartilage — see Sprain, knee, specified site — continued
    with current tear — see Tear, meniscus — continued
      old — see Derangement, knee, meniscus, due to old tear
  shoulder joint S43.40- ☑
    acromioclavicular joint (ligament) — see Sprain, acromioclavicular joint
    blade — see Sprain, shoulder, girdle, specified site NEC
    coracoclavicular joint (ligament) — see Sprain, coracoclavicular joint
    coracohumeral ligament — see Sprain, coracohumeral joint
    girdle S43.9- ☑
      specified site NEC S43.8- ☑
    rotator cuff — see Sprain, rotator cuff
    specified site NEC S43.49- ☑
    sternoclavicular joint (ligament) — see Sprain, sternoclavicular joint
  spine
    cervical S13.4- ☑
    lumbar S33.5- ☑
    thoracic S23.3- ☑
  sternoclavicular joint S43.6- ☑
  sternum S23.429-
    chondrosternal joint S23.421- ☑
    specified site NEC S23.428- ☑
    sternoclavicular (joint) (ligament) S43.6- ☑
  symphysis
    jaw S03.4- ☑
      old M26.69
    mandibular S03.4- ☑
      old M26.69
  talofibular — see Sprain, ankle
  tarsal — see Sprain, foot, specified site NEC
  tarsometatarsal — see Sprain, foot, specified site NEC
  temporomandibular S03.4- ☑
    old M26.69
  thorax S23.9- ☑
    ribs S23.41- ☑
    specified site NEC S23.8- ☑
    spine S23.3- ☑
    sternum — see Sprain, sternum
  thumb S63.60- ☑
    interphalangeal (joint) S63.62- ☑
    metacarpophalangeal (joint) S63.64- ☑
    specified site NEC S63.68- ☑
  thyroid cartilage or region S13.5- ☑
  tibia (proximal end) — see Sprain, knee, specified site NEC
  tibial collateral, knee — see Sprain, knee, collateral
  tibiofibular
    distal — see Sprain, ankle
    superior — see Sprain, knee, specified site NEC
  toe(s) S93.50- ☑
    great S93.50- ☑
    interphalangeal joint S93.51- ☑
      great S93.51- ☑
      lesser S93.51- ☑
    lesser S93.50- ☑
    metatarsophalangeal joint S93.52- ☑
      great S93.52- ☑
      lesser S93.52- ☑
  ulna, collateral — see Rupture, traumatic, ligament, ulnar collateral
  ulnohumeral — see Sprain, elbow
  wrist S63.50- ☑
    carpal S63.51- ☑
    radiocarpal S63.52- ☑
    specified site NEC S63.59- ☑
  xiphoid cartilage — see Sprain, sternum
Sprengel's deformity (congenital) Q74.0
Sprue (tropical) K90.1
  celiac K90.0
  idiopathic K90.49
  meaning thrush B37.0
  nontropical K90.0
Spur, bone — see also Enthesopathy
  calcaneal M77.3- ☑
  iliac crest M76.2- ☑
  nose (septum) J34.89
Spurway's syndrome Q78.0
Sputum
  abnormal (amount) (color) (odor) (purulent) R09.3

Sputum — continued
  blood-stained R04.2
  excessive (cause unknown) R09.3
Squamous — see also condition
  epithelium in
    cervical canal (congenital) Q51.828
    uterine mucosa (congenital) Q51.818
Squashed nose M95.0
  congenital Q67.4
Squeeze, diver's T70.3- ☑
Squint — see also Strabismus
  accommodative — see Strabismus, convergent concomitant
SSADHD (succinic semialdehyde dehydrogenase deficiency) E72.81
St. Hubert's disease A82.9
Stab — see also Laceration
  internal organs — see Injury, by site
Stafne's cyst or cavity M27.0
Staggering gait R26.0
  hysterical F44.4
Staghorn calculus — see Calculus, kidney
Stahli's line (cornea) (pigment) — see Pigmentation, cornea, anterior
Stain, staining
  meconium (newborn) P96.83
  port wine Q82.5
  tooth, teeth (hard tissues) (extrinsic) K03.6
    due to
      accretions K03.6
      deposits (betel) (black) (green) (materia alba) (orange) (soft) (tobacco) K03.6
      metals (copper) (silver) K03.7
      nicotine K03.6
      pulpal bleeding K03.7
      tobacco K03.6
    intrinsic K00.8
Stammering — see also Disorder, fluency F80.81
Standstill
  auricular I45.5
  cardiac — see Arrest, cardiac
  sinoatrial I45.5
  ventricular — see Arrest, cardiac
Stannosis J63.5
Stanton's disease — see Melioidosis
Staphylitis (acute) (catarrhal) (chronic) (gangrenous) (membranous) (suppurative) (ulcerative) K12.2
Staphylococcal scalded skin syndrome L00
Staphylococcemia A41.2
Staphylococcus, staphylococcal — see also condition
  as cause of disease classified elsewhere B95.8
    aureus (methicillin susceptible) (MSSA) B95.61
      methicillin resistant (MRSA) B95.62
    specified NEC, as cause of disease classified elsewhere B95.7
Staphyloma (sclera)
  cornea H18.72- ☑
  equatorial H15.81- ☑
  localized (anterior) H15.82- ☑
  posticum H15.83- ☑
  ring H15.85- ☑
Stargardt's disease — see Dystrophy, retina
Starvation (inanition) (due to lack of food) T73.0- ☑
  edema — see Malnutrition, severe
Stasis
  bile (noncalculous) K83.1
  bronchus J98.09
    with infection — see Bronchitis
  cardiac — see Failure, heart, congestive
  cecum K59.89
  colon K59.89
  dermatitis I87.2
    with
      varicose ulcer — see Varix, leg, with ulcer, with inflammation
      varicose veins — see Varix, leg, with, inflammation
    due to postthrombotic syndrome — see Syndrome, postthrombotic
  duodenal K31.5
  eczema — see Varix, leg, with, inflammation
  edema — see Hypertension, venous (chronic), idiopathic
  foot T69.02- ☑
  ileocecal coil K59.89
  ileum K59.89
  intestinal K59.89
  jejunum K59.89
  kidney N19
  liver (cirrhotic) K76.1

Stasis — continued
  lymphatic I89.8
  pneumonia J18.2
  pulmonary — see Edema, lung
  rectal K59.89
  renal N19
    tubular N17.0
  ulcer — see Varix, leg, with, ulcer
    without varicose veins — see also Ulcer, by site I87.2
  urine — see Retention, urine
  venous I87.8
State (of)
  affective and paranoid, mixed, organic psychotic F06.8
  agitated R45.1
    acute reaction to stress F43.0
  anxiety (neurotic) F41.1
  apprehension F41.1
  burn-out Z73.0
  climacteric, female Z78.0
    symptomatic N95.1
  compulsive F42.8
    mixed with obsessional thoughts F42.2
  confusional (psychogenic) F44.89
    acute — see also Delirium
      with
        arteriosclerotic dementia — see also Dementia, vascular F01.50
          with behavioral disturbance — see Dementia, vascular
        senility or dementia F05
    alcoholic F10.231
    epileptic F05
    reactive (from emotional stress, psychological trauma) F44.89
    subacute — see Delirium
  convulsive — see Convulsions
  crisis F43.0
  depressive F32.A
    neurotic F34.1
  dissociative F44.9
  emotional shock (stress) R45.7
  hypercoagulation — see Hypercoagulable
  locked-in G83.5
  menopausal Z78.0
    symptomatic N95.1
  neurotic F48.9
    with depersonalization F48.1
  obsessional F42.8
  oneiroid (schizophrenia-like) F23
  organic
    hallucinatory (nonalcoholic) F06.0
    paranoid (-hallucinatory) F06.2
  panic F41.0
  paranoid F22
    climacteric F22
    involutional F22
    menopausal F22
    organic F06.2
    senile F03.- ☑
    simple F22
  persistent vegetative R40.3
  phobic F40.9
  postleukotomy F07.0
  pregnant
    gestational carrier Z33.3
    incidental Z33.1
  psychogenic, twilight F44.89
  psychopathic (constitutional) F60.2
  psychotic, organic — see also Psychosis, organic
    mixed paranoid and affective F06.8
    senile or presenile F03.- ☑
    transient NEC F06.8
      with
        depression F06.31
        hallucinations F06.0
  residual schizophrenic F20.5
  restlessness R45.1
  stress (emotional) R45.7
  tension (mental) F48.9
    specified NEC F48.8
  transient organic psychotic NEC F06.8
    depressive type F06.31
    hallucinatory type F06.0
  twilight
    epileptic F05
    psychogenic F44.89
  vegetative, persistent R40.3
  vital exhaustion Z73.0
  withdrawal, — see Withdrawal, state

Status (post) — see also Presence (of)
- absence, epileptic — see Epilepsy, by type, with status epilepticus
- administration of tPA (rtPA) in a different facility within the last 24 hours prior to admission to current facility Z92.82
- adrenalectomy (unilateral) (bilateral) E89.6
- anastomosis Z98.0
- anginosus I20.9
- angioplasty (peripheral) Z98.62
  - with implant Z95.820
    - coronary artery Z98.61
      - with implant Z95.5
- aortocoronary bypass Z95.1
- arthrodesis Z98.1
- artificial opening (of) Z93.9
  - gastrointestinal tract Z93.4
  - specified NEC Z93.8
  - urinary tract Z93.6
  - vagina Z93.8
- asthmaticus — see Asthma, by type, with status asthmaticus
- awaiting organ transplant Z76.82
- bariatric surgery Z98.84
- bed confinement Z74.01
- bleb, filtering (vitreous), after glaucoma surgery Z98.83
- breast implant Z98.82
  - removal Z98.86
- cataract extraction Z98.4- ☑
- cholecystectomy Z90.49
- clitorectomy N90.811
  - with excision of labia minora N90.812
- colectomy (complete) (partial) Z90.49
- colonization — see Carrier (suspected) of
- colostomy Z93.3
- combined receptor
  - negative
    - hormone receptor negative with human epidermal growth factor receptor 2 negative Z17.421
    - hormone receptor negative with human epidermal growth factor receptor 2 positive Z17.420
  - positive
    - hormone receptor positive with human epidermal growth factor receptor 2 negative Z17.411
    - hormone receptor positive with human epidermal growth factor receptor 2 positive Z17.410
- convulsivus idiopathicus — see Epilepsy, by type, with status epilepticus
- coronary artery angioplasty — see Status, angioplasty, coronary artery
- coronary artery bypass graft Z95.1
- cystectomy (urinary bladder) Z90.6
- cystostomy Z93.50
  - appendico-vesicostomy Z93.52
  - cutaneous Z93.51
  - specified NEC Z93.59
- delinquent immunization Z28.39
  - COVID-19 Z28.31- ☑
- dental Z98.818
  - crown Z98.811
  - fillings Z98.811
  - restoration Z98.811
  - sealant Z98.810
  - specified NEC Z98.818
- deployment (current) (military) Z56.82
- dialysis (hemodialysis) (peritoneal) Z99.2
- do not resuscitate (DNR) Z66
- donor — see Donor
- embedded fragments — see Retained, foreign body fragments (type of)
- embedded splinter — see Retained, foreign body fragments (type of)
- enterostomy Z93.4
- epileptic, epilepticus — see also Epilepsy, by type, with status epilepticus G40.901
- estrogen receptor
  - negative Z17.1
  - positive Z17.0
- female genital cutting — see Female genital mutilation status
- female genital mutilation — see Female genital mutilation status
- filtering (vitreous) bleb after glaucoma surgery Z98.83
- gastrectomy (complete) (partial) Z90.3
- gastric banding Z98.84
- gastric bypass for obesity Z98.84
- gastrostomy Z93.1
- human epidermal growth factor 2 receptor
  - negative Z17.32

Status — continued
- human epidermal growth factor 2 receptor — continued
  - positive Z17.31
- human immunodeficiency virus (HIV) infection, asymptomatic Z21
- hysterectomy (complete) (total) Z90.710
  - partial (with remaining cervical stump) Z90.711
- ileostomy (ileal pouch) (Kock pouch) Z93.2
- implant
  - breast Z98.82
- infibulation N90.813
- intestinal bypass Z98.0
- jejunostomy Z93.4
- lapsed immunization schedule Z28.39
- laryngectomy Z90.02
- lymphaticus E32.8
- malignancy
  - castrate resistant prostate Z19.2
  - hormone resistant Z19.2
  - hormone sensitive Z19.1
- marmoratus G80.3
- mastectomy (unilateral) (bilateral) Z90.1- ☑
- military deployment status (current) Z56.82
  - in theater or in support of military war, peacekeeping and humanitarian operations Z56.82
- nephrectomy (unilateral) (bilateral) Z90.5
- nephrostomy Z93.6
- obesity surgery Z98.84
- oophorectomy
  - bilateral Z90.722
  - unilateral Z90.721
- organ replacement
  - by artificial or mechanical device or prosthesis of
    - artery Z95.828
    - bladder Z96.0
    - blood vessel Z95.828
    - breast Z97.8
    - eye globe Z97.0
    - heart Z95.812
      - valve Z95.2
    - intestine Z97.8
    - joint Z96.60
      - hip — see Presence, hip joint implant
      - knee — see Presence, knee joint implant
      - specified site NEC Z96.698
    - kidney Z97.8
    - larynx Z96.3
    - lens Z96.1
    - limbs — see Presence, artificial, limb
    - liver Z97.8
    - lung Z97.8
    - pancreas Z97.8
  - by organ transplant (heterologous) (homologous) — see Transplant
- pacemaker
  - brain Z96.89
  - cardiac Z95.0
  - specified NEC Z96.89
- pancreatectomy Z90.410
  - complete Z90.410
  - partial Z90.411
  - total Z90.410
- physical restraint Z78.1
- pneumonectomy (complete) (partial) Z90.2
- pneumothorax, therapeutic Z98.3
- postcommotio cerebri F07.81
- postoperative (postprocedural) NEC Z98.890
  - breast implant Z98.82
  - dental Z98.818
    - crown Z98.811
    - fillings Z98.811
    - restoration Z98.811
    - sealant Z98.810
    - specified NEC Z98.818
  - pneumothorax, therapeutic Z98.3
  - uterine scar Z98.891
- postpartum (routine follow-up) Z39.2
  - care immediately after delivery Z39.0
- postsurgical (postprocedural) NEC Z98.890
  - pneumothorax, therapeutic Z98.3
- pregnancy, incidental Z33.1
- progesterone receptor
  - negative Z17.22
  - positive Z17.21
- prosthesis coronary angioplasty Z95.5
- pseudophakia Z96.1
- renal dialysis (hemodialysis) (peritoneal) Z99.2

Status — continued
- retained foreign body — see Retained, foreign body fragments (type of)
- reversed jejunal transposition (for bypass) Z98.0
- salpingo-oophorectomy
  - bilateral Z90.722
  - unilateral Z90.721
- sex reassignment surgery status Z87.890
- shunt
  - arteriovenous (for dialysis) Z99.2
  - cerebrospinal fluid Z98.2
  - ventricular (communicating) (for drainage) Z98.2
- splenectomy Z90.81
- thymicolymphaticus E32.8
- thymicus E32.8
- thymolymphaticus E32.8
- thyroidectomy (hypothyroidism) E89.0
- tooth (teeth) extraction — see also Absence, teeth, acquired K08.409
- tPA (rtPA) administration in a different facility within the last 24 hours prior to admission to current facility Z92.82
- tracheostomy Z93.0
- transplant — see Transplant
  - organ removed Z98.85
- tubal ligation Z98.51
- underimmunization Z28.39
  - COVID-19 Z28.31- ☑
    - partially vaccinated (for) Z28.311
    - unvaccinated (for) Z28.310
- ureterostomy Z93.6
- urethrostomy Z93.6
- vagina, artificial Z93.8
- vasectomy Z98.52
- ventilator Z99.11
- wheelchair confinement Z99.3

Stealing
- child problem F91.8
- in company with others Z72.810
- pathological (compulsive) F63.2

Steam burn — see Burn

Steatocystoma multiplex L72.2

Steatohepatitis (nonalcoholic) (NASH) K75.81
- metabolic dysfunction-associated steatohepatitis (MASH) K75.81

Steatoma L72.3
- eyelid (cystic) — see Dermatosis, eyelid
- infected — see Hordeolum

Steatorrhea (chronic) K90.9
- with lacteal obstruction K90.2
- idiopathic (adult) (infantile) K90.9
- pancreatic K90.3
- primary K90.0
- tropical K90.1

Steatosis E88.89
- heart — see Degeneration, myocardial
- kidney N28.89
- liver NEC K76.0

Steele-Richardson-Olszewski disease or syndrome G23.1

Stein-Leventhal syndrome E28.2

Steinbrocker's syndrome G90.89

Steinert's disease G71.11

Stein's syndrome E28.2

STEMI — see also Infarct, myocardium, ST elevation I21.3

Stenocardia I20.89

Stenocephaly Q75.8

Stenosis, stenotic (cicatricial) — see also Stricture
- ampulla of Vater K83.1
- anus, anal (canal) (sphincter) K62.4
  - and rectum K62.4
  - congenital Q42.3
    - with fistula Q42.2
- aorta (ascending) (supravalvular) (congenital) Q25.1
  - arteriosclerotic I70.0
  - calcified I70.0
  - supravalvular Q25.3
- aortic (valve) I35.0
  - with insufficiency I35.2
  - congenital Q23.0
  - rheumatic I06.0
    - with
      - incompetency, insufficiency or regurgitation I06.2
        - with mitral (valve) disease I08.0
          - with tricuspid (valve) disease I08.3
      - mitral (valve) disease I08.0
        - with tricuspid (valve) disease I08.3
      - tricuspid (valve) disease I08.2
        - with mitral (valve) disease I08.3

Stenosis, stenotic — continued
- aortic — continued
  - specified cause NEC I35.0
  - syphilitic A52.03
- aqueduct of Sylvius (congenital) Q03.0
  - with spina bifida — see Spina bifida, by site, with hydrocephalus
  - acquired G91.1
- artery NEC — see also Arteriosclerosis I77.1
  - celiac (compression) I77.4
    - arteriosclerotic I70.8
    - atherosclerosis I70.8
  - cerebral — see Occlusion, artery, cerebral
  - extremities — see Arteriosclerosis, extremities
  - precerebral — see Occlusion, artery, precerebral
  - pulmonary (congenital) Q25.6
    - acquired I28.8
  - renal I70.1
  - stent
    - coronary T82.855- ☑
    - peripheral T82.856- ☑
- bile duct (common) (hepatic) K83.1
  - congenital Q44.3
- bladder-neck (acquired) N32.0
  - congenital Q64.31
- brain G93.89
- bronchus J98.09
  - congenital Q32.3
  - syphilitic A52.72
- cardia (stomach) K22.2
  - congenital Q39.3
- cardiovascular — see Disease, cardiovascular
- caudal M48.08
- cervix, cervical (canal) N88.2
  - congenital Q51.828
  - in pregnancy or childbirth — see Pregnancy, complicated by, abnormal cervix
- colon — see also Obstruction, intestine
  - congenital Q42.9
    - specified NEC Q42.8
- colostomy K94.03
- common (bile) duct K83.1
  - congenital Q44.3
- coronary (artery) — see Disease, heart, ischemic, atherosclerotic
- cystic duct — see Obstruction, gallbladder
- due to presence of device, implant or graft — see also Complications, by site and type, specified NEC T85.858- ☑
  - arterial graft NEC T82.858- ☑
  - breast (implant) T85.858- ☑
  - catheter T85.858- ☑
    - dialysis (renal) T82.858- ☑
      - intraperitoneal T85.858- ☑
    - infusion NEC T82.858- ☑
      - spinal (epidural) (subdural) T85.850- ☑
    - urinary (indwelling) T83.85- ☑
  - fixation, internal (orthopedic) NEC T84.85- ☑
  - gastrointestinal (bile duct) (esophagus) T85.858- ☑
  - genital NEC T83.85- ☑
  - heart NEC T82.857- ☑
  - joint prosthesis T84.85- ☑
  - ocular (corneal graft) (orbital implant) NEC T85.858- ☑
  - orthopedic NEC T84.85- ☑
  - specified NEC T85.858- ☑
  - urinary NEC T83.85- ☑
  - vascular NEC T82.858- ☑
  - ventricular intracranial shunt T85.850- ☑
- duodenum K31.5
  - congenital Q41.0
- ejaculatory duct NEC N50.89
  - stent
    - vascular
      - end stent
        - adjacent to stent — see Arteriosclerosis
        - within the stent
          - coronary T82.855- ☑
          - peripheral T82.856- ☑
      - in stent
        - coronary vessel T82.855- ☑
        - peripheral vessel T82.856- ☑
- endocervical os — see Stenosis, cervix
- enterostomy K94.13
- esophagus K22.2
  - congenital Q39.3
  - syphilitic A52.79
    - congenital A50.59 [K23]

Stenosis, stenotic — continued
- eustachian tube — see Obstruction, eustachian tube
- external ear canal (acquired) H61.30- ☑
  - congenital Q16.1
  - due to
    - inflammation H61.32- ☑
    - trauma H61.31- ☑
  - postprocedural H95.81- ☑
  - specified cause NEC H61.39- ☑
- gallbladder — see Obstruction, gallbladder
- glottis J38.6
- heart valve — see also Endocarditis I38
  - aortic — see Stenosis, aortic
  - congenital Q24.8
  - mitral — see Stenosis, mitral
  - pulmonary — see Stenosis, pulmonary valve
  - tricuspid — see Stenosis, tricuspid
- hepatic duct K83.1
- hymen N89.6
- hypertrophic subaortic (idiopathic) I42.1
- ileum — see also Obstruction, intestine, specified NEC K56.699
  - congenital Q41.2
- infundibulum cardia Q24.3
- intervertebral foramina — see also Lesion, biomechanical, specified NEC
  - connective tissue M99.79
    - abdomen M99.79
    - cervical region M99.71
    - cervicothoracic M99.71
    - head region M99.70
    - lumbar region M99.73
    - lumbosacral M99.73
    - occipitocervical M99.70
    - sacral region M99.74
    - sacrococcygeal M99.74
    - sacroiliac M99.74
    - specified NEC M99.79
    - thoracic region M99.72
    - thoracolumbar M99.72
  - disc M99.79
    - abdomen M99.79
    - cervical region M99.71
    - cervicothoracic M99.71
    - head region M99.70
    - lower extremity M99.76
    - lumbar region M99.73
    - lumbosacral M99.73
    - occipitocervical M99.70
    - pelvic M99.75
    - rib cage M99.78
    - sacral region M99.74
    - sacrococcygeal M99.74
    - sacroiliac M99.74
    - specified NEC M99.79
    - thoracic region M99.72
    - thoracolumbar M99.72
    - upper extremity M99.77
  - osseous M99.69
    - abdomen M99.69
    - cervical region M99.61
    - cervicothoracic M99.61
    - head region M99.60
    - lower extremity M99.66
    - lumbar region M99.63
    - lumbosacral M99.63
    - occipitocervical M99.60
    - pelvic M99.65
    - rib cage M99.68
    - sacral region M99.64
    - sacrococcygeal M99.64
    - sacroiliac M99.64
    - specified NEC M99.69
    - thoracic region M99.62
    - thoracolumbar M99.62
    - upper extremity M99.67
  - subluxation — see Stenosis, intervertebral foramina, osseous
- intestine — see also Obstruction, intestine
  - congenital (small) Q41.9
    - large Q42.9
      - specified NEC Q42.8
    - specified NEC Q41.8
- jejunum — see also Obstruction, intestine, specified NEC K56.699
  - congenital Q41.1
- lacrimal (passage)
  - canaliculi H04.54- ☑

Stenosis, stenotic — continued
- lacrimal — continued
  - congenital Q10.5
  - duct H04.55- ☑
  - punctum H04.56- ☑
  - sac H04.57- ☑
- lacrimonasal duct — see Stenosis, lacrimal, duct
  - congenital Q10.5
- larynx J38.6
  - congenital NEC Q31.8
    - subglottic Q31.1
  - syphilitic A52.73
    - congenital A50.59 [J99]
- mitral (chronic) (inactive) (valve) I05.0
  - with
    - aortic valve disease I08.0
    - incompetency, insufficiency or regurgitation I05.2
      - active or acute I01.1
        - with rheumatic or Sydenham's chorea I02.0
  - congenital Q23.2
  - specified cause, except rheumatic I34.2
  - syphilitic A52.03
- myocardium, myocardial — see also Degeneration, myocardial
  - hypertrophic subaortic (idiopathic) I42.1
- nares (anterior) (posterior) J34.89
  - congenital Q30.0
- nasal duct — see also Stenosis, lacrimal, duct
  - congenital Q10.5
- nasolacrimal duct — see also Stenosis, lacrimal, duct
  - congenital Q10.5
- neural canal — see also Lesion, biomechanical, specified NEC
  - connective tissue M99.49
    - abdomen M99.49
    - cervical region M99.41
    - cervicothoracic M99.41
    - head region M99.40
    - lower extremity M99.46
    - lumbar region M99.43
    - lumbosacral M99.43
    - occipitocervical M99.40
    - pelvic M99.45
    - rib cage M99.48
    - sacral region M99.44
    - sacrococcygeal M99.44
    - sacroiliac M99.44
    - specified NEC M99.49
    - thoracic region M99.42
    - thoracolumbar M99.42
    - upper extremity M99.47
  - intervertebral disc M99.59
    - abdomen M99.59
    - cervical region M99.51
    - cervicothoracic M99.51
    - head region M99.50
    - lower extremity M99.56
    - lumbar region M99.53
    - lumbosacral M99.53
    - occipitocervical M99.50
    - pelvic M99.55
    - rib cage M99.58
    - sacral region M99.54
    - sacrococcygeal M99.54
    - sacroiliac M99.54
    - specified NEC M99.59
    - thoracic region M99.52
    - thoracolumbar M99.52
    - upper extremity M99.57
  - osseous M99.39
    - abdomen M99.39
    - cervical region M99.31
    - cervicothoracic M99.31
    - head region M99.30
    - lower extremity M99.36
    - lumbar region M99.33
    - lumbosacral M99.33
    - occipitocervical M99.30
    - pelvic M99.35
    - rib cage M99.38
    - sacral region M99.34
    - sacrococcygeal M99.34
    - sacroiliac M99.34
    - specified NEC M99.39
    - thoracic region M99.32
    - thoracolumbar M99.32
    - upper extremity M99.37
  - subluxation M99.29
    - cervical region M99.21

☑ Additional Character Required — Refer to the Tabular List for Character Selection

Stenosis, stenotic — continued
- neural canal — see also Lesion, biomechanical, specified — continued
  - subluxation — continued
    - cervicothoracic M99.21
    - head region M99.20
    - lower extremity M99.26
    - lumbar region M99.23
    - lumbosacral M99.23
    - occipitocervical M99.20
    - pelvic M99.25
    - rib cage M99.28
    - sacral region M99.24
    - sacrococcygeal M99.24
    - sacroiliac M99.24
    - specified NEC M99.29
    - thoracic region M99.22
    - thoracolumbar M99.22
    - upper extremity M99.27
- organ or site, congenital NEC — see Atresia, by site
- papilla of Vater K83.1
- pulmonary (artery) (congenital) Q25.6
  - with ventricular septal defect, transposition of aorta, and hypertrophy of right ventricle Q21.3
  - acquired I28.8
  - in tetralogy of Fallot Q21.3
  - infundibular Q24.3
  - subvalvular Q24.3
  - supravalvular Q25.6
  - valve I37.0
    - with insufficiency I37.2
    - congenital Q22.1
    - rheumatic I09.89
      - with aortic, mitral or tricuspid (valve) disease I08.8
  - vein, acquired I28.8
  - vessel NEC I28.8
- pulmonic (congenital) Q22.1
  - infundibular Q24.3
  - subvalvular Q24.3
- pylorus (hypertrophic) (acquired) K31.1
  - adult K31.1
  - congenital Q40.0
  - infantile Q40.0
- rectum (sphincter) — see Stricture, rectum
- renal artery I70.1
  - congenital Q27.1
- salivary duct (any) K11.8
- sphincter of Oddi K83.1
- spinal M48.00
  - cervical region M48.02
  - cervicothoracic region M48.03
  - lumbar region (NOS) (without neurogenic claudication) M48.061
    - with neurogenic claudication M48.062
  - lumbosacral region M48.07
  - occipito-atlanto-axial region M48.01
  - sacrococcygeal region M48.08
  - thoracic region M48.04
  - thoracolumbar region M48.05
- stomach, hourglass K31.2
- subaortic (congenital) Q24.4
  - hypertrophic (idiopathic) I42.1
- subglottic J38.6
  - congenital Q31.1
  - postprocedural J95.5
- trachea J39.8
  - congenital Q32.1
  - syphilitic A52.73
  - tuberculous NEC A15.5
- tracheostomy J95.03
- tricuspid (valve) I07.0
  - with
    - aortic (valve) disease I08.2
      - incompetency, insufficiency or regurgitation I07.2
        - with aortic (valve) disease I08.2
          - with mitral (valve) disease I08.3
    - mitral (valve) disease I08.1
      - with aortic (valve) disease I08.3
  - congenital Q22.4
  - nonrheumatic I36.0
    - with insufficiency I36.2
- tubal N97.1
- ureter — see Atresia, ureter
- ureteropelvic junction, congenital Q62.11
- ureterovesical orifice, congenital Q62.12
- urethra (valve) see also Stricture, urethra
  - congenital Q64.32
- urinary meatus, congenital Q64.33

Stenosis, stenotic — continued
- vagina N89.5
  - congenital Q52.4
  - in pregnancy — see Pregnancy, complicated by, abnormal vagina
    - causing obstructed labor O65.5
- valve (cardiac) (heart) — see also Endocarditis I38
  - congenital Q24.8
    - aortic Q23.0
    - mitral Q23.2
    - pulmonary Q22.1
    - tricuspid Q22.4
- vena cava (inferior) (superior) I87.1
  - congenital Q26.0
- vesicourethral orifice Q64.31
- vulva N90.5

Stent jail T82.897- ☑
Stercolith (impaction) K56.41
- appendix K38.1

Stercoraceous, stercoral ulcer K63.3
- anus or rectum K62.6

Stereotypies NEC F98.4
Sterility — see Infertility
Sterilization — see Encounter (for), sterilization
Sternalgia — see Angina
Sternopagus Q89.4
Sternum bifidum Q76.7
Steroid
- effects (adverse) (adrenocortical) (iatrogenic)
  - cushingoid E24.2
    - correct substance properly administered — see Table of Drugs and Chemicals, by drug, adverse effect
    - overdose or wrong substance given or taken — see Table of Drugs and Chemicals, by drug, poisoning
  - diabetes — see subcategory E09.-
    - correct substance properly administered — see Table of Drugs and Chemicals, by drug, adverse effect
    - overdose or wrong substance given or taken — see Table of Drugs and Chemicals, by drug, poisoning
  - fever R50.2
  - insufficiency E27.3
    - correct substance properly administered — see Table of Drugs and Chemicals, by drug, adverse effect
    - overdose or wrong substance given or taken — see Table of Drugs and Chemicals, by drug, poisoning
- responder H40.04- ☑

Stevens-Johnson disease or syndrome L51.1
- toxic epidermal necrolysis overlap L51.3

Stewart-Morel syndrome M85.2
Sticker's disease B08.3
Sticky eye — see Conjunctivitis, acute, mucopurulent
Stieda's disease — see Bursitis, tibial collateral
Stiff-man syndrome G25.82
Stiff neck — see Torticollis
Stiffness, joint NEC M25.60
- ankle M25.67- ☑
- ankylosis — see Ankylosis, joint
- contracture — see Contraction, joint
- elbow M25.62- ☑
- foot M25.67- ☑
- hand M25.64- ☑
- hip M25.65- ☑
- knee M25.66- ☑
- shoulder M25.61- ☑
- specified site NEC M25.69
- wrist M25.63- ☑

Stigmata congenital syphilis A50.59
Still-Felty syndrome — see Felty's syndrome
Stillbirth P95
Still's disease or syndrome (juvenile) M08.20
- adult-onset M06.1
- ankle M08.27- ☑
- elbow M08.22- ☑
- foot joint M08.27- ☑
- hand joint M08.24- ☑
- hip M08.25- ☑
- knee M08.26- ☑
- multiple site M08.29
- shoulder M08.21- ☑
- specified site NEC M08.2A
- vertebra M08.28
- wrist M08.23- ☑

Stimulation, ovary E28.1
Sting (venomous) (with allergic or anaphylactic shock) — see Table of Drugs and Chemicals, by animal or substance, poisoning
Stippled epiphyses Q78.8
Stitch
- abscess T81.41- ☑
- burst (in operation wound) — see Disruption, wound, operation

Stokes-Adams disease or syndrome I45.9
Stokes' disease E05.00
- with thyroid storm E05.01

Stokvis (-Talma) **disease** D74.8
Stoma malfunction
- colostomy K94.03
- enterostomy K94.13
- gastrostomy K94.23
- ileostomy K94.13
- tracheostomy J95.03

Stomach — see condition
Stomatitis (denture) (ulcerative) K12.1
- angular K13.0
  - due to dietary or vitamin deficiency E53.0
- aphthous K12.0
- bovine B08.61
- candidal B37.0
- catarrhal K12.1
- diphtheritic A36.89
- due to
  - dietary deficiency E53.0
  - thrush B37.0
  - vitamin deficiency
    - B group NEC E53.9
    - B2 (riboflavin) E53.0
- epidemic B08.8
- epizootic B08.8
- follicular K12.1
- gangrenous A69.0
- Geotrichum B48.3
- herpesviral, herpetic B00.2
- herpetiformis K12.0
- malignant K12.1
- membranous acute K12.1
- monilial B37.0
- mycotic B37.0
- necrotizing ulcerative A69.0
- parasitic B37.0
- septic K12.1
- spirochetal A69.1
- suppurative (acute) K12.2
- ulceromembranous A69.1
- vesicular K12.1
  - with exanthem (enteroviral) B08.4
  - virus disease A93.8
- Vincent's A69.1

Stomatocytosis D58.8
Stomatomycosis B37.0
Stomatorrhagia K13.79
Stone(s) — see also Calculus
- bladder (diverticulum) N21.0
- cystine E72.09
- heart syndrome I50.1
- kidney N20.0
- prostate N42.0
- pulpal (dental) K04.2
- renal N20.0
- salivary gland or duct (any) K11.5
- urethra (impacted) N21.1
- urinary (duct) (impacted) (passage) N20.9
  - bladder (diverticulum) N21.0
  - lower tract N21.9
  - specified NEC N21.8
- xanthine E79.82 [N22]

Stonecutter's lung J62.8
Stonemason's asthma, disease, lung or pneumoconiosis J62.8
Stoppage
- heart — see Arrest, cardiac
- urine — see Retention, urine

Storm, thyroid — see Thyrotoxicosis
Strabismus (congenital) (nonparalytic) H50.9
- concomitant H50.40
  - convergent — see Strabismus, convergent concomitant
  - divergent — see Strabismus, divergent concomitant
- convergent concomitant H50.00
  - accommodative component H50.43
  - alternating H50.05

Strabismus — continued
  convergent concomitant — continued
    alternating — continued
      with
        A pattern H50.06
        specified nonconcomitances NEC H50.08
        V pattern H50.07
      monocular H50.01- ☑
        with
          A pattern H50.02- ☑
          specified nonconcomitances NEC H50.04- ☑
          V pattern H50.03- ☑
        intermittent H50.31- ☑
          alternating H50.32
  cyclotropia H50.41- ☑
  divergent concomitant H50.10
    alternating H50.15
      with
        A pattern H50.16
        specified noncomitances NEC H50.18
        V pattern H50.17
      monocular H50.11- ☑
        with
          A pattern H50.12- ☑
          specified nonconcomitances NEC H50.14- ☑
          V pattern H50.13- ☑
        intermittent H50.33- ☑
          alternating H50.34
  Duane's syndrome H50.81- ☑
  due to adhesions, scars H50.69
  heterophoria H50.50
    alternating H50.55
    cyclophoria H50.54
    esophoria H50.51
    exophoria H50.52
    vertical H50.53
  heterotropia H50.40
    intermittent H50.30
  hypertropia H50.2- ☑
  hypotropia — see Hypertropia
  latent H50.50
  mechanical H50.60
    Brown's sheath syndrome H50.61- ☑
    specified type NEC H50.69
  monofixation syndrome H50.42
  paralytic H49.9
    abducens nerve H49.2- ☑
    fourth nerve H49.1- ☑
    Kearns-Sayre syndrome H49.81- ☑
    ophthalmoplegia (external)
      progressive H49.4- ☑
        with pigmentary retinopathy H49.81- ☑
      total H49.3- ☑
    sixth nerve H49.2- ☑
    specified type NEC H49.88- ☑
    third nerve H49.0- ☑
    trochlear nerve H49.1- ☑
  specified type NEC H50.89
  vertical H50.2- ☑
Strain
  back S39.012- ☑
  cervical S16.1- ☑
  eye NEC — see Disturbance, vision, subjective
  heart — see Disease, heart
  low back S39.012- ☑
  mental NOS Z73.3
    work-related Z56.6
  muscle (tendon) — see Injury, muscle, by site, strain
  neck S16.1- ☑
  physical NOS Z73.3
    work-related Z56.6
  postural — see also Disorder, soft tissue, due to use
  psychological NEC Z73.3
  tendon — see Injury, muscle, by site, strain
Straining, on urination R39.16
Strand, vitreous — see Opacity, vitreous, membranes and strands
Strangulation, strangulated — see also Asphyxia, traumatic
  appendix K38.8
  bladder-neck N32.0
  bowel or colon K56.2
  food or foreign body — see Foreign body, by site
  hemorrhoids — see Hemorrhoids, with complication
  hernia — see also Hernia, by site, with obstruction
    with gangrene — see Hernia, by site, with gangrene
  intestine (large) (small) K56.2

Strangulation, strangulated — continued
  intestine — continued
    with hernia — see also Hernia, by site, with obstruction
      with gangrene — see Hernia, by site, with gangrene
  mesentery K56.2
  mucus — see Asphyxia, mucus
  omentum K56.2
  organ or site, congenital NEC — see Atresia, by site
  ovary — see Torsion, ovary
  penis N48.89
    foreign body T19.4- ☑
  rupture — see Hernia, by site, with obstruction
  stomach due to hernia — see also Hernia, by site, with obstruction
    with gangrene — see Hernia, by site, with gangrene
  vesicourethral orifice N32.0
Strangury R30.0
Straw itch B88.09
Strawberry
  gallbladder K82.4
  mark Q82.5
  tongue (red) (white) K14.3
Streak(s)
  macula, angioid H35.33
  ovarian Q50.32
Strephosymbolia F81.0
  secondary to organic lesion R48.8
Streptobacillary fever A25.1
Streptobacillosis A25.1
Streptobacillus moniliformis A25.1
Streptococcus, streptococcal — see also condition
  as cause of disease classified elsewhere B95.5
  group
    A, as cause of disease classified elsewhere B95.0
    B, as cause of disease classified elsewhere B95.1
    D, as cause of disease classified elsewhere B95.2
  pneumoniae, as cause of disease classified elsewhere B95.3
  specified NEC, as cause of disease classified elsewhere B95.4
Streptomycosis B47.1
Streptotrichosis A48.8
Stress F43.9
  family — see Disruption, family
  fetal P84
    complicating pregnancy O77.9
      due to drug administration O77.1
  mental NEC Z73.3
    work-related Z56.6
  physical NEC Z73.3
    work-related Z56.6
  polycythemia D75.1
  reaction — see also Reaction, stress F43.9
  work schedule Z56.3
  workplace Z56.6
Stretching, nerve — see Injury, nerve
Striae albicantes, atrophicae or distensae (cutis) L90.6
Stricture — see also Stenosis
  ampulla of Vater K83.1
  anus (sphincter) K62.4
    congenital Q42.3
      with fistula Q42.2
    infantile Q42.3
      with fistula Q42.2
  aorta (ascending) (congenital) Q25.1
    arteriosclerotic I70.0
    calcified I70.0
    supravalvular, congenital Q25.3
  aortic (valve) — see Stenosis, aortic
  aqueduct of Sylvius (congenital) Q03.0
    with spina bifida — see Spina bifida, by site, with hydrocephalus
    acquired G91.1
  artery I77.1
    basilar — see Occlusion, artery, basilar
    carotid — see Occlusion, artery, carotid
    celiac (compression) I77.4
      arteriosclerotic I70.0
      atherosclerosis I70.0
    congenital (peripheral) Q27.8
      cerebral Q28.3
      coronary Q24.5
      digestive system Q27.8
      lower limb Q27.8
      retinal Q14.1
      specified site NEC Q27.8
      umbilical Q27.0

Stricture — continued
  artery — continued
    congenital — continued
      upper limb Q27.8
    coronary — see Disease, heart, ischemic, atherosclerotic
      congenital Q24.5
    precerebral — see Occlusion, artery, precerebral
    pulmonary (congenital) Q25.6
      acquired I28.8
    renal I70.1
    vertebral — see Occlusion, artery, vertebral
  auditory canal (external) (congenital)
    acquired — see Stenosis, external ear canal
  bile duct (common) (hepatic) K83.1
    congenital Q44.3
    postoperative K91.89
  bladder N32.89
    neck N32.0
  bowel — see Obstruction, intestine
  brain G93.89
  bronchus J98.09
    congenital Q32.3
    syphilitic A52.72
  cardia (stomach) K22.2
    congenital Q39.3
  cardiac — see also Disease, heart
    orifice (stomach) K22.2
  cecum — see Obstruction, intestine
  cervix, cervical (canal) N88.2
    congenital Q51.828
    in pregnancy — see Pregnancy, complicated by, abnormal cervix
      causing obstructed labor O65.5
  colon — see also Obstruction, intestine
    congenital Q42.9
    specified NEC Q42.8
  colostomy K94.03
  common (bile) duct K83.1
  coronary (artery) — see Disease, heart, ischemic, atherosclerotic
  cystic duct — see Obstruction, gallbladder
  digestive organs NEC, congenital Q45.8
  duodenum K31.5
    congenital Q41.0
  ear canal (external) (congenital) Q16.1
    acquired — see Stricture, auditory canal, acquired
  ejaculatory duct N50.89
  enterostomy K94.13
  esophagus K22.2
    congenital Q39.3
    syphilitic A52.79
      congenital A50.59 [K23]
  eustachian tube — see also Obstruction, eustachian tube
    congenital Q17.8
  fallopian tube N97.1
    gonococcal A54.24
    tuberculous A18.17
  gallbladder — see Obstruction, gallbladder
  glottis J38.6
  heart — see also Disease, heart
    valve — see also Endocarditis I38
      aortic Q23.0
      mitral Q23.2
      pulmonary Q22.1
      tricuspid Q22.4
  hepatic duct K83.1
  hourglass, of stomach K31.2
  hymen N89.6
  hypopharynx J39.2
  ileum — see also Obstruction, intestine, specified NEC K56.699
    congenital Q41.2
  intestine — see also Obstruction, intestine
    congenital (small) Q41.9
      large Q42.9
        specified NEC Q42.8
      specified NEC Q41.8
    ischemic K55.1
  jejunum — see also Obstruction, intestine, specified NEC K56.699
    congenital Q41.1
  lacrimal passages — see also Stenosis, lacrimal
    congenital Q10.5
  larynx J38.6
    congenital NEC Q31.8
      subglottic Q31.1
    syphilitic A52.73
      congenital A50.59 [J99]

☑ Additional Character Required — Refer to the Tabular List for Character Selection

Stricture — continued
- meatus
  - ear (congenital) Q16.1
    - acquired — see Stricture, auditory canal, acquired
  - osseous (ear) (congenital) Q16.1
    - acquired — see Stricture, auditory canal, acquired
  - urinarius — see also Stricture, urethra
    - congenital Q64.33
- mitral (valve) — see Stenosis, mitral
- myocardium, myocardial I51.5
  - hypertrophic subaortic (idiopathic) I42.1
- nares (anterior) (posterior) J34.89
  - congenital Q30.0
- nasal duct — see also Stenosis, lacrimal, duct
  - congenital Q10.5
- nasolacrimal duct — see also Stenosis, lacrimal, duct
  - congenital Q10.5
- nasopharynx J39.2
  - syphilitic A52.73
- nose J34.89
  - congenital Q30.0
- nostril (anterior) (posterior) J34.89
  - congenital Q30.0
  - syphilitic A52.73
    - congenital A50.59 [J99]
- organ or site, congenital NEC — see Atresia, by site
- os uteri — see Stricture, cervix
- osseous meatus (ear) (congenital) Q16.1
  - acquired — see Stricture, auditory canal, acquired
- oviduct — see Stricture, fallopian tube
- pelviureteric junction (congenital) Q62.11
  - acquired, with hydronephrosis N13.0
- penis, by foreign body T19.4- ☑
- pharynx J39.2
- prostate N42.89
- pulmonary, pulmonic
  - artery (congenital) Q25.6
    - acquired I28.8
    - noncongenital I28.8
  - infundibulum (congenital) Q24.3
  - valve I37.0
    - congenital Q22.1
  - vein, acquired I28.8
  - vessel NEC I28.8
- punctum lacrimale — see also Stenosis, lacrimal, punctum
  - congenital Q10.5
- pylorus (hypertrophic) K31.1
  - adult K31.1
  - congenital Q40.0
  - infantile Q40.0
- rectosigmoid — see also Obstruction, intestine, specified NEC K56.699
- rectum (sphincter) K62.4
  - congenital Q42.1
    - with fistula Q42.0
  - due to
    - chlamydial lymphogranuloma A55
    - irradiation K91.89
    - lymphogranuloma venereum A55
  - gonococcal A54.6
  - inflammatory (chlamydial) A55
  - syphilitic A52.74
  - tuberculous A18.32
- renal artery I70.1
  - congenital Q27.1
- salivary duct or gland (any) K11.8
- sigmoid (flexure) — see Obstruction, intestine
- spermatic cord N50.89
- stoma (following) (of)
  - colostomy K94.03
  - enterostomy K94.13
  - gastrostomy K94.23
  - ileostomy K94.13
  - tracheostomy J95.03
- stomach K31.89
  - congenital Q40.2
  - hourglass K31.2
- subaortic Q24.4
  - hypertrophic (acquired) (idiopathic) I42.1
- subglottic J38.6
- syphilitic NEC A52.79
- trachea J39.8
  - congenital Q32.1
  - syphilitic A52.73
  - tuberculous NEC A15.5
- tracheostomy J95.03
- tricuspid (valve) — see Stenosis, tricuspid
- tunica vaginalis N50.89

Stricture — continued
- ureter (postoperative) N13.5
  - with
    - hydronephrosis N13.1
      - with infection N13.6
    - pyelonephritis (chronic) N11.1
  - congenital — see Atresia, ureter
  - tuberculous A18.11
- ureteropelvic junction (congenital) Q62.11
  - acquired, with hydronephrosis N13.0
- ureterovesical orifice N13.5
  - with infection N13.6
- urethra (organic) (spasmodic) — see also Stricture, urethra, male N35.919
  - associated with schistosomiasis B65.0 [N37]
  - congenital Q64.39
    - valvular (posterior) Q64.2
  - due to
    - infection — see Stricture, urethra, postinfective
    - trauma — see Stricture, urethra, post-traumatic
  - female N35.92
    - gonococcal, gonorrheal A54.01
  - infective NEC — see Stricture, urethra, postinfective
  - late effect (sequelae) of injury — see Stricture, urethra, post-traumatic
  - male N35.919
    - anterior urethra N35.914
    - bulbous urethra N35.912
    - meatal N35.911
    - membranous urethra N35.913
    - overlapping sites N35.916
  - postcatheterization — see Stricture, urethra, postprocedural
  - postinfective NEC
    - female N35.12
    - male N35.119
      - anterior urethra N35.114
      - bulbous urethra N35.112
      - meatal N35.111
      - membranous urethra N35.113
      - overlapping sites N35.116
  - postobstetric N35.021
  - postoperative — see Stricture, urethra, postprocedural
  - postprocedural
    - female N99.12
    - male N99.114
      - anterior bulbous urethra N99.113
      - bulbous urethra N99.111
      - fossa navicularis N99.115
      - meatal N99.110
      - membranous urethra N99.112
      - overlapping sites N99.116
  - post-traumatic
    - female N35.028
      - due to childbirth N35.021
    - male N35.014
      - anterior urethra N35.013
      - bulbous urethra N35.011
      - meatal N35.010
      - membranous urethra N35.012
      - overlapping sites N35.016
  - sequela (late effect) of
    - childbirth N35.021
    - injury — see Stricture, urethra, post-traumatic
  - specified cause NEC
    - female N35.82
    - male N35.819
      - anterior urethra N35.814
      - bulbous urethra N35.812
      - meatal N35.811
      - membranous urethra N35.813
      - overlapping sites N35.816
  - syphilitic A52.76
  - traumatic — see Stricture, urethra, post-traumatic
  - valvular (posterior), congenital Q64.2
- urinary meatus — see Stricture, urethra
- uterus, uterine (synechiae) N85.6
  - os (external) (internal) — see Stricture, cervix
- vagina (outlet) — see Stenosis, vagina
- valve (cardiac) (heart) — see also Endocarditis
  - congenital
    - aortic Q23.0
    - mitral Q23.2
    - pulmonary Q22.1
    - tricuspid Q22.4
- vas deferens N50.89
  - congenital Q55.4
- vein I87.1
- vena cava (inferior) (superior) NEC I87.1

Stricture — continued
- vena cava — continued
  - congenital Q26.0
- vesicourethral orifice N32.0
  - congenital Q64.31
- vulva (acquired) N90.5

Stridor R06.1
- congenital (larynx) P28.89

Stridulous — see condition

Stroke (apoplectic) (brain) (ischemic) (paralytic) I63.9
- cerebral, perinatal P91.82- ☑
- cerebrovascular (ischemic) I63.9
  - chronic (old) (remote) (imaging) (without sequelae) Z86.73
    - with residual defects — see Sequelae, disease, cerebrovascular
  - embolic I63.- ☑
  - thrombotic I63.- ☑
- cryptogenic — see also infarction, cerebral I63.9
- epileptic — see Epilepsy
- heat T67.01- ☑
  - exertional T67.02- ☑
  - specified NEC T67.09- ☑
- in evolution I63.9
- intraoperative
  - during cardiac surgery I97.810
  - during other surgery I97.811
- ischemic, perinatal arterial P91.82- ☑
- lightning — see Lightning
- meaning
  - cerebral hemorrhage — code to Hemorrhage, intracranial
  - cerebral infarction — code to Infarction, cerebral
- neonatal P91.82- ☑
- postprocedural
  - following cardiac surgery I97.820
  - following other surgery I97.821
- sun T67.01- ☑
  - specified NEC T67.09- ☑
- unspecified (NOS) I63.9

Stromatosis, endometrial D39.0
Strongyloidiasis, strongyloidosis B78.9
- cutaneous B78.1
- disseminated B78.7
- intestinal B78.0

Strophulus pruriginosus L28.2
Struck by lightning — see Lightning
Struma — see also Goiter
- Hashimoto E06.3
- lymphomatosa E06.3
- nodosa (simplex) E04.9
  - endemic E01.2
    - multinodular E01.1
  - multinodular E04.2
    - iodine-deficiency related E01.1
  - toxic or with hyperthyroidism E05.20
    - with thyroid storm E05.21
    - multinodular E05.20
      - with thyroid storm E05.21
    - uninodular E05.10
      - with thyroid storm E05.11
  - toxicosa E05.20
    - with thyroid storm E05.21
    - multinodular E05.20
      - with thyroid storm E05.21
    - uninodular E05.10
      - with thyroid storm E05.11
  - uninodular E04.1
- ovarii D27.- ☑
- Riedel's E06.5

Strumipriva cachexia E03.4
Strumpell-Marie spine — see Spondylitis, ankylosing
Strumpell-Westphal pseudosclerosis E83.01
Stuart deficiency disease (factor X) D68.2
Stuart-Prower factor deficiency (factor X) D68.2
Student's elbow — see Bursitis, elbow, olecranon
Stump — see Amputation
Stunting, nutritional E45
Stupor (catatonic) R40.1
- depressive (single episode) F32.89
  - recurrent episode F33.8
- dissociative F44.2
- manic F30.2
- manic-depressive F31.89
- psychogenic (anergic) F44.2
- reaction to exceptional stress (transient) F43.0

Sturge (-Weber) (-Dimitri) (-Kalischer) **disease or syndrome** Q85.89

Stuttering F80.81
  adult onset F98.5
  childhood onset F80.81
  following cerebrovascular disease — *see* Disorder, fluency, following cerebrovascular disease
  in conditions classified elsewhere R47.82
Sty, stye (external) (internal) (meibomian) (zeisian) — *see* Hordeolum
Subacidity, gastric K31.89
  psychogenic F45.8
Subacute — *see* condition
Subarachnoid — *see* condition
Subcortical — *see* condition
Subcostal syndrome, nerve compression — *see* Mononeuropathy, upper limb, specified site NEC
Subcutaneous, subcuticular — *see* condition
Subdural — *see* condition
Subendocardium — *see* condition
Subependymoma
  specified site — *see* Neoplasm, uncertain behavior, by site
  unspecified site D43.2
Suberosis J67.3
Subglossitis — *see* Glossitis
Subhemophilia D66
Subinvolution
  breast (postlactational) (postpuerperal) N64.89
  puerperal O90.89
  uterus (chronic) (nonpuerperal) N85.3
    puerperal O90.89
Sublingual — *see* condition
Sublinguitis — *see* Sialoadenitis
Subluxatable hip Q65.6
Subluxation — *see also* Dislocation
  acromioclavicular S43.11- ☑
  ankle S93.0- ☑
  atlantoaxial, recurrent M43.4
    with myelopathy M43.3
  carpometacarpal (joint) NEC S63.05- ☑
    thumb S63.04- ☑
  complex, vertebral — *see* Complex, subluxation
  congenital — *see also* Malposition, congenital
    hip — *see* Dislocation, hip, congenital, partial
    joint (excluding hip)
      lower limb Q68.8
      shoulder Q68.8
      upper limb Q68.8
  elbow (traumatic) S53.10- ☑
    anterior S53.11- ☑
    lateral S53.14- ☑
    medial S53.13- ☑
    posterior S53.12- ☑
    specified type NEC S53.19- ☑
  finger S63.20- ☑
    index S63.20- ☑
    interphalangeal S63.22- ☑
      distal S63.24- ☑
        index S63.24- ☑
        little S63.24- ☑
        middle S63.24- ☑
        ring S63.24- ☑
      index S63.22- ☑
      little S63.22- ☑
      middle S63.22- ☑
      proximal S63.23- ☑
        index S63.23- ☑
        little S63.23- ☑
        middle S63.23- ☑
        ring S63.23- ☑
      ring S63.22- ☑
    little S63.20- ☑
    metacarpophalangeal S63.21- ☑
      index S63.21- ☑
      little S63.21- ☑
      middle S63.21- ☑
      ring S63.21- ☑
    middle S63.20- ☑
    ring S63.20- ☑
  foot S93.30- ☑
    specified site NEC S93.33- ☑
    tarsal joint S93.31- ☑
    tarsometatarsal joint S93.32- ☑
    toe — *see* Subluxation, toe
  hip S73.00- ☑
    anterior S73.03- ☑
      obturator S73.02- ☑
    central S73.04- ☑

Subluxation — *continued*
  hip — *continued*
    posterior S73.01- ☑
  interphalangeal (joint)
    finger S63.22- ☑
      distal joint S63.24- ☑
        index S63.24- ☑
        little S63.24- ☑
        middle S63.24- ☑
        ring S63.24- ☑
      index S63.22- ☑
      little S63.22- ☑
      middle S63.22- ☑
      proximal joint S63.23- ☑
        index S63.23- ☑
        little S63.23- ☑
        middle S63.23- ☑
        ring S63.23- ☑
      ring S63.22- ☑
    thumb S63.12- ☑
    toe S93.13- ☑
      great S93.13- ☑
      lesser S93.13- ☑
  joint prosthesis — *see* Complications, joint prosthesis, mechanical, displacement, by site
  knee S83.10- ☑
    cap — *see* Subluxation, patella
    patella — *see* Subluxation, patella
    proximal tibia
      anteriorly S83.11- ☑
      laterally S83.14- ☑
      medially S83.13- ☑
      posteriorly S83.12- ☑
    specified type NEC S83.19- ☑
  lens — *see* Dislocation, lens, partial
  ligament, traumatic — *see* Sprain, by site
  metacarpal (bone)
    proximal end S63.06- ☑
  metacarpophalangeal (joint)
    finger S63.21- ☑
      index S63.21- ☑
      little S63.21- ☑
      middle S63.21- ☑
      ring S63.21- ☑
    thumb S63.11- ☑
  metatarsophalangeal joint S93.14- ☑
    great toe S93.14- ☑
    lesser toe S93.14- ☑
  midcarpal (joint) S63.03- ☑
  patella S83.00- ☑
    lateral S83.01- ☑
    recurrent (nontraumatic) — *see* Dislocation, patella, recurrent, incomplete
    specified type NEC S83.09- ☑
  pathological — *see* Dislocation, pathological
  radial head S53.00- ☑
    anterior S53.01- ☑
    nursemaid's elbow S53.03- ☑
    posterior S53.02- ☑
    specified type NEC S53.09- ☑
  radiocarpal (joint) S63.02- ☑
  radioulnar (joint)
    distal S63.01- ☑
    proximal — *see* Subluxation, elbow
  shoulder
    congenital Q68.8
    girdle S43.30- ☑
      scapula S43.31- ☑
      specified site NEC S43.39- ☑
    traumatic S43.00- ☑
      anterior S43.01- ☑
      inferior S43.03- ☑
      posterior S43.02- ☑
      specified type NEC S43.08- ☑
  sternoclavicular (joint) S43.20- ☑
    anterior S43.21- ☑
    posterior S43.22- ☑
  symphysis (pubis) — *see also* Dislocation, symphysis pubis
  thumb S63.103- ☑
    interphalangeal joint — *see* Subluxation, interphalangeal (joint), thumb
    metacarpophalangeal joint — *see* Subluxation, metacarpophalangeal (joint), thumb
  toe(s) S93.10- ☑
    great S93.10- ☑

Subluxation — *continued*
  toe(s) — *continued*
    great — *continued*
      interphalangeal joint S93.13- ☑
      metatarsophalangeal joint S93.14- ☑
    interphalangeal joint S93.13- ☑
    lesser S93.10- ☑
      interphalangeal joint S93.13- ☑
      metatarsophalangeal joint S93.14- ☑
    metatarsophalangeal joint S93.149- ☑
  ulna
    distal end S63.07- ☑
    proximal end — *see* Subluxation, elbow
  ulnohumeral joint — *see* Subluxation, elbow
  vertebral
    recurrent NEC — *see* subcategory M43.5- ☑
    traumatic
      cervical S13.100- ☑
        atlantoaxial joint S13.120- ☑
        atlantooccipital joint S13.110- ☑
        atloidooccipital joint S13.110- ☑
        joint between
          C0 and C1 S13.110- ☑
          C1 and C2 S13.120- ☑
          C2 and C3 S13.130- ☑
          C3 and C4 S13.140- ☑
          C4 and C5 S13.150- ☑
          C5 and C6 S13.160- ☑
          C6 and C7 S13.170- ☑
          C7 and T1 S13.180- ☑
        occipitoatloid joint S13.110- ☑
      lumbar S33.100- ☑
        joint between
          L1 and L2 S33.110- ☑
          L2 and L3 S33.120- ☑
          L3 and L4 S33.130- ☑
          L4 and L5 S33.140- ☑
      thoracic S23.100- ☑
        joint between
          T1 and T2 S23.110- ☑
          T2 and T3 S23.120- ☑
          T3 and T4 S23.122- ☑
          T4 and T5 S23.130- ☑
          T5 and T6 S23.132- ☑
          T6 and T7 S23.140- ☑
          T7 and T8 S23.142- ☑
          T8 and T9 S23.150- ☑
          T9 and T10 S23.152- ☑
          T10 and T11 S23.160- ☑
          T11 and T12 S23.162- ☑
          T12 and L1 S23.170- ☑
  wrist (carpal bone) S63.00- ☑
    carpometacarpal joint — *see* Subluxation, carpometacarpal (joint)
    distal radioulnar joint — *see* Subluxation, radioulnar (joint), distal
    metacarpal bone, proximal — *see* Subluxation, metacarpal (bone), proximal end
    midcarpal — *see* Subluxation, midcarpal (joint)
    radiocarpal joint — *see* Subluxation, radiocarpal (joint)
    recurrent — *see* Dislocation, recurrent, wrist
    specified site NEC S63.09- ☑
    ulna — *see* Subluxation, ulna, distal end
Submaxillary — *see* condition
Submersion (fatal) (nonfatal) T75.1- ☑
Submucous — *see* condition
Subnormal, subnormality
  accommodation (old age) H52.4
  mental — *see* Disability, intellectual
  temperature (accidental) T68.- ☑
Subphrenic — *see* condition
Subscapular nerve — *see* condition
Subseptus uterus Q51.28
Subsiding appendicitis K36
Substance (other psychoactive) **-induced**
  anxiety disorder F19.980
  bipolar and related disorder F19.94
  delirium F19.921
  depressive disorder F19.94
  major neurocognitive disorder F19.97
  mild neurocognitive disorder F19.988
  obsessive-compulsive and related disorder F19.988
  psychotic disorder F19.959
  sexual dysfunction F19.981
  sleep disorder F19.982
Substernal thyroid E04.9
  congenital Q89.2

Substitution disorder F44.9
Subtentorial — see condition
Subthyroidism (acquired) — see also Hypothyroidism
  congenital E03.1
Succenturiate placenta O43.19- ☑
Sucking thumb, child (excessive) F98.8
Sudamen, sudamina L74.1
Sudanese kala-azar B55.0
Sudden
  hearing loss — see Deafness, sudden
  heart failure — see Failure, heart
Sudden infant death syndrome (SIDS) R99
Sudeck's atrophy, disease, or syndrome — see Algoneurodystrophy
Suffocation — see Asphyxia, traumatic
Sugar
  blood
    high (transient) R73.9
    low (transient) E16.2
  in urine R81
Suicide, suicidal (attempted) T14.91- ☑
  by poisoning — see Table of Drugs and Chemicals
  history of (personal) Z91.51
    in family Z81.8
  ideation — see Ideation, suicidal
  risk
    meaning personal history of attempted suicide Z91.51
    meaning suicidal ideation — see Ideation, suicidal
  tendencies
    meaning personal history of attempted suicide Z91.51
    meaning suicidal ideation — see Ideation, suicidal
  trauma — see nature of injury by site
Suipestifer infection — see Infection, salmonella
Sulfhemoglobinemia, sulphemoglobinemia (acquired) (with methemoglobinemia) D74.8
Sumatran mite fever A75.3
Summer — see condition
Sunburn L55.9
  due to
    tanning bed (acute) L56.8
      chronic L57.8
    ultraviolet radiation (acute) L56.8
      chronic L57.8
  first degree L55.0
  second degree L55.1
  third degree L55.2
SUNCT (short lasting unilateral neuralgiform headache with conjunctival injection and tearing) G44.059
  intractable G44.051
  not intractable G44.059
Sundowning F05
Sunken acetabulum — see Derangement, joint, specified type NEC, hip
Sunstroke T67.01- ☑
  specified NEC T67.09- ☑
Superfecundation — see Pregnancy, multiple
Superfetation — see Pregnancy, multiple
Superinvolution (uterus) N85.8
Supernumerary (congenital)
  aortic cusps Q23.88
  auditory ossicles Q16.3
  bone Q79.8
  breast Q83.1
  carpal bones Q74.0
  cusps, heart valve NEC Q24.8
    aortic Q23.88
    mitral Q23.2
    pulmonary Q22.3
  digit(s) Q69.9
  ear (lobule) Q17.0
  fallopian tube Q50.6
  finger Q69.0
  hymen Q52.4
  kidney Q63.0
  lacrimonasal duct Q10.6
  lobule (ear) Q17.0
  mitral cusps Q23.2
  muscle Q79.8
  nipple(s) Q83.3
  organ or site not listed — see Accessory
  ossicles, auditory Q16.3
  ovary Q50.31
  oviduct Q50.6
  pulmonary, pulmonic cusps Q22.3
  rib Q76.6
    cervical or first (syndrome) Q76.5
  roots (of teeth) K00.2
  spleen Q89.09
  tarsal bones Q74.2

Supernumerary — continued
  teeth K00.1
  testis Q55.29
  thumb Q69.1
  toe Q69.2
  uterus Q51.28
  vagina Q52.1- ☑
  vertebra Q76.49
Supervision (of)
  contraceptive — see Prescription, contraceptives
  dietary (for) Z71.3
    allergy (food) Z71.3
    colitis Z71.3
    diabetes mellitus Z71.3
    food allergy or intolerance Z71.3
    gastritis Z71.3
    hypercholesterolemia Z71.3
    hypoglycemia Z71.3
    intolerance (food) Z71.3
    obesity Z71.3
    specified NEC Z71.3
  healthy infant or child Z76.2
    foundling Z76.1
  high-risk pregnancy — see Pregnancy, supervision of, high-risk
  lactation Z39.1
  pregnancy — see Pregnancy, supervision of
Supplemental teeth K00.1
Suppression
  binocular vision H53.34
  lactation O92.5
  menstruation N94.89
  ovarian secretion E28.39
  renal N28.9
  urine, urinary secretion R34
Suppuration, suppurative — see also condition
  accessory sinus (chronic) — see Sinusitis
  adrenal gland
  antrum (chronic) — see Sinusitis, maxillary
  bladder — see Cystitis
  brain G06.0
    sequelae G09
  breast N61.1
    puerperal, postpartum or gestational — see Mastitis, obstetric, purulent
  dental periosteum M27.3
  ear (middle) — see also Otitis, media
    external NEC — see Otitis, externa, infective
    internal — see subcategory H83.0- ☑
  ethmoidal (chronic) (sinus) — see Sinusitis, ethmoidal
  fallopian tube — see Salpingo-oophoritis
  frontal (chronic) (sinus) — see Sinusitis, frontal
  gallbladder (acute) K81.0
  gum K05.20
    generalized — see Periodontitis, aggressive, generalized
    localized — see Periodontitis, aggressive, localized
  intracranial G06.0
  joint — see Arthritis, pyogenic or pyemic
  labyrinthine — see subcategory H83.0- ☑
  lung — see Abscess, lung
  mammary gland N61.1
    puerperal, postpartum O91.12
      associated with lactation O91.13
  maxilla, maxillary M27.2
    sinus (chronic) — see Sinusitis, maxillary
  muscle — see Myositis, infective
  nasal sinus (chronic) — see Sinusitis
  pancreas, acute — see also Pancreatitis, acute K85.80
  parotid gland — see Sialoadenitis
  pelvis, pelvic
    female — see Disease, pelvis, inflammatory
    male K65.0
  pericranial — see Osteomyelitis
  salivary duct or gland (any) — see Sialoadenitis
  sinus (accessory) (chronic) (nasal) — see Sinusitis
  sphenoidal sinus (chronic) — see Sinusitis, sphenoidal
  thymus (gland) E32.1
  thyroid (gland) E06.0
  tonsil — see Tonsillitis
  uterus — see Endometritis
Supraeruption of tooth (teeth) M26.34
Supraglottitis J04.30
  with obstruction J04.31
Suprarenal (gland) — see condition
Suprascapular nerve — see condition
Suprasellar — see condition
Surfer's knots or nodules S89.8- ☑

Surgical
  emphysema T81.82- ☑
  procedures, complication or misadventure — see Complications, surgical procedures
  shock T81.10- ☑
Surveillance (of) (for) — see also Observation
  alcohol abuse Z71.41
  contraceptive — see Prescription, contraceptives
  dietary Z71.3
  drug abuse Z71.51
  neoplasm — see Screening, neoplasm
Susceptibility to disease, genetic Z15.89
  malignant neoplasm Z15.09
    breast Z15.01
    endometrium Z15.04
    fallopian tube(s) Z15.05
    ovary Z15.02
    prostate Z15.03
    specified NEC Z15.09
  multiple endocrine neoplasia Z15.81
Suspected condition, ruled out — see also Observation, suspected
  amniotic cavity and membrane Z03.71
  cervical shortening Z03.75
  fetal anomaly Z03.73
  fetal growth Z03.74
  maternal and fetal conditions NEC Z03.79
  newborn — see also Observation, newborn, suspected condition ruled out Z05.9
  oligohydramnios Z03.71
  placental problem Z03.72
  polyhydramnios Z03.71
Suspended uterus
  in pregnancy or childbirth — see Pregnancy, complicated by, abnormal uterus
Sutton's nevus D22.9
Suture
  burst (in operation wound) T81.31- ☑
    external operation wound T81.31- ☑
    internal operation wound T81.329- ☑
  inadvertently left in operation wound — see Foreign body, accidentally left during a procedure
  removal Z48.02
Swab inadvertently left in operation wound — see Foreign body, accidentally left during a procedure
Swallowed, swallowing
  difficulty — see Dysphagia
  foreign body — see Foreign body, alimentary tract
Swan-neck deformity (finger) — see Deformity, finger, swan-neck
Swearing, compulsive F42.8
  in Gilles de la Tourette's syndrome F95.2
Sweat, sweats
  fetid L75.0
  night R61
Sweating, excessive R61
Sweeley-Klionsky disease E75.21
Sweet's disease or dermatosis L98.2
Swelling (of) R60.9
  abdomen, abdominal (not referable to any particular organ) — see Mass, abdominal
  ankle — see Effusion, joint, ankle
  arm M79.89
    forearm M79.89
  breast — see also Lump, breast N63.0
  Calabar B74.3
  cervical gland R59.0
  chest, localized R22.2
  ear H93.8- ☑
  extremity (lower) (upper) — see Disorder, soft tissue, specified type NEC
  finger M79.89
  foot M79.89
  glands R59.9
    generalized R59.1
    localized R59.0
  hand M79.89
  head (localized) R22.0
  inflammatory — see Inflammation
  intra-abdominal — see Mass, abdominal
  joint — see Effusion, joint
  leg M79.89
    lower M79.89
  limb — see Disorder, soft tissue, specified type NEC
  localized (skin) R22.9
    chest R22.2
    head R22.0

Swelling — continued
  localized — continued
    limb
      lower — see Mass, localized, limb, lower
      upper — see Mass, localized, limb, upper
    neck R22.1
    trunk R22.2
  neck (localized) R22.1
  pelvic — see Mass, abdominal
  scrotum N50.89
  splenic — see Splenomegaly
  testis N50.89
  toe M79.89
  umbilical R19.09
  wandering, due to Gnathostoma (spinigerum) B83.1
  white — see Tuberculosis, arthritis
Swift (-Feer) disease
  overdose or wrong substance given or taken — see Table of Drugs and Chemicals, by drug, poisoning
Swimmer's
  cramp T75.1- ☑
  ear H60.33- ☑
  itch B65.3
Swimming in the head R42
Swollen — see Swelling
Swyer syndrome Q99.1
Sycosis L73.8
  barbae (not parasitic) L73.8
  contagiosa (mycotic) B35.0
  lupoides L73.8
  mycotic B35.0
  parasitic B35.0
  vulgaris L73.8
Sydenham's chorea — see Chorea, Sydenham's
Sylvatic yellow fever A95.0
Sylvest's disease B33.0
Symblepharon H11.23- ☑
  congenital Q10.3
Symond's syndrome G93.2
Sympathetic — see condition
Sympatheticotonia G90.89
Sympathicoblastoma
  specified site — see Neoplasm, malignant, by site
  unspecified site C74.90
Sympathogonioma — see Sympathicoblastoma
Symphalangy (fingers) (toes) Q70.9
Symptoms NEC R68.89
  breast NEC N64.59
  cold J00
  development NEC R63.8
  factitious, self-induced — see Disorder, factitious
  genital organs, female R10.20
  involving
    abdomen NEC R19.8
    appearance NEC R46.89
    awareness R41.9
      altered mental status R41.82
      amnesia — see Amnesia
      borderline intellectual functioning R41.83
      coma — see Coma
      disorientation R41.0
      neurologic neglect syndrome R41.4
      senile cognitive decline R41.81
      specified symptom NEC R41.89
    behavior NEC R46.89
    cardiovascular system NEC R09.89
    chest NEC R09.89
    circulatory system NEC R09.89
    cognitive functions R41.9
      altered mental status R41.82
      amnesia — see Amnesia
      borderline intellectual functioning R41.83
      coma — see Coma
      disorientation R41.0
      neurologic neglect syndrome R41.4
      senile cognitive decline R41.81
      specified symptom NEC R41.89
    development NEC R62.50
    digestive system NEC R19.8
    emotional state NEC R45.89
      emotional lability R45.86
    food and fluid intake R63.8
    general perceptions and sensations R44.9
      specified NEC R44.8
    musculoskeletal system R29.91
      specified NEC R29.898
    nervous system R29.90
      specified NEC R29.818
    pelvis NEC R19.8

Symptoms — continued
  involving — continued
    respiratory system NEC R09.89
    skin and integument R23.9
    urinary system R39.9
  menopausal N95.1
  metabolism NEC R63.8
  neurotic F48.8
  of infancy R68.19
  pelvis NEC, female R10.20
  skin and integument NEC R23.9
  subcutaneous tissue NEC R23.9
  viral cold J00
Sympus Q74.2
Synaptopathy
  DLG4-related QA0.0142
  specified NEC QA0.0149
Syncephalus Q89.4
Synchondrosis
  abnormal (congenital) Q78.8
  ischiopubic M91.0
Synchysis (scintillans) (senile) (vitreous body) H43.89
Syncope (near) (pre-) R55
  anginosa I20.89
  bradycardia R00.1
  cardiac R55
  carotid sinus G90.01
  due to spinal (lumbar) puncture G97.1
  heart R55
  heat T67.1- ☑
  laryngeal R05.4
  psychogenic F48.8
  tussive R05.8
  vasoconstriction R55
  vasodepressor R55
  vasomotor R55
  vasovagal R55
Syndactylism, syndactyly Q70.9
  complex (with synostosis)
    fingers Q70.0- ☑
    toes Q70.2- ☑
  simple (without synostosis)
    fingers Q70.1- ☑
    toes Q70.3- ☑
Syndrome — see also Disease
  22q13.3 deletion Q93.52
  48,XXXX Q97.1
  49,XXXXX Q97.1
  4H G11.5
  5q minus NOS D46.C (following D46.2)
  abdominal
    acute R10.0
    muscle deficiency Q79.4
  abnormal innervation H02.519
    left H02.516
      lower H02.515
      upper H02.514
    right H02.513
      lower H02.512
      upper H02.511
  abstinence, neonatal P96.1
  acid pulmonary aspiration, obstetric O74.0
  acquired immunodeficiency — see Human, immunodeficiency virus (HIV) disease
  activated phosphoinositide 3-kinase delta syndrome [APDS] D81.82
  acute abdominal R10.0
  acute respiratory distress (adult) (child) J80
    idiopathic J84.114
  Adair-Dighton Q78.0
  Adams-Stokes (-Morgagni) I45.9
  adiposogenital E23.6
  adrenal
    hemorrhage (meningococcal) A39.1
    meningococcic A39.1
  adrenocortical — see Cushing's, syndrome
  adrenogenital E25.9
    congenital, associated with enzyme deficiency E25.0
  afferent loop NEC K91.89
  Aicardi-Goutières E79.81
  Alagille (-Watson) Q44.71
  alcohol withdrawal (without convulsions) — see Dependence, alcohol, with, withdrawal
  Alder's D72.0
  Aldrich (-Wiskott) D82.0
  alien hand R41.4
  Alport Q87.81
  alveolar hypoventilation E66.2

Syndrome — continued
  alveolocapillary block J84.10
  amnesic, amnestic (confabulatory) (due to) — see Disorder, amnesic
  amyostatic (Wilson's disease) E83.01
  androgen insensitivity E34.50
    complete E34.51
    partial E34.52
  androgen resistance — see also Syndrome, androgen insensitivity E34.50
  Angelman Q93.51
  anginal — see Angina
  ankyloglossia superior Q38.1
  anterior
    chest wall R07.89
    cord G83.82
    spinal artery G95.19
      compression M47.019
        cervical region M47.012
        cervicothoracic region M47.013
        lumbar region M47.016
        occipito-atlanto-axial region M47.011
        thoracic region M47.014
        thoracolumbar region M47.015
    tibial M76.81- ☑
  antibody deficiency D80.9
    agammaglobulinemic D80.1
      hereditary D80.0
    congenital D80.0
    hypogammaglobulinemic D80.1
      hereditary D80.0
  anticardiolipin (-antibody) D68.61
  antidepressant discontinuation T43.205- ☑
  antiphospholipid (-antibody) D68.61
  aortic
    arch M31.4
    bifurcation I74.09
  aortomesenteric duodenum occlusion K31.5
  apical ballooning (transient left ventricular) I51.81
  arcuate ligament I77.4
  argentaffin, argintaffinoma E34.09
  Arnold-Chiari — see Arnold-Chiari disease
  Arrillaga-Ayerza I27.0
  arterial tortuosity Q87.82
  arteriovenous steal T82.898- ☑
  Asherman's N85.6
  aspiration, of newborn — see Aspiration, by substance, with pneumonia
    meconium P24.01
  ataxia-telangiectasia G11.3
  auriculotemporal G50.8
  autoerythrocyte sensitization (Gardner-Diamond) D69.2
  autoimmune lymphoproliferative [ALPS] D89.82
  autoimmune polyglandular E31.0
  autoinflammatory M04.9
    specified type NEC M04.8
  autosomal — see Abnormal, autosomes
  Avellis' G46.8
  Axenfeld-Rieger Q13.81
  Ayerza (-Arrillaga) I27.0
  Babinski-Nageotte G83.89
  Bakwin-Krida Q78.5
  Bardet-Biedl Q87.83
  bare lymphocyte D81.6
  Barre-Guillain G61.0
  Barre-Lieou M53.0
  Barrett's — see Barrett's, esophagus
  Barsony-Polgar K22.4
  Barsony-Teschendorf K22.4
  Barth E78.71
  Bartter's E26.81
  basal cell nevus Q87.89
  Basedow's E05.00
    with thyroid storm E05.01
  basilar artery G45.0
  Batten-Steinert G71.11
  battered
    baby or child — see Maltreatment, child, physical abuse
    spouse — see Maltreatment, adult, physical abuse
  Beals Q87.40
  Beau's I51.5
  Beck's I65.8
  Benedikt's G46.3
  Bequez Cesar (-Steinbrinck-Chediak-Higashi) E70.330
  Berardinelli-Siep E88.12
  Bernhardt-Roth — see Meralgia paresthetica
  Bernheim's — see Failure, heart, right
  big spleen D73.1

Syndrome — *continued*
- bilateral polycystic ovarian E28.2
- Bing-Horton's — *see* Horton's headache
- Birt-Hogg-Dube syndrome Q87.89
- Bjorck (-Thorsen) E34.09
- black
  - lung J60
  - widow spider bite — *see* Toxicity, venom, spider, black widow
- Blackfan-Diamond D61.01
- Blau M04.8
- blind loop K90.2
  - congenital Q43.8
  - postsurgical K91.2
- blue sclera Q78.0
- blue toe I75.02- ☑
- Boder-Sedgewick G11.3
- Boerhaave's K22.3
- Borjeson Forssman Lehmann Q89.89
- Bouillaud's I01.9
- Bourneville (-Pringle) Q85.1
- Bouveret (-Hoffman) I47.9
- brachial plexus G54.0
- bradycardia-tachycardia I49.5
- brain (nonpsychotic) F09
  - with psychosis, psychotic reaction F09
  - acute or subacute — *see* Delirium
  - congenital — *see* Disability, intellectual
  - organic F09
    - post-traumatic (nonpsychotic) F07.81
      - psychotic F09
    - personality change F07.0
    - postcontusional F07.81
    - post-traumatic, nonpsychotic F07.81
    - psycho-organic F09
    - psychotic F06.8
- brain stem stroke G46.3
- Brandt's (acrodermatitis enteropathica) E83.2
- broad ligament laceration N83.8
- Brock's J98.11
- bronchiolitis obliterans — *see also* Bronchiolitis, obliterative J44.81
- bronze baby P83.88
- Brown-Sequard G83.81
- Brugada I49.8
- bubbly lung P27.0
- Buchem's M85.2
- Budd-Chiari I82.0
- bulbar (progressive) G12.22
- Burger-Grutz E78.3
- Burke's K86.89
- Burnett's (milk-alkali) E83.52
- burning feet E53.9
- Bywaters' T79.5- ☑
- Call-Fleming I67.841
- cannabinoid hyperemesis R11.16
- cannabis hyperemesis R11.16
- carbohydrate-deficient glycoprotein (CDGS) E77.8
- carcinogenic thrombophlebitis I82.1
- carcinoid E34.00
  - heart E34.01
  - specified NEC E34.09
- cardiac asthma I50.1
- cardiacos negros I27.0
- cardiofaciocutaneous Q87.89
- cardiopulmonary-obesity E66.2
- cardiorenal — *see* Failure, heart; *also see* Failure, renal
- cardiorespiratory distress (idiopathic), newborn P22.0
- cardiovascular renal — *see* Failure, heart; *also see* Failure, renal
- carotid
  - artery (hemispheric) (internal) G45.1
    - body G90.01
    - sinus G90.01
- carpal tunnel G56.0- ☑
- Cassidy (-Scholte) E34.09
- cat cry Q93.4
- cat eye Q92.8
- cauda equina G83.4
- causalgia — *see* Causalgia
- celiac K90.0
  - artery compression I77.4
  - axis I77.4
- central pain G89.0
- cerebellar
  - hereditary G11.9
  - stroke G46.4
- cerebellomedullary malformation — *see* Spina bifida

Syndrome — *continued*
- cerebral
  - artery
    - anterior G46.1
    - middle G46.0
    - posterior G46.2
  - gigantism E22.0
- cervical (root) M53.1
  - disc — *see* Disorder, disc, cervical, with neuritis
  - fusion Q76.1
  - posterior, sympathicus M53.0
  - rib Q76.5
  - sympathetic paralysis G90.2
- cervicobrachial (diffuse) M53.1
- cervicocranial M53.0
- cervicodorsal outlet G54.2
- cervicothoracic outlet — *see also* Syndrome, thoracic outlet G54.0
- Cestan (-Raymond) I65.8
- Charcot-Weiss-Baker G90.09
- Charcot's (angina cruris) (intermittent claudication) I73.9
- CHARGE Q89.89
- Chediak-Higashi (-Steinbrinck) E70.330
- chest wall R07.1
- Chiari's (hepatic vein thrombosis) I82.0
- Chilaiditi's Q43.3
- child maltreatment — *see* Maltreatment, child
- chondrocostal junction M94.0
- chondroectodermal dysplasia Q77.6
- chromosome 4 short arm deletion Q93.3
- chromosome 5 short arm deletion Q93.4
- chronic
  - infantile neurological, cutaneous and articular (CINCA) M04.2
  - pain G89.4
    - personality F68.8
- Churg-Strauss M30.1
- Clarke-Hadfield K86.89
- Clerambault's automatism G93.89
- clinically isolated G37.9
- Clouston's (hidrotic ectodermal dysplasia) Q82.4
- clumsiness, clumsy child F82
- cluster headache G44.009
  - intractable G44.001
  - not intractable G44.009
- Coffin-Lowry Q89.89
- cold injury (newborn) P80.0
- combined immunity deficiency D81.9
- compartment (deep) (posterior) (traumatic) T79.A0- ☑ (*following* T79.7)
  - abdomen T79.A3- ☑ (*following* T79.7)
  - lower extremity (hip, buttock, thigh, leg, foot, toes) T79.A2- ☑ (*following* T79.7)
  - nontraumatic
    - abdomen M79.A3 (*following* M79.7)
    - lower extremity (hip, buttock, thigh, leg, foot, toes) M79.A2- ☑ (*following* M79.7)
    - specified site NEC M79.A9 (*following* M79.7)
    - upper extremity (shoulder, arm, forearm, wrist, hand, fingers) M79.A1- ☑ (*following* M79.7)
  - postprocedural — *see* Syndrome, compartment, nontraumatic
  - specified site NEC T79.A9- ☑ (*following* T79.7)
  - upper extremity (shoulder, arm, forearm, wrist, hand, fingers) T79.A1- ☑ (*following* T79.7)
- complex regional pain — *see* Syndrome, pain, complex regional
- compression T79.5- ☑
  - anterior spinal — *see* Syndrome, anterior, spinal artery, compression
  - cauda equina G83.4
  - celiac artery I77.4
  - vertebral artery M47.029
    - cervical region M47.022
    - occipito-atlanto-axial region M47.021
- concussion F07.81
- congenital
  - affecting multiple systems NEC Q87.89
  - central alveolar hypoventilation G47.35
  - facial diplegia Q87.0
  - muscular hypertrophy-cerebral Q87.89
  - oculo-auriculovertebral Q87.0
  - oculofacial diplegia (Moebius) Q87.0
  - rubella (manifest) P35.0
- congestion-fibrosis (pelvic), female N94.89
- congestive dysmenorrhea N94.6
- connective tissue M35.9
  - overlap NEC M35.1

Syndrome — *continued*
- Conn's E26.01
- conus medullaris G95.81
- cord
  - anterior G83.82
  - posterior G83.83
- coronary
  - acute NEC I24.9
  - insufficiency or intermediate I20.0
  - slow flow I20.89
- Costen's (complex) M26.69
- costochondral junction M94.0
- costoclavicular G54.0
- costovertebral E22.0
- Cowden
  - PTEN related Q85.81
  - specified NEC Q85.82
- craniovertebral M53.0
- Creutzfeldt-Jakob — *see* Creutzfeldt-Jakob disease or syndrome
- cri-du-chat Q93.4
- crib death R99
- cricopharyngeal — *see* Dysphagia
- croup J05.0
- CRPS I — *see* Syndrome, pain, complex regional I
- crush T79.5- ☑
- cryopyrin-associated perodic M04.2
- cryptophthalmos Q87.0
- CTNNB1 Q87.88
- cubital tunnel — *see* Lesion, nerve, ulnar
- Curschmann (-Batten) (-Steinert) G71.11
- Cushing's E24.9
  - alcohol-induced E24.4
  - due to
    - alcohol
      - drugs E24.2
    - ectopic ACTH E24.3
    - overproduction of pituitary ACTH E24.0
  - drug-induced E24.2
  - overdose or wrong substance given or taken — *see* Table of Drugs and Chemicals, by drug, poisoning
  - pituitary-dependent E24.0
  - specified type NEC E24.8
- cystic duct stump K91.5
- cytokine release D89.839
  - grade 1 D89.831
  - grade 2 D89.832
  - grade 3 D89.833
  - grade 4 D89.834
  - grade 5 D89.835
- Dana-Putnam D51.0
- Danbolt (-Cross) (acrodermatitis enteropathica) E83.2
- Dandy-Walker Q03.1
  - with spina bifida Q07.01
- Danlos' — *see also* Syndrome, Ehlers-Danlos Q79.60
- De Quervain E34.51
- de Toni-Fanconi (-Debre) E72.09
  - with cystinosis E72.04
- de Vivo syndrome E74.810
- defibrination — *see also* Fibrinolysis
  - with
    - antepartum hemorrhage — *see* Hemorrhage, antepartum, with coagulation defect
    - intrapartum hemorrhage — *see* Hemorrhage, complicating, delivery
  - newborn P60
  - postpartum O72.3
- Degos' I77.89
- Dejerine-Roussy G89.0
- delayed sleep phase G47.21
- demyelinating G37.9
- dependence — *see* F10-F19 with fourth character .2
- depersonalization (-derealization) F48.1
- di George's D82.1
- diabetes mellitus-hypertension-nephrosis — *see* Diabetes, nephrosis
- diabetes mellitus in newborn infant P70.2
- diabetes-nephrosis — *see* Diabetes, nephrosis
- diabetic amyotrophy — *see* Diabetes, amyotrophy
- dialysis associated steal T82.898- ☑
- Diamond-Blackfan D61.01
- Diamond-Gardener D69.2
- DIC (diffuse or disseminated intravascular coagulopathy) D65
- Dighton's Q78.0
- disequilibrium E87.8
- Dohle body-panmyelopathic D72.0
- dorsolateral medullary G46.4

Syndrome — *continued*
- double athetosis G80.3
- Down — *see also* Down syndrome Q90.9
- Dravet (intractable) G40.834
  - with status epilepticus G40.833
  - without status epilepticus G40.834
- Dresbach's (elliptocytosis) D58.1
- DRESS (drug rash with eosinophilia and systemic symptoms) D72.12
- Dressler's (postmyocardial infarction) I24.1
  - postcardiotomy I97.0
- drug rash with eosinophilia and systemic symptoms (DRESS) D72.12
- drug withdrawal, infant of dependent mother P96.1
- dry eye H04.12- ☑
- due to abnormality
  - chromosomal Q99.9
    - sex
      - female phenotype Q97.9
      - male phenotype Q98.9
    - specified NEC Q99.8- ☑
- dumping (postgastrectomy) K91.1
  - nonsurgical K31.89
- Dupre's (meningism) R29.1
- dysmetabolic X E88.810
- dyspraxia, developmental F82
- Eagle-Barrett Q79.4
- Eaton-Lambert — *see* Syndrome, Lambert-Eaton
- Ebstein's Q22.5
- ectopic ACTH E24.3
- eczema-thrombocytopenia D82.0
- Eddowes' Q78.0
- effort (psychogenic) F45.8
- Ehlers-Danlos Q79.60
  - classical (cEDS) (classical EDS) Q79.61
  - hypermobile (hEDS) (hypermobile EDS) Q79.62
  - specified NEC Q79.69
  - vascular (vascular EDS) (vEDS) Q79.63
- Eisenmenger's I27.83
- Ekman's Q78.0
- electric feet E53.8
- Ellis-van Creveld Q77.6
- empty nest Z60.0
- endocrine-hypertensive E27.0
- entrapment — *see* Neuropathy, entrapment
- eosinophilia-myalgia M35.89
- epileptic — *see also* Epilepsy, by type
  - absence G40.A09 (*following* G40.3)
    - intractable G40.A19 (*following* G40.3)
      - with status epilepticus G40.A11 (*following* G40.3)
      - without status epilepticus G40.A19 (*following* G40.3)
    - not intractable G40.A09 (*following* G40.3)
      - with status epilepticus G40.A01 (*following* G40.3)
      - without status epilepticus G40.A09 (*following* G40.3)
- Erdheim-Chester (ECD) E88.89
- Erdheim's E22.0
- erythrocyte fragmentation D59.4
- Evans D69.41
- exhaustion F48.8
- extrapyramidal G25.9
  - specified NEC G25.89
- eye retraction — *see* Strabismus
- eyelid-malar-mandible Q87.0
- Faber's D50.9
- facet M47.89- ☑
- facet joint — *see also* Spondylosis M47.819
- facial pain, paroxysmal G50.0
- Fallot's Q21.3
- familial cold autoinflammatory M04.2
- familial eczema-thrombocytopenia (Wiskott-Aldrich) D82.0
- Fanconi (-de Toni) (-Debre) E72.09
  - with cystinosis E72.04
- fatigue
  - chronic G93.32
  - postviral G93.31
  - psychogenic F48.8
- faulty bowel habit K59.39
- Feil-Klippel (brevicollis) Q76.1
- Felty's — *see* Felty's syndrome
- fertile eunuch E23.0
- fetal
  - alcohol (dysmorphic) Q86.0
  - hydantoin Q86.1
- Fiedler's I40.1

Syndrome — *continued*
- first arch Q87.0
- fish odor E72.89
- Fisher's G61.0
- Fitzhugh-Curtis
  - due to
    - Chlamydia trachomatis A74.81
    - Neisseria gonorrhea (gonococcal peritonitis) A54.85
- Fitz's — *see also* Pancreatitis, acute K85.80
- Flajani (-Basedow) E05.00
  - with thyroid storm E05.01
- flatback — *see* Flatback syndrome
- floppy
  - baby P94.2
  - iris (intraoperative) (IFIS) H21.81
  - mitral valve I34.1
- flush E34.09
- Foix-Alajouanine G95.19
- Fong's Q87.2
- food protein-induced enterocolitis (FPIES) K52.21
- foramen magnum G93.5
- Foster-Kennedy H47.14- ☑
- Foville's (peduncular) G46.3
- FOXG1 QA0.0151
- fragile X Q99.2
- Franceschetti Q75.4
- Frey's
  - auriculotemporal G50.8
  - hyperhidrosis L74.52
- Friderichsen-Waterhouse A39.1
- Froin's G95.89
- frontal lobe F07.0
- Fukuhara E88.49
- functional
  - bowel K59.9
  - prepubertal castrate E29.1
- Gaisbock's D75.1
- ganglion (basal ganglia brain) G25.9
  - geniculi G51.1
- Gardner-Diamond D69.2
- gastroesophageal
  - junction K22.0
  - laceration-hemorrhage K22.6
- gastrojejunal loop obstruction K91.89
- Gee-Herter-Heubner K90.0
- Gelineau's G47.419
  - with cataplexy G47.411
- genito-anorectal A55
- Gerstmann-Straussler-Scheinker (GSS) A81.82
- Gianotti-Crosti L44.4
- giant platelet (Bernard-Soulier) D69.1
- Gilles de la Tourette's F95.2
- Glass Q87.89
- Gleich's D72.118
- goiter-deafness E07.1
- Goldberg Q89.89
- Goldberg-Maxwell E34.51
- Good's D83.8
- Gopalan's (burning feet) E53.8
- Gorlin's Q87.89
- Gougerot-Blum L81.7
- Gouley's I31.1
- Gower's R55
- gray or grey (newborn) P93.0
  - platelet D69.1
- Gubler-Millard G46.3
- Guillain-Barre (-Strohl) G61.0
- Gulf war T75.830- ☑
- gustatory sweating G50.8
- Hadfield-Clarke K86.89
- hair tourniquet — *see* Constriction, external, by site
- Hamman's J98.19
- hand-foot L27.1
- hand-shoulder G90.89
- hantavirus (cardio)-pulmonary (HPS) (HCPS) B33.4
- Hao-Fountain (HAFOUS) Q87.87
- happy puppet Q93.51
- Harada's H30.81- ☑
- Hayem-Faber D50.9
- headache NEC G44.89
  - complicated NEC G44.59
- Heberden's I20.89
- Hedinger's E34.01
- Hegglin's D72.0
- HELLP (hemolysis, elevated liver enzymes and low platelet count) O14.2- ☑
  - complicating
    - childbirth O14.24

Syndrome — *continued*
- HELLP — *continued*
  - complicating — *continued*
    - puerperium O14.25
- hemolytic-uremic D59.30
  - atypical D59.39
    - genetic D59.32
    - hereditary D59.32
    - infection-associated D59.31
    - secondary D59.39
    - specified NEC D59.39
  - due to genetic disorder D59.32
  - familial D59.32
  - hereditary D59.32
  - infection-associated D59.31
  - secondary D59.39
  - Shiga toxin-producing E. coli [STEC] related D59.31
  - specified NEC D59.39
  - typical D59.31
- hemophagocytic, infection-associated D76.2
- Henoch-Schonlein D69.0
- hepatic flexure K59.89
- hepatopulmonary K76.81
- hepatorenal K76.7
  - following delivery O90.41
  - postoperative or postprocedural K91.83
  - postpartum, puerperal O90.41
- hepatourologic K76.7
- hereditary alpha tryptasemia D89.44
- Herter (-Gee) (nontropical sprue) K90.0
- Heubner-Herter K90.0
- Heyd's K76.7
- Hilger's G90.09
- histamine-like (fish poisoning) — *see* Poisoning, fish
- histiocytic D76.3
- histiocytosis NEC D76.3
- HIV infection, acute B20
- Hoffmann-Werdnig G12.0
- Hollander-Simons E88.19
- Hoppe-Goldflam G70.00
  - with exacerbation (acute) G70.01
  - in crisis G70.01
- Horner's G90.2
- hungry bone E83.81
- hunterian glossitis D51.0
- Hunt's (herpetic geniculate ganglionitis) (neuralgia) B02.21
  - dyssynergia cerebellaris myoclonica G11.19
- Hutchinson's triad A50.53
- hyperabduction G54.0
- hyperammonemia-hyperornithinemia-homocitrullinemia E72.4
- hypereosinophilic (HES) D72.119
  - idiopathic (IHES) D72.110
  - lymphocytic variant (LHES) D72.111
  - myeloid D72.118
  - specified NEC D72.118
- hyperimmunoglobulin D M04.1
- hyperimmunoglobulin E (IgE) D82.4
- hyperkalemic E87.5
- hyperkinetic — *see* Hyperkinesia
- hypermobility M35.7
- hypernatremia E87.0
- hyperosmolarity — *see also* Diabetes, by type, with hyperosmolarity E87.0
- hyperperfusion G97.82
- hypersplenic D73.1
- hypertransfusion, newborn P61.1
- hyperventilation F45.8
- hyperviscosity (of serum)
  - polycythemic D75.1
  - sclerothymic D58.8
- hypoglycemic (familial) (neonatal) E16.2
- hypokalemic E87.6
- hyponatremic E87.1
- hypopituitarism E23.0
- hypoplastic left-heart Q23.4
- hypopotassemia E87.6
- hyposmolality E87.1
- hypotension, maternal O26.5- ☑
- hypothenar hammer I73.89
- hypoventilation, obesity (OHS) E66.2
- ICF (intravascular coagulation-fibrinolysis) D65
- idiopathic
  - cardiorespiratory distress, newborn P22.0
  - nephrotic (infantile) N04.9
- iliotibial band M76.3- ☑
- immobility, immobilization (paraplegic) M62.3

☑ Additional Character Required — Refer to the Tabular List for Character Selection

Syndrome — continued
- immune effector cell-associated neurotoxicity (ICANS) G92.00
  - grade
    - 1 G92.01
    - 2 G92.02
    - 3 G92.03
    - 4 G92.04
    - 5 G92.05
  - unspecified G92.00
- immune reconstitution D89.3
- immune reconstitution inflammatory [IRIS] D89.3
- immunity deficiency, combined D81.9
- immunodeficiency
  - acquired — see Human, immunodeficiency virus (HIV) disease
  - combined D81.9
- impending coronary I20.0
- impingement, shoulder M75.4- ☑
- inappropriate secretion of antidiuretic hormone E22.2
- infant
  - gestational diabetes P70.0
  - of diabetic mother P70.1
- infantilism (pituitary) E23.0
- inferior vena cava I87.1
- inspissated bile (newborn) P59.1
- institutional (childhood) F94.2
- insufficient sleep F51.12
- insulin resistance
  - type A E88.811
  - type B E88.818
- intermediate coronary (artery) I20.0
- interspinous ligament — see Spondylopathy, specified NEC
- intestinal
  - carcinoid E34.09
  - knot K56.2
- intravascular coagulation-fibrinolysis (ICF) D65
- iodine-deficiency, congenital E00.9
  - type
    - mixed E00.2
    - myxedematous E00.1
    - neurological E00.0
- IRDS (idiopathic respiratory distress, newborn) P22.0
- irritable
  - bowel K58.9
    - with
      - constipation K58.1
      - diarrhea K58.0
    - mixed K58.2
    - psychogenic F45.8
    - specified NEC K58.8
  - heart (psychogenic) F45.8
  - weakness F48.8
- ischemic
  - bowel (transient) K55.9
    - chronic K55.1
    - due to mesenteric artery insufficiency K55.1
  - steal T82.898- ☑
- IVC (intravascular coagulopathy) D65
- Ivemark's Q89.01
- Jaccoud's — see Arthropathy, postrheumatic, chronic
- Jackson's G83.89
- Jakob-Creutzfeldt — see Creutzfeldt-Jakob disease or syndrome
- jaw-winking Q07.8
- Jervell-Lange-Nielsen I45.81
- jet lag G47.25
- Job's D71.8
- Joseph-Diamond-Blackfan D61.01
- jugular foramen G52.7
- Kabuki (type 1, due to KMT2D mutation) (type 2, due to KDM6A mutation) Q89.81
- Kanner's (autism) F84.0
- Kartagener's Q89.3
- Kelly's D50.1
- Kimmelstiel-Wilson — see Diabetes, specified type, with Kimmelstiel-Wilson disease
- Kleefstra Q87.86
- Klein (e)-Levine G47.13
- Klippel-Feil (brevicollis) Q76.1
- Kohler-Pellegrini-Stieda — see Bursitis, tibial collateral
- Konig's K59.89
- Korsakoff (-Wernicke) (nonalcoholic) F04
  - alcoholic F10.26
- Kostmann's D70.0
- Krabbe's congenital muscle hypoplasia Q79.8
- labyrinthine — see subcategory H83.2- ☑
- lacunar NEC G46.7

Syndrome — continued
- Lambert-Eaton G70.80
  - in
    - neoplastic disease G73.1
    - specified disease NEC G70.81
- Landau-Kleffner — see Epilepsy, specified NEC
- Larsen's Q74.8
- Lassueur Graham-Little Piccardi L66.19
- lateral
  - cutaneous nerve of thigh G57.1- ☑
  - medullary G46.4
- Launois' E22.0
- Laurence-Moon Q87.84
- Lawrence E88.12
- lazy
  - leukocyte D70.8
  - posture M62.3
- Lemierre I80.8
- Lennox-Gastaut G40.812
  - intractable G40.814
    - with status epilepticus G40.813
    - without status epilepticus G40.814
  - not intractable G40.812
    - with status epilepticus G40.811
    - without status epilepticus G40.812
- lenticular, progressive E83.01
- Leopold-Levi's E05.90
- Lev's I44.2
- Li-Fraumeni Z15.01
- Lichtheim's D51.0
- Lightwood's N25.89
- Lignac (de Toni) (-Fanconi) (-Debre) E72.09
  - with cystinosis E72.04
- Likoff's I20.89
- limbic epilepsy personality F07.0
- liver-kidney K76.7
- lobotomy F07.0
- Loffler's J82.89
- long arm 18 or 21 deletion Q93.89
- long QT I45.81
- Louis-Barre G11.3
- low
  - atmospheric pressure T70.29- ☑
  - back M54.50
  - output (cardiac) I50.9
- lower radicular, newborn (birth injury) P14.8
- Luetscher's (dehydration) E86.0
- Lupus anticoagulant D68.62
- Lutembacher's Q21.19
- macrophage activation D76.1
  - due to infection D76.2
- magnesium-deficiency R29.0
- Majeed M04.8
- Mal de Debarquement R42
- malabsorption K90.9
  - postsurgical K91.2
- malformation, congenital, due to
  - alcohol Q86.0
  - exogenous cause NEC Q86.8
  - hydantoin Q86.1
  - warfarin Q86.2
- malignant
  - carcinoid E34.00
  - neuroleptic G21.0
- Mallory-Weiss K22.6
- mandibulofacial dysostosis Q75.4
- manic-depressive — see Disorder, bipolar
- maple-syrup-urine E71.0
- Marable's I77.4
- Marfan Q87.40
  - with
    - cardiovascular manifestations Q87.418
      - aortic dilation Q87.410
    - ocular manifestations Q87.42
    - skeletal manifestations Q87.43
- Marie's (acromegaly) E22.0
- mast cell activation — see Activation, mast cell
- maternal hypotension — see Syndrome, hypotension, maternal
- May (-Hegglin) D72.0
- McArdle (-Schmidt) (-Pearson) E74.04
- McQuarrie's E16.2
- meconium plug (newborn) P76.0
- MED13L (mediator complex subunit 13L) Q87.85
- median arcuate ligament I77.4
- mediator complex subunit 13L (MED13L) Q87.85
- Meekeren-Ehlers-Danlos Q79.6- ☑
- megavitamin-B6 E67.2
- Meige G24.4

Syndrome — continued
- MELAS E88.41
- Mendelson's O74.0
- MERRF (myoclonic epilepsy associated with ragged-red fibers) E88.42
- mesenteric
  - artery (superior) K55.1
  - vascular insufficiency K55.1
- metabolic E88.810
- metastatic carcinoid E34.00
- micrognathia-glossoptosis Q87.0
- midbrain NEC G93.89
- middle lobe (lung) J98.19
- middle radicular G54.0
- migraine — see also Migraine G43.909
- Mikulicz' K11.8
- milk-alkali E83.52
- Millard-Gubler G46.3
- Miller-Dieker Q93.88
- Miller-Fisher G61.0
- Minkowski-Chauffard D58.0
- Mirizzi's K83.1
- MNGIE (Mitochondrial Neurogastrointestinal Encephalopathy) E88.49
- Mobius, ophthalmoplegic migraine — see Migraine, ophthalmoplegic
- monofixation H50.42
- Morel-Moore M85.2
- Morel-Morgagni M85.2
- Morgagni (-Morel) (-Stewart) M85.2
- Morgagni-Adams-Stokes I45.9
- Mounier-Kuhn Q32.4
  - with bronchiectasis J47.9
    - with
      - exacerbation (acute) J47.1
      - lower respiratory infection J47.0
  - acquired J98.09
    - with bronchiectasis J47.9
      - with
        - exacerbation (acute) J47.1
        - lower respiratory infection J47.0
- Muckle-Wells M04.2
- mucocutaneous lymph node (acute febrile) (MCLS) M30.3
- multiple endocrine neoplasia (MEN) — see Neoplasia, endocrine, multiple (MEN)
- multiple operations — see Disorder, factitious
- multisystem inflammatory (in adults) (in children) M35.81
- myasthenic G70.9
  - in
    - diabetes mellitus — see Diabetes, amyotrophy
    - endocrine disease NEC E34.9 [G73.3]
    - neoplastic disease — see also Neoplasm D49.9 [G73.3]
    - thyrotoxicosis (hyperthyroidism) E05.90 [G73.3]
      - with thyroid storm E05.91 [G73.3]
- myelodysplastic D46.9
  - with
    - 5q deletion D46.C (following D46.2)
    - isolated del (5q) chromosomal abnormality D46.C (following D46.2)
    - multilineage dysplasia D46.A (following D46.2)
      - with ringed sideroblasts D46.B (following D46.2)
  - lesions, low grade D46.20
  - specified NEC D46.Z (following D46.4)
- myeloid hypereosinophilic D72.118
- myelopathic pain G89.0
- myeloproliferative (chronic) D47.1
- myofascial pain M79.18
- Naffziger's G54.0
- nail patella Q87.2
- NARP (Neuropathy, Ataxia and Retinitis pigmentosa) E88.49
- neonatal abstinence P96.1
- nephritic — see also Nephritis
  - with edema — see Nephrosis
  - acute N00.9
  - chronic N03.9
  - rapidly progressive N01.9
- nephrotic (congenital) — see also Nephrosis N04.9
  - with
    - C3
      - glomerulonephritis N04.A
      - glomerulopathy N04.A
        - with dense deposit disease N04.6
    - dense deposit disease N04.6
    - diffuse
      - crescentic glomerulonephritis N04.7
      - endocapillary proliferative glomerulonephritis N04.4

Syndrome — *continued*
- nephrotic — *see also* Nephrosis — *continued*
  - with — *continued*
    - diffuse — *continued*
      - membranous glomerulonephritis N04.20
      - mesangial proliferative glomerulonephritis N04.3
      - mesangiocapillary glomerulonephritis N04.5
      - focal and segmental glomerular lesions N04.1
      - minor glomerular abnormality N04.0
      - specified morphological changes NEC N04.8
  - diabetic — *see* Diabetes, nephrosis
  - specified type NEC with diffuse membranous glomerulonephritis N04.29
- neurologic neglect R41.4
- Nezelof's D81.4
- Niikawa-Kuroki Q89.81
- Nonne-Milroy-Meige Q82.0
- Nothnagel's vasomotor acroparesthesia I73.89
- obesity hypoventilation (OHS) E66.2
- obliterans
  - bronchiolitis — *see also* Bronchiolitis, obliterative J44.81
- oculomotor H51.9
- Ogilvie K59.81
- Oliver-McFarlane Q87.89
- ophthalmoplegia-cerebellar ataxia — *see* Strabismus, paralytic, third nerve
- oral allergy T78.19-
- oral-facial-digital Q87.0
- organic
  - affective F06.30
  - amnesic (not alcohol- or drug-induced) F04
  - brain F09
  - depressive F06.31
  - hallucinosis F06.0
  - personality F07.0
- Ormond's N13.5
- oro-facial-digital Q87.0
- os trigonum Q68.8
- Osler-Weber-Rendu I78.0
- osteoporosis-osteomalacia M83.8
- Ostereicher-Turner Q87.2
- oto-palato-digital Q87.0
- otolith — *see* subcategory H81.8- ☑
- outlet (thoracic) — *see also* Syndrome, thoracic outlet G54.0
- ovary
  - polycystic E28.2
  - resistant E28.39
  - sclerocystic E28.2
- Owren's D68.2
- Paget-Schroetter I82.890
- pain — *see also* Pain
  - complex regional I G90.50
    - lower limb G90.52- ☑
    - specified site NEC G90.59
    - upper limb G90.51- ☑
  - complex regional II — *see* Causalgia
- painful
  - bruising D69.2
  - feet E53.8
  - prostate N42.81
- paralysis agitans — *see* Parkinsonism
- paralytic G83.9
  - specified NEC G83.89
- Parinaud's H51.0
- parkinsonian — *see* Parkinsonism
- Parkinson's — *see* Parkinsonism
- paroxysmal facial pain G50.0
- Parry's E05.00
  - with thyroid storm E05.01
- Parsonage (-Aldren)-Turner G54.5
- patella clunk M25.86- ☑
- Paterson (-Brown) (-Kelly) D50.1
- pectoral girdle I77.89
- pectoralis minor I77.89
- pediatric autoimmune neuropsychiatric disorders associated with streptococcal infections (PANDAS) D89.89
- pediatric inflammatory multisystem M35.81
- Pelger-Huet D72.0
- pellagra-cerebellar ataxia-renal aminoaciduria E72.02
- pellagroid E52
- Pellegrini-Stieda — *see* Bursitis, tibial collateral
- pelvic congestion-fibrosis, female N94.89
- penta X Q97.1
- peptic ulcer — *see* Ulcer, peptic

Syndrome — *continued*
- perabduction I77.89
- periodic fever M04.1
- periodic fever, aphthous stomatitis, pharyngitis, and adenopathy [PFAPA] M04.8
- periodic headache, in adults and children — *see* Headache, periodic syndromes in adults and children
- periurethral fibrosis N13.5
- Peutz-Jeghers Q85.89
- phantom limb (without pain) G54.7
  - with pain G54.6
- pharyngeal pouch D82.1
- Phelan-McDermid Q93.52
- Pick's — *see* Disease, Pick's
- Pickwickian E66.2
- PIE (pulmonary infiltration with eosinophilia) — *see also* Eosinophilia, pulmonary J82.89
- pigmentary pallidal degeneration (progressive) G23.0
- pineal E34.8
- pituitary E22.0
- placental transfusion — *see* Pregnancy, complicated by, placental transfusion syndromes
- plantar fascia M72.2
- plateau iris (post-iridectomy) (postprocedural) H21.82
- Plummer-Vinson D50.1
- pluricarential of infancy E40
- plurideficiency E40
- pluriglandular (compensatory) E31.8
  - autoimmune E31.0
- pneumatic hammer T75.21- ☑
- polyangiitis overlap M30.8
- polycarential of infancy E40
- polyglandular E31.8
  - autoimmune E31.0
- polysplenia Q89.09
- pontine NEC G93.89
- popliteal
  - artery entrapment I77.89
  - web Q87.89
- post chemoembolization — *code to* associated conditions
- post endometrial ablation N99.85
- postbacterial fatigue G93.39
- postcardiac injury
  - postcardiotomy I97.0
  - postmyocardial infarction I24.1
- postcardiotomy I97.0
- postcholecystectomy K91.5
- postcommissurotomy I97.0
- postconcussional F07.81
- postcontusional F07.81
- post-COVID (-19) U09.9
- postencephalitic F07.89
- posterior
  - cervical sympathetic M53.0
  - cord G83.83
  - fossa compression G93.5
  - reversible encephalopathy (PRES) I67.83
- postgastrectomy (dumping) K91.1
- postgastric surgery K91.1
- postinfarction I24.1
- postinfectious fatigue G93.39
- postlaminectomy NEC M96.1
- postleukotomy F07.0
- postmastectomy lymphedema I97.2
- postmyocardial infarction I24.1
- postoperative NEC T81.9- ☑
  - blind loop K90.2
- postpartum panhypopituitary (Sheehan) E23.0
- postpolio (myelitic) G14
- postthrombotic I87.009
  - with
    - inflammation I87.02- ☑
      - with ulcer I87.03- ☑
    - specified complication NEC I87.09- ☑
    - ulcer I87.01- ☑
      - with inflammation I87.03- ☑
  - asymptomatic I87.00- ☑
- postural
  - orthostatic tachycardia [POTS] G90.A
  - tachycardia G90.A
- postvagotomy K91.1
- postvalvulotomy I97.0
- postviral NEC G93.31
  - fatigue G93.31
- Potain's K31.0
- potassium intoxication E87.5
- Prader-Willi Q87.11

Syndrome — *continued*
- Prader-Willi-like Q87.19
- precerebral artery (multiple) (bilateral) G45.2
- preinfarction I20.0
- preleukemic D46.9
- premature senility E34.8
- premenstrual dysphoric F32.81
- premenstrual tension N94.3
- Prinzmetal-Massumi R07.1
- prune belly Q79.4
- pseudo -Turner's Q87.19
- pseudocarpal tunnel (sublimis) — *see* Syndrome, carpal tunnel
- pseudoparalytica G70.00
  - with exacerbation (acute) G70.01
  - in crisis G70.01
- psycho-organic (nonpsychotic severity) F07.9
  - acute or subacute F05
  - depressive type F06.31
  - hallucinatory type F06.0
  - nonpsychotic severity F07.0
  - specified NEC F07.89
- PTEN (hamartoma) tumor Q85.81
- pulmonary
  - arteriosclerosis I27.0
  - dysmaturity (Wilson-Mikity) P27.0
  - hypoperfusion (idiopathic) P22.0
  - renal (hemorrhagic) (Goodpasture's) M31.0
- pure
  - motor lacunar G46.5
  - sensory lacunar G46.6
- Putnam-Dana D51.0
- pyogenic arthritis, pyoderma gangrenosum, and acne [PAPA] M04.8
- pyramidopallidonigral G20.C
- pyriformis — *see* Lesion, nerve, sciatic
- QT interval prolongation I45.81
- radicular NEC — *see* Radiculopathy
  - upper limbs, newborn (birth injury) P14.3
- rapid time-zone change G47.25
- Rasmussen G04.81
- Raymond (-Cestan) I65.8
- Raynaud's I73.00
  - with gangrene I73.01
- RDS (respiratory distress syndrome, newborn) P22.0
- reactive airways dysfunction J68.3
- Refsum's G60.1
- Reifenstein E34.52
- renal glomerulohyalinosis-diabetic — *see* Diabetes, nephrosis
- Rendu-Osler-Weber I78.0
- residual ovary N99.83
- resistant ovary E28.39
- respiratory
  - distress
    - acute J80
      - adult J80
      - child J80
      - idiopathic J84.114
    - newborn (idiopathic) (type I) P22.0
      - type II P22.1
- restless legs G25.81
- restrictive allograft J4A.0
- retinoblastoma (familial) C69.2- ☑
- retroperitoneal fibrosis K68.2
- retroviral seroconversion (acute) Z21
- Reye's G93.7
- Richter — *see* Leukemia, chronic lymphocytic, B-cell type
- Ridley's I50.1
- right
  - heart, hypoplastic Q22.6
  - ventricular obstruction — *see* Failure, heart, right
- Romano-Ward (prolonged QT interval) I45.81
- rotator cuff, shoulder — *see also* Tear, rotator cuff M75.10- ☑
- Rotes Querol — *see* Hyperostosis, ankylosing
- Roth — *see* Meralgia paresthetica
- rubella (congenital) P35.0
- Ruvalcaba-Myhre-Smith E71.440
- Rytand-Lipsitch I44.2
- salt
  - depletion E87.1
    - due to heat NEC T67.8- ☑
      - causing heat exhaustion or prostration T67.4- ☑
  - low E87.1
- salt-losing N28.89
- SATB2-associated Q87.89
- Scaglietti-Dagnini E22.0

Syndrome — *continued*
- scalenus anticus (anterior) G54.0
- scapulocostal — *see* Mononeuropathy, upper limb, specified site NEC
- scapuloperoneal G71.09
- schizophrenic, of childhood NEC F20.9
- Schnitzler D47.2
- Scholte's E34.09
- Schroeder's E27.0
- Schuller-Christian C96.5
- Schwachman (-Diamond) D61.02
- Schwartz (-Jampel) G71.13
- Schwartz-Bartter E22.2
- scimitar Q26.8
- sclerocystic ovary E28.2
- Seitelberger's G31.89
- septicemic adrenal hemorrhage A39.1
- seroconversion, retroviral (acute) Z21
- serotonin G90.81
- serous meningitis G93.2
- severe acute respiratory (SARS) J12.81
  - coronavirus 2 (*see also* COVID-19) U07.1
    - pneumonia J12.82
- shaken infant T74.4- ☑
- shock (traumatic) T79.4- ☑
  - kidney N17.0
    - following crush injury T79.5- ☑
  - toxic A48.3
- shock-lung J80
- Shone's — *code to* specific anomalies
- short
  - bowel K90.829
    - with
      - colon in continuity K90.821
        - iliocolonic anastomosis K90.821
      - without colon in continuity K90.822
  - gut — *see* Syndrome, short, bowel
  - rib Q77.2
- shoulder-hand — *see* Algoneurodystrophy
- Shwachman (-Diamond) D61.02
- sicca — *see* Syndrome, Sjogren
- sick
  - cell E87.1
  - sinus I49.5
- sick-euthyroid E07.81
- sideropenic D50.1
- Siemens' ectodermal dysplasia Q82.4
- Silfverskold's Q78.9
- Simons' E88.11
- sinus tarsi M25.57- ☑
- sinusitis-bronchiectasis-situs inversus Q89.3
- Sipple's E31.22
- sirenomelia Q87.2
- Sjogren M35.00
  - with
    - central nervous system involvement M35.07
    - dental involvement M35.0C
    - gastrointestinal involvement M35.08
    - glomerular disease M35.0A
    - inflammatory arthritis M35.05
    - keratoconjunctivitis M35.01
    - lung involvement M35.02
    - myopathy M35.03
    - peripheral nervous system involvement M35.06
    - renal tubular acidosis M35.04
    - specified organ involvement, NEC M35.09
    - tubulo-interstitial nephropathy M35.04
    - vasculitis M35.0B
- Slocumb's E27.0
- slow flow, coronary I20.89
- Sluder's G44.89
- Smith-Magenis Q93.88
- Sneddon-Wilkinson L13.1
- Snyder-Robinson Q87.89
- Sotos' Q87.3
- South African cardiomyopathy I42.8
- spasmodic
  - upward movement, eyes H51.8
  - winking F95.8
- Spen's I45.9
- splenic
  - agenesis Q89.01
  - flexure K59.89
  - neutropenia D73.81
- Spurway's Q78.0
- staphylococcal scalded skin L00
- steal
  - arteriovenous T82.898- ☑

Syndrome — *continued*
- steal — *continued*
  - ischemic T82.898- ☑
  - subclavian G45.8
- Stein-Leventhal E28.2
- Stein's E28.2
- Stevens-Johnson syndrome L51.1
  - toxic epidermal necrolysis overlap L51.3
- Stewart-Morel M85.2
- Stickler Q89.89
- stiff baby Q89.89
- stiff man G25.82
- Still-Felty — *see* Felty's syndrome
- Stokes (-Adams) I45.9
- stone heart I50.1
- straight back, congenital Q76.49
- Sturge-Weber (-Dimitri) Q85.89
- subclavian steal G45.8
- subcoracoid-pectoralis minor G54.0
- subcostal nerve compression I77.89
- subphrenic interposition Q43.3
- superior
  - cerebellar artery I63.89
  - mesenteric artery K55.1
  - semi-circular canal dehiscence H83.8X- ☑
  - vena cava I87.1
- supine hypotensive (maternal) — *see* Syndrome, hypotension, maternal
- suprarenal cortical E27.0
- supraspinatus — *see also* Tear, rotator cuff M75.10- ☑
- Susac G93.49
- swallowed blood P78.2
- sweat retention L74.0
- Swyer Q99.1
- Symond's G93.2
- sympathetic
  - cervical paralysis G90.2
  - pelvic, female N94.89
- systemic inflammatory response (SIRS), of non-infectious origin (without organ dysfunction) R65.10
  - with acute organ dysfunction R65.11
- tachycardia-bradycardia I49.5
- takotsubo I51.81
- TAR (thrombocytopenia with absent radius) Q87.2
- tarsal tunnel G57.5- ☑
- teething K00.7
- tegmental G93.89
- telangiectasic-pigmentation-cataract Q82.8
- temporal pyramidal apex — *see* Otitis, media, suppurative, acute
- temporomandibular joint-pain-dysfunction M26.62- ☑
- Terry's — *see also* Myopia, degenerative H44.2- ☑
- testicular feminization — *see also* Syndrome, androgen insensitivity E34.51
- thalamic pain (hyperesthetic) G89.0
- thoracic outlet (compression) G54.0
  - arterial I77.89
  - neurogenic G54.0
  - venous I87.1
- Thorson-Bjorck E34.09
- thrombocytopenia with absent radius (TAR) Q87.2
- thrombosis with thrombocytopenia D75.84
- thyroid-adrenocortical insufficiency E31.0
- tibial
  - anterior M76.81- ☑
  - posterior M76.82- ☑
- Tietze's M94.0
- time-zone (rapid) G47.25
- Toni-Fanconi E72.09
  - with cystinosis E72.04
- Touraine's Q79.8
- tourniquet — *see* Constriction, external, by site
- toxic shock A48.3
- transient left ventricular apical ballooning I51.81
- traumatic vasospastic T75.22- ☑
- Treacher Collins Q75.4
- triple X, female Q97.0
- trisomy Q92.9
  - 13 Q91.7
    - meiotic nondisjunction Q91.4
    - mitotic nondisjunction Q91.5
    - mosaicism Q91.5
    - translocation Q91.6
  - 18 Q91.3
    - meiotic nondisjunction Q91.0
    - mitotic nondisjunction Q91.1
    - mosaicism Q91.1
    - translocation Q91.2

Syndrome — *continued*
- trisomy — *continued*
  - 20 (q)(p) Q92.8
  - 21 Q90.9
    - meiotic nondisjunction Q90.0
    - mitotic nondisjunction Q90.1
    - mosaicism Q90.1
    - translocation Q90.2
  - 22 Q92.8
- tropical wet feet T69.02- ☑
- Trousseau's I82.1
- tumor lysis (following antineoplastic chemotherapy) (spontaneous) NEC E88.3
- tumor necrosis factor receptor associated periodic (TRAPS) M04.1
- Twiddler's (due to)
  - automatic implantable defibrillator T82.198- ☑
  - cardiac pacemaker T82.198- ☑
- Unverricht (-Lundborg) — *see* Epilepsy, generalized, idiopathic
- upward gaze H51.8
- uremia, chronic — *see also* Disease, kidney, chronic N18.9
- urethral N34.3
- urethro-oculo-articular — *see* Reiter's disease
- urohepatic K76.7
- usher Q99.819
  - specified NEC Q99.818
  - type 1 Q99.811
  - type 2 Q99.812
  - type 3 Q99.813
  - type 4 Q99.818
- vago-hypoglossal G52.7
- van Buchem's M85.2
- van der Hoeve's Q78.0
- vascular NEC in cerebrovascular disease G46.8
- vasoconstriction, reversible cerebrovascular I67.841
- vasomotor I73.9
- vasospastic (traumatic) T75.22- ☑
- vasovagal R55
- VATER Q87.2
- velo-cardio-facial Q93.81
- vena cava (inferior) (superior) (obstruction) I87.1
- vertebral
  - artery G45.0
    - compression — *see* Syndrome, anterior, spinal artery, compression
  - steal G45.0
- vertebro-basilar artery G45.0
- vertebrogenic (pain) — *see also* Pain, vertebrogenic M54.89
- vertiginous — *see* Disorder, vestibular function
- Vinson-Plummer D50.1
- virus B34.9
- visceral larva migrans B83.0
- visual disorientation H53.8
- vitamin B6 deficiency E53.1
- vitreal corneal H59.01- ☑
- vitreous (touch) H59.01- ☑
- Vogt-Koyanagi H20.82- ☑
- Volkmann's T79.6- ☑
- von Hippel-Lindau Q85.83
- von Schroetter's I82.890
- von Willebrand (-Jurgen) — *see* Disease, von Willebrand
  - acquired — *see also* Disease, von Willebrand D68.04
- Waldenstrom-Kjellberg D50.1
- Wallenberg's G46.3
- wasting (syndrome) due to underlying condition E88.A
- water retention E87.79
- Waterhouse (-Friderichsen) A39.1
- Weber-Gubler G46.3
- Weber-Leyden G46.3
- Weber's G46.3
- Wegener's M31.30
  - with
    - kidney involvement M31.31
    - lung involvement M31.30
      - with kidney involvement M31.31
- Weingarten's (tropical eosinophilia) J82.89
- Weiss-Baker G90.09
- Werdnig-Hoffman G12.0
- Werner's E31.21
- Werner's E34.8
- Wernicke-Korsakoff (nonalcoholic) F04
  - alcoholic F10.26
- Westphal-Strumpell E83.01
- West's — *see* Epilepsy, spasms
- wet
  - feet (maceration) (tropical) T69.02- ☑

Syndrome — continued
- wet — continued
  - lung, newborn P22.1
- whiplash S13.4- ☑
- whistling face Q87.0
- Wilkie's K55.1
- Wilkinson-Sneddon L13.1
- Willebrand (-Jurgens) — see Disease, von Willebrand
- Williams Q93.82
- Wilson's (hepatolenticular degeneration) E83.01
- Wiskott-Aldrich D82.0
- withdrawal — see Withdrawal, state
  - drug
    - infant of dependent mother P96.1
    - therapeutic use, newborn P96.2
- Woakes' (ethmoiditis) J33.1
- Wright's (hyperabduction) G54.0
- X I20.9
- XXXX Q97.1
- XXXXX Q97.1
- XXXXY Q98.1
- XXY Q98.0
- Yao M04.8
- yellow nail L60.5
- Zahorsky's B08.5
- Zellweger-like syndrome E71.541
- Zellweger syndrome E71.510

Synechia (anterior) (iris) (posterior) (pupil) — see also Adhesions, iris
- intra-uterine (traumatic) N85.6

Synesthesia R20.8

Syngamiasis, syngamosis B83.3

Synodontia K00.2

Synorchidism, synorchism Q55.1

Synostosis (congenital) Q78.8
- astragalo-scaphoid Q74.2
- radioulnar Q74.0

Synovial sarcoma — see Neoplasm, connective tissue, malignant

Synovioma (malignant) — see also Neoplasm, connective tissue, malignant
- benign — see Neoplasm, connective tissue, benign

Synoviosarcoma — see Neoplasm, connective tissue, malignant

Synovitis — see also Tenosynovitis M65.90
- ankle and foot M65.97- ☑
- arm, upper M65.92- ☑
- crepitant
  - hand M70.04- ☑
  - wrist M70.03- ☑
- forearm M65.93- ☑
- gonococcal A54.49
- gouty — see Gout
- hand M65.94- ☑
- in (due to)
  - crystals M65.8- ☑
  - gonorrhea A54.49
  - syphilis (late) A52.78
  - use, overuse, pressure — see Disorder, soft tissue, due to use
- infective NEC — see Tenosynovitis, infective NEC
- leg, lower M65.96- ☑
- multiple sites, unspecified type M65.99
- shoulder M65.91- ☑
- specified NEC — see Tenosynovitis, specified type NEC
- specified site, unspecified type M65.98
- syphilitic A52.78
  - congenital (early) A50.02
- thigh M65.95- ☑
- toxic — see Synovitis, transient
- transient M67.3- ☑
  - ankle M67.37- ☑
  - elbow M67.32- ☑
  - foot joint M67.37- ☑
  - hand joint M67.34- ☑
  - hip M67.35- ☑
  - knee M67.36- ☑
  - multiple site M67.39
  - pelvic region M67.35- ☑
  - shoulder M67.31- ☑
  - specified joint NEC M67.38
  - wrist M67.33- ☑
- traumatic, current — see Sprain
- tuberculous — see Tuberculosis, synovitis
- villonodular (pigmented) M12.2- ☑
  - ankle M12.27- ☑
  - elbow M12.22- ☑
  - foot joint M12.27- ☑

Synovitis — continued
- villonodular — continued
  - hand joint M12.24- ☑
  - hip M12.25- ☑
  - knee M12.26- ☑
  - multiple site M12.29
  - pelvic region M12.25- ☑
  - shoulder M12.21- ☑
  - specified joint NEC M12.28
  - vertebrae M12.28
  - wrist M12.23- ☑

Syphilid A51.39
- congenital A50.06
- newborn A50.06
- tubercular (late) A52.79

Syphilis, syphilitic (acquired) A53.9
- abdomen (late) A52.79
- acoustic nerve A52.15
- adenopathy (secondary) A51.49
- adrenal (gland) (with cortical hypofunction) A52.79
- age under 2 years NOS — see also Syphilis, congenital, early
  - acquired A51.9
- alopecia (secondary) A51.32
- anemia (late) A52.79 [D63.8]
- aneurysm (aorta) (ruptured) A52.01
  - central nervous system A52.05
  - congenital A50.54 [I79.0]
- anus (late) A52.74
  - primary A51.1
  - secondary A51.39
- aorta (arch) (abdominal) (thoracic) A52.02
  - aneurysm A52.01
- aortic (insufficiency) (regurgitation) (stenosis) A52.03
  - aneurysm A52.01
- arachnoid (adhesive) (cerebral) (spinal) A52.13
- asymptomatic — see Syphilis, latent
- ataxia (locomotor) A52.11
- atrophoderma maculatum A51.39
- auricular fibrillation A52.06
- bladder (late) A52.76
- bone A52.77
  - secondary A51.46
- brain A52.17
- breast (late) A52.79
- bronchus (late) A52.72
- bubo (primary) A51.0
- bulbar palsy A52.19
- bursa (late) A52.78
- cardiac decompensation A52.06
- cardiovascular A52.00
- central nervous system (late) (recurrent) (relapse) (tertiary) A52.3
  - with
    - ataxia A52.11
    - general paralysis A52.17
      - juvenile A50.45
    - paresis (general) A52.17
      - juvenile A50.45
    - tabes (dorsalis) A52.11
      - juvenile A50.45
    - taboparesis A52.17
      - juvenile A50.45
  - aneurysm A52.05
  - congenital A50.40
    - juvenile A50.40
  - remission in (sustained) A52.3
  - serology doubtful, negative, or positive A52.3
  - specified nature or site NEC A52.19
  - vascular A52.05
- cerebral A52.17
  - meningovascular A52.13
  - nerves (multiple palsies) A52.15
  - sclerosis A52.17
  - thrombosis A52.05
- cerebrospinal (tabetic type) A52.12
- cerebrovascular A52.05
- cervix (late) A52.76
- chancre (multiple) A51.0
  - extragenital A51.2
  - Rollet's A51.0
- Charcot's joint A52.16
- chorioretinitis A51.43
  - congenital A50.01
  - late A52.71
  - prenatal A50.01
- choroiditis — see Syphilitic chorioretinitis
- choroidoretinitis — see Syphilitic chorioretinitis

Syphilis, syphilitic — continued
- ciliary body (secondary) A51.43
  - late A52.71
- colon (late) A52.74
- combined spinal sclerosis A52.11
- condyloma (latum) A51.31
- congenital A50.9
  - with
    - paresis (general) A50.45
    - tabes (dorsalis) A50.45
    - taboparesis A50.45
  - chorioretinitis, choroiditis A50.01 [H32]
  - early, or less than 2 years after birth NEC A50.2
    - with manifestations — see Syphilis, congenital, early, symptomatic
    - latent (without manifestations) A50.1
      - negative spinal fluid test A50.1
      - serology positive A50.1
    - symptomatic A50.09
      - cutaneous A50.06
      - mucocutaneous A50.07
      - oculopathy A50.01
      - osteochondropathy A50.02
      - pharyngitis A50.03
      - pneumonia A50.04
      - rhinitis A50.05
      - visceral A50.08
  - interstitial keratitis A50.31
  - juvenile neurosyphilis A50.45
  - late, or 2 years or more after birth NEC A50.7
    - chorioretinitis, choroiditis A50.32
    - interstitial keratitis A50.31
    - juvenile neurosyphilis A50.45
    - latent (without manifestations) A50.6
      - negative spinal fluid test A50.6
      - serology positive A50.6
    - symptomatic or with manifestations NEC A50.59
      - arthropathy A50.55
      - cardiovascular A50.54
      - Clutton's joints A50.51
      - Hutchinson's teeth A50.52
      - Hutchinson's triad A50.53
      - osteochondropathy A50.56
      - saddle nose A50.57
- conjugal A53.9
  - tabes A52.11
- conjunctiva (late) A52.71
- contact Z20.2
- cord bladder A52.19
- cornea, late A52.71
- coronary (artery) (sclerosis) A52.06
- coryza, congenital A50.05
- cranial nerve A52.15
  - multiple palsies A52.15
- cutaneous — see Syphilis, skin
- dacryocystitis (late) A52.71
- degeneration, spinal cord A52.12
- dementia paralytica A52.17
  - juvenilis A50.45
- destruction of bone A52.77
- dilatation, aorta A52.01
- due to blood transfusion A53.9
- dura mater A52.13
- ear A52.79
  - inner A52.79
    - nerve (eighth) A52.15
    - neurorecurrence A52.15
- early A51.9
  - cardiovascular A52.00
  - central nervous system A52.3
  - latent (without manifestations) (less than 2 years after infection) A51.5
    - negative spinal fluid test A51.5
    - serological relapse after treatment A51.5
    - serology positive A51.5
  - relapse (treated, untreated) A51.9
  - skin A51.39
  - symptomatic A51.9
    - extragenital chancre A51.2
    - primary, except extragenital chancre A51.0
    - secondary — see also Syphilis, secondary A51.39
      - relapse (treated, untreated) A51.49
  - ulcer A51.39
- eighth nerve (neuritis) A52.15
- endemic A65
- endocarditis A52.03
  - aortic A52.03
  - pulmonary A52.03
- epididymis (late) A52.76

Syphilis, syphilitic — continued
　epiglottis (late) A52.73
　epiphysitis (congenital) (early) A50.02
　episcleritis (late) A52.71
　esophagus A52.79
　eustachian tube A52.73
　exposure to Z20.2
　eye A52.71
　eyelid (late) (with gumma) A52.71
　fallopian tube (late) A52.76
　fracture A52.77
　gallbladder (late) A52.74
　gastric (polyposis) (late) A52.74
　general A53.9
　　paralysis A52.17
　　　juvenile A50.45
　genital (primary) A51.0
　glaucoma A52.71
　gumma NEC A52.79
　　cardiovascular system A52.00
　　central nervous system A52.3
　　congenital A50.59
　heart (block) (decompensation) (disease) (failure) A52.06 [I52]
　　valve NEC A52.03
　hemianesthesia A52.19
　hemianopsia A52.71
　hemiparesis A52.17
　hemiplegia A52.17
　hepatic artery A52.09
　hepatis A52.74
　hepatomegaly, congenital A50.08
　hereditaria tarda — see Syphilis, congenital, late
　hereditary — see Syphilis, congenital
　Hutchinson's teeth A50.52
　hyalitis A52.71
　inactive — see Syphilis, latent
　infantum — see Syphilis, congenital
　inherited — see Syphilis, congenital
　internal ear A52.79
　intestine (late) A52.74
　iris, iritis (secondary) A51.43
　　late A52.71
　joint (late) A52.77
　keratitis (congenital) (interstitial) (late) A50.31
　kidney (late) A52.75
　lacrimal passages (late) A52.71
　larynx (late) A52.73
　late A52.9
　　cardiovascular A52.00
　　central nervous system A52.3
　　kidney A52.75
　　latent or 2 years or more after infection (without manifestations) A52.8
　　　negative spinal fluid test A52.8
　　　serology positive A52.8
　　paresis A52.17
　　specified site NEC A52.79
　　symptomatic or with manifestations A52.79
　　tabes A52.11
　latent A53.0
　　with signs or symptoms — code by site and stage under Syphilis
　　central nervous system A52.2
　　date of infection unspecified A53.0
　　early, or less than 2 years after infection A51.5
　　follow-up of latent syphilis A53.0
　　　date of infection unspecified A53.0
　　　late, or 2 years or more after infection A52.8
　　late, or 2 years or more after infection A52.8
　　positive serology (only finding) A53.0
　　　date of infection unspecified A53.0
　　　early, or less than 2 years after infection A51.5
　　　late, or 2 years or more after infection A52.8
　lens (late) A52.71
　leukoderma A51.39
　　late A52.79
　lienitis A52.79
　lip A51.39
　　chancre (primary) A51.2
　　late A52.79
　Lissauer's paralysis A52.17
　liver A52.74
　locomotor ataxia A52.11
　lung A52.72
　lymph gland (early) (secondary) A51.49
　　late A52.79
　lymphadenitis (secondary) A51.49
　macular atrophy of skin A51.39

Syphilis, syphilitic — continued
　macular atrophy of skin — continued
　　striated A52.79
　mediastinum (late) A52.73
　meninges (adhesive) (brain) (spinal cord) A52.13
　meningitis A52.13
　　acute (secondary) A51.41
　　congenital A50.41
　meningoencephalitis A52.14
　meningovascular A52.13
　　congenital A50.41
　mesarteritis A52.09
　　brain A52.04
　middle ear A52.77
　mitral stenosis A52.03
　monoplegia A52.17
　mouth (secondary) A51.39
　　late A52.79
　mucocutaneous (secondary) A51.39
　　late A52.79
　mucous
　　membrane (secondary) A51.39
　　　late A52.79
　　patches A51.39
　　　congenital A50.07
　mulberry molars A50.52
　muscle A52.78
　myocardium A52.06
　nasal sinus (late) A52.73
　neonatorum — see Syphilis, congenital
　nephrotic syndrome (secondary) A51.44
　nerve palsy (any cranial nerve) A52.15
　　multiple A52.15
　nervous system, central A52.3
　neuritis A52.15
　　acoustic A52.15
　neurorecidive of retina A52.19
　neuroretinitis A52.19
　newborn — see Syphilis, congenital
　nodular superficial (late) A52.79
　nonvenereal A65
　nose (late) A52.73
　　saddle back deformity A50.57
　occlusive arterial disease A52.09
　oculopathy A52.71
　ophthalmic (late) A52.71
　optic nerve (atrophy) (neuritis) (papilla) A52.15
　orbit (late) A52.71
　organic A53.9
　osseous (late) A52.77
　osteochondritis (congenital) (early) A50.02 [M90.80]
　osteoporosis A52.77
　ovary (late) A52.76
　oviduct (late) A52.76
　palate (late) A52.79
　pancreas (late) A52.74
　paralysis A52.17
　　general A52.17
　　　juvenile A50.45
　paresis (general) A52.17
　　juvenile A50.45
　paresthesia A52.19
　Parkinson's disease or syndrome A52.19
　paroxysmal tachycardia A52.06
　pemphigus (congenital) A50.06
　penis (chancre) A51.0
　　late A52.76
　pericardium A52.06
　perichondritis, larynx (late) A52.73
　periosteum (late) A52.77
　　congenital (early) A50.02 [M90.80]
　　early (secondary) A51.46
　peripheral nerve A52.79
　petrous bone (late) A52.77
　pharynx (late) A52.73
　　secondary A51.39
　pituitary (gland) A52.79
　pleura (late) A52.73
　pneumonia, white A50.04
　pontine lesion A52.17
　portal vein A52.09
　primary A51.0
　　anal A51.1
　　and secondary — see Syphilis, secondary
　　central nervous system A52.3
　　extragenital chancre NEC A51.2
　　fingers A51.2
　　genital A51.0
　　lip A51.2

Syphilis, syphilitic — continued
　primary — continued
　　specified site NEC A51.2
　　tonsils A51.2
　prostate (late) A52.76
　ptosis (eyelid) A52.71
　pulmonary (late) A52.72
　　artery A52.09
　pyelonephritis (late) A52.75
　recently acquired, symptomatic A51.9
　rectum (late) A52.74
　respiratory tract (late) A52.73
　retina, late A52.71
　retrobulbar neuritis A52.15
　salpingitis A52.76
　sclera (late) A52.71
　sclerosis
　　cerebral A52.17
　　coronary A52.06
　　multiple A52.11
　scotoma (central) A52.71
　scrotum (late) A52.76
　secondary (and primary) A51.49
　　adenopathy A51.49
　　anus A51.39
　　bone A51.46
　　chorioretinitis, choroiditis A51.43
　　hepatitis A51.45
　　liver A51.45
　　lymphadenitis A51.49
　　meningitis (acute) A51.41
　　mouth A51.39
　　mucous membranes A51.39
　　periosteum, periostitis A51.46
　　pharynx A51.39
　　relapse (treated, untreated) A51.49
　　skin A51.39
　　specified form NEC A51.49
　　tonsil A51.39
　　ulcer A51.39
　　viscera NEC A51.49
　　vulva A51.39
　seminal vesicle (late) A52.76
　seronegative with signs or symptoms — code by site and stage under Syphilis
　seropositive
　　with signs or symptoms — code by site and stage under Syphilis
　　follow-up of latent syphilis — see Syphilis, latent
　　only finding — see Syphilis, latent
　seventh nerve (paralysis) A52.15
　sinus, sinusitis (late) A52.73
　skeletal system A52.77
　skin (with ulceration) (early) (secondary) A51.39
　　late or tertiary A52.79
　small intestine A52.74
　spastic spinal paralysis A52.17
　spermatic cord (late) A52.76
　spinal (cord) A52.12
　spleen A52.79
　splenomegaly A52.79
　spondylitis A52.77
　staphyloma A52.71
　stigmata (congenital) A50.59
　stomach A52.74
　synovium A52.78
　tabes dorsalis (late) A52.11
　　juvenile A50.45
　tabetic type A52.11
　　juvenile A50.45
　taboparesis A52.17
　　juvenile A50.45
　tachycardia A52.06
　tendon (late) A52.78
　tertiary A52.9
　　with symptoms NEC A52.79
　　cardiovascular A52.00
　　central nervous system A52.3
　　multiple NEC A52.79
　　specified site NEC A52.79
　testis A52.76
　thorax A52.73
　throat A52.73
　thymus (gland) (late) A52.79
　thyroid (late) A52.79
　tongue (late) A52.79
　tonsil (lingual) (late) A52.73
　　primary A51.2
　　secondary A51.39

Syphilis, syphilitic — *continued*
- trachea (late) A52.73
- tunica vaginalis (late) A52.76
- ulcer (any site) (early) (secondary) A51.39
  - late A52.79
    - perforating A52.79
      - foot A52.11
- urethra (late) A52.76
- urogenital (late) A52.76
- uterus (late) A52.76
- uveal tract (secondary) A51.43
  - late A52.71
- uveitis (secondary) A51.43
  - late A52.71
- uvula (late) (perforated) A52.79
- vagina A51.0
  - late A52.76
- valvulitis NEC A52.03
- vascular A52.00

Syphilis, syphilitic — *continued*
- vascular — *continued*
  - brain (cerebral) A52.05
- ventriculi A52.74
- vesicae urinariae (late) A52.76
- viscera (abdominal) (late) A52.74
  - secondary A51.49
- vitreous (opacities) (late) A52.71
  - hemorrhage A52.71
- vulva A51.0
  - late A52.76
  - secondary A51.39

Syphiloma A52.79
- cardiovascular system A52.00
- central nervous system A52.3
- circulatory system A52.00
- congenital A50.59

Syphilophobia F45.29

Syringadenoma — *see also* Neoplasm, skin, benign

Syringadenoma — *continued*
- papillary — *see* Neoplasm, skin, benign

Syringobulbia G95.0

Syringocystadenoma — *see* Neoplasm, skin, benign
- papillary — *see* Neoplasm, skin, benign

Syringoma — *see also* Neoplasm, skin, benign
- chondroid — *see* Neoplasm, skin, benign

Syringomyelia G95.0

Syringomyelitis — *see* Encephalitis

Syringomyelocele — *see* Spina bifida

Syringopontia G95.0

System, systemic — *see also* condition
- disease, combined — *see* Degeneration, combined
- inflammatory response syndrome (SIRS) of non-infectious origin (without organ dysfunction) R65.10
  - with acute organ dysfunction R65.11
- lupus erythematosus M32.9
  - inhibitor present D68.62

Systemic exertion intolerance disease [SEID] G93.32

T

T-shaped incisors K00.2
Tabacism, tabacosis, tabagism — see also Poisoning, tobacco
    meaning dependence (without remission) — see Dependence, drug, nicotine
Tabardillo A75.9
    flea-borne A75.2
    louse-borne A75.0
Tabes, tabetic A52.10
    with
        central nervous system syphilis A52.10
        Charcot's joint A52.16
        cord bladder A52.19
        crisis, viscera (any) A52.19
        paralysis, general A52.17
        paresis (general) A52.17
        perforating ulcer (foot) A52.19
    arthropathy (Charcot) A52.16
    bladder A52.19
    bone A52.11
    cerebrospinal A52.12
    congenital A50.45
    conjugal A52.10
    dorsalis A52.11
        juvenile A50.49
    juvenile A50.49
    latent A52.19
    mesenterica A18.39
    paralysis, insane, general A52.17
    spasmodic A52.17
    syphilis (cerebrospinal) A52.12
Taboparalysis A52.17
Taboparesis (remission) A52.17
    juvenile A50.45
TAC (trigeminal autonomic cephalgia) **NEC** G44.099
    intractable G44.091
    not intractable G44.099
Tache noir S60.22- ☑
Tachyalimentation K91.2
Tachyarrhythmia, tachyrhythmia — see Tachycardia
Tachycardia R00.0
    atrial (paroxysmal) I47.19
    auricular I47.19
    AV nodal re-entry (re-entrant) I47.19
    junctional (paroxysmal) I47.19
    newborn P29.11
    nodal (paroxysmal) I47.19
    non-paroxysmal AV nodal I45.89
    paroxysmal (sustained) (nonsustained) I47.9
        with sinus bradycardia I49.5
        atrial (PAT) I47.19
        atrioventricular (AV) (re-entrant) I47.19
            psychogenic F54
        junctional I47.19
            ectopic I47.19
        nodal I47.19
        psychogenic (atrial) (supraventricular) (ventricular) F54
        supraventricular (sustained) I47.10
            psychogenic F54
        ventricular I47.20
            psychogenic F54
            specified type NEC I47.29
    psychogenic F45.8
    sick sinus I49.5
    sinoauricular NOS R00.0
        paroxysmal I47.19
    sinus [sinusal] NOS R00.0
        inappropriate, so stated (IST) I47.11
        paroxysmal I47.19
    supraventricular I47.10
    ventricular (paroxysmal) (sustained) I47.20
        psychogenic F54
        specified NEC I47.29
Tachygastria K31.89
Tachypnea R06.82
    hysterical F45.8
    newborn (idiopathic) (transitory) P22.1
    psychogenic F45.8
    transitory, of newborn P22.1
TACO (transfusion associated circulatory overload) E87.71
TAD (transfusion-associated dyspnea) J95.87
Taenia (infection) (infestation) B68.9
    diminuta B71.0
    echinococcal infestation B67.90
    mediocanellata B68.1

Taenia — continued
    nana B71.0
    saginata B68.1
    solium (intestinal form) B68.0
        larval form — see Cysticercosis
Taeniasis (intestine) — see Taenia
Tag (hypertrophied skin) (infected) L91.8
    adenoid J35.8
    anus K64.4
    hemorrhoidal K64.4
    hymen N89.8
    perineal N90.89
    preauricular Q17.0
    sentinel K64.4
    skin L91.8
        accessory (congenital) Q82.8
        anus K64.4
        congenital Q82.8
        preauricular Q17.0
    tonsil J35.8
    urethra, urethral N36.8
    vulva N90.89
Tahyna fever B33.8
Takahara's disease E80.3
Takayasu's disease or syndrome M31.4
Talaromycosis B48.4
Talcosis (pulmonary) J62.0
Talipes (congenital) Q66.89
    acquired, planus — see Deformity, limb, flat foot
    asymmetric Q66.89
    calcaneovalgus Q66.4- ☑
    calcaneovarus Q66.1- ☑
    calcaneus Q66.89
    cavus Q66.7- ☑
    equinovalgus Q66.6
    equinovarus Q66.0- ☑
    equinus Q66.89
    percavus Q66.7- ☑
    planovalgus Q66.6
    planus (acquired) (any degree) — see also Deformity, limb, flat foot
        congenital Q66.5- ☑
        due to rickets (sequelae) E64.3
    valgus Q66.6
    varus Q66.3- ☑
Tall stature, constitutional E34.4
Talma's disease M62.89
Talon noir S90.3- ☑
    hand S60.22- ☑
    heel S90.3- ☑
    toe S90.1- ☑
Tamponade, heart I31.4
Tanapox (virus disease) B08.71
Tangier disease E78.6
Tantrum, child problem F91.8
Tapeworm (infection) (infestation) — see Infestation, tapeworm
Tapia's syndrome G52.7
TAR (thrombocytopenia with absent radius) **syndrome** Q87.2
Tarral-Besnier disease L44.0
Tarsal tunnel syndrome — see Syndrome, tarsal tunnel
Tarsalgia — see Pain, limb, lower
Tarsitis (eyelid) H01.8- ☑
    syphilitic A52.71
    tuberculous A18.4
Tartar (teeth) (dental calculus) K03.6
Tattoo (mark) L81.8
Tauri's disease E74.09
Taurodontism K00.2
Taussig-Bing syndrome Q20.1
Tay-Sachs amaurotic familial idiocy or disease E75.02
Taybi's syndrome Q87.2
TBI (traumatic brain injury) S06.9- ☑
Teacher's node or nodule J38.2
Tear-stone — see Dacryolith
Tear, torn (traumatic) — see also Laceration
    with abortion — see Abortion
    annular fibrosis M51.35
    anus, anal (sphincter) S31.831- ☑
        complicating delivery
            with third degree perineal laceration — see also Delivery, complicated, by, laceration, perineum, third degree O70.20
                with mucosa O70.3
            without third degree perineal laceration O70.4
    nontraumatic (healed) (old) K62.81

Tear, torn — continued
    articular cartilage, old — see Derangement, joint, articular cartilage, by site
    bladder
        with ectopic or molar pregnancy O08.6
        following ectopic or molar pregnancy O08.6
        obstetrical O71.5
        traumatic — see Injury, bladder
    bowel
        with ectopic or molar pregnancy O08.6
        following ectopic or molar pregnancy O08.6
        obstetrical trauma O71.5
    broad ligament
        with ectopic or molar pregnancy O08.6
        following ectopic or molar pregnancy O08.6
        obstetrical trauma O71.6
    bucket handle (knee) (meniscus) — see Tear, meniscus
    capsule, joint — see Sprain
    cartilage — see also Sprain
        articular, old — see Derangement, joint, articular cartilage, by site
    cervix
        with ectopic or molar pregnancy O08.6
        following ectopic or molar pregnancy O08.6
        obstetrical trauma (current) O71.3
        old N88.1
        traumatic — see Injury, uterus
    dural G97.41
        nontraumatic G96.11
    internal organ — see Injury, by site
    knee cartilage
        articular (current) S83.3- ☑
        old — see Derangement, knee, meniscus, due to old tear
    ligament — see Sprain
    meniscus (knee) (current injury) S83.209- ☑
        bucket-handle S83.20- ☑
        lateral
            bucket-handle S83.25- ☑
            complex S83.27- ☑
            peripheral S83.26- ☑
            specified type NEC S83.28- ☑
        medial
            bucket-handle S83.21- ☑
            complex S83.23- ☑
            peripheral S83.22- ☑
            specified type NEC S83.24- ☑
        old — see Derangement, knee, meniscus, due to old tear
        site other than knee — code as Sprain
        specified type NEC S83.20- ☑
    muscle — see Strain
    pelvic
        floor, complicating delivery O70.1
        organ NEC, obstetrical trauma O71.5
            with ectopic or molar pregnancy O08.6
            following ectopic or molar pregnancy O08.6
    perineal, secondary O90.1
    periurethral tissue, obstetrical trauma O71.82
        with ectopic or molar pregnancy O08.6
        following ectopic or molar pregnancy O08.6
    rectovaginal septum — see Laceration, vagina
    retina, retinal (without detachment) (horseshoe) — see also Break, retina, horseshoe
        with detachment — see Detachment, retina, with retinal, break
    rotator cuff (nontraumatic) M75.10- ☑
        complete M75.12- ☑
        incomplete M75.11- ☑
        traumatic S46.01- ☑
            capsule S43.42- ☑
    semilunar cartilage, knee — see Tear, meniscus
    supraspinatus (complete) (incomplete) (nontraumatic) — see also Tear, rotator cuff M75.10- ☑
    tendon — see Strain
    tentorial, at birth P10.4
    umbilical cord
        complicating delivery O69.89- ☑
    urethra
        with ectopic or molar pregnancy O08.6
        following ectopic or molar pregnancy O08.6
        obstetrical trauma O71.5
    uterus — see Injury, uterus
    vagina — see Laceration, vagina
    vessel, from catheter — see Puncture, accidental complicating surgery
    vulva, complicating delivery O70.0
Teeth — see also condition

Teeth — continued
  grinding
    psychogenic F45.8
    sleep related G47.63
Teething (syndrome) K00.7
Telangiectasia, telangiectasis (verrucous) I78.1
  ataxic (cerebellar) (Louis-Bar) G11.3
  familial I78.0
  hemorrhagic, hereditary (congenital) (senile) I78.0
  hereditary, hemorrhagic (congenital) (senile) I78.0
  juxtafoveal H35.07- ☑
  macular H35.07- ☑
  macularis eruptiva perstans D47.01
  parafoveal H35.07- ☑
  retinal (idiopathic) (juxtafoveal) (macular) (parafoveal) H35.07- ☑
  spider I78.1
Telephone scatologia F65.89
Telescoped bowel or intestine K56.1
  congenital Q43.8
Temperature
  body, high (of unknown origin) R50.9
  cold, trauma from T69.9- ☑
    newborn P80.0
    specified effect NEC T69.8- ☑
Temple — see condition
Temporal — see condition
Temporomandibular joint pain-dysfunction syndrome M26.62- ☑
Temporosphenoidal — see condition
Tendency
  bleeding — see Defect, coagulation
  suicide
    meaning personal history of attempted suicide Z91.51
    meaning suicidal ideation — see Ideation, suicidal
    to fall R29.6
Tenderness, abdominal R10.819
  costovertebral (angle) R39.859
    bilateral R39.853
    left R39.852
    right R39.851
  epigastric R10.816
  flank R10.8A9
    left R10.8A2
    right R10.8A1
  generalized R10.817
  left lower quadrant R10.814
  left upper quadrant R10.812
  periumbilic R10.815
  rebound R10.829
    epigastric R10.826
    generalized R10.827
    left lower quadrant R10.824
    left upper quadrant R10.822
    periumbilic R10.825
    right lower quadrant R10.823
    right upper quadrant R10.821
  right lower quadrant R10.813
  right upper quadrant R10.811
  suprapubic R10.8A3
Tendinitis, tendonitis — see also Enthesopathy
  Achilles M76.6- ☑
  adhesive — see Tenosynovitis, specified type NEC
    shoulder — see Capsulitis, adhesive
  bicipital M75.2- ☑
  calcific M65.2- ☑
    ankle M65.27- ☑
    foot M65.27- ☑
    forearm M65.23- ☑
    hand M65.24- ☑
    lower leg M65.26- ☑
    multiple sites M65.29
    pelvic region M65.25- ☑
    shoulder M75.3- ☑
    specified site NEC M65.28
    thigh M65.25- ☑
    upper arm M65.22- ☑
  due to use, overuse, pressure — see also Disorder, soft tissue, due to use
    specified NEC — see Disorder, soft tissue, due to use, specified NEC
  gluteal M76.0- ☑
  patellar M76.5- ☑
  peroneal M76.7- ☑
  psoas M76.1- ☑
  tibial (posterior) M76.82- ☑
    anterior M76.81- ☑
  trochanteric — see Bursitis, hip, trochanteric

Tendon — see condition
Tendosynovitis — see Tenosynovitis
Tenesmus (rectal) R19.8
  vesical R30.1
Tennis elbow — see Epicondylitis, lateral
Tenonitis — see also Tenosynovitis
  eye (capsule) H05.04- ☑
Tenontosynovitis — see Tenosynovitis
Tenontothecitis — see Tenosynovitis
Tenophyte — see Disorder, synovium, specified type NEC
Tenosynovitis — see also Synovitis M65.90
  adhesive — see Tenosynovitis, specified type NEC
    shoulder — see Capsulitis, adhesive
  bicipital (calcifying) — see Tendinitis, bicipital
  gonococcal A54.49
  in (due to)
    crystals M65.8- ☑
    gonorrhea A54.49
    syphilis (late) A52.78
    use, overuse, pressure — see also Disorder, soft tissue, due to use
      specified NEC — see Disorder, soft tissue, due to use, specified NEC
  infective NEC M65.1- ☑
    ankle M65.17- ☑
    foot M65.17- ☑
    forearm M65.13- ☑
    hand M65.14- ☑
    lower leg M65.16- ☑
    multiple sites M65.19
    pelvic region M65.15- ☑
    shoulder region M65.11- ☑
    specified site NEC M65.18
    thigh M65.15- ☑
    upper arm M65.12- ☑
  radial styloid M65.4
  shoulder region M65.81- ☑
    adhesive — see Capsulitis, adhesive
  specified type NEC M65.88
    ankle M65.87- ☑
    foot M65.87- ☑
    forearm M65.83- ☑
    hand M65.84- ☑
    lower leg M65.86- ☑
    multiple sites M65.89
    pelvic region M65.85- ☑
    shoulder region M65.81- ☑
    specified site NEC M65.88
    thigh M65.85- ☑
    upper arm M65.82- ☑
  tuberculous — see Tuberculosis, tenosynovitis
Tenovaginitis — see Tenosynovitis
Tension
  arterial, high — see also Hypertension
    without diagnosis of hypertension R03.0
  headache G44.209
    intractable G44.201
    not intractable G44.209
  nervous R45.0
  pneumothorax J93.0
  premenstrual N94.3
  state (mental) F48.9
Tentorium — see condition
Teratencephalus Q89.89
Teratism Q89.7
Teratoblastoma (malignant) — see Neoplasm, malignant, by site
Teratocarcinoma — see also Neoplasm, malignant, by site
  liver C22.7
Teratoma (solid) — see also Neoplasm, uncertain behavior, by site
  with embryonal carcinoma, mixed — see Neoplasm, malignant, by site
  with malignant transformation — see Neoplasm, malignant, by site
  adult (cystic) — see Neoplasm, benign, by site
  benign — see Neoplasm, benign, by site
  combined with choriocarcinoma — see Neoplasm, malignant, by site
  cystic (adult) — see Neoplasm, benign, by site
  differentiated — see Neoplasm, benign, by site
  embryonal — see also Neoplasm, malignant, by site
    liver C22.7
  immature — see Neoplasm, malignant, by site
    liver C22.7
    adult, benign, cystic, differentiated or mature D13.4
  malignant — see also Neoplasm, malignant, by site

Teratoma — continued
  malignant — see also Neoplasm, malignant, by site — continued
    anaplastic — see Neoplasm, malignant, by site
    intermediate — see Neoplasm, malignant, by site
    specified site — see Neoplasm, malignant, by site
    unspecified site C62.90
    undifferentiated — see Neoplasm, malignant, by site
  mature — see Neoplasm, uncertain behavior, by site
    malignant — see Neoplasm, by site, malignant, by site
  ovary D27.- ☑
    embryonal, immature or malignant C56.- ☑
  solid — see Neoplasm, uncertain behavior, by site
  testis C62.9- ☑
    adult, benign, cystic, differentiated type or mature D29.2- ☑
    scrotal C62.1- ☑
    undescended C62.0- ☑
Termination
  anomalous — see also Malposition, congenital
    right pulmonary vein Q26.3
  pregnancy, elective Z33.2
Ternidens diminutus infestation B81.8
Ternidensiasis B81.8
Terror(s) night (child) F51.4
Terrorism, victim of Z65.4
Terry's syndrome — see also Myopia, degenerative H44.2- ☑
Tertiary — see condition
Test, tests, testing (for)
  adequacy (for dialysis)
    hemodialysis Z49.31
    peritoneal Z49.32
  blood-alcohol Z02.83
    positive — see Findings, abnormal, in blood
  blood-drug Z02.83
    positive — see Findings, abnormal, in blood
  blood pressure Z01.30
    abnormal reading — see Blood, pressure
  blood typing Z01.83
    Rh typing Z01.83
  cardiac pulse generator (battery) Z45.010
  fertility Z31.41
  genetic
    disease carrier status for procreative management
      female Z31.430
      male Z31.440
    male partner of patient with recurrent pregnancy loss Z31.441
    procreative management NEC
      female Z31.438
      male Z31.448
  hearing Z01.10
    with abnormal findings NEC Z01.118
    infant or child (over 28 days old) Z00.129
      with abnormal findings Z00.121
  HIV (human immunodeficiency virus)
    nonconclusive (in infants) R75
    positive Z21
    seropositive Z21
  immunity status Z01.84
  intelligence NEC Z01.89
  laboratory (as part of a general medical examination) Z00.00
    with abnormal finding Z00.01
    for medicolegal reason NEC Z04.89
  male partner of patient with recurrent pregnancy loss Z31.441
  Mantoux (for tuberculosis) Z11.1
    abnormal result R76.11
  pregnancy, positive first pregnancy — see Pregnancy, normal, first
  procreative Z31.49
    fertility Z31.41
  skin, diagnostic
    allergy Z01.82
    special screening examination — see Screening, by name of disease
    Mantoux Z11.1
    tuberculin Z11.1
  specified NEC Z01.89
  tuberculin Z11.1
    abnormal result R76.11
  vision Z01.00
    with abnormal findings Z01.01
    following failed vision screening Z01.020
      with abnormal findings Z01.021

Test, tests, testing — continued
- vision — continued
  - infant or child (over 28 days old) Z00.129
    - with abnormal findings Z00.121
  - Wassermann Z11.3
    - positive — see Serology for syphilis, positive

Testicle, testicular, testis — see also condition
- feminization syndrome — see also Syndrome, androgen insensitivity E34.51
- migrans Q55.29

Tetanus, tetanic (cephalic) (convulsions) A35
- with
  - abortion A34
  - ectopic or molar pregnancy O08.0
- following ectopic or molar pregnancy O08.0
- inoculation reaction (due to serum) — see Complications, vaccination
- neonatorum A33
- obstetrical A34
- puerperal, postpartum, childbirth A34

Tetany (due to) R29.0
- alkalosis E87.3
- associated with rickets E55.0
- convulsions R29.0
  - hysterical F44.5
- functional (hysterical) F44.5
- hyperkinetic R29.0
  - hysterical F44.5
- hyperpnea R06.4
  - hysterical F44.5
  - psychogenic F45.8
- hyperventilation — see also Hyperventilation R06.4
  - hysterical F44.5
- neonatal (without calcium or magnesium deficiency) P71.3
- parathyroid (gland) E20.9
- parathyroprival E89.2
- post- (para)thyroidectomy E89.2
- postoperative E89.2
- pseudotetany R29.0
- psychogenic (conversion reaction) F44.5

Tetralogy of Fallot Q21.3
Tetraplegia (chronic) — see also Quadriplegia G82.50
Thailand hemorrhagic fever A91
Thalassanemia — see Thalassemia
Thalassemia (anemia) (disease) D56.9
- with other hemoglobinopathy D56.8
- alpha (major) (severe) (triple gene defect) D56.0
  - minor D56.3
  - silent carrier D56.3
  - trait D56.3
- beta (severe) D56.1
  - homozygous D56.1
  - major D56.1
  - minor D56.3
  - trait D56.3
- delta-beta (homozygous) D56.2
  - minor D56.3
  - trait D56.3
- dominant D56.8
- hemoglobin
  - C D56.8
  - E-beta D56.5
- intermedia D56.1
- major D56.1
- minor D56.3
- mixed D56.8
- sickle-cell — see Disease, sickle-cell, thalassemia
- specified type NEC D56.8
- trait D56.3
- variants D56.8

Thanatophoric dwarfism or short stature Q77.1
Thaysen-Gee disease (nontropical sprue) K90.0
Thaysen's disease K90.0
Thecoma D27.-
- luteinized D27.-
- malignant C56.-

Thelarche, premature E30.8
Thelaziasis B83.8
Thelitis N61.0
- puerperal, postpartum or gestational — see Infection, nipple

Therapeutic — see condition
Therapy
- drug, long-term (current) (prophylactic)
  - agents affecting estrogen receptors and estrogen levels NEC Z79.818
  - anastrozole (Arimidex) Z79.811
  - anti-inflammatory Z79.1

Therapy — continued
- drug, long-term — continued
  - antibiotics Z79.2
    - short-term use — omit code
  - anticoagulants Z79.01
  - antiplatelet Z79.02
  - antithrombotics Z79.02
  - aromatase inhibitors Z79.811
  - aspirin Z79.82
  - birth control pill or patch Z79.3
  - bisphosphonates Z79.83
  - contraceptive, oral Z79.3
  - drug, specified NEC Z79.899
  - estrogen receptor downregulators Z79.818
  - Evista Z79.810
  - exemestane (Aromasin) Z79.811
  - Fareston Z79.810
  - fulvestrant (Faslodex) Z79.818
  - gonadotropin-releasing hormone (GnRH) agonist Z79.818
  - goserelin acetate (Zoladex) Z79.818
  - hormone replacement Z79.890
  - insulin Z79.4
  - letrozole (Femara) Z79.811
  - leuprolide acetate (leuprorelin) (Lupron) Z79.818
  - megestrol acetate (Megace) Z79.818
  - methadone
    - for pain management Z79.891
    - maintenance therapy F11.20
  - Nolvadex Z79.810
  - opiate analgesic Z79.891
  - oral antidiabetic Z79.84
  - oral contraceptive Z79.3
  - oral hypoglycemic Z79.84
  - raloxifene (Evista) Z79.810
  - selective estrogen receptor modulators (SERMs) Z79.810
  - short term — omit code
  - steroids
    - inhaled Z79.51
    - systemic Z79.52
  - tamoxifen (Nolvadex) Z79.810
  - toremifene (Fareston) Z79.810

Thermic — see condition
Thermography (abnormal) — see also Abnormal, diagnostic imaging R93.89
- breast R92.8

Thermoplegia T67.01- ☑
Thesaurismosis, glycogen — see Disease, glycogen storage
Thiamin deficiency E51.9
- specified NEC E51.8

Thiaminic deficiency with beriberi E51.11
Thibierge-Weissenbach syndrome — see Sclerosis, systemic
Thickening
- bone — see Hypertrophy, bone
- breast N64.59
- endometrium R93.89
- epidermal L85.9
  - specified NEC L85.8
- hymen N89.6
- larynx J38.7
- nail L60.2
  - congenital Q84.5
- periosteal — see Hypertrophy, bone
- pleura J92.9
  - with asbestos J92.0
- skin R23.4
- subepiglottic J38.7
- tongue K14.8
- valve, heart — see Endocarditis

Thigh — see condition
Thinning vertebra — see Spondylopathy, specified NEC
Thirst, excessive R63.1
- due to deprivation of water T73.1- ☑

Thomsen disease G71.12
Thoracic — see also condition
- kidney Q63.2
- outlet syndrome — see also Syndrome, thoracic outlet G54.0

Thoracogastroschisis (congenital) Q79.8
Thoracopagus Q89.4
Thorax — see condition
Thorn's syndrome N28.89
Thorson-Bjorck syndrome E34.09
Threadworm (infection) (infestation) B80
Threatened
- abortion O20.0
  - with subsequent abortion O03.9

Threatened — continued
- abuse (harm)
  - adult — see Maltreatment, adult, threatened abuse
  - child — see Maltreatment, child, threatened abuse
- job loss, anxiety concerning Z56.2
- labor (without delivery) O47.9
  - at or after 37 completed weeks of gestation O47.1
  - before 37 completed weeks of gestation O47.0- ☑
- loss of job, anxiety concerning Z56.2
- miscarriage O20.0
- unemployment, anxiety concerning Z56.2

Three-day fever A93.1
Threshers' lung J67.0
Thrix annulata (congenital) Q84.1
Throat — see condition
Thrombasthenia (Glanzmann) (hemorrhagic) (hereditary) D69.1
Thromboangiitis I73.1
- obliterans (general) I73.1
  - cerebral I67.89
  - vessels
    - brain I67.89
    - spinal cord I67.89

Thromboarteritis — see Arteritis
Thromboasthenia (Glanzmann) (hemorrhagic) (hereditary) D69.1
Thrombocytasthenia (Glanzmann) D69.1
Thrombocythemia (hemorrhagic) see also Thrombocytosis D75.839
- essential D47.3
- idiopathic D47.3
- primary D47.3

Thrombocytopathy (dystrophic) (granulopenic) D69.1
Thrombocytopenia, thrombocytopenic D69.6
- with absent radius (TAR) Q87.2
- congenital D69.42
- dilutional D69.59
- due to
  - (massive) blood transfusion D69.59
  - drugs D69.59
  - extracorporeal circulation of blood D69.59
  - platelet alloimmunization D69.59
- essential D69.3
- heparin-associated D75.821
- heparin induced (HIT) D75.829
  - delayed-onset D75.828
  - immune-mediated D75.822
  - non-immune D75.821
  - persisting D75.828
  - syndrome
    - autoimmune D75.828
    - specified NEC D75.828
    - spontaneous (without heparin exposure) D75.84
  - type 1 D75.821
  - type 2 D75.822
- hereditary D69.42
- idiopathic D69.3
- neonatal, transitory P61.0
  - due to
    - exchange transfusion P61.0
    - idiopathic maternal thrombocytopenia P61.0
    - isoimmunization P61.0
- primary NEC D69.49
  - idiopathic D69.3
- puerperal, postpartum O72.3
- secondary D69.59
- transient neonatal P61.0
- vaccine-induced thrombotic D75.84

Thrombocytosis D75.839
- essential D47.3
- idiopathic D47.3
- primary D47.3
- reactive D75.838
- secondary D75.838
- specified NEC D75.838

Thromboembolism — see Embolism
Thrombopathy (Bernard-Soulier) D69.1
- constitutional — see Disease, von Willebrand
- Willebrand-Jurgens — see Disease, von Willebrand

Thrombopenia — see Thrombocytopenia
Thrombophilia D68.59
- primary NEC D68.59
- secondary NEC D68.69
- specified NEC D68.69

Thrombophlebitis I80.9
- antepartum O22.2- ☑
  - deep O22.3- ☑
  - superficial O22.2- ☑

Thrombophlebitis — continued
- calf muscular vein (NOS) I80.25- ☑
- cavernous (venous) sinus G08
  - complicating pregnancy O22.5- ☑
  - nonpyogenic I67.6
- cerebral (sinus) (vein) G08
  - nonpyogenic I67.6
  - sequelae G09
- due to implanted device — see Complications, by site and type, specified NEC
- during or resulting from a procedure NEC T81.72- ☑
- femoral vein (superficial) I80.1- ☑
- femoropopliteal vein I80.0- ☑
- gastrocnemial vein I80.25- ☑
- hepatic (vein) I80.8
- idiopathic, recurrent I82.1
- iliac vein (common) (external) (internal) I80.21- ☑
- iliofemoral I80.1- ☑
- intracranial venous sinus (any) G08
  - nonpyogenic I67.6
  - sequelae G09
- intraspinal venous sinuses and veins G08
  - nonpyogenic G95.19
- lateral (venous) sinus G08
  - nonpyogenic I67.6
- leg I80.3
  - superficial I80.0- ☑
- longitudinal (venous) sinus G08
  - nonpyogenic I67.6
- lower extremity I80.299
- migrans, migrating I82.1
- pelvic
  - with ectopic or molar pregnancy O08.0
  - following ectopic or molar pregnancy O08.0
  - puerperal O87.1
- peroneal vein I80.24- ☑
- popliteal vein — see Phlebitis, leg, deep, popliteal
- portal (vein) K75.1
- postoperative T81.72- ☑
- pregnancy — see Thrombophlebitis, antepartum
- puerperal, postpartum, childbirth O87.0
  - deep O87.1
  - pelvic O87.1
  - septic O86.81
  - superficial O87.0
- saphenous (greater) (lesser) I80.0- ☑
- sinus (intracranial) G08
  - nonpyogenic I67.6
- soleal vein I80.25- ☑
- specified site NEC I80.8
- tibial vein (anterior) (posterior) I80.23- ☑

Thrombosis, thrombotic (bland) (multiple) (progressive) (silent) (vessel) I82.90
- anal K64.5
- antepartum — see Thrombophlebitis, antepartum
- aorta, aortic I74.10
  - abdominal I74.09
    - saddle I74.01
  - bifurcation I74.09
  - saddle I74.01
  - specified site NEC I74.19
  - terminal I74.09
  - thoracic I74.11
  - valve — see Endocarditis, aortic
- apoplexy I63.3- ☑
- artery, arteries (postinfectional) I74.9
  - auditory, internal — see Occlusion, artery, precerebral, specified NEC
  - basilar — see Occlusion, artery, basilar
  - carotid (common) (internal) — see Occlusion, artery, carotid
  - cerebellar (anterior inferior) (posterior inferior) (superior) — see Occlusion, artery, cerebellar
  - cerebral — see Occlusion, artery, cerebral
  - choroidal (anterior) — see Occlusion, artery, precerebral, specified NEC
  - communicating, posterior — see Occlusion, artery, precerebral, specified NEC
  - coronary — see also Infarct, myocardium
    - not resulting in infarction I24.0
  - hepatic I74.8
  - hypophyseal — see Occlusion, artery, precerebral, specified NEC
  - iliac I74.5
  - limb I74.4
    - lower I74.3
    - upper I74.2

Thrombosis, thrombotic — continued
- artery, arteries — continued
  - meningeal, anterior or posterior — see Occlusion, artery, cerebral, specified NEC
  - mesenteric (with gangrene) — see also Infarct, intestine K55.069
  - ophthalmic — see Occlusion, artery, retina
  - pontine — see Occlusion, artery, precerebral, specified NEC
  - precerebral — see Occlusion, artery, precerebral
  - pulmonary (iatrogenic) — see Embolism, pulmonary
  - renal N28.0
  - retinal — see Occlusion, artery, retina
  - spinal, anterior or posterior G95.11
  - traumatic NEC T14.8- ☑
  - vertebral — see Occlusion, artery, vertebral
- atrium, auricular — see also Infarct, myocardium
  - following acute myocardial infarction (current complication) I23.6
  - not resulting in infarction I51.3
  - old I51.3
- basilar (artery) — see Occlusion, artery, basilar
- brain (artery) (stem) — see also Occlusion, artery, cerebral
  - due to syphilis A52.05
  - puerperal O99.43
  - sinus — see Thrombosis, intracranial, venous sinus
- capillary I78.8
- cardiac — see also Infarct, myocardium
  - not resulting in infarction I51.3
  - old I51.3
  - valve — see Endocarditis
- carotid (artery) (common) (internal) — see Occlusion, artery, carotid
- cavernous (venous) sinus — see Thrombosis, intracranial, venous sinus
- cerebellar artery (anterior inferior) (posterior inferior) (superior) I66.3
- cerebral (artery) — see Occlusion, artery, cerebral
- cerebrovenous sinus — see also Thrombosis, intracranial, venous sinus
  - puerperium O87.3
- chronic I82.91
- coronary (artery) (vein) — see also Infarct, myocardium
  - not resulting in infarction I24.0
- corpus cavernosum N48.89
- cortical I66.9
- deep — see Embolism, vein, lower extremity
- due to device, implant or graft — see also Complications, by site and type, specified NEC T85.868- ☑
  - arterial graft NEC T82.868- ☑
  - breast (implant) T85.868- ☑
  - catheter NEC T85.868- ☑
    - dialysis (renal) T82.868- ☑
      - intraperitoneal T85.868- ☑
    - infusion NEC T82.868- ☑
      - spinal (epidural) (subdural) T85.860- ☑
    - urinary (indwelling) T83.86- ☑
  - electronic (electrode) (pulse generator) (stimulator)
    - bone T84.86- ☑
    - cardiac T82.867- ☑
    - nervous system (brain) (peripheral nerve) (spinal) T85.860- ☑
    - urinary T83.86- ☑
  - fixation, internal (orthopedic) NEC T84.86- ☑
  - gastrointestinal (bile duct) (esophagus) T85.868- ☑
  - genital NEC T83.86- ☑
  - heart T82.867- ☑
  - joint prosthesis T84.86- ☑
  - ocular (corneal graft) (orbital implant) NEC T85.868- ☑
  - orthopedic NEC T84.86- ☑
  - specified NEC T85.868- ☑
  - urinary NEC T83.86- ☑
  - vascular NEC T82.868- ☑
  - ventricular intracranial shunt T85.860- ☑
- during the puerperium — see Thrombosis, puerperal
- endocardial — see also Infarct, myocardium
  - not resulting in infarction I51.3
- eye — see Occlusion, retina
- genital organ
  - female NEC N94.89
    - pregnancy — see Thrombophlebitis, antepartum
  - male N50.1
- gestational — see Phlebopathy, gestational
- heart (chamber) — see also Infarct, myocardium
  - not resulting in infarction I51.3
  - old I51.3
- hepatic (vein) I82.0

Thrombosis, thrombotic — continued
- hepatic — continued
  - artery I74.8
- history (of) Z86.718
- intestine (with gangrene) — see also Infarct, intestine K55.069
- intracardiac NEC (apical) (atrial) (auricular) (ventricular) (old) I51.3
- intracranial (arterial) I66.9
  - venous sinus (any) G08
    - nonpyogenic I67.6
    - nonpyogenic origin I67.6
    - puerperium O87.3
- intramural — see also Infarct, myocardium
  - not resulting in infarction I51.3
  - old I51.3
- intraspinal venous sinuses and veins G08
  - nonpyogenic G95.19
- kidney (artery) N28.0
- lateral (venous) sinus — see Thrombosis, intracranial, venous sinus
- leg — see Thrombosis, vein, lower extremity
  - arterial I74.3
- liver (venous) I82.0
  - artery I74.8
  - portal vein I81
- longitudinal (venous) sinus — see Thrombosis, intracranial, venous sinus
- lower limb — see Thrombosis, vein, lower extremity
- lung (iatrogenic) (postoperative) — see Embolism, pulmonary
- meninges (brain) (arterial) I66.8
- mesenteric (artery) (with gangrene) — see also Infarct, intestine K55.069
  - vein (inferior) (superior) K55.0- ☑
- mitral I34.89
- mural — see also Infarct, myocardium
  - due to syphilis A52.06
  - not resulting in infarction I51.3
  - old I51.3
- omentum (with gangrene) — see also Infarct, intestine K55.069
- ophthalmic — see Occlusion, retina
- pampiniform plexus (male) N50.1
- parietal — see also Infarct, myocardium
  - not resulting in infarction I24.0
- penis, superficial vein N48.81
- perianal venous K64.5
- peripheral arteries I74.4
  - upper I74.2
- personal history (of) Z86.718
- portal I81
  - due to syphilis A52.09
- precerebral artery — see Occlusion, artery, precerebral
- puerperal, postpartum O87.0
  - brain (artery) O99.43
    - venous (sinus) O87.3
  - cardiac O99.43
  - cerebral (artery) O99.43
    - venous (sinus) O87.3
  - superficial O87.0
- pulmonary (artery) (iatrogenic) (postoperative) (vein) — see Embolism, pulmonary
- renal (artery) N28.0
  - vein I82.3
- resulting from presence of device, implant or graft — see Complications, by site and type, specified NEC
- retina, retinal — see Occlusion, retina
- scrotum N50.1
- seminal vesicle N50.1
- sigmoid (venous) sinus — see Thrombosis, intracranial, venous sinus
- sinus, intracranial (any) — see Thrombosis, intracranial, venous sinus
- specified site NEC I82.890
  - chronic I82.891
- spermatic cord N50.1
- spinal cord (arterial) G95.11
  - due to syphilis A52.09
  - pyogenic origin G06.1
- spleen, splenic D73.5
  - artery I74.8
- testis N50.1
- traumatic NEC T14.8- ☑
- tricuspid I07.8
- tumor — see Neoplasm, unspecified behavior, by site
- tunica vaginalis N50.1
- umbilical cord (vessels), complicating delivery O69.5- ☑
- vas deferens N50.1

☑ Additional Character Required — Refer to the Tabular List for Character Selection

Thrombosis, thrombotic — *continued*
  vein (acute) I82.90
    antecubital I82.61- ☑
      chronic I82.71- ☑
    axillary I82.A1- ☑ (*following* I82.7)
      chronic I82.A2- ☑ (*following* I82.7)
    basilic I82.61- ☑
      chronic I82.71- ☑
    brachial I82.62- ☑
      chronic I82.72- ☑
    brachiocephalic (innominate) I82.290
      chronic I82.291
    calf muscular I82.46- ☑
      chronic I82.56- ☑
    cephalic I82.61- ☑
      chronic I82.71- ☑
    cerebral, nonpyogenic I67.6
    chronic I82.91
    deep (DVT) I82.40- ☑
      calf I82.4Z- ☑
        chronic I82.5Z- ☑
      lower leg I82.4Z- ☑
        chronic I82.5Z- ☑
      thigh I82.4Y- ☑
        chronic I82.5Y- ☑
      upper leg I82.4Y- ☑
        chronic I82.5Y- ☑
    femoral I82.41- ☑
      chronic I82.51- ☑
    iliac (iliofemoral) I82.42- ☑
      chronic I82.52- ☑
    innominate I82.290
      chronic I82.291
    internal jugular I82.C1- ☑ (*following* I82.7)
      chronic I82.C2- ☑ (*following* I82.7)
    lower extremity
      deep I82.40- ☑
        chronic I82.50- ☑
        specified NEC I82.49- ☑
          chronic NEC I82.59- ☑
      distal
        deep I82.4Z- ☑
      proximal
        deep I82.4Y- ☑
          chronic I82.5Y- ☑
      superficial I82.81- ☑
    perianal K64.5
    peroneal I82.45- ☑
      chronic I82.55- ☑
    popliteal I82.43- ☑
      chronic I82.53- ☑
    radial I82.62- ☑
      chronic I82.72- ☑
    renal I82.3
    saphenous (greater) (lesser) I82.81- ☑
    specified NEC I82.890
      chronic NEC I82.891
    subclavian I82.B1- ☑ (*following* I82.7)
      chronic I82.B2- ☑ (*following* I82.7)
    thoracic NEC I82.290
      chronic I82.291
    tibial I82.44- ☑
      chronic I82.54- ☑
    ulnar I82.62- ☑
      chronic I82.72- ☑
    upper extremity I82.60- ☑
      chronic I82.70- ☑
      deep I82.62- ☑
        chronic I82.72- ☑
      superficial I82.61- ☑
        chronic I82.71- ☑
  vena cava
    inferior I82.220
      chronic I82.221
    superior I82.210
      chronic I82.211
  venous, perianal K64.5
  ventricle — *see also* Infarct, myocardium
    following acute myocardial infarction (current complication) I23.6
    not resulting in infarction I24.0
    old I51.3
Thrombus — *see* Thrombosis
Thrush — *see also* Candidiasis
  newborn P37.5
  oral B37.0

Thrush — *continued*
  vaginal (acute) B37.31
    chronic (recurrent) B37.32
Thumb — *see also* condition
  sucking (child problem) F98.8
Thymitis E32.8
Thymoma — *see also* Neoplasm, thymus, by type
  malignant C37
  metaplastic C37
  microscopic D15.0
  sclerosing C37
  type A C37
  type AB C37
  type B1 C37
  type B2 C37
  type B3 C37
Thymus, thymic (gland) — *see* condition
Thyrocele — *see* Goiter
Thyroglossal — *see also* condition
  cyst Q89.2
  duct, persistent Q89.2
Thyroid (gland) (body) — *see also* condition
  hormone resistance E07.89
  lingual Q89.2
  nodule (cystic) (nontoxic) (single) E04.1
Thyroiditis E06.9
  acute (nonsuppurative) (pyogenic) (suppurative) E06.0
  autoimmune E06.3
  chronic (nonspecific) (sclerosing) E06.5
    with thyrotoxicosis, transient E06.2
    fibrous E06.5
    lymphadenoid E06.3
    lymphocytic E06.3
    lymphoid E06.3
  de Quervain's E06.1
  drug-induced E06.4
  fibrous (chronic) E06.5
  giant-cell (follicular) E06.1
  granulomatous (de Quervain) (subacute) E06.1
  Hashimoto's (struma lymphomatosa) E06.3
  iatrogenic E06.4
  ligneous E06.5
  lymphocytic (chronic) E06.3
  lymphoid E06.3
  lymphomatous E06.3
  nonsuppurative E06.1
  postpartum, puerperal O90.5
  pseudotuberculous E06.1
  pyogenic E06.0
  radiation E06.4
  Riedel's E06.5
  subacute (granulomatous) E06.1
  suppurative E06.0
  tuberculous A18.81
  viral E06.1
  woody E06.5
Thyrolingual duct, persistent Q89.2
Thyromegaly E01.0
Thyrotoxic
  crisis — *see* Thyrotoxicosis
  heart disease or failure — *see also* Thyrotoxicosis E05.90 [I43]
    with thyroid storm E05.91 [I43]
  storm — *see* Thyrotoxicosis
Thyrotoxicosis (recurrent) E05.90
  with
    goiter (diffuse) E05.00
      with thyroid storm E05.01
      adenomatous uninodular E05.10
        with thyroid storm E05.11
      multinodular E05.20
        with thyroid storm E05.21
      nodular E05.20
        with thyroid storm E05.21
      uninodular E05.10
        with thyroid storm E05.11
    infiltrative
      dermopathy E05.00
        with thyroid storm E05.01
      ophthalmopathy E05.00
        with thyroid storm E05.01
    single thyroid nodule E05.10
      with thyroid storm E05.11
    thyroid storm E05.91
  due to
    ectopic thyroid nodule or tissue E05.30
      with thyroid storm E05.31
    ingestion of (excessive) thyroid material E05.40
      with thyroid storm E05.41

Thyrotoxicosis — *continued*
  due to — *continued*
    overproduction of thyroid-stimulating hormone E05.80
      with thyroid storm E05.81
    specified cause NEC E05.80
      with thyroid storm E05.81
  factitia E05.40
    with thyroid storm E05.41
  heart — *see also* Failure, heart, high-output E05.90 [I43]
    with thyroid storm — *see also* Failure, heart, high-output E05.91 [I43]
    failure — *see also* Failure, heart, high-output E05.90 [I43]
  neonatal (transient) P72.1
  transient with chronic thyroiditis E06.2
Tibia vara M92.51- ☑
Tic (disorder) F95.9
  breathing F95.8
  child problem F95.0
  compulsive F95.1
  de la Tourette F95.2
  degenerative (generalized) (localized) G25.69
    facial G25.69
  disorder
    chronic
      motor F95.1
      vocal F95.1
    combined vocal and multiple motor F95.2
    transient F95.0
  douloureux G50.0
    atypical G50.1
    postherpetic, postzoster B02.22
  drug-induced G25.61
  eyelid F95.8
  habit F95.9
    chronic F95.1
    transient of childhood F95.0
  lid, transient of childhood F95.0
  motor-verbal F95.2
  occupational F48.8
  orbicularis F95.8
    transient of childhood F95.0
  organic origin G25.69
  postchoreic G25.69
  provisional F95.0
  psychogenic, compulsive F95.1
  salaam R25.8
  spasm (motor or vocal) F95.9
    chronic F95.1
    transient of childhood F95.0
  specified NEC F95.8
Tick-borne — *see* condition
Tietze's disease or syndrome M94.0
Tight, tightness
  anus K62.89
  chest R07.89
  fascia (lata) M62.89
  foreskin (congenital) N47.1
  hymen, hymenal ring N89.6
  introitus (acquired) (congenital) N89.6
  rectal sphincter K62.89
  tendon — *see* Short, tendon
  urethral sphincter N35.919
Tilting vertebra — *see* Dorsopathy, deforming, specified NEC
Timidity, child F93.8
Tin-miner's lung J63.5
Tinea (intersecta) (tarsi) B35.9
  amiantacea L44.8
  asbestina B35.0
  barbae B35.0
  beard B35.0
  black dot B35.0
  blanca B36.2
  capitis B35.0
  corporis B35.4
  cruris B35.6
  flava B36.0
  foot B35.3
  furfuracea B36.0
  imbricata (Tokelau) B35.5
  kerion B35.0
  manuum B35.2
  microsporic — *see* Dermatophytosis
  nigra B36.1
  nodosa — *see* Piedra
  pedis B35.3
  scalp B35.0

Tinea — *continued*
  specified NEC B35.8
  sycosis B35.0
  tonsurans B35.0
  trichophytic — *see* Dermatophytosis
  unguium B35.1
  versicolor B36.0
Tingling sensation (skin) R20.2
Tinnitus NOS H93.1- ☑
  audible H93.1- ☑
  aurium H93.1- ☑
  pulsatile H93.A- ☑
  subjective H93.1- ☑
Tipped tooth (teeth) M26.33
Tipping
  pelvis M95.5
    with disproportion (fetopelvic) O33.0
      causing obstructed labor O65.0
  tooth (teeth), fully erupted M26.33
Tiredness R53.83
Tissue — *see* condition
Tobacco (nicotine)
  abuse — *see* Tobacco, use
  dependence — *see* Dependence, drug, nicotine
  harmful use Z72.0
  heart — *see* Tobacco, toxic effect
  maternal use, affecting newborn P04.2
  toxic effect — *see* Table of Drugs and Chemicals, by substance, poisoning
    chewing tobacco — *see* Table of Drugs and Chemicals, by substance, poisoning
    cigarettes — *see* Table of Drugs and Chemicals, by substance, poisoning
  use Z72.0
    complicating
      childbirth O99.334
      pregnancy O99.33- ☑
      puerperium O99.335
    counseling and surveillance Z71.6
    history Z87.891
    withdrawal state — *see also* Dependence, drug, nicotine F17.203
Tocopherol deficiency E56.0
Todd's
  cirrhosis K74.3
  paralysis (postepileptic) (transitory) G83.84
Toe — *see* condition
Toilet, artificial opening — *see* Attention to, artificial, opening
Tokelau (ringworm) B35.5
Tollwut — *see* Rabies
Tommaselli's disease R31.9
  correct substance properly administered — *see* Table of Drugs and Chemicals, by drug, adverse effect
  overdose or wrong substance given or taken — *see* Table of Drugs and Chemicals, by drug, poisoning
Tongue — *see also* condition
  tie Q38.1
Toni-Fanconi syndrome (cystinosis) E72.09
  with cystinosis E72.04
Tonic pupil — *see* Anomaly, pupil, function, tonic pupil
Tonsil — *see* condition
Tonsillitis (acute) (catarrhal) (croupous) (follicular) (gangrenous) (infective) (lacunar) (lingual) (malignant) (membranous) (parenchymatous) (phlegmonous) (pseudomembranous) (purulent) (septic) (subacute) (suppurative) (toxic) (ulcerative) (vesicular) (viral) J03.90
  chronic J35.01
    with adenoiditis J35.03
  diphtheritic A36.0
  hypertrophic J35.01
    with adenoiditis J35.03
  recurrent J03.91
  specified organism NEC J03.80
    recurrent J03.81
  staphylococcal J03.80
    recurrent J03.81
  streptococcal J03.00
    recurrent J03.01
  tuberculous A15.8
  Vincent's A69.1
Tooth, teeth — *see* condition
Toothache K08.89
Topagnosis R20.8
Tophi — *see* Gout, chronic
TORCH infection — *see* Infection, congenital
  without active infection P00.2

Torn — *see* Tear
Tornwaldt's cyst or disease J39.2
Torsades de pointes I47.21
Torsion
  accessory tube — *see* Torsion, fallopian tube
  adnexa (female) — *see* Torsion, fallopian tube
  aorta, acquired I77.1
  appendix epididymis N44.04
  appendix testis N44.03
  bile duct (common) (hepatic) K83.8
    congenital Q44.5
  bowel, colon or intestine K56.2
  cervix — *see* Malposition, uterus
  cystic duct K82.8
  dystonia — *see* Dystonia, torsion
  epididymis (appendix) N44.04
  fallopian tube N83.52- ☑
    with ovary N83.53
  gallbladder K82.8
    congenital Q44.1
  hydatid of Morgagni
    female N83.52- ☑
    male N44.03
  kidney (pedicle) (leading to infarction) N28.0
  Meckel's diverticulum (congenital) Q43.0
    malignant — *see* Table of Neoplasms, small intestine, malignant
  mesentery K56.2
  omentum K56.2
  organ or site, congenital NEC — *see* Anomaly, by site
  ovary (pedicle) N83.51- ☑
    with fallopian tube N83.53
    congenital Q50.2
  oviduct — *see* Torsion, fallopian tube
  penis (acquired) N48.82
    congenital Q55.63
  spasm — *see* Dystonia, torsion
  spermatic cord N44.02
    extravaginal N44.01
    intravaginal N44.02
  spleen D73.5
  testis, testicle N44.00
    appendix N44.03
  tibia — *see* Deformity, limb, specified type NEC, lower leg
  uterus — *see* Malposition, uterus
Torticollis (intermittent) (spastic) M43.6
  congenital (sternomastoid) Q68.0
  due to birth injury P15.8
  hysterical F44.4
  ocular R29.891
  psychogenic F45.8
    conversion reaction F44.4
  rheumatic M43.6
  rheumatoid M06.88
  spasmodic G24.3
  traumatic, current S13.4- ☑
Tortipelvis G24.1
Tortuous
  aortic arch Q25.46
  artery I77.1
  organ or site, congenital NEC — *see* Distortion
  retinal vessel, congenital Q14.1
  ureter N13.8
  urethra N36.8
  vein — *see* Varix
Torture, victim of Z65.4
Torula, torular (histolytica) (infection) — *see* Cryptococcosis
Torulosis — *see* Cryptococcosis
Torus (mandibularis) (palatinus) M27.0
  fracture — *see* Fracture, by site, torus
Touraine's syndrome Q79.8
Tourette's syndrome F95.2
Tourniquet syndrome — *see* Constriction, external, by site
Tower skull Q75.058
  with exophthalmos Q87.0
Toxemia R68.89
  bacterial — *see* Sepsis
  burn — *see* Burn
  eclamptic (with pre-existing hypertension) — *see* Eclampsia
  erysipelatous — *see* Erysipelas
  fatigue R68.89
  food — *see* Poisoning, food
  gastrointestinal K52.1
  intestinal K52.1
  kidney — *see* Uremia
  malarial — *see* Malaria
  myocardial — *see* Myocarditis, toxic

Toxemia — *continued*
  of pregnancy — *see* Pre-eclampsia
  pre-eclamptic — *see* Pre-eclampsia
  small intestine K52.1
  staphylococcal, due to food A05.0
  stasis R68.89
  uremic — *see* Uremia
  urinary — *see* Uremia
Toxemica cerebropathia psychica (nonalcoholic) F04
  alcoholic — *see* Alcohol, amnestic disorder
Toxic (poisoning) — *see also* condition T65.91- ☑
  effect — *see* Table of Drugs and Chemicals, by substance, poisoning
  shock syndrome A48.3
  thyroid (gland) — *see* Thyrotoxicosis
Toxicemia — *see* Toxemia
Toxicity — *see* Table of Drugs and Chemicals, by substance, poisoning
  fava bean D55.0
  food, noxious — *see* Poisoning, food
  from drug or nonmedicinal substance — *see* Table of Drugs and Chemicals, by drug
Toxicosis — *see also* Toxemia
  capillary, hemorrhagic D69.0
Toxinfection, gastrointestinal K52.1
Toxocariasis B83.0
Toxoplasma, toxoplasmosis (acquired) B58.9
  with
    hepatitis B58.1
    meningoencephalitis B58.2
    ocular involvement B58.00
    other organ involvement B58.89
    pneumonia, pneumonitis B58.3
  congenital (acute) (subacute) (chronic) P37.1
  maternal, manifest toxoplasmosis in infant (acute) (subacute) (chronic) P37.1
tPA (rtPA) **administration in a different facility within the last 24 hours prior to admission to current facility** Z92.82
Trabeculation, bladder N32.89
Trachea — *see* condition
Tracheitis (catarrhal) (infantile) (membranous) (plastic) (septal) (suppurative) (viral) J04.10
  with
    bronchitis (15 years of age and above) J40
      acute or subacute — *see* Bronchitis, acute
      chronic J42
      tuberculous NEC A15.5
      under 15 years of age J20.9
    laryngitis (acute) J04.2
      chronic J37.1
      tuberculous NEC A15.5
  acute J04.10
    with obstruction J04.11
  chronic J42
    with
      bronchitis (chronic) J42
      laryngitis (chronic) J37.1
  diphtheritic (membranous) A36.89
  due to external agent — *see* Inflammation, respiratory, upper, due to
  syphilitic A52.73
  tuberculous A15.5
Trachelitis (nonvenereal) — *see* Cervicitis
Tracheobronchial — *see* condition
Tracheobronchitis (15 years of age and above) — *see also* Bronchitis
  due to
    Bordetella bronchiseptica A37.80
      with pneumonia A37.81
    Francisella tularensis A21.8
Tracheobronchomegaly Q32.4
  with bronchiectasis J47.9
    with
      exacerbation (acute) J47.1
      lower respiratory infection J47.0
  acquired J98.09
    with bronchiectasis J47.9
      with
        exacerbation (acute) J47.1
        lower respiratory infection J47.0
Tracheobronchopneumonitis — *see* Pneumonia, broncho-
Tracheocele (external) (internal) J39.8
  congenital Q32.1
Tracheomalacia J39.8
  congenital Q32.0
Tracheopharyngitis (acute) J06.9
  chronic J42

Tracheopharyngitis — continued
- due to external agent — see Inflammation, respiratory, upper, due to

Tracheostenosis J39.8

Tracheostomy
- complication — see Complication, tracheostomy
- status Z93.0
  - attention to Z43.0
  - malfunctioning J95.03

Trachoma, trachomatous A71.9
- active (stage) A71.1
- contraction of conjunctiva A71.1
- dubium A71.0
- healed or sequelae B94.0
- initial (stage) A71.0
- pannus A71.1
- Türck's J37.0

Traction, vitreomacular H43.82- ☑

Train sickness T75.3- ☑

Trait(s)
- Hb-S D57.3
- hemoglobin
  - abnormal NEC D58.2
    - with thalassemia D56.3
  - C — see Disease, hemoglobin C
  - S (Hb-S) D57.3
  - Lepore D56.3
- personality, accentuated Z73.1
- sickle-cell D57.3
  - with elliptocytosis or spherocytosis D57.3
- type A personality Z73.1

Tramp Z59.00

Trance R41.89
- hysterical F44.89

Transaminasemia R74.01

Transection
- abdomen (partial) S38.3- ☑
- aorta (incomplete) — see also Injury, aorta
  - complete — see Injury, aorta, laceration, major
- carotid artery (incomplete) — see also Injury, blood vessel, carotid, laceration
  - complete — see Injury, blood vessel, carotid, laceration, major
- celiac artery (incomplete) S35.211- ☑
  - branch (incomplete) S35.291- ☑
    - complete S35.292- ☑
  - complete S35.212- ☑
- innominate
  - artery (incomplete) — see also Injury, blood vessel, thoracic, innominate, artery, laceration
    - complete — see Injury, blood vessel, thoracic, innominate, artery, laceration, major
  - vein (incomplete) — see also Injury, blood vessel, thoracic, innominate, vein, laceration
    - complete — see Injury, blood vessel, thoracic, innominate, vein, laceration, major
- jugular vein (external) (incomplete) — see also Injury, blood vessel, jugular vein, laceration
  - complete — see Injury, blood vessel, jugular vein, laceration, major
  - internal (incomplete) — see also Injury, blood vessel, jugular vein, internal, laceration
    - complete — see Injury, blood vessel, jugular vein, internal, laceration, major
- mesenteric artery (incomplete) — see also Injury, mesenteric, artery, laceration
  - complete — see Injury, mesenteric artery, laceration, major
- pulmonary vessel (incomplete) — see also Injury, blood vessel, thoracic, pulmonary, laceration
  - complete — see Injury, blood vessel, thoracic, pulmonary, laceration, major
- subclavian — see Transection, innominate
- vena cava (incomplete) — see also Injury, vena cava
  - complete — see Injury, vena cava, laceration, major
- vertebral artery (incomplete) — see also Injury, blood vessel, vertebral, laceration
  - complete — see Injury, blood vessel, vertebral, laceration, major

Transfusion
- associated (red blood cell) hemochromatosis E83.111
- blood
  - ABO incompatible — see Complication(s), transfusion, incompatibility reaction, ABO
  - minor blood group (Duffy) (E) (K) (Kell) (Kidd) (Lewis) (M) (N) (P) (S) T80.89- ☑
  - reaction or complication — see Complications, transfusion

Transfusion — continued
- fetomaternal (mother) — see Pregnancy, complicated by, placenta, transfusion syndrome
- maternofetal (mother) — see Pregnancy, complicated by, placenta, transfusion syndrome
- placental (syndrome) (mother) — see Pregnancy, complicated by, placenta, transfusion syndrome
- reaction (adverse) — see Complications, transfusion
- related acute lung injury (TRALI) J95.84
- twin-to-twin — see Pregnancy, complicated by, placenta, transfusion syndrome, fetus to fetus

Transgender F64.0

Transient (meaning homeless) — see also condition Z59.00

Translocation
- balanced autosomal Q95.9
  - in normal individual Q95.0
- chromosomes NEC Q99.8- ☑
  - balanced and insertion in normal individual Q95.0
- Down syndrome Q90.2
- trisomy
  - 13 Q91.6
  - 18 Q91.2
  - 21 Q90.2

Translucency, iris — see Degeneration, iris

Transmission of chemical substances through the placenta — see Absorption, chemical, through placenta

Transparency, lung, unilateral J43.0

Transplant (ed) (status) Z94.9
- awaiting organ Z76.82
- bone Z94.6
  - marrow Z94.81
- candidate Z76.82
- complication — see Complication, transplant
- cornea Z94.7
- heart Z94.1
  - and lung(s) Z94.3
  - valve Z95.2
    - prosthetic Z95.2
    - specified NEC Z95.4
    - xenogenic Z95.3
- intestine Z94.82
- kidney Z94.0
- liver Z94.4
- lung(s) Z94.2
  - and heart Z94.3
- organ (failure) (infection) (rejection) Z94.9
  - removal status Z98.85
- pancreas Z94.83
- skin Z94.5
- social Z60.3
- specified organ or tissue NEC Z94.89
- stem cells Z94.84
- tissue Z94.9

Transplants, ovarian, endometrial N80.10- ☑

Transposed — see Transposition

Transposition (congenital) — see also Malposition, congenital
- abdominal viscera Q89.3
- aorta (dextra) Q20.3
- appendix Q43.8
- colon Q43.8
- corrected Q20.5
- great vessels (complete) (partial) Q20.3
- heart Q24.0
  - with complete transposition of viscera Q89.3
- intestine (large) (small) Q43.8
- reversed jejunal (for bypass) (status) Z98.0
- scrotum Q55.23
- stomach Q40.2
  - with general transposition of viscera Q89.3
- tooth, teeth, fully erupted M26.30
- vessels, great (complete) (partial) Q20.3
- viscera (abdominal) (thoracic) Q89.3

Transsexualism F64.0

Transverse — see also condition
- arrest (deep), in labor O64.0- ☑
- lie (mother) O32.2- ☑
  - causing obstructed labor O64.8- ☑

Transvestism, transvestitism (dual-role) F64.1
- fetishistic F65.1

Trapped placenta (with hemorrhage) O72.0
- without hemorrhage O73.0

TRAPS (tumor necrosis factor receptor associated periodic syndrome) M04.1

Trauma, traumatism — see also Injury
- acoustic — see subcategory H83.3- ☑
- birth — see Birth, injury
- complicating ectopic or molar pregnancy O08.6

Trauma, traumatism — continued
- during delivery O71.9
- following ectopic or molar pregnancy O08.6
- non-accidental — see Abuse, physical
- obstetric O71.9
  - specified NEC O71.89
- occusal
  - primary K08.81
  - secondary K08.82

Traumatic — see also condition
- brain injury S06.9- ☑

Treacher Collins syndrome Q75.4

Treitz's hernia — see Hernia, abdomen, specified site NEC

Trematode infestation — see Infestation, fluke

Trematodiasis — see Infestation, fluke

Trembling paralysis — see Parkinsonism

Tremor(s) R25.1
- drug induced G25.1
- essential (benign) G25.0
- familial G25.0
- hereditary G25.0
- hysterical F44.4
- intention G25.2
- medication induced postural G25.1
- mercurial — see subcategory T56.1- ☑
- Parkinson's — see Parkinsonism
- psychogenic (conversion reaction) F44.4
- senilis R54
- specified type NEC G25.2

Trench
- fever A79.0
- foot — see Immersion, foot
- mouth A69.1

Treponema pallidum infection — see Syphilis

Treponematosis
- due to
  - T. pallidum — see Syphilis
  - T. pertenue — see Yaws

Triad
- Hutchinson's (congenital syphilis) A50.53
- Kartagener's Q89.3
- Saint's — see Hernia, diaphragm

Trichiasis (eyelid) H02.059
- with entropion — see Entropion
- left H02.056
  - lower H02.055
  - upper H02.054
- right H02.053
  - lower H02.052
  - upper H02.051

Trichinella spiralis (infection) (infestation) B75

Trichinellosis, trichiniasis, trichinelliasis, trichinosis B75
- with muscle disorder B75 [M63.80]
  - ankle B75 [M63.87-] ☑
  - foot B75 [M63.87-] ☑
  - forearm B75 [M63.83-] ☑
  - hand B75 [M63.84-] ☑
  - lower leg B75 [M63.86-] ☑
  - multiple sites B75 [M63.89]
  - pelvic region B75 [M63.85-] ☑
  - shoulder region B75 [M63.81-] ☑
  - specified site NEC B75 [M63.88]
  - thigh B75 [M63.85-] ☑
  - upper arm B75 [M63.82-] ☑

Trichobezoar T18.9- ☑
- intestine T18.3- ☑
- stomach T18.2- ☑

Trichocephaliasis, trichocephalosis B79

Trichocephalus infestation B79

Trichoclasis L67.8

Trichoepithelioma — see also Neoplasm, skin, benign
- malignant — see Neoplasm, skin, malignant

Trichofolliculoma — see Neoplasm, skin, benign

Tricholemmoma — see Neoplasm, skin, benign

Trichomoniasis A59.9
- bladder A59.03
- cervix A59.09
- intestinal A07.8
- prostate A59.02
- seminal vesicles A59.09
- specified site NEC A59.8
- urethra A59.03
- urogenitalis A59.00
- vagina A59.01
- vulva A59.01

Trichomycosis
- axillaris A48.8
- nodosa, nodularis B36.8

Trichonodosis L67.8
Trichophytid, trichophyton infection — see Dermatophytosis
Trichophytobezoar T18.9- ☑
  intestine T18.3- ☑
  stomach T18.2- ☑
Trichophytosis — see Dermatophytosis
Trichoptilosis L67.8
Trichorrhexis (nodosa) (invaginata) L67.0
Trichosis axillaris A48.8
Trichosporosis nodosa B36.2
Trichostasis spinulosa (congenital) Q84.1
Trichostrongyliasis, trichostrongylosis (small intestine) B81.2
Trichostrongylus infection B81.2
Trichotillomania F63.3
Trichromat, trichromatopsia, anomalous (congenital) H53.55
Trichuriasis B79
Trichuris trichiura (infection) (infestation) (any site) B79
Tricuspid (valve) — see condition
Trifid — see also Accessory
  kidney (pelvis) Q63.8
  tongue Q38.3
Trigeminal neuralgia — see Neuralgia, trigeminal
Trigeminy R00.8
Trigger finger (acquired) M65.30
  congenital Q74.0
  index finger M65.32- ☑
  little finger M65.35- ☑
  middle finger M65.33- ☑
  ring finger M65.34- ☑
  thumb M65.31- ☑
Trigonitis (bladder) (chronic) (pseudomembranous) N30.30
  with hematuria N30.31
Trigonocephaly Q75.03
Trilocular heart — see Cor triloculare
Trimethylaminuria E72.52
Tripartite placenta O43.19- ☑
Triphalangeal thumb Q74.0
Triple — see also Accessory
  kidneys Q63.0
  negative breast cancer (TNBC) Z17.421
  uteri Q51.818
  X, female Q97.0
Triple I O41.12- ☑
Triplegia G83.89
  congenital G80.8
Triplet (newborn) — see also Newborn, triplet
  complicating pregnancy — see Pregnancy, triplet
Triplication — see Accessory
Triploidy Q92.7
Trismus R25.2
  neonatorum A33
  newborn A33
Trisomy (syndrome) Q92.9
  13 (partial) Q91.7
    meiotic nondisjunction Q91.4
    mitotic nondisjunction Q91.5
    mosaicism Q91.5
    translocation Q91.6
  18 (partial) Q91.3
    meiotic nondisjunction Q91.0
    mitotic nondisjunction Q91.1
    mosaicism Q91.1
    translocation Q91.2
  20 Q92.8
  21 (partial) Q90.9
    meiotic nondisjunction Q90.0
    mitotic nondisjunction Q90.1
    mosaicism Q90.1
    translocation Q90.2
  22 Q92.8
  autosomes Q92.9
  chromosome specified NEC Q92.8
    partial Q92.2
      due to unbalanced translocation Q92.5
    specified NEC Q92.8
    whole (nonsex chromosome)
      meiotic nondisjunction Q92.0
      mitotic nondisjunction Q92.1
      mosaicism Q92.1
  due to
    dicentrics — see Extra, marker chromosomes
    extra rings — see Extra, marker chromosomes
    isochromosomes — see Extra, marker chromosomes
  specified NEC Q92.8
  whole chromosome Q92.9

Trisomy — continued
  whole chromosome — continued
    meiotic nondisjunction Q92.0
    mitotic nondisjunction Q92.1
    mosaicism Q92.1
    partial Q92.9
    specified NEC Q92.8
Tritanomaly, tritanopia H53.55
Trombiculosis, trombiculiasis, trombidiosis B88.09
Trophedema (congenital) (hereditary) Q82.0
Trophoblastic disease — see also Mole, hydatidiform O01.9
Tropholymphedema Q82.0
Trophoneurosis NEC G96.89
  disseminated M34.9
Tropical — see condition
Trouble — see also Disease
  heart — see Disease, heart
  kidney — see Disease, renal
  nervous R45.0
  sinus — see Sinusitis
Trousseau's syndrome (thrombophlebitis migrans) I82.1
Truancy, childhood
  from school Z72.810
Truncus
  arteriosus (persistent) Q20.0
  communis Q20.0
Trunk — see condition
Trypanosomiasis
  African B56.9
    by Trypanosoma brucei
      gambiense B56.0
      rhodesiense B56.1
  American — see Chagas' disease
  Brazilian — see Chagas' disease
  by Trypanosoma
    brucei gambiense B56.0
    brucei rhodesiense B56.1
    cruzi — see Chagas' disease
  gambiensis, Gambian B56.0
  rhodesiensis, Rhodesian B56.1
  South American — see Chagas' disease
  where
    African trypanosomiasis is prevalent B56.9
    Chagas' disease is prevalent B57.2
Tryptasemia, hereditary alpha D89.44
Tsutsugamushi (disease) (fever) A75.3
Tube, tubal, tubular — see condition
Tubercle — see also Tuberculosis
  brain, solitary A17.81
  Darwin's Q17.8
  Ghon, primary infection A15.7
Tuberculid, tuberculide (indurating, subcutaneous) (lichenoid) (miliary) (papulonecrotic) (primary) (skin) A18.4
Tuberculoma — see also Tuberculosis
  brain A17.81
  meninges (cerebral) (spinal) A17.1
  spinal cord A17.81
Tuberculosis, tubercular, tuberculous (calcification) (calcified) (caseous) (chromogenic acid-fast bacilli) (degeneration) (fibrocaseous) (fistula) (interstitial) (isolated circumscribed lesions) (necrosis) (parenchymatous) (ulcerative) A15.9
  with pneumoconiosis (any condition in J60-J64) J65
  abdomen (lymph gland) A18.39
  abscess (respiratory) A15.9
    bone A18.03
      hip A18.02
      knee A18.02
      sacrum A18.01
      specified site NEC A18.03
      spinal A18.01
      vertebra A18.01
    brain A17.81
    breast A18.89
    Cowper's gland A18.15
    dura (mater) (cerebral) (spinal) A17.81
    epidural (cerebral) (spinal) A17.81
    female pelvis A18.17
    frontal sinus A15.8
    genital organs NEC A18.10
    genitourinary A18.10
    gland (lymphatic) — see Tuberculosis, lymph gland
    hip A18.02
    intestine A18.32
    ischiorectal A18.32
    joint NEC A18.02
      hip A18.02
      knee A18.02

Tuberculosis, tubercular, tuberculous — continued
  abscess — continued
    joint — continued
      specified NEC A18.02
      vertebral A18.01
    kidney A18.11
    knee A18.02
    latent Z22.7
    lumbar (spine) A18.01
    lung — see Tuberculosis, pulmonary
    meninges (cerebral) (spinal) A17.0
    muscle A18.09
    perianal (fistula) A18.32
    perinephritic A18.11
    perirectal A18.32
    rectum A18.32
    retropharyngeal A15.8
    sacrum A18.01
    scrofulous A18.2
    scrotum A18.15
    skin (primary) A18.4
    spinal cord A17.81
    spine or vertebra (column) A18.01
    subdiaphragmatic A18.31
    testis A18.15
    urinary A18.13
    uterus A18.17
  accessory sinus — see Tuberculosis, sinus
  Addison's disease A18.7
  adenitis — see Tuberculosis, lymph gland
  adenoids A15.8
  adenopathy — see Tuberculosis, lymph gland
  adherent pericardium A18.84
  adnexa (uteri) A18.17
  adrenal (capsule) (gland) A18.7
  alimentary canal A18.32
  anemia A18.89
  ankle (joint) (bone) A18.02
  anus A18.32
  apex, apical — see Tuberculosis, pulmonary
  appendicitis, appendix A18.32
  arachnoid A17.0
  artery, arteritis A18.89
    cerebral A18.89
  arthritis (chronic) (synovial) A18.02
    spine or vertebra (column) A18.01
  articular — see Tuberculosis, joint
  ascites A18.31
  asthma — see Tuberculosis, pulmonary
  axilla, axillary (gland) A18.2
  bladder A18.12
  bone A18.03
    hip A18.02
    knee A18.02
    limb NEC A18.03
    sacrum A18.01
    spine or vertebral column A18.01
  bowel (miliary) A18.32
  brain A17.81
  breast A18.89
  broad ligament A18.17
  bronchi, bronchial, bronchus A15.5
    ectasia, ectasis (bronchiectasis) — see Tuberculosis, pulmonary
    fistula A15.5
      primary (progressive) A15.7
    gland or node A15.4
      primary (progressive) A15.7
    lymph gland or node A15.4
      primary (progressive) A15.7
  bronchiectasis — see Tuberculosis, pulmonary
  bronchitis A15.5
  bronchopleural A15.6
  bronchopneumonia, bronchopneumonic — see Tuberculosis, pulmonary
  bronchorrhagia A15.5
  bronchotracheal A15.5
  bronze disease A18.7
  buccal cavity A18.83
  bulbourethral gland A18.15
  bursa A18.09
  cachexia A15.9
  cardiomyopathy A18.84
  caries — see Tuberculosis, bone
  cartilage A18.02
    intervertebral A18.01
  catarrhal — see Tuberculosis, respiratory
  cecum A18.32
  cellulitis (primary) A18.4

Tuberculosis, tubercular, tuberculous — continued
cerebellum A17.81
cerebral, cerebrum A17.81
cerebrospinal A17.81
  meninges A17.0
cervical (lymph gland or node) A18.2
cervicitis, cervix (uteri) A18.16
chest — see Tuberculosis, respiratory
chorioretinitis A18.53
choroid, choroiditis A18.53
ciliary body A18.54
colitis A18.32
collier's J65
colliquativa (primary) A18.4
colon A18.32
complex, primary A15.7
congenital P37.0
conjunctiva A18.59
connective tissue (systemic) A18.89
contact Z20.1
cornea (ulcer) A18.52
Cowper's gland A18.15
coxae A18.02
coxalgia A18.02
cul-de-sac of Douglas A18.17
curvature, spine A18.01
cutis (colliquativa) (primary) A18.4
cyst, ovary A18.18
cystitis A18.12
dactylitis A18.03
diarrhea A18.32
diffuse — see Tuberculosis, miliary
digestive tract A18.32
disseminated — see Tuberculosis, miliary
duodenum A18.32
dura (mater) (cerebral) (spinal) A17.0
  abscess (cerebral) (spinal) A17.81
dysentery A18.32
ear (inner) (middle) A18.6
  bone A18.03
  external (primary) A18.4
  skin (primary) A18.4
elbow A18.02
emphysema — see Tuberculosis, pulmonary
empyema A15.6
encephalitis A17.82
endarteritis A18.89
endocarditis A18.84
  aortic A18.84
  mitral A18.84
  pulmonary A18.84
  tricuspid A18.84
endocrine glands NEC A18.82
endometrium A18.17
enteric, enterica, enteritis A18.32
enterocolitis A18.32
epididymis, epididymitis A18.15
epidural abscess (cerebral) (spinal) A17.81
epiglottis A15.5
episcleritis A18.51
erythema (induratum) (nodosum) (primary) A18.4
esophagus A18.83
eustachian tube A18.6
exposure (to) Z20.1
exudative — see Tuberculosis, pulmonary
eye A18.50
eyelid (primary) (lupus) A18.4
fallopian tube (acute) (chronic) A18.17
fascia A18.09
fauces A15.8
female pelvic inflammatory disease A18.17
finger A18.03
first infection A15.7
gallbladder A18.83
ganglion A18.09
gastritis A18.83
gastrocolic fistula A18.32
gastroenteritis A18.32
gastrointestinal tract A18.32
general, generalized — see Tuberculosis, miliary
genital organs A18.10
genitourinary A18.10
genu A18.02
glandula suprarenalis A18.7
glandular, general A18.2
glottis A15.5
grinder's J65
gum A18.83
hand A18.03

Tuberculosis, tubercular, tuberculous — continued
heart A18.84
hematogenous — see Tuberculosis, miliary
hemoptysis — see Tuberculosis, pulmonary
hemorrhage NEC — see Tuberculosis, pulmonary
hemothorax A15.6
hepatitis A18.83
hilar lymph nodes A15.4
  primary (progressive) A15.7
hip (joint) (disease) (bone) A18.02
hydropneumothorax A15.6
hydrothorax A15.6
hypoadrenalism A18.7
hypopharynx A15.8
ileocecal (hyperplastic) A18.32
ileocolitis A18.32
ileum A18.32
iliac spine (superior) A18.03
immunological findings only A15.7
indurativa (primary) A18.4
infantile A15.7
infection A15.9
  without clinical manifestations A15.7
infraclavicular gland A18.2
inguinal gland A18.2
inguinalis A18.2
intestine (any part) A18.32
iridocyclitis A18.54
iris, iritis A18.54
ischiorectal A18.32
jaw A18.03
jejunum A18.32
joint A18.02
  vertebral A18.01
keratitis (interstitial) A18.52
keratoconjunctivitis A18.52
kidney A18.11
knee (joint) A18.02
kyphosis, kyphoscoliosis A18.01
laryngitis A15.5
larynx A15.5
latent Z22.7
leptomeninges, leptomeningitis (cerebral) (spinal) A17.0
lichenoides (primary) A18.4
linguae A18.83
lip A18.83
liver A18.83
lordosis A18.01
lung — see Tuberculosis, pulmonary
lupus vulgaris A18.4
lymph gland or node (peripheral) A18.2
  abdomen A18.39
  bronchial A15.4
    primary (progressive) A15.7
  cervical A18.2
  hilar A15.4
    primary (progressive) A15.7
  intrathoracic A15.4
    primary (progressive) A15.7
  mediastinal A15.4
    primary (progressive) A15.7
  mesenteric A18.39
  retroperitoneal A18.39
  tracheobronchial A15.4
    primary (progressive) A15.7
lymphadenitis — see Tuberculosis, lymph gland
lymphangitis — see Tuberculosis, lymph gland
lymphatic (gland) (vessel) — see Tuberculosis, lymph gland
mammary gland A18.89
marasmus A15.9
mastoiditis A18.03
mediastinal lymph gland or node A15.4
  primary (progressive) A15.7
mediastinitis A15.8
  primary (progressive) A15.7
mediastinum A15.8
  primary (progressive) A15.7
medulla A17.81
melanosis, Addisonian A18.7
meninges, meningitis (basilar) (cerebral) (cerebrospinal) (spinal) A17.0
meningoencephalitis A17.82
mesentery, mesenteric (gland or node) A18.39
miliary A19.9
  acute A19.2
    multiple sites A19.1
    single specified site A19.0
  chronic A19.8

Tuberculosis, tubercular, tuberculous — continued
miliary — continued
  specified NEC A19.8
millstone makers' J65
miner's J65
molder's J65
mouth A18.83
multiple A19.9
  acute A19.1
  chronic A19.8
muscle A18.09
myelitis A17.82
myocardium, myocarditis A18.84
nasal (passage) (sinus) A15.8
nasopharynx A15.8
neck gland A18.2
nephritis A18.11
nerve (mononeuropathy) A17.83
nervous system A17.9
nose (septum) A15.8
ocular A18.50
omentum A18.31
oophoritis (acute) (chronic) A18.17
optic (nerve trunk) (papilla) A18.59
orbit A18.59
orchitis A18.15
organ, specified NEC A18.89
osseous — see Tuberculosis, bone
osteitis — see Tuberculosis, bone
osteomyelitis — see Tuberculosis, bone
otitis media A18.6
ovary, ovaritis (acute) (chronic) A18.17
oviduct (acute) (chronic) A18.17
pachymeningitis A17.0
palate (soft) A18.83
pancreas A18.83
papulonecrotic (a) (primary) A18.4
parathyroid glands A18.82
paronychia (primary) A18.4
parotid gland or region A18.83
pelvis (bony) A18.03
penis A18.15
peribronchitis A15.5
pericardium, pericarditis A18.84
perichondritis, larynx A15.5
periostitis — see Tuberculosis, bone
perirectal fistula A18.32
peritoneum NEC A18.31
peritonitis A18.31
pharynx, pharyngitis A15.8
phlyctenulosis (keratoconjunctivitis) A18.52
phthisis NEC — see Tuberculosis, pulmonary
pituitary gland A18.82
pleura, pleural, pleurisy, pleuritis (fibrinous) (obliterative) (purulent) (simple plastic) (with effusion) A15.6
  primary (progressive) A15.7
pneumonia, pneumonic — see Tuberculosis, pulmonary
pneumothorax (spontaneous) (tense valvular) — see Tuberculosis, pulmonary
polyneuropathy A17.89
polyserositis A19.9
  acute A19.1
  chronic A19.8
potter's J65
prepuce A18.15
primary (complex) A15.7
proctitis A18.32
prostate, prostatitis A18.14
pulmonalis — see Tuberculosis, pulmonary
pulmonary (cavitated) (fibrotic) (infiltrative) (nodular) A15.0
  childhood type or first infection A15.7
  primary (complex) A15.7
pyelitis A18.11
pyelonephritis A18.11
pyemia — see Tuberculosis, miliary
pyonephrosis A18.11
pyopneumothorax A15.6
pyothorax A15.6
rectum (fistula) (with abscess) A18.32
reinfection stage — see Tuberculosis, pulmonary
renal A18.11
renis A18.11
respiratory A15.9
  primary A15.7
  specified site NEC A15.8
retina, retinitis A18.53
retroperitoneal (lymph gland or node) A18.39
rheumatism NEC A18.09

Tuberculosis, tubercular, tuberculous — *continued*
- rhinitis A15.8
- sacroiliac (joint) A18.01
- sacrum A18.01
- salivary gland A18.83
- salpingitis (acute) (chronic) A18.17
- sandblaster's J65
- sclera A18.51
- scoliosis A18.01
- scrofulous A18.2
- scrotum A18.15
- seminal tract or vesicle A18.15
- senile A15.9
- septic — *see* Tuberculosis, miliary
- shoulder (joint) A18.02
  - blade A18.03
- sigmoid A18.32
- sinus (any nasal) A15.8
  - bone A18.03
  - epididymis A18.15
- skeletal NEC A18.03
- skin (any site) (primary) A18.4
- small intestine A18.32
- soft palate A18.83
- spermatic cord A18.15
- spine, spinal (column) A18.01
  - cord A17.81
  - medulla A17.81
  - membrane A17.0
  - meninges A17.0
- spleen, splenitis A18.85
- spondylitis A18.01
- sternoclavicular joint A18.02
- stomach A18.83
- stonemason's J65
- subcutaneous tissue (cellular) (primary) A18.4
- subcutis (primary) A18.4
- subdeltoid bursa A18.83
- submaxillary (region) A18.83
- supraclavicular gland A18.2
- suprarenal (capsule) (gland) A18.7
- swelling, joint (*see also* category M01) — *see also* Tuberculosis, joint A18.02
- symphysis pubis A18.02
- synovitis A18.09
  - articular A18.02
  - spine or vertebra A18.01
- systemic — *see* Tuberculosis, miliary
- tarsitis A18.4
- tendon (sheath) — *see* Tuberculosis, tenosynovitis
- tenosynovitis A18.09
  - spine or vertebra A18.01
- testis A18.15
- throat A15.8
- thymus gland A18.82
- thyroid gland A18.81
- tongue A18.83
- tonsil, tonsillitis A15.8
- trachea, tracheal A15.5
  - lymph gland or node A15.4
    - primary (progressive) A15.7
- tracheobronchial A15.5
  - lymph gland or node A15.4
    - primary (progressive) A15.7
- tubal (acute) (chronic) A18.17
- tunica vaginalis A18.15
- ulcer (skin) (primary) A18.4
  - bowel or intestine A18.32
  - specified NEC — *see* Tuberculosis, by site
- unspecified site A15.9
- ureter A18.11
- urethra, urethral (gland) A18.13
- urinary organ or tract A18.13
- uterus A18.17
- uveal tract A18.54
- uvula A18.83
- vagina A18.18
- vas deferens A18.15
- verruca, verrucosa (cutis) (primary) A18.4
- vertebra (column) A18.01
- vesiculitis A18.15
- vulva A18.18
- wrist (joint) A18.02

Tuberculum
- Carabelli — *see* Excludes Note at K00.2
- occlusal — *see* Excludes Note at K00.2
- paramolare K00.2

Tuberosity, entire maxillary M26.07
Tuberous sclerosis (brain) Q85.1

Tubo-ovarian — *see* condition
Tuboplasty, after previous sterilization Z31.0
- aftercare Z31.42

Tubotympanitis, catarrhal (chronic) — *see* Otitis, media, nonsuppurative, chronic, serous

Tularemia A21.9
- with
  - conjunctivitis A21.1
  - pneumonia A21.2
- abdominal A21.3
- bronchopneumonic A21.2
- conjunctivitis A21.1
- cryptogenic A21.3
- enteric A21.3
- gastrointestinal A21.3
- generalized A21.7
- ingestion A21.3
- intestinal A21.3
- oculoglandular A21.1
- ophthalmic A21.1
- pneumonia (any), pneumonic A21.2
- pulmonary A21.2
- sepsis A21.7
- specified NEC A21.8
- typhoidal A21.7
- ulceroglandular A21.0

Tularensis conjunctivitis A21.1
Tumefaction — *see also* Swelling
- liver — *see* Hypertrophy, liver

Tumor — *see also* Neoplasm, unspecified behavior, by site
- acinar cell — *see* Neoplasm, uncertain behavior, by site
- acinic cell — *see* Neoplasm, uncertain behavior, by site
- adenocarcinoid — *see* Neoplasm, malignant, by site
- adenomatoid — *see also* Neoplasm, benign, by site
  - odontogenic — *see* Cyst, calcifying odontogenic
- adnexal (skin) — *see* Neoplasm, skin, benign, by site
- adrenal
  - cortical (benign) D35.0- ☑
    - malignant C74.0- ☑
  - rest — *see* Neoplasm, benign, by site
- alpha-cell
  - malignant
    - pancreas C25.4
    - specified site NEC — *see* Neoplasm, malignant, by site
    - unspecified site C25.4
  - pancreas D13.7
  - specified site NEC — *see* Neoplasm, benign, by site
  - unspecified site D13.7
- aneurysmal — *see* Aneurysm
- aortic body D44.7
  - malignant C75.5
- Askin's — *see* Neoplasm, connective tissue, malignant
- basal cell — *see also* Neoplasm, skin, uncertain behavior D48.5
- Bednar — *see* Neoplasm, skin, malignant
- benign (unclassified) — *see* Neoplasm, benign, by site
- beta-cell
  - malignant
    - pancreas C25.4
    - specified site NEC — *see* Neoplasm, malignant, by site
    - unspecified site C25.4
  - pancreas D13.7
  - specified site NEC — *see* Neoplasm, benign, by site
  - unspecified site D13.7
- Brenner D27.9
  - borderline malignancy D39.1- ☑
  - malignant C56.- ☑
  - proliferating D39.1- ☑
- bronchial alveolar, intravascular D38.1
- Brooke's — *see* Neoplasm, skin, benign
- brown fat — *see* Lipoma
- Burkitt — *see* Lymphoma, Burkitt
- calcifying epithelial odontogenic — *see* Cyst, calcifying odontogenic
- carcinoid D3A.00 (*following* D36)
  - benign D3A.00 (*following* D36)
    - appendix D3A.020 (*following* D36)
    - ascending colon D3A.022 (*following* D36)
    - bronchus (lung) D3A.090 (*following* D36)
    - cecum D3A.021 (*following* D36)
    - colon D3A.029 (*following* D36)
    - descending colon D3A.024 (*following* D36)
    - duodenum D3A.010 (*following* D36)
    - foregut NOS D3A.094 (*following* D36)
    - hindgut NOS D3A.096 (*following* D36)
    - ileum D3A.012 (*following* D36)

Tumor — *continued*
- carcinoid — *continued*
  - benign — *continued*
    - jejunum D3A.011 (*following* D36)
    - kidney D3A.093 (*following* D36)
    - large intestine D3A.029 (*following* D36)
    - lung (bronchus) D3A.090 (*following* D36)
    - midgut NOS D3A.095 (*following* D36)
    - rectum D3A.026 (*following* D36)
    - sigmoid colon D3A.025 (*following* D36)
    - small intestine D3A.019 (*following* D36)
    - specified NEC D3A.098 (*following* D36)
    - stomach D3A.092 (*following* D36)
    - thymus D3A.091 (*following* D36)
    - transverse colon D3A.023 (*following* D36)
  - malignant C7A.00 (*following* C75)
    - appendix C7A.020 (*following* C75)
    - ascending colon C7A.022 (*following* C75)
    - bronchus (lung) C7A.090 (*following* C75)
    - cecum C7A.021 (*following* C75)
    - colon C7A.029 (*following* C75)
    - descending colon C7A.024 (*following* C75)
    - duodenum C7A.010 (*following* C75)
    - foregut NOS C7A.094 (*following* C75)
    - hindgut NOS C7A.096 (*following* C75)
    - ileum C7A.012 (*following* C75)
    - jejunum C7A.011 (*following* C75)
    - kidney C7A.093 (*following* C75)
    - large intestine C7A.029 (*following* C75)
    - lung (bronchus) C7A.090 (*following* C75)
    - midgut NOS C7A.095 (*following* C75)
    - rectum C7A.026 (*following* C75)
    - sigmoid colon C7A.025 (*following* C75)
    - small intestine C7A.019 (*following* C75)
    - specified NEC C7A.098 (*following* C75)
    - stomach C7A.092 (*following* C75)
    - thymus C7A.091 (*following* C75)
    - transverse colon C7A.023 (*following* C75)
  - mesentery metastasis C7B.04 (*following* C75)
  - secondary C7B.00 (*following* C75)
    - bone C7B.03 (*following* C75)
    - distant lymph nodes C7B.01 (*following* C75)
    - liver C7B.02 (*following* C75)
    - peritoneum C7B.04 (*following* C75)
    - specified NEC C7B.09 (*following* C75)
- carotid body D44.6
  - malignant C75.4
- cells — *see also* Neoplasm, unspecified behavior, by site
  - benign — *see* Neoplasm, benign, by site
  - malignant — *see* Neoplasm, malignant, by site
  - uncertain whether benign or malignant — *see* Neoplasm, uncertain behavior, by site
- cervix, in pregnancy or childbirth — *see* Pregnancy, complicated by, tumor, cervix
- chondromatous giant cell — *see* Neoplasm, bone, benign
- chromaffin — *see also* Neoplasm, benign, by site
  - malignant — *see* Neoplasm, malignant, by site
- Cock's peculiar L72.3
- Codman's — *see* Neoplasm, bone, benign
- dentigerous, mixed — *see* Cyst, calcifying odontogenic
- dermoid — *see also* Neoplasm, benign, by site
  - with malignant transformation C56.- ☑
- desmoid (extra-abdominal) — *see also* Neoplasm, connective tissue, uncertain behavior
  - abdominal — *see* Neoplasm, connective tissue, uncertain behavior
- embolus — *see* Neoplasm, secondary, by site
- embryonal (mixed) — *see also* Neoplasm, uncertain behavior, by site
  - liver C22.7
- endodermal sinus
  - specified site — *see* Neoplasm, malignant, by site
  - unspecified site
    - female C56.- ☑
    - male C62.90
- epithelial
  - benign — *see* Neoplasm, benign, by site
  - malignant — *see* Neoplasm, malignant, by site
- Ewing's — *see* Neoplasm, bone, malignant, by site
- fatty — *see* Lipoma
- fibroid — *see* Leiomyoma
- G cell
  - malignant
    - pancreas C25.4
    - specified site NEC — *see* Neoplasm, malignant, by site
    - unspecified site C25.4
  - specified site — *see* Neoplasm, uncertain behavior, by site

☑ Additional Character Required — Refer to the Tabular List for Character Selection

Tumor

Tumor — continued
- G cell — continued
  - unspecified site D37.8
- germ cell — see also Neoplasm, malignant, by site
  - mixed — see Neoplasm, malignant, by site
- ghost cell, odontogenic — see Cyst, calcifying odontogenic
- giant cell — see also Neoplasm, uncertain behavior, by site
  - bone D48.0
    - malignant — see Neoplasm, bone, malignant
  - chondromatous — see Neoplasm, bone, benign
  - malignant — see Neoplasm, malignant, by site
  - soft parts — see Neoplasm, connective tissue, uncertain behavior
    - malignant — see Neoplasm, connective tissue, malignant
- glomus D18.00
  - intra-abdominal D18.03
  - intracranial D18.02
  - jugulare D44.7
    - malignant C75.5
  - skin D18.01
  - specified site NEC D18.09
- gonadal stromal — see Neoplasm, uncertain behavior, by site
- granular cell — see also Neoplasm, connective tissue, benign
  - malignant — see Neoplasm, connective tissue, malignant
- granulosa cell D39.1- ☑
  - juvenile D39.1- ☑
  - malignant C56.- ☑
- granulosa cell-theca cell D39.1- ☑
  - malignant C56.- ☑
- Grawitz's C64.- ☑
- hemorrhoidal — see Hemorrhoids
- hilar cell D27.- ☑
- hilus cell D27.- ☑
- Hurthle cell (benign) D34
  - malignant C73
- hydatid — see Echinococcus
- hypernephroid — see also Neoplasm, uncertain behavior, by site
- interstitial cell — see also Neoplasm, uncertain behavior, by site
  - benign — see Neoplasm, benign, by site
  - malignant — see Neoplasm, malignant, by site
- intravascular bronchial alveolar D38.1
- islet cell — see Neoplasm, benign, by site
  - malignant — see Neoplasm, malignant, by site
    - pancreas C25.4
    - specified site NEC — see Neoplasm, malignant, by site
    - unspecified site C25.4
  - pancreas D13.7
  - specified site NEC — see Neoplasm, benign, by site
  - unspecified site D13.7
- juxtaglomerular D41.0- ☑
- Klatskin's C22.1
- Krukenberg's C79.6- ☑
- Leydig cell — see Neoplasm, uncertain behavior, by site
  - benign — see Neoplasm, benign, by site
    - specified site — see Neoplasm, benign, by site
    - unspecified site
      - female D27.9
      - male D29.20
  - malignant — see Neoplasm, malignant, by site
    - specified site — see Neoplasm, malignant, by site
    - unspecified site
      - female C56.9
      - male C62.90
  - specified site — see Neoplasm, uncertain behavior, by site
  - unspecified site
    - female D39.10
    - male D40.10
- lipid cell, ovary D27.- ☑
- lipoid cell, ovary D27.- ☑
- malignant — see also Neoplasm, malignant, by site C80.1
  - fusiform cell (type) C80.1
  - giant cell (type) C80.1
  - localized, plasma cell — see Plasmacytoma, solitary
  - mixed NEC C80.1
  - small cell (type) C80.1
  - spindle cell (type) C80.1
  - unclassified C80.1
- mast cell D47.09

Tumor — continued
- melanotic, neuroectodermal — see Neoplasm, benign, by site
- Merkel cell — see Carcinoma, Merkel cell
- mesenchymal
  - malignant — see Neoplasm, connective tissue, malignant
  - mixed — see Neoplasm, connective tissue, uncertain behavior
- mesodermal, mixed — see also Neoplasm, malignant, by site
  - liver C22.4
- mesonephric — see also Neoplasm, uncertain behavior, by site
  - malignant — see Neoplasm, malignant, by site
- metastatic
  - from specified site — see Neoplasm, malignant, by site
  - of specified site — see Neoplasm, malignant, by site
  - to specified site — see Neoplasm, secondary, by site
- mixed NEC — see also Neoplasm, benign, by site
  - malignant — see Neoplasm, malignant, by site
- mucinous of low malignant potential
  - specified site — see Neoplasm, malignant, by site
  - unspecified site C56.9
- mucocarcinoid
  - specified site — see Neoplasm, malignant, by site
  - unspecified site C18.1
- mucoepidermoid — see Neoplasm, uncertain behavior, by site
- Mullerian, mixed
  - specified site — see Neoplasm, malignant, by site
  - unspecified site C54.9
- myoepithelial — see Neoplasm, benign, by site
- neuroectodermal (peripheral) — see Neoplasm, malignant, by site
  - primitive
    - specified site — see Neoplasm, malignant, by site
    - unspecified site C71.9
- neuroendocrine D3A.8 (following D36)
  - malignant poorly differentiated C7A.1 (following C75)
  - secondary NEC C7B.8 (following C75)
  - specified NEC C7A.8 (following C75)
- neurogenic olfactory C30.0
- nonencapsulated sclerosing C73
- odontogenic (adenomatoid) (benign) (calcifying epithelial) (keratocystic) (squamous) — see Cyst, calcifying odontogenic
  - malignant C41.1
    - upper jaw (bone) C41.0
- ovarian stromal D39.1- ☑
- ovary, in pregnancy — see Pregnancy, complicated by
- pacinian — see Neoplasm, skin, benign
- Pancoast's — see Pancoast's syndrome
- papillary — see also Papilloma
  - cystic D37.9
  - mucinous of low malignant potential C56.- ☑
    - specified site — see Neoplasm, malignant, by site
    - unspecified site C56.9
  - serous of low malignant potential
    - specified site — see Neoplasm, malignant, by site
    - unspecified site C56.9
- pelvic, in pregnancy or childbirth — see Pregnancy, complicated by
- phantom F45.8
- phyllodes D48.6- ☑
  - benign D24.- ☑
  - malignant — see Neoplasm, breast, malignant
- Pindborg — see Cyst, calcifying odontogenic
- placental site trophoblastic D39.2
- plasma cell (malignant) (localized) — see Plasmacytoma, solitary
- polyvesicular vitelline
  - specified site — see Neoplasm, malignant, by site
  - unspecified site
    - female C56.9
    - male C62.90
- Pott's puffy — see Osteomyelitis, specified NEC
- Rathke's pouch D44.3
- retinal anlage — see Neoplasm, benign, by site
- salivary gland or duct type, mixed — see Neoplasm, salivary gland or duct, benign
  - malignant — see Neoplasm, salivary gland or duct, malignant
- Sampson's N80.10- ☑
- Schmincke's — see Neoplasm, nasopharynx, malignant
- sclerosing stromal D27.- ☑
- sebaceous — see Cyst, sebaceous

Tumor — continued
- secondary — see Neoplasm, secondary, by site
  - carcinoid C7B.00 (following C75)
    - bone C7B.03 (following C75)
    - distant lymph nodes C7B.01 (following C75)
    - liver C7B.02 (following C75)
    - peritoneum C7B.04 (following C75)
    - specified NEC C7B.09 (following C75)
  - neuroendocrine NEC C7B.8 (following C75)
- serous of low malignant potential
  - specified site — see Neoplasm, malignant, by site
  - unspecified site C56.9
- Sertoli cell — see Neoplasm, benign, by site
  - with lipid storage
    - specified site — see Neoplasm, benign, by site
    - unspecified site
      - female D27.9
      - male D29.20
  - specified site — see Neoplasm, benign, by site
  - unspecified site
    - female D27.9
    - male D29.20
- Sertoli-Leydig cell — see Neoplasm, benign, by site
  - specified site — see Neoplasm, benign, by site
  - unspecified site
    - female D27.9
    - male D29.20
- sex cord (-stromal) — see Neoplasm, uncertain behavior, by site
  - with annular tubules D39.1- ☑
- skin appendage — see Neoplasm, skin, benign
- smooth muscle — see Neoplasm, connective tissue, uncertain behavior
- soft tissue
  - benign — see Neoplasm, connective tissue, benign
  - malignant — see Neoplasm, connective tissue, malignant
- sternomastoid (congenital) Q68.0
- stromal
  - endometrial D39.0
  - gastric D48.19
    - benign D21.4
    - malignant C49.A2
    - uncertain behavior D48.19
  - gastrointestinal C49.A- ☑
    - benign D21.4
    - esophagus C49.A1
    - malignant C49.A0
      - colon C49.A4
      - duodenum C49.A3
      - esophagus C49.A1
      - ileum C49.A3
      - jejunum C49.A3
      - large intestine C49.A4
      - Meckel diverticulum C49.A3
      - omentum C49.A9
      - peritoneum C49.A9
      - rectum C49.A5
      - small intestine C49.A3
      - specified site NEC C49.A9
      - stomach C49.A2
    - rectum C49.A5
    - small intestine C49.A3
    - specified site NEC C49.A9
    - stomach C49.A2
    - uncertain behavior D48.19
  - intestine
    - benign D21.4
    - malignant C49.4
      - large C49.A4
      - small C49.A3
    - uncertain behavior D48.19
  - ovarian D39.1- ☑
  - stomach C49.A2
    - benign D21.4
    - malignant C49.A2
    - uncertain behavior D48.19
- sweat gland — see also Neoplasm, skin, uncertain behavior
  - benign — see Neoplasm, skin, benign
  - malignant — see Neoplasm, skin, malignant
- syphilitic, brain A52.17
- testicular D40.10
- testicular stromal D40.1- ☑
- theca cell D27.- ☑
- theca cell-granulosa cell D39.1- ☑
- Triton, malignant — see Neoplasm, nerve, malignant
- trophoblastic, placental site D39.2

Tumor — *continued*
- turban D23.4
- uterus (body), in pregnancy or childbirth — *see* Pregnancy, complicated by, tumor, uterus
- vagina, in pregnancy or childbirth — *see* Pregnancy, complicated by
- varicose — *see* Varix
- von Recklinghausen's — *see* Neurofibromatosis
- vulva or perineum, in pregnancy or childbirth — *see* Pregnancy, complicated by
  - causing obstructed labor O65.5
- Warthin's — *see* Neoplasm, salivary gland or duct, benign
- Wilms' C64.- ☑
- yolk sac — *see* Neoplasm, malignant, by site
  - specified site — *see* Neoplasm, malignant, by site
  - unspecified site
    - female C56.9
    - male C62.90

Tumor lysis syndrome (following antineoplastic chemotherapy) (spontaneous) NEC E88.3
Tumorlet — *see* Neoplasm, uncertain behavior, by site
Tungiasis B88.1
Tunica vasculosa lentis Q12.2
Turban tumor D23.4
Türck's trachoma J37.0
Turner-Kieser syndrome Q87.2
Turner-like syndrome Q87.19
Turner-Ullrich syndrome Q96.9
Turner's
- hypoplasia (tooth) K00.4
- syndrome Q96.9
  - specified NEC Q96.8
- tooth K00.4

Tussis convulsiva — *see* Whooping cough
Twiddler's syndrome (due to)
- automatic implantable defibrillator T82.198
- cardiac pacemaker T82.198- ☑

Twilight state
- epileptic F05
- psychogenic F44.89

Twin (newborn) — *see also* Newborn, twin
- conjoined Q89.4
- pregnancy — *see* Pregnancy, twin

Twinning, teeth K00.2
Twist, twisted
- bowel, colon or intestine K56.2
- hair (congenital) Q84.1
- mesentery K56.2
- omentum K56.2
- organ or site, congenital NEC — *see* Anomaly, by site
- ovarian pedicle — *see* Torsion, ovary

Twitching R25.3
Tylosis (acquired) L84
- buccalis K13.29
- linguae K13.29
- palmaris et plantaris (congenital) (inherited) Q82.8
  - acquired L85.1

Tympanism R14.0
Tympanites (abdominal) (intestinal) R14.0
Tympanitis — *see* Myringitis
Tympanosclerosis H74.0- ☑
Tympanum — *see* condition
Tympany
- abdomen R14.0
- chest R09.89

Type A behavior pattern Z73.1
Typhlitis — *see* Cecitis
Typhoenteritis — *see* Typhoid
Typhoid (abortive) (ambulant) (any site) (clinical) (fever) (hemorrhagic) (infection) (intermittent) (malignant) (rheumatic) (Widal negative) A01.00
- with pneumonia A01.03
- abdominal A01.09
- arthritis A01.04
- carrier (suspected) of Z22.0
- cholecystitis (current) A01.09
- endocarditis A01.02
- heart involvement A01.02
- inoculation reaction — *see* Complications, vaccination
- meningitis A01.01
- mesenteric lymph nodes A01.09
- myocarditis A01.02
- osteomyelitis A01.05
- perichondritis, larynx A01.09
- pneumonia A01.03
- specified NEC A01.09
- spine A01.05
- ulcer (perforating) A01.09

Typhomalaria (fever) — *see* Malaria

Typhomania A01.00
Typhoperitonitis A01.09
Typhus (fever) A75.9
- abdominal, abdominalis — *see* Typhoid
- African tick A77.1
- amarillic A95.9
- brain A75.9 [G94]
- cerebral A75.9 [G94]
- classical A75.0
- due to Rickettsia
  - prowazekii A75.0
    - recrudescent A75.1
  - tsutsugamushi A75.3
  - typhi A75.2
- endemic (flea-borne) A75.2
- epidemic (louse-borne) A75.0
- exanthematic NEC A75.0
- exanthematicus SAI A75.0
  - brillii SAI A75.1
  - mexicanus SAI A75.2
  - typhus murinus A75.2
- flea-borne A75.2
- India tick A77.1
- Kenya (tick) A77.1
- louse-borne A75.0
- Mexican A75.2
- mite-borne A75.3
- murine A75.2
- North Asian tick-borne A77.2
- Orientia Tsutsugamushi (scrub typhus) A75.3
- petechial A75.9
- Queensland tick A77.3
- rat A75.2
- recrudescent A75.1
- recurrens — *see* Fever, relapsing
- Sao Paulo A77.0
- scrub (China) (India) (Malaysia) (New Guinea) A75.3
- shop (of Malaysia) A75.2
- Siberian tick A77.2
- tick-borne A77.9
- tropical (mite-borne) A75.3

Tyrosinemia E70.21
- newborn, transitory P74.5

Tyrosinosis E70.21
Tyrosinuria E70.29

U

Uhl's anomaly or disease Q24.8
Ulcer, ulcerated, ulcerating, ulceration, ulcerative
- abdomen L98.439
  - with
    - bone involvement without evidence of necrosis L98.436
    - bone necrosis L98.434
    - exposed fat layer L98.432
    - muscle involvement without evidence of necrosis L98.435
    - muscle necrosis L98.433
    - skin breakdown only L98.431
    - specified severity NEC L98.438
- alveolar process M27.3
- amebic (intestine) A06.1
  - skin A06.7
- anastomotic — *see* Ulcer, gastrojejunal
- anorectal K62.6
- antral — *see* Ulcer, stomach
- anus (sphincter) (solitary) K62.6
- aorta — *see* Aneurysm
- aphthous (oral) (recurrent) K12.0
  - genital organ(s)
    - female N76.6
    - male N50.89
- artery I77.2
- atrophic — *see* Ulcer, skin
  - decubitus — *see* Ulcer, pressure, by site
- back L98.429
  - with
    - bone involvement without evidence of necrosis L98.426
    - bone necrosis L98.424
    - exposed fat layer L98.422
    - muscle involvement without evidence of necrosis L98.425
    - muscle necrosis L98.423
    - skin breakdown only L98.421
    - specified severity NEC L98.428
- Barrett's (esophagus) K22.10
  - with bleeding K22.11

Ulcer, ulcerated, ulcerating, ulceration, ulcerative — *continued*
- bile duct (common) (hepatic) K83.8
- bladder (solitary) (sphincter) NEC N32.89
  - bilharzial B65.9 [N33]
  - in schistosomiasis (bilharzial) B65.9 [N33]
  - submucosal — *see* Cystitis, interstitial
  - tuberculous A18.12
- bleeding K27.4
- bone — *see* Osteomyelitis, specified type NEC
- bowel — *see* Ulcer, intestine
- breast N61.1
- bronchus J98.09
- buccal (cavity) (traumatic) K12.1
- Buruli A31.1
- buttock L98.419
  - with
    - bone involvement without evidence of necrosis L98.416
    - bone necrosis L98.414
    - exposed fat layer L98.412
    - muscle involvement without evidence of necrosis L98.415
    - muscle necrosis L98.413
    - skin breakdown only L98.411
    - specified severity NEC L98.418
- cameron *see* Ulcer, stomach
- cancerous — *see* Neoplasm, malignant, by site
- cardia K22.10
  - with bleeding K22.11
- cardioesophageal (peptic) K22.10
  - with bleeding K22.11
- cecum — *see* Ulcer, intestine
- cervix (uteri) (decubitus) (trophic) N86
  - with cervicitis N72
- chancroidal A57
- chest L98.449
  - with
    - bone involvement without evidence of necrosis L98.446
    - bone necrosis L98.444
    - exposed fat layer L98.442
    - muscle involvement without evidence of necrosis L98.445
    - muscle necrosis L98.443
    - skin breakdown only L98.441
    - specified severity NEC L98.448
- chiclero B55.1
- chronic (cause unknown) — *see* Ulcer, skin
- Cochin-China B55.1
- colon — *see* Ulcer, intestine
- conjunctiva H10.89
- cornea H16.00- ☑
  - with hypopyon H16.03- ☑
  - central H16.01- ☑
  - dendritic (herpes simplex) B00.52
  - marginal H16.04- ☑
  - Mooren's H16.05- ☑
  - mycotic H16.06- ☑
  - perforated H16.07- ☑
  - ring H16.02- ☑
  - tuberculous (phlyctenular) A18.52
- corpus cavernosum (chronic) N48.5
- crural — *see* Ulcer, lower limb
- Curling's — *see* Ulcer, peptic, acute
- Cushing's — *see* Ulcer, peptic, acute
- cystic duct K82.8
- cystitis (interstitial) — *see* Cystitis, interstitial
- decubitus — *see* Ulcer, pressure, by site
- dendritic, cornea (herpes simplex) B00.52
- diabetes, diabetic — *see* Diabetes, ulcer
- Dieulafoy's K25.0
- due to
  - infection NEC — *see* Ulcer, skin
  - radiation NEC L59.8
  - trophic disturbance (any region) — *see* Ulcer, skin
  - X-ray L58.1
- duodenum, duodenal (eroded) (peptic) K26.9
  - with
    - hemorrhage K26.4
      - and perforation K26.6
    - perforation K26.5
  - acute K26.3
    - with
      - hemorrhage K26.0
        - and perforation K26.2
      - perforation K26.1
  - chronic (erosive) K26.7

Ulcer, ulcerated, ulcerating, ulceration, ulcerative — continued
- duodenum, duodenal — continued
  - chronic — continued
    - with
      - hemorrhage K26.4
        - and perforation K26.6
      - perforation K26.5
  - dysenteric A09
  - elusive — see Cystitis, interstitial
  - endocarditis (acute) (chronic) (subacute) I28.8
  - epiglottis J38.7
  - esophagus (peptic) K22.10
    - with bleeding K22.11
    - due to
      - aspirin K22.10
        - with bleeding K22.11
      - gastrointestinal reflux disease (without bleeding) K21.00
        - with bleeding K21.01
      - ingestion of chemical or medicament K22.10
        - with bleeding K22.11
    - fungal K22.10
      - with bleeding K22.11
    - infective K22.10
      - with bleeding K22.11
    - varicose — see Varix, esophagus
  - eyelid (region) H01.8- ☑
  - face L98.469
    - with
      - bone involvement without evidence of necrosis L98.466
      - bone necrosis L98.464
      - exposed fat layer L98.462
      - muscle involvement without evidence of necrosis L98.465
      - muscle necrosis L98.463
      - skin breakdown only L98.461
      - specified severity NEC L98.468
  - fauces J39.2
  - Fenwick (-Hunner) (solitary) — see Cystitis, interstitial
  - fistulous — see Ulcer, skin
  - foot (indolent) (trophic) — see Ulcer, lower limb
  - forearm L98.A299
    - with
      - bone involvement without evidence of necrosis L98.A296
      - bone necrosis L98.A294
      - exposed fat layer L98.A292
      - muscle involvement without evidence of necrosis L98.A295
      - muscle necrosis L98.A293
      - skin breakdown only L98.A291
      - specified severity NEC L98.A298
    - left L98.A229
      - with
        - bone involvement without evidence of necrosis L98.A226
        - bone necrosis L98.A224
        - exposed fat layer L98.A222
        - muscle involvement without evidence of necrosis L98.A225
        - muscle necrosis L98.A223
        - skin breakdown only L98.A221
        - specified severity NEC L98.A228
    - right L98.A219
      - with
        - bone involvement without evidence of necrosis L98.A216
        - bone necrosis L98.A214
        - exposed fat layer L98.A212
        - muscle involvement without evidence of necrosis L98.A215
        - muscle necrosis L98.A213
        - skin breakdown only L98.A211
        - specified severity NEC L98.A218
  - frambesial, initial A66.0
  - frenum (tongue) K14.0
  - gallbladder or duct K82.8
  - gangrenous — see Gangrene
  - gastric — see Ulcer, stomach
  - gastrocolic — see Ulcer, gastrojejunal
  - gastroduodenal — see Ulcer, peptic
  - gastroesophageal — see Ulcer, stomach
  - gastrointestinal — see Ulcer, gastrojejunal
  - gastrojejunal (peptic) K28.9
    - with
      - hemorrhage K28.4
        - and perforation K28.6

Ulcer, ulcerated, ulcerating, ulceration, ulcerative — continued
- gastrojejunal — continued
  - with — continued
    - perforation K28.5
  - acute K28.3
    - with
      - hemorrhage K28.0
        - and perforation K28.2
      - perforation K28.1
  - chronic K28.7
    - with
      - hemorrhage K28.4
        - and perforation K28.6
      - perforation K28.5
- gastrojejunocolic — see Ulcer, gastrojejunal
- gingiva K06.8
- gingivitis K05.10
  - nonplaque induced K05.11
  - plaque induced K05.10
- glottis J38.7
- granuloma of pudenda A58
- groin L98.479
  - with
    - bone involvement without evidence of necrosis L98.476
    - bone necrosis L98.474
    - exposed fat layer L98.472
    - muscle involvement without evidence of necrosis L98.475
    - muscle necrosis L98.473
    - skin breakdown only L98.471
    - specified severity NEC L98.478
- gum K06.8
- gumma, due to yaws A66.4
- hand L98.A399
  - with
    - bone involvement without evidence of necrosis L98.A396
    - bone necrosis L98.A394
    - exposed fat layer L98.A392
    - muscle involvement without evidence of necrosis L98.A395
    - muscle necrosis L98.A393
    - skin breakdown only L98.A391
    - specified severity NEC L98.A398
  - left L98.A329
    - with
      - bone involvement without evidence of necrosis L98.A326
      - bone necrosis L98.A324
      - exposed fat layer L98.A322
      - muscle involvement without evidence of necrosis L98.A325
      - muscle necrosis L98.A323
      - skin breakdown only L98.A321
      - specified severity NEC L98.A328
  - right L98.A319
    - with
      - bone involvement without evidence of necrosis L98.A316
      - bone necrosis L98.A314
      - exposed fat layer L98.A312
      - muscle involvement without evidence of necrosis L98.A315
      - muscle necrosis L98.A313
      - skin breakdown only L98.A311
      - specified severity NEC L98.A318
- heel — see Ulcer, lower limb
- hemorrhoid — see also Hemorrhoids, by degree K64.8
- Hunner's — see Cystitis, interstitial
- hypopharynx J39.2
- hypopyon (chronic) (subacute) — see Ulcer, cornea, with hypopyon
- hypostaticum — see Ulcer, varicose
- ileum — see Ulcer, intestine
- intestine, intestinal K63.3
  - with perforation K63.1
  - amebic A06.1
  - duodenal — see Ulcer, duodenum
  - granulocytopenic (with hemorrhage) — see Neutropenia
  - marginal — see Ulcer, gastrojejunal
  - perforating K63.1
    - newborn P78.0
  - primary, small intestine K63.3
  - rectum K62.6
  - stercoraceous, stercoral K63.3
  - tuberculous A18.32

Ulcer, ulcerated, ulcerating, ulceration, ulcerative — continued
- intestine, intestinal — continued
  - typhoid (fever) — see Typhoid
  - varicose I86.8
- jejunum, jejunal — see Ulcer, gastrojejunal
- keratitis — see Ulcer, cornea
- knee — see Ulcer, lower limb
- labium (majus) (minus) N76.6
- laryngitis — see Laryngitis
- larynx (aphthous) (contact) J38.7
  - diphtheritic A36.2
- leg — see Ulcer, lower limb
- lip K13.0
- Lipschütz's N76.6
- lower limb (atrophic) (chronic) (neurogenic) (perforating) (pyogenic) (trophic) (tropical) L97.909
  - with
    - bone involvement without evidence of necrosis L97.906
    - bone necrosis L97.904
    - exposed fat layer L97.902
    - muscle involvement without evidence of necrosis L97.905
    - muscle necrosis L97.903
    - skin breakdown only L97.901
    - specified severity NEC L97.908
  - ankle L97.309
    - with
      - bone involvement without evidence of necrosis L97.306
      - bone necrosis L97.304
      - exposed fat layer L97.302
      - muscle involvement without evidence of necrosis L97.305
      - muscle necrosis L97.303
      - skin breakdown only L97.301
      - specified severity NEC L97.308
    - left L97.329
      - with
        - bone involvement without evidence of necrosis L97.326
        - bone necrosis L97.324
        - exposed fat layer L97.322
        - muscle involvement without evidence of necrosis L97.325
        - muscle necrosis L97.323
        - skin breakdown only L97.321
        - specified severity NEC L97.328
    - right L97.319
      - with
        - bone involvement without evidence of necrosis L97.316
        - bone necrosis L97.314
        - exposed fat layer L97.312
        - muscle involvement without evidence of necrosis L97.315
        - muscle necrosis L97.313
        - skin breakdown only L97.311
        - specified severity NEC L97.318
  - calf L97.209
    - with
      - bone involvement without evidence of necrosis L97.206
      - bone necrosis L97.204
      - exposed fat layer L97.202
      - muscle involvement without evidence of necrosis L97.205
      - muscle necrosis L97.203
      - skin breakdown only L97.201
      - specified severity NEC L97.208
    - left L97.229
      - with
        - bone involvement without evidence of necrosis L97.226
        - bone necrosis L97.224
        - exposed fat layer L97.222
        - muscle involvement without evidence of necrosis L97.225
        - muscle necrosis L97.223
        - skin breakdown only L97.221
        - specified severity NEC L97.228
    - right L97.219
      - with
        - bone involvement without evidence of necrosis L97.216
        - bone necrosis L97.214
        - exposed fat layer L97.212

Ulcer, ulcerated, ulcerating, ulceration, ulcerative — *continued*
- lower limb — *continued*
  - calf — *continued*
    - right — *continued*
      - with — *continued*
        - muscle involvement without evidence of necrosis L97.215
        - muscle necrosis L97.213
        - skin breakdown only L97.211
        - specified severity NEC L97.218
  - decubitus — *see* Ulcer, pressure, by site
  - foot specified NEC L97.509
    - with
      - bone involvement without evidence of necrosis L97.506
      - bone necrosis L97.504
      - exposed fat layer L97.502
      - muscle involvement without evidence of necrosis L97.505
      - muscle necrosis L97.503
      - skin breakdown only L97.501
      - specified severity NEC L97.508
    - left L97.529
      - with
        - bone involvement without evidence of necrosis L97.526
        - bone necrosis L97.524
        - exposed fat layer L97.522
        - muscle involvement without evidence of necrosis L97.525
        - muscle necrosis L97.523
        - skin breakdown only L97.521
        - specified severity NEC L97.528
    - right L97.519
      - with
        - bone involvement without evidence of necrosis L97.516
        - bone necrosis L97.514
        - exposed fat layer L97.512
        - muscle involvement without evidence of necrosis L97.515
        - muscle necrosis L97.513
        - skin breakdown only L97.511
        - specified severity NEC L97.518
  - heel L97.409
    - with
      - bone involvement without evidence of necrosis L97.406
      - bone necrosis L97.404
      - exposed fat layer L97.402
      - muscle involvement without evidence of necrosis L97.405
      - muscle necrosis L97.403
      - skin breakdown only L97.401
      - specified severity NEC L97.408
    - left L97.429
      - with
        - bone involvement without evidence of necrosis L97.426
        - bone necrosis L97.424
        - exposed fat layer L97.422
        - muscle involvement without evidence of necrosis L97.425
        - muscle necrosis L97.423
        - skin breakdown only L97.421
        - specified severity NEC L97.428
    - right L97.419
      - with
        - bone involvement without evidence of necrosis L97.416
        - bone necrosis L97.414
        - exposed fat layer L97.412
        - muscle involvement without evidence of necrosis L97.415
        - muscle necrosis L97.413
        - skin breakdown only L97.411
        - specified severity NEC L97.418
    - left L97.929
      - with
        - bone involvement without evidence of necrosis L97.926
        - bone necrosis L97.924
        - exposed fat layer L97.922
        - muscle involvement without evidence of necrosis L97.925
        - muscle necrosis L97.923
        - skin breakdown only L97.921
        - specified severity NEC L97.928

Ulcer, ulcerated, ulcerating, ulceration, ulcerative — *continued*
- lower limb — *continued*
  - leprous A30.1
  - lower leg NOS L97.909
    - with
      - bone involvement without evidence of necrosis L97.906
      - bone necrosis L97.904
      - exposed fat layer L97.902
      - muscle involvement without evidence of necrosis L97.905
      - muscle necrosis L97.903
      - skin breakdown only L97.901
      - specified severity NEC L97.908
    - left L97.929
      - with
        - bone involvement without evidence of necrosis L97.926
        - bone necrosis L97.924
        - exposed fat layer L97.922
        - muscle involvement without evidence of necrosis L97.925
        - muscle necrosis L97.923
        - skin breakdown only L97.921
        - specified severity NEC L97.928
    - right L97.919
      - with
        - bone involvement without evidence of necrosis L97.916
        - bone necrosis L97.914
        - exposed fat layer L97.912
        - muscle involvement without evidence of necrosis L97.915
        - muscle necrosis L97.913
        - skin breakdown only L97.911
        - specified severity NEC L97.918
  - specified site NEC L97.809
    - with
      - bone involvement without evidence of necrosis L97.806
      - bone necrosis L97.804
      - exposed fat layer L97.802
      - muscle involvement without evidence of necrosis L97.805
      - muscle necrosis L97.803
      - skin breakdown only L97.801
      - specified severity NEC L97.808
    - left L97.829
      - with
        - bone involvement without evidence of necrosis L97.826
        - bone necrosis L97.824
        - exposed fat layer L97.822
        - muscle involvement without evidence of necrosis L97.825
        - muscle necrosis L97.823
        - skin breakdown only L97.821
        - specified severity NEC L97.828
    - right L97.819
      - with
        - bone involvement without evidence of necrosis L97.816
        - bone necrosis L97.814
        - exposed fat layer L97.812
        - muscle involvement without evidence of necrosis L97.815
        - muscle necrosis L97.813
        - skin breakdown only L97.811
        - specified severity NEC L97.818
  - midfoot L97.409
    - with
      - bone involvement without evidence of necrosis L97.406
      - bone necrosis L97.404
      - exposed fat layer L97.402
      - muscle involvement without evidence of necrosis L97.405
      - muscle necrosis L97.403
      - skin breakdown only L97.401
      - specified severity NEC L97.408
    - left L97.429
      - with
        - bone involvement without evidence of necrosis L97.426
        - bone necrosis L97.424
        - exposed fat layer L97.422
        - muscle involvement without evidence of necrosis L97.425

Ulcer, ulcerated, ulcerating, ulceration, ulcerative — *continued*
- lower limb — *continued*
  - midfoot — *continued*
    - left — *continued*
      - with — *continued*
        - muscle necrosis L97.423
        - skin breakdown only L97.421
        - specified severity NEC L97.428
    - right L97.419
      - with
        - bone involvement without evidence of necrosis L97.416
        - bone necrosis L97.414
        - exposed fat layer L97.412
        - muscle involvement without evidence of necrosis L97.415
        - muscle necrosis L97.413
        - skin breakdown only L97.411
        - specified severity NEC L97.418
    - right L97.919
      - with
        - bone involvement without evidence of necrosis L97.916
        - bone necrosis L97.914
        - exposed fat layer L97.912
        - muscle involvement without evidence of necrosis L97.915
        - muscle necrosis L97.913
        - skin breakdown only L97.911
        - specified severity NEC L97.918
  - shin — *see also* Ulcer, lower limb, calf L97.209
  - syphilitic A52.19
  - thigh L97.109
    - with
      - bone involvement without evidence of necrosis L97.106
      - bone necrosis L97.104
      - exposed fat layer L97.102
      - muscle involvement without evidence of necrosis L97.105
      - muscle necrosis L97.103
      - skin breakdown only L97.101
      - specified severity NEC L97.108
    - left L97.129
      - with
        - bone involvement without evidence of necrosis L97.126
        - bone necrosis L97.124
        - exposed fat layer L97.122
        - muscle involvement without evidence of necrosis L97.125
        - muscle necrosis L97.123
        - skin breakdown only L97.121
        - specified severity NEC L97.128
    - right L97.119
      - with
        - bone involvement without evidence of necrosis L97.116
        - bone necrosis L97.114
        - exposed fat layer L97.112
        - muscle involvement without evidence of necrosis L97.115
        - muscle necrosis L97.113
        - skin breakdown only L97.111
        - specified severity NEC L97.118
  - toe L97.509
    - with
      - bone involvement without evidence of necrosis L97.506
      - bone necrosis L97.504
      - exposed fat layer L97.502
      - muscle involvement without evidence of necrosis L97.505
      - muscle necrosis L97.503
      - skin breakdown only L97.501
      - specified severity NEC L97.508
    - left L97.529
      - with
        - bone involvement without evidence of necrosis L97.526
        - bone necrosis L97.524
        - exposed fat layer L97.522
        - muscle involvement without evidence of necrosis L97.525
        - muscle necrosis L97.523
        - skin breakdown only L97.521
        - specified severity NEC L97.528
    - right L97.519

Ulcer, ulcerated, ulcerating, ulceration, ulcerative — *continued*
- lower limb — *continued*
  - toe — *continued*
    - right — *continued*
      - with
        - bone involvement without evidence of necrosis L97.516
        - bone necrosis L97.514
        - exposed fat layer L97.512
        - muscle involvement without evidence of necrosis L97.515
        - muscle necrosis L97.513
        - skin breakdown only L97.511
        - specified severity NEC L97.518
- varicose — *see* Varix, leg, with, ulcer
- luetic — *see* Ulcer, syphilitic
- lung J98.4
  - tuberculous — *see* Tuberculosis, pulmonary
- malignant — *see* Neoplasm, malignant, by site
- marginal NEC — *see* Ulcer, gastrojejunal
- meatus (urinarius) N34.2
- Meckel's diverticulum Q43.0
  - malignant — *see* Table of Neoplasms, small intestine, malignant
- Meleney's (chronic undermining) — *see* Ulcer, skin
- Mooren's (cornea) — *see* Ulcer, cornea, Mooren's
- mycobacterial (skin) A31.1
- nasopharynx J39.2
- neck L98.459
  - with
    - bone involvement without evidence of necrosis L98.456
    - bone necrosis L98.454
    - exposed fat layer L98.452
    - muscle involvement without evidence of necrosis L98.455
    - muscle necrosis L98.453
    - skin breakdown only L98.451
    - specified severity NEC L98.458
- uterus N86
- neurogenic NEC — *see* Ulcer, skin
- nose, nasal (passage) (infective) (septum) J34.0
  - skin — *see* Ulcer, skin
  - spirochetal A69.8
  - varicose (bleeding) I86.8
- oral mucosa (traumatic) K12.1
- palate (soft) K12.1
- penis (chronic) N48.5
- peptic (site unspecified) K27.9
  - with
    - hemorrhage K27.4
      - and perforation K27.6
    - perforation K27.5
  - acute K27.3
    - with
      - hemorrhage K27.0
        - and perforation K27.2
      - perforation K27.1
  - chronic K27.7
    - with
      - hemorrhage K27.4
        - and perforation K27.6
      - perforation K27.5
  - esophagus K22.10
    - with bleeding K22.11
  - newborn P78.82
- perforating K27.5
  - skin — *see* Ulcer, skin
- peritonsillar J35.8
- phagedenic (tropical) — *see* Ulcer, skin
- pharynx J39.2
- phlebitis — *see* Phlebitis
- plaster — *see* Ulcer, pressure, by site
- popliteal space — *see* Ulcer, lower limb
- postpyloric — *see* Ulcer, duodenum
- prepuce N47.7
- prepyloric — *see* Ulcer, stomach
- pressure (pressure area) L89.9- ☑
  - ankle L89.5- ☑
  - back L89.1- ☑
  - buttock L89.3- ☑
  - coccyx L89.15- ☑
  - contiguous site of back, buttock, hip L89.4- ☑
  - elbow L89.0- ☑
  - face L89.81- ☑
  - head L89.81- ☑
  - heel L89.6- ☑

Ulcer, ulcerated, ulcerating, ulceration, ulcerative — *continued*
- pressure — *continued*
  - hip L89.2- ☑
  - sacral region (tailbone) L89.15- ☑
  - specified site NEC L89.89- ☑
  - stage 1 (healing) (pre-ulcer skin changes limited to persistent focal edema)
    - ankle L89.5- ☑
    - back L89.1- ☑
    - buttock L89.3- ☑
    - coccyx L89.15- ☑
    - contiguous site of back, buttock, hip L89.4- ☑
    - elbow L89.0- ☑
    - face L89.81- ☑
    - head L89.81- ☑
    - heel L89.6- ☑
    - hip L89.2- ☑
    - sacral region (tailbone) L89.15- ☑
    - specified site NEC L89.89- ☑
  - stage 2 (healing) (abrasion, blister, partial thickness skin loss involving epidermis and/or dermis)
    - ankle L89.5- ☑
    - back L89.1- ☑
    - buttock L89.3- ☑
    - coccyx L89.15- ☑
    - contiguous site of back, buttock, hip L89.4- ☑
    - elbow L89.0- ☑
    - face L89.81- ☑
    - head L89.81- ☑
    - heel L89.6- ☑
    - hip L89.2- ☑
    - sacral region (tailbone) L89.15- ☑
    - specified site NEC L89.89- ☑
  - stage 3 (healing) (full thickness skin loss involving damage or necrosis of subcutaneous tissue)
    - ankle L89.5- ☑
    - back L89.1- ☑
    - buttock L89.3- ☑
    - coccyx L89.15- ☑
    - contiguous site of back, buttock, hip L89.4- ☑
    - elbow L89.0- ☑
    - face L89.81- ☑
    - head L89.81- ☑
    - heel L89.6- ☑
    - hip L89.2- ☑
    - sacral region (tailbone) L89.15- ☑
    - specified site NEC L89.89- ☑
  - stage 4 (healing) (necrosis of soft tissues through to underlying muscle, tendon, or bone)
    - ankle L89.5- ☑
    - back L89.1- ☑
    - buttock L89.3- ☑
    - coccyx L89.15- ☑
    - contiguous site of back, buttock, hip L89.4- ☑
    - elbow L89.0- ☑
    - face L89.81- ☑
    - head L89.81- ☑
    - heel L89.6- ☑
    - hip L89.2- ☑
    - sacral region (tailbone) L89.15- ☑
    - specified site NEC L89.89- ☑
  - unspecified stage
    - ankle L89.5- ☑
    - back L89.1- ☑
    - buttock L89.3- ☑
    - coccyx L89.15- ☑
    - contiguous site of back, buttock, hip L89.4- ☑
    - elbow L89.0- ☑
    - face L89.81- ☑
    - head L89.81- ☑
    - heel L89.6- ☑
    - hip L89.2- ☑
    - sacral region (tailbone) L89.15- ☑
    - specified site NEC L89.89- ☑
  - unstageable
    - ankle L89.5- ☑
    - back L89.1- ☑
    - buttock L89.3- ☑
    - coccyx L89.15- ☑
    - contiguous site of back, buttock, hip L89.4- ☑
    - elbow L89.0- ☑
    - face L89.81- ☑
    - head L89.81- ☑
    - heel L89.6- ☑

Ulcer, ulcerated, ulcerating, ulceration, ulcerative — *continued*
- pressure — *continued*
  - unstageable — *continued*
    - hip L89.2- ☑
    - sacral region (tailbone) L89.15- ☑
    - specified site NEC L89.89- ☑
- primary of intestine K63.3
  - with perforation K63.1
- prostate N41.9
- pyloric — *see* Ulcer, stomach
- rectosigmoid K63.3
  - with perforation K63.1
- rectum (sphincter) (solitary) K62.6
  - stercoraceous, stercoral K62.6
- retina — *see* Inflammation, chorioretinal
- rodent — *see also* Neoplasm, skin, malignant
- sclera — *see* Scleritis
- scrofulous (tuberculous) A18.2
- scrotum N50.89
  - tuberculous A18.15
  - varicose I86.1
- seminal vesicle N50.89
- sigmoid — *see* Ulcer, intestine
- skin (atrophic) (chronic) (neurogenic) (non-healing) (perforating) (pyogenic) (trophic) (tropical) L98.499
  - with gangrene — *see* Gangrene
  - amebic A06.7
  - back — *see* Ulcer, back
  - buttock — *see* Ulcer, buttock
  - decubitus — *see* Ulcer, pressure
  - lower limb — *see* Ulcer, lower limb
  - mycobacterial A31.1
  - specified site NEC L98.499
    - with
      - bone involvement without evidence of necrosis L98.496
      - bone necrosis L98.494
      - exposed fat layer L98.492
      - muscle involvement without evidence of necrosis L98.495
      - muscle necrosis L98.493
      - skin breakdown only L98.491
      - specified severity NEC L98.498
  - tuberculous (primary) A18.4
  - upper limb — *see* Ulcer, upper limb
  - varicose — *see* Ulcer, varicose
- sloughing — *see* Ulcer, skin
- solitary, anus or rectum (sphincter) K62.6
- sore throat J02.9
  - streptococcal J02.0
- spermatic cord N50.89
- spine (tuberculous) A18.01
- stasis (venous) — *see* Varix, leg, with, ulcer
  - without varicose veins — *see also* Ulcer, by site I87.2
- stercoraceous, stercoral K63.3
  - with perforation K63.1
  - anus or rectum K62.6
- stoma, stomal — *see* Ulcer, gastrojejunal
- stomach (eroded) (peptic) (round) K25.9
  - with
    - hemorrhage K25.4
      - and perforation K25.6
    - perforation K25.5
  - acute K25.3
    - with
      - hemorrhage K25.0
        - and perforation K25.2
      - perforation K25.1
  - chronic K25.7
    - with
      - hemorrhage K25.4
        - and perforation K25.6
      - perforation K25.5
- stomal — *see* Ulcer, gastrojejunal
- stomatitis K12.1
- stress — *see* Ulcer, peptic
- strumous (tuberculous) A18.2
- submucosal, bladder — *see* Cystitis, interstitial
- syphilitic (any site) (early) (secondary) A51.39
  - late A52.79
    - perforating A52.79
      - foot A52.11
- testis N50.89
- thigh — *see* Ulcer, lower limb
- throat J39.2
  - diphtheritic A36.0
- toe — *see* Ulcer, lower limb
- tongue (traumatic) K14.0

Ulcer, ulcerated, ulcerating, ulceration, ulcerative — continued
- tonsil J35.8
- diphtheritic A36.0
- trachea J39.8
- trophic — see Ulcer, skin
- tropical — see Ulcer, skin
- tuberculous — see Tuberculosis, ulcer
- tunica vaginalis N50.89
- turbinate J34.89
- typhoid (perforating) — see Typhoid
- unspecified site — see Ulcer, skin
- upper limb (chronic)
  - upper arm L98.A199
    - with
      - bone involvement without evidence of necrosis L98.A196
      - bone necrosis L98.A194
      - exposed fat layer L98.A192
      - muscle involvement without evidence of necrosis L98.A195
      - muscle necrosis L98.A193
      - skin breakdown only L98.A191
      - specified severity NEC L98.A198
    - left L98.A129
      - with
        - bone involvement without evidence of necrosis L98.A126
        - bone necrosis L98.A124
        - exposed fat layer L98.A122
        - muscle involvement without evidence of necrosis L98.A125
        - muscle necrosis L98.A123
        - skin breakdown only L98.A121
        - specified severity NEC L98.A128
    - right L98.A119
      - with
        - bone involvement without evidence of necrosis L98.A116
        - bone necrosis L98.A114
        - exposed fat layer L98.A112
        - muscle involvement without evidence of necrosis L98.A115
        - muscle necrosis L98.A113
        - skin breakdown only L98.A111
        - specified severity NEC L98.A118
- urethra (meatus) — see Urethritis
- uterus N85.8
  - cervix N86
    - with cervicitis N72
  - neck N86
    - with cervicitis N72
  - vagina N76.5
    - in Behcet's disease M35.2 [N77.0]
  - pessary N89.8
- valve, heart I33.0
- varicose (lower limb, any part) — see also Varix, leg, with, ulcer
  - broad ligament I86.2
  - esophagus — see Varix, esophagus
  - inflamed or infected — see Varix, leg, with ulcer, with inflammation
  - nasal septum J86.8
  - perineum I86.3
  - scrotum I86.1
  - specified site NEC I86.8
  - sublingual I86.0
  - vulva I86.3
- vas deferens N50.89
- vulva (acute) (infectional) N76.6
  - in (due to)
    - Behcet's disease M35.2 [N77.0]
    - herpesviral (herpes simplex) infection A60.04
    - tuberculosis A18.18
- vulvobuccal, recurring N76.6
- X-ray L58.1
- yaws A66.4

Ulcerosa scarlatina A38.8
Ulcus — see also Ulcer
- cutis tuberculosum A18.4
- duodeni — see Ulcer, duodenum
- durum (syphilitic) A51.0
  - extragenital A51.2
- gastrojejunale — see Ulcer, gastrojejunal
- hypostaticum — see Ulcer, varicose
- molle (cutis) (skin) A57
- serpens corneae — see Ulcer, cornea, central
- ventriculi — see Ulcer, stomach

Ulegyria Q04.8

Ulerythema
- ophryogenes, congenital Q84.2
- sycosiforme L73.8

Ullrich-Feichtiger syndrome Q87.0
Ullrich (-Bonnevie) (-Turner) **syndrome** — see also Turner's syndrome Q87.19
Ulnar — see condition
Ulorrhagia, ulorrhea K06.8
Umbilicus, umbilical — see condition
Unable to
- make ends meet Z59.868
- obtain
  - adequate
    - childcare due to limited financial resources, specified NEC Z59.87
    - clothing due to limited financial resources, specified NEC Z59.87
    - utilities due to limited financial resources, specified NEC Z59.861
  - basic
    - needs due to limited financial resources, specified NEC Z59.87
    - services in physical environment Z58.81
  - internet service, due to unavailability in geographic area Z58.81
  - telephone service, due to unavailability in geographic area Z58.81
  - utilities, due to inadequate physical environment Z58.81

Unacceptable
- contours of tooth K08.54
- morphology of tooth K08.54

Unaffordable transportation Z59.82
Unavailability (of)
- bed at medical facility Z75.1
- health service-related agencies Z75.4
- medical facilities (at) Z75.3
  - due to
    - investigation by social service agency Z75.2
    - lack of services at home Z75.0
    - remoteness from facility Z75.3
    - waiting list Z75.1
- home Z75.0
- outpatient clinic Z75.3
- schooling Z55.1
- social service agencies Z75.4

Uncinaria americana infestation B76.1
Uncinariasis B76.9
Uncongenial work Z56.5
Unconscious (ness) — see Coma
Under observation — see Observation
Underachievement in school Z55.3
Underdevelopment — see also Undeveloped
- nose Q30.1
- sexual E30.0

Underdosing — see also Table of Drugs and Chemicals, categories T36-T50, with final character 6 Z91.14- ☑
- intentional NEC Z91.128
  - due to financial hardship of patient Z91.120
- unintentional NEC Z91.138
  - due to patient's age related debility Z91.130

Underemployed Z56.89
Underfeeding, newborn P92.3
Underfill, endodontic M27.53
Underimmunization status Z28.39
- COVID-19 Z28.31- ☑
  - partially vaccinated (for) Z28.311
  - unvaccinated (for) Z28.310

Undernourishment — see Malnutrition
Undernutrition — see Malnutrition
Underweight R63.6
- for gestational age — see Light for dates

Underwood's disease P83.0
Undescended — see also Malposition, congenital
- cecum Q43.3
- colon Q43.3
- testicle — see Cryptorchid

Undeveloped, undevelopment — see also Hypoplasia
- brain (congenital) Q02
- cerebral (congenital) Q02
- heart Q24.8
- lung Q33.6
- testis E29.1
- uterus E30.0

Undiagnosed (disease) R69
Undulant fever — see Brucellosis
Unemployment, anxiety concerning Z56.0
- threatened Z56.2

Unequal length (acquired) (limb) — see also Deformity, limb, unequal length
- leg — see also Deformity, limb, unequal length
- congenital Q72.9- ☑

Unextracted dental root K08.3
Unguis incarnatus L60.0
Unhappiness R45.2
Unicornate uterus Q51.4
- in pregnancy or childbirth O34.00

Unicuspid aortic valve (at birth) (congenital) Q23.81
Unilateral — see also condition
- development, breast N64.89
- organ or site, congenital NEC — see Agenesis, by site

Unilocular heart Q20.8
Unimmunized — see also Underimmunization status
- for COVID-19 Z28.310

Union, abnormal — see also Fusion
- larynx and trachea Q34.8

Universal mesentery Q43.3
Unreliable transportation Z59.82
Unrepairable overhanging of dental restorative materials K08.52
Unroofed coronary sinus Q21.13
Unsafe transportation Z59.82
Unsatisfactory
- restoration of tooth K08.50
  - specified NEC K08.59
- sample of cytologic smear
  - anus R85.615
  - cervix R87.615
  - vagina R87.625
- surroundings Z59.19
- work Z56.5

Unsoundness of mind — see Psychosis
Unstable
- back NEC — see Instability, joint, spine
- hip (congenital) Q65.6
  - acquired — see Derangement, joint, specified type NEC, hip
- joint — see Instability, joint
  - secondary to removal of joint prosthesis M96.89
- lie (mother) O32.0- ☑
- lumbosacral joint (congenital) — see subcategory M53.2
- sacroiliac — see subcategory M53.2- ☑
- spine NEC — see Instability, joint, spine

Unsteadiness on feet R26.81
Untruthfulness, child problem F91.8
Unvaccinated — see also Underimmunization status
- for COVID-19 Z28.310

Unverricht (-Lundborg) **disease or epilepsy** — see Epilepsy, generalized, idiopathic

Unwanted
- multiple moves in the last 12 months Z59.81- ☑
- pregnancy Z64.0

Upbringing, institutional Z62.22
- away from parents NEC Z62.29
- in care of non-parental family member Z62.21
- in foster care Z62.21
- in orphanage or group home Z62.22
- in welfare custody Z62.21

Upper respiratory — see condition
Upset
- gastric K30
- gastrointestinal K30
  - psychogenic F45.8
- intestinal (large) (small) K59.9
  - psychogenic F45.8
- menstruation N93.9
- mental F48.9
- stomach K30
  - psychogenic F45.8

Urachus — see also condition
- patent or persistent Q64.4

Urbach-Oppenheim disease (necrobiosis lipoidica diabeticorum) — see E08-E13 with .620
Urbach-Wiethe disease E78.89
Urbach's lipoid proteinosis E78.89
Urban yellow fever A95.1
Urea
- blood, high — see Uremia
- cycle metabolism disorder — see Disorder, urea cycle metabolism

Uremia, uremic N19
- with
  - ectopic or molar pregnancy O08.4
  - polyneuropathy N18.9 [G63]
- chronic NOS — see also Disease, kidney, chronic N18.9
  - due to hypertension — see Hypertensive, kidney

☑ **Additional Character Required** — Refer to the Tabular List for Character Selection

Uremia, uremic — continued
　complicating
　　ectopic or molar pregnancy O08.4
　congenital P96.0
　extrarenal R39.2
　following ectopic or molar pregnancy O08.4
　newborn P96.0
　prerenal R39.2
Ureter, ureteral — see condition
Ureteralgia N23
Ureterectasis — see Hydroureter
Ureteritis N28.89
　cystica N28.86
　due to calculus N20.1
　　with calculus, kidney N20.2
　　　with hydronephrosis N13.2
　gonococcal (acute) (chronic) A54.21
　nonspecific N28.89
Ureterocele N28.89
　congenital (orthotopic) Q62.31
　　ectopic Q62.32
Ureterolith, ureterolithiasis — see Calculus, ureter
Ureterostomy
　attention to Z43.6
　status Z93.6
Urethra, urethral — see condition
Urethralgia R39.89
Urethritis (anterior) (posterior) N34.2
　calculous N21.1
　candidal B37.41
　chlamydial A56.01
　diplococcal (gonococcal) A54.01
　　with abscess (accessory gland) (periurethral) A54.1
　gonococcal A54.01
　　with abscess (accessory gland) (periurethral) A54.1
　nongonococcal N34.1
　　Reiter's — see Reiter's disease
　nonspecific N34.1
　nonvenereal N34.1
　postmenopausal N34.2
　puerperal O86.22
　Reiter's — see Reiter's disease
　specified NEC N34.2
　trichomonal or due to Trichomonas (vaginalis) A59.03
Urethrocele N81.0
　with
　　cystocele — see Cystocele
　　prolapse of uterus — see Prolapse, uterus
Urethrolithiasis (with colic or infection) N21.1
Urethrorectal — see condition
Urethrorrhagia N36.8
Urethrorrhea R36.9
Urethrostomy
　attention to Z43.6
　status Z93.6
Urethrotrigonitis — see Trigonitis
Urethrovaginal — see condition
Urgency
　fecal R15.2
　hypertensive — see Hypertension
　urinary R39.15
Urhidrosis, uridrosis L74.8
Uric acid in blood (increased) E79.0
Uricacidemia (asymptomatic) E79.0
Uricemia (asymptomatic) E79.0
Uricosuria R82.998
Urinary — see condition
Urination
　frequent R35.0
　painful R30.9
Urine
　blood in — see Hematuria
　discharge, excessive R35.89
　enuresis, nonorganic origin F98.0
　extravasation R39.0
　frequency R35.0
　incontinence R32
　　nonorganic origin F98.0
　intermittent stream R39.198
　pus in N39.0
　retention or stasis R33.9
　　organic R33.8
　　　drug-induced R33.0
　　psychogenic F45.8
　secretion
　　deficient R34
　　excessive R35.89
　　frequency R35.0

Urine — continued
　stream
　　intermittent R39.198
　　slowing R39.198
　　splitting R39.13
　　weak R39.12
Urinemia — see Uremia
Urinoma, urethra N36.8
Uroarthritis, infectious (Reiter's) — see Reiter's disease
Urodialysis R34
Urolithiasis — see Calculus, urinary
Uronephrosis — see Hydronephrosis
Uropathy N39.9
　obstructive N13.9
　　specified NEC N13.8
　reflux N13.9
　　specified NEC N13.8
　vesicoureteral reflux-associated — see Reflux, vesicoureteral
Urosepsis — code to condition
Urticaria L50.9
　with angioneurotic edema T78.3- ☑
　　hereditary D84.1
　allergic L50.0
　cholinergic L50.5
　chronic L50.8
　cold, familial L50.2
　contact L50.6
　dermatographic L50.3
　due to
　　cold or heat L50.2
　　drugs L50.0
　　food L50.0
　　inhalants L50.0
　　plants L50.6
　　serum — see also Reaction, serum T80.69- ☑
　factitial L50.3
　familial cold M04.2
　giant T78.3- ☑
　　hereditary D84.1
　gigantea T78.3- ☑
　idiopathic L50.1
　larynx T78.3- ☑
　　hereditary D84.1
　neonatorum P83.88
　nonallergic L50.1
　papulosa (Hebra) L28.2
　pigmentosa D47.01
　　congenital Q82.2
　　of neonatal onset Q82.2
　　of newborn onset Q82.2
　recurrent periodic L50.8
　serum — see also Reaction, serum T80.69- ☑
　solar L56.3
　specified type NEC L50.8
　thermal (cold) (heat) L50.2
　vibratory L50.4
　xanthelasmoidea — see Urticaria pigmentosa
Use (of)
　alcohol — see also Alcohol, alcoholic, by disorder F10.90
　　with
　　　anxiety disorder F10.980
　　　intoxication F10.929
　　　sleep disorder F10.982
　　　withdrawal F10.939
　　　　with
　　　　　perceptual disturbance F10.932
　　　　　delirium F10.931
　　　　uncomplicated F10.930
　　harmful — see Abuse, alcohol
　　in remission F10.91
　amphetamines — see Use, stimulant NEC
　caffeine — see Use, stimulant NEC
　cannabis F12.90
　　with
　　　anxiety disorder F12.980
　　　intoxication F12.929
　　　　with
　　　　　delirium F12.921
　　　　　perceptual disturbance F12.922
　　　　uncomplicated F12.920
　　　other specified disorder F12.988
　　　psychosis F12.959
　　　　delusions F12.950
　　　　hallucinations F12.951
　　　unspecified disorder F12.99
　　　withdrawal F12.93
　　in remission F12.91

Use — continued
　cocaine F14.90
　　with
　　　anxiety disorder F14.980
　　　intoxication F14.929
　　　　with
　　　　　delirium F14.921
　　　　　perceptual disturbance F14.922
　　　　uncomplicated F14.920
　　　other specified disorder F14.988
　　　psychosis F14.959
　　　　delusions F14.950
　　　　hallucinations F14.951
　　　sexual dysfunction F14.981
　　　sleep disorder F14.982
　　　unspecified disorder F14.99
　　　withdrawal F14.93
　　harmful — see Abuse, drug, cocaine
　　in remission F14.91
　drug(s) NEC F19.90
　　with sleep disorder F19.982
　　harmful — see Abuse, drug, by type
　hallucinogen NEC F16.90
　　with
　　　anxiety disorder F16.980
　　　intoxication F16.929
　　　　with
　　　　　delirium F16.921
　　　　uncomplicated F16.920
　　　mood disorder F16.94
　　　other specified disorder F16.988
　　　perception disorder (flashbacks) F16.983
　　　psychosis F16.959
　　　　delusions F16.950
　　　　hallucinations F16.951
　　　unspecified disorder F16.99
　　harmful — see Abuse, drug, hallucinogen NEC
　　in remission F16.91
　inhalants F18.90
　　with
　　　anxiety disorder F18.980
　　　intoxication F18.929
　　　　with delirium F18.921
　　　　uncomplicated F18.920
　　　mood disorder F18.94
　　　other specified disorder F18.988
　　　persisting dementia F18.97
　　　psychosis F18.959
　　　　delusions F18.950
　　　　hallucinations F18.951
　　　unspecified disorder F18.99
　　harmful — see Abuse, drug, inhalant
　　in remission F18.91
　methadone — see Use, opioid
　nonprescribed drugs F19.90
　　harmful — see Abuse, non-psychoactive substance
　opioid F11.90
　　with
　　　disorder F11.99
　　　　mood F11.94
　　　　sleep F11.982
　　　　specified type NEC F11.988
　　　intoxication F11.929
　　　　with
　　　　　delirium F11.921
　　　　　perceptual disturbance F11.922
　　　　uncomplicated F11.920
　　　opioid-associated amnestic syndrome F11.988
　　　withdrawal F11.93
　　harmful — see Abuse, drug, opioid
　　in remission F11.91
　patent medicines F19.90
　　harmful — see Abuse, non-psychoactive substance
　psychoactive drug NEC F19.90
　　with
　　　anxiety disorder F19.980
　　　intoxication F19.929
　　　　with
　　　　　delirium F19.921
　　　　　perceptual disturbance F19.922
　　　　uncomplicated F19.920
　　　mood disorder F19.94
　　　other specified disorder F19.988
　　　persisting
　　　　amnestic disorder F19.96
　　　　dementia F19.97
　　　psychosis F19.959
　　　　delusions F19.950
　　　　hallucinations F19.951

Use — continued
  psychoactive drug — continued
    with — continued
      sexual dysfunction F19.981
      sleep disorder F19.982
      unspecified disorder F19.99
      withdrawal F19.939
        with
          delirium F19.931
          perceptual disturbance F19.932
        uncomplicated F19.930
      harmful — see Abuse, drug NEC, psychoactive NEC
    in remission F19.91
  sedative, hypnotic, or anxiolytic F13.90
    with
      anxiety disorder F13.980
      intoxication F13.929
        with
          delirium F13.921
        uncomplicated F13.920
      other specified disorder F13.988
      persisting
        amnestic disorder F13.96
        dementia F13.97
      psychosis F13.959
        delusions F13.950
        hallucinations F13.951
      sexual dysfunction F13.981
      sleep disorder F13.982
      unspecified disorder F13.99
    harmful — see Abuse, drug, sedative, hypnotic, or anxiolytic
    in remission F13.91
  stimulant NEC F15.90
    with
      anxiety disorder F15.980
      intoxication F15.929
        with
          delirium F15.921
          perceptual disturbance F15.922
        uncomplicated F15.920
      mood disorder F15.94
      other specified disorder F15.988
      psychosis F15.959
        delusions F15.950
        hallucinations F15.951
      sexual dysfunction F15.981
      sleep disorder F15.982
      unspecified disorder F15.99
      withdrawal F15.93
    harmful — see Abuse, drug, stimulant NEC
    in remission F15.91
  tobacco Z72.0
    with dependence — see Dependence, drug, nicotine
  volatile solvents — see also Use, inhalant F18.90
    harmful — see Abuse, drug, inhalant
Usher-Senear disease or syndrome L10.4
Uta B55.1
Uteromegaly N85.2
Uterovaginal — see condition
Uterovesical — see condition
Uveal — see condition
Uveitis (anterior) — see also Iridocyclitis
  acute — see Iridocyclitis, acute
  chronic — see Iridocyclitis, chronic
  due to toxoplasmosis (acquired) B58.09
    congenital P37.1
  granulomatous — see Iridocyclitis, chronic
  heterochromic — see Cyclitis, Fuchs' heterochromic
  lens-induced — see Iridocyclitis, lens-induced
  posterior — see Chorioretinitis
  sympathetic H44.13- ☑
  syphilitic (secondary) A51.43
    congenital (early) A50.01
    late A52.71
  tuberculous A18.54
Uveoencephalitis — see Inflammation, chorioretinal
Uveokeratitis — see Iridocyclitis
Uveoparotitis D86.89
Uvula — see condition
Uvulitis (acute) (catarrhal) (chronic) (membranous) (suppurative) (ulcerative) K12.2

V

Vaccination (prophylactic)
  complication or reaction — see Complications, vaccination

Vaccination — continued
  delayed Z28.9
  encounter for Z23
  not done — see Immunization, not done
  partial — see also Underimmunization status
    for COVID-19 Z28.311
Vaccinia (generalized) (localized) T88.1- ☑
  congenital P35.8
  without vaccination B08.011
Vacuum, in sinus (accessory) (nasal) J34.89
Vagabond, vagabondage Z59.00
Vagabond's disease B85.1
Vagina, vaginal — see condition
Vaginalitis (tunica) (testis) N49.1
Vaginismus (reflex) N94.2
  functional F52.5
  nonorganic F52.5
  psychogenic F52.5
  secondary N94.2
Vaginitis (acute) (circumscribed) (diffuse) (emphysematous) (nonvenereal) (ulcerative) N76.0
  with ectopic or molar pregnancy O08.0
  amebic A06.82
  atrophic, postmenopausal N95.2
  bacterial N76.0
  blennorrhagic (gonococcal) A54.02
  candidal (acute) B37.31
    chronic (recurrent) B37.32
  chlamydial A56.02
  chronic N76.1
  due to Trichomonas (vaginalis) A59.01
  following ectopic or molar pregnancy O08.0
  gonococcal A54.02
    with abscess (accessory gland) (periurethral) A54.1
  granuloma A58
  in (due to)
    candidiasis (acute) B37.31
      chronic (recurrent) B37.32
    herpesviral (herpes simplex) infection A60.04
    pinworm infection B80 [N77.1]
  monilial (acute) B37.31
    chronic (recurrent) B37.32
  mycotic (candidal) (acute) B37.31
    chronic (recurrent) B37.32
  postmenopausal atrophic N95.2
  puerperal (postpartum) O86.13
  senile (atrophic) N95.2
  subacute or chronic N76.1
  syphilitic (early) A51.0
    late A52.76
  trichomonal A59.01
  tuberculous A18.18
Vaginosis — see Vaginitis
Vagotonia G52.2
Vagrancy Z59.00
VAIN — see Neoplasia, intraepithelial, vagina
Vallecula — see condition
Valley fever B38.0
Valsuani's disease O99.03
Valve, valvular (formation) — see also condition
  cerebral ventricle (communicating) in situ Z98.2
  cervix, internal os Q51.828
  congenital NEC — see Atresia, by site
  ureter (pelvic junction) (vesical orifice) Q62.39
  urethra (congenital) (posterior) Q64.2
Valvulitis (chronic) — see Endocarditis
Valvulopathy — see Endocarditis
Van Bogaert-Scherer-Epstein disease or syndrome E75.5
Van Bogaert's leukoencephalopathy (sclerosing) (subacute) A81.1
Van Buchem's syndrome M85.2
Van Creveld-von Gierke disease E74.01
Van der Hoeve (-de Kleyn) **syndrome** Q78.0
Van der Woude's syndrome Q38.0
Van Neck's disease or osteochondrosis M91.0
Vanishing lung J44.89
Vapor asphyxia or suffocation T59.9- ☑
  specified agent — see Table of Drugs and Chemicals
Variance, lethal ball, prosthetic heart valve T82.09- ☑
Variants, thalassemic D56.8
Variations in hair color L67.1
Varicella B01.9
  with
    complications NEC B01.89
    encephalitis B01.11
    encephalomyelitis B01.11
    meningitis B01.0
    myelitis B01.12
    pneumonia B01.2

Varicella — continued
  congenital P35.8
Varices — see Varix
Varicocele (scrotum) (thrombosed) I86.1
  ovary I86.2
  perineum I86.3
  spermatic cord (ulcerated) I86.1
Varicose
  aneurysm (ruptured) I77.0
  dermatitis — see Varix, leg, with, inflammation
  eczema — see Varix, leg, with, inflammation
  phlebitis — see Varix, with, inflammation
  tumor — see Varix
  ulcer (lower limb, any part) — see also Varix, leg, with, ulcer
    anus — see also Hemorrhoids K64.8
    esophagus — see Varix, esophagus
    inflamed or infected — see Varix, leg, with ulcer, with inflammation
    nasal septum I86.8
    perineum I86.3
    scrotum I86.1
    specified site NEC I86.8
  vein — see Varix
  vessel — see Varix, leg
Varicosis, varicosities, varicosity — see Varix
Variola (major) (minor) B03
Varioloid B03
Varix (lower limb) I83.90
  with
    bleeding I83.899
    edema I83.899
    inflammation I83.10
      with ulcer (venous) I83.209
    pain I83.819
    rupture I83.899
    specified complication NEC I83.899
    stasis dermatitis I83.10
      with ulcer (venous) I83.209
    swelling I83.899
    ulcer I83.009
      with inflammation I83.209
  aneurysmal I77.0
  asymptomatic I83.9- ☑
  bladder I86.2
  broad ligament I86.2
  complicating
    childbirth (lower extremity) O87.4
      anus or rectum O87.2
      genital (vagina, vulva or perineum) O87.8
    pregnancy (lower extremity) O22.0- ☑
      anus or rectum O22.4- ☑
      genital (vagina, vulva or perineum) O22.1- ☑
    puerperium (lower extremity) O87.4
      anus or rectum O87.2
      genital (vagina, vulva, perineum) O87.8
  congenital (any site) Q27.8
  esophagus (idiopathic) (primary) (ulcerated) I85.00
    bleeding I85.01
    congenital Q27.8
    in (due to)
      alcoholic liver disease I85.10
        bleeding I85.11
      cirrhosis of liver I85.10
        bleeding I85.11
      portal hypertension I85.10
        bleeding I85.11
      schistosomiasis I85.10
        bleeding I85.11
      toxic liver disease I85.10
        bleeding I85.11
    secondary I85.10
      bleeding I85.11
  gastric I86.4
  inflamed or infected I83.10
    ulcerated I83.209
  labia (majora) I86.3
  leg (asymptomatic) I83.9- ☑
    with
      edema I83.899
      inflammation I83.10
        with ulcer — see Varix, leg, with, ulcer, with inflammation by site
      pain I83.819
      specified complication NEC I83.899
      swelling I83.899
      ulcer I83.0- ☑
        with inflammation I83.2- ☑

Varix — *continued*
  leg — *continued*
    with — *continued*
      ulcer — *continued*
        ankle I83.003
          with inflammation I83.203
        calf I83.002
          with inflammation I83.202
        foot NEC I83.005
          with inflammation I83.205
        heel I83.004
          with inflammation I83.204
        lower leg NEC I83.008
          with inflammation I83.208
        midfoot I83.004
          with inflammation I83.204
        thigh I83.001
          with inflammation I83.201
  bilateral (asymptomatic) I83.93
    with
      edema I83.893
      pain I83.813
      specified complication NEC I83.893
      swelling I83.893
      ulcer I83.0- ☑
        with inflammation I83.209
  left (asymptomatic) I83.92
    with
      edema I83.892
      inflammation I83.12
        with ulcer — *see* Varix, leg, with, ulcer, with inflammation by site
      pain I83.812
      specified complication NEC I83.892
      swelling I83.892
      ulcer I83.029
        with inflammation I83.229
        ankle I83.023
          with inflammation I83.223
        calf I83.022
          with inflammation I83.222
        foot NEC I83.025
          with inflammation I83.225
        heel I83.024
          with inflammation I83.224
        lower leg NEC I83.028
          with inflammation I83.228
        midfoot I83.024
          with inflammation I83.224
        thigh I83.021
          with inflammation I83.221
  right (asymptomatic) I83.91
    with
      edema I83.891
      inflammation I83.11
        with ulcer — *see* Varix, leg, with, ulcer, with inflammation by site
      pain I83.811
      specified complication NEC I83.891
      swelling I83.891
      ulcer I83.019
        with inflammation I83.219
        ankle I83.013
          with inflammation I83.213
        calf I83.012
          with inflammation I83.212
        foot NEC I83.015
          with inflammation I83.215
        heel I83.014
          with inflammation I83.214
        lower leg NEC I83.018
          with inflammation I83.218
        midfoot I83.014
          with inflammation I83.214
        thigh I83.011
          with inflammation I83.211
  nasal septum I86.8
  orbit I86.8
    congenital Q27.8
  ovary I86.2
  papillary I78.1
  pelvis I86.2
  perineum I86.3
  pharynx I86.8
  placenta O43.89- ☑
  renal papilla I86.8
  retina H35.09
  scrotum (ulcerated) I86.1
  sigmoid colon I86.8

Varix — *continued*
  specified site NEC I86.8
  spinal (cord) (vessels) I86.8
  spleen, splenic (vein) (with phlebolith) I86.8
  stomach I86.4
  sublingual I86.0
  ulcerated I83.009
    inflamed or infected I83.209
  uterine ligament I86.2
  vagina I86.8
  vocal cord I86.8
  vulva I86.3
Vas deferens — *see* condition
Vas deferentitis N49.1
Vasa previa O69.4- ☑
  hemorrhage from, affecting newborn P50.0
Vascular — *see also* condition
  loop on optic papilla Q14.2
  spasm I73.9
  spider I78.1
Vascularization, cornea — *see* Neovascularization, cornea
Vasculitis I77.6
  allergic D69.0
  ANCA (antineutrophilic cytoplasmic antibody) associated I77.82
  ANCA (antineutrophilic cytoplasmic antibody) positive I77.82
  antineutrophilic cytoplasmic antibody [ANCA] I77.82
  cryoglobulinemic D89.1
  disseminated I77.6
  hypocomplementemic M31.8
  kidney I77.89
  leukocytoclastic M31.0
  livedoid L95.0
  nodular L95.8
  retina H35.06- ☑
  rheumatic — *see* Fever, rheumatic
  rheumatoid — *see* Rheumatoid, vasculitis
  skin (limited to) L95.9
    specified NEC L95.8
  systemic M31.8
Vasculopathy, necrotizing M31.9
  cardiac allograft T86.290
  specified NEC M31.8
Vasitis (nodosa) N49.1
  tuberculous A18.15
Vasodilation I73.9
Vasomotor — *see* condition
Vasoplasty, after previous sterilization Z31.0
  aftercare Z31.42
Vasospasm (vasoconstriction) — *see also* Angiospasm I73.9
  cerebral (cerebrovascular) (artery) I67.848
    reversible I67.841
  coronary I20.1
  nerve
    arm — *see* Mononeuropathy, upper limb
    brachial plexus G54.0
    cervical plexus G54.2
    leg — *see* Mononeuropathy, lower limb
  peripheral NOS I73.9
  retina (artery) — *see* Occlusion, artery, retina
Vasospastic — *see* condition
Vasovagal attack (paroxysmal) R55
  psychogenic F45.8
VATER syndrome Q87.2
Vater's ampulla — *see* condition
Vegetation, vegetative
  adenoid (nasal fossa) J35.8
  endocarditis (acute) (any valve) (subacute) I33.0
  heart (mycotic) (valve) I33.0
Veil
  Jackson's Q43.3
Vein, venous — *see* condition
Veldt sore — *see* Ulcer, skin
Velpeau's hernia — *see* Hernia, femoral
Venereal
  bubo A55
  disease A64
  granuloma inguinale A58
  lymphogranuloma (Durand-Nicolas-Favre) A55
Venofibrosis I87.8
Venom, venomous — *see* Table of Drugs and Chemicals, by animal or substance, poisoning
Venous — *see* condition
Ventilator lung, newborn P27.8
Ventral — *see* condition
Ventricle, ventricular — *see also* condition
  escape I49.3
  inversion Q20.5

Ventriculitis (cerebral) — *see also* Encephalitis G04.90
Ventriculostomy status Z98.2
Vernet's syndrome G52.7
Verneuil's disease (syphilitic bursitis) A52.78
Verruca (due to HPV) (filiformis) (simplex) (viral) (vulgaris) B07.9
  acuminata A63.0
  necrogenica (primary) (tuberculosa) A18.4
  plana B07.8
  plantaris B07.0
  seborrheica L82.1
    inflamed L82.0
  senile (seborrheic) L82.1
    inflamed L82.0
  tuberculosa (primary) A18.4
  venereal A63.0
Verrucosities — *see* Verruca
Verruga peruana, peruviana A44.1
Version
  cervix — *see* Malposition, uterus
  uterus (postinfectional) (postpartal, old) — *see* Malposition, uterus
Vertebra, vertebral — *see* condition
Vertical talus (congenital) Q66.80
  left foot Q66.82
  right foot Q66.81
Vertigo R42
  auditory — *see* Vertigo, aural
  aural H81.31- ☑
  benign paroxysmal (positional) H81.1- ☑
  central (origin) H81.4
  cerebral H81.4
  Dix and Hallpike (epidemic) — *see* Neuronitis, vestibular
  due to infrasound T75.23- ☑
  epidemic A88.1
    Dix and Hallpike — *see* Neuronitis, vestibular
    Pedersen's — *see* Neuronitis, vestibular
    vestibular neuronitis — *see* Neuronitis, vestibular
  hysterical F44.89
  infrasound T75.23- ☑
  labyrinthine — *see* subcategory H81.0- ☑
  laryngeal R05.4
  malignant positional H81.4
  Meniere's — *see* subcategory H81.0- ☑
  menopausal N95.1
  otogenic — *see* Vertigo, aural
  paroxysmal positional, benign — *see* Vertigo, benign paroxysmal
  Pedersen's (epidemic) — *see* Neuronitis, vestibular
  peripheral NEC H81.39- ☑
  positional
    benign paroxysmal — *see* Vertigo, benign paroxysmal
    malignant H81.4
Very-low-density-lipoprotein-type (VLDL) **hyperlipoproteinemia** E78.1
Vesania — *see* Psychosis
Vesical — *see* condition
Vesicle
  cutaneous R23.8
  seminal — *see* condition
  skin R23.8
Vesicocolic — *see* condition
Vesicoperineal — *see* condition
Vesicorectal — *see* condition
Vesicourethrorectal — *see* condition
Vesicovaginal — *see* condition
Vesicular — *see* condition
Vesiculitis (seminal) N49.0
  amebic A06.82
  gonorrheal (acute) (chronic) A54.23
  trichomonal A59.09
  tuberculous A18.15
Vestibulitis (ear) — *see also* subcategory H83.0- ☑
  nose (external) J34.89
  vulvar N94.810
Vestibulopathy, acute peripheral (recurrent) — *see* Neuronitis, vestibular
Vestige, vestigial — *see also* Persistence
  branchial Q18.0
  structures in vitreous Q14.0
Vibration
  adverse effects T75.20- ☑
    pneumatic hammer syndrome T75.21- ☑
    specified effect NEC T75.29- ☑
    vasospastic syndrome T75.22- ☑
    vertigo from infrasound T75.23- ☑
  exposure (occupational) Z57.7
  vertigo T75.23- ☑

Vibriosis A28.9
Victim (of)
  crime Z65.4
  disaster Z65.5
  terrorism Z65.4
  torture Z65.4
  war Z65.5
Vidal's disease L28.0
Villaret's syndrome G52.7
Villous — see condition
VIN — see Neoplasia, intraepithelial, vulva
Vincent's infection (angina) (gingivitis) A69.1
  stomatitis NEC A69.1
Vinson-Plummer syndrome D50.1
Violence, physical R45.6
Viosterol deficiency — see Deficiency, calciferol
Vipoma — see Neoplasm, malignant, by site
Viremia B34.9
Virilism (adrenal) E25.9
  congenital E25.0
Virilization (female) (suprarenal) E25.9
  congenital E25.0
  isosexual E28.2
Virulent bubo A57
Virus, viral — see also condition
  as cause of disease classified elsewhere B97.89
    respiratory syncytial virus (RSV) — see Virus, respiratory syncytial (RSV)
  cytomegalovirus B25.9
  human immunodeficiency (HIV) — see Human, immunodeficiency virus (HIV) disease
  infection — see Infection, virus
  respiratory syncytial (RSV)
    as cause of disease classified elsewhere B97.4
    bronchiolitis J21.0
    bronchitis J20.5
    bronchopneumonia J12.1
    otitis media H65.- ☑ [B97.4]
    pneumonia J12.1
    upper respiratory infection J06.9 [B97.4]
  specified NEC B34.8
  swine influenza (viruses that normally cause infections in pigs) — see also Influenza, due to, identified novel influenza A virus J09.X2
  West Nile (fever) A92.30
    with
      complications NEC A92.39
      cranial nerve disorders A92.32
      encephalitis A92.31
      encephalomyelitis A92.31
      neurologic manifestation NEC A92.32
      optic neuritis A92.32
      polyradiculitis A92.32
Viscera, visceral — see condition
Visceroptosis K63.4
Visible peristalsis R19.2
Vision, visual
  binocular, suppression H53.34
  blurred, blurring H53.8
    hysterical F44.6
  defect, defective NEC H54.7
  disorientation (syndrome) H53.8
  disturbance H53.9
    hysterical F44.6
  double H53.2
  examination Z01.00
    with abnormal findings Z01.01
    following failed vision screening Z01.020
      with abnormal findings Z01.021
  field, limitation (defect) — see Defect, visual field
  hallucinations R44.1
  halos H53.19
  loss — see Loss, vision
    sudden — see Disturbance, vision, subjective, loss, sudden
  low (both eyes) — see Low, vision
  perception, simultaneous without fusion H53.33
Vitality, lack or want of R53.83
  newborn P96.89
Vitamin deficiency — see Deficiency, vitamin
Vitelline duct, persistent Q43.0
Vitiligo L80
  eyelid H02.739
    left H02.736
      lower H02.735
      upper H02.734
    right H02.733
      lower H02.732
      upper H02.731

Vitiligo — continued
  pinta A67.2
  vulva N90.89
Vitreal corneal syndrome H59.01- ☑
Vitreoretinopathy, proliferative — see also Retinopathy, proliferative
  with retinal detachment — see Detachment, retina, traction
Vitreous — see also condition
  touch syndrome — see Complication, postprocedural, following cataract surgery
Vocal cord — see condition
Vogt-Koyanagi syndrome H20.82- ☑
Vogt-Spielmeyer amaurotic idiocy or disease E75.4
Vogt's disease or syndrome G80.3
Voice
  change R49.9
    specified NEC R49.8
  loss — see Aphonia
Volhynian fever A79.0
Volkmann's ischemic contracture or paralysis (complicating trauma) T79.6- ☑
Volvulus (bowel) (colon) (intestine) K56.2
  with perforation K56.2
  congenital Q43.8
  duodenum K31.5
  fallopian tube — see Torsion, fallopian tube
  oviduct — see Torsion, fallopian tube
  stomach (due to absence of gastrocolic ligament) K31.89
Vomiting R11.10
  with nausea R11.2
  asphyxia — see Foreign body, by site, causing asphyxia, gastric contents
  bilious (cause unknown) R11.14
    following gastro-intestinal surgery K91.0
    in newborn P92.01
  blood — see Hematemesis
  causing asphyxia, choking, or suffocation — see Foreign body, by site
  cyclical, in migraine G43.A0 (following G43.7)
    with refractory migraine G43.A1 (following G43.7)
    intractable G43.A1 (following G43.7)
    not intractable G43.A0 (following G43.7)
    psychogenic F50.89
    without refractory migraine G43.A0 (following G43.7)
  cyclical syndrome NOS (unrelated to migraine) R11.15
  fecal matter R11.13
  following gastrointestinal surgery K91.0
    psychogenic F50.89
  functional K31.89
  hysterical F50.89
  nervous F50.89
  neurotic F50.89
  newborn NEC P92.09
    bilious P92.01
  periodic R11.10
    psychogenic F50.89
  persistent R11.15
  projectile R11.12
  psychogenic F50.89
  uremic — see Uremia
  without nausea R11.11
Vomito negro — see Fever, yellow
Von Bezold's abscess — see Mastoiditis, acute
Von Economo-Cruchet disease A85.8
Von Eulenburg's disease G71.19
Von Gierke's disease E74.01
Von Hippel (-Lindau) **disease or syndrome** Q85.83
Von Jaksch's anemia or disease D64.89
Von Recklinghausen
  disease (neurofibromatosis) Q85.01
  bones E21.0
Von Schroetter's syndrome I82.890
Von Willebrand (-Jurgens) (-Minot) **disease or syndrome** — see Disease, von Willebrand
Von Zumbusch's disease L40.1
Voyeurism F65.3
Vrolik's disease Q78.0
Vulva — see condition
Vulvismus N94.2
Vulvitis (acute) (allergic) (atrophic) (hypertrophic) (intertriginous) (senile) N76.2
  with ectopic or molar pregnancy O08.0
  adhesive, congenital Q52.79
  blennorrhagic (gonococcal) A54.02
  candidal (acute) B37.31
    chronic (recurrent) B37.32
  chlamydial A56.02
  due to Haemophilus ducreyi A57

Vulvitis — continued
  following ectopic or molar pregnancy O08.0
  gonococcal A54.02
    with abscess (accessory gland) (periurethral) A54.1
  herpesviral A60.04
  leukoplakic N90.4
  monilial (acute) B37.31
    chronic (recurrent) B37.32
  puerperal (postpartum) O86.19
  subacute or chronic N76.3
  syphilitic (early) A51.0
    late A52.76
  trichomonal A59.01
  tuberculous A18.18
Vulvodynia N94.819
  specified NEC N94.818
Vulvorectal — see condition
Vulvovaginitis (acute) — see Vaginitis

W

Waiting list, person on Z75.1
  for organ transplant Z76.82
  undergoing social agency investigation Z75.2
Waldenstrom
  hypergammaglobulinemia D89.0
  syndrome or macroglobulinemia C88.0- ☑
Waldenstrom-Kjellberg syndrome D50.1
Walking
  difficulty R26.2
    psychogenic F44.4
  sleep F51.3
    hysterical F44.89
Wall, abdominal — see condition
Wallenberg's disease or syndrome G46.3
Wallgren's disease I87.8
Wandering
  gallbladder, congenital Q44.1
  in diseases classified elsewhere Z91.83
  kidney, congenital Q63.8
  organ or site, congenital NEC — see Malposition, congenital, by site
  pacemaker (heart) I49.8
  spleen D73.89
War neurosis F48.8
Wart (due to HPV) (filiform) (infectious) (viral) B07.9
  anogenital region (venereal) A63.0
  common B07.8
  external genital organs (venereal) A63.0
  flat B07.8
  Hassal-Henle's (of cornea) H18.49
  Peruvian A44.1
  plantar B07.0
  prosector (tuberculous) A18.4
  seborrheic L82.1
    inflamed L82.0
  senile (seborrheic) L82.1
    inflamed L82.0
  tuberculous A18.4
  venereal A63.0
Warthin's tumor — see Neoplasm, salivary gland or duct, benign
Wassilieff's disease A27.0
Wasting
  disease (syndrome) E88.A
    due to
      malnutrition E43
        with marasmus E41
      underlying condition E88.A
  extreme (due to malnutrition) E43
    with marasmus E41
  muscle NEC — see Atrophy, muscle
Water
  clefts (senile cataract) — see Cataract, senile, incipient
  deprivation of T73.1- ☑
  intoxication E87.79
  itch B76.9
  lack of T73.1- ☑
  safe drinking Z58.6
  loading E87.70
  on
    brain — see Hydrocephalus
    chest J94.8
  poisoning E87.79
Water-losing nephritis N25.89
Waterbrash R12
Waterhouse (-Friderichsen) **syndrome or disease** (meningococcal) A39.1

Watermelon stomach K31.819
- with hemorrhage K31.811
- without hemorrhage K31.819

Watsoniasis B66.8

Wax in ear — *see* Impaction, cerumen

Weak, weakening, weakness (generalized) R53.1
- arches (acquired) — *see also* Deformity, limb, flat foot
- bladder (sphincter) R32
- facial R29.810
  - following
    - cerebrovascular disease I69.992
      - cerebral infarction I69.392
      - intracerebral hemorrhage I69.192
      - nontraumatic intracranial hemorrhage NEC I69.292
      - specified disease NEC I69.892
      - stroke I69.392
      - subarachnoid hemorrhage I69.092
- foot (double) — *see also* Weak, arches
- heart, cardiac — *see* Failure, heart
- mind F70
- muscle M62.81
- myocardium — *see* Failure, heart
- newborn P96.89
- pelvic fundus N81.89
- pubocervical tissue N81.82
- rectovaginal tissue N81.83
- senile R54
- urinary stream R39.12
- valvular — *see* Endocarditis

Wear, worn (with normal or routine use)
- articular bearing surface of internal joint prosthesis — *see* Complications, joint prosthesis, mechanical, wear of articular bearing surfaces, by site
- device, implant or graft — *see* Complications, by site, mechanical complication
- tooth, teeth (approximal) (hard tissues) (interproximal) (occlusal) K03.0

Weather, weathered
- effects of
  - cold T69.9- ☑
    - specified effect NEC T69.8- ☑
  - hot — *see* Heat
- skin L57.8

Weaver's syndrome Q87.3

Web, webbed (congenital)
- duodenal Q43.8
- esophagus Q39.4
- fingers Q70.1- ☑
- larynx (glottic) (subglottic) Q31.0
- neck (pterygium colli) Q18.3
- Paterson-Kelly D50.1
- popliteal syndrome Q87.89
- toes Q70.3- ☑

Weber-Christian disease M35.6
Weber-Cockayne syndrome (epidermolysis bullosa) Q81.8
Weber-Gubler syndrome G46.3
Weber-Leyden syndrome G46.3
Weber-Osler syndrome I78.0
Weber's paralysis or syndrome G46.3
Wedge-shaped or wedging vertebra — *see* Collapse, vertebra NEC
Wegener's granulomatosis or syndrome M31.30
- with
  - kidney involvement M31.31
  - lung involvement M31.30
    - with kidney involvement M31.31

Wegner's disease A50.02

Weight
- 1000-2499 grams at birth (low) — *see* Low, birthweight
- 999 grams or less at birth (extremely low) — *see* Low, birthweight, extreme
- and length below 10th percentile for gestational age P05.1- ☑
- below but length above 10th percentile for gestational age P05.0- ☑
- gain (abnormal) (excessive) R63.5
  - in pregnancy — *see* Pregnancy, complicated by, excessive weight gain
  - low — *see* Pregnancy, complicated by, insufficient, weight gain
- loss (abnormal) (cause unknown) R63.4

Weightlessness (effect of) T75.82- ☑
Weil (I)**-Marchesani syndrome** Q87.19
Weil's disease A27.0
Weingarten's syndrome J82.89
Weir Mitchell's disease I73.81
Weiss-Baker syndrome G90.09

Wells' disease L98.3
Wen — *see* Cyst, sebaceous
Wenckebach's block or phenomenon I44.1
Werdnig-Hoffmann syndrome (muscular atrophy) G12.0
Werlhof's disease D69.3
Wermer's disease or syndrome E31.21
Werner-His disease A79.0
Werner's disease or syndrome E34.8
Wernicke-Korsakoff's syndrome or psychosis (alcoholic) F10.96
- with dependence F10.26
- drug-induced
  - due to drug abuse — *see* Abuse, drug, by type, with amnestic disorder
  - due to drug dependence — *see* Dependence, drug, by type, with amnestic disorder
- nonalcoholic F04

Wernicke-Posadas disease B38.9

Wernicke's
- developmental aphasia F80.2
- disease or syndrome E51.2
- encephalopathy E51.2
- polioencephalitis, superior E51.2

West African fever B50.8
Westphal-Strumpell syndrome E83.01
West's syndrome — *see* Epilepsy, spasms
Wet
- feet, tropical (maceration) (syndrome) — *see* Immersion, foot
- lung (syndrome), newborn P22.1

Wharton's duct — *see* condition
Wheal — *see* Urticaria
Wheezing R06.2
Whiplash injury S13.4- ☑
Whipple's disease — *see also* subcategory M14.8- K90.81
Whipworm (disease) (infection) (infestation) B79
Whistling face Q87.0
White — *see also* condition
- kidney, small N03.9
- leg, puerperal, postpartum, childbirth O87.1
- mouth B37.0
- patches of mouth K13.29
- spot lesions, teeth
  - chewing surface K02.51
  - pit and fissure surface K02.51
  - smooth surface K02.61

Whitehead L70.0
Whitlow — *see also* Cellulitis, digit
- with lymphangitis — *see* Lymphangitis, acute, digit
- herpesviral B00.89

Whitmore's disease or fever — *see* Melioidosis
Whooping cough A37.90
- with pneumonia A37.91
  - due to Bordetella
    - bronchiseptica A37.81
    - parapertussis A37.11
    - pertussis A37.01
  - specified organism NEC A37.81
- due to
  - Bordetella
    - bronchiseptica A37.80
      - with pneumonia A37.81
    - parapertussis A37.10
      - with pneumonia A37.11
    - pertussis A37.00
      - with pneumonia A37.01
  - specified NEC A37.80
    - with pneumonia A37.81

Wichman's asthma J38.5
Wide cranial sutures, newborn P96.3
Widening aorta — *see* Ectasia, aorta
- with aneurysm — *see* Aneurysm, aorta

Wilkie's disease or syndrome K55.1
Wilkinson-Sneddon disease or syndrome L13.1
Willebrand (-Jurgens) **thrombopathy** — *see* Disease, von Willebrand
Williams syndrome Q93.82
Willige-Hunt disease or syndrome G23.1
Wilms' tumor C64.- ☑
Wilson-Mikity syndrome P27.0
Wilson's
- disease or syndrome E83.01
- hepatolenticular degeneration E83.01
- lichen ruber L43.7

Window — *see also* Imperfect, closure
- aorticopulmonary Q21.4

Winter — *see* condition
Wiskott-Aldrich syndrome D82.0

Withdrawal state — *see also* Dependence, drug by type, with withdrawal
- alcohol
  - with perceptual disturbances F10.232
    - due to alcohol abuse F10.132
    - due to alcohol use F10.932
  - abuse — *see* Abuse, alcohol, with, withdrawal
  - dependence — *see* Dependence, alcohol, with, withdrawal
  - use — *see* Use, alcohol, with, withdrawal
  - without perceptual disturbances F10.239
    - due to alcohol abuse F10.139
    - due to alcohol use F10.939
- caffeine F15.93
- cannabis F12.23
- newborn
  - correct therapeutic substance properly administered P96.2
  - infant of dependent mother P96.1
- therapeutic substance, neonatal P96.2

Witts' anemia D50.8
Witzelsucht F07.0
Woakes' ethmoiditis or syndrome J33.1
Wolff-Hirschhorn syndrome Q93.3
Wolff-Parkinson-White syndrome I45.6
Wolhynian fever A79.0
Wolman's disease E75.5
Wood lung or pneumonitis J67.8
Woolly, wooly hair (congenital) (nevus) Q84.1
Woolsorter's disease A22.1
Word
- blindness (congenital) (developmental) F81.0
- deafness (congenital) (developmental) H93.25

Worm(s) (infection) (infestation) — *see also* Infestation, helminth
- guinea B72
- in intestine NEC B82.0

Worm-eaten soles A66.3
Worn out — *see* Exhaustion
- cardiac
  - defibrillator (with synchronous cardiac pacemaker) Z45.02
  - pacemaker
    - battery Z45.010
    - lead Z45.018
- device, implant or graft — *see* Complications, by site, mechanical

Worried well Z71.1
Worries R45.82
Wound check Z48.0- ☑
- due to injury — *code to* Injury, by site, using appropriate seventh character for subsequent encounter
- postoperative — *see* Aftercare

Wound, open T14.8- ☑
- abdomen, abdominal
  - wall S31.109- ☑
    - with penetration into peritoneal cavity S31.609- ☑
    - bite — *see* Bite, abdomen, wall
    - epigastric region S31.102- ☑
      - with penetration into peritoneal cavity S31.602- ☑
      - bite — *see* Bite, abdomen, wall, epigastric region
      - laceration — *see* Laceration, abdomen, wall, epigastric region
      - puncture — *see* Puncture, abdomen, wall, epigastric region
    - laceration — *see* Laceration, abdomen, wall
    - left
      - lower quadrant S31.104- ☑
        - with penetration into peritoneal cavity S31.604- ☑
        - bite — *see* Bite, abdomen, wall, left, lower quadrant
        - laceration — *see* Laceration, abdomen, wall, left, lower quadrant
        - puncture — *see* Puncture, abdomen, wall, left, lower quadrant
      - upper quadrant S31.101- ☑
        - with penetration into peritoneal cavity S31.601- ☑
        - bite — *see* Bite, abdomen, wall, left, upper quadrant
        - laceration — *see* Laceration, abdomen, wall, left, upper quadrant
        - puncture — *see* Puncture, abdomen, wall, left, upper quadrant
    - periumbilic region S31.105- ☑

Wound, open — continued
    abdomen, abdominal — continued
        wall — continued
            periumbilic region — continued
                with penetration into peritoneal cavity S31.605- ☑
                bite — see Bite, abdomen, wall, periumbilic region
                laceration — see Laceration, abdomen, wall, periumbilic region
                puncture — see Puncture, abdomen, wall, periumbilic region
            puncture — see Puncture, abdomen, wall
            right
                lower quadrant S31.103- ☑
                    with penetration into peritoneal cavity S31.603- ☑
                    bite — see Bite, abdomen, wall, right, lower quadrant
                    laceration — see Laceration, abdomen, wall, right, lower quadrant
                    puncture — see Puncture, abdomen, wall, right, lower quadrant
                upper quadrant S31.100- ☑
                    with penetration into peritoneal cavity S31.600- ☑
                    bite — see Bite, abdomen, wall, right, upper quadrant
                    laceration — see Laceration, abdomen, wall, right, upper quadrant
                    puncture — see Puncture, abdomen, wall, right, upper quadrant
    alveolar (process) — see Wound, open, oral cavity
    ankle S91.00- ☑
        bite — see Bite, ankle
        laceration — see Laceration, ankle
        puncture — see Puncture, ankle
    antecubital space — see Wound, open, elbow
    anterior chamber, eye — see Wound, open, ocular
    anus S31.839- ☑
        bite S31.835- ☑
        laceration — see Laceration, anus
        puncture — see Puncture, anus
    arm (upper) S41.10- ☑
        with amputation — see Amputation, traumatic, arm
        bite — see Bite, arm
        forearm — see Wound, open, forearm
        laceration — see Laceration, arm
        puncture — see Puncture, arm
    auditory canal (external) (meatus) — see Wound, open, ear
    auricle, ear — see Wound, open, ear
    axilla — see Wound, open, arm
    back — see also Wound, open, thorax, back
        lower S31.000- ☑
            with penetration into retroperitoneal space S31.001- ☑
            bite — see Bite, back, lower
            laceration — see Laceration, back, lower
            puncture — see Puncture, back, lower
    bite — see Bite
    blood vessel — see Injury, blood vessel
    breast S21.00- ☑
        with amputation — see Amputation, traumatic, breast
        bite — see Bite, breast
        laceration — see Laceration, breast
        puncture — see Puncture, breast
    buttock S31.809- ☑
        bite — see Bite, buttock
        laceration — see Laceration, buttock
        left S31.829- ☑
        puncture — see Puncture, buttock
        right S31.819- ☑
    calf — see Wound, open, leg
    canaliculus lacrimalis — see Wound, open, eyelid
    canthus, eye — see Wound, open, eyelid
    cervical esophagus S11.20- ☑
        bite S11.25- ☑
        laceration — see Laceration, esophagus, traumatic, cervical
        puncture — see Puncture, cervical esophagus
    cheek (external) S01.40- ☑
        bite — see Bite, cheek
        internal — see Wound, open, oral cavity
        laceration — see Laceration, cheek
        puncture — see Puncture, cheek
    chest wall — see Wound, open, thorax
    chin — see Wound, open, head, specified site NEC

Wound, open — continued
    choroid — see Wound, open, ocular
    ciliary body (eye) — see Wound, open, ocular
    clitoris S31.40- ☑
        with amputation — see Amputation, traumatic, clitoris
        bite S31.45- ☑
        laceration — see Laceration, vulva
        puncture — see Puncture, vulva
    conjunctiva — see Wound, open, ocular
    cornea — see Wound, open, ocular
    costal region — see Wound, open, thorax
    Descemet's membrane — see Wound, open, ocular
    digit(s)
        foot — see Wound, open, toe
        hand — see Wound, open, finger
    ear (canal) (external) S01.30- ☑
        with amputation — see Amputation, traumatic, ear
        bite — see Bite, ear
        drum S09.2- ☑
        laceration — see Laceration, ear
        puncture — see Puncture, ear
    elbow S51.00- ☑
        bite — see Bite, elbow
        laceration — see Laceration, elbow
        puncture — see Puncture, elbow
    epididymis — see Wound, open, testis
    epigastric region S31.102- ☑
        with penetration into peritoneal cavity S31.602- ☑
        bite — see Bite, abdomen, wall, epigastric region
        laceration — see Laceration, abdomen, wall, epigastric region
        puncture — see Puncture, abdomen, wall, epigastric region
    epiglottis — see Wound, open, neck, specified site NEC
    esophagus (thoracic) S27.819- ☑
        cervical — see Wound, open, cervical esophagus
        laceration S27.813- ☑
        specified type NEC S27.818- ☑
    eye — see Wound, open, ocular
    eyeball — see Wound, open, ocular
    eyebrow — see Wound, open, eyelid
    eyelid S01.10- ☑
        bite — see Bite, eyelid
        laceration — see Laceration, eyelid
        puncture — see Puncture, eyelid
    face NEC — see Wound, open, head, specified site NEC
    finger(s) S61.209- ☑
        with
            amputation — see Amputation, traumatic, finger
            damage to nail S61.309- ☑
        bite — see Bite, finger
        index S61.208- ☑
            with
                damage to nail S61.308- ☑
            left S61.201- ☑
                with
                    damage to nail S61.301- ☑
            right S61.200- ☑
                with
                    damage to nail S61.300- ☑
        laceration — see Laceration, finger
        little S61.208- ☑
            with
                damage to nail S61.308- ☑
            left S61.207- ☑
                with damage to nail S61.307- ☑
            right S61.206- ☑
                with damage to nail S61.306- ☑
        middle S61.208- ☑
            with
                damage to nail S61.308- ☑
            left S61.203- ☑
                with damage to nail S61.303- ☑
            right S61.202- ☑
                with damage to nail S61.302- ☑
        puncture — see Puncture, finger
        ring S61.208- ☑
            with
                damage to nail S61.308- ☑
            left S61.205- ☑
                with damage to nail S61.305- ☑
            right S61.204- ☑
                with damage to nail S61.304- ☑
    flank S31.10A- ☑
        with penetration into peritoneal cavity S31.60A- ☑
        left S31.107- ☑
            with penetration into peritoneal cavity S31.607

Wound, open — continued
    flank — continued
        right S31.106- ☑
            with penetration into peritoneal cavity S31.606- ☑
    foot (except toe(s) alone) S91.30- ☑
        with amputation — see Amputation, traumatic, foot
        bite — see Bite, foot
        laceration — see Laceration, foot
        puncture — see Puncture, foot
        toe — see Wound, open, toe
    forearm S51.80- ☑
        with
            amputation — see Amputation, traumatic, forearm
        bite — see Bite, forearm
        elbow only — see Wound, open, elbow
        laceration — see Laceration, forearm
        puncture — see Puncture, forearm
    forehead — see Wound, open, head, specified site NEC
    genital organs, external
        with amputation — see Amputation, traumatic, genital organs
        bite — see Bite, genital organ
        female S31.502- ☑
            vagina S31.40- ☑
            vulva S31.40- ☑
        laceration — see Laceration, genital organ
        male S31.501- ☑
            penis S31.20- ☑
            scrotum S31.30- ☑
            testes S31.30- ☑
        puncture — see Puncture, genital organ
    globe (eye) — see Wound, open, ocular
    groin — see Wound, open, abdomen, wall
    gum — see Wound, open, oral cavity
    hand S61.40- ☑
        with
            amputation — see Amputation, traumatic, hand
        bite — see Bite, hand
        finger(s) — see Wound, open, finger
        laceration — see Laceration, hand
        puncture — see Puncture, hand
        thumb — see Wound, open, thumb
    head S01.90- ☑
        bite — see Bite, head
        cheek — see Wound, open, cheek
        ear — see Wound, open, ear
        eyelid — see Wound, open, eyelid
        laceration — see Laceration, head
        lip — see Wound, open, lip
        nose S01.20- ☑
        oral cavity — see Wound, open, oral cavity
        puncture — see Puncture, head
        scalp — see Wound, open, scalp
        specified site NEC S01.80- ☑
        temporomandibular area — see Wound, open, cheek
    heel — see Wound, open, foot
    hip S71.00- ☑
        with amputation — see Amputation, traumatic, hip
        bite — see Bite, hip
        laceration — see Laceration, hip
        puncture — see Puncture, hip
    hymen S31.40- ☑
        bite — see Bite, vulva
        laceration — see Laceration, vagina
        puncture — see Puncture, vagina
    hypochondrium S31.109- ☑
        bite — see Bite, hypochondrium
        laceration — see Laceration, hypochondrium
        puncture — see Puncture, hypochondrium
    hypogastric region S31.109- ☑
        bite — see Bite, hypogastric region
        laceration — see Laceration, hypogastric region
        puncture — see Puncture, hypogastric region
    iliac (region) — see Wound, open, inguinal region
    inguinal region S31.109- ☑
        bite — see Bite, abdomen, wall, lower quadrant
        laceration — see Laceration, inguinal region
        puncture — see Puncture, inguinal region
    instep — see Wound, open, foot
    interscapular region — see Wound, open, thorax, back
    intraocular — see Wound, open, ocular
    iris — see Wound, open, ocular
    jaw — see Wound, open, head, specified site NEC
    knee S81.00- ☑
        bite — see Bite, knee
        laceration — see Laceration, knee
        puncture — see Puncture, knee
    labium (majus) (minus) — see Wound, open, vulva

☑ Additional Character Required — Refer to the Tabular List for Character Selection

Wound, open — continued
    laceration — see Laceration, by site
    lacrimal duct — see Wound, open, eyelid
    larynx S11.019- ☑
        bite — see Bite, larynx
        laceration — see Laceration, larynx
        puncture — see Puncture, larynx
    left
        lower quadrant S31.104- ☑
            with penetration into peritoneal cavity S31.604- ☑
            bite — see Bite, abdomen, wall, left, lower quadrant
            laceration — see Laceration, abdomen, wall, left, lower quadrant
            puncture — see Puncture, abdomen, wall, left, lower quadrant
        upper quadrant S31.101- ☑
            with penetration into peritoneal cavity S31.601- ☑
            bite — see Bite, abdomen, wall, left, upper quadrant
            laceration — see Laceration, abdomen, wall, left, upper quadrant
            puncture — see Puncture, abdomen, wall, left, upper quadrant
    leg (lower) S81.80- ☑
        with amputation — see Amputation, traumatic, leg
        ankle — see Wound, open, ankle
        bite — see Bite, leg
        foot — see Wound, open, foot
        knee — see Wound, open, knee
        laceration — see Laceration, leg
        puncture — see Puncture, leg
        toe — see Wound, open, toe
        upper — see Wound, open, thigh
    lip S01.501- ☑
        bite — see Bite, lip
        laceration — see Laceration, lip
        puncture — see Puncture, lip
    loin S31.109- ☑
        bite — see Bite, abdomen, wall
        laceration — see Laceration, loin
        puncture — see Puncture, loin
    lower back — see Wound, open, back, lower
    lumbar region — see Wound, open, back, lower
    malar region — see Wound, open, head, specified site NEC
    mammary — see Wound, open, breast
    mastoid region — see Wound, open, head, specified site NEC
    mouth — see Wound, open, oral cavity
    nail
        finger — see Wound, open, finger, with damage to nail
        toe — see Wound, open, toe, with damage to nail
    nape (neck) — see Wound, open, neck
    nasal (septum) (sinus) — see Wound, open, nose
    nasopharynx — see Wound, open, head, specified site NEC
    neck S11.90- ☑
        bite — see Bite, neck
        involving
            cervical esophagus S11.20- ☑
            larynx — see Wound, open, larynx
            pharynx S11.20- ☑
            thyroid S11.10- ☑
            trachea (cervical) S11.029- ☑
                bite — see Bite, trachea
                laceration S11.021- ☑
                    with foreign body S11.022- ☑
                puncture S11.023- ☑
                    with foreign body S11.024- ☑
        laceration — see Laceration, neck
        puncture — see Puncture, neck
        specified site NEC S11.80- ☑
        specified type NEC S11.89- ☑
    nose (septum) (sinus) S01.20- ☑
        with amputation — see Amputation, traumatic, nose
        bite — see Bite, nose
        laceration — see Laceration, nose
        puncture — see Puncture, nose
    ocular S05.90- ☑
        avulsion (traumatic enucleation) S05.7- ☑
        eyeball S05.6- ☑
            with foreign body S05.5- ☑
        eyelid — see Wound, open, eyelid
        laceration and rupture S05.3- ☑
            with prolapse or loss of intraocular tissue S05.2- ☑

Wound, open — continued
    ocular — continued
        orbit (penetrating) (with or without foreign body) S05.4- ☑
        periocular area — see Wound, open, eyelid
        specified NEC S05.8X- ☑
    oral cavity S01.502- ☑
        bite S01.552- ☑
        laceration — see Laceration, oral cavity
        puncture — see Puncture, oral cavity
    orbit — see Wound, open, ocular, orbit
    palate — see Wound, open, oral cavity
    palm — see Wound, open, hand
    pelvis, pelvic — see also Wound, open, back, lower
        girdle — see Wound, open, hip
    penetrating — see Puncture, by site
    penis S31.20- ☑
        with amputation — see Amputation, traumatic, penis
        bite S31.25- ☑
        laceration — see Laceration, penis
        puncture — see Puncture, penis
    perineum
        bite — see Bite, perineum
        female S31.502- ☑
        laceration — see Laceration, perineum
        male S31.501- ☑
        puncture — see Puncture, perineum
    periocular area (with or without lacrimal passages) — see Wound, open, eyelid
    periumbilic region S31.105- ☑
        with penetration into peritoneal cavity S31.605- ☑
        bite — see Bite, abdomen, wall, periumbilic region
        laceration — see Laceration, abdomen, wall, periumbilic region
        puncture — see Puncture, abdomen, wall, periumbilic region
    phalanges
        finger — see Wound, open, finger
        toe — see Wound, open, toe
    pharynx S11.20- ☑
    pinna — see Wound, open, ear
    popliteal space — see Wound, open, knee
    prepuce — see Wound, open, penis
    pubic region — see Wound, open, back, lower
    pudendum — see Wound, open, genital organs, external
    puncture wound — see Puncture
    rectovaginal septum — see Wound, open, vagina
    right
        lower quadrant S31.103- ☑
            with penetration into peritoneal cavity S31.603- ☑
            bite — see Bite, abdomen, wall, right, lower quadrant
            laceration — see Laceration, abdomen, wall, right, lower quadrant
            puncture — see Puncture, abdomen, wall, right, lower quadrant
        upper quadrant S31.100- ☑
            with penetration into peritoneal cavity S31.600- ☑
            bite — see Bite, abdomen, wall, right, upper quadrant
            laceration — see Laceration, abdomen, wall, right, upper quadrant
            puncture — see Puncture, abdomen, wall, right, upper quadrant
    sacral region — see Wound, open, back, lower
    sacroiliac region — see Wound, open, back, lower
    salivary gland — see Wound, open, oral cavity
    scalp S01.00- ☑
        bite S01.05- ☑
        laceration — see Laceration, scalp
        puncture — see Puncture, scalp
    scalpel, newborn (birth injury) P15.8
    scapular region — see Wound, open, shoulder
    sclera — see Wound, open, ocular
    scrotum S31.30- ☑
        with amputation — see Amputation, traumatic, scrotum
        bite S31.35- ☑
        laceration — see Laceration, scrotum
        puncture — see Puncture, scrotum
    shin — see Wound, open, leg
    shoulder S41.00- ☑
        with amputation — see Amputation, traumatic, arm
        bite — see Bite, shoulder
        laceration — see Laceration, shoulder
        puncture — see Puncture, shoulder
    skin NOS T14.8- ☑
    spermatic cord — see Wound, open, testis

Wound, open — continued
    sternal region — see Wound, open, thorax, front wall
    submaxillary region — see Wound, open, head, specified site NEC
    submental region — see Wound, open, head, specified site NEC
    subungual
        finger(s) — see Wound, open, finger
        toe(s) — see Wound, open, toe
    supraclavicular region — see Wound, open, neck, specified site NEC
    temple, temporal region — see Wound, open, head, specified site NEC
    temporomandibular area — see Wound, open, cheek
    testis S31.30- ☑
        with amputation — see Amputation, traumatic, testes
        bite S31.35- ☑
        laceration — see Laceration, testis
        puncture — see Puncture, testis
    thigh S71.10- ☑
        with amputation — see Amputation, traumatic, hip
        bite — see Bite, thigh
        laceration — see Laceration, thigh
        puncture — see Puncture, thigh
    thorax, thoracic (wall) S21.90- ☑
        back S21.20- ☑
            with penetration S21.40- ☑
        bite — see Bite, thorax
        breast — see Wound, open, breast
        front S21.10- ☑
            with penetration S21.30- ☑
        laceration — see Laceration, thorax
        puncture — see Puncture, thorax
    throat — see Wound, open, neck
    thumb S61.009- ☑
        with
            amputation — see Amputation, traumatic, thumb
            damage to nail S61.109- ☑
        bite — see Bite, thumb
        laceration — see Laceration, thumb
        left S61.002- ☑
            with
                damage to nail S61.102- ☑
        puncture — see Puncture, thumb
        right S61.001- ☑
            with
                damage to nail S61.101- ☑
    thyroid (gland) — see Wound, open, neck, thyroid
    toe(s) S91.109- ☑
        with
            amputation — see Amputation, traumatic, toe
            damage to nail S91.209- ☑
        bite — see Bite, toe
        great S91.103- ☑
            with
                damage to nail S91.203- ☑
            left S91.102- ☑
                with
                    damage to nail S91.202- ☑
            right S91.101- ☑
                with
                    damage to nail S91.201- ☑
        laceration — see Laceration, toe
        lesser S91.106- ☑
            with
                damage to nail S91.206- ☑
            left S91.105- ☑
                with
                    damage to nail S91.205- ☑
            right S91.104- ☑
                with
                    damage to nail S91.204- ☑
        puncture — see Puncture, toe
    tongue — see Wound, open, oral cavity
    trachea (cervical region) — see Wound, open, neck, trachea
    tunica vaginalis — see Wound, open, testis
    tympanum, tympanic membrane S09.2- ☑
        laceration — see Laceration, ear, drum
        puncture — see Puncture, tympanum
    umbilical region — see Wound, open, abdomen, wall, periumbilic region
    uvula — see Wound, open, oral cavity
    vagina S31.40- ☑
        bite S31.45- ☑
        laceration — see Laceration, vagina
        puncture — see Puncture, vagina

☑ Additional Character Required — Refer to the Tabular List for Character Selection

Wound, open — *continued*
  vitreous (humor) — *see* Wound, open, ocular
  vocal cord S11.039- ☑
    bite — *see* Bite, vocal cord
    laceration S11.031- ☑
      with foreign body S11.032- ☑
    puncture S11.033- ☑
      with foreign body S11.034- ☑
  vulva S31.40- ☑
    with amputation — *see* Amputation, traumatic, vulva
    bite S31.45- ☑
    laceration — *see* Laceration, vulva
    puncture — *see* Puncture, vulva
  wrist S61.50- ☑
    bite — *see* Bite, wrist
    laceration — *see* Laceration, wrist
    puncture — *see* Puncture, wrist
Wound, superficial — *see* Injury — *see also* specified injury type
Wright's syndrome G54.0
Wrist — *see* condition
Wrong drug (by accident) (given in error) — *see* Table of Drugs and Chemicals, by drug, poisoning
Wry neck — *see* Torticollis
Wuchereria (bancrofti) **infestation** B74.0
Wuchereriasis B74.0
Wuchernde Struma Langhans C73

X

X-ray (of)
  abnormal findings — *see* Abnormal, diagnostic imaging
  breast (mammogram) (routine) Z12.31
  chest
    routine (as part of a general medical examination) Z00.00
      with abnormal findings Z00.01
  routine (as part of a general medical examination) Z00.00
    with abnormal findings Z00.01
Xanthelasma (eyelid) (palpebrarum) H02.60
  left H02.66
    lower H02.65
    upper H02.64
  right H02.63
    lower H02.62
    upper H02.61
Xanthelasmatosis (essential) E78.2
Xanthinuria, hereditary E79.82
Xanthoastrocytoma
  specified site — *see* Neoplasm, malignant, by site
  unspecified site C71.9
Xanthofibroma — *see* Neoplasm, connective tissue, benign
Xanthogranuloma D76.3
Xanthoma(s), xanthomatosis (primary) (familial) (hereditary) E78.2
  with
    hyperlipoproteinemia
      Type I E78.3
      Type III E78.2
      Type IV E78.1
      Type V E78.3
  bone (generalisata) C96.5

Xanthoma(s), xanthomatosis — *continued*
  cerebrotendinous E75.5
  cutaneotendinous E75.5
  disseminatum (skin) E78.2
  eruptive E78.2
  hypercholesterinemic E78.00
  hypercholesterolemic E78.00
  hyperlipidemic E78.5
  joint E75.5
  multiple (skin) E78.2
  tendon (sheath) E75.5
  tuberosum E78.2
  tuberous E78.2
  tubo-eruptive E78.2
  verrucous, oral mucosa K13.4
Xanthosis R23.8
Xenophobia F40.10
Xeroderma — *see also* Ichthyosis
  acquired L85.0
    eyelid H01.149
      left H01.146
        lower H01.145
        upper H01.144
      right H01.143
        lower H01.142
        upper H01.141
  pigmentosum Q82.1
  vitamin A deficiency E50.8
Xerophthalmia (vitamin A deficiency) E50.7
  unrelated to vitamin A deficiency — *see* Keratoconjunctivitis
Xerosis
  conjunctiva H11.14- ☑
    with Bitot's spots — *see also* Pigmentation, conjunctiva
      vitamin A deficiency E50.1
    vitamin A deficiency E50.0
  cornea H18.89- ☑
    with ulceration — *see* Ulcer, cornea
    vitamin A deficiency E50.3
    vitamin A deficiency E50.2
  cutis (dry skin) L85.3
  skin L85.3
Xerostomia K11.7
Xiphopagus Q89.4
XO syndrome Q96.9
XXXXY syndrome Q98.1
XXY syndrome Q98.0

Y

Yaba pox (virus disease) B08.72
Yatapoxvirus B08.70
  specified NEC B08.79
Yawning R06.89
  psychogenic F45.8
Yaws A66.9
  bone lesions A66.6
  butter A66.1
  chancre A66.0
  cutaneous, less than five years after infection A66.2

Yaws — *continued*
  early (cutaneous) (macular) (maculopapular) (micropapular) (papular) A66.2
    frambeside A66.2
    skin lesions NEC A66.2
  eyelid A66.2
  ganglion A66.6
  gangosis, gangosa A66.5
  gumma, gummata A66.4
    bone A66.6
  gummatous
    frambeside A66.4
    osteitis A66.6
    periostitis A66.6
  hydrarthrosis — *see also* subcategory M14.8- A66.6
  hyperkeratosis (early) (late) A66.3
  initial lesions A66.0
  joint lesions — *see also* subcategory M14.8- A66.6
  juxta-articular nodules A66.7
  late nodular (ulcerated) A66.4
  latent (without clinical manifestations) (with positive serology) A66.8
  mother A66.0
  mucosal A66.7
  multiple papillomata A66.1
  nodular, late (ulcerated) A66.4
  osteitis A66.6
  papilloma, plantar or palmar A66.1
  periostitis (hypertrophic) A66.6
  specified NEC A66.7
  ulcers A66.4
  wet crab A66.1
Yeast infection — *see also* Candidiasis B37.9
Yellow
  atrophy (liver) — *see* Failure, hepatic
  fever — *see* Fever, yellow
  jack — *see* Fever, yellow
  jaundice — *see* Jaundice
  nail syndrome L60.5
Yersiniosis — *see also* Infection, Yersinia
  extraintestinal A28.2
  intestinal A04.6

Z

Zahorsky's syndrome (herpangina) B08.5
Zellweger's syndrome E71.510
Zenker's diverticulum (esophagus) K22.5
Ziehen-Oppenheim disease G24.1
Zieve's syndrome K70.0
Zika NOS A92.5
  congenital P35.4
Zinc
  deficiency, dietary E60
  metabolism disorder E83.2
Zollinger-Ellison syndrome E16.4
Zona — *see* Herpes, zoster
Zoophobia F40.218
Zoster (herpes) — *see* Herpes, zoster
Zygomycosis B46.9
  specified NEC B46.8
Zymotic — *see* condition

Note: The list below gives the code number for neoplasms by anatomical site. For each site there are six possible code numbers according to whether the neoplasm in question is malignant, benign, in situ, of uncertain behavior, or of unspecified nature. The description of the neoplasm will often indicate which of the six columns is appropriate; e.g., malignant melanoma of skin, benign fibroadenoma of breast, carcinoma in situ of cervix uteri. Where such descriptors are not present, the remainder of the Index should be consulted where guidance is given to the appropriate column for each morphological (histological) variety listed; e.g., Mesonephroma – see Neoplasm, malignant; Embryoma — see also Neoplasm, uncertain behavior; Disease, Bowen's – see Neoplasm, skin, in situ. However, the guidance in the Index can be overridden if one of the descriptors mentioned above is present; e.g., malignant adenoma of colon is coded to C18.9 and not to D12.6 as the adjective "malignant" overrides the Index entry "Adenoma — see also Neoplasm, benign, by site." Codes listed with a dash -, following the code have a required additional character for laterality. The tabular list must be reviewed for the complete code.

	Malignant Primary	Malignant Secondary	Ca in situ	Benign	Uncertain Behavior	Unspecified Behavior
Neoplasm, neoplastic	C80.1	C79.9	D09.9	D36.9	D48.9	D49.9
abdomen, abdominal	C76.2	C79.8-☑	D09.8	D36.7	D48.7	D49.89
cavity	C76.2	C79.8-☑	D09.8	D36.7	D48.7	D49.89
organ	C76.2	C79.8-☑	D09.8	D36.7	D48.7	D49.89
viscera	C76.2	C79.8-☑	D09.8	D36.7	D48.7	D49.89
wall — see also Neoplasm, abdomen, wall, skin	C44.509	C79.2	D04.5	D23.5	D48.5	D49.2
connective tissue	C49.4	C79.8-☑	—	D21.4	D48.1-☑	D49.2
skin	C44.509	—	—	—	—	—
basal cell carcinoma	C44.519	—	—	—	—	—
specified type NEC	C44.599	—	—	—	—	—
squamous cell carcinoma	C44.529	—	—	—	—	—
abdominopelvic	C76.8	C79.8-☑	—	D36.7	D48.7	D49.89
accessory sinus — see Neoplasm, sinus						
acoustic nerve	C72.4-☑	C79.49	—	D33.3	D43.3	D49.7
adenoid (pharynx) (tissue)	C11.1	C79.89	D00.08	D10.6	D37.05	D49.0
adipose tissue — see also Neoplasm, connective tissue	C49.4	C79.89	—	D21.9	D48.1-☑	D49.2
adnexa (uterine)	C57.4	C79.89	D07.39	D28.7	D39.8	D49.59
adrenal	C74.9-☑	C79.7-☑	D09.3	D35.0-☑	D44.1-☑	D49.7
capsule	C74.9-☑	C79.7-☑	D09.3	D35.0-☑	D44.1-☑	D49.7
cortex	C74.0-☑	C79.7-☑	D09.3	D35.0-☑	D44.1-☑	D49.7
gland	C74.9-☑	C79.7-☑	D09.3	D35.0-☑	D44.1-☑	D49.7
medulla	C74.1-☑	C79.7-☑	D09.3	D35.0-☑	D44.1-☑	D49.7
ala nasi (external) — see also Neoplasm, skin, nose	C44.301	C79.2	D04.39	D23.39	D48.5	D49.2
alimentary canal or tract NEC	C26.9	C78.80	D01.9	D13.99	D37.9	D49.0
alveolar	C03.9	C79.89	D00.03	D10.39	D37.09	D49.0
mucosa	C03.9	C79.89	D00.03	D10.39	D37.09	D49.0
lower	C03.1	C79.89	D00.03	D10.39	D37.09	D49.0
upper	C03.0	C79.89	D00.03	D10.39	D37.09	D49.0
ridge or process	C41.1	C79.51	—	D16.5	D48.0	D49.2
carcinoma	C03.9	C79.8-☑	—	—	—	—
lower	C03.1	C79.8-☑	—	—	—	—
upper	C03.0	C79.8-☑	—	—	—	—
lower	C41.1	C79.51	—	D16.5	D48.0	D49.2
mucosa	C03.9	C79.89	D00.03	D10.39	D37.09	D49.0
lower	C03.1	C79.89	D00.03	D10.39	D37.09	D49.0
upper	C03.0	C79.89	D00.03	D10.39	D37.09	D49.0
upper	C41.0	C79.51	—	D16.4	D48.0	D49.2
sulcus	C06.1	C79.89	D00.02	D10.39	D37.09	D49.0
alveolus	C03.9	C79.89	D00.03	D10.39	D37.09	D49.0
lower	C03.1	C79.89	D00.03	D10.39	D37.09	D49.0
upper	C03.0	C79.89	D00.03	D10.39	D37.09	D49.0
ampulla of Vater	C24.1	C78.89	D01.5	D13.5	D37.6	D49.0
ankle NEC	C76.5-☑	C79.89	D04.7-☑	D36.7	D48.7	D49.89
anorectum, anorectal (junction)	C21.8	C78.5	D01.3	D12.9	D37.8	D49.0
antecubital fossa or space	C76.4-☑	C79.89	D04.6-☑	D36.7	D48.7	D49.89

	Malignant Primary	Malignant Secondary	Ca in situ	Benign	Uncertain Behavior	Unspecified Behavior
Neoplasm, neoplastic — continued						
antrum (Highmore) (maxillary)	C31.0	C78.39	D02.3	D14.0	D38.5	D49.1
pyloric	C16.3	C78.89	D00.2	D13.1	D37.1	D49.0
tympanicum	C30.1	C78.39	D02.3	D14.0	D38.5	D49.1
anus, anal	C21.0	C78.5	D01.3	D12.9	D37.8	D49.0
canal	C21.1	C78.5	D01.3	D12.9	D37.8	D49.0
cloacogenic zone	C21.2	C78.5	D01.3	D12.9	D37.8	D49.0
margin — see also Neoplasm, anus, skin	C44.500	C79.2	D04.5	D23.5	D48.5	D49.2
overlapping lesion with rectosigmoid junction or rectum	C21.8	—	—	—	—	—
skin	C44.500	C79.2	D04.5	D23.5	D48.5	D49.2
basal cell carcinoma	C44.510	—	—	—	—	—
specified type NEC	C44.590	—	—	—	—	—
squamous cell carcinoma	C44.520	—	—	—	—	—
sphincter	C21.1	C78.5	D01.3	D12.9	D37.8	D49.0
aorta (thoracic)	C49.3	C79.89	—	D21.3	D48.1-☑	D49.2
abdominal	C49.4	C79.89	—	D21.4	D48.1-☑	D49.2
aortic body	C75.5	C79.89	—	D35.6	D44.7	D49.7
aponeurosis	C49.9	C79.89	—	D21.9	D48.1-☑	D49.2
palmar	C49.1-☑	C79.89	—	D21.1-☑	D48.1-☑	D49.2
plantar	C49.2-☑	C79.89	—	D21.2-☑	D48.1-☑	D49.2
appendix	C18.1	C78.5	D01.0	D12.1	D37.3	D49.0
arachnoid	C70.9	C79.49	—	D32.9	D42.9	D49.7
cerebral	C70.0	C79.32	—	D32.0	D42.0	D49.7
spinal	C70.1	C79.49	—	D32.1	D42.1	D49.7
areola	C50.0-☑	C79.81	D05.-☑	D24.-☑	D48.6-☑	D49.3
arm NEC	C76.4-☑	C79.89	D04.6-☑	D36.7	D48.7	D49.89
artery — see Neoplasm, connective tissue						
aryepiglottic fold	C13.1	C79.89	D00.08	D10.7	D37.05	D49.0
hypopharyngeal aspect	C13.1	C79.89	D00.08	D10.7	D37.05	D49.0
laryngeal aspect	C32.1	C78.39	D02.0	D14.1	D38.0	D49.1
marginal zone	C13.1	C79.89	D00.08	D10.7	D37.05	D49.0
arytenoid (cartilage)	C32.3	C78.39	D02.0	D14.1	D38.0	D49.1
fold — see Neoplasm, aryepiglottic						
associated with transplanted organ	C80.2	—	—	—	—	—
atlas	C41.2	C79.51	—	D16.6	D48.0	D49.2
atrium, cardiac	C38.0	C79.89	—	D15.1	D48.7	D49.89
auditory						
canal (external) (skin)	C44.20-☑	C79.2	D04.2-☑	D23.2-☑	D48.5	D49.2
internal	C30.1	C78.39	D02.3	D14.0	D38.5	D49.1
nerve	C72.4-☑	C79.49	—	D33.3	D43.3	D49.7
tube	C30.1	C78.39	D02.3	D14.0	D38.5	D49.1
opening	C11.2	C79.89	D00.08	D10.6	D37.05	D49.0
auricle, ear — see also Neoplasm, skin, ear	C44.20-☑	C79.2	D04.2-☑	D23.2-☑	D48.5	D49.2
auricular canal (external) — see also Neoplasm, skin, ear	C44.20-☑	C79.2	D04.2-☑	D23.2-☑	D48.5	D49.2
internal	C30.1	C78.39	D02.3	D14.0	D38.5	D49.2
autonomic nerve or nervous system NEC (see Neoplasm, nerve, peripheral)						
axilla, axillary	C76.1	C79.89	D09.8	D36.7	D48.7	D49.89
fold — see also Neoplasm, skin, trunk	C44.509	C79.2	D04.5	D23.5	D48.5	D49.2
back NEC	C76.8	C79.89	D04.5	D36.7	D48.5	D49.89
Bartholin's gland	C51.0	C79.82	D07.1	D28.0	D39.8	D49.59
basal ganglia	C71.0	C79.31	—	D33.0	D43.0	D49.6
basis pedunculi	C71.7	C79.31	—	D33.1	D43.1	D49.6
bile or biliary (tract)	C24.9	C78.89	D01.5	D13.5	D37.6	D49.0

☑ **Additional Character Required** — Refer to the Tabular List for Character Selection

Neoplasm, neoplastic	Malignant Primary	Malignant Secondary	Ca in situ	Benign	Uncertain Behavior	Unspecified Behavior
— continued						
bile or biliary — continued						
canaliculi (biliferi) (intrahepatic)	C22.1	C78.7	D01.5	D13.4	D37.6	D49.0
canals, interlobular	C22.1	C78.89	D01.5	D13.4	D37.6	D49.0
duct or passage (common) (cystic) (extrahepatic)	C24.0	C78.89	D01.5	D13.5	D37.6	D49.0
interlobular	C22.1	C78.89	D01.5	D13.4	D37.6	D49.0
intrahepatic and extrahepatic	C24.8	C78.89	D01.5	D13.5	D37.6	D49.0
bladder (urinary)	C67.9	C79.11	D09.0	D30.3	D41.4	D49.4
dome	C67.1	C79.11	D09.0	D30.3	D41.4	D49.4
neck	C67.5	C79.11	D09.0	D30.3	D41.4	D49.4
orifice	C67.9	C79.11	D09.0	D30.3	D41.4	D49.4
ureteric	C67.6	C79.11	D09.0	D30.3	D41.4	D49.4
urethral	C67.5	C79.11	D09.0	D30.3	D41.4	D49.4
overlapping lesion	C67.8	—	—	—	—	—
sphincter	C67.8	C79.11	D09.0	D30.3	D41.4	D49.4
trigone	C67.0	C79.11	D09.0	D30.3	D41.4	D49.4
urachus	C67.7	C79.11	D09.0	D30.3	D41.4	D49.4
wall	C67.9	C79.11	D09.0	D30.3	D41.4	D49.4
anterior	C67.3	C79.11	D09.0	D30.3	D41.4	D49.4
lateral	C67.2	C79.11	D09.0	D30.3	D41.4	D49.4
posterior	C67.4	C79.11	D09.0	D30.3	D41.4	D49.4
blood vessel — see Neoplasm, connective tissue						
bone (periosteum)	C41.9	C79.51	—	D16.9	D48.0	D49.2
acetabulum						
ankle	C40.3-☑	C79.51	—	D16.3-☑	—	—
arm NEC	C40.0-☑	C79.51	—	D16.0-☑	—	—
astragalus	C40.3-☑	C79.51	—	D16.3-☑	—	—
atlas	C41.2	C79.51	—	D16.6	D48.0	D49.2
axis	C41.2	C79.51	—	D16.6	D48.0	D49.2
back NEC	C41.2	C79.51	—	D16.6	D48.0	D49.2
calcaneus	C40.3-☑	C79.51	—	D16.3-☑	—	—
calvarium	C41.0	C79.51	—	D16.4	D48.0	D49.2
carpus (any)	C40.1-☑	C79.51	—	D16.1-☑	—	—
cartilage NEC	C41.9	C79.51	—	D16.9	D48.0	D49.2
clavicle	C41.3	C79.51	—	D16.7	D48.0	D49.2
clivus	C41.0	C79.51	—	D16.4	D48.0	D49.2
coccygeal vertebra	C41.4	C79.51	—	D16.8	D48.0	D49.2
coccyx	C41.4	C79.51	—	D16.8	D48.0	D49.2
costal cartilage	C41.3	C79.51	—	D16.7	D48.0	D49.2
costovertebral joint	C41.3	C79.51	—	D16.7	D48.0	D49.2
cranial	C41.0	C79.51	—	D16.4	D48.0	D49.2
cuboid	C40.3-☑	C79.51	—	D16.3-☑	—	—
cuneiform	C41.9	C79.51	—	D16.9	D48.0	D49.2
elbow	C40.0-☑	C79.51	—	D16.0-☑	—	—
ethmoid (labyrinth)	C41.0	C79.51	—	D16.4	D48.0	D49.2
face	C41.0	C79.51	—	D16.4	D48.0	D49.2
femur (any part)	C40.2-☑	C79.51	—	D16.2-☑	—	—
fibula (any part)	C40.2-☑	C79.51	—	D16.2-☑	—	—
finger (any)	C40.1-☑	C79.51	—	D16.1-☑	—	—
foot	C40.3-☑	C79.51	—	D16.3-☑	—	—
forearm	C40.0-☑	C79.51	—	D16.0-☑	—	—
frontal	C41.0	C79.51	—	D16.4	D48.0	D49.2
hand	C40.1-☑	C79.51	—	D16.1-☑	—	—
heel	C40.3-☑	C79.51	—	D16.3-☑	—	—
hip	C41.4	C79.51	—	D16.8	D48.0	D49.2
humerus (any part)	C40.0-☑	C79.51	—	D16.0-☑	—	—
hyoid	C41.0	C79.51	—	D16.4	D48.0	D49.2
ilium	C41.4	C79.51	—	D16.8	D48.0	D49.2
innominate	C41.4	C79.51	—	D16.8	D48.0	D49.2
intervertebral cartilage or disc	C41.2	C79.51	—	D16.6	D48.0	D49.2
ischium	C41.4	C79.51	—	D16.8	D48.0	D49.2
jaw (lower)	C41.1	C79.51	—	D16.5	D48.0	D49.2
knee	C40.2-☑	C79.51	—	D16.2-☑	—	—
leg NEC	C40.2-☑	C79.51	—	D16.2-☑	—	—
limb NEC	C40.9-☑	C79.51	—	D16.9	—	—
lower (long bones)	C40.2-☑	C79.51	—	D16.2-☑	—	—
short bones	C40.3-☑	C79.51	—	D16.3-☑	—	—
upper (long bones)	C40.0-☑	C79.51	—	D16.0-☑	—	—
short bones	C40.1-☑	C79.51	—	D16.1-☑	—	—
malar	C41.0	C79.51	—	D16.4	D48.0	D49.2
mandible	C41.1	C79.51	—	D16.5	D48.0	D49.2
marrow NEC (any bone)	C96.9	C79.52	—	—	D47.9	D49.89
mastoid	C41.0	C79.51	—	D16.4	D48.0	D49.2
maxilla, maxillary (superior)	C41.0	C79.51	—	D16.4	D48.0	D49.2
inferior	C41.1	C79.51	—	D16.5	D48.0	D49.2
metacarpus (any)	C40.1-☑	C79.51	—	D16.1-☑	—	—
metatarsus (any)	C40.3-☑	C79.51	—	D16.3-☑	—	—
navicular						
ankle	C40.3-☑	C79.51	—	—	—	—
hand	C40.1-☑	C79.51	—	—	—	—
nose, nasal	C41.0	C79.51	—	D16.4	D48.0	D49.2
occipital	C41.0	C79.51	—	D16.4	D48.0	D49.2
orbit	C41.0	C79.51	—	D16.4	D48.0	D49.2
overlapping sites	C40.8-☑	—	—	—	—	—
parietal	C41.0	C79.51	—	D16.4	D48.0	D49.2
patella	C40.2-☑	C79.51	—	—	—	—
pelvic	C41.4	C79.51	—	D16.8	D48.0	D49.2
phalanges						
foot	C40.3-☑	C79.51	—	—	—	—
hand	C40.1-☑	C79.51	—	—	—	—
pubic	C41.4	C79.51	—	D16.8	D48.0	D49.2
radius (any part)	C40.0-☑	C79.51	—	D16.0-☑	—	—
rib	C41.3	C79.51	—	D16.7	D48.0	D49.2
sacral vertebra	C41.4	C79.51	—	D16.8	D48.0	D49.2
sacrum	C41.4	C79.51	—	D16.8	D48.0	D49.2
scaphoid						
of ankle	C40.3-☑	C79.51	—	—	—	—
of hand	C40.1-☑	C79.51	—	—	—	—
scapula (any part)	C40.0-☑	C79.51	—	D16.0-☑	—	—
sella turcica	C41.0	C79.51	—	D16.4	D48.0	D49.2
shoulder	C40.0-☑	C79.51	—	D16.0-☑	—	—
skull	C41.0	C79.51	—	D16.4	D48.0	D49.2
sphenoid	C41.0	C79.51	—	D16.4	D48.0	D49.2
spine, spinal (column)	C41.2	C79.51	—	D16.6	D48.0	D49.2
coccyx	C41.4	C79.51	—	D16.8	D48.0	D49.2
sacrum	C41.4	C79.51	—	D16.8	D48.0	D49.2
sternum	C41.3	C79.51	—	D16.7	D48.0	D49.2
tarsus (any)	C40.3-☑	C79.51	—	—	—	—
temporal	C41.0	C79.51	—	D16.4	D48.0	D49.2
thumb	C40.1-☑	C79.51	—	—	—	—
tibia (any part)	C40.2-☑	C79.51	—	—	—	—
toe (any)	C40.3-☑	C79.51	—	—	—	—
trapezium	C40.1-☑	C79.51	—	—	—	—
trapezoid	C40.1-☑	C79.51	—	—	—	—
turbinate	C41.0	C79.51	—	D16.4	D48.0	D49.2
ulna (any part)	C40.0-☑	C79.51	—	D16.0-☑	—	—
unciform	C40.1-☑	C79.51	—	—	—	—
vertebra (column)	C41.2	C79.51	—	D16.6	D48.0	D49.2
coccyx	C41.4	C79.51	—	D16.8	D48.0	D49.2
sacrum	C41.4	C79.51	—	D16.8	D48.0	D49.2
vomer	C41.0	C79.51	—	D16.4	D48.0	D49.2
wrist	C40.1-☑	C79.51	—	—	—	—
xiphoid process	C41.3	C79.51	—	D16.7	D48.0	D49.2
zygomatic	C41.0	C79.51	—	D16.4	D48.0	D49.2
book-leaf (mouth) — ventral surface of tongue and floor of mouth	C06.89	C79.89	D00.00	D10.39	D37.09	D49.0
bowel — see Neoplasm, intestine						
brachial plexus	C47.1-☑	C79.89	—	D36.12	D48.2	D49.2
brain NEC	C71.9	C79.31	—	D33.2	D43.2	D49.6

☑ Additional Character Required — Refer to the Tabular List for Character Selection

Neoplasm, brain NEC

	Malignant Primary	Malignant Secondary	Ca in situ	Benign	Uncertain Behavior	Unspecified Behavior
Neoplasm, neoplastic — *continued*						
brain — *continued*						
basal ganglia	C71.0	C79.31	—	D33.0	D43.0	D49.6
cerebellopontine angle	C71.6	C79.31	—	D33.1	D43.1	D49.6
cerebellum NOS	C71.6	C79.31	—	D33.1	D43.1	D49.6
cerebrum	C71.0	C79.31	—	D33.0	D43.0	D49.6
choroid plexus	C71.7	C79.31	—	D33.1	D43.1	D49.6
corpus callosum	C71.8	C79.31	—	D33.2	D43.2	D49.6
corpus striatum	C71.0	C79.31	—	D33.0	D43.0	D49.6
cortex (cerebral)	C71.0	C79.31	—	D33.0	D43.0	D49.6
frontal lobe	C71.1	C79.31	—	D33.0	D43.0	D49.6
globus pallidus	C71.0	C79.31	—	D33.0	D43.0	D49.6
hippocampus	C71.2	C79.31	—	D33.0	D43.0	D49.6
hypothalamus	C71.0	C79.31	—	D33.0	D43.0	D49.6
internal capsule	C71.0	C79.31	—	D33.0	D43.0	D49.6
medulla oblongata	C71.7	C79.31	—	D33.1	D43.1	D49.6
meninges	C70.0	C79.32	—	D32.0	D42.0	D49.7
midbrain	C71.7	C79.31	—	D33.1	D43.1	D49.6
occipital lobe	C71.4	C79.31	—	D33.0	D43.0	D49.6
overlapping lesion	C71.8	C79.31	—	—	—	—
parietal lobe	C71.3	C79.31	—	D33.0	D43.0	D49.6
peduncle	C71.7	C79.31	—	D33.1	D43.1	D49.6
pons	C71.7	C79.31	—	D33.1	D43.1	D49.6
stem	C71.7	C79.31	—	D33.1	D43.1	D49.6
tapetum	C71.8	C79.31	—	D33.2	D43.2	D49.6
temporal lobe	C71.2	C79.31	—	D33.0	D43.0	D49.6
thalamus	C71.0	C79.31	—	D33.0	D43.0	D49.6
uncus	C71.2	C79.31	—	D33.0	D43.0	D49.6
ventricle (floor)	C71.5	C79.31	—	D33.0	D43.0	D49.6
fourth	C71.7	C79.31	—	D33.1	D43.1	D49.6
branchial (cleft) (cyst) (vestiges)	C10.4	C79.89	D00.08	D10.5	D37.05	D49.0
breast (connective tissue) (glandular tissue) (soft parts)	C50.9-☑	C79.81	D05.-☑	D24.-☑	D48.6-☑	D49.3
areola	C50.0-☑	C79.81	D05.-☑	D24.-☑	D48.6-☑	D49.3
axillary tail	C50.6-☑	C79.81	D05.-☑	D24.-☑	D48.6-☑	D49.3
central portion	C50.1-☑	C79.81	D05.-☑	D24.-☑	D48.6-☑	D49.3
inflammatory	C50.A-☑	—	—	—	—	—
inner	C50.8-☑	C79.81	D05.-☑	D24.-☑	D48.6-☑	D49.3
lower	C50.8-☑	C79.81	D05.-☑	D24.-☑	D48.6-☑	D49.3
lower-inner quadrant	C50.3-☑	C79.81	D05.-☑	D24.-☑	D48.6-☑	D49.3
lower-outer quadrant	C50.5-☑	C79.81	D05.-☑	D24.-☑	D48.6-☑	D49.3
mastectomy site (skin) — *see also* Neoplasm, breast, skin	C44.501	C79.2	—	—	—	—
specified as breast tissue	C50.8-☑	C79.81	—	—	—	—
midline	C50.8-☑	C79.81	D05.-☑	D24.-☑	D48.6-☑	D49.3
nipple	C50.0-☑	C79.81	D05.-☑	D24.-☑	D48.6-☑	D49.3
outer	C50.8-☑	C79.81	D05.-☑	D24.-☑	D48.6-☑	D49.3
overlapping lesion	C50.8-☑	—	—	—	—	—
skin	C44.501	C79.2	D04.5	D23.5	D48.5	D49.2
basal cell carcinoma	C44.511	—	—	—	—	—
specified type NEC	C44.591	—	—	—	—	—
squamous cell carcinoma	C44.521	—	—	—	—	—
tail (axillary)	C50.6-☑	C79.81	D05.-☑	D24.-☑	D48.6-☑	D49.3
upper	C50.8-☑	C79.81	D05.-☑	D24.-☑	D48.6-☑	D49.3
upper-inner quadrant	C50.2-☑	C79.81	D05.-☑	D24.-☑	D48.6-☑	D49.3
upper-outer quadrant	C50.4-☑	C79.81	D05.-☑	D24.-☑	D48.6-☑	D49.3
broad ligament	C57.1-☑	C79.82	D07.39	D28.2	D39.8	D49.59
bronchiogenic, bronchogenic (lung)	C34.9-☑	C78.0-☑	D02.2-☑	D14.3-☑	D38.1	D49.1
bronchiole	C34.9-☑	C78.0-☑	D02.2-☑	D14.3-☑	D38.1	D49.1
bronchus	C34.9-☑	C78.0-☑	D02.2-☑	D14.3-☑	D38.1	D49.1
carina	C34.0-☑	C78.0-☑	D02.2-☑	D14.3-☑	D38.1	D49.1

	Malignant Primary	Malignant Secondary	Ca in situ	Benign	Uncertain Behavior	Unspecified Behavior
Neoplasm, neoplastic — *continued*						
bronchus — *continued*						
lower lobe of lung	C34.3-☑	C78.0-☑	D02.2-☑	D14.3-☑	D38.1	D49.1
main	C34.0-☑	C78.0-☑	D02.2-☑	D14.3-☑	D38.1	D49.1
middle lobe of lung	C34.2	C78.0-☑	D02.21	D14.31	D38.1	D49.1
overlapping lesion	C34.8-☑	—	—	—	—	—
upper lobe of lung	C34.1-☑	C78.0-☑	D02.2-☑	D14.3-☑	D38.1	D49.1
brow	C44.309	C79.2	D04.39	D23.39	D48.5	D49.2
basal cell carcinoma	C44.319	—	—	—	—	—
specified type NEC	C44.399	—	—	—	—	—
squamous cell carcinoma	C44.329	—	—	—	—	—
buccal (cavity)	C06.9	C79.89	D00.00	D10.39	D37.09	D49.0
commissure	C06.0	C79.89	D00.02	D10.39	D37.09	D49.0
groove (lower) (upper)	C06.1	C79.89	D00.02	D10.39	D37.09	D49.0
mucosa	C06.0	C79.89	D00.02	D10.39	D37.09	D49.0
sulcus (lower) (upper)	C06.1	C79.89	D00.02	D10.39	D37.09	D49.0
bulbourethral gland	C68.0	C79.19	D09.19	D30.4	D41.3	D49.59
bursa — *see* Neoplasm, connective tissue						
buttock NEC	C76.3	C79.89	D04.5	D36.7	D48.7	D49.89
calf	C76.5-☑	C79.89	D04.7-☑	D36.7	D48.7	D49.89
calvarium	C41.0	C79.51	—	D16.4	D48.0	D49.2
calyx, renal	C65.-☑	C79.0-☑	D09.19	D30.1-☑	D41.1-☑	D49.51-☑
canal						
anal	C21.1	C78.5	D01.3	D12.9	D37.8	D49.0
auditory (external) — *see also* Neoplasm, skin, ear	C44.20-☑	C79.2	D04.2-☑	D23.2-☑	D48.5	D49.2
auricular (external) — *see also* Neoplasm, skin, ear	C44.20-☑	C79.2	D04.2-☑	D23.2-☑	D48.5	D49.2
canaliculi, biliary (biliferi) (intrahepatic)	C22.1	C78.7	D01.5	D13.4	D37.6	D49.0
canthus (eye) (inner) (outer)	C44.10-☑	C79.2	D04.1-☑	D23.1-☑	D48.5	D49.2
basal cell carcinoma	C44.11-☑	—	—	—	—	—
sebaceous cell	C44.13-☑	—	—	—	—	—
specified type NEC	C44.19-☑	—	—	—	—	—
squamous cell carcinoma	C44.12-☑	—	—	—	—	—
capillary — *see* Neoplasm, connective tissue						
caput coli	C18.0	C78.5	D01.0	D12.0	D37.4	D49.0
carcinoid — *see* Tumor, carcinoid						
cardia (gastric)	C16.0	C78.89	D00.2	D13.1	D37.1	D49.0
cardiac orifice (stomach)	C16.0	C78.89	D00.2	D13.1	D37.1	D49.0
cardio-esophageal junction	C16.0	C78.89	D00.2	D13.1	D37.1	D49.0
cardio-esophagus	C16.0	C78.89	D00.2	D13.1	D37.1	D49.0
carina (bronchus)	C34.0-☑	C78.0-☑	D02.2-☑	D14.3-☑	D38.1	D49.1
carotid (artery)	C49.0	C79.89	—	D21.0	D48.1-☑	D49.2
body	C75.4	C79.89	—	D35.5	D44.6	D49.7
carpus (any bone)	C40.1-☑	C79.51	—	D16.1-☑	—	—
cartilage (articular) (joint) NEC — *see also* Neoplasm, bone	C41.9	C79.51	—	D16.9	D48.0	D49.2
arytenoid	C32.3	C78.39	D02.0	D14.1	D38.0	D49.1
auricular	C49.0	C79.89	—	D21.0	D48.1-☑	D49.2
bronchi	C34.0-☑	C78.0-☑	—	D14.3-☑	D38.1	D49.1
costal	C41.3	C79.51	—	D16.7	D48.0	D49.2
cricoid	C32.3	C78.39	D02.0	D14.1	D38.0	D49.1
cuneiform	C32.3	C78.39	D02.0	D14.1	D38.0	D49.1
ear (external)	C49.0	C79.89	—	D21.0	D48.1-☑	D49.2

Neoplasm, connective tissue NEC

	Malignant Primary	Malignant Secondary	Ca in situ	Benign	Uncertain Behavior	Unspecified Behavior
Neoplasm, neoplastic — continued						
cartilage — see also Neoplasm, bone — continued						
ensiform	C41.3	C79.51	—	D16.7	D48.0	D49.2
epiglottis	C32.1	C78.39	D02.0	D14.1	D38.0	D49.1
anterior surface	C10.1	C79.89	D00.08	D10.5	D37.05	D49.0
eyelid	C49.0	C79.89	—	D21.0	D48.1-✓	D49.2
intervertebral	C41.2	C79.51	—	D16.6	D48.0	D49.2
larynx, laryngeal	C32.3	C78.39	D02.0	D14.1	D38.0	D49.1
nose, nasal	C30.0	C78.39	D02.3	D14.0	D38.5	D49.1
pinna	C49.0	C79.89	—	D21.0	D48.1-✓	D49.2
rib	C41.3	C79.51	—	D16.7	D48.0	D49.2
semilunar (knee)	C40.2-✓	C79.51	—	D16.2-✓	D48.0	D49.2
thyroid	C32.3	C78.39	D02.0	D14.1	D38.0	D49.1
trachea	C33	C78.39	D02.1	D14.2	D38.1	D49.1
cauda equina	C72.1	C79.49	—	D33.4	D43.4	D49.7
cavity						
buccal	C06.9	C79.89	D00.00	D10.30	D37.09	D49.0
nasal	C30.0	C78.39	D02.3	D14.0	D38.5	D49.1
oral	C06.9	C79.89	D00.00	D10.30	D37.09	D49.0
peritoneal	C48.2	C78.6	—	D20.1	D48.4	D49.0
tympanic	C30.1	C78.39	D02.3	D14.0	D38.5	D49.1
cecum	C18.0	C78.5	D01.0	D12.0	D37.4	D49.0
central nervous system	C72.9	C79.40	—	—	—	—
cerebellopontine (angle)	C71.6	C79.31	—	D33.1	D43.1	D49.6
cerebellum, cerebellar	C71.6	C79.31	—	D33.1	D43.1	D49.6
cerebrum, cerebral (cortex) (hemisphere) (white matter)	C71.0	C79.31	—	D33.0	D43.0	D49.6
meninges	C70.0	C79.32	—	D32.0	D42.0	D49.7
peduncle	C71.7	C79.31	—	D33.1	D43.1	D49.6
ventricle	C71.5	C79.31	—	D33.0	D43.0	D49.6
fourth	C71.7	C79.31	—	D33.1	D43.1	D49.6
cervical region	C76.0	C79.89	D09.8	D36.7	D48.7	D49.89
cervix (cervical) (uteri) (uterus)	C53.9	C79.82	D06.9	D26.0	D39.0	D49.59
canal	C53.0	C79.82	D06.0	D26.0	D39.0	D49.59
endocervix (canal) (gland)	C53.0	C79.82	D06.0	D26.0	D39.0	D49.59
exocervix	C53.1	C79.82	D06.1	D26.0	D39.0	D49.59
external os	C53.1	C79.82	D06.1	D26.0	D39.0	D49.59
internal os	C53.0	C79.82	D06.0	D26.0	D39.0	D49.59
nabothian gland	C53.0	C79.82	D06.0	D26.0	D39.0	D49.59
overlapping lesion	C53.8	—	—	—	—	—
squamocolumnar junction	C53.8	C79.82	D06.7	D26.0	D39.0	D49.59
stump	C53.8	C79.82	D06.7	D26.0	D39.0	D49.59
cheek	C76.0	C79.89	D09.8	D36.7	D48.7	D49.89
external	C44.309	C79.2	D04.39	D23.39	D48.5	D49.2
basal cell carcinoma	C44.319	—	—	—	—	—
specified type NEC	C44.399	—	—	—	—	—
squamous cell carcinoma	C44.329	—	—	—	—	—
inner aspect	C06.0	C79.89	D00.02	D10.39	D37.09	D49.0
internal	C06.0	C79.89	D00.02	D10.39	D37.09	D49.0
mucosa	C06.0	C79.89	D00.02	D10.39	D37.09	D49.0
chest (wall) NEC	C76.1	C79.89	D09.8	D36.7	D48.7	D49.89
chiasma opticum	C72.3-✓	C79.49	—	D33.3	D43.3	D49.7
chin	C44.309	C79.2	D04.39	D23.39	D48.5	D49.2
basal cell carcinoma	C44.319	—	—	—	—	—
specified type NEC	C44.399	—	—	—	—	—
squamous cell carcinoma	C44.329	—	—	—	—	—
choana	C11.3	C79.89	D00.08	D10.6	D37.05	D49.0
cholangiole	C22.1	C78.89	D01.5	D13.4	D37.6	D49.0
choledochal duct	C24.0	C78.89	D01.5	D13.5	D37.6	D49.0
choroid	C69.3-✓	C79.49	D09.2-✓	D31.3-✓	D48.7	D49.81
plexus	C71.5	C79.31	—	D33.0	D43.0	D49.6
ciliary body	C69.4-✓	C79.49	D09.2-✓	D31.4-✓	D48.7	D49.89
clavicle	C41.3	C79.51	—	D16.7	D48.0	D49.2
clitoris	C51.2	C79.82	D07.1	D28.0	D39.8	D49.59
clivus	C41.0	C79.51	—	D16.4	D48.0	D49.2
cloacogenic zone	C21.2	C78.5	D01.3	D12.9	D37.8	D49.0
coccygeal body or glomus	C49.5	C79.89	—	D21.5	D48.1-✓	D49.2
vertebra	C41.4	C79.51	—	D16.8	D48.0	D49.2
coccyx	C41.4	C79.51	—	D16.8	D48.0	D49.2
colon — see also Neoplasm, intestine, large	C18.9	C78.5	—	—	—	—
with rectum	C19	C78.5	D01.1	D12.7	D37.5	D49.0
column, spinal — see Neoplasm, spine						
columnella — see also Neoplasm, skin, face	C44.390	C79.2	D04.39	D23.39	D48.5	D49.2
commissure						
labial, lip	C00.6	C79.89	D00.01	D10.39	D37.01	D49.0
laryngeal	C32.0	C78.39	D02.0	D14.1	D38.0	D49.1
common (bile) duct	C24.0	C78.89	D01.5	D13.5	D37.6	D49.0
concha — see also Neoplasm, skin, ear	C44.20-✓	C79.2	D04.2-✓	D23.2-✓	D48.5	D49.2
nose	C30.0	C78.39	D02.3	D14.0	D38.5	D49.1
conjunctiva	C69.0-✓	C79.49	D09.2-✓	D31.0-✓	D48.7	D49.89
connective tissue NEC	C49.9	C79.89	—	D21.9	D48.1-✓	D49.2

Note: For neoplasms of connective tissue (blood vessel, bursa, fascia, ligament, muscle, peripheral nerves, sympathetic and parasympathetic nerves and ganglia, synovia, tendon, etc.) or of morphological types that indicate connective tissue, code according to the list under "Neoplasm, connective tissue". For sites that do not appear in this list, code to neoplasm of that site; e.g., fibrosarcoma, pancreas (C25.9)

Note: Morphological types that indicate connective tissue appear in their proper place in the alphabetic index with the instruction "see Neoplasm, connective tissue ...."

	Malignant Primary	Malignant Secondary	Ca in situ	Benign	Uncertain Behavior	Unspecified Behavior
abdomen	C49.4	C79.89	—	D21.4	D48.1-✓	D49.2
abdominal wall	C49.4	C79.89	—	D21.4	D48.1-✓	D49.2
ankle	C49.2-✓	C79.89	—	D21.2-✓	D48.1-✓	D49.2
antecubital fossa or space	C49.1-✓	C79.89	—	D21.1-✓	D48.1-✓	D49.2
arm	C49.1-✓	C79.89	—	D21.1-✓	D48.1-✓	D49.2
auricle (ear)	C49.0	C79.89	—	D21.0	D48.1-✓	D49.2
axilla	C49.3	C79.89	—	D21.3	D48.1-✓	D49.2
back	C49.6	C79.89	—	D21.6	D48.1-✓	D49.2
breast — see Neoplasm, breast						
buttock	C49.5	C79.89	—	D21.5	D48.1-✓	D49.2
calf	C49.2-✓	C79.89	—	D21.2-✓	D48.1-✓	D49.2
cervical region	C49.0	C79.89	—	D21.0	D48.1-✓	D49.2
cheek	C49.0	C79.89	—	D21.0	D48.1-✓	D49.2
chest (wall)	C49.3	C79.89	—	D21.3	D48.1-✓	D49.2
chin	C49.0	C79.89	—	D21.0	D48.1-✓	D49.2
diaphragm	C49.3	C79.89	—	D21.3	D48.1-✓	D49.2
ear (external)	C49.0	C79.89	—	D21.0	D48.1-✓	D49.2
elbow	C49.1-✓	C79.89	—	D21.1-✓	D48.1-✓	D49.2
extrarectal	C49.5	C79.89	—	D21.5	D48.1-✓	D49.2
extremity	C49.9	C79.89	—	D21.9	D48.1-✓	D49.2
lower	C49.2-✓	C79.89	—	D21.2-✓	D48.1-✓	D49.2
upper	C49.1-✓	C79.89	—	D21.1-✓	D48.1-✓	D49.2
eyelid	C49.0	C79.89	—	D21.0	D48.1-✓	D49.2
face	C49.0	C79.89	—	D21.0	D48.1-✓	D49.2
finger	C49.1-✓	C79.89	—	D21.1-✓	D48.1-✓	D49.2
flank	C49.6	C79.89	—	D21.6	D48.1-✓	D49.2
foot	C49.2-✓	C79.89	—	D21.2-✓	D48.1-✓	D49.2
forearm	C49.1-✓	C79.89	—	D21.1-✓	D48.1-✓	D49.2
forehead	C49.0	C79.89	—	D21.0	D48.1-✓	D49.2
gastric	C49.4	C79.89	—	D21.4	D48.1-✓	D49.2
gastrointestinal	C49.4	C79.89	—	D21.4	D48.1-✓	D49.2
gluteal region	C49.5	C79.89	—	D21.5	D48.1-✓	D49.2
great vessels NEC	C49.3	C79.89	—	D21.3	D48.1-✓	D49.2
groin	C49.5	C79.89	—	D21.5	D48.1-✓	D49.2

✓ Additional Character Required — Refer to the Tabular List for Character Selection

Neoplasm, connective tissue NEC

Neoplasm, neoplastic — continued	Malignant Primary	Malignant Secondary	Ca in situ	Benign	Uncertain Behavior	Unspecified Behavior
connective tissue — continued						
hand	C49.1-☑	C79.89	—	D21.1-☑	D48.1-☑	D49.2
head	C49.0	C79.89	—	D21.0	D48.1-☑	D49.2
heel	C49.2-☑	C79.89	—	D21.2-☑	D48.1-☑	D49.2
hip	C49.2-☑	C79.89	—	D21.2-☑	D48.1-☑	D49.2
hypochondrium	C49.4	C79.89	—	D21.4	D48.1-☑	D49.2
iliopsoas muscle	C49.5	C79.89	—	D21.5	D48.1-☑	D49.2
infraclavicular region	C49.3	C79.89	—	D21.3	D48.1-☑	D49.2
inguinal (canal) (region)	C49.5	C79.89	—	D21.5	D48.1-☑	D49.2
intestinal	C49.4	C79.89	—	D21.4	D48.1-☑	D49.2
intrathoracic	C49.3	C79.89	—	D21.3	D48.1-☑	D49.2
ischiorectal fossa	C49.5	C79.89	—	D21.5	D48.1-☑	D49.2
jaw	C03.9	C79.89	D00.03	D10.39	D48.1-☑	D49.0
knee	C49.2-☑	C79.89	—	D21.2-☑	D48.1-☑	D49.2
leg	C49.2-☑	C79.89	—	D21.2-☑	D48.1-☑	D49.2
limb NEC	C49.9	C79.89	—	D21.9	D48.1-☑	D49.2
lower	C49.2-☑	C79.89	—	D21.2-☑	D48.1-☑	D49.2
upper	C49.1-☑	C79.89	—	D21.1-☑	D48.1-☑	D49.2
nates	C49.5	C79.89	—	D21.5	D48.1-☑	D49.2
neck	C49.0	C79.89	—	D21.0	D48.1-☑	D49.2
orbit	C69.6-☑	C79.49	D09.2-☑	D31.6-☑	D48.1-☑	D49.89
overlapping lesion	C49.8	—	—	—	—	—
para-urethral	C49.5	C79.89	—	D21.5	D48.1-☑	D49.2
pararectal	C49.5	C79.89	—	D21.5	D48.1-☑	D49.2
paravaginal	C49.5	C79.89	—	D21.5	D48.1-☑	D49.2
pelvis (floor)	C49.5	C79.89	—	D21.5	D48.1-☑	D49.2
pelvo-abdominal	C49.8	C79.89	—	D21.6	D48.1-☑	D49.2
perineum	C49.5	C79.89	—	D21.5	D48.1-☑	D49.2
perirectal (tissue)	C49.5	C79.89	—	D21.5	D48.1-☑	D49.2
periurethral (tissue)	C49.5	C79.89	—	D21.5	D48.1-☑	D49.2
popliteal fossa or space	C49.2-☑	C79.89	—	D21.2-☑	D48.1-☑	D49.2
presacral	C49.5	C79.89	—	D21.5	D48.1-☑	D49.2
psoas muscle	C49.4	C79.89	—	D21.4	D48.1-☑	D49.2
pterygoid fossa	C49.0	C79.89	—	D21.0	D48.1-☑	D49.2
rectovaginal septum or wall	C49.5	C79.89	—	D21.5	D48.1-☑	D49.2
rectovesical	C49.5	C79.89	—	D21.5	D48.1-☑	D49.2
retroperitoneum	C48.0	C78.6	—	D20.0	D48.3	D49.0
sacrococcygeal region	C49.5	C79.89	—	D21.5	D48.1-☑	D49.2
scalp	C49.0	C79.89	—	D21.0	D48.1-☑	D49.2
scapular region	C49.3	C79.89	—	D21.3	D48.1-☑	D49.2
shoulder	C49.1-☑	C79.89	—	D21.1-☑	D48.1-☑	D49.2
skin (dermis) NEC — see also Neoplasm, skin, by site	C44.90	C79.2	D04.9	D23.9	D48.5	D49.2
stomach	C49.4	C79.89	—	D21.4	D48.1-☑	D49.2
submental	C49.0	C79.89	—	D21.0	D48.1-☑	D49.2
supraclavicular region	C49.0	C79.89	—	D21.0	D48.1-☑	D49.2
temple	C49.0	C79.89	—	D21.0	D48.1-☑	D49.2
temporal region	C49.0	C79.89	—	D21.0	D48.1-☑	D49.2
thigh	C49.2-☑	C79.89	—	D21.2-☑	D48.1-☑	D49.2
thoracic (duct) (wall)	C49.3	C79.89	—	D21.3	D48.1-☑	D49.2
thorax	C49.3	C79.89	—	D21.3	D48.1-☑	D49.2
thumb	C49.1-☑	C79.89	—	D21.1-☑	D48.1-☑	D49.2
toe	C49.2-☑	C79.89	—	D21.2-☑	D48.1-☑	D49.2
trunk	C49.6	C79.89	—	D21.6	D48.1-☑	D49.2
umbilicus	C49.4	C79.89	—	D21.4	D48.1-☑	D49.2
vesicorectal	C49.5	C79.89	—	D21.5	D48.1-☑	D49.2
wrist	C49.1-☑	C79.89	—	D21.1-☑	D48.1-☑	D49.2
conus medullaris	C72.0	C79.49	—	D33.4	D43.4	D49.7
cord (true) (vocal)	C32.0	C78.39	D02.0	D14.1	D38.0	D49.1
false	C32.1	C78.39	D02.0	D14.1	D38.0	D49.1
spermatic	C63.1-☑	C79.82	D07.69	D29.8	D40.8	D49.59
spinal (cervical) (lumbar) (thoracic)	C72.0	C79.49	—	D33.4	D43.4	D49.7
cornea (limbus)	C69.1-☑	C79.49	D09.2-☑	D31.1-☑	D48.7	D49.89
corpus						
albicans	C56.-☑	C79.6-☑	D07.39	D27.-☑	D39.1-☑	D49.59
callosum, brain	C71.0	C79.31	—	D33.2	D43.0	D49.6
cavernosum	C60.2	C79.82	D07.4	D29.0	D40.8	D49.59
gastric	C16.2	C78.89	D00.2	D13.1	D37.1	D49.0
overlapping sites	C54.8	—	—	—	—	—
penis	C60.2	C79.82	D07.4	D29.0	D40.8	D49.59
striatum, cerebrum	C71.0	C79.31	—	D33.0	D43.0	D49.6
uteri	C54.9	C79.82	D07.0	D26.1	D39.0	D49.59
isthmus	C54.0	C79.82	D07.0	D26.1	D39.0	D49.59
cortex						
adrenal	C74.0-☑	C79.7-☑	D09.3	D35.0-☑	D44.1-☑	D49.7
cerebral	C71.0	C79.31	—	D33.0	D43.0	D49.6
costal cartilage	C41.3	C79.51	—	D16.7	D48.0	D49.2
costovertebral joint	C41.3	C79.51	—	D16.7	D48.0	D49.2
Cowper's gland	C68.0	C79.19	D09.19	D30.4	D41.3	D49.59
cranial (fossa, any)	C71.9	C79.31	—	D33.2	D43.2	D49.7
meninges	C70.0	C79.32	—	D32.0	D42.0	D49.7
nerve	C72.50	C79.49	—	D33.3	D43.3	D49.7
specified NEC	C72.59	C79.49	—	D33.3	D43.3	D49.7
craniobuccal pouch	C75.2	C79.89	D09.3	D35.2	D44.3	D49.7
craniopharyngeal (duct) (pouch)	C75.2	C79.89	D09.3	D35.3	D44.4	D49.7
cricoid	C13.0	C79.89	D00.08	D10.7	D37.05	D49.0
cartilage	C32.3	C79.89	D02.0	D14.1	D38.0	D49.1
cricopharynx	C13.0	C79.89	D00.08	D10.7	D37.05	D49.0
crypt of Morgagni	C21.8	C78.5	D01.3	D12.9	D37.8	D49.0
crystalline lens	C69.4-☑	C79.49	D09.2-☑	D31.4-☑	D48.7	D49.89
cul-de-sac (Douglas')	C48.1	C78.6	—	D20.1	D48.4	D49.0
cuneiform cartilage	C32.3	C78.39	D02.0	D14.1	D38.0	D49.1
cutaneous — see Neoplasm, skin						
cutis — see Neoplasm, skin						
cystic (bile) duct (common)	C24.0	C78.89	D01.5	D13.5	D37.6	D49.0
dermis — see Neoplasm, skin						
diaphragm	C49.3	C79.89	—	D21.3	D48.1-☑	D49.2
digestive organs, system, tube, or tract NEC	C26.9	C78.89	D01.9	D13.99	D37.9	D49.0
disc, intervertebral	C41.2	C79.51	—	D16.6	D48.0	D49.2
disease, generalized	C80.0	—	—	—	—	—
disseminated	C80.0	—	—	—	—	—
Douglas' cul-de-sac or pouch	C48.1	C78.6	—	D20.1	D48.4	D49.0
duodenojejunal junction	C17.8	C78.4	D01.49	D13.39	D37.2	D49.0
duodenum	C17.0	C78.4	D01.49	D13.2	D37.2	D49.0
dura (cranial) (mater)	C70.9	C79.49	—	D32.9	D42.9	D49.7
cerebral	C70.0	C79.32	—	D32.0	D42.0	D49.7
spinal	C70.1	C79.49	—	D32.1	D42.1	D49.7
ear (external) — see also Neoplasm, skin, ear	C44.20-☑	C79.2	D04.2-☑	D23.2-☑	D48.5	D49.2
auricle or auris — see also Neoplasm, skin, ear	C44.20-☑	C79.2	D04.2-☑	D23.2-☑	D48.5	D49.2
canal, external — see also Neoplasm, skin, ear	C44.20-☑	C79.2	D04.2-☑	D23.2-☑	D48.5	D49.2
cartilage	C49.0	C79.89	—	D21.0	D48.1-☑	D49.2
external meatus — see also Neoplasm, skin, ear	C44.20-☑	C79.2	D04.2-☑	D23.2-☑	D48.5	D49.2
inner	C30.1	C78.39	D02.3	D14.0	D38.5	D49.1
lobule — see also Neoplasm, skin, ear	C44.20-☑	C79.2	D04.2-☑	D23.2-☑	D48.5	D49.2

☑ Additional Character Required — Refer to the Tabular List for Character Selection

Neoplasm, neoplastic — continued	Malignant Primary	Malignant Secondary	Ca in situ	Benign	Uncertain Behavior	Unspecified Behavior
ear — see also Neoplasm, skin, ear — continued						
middle	C30.1	C78.39	D02.3	D14.0	D38.5	D49.1
overlapping lesion with accessory sinuses	C31.8	—	—	—	—	—
skin	C44.20-☑	C79.2	D04.2-☑	D23.2-☑	D48.5	D49.2
basal cell carcinoma	C44.21-☑	—	—	—	—	—
specified type NEC	C44.29-☑	—	—	—	—	—
squamous cell carcinoma	C44.22-☑	—	—	—	—	—
earlobe	C44.20-☑	C79.2	D04.2-☑	D23.2-☑	D48.5	D49.2
basal cell carcinoma	C44.21-☑	—	—	—	—	—
specified type NEC	C44.29-☑	—	—	—	—	—
squamous cell carcinoma	C44.22-☑	—	—	—	—	—
ejaculatory duct	C63.7	C79.82	D07.69	D29.8	D40.8	D49.59
elbow NEC	C76.4-☑	C79.89	D04.6-☑	D36.7	D48.7	D49.89
endocardium	C38.0	C79.89	—	D15.1	D48.7	D49.89
endocervix (canal) (gland)	C53.0	C79.82	D06.0	D26.0	D39.0	D49.59
endocrine gland NEC	C75.9	C79.89	D09.3	D35.9	D44.9	D49.7
pluriglandular	C75.8	C79.89	D09.3	D35.7	D44.9	D49.7
endometrium (gland) (stroma)	C54.1	C79.82	D07.0	D26.1	D39.0	D49.59
ensiform cartilage	C41.3	C79.51	—	D16.7	D48.0	D49.2
enteric — see Neoplasm, intestine						
ependyma (brain)	C71.5	C79.31	—	D33.0	D43.0	D49.6
fourth ventricle	C71.7	C79.31	—	D33.1	D43.1	D49.6
epicardium	C38.0	C79.89	—	D15.1	D48.7	D49.89
epididymis	C63.0-☑	C79.82	D07.69	D29.3-☑	D40.8	D49.59
epidural	C72.9	C79.49	—	D33.9	D43.9	D49.7
epiglottis	C32.1	C78.39	D02.0	D14.1	D38.0	D49.1
anterior aspect or surface	C10.1	C79.89	D00.08	D10.5	D37.05	D49.0
cartilage	C32.3	C78.39	D02.0	D14.1	D38.0	D49.1
free border (margin)	C10.1	C79.89	D00.08	D10.5	D37.05	D49.0
junctional region	C10.8	C79.89	D00.08	D10.5	D37.05	D49.0
posterior (laryngeal) surface	C32.1	C78.39	D02.0	D14.1	D38.0	D49.1
suprahyoid portion	C32.1	C78.39	D02.0	D14.1	D38.0	D49.1
esophagogastric junction	C16.0	C78.89	D00.2	D13.1	D37.1	D49.0
esophagus	C15.9	C78.89	D00.1	D13.0	D37.8	D49.0
abdominal	C15.5	C78.89	D00.1	D13.0	D37.8	D49.0
cervical	C15.3	C78.89	D00.1	D13.0	D37.8	D49.0
distal (third)	C15.5	C78.89	D00.1	D13.0	D37.8	D49.0
lower (third)	C15.5	C78.89	D00.1	D13.0	D37.8	D49.0
middle (third)	C15.4	C78.89	D00.1	D13.0	D37.8	D49.0
overlapping lesion	C15.8	—	—	—	—	—
proximal (third)	C15.3	C78.89	D00.1	D13.0	D37.8	D49.0
thoracic	C15.4	C78.89	D00.1	D13.0	D37.8	D49.0
upper (third)	C15.3	C78.89	D00.1	D13.0	D37.8	D49.0
ethmoid (sinus)	C31.1	C78.39	D02.3	D14.0	D38.5	D49.1
bone or labyrinth	C41.0	C79.51	—	D16.4	D48.0	D49.2
eustachian tube	C30.1	C78.39	D02.3	D14.0	D38.5	D49.1
exocervix	C53.1	C79.82	D06.1	D26.0	D39.0	D49.59
external						
meatus (ear) — see also Neoplasm, skin, ear	C44.20-☑	C79.2	D04.2-☑	D23.2-☑	D48.5	D49.2
os, cervix uteri	C53.1	C79.82	D06.1	D26.0	D39.0	D49.59
extradural	C72.9	C79.49	—	D33.9	D43.9	D49.7
extrahepatic (bile) duct	C24.0	C78.89	D01.5	D13.5	D37.6	D49.0
overlapping lesion with gallbladder	C24.8	—	—	—	—	—

Neoplasm, neoplastic — continued	Malignant Primary	Malignant Secondary	Ca in situ	Benign	Uncertain Behavior	Unspecified Behavior
extraocular muscle	C69.6-☑	C79.49	D09.2-☑	D31.6-☑	D48.7	D49.89
extrarectal	C76.3	C79.89	D09.8	D36.7	D48.7	D49.89
extremity	C76.8	C79.89	D04.8	D36.7	D48.7	D49.89
lower	C76.5-☑	C79.89	D04.7-☑	D36.7	D48.7	D49.89
upper	C76.4-☑	C79.89	D04.6-☑	D36.7	D48.7	D49.89
eye NEC	C69.9-☑	C79.49	D09.2-☑	D31.9-☑	D48.7	D49.89
overlapping sites	C69.8-☑	—	—	—	—	—
eyeball	C69.9-☑	C79.49	D09.2-☑	D31.9-☑	D48.7	D49.89
eyebrow	C44.309	C79.2	D04.39	D23.39	D48.5	D49.2
basal cell carcinoma	C44.319	—	—	—	—	—
specified type NEC	C44.399	—	—	—	—	—
squamous cell carcinoma	C44.329	—	—	—	—	—
eyelid (lower) (skin) (upper)	C44.10-☑	—	—	—	—	—
basal cell carcinoma	C44.11-☑	—	—	—	—	—
cartilage	C49.0	C79.89	—	D21.0	D48.1-☑	D49.2
sebaceous cell	C44.13-☑	—	—	—	—	—
specified type NEC	C44.19-☑	—	—	—	—	—
squamous cell carcinoma	C44.12-☑	—	—	—	—	—
face NEC	C76.0	C79.89	D04.39	D36.7	D48.7	D49.89
fallopian tube (accessory)	C57.0-☑	C79.82	D07.39	D28.2	D39.8	D49.59
falx (cerebella) (cerebri)	C70.0	C79.32	—	D32.0	D42.0	D49.7
fascia — see also Neoplasm, connective tissue						
palmar	C49.1-☑	C79.89	—	D21.1-☑	D48.1-☑	D49.2
plantar	C49.2-☑	C79.89	—	D21.2-☑	D48.1-☑	D49.2
fatty tissue — see Neoplasm, connective tissue						
fauces, faucial NEC	C10.9	C79.89	D00.08	D10.5	D37.05	D49.0
pillars	C09.1	C79.89	D00.08	D10.5	D37.05	D49.0
tonsil	C09.9	C79.89	D00.08	D10.4	D37.05	D49.0
femur (any part)	C40.2-☑	C79.5-☑	—	D16.2-☑	—	—
fetal membrane	C58	C79.82	D07.0	D26.7	D39.2	D49.59
fibrous tissue — see Neoplasm, connective tissue						
fibula (any part)	C40.2-☑	C79.51	—	D16.2-☑	—	—
filum terminale	C72.0	C79.49	—	D33.4	D43.4	D49.7
finger NEC	C76.4-☑	C79.89	D04.6-☑	D36.7	D48.7	D49.89
flank NEC	C76.8	C79.89	D04.5	D36.7	D48.7	D49.89
follicle, nabothian	C53.0	C79.82	D06.0	D26.0	D39.0	D49.59
foot NEC	C76.5-☑	C79.89	D04.7-☑	D36.7	D48.7	D49.89
forearm NEC	C76.4-☑	C79.89	D04.6-☑	D36.7	D48.7	D49.89
forehead (skin)	C44.309	C79.2	D04.39	D23.39	D48.5	D49.2
basal cell carcinoma	C44.319	—	—	—	—	—
specified type NEC	C44.399	—	—	—	—	—
squamous cell carcinoma	C44.329	—	—	—	—	—
foreskin	C60.0	C79.82	D07.4	D29.0	D40.8	D49.59
fornix						
pharyngeal	C11.3	C79.89	D00.08	D10.6	D37.05	D49.0
vagina	C52	C79.82	D07.2	D28.1	D39.8	D49.59
fossa (of)						
anterior (cranial)	C71.9	C79.31	—	D33.2	D43.2	D49.6
cranial	C71.9	C79.31	—	D33.2	D43.2	D49.6
ischiorectal	C76.3	C79.89	D09.8	D36.7	D48.7	D49.89
middle (cranial)	C71.9	C79.31	—	D33.2	D43.2	D49.6
piriform	C12	C79.89	D00.08	D10.7	D37.05	D49.0
pituitary	C75.1	C79.89	D09.3	D35.2	D44.3	D49.7
posterior (cranial)	C71.9	C79.31	—	D33.2	D43.2	D49.6
pterygoid	C49.0	C79.89	—	D21.0	D48.1-☑	D49.2
pyriform	C12	C79.89	D00.08	D10.7	D37.05	D49.0
Rosenmuller	C11.2	C79.89	D00.08	D10.6	D37.05	D49.0
tonsillar	C09.0	C79.89	D00.08	D10.5	D37.05	D49.0
fourchette	C51.9	C79.82	D07.1	D28.0	D39.8	D49.59

☑ Additional Character Required — Refer to the Tabular List for Character Selection

Neoplasm, frenulum

Neoplasm, neoplastic — continued	Malignant Primary	Malignant Secondary	Ca in situ	Benign	Uncertain Behavior	Unspecified Behavior
frenulum						
labii — see Neoplasm, lip, internal						
linguae	C02.2	C79.89	D00.07	D10.1	D37.02	D49.0
frontal						
bone	C41.0	C79.51	—	D16.4	D48.0	D49.2
lobe, brain	C71.1	C79.31	—	D33.0	D43.0	D49.6
pole	C71.1	C79.31	—	D33.0	D43.0	D49.6
sinus	C31.2	C78.39	D02.3	D14.0	D38.5	D49.1
fundus						
stomach	C16.1	C78.89	D00.2	D13.1	D37.1	D49.0
uterus	C54.3	C79.82	D07.0	D26.1	D39.0	D49.59
gall duct (extrahepatic)	C24.0	C78.89	D01.5	D13.5	D37.6	D49.0
intrahepatic	C22.1	C78.7	D01.5	D13.4	D37.6	D49.0
gallbladder	C23	C78.89	D01.5	D13.5	D37.6	D49.0
overlapping lesion with extrahepatic bile ducts	C24.8	—	—	—	—	—
ganglia — see also Neoplasm, nerve, peripheral	C47.9	C79.89	—	D36.10	D48.2	D49.2
basal	C71.0	C79.31	—	D33.0	D43.0	D49.6
cranial nerve	C72.50	C79.49	—	D33.3	D43.3	D49.7
Gartner's duct	C52	C79.82	D07.2	D28.1	D39.8	D49.59
gastric — see Neoplasm, stomach						
gastrocolic	C26.9	C78.89	D01.9	D13.99	D37.9	D49.0
gastroesophageal junction	C16.0	C78.89	D00.2	D13.1	D37.1	D49.0
gastrointestinal (tract) NEC	C26.9	C78.89	D01.9	D13.99	D37.9	D49.0
generalized	C80.0	—	—	—	—	—
genital organ or tract						
female NEC	C57.9	C79.82	D07.30	D28.9	D39.9	D49.59
overlapping lesion	C57.8	—	—	—	—	—
specified site NEC	C57.7	C79.82	D07.39	D28.7	D39.8	D49.59
male NEC	C63.9	C79.82	D07.60	D29.9	D40.9	D49.59
overlapping lesion	C63.8	—	—	—	—	—
specified site NEC	C63.7	C79.82	D07.69	D29.8	D40.8	D49.59
genitourinary tract						
female	C57.9	C79.82	D07.30	D28.9	D39.9	D49.59
male	C63.9	C79.82	D07.60	D29.9	D40.9	D49.59
gingiva (alveolar) (marginal)	C03.9	C79.89	D00.03	D10.39	D37.09	D49.0
lower	C03.1	C79.89	D00.03	D10.39	D37.09	D49.0
mandibular	C03.1	C79.89	D00.03	D10.39	D37.09	D49.0
maxillary	C03.0	C79.89	D00.03	D10.39	D37.09	D49.0
upper	C03.0	C79.89	D00.03	D10.39	D37.09	D49.0
gland, glandular (lymphatic) (system) — see also Neoplasm, lymph gland						
endocrine NEC	C75.9	C79.89	D09.3	D35.9	D44.9	D49.7
salivary — see Neoplasm, salivary gland						
glans penis	C60.1	C79.82	D07.4	D29.0	D40.8	D49.59
globus pallidus	C71.0	C79.31	—	D33.0	D43.0	D49.6
glomus						
coccygeal	C49.5	C79.89	—	D21.5	D48.1-☑	D49.2
jugularis	C75.5	C79.89	—	D35.6	D44.7	D49.7
glosso-epiglottic fold(s)	C10.1	C79.89	D00.08	D10.5	D37.05	D49.0
glossopalatine fold	C09.1	C79.89	D00.08	D10.5	D37.05	D49.0
glossopharyngeal sulcus	C09.0	C79.89	D00.08	D10.5	D37.05	D49.0
glottis	C32.0	C78.39	D02.0	D14.1	D38.0	D49.1
gluteal region	C76.3	C79.89	D04.5	D36.7	D48.7	D49.89
great vessels NEC	C49.3	C79.89	—	D21.3	D48.1-☑	D49.2
groin NEC	C76.3	C79.89	D04.5	D36.7	D48.7	D49.89
gum	C03.9	C79.89	D00.03	D10.39	D37.09	D49.0
lower	C03.1	C79.89	D00.03	D10.39	D37.09	D49.0
upper	C03.0	C79.89	D00.03	D10.39	D37.09	D49.0

Neoplasm, neoplastic — continued	Malignant Primary	Malignant Secondary	Ca in situ	Benign	Uncertain Behavior	Unspecified Behavior
hand NEC	C76.4-☑	C79.89	D04.6-☑	D36.7	D48.7	D49.89
head NEC	C76.0	C79.89	D04.4	D36.7	D48.7	D49.89
heart	C38.0	C79.89	—	D15.1	D48.7	D49.89
heel NEC	C76.5-☑	C79.89	D04.7-☑	D36.7	D48.7	D49.89
helix — see also Neoplasm, skin, ear	C44.20-☑	C79.2	D04.2-☑	D23.2-☑	D48.5	D49.2
hematopoietic, hemopoietic tissue NEC	C96.9	—	—	—	—	—
specified NEC	C96.Z	—	—	—	—	—
hemisphere, cerebral	C71.0	C79.31	—	D33.0	D43.0	D49.6
hemorrhoidal zone	C21.1	C78.5	D01.3	D12.9	D37.8	D49.0
hepatic — see also Index to disease, by histology	C22.9	C78.7	D01.5	D13.4	D37.6	D49.0
duct (bile)	C24.0	C78.89	D01.5	D13.5	D37.6	D49.0
flexure (colon)	C18.3	C78.5	D01.0	D12.3	D37.4	D49.0
primary	C22.8	C78.7	D01.5	D13.4	D37.6	D49.0
hepatobiliary	C24.9	C78.89	D01.5	D13.5	D37.6	D49.0
hepatoblastoma	C22.2	C78.7	D01.5	D13.4	D37.6	D49.0
hepatoma	C22.0	C78.7	D01.5	D13.4	D37.6	D49.0
hilus of lung	C34.0-☑	C78.0-☑	D02.2-☑	D14.3-☑	D38.1	D49.1
hip NEC	C76.5-☑	C79.89	D04.7-☑	D36.7	D48.7	D49.89
hippocampus, brain	C71.2	C79.31	—	D33.0	D43.0	D49.6
humerus (any part)	C40.0-☑	C79.51	—	D16.0-☑	—	—
hymen	C52	C79.82	D07.2	D28.1	D39.8	D49.59
hypopharynx, hypopharyngeal NEC	C13.9	C79.89	D00.08	D10.7	D37.05	D49.0
overlapping lesion	C13.8	—	—	—	—	—
postcricoid region	C13.0	C79.89	D00.08	D10.7	D37.05	D49.0
posterior wall	C13.2	C79.89	D00.08	D10.7	D37.05	D49.0
pyriform fossa (sinus)	C12	C79.89	D00.08	D10.7	D37.05	D49.0
hypophysis	C75.1	C79.89	D09.3	D35.2	D44.3	D49.7
hypothalamus	C71.0	C79.31	—	D33.0	D43.0	D49.6
ileocecum, ileocecal (coil) (junction) (valve)	C18.0	C78.5	D01.0	D12.0	D37.4	D49.0
ileum	C17.2	C78.4	D01.49	D13.39	D37.2	D49.0
ilium	C41.4	C79.51	—	D16.8	D48.0	D49.2
immunoproliferative NEC	C88.9-☑	—	—	—	—	—
infraclavicular (region)	C76.1	C79.89	D04.5	D36.7	D48.7	D49.89
inguinal (region)	C76.3	C79.89	D04.5	D36.7	D48.7	D49.89
insula	C71.0	C79.31	—	D33.0	D43.0	D49.6
insular tissue (pancreas)	C25.4	C78.89	D01.7	D13.7	D37.8	D49.0
brain	C71.0	C79.31	—	D33.0	D43.0	D49.6
interarytenoid fold	C13.1	C78.39	D00.08	D10.7	D37.05	D49.0
hypopharyngeal aspect	C13.1	C79.89	D00.08	D10.7	D37.05	D49.0
laryngeal aspect	C32.1	C79.89	D02.0	D14.1	D38.0	D49.1
marginal zone	C13.1	C79.89	D00.08	D10.7	D37.05	D49.0
interdental papillae	C03.9	C79.89	D00.03	D10.39	D37.09	D49.0
lower	C03.1	C79.89	D00.03	D10.39	D37.09	D49.0
upper	C03.0	C79.89	D00.03	D10.39	D37.09	D49.0
internal						
capsule	C71.0	C79.31	—	D33.0	D43.0	D49.6
os (cervix)	C53.0	C79.82	D06.0	D26.0	D39.0	D49.59
intervertebral cartilage or disc	C41.2	C79.51	—	D16.6	D48.0	D49.2
intestine, intestinal	C26.0	C78.80	D01.40	D13.99	D37.8	D49.0
large	C18.9	C78.5	D01.0	D12.6	D37.4	D49.0
appendix	C18.1	C78.5	D01.0	D12.1	D37.3	D49.0
caput coli	C18.0	C78.5	D01.0	D12.0	D37.4	D49.0
cecum	C18.0	C78.5	D01.0	D12.0	D37.4	D49.0
colon	C18.9	C78.5	D01.0	D12.6	D37.4	D49.0
and rectum	C19	C78.5	D01.1	D12.7	D37.5	D49.0
ascending	C18.2	C78.5	D01.0	D12.2	D37.4	D49.0

☑ Additional Character Required — Refer to the Tabular List for Character Selection

Neoplasm, neoplastic — continued	Malignant Primary	Malignant Secondary	Ca in situ	Benign	Uncertain Behavior	Unspecified Behavior
intestine, intestinal — continued						
large — continued						
colon — continued						
caput	C18.0	C78.5	D01.0	D12.0	D37.4	D49.0
descending	C18.6	C78.5	D01.0	D12.4	D37.4	D49.0
distal	C18.6	C78.5	D01.0	D12.4	D37.4	D49.0
left	C18.6	C78.5	D01.0	D12.4	D37.4	D49.0
overlapping lesion	C18.8	—	—	—	—	—
pelvic	C18.7	C78.5	D01.0	D12.5	D37.4	D49.0
right	C18.2	C78.5	D01.0	D12.2	D37.4	D49.0
sigmoid (flexure)	C18.7	C78.5	D01.0	D12.5	D37.4	D49.0
transverse	C18.4	C78.5	D01.0	D12.3	D37.4	D49.0
hepatic flexure	C18.3	C78.5	D01.0	D12.3	D37.4	D49.0
ileocecum, ileocecal (coil) (valve)	C18.0	C78.5	D01.0	D12.0	D37.4	D49.0
overlapping lesion	C18.8	—	—	—	—	—
sigmoid flexure (lower) (upper)	C18.7	C78.5	D01.0	D12.5	D37.4	D49.0
splenic flexure	C18.5	C78.5	D01.0	D12.3	D37.4	D49.0
small	C17.9	C78.4	D01.40	D13.30	D37.2	D49.0
duodenum	C17.0	C78.4	D01.49	D13.2	D37.2	D49.0
ileum	C17.2	C78.4	D01.49	D13.39	D37.2	D49.0
jejunum	C17.1	C78.4	D01.49	D13.39	D37.2	D49.0
overlapping lesion	C17.8	—	—	—	—	—
tract NEC	C26.0	C78.89	D01.40	D13.99	D37.8	D49.0
intra-abdominal	C76.2	C79.89	D09.8	D36.7	D48.7	D49.89
intracranial NEC	C71.9	C79.31	—	D33.2	D43.2	D49.6
intrahepatic (bile) duct	C22.1	C78.7	D01.5	D13.4	D37.6	D49.0
intraocular	C69.9-✓	C79.49	D09.2-✓	D31.9-✓	D48.7	D49.89
intraorbital	C69.6-✓	C79.49	D09.2-✓	D31.6-✓	D48.7	D49.89
intrasellar	C75.1	C79.89	D09.3	D35.2	D44.3	D49.7
intrathoracic (cavity) (organs)	C76.1	C79.89	D09.8	D15.9	D48.7	D49.89
specified NEC	C76.1	C79.89	D09.8	D15.7	—	—
iris	C69.4-✓	C79.49	D09.2-✓	D31.4-✓	D48.7	D49.89
ischiorectal (fossa)	C76.3	C79.89	D09.8	D36.7	D48.7	D49.89
ischium	C41.4	C79.51	—	D16.8	D48.0	D49.2
island of Reil	C71.0	C79.31	—	D33.0	D43.0	D49.6
islands or islets of Langerhans	C25.4	C78.89	D01.7	D13.7	D37.8	D49.0
isthmus uteri	C54.0	C79.82	D07.0	D26.1	D39.0	D49.59
jaw	C76.0	C79.89	D09.8	D36.7	D48.7	D49.89
bone	C41.1	C79.51	—	D16.5	D48.0	D49.2
lower	C41.1	C79.51	—	D16.5	—	—
upper	C41.0	C79.51	—	D16.4	—	—
carcinoma (any type) (lower) (upper)	C76.0	C79.89	—	—	—	—
skin — see also Neoplasm, skin, face	C44.309	C79.2	D04.39	D23.39	D48.5	D49.2
soft tissues	C03.9	C79.89	D00.03	D10.39	D37.09	D49.0
lower	C03.1	C79.89	D00.03	D10.39	D37.09	D49.0
upper	C03.0	C79.89	D00.03	D10.39	D37.09	D49.0
jejunum	C17.1	C78.4	D01.49	D13.39	D37.2	D49.0
joint NEC — see also Neoplasm, bone	C41.9	C79.51	—	D16.9	D48.0	D49.2
acromioclavicular	C40.0-✓	C79.51	—	D16.0-✓	—	—
bursa or synovial membrane — see Neoplasm, connective tissue						
costovertebral	C41.3	C79.51	—	D16.7	D48.0	D49.2
sternocostal	C41.3	C79.51	—	D16.7	D48.0	D49.2
temporomandibular	C41.1	C79.51	—	D16.5	D48.0	D49.2
junction						
anorectal	C21.8	C78.5	D01.3	D12.9	D37.8	D49.0
cardioesophageal	C16.0	C78.89	D00.2	D13.1	D37.1	D49.0
esophagogastric	C16.0	C78.89	D00.2	D13.1	D37.1	D49.0
gastroesophageal	C16.0	C78.89	D00.2	D13.1	D37.1	D49.0

Neoplasm, neoplastic — continued	Malignant Primary	Malignant Secondary	Ca in situ	Benign	Uncertain Behavior	Unspecified Behavior
junction — continued						
hard and soft palate	C05.9	C79.89	D00.00	D10.39	D37.09	D49.0
ileocecal	C18.0	C78.5	D01.0	D12.0	D37.4	D49.0
pelvirectal	C19	C78.5	D01.1	D12.7	D37.5	D49.0
pelviureteric	C65.-✓	C79.0-✓	D09.19	D30.1-✓	D41.1-✓	D49.59
rectosigmoid	C19	C78.5	D01.1	D12.7	D37.5	D49.0
squamocolumnar, of cervix	C53.8	C79.82	D06.7	D26.0	D39.0	D49.59
Kaposi's sarcoma — see Kaposi's, sarcoma						
kidney (parenchymal)	C64.-✓	C79.0-✓	D09.19	D30.0-✓	D41.0-✓	D49.51-✓
calyx	C65.-✓	C79.0-✓	D09.19	D30.1-✓	D41.1-✓	D49.51-✓
hilus	C65.-✓	C79.0-✓	D09.19	D30.1-✓	D41.1-✓	D49.51-✓
pelvis	C65.-✓	C79.0-✓	D09.19	D30.1-✓	D41.1-✓	D49.51-✓
knee NEC	C76.5-✓	C79.89	D04.7-✓	D36.7	D48.7	D49.89
labia (skin)	C51.9	C79.82	D07.1	D28.0	D39.8	D49.59
majora	C51.0	C79.82	D07.1	D28.0	D39.8	D49.59
minora	C51.1	C79.82	D07.1	D28.0	D39.8	D49.59
labial — see also Neoplasm, lip	C00.9	C79.89	D00.01	D10.0	D37.01	D49.0
sulcus (lower) (upper)	C06.1	C79.89	D00.02	D10.39	D37.09	D49.0
labium (skin)	C51.9	C79.82	D07.1	D28.0	D39.8	D49.59
majus	C51.0	C79.82	D07.1	D28.0	D39.8	D49.59
minus	C51.1	C79.82	D07.1	D28.0	D39.8	D49.59
lacrimal						
canaliculi	C69.5-✓	C79.49	D09.2-✓	D31.5-✓	D48.7	D49.89
duct (nasal)	C69.5-✓	C79.49	D09.2-✓	D31.5-✓	D48.7	D49.89
gland	C69.5-✓	C79.49	D09.2-✓	D31.5-✓	D48.7	D49.89
punctum	C69.5-✓	C79.49	D09.2-✓	D31.5-✓	D48.7	D49.89
sac	C69.5-✓	C79.49	D09.2-✓	D31.5-✓	D48.7	D49.89
Langerhans, islands or islets	C25.4	C78.89	D01.7	D13.7	D37.8	D49.0
laryngopharynx	C13.9	C79.89	D00.08	D10.7	D37.05	D49.0
larynx, laryngeal NEC	C32.9	C78.39	D02.0	D14.1	D38.0	D49.1
aryepiglottic fold	C32.1	C78.39	D02.0	D14.1	D38.0	D49.1
cartilage (arytenoid) (cricoid) (cuneiform) (thyroid)	C32.3	C78.39	D02.0	D14.1	D38.0	D49.1
commissure (anterior) (posterior)	C32.0	C78.39	D02.0	D14.1	D38.0	D49.1
extrinsic NEC	C32.1	C78.39	D02.0	D14.1	D38.0	D49.1
meaning hypopharynx	C13.9	C79.89	D00.08	D10.7	D37.05	D49.0
interarytenoid fold	C32.1	C78.39	D02.0	D14.1	D38.0	D49.1
intrinsic	C32.0	C78.39	D02.0	D14.1	D38.0	D49.1
overlapping lesion	C32.8	—	—	—	—	—
ventricular band	C32.1	C78.39	D02.0	D14.1	D38.0	D49.1
leg NEC	C76.5-✓	C79.89	D04.7-✓	D36.7	D48.7	D49.89
lens, crystalline	C69.4-✓	C79.49	D09.2-✓	D31.4-✓	D48.7	D49.89
lid (lower) (upper)	C44.10-✓	C79.2	D04.1-✓	D23.1-✓	D48.5	D49.2
basal cell carcinoma	C44.11-✓	—	—	—	—	—
sebaceous cell	C44.13-✓	—	—	—	—	—
specified type NEC	C44.19-✓	—	—	—	—	—
squamous cell carcinoma	C44.12-✓	—	—	—	—	—
ligament — see also Neoplasm, connective tissue						
broad	C57.1-✓	C79.82	D07.39	D28.2	D39.8	D49.59
Mackenrodt's	C57.7	C79.82	D07.39	D28.7	D39.8	D49.59
non-uterine — see Neoplasm, connective tissue						
round	C57.2-✓	C79.82	—	D28.2	D39.8	D49.59
sacro-uterine	C57.3	C79.82	—	D28.2	D39.8	D49.59
uterine	C57.3	C79.82	—	D28.2	D39.8	D49.59
utero-ovarian	C57.7	C79.82	D07.39	D28.2	D39.8	D49.59
uterosacral	C57.3	C79.82	—	D28.2	D39.8	D49.59
limb	C76.8	C79.89	D04.8	D36.7	D48.7	D49.89

✓ Additional Character Required — Refer to the Tabular List for Character Selection

Neoplasm, limb

	Malignant Primary	Malignant Secondary	Ca in situ	Benign	Uncertain Behavior	Unspecified Behavior
Neoplasm, neoplastic — *continued*						
limb — *continued*						
lower	C76.5-☑	C79.89	D04.7-☑	D36.7	D48.7	D49.89
upper	C76.4-☑	C79.89	D04.6-☑	D36.7	D48.7	D49.89
limbus of cornea	C69.1-☑	C79.49	D09.2-☑	D31.1-☑	D48.7	D49.89
lingual NEC — *see also Neoplasm, tongue*	C02.9	C79.89	D00.07	D10.1	D37.02	D49.0
lingula, lung	C34.1-☑	C78.0-☑	D02.2-☑	D14.3-☑	D38.1	D49.1
lip	C00.9	C79.89	D00.01	D10.0	D37.01	D49.0
buccal aspect — *see Neoplasm, lip, internal*						
commissure	C00.6	C79.89	D00.01	D10.0	D37.01	D49.0
external	C00.2	C79.89	D00.01	D10.0	D37.01	D49.0
lower	C00.1	C79.89	D00.01	D10.0	D37.01	D49.0
upper	C00.0	C79.89	D00.01	D10.0	D37.01	D49.0
frenulum — *see Neoplasm, lip, internal*						
inner aspect — *see Neoplasm, lip, internal*						
internal	C00.5	C79.89	D00.01	D10.0	D37.01	D49.0
lower	C00.4	C79.89	D00.01	D10.0	D37.01	D49.0
upper	C00.3	C79.89	D00.01	D10.0	D37.01	D49.0
lipstick area	C00.2	C79.89	D00.01	D10.0	D37.01	D49.0
lower	C00.1	C79.89	D00.01	D10.0	D37.01	D49.0
upper	C00.0	C79.89	D00.01	D10.0	D37.01	D49.0
lower	C00.1	C79.89	D00.01	D10.0	D37.01	D49.0
internal	C00.4	C79.89	D00.01	D10.0	D37.01	D49.0
mucosa — *see Neoplasm, lip, internal*						
oral aspect — *see Neoplasm, lip, internal*						
overlapping lesion	C00.8	—	—	—	—	—
with oral cavity or pharynx	C14.8	—	—	—	—	—
skin (commissure) (lower) (upper)	C44.00	C79.2	D04.0	D23.0	D48.5	D49.2
basal cell carcinoma	C44.01	—	—	—	—	—
specified type NEC	C44.09	—	—	—	—	—
squamous cell carcinoma	C44.02	—	—	—	—	—
upper	C00.0	C79.89	D00.01	D10.0	D37.01	D49.0
internal	C00.3	C79.89	D00.01	D10.0	D37.01	D49.0
vermilion border	C00.2	C79.89	D00.01	D10.0	D37.01	D49.0
lower	C00.1	C79.89	D00.01	D10.0	D37.01	D49.0
upper	C00.0	C79.89	D00.01	D10.0	D37.01	D49.0
lipomatous — *see Lipoma, by site*						
liver — *see also Index to disease, by histology*	C22.9	C78.7	D01.5	D13.4	D37.6	D49.0
primary	C22.8	C78.7	D01.5	D13.4	D37.6	D49.0
lumbosacral plexus	C47.5	C79.89	—	D36.16	D48.2	D49.2
lung	C34.9-☑	C78.0-☑	D02.2-☑	D14.3-☑	D38.1	D49.1
azygos lobe	C34.1-☑	C78.0-☑	D02.2-☑	D14.3-☑	D38.1	D49.1
carina	C34.0-☑	C78.0-☑	D02.2-☑	D14.3-☑	D38.1	D49.1
hilus	C34.0-☑	C78.0-☑	D02.2-☑	D14.3-☑	D38.1	D49.1
lingula	C34.1-☑	C78.0-☑	D02.2-☑	D14.3-☑	D38.1	D49.1
lobe NEC	C34.9-☑	C78.0-☑	D02.2-☑	D14.3-☑	D38.1	D49.1
lower lobe	C34.3-☑	C78.0-☑	D02.2-☑	D14.3-☑	D38.1	D49.1
main bronchus	C34.0-☑	C78.0-☑	D02.2-☑	D14.3-☑	D38.1	D49.1
mesothelioma — *see Mesothelioma*						
middle lobe	C34.2	C78.0-☑	D02.21	D14.31	D38.1	D49.1
overlapping lesion	C34.8-☑	—	—	—	—	—
upper lobe	C34.1-☑	C78.0-☑	D02.2-☑	D14.3-☑	D38.1	D49.1
lymph, lymphatic channel NEC	C49.9	C79.89	—	D21.9	D48.1-☑	D49.2

	Malignant Primary	Malignant Secondary	Ca in situ	Benign	Uncertain Behavior	Unspecified Behavior
Neoplasm, neoplastic — *continued*						
lymph, lymphatic channel — *continued*						
gland (secondary)	—	C77.9	—	D36.0	D48.7	D49.89
abdominal	—	C77.2	—	D36.0	D48.7	D49.89
aortic	—	C77.2	—	D36.0	D48.7	D49.89
arm	—	C77.3	—	D36.0	D48.7	D49.89
auricular (anterior) (posterior)	—	C77.0	—	D36.0	D48.7	D49.89
axilla, axillary	—	C77.3	—	D36.0	D48.7	D49.89
brachial	—	C77.3	—	D36.0	D48.7	D49.89
bronchial	—	C77.1	—	D36.0	D48.7	D49.89
bronchopulmonary	—	C77.1	—	D36.0	D48.7	D49.89
celiac	—	C77.2	—	D36.0	D48.7	D49.89
cervical	—	C77.0	—	D36.0	D48.7	D49.89
cervicofacial	—	C77.0	—	D36.0	D48.7	D49.89
Cloquet	—	C77.4	—	D36.0	D48.7	D49.89
colic	—	C77.2	—	D36.0	D48.7	D49.89
common duct	—	C77.2	—	D36.0	D48.7	D49.89
cubital	—	C77.3	—	D36.0	D48.7	D49.89
diaphragmatic	—	C77.1	—	D36.0	D48.7	D49.89
epigastric, inferior	—	C77.1	—	D36.0	D48.7	D49.89
epitrochlear	—	C77.3	—	D36.0	D48.7	D49.89
esophageal	—	C77.1	—	D36.0	D48.7	D49.89
face	—	C77.0	—	D36.0	D48.7	D49.89
femoral	—	C77.4	—	D36.0	D48.7	D49.89
gastric	—	C77.2	—	D36.0	D48.7	D49.89
groin	—	C77.4	—	D36.0	D48.7	D49.89
head	—	C77.0	—	D36.0	D48.7	D49.89
hepatic	—	C77.2	—	D36.0	D48.7	D49.89
hilar (pulmonary)	—	C77.1	—	D36.0	D48.7	D49.89
splenic	—	C77.2	—	D36.0	D48.7	D49.89
hypogastric	—	C77.5	—	D36.0	D48.7	D49.89
ileocolic	—	C77.2	—	D36.0	D48.7	D49.89
iliac	—	C77.5	—	D36.0	D48.7	D49.89
infraclavicular	—	C77.3	—	D36.0	D48.7	D49.89
inguina, inguinal	—	C77.4	—	D36.0	D48.7	D49.89
innominate	—	C77.1	—	D36.0	D48.7	D49.89
intercostal	—	C77.1	—	D36.0	D48.7	D49.89
intestinal	—	C77.2	—	D36.0	D48.7	D49.89
intrabdominal	—	C77.2	—	D36.0	D48.7	D49.89
intrapelvic	—	C77.5	—	D36.0	D48.7	D49.89
intrathoracic	—	C77.1	—	D36.0	D48.7	D49.89
jugular	—	C77.0	—	D36.0	D48.7	D49.89
leg	—	C77.4	—	D36.0	D48.7	D49.89
limb						
lower	—	C77.4	—	D36.0	D48.7	D49.89
upper	—	C77.3	—	D36.0	D48.7	D49.89
lower limb	—	C77.4	—	D36.0	D48.7	D49.89
lumbar	—	C77.2	—	D36.0	D48.7	D49.89
mandibular	—	C77.0	—	D36.0	D48.7	D49.89
mediastinal	—	C77.1	—	D36.0	D48.7	D49.89
mesenteric (inferior) (superior)	—	C77.2	—	D36.0	D48.7	D49.89
midcolic	—	C77.2	—	D36.0	D48.7	D49.89
multiple sites in categories C77.0 - C77.5	—	C77.8	—	D36.0	D48.7	D49.89
neck	—	C77.0	—	D36.0	D48.7	D49.89
obturator	—	C77.5	—	D36.0	D48.7	D49.89
occipital	—	C77.0	—	D36.0	D48.7	D49.89
pancreatic	—	C77.2	—	D36.0	D48.7	D49.89
para-aortic	—	C77.2	—	D36.0	D48.7	D49.89
paracervical	—	C77.5	—	D36.0	D48.7	D49.89
parametrial	—	C77.5	—	D36.0	D48.7	D49.89
parasternal	—	C77.1	—	D36.0	D48.7	D49.89
parotid	—	C77.0	—	D36.0	D48.7	D49.89
pectoral	—	C77.3	—	D36.0	D48.7	D49.89
pelvic	—	C77.5	—	D36.0	D48.7	D49.89
peri-aortic	—	C77.2	—	D36.0	D48.7	D49.89
peripancreatic	—	C77.2	—	D36.0	D48.7	D49.89
popliteal	—	C77.4	—	D36.0	D48.7	D49.89
porta hepatis	—	C77.2	—	D36.0	D48.7	D49.89
portal	—	C77.2	—	D36.0	D48.7	D49.89
preauricular	—	C77.0	—	D36.0	D48.7	D49.89
prelaryngeal	—	C77.0	—	D36.0	D48.7	D49.89

☑ Additional Character Required — Refer to the Tabular List for Character Selection

	Malignant Primary	Malignant Secondary	Ca in situ	Benign	Uncertain Behavior	Unspecified Behavior		Malignant Primary	Malignant Secondary	Ca in situ	Benign	Uncertain Behavior	Unspecified Behavior
Neoplasm, neoplastic — *continued*							**Neoplasm, neoplastic** — *continued*						
lymph, lymphatic channel — *continued*							Meckel diverticulum, malignant	C17.3	C78.4	D01.49	D13.39	D37.2	D49.0
gland — *continued*							mediastinum, mediastinal	C38.3	C78.1	—	D15.2	D38.3	D49.89
presymphysial	—	C77.5	—	D36.0	D48.7	D49.89	anterior	C38.1	C78.1	—	D15.2	D38.3	D49.89
pretracheal	—	C77.0	—	D36.0	D48.7	D49.89	posterior	C38.2	C78.1	—	D15.2	D38.3	D49.89
primary (any site) NEC	C96.9	—	—	—	—	—	medulla						
pulmonary (hiler)	—	C77.1	—	D36.0	D48.7	D49.89	adrenal	C74.1-☑	C79.7-☑	D09.3	D35.0-☑	D44.1-☑	D49.7
pyloric	—	C77.2	—	D36.0	D48.7	D49.89	oblongata	C71.7	C79.31	—	D33.1	D43.1	D49.6
retroperitoneal	—	C77.2	—	D36.0	D48.7	D49.89	meibomian gland	C44.10-☑	C79.2	D04.1-☑	D23.1-☑	D48.5	D49.2
retropharyngeal	—	C77.0	—	D36.0	D48.7	D49.89	basal cell carcinoma	C44.11-☑	—	—	—	—	—
Rosenmuller's	—	C77.4	—	D36.0	D48.7	D49.89	sebaceous cell	C44.13-☑	—	—	—	—	—
sacral	—	C77.5	—	D36.0	D48.7	D49.89	specified type NEC	C44.19-☑	—	—	—	—	—
scalene	—	C77.0	—	D36.0	D48.7	D49.89	squamous cell carcinoma	C44.12-☑	—	—	—	—	—
site NEC	—	C77.9	—	D36.0	D48.7	D49.89	melanoma — *see* Melanoma						
splenic (hilar)	—	C77.2	—	D36.0	D48.7	D49.89	meninges	C70.9	C79.49	—	D32.9	D42.9	D49.7
subclavicular	—	C77.3	—	D36.0	D48.7	D49.89	brain	C70.0	C79.32	—	D32.0	D42.0	D49.7
subinguinal	—	C77.4	—	D36.0	D48.7	D49.89	cerebral	C70.0	C79.32	—	D32.0	D42.0	D49.7
sublingual	—	C77.0	—	D36.0	D48.7	D49.89	cranial	C70.0	C79.32	—	D32.0	D42.0	D49.7
submandibular	—	C77.0	—	D36.0	D48.7	D49.89	intracranial	C70.0	C79.32	—	D32.0	D42.0	D49.7
submaxillary	—	C77.0	—	D36.0	D48.7	D49.89	spinal (cord)	C70.1	C79.49	—	D32.1	D42.1	D49.7
submental	—	C77.0	—	D36.0	D48.7	D49.89	meniscus, knee joint (lateral)						
subscapular	—	C77.3	—	D36.0	D48.7	D49.89	(medial)	C40.2-☑	C79.51	—	D16.2-☑	D48.0	D49.2
supraclavicular	—	C77.0	—	D36.0	D48.7	D49.89	Merkel cell — *see* Carcinoma, Merkel cell						
thoracic	—	C77.1	—	D36.0	D48.7	D49.89							
tibial	—	C77.4	—	D36.0	D48.7	D49.89	mesentery, mesenteric	C48.1	C78.6	—	D20.1	D48.4	D49.0
tracheal	—	C77.1	—	D36.0	D48.7	D49.89	mesoappendix	C48.1	C78.6	—	D20.1	D48.4	D49.0
tracheobronchial	—	C77.1	—	D36.0	D48.7	D49.89	mesocolon	C48.1	C78.6	—	D20.1	D48.4	D49.0
upper limb	—	C77.3	—	D36.0	D48.7	D49.89	mesopharynx — *see* Neoplasm, oropharynx						
Virchow's	—	C77.0	—	D36.0	D48.7	D49.89	mesosalpinx	C57.1-☑	C79.82	D07.39	D28.2	D39.8	D49.59
node — *see also* Neoplasm, lymph gland							mesothelial tissue — *see* Mesothelioma						
primary NEC	C96.9	—	—	—	—	—	mesothelioma — *see* Mesothelioma						
vessel — *see also* Neoplasm, connective tissue	C49.9	C79.89	—	D21.9	D48.1-☑	D49.2	mesovarium	C57.1-☑	C79.82	D07.39	D28.2	D39.8	D49.59
Mackenrodt's ligament	C57.7	C79.82	D07.39	D28.7	D39.8	D49.59	metacarpus (any bone)	C40.1-☑	C79.51	—	D16.1-☑	—	—
malar	C41.0	C79.51	—	D16.4	D48.0	D49.2	metastatic NEC — *see also* Neoplasm, by site, secondary	—	C79.9	—	—	—	—
region — *see* Neoplasm, cheek													
mammary gland — *see* Neoplasm, breast							metatarsus (any bone)	C40.3-☑	C79.51	—	D16.3-☑	—	—
mandible	C41.1	C79.51	—	D16.5	D48.0	D49.2	midbrain	C71.7	C79.31	—	D33.1	D43.1	D49.6
alveolar mucosa (carcinoma)	C03.1	C79.89	D00.03	D10.39	D37.09	D49.0	milk duct — *see* Neoplasm, breast						
ridge or process	C41.1	C79.51	—	D16.5	D48.0	D49.2	mons pubis	C51.9	C79.82	D07.1	D28.0	D39.8	D49.59
marrow (bone) NEC	C96.9	C79.52	—	—	D47.9	D49.89	veneris	C51.9	C79.82	D07.1	D28.0	D39.8	D49.59
mastectomy site (skin) — *see also* Neoplasm, breast, skin	C44.501	C79.2	—	—	—	—	motor tract	C72.9	C79.49	—	D33.9	D43.9	D49.7
							brain	C71.9	C79.31	—	D33.2	D43.2	D49.6
specified as breast tissue	C50.8-☑	C79.81	—	—	—	—	cauda equina	C72.1	C79.49	—	D33.4	D43.4	D49.7
mastoid (air cells) (antrum) (cavity)	C30.1	C78.39	D02.3	D14.0	D38.5	D49.1	spinal	C72.0	C79.49	—	D33.4	D43.4	D49.7
							mouth	C06.9	C79.89	D00.00	D10.30	D37.09	D49.0
bone or process	C41.0	C79.51	—	D16.4	D48.0	D49.2	book-leaf	C06.89	C79.89	—	—	—	—
maxilla, maxillary (superior)	C41.0	C79.51	—	D16.4	D48.0	D49.2	floor	C04.9	C79.89	D00.06	D10.2	D37.09	D49.0
alveolar mucosa	C03.0	C79.89	D00.03	D10.39	D37.09	D49.0	anterior portion	C04.0	C79.89	D00.06	D10.2	D37.09	D49.0
							lateral portion	C04.1	C79.89	D00.06	D10.2	D37.09	D49.0
ridge or process (carcinoma)	C41.0	C79.51	—	D16.4	D48.0	D49.2	overlapping lesion	C04.8	—	—	—	—	—
antrum	C31.0	C78.39	D02.3	D14.0	D38.5	D49.1	overlapping NEC	C06.80	—	—	—	—	—
carcinoma	C03.0	C79.51	—	—	—	—	roof	C05.9	C79.89	D00.00	D10.39	D37.09	D49.0
inferior — *see* Neoplasm, mandible							specified part NEC	C06.89	C79.89	D00.00	D10.39	D37.09	D49.0
sinus	C31.0	C78.39	D02.3	D14.0	D38.5	D49.1	vestibule	C06.1	C79.89	D00.00	D10.39	D37.09	D49.0
meatus external (ear) — *see also* Neoplasm, skin, ear	C44.20-☑	C79.2	D04.2-☑	D23.2-☑	D48.5	D49.2	mucosa						
							alveolar (ridge or process)	C03.9	C79.89	D00.03	D10.39	D37.09	D49.0
							lower	C03.1	C79.89	D00.03	D10.39	D37.09	D49.0
							upper	C03.0	C79.89	D00.03	D10.39	D37.09	D49.0

☑ **Additional Character Required** — Refer to the Tabular List for Character Selection

Neoplasm, mucosa

	Malignant Primary	Malignant Secondary	Ca in situ	Benign	Uncertain Behavior	Unspecified Behavior
Neoplasm, neoplastic						
— continued						
mucosa — continued						
buccal	C06.0	C79.89	D00.02	D10.39	D37.09	D49.0
cheek	C06.0	C79.89	D00.02	D10.39	D37.09	D49.0
lip — see Neoplasm, lip, internal						
nasal	C30.0	C78.39	D02.3	D14.0	D38.5	D49.1
oral	C06.0	C79.89	D00.02	D10.39	D37.09	D49.0
Mullerian duct						
female	C57.7	C79.82	D07.39	D28.7	D39.8	D49.59
male	C63.7	C79.82	D07.69	D29.8	D40.8	D49.59
muscle — see also Neoplasm, connective tissue						
extraocular	C69.6-☑	C79.49	D09.2-☑	D31.6-☑	D48.7	D49.89
myocardium	C38.0	C79.89	—	D15.1	D48.7	D49.89
myometrium	C54.2	C79.82	D07.0	D26.1	D39.0	D49.59
myopericardium	C38.0	C79.89	—	D15.1	D48.7	D49.89
nabothian gland (follicle)	C53.0	C79.82	D06.0	D26.0	D39.0	D49.59
nail — see also Neoplasm, skin, limb	C44.90	C79.2	D04.9	D23.9	D48.5	D49.2
finger — see also Neoplasm, skin, limb, upper	C44.60-☑	C79.2	D04.6-☑	D23.6-☑	D48.5	D49.2
toe — see also Neoplasm, skin, limb, lower	C44.70-☑	C79.2	D04.7-☑	D23.7-☑	D48.5	D49.2
nares, naris (anterior) (posterior)	C30.0	C78.39	D02.3	D14.0	D38.5	D49.1
nasal — see Neoplasm, nose						
nasolabial groove — see also Neoplasm, skin, face	C44.309	C79.2	D04.39	D23.39	D48.5	D49.2
nasolacrimal duct	C69.5-☑	C79.49	D09.2-☑	D31.5-☑	D48.7	D49.89
nasopharynx, nasopharyngeal	C11.9	C79.89	D00.08	D10.6	D37.05	D49.0
floor	C11.3	C79.89	D00.08	D10.6	D37.05	D49.0
overlapping lesion	C11.8	—	—	—	—	—
roof	C11.0	C79.89	D00.08	D10.6	D37.05	D49.0
wall	C11.9	C79.89	D00.08	D10.6	D37.05	D49.0
anterior	C11.3	C79.89	D00.08	D10.6	D37.05	D49.0
lateral	C11.2	C79.89	D00.08	D10.6	D37.05	D49.0
posterior	C11.1	C79.89	D00.08	D10.6	D37.05	D49.0
superior	C11.0	C79.89	D00.08	D10.6	D37.05	D49.0
nates — see also Neoplasm, skin, trunk	C44.509	C79.2	D04.5	D23.5	D48.5	D49.2
neck NEC	C76.0	C79.89	D09.8	D36.7	D48.7	D49.89
skin	C44.40	—	—	—	—	—
basal cell carcinoma	C44.41	—	—	—	—	—
specified type NEC	C44.49	—	—	—	—	—
squamous cell carcinoma	C44.42	—	—	—	—	—
nerve (ganglion)	C47.9	C79.89	—	D36.10	D48.2	D49.2
abducens	C72.59	C79.49	—	D33.3	D43.3	D49.7
accessory (spinal)	C72.59	C79.49	—	D33.3	D43.3	D49.7
acoustic	C72.4-☑	C79.49	—	D33.3	D43.3	D49.7
auditory	C72.4-☑	C79.49	—	D33.3	D43.3	D49.7
autonomic NEC — see also Neoplasm, nerve, peripheral	C47.9	C79.89	—	D36.10	D48.2	D49.2
brachial	C47.1-☑	C79.89	—	D36.12	D48.2	D49.2
cranial	C72.50	C79.49	—	D33.3	D43.3	D49.7
specified NEC	C72.59	C79.49	—	D33.3	D43.3	D49.7
facial	C72.59	C79.49	—	D33.3	D43.3	D49.7
femoral	C47.2-☑	C79.89	—	D36.13	D48.2	D49.2
ganglion NEC — see also Neoplasm, nerve, peripheral	C47.9	C79.89	—	D36.10	D48.2	D49.2
glossopharyngeal	C72.59	C79.49	—	D33.3	D43.3	D49.7
hypoglossal	C72.59	C79.49	—	D33.3	D43.3	D49.7
intercostal	C47.3	C79.89	—	D36.14	D48.2	D49.2
lumbar	C47.6	C79.89	—	D36.17	D48.2	D49.2
Neoplasm, neoplastic						
— continued						
nerve — continued						
median	C47.1-☑	C79.89	—	D36.12	D48.2	D49.2
obturator	C47.2-☑	C79.89	—	D36.13	D48.2	D49.2
oculomotor	C72.59	C79.49	—	D33.3	D43.3	D49.7
olfactory	C47.2-☑	C79.49	—	D33.3	D43.3	D49.7
optic	C72.3-☑	C79.49	—	D33.3	D43.3	D49.7
parasympathetic NEC	C47.9	C79.89	—	D36.10	D48.2	D49.2
peripheral NEC	C47.9	C79.89	—	D36.10	D48.2	D49.2
abdomen	C47.4	C79.89	—	D36.15	D48.2	D49.2
abdominal wall	C47.4	C79.89	—	D36.15	D48.2	D49.2
ankle	C47.2-☑	C79.89	—	D36.13	D48.2	D49.2
antecubital fossa or space	C47.1-☑	C79.89	—	D36.12	D48.2	D49.2
arm	C47.1-☑	C79.89	—	D36.12	D48.2	D49.2
auricle (ear)	C47.0	C79.89	—	D36.11	D48.2	D49.2
axilla	C47.3	C79.89	—	D36.12	D48.2	D49.2
back	C47.6	C79.89	—	D36.17	D48.2	D49.2
buttock	C47.5	C79.89	—	D36.16	D48.2	D49.2
calf	C47.2-☑	C79.89	—	D36.13	D48.2	D49.2
cervical region	C47.0	C79.89	—	D36.11	D48.2	D49.2
cheek	C47.0	C79.89	—	D36.11	D48.2	D49.2
chest (wall)	C47.3	C79.89	—	D36.14	D48.2	D49.2
chin	C47.0	C79.89	—	D36.11	D48.2	D49.2
ear (external)	C47.0	C79.89	—	D36.11	D48.2	D49.2
elbow	C47.1-☑	C79.89	—	D36.12	D48.2	D49.2
extrarectal	C47.5	C79.89	—	D36.16	D48.2	D49.2
extremity	C47.9	C79.89	—	D36.10	D48.2	D49.2
lower	C47.2-☑	C79.89	—	D36.13	D48.2	D49.2
upper	C47.1-☑	C79.89	—	D36.12	D48.2	D49.2
eyelid	C47.0	C79.89	—	D36.11	D48.2	D49.2
face	C47.0	C79.89	—	D36.11	D48.2	D49.2
finger	C47.1-☑	C79.89	—	D36.12	D48.2	D49.2
flank	C47.6	C79.89	—	D36.17	D48.2	D49.2
foot	C47.2-☑	C79.89	—	D36.13	D48.2	D49.2
forearm	C47.1-☑	C79.89	—	D36.12	D48.2	D49.2
forehead	C47.0	C79.89	—	D36.11	D48.2	D49.2
gluteal region	C47.5	C79.89	—	D36.16	D48.2	D49.2
groin	C47.5	C79.89	—	D36.16	D48.2	D49.2
hand	C47.1-☑	C79.89	—	D36.12	D48.2	D49.2
head	C47.0	C79.89	—	D36.11	D48.2	D49.2
heel	C47.2-☑	C79.89	—	D36.13	D48.2	D49.2
hip	C47.2-☑	C79.89	—	D36.13	D48.2	D49.2
infraclavicular region	C47.3	C79.89	—	D36.14	D48.2	D49.2
inguinal (canal) (region)	C47.5	C79.89	—	D36.16	D48.2	D49.2
intrathoracic	C47.3	C79.89	—	D36.14	D48.2	D49.2
ischiorectal fossa	C47.5	C79.89	—	D36.16	D48.2	D49.2
knee	C47.2-☑	C79.89	—	D36.13	D48.2	D49.2
leg	C47.2-☑	C79.89	—	D36.13	D48.2	D49.2
limb NEC	C47.9	C79.89	—	D36.10	D48.2	D49.2
lower	C47.2-☑	C79.89	—	D36.13	D48.2	D49.2
upper	C47.1-☑	C79.89	—	D36.12	D48.2	D49.2
nates	C47.5	C79.89	—	D36.16	D48.2	D49.2
neck	C47.0	C79.89	—	D36.11	D48.2	D49.2
orbit	C69.6-☑	C79.49	—	D31.6-☑	D48.7	D49.2
pararectal	C47.5	C79.89	—	D36.16	D48.2	D49.2
paraurethral	C47.5	C79.89	—	D36.16	D48.2	D49.2
paravaginal	C47.5	C79.89	—	D36.16	D48.2	D49.2
pelvis (floor)	C47.5	C79.89	—	D36.16	D48.2	D49.2
pelvoabdominal	C47.8	C79.89	—	D36.17	D48.2	D49.2
perineum	C47.5	C79.89	—	D36.16	D48.2	D49.2
perirectal (tissue)	C47.5	C79.89	—	D36.16	D48.2	D49.2
periurethral (tissue)	C47.5	C79.89	—	D36.16	D48.2	D49.2
popliteal fossa or space	C47.2-☑	C79.89	—	D36.13	D48.2	D49.2
presacral	C47.5	C79.89	—	D36.16	D48.2	D49.2
pterygoid fossa	C47.0	C79.89	—	D36.11	D48.2	D49.2
rectovaginal septum or wall	C47.5	C79.89	—	D36.16	D48.2	D49.2
rectovesical	C47.5	C79.89	—	D36.16	D48.2	D49.2
sacrococcygeal region	C47.5	C79.89	—	D36.16	D48.2	D49.2

☑ Additional Character Required — Refer to the Tabular List for Character Selection

Neoplasm, neoplastic	Malignant Primary	Malignant Secondary	Ca in situ	Benign	Uncertain Behavior	Unspecified Behavior
— continued						
nerve — continued						
peripheral — continued						
scalp	C47.0	C79.89	—	D36.11	D48.2	D49.2
scapular region	C47.3	C79.89	—	D36.14	D48.2	D49.2
shoulder	C47.1-✓	C79.89	—	D36.12	D48.2	D49.2
submental	C47.0	C79.89	—	D36.11	D48.2	D49.2
supraclavicular region	C47.0	C79.89	—	D36.11	D48.2	D49.2
temple	C47.0	C79.89	—	D36.11	D48.2	D49.2
temporal region	C47.0	C79.89	—	D36.11	D48.2	D49.2
thigh	C47.2-✓	C79.89	—	D36.13	D48.2	D49.2
thoracic (duct) (wall)	C47.3	C79.89	—	D36.14	D48.2	D49.2
thorax	C47.3	C79.89	—	D36.14	D48.2	D49.2
thumb	C47.1-✓	C79.89	—	D36.12	D48.2	D49.2
toe	C47.2-✓	C79.89	—	D36.13	D48.2	D49.2
trunk	C47.6	C79.89	—	D36.17	D48.2	D49.2
umbilicus	C47.4	C79.89	—	D36.15	D48.2	D49.2
vesicorectal	C47.5	C79.89	—	D36.16	D48.2	D49.2
wrist	C47.1-✓	C79.89	—	D36.12	D48.2	D49.2
radial	C47.1-✓	C79.89	—	D36.12	D48.2	D49.2
sacral	C47.5	C79.89	—	D36.16	D48.2	D49.2
sciatic	C47.2-✓	C79.89	—	D36.13	D48.2	D49.2
spinal NEC	C47.9	C79.89	—	D36.10	D48.2	D49.2
accessory	C72.59	C79.49	—	D33.3	D43.3	D49.7
sympathetic NEC — see also Neoplasm, nerve, peripheral	C47.9	C79.89	—	D36.10	D48.2	D49.2
trigeminal	C72.59	C79.49	—	D33.3	D43.3	D49.7
trochlear	C72.59	C79.49	—	D33.3	D43.3	D49.7
ulnar	C47.1-✓	C79.89	—	D36.12	D48.2	D49.2
vagus	C72.59	C79.49	—	D33.3	D43.3	D49.7
nervous system (central)	C72.9	C79.40	—	D33.9	D43.9	D49.7
autonomic — see Neoplasm, nerve, peripheral						
parasympathetic — see Neoplasm, nerve, peripheral						
specified site NEC	—	C79.49	—	D33.7	D43.8	—
sympathetic — see Neoplasm, nerve, peripheral						
nevus — see Nevus						
nipple	C50.0-✓	C79.81	D05.-✓	D24.-✓	—	—
nose, nasal	C76.0	C79.89	D09.8	D36.7	D48.7	D49.89
ala (external) (nasi) — see also Neoplasm, nose, skin	C44.301	C79.2	D04.39	D23.39	D48.5	D49.2
bone	C41.0	C79.51	—	D16.4	D48.0	D49.2
cartilage	C30.0	C78.39	D02.3	D14.0	D38.5	D49.1
cavity	C30.0	C78.39	D02.3	D14.0	D38.5	D49.1
choana	C11.3	C79.89	D00.08	D10.6	D37.05	D49.0
external (skin) — see also Neoplasm, nose, skin	C44.301	C79.2	D04.39	D23.39	D48.5	D49.2
fossa	C30.0	C78.39	D02.3	D14.0	D38.5	D49.1
internal	C30.0	C78.39	D02.3	D14.0	D38.5	D49.1
mucosa	C30.0	C78.39	D02.3	D14.0	D38.5	D49.1
septum	C30.0	C78.39	D02.3	D14.0	D38.5	D49.1
posterior margin	C11.3	C79.89	D00.08	D10.6	D37.05	D49.0
sinus — see Neoplasm, sinus						
skin	C44.301	C79.2	D04.39	D23.39	D48.5	D49.2
basal cell carcinoma	C44.311	—	—	—	—	—
specified type NEC	C44.391	—	—	—	—	—
squamous cell carcinoma	C44.321	—	—	—	—	—
turbinate (mucosa)	C30.0	C78.39	D02.3	D14.0	D38.5	D49.1
bone	C41.0	C79.51	—	D16.4	D48.0	D49.2
vestibule	C30.0	C78.39	D02.3	D14.0	D38.5	D49.1
nostril	C30.0	C78.39	D02.3	D14.0	D38.5	D49.1
nucleus pulposus	C41.2	C79.51	—	D16.6	D48.0	D49.2
occipital bone	C41.0	C79.51	—	D16.4	D48.0	D49.2
lobe or pole, brain	C71.4	C79.31	—	D33.0	D43.0	D49.6
odontogenic — see Neoplasm, jaw, bone						
olfactory nerve or bulb	C72.2-✓	C79.49	—	D33.3	D43.3	D49.7
olive (brain)	C71.7	C79.31	—	D33.1	D43.1	D49.6
omentum	C48.1	C78.6	—	D20.1	D48.4	D49.0
operculum (brain)	C71.0	C79.31	—	D33.0	D43.0	D49.6
optic nerve, chiasm, or tract	C72.3-✓	C79.49	—	D33.3	D43.3	D49.7
oral (cavity)	C06.9	C79.89	D00.00	D10.30	D37.09	D49.0
ill-defined	C14.8	C79.89	D00.00	D10.30	D37.09	D49.0
mucosa	C06.0	C79.89	D00.02	D10.39	D37.09	D49.0
orbit	C69.6-✓	C79.49	D09.2-✓	D31.6-✓	D48.7	D49.89
autonomic nerve	C69.6-✓	C79.49	—	D31.6-✓	D48.7	D49.2
bone	C41.0	C79.51	—	D16.4	D48.0	D49.2
eye	C69.6-✓	C79.49	D09.2-✓	D31.6-✓	D48.7	D49.89
peripheral nerves	C69.6-✓	C79.49	—	D31.6-✓	D48.7	D49.2
soft parts	C69.6-✓	C79.49	D09.2-✓	D31.6-✓	D48.7	D49.89
organ of Zuckerkandl	C75.5	C79.89	—	D35.6	D44.7	D49.7
oropharynx	C10.9	C79.89	D00.08	D10.5	D37.05	D49.0
branchial cleft (vestige)	C10.4	C79.89	D00.08	D10.5	D37.05	D49.0
junctional region	C10.8	C79.89	D00.08	D10.5	D37.05	D49.0
lateral wall	C10.2	C79.89	D00.08	D10.5	D37.05	D49.0
overlapping lesion	C10.8	—	—	—	—	—
pillars or fauces	C09.1	C79.89	D00.08	D10.5	D37.05	D49.0
posterior wall	C10.3	C79.89	D00.08	D10.5	D37.05	D49.0
vallecula	C10.0	C79.89	D00.08	D10.5	D37.05	D49.0
os						
external	C53.1	C79.82	D06.1	D26.0	D39.0	D49.59
internal	C53.0	C79.82	D06.0	D26.0	D39.0	D49.59
ovary	C56.-✓	C79.6-✓	D07.39	D27.-✓	D39.1-✓	D49.59
oviduct	C57.0-✓	C79.82	D07.39	D28.2	D39.8	D49.59
palate	C05.9	C79.89	D00.00	D10.39	D37.09	D49.0
hard	C05.0	C79.89	D00.05	D10.39	D37.09	D49.0
junction of hard and soft palate	C05.9	C79.89	D00.00	D10.39	D37.09	D49.0
overlapping lesions	C05.8	—	—	—	—	—
soft	C05.1	C79.89	D00.04	D10.39	D37.09	D49.0
nasopharyngeal surface	C11.3	C79.89	D00.08	D10.6	D37.05	D49.0
posterior surface	C11.3	C79.89	D00.08	D10.6	D37.05	D49.0
superior surface	C11.3	C79.89	D00.08	D10.6	D37.05	D49.0
palatoglossal arch	C09.1	C79.89	D00.08	D10.5	D37.05	D49.0
palatopharyngeal arch	C09.1	C79.89	D00.00	D10.5	D37.09	D49.0
pallium	C71.0	C79.31	—	D33.0	D43.0	D49.6
palpebra	C44.10-✓	C79.2	D04.1-✓	D23.1-✓	D48.5	D49.2
basal cell carcinoma	C44.11-✓	—	—	—	—	—
sebaceous cell	C44.13-✓	—	—	—	—	—
specified type NEC	C44.19-✓	—	—	—	—	—
squamous cell carcinoma	C44.12-✓	—	—	—	—	—
pancreas	C25.9	C78.89	D01.7	D13.6	D37.8	D49.0
body	C25.1	C78.89	D01.7	D13.6	D37.8	D49.0
duct (of Santorini) (of Wirsung)	C25.3	C78.89	D01.7	D13.6	D37.8	D49.0
ectopic tissue	C25.7	C78.89	—	D13.6	D37.8	D49.0
head	C25.0	C78.89	D01.7	D13.6	D37.8	D49.0
islet cells	C25.4	C78.89	D01.7	D13.7	D37.8	D49.0
neck	C25.7	C78.89	D01.7	D13.6	D37.8	D49.0

✓ Additional Character Required — Refer to the Tabular List for Character Selection

Neoplasm, pancreas

Neoplasm, neoplastic	Malignant Primary	Malignant Secondary	Ca in situ	Benign	Uncertain Behavior	Unspecified Behavior
pancreas — *continued*						
overlapping lesion	C25.8	—	—	—	—	—
tail	C25.2	C78.89	D01.7	D13.6	D37.8	D49.0
para-aortic body	C75.5	C79.89	—	D35.6	D44.7	D49.7
paraganglion NEC	C75.5	C79.89	—	D35.6	D44.7	D49.7
parametrium	C57.3	C79.82	—	D28.2	D39.8	D49.59
paranephric	C48.0	C78.6	—	D20.0	D48.3	D49.0
pararectal	C76.3	C79.89	—	D36.7	D48.7	D49.89
parasagittal (region)	C76.0	C79.89	D09.8	D36.7	D48.7	D49.89
parasellar	C72.9	C79.49	—	D33.9	D43.8	D49.7
parathyroid (gland)	C75.0	C79.89	D09.3	D35.1	D44.2	D49.7
paraurethral	C76.3	C79.89	—	D36.7	D48.7	D49.89
gland	C68.1	C79.19	D09.19	D30.8	D41.8	D49.59
paravaginal	C76.3	C79.89	—	D36.7	D48.7	D49.89
parenchyma, kidney	C64.- ☑	C79.0- ☑	D09.19	D30.0- ☑	D41.0- ☑	D49.51- ☑
parietal						
bone	C41.0	C79.51	—	D16.4	D48.0	D49.2
lobe, brain	C71.3	C79.31	—	D33.0	D43.0	D49.6
paroophoron	C57.1- ☑	C79.82	D07.39	D28.2	D39.8	D49.59
parotid (duct) (gland)	C07	C79.89	D00.00	D11.0	D37.030	D49.0
parovarium	C57.1- ☑	C79.82	D07.39	D28.2	D39.8	D49.59
patella	C40.2- ☑	C79.51	—	—	—	—
peduncle, cerebral	C71.7	C79.31	—	D33.1	D43.1	D49.6
pelvirectal junction	C19	C78.5	D01.1	D12.7	D37.5	D49.0
pelvis, pelvic	C76.3	C79.89	D09.8	D36.7	D48.7	D49.89
bone	C41.4	C79.51	—	D16.8	D48.0	D49.2
floor	C76.3	C79.89	D09.8	D36.7	D48.7	D49.89
renal	C65.- ☑	C79.0- ☑	D09.19	D30.1- ☑	D41.1- ☑	D49.51- ☑
viscera	C76.3	C79.89	D09.8	D36.7	D48.7	D49.89
wall	C76.3	C79.89	D09.8	D36.7	D48.7	D49.89
pelvo-abdominal	C76.8	C79.89	D09.8	D36.7	D48.7	D49.89
penis	C60.9	C79.82	D07.4	D29.0	D40.8	D49.59
body	C60.2	C79.82	D07.4	D29.0	D40.8	D49.59
corpus (cavernosum)	C60.2	C79.82	D07.4	D29.0	D40.8	D49.59
glans	C60.1	C79.82	D07.4	D29.0	D40.8	D49.59
overlapping sites	C60.8	—	—	—	—	—
skin NEC	C60.9	C79.82	D07.4	D29.0	D40.8	D49.59
periadrenal (tissue)	C48.0	C78.6	—	D20.0	D48.3	D49.0
perianal (skin) — *see also* Neoplasm, anus, skin	C44.500	C79.2	D04.5	D23.5	D48.5	D49.2
pericardium	C38.0	C79.89	—	D15.1	D48.7	D49.89
perinephric	C48.0	C78.6	—	D20.0	D48.3	D49.0
perineum	C76.3	C79.89	D09.8	D36.7	D48.7	D49.89
periodontal tissue NEC	C03.9	C79.89	D00.03	D10.39	D37.09	D49.0
periosteum — *see* Neoplasm, bone						
peripancreatic	C48.0	C78.6	—	D20.0	D48.3	D49.0
peripheral nerve NEC	C47.9	C79.89	—	D36.10	D48.2	D49.2
perirectal (tissue)	C76.3	C79.89	—	D36.7	D48.7	D49.89
perirenal (tissue)	C48.0	C78.6	—	D20.0	D48.3	D49.0
peritoneum, peritoneal (cavity)	C48.2	C78.6	—	D20.1	D48.4	D49.0
benign mesothelial tissue — *see* Mesothelioma, benign						
overlapping lesion with digestive organs	C48.8	—	—	—	—	—
	C26.9	—	—	—	—	—
parietal	C48.1	C78.6	—	D20.1	D48.4	D49.0
pelvic	C48.1	C78.6	—	D20.1	D48.4	D49.0
specified part NEC	C48.1	C78.6	—	D20.1	D48.4	D49.0
peritonsillar (tissue)	C76.0	C79.89	D09.8	D36.7	D48.7	D49.89
periurethral tissue	C76.3	C79.89	—	D36.7	D48.7	D49.89
phalanges						
foot	C40.3- ☑	C79.51	—	D16.3- ☑	—	—

Neoplasm, neoplastic	Malignant Primary	Malignant Secondary	Ca in situ	Benign	Uncertain Behavior	Unspecified Behavior
phalanges — *continued*						
hand	C40.1- ☑	C79.51	—	D16.1- ☑	—	—
pharynx, pharyngeal	C14.0	C79.89	D00.08	D10.9	D37.05	D49.0
bursa	C11.1	C79.89	D00.08	D10.6	D37.05	D49.0
fornix	C11.3	C79.89	D00.08	D10.6	D37.05	D49.0
recess	C11.2	C79.89	D00.08	D10.6	D37.05	D49.0
region	C14.0	C79.89	D00.08	D10.9	D37.05	D49.0
tonsil	C11.1	C79.89	D00.08	D10.6	D37.05	D49.0
wall (lateral) (posterior)	C14.0	C79.89	D00.08	D10.9	D37.05	D49.0
pia mater	C70.9	C79.40	—	D32.9	D42.9	D49.7
cerebral	C70.0	C79.32	—	D32.0	D42.0	D49.7
cranial	C70.0	C79.32	—	D32.0	D42.0	D49.7
spinal	C70.1	C79.49	—	D32.1	D42.1	D49.7
pillars of fauces	C09.1	C79.89	D00.08	D10.5	D37.05	D49.0
pineal (body) (gland)	C75.3	C79.89	D09.3	D35.4	D44.5	D49.7
pinna (ear) NEC — *see also* Neoplasm, skin, ear	C44.20- ☑	C79.2	D04.2- ☑	D23.2- ☑	D48.5	D49.2
piriform fossa or sinus	C12	C79.89	D00.08	D10.7	D37.05	D49.0
pituitary (body) (fossa) (gland) (lobe)	C75.1	C79.89	D09.3	D35.2	D44.3	D49.7
placenta	C58	C79.82	D07.0	D26.7	D39.2	D49.59
pleura, pleural (cavity)	C38.4	C78.2	—	D19.0	D38.2	D49.1
overlapping lesion with heart or mediastinum	C38.8	—	—	—	—	—
parietal	C38.4	C78.2	—	D19.0	D38.2	D49.1
visceral	C38.4	C78.2	—	D19.0	D38.2	D49.1
plexus						
brachial	C47.1- ☑	C79.89	—	D36.12	D48.2	D49.2
cervical	C47.0	C79.89	—	D36.11	D48.2	D49.2
choroid	C71.5	C79.31	—	D33.0	D43.0	D49.6
lumbosacral	C47.5	C79.89	—	D36.16	D48.2	D49.2
sacral	C47.5	C79.89	—	D36.16	D48.2	D49.2
pluriendocrine	C75.8	C79.89	D09.3	D35.7	D44.9	D49.7
pole						
frontal	C71.1	C79.31	—	D33.0	D43.0	D49.6
occipital	C71.4	C79.31	—	D33.0	D43.0	D49.6
pons (varolii)	C71.7	C79.31	—	D33.1	D43.1	D49.6
popliteal fossa or space	C76.5- ☑	C79.89	D04.7- ☑	D36.7	D48.7	D49.89
postcricoid (region)	C13.0	C79.89	D00.08	D10.7	D37.05	D49.0
posterior fossa (cranial)	C71.9	C79.31	—	D33.2	D43.2	D49.6
postnasal space	C11.9	C79.89	D00.08	D10.6	D37.05	D49.0
prepuce	C60.0	C79.82	D07.4	D29.0	D40.8	D49.59
prepylorus	C16.4	C78.89	D00.2	D13.1	D37.1	D49.0
presacral (region)	C76.3	C79.89	—	D36.7	D48.7	D49.89
prostate (gland)	C61	C79.82	D07.5	D29.1	D40.0	D49.59
utricle	C68.0	C79.19	D09.19	D30.4	D41.3	D49.59
pterygoid fossa	C49.0	C79.89	—	D21.0	D48.1- ☑	D49.2
pubic bone	C41.4	C79.51	—	D16.8	D48.0	D49.2
pudenda, pudendum (female)	C51.9	C79.82	D07.1	D28.0	D39.8	D49.59
pulmonary — *see also* Neoplasm, lung	C34.9- ☑	C78.0- ☑	D02.2- ☑	D14.3- ☑	D38.1	D49.1
putamen	C71.0	C79.31	—	D33.0	D43.0	D49.6
pyloric						
antrum	C16.3	C78.89	D00.2	D13.1	D37.1	D49.0
canal	C16.4	C78.89	D00.2	D13.1	D37.1	D49.0
pylorus	C16.4	C78.89	D00.2	D13.1	D37.1	D49.0
pyramid (brain)	C71.7	C79.31	—	D33.1	D43.1	D49.6
pyriform fossa or sinus	C12	C79.89	D00.08	D10.7	D37.05	D49.0
radius (any part)	C40.0- ☑	C79.51	—	D16.0- ☑	—	—
Rathke's pouch	C75.1	C79.89	D09.3	D35.2	D44.3	D49.7
rectosigmoid (junction)	C19	C78.5	D01.1	D12.7	D37.5	D49.0
overlapping lesion with anus or rectum	C21.8	—	—	—	—	—
rectouterine pouch	C48.1	C78.6	—	D20.1	D48.4	D49.0

☑ **Additional Character Required** — Refer to the Tabular List for Character Selection

Neoplasm, neoplastic — continued	Malignant Primary	Malignant Secondary	Ca in situ	Benign	Uncertain Behavior	Unspecified Behavior
rectovaginal septum or wall	C76.3	C79.89	D09.8	D36.7	D48.7	D49.89
rectovesical septum	C76.3	C79.89	D09.8	D36.7	D48.7	D49.89
rectum (ampulla)	C20	C78.5	D01.2	D12.8	D37.5	D49.0
and colon	C19	C78.5	D01.1	D12.7	D37.5	D49.0
overlapping lesion with anus or rectosigmoid junction	C21.8	—	—	—	—	—
renal	C64.-☑	C79.0-☑	D09.19	D30.0-☑	D41.0-☑	D49.51-☑
calyx	C65.-☑	C79.0-☑	D09.19	D30.1-☑	D41.1-☑	D49.51-☑
hilus	C65.-☑	C79.0-☑	D09.19	D30.1-☑	D41.1-☑	D49.51-☑
parenchyma	C64.-☑	C79.0-☑	D09.19	D30.0-☑	D41.0-☑	D49.51-☑
pelvis	C65.-☑	C79.0-☑	D09.19	D30.1-☑	D41.1-☑	D49.51-☑
respiratory organs or system NEC	C39.9	C78.30	D02.4	D14.4	D38.6	D49.1
tract NEC	C39.9	C78.30	D02.4	D14.4	D38.5	D49.1
upper	C39.0	C78.30	D02.4	D14.4	D38.5	D49.1
retina	C69.2-☑	C79.49	D09.2-☑	D31.2-☑	D48.7	D49.81
retro-orbital	C76.0	C79.49	D09.8	D36.7	D48.7	D49.89
retrobulbar	C69.6-☑	C79.49	—	D31.6-☑	D48.7	D49.89
retrocecal	C48.0	C78.6	—	D20.0	D48.3	D49.0
retromolar (area) (triangle) (trigone)	C06.2	C79.89	D00.00	D10.39	D37.09	D49.0
retroperitoneal (space) (tissue)	C48.0	C78.6	—	D20.0	D48.3	D49.0
retroperitoneum	C48.0	C78.6	—	D20.0	D48.3	D49.0
retropharyngeal	C14.0	C79.89	D00.08	D10.9	D37.05	D49.0
retrovesical (septum)	C76.3	C79.89	D09.8	D36.7	D48.7	D49.89
rhinencephalon	C71.0	C79.31	—	D33.0	D43.0	D49.6
rib	C41.3	C79.51	—	D16.7	D48.0	D49.2
Rosenmuller's fossa	C11.2	C79.89	D00.08	D10.6	D37.05	D49.0
round ligament	C57.2-☑	C79.82	—	D28.2	D39.8	D49.59
sacrococcyx, sacrococcygeal region	C41.4	C79.51	—	D16.8	D48.0	D49.2
	C76.3	C79.89	D09.8	D36.7	D48.7	D49.89
sacrouterine ligament	C57.3	C79.82	—	D28.2	D39.8	D49.59
sacrum, sacral (vertebra)	C41.4	C79.51	—	D16.8	D48.0	D49.2
salivary gland or duct (major)	C08.9	C79.89	D00.00	D11.9	D37.039	D49.0
minor NEC	C06.9	C79.89	D00.00	D10.39	D37.04	D49.0
overlapping lesion	C08.9	—	—	—	—	—
parotid	C07	C79.89	D00.00	D11.0	D37.030	D49.0
pluriglandular	C08.9	C79.89	D00.00	D11.9	D37.039	D49.0
sublingual	C08.1	C79.89	D00.00	D11.7	D37.031	D49.0
submandibular	C08.0	C79.89	D00.00	D11.7	D37.032	D49.0
submaxillary	C08.0	C79.89	D00.00	D11.7	D37.032	D49.0
salpinx (uterine)	C57.0-☑	C79.82	D07.39	D28.2	D39.8	D49.59
Santorini's duct	C25.3	C78.89	D01.7	D13.6	D37.8	D49.0
scalp	C44.40	C79.2	D04.4	D23.4	D48.5	D49.2
basal cell carcinoma	C44.41	—	—	—	—	—
specified type NEC	C44.49	—	—	—	—	—
squamous cell carcinoma	C44.42	—	—	—	—	—
scapula (any part)	C40.0-☑	C79.51	—	D16.0-☑	—	—
scapular region	C76.1	C79.89	D09.8	D36.7	D48.7	D49.89
scar NEC — see also Neoplasm, skin, by site	C44.90	C79.2	D04.9	D23.9	D48.5	D49.2
sciatic nerve	C47.2-☑	C79.89	—	D36.13	D48.2	D49.2
sclera	C69.4-☑	C79.49	D09.2-☑	D31.4-☑	D48.7	D49.89
scrotum (skin)	C63.2	C79.82	D07.61	D29.4	D40.8	D49.59
sebaceous gland — see Neoplasm, skin						
sella turcica	C75.1	C79.89	D09.3	D35.2	D44.3	D49.7
bone	C41.0	C79.51	—	D16.4	D48.0	D49.2
semilunar cartilage (knee)	C40.2-☑	C79.51	—	D16.2-☑	D48.0	D49.2
seminal vesicle	C63.7	C79.82	D07.69	D29.8	D40.8	D49.59
septum nasal	C30.0	C78.39	D02.3	D14.0	D38.5	D49.1

Neoplasm, neoplastic — continued	Malignant Primary	Malignant Secondary	Ca in situ	Benign	Uncertain Behavior	Unspecified Behavior
septum — continued nasal — continued posterior margin	C11.3	C79.89	D00.08	D10.6	D37.05	D49.0
rectovaginal	C76.3	C79.89	D09.8	D36.7	D48.7	D49.89
rectovesical	C76.3	C79.89	D09.8	D36.7	D48.7	D49.89
urethrovaginal	C57.9	C79.82	D07.30	D28.9	D39.9	D49.59
vesicovaginal	C57.9	C79.82	D07.30	D28.9	D39.9	D49.59
shoulder NEC	C76.4-☑	C79.89	D04.6-☑	D36.7	D48.7	D49.89
sigmoid flexure (lower) (upper)	C18.7	C78.5	D01.0	D12.5	D37.4	D49.0
sinus (accessory)	C31.9	C78.39	D02.3	D14.0	D38.5	D49.1
bone (any)	C41.0	C79.51	—	D16.4	D48.0	D49.2
ethmoidal	C31.1	C78.39	D02.3	D14.0	D38.5	D49.1
frontal	C31.2	C78.39	D02.3	D14.0	D38.5	D49.1
maxillary	C31.0	C78.39	D02.3	D14.0	D38.5	D49.1
nasal, paranasal NEC	C31.9	C78.39	D02.3	D14.0	D38.5	D49.1
overlapping lesion	C31.8	—	—	—	—	—
pyriform	C12	C79.89	D00.08	D10.7	D37.05	D49.0
sphenoid	C31.3	C78.39	D02.3	D14.0	D38.5	D49.1
skeleton, skeletal NEC	C41.9	C79.51	—	D16.9	D48.0	D49.2
Skene's gland	C68.1	C79.19	D09.19	D30.8	D41.8	D49.59
skin NOS	C44.90	C79.2	D04.9	D23.9	D48.5	D49.2
abdominal wall	C44.509	C79.2	D04.5	D23.5	D48.5	D49.2
basal cell carcinoma	C44.519	—	—	—	—	—
specified type NEC	C44.599	—	—	—	—	—
squamous cell carcinoma	C44.529	—	—	—	—	—
ala nasi — see also Neoplasm, nose, skin	C44.301	C79.2	D04.39	D23.39	D48.5	D49.2
ankle — see also Neoplasm, skin, limb, lower	C44.70-☑	C79.2	D04.7-☑	D23.7-☑	D48.5	D49.2
antecubital space — see also Neoplasm, skin, limb, upper	C44.60-☑	C79.2	D04.6-☑	D23.6-☑	D48.5	D49.2
anus	C44.500	C79.2	D04.5	D23.5	D48.5	D49.2
basal cell carcinoma	C44.510	—	—	—	—	—
specified type NEC	C44.590	—	—	—	—	—
squamous cell carcinoma	C44.520	—	—	—	—	—
arm — see also Neoplasm, skin, limb, upper	C44.60-☑	C79.2	D04.6-☑	D23.6-☑	D48.5	D49.2
auditory canal (external) — see also Neoplasm, skin, ear	C44.20-☑	C79.2	D04.2-☑	D23.2-☑	D48.5	D49.2
auricle (ear) — see also Neoplasm, skin, ear	C44.20-☑	C79.2	D04.2-☑	D23.2-☑	D48.5	D49.2
auricular canal (external) — see also Neoplasm, skin, ear	C44.20-☑	C79.2	D04.2-☑	D23.2-☑	D48.5	D49.2
axilla, axillary fold — see also Neoplasm, skin, trunk	C44.509	C79.2	D04.5	D23.5	D48.5	D49.2
back — see also Neoplasm, skin, trunk	C44.509	C79.2	D04.5	D23.5	D48.5	D49.2
basal cell carcinoma	C44.91	—	—	—	—	—
breast	C44.501	C79.2	D04.5	D23.5	D48.5	D49.2
basal cell carcinoma	C44.511	—	—	—	—	—
specified type NEC	C44.591	—	—	—	—	—
squamous cell carcinoma	C44.521	—	—	—	—	—

☑ Additional Character Required — Refer to the Tabular List for Character Selection

Neoplasm, skin NOS

	Malignant Primary	Malignant Secondary	Ca in situ	Benign	Uncertain Behavior	Unspecified Behavior
Neoplasm, neoplastic — *continued*						
skin — *continued*						
brow — *see also* Neoplasm, skin, face	C44.309	C79.2	D04.39	D23.39	D48.5	D49.2
buttock — *see also* Neoplasm, skin, trunk	C44.509	C79.2	D04.5	D23.5	D48.5	D49.2
calf — *see also* Neoplasm, skin, limb, lower	C44.70-☑	C79.2	D04.7-☑	D23.7-☑	D48.5	D49.2
canthus (eye) (inner) (outer)	C44.10-☑	C79.2	D04.1-☑	D23.1-☑	D48.5	D49.2
basal cell carcinoma	C44.11-☑	—	—	—	—	—
sebaceous cell	C44.13-☑	—	—	—	—	—
specified type NEC	C44.19-☑	—	—	—	—	—
squamous cell carcinoma	C44.12-☑	—	—	—	—	—
cervical region — *see also* Neoplasm, skin, neck	C44.40	C79.2	D04.4	D23.4	D48.5	D49.2
cheek (external) — *see also* Neoplasm, skin, face	C44.309	C79.2	D04.39	D23.39	D48.5	D49.2
chest (wall) — *see also* Neoplasm, skin, trunk	C44.509	C79.2	D04.5	D23.5	D48.5	D49.2
chin — *see also* Neoplasm, skin, face	C44.309	C79.2	D04.39	D23.39	D48.5	D49.2
clavicular area — *see also* Neoplasm, skin, trunk	C44.509	C79.2	D04.5	D23.5	D48.5	D49.2
clitoris	C51.2	C79.82	D07.1	D28.0	D39.8	D49.59
columnella — *see also* Neoplasm, skin, face	C44.309	C79.2	D04.39	D23.39	D48.5	D49.2
concha — *see also* Neoplasm, skin, ear	C44.20-☑	C79.2	D04.2-☑	D23.2-☑	D48.5	D49.2
ear (external)	C44.20-☑	C79.2	D04.2-☑	D23.2-☑	D48.5	D49.2
basal cell carcinoma	C44.21-☑	—	—	—	—	—
specified type NEC	C44.29-☑	—	—	—	—	—
squamous cell carcinoma	C44.22-☑	—	—	—	—	—
elbow — *see also* Neoplasm, skin, limb, upper	C44.60-☑	C79.2	D04.6-☑	D23.6-☑	D48.5	D49.2
eyebrow — *see also* Neoplasm, skin, face	C44.309	C79.2	D04.39	D23.39	D48.5	D49.2
eyelid	C44.10-☑	C79.2	D04.1-☑	D23.1-☑	D48.5	D49.2
basal cell carcinoma	C44.11-☑	—	—	—	—	—
sebaceous cell	C44.13-☑	—	—	—	—	—
specified type NEC	C44.19-☑	—	—	—	—	—
squamous cell carcinoma	C44.12-☑	—	—	—	—	—
face NOS	C44.300	C79.2	D04.30	D23.30	D48.5	D49.2
basal cell carcinoma	C44.310	—	—	—	—	—
specified type NEC	C44.390	—	—	—	—	—
squamous cell carcinoma	C44.320	—	—	—	—	—
female genital organs (external)	C51.9	C79.82	D07.1	D28.0	D39.8	D49.59
clitoris	C51.2	C79.82	D07.1	D28.0	D39.8	D49.59
labium NEC	C51.9	C79.82	D07.1	D28.0	D39.8	D49.59
majus	C51.0	C79.82	D07.1	D28.0	D39.8	D49.59
minus	C51.1	C79.82	D07.1	D28.0	D39.8	D49.59
pudendum	C51.9	C79.82	D07.1	D28.0	D39.8	D49.59
vulva	C51.9	C79.82	D07.1	D28.0	D39.8	D49.59
finger — *see also* Neoplasm, skin, limb, upper	C44.60-☑	C79.2	D04.6-☑	D23.6-☑	D48.5	D49.2

	Malignant Primary	Malignant Secondary	Ca in situ	Benign	Uncertain Behavior	Unspecified Behavior
Neoplasm, neoplastic — *continued*						
skin — *continued*						
flank — *see also* Neoplasm, skin, trunk	C44.509	C79.2	D04.5	D23.5	D48.5	D49.2
foot — *see also* Neoplasm, skin, limb, lower	C44.70-☑	C79.2	D04.7-☑	D23.7-☑	D48.5	D49.2
forearm — *see also* Neoplasm, skin, limb, upper	C44.60-☑	C79.2	D04.6-☑	D23.6-☑	D48.5	D49.2
forehead — *see also* Neoplasm, skin, face	C44.309	C79.2	D04.39	D23.39	D48.5	D49.2
glabella — *see also* Neoplasm, skin, face	C44.309	C79.2	D04.39	D23.39	D48.5	D49.2
gluteal region — *see also* Neoplasm, skin, trunk	C44.509	C79.2	D04.5	D23.5	D48.5	D49.2
groin — *see also* Neoplasm, skin, trunk	C44.509	C79.2	D04.5	D23.5	D48.5	D49.2
hand — *see also* Neoplasm, skin, limb, upper	C44.60-☑	C79.2	D04.6-☑	D23.6-☑	D48.5	D49.2
head NEC — *see also* Neoplasm, skin, scalp	C44.40	C79.2	D04.4	D23.4	D48.5	D49.2
heel — *see also* Neoplasm, skin, limb, lower	C44.70-☑	C79.2	D04.7-☑	D23.7-☑	D48.5	D49.2
helix — *see also* Neoplasm, skin, ear	C44.20-☑	C79.2	D04.2-☑	D23.2-☑	D48.5	D49.2
hip — *see also* Neoplasm, skin, limb, lower	C44.70-☑	C79.2	D04.7-☑	D23.7-☑	D48.5	D49.2
infraclavicular region — *see also* Neoplasm, skin, trunk	C44.509	C79.2	D04.5	D23.5	D48.5	D49.2
inguinal region — *see also* Neoplasm, skin, trunk	C44.509	C79.2	D04.5	D23.5	D48.5	D49.2
jaw — *see also* Neoplasm, skin, face	C44.309	C79.2	D04.39	D23.39	D48.5	D49.2
Kaposi's sarcoma — *see* Kaposi's, sarcoma, skin						
knee — *see also* Neoplasm, skin, limb, lower	C44.70-☑	C79.2	D04.7-☑	D23.7-☑	D48.5	D49.2
labia						
majora	C51.0	C79.82	D07.1	D28.0	D39.8	D49.59
minora	C51.1	C79.82	D07.1	D28.0	D39.8	D49.59
leg — *see also* Neoplasm, skin, limb, lower	C44.70-☑	C79.2	D04.7-☑	D23.7-☑	D48.5	D49.2
lid (lower) (upper)	C44.10-☑	C79.2	D04.1-☑	D23.1-☑	D48.5	D49.2
basal cell carcinoma	C44.11-☑	—	—	—	—	—
sebaceous cell	C44.13-☑	—	—	—	—	—
specified type NEC	C44.19-☑	—	—	—	—	—
squamous cell carcinoma	C44.12-☑	—	—	—	—	—
limb NEC	C44.90	C79.2	D04.9	D23.9	D48.5	D49.2
basal cell carcinoma	C44.91	—	—	—	—	—
lower	C44.70-☑	C79.2	D04.7-☑	D23.7-☑	D48.5	D49.2
basal cell carcinoma	C44.71-☑	—	—	—	—	—
specified type NEC	C44.79-☑	—	—	—	—	—
squamous cell carcinoma	C44.72-☑	—	—	—	—	—
upper	C44.60-☑	C79.2	D04.6-☑	D23.6-☑	D48.5	D49.2
basal cell carcinoma	C44.61-☑	—	—	—	—	—

☑ **Additional Character Required** — Refer to the Tabular List for Character Selection

Neoplasm, neoplastic — continued	Malignant Primary	Malignant Secondary	Ca in situ	Benign	Uncertain Behavior	Unspecified Behavior
skin — continued						
limb — continued						
upper — continued						
specified type NEC	C44.69-☑	—	—	—	—	—
squamous cell carcinoma	C44.62-☑	—	—	—	—	—
lip (lower) (upper)	C44.00	C79.2	D04.0	D23.0	D48.5	D49.2
basal cell carcinoma	C44.01	—	—	—	—	—
specified type NEC	C44.09	—	—	—	—	—
squamous cell carcinoma	C44.02	—	—	—	—	—
male genital organs	C63.9	C79.82	D07.60	D29.9	D40.8	D49.59
penis	C60.9	C79.82	D07.4	D29.0	D40.8	D49.59
prepuce	C60.0	C79.82	D07.4	D29.0	D40.8	D49.59
scrotum	C63.2	C79.82	D07.61	D29.4	D40.8	D49.59
mastectomy site (skin) — see also Neoplasm, skin, breast	C44.501	C79.2	—	—	—	—
specified as breast tissue	C50.8-☑	C79.81	—	—	—	—
meatus, acoustic (external) — see also Neoplasm, skin, ear	C44.20-☑	C79.2	D04.2-☑	D23.2-☑	D48.5	D49.2
melanotic — see Melanoma						
Merkel cell — see Carcinoma, Merkel cell						
nates — see also Neoplasm, skin, trunk	C44.509	C79.2	D04.5	D23.5	D48.5	D49.2
neck	C44.40	C79.2	D04.4	D23.4	D48.5	D49.2
basal cell carcinoma	C44.41	—	—	—	—	—
specified type NEC	C44.49	—	—	—	—	—
squamous cell carcinoma	C44.42	—	—	—	—	—
nevus — see Nevus, skin						
nose (external) — see also Neoplasm, nose, skin	C44.301	C79.2	D04.39	D23.39	D48.5	D49.2
overlapping lesion	C44.80	—	—	—	—	—
basal cell carcinoma	C44.81	—	—	—	—	—
specified type NEC	C44.89	—	—	—	—	—
squamous cell carcinoma	C44.82	—	—	—	—	—
palm — see also Neoplasm, skin, limb, upper	C44.60-☑	C79.2	D04.6-☑	D23.6-☑	D48.5	D49.2
palpebra	C44.10-☑	C79.2	D04.1-☑	D23.1-☑	D48.5	D49.2
basal cell carcinoma	C44.11-☑	—	—	—	—	—
sebaceous cell	C44.13-☑	—	—	—	—	—
specified type NEC	C44.19-☑	—	—	—	—	—
squamous cell carcinoma	C44.12-☑	—	—	—	—	—
penis NEC	C60.9	C79.82	D07.4	D29.0	D40.8	D49.59
perianal — see also Neoplasm, skin, anus	C44.500	C79.2	D04.5	D23.5	D48.5	D49.2
perineum — see also Neoplasm, skin, anus	C44.500	C79.2	D04.5	D23.5	D48.5	D49.2
pinna — see also Neoplasm, skin, ear	C44.20-☑	C79.2	D04.2-☑	D23.2-☑	D48.5	D49.2
plantar — see also Neoplasm, skin, limb, lower	C44.70-☑	C79.2	D04.7-☑	D23.7-☑	D48.5	D49.2
popliteal fossa or space — see also Neoplasm, skin, limb, lower	C44.70-☑	C79.2	D04.7-☑	D23.7-☑	D48.5	D49.2
prepuce	C60.0	C79.82	D07.4	D29.0	D40.8	D49.59
pubes — see also Neoplasm, skin, trunk	C44.509	C79.2	D04.5	D23.5	D48.5	D49.2
sacrococcygeal region — see also Neoplasm, skin, trunk	C44.509	C79.2	D04.5	D23.5	D48.5	D49.2
scalp	C44.40	C79.2	D04.4	D23.4	D48.5	D49.2
basal cell carcinoma	C44.41	—	—	—	—	—
specified type NEC	C44.49	—	—	—	—	—
squamous cell carcinoma	C44.42	—	—	—	—	—
scapular region — see also Neoplasm, skin, trunk	C44.509	C79.2	D04.5	D23.5	D48.5	D49.2
scrotum	C63.2	C79.82	D07.61	D29.4	D40.8	D49.59
shoulder — see also Neoplasm, skin, limb, upper	C44.60-☑	C79.2	D04.6-☑	D23.6-☑	D48.5	D49.2
sole (foot) — see also Neoplasm, skin, limb, lower	C44.70-☑	C79.2	D04.7-☑	D23.7-☑	D48.5	D49.2
specified sites NEC	C44.80	C79.2	D04.8	D23.9	D48.5	D49.2
basal cell carcinoma	C44.81	—	—	—	—	—
specified type NEC	C44.89	—	—	—	—	—
squamous cell carcinoma	C44.82	—	—	—	—	—
specified type NEC	C44.99	—	—	—	—	—
squamous cell carcinoma	C44.92	—	—	—	—	—
submammary fold — see also Neoplasm, skin, trunk	C44.509	C79.2	D04.5	D23.5	D48.5	D49.2
supraclavicular region — see also Neoplasm, skin, neck	C44.40	C79.2	D04.4	D23.4	D48.5	D49.2
temple — see also Neoplasm, skin, face	C44.309	C79.2	D04.39	D23.39	D48.5	D49.2
thigh — see also Neoplasm, skin, limb, lower	C44.70-☑	C79.2	D04.7-☑	D23.7-☑	D48.5	D49.2
thoracic wall — see also Neoplasm, skin, trunk	C44.509	C79.2	D04.5	D23.5	D48.5	D49.2
thumb — see also Neoplasm, skin, limb, upper	C44.60-☑	C79.2	D04.6-☑	D23.6-☑	D48.5	D49.2
toe — see also Neoplasm, skin, limb, lower	C44.70-☑	C79.2	D04.7-☑	D23.7-☑	D48.5	D49.2
tragus — see also Neoplasm, skin, ear	C44.20-☑	C79.2	D04.2-☑	D23.2-☑	D48.5	D49.2
trunk	C44.509	C79.2	D04.5	D23.5	D48.5	D49.2
basal cell carcinoma	C44.519	—	—	—	—	—
specified type NEC	C44.599	—	—	—	—	—
squamous cell carcinoma	C44.529	—	—	—	—	—
umbilicus — see also Neoplasm, skin, trunk	C44.509	C79.2	D04.5	D23.5	D48.5	D49.2
vulva	C51.9	C79.82	D07.1	D28.0	D39.8	D49.59
overlapping lesion	C51.8	—	—	—	—	—

☑ Additional Character Required — Refer to the Tabular List for Character Selection

Neoplasm, skin NOS

	Malignant Primary	Malignant Secondary	Ca in situ	Benign	Uncertain Behavior	Unspecified Behavior
Neoplasm, neoplastic — continued						
skin — continued						
wrist — see also Neoplasm, skin, limb, upper	C44.60-☑	C79.2	D04.6-☑	D23.6-☑	D48.5	D49.2
skull	C41.0	C79.51	—	D16.4	D48.0	D49.2
soft parts or tissues — see Neoplasm, connective tissue						
specified site NEC	C76.8	C79.89	D09.8	D36.7	D48.7	D49.89
spermatic cord	C63.1-☑	C79.82	D07.69	D29.8	D40.8	D49.59
sphenoid	C31.3	C78.39	D02.3	D14.0	D38.5	D49.1
bone	C41.0	C79.51	—	D16.4	D48.0	D49.2
sinus	C31.3	C78.39	D02.3	D14.0	D38.5	D49.1
sphincter						
anal	C21.1	C78.5	D01.3	D12.9	D37.8	D49.0
of Oddi	C24.0	C78.89	D01.5	D13.5	D37.6	D49.0
spine, spinal (column)	C41.2	C79.51	—	D16.6	D48.0	D49.2
bulb	C71.7	C79.31	—	D33.1	D43.1	D49.6
coccyx	C41.4	C79.51	—	D16.8	D48.0	D49.2
cord (cervical) (lumbar) (sacral) (thoracic)	C72.0	C79.49	—	D33.4	D43.4	D49.7
dura mater	C70.1	C79.49	—	D32.1	D42.1	D49.7
lumbosacral	C41.2	C79.51	—	D16.6	D48.0	D49.2
marrow NEC	C96.9	C79.52	—	—	D47.9	D49.89
membrane	C70.1	C79.49	—	D32.1	D42.1	D49.7
meninges	C70.1	C79.49	—	D32.1	D42.1	D49.7
nerve (root)	C47.9	C79.89	—	D36.10	D48.2	D49.2
pia mater	C70.1	C79.49	—	D32.1	D42.1	D49.7
root	C47.9	C79.89	—	D36.10	D48.2	D49.2
sacrum	C41.4	C79.51	—	D16.8	D48.0	D49.2
spleen, splenic NEC	C26.1	C78.89	D01.7	D13.99	D37.8	D49.0
flexure (colon)	C18.5	C78.5	D01.0	D12.3	D37.4	D49.0
stem, brain	C71.7	C79.31	—	D33.1	D43.1	D49.6
Stensen's duct	C07	C79.89	D00.00	D11.0	D37.030	D49.0
sternum	C41.3	C79.51	—	D16.7	D48.0	D49.2
stomach	C16.9	C78.89	D00.2	D13.1	D37.1	D49.0
antrum (pyloric)	C16.3	C78.89	D00.2	D13.1	D37.1	D49.0
body	C16.2	C78.89	D00.2	D13.1	D37.1	D49.0
cardia	C16.0	C78.89	D00.2	D13.1	D37.1	D49.0
cardiac orifice	C16.0	C78.89	D00.2	D13.1	D37.1	D49.0
corpus	C16.2	C78.89	D00.2	D13.1	D37.1	D49.0
fundus	C16.1	C78.89	D00.2	D13.1	D37.1	D49.0
greater curvature NEC	C16.6	C78.89	D00.2	D13.1	D37.1	D49.0
lesser curvature NEC	C16.5	C78.89	D00.2	D13.1	D37.1	D49.0
overlapping lesion	C16.8	—	—	—	—	—
prepylorus	C16.4	C78.89	D00.2	D13.1	D37.1	D49.0
pylorus	C16.4	C78.89	D00.2	D13.1	D37.1	D49.0
wall NEC	C16.9	C78.89	D00.2	D13.1	D37.1	D49.0
anterior NEC	C16.8	C78.89	D00.2	D13.1	D37.1	D49.0
posterior NEC	C16.8	C78.89	D00.2	D13.1	D37.1	D49.0
stroma, endometrial	C54.1	C79.82	D07.0	D26.1	D39.0	D49.59
stump, cervical	C53.8	C79.82	D06.7	D26.0	D39.0	D49.59
subcutaneous (nodule) (tissue) NEC — see Neoplasm, connective tissue						
subdural	C70.9	C79.32	—	D32.9	D42.9	D49.7
subglottis, subglottic	C32.2	C78.39	D02.0	D14.1	D38.0	D49.1
sublingual	C04.9	C79.89	D00.06	D10.2	D37.09	D49.0
gland or duct	C08.1	C79.89	D00.00	D11.7	D37.031	D49.0
submandibular gland	C08.0	C79.89	D00.00	D11.7	D37.032	D49.0
submaxillary gland or duct	C08.0	C79.89	D00.00	D11.7	D37.032	D49.0
submental	C76.0	C79.89	D09.8	D36.7	D48.7	D49.89
subpleural	C34.9-☑	C78.0-☑	D02.2-☑	D14.3-☑	D38.1	D49.1
substernal	C38.1	C78.1	—	D15.2	D38.3	D49.89
sudoriferous, sudoriparous gland, site unspecified	C44.90	C79.2	D04.9	D23.9	D48.5	D49.2
specified site — see Neoplasm, skin						

	Malignant Primary	Malignant Secondary	Ca in situ	Benign	Uncertain Behavior	Unspecified Behavior
Neoplasm, neoplastic — continued						
supraclavicular region	C76.0	C79.89	D09.8	D36.7	D48.7	D49.89
supraglottis	C32.1	C78.39	D02.0	D14.1	D38.0	D49.1
suprarenal	C74.9-☑	C79.7-☑	D09.3	D35.0-☑	D44.1-☑	D49.7
capsule	C74.9-☑	C79.7-☑	D09.3	D35.0-☑	D44.1-☑	D49.7
cortex	C74.0-☑	C79.7-☑	D09.3	D35.0-☑	D44.1-☑	D49.7
gland	C74.9-☑	C79.7-☑	D09.3	D35.0-☑	D44.1-☑	D49.7
medulla	C74.1-☑	C79.7-☑	D09.3	D35.0-☑	D44.1-☑	D49.7
suprasellar (region)	C71.9	C79.31	—	D33.2	D43.2	D49.6
supratentorial (brain) NEC	C71.0	C79.31	—	D33.0	D43.0	D49.6
sweat gland (apocrine) (eccrine), site unspecified	C44.90	C79.2	D04.9	D23.9	D48.5	D49.2
specified site — see Neoplasm, skin						
sympathetic nerve or nervous system NEC	C47.9	C79.89	—	D36.10	D48.2	D49.2
symphysis pubis	C41.4	C79.51	—	D16.8	D48.0	D49.2
synovial membrane — see Neoplasm, connective tissue						
tapetum, brain	C71.8	C79.31	—	D33.2	D43.2	D49.6
tarsus (any bone)	C40.3-☑	C79.51	—	D16.3-☑	—	—
temple (skin) — see also Neoplasm, skin, face	C44.309	C79.2	D04.39	D23.39	D48.5	D49.2
temporal						
bone	C41.0	C79.51	—	D16.4	D48.0	D49.2
lobe or pole	C71.2	C79.31	—	D33.0	D43.0	D49.6
region	C76.0	C79.89	D09.8	D36.7	D48.7	D49.89
skin — see also Neoplasm, skin, face	C44.309	C79.2	D04.39	D23.39	D48.5	D49.2
tendon (sheath) — see Neoplasm, connective tissue						
tentorium (cerebelli)	C70.0	C79.32	—	D32.0	D42.0	D49.7
testis, testes	C62.9-☑	C79.82	D07.69	D29.2-☑	D40.1-☑	D49.59
descended	C62.1-☑	C79.82	D07.69	D29.2-☑	D40.1-☑	D49.59
ectopic	C62.0-☑	C79.82	D07.69	D29.2-☑	D40.1-☑	D49.59
retained	C62.0-☑	C79.82	D07.69	D29.2-☑	D40.1-☑	D49.59
scrotal	C62.1-☑	C79.82	D07.69	D29.2-☑	D40.1-☑	D49.59
undescended	C62.0-☑	C79.82	D07.69	D29.2-☑	D40.1-☑	D49.59
unspecified whether descended or undescended	C62.9-☑	C79.82	D07.69	D29.2-☑	D40.1-☑	D49.59
thalamus	C71.0	C79.31	—	D33.0	D43.0	D49.6
thigh NEC	C76.5-☑	C79.89	D04.7-☑	D36.7	D48.7	D49.89
thorax, thoracic (cavity) (organs NEC)	C76.1	C79.89	D09.8	D36.7	D48.7	D49.89
duct	C49.3	C79.89	—	D21.3	D48.1-☑	D49.2
wall NEC	C76.1	C79.89	D09.8	D36.7	D48.7	D49.89
throat	C14.0	C79.89	D00.08	D10.9	D37.05	D49.0
thumb NEC	C76.4-☑	C79.89	D04.6-☑	D36.7	D48.7	D49.89
thymus (gland)	C37	C79.89	D09.3	D15.0	D38.4	D49.89
thyroglossal duct	C73	C79.89	D09.3	D34	D44.0	D49.7
thyroid (gland)	C73	C79.89	D09.3	D34	D44.0	D49.7
cartilage	C32.3	C78.39	D02.0	D14.1	D38.0	D49.1
tibia (any part)	C40.2-☑	C79.51	—	D16.2-☑	—	—
toe NEC	C76.5-☑	C79.89	D04.7-☑	D36.7	D48.7	D49.89
tongue	C02.9	C79.89	D00.07	D10.1	D37.02	D49.0
anterior (two-thirds) NEC	C02.3	C79.89	D00.07	D10.1	D37.02	D49.0
dorsal surface	C02.0	C79.89	D00.07	D10.1	D37.02	D49.0
ventral surface	C02.2	C79.89	D00.07	D10.1	D37.02	D49.0
base (dorsal surface)	C01	C79.89	D00.07	D10.1	D37.02	D49.0
border (lateral)	C02.1	C79.89	D00.07	D10.1	D37.02	D49.0
dorsal surface NEC	C02.0	C79.89	D00.07	D10.1	D37.02	D49.0
fixed part NEC	C01	C79.89	D00.07	D10.1	D37.02	D49.0
foramen cecum	C02.0	C79.89	D00.07	D10.1	D37.02	D49.0
frenulum linguae	C02.2	C79.89	D00.07	D10.1	D37.02	D49.0
junctional zone	C02.8	C79.89	D00.07	D10.1	D37.02	D49.0
margin (lateral)	C02.1	C79.89	D00.07	D10.1	D37.02	D49.0

Neoplasm, neoplastic — continued	Malignant Primary	Malignant Secondary	Ca in situ	Benign	Uncertain Behavior	Unspecified Behavior
tongue — continued						
midline NEC	C02.0	C79.89	D00.07	D10.1	D37.02	D49.0
mobile part NEC	C02.3	C79.89	D00.07	D10.1	D37.02	D49.0
overlapping lesion	C02.8	—	—	—	—	—
posterior (third)	C01	C79.89	D00.07	D10.1	D37.02	D49.0
root	C01	C79.89	D00.07	D10.1	D37.02	D49.0
surface (dorsal)	C02.0	C79.89	D00.07	D10.1	D37.02	D49.0
base	C01	C79.89	D00.07	D10.1	D37.02	D49.0
ventral	C02.2	C79.89	D00.07	D10.1	D37.02	D49.0
tip	C02.1	C79.89	D00.07	D10.1	D37.02	D49.0
tonsil	C02.4	C79.89	D00.07	D10.1	D37.02	D49.0
tonsil	C09.9	C79.89	D00.08	D10.4	D37.05	D49.0
fauces, faucial	C09.9	C79.89	D00.08	D10.4	D37.05	D49.0
lingual	C02.4	C79.89	D00.07	D10.1	D37.02	D49.0
overlapping sites	C09.8	—	—	—	—	—
palatine	C09.9	C79.89	D00.08	D10.4	D37.05	D49.0
pharyngeal	C11.1	C79.89	D00.08	D10.6	D37.05	D49.0
pillar (anterior) (posterior)	C09.1	C79.89	D00.08	D10.5	D37.05	D49.0
tonsillar fossa	C09.0	C79.89	D00.08	D10.5	D37.05	D49.0
tooth socket NEC	C03.9	C79.89	D00.03	D10.39	D37.09	D49.0
trachea (cartilage) (mucosa)	C33	C78.39	D02.1	D14.2	D38.1	D49.1
overlapping lesion with bronchus or lung	C34.8-☑	—	—	—	—	—
tracheobronchial	C34.8-☑	C78.39	D02.1	D14.2	D38.1	D49.1
overlapping lesion with lung	C34.8-☑	—	—	—	—	—
tragus — see also Neoplasm, skin, ear	C44.20-☑	C79.2	D04.2-☑	D23.2-☑	D48.5	D49.2
trunk NEC	C76.8	C79.89	D04.5	D36.7	D48.7	D49.89
tubo-ovarian	C57.8	C79.82	D07.39	D28.7	D39.8	D49.59
tunica vaginalis	C63.7	C79.82	D07.69	D29.8	D40.8	D49.59
turbinate (bone)	C41.0	C79.51	—	D16.4	D48.0	D49.2
nasal	C30.0	C78.39	D02.3	D14.0	D38.5	D49.1
tympanic cavity	C30.1	C78.39	D02.3	D14.0	D38.5	D49.1
ulna (any part)	C40.0-☑	C79.51	—	D16.0-☑	—	—
umbilicus, umbilical — see also Neoplasm, skin, trunk	C44.509	C79.2	D04.5	D23.5	D48.5	D49.2
uncus, brain	C71.2	C79.31	—	D33.0	D43.0	D49.6
unknown site or unspecified	C80.1	C79.9	D09.9	D36.9	D48.9	D49.9
urachus	C67.7	C79.11	D09.0	D30.3	D41.4	D49.4
ureter-bladder (junction)	C67.6	C79.11	D09.0	D30.3	D41.4	D49.4
ureter, ureteral	C66.-☑	C79.19	D09.19	D30.2-☑	D41.2-☑	D49.59
orifice (bladder)	C67.6	C79.11	D09.0	D30.3	D41.4	D49.4
urethra, urethral (gland)	C68.0	C79.19	D09.19	D30.4	D41.3	D49.59
orifice, internal	C67.5	C79.11	D09.0	D30.3	D41.4	D49.4
urethrovaginal (septum)	C57.9	C79.82	D07.30	D28.9	D39.8	D49.59
urinary organ or system	C68.9	C79.10	D09.10	D30.9	D41.9	D49.59
bladder — see Neoplasm, bladder						
overlapping lesion	C68.8	—	—	—	—	—
specified sites NEC	C68.8	C79.19	D09.19	D30.8	D41.8	D49.59
utero-ovarian	C57.8	C79.82	D07.39	D28.7	D39.8	D49.59
ligament	C57.1-☑	C79.82	D07.39	D28.2	D39.8	D49.59
uterosacral ligament	C57.3	C79.82	—	D28.2	D39.8	D49.59
uterus, uteri, uterine	C55	C79.82	D07.0	D26.9	D39.0	D49.59
adnexa NEC	C57.4	C79.82	D07.39	D28.7	D39.8	D49.59
body	C54.9	C79.82	D07.0	D26.1	D39.0	D49.59
cervix	C53.9	C79.82	D06.9	D26.0	D39.0	D49.59
cornu	C54.9	C79.82	D07.0	D26.1	D39.0	D49.59
corpus	C54.9	C79.82	D07.0	D26.1	D39.0	D49.59
endocervix (canal) (gland)	C53.0	C79.82	D06.0	D26.0	D39.0	D49.59
endometrium	C54.1	C79.82	D07.0	D26.1	D39.0	D49.59
exocervix	C53.1	C79.82	D06.1	D26.0	D39.0	D49.59

Neoplasm, neoplastic — continued	Malignant Primary	Malignant Secondary	Ca in situ	Benign	Uncertain Behavior	Unspecified Behavior
uterus, uteri, uterine — continued						
external os	C53.1	C79.82	D06.1	D26.0	D39.0	D49.59
fundus	C54.3	C79.82	D07.0	D26.1	D39.0	D49.59
internal os	C53.0	C79.82	D06.0	D26.0	D39.0	D49.59
isthmus	C54.0	C79.82	D07.0	D26.1	D39.0	D49.59
ligament	C57.3	C79.82	—	D28.2	D39.8	D49.59
broad	C57.1-☑	C79.82	D07.39	D28.2	D39.8	D49.59
round	C57.2-☑	C79.82	—	D28.2	D39.8	D49.59
lower segment	C54.0	C79.82	D07.0	D26.1	D39.0	D49.59
myometrium	C54.2	C79.82	D07.0	D26.1	D39.0	D49.59
overlapping sites	C54.8	—	—	—	—	—
squamocolumnar junction	C53.8	C79.82	D06.7	D26.0	D39.0	D49.59
tube	C57.0-☑	C79.82	D07.39	D28.2	D39.8	D49.59
utricle, prostatic	C68.0	C79.19	D09.19	D30.4	D41.3	D49.59
uveal tract	C69.4-☑	C79.49	D09.2-☑	D31.4-☑	D48.7	D49.89
uvula	C05.2	C79.89	D00.04	D10.39	D37.09	D49.0
vagina, vaginal (fornix) (vault) (wall)	C52	C79.82	D07.2	D28.1	D39.8	D49.59
vaginovesical	C57.9	C79.82	D07.30	D28.9	D39.9	D49.59
septum	C57.9	C79.82	D07.30	D28.9	D39.9	D49.59
vallecula (epiglottis)	C10.0	C79.89	D00.08	D10.5	D37.05	D49.0
vas deferens	C63.1-☑	C79.82	D07.69	D29.8	D40.8	D49.59
vascular — see Neoplasm, connective tissue						
Vater's ampulla	C24.1	C78.89	D01.5	D13.5	D37.6	D49.0
vein, venous — see Neoplasm, connective tissue						
vena cava (abdominal) (inferior)	C49.4	C79.89	—	D21.4	D48.1-☑	D49.2
superior	C49.3	C79.89	—	D21.3	D48.1-☑	D49.2
ventricle (cerebral) (floor) (lateral) (third)	C71.5	C79.31	—	D33.0	D43.0	D49.6
cardiac (left) (right)	C38.0	C79.89	—	D15.1	D48.7	D49.89
fourth	C71.7	C79.31	—	D33.1	D43.1	D49.6
ventricular band of larynx	C32.1	C78.39	D02.0	D14.1	D38.0	D49.1
ventriculus — see Neoplasm, stomach						
vermillion border — see Neoplasm, lip						
vermis, cerebellum	C71.6	C79.31	—	D33.1	D43.1	D49.6
vertebra (column)	C41.2	C79.51	—	D16.6	D48.0	D49.2
coccyx	C41.4	C79.51	—	D16.8	D48.0	D49.2
marrow NEC	C96.9	C79.52	—	—	D47.9	D49.89
sacrum	C41.4	C79.51	—	D16.8	D48.0	D49.2
vesical — see Neoplasm, bladder						
vesicle, seminal	C63.7	C79.82	D07.69	D29.8	D40.8	D49.59
vesicocervical tissue	C57.9	C79.82	D07.30	D28.9	D39.9	D49.59
vesicorectal	C76.3	C79.82	D09.8	D36.7	D48.7	D49.89
vesicovaginal	C57.9	C79.82	D07.30	D28.9	D39.9	D49.59
septum	C57.9	C79.82	D07.30	D28.9	D39.8	D49.59
vessel (blood) — see Neoplasm, connective tissue						
vestibular gland, greater	C51.0	C79.82	D07.1	D28.0	D39.8	D49.59
vestibule						
mouth	C06.1	C79.89	D00.00	D10.39	D37.09	D49.0
nose	C30.0	C78.39	D02.3	D14.0	D38.5	D49.1
Virchow's gland	C77.0	C77.0	—	D36.0	D48.7	D49.89
viscera NEC	C76.8	C79.89	D09.8	D36.7	D48.7	D49.89
vocal cords (true)	C32.0	C78.39	D02.0	D14.1	D38.0	D49.1
false	C32.1	C78.39	D02.0	D14.1	D38.0	D49.1
vomer	C41.0	C79.51	—	D16.4	D48.0	D49.2
vulva	C51.9	C79.82	D07.1	D28.0	D39.8	D49.59
vulvovaginal gland	C51.0	C79.82	D07.1	D28.0	D39.8	D49.59
Waldeyer's ring	C14.2	C79.89	D00.08	D10.9	D37.05	D49.0
Wharton's duct	C08.0	C79.89	D00.00	D11.7	D37.032	D49.0

☑ **Additional Character Required** — Refer to the Tabular List for Character Selection

	Malignant Primary	Malignant Secondary	Ca in situ	Benign	Uncertain Behavior	Unspecified Behavior
Neoplasm, neoplastic — *continued*						
white matter (central) (cerebral)	C71.0	C79.31	—	D33.0	D43.0	D49.6
windpipe	C33	C78.39	D02.1	D14.2	D38.1	D49.1
Wirsung's duct	C25.3	C78.89	D01.7	D13.6	D37.8	D49.0
wolffian (body) (duct)						
female	C57.7	C79.82	D07.39	D28.7	D39.8	D49.59
male	C63.7	C79.82	D07.69	D29.8	D40.8	D49.59
womb — *see* Neoplasm, uterus						
wrist NEC	C76.4-☑	C79.89	D04.6-☑	D36.7	D48.7	D49.89
xiphoid process	C41.3	C79.51	—	D16.7	D48.0	D49.2
Zuckerkandl organ	C75.5	C79.89	—	D35.6	D44.7	D49.7

Substance	Poisoning, Accidental (unintentional)	Poisoning, Intentional Self-harm	Poisoning, Assault	Poisoning, Undetermined	Adverse Effect	Under-dosing
1-Propanol	T51.3X1	T51.3X2	T51.3X3	T51.3X4	—	—
14-hydroxydihydro-morphinone	T40.2X1	T40.2X2	T40.2X3	T40.2X4	T40.2X5	T40.2X6
2-Deoxy-5-fluorouridine	T45.1X1	T45.1X2	T45.1X3	T45.1X4	T45.1X5	T45.1X6
2-Ethoxyethanol	T52.3X1	T52.3X2	T52.3X3	T52.3X4	—	—
2-Methoxyethanol	T52.3X1	T52.3X2	T52.3X3	T52.3X4	—	—
2-Propanol	T51.2X1	T51.2X2	T51.2X3	T51.2X4	—	—
2,3,7,8-Tetrachlorodibenzo-p-dioxin	T53.7X1	T53.7X2	T53.7X3	T53.7X4	—	—
2,4-D (dichlorophen-oxyacetic acid)	T60.3X1	T60.3X2	T60.3X3	T60.3X4	—	—
2,4-Toluene diisocyanate	T65.0X1	T65.0X2	T65.0X3	T65.0X4	—	—
2,4,5-T (trichloro-phenoxyacetic acid)	T60.1X1	T60.1X2	T60.1X3	T60.1X4	—	—
2,4,5-Trichlorophen-oxyacetic acid	T60.3X1	T60.3X2	T60.3X3	T60.3X4	—	—
3,4-methylenedioxymeth-amphetamine	T43.641	T43.642	T43.643	T43.644	—	—
4-Aminobutyric acid	T43.8X1	T43.8X2	T43.8X3	T43.8X4	T43.8X5	T43.8X6
4-Aminophenol derivatives	T39.1X1	T39.1X2	T39.1X3	T39.1X4	T39.1X5	T39.1X6
5-Deoxy-5-fluorouridine	T45.1X1	T45.1X2	T45.1X3	T45.1X4	T45.1X5	T45.1X6
5-Methoxypsoralen (5-MOP)	T50.991	T50.992	T50.993	T50.994	T50.995	T50.996
8-Aminoquinoline drugs	T37.2X1	T37.2X2	T37.2X3	T37.2X4	T37.2X5	T37.2X6
8-Methoxypsoralen (8-MOP)	T50.991	T50.992	T50.993	T50.994	T50.995	T50.996
9-hydoxyrisperidone*	T43.591	T43.592	T43.593	T43.594	T43.595	T43.596
ABOB	T37.5X1	T37.5X2	T37.5X3	T37.5X4	T37.5X5	T37.5X6
Abrine	T62.2X1	T62.2X2	T62.2X3	T62.2X4	—	—
Abrus (seed)	T62.2X1	T62.2X2	T62.2X3	T62.2X4	—	—
Absinthe	T51.0X1	T51.0X2	T51.0X3	T51.0X4	—	—
beverage	T51.0X1	T51.0X2	T51.0X3	T51.0X4	—	—
Acaricide	T60.8X1	T60.8X2	T60.8X3	T60.8X4	—	—
Acebutolol	T44.7X1	T44.7X2	T44.7X3	T44.7X4	T44.7X5	T44.7X6
Acecarbromal	T42.6X1	T42.6X2	T42.6X3	T42.6X4	T42.6X5	T42.6X6
Aceclidine	T44.1X1	T44.1X2	T44.1X3	T44.1X4	T44.1X5	T44.1X6
Acedapsone	T37.0X1	T37.0X2	T37.0X3	T37.0X4	T37.0X5	T37.0X6
Acefylline piperazine	T48.6X1	T48.6X2	T48.6X3	T48.6X4	T48.6X5	T48.6X6
Acemorphan	T40.2X1	T40.2X2	T40.2X3	T40.2X4	T40.2X5	T40.2X6
Acenocoumarin	T45.511	T45.512	T45.513	T45.514	T45.515	T45.516
Acenocoumarol	T45.511	T45.512	T45.513	T45.514	T45.515	T45.516
Aceon*	T46.4X1	T46.4X2	T46.4X3	T46.4X4	T46.4X5	T46.4X6
Acepifylline	T48.6X1	T48.6X2	T48.6X3	T48.6X4	T48.6X5	T48.6X6
Acepromazine	T43.3X1	T43.3X2	T43.3X3	T43.3X4	T43.3X5	T43.3X6
Acesulfamethoxypyridazine	T37.0X1	T37.0X2	T37.0X3	T37.0X4	T37.0X5	T37.0X6
Acetal	T52.8X1	T52.8X2	T52.8X3	T52.8X4	—	—
Acetaldehyde (vapor)	T52.8X1	T52.8X2	T52.8X3	T52.8X4	—	—
liquid	T65.891	T65.892	T65.893	T65.894	—	—
Acetaminophen	T39.1X1	T39.1X2	T39.1X3	T39.1X4	T39.1X5	T39.1X6
Acetaminosalol	T39.1X1	T39.1X2	T39.1X3	T39.1X4	T39.1X5	T39.1X6
Acetanilide	T39.1X1	T39.1X2	T39.1X3	T39.1X4	T39.1X5	T39.1X6
Acetarsol	T37.3X1	T37.3X2	T37.3X3	T37.3X4	T37.3X5	T37.3X6
Acetazolamide	T50.2X1	T50.2X2	T50.2X3	T50.2X4	T50.2X5	T50.2X6
Acetiamine	T45.2X1	T45.2X2	T45.2X3	T45.2X4	T45.2X5	T45.2X6
Acetic						
acid	T54.2X1	T54.2X2	T54.2X3	T54.2X4	—	—
with sodium acetate (ointment)	T49.3X1	T49.3X2	T49.3X3	T49.3X4	T49.3X5	T49.3X6
ester (solvent)(vapor)	T52.8X1	T52.8X2	T52.8X3	T52.8X4	—	—
irrigating solution	T50.3X1	T50.3X2	T50.3X3	T50.3X4	T50.3X5	T50.3X6
medicinal (lotion)	T49.2X1	T49.2X2	T49.2X3	T49.2X4	T49.2X5	T49.2X6
anhydride	T65.891	T65.892	T65.893	T65.894	—	—
ether (vapor)	T52.8X1	T52.8X2	T52.8X3	T52.8X4	—	—
Acetohexamide	T38.3X1	T38.3X2	T38.3X3	T38.3X4	T38.3X5	T38.3X6
Acetohydroxamic acid	T50.991	T50.992	T50.993	T50.994	T50.995	T50.996
Acetomenaphthone	T45.7X1	T45.7X2	T45.7X3	T45.7X4	T45.7X5	T45.7X6
Acetomorphine	T40.1X1	T40.1X2	T40.1X3	T40.1X4	—	—
Acetone (oils)	T52.4X1	T52.4X2	T52.4X3	T52.4X4	—	—
chlorinated	T52.4X1	T52.4X2	T52.4X3	T52.4X4	—	—
vapor	T52.4X1	T52.4X2	T52.4X3	T52.4X4	—	—
Acetonitrile	T52.8X1	T52.8X2	T52.8X3	T52.8X4	—	—
Acetophenazine	T43.3X1	T43.3X2	T43.3X3	T43.3X4	T43.3X5	T43.3X6
Acetophenetedin	T39.1X1	T39.1X2	T39.1X3	T39.1X4	T39.1X5	T39.1X6
Acetophenone	T52.4X1	T52.4X2	T52.4X3	T52.4X4	—	—
Acetorphine	T40.2X1	T40.2X2	T40.2X3	T40.2X4	—	—
Acetosulfone (sodium)	T37.1X1	T37.1X2	T37.1X3	T37.1X4	T37.1X5	T37.1X6
Acetrizoate (sodium)	T50.8X1	T50.8X2	T50.8X3	T50.8X4	T50.8X5	T50.8X6
Acetrizoic acid	T50.8X1	T50.8X2	T50.8X3	T50.8X4	T50.8X5	T50.8X6
Acetyl						
bromide	T53.6X1	T53.6X2	T53.6X3	T53.6X4	—	—
chloride	T53.6X1	T53.6X2	T53.6X3	T53.6X4	—	—
Acetylcarbromal	T42.6X1	T42.6X2	T42.6X3	T42.6X4	T42.6X5	T42.6X6
Acetylcholine						

Substance	Poisoning, Accidental (unintentional)	Poisoning, Intentional Self-harm	Poisoning, Assault	Poisoning, Undetermined	Adverse Effect	Under-dosing
Acetylcholine — continued						
chloride	T44.1X1	T44.1X2	T44.1X3	T44.1X4	T44.1X5	T44.1X6
derivative	T44.1X1	T44.1X2	T44.1X3	T44.1X4	T44.1X5	T44.1X6
Acetylcysteine	T48.4X1	T48.4X2	T48.4X3	T48.4X4	T48.4X5	T48.4X6
Acetyldigitoxin	T46.0X1	T46.0X2	T46.0X3	T46.0X4	T46.0X5	T46.0X6
Acetyldigoxin	T46.0X1	T46.0X2	T46.0X3	T46.0X4	T46.0X5	T46.0X6
Acetyldihydrocodeine	T40.2X1	T40.2X2	T40.2X3	T40.2X4	—	—
Acetyldihydrocodeinone	T40.2X1	T40.2X2	T40.2X3	T40.2X4	—	—
Acetylene (gas)	T59.891	T59.892	T59.893	T59.894	—	—
dichloride	T53.6X1	T53.6X2	T53.6X3	T53.6X4	—	—
incomplete combustion of	T58.11	T58.12	T58.13	T58.14	—	—
industrial	T59.891	T59.892	T59.893	T59.894	—	—
tetrachloride	T53.6X1	T53.6X2	T53.6X3	T53.6X4	—	—
vapor	T53.6X1	T53.6X2	T53.6X3	T53.6X4	—	—
Acetylpheneturide	T42.6X1	T42.6X2	T42.6X3	T42.6X4	T42.6X5	T42.6X6
Acetylphenylhydrazine	T39.8X1	T39.8X2	T39.8X3	T39.8X4	T39.8X5	T39.8X6
Acetylsalicylic acid (salts)	T39.011	T39.012	T39.013	T39.014	T39.015	T39.016
enteric coated	T39.011	T39.012	T39.013	T39.014	T39.015	T39.016
Acetylsulfamethoxypyridazine	T37.0X1	T37.0X2	T37.0X3	T37.0X4	T37.0X5	T37.0X6
Achromycin	T36.4X1	T36.4X2	T36.4X3	T36.4X4	T36.4X5	T36.4X6
ophthalmic preparation	T49.5X1	T49.5X2	T49.5X3	T49.5X4	T49.5X5	T49.5X6
topical NEC	T49.0X1	T49.0X2	T49.0X3	T49.0X4	T49.0X5	T49.0X6
Aciclovir	T37.5X1	T37.5X2	T37.5X3	T37.5X4	T37.5X5	T37.5X6
Acid (corrosive) NEC	T54.2X1	T54.2X2	T54.2X3	T54.2X4	—	—
Acidifying agent NEC	T50.901	T50.902	T50.903	T50.904	T50.905	T50.906
AcipHex*	T47.1X1	T47.1X2	T47.1X3	T47.1X4	T47.1X5	T47.1X6
Acipimox	T46.6X1	T46.6X2	T46.6X3	T46.6X4	T46.6X5	T46.6X6
Acitretin	T50.991	T50.992	T50.993	T50.994	T50.995	T50.996
Aclarubicin	T45.1X1	T45.1X2	T45.1X3	T45.1X4	T45.1X5	T45.1X6
Aclatonium napadisilate	T48.1X1	T48.1X2	T48.1X3	T48.1X4	T48.1X5	T48.1X6
Aconite (wild)	T46.991	T46.992	T46.993	T46.994	T46.995	T46.996
Aconitine	T46.991	T46.992	T46.993	T46.994	T46.995	T46.996
Aconitum ferox	T46.991	T46.992	T46.993	T46.994	T46.995	T46.996
Acridine	T65.6X1	T65.6X2	T65.6X3	T65.6X4	—	—
vapor	T59.891	T59.892	T59.893	T59.894	—	—
Acriflavine	T37.91	T37.92	T37.93	T37.94	T37.95	T37.96
Acriflavinium chloride	T49.0X1	T49.0X2	T49.0X3	T49.0X4	T49.0X5	T49.0X6
Acrinol	T49.0X1	T49.0X2	T49.0X3	T49.0X4	T49.0X5	T49.0X6
Acrisorcin	T49.0X1	T49.0X2	T49.0X3	T49.0X4	T49.0X5	T49.0X6
Acrivastine	T45.0X1	T45.0X2	T45.0X3	T45.0X4	T45.0X5	T45.0X6
Acrolein (gas)	T59.891	T59.892	T59.893	T59.894	—	—
liquid	T54.1X1	T54.1X2	T54.1X3	T54.1X4	—	—
Acrylamide	T65.891	T65.892	T65.893	T65.894	—	—
Acrylic resin	T49.3X1	T49.3X2	T49.3X3	T49.3X4	T49.3X5	T49.3X6
Acrylonitrile	T65.891	T65.892	T65.893	T65.894	—	—
Actaea spicata	T62.2X1	T62.2X2	T62.2X3	T62.2X4	—	—
berry	T62.1X1	T62.1X2	T62.1X3	T62.1X4	—	—
Acterol	T37.3X1	T37.3X2	T37.3X3	T37.3X4	T37.3X5	T37.3X6
ACTH	T38.811	T38.812	T38.813	T38.814	T38.815	T38.816
Acticlate*	T36.4X1	T36.4X2	T36.4X3	T36.4X4	T36.4X5	T36.4X6
Actinomycin C	T45.1X1	T45.1X2	T45.1X3	T45.1X4	T45.1X5	T45.1X6
Actinomycin D	T45.1X1	T45.1X2	T45.1X3	T45.1X4	T45.1X5	T45.1X6
Activated charcoal — see also Charcoal, medicinal	T47.6X1	T47.6X2	T47.6X3	T47.6X4	T47.6X5	T47.6X6
Activella*	T38.5X1	T38.5X2	T38.5X3	T38.5X4	T38.5X5	T38.5X6
Acyclovir	T37.5X1	T37.5X2	T37.5X3	T37.5X4	T37.5X5	T37.5X6
Adenine	T45.2X1	T45.2X2	T45.2X3	T45.2X4	T45.2X5	T45.2X6
arabinoside	T37.5X1	T37.5X2	T37.5X3	T37.5X4	T37.5X5	T37.5X6
Adenosine (phosphate)	T46.2X1	T46.2X2	T46.2X3	T46.2X4	T46.2X5	T46.2X6
ADH	T38.891	T38.892	T38.893	T38.894	T38.895	T38.896
Adhesive NEC	T65.891	T65.892	T65.893	T65.894	—	—
Adicillin	T36.0X1	T36.0X2	T36.0X3	T36.0X4	T36.0X5	T36.0X6
Adiphenine	T44.3X1	T44.3X2	T44.3X3	T44.3X4	T44.3X5	T44.3X6
Adipiodone	T50.8X1	T50.8X2	T50.8X3	T50.8X4	T50.8X5	T50.8X6
Adjunct, pharmaceutical	T50.901	T50.902	T50.903	T50.904	T50.905	T50.906
Adrenal (extract, cortex or medulla) (glucocorticoids) (hormones) (mineralocorticoids)	T38.0X1	T38.0X2	T38.0X3	T38.0X4	T38.0X5	T38.0X6
ENT agent	T49.6X1	T49.6X2	T49.6X3	T49.6X4	T49.6X5	T49.6X6
ophthalmic preparation	T49.5X1	T49.5X2	T49.5X3	T49.5X4	T49.5X5	T49.5X6
topical NEC	T49.0X1	T49.0X2	T49.0X3	T49.0X4	T49.0X5	T49.0X6
Adrenalin — see Adrenaline						
Adrenaline	T44.5X1	T44.5X2	T44.5X3	T44.5X4	T44.5X5	T44.5X6
Adrenergic NEC	T44.901	T44.902	T44.903	T44.904	T44.905	T44.906
blocking agent NEC	T44.8X1	T44.8X2	T44.8X3	T44.8X4	T44.8X5	T44.8X6
beta, heart	T44.7X1	T44.7X2	T44.7X3	T44.7X4	T44.7X5	T44.7X6
specified NEC	T44.991	T44.992	T44.993	T44.994	T44.995	T44.996
Adrenochrome (mono) semicarbazone	T46.991	T46.992	T46.993	T46.994	T46.995	T46.996
derivative	T46.991	T46.992	T46.993	T46.994	T46.995	T46.996
Adrenocorticotrophic hormone	T38.811	T38.812	T38.813	T38.814	T38.815	T38.816

*Optum Value-Add

Substance	Poisoning, Accidental (unintentional)	Poisoning, Intentional Self-harm	Poisoning, Assault	Poisoning, Undetermined	Adverse Effect	Under-dosing
Adrenocorticotrophin	T38.811	T38.812	T38.813	T38.814	T38.815	T38.816
Adriamycin	T45.1X1	T45.1X2	T45.1X3	T45.1X4	T45.1X5	T45.1X6
Adrucil*	T45.1X1	T45.1X2	T45.1X3	T45.1X4	T45.1X5	T45.1X6
Aerosol spray NEC	T65.91	T65.92	T65.93	T65.94	—	—
Aerosporin	T36.8X1	T36.8X2	T36.8X3	T36.8X4	T36.8X5	T36.8X6
ENT agent	T49.6X1	T49.6X2	T49.6X3	T49.6X4	T49.6X5	T49.6X6
ophthalmic preparation	T49.5X1	T49.5X2	T49.5X3	T49.5X4	T49.5X5	T49.5X6
topical NEC	T49.ØX1	T49.ØX2	T49.ØX3	T49.ØX4	T49.ØX5	T49.ØX6
Aethusa cynapium	T62.2X1	T62.2X2	T62.2X3	T62.2X4	—	—
Afghanistan black	T4Ø.711	T4Ø.712	T4Ø.713	T4Ø.714	T4Ø.715	T4Ø.716
Aflatoxin	T64.Ø1	T64.Ø2	T64.Ø3	T64.Ø4	—	—
Afloqualone	T42.8X1	T42.8X2	T42.8X3	T42.8X4	T42.8X5	T42.8X6
African boxwood	T62.2X1	T62.2X2	T62.2X3	T62.2X4	—	—
Agar	T47.4X1	T47.4X2	T47.4X3	T47.4X4	T47.4X5	T47.4X6
Agonist						
predominantly						
alpha-adrenoreceptor	T44.4X1	T44.4X2	T44.4X3	T44.4X4	T44.4X5	T44.4X6
beta-adrenoreceptor	T44.5X1	T44.5X2	T44.5X3	T44.5X4	T44.5X5	T44.5X6
Agricultural agent NEC	T65.91	T65.92	T65.93	T65.94	—	—
Agrypnal	T42.3X1	T42.3X2	T42.3X3	T42.3X4	T42.3X5	T42.3X6
AHLG	T5Ø.Z11	T5Ø.Z12	T5Ø.Z13	T5Ø.Z14	T5Ø.Z15	T5Ø.Z16
Air contaminant(s), **source/type NOS**	T65.91	T65.92	T65.93	T65.94	—	—
Ajmaline	T46.2X1	T46.2X2	T46.2X3	T46.2X4	T46.2X5	T46.2X6
Akee	T62.1X1	T62.1X2	T62.1X3	T62.1X4	—	—
Akne-Mycin*	T49.ØX1	T49.ØX2	T49.ØX3	T49.ØX4	T49.ØX5	T49.ØX6
Akrinol	T49.ØX1	T49.ØX2	T49.ØX3	T49.ØX4	T49.ØX5	T49.ØX6
Akritoin	T37.8X1	T37.8X2	T37.8X3	T37.8X4	T37.8X5	T37.8X6
Alacepril	T46.4X1	T46.4X2	T46.4X3	T46.4X4	T46.4X5	T46.4X6
Alantolactone	T37.4X1	T37.4X2	T37.4X3	T37.4X4	T37.4X5	T37.4X6
Albamycin	T36.8X1	T36.8X2	T36.8X3	T36.8X4	T36.8X5	T36.8X6
Albendazole	T37.4X1	T37.4X2	T37.4X3	T37.4X4	T37.4X5	T37.4X6
Albigutide*	T38.3X1	T38.3X2	T38.3X3	T38.3X4	T38.3X5	T38.3X6
Albumin						
bovine	T45.8X1	T45.8X2	T45.8X3	T45.8X4	T45.8X5	T45.8X6
human serum	T45.8X1	T45.8X2	T45.8X3	T45.8X4	T45.8X5	T45.8X6
salt-poor	T45.8X1	T45.8X2	T45.8X3	T45.8X4	T45.8X5	T45.8X6
normal human serum	T45.8X1	T45.8X2	T45.8X3	T45.8X4	T45.8X5	T45.8X6
Albuterol	T48.6X1	T48.6X2	T48.6X3	T48.6X4	T48.6X5	T48.6X6
Albutoin	T42.ØX1	T42.ØX2	T42.ØX3	T42.ØX4	T42.ØX5	T42.ØX6
Alclometasone	T49.ØX1	T49.ØX2	T49.ØX3	T49.ØX4	T49.ØX5	T49.ØX6
Alcohol	T51.91	T51.92	T51.93	T51.94	—	—
absolute	T51.ØX1	T51.ØX2	T51.ØX3	T51.ØX4	—	—
beverage	T51.ØX1	T51.ØX2	T51.ØX3	T51.ØX4	—	—
allyl	T51.8X1	T51.8X2	T51.8X3	T51.8X4	—	—
amyl	T51.3X1	T51.3X2	T51.3X3	T51.3X4	—	—
antifreeze	T51.1X1	T51.1X2	T51.1X3	T51.1X4	—	—
beverage	T51.ØX1	T51.ØX2	T51.ØX3	T51.ØX4	—	—
butyl	T51.3X1	T51.3X2	T51.3X3	T51.3X4	—	—
dehydrated	T51.ØX1	T51.ØX2	T51.ØX3	T51.ØX4	—	—
beverage	T51.ØX1	T51.ØX2	T51.ØX3	T51.ØX4	—	—
denatured	T51.ØX1	T51.ØX2	T51.ØX3	T51.ØX4	—	—
deterrent NEC	T5Ø.6X1	T5Ø.6X2	T5Ø.6X3	T5Ø.6X4	T5Ø.6X5	T5Ø.6X6
diagnostic (gastric function)	T5Ø.8X1	T5Ø.8X2	T5Ø.8X3	T5Ø.8X4	T5Ø.8X5	T5Ø.8X6
ethyl	T51.ØX1	T51.ØX2	T51.ØX3	T51.ØX4	—	—
beverage	T51.ØX1	T51.ØX2	T51.ØX3	T51.ØX4	—	—
grain	T51.ØX1	T51.ØX2	T51.ØX3	T51.ØX4	—	—
beverage	T51.ØX1	T51.ØX2	T51.ØX3	T51.ØX4	—	—
industrial	T51.ØX1	T51.ØX2	T51.ØX3	T51.ØX4	—	—
isopropyl	T51.2X1	T51.2X2	T51.2X3	T51.2X4	—	—
methyl	T51.1X1	T51.1X2	T51.1X3	T51.1X4	—	—
preparation for consumption	T51.ØX1	T51.ØX2	T51.ØX3	T51.ØX4	—	—
propyl	T51.3X1	T51.3X2	T51.3X3	T51.3X4	—	—
secondary	T51.2X1	T51.2X2	T51.2X3	T51.2X4	—	—
radiator	T51.1X1	T51.1X2	T51.1X3	T51.1X4	—	—
rubbing	T51.2X1	T51.2X2	T51.2X3	T51.2X4	—	—
specified type NEC	T51.8X1	T51.8X2	T51.8X3	T51.8X4	—	—
surgical	T51.ØX1	T51.ØX2	T51.ØX3	T51.ØX4	—	—
vapor (from any type of Alcohol)	T59.891	T59.892	T59.893	T59.894	—	—
wood	T51.1X1	T51.1X2	T51.1X3	T51.1X4	—	—
Alcuronium (chloride)	T48.1X1	T48.1X2	T48.1X3	T48.1X4	T48.1X5	T48.1X6
Aldactone	T5Ø.ØX1	T5Ø.ØX2	T5Ø.ØX3	T5Ø.ØX4	T5Ø.ØX5	T5Ø.ØX6
Aldesulfone sodium	T37.1X1	T37.1X2	T37.1X3	T37.1X4	T37.1X5	T37.1X6
Aldicarb	T6Ø.ØX1	T6Ø.ØX2	T6Ø.ØX3	T6Ø.ØX4	—	—
Aldomet	T46.5X1	T46.5X2	T46.5X3	T46.5X4	T46.5X5	T46.5X6
Aldosterone	T5Ø.ØX1	T5Ø.ØX2	T5Ø.ØX3	T5Ø.ØX4	T5Ø.ØX5	T5Ø.ØX6
Aldrin (dust)	T6Ø.1X1	T6Ø.1X2	T6Ø.1X3	T6Ø.1X4	—	—
Aleve — *see* Naproxen						
Alexitol sodium	T47.1X1	T47.1X2	T47.1X3	T47.1X4	T47.1X5	T47.1X6
Alfacalcidol	T45.2X1	T45.2X2	T45.2X3	T45.2X4	T45.2X5	T45.2X6
Alfadolone	T41.1X1	T41.1X2	T41.1X3	T41.1X4	T41.1X5	T41.1X6
Alfaxalone	T41.1X1	T41.1X2	T41.1X3	T41.1X4	T41.1X5	T41.1X6
Alfentanil	T4Ø.411	T4Ø.412	T4Ø.413	T4Ø.414	T4Ø.415	T4Ø.416
Alfuzosin (hydrochloride)	T44.8X1	T44.8X2	T44.8X3	T44.8X4	T44.8X5	T44.8X6
Algae (harmful) (toxin)	T65.821	T65.822	T65.823	T65.824	—	—
Algeldrate	T47.1X1	T47.1X2	T47.1X3	T47.1X4	T47.1X5	T47.1X6
Algin	T47.8X1	T47.8X2	T47.8X3	T47.8X4	T47.8X5	T47.8X6
Alglucerase	T45.3X1	T45.3X2	T45.3X3	T45.3X4	T45.3X5	T45.3X6
Alidase	T45.3X1	T45.3X2	T45.3X3	T45.3X4	T45.3X5	T45.3X6
Alimemazine	T43.3X1	T43.3X2	T43.3X3	T43.3X4	T43.3X5	T43.3X6
Aliphatic thiocyanates	T65.ØX1	T65.ØX2	T65.ØX3	T65.ØX4	—	—
Alitretinoin*	T49.ØX1	T49.ØX2	T49.ØX3	T49.ØX4	T49.ØX5	T49.ØX6
Alizapride	T45.ØX1	T45.ØX2	T45.ØX3	T45.ØX4	T45.ØX5	T45.ØX6
Alka-seltzer	T39.Ø11	T39.Ø12	T39.Ø13	T39.Ø14	T39.Ø15	T39.Ø16
Alkali (caustic)	T54.3X1	T54.3X2	T54.3X3	T54.3X4	—	—
Alkaline antiseptic solution (aromatic)	T49.6X1	T49.6X2	T49.6X3	T49.6X4	T49.6X5	T49.6X6
Alkalinizing agents (medicinal)	T5Ø.9Ø1	T5Ø.9Ø2	T5Ø.9Ø3	T5Ø.9Ø4	T5Ø.9Ø5	T5Ø.9Ø6
Alkalizing agent NEC	T5Ø.9Ø1	T5Ø.9Ø2	T5Ø.9Ø3	T5Ø.9Ø4	T5Ø.9Ø5	T5Ø.9Ø6
Alkavervir	T46.5X1	T46.5X2	T46.5X3	T46.5X4	T46.5X5	T46.5X6
Alkeran*	T45.1X1	T45.1X2	T45.1X3	T45.1X4	T45.1X5	T45.1X6
Alkonium (bromide)	T49.ØX1	T49.ØX2	T49.ØX3	T49.ØX4	T49.ØX5	T49.ØX6
Alkylating drug NEC	T45.1X1	T45.1X2	T45.1X3	T45.1X4	T45.1X5	T45.1X6
antimyeloproliferative	T45.1X1	T45.1X2	T45.1X3	T45.1X4	T45.1X5	T45.1X6
lymphatic	T45.1X1	T45.1X2	T45.1X3	T45.1X4	T45.1X5	T45.1X6
Alkylisocyanate	T65.ØX1	T65.ØX2	T65.ØX3	T65.ØX4	—	—
Allantoin	T49.4X1	T49.4X2	T49.4X3	T49.4X4	T49.4X5	T49.4X6
Allegron	T43.Ø11	T43.Ø12	T43.Ø13	T43.Ø14	T43.Ø15	T43.Ø16
Allethrin	T49.ØX1	T49.ØX2	T49.ØX3	T49.ØX4	T49.ØX5	T49.ØX6
Allobarbital	T42.3X1	T42.3X2	T42.3X3	T42.3X4	T42.3X5	T42.3X6
Allopurinol	T5Ø.4X1	T5Ø.4X2	T5Ø.4X3	T5Ø.4X4	T5Ø.4X5	T5Ø.4X6
Allyl						
alcohol	T51.8X1	T51.8X2	T51.8X3	T51.8X4	—	—
disulfide	T46.6X1	T46.6X2	T46.6X3	T46.6X4	T46.6X5	T46.6X6
Allylestrenol	T38.5X1	T38.5X2	T38.5X3	T38.5X4	T38.5X5	T38.5X6
Allylisopropylacetylurea	T42.6X1	T42.6X2	T42.6X3	T42.6X4	T42.6X5	T42.6X6
Allylisopropylmalonylurea	T42.3X1	T42.3X2	T42.3X3	T42.3X4	T42.3X5	T42.3X6
Allylthiourea	T49.3X1	T49.3X2	T49.3X3	T49.3X4	T49.3X5	T49.3X6
Allyltribromide	T42.6X1	T42.6X2	T42.6X3	T42.6X4	T42.6X5	T42.6X6
Allypropymal	T42.3X1	T42.3X2	T42.3X3	T42.3X4	T42.3X5	T42.3X6
Almagate	T47.1X1	T47.1X2	T47.1X3	T47.1X4	T47.1X5	T47.1X6
Almasilate	T47.1X1	T47.1X2	T47.1X3	T47.1X4	T47.1X5	T47.1X6
Almitrine	T5Ø.7X1	T5Ø.7X2	T5Ø.7X3	T5Ø.7X4	T5Ø.7X5	T5Ø.7X6
Aloes	T47.2X1	T47.2X2	T47.2X3	T47.2X4	T47.2X5	T47.2X6
Aloglutamol	T47.1X1	T47.1X2	T47.1X3	T47.1X4	T47.1X5	T47.1X6
Aloin	T47.2X1	T47.2X2	T47.2X3	T47.2X4	T47.2X5	T47.2X6
Aloxidone	T42.2X1	T42.2X2	T42.2X3	T42.2X4	T42.2X5	T42.2X6
Alpha						
acetyldigoxin	T46.ØX1	T46.ØX2	T46.ØX3	T46.ØX4	T46.ØX5	T46.ØX6
adrenergic blocking drug	T44.6X1	T44.6X2	T44.6X3	T44.6X4	T44.6X5	T44.6X6
amylase	T45.3X1	T45.3X2	T45.3X3	T45.3X4	T45.3X5	T45.3X6
tocoferol (acetate)	T45.2X1	T45.2X2	T45.2X3	T45.2X4	T45.2X5	T45.2X6
tocopherol	T45.2X1	T45.2X2	T45.2X3	T45.2X4	T45.2X5	T45.2X6
Alphadolone	T41.1X1	T41.1X2	T41.1X3	T41.1X4	T41.1X5	T41.1X6
Alphaprodine	T4Ø.491	T4Ø.492	T4Ø.493	T4Ø.494	T4Ø.495	T4Ø.496
Alphaxalone	T41.1X1	T41.1X2	T41.1X3	T41.1X4	T41.1X5	T41.1X6
Alprazolam	T42.4X1	T42.4X2	T42.4X3	T42.4X4	T42.4X5	T42.4X6
Alprenolol	T44.7X1	T44.7X2	T44.7X3	T44.7X4	T44.7X5	T44.7X6
Alprostadil	T46.7X1	T46.7X2	T46.7X3	T46.7X4	T46.7X5	T46.7X6
Alsactide	T38.811	T38.812	T38.813	T38.814	T38.815	T38.816
Alseroxylon	T46.5X1	T46.5X2	T46.5X3	T46.5X4	T46.5X5	T46.5X6
Alteplase	T45.611	T45.612	T45.613	T45.614	T45.615	T45.616
Altizide	T5Ø.2X1	T5Ø.2X2	T5Ø.2X3	T5Ø.2X4	T5Ø.2X5	T5Ø.2X6
Altoprev*	T46.6X1	T46.6X2	T46.6X3	T46.6X4	T46.6X5	T46.6X6
Altretamine	T45.1X1	T45.1X2	T45.1X3	T45.1X4	T45.1X5	T45.1X6
Alum (medicinal)	T49.4X1	T49.4X2	T49.4X3	T49.4X4	T49.4X5	T49.4X6
nonmedicinal (ammonium) (potassium)	T56.891	T56.892	T56.893	T56.894	—	—
Aluminium, aluminum						
acetate	T49.2X1	T49.2X2	T49.2X3	T49.2X4	T49.2X5	T49.2X6
solution	T49.ØX1	T49.ØX2	T49.ØX3	T49.ØX4	T49.ØX5	T49.ØX6
aspirin	T39.Ø11	T39.Ø12	T39.Ø13	T39.Ø14	T39.Ø15	T39.Ø16
bis (acetylsalicylate)	T39.Ø11	T39.Ø12	T39.Ø13	T39.Ø14	T39.Ø15	T39.Ø16
carbonate (gel, basic)	T47.1X1	T47.1X2	T47.1X3	T47.1X4	T47.1X5	T47.1X6
chlorhydroxide-complex	T47.1X1	T47.1X2	T47.1X3	T47.1X4	T47.1X5	T47.1X6
chloride	T49.2X1	T49.2X2	T49.2X3	T49.2X4	T49.2X5	T49.2X6
clofibrate	T46.6X1	T46.6X2	T46.6X3	T46.6X4	T46.6X5	T46.6X6
diacetate	T49.2X1	T49.2X2	T49.2X3	T49.2X4	T49.2X5	T49.2X6
glycinate	T47.1X1	T47.1X2	T47.1X3	T47.1X4	T47.1X5	T47.1X6
hydroxide (gel)	T47.1X1	T47.1X2	T47.1X3	T47.1X4	T47.1X5	T47.1X6
hydroxide-magnesium carb. gel	T47.1X1	T47.1X2	T47.1X3	T47.1X4	T47.1X5	T47.1X6

362 ☑ Additional Character May Be Required — Refer to the Tabular List for Character Selection *Optum Value-Add

Substance	Poisoning, Accidental (unintentional)	Poisoning, Intentional Self-harm	Poisoning, Assault	Poisoning, Undetermined	Adverse Effect	Under-dosing
Aluminium, aluminum — *continued*						
magnesium silicate	T47.1X1	T47.1X2	T47.1X3	T47.1X4	T47.1X5	T47.1X6
nicotinate	T46.7X1	T46.7X2	T46.7X3	T46.7X4	T46.7X5	T46.7X6
ointment (surgical) (topical)	T49.3X1	T49.3X2	T49.3X3	T49.3X4	T49.3X5	T49.3X6
phosphate	T47.1X1	T47.1X2	T47.1X3	T47.1X4	T47.1X5	T47.1X6
salicylate	T39.091	T39.092	T39.093	T39.094	T39.095	T39.096
silicate	T47.1X1	T47.1X2	T47.1X3	T47.1X4	T47.1X5	T47.1X6
sodium silicate	T47.1X1	T47.1X2	T47.1X3	T47.1X4	T47.1X5	T47.1X6
subacetate	T49.2X1	T49.2X2	T49.2X3	T49.2X4	T49.2X5	T49.2X6
sulfate	T49.0X1	T49.0X2	T49.0X3	T49.0X4	T49.0X5	T49.0X6
tannate	T47.6X1	T47.6X2	T47.6X3	T47.6X4	T47.6X5	T47.6X6
topical NEC	T49.3X1	T49.3X2	T49.3X3	T49.3X4	T49.3X5	T49.3X6
Alurate	T42.3X1	T42.3X2	T42.3X3	T42.3X4	T42.3X5	T42.3X6
Alverine	T44.3X1	T44.3X2	T44.3X3	T44.3X4	T44.3X5	T44.3X6
Alvodine	T40.2X1	T40.2X2	T40.2X3	T40.2X4	T40.2X5	T40.2X6
Amanita phalloides	T62.0X1	T62.0X2	T62.0X3	T62.0X4	—	—
Amanitine	T62.0X1	T62.0X2	T62.0X3	T62.0X4	—	—
Amantadine	T42.8X1	T42.8X2	T42.8X3	T42.8X4	T42.8X5	T42.8X6
Ambazone	T49.6X1	T49.6X2	T49.6X3	T49.6X4	T49.6X5	T49.6X6
Ambenonium (chloride)	T44.0X1	T44.0X2	T44.0X3	T44.0X4	T44.0X5	T44.0X6
Ambien*	T42.6X1	T42.6X2	T42.6X3	T42.6X4	T42.6X5	T42.6X6
Ambroxol	T48.4X1	T48.4X2	T48.4X3	T48.4X4	T48.4X5	T48.4X6
Ambuphylline	T48.6X1	T48.6X2	T48.6X3	T48.6X4	T48.6X5	T48.6X6
Ambutonium bromide	T44.3X1	T44.3X2	T44.3X3	T44.3X4	T44.3X5	T44.3X6
Amcinonide	T49.0X1	T49.0X2	T49.0X3	T49.0X4	T49.0X5	T49.0X6
Amdinocilline	T36.0X1	T36.0X2	T36.0X3	T36.0X4	T36.0X5	T36.0X6
Americaine*	T41.3X1	T41.3X2	T41.3X3	T41.3X4	T41.3X5	T41.3X6
Ametazole	T50.8X1	T50.8X2	T50.8X3	T50.8X4	T50.8X5	T50.8X6
Amethocaine	T41.3X1	T41.3X2	T41.3X3	T41.3X4	T41.3X5	T41.3X6
regional	T41.3X1	T41.3X2	T41.3X3	T41.3X4	T41.3X5	T41.3X6
spinal	T41.3X1	T41.3X2	T41.3X3	T41.3X4	T41.3X5	T41.3X6
Amethopterin	T45.1X1	T45.1X2	T45.1X3	T45.1X4	T45.1X5	T45.1X6
Amezinium metilsulfate	T44.991	T44.992	T44.993	T44.994	T44.995	T44.996
Amfebutamone	T43.291	T43.292	T43.293	T43.294	T43.295	T43.296
Amfepramone	T50.5X1	T50.5X2	T50.5X3	T50.5X4	T50.5X5	T50.5X6
Amfetamine	T43.621	T43.622	T43.623	T43.624	T43.625	T43.626
Amfetaminil	T43.621	T43.622	T43.623	T43.624	T43.625	T43.626
Amfomycin	T36.8X1	T36.8X2	T36.8X3	T36.8X4	T36.8X5	T36.8X6
Amidefrine mesilate	T48.5X1	T48.5X2	T48.5X3	T48.5X4	T48.5X5	T48.5X6
Amidone	T40.3X1	T40.3X2	T40.3X3	T40.3X4	T40.3X5	T40.3X6
Amidopyrine	T39.2X1	T39.2X2	T39.2X3	T39.2X4	T39.2X5	T39.2X6
Amidotrizoate	T50.8X1	T50.8X2	T50.8X3	T50.8X4	T50.8X5	T50.8X6
Amiflamine	T43.1X1	T43.1X2	T43.1X3	T43.1X4	T43.1X5	T43.1X6
Amikacin	T36.5X1	T36.5X2	T36.5X3	T36.5X4	T36.5X5	T36.5X6
Amikhelline	T46.3X1	T46.3X2	T46.3X3	T46.3X4	T46.3X5	T46.3X6
Amiloride	T50.2X1	T50.2X2	T50.2X3	T50.2X4	T50.2X5	T50.2X6
Aminacrine	T49.0X1	T49.0X2	T49.0X3	T49.0X4	T49.0X5	T49.0X6
Amineptine	T43.011	T43.012	T43.013	T43.014	T43.015	T43.016
Aminitrozole	T37.3X1	T37.3X2	T37.3X3	T37.3X4	T37.3X5	T37.3X6
Amino acids	T50.3X1	T50.3X2	T50.3X3	T50.3X4	T50.3X5	T50.3X6
Aminoacetic acid (derivatives)	T50.3X1	T50.3X2	T50.3X3	T50.3X4	T50.3X5	T50.3X6
Aminoacridine	T49.0X1	T49.0X2	T49.0X3	T49.0X4	T49.0X5	T49.0X6
Aminobenzoic acid (-p)	T49.3X1	T49.3X2	T49.3X3	T49.3X4	T49.3X5	T49.3X6
Aminocaproic acid	T45.621	T45.622	T45.623	T45.624	T45.625	T45.626
Aminoethylisothiourium	T45.8X1	T45.8X2	T45.8X3	T45.8X4	T45.8X5	T45.8X6
Aminofenazone	T39.2X1	T39.2X2	T39.2X3	T39.2X4	T39.2X5	T39.2X6
Aminoglutethimide	T45.1X1	T45.1X2	T45.1X3	T45.1X4	T45.1X5	T45.1X6
Aminoglycosides*	T36.5X1	T36.5X2	T36.5X3	T36.5X4	T36.5X5	T36.5X6
Aminohippuric acid	T50.8X1	T50.8X2	T50.8X3	T50.8X4	T50.8X5	T50.8X6
Aminomethylbenzoic acid	T45.691	T45.692	T45.693	T45.694	T45.695	T45.696
Aminometradine	T50.2X1	T50.2X2	T50.2X3	T50.2X4	T50.2X5	T50.2X6
Aminopentamide	T44.3X1	T44.3X2	T44.3X3	T44.3X4	T44.3X5	T44.3X6
Aminophenazone	T39.2X1	T39.2X2	T39.2X3	T39.2X4	T39.2X5	T39.2X6
Aminophenol	T54.0X1	T54.0X2	T54.0X3	T54.0X4	—	—
Aminophenylpyridone	T43.591	T43.592	T43.593	T43.594	T43.595	T43.596
Aminophylline	T48.6X1	T48.6X2	T48.6X3	T48.6X4	T48.6X5	T48.6X6
Aminopterin sodium	T45.1X1	T45.1X2	T45.1X3	T45.1X4	T45.1X5	T45.1X6
Aminopyrine	T39.2X1	T39.2X2	T39.2X3	T39.2X4	T39.2X5	T39.2X6
Aminorex	T50.5X1	T50.5X2	T50.5X3	T50.5X4	T50.5X5	T50.5X6
Aminosalicylic acid	T37.1X1	T37.1X2	T37.1X3	T37.1X4	T37.1X5	T37.1X6
Aminosalylum	T37.1X1	T37.1X2	T37.1X3	T37.1X4	T37.1X5	T37.1X6
Amiodarone	T46.2X1	T46.2X2	T46.2X3	T46.2X4	T46.2X5	T46.2X6
Amiphenazole	T50.7X1	T50.7X2	T50.7X3	T50.7X4	T50.7X5	T50.7X6
Amiquinsin	T46.5X1	T46.5X2	T46.5X3	T46.5X4	T46.5X5	T46.5X6
Amisometradine	T50.2X1	T50.2X2	T50.2X3	T50.2X4	T50.2X5	T50.2X6
Amisulpride	T43.591	T43.592	T43.593	T43.594	T43.595	T43.596
Amitriptyline	T43.011	T43.012	T43.013	T43.014	T43.015	T43.016
Amitriptylinoxide	T43.011	T43.012	T43.013	T43.014	T43.015	T43.016
Amlexanox	T48.6X1	T48.6X2	T48.6X3	T48.6X4	T48.6X5	T48.6X6
Amlodipine*	T46.1X1	T46.1X2	T46.1X3	T46.1X4	T46.1X5	T46.1X6

Substance	Poisoning, Accidental (unintentional)	Poisoning, Intentional Self-harm	Poisoning, Assault	Poisoning, Undetermined	Adverse Effect	Under-dosing
Ammonia (fumes) (gas) (vapor)	T59.891	T59.892	T59.893	T59.894	—	—
aromatic spirit	T48.991	T48.992	T48.993	T48.994	T48.995	T48.996
liquid (household)	T54.3X1	T54.3X2	T54.3X3	T54.3X4	—	—
Ammoniated mercury	T49.0X1	T49.0X2	T49.0X3	T49.0X4	T49.0X5	T49.0X6
Ammonium						
acid tartrate	T49.5X1	T49.5X2	T49.5X3	T49.5X4	T49.5X5	T49.5X6
bromide	T42.6X1	T42.6X2	T42.6X3	T42.6X4	T42.6X5	T42.6X6
carbonate	T54.3X1	T54.3X2	T54.3X3	T54.3X4	—	—
chloride	T50.991	T50.992	T50.993	T50.994	T50.995	T50.996
expectorant	T48.4X1	T48.4X2	T48.4X3	T48.4X4	T48.4X5	T48.4X6
compounds (household) NEC	T54.3X1	T54.3X2	T54.3X3	T54.3X4	—	—
fumes (any usage)	T59.891	T59.892	T59.893	T59.894	—	—
industrial	T54.3X1	T54.3X2	T54.3X3	T54.3X4	—	—
ichthyosulronate	T49.4X1	T49.4X2	T49.4X3	T49.4X4	T49.4X5	T49.4X6
mandelate	T37.91	T37.92	T37.93	T37.94	T37.95	T37.96
sulfamate	T60.3X1	T60.3X2	T60.3X3	T60.3X4	—	—
sulfonate resin	T47.8X1	T47.8X2	T47.8X3	T47.8X4	T47.8X5	T47.8X6
Amobarbital (sodium)	T42.3X1	T42.3X2	T42.3X3	T42.3X4	T42.3X5	T42.3X6
Amodiaquine	T37.2X1	T37.2X2	T37.2X3	T37.2X4	T37.2X5	T37.2X6
Amopyroquin (e)	T37.2X1	T37.2X2	T37.2X3	T37.2X4	T37.2X5	T37.2X6
Amoxapine	T43.011	T43.012	T43.013	T43.014	T43.015	T43.016
Amoxicillin	T36.0X1	T36.0X2	T36.0X3	T36.0X4	T36.0X5	T36.0X6
Amperozide	T43.591	T43.592	T43.593	T43.594	T43.595	T43.596
Amphenidone	T43.591	T43.592	T43.593	T43.594	T43.595	T43.596
Amphetamine NEC	T43.621	T43.622	T43.623	T43.624	T43.625	T43.626
Amphogel*	T47.1X1	T47.1X2	T47.1X3	T47.1X4	T47.1X5	T47.1X6
Amphomycin	T36.8X1	T36.8X2	T36.8X3	T36.8X4	T36.8X5	T36.8X6
Amphotalide	T37.4X1	T37.4X2	T37.4X3	T37.4X4	T37.4X5	T37.4X6
Amphotericin B	T36.7X1	T36.7X2	T36.7X3	T36.7X4	T36.7X5	T36.7X6
topical	T49.0X1	T49.0X2	T49.0X3	T49.0X4	T49.0X5	T49.0X6
Ampicillin	T36.0X1	T36.0X2	T36.0X3	T36.0X4	T36.0X5	T36.0X6
Amprotropine	T44.3X1	T44.3X2	T44.3X3	T44.3X4	T44.3X5	T44.3X6
Amsacrine	T45.1X1	T45.1X2	T45.1X3	T45.1X4	T45.1X5	T45.1X6
Amygdaline	T62.2X1	T62.2X2	T62.2X3	T62.2X4	—	—
Amyl						
acetate	T52.8X1	T52.8X2	T52.8X3	T52.8X4	—	—
vapor	T59.891	T59.892	T59.893	T59.894	—	—
alcohol	T51.3X1	T51.3X2	T51.3X3	T51.3X4	—	—
chloride	T53.6X1	T53.6X2	T53.6X3	T53.6X4	—	—
formate	T52.8X1	T52.8X2	T52.8X3	T52.8X4	—	—
nitrite	T46.3X1	T46.3X2	T46.3X3	T46.3X4	T46.3X5	T46.3X6
propionate	T65.891	T65.892	T65.893	T65.894	—	—
Amylase	T47.5X1	T47.5X2	T47.5X3	T47.5X4	T47.5X5	T47.5X6
Amyleine, regional	T41.3X1	T41.3X2	T41.3X3	T41.3X4	T41.3X5	T41.3X6
Amylene						
dichloride	T53.6X1	T53.6X2	T53.6X3	T53.6X4	—	—
hydrate	T51.3X1	T51.3X2	T51.3X3	T51.3X4	—	—
Amylmetacresol	T49.6X1	T49.6X2	T49.6X3	T49.6X4	T49.6X5	T49.6X6
Amylobarbitone	T42.3X1	T42.3X2	T42.3X3	T42.3X4	T42.3X5	T42.3X6
Amylocaine, regional	T41.3X1	T41.3X2	T41.3X3	T41.3X4	T41.3X5	T41.3X6
infiltration (subcutaneous)	T41.3X1	T41.3X2	T41.3X3	T41.3X4	T41.3X5	T41.3X6
nerve block (peripheral) (plexus)	T41.3X1	T41.3X2	T41.3X3	T41.3X4	T41.3X5	T41.3X6
spinal	T41.3X1	T41.3X2	T41.3X3	T41.3X4	T41.3X5	T41.3X6
topical (surface)	T41.3X1	T41.3X2	T41.3X3	T41.3X4	T41.3X5	T41.3X6
Amylopectin	T47.6X1	T47.6X2	T47.6X3	T47.6X4	T47.6X5	T47.6X6
Amytal (sodium)	T42.3X1	T42.3X2	T42.3X3	T42.3X4	T42.3X5	T42.3X6
Anabolic steroid	T38.7X1	T38.7X2	T38.7X3	T38.7X4	T38.7X5	T38.7X6
Anacaine*	T41.3X1	T41.3X2	T41.3X3	T41.3X4	T41.3X5	T41.3X6
Analeptic NEC	T50.7X1	T50.7X2	T50.7X3	T50.7X4	T50.7X5	T50.7X6
Analgesic	T39.91	T39.92	T39.93	T39.94	T39.95	T39.96
anti-inflammatory NEC	T39.91	T39.92	T39.93	T39.94	T39.95	T39.96
propionic acid derivative	T39.311	T39.312	T39.313	T39.314	T39.315	T39.316
antirheumatic NEC	T39.4X1	T39.4X2	T39.4X3	T39.4X4	T39.4X5	T39.4X6
aromatic NEC	T39.1X1	T39.1X2	T39.1X3	T39.1X4	T39.1X5	T39.1X6
narcotic NEC	T40.601	T40.602	T40.603	T40.604	T40.605	T40.606
combination	T40.601	T40.602	T40.603	T40.604	T40.605	T40.606
obstetric	T40.601	T40.602	T40.603	T40.604	T40.605	T40.606
non-narcotic NEC	T39.91	T39.92	T39.93	T39.94	T39.95	T39.96
combination	T39.91	T39.92	T39.93	T39.94	T39.95	T39.96
pyrazole	T39.2X1	T39.2X2	T39.2X3	T39.2X4	T39.2X5	T39.2X6
specified NEC	T39.8X1	T39.8X2	T39.8X3	T39.8X4	T39.8X5	T39.8X6
Analgin	T39.2X1	T39.2X2	T39.2X3	T39.2X4	T39.2X5	T39.2X6
Anamirta cocculus	T62.1X1	T62.1X2	T62.1X3	T62.1X4	—	—
Ancillin	T36.0X1	T36.0X2	T36.0X3	T36.0X4	T36.0X5	T36.0X6
Ancrod	T45.691	T45.692	T45.693	T45.694	T45.695	T45.696
Androgen	T38.7X1	T38.7X2	T38.7X3	T38.7X4	T38.7X5	T38.7X6
Androgen-estrogen mixture	T38.7X1	T38.7X2	T38.7X3	T38.7X4	T38.7X5	T38.7X6
Androstalone	T38.7X1	T38.7X2	T38.7X3	T38.7X4	T38.7X5	T38.7X6
Androstanolone	T38.7X1	T38.7X2	T38.7X3	T38.7X4	T38.7X5	T38.7X6

*Optum Value-Add

☑ Additional Character May Be Required — Refer to the Tabular List for Character Selection

363

Substance	Poisoning, Accidental (unintentional)	Poisoning, Intentional Self-harm	Poisoning, Assault	Poisoning, Undetermined	Adverse Effect	Under-dosing
Androsterone	T38.7X1	T38.7X2	T38.7X3	T38.7X4	T38.7X5	T38.7X6
Anemone pulsatilla	T62.2X1	T62.2X2	T62.2X3	T62.2X4	—	—
Anesthesia						
caudal	T41.3X1	T41.3X2	T41.3X3	T41.3X4	T41.3X5	T41.3X6
endotracheal	T41.ØX1	T41.ØX2	T41.ØX3	T41.ØX4	T41.ØX5	T41.ØX6
epidural	T41.3X1	T41.3X2	T41.3X3	T41.3X4	T41.3X5	T41.3X6
inhalation	T41.ØX1	T41.ØX2	T41.ØX3	T41.ØX4	T41.ØX5	T41.ØX6
local	T41.3X1	T41.3X2	T41.3X3	T41.3X4	T41.3X5	T41.3X6
mucosal	T41.3X1	T41.3X2	T41.3X3	T41.3X4	T41.3X5	T41.3X6
muscle relaxation	T48.1X1	T48.1X2	T48.1X3	T48.1X4	T48.1X5	T48.1X6
nerve blocking	T41.3X1	T41.3X2	T41.3X3	T41.3X4	T41.3X5	T41.3X6
plexus blocking	T41.3X1	T41.3X2	T41.3X3	T41.3X4	T41.3X5	T41.3X6
potentiated	T41.2Ø1	T41.2Ø2	T41.2Ø3	T41.2Ø4	T41.2Ø5	T41.2Ø6
rectal	T41.2Ø1	T41.2Ø2	T41.2Ø3	T41.2Ø4	T41.2Ø5	T41.2Ø6
general	T41.2Ø1	T41.2Ø2	T41.2Ø3	T41.2Ø4	T41.2Ø5	T41.2Ø6
local	T41.3X1	T41.3X2	T41.3X3	T41.3X4	T41.3X5	T41.3X6
regional	T41.3X1	T41.3X2	T41.3X3	T41.3X4	T41.3X5	T41.3X6
surface	T41.3X1	T41.3X2	T41.3X3	T41.3X4	T41.3X5	T41.3X6
Anesthetic NEC — *see also* Anesthesia	T41.41	T41.42	T41.43	T41.44	T41.45	T41.46
gaseous NEC	T41.ØX1	T41.ØX2	T41.ØX3	T41.ØX4	T41.ØX5	T41.ØX6
general NEC	T41.2Ø1	T41.2Ø2	T41.2Ø3	T41.2Ø4	T41.2Ø5	T41.2Ø6
halogenated hydrocarbon derivatives NEC	T41.ØX1	T41.ØX2	T41.ØX3	T41.ØX4	T41.ØX5	T41.ØX6
infiltration NEC	T41.3X1	T41.3X2	T41.3X3	T41.3X4	T41.3X5	T41.3X6
intravenous NEC	T41.1X1	T41.1X2	T41.1X3	T41.1X4	T41.1X5	T41.1X6
local NEC	T41.3X1	T41.3X2	T41.3X3	T41.3X4	T41.3X5	T41.3X6
rectal	T41.2Ø1	T41.2Ø2	T41.2Ø3	T41.2Ø4	T41.2Ø5	T41.2Ø6
general	T41.2Ø1	T41.2Ø2	T41.2Ø3	T41.2Ø4	T41.2Ø5	T41.2Ø6
local	T41.3X1	T41.3X2	T41.3X3	T41.3X4	T41.3X5	T41.3X6
regional NEC	T41.3X1	T41.3X2	T41.3X3	T41.3X4	T41.3X5	T41.3X6
spinal NEC	T41.3X1	T41.3X2	T41.3X3	T41.3X4	T41.3X5	T41.3X6
thiobarbiturate	T41.1X1	T41.1X2	T41.1X3	T41.1X4	T41.1X5	T41.1X6
topical	T41.3X1	T41.3X2	T41.3X3	T41.3X4	T41.3X5	T41.3X6
with muscle relaxant	T41.2Ø1	T41.2Ø2	T41.2Ø3	T41.2Ø4	T41.2Ø5	T41.2Ø6
general	T41.2Ø1	T41.2Ø2	T41.2Ø3	T41.2Ø4	T41.2Ø5	T41.2Ø6
local	T41.3X1	T41.3X2	T41.3X3	T41.3X4	T41.3X5	T41.3X6
Aneurine	T45.2X1	T45.2X2	T45.2X3	T45.2X4	T45.2X5	T45.2X6
Angeliq*	T38.5X1	T38.5X2	T38.5X3	T38.5X4	T38.5X5	T38.5X6
Angio-Conray	T5Ø.8X1	T5Ø.8X2	T5Ø.8X3	T5Ø.8X4	T5Ø.8X5	T5Ø.8X6
Angiotensin	T44.5X1	T44.5X2	T44.5X3	T44.5X4	T44.5X5	T44.5X6
Angiotensinamide	T44.991	T44.992	T44.993	T44.994	T44.995	T44.996
Anhydrohydroxy-progesterone	T38.5X1	T38.5X2	T38.5X3	T38.5X4	T38.5X5	T38.5X6
Anhydron	T5Ø.2X1	T5Ø.2X2	T5Ø.2X3	T5Ø.2X4	T5Ø.2X5	T5Ø.2X6
Anileridine	T4Ø.491	T4Ø.492	T4Ø.493	T4Ø.494	T4Ø.495	T4Ø.496
Aniline (dye) (liquid)	T65.3X1	T65.3X2	T65.3X3	T65.3X4	—	—
analgesic	T39.1X1	T39.1X2	T39.1X3	T39.1X4	T39.1X5	T39.1X6
derivatives, therapeutic NEC	T39.1X1	T39.1X2	T39.1X3	T39.1X4	T39.1X5	T39.1X6
vapor	T65.3X1	T65.3X2	T65.3X3	T65.3X4	—	—
Aniscoropine	T44.3X1	T44.3X2	T44.3X3	T44.3X4	T44.3X5	T44.3X6
Anise oil	T47.5X1	T47.5X2	T47.5X3	T47.5X4	T47.5X5	T47.5X6
Anisidine	T65.3X1	T65.3X2	T65.3X3	T65.3X4	—	—
Anisindione	T45.511	T45.512	T45.513	T45.514	T45.515	T45.516
Anisotropine methyl-bromide	T44.3X1	T44.3X2	T44.3X3	T44.3X4	T44.3X5	T44.3X6
Anistreplase	T45.611	T45.612	T45.613	T45.614	T45.615	T45.616
Anorexiant (central)	T5Ø.5X1	T5Ø.5X2	T5Ø.5X3	T5Ø.5X4	T5Ø.5X5	T5Ø.5X6
Anorexic agents	T5Ø.5X1	T5Ø.5X2	T5Ø.5X3	T5Ø.5X4	T5Ø.5X5	T5Ø.5X6
Ansaid*	T39.311	T39.312	T39.313	T39.314	T39.315	T39.316
Ansamycin	T36.6X1	T36.6X2	T36.6X3	T36.6X4	T36.6X5	T36.6X6
Ant (bite) (sting)	T63.421	T63.422	T63.423	T63.424	—	—
Ant poison — *see* Insecticide						
Antabuse	T5Ø.6X1	T5Ø.6X2	T5Ø.6X3	T5Ø.6X4	T5Ø.6X5	T5Ø.6X6
Antacid NEC	T47.1X1	T47.1X2	T47.1X3	T47.1X4	T47.1X5	T47.1X6
Antagonist						
Aldosterone	T5Ø.ØX1	T5Ø.ØX2	T5Ø.ØX3	T5Ø.ØX4	T5Ø.ØX5	T5Ø.ØX6
alpha-adrenoreceptor	T44.6X1	T44.6X2	T44.6X3	T44.6X4	T44.6X5	T44.6X6
anticoagulant	T45.7X1	T45.7X2	T45.7X3	T45.7X4	T45.7X5	T45.7X6
beta-adrenoreceptor	T44.7X1	T44.7X2	T44.7X3	T44.7X4	T44.7X5	T44.7X6
extrapyramidal NEC	T44.3X1	T44.3X2	T44.3X3	T44.3X4	T44.3X5	T44.3X6
folic acid	T45.1X1	T45.1X2	T45.1X3	T45.1X4	T45.1X5	T45.1X6
H2 receptor	T47.ØX1	T47.ØX2	T47.ØX3	T47.ØX4	T47.ØX5	T47.ØX6
heavy metal	T45.8X1	T45.8X2	T45.8X3	T45.8X4	T45.8X5	T45.8X6
narcotic analgesic	T5Ø.7X1	T5Ø.7X2	T5Ø.7X3	T5Ø.7X4	T5Ø.7X5	T5Ø.7X6
opiate	T5Ø.7X1	T5Ø.7X2	T5Ø.7X3	T5Ø.7X4	T5Ø.7X5	T5Ø.7X6
pyrimidine	T45.1X1	T45.1X2	T45.1X3	T45.1X4	T45.1X5	T45.1X6
serotonin	T46.5X1	T46.5X2	T46.5X3	T46.5X4	T46.5X5	T46.5X6
Antazolin (e)	T45.ØX1	T45.ØX2	T45.ØX3	T45.ØX4	T45.ØX5	T45.ØX6
Anterior pituitary hormone NEC	T38.811	T38.812	T38.813	T38.814	T38.815	T38.816
Anthelmintic NEC	T37.4X1	T37.4X2	T37.4X3	T37.4X4	T37.4X5	T37.4X6
Anthiolimine	T37.4X1	T37.4X2	T37.4X3	T37.4X4	T37.4X5	T37.4X6
Anthralin	T49.4X1	T49.4X2	T49.4X3	T49.4X4	T49.4X5	T49.4X6
Anthramycin	T45.1X1	T45.1X2	T45.1X3	T45.1X4	T45.1X5	T45.1X6
Anti-anemic (drug) (preparation)	T45.8X1	T45.8X2	T45.8X3	T45.8X4	T45.8X5	T45.8X6
Anti-common-cold drug NEC	T48.5X1	T48.5X2	T48.5X3	T48.5X4	T48.5X5	T48.5X6
Anti-D immunoglobulin (human)	T5Ø.Z11	T5Ø.Z12	T5Ø.Z13	T5Ø.Z14	T5Ø.Z15	T5Ø.Z16
Anti-gastric-secretion drug NEC	T47.1X1	T47.1X2	T47.1X3	T47.1X4	T47.1X5	T47.1X6
Anti-human lymphocytic globulin	T5Ø.Z11	T5Ø.Z12	T5Ø.Z13	T5Ø.Z14	T5Ø.Z15	T5Ø.Z16
Anti-infective NEC	T37.91	T37.92	T37.93	T37.94	T37.95	T37.96
anthelmintic	T37.4X1	T37.4X2	T37.4X3	T37.4X4	T37.4X5	T37.4X6
antibiotics	T36.91	T36.92	T36.93	T36.94	T36.95	T36.96
specified NEC	T36.8X1	T36.8X2	T36.8X3	T36.8X4	T36.8X5	T36.8X6
antimalarial	T37.2X1	T37.2X2	T37.2X3	T37.2X4	T37.2X5	T37.2X6
antimycobacterial NEC	T37.1X1	T37.1X2	T37.1X3	T37.1X4	T37.1X5	T37.1X6
antibiotics	T36.5X1	T36.5X2	T36.5X3	T36.5X4	T36.5X5	T36.5X6
antiprotozoal NEC	T37.3X1	T37.3X2	T37.3X3	T37.3X4	T37.3X5	T37.3X6
blood	T37.2X1	T37.2X2	T37.2X3	T37.2X4	T37.2X5	T37.2X6
antiviral	T37.5X1	T37.5X2	T37.5X3	T37.5X4	T37.5X5	T37.5X6
arsenical	T37.8X1	T37.8X2	T37.8X3	T37.8X4	T37.8X5	T37.8X6
bismuth, local	T49.ØX1	T49.ØX2	T49.ØX3	T49.ØX4	T49.ØX5	T49.ØX6
ENT	T49.6X1	T49.6X2	T49.6X3	T49.6X4	T49.6X5	T49.6X6
eye NEC	T49.5X1	T49.5X2	T49.5X3	T49.5X4	T49.5X5	T49.5X6
heavy metals NEC	T37.8X1	T37.8X2	T37.8X3	T37.8X4	T37.8X5	T37.8X6
local NEC	T49.ØX1	T49.ØX2	T49.ØX3	T49.ØX4	T49.ØX5	T49.ØX6
specified NEC	T49.ØX1	T49.ØX2	T49.ØX3	T49.ØX4	T49.ØX5	T49.ØX6
mixed	T37.91	T37.92	T37.93	T37.94	T37.95	T37.96
ophthalmic preparation	T49.5X1	T49.5X2	T49.5X3	T49.5X4	T49.5X5	T49.5X6
topical NEC	T49.ØX1	T49.ØX2	T49.ØX3	T49.ØX4	T49.ØX5	T49.ØX6
Anti-inflammatory drug NEC	T39.391	T39.392	T39.393	T39.394	T39.395	T39.396
local	T49.ØX1	T49.ØX2	T49.ØX3	T49.ØX4	T49.ØX5	T49.ØX6
nonsteroidal NEC	T39.391	T39.392	T39.393	T39.394	T39.395	T39.396
propionic acid derivative	T39.311	T39.312	T39.313	T39.314	T39.315	T39.316
specified NEC	T39.391	T39.392	T39.393	T39.394	T39.395	T39.396
Antiadrenergic NEC	T44.8X1	T44.8X2	T44.8X3	T44.8X4	T44.8X5	T44.8X6
Antiallergic NEC	T45.ØX1	T45.ØX2	T45.ØX3	T45.ØX4	T45.ØX5	T45.ØX6
Antiandrogen NEC	T38.6X1	T38.6X2	T38.6X3	T38.6X4	T38.6X5	T38.6X6
Antianxiety drug NEC	T43.5Ø1	T43.5Ø2	T43.5Ø3	T43.5Ø4	T43.5Ø5	T43.5Ø6
Antiaris toxicaria	T65.891	T65.892	T65.893	T65.894	—	—
Antiarteriosclerotic drug	T46.6X1	T46.6X2	T46.6X3	T46.6X4	T46.6X5	T46.6X6
Antiasthmatic drug NEC	T48.6X1	T48.6X2	T48.6X3	T48.6X4	T48.6X5	T48.6X6
Antibiotic NEC	T36.91	T36.92	T36.93	T36.94	T36.95	T36.96
aminoglycoside	T36.5X1	T36.5X2	T36.5X3	T36.5X4	T36.5X5	T36.5X6
anticancer	T45.1X1	T45.1X2	T45.1X3	T45.1X4	T45.1X5	T45.1X6
antifungal	T36.7X1	T36.7X2	T36.7X3	T36.7X4	T36.7X5	T36.7X6
antimycobacterial	T36.5X1	T36.5X2	T36.5X3	T36.5X4	T36.5X5	T36.5X6
antineoplastic	T45.1X1	T45.1X2	T45.1X3	T45.1X4	T45.1X5	T45.1X6
b-lactam NEC	T36.1X1	T36.1X2	T36.1X3	T36.1X4	T36.1X5	T36.1X6
cephalosporin (group)	T36.1X1	T36.1X2	T36.1X3	T36.1X4	T36.1X5	T36.1X6
chloramphenicol (group)	T36.2X1	T36.2X2	T36.2X3	T36.2X4	T36.2X5	T36.2X6
ENT	T49.6X1	T49.6X2	T49.6X3	T49.6X4	T49.6X5	T49.6X6
eye	T49.5X1	T49.5X2	T49.5X3	T49.5X4	T49.5X5	T49.5X6
fungicidal (local)	T49.ØX1	T49.ØX2	T49.ØX3	T49.ØX4	T49.ØX5	T49.ØX6
intestinal	T36.8X1	T36.8X2	T36.8X3	T36.8X4	T36.8X5	T36.8X6
local	T49.ØX1	T49.ØX2	T49.ØX3	T49.ØX4	T49.ØX5	T49.ØX6
macrolides	T36.3X1	T36.3X2	T36.3X3	T36.3X4	T36.3X5	T36.3X6
polypeptide	T36.8X1	T36.8X2	T36.8X3	T36.8X4	T36.8X5	T36.8X6
specified NEC	T36.8X1	T36.8X2	T36.8X3	T36.8X4	T36.8X5	T36.8X6
tetracycline (group)	T36.4X1	T36.4X2	T36.4X3	T36.4X4	T36.4X5	T36.4X6
throat	T49.6X1	T49.6X2	T49.6X3	T49.6X4	T49.6X5	T49.6X6
Antibiotic Otic Suspension (Solution)*	T49.6X1	T49.6X2	T49.6X3	T49.6X4	T49.6X5	T49.6X6
Anticancer agents NEC	T45.1X1	T45.1X2	T45.1X3	T45.1X4	T45.1X5	T45.1X6
Anticholesterolemic drug NEC	T46.6X1	T46.6X2	T46.6X3	T46.6X4	T46.6X5	T46.6X6
Anticholinergic NEC	T44.3X1	T44.3X2	T44.3X3	T44.3X4	T44.3X5	T44.3X6
Anticholinesterase	T44.ØX1	T44.ØX2	T44.ØX3	T44.ØX4	T44.ØX5	T44.ØX6
organophosphorus	T44.ØX1	T44.ØX2	T44.ØX3	T44.ØX4	T44.ØX5	T44.ØX6
insecticide	T6Ø.ØX1	T6Ø.ØX2	T6Ø.ØX3	T6Ø.ØX4	—	—
nerve gas	T59.891	T59.892	T59.893	T59.894	—	—
reversible	T44.ØX1	T44.ØX2	T44.ØX3	T44.ØX4	T44.ØX5	T44.ØX6
ophthalmological	T49.5X1	T49.5X2	T49.5X3	T49.5X4	T49.5X5	T49.5X6
Anticoagulant NEC	T45.511	T45.512	T45.513	T45.514	T45.515	T45.516
Antagonist	T45.7X1	T45.7X2	T45.7X3	T45.7X4	T45.7X5	T45.7X6
Anticonvulsant	T42.71	T42.72	T42.73	T42.74	T42.75	T42.76
barbiturate	T42.3X1	T42.3X2	T42.3X3	T42.3X4	T42.3X5	T42.3X6
combination (with barbiturate)	T42.3X1	T42.3X2	T42.3X3	T42.3X4	T42.3X5	T42.3X6
hydantoin	T42.ØX1	T42.ØX2	T42.ØX3	T42.ØX4	T42.ØX5	T42.ØX6

Substance	Poisoning, Accidental (unintentional)	Poisoning, Intentional Self-harm	Poisoning, Assault	Poisoning, Undetermined	Adverse Effect	Under-dosing
Anticonvulsant — *continued*						
hypnotic NEC	T42.6X1	T42.6X2	T42.6X3	T42.6X4	T42.6X5	T42.6X6
oxazolidinedione	T42.2X1	T42.2X2	T42.2X3	T42.2X4	T42.2X5	T42.2X6
pyrimidinedione	T42.6X1	T42.6X2	T42.6X3	T42.6X4	T42.6X5	T42.6X6
specified NEC	T42.6X1	T42.6X2	T42.6X3	T42.6X4	T42.6X5	T42.6X6
succinimide	T42.2X1	T42.2X2	T42.2X3	T42.2X4	T42.2X5	T42.2X6
Antidepressant	T43.2Ø1	T43.2Ø2	T43.2Ø3	T43.2Ø4	T43.2Ø5	T43.2Ø6
monoamine oxidase inhibitor	T43.1X1	T43.1X2	T43.1X3	T43.1X4	T43.1X5	T43.1X6
selective serotonin norepinephrine reuptake inhibitor	T43.211	T43.212	T43.213	T43.214	T43.215	T43.216
selective serotonin reuptake inhibitor	T43.221	T43.222	T43.223	T43.224	T43.225	T43.226
specified NEC	T43.291	T43.292	T43.293	T43.294	T43.295	T43.296
tetracyclic	T43.Ø21	T43.Ø22	T43.Ø23	T43.Ø24	T43.Ø25	T43.Ø26
triazolopyridine	T43.211	T43.212	T43.213	T43.214	T43.215	T43.216
tricyclic	T43.Ø11	T43.Ø12	T43.Ø13	T43.Ø14	T43.Ø15	T43.Ø16
Antidiabetic NEC	T38.3X1	T38.3X2	T38.3X3	T38.3X4	T38.3X5	T38.3X6
biguanide	T38.3X1	T38.3X2	T38.3X3	T38.3X4	T38.3X5	T38.3X6
and sulfonyl combined	T38.3X1	T38.3X2	T38.3X3	T38.3X4	T38.3X5	T38.3X6
combined	T38.3X1	T38.3X2	T38.3X3	T38.3X4	T38.3X5	T38.3X6
sulfonylurea	T38.3X1	T38.3X2	T38.3X3	T38.3X4	T38.3X5	T38.3X6
Antidiarrheal drug NEC	T47.6X1	T47.6X2	T47.6X3	T47.6X4	T47.6X5	T47.6X6
absorbent	T47.6X1	T47.6X2	T47.6X3	T47.6X4	T47.6X5	T47.6X6
Antidiphtheria serum	T5Ø.Z11	T5Ø.Z12	T5Ø.Z13	T5Ø.Z14	T5Ø.Z15	T5Ø.Z16
Antidiuretic hormone	T38.891	T38.892	T38.893	T38.894	T38.895	T38.896
Antidote NEC	T5Ø.6X1	T5Ø.6X2	T5Ø.6X3	T5Ø.6X4	T5Ø.6X5	T5Ø.6X6
heavy metal	T45.8X1	T45.8X2	T45.8X3	T45.8X4	T45.8X5	T45.8X6
Antidysrhythmic NEC	T46.2X1	T46.2X2	T46.2X3	T46.2X4	T46.2X5	T46.2X6
Antiemetic drug	T45.ØX1	T45.ØX2	T45.ØX3	T45.ØX4	T45.ØX5	T45.ØX6
Antiepilepsy agent	T42.71	T42.72	T42.73	T42.74	T42.75	T42.76
combination	T42.5X1	T42.5X2	T42.5X3	T42.5X4	T42.5X5	T42.5X6
mixed	T42.5X1	T42.5X2	T42.5X3	T42.5X4	T42.5X5	T42.5X6
specified, NEC	T42.6X1	T42.6X2	T42.6X3	T42.6X4	T42.6X5	T42.6X6
Antiestrogen NEC	T38.6X1	T38.6X2	T38.6X3	T38.6X4	T38.6X5	T38.6X6
Antifertility pill	T38.4X1	T38.4X2	T38.4X3	T38.4X4	T38.4X5	T38.4X6
Antifibrinolytic drug	T45.621	T45.622	T45.623	T45.624	T45.625	T45.626
Antifilarial drug	T37.4X1	T37.4X2	T37.4X3	T37.4X4	T37.4X5	T37.4X6
Antiflatulent	T47.5X1	T47.5X2	T47.5X3	T47.5X4	T47.5X5	T47.5X6
Antifreeze	T65.91	T65.92	T65.93	T65.94	—	—
alcohol	T51.1X1	T51.1X2	T51.1X3	T51.1X4	—	—
ethylene glycol	T51.8X1	T51.8X2	T51.8X3	T51.8X4	—	—
Antifungal						
anti-infective NEC	T37.91	T37.92	T37.93	T37.94	T37.95	T37.96
antibiotic (systemic)	T36.7X1	T36.7X2	T36.7X3	T36.7X4	T36.7X5	T36.7X6
disinfectant, local	T49.ØX1	T49.ØX2	T49.ØX3	T49.ØX4	T49.ØX5	T49.ØX6
nonmedicinal (spray)	T6Ø.3X1	T6Ø.3X2	T6Ø.3X3	T6Ø.3X4	—	—
topical	T49.ØX1	T49.ØX2	T49.ØX3	T49.ØX4	T49.ØX5	T49.ØX6
Antigonadotrophin NEC	T38.6X1	T38.6X2	T38.6X3	T38.6X4	T38.6X5	T38.6X6
Antihallucinogen	T43.5Ø1	T43.5Ø2	T43.5Ø3	T43.5Ø4	T43.5Ø5	T43.5Ø6
Antihelmintics	T37.4X1	T37.4X2	T37.4X3	T37.4X4	T37.4X5	T37.4X6
Antihemophilic						
factor	T45.8X1	T45.8X2	T45.8X3	T45.8X4	T45.8X5	T45.8X6
fraction	T45.8X1	T45.8X2	T45.8X3	T45.8X4	T45.8X5	T45.8X6
globulin concentrate	T45.7X1	T45.7X2	T45.7X3	T45.7X4	T45.7X5	T45.7X6
human plasma	T45.8X1	T45.8X2	T45.8X3	T45.8X4	T45.8X5	T45.8X6
plasma, dried	T45.7X1	T45.7X2	T45.7X3	T45.7X4	T45.7X5	T45.7X6
Antihemorrhoidal preparation	T49.2X1	T49.2X2	T49.2X3	T49.2X4	T49.2X5	T49.2X6
Antiheparin drug	T45.7X1	T45.7X2	T45.7X3	T45.7X4	T45.7X5	T45.7X6
Antihistamine	T45.ØX1	T45.ØX2	T45.ØX3	T45.ØX4	T45.ØX5	T45.ØX6
Antihookworm drug	T37.4X1	T37.4X2	T37.4X3	T37.4X4	T37.4X5	T37.4X6
Antihyperlipidemic drug	T46.6X1	T46.6X2	T46.6X3	T46.6X4	T46.6X5	T46.6X6
Antihypertensive drug NEC	T46.5X1	T46.5X2	T46.5X3	T46.5X4	T46.5X5	T46.5X6
Antikaluretic	T5Ø.3X1	T5Ø.3X2	T5Ø.3X3	T5Ø.3X4	T5Ø.3X5	T5Ø.3X6
Antiknock (tetraethyl lead)	T56.ØX1	T56.ØX2	T56.ØX3	T56.ØX4	—	—
Antilipemic drug NEC	T46.6X1	T46.6X2	T46.6X3	T46.6X4	T46.6X5	T46.6X6
Antilysin*	T45.621	T45.622	T45.623	T45.624	T45.625	T45.626
Antimalarial	T37.2X1	T37.2X2	T37.2X3	T37.2X4	T37.2X5	T37.2X6
prophylactic NEC	T37.2X1	T37.2X2	T37.2X3	T37.2X4	T37.2X5	T37.2X6
pyrimidine derivative	T37.2X1	T37.2X2	T37.2X3	T37.2X4	T37.2X5	T37.2X6
Antimetabolite	T45.1X1	T45.1X2	T45.1X3	T45.1X4	T45.1X5	T45.1X6
Antimitotic agent	T45.1X1	T45.1X2	T45.1X3	T45.1X4	T45.1X5	T45.1X6
Antimony (compounds) (vapor) **NEC**	T56.891	T56.892	T56.893	T56.894	—	—
anti-infectives	T37.8X1	T37.8X2	T37.8X3	T37.8X4	T37.8X5	T37.8X6
dimercaptosuccinate	T37.3X1	T37.3X2	T37.3X3	T37.3X4	T37.3X5	T37.3X6
hydride	T56.891	T56.892	T56.893	T56.894	—	—
sodium dimercaptosuccinate	T37.3X1	T37.3X2	T37.3X3	T37.3X4	T37.3X5	T37.3X6
tartrated	T37.8X1	T37.8X2	T37.8X3	T37.8X4	T37.8X5	T37.8X6

Substance	Poisoning, Accidental (unintentional)	Poisoning, Intentional Self-harm	Poisoning, Assault	Poisoning, Undetermined	Adverse Effect	Under-dosing
Antimony (compounds) (vapor) **NEC** — *continued*						
pesticide (vapor)	T6Ø.8X1	T6Ø.8X2	T6Ø.8X3	T6Ø.8X4	—	—
potassium (sodium) tartrate	T37.8X1	T37.8X2	T37.8X3	T37.8X4	T37.8X5	T37.8X6
Antimuscarinic NEC	T44.3X1	T44.3X2	T44.3X3	T44.3X4	T44.3X5	T44.3X6
Antimycobacterial drug NEC	T37.1X1	T37.1X2	T37.1X3	T37.1X4	T37.1X5	T37.1X6
antibiotics	T36.5X1	T36.5X2	T36.5X3	T36.5X4	T36.5X5	T36.5X6
combination	T37.1X1	T37.1X2	T37.1X3	T37.1X4	T37.1X5	T37.1X6
Antinausea drug	T45.ØX1	T45.ØX2	T45.ØX3	T45.ØX4	T45.ØX5	T45.ØX6
Antinematode drug	T37.4X1	T37.4X2	T37.4X3	T37.4X4	T37.4X5	T37.4X6
Antineoplastic NEC	T45.1X1	T45.1X2	T45.1X3	T45.1X4	T45.1X5	T45.1X6
alkaloidal	T45.1X1	T45.1X2	T45.1X3	T45.1X4	T45.1X5	T45.1X6
antibiotics	T45.1X1	T45.1X2	T45.1X3	T45.1X4	T45.1X5	T45.1X6
combination	T45.1X1	T45.1X2	T45.1X3	T45.1X4	T45.1X5	T45.1X6
estrogen	T38.5X1	T38.5X2	T38.5X3	T38.5X4	T38.5X5	T38.5X6
steroid	T38.7X1	T38.7X2	T38.7X3	T38.7X4	T38.7X5	T38.7X6
Antiparasitic drug (systemic)	T37.91	T37.92	T37.93	T37.94	T37.95	T37.96
local	T49.ØX1	T49.ØX2	T49.ØX3	T49.ØX4	T49.ØX5	T49.ØX6
specified NEC	T37.8X1	T37.8X2	T37.8X3	T37.8X4	T37.8X5	T37.8X6
Antiparkinsonism drug NEC	T42.8X1	T42.8X2	T42.8X3	T42.8X4	T42.8X5	T42.8X6
Antiperspirant NEC	T49.2X1	T49.2X2	T49.2X3	T49.2X4	T49.2X5	T49.2X6
Antiphlogistic NEC	T39.4X1	T39.4X2	T39.4X3	T39.4X4	T39.4X5	T39.4X6
Antiplatyhelmintic drug	T37.4X1	T37.4X2	T37.4X3	T37.4X4	T37.4X5	T37.4X6
Antiprotozoal drug NEC	T37.3X1	T37.3X2	T37.3X3	T37.3X4	T37.3X5	T37.3X6
blood	T37.2X1	T37.2X2	T37.2X3	T37.2X4	T37.2X5	T37.2X6
local	T49.ØX1	T49.ØX2	T49.ØX3	T49.ØX4	T49.ØX5	T49.ØX6
Antipruritic drug NEC	T49.1X1	T49.1X2	T49.1X3	T49.1X4	T49.1X5	T49.1X6
Antipsychotic drug	T43.5Ø1	T43.5Ø2	T43.5Ø3	T43.5Ø4	T43.5Ø5	T43.5Ø6
specified NEC	T43.591	T43.592	T43.593	T43.594	T43.595	T43.596
Antipyretic	T39.91	T39.92	T39.93	T39.94	T39.95	T39.96
specified NEC	T39.8X1	T39.8X2	T39.8X3	T39.8X4	T39.8X5	T39.8X6
Antipyrine	T39.2X1	T39.2X2	T39.2X3	T39.2X4	T39.2X5	T39.2X6
Antirabies hyperimmune serum	T5Ø.Z11	T5Ø.Z12	T5Ø.Z13	T5Ø.Z14	T5Ø.Z15	T5Ø.Z16
Antirheumatic NEC	T39.4X1	T39.4X2	T39.4X3	T39.4X4	T39.4X5	T39.4X6
Antirigidity drug NEC	T42.8X1	T42.8X2	T42.8X3	T42.8X4	T42.8X5	T42.8X6
Antischistosomal drug	T37.4X1	T37.4X2	T37.4X3	T37.4X4	T37.4X5	T37.4X6
Antiscorpion sera	T5Ø.Z11	T5Ø.Z12	T5Ø.Z13	T5Ø.Z14	T5Ø.Z15	T5Ø.Z16
Antiseborrheics	T49.4X1	T49.4X2	T49.4X3	T49.4X4	T49.4X5	T49.4X6
Antiseptics (external) (medicinal)	T49.ØX1	T49.ØX2	T49.ØX3	T49.ØX4	T49.ØX5	T49.ØX6
Antistine	T45.ØX1	T45.ØX2	T45.ØX3	T45.ØX4	T45.ØX5	T45.ØX6
Antitapeworm drug	T37.4X1	T37.4X2	T37.4X3	T37.4X4	T37.4X5	T37.4X6
Antitetanus immunoglobulin	T5Ø.Z11	T5Ø.Z12	T5Ø.Z13	T5Ø.Z14	T5Ø.Z15	T5Ø.Z16
Antithrombin III*	T45.511	T45.512	T45.513	T45.514	T45.515	T45.516
Antithrombotic	T45.521	T45.522	T45.523	T45.524	T45.525	T45.526
Antithyroid drug NEC	T38.2X1	T38.2X2	T38.2X3	T38.2X4	T38.2X5	T38.2X6
Antitoxin	T5Ø.Z11	T5Ø.Z12	T5Ø.Z13	T5Ø.Z14	T5Ø.Z15	T5Ø.Z16
diphtheria	T5Ø.Z11	T5Ø.Z12	T5Ø.Z13	T5Ø.Z14	T5Ø.Z15	T5Ø.Z16
gas gangrene	T5Ø.Z11	T5Ø.Z12	T5Ø.Z13	T5Ø.Z14	T5Ø.Z15	T5Ø.Z16
tetanus	T5Ø.Z11	T5Ø.Z12	T5Ø.Z13	T5Ø.Z14	T5Ø.Z15	T5Ø.Z16
Antitrichomonal drug	T37.3X1	T37.3X2	T37.3X3	T37.3X4	T37.3X5	T37.3X6
Antituberculars	T37.1X1	T37.1X2	T37.1X3	T37.1X4	T37.1X5	T37.1X6
antibiotics	T36.5X1	T36.5X2	T36.5X3	T36.5X4	T36.5X5	T36.5X6
Antitussive NEC	T48.3X1	T48.3X2	T48.3X3	T48.3X4	T48.3X5	T48.3X6
codeine mixture	T4Ø.2X1	T4Ø.2X2	T4Ø.2X3	T4Ø.2X4	T4Ø.2X5	T4Ø.2X6
opiate	T4Ø.2X1	T4Ø.2X2	T4Ø.2X3	T4Ø.2X4	T4Ø.2X5	T4Ø.2X6
Antivaricose drug	T46.8X1	T46.8X2	T46.8X3	T46.8X4	T46.8X5	T46.8X6
Antivenin, antivenom (sera)	T5Ø.Z11	T5Ø.Z12	T5Ø.Z13	T5Ø.Z14	T5Ø.Z15	T5Ø.Z16
crotaline	T5Ø.Z11	T5Ø.Z12	T5Ø.Z13	T5Ø.Z14	T5Ø.Z15	T5Ø.Z16
spider bite	T5Ø.Z11	T5Ø.Z12	T5Ø.Z13	T5Ø.Z14	T5Ø.Z15	T5Ø.Z16
Antivert*	T45.ØX1	T45.ØX2	T45.ØX3	T45.ØX4	T45.ØX5	T45.ØX6
Antivertigo drug	T45.ØX1	T45.ØX2	T45.ØX3	T45.ØX4	T45.ØX5	T45.ØX6
Antiviral drug NEC	T37.5X1	T37.5X2	T37.5X3	T37.5X4	T37.5X5	T37.5X6
eye	T49.5X1	T49.5X2	T49.5X3	T49.5X4	T49.5X5	T49.5X6
Antiwhipworm drug	T37.4X1	T37.4X2	T37.4X3	T37.4X4	T37.4X5	T37.4X6
Antrol — *see also* by specific chemical substance	T6Ø.91	T6Ø.92	T6Ø.93	T6Ø.94	—	—
fungicide	T6Ø.91	T6Ø.92	T6Ø.93	T6Ø.94	—	—
ANTU (alpha naphthylthiourea)	T6Ø.4X1	T6Ø.4X2	T6Ø.4X3	T6Ø.4X4	—	—
Apalcillin	T36.ØX1	T36.ØX2	T36.ØX3	T36.ØX4	T36.ØX5	T36.ØX6
APC	T48.5X1	T48.5X2	T48.5X3	T48.5X4	T48.5X5	T48.5X6
Aplonidine	T44.4X1	T44.4X2	T44.4X3	T44.4X4	T44.4X5	T44.4X6
Apomorphine	T47.7X1	T47.7X2	T47.7X3	T47.7X4	T47.7X5	T47.7X6
Appetite depressants, central	T5Ø.5X1	T5Ø.5X2	T5Ø.5X3	T5Ø.5X4	T5Ø.5X5	T5Ø.5X6

*Optum Value-Add
☑ Additional Character May Be Required — Refer to the Tabular List for Character Selection
365

Substance	Poisoning, Accidental (unintentional)	Poisoning, Intentional Self-harm	Poisoning, Assault	Poisoning, Undetermined	Adverse Effect	Under-dosing
Apraclonidine (hydrochloride)	T44.4X1	T44.4X2	T44.4X3	T44.4X4	T44.4X5	T44.4X6
Apresoline	T46.5X1	T46.5X2	T46.5X3	T46.5X4	T46.5X5	T46.5X6
Apri*	T38.4X1	T38.4X2	T38.4X3	T38.4X4	T38.4X5	T38.4X6
Aprindine	T46.2X1	T46.2X2	T46.2X3	T46.2X4	T46.2X5	T46.2X6
Aprobarbital	T42.3X1	T42.3X2	T42.3X3	T42.3X4	T42.3X5	T42.3X6
Apronalide	T42.6X1	T42.6X2	T42.6X3	T42.6X4	T42.6X5	T42.6X6
Aprotinin	T45.621	T45.622	T45.623	T45.624	T45.625	T45.626
Aptocaine	T41.3X1	T41.3X2	T41.3X3	T41.3X4	T41.3X5	T41.3X6
Aqua fortis	T54.2X1	T54.2X2	T54.2X3	T54.2X4	—	—
Ara-A	T37.5X1	T37.5X2	T37.5X3	T37.5X4	T37.5X5	T37.5X6
Ara-C	T45.1X1	T45.1X2	T45.1X3	T45.1X4	T45.1X5	T45.1X6
Arachis oil	T49.3X1	T49.3X2	T49.3X3	T49.3X4	T49.3X5	T49.3X6
cathartic	T47.4X1	T47.4X2	T47.4X3	T47.4X4	T47.4X5	T47.4X6
Aralen	T37.2X1	T37.2X2	T37.2X3	T37.2X4	T37.2X5	T37.2X6
Arecoline	T44.1X1	T44.1X2	T44.1X3	T44.1X4	T44.1X5	T44.1X6
Arginine	T5Ø.991	T5Ø.992	T5Ø.993	T5Ø.994	T5Ø.995	T5Ø.996
glutamate	T5Ø.991	T5Ø.992	T5Ø.993	T5Ø.994	T5Ø.995	T5Ø.996
Argyrol	T49.ØX1	T49.ØX2	T49.ØX3	T49.ØX4	T49.ØX5	T49.ØX6
ENT agent	T49.6X1	T49.6X2	T49.6X3	T49.6X4	T49.6X5	T49.6X6
ophthalmic preparation	T49.5X1	T49.5X2	T49.5X3	T49.5X4	T49.5X5	T49.5X6
Aristocort	T38.ØX1	T38.ØX2	T38.ØX3	T38.ØX4	T38.ØX5	T38.ØX6
ENT agent	T49.6X1	T49.6X2	T49.6X3	T49.6X4	T49.6X5	T49.6X6
ophthalmic preparation	T49.5X1	T49.5X2	T49.5X3	T49.5X4	T49.5X5	T49.5X6
topical NEC	T49.ØX1	T49.ØX2	T49.ØX3	T49.ØX4	T49.ØX5	T49.ØX6
Armour*	T38.1X1	T38.1X2	T38.1X3	T38.1X4	T38.1X5	T38.1X6
Aromatics, corrosive	T54.1X1	T54.1X2	T54.1X3	T54.1X4	—	—
disinfectants	T54.1X1	T54.1X2	T54.1X3	T54.1X4	—	—
Arsenate of lead	T57.ØX1	T57.ØX2	T57.ØX3	T57.ØX4	—	—
herbicide	T57.ØX1	T57.ØX2	T57.ØX3	T57.ØX4	—	—
Arsenic, arsenicals (compounds) (dust) (vapor) **NEC**	T57.ØX1	T57.ØX2	T57.ØX3	T57.ØX4	—	—
anti-infectives	T37.8X1	T37.8X2	T37.8X3	T37.8X4	T37.8X5	T37.8X6
pesticide (dust) (fumes)	T57.ØX1	T57.ØX2	T57.ØX3	T57.ØX4	—	—
Arsine (gas)	T57.ØX1	T57.ØX2	T57.ØX3	T57.ØX4	—	—
Arsobal*	T37.3X1	T37.3X2	T37.3X3	T37.3X4	T37.3X5	T37.3X6
Arsphenamine (silver)	T37.8X1	T37.8X2	T37.8X3	T37.8X4	T37.8X5	T37.8X6
Arsthinol	T37.3X1	T37.3X2	T37.3X3	T37.3X4	T37.3X5	T37.3X6
Artane	T44.3X1	T44.3X2	T44.3X3	T44.3X4	T44.3X5	T44.3X6
Arthropod (venomous) **NEC**	T63.481	T63.482	T63.483	T63.484	—	—
Articaine	T41.3X1	T41.3X2	T41.3X3	T41.3X4	T41.3X5	T41.3X6
Asbestos	T57.8X1	T57.8X2	T57.8X3	T57.8X4	—	—
Ascaridole	T37.4X1	T37.4X2	T37.4X3	T37.4X4	T37.4X5	T37.4X6
Ascorbic acid	T45.2X1	T45.2X2	T45.2X3	T45.2X4	T45.2X5	T45.2X6
Asiaticoside	T49.ØX1	T49.ØX2	T49.ØX3	T49.ØX4	T49.ØX5	T49.ØX6
Asparaginase	T45.1X1	T45.1X2	T45.1X3	T45.1X4	T45.1X5	T45.1X6
Aspidium (oleoresin)	T37.4X1	T37.4X2	T37.4X3	T37.4X4	T37.4X5	T37.4X6
Aspirin (aluminum) (soluble)	T39.Ø11	T39.Ø12	T39.Ø13	T39.Ø14	T39.Ø15	T39.Ø16
Aspoxicillin	T36.ØX1	T36.ØX2	T36.ØX3	T36.ØX4	T36.ØX5	T36.ØX6
Astemizole	T45.ØX1	T45.ØX2	T45.ØX3	T45.ØX4	T45.ØX5	T45.ØX6
Astringent (local)	T49.2X1	T49.2X2	T49.2X3	T49.2X4	T49.2X5	T49.2X6
specified NEC	T49.2X1	T49.2X2	T49.2X3	T49.2X4	T49.2X5	T49.2X6
Astromicin	T36.5X1	T36.5X2	T36.5X3	T36.5X4	T36.5X5	T36.5X6
Ataractic drug NEC	T43.5Ø1	T43.5Ø2	T43.5Ø3	T43.5Ø4	T43.5Ø5	T43.5Ø6
Atenolol	T44.7X1	T44.7X2	T44.7X3	T44.7X4	T44.7X5	T44.7X6
Atonia drug, intestinal	T47.4X1	T47.4X2	T47.4X3	T47.4X4	T47.4X5	T47.4X6
Atophan	T5Ø.4X1	T5Ø.4X2	T5Ø.4X3	T5Ø.4X4	T5Ø.4X5	T5Ø.4X6
Atorvastatin*	T46.6X1	T46.6X2	T46.6X3	T46.6X4	T46.6X5	T46.6X6
Atracurium besilate	T48.1X1	T48.1X2	T48.1X3	T48.1X4	T48.1X5	T48.1X6
Atropine	T44.3X1	T44.3X2	T44.3X3	T44.3X4	T44.3X5	T44.3X6
derivative	T44.3X1	T44.3X2	T44.3X3	T44.3X4	T44.3X5	T44.3X6
methonitrate	T44.3X1	T44.3X2	T44.3X3	T44.3X4	T44.3X5	T44.3X6
Atrovent*	T48.6X1	T48.6X2	T48.6X3	T48.6X4	T48.6X5	T48.6X6
Attapulgite	T47.6X1	T47.6X2	T47.6X3	T47.6X4	T47.6X5	T47.6X6
Augmentin (ES-600) (XR)*	T36.ØX1	T36.ØX2	T36.ØX3	T36.ØX4	T36.ØX5	T36.ØX6
Auramine	T65.891	T65.892	T65.893	T65.894	—	—
dye	T65.6X1	T65.6X2	T65.6X3	T65.6X4	—	—
fungicide	T6Ø.3X1	T6Ø.3X2	T6Ø.3X3	T6Ø.3X4	—	—
Auranofin	T39.4X1	T39.4X2	T39.4X3	T39.4X4	T39.4X5	T39.4X6
Aurantiin	T46.991	T46.992	T46.993	T46.994	T46.995	T46.996
Aureomycin	T36.4X1	T36.4X2	T36.4X3	T36.4X4	T36.4X5	T36.4X6
ophthalmic preparation	T49.5X1	T49.5X2	T49.5X3	T49.5X4	T49.5X5	T49.5X6
topical NEC	T49.ØX1	T49.ØX2	T49.ØX3	T49.ØX4	T49.ØX5	T49.ØX6
Aurothioglucose	T39.4X1	T39.4X2	T39.4X3	T39.4X4	T39.4X5	T39.4X6
Aurothioglycanide	T39.4X1	T39.4X2	T39.4X3	T39.4X4	T39.4X5	T39.4X6
Aurothiomalate sodium	T39.4X1	T39.4X2	T39.4X3	T39.4X4	T39.4X5	T39.4X6
Aurotioprol	T39.4X1	T39.4X2	T39.4X3	T39.4X4	T39.4X5	T39.4X6
Automobile fuel	T52.ØX1	T52.ØX2	T52.ØX3	T52.ØX4	—	—
Autonomic nervous system agent NEC	T44.9Ø1	T44.9Ø2	T44.9Ø3	T44.9Ø4	T44.9Ø5	T44.9Ø6
Avelox*	T36.8X1	T36.8X2	T36.8X3	T36.8X4	T36.8X5	T36.8X6
Avlosulfon	T37.1X1	T37.1X2	T37.1X3	T37.1X4	T37.1X5	T37.1X6

Substance	Poisoning, Accidental (unintentional)	Poisoning, Intentional Self-harm	Poisoning, Assault	Poisoning, Undetermined	Adverse Effect	Under-dosing
Avomine	T42.6X1	T42.6X2	T42.6X3	T42.6X4	T42.6X5	T42.6X6
Axerophthol	T45.2X1	T45.2X2	T45.2X3	T45.2X4	T45.2X5	T45.2X6
Azacitidine	T45.1X1	T45.1X2	T45.1X3	T45.1X4	T45.1X5	T45.1X6
Azacyclonol	T43.591	T43.592	T43.593	T43.594	T43.595	T43.596
Azadirachta	T6Ø.2X1	T6Ø.2X2	T6Ø.2X3	T6Ø.2X4	—	—
Azanidazole	T37.3X1	T37.3X2	T37.3X3	T37.3X4	T37.3X5	T37.3X6
Azapetine	T46.7X1	T46.7X2	T46.7X3	T46.7X4	T46.7X5	T46.7X6
Azapropazone	T39.2X1	T39.2X2	T39.2X3	T39.2X4	T39.2X5	T39.2X6
Azaribine	T45.1X1	T45.1X2	T45.1X3	T45.1X4	T45.1X5	T45.1X6
Azaserine	T45.1X1	T45.1X2	T45.1X3	T45.1X4	T45.1X5	T45.1X6
Azatadine	T45.ØX1	T45.ØX2	T45.ØX3	T45.ØX4	T45.ØX5	T45.ØX6
Azatepa	T45.1X1	T45.1X2	T45.1X3	T45.1X4	T45.1X5	T45.1X6
Azathioprine	T45.1X1	T45.1X2	T45.1X3	T45.1X4	T45.1X5	T45.1X6
Azelaic acid	T49.ØX1	T49.ØX2	T49.ØX3	T49.ØX4	T49.ØX5	T49.ØX6
Azelastine	T45.ØX1	T45.ØX2	T45.ØX3	T45.ØX4	T45.ØX5	T45.ØX6
Azidocillin	T36.ØX1	T36.ØX2	T36.ØX3	T36.ØX4	T36.ØX5	T36.ØX6
Azidothymidine	T37.5X1	T37.5X2	T37.5X3	T37.5X4	T37.5X5	T37.5X6
Azinphos (ethyl) (methyl)	T6Ø.ØX1	T6Ø.ØX2	T6Ø.ØX3	T6Ø.ØX4	—	—
Aziridine (chelating)	T54.1X1	T54.1X2	T54.1X3	T54.1X4	—	—
Azithromycin	T36.3X1	T36.3X2	T36.3X3	T36.3X4	T36.3X5	T36.3X6
Azlocillin	T36.ØX1	T36.ØX2	T36.ØX3	T36.ØX4	T36.ØX5	T36.ØX6
Azo-Standard*	T49.ØX1	T49.ØX2	T49.ØX3	T49.ØX4	T49.ØX5	T49.ØX6
Azobenzene smoke	T65.3X1	T65.3X2	T65.3X3	T65.3X4	—	—
acaricide	T6Ø.8X1	T6Ø.8X2	T6Ø.8X3	T6Ø.8X4	—	—
Azosulfamide	T37.ØX1	T37.ØX2	T37.ØX3	T37.ØX4	T37.ØX5	T37.ØX6
AZT	T37.5X1	T37.5X2	T37.5X3	T37.5X4	T37.5X5	T37.5X6
Aztreonam	T36.1X1	T36.1X2	T36.1X3	T36.1X4	T36.1X5	T36.1X6
Azulfidine	T37.ØX1	T37.ØX2	T37.ØX3	T37.ØX4	T37.ØX5	T37.ØX6
Azuresin	T5Ø.8X1	T5Ø.8X2	T5Ø.8X3	T5Ø.8X4	T5Ø.8X5	T5Ø.8X6
b-acetyldigoxin	T46.ØX1	T46.ØX2	T46.ØX3	T46.ØX4	T46.ØX5	T46.ØX6
b-benzalbutyramide	T46.6X1	T46.6X2	T46.6X3	T46.6X4	T46.6X5	T46.6X6
b-eucaine	T49.1X1	T49.1X2	T49.1X3	T49.1X4	T49.1X5	T49.1X6
b-Galactosidase	T47.5X1	T47.5X2	T47.5X3	T47.5X4	T47.5X5	T47.5X6
b-sitosterol(s)	T46.6X1	T46.6X2	T46.6X3	T46.6X4	T46.6X5	T46.6X6
Bacampicillin	T36.ØX1	T36.ØX2	T36.ØX3	T36.ØX4	T36.ØX5	T36.ØX6
Bacillus						
lactobacillus	T47.8X1	T47.8X2	T47.8X3	T47.8X4	T47.8X5	T47.8X6
subtilis	T47.6X1	T47.6X2	T47.6X3	T47.6X4	T47.6X5	T47.6X6
Bacimycin	T49.ØX1	T49.ØX2	T49.ØX3	T49.ØX4	T49.ØX5	T49.ØX6
ophthalmic preparation	T49.5X1	T49.5X2	T49.5X3	T49.5X4	T49.5X5	T49.5X6
Bacitracin zinc	T49.ØX1	T49.ØX2	T49.ØX3	T49.ØX4	T49.ØX5	T49.ØX6
ENT agent	T49.6X1	T49.6X2	T49.6X3	T49.6X4	T49.6X5	T49.6X6
ophthalmic preparation	T49.5X1	T49.5X2	T49.5X3	T49.5X4	T49.5X5	T49.5X6
topical NEC	T49.ØX1	T49.ØX2	T49.ØX3	T49.ØX4	T49.ØX5	T49.ØX6
with neomycin	T49.ØX1	T49.ØX2	T49.ØX3	T49.ØX4	T49.ØX5	T49.ØX6
Baclofen	T42.8X1	T42.8X2	T42.8X3	T42.8X4	T42.8X5	T42.8X6
Bactrim*	T36.8X1	T36.8X2	T36.8X3	T36.8X4	T36.8X5	T36.8X6
Baking soda	T5Ø.991	T5Ø.992	T5Ø.993	T5Ø.994	T5Ø.995	T5Ø.996
BAL	T45.8X1	T45.8X2	T45.8X3	T45.8X4	T45.8X5	T45.8X6
Bambuterol	T48.6X1	T48.6X2	T48.6X3	T48.6X4	T48.6X5	T48.6X6
Bamethan (sulfate)	T46.7X1	T46.7X2	T46.7X3	T46.7X4	T46.7X5	T46.7X6
Bamifylline	T48.6X1	T48.6X2	T48.6X3	T48.6X4	T48.6X5	T48.6X6
Bamipine	T45.ØX1	T45.ØX2	T45.ØX3	T45.ØX4	T45.ØX5	T45.ØX6
Baneberry — *see* Actaea spicata						
Banewort — *see* Belladonna						
Barbenyl	T42.3X1	T42.3X2	T42.3X3	T42.3X4	T42.3X5	T42.3X6
Barbexaclone	T42.6X1	T42.6X2	T42.6X3	T42.6X4	T42.6X5	T42.6X6
Barbital	T42.3X1	T42.3X2	T42.3X3	T42.3X4	T42.3X5	T42.3X6
sodium	T42.3X1	T42.3X2	T42.3X3	T42.3X4	T42.3X5	T42.3X6
Barbitone	T42.3X1	T42.3X2	T42.3X3	T42.3X4	T42.3X5	T42.3X6
Barbiturate NEC	T42.3X1	T42.3X2	T42.3X3	T42.3X4	T42.3X5	T42.3X6
anesthetic (intravenous)	T41.1X1	T41.1X2	T41.1X3	T41.1X4	T41.1X5	T41.1X6
with tranquilizer	T42.3X1	T42.3X2	T42.3X3	T42.3X4	T42.3X5	T42.3X6
Barium (carbonate) (chloride) (sulfite)	T57.8X1	T57.8X2	T57.8X3	T57.8X4	—	—
diagnostic agent	T5Ø.8X1	T5Ø.8X2	T5Ø.8X3	T5Ø.8X4	T5Ø.8X5	T5Ø.8X6
pesticide	T6Ø.4X1	T6Ø.4X2	T6Ø.4X3	T6Ø.4X4	—	—
rodenticide	T6Ø.4X1	T6Ø.4X2	T6Ø.4X3	T6Ø.4X4	—	—
sulfate (medicinal)	T5Ø.8X1	T5Ø.8X2	T5Ø.8X3	T5Ø.8X4	T5Ø.8X5	T5Ø.8X6
Barrier cream	T49.3X1	T49.3X2	T49.3X3	T49.3X4	T49.3X5	T49.3X6
Basic fuchsin	T49.ØX1	T49.ØX2	T49.ØX3	T49.ØX4	T49.ØX5	T49.ØX6
Basiliximab*	T45.1X1	T45.1X2	T45.1X3	T45.1X4	T45.1X5	T45.1X6
Battery acid or fluid	T54.2X1	T54.2X2	T54.2X3	T54.2X4	—	—
Bay rum	T51.8X1	T51.8X2	T51.8X3	T51.8X4	—	—
BCG (vaccine)	T5Ø.A91	T5Ø.A92	T5Ø.A93	T5Ø.A94	T5Ø.A95	T5Ø.A96
BCNU	T45.1X1	T45.1X2	T45.1X3	T45.1X4	T45.1X5	T45.1X6
Bearsfoot	T62.2X1	T62.2X2	T62.2X3	T62.2X4	—	—
Beclamide	T42.6X1	T42.6X2	T42.6X3	T42.6X4	T42.6X5	T42.6X6
Beclomethasone	T44.5X1	T44.5X2	T44.5X3	T44.5X4	T44.5X5	T44.5X6
Bee (sting) (venom)	T63.441	T63.442	T63.443	T63.444	—	—
Befunolol	T49.5X1	T49.5X2	T49.5X3	T49.5X4	T49.5X5	T49.5X6
Bekanamycin	T36.5X1	T36.5X2	T36.5X3	T36.5X4	T36.5X5	T36.5X6

Substance	Poisoning, Accidental (unintentional)	Poisoning, Intentional Self-harm	Poisoning, Assault	Poisoning, Undetermined	Adverse Effect	Under-dosing
Belladonna — *see also* Nightshade						
alkaloids	T44.3X1	T44.3X2	T44.3X3	T44.3X4	T44.3X5	T44.3X6
extract	T44.3X1	T44.3X2	T44.3X3	T44.3X4	T44.3X5	T44.3X6
herb	T44.3X1	T44.3X2	T44.3X3	T44.3X4	T44.3X5	T44.3X6
Belviq*	T50.5X1	T50.5X2	T50.5X3	T50.5X4	T50.5X5	T50.5X6
Bemegride	T50.7X1	T50.7X2	T50.7X3	T50.7X4	T50.7X5	T50.7X6
Benactyzine	T44.3X1	T44.3X2	T44.3X3	T44.3X4	T44.3X5	T44.3X6
Benadryl	T45.ØX1	T45.ØX2	T45.ØX3	T45.ØX4	T45.ØX5	T45.ØX6
Benaprizine	T44.3X1	T44.3X2	T44.3X3	T44.3X4	T44.3X5	T44.3X6
Benazepril	T46.4X1	T46.4X2	T46.4X3	T46.4X4	T46.4X5	T46.4X6
Bencyclane	T46.7X1	T46.7X2	T46.7X3	T46.7X4	T46.7X5	T46.7X6
Bendazol	T46.3X1	T46.3X2	T46.3X3	T46.3X4	T46.3X5	T46.3X6
Bendrofluazide	T50.2X1	T50.2X2	T50.2X3	T50.2X4	T50.2X5	T50.2X6
Bendroflumethiazide	T50.2X1	T50.2X2	T50.2X3	T50.2X4	T50.2X5	T50.2X6
Benemid	T50.4X1	T50.4X2	T50.4X3	T50.4X4	T50.4X5	T50.4X6
Benethamine penicillin	T36.ØX1	T36.ØX2	T36.ØX3	T36.ØX4	T36.ØX5	T36.ØX6
Benexate	T47.1X1	T47.1X2	T47.1X3	T47.1X4	T47.1X5	T47.1X6
Benfluorex	T46.6X1	T46.6X2	T46.6X3	T46.6X4	T46.6X5	T46.6X6
Benfotiamine	T45.2X1	T45.2X2	T45.2X3	T45.2X4	T45.2X5	T45.2X6
Benisone	T49.ØX1	T49.ØX2	T49.ØX3	T49.ØX4	T49.ØX5	T49.ØX6
Benomyl	T60.ØX1	T60.ØX2	T60.ØX3	T60.ØX4	—	—
Benoquin	T49.8X1	T49.8X2	T49.8X3	T49.8X4	T49.8X5	T49.8X6
Benoxinate	T41.3X1	T41.3X2	T41.3X3	T41.3X4	T41.3X5	T41.3X6
Benperidol	T43.4X1	T43.4X2	T43.4X3	T43.4X4	T43.4X5	T43.4X6
Benproperine	T48.3X1	T48.3X2	T48.3X3	T48.3X4	T48.3X5	T48.3X6
Benserazide	T42.8X1	T42.8X2	T42.8X3	T42.8X4	T42.8X5	T42.8X6
Bentazepam	T42.4X1	T42.4X2	T42.4X3	T42.4X4	T42.4X5	T42.4X6
Bentiromide	T50.8X1	T50.8X2	T50.8X3	T50.8X4	T50.8X5	T50.8X6
Bentonite	T49.3X1	T49.3X2	T49.3X3	T49.3X4	T49.3X5	T49.3X6
Benzalbutyramide	T46.6X1	T46.6X2	T46.6X3	T46.6X4	T46.6X5	T46.6X6
Benzalkonium (chloride)	T49.ØX1	T49.ØX2	T49.ØX3	T49.ØX4	T49.ØX5	T49.ØX6
ophthalmic preparation	T49.5X1	T49.5X2	T49.5X3	T49.5X4	T49.5X5	T49.5X6
Benzamidosalicylate (calcium)	T37.1X1	T37.1X2	T37.1X3	T37.1X4	T37.1X5	T37.1X6
Benzamine	T41.3X1	T41.3X2	T41.3X3	T41.3X4	T41.3X5	T41.3X6
lactate	T49.1X1	T49.1X2	T49.1X3	T49.1X4	T49.1X5	T49.1X6
Benzamphetamine	T50.5X1	T50.5X2	T50.5X3	T50.5X4	T50.5X5	T50.5X6
Benzapril hydrochloride	T46.5X1	T46.5X2	T46.5X3	T46.5X4	T46.5X5	T46.5X6
Benzathine benzylpenicillin	T36.ØX1	T36.ØX2	T36.ØX3	T36.ØX4	T36.ØX5	T36.ØX6
Benzathine penicillin	T36.ØX1	T36.ØX2	T36.ØX3	T36.ØX4	T36.ØX5	T36.ØX6
Benzatropine	T42.8X1	T42.8X2	T42.8X3	T42.8X4	T42.8X5	T42.8X6
Benzbromarone	T50.4X1	T50.4X2	T50.4X3	T50.4X4	T50.4X5	T50.4X6
Benzcarbimine	T45.1X1	T45.1X2	T45.1X3	T45.1X4	T45.1X5	T45.1X6
Benzedrex	T44.991	T44.992	T44.993	T44.994	T44.995	T44.996
Benzedrine (amphetamine)	T43.621	T43.622	T43.623	T43.624	T43.625	T43.626
Benzenamine	T65.3X1	T65.3X2	T65.3X3	T65.3X4	—	—
Benzene	T52.1X1	T52.1X2	T52.1X3	T52.1X4	—	—
homologues (acetyl) (dimethyl) (methyl) (solvent)	T52.2X1	T52.2X2	T52.2X3	T52.2X4	—	—
Benzethonium (chloride)	T49.ØX1	T49.ØX2	T49.ØX3	T49.ØX4	T49.ØX5	T49.ØX6
Benzfetamine	T50.5X1	T50.5X2	T50.5X3	T50.5X4	T50.5X5	T50.5X6
Benzhexol	T44.3X1	T44.3X2	T44.3X3	T44.3X4	T44.3X5	T44.3X6
Benzhydramine (chloride)	T45.ØX1	T45.ØX2	T45.ØX3	T45.ØX4	T45.ØX5	T45.ØX6
Benzidine	T65.891	T65.892	T65.893	T65.894	—	—
Benzilonium bromide	T44.3X1	T44.3X2	T44.3X3	T44.3X4	T44.3X5	T44.3X6
Benzimidazole	T60.3X1	T60.3X2	T60.3X3	T60.3X4	—	—
Benzin (e) — *see* Ligroin						
Benziodarone	T46.3X1	T46.3X2	T46.3X3	T46.3X4	T46.3X5	T46.3X6
Benznidazole	T37.3X1	T37.3X2	T37.3X3	T37.3X4	T37.3X5	T37.3X6
Benzocaine	T41.3X1	T41.3X2	T41.3X3	T41.3X4	T41.3X5	T41.3X6
Benzocol*	T41.3X1	T41.3X2	T41.3X3	T41.3X4	T41.3X5	T41.3X6
Benzodiapin	T42.4X1	T42.4X2	T42.4X3	T42.4X4	T42.4X5	T42.4X6
Benzodiazepine NEC	T42.4X1	T42.4X2	T42.4X3	T42.4X4	T42.4X5	T42.4X6
Benzoic acid	T49.ØX1	T49.ØX2	T49.ØX3	T49.ØX4	T49.ØX5	T49.ØX6
with salicylic acid	T49.ØX1	T49.ØX2	T49.ØX3	T49.ØX4	T49.ØX5	T49.ØX6
Benzoin (tincture)	T48.5X1	T48.5X2	T48.5X3	T48.5X4	T48.5X5	T48.5X6
Benzol (benzene)	T52.1X1	T52.1X2	T52.1X3	T52.1X4	—	—
vapor	T52.ØX1	T52.ØX2	T52.ØX3	T52.ØX4	—	—
Benzomorphan	T40.2X1	T40.2X2	T40.2X3	T40.2X4	T40.2X5	T40.2X6
Benzonatate	T48.3X1	T48.3X2	T48.3X3	T48.3X4	T48.3X5	T48.3X6
Benzophenones	T49.3X1	T49.3X2	T49.3X3	T49.3X4	T49.3X5	T49.3X6
Benzopyrone	T46.991	T46.992	T46.993	T46.994	T46.995	T46.996
Benzothiadiazides	T50.2X1	T50.2X2	T50.2X3	T50.2X4	T50.2X5	T50.2X6
Benzoxonium chloride	T49.ØX1	T49.ØX2	T49.ØX3	T49.ØX4	T49.ØX5	T49.ØX6
Benzoyl peroxide	T49.ØX1	T49.ØX2	T49.ØX3	T49.ØX4	T49.ØX5	T49.ØX6
Benzoylpas calcium	T37.1X1	T37.1X2	T37.1X3	T37.1X4	T37.1X5	T37.1X6
Benzperidin	T43.591	T43.592	T43.593	T43.594	T43.595	T43.596
Benzperidol	T43.591	T43.592	T43.593	T43.594	T43.595	T43.596
Benzphetamine	T50.5X1	T50.5X2	T50.5X3	T50.5X4	T50.5X5	T50.5X6
Benzpyrinium bromide	T44.1X1	T44.1X2	T44.1X3	T44.1X4	T44.1X5	T44.1X6
Benzquinamide	T45.ØX1	T45.ØX2	T45.ØX3	T45.ØX4	T45.ØX5	T45.ØX6

Substance	Poisoning, Accidental (unintentional)	Poisoning, Intentional Self-harm	Poisoning, Assault	Poisoning, Undetermined	Adverse Effect	Under-dosing
Benzthiazide	T50.2X1	T50.2X2	T50.2X3	T50.2X4	T50.2X5	T50.2X6
Benztropine						
anticholinergic	T44.3X1	T44.3X2	T44.3X3	T44.3X4	T44.3X5	T44.3X6
antiparkinson	T42.8X1	T42.8X2	T42.8X3	T42.8X4	T42.8X5	T42.8X6
Benzydamine	T49.ØX1	T49.ØX2	T49.ØX3	T49.ØX4	T49.ØX5	T49.ØX6
Benzyl						
acetate	T52.8X1	T52.8X2	T52.8X3	T52.8X4	—	—
alcohol	T49.ØX1	T49.ØX2	T49.ØX3	T49.ØX4	T49.ØX5	T49.ØX6
benzoate	T49.ØX1	T49.ØX2	T49.ØX3	T49.ØX4	T49.ØX5	T49.ØX6
Benzoic acid	T49.ØX1	T49.ØX2	T49.ØX3	T49.ØX4	T49.ØX5	T49.ØX6
hydroquinone*	T49.4X1	T49.4X2	T49.4X3	T49.4X4	T49.4X5	T49.4X6
morphine	T40.2X1	T40.2X2	T40.2X3	T40.2X4	—	—
nicotinate	T46.6X1	T46.6X2	T46.6X3	T46.6X4	T46.6X5	T46.6X6
penicillin	T36.ØX1	T36.ØX2	T36.ØX3	T36.ØX4	T36.ØX5	T36.ØX6
Benzylhydrochlorothiazide	T50.2X1	T50.2X2	T50.2X3	T50.2X4	T50.2X5	T50.2X6
Benzylpenicillin	T36.ØX1	T36.ØX2	T36.ØX3	T36.ØX4	T36.ØX5	T36.ØX6
Benzylthiouracil	T38.2X1	T38.2X2	T38.2X3	T38.2X4	T38.2X5	T38.2X6
Bephenium hydroxynaphthoate	T37.4X1	T37.4X2	T37.4X3	T37.4X4	T37.4X5	T37.4X6
Bepridil	T46.1X1	T46.1X2	T46.1X3	T46.1X4	T46.1X5	T46.1X6
Bergamot oil	T65.891	T65.892	T65.893	T65.894	—	—
Bergapten	T50.991	T50.992	T50.993	T50.994	T50.995	T50.996
Berries, poisonous	T62.1X1	T62.1X2	T62.1X3	T62.1X4	—	—
Beryllium (compounds)	T56.7X1	T56.7X2	T56.7X3	T56.7X4	—	—
beta adrenergic blocking agent, heart	T44.7X1	T44.7X2	T44.7X3	T44.7X4	T44.7X5	T44.7X6
Beta-Chlor	T42.6X1	T42.6X2	T42.6X3	T42.6X4	T42.6X5	T42.6X6
Betacarotene	T45.2X1	T45.2X2	T45.2X3	T45.2X4	T45.2X5	T45.2X6
Betahistine	T46.7X1	T46.7X2	T46.7X3	T46.7X4	T46.7X5	T46.7X6
Betaine	T47.5X1	T47.5X2	T47.5X3	T47.5X4	T47.5X5	T47.5X6
Betamethasone	T49.ØX1	T49.ØX2	T49.ØX3	T49.ØX4	T49.ØX5	T49.ØX6
topical	T49.ØX1	T49.ØX2	T49.ØX3	T49.ØX4	T49.ØX5	T49.ØX6
Betamicin	T36.8X1	T36.8X2	T36.8X3	T36.8X4	T36.8X5	T36.8X6
Betanidine	T46.5X1	T46.5X2	T46.5X3	T46.5X4	T46.5X5	T46.5X6
Betaxolol	T44.7X1	T44.7X2	T44.7X3	T44.7X4	T44.7X5	T44.7X6
Betazole	T50.8X1	T50.8X2	T50.8X3	T50.8X4	T50.8X5	T50.8X6
Bethanechol	T44.1X1	T44.1X2	T44.1X3	T44.1X4	T44.1X5	T44.1X6
chloride	T44.1X1	T44.1X2	T44.1X3	T44.1X4	T44.1X5	T44.1X6
Bethanidine	T46.5X1	T46.5X2	T46.5X3	T46.5X4	T46.5X5	T46.5X6
Betoxycaine	T41.3X1	T41.3X2	T41.3X3	T41.3X4	T41.3X5	T41.3X6
Betula oil	T49.3X1	T49.3X2	T49.3X3	T49.3X4	T49.3X5	T49.3X6
Bevantolol	T44.7X1	T44.7X2	T44.7X3	T44.7X4	T44.7X5	T44.7X6
Bevonium metilsulfate	T44.3X1	T44.3X2	T44.3X3	T44.3X4	T44.3X5	T44.3X6
Bezafibrate	T46.6X1	T46.6X2	T46.6X3	T46.6X4	T46.6X5	T46.6X6
Bezitramide	T40.491	T40.492	T40.493	T40.494	T40.495	T40.496
BHA	T50.991	T50.992	T50.993	T50.994	T50.995	T50.996
Bhang	T40.711	T40.712	T40.713	T40.714	T40.715	T40.716
BHC (medicinal)	T49.ØX1	T49.ØX2	T49.ØX3	T49.ØX4	T49.ØX5	T49.ØX6
nonmedicinal (vapor)	T53.6X1	T53.6X2	T53.6X3	T53.6X4	—	—
Bialamicol	T37.3X1	T37.3X2	T37.3X3	T37.3X4	T37.3X5	T37.3X6
Bibenzonium bromide	T48.3X1	T48.3X2	T48.3X3	T48.3X4	T48.3X5	T48.3X6
Bibrocathol	T49.5X1	T49.5X2	T49.5X3	T49.5X4	T49.5X5	T49.5X6
Bichloride of mercury — *see* Mercury, chloride						
Bichromates (calcium) (potassium)(sodium) (crystals)	T57.8X1	T57.8X2	T57.8X3	T57.8X4	—	—
fumes	T56.2X1	T56.2X2	T56.2X3	T56.2X4	—	—
Biclotymol	T49.6X1	T49.6X2	T49.6X3	T49.6X4	T49.6X5	T49.6X6
BiCNU*	T45.1X1	T45.1X2	T45.1X3	T45.1X4	T45.1X5	T45.1X6
Bicucculine	T50.7X1	T50.7X2	T50.7X3	T50.7X4	T50.7X5	T50.7X6
Bifemelane	T43.291	T43.292	T43.293	T43.294	T43.295	T43.296
Biguanide derivatives, oral	T38.3X1	T38.3X2	T38.3X3	T38.3X4	T38.3X5	T38.3X6
Bile salts	T47.5X1	T47.5X2	T47.5X3	T47.5X4	T47.5X5	T47.5X6
Biligrafin	T50.8X1	T50.8X2	T50.8X3	T50.8X4	T50.8X5	T50.8X6
Bilopaque	T50.8X1	T50.8X2	T50.8X3	T50.8X4	T50.8X5	T50.8X6
Binifibrate	T46.6X1	T46.6X2	T46.6X3	T46.6X4	T46.6X5	T46.6X6
Binitrobenzol	T65.3X1	T65.3X2	T65.3X3	T65.3X4	—	—
Bioflavonoid(s)	T46.991	T46.992	T46.993	T46.994	T46.995	T46.996
Biological substance NEC	T50.901	T50.902	T50.903	T50.904	T50.905	T50.906
Biotin	T45.2X1	T45.2X2	T45.2X3	T45.2X4	T45.2X5	T45.2X6
Biperiden	T44.3X1	T44.3X2	T44.3X3	T44.3X4	T44.3X5	T44.3X6
Bisacodyl	T47.2X1	T47.2X2	T47.2X3	T47.2X4	T47.2X5	T47.2X6
Bisbentiamine	T45.2X1	T45.2X2	T45.2X3	T45.2X4	T45.2X5	T45.2X6
Bisbutiamine	T45.2X1	T45.2X2	T45.2X3	T45.2X4	T45.2X5	T45.2X6
Bisdequalinium (salts) (diacetate)	T49.6X1	T49.6X2	T49.6X3	T49.6X4	T49.6X5	T49.6X6
Bishydroxycoumarin	T45.511	T45.512	T45.513	T45.514	T45.515	T45.516
Bismarsen	T37.8X1	T37.8X2	T37.8X3	T37.8X4	T37.8X5	T37.8X6
Bismuth salts	T47.6X1	T47.6X2	T47.6X3	T47.6X4	T47.6X5	T47.6X6
aluminate	T47.1X1	T47.1X2	T47.1X3	T47.1X4	T47.1X5	T47.1X6
anti-infectives	T37.8X1	T37.8X2	T37.8X3	T37.8X4	T37.8X5	T37.8X6

Belladonna — Bismuth salts

*Optum Value-Add

☑ Additional Character May Be Required — Refer to the Tabular List for Character Selection

367

Substance	Poisoning, Accidental (unintentional)	Poisoning, Intentional Self-harm	Poisoning, Assault	Poisoning, Undetermined	Adverse Effect	Under-dosing
Bismuth salts — *continued*						
formic iodide	T49.ØX1	T49.ØX2	T49.ØX3	T49.ØX4	T49.ØX5	T49.ØX6
glycolylarsenate	T49.ØX1	T49.ØX2	T49.ØX3	T49.ØX4	T49.ØX5	T49.ØX6
nonmedicinal (compounds) NEC	T65.91	T65.92	T65.93	T65.94	—	—
subcarbonate	T47.6X1	T47.6X2	T47.6X3	T47.6X4	T47.6X5	T47.6X6
subsalicylate	T37.8X1	T37.8X2	T37.8X3	T37.8X4	T37.8X5	T37.8X6
sulfarsphenamine	T37.8X1	T37.8X2	T37.8X3	T37.8X4	T37.8X5	T37.8X6
Bisoprolol	T44.7X1	T44.7X2	T44.7X3	T44.7X4	T44.7X5	T44.7X6
Bisoxatin	T47.2X1	T47.2X2	T47.2X3	T47.2X4	T47.2X5	T47.2X6
Bisulepin (hydrochloride)	T45.ØX1	T45.ØX2	T45.ØX3	T45.ØX4	T45.ØX5	T45.ØX6
Bithionol	T37.8X1	T37.8X2	T37.8X3	T37.8X4	T37.8X5	T37.8X6
anthelmintic	T37.4X1	T37.4X2	T37.4X3	T37.4X4	T37.4X5	T37.4X6
Bitolterol	T48.6X1	T48.6X2	T48.6X3	T48.6X4	T48.6X5	T48.6X6
Bitoscanate	T37.4X1	T37.4X2	T37.4X3	T37.4X4	T37.4X5	T37.4X6
Bitter almond oil	T62.8X1	T62.8X2	T62.8X3	T62.8X4	—	—
Bittersweet	T62.2X1	T62.2X2	T62.2X3	T62.2X4	—	—
Bivalirudin*	T45.511	T45.512	T45.513	T45.514	T45.515	T45.516
Black						
flag	T6Ø.91	T6Ø.92	T6Ø.93	T6Ø.94	—	—
henbane	T62.2X1	T62.2X2	T62.2X3	T62.2X4	—	—
leaf (40)	T6Ø.91	T6Ø.92	T6Ø.93	T6Ø.94	—	—
widow spider (bite)	T63.311	T63.312	T63.313	T63.314	—	—
antivenin	T5Ø.Z11	T5Ø.Z12	T5Ø.Z13	T5Ø.Z14	T5Ø.Z15	T5Ø.Z16
Blast furnace gas (carbon monoxide from)	T58.8X1	T58.8X2	T58.8X3	T58.8X4	—	—
Bleach	T54.91	T54.92	T54.93	T54.94	—	—
Bleaching agent (medicinal)	T49.4X1	T49.4X2	T49.4X3	T49.4X4	T49.4X5	T49.4X6
Bleomycin	T45.1X1	T45.1X2	T45.1X3	T45.1X4	T45.1X5	T45.1X6
Blockain	T41.3X1	T41.3X2	T41.3X3	T41.3X4	T41.3X5	T41.3X6
infiltration (subcutaneous)	T41.3X1	T41.3X2	T41.3X3	T41.3X4	T41.3X5	T41.3X6
nerve block (peripheral) (plexus)	T41.3X1	T41.3X2	T41.3X3	T41.3X4	T41.3X5	T41.3X6
topical (surface)	T41.3X1	T41.3X2	T41.3X3	T41.3X4	T41.3X5	T41.3X6
Blockers, calcium channel	T46.1X1	T46.1X2	T46.1X3	T46.1X4	T46.1X5	T46.1X6
Blood (derivatives) (natural) (plasma) (whole)	T45.8X1	T45.8X2	T45.8X3	T45.8X4	T45.8X5	T45.8X6
dried	T45.8X1	T45.8X2	T45.8X3	T45.8X4	T45.8X5	T45.8X6
drug affecting NEC	T45.91	T45.92	T45.93	T45.94	T45.95	T45.96
expander NEC	T45.8X1	T45.8X2	T45.8X3	T45.8X4	T45.8X5	T45.8X6
fraction NEC	T45.8X1	T45.8X2	T45.8X3	T45.8X4	T45.8X5	T45.8X6
substitute (macromolecular)	T45.8X1	T45.8X2	T45.8X3	T45.8X4	T45.8X5	T45.8X6
Blue velvet	T4Ø.2X1	T4Ø.2X2	T4Ø.2X3	T4Ø.2X4	—	—
Bone meal	T62.8X1	T62.8X2	T62.8X3	T62.8X4	—	—
Bonine	T45.ØX1	T45.ØX2	T45.ØX3	T45.ØX4	T45.ØX5	T45.ØX6
Bontril*	T5Ø.5X1	T5Ø.5X2	T5Ø.5X3	T5Ø.5X4	T5Ø.5X5	T5Ø.5X6
Bopindolol	T44.7X1	T44.7X2	T44.7X3	T44.7X4	T44.7X5	T44.7X6
Boracic acid	T49.ØX1	T49.ØX2	T49.ØX3	T49.ØX4	T49.ØX5	T49.ØX6
ENT agent	T49.6X1	T49.6X2	T49.6X3	T49.6X4	T49.6X5	T49.6X6
ophthalmic preparation	T49.5X1	T49.5X2	T49.5X3	T49.5X4	T49.5X5	T49.5X6
Borane complex	T57.8X1	T57.8X2	T57.8X3	T57.8X4	—	—
Borate(s)	T57.8X1	T57.8X2	T57.8X3	T57.8X4	—	—
buffer	T5Ø.991	T5Ø.992	T5Ø.993	T5Ø.994	T5Ø.995	T5Ø.996
cleanser	T54.91	T54.92	T54.93	T54.94	—	—
sodium	T57.8X1	T57.8X2	T57.8X3	T57.8X4	—	—
Borax (cleanser)	T54.91	T54.92	T54.93	T54.94	—	—
Bordeaux mixture	T6Ø.3X1	T6Ø.3X2	T6Ø.3X3	T6Ø.3X4	—	—
Boric acid	T49.ØX1	T49.ØX2	T49.ØX3	T49.ØX4	T49.ØX5	T49.ØX6
ENT agent	T49.6X1	T49.6X2	T49.6X3	T49.6X4	T49.6X5	T49.6X6
ophthalmic preparation	T49.5X1	T49.5X2	T49.5X3	T49.5X4	T49.5X5	T49.5X6
Bornaprine	T44.3X1	T44.3X2	T44.3X3	T44.3X4	T44.3X5	T44.3X6
Boron	T57.8X1	T57.8X2	T57.8X3	T57.8X4	—	—
hydride NEC	T57.8X1	T57.8X2	T57.8X3	T57.8X4	—	—
fumes or gas	T57.8X1	T57.8X2	T57.8X3	T57.8X4	—	—
trifluoride	T59.891	T59.892	T59.893	T59.894	—	—
Botox	T48.291	T48.292	T48.293	T48.294	T48.295	T48.296
Botulinus anti-toxin (type A, B)	T5Ø.Z11	T5Ø.Z12	T5Ø.Z13	T5Ø.Z14	T5Ø.Z15	T5Ø.Z16
Brake fluid vapor	T59.891	T59.892	T59.893	T59.894	—	—
Brallobarbital	T42.3X1	T42.3X2	T42.3X3	T42.3X4	T42.3X5	T42.3X6
Bran (wheat)	T47.4X1	T47.4X2	T47.4X3	T47.4X4	T47.4X5	T47.4X6
Brass (fumes)	T56.891	T56.892	T56.893	T56.894	—	—
Brasso	T52.ØX1	T52.ØX2	T52.ØX3	T52.ØX4	—	—
Bretylium tosilate	T46.2X1	T46.2X2	T46.2X3	T46.2X4	T46.2X5	T46.2X6
Brevital (sodium)	T41.1X1	T41.1X2	T41.1X3	T41.1X4	T41.1X5	T41.1X6
Brinase	T45.3X1	T45.3X2	T45.3X3	T45.3X4	T45.3X5	T45.3X6
British antilewisite	T45.8X1	T45.8X2	T45.8X3	T45.8X4	T45.8X5	T45.8X6
Brodalumab*	T5Ø.991	T5Ø.992	T5Ø.993	T5Ø.994	T5Ø.995	T5Ø.996
Brodifacoum	T6Ø.4X1	T6Ø.4X2	T6Ø.4X3	T6Ø.4X4	—	—
Bromal (hydrate)	T42.6X1	T42.6X2	T42.6X3	T42.6X4	T42.6X5	T42.6X6
Bromazepam	T42.4X1	T42.4X2	T42.4X3	T42.4X4	T42.4X5	T42.4X6

Substance	Poisoning, Accidental (unintentional)	Poisoning, Intentional Self-harm	Poisoning, Assault	Poisoning, Undetermined	Adverse Effect	Under-dosing
Bromazine	T45.ØX1	T45.ØX2	T45.ØX3	T45.ØX4	T45.ØX5	T45.ØX6
Brombenzylcyanide	T59.3X1	T59.3X2	T59.3X3	T59.3X4	—	—
Bromelains	T45.3X1	T45.3X2	T45.3X3	T45.3X4	T45.3X5	T45.3X6
Bromethalin	T6Ø.4X1	T6Ø.4X2	T6Ø.4X3	T6Ø.4X4	—	—
Bromhexine	T48.4X1	T48.4X2	T48.4X3	T48.4X4	T48.4X5	T48.4X6
Bromide salts	T42.6X1	T42.6X2	T42.6X3	T42.6X4	T42.6X5	T42.6X6
Bromindione	T45.511	T45.512	T45.513	T45.514	T45.515	T45.516
Bromine						
compounds (medicinal)	T42.6X1	T42.6X2	T42.6X3	T42.6X4	T42.6X5	T42.6X6
sedative	T42.6X1	T42.6X2	T42.6X3	T42.6X4	T42.6X5	T42.6X6
vapor	T59.891	T59.892	T59.893	T59.894	—	—
Bromisoval	T42.6X1	T42.6X2	T42.6X3	T42.6X4	T42.6X5	T42.6X6
Bromisovalum	T42.6X1	T42.6X2	T42.6X3	T42.6X4	T42.6X5	T42.6X6
Bromo-seltzer	T39.1X1	T39.1X2	T39.1X3	T39.1X4	T39.1X5	T39.1X6
Bromobenzylcyanide	T59.3X1	T59.3X2	T59.3X3	T59.3X4	—	—
Bromochlorosalicylanilide	T49.ØX1	T49.ØX2	T49.ØX3	T49.ØX4	T49.ØX5	T49.ØX6
Bromocriptine	T42.8X1	T42.8X2	T42.8X3	T42.8X4	T42.8X5	T42.8X6
Bromodiphenhydramine	T45.ØX1	T45.ØX2	T45.ØX3	T45.ØX4	T45.ØX5	T45.ØX6
Bromoform	T42.6X1	T42.6X2	T42.6X3	T42.6X4	T42.6X5	T42.6X6
Bromophenol blue reagent	T5Ø.991	T5Ø.992	T5Ø.993	T5Ø.994	T5Ø.995	T5Ø.996
Bromopride	T47.8X1	T47.8X2	T47.8X3	T47.8X4	T47.8X5	T47.8X6
Bromosalicylchloranitide	T49.ØX1	T49.ØX2	T49.ØX3	T49.ØX4	T49.ØX5	T49.ØX6
Bromosalicylhydroxamic acid	T37.1X1	T37.1X2	T37.1X3	T37.1X4	T37.1X5	T37.1X6
Bromoxynil	T6Ø.3X1	T6Ø.3X2	T6Ø.3X3	T6Ø.3X4	—	—
Bromperidol	T43.4X1	T43.4X2	T43.4X3	T43.4X4	T43.4X5	T43.4X6
Brompheniramine	T45.ØX1	T45.ØX2	T45.ØX3	T45.ØX4	T45.ØX5	T45.ØX6
Bromsulfophthalein	T5Ø.8X1	T5Ø.8X2	T5Ø.8X3	T5Ø.8X4	T5Ø.8X5	T5Ø.8X6
Bromural	T42.6X1	T42.6X2	T42.6X3	T42.6X4	T42.6X5	T42.6X6
Bromvaletone	T42.6X1	T42.6X2	T42.6X3	T42.6X4	T42.6X5	T42.6X6
Bronchodilator NEC	T48.6X1	T48.6X2	T48.6X3	T48.6X4	T48.6X5	T48.6X6
Brotizolam	T42.4X1	T42.4X2	T42.4X3	T42.4X4	T42.4X5	T42.4X6
Brovincamine	T46.7X1	T46.7X2	T46.7X3	T46.7X4	T46.7X5	T46.7X6
Brown recluse spider (bite) (venom)	T63.331	T63.332	T63.333	T63.334	—	—
Brown spider (bite) (venom)	T63.391	T63.392	T63.393	T63.394	—	—
Broxaterol	T48.6X1	T48.6X2	T48.6X3	T48.6X4	T48.6X5	T48.6X6
Broxuridine	T45.1X1	T45.1X2	T45.1X3	T45.1X4	T45.1X5	T45.1X6
Broxyquinoline	T37.8X1	T37.8X2	T37.8X3	T37.8X4	T37.8X5	T37.8X6
Bruceine	T48.291	T48.292	T48.293	T48.294	T48.295	T48.296
Brucia	T62.2X1	T62.2X2	T62.2X3	T62.2X4	—	—
Brucine	T65.1X1	T65.1X2	T65.1X3	T65.1X4	—	—
Brunswick green — *see* Copper						
Bruten — *see* Ibuprofen						
Bryonia	T47.2X1	T47.2X2	T47.2X3	T47.2X4	T47.2X5	T47.2X6
Buclizine	T45.ØX1	T45.ØX2	T45.ØX3	T45.ØX4	T45.ØX5	T45.ØX6
Buclosamide	T49.ØX1	T49.ØX2	T49.ØX3	T49.ØX4	T49.ØX5	T49.ØX6
Budesonide	T44.5X1	T44.5X2	T44.5X3	T44.5X4	T44.5X5	T44.5X6
Budralazine	T46.5X1	T46.5X2	T46.5X3	T46.5X4	T46.5X5	T46.5X6
Bufferin	T39.Ø11	T39.Ø12	T39.Ø13	T39.Ø14	T39.Ø15	T39.Ø16
Buflomedil	T46.7X1	T46.7X2	T46.7X3	T46.7X4	T46.7X5	T46.7X6
Buformin	T38.3X1	T38.3X2	T38.3X3	T38.3X4	T38.3X5	T38.3X6
Bufotenine	T4Ø.991	T4Ø.992	T4Ø.993	T4Ø.994	—	—
Bufrolin	T48.6X1	T48.6X2	T48.6X3	T48.6X4	T48.6X5	T48.6X6
Bufylline	T48.6X1	T48.6X2	T48.6X3	T48.6X4	T48.6X5	T48.6X6
Bulgaricum IB*	T47.6X1	T47.6X2	T47.6X3	T47.6X4	T47.6X5	T47.6X6
Bulk filler	T5Ø.5X1	T5Ø.5X2	T5Ø.5X3	T5Ø.5X4	T5Ø.5X5	T5Ø.5X6
cathartic	T47.4X1	T47.4X2	T47.4X3	T47.4X4	T47.4X5	T47.4X6
Bumetanide	T5Ø.1X1	T5Ø.1X2	T5Ø.1X3	T5Ø.1X4	T5Ø.1X5	T5Ø.1X6
Bunaftine	T46.2X1	T46.2X2	T46.2X3	T46.2X4	T46.2X5	T46.2X6
Bunamiodyl	T5Ø.8X1	T5Ø.8X2	T5Ø.8X3	T5Ø.8X4	T5Ø.8X5	T5Ø.8X6
Bunazosin	T44.6X1	T44.6X2	T44.6X3	T44.6X4	T44.6X5	T44.6X6
Bunitrolol	T44.7X1	T44.7X2	T44.7X3	T44.7X4	T44.7X5	T44.7X6
Buphenine	T46.7X1	T46.7X2	T46.7X3	T46.7X4	T46.7X5	T46.7X6
Bupivacaine	T41.3X1	T41.3X2	T41.3X3	T41.3X4	T41.3X5	T41.3X6
infiltration (subcutaneous)	T41.3X1	T41.3X2	T41.3X3	T41.3X4	T41.3X5	T41.3X6
nerve block (peripheral) (plexus)	T41.3X1	T41.3X2	T41.3X3	T41.3X4	T41.3X5	T41.3X6
spinal	T41.3X1	T41.3X2	T41.3X3	T41.3X4	T41.3X5	T41.3X6
Bupranolol	T44.7X1	T44.7X2	T44.7X3	T44.7X4	T44.7X5	T44.7X6
Buprenorphine	T4Ø.491	T4Ø.492	T4Ø.493	T4Ø.494	T4Ø.495	T4Ø.496
Bupropion	T43.291	T43.292	T43.293	T43.294	T43.295	T43.296
Burimamide	T47.1X1	T47.1X2	T47.1X3	T47.1X4	T47.1X5	T47.1X6
Buserelin	T38.891	T38.892	T38.893	T38.894	T38.895	T38.896
Buspirone	T43.591	T43.592	T43.593	T43.594	T43.595	T43.596
Busulfan, busulphan	T45.1X1	T45.1X2	T45.1X3	T45.1X4	T45.1X5	T45.1X6
Busulfex*	T45.1X1	T45.1X2	T45.1X3	T45.1X4	T45.1X5	T45.1X6
Butabarbital (sodium)	T42.3X1	T42.3X2	T42.3X3	T42.3X4	T42.3X5	T42.3X6
Butabarbitone	T42.3X1	T42.3X2	T42.3X3	T42.3X4	T42.3X5	T42.3X6
Butabarpal	T42.3X1	T42.3X2	T42.3X3	T42.3X4	T42.3X5	T42.3X6
Butacaine	T41.3X1	T41.3X2	T41.3X3	T41.3X4	T41.3X5	T41.3X6

Substance	Poisoning, Accidental (unintentional)	Poisoning, Intentional Self-harm	Poisoning, Assault	Poisoning, Undetermined	Adverse Effect	Under-dosing
Butalamine	T46.7X1	T46.7X2	T46.7X3	T46.7X4	T46.7X5	T46.7X6
Butalbital	T42.3X1	T42.3X2	T42.3X3	T42.3X4	T42.3X5	T42.3X6
Butallylonal	T42.3X1	T42.3X2	T42.3X3	T42.3X4	T42.3X5	T42.3X6
Butamben	T41.3X1	T41.3X2	T41.3X3	T41.3X4	T41.3X5	T41.3X6
Butamirate	T48.3X1	T48.3X2	T48.3X3	T48.3X4	T48.3X5	T48.3X6
Butane (distributed in mobile container)	T59.891	T59.892	T59.893	T59.894	—	—
distributed through pipes	T59.891	T59.892	T59.893	T59.894	—	—
incomplete combustion	T58.11	T58.12	T58.13	T58.14	—	—
Butanilicaine	T41.3X1	T41.3X2	T41.3X3	T41.3X4	T41.3X5	T41.3X6
Butanol	T51.3X1	T51.3X2	T51.3X3	T51.3X4	—	—
Butanone, 2-butanone	T52.4X1	T52.4X2	T52.4X3	T52.4X4	—	—
Butantrone	T49.4X1	T49.4X2	T49.4X3	T49.4X4	T49.4X5	T49.4X6
Butaperazine	T43.3X1	T43.3X2	T43.3X3	T43.3X4	T43.3X5	T43.3X6
Butazolidin	T39.2X1	T39.2X2	T39.2X3	T39.2X4	T39.2X5	T39.2X6
Butetamate	T48.6X1	T48.6X2	T48.6X3	T48.6X4	T48.6X5	T48.6X6
Butethal	T42.3X1	T42.3X2	T42.3X3	T42.3X4	T42.3X5	T42.3X6
Butethamate	T44.3X1	T44.3X2	T44.3X3	T44.3X4	T44.3X5	T44.3X6
Buthalitone (sodium)	T41.1X1	T41.1X2	T41.1X3	T41.1X4	T41.1X5	T41.1X6
Butisol (sodium)	T42.3X1	T42.3X2	T42.3X3	T42.3X4	T42.3X5	T42.3X6
Butizide	T50.2X1	T50.2X2	T50.2X3	T50.2X4	T50.2X5	T50.2X6
Butobarbital	T42.3X1	T42.3X2	T42.3X3	T42.3X4	T42.3X5	T42.3X6
sodium	T42.3X1	T42.3X2	T42.3X3	T42.3X4	T42.3X5	T42.3X6
Butobarbitone	T42.3X1	T42.3X2	T42.3X3	T42.3X4	T42.3X5	T42.3X6
Butoconazole (nitrate)	T49.0X1	T49.0X2	T49.0X3	T49.0X4	T49.0X5	T49.0X6
Butorphanol	T40.491	T40.492	T40.493	T40.494	T40.495	T40.496
Butriptyline	T43.011	T43.012	T43.013	T43.014	T43.015	T43.016
Butropium bromide	T44.3X1	T44.3X2	T44.3X3	T44.3X4	T44.3X5	T44.3X6
Butter of antimony — *see* Antimony						
Buttercups	T62.2X1	T62.2X2	T62.2X3	T62.2X4	—	—
Butyl						
acetate (secondary)	T52.8X1	T52.8X2	T52.8X3	T52.8X4	—	—
alcohol	T51.3X1	T51.3X2	T51.3X3	T51.3X4	—	—
aminobenzoate	T41.3X1	T41.3X2	T41.3X3	T41.3X4	T41.3X5	T41.3X6
butyrate	T52.8X1	T52.8X2	T52.8X3	T52.8X4	—	—
carbinol	T51.3X1	T51.3X2	T51.3X3	T51.3X4	—	—
carbitol	T52.3X1	T52.3X2	T52.3X3	T52.3X4	—	—
cellosolve	T52.3X1	T52.3X2	T52.3X3	T52.3X4	—	—
chloral (hydrate)	T42.6X1	T42.6X2	T42.6X3	T42.6X4	T42.6X5	T42.6X6
formate	T52.8X1	T52.8X2	T52.8X3	T52.8X4	—	—
lactate	T52.8X1	T52.8X2	T52.8X3	T52.8X4	—	—
propionate	T52.8X1	T52.8X2	T52.8X3	T52.8X4	—	—
scopolamine bromide	T44.3X1	T44.3X2	T44.3X3	T44.3X4	T44.3X5	T44.3X6
thiobarbital sodium	T41.1X1	T41.1X2	T41.1X3	T41.1X4	T41.1X5	T41.1X6
Butylated hydroxyanisole	T50.991	T50.992	T50.993	T50.994	T50.995	T50.996
Butylchloral hydrate	T42.6X1	T42.6X2	T42.6X3	T42.6X4	T42.6X5	T42.6X6
Butyltoluene	T52.2X1	T52.2X2	T52.2X3	T52.2X4	—	—
Butyn	T41.3X1	T41.3X2	T41.3X3	T41.3X4	T41.3X5	T41.3X6
Butyrophenone (-based tranquilizers)	T43.4X1	T43.4X2	T43.4X3	T43.4X4	T43.4X5	T43.4X6
Cabazitaxel*	T45.1X1	T45.1X2	T45.1X3	T45.1X4	T45.1X5	T45.1X6
Cabergoline	T42.8X1	T42.8X2	T42.8X3	T42.8X4	T42.8X5	T42.8X6
Cacodyl, cacodylic acid	T57.0X1	T57.0X2	T57.0X3	T57.0X4	—	—
Cactinomycin	T45.1X1	T45.1X2	T45.1X3	T45.1X4	T45.1X5	T45.1X6
Cade oil	T49.4X1	T49.4X2	T49.4X3	T49.4X4	T49.4X5	T49.4X6
Cadexomer iodine	T49.0X1	T49.0X2	T49.0X3	T49.0X4	T49.0X5	T49.0X6
Cadmium (chloride) (fumes) (oxide)	T56.3X1	T56.3X2	T56.3X3	T56.3X4	—	—
sulfide (medicinal) NEC	T49.4X1	T49.4X2	T49.4X3	T49.4X4	T49.4X5	T49.4X6
Cadralazine	T46.5X1	T46.5X2	T46.5X3	T46.5X4	T46.5X5	T46.5X6
Caffeine	T43.611	T43.612	T43.613	T43.614	T43.615	T43.616
Calabar bean	T62.2X1	T62.2X2	T62.2X3	T62.2X4	—	—
Caladium seguinum	T62.2X1	T62.2X2	T62.2X3	T62.2X4	—	—
Calamine (lotion)	T49.3X1	T49.3X2	T49.3X3	T49.3X4	T49.3X5	T49.3X6
Calcifediol	T45.2X1	T45.2X2	T45.2X3	T45.2X4	T45.2X5	T45.2X6
Calciferol	T45.2X1	T45.2X2	T45.2X3	T45.2X4	T45.2X5	T45.2X6
Calcijex*	T45.2X1	T45.2X2	T45.2X3	T45.2X4	T45.2X5	T45.2X6
Calcitonin	T50.991	T50.992	T50.993	T50.994	T50.995	T50.996
Calcitriol	T45.2X1	T45.2X2	T45.2X3	T45.2X4	T45.2X5	T45.2X6
Calcium	T50.3X1	T50.3X2	T50.3X3	T50.3X4	T50.3X5	T50.3X6
actylsalicylate	T39.011	T39.012	T39.013	T39.014	T39.015	T39.016
benzamidosalicylate	T37.1X1	T37.1X2	T37.1X3	T37.1X4	T37.1X5	T37.1X6
bromide	T42.6X1	T42.6X2	T42.6X3	T42.6X4	T42.6X5	T42.6X6
bromolactobionate	T42.6X1	T42.6X2	T42.6X3	T42.6X4	T42.6X5	T42.6X6
carbaspirin	T39.011	T39.012	T39.013	T39.014	T39.015	T39.016
carbimide	T50.6X1	T50.6X2	T50.6X3	T50.6X4	T50.6X5	T50.6X6
carbonate	T47.1X1	T47.1X2	T47.1X3	T47.1X4	T47.1X5	T47.1X6
chloride	T50.991	T50.992	T50.993	T50.994	T50.995	T50.996
anhydrous	T50.991	T50.992	T50.993	T50.994	T50.995	T50.996
cyanide	T57.8X1	T57.8X2	T57.8X3	T57.8X4	—	—
dioctyl sulfosuccinate	T47.4X1	T47.4X2	T47.4X3	T47.4X4	T47.4X5	T47.4X6
disodium edathamil	T45.8X1	T45.8X2	T45.8X3	T45.8X4	T45.8X5	T45.8X6

Substance	Poisoning, Accidental (unintentional)	Poisoning, Intentional Self-harm	Poisoning, Assault	Poisoning, Undetermined	Adverse Effect	Under-dosing
Calcium — *continued*						
disodium edetate	T45.8X1	T45.8X2	T45.8X3	T45.8X4	T45.8X5	T45.8X6
dobesilate	T46.991	T46.992	T46.993	T46.994	T46.995	T46.996
EDTA	T45.8X1	T45.8X2	T45.8X3	T45.8X4	T45.8X5	T45.8X6
ferrous citrate	T45.4X1	T45.4X2	T45.4X3	T45.4X4	T45.4X5	T45.4X6
folinate	T45.8X1	T45.8X2	T45.8X3	T45.8X4	T45.8X5	T45.8X6
glubionate	T50.3X1	T50.3X2	T50.3X3	T50.3X4	T50.3X5	T50.3X6
gluconate	T50.3X1	T50.3X2	T50.3X3	T50.3X4	T50.3X5	T50.3X6
gluconogalactogluconate	T50.3X1	T50.3X2	T50.3X3	T50.3X4	T50.3X5	T50.3X6
hydrate, hydroxide	T54.3X1	T54.3X2	T54.3X3	T54.3X4	—	—
hypochlorite	T54.3X1	T54.3X2	T54.3X3	T54.3X4	—	—
iodide	T48.4X1	T48.4X2	T48.4X3	T48.4X4	T48.4X5	T48.4X6
ipodate	T50.8X1	T50.8X2	T50.8X3	T50.8X4	T50.8X5	T50.8X6
lactate	T50.3X1	T50.3X2	T50.3X3	T50.3X4	T50.3X5	T50.3X6
leucovorin	T45.8X1	T45.8X2	T45.8X3	T45.8X4	T45.8X5	T45.8X6
mandelate	T37.91	T37.92	T37.93	T37.94	T37.95	T37.96
oxide	T54.3X1	T54.3X2	T54.3X3	T54.3X4	—	—
pantothenate	T45.2X1	T45.2X2	T45.2X3	T45.2X4	T45.2X5	T45.2X6
phosphate	T50.3X1	T50.3X2	T50.3X3	T50.3X4	T50.3X5	T50.3X6
salicylate	T39.091	T39.092	T39.093	T39.094	T39.095	T39.096
salts	T50.3X1	T50.3X2	T50.3X3	T50.3X4	T50.3X5	T50.3X6
Calculus-dissolving drug	T50.991	T50.992	T50.993	T50.994	T50.995	T50.996
Calomel	T49.0X1	T49.0X2	T49.0X3	T49.0X4	T49.0X5	T49.0X6
Caloric agent	T50.3X1	T50.3X2	T50.3X3	T50.3X4	T50.3X5	T50.3X6
Calusterone	T38.7X1	T38.7X2	T38.7X3	T38.7X4	T38.7X5	T38.7X6
Camazepam	T42.4X1	T42.4X2	T42.4X3	T42.4X4	T42.4X5	T42.4X6
Camomile	T49.0X1	T49.0X2	T49.0X3	T49.0X4	T49.0X5	T49.0X6
Camoquin	T37.2X1	T37.2X2	T37.2X3	T37.2X4	T37.2X5	T37.2X6
Camphor						
insecticide	T60.2X1	T60.2X2	T60.2X3	T60.2X4	—	—
medicinal	T49.8X1	T49.8X2	T49.8X3	T49.8X4	T49.8X5	T49.8X6
Camylofin	T44.3X1	T44.3X2	T44.3X3	T44.3X4	T44.3X5	T44.3X6
Cancer chemotherapy drug regimen	T45.1X1	T45.1X2	T45.1X3	T45.1X4	T45.1X5	T45.1X6
Candeptin	T49.0X1	T49.0X2	T49.0X3	T49.0X4	T49.0X5	T49.0X6
Candicidin	T49.0X1	T49.0X2	T49.0X3	T49.0X4	T49.0X5	T49.0X6
Cankaid*	T49.6X1	T49.6X2	T49.6X3	T49.6X4	T49.6X5	T49.6X6
Cannabinoids, synthetic	T40.721	T40.722	T40.723	T40.724	T40.725	T40.726
Cannabinol	T40.711	T40.712	T40.713	T40.714	T40.715	T40.716
Cannabis (derivatives)	T40.711	T40.712	T40.713	T40.714	T40.715	T40.716
Canned heat	T51.1X1	T51.1X2	T51.1X3	T51.1X4	—	—
Canrenoic acid	T50.0X1	T50.0X2	T50.0X3	T50.0X4	T50.0X5	T50.0X6
Canrenone	T50.0X1	T50.0X2	T50.0X3	T50.0X4	T50.0X5	T50.0X6
Cantharides, cantharidin, cantharis	T49.8X1	T49.8X2	T49.8X3	T49.8X4	T49.8X5	T49.8X6
Canthaxanthin	T50.991	T50.992	T50.993	T50.994	T50.995	T50.996
Capillary-active drug NEC	T46.901	T46.902	T46.903	T46.904	T46.905	T46.906
Capreomycin	T36.8X1	T36.8X2	T36.8X3	T36.8X4	T36.8X5	T36.8X6
Capresla*	T45.1X1	T45.1X2	T45.1X3	T45.1X4	T45.1X5	T45.1X6
Capsicum	T49.4X1	T49.4X2	T49.4X3	T49.4X4	T49.4X5	T49.4X6
Captafol	T60.3X1	T60.3X2	T60.3X3	T60.3X4	—	—
Captan	T60.3X1	T60.3X2	T60.3X3	T60.3X4	—	—
Captodiame, captodiamine	T43.591	T43.592	T43.593	T43.594	T43.595	T43.596
Captopril	T46.4X1	T46.4X2	T46.4X3	T46.4X4	T46.4X5	T46.4X6
Caramiphen	T44.3X1	T44.3X2	T44.3X3	T44.3X4	T44.3X5	T44.3X6
Carazolol	T44.7X1	T44.7X2	T44.7X3	T44.7X4	T44.7X5	T44.7X6
Carbachol	T44.1X1	T44.1X2	T44.1X3	T44.1X4	T44.1X5	T44.1X6
Carbacrylamine (resin)	T50.3X1	T50.3X2	T50.3X3	T50.3X4	T50.3X5	T50.3X6
Carbamate (insecticide)	T60.0X1	T60.0X2	T60.0X3	T60.0X4	—	—
Carbamate (sedative)	T42.6X1	T42.6X2	T42.6X3	T42.6X4	T42.6X5	T42.6X6
herbicide	T60.0X1	T60.0X2	T60.0X3	T60.0X4	—	—
insecticide	T60.0X1	T60.0X2	T60.0X3	T60.0X4	—	—
Carbamazepine	T42.1X1	T42.1X2	T42.1X3	T42.1X4	T42.1X5	T42.1X6
Carbamide	T47.3X1	T47.3X2	T47.3X3	T47.3X4	T47.3X5	T47.3X6
peroxide	T49.0X1	T49.0X2	T49.0X3	T49.0X4	T49.0X5	T49.0X6
topical	T49.8X1	T49.8X2	T49.8X3	T49.8X4	T49.8X5	T49.8X6
Carbamylcholine chloride	T44.1X1	T44.1X2	T44.1X3	T44.1X4	T44.1X5	T44.1X6
Carbaril	T60.0X1	T60.0X2	T60.0X3	T60.0X4	—	—
Carbarsone	T37.3X1	T37.3X2	T37.3X3	T37.3X4	T37.3X5	T37.3X6
Carbaryl	T60.0X1	T60.0X2	T60.0X3	T60.0X4	—	—
Carbaspirin	T39.011	T39.012	T39.013	T39.014	T39.015	T39.016
Carbastat*	T49.5X1	T49.5X2	T49.5X3	T49.5X4	T49.5X5	T49.5X6
Carbazochrome (salicylate) (sodium sulfonate)	T49.4X1	T49.4X2	T49.4X3	T49.4X4	T49.4X5	T49.4X6
Carbenicillin	T36.0X1	T36.0X2	T36.0X3	T36.0X4	T36.0X5	T36.0X6
Carbenoxolone	T47.1X1	T47.1X2	T47.1X3	T47.1X4	T47.1X5	T47.1X6
Carbetapentane	T48.3X1	T48.3X2	T48.3X3	T48.3X4	T48.3X5	T48.3X6
Carbethyl salicylate	T39.091	T39.092	T39.093	T39.094	T39.095	T39.096
Carbidopa (with levodopa)	T42.8X1	T42.8X2	T42.8X3	T42.8X4	T42.8X5	T42.8X6
Carbimazole	T38.2X1	T38.2X2	T38.2X3	T38.2X4	T38.2X5	T38.2X6
Carbinol	T51.1X1	T51.1X2	T51.1X3	T51.1X4	—	—
Carbinoxamine	T45.0X1	T45.0X2	T45.0X3	T45.0X4	T45.0X5	T45.0X6

*Optum Value-Add
☑ Additional Character May Be Required — Refer to the Tabular List for Character Selection
369

Substance	Poisoning, Accidental (unintentional)	Poisoning, Intentional Self-harm	Poisoning, Assault	Poisoning, Undetermined	Adverse Effect	Underdosing
Carbiphene	T39.8X1	T39.8X2	T39.8X3	T39.8X4	T39.8X5	T39.8X6
Carbitol	T52.3X1	T52.3X2	T52.3X3	T52.3X4	—	—
Carbo medicinalis	T47.6X1	T47.6X2	T47.6X3	T47.6X4	T47.6X5	T47.6X6
Carbocaine	T41.3X1	T41.3X2	T41.3X3	T41.3X4	T41.3X5	T41.3X6
infiltration (subcutaneous)	T41.3X1	T41.3X2	T41.3X3	T41.3X4	T41.3X5	T41.3X6
nerve block (peripheral) (plexus)	T41.3X1	T41.3X2	T41.3X3	T41.3X4	T41.3X5	T41.3X6
topical (surface)	T41.3X1	T41.3X2	T41.3X3	T41.3X4	T41.3X5	T41.3X6
Carbocisteine	T48.4X1	T48.4X2	T48.4X3	T48.4X4	T48.4X5	T48.4X6
Carbocromen	T46.3X1	T46.3X2	T46.3X3	T46.3X4	T46.3X5	T46.3X6
Carbol fuchsin	T49.0X1	T49.0X2	T49.0X3	T49.0X4	T49.0X5	—
Carbolic acid — see also Phenol	T54.0X1	T54.0X2	T54.0X3	T54.0X4	—	—
Carbolonium (bromide)	T48.1X1	T48.1X2	T48.1X3	T48.1X4	T48.1X5	T48.1X6
Carbomycin	T36.8X1	T36.8X2	T36.8X3	T36.8X4	T36.8X5	T36.8X6
Carbon						
bisulfide (liquid)	T65.4X1	T65.4X2	T65.4X3	T65.4X4	—	—
vapor	T65.4X1	T65.4X2	T65.4X3	T65.4X4	—	—
dioxide (gas)	T59.7X1	T59.7X2	T59.7X3	T59.7X4	—	—
medicinal	T41.5X1	T41.5X2	T41.5X3	T41.5X4	T41.5X5	T41.5X6
nonmedicinal	T59.7X1	T59.7X2	T59.7X3	T59.7X4	—	—
snow	T49.4X1	T49.4X2	T49.4X3	T49.4X4	T49.4X5	T49.4X6
disulfide (liquid)	T65.4X1	T65.4X2	T65.4X3	T65.4X4	—	—
vapor	T65.4X1	T65.4X2	T65.4X3	T65.4X4	—	—
monoxide (from incomplete combustion)	T58.91	T58.92	T58.93	T58.94	—	—
blast furnace gas	T58.8X1	T58.8X2	T58.8X3	T58.8X4	—	—
butane (distributed in mobile container)	T58.11	T58.12	T58.13	T58.14	—	—
distributed through pipes	T58.11	T58.12	T58.13	T58.14	—	—
charcoal fumes	T58.2X1	T58.2X2	T58.2X3	T58.2X4	—	—
coal	T58.2X1	T58.2X2	T58.2X3	T58.2X4	—	—
coke (in domestic stoves, fireplaces)	T58.2X1	T58.2X2	T58.2X3	T58.2X4	—	—
exhaust gas (motor) not in transit	T58.01	T58.02	T58.03	T58.04	—	—
combustion engine, any not in watercraft	T58.01	T58.02	T58.03	T58.04	—	—
farm tractor, not in transit	T58.01	T58.02	T58.03	T58.04	—	—
gas engine	T58.01	T58.02	T58.03	T58.04	—	—
motor pump	T58.01	T58.02	T58.03	T58.04	—	—
motor vehicle, not in transit	T58.01	T58.02	T58.03	T58.04	—	—
fuel (in domestic use)	T58.2X1	T58.2X2	T58.2X3	T58.2X4	—	—
gas (piped)	T58.11	T58.12	T58.13	T58.14	—	—
in mobile container	T58.11	T58.12	T58.13	T58.14	—	—
piped (natural)	T58.11	T58.12	T58.13	T58.14	—	—
utility	T58.11	T58.12	T58.13	T58.14	—	—
in mobile container	T58.11	T58.12	T58.13	T58.14	—	—
gas (piped)	T58.11	T58.12	T58.13	T58.14	—	—
illuminating gas	T58.11	T58.12	T58.13	T58.14	—	—
industrial fuels or gases, any	T58.8X1	T58.8X2	T58.8X3	T58.8X4	—	—
kerosene (in domestic stoves, fireplaces)	T58.2X1	T58.2X2	T58.2X3	T58.2X4	—	—
kiln gas or vapor	T58.8X1	T58.8X2	T58.8X3	T58.8X4	—	—
motor exhaust gas, not in transit	T58.01	T58.02	T58.03	T58.04	—	—
piped gas (manufactured) (natural)	T58.11	T58.12	T58.13	T58.14	—	—
producer gas	T58.8X1	T58.8X2	T58.8X3	T58.8X4	—	—
propane (distributed in mobile container)	T58.11	T58.12	T58.13	T58.14	—	—
distributed through pipes	T58.11	T58.12	T58.13	T58.14	—	—
solid (in domestic stoves, fireplaces)	T58.2X1	T58.2X2	T58.2X3	T58.2X4	—	—
specified source NEC	T58.8X1	T58.8X2	T58.8X3	T58.8X4	—	—
stove gas	T58.11	T58.12	T58.13	T58.14	—	—
piped	T58.11	T58.12	T58.13	T58.14	—	—
utility gas	T58.11	T58.12	T58.13	T58.14	—	—
piped	T58.11	T58.12	T58.13	T58.14	—	—
water gas	T58.11	T58.12	T58.13	T58.14	—	—
wood (in domestic stoves, fireplaces)	T58.2X1	T58.2X2	T58.2X3	T58.2X4	—	—
tetrachloride (vapor) NEC	T53.0X1	T53.0X2	T53.0X3	T53.0X4	—	—
liquid (cleansing agent) NEC	T53.0X1	T53.0X2	T53.0X3	T53.0X4	—	—
solvent	T53.0X1	T53.0X2	T53.0X3	T53.0X4	—	—
Carbonic acid gas	T59.7X1	T59.7X2	T59.7X3	T59.7X4	—	—
anhydrase inhibitor NEC	T50.2X1	T50.2X2	T50.2X3	T50.2X4	T50.2X5	T50.2X6
Carbophenothion	T60.0X1	T60.0X2	T60.0X3	T60.0X4	—	—
Carboplatin	T45.1X1	T45.1X2	T45.1X3	T45.1X4	T45.1X5	T45.1X6
Carboprost	T48.0X1	T48.0X2	T48.0X3	T48.0X4	T48.0X5	T48.0X6
Carboquone	T45.1X1	T45.1X2	T45.1X3	T45.1X4	T45.1X5	T45.1X6
Carbowax	T49.3X1	T49.3X2	T49.3X3	T49.3X4	T49.3X5	T49.3X6
Carboxymethylcellulose	T47.4X1	T47.4X2	T47.4X3	T47.4X4	T47.4X5	T47.4X6
Carbrital	T42.3X1	T42.3X2	T42.3X3	T42.3X4	T42.3X5	T42.3X6
Carbromal	T42.6X1	T42.6X2	T42.6X3	T42.6X4	T42.6X5	T42.6X6
Carbutamide	T38.3X1	T38.3X2	T38.3X3	T38.3X4	T38.3X5	T38.3X6
Carbuterol	T48.6X1	T48.6X2	T48.6X3	T48.6X4	T48.6X5	T48.6X6
Cardiac						
depressants	T46.2X1	T46.2X2	T46.2X3	T46.2X4	T46.2X5	T46.2X6
rhythm regulator	T46.2X1	T46.2X2	T46.2X3	T46.2X4	T46.2X5	T46.2X6
specified NEC	T46.2X1	T46.2X2	T46.2X3	T46.2X4	T46.2X5	T46.2X6
Cardiografin	T50.8X1	T50.8X2	T50.8X3	T50.8X4	T50.8X5	T50.8X6
Cardiogreen	T50.8X1	T50.8X2	T50.8X3	T50.8X4	T50.8X5	T50.8X6
Cardiotonic (glycoside) NEC	T46.0X1	T46.0X2	T46.0X3	T46.0X4	T46.0X5	T46.0X6
Cardiovascular drug NEC	T46.901	T46.902	T46.903	T46.904	T46.905	T46.906
Cardizem*	T46.1X1	T46.1X2	T46.1X3	T46.1X4	T46.1X5	T46.1X6
Cardrase	T50.2X1	T50.2X2	T50.2X3	T50.2X4	T50.2X5	T50.2X6
Carfecillin	T36.0X1	T36.0X2	T36.0X3	T36.0X4	T36.0X5	T36.0X6
Carfenazine	T43.3X1	T43.3X2	T43.3X3	T43.3X4	T43.3X5	T43.3X6
Carfusin	T49.0X1	T49.0X2	T49.0X3	T49.0X4	T49.0X5	T49.0X6
Carindacillin	T36.0X1	T36.0X2	T36.0X3	T36.0X4	T36.0X5	T36.0X6
Carisoprodol	T42.8X1	T42.8X2	T42.8X3	T42.8X4	T42.8X5	T42.8X6
Carmellose	T47.4X1	T47.4X2	T47.4X3	T47.4X4	T47.4X5	T47.4X6
Carminative	T47.5X1	T47.5X2	T47.5X3	T47.5X4	T47.5X5	T47.5X6
Carmofur	T45.1X1	T45.1X2	T45.1X3	T45.1X4	T45.1X5	T45.1X6
Carmustine	T45.1X1	T45.1X2	T45.1X3	T45.1X4	T45.1X5	T45.1X6
Carotene	T45.2X1	T45.2X2	T45.2X3	T45.2X4	T45.2X5	T45.2X6
Carphenazine	T43.3X1	T43.3X2	T43.3X3	T43.3X4	T43.3X5	T43.3X6
Carpipramine	T42.4X1	T42.4X2	T42.4X3	T42.4X4	T42.4X5	T42.4X6
Carprofen	T39.311	T39.312	T39.313	T39.314	T39.315	T39.316
Carpronium chloride	T44.3X1	T44.3X2	T44.3X3	T44.3X4	T44.3X5	T44.3X6
Carrageenan	T47.8X1	T47.8X2	T47.8X3	T47.8X4	T47.8X5	T47.8X6
Carteolol	T44.7X1	T44.7X2	T44.7X3	T44.7X4	T44.7X5	T44.7X6
Carter's Little Pills	T47.2X1	T47.2X2	T47.2X3	T47.2X4	T47.2X5	T47.2X6
Cartia*	T46.1X1	T46.1X2	T46.1X3	T46.1X4	T46.1X5	T46.1X6
Cascara (sagrada)	T47.2X1	T47.2X2	T47.2X3	T47.2X4	T47.2X5	T47.2X6
Cassava	T62.2X1	T62.2X2	T62.2X3	T62.2X4	—	—
Castellani's paint	T49.0X1	T49.0X2	T49.0X3	T49.0X4	T49.0X5	T49.0X6
Castor						
bean	T62.2X1	T62.2X2	T62.2X3	T62.2X4	—	—
oil	T47.2X1	T47.2X2	T47.2X3	T47.2X4	T47.2X5	T47.2X6
Catalase	T45.3X1	T45.3X2	T45.3X3	T45.3X4	T45.3X5	T45.3X6
Caterpillar (sting)	T63.431	T63.432	T63.433	T63.434	—	—
Catha (edulis) (tea)	T43.691	T43.692	T43.693	T43.694	—	—
Cathartic NEC	T47.4X1	T47.4X2	T47.4X3	T47.4X4	T47.4X5	T47.4X6
anthacene derivative	T47.2X1	T47.2X2	T47.2X3	T47.2X4	T47.2X5	T47.2X6
bulk	T47.4X1	T47.4X2	T47.4X3	T47.4X4	T47.4X5	T47.4X6
contact	T47.2X1	T47.2X2	T47.2X3	T47.2X4	T47.2X5	T47.2X6
emollient NEC	T47.4X1	T47.4X2	T47.4X3	T47.4X4	T47.4X5	T47.4X6
irritant NEC	T47.2X1	T47.2X2	T47.2X3	T47.2X4	T47.2X5	T47.2X6
mucilage	T47.4X1	T47.4X2	T47.4X3	T47.4X4	T47.4X5	T47.4X6
saline	T47.3X1	T47.3X2	T47.3X3	T47.3X4	T47.3X5	T47.3X6
vegetable	T47.2X1	T47.2X2	T47.2X3	T47.2X4	T47.2X5	T47.2X6
Cathine	T50.5X1	T50.5X2	T50.5X3	T50.5X4	T50.5X5	T50.5X6
Cathomycin	T36.8X1	T36.8X2	T36.8X3	T36.8X4	T36.8X5	T36.8X6
Cation exchange resin	T50.3X1	T50.3X2	T50.3X3	T50.3X4	T50.3X5	T50.3X6
Caustic(s) NEC	T54.91	T54.92	T54.93	T54.94		
alkali	T54.3X1	T54.3X2	T54.3X3	T54.3X4	—	—
hydroxide	T54.3X1	T54.3X2	T54.3X3	T54.3X4	—	—
potash	T54.3X1	T54.3X2	T54.3X3	T54.3X4	—	—
soda	T54.3X1	T54.3X2	T54.3X3	T54.3X4	—	—
specified NEC	T54.91	T54.92	T54.93	T54.94		
Ceepryn	T49.0X1	T49.0X2	T49.0X3	T49.0X4	T49.0X5	T49.0X6
ENT agent	T49.6X1	T49.6X2	T49.6X3	T49.6X4	T49.6X5	T49.6X6
lozenges	T49.6X1	T49.6X2	T49.6X3	T49.6X4	T49.6X5	T49.6X6
Cefacetrile	T36.1X1	T36.1X2	T36.1X3	T36.1X4	T36.1X5	T36.1X6
Cefaclor	T36.1X1	T36.1X2	T36.1X3	T36.1X4	T36.1X5	T36.1X6
Cefadroxil	T36.1X1	T36.1X2	T36.1X3	T36.1X4	T36.1X5	T36.1X6
Cefalexin	T36.1X1	T36.1X2	T36.1X3	T36.1X4	T36.1X5	T36.1X6
Cefaloglycin	T36.1X1	T36.1X2	T36.1X3	T36.1X4	T36.1X5	T36.1X6
Cefaloridine	T36.1X1	T36.1X2	T36.1X3	T36.1X4	T36.1X5	T36.1X6
Cefalosporins	T36.1X1	T36.1X2	T36.1X3	T36.1X4	T36.1X5	T36.1X6
Cefalotin	T36.1X1	T36.1X2	T36.1X3	T36.1X4	T36.1X5	T36.1X6
Cefamandole	T36.1X1	T36.1X2	T36.1X3	T36.1X4	T36.1X5	T36.1X6
Cefamycin antibiotic	T36.1X1	T36.1X2	T36.1X3	T36.1X4	T36.1X5	T36.1X6
Cefapirin	T36.1X1	T36.1X2	T36.1X3	T36.1X4	T36.1X5	T36.1X6
Cefatrizine	T36.1X1	T36.1X2	T36.1X3	T36.1X4	T36.1X5	T36.1X6
Cefazedone	T36.1X1	T36.1X2	T36.1X3	T36.1X4	T36.1X5	T36.1X6
Cefazolin	T36.1X1	T36.1X2	T36.1X3	T36.1X4	T36.1X5	T36.1X6
Cefbuperazone	T36.1X1	T36.1X2	T36.1X3	T36.1X4	T36.1X5	T36.1X6

Substance	Poisoning, Accidental (unintentional)	Poisoning, Intentional Self-harm	Poisoning, Assault	Poisoning, Undetermined	Adverse Effect	Under-dosing
Cefetamet	T36.1X1	T36.1X2	T36.1X3	T36.1X4	T36.1X5	T36.1X6
Cefixime	T36.1X1	T36.1X2	T36.1X3	T36.1X4	T36.1X5	T36.1X6
Cefmenoxime	T36.1X1	T36.1X2	T36.1X3	T36.1X4	T36.1X5	T36.1X6
Cefmetazole	T36.1X1	T36.1X2	T36.1X3	T36.1X4	T36.1X5	T36.1X6
Cefminox	T36.1X1	T36.1X2	T36.1X3	T36.1X4	T36.1X5	T36.1X6
Cefonicid	T36.1X1	T36.1X2	T36.1X3	T36.1X4	T36.1X5	T36.1X6
Cefoperazone	T36.1X1	T36.1X2	T36.1X3	T36.1X4	T36.1X5	T36.1X6
Ceforanide	T36.1X1	T36.1X2	T36.1X3	T36.1X4	T36.1X5	T36.1X6
Cefotaxime	T36.1X1	T36.1X2	T36.1X3	T36.1X4	T36.1X5	T36.1X6
Cefotetan	T36.1X1	T36.1X2	T36.1X3	T36.1X4	T36.1X5	T36.1X6
Cefotiam	T36.1X1	T36.1X2	T36.1X3	T36.1X4	T36.1X5	T36.1X6
Cefoxitin	T36.1X1	T36.1X2	T36.1X3	T36.1X4	T36.1X5	T36.1X6
Cefpimizole	T36.1X1	T36.1X2	T36.1X3	T36.1X4	T36.1X5	T36.1X6
Cefpiramide	T36.1X1	T36.1X2	T36.1X3	T36.1X4	T36.1X5	T36.1X6
Cefradine	T36.1X1	T36.1X2	T36.1X3	T36.1X4	T36.1X5	T36.1X6
Cefroxadine	T36.1X1	T36.1X2	T36.1X3	T36.1X4	T36.1X5	T36.1X6
Cefsulodin	T36.1X1	T36.1X2	T36.1X3	T36.1X4	T36.1X5	T36.1X6
Ceftazidime	T36.1X1	T36.1X2	T36.1X3	T36.1X4	T36.1X5	T36.1X6
Cefteram	T36.1X1	T36.1X2	T36.1X3	T36.1X4	T36.1X5	T36.1X6
Ceftezole	T36.1X1	T36.1X2	T36.1X3	T36.1X4	T36.1X5	T36.1X6
Ceftin*	T36.1X1	T36.1X2	T36.1X3	T36.1X4	T36.1X5	T36.1X6
Ceftizoxime	T36.1X1	T36.1X2	T36.1X3	T36.1X4	T36.1X5	T36.1X6
Ceftriaxone	T36.1X1	T36.1X2	T36.1X3	T36.1X4	T36.1X5	T36.1X6
Cefuroxime	T36.1X1	T36.1X2	T36.1X3	T36.1X4	T36.1X5	T36.1X6
Cefuzonam	T36.1X1	T36.1X2	T36.1X3	T36.1X4	T36.1X5	T36.1X6
Celestone	T38.ØX1	T38.ØX2	T38.ØX3	T38.ØX4	T38.ØX5	T38.ØX6
topical	T49.ØX1	T49.ØX2	T49.ØX3	T49.ØX4	T49.ØX5	T49.ØX6
Celexa*	T43.221	T43.222	T43.223	T43.224	T43.225	T43.226
Celiprolol	T44.7X1	T44.7X2	T44.7X3	T44.7X4	T44.7X5	T44.7X6
Cell stimulants and proliferants	T49.8X1	T49.8X2	T49.8X3	T49.8X4	T49.8X5	T49.8X6
Cellosolve	T52.91	T52.92	T52.93	T52.94	—	—
Cellulose						
cathartic	T47.4X1	T47.4X2	T47.4X3	T47.4X4	T47.4X5	T47.4X6
hydroxyethyl	T47.4X1	T47.4X2	T47.4X3	T47.4X4	T47.4X5	T47.4X6
nitrates (topical)	T49.3X1	T49.3X2	T49.3X3	T49.3X4	T49.3X5	T49.3X6
oxidized	T49.4X1	T49.4X2	T49.4X3	T49.4X4	T49.4X5	T49.4X6
Centipede (bite)	T63.411	T63.412	T63.413	T63.414	—	—
Central nervous system						
depressants	T42.71	T42.72	T42.73	T42.74	T42.75	T42.76
anesthetic (general) NEC	T41.2Ø1	T41.2Ø2	T41.2Ø3	T41.2Ø4	T41.2Ø5	T41.2Ø6
gases NEC	T41.ØX1	T41.ØX2	T41.ØX3	T41.ØX4	T41.ØX5	T41.ØX6
intravenous	T41.1X1	T41.1X2	T41.1X3	T41.1X4	T41.1X5	T41.1X6
barbiturates	T42.3X1	T42.3X2	T42.3X3	T42.3X4	T42.3X5	T42.3X6
benzodiazepines	T42.4X1	T42.4X2	T42.4X3	T42.4X4	T42.4X5	T42.4X6
bromides	T42.6X1	T42.6X2	T42.6X3	T42.6X4	T42.6X5	T42.6X6
cannabis sativa	T4Ø.711	T4Ø.712	T4Ø.713	T4Ø.714	T4Ø.715	T4Ø.716
chloral hydrate	T42.6X1	T42.6X2	T42.6X3	T42.6X4	T42.6X5	T42.6X6
ethanol	T51.ØX1	T51.ØX2	T51.ØX3	T51.ØX4	—	—
hallucinogenics	T4Ø.9Ø1	T4Ø.9Ø2	T4Ø.9Ø3	T4Ø.9Ø4	T4Ø.9Ø5	T4Ø.9Ø6
hypnotics	T42.71	T42.72	T42.73	T42.74	T42.75	T42.76
specified NEC	T42.6X1	T42.6X2	T42.6X3	T42.6X4	T42.6X5	T42.6X6
muscle relaxants	T42.8X1	T42.8X2	T42.8X3	T42.8X4	T42.8X5	T42.8X6
paraldehyde	T42.6X1	T42.6X2	T42.6X3	T42.6X4	T42.6X5	T42.6X6
sedatives; sedative-hypnotics	T42.71	T42.72	T42.73	T42.74	T42.75	T42.76
mixed NEC	T42.6X1	T42.6X2	T42.6X3	T42.6X4	T42.6X5	T42.6X6
specified NEC	T42.6X1	T42.6X2	T42.6X3	T42.6X4	T42.6X5	T42.6X6
muscle-tone depressants	T42.8X1	T42.8X2	T42.8X3	T42.8X4	T42.8X5	T42.8X6
stimulants	T43.6Ø1	T43.6Ø2	T43.6Ø3	T43.6Ø4	T43.6Ø5	T43.6Ø6
amphetamines	T43.621	T43.622	T43.623	T43.624	T43.625	T43.626
analeptics	T5Ø.7X1	T5Ø.7X2	T5Ø.7X3	T5Ø.7X4	T5Ø.7X5	T5Ø.7X6
antidepressants	T43.2Ø1	T43.2Ø2	T43.2Ø3	T43.2Ø4	T43.2Ø5	T43.2Ø6
opiate antagonists	T5Ø.7X1	T5Ø.7X2	T5Ø.7X3	T5Ø.7X4	T5Ø.7X5	T5Ø.7X6
specified NEC	T43.691	T43.692	T43.693	T43.694	T43.695	T43.696
Cepacol*	T41.3X1	T41.3X2	T41.3X3	T41.3X4	T41.3X5	T41.3X6
Cephalexin	T36.1X1	T36.1X2	T36.1X3	T36.1X4	T36.1X5	T36.1X6
Cephaloglycin	T36.1X1	T36.1X2	T36.1X3	T36.1X4	T36.1X5	T36.1X6
Cephaloridine	T36.1X1	T36.1X2	T36.1X3	T36.1X4	T36.1X5	T36.1X6
Cephalosporins	T36.1X1	T36.1X2	T36.1X3	T36.1X4	T36.1X5	T36.1X6
N (adicillin)	T36.ØX1	T36.ØX2	T36.ØX3	T36.ØX4	T36.ØX5	T36.ØX6
Cephalothin	T36.1X1	T36.1X2	T36.1X3	T36.1X4	T36.1X5	T36.1X6
Cephalotin	T36.1X1	T36.1X2	T36.1X3	T36.1X4	T36.1X5	T36.1X6
Cephradine	T36.1X1	T36.1X2	T36.1X3	T36.1X4	T36.1X5	T36.1X6
Cerbera (odallam)	T62.2X1	T62.2X2	T62.2X3	T62.2X4	—	—
Cerberin	T46.ØX1	T46.ØX2	T46.ØX3	T46.ØX4	T46.ØX5	T46.ØX6
Cerebral stimulants	T43.6Ø1	T43.6Ø2	T43.6Ø3	T43.6Ø4	T43.6Ø5	T43.6Ø6
psychotherapeutic	T43.6Ø1	T43.6Ø2	T43.6Ø3	T43.6Ø4	T43.6Ø5	T43.6Ø6
specified NEC	T43.691	T43.692	T43.693	T43.694	T43.695	T43.696
Cerium oxalate	T45.ØX1	T45.ØX2	T45.ØX3	T45.ØX4	T45.ØX5	T45.ØX6
Cerous oxalate	T45.ØX1	T45.ØX2	T45.ØX3	T45.ØX4	T45.ØX5	T45.ØX6
Ceruletide	T5Ø.8X1	T5Ø.8X2	T5Ø.8X3	T5Ø.8X4	T5Ø.8X5	T5Ø.8X6
Cetacort*	T49.ØX1	T49.ØX2	T49.ØX3	T49.ØX4	T49.ØX5	T49.ØX6

Substance	Poisoning, Accidental (unintentional)	Poisoning, Intentional Self-harm	Poisoning, Assault	Poisoning, Undetermined	Adverse Effect	Under-dosing
Cetalkonium (chloride)	T49.ØX1	T49.ØX2	T49.ØX3	T49.ØX4	T49.ØX5	T49.ØX6
Cethexonium chloride	T49.ØX1	T49.ØX2	T49.ØX3	T49.ØX4	T49.ØX5	T49.ØX6
Cetiedil	T46.7X1	T46.7X2	T46.7X3	T46.7X4	T46.7X5	T46.7X6
Cetirizine	T45.ØX1	T45.ØX2	T45.ØX3	T45.ØX4	T45.ØX5	T45.ØX6
Cetomacrogol	T5Ø.991	T5Ø.992	T5Ø.993	T5Ø.994	T5Ø.995	T5Ø.996
Cetotiamine	T45.2X1	T45.2X2	T45.2X3	T45.2X4	T45.2X5	T45.2X6
Cetoxime	T45.ØX1	T45.ØX2	T45.ØX3	T45.ØX4	T45.ØX5	T45.ØX6
Cetraxate	T47.1X1	T47.1X2	T47.1X3	T47.1X4	T47.1X5	T47.1X6
Cetrimide	T49.ØX1	T49.ØX2	T49.ØX3	T49.ØX4	T49.ØX5	T49.ØX6
Cetrimonium (bromide)	T49.ØX1	T49.ØX2	T49.ØX3	T49.ØX4	T49.ØX5	T49.ØX6
Cetylpyridinium chloride	T49.ØX1	T49.ØX2	T49.ØX3	T49.ØX4	T49.ØX5	T49.ØX6
ENT agent	T49.6X1	T49.6X2	T49.6X3	T49.6X4	T49.6X5	T49.6X6
lozenges	T49.6X1	T49.6X2	T49.6X3	T49.6X4	T49.6X5	T49.6X6
Cevadilla — *see* Sabadilla						
Cevitamic acid	T45.2X1	T45.2X2	T45.2X3	T45.2X4	T45.2X5	T45.2X6
Chalk, precipitated	T47.1X1	T47.1X2	T47.1X3	T47.1X4	T47.1X5	T47.1X6
Chamomile	T49.ØX1	T49.ØX2	T49.ØX3	T49.ØX4	T49.ØX5	T49.ØX6
Ch'an su	T46.ØX1	T46.ØX2	T46.ØX3	T46.ØX4	T46.ØX5	T46.ØX6
Charcoal	T47.6X1	T47.6X2	T47.6X3	T47.6X4	T47.6X5	T47.6X6
activated — *see also* Charcoal, medicinal	T47.6X1	T47.6X2	T47.6X3	T47.6X4	T47.6X5	T47.6X6
fumes (Carbon monoxide)	T58.2X1	T58.2X2	T58.2X3	T58.2X4	—	—
industrial	T58.8X1	T58.8X2	T58.8X3	T58.8X4	—	—
medicinal (activated)	T47.6X1	T47.6X2	T47.6X3	T47.6X4	T47.6X5	T47.6X6
antidiarrheal	T47.6X1	T47.6X2	T47.6X3	T47.6X4	T47.6X5	T47.6X6
poison control	T47.8X1	T47.8X2	T47.8X3	T47.8X4	T47.8X5	T47.8X6
specified use other than for diarrhea	T47.8X1	T47.8X2	T47.8X3	T47.8X4	T47.8X5	T47.8X6
topical	T49.8X1	T49.8X2	T49.8X3	T49.8X4	T49.8X5	T49.8X6
Chaulmosulfone	T37.1X1	T37.1X2	T37.1X3	T37.1X4	T37.1X5	T37.1X6
Chelating agent NEC	T5Ø.6X1	T5Ø.6X2	T5Ø.6X3	T5Ø.6X4	T5Ø.6X5	T5Ø.6X6
Chelidonium majus	T62.2X1	T62.2X2	T62.2X3	T62.2X4	—	—
Chemical substance NEC	T65.91	T65.92	T65.93	T65.94	—	—
Chenodeoxycholic acid	T47.5X1	T47.5X2	T47.5X3	T47.5X4	T47.5X5	T47.5X6
Chenodiol	T47.5X1	T47.5X2	T47.5X3	T47.5X4	T47.5X5	T47.5X6
Chenopodium	T37.4X1	T37.4X2	T37.4X3	T37.4X4	T37.4X5	T37.4X6
Cherry laurel	T62.2X1	T62.2X2	T62.2X3	T62.2X4	—	—
Chiggertox*	T41.3X1	T41.3X2	T41.3X3	T41.3X4	T41.3X5	T41.3X6
Chinidin (e)	T46.2X1	T46.2X2	T46.2X3	T46.2X4	T46.2X5	T46.2X6
Chiniofon	T37.8X1	T37.8X2	T37.8X3	T37.8X4	T37.8X5	T37.8X6
Chlophedianol	T48.3X1	T48.3X2	T48.3X3	T48.3X4	T48.3X5	T48.3X6
Chlor-Trimeton	T45.ØX1	T45.ØX2	T45.ØX3	T45.ØX4	T45.ØX5	T45.ØX6
Chloral	T42.6X1	T42.6X2	T42.6X3	T42.6X4	T42.6X5	T42.6X6
derivative	T42.6X1	T42.6X2	T42.6X3	T42.6X4	T42.6X5	T42.6X6
hydrate	T42.6X1	T42.6X2	T42.6X3	T42.6X4	T42.6X5	T42.6X6
Chloralamide	T42.6X1	T42.6X2	T42.6X3	T42.6X4	T42.6X5	T42.6X6
Chloralodol	T42.6X1	T42.6X2	T42.6X3	T42.6X4	T42.6X5	T42.6X6
Chloralose	T6Ø.4X1	T6Ø.4X2	T6Ø.4X3	T6Ø.4X4	—	—
Chlorambucil	T45.1X1	T45.1X2	T45.1X3	T45.1X4	T45.1X5	T45.1X6
Chloramine	T57.8X1	T57.8X2	T57.8X3	T57.8X4	—	—
T	T49.ØX1	T49.ØX2	T49.ØX3	T49.ØX4	T49.ØX5	T49.ØX6
topical	T49.ØX1	T49.ØX2	T49.ØX3	T49.ØX4	T49.ØX5	T49.ØX6
Chloramphenicol	T36.2X1	T36.2X2	T36.2X3	T36.2X4	T36.2X5	T36.2X6
ENT agent	T49.6X1	T49.6X2	T49.6X3	T49.6X4	T49.6X5	T49.6X6
ophthalmic preparation	T49.5X1	T49.5X2	T49.5X3	T49.5X4	T49.5X5	T49.5X6
topical NEC	T49.ØX1	T49.ØX2	T49.ØX3	T49.ØX4	T49.ØX5	T49.ØX6
Chlorate (potassium) (sodium) **NEC**	T6Ø.3X1	T6Ø.3X2	T6Ø.3X3	T6Ø.3X4	—	—
herbicide	T6Ø.3X1	T6Ø.3X2	T6Ø.3X3	T6Ø.3X4	—	—
Chlorazanil	T5Ø.2X1	T5Ø.2X2	T5Ø.2X3	T5Ø.2X4	T5Ø.2X5	T5Ø.2X6
Chlorbenzene, chlorbenzol	T53.7X1	T53.7X2	T53.7X3	T53.7X4	—	—
Chlorbenzoxamine	T44.3X1	T44.3X2	T44.3X3	T44.3X4	T44.3X5	T44.3X6
Chlorbutol	T42.6X1	T42.6X2	T42.6X3	T42.6X4	T42.6X5	T42.6X6
Chlorcyclizine	T45.ØX1	T45.ØX2	T45.ØX3	T45.ØX4	T45.ØX5	T45.ØX6
Chlordan (e) (dust)	T6Ø.1X1	T6Ø.1X2	T6Ø.1X3	T6Ø.1X4	—	—
Chlordantoin	T49.ØX1	T49.ØX2	T49.ØX3	T49.ØX4	T49.ØX5	T49.ØX6
Chlordiazepoxide	T42.4X1	T42.4X2	T42.4X3	T42.4X4	T42.4X5	T42.4X6
Chlordiethyl benzamide	T49.3X1	T49.3X2	T49.3X3	T49.3X4	T49.3X5	T49.3X6
Chloresium	T49.8X1	T49.8X2	T49.8X3	T49.8X4	T49.8X5	T49.8X6
Chlorethiazol	T42.6X1	T42.6X2	T42.6X3	T42.6X4	T42.6X5	T42.6X6
Chlorethyl — *see* Ethyl, chloride						
Chloretone	T42.6X1	T42.6X2	T42.6X3	T42.6X4	T42.6X5	T42.6X6
Chlorex	T53.6X1	T53.6X2	T53.6X3	T53.6X4	—	—
insecticide	T6Ø.1X1	T6Ø.1X2	T6Ø.1X3	T6Ø.1X4	—	—
Chlorfenvinphos	T6Ø.ØX1	T6Ø.ØX2	T6Ø.ØX3	T6Ø.ØX4	—	—
Chlorhexadol	T42.6X1	T42.6X2	T42.6X3	T42.6X4	T42.6X5	T42.6X6
Chlorhexamide	T45.1X1	T45.1X2	T45.1X3	T45.1X4	T45.1X5	T45.1X6
Chlorhexidine	T49.ØX1	T49.ØX2	T49.ØX3	T49.ØX4	T49.ØX5	T49.ØX6
Chlorhexidine Gluconate Oral Rinse*	T49.6X1	T49.6X2	T49.6X3	T49.6X4	T49.6X5	T49.6X6
Chlorhydroxyquinolin	T49.ØX1	T49.ØX2	T49.ØX3	T49.ØX4	T49.ØX5	T49.ØX6
Chloride of lime (bleach)	T54.3X1	T54.3X2	T54.3X3	T54.3X4	—	—

Substance	Poisoning, Accidental (unintentional)	Poisoning, Intentional Self-harm	Poisoning, Assault	Poisoning, Undetermined	Adverse Effect	Under-dosing
Chlorimipramine	T43.Ø11	T43.Ø12	T43.Ø13	T43.Ø14	T43.Ø15	T43.Ø16
Chlorinated						
camphene	T53.6X1	T53.6X2	T53.6X3	T53.6X4	—	—
diphenyl	T53.7X1	T53.7X2	T53.7X3	T53.7X4	—	—
hydrocarbons NEC	T53.91	T53.92	T53.93	T53.94	—	—
solvents	T53.91	T53.92	T53.93	T53.94	—	—
lime (bleach)	T54.3X1	T54.3X2	T54.3X3	T54.3X4	—	—
and boric acid solution	T49.ØX1	T49.ØX2	T49.ØX3	T49.ØX4	T49.ØX5	T49.ØX6
naphthalene (insecticide)	T6Ø.1X1	T6Ø.1X2	T6Ø.1X3	T6Ø.1X4	—	—
industrial (non-pesticide)	T53.7X1	T53.7X2	T53.7X3	T53.7X4	—	—
pesticide NEC	T6Ø.8X1	T6Ø.8X2	T6Ø.8X3	T6Ø.8X4	—	—
soda — *see also* sodium hypochlorite						
solution	T49.ØX1	T49.ØX2	T49.ØX3	T49.ØX4	T49.ØX5	T49.ØX6
Chlorine (fumes) (gas)	T59.4X1	T59.4X2	T59.4X3	T59.4X4	—	—
bleach	T54.3X1	T54.3X2	T54.3X3	T54.3X4	—	—
compound gas NEC	T59.4X1	T59.4X2	T59.4X3	T59.4X4	—	—
disinfectant	T59.4X1	T59.4X2	T59.4X3	T59.4X4	—	—
releasing agents NEC	T59.4X1	T59.4X2	T59.4X3	T59.4X4	—	—
Chlorisondamine chloride	T46.991	T46.992	T46.993	T46.994	T46.995	T46.996
Chlormadinone	T38.5X1	T38.5X2	T38.5X3	T38.5X4	T38.5X5	T38.5X6
Chlormephos	T6Ø.ØX1	T6Ø.ØX2	T6Ø.ØX3	T6Ø.ØX4	—	—
Chlormerodrin	T5Ø.2X1	T5Ø.2X2	T5Ø.2X3	T5Ø.2X4	T5Ø.2X5	T5Ø.2X6
Chlormethiazole	T42.6X1	T42.6X2	T42.6X3	T42.6X4	T42.6X5	T42.6X6
Chlormethine	T45.1X1	T45.1X2	T45.1X3	T45.1X4	T45.1X5	T45.1X6
Chlormethylenecycline	T36.4X1	T36.4X2	T36.4X3	T36.4X4	T36.4X5	T36.4X6
Chlormezanone	T42.6X1	T42.6X2	T42.6X3	T42.6X4	T42.6X5	T42.6X6
Chloroacetic acid	T6Ø.3X1	T6Ø.3X2	T6Ø.3X3	T6Ø.3X4	—	—
Chloroacetone	T59.3X1	T59.3X2	T59.3X3	T59.3X4	—	—
Chloroacetophenone	T59.3X1	T59.3X2	T59.3X3	T59.3X4	—	—
Chloroaniline	T53.7X1	T53.7X2	T53.7X3	T53.7X4	—	—
Chlorobenzene, chlorobenzol	T53.7X1	T53.7X2	T53.7X3	T53.7X4	—	—
Chlorobromomethane (fire extinguisher)	T53.6X1	T53.6X2	T53.6X3	T53.6X4	—	—
Chlorobutanol	T49.ØX1	T49.ØX2	T49.ØX3	T49.ØX4	T49.ØX5	T49.ØX6
Chlorocresol	T49.ØX1	T49.ØX2	T49.ØX3	T49.ØX4	T49.ØX5	T49.ØX6
Chlorodehydromethyltestosterone	T38.7X1	T38.7X2	T38.7X3	T38.7X4	T38.7X5	T38.7X6
Chlorodeoxyadenosine*	T45.1X1	T45.1X2	T45.1X3	T45.1X4	T45.1X5	T45.1X6
Chlorodinitrobenzene	T53.7X1	T53.7X2	T53.7X3	T53.7X4	—	—
dust or vapor	T53.7X1	T53.7X2	T53.7X3	T53.7X4	—	—
Chlorodiphenyl	T53.7X1	T53.7X2	T53.7X3	T53.7X4	—	—
Chloroethane — *see* Ethyl, chloride						
Chloroethylene	T53.6X1	T53.6X2	T53.6X3	T53.6X4	—	—
Chlorofluorocarbons	T53.5X1	T53.5X2	T53.5X3	T53.5X4	—	—
Chloroform (fumes) (vapor)	T53.1X1	T53.1X2	T53.1X3	T53.1X4	—	—
anesthetic	T41.ØX1	T41.ØX2	T41.ØX3	T41.ØX4	T41.ØX5	T41.ØX6
solvent	T53.1X1	T53.1X2	T53.1X3	T53.1X4	—	—
water, concentrated	T41.ØX1	T41.ØX2	T41.ØX3	T41.ØX4	T41.ØX5	T41.ØX6
Chloroguanide	T37.2X1	T37.2X2	T37.2X3	T37.2X4	T37.2X5	T37.2X6
Chloromycetin	T36.2X1	T36.2X2	T36.2X3	T36.2X4	T36.2X5	T36.2X6
ENT agent	T49.6X1	T49.6X2	T49.6X3	T49.6X4	T49.6X5	T49.6X6
ophthalmic preparation	T49.5X1	T49.5X2	T49.5X3	T49.5X4	T49.5X5	T49.5X6
otic solution	T49.6X1	T49.6X2	T49.6X3	T49.6X4	T49.6X5	T49.6X6
topical NEC	T49.ØX1	T49.ØX2	T49.ØX3	T49.ØX4	T49.ØX5	T49.ØX6
Chloronitrobenzene	T53.7X1	T53.7X2	T53.7X3	T53.7X4	—	—
dust or vapor	T53.7X1	T53.7X2	T53.7X3	T53.7X4	—	—
Chlorophacinone	T6Ø.4X1	T6Ø.4X2	T6Ø.4X3	T6Ø.4X4	—	—
Chlorophenol	T53.7X1	T53.7X2	T53.7X3	T53.7X4	—	—
Chlorophenothane	T6Ø.1X1	T6Ø.1X2	T6Ø.1X3	T6Ø.1X4	—	—
Chlorophyll	T5Ø.991	T5Ø.992	T5Ø.993	T5Ø.994	T5Ø.995	T5Ø.996
Chloropicrin (fumes)	T53.6X1	T53.6X2	T53.6X3	T53.6X4	—	—
fumigant	T6Ø.8X1	T6Ø.8X2	T6Ø.8X3	T6Ø.8X4	—	—
fungicide	T6Ø.3X1	T6Ø.3X2	T6Ø.3X3	T6Ø.3X4	—	—
pesticide	T6Ø.8X1	T6Ø.8X2	T6Ø.8X3	T6Ø.8X4	—	—
Chloroprocaine	T41.3X1	T41.3X2	T41.3X3	T41.3X4	T41.3X5	T41.3X6
infiltration (subcutaneous)	T41.3X1	T41.3X2	T41.3X3	T41.3X4	T41.3X5	T41.3X6
nerve block (peripheral) (plexus)	T41.3X1	T41.3X2	T41.3X3	T41.3X4	T41.3X5	T41.3X6
spinal	T41.3X1	T41.3X2	T41.3X3	T41.3X4	T41.3X5	T41.3X6
Chloroptic	T49.5X1	T49.5X2	T49.5X3	T49.5X4	T49.5X5	T49.5X6
Chloropurine	T45.1X1	T45.1X2	T45.1X3	T45.1X4	T45.1X5	T45.1X6
Chloropyramine	T45.ØX1	T45.ØX2	T45.ØX3	T45.ØX4	T45.ØX5	T45.ØX6
Chloropyrifos	T6Ø.ØX1	T6Ø.ØX2	T6Ø.ØX3	T6Ø.ØX4	—	—
Chloropyrilene	T45.ØX1	T45.ØX2	T45.ØX3	T45.ØX4	T45.ØX5	T45.ØX6
Chloroquine	T37.2X1	T37.2X2	T37.2X3	T37.2X4	T37.2X5	T37.2X6
Chlorostat*	T49.ØX1	T49.ØX2	T49.ØX3	T49.ØX4	T49.ØX5	T49.ØX6
Chlorothalonil	T6Ø.3X1	T6Ø.3X2	T6Ø.3X3	T6Ø.3X4	—	—
Chlorothen	T45.ØX1	T45.ØX2	T45.ØX3	T45.ØX4	T45.ØX5	T45.ØX6
Chlorothiazide	T5Ø.2X1	T5Ø.2X2	T5Ø.2X3	T5Ø.2X4	T5Ø.2X5	T5Ø.2X6

Substance	Poisoning, Accidental (unintentional)	Poisoning, Intentional Self-harm	Poisoning, Assault	Poisoning, Undetermined	Adverse Effect	Under-dosing
Chlorothymol	T49.4X1	T49.4X2	T49.4X3	T49.4X4	T49.4X5	T49.4X6
Chlorotrianisene	T38.5X1	T38.5X2	T38.5X3	T38.5X4	T38.5X5	T38.5X6
Chlorovinyldichloroarsine, not in war	T57.ØX1	T57.ØX2	T57.ØX3	T57.ØX4	—	—
Chloroxine	T49.4X1	T49.4X2	T49.4X3	T49.4X4	T49.4X5	T49.4X6
Chloroxylenol	T49.ØX1	T49.ØX2	T49.ØX3	T49.ØX4	T49.ØX5	T49.ØX6
Chlorphenamine	T45.ØX1	T45.ØX2	T45.ØX3	T45.ØX4	T45.ØX5	T45.ØX6
Chlorphenesin	T42.8X1	T42.8X2	T42.8X3	T42.8X4	T42.8X5	T42.8X6
topical (antifungal)	T49.ØX1	T49.ØX2	T49.ØX3	T49.ØX4	T49.ØX5	T49.ØX6
Chlorpheniramine	T45.ØX1	T45.ØX2	T45.ØX3	T45.ØX4	T45.ØX5	T45.ØX6
Chlorphenoxamine	T45.ØX1	T45.ØX2	T45.ØX3	T45.ØX4	T45.ØX5	T45.ØX6
Chlorphentermine	T5Ø.5X1	T5Ø.5X2	T5Ø.5X3	T5Ø.5X4	T5Ø.5X5	T5Ø.5X6
Chlorprocaine — *see* Chloroprocaine						
Chlorproguanil	T37.2X1	T37.2X2	T37.2X3	T37.2X4	T37.2X5	T37.2X6
Chlorpromazine	T43.3X1	T43.3X2	T43.3X3	T43.3X4	T43.3X5	T43.3X6
Chlorpropamide	T38.3X1	T38.3X2	T38.3X3	T38.3X4	T38.3X5	T38.3X6
Chlorprothixene	T43.4X1	T43.4X2	T43.4X3	T43.4X4	T43.4X5	T43.4X6
Chlorquinaldol	T49.ØX1	T49.ØX2	T49.ØX3	T49.ØX4	T49.ØX5	T49.ØX6
Chlorquinol	T49.ØX1	T49.ØX2	T49.ØX3	T49.ØX4	T49.ØX5	T49.ØX6
Chlortalidone	T5Ø.2X1	T5Ø.2X2	T5Ø.2X3	T5Ø.2X4	T5Ø.2X5	T5Ø.2X6
Chlortetracycline	T36.4X1	T36.4X2	T36.4X3	T36.4X4	T36.4X5	T36.4X6
Chlorthalidone	T5Ø.2X1	T5Ø.2X2	T5Ø.2X3	T5Ø.2X4	T5Ø.2X5	T5Ø.2X6
Chlorthion	T6Ø.ØX1	T6Ø.ØX2	T6Ø.ØX3	T6Ø.ØX4	—	—
Chlorthiophos	T6Ø.ØX1	T6Ø.ØX2	T6Ø.ØX3	T6Ø.ØX4	—	—
Chlortrianisene	T38.5X1	T38.5X2	T38.5X3	T38.5X4	T38.5X5	T38.5X6
Chlorzoxazone	T42.8X1	T42.8X2	T42.8X3	T42.8X4	T42.8X5	T42.8X6
Choke damp	T59.7X1	T59.7X2	T59.7X3	T59.7X4	—	—
Cholagogues	T47.5X1	T47.5X2	T47.5X3	T47.5X4	T47.5X5	T47.5X6
Cholebrine	T5Ø.8X1	T5Ø.8X2	T5Ø.8X3	T5Ø.8X4	T5Ø.8X5	T5Ø.8X6
Cholecalciferol	T45.2X1	T45.2X2	T45.2X3	T45.2X4	T45.2X5	T45.2X6
Cholecystokinin	T5Ø.8X1	T5Ø.8X2	T5Ø.8X3	T5Ø.8X4	T5Ø.8X5	T5Ø.8X6
Cholera vaccine	T5Ø.A91	T5Ø.A92	T5Ø.A93	T5Ø.A94	T5Ø.A95	T5Ø.A96
Choleretic	T47.5X1	T47.5X2	T47.5X3	T47.5X4	T47.5X5	T47.5X6
Cholesterol-lowering agents	T46.6X1	T46.6X2	T46.6X3	T46.6X4	T46.6X5	T46.6X6
Cholestyramine (resin)	T46.6X1	T46.6X2	T46.6X3	T46.6X4	T46.6X5	T46.6X6
Cholic acid	T47.5X1	T47.5X2	T47.5X3	T47.5X4	T47.5X5	T47.5X6
Choline	T48.6X1	T48.6X2	T48.6X3	T48.6X4	T48.6X5	T48.6X6
chloride	T5Ø.991	T5Ø.992	T5Ø.993	T5Ø.994	T5Ø.995	T5Ø.996
dihydrogen citrate	T5Ø.991	T5Ø.992	T5Ø.993	T5Ø.994	T5Ø.995	T5Ø.996
salicylate	T39.Ø91	T39.Ø92	T39.Ø93	T39.Ø94	T39.Ø95	T39.Ø96
theophyllinate	T48.6X1	T48.6X2	T48.6X3	T48.6X4	T48.6X5	T48.6X6
Cholinergic (drug) **NEC**	T44.1X1	T44.1X2	T44.1X3	T44.1X4	T44.1X5	T44.1X6
muscle tone enhancer	T44.1X1	T44.1X2	T44.1X3	T44.1X4	T44.1X5	T44.1X6
organophosphorus	T44.ØX1	T44.ØX2	T44.ØX3	T44.ØX4	T44.ØX5	T44.ØX6
insecticide	T6Ø.ØX1	T6Ø.ØX2	T6Ø.ØX3	T6Ø.ØX4	—	—
nerve gas	T59.891	T59.892	T59.893	T59.894	—	—
trimethyl ammonium propanediol	T44.1X1	T44.1X2	T44.1X3	T44.1X4	T44.1X5	T44.1X6
Cholinesterase reactivator	T5Ø.6X1	T5Ø.6X2	T5Ø.6X3	T5Ø.6X4	T5Ø.6X5	T5Ø.6X6
Chografin	T5Ø.8X1	T5Ø.8X2	T5Ø.8X3	T5Ø.8X4	T5Ø.8X5	T5Ø.8X6
Chorionic gonadotropin	T38.891	T38.892	T38.893	T38.894	T38.895	T38.896
Chromate	T56.2X1	T56.2X2	T56.2X3	T56.2X4	—	—
dust or mist	T56.2X1	T56.2X2	T56.2X3	T56.2X4	—	—
lead — *see also* lead	T56.ØX1	T56.ØX2	T56.ØX3	T56.ØX4	—	—
paint	T56.ØX1	T56.ØX2	T56.ØX3	T56.ØX4	—	—
Chromelin*	T49.3X1	T49.3X2	T49.3X3	T49.3X4	T49.3X5	T49.3X6
Chromic						
acid	T56.2X1	T56.2X2	T56.2X3	T56.2X4	—	—
dust or mist	T56.2X1	T56.2X2	T56.2X3	T56.2X4	—	—
phosphate 32P	T45.1X1	T45.1X2	T45.1X3	T45.1X4	T45.1X5	T45.1X6
Chromium	T56.2X1	T56.2X2	T56.2X3	T56.2X4	—	—
compounds — *see* Chromate						
sesquioxide	T5Ø.8X1	T5Ø.8X2	T5Ø.8X3	T5Ø.8X4	T5Ø.8X5	T5Ø.8X6
Chromomycin A3	T45.1X1	T45.1X2	T45.1X3	T45.1X4	T45.1X5	T45.1X6
Chromonar	T46.3X1	T46.3X2	T46.3X3	T46.3X4	T46.3X5	T46.3X6
Chromyl chloride	T56.2X1	T56.2X2	T56.2X3	T56.2X4	—	—
Chrysarobin	T49.4X1	T49.4X2	T49.4X3	T49.4X4	T49.4X5	T49.4X6
Chrysazin	T47.2X1	T47.2X2	T47.2X3	T47.2X4	T47.2X5	T47.2X6
Chymar	T45.3X1	T45.3X2	T45.3X3	T45.3X4	T45.3X5	T45.3X6
ophthalmic preparation	T49.5X1	T49.5X2	T49.5X3	T49.5X4	T49.5X5	T49.5X6
Chymopapain	T45.3X1	T45.3X2	T45.3X3	T45.3X4	T45.3X5	T45.3X6
Chymotrypsin	T45.3X1	T45.3X2	T45.3X3	T45.3X4	T45.3X5	T45.3X6
ophthalmic preparation	T49.5X1	T49.5X2	T49.5X3	T49.5X4	T49.5X5	T49.5X6
Cialis*	T46.7X1	T46.7X2	T46.7X3	T46.7X4	T46.7X5	T46.7X6
Cianidanol	T5Ø.991	T5Ø.992	T5Ø.993	T5Ø.994	T5Ø.995	T5Ø.996
Cianopramine	T43.Ø11	T43.Ø12	T43.Ø13	T43.Ø14	T43.Ø15	T43.Ø16
Cibenzoline	T46.2X1	T46.2X2	T46.2X3	T46.2X4	T46.2X5	T46.2X6
Ciclacillin	T36.ØX1	T36.ØX2	T36.ØX3	T36.ØX4	T36.ØX5	T36.ØX6
Ciclobarbital — *see* Hexobarbital						
Ciclonicate	T46.7X1	T46.7X2	T46.7X3	T46.7X4	T46.7X5	T46.7X6

Substance	Poisoning, Accidental (unintentional)	Poisoning, Intentional Self-harm	Poisoning, Assault	Poisoning, Undetermined	Adverse Effect	Under-dosing
Ciclopirox (olamine)	T49.ØX1	T49.ØX2	T49.ØX3	T49.ØX4	T49.ØX5	T49.ØX6
Ciclosporin	T45.1X1	T45.1X2	T45.1X3	T45.1X4	T45.1X5	T45.1X6
Cicuta maculata or virosa	T62.2X1	T62.2X2	T62.2X3	T62.2X4	—	—
Cicutoxin	T62.2X1	T62.2X2	T62.2X3	T62.2X4	—	—
Cigarette lighter fluid	T52.ØX1	T52.ØX2	T52.ØX3	T52.ØX4	—	—
Cigarettes (tobacco)	T65.221	T65.222	T65.223	T65.224	—	—
Ciguatoxin	T61.Ø1	T61.Ø2	T61.Ø3	T61.Ø4	—	—
Cilazapril	T46.4X1	T46.4X2	T46.4X3	T46.4X4	T46.4X5	T46.4X6
Cimetidine	T47.ØX1	T47.ØX2	T47.ØX3	T47.ØX4	T47.ØX5	T47.ØX6
Cimetropium bromide	T44.3X1	T44.3X2	T44.3X3	T44.3X4	T44.3X5	T44.3X6
Cinchocaine	T41.3X1	T41.3X2	T41.3X3	T41.3X4	T41.3X5	T41.3X6
topical (surface)	T41.3X1	T41.3X2	T41.3X3	T41.3X4	T41.3X5	T41.3X6
Cinchona	T37.2X1	T37.2X2	T37.2X3	T37.2X4	T37.2X5	T37.2X6
Cinchonine alkaloids	T37.2X1	T37.2X2	T37.2X3	T37.2X4	T37.2X5	T37.2X6
Cinchophen	T5Ø.4X1	T5Ø.4X2	T5Ø.4X3	T5Ø.4X4	T5Ø.4X5	T5Ø.4X6
Cinepazide	T46.7X1	T46.7X2	T46.7X3	T46.7X4	T46.7X5	T46.7X6
Cinnamedrine	T48.5X1	T48.5X2	T48.5X3	T48.5X4	T48.5X5	T48.5X6
Cinnarizine	T45.ØX1	T45.ØX2	T45.ØX3	T45.ØX4	T45.ØX5	T45.ØX6
Cinoxacin	T37.8X1	T37.8X2	T37.8X3	T37.8X4	T37.8X5	T37.8X6
Ciprofibrate	T46.6X1	T46.6X2	T46.6X3	T46.6X4	T46.6X5	T46.6X6
Ciprofloxacin	T36.8X1	T36.8X2	T36.8X3	T36.8X4	T36.8X5	T36.8X6
Cisapride	T47.8X1	T47.8X2	T47.8X3	T47.8X4	T47.8X5	T47.8X6
Cisplatin	T45.1X1	T45.1X2	T45.1X3	T45.1X4	T45.1X5	T45.1X6
Citalopram	T43.221	T43.222	T43.223	T43.224	T43.225	T43.226
Citanest	T41.3X1	T41.3X2	T41.3X3	T41.3X4	T41.3X5	T41.3X6
infiltration (subcutaneous)	T41.3X1	T41.3X2	T41.3X3	T41.3X4	T41.3X5	T41.3X6
nerve block (peripheral) (plexus)	T41.3X1	T41.3X2	T41.3X3	T41.3X4	T41.3X5	T41.3X6
Citracel*	T5Ø.3X1	T5Ø.3X2	T5Ø.3X3	T5Ø.3X4	T5Ø.3X5	T5Ø.3X6
Citric acid	T47.5X1	T47.5X2	T47.5X3	T47.5X4	T47.5X5	T47.5X6
Citrovorum (factor)	T45.8X1	T45.8X2	T45.8X3	T45.8X4	T45.8X5	T45.8X6
Claviceps purpurea	T62.2X1	T62.2X2	T62.2X3	T62.2X4	—	—
Clavulanic acid	T36.1X1	T36.1X2	T36.1X3	T36.1X4	T36.1X5	T36.1X6
Cleaner, cleansing agent, type not specified	T65.891	T65.892	T65.893	T65.894	—	—
of paint or varnish	T52.91	T52.92	T52.93	T52.94	—	—
specified type NEC	T65.891	T65.892	T65.893	T65.894	—	—
Clebopride	T47.8X1	T47.8X2	T47.8X3	T47.8X4	T47.8X5	T47.8X6
Clefamide	T37.3X1	T37.3X2	T37.3X3	T37.3X4	T37.3X5	T37.3X6
Clemastine	T45.ØX1	T45.ØX2	T45.ØX3	T45.ØX4	T45.ØX5	T45.ØX6
Clematis vitalba	T62.2X1	T62.2X2	T62.2X3	T62.2X4	—	—
Clemizole	T45.ØX1	T45.ØX2	T45.ØX3	T45.ØX4	T45.ØX5	T45.ØX6
penicillin	T36.ØX1	T36.ØX2	T36.ØX3	T36.ØX4	T36.ØX5	T36.ØX6
Clenbuterol	T48.6X1	T48.6X2	T48.6X3	T48.6X4	T48.6X5	T48.6X6
Clidinium bromide	T44.3X1	T44.3X2	T44.3X3	T44.3X4	T44.3X5	T44.3X6
Climara*	T38.5X1	T38.5X2	T38.5X3	T38.5X4	T38.5X5	T38.5X6
Clinda-Derm*	T49.ØX1	T49.ØX2	T49.ØX3	T49.ØX4	T49.ØX5	T49.ØX6
Clindamycin	T36.8X1	T36.8X2	T36.8X3	T36.8X4	T36.8X5	T36.8X6
Clinofibrate	T46.6X1	T46.6X2	T46.6X3	T46.6X4	T46.6X5	T46.6X6
Clioquinol	T37.8X1	T37.8X2	T37.8X3	T37.8X4	T37.8X5	T37.8X6
Cliradon	T4Ø.2X1	T4Ø.2X2	T4Ø.2X3	T4Ø.2X4	—	—
Clobazam	T42.4X1	T42.4X2	T42.4X3	T42.4X4	T42.4X5	T42.4X6
Clobenzorex	T5Ø.5X1	T5Ø.5X2	T5Ø.5X3	T5Ø.5X4	T5Ø.5X5	T5Ø.5X6
Clobetasol	T49.ØX1	T49.ØX2	T49.ØX3	T49.ØX4	T49.ØX5	T49.ØX6
Clobetasone	T49.ØX1	T49.ØX2	T49.ØX3	T49.ØX4	T49.ØX5	T49.ØX6
Clobutinol	T48.3X1	T48.3X2	T48.3X3	T48.3X4	T48.3X5	T48.3X6
Clocortolone	T38.ØX1	T38.ØX2	T38.ØX3	T38.ØX4	T38.ØX5	T38.ØX6
Clodantoin	T49.ØX1	T49.ØX2	T49.ØX3	T49.ØX4	T49.ØX5	T49.ØX6
Clodronic acid	T5Ø.991	T5Ø.992	T5Ø.993	T5Ø.994	T5Ø.995	T5Ø.996
Clofazimine	T37.1X1	T37.1X2	T37.1X3	T37.1X4	T37.1X5	T37.1X6
Clofedanol	T48.3X1	T48.3X2	T48.3X3	T48.3X4	T48.3X5	T48.3X6
Clofenamide	T5Ø.2X1	T5Ø.2X2	T5Ø.2X3	T5Ø.2X4	T5Ø.2X5	T5Ø.2X6
Clofenotane	T49.ØX1	T49.ØX2	T49.ØX3	T49.ØX4	T49.ØX5	T49.ØX6
Clofezone	T39.2X1	T39.2X2	T39.2X3	T39.2X4	T39.2X5	T39.2X6
Clofibrate	T46.6X1	T46.6X2	T46.6X3	T46.6X4	T46.6X5	T46.6X6
Clofibride	T46.6X1	T46.6X2	T46.6X3	T46.6X4	T46.6X5	T46.6X6
Cloforex	T5Ø.5X1	T5Ø.5X2	T5Ø.5X3	T5Ø.5X4	T5Ø.5X5	T5Ø.5X6
Clomethiazole	T42.6X1	T42.6X2	T42.6X3	T42.6X4	T42.6X5	T42.6X6
Clometocillin	T36.ØX1	T36.ØX2	T36.ØX3	T36.ØX4	T36.ØX5	T36.ØX6
Clomifene	T38.5X1	T38.5X2	T38.5X3	T38.5X4	T38.5X5	T38.5X6
Clomiphene	T38.5X1	T38.5X2	T38.5X3	T38.5X4	T38.5X5	T38.5X6
Clomipramine	T43.Ø11	T43.Ø12	T43.Ø13	T43.Ø14	T43.Ø15	T43.Ø16
Clomocycline	T36.4X1	T36.4X2	T36.4X3	T36.4X4	T36.4X5	T36.4X6
Clonazepam	T42.4X1	T42.4X2	T42.4X3	T42.4X4	T42.4X5	T42.4X6
Clonidine	T46.5X1	T46.5X2	T46.5X3	T46.5X4	T46.5X5	T46.5X6
Clonixin	T39.8X1	T39.8X2	T39.8X3	T39.8X4	T39.8X5	T39.8X6
Clopamide	T5Ø.2X1	T5Ø.2X2	T5Ø.2X3	T5Ø.2X4	T5Ø.2X5	T5Ø.2X6
Clopenthixol	T43.4X1	T43.4X2	T43.4X3	T43.4X4	T43.4X5	T43.4X6
Cloperastine	T48.3X1	T48.3X2	T48.3X3	T48.3X4	T48.3X5	T48.3X6
Clophedianol	T48.3X1	T48.3X2	T48.3X3	T48.3X4	T48.3X5	T48.3X6
Cloponone	T36.2X1	T36.2X2	T36.2X3	T36.2X4	T36.2X5	T36.2X6
Cloprednol	T38.ØX1	T38.ØX2	T38.ØX3	T38.ØX4	T38.ØX5	T38.ØX6
Cloral betaine	T42.6X1	T42.6X2	T42.6X3	T42.6X4	T42.6X5	T42.6X6
Cloramfenicol	T36.2X1	T36.2X2	T36.2X3	T36.2X4	T36.2X5	T36.2X6
Clorazepate (dipotassium)	T42.4X1	T42.4X2	T42.4X3	T42.4X4	T42.4X5	T42.4X6
Clorexolone	T5Ø.2X1	T5Ø.2X2	T5Ø.2X3	T5Ø.2X4	T5Ø.2X5	T5Ø.2X6
Clorfenamine	T45.ØX1	T45.ØX2	T45.ØX3	T45.ØX4	T45.ØX5	T45.ØX6
Clorgiline	T43.1X1	T43.1X2	T43.1X3	T43.1X4	T43.1X5	T43.1X6
Clorotepine	T44.3X1	T44.3X2	T44.3X3	T44.3X4	T44.3X5	T44.3X6
Clorox (bleach)	T54.91	T54.92	T54.93	T54.94	—	—
Clorprenaline	T48.6X1	T48.6X2	T48.6X3	T48.6X4	T48.6X5	T48.6X6
Clortermine	T5Ø.5X1	T5Ø.5X2	T5Ø.5X3	T5Ø.5X4	T5Ø.5X5	T5Ø.5X6
Clotiapine	T43.591	T43.592	T43.593	T43.594	T43.595	T43.596
Clotiazepam	T42.4X1	T42.4X2	T42.4X3	T42.4X4	T42.4X5	T42.4X6
Clotibric acid	T46.6X1	T46.6X2	T46.6X3	T46.6X4	T46.6X5	T46.6X6
Clotrimazole	T49.ØX1	T49.ØX2	T49.ØX3	T49.ØX4	T49.ØX5	T49.ØX6
Cloxacillin	T36.ØX1	T36.ØX2	T36.ØX3	T36.ØX4	T36.ØX5	T36.ØX6
Cloxazolam	T42.4X1	T42.4X2	T42.4X3	T42.4X4	T42.4X5	T42.4X6
Cloxiquine	T49.ØX1	T49.ØX2	T49.ØX3	T49.ØX4	T49.ØX5	T49.ØX6
Clozapine	T42.4X1	T42.4X2	T42.4X3	T42.4X4	T42.4X5	T42.4X6
Coagulant NEC	T45.7X1	T45.7X2	T45.7X3	T45.7X4	T45.7X5	T45.7X6
Coal (carbon monoxide from) — *see also* Carbon, monoxide, coal	T58.2X1	T58.2X2	T58.2X3	T58.2X4	—	—
oil — *see* Kerosene						
tar	T49.1X1	T49.1X2	T49.1X3	T49.1X4	T49.1X5	T49.1X6
fumes	T59.891	T59.892	T59.893	T59.894	—	—
medicinal (ointment)	T49.4X1	T49.4X2	T49.4X3	T49.4X4	T49.4X5	T49.4X6
analgesics NEC	T39.2X1	T39.2X2	T39.2X3	T39.2X4	T39.2X5	T39.2X6
naphtha (solvent)	T52.ØX1	T52.ØX2	T52.ØX3	T52.ØX4	—	—
Coartem*	T37.2X1	T37.2X2	T37.2X3	T37.2X4	T37.2X5	T37.2X6
Cobalamine	T45.2X1	T45.2X2	T45.2X3	T45.2X4	T45.2X5	T45.2X6
Cobalt (nonmedicinal) (fumes) (industrial)	T56.891	T56.892	T56.893	T56.894	—	—
medicinal (trace) (chloride)	T45.8X1	T45.8X2	T45.8X3	T45.8X4	T45.8X5	T45.8X6
Cobra (venom)	T63.Ø41	T63.Ø42	T63.Ø43	T63.Ø44	—	—
Coca (leaf)	T4Ø.5X1	T4Ø.5X2	T4Ø.5X3	T4Ø.5X4	T4Ø.5X5	T4Ø.5X6
Cocaine	T4Ø.5X1	T4Ø.5X2	T4Ø.5X3	T4Ø.5X4	T4Ø.5X5	T4Ø.5X6
topical anesthetic	T41.3X1	T41.3X2	T41.3X3	T41.3X4	T41.3X5	T41.3X6
Cocarboxylase	T45.3X1	T45.3X2	T45.3X3	T45.3X4	T45.3X5	T45.3X6
Coccidioidin	T5Ø.8X1	T5Ø.8X2	T5Ø.8X3	T5Ø.8X4	T5Ø.8X5	T5Ø.8X6
Cocculus indicus	T62.1X1	T62.1X2	T62.1X3	T62.1X4	—	—
Cochineal	T65.6X1	T65.6X2	T65.6X3	T65.6X4	—	—
medicinal products	T5Ø.991	T5Ø.992	T5Ø.993	T5Ø.994	T5Ø.995	T5Ø.996
Cod-liver oil	T45.2X1	T45.2X2	T45.2X3	T45.2X4	T45.2X5	T45.2X6
Codeine	T4Ø.2X1	T4Ø.2X2	T4Ø.2X3	T4Ø.2X4	T4Ø.2X5	T4Ø.2X6
Coenzyme A	T5Ø.991	T5Ø.992	T5Ø.993	T5Ø.994	T5Ø.995	T5Ø.996
Coffee	T62.8X1	T62.8X2	T62.8X3	T62.8X4	—	—
Cogalactoisomerase	T5Ø.991	T5Ø.992	T5Ø.993	T5Ø.994	T5Ø.995	T5Ø.996
Cogentin	T44.3X1	T44.3X2	T44.3X3	T44.3X4	T44.3X5	T44.3X6
Coke fumes or gas (carbon monoxide)	T58.2X1	T58.2X2	T58.2X3	T58.2X4	—	—
industrial use	T58.8X1	T58.8X2	T58.8X3	T58.8X4	—	—
Colace	T47.4X1	T47.4X2	T47.4X3	T47.4X4	T47.4X5	T47.4X6
Colaspase	T45.1X1	T45.1X2	T45.1X3	T45.1X4	T45.1X5	T45.1X6
Colazal*	T47.8X1	T47.8X2	T47.8X3	T47.8X4	T47.8X5	T47.8X6
Colchicine	T5Ø.4X1	T5Ø.4X2	T5Ø.4X3	T5Ø.4X4	T5Ø.4X5	T5Ø.4X6
Colchicum	T62.2X1	T62.2X2	T62.2X3	T62.2X4	—	—
Cold cream	T49.3X1	T49.3X2	T49.3X3	T49.3X4	T49.3X5	T49.3X6
Colecalciferol	T45.2X1	T45.2X2	T45.2X3	T45.2X4	T45.2X5	T45.2X6
Colestipol	T46.6X1	T46.6X2	T46.6X3	T46.6X4	T46.6X5	T46.6X6
Colestyramine	T46.6X1	T46.6X2	T46.6X3	T46.6X4	T46.6X5	T46.6X6
Colimycin	T36.8X1	T36.8X2	T36.8X3	T36.8X4	T36.8X5	T36.8X6
Colistimethate	T36.8X1	T36.8X2	T36.8X3	T36.8X4	T36.8X5	T36.8X6
Colistin	T36.8X1	T36.8X2	T36.8X3	T36.8X4	T36.8X5	T36.8X6
sulfate (eye preparation)	T49.5X1	T49.5X2	T49.5X3	T49.5X4	T49.5X5	T49.5X6
Collagen	T5Ø.991	T5Ø.992	T5Ø.993	T5Ø.994	T5Ø.995	T5Ø.996
Collagenase	T49.4X1	T49.4X2	T49.4X3	T49.4X4	T49.4X5	T49.4X6
Collodion	T49.3X1	T49.3X2	T49.3X3	T49.3X4	T49.3X5	T49.3X6
Colocynth	T47.2X1	T47.2X2	T47.2X3	T47.2X4	T47.2X5	T47.2X6
Colophony adhesive	T49.3X1	T49.3X2	T49.3X3	T49.3X4	T49.3X5	T49.3X6
Colorant — *see also* Dye	T5Ø.991	T5Ø.992	T5Ø.993	T5Ø.994	T5Ø.995	T5Ø.996
Coloring matter — *see* Dye(s)						
Combustion gas (after combustion) — *see* Carbon, monoxide						
prior to combustion	T59.891	T59.892	T59.893	T59.894	—	—
Cometriq*	T45.1X1	T45.1X2	T45.1X3	T45.1X4	T45.1X5	T45.1X6
Compazine	T43.3X1	T43.3X2	T43.3X3	T43.3X4	T43.3X5	T43.3X6
Compound						
1080 (sodium fluoroacetate)	T6Ø.4X1	T6Ø.4X2	T6Ø.4X3	T6Ø.4X4	—	—
269 (endrin)	T6Ø.1X1	T6Ø.1X2	T6Ø.1X3	T6Ø.1X4	—	—
3422 (parathion)	T6Ø.ØX1	T6Ø.ØX2	T6Ø.ØX3	T6Ø.ØX4	—	—
3911 (phorate)	T6Ø.ØX1	T6Ø.ØX2	T6Ø.ØX3	T6Ø.ØX4	—	—
3956 (toxaphene)	T6Ø.1X1	T6Ø.1X2	T6Ø.1X3	T6Ø.1X4	—	—

*Optum Value-Add

☑ Additional Character May Be Required — Refer to the Tabular List for Character Selection 373

Substance	Poisoning, Accidental (unintentional)	Poisoning, Intentional Self-harm	Poisoning, Assault	Poisoning, Undetermined	Adverse Effect	Under-dosing
Compound — *continued*						
4049 (malathion)	T6Ø.ØX1	T6Ø.ØX2	T6Ø.ØX3	T6Ø.ØX4	—	—
4069 (malathion)	T6Ø.ØX1	T6Ø.ØX2	T6Ø.ØX3	T6Ø.ØX4	—	—
4124 (dicapthon)	T6Ø.ØX1	T6Ø.ØX2	T6Ø.ØX3	T6Ø.ØX4	—	—
42 (warfarin)	T6Ø.4X1	T6Ø.4X2	T6Ø.4X3	T6Ø.4X4	—	—
497 (dieldrin)	T6Ø.1X1	T6Ø.1X2	T6Ø.1X3	T6Ø.1X4	—	—
E (cortisone)	T38.ØX1	T38.ØX2	T38.ØX3	T38.ØX4	T38.ØX5	T38.ØX6
F (hydrocortisone)	T38.ØX1	T38.ØX2	T38.ØX3	T38.ØX4	T38.ØX5	T38.ØX6
Comvax*	T5Ø.A21	T5Ø.A22	T5Ø.A23	T5Ø.A24	T5Ø.A25	T5Ø.A26
Congener, anabolic	T38.7X1	T38.7X2	T38.7X3	T38.7X4	T38.7X5	T38.7X6
Congo red	T5Ø.8X1	T5Ø.8X2	T5Ø.8X3	T5Ø.8X4	T5Ø.8X5	T5Ø.8X6
Coniine, conine	T62.2X1	T62.2X2	T62.2X3	T62.2X4	—	—
Conium (maculatum)	T62.2X1	T62.2X2	T62.2X3	T62.2X4	—	—
Conjugated estrogenic substances	T38.5X1	T38.5X2	T38.5X3	T38.5X4	T38.5X5	T38.5X6
Contac	T48.5X1	T48.5X2	T48.5X3	T48.5X4	T48.5X5	T48.5X6
Contact lens solution	T49.5X1	T49.5X2	T49.5X3	T49.5X4	T49.5X5	T49.5X6
Contraceptive (oral)	T38.4X1	T38.4X2	T38.4X3	T38.4X4	T38.4X5	T38.4X6
vaginal	T49.8X1	T49.8X2	T49.8X3	T49.8X4	T49.8X5	T49.8X6
Contrast medium, radiography	T5Ø.8X1	T5Ø.8X2	T5Ø.8X3	T5Ø.8X4	T5Ø.8X5	T5Ø.8X6
Convallaria glycosides	T46.ØX1	T46.ØX2	T46.ØX3	T46.ØX4	T46.ØX5	T46.ØX6
Convallaria majalis	T62.2X1	T62.2X2	T62.2X3	T62.2X4	—	—
berry	T62.1X1	T62.1X2	T62.1X3	T62.1X4	—	—
Copper (dust) (fumes) (nonmedicinal) **NEC**	T56.4X1	T56.4X2	T56.4X3	T56.4X4	—	—
arsenate, arsenite	T57.ØX1	T57.ØX2	T57.ØX3	T57.ØX4	—	—
insecticide	T6Ø.2X1	T6Ø.2X2	T6Ø.2X3	T6Ø.2X4	—	—
emetic	T47.7X1	T47.7X2	T47.7X3	T47.7X4	T47.7X5	T47.7X6
fungicide	T6Ø.3X1	T6Ø.3X2	T6Ø.3X3	T6Ø.3X4	—	—
gluconate	T49.ØX1	T49.ØX2	T49.ØX3	T49.ØX4	T49.ØX5	T49.ØX6
insecticide	T6Ø.2X1	T6Ø.2X2	T6Ø.2X3	T6Ø.2X4	—	—
oleate	T49.ØX1	T49.ØX2	T49.ØX3	T49.ØX4	T49.ØX5	T49.ØX6
sulfate	T56.4X1	T56.4X2	T56.4X3	T56.4X4	—	—
cupric	T56.4X1	T56.4X2	T56.4X3	T56.4X4	—	—
fungicide	T6Ø.3X1	T6Ø.3X2	T6Ø.3X3	T6Ø.3X4	—	—
medicinal						
ear	T49.6X1	T49.6X2	T49.6X3	T49.6X4	T49.6X5	T49.6X6
emetic	T47.7X1	T47.7X2	T47.7X3	T47.7X4	T47.7X5	T47.7X6
eye	T49.5X1	T49.5X2	T49.5X3	T49.5X4	T49.5X5	T49.5X6
cuprous	T56.4X1	T56.4X2	T56.4X3	T56.4X4	—	—
fungicide	T6Ø.3X1	T6Ø.3X2	T6Ø.3X3	T6Ø.3X4	—	—
medicinal						
ear	T49.6X1	T49.6X2	T49.6X3	T49.6X4	T49.6X5	T49.6X6
emetic	T47.7X1	T47.7X2	T47.7X3	T47.7X4	T47.7X5	T47.7X6
eye	T49.5X1	T49.5X2	T49.5X3	T49.5X4	T49.5X5	T49.5X6
medicinal (trace)	T45.8X1	T45.8X2	T45.8X3	T45.8X4	T45.8X5	T45.8X6
Copperhead snake (bite) (venom)	T63.Ø61	T63.Ø62	T63.Ø63	T63.Ø64	—	—
Coral (sting)	T63.691	T63.692	T63.693	T63.694	—	—
snake (bite) (venom)	T63.Ø21	T63.Ø22	T63.Ø23	T63.Ø24	—	—
Corbadrine	T49.6X1	T49.6X2	T49.6X3	T49.6X4	T49.6X5	T49.6X6
Cordite	T65.891	T65.892	T65.893	T65.894	—	—
vapor	T59.891	T59.892	T59.893	T59.894	—	—
Cordran	T49.ØX1	T49.ØX2	T49.ØX3	T49.ØX4	T49.ØX5	T49.ØX6
Coreg*	T44.7X1	T44.7X2	T44.7X3	T44.7X4	T44.7X5	T44.7X6
Cormax*	T49.ØX1	T49.ØX2	T49.ØX3	T49.ØX4	T49.ØX5	T49.ØX6
Corn cures	T49.4X1	T49.4X2	T49.4X3	T49.4X4	T49.4X5	T49.4X6
Corn starch	T49.3X1	T49.3X2	T49.3X3	T49.3X4	T49.3X5	T49.3X6
Cornhusker's lotion	T49.3X1	T49.3X2	T49.3X3	T49.3X4	T49.3X5	T49.3X6
Coronary vasodilator NEC	T46.3X1	T46.3X2	T46.3X3	T46.3X4	T46.3X5	T46.3X6
Corrosive NEC	T54.91	T54.92	T54.93	T54.94	—	—
acid NEC	T54.2X1	T54.2X2	T54.2X3	T54.2X4	—	—
aromatics	T54.1X1	T54.1X2	T54.1X3	T54.1X4	—	—
disinfectant	T54.1X1	T54.1X2	T54.1X3	T54.1X4	—	—
fumes NEC	T54.91	T54.92	T54.93	T54.94	—	—
specified NEC	T54.91	T54.92	T54.93	T54.94	—	—
sublimate	T56.1X1	T56.1X2	T56.1X3	T56.1X4	—	—
Cort-Dome	T38.ØX1	T38.ØX2	T38.ØX3	T38.ØX4	T38.ØX5	T38.ØX6
ENT agent	T49.6X1	T49.6X2	T49.6X3	T49.6X4	T49.6X5	T49.6X6
ophthalmic preparation	T49.5X1	T49.5X2	T49.5X3	T49.5X4	T49.5X5	T49.5X6
topical NEC	T49.ØX1	T49.ØX2	T49.ØX3	T49.ØX4	T49.ØX5	T49.ØX6
Cortate	T38.ØX1	T38.ØX2	T38.ØX3	T38.ØX4	T38.ØX5	T38.ØX6
Cortef	T38.ØX1	T38.ØX2	T38.ØX3	T38.ØX4	T38.ØX5	T38.ØX6
ENT agent	T49.6X1	T49.6X2	T49.6X3	T49.6X4	T49.6X5	T49.6X6
ophthalmic preparation	T49.5X1	T49.5X2	T49.5X3	T49.5X4	T49.5X5	T49.5X6
topical NEC	T49.ØX1	T49.ØX2	T49.ØX3	T49.ØX4	T49.ØX5	T49.ØX6
Corticosteroid	T38.ØX1	T38.ØX2	T38.ØX3	T38.ØX4	T38.ØX5	T38.ØX6
ENT agent	T49.6X1	T49.6X2	T49.6X3	T49.6X4	T49.6X5	T49.6X6
mineral	T5Ø.ØX1	T5Ø.ØX2	T5Ø.ØX3	T5Ø.ØX4	T5Ø.ØX5	T5Ø.ØX6
ophthalmic	T49.5X1	T49.5X2	T49.5X3	T49.5X4	T49.5X5	T49.5X6
topical NEC	T49.ØX1	T49.ØX2	T49.ØX3	T49.ØX4	T49.ØX5	T49.ØX6
Corticotropin	T38.811	T38.812	T38.813	T38.814	T38.815	T38.816
Cortisol	T49.ØX1	T49.ØX2	T49.ØX3	T49.ØX4	T49.ØX5	T49.ØX6
ENT agent	T49.6X1	T49.6X2	T49.6X3	T49.6X4	T49.6X5	T49.6X6
ophthalmic preparation	T49.5X1	T49.5X2	T49.5X3	T49.5X4	T49.5X5	T49.5X6
topical NEC	T49.ØX1	T49.ØX2	T49.ØX3	T49.ØX4	T49.ØX5	T49.ØX6
Cortisone (acetate)	T38.ØX1	T38.ØX2	T38.ØX3	T38.ØX4	T38.ØX5	T38.ØX6
ENT agent	T49.6X1	T49.6X2	T49.6X3	T49.6X4	T49.6X5	T49.6X6
ophthalmic preparation	T49.5X1	T49.5X2	T49.5X3	T49.5X4	T49.5X5	T49.5X6
topical NEC	T49.ØX1	T49.ØX2	T49.ØX3	T49.ØX4	T49.ØX5	T49.ØX6
Cortisporin*	T49.ØX1	T49.ØX2	T49.ØX3	T49.ØX4	T49.ØX5	T49.ØX6
Cortivazol	T38.ØX1	T38.ØX2	T38.ØX3	T38.ØX4	T38.ØX5	T38.ØX6
Cortogen	T38.ØX1	T38.ØX2	T38.ØX3	T38.ØX4	T38.ØX5	T38.ØX6
ENT agent	T49.6X1	T49.6X2	T49.6X3	T49.6X4	T49.6X5	T49.6X6
ophthalmic preparation	T49.5X1	T49.5X2	T49.5X3	T49.5X4	T49.5X5	T49.5X6
Cortone	T38.ØX1	T38.ØX2	T38.ØX3	T38.ØX4	T38.ØX5	T38.ØX6
ENT agent	T49.6X1	T49.6X2	T49.6X3	T49.6X4	T49.6X5	T49.6X6
ophthalmic preparation	T49.5X1	T49.5X2	T49.5X3	T49.5X4	T49.5X5	T49.5X6
Cortril	T38.ØX1	T38.ØX2	T38.ØX3	T38.ØX4	T38.ØX5	T38.ØX6
ENT agent	T49.6X1	T49.6X2	T49.6X3	T49.6X4	T49.6X5	T49.6X6
ophthalmic preparation	T49.5X1	T49.5X2	T49.5X3	T49.5X4	T49.5X5	T49.5X6
topical NEC	T49.ØX1	T49.ØX2	T49.ØX3	T49.ØX4	T49.ØX5	T49.ØX6
Corynebacterium parvum	T45.1X1	T45.1X2	T45.1X3	T45.1X4	T45.1X5	T45.1X6
Cosmetic preparation	T49.8X1	T49.8X2	T49.8X3	T49.8X4	T49.8X5	T49.8X6
Cosmetics	T49.8X1	T49.8X2	T49.8X3	T49.8X4	T49.8X5	T49.8X6
Cosyntropin	T38.811	T38.812	T38.813	T38.814	T38.815	T38.816
Cotarnine	T45.7X1	T45.7X2	T45.7X3	T45.7X4	T45.7X5	T45.7X6
Co-trimoxazole	T36.8X1	T36.8X2	T36.8X3	T36.8X4	T36.8X5	T36.8X6
Cottonseed oil	T49.3X1	T49.3X2	T49.3X3	T49.3X4	T49.3X5	T49.3X6
Cough mixture (syrup)	T48.4X1	T48.4X2	T48.4X3	T48.4X4	T48.4X5	T48.4X6
containing opiates	T4Ø.2X1	T4Ø.2X2	T4Ø.2X3	T4Ø.2X4	T4Ø.2X5	T4Ø.2X6
expectorants	T48.4X1	T48.4X2	T48.4X3	T48.4X4	T48.4X5	T48.4X6
Coumadin	T45.511	T45.512	T45.513	T45.514	T45.515	T45.516
rodenticide	T6Ø.4X1	T6Ø.4X2	T6Ø.4X3	T6Ø.4X4	—	—
Coumaphos	T6Ø.ØX1	T6Ø.ØX2	T6Ø.ØX3	T6Ø.ØX4	—	—
Coumarin	T45.511	T45.512	T45.513	T45.514	T45.515	T45.516
Coumetarol	T45.511	T45.512	T45.513	T45.514	T45.515	T45.516
Cowbane	T62.2X1	T62.2X2	T62.2X3	T62.2X4	—	—
Cozaar*	T46.5X1	T46.5X2	T46.5X3	T46.5X4	T46.5X5	T46.5X6
Cozyme	T45.2X1	T45.2X2	T45.2X3	T45.2X4	T45.2X5	T45.2X6
Crack	T4Ø.5X1	T4Ø.5X2	T4Ø.5X3	T4Ø.5X4	—	—
Crataegus extract	T46.ØX1	T46.ØX2	T46.ØX3	T46.ØX4	T46.ØX5	T46.ØX6
Creolin	T54.1X1	T54.1X2	T54.1X3	T54.1X4	—	—
disinfectant	T54.1X1	T54.1X2	T54.1X3	T54.1X4	—	—
Creosol (compound)	T49.ØX1	T49.ØX2	T49.ØX3	T49.ØX4	T49.ØX5	T49.ØX6
Creosote (coal tar) (beechwood)	T49.ØX1	T49.ØX2	T49.ØX3	T49.ØX4	T49.ØX5	T49.ØX6
medicinal (expectorant)	T48.4X1	T48.4X2	T48.4X3	T48.4X4	T48.4X5	T48.4X6
syrup	T48.4X1	T48.4X2	T48.4X3	T48.4X4	T48.4X5	T48.4X6
Cresol(s)	T49.ØX1	T49.ØX2	T49.ØX3	T49.ØX4	T49.ØX5	T49.ØX6
and soap solution	T49.ØX1	T49.ØX2	T49.ØX3	T49.ØX4	T49.ØX5	T49.ØX6
Crestor*	T46.6X1	T46.6X2	T46.6X3	T46.6X4	T46.6X5	T46.6X6
Cresyl acetate	T49.ØX1	T49.ØX2	T49.ØX3	T49.ØX4	T49.ØX5	T49.ØX6
Cresylic acid	T49.ØX1	T49.ØX2	T49.ØX3	T49.ØX4	T49.ØX5	T49.ØX6
Crimidine	T6Ø.4X1	T6Ø.4X2	T6Ø.4X3	T6Ø.4X4	—	—
Croconazole	T37.8X1	T37.8X2	T37.8X3	T37.8X4	T37.8X5	T37.8X6
Cromoglicic acid	T48.6X1	T48.6X2	T48.6X3	T48.6X4	T48.6X5	T48.6X6
Cromolyn	T48.6X1	T48.6X2	T48.6X3	T48.6X4	T48.6X5	T48.6X6
Cromonar	T46.3X1	T46.3X2	T46.3X3	T46.3X4	T46.3X5	T46.3X6
Cropropamide	T39.8X1	T39.8X2	T39.8X3	T39.8X4	T39.8X5	T39.8X6
with crotethamide	T5Ø.7X1	T5Ø.7X2	T5Ø.7X3	T5Ø.7X4	T5Ø.7X5	T5Ø.7X6
Crotamiton	T49.ØX1	T49.ØX2	T49.ØX3	T49.ØX4	T49.ØX5	T49.ØX6
Crotethamide	T39.8X1	T39.8X2	T39.8X3	T39.8X4	T39.8X5	T39.8X6
with cropropamide	T5Ø.7X1	T5Ø.7X2	T5Ø.7X3	T5Ø.7X4	T5Ø.7X5	T5Ø.7X6
Croton (oil)	T47.2X1	T47.2X2	T47.2X3	T47.2X4	T47.2X5	T47.2X6
chloral	T42.6X1	T42.6X2	T42.6X3	T42.6X4	T42.6X5	T42.6X6
Crude oil	T52.ØX1	T52.ØX2	T52.ØX3	T52.ØX4	—	—
Cryogenine	T39.8X1	T39.8X2	T39.8X3	T39.8X4	T39.8X5	T39.8X6
Cryolite (vapor)	T6Ø.1X1	T6Ø.1X2	T6Ø.1X3	T6Ø.1X4	—	—
insecticide	T6Ø.1X1	T6Ø.1X2	T6Ø.1X3	T6Ø.1X4	—	—
Cryptenamine (tannates)	T46.5X1	T46.5X2	T46.5X3	T46.5X4	T46.5X5	T46.5X6
Crystal violet	T49.ØX1	T49.ØX2	T49.ØX3	T49.ØX4	T49.ØX5	T49.ØX6
Cuckoopint	T62.2X1	T62.2X2	T62.2X3	T62.2X4	—	—
Cumetharol	T45.511	T45.512	T45.513	T45.514	T45.515	T45.516
Cupric						
acetate	T6Ø.3X1	T6Ø.3X2	T6Ø.3X3	T6Ø.3X4	—	—
acetoarsenite	T57.ØX1	T57.ØX2	T57.ØX3	T57.ØX4	—	—
arsenate	T57.ØX1	T57.ØX2	T57.ØX3	T57.ØX4	—	—
gluconate	T49.ØX1	T49.ØX2	T49.ØX3	T49.ØX4	T49.ØX5	T49.ØX6
oleate	T49.ØX1	T49.ØX2	T49.ØX3	T49.ØX4	T49.ØX5	T49.ØX6
sulfate	T56.4X1	T56.4X2	T56.4X3	T56.4X4	—	—
Cuprimine*	T5Ø.6X1	T5Ø.6X2	T5Ø.6X3	T5Ø.6X4	T5Ø.6X5	T5Ø.6X6
Cuprous sulfate — *see also* Copper, sulfate	T56.4X1	T56.4X2	T56.4X3	T56.4X4	—	—
Curare, curarine	T48.1X1	T48.1X2	T48.1X3	T48.1X4	T48.1X5	T48.1X6

Substance	Poisoning, Accidental (unintentional)	Poisoning, Intentional Self-harm	Poisoning, Assault	Poisoning, Undetermined	Adverse Effect	Under-dosing
Cyamemazine	T43.3X1	T43.3X2	T43.3X3	T43.3X4	T43.3X5	T43.3X6
Cyamopsis tetragonoloba	T46.6X1	T46.6X2	T46.6X3	T46.6X4	T46.6X5	T46.6X6
Cyanacetyl hydrazide	T37.1X1	T37.1X2	T37.1X3	T37.1X4	T37.1X5	T37.1X6
Cyanic acid (gas)	T59.891	T59.892	T59.893	T59.894	—	—
Cyanide(s) (compounds) (potassium) (sodium) NEC	T65.0X1	T65.0X2	T65.0X3	T65.0X4	—	—
fumigant	T65.0X1	T65.0X2	T65.0X3	T65.0X4	—	—
hydrogen	T57.3X1	T57.3X2	T57.3X3	T57.3X4	—	—
mercuric — see Mercury						
dust or gas (inhalation) NEC	T57.3X1	T57.3X2	T57.3X3	T57.3X4	—	—
pesticide (dust) (fumes)	T65.0X1	T65.0X2	T65.0X3	T65.0X4	—	—
Cyanoacrylate adhesive	T49.3X1	T49.3X2	T49.3X3	T49.3X4	T49.3X5	T49.3X6
Cyanocobalamin	T45.8X1	T45.8X2	T45.8X3	T45.8X4	T45.8X5	T45.8X6
Cyanogen (chloride) (gas) NEC	T59.891	T59.892	T59.893	T59.894	—	—
Cyclacillin	T36.0X1	T36.0X2	T36.0X3	T36.0X4	T36.0X5	T36.0X6
Cyclaine	T41.3X1	T41.3X2	T41.3X3	T41.3X4	T41.3X5	T41.3X6
Cyclamate	T50.991	T50.992	T50.993	T50.994	T50.995	T50.996
Cyclamen europaeum	T62.2X1	T62.2X2	T62.2X3	T62.2X4	—	—
Cyclandelate	T46.7X1	T46.7X2	T46.7X3	T46.7X4	T46.7X5	T46.7X6
Cyclazocine	T50.7X1	T50.7X2	T50.7X3	T50.7X4	T50.7X5	T50.7X6
Cyclizine	T45.0X1	T45.0X2	T45.0X3	T45.0X4	T45.0X5	T45.0X6
Cyclobarbital	T42.3X1	T42.3X2	T42.3X3	T42.3X4	T42.3X5	T42.3X6
Cyclobarbitone	T42.3X1	T42.3X2	T42.3X3	T42.3X4	T42.3X5	T42.3X6
Cyclobenzaprine	T48.1X1	T48.1X2	T48.1X3	T48.1X4	T48.1X5	T48.1X6
Cyclodrine	T44.3X1	T44.3X2	T44.3X3	T44.3X4	T44.3X5	T44.3X6
Cycloguanil embonate	T37.2X1	T37.2X2	T37.2X3	T37.2X4	T37.2X5	T37.2X6
Cyclohexane	T52.8X1	T52.8X2	T52.8X3	T52.8X4	—	—
Cyclohexanol	T51.8X1	T51.8X2	T51.8X3	T51.8X4	—	—
Cyclohexanone	T52.4X1	T52.4X2	T52.4X3	T52.4X4	—	—
Cycloheximide	T60.3X1	T60.3X2	T60.3X3	T60.3X4	—	—
Cyclohexyl acetate	T52.8X1	T52.8X2	T52.8X3	T52.8X4	—	—
Cycloleucin	T45.1X1	T45.1X2	T45.1X3	T45.1X4	T45.1X5	T45.1X6
Cyclomethycaine	T41.3X1	T41.3X2	T41.3X3	T41.3X4	T41.3X5	T41.3X6
Cyclopentamine	T44.4X1	T44.4X2	T44.4X3	T44.4X4	T44.4X5	T44.4X6
Cyclopenthiazide	T50.2X1	T50.2X2	T50.2X3	T50.2X4	T50.2X5	T50.2X6
Cyclopentolate	T44.3X1	T44.3X2	T44.3X3	T44.3X4	T44.3X5	T44.3X6
Cyclophosphamide	T45.1X1	T45.1X2	T45.1X3	T45.1X4	T45.1X5	T45.1X6
Cycloplegic drug	T49.5X1	T49.5X2	T49.5X3	T49.5X4	T49.5X5	T49.5X6
Cyclopropane	T41.291	T41.292	T41.293	T41.294	T41.295	T41.296
Cyclopyrabital	T39.8X1	T39.8X2	T39.8X3	T39.8X4	T39.8X5	T39.8X6
Cycloserine	T37.1X1	T37.1X2	T37.1X3	T37.1X4	T37.1X5	T37.1X6
Cyclosporin	T45.1X1	T45.1X2	T45.1X3	T45.1X4	T45.1X5	T45.1X6
Cyclothiazide	T50.2X1	T50.2X2	T50.2X3	T50.2X4	T50.2X5	T50.2X6
Cycrimine	T44.3X1	T44.3X2	T44.3X3	T44.3X4	T44.3X5	T44.3X6
Cyhalothrin	T60.1X1	T60.1X2	T60.1X3	T60.1X4	—	—
Cymarin	T46.0X1	T46.0X2	T46.0X3	T46.0X4	T46.0X5	T46.0X6
Cymbalta*	T43.221	T43.222	T43.223	T43.224	T43.225	T43.226
Cypermethrin	T60.1X1	T60.1X2	T60.1X3	T60.1X4	—	—
Cyphenothrin	T60.2X1	T60.2X2	T60.2X3	T60.2X4	—	—
Cyproheptadine	T45.0X1	T45.0X2	T45.0X3	T45.0X4	T45.0X5	T45.0X6
Cyproterone	T38.6X1	T38.6X2	T38.6X3	T38.6X4	T38.6X5	T38.6X6
Cystaran*	T49.5X1	T49.5X2	T49.5X3	T49.5X4	T49.5X5	T49.5X6
Cysteamine	T50.6X1	T50.6X2	T50.6X3	T50.6X4	T50.6X5	T50.6X6
Cytarabine	T45.1X1	T45.1X2	T45.1X3	T45.1X4	T45.1X5	T45.1X6
Cytisus						
laburnum	T62.2X1	T62.2X2	T62.2X3	T62.2X4	—	—
scoparius	T62.2X1	T62.2X2	T62.2X3	T62.2X4	—	—
Cytochrome C	T47.5X1	T47.5X2	T47.5X3	T47.5X4	T47.5X5	T47.5X6
Cytomel	T38.1X1	T38.1X2	T38.1X3	T38.1X4	T38.1X5	T38.1X6
Cytosine arabinoside	T45.1X1	T45.1X2	T45.1X3	T45.1X4	T45.1X5	T45.1X6
Cytoxan	T45.1X1	T45.1X2	T45.1X3	T45.1X4	T45.1X5	T45.1X6
Cytozyme	T45.7X1	T45.7X2	T45.7X3	T45.7X4	T45.7X5	T45.7X6
D-Con	T60.91	T60.92	T60.93	T60.94	—	—
insecticide	T60.2X1	T60.2X2	T60.2X3	T60.2X4	—	—
rodenticide	T60.4X1	T60.4X2	T60.4X3	T60.4X4	—	—
D-lysergic acid diethylamide	T40.8X1	T40.8X2	T40.8X3	T40.8X4	—	—
Dabigatran*	T45.511	T45.512	T45.513	T45.514	T45.515	T45.516
Dacarbazine	T45.1X1	T45.1X2	T45.1X3	T45.1X4	T45.1X5	T45.1X6
Dactinomycin	T45.1X1	T45.1X2	T45.1X3	T45.1X4	T45.1X5	T45.1X6
DADPS	T37.1X1	T37.1X2	T37.1X3	T37.1X4	T37.1X5	T37.1X6
Dakin's solution	T49.0X1	T49.0X2	T49.0X3	T49.0X4	T49.0X5	T49.0X6
Dalapon (sodium)	T60.3X1	T60.3X2	T60.3X3	T60.3X4	—	—
Dalmane	T42.4X1	T42.4X2	T42.4X3	T42.4X4	T42.4X5	T42.4X6
Danazol	T38.6X1	T38.6X2	T38.6X3	T38.6X4	T38.6X5	T38.6X6
Danilone	T45.511	T45.512	T45.513	T45.514	T45.515	T45.516
Danthron	T47.2X1	T47.2X2	T47.2X3	T47.2X4	T47.2X5	T47.2X6
Dantrolene	T42.8X1	T42.8X2	T42.8X3	T42.8X4	T42.8X5	T42.8X6
Dantron	T47.2X1	T47.2X2	T47.2X3	T47.2X4	T47.2X5	T47.2X6
Daphne (gnidium) (mezereum)	T62.2X1	T62.2X2	T62.2X3	T62.2X4	—	—
berry	T62.1X1	T62.1X2	T62.1X3	T62.1X4	—	—
Dapsone	T37.1X1	T37.1X2	T37.1X3	T37.1X4	T37.1X5	T37.1X6
Daraprim	T37.2X1	T37.2X2	T37.2X3	T37.2X4	T37.2X5	T37.2X6
Darnel	T62.2X1	T62.2X2	T62.2X3	T62.2X4	—	—
Darvon	T39.8X1	T39.8X2	T39.8X3	T39.8X4	T39.8X5	T39.8X6
Daunomycin	T45.1X1	T45.1X2	T45.1X3	T45.1X4	T45.1X5	T45.1X6
Daunorubicin	T45.1X1	T45.1X2	T45.1X3	T45.1X4	T45.1X5	T45.1X6
DBI	T38.3X1	T38.3X2	T38.3X3	T38.3X4	T38.3X5	T38.3X6
DDAVP	T38.891	T38.892	T38.893	T38.894	T38.895	T38.896
DDE (bis(chlorophenyl)-dichloroethylene)	T60.2X1	T60.2X2	T60.2X3	T60.2X4	—	—
DDS	T37.1X1	T37.1X2	T37.1X3	T37.1X4	T37.1X5	T37.1X6
DDT (dust)	T60.1X1	T60.1X2	T60.1X3	T60.1X4	—	—
Deadly nightshade — see also Belladonna	T62.2X1	T62.2X2	T62.2X3	T62.2X4	—	—
berry	T62.1X1	T62.1X2	T62.1X3	T62.1X4	—	—
Deamino-D-arginine vasopressin	T38.891	T38.892	T38.893	T38.894	T38.895	T38.896
Deanol (aceglumate)	T50.991	T50.992	T50.993	T50.994	T50.995	T50.996
Debrisoquine	T46.5X1	T46.5X2	T46.5X3	T46.5X4	T46.5X5	T46.5X6
Decaborane	T57.8X1	T57.8X2	T57.8X3	T57.8X4	—	—
fumes	T59.891	T59.892	T59.893	T59.894	—	—
Decadron	T38.0X1	T38.0X2	T38.0X3	T38.0X4	T38.0X5	T38.0X6
ENT agent	T49.6X1	T49.6X2	T49.6X3	T49.6X4	T49.6X5	T49.6X6
ophthalmic preparation	T49.5X1	T49.5X2	T49.5X3	T49.5X4	T49.5X5	T49.5X6
topical NEC	T49.0X1	T49.0X2	T49.0X3	T49.0X4	T49.0X5	T49.0X6
Decahydronaphthalene	T52.8X1	T52.8X2	T52.8X3	T52.8X4	—	—
Decalin	T52.8X1	T52.8X2	T52.8X3	T52.8X4	—	—
Decamethonium (bromide)	T48.1X1	T48.1X2	T48.1X3	T48.1X4	T48.1X5	T48.1X6
Decholin	T47.5X1	T47.5X2	T47.5X3	T47.5X4	T47.5X5	T47.5X6
Declomycin	T36.4X1	T36.4X2	T36.4X3	T36.4X4	T36.4X5	T36.4X6
Decongestant, nasal (mucosa)	T48.5X1	T48.5X2	T48.5X3	T48.5X4	T48.5X5	T48.5X6
combination	T48.5X1	T48.5X2	T48.5X3	T48.5X4	T48.5X5	T48.5X6
Deet	T60.8X1	T60.8X2	T60.8X3	T60.8X4	—	—
Deferoxamine	T45.8X1	T45.8X2	T45.8X3	T45.8X4	T45.8X5	T45.8X6
Deflazacort	T38.0X1	T38.0X2	T38.0X3	T38.0X4	T38.0X5	T38.0X6
Deglycyrrhizinized extract of licorice	T48.4X1	T48.4X2	T48.4X3	T48.4X4	T48.4X5	T48.4X6
Dehydrocholic acid	T47.5X1	T47.5X2	T47.5X3	T47.5X4	T47.5X5	T47.5X6
Dehydroemetine	T37.3X1	T37.3X2	T37.3X3	T37.3X4	T37.3X5	T37.3X6
Dekalin	T52.8X1	T52.8X2	T52.8X3	T52.8X4	—	—
Delafloxacin*	T36.8X1	T36.8X2	T36.8X3	T36.8X4	T36.8X5	T36.8X6
Delalutin	T38.5X1	T38.5X2	T38.5X3	T38.5X4	T38.5X5	T38.5X6
Delorazepam	T42.4X1	T42.4X2	T42.4X3	T42.4X4	T42.4X5	T42.4X6
Delphinium	T62.2X1	T62.2X2	T62.2X3	T62.2X4	—	—
Deltacortisone*	T38.0X1	T38.0X2	T38.0X3	T38.0X4	T38.0X5	T38.0X6
Deltamethrin	T60.1X1	T60.1X2	T60.1X3	T60.1X4	—	—
Deltasone	T38.0X1	T38.0X2	T38.0X3	T38.0X4	T38.0X5	T38.0X6
Deltra	T38.0X1	T38.0X2	T38.0X3	T38.0X4	T38.0X5	T38.0X6
Delvinal	T42.3X1	T42.3X2	T42.3X3	T42.3X4	T42.3X5	T42.3X6
Demecarium (bromide)	T49.5X1	T49.5X2	T49.5X3	T49.5X4	T49.5X5	T49.5X6
Demeclocycline	T36.4X1	T36.4X2	T36.4X3	T36.4X4	T36.4X5	T36.4X6
Demecolcine	T45.1X1	T45.1X2	T45.1X3	T45.1X4	T45.1X5	T45.1X6
Demegestone	T38.5X1	T38.5X2	T38.5X3	T38.5X4	T38.5X5	T38.5X6
Demelanizing agents	T49.8X1	T49.8X2	T49.8X3	T49.8X4	T49.8X5	T49.8X6
Demephion -O and -S	T60.0X1	T60.0X2	T60.0X3	T60.0X4	—	—
Demerol	T40.2X1	T40.2X2	T40.2X3	T40.2X4	T40.2X5	T40.2X6
Demethylchlortetracycline	T36.4X1	T36.4X2	T36.4X3	T36.4X4	T36.4X5	T36.4X6
Demethyltetracycline	T36.4X1	T36.4X2	T36.4X3	T36.4X4	T36.4X5	T36.4X6
Demeton -O and -S	T60.0X1	T60.0X2	T60.0X3	T60.0X4	—	—
Demulcent (external)	T49.3X1	T49.3X2	T49.3X3	T49.3X4	T49.3X5	T49.3X6
specified NEC	T49.3X1	T49.3X2	T49.3X3	T49.3X4	T49.3X5	T49.3X6
Demulen	T38.4X1	T38.4X2	T38.4X3	T38.4X4	T38.4X5	T38.4X6
Denatured alcohol	T51.0X1	T51.0X2	T51.0X3	T51.0X4	—	—
Dendrid	T49.5X1	T49.5X2	T49.5X3	T49.5X4	T49.5X5	T49.5X6
Dental drug, topical application NEC	T49.7X1	T49.7X2	T49.7X3	T49.7X4	T49.7X5	T49.7X6
Dentifrice	T49.7X1	T49.7X2	T49.7X3	T49.7X4	T49.7X5	T49.7X6
Deodorant spray (feminine hygiene)	T49.8X1	T49.8X2	T49.8X3	T49.8X4	T49.8X5	T49.8X6
Deoxycortone	T50.0X1	T50.0X2	T50.0X3	T50.0X4	T50.0X5	T50.0X6
Deoxyribonuclease (pancreatic)	T45.3X1	T45.3X2	T45.3X3	T45.3X4	T45.3X5	T45.3X6
Depilatory	T49.4X1	T49.4X2	T49.4X3	T49.4X4	T49.4X5	T49.4X6
Deprenalin	T42.8X1	T42.8X2	T42.8X3	T42.8X4	T42.8X5	T42.8X6
Deprenyl	T42.8X1	T42.8X2	T42.8X3	T42.8X4	T42.8X5	T42.8X6
Depressant						
appetite (central)	T50.5X1	T50.5X2	T50.5X3	T50.5X4	T50.5X5	T50.5X6
cardiac	T46.2X1	T46.2X2	T46.2X3	T46.2X4	T46.2X5	T46.2X6

*Optum Value-Add

Substance	Poisoning, Accidental (unintentional)	Poisoning, Intentional Self-harm	Poisoning, Assault	Poisoning, Undetermined	Adverse Effect	Under-dosing
Depressant — *continued*						
central nervous system (anesthetic) — *see also* Central nervous system, depressants	T42.71	T42.72	T42.73	T42.74	T42.75	T42.76
general anesthetic	T41.2Ø1	T41.2Ø2	T41.2Ø3	T41.2Ø4	T41.2Ø5	T41.2Ø6
muscle tone	T42.8X1	T42.8X2	T42.8X3	T42.8X4	T42.8X5	T42.8X6
muscle tone, central	T42.8X1	T42.8X2	T42.8X3	T42.8X4	T42.8X5	T42.8X6
psychotherapeutic	T43.5Ø1	T43.5Ø2	T43.5Ø3	T43.5Ø4	T43.5Ø5	T43.5Ø6
Depressant, appetite	T5Ø.5X1	T5Ø.5X2	T5Ø.5X3	T5Ø.5X4	T5Ø.5X5	T5Ø.5X6
Deptropine	T45.ØX1	T45.ØX2	T45.ØX3	T45.ØX4	T45.ØX5	T45.ØX6
Dequalinium (chloride)	T49.ØX1	T49.ØX2	T49.ØX3	T49.ØX4	T49.ØX5	T49.ØX6
Derris root	T6Ø.2X1	T6Ø.2X2	T6Ø.2X3	T6Ø.2X4	—	—
Deserpidine	T46.5X1	T46.5X2	T46.5X3	T46.5X4	T46.5X5	T46.5X6
Desferrioxamine	T45.8X1	T45.8X2	T45.8X3	T45.8X4	T45.8X5	T45.8X6
Desipramine	T43.Ø11	T43.Ø12	T43.Ø13	T43.Ø14	T43.Ø15	T43.Ø16
Deslanoside	T46.ØX1	T46.ØX2	T46.ØX3	T46.ØX4	T46.ØX5	T46.ØX6
Desloughing agent	T49.4X1	T49.4X2	T49.4X3	T49.4X4	T49.4X5	T49.4X6
Desmethylimipramine	T43.Ø11	T43.Ø12	T43.Ø13	T43.Ø14	T43.Ø15	T43.Ø16
Desmopressin	T38.891	T38.892	T38.893	T38.894	T38.895	T38.896
Desocodeine	T4Ø.2X1	T4Ø.2X2	T4Ø.2X3	T4Ø.2X4	T4Ø.2X5	T4Ø.2X6
Desogestrel	T38.5X1	T38.5X2	T38.5X3	T38.5X4	T38.5X5	T38.5X6
Desomorphine	T4Ø.2X1	T4Ø.2X2	T4Ø.2X3	T4Ø.2X4	—	—
Desonide	T49.ØX1	T49.ØX2	T49.ØX3	T49.ØX4	T49.ØX5	T49.ØX6
Desoximetasone	T49.ØX1	T49.ØX2	T49.ØX3	T49.ØX4	T49.ØX5	T49.ØX6
Desoxycorticosteroid	T5Ø.ØX1	T5Ø.ØX2	T5Ø.ØX3	T5Ø.ØX4	T5Ø.ØX5	T5Ø.ØX6
Desoxycortone	T5Ø.ØX1	T5Ø.ØX2	T5Ø.ØX3	T5Ø.ØX4	T5Ø.ØX5	T5Ø.ØX6
Desoxyephedrine	T43.651	T43.652	T43.653	T43.654	T43.655	T43.656
Dessicated thyroid*	T38.1X1	T38.1X2	T38.1X3	T38.1X4	T38.1X5	T38.1X6
Detaxtran	T46.6X1	T46.6X2	T46.6X3	T46.6X4	T46.6X5	T46.6X6
Detergent	T49.2X1	T49.2X2	T49.2X3	T49.2X4	T49.2X5	T49.2X6
external medication	T49.2X1	T49.2X2	T49.2X3	T49.2X4	T49.2X5	T49.2X6
local	T49.2X1	T49.2X2	T49.2X3	T49.2X4	T49.2X5	T49.2X6
medicinal	T49.2X1	T49.2X2	T49.2X3	T49.2X4	T49.2X5	T49.2X6
nonmedicinal	T55.1X1	T55.1X2	T55.1X3	T55.1X4	—	—
specified NEC	T55.1X1	T55.1X2	T55.1X3	T55.1X4	—	—
Deterrent, alcohol	T5Ø.6X1	T5Ø.6X2	T5Ø.6X3	T5Ø.6X4	T5Ø.6X5	T5Ø.6X6
Detoxifying agent	T5Ø.6X1	T5Ø.6X2	T5Ø.6X3	T5Ø.6X4	T5Ø.6X5	T5Ø.6X6
Detrothyronine	T38.1X1	T38.1X2	T38.1X3	T38.1X4	T38.1X5	T38.1X6
Dettol (external medication)	T49.ØX1	T49.ØX2	T49.ØX3	T49.ØX4	T49.ØX5	T49.ØX6
Dexamethasone	T38.ØX1	T38.ØX2	T38.ØX3	T38.ØX4	T38.ØX5	T38.ØX6
ENT agent	T49.6X1	T49.6X2	T49.6X3	T49.6X4	T49.6X5	T49.6X6
ophthalmic preparation	T49.5X1	T49.5X2	T49.5X3	T49.5X4	T49.5X5	T49.5X6
topical NEC	T49.ØX1	T49.ØX2	T49.ØX3	T49.ØX4	T49.ØX5	T49.ØX6
Dexamfetamine	T43.621	T43.622	T43.623	T43.624	T43.625	T43.626
Dexamphetamine	T43.621	T43.622	T43.623	T43.624	T43.625	T43.626
Dexbrompheniramine	T45.ØX1	T45.ØX2	T45.ØX3	T45.ØX4	T45.ØX5	T45.ØX6
Dexchlorpheniramine	T45.ØX1	T45.ØX2	T45.ØX3	T45.ØX4	T45.ØX5	T45.ØX6
Dexedrine	T43.621	T43.622	T43.623	T43.624	T43.625	T43.626
Dexetimide	T44.3X1	T44.3X2	T44.3X3	T44.3X4	T44.3X5	T44.3X6
Dexfenfluramine	T5Ø.5X1	T5Ø.5X2	T5Ø.5X3	T5Ø.5X4	T5Ø.5X5	T5Ø.5X6
Dexpanthenol	T45.2X1	T45.2X2	T45.2X3	T45.2X4	T45.2X5	T45.2X6
Dextran (40) (70) (150)	T45.8X1	T45.8X2	T45.8X3	T45.8X4	T45.8X5	T45.8X6
Dextriferron	T45.4X1	T45.4X2	T45.4X3	T45.4X4	T45.4X5	T45.4X6
Dextro calcium pantothenate	T45.2X1	T45.2X2	T45.2X3	T45.2X4	T45.2X5	T45.2X6
Dextro pantothenyl alcohol	T45.2X1	T45.2X2	T45.2X3	T45.2X4	T45.2X5	T45.2X6
Dextroamphetamine	T43.621	T43.622	T43.623	T43.624	T43.625	T43.626
Dextromethorphan	T48.3X1	T48.3X2	T48.3X3	T48.3X4	T48.3X5	T48.3X6
Dextromoramide	T4Ø.491	T4Ø.492	T4Ø.493	T4Ø.494	—	—
topical	T49.8X1	T49.8X2	T49.8X3	T49.8X4	T49.8X5	T49.8X6
Dextropropoxyphene	T4Ø.491	T4Ø.492	T4Ø.493	T4Ø.494	T4Ø.495	T4Ø.496
Dextrorphan	T4Ø.2X1	T4Ø.2X2	T4Ø.2X3	T4Ø.2X4	T4Ø.2X5	T4Ø.2X6
Dextrose	T5Ø.3X1	T5Ø.3X2	T5Ø.3X3	T5Ø.3X4	T5Ø.3X5	T5Ø.3X6
concentrated solution, intravenous	T46.8X1	T46.8X2	T46.8X3	T46.8X4	T46.8X5	T46.8X6
Dextrothyroxin	T38.1X1	T38.1X2	T38.1X3	T38.1X4	T38.1X5	T38.1X6
Dextrothyroxine sodium	T38.1X1	T38.1X2	T38.1X3	T38.1X4	T38.1X5	T38.1X6
DFP	T44.ØX1	T44.ØX2	T44.ØX3	T44.ØX4	T44.ØX5	T44.ØX6
DHE	T37.3X1	T37.3X2	T37.3X3	T37.3X4	T37.3X5	T37.3X6
45	T46.5X1	T46.5X2	T46.5X3	T46.5X4	T46.5X5	T46.5X6
DiaBeta*	T38.3X1	T38.3X2	T38.3X3	T38.3X4	T38.3X5	T38.3X6
Diabinese	T38.3X1	T38.3X2	T38.3X3	T38.3X4	T38.3X5	T38.3X6
Diacetone alcohol	T52.4X1	T52.4X2	T52.4X3	T52.4X4	—	—
Diacetyl monoxime	T5Ø.991	T5Ø.992	T5Ø.993	T5Ø.994	—	—
Diacetylmorphine	T4Ø.1X1	T4Ø.1X2	T4Ø.1X3	T4Ø.1X4	—	—
Diachylon plaster	T49.4X1	T49.4X2	T49.4X3	T49.4X4	T49.4X5	T49.4X6
Diaethylstilboestrolum	T38.5X1	T38.5X2	T38.5X3	T38.5X4	T38.5X5	T38.5X6
Diagnostic agent NEC	T5Ø.8X1	T5Ø.8X2	T5Ø.8X3	T5Ø.8X4	T5Ø.8X5	T5Ø.8X6
Dial (soap)	T49.2X1	T49.2X2	T49.2X3	T49.2X4	T49.2X5	T49.2X6
sedative	T42.3X1	T42.3X2	T42.3X3	T42.3X4	T42.3X5	T42.3X6
Dialkyl carbonate	T52.91	T52.92	T52.93	T52.94	—	—

Substance	Poisoning, Accidental (unintentional)	Poisoning, Intentional Self-harm	Poisoning, Assault	Poisoning, Undetermined	Adverse Effect	Under-dosing
Diallylbarbituric acid	T42.3X1	T42.3X2	T42.3X3	T42.3X4	T42.3X5	T42.3X6
Diallymal	T42.3X1	T42.3X2	T42.3X3	T42.3X4	T42.3X5	T42.3X6
Dialysis solution (intraperitoneal)	T5Ø.3X1	T5Ø.3X2	T5Ø.3X3	T5Ø.3X4	T5Ø.3X5	T5Ø.3X6
Diaminodiphenylsulfone	T37.1X1	T37.1X2	T37.1X3	T37.1X4	T37.1X5	T37.1X6
Diamorphine	T4Ø.1X1	T4Ø.1X2	T4Ø.1X3	T4Ø.1X4	—	—
Diamox	T5Ø.2X1	T5Ø.2X2	T5Ø.2X3	T5Ø.2X4	T5Ø.2X5	T5Ø.2X6
Diamthazole	T49.ØX1	T49.ØX2	T49.ØX3	T49.ØX4	T49.ØX5	T49.ØX6
Dianthone	T47.2X1	T47.2X2	T47.2X3	T47.2X4	T47.2X5	T47.2X6
Diaphenylsulfone	T37.ØX1	T37.ØX2	T37.ØX3	T37.ØX4	T37.ØX5	T37.ØX6
Diasone (sodium)	T37.1X1	T37.1X2	T37.1X3	T37.1X4	T37.1X5	T37.1X6
Diastase	T47.5X1	T47.5X2	T47.5X3	T47.5X4	T47.5X5	T47.5X6
Diastat*	T42.4X1	T42.4X2	T42.4X3	T42.4X4	T42.4X5	T42.4X6
Diatrizoate	T5Ø.8X1	T5Ø.8X2	T5Ø.8X3	T5Ø.8X4	T5Ø.8X5	T5Ø.8X6
Diazepam	T42.4X1	T42.4X2	T42.4X3	T42.4X4	T42.4X5	T42.4X6
Diazinon	T6Ø.ØX1	T6Ø.ØX2	T6Ø.ØX3	T6Ø.ØX4	—	—
Diazomethane (gas)	T59.891	T59.892	T59.893	T59.894	—	—
Diazoxide	T46.5X1	T46.5X2	T46.5X3	T46.5X4	T46.5X5	T46.5X6
Dibekacin	T36.5X1	T36.5X2	T36.5X3	T36.5X4	T36.5X5	T36.5X6
Dibenamine	T44.6X1	T44.6X2	T44.6X3	T44.6X4	T44.6X5	T44.6X6
Dibenzepin	T43.Ø11	T43.Ø12	T43.Ø13	T43.Ø14	T43.Ø15	T43.Ø16
Dibenzheptropine	T45.ØX1	T45.ØX2	T45.ØX3	T45.ØX4	T45.ØX5	T45.ØX6
Dibenzyline	T44.6X1	T44.6X2	T44.6X3	T44.6X4	T44.6X5	T44.6X6
Diborane (gas)	T59.891	T59.892	T59.893	T59.894	—	—
Dibromochloropropane	T6Ø.8X1	T6Ø.8X2	T6Ø.8X3	T6Ø.8X4	—	—
Dibromodulcitol	T45.1X1	T45.1X2	T45.1X3	T45.1X4	T45.1X5	T45.1X6
Dibromoethane	T53.6X1	T53.6X2	T53.6X3	T53.6X4	—	—
Dibromomannitol	T45.1X1	T45.1X2	T45.1X3	T45.1X4	T45.1X5	T45.1X6
Dibromopropamidine isethionate	T49.ØX1	T49.ØX2	T49.ØX3	T49.ØX4	T49.ØX5	T49.ØX6
Dibrompropamidine	T49.ØX1	T49.ØX2	T49.ØX3	T49.ØX4	T49.ØX5	T49.ØX6
Dibucaine	T41.3X1	T41.3X2	T41.3X3	T41.3X4	T41.3X5	T41.3X6
topical (surface)	T41.3X1	T41.3X2	T41.3X3	T41.3X4	T41.3X5	T41.3X6
Dibunate sodium	T48.3X1	T48.3X2	T48.3X3	T48.3X4	T48.3X5	T48.3X6
Dibutoline sulfate	T44.3X1	T44.3X2	T44.3X3	T44.3X4	T44.3X5	T44.3X6
Dicamba	T6Ø.3X1	T6Ø.3X2	T6Ø.3X3	T6Ø.3X4	—	—
Dicapthon	T6Ø.ØX1	T6Ø.ØX2	T6Ø.ØX3	T6Ø.ØX4	—	—
Dichlobenil	T6Ø.3X1	T6Ø.3X2	T6Ø.3X3	T6Ø.3X4	—	—
Dichlone	T6Ø.3X1	T6Ø.3X2	T6Ø.3X3	T6Ø.3X4	—	—
Dichloralphenozone	T42.6X1	T42.6X2	T42.6X3	T42.6X4	T42.6X5	T42.6X6
Dichlorbenzidine	T65.3X1	T65.3X2	T65.3X3	T65.3X4	—	—
Dichlorhydrin	T52.8X1	T52.8X2	T52.8X3	T52.8X4	—	—
Dichlorhydroxyquinoline	T37.8X1	T37.8X2	T37.8X3	T37.8X4	T37.8X5	T37.8X6
Dichlorobenzene	T53.7X1	T53.7X2	T53.7X3	T53.7X4	—	—
Dichlorobenzyl alcohol	T49.6X1	T49.6X2	T49.6X3	T49.6X4	T49.6X5	T49.6X6
Dichlorodifluoromethane	T53.5X1	T53.5X2	T53.5X3	T53.5X4	—	—
Dichloroethane	T52.8X1	T52.8X2	T52.8X3	T52.8X4	—	—
Dichloroethyl sulfide, not in war	T59.891	T59.892	T59.893	T59.894	—	—
Dichloroethylene	T53.6X1	T53.6X2	T53.6X3	T53.6X4	—	—
Dichloroformoxine, not in war	T59.891	T59.892	T59.893	T59.894	—	—
Dichlorohydrin, alpha-dichlorohydrin	T52.8X1	T52.8X2	T52.8X3	T52.8X4	—	—
Dichloromethane (solvent)	T53.4X1	T53.4X2	T53.4X3	T53.4X4	—	—
vapor	T53.4X1	T53.4X2	T53.4X3	T53.4X4	—	—
Dichloronaphthoquinone	T6Ø.3X1	T6Ø.3X2	T6Ø.3X3	T6Ø.3X4	—	—
Dichlorophen	T37.4X1	T37.4X2	T37.4X3	T37.4X4	T37.4X5	T37.4X6
Dichloropropene	T6Ø.3X1	T6Ø.3X2	T6Ø.3X3	T6Ø.3X4	—	—
Dichloropropionic acid	T6Ø.3X1	T6Ø.3X2	T6Ø.3X3	T6Ø.3X4	—	—
Dichlorphenamide	T5Ø.2X1	T5Ø.2X2	T5Ø.2X3	T5Ø.2X4	T5Ø.2X5	T5Ø.2X6
Dichlorvos	T6Ø.ØX1	T6Ø.ØX2	T6Ø.ØX3	T6Ø.ØX4	—	—
Dichysterol*	T45.2X1	T45.2X2	T45.2X3	T45.2X4	T45.2X5	T45.2X6
Diclofenac	T39.391	T39.392	T39.393	T39.394	T39.395	T39.396
Diclofenamide	T5Ø.2X1	T5Ø.2X2	T5Ø.2X3	T5Ø.2X4	T5Ø.2X5	T5Ø.2X6
Diclofensine	T43.291	T43.292	T43.293	T43.294	T43.295	T43.296
Diclonixine	T39.8X1	T39.8X2	T39.8X3	T39.8X4	T39.8X5	T39.8X6
Dicloxacillin	T36.ØX1	T36.ØX2	T36.ØX3	T36.ØX4	T36.ØX5	T36.ØX6
Dicophane	T49.ØX1	T49.ØX2	T49.ØX3	T49.ØX4	T49.ØX5	T49.ØX6
Dicoumarol, dicoumarin, dicumarol	T45.511	T45.512	T45.513	T45.514	T45.515	T45.516
Dicrotophos	T6Ø.ØX1	T6Ø.ØX2	T6Ø.ØX3	T6Ø.ØX4	—	—
Dicyanogen (gas)	T65.ØX1	T65.ØX2	T65.ØX3	T65.ØX4	—	—
Dicyclomine	T44.3X1	T44.3X2	T44.3X3	T44.3X4	T44.3X5	T44.3X6
Dicycloverine	T44.3X1	T44.3X2	T44.3X3	T44.3X4	T44.3X5	T44.3X6
Didanosine*	T37.5X1	T37.5X2	T37.5X3	T37.5X4	T37.5X5	T37.5X6
Dideoxycytidine	T37.5X1	T37.5X2	T37.5X3	T37.5X4	T37.5X5	T37.5X6
Dideoxyinosine	T37.5X1	T37.5X2	T37.5X3	T37.5X4	T37.5X5	T37.5X6
Dieldrin (vapor)	T6Ø.1X1	T6Ø.1X2	T6Ø.1X3	T6Ø.1X4	—	—
Diemal	T42.3X1	T42.3X2	T42.3X3	T42.3X4	T42.3X5	T42.3X6
Dienestrol	T38.5X1	T38.5X2	T38.5X3	T38.5X4	T38.5X5	T38.5X6
Dienoestrol	T38.5X1	T38.5X2	T38.5X3	T38.5X4	T38.5X5	T38.5X6
Dietetic drug NEC	T5Ø.9Ø1	T5Ø.9Ø2	T5Ø.9Ø3	T5Ø.9Ø4	T5Ø.9Ø5	T5Ø.9Ø6

Substance	Poisoning, Accidental (unintentional)	Poisoning, Intentional Self-harm	Poisoning, Assault	Poisoning, Undetermined	Adverse Effect	Under-dosing
Diethazine	T42.8X1	T42.8X2	T42.8X3	T42.8X4	T42.8X5	T42.8X6
Diethyl						
barbituric acid	T42.3X1	T42.3X2	T42.3X3	T42.3X4	T42.3X5	T42.3X6
carbamazine	T37.4X1	T37.4X2	T37.4X3	T37.4X4	T37.4X5	T37.4X6
carbinol	T51.3X1	T51.3X2	T51.3X3	T51.3X4	—	—
carbonate	T52.8X1	T52.8X2	T52.8X3	T52.8X4	—	—
ether (vapor) — see also ether	T41.0X1	T41.0X2	T41.0X3	T41.0X4	T41.0X5	T41.0X6
oxide	T52.8X1	T52.8X2	T52.8X3	T52.8X4	—	—
propion	T50.5X1	T50.5X2	T50.5X3	T50.5X4	T50.5X5	T50.5X6
stilbestrol	T38.5X1	T38.5X2	T38.5X3	T38.5X4	T38.5X5	T38.5X6
toluamide (nonmedicinal)	T60.8X1	T60.8X2	T60.8X3	T60.8X4	—	—
medicinal	T49.3X1	T49.3X2	T49.3X3	T49.3X4	T49.3X5	T49.3X6
Diethylcarbamazine	T37.4X1	T37.4X2	T37.4X3	T37.4X4	T37.4X5	T37.4X6
Diethylene						
dioxide	T52.8X1	T52.8X2	T52.8X3	T52.8X4	—	—
glycol (monoacetate) (monobutyl ether) (monoethyl ether)	T52.3X1	T52.3X2	T52.3X3	T52.3X4	—	—
Diethylhexylphthalate	T65.891	T65.892	T65.893	T65.894	—	—
Diethylpropion	T50.5X1	T50.5X2	T50.5X3	T50.5X4	T50.5X5	T50.5X6
Diethylstilbestrol	T38.5X1	T38.5X2	T38.5X3	T38.5X4	T38.5X5	T38.5X6
Diethylstilboestrol	T38.5X1	T38.5X2	T38.5X3	T38.5X4	T38.5X5	T38.5X6
Diethylsulfone-diethyl-methane	T42.6X1	T42.6X2	T42.6X3	T42.6X4	T42.6X5	T42.6X6
Diethyltoluamide	T49.0X1	T49.0X2	T49.0X3	T49.0X4	T49.0X5	T49.0X6
Diethyltryptamine (DET)	T40.991	T40.992	T40.993	T40.994	—	—
Difebarbamate	T42.3X1	T42.3X2	T42.3X3	T42.3X4	T42.3X5	T42.3X6
Difencloxazine	T40.2X1	T40.2X2	T40.2X3	T40.2X4	T40.2X5	T40.2X6
Difenidol	T45.0X1	T45.0X2	T45.0X3	T45.0X4	T45.0X5	T45.0X6
Difenoxin	T47.6X1	T47.6X2	T47.6X3	T47.6X4	T47.6X5	T47.6X6
Difetarsone	T37.3X1	T37.3X2	T37.3X3	T37.3X4	T37.3X5	T37.3X6
Diffusin	T45.3X1	T45.3X2	T45.3X3	T45.3X4	T45.3X5	T45.3X6
Diflorasone	T49.0X1	T49.0X2	T49.0X3	T49.0X4	T49.0X5	T49.0X6
Diflos	T44.0X1	T44.0X2	T44.0X3	T44.0X4	T44.0X5	T44.0X6
Diflubenzuron	T60.1X1	T60.1X2	T60.1X3	T60.1X4	—	—
Diflucan*	T37.8X1	T37.8X2	T37.8X3	T37.8X4	T37.8X5	T37.8X6
Diflucortolone	T49.0X1	T49.0X2	T49.0X3	T49.0X4	T49.0X5	T49.0X6
Diflunisal	T39.091	T39.092	T39.093	T39.094	T39.095	T39.096
Difluoromethyldopa	T42.8X1	T42.8X2	T42.8X3	T42.8X4	T42.8X5	T42.8X6
Difluorophate	T44.0X1	T44.0X2	T44.0X3	T44.0X4	T44.0X5	T44.0X6
Digestant NEC	T47.5X1	T47.5X2	T47.5X3	T47.5X4	T47.5X5	T47.5X6
Digitalin (e)	T46.0X1	T46.0X2	T46.0X3	T46.0X4	T46.0X5	T46.0X6
Digitalis (leaf)(glycoside)	T46.0X1	T46.0X2	T46.0X3	T46.0X4	T46.0X5	T46.0X6
lanata	T46.0X1	T46.0X2	T46.0X3	T46.0X4	T46.0X5	T46.0X6
purpurea	T46.0X1	T46.0X2	T46.0X3	T46.0X4	T46.0X5	T46.0X6
Digitoxin	T46.0X1	T46.0X2	T46.0X3	T46.0X4	T46.0X5	T46.0X6
Digitoxose	T46.0X1	T46.0X2	T46.0X3	T46.0X4	T46.0X5	T46.0X6
Digoxin	T46.0X1	T46.0X2	T46.0X3	T46.0X4	T46.0X5	T46.0X6
Digoxine	T46.0X1	T46.0X2	T46.0X3	T46.0X4	T46.0X5	T46.0X6
Dihydralazine	T46.5X1	T46.5X2	T46.5X3	T46.5X4	T46.5X5	T46.5X6
Dihydrazine	T46.5X1	T46.5X2	T46.5X3	T46.5X4	T46.5X5	T46.5X6
Dihydrocodeine	T40.2X1	T40.2X2	T40.2X3	T40.2X4	T40.2X5	T40.2X6
Dihydrocodeinone	T40.2X1	T40.2X2	T40.2X3	T40.2X4	T40.2X5	T40.2X6
Dihydroergocornine	T46.7X1	T46.7X2	T46.7X3	T46.7X4	T46.7X5	T46.7X6
Dihydroergocristine (mesilate)	T46.7X1	T46.7X2	T46.7X3	T46.7X4	T46.7X5	T46.7X6
Dihydroergokryptine	T46.7X1	T46.7X2	T46.7X3	T46.7X4	T46.7X5	T46.7X6
Dihydroergotamine	T46.5X1	T46.5X2	T46.5X3	T46.5X4	T46.5X5	T46.5X6
Dihydroergotoxine	T46.7X1	T46.7X2	T46.7X3	T46.7X4	T46.7X5	T46.7X6
mesilate	T46.7X1	T46.7X2	T46.7X3	T46.7X4	T46.7X5	T46.7X6
Dihydrohydroxycodeinone	T40.2X1	T40.2X2	T40.2X3	T40.2X4	T40.2X5	T40.2X6
Dihydrohydroxymorphinone	T40.2X1	T40.2X2	T40.2X3	T40.2X4	T40.2X5	T40.2X6
Dihydroisocodeine	T40.2X1	T40.2X2	T40.2X3	T40.2X4	T40.2X5	T40.2X6
Dihydromorphine	T40.2X1	T40.2X2	T40.2X3	T40.2X4	—	T40.2X6
Dihydromorphinone	T40.2X1	T40.2X2	T40.2X3	T40.2X4	T40.2X5	T40.2X6
Dihydrostreptomycin	T36.5X1	T36.5X2	T36.5X3	T36.5X4	T36.5X5	T36.5X6
Dihydrotachysterol	T45.2X1	T45.2X2	T45.2X3	T45.2X4	T45.2X5	T45.2X6
Dihydroxyacetone*	T49.3X1	T49.3X2	T49.3X3	T49.3X4	T49.3X5	T49.3X6
Dihydroxyaluminum aminoacetate	T47.1X1	T47.1X2	T47.1X3	T47.1X4	T47.1X5	T47.1X6
Dihydroxyaluminum sodium carbonate	T47.1X1	T47.1X2	T47.1X3	T47.1X4	T47.1X5	T47.1X6
Dihydroxyanthraquinone	T47.2X1	T47.2X2	T47.2X3	T47.2X4	T47.2X5	T47.2X6
Dihydroxycodeinone	T40.2X1	T40.2X2	T40.2X3	T40.2X4	T40.2X5	T40.2X6
Dihydroxypropyl theophylline	T50.2X1	T50.2X2	T50.2X3	T50.2X4	T50.2X5	T50.2X6
Diiodohydroxyquin	T37.8X1	T37.8X2	T37.8X3	T37.8X4	T37.8X5	T37.8X6
topical	T49.0X1	T49.0X2	T49.0X3	T49.0X4	T49.0X5	T49.0X6
Diiodohydroxyquinoline	T37.8X1	T37.8X2	T37.8X3	T37.8X4	T37.8X5	T37.8X6
Diiodotyrosine	T38.2X1	T38.2X2	T38.2X3	T38.2X4	T38.2X5	T38.2X6
Diisopromine	T44.3X1	T44.3X2	T44.3X3	T44.3X4	T44.3X5	T44.3X6
Diisopropylamine	T46.3X1	T46.3X2	T46.3X3	T46.3X4	T46.3X5	T46.3X6
Diisopropylfluorophosphonate	T44.0X1	T44.0X2	T44.0X3	T44.0X4	T44.0X5	T44.0X6
Dilantin	T42.0X1	T42.0X2	T42.0X3	T42.0X4	T42.0X5	T42.0X6
Dilatrate*	T46.3X1	T46.3X2	T46.3X3	T46.3X4	T46.3X5	T46.3X6
Dilaudid	T40.2X1	T40.2X2	T40.2X3	T40.2X4	T40.2X5	T40.2X6
Dilazep	T46.3X1	T46.3X2	T46.3X3	T46.3X4	T46.3X5	T46.3X6
Dill	T47.5X1	T47.5X2	T47.5X3	T47.5X4	T47.5X5	T47.5X6
Diloxanide	T37.3X1	T37.3X2	T37.3X3	T37.3X4	T37.3X5	T37.3X6
Diltiazem	T46.1X1	T46.1X2	T46.1X3	T46.1X4	T46.1X5	T46.1X6
Dimazole	T49.0X1	T49.0X2	T49.0X3	T49.0X4	T49.0X5	T49.0X6
Dimefline	T50.7X1	T50.7X2	T50.7X3	T50.7X4	T50.7X5	T50.7X6
Dimefox	T60.0X1	T60.0X2	T60.0X3	T60.0X4	—	—
Dimemorfan	T48.3X1	T48.3X2	T48.3X3	T48.3X4	T48.3X5	T48.3X6
Dimenhydrinate	T45.0X1	T45.0X2	T45.0X3	T45.0X4	T45.0X5	T45.0X6
Dimercaprol (British anti-lewisite)	T45.8X1	T45.8X2	T45.8X3	T45.8X4	T45.8X5	T45.8X6
Dimercaptopropanol	T45.8X1	T45.8X2	T45.8X3	T45.8X4	T45.8X5	T45.8X6
Dimestrol	T38.5X1	T38.5X2	T38.5X3	T38.5X4	T38.5X5	T38.5X6
Dimetane	T45.0X1	T45.0X2	T45.0X3	T45.0X4	T45.0X5	T45.0X6
Dimethicone	T47.1X1	T47.1X2	T47.1X3	T47.1X4	T47.1X5	T47.1X6
Dimethindene	T45.0X1	T45.0X2	T45.0X3	T45.0X4	T45.0X5	T45.0X6
Dimethisoquin	T49.1X1	T49.1X2	T49.1X3	T49.1X4	T49.1X5	T49.1X6
Dimethisterone	T38.5X1	T38.5X2	T38.5X3	T38.5X4	T38.5X5	T38.5X6
Dimethoate	T60.0X1	T60.0X2	T60.0X3	T60.0X4	—	—
Dimethocaine	T41.3X1	T41.3X2	T41.3X3	T41.3X4	T41.3X5	T41.3X6
Dimethoxanate	T48.3X1	T48.3X2	T48.3X3	T48.3X4	T48.3X5	T48.3X6
Dimethyl						
arsine, arsinic acid	T57.0X1	T57.0X2	T57.0X3	T57.0X4	—	—
carbinol	T51.2X1	T51.2X2	T51.2X3	T51.2X4	—	—
carbonate	T52.8X1	T52.8X2	T52.8X3	T52.8X4	—	—
diguanide	T38.3X1	T38.3X2	T38.3X3	T38.3X4	T38.3X5	T38.3X6
ketone	T52.4X1	T52.4X2	T52.4X3	T52.4X4	—	—
vapor	T52.4X1	T52.4X2	T52.4X3	T52.4X4	—	—
meperidine	T40.2X1	T40.2X2	T40.2X3	T40.2X4	T40.2X5	T40.2X6
parathion	T60.0X1	T60.0X2	T60.0X3	T60.0X4	—	—
phthlate	T49.3X1	T49.3X2	T49.3X3	T49.3X4	T49.3X5	T49.3X6
polysiloxane	T47.8X1	T47.8X2	T47.8X3	T47.8X4	T47.8X5	T47.8X6
sulfate (fumes)	T59.891	T59.892	T59.893	T59.894	—	—
liquid	T65.891	T65.892	T65.893	T65.894	—	—
sulfoxide (nonmedicinal)	T52.8X1	T52.8X2	T52.8X3	T52.8X4	—	—
medicinal	T49.4X1	T49.4X2	T49.4X3	T49.4X4	T49.4X5	T49.4X6
tryptamine	T40.991	T40.992	T40.993	T40.994	—	—
tubocurarine	T48.1X1	T48.1X2	T48.1X3	T48.1X4	T48.1X5	T48.1X6
Dimethylamine sulfate	T49.4X1	T49.4X2	T49.4X3	T49.4X4	T49.4X5	T49.4X6
Dimethylcysteine*	T50.6X1	T50.6X2	T50.6X3	T50.6X4	T50.6X5	T50.6X6
Dimethylformamide	T52.8X1	T52.8X2	T52.8X3	T52.8X4	—	—
Dimethyltubocurarinium chloride	T48.1X1	T48.1X2	T48.1X3	T48.1X4	T48.1X5	T48.1X6
Dimeticone	T47.1X1	T47.1X2	T47.1X3	T47.1X4	T47.1X5	T47.1X6
Dimetilan	T60.0X1	T60.0X2	T60.0X3	T60.0X4	—	—
Dimetindene	T45.0X1	T45.0X2	T45.0X3	T45.0X4	T45.0X5	T45.0X6
Dimetotiazine	T43.3X1	T43.3X2	T43.3X3	T43.3X4	T43.3X5	T43.3X6
Dimorpholamine	T50.7X1	T50.7X2	T50.7X3	T50.7X4	T50.7X5	T50.7X6
Dimoxyline	T46.3X1	T46.3X2	T46.3X3	T46.3X4	T46.3X5	T46.3X6
Dinitro (-ortho-)cresol (pesticide) (spray)	T65.3X1	T65.3X2	T65.3X3	T65.3X4	—	—
Dinitrobenzene	T65.3X1	T65.3X2	T65.3X3	T65.3X4	—	—
vapor	T59.891	T59.892	T59.893	T59.894	—	—
Dinitrobenzol	T65.3X1	T65.3X2	T65.3X3	T65.3X4	—	—
vapor	T59.891	T59.892	T59.893	T59.894	—	—
Dinitrobutylphenol	T65.3X1	T65.3X2	T65.3X3	T65.3X4	—	—
Dinitrocyclohexylphenol	T65.3X1	T65.3X2	T65.3X3	T65.3X4	—	—
Dinitrophenol	T65.3X1	T65.3X2	T65.3X3	T65.3X4	—	—
Dinoprost	T48.0X1	T48.0X2	T48.0X3	T48.0X4	T48.0X5	T48.0X6
Dinoprostone	T48.0X1	T48.0X2	T48.0X3	T48.0X4	T48.0X5	T48.0X6
Dinoseb	T60.3X1	T60.3X2	T60.3X3	T60.3X4	—	—
Dioctyl sulfosuccinate (calcium) (sodium)	T47.4X1	T47.4X2	T47.4X3	T47.4X4	T47.4X5	T47.4X6
Diodone	T50.8X1	T50.8X2	T50.8X3	T50.8X4	T50.8X5	T50.8X6
Diodoquin	T37.8X1	T37.8X2	T37.8X3	T37.8X4	T37.8X5	T37.8X6
Dionin	T40.2X1	T40.2X2	T40.2X3	T40.2X4	T40.2X5	T40.2X6
Diosmin	T46.991	T46.992	T46.993	T46.994	T46.995	T46.996
Diovan*	T46.5X1	T46.5X2	T46.5X3	T46.5X4	T46.5X5	T46.5X6
Dioxane	T52.8X1	T52.8X2	T52.8X3	T52.8X4	—	—
Dioxathion	T60.0X1	T60.0X2	T60.0X3	T60.0X4	—	—
Dioxin	T53.7X1	T53.7X2	T53.7X3	T53.7X4	—	—
Dioxopromethazine	T43.3X1	T43.3X2	T43.3X3	T43.3X4	T43.3X5	T43.3X6
Dioxyline	T46.3X1	T46.3X2	T46.3X3	T46.3X4	T46.3X5	T46.3X6
Dipentene	T52.8X1	T52.8X2	T52.8X3	T52.8X4	—	—
Diperodon	T41.3X1	T41.3X2	T41.3X3	T41.3X4	T41.3X5	T41.3X6
Diphacinone	T60.4X1	T60.4X2	T60.4X3	T60.4X4	—	—
Diphemanil	T44.3X1	T44.3X2	T44.3X3	T44.3X4	T44.3X5	T44.3X6
metilsulfate	T44.3X1	T44.3X2	T44.3X3	T44.3X4	T44.3X5	T44.3X6
Diphenadione	T45.511	T45.512	T45.513	T45.514	T45.515	T45.516

*Optum Value-Add

Substance	Poisoning, Accidental (unintentional)	Poisoning, Intentional Self-harm	Poisoning, Assault	Poisoning, Undetermined	Adverse Effect	Under-dosing
Diphenadione — *continued*						
rodenticide	T6Ø.4X1	T6Ø.4X2	T6Ø.4X3	T6Ø.4X4	—	—
Diphenhydramine	T45.ØX1	T45.ØX2	T45.ØX3	T45.ØX4	T45.ØX5	T45.ØX6
Diphenidol	T45.ØX1	T45.ØX2	T45.ØX3	T45.ØX4	T45.ØX5	T45.ØX6
Diphenoxylate	T47.6X1	T47.6X2	T47.6X3	T47.6X4	T47.6X5	T47.6X6
Diphenylamine	T65.3X1	T65.3X2	T65.3X3	T65.3X4	—	—
Diphenylbutazone	T39.2X1	T39.2X2	T39.2X3	T39.2X4	T39.2X5	T39.2X6
Diphenylchloroarsine, not in war	T57.ØX1	T57.ØX2	T57.ØX3	T57.ØX4	—	—
Diphenylhydantoin	T42.ØX1	T42.ØX2	T42.ØX3	T42.ØX4	T42.ØX5	T42.ØX6
Diphenylmethane dye	T52.1X1	T52.1X2	T52.1X3	T52.1X4	—	—
Diphenylpyraline	T45.ØX1	T45.ØX2	T45.ØX3	T45.ØX4	T45.ØX5	T45.ØX6
Diphtheria						
antitoxin	T5Ø.Z11	T5Ø.Z12	T5Ø.Z13	T5Ø.Z14	T5Ø.Z15	T5Ø.Z16
toxoid	T5Ø.A91	T5Ø.A92	T5Ø.A93	T5Ø.A94	T5Ø.A95	T5Ø.A96
with tetanus toxoid	T5Ø.A21	T5Ø.A22	T5Ø.A23	T5Ø.A24	T5Ø.A25	T5Ø.A26
with pertussis component	T5Ø.A11	T5Ø.A12	T5Ø.A13	T5Ø.A14	T5Ø.A15	T5Ø.A16
vaccine	T5Ø.A91	T5Ø.A92	T5Ø.A93	T5Ø.A94	T5Ø.A95	T5Ø.A96
combination						
including pertussis	T5Ø.A11	T5Ø.A12	T5Ø.A13	T5Ø.A14	T5Ø.A15	T5Ø.A16
without pertussis	T5Ø.A21	T5Ø.A22	T5Ø.A23	T5Ø.A24	T5Ø.A25	T5Ø.A26
Diphylline	T5Ø.2X1	T5Ø.2X2	T5Ø.2X3	T5Ø.2X4	T5Ø.2X5	T5Ø.2X6
Dipipanone	T4Ø.491	T4Ø.492	T4Ø.493	T4Ø.494	—	—
Dipivefrine	T49.5X1	T49.5X2	T49.5X3	T49.5X4	T49.5X5	T49.5X6
Diplovax	T5Ø.B91	T5Ø.B92	T5Ø.B93	T5Ø.B94	T5Ø.B95	T5Ø.B96
Diprophylline	T5Ø.2X1	T5Ø.2X2	T5Ø.2X3	T5Ø.2X4	T5Ø.2X5	T5Ø.2X6
Dipropyline	T48.291	T48.292	T48.293	T48.294	T48.295	T48.296
Dipyridamole	T46.3X1	T46.3X2	T46.3X3	T46.3X4	T46.3X5	T46.3X6
Dipyrone	T39.2X1	T39.2X2	T39.2X3	T39.2X4	T39.2X5	T39.2X6
Diquat (dibromide)	T6Ø.3X1	T6Ø.3X2	T6Ø.3X3	T6Ø.3X4	—	—
Disinfectant	T65.891	T65.892	T65.893	T65.894	—	—
alkaline	T54.3X1	T54.3X2	T54.3X3	T54.3X4	—	—
aromatic	T54.1X1	T54.1X2	T54.1X3	T54.1X4	—	—
intestinal	T37.8X1	T37.8X2	T37.8X3	T37.8X4	T37.8X5	T37.8X6
Disipal	T42.8X1	T42.8X2	T42.8X3	T42.8X4	T42.8X5	T42.8X6
Disodium edetate	T5Ø.6X1	T5Ø.6X2	T5Ø.6X3	T5Ø.6X4	T5Ø.6X5	T5Ø.6X6
Disoprofol	T41.291	T41.292	T41.293	T41.294	T41.295	T41.296
Disopyramide*	T46.2X1	T46.2X2	T46.2X3	T46.2X4	T46.2X5	T46.2X6
Distigmine (bromide)	T44.ØX1	T44.ØX2	T44.ØX3	T44.ØX4	T44.ØX5	T44.ØX6
Disulfamide	T5Ø.2X1	T5Ø.2X2	T5Ø.2X3	T5Ø.2X4	T5Ø.2X5	T5Ø.2X6
Disulfanilamide	T37.ØX1	T37.ØX2	T37.ØX3	T37.ØX4	T37.ØX5	T37.ØX6
Disulfiram	T5Ø.6X1	T5Ø.6X2	T5Ø.6X3	T5Ø.6X4	T5Ø.6X5	T5Ø.6X6
Disulfoton	T6Ø.ØX1	T6Ø.ØX2	T6Ø.ØX3	T6Ø.ØX4	—	—
Dithiazanine iodide	T37.4X1	T37.4X2	T37.4X3	T37.4X4	T37.4X5	T37.4X6
Dithiocarbamate	T6Ø.ØX1	T6Ø.ØX2	T6Ø.ØX3	T6Ø.ØX4	—	—
Dithranol	T49.4X1	T49.4X2	T49.4X3	T49.4X4	T49.4X5	T49.4X6
Diucardin	T5Ø.2X1	T5Ø.2X2	T5Ø.2X3	T5Ø.2X4	T5Ø.2X5	T5Ø.2X6
Diupres	T5Ø.2X1	T5Ø.2X2	T5Ø.2X3	T5Ø.2X4	T5Ø.2X5	T5Ø.2X6
Diuretic NEC	T5Ø.2X1	T5Ø.2X2	T5Ø.2X3	T5Ø.2X4	T5Ø.2X5	T5Ø.2X6
benzothiadiazine	T5Ø.2X1	T5Ø.2X2	T5Ø.2X3	T5Ø.2X4	T5Ø.2X5	T5Ø.2X6
carbonic acid anhydrase inhibitors	T5Ø.2X1	T5Ø.2X2	T5Ø.2X3	T5Ø.2X4	T5Ø.2X5	T5Ø.2X6
furfuryl NEC	T5Ø.2X1	T5Ø.2X2	T5Ø.2X3	T5Ø.2X4	T5Ø.2X5	T5Ø.2X6
loop (high-ceiling)	T5Ø.1X1	T5Ø.1X2	T5Ø.1X3	T5Ø.1X4	T5Ø.1X5	T5Ø.1X6
mercurial NEC	T5Ø.2X1	T5Ø.2X2	T5Ø.2X3	T5Ø.2X4	T5Ø.2X5	T5Ø.2X6
osmotic	T5Ø.2X1	T5Ø.2X2	T5Ø.2X3	T5Ø.2X4	T5Ø.2X5	T5Ø.2X6
purine NEC	T5Ø.2X1	T5Ø.2X2	T5Ø.2X3	T5Ø.2X4	T5Ø.2X5	T5Ø.2X6
saluretic NEC	T5Ø.2X1	T5Ø.2X2	T5Ø.2X3	T5Ø.2X4	T5Ø.2X5	T5Ø.2X6
sulfonamide	T5Ø.2X1	T5Ø.2X2	T5Ø.2X3	T5Ø.2X4	T5Ø.2X5	T5Ø.2X6
thiazide NEC	T5Ø.2X1	T5Ø.2X2	T5Ø.2X3	T5Ø.2X4	T5Ø.2X5	T5Ø.2X6
xanthine	T5Ø.2X1	T5Ø.2X2	T5Ø.2X3	T5Ø.2X4	T5Ø.2X5	T5Ø.2X6
Diurgin	T5Ø.2X1	T5Ø.2X2	T5Ø.2X3	T5Ø.2X4	T5Ø.2X5	T5Ø.2X6
Diuril	T5Ø.2X1	T5Ø.2X2	T5Ø.2X3	T5Ø.2X4	T5Ø.2X5	T5Ø.2X6
Diuron	T6Ø.3X1	T6Ø.3X2	T6Ø.3X3	T6Ø.3X4	—	—
Divalproex	T42.6X1	T42.6X2	T42.6X3	T42.6X4	T42.6X5	T42.6X6
Divinyl ether	T41.ØX1	T41.ØX2	T41.ØX3	T41.ØX4	T41.ØX5	T41.ØX6
Dixanthogen	T49.ØX1	T49.ØX2	T49.ØX3	T49.ØX4	T49.ØX5	T49.ØX6
Dixyrazine	T43.3X1	T43.3X2	T43.3X3	T43.3X4	T43.3X5	T43.3X6
DMCT	T36.4X1	T36.4X2	T36.4X3	T36.4X4	T36.4X5	T36.4X6
DMSO — *see* Dimethyl, sulfoxide						
DNBP	T6Ø.3X1	T6Ø.3X2	T6Ø.3X3	T6Ø.3X4	—	—
DNOC	T65.3X1	T65.3X2	T65.3X3	T65.3X4	—	—
Dobutamine	T44.5X1	T44.5X2	T44.5X3	T44.5X4	T44.5X5	T44.5X6
DOCA	T38.ØX1	T38.ØX2	T38.ØX3	T38.ØX4	T38.ØX5	T38.ØX6
Docusate sodium	T47.4X1	T47.4X2	T47.4X3	T47.4X4	T47.4X5	T47.4X6
Dodicin	T49.ØX1	T49.ØX2	T49.ØX3	T49.ØX4	T49.ØX5	T49.ØX6
Dofamium chloride	T49.ØX1	T49.ØX2	T49.ØX3	T49.ØX4	T49.ØX5	T49.ØX6
Dolophine	T4Ø.3X1	T4Ø.3X2	T4Ø.3X3	T4Ø.3X4	T4Ø.3X5	T4Ø.3X6
Doloxene	T39.8X1	T39.8X2	T39.8X3	T39.8X4	T39.8X5	T39.8X6
Domestic gas (after combustion) — *see* Gas, utility						
prior to combustion	T59.891	T59.892	T59.893	T59.894	—	—

Substance	Poisoning, Accidental (unintentional)	Poisoning, Intentional Self-harm	Poisoning, Assault	Poisoning, Undetermined	Adverse Effect	Under-dosing
Domiodol	T48.4X1	T48.4X2	T48.4X3	T48.4X4	T48.4X5	T48.4X6
Domiphen (bromide)	T49.ØX1	T49.ØX2	T49.ØX3	T49.ØX4	T49.ØX5	T49.ØX6
Domperidone	T45.ØX1	T45.ØX2	T45.ØX3	T45.ØX4	T45.ØX5	T45.ØX6
Donepezil*	T44.ØX1	T44.ØX2	T44.ØX3	T44.ØX4	T44.ØX5	T44.ØX6
Dopa	T42.8X1	T42.8X2	T42.8X3	T42.8X4	T42.8X5	T42.8X6
Dopamine	T44.991	T44.992	T44.993	T44.994	T44.995	T44.996
Doriden	T42.6X1	T42.6X2	T42.6X3	T42.6X4	T42.6X5	T42.6X6
Dormiral	T42.3X1	T42.3X2	T42.3X3	T42.3X4	T42.3X5	T42.3X6
Dormison	T42.6X1	T42.6X2	T42.6X3	T42.6X4	T42.6X5	T42.6X6
Dornase	T48.4X1	T48.4X2	T48.4X3	T48.4X4	T48.4X5	T48.4X6
Dorsacaine	T41.3X1	T41.3X2	T41.3X3	T41.3X4	T41.3X5	T41.3X6
Dosulepin	T43.Ø11	T43.Ø12	T43.Ø13	T43.Ø14	T43.Ø15	T43.Ø16
Dothiepin	T43.Ø11	T43.Ø12	T43.Ø13	T43.Ø14	T43.Ø15	T43.Ø16
Doxantrazole	T48.6X1	T48.6X2	T48.6X3	T48.6X4	T48.6X5	T48.6X6
Doxapram	T5Ø.7X1	T5Ø.7X2	T5Ø.7X3	T5Ø.7X4	T5Ø.7X5	T5Ø.7X6
Doxazosin	T44.6X1	T44.6X2	T44.6X3	T44.6X4	T44.6X5	T44.6X6
Doxepin	T43.Ø11	T43.Ø12	T43.Ø13	T43.Ø14	T43.Ø15	T43.Ø16
Doxifluridine	T45.1X1	T45.1X2	T45.1X3	T45.1X4	T45.1X5	T45.1X6
Doxil*	T45.1X1	T45.1X2	T45.1X3	T45.1X4	T45.1X5	T45.1X6
Doxorubicin	T45.1X1	T45.1X2	T45.1X3	T45.1X4	T45.1X5	T45.1X6
Doxycycline	T36.4X1	T36.4X2	T36.4X3	T36.4X4	T36.4X5	T36.4X6
Doxylamine	T45.ØX1	T45.ØX2	T45.ØX3	T45.ØX4	T45.ØX5	T45.ØX6
Dramamine	T45.ØX1	T45.ØX2	T45.ØX3	T45.ØX4	T45.ØX5	T45.ØX6
Drano (drain cleaner)	T54.3X1	T54.3X2	T54.3X3	T54.3X4	—	—
Dressing, live pulp	T49.7X1	T49.7X2	T49.7X3	T49.7X4	T49.7X5	T49.7X6
Drocode	T4Ø.2X1	T4Ø.2X2	T4Ø.2X3	T4Ø.2X4	T4Ø.2X5	T4Ø.2X6
Dromoran	T4Ø.2X1	T4Ø.2X2	T4Ø.2X3	T4Ø.2X4	T4Ø.2X5	T4Ø.2X6
Dromostanolone	T38.7X1	T38.7X2	T38.7X3	T38.7X4	T38.7X5	T38.7X6
Dronabinol	T4Ø.711	T4Ø.712	T4Ø.713	T4Ø.714	T4Ø.715	T4Ø.716
Droperidol	T43.591	T43.592	T43.593	T43.594	T43.595	T43.596
Dropropizine	T48.3X1	T48.3X2	T48.3X3	T48.3X4	T48.3X5	T48.3X6
Drostanolone	T38.7X1	T38.7X2	T38.7X3	T38.7X4	T38.7X5	T38.7X6
Drotaverine	T44.3X1	T44.3X2	T44.3X3	T44.3X4	T44.3X5	T44.3X6
Drotrecogin alfa	T45.511	T45.512	T45.513	T45.514	T45.515	T45.516
Drug NEC	T5Ø.9Ø1	T5Ø.9Ø2	T5Ø.9Ø3	T5Ø.9Ø4	T5Ø.9Ø5	T5Ø.9Ø6
specified NEC	T5Ø.991	T5Ø.992	T5Ø.993	T5Ø.994	T5Ø.995	T5Ø.996
DTIC	T45.1X1	T45.1X2	T45.1X3	T45.1X4	T45.1X5	T45.1X6
Duboisine	T44.3X1	T44.3X2	T44.3X3	T44.3X4	T44.3X5	T44.3X6
Dulcolax	T47.2X1	T47.2X2	T47.2X3	T47.2X4	T47.2X5	T47.2X6
Duponol (C) (EP)	T49.2X1	T49.2X2	T49.2X3	T49.2X4	T49.2X5	T49.2X6
Durabolin	T38.7X1	T38.7X2	T38.7X3	T38.7X4	T38.7X5	T38.7X6
Durezol*	T49.5X1	T49.5X2	T49.5X3	T49.5X4	T49.5X5	T49.5X6
Dyclone	T41.3X1	T41.3X2	T41.3X3	T41.3X4	T41.3X5	T41.3X6
Dyclonine	T41.3X1	T41.3X2	T41.3X3	T41.3X4	T41.3X5	T41.3X6
Dydrogesterone	T38.5X1	T38.5X2	T38.5X3	T38.5X4	T38.5X5	T38.5X6
Dye NEC	T65.6X1	T65.6X2	T65.6X3	T65.6X4	—	—
antiseptic	T49.ØX1	T49.ØX2	T49.ØX3	T49.ØX4	T49.ØX5	T49.ØX6
diagnostic agents	T5Ø.8X1	T5Ø.8X2	T5Ø.8X3	T5Ø.8X4	T5Ø.8X5	T5Ø.8X6
pharmaceutical NEC	T5Ø.9Ø1	T5Ø.9Ø2	T5Ø.9Ø3	T5Ø.9Ø4	T5Ø.9Ø5	T5Ø.9Ø6
Dyflos	T44.ØX1	T44.ØX2	T44.ØX3	T44.ØX4	T44.ØX5	T44.ØX6
Dymelor	T38.3X1	T38.3X2	T38.3X3	T38.3X4	T38.3X5	T38.3X6
Dynamite	T65.3X1	T65.3X2	T65.3X3	T65.3X4	—	—
fumes	T59.891	T59.892	T59.893	T59.894	—	—
Dyphylline	T44.3X1	T44.3X2	T44.3X3	T44.3X4	T44.3X5	T44.3X6
Ear drug NEC	T49.6X1	T49.6X2	T49.6X3	T49.6X4	T49.6X5	T49.6X6
Ear preparations	T49.6X1	T49.6X2	T49.6X3	T49.6X4	T49.6X5	T49.6X6
Echothiophate, echothiopate, ecothiopate	T49.5X1	T49.5X2	T49.5X3	T49.5X4	T49.5X5	T49.5X6
Econazole	T49.ØX1	T49.ØX2	T49.ØX3	T49.ØX4	T49.ØX5	T49.ØX6
Ecothiopate iodide	T49.5X1	T49.5X2	T49.5X3	T49.5X4	T49.5X5	T49.5X6
Ecstasy	T43.641	T43.642	T43.643	T43.644	—	—
Ectylurea	T42.6X1	T42.6X2	T42.6X3	T42.6X4	T42.6X5	T42.6X6
Edathamil disodium	T45.8X1	T45.8X2	T45.8X3	T45.8X4	T45.8X5	T45.8X6
Edecrin	T5Ø.1X1	T5Ø.1X2	T5Ø.1X3	T5Ø.1X4	T5Ø.1X5	T5Ø.1X6
Edetate, disodium (calcium)	T45.8X1	T45.8X2	T45.8X3	T45.8X4	T45.8X5	T45.8X6
Edoxudine	T49.5X1	T49.5X2	T49.5X3	T49.5X4	T49.5X5	T49.5X6
Edrophonium	T44.ØX1	T44.ØX2	T44.ØX3	T44.ØX4	T44.ØX5	T44.ØX6
chloride	T44.ØX1	T44.ØX2	T44.ØX3	T44.ØX4	T44.ØX5	T44.ØX6
EDTA	T5Ø.6X1	T5Ø.6X2	T5Ø.6X3	T5Ø.6X4	T5Ø.6X5	T5Ø.6X6
Effexor*	T43.221	T43.222	T43.223	T43.224	T43.225	T43.226
Eflornithine	T37.2X1	T37.2X2	T37.2X3	T37.2X4	T37.2X5	T37.2X6
Efloxate	T46.3X1	T46.3X2	T46.3X3	T46.3X4	T46.3X5	T46.3X6
Elase	T49.8X1	T49.8X2	T49.8X3	T49.8X4	T49.8X5	T49.8X6
Elastase	T47.5X1	T47.5X2	T47.5X3	T47.5X4	T47.5X5	T47.5X6
Elaterium	T47.2X1	T47.2X2	T47.2X3	T47.2X4	T47.2X5	T47.2X6
Elcatonin	T5Ø.991	T5Ø.992	T5Ø.993	T5Ø.994	T5Ø.995	T5Ø.996
Elder	T62.2X1	T62.2X2	T62.2X3	T62.2X4	—	—
berry, (unripe)	T62.1X1	T62.1X2	T62.1X3	T62.1X4	—	—
Electrolyte balance drug	T5Ø.3X1	T5Ø.3X2	T5Ø.3X3	T5Ø.3X4	T5Ø.3X5	T5Ø.3X6
Electrolytes NEC	T5Ø.3X1	T5Ø.3X2	T5Ø.3X3	T5Ø.3X4	T5Ø.3X5	T5Ø.3X6
Electrolytic agent NEC	T5Ø.3X1	T5Ø.3X2	T5Ø.3X3	T5Ø.3X4	T5Ø.3X5	T5Ø.3X6
Elemental diet	T5Ø.9Ø1	T5Ø.9Ø2	T5Ø.9Ø3	T5Ø.9Ø4	T5Ø.9Ø5	T5Ø.9Ø6

Substance	Poisoning, Accidental (unintentional)	Poisoning, Intentional Self-harm	Poisoning, Assault	Poisoning, Undetermined	Adverse Effect	Under-dosing
Elliptinium acetate	T45.1X1	T45.1X2	T45.1X3	T45.1X4	T45.1X5	T45.1X6
Elocon*	T49.ØX1	T49.ØX2	T49.ØX3	T49.ØX4	T49.ØX5	T49.ØX6
Embramine	T45.ØX1	T45.ØX2	T45.ØX3	T45.ØX4	T45.ØX5	T45.ØX6
Emepronium (salts)	T44.3X1	T44.3X2	T44.3X3	T44.3X4	T44.3X5	T44.3X6
bromide	T44.3X1	T44.3X2	T44.3X3	T44.3X4	T44.3X5	T44.3X6
Emetic NEC	T47.7X1	T47.7X2	T47.7X3	T47.7X4	T47.7X5	T47.7X6
Emetine	T37.3X1	T37.3X2	T37.3X3	T37.3X4	T37.3X5	T37.3X6
Emollient NEC	T49.3X1	T49.3X2	T49.3X3	T49.3X4	T49.3X5	T49.3X6
Emorfazone	T39.8X1	T39.8X2	T39.8X3	T39.8X4	T39.8X5	T39.8X6
Emylcamate	T43.591	T43.592	T43.593	T43.594	T43.595	T43.596
Enalapril	T46.4X1	T46.4X2	T46.4X3	T46.4X4	T46.4X5	T46.4X6
Enalaprilat	T46.4X1	T46.4X2	T46.4X3	T46.4X4	T46.4X5	T46.4X6
Enbrel*	T39.4X1	T39.4X2	T39.4X3	T39.4X4	T39.4X5	T39.4X6
Encainide	T46.2X1	T46.2X2	T46.2X3	T46.2X4	T46.2X5	T46.2X6
Endocaine	T41.3X1	T41.3X2	T41.3X3	T41.3X4	T41.3X5	T41.3X6
Endosulfan	T6Ø.2X1	T6Ø.2X2	T6Ø.2X3	T6Ø.2X4	—	—
Endothall	T6Ø.3X1	T6Ø.3X2	T6Ø.3X3	T6Ø.3X4	—	—
Endralazine	T46.5X1	T46.5X2	T46.5X3	T46.5X4	T46.5X5	T46.5X6
Endrin	T6Ø.1X1	T6Ø.1X2	T6Ø.1X3	T6Ø.1X4	—	—
Enflurane	T41.ØX1	T41.ØX2	T41.ØX3	T41.ØX4	T41.ØX5	T41.ØX6
Enfuvirtide*	T37.5X1	T37.5X2	T37.5X3	T37.5X4	T37.5X5	T37.5X6
Enhexymal	T42.3X1	T42.3X2	T42.3X3	T42.3X4	T42.3X5	T42.3X6
Enocitabine	T45.1X1	T45.1X2	T45.1X3	T45.1X4	T45.1X5	T45.1X6
Enovid	T38.4X1	T38.4X2	T38.4X3	T38.4X4	T38.4X5	T38.4X6
Enoxacin	T36.8X1	T36.8X2	T36.8X3	T36.8X4	T36.8X5	T36.8X6
Enoxaparin (sodium)	T45.511	T45.512	T45.513	T45.514	T45.515	T45.516
Enpiprazole	T43.591	T43.592	T43.593	T43.594	T43.595	T43.596
Enprofylline	T48.6X1	T48.6X2	T48.6X3	T48.6X4	T48.6X5	T48.6X6
Enprostil	T47.1X1	T47.1X2	T47.1X3	T47.1X4	T47.1X5	T47.1X6
ENT preparations (anti-infectives)	T49.6X1	T49.6X2	T49.6X3	T49.6X4	T49.6X5	T49.6X6
Enterogastrone	T38.891	T38.892	T38.893	T38.894	T38.895	T38.896
Enviomycin	T36.8X1	T36.8X2	T36.8X3	T36.8X4	T36.8X5	T36.8X6
Enzodase	T45.3X1	T45.3X2	T45.3X3	T45.3X4	T45.3X5	T45.3X6
Enzyme NEC	T45.3X1	T45.3X2	T45.3X3	T45.3X4	T45.3X5	T45.3X6
depolymerizing	T49.8X1	T49.8X2	T49.8X3	T49.8X4	T49.8X5	T49.8X6
fibrolytic	T45.3X1	T45.3X2	T45.3X3	T45.3X4	T45.3X5	T45.3X6
gastric	T47.5X1	T47.5X2	T47.5X3	T47.5X4	T47.5X5	T47.5X6
intestinal	T47.5X1	T47.5X2	T47.5X3	T47.5X4	T47.5X5	T47.5X6
local action	T49.4X1	T49.4X2	T49.4X3	T49.4X4	T49.4X5	T49.4X6
proteolytic	T49.4X1	T49.4X2	T49.4X3	T49.4X4	T49.4X5	T49.4X6
thrombolytic	T45.3X1	T45.3X2	T45.3X3	T45.3X4	T45.3X5	T45.3X6
EPAB	T41.3X1	T41.3X2	T41.3X3	T41.3X4	T41.3X5	T41.3X6
Epanutin	T42.ØX1	T42.ØX2	T42.ØX3	T42.ØX4	T42.ØX5	T42.ØX6
Ephedra	T44.991	T44.992	T44.993	T44.994	T44.995	T44.996
Ephedrine	T44.991	T44.992	T44.993	T44.994	T44.995	T44.996
Epichlorhydrin, epichlorohydrin	T52.8X1	T52.8X2	T52.8X3	T52.8X4	—	—
Epicillin	T36.ØX1	T36.ØX2	T36.ØX3	T36.ØX4	T36.ØX5	T36.ØX6
Epiestriol	T38.5X1	T38.5X2	T38.5X3	T38.5X4	T38.5X5	T38.5X6
Epilim — *see* Sodium, valproate						
Epimestrol	T38.5X1	T38.5X2	T38.5X3	T38.5X4	T38.5X5	T38.5X6
Epinephrine	T44.5X1	T44.5X2	T44.5X3	T44.5X4	T44.5X5	T44.5X6
EpiPen*	T44.5X1	T44.5X2	T44.5X3	T44.5X4	T44.5X5	T44.5X6
Epirubicin	T45.1X1	T45.1X2	T45.1X3	T45.1X4	T45.1X5	T45.1X6
Epitiostanol	T38.7X1	T38.7X2	T38.7X3	T38.7X4	T38.7X5	T38.7X6
Epitizide	T5Ø.2X1	T5Ø.2X2	T5Ø.2X3	T5Ø.2X4	T5Ø.2X5	T5Ø.2X6
EPN	T6Ø.ØX1	T6Ø.ØX2	T6Ø.ØX3	T6Ø.ØX4	—	—
EPO	T45.8X1	T45.8X2	T45.8X3	T45.8X4	T45.8X5	T45.8X6
Epoetin alpha	T45.8X1	T45.8X2	T45.8X3	T45.8X4	T45.8X5	T45.8X6
Epomediol	T5Ø.991	T5Ø.992	T5Ø.993	T5Ø.994	T5Ø.995	T5Ø.996
Epoprostenol	T45.521	T45.522	T45.523	T45.524	T45.525	T45.526
Epoxy resin	T65.891	T65.892	T65.893	T65.894	—	—
Eprazinone	T48.4X1	T48.4X2	T48.4X3	T48.4X4	T48.4X5	T48.4X6
Epsilon aminocaproic acid	T45.621	T45.622	T45.623	T45.624	T45.625	T45.626
Epsom salt	T47.3X1	T47.3X2	T47.3X3	T47.3X4	T47.3X5	T47.3X6
Eptazocine	T4Ø.491	T4Ø.492	T4Ø.493	T4Ø.494	T4Ø.495	T4Ø.496
Equanil	T43.591	T43.592	T43.593	T43.594	T43.595	T43.596
Equisetum	T62.2X1	T62.2X2	T62.2X3	T62.2X4	—	—
diuretic	T5Ø.2X1	T5Ø.2X2	T5Ø.2X3	T5Ø.2X4	T5Ø.2X5	T5Ø.2X6
Ergobasine	T48.ØX1	T48.ØX2	T48.ØX3	T48.ØX4	T48.ØX5	T48.ØX6
Ergocalciferol	T45.2X1	T45.2X2	T45.2X3	T45.2X4	T45.2X5	T45.2X6
Ergoloid mesylates	T46.7X1	T46.7X2	T46.7X3	T46.7X4	T46.7X5	T46.7X6
Ergometrine	T48.ØX1	T48.ØX2	T48.ØX3	T48.ØX4	T48.ØX5	T48.ØX6
Ergonovine	T48.ØX1	T48.ØX2	T48.ØX3	T48.ØX4	T48.ØX5	T48.ØX6
Ergot NEC	T64.81	T64.82	T64.83	T64.84	—	—
derivative	T48.ØX1	T48.ØX2	T48.ØX3	T48.ØX4	T48.ØX5	T48.ØX6
medicinal (alkaloids)	T48.ØX1	T48.ØX2	T48.ØX3	T48.ØX4	T48.ØX5	T48.ØX6
prepared	T48.ØX1	T48.ØX2	T48.ØX3	T48.ØX4	T48.ØX5	T48.ØX6
Ergotamine	T46.5X1	T46.5X2	T46.5X3	T46.5X4	T46.5X5	T46.5X6
Ergotocine	T48.ØX1	T48.ØX2	T48.ØX3	T48.ØX4	T48.ØX5	T48.ØX6
Ergotrate	T48.ØX1	T48.ØX2	T48.ØX3	T48.ØX4	T48.ØX5	T48.ØX6
Eritrityl tetranitrate	T46.3X1	T46.3X2	T46.3X3	T46.3X4	T46.3X5	T46.3X6
Erythrityl tetranitrate	T46.3X1	T46.3X2	T46.3X3	T46.3X4	T46.3X5	T46.3X6
Erythrol tetranitrate	T46.3X1	T46.3X2	T46.3X3	T46.3X4	T46.3X5	T46.3X6
Erythromycin (salts)	T36.3X1	T36.3X2	T36.3X3	T36.3X4	T36.3X5	T36.3X6
ophthalmic preparation	T49.5X1	T49.5X2	T49.5X3	T49.5X4	T49.5X5	T49.5X6
topical NEC	T49.ØX1	T49.ØX2	T49.ØX3	T49.ØX4	T49.ØX5	T49.ØX6
Erythropoietin	T45.8X1	T45.8X2	T45.8X3	T45.8X4	T45.8X5	T45.8X6
human	T45.8X1	T45.8X2	T45.8X3	T45.8X4	T45.8X5	T45.8X6
Esbriet*	T48.991	T48.992	T48.993	T48.994	T48.995	T48.996
Escin	T46.991	T46.992	T46.993	T46.994	T46.995	T46.996
Escitalopram*	T43.221	T43.222	T43.223	T43.224	T43.225	T43.226
Esculin	T45.2X1	T45.2X2	T45.2X3	T45.2X4	T45.2X5	T45.2X6
Esculoside	T45.2X1	T45.2X2	T45.2X3	T45.2X4	T45.2X5	T45.2X6
ESDT (ether-soluble tar distillate)	T49.1X1	T49.1X2	T49.1X3	T49.1X4	T49.1X5	T49.1X6
Eserine	T49.5X1	T49.5X2	T49.5X3	T49.5X4	T49.5X5	T49.5X6
Esflurbiprofen	T39.311	T39.312	T39.313	T39.314	T39.315	T39.316
Eskabarb	T42.3X1	T42.3X2	T42.3X3	T42.3X4	T42.3X5	T42.3X6
Eskalith	T43.8X1	T43.8X2	T43.8X3	T43.8X4	T43.8X5	T43.8X6
Esmolol	T44.7X1	T44.7X2	T44.7X3	T44.7X4	T44.7X5	T44.7X6
Estanozolol	T38.7X1	T38.7X2	T38.7X3	T38.7X4	T38.7X5	T38.7X6
Estazolam	T42.4X1	T42.4X2	T42.4X3	T42.4X4	T42.4X5	T42.4X6
Estradiol	T38.5X1	T38.5X2	T38.5X3	T38.5X4	T38.5X5	T38.5X6
benzoate	T38.5X1	T38.5X2	T38.5X3	T38.5X4	T38.5X5	T38.5X6
with testosterone	T38.7X1	T38.7X2	T38.7X3	T38.7X4	T38.7X5	T38.7X6
Estramustine	T45.1X1	T45.1X2	T45.1X3	T45.1X4	T45.1X5	T45.1X6
Estriol	T38.5X1	T38.5X2	T38.5X3	T38.5X4	T38.5X5	T38.5X6
Estrogen	T38.5X1	T38.5X2	T38.5X3	T38.5X4	T38.5X5	T38.5X6
conjugated	T38.5X1	T38.5X2	T38.5X3	T38.5X4	T38.5X5	T38.5X6
with progesterone	T38.5X1	T38.5X2	T38.5X3	T38.5X4	T38.5X5	T38.5X6
Estrone	T38.5X1	T38.5X2	T38.5X3	T38.5X4	T38.5X5	T38.5X6
Estropipate	T38.5X1	T38.5X2	T38.5X3	T38.5X4	T38.5X5	T38.5X6
Etacrynate sodium	T5Ø.1X1	T5Ø.1X2	T5Ø.1X3	T5Ø.1X4	T5Ø.1X5	T5Ø.1X6
Etacrynic acid	T5Ø.1X1	T5Ø.1X2	T5Ø.1X3	T5Ø.1X4	T5Ø.1X5	T5Ø.1X6
Etafedrine	T48.6X1	T48.6X2	T48.6X3	T48.6X4	T48.6X5	T48.6X6
Etafenone	T46.3X1	T46.3X2	T46.3X3	T46.3X4	T46.3X5	T46.3X6
Etambutol	T37.1X1	T37.1X2	T37.1X3	T37.1X4	T37.1X5	T37.1X6
Etamiphyllin	T48.6X1	T48.6X2	T48.6X3	T48.6X4	T48.6X5	T48.6X6
Etamivan	T5Ø.7X1	T5Ø.7X2	T5Ø.7X3	T5Ø.7X4	T5Ø.7X5	T5Ø.7X6
Etamsylate	T45.7X1	T45.7X2	T45.7X3	T45.7X4	T45.7X5	T45.7X6
Etebenecid	T5Ø.4X1	T5Ø.4X2	T5Ø.4X3	T5Ø.4X4	T5Ø.4X5	T5Ø.4X6
Ethacridine	T49.ØX1	T49.ØX2	T49.ØX3	T49.ØX4	T49.ØX5	T49.ØX6
Ethacrynate*	T5Ø.1X1	T5Ø.1X2	T5Ø.1X3	T5Ø.1X4	T5Ø.1X5	T5Ø.1X6
Ethacrynic acid	T5Ø.1X1	T5Ø.1X2	T5Ø.1X3	T5Ø.1X4	T5Ø.1X5	T5Ø.1X6
Ethadione	T42.2X1	T42.2X2	T42.2X3	T42.2X4	T42.2X5	T42.2X6
Ethambutol	T37.1X1	T37.1X2	T37.1X3	T37.1X4	T37.1X5	T37.1X6
Ethamide	T5Ø.2X1	T5Ø.2X2	T5Ø.2X3	T5Ø.2X4	T5Ø.2X5	T5Ø.2X6
Ethamivan	T5Ø.7X1	T5Ø.7X2	T5Ø.7X3	T5Ø.7X4	T5Ø.7X5	T5Ø.7X6
Ethamsylate	T45.7X1	T45.7X2	T45.7X3	T45.7X4	T45.7X5	T45.7X6
Ethanol	T51.ØX1	T51.ØX2	T51.ØX3	T51.ØX4	—	—
beverage	T51.ØX1	T51.ØX2	T51.ØX3	T51.ØX4	—	—
Ethanolamine oleate	T46.8X1	T46.8X2	T46.8X3	T46.8X4	T46.8X5	T46.8X6
Ethaverine	T44.3X1	T44.3X2	T44.3X3	T44.3X4	T44.3X5	T44.3X6
Ethchlorvynol	T42.6X1	T42.6X2	T42.6X3	T42.6X4	T42.6X5	T42.6X6
Ethebenecid	T5Ø.4X1	T5Ø.4X2	T5Ø.4X3	T5Ø.4X4	T5Ø.4X5	T5Ø.4X6
Ether (vapor)	T41.ØX1	T41.ØX2	T41.ØX3	T41.ØX4	T41.ØX5	T41.ØX6
anesthetic	T41.ØX1	T41.ØX2	T41.ØX3	T41.ØX4	T41.ØX5	T41.ØX6
divinyl	T41.ØX1	T41.ØX2	T41.ØX3	T41.ØX4	T41.ØX5	T41.ØX6
ethyl (medicinal)	T41.ØX1	T41.ØX2	T41.ØX3	T41.ØX4	T41.ØX5	T41.ØX6
nonmedicinal	T52.8X1	T52.8X2	T52.8X3	T52.8X4	—	—
petroleum — *see* Ligroin						
solvent	T52.8X1	T52.8X2	T52.8X3	T52.8X4	—	—
Ethiazide	T5Ø.2X1	T5Ø.2X2	T5Ø.2X3	T5Ø.2X4	T5Ø.2X5	T5Ø.2X6
Ethidium chloride (vapor)	T59.891	T59.892	T59.893	T59.894	—	—
Ethinamate	T42.6X1	T42.6X2	T42.6X3	T42.6X4	T42.6X5	T42.6X6
Ethinylestradiol, ethinyloestradiol	T38.5X1	T38.5X2	T38.5X3	T38.5X4	T38.5X5	T38.5X6
with						
levonorgestrel	T38.4X1	T38.4X2	T38.4X3	T38.4X4	T38.4X5	T38.4X6
norethisterone	T38.4X1	T38.4X2	T38.4X3	T38.4X4	T38.4X5	T38.4X6
Ethiodized oil (131 I)	T5Ø.8X1	T5Ø.8X2	T5Ø.8X3	T5Ø.8X4	T5Ø.8X5	T5Ø.8X6
Ethiofos*	T5Ø.991	T5Ø.992	T5Ø.993	T5Ø.994	T5Ø.995	T5Ø.996
Ethion	T6Ø.ØX1	T6Ø.ØX2	T6Ø.ØX3	T6Ø.ØX4	—	—
Ethionamide	T37.1X1	T37.1X2	T37.1X3	T37.1X4	T37.1X5	T37.1X6
Ethioniamide	T37.1X1	T37.1X2	T37.1X3	T37.1X4	T37.1X5	T37.1X6
Ethisterone	T38.5X1	T38.5X2	T38.5X3	T38.5X4	T38.5X5	T38.5X6
Ethobral	T42.3X1	T42.3X2	T42.3X3	T42.3X4	T42.3X5	T42.3X6
Ethocaine (infiltration) (topical)	T41.3X1	T41.3X2	T41.3X3	T41.3X4	T41.3X5	T41.3X6
nerve block (peripheral) (plexus)	T41.3X1	T41.3X2	T41.3X3	T41.3X4	T41.3X5	T41.3X6
spinal	T41.3X1	T41.3X2	T41.3X3	T41.3X4	T41.3X5	T41.3X6
Ethoheptazine	T4Ø.491	T4Ø.492	T4Ø.493	T4Ø.494	T4Ø.495	T4Ø.496
Ethopropazine	T44.3X1	T44.3X2	T44.3X3	T44.3X4	T44.3X5	T44.3X6

Ethosuximide ICD-10-CM 2026

Table of Drugs and Chemicals

Substance	Poisoning, Accidental (unintentional)	Poisoning, Intentional Self-harm	Poisoning, Assault	Poisoning, Undetermined	Adverse Effect	Under-dosing
Ethosuximide	T42.2X1	T42.2X2	T42.2X3	T42.2X4	T42.2X5	T42.2X6
Ethotoin	T42.ØX1	T42.ØX2	T42.ØX3	T42.ØX4	T42.ØX5	T42.ØX6
Ethoxazene	T37.91	T37.92	T37.93	T37.94	T37.95	T37.96
Ethoxazorutoside	T46.991	T46.992	T46.993	T46.994	T46.995	T46.996
Ethoxzolamide	T5Ø.2X1	T5Ø.2X2	T5Ø.2X3	T5Ø.2X4	T5Ø.2X5	T5Ø.2X6
Ethyl						
acetate	T52.8X1	T52.8X2	T52.8X3	T52.8X4	—	—
alcohol	T51.ØX1	T51.ØX2	T51.ØX3	T51.ØX4	—	—
beverage	T51.ØX1	T51.ØX2	T51.ØX3	T51.ØX4	—	—
aldehyde (vapor)	T59.891	T59.892	T59.893	T59.894	—	—
liquid	T52.8X1	T52.8X2	T52.8X3	T52.8X4	—	—
aminobenzoate	T41.3X1	T41.3X2	T41.3X3	T41.3X4	T41.3X5	T41.3X6
aminophenothiazine	T43.3X1	T43.3X2	T43.3X3	T43.3X4	T43.3X5	T43.3X6
benzoate	T52.8X1	T52.8X2	T52.8X3	T52.8X4	—	—
biscoumacetate	T45.511	T45.512	T45.513	T45.514	T45.515	T45.516
bromide (anesthetic)	T41.ØX1	T41.ØX2	T41.ØX3	T41.ØX4	T41.ØX5	T41.ØX6
carbamate	T45.1X1	T45.1X2	T45.1X3	T45.1X4	T45.1X5	T45.1X6
carbinol	T51.3X1	T51.3X2	T51.3X3	T51.3X4	—	—
carbonate	T52.8X1	T52.8X2	T52.8X3	T52.8X4	—	—
chaulmoograte	T37.1X1	T37.1X2	T37.1X3	T37.1X4	T37.1X5	T37.1X6
chloride (anesthetic)	T41.ØX1	T41.ØX2	T41.ØX3	T41.ØX4	T41.ØX5	T41.ØX6
anesthetic (local)	T41.3X1	T41.3X2	T41.3X3	T41.3X4	T41.3X5	T41.3X6
inhaled	T41.ØX1	T41.ØX2	T41.ØX3	T41.ØX4	T41.ØX5	T41.ØX6
local	T49.4X1	T49.4X2	T49.4X3	T49.4X4	T49.4X5	T49.4X6
solvent	T53.6X1	T53.6X2	T53.6X3	T53.6X4	—	—
dibunate	T48.3X1	T48.3X2	T48.3X3	T48.3X4	T48.3X5	T48.3X6
dichloroarsine (vapor)	T57.ØX1	T57.ØX2	T57.ØX3	T57.ØX4	—	—
estranol	T38.7X1	T38.7X2	T38.7X3	T38.7X4	T38.7X5	T38.7X6
ether — *see also* ether	T52.8X1	T52.8X2	T52.8X3	T52.8X4	—	—
formate NEC (solvent)	T52.ØX1	T52.ØX2	T52.ØX3	T52.ØX4	—	—
fumarate	T49.4X1	T49.4X2	T49.4X3	T49.4X4	T49.4X5	T49.4X6
hydroxyisobutyrate NEC (solvent)	T52.8X1	T52.8X2	T52.8X3	T52.8X4	—	—
iodoacetate	T59.3X1	T59.3X2	T59.3X3	T59.3X4	—	—
lactate NEC (solvent)	T52.8X1	T52.8X2	T52.8X3	T52.8X4	—	—
loflazepate	T42.4X1	T42.4X2	T42.4X3	T42.4X4	T42.4X5	T42.4X6
mercuric chloride	T56.1X1	T56.1X2	T56.1X3	T56.1X4	—	—
methylcarbinol	T51.8X1	T51.8X2	T51.8X3	T51.8X4	—	—
morphine	T4Ø.2X1	T4Ø.2X2	T4Ø.2X3	T4Ø.2X4	T4Ø.2X5	T4Ø.2X6
noradrenaline	T48.6X1	T48.6X2	T48.6X3	T48.6X4	T48.6X5	T48.6X6
oxybutyrate NEC (solvent)	T52.8X1	T52.8X2	T52.8X3	T52.8X4	—	—
Ethylene (gas)	T59.891	T59.892	T59.893	T59.894	—	—
anesthetic (general)	T41.ØX1	T41.ØX2	T41.ØX3	T41.ØX4	T41.ØX5	T41.ØX6
chlorohydrin	T52.8X1	T52.8X2	T52.8X3	T52.8X4	—	—
vapor	T53.6X1	T53.6X2	T53.6X3	T53.6X4	—	—
dichloride	T52.8X1	T52.8X2	T52.8X3	T52.8X4	—	—
vapor	T53.6X1	T53.6X2	T53.6X3	T53.6X4	—	—
dinitrate	T52.3X1	T52.3X2	T52.3X3	T52.3X4	—	—
glycol(s)	T52.8X1	T52.8X2	T52.8X3	T52.8X4	—	—
dinitrate	T52.3X1	T52.3X2	T52.3X3	T52.3X4	—	—
monobutyl ether	T52.3X1	T52.3X2	T52.3X3	T52.3X4	—	—
imine	T54.1X1	T54.1X2	T54.1X3	T54.1X4	—	—
oxide (fumigant) (nonmedicinal)	T59.891	T59.892	T59.893	T59.894	—	—
medicinal	T49.ØX1	T49.ØX2	T49.ØX3	T49.ØX4	T49.ØX5	T49.ØX6
Ethylenediamine theophylline	T48.6X1	T48.6X2	T48.6X3	T48.6X4	T48.6X5	T48.6X6
Ethylenediaminetetra-acetic acid	T5Ø.6X1	T5Ø.6X2	T5Ø.6X3	T5Ø.6X4	T5Ø.6X5	T5Ø.6X6
Ethylenedinitrilotetra-acetate	T5Ø.6X1	T5Ø.6X2	T5Ø.6X3	T5Ø.6X4	T5Ø.6X5	T5Ø.6X6
Ethylestrenol	T38.7X1	T38.7X2	T38.7X3	T38.7X4	T38.7X5	T38.7X6
Ethylhydroxycellulose	T47.4X1	T47.4X2	T47.4X3	T47.4X4	T47.4X5	T47.4X6
Ethylidene						
chloride NEC	T53.6X1	T53.6X2	T53.6X3	T53.6X4	—	—
diacetate	T6Ø.3X1	T6Ø.3X2	T6Ø.3X3	T6Ø.3X4	—	—
dicoumarin	T45.511	T45.512	T45.513	T45.514	T45.515	T45.516
dicoumarol	T45.511	T45.512	T45.513	T45.514	T45.515	T45.516
diethyl ether	T52.ØX1	T52.ØX2	T52.ØX3	T52.ØX4	—	—
Ethylmorphine	T4Ø.2X1	T4Ø.2X2	T4Ø.2X3	T4Ø.2X4	T4Ø.2X5	T4Ø.2X6
Ethylnorepinephrine	T48.6X1	T48.6X2	T48.6X3	T48.6X4	T48.6X5	T48.6X6
Ethylparachlorophen-oxyisobutyrate	T46.6X1	T46.6X2	T46.6X3	T46.6X4	T46.6X5	T46.6X6
Ethynodiol	T38.4X1	T38.4X2	T38.4X3	T38.4X4	T38.4X5	T38.4X6
with mestranol diacetate	T38.4X1	T38.4X2	T38.4X3	T38.4X4	T38.4X5	T38.4X6
Ethyol*	T5Ø.991	T5Ø.992	T5Ø.993	T5Ø.994	T5Ø.995	T5Ø.996
Etidocaine	T41.3X1	T41.3X2	T41.3X3	T41.3X4	T41.3X5	T41.3X6
infiltration (subcutaneous)	T41.3X1	T41.3X2	T41.3X3	T41.3X4	T41.3X5	T41.3X6
nerve (peripheral) (plexus)	T41.3X1	T41.3X2	T41.3X3	T41.3X4	T41.3X5	T41.3X6
Etidronate	T5Ø.991	T5Ø.992	T5Ø.993	T5Ø.994	T5Ø.995	T5Ø.996
Etidronic acid (disodium salt)	T5Ø.991	T5Ø.992	T5Ø.993	T5Ø.994	T5Ø.995	T5Ø.996
Etifoxine	T42.6X1	T42.6X2	T42.6X3	T42.6X4	T42.6X5	T42.6X6
Etilefrine	T44.4X1	T44.4X2	T44.4X3	T44.4X4	T44.4X5	T44.4X6

Substance	Poisoning, Accidental (unintentional)	Poisoning, Intentional Self-harm	Poisoning, Assault	Poisoning, Undetermined	Adverse Effect	Under-dosing
Etilfen	T42.3X1	T42.3X2	T42.3X3	T42.3X4	T42.3X5	T42.3X6
Etinodiol	T38.4X1	T38.4X2	T38.4X3	T38.4X4	T38.4X5	T38.4X6
Etiroxate	T46.6X1	T46.6X2	T46.6X3	T46.6X4	T46.6X5	T46.6X6
Etizolam	T42.4X1	T42.4X2	T42.4X3	T42.4X4	T42.4X5	T42.4X6
Etodolac	T39.391	T39.392	T39.393	T39.394	T39.395	T39.396
Etofamide	T37.3X1	T37.3X2	T37.3X3	T37.3X4	T37.3X5	T37.3X6
Etofibrate	T46.6X1	T46.6X2	T46.6X3	T46.6X4	T46.6X5	T46.6X6
Etofylline	T46.7X1	T46.7X2	T46.7X3	T46.7X4	T46.7X5	T46.7X6
clofibrate	T46.6X1	T46.6X2	T46.6X3	T46.6X4	T46.6X5	T46.6X6
Etoglucid	T45.1X1	T45.1X2	T45.1X3	T45.1X4	T45.1X5	T45.1X6
Etomidate	T41.1X1	T41.1X2	T41.1X3	T41.1X4	T41.1X5	T41.1X6
Etomide	T39.8X1	T39.8X2	T39.8X3	T39.8X4	T39.8X5	T39.8X6
Etomidoline	T44.3X1	T44.3X2	T44.3X3	T44.3X4	T44.3X5	T44.3X6
Etoposide	T45.1X1	T45.1X2	T45.1X3	T45.1X4	T45.1X5	T45.1X6
Etorphine	T4Ø.2X1	T4Ø.2X2	T4Ø.2X3	T4Ø.2X4	T4Ø.2X5	T4Ø.2X6
Etoval	T42.3X1	T42.3X2	T42.3X3	T42.3X4	T42.3X5	T42.3X6
Etozolin	T5Ø.1X1	T5Ø.1X2	T5Ø.1X3	T5Ø.1X4	T5Ø.1X5	T5Ø.1X6
Etravirine*	T37.5X1	T37.5X2	T37.5X3	T37.5X4	T37.5X5	T37.5X6
Etretinate	T5Ø.991	T5Ø.992	T5Ø.993	T5Ø.994	T5Ø.995	T5Ø.996
Etryptamine	T43.691	T43.692	T43.693	T43.694	T43.695	T43.696
Etybenzatropine	T44.3X1	T44.3X2	T44.3X3	T44.3X4	T44.3X5	T44.3X6
Etynodiol	T38.4X1	T38.4X2	T38.4X3	T38.4X4	T38.4X5	T38.4X6
Eucaine	T41.3X1	T41.3X2	T41.3X3	T41.3X4	T41.3X5	T41.3X6
Eucalyptus oil	T49.7X1	T49.7X2	T49.7X3	T49.7X4	T49.7X5	T49.7X6
Eucatropine	T49.5X1	T49.5X2	T49.5X3	T49.5X4	T49.5X5	T49.5X6
Eucodal	T4Ø.2X1	T4Ø.2X2	T4Ø.2X3	T4Ø.2X4	T4Ø.2X5	T4Ø.2X6
Euneryl	T42.3X1	T42.3X2	T42.3X3	T42.3X4	T42.3X5	T42.3X6
Euphthalmine	T44.3X1	T44.3X2	T44.3X3	T44.3X4	T44.3X5	T44.3X6
Eurax	T49.ØX1	T49.ØX2	T49.ØX3	T49.ØX4	T49.ØX5	T49.ØX6
Euresol	T49.4X1	T49.4X2	T49.4X3	T49.4X4	T49.4X5	T49.4X6
Euthroid	T38.1X1	T38.1X2	T38.1X3	T38.1X4	T38.1X5	T38.1X6
Evans blue	T5Ø.8X1	T5Ø.8X2	T5Ø.8X3	T5Ø.8X4	T5Ø.8X5	T5Ø.8X6
Evipal	T42.3X1	T42.3X2	T42.3X3	T42.3X4	T42.3X5	T42.3X6
sodium	T41.1X1	T41.1X2	T41.1X3	T41.1X4	T41.1X5	T41.1X6
Evipan	T42.3X1	T42.3X2	T42.3X3	T42.3X4	T42.3X5	T42.3X6
sodium	T41.1X1	T41.1X2	T41.1X3	T41.1X4	T41.1X5	T41.1X6
Ex-Lax (phenolphthalein)	T47.2X1	T47.2X2	T47.2X3	T47.2X4	T47.2X5	T47.2X6
Exalamide	T49.ØX1	T49.ØX2	T49.ØX3	T49.ØX4	T49.ØX5	T49.ØX6
Exalgin	T39.1X1	T39.1X2	T39.1X3	T39.1X4	T39.1X5	T39.1X6
Excipients, pharmaceutical	T5Ø.9Ø1	T5Ø.9Ø2	T5Ø.9Ø3	T5Ø.9Ø4	T5Ø.9Ø5	T5Ø.9Ø6
Exhaust gas (engine) (motor vehicle)	T58.Ø1	T58.Ø2	T58.Ø3	T58.Ø4	—	—
Expectorant NEC	T48.4X1	T48.4X2	T48.4X3	T48.4X4	T48.4X5	T48.4X6
Extended insulin zinc suspension	T38.3X1	T38.3X2	T38.3X3	T38.3X4	T38.3X5	T38.3X6
External medications (skin) (mucous membrane)	T49.91	T49.92	T49.93	T49.94	T49.95	T49.96
dental agent	T49.7X1	T49.7X2	T49.7X3	T49.7X4	T49.7X5	T49.7X6
ENT agent	T49.6X1	T49.6X2	T49.6X3	T49.6X4	T49.6X5	T49.6X6
ophthalmic preparation	T49.5X1	T49.5X2	T49.5X3	T49.5X4	T49.5X5	T49.5X6
specified NEC	T49.8X1	T49.8X2	T49.8X3	T49.8X4	T49.8X5	T49.8X6
Extina*	T49.ØX1	T49.ØX2	T49.ØX3	T49.ØX4	T49.ØX5	T49.ØX6
Extrapyramidal antagonist NEC	T44.3X1	T44.3X2	T44.3X3	T44.3X4	T44.3X5	T44.3X6
Eye agents (anti-infective)	T49.5X1	T49.5X2	T49.5X3	T49.5X4	T49.5X5	T49.5X6
Eye drug NEC	T49.5X1	T49.5X2	T49.5X3	T49.5X4	T49.5X5	T49.5X6
FAC (fluorouracil + doxorubicin + cyclophosphamide)	T45.1X1	T45.1X2	T45.1X3	T45.1X4	T45.1X5	T45.1X6
Factor						
I (fibrinogen)	T45.8X1	T45.8X2	T45.8X3	T45.8X4	T45.8X5	T45.8X6
III (thromboplastin)	T45.8X1	T45.8X2	T45.8X3	T45.8X4	T45.8X5	T45.8X6
IX complex	T45.7X1	T45.7X2	T45.7X3	T45.7X4	T45.7X5	T45.7X6
human	T45.8X1	T45.8X2	T45.8X3	T45.8X4	T45.8X5	T45.8X6
VIII (antihemophilic Factor) (concentrate)	T45.8X1	T45.8X2	T45.8X3	T45.8X4	T45.8X5	T45.8X6
Famotidine	T47.ØX1	T47.ØX2	T47.ØX3	T47.ØX4	T47.ØX5	T47.ØX6
Fat suspension, intravenous	T5Ø.991	T5Ø.992	T5Ø.993	T5Ø.994	T5Ø.995	T5Ø.996
Fazadinium bromide	T48.1X1	T48.1X2	T48.1X3	T48.1X4	T48.1X5	T48.1X6
Febarbamate	T42.3X1	T42.3X2	T42.3X3	T42.3X4	T42.3X5	T42.3X6
Fecal softener	T47.4X1	T47.4X2	T47.4X3	T47.4X4	T47.4X5	T47.4X6
Fedrilate	T48.3X1	T48.3X2	T48.3X3	T48.3X4	T48.3X5	T48.3X6
Felodipine	T46.1X1	T46.1X2	T46.1X3	T46.1X4	T46.1X5	T46.1X6
Felypressin	T38.891	T38.892	T38.893	T38.894	T38.895	T38.896
Femizol*	T49.ØX1	T49.ØX2	T49.ØX3	T49.ØX4	T49.ØX5	T49.ØX6
Femoxetine	T43.221	T43.222	T43.223	T43.224	T43.225	T43.226
Fenalcomine	T46.3X1	T46.3X2	T46.3X3	T46.3X4	T46.3X5	T46.3X6
Fenamisal	T37.1X1	T37.1X2	T37.1X3	T37.1X4	T37.1X5	T37.1X6
Fenazone	T39.2X1	T39.2X2	T39.2X3	T39.2X4	T39.2X5	T39.2X6
Fenbendazole	T37.4X1	T37.4X2	T37.4X3	T37.4X4	T37.4X5	T37.4X6
Fenbutrazate	T5Ø.5X1	T5Ø.5X2	T5Ø.5X3	T5Ø.5X4	T5Ø.5X5	T5Ø.5X6
Fencamfamine	T43.691	T43.692	T43.693	T43.694	T43.695	T43.696

Ethosuximide — Fencamfamine

380 ☑ Additional Character May Be Required — Refer to the Tabular List for Character Selection *Optum Value-Add

Substance	Poisoning, Accidental (unintentional)	Poisoning, Intentional Self-harm	Poisoning, Assault	Poisoning, Undetermined	Adverse Effect	Under-dosing
Fendiline	T46.1X1	T46.1X2	T46.1X3	T46.1X4	T46.1X5	T46.1X6
Fenetylline	T43.691	T43.692	T43.693	T43.694	T43.695	T43.696
Fenflumizole	T39.391	T39.392	T39.393	T39.394	T39.395	T39.396
Fenfluramine	T5Ø.5X1	T5Ø.5X2	T5Ø.5X3	T5Ø.5X4	T5Ø.5X5	T5Ø.5X6
Fenobarbital	T42.3X1	T42.3X2	T42.3X3	T42.3X4	T42.3X5	T42.3X6
Fenofibrate	T46.6X1	T46.6X2	T46.6X3	T46.6X4	T46.6X5	T46.6X6
Fenoprofen	T39.311	T39.312	T39.313	T39.314	T39.315	T39.316
Fenoterol	T48.6X1	T48.6X2	T48.6X3	T48.6X4	T48.6X5	T48.6X6
Fenoverine	T44.3X1	T44.3X2	T44.3X3	T44.3X4	T44.3X5	T44.3X6
Fenoxazoline	T48.5X1	T48.5X2	T48.5X3	T48.5X4	T48.5X5	T48.5X6
Fenproporex	T5Ø.5X1	T5Ø.5X2	T5Ø.5X3	T5Ø.5X4	T5Ø.5X5	T5Ø.5X6
Fenquizone	T5Ø.2X1	T5Ø.2X2	T5Ø.2X3	T5Ø.2X4	T5Ø.2X5	T5Ø.2X6
Fentanyl (analogs)	T4Ø.411	T4Ø.412	T4Ø.413	T4Ø.414	T4Ø.415	T4Ø.416
Fentazin	T43.3X1	T43.3X2	T43.3X3	T43.3X4	T43.3X5	T43.3X6
Fenthion	T6Ø.ØX1	T6Ø.ØX2	T6Ø.ØX3	T6Ø.ØX4	—	—
Fenticlor	T49.ØX1	T49.ØX2	T49.ØX3	T49.ØX4	T49.ØX5	T49.ØX6
Fenylbutazone	T39.2X1	T39.2X2	T39.2X3	T39.2X4	T39.2X5	T39.2X6
Feprazone	T39.2X1	T39.2X2	T39.2X3	T39.2X4	T39.2X5	T39.2X6
Fer de lance (bite) (venom)	T63.Ø61	T63.Ø62	T63.Ø63	T63.Ø64	—	—
Ferrex*	T45.4X1	T45.4X2	T45.4X3	T45.4X4	T45.4X5	T45.4X6
Ferric — *see also* Iron						
chloride	T45.4X1	T45.4X2	T45.4X3	T45.4X4	T45.4X5	T45.4X6
citrate	T45.4X1	T45.4X2	T45.4X3	T45.4X4	T45.4X5	T45.4X6
hydroxide						
colloidal	T45.4X1	T45.4X2	T45.4X3	T45.4X4	T45.4X5	T45.4X6
polymaltose	T45.4X1	T45.4X2	T45.4X3	T45.4X4	T45.4X5	T45.4X6
pyrophosphate	T45.4X1	T45.4X2	T45.4X3	T45.4X4	T45.4X5	T45.4X6
Ferritin	T45.4X1	T45.4X2	T45.4X3	T45.4X4	T45.4X5	T45.4X6
Ferrocholinate	T45.4X1	T45.4X2	T45.4X3	T45.4X4	T45.4X5	T45.4X6
Ferrodextrane	T45.4X1	T45.4X2	T45.4X3	T45.4X4	T45.4X5	T45.4X6
Ferropolimaler	T45.4X1	T45.4X2	T45.4X3	T45.4X4	T45.4X5	T45.4X6
Ferrous — *see also* Iron						
phosphate	T45.4X1	T45.4X2	T45.4X3	T45.4X4	T45.4X5	T45.4X6
salt	T45.4X1	T45.4X2	T45.4X3	T45.4X4	T45.4X5	T45.4X6
with folic acid	T45.4X1	T45.4X2	T45.4X3	T45.4X4	T45.4X5	T45.4X6
Ferrous fumerate, gluconate, lactate, salt NEC, sulfate (medicinal)	T45.4X1	T45.4X2	T45.4X3	T45.4X4	T45.4X5	T45.4X6
Ferrovanadium (fumes)	T59.891	T59.892	T59.893	T59.894	—	—
Ferrum — *see* Iron						
Fertilizers NEC	T65.891	T65.892	T65.893	T65.894	—	—
with herbicide mixture	T6Ø.3X1	T6Ø.3X2	T6Ø.3X3	T6Ø.3X4	—	—
Fetoxilate	T47.6X1	T47.6X2	T47.6X3	T47.6X4	T47.6X5	T47.6X6
Fiber, dietary	T47.4X1	T47.4X2	T47.4X3	T47.4X4	T47.4X5	T47.4X6
Fiberglass	T65.831	T65.832	T65.833	T65.834	—	—
Fibrinogen (human)	T45.8X1	T45.8X2	T45.8X3	T45.8X4	T45.8X5	T45.8X6
Fibrinolysin (human)	T45.691	T45.692	T45.693	T45.694	T45.695	T45.696
Fibrinolysis						
affecting drug	T45.6Ø1	T45.6Ø2	T45.6Ø3	T45.6Ø4	T45.6Ø5	T45.6Ø6
inhibitor NEC	T45.621	T45.622	T45.623	T45.624	T45.625	T45.626
Fibrinolytic drug	T45.611	T45.612	T45.613	T45.614	T45.615	T45.616
Filix mas	T37.4X1	T37.4X2	T37.4X3	T37.4X4	T37.4X5	T37.4X6
Filtering cream	T49.3X1	T49.3X2	T49.3X3	T49.3X4	T49.3X5	T49.3X6
Finacea*	T49.ØX1	T49.ØX2	T49.ØX3	T49.ØX4	T49.ØX5	T49.ØX6
Fiorinal	T39.Ø11	T39.Ø12	T39.Ø13	T39.Ø14	T39.Ø15	T39.Ø16
Firedamp	T59.891	T59.892	T59.893	T59.894	—	—
Fish, noxious, nonbacterial	T61.91	T61.92	T61.93	T61.94	—	—
ciguatera	T61.Ø1	T61.Ø2	T61.Ø3	T61.Ø4	—	—
scombroid	T61.11	T61.12	T61.13	T61.14	—	—
shell	T61.781	T61.782	T61.783	T61.784	—	—
specified NEC	T61.771	T61.772	T61.773	T61.774	—	—
Flagyl	T37.3X1	T37.3X2	T37.3X3	T37.3X4	T37.3X5	T37.3X6
Flavine adenine dinucleotide	T45.2X1	T45.2X2	T45.2X3	T45.2X4	T45.2X5	T45.2X6
Flavodic acid	T46.991	T46.992	T46.993	T46.994	T46.995	T46.996
Flavoxate	T44.3X1	T44.3X2	T44.3X3	T44.3X4	T44.3X5	T44.3X6
Flaxedil	T48.1X1	T48.1X2	T48.1X3	T48.1X4	T48.1X5	T48.1X6
Flaxseed (medicinal)	T49.3X1	T49.3X2	T49.3X3	T49.3X4	T49.3X5	T49.3X6
Flecainide	T46.2X1	T46.2X2	T46.2X3	T46.2X4	T46.2X5	T46.2X6
Fleroxacin	T36.8X1	T36.8X2	T36.8X3	T36.8X4	T36.8X5	T36.8X6
Floctafenine	T39.8X1	T39.8X2	T39.8X3	T39.8X4	T39.8X5	T39.8X6
Flomax	T44.6X1	T44.6X2	T44.6X3	T44.6X4	T44.6X5	T44.6X6
Flomoxef	T36.1X1	T36.1X2	T36.1X3	T36.1X4	T36.1X5	T36.1X6
Flonase*	T49.6X1	T49.6X2	T49.6X3	T49.6X4	T49.6X5	T49.6X6
Flopropione	T44.3X1	T44.3X2	T44.3X3	T44.3X4	T44.3X5	T44.3X6
FLORAjen*	T47.6X1	T47.6X2	T47.6X3	T47.6X4	T47.6X5	T47.6X6
Florantyrone	T47.5X1	T47.5X2	T47.5X3	T47.5X4	T47.5X5	T47.5X6
Floraquin	T37.8X1	T37.8X2	T37.8X3	T37.8X4	T37.8X5	T37.8X6
Florinef	T38.ØX1	T38.ØX2	T38.ØX3	T38.ØX4	T38.ØX5	T38.ØX6
ENT agent	T49.6X1	T49.6X2	T49.6X3	T49.6X4	T49.6X5	T49.6X6
ophthalmic preparation	T49.5X1	T49.5X2	T49.5X3	T49.5X4	T49.5X5	T49.5X6
topical NEC	T49.ØX1	T49.ØX2	T49.ØX3	T49.ØX4	T49.ØX5	T49.ØX6
Flovent*	T38.ØX1	T38.ØX2	T38.ØX3	T38.ØX4	T38.ØX5	T38.ØX6
Flowers of sulfur	T49.4X1	T49.4X2	T49.4X3	T49.4X4	T49.4X5	T49.4X6
Floxuridine	T45.1X1	T45.1X2	T45.1X3	T45.1X4	T45.1X5	T45.1X6
Fluanisone	T43.4X1	T43.4X2	T43.4X3	T43.4X4	T43.4X5	T43.4X6
Flubendazole	T37.4X1	T37.4X2	T37.4X3	T37.4X4	T37.4X5	T37.4X6
Fluclorolone acetonide	T49.ØX1	T49.ØX2	T49.ØX3	T49.ØX4	T49.ØX5	T49.ØX6
Flucloxacillin	T36.ØX1	T36.ØX2	T36.ØX3	T36.ØX4	T36.ØX5	T36.ØX6
Fluconazole	T37.8X1	T37.8X2	T37.8X3	T37.8X4	T37.8X5	T37.8X6
Flucytosine	T37.8X1	T37.8X2	T37.8X3	T37.8X4	T37.8X5	T37.8X6
Fludeoxyglucose (18F)	T5Ø.8X1	T5Ø.8X2	T5Ø.8X3	T5Ø.8X4	T5Ø.8X5	T5Ø.8X6
Fludiazepam	T42.4X1	T42.4X2	T42.4X3	T42.4X4	T42.4X5	T42.4X6
Fludrocortisone	T5Ø.ØX1	T5Ø.ØX2	T5Ø.ØX3	T5Ø.ØX4	T5Ø.ØX5	T5Ø.ØX6
ENT agent	T49.6X1	T49.6X2	T49.6X3	T49.6X4	T49.6X5	T49.6X6
ophthalmic preparation	T49.5X1	T49.5X2	T49.5X3	T49.5X4	T49.5X5	T49.5X6
topical NEC	T49.ØX1	T49.ØX2	T49.ØX3	T49.ØX4	T49.ØX5	T49.ØX6
Fludroxycortide	T49.ØX1	T49.ØX2	T49.ØX3	T49.ØX4	T49.ØX5	T49.ØX6
Flufenamic acid	T39.391	T39.392	T39.393	T39.394	T39.395	T39.396
Fluindione	T45.511	T45.512	T45.513	T45.514	T45.515	T45.516
Flumequine	T37.8X1	T37.8X2	T37.8X3	T37.8X4	T37.8X5	T37.8X6
Flumethasone	T49.ØX1	T49.ØX2	T49.ØX3	T49.ØX4	T49.ØX5	T49.ØX6
Flumethiazide	T5Ø.2X1	T5Ø.2X2	T5Ø.2X3	T5Ø.2X4	T5Ø.2X5	T5Ø.2X6
Flumidin	T37.5X1	T37.5X2	T37.5X3	T37.5X4	T37.5X5	T37.5X6
Flunarizine	T46.7X1	T46.7X2	T46.7X3	T46.7X4	T46.7X5	T46.7X6
Flunidazole	T37.8X1	T37.8X2	T37.8X3	T37.8X4	T37.8X5	T37.8X6
Flunisolide	T48.6X1	T48.6X2	T48.6X3	T48.6X4	T48.6X5	T48.6X6
Flunitrazepam	T42.4X1	T42.4X2	T42.4X3	T42.4X4	T42.4X5	T42.4X6
Fluocinolone (acetonide)	T49.ØX1	T49.ØX2	T49.ØX3	T49.ØX4	T49.ØX5	T49.ØX6
Fluocinonide	T49.ØX1	T49.ØX2	T49.ØX3	T49.ØX4	T49.ØX5	T49.ØX6
Fluocortin (butyl)	T49.ØX1	T49.ØX2	T49.ØX3	T49.ØX4	T49.ØX5	T49.ØX6
Fluocortolone	T49.ØX1	T49.ØX2	T49.ØX3	T49.ØX4	T49.ØX5	T49.ØX6
Fluohydrocortisone	T38.ØX1	T38.ØX2	T38.ØX3	T38.ØX4	T38.ØX5	T38.ØX6
ENT agent	T49.6X1	T49.6X2	T49.6X3	T49.6X4	T49.6X5	T49.6X6
ophthalmic preparation	T49.5X1	T49.5X2	T49.5X3	T49.5X4	T49.5X5	T49.5X6
topical NEC	T49.ØX1	T49.ØX2	T49.ØX3	T49.ØX4	T49.ØX5	T49.ØX6
Fluonid	T49.ØX1	T49.ØX2	T49.ØX3	T49.ØX4	T49.ØX5	T49.ØX6
Fluopromazine	T43.3X1	T43.3X2	T43.3X3	T43.3X4	T43.3X5	T43.3X6
Fluoracetate	T6Ø.8X1	T6Ø.8X2	T6Ø.8X3	T6Ø.8X4	—	—
Fluorescein	T5Ø.8X1	T5Ø.8X2	T5Ø.8X3	T5Ø.8X4	T5Ø.8X5	T5Ø.8X6
Fluorhydrocortisone	T5Ø.ØX1	T5Ø.ØX2	T5Ø.ØX3	T5Ø.ØX4	T5Ø.ØX5	T5Ø.ØX6
Fluoride (nonmedicinal) (pesticide) (sodium) **NEC**	T6Ø.8X1	T6Ø.8X2	T6Ø.8X3	T6Ø.8X4	—	—
hydrogen — *see* Hydrofluoric acid						
medicinal NEC	T5Ø.991	T5Ø.992	T5Ø.993	T5Ø.994	T5Ø.995	T5Ø.996
dental use	T49.7X1	T49.7X2	T49.7X3	T49.7X4	T49.7X5	T49.7X6
not pesticide NEC	T54.91	T54.92	T54.93	T54.94	—	—
stannous	T49.7X1	T49.7X2	T49.7X3	T49.7X4	T49.7X5	T49.7X6
Fluorigard*	T47.7X1	T47.7X2	T47.7X3	T47.7X4	T47.7X5	T47.7X6
Fluorinated corticosteroids	T38.ØX1	T38.ØX2	T38.ØX3	T38.ØX4	T38.ØX5	T38.ØX6
Fluorine (gas)	T59.5X1	T59.5X2	T59.5X3	T59.5X4	—	—
salt — *see* Fluoride(s)						
Fluoristan	T49.7X1	T49.7X2	T49.7X3	T49.7X4	T49.7X5	T49.7X6
Fluormetholone	T49.ØX1	T49.ØX2	T49.ØX3	T49.ØX4	T49.ØX5	T49.ØX6
Fluoroacetate	T6Ø.8X1	T6Ø.8X2	T6Ø.8X3	T6Ø.8X4	—	—
Fluorocarbon monomer	T53.6X1	T53.6X2	T53.6X3	T53.6X4	—	—
Fluorocytosine	T37.8X1	T37.8X2	T37.8X3	T37.8X4	T37.8X5	T37.8X6
Fluorodeoxyuridine	T45.1X1	T45.1X2	T45.1X3	T45.1X4	T45.1X5	T45.1X6
Fluorometholone	T49.ØX1	T49.ØX2	T49.ØX3	T49.ØX4	T49.ØX5	T49.ØX6
ophthalmic preparation	T49.5X1	T49.5X2	T49.5X3	T49.5X4	T49.5X5	T49.5X6
Fluorophosphate insecticide	T6Ø.ØX1	T6Ø.ØX2	T6Ø.ØX3	T6Ø.ØX4	—	—
Fluoroquinolone antibiotics	T36.AX1	T36.AX2	T36.AX3	T36.AX4	T36.AX5	T36.AX6
Fluorosol	T46.3X1	T46.3X2	T46.3X3	T46.3X4	T46.3X5	T46.3X6
Fluorouracil	T45.1X1	T45.1X2	T45.1X3	T45.1X4	T45.1X5	T45.1X6
Fluorphenylalanine	T49.5X1	T49.5X2	T49.5X3	T49.5X4	T49.5X5	T49.5X6
Fluothane	T41.ØX1	T41.ØX2	T41.ØX3	T41.ØX4	T41.ØX5	T41.ØX6
Fluoxetine	T43.221	T43.222	T43.223	T43.224	T43.225	T43.226
Fluoxymesterone	T38.7X1	T38.7X2	T38.7X3	T38.7X4	T38.7X5	T38.7X6
Flupenthixol	T43.4X1	T43.4X2	T43.4X3	T43.4X4	T43.4X5	T43.4X6
Flupentixol	T43.4X1	T43.4X2	T43.4X3	T43.4X4	T43.4X5	T43.4X6
Fluphenazine	T43.3X1	T43.3X2	T43.3X3	T43.3X4	T43.3X5	T43.3X6
Fluprednidene	T49.ØX1	T49.ØX2	T49.ØX3	T49.ØX4	T49.ØX5	T49.ØX6
Fluprednisolone	T38.ØX1	T38.ØX2	T38.ØX3	T38.ØX4	T38.ØX5	T38.ØX6
Fluradoline	T39.8X1	T39.8X2	T39.8X3	T39.8X4	T39.8X5	T39.8X6
Flurandrenolide	T49.ØX1	T49.ØX2	T49.ØX3	T49.ØX4	T49.ØX5	T49.ØX6
Flurandrenolone	T49.ØX1	T49.ØX2	T49.ØX3	T49.ØX4	T49.ØX5	T49.ØX6
Flurazepam	T42.4X1	T42.4X2	T42.4X3	T42.4X4	T42.4X5	T42.4X6
Flurbiprofen	T39.311	T39.312	T39.313	T39.314	T39.315	T39.316
Flurobate	T49.ØX1	T49.ØX2	T49.ØX3	T49.ØX4	T49.ØX5	T49.ØX6
Fluroxene	T41.ØX1	T41.ØX2	T41.ØX3	T41.ØX4	T41.ØX5	T41.ØX6
Fluspirilene	T43.591	T43.592	T43.593	T43.594	T43.595	T43.596

*Optum Value-Add

☑ Additional Character May Be Required — Refer to the Tabular List for Character Selection 381

Substance	Poisoning, Accidental (unintentional)	Poisoning, Intentional Self-harm	Poisoning, Assault	Poisoning, Undetermined	Adverse Effect	Underdosing
Flutamide	T38.6X1	T38.6X2	T38.6X3	T38.6X4	T38.6X5	T38.6X6
Flutazolam	T38.0X1	T38.0X2	T38.0X3	T38.0X4	T38.0X5	T38.0X6
Fluticasone propionate	T38.0X1	T38.0X2	T38.0X3	T38.0X4	T38.0X5	T38.0X6
Flutoprazepam	T42.4X1	T42.4X2	T42.4X3	T42.4X4	T42.4X5	T42.4X6
Flutropium bromide	T48.6X1	T48.6X2	T48.6X3	T48.6X4	T48.6X5	T48.6X6
Fluvoxamine	T43.221	T43.222	T43.223	T43.224	T43.225	T43.226
Folacin	T45.8X1	T45.8X2	T45.8X3	T45.8X4	T45.8X5	T45.8X6
Folic acid	T45.8X1	T45.8X2	T45.8X3	T45.8X4	T45.8X5	T45.8X6
antagonist	T45.1X1	T45.1X2	T45.1X3	T45.1X4	T45.1X5	T45.1X6
with ferrous salt	T45.2X1	T45.2X2	T45.2X3	T45.2X4	T45.2X5	T45.2X6
Folinic acid	T45.8X1	T45.8X2	T45.8X3	T45.8X4	T45.8X5	T45.8X6
Folium stramoniae	T48.6X1	T48.6X2	T48.6X3	T48.6X4	T48.6X5	T48.6X6
Follicle-stimulating hormone, human	T38.811	T38.812	T38.813	T38.814	T38.815	T38.816
Folpet	T60.3X1	T60.3X2	T60.3X3	T60.3X4	—	—
Fomepizole*	T50.6X1	T50.6X2	T50.6X3	T50.6X4	T50.6X5	T50.6X6
Fominoben	T48.3X1	T48.3X2	T48.3X3	T48.3X4	T48.3X5	T48.3X6
Food, foodstuffs, noxious, nonbacterial, NEC	T62.91	T62.92	T62.93	T62.94	—	—
berries	T62.1X1	T62.1X2	T62.1X3	T62.1X4	—	—
fish — *see also* Fish	T61.91	T61.92	T61.93	T61.94	—	—
mushrooms	T62.0X1	T62.0X2	T62.0X3	T62.0X4	—	—
plants	T62.2X1	T62.2X2	T62.2X3	T62.2X4	—	—
seafood	T61.91	T61.92	T61.93	T61.94	—	—
specified NEC	T61.8X1	T61.8X2	T61.8X3	T61.8X4	—	—
seeds	T62.2X1	T62.2X2	T62.2X3	T62.2X4	—	—
shellfish	T61.781	T61.782	T61.783	T61.784	—	—
specified NEC	T62.8X1	T62.8X2	T62.8X3	T62.8X4	—	—
Fool's parsley	T62.2X1	T62.2X2	T62.2X3	T62.2X4	—	—
Formaldehyde (solution), gas or vapor	T59.2X1	T59.2X2	T59.2X3	T59.2X4	—	—
fungicide	T60.3X1	T60.3X2	T60.3X3	T60.3X4	—	—
Formalin	T59.2X1	T59.2X2	T59.2X3	T59.2X4	—	—
fungicide	T60.3X1	T60.3X2	T60.3X3	T60.3X4	—	—
vapor	T59.2X1	T59.2X2	T59.2X3	T59.2X4	—	—
Formic acid	T54.2X1	T54.2X2	T54.2X3	T54.2X4	—	—
vapor	T59.891	T59.892	T59.893	T59.894	—	—
Formoterol*	T48.6X1	T48.6X2	T48.6X3	T48.6X4	T48.6X5	T48.6X6
Fortaz*	T36.1X1	T36.1X2	T36.1X3	T36.1X4	T36.1X5	T36.1X6
Foscarnet sodium	T37.5X1	T37.5X2	T37.5X3	T37.5X4	T37.5X5	T37.5X6
Fosfestrol	T38.5X1	T38.5X2	T38.5X3	T38.5X4	T38.5X5	T38.5X6
Fosfomycin	T36.8X1	T36.8X2	T36.8X3	T36.8X4	T36.8X5	T36.8X6
Fosfonet sodium	T37.5X1	T37.5X2	T37.5X3	T37.5X4	T37.5X5	T37.5X6
Fosinopril	T46.4X1	T46.4X2	T46.4X3	T46.4X4	T46.4X5	T46.4X6
sodium	T46.4X1	T46.4X2	T46.4X3	T46.4X4	T46.4X5	T46.4X6
Fowler's solution	T57.0X1	T57.0X2	T57.0X3	T57.0X4	—	—
Foxglove	T62.2X1	T62.2X2	T62.2X3	T62.2X4	—	—
Framycetin	T36.5X1	T36.5X2	T36.5X3	T36.5X4	T36.5X5	T36.5X6
Frangula	T47.2X1	T47.2X2	T47.2X3	T47.2X4	T47.2X5	T47.2X6
extract	T47.2X1	T47.2X2	T47.2X3	T47.2X4	T47.2X5	T47.2X6
Frei antigen	T50.8X1	T50.8X2	T50.8X3	T50.8X4	T50.8X5	T50.8X6
Freon	T53.5X1	T53.5X2	T53.5X3	T53.5X4	—	—
Fructose	T50.3X1	T50.3X2	T50.3X3	T50.3X4	T50.3X5	T50.3X6
Frusemide	T50.1X1	T50.1X2	T50.1X3	T50.1X4	T50.1X5	T50.1X6
FSH	T38.811	T38.812	T38.813	T38.814	T38.815	T38.816
Ftorafur	T45.1X1	T45.1X2	T45.1X3	T45.1X4	T45.1X5	T45.1X6
Fuel						
automobile	T52.0X1	T52.0X2	T52.0X3	T52.0X4	—	—
exhaust gas, not in transit	T58.01	T58.02	T58.03	T58.04	—	—
vapor NEC	T52.0X1	T52.0X2	T52.0X3	T52.0X4	—	—
gas (domestic use) — *see also* Carbon, monoxide, fuel, utility	T59.891	T59.892	T59.893	T59.894	—	—
utility	T59.891	T59.892	T59.893	T59.894	—	—
in mobile container	T59.891	T59.892	T59.893	T59.894	—	—
incomplete combustion of — *see* Carbon, monoxide, fuel, utility						
piped (natural)	T59.891	T59.892	T59.893	T59.894	—	—
industrial, incomplete combustion	T58.8X1	T58.8X2	T58.8X3	T58.8X4	—	—
Fugillin	T36.8X1	T36.8X2	T36.8X3	T36.8X4	T36.8X5	T36.8X6
Fulminate of mercury	T56.1X1	T56.1X2	T56.1X3	T56.1X4	—	—
Fulvicin	T36.7X1	T36.7X2	T36.7X3	T36.7X4	T36.7X5	T36.7X6
Fumadil	T36.8X1	T36.8X2	T36.8X3	T36.8X4	T36.8X5	T36.8X6
Fumagillin	T36.8X1	T36.8X2	T36.8X3	T36.8X4	T36.8X5	T36.8X6
Fumaric acid	T49.4X1	T49.4X2	T49.4X3	T49.4X4	T49.4X5	T49.4X6
Fumes (from)	T59.91	T59.92	T59.93	T59.94	—	—
carbon monoxide — *see* Carbon, monoxide						
charcoal (domestic use) — *see* Charcoal, fumes						
Fumes — *continued*						
chloroform — *see* Chloroform						
coke (in domestic stoves, fireplaces) — *see* Coke fumes						
corrosive NEC	T54.91	T54.92	T54.93	T54.94	—	—
ether — *see* ether						
freons	T53.5X1	T53.5X2	T53.5X3	T53.5X4	—	—
hydrocarbons	T59.891	T59.892	T59.893	T59.894	—	—
petroleum (liquefied)	T59.891	T59.892	T59.893	T59.894	—	—
distributed through pipes (pure or mixed with air)	T59.891	T59.892	T59.893	T59.894	—	—
lead — *see* lead						
metal — *see* Metals, or the specified metal						
nitrogen dioxide	T59.0X1	T59.0X2	T59.0X3	T59.0X4	—	—
pesticides — *see* Pesticides						
petroleum (liquefied)	T59.891	T59.892	T59.893	T59.894	—	—
distributed through pipes (pure or mixed with air)	T59.891	T59.892	T59.893	T59.894	—	—
polyester	T59.891	T59.892	T59.893	T59.894	—	—
specified source NEC — *see also* substance specified	T59.891	T59.892	T59.893	T59.894	—	—
sulfur dioxide	T59.1X1	T59.1X2	T59.1X3	T59.1X4	—	—
Fumigant NEC	T60.91	T60.92	T60.93	T60.94	—	—
Fungi, noxious, used as food	T62.0X1	T62.0X2	T62.0X3	T62.0X4	—	—
Fungicide NEC (nonmedicinal)	T60.3X1	T60.3X2	T60.3X3	T60.3X4	—	—
Fungizone	T36.7X1	T36.7X2	T36.7X3	T36.7X4	T36.7X5	T36.7X6
topical	T49.0X1	T49.0X2	T49.0X3	T49.0X4	T49.0X5	T49.0X6
Fungoid*	T49.0X1	T49.0X2	T49.0X3	T49.0X4	T49.0X5	T49.0X6
Furacin	T49.0X1	T49.0X2	T49.0X3	T49.0X4	T49.0X5	T49.0X6
Furadantin	T37.91	T37.92	T37.93	T37.94	T37.95	T37.96
Furazolidone	T37.8X1	T37.8X2	T37.8X3	T37.8X4	T37.8X5	T37.8X6
Furazolium chloride	T49.0X1	T49.0X2	T49.0X3	T49.0X4	T49.0X5	T49.0X6
Furfural	T52.8X1	T52.8X2	T52.8X3	T52.8X4	—	—
Furnace (coal burning) (domestic), gas from	T58.2X1	T58.2X2	T58.2X3	T58.2X4	—	—
industrial	T58.8X1	T58.8X2	T58.8X3	T58.8X4	—	—
Furniture polish	T65.891	T65.892	T65.893	T65.894	—	—
Furosemide	T50.1X1	T50.1X2	T50.1X3	T50.1X4	T50.1X5	T50.1X6
Furoxone	T37.91	T37.92	T37.93	T37.94	T37.95	T37.96
Fursultiamine	T45.2X1	T45.2X2	T45.2X3	T45.2X4	T45.2X5	T45.2X6
Fusafungine	T36.8X1	T36.8X2	T36.8X3	T36.8X4	T36.8X5	T36.8X6
Fusel oil (any) (amyl) (butyl) (propyl), vapor	T51.3X1	T51.3X2	T51.3X3	T51.3X4	—	—
Fusidate (ethanolamine) (sodium)	T36.8X1	T36.8X2	T36.8X3	T36.8X4	T36.8X5	T36.8X6
Fusidic acid	T36.8X1	T36.8X2	T36.8X3	T36.8X4	T36.8X5	T36.8X6
Fytic acid, nonasodium	T50.6X1	T50.6X2	T50.6X3	T50.6X4	T50.6X5	T50.6X6
GABA	T43.8X1	T43.8X2	T43.8X3	T43.8X4	T43.8X5	T43.8X6
Gabapentin*	T42.6X1	T42.6X2	T42.6X3	T42.6X4	T42.6X5	T42.6X6
Gabitril*	T42.6X1	T42.6X2	T42.6X3	T42.6X4	T42.6X5	T42.6X6
Gadolinium	T56.821	T56.822	T56.823	T56.824	—	—
Gadopentetic acid	T50.8X1	T50.8X2	T50.8X3	T50.8X4	T50.8X5	T50.8X6
Galactose	T50.3X1	T50.3X2	T50.3X3	T50.3X4	T50.3X5	T50.3X6
Galantamine	T44.0X1	T44.0X2	T44.0X3	T44.0X4	T44.0X5	T44.0X6
Gallamine (triethiodide)	T48.1X1	T48.1X2	T48.1X3	T48.1X4	T48.1X5	T48.1X6
Gallium citrate	T50.991	T50.992	T50.993	T50.994	T50.995	T50.996
Gallopamil	T46.1X1	T46.1X2	T46.1X3	T46.1X4	T46.1X5	T46.1X6
Gamboge	T47.2X1	T47.2X2	T47.2X3	T47.2X4	T47.2X5	T47.2X6
Gamimune	T50.Z11	T50.Z12	T50.Z13	T50.Z14	T50.Z15	T50.Z16
Gamma-aminobutyric acid	T43.8X1	T43.8X2	T43.8X3	T43.8X4	T43.8X5	T43.8X6
Gamma-benzene hexachloride (medicinal)	T49.0X1	T49.0X2	T49.0X3	T49.0X4	T49.0X5	T49.0X6
nonmedicinal, vapor	T53.6X1	T53.6X2	T53.6X3	T53.6X4	—	—
Gamma-BHC (medicinal) — *see also* Gamma-benzene hexachloride	T49.0X1	T49.0X2	T49.0X3	T49.0X4	T49.0X5	T49.0X6
Gamma globulin	T50.Z11	T50.Z12	T50.Z13	T50.Z14	T50.Z15	T50.Z16
Gamulin	T50.Z11	T50.Z12	T50.Z13	T50.Z14	T50.Z15	T50.Z16
Ganciclovir (sodium)	T37.5X1	T37.5X2	T37.5X3	T37.5X4	T37.5X5	T37.5X6
Ganglionic blocking drug NEC	T44.2X1	T44.2X2	T44.2X3	T44.2X4	T44.2X5	T44.2X6
specified NEC	T44.2X1	T44.2X2	T44.2X3	T44.2X4	T44.2X5	T44.2X6
Ganja	T40.711	T40.712	T40.713	T40.714	T40.715	T40.716
Garamycin	T36.5X1	T36.5X2	T36.5X3	T36.5X4	T36.5X5	T36.5X6
ophthalmic preparation	T49.5X1	T49.5X2	T49.5X3	T49.5X4	T49.5X5	T49.5X6
topical NEC	T49.0X1	T49.0X2	T49.0X3	T49.0X4	T49.0X5	T49.0X6
Gardenal	T42.3X1	T42.3X2	T42.3X3	T42.3X4	T42.3X5	T42.3X6

Substance	Poisoning, Accidental (unintentional)	Poisoning, Intentional Self-harm	Poisoning, Assault	Poisoning, Undetermined	Adverse Effect	Under-dosing
Gardepanyl	T42.3X1	T42.3X2	T42.3X3	T42.3X4	T42.3X5	T42.3X6
Gas NEC	T59.91	T59.92	T59.93	T59.94	—	—
acetylene	T59.891	T59.892	T59.893	T59.894	—	—
incomplete combustion of	T58.11	T58.12	T58.13	T58.14	—	—
air contaminants, source or type not specified	T59.91	T59.92	T59.93	T59.94	—	—
anesthetic	T41.0X1	T41.0X2	T41.0X3	T41.0X4	T41.0X5	T41.0X6
blast furnace	T58.8X1	T58.8X2	T58.8X3	T58.8X4	—	—
butane — see butane						
carbon monoxide — see Carbon, monoxide						
chlorine	T59.4X1	T59.4X2	T59.4X3	T59.4X4	—	—
coal	T58.2X1	T58.2X2	T58.2X3	T58.2X4	—	—
cyanide	T57.3X1	T57.3X2	T57.3X3	T57.3X4	—	—
dicyanogen	T65.0X1	T65.0X2	T65.0X3	T65.0X4	—	—
domestic — see Domestic gas						
exhaust	T58.01	T58.02	T58.03	T58.04	—	—
from utility (for cooking, heating, or lighting) (after combustion) — see Carbon, monoxide, fuel, utility						
prior to combustion	T59.891	T59.892	T59.893	T59.894	—	—
from wood- or coal-burning stove or fireplace	T58.2X1	T58.2X2	T58.2X3	T58.2X4	—	—
fuel (domestic use) (after combustion) — see also Carbon, monoxide, fuel						
industrial use	T58.8X1	T58.8X2	T58.8X3	T58.8X4	—	—
prior to combustion	T59.891	T59.892	T59.893	T59.894	—	—
utility	T59.891	T59.892	T59.893	T59.894	—	—
in mobile container	T59.891	T59.892	T59.893	T59.894	—	—
incomplete combustion of — see Carbon, monoxide, fuel, utility						
piped (natural)	T59.891	T59.892	T59.893	T59.894	—	—
garage	T58.01	T58.02	T58.03	T58.04	—	—
hydrocarbon NEC	T59.891	T59.892	T59.893	T59.894	—	—
incomplete combustion of — see Carbon, monoxide, fuel, utility						
liquefied — see butane						
piped	T59.891	T59.892	T59.893	T59.894	—	—
hydrocyanic acid	T65.0X1	T65.0X2	T65.0X3	T65.0X4	—	—
illuminating (after combustion)	T58.11	T58.12	T58.13	T58.14	—	—
prior to combustion	T59.891	T59.892	T59.893	T59.894	—	—
incomplete combustion, any — see Carbon, monoxide						
kiln	T58.8X1	T58.8X2	T58.8X3	T58.8X4	—	—
lacrimogenic	T59.3X1	T59.3X2	T59.3X3	T59.3X4	—	—
liquefied petroleum — see butane						
marsh	T59.891	T59.892	T59.893	T59.894	—	—
motor exhaust, not in transit	T58.01	T58.02	T58.03	T58.04	—	—
mustard, not in war	T59.891	T59.892	T59.893	T59.894	—	—
natural	T59.891	T59.892	T59.893	T59.894	—	—
nerve, not in war	T59.91	T59.92	T59.93	T59.94	—	—
oil	T52.0X1	T52.0X2	T52.0X3	T52.0X4	—	—
petroleum (liquefied) (distributed in mobile containers)	T59.891	T59.892	T59.893	T59.894	—	—
piped (pure or mixed with air)	T59.891	T59.892	T59.893	T59.894	—	—
piped (manufactured) (natural) NEC	T59.891	T59.892	T59.893	T59.894	—	—
producer	T58.8X1	T58.8X2	T58.8X3	T58.8X4	—	—
propane — see propane						
refrigerant	T53.5X1	T53.5X2	T53.5X3	T53.5X4	—	—
(chlorofluoro-carbon)						
not chlorofluoro-carbon	T59.891	T59.892	T59.893	T59.894	—	—
sewer	T59.91	T59.92	T59.93	T59.94	—	—
specified source NEC	T59.91	T59.92	T59.93	T59.94	—	—
stove (after combustion)	T58.11	T58.12	T58.13	T58.14	—	—
prior to combustion	T59.891	T59.892	T59.893	T59.894	—	—
tear	T59.3X1	T59.3X2	T59.3X3	T59.3X4	—	—
therapeutic	T41.5X1	T41.5X2	T41.5X3	T41.5X4	T41.5X5	T41.5X6
utility (for cooking, heating, or lighting) (piped) NEC	T59.891	T59.892	T59.893	T59.894	—	—
in mobile container	T59.891	T59.892	T59.893	T59.894	—	—
Gas — continued						
utility — continued						
incomplete combustion of — see Carbon, monoxide, fuel, utility						
piped (natural)	T59.891	T59.892	T59.893	T59.894	—	—
water	T58.11	T58.12	T58.13	T58.14	—	—
incomplete combustion of — see Carbon, monoxide, fuel, utility						
Gaseous substance — see Gas						
Gasoline	T52.0X1	T52.0X2	T52.0X3	T52.0X4	—	—
vapor	T52.0X1	T52.0X2	T52.0X3	T52.0X4	—	—
Gastric enzymes	T47.5X1	T47.5X2	T47.5X3	T47.5X4	T47.5X5	T47.5X6
Gastrografin	T50.8X1	T50.8X2	T50.8X3	T50.8X4	T50.8X5	T50.8X6
Gastrointestinal drug	T47.91	T47.92	T47.93	T47.94	T47.95	T47.96
biological	T47.8X1	T47.8X2	T47.8X3	T47.8X4	T47.8X5	T47.8X6
specified NEC	T47.8X1	T47.8X2	T47.8X3	T47.8X4	T47.8X5	T47.8X6
Gaultheria procumbens	T62.2X1	T62.2X2	T62.2X3	T62.2X4	—	—
Gaviscon*	T47.1X1	T47.1X2	T47.1X3	T47.1X4	T47.1X5	T47.1X6
Gefarnate	T44.3X1	T44.3X2	T44.3X3	T44.3X4	T44.3X5	T44.3X6
Gelatin (intravenous)	T45.8X1	T45.8X2	T45.8X3	T45.8X4	T45.8X5	T45.8X6
absorbable (sponge)	T45.7X1	T45.7X2	T45.7X3	T45.7X4	T45.7X5	T45.7X6
Gelfilm	T49.8X1	T49.8X2	T49.8X3	T49.8X4	T49.8X5	T49.8X6
Gelfoam	T45.7X1	T45.7X2	T45.7X3	T45.7X4	T45.7X5	T45.7X6
Gelsemine	T50.991	T50.992	T50.993	T50.994	T50.995	T50.996
Gelsemium (sempervirens)	T62.2X1	T62.2X2	T62.2X3	T62.2X4	—	—
Gemeprost	T48.0X1	T48.0X2	T48.0X3	T48.0X4	T48.0X5	T48.0X6
Gemfibrozil	T46.6X1	T46.6X2	T46.6X3	T46.6X4	T46.6X5	T46.6X6
Gemonil	T42.3X1	T42.3X2	T42.3X3	T42.3X4	T42.3X5	T42.3X6
Gentamicin	T36.5X1	T36.5X2	T36.5X3	T36.5X4	T36.5X5	T36.5X6
ophthalmic preparation	T49.5X1	T49.5X2	T49.5X3	T49.5X4	T49.5X5	T49.5X6
topical NEC	T49.0X1	T49.0X2	T49.0X3	T49.0X4	T49.0X5	T49.0X6
Gentasol*	T49.5X1	T49.5X2	T49.5X3	T49.5X4	T49.5X5	T49.5X6
Gentian	T47.5X1	T47.5X2	T47.5X3	T47.5X4	T47.5X5	T47.5X6
violet	T49.0X1	T49.0X2	T49.0X3	T49.0X4	T49.0X5	T49.0X6
Gepefrine	T44.4X1	T44.4X2	T44.4X3	T44.4X4	T44.4X5	T44.4X6
Gestonorone caproate	T38.5X1	T38.5X2	T38.5X3	T38.5X4	T38.5X5	T38.5X6
Gexane	T49.0X1	T49.0X2	T49.0X3	T49.0X4	T49.0X5	T49.0X6
Gila monster (venom)	T63.111	T63.112	T63.113	T63.114	—	—
Ginger	T47.5X1	T47.5X2	T47.5X3	T47.5X4	T47.5X5	T47.5X6
Jamaica — see Jamaica, ginger						
Gitalin	T46.0X1	T46.0X2	T46.0X3	T46.0X4	T46.0X5	T46.0X6
amorphous	T46.0X1	T46.0X2	T46.0X3	T46.0X4	T46.0X5	T46.0X6
Gitaloxin	T46.0X1	T46.0X2	T46.0X3	T46.0X4	T46.0X5	T46.0X6
Gitoxin	T46.0X1	T46.0X2	T46.0X3	T46.0X4	T46.0X5	T46.0X6
Glafenine	T39.8X1	T39.8X2	T39.8X3	T39.8X4	T39.8X5	T39.8X6
Glandular extract (medicinal) NEC	T50.Z91	T50.Z92	T50.Z93	T50.Z94	T50.Z95	T50.Z96
Glaucarubin	T37.3X1	T37.3X2	T37.3X3	T37.3X4	T37.3X5	T37.3X6
Glibenclamide	T38.3X1	T38.3X2	T38.3X3	T38.3X4	T38.3X5	T38.3X6
Glibornuride	T38.3X1	T38.3X2	T38.3X3	T38.3X4	T38.3X5	T38.3X6
Gliclazide	T38.3X1	T38.3X2	T38.3X3	T38.3X4	T38.3X5	T38.3X6
Glimidine	T38.3X1	T38.3X2	T38.3X3	T38.3X4	T38.3X5	T38.3X6
Glipizide	T38.3X1	T38.3X2	T38.3X3	T38.3X4	T38.3X5	T38.3X6
Gliquidone	T38.3X1	T38.3X2	T38.3X3	T38.3X4	T38.3X5	T38.3X6
Glisolamide	T38.3X1	T38.3X2	T38.3X3	T38.3X4	T38.3X5	T38.3X6
Glisoxepide	T38.3X1	T38.3X2	T38.3X3	T38.3X4	T38.3X5	T38.3X6
Globin zinc insulin	T38.3X1	T38.3X2	T38.3X3	T38.3X4	T38.3X5	T38.3X6
Globulin						
antilymphocytic	T50.Z11	T50.Z12	T50.Z13	T50.Z14	T50.Z15	T50.Z16
antirhesus	T50.Z11	T50.Z12	T50.Z13	T50.Z14	T50.Z15	T50.Z16
antivenin	T50.Z11	T50.Z12	T50.Z13	T50.Z14	T50.Z15	T50.Z16
antiviral	T50.Z11	T50.Z12	T50.Z13	T50.Z14	T50.Z15	T50.Z16
Glucagon	T38.3X1	T38.3X2	T38.3X3	T38.3X4	T38.3X5	T38.3X6
Glucocorticoids	T38.0X1	T38.0X2	T38.0X3	T38.0X4	T38.0X5	T38.0X6
Glucocorticosteroid	T38.0X1	T38.0X2	T38.0X3	T38.0X4	T38.0X5	T38.0X6
Gluconic acid	T50.991	T50.992	T50.993	T50.994	T50.995	T50.996
Glucosamine sulfate	T39.4X1	T39.4X2	T39.4X3	T39.4X4	T39.4X5	T39.4X6
Glucose	T50.3X1	T50.3X2	T50.3X3	T50.3X4	T50.3X5	T50.3X6
with sodium chloride	T50.3X1	T50.3X2	T50.3X3	T50.3X4	T50.3X5	T50.3X6
Glucosulfone sodium	T37.1X1	T37.1X2	T37.1X3	T37.1X4	T37.1X5	T37.1X6
Glucotrol*	T38.3X1	T38.3X2	T38.3X3	T38.3X4	T38.3X5	T38.3X6
Glucurolactone	T47.8X1	T47.8X2	T47.8X3	T47.8X4	T47.8X5	T47.8X6
Glue NEC	T52.8X1	T52.8X2	T52.8X3	T52.8X4	—	—
Glutamic acid	T47.5X1	T47.5X2	T47.5X3	T47.5X4	T47.5X5	T47.5X6
Glutaral (medicinal)	T49.0X1	T49.0X2	T49.0X3	T49.0X4	T49.0X5	T49.0X6
nonmedicinal	T65.891	T65.892	T65.893	T65.894	—	—
Glutaraldehyde (nonmedicinal)	T65.891	T65.892	T65.893	T65.894	—	—
medicinal	T49.0X1	T49.0X2	T49.0X3	T49.0X4	T49.0X5	T49.0X6
Glutathione	T50.6X1	T50.6X2	T50.6X3	T50.6X4	T50.6X5	T50.6X6
Glutethimide	T42.6X1	T42.6X2	T42.6X3	T42.6X4	T42.6X5	T42.6X6

*Optum Value-Add

Substance	Poisoning, Accidental (unintentional)	Poisoning, Intentional Self-harm	Poisoning, Assault	Poisoning, Undetermined	Adverse Effect	Under-dosing
Glyburide	T38.3X1	T38.3X2	T38.3X3	T38.3X4	T38.3X5	T38.3X6
Glycerin	T47.4X1	T47.4X2	T47.4X3	T47.4X4	T47.4X5	T47.4X6
Glycerol	T47.4X1	T47.4X2	T47.4X3	T47.4X4	T47.4X5	T47.4X6
borax	T49.6X1	T49.6X2	T49.6X3	T49.6X4	T49.6X5	T49.6X6
intravenous	T50.3X1	T50.3X2	T50.3X3	T50.3X4	T50.3X5	T50.3X6
iodinated	T48.4X1	T48.4X2	T48.4X3	T48.4X4	T48.4X5	T48.4X6
Glycerophosphate	T50.991	T50.992	T50.993	T50.994	T50.995	T50.996
Glyceryl						
gualacolate	T48.4X1	T48.4X2	T48.4X3	T48.4X4	T48.4X5	T48.4X6
nitrate	T46.3X1	T46.3X2	T46.3X3	T46.3X4	T46.3X5	T46.3X6
triacetate (topical)	T49.0X1	T49.0X2	T49.0X3	T49.0X4	T49.0X5	T49.0X6
trinitrate	T46.3X1	T46.3X2	T46.3X3	T46.3X4	T46.3X5	T46.3X6
Glycine	T50.3X1	T50.3X2	T50.3X3	T50.3X4	T50.3X5	T50.3X6
Glyclopyramide	T38.3X1	T38.3X2	T38.3X3	T38.3X4	T38.3X5	T38.3X6
Glycobiarsol	T37.3X1	T37.3X2	T37.3X3	T37.3X4	T37.3X5	T37.3X6
Glycols (ether)	T52.3X1	T52.3X2	T52.3X3	T52.3X4	—	—
Glyconiazide	T37.1X1	T37.1X2	T37.1X3	T37.1X4	T37.1X5	T37.1X6
Glycopyrrolate	T44.3X1	T44.3X2	T44.3X3	T44.3X4	T44.3X5	T44.3X6
Glycopyrronium	T44.3X1	T44.3X2	T44.3X3	T44.3X4	T44.3X5	T44.3X6
bromide	T44.3X1	T44.3X2	T44.3X3	T44.3X4	T44.3X5	T44.3X6
Glycoside, cardiac (stimulant)	T46.0X1	T46.0X2	T46.0X3	T46.0X4	T46.0X5	T46.0X6
Glycyclamide	T38.3X1	T38.3X2	T38.3X3	T38.3X4	T38.3X5	T38.3X6
Glycyrrhiza extract	T48.4X1	T48.4X2	T48.4X3	T48.4X4	T48.4X5	T48.4X6
Glycyrrhizic acid	T48.4X1	T48.4X2	T48.4X3	T48.4X4	T48.4X5	T48.4X6
Glycyrrhizinate potassium	T48.4X1	T48.4X2	T48.4X3	T48.4X4	T48.4X5	T48.4X6
Glymidine sodium	T38.3X1	T38.3X2	T38.3X3	T38.3X4	T38.3X5	T38.3X6
Glyphosate	T60.3X1	T60.3X2	T60.3X3	T60.3X4	—	—
Glyphylline	T48.6X1	T48.6X2	T48.6X3	T48.6X4	T48.6X5	T48.6X6
Gold						
colloidal (198Au)	T45.1X1	T45.1X2	T45.1X3	T45.1X4	T45.1X5	T45.1X6
salts	T39.4X1	T39.4X2	T39.4X3	T39.4X4	T39.4X5	T39.4X6
Golden sulfide of antimony	T56.891	T56.892	T56.893	T56.894	—	—
Goldylocks	T62.2X1	T62.2X2	T62.2X3	T62.2X4	—	—
Gonadal tissue extract	T38.901	T38.902	T38.903	T38.904	T38.905	T38.906
female	T38.5X1	T38.5X2	T38.5X3	T38.5X4	T38.5X5	T38.5X6
male	T38.7X1	T38.7X2	T38.7X3	T38.7X4	T38.7X5	T38.7X6
Gonadorelin	T38.891	T38.892	T38.893	T38.894	T38.895	T38.896
Gonadotropin	T38.891	T38.892	T38.893	T38.894	T38.895	T38.896
chorionic	T38.891	T38.892	T38.893	T38.894	T38.895	T38.896
pituitary	T38.811	T38.812	T38.813	T38.814	T38.815	T38.816
Goserelin	T45.1X1	T45.1X2	T45.1X3	T45.1X4	T45.1X5	T45.1X6
Grain alcohol	T51.0X1	T51.0X2	T51.0X3	T51.0X4	—	—
Gralise*	T42.6X1	T42.6X2	T42.6X3	T42.6X4	T42.6X5	T42.6X6
Gramicidin	T49.0X1	T49.0X2	T49.0X3	T49.0X4	T49.0X5	T49.0X6
Granisetron	T45.0X1	T45.0X2	T45.0X3	T45.0X4	T45.0X5	T45.0X6
Gratiola officinalis	T62.2X1	T62.2X2	T62.2X3	T62.2X4	—	—
Grease	T65.891	T65.892	T65.893	T65.894	—	—
Green hellebore	T62.2X1	T62.2X2	T62.2X3	T62.2X4	—	—
Green soap	T49.2X1	T49.2X2	T49.2X3	T49.2X4	T49.2X5	T49.2X6
Grifulvin	T36.7X1	T36.7X2	T36.7X3	T36.7X4	T36.7X5	T36.7X6
Griseofulvin	T36.7X1	T36.7X2	T36.7X3	T36.7X4	T36.7X5	T36.7X6
Growth hormone	T38.811	T38.812	T38.813	T38.814	T38.815	T38.816
Guaiac reagent	T50.991	T50.992	T50.993	T50.994	T50.995	T50.996
Guaiacol derivatives	T48.4X1	T48.4X2	T48.4X3	T48.4X4	T48.4X5	T48.4X6
Guaifenesin	T48.4X1	T48.4X2	T48.4X3	T48.4X4	T48.4X5	T48.4X6
Guaimesal	T48.4X1	T48.4X2	T48.4X3	T48.4X4	T48.4X5	T48.4X6
Guaiphenesin	T48.4X1	T48.4X2	T48.4X3	T48.4X4	T48.4X5	T48.4X6
Guaituss*	T48.4X1	T48.4X2	T48.4X3	T48.4X4	T48.4X5	T48.4X6
Guamecycline	T36.4X1	T36.4X2	T36.4X3	T36.4X4	T36.4X5	T36.4X6
Guanabenz	T46.5X1	T46.5X2	T46.5X3	T46.5X4	T46.5X5	T46.5X6
Guanacline	T46.5X1	T46.5X2	T46.5X3	T46.5X4	T46.5X5	T46.5X6
Guanadrel	T46.5X1	T46.5X2	T46.5X3	T46.5X4	T46.5X5	T46.5X6
Guanatol	T37.2X1	T37.2X2	T37.2X3	T37.2X4	T37.2X5	T37.2X6
Guanethidine	T46.5X1	T46.5X2	T46.5X3	T46.5X4	T46.5X5	T46.5X6
Guanfacine	T46.5X1	T46.5X2	T46.5X3	T46.5X4	T46.5X5	T46.5X6
Guano	T65.891	T65.892	T65.893	T65.894	—	—
Guanochlor	T46.5X1	T46.5X2	T46.5X3	T46.5X4	T46.5X5	T46.5X6
Guanoclor	T46.5X1	T46.5X2	T46.5X3	T46.5X4	T46.5X5	T46.5X6
Guanoctine	T46.5X1	T46.5X2	T46.5X3	T46.5X4	T46.5X5	T46.5X6
Guanoxabenz	T46.5X1	T46.5X2	T46.5X3	T46.5X4	T46.5X5	T46.5X6
Guanoxan	T46.5X1	T46.5X2	T46.5X3	T46.5X4	T46.5X5	T46.5X6
Guar gum (medicinal)	T46.6X1	T46.6X2	T46.6X3	T46.6X4	T46.6X5	T46.6X6
Hachimycin	T36.7X1	T36.7X2	T36.7X3	T36.7X4	T36.7X5	T36.7X6
Hair						
dye	T49.4X1	T49.4X2	T49.4X3	T49.4X4	T49.4X5	T49.4X6
preparation NEC	T49.4X1	T49.4X2	T49.4X3	T49.4X4	T49.4X5	T49.4X6
Halazepam	T42.4X1	T42.4X2	T42.4X3	T42.4X4	T42.4X5	T42.4X6
Halcinolone	T49.0X1	T49.0X2	T49.0X3	T49.0X4	T49.0X5	T49.0X6
Halcinonide	T49.0X1	T49.0X2	T49.0X3	T49.0X4	T49.0X5	T49.0X6
Halethazole	T49.0X1	T49.0X2	T49.0X3	T49.0X4	T49.0X5	T49.0X6
Hallucinogen NOS	T40.901	T40.902	T40.903	T40.904	T40.905	T40.906

Substance	Poisoning, Accidental (unintentional)	Poisoning, Intentional Self-harm	Poisoning, Assault	Poisoning, Undetermined	Adverse Effect	Under-dosing
Hallucinogen — *continued*						
specified NEC	T40.991	T40.992	T40.993	T40.994	T40.995	T40.996
Halofantrine	T37.2X1	T37.2X2	T37.2X3	T37.2X4	T37.2X5	T37.2X6
Halofenate	T46.6X1	T46.6X2	T46.6X3	T46.6X4	T46.6X5	T46.6X6
Halometasone	T49.0X1	T49.0X2	T49.0X3	T49.0X4	T49.0X5	T49.0X6
Haloperidol	T43.4X1	T43.4X2	T43.4X3	T43.4X4	T43.4X5	T43.4X6
Haloprogin	T49.0X1	T49.0X2	T49.0X3	T49.0X4	T49.0X5	T49.0X6
Halotex	T49.0X1	T49.0X2	T49.0X3	T49.0X4	T49.0X5	T49.0X6
Halothane	T41.0X1	T41.0X2	T41.0X3	T41.0X4	T41.0X5	T41.0X6
Haloxazolam	T42.4X1	T42.4X2	T42.4X3	T42.4X4	T42.4X5	T42.4X6
Halquinols	T49.0X1	T49.0X2	T49.0X3	T49.0X4	T49.0X5	T49.0X6
Hamamelis	T49.2X1	T49.2X2	T49.2X3	T49.2X4	T49.2X5	T49.2X6
Haptendextran	T45.8X1	T45.8X2	T45.8X3	T45.8X4	T45.8X5	T45.8X6
Harmonyl	T46.5X1	T46.5X2	T46.5X3	T46.5X4	T46.5X5	T46.5X6
Hartmann's solution	T50.3X1	T50.3X2	T50.3X3	T50.3X4	T50.3X5	T50.3X6
Hashish	T40.711	T40.712	T40.713	T40.714	T40.715	T40.716
Havrix*	T50.B91	T50.B92	T50.B93	T50.B94	T50.B95	T50.B96
Hawaiian Woodrose seeds	T40.991	T40.992	T40.993	T40.994	—	—
HCB	T60.3X1	T60.3X2	T60.3X3	T60.3X4	—	—
HCH	T53.6X1	T53.6X2	T53.6X3	T53.6X4	—	—
medicinal	T49.0X1	T49.0X2	T49.0X3	T49.0X4	T49.0X5	T49.0X6
HCN	T57.3X1	T57.3X2	T57.3X3	T57.3X4	—	—
Headache cures, drugs, powders NEC	T50.901	T50.902	T50.903	T50.904	T50.905	T50.906
Heavenly Blue (morning glory)	T40.991	T40.992	T40.993	T40.994	—	—
Heavy metal antidote	T45.8X1	T45.8X2	T45.8X3	T45.8X4	T45.8X5	T45.8X6
Hedaquinium	T49.0X1	T49.0X2	T49.0X3	T49.0X4	T49.0X5	T49.0X6
Hedge hyssop	T62.2X1	T62.2X2	T62.2X3	T62.2X4	—	—
Heet	T49.8X1	T49.8X2	T49.8X3	T49.8X4	T49.8X5	T49.8X6
Helenin	T37.4X1	T37.4X2	T37.4X3	T37.4X4	T37.4X5	T37.4X6
Helium (nonmedicinal) **NEC**	T59.891	T59.892	T59.893	T59.894	—	—
medicinal	T48.991	T48.992	T48.993	T48.994	T48.995	T48.996
Hellebore (black) (green) (white)	T62.2X1	T62.2X2	T62.2X3	T62.2X4	—	—
Hematin	T45.8X1	T45.8X2	T45.8X3	T45.8X4	T45.8X5	T45.8X6
Hematinic preparation	T45.8X1	T45.8X2	T45.8X3	T45.8X4	T45.8X5	T45.8X6
Hematological agent	T45.91	T45.92	T45.93	T45.94	T45.95	T45.96
specified NEC	T45.8X1	T45.8X2	T45.8X3	T45.8X4	T45.8X5	T45.8X6
Hemlock	T62.2X1	T62.2X2	T62.2X3	T62.2X4	—	—
Hemostatic	T45.621	T45.622	T45.623	T45.624	T45.625	T45.626
drug, systemic	T45.621	T45.622	T45.623	T45.624	T45.625	T45.626
Hemostyptic	T49.4X1	T49.4X2	T49.4X3	T49.4X4	T49.4X5	T49.4X6
Henbane	T62.2X1	T62.2X2	T62.2X3	T62.2X4	—	—
Heparin (sodium)	T45.511	T45.512	T45.513	T45.514	T45.515	T45.516
action reverser	T45.7X1	T45.7X2	T45.7X3	T45.7X4	T45.7X5	T45.7X6
Heparin-fraction	T45.511	T45.512	T45.513	T45.514	T45.515	T45.516
Heparinoid (systemic)	T45.511	T45.512	T45.513	T45.514	T45.515	T45.516
Hepatic secretion stimulant	T47.8X1	T47.8X2	T47.8X3	T47.8X4	T47.8X5	T47.8X6
Hepatitis A vaccine*	T50.B91	T50.B92	T50.B93	T50.B94	T50.B95	T50.B96
Hepatitis B						
immune globulin	T50.Z11	T50.Z12	T50.Z13	T50.Z14	T50.Z15	T50.Z16
vaccine	T50.B91	T50.B92	T50.B93	T50.B94	T50.B95	T50.B96
Hepronicate	T46.7X1	T46.7X2	T46.7X3	T46.7X4	T46.7X5	T46.7X6
Heptabarb	T42.3X1	T42.3X2	T42.3X3	T42.3X4	T42.3X5	T42.3X6
Heptabarbital	T42.3X1	T42.3X2	T42.3X3	T42.3X4	T42.3X5	T42.3X6
Heptabarbitone	T42.3X1	T42.3X2	T42.3X3	T42.3X4	T42.3X5	T42.3X6
Heptachlor	T60.1X1	T60.1X2	T60.1X3	T60.1X4	—	—
Heptalgin	T40.2X1	T40.2X2	T40.2X3	T40.2X4	T40.2X5	T40.2X6
Heptaminol	T46.3X1	T46.3X2	T46.3X3	T46.3X4	T46.3X5	T46.3X6
Herbicide NEC	T60.3X1	T60.3X2	T60.3X3	T60.3X4	—	—
Heroin	T40.1X1	T40.1X2	T40.1X3	T40.1X4	—	—
Herplex	T49.5X1	T49.5X2	T49.5X3	T49.5X4	T49.5X5	T49.5X6
HES	T45.8X1	T45.8X2	T45.8X3	T45.8X4	T45.8X5	T45.8X6
Hesperidin	T46.991	T46.992	T46.993	T46.994	T46.995	T46.996
Hetacillin	T36.0X1	T36.0X2	T36.0X3	T36.0X4	T36.0X5	T36.0X6
Hetastarch	T45.8X1	T45.8X2	T45.8X3	T45.8X4	T45.8X5	T45.8X6
HETP	T60.0X1	T60.0X2	T60.0X3	T60.0X4	—	—
Hexa-germ	T49.2X1	T49.2X2	T49.2X3	T49.2X4	T49.2X5	T49.2X6
Hexachlorobenzene (vapor)	T60.3X1	T60.3X2	T60.3X3	T60.3X4	—	—
Hexachlorocyclohexane	T53.6X1	T53.6X2	T53.6X3	T53.6X4	—	—
Hexachlorophene	T49.0X1	T49.0X2	T49.0X3	T49.0X4	T49.0X5	T49.0X6
Hexadiline	T46.3X1	T46.3X2	T46.3X3	T46.3X4	T46.3X5	T46.3X6
Hexadimethrine (bromide)	T45.7X1	T45.7X2	T45.7X3	T45.7X4	T45.7X5	T45.7X6
Hexadylamine	T46.3X1	T46.3X2	T46.3X3	T46.3X4	T46.3X5	T46.3X6
Hexaethyl tetraphosphate	T60.0X1	T60.0X2	T60.0X3	T60.0X4	—	—
Hexafluorenium bromide	T48.1X1	T48.1X2	T48.1X3	T48.1X4	T48.1X5	T48.1X6
Hexafluronium (bromide)	T48.1X1	T48.1X2	T48.1X3	T48.1X4	T48.1X5	T48.1X6
Hexahydrobenzol	T52.8X1	T52.8X2	T52.8X3	T52.8X4	—	—
Hexahydrocresol(s)	T51.8X1	T51.8X2	T51.8X3	T51.8X4	—	—
arsenide	T57.0X1	T57.0X2	T57.0X3	T57.0X4	—	—

Substance	Poisoning, Accidental (unintentional)	Poisoning, Intentional Self-harm	Poisoning, Assault	Poisoning, Undetermined	Adverse Effect	Underdosing
Hexahydrocresol(s) — continued						
arseniurated	T57.0X1	T57.0X2	T57.0X3	T57.0X4	—	—
cyanide	T57.3X1	T57.3X2	T57.3X3	T57.3X4	—	—
gas	T59.891	T59.892	T59.893	T59.894	—	—
Fluoride (liquid)	T57.8X1	T57.8X2	T57.8X3	T57.8X4	—	—
vapor	T59.891	T59.892	T59.893	T59.894	—	—
phophorated	T60.0X1	T60.0X2	T60.0X3	T60.0X4	—	—
sulfate	T57.8X1	T57.8X2	T57.8X3	T57.8X4	—	—
sulfide (gas)	T59.6X1	T59.6X2	T59.6X3	T59.6X4	—	—
arseniurated	T57.0X1	T57.0X2	T57.0X3	T57.0X4	—	—
sulfurated	T57.8X1	T57.8X2	T57.8X3	T57.8X4	—	—
Hexahydrophenol	T51.8X1	T51.8X2	T51.8X3	T51.8X4	—	—
Hexalen	T51.8X1	T51.8X2	T51.8X3	T51.8X4	—	—
Hexamethonium bromide	T44.2X1	T44.2X2	T44.2X3	T44.2X4	T44.2X5	T44.2X6
Hexamethylene	T52.8X1	T52.8X2	T52.8X3	T52.8X4	—	—
Hexamethylmelamine	T45.1X1	T45.1X2	T45.1X3	T45.1X4	T45.1X5	T45.1X6
Hexamidine	T49.0X1	T49.0X2	T49.0X3	T49.0X4	T49.0X5	T49.0X6
Hexamine (mandelate)	T37.8X1	T37.8X2	T37.8X3	T37.8X4	T37.8X5	T37.8X6
Hexanone, 2-hexanone	T52.4X1	T52.4X2	T52.4X3	T52.4X4	—	—
Hexanuorenium	T48.1X1	T48.1X2	T48.1X3	T48.1X4	T48.1X5	T48.1X6
Hexapropymate	T42.6X1	T42.6X2	T42.6X3	T42.6X4	T42.6X5	T42.6X6
Hexasonium iodide	T44.3X1	T44.3X2	T44.3X3	T44.3X4	T44.3X5	T44.3X6
Hexcarbacholine bromide	T48.1X1	T48.1X2	T48.1X3	T48.1X4	T48.1X5	T48.1X6
Hexemal	T42.3X1	T42.3X2	T42.3X3	T42.3X4	T42.3X5	T42.3X6
Hexestrol	T38.5X1	T38.5X2	T38.5X3	T38.5X4	T38.5X5	T38.5X6
Hexethal (sodium)	T42.3X1	T42.3X2	T42.3X3	T42.3X4	T42.3X5	T42.3X6
Hexetidine	T37.8X1	T37.8X2	T37.8X3	T37.8X4	T37.8X5	T37.8X6
Hexobarbital	T42.3X1	T42.3X2	T42.3X3	T42.3X4	T42.3X5	T42.3X6
rectal	T41.291	T41.292	T41.293	T41.294	T41.295	T41.296
sodium	T41.1X1	T41.1X2	T41.1X3	T41.1X4	T41.1X5	T41.1X6
Hexobendine	T46.3X1	T46.3X2	T46.3X3	T46.3X4	T46.3X5	T46.3X6
Hexocyclium	T44.3X1	T44.3X2	T44.3X3	T44.3X4	T44.3X5	T44.3X6
metilsulfate	T44.3X1	T44.3X2	T44.3X3	T44.3X4	T44.3X5	T44.3X6
Hexoestrol	T38.5X1	T38.5X2	T38.5X3	T38.5X4	T38.5X5	T38.5X6
Hexone	T52.4X1	T52.4X2	T52.4X3	T52.4X4	—	—
Hexoprenaline	T48.6X1	T48.6X2	T48.6X3	T48.6X4	T48.6X5	T48.6X6
Hexylcaine	T41.3X1	T41.3X2	T41.3X3	T41.3X4	T41.3X5	T41.3X6
Hexylresorcinol	T52.2X1	T52.2X2	T52.2X3	T52.2X4	—	—
HGH (human growth hormone)	T38.811	T38.812	T38.813	T38.814	T38.815	T38.816
Hibistat*	T49.0X1	T49.0X2	T49.0X3	T49.0X4	T49.0X5	T49.0X6
Hinkle's pills	T47.2X1	T47.2X2	T47.2X3	T47.2X4	T47.2X5	T47.2X6
Histalog	T50.8X1	T50.8X2	T50.8X3	T50.8X4	T50.8X5	T50.8X6
Histamine (phosphate)	T50.8X1	T50.8X2	T50.8X3	T50.8X4	T50.8X5	T50.8X6
Histolyn*	T50.8X1	T50.8X2	T50.8X3	T50.8X4	T50.8X5	T50.8X6
Histoplasmin	T50.8X1	T50.8X2	T50.8X3	T50.8X4	T50.8X5	T50.8X6
Holly berries	T62.2X1	T62.2X2	T62.2X3	T62.2X4	—	—
Homatropine	T44.3X1	T44.3X2	T44.3X3	T44.3X4	T44.3X5	T44.3X6
methylbromide	T44.3X1	T44.3X2	T44.3X3	T44.3X4	T44.3X5	T44.3X6
Homo-tet	T50.Z11	T50.Z12	T50.Z13	T50.Z14	T50.Z15	T50.Z16
Homochlorcyclizine	T45.0X1	T45.0X2	T45.0X3	T45.0X4	T45.0X5	T45.0X6
Homosalate	T49.3X1	T49.3X2	T49.3X3	T49.3X4	T49.3X5	T49.3X6
Hormone	T38.801	T38.802	T38.803	T38.804	T38.805	T38.806
adrenal cortical steroids	T38.0X1	T38.0X2	T38.0X3	T38.0X4	T38.0X5	T38.0X6
androgenic	T38.7X1	T38.7X2	T38.7X3	T38.7X4	T38.7X5	T38.7X6
anterior pituitary NEC	T38.811	T38.812	T38.813	T38.814	T38.815	T38.816
antidiabetic agents	T38.3X1	T38.3X2	T38.3X3	T38.3X4	T38.3X5	T38.3X6
antidiuretic	T38.891	T38.892	T38.893	T38.894	T38.895	T38.896
cancer therapy	T45.1X1	T45.1X2	T45.1X3	T45.1X4	T45.1X5	T45.1X6
follicle stimulating	T38.811	T38.812	T38.813	T38.814	T38.815	T38.816
gonadotropic	T38.891	T38.892	T38.893	T38.894	T38.895	T38.896
pituitary	T38.811	T38.812	T38.813	T38.814	T38.815	T38.816
growth	T38.811	T38.812	T38.813	T38.814	T38.815	T38.816
luteinizing	T38.811	T38.812	T38.813	T38.814	T38.815	T38.816
ovarian	T38.5X1	T38.5X2	T38.5X3	T38.5X4	T38.5X5	T38.5X6
oxytocic	T48.0X1	T48.0X2	T48.0X3	T48.0X4	T48.0X5	T48.0X6
parathyroid (derivatives)	T50.991	T50.992	T50.993	T50.994	T50.995	T50.996
pituitary (posterior) NEC	T38.891	T38.892	T38.893	T38.894	T38.895	T38.896
anterior	T38.811	T38.812	T38.813	T38.814	T38.815	T38.816
specified, NEC	T38.891	T38.892	T38.893	T38.894	T38.895	T38.896
thyroid	T38.1X1	T38.1X2	T38.1X3	T38.1X4	T38.1X5	T38.1X6
Hornet (sting)	T63.451	T63.452	T63.453	T63.454	—	—
Horse anti-human lymphocytic serum	T50.Z11	T50.Z12	T50.Z13	T50.Z14	T50.Z15	T50.Z16
Horticulture agent NEC	T65.91	T65.92	T65.93	T65.94	—	—
with pesticide	T60.91	T60.92	T60.93	T60.94	—	—
Human						
albumin	T45.8X1	T45.8X2	T45.8X3	T45.8X4	T45.8X5	T45.8X6
growth hormone (HGH)	T38.811	T38.812	T38.813	T38.814	T38.815	T38.816
immune serum	T50.Z11	T50.Z12	T50.Z13	T50.Z14	T50.Z15	T50.Z16
Hyaluronidase	T45.3X1	T45.3X2	T45.3X3	T45.3X4	T45.3X5	T45.3X6
Hyazyme	T45.3X1	T45.3X2	T45.3X3	T45.3X4	T45.3X5	T45.3X6
Hycodan	T40.2X1	T40.2X2	T40.2X3	T40.2X4	T40.2X5	T40.2X6
Hydantoin derivative NEC	T42.0X1	T42.0X2	T42.0X3	T42.0X4	T42.0X5	T42.0X6
Hydeltra	T38.0X1	T38.0X2	T38.0X3	T38.0X4	T38.0X5	T38.0X6
Hydergine	T44.6X1	T44.6X2	T44.6X3	T44.6X4	T44.6X5	T44.6X6
Hydrabamine penicillin	T36.0X1	T36.0X2	T36.0X3	T36.0X4	T36.0X5	T36.0X6
Hydralazine	T46.5X1	T46.5X2	T46.5X3	T46.5X4	T46.5X5	T46.5X6
Hydrargaphen	T49.0X1	T49.0X2	T49.0X3	T49.0X4	T49.0X5	T49.0X6
Hydrargyri aminochloridum	T49.0X1	T49.0X2	T49.0X3	T49.0X4	T49.0X5	T49.0X6
Hydrastine	T48.291	T48.292	T48.293	T48.294	T48.295	T48.296
Hydrazine	T54.1X1	T54.1X2	T54.1X3	T54.1X4	—	—
monoamine oxidase inhibitors	T43.1X1	T43.1X2	T43.1X3	T43.1X4	T43.1X5	T43.1X6
Hydrazoic acid, azides	T54.2X1	T54.2X2	T54.2X3	T54.2X4	—	—
Hydriodic acid	T48.4X1	T48.4X2	T48.4X3	T48.4X4	T48.4X5	T48.4X6
Hydrisalic*	T49.4X1	T49.4X2	T49.4X3	T49.4X4	T49.4X5	T49.4X6
Hydro-ride*	T50.2X1	T50.2X2	T50.2X3	T50.2X4	T50.2X5	T50.2X6
Hydrocarbon gas	T59.891	T59.892	T59.893	T59.894	—	—
incomplete combustion of — see Carbon, monoxide, fuel, utility						
liquefied (mobile container)	T59.891	T59.892	T59.893	T59.894	—	—
piped (natural)	T59.891	T59.892	T59.893	T59.894	—	—
Hydrochloric acid (liquid)	T54.2X1	T54.2X2	T54.2X3	T54.2X4	—	—
medicinal (digestant)	T47.5X1	T47.5X2	T47.5X3	T47.5X4	T47.5X5	T47.5X6
vapor	T59.891	T59.892	T59.893	T59.894	—	—
Hydrochlorothiazide	T50.2X1	T50.2X2	T50.2X3	T50.2X4	T50.2X5	T50.2X6
Hydrocodone	T40.2X1	T40.2X2	T40.2X3	T40.2X4	T40.2X5	T40.2X6
Hydrocortisone (derivatives)	T38.0X1	T38.0X2	T38.0X3	T38.0X4	T38.0X5	T38.0X6
aceponate	T49.0X1	T49.0X2	T49.0X3	T49.0X4	T49.0X5	T49.0X6
ENT agent	T49.6X1	T49.6X2	T49.6X3	T49.6X4	T49.6X5	T49.6X6
ophthalmic preparation	T49.5X1	T49.5X2	T49.5X3	T49.5X4	T49.5X5	T49.5X6
topical NEC	T49.0X1	T49.0X2	T49.0X3	T49.0X4	T49.0X5	T49.0X6
Hydrocortone	T38.0X1	T38.0X2	T38.0X3	T38.0X4	T38.0X5	T38.0X6
ENT agent	T49.6X1	T49.6X2	T49.6X3	T49.6X4	T49.6X5	T49.6X6
ophthalmic preparation	T49.5X1	T49.5X2	T49.5X3	T49.5X4	T49.5X5	T49.5X6
topical NEC	T49.0X1	T49.0X2	T49.0X3	T49.0X4	T49.0X5	T49.0X6
Hydrocyanic acid (liquid)	T57.3X1	T57.3X2	T57.3X3	T57.3X4	—	—
gas	T65.0X1	T65.0X2	T65.0X3	T65.0X4	—	—
Hydroflumethiazide	T50.2X1	T50.2X2	T50.2X3	T50.2X4	T50.2X5	T50.2X6
Hydrofluoric acid (liquid)	T54.2X1	T54.2X2	T54.2X3	T54.2X4	—	—
vapor	T59.891	T59.892	T59.893	T59.894	—	—
Hydrogen	T59.891	T59.892	T59.893	T59.894	—	—
arsenide	T57.0X1	T57.0X2	T57.0X3	T57.0X4	—	—
arseniureted	T57.0X1	T57.0X2	T57.0X3	T57.0X4	—	—
chloride	T57.8X1	T57.8X2	T57.8X3	T57.8X4	—	—
cyanide (salts)	T57.3X1	T57.3X2	T57.3X3	T57.3X4	—	—
gas	T57.3X1	T57.3X2	T57.3X3	T57.3X4	—	—
Fluoride	T59.5X1	T59.5X2	T59.5X3	T59.5X4	—	—
vapor	T59.5X1	T59.5X2	T59.5X3	T59.5X4	—	—
peroxide	T49.0X1	T49.0X2	T49.0X3	T49.0X4	T49.0X5	T49.0X6
phosphureted	T57.1X1	T57.1X2	T57.1X3	T57.1X4	—	—
sulfide	T59.6X1	T59.6X2	T59.6X3	T59.6X4	—	—
arseniureted	T57.0X1	T57.0X2	T57.0X3	T57.0X4	—	—
sulfureted	T59.6X1	T59.6X2	T59.6X3	T59.6X4	—	—
Hydromethylpyridine	T46.7X1	T46.7X2	T46.7X3	T46.7X4	T46.7X5	T46.7X6
Hydromorphinol	T40.2X1	T40.2X2	T40.2X3	T40.2X4	—	—
Hydromorphinone	T40.2X1	T40.2X2	T40.2X3	T40.2X4	T40.2X5	T40.2X6
Hydromorphone	T40.2X1	T40.2X2	T40.2X3	T40.2X4	T40.2X5	T40.2X6
Hydromox	T50.2X1	T50.2X2	T50.2X3	T50.2X4	T50.2X5	T50.2X6
Hydrophilic lotion	T49.3X1	T49.3X2	T49.3X3	T49.3X4	T49.3X5	T49.3X6
Hydroquinidine	T46.2X1	T46.2X2	T46.2X3	T46.2X4	T46.2X5	T46.2X6
Hydroquinone	T52.2X1	T52.2X2	T52.2X3	T52.2X4	—	—
vapor	T59.891	T59.892	T59.893	T59.894	—	—
Hydrosulfuric acid (gas)	T59.6X1	T59.6X2	T59.6X3	T59.6X4	—	—
Hydrotalcite	T47.1X1	T47.1X2	T47.1X3	T47.1X4	T47.1X5	T47.1X6
Hydrous wool fat	T49.3X1	T49.3X2	T49.3X3	T49.3X4	T49.3X5	T49.3X6
Hydroxide, caustic	T54.3X1	T54.3X2	T54.3X3	T54.3X4	—	—
Hydroxocobalamin	T45.8X1	T45.8X2	T45.8X3	T45.8X4	T45.8X5	T45.8X6
Hydroxyamphetamine	T49.5X1	T49.5X2	T49.5X3	T49.5X4	T49.5X5	T49.5X6
Hydroxycarbamide	T45.1X1	T45.1X2	T45.1X3	T45.1X4	T45.1X5	T45.1X6
Hydroxychloroquine	T37.8X1	T37.8X2	T37.8X3	T37.8X4	T37.8X5	T37.8X6
Hydroxydaunorubicin*	T45.1X1	T45.1X2	T45.1X3	T45.1X4	T45.1X5	T45.1X6
Hydroxydihydrocodeinone	T40.2X1	T40.2X2	T40.2X3	T40.2X4	T40.2X5	T40.2X6
Hydroxyestrone	T38.5X1	T38.5X2	T38.5X3	T38.5X4	T38.5X5	T38.5X6
Hydroxyethyl starch	T45.8X1	T45.8X2	T45.8X3	T45.8X4	T45.8X5	T45.8X6
Hydroxymethylpentanone	T52.4X1	T52.4X2	T52.4X3	T52.4X4	—	—
Hydroxyphenamate	T43.591	T43.592	T43.593	T43.594	T43.595	T43.596
Hydroxyphenylbutazone	T39.2X1	T39.2X2	T39.2X3	T39.2X4	T39.2X5	T39.2X6
Hydroxyprogesterone	T38.5X1	T38.5X2	T38.5X3	T38.5X4	T38.5X5	T38.5X6
caproate	T38.5X1	T38.5X2	T38.5X3	T38.5X4	T38.5X5	T38.5X6

*Optum Value-Add

Substance	Poisoning, Accidental (unintentional)	Poisoning, Intentional Self-harm	Poisoning, Assault	Poisoning, Undetermined	Adverse Effect	Under-dosing
Hydroxyquinoline (derivatives) NEC	T37.8X1	T37.8X2	T37.8X3	T37.8X4	T37.8X5	T37.8X6
Hydroxystilbamidine	T37.3X1	T37.3X2	T37.3X3	T37.3X4	T37.3X5	T37.3X6
Hydroxytoluene	T54.0X1	T54.0X2	T54.0X3	T54.0X4	—	—
(nonmedicinal)						
medicinal	T49.0X1	T49.0X2	T49.0X3	T49.0X4	T49.0X5	T49.0X6
Hydroxyurea	T45.1X1	T45.1X2	T45.1X3	T45.1X4	T45.1X5	T45.1X6
Hydroxyzine	T43.591	T43.592	T43.593	T43.594	T43.595	T43.596
antiallergic	T45.0X1	T45.0X2	T45.0X3	T45.0X4	T45.0X5	T45.0X6
Hyoscine	T44.3X1	T44.3X2	T44.3X3	T44.3X4	T44.3X5	T44.3X6
Hyoscyamine	T44.3X1	T44.3X2	T44.3X3	T44.3X4	T44.3X5	T44.3X6
Hyoscyamus	T44.3X1	T44.3X2	T44.3X3	T44.3X4	T44.3X5	T44.3X6
dry extract	T44.3X1	T44.3X2	T44.3X3	T44.3X4	T44.3X5	T44.3X6
Hypaque	T50.8X1	T50.8X2	T50.8X3	T50.8X4	T50.8X5	T50.8X6
HyperRAB*	T50.Z11	T50.Z12	T50.Z13	T50.Z14	T50.Z15	T50.Z16
Hypertussis	T50.Z11	T50.Z12	T50.Z13	T50.Z14	T50.Z15	T50.Z16
Hypnotic	T42.71	T42.72	T42.73	T42.74	T42.75	T42.76
anticonvulsant	T42.71	T42.72	T42.73	T42.74	T42.75	T42.76
specified NEC	T42.6X1	T42.6X2	T42.6X3	T42.6X4	T42.6X5	T42.6X6
Hypochlorite	T49.0X1	T49.0X2	T49.0X3	T49.0X4	T49.0X5	T49.0X6
Hypophysis, posterior	T38.891	T38.892	T38.893	T38.894	T38.895	T38.896
Hypotensive NEC	T46.5X1	T46.5X2	T46.5X3	T46.5X4	T46.5X5	T46.5X6
Hypromellose	T49.5X1	T49.5X2	T49.5X3	T49.5X4	T49.5X5	T49.5X6
I-thyroxine sodium	T38.1X1	T38.1X2	T38.1X3	T38.1X4	T38.1X5	T38.1X6
Ibacitabine	T37.5X1	T37.5X2	T37.5X3	T37.5X4	T37.5X5	T37.5X6
Ibopamine	T44.991	T44.992	T44.993	T44.994	T44.995	T44.996
Ibufenac	T39.311	T39.312	T39.313	T39.314	T39.315	T39.316
Ibuprofen	T39.311	T39.312	T39.313	T39.314	T39.315	T39.316
Ibuproxam	T39.311	T39.312	T39.313	T39.314	T39.315	T39.316
Ibuterol	T48.6X1	T48.6X2	T48.6X3	T48.6X4	T48.6X5	T48.6X6
Ichthammol	T49.0X1	T49.0X2	T49.0X3	T49.0X4	T49.0X5	T49.0X6
Ichthyol	T49.4X1	T49.4X2	T49.4X3	T49.4X4	T49.4X5	T49.4X6
Idarubicin	T45.1X1	T45.1X2	T45.1X3	T45.1X4	T45.1X5	T45.1X6
Idrocilamide	T42.8X1	T42.8X2	T42.8X3	T42.8X4	T42.8X5	T42.8X6
Ifenprodil	T46.7X1	T46.7X2	T46.7X3	T46.7X4	T46.7X5	T46.7X6
Ifosfamide	T45.1X1	T45.1X2	T45.1X3	T45.1X4	T45.1X5	T45.1X6
Iletin	T38.3X1	T38.3X2	T38.3X3	T38.3X4	T38.3X5	T38.3X6
Ilex	T62.2X1	T62.2X2	T62.2X3	T62.2X4	—	—
Illuminating gas (after combustion)	T58.11	T58.12	T58.13	T58.14	—	—
prior to combustion	T59.891	T59.892	T59.893	T59.894	—	—
Ilopan	T45.2X1	T45.2X2	T45.2X3	T45.2X4	T45.2X5	T45.2X6
Iloprost	T46.7X1	T46.7X2	T46.7X3	T46.7X4	T46.7X5	T46.7X6
Ilotycin	T36.3X1	T36.3X2	T36.3X3	T36.3X4	T36.3X5	T36.3X6
ophthalmic preparation	T49.5X1	T49.5X2	T49.5X3	T49.5X4	T49.5X5	T49.5X6
topical NEC	T49.0X1	T49.0X2	T49.0X3	T49.0X4	T49.0X5	T49.0X6
Imdur*	T46.3X1	T46.3X2	T46.3X3	T46.3X4	T46.3X5	T46.3X6
Imidazole-4-carboxamide	T45.1X1	T45.1X2	T45.1X3	T45.1X4	T45.1X5	T45.1X6
Iminostilbene	T42.1X1	T42.1X2	T42.1X3	T42.1X4	T42.1X5	T42.1X6
Imipenem	T36.0X1	T36.0X2	T36.0X3	T36.0X4	T36.0X5	T36.0X6
Imipramine	T43.011	T43.012	T43.013	T43.014	T43.015	T43.016
Immu-G	T50.Z11	T50.Z12	T50.Z13	T50.Z14	T50.Z15	T50.Z16
Immu-tetanus	T50.Z11	T50.Z12	T50.Z13	T50.Z14	T50.Z15	T50.Z16
Immuglobin	T50.Z11	T50.Z12	T50.Z13	T50.Z14	T50.Z15	T50.Z16
Immune						
checkpoint inhibitors	T45.AX1	T45.AX2	T45.AX3	T45.AX4	T45.AX5	T45.AX6
globulin	T50.Z11	T50.Z12	T50.Z13	T50.Z14	T50.Z15	T50.Z16
serum globulin	T50.Z11	T50.Z12	T50.Z13	T50.Z14	T50.Z15	T50.Z16
Immunoglobin human	T50.Z11	T50.Z12	T50.Z13	T50.Z14	T50.Z15	T50.Z16
(intravenous) (normal)						
unmodified	T50.Z11	T50.Z12	T50.Z13	T50.Z14	T50.Z15	T50.Z16
Immunostimulant drug	T45.AX1	T45.AX2	T45.AX3	T45.AX4	T45.AX5	T45.AX6
Immunosuppressive drug	T45.1X1	T45.1X2	T45.1X3	T45.1X4	T45.1X5	T45.1X6
Indalpine	T43.221	T43.222	T43.223	T43.224	T43.225	T43.226
Indanazoline	T48.5X1	T48.5X2	T48.5X3	T48.5X4	T48.5X5	T48.5X6
Indandione (derivatives)	T45.511	T45.512	T45.513	T45.514	T45.515	T45.516
Indapamide	T46.5X1	T46.5X2	T46.5X3	T46.5X4	T46.5X5	T46.5X6
Indendione (derivatives)	T45.511	T45.512	T45.513	T45.514	T45.515	T45.516
Indenolol	T44.7X1	T44.7X2	T44.7X3	T44.7X4	T44.7X5	T44.7X6
Inderal	T44.7X1	T44.7X2	T44.7X3	T44.7X4	T44.7X5	T44.7X6
Indian						
hemp	T40.711	T40.712	T40.713	T40.714	T40.715	T40.716
tobacco	T62.2X1	T62.2X2	T62.2X3	T62.2X4	—	—
Indigo carmine	T50.8X1	T50.8X2	T50.8X3	T50.8X4	T50.8X5	T50.8X6
Indobufen	T45.521	T45.522	T45.523	T45.524	T45.525	T45.526
Indocin	T39.2X1	T39.2X2	T39.2X3	T39.2X4	T39.2X5	T39.2X6
Indocyanine green	T50.8X1	T50.8X2	T50.8X3	T50.8X4	T50.8X5	T50.8X6
Indometacin	T39.391	T39.392	T39.393	T39.394	T39.395	T39.396
Indomethacin	T39.391	T39.392	T39.393	T39.394	T39.395	T39.396
farnesil	T39.4X1	T39.4X2	T39.4X3	T39.4X4	T39.4X5	T39.4X6
Indoramin	T44.6X1	T44.6X2	T44.6X3	T44.6X4	T44.6X5	T44.6X6
Industrial						
alcohol	T51.0X1	T51.0X2	T51.0X3	T51.0X4	—	—
Industrial — continued						
fumes	T59.891	T59.892	T59.893	T59.894	—	—
solvents (fumes) (vapors)	T52.91	T52.92	T52.93	T52.94	—	—
Inflectra*	T39.4X1	T39.4X2	T39.4X3	T39.4X4	T39.4X5	T39.4X6
Influenza vaccine	T50.B91	T50.B92	T50.B93	T50.B94	T50.B95	T50.B96
Ingested substance NEC	T65.91	T65.92	T65.93	T65.94	—	—
INH	T37.1X1	T37.1X2	T37.1X3	T37.1X4	T37.1X5	T37.1X6
Inhalation, gas (noxious) — see Gas						
Inhibitor						
angiotensin-converting enzyme	T46.4X1	T46.4X2	T46.4X3	T46.4X4	T46.4X5	T46.4X6
carbonic anhydrase	T50.2X1	T50.2X2	T50.2X3	T50.2X4	T50.2X5	T50.2X6
fibrinolysis	T45.621	T45.622	T45.623	T45.624	T45.625	T45.626
monoamine oxidase NEC	T43.1X1	T43.1X2	T43.1X3	T43.1X4	T43.1X5	T43.1X6
hydrazine	T43.1X1	T43.1X2	T43.1X3	T43.1X4	T43.1X5	T43.1X6
postsynaptic	T43.8X1	T43.8X2	T43.8X3	T43.8X4	T43.8X5	T43.8X6
prothrombin synthesis	T45.511	T45.512	T45.513	T45.514	T45.515	T45.516
Ink	T65.891	T65.892	T65.893	T65.894	—	—
Innopran*	T44.7X1	T44.7X2	T44.7X3	T44.7X4	T44.7X5	T44.7X6
Inorganic substance NEC	T57.91	T57.92	T57.93	T57.94	—	—
Inosine pranobex	T37.5X1	T37.5X2	T37.5X3	T37.5X4	T37.5X5	T37.5X6
Inositol	T50.991	T50.992	T50.993	T50.994	T50.995	T50.996
nicotinate	T46.7X1	T46.7X2	T46.7X3	T46.7X4	T46.7X5	T46.7X6
Inproquone	T45.1X1	T45.1X2	T45.1X3	T45.1X4	T45.1X5	T45.1X6
Insect (sting), venomous	T63.481	T63.482	T63.483	T63.484	—	—
ant	T63.421	T63.422	T63.423	T63.424	—	—
bee	T63.441	T63.442	T63.443	T63.444	—	—
caterpillar	T63.431	T63.432	T63.433	T63.434	—	—
hornet	T63.451	T63.452	T63.453	T63.454	—	—
wasp	T63.461	T63.462	T63.463	T63.464	—	—
Insecticide NEC	T60.91	T60.92	T60.93	T60.94		
carbamate	T60.0X1	T60.0X2	T60.0X3	T60.0X4		
chlorinated	T60.1X1	T60.1X2	T60.1X3	T60.1X4		
mixed	T60.91	T60.92	T60.93	T60.94		
organochlorine	T60.1X1	T60.1X2	T60.1X3	T60.1X4		
organophosphorus	T60.0X1	T60.0X2	T60.0X3	T60.0X4		
Insular tissue extract	T38.3X1	T38.3X2	T38.3X3	T38.3X4	T38.3X5	T38.3X6
Insulin (amorphous) (globin) (isophane) (Lente) (NPH) (Semilente) (Ultralente)	T38.3X1	T38.3X2	T38.3X3	T38.3X4	T38.3X5	T38.3X6
defalan	T38.3X1	T38.3X2	T38.3X3	T38.3X4	T38.3X5	T38.3X6
human	T38.3X1	T38.3X2	T38.3X3	T38.3X4	T38.3X5	T38.3X6
injection, soluble	T38.3X1	T38.3X2	T38.3X3	T38.3X4	T38.3X5	T38.3X6
biphasic	T38.3X1	T38.3X2	T38.3X3	T38.3X4	T38.3X5	T38.3X6
intermediate acting	T38.3X1	T38.3X2	T38.3X3	T38.3X4	T38.3X5	T38.3X6
protamine zinc	T38.3X1	T38.3X2	T38.3X3	T38.3X4	T38.3X5	T38.3X6
slow acting	T38.3X1	T38.3X2	T38.3X3	T38.3X4	T38.3X5	T38.3X6
zinc						
protamine injection	T38.3X1	T38.3X2	T38.3X3	T38.3X4	T38.3X5	T38.3X6
suspension (amorphous) (crystalline)	T38.3X1	T38.3X2	T38.3X3	T38.3X4	T38.3X5	T38.3X6
Interferon (alpha) (beta) (gamma)	T37.5X1	T37.5X2	T37.5X3	T37.5X4	T37.5X5	T37.5X6
Intestinal motility control drug	T47.6X1	T47.6X2	T47.6X3	T47.6X4	T47.6X5	T47.6X6
biological	T47.8X1	T47.8X2	T47.8X3	T47.8X4	T47.8X5	T47.8X6
Intranarcon	T41.1X1	T41.1X2	T41.1X3	T41.1X4	T41.1X5	T41.1X6
Intravenous						
amino acids	T50.991	T50.992	T50.993	T50.994	T50.995	T50.996
fat suspension	T50.991	T50.992	T50.993	T50.994	T50.995	T50.996
Inulin	T50.8X1	T50.8X2	T50.8X3	T50.8X4	T50.8X5	T50.8X6
Invanz*	T36.1X1	T36.1X2	T36.1X3	T36.1X4	T36.1X5	T36.1X6
Invert sugar	T50.3X1	T50.3X2	T50.3X3	T50.3X4	T50.3X5	T50.3X6
Inza — see Naproxen						
Iobenzamic acid	T50.8X1	T50.8X2	T50.8X3	T50.8X4	T50.8X5	T50.8X6
Iocarmic acid	T50.8X1	T50.8X2	T50.8X3	T50.8X4	T50.8X5	T50.8X6
Iocetamic acid	T50.8X1	T50.8X2	T50.8X3	T50.8X4	T50.8X5	T50.8X6
Iodamide	T50.8X1	T50.8X2	T50.8X3	T50.8X4	T50.8X5	T50.8X6
Iodide NEC — see also Iodine	T49.0X1	T49.0X2	T49.0X3	T49.0X4	T49.0X5	T49.0X6
mercury (ointment)	T49.0X1	T49.0X2	T49.0X3	T49.0X4	T49.0X5	T49.0X6
methylate	T49.0X1	T49.0X2	T49.0X3	T49.0X4	T49.0X5	T49.0X6
potassium (expectorant) NEC	T48.4X1	T48.4X2	T48.4X3	T48.4X4	T48.4X5	T48.4X6
Iodinated						
contrast medium	T50.8X1	T50.8X2	T50.8X3	T50.8X4	T50.8X5	T50.8X6
glycerol	T48.4X1	T48.4X2	T48.4X3	T48.4X4	T48.4X5	T48.4X6
human serum albumin (131I)	T50.8X1	T50.8X2	T50.8X3	T50.8X4	T50.8X5	T50.8X6
Iodine (antiseptic, external) (tincture) NEC	T49.0X1	T49.0X2	T49.0X3	T49.0X4	T49.0X5	T49.0X6

Substance	Poisoning, Accidental (unintentional)	Poisoning, Intentional Self-harm	Poisoning, Assault	Poisoning, Undetermined	Adverse Effect	Under-dosing
Iodine (antiseptic, external) (tincture) **NEC** — *continued*						
125 — *see also* Radiation sickness, and exposure to radioactive isotopes	T5Ø.8X1	T5Ø.8X2	T5Ø.8X3	T5Ø.8X4	T5Ø.8X5	T5Ø.8X6
therapeutic	T5Ø.991	T5Ø.992	T5Ø.993	T5Ø.994	T5Ø.995	T5Ø.996
131 — *see also* Radiation sickness, and exposure to radioactive isotopes	T5Ø.8X1	T5Ø.8X2	T5Ø.8X3	T5Ø.8X4	T5Ø.8X5	T5Ø.8X6
therapeutic	T38.2X1	T38.2X2	T38.2X3	T38.2X4	T38.2X5	T38.2X6
diagnostic	T5Ø.8X1	T5Ø.8X2	T5Ø.8X3	T5Ø.8X4	T5Ø.8X5	T5Ø.8X6
solution	T49.ØX1	T49.ØX2	T49.ØX3	T49.ØX4	T49.ØX5	T49.ØX6
vapor	T59.891	T59.892	T59.893	T59.894	—	—
for thyroid conditions (antithyroid)	T38.2X1	T38.2X2	T38.2X3	T38.2X4	T38.2X5	T38.2X6
Iodipamide	T5Ø.8X1	T5Ø.8X2	T5Ø.8X3	T5Ø.8X4	T5Ø.8X5	T5Ø.8X6
Iodized (poppy seed) oil	T5Ø.8X1	T5Ø.8X2	T5Ø.8X3	T5Ø.8X4	T5Ø.8X5	T5Ø.8X6
Iodobismitol	T37.8X1	T37.8X2	T37.8X3	T37.8X4	T37.8X5	T37.8X6
Iodochlorhydroxyquin	T37.8X1	T37.8X2	T37.8X3	T37.8X4	T37.8X5	T37.8X6
topical	T49.ØX1	T49.ØX2	T49.ØX3	T49.ØX4	T49.ØX5	T49.ØX6
Iodochlorhydroxyquinoline	T37.8X1	T37.8X2	T37.8X3	T37.8X4	T37.8X5	T37.8X6
Iodocholesterol (131I)	T5Ø.8X1	T5Ø.8X2	T5Ø.8X3	T5Ø.8X4	T5Ø.8X5	T5Ø.8X6
Iodoform	T49.ØX1	T49.ØX2	T49.ØX3	T49.ØX4	T49.ØX5	T49.ØX6
Iodohippuric acid	T5Ø.8X1	T5Ø.8X2	T5Ø.8X3	T5Ø.8X4	T5Ø.8X5	T5Ø.8X6
Iodopanoic acid	T5Ø.8X1	T5Ø.8X2	T5Ø.8X3	T5Ø.8X4	T5Ø.8X5	T5Ø.8X6
Iodophthalein (sodium)	T5Ø.8X1	T5Ø.8X2	T5Ø.8X3	T5Ø.8X4	T5Ø.8X5	T5Ø.8X6
Iodopyracet	T5Ø.8X1	T5Ø.8X2	T5Ø.8X3	T5Ø.8X4	T5Ø.8X5	T5Ø.8X6
Iodoquinol	T37.8X1	T37.8X2	T37.8X3	T37.8X4	T37.8X5	T37.8X6
Iodoxamic acid	T5Ø.8X1	T5Ø.8X2	T5Ø.8X3	T5Ø.8X4	T5Ø.8X5	T5Ø.8X6
Iofendylate	T5Ø.8X1	T5Ø.8X2	T5Ø.8X3	T5Ø.8X4	T5Ø.8X5	T5Ø.8X6
Ioglycamic acid	T5Ø.8X1	T5Ø.8X2	T5Ø.8X3	T5Ø.8X4	T5Ø.8X5	T5Ø.8X6
Iohexol	T5Ø.8X1	T5Ø.8X2	T5Ø.8X3	T5Ø.8X4	T5Ø.8X5	T5Ø.8X6
Ion exchange resin						
anion	T47.8X1	T47.8X2	T47.8X3	T47.8X4	T47.8X5	T47.8X6
cation	T5Ø.3X1	T5Ø.3X2	T5Ø.3X3	T5Ø.3X4	T5Ø.3X5	T5Ø.3X6
cholestyramine	T46.6X1	T46.6X2	T46.6X3	T46.6X4	T46.6X5	T46.6X6
intestinal	T47.8X1	T47.8X2	T47.8X3	T47.8X4	T47.8X5	T47.8X6
Iopamidol	T5Ø.8X1	T5Ø.8X2	T5Ø.8X3	T5Ø.8X4	T5Ø.8X5	T5Ø.8X6
Iopanoic acid	T5Ø.8X1	T5Ø.8X2	T5Ø.8X3	T5Ø.8X4	T5Ø.8X5	T5Ø.8X6
Iophenoic acid	T5Ø.8X1	T5Ø.8X2	T5Ø.8X3	T5Ø.8X4	T5Ø.8X5	T5Ø.8X6
Iopodate, sodium	T5Ø.8X1	T5Ø.8X2	T5Ø.8X3	T5Ø.8X4	T5Ø.8X5	T5Ø.8X6
Iopodic acid	T5Ø.8X1	T5Ø.8X2	T5Ø.8X3	T5Ø.8X4	T5Ø.8X5	T5Ø.8X6
Iopromide	T5Ø.8X1	T5Ø.8X2	T5Ø.8X3	T5Ø.8X4	T5Ø.8X5	T5Ø.8X6
Iopydol	T5Ø.8X1	T5Ø.8X2	T5Ø.8X3	T5Ø.8X4	T5Ø.8X5	T5Ø.8X6
Iotalamic acid	T5Ø.8X1	T5Ø.8X2	T5Ø.8X3	T5Ø.8X4	T5Ø.8X5	T5Ø.8X6
Iothalamate	T5Ø.8X1	T5Ø.8X2	T5Ø.8X3	T5Ø.8X4	T5Ø.8X5	T5Ø.8X6
Iothiouracil	T38.2X1	T38.2X2	T38.2X3	T38.2X4	T38.2X5	T38.2X6
Iotrol	T5Ø.8X1	T5Ø.8X2	T5Ø.8X3	T5Ø.8X4	T5Ø.8X5	T5Ø.8X6
Iotrolan	T5Ø.8X1	T5Ø.8X2	T5Ø.8X3	T5Ø.8X4	T5Ø.8X5	T5Ø.8X6
Iotroxate	T5Ø.8X1	T5Ø.8X2	T5Ø.8X3	T5Ø.8X4	T5Ø.8X5	T5Ø.8X6
Iotroxic acid	T5Ø.8X1	T5Ø.8X2	T5Ø.8X3	T5Ø.8X4	T5Ø.8X5	T5Ø.8X6
Ioversol	T5Ø.8X1	T5Ø.8X2	T5Ø.8X3	T5Ø.8X4	T5Ø.8X5	T5Ø.8X6
Ioxaglate	T5Ø.8X1	T5Ø.8X2	T5Ø.8X3	T5Ø.8X4	T5Ø.8X5	T5Ø.8X6
Ioxaglic acid	T5Ø.8X1	T5Ø.8X2	T5Ø.8X3	T5Ø.8X4	T5Ø.8X5	T5Ø.8X6
Ioxitalamic acid	T5Ø.8X1	T5Ø.8X2	T5Ø.8X3	T5Ø.8X4	T5Ø.8X5	T5Ø.8X6
Ipecac	T47.7X1	T47.7X2	T47.7X3	T47.7X4	T47.7X5	T47.7X6
Ipecacuanha	T48.4X1	T48.4X2	T48.4X3	T48.4X4	T48.4X5	T48.4X6
Ipodate, calcium	T5Ø.8X1	T5Ø.8X2	T5Ø.8X3	T5Ø.8X4	T5Ø.8X5	T5Ø.8X6
IPOL*	T5Ø.B91	T5Ø.B92	T5Ø.B93	T5Ø.B94	T5Ø.B95	T5Ø.B96
Ipral	T42.3X1	T42.3X2	T42.3X3	T42.3X4	T42.3X5	T42.3X6
Ipratropium (bromide)	T48.6X1	T48.6X2	T48.6X3	T48.6X4	T48.6X5	T48.6X6
Ipriflavone	T46.3X1	T46.3X2	T46.3X3	T46.3X4	T46.3X5	T46.3X6
Iprindole	T43.Ø11	T43.Ø12	T43.Ø13	T43.Ø14	T43.Ø15	T43.Ø16
Iproclozide	T43.1X1	T43.1X2	T43.1X3	T43.1X4	T43.1X5	T43.1X6
Iprofenin	T5Ø.8X1	T5Ø.8X2	T5Ø.8X3	T5Ø.8X4	T5Ø.8X5	T5Ø.8X6
Iproheptine	T49.2X1	T49.2X2	T49.2X3	T49.2X4	T49.2X5	T49.2X6
Iproniazid	T43.1X1	T43.1X2	T43.1X3	T43.1X4	T43.1X5	T43.1X6
Iproplatin	T45.1X1	T45.1X2	T45.1X3	T45.1X4	T45.1X5	T45.1X6
Iproveratril	T46.1X1	T46.1X2	T46.1X3	T46.1X4	T46.1X5	T46.1X6
Irinotecan*	T45.1X1	T45.1X2	T45.1X3	T45.1X4	T45.1X5	T45.1X6
Iron (compounds) (medicinal) **NEC**	T45.4X1	T45.4X2	T45.4X3	T45.4X4	T45.4X5	T45.4X6
ammonium	T45.4X1	T45.4X2	T45.4X3	T45.4X4	T45.4X5	T45.4X6
dextran injection	T45.4X1	T45.4X2	T45.4X3	T45.4X4	T45.4X5	T45.4X6
nonmedicinal	T56.891	T56.892	T56.893	T56.894	—	—
salts	T45.4X1	T45.4X2	T45.4X3	T45.4X4	T45.4X5	T45.4X6
sorbitex	T45.4X1	T45.4X2	T45.4X3	T45.4X4	T45.4X5	T45.4X6
sorbitol citric acid complex	T45.4X1	T45.4X2	T45.4X3	T45.4X4	T45.4X5	T45.4X6
Irrigating fluid (vaginal)	T49.8X1	T49.8X2	T49.8X3	T49.8X4	T49.8X5	T49.8X6
eye	T49.5X1	T49.5X2	T49.5X3	T49.5X4	T49.5X5	T49.5X6
Isepamicin	T36.5X1	T36.5X2	T36.5X3	T36.5X4	T36.5X5	T36.5X6
Isoaminile (citrate)	T48.3X1	T48.3X2	T48.3X3	T48.3X4	T48.3X5	T48.3X6
Isoamyl nitrite	T46.3X1	T46.3X2	T46.3X3	T46.3X4	T46.3X5	T46.3X6

Substance	Poisoning, Accidental (unintentional)	Poisoning, Intentional Self-harm	Poisoning, Assault	Poisoning, Undetermined	Adverse Effect	Under-dosing
Isobenzan	T6Ø.1X1	T6Ø.1X2	T6Ø.1X3	T6Ø.1X4	—	—
Isobutyl acetate	T52.8X1	T52.8X2	T52.8X3	T52.8X4	—	—
Isocarboxazid	T43.1X1	T43.1X2	T43.1X3	T43.1X4	T43.1X5	T43.1X6
Isoconazole	T49.ØX1	T49.ØX2	T49.ØX3	T49.ØX4	T49.ØX5	T49.ØX6
Isocyanate	T65.ØX1	T65.ØX2	T65.ØX3	T65.ØX4	—	—
Isoephedrine	T44.991	T44.992	T44.993	T44.994	T44.995	T44.996
Isoetarine	T48.6X1	T48.6X2	T48.6X3	T48.6X4	T48.6X5	T48.6X6
Isoethadione	T42.2X1	T42.2X2	T42.2X3	T42.2X4	T42.2X5	T42.2X6
Isoetharine	T44.5X1	T44.5X2	T44.5X3	T44.5X4	T44.5X5	T44.5X6
Isoflurane	T41.ØX1	T41.ØX2	T41.ØX3	T41.ØX4	T41.ØX5	T41.ØX6
Isoflurophate	T44.ØX1	T44.ØX2	T44.ØX3	T44.ØX4	T44.ØX5	T44.ØX6
Isomaltose, ferric complex	T45.4X1	T45.4X2	T45.4X3	T45.4X4	T45.4X5	T45.4X6
Isometheptene	T44.3X1	T44.3X2	T44.3X3	T44.3X4	T44.3X5	T44.3X6
Isoniazid	T37.1X1	T37.1X2	T37.1X3	T37.1X4	T37.1X5	T37.1X6
with						
rifampicin	T36.6X1	T36.6X2	T36.6X3	T36.6X4	T36.6X5	T36.6X6
thioacetazone	T37.1X1	T37.1X2	T37.1X3	T37.1X4	T37.1X5	T37.1X6
Isonicotinic acid hydrazide	T37.1X1	T37.1X2	T37.1X3	T37.1X4	T37.1X5	T37.1X6
Isonipecaine	T4Ø.491	T4Ø.492	T4Ø.493	T4Ø.494	T4Ø.495	T4Ø.496
Isopentaquine	T37.2X1	T37.2X2	T37.2X3	T37.2X4	T37.2X5	T37.2X6
Isophane insulin	T38.3X1	T38.3X2	T38.3X3	T38.3X4	T38.3X5	T38.3X6
Isophorone	T65.891	T65.892	T65.893	T65.894	—	—
Isophosphamide	T45.1X1	T45.1X2	T45.1X3	T45.1X4	T45.1X5	T45.1X6
Isopregnenone	T38.5X1	T38.5X2	T38.5X3	T38.5X4	T38.5X5	T38.5X6
Isoprenaline	T48.6X1	T48.6X2	T48.6X3	T48.6X4	T48.6X5	T48.6X6
Isopromethazine	T43.3X1	T43.3X2	T43.3X3	T43.3X4	T43.3X5	T43.3X6
Isopropamide	T44.3X1	T44.3X2	T44.3X3	T44.3X4	T44.3X5	T44.3X6
iodide	T44.3X1	T44.3X2	T44.3X3	T44.3X4	T44.3X5	T44.3X6
Isopropanol	T51.2X1	T51.2X2	T51.2X3	T51.2X4	—	—
Isopropyl						
acetate	T52.8X1	T52.8X2	T52.8X3	T52.8X4	—	—
alcohol	T51.2X1	T51.2X2	T51.2X3	T51.2X4	—	—
medicinal	T49.4X1	T49.4X2	T49.4X3	T49.4X4	T49.4X5	T49.4X6
ether	T52.8X1	T52.8X2	T52.8X3	T52.8X4	—	—
Isopropylaminophenazone	T39.2X1	T39.2X2	T39.2X3	T39.2X4	T39.2X5	T39.2X6
Isoproterenol	T48.6X1	T48.6X2	T48.6X3	T48.6X4	T48.6X5	T48.6X6
Isosorbide dinitrate	T46.3X1	T46.3X2	T46.3X3	T46.3X4	T46.3X5	T46.3X6
Isothipendyl	T45.ØX1	T45.ØX2	T45.ØX3	T45.ØX4	T45.ØX5	T45.ØX6
Isotretinoin	T5Ø.991	T5Ø.992	T5Ø.993	T5Ø.994	T5Ø.995	T5Ø.996
Isoxazolyl penicillin	T36.ØX1	T36.ØX2	T36.ØX3	T36.ØX4	T36.ØX5	T36.ØX6
Isoxicam	T39.391	T39.392	T39.393	T39.394	T39.395	T39.396
Isoxsuprine	T46.7X1	T46.7X2	T46.7X3	T46.7X4	T46.7X5	T46.7X6
Ispagula	T47.4X1	T47.4X2	T47.4X3	T47.4X4	T47.4X5	T47.4X6
husk	T47.4X1	T47.4X2	T47.4X3	T47.4X4	T47.4X5	T47.4X6
Isradipine	T46.1X1	T46.1X2	T46.1X3	T46.1X4	T46.1X5	T46.1X6
Itraconazole	T37.8X1	T37.8X2	T37.8X3	T37.8X4	T37.8X5	T37.8X6
Itramin tosilate	T46.3X1	T46.3X2	T46.3X3	T46.3X4	T46.3X5	T46.3X6
Ivarest*	T41.3X1	T41.3X2	T41.3X3	T41.3X4	T41.3X5	T41.3X6
Ivermectin	T37.4X1	T37.4X2	T37.4X3	T37.4X4	T37.4X5	T37.4X6
Izoniazid	T37.1X1	T37.1X2	T37.1X3	T37.1X4	T37.1X5	T37.1X6
with thioacetazone	T37.1X1	T37.1X2	T37.1X3	T37.1X4	T37.1X5	T37.1X6
Jalap	T47.2X1	T47.2X2	T47.2X3	T47.2X4	T47.2X5	T47.2X6
Jamaica						
dogwood (bark)	T39.8X1	T39.8X2	T39.8X3	T39.8X4	T39.8X5	T39.8X6
ginger	T65.891	T65.892	T65.893	T65.894	—	—
root	T62.2X1	T62.2X2	T62.2X3	T62.2X4	—	—
Jantoven*	T45.511	T45.512	T45.513	T45.514	T45.515	T45.516
Jatropha	T62.2X1	T62.2X2	T62.2X3	T62.2X4	—	—
curcas	T62.2X1	T62.2X2	T62.2X3	T62.2X4	—	—
Jectofer	T45.4X1	T45.4X2	T45.4X3	T45.4X4	T45.4X5	T45.4X6
Jellyfish (sting)	T63.621	T63.622	T63.623	T63.624	—	—
Jequirity (bean)	T62.2X1	T62.2X2	T62.2X3	T62.2X4	—	—
Jimson weed (stramonium)	T62.2X1	T62.2X2	T62.2X3	T62.2X4	—	—
seeds	T62.2X1	T62.2X2	T62.2X3	T62.2X4	—	—
Josamycin	T36.3X1	T36.3X2	T36.3X3	T36.3X4	T36.3X5	T36.3X6
Juniper tar	T49.1X1	T49.1X2	T49.1X3	T49.1X4	T49.1X5	T49.1X6
Kaletra*	T37.5X1	T37.5X2	T37.5X3	T37.5X4	T37.5X5	T37.5X6
Kallidinogenase	T46.7X1	T46.7X2	T46.7X3	T46.7X4	T46.7X5	T46.7X6
Kallikrein	T46.7X1	T46.7X2	T46.7X3	T46.7X4	T46.7X5	T46.7X6
Kanamycin	T36.5X1	T36.5X2	T36.5X3	T36.5X4	T36.5X5	T36.5X6
Kantrex	T36.5X1	T36.5X2	T36.5X3	T36.5X4	T36.5X5	T36.5X6
Kaolin	T47.6X1	T47.6X2	T47.6X3	T47.6X4	T47.6X5	T47.6X6
light	T47.6X1	T47.6X2	T47.6X3	T47.6X4	T47.6X5	T47.6X6
Karaya (gum)	T47.4X1	T47.4X2	T47.4X3	T47.4X4	T47.4X5	T47.4X6
Kebuzone	T39.2X1	T39.2X2	T39.2X3	T39.2X4	T39.2X5	T39.2X6
Keflex*	T36.1X1	T36.1X2	T36.1X3	T36.1X4	T36.1X5	T36.1X6
Kelevan	T6Ø.1X1	T6Ø.1X2	T6Ø.1X3	T6Ø.1X4	—	—
Kemithal	T41.1X1	T41.1X2	T41.1X3	T41.1X4	T41.1X5	T41.1X6
Kenacort	T38.ØX1	T38.ØX2	T38.ØX3	T38.ØX4	T38.ØX5	T38.ØX6
Keratolytic drug NEC	T49.4X1	T49.4X2	T49.4X3	T49.4X4	T49.4X5	T49.4X6
anthracene	T49.4X1	T49.4X2	T49.4X3	T49.4X4	T49.4X5	T49.4X6
Keratoplastic NEC	T49.4X1	T49.4X2	T49.4X3	T49.4X4	T49.4X5	T49.4X6

Substance	Poisoning, Accidental (unintentional)	Poisoning, Intentional Self-harm	Poisoning, Assault	Poisoning, Undetermined	Adverse Effect	Under-dosing
Kerosene, kerosine (fuel) (solvent) **NEC**	T52.0X1	T52.0X2	T52.0X3	T52.0X4	—	—
insecticide	T52.0X1	T52.0X2	T52.0X3	T52.0X4	—	—
vapor	T52.0X1	T52.0X2	T52.0X3	T52.0X4	—	—
Ketamine	T41.291	T41.292	T41.293	T41.294	T41.295	T41.296
Ketazolam	T42.4X1	T42.4X2	T42.4X3	T42.4X4	T42.4X5	T42.4X6
Ketazon	T39.2X1	T39.2X2	T39.2X3	T39.2X4	T39.2X5	T39.2X6
Ketobemidone	T40.491	T40.492	T40.493	T40.494		
Ketoconazole	T49.0X1	T49.0X2	T49.0X3	T49.0X4	T49.0X5	T49.0X6
Ketols	T52.4X1	T52.4X2	T52.4X3	T52.4X4	—	—
Ketone oils	T52.4X1	T52.4X2	T52.4X3	T52.4X4	—	—
Ketoprofen	T39.311	T39.312	T39.313	T39.314	T39.315	T39.316
Ketorolac	T39.8X1	T39.8X2	T39.8X3	T39.8X4	T39.8X5	T39.8X6
Ketotifen	T45.0X1	T45.0X2	T45.0X3	T45.0X4	T45.0X5	T45.0X6
Keytruda*	T45.1X1	T45.1X2	T45.1X3	T45.1X4	T45.1X5	T45.1X6
Khat	T43.691	T43.692	T43.693	T43.694		
Khellin	T46.3X1	T46.3X2	T46.3X3	T46.3X4	T46.3X5	T46.3X6
Khelloside	T46.3X1	T46.3X2	T46.3X3	T46.3X4	T46.3X5	T46.3X6
Kiln gas or vapor (carbon monoxide)	T58.8X1	T58.8X2	T58.8X3	T58.8X4	—	—
Kineret*	T39.4X1	T39.4X2	T39.4X3	T39.4X4	T39.4X5	T39.4X6
Kitasamycin	T36.3X1	T36.3X2	T36.3X3	T36.3X4	T36.3X5	T36.3X6
Klonopin*	T42.4X1	T42.4X2	T42.4X3	T42.4X4	T42.4X5	T42.4X6
Komgiblyze*	T38.3X1	T38.3X2	T38.3X3	T38.3X4	T38.3X5	T38.3X6
Konsyl	T47.4X1	T47.4X2	T47.4X3	T47.4X4	T47.4X5	T47.4X6
Kosam seed	T62.2X1	T62.2X2	T62.2X3	T62.2X4		
Krait (venom)	T63.091	T63.092	T63.093	T63.094	—	—
Kwell (insecticide)	T60.1X1	T60.1X2	T60.1X3	T60.1X4		
anti-infective (topical)	T49.0X1	T49.0X2	T49.0X3	T49.0X4	T49.0X5	T49.0X6
L-dopa	T42.8X1	T42.8X2	T42.8X3	T42.8X4	T42.8X5	T42.8X6
L-Tryptophan — see amino acid						
Labetalol	T44.8X1	T44.8X2	T44.8X3	T44.8X4	T44.8X5	T44.8X6
Laburnum (seeds)	T62.2X1	T62.2X2	T62.2X3	T62.2X4	—	—
leaves	T62.2X1	T62.2X2	T62.2X3	T62.2X4		
Lachesine	T49.5X1	T49.5X2	T49.5X3	T49.5X4	T49.5X5	T49.5X6
Lacidipine	T46.5X1	T46.5X2	T46.5X3	T46.5X4	T46.5X5	T46.5X6
Lacquer	T65.6X1	T65.6X2	T65.6X3	T65.6X4	—	—
Lacrimogenic gas	T59.3X1	T59.3X2	T59.3X3	T59.3X4		
Lactated potassic saline	T50.3X1	T50.3X2	T50.3X3	T50.3X4	T50.3X5	T50.3X6
Lactic acid	T49.8X1	T49.8X2	T49.8X3	T49.8X4	T49.8X5	T49.8X6
Lactobacillus						
acidophilus	T47.6X1	T47.6X2	T47.6X3	T47.6X4	T47.6X5	T47.6X6
compound	T47.6X1	T47.6X2	T47.6X3	T47.6X4	T47.6X5	T47.6X6
bifidus, lyophilized	T47.6X1	T47.6X2	T47.6X3	T47.6X4	T47.6X5	T47.6X6
bulgaricus	T47.6X1	T47.6X2	T47.6X3	T47.6X4	T47.6X5	T47.6X6
sporogenes	T47.6X1	T47.6X2	T47.6X3	T47.6X4	T47.6X5	T47.6X6
Lactoflavin	T45.2X1	T45.2X2	T45.2X3	T45.2X4	T45.2X5	T45.2X6
Lactose (as excipient)	T50.901	T50.902	T50.903	T50.904	T50.905	T50.906
Lactuca (virosa) (extract)	T42.6X1	T42.6X2	T42.6X3	T42.6X4	T42.6X5	T42.6X6
Lactucarium	T42.6X1	T42.6X2	T42.6X3	T42.6X4	T42.6X5	T42.6X6
Lactulose	T47.3X1	T47.3X2	T47.3X3	T47.3X4	T47.3X5	T47.3X6
Laevo — see Levo-						
Lanatosides	T46.0X1	T46.0X2	T46.0X3	T46.0X4	T46.0X5	T46.0X6
Lanolin	T49.3X1	T49.3X2	T49.3X3	T49.3X4	T49.3X5	T49.3X6
Lanoxin*	T46.0X1	T46.0X2	T46.0X3	T46.0X4	T46.0X5	T46.0X6
Largactil	T43.3X1	T43.3X2	T43.3X3	T43.3X4	T43.3X5	T43.3X6
Larkspur	T62.2X1	T62.2X2	T62.2X3	T62.2X4	—	—
Laroxyl	T43.012	T43.012	T43.013	T43.014	T43.015	T43.016
Lasix	T50.1X1	T50.1X2	T50.1X3	T50.1X4	T50.1X5	T50.1X6
Lassar's paste	T49.4X1	T49.4X2	T49.4X3	T49.4X4	T49.4X5	T49.4X6
Latamoxef	T36.1X1	T36.1X2	T36.1X3	T36.1X4	T36.1X5	T36.1X6
Latex	T65.811	T65.812	T65.813	T65.814	—	—
Lathyrus (seed)	T62.2X1	T62.2X2	T62.2X3	T62.2X4	—	—
Laudanum	T40.0X1	T40.0X2	T40.0X3	T40.0X4	T40.0X5	T40.0X6
Laudexium	T48.1X1	T48.1X2	T48.1X3	T48.1X4	T48.1X5	T48.1X6
Laughing gas	T41.0X1	T41.0X2	T41.0X3	T41.0X4	T41.0X5	T41.0X6
Laurel, black or cherry	T62.2X1	T62.2X2	T62.2X3	T62.2X4		
Laurolinium	T49.0X1	T49.0X2	T49.0X3	T49.0X4	T49.0X5	T49.0X6
Lauryl sulfoacetate	T49.2X1	T49.2X2	T49.2X3	T49.2X4	T49.2X5	T49.2X6
Laxative NEC	T47.4X1	T47.4X2	T47.4X3	T47.4X4	T47.4X5	T47.4X6
osmotic	T47.3X1	T47.3X2	T47.3X3	T47.3X4	T47.3X5	T47.3X6
saline	T47.3X1	T47.3X2	T47.3X3	T47.3X4	T47.3X5	T47.3X6
stimulant	T47.2X1	T47.2X2	T47.2X3	T47.2X4	T47.2X5	T47.2X6
Lead (dust) (fumes) (vapor) **NEC**	T56.0X1	T56.0X2	T56.0X3	T56.0X4	—	—
acetate	T49.2X1	T49.2X2	T49.2X3	T49.2X4	T49.2X5	T49.2X6
anti-infectives	T37.8X1	T37.8X2	T37.8X3	T37.8X4	T37.8X5	T37.8X6
carbonate	T56.0X1	T56.0X2	T56.0X3	T56.0X4	—	—
paint	T56.0X1	T56.0X2	T56.0X3	T56.0X4		
chromate	T56.0X1	T56.0X2	T56.0X3	T56.0X4		
paint	T56.0X1	T56.0X2	T56.0X3	T56.0X4		
dioxide	T56.0X1	T56.0X2	T56.0X3	T56.0X4		
inorganic	T56.0X1	T56.0X2	T56.0X3	T56.0X4		

Substance	Poisoning, Accidental (unintentional)	Poisoning, Intentional Self-harm	Poisoning, Assault	Poisoning, Undetermined	Adverse Effect	Under-dosing
Lead (dust) (fumes) (vapor) **NEC** — continued						
iodide	T56.0X1	T56.0X2	T56.0X3	T56.0X4	—	—
organic	T56.0X1	T56.0X2	T56.0X3	T56.0X4	—	—
oxide	T56.0X1	T56.0X2	T56.0X3	T56.0X4		
paint	T56.0X1	T56.0X2	T56.0X3	T56.0X4		
salts	T56.0X1	T56.0X2	T56.0X3	T56.0X4		
specified compound NEC	T56.0X1	T56.0X2	T56.0X3	T56.0X4		
tetra-ethyl	T56.0X1	T56.0X2	T56.0X3	T56.0X4		
alkyl (fuel additive)	T56.0X1	T56.0X2	T56.0X3	T56.0X4		
antiknock compound (tetraethyl)	T56.0X1	T56.0X2	T56.0X3	T56.0X4		
arsenate, arsenite (dust)(herbicide) (insecticide) (vapor)	T57.0X1	T57.0X2	T57.0X3	T57.0X4		
pigment (paint)	T56.0X1	T56.0X2	T56.0X3	T56.0X4		
monoxide (dust)	T56.0X1	T56.0X2	T56.0X3	T56.0X4		
paint	T56.0X1	T56.0X2	T56.0X3	T56.0X4		
Lebanese red	T40.711	T40.712	T40.713	T40.714	T40.715	T40.716
Lefetamine	T39.8X1	T39.8X2	T39.8X3	T39.8X4	T39.8X5	T39.8X6
Lenperone	T43.4X1	T43.4X2	T43.4X3	T43.4X4	T43.4X5	T43.4X6
Lente Iletin (insulin)	T38.3X1	T38.3X2	T38.3X3	T38.3X4	T38.3X5	T38.3X6
Leptazol	T50.7X1	T50.7X2	T50.7X3	T50.7X4	T50.7X5	T50.7X6
Leptophos	T60.0X1	T60.0X2	T60.0X3	T60.0X4	—	—
Leritine	T40.2X1	T40.2X2	T40.2X3	T40.2X4	T40.2X5	T40.2X6
Lescol*	T46.6X1	T46.6X2	T46.6X3	T46.6X4	T46.6X5	T46.6X6
Letosteine	T48.4X1	T48.4X2	T48.4X3	T48.4X4	T48.4X5	T48.4X6
Letter	T38.1X1	T38.1X2	T38.1X3	T38.1X4	T38.1X5	T38.1X6
Lettuce opium	T42.6X1	T42.6X2	T42.6X3	T42.6X4	T42.6X5	T42.6X6
Leucinocaine	T41.3X1	T41.3X2	T41.3X3	T41.3X4	T41.3X5	T41.3X6
Leucocianidol	T46.991	T46.992	T46.993	T46.994	T46.995	T46.996
Leucovorin (factor)	T45.8X1	T45.8X2	T45.8X3	T45.8X4	T45.8X5	T45.8X6
Leukeran	T45.1X1	T45.1X2	T45.1X3	T45.1X4	T45.1X5	T45.1X6
Leuprolide	T38.891	T38.892	T38.893	T38.894	T38.895	T38.896
Levalbuterol	T48.6X1	T48.6X2	T48.6X3	T48.6X4	T48.6X5	T48.6X6
Levallorphan	T50.7X1	T50.7X2	T50.7X3	T50.7X4	T50.7X5	T50.7X6
Levamisole	T37.4X1	T37.4X2	T37.4X3	T37.4X4	T37.4X5	T37.4X6
Levanil	T42.6X1	T42.6X2	T42.6X3	T42.6X4	T42.6X5	T42.6X6
Levarterenol	T44.4X1	T44.4X2	T44.4X3	T44.4X4	T44.4X5	T44.4X6
Levdropropizine	T48.3X1	T48.3X2	T48.3X3	T48.3X4	T48.3X5	T48.3X6
Levo-dromoran	T40.2X1	T40.2X2	T40.2X3	T40.2X4	T40.2X5	T40.2X6
Levo-isomethadone	T40.3X1	T40.3X2	T40.3X3	T40.3X4	T40.3X5	T40.3X6
Levobunolol	T49.5X1	T49.5X2	T49.5X3	T49.5X4	T49.5X5	T49.5X6
Levocabastine (hydrochloride)	T45.0X1	T45.0X2	T45.0X3	T45.0X4	T45.0X5	T45.0X6
Levocarnitine	T50.991	T50.992	T50.993	T50.994	T50.995	T50.996
Levodopa	T42.8X1	T42.8X2	T42.8X3	T42.8X4	T42.8X5	T42.8X6
with carbidopa	T42.8X1	T42.8X2	T42.8X3	T42.8X4	T42.8X5	T42.8X6
Levoglutamide	T50.991	T50.992	T50.993	T50.994	T50.995	T50.996
Levoid	T38.1X1	T38.1X2	T38.1X3	T38.1X4	T38.1X5	T38.1X6
Levomepromazine	T43.3X1	T43.3X2	T43.3X3	T43.3X4	T43.3X5	T43.3X6
Levonordefrin	T49.6X1	T49.6X2	T49.6X3	T49.6X4	T49.6X5	T49.6X6
Levonorgestrel	T38.4X1	T38.4X2	T38.4X3	T38.4X4	T38.4X5	T38.4X6
with ethinylestradiol	T38.5X1	T38.5X2	T38.5X3	T38.5X4	T38.5X5	T38.5X6
Levopromazine	T43.3X1	T43.3X2	T43.3X3	T43.3X4	T43.3X5	T43.3X6
Levoprome	T42.6X1	T42.6X2	T42.6X3	T42.6X4	T42.6X5	T42.6X6
Levopropoxyphene	T40.491	T40.492	T40.493	T40.494	T40.495	T40.496
Levopropylhexedrine	T50.5X1	T50.5X2	T50.5X3	T50.5X4	T50.5X5	T50.5X6
Levoproxyphylline	T48.6X1	T48.6X2	T48.6X3	T48.6X4	T48.6X5	T48.6X6
Levorphanol	T40.491	T40.492	T40.493	T40.494	T40.495	T40.496
Levothroid*	T38.1X1	T38.1X2	T38.1X3	T38.1X4	T38.1X5	T38.1X6
Levothyroxine	T38.1X1	T38.1X2	T38.1X3	T38.1X4	T38.1X5	T38.1X6
sodium	T38.1X1	T38.1X2	T38.1X3	T38.1X4	T38.1X5	T38.1X6
Levoxyl*	T38.1X1	T38.1X2	T38.1X3	T38.1X4	T38.1X5	T38.1X6
Levsin	T44.3X1	T44.3X2	T44.3X3	T44.3X4	T44.3X5	T44.3X6
Levulose	T50.3X1	T50.3X2	T50.3X3	T50.3X4	T50.3X5	T50.3X6
Lewisite (gas), not in war	T57.0X1	T57.0X2	T57.0X3	T57.0X4	—	—
Lexapro*	T43.221	T43.222	T43.223	T43.224	T43.225	T43.226
Librium	T42.4X1	T42.4X2	T42.4X3	T42.4X4	T42.4X5	T42.4X6
Lidex	T49.0X1	T49.0X2	T49.0X3	T49.0X4	T49.0X5	T49.0X6
Lidocaine	T41.3X1	T41.3X2	T41.3X3	T41.3X4	T41.3X5	T41.3X6
regional	T41.3X1	T41.3X2	T41.3X3	T41.3X4	T41.3X5	T41.3X6
spinal	T41.3X1	T41.3X2	T41.3X3	T41.3X4	T41.3X5	T41.3X6
Lidofenin	T50.8X1	T50.8X2	T50.8X3	T50.8X4	T50.8X5	T50.8X6
Lidoflazine	T46.1X1	T46.1X2	T46.1X3	T46.1X4	T46.1X5	T46.1X6
Lighter fluid	T52.0X1	T52.0X2	T52.0X3	T52.0X4	—	—
Lignin hemicellulose	T47.6X1	T47.6X2	T47.6X3	T47.6X4	T47.6X5	T47.6X6
Lignocaine	T41.3X1	T41.3X2	T41.3X3	T41.3X4	T41.3X5	T41.3X6
regional	T41.3X1	T41.3X2	T41.3X3	T41.3X4	T41.3X5	T41.3X6
spinal	T41.3X1	T41.3X2	T41.3X3	T41.3X4	T41.3X5	T41.3X6
Ligroin (e) (solvent)	T52.0X1	T52.0X2	T52.0X3	T52.0X4	—	—
vapor	T59.891	T59.892	T59.893	T59.894		

Substance	Poisoning, Accidental (unintentional)	Poisoning, Intentional Self-harm	Poisoning, Assault	Poisoning, Undetermined	Adverse Effect	Under-dosing
Ligustrum vulgare	T62.2X1	T62.2X2	T62.2X3	T62.2X4	—	—
Lily of the valley	T62.2X1	T62.2X2	T62.2X3	T62.2X4	—	—
Lime (chloride)	T54.3X1	T54.3X2	T54.3X3	T54.3X4	—	—
Limonene	T52.8X1	T52.8X2	T52.8X3	T52.8X4	—	—
Lincomycin	T36.8X1	T36.8X2	T36.8X3	T36.8X4	T36.8X5	T36.8X6
Lindane (insecticide)	T53.6X1	T53.6X2	T53.6X3	T53.6X4	—	—
(nonmedicinal) (vapor)						
medicinal	T49.0X1	T49.0X2	T49.0X3	T49.0X4	T49.0X5	T49.0X6
Liniments NEC	T49.91	T49.92	T49.93	T49.94	T49.95	T49.96
Linoleic acid	T46.6X1	T46.6X2	T46.6X3	T46.6X4	T46.6X5	T46.6X6
Linolenic acid	T46.6X1	T46.6X2	T46.6X3	T46.6X4	T46.6X5	T46.6X6
Linseed	T47.4X1	T47.4X2	T47.4X3	T47.4X4	T47.4X5	T47.4X6
Liothyronine	T38.1X1	T38.1X2	T38.1X3	T38.1X4	T38.1X5	T38.1X6
Liotrix	T38.1X1	T38.1X2	T38.1X3	T38.1X4	T38.1X5	T38.1X6
Lipancreatin	T47.5X1	T47.5X2	T47.5X3	T47.5X4	T47.5X5	T47.5X6
Lipitor*	T46.6X1	T46.6X2	T46.6X3	T46.6X4	T46.6X5	T46.6X6
Lipo-alprostadil	T46.7X1	T46.7X2	T46.7X3	T46.7X4	T46.7X5	T46.7X6
Lipo-Lutin	T38.5X1	T38.5X2	T38.5X3	T38.5X4	T38.5X5	T38.5X6
Lipotropic drug NEC	T50.901	T50.902	T50.903	T50.904	T50.905	T50.906
Liquefied petroleum gases	T59.891	T59.892	T59.893	T59.894	—	—
piped (pure or mixed with air)	T59.891	T59.892	T59.893	T59.894	—	—
Liquid						
paraffin	T47.4X1	T47.4X2	T47.4X3	T47.4X4	T47.4X5	T47.4X6
petrolatum	T47.4X1	T47.4X2	T47.4X3	T47.4X4	T47.4X5	T47.4X6
topical	T49.3X1	T49.3X2	T49.3X3	T49.3X4	T49.3X5	T49.3X6
specified NEC	T65.891	T65.892	T65.893	T65.894	—	—
substance	T65.91	T65.92	T65.93	T65.94	—	—
Liquor creosolis compositus	T65.891	T65.892	T65.893	T65.894	—	—
Liquorice	T48.4X1	T48.4X2	T48.4X3	T48.4X4	T48.4X5	T48.4X6
extract	T47.8X1	T47.8X2	T47.8X3	T47.8X4	T47.8X5	T47.8X6
Liraglutide*	T38.3X1	T38.3X2	T38.3X3	T38.3X4	T38.3X5	T38.3X6
Lisinopril	T46.4X1	T46.4X2	T46.4X3	T46.4X4	T46.4X5	T46.4X6
Lisuride	T42.8X1	T42.8X2	T42.8X3	T42.8X4	T42.8X5	T42.8X6
Lithane	T43.8X1	T43.8X2	T43.8X3	T43.8X4	T43.8X5	T43.8X6
Lithium	T56.891	T56.892	T56.893	T56.894	—	—
gluconate	T43.591	T43.592	T43.593	T43.594	T43.595	T43.596
salts (carbonate)	T43.591	T43.592	T43.593	T43.594	T43.595	T43.596
Lithonate	T43.8X1	T43.8X2	T43.8X3	T43.8X4	T43.8X5	T43.8X6
Liver						
extract	T45.8X1	T45.8X2	T45.8X3	T45.8X4	T45.8X5	T45.8X6
for parenteral use	T45.8X1	T45.8X2	T45.8X3	T45.8X4	T45.8X5	T45.8X6
fraction 1	T45.8X1	T45.8X2	T45.8X3	T45.8X4	T45.8X5	T45.8X6
hydrolysate	T45.8X1	T45.8X2	T45.8X3	T45.8X4	T45.8X5	T45.8X6
Lizard (bite) (venom)	T63.121	T63.122	T63.123	T63.124	—	—
LMD	T45.8X1	T45.8X2	T45.8X3	T45.8X4	T45.8X5	T45.8X6
Lobelia	T62.2X1	T62.2X2	T62.2X3	T62.2X4	—	—
Lobeline	T50.7X1	T50.7X2	T50.7X3	T50.7X4	T50.7X5	T50.7X6
Local action drug NEC	T49.8X1	T49.8X2	T49.8X3	T49.8X4	T49.8X5	T49.8X6
Locorten	T49.0X1	T49.0X2	T49.0X3	T49.0X4	T49.0X5	T49.0X6
Lofepramine	T43.011	T43.012	T43.013	T43.014	T43.015	T43.016
Lolium temulentum	T62.2X1	T62.2X2	T62.2X3	T62.2X4	—	—
Lomotil	T47.6X1	T47.6X2	T47.6X3	T47.6X4	T47.6X5	T47.6X6
Lomustine	T45.1X1	T45.1X2	T45.1X3	T45.1X4	T45.1X5	T45.1X6
Lonidamine	T45.1X1	T45.1X2	T45.1X3	T45.1X4	T45.1X5	T45.1X6
LoOvral*	T38.4X1	T38.4X2	T38.4X3	T38.4X4	T38.4X5	T38.4X6
Loperamide	T47.6X1	T47.6X2	T47.6X3	T47.6X4	T47.6X5	T47.6X6
Loprazolam	T42.4X1	T42.4X2	T42.4X3	T42.4X4	T42.4X5	T42.4X6
Lopressor*	T44.7X1	T44.7X2	T44.7X3	T44.7X4	T44.7X5	T44.7X6
Lorajmine	T46.2X1	T46.2X2	T46.2X3	T46.2X4	T46.2X5	T46.2X6
Loratidine	T45.0X1	T45.0X2	T45.0X3	T45.0X4	T45.0X5	T45.0X6
Lorazepam	T42.4X1	T42.4X2	T42.4X3	T42.4X4	T42.4X5	T42.4X6
Lorcainide	T46.2X1	T46.2X2	T46.2X3	T46.2X4	T46.2X5	T46.2X6
Lormetazepam	T42.4X1	T42.4X2	T42.4X3	T42.4X4	T42.4X5	T42.4X6
Losartan*	T46.5X1	T46.5X2	T46.5X3	T46.5X4	T46.5X5	T46.5X6
Lotions NEC	T49.91	T49.92	T49.93	T49.94	T49.95	T49.96
Lotrimin*	T49.0X1	T49.0X2	T49.0X3	T49.0X4	T49.0X5	T49.0X6
Lotusate	T42.3X1	T42.3X2	T42.3X3	T42.3X4	T42.3X5	T42.3X6
Lovastatin	T46.6X1	T46.6X2	T46.6X3	T46.6X4	T46.6X5	T46.6X6
Lowila	T49.2X1	T49.2X2	T49.2X3	T49.2X4	T49.2X5	T49.2X6
Loxapine	T43.591	T43.592	T43.593	T43.594	T43.595	T43.596
Lozenges (throat)	T49.6X1	T49.6X2	T49.6X3	T49.6X4	T49.6X5	T49.6X6
LSD	T40.8X1	T40.8X2	T40.8X3	T40.8X4	—	—
Lubricant, eye	T49.5X1	T49.5X2	T49.5X3	T49.5X4	T49.5X5	T49.5X6
Lubricating oil NEC	T52.0X1	T52.0X2	T52.0X3	T52.0X4	—	—
Lucanthone	T37.4X1	T37.4X2	T37.4X3	T37.4X4	T37.4X5	T37.4X6
Luminal	T42.3X1	T42.3X2	T42.3X3	T42.3X4	T42.3X5	T42.3X6
Lung irritant (gas) NEC	T59.91	T59.92	T59.93	T59.94	—	—
Luteinizing hormone	T38.811	T38.812	T38.813	T38.814	T38.815	T38.816
Lutocylol	T38.5X1	T38.5X2	T38.5X3	T38.5X4	T38.5X5	T38.5X6
Lutromone	T38.5X1	T38.5X2	T38.5X3	T38.5X4	T38.5X5	T38.5X6
Lututrin	T48.291	T48.292	T48.293	T48.294	T48.295	T48.296
Luveris*	T38.891	T38.892	T38.893	T38.894	T38.895	T38.896
Lye (concentrated)	T54.3X1	T54.3X2	T54.3X3	T54.3X4	—	—
Lygranum (skin test)	T50.8X1	T50.8X2	T50.8X3	T50.8X4	T50.8X5	T50.8X6
Lymecycline	T36.4X1	T36.4X2	T36.4X3	T36.4X4	T36.4X5	T36.4X6
Lymphogranuloma venereum antigen	T50.8X1	T50.8X2	T50.8X3	T50.8X4	T50.8X5	T50.8X6
Lynestrenol	T38.4X1	T38.4X2	T38.4X3	T38.4X4	T38.4X5	T38.4X6
Lyovac Sodium Edecrin	T50.1X1	T50.1X2	T50.1X3	T50.1X4	T50.1X5	T50.1X6
Lypressin	T38.891	T38.892	T38.893	T38.894	T38.895	T38.896
Lysergic acid diethylamide	T40.8X1	T40.8X2	T40.8X3	T40.8X4	—	—
Lysergide	T40.8X1	T40.8X2	T40.8X3	T40.8X4	—	—
Lysine vasopressin	T38.891	T38.892	T38.893	T38.894	T38.895	T38.896
Lysol	T54.1X1	T54.1X2	T54.1X3	T54.1X4	—	—
Lysozyme	T49.0X1	T49.0X2	T49.0X3	T49.0X4	T49.0X5	T49.0X6
Lytta (vitatta)	T49.8X1	T49.8X2	T49.8X3	T49.8X4	T49.8X5	T49.8X6
M-AMSA	T45.1X1	T45.1X2	T45.1X3	T45.1X4	T45.1X5	T45.1X6
M-vac	T45.1X1	T45.1X2	T45.1X3	T45.1X4	T45.1X5	T45.1X6
Mace	T59.3X1	T59.3X2	T59.3X3	T59.3X4	—	—
Macrogol	T50.991	T50.992	T50.993	T50.994	T50.995	T50.996
Macrolide						
anabolic drug	T38.7X1	T38.7X2	T38.7X3	T38.7X4	T38.7X5	T38.7X6
antibiotic	T36.3X1	T36.3X2	T36.3X3	T36.3X4	T36.3X5	T36.3X6
Mafenide	T49.0X1	T49.0X2	T49.0X3	T49.0X4	T49.0X5	T49.0X6
Magaldrate	T47.1X1	T47.1X2	T47.1X3	T47.1X4	T47.1X5	T47.1X6
Magic mushroom	T40.991	T40.992	T40.993	T40.994	—	—
Magnamycin	T36.8X1	T36.8X2	T36.8X3	T36.8X4	T36.8X5	T36.8X6
Magnesia magma	T47.1X1	T47.1X2	T47.1X3	T47.1X4	T47.1X5	T47.1X6
Magnesium NEC	T56.891	T56.892	T56.893	T56.894	—	—
carbonate	T47.1X1	T47.1X2	T47.1X3	T47.1X4	T47.1X5	T47.1X6
citrate	T47.4X1	T47.4X2	T47.4X3	T47.4X4	T47.4X5	T47.4X6
hydroxide	T47.1X1	T47.1X2	T47.1X3	T47.1X4	T47.1X5	T47.1X6
oxide	T47.1X1	T47.1X2	T47.1X3	T47.1X4	T47.1X5	T47.1X6
peroxide	T49.0X1	T49.0X2	T49.0X3	T49.0X4	T49.0X5	T49.0X6
salicylate	T39.091	T39.092	T39.093	T39.094	T39.095	T39.096
silicofluoride	T50.3X1	T50.3X2	T50.3X3	T50.3X4	T50.3X5	T50.3X6
sulfate	T47.4X1	T47.4X2	T47.4X3	T47.4X4	T47.4X5	T47.4X6
thiosulfate	T45.0X1	T45.0X2	T45.0X3	T45.0X4	T45.0X5	T45.0X6
trisilicate	T47.1X1	T47.1X2	T47.1X3	T47.1X4	T47.1X5	T47.1X6
Malathion (medicinal)	T49.0X1	T49.0X2	T49.0X3	T49.0X4	T49.0X5	T49.0X6
insecticide	T60.0X1	T60.0X2	T60.0X3	T60.0X4	—	—
Male fern extract	T37.4X1	T37.4X2	T37.4X3	T37.4X4	T37.4X5	T37.4X6
Mandelic acid	T37.8X1	T37.8X2	T37.8X3	T37.8X4	T37.8X5	T37.8X6
Manganese (dioxide) (salts)	T57.2X1	T57.2X2	T57.2X3	T57.2X4	—	—
medicinal	T50.991	T50.992	T50.993	T50.994	T50.995	T50.996
Mannitol	T47.3X1	T47.3X2	T47.3X3	T47.3X4	T47.3X5	T47.3X6
hexanitrate	T46.3X1	T46.3X2	T46.3X3	T46.3X4	T46.3X5	T46.3X6
Mannomustine	T45.1X1	T45.1X2	T45.1X3	T45.1X4	T45.1X5	T45.1X6
MAO inhibitors	T43.1X1	T43.1X2	T43.1X3	T43.1X4	T43.1X5	T43.1X6
Mapharsen	T37.8X1	T37.8X2	T37.8X3	T37.8X4	T37.8X5	T37.8X6
Maphenide	T49.0X1	T49.0X2	T49.0X3	T49.0X4	T49.0X5	T49.0X6
Maprotiline	T43.021	T43.022	T43.023	T43.024	T43.025	T43.026
Marcaine	T41.3X1	T41.3X2	T41.3X3	T41.3X4	T41.3X5	T41.3X6
infiltration (subcutaneous)	T41.3X1	T41.3X2	T41.3X3	T41.3X4	T41.3X5	T41.3X6
nerve block (peripheral) (plexus)	T41.3X1	T41.3X2	T41.3X3	T41.3X4	T41.3X5	T41.3X6
Marezine	T45.0X1	T45.0X2	T45.0X3	T45.0X4	T45.0X5	T45.0X6
Marihuana	T40.711	T40.712	T40.713	T40.714	T40.715	T40.716
Marijuana	T40.711	T40.712	T40.713	T40.714	T40.715	T40.716
Marine (sting)	T63.691	T63.692	T63.693	T63.694		
animals (sting)	T63.691	T63.692	T63.693	T63.694	—	—
plants (sting)	T63.711	T63.712	T63.713	T63.714	—	—
Marplan	T43.1X1	T43.1X2	T43.1X3	T43.1X4	T43.1X5	T43.1X6
Marsh gas	T59.891	T59.892	T59.893	T59.894	—	—
Marsilid	T43.1X1	T43.1X2	T43.1X3	T43.1X4	T43.1X5	T43.1X6
Massengill*	T49.0X1	T49.0X2	T49.0X3	T49.0X4	T49.0X5	T49.0X6
Matulane	T45.1X1	T45.1X2	T45.1X3	T45.1X4	T45.1X5	T45.1X6
Mazindol	T50.5X1	T50.5X2	T50.5X3	T50.5X4	T50.5X5	T50.5X6
MCPA	T60.3X1	T60.3X2	T60.3X3	T60.3X4	—	—
MDMA	T43.641	T43.642	T43.643	T43.644	—	—
Meadow saffron	T62.2X1	T62.2X2	T62.2X3	T62.2X4	—	—
Measles virus vaccine (attenuated)	T50.B91	T50.B92	T50.B93	T50.B94	T50.B95	T50.B96
Meat, noxious	T62.8X1	T62.8X2	T62.8X3	T62.8X4	—	—
Meballymal	T42.3X1	T42.3X2	T42.3X3	T42.3X4	T42.3X5	T42.3X6
Mebanazine	T43.1X1	T43.1X2	T43.1X3	T43.1X4	T43.1X5	T43.1X6
Mebaral	T42.3X1	T42.3X2	T42.3X3	T42.3X4	T42.3X5	T42.3X6
Mebendazole	T37.4X1	T37.4X2	T37.4X3	T37.4X4	T37.4X5	T37.4X6
Mebeverine	T44.3X1	T44.3X2	T44.3X3	T44.3X4	T44.3X5	T44.3X6
Mebhydrolin	T45.0X1	T45.0X2	T45.0X3	T45.0X4	T45.0X5	T45.0X6
Mebumal	T42.3X1	T42.3X2	T42.3X3	T42.3X4	T42.3X5	T42.3X6
Mebutamate	T43.591	T43.592	T43.593	T43.594	T43.595	T43.596
Mecamylamine	T44.2X1	T44.2X2	T44.2X3	T44.2X4	T44.2X5	T44.2X6
Mechlorethamine	T45.1X1	T45.1X2	T45.1X3	T45.1X4	T45.1X5	T45.1X6

Substance	Poisoning, Accidental (unintentional)	Poisoning, Intentional Self-harm	Poisoning, Assault	Poisoning, Undetermined	Adverse Effect	Under-dosing
Mecillinam	T36.ØX1	T36.ØX2	T36.ØX3	T36.ØX4	T36.ØX5	T36.ØX6
Meclizine (hydrochloride)	T45.ØX1	T45.ØX2	T45.ØX3	T45.ØX4	T45.ØX5	T45.ØX6
Meclocycline	T36.4X1	T36.4X2	T36.4X3	T36.4X4	T36.4X5	T36.4X6
Meclofenamate	T39.391	T39.392	T39.393	T39.394	T39.395	T39.396
Meclofenamic acid	T39.391	T39.392	T39.393	T39.394	T39.395	T39.396
Meclofenoxate	T43.691	T43.692	T43.693	T43.694	T43.695	T43.696
Meclozine	T45.ØX1	T45.ØX2	T45.ØX3	T45.ØX4	T45.ØX5	T45.ØX6
Mecobalamin	T45.8X1	T45.8X2	T45.8X3	T45.8X4	T45.8X5	T45.8X6
Mecoprop	T6Ø.3X1	T6Ø.3X2	T6Ø.3X3	T6Ø.3X4	—	—
Mecrilate	T49.3X1	T49.3X2	T49.3X3	T49.3X4	T49.3X5	T49.3X6
Mecysteine	T48.4X1	T48.4X2	T48.4X3	T48.4X4	T48.4X5	T48.4X6
Medazepam	T42.4X1	T42.4X2	T42.4X3	T42.4X4	T42.4X5	T42.4X6
Medicament NEC	T5Ø.9Ø1	T5Ø.9Ø2	T5Ø.9Ø3	T5Ø.9Ø4	T5Ø.9Ø5	T5Ø.9Ø6
Medinal	T42.3X1	T42.3X2	T42.3X3	T42.3X4	T42.3X5	T42.3X6
Medomin	T42.3X1	T42.3X2	T42.3X3	T42.3X4	T42.3X5	T42.3X6
Medrogestone	T38.5X1	T38.5X2	T38.5X3	T38.5X4	T38.5X5	T38.5X6
Medrol*	T38.ØX1	T38.ØX2	T38.ØX3	T38.ØX4	T38.ØX5	T38.ØX6
Medroxalol	T44.8X1	T44.8X2	T44.8X3	T44.8X4	T44.8X5	T44.8X6
Medroxyprogesterone acetate (depot)	T38.5X1	T38.5X2	T38.5X3	T38.5X4	T38.5X5	T38.5X6
Medrysone	T49.ØX1	T49.ØX2	T49.ØX3	T49.ØX4	T49.ØX5	T49.ØX6
Mefenamic acid	T39.391	T39.392	T39.393	T39.394	T39.395	T39.396
Mefenorex	T5Ø.5X1	T5Ø.5X2	T5Ø.5X3	T5Ø.5X4	T5Ø.5X5	T5Ø.5X6
Mefloquine	T37.2X1	T37.2X2	T37.2X3	T37.2X4	T37.2X5	T37.2X6
Mefoxin*	T36.1X1	T36.1X2	T36.1X3	T36.1X4	T36.1X5	T36.1X6
Mefruside	T5Ø.2X1	T5Ø.2X2	T5Ø.2X3	T5Ø.2X4	T5Ø.2X5	T5Ø.2X6
Megahallucinogen	T4Ø.9Ø1	T4Ø.9Ø2	T4Ø.9Ø3	T4Ø.9Ø4	T4Ø.9Ø5	T4Ø.9Ø6
Megestrol	T38.5X1	T38.5X2	T38.5X3	T38.5X4	T38.5X5	T38.5X6
Meglumine						
antimoniate	T37.8X1	T37.8X2	T37.8X3	T37.8X4	T37.8X5	T37.8X6
diatrizoate	T5Ø.8X1	T5Ø.8X2	T5Ø.8X3	T5Ø.8X4	T5Ø.8X5	T5Ø.8X6
iodipamide	T5Ø.8X1	T5Ø.8X2	T5Ø.8X3	T5Ø.8X4	T5Ø.8X5	T5Ø.8X6
iotroxate	T5Ø.8X1	T5Ø.8X2	T5Ø.8X3	T5Ø.8X4	T5Ø.8X5	T5Ø.8X6
MEK (methyl ethyl ketone)	T52.4X1	T52.4X2	T52.4X3	T52.4X4	—	—
Meladinin	T49.3X1	T49.3X2	T49.3X3	T49.3X4	T49.3X5	T49.3X6
Meladrazine	T44.3X1	T44.3X2	T44.3X3	T44.3X4	T44.3X5	T44.3X6
Melaleuca alternifolia oil	T49.ØX1	T49.ØX2	T49.ØX3	T49.ØX4	T49.ØX5	T49.ØX6
Melanizing agents	T49.3X1	T49.3X2	T49.3X3	T49.3X4	T49.3X5	T49.3X6
Melanocyte-stimulating hormone	T38.891	T38.892	T38.893	T38.894	T38.895	T38.896
Melarsonyl potassium	T37.3X1	T37.3X2	T37.3X3	T37.3X4	T37.3X5	T37.3X6
Melarsoprol	T37.3X1	T37.3X2	T37.3X3	T37.3X4	T37.3X5	T37.3X6
Melia azedarach	T62.2X1	T62.2X2	T62.2X3	T62.2X4	—	—
Melitracen	T43.Ø11	T43.Ø12	T43.Ø13	T43.Ø14	T43.Ø15	T43.Ø16
Mellaril	T43.3X1	T43.3X2	T43.3X3	T43.3X4	T43.3X5	T43.3X6
Meloxicam*	T39.391	T39.392	T39.393	T39.394	T39.395	T39.396
Meloxine	T49.3X1	T49.3X2	T49.3X3	T49.3X4	T49.3X5	T49.3X6
Melperone	T43.4X1	T43.4X2	T43.4X3	T43.4X4	T43.4X5	T43.4X6
Melphalan	T45.1X1	T45.1X2	T45.1X3	T45.1X4	T45.1X5	T45.1X6
Memantine	T43.8X1	T43.8X2	T43.8X3	T43.8X4	T43.8X5	T43.8X6
Menadiol	T45.7X1	T45.7X2	T45.7X3	T45.7X4	T45.7X5	T45.7X6
sodium sulfate	T45.7X1	T45.7X2	T45.7X3	T45.7X4	T45.7X5	T45.7X6
Menadione	T45.7X1	T45.7X2	T45.7X3	T45.7X4	T45.7X5	T45.7X6
sodium bisulfite	T45.7X1	T45.7X2	T45.7X3	T45.7X4	T45.7X5	T45.7X6
Menaphthone	T45.7X1	T45.7X2	T45.7X3	T45.7X4	T45.7X5	T45.7X6
Menaquinone	T45.7X1	T45.7X2	T45.7X3	T45.7X4	T45.7X5	T45.7X6
Menatetrenone	T45.7X1	T45.7X2	T45.7X3	T45.7X4	T45.7X5	T45.7X6
Meningococcal vaccine	T5Ø.A91	T5Ø.A92	T5Ø.A93	T5Ø.A94	T5Ø.A95	T5Ø.A96
Menningovax (-AC) (-C)	T5Ø.A91	T5Ø.A92	T5Ø.A93	T5Ø.A94	T5Ø.A95	T5Ø.A96
Menotropins	T38.811	T38.812	T38.813	T38.814	T38.815	T38.816
Menthol	T48.5X1	T48.5X2	T48.5X3	T48.5X4	T48.5X5	T48.5X6
Mepacrine	T37.2X1	T37.2X2	T37.2X3	T37.2X4	T37.2X5	T37.2X6
Meparfynol	T42.6X1	T42.6X2	T42.6X3	T42.6X4	T42.6X5	T42.6X6
Mepartricin	T36.7X1	T36.7X2	T36.7X3	T36.7X4	T36.7X5	T36.7X6
Mepazine	T43.3X1	T43.3X2	T43.3X3	T43.3X4	T43.3X5	T43.3X6
Mepenzolate	T44.3X1	T44.3X2	T44.3X3	T44.3X4	T44.3X5	T44.3X6
bromide	T44.3X1	T44.3X2	T44.3X3	T44.3X4	T44.3X5	T44.3X6
Meperidine	T4Ø.491	T4Ø.492	T4Ø.493	T4Ø.494	T4Ø.495	T4Ø.496
Mephebarbital	T42.3X1	T42.3X2	T42.3X3	T42.3X4	T42.3X5	T42.3X6
Mephenamin (e)	T42.8X1	T42.8X2	T42.8X3	T42.8X4	T42.8X5	T42.8X6
Mephenesin	T42.8X1	T42.8X2	T42.8X3	T42.8X4	T42.8X5	T42.8X6
Mephenhydramine	T45.ØX1	T45.ØX2	T45.ØX3	T45.ØX4	T45.ØX5	T45.ØX6
Mephenoxalone	T42.8X1	T42.8X2	T42.8X3	T42.8X4	T42.8X5	T42.8X6
Mephentermine	T44.991	T44.992	T44.993	T44.994	T44.995	T44.996
Mephenytoin	T42.ØX1	T42.ØX2	T42.ØX3	T42.ØX4	T42.ØX5	T42.ØX6
with phenobarbital	T42.3X1	T42.3X2	T42.3X3	T42.3X4	T42.3X5	T42.3X6
Mephobarbital	T42.3X1	T42.3X2	T42.3X3	T42.3X4	T42.3X5	T42.3X6
Mephosfolan	T6Ø.ØX1	T6Ø.ØX2	T6Ø.ØX3	T6Ø.ØX4	—	—
Mepindolol	T44.7X1	T44.7X2	T44.7X3	T44.7X4	T44.7X5	T44.7X6
Mepiperphenidol	T44.3X1	T44.3X2	T44.3X3	T44.3X4	T44.3X5	T44.3X6
Mepitiostane	T38.7X1	T38.7X2	T38.7X3	T38.7X4	T38.7X5	T38.7X6
Mepivacaine	T41.3X1	T41.3X2	T41.3X3	T41.3X4	T41.3X5	T41.3X6
epidural	T41.3X1	T41.3X2	T41.3X3	T41.3X4	T41.3X5	T41.3X6

Substance	Poisoning, Accidental (unintentional)	Poisoning, Intentional Self-harm	Poisoning, Assault	Poisoning, Undetermined	Adverse Effect	Under-dosing
Meprednisone	T38.ØX1	T38.ØX2	T38.ØX3	T38.ØX4	T38.ØX5	T38.ØX6
Meprobam	T43.591	T43.592	T43.593	T43.594	T43.595	T43.596
Meprobamate	T43.591	T43.592	T43.593	T43.594	T43.595	T43.596
Meproscillarin	T46.ØX1	T46.ØX2	T46.ØX3	T46.ØX4	T46.ØX5	T46.ØX6
Meprylcaine	T41.3X1	T41.3X2	T41.3X3	T41.3X4	T41.3X5	T41.3X6
Meptazinol	T39.8X1	T39.8X2	T39.8X3	T39.8X4	T39.8X5	T39.8X6
Mepyramine	T45.ØX1	T45.ØX2	T45.ØX3	T45.ØX4	T45.ØX5	T45.ØX6
Mequinol*	T49.8X1	T49.8X2	T49.8X3	T49.8X4	T49.8X5	T49.8X6
Mequitazine	T43.3X1	T43.3X2	T43.3X3	T43.3X4	T43.3X5	T43.3X6
Meralluride	T5Ø.2X1	T5Ø.2X2	T5Ø.2X3	T5Ø.2X4	T5Ø.2X5	T5Ø.2X6
Merbaphen	T5Ø.2X1	T5Ø.2X2	T5Ø.2X3	T5Ø.2X4	T5Ø.2X5	T5Ø.2X6
Merbromin	T49.ØX1	T49.ØX2	T49.ØX3	T49.ØX4	T49.ØX5	T49.ØX6
Mercaptobenzothiazole salts	T49.ØX1	T49.ØX2	T49.ØX3	T49.ØX4	T49.ØX5	T49.ØX6
Mercaptomerin	T5Ø.2X1	T5Ø.2X2	T5Ø.2X3	T5Ø.2X4	T5Ø.2X5	T5Ø.2X6
Mercaptopurine	T45.1X1	T45.1X2	T45.1X3	T45.1X4	T45.1X5	T45.1X6
Mercumatilin	T5Ø.2X1	T5Ø.2X2	T5Ø.2X3	T5Ø.2X4	T5Ø.2X5	T5Ø.2X6
Mercuramide	T5Ø.2X1	T5Ø.2X2	T5Ø.2X3	T5Ø.2X4	T5Ø.2X5	T5Ø.2X6
Mercurochrome	T49.ØX1	T49.ØX2	T49.ØX3	T49.ØX4	T49.ØX5	T49.ØX6
Mercurophylline	T5Ø.2X1	T5Ø.2X2	T5Ø.2X3	T5Ø.2X4	T5Ø.2X5	T5Ø.2X6
Mercury, mercurial, mercuric, mercurous (compounds) (cyanide) (fumes) (nonmedicinal) (vapor) **NEC**	T56.1X1	T56.1X2	T56.1X3	T56.1X4	—	—
ammoniated	T49.ØX1	T49.ØX2	T49.ØX3	T49.ØX4	T49.ØX5	T49.ØX6
anti-infective						
local	T49.ØX1	T49.ØX2	T49.ØX3	T49.ØX4	T49.ØX5	T49.ØX6
systemic	T37.8X1	T37.8X2	T37.8X3	T37.8X4	T37.8X5	T37.8X6
topical	T49.ØX1	T49.ØX2	T49.ØX3	T49.ØX4	T49.ØX5	T49.ØX6
chloride (ammoniated)	T49.ØX1	T49.ØX2	T49.ØX3	T49.ØX4	T49.ØX5	T49.ØX6
fungicide	T56.1X1	T56.1X2	T56.1X3	T56.1X4	—	—
diuretic NEC	T5Ø.2X1	T5Ø.2X2	T5Ø.2X3	T5Ø.2X4	T5Ø.2X5	T5Ø.2X6
fungicide	T56.1X1	T56.1X2	T56.1X3	T56.1X4	—	—
organic (fungicide)	T56.1X1	T56.1X2	T56.1X3	T56.1X4	—	—
oxide, yellow	T49.ØX1	T49.ØX2	T49.ØX3	T49.ØX4	T49.ØX5	T49.ØX6
Mersalyl	T5Ø.2X1	T5Ø.2X2	T5Ø.2X3	T5Ø.2X4	T5Ø.2X5	T5Ø.2X6
Merthiolate	T49.ØX1	T49.ØX2	T49.ØX3	T49.ØX4	T49.ØX5	T49.ØX6
ophthalmic preparation	T49.5X1	T49.5X2	T49.5X3	T49.5X4	T49.5X5	T49.5X6
Meruvax	T5Ø.B91	T5Ø.B92	T5Ø.B93	T5Ø.B94	T5Ø.B95	T5Ø.B96
Mesalazine	T47.8X1	T47.8X2	T47.8X3	T47.8X4	T47.8X5	T47.8X6
Mescal buttons	T4Ø.991	T4Ø.992	T4Ø.993	T4Ø.994	—	—
Mescaline	T4Ø.991	T4Ø.992	T4Ø.993	T4Ø.994	—	—
Mesna	T48.4X1	T48.4X2	T48.4X3	T48.4X4	T48.4X5	T48.4X6
Mesoglycan	T46.6X1	T46.6X2	T46.6X3	T46.6X4	T46.6X5	T46.6X6
Mesoridazine	T43.3X1	T43.3X2	T43.3X3	T43.3X4	T43.3X5	T43.3X6
Mestanolone	T38.7X1	T38.7X2	T38.7X3	T38.7X4	T38.7X5	T38.7X6
Mesterolone	T38.7X1	T38.7X2	T38.7X3	T38.7X4	T38.7X5	T38.7X6
Mestranol	T38.5X1	T38.5X2	T38.5X3	T38.5X4	T38.5X5	T38.5X6
Mesulergine	T42.8X1	T42.8X2	T42.8X3	T42.8X4	T42.8X5	T42.8X6
Mesulfen	T49.ØX1	T49.ØX2	T49.ØX3	T49.ØX4	T49.ØX5	T49.ØX6
Mesuximide	T42.2X1	T42.2X2	T42.2X3	T42.2X4	T42.2X5	T42.2X6
Metabutethamine	T41.3X1	T41.3X2	T41.3X3	T41.3X4	T41.3X5	T41.3X6
Metactesylacetate	T49.ØX1	T49.ØX2	T49.ØX3	T49.ØX4	T49.ØX5	T49.ØX6
Metacycline	T36.4X1	T36.4X2	T36.4X3	T36.4X4	T36.4X5	T36.4X6
Metaldehyde (snail killer) **NEC**	T6Ø.8X1	T6Ø.8X2	T6Ø.8X3	T6Ø.8X4	—	—
Metals (heavy) (nonmedicinal)	T56.91	T56.92	T56.93	T56.94	—	—
dust, fumes, or vapor NEC	T56.91	T56.92	T56.93	T56.94	—	—
gadolinium	T56.821	T56.822	T56.823	T56.824	—	—
light NEC	T56.91	T56.92	T56.93	T56.94	—	—
dust, fumes, or vapor NEC	T56.91	T56.92	T56.93	T56.94	—	—
specified NEC	T56.891	T56.892	T56.893	T56.894	—	—
thallium	T56.811	T56.812	T56.813	T56.814	—	—
Metamfetamine	T43.651	T43.652	T43.653	T43.654	T43.655	T43.656
Metamizole sodium	T39.2X1	T39.2X2	T39.2X3	T39.2X4	T39.2X5	T39.2X6
Metampicillin	T36.ØX1	T36.ØX2	T36.ØX3	T36.ØX4	T36.ØX5	T36.ØX6
Metamucil	T47.4X1	T47.4X2	T47.4X3	T47.4X4	T47.4X5	T47.4X6
Metandienone	T38.7X1	T38.7X2	T38.7X3	T38.7X4	T38.7X5	T38.7X6
Metandrostenolone	T38.7X1	T38.7X2	T38.7X3	T38.7X4	T38.7X5	T38.7X6
Metaphen	T49.ØX1	T49.ØX2	T49.ØX3	T49.ØX4	T49.ØX5	T49.ØX6
Metaphos	T6Ø.ØX1	T6Ø.ØX2	T6Ø.ØX3	T6Ø.ØX4	—	—
Metapramine	T43.Ø11	T43.Ø12	T43.Ø13	T43.Ø14	T43.Ø15	T43.Ø16
Metaproterenol	T48.291	T48.292	T48.293	T48.294	T48.295	T48.296
Metaraminol	T44.4X1	T44.4X2	T44.4X3	T44.4X4	T44.4X5	T44.4X6
Metaxalone	T42.8X1	T42.8X2	T42.8X3	T42.8X4	T42.8X5	T42.8X6
Meted*	T49.4X1	T49.4X2	T49.4X3	T49.4X4	T49.4X5	T49.4X6
Metenolone	T38.7X1	T38.7X2	T38.7X3	T38.7X4	T38.7X5	T38.7X6
Metergoline	T42.8X1	T42.8X2	T42.8X3	T42.8X4	T42.8X5	T42.8X6
Metescufylline	T46.991	T46.992	T46.993	T46.994	T46.995	T46.996
Metetoin	T42.ØX1	T42.ØX2	T42.ØX3	T42.ØX4	T42.ØX5	T42.ØX6

Substance	Poisoning, Accidental (unintentional)	Poisoning, Intentional Self-harm	Poisoning, Assault	Poisoning, Undetermined	Adverse Effect	Under-dosing
Metformin	T38.3X1	T38.3X2	T38.3X3	T38.3X4	T38.3X5	T38.3X6
Methacholine	T44.1X1	T44.1X2	T44.1X3	T44.1X4	T44.1X5	T44.1X6
Methacycline	T36.4X1	T36.4X2	T36.4X3	T36.4X4	T36.4X5	T36.4X6
Methadone	T4Ø.3X1	T4Ø.3X2	T4Ø.3X3	T4Ø.3X4	T4Ø.3X5	T4Ø.3X6
Methadose*	T4Ø.3X1	T4Ø.3X2	T4Ø.3X3	T4Ø.3X4	T4Ø.3X5	T4Ø.3X6
Methallenestril	T38.5X1	T38.5X2	T38.5X3	T38.5X4	T38.5X5	T38.5X6
Methallenoestril	T38.5X1	T38.5X2	T38.5X3	T38.5X4	T38.5X5	T38.5X6
Methamphetamine	T43.651	T43.652	T43.653	T43.654	T43.655	T43.656
Methampyrone	T39.2X1	T39.2X2	T39.2X3	T39.2X4	T39.2X5	T39.2X6
Methandienone	T38.7X1	T38.7X2	T38.7X3	T38.7X4	T38.7X5	T38.7X6
Methandriol	T38.7X1	T38.7X2	T38.7X3	T38.7X4	T38.7X5	T38.7X6
Methandrostenolone	T38.7X1	T38.7X2	T38.7X3	T38.7X4	T38.7X5	T38.7X6
Methane	T59.891	T59.892	T59.893	T59.894	—	—
Methanethiol	T59.891	T59.892	T59.893	T59.894	—	—
Methaniazide	T37.1X1	T37.1X2	T37.1X3	T37.1X4	T37.1X5	T37.1X6
Methanol (vapor)	T51.1X1	T51.1X2	T51.1X3	T51.1X4	—	—
Methantheline	T44.3X1	T44.3X2	T44.3X3	T44.3X4	T44.3X5	T44.3X6
Methanthelinium bromide	T44.3X1	T44.3X2	T44.3X3	T44.3X4	T44.3X5	T44.3X6
Methaphenilene	T45.ØX1	T45.ØX2	T45.ØX3	T45.ØX4	T45.ØX5	T45.ØX6
Methapyrilene	T45.ØX1	T45.ØX2	T45.ØX3	T45.ØX4	T45.ØX5	T45.ØX6
Methaqualone (compound)	T42.6X1	T42.6X2	T42.6X3	T42.6X4	T42.6X5	T42.6X6
Metharbital	T42.3X1	T42.3X2	T42.3X3	T42.3X4	T42.3X5	T42.3X6
Methazolamide	T5Ø.2X1	T5Ø.2X2	T5Ø.2X3	T5Ø.2X4	T5Ø.2X5	T5Ø.2X6
Methdilazine	T43.3X1	T43.3X2	T43.3X3	T43.3X4	T43.3X5	T43.3X6
Methedrine	T43.651	T43.652	T43.653	T43.654	T43.655	T43.656
Methenamine (mandelate)	T37.8X1	T37.8X2	T37.8X3	T37.8X4	T37.8X5	T37.8X6
Methenolone	T38.7X1	T38.7X2	T38.7X3	T38.7X4	T38.7X5	T38.7X6
Methergine	T48.ØX1	T48.ØX2	T48.ØX3	T48.ØX4	T48.ØX5	T48.ØX6
Methetoin	T42.ØX1	T42.ØX2	T42.ØX3	T42.ØX4	T42.ØX5	T42.ØX6
Methiacil	T38.2X1	T38.2X2	T38.2X3	T38.2X4	T38.2X5	T38.2X6
Methicillin	T36.ØX1	T36.ØX2	T36.ØX3	T36.ØX4	T36.ØX5	T36.ØX6
Methimazole	T38.2X1	T38.2X2	T38.2X3	T38.2X4	T38.2X5	T38.2X6
Methiodal sodium	T5Ø.8X1	T5Ø.8X2	T5Ø.8X3	T5Ø.8X4	T5Ø.8X5	T5Ø.8X6
Methionine	T5Ø.991	T5Ø.992	T5Ø.993	T5Ø.994	T5Ø.995	T5Ø.996
Methisazone	T37.5X1	T37.5X2	T37.5X3	T37.5X4	T37.5X5	T37.5X6
Methisoprinol	T37.5X1	T37.5X2	T37.5X3	T37.5X4	T37.5X5	T37.5X6
Methitural	T42.3X1	T42.3X2	T42.3X3	T42.3X4	T42.3X5	T42.3X6
Methixene	T44.3X1	T44.3X2	T44.3X3	T44.3X4	T44.3X5	T44.3X6
Methobarbital, methobarbitone	T42.3X1	T42.3X2	T42.3X3	T42.3X4	T42.3X5	T42.3X6
Methocarbamol	T42.8X1	T42.8X2	T42.8X3	T42.8X4	T42.8X5	T42.8X6
skeletal muscle relaxant	T48.1X1	T48.1X2	T48.1X3	T48.1X4	T48.1X5	T48.1X6
Methohexital	T41.1X1	T41.1X2	T41.1X3	T41.1X4	T41.1X5	T41.1X6
Methohexitone	T41.1X1	T41.1X2	T41.1X3	T41.1X4	T41.1X5	T41.1X6
Methoin	T42.ØX1	T42.ØX2	T42.ØX3	T42.ØX4	T42.ØX5	T42.ØX6
Methopholine	T39.8X1	T39.8X2	T39.8X3	T39.8X4	T39.8X5	T39.8X6
Methopromazine	T43.3X1	T43.3X2	T43.3X3	T43.3X4	T43.3X5	T43.3X6
Methorate	T48.3X1	T48.3X2	T48.3X3	T48.3X4	T48.3X5	T48.3X6
Methoserpidine	T46.5X1	T46.5X2	T46.5X3	T46.5X4	T46.5X5	T46.5X6
Methotrexate	T45.1X1	T45.1X2	T45.1X3	T45.1X4	T45.1X5	T45.1X6
Methotrimeprazine	T43.3X1	T43.3X2	T43.3X3	T43.3X4	T43.3X5	T43.3X6
Methoxa-Dome	T49.3X1	T49.3X2	T49.3X3	T49.3X4	T49.3X5	T49.3X6
Methoxamine	T44.4X1	T44.4X2	T44.4X3	T44.4X4	T44.4X5	T44.4X6
Methoxsalen	T5Ø.991	T5Ø.992	T5Ø.993	T5Ø.994	T5Ø.995	T5Ø.996
Methoxy-DDT	T53.7X1	T53.7X2	T53.7X3	T53.7X4	—	—
Methoxyaniline	T65.3X1	T65.3X2	T65.3X3	T65.3X4	—	—
Methoxybenzyl penicillin	T36.ØX1	T36.ØX2	T36.ØX3	T36.ØX4	T36.ØX5	T36.ØX6
Methoxychlor	T53.7X1	T53.7X2	T53.7X3	T53.7X4	—	—
Methoxyflurane	T41.ØX1	T41.ØX2	T41.ØX3	T41.ØX4	T41.ØX5	T41.ØX6
Methoxyphenamine	T48.6X1	T48.6X2	T48.6X3	T48.6X4	T48.6X5	T48.6X6
Methoxypromazine	T43.3X1	T43.3X2	T43.3X3	T43.3X4	T43.3X5	T43.3X6
Methscopolamine bromide	T44.3X1	T44.3X2	T44.3X3	T44.3X4	T44.3X5	T44.3X6
Methsuximide	T42.2X1	T42.2X2	T42.2X3	T42.2X4	T42.2X5	T42.2X6
Methyclothiazide	T5Ø.2X1	T5Ø.2X2	T5Ø.2X3	T5Ø.2X4	T5Ø.2X5	T5Ø.2X6
Methyl						
acetate	T52.4X1	T52.4X2	T52.4X3	T52.4X4	—	—
acetone	T52.4X1	T52.4X2	T52.4X3	T52.4X4	—	—
acrylate	T65.891	T65.892	T65.893	T65.894	—	—
alcohol	T51.1X1	T51.1X2	T51.1X3	T51.1X4	—	—
aminophenol	T65.3X1	T65.3X2	T65.3X3	T65.3X4	—	—
amphetamine	T43.651	T43.652	T43.653	T43.654	T43.655	T43.656
androstanolone	T38.7X1	T38.7X2	T38.7X3	T38.7X4	T38.7X5	T38.7X6
atropine	T44.3X1	T44.3X2	T44.3X3	T44.3X4	T44.3X5	T44.3X6
benzene	T52.2X1	T52.2X2	T52.2X3	T52.2X4	—	—
benzoate	T52.8X1	T52.8X2	T52.8X3	T52.8X4	—	—
benzol	T52.2X1	T52.2X2	T52.2X3	T52.2X4	—	—
bromide (gas)	T59.891	T59.892	T59.893	T59.894	—	—
fumigant	T6Ø.8X1	T6Ø.8X2	T6Ø.8X3	T6Ø.8X4	—	—
butanol	T51.3X1	T51.3X2	T51.3X3	T51.3X4	—	—
carbinol	T51.1X1	T51.1X2	T51.1X3	T51.1X4	—	—
carbonate	T52.8X1	T52.8X2	T52.8X3	T52.8X4	—	—
CCNU	T45.1X1	T45.1X2	T45.1X3	T45.1X4	T45.1X5	T45.1X6

Substance	Poisoning, Accidental (unintentional)	Poisoning, Intentional Self-harm	Poisoning, Assault	Poisoning, Undetermined	Adverse Effect	Under-dosing
Methyl — *continued*						
cellosolve	T52.91	T52.92	T52.93	T52.94	—	—
cellulose	T47.4X1	T47.4X2	T47.4X3	T47.4X4	T47.4X5	T47.4X6
chloride (gas)	T59.891	T59.892	T59.893	T59.894	—	—
chloroformate	T59.3X1	T59.3X2	T59.3X3	T59.3X4	—	—
cyclohexane	T52.8X1	T52.8X2	T52.8X3	T52.8X4	—	—
cyclohexanol	T51.8X1	T51.8X2	T51.8X3	T51.8X4	—	—
cyclohexanone	T52.8X1	T52.8X2	T52.8X3	T52.8X4	—	—
cyclohexyl acetate	T52.8X1	T52.8X2	T52.8X3	T52.8X4	—	—
demeton	T6Ø.ØX1	T6Ø.ØX2	T6Ø.ØX3	T6Ø.ØX4	—	—
dihydromorphinone	T4Ø.2X1	T4Ø.2X2	T4Ø.2X3	T4Ø.2X4	T4Ø.2X5	T4Ø.2X6
ergometrine	T48.ØX1	T48.ØX2	T48.ØX3	T48.ØX4	T48.ØX5	T48.ØX6
ergonovine	T48.ØX1	T48.ØX2	T48.ØX3	T48.ØX4	T48.ØX5	T48.ØX6
ethyl ketone	T52.4X1	T52.4X2	T52.4X3	T52.4X4	—	—
glucamine antimonate	T37.8X1	T37.8X2	T37.8X3	T37.8X4	T37.8X5	T37.8X6
hydrazine	T65.891	T65.892	T65.893	T65.894	—	—
iodide	T65.891	T65.892	T65.893	T65.894	—	—
isobutyl ketone	T52.4X1	T52.4X2	T52.4X3	T52.4X4	—	—
isothiocyanate	T6Ø.3X1	T6Ø.3X2	T6Ø.3X3	T6Ø.3X4	—	—
mercaptan	T59.891	T59.892	T59.893	T59.894	—	—
morphine NEC	T4Ø.2X1	T4Ø.2X2	T4Ø.2X3	T4Ø.2X4	T4Ø.2X5	T4Ø.2X6
nicotinate	T49.4X1	T49.4X2	T49.4X3	T49.4X4	T49.4X5	T49.4X6
paraben	T49.ØX1	T49.ØX2	T49.ØX3	T49.ØX4	T49.ØX5	T49.ØX6
parafynol	T42.6X1	T42.6X2	T42.6X3	T42.6X4	T42.6X5	T42.6X6
parathion	T6Ø.ØX1	T6Ø.ØX2	T6Ø.ØX3	T6Ø.ØX4	—	—
peridol	T43.4X1	T43.4X2	T43.4X3	T43.4X4	T43.4X5	T43.4X6
phenidate	T43.631	T43.632	T43.633	T43.634	T43.635	T43.636
prednisolone	T38.ØX1	T38.ØX2	T38.ØX3	T38.ØX4	T38.ØX5	T38.ØX6
ENT agent	T49.6X1	T49.6X2	T49.6X3	T49.6X4	T49.6X5	T49.6X6
ophthalmic preparation	T49.5X1	T49.5X2	T49.5X3	T49.5X4	T49.5X5	T49.5X6
topical NEC	T49.ØX1	T49.ØX2	T49.ØX3	T49.ØX4	T49.ØX5	T49.ØX6
propylcarbinol	T51.3X1	T51.3X2	T51.3X3	T51.3X4	—	—
rosaniline NEC	T49.ØX1	T49.ØX2	T49.ØX3	T49.ØX4	T49.ØX5	T49.ØX6
salicylate	T49.2X1	T49.2X2	T49.2X3	T49.2X4	T49.2X5	T49.2X6
sulfate (fumes)	T59.891	T59.892	T59.893	T59.894	—	—
liquid	T52.8X1	T52.8X2	T52.8X3	T52.8X4	—	—
sulfonal	T42.6X1	T42.6X2	T42.6X3	T42.6X4	T42.6X5	T42.6X6
testosterone	T38.7X1	T38.7X2	T38.7X3	T38.7X4	T38.7X5	T38.7X6
thiouracil	T38.2X1	T38.2X2	T38.2X3	T38.2X4	T38.2X5	T38.2X6
Methylacetoxyprogesterone*	T38.5X1	T38.5X2	T38.5X3	T38.5X4	T38.5X5	T38.5X6
Methylamphetamine	T43.651	T43.652	T43.653	T43.654	T43.655	T43.656
Methylated spirit	T51.1X1	T51.1X2	T51.1X3	T51.1X4	—	—
Methylatropine nitrate	T44.3X1	T44.3X2	T44.3X3	T44.3X4	T44.3X5	T44.3X6
Methylbenactyzium bromide	T44.3X1	T44.3X2	T44.3X3	T44.3X4	T44.3X5	T44.3X6
Methylbenzethonium chloride	T49.ØX1	T49.ØX2	T49.ØX3	T49.ØX4	T49.ØX5	T49.ØX6
Methylcellulose	T47.4X1	T47.4X2	T47.4X3	T47.4X4	T47.4X5	T47.4X6
laxative	T47.4X1	T47.4X2	T47.4X3	T47.4X4	T47.4X5	T47.4X6
Methylchlorophenoxyacetic acid	T6Ø.3X1	T6Ø.3X2	T6Ø.3X3	T6Ø.3X4	—	—
Methyldopa	T46.5X1	T46.5X2	T46.5X3	T46.5X4	T46.5X5	T46.5X6
Methyldopate	T46.5X1	T46.5X2	T46.5X3	T46.5X4	T46.5X5	T46.5X6
Methylene						
blue	T5Ø.6X1	T5Ø.6X2	T5Ø.6X3	T5Ø.6X4	T5Ø.6X5	T5Ø.6X6
chloride or dichloride (solvent) NEC	T53.4X1	T53.4X2	T53.4X3	T53.4X4	—	—
Methylenedioxyamphetamine	T43.621	T43.622	T43.623	T43.624	T43.625	T43.626
Methylenedioxymeth-amphetamine	T43.641	T43.642	T43.643	T43.644	—	—
Methylergometrine	T48.ØX1	T48.ØX2	T48.ØX3	T48.ØX4	T48.ØX5	T48.ØX6
Methylergonovine	T48.ØX1	T48.ØX2	T48.ØX3	T48.ØX4	T48.ØX5	T48.ØX6
Methylestrenolone	T38.5X1	T38.5X2	T38.5X3	T38.5X4	T38.5X5	T38.5X6
Methylethyl cellulose	T5Ø.991	T5Ø.992	T5Ø.993	T5Ø.994	T5Ø.995	T5Ø.996
Methylhexabital	T42.3X1	T42.3X2	T42.3X3	T42.3X4	T42.3X5	T42.3X6
Methylmorphine	T4Ø.2X1	T4Ø.2X2	T4Ø.2X3	T4Ø.2X4	T4Ø.2X5	T4Ø.2X6
Methylparaben (ophthalmic)	T49.5X1	T49.5X2	T49.5X3	T49.5X4	T49.5X5	T49.5X6
Methylparafynol	T42.6X1	T42.6X2	T42.6X3	T42.6X4	T42.6X5	T42.6X6
Methylpentynol, methylpenthynol	T42.6X1	T42.6X2	T42.6X3	T42.6X4	T42.6X5	T42.6X6
Methylphenidate	T43.631	T43.632	T43.633	T43.634	T43.635	T43.636
Methylphenobarbital	T42.3X1	T42.3X2	T42.3X3	T42.3X4	T42.3X5	T42.3X6
Methylpolysiloxane	T47.1X1	T47.1X2	T47.1X3	T47.1X4	T47.1X5	T47.1X6
Methylprednisolone — *see* Methyl, prednisolone						
Methylrosaniline	T49.ØX1	T49.ØX2	T49.ØX3	T49.ØX4	T49.ØX5	T49.ØX6
Methylrosanilinium chloride	T49.ØX1	T49.ØX2	T49.ØX3	T49.ØX4	T49.ØX5	T49.ØX6
Methyltestosterone	T38.7X1	T38.7X2	T38.7X3	T38.7X4	T38.7X5	T38.7X6
Methylthionine chloride	T5Ø.6X1	T5Ø.6X2	T5Ø.6X3	T5Ø.6X4	T5Ø.6X5	T5Ø.6X6
Methylthioninium chloride	T5Ø.6X1	T5Ø.6X2	T5Ø.6X3	T5Ø.6X4	T5Ø.6X5	T5Ø.6X6

Table of Drugs and Chemicals

Substance	Poisoning, Accidental (unintentional)	Poisoning, Intentional Self-harm	Poisoning, Assault	Poisoning, Undetermined	Adverse Effect	Under-dosing
Methylthiouracil	T38.2X1	T38.2X2	T38.2X3	T38.2X4	T38.2X5	T38.2X6
Methyprylon	T42.6X1	T42.6X2	T42.6X3	T42.6X4	T42.6X5	T42.6X6
Methysergide	T46.5X1	T46.5X2	T46.5X3	T46.5X4	T46.5X5	T46.5X6
Metiamide	T47.1X1	T47.1X2	T47.1X3	T47.1X4	T47.1X5	T47.1X6
Meticillin	T36.0X1	T36.0X2	T36.0X3	T36.0X4	T36.0X5	T36.0X6
Meticrane	T50.2X1	T50.2X2	T50.2X3	T50.2X4	T50.2X5	T50.2X6
Metildigoxin	T46.0X1	T46.0X2	T46.0X3	T46.0X4	T46.0X5	T46.0X6
Metipranolol	T49.5X1	T49.5X2	T49.5X3	T49.5X4	T49.5X5	T49.5X6
Metirosine	T46.5X1	T46.5X2	T46.5X3	T46.5X4	T46.5X5	T46.5X6
Metisazone	T37.5X1	T37.5X2	T37.5X3	T37.5X4	T37.5X5	T37.5X6
Metixene	T44.3X1	T44.3X2	T44.3X3	T44.3X4	T44.3X5	T44.3X6
Metizoline	T48.5X1	T48.5X2	T48.5X3	T48.5X4	T48.5X5	T48.5X6
Metoclopramide	T45.0X1	T45.0X2	T45.0X3	T45.0X4	T45.0X5	T45.0X6
Metofenazate	T43.3X1	T43.3X2	T43.3X3	T43.3X4	T43.3X5	T43.3X6
Metofoline	T39.8X1	T39.8X2	T39.8X3	T39.8X4	T39.8X5	T39.8X6
Metolazone	T50.2X1	T50.2X2	T50.2X3	T50.2X4	T50.2X5	T50.2X6
Metopon	T40.2X1	T40.2X2	T40.2X3	T40.2X4	T40.2X5	T40.2X6
Metoprine	T45.1X1	T45.1X2	T45.1X3	T45.1X4	T45.1X5	T45.1X6
Metoprolol	T44.7X1	T44.7X2	T44.7X3	T44.7X4	T44.7X5	T44.7X6
Metrifonate	T60.0X1	T60.0X2	T60.0X3	T60.0X4	—	—
Metrizamide	T50.8X1	T50.8X2	T50.8X3	T50.8X4	T50.8X5	T50.8X6
Metrizoic acid	T50.8X1	T50.8X2	T50.8X3	T50.8X4	T50.8X5	T50.8X6
MetroGel*	T49.0X1	T49.0X2	T49.0X3	T49.0X4	T49.0X5	T49.0X6
Metronidazole	T37.8X1	T37.8X2	T37.8X3	T37.8X4	T37.8X5	T37.8X6
Metycaine	T41.3X1	T41.3X2	T41.3X3	T41.3X4	T41.3X5	T41.3X6
infiltration (subcutaneous)	T41.3X1	T41.3X2	T41.3X3	T41.3X4	T41.3X5	T41.3X6
nerve block (peripheral) (plexus)	T41.3X1	T41.3X2	T41.3X3	T41.3X4	T41.3X5	T41.3X6
topical (surface)	T41.3X1	T41.3X2	T41.3X3	T41.3X4	T41.3X5	T41.3X6
Metyrapone	T50.8X1	T50.8X2	T50.8X3	T50.8X4	T50.8X5	T50.8X6
Mevacor*	T46.6X1	T46.6X2	T46.6X3	T46.6X4	T46.6X5	T46.6X6
Mevinphos	T60.0X1	T60.0X2	T60.0X3	T60.0X4	—	—
Mexazolam	T42.4X1	T42.4X2	T42.4X3	T42.4X4	T42.4X5	T42.4X6
Mexenone	T49.3X1	T49.3X2	T49.3X3	T49.3X4	T49.3X5	T49.3X6
Mexiletine	T46.2X1	T46.2X2	T46.2X3	T46.2X4	T46.2X5	T46.2X6
Mezereon	T62.2X1	T62.2X2	T62.2X3	T62.2X4	—	—
berries	T62.1X1	T62.1X2	T62.1X3	T62.1X4	—	—
Mezlocillin	T36.0X1	T36.0X2	T36.0X3	T36.0X4	T36.0X5	T36.0X6
Mianserin	T43.021	T43.022	T43.023	T43.024	T43.025	T43.026
Micatin	T49.0X1	T49.0X2	T49.0X3	T49.0X4	T49.0X5	T49.0X6
Miconazole	T49.0X1	T49.0X2	T49.0X3	T49.0X4	T49.0X5	T49.0X6
Micronomicin	T36.5X1	T36.5X2	T36.5X3	T36.5X4	T36.5X5	T36.5X6
Microzide*	T50.2X1	T50.2X2	T50.2X3	T50.2X4	T50.2X5	T50.2X6
Midazolam	T42.4X1	T42.4X2	T42.4X3	T42.4X4	T42.4X5	T42.4X6
Midecamycin	T36.3X1	T36.3X2	T36.3X3	T36.3X4	T36.3X5	T36.3X6
Mifepristone	T38.6X1	T38.6X2	T38.6X3	T38.6X4	T38.6X5	T38.6X6
Milk of magnesia	T47.1X1	T47.1X2	T47.1X3	T47.1X4	T47.1X5	T47.1X6
Millipede (tropical) (venomous)	T63.411	T63.412	T63.413	T63.414	—	—
Miltown	T43.591	T43.592	T43.593	T43.594	T43.595	T43.596
Milverine	T44.3X1	T44.3X2	T44.3X3	T44.3X4	T44.3X5	T44.3X6
Minaprine	T43.291	T43.292	T43.293	T43.294	T43.295	T43.296
Minaxolone	T41.291	T41.292	T41.293	T41.294	T41.295	T41.296
Mineral						
acids	T54.2X1	T54.2X2	T54.2X3	T54.2X4	—	—
oil (laxative)(medicinal)	T47.4X1	T47.4X2	T47.4X3	T47.4X4	T47.4X5	T47.4X6
emulsion	T47.2X1	T47.2X2	T47.2X3	T47.2X4	T47.2X5	T47.2X6
nonmedicinal	T52.0X1	T52.0X2	T52.0X3	T52.0X4	—	—
topical	T49.3X1	T49.3X2	T49.3X3	T49.3X4	T49.3X5	T49.3X6
salt NEC	T50.3X1	T50.3X2	T50.3X3	T50.3X4	T50.3X5	T50.3X6
spirits	T52.0X1	T52.0X2	T52.0X3	T52.0X4	—	—
Mineralocorticosteroid	T50.0X1	T50.0X2	T50.0X3	T50.0X4	T50.0X5	T50.0X6
Minocycline	T36.4X1	T36.4X2	T36.4X3	T36.4X4	T36.4X5	T36.4X6
Minoxidil	T46.7X1	T46.7X2	T46.7X3	T46.7X4	T46.7X5	T46.7X6
Miokamycin	T36.3X1	T36.3X2	T36.3X3	T36.3X4	T36.3X5	T36.3X6
Miotic drug	T49.5X1	T49.5X2	T49.5X3	T49.5X4	T49.5X5	T49.5X6
Mipafox	T60.0X1	T60.0X2	T60.0X3	T60.0X4	—	—
Mipomerson*	T46.6X1	T46.6X2	T46.6X3	T46.6X4	T46.6X5	T46.6X6
Mirex	T60.1X1	T60.1X2	T60.1X3	T60.1X4	—	—
Mirtazapine	T43.021	T43.022	T43.023	T43.024	T43.025	T43.026
Misonidazole	T37.3X1	T37.3X2	T37.3X3	T37.3X4	T37.3X5	T37.3X6
Misoprostol	T47.1X1	T47.1X2	T47.1X3	T47.1X4	T47.1X5	T47.1X6
Mithramycin	T45.1X1	T45.1X2	T45.1X3	T45.1X4	T45.1X5	T45.1X6
Mitobronitol	T45.1X1	T45.1X2	T45.1X3	T45.1X4	T45.1X5	T45.1X6
Mitoguazone	T45.1X1	T45.1X2	T45.1X3	T45.1X4	T45.1X5	T45.1X6
Mitolactol	T45.1X1	T45.1X2	T45.1X3	T45.1X4	T45.1X5	T45.1X6
Mitomycin	T45.1X1	T45.1X2	T45.1X3	T45.1X4	T45.1X5	T45.1X6
Mitopodozide	T45.1X1	T45.1X2	T45.1X3	T45.1X4	T45.1X5	T45.1X6
Mitotane	T45.1X1	T45.1X2	T45.1X3	T45.1X4	T45.1X5	T45.1X6
Mitoxantrone	T45.1X1	T45.1X2	T45.1X3	T45.1X4	T45.1X5	T45.1X6
Mivacurium chloride	T48.1X1	T48.1X2	T48.1X3	T48.1X4	T48.1X5	T48.1X6
Miyari bacteria	T47.6X1	T47.6X2	T47.6X3	T47.6X4	T47.6X5	T47.6X6
Mobic*	T39.391	T39.392	T39.393	T39.394	T39.395	T39.396
Moclobemide	T43.1X1	T43.1X2	T43.1X3	T43.1X4	T43.1X5	T43.1X6
Moderil	T46.5X1	T46.5X2	T46.5X3	T46.5X4	T46.5X5	T46.5X6
Mofebutazone	T39.2X1	T39.2X2	T39.2X3	T39.2X4	T39.2X5	T39.2X6
Mogadon — see Nitrazepam						
Molindone	T43.591	T43.592	T43.593	T43.594	T43.595	T43.596
Molsidomine	T46.3X1	T46.3X2	T46.3X3	T46.3X4	T46.3X5	T46.3X6
Mometasone	T49.0X1	T49.0X2	T49.0X3	T49.0X4	T49.0X5	T49.0X6
Monistat	T49.0X1	T49.0X2	T49.0X3	T49.0X4	T49.0X5	T49.0X6
Monkshood	T62.2X1	T62.2X2	T62.2X3	T62.2X4	—	—
Monoamine oxidase inhibitor NEC	T43.1X1	T43.1X2	T43.1X3	T43.1X4	T43.1X5	T43.1X6
hydrazine	T43.1X1	T43.1X2	T43.1X3	T43.1X4	T43.1X5	T43.1X6
Monobenzone	T49.4X1	T49.4X2	T49.4X3	T49.4X4	T49.4X5	T49.4X6
Monochloroacetic acid	T60.3X1	T60.3X2	T60.3X3	T60.3X4	—	—
Monochlorobenzene	T53.7X1	T53.7X2	T53.7X3	T53.7X4	—	—
Monoethanolamine	T46.8X1	T46.8X2	T46.8X3	T46.8X4	T46.8X5	T46.8X6
oleate	T46.8X1	T46.8X2	T46.8X3	T46.8X4	T46.8X5	T46.8X6
Monooctanoin	T50.991	T50.992	T50.993	T50.994	T50.995	T50.996
Monophenylbutazone	T39.2X1	T39.2X2	T39.2X3	T39.2X4	T39.2X5	T39.2X6
Monopril*	T46.4X1	T46.4X2	T46.4X3	T46.4X4	T46.4X5	T46.4X6
Monosodium glutamate	T65.891	T65.892	T65.893	T65.894	—	—
Monosulfiram	T49.0X1	T49.0X2	T49.0X3	T49.0X4	—	T49.0X6
Monoxide, carbon — see Carbon, monoxide						
Monoxidine hydrochloride	T46.1X1	T46.1X2	T46.1X3	T46.1X4	T46.1X5	T46.1X6
Montelukast*	T48.6X1	T48.6X2	T48.6X3	T48.6X4	T48.6X5	T48.6X6
Monuron	T60.3X1	T60.3X2	T60.3X3	T60.3X4	—	—
Moperone	T43.4X1	T43.4X2	T43.4X3	T43.4X4	T43.4X5	T43.4X6
Mopidamol	T45.1X1	T45.1X2	T45.1X3	T45.1X4	T45.1X5	T45.1X6
MOPP (mechlorethamine + vincristine + prednisone + procarbazine)	T45.1X1	T45.1X2	T45.1X3	T45.1X4	T45.1X5	T45.1X6
Morfin	T40.2X1	T40.2X2	T40.2X3	T40.2X4	T40.2X5	T40.2X6
Morinamide	T37.1X1	T37.1X2	T37.1X3	T37.1X4	T37.1X5	T37.1X6
Morning glory seeds	T40.991	T40.992	T40.993	T40.994	—	—
Moroxydine	T37.5X1	T37.5X2	T37.5X3	T37.5X4	T37.5X5	T37.5X6
Morphazinamide	T37.1X1	T37.1X2	T37.1X3	T37.1X4	T37.1X5	T37.1X6
Morphine	T40.2X1	T40.2X2	T40.2X3	T40.2X4	T40.2X5	T40.2X6
antagonist	T50.7X1	T50.7X2	T50.7X3	T50.7X4	T50.7X5	T50.7X6
Morpholinylethylmorphine	T40.2X1	T40.2X2	T40.2X3	T40.2X4	—	—
Morsuximide	T42.2X1	T42.2X2	T42.2X3	T42.2X4	T42.2X5	T42.2X6
Mosapramine	T43.591	T43.592	T43.593	T43.594	T43.595	T43.596
Moth balls — see also Pesticide	T60.2X1	T60.2X2	T60.2X3	T60.2X4	—	—
naphthalene	T60.2X1	T60.2X2	T60.2X3	T60.2X4	—	—
paradichlorobenzene	T60.1X1	T60.1X2	T60.1X3	T60.1X4	—	—
Motor exhaust gas	T58.01	T58.02	T58.03	T58.04	—	—
Motrin*	T39.311	T39.312	T39.313	T39.314	T39.315	T39.316
Mouthwash (antiseptic) (zinc chloride)	T49.6X1	T49.6X2	T49.6X3	T49.6X4	T49.6X5	T49.6X6
Moxastine	T45.0X1	T45.0X2	T45.0X3	T45.0X4	T45.0X5	T45.0X6
Moxaverine	T44.3X1	T44.3X2	T44.3X3	T44.3X4	T44.3X5	T44.3X6
Moxisylyte	T46.7X1	T46.7X2	T46.7X3	T46.7X4	T46.7X5	T46.7X6
Mucilage, plant	T47.4X1	T47.4X2	T47.4X3	T47.4X4	T47.4X5	T47.4X6
Mucolytic drug	T48.4X1	T48.4X2	T48.4X3	T48.4X4	T48.4X5	T48.4X6
Mucomyst	T48.4X1	T48.4X2	T48.4X3	T48.4X4	T48.4X5	T48.4X6
Mucous membrane agents (external)	T49.91	T49.92	T49.93	T49.94	T49.95	T49.96
specified NEC	T49.8X1	T49.8X2	T49.8X3	T49.8X4	T49.8X5	T49.8X6
Multaq*	T46.2X1	T46.2X2	T46.2X3	T46.2X4	T46.2X5	T46.2X6
Multiple unspecified drugs, medicaments and biological substances	T50.911	T50.912	T50.913	T50.914	T50.915	T50.916
Mumps						
immune globulin (human)	T50.Z11	T50.Z12	T50.Z13	T50.Z14	T50.Z15	T50.Z16
skin test antigen	T50.8X1	T50.8X2	T50.8X3	T50.8X4	T50.8X5	T50.8X6
vaccine	T50.B91	T50.B92	T50.B93	T50.B94	T50.B95	T50.B96
Mumpsvax	T50.B91	T50.B92	T50.B93	T50.B94	T50.B95	T50.B96
Mupirocin	T49.0X1	T49.0X2	T49.0X3	T49.0X4	T49.0X5	T49.0X6
Muriatic acid — see Hydrochloric acid						
Muromonab-CD3	T45.1X1	T45.1X2	T45.1X3	T45.1X4	T45.1X5	T45.1X6
Muscle-action drug NEC	T48.201	T48.202	T48.203	T48.204	T48.205	T48.206
Muscle affecting agents NEC	T48.201	T48.202	T48.203	T48.204	T48.205	T48.206
oxytocic	T48.0X1	T48.0X2	T48.0X3	T48.0X4	T48.0X5	T48.0X6
relaxants	T48.201	T48.202	T48.203	T48.204	T48.205	T48.206
central nervous system	T42.8X1	T42.8X2	T42.8X3	T42.8X4	T42.8X5	T42.8X6
skeletal	T48.1X1	T48.1X2	T48.1X3	T48.1X4	T48.1X5	T48.1X6
smooth	T44.3X1	T44.3X2	T44.3X3	T44.3X4	T44.3X5	T44.3X6
Muscle relaxant — see Relaxant, muscle						

Substance	Poisoning, Accidental (unintentional)	Poisoning, Intentional Self-harm	Poisoning, Assault	Poisoning, Undetermined	Adverse Effect	Under-dosing
Muscle-tone depressant, central NEC	T42.8X1	T42.8X2	T42.8X3	T42.8X4	T42.8X5	T42.8X6
specified NEC	T42.8X1	T42.8X2	T42.8X3	T42.8X4	T42.8X5	T42.8X6
Mushroom, noxious	T62.0X1	T62.0X2	T62.0X3	T62.0X4	—	—
Mussel, noxious	T61.781	T61.782	T61.783	T61.784	—	—
Mustard (emetic)	T47.7X1	T47.7X2	T47.7X3	T47.7X4	T47.7X5	T47.7X6
black	T47.7X1	T47.7X2	T47.7X3	T47.7X4	T47.7X5	T47.7X6
gas, not in war	T59.91	T59.92	T59.93	T59.94	—	—
nitrogen	T45.1X1	T45.1X2	T45.1X3	T45.1X4	T45.1X5	T45.1X6
Mustine	T45.1X1	T45.1X2	T45.1X3	T45.1X4	T45.1X5	T45.1X6
Mycifradin	T36.5X1	T36.5X2	T36.5X3	T36.5X4	T36.5X5	T36.5X6
topical	T49.0X1	T49.0X2	T49.0X3	T49.0X4	T49.0X5	T49.0X6
Mycitracin	T36.8X1	T36.8X2	T36.8X3	T36.8X4	T36.8X5	T36.8X6
ophthalmic preparation	T49.5X1	T49.5X2	T49.5X3	T49.5X4	T49.5X5	T49.5X6
Mycostatin	T36.7X1	T36.7X2	T36.7X3	T36.7X4	T36.7X5	T36.7X6
topical	T49.0X1	T49.0X2	T49.0X3	T49.0X4	T49.0X5	T49.0X6
Mycotoxins	T64.81	T64.82	T64.83	T64.84	—	—
aflatoxin	T64.01	T64.02	T64.03	T64.04	—	—
specified NEC	T64.81	T64.82	T64.83	T64.84	—	—
Mydriacyl	T44.3X1	T44.3X2	T44.3X3	T44.3X4	T44.3X5	T44.3X6
Mydriatic drug	T49.5X1	T49.5X2	T49.5X3	T49.5X4	T49.5X5	T49.5X6
Myelobromal	T45.1X1	T45.1X2	T45.1X3	T45.1X4	T45.1X5	T45.1X6
Myleran	T45.1X1	T45.1X2	T45.1X3	T45.1X4	T45.1X5	T45.1X6
Myochrysin (e)	T39.2X1	T39.2X2	T39.2X3	T39.2X4	T39.2X5	T39.2X6
Myoneural blocking agents	T48.1X1	T48.1X2	T48.1X3	T48.1X4	T48.1X5	T48.1X6
Myrac*	T36.4X1	T36.4X2	T36.4X3	T36.4X4	T36.4X5	T36.4X6
Myralact	T49.0X1	T49.0X2	T49.0X3	T49.0X4	T49.0X5	T49.0X6
Myristica fragrans	T62.2X1	T62.2X2	T62.2X3	T62.2X4	—	—
Myristicin	T65.891	T65.892	T65.893	T65.894	—	—
Mysoline	T42.3X1	T42.3X2	T42.3X3	T42.3X4	T42.3X5	T42.3X6
Nabilone	T40.711	T40.712	T40.713	T40.714	T40.715	T40.716
Nabumetone	T39.391	T39.392	T39.393	T39.394	T39.395	T39.396
Nadolol	T44.7X1	T44.7X2	T44.7X3	T44.7X4	T44.7X5	T44.7X6
Nafcillin	T36.0X1	T36.0X2	T36.0X3	T36.0X4	T36.0X5	T36.0X6
Nafoxidine	T38.6X1	T38.6X2	T38.6X3	T38.6X4	T38.6X5	T38.6X6
Naftazone	T46.991	T46.992	T46.993	T46.994	T46.995	T46.996
Naftidrofuryl (oxalate)	T46.7X1	T46.7X2	T46.7X3	T46.7X4	T46.7X5	T46.7X6
Naftifine	T49.0X1	T49.0X2	T49.0X3	T49.0X4	T49.0X5	T49.0X6
Nail polish remover	T52.91	T52.92	T52.93	T52.94	—	—
Nalbuphine	T40.491	T40.492	T40.493	T40.494	T40.495	T40.496
Naled	T60.0X1	T60.0X2	T60.0X3	T60.0X4	—	—
Nalidixic acid	T37.8X1	T37.8X2	T37.8X3	T37.8X4	T37.8X5	T37.8X6
Nalorphine	T50.7X1	T50.7X2	T50.7X3	T50.7X4	T50.7X5	T50.7X6
Naloxone	T50.7X1	T50.7X2	T50.7X3	T50.7X4	T50.7X5	T50.7X6
Naltrexone	T50.7X1	T50.7X2	T50.7X3	T50.7X4	T50.7X5	T50.7X6
Namenda	T43.8X1	T43.8X2	T43.8X3	T43.8X4	T43.8X5	T43.8X6
Nandrolone	T38.7X1	T38.7X2	T38.7X3	T38.7X4	T38.7X5	T38.7X6
Naphazoline	T48.5X1	T48.5X2	T48.5X3	T48.5X4	T48.5X5	T48.5X6
Naphtha (painters') (petroleum)	T52.0X1	T52.0X2	T52.0X3	T52.0X4	—	—
solvent	T52.0X1	T52.0X2	T52.0X3	T52.0X4	—	—
vapor	T52.0X1	T52.0X2	T52.0X3	T52.0X4	—	—
Naphthalene (non-chlorinated)	T60.2X1	T60.2X2	T60.2X3	T60.2X4	—	—
chlorinated	T60.1X1	T60.1X2	T60.1X3	T60.1X4	—	—
vapor	T60.1X1	T60.1X2	T60.1X3	T60.1X4	—	—
insecticide or moth repellent	T60.2X1	T60.2X2	T60.2X3	T60.2X4	—	—
chlorinated	T60.1X1	T60.1X2	T60.1X3	T60.1X4	—	—
vapor	T60.2X1	T60.2X2	T60.2X3	T60.2X4	—	—
chlorinated	T60.1X1	T60.1X2	T60.1X3	T60.1X4	—	—
Naphthol	T65.891	T65.892	T65.893	T65.894	—	—
Naphthylamine	T65.891	T65.892	T65.893	T65.894	—	—
Naphthylthiourea (ANTU)	T60.4X1	T60.4X2	T60.4X3	T60.4X4	—	—
Naprosyn — *see* Naproxen						
Naproxen	T39.311	T39.312	T39.313	T39.314	T39.315	T39.316
Narcotic (drug)	T40.601	T40.602	T40.603	T40.604	T40.605	T40.606
analgesic NEC	T40.601	T40.602	T40.603	T40.604	T40.605	T40.606
antagonist	T50.7X1	T50.7X2	T50.7X3	T50.7X4	T50.7X5	T50.7X6
specified NEC	T40.691	T40.692	T40.693	T40.694	T40.695	T40.696
synthetic	T40.491	T40.492	T40.493	T40.494	T40.495	T40.496
Narcotine	T48.3X1	T48.3X2	T48.3X3	T48.3X4	T48.3X5	T48.3X6
Nardil	T43.1X1	T43.1X2	T43.1X3	T43.1X4	T43.1X5	T43.1X6
Nasacort*	T49.5X1	T49.5X2	T49.5X3	T49.5X4	T49.5X5	T49.5X6
Nasal drug NEC	T49.6X1	T49.6X2	T49.6X3	T49.6X4	T49.6X5	T49.6X6
Natamycin	T49.0X1	T49.0X2	T49.0X3	T49.0X4	T49.0X5	T49.0X6
Natrium cyanide — *see* Cyanide(s)						
Natural						
blood (product)	T45.8X1	T45.8X2	T45.8X3	T45.8X4	T45.8X5	T45.8X6
gas (piped)	T59.891	T59.892	T59.893	T59.894	—	—
incomplete combustion	T58.11	T58.12	T58.13	T58.14	—	—

Substance	Poisoning, Accidental (unintentional)	Poisoning, Intentional Self-harm	Poisoning, Assault	Poisoning, Undetermined	Adverse Effect	Under-dosing
Nealbarbital	T42.3X1	T42.3X2	T42.3X3	T42.3X4	T42.3X5	T42.3X6
Nectadon	T48.3X1	T48.3X2	T48.3X3	T48.3X4	T48.3X5	T48.3X6
Nedocromil	T48.6X1	T48.6X2	T48.6X3	T48.6X4	T48.6X5	T48.6X6
Nefopam	T39.8X1	T39.8X2	T39.8X3	T39.8X4	T39.8X5	T39.8X6
Nematocyst (sting)	T63.691	T63.692	T63.693	T63.694	—	—
Nembutal	T42.3X1	T42.3X2	T42.3X3	T42.3X4	T42.3X5	T42.3X6
Nemonapride	T43.591	T43.592	T43.593	T43.594	T43.595	T43.596
Neoarsphenamine	T37.8X1	T37.8X2	T37.8X3	T37.8X4	T37.8X5	T37.8X6
Neocinchophen	T50.4X1	T50.4X2	T50.4X3	T50.4X4	T50.4X5	T50.4X6
Neomycin (derivatives)	T36.5X1	T36.5X2	T36.5X3	T36.5X4	T36.5X5	T36.5X6
ENT agent	T49.6X1	T49.6X2	T49.6X3	T49.6X4	T49.6X5	T49.6X6
ophthalmic preparation	T49.5X1	T49.5X2	T49.5X3	T49.5X4	T49.5X5	T49.5X6
topical NEC	T49.0X1	T49.0X2	T49.0X3	T49.0X4	T49.0X5	T49.0X6
with						
bacitracin	T49.0X1	T49.0X2	T49.0X3	T49.0X4	T49.0X5	T49.0X6
neostigmine	T44.0X1	T44.0X2	T44.0X3	T44.0X4	T44.0X5	T44.0X6
Neonal	T42.3X1	T42.3X2	T42.3X3	T42.3X4	T42.3X5	T42.3X6
Neopham*	T50.3X1	T50.3X2	T50.3X3	T50.3X4	T50.3X5	T50.3X6
Neoprontosil	T37.0X1	T37.0X2	T37.0X3	T37.0X4	T37.0X5	T37.0X6
Neosalvarsan	T37.8X1	T37.8X2	T37.8X3	T37.8X4	T37.8X5	T37.8X6
Neosilversalvarsan	T37.8X1	T37.8X2	T37.8X3	T37.8X4	T37.8X5	T37.8X6
Neosporin	T36.8X1	T36.8X2	T36.8X3	T36.8X4	T36.8X5	T36.8X6
ENT agent	T49.6X1	T49.6X2	T49.6X3	T49.6X4	T49.6X5	T49.6X6
ophthalmic preparation	T49.5X1	T49.5X2	T49.5X3	T49.5X4	T49.5X5	T49.5X6
topical NEC	T49.0X1	T49.0X2	T49.0X3	T49.0X4	T49.0X5	T49.0X6
Neostigmine bromide	T44.0X1	T44.0X2	T44.0X3	T44.0X4	T44.0X5	T44.0X6
Neraval	T42.3X1	T42.3X2	T42.3X3	T42.3X4	T42.3X5	T42.3X6
Neravan	T42.3X1	T42.3X2	T42.3X3	T42.3X4	T42.3X5	T42.3X6
Nerium oleander	T62.2X1	T62.2X2	T62.2X3	T62.2X4	—	—
Nerlynx*	T45.1X1	T45.1X2	T45.1X3	T45.1X4	T45.1X5	T45.1X6
Nerve gas, not in war	T59.91	T59.92	T59.93	T59.94	—	—
Nesacaine	T41.3X1	T41.3X2	T41.3X3	T41.3X4	T41.3X5	T41.3X6
infiltration (subcutaneous)	T41.3X1	T41.3X2	T41.3X3	T41.3X4	T41.3X5	T41.3X6
nerve block (peripheral) (plexus)	T41.3X1	T41.3X2	T41.3X3	T41.3X4	T41.3X5	T41.3X6
Netilmicin	T36.5X1	T36.5X2	T36.5X3	T36.5X4	T36.5X5	T36.5X6
Neurobarb	T42.3X1	T42.3X2	T42.3X3	T42.3X4	T42.3X5	T42.3X6
Neuroleptic drug NEC	T43.501	T43.502	T43.503	T43.504	T43.505	T43.506
Neuromuscular blocking drug	T48.1X1	T48.1X2	T48.1X3	T48.1X4	T48.1X5	T48.1X6
Neurontin*	T42.6X1	T42.6X2	T42.6X3	T42.6X4	T42.6X5	T42.6X6
Neutral insulin injection	T38.3X1	T38.3X2	T38.3X3	T38.3X4	T38.3X5	T38.3X6
Neutral spirits	T51.0X1	T51.0X2	T51.0X3	T51.0X4	—	—
beverage	T51.0X1	T51.0X2	T51.0X3	T51.0X4	—	—
Niacin	T46.7X1	T46.7X2	T46.7X3	T46.7X4	T46.7X5	T46.7X6
Niacinamide	T45.2X1	T45.2X2	T45.2X3	T45.2X4	T45.2X5	T45.2X6
Nialamide	T43.1X1	T43.1X2	T43.1X3	T43.1X4	T43.1X5	T43.1X6
Niaprazine	T42.6X1	T42.6X2	T42.6X3	T42.6X4	T42.6X5	T42.6X6
Nicametate	T46.7X1	T46.7X2	T46.7X3	T46.7X4	T46.7X5	T46.7X6
Nicardipine	T46.1X1	T46.1X2	T46.1X3	T46.1X4	T46.1X5	T46.1X6
Nicergoline	T46.7X1	T46.7X2	T46.7X3	T46.7X4	T46.7X5	T46.7X6
Nickel (carbonyl) (tetra-carbonyl) (fumes) (vapor)	T56.891	T56.892	T56.893	T56.894	—	—
Nickelocene	T56.891	T56.892	T56.893	T56.894	—	—
Niclosamide	T37.4X1	T37.4X2	T37.4X3	T37.4X4	T37.4X5	T37.4X6
Nicofuranose	T46.7X1	T46.7X2	T46.7X3	T46.7X4	T46.7X5	T46.7X6
Nicomorphine	T40.2X1	T40.2X2	T40.2X3	T40.2X4	—	—
Nicorandil	T46.3X1	T46.3X2	T46.3X3	T46.3X4	T46.3X5	T46.3X6
Nicotiana (plant)	T62.2X1	T62.2X2	T62.2X3	T62.2X4	—	—
Nicotinamide	T45.2X1	T45.2X2	T45.2X3	T45.2X4	T45.2X5	T45.2X6
Nicotine (insecticide) (spray) (sulfate) **NEC**	T60.2X1	T60.2X2	T60.2X3	T60.2X4	—	—
from tobacco	T65.291	T65.292	T65.293	T65.294	—	—
cigarettes	T65.221	T65.222	T65.223	T65.224	—	—
not insecticide	T65.291	T65.292	T65.293	T65.294	—	—
Nicotinic acid	T46.7X1	T46.7X2	T46.7X3	T46.7X4	T46.7X5	T46.7X6
Nicotinyl alcohol	T46.7X1	T46.7X2	T46.7X3	T46.7X4	T46.7X5	T46.7X6
Nicoumalone	T45.511	T45.512	T45.513	T45.514	T45.515	T45.516
Nifedipine	T46.1X1	T46.1X2	T46.1X3	T46.1X4	T46.1X5	T46.1X6
Nifenazone	T39.2X1	T39.2X2	T39.2X3	T39.2X4	T39.2X5	T39.2X6
Nifuraldezone	T37.91	T37.92	T37.93	T37.94	T37.95	T37.96
Nifuratel	T37.8X1	T37.8X2	T37.8X3	T37.8X4	T37.8X5	T37.8X6
Nifurtimox	T37.3X1	T37.3X2	T37.3X3	T37.3X4	T37.3X5	T37.3X6
Nifurtoinol	T37.8X1	T37.8X2	T37.8X3	T37.8X4	T37.8X5	T37.8X6
Nightshade, deadly (solanum) — *see also* Belladonna	T62.2X1	T62.2X2	T62.2X3	T62.2X4	—	—
berry	T62.1X1	T62.1X2	T62.1X3	T62.1X4	—	—
Nikethamide	T50.7X1	T50.7X2	T50.7X3	T50.7X4	T50.7X5	T50.7X6
Nilstat	T36.7X1	T36.7X2	T36.7X3	T36.7X4	T36.7X5	T36.7X6
topical	T49.0X1	T49.0X2	T49.0X3	T49.0X4	T49.0X5	T49.0X6
Nilutamide	T38.6X1	T38.6X2	T38.6X3	T38.6X4	T38.6X5	T38.6X6
Nimesulide	T39.391	T39.392	T39.393	T39.394	T39.395	T39.396
Nimetazepam	T42.4X1	T42.4X2	T42.4X3	T42.4X4	T42.4X5	T42.4X6

*Optum Value-Add

☑ Additional Character May Be Required — Refer to the Tabular List for Character Selection

393

Substance	Poisoning, Accidental (unintentional)	Poisoning, Intentional Self-harm	Poisoning, Assault	Poisoning, Undetermined	Adverse Effect	Under-dosing
Nimodipine	T46.1X1	T46.1X2	T46.1X3	T46.1X4	T46.1X5	T46.1X6
Nimorazole	T37.3X1	T37.3X2	T37.3X3	T37.3X4	T37.3X5	T37.3X6
Nimustine	T45.1X1	T45.1X2	T45.1X3	T45.1X4	T45.1X5	T45.1X6
Nipent*	T45.1X1	T45.1X2	T45.1X3	T45.1X4	T45.1X5	T45.1X6
Niridazole	T37.4X1	T37.4X2	T37.4X3	T37.4X4	T37.4X5	T37.4X6
Nisentil	T40.2X1	T40.2X2	T40.2X3	T40.2X4	T40.2X5	T40.2X6
Nisoldipine	T46.1X1	T46.1X2	T46.1X3	T46.1X4	T46.1X5	T46.1X6
Nitramine	T65.3X1	T65.3X2	T65.3X3	T65.3X4	—	—
Nitrate, organic	T46.3X1	T46.3X2	T46.3X3	T46.3X4	T46.3X5	T46.3X6
Nitrazepam	T42.4X1	T42.4X2	T42.4X3	T42.4X4	T42.4X5	T42.4X6
Nitrefazole	T50.6X1	T50.6X2	T50.6X3	T50.6X4	T50.6X5	T50.6X6
Nitrendipine	T46.1X1	T46.1X2	T46.1X3	T46.1X4	T46.1X5	T46.1X6
Nitric						
acid (liquid)	T54.2X1	T54.2X2	T54.2X3	T54.2X4	—	—
vapor	T59.891	T59.892	T59.893	T59.894	—	—
oxide (gas)	T59.0X1	T59.0X2	T59.0X3	T59.0X4	—	—
Nitrimidazine	T37.3X1	T37.3X2	T37.3X3	T37.3X4	T37.3X5	T37.3X6
Nitrite, amyl (medicinal)	T46.3X1	T46.3X2	T46.3X3	T46.3X4	T46.3X5	T46.3X6
(vapor)						
Nitroaniline	T65.3X1	T65.3X2	T65.3X3	T65.3X4	—	—
vapor	T59.891	T59.892	T59.893	T59.894	—	—
Nitrobenzene, nitrobenzol	T65.3X1	T65.3X2	T65.3X3	T65.3X4	—	—
vapor	T65.3X1	T65.3X2	T65.3X3	T65.3X4	—	—
Nitrocellulose	T65.891	T65.892	T65.893	T65.894	—	—
lacquer	T65.891	T65.892	T65.893	T65.894	—	—
Nitrodiphenyl	T65.3X1	T65.3X2	T65.3X3	T65.3X4	—	—
Nitrofural	T49.0X1	T49.0X2	T49.0X3	T49.0X4	T49.0X5	T49.0X6
Nitrofurantoin	T37.8X1	T37.8X2	T37.8X3	T37.8X4	T37.8X5	T37.8X6
Nitrofurazone	T49.0X1	T49.0X2	T49.0X3	T49.0X4	T49.0X5	T49.0X6
Nitrogen	T59.0X1	T59.0X2	T59.0X3	T59.0X4	—	—
mustard	T45.1X1	T45.1X2	T45.1X3	T45.1X4	T45.1X5	T45.1X6
Nitroglycerin, nitroglycerol	T46.3X1	T46.3X2	T46.3X3	T46.3X4	T46.3X5	T46.3X6
(medicinal)						
nonmedicinal	T65.5X1	T65.5X2	T65.5X3	T65.5X4	—	—
fumes	T65.5X1	T65.5X2	T65.5X3	T65.5X4	—	—
Nitroglycol	T52.3X1	T52.3X2	T52.3X3	T52.3X4	—	—
Nitrohydrochloric acid	T54.2X1	T54.2X2	T54.2X3	T54.2X4	—	—
Nitromersol	T49.0X1	T49.0X2	T49.0X3	T49.0X4	T49.0X5	T49.0X6
Nitronaphthalene	T65.891	T65.892	T65.893	T65.894	—	—
Nitrophenol	T54.0X1	T54.0X2	T54.0X3	T54.0X4	—	—
Nitropropane	T52.8X1	T52.8X2	T52.8X3	T52.8X4	—	—
Nitroprusside	T46.5X1	T46.5X2	T46.5X3	T46.5X4	T46.5X5	T46.5X6
Nitrosodimethylamine	T65.3X1	T65.3X2	T65.3X3	T65.3X4	—	—
Nitrothiazol	T37.4X1	T37.4X2	T37.4X3	T37.4X4	T37.4X5	T37.4X6
Nitrotoluene, nitrotoluol	T65.3X1	T65.3X2	T65.3X3	T65.3X4	—	—
vapor	T65.3X1	T65.3X2	T65.3X3	T65.3X4	—	—
Nitrous						
acid (liquid)	T54.2X1	T54.2X2	T54.2X3	T54.2X4	—	—
fumes	T59.891	T59.892	T59.893	T59.894	—	—
ether spirit	T46.3X1	T46.3X2	T46.3X3	T46.3X4	T46.3X5	T46.3X6
oxide	T41.0X1	T41.0X2	T41.0X3	T41.0X4	T41.0X5	T41.0X6
Nitroxoline	T37.8X1	T37.8X2	T37.8X3	T37.8X4	T37.8X5	T37.8X6
Nitrozone	T49.0X1	T49.0X2	T49.0X3	T49.0X4	T49.0X5	T49.0X6
Nizatidine	T47.0X1	T47.0X2	T47.0X3	T47.0X4	T47.0X5	T47.0X6
Nizofenone	T43.8X1	T43.8X2	T43.8X3	T43.8X4	T43.8X5	T43.8X6
No Doz*	T43.611	T43.612	T43.613	T43.614	T43.615	T43.616
Noctec	T42.6X1	T42.6X2	T42.6X3	T42.6X4	T42.6X5	T42.6X6
Noludar	T42.6X1	T42.6X2	T42.6X3	T42.6X4	T42.6X5	T42.6X6
Nomegestrol	T38.5X1	T38.5X2	T38.5X3	T38.5X4	T38.5X5	T38.5X6
Nomifensine	T43.291	T43.292	T43.293	T43.294	T43.295	T43.296
Nonoxinol	T49.8X1	T49.8X2	T49.8X3	T49.8X4	T49.8X5	T49.8X6
Nonylphenoxy	T49.8X1	T49.8X2	T49.8X3	T49.8X4	T49.8X5	T49.8X6
(polyethoxyethanol)						
Noptil	T42.3X1	T42.3X2	T42.3X3	T42.3X4	T42.3X5	T42.3X6
Noradrenaline	T44.4X1	T44.4X2	T44.4X3	T44.4X4	T44.4X5	T44.4X6
Noramidopyrine	T39.2X1	T39.2X2	T39.2X3	T39.2X4	T39.2X5	T39.2X6
methanesulfonate sodium	T39.2X1	T39.2X2	T39.2X3	T39.2X4	T39.2X5	T39.2X6
Norbormide	T60.4X1	T60.4X2	T60.4X3	T60.4X4	—	—
Nordazepam	T42.4X1	T42.4X2	T42.4X3	T42.4X4	T42.4X5	T42.4X6
Norepinephrine	T44.4X1	T44.4X2	T44.4X3	T44.4X4	T44.4X5	T44.4X6
Norethandrolone	T38.7X1	T38.7X2	T38.7X3	T38.7X4	T38.7X5	T38.7X6
Norethindrone	T38.4X1	T38.4X2	T38.4X3	T38.4X4	T38.4X5	T38.4X6
Norethisterone (acetate)	T38.4X1	T38.4X2	T38.4X3	T38.4X4	T38.4X5	T38.4X6
(enantate)						
with ethinylestradiol	T38.5X1	T38.5X2	T38.5X3	T38.5X4	T38.5X5	T38.5X6
Noretynodrel	T38.5X1	T38.5X2	T38.5X3	T38.5X4	T38.5X5	T38.5X6
Norfenefrine	T44.4X1	T44.4X2	T44.4X3	T44.4X4	T44.4X5	T44.4X6
Norfloxacin	T36.8X1	T36.8X2	T36.8X3	T36.8X4	T36.8X5	T36.8X6
Norgestrel	T38.4X1	T38.4X2	T38.4X3	T38.4X4	T38.4X5	T38.4X6
Norgestrienone	T38.4X1	T38.4X2	T38.4X3	T38.4X4	T38.4X5	T38.4X6
Norlestrin	T38.4X1	T38.4X2	T38.4X3	T38.4X4	T38.4X5	T38.4X6
Norlutin	T38.4X1	T38.4X2	T38.4X3	T38.4X4	T38.4X5	T38.4X6

Substance	Poisoning, Accidental (unintentional)	Poisoning, Intentional Self-harm	Poisoning, Assault	Poisoning, Undetermined	Adverse Effect	Under-dosing
Normal serum albumin (human), salt-poor	T45.8X1	T45.8X2	T45.8X3	T45.8X4	T45.8X5	T45.8X6
Normethandrone	T38.5X1	T38.5X2	T38.5X3	T38.5X4	T38.5X5	T38.5X6
Normison — see Benzodiazepines						
Normorphine	T40.2X1	T40.2X2	T40.2X3	T40.2X4	—	—
Norpseudoephedrine	T50.5X1	T50.5X2	T50.5X3	T50.5X4	T50.5X5	T50.5X6
Nortestosterone (furanpropionate)	T38.7X1	T38.7X2	T38.7X3	T38.7X4	T38.7X5	T38.7X6
Nortriptyline	T43.011	T43.012	T43.013	T43.014	T43.015	T43.016
Norvasc*	T46.1X1	T46.1X2	T46.1X3	T46.1X4	T46.1X5	T46.1X6
Noscapine	T48.3X1	T48.3X2	T48.3X3	T48.3X4	T48.3X5	T48.3X6
Nose preparations	T49.6X1	T49.6X2	T49.6X3	T49.6X4	T49.6X5	T49.6X6
Novobiocin	T36.5X1	T36.5X2	T36.5X3	T36.5X4	T36.5X5	T36.5X6
Novocain (infiltration) (topical)	T41.3X1	T41.3X2	T41.3X3	T41.3X4	T41.3X5	T41.3X6
nerve block (peripheral) (plexus)	T41.3X1	T41.3X2	T41.3X3	T41.3X4	T41.3X5	T41.3X6
spinal	T41.3X1	T41.3X2	T41.3X3	T41.3X4	T41.3X5	T41.3X6
Noxious foodstuff	T62.91	T62.92	T62.93	T62.94	—	—
specified NEC	T62.8X1	T62.8X2	T62.8X3	T62.8X4	—	—
Noxiptiline	T43.011	T43.012	T43.013	T43.014	T43.015	T43.016
Noxytiolin	T49.0X1	T49.0X2	T49.0X3	T49.0X4	T49.0X5	T49.0X6
NPH Iletin (insulin)	T38.3X1	T38.3X2	T38.3X3	T38.3X4	T38.3X5	T38.3X6
Numorphan	T40.2X1	T40.2X2	T40.2X3	T40.2X4	T40.2X5	T40.2X6
Nunol	T42.3X1	T42.3X2	T42.3X3	T42.3X4	T42.3X5	T42.3X6
Nupercaine (spinal anesthetic)	T41.3X1	T41.3X2	T41.3X3	T41.3X4	T41.3X5	T41.3X6
topical (surface)	T41.3X1	T41.3X2	T41.3X3	T41.3X4	T41.3X5	T41.3X6
Nutmeg oil (liniment)	T49.3X1	T49.3X2	T49.3X3	T49.3X4	T49.3X5	T49.3X6
Nutrilipid*	T50.991	T50.992	T50.993	T50.994	T50.995	T50.996
Nutritional supplement	T50.901	T50.902	T50.903	T50.904	T50.905	T50.906
Nux vomica	T65.1X1	T65.1X2	T65.1X3	T65.1X4	—	—
Nydrazid	T37.1X1	T37.1X2	T37.1X3	T37.1X4	T37.1X5	T37.1X6
Nylidrin	T46.7X1	T46.7X2	T46.7X3	T46.7X4	T46.7X5	T46.7X6
Nystatin	T36.7X1	T36.7X2	T36.7X3	T36.7X4	T36.7X5	T36.7X6
topical	T49.0X1	T49.0X2	T49.0X3	T49.0X4	T49.0X5	T49.0X6
Nytol	T45.0X1	T45.0X2	T45.0X3	T45.0X4	T45.0X5	T45.0X6
Obidoxime chloride	T50.6X1	T50.6X2	T50.6X3	T50.6X4	T50.6X5	T50.6X6
Octafonium (chloride)	T49.3X1	T49.3X2	T49.3X3	T49.3X4	T49.3X5	T49.3X6
Octamethyl pyrophosphoramide	T60.0X1	T60.0X2	T60.0X3	T60.0X4	—	—
Octanoin	T50.991	T50.992	T50.993	T50.994	T50.995	T50.996
Octatropine methylbromide	T44.3X1	T44.3X2	T44.3X3	T44.3X4	T44.3X5	T44.3X6
Octotiamine	T45.2X1	T45.2X2	T45.2X3	T45.2X4	T45.2X5	T45.2X6
Octoxinol (9)	T49.8X1	T49.8X2	T49.8X3	T49.8X4	T49.8X5	T49.8X6
Octreotide	T38.991	T38.992	T38.993	T38.994	T38.995	T38.996
Octyl nitrite	T46.3X1	T46.3X2	T46.3X3	T46.3X4	T46.3X5	T46.3X6
Oestradiol	T38.5X1	T38.5X2	T38.5X3	T38.5X4	T38.5X5	T38.5X6
Oestriol	T38.5X1	T38.5X2	T38.5X3	T38.5X4	T38.5X5	T38.5X6
Oestrogen	T38.5X1	T38.5X2	T38.5X3	T38.5X4	T38.5X5	T38.5X6
Oestrone	T38.5X1	T38.5X2	T38.5X3	T38.5X4	T38.5X5	T38.5X6
Ofloxacin	T36.8X1	T36.8X2	T36.8X3	T36.8X4	T36.8X5	T36.8X6
Oil (of)	T65.891	T65.892	T65.893	T65.894	—	—
bitter almond	T62.8X1	T62.8X2	T62.8X3	T62.8X4	—	—
cloves	T49.7X1	T49.7X2	T49.7X3	T49.7X4	T49.7X5	T49.7X6
colors	T65.6X1	T65.6X2	T65.6X3	T65.6X4	—	—
fumes	T59.891	T59.892	T59.893	T59.894	—	—
lubricating	T52.0X1	T52.0X2	T52.0X3	T52.0X4	—	—
Niobe	T52.8X1	T52.8X2	T52.8X3	T52.8X4	—	—
vitriol (liquid)	T54.2X1	T54.2X2	T54.2X3	T54.2X4	—	—
fumes	T54.2X1	T54.2X2	T54.2X3	T54.2X4	—	—
wintergreen (bitter) NEC	T49.3X1	T49.3X2	T49.3X3	T49.3X4	T49.3X5	T49.3X6
Oily preparation (for skin)	T49.3X1	T49.3X2	T49.3X3	T49.3X4	T49.3X5	T49.3X6
Ointment NEC	T49.3X1	T49.3X2	T49.3X3	T49.3X4	T49.3X5	T49.3X6
Olanzapine	T43.591	T43.592	T43.593	T43.594	T43.595	T43.596
Oleander	T62.2X1	T62.2X2	T62.2X3	T62.2X4	—	—
Oleandomycin	T36.3X1	T36.3X2	T36.3X3	T36.3X4	T36.3X5	T36.3X6
Oleandrin	T46.0X1	T46.0X2	T46.0X3	T46.0X4	T46.0X5	T46.0X6
Oleic acid	T46.6X1	T46.6X2	T46.6X3	T46.6X4	T46.6X5	T46.6X6
Oleovitamin A	T45.2X1	T45.2X2	T45.2X3	T45.2X4	T45.2X5	T45.2X6
Oleum ricini	T47.2X1	T47.2X2	T47.2X3	T47.2X4	T47.2X5	T47.2X6
Olive oil (medicinal) NEC	T47.4X1	T47.4X2	T47.4X3	T47.4X4	T47.4X5	T47.4X6
Olivomycin	T45.1X1	T45.1X2	T45.1X3	T45.1X4	T45.1X5	T45.1X6
Olodaterol*	T48.6X1	T48.6X2	T48.6X3	T48.6X4	T48.6X5	T48.6X6
Olsalazine	T47.8X1	T47.8X2	T47.8X3	T47.8X4	T47.8X5	T47.8X6
Omeprazole	T47.1X1	T47.1X2	T47.1X3	T47.1X4	T47.1X5	T47.1X6
OMPA	T60.0X1	T60.0X2	T60.0X3	T60.0X4	—	—
Oncovin	T45.1X1	T45.1X2	T45.1X3	T45.1X4	T45.1X5	T45.1X6
Ondansetron	T45.0X1	T45.0X2	T45.0X3	T45.0X4	T45.0X5	T45.0X6
Ophthaine	T41.3X1	T41.3X2	T41.3X3	T41.3X4	T41.3X5	T41.3X6
Ophthetic	T41.3X1	T41.3X2	T41.3X3	T41.3X4	T41.3X5	T41.3X6

Substance	Poisoning, Accidental (unintentional)	Poisoning, Intentional Self-harm	Poisoning, Assault	Poisoning, Undetermined	Adverse Effect	Under- dosing
Opiate NEC	T40.601	T40.602	T40.603	T40.604	T40.605	T40.606
antagonists	T50.7X1	T50.7X2	T50.7X3	T50.7X4	T50.7X5	T50.7X6
Opioid NEC	T40.2X1	T40.2X2	T40.2X3	T40.2X4	T40.2X5	T40.2X6
Opipramol	T43.011	T43.012	T43.013	T43.014	T43.015	T43.016
Opium alkaloids (total)	T40.0X1	T40.0X2	T40.0X3	T40.0X4	T40.0X5	T40.0X6
standardized powdered	T40.0X1	T40.0X2	T40.0X3	T40.0X4	T40.0X5	T40.0X6
tincture (camphorated)	T40.0X1	T40.0X2	T40.0X3	T40.0X4	T40.0X5	T40.0X6
Optivar*	T49.5X1	T49.5X2	T49.5X3	T49.5X4	T49.5X5	T49.5X6
Oracon	T38.4X1	T38.4X2	T38.4X3	T38.4X4	T38.4X5	T38.4X6
Oragrafin	T50.8X1	T50.8X2	T50.8X3	T50.8X4	T50.8X5	T50.8X6
Oral contraceptives	T38.4X1	T38.4X2	T38.4X3	T38.4X4	T38.4X5	T38.4X6
Oral rehydration salts	T50.3X1	T50.3X2	T50.3X3	T50.3X4	T50.3X5	T50.3X6
Orazamide	T50.991	T50.992	T50.993	T50.994	T50.995	T50.996
Orciprenaline	T48.291	T48.292	T48.293	T48.294	T48.295	T48.296
Organidin	T48.4X1	T48.4X2	T48.4X3	T48.4X4	T48.4X5	T48.4X6
Organonitrate NEC	T46.3X1	T46.3X2	T46.3X3	T46.3X4	T46.3X5	T46.3X6
Organophosphates	T60.0X1	T60.0X2	T60.0X3	T60.0X4	—	—
Orimune	T50.B91	T50.B92	T50.B93	T50.B94	T50.B95	T50.B96
Orinase	T38.3X1	T38.3X2	T38.3X3	T38.3X4	T38.3X5	T38.3X6
Ormeloxifene	T38.6X1	T38.6X2	T38.6X3	T38.6X4	T38.6X5	T38.6X6
Ornidazole	T37.3X1	T37.3X2	T37.3X3	T37.3X4	T37.3X5	T37.3X6
Ornithine aspartate	T50.991	T50.992	T50.993	T50.994	T50.995	T50.996
Ornoprostil	T47.1X1	T47.1X2	T47.1X3	T47.1X4	T47.1X5	T47.1X6
Orphenadrine	T42.8X1	T42.8X2	T42.8X3	T42.8X4	T42.8X5	T42.8X6
(hydrochloride)						
Ortal (sodium)	T42.3X1	T42.3X2	T42.3X3	T42.3X4	T42.3X5	T42.3X6
Ortho-Novum	T38.4X1	T38.4X2	T38.4X3	T38.4X4	T38.4X5	T38.4X6
Orthoboric acid	T49.0X1	T49.0X2	T49.0X3	T49.0X4	T49.0X5	T49.0X6
ENT agent	T49.6X1	T49.6X2	T49.6X3	T49.6X4	T49.6X5	T49.6X6
ophthalmic preparation	T49.5X1	T49.5X2	T49.5X3	T49.5X4	T49.5X5	T49.5X6
Orthocaine	T41.3X1	T41.3X2	T41.3X3	T41.3X4	T41.3X5	T41.3X6
Orthodichlorobenzene	T53.7X1	T53.7X2	T53.7X3	T53.7X4	—	—
Orthotolidine (reagent)	T54.2X1	T54.2X2	T54.2X3	T54.2X4	—	—
Osmic acid (liquid)	T54.2X1	T54.2X2	T54.2X3	T54.2X4	—	—
fumes	T54.2X1	T54.2X2	T54.2X3	T54.2X4	—	—
Osmotic diuretics	T50.2X1	T50.2X2	T50.2X3	T50.2X4	T50.2X5	T50.2X6
Otilonium bromide	T44.3X1	T44.3X2	T44.3X3	T44.3X4	T44.3X5	T44.3X6
Otorhinolaryngological drug NEC	T49.6X1	T49.6X2	T49.6X3	T49.6X4	T49.6X5	T49.6X6
Ouabain (e)	T46.0X1	T46.0X2	T46.0X3	T46.0X4	T46.0X5	T46.0X6
Ovarian						
hormone	T38.5X1	T38.5X2	T38.5X3	T38.5X4	T38.5X5	T38.5X6
stimulant	T38.5X1	T38.5X2	T38.5X3	T38.5X4	T38.5X5	T38.5X6
Ovide*	T49.0X1	T49.0X2	T49.0X3	T49.0X4	T49.0X5	T49.0X6
Ovral	T38.4X1	T38.4X2	T38.4X3	T38.4X4	T38.4X5	T38.4X6
Ovulen	T38.4X1	T38.4X2	T38.4X3	T38.4X4	T38.4X5	T38.4X6
Ox bile extract	T47.5X1	T47.5X2	T47.5X3	T47.5X4	T47.5X5	T47.5X6
Oxacillin	T36.0X1	T36.0X2	T36.0X3	T36.0X4	T36.0X5	T36.0X6
Oxalic acid	T54.2X1	T54.2X2	T54.2X3	T54.2X4	—	—
ammonium salt	T50.991	T50.992	T50.993	T50.994	T50.995	T50.996
Oxamniquine	T37.4X1	T37.4X2	T37.4X3	T37.4X4	T37.4X5	T37.4X6
Oxanamide	T43.591	T43.592	T43.593	T43.594	T43.595	T43.596
Oxandrolone	T38.7X1	T38.7X2	T38.7X3	T38.7X4	T38.7X5	T38.7X6
Oxantel	T37.4X1	T37.4X2	T37.4X3	T37.4X4	T37.4X5	T37.4X6
Oxapium iodide	T44.3X1	T44.3X2	T44.3X3	T44.3X4	T44.3X5	T44.3X6
Oxaprotiline	T43.021	T43.022	T43.023	T43.024	T43.025	T43.026
Oxaprozin	T39.311	T39.312	T39.313	T39.314	T39.315	T39.316
Oxatomide	T45.0X1	T45.0X2	T45.0X3	T45.0X4	T45.0X5	T45.0X6
Oxazepam	T42.4X1	T42.4X2	T42.4X3	T42.4X4	T42.4X5	T42.4X6
Oxazimedrine	T50.5X1	T50.5X2	T50.5X3	T50.5X4	T50.5X5	T50.5X6
Oxazolam	T42.4X1	T42.4X2	T42.4X3	T42.4X4	T42.4X5	T42.4X6
Oxazolidine derivatives	T42.2X1	T42.2X2	T42.2X3	T42.2X4	T42.2X5	T42.2X6
Oxazolidinedione (derivative)	T42.2X1	T42.2X2	T42.2X3	T42.2X4	T42.2X5	T42.2X6
Oxcarbazepine	T42.1X1	T42.1X2	T42.1X3	T42.1X4	T42.1X5	T42.1X6
Oxedrine	T44.4X1	T44.4X2	T44.4X3	T44.4X4	T44.4X5	T44.4X6
Oxeladin (citrate)	T48.3X1	T48.3X2	T48.3X3	T48.3X4	T48.3X5	T48.3X6
Oxendolone	T38.5X1	T38.5X2	T38.5X3	T38.5X4	T38.5X5	T38.5X6
Oxetacaine	T41.3X1	T41.3X2	T41.3X3	T41.3X4	T41.3X5	T41.3X6
Oxethazine	T41.3X1	T41.3X2	T41.3X3	T41.3X4	T41.3X5	T41.3X6
Oxetorone	T39.8X1	T39.8X2	T39.8X3	T39.8X4	T39.8X5	T39.8X6
Oxiconazole	T49.0X1	T49.0X2	T49.0X3	T49.0X4	T49.0X5	T49.0X6
Oxidizing agent NEC	T54.91	T54.92	T54.93	T54.94	—	—
Oxipurinol	T50.4X1	T50.4X2	T50.4X3	T50.4X4	T50.4X5	T50.4X6
Oxitriptan	T43.291	T43.292	T43.293	T43.294	T43.295	T43.296
Oxitropium bromide	T48.6X1	T48.6X2	T48.6X3	T48.6X4	T48.6X5	T48.6X6
Oxodipine	T46.1X1	T46.1X2	T46.1X3	T46.1X4	T46.1X5	T46.1X6
Oxolamine	T48.3X1	T48.3X2	T48.3X3	T48.3X4	T48.3X5	T48.3X6
Oxolinic acid	T37.8X1	T37.8X2	T37.8X3	T37.8X4	T37.8X5	T37.8X6
Oxomemazine	T43.3X1	T43.3X2	T43.3X3	T43.3X4	T43.3X5	T43.3X6
Oxophenarsine	T37.3X1	T37.3X2	T37.3X3	T37.3X4	T37.3X5	T37.3X6
Oxprenolol	T44.7X1	T44.7X2	T44.7X3	T44.7X4	T44.7X5	T44.7X6
Oxsoralen	T49.3X1	T49.3X2	T49.3X3	T49.3X4	T49.3X5	T49.3X6

Substance	Poisoning, Accidental (unintentional)	Poisoning, Intentional Self-harm	Poisoning, Assault	Poisoning, Undetermined	Adverse Effect	Under- dosing
Oxtriphylline	T48.6X1	T48.6X2	T48.6X3	T48.6X4	T48.6X5	T48.6X6
Oxybate sodium	T41.291	T41.292	T41.293	T41.294	T41.295	T41.296
Oxybuprocaine	T41.3X1	T41.3X2	T41.3X3	T41.3X4	T41.3X5	T41.3X6
Oxybutynin	T44.3X1	T44.3X2	T44.3X3	T44.3X4	T44.3X5	T44.3X6
Oxychlorosene	T49.0X1	T49.0X2	T49.0X3	T49.0X4	T49.0X5	T49.0X6
Oxycodone	T40.2X1	T40.2X2	T40.2X3	T40.2X4	T40.2X5	T40.2X6
OxyContin*	T40.2X1	T40.2X2	T40.2X3	T40.2X4	T40.2X5	T40.2X6
Oxyfedrine	T46.3X1	T46.3X2	T46.3X3	T46.3X4	T46.3X5	T46.3X6
Oxygen	T41.5X1	T41.5X2	T41.5X3	T41.5X4	T41.5X5	T41.5X6
Oxylone	T49.0X1	T49.0X2	T49.0X3	T49.0X4	T49.0X5	T49.0X6
ophthalmic preparation	T49.5X1	T49.5X2	T49.5X3	T49.5X4	T49.5X5	T49.5X6
Oxymesterone	T38.7X1	T38.7X2	T38.7X3	T38.7X4	T38.7X5	T38.7X6
Oxymetazoline	T48.5X1	T48.5X2	T48.5X3	T48.5X4	T48.5X5	T48.5X6
Oxymetholone	T38.7X1	T38.7X2	T38.7X3	T38.7X4	T38.7X5	T38.7X6
Oxymorphone	T40.2X1	T40.2X2	T40.2X3	T40.2X4	T40.2X5	T40.2X6
Oxypertine	T43.591	T43.592	T43.593	T43.594	T43.595	T43.596
Oxyphenbutazone	T39.2X1	T39.2X2	T39.2X3	T39.2X4	T39.2X5	T39.2X6
Oxyphencyclimine	T44.3X1	T44.3X2	T44.3X3	T44.3X4	T44.3X5	T44.3X6
Oxyphenisatine	T47.2X1	T47.2X2	T47.2X3	T47.2X4	T47.2X5	T47.2X6
Oxyphenonium bromide	T44.3X1	T44.3X2	T44.3X3	T44.3X4	T44.3X5	T44.3X6
Oxypolygelatin	T45.8X1	T45.8X2	T45.8X3	T45.8X4	T45.8X5	T45.8X6
Oxyquinoline (derivatives)	T37.8X1	T37.8X2	T37.8X3	T37.8X4	T37.8X5	T37.8X6
Oxytetracycline	T36.4X1	T36.4X2	T36.4X3	T36.4X4	T36.4X5	T36.4X6
Oxytocic drug NEC	T48.0X1	T48.0X2	T48.0X3	T48.0X4	T48.0X5	T48.0X6
Oxytocin (synthetic)	T48.0X1	T48.0X2	T48.0X3	T48.0X4	T48.0X5	T48.0X6
Oxytrol*	T44.3X1	T44.3X2	T44.3X3	T44.3X4	T44.3X5	T44.3X6
Ozone	T59.891	T59.892	T59.893	T59.894	—	—
P-Acetamidophenol	T39.1X1	T39.1X2	T39.1X3	T39.1X4	T39.1X5	T39.1X6
PABA	T49.3X1	T49.3X2	T49.3X3	T49.3X4	T49.3X5	T49.3X6
Packed red cells	T45.8X1	T45.8X2	T45.8X3	T45.8X4	T45.8X5	T45.8X6
Padimate	T49.3X1	T49.3X2	T49.3X3	T49.3X4	T49.3X5	T49.3X6
Paint NEC	T65.6X1	T65.6X2	T65.6X3	T65.6X4	—	—
cleaner	T52.91	T52.92	T52.93	T52.94	—	—
fumes NEC	T59.891	T59.892	T59.893	T59.894	—	—
lead (fumes)	T56.0X1	T56.0X2	T56.0X3	T56.0X4	—	—
solvent NEC	T52.8X1	T52.8X2	T52.8X3	T52.8X4	—	—
stripper	T52.8X1	T52.8X2	T52.8X3	T52.8X4	—	—
Palfium	T40.2X1	T40.2X2	T40.2X3	T40.2X4	—	—
Palm kernel oil	T50.991	T50.992	T50.993	T50.994	T50.995	T50.996
Paludrine	T37.2X1	T37.2X2	T37.2X3	T37.2X4	T37.2X5	T37.2X6
PAM (pralidoxime)	T50.6X1	T50.6X2	T50.6X3	T50.6X4	T50.6X5	T50.6X6
Pamaquine (naphthoute)	T37.2X1	T37.2X2	T37.2X3	T37.2X4	T37.2X5	T37.2X6
Panadol	T39.1X1	T39.1X2	T39.1X3	T39.1X4	T39.1X5	T39.1X6
Pancreatic						
digestive secretion stimulant	T47.8X1	T47.8X2	T47.8X3	T47.8X4	T47.8X5	T47.8X6
dornase	T45.3X1	T45.3X2	T45.3X3	T45.3X4	T45.3X5	T45.3X6
Pancreatin	T47.5X1	T47.5X2	T47.5X3	T47.5X4	T47.5X5	T47.5X6
Pancrelipase	T47.5X1	T47.5X2	T47.5X3	T47.5X4	T47.5X5	T47.5X6
Pancuronium (bromide)	T48.1X1	T48.1X2	T48.1X3	T48.1X4	T48.1X5	T48.1X6
Pangamic acid	T45.2X1	T45.2X2	T45.2X3	T45.2X4	T45.2X5	T45.2X6
Panthenol	T45.2X1	T45.2X2	T45.2X3	T45.2X4	T45.2X5	T45.2X6
topical	T49.8X1	T49.8X2	T49.8X3	T49.8X4	T49.8X5	T49.8X6
Pantopon	T40.0X1	T40.0X2	T40.0X3	T40.0X4	T40.0X5	T40.0X6
Pantoprazole*	T47.1X1	T47.1X2	T47.1X3	T47.1X4	T47.1X5	T47.1X6
Pantothenic acid	T45.2X1	T45.2X2	T45.2X3	T45.2X4	T45.2X5	T45.2X6
Panwarfin	T45.511	T45.512	T45.513	T45.514	T45.515	T45.516
Papain	T47.5X1	T47.5X2	T47.5X3	T47.5X4	T47.5X5	T47.5X6
digestant	T47.5X1	T47.5X2	T47.5X3	T47.5X4	T47.5X5	T47.5X6
Papaveretum	T40.0X1	T40.0X2	T40.0X3	T40.0X4	T40.0X5	T40.0X6
Papaverine	T44.3X1	T44.3X2	T44.3X3	T44.3X4	T44.3X5	T44.3X6
Para-acetamidophenol	T39.1X1	T39.1X2	T39.1X3	T39.1X4	T39.1X5	T39.1X6
Para-aminobenzoic acid	T49.3X1	T49.3X2	T49.3X3	T49.3X4	T49.3X5	T49.3X6
Para-aminophenol derivatives	T39.1X1	T39.1X2	T39.1X3	T39.1X4	T39.1X5	T39.1X6
Para-aminosalicylic acid	T37.1X1	T37.1X2	T37.1X3	T37.1X4	T37.1X5	T37.1X6
Paracetaldehyde	T42.6X1	T42.6X2	T42.6X3	T42.6X4	T42.6X5	T42.6X6
Paracetamol	T39.1X1	T39.1X2	T39.1X3	T39.1X4	T39.1X5	T39.1X6
Parachlorophenol (camphorated)	T49.0X1	T49.0X2	T49.0X3	T49.0X4	T49.0X5	T49.0X6
Paracodin	T40.2X1	T40.2X2	T40.2X3	T40.2X4	T40.2X5	T40.2X6
Paradione	T42.2X1	T42.2X2	T42.2X3	T42.2X4	T42.2X5	T42.2X6
Paraffin(s) (wax)	T52.0X1	T52.0X2	T52.0X3	T52.0X4	—	—
liquid (medicinal)	T47.4X1	T47.4X2	T47.4X3	T47.4X4	T47.4X5	T47.4X6
nonmedicinal	T52.0X1	T52.0X2	T52.0X3	T52.0X4	—	—
Paraformaldehyde	T60.3X1	T60.3X2	T60.3X3	T60.3X4	—	—
Paraldehyde	T42.6X1	T42.6X2	T42.6X3	T42.6X4	T42.6X5	T42.6X6
Paramethadione	T42.2X1	T42.2X2	T42.2X3	T42.2X4	T42.2X5	T42.2X6
Paramethasone	T38.0X1	T38.0X2	T38.0X3	T38.0X4	T38.0X5	T38.0X6
acetate	T49.0X1	T49.0X2	T49.0X3	T49.0X4	T49.0X5	T49.0X6
Paraoxon	T60.0X1	T60.0X2	T60.0X3	T60.0X4	—	—
Paraquat	T60.3X1	T60.3X2	T60.3X3	T60.3X4	—	—
Parasympatholytic NEC	T44.3X1	T44.3X2	T44.3X3	T44.3X4	T44.3X5	T44.3X6

*Optum Value-Add ☑ Additional Character May Be Required — Refer to the Tabular List for Character Selection

Substance	Poisoning, Accidental (unintentional)	Poisoning, Intentional Self-harm	Poisoning, Assault	Poisoning, Undetermined	Adverse Effect	Under-dosing
Parasympathomimetic drug NEC	T44.1X1	T44.1X2	T44.1X3	T44.1X4	T44.1X5	T44.1X6
Parathion	T6Ø.ØX1	T6Ø.ØX2	T6Ø.ØX3	T6Ø.ØX4	—	—
Parathormone	T5Ø.991	T5Ø.992	T5Ø.993	T5Ø.994	T5Ø.995	T5Ø.996
Parathyroid extract	T5Ø.991	T5Ø.992	T5Ø.993	T5Ø.994	T5Ø.995	T5Ø.996
Paratyphoid vaccine	T5Ø.A91	T5Ø.A92	T5Ø.A93	T5Ø.A94	T5Ø.A95	T5Ø.A96
Paredrine	T44.4X1	T44.4X2	T44.4X3	T44.4X4	T44.4X5	T44.4X6
Paregoric	T4Ø.ØX1	T4Ø.ØX2	T4Ø.ØX3	T4Ø.ØX4	T4Ø.ØX5	T4Ø.ØX6
Pargyline	T46.5X1	T46.5X2	T46.5X3	T46.5X4	T46.5X5	T46.5X6
Paris green	T57.ØX1	T57.ØX2	T57.ØX3	T57.ØX4	—	—
insecticide	T57.ØX1	T57.ØX2	T57.ØX3	T57.ØX4	—	—
Parnate	T43.1X1	T43.1X2	T43.1X3	T43.1X4	T43.1X5	T43.1X6
Paromomycin	T36.5X1	T36.5X2	T36.5X3	T36.5X4	T36.5X5	T36.5X6
Paroxypropione	T45.1X1	T45.1X2	T45.1X3	T45.1X4	T45.1X5	T45.1X6
Parsabiv*	T5Ø.991	T5Ø.992	T5Ø.993	T5Ø.994	T5Ø.995	T5Ø.996
Parzone	T4Ø.2X1	T4Ø.2X2	T4Ø.2X3	T4Ø.2X4	T4Ø.2X5	T4Ø.2X6
PAS	T37.1X1	T37.1X2	T37.1X3	T37.1X4	T37.1X5	T37.1X6
Pasiniazid	T37.1X1	T37.1X2	T37.1X3	T37.1X4	T37.1X5	T37.1X6
PBB (polybrominated biphenyls)	T65.891	T65.892	T65.893	T65.894	—	—
PCB	T65.891	T65.892	T65.893	T65.894	—	—
PCP						
meaning pentachlorophenol	T6Ø.1X1	T6Ø.1X2	T6Ø.1X3	T6Ø.1X4	—	—
fungicide	T6Ø.3X1	T6Ø.3X2	T6Ø.3X3	T6Ø.3X4	—	—
herbicide	T6Ø.3X1	T6Ø.3X2	T6Ø.3X3	T6Ø.3X4	—	—
insecticide	T6Ø.1X1	T6Ø.1X2	T6Ø.1X3	T6Ø.1X4	—	—
meaning phencyclidine	T4Ø.991	T4Ø.992	T4Ø.993	T4Ø.994	—	—
Peach kernel oil (emulsion)	T47.4X1	T47.4X2	T47.4X3	T47.4X4	T47.4X5	T47.4X6
Peanut oil (emulsion) **NEC**	T47.4X1	T47.4X2	T47.4X3	T47.4X4	T47.4X5	T47.4X6
topical	T49.3X1	T49.3X2	T49.3X3	T49.3X4	T49.3X5	T49.3X6
Pearly Gates (morning glory seeds)	T4Ø.991	T4Ø.992	T4Ø.993	T4Ø.994	—	—
Pecazine	T43.3X1	T43.3X2	T43.3X3	T43.3X4	T43.3X5	T43.3X6
Pectin	T47.6X1	T47.6X2	T47.6X3	T47.6X4	T47.6X5	T47.6X6
Pediaflor*	T49.7X1	T49.7X2	T49.7X3	T49.7X4	T49.7X5	T49.7X6
Pefloxacin	T37.8X1	T37.8X2	T37.8X3	T37.8X4	T37.8X5	T37.8X6
Pegademase, bovine	T5Ø.Z91	T5Ø.Z92	T5Ø.Z93	T5Ø.Z94	T5Ø.Z95	T5Ø.Z96
Pelletierine tannate	T37.4X1	T37.4X2	T37.4X3	T37.4X4	T37.4X5	T37.4X6
Pemirolast (potassium)	T48.6X1	T48.6X2	T48.6X3	T48.6X4	T48.6X5	T48.6X6
Pemoline	T5Ø.7X1	T5Ø.7X2	T5Ø.7X3	T5Ø.7X4	T5Ø.7X5	T5Ø.7X6
Pempidine	T44.2X1	T44.2X2	T44.2X3	T44.2X4	T44.2X5	T44.2X6
Penamecillin	T36.ØX1	T36.ØX2	T36.ØX3	T36.ØX4	T36.ØX5	T36.ØX6
Penbutolol	T44.7X1	T44.7X2	T44.7X3	T44.7X4	T44.7X5	T44.7X6
Penethamate	T36.ØX1	T36.ØX2	T36.ØX3	T36.ØX4	T36.ØX5	T36.ØX6
Penfluridol	T43.591	T43.592	T43.593	T43.594	T43.595	T43.596
Penflutizide	T5Ø.2X1	T5Ø.2X2	T5Ø.2X3	T5Ø.2X4	T5Ø.2X5	T5Ø.2X6
Pengitoxin	T46.ØX1	T46.ØX2	T46.ØX3	T46.ØX4	T46.ØX5	T46.ØX6
Penicillamine	T5Ø.6X1	T5Ø.6X2	T5Ø.6X3	T5Ø.6X4	T5Ø.6X5	T5Ø.6X6
Penicillin (any)	T36.ØX1	T36.ØX2	T36.ØX3	T36.ØX4	T36.ØX5	T36.ØX6
Penicillinase	T45.3X1	T45.3X2	T45.3X3	T45.3X4	T45.3X5	T45.3X6
Penicilloyl polylysine	T5Ø.8X1	T5Ø.8X2	T5Ø.8X3	T5Ø.8X4	T5Ø.8X5	T5Ø.8X6
Penimepicycline	T36.4X1	T36.4X2	T36.4X3	T36.4X4	T36.4X5	T36.4X6
Pentacel*	T5Ø.A11	T5Ø.A12	T5Ø.A13	T5Ø.A14	T5Ø.A15	T5Ø.A16
Pentachloroethane	T53.6X1	T53.6X2	T53.6X3	T53.6X4	—	—
Pentachloronaphthalene	T53.7X1	T53.7X2	T53.7X3	T53.7X4	—	—
Pentachlorophenol (pesticide)	T6Ø.1X1	T6Ø.1X2	T6Ø.1X3	T6Ø.1X4	—	—
fungicide	T6Ø.3X1	T6Ø.3X2	T6Ø.3X3	T6Ø.3X4	—	—
herbicide	T6Ø.3X1	T6Ø.3X2	T6Ø.3X3	T6Ø.3X4	—	—
insecticide	T6Ø.1X1	T6Ø.1X2	T6Ø.1X3	T6Ø.1X4	—	—
Pentaerythritol	T46.3X1	T46.3X2	T46.3X3	T46.3X4	T46.3X5	T46.3X6
chloral	T42.6X1	T42.6X2	T42.6X3	T42.6X4	T42.6X5	T42.6X6
tetranitrate NEC	T46.3X1	T46.3X2	T46.3X3	T46.3X4	T46.3X5	T46.3X6
Pentaerythrityl tetranitrate	T46.3X1	T46.3X2	T46.3X3	T46.3X4	T46.3X5	T46.3X6
Pentagastrin	T5Ø.8X1	T5Ø.8X2	T5Ø.8X3	T5Ø.8X4	T5Ø.8X5	T5Ø.8X6
Pentalin	T53.6X1	T53.6X2	T53.6X3	T53.6X4	—	—
Pentamethonium bromide	T44.2X1	T44.2X2	T44.2X3	T44.2X4	T44.2X5	T44.2X6
Pentamidine	T37.3X1	T37.3X2	T37.3X3	T37.3X4	T37.3X5	T37.3X6
Pentanol	T51.3X1	T51.3X2	T51.3X3	T51.3X4	—	—
Pentapyrrolinium (bitartrate)	T44.2X1	T44.2X2	T44.2X3	T44.2X4	T44.2X5	T44.2X6
Pentaquine	T37.2X1	T37.2X2	T37.2X3	T37.2X4	T37.2X5	T37.2X6
Pentazocine	T4Ø.491	T4Ø.492	T4Ø.493	T4Ø.494	T4Ø.495	T4Ø.496
Pentetrazole	T5Ø.7X1	T5Ø.7X2	T5Ø.7X3	T5Ø.7X4	T5Ø.7X5	T5Ø.7X6
Penthienate bromide	T44.3X1	T44.3X2	T44.3X3	T44.3X4	T44.3X5	T44.3X6
Pentifylline	T46.7X1	T46.7X2	T46.7X3	T46.7X4	T46.7X5	T46.7X6
Pentobarbital	T42.3X1	T42.3X2	T42.3X3	T42.3X4	T42.3X5	T42.3X6
sodium	T42.3X1	T42.3X2	T42.3X3	T42.3X4	T42.3X5	T42.3X6
Pentobarbitone	T42.3X1	T42.3X2	T42.3X3	T42.3X4	T42.3X5	T42.3X6
Pentolonium tartrate	T44.2X1	T44.2X2	T44.2X3	T44.2X4	T44.2X5	T44.2X6

Substance	Poisoning, Accidental (unintentional)	Poisoning, Intentional Self-harm	Poisoning, Assault	Poisoning, Undetermined	Adverse Effect	Under-dosing
Pentosan polysulfate (sodium)	T39.8X1	T39.8X2	T39.8X3	T39.8X4	T39.8X5	T39.8X6
Pentostatin	T45.1X1	T45.1X2	T45.1X3	T45.1X4	T45.1X5	T45.1X6
Pentothal	T41.1X1	T41.1X2	T41.1X3	T41.1X4	T41.1X5	T41.1X6
Pentoxifylline	T46.7X1	T46.7X2	T46.7X3	T46.7X4	T46.7X5	T46.7X6
Pentoxyverine	T48.3X1	T48.3X2	T48.3X3	T48.3X4	T48.3X5	T48.3X6
Pentrinat	T46.3X1	T46.3X2	T46.3X3	T46.3X4	T46.3X5	T46.3X6
Pentylenetetrazole	T5Ø.7X1	T5Ø.7X2	T5Ø.7X3	T5Ø.7X4	T5Ø.7X5	T5Ø.7X6
Pentylsalicylamide	T37.1X1	T37.1X2	T37.1X3	T37.1X4	T37.1X5	T37.1X6
Pentymal	T42.3X1	T42.3X2	T42.3X3	T42.3X4	T42.3X5	T42.3X6
Pepcid*	T47.ØX1	T47.ØX2	T47.ØX3	T47.ØX4	T47.ØX5	T47.ØX6
Peplomycin	T45.1X1	T45.1X2	T45.1X3	T45.1X4	T45.1X5	T45.1X6
Peppermint (oil)	T47.5X1	T47.5X2	T47.5X3	T47.5X4	T47.5X5	T47.5X6
Pepsin	T47.5X1	T47.5X2	T47.5X3	T47.5X4	T47.5X5	T47.5X6
digestant	T47.5X1	T47.5X2	T47.5X3	T47.5X4	T47.5X5	T47.5X6
Pepstatin	T47.1X1	T47.1X2	T47.1X3	T47.1X4	T47.1X5	T47.1X6
Peptavlon	T5Ø.8X1	T5Ø.8X2	T5Ø.8X3	T5Ø.8X4	T5Ø.8X5	T5Ø.8X6
Perazine	T43.3X1	T43.3X2	T43.3X3	T43.3X4	T43.3X5	T43.3X6
Percaine (spinal)	T41.3X1	T41.3X2	T41.3X3	T41.3X4	T41.3X5	T41.3X6
topical (surface)	T41.3X1	T41.3X2	T41.3X3	T41.3X4	T41.3X5	T41.3X6
Perchloroethylene	T53.3X1	T53.3X2	T53.3X3	T53.3X4	—	—
medicinal	T37.4X1	T37.4X2	T37.4X3	T37.4X4	T37.4X5	T37.4X6
vapor	T53.3X1	T53.3X2	T53.3X3	T53.3X4	—	—
Percodan	T4Ø.2X1	T4Ø.2X2	T4Ø.2X3	T4Ø.2X4	T4Ø.2X5	T4Ø.2X6
Percogesic — *see also* acetaminophen	T45.ØX1	T45.ØX2	T45.ØX3	T45.ØX4	T45.ØX5	T45.ØX6
Percorten	T38.ØX1	T38.ØX2	T38.ØX3	T38.ØX4	T38.ØX5	T38.ØX6
Pergolide	T42.8X1	T42.8X2	T42.8X3	T42.8X4	T42.8X5	T42.8X6
Pergonal	T38.811	T38.812	T38.813	T38.814	T38.815	T38.816
Perhexilene	T46.3X1	T46.3X2	T46.3X3	T46.3X4	T46.3X5	T46.3X6
Perhexiline (maleate)	T46.3X1	T46.3X2	T46.3X3	T46.3X4	T46.3X5	T46.3X6
Periactin	T45.ØX1	T45.ØX2	T45.ØX3	T45.ØX4	T45.ØX5	T45.ØX6
Periciazine	T43.3X1	T43.3X2	T43.3X3	T43.3X4	T43.3X5	T43.3X6
Periclor	T42.6X1	T42.6X2	T42.6X3	T42.6X4	T42.6X5	T42.6X6
Perindopril	T46.4X1	T46.4X2	T46.4X3	T46.4X4	T46.4X5	T46.4X6
Perisoxal	T39.8X1	T39.8X2	T39.8X3	T39.8X4	T39.8X5	T39.8X6
Peritoneal dialysis solution	T5Ø.3X1	T5Ø.3X2	T5Ø.3X3	T5Ø.3X4	T5Ø.3X5	T5Ø.3X6
Peritrate	T46.3X1	T46.3X2	T46.3X3	T46.3X4	T46.3X5	T46.3X6
Perlapine	T42.4X1	T42.4X2	T42.4X3	T42.4X4	T42.4X5	T42.4X6
Permanganate	T65.891	T65.892	T65.893	T65.894	—	—
Permapen*	T36.ØX1	T36.ØX2	T36.ØX3	T36.ØX4	T36.ØX5	T36.ØX6
Permethrin	T6Ø.1X1	T6Ø.1X2	T6Ø.1X3	T6Ø.1X4	—	—
Pernocton	T42.3X1	T42.3X2	T42.3X3	T42.3X4	T42.3X5	T42.3X6
Pernoston	T42.3X1	T42.3X2	T42.3X3	T42.3X4	T42.3X5	T42.3X6
Peronine	T4Ø.2X1	T4Ø.2X2	T4Ø.2X3	T4Ø.2X4	—	—
Perphenazine	T43.3X1	T43.3X2	T43.3X3	T43.3X4	T43.3X5	T43.3X6
Pertofrane	T43.Ø11	T43.Ø12	T43.Ø13	T43.Ø14	T43.Ø15	T43.Ø16
Pertussis						
immune serum (human)	T5Ø.Z11	T5Ø.Z12	T5Ø.Z13	T5Ø.Z14	T5Ø.Z15	T5Ø.Z16
vaccine (with diphtheria toxoid) (with tetanus toxoid)	T5Ø.A11	T5Ø.A12	T5Ø.A13	T5Ø.A14	T5Ø.A15	T5Ø.A16
Peruvian balsam	T49.ØX1	T49.ØX2	T49.ØX3	T49.ØX4	T49.ØX5	T49.ØX6
Peruvoside	T46.ØX1	T46.ØX2	T46.ØX3	T46.ØX4	T46.ØX5	T46.ØX6
Pesticide (dust) (fumes) (vapor) **NEC**	T6Ø.91	T6Ø.92	T6Ø.93	T6Ø.94	—	—
arsenic	T57.ØX1	T57.ØX2	T57.ØX3	T57.ØX4	—	—
chlorinated	T6Ø.1X1	T6Ø.1X2	T6Ø.1X3	T6Ø.1X4	—	—
cyanide	T65.ØX1	T65.ØX2	T65.ØX3	T65.ØX4	—	—
kerosene	T52.ØX1	T52.ØX2	T52.ØX3	T52.ØX4	—	—
naphthalene	T6Ø.2X1	T6Ø.2X2	T6Ø.2X3	T6Ø.2X4	—	—
specified ingredient NEC	T6Ø.8X1	T6Ø.8X2	T6Ø.8X3	T6Ø.8X4	—	—
strychnine	T65.1X1	T65.1X2	T65.1X3	T65.1X4	—	—
thallium	T6Ø.4X1	T6Ø.4X2	T6Ø.4X3	T6Ø.4X4	—	—
mixture (of compounds)	T6Ø.91	T6Ø.92	T6Ø.93	T6Ø.94	—	—
organochlorine (compounds)	T6Ø.1X1	T6Ø.1X2	T6Ø.1X3	T6Ø.1X4	—	—
petroleum (distillate) (products) NEC	T6Ø.8X1	T6Ø.8X2	T6Ø.8X3	T6Ø.8X4	—	—
Pethidine	T4Ø.491	T4Ø.492	T4Ø.493	T4Ø.494	T4Ø.495	T4Ø.496
Petrichloral	T42.6X1	T42.6X2	T42.6X3	T42.6X4	T42.6X5	T42.6X6
Petrol	T52.ØX1	T52.ØX2	T52.ØX3	T52.ØX4	—	—
vapor	T52.ØX1	T52.ØX2	T52.ØX3	T52.ØX4	—	—
Petrolatum	T49.3X1	T49.3X2	T49.3X3	T49.3X4	T49.3X5	T49.3X6
hydrophilic	T49.3X1	T49.3X2	T49.3X3	T49.3X4	T49.3X5	T49.3X6
liquid	T47.4X1	T47.4X2	T47.4X3	T47.4X4	T47.4X5	T47.4X6
topical	T49.3X1	T49.3X2	T49.3X3	T49.3X4	T49.3X5	T49.3X6
nonmedicinal	T52.ØX1	T52.ØX2	T52.ØX3	T52.ØX4	—	—
red veterinary	T49.3X1	T49.3X2	T49.3X3	T49.3X4	T49.3X5	T49.3X6
white	T49.3X1	T49.3X2	T49.3X3	T49.3X4	T49.3X5	T49.3X6
Petroleum (products) **NEC**	T52.ØX1	T52.ØX2	T52.ØX3	T52.ØX4	—	—
benzine(s) — *see* Ligroin						
ether — *see* Ligroin						

Substance	Poisoning, Accidental (unintentional)	Poisoning, Intentional Self-harm	Poisoning, Assault	Poisoning, Undetermined	Adverse Effect	Under-dosing
Petroleum (products) **NEC** — *continued*						
jelly — *see* Petrolatum						
naphtha — *see* Ligroin						
pesticide	T6Ø.8X1	T6Ø.8X2	T6Ø.8X3	T6Ø.8X4	—	—
solids	T52.ØX1	T52.ØX2	T52.ØX3	T52.ØX4	—	—
solvents	T52.ØX1	T52.ØX2	T52.ØX3	T52.ØX4	—	—
vapor	T52.ØX1	T52.ØX2	T52.ØX3	T52.ØX4	—	—
Peyote	T4Ø.991	T4Ø.992	T4Ø.993	T4Ø.994	—	—
Phanodorm, phanodorn	T42.3X1	T42.3X2	T42.3X3	T42.3X4	T42.3X5	T42.3X6
Phanquinone	T37.3X1	T37.3X2	T37.3X3	T37.3X4	T37.3X5	T37.3X6
Phanquone	T37.3X1	T37.3X2	T37.3X3	T37.3X4	T37.3X5	T37.3X6
Pharmaceutical						
adjunct NEC	T5Ø.9Ø1	T5Ø.9Ø2	T5Ø.9Ø3	T5Ø.9Ø4	T5Ø.9Ø5	T5Ø.9Ø6
excipient NEC	T5Ø.9Ø1	T5Ø.9Ø2	T5Ø.9Ø3	T5Ø.9Ø4	T5Ø.9Ø5	T5Ø.9Ø6
sweetener	T5Ø.9Ø1	T5Ø.9Ø2	T5Ø.9Ø3	T5Ø.9Ø4	T5Ø.9Ø5	T5Ø.9Ø6
viscous agent	T5Ø.9Ø1	T5Ø.9Ø2	T5Ø.9Ø3	T5Ø.9Ø4	T5Ø.9Ø5	T5Ø.9Ø6
Phazyme*	T47.1X1	T47.1X2	T47.1X3	T47.1X4	T47.1X5	T47.1X6
Phemitone	T42.3X1	T42.3X2	T42.3X3	T42.3X4	T42.3X5	T42.3X6
Phenacaine	T41.3X1	T41.3X2	T41.3X3	T41.3X4	T41.3X5	T41.3X6
Phenacemide	T42.6X1	T42.6X2	T42.6X3	T42.6X4	T42.6X5	T42.6X6
Phenacetin	T39.1X1	T39.1X2	T39.1X3	T39.1X4	T39.1X5	T39.1X6
Phenadoxone	T4Ø.2X1	T4Ø.2X2	T4Ø.2X3	T4Ø.2X4	—	—
Phenaglycodol	T43.591	T43.592	T43.593	T43.594	T43.595	T43.596
Phenantoin	T42.ØX1	T42.ØX2	T42.ØX3	T42.ØX4	T42.ØX5	T42.ØX6
Phenaphthazine reagent	T5Ø.991	T5Ø.992	T5Ø.993	T5Ø.994	T5Ø.995	T5Ø.996
Phenazocine	T4Ø.491	T4Ø.492	T4Ø.493	T4Ø.494	T4Ø.495	T4Ø.496
Phenazone	T39.2X1	T39.2X2	T39.2X3	T39.2X4	T39.2X5	T39.2X6
Phenazopyridine	T39.8X1	T39.8X2	T39.8X3	T39.8X4	T39.8X5	T39.8X6
Phenbenicillin	T36.ØX1	T36.ØX2	T36.ØX3	T36.ØX4	T36.ØX5	T36.ØX6
Phenbutrazate	T5Ø.5X1	T5Ø.5X2	T5Ø.5X3	T5Ø.5X4	T5Ø.5X5	T5Ø.5X6
Phencyclidine	T4Ø.991	T4Ø.992	T4Ø.993	T4Ø.994	T4Ø.995	T4Ø.996
Phendimetrazine	T5Ø.5X1	T5Ø.5X2	T5Ø.5X3	T5Ø.5X4	T5Ø.5X5	T5Ø.5X6
Phenelzine	T43.1X1	T43.1X2	T43.1X3	T43.1X4	T43.1X5	T43.1X6
Phenemal	T42.3X1	T42.3X2	T42.3X3	T42.3X4	T42.3X5	T42.3X6
Phenergan	T42.6X1	T42.6X2	T42.6X3	T42.6X4	T42.6X5	T42.6X6
Pheneticillin	T36.ØX1	T36.ØX2	T36.ØX3	T36.ØX4	T36.ØX5	T36.ØX6
Pheneturide	T42.6X1	T42.6X2	T42.6X3	T42.6X4	T42.6X5	T42.6X6
Phenformin	T38.3X1	T38.3X2	T38.3X3	T38.3X4	T38.3X5	T38.3X6
Phenglutarimide	T44.3X1	T44.3X2	T44.3X3	T44.3X4	T44.3X5	T44.3X6
Phenicarbazide	T39.8X1	T39.8X2	T39.8X3	T39.8X4	T39.8X5	T39.8X6
Phenindamine	T45.ØX1	T45.ØX2	T45.ØX3	T45.ØX4	T45.ØX5	T45.ØX6
Phenindione	T45.511	T45.512	T45.513	T45.514	T45.515	T45.516
Pheniprazine	T43.1X1	T43.1X2	T43.1X3	T43.1X4	T43.1X5	T43.1X6
Pheniramine	T45.ØX1	T45.ØX2	T45.ØX3	T45.ØX4	T45.ØX5	T45.ØX6
Phenisatin	T47.2X1	T47.2X2	T47.2X3	T47.2X4	T47.2X5	T47.2X6
Phenmetrazine	T5Ø.5X1	T5Ø.5X2	T5Ø.5X3	T5Ø.5X4	T5Ø.5X5	T5Ø.5X6
Phenobal	T42.3X1	T42.3X2	T42.3X3	T42.3X4	T42.3X5	T42.3X6
Phenobarbital	T42.3X1	T42.3X2	T42.3X3	T42.3X4	T42.3X5	T42.3X6
sodium	T42.3X1	T42.3X2	T42.3X3	T42.3X4	T42.3X5	T42.3X6
with						
mephenytoin	T42.3X1	T42.3X2	T42.3X3	T42.3X4	T42.3X5	T42.3X6
phenytoin	T42.3X1	T42.3X2	T42.3X3	T42.3X4	T42.3X5	T42.3X6
Phenobarbitone	T42.3X1	T42.3X2	T42.3X3	T42.3X4	T42.3X5	T42.3X6
Phenobutiodil	T5Ø.8X1	T5Ø.8X2	T5Ø.8X3	T5Ø.8X4	T5Ø.8X5	T5Ø.8X6
Phenoctide	T49.ØX1	T49.ØX2	T49.ØX3	T49.ØX4	T49.ØX5	T49.ØX6
Phenol	T49.ØX1	T49.ØX2	T49.ØX3	T49.ØX4	T49.ØX5	T49.ØX6
disinfectant	T54.ØX1	T54.ØX2	T54.ØX3	T54.ØX4	—	—
in oil injection	T46.8X1	T46.8X2	T46.8X3	T46.8X4	T46.8X5	T46.8X6
medicinal	T49.1X1	T49.1X2	T49.1X3	T49.1X4	T49.1X5	T49.1X6
nonmedicinal NEC	T54.ØX1	T54.ØX2	T54.ØX3	T54.ØX4	—	—
pesticide	T6Ø.8X1	T6Ø.8X2	T6Ø.8X3	T6Ø.8X4	—	—
red	T5Ø.8X1	T5Ø.8X2	T5Ø.8X3	T5Ø.8X4	T5Ø.8X5	T5Ø.8X6
Phenolic preparation	T49.1X1	T49.1X2	T49.1X3	T49.1X4	T49.1X5	T49.1X6
Phenolphthalein	T47.2X1	T47.2X2	T47.2X3	T47.2X4	T47.2X5	T47.2X6
Phenolsulfonphthalein	T5Ø.8X1	T5Ø.8X2	T5Ø.8X3	T5Ø.8X4	T5Ø.8X5	T5Ø.8X6
Phenomorphan	T4Ø.2X1	T4Ø.2X2	T4Ø.2X3	T4Ø.2X4	—	—
Phenonyl	T42.3X1	T42.3X2	T42.3X3	T42.3X4	T42.3X5	T42.3X6
Phenoperidine	T4Ø.491	T4Ø.492	T4Ø.493	T4Ø.494	—	—
Phenopyrazone	T46.991	T46.992	T46.993	T46.994	T46.995	T46.996
Phenoquin	T5Ø.4X1	T5Ø.4X2	T5Ø.4X3	T5Ø.4X4	T5Ø.4X5	T5Ø.4X6
Phenothiazine (psychotropic) **NEC**	T43.3X1	T43.3X2	T43.3X3	T43.3X4	T43.3X5	T43.3X6
insecticide	T6Ø.2X1	T6Ø.2X2	T6Ø.2X3	T6Ø.2X4	—	—
Phenothrin	T49.ØX1	T49.ØX2	T49.ØX3	T49.ØX4	T49.ØX5	T49.ØX6
Phenoxybenzamine	T46.7X1	T46.7X2	T46.7X3	T46.7X4	T46.7X5	T46.7X6
Phenoxyethanol	T49.ØX1	T49.ØX2	T49.ØX3	T49.ØX4	T49.ØX5	T49.ØX6
Phenoxymethyl penicillin	T36.ØX1	T36.ØX2	T36.ØX3	T36.ØX4	T36.ØX5	T36.ØX6
Phenprobamate	T42.8X1	T42.8X2	T42.8X3	T42.8X4	T42.8X5	T42.8X6
Phenprocoumon	T45.511	T45.512	T45.513	T45.514	T45.515	T45.516
Phensuximide	T42.2X1	T42.2X2	T42.2X3	T42.2X4	T42.2X5	T42.2X6
Phentermine	T5Ø.5X1	T5Ø.5X2	T5Ø.5X3	T5Ø.5X4	T5Ø.5X5	T5Ø.5X6
Phenthicillin	T36.ØX1	T36.ØX2	T36.ØX3	T36.ØX4	T36.ØX5	T36.ØX6

Substance	Poisoning, Accidental (unintentional)	Poisoning, Intentional Self-harm	Poisoning, Assault	Poisoning, Undetermined	Adverse Effect	Under-dosing
Phentolamine	T46.7X1	T46.7X2	T46.7X3	T46.7X4	T46.7X5	T46.7X6
Phenyl						
butazone	T39.2X1	T39.2X2	T39.2X3	T39.2X4	T39.2X5	T39.2X6
enediamine	T65.3X1	T65.3X2	T65.3X3	T65.3X4	—	—
hydrazine	T65.3X1	T65.3X2	T65.3X3	T65.3X4		
antineoplastic	T45.1X1	T45.1X2	T45.1X3	T45.1X4	T45.1X5	T45.1X6
mercuric compounds — *see* Mercury						
salicylate	T49.3X1	T49.3X2	T49.3X3	T49.3X4	T49.3X5	T49.3X6
Phenylalanine mustard	T45.1X1	T45.1X2	T45.1X3	T45.1X4	T45.1X5	T45.1X6
Phenylbutazone	T39.2X1	T39.2X2	T39.2X3	T39.2X4	T39.2X5	T39.2X6
Phenylenediamine	T65.3X1	T65.3X2	T65.3X3	T65.3X4	—	—
Phenylephrine	T44.4X1	T44.4X2	T44.4X3	T44.4X4	T44.4X5	T44.4X6
Phenylethylbiguanide	T38.3X1	T38.3X2	T38.3X3	T38.3X4	T38.3X5	T38.3X6
Phenylmercuric						
acetate	T49.ØX1	T49.ØX2	T49.ØX3	T49.ØX4	T49.ØX5	T49.ØX6
borate	T49.ØX1	T49.ØX2	T49.ØX3	T49.ØX4	T49.ØX5	T49.ØX6
nitrate	T49.ØX1	T49.ØX2	T49.ØX3	T49.ØX4	T49.ØX5	T49.ØX6
Phenylmethylbarbitone	T42.3X1	T42.3X2	T42.3X3	T42.3X4	T42.3X5	T42.3X6
Phenylpropanol	T47.5X1	T47.5X2	T47.5X3	T47.5X4	T47.5X5	T47.5X6
Phenylpropanolamine	T44.991	T44.992	T44.993	T44.994	T44.995	T44.996
Phenylsulfthion	T6Ø.ØX1	T6Ø.ØX2	T6Ø.ØX3	T6Ø.ØX4	—	—
Phenyltoloxamine	T45.ØX1	T45.ØX2	T45.ØX3	T45.ØX4	T45.ØX5	T45.ØX6
Phenyramidol, phenyramidon	T39.8X1	T39.8X2	T39.8X3	T39.8X4	T39.8X5	T39.8X6
Phenytek*	T42.ØX1	T42.ØX2	T42.ØX3	T42.ØX4	T42.ØX5	T42.ØX6
Phenytoin	T42.ØX1	T42.ØX2	T42.ØX3	T42.ØX4	T42.ØX5	T42.ØX6
with Phenobarbital	T42.3X1	T42.3X2	T42.3X3	T42.3X4	T42.3X5	T42.3X6
pHisoHex	T49.2X1	T49.2X2	T49.2X3	T49.2X4	T49.2X5	T49.2X6
Pholcodine	T48.3X1	T48.3X2	T48.3X3	T48.3X4	T48.3X5	T48.3X6
Pholedrine	T46.991	T46.992	T46.993	T46.994	T46.995	T46.996
Phorate	T6Ø.ØX1	T6Ø.ØX2	T6Ø.ØX3	T6Ø.ØX4	—	—
Phosdrin	T6Ø.ØX1	T6Ø.ØX2	T6Ø.ØX3	T6Ø.ØX4	—	—
Phosfolan	T6Ø.ØX1	T6Ø.ØX2	T6Ø.ØX3	T6Ø.ØX4	—	—
Phosgene (gas)	T59.891	T59.892	T59.893	T59.894	—	—
Phosphamidon	T6Ø.ØX1	T6Ø.ØX2	T6Ø.ØX3	T6Ø.ØX4	—	—
Phosphate	T65.891	T65.892	T65.893	T65.894	—	—
laxative	T47.4X1	T47.4X2	T47.4X3	T47.4X4	T47.4X5	T47.4X6
organic	T6Ø.ØX1	T6Ø.ØX2	T6Ø.ØX3	T6Ø.ØX4	—	—
solvent	T52.91	T52.92	T52.93	T52.94	—	—
tricresyl	T65.891	T65.892	T65.893	T65.894	—	—
Phosphine	T57.1X1	T57.1X2	T57.1X3	T57.1X4	—	—
fumigant	T57.1X1	T57.1X2	T57.1X3	T57.1X4	—	—
Phospholine	T49.5X1	T49.5X2	T49.5X3	T49.5X4	T49.5X5	T49.5X6
Phosphoric acid	T54.2X1	T54.2X2	T54.2X3	T54.2X4	—	—
Phosphorus (compound) **NEC**	T57.1X1	T57.1X2	T57.1X3	T57.1X4	—	—
pesticide	T6Ø.ØX1	T6Ø.ØX2	T6Ø.ØX3	T6Ø.ØX4	—	—
Photrexa*	T49.5X1	T49.5X2	T49.5X3	T49.5X4	T49.5X5	T49.5X6
Phthalates	T65.891	T65.892	T65.893	T65.894	—	—
Phthalic anhydride	T65.891	T65.892	T65.893	T65.894	—	—
Phthalimidoglutarimide	T42.6X1	T42.6X2	T42.6X3	T42.6X4	T42.6X5	T42.6X6
Phthalylsulfathiazole	T37.ØX1	T37.ØX2	T37.ØX3	T37.ØX4	T37.ØX5	T37.ØX6
Phylloquinone	T45.7X1	T45.7X2	T45.7X3	T45.7X4	T45.7X5	T45.7X6
Physeptone	T4Ø.3X1	T4Ø.3X2	T4Ø.3X3	T4Ø.3X4	T4Ø.3X5	T4Ø.3X6
Physostigma venenosum	T62.2X1	T62.2X2	T62.2X3	T62.2X4	—	—
Physostigmine	T49.5X1	T49.5X2	T49.5X3	T49.5X4	T49.5X5	T49.5X6
Phytolacca decandra	T62.2X1	T62.2X2	T62.2X3	T62.2X4	—	—
berries	T62.1X1	T62.1X2	T62.1X3	T62.1X4	—	—
Phytomenadione	T45.7X1	T45.7X2	T45.7X3	T45.7X4	T45.7X5	T45.7X6
Phytonadione	T45.7X1	T45.7X2	T45.7X3	T45.7X4	T45.7X5	T45.7X6
Picoperine	T48.3X1	T48.3X2	T48.3X3	T48.3X4	T48.3X5	T48.3X6
Picosulfate (sodium)	T47.2X1	T47.2X2	T47.2X3	T47.2X4	T47.2X5	T47.2X6
Picric (acid)	T54.2X1	T54.2X2	T54.2X3	T54.2X4	—	—
Picrotoxin	T5Ø.7X1	T5Ø.7X2	T5Ø.7X3	T5Ø.7X4	T5Ø.7X5	T5Ø.7X6
Piketoprofen	T49.ØX1	T49.ØX2	T49.ØX3	T49.ØX4	T49.ØX5	T49.ØX6
Pilocarpine	T44.1X1	T44.1X2	T44.1X3	T44.1X4	T44.1X5	T44.1X6
Pilocarpus (jaborandi) extract	T44.1X1	T44.1X2	T44.1X3	T44.1X4	T44.1X5	T44.1X6
Pilsicainide (hydrochloride)	T46.2X1	T46.2X2	T46.2X3	T46.2X4	T46.2X5	T46.2X6
Pimaricin	T36.7X1	T36.7X2	T36.7X3	T36.7X4	T36.7X5	T36.7X6
Pimeclone	T5Ø.7X1	T5Ø.7X2	T5Ø.7X3	T5Ø.7X4	T5Ø.7X5	T5Ø.7X6
Pimelic ketone	T52.8X1	T52.8X2	T52.8X3	T52.8X4	—	—
Pimethixene	T45.ØX1	T45.ØX2	T45.ØX3	T45.ØX4	T45.ØX5	T45.ØX6
Piminodine	T4Ø.2X1	T4Ø.2X2	T4Ø.2X3	T4Ø.2X4	T4Ø.2X5	T4Ø.2X6
Pimozide	T43.591	T43.592	T43.593	T43.594	T43.595	T43.596
Pinacidil	T46.5X1	T46.5X2	T46.5X3	T46.5X4	T46.5X5	T46.5X6
Pinaverium bromide	T44.3X1	T44.3X2	T44.3X3	T44.3X4	T44.3X5	T44.3X6
Pinazepam	T42.4X1	T42.4X2	T42.4X3	T42.4X4	T42.4X5	T42.4X6
Pindolol	T44.7X1	T44.7X2	T44.7X3	T44.7X4	T44.7X5	T44.7X6
Pindone	T6Ø.4X1	T6Ø.4X2	T6Ø.4X3	T6Ø.4X4	—	—
Pine oil (disinfectant)	T65.891	T65.892	T65.893	T65.894	—	—
Pinkroot	T37.4X1	T37.4X2	T37.4X3	T37.4X4	T37.4X5	T37.4X6

*Optum Value-Add

Substance	Poisoning, Accidental (unintentional)	Poisoning, Intentional Self-harm	Poisoning, Assault	Poisoning, Undetermined	Adverse Effect	Underdosing
Pipadone	T40.2X1	T40.2X2	T40.2X3	T40.2X4	—	—
Pipamazine	T45.0X1	T45.0X2	T45.0X3	T45.0X4	T45.0X5	T45.0X6
Pipamperone	T43.4X1	T43.4X2	T43.4X3	T43.4X4	T43.4X5	T43.4X6
Pipazetate	T48.3X1	T48.3X2	T48.3X3	T48.3X4	T48.3X5	T48.3X6
Pipemidic acid	T37.8X1	T37.8X2	T37.8X3	T37.8X4	T37.8X5	T37.8X6
Pipenzolate bromide	T44.3X1	T44.3X2	T44.3X3	T44.3X4	T44.3X5	T44.3X6
Piper cubeba	T62.2X1	T62.2X2	T62.2X3	T62.2X4	—	—
Piperacetazine	T43.3X1	T43.3X2	T43.3X3	T43.3X4	T43.3X5	T43.3X6
Piperacillin	T36.0X1	T36.0X2	T36.0X3	T36.0X4	T36.0X5	T36.0X6
Piperazine	T37.4X1	T37.4X2	T37.4X3	T37.4X4	T37.4X5	T37.4X6
estrone sulfate	T38.5X1	T38.5X2	T38.5X3	T38.5X4	T38.5X5	T38.5X6
Piperidione	T48.3X1	T48.3X2	T48.3X3	T48.3X4	T48.3X5	T48.3X6
Piperidolate	T44.3X1	T44.3X2	T44.3X3	T44.3X4	T44.3X5	T44.3X6
Piperocaine	T41.3X1	T41.3X2	T41.3X3	T41.3X4	T41.3X5	T41.3X6
infiltration (subcutaneous)	T41.3X1	T41.3X2	T41.3X3	T41.3X4	T41.3X5	T41.3X6
nerve block (peripheral) (plexus)	T41.3X1	T41.3X2	T41.3X3	T41.3X4	T41.3X5	T41.3X6
topical (surface)	T41.3X1	T41.3X2	T41.3X3	T41.3X4	T41.3X5	T41.3X6
Piperonyl butoxide	T60.8X1	T60.8X2	T60.8X3	T60.8X4	—	—
Pipethanate	T44.3X1	T44.3X2	T44.3X3	T44.3X4	T44.3X5	T44.3X6
Pipobroman	T45.1X1	T45.1X2	T45.1X3	T45.1X4	T45.1X5	T45.1X6
Pipotiazine	T43.3X1	T43.3X2	T43.3X3	T43.3X4	T43.3X5	T43.3X6
Pipoxizine	T45.0X1	T45.0X2	T45.0X3	T45.0X4	T45.0X5	T45.0X6
Pipradrol	T43.691	T43.692	T43.693	T43.694	T43.695	T43.696
Piprinhydrinate	T45.0X1	T45.0X2	T45.0X3	T45.0X4	T45.0X5	T45.0X6
Pirarubicin	T45.1X1	T45.1X2	T45.1X3	T45.1X4	T45.1X5	T45.1X6
Pirazinamide	T37.1X1	T37.1X2	T37.1X3	T37.1X4	T37.1X5	T37.1X6
Pirbuterol	T48.6X1	T48.6X2	T48.6X3	T48.6X4	T48.6X5	T48.6X6
Pirenzepine	T47.1X1	T47.1X2	T47.1X3	T47.1X4	T47.1X5	T47.1X6
Piretanide	T50.1X1	T50.1X2	T50.1X3	T50.1X4	T50.1X5	T50.1X6
Pirfenidone*	T48.991	T48.992	T48.993	T48.994	T48.995	T48.996
Piribedil	T42.8X1	T42.8X2	T42.8X3	T42.8X4	T42.8X5	T42.8X6
Piridoxilate	T46.3X1	T46.3X2	T46.3X3	T46.3X4	T46.3X5	T46.3X6
Piritramide	T40.491	T40.492	T40.493	T40.494	—	—
Piromidic acid	T37.8X1	T37.8X2	T37.8X3	T37.8X4	T37.8X5	T37.8X6
Piroxicam	T39.391	T39.392	T39.393	T39.394	T39.395	T39.396
beta-cyclodextrin complex	T39.8X1	T39.8X2	T39.8X3	T39.8X4	T39.8X5	T39.8X6
Pirozadil	T46.6X1	T46.6X2	T46.6X3	T46.6X4	T46.6X5	T46.6X6
Piscidia (bark) (erythrina)	T39.8X1	T39.8X2	T39.8X3	T39.8X4	T39.8X5	T39.8X6
Pitch	T65.891	T65.892	T65.893	T65.894	—	—
Pitkin's solution	T41.3X1	T41.3X2	T41.3X3	T41.3X4	T41.3X5	T41.3X6
Pitocin	T48.0X1	T48.0X2	T48.0X3	T48.0X4	T48.0X5	T48.0X6
Pitressin (tannate)	T38.891	T38.892	T38.893	T38.894	T38.895	T38.896
Pituitary extracts (posterior)	T38.891	T38.892	T38.893	T38.894	T38.895	T38.896
anterior	T38.811	T38.812	T38.813	T38.814	T38.815	T38.816
Pituitrin	T38.891	T38.892	T38.893	T38.894	T38.895	T38.896
Pivampicillin	T36.0X1	T36.0X2	T36.0X3	T36.0X4	T36.0X5	T36.0X6
Pivmecillinam	T36.0X1	T36.0X2	T36.0X3	T36.0X4	T36.0X5	T36.0X6
Placental hormone	T38.891	T38.892	T38.893	T38.894	T38.895	T38.896
Placidyl	T42.6X1	T42.6X2	T42.6X3	T42.6X4	T42.6X5	T42.6X6
Plague vaccine	T50.A91	T50.A92	T50.A93	T50.A94	T50.A95	T50.A96
Plant						
food or fertilizer NEC	T65.891	T65.892	T65.893	T65.894	—	—
containing herbicide	T60.3X1	T60.3X2	T60.3X3	T60.3X4	—	—
noxious, used as food	T62.2X1	T62.2X2	T62.2X3	T62.2X4	—	—
berries	T62.1X1	T62.1X2	T62.1X3	T62.1X4	—	—
seeds	T62.2X1	T62.2X2	T62.2X3	T62.2X4	—	—
specified type NEC	T62.2X1	T62.2X2	T62.2X3	T62.2X4	—	—
Plasma	T45.8X1	T45.8X2	T45.8X3	T45.8X4	T45.8X5	T45.8X6
expander NEC	T45.8X1	T45.8X2	T45.8X3	T45.8X4	T45.8X5	T45.8X6
protein fraction (human)	T45.8X1	T45.8X2	T45.8X3	T45.8X4	T45.8X5	T45.8X6
Plasmanate	T45.8X1	T45.8X2	T45.8X3	T45.8X4	T45.8X5	T45.8X6
Plasminogen (tissue) activator	T45.611	T45.612	T45.613	T45.614	T45.615	T45.616
Plaster dressing	T49.3X1	T49.3X2	T49.3X3	T49.3X4	T49.3X5	T49.3X6
Plastic dressing	T49.3X1	T49.3X2	T49.3X3	T49.3X4	T49.3X5	T49.3X6
Plavix*	T45.521	T45.522	T45.523	T45.524	T45.525	T45.526
Plegicil	T43.3X1	T43.3X2	T43.3X3	T43.3X4	T43.3X5	T43.3X6
Plicamycin	T45.1X1	T45.1X2	T45.1X3	T45.1X4	T45.1X5	T45.1X6
Podophyllotoxin	T49.8X1	T49.8X2	T49.8X3	T49.8X4	T49.8X5	T49.8X6
Podophyllum (resin)	T49.4X1	T49.4X2	T49.4X3	T49.4X4	T49.4X5	T49.4X6
Poison NEC	T65.91	T65.92	T65.93	T65.94	—	—
Poisonous berries	T62.1X1	T62.1X2	T62.1X3	T62.1X4	—	—
Pokeweed (any part)	T62.2X1	T62.2X2	T62.2X3	T62.2X4	—	—
Poldine metilsulfate	T44.3X1	T44.3X2	T44.3X3	T44.3X4	T44.3X5	T44.3X6
Polidexide (sulfate)	T46.6X1	T46.6X2	T46.6X3	T46.6X4	T46.6X5	T46.6X6
Polidocanol	T46.8X1	T46.8X2	T46.8X3	T46.8X4	T46.8X5	T46.8X6
Poliomyelitis vaccine	T50.B91	T50.B92	T50.B93	T50.B94	T50.B95	T50.B96
Polish (car) (floor) (furniture)	T65.891	T65.892	T65.893	T65.894	—	—
(metal) (porcelain) (silver)						
abrasive	T65.891	T65.892	T65.893	T65.894	—	—
Polish — continued						
porcelain	T65.891	T65.892	T65.893	T65.894	—	—
Poloxalkol	T47.4X1	T47.4X2	T47.4X3	T47.4X4	T47.4X5	T47.4X6
Poloxamer	T47.4X1	T47.4X2	T47.4X3	T47.4X4	T47.4X5	T47.4X6
Poly-Pred*	T49.5X1	T49.5X2	T49.5X3	T49.5X4	T49.5X5	T49.5X6
Polyaminostyrene resins	T50.3X1	T50.3X2	T50.3X3	T50.3X4	T50.3X5	T50.3X6
Polycarbophil	T47.4X1	T47.4X2	T47.4X3	T47.4X4	T47.4X5	T47.4X6
Polychlorinated biphenyl	T65.891	T65.892	T65.893	T65.894	—	—
Polycycline	T36.4X1	T36.4X2	T36.4X3	T36.4X4	T36.4X5	T36.4X6
Polyester fumes	T59.891	T59.892	T59.893	T59.894	—	—
Polyester resin hardener	T52.91	T52.92	T52.93	T52.94	—	—
fumes	T59.891	T59.892	T59.893	T59.894	—	—
Polyestradiol phosphate	T38.5X1	T38.5X2	T38.5X3	T38.5X4	T38.5X5	T38.5X6
Polyethanolamine alkyl sulfate	T49.2X1	T49.2X2	T49.2X3	T49.2X4	T49.2X5	T49.2X6
Polyethylene adhesive	T49.3X1	T49.3X2	T49.3X3	T49.3X4	T49.3X5	T49.3X6
Polyferose	T45.4X1	T45.4X2	T45.4X3	T45.4X4	T45.4X5	T45.4X6
Polygeline	T45.8X1	T45.8X2	T45.8X3	T45.8X4	T45.8X5	T45.8X6
Polymyxin	T36.8X1	T36.8X2	T36.8X3	T36.8X4	T36.8X5	T36.8X6
B	T36.8X1	T36.8X2	T36.8X3	T36.8X4	T36.8X5	T36.8X6
ENT agent	T49.6X1	T49.6X2	T49.6X3	T49.6X4	T49.6X5	T49.6X6
ophthalmic preparation	T49.5X1	T49.5X2	T49.5X3	T49.5X4	T49.5X5	T49.5X6
topical NEC	T49.0X1	T49.0X2	T49.0X3	T49.0X4	T49.0X5	T49.0X6
E sulfate (eye preparation)	T49.5X1	T49.5X2	T49.5X3	T49.5X4	T49.5X5	T49.5X6
Polynoxylin	T49.0X1	T49.0X2	T49.0X3	T49.0X4	T49.0X5	T49.0X6
Polyoestradiol phosphate	T38.5X1	T38.5X2	T38.5X3	T38.5X4	T38.5X5	T38.5X6
Polyoxymethyleneurea	T49.0X1	T49.0X2	T49.0X3	T49.0X4	T49.0X5	T49.0X6
Polysilane	T47.8X1	T47.8X2	T47.8X3	T47.8X4	T47.8X5	T47.8X6
Polytetrafluoroethylene (inhaled)	T59.891	T59.892	T59.893	T59.894	—	—
Polythiazide	T50.2X1	T50.2X2	T50.2X3	T50.2X4	T50.2X5	T50.2X6
Polyvidone	T45.8X1	T45.8X2	T45.8X3	T45.8X4	T45.8X5	T45.8X6
Polyvinylpyrrolidone	T45.8X1	T45.8X2	T45.8X3	T45.8X4	T45.8X5	T45.8X6
Pontocaine (hydrochloride) (infiltration) (topical)	T41.3X1	T41.3X2	T41.3X3	T41.3X4	T41.3X5	T41.3X6
nerve block (peripheral) (plexus)	T41.3X1	T41.3X2	T41.3X3	T41.3X4	T41.3X5	T41.3X6
spinal	T41.3X1	T41.3X2	T41.3X3	T41.3X4	T41.3X5	T41.3X6
Porfiromycin	T45.1X1	T45.1X2	T45.1X3	T45.1X4	T45.1X5	T45.1X6
Portactant alfa*	T48.991	T48.992	T48.993	T48.994	T48.995	T48.996
Posterior pituitary hormone NEC	T38.891	T38.892	T38.893	T38.894	T38.895	T38.896
Pot	T40.711	T40.712	T40.713	T40.714	T40.715	T40.716
Potash (caustic)	T54.3X1	T54.3X2	T54.3X3	T54.3X4	—	—
Potassic saline injection (lactated)	T50.3X1	T50.3X2	T50.3X3	T50.3X4	T50.3X5	T50.3X6
Potassium (salts) NEC	T50.3X1	T50.3X2	T50.3X3	T50.3X4	T50.3X5	T50.3X6
aminobenzoate	T45.8X1	T45.8X2	T45.8X3	T45.8X4	T45.8X5	T45.8X6
aminosalicylate	T37.1X1	T37.1X2	T37.1X3	T37.1X4	T37.1X5	T37.1X6
antimony 'tartrate'	T37.8X1	T37.8X2	T37.8X3	T37.8X4	T37.8X5	T37.8X6
arsenite (solution)	T57.0X1	T57.0X2	T57.0X3	T57.0X4	—	—
bichromate	T56.2X1	T56.2X2	T56.2X3	T56.2X4	—	—
bisulfate	T47.3X1	T47.3X2	T47.3X3	T47.3X4	T47.3X5	T47.3X6
bromide	T42.6X1	T42.6X2	T42.6X3	T42.6X4	T42.6X5	T42.6X6
canrenoate	T50.0X1	T50.0X2	T50.0X3	T50.0X4	T50.0X5	T50.0X6
carbonate	T54.3X1	T54.3X2	T54.3X3	T54.3X4	—	—
chlorate NEC	T65.891	T65.892	T65.893	T65.894	—	—
chloride	T50.3X1	T50.3X2	T50.3X3	T50.3X4	T50.3X5	T50.3X6
citrate	T50.991	T50.992	T50.993	T50.994	T50.995	T50.996
cyanide	T65.0X1	T65.0X2	T65.0X3	T65.0X4	—	—
ferric hexacyanoferrate (medicinal)	T50.6X1	T50.6X2	T50.6X3	T50.6X4	T50.6X5	T50.6X6
nonmedicinal	T65.891	T65.892	T65.893	T65.894	—	—
Fluoride	T57.8X1	T57.8X2	T57.8X3	T57.8X4	—	—
glucaldrate	T47.1X1	T47.1X2	T47.1X3	T47.1X4	T47.1X5	T47.1X6
hydroxide	T54.3X1	T54.3X2	T54.3X3	T54.3X4	—	—
iodate	T49.0X1	T49.0X2	T49.0X3	T49.0X4	T49.0X5	T49.0X6
iodide	T48.4X1	T48.4X2	T48.4X3	T48.4X4	T48.4X5	T48.4X6
nitrate	T57.8X1	T57.8X2	T57.8X3	T57.8X4	—	—
oxalate	T65.891	T65.892	T65.893	T65.894	—	—
perchlorate (nonmedicinal) NEC	T65.891	T65.892	T65.893	T65.894	—	—
antithyroid	T38.2X1	T38.2X2	T38.2X3	T38.2X4	T38.2X5	T38.2X6
medicinal	T38.2X1	T38.2X2	T38.2X3	T38.2X4	T38.2X5	T38.2X6
Permanganate (nonmedicinal)	T65.891	T65.892	T65.893	T65.894	—	—
medicinal	T49.0X1	T49.0X2	T49.0X3	T49.0X4	T49.0X5	T49.0X6
sulfate	T47.2X1	T47.2X2	T47.2X3	T47.2X4	T47.2X5	T47.2X6
Potassium-removing resin	T50.3X1	T50.3X2	T50.3X3	T50.3X4	T50.3X5	T50.3X6
Potassium-retaining drug	T50.3X1	T50.3X2	T50.3X3	T50.3X4	T50.3X5	T50.3X6
Povidone	T45.8X1	T45.8X2	T45.8X3	T45.8X4	T45.8X5	T45.8X6
iodine	T49.0X1	T49.0X2	T49.0X3	T49.0X4	T49.0X5	T49.0X6
Practolol	T44.7X1	T44.7X2	T44.7X3	T44.7X4	T44.7X5	T44.7X6

Substance	Poisoning, Accidental (unintentional)	Poisoning, Intentional Self-harm	Poisoning, Assault	Poisoning, Undetermined	Adverse Effect	Under-dosing
Prajmalium bitartrate	T46.2X1	T46.2X2	T46.2X3	T46.2X4	T46.2X5	T46.2X6
Pralidoxime (iodide)	T5Ø.6X1	T5Ø.6X2	T5Ø.6X3	T5Ø.6X4	T5Ø.6X5	T5Ø.6X6
chloride	T5Ø.6X1	T5Ø.6X2	T5Ø.6X3	T5Ø.6X4	T5Ø.6X5	T5Ø.6X6
Pramiverine	T44.3X1	T44.3X2	T44.3X3	T44.3X4	T44.3X5	T44.3X6
Pramlintide*	T38.3X1	T38.3X2	T38.3X3	T38.3X4	T38.3X5	T38.3X6
Pramocaine	T49.1X1	T49.1X2	T49.1X3	T49.1X4	T49.1X5	T49.1X6
Pramoxine	T49.1X1	T49.1X2	T49.1X3	T49.1X4	T49.1X5	T49.1X6
Prasterone	T38.7X1	T38.7X2	T38.7X3	T38.7X4	T38.7X5	T38.7X6
Pravachol*	T46.6X1	T46.6X2	T46.6X3	T46.6X4	T46.6X5	T46.6X6
Pravastatin	T46.6X1	T46.6X2	T46.6X3	T46.6X4	T46.6X5	T46.6X6
Prazepam	T42.4X1	T42.4X2	T42.4X3	T42.4X4	T42.4X5	T42.4X6
Praziquantel	T37.4X1	T37.4X2	T37.4X3	T37.4X4	T37.4X5	T37.4X6
Prazitone	T43.291	T43.292	T43.293	T43.294	T43.295	T43.296
Prazosin	T44.6X1	T44.6X2	T44.6X3	T44.6X4	T44.6X5	T44.6X6
Prednicarbate	T49.ØX1	T49.ØX2	T49.ØX3	T49.ØX4	T49.ØX5	T49.ØX6
Prednimustine	T45.1X1	T45.1X2	T45.1X3	T45.1X4	T45.1X5	T45.1X6
Prednisolone	T38.ØX1	T38.ØX2	T38.ØX3	T38.ØX4	T38.ØX5	T38.ØX6
ENT agent	T49.6X1	T49.6X2	T49.6X3	T49.6X4	T49.6X5	T49.6X6
ophthalmic preparation	T49.5X1	T49.5X2	T49.5X3	T49.5X4	T49.5X5	T49.5X6
steaglate	T49.ØX1	T49.ØX2	T49.ØX3	T49.ØX4	T49.ØX5	T49.ØX6
topical NEC	T49.ØX1	T49.ØX2	T49.ØX3	T49.ØX4	T49.ØX5	T49.ØX6
Prednisone	T38.ØX1	T38.ØX2	T38.ØX3	T38.ØX4	T38.ØX5	T38.ØX6
Prednylidene	T38.ØX1	T38.ØX2	T38.ØX3	T38.ØX4	T38.ØX5	T38.ØX6
Pregnandiol	T38.5X1	T38.5X2	T38.5X3	T38.5X4	T38.5X5	T38.5X6
Pregneninolone	T38.5X1	T38.5X2	T38.5X3	T38.5X4	T38.5X5	T38.5X6
Preludin	T43.691	T43.692	T43.693	T43.694	T43.695	T43.696
Premarin	T38.5X1	T38.5X2	T38.5X3	T38.5X4	T38.5X5	T38.5X6
Premedication anesthetic	T41.2Ø1	T41.2Ø2	T41.2Ø3	T41.2Ø4	T41.2Ø5	T41.2Ø6
Prenalterol	T44.5X1	T44.5X2	T44.5X3	T44.5X4	T44.5X5	T44.5X6
Prenoxdiazine	T48.3X1	T48.3X2	T48.3X3	T48.3X4	T48.3X5	T48.3X6
Prenylamine	T46.3X1	T46.3X2	T46.3X3	T46.3X4	T46.3X5	T46.3X6
Preparation H	T49.8X1	T49.8X2	T49.8X3	T49.8X4	T49.8X5	T49.8X6
Preparation, local	T49.4X1	T49.4X2	T49.4X3	T49.4X4	T49.4X5	T49.4X6
Preservative (nonmedicinal)	T65.891	T65.892	T65.893	T65.894	—	—
medicinal	T5Ø.9Ø1	T5Ø.9Ø2	T5Ø.9Ø3	T5Ø.9Ø4	T5Ø.9Ø5	T5Ø.9Ø6
wood	T6Ø.91	T6Ø.92	T6Ø.93	T6Ø.94	—	—
Prethcamide	T5Ø.7X1	T5Ø.7X2	T5Ø.7X3	T5Ø.7X4	T5Ø.7X5	T5Ø.7X6
Prevacid*	T47.1X1	T47.1X2	T47.1X3	T47.1X4	T47.1X5	T47.1X6
Pride of China	T62.2X1	T62.2X2	T62.2X3	T62.2X4	—	—
Pridinol	T44.3X1	T44.3X2	T44.3X3	T44.3X4	T44.3X5	T44.3X6
Prifinium bromide	T44.3X1	T44.3X2	T44.3X3	T44.3X4	T44.3X5	T44.3X6
Prilocaine	T41.3X1	T41.3X2	T41.3X3	T41.3X4	T41.3X5	T41.3X6
infiltration (subcutaneous)	T41.3X1	T41.3X2	T41.3X3	T41.3X4	T41.3X5	T41.3X6
nerve block (peripheral) (plexus)	T41.3X1	T41.3X2	T41.3X3	T41.3X4	T41.3X5	T41.3X6
regional	T41.3X1	T41.3X2	T41.3X3	T41.3X4	T41.3X5	T41.3X6
Prilosec*	T47.1X1	T47.1X2	T47.1X3	T47.1X4	T47.1X5	T47.1X6
Primaquine	T37.2X1	T37.2X2	T37.2X3	T37.2X4	T37.2X5	T37.2X6
Primidone	T42.6X1	T42.6X2	T42.6X3	T42.6X4	T42.6X5	T42.6X6
Primula (veris)	T62.2X1	T62.2X2	T62.2X3	T62.2X4	—	—
Prinadol	T4Ø.2X1	T4Ø.2X2	T4Ø.2X3	T4Ø.2X4	T4Ø.2X5	T4Ø.2X6
Prinivil*	T46.4X1	T46.4X2	T46.4X3	T46.4X4	T46.4X5	T46.4X6
Priscol, Priscoline	T44.6X1	T44.6X2	T44.6X3	T44.6X4	T44.6X5	T44.6X6
Pristinamycin	T36.3X1	T36.3X2	T36.3X3	T36.3X4	T36.3X5	T36.3X6
Pristiq*	T43.211	T43.212	T43.213	T43.214	T43.215	T43.216
Privet	T62.2X1	T62.2X2	T62.2X3	T62.2X4	—	—
berries	T62.1X1	T62.1X2	T62.1X3	T62.1X4	—	—
Privine	T44.4X1	T44.4X2	T44.4X3	T44.4X4	T44.4X5	T44.4X6
Pro-Banthine	T44.3X1	T44.3X2	T44.3X3	T44.3X4	T44.3X5	T44.3X6
Probarbital	T42.3X1	T42.3X2	T42.3X3	T42.3X4	T42.3X5	T42.3X6
Probenecid	T5Ø.4X1	T5Ø.4X2	T5Ø.4X3	T5Ø.4X4	T5Ø.4X5	T5Ø.4X6
Probucol	T46.6X1	T46.6X2	T46.6X3	T46.6X4	T46.6X5	T46.6X6
Procainamide	T46.2X1	T46.2X2	T46.2X3	T46.2X4	T46.2X5	T46.2X6
Procaine	T41.3X1	T41.3X2	T41.3X3	T41.3X4	T41.3X5	T41.3X6
benzylpenicillin	T36.ØX1	T36.ØX2	T36.ØX3	T36.ØX4	T36.ØX5	T36.ØX6
nerve block (periphreal) (plexus)	T41.3X1	T41.3X2	T41.3X3	T41.3X4	T41.3X5	T41.3X6
penicillin G	T36.ØX1	T36.ØX2	T36.ØX3	T36.ØX4	T36.ØX5	T36.ØX6
regional	T41.3X1	T41.3X2	T41.3X3	T41.3X4	T41.3X5	T41.3X6
spinal	T41.3X1	T41.3X2	T41.3X3	T41.3X4	T41.3X5	T41.3X6
Procalmidol	T43.591	T43.592	T43.593	T43.594	T43.595	T43.596
Procarbazine	T45.1X1	T45.1X2	T45.1X3	T45.1X4	T45.1X5	T45.1X6
Procaterol	T44.5X1	T44.5X2	T44.5X3	T44.5X4	T44.5X5	T44.5X6
Prochlorperazine	T43.3X1	T43.3X2	T43.3X3	T43.3X4	T43.3X5	T43.3X6
Procyclidine	T44.3X1	T44.3X2	T44.3X3	T44.3X4	T44.3X5	T44.3X6
Producer gas	T58.8X1	T58.8X2	T58.8X3	T58.8X4	—	—
Profadol	T4Ø.491	T4Ø.492	T4Ø.493	T4Ø.494	T4Ø.495	T4Ø.496
Profenamine	T44.3X1	T44.3X2	T44.3X3	T44.3X4	T44.3X5	T44.3X6
Profenil	T44.3X1	T44.3X2	T44.3X3	T44.3X4	T44.3X5	T44.3X6
Proflavine	T49.ØX1	T49.ØX2	T49.ØX3	T49.ØX4	T49.ØX5	T49.ØX6
Progabide	T42.6X1	T42.6X2	T42.6X3	T42.6X4	T42.6X5	T42.6X6
Progesterone	T38.5X1	T38.5X2	T38.5X3	T38.5X4	T38.5X5	T38.5X6

Substance	Poisoning, Accidental (unintentional)	Poisoning, Intentional Self-harm	Poisoning, Assault	Poisoning, Undetermined	Adverse Effect	Under-dosing
Progestin	T38.5X1	T38.5X2	T38.5X3	T38.5X4	T38.5X5	T38.5X6
oral contraceptive	T38.4X1	T38.4X2	T38.4X3	T38.4X4	T38.4X5	T38.4X6
Progestogen NEC	T38.5X1	T38.5X2	T38.5X3	T38.5X4	T38.5X5	T38.5X6
Progestone	T38.5X1	T38.5X2	T38.5X3	T38.5X4	T38.5X5	T38.5X6
Proglumide	T47.1X1	T47.1X2	T47.1X3	T47.1X4	T47.1X5	T47.1X6
Prograf*	T45.1X1	T45.1X2	T45.1X3	T45.1X4	T45.1X5	T45.1X6
Proguanil	T37.2X1	T37.2X2	T37.2X3	T37.2X4	T37.2X5	T37.2X6
Prolactin	T38.811	T38.812	T38.813	T38.814	T38.815	T38.816
Prolintane	T43.691	T43.692	T43.693	T43.694	T43.695	T43.696
Proloid	T38.1X1	T38.1X2	T38.1X3	T38.1X4	T38.1X5	T38.1X6
Proluton	T38.5X1	T38.5X2	T38.5X3	T38.5X4	T38.5X5	T38.5X6
Promacetin	T37.1X1	T37.1X2	T37.1X3	T37.1X4	T37.1X5	T37.1X6
Promazine	T43.3X1	T43.3X2	T43.3X3	T43.3X4	T43.3X5	T43.3X6
Promedol	T4Ø.2X1	T4Ø.2X2	T4Ø.2X3	T4Ø.2X4	—	—
Promegestone	T38.5X1	T38.5X2	T38.5X3	T38.5X4	T38.5X5	T38.5X6
Promethazine (teoclate)	T43.3X1	T43.3X2	T43.3X3	T43.3X4	T43.3X5	T43.3X6
Promin	T37.1X1	T37.1X2	T37.1X3	T37.1X4	T37.1X5	T37.1X6
Pronase	T45.3X1	T45.3X2	T45.3X3	T45.3X4	T45.3X5	T45.3X6
Pronestyl (hydrochloride)	T46.2X1	T46.2X2	T46.2X3	T46.2X4	T46.2X5	T46.2X6
Pronetalol	T44.7X1	T44.7X2	T44.7X3	T44.7X4	T44.7X5	T44.7X6
Prontosil	T37.ØX1	T37.ØX2	T37.ØX3	T37.ØX4	T37.ØX5	T37.ØX6
Propachlor	T6Ø.3X1	T6Ø.3X2	T6Ø.3X3	T6Ø.3X4	—	—
Propafenone	T46.2X1	T46.2X2	T46.2X3	T46.2X4	T46.2X5	T46.2X6
Propallylonal	T42.3X1	T42.3X2	T42.3X3	T42.3X4	T42.3X5	T42.3X6
Propamidine	T49.ØX1	T49.ØX2	T49.ØX3	T49.ØX4	T49.ØX5	T49.ØX6
Propane (distributed in mobile container)	T59.891	T59.892	T59.893	T59.894	—	—
distributed through pipes	T59.891	T59.892	T59.893	T59.894	—	—
incomplete combustion	T58.11	T58.12	T58.13	T58.14	—	—
Propanidid	T41.291	T41.292	T41.293	T41.294	T41.295	T41.296
Propanil	T6Ø.3X1	T6Ø.3X2	T6Ø.3X3	T6Ø.3X4	—	—
Propantheline	T44.3X1	T44.3X2	T44.3X3	T44.3X4	T44.3X5	T44.3X6
bromide	T44.3X1	T44.3X2	T44.3X3	T44.3X4	T44.3X5	T44.3X6
Proparacaine	T41.3X1	T41.3X2	T41.3X3	T41.3X4	T41.3X5	T41.3X6
Propatylnitrate	T46.3X1	T46.3X2	T46.3X3	T46.3X4	T46.3X5	T46.3X6
Propicillin	T36.ØX1	T36.ØX2	T36.ØX3	T36.ØX4	T36.ØX5	T36.ØX6
Propine*	T49.5X1	T49.5X2	T49.5X3	T49.5X4	T49.5X5	T49.5X6
Propiolactone	T49.ØX1	T49.ØX2	T49.ØX3	T49.ØX4	T49.ØX5	T49.ØX6
Propiomazine	T45.ØX1	T45.ØX2	T45.ØX3	T45.ØX4	T45.ØX5	T45.ØX6
Propion gel	T49.ØX1	T49.ØX2	T49.ØX3	T49.ØX4	T49.ØX5	T49.ØX6
Propionaldehyde (medicinal)	T42.6X1	T42.6X2	T42.6X3	T42.6X4	T42.6X5	T42.6X6
Propionate (calcium) (sodium)	T49.ØX1	T49.ØX2	T49.ØX3	T49.ØX4	T49.ØX5	T49.ØX6
Propitocaine	T41.3X1	T41.3X2	T41.3X3	T41.3X4	T41.3X5	T41.3X6
infiltration (subcutaneous)	T41.3X1	T41.3X2	T41.3X3	T41.3X4	T41.3X5	T41.3X6
nerve block (peripheral) (plexus)	T41.3X1	T41.3X2	T41.3X3	T41.3X4	T41.3X5	T41.3X6
Propofol	T41.291	T41.292	T41.293	T41.294	T41.295	T41.296
Propoxur	T6Ø.ØX1	T6Ø.ØX2	T6Ø.ØX3	T6Ø.ØX4	—	—
Propoxycaine	T41.3X1	T41.3X2	T41.3X3	T41.3X4	T41.3X5	T41.3X6
infiltration (subcutaneous)	T41.3X1	T41.3X2	T41.3X3	T41.3X4	T41.3X5	T41.3X6
nerve block (peripheral) (plexus)	T41.3X1	T41.3X2	T41.3X3	T41.3X4	T41.3X5	T41.3X6
topical (surface)	T41.3X1	T41.3X2	T41.3X3	T41.3X4	T41.3X5	T41.3X6
Propoxyphene	T4Ø.491	T4Ø.492	T4Ø.493	T4Ø.494	T4Ø.495	T4Ø.496
Propranolol	T44.7X1	T44.7X2	T44.7X3	T44.7X4	T44.7X5	T44.7X6
Propyl						
alcohol	T51.3X1	T51.3X2	T51.3X3	T51.3X4	—	—
carbinol	T51.3X1	T51.3X2	T51.3X3	T51.3X4	—	—
hexadrine	T44.4X1	T44.4X2	T44.4X3	T44.4X4	T44.4X5	T44.4X6
iodone	T5Ø.8X1	T5Ø.8X2	T5Ø.8X3	T5Ø.8X4	T5Ø.8X5	T5Ø.8X6
thiouracil	T38.2X1	T38.2X2	T38.2X3	T38.2X4	T38.2X5	T38.2X6
Propylaminophenothiazine	T43.3X1	T43.3X2	T43.3X3	T43.3X4	T43.3X5	T43.3X6
Propylene	T59.891	T59.892	T59.893	T59.894	—	—
Propylhexedrine	T48.5X1	T48.5X2	T48.5X3	T48.5X4	T48.5X5	T48.5X6
Propyliodone	T5Ø.8X1	T5Ø.8X2	T5Ø.8X3	T5Ø.8X4	T5Ø.8X5	T5Ø.8X6
Propylparaben (ophthalmic)	T49.5X1	T49.5X2	T49.5X3	T49.5X4	T49.5X5	T49.5X6
Propylthiouracil	T38.2X1	T38.2X2	T38.2X3	T38.2X4	T38.2X5	T38.2X6
Propyphenazone	T39.2X1	T39.2X2	T39.2X3	T39.2X4	T39.2X5	T39.2X6
Proquazone	T39.391	T39.392	T39.393	T39.394	T39.395	T39.396
Proscar*	T38.6X1	T38.6X2	T38.6X3	T38.6X4	T38.6X5	T38.6X6
Proscillaridin	T46.ØX1	T46.ØX2	T46.ØX3	T46.ØX4	T46.ØX5	T46.ØX6
Prostacyclin	T45.521	T45.522	T45.523	T45.524	T45.525	T45.526
Prostaglandin (I2)	T45.521	T45.522	T45.523	T45.524	T45.525	T45.526
E1	T46.7X1	T46.7X2	T46.7X3	T46.7X4	T46.7X5	T46.7X6
E2	T48.ØX1	T48.ØX2	T48.ØX3	T48.ØX4	T48.ØX5	T48.ØX6
F2 alpha	T48.ØX1	T48.ØX2	T48.ØX3	T48.ØX4	T48.ØX5	T48.ØX6
Prostigmin	T44.ØX1	T44.ØX2	T44.ØX3	T44.ØX4	T44.ØX5	T44.ØX6
Prosultiamine	T45.2X1	T45.2X2	T45.2X3	T45.2X4	T45.2X5	T45.2X6
Protamine sulfate	T45.7X1	T45.7X2	T45.7X3	T45.7X4	T45.7X5	T45.7X6
zinc insulin	T38.3X1	T38.3X2	T38.3X3	T38.3X4	T38.3X5	T38.3X6

Substance	Poisoning, Accidental (unintentional)	Poisoning, Intentional Self-harm	Poisoning, Assault	Poisoning, Undetermined	Adverse Effect	Under-dosing
Protease	T47.5X1	T47.5X2	T47.5X3	T47.5X4	T47.5X5	T47.5X6
Protectant, skin NEC	T49.3X1	T49.3X2	T49.3X3	T49.3X4	T49.3X5	T49.3X6
Protein hydrolysate	T5Ø.991	T5Ø.992	T5Ø.993	T5Ø.994	T5Ø.995	T5Ø.996
Prothiaden — *see* Dothiepin hydrochloride						
Prothionamide	T37.1X1	T37.1X2	T37.1X3	T37.1X4	T37.1X5	T37.1X6
Prothipendyl	T43.591	T43.592	T43.593	T43.594	T43.595	T43.596
Prothoate	T6Ø.ØX1	T6Ø.ØX2	T6Ø.ØX3	T6Ø.ØX4	—	—
Prothrombin						
activator	T45.7X1	T45.7X2	T45.7X3	T45.7X4	T45.7X5	T45.7X6
synthesis inhibitor	T45.511	T45.512	T45.513	T45.514	T45.515	T45.516
Protionamide	T37.1X1	T37.1X2	T37.1X3	T37.1X4	T37.1X5	T37.1X6
Protirelin	T38.891	T38.892	T38.893	T38.894	T38.895	T38.896
Protokylol	T48.6X1	T48.6X2	T48.6X3	T48.6X4	T48.6X5	T48.6X6
Protonix*	T47.1X1	T47.1X2	T47.1X3	T47.1X4	T47.1X5	T47.1X6
Protopam	T5Ø.6X1	T5Ø.6X2	T5Ø.6X3	T5Ø.6X4	T5Ø.6X5	T5Ø.6X6
Protoveratrine(s) (A) (B)	T46.5X1	T46.5X2	T46.5X3	T46.5X4	T46.5X5	T46.5X6
Protriptyline	T43.Ø11	T43.Ø12	T43.Ø13	T43.Ø14	T43.Ø15	T43.Ø16
Proventil*	T48.6X1	T48.6X2	T48.6X3	T48.6X4	T48.6X5	T48.6X6
Provera	T38.5X1	T38.5X2	T38.5X3	T38.5X4	T38.5X5	T38.5X6
Provitamin A	T45.2X1	T45.2X2	T45.2X3	T45.2X4	T45.2X5	T45.2X6
Proxibarbal	T42.3X1	T42.3X2	T42.3X3	T42.3X4	T42.3X5	T42.3X6
Proxymetacaine	T41.3X1	T41.3X2	T41.3X3	T41.3X4	T41.3X5	T41.3X6
Proxyphylline	T48.6X1	T48.6X2	T48.6X3	T48.6X4	T48.6X5	T48.6X6
Prozac — *see* Fluoxetine hydrochloride						
Prunus						
laurocerasus	T62.2X1	T62.2X2	T62.2X3	T62.2X4	—	—
virginiana	T62.2X1	T62.2X2	T62.2X3	T62.2X4	—	—
Prussian blue						
commercial	T65.891	T65.892	T65.893	T65.894	—	—
therapeutic	T5Ø.6X1	T5Ø.6X2	T5Ø.6X3	T5Ø.6X4	T5Ø.6X5	T5Ø.6X6
Prussic acid	T65.ØX1	T65.ØX2	T65.ØX3	T65.ØX4	—	—
vapor	T57.3X1	T57.3X2	T57.3X3	T57.3X4	—	—
Pseudoephedrine	T44.991	T44.992	T44.993	T44.994	T44.995	T44.996
Psilocin	T4Ø.991	T4Ø.992	T4Ø.993	T4Ø.994	—	—
Psilocybin	T4Ø.991	T4Ø.992	T4Ø.993	T4Ø.994	—	—
Psilocybine	T4Ø.991	T4Ø.992	T4Ø.993	T4Ø.994	—	—
Psoralene (nonmedicinal)	T65.891	T65.892	T65.893	T65.894	—	—
Psoralens (medicinal)	T5Ø.991	T5Ø.992	T5Ø.993	T5Ø.994	T5Ø.995	T5Ø.996
PSP (phenolsulfonphthalein)	T5Ø.8X1	T5Ø.8X2	T5Ø.8X3	T5Ø.8X4	T5Ø.8X5	T5Ø.8X6
Psychodysleptic drug NOS	T4Ø.9Ø1	T4Ø.9Ø2	T4Ø.9Ø3	T4Ø.9Ø4	T4Ø.9Ø5	T4Ø.9Ø6
specified NEC	T4Ø.991	T4Ø.992	T4Ø.993	T4Ø.994	T4Ø.995	T4Ø.996
Psychostimulant	T43.6Ø1	T43.6Ø2	T43.6Ø3	T43.6Ø4	T43.6Ø5	T43.6Ø6
amphetamine	T43.621	T43.622	T43.623	T43.624	T43.625	T43.626
caffeine	T43.611	T43.612	T43.613	T43.614	T43.615	T43.616
methylphenidate	T43.631	T43.632	T43.633	T43.634	T43.635	T43.636
specified NEC	T43.691	T43.692	T43.693	T43.694	T43.695	T43.696
Psychotherapeutic drug NEC	T43.91	T43.92	T43.93	T43.94	T43.95	T43.96
antidepressants — *see also* Antidepressant	T43.2Ø1	T43.2Ø2	T43.2Ø3	T43.2Ø4	T43.2Ø5	T43.2Ø6
specified NEC	T43.8X1	T43.8X2	T43.8X3	T43.8X4	T43.8X5	T43.8X6
tranquilizers NEC	T43.5Ø1	T43.5Ø2	T43.5Ø3	T43.5Ø4	T43.5Ø5	T43.5Ø6
Psychotomimetic agents	T4Ø.9Ø1	T4Ø.9Ø2	T4Ø.9Ø3	T4Ø.9Ø4	T4Ø.9Ø5	T4Ø.9Ø6
Psychotropic drug NEC	T43.91	T43.92	T43.93	T43.94	T43.95	T43.96
specified NEC	T43.8X1	T43.8X2	T43.8X3	T43.8X4	T43.8X5	T43.8X6
Psyllium hydrophilic mucilloid	T47.4X1	T47.4X2	T47.4X3	T47.4X4	T47.4X5	T47.4X6
Pteroylglutamic acid	T45.8X1	T45.8X2	T45.8X3	T45.8X4	T45.8X5	T45.8X6
Pteroyltriglutamate	T45.1X1	T45.1X2	T45.1X3	T45.1X4	T45.1X5	T45.1X6
PTFE — *see* Polytetrafluoroethylene						
Pulmicort*	T44.5X1	T44.5X2	T44.5X3	T44.5X4	T44.5X5	T44.5X6
Pulp						
devitalizing paste	T49.7X1	T49.7X2	T49.7X3	T49.7X4	T49.7X5	T49.7X6
dressing	T49.7X1	T49.7X2	T49.7X3	T49.7X4	T49.7X5	T49.7X6
Pulsatilla	T62.2X1	T62.2X2	T62.2X3	T62.2X4	—	—
Pumpkin seed extract	T37.4X1	T37.4X2	T37.4X3	T37.4X4	T37.4X5	T37.4X6
Purex (bleach)	T54.91	T54.92	T54.93	T54.94	—	—
Purgative NEC — *see also* Cathartic	T47.4X1	T47.4X2	T47.4X3	T47.4X4	T47.4X5	T47.4X6
Purine analogue (antineoplastic)	T45.1X1	T45.1X2	T45.1X3	T45.1X4	T45.1X5	T45.1X6
Purine diuretics	T5Ø.2X1	T5Ø.2X2	T5Ø.2X3	T5Ø.2X4	T5Ø.2X5	T5Ø.2X6
Purinethol	T45.1X1	T45.1X2	T45.1X3	T45.1X4	T45.1X5	T45.1X6
PVP	T45.8X1	T45.8X2	T45.8X3	T45.8X4	T45.8X5	T45.8X6
Pyrabital	T39.8X1	T39.8X2	T39.8X3	T39.8X4	T39.8X5	T39.8X6
Pyramidon	T39.2X1	T39.2X2	T39.2X3	T39.2X4	T39.2X5	T39.2X6
Pyrantel	T37.4X1	T37.4X2	T37.4X3	T37.4X4	T37.4X5	T37.4X6
Pyrathiazine	T45.ØX1	T45.ØX2	T45.ØX3	T45.ØX4	T45.ØX5	T45.ØX6
Pyrazinamide	T37.1X1	T37.1X2	T37.1X3	T37.1X4	T37.1X5	T37.1X6

Substance	Poisoning, Accidental (unintentional)	Poisoning, Intentional Self-harm	Poisoning, Assault	Poisoning, Undetermined	Adverse Effect	Under-dosing
Pyrazinoic acid (amide)	T37.1X1	T37.1X2	T37.1X3	T37.1X4	T37.1X5	T37.1X6
Pyrazole (derivatives)	T39.2X1	T39.2X2	T39.2X3	T39.2X4	T39.2X5	T39.2X6
Pyrazolone analgesic NEC	T39.2X1	T39.2X2	T39.2X3	T39.2X4	T39.2X5	T39.2X6
Pyrethrin, pyrethrum (nonmedicinal)	T6Ø.2X1	T6Ø.2X2	T6Ø.2X3	T6Ø.2X4	—	—
Pyrethrum extract	T49.ØX1	T49.ØX2	T49.ØX3	T49.ØX4	T49.ØX5	T49.ØX6
Pyribenzamine	T45.ØX1	T45.ØX2	T45.ØX3	T45.ØX4	T45.ØX5	T45.ØX6
Pyridine	T52.8X1	T52.8X2	T52.8X3	T52.8X4	—	—
aldoxime methiodide	T5Ø.6X1	T5Ø.6X2	T5Ø.6X3	T5Ø.6X4	T5Ø.6X5	T5Ø.6X6
aldoxime methyl chloride	T5Ø.6X1	T5Ø.6X2	T5Ø.6X3	T5Ø.6X4	T5Ø.6X5	T5Ø.6X6
vapor	T59.891	T59.892	T59.893	T59.894	—	—
Pyridium	T39.8X1	T39.8X2	T39.8X3	T39.8X4	T39.8X5	T39.8X6
Pyridostigmine bromide	T44.ØX1	T44.ØX2	T44.ØX3	T44.ØX4	T44.ØX5	T44.ØX6
Pyridoxal phosphate	T45.2X1	T45.2X2	T45.2X3	T45.2X4	T45.2X5	T45.2X6
Pyridoxine	T45.2X1	T45.2X2	T45.2X3	T45.2X4	T45.2X5	T45.2X6
Pyrilamine	T45.ØX1	T45.ØX2	T45.ØX3	T45.ØX4	T45.ØX5	T45.ØX6
Pyrimethamine	T37.2X1	T37.2X2	T37.2X3	T37.2X4	T37.2X5	T37.2X6
with sulfadoxine	T37.2X1	T37.2X2	T37.2X3	T37.2X4	T37.2X5	T37.2X6
Pyrimidine antagonist	T45.1X1	T45.1X2	T45.1X3	T45.1X4	T45.1X5	T45.1X6
Pyriminil	T6Ø.4X1	T6Ø.4X2	T6Ø.4X3	T6Ø.4X4	—	—
Pyrithione zinc	T49.4X1	T49.4X2	T49.4X3	T49.4X4	T49.4X5	T49.4X6
Pyrithyldione	T42.6X1	T42.6X2	T42.6X3	T42.6X4	T42.6X5	T42.6X6
Pyrogallic acid	T49.ØX1	T49.ØX2	T49.ØX3	T49.ØX4	T49.ØX5	T49.ØX6
Pyrogallol	T49.ØX1	T49.ØX2	T49.ØX3	T49.ØX4	T49.ØX5	T49.ØX6
Pyroxylin	T49.3X1	T49.3X2	T49.3X3	T49.3X4	T49.3X5	T49.3X6
Pyrrobutamine	T45.ØX1	T45.ØX2	T45.ØX3	T45.ØX4	T45.ØX5	T45.ØX6
Pyrrolizidine alkaloids	T62.8X1	T62.8X2	T62.8X3	T62.8X4	—	—
Pyrvinium chloride	T37.4X1	T37.4X2	T37.4X3	T37.4X4	T37.4X5	T37.4X6
PZI	T38.3X1	T38.3X2	T38.3X3	T38.3X4	T38.3X5	T38.3X6
Qbrelis*	T46.4X1	T46.4X2	T46.4X3	T46.4X4	T46.4X5	T46.4X6
Quaalude	T42.6X1	T42.6X2	T42.6X3	T42.6X4	T42.6X5	T42.6X6
Quarternary ammonium						
anti-infective	T49.ØX1	T49.ØX2	T49.ØX3	T49.ØX4	T49.ØX5	T49.ØX6
ganglion blocking	T44.2X1	T44.2X2	T44.2X3	T44.2X4	T44.2X5	T44.2X6
parasympatholytic	T44.3X1	T44.3X2	T44.3X3	T44.3X4	T44.3X5	T44.3X6
Quazepam	T42.4X1	T42.4X2	T42.4X3	T42.4X4	T42.4X5	T42.4X6
Quicklime	T54.3X1	T54.3X2	T54.3X3	T54.3X4	—	—
Quilbron-T*	T48.6X1	T48.6X2	T48.6X3	T48.6X4	T48.6X5	T48.6X6
Quillaja extract	T48.4X1	T48.4X2	T48.4X3	T48.4X4	T48.4X5	T48.4X6
Quinacrine	T37.2X1	T37.2X2	T37.2X3	T37.2X4	T37.2X5	T37.2X6
Quinaglute	T46.2X1	T46.2X2	T46.2X3	T46.2X4	T46.2X5	T46.2X6
Quinalbarbital	T42.3X1	T42.3X2	T42.3X3	T42.3X4	T42.3X5	T42.3X6
Quinalbarbitone sodium	T42.3X1	T42.3X2	T42.3X3	T42.3X4	T42.3X5	T42.3X6
Quinalphos	T6Ø.ØX1	T6Ø.ØX2	T6Ø.ØX3	T6Ø.ØX4	—	—
Quinapril	T46.4X1	T46.4X2	T46.4X3	T46.4X4	T46.4X5	T46.4X6
Quinestradiol	T38.5X1	T38.5X2	T38.5X3	T38.5X4	T38.5X5	T38.5X6
Quinestradol	T38.5X1	T38.5X2	T38.5X3	T38.5X4	T38.5X5	T38.5X6
Quinestrol	T38.5X1	T38.5X2	T38.5X3	T38.5X4	T38.5X5	T38.5X6
Quinethazone	T5Ø.2X1	T5Ø.2X2	T5Ø.2X3	T5Ø.2X4	T5Ø.2X5	T5Ø.2X6
Quingestanol	T38.4X1	T38.4X2	T38.4X3	T38.4X4	T38.4X5	T38.4X6
Quinidine	T46.2X1	T46.2X2	T46.2X3	T46.2X4	T46.2X5	T46.2X6
Quinine	T37.2X1	T37.2X2	T37.2X3	T37.2X4	T37.2X5	T37.2X6
Quiniobine	T37.8X1	T37.8X2	T37.8X3	T37.8X4	T37.8X5	T37.8X6
Quinisocaine	T49.1X1	T49.1X2	T49.1X3	T49.1X4	T49.1X5	T49.1X6
Quinocide	T37.2X1	T37.2X2	T37.2X3	T37.2X4	T37.2X5	T37.2X6
Quinoline (derivatives) **NEC**	T37.8X1	T37.8X2	T37.8X3	T37.8X4	T37.8X5	T37.8X6
Quinupramine	T43.Ø11	T43.Ø12	T43.Ø13	T43.Ø14	T43.Ø15	T43.Ø16
Quixin*	T49.5X1	T49.5X2	T49.5X3	T49.5X4	T49.5X5	T49.5X6
Quotane	T41.3X1	T41.3X2	T41.3X3	T41.3X4	T41.3X5	T41.3X6
Rabies						
immune globulin (human)	T5Ø.Z11	T5Ø.Z12	T5Ø.Z13	T5Ø.Z14	T5Ø.Z15	T5Ø.Z16
vaccine	T5Ø.B91	T5Ø.B92	T5Ø.B93	T5Ø.B94	T5Ø.B95	T5Ø.B96
Racemoramide	T4Ø.2X1	T4Ø.2X2	T4Ø.2X3	T4Ø.2X4	—	—
Racemorphan	T4Ø.2X1	T4Ø.2X2	T4Ø.2X3	T4Ø.2X4	T4Ø.2X5	T4Ø.2X6
Racepinefrin	T44.5X1	T44.5X2	T44.5X3	T44.5X4	T44.5X5	T44.5X6
Raclopride	T43.591	T43.592	T43.593	T43.594	T43.595	T43.596
Radiator alcohol	T51.1X1	T51.1X2	T51.1X3	T51.1X4	—	—
Radio-opaque (drugs) (materials)	T5Ø.8X1	T5Ø.8X2	T5Ø.8X3	T5Ø.8X4	T5Ø.8X5	T5Ø.8X6
Radioactive drug NEC	T5Ø.8X1	T5Ø.8X2	T5Ø.8X3	T5Ø.8X4	T5Ø.8X5	T5Ø.8X6
Ramifenazone	T39.2X1	T39.2X2	T39.2X3	T39.2X4	T39.2X5	T39.2X6
Ramipril	T46.4X1	T46.4X2	T46.4X3	T46.4X4	T46.4X5	T46.4X6
Ranitidine	T47.ØX1	T47.ØX2	T47.ØX3	T47.ØX4	T47.ØX5	T47.ØX6
Ranunculus	T62.2X1	T62.2X2	T62.2X3	T62.2X4	—	—
Rat poison NEC	T6Ø.4X1	T6Ø.4X2	T6Ø.4X3	T6Ø.4X4	—	—
Rattlesnake (venom)	T63.Ø11	T63.Ø12	T63.Ø13	T63.Ø14	—	—
Raubasine	T46.7X1	T46.7X2	T46.7X3	T46.7X4	T46.7X5	T46.7X6
Raudixin	T46.5X1	T46.5X2	T46.5X3	T46.5X4	T46.5X5	T46.5X6
Rautensin	T46.5X1	T46.5X2	T46.5X3	T46.5X4	T46.5X5	T46.5X6
Rautina	T46.5X1	T46.5X2	T46.5X3	T46.5X4	T46.5X5	T46.5X6
Rautotal	T46.5X1	T46.5X2	T46.5X3	T46.5X4	T46.5X5	T46.5X6
Rauwiloid	T46.5X1	T46.5X2	T46.5X3	T46.5X4	T46.5X5	T46.5X6
Rauwoldin	T46.5X1	T46.5X2	T46.5X3	T46.5X4	T46.5X5	T46.5X6

Substance	Poisoning, Accidental (unintentional)	Poisoning, Intentional Self-harm	Poisoning, Assault	Poisoning, Undetermined	Adverse Effect	Under-dosing
Rauwolfia (alkaloids)	T46.5X1	T46.5X2	T46.5X3	T46.5X4	T46.5X5	T46.5X6
Razadyne*	T44.ØX1	T44.ØX2	T44.ØX3	T44.ØX4	T44.ØX5	T44.ØX6
Razoxane	T45.1X1	T45.1X2	T45.1X3	T45.1X4	T45.1X5	T45.1X6
Realgar	T57.ØX1	T57.ØX2	T57.ØX3	T57.ØX4	—	—
Recombinant (R) — *see* specific protein						
Red blood cells, packed	T45.8X1	T45.8X2	T45.8X3	T45.8X4	T45.8X5	T45.8X6
Red squill (scilliroside)	T6Ø.4X1	T6Ø.4X2	T6Ø.4X3	T6Ø.4X4	—	—
Reducing agent, industrial NEC	T65.891	T65.892	T65.893	T65.894	—	—
Refrigerant gas (chlorofluorocarbon)	T53.5X1	T53.5X2	T53.5X3	T53.5X4	—	—
not chlorofluorocarbon	T59.891	T59.892	T59.893	T59.894	—	—
Regroton	T5Ø.2X1	T5Ø.2X2	T5Ø.2X3	T5Ø.2X4	T5Ø.2X5	T5Ø.2X6
Rehydration salts (oral)	T5Ø.3X1	T5Ø.3X2	T5Ø.3X3	T5Ø.3X4	T5Ø.3X5	T5Ø.3X6
Rela	T42.8X1	T42.8X2	T42.8X3	T42.8X4	T42.8X5	T42.8X6
Relaxant, muscle						
anesthetic	T48.1X1	T48.1X2	T48.1X3	T48.1X4	T48.1X5	T48.1X6
central nervous system	T42.8X1	T42.8X2	T42.8X3	T42.8X4	T42.8X5	T42.8X6
skeletal NEC	T48.1X1	T48.1X2	T48.1X3	T48.1X4	T48.1X5	T48.1X6
smooth NEC	T44.3X1	T44.3X2	T44.3X3	T44.3X4	T44.3X5	T44.3X6
Remoxipride	T43.591	T43.592	T43.593	T43.594	T43.595	T43.596
Renese	T5Ø.2X1	T5Ø.2X2	T5Ø.2X3	T5Ø.2X4	T5Ø.2X5	T5Ø.2X6
Renografin	T5Ø.8X1	T5Ø.8X2	T5Ø.8X3	T5Ø.8X4	T5Ø.8X5	T5Ø.8X6
Replacement solution	T5Ø.3X1	T5Ø.3X2	T5Ø.3X3	T5Ø.3X4	T5Ø.3X5	T5Ø.3X6
Reproterol	T48.6X1	T48.6X2	T48.6X3	T48.6X4	T48.6X5	T48.6X6
Rescinnamine	T46.5X1	T46.5X2	T46.5X3	T46.5X4	T46.5X5	T46.5X6
Reserpin (e)	T46.5X1	T46.5X2	T46.5X3	T46.5X4	T46.5X5	T46.5X6
Resorcin, resorcinol (nonmedicinal)	T65.891	T65.892	T65.893	T65.894	—	—
medicinal	T49.4X1	T49.4X2	T49.4X3	T49.4X4	T49.4X5	T49.4X6
Respaire	T48.4X1	T48.4X2	T48.4X3	T48.4X4	T48.4X5	T48.4X6
Respiratory drug NEC	T48.9Ø1	T48.9Ø2	T48.9Ø3	T48.9Ø4	T48.9Ø5	T48.9Ø6
anti-common-cold NEC	T48.5X1	T48.5X2	T48.5X3	T48.5X4	T48.5X5	T48.5X6
antiasthmatic NEC	T48.6X1	T48.6X2	T48.6X3	T48.6X4	T48.6X5	T48.6X6
expectorant NEC	T48.4X1	T48.4X2	T48.4X3	T48.4X4	T48.4X5	T48.4X6
stimulant	T48.9Ø1	T48.9Ø2	T48.9Ø3	T48.9Ø4	T48.9Ø5	T48.9Ø6
Restoril*	T42.4X1	T42.4X2	T42.4X3	T42.4X4	T42.4X5	T42.4X6
Retinoic acid	T49.ØX1	T49.ØX2	T49.ØX3	T49.ØX4	T49.ØX5	T49.ØX6
Retinol	T45.2X1	T45.2X2	T45.2X3	T45.2X4	T45.2X5	T45.2X6
Revatio*	T46.7X1	T46.7X2	T46.7X3	T46.7X4	T46.7X5	T46.7X6
Rh (D) **immune globulin** (human)	T5Ø.Z11	T5Ø.Z12	T5Ø.Z13	T5Ø.Z14	T5Ø.Z15	T5Ø.Z16
Rhodine	T39.Ø11	T39.Ø12	T39.Ø13	T39.Ø14	T39.Ø15	T39.Ø16
RhoGAM	T5Ø.Z11	T5Ø.Z12	T5Ø.Z13	T5Ø.Z14	T5Ø.Z15	T5Ø.Z16
Rhubarb						
dry extract	T47.2X1	T47.2X2	T47.2X3	T47.2X4	T47.2X5	T47.2X6
tincture, compound	T47.2X1	T47.2X2	T47.2X3	T47.2X4	T47.2X5	T47.2X6
Ribavirin	T37.5X1	T37.5X2	T37.5X3	T37.5X4	T37.5X5	T37.5X6
Riboflavin	T45.2X1	T45.2X2	T45.2X3	T45.2X4	T45.2X5	T45.2X6
Ribostamycin	T36.5X1	T36.5X2	T36.5X3	T36.5X4	T36.5X5	T36.5X6
Ricin	T62.2X1	T62.2X2	T62.2X3	T62.2X4	—	—
Ricinus communis	T62.2X1	T62.2X2	T62.2X3	T62.2X4	—	—
Rickettsial vaccine NEC	T5Ø.A91	T5Ø.A92	T5Ø.A93	T5Ø.A94	T5Ø.A95	T5Ø.A96
Rifabutin	T36.6X1	T36.6X2	T36.6X3	T36.6X4	T36.6X5	T36.6X6
Rifamide	T36.6X1	T36.6X2	T36.6X3	T36.6X4	T36.6X5	T36.6X6
Rifampicin	T36.6X1	T36.6X2	T36.6X3	T36.6X4	T36.6X5	T36.6X6
with isoniazid	T37.1X1	T37.1X2	T37.1X3	T37.1X4	T37.1X5	T37.1X6
Rifampin	T36.6X1	T36.6X2	T36.6X3	T36.6X4	T36.6X5	T36.6X6
Rifamycin	T36.6X1	T36.6X2	T36.6X3	T36.6X4	T36.6X5	T36.6X6
Rifaximin	T36.6X1	T36.6X2	T36.6X3	T36.6X4	T36.6X5	T36.6X6
Rimantadine	T37.5X1	T37.5X2	T37.5X3	T37.5X4	T37.5X5	T37.5X6
Rimazolium metilsulfate	T39.8X1	T39.8X2	T39.8X3	T39.8X4	T39.8X5	T39.8X6
Rimifon	T37.1X1	T37.1X2	T37.1X3	T37.1X4	T37.1X5	T37.1X6
Rimiterol	T48.6X1	T48.6X2	T48.6X3	T48.6X4	T48.6X5	T48.6X6
Ringer (lactate) **solution**	T5Ø.3X1	T5Ø.3X2	T5Ø.3X3	T5Ø.3X4	T5Ø.3X5	T5Ø.3X6
Riomet*	T38.3X1	T38.3X2	T38.3X3	T38.3X4	T38.3X5	T38.3X6
Risperdal*	T43.591	T43.592	T43.593	T43.594	T43.595	T43.596
Ristocetin	T36.8X1	T36.8X2	T36.8X3	T36.8X4	T36.8X5	T36.8X6
Ritalin	T43.631	T43.632	T43.633	T43.634	T43.635	T43.636
Ritodrine	T44.5X1	T44.5X2	T44.5X3	T44.5X4	T44.5X5	T44.5X6
Roach killer — *see* Insecticide						
Robaxin*	T48.1X1	T48.1X2	T48.1X3	T48.1X4	T48.1X5	T48.1X6
Robitussin*	T48.3X1	T48.3X2	T48.3X3	T48.3X4	T48.3X5	T48.3X6
Rociverine	T44.3X1	T44.3X2	T44.3X3	T44.3X4	T44.3X5	T44.3X6
Rocky Mountain spotted fever vaccine	T5Ø.A91	T5Ø.A92	T5Ø.A93	T5Ø.A94	T5Ø.A95	T5Ø.A96
Rodenticide NEC	T6Ø.4X1	T6Ø.4X2	T6Ø.4X3	T6Ø.4X4	—	—
Rohypnol	T42.4X1	T42.4X2	T42.4X3	T42.4X4	T42.4X5	T42.4X6
Rokitamycin	T36.3X1	T36.3X2	T36.3X3	T36.3X4	T36.3X5	T36.3X6
Rolaids	T47.1X1	T47.1X2	T47.1X3	T47.1X4	T47.1X5	T47.1X6
Rolitetracycline	T36.4X1	T36.4X2	T36.4X3	T36.4X4	T36.4X5	T36.4X6
Romilar	T48.3X1	T48.3X2	T48.3X3	T48.3X4	T48.3X5	T48.3X6

Substance	Poisoning, Accidental (unintentional)	Poisoning, Intentional Self-harm	Poisoning, Assault	Poisoning, Undetermined	Adverse Effect	Under-dosing
Ronifibrate	T46.6X1	T46.6X2	T46.6X3	T46.6X4	T46.6X5	T46.6X6
Rosaprostol	T47.1X1	T47.1X2	T47.1X3	T47.1X4	T47.1X5	T47.1X6
Rose bengal sodium (131I)	T5Ø.8X1	T5Ø.8X2	T5Ø.8X3	T5Ø.8X4	T5Ø.8X5	T5Ø.8X6
Rose water ointment	T49.3X1	T49.3X2	T49.3X3	T49.3X4	T49.3X5	T49.3X6
Rosoxacin	T37.8X1	T37.8X2	T37.8X3	T37.8X4	T37.8X5	T37.8X6
Rotenone	T6Ø.2X1	T6Ø.2X2	T6Ø.2X3	T6Ø.2X4	—	—
Rotoxamine	T45.ØX1	T45.ØX2	T45.ØX3	T45.ØX4	T45.ØX5	T45.ØX6
Rough-on-rats	T6Ø.4X1	T6Ø.4X2	T6Ø.4X3	T6Ø.4X4	—	—
Roxatidine	T47.ØX1	T47.ØX2	T47.ØX3	T47.ØX4	T47.ØX5	T47.ØX6
Roxithromycin	T36.3X1	T36.3X2	T36.3X3	T36.3X4	T36.3X5	T36.3X6
Rt-PA	T45.611	T45.612	T45.613	T45.614	T45.615	T45.616
Rubbing alcohol	T51.2X1	T51.2X2	T51.2X3	T51.2X4	—	—
Rubefacient	T49.4X1	T49.4X2	T49.4X3	T49.4X4	T49.4X5	T49.4X6
Rubella vaccine	T5Ø.B91	T5Ø.B92	T5Ø.B93	T5Ø.B94	T5Ø.B95	T5Ø.B96
Rubeola vaccine	T5Ø.B91	T5Ø.B92	T5Ø.B93	T5Ø.B94	T5Ø.B95	T5Ø.B96
Rubidium chloride Rb82	T5Ø.8X1	T5Ø.8X2	T5Ø.8X3	T5Ø.8X4	T5Ø.8X5	T5Ø.8X6
Rubidomycin	T45.1X1	T45.1X2	T45.1X3	T45.1X4	T45.1X5	T45.1X6
Rue	T62.2X1	T62.2X2	T62.2X3	T62.2X4	—	—
Rufocromomycin	T45.1X1	T45.1X2	T45.1X3	T45.1X4	T45.1X5	T45.1X6
Russel's viper venin	T45.7X1	T45.7X2	T45.7X3	T45.7X4	T45.7X5	T45.7X6
Ruta (graveolens)	T62.2X1	T62.2X2	T62.2X3	T62.2X4	—	—
Rutinum	T46.991	T46.992	T46.993	T46.994	T46.995	T46.996
Rutoside	T46.991	T46.992	T46.993	T46.994	T46.995	T46.996
S-Carboxymethylcysteine	T48.4X1	T48.4X2	T48.4X3	T48.4X4	T48.4X5	T48.4X6
Sabadilla (plant)	T62.2X1	T62.2X2	T62.2X3	T62.2X4	—	—
pesticide	T6Ø.2X1	T6Ø.2X2	T6Ø.2X3	T6Ø.2X4	—	—
Sabril*	T42.6X1	T42.6X2	T42.6X3	T42.6X4	T42.6X5	T42.6X6
Saccharated iron oxide	T45.8X1	T45.8X2	T45.8X3	T45.8X4	T45.8X5	T45.8X6
Saccharin	T5Ø.9Ø1	T5Ø.9Ø2	T5Ø.9Ø3	T5Ø.9Ø4	T5Ø.9Ø5	T5Ø.9Ø6
Saccharomyces boulardii	T47.6X1	T47.6X2	T47.6X3	T47.6X4	T47.6X5	T47.6X6
Safflower oil	T46.6X1	T46.6X2	T46.6X3	T46.6X4	T46.6X5	T46.6X6
Safrazine	T43.1X1	T43.1X2	T43.1X3	T43.1X4	T43.1X5	T43.1X6
Salazosulfapyridine	T37.ØX1	T37.ØX2	T37.ØX3	T37.ØX4	T37.ØX5	T37.ØX6
Salbutamol	T48.6X1	T48.6X2	T48.6X3	T48.6X4	T48.6X5	T48.6X6
Salicylamide	T39.Ø91	T39.Ø92	T39.Ø93	T39.Ø94	T39.Ø95	T39.Ø96
Salicylate NEC	T39.Ø91	T39.Ø92	T39.Ø93	T39.Ø94	T39.Ø95	T39.Ø96
methyl	T49.3X1	T49.3X2	T49.3X3	T49.3X4	T49.3X5	T49.3X6
theobromine calcium	T5Ø.2X1	T5Ø.2X2	T5Ø.2X3	T5Ø.2X4	T5Ø.2X5	T5Ø.2X6
Salicylazosulfapyridine	T37.ØX1	T37.ØX2	T37.ØX3	T37.ØX4	T37.ØX5	T37.ØX6
Salicylhydroxamic acid	T49.ØX1	T49.ØX2	T49.ØX3	T49.ØX4	T49.ØX5	T49.ØX6
Salicylic acid	T49.4X1	T49.4X2	T49.4X3	T49.4X4	T49.4X5	T49.4X6
congeners	T39.Ø91	T39.Ø92	T39.Ø93	T39.Ø94	T39.Ø95	T39.Ø96
derivative	T39.Ø91	T39.Ø92	T39.Ø93	T39.Ø94	T39.Ø95	T39.Ø96
salts	T39.Ø91	T39.Ø92	T39.Ø93	T39.Ø94	T39.Ø95	T39.Ø96
with benzoic acid	T49.4X1	T49.4X2	T49.4X3	T49.4X4	T49.4X5	T49.4X6
Salinazid	T37.1X1	T37.1X2	T37.1X3	T37.1X4	T37.1X5	T37.1X6
Salmeterol	T48.6X1	T48.6X2	T48.6X3	T48.6X4	T48.6X5	T48.6X6
Salol	T49.3X1	T49.3X2	T49.3X3	T49.3X4	T49.3X5	T49.3X6
Salsalate	T39.Ø91	T39.Ø92	T39.Ø93	T39.Ø94	T39.Ø95	T39.Ø96
Salt-replacing drug	T5Ø.9Ø1	T5Ø.9Ø2	T5Ø.9Ø3	T5Ø.9Ø4	T5Ø.9Ø5	T5Ø.9Ø6
Salt-retaining mineralocorticoid	T5Ø.ØX1	T5Ø.ØX2	T5Ø.ØX3	T5Ø.ØX4	T5Ø.ØX5	T5Ø.ØX6
Salt substitute	T5Ø.9Ø1	T5Ø.9Ø2	T5Ø.9Ø3	T5Ø.9Ø4	T5Ø.9Ø5	T5Ø.9Ø6
Saluretic NEC	T5Ø.2X1	T5Ø.2X2	T5Ø.2X3	T5Ø.2X4	T5Ø.2X5	T5Ø.2X6
Saluron	T5Ø.2X1	T5Ø.2X2	T5Ø.2X3	T5Ø.2X4	T5Ø.2X5	T5Ø.2X6
Salvarsan 606 (neosilver) (silver)	T37.8X1	T37.8X2	T37.8X3	T37.8X4	T37.8X5	T37.8X6
Sambucus canadensis	T62.2X1	T62.2X2	T62.2X3	T62.2X4	—	—
berry	T62.1X1	T62.1X2	T62.1X3	T62.1X4	—	—
Sandril	T46.5X1	T46.5X2	T46.5X3	T46.5X4	T46.5X5	T46.5X6
Sanguinaria canadensis	T62.2X1	T62.2X2	T62.2X3	T62.2X4	—	—
Saniflush (cleaner)	T54.2X1	T54.2X2	T54.2X3	T54.2X4	—	—
Santonin	T37.4X1	T37.4X2	T37.4X3	T37.4X4	T37.4X5	T37.4X6
Santyl	T49.8X1	T49.8X2	T49.8X3	T49.8X4	T49.8X5	T49.8X6
Saralasin	T46.5X1	T46.5X2	T46.5X3	T46.5X4	T46.5X5	T46.5X6
Sarcolysin	T45.1X1	T45.1X2	T45.1X3	T45.1X4	T45.1X5	T45.1X6
Sarilumab*	T39.4X1	T39.4X2	T39.4X3	T39.4X4	T39.4X5	T39.4X6
Sarkomycin	T45.1X1	T45.1X2	T45.1X3	T45.1X4	T45.1X5	T45.1X6
Saroten	T43.Ø11	T43.Ø12	T43.Ø13	T43.Ø14	T43.Ø15	T43.Ø16
Saturnine — *see* Lead						
Savin (oil)	T49.4X1	T49.4X2	T49.4X3	T49.4X4	T49.4X5	T49.4X6
Scammony	T47.2X1	T47.2X2	T47.2X3	T47.2X4	T47.2X5	T47.2X6
Scarlet red	T49.8X1	T49.8X2	T49.8X3	T49.8X4	T49.8X5	T49.8X6
Scheele's green	T57.ØX1	T57.ØX2	T57.ØX3	T57.ØX4	—	—
insecticide	T57.ØX1	T57.ØX2	T57.ØX3	T57.ØX4	—	—
Schizontozide (blood) (tissue)	T37.2X1	T37.2X2	T37.2X3	T37.2X4	T37.2X5	T37.2X6
Schradan	T6Ø.ØX1	T6Ø.ØX2	T6Ø.ØX3	T6Ø.ØX4	—	—
Schweinfurth green	T57.ØX1	T57.ØX2	T57.ØX3	T57.ØX4	—	—
insecticide	T57.ØX1	T57.ØX2	T57.ØX3	T57.ØX4	—	—
Scilla, rat poison	T6Ø.4X1	T6Ø.4X2	T6Ø.4X3	T6Ø.4X4	—	—
Scillaren	T6Ø.4X1	T6Ø.4X2	T6Ø.4X3	T6Ø.4X4	—	—
Sclerosing agent	T46.8X1	T46.8X2	T46.8X3	T46.8X4	T46.8X5	T46.8X6

*Optum Value-Add ☑ Additional Character May Be Required — Refer to the Tabular List for Character Selection 401

Substance	Poisoning, Accidental (unintentional)	Poisoning, Intentional Self-harm	Poisoning, Assault	Poisoning, Undetermined	Adverse Effect	Under-dosing
Scombrotoxin	T61.11	T61.12	T61.13	T61.14	—	—
Scopolamine	T44.3X1	T44.3X2	T44.3X3	T44.3X4	T44.3X5	T44.3X6
Scopolia extract	T44.3X1	T44.3X2	T44.3X3	T44.3X4	T44.3X5	T44.3X6
Scouring powder	T65.891	T65.892	T65.893	T65.894	—	—
Sea						
anemone (sting)	T63.631	T63.632	T63.633	T63.634	—	—
cucumber (sting)	T63.691	T63.692	T63.693	T63.694	—	—
snake (bite) (venom)	T63.Ø91	T63.Ø92	T63.Ø93	T63.Ø94	—	—
urchin spine (puncture)	T63.691	T63.692	T63.693	T63.694	—	—
Seafood	T61.91	T61.92	T61.93	T61.94	—	—
specified NEC	T61.8X1	T61.8X2	T61.8X3	T61.8X4	—	—
Secbutabarbital	T42.3X1	T42.3X2	T42.3X3	T42.3X4	T42.3X5	T42.3X6
Secbutabarbitone	T42.3X1	T42.3X2	T42.3X3	T42.3X4	T42.3X5	T42.3X6
Secnidazole	T37.3X1	T37.3X2	T37.3X3	T37.3X4	T37.3X5	T37.3X6
Secobarbital	T42.3X1	T42.3X2	T42.3X3	T42.3X4	T42.3X5	T42.3X6
Seconal	T42.3X1	T42.3X2	T42.3X3	T42.3X4	T42.3X5	T42.3X6
Secretin	T5Ø.8X1	T5Ø.8X2	T5Ø.8X3	T5Ø.8X4	T5Ø.8X5	T5Ø.8X6
Sectral*	T44.7X1	T44.7X2	T44.7X3	T44.7X4	T44.7X5	T44.7X6
Sedative NEC	T42.71	T42.72	T42.73	T42.74	T42.75	T42.76
mixed NEC	T42.6X1	T42.6X2	T42.6X3	T42.6X4	T42.6X5	T42.6X6
Sedormid	T42.6X1	T42.6X2	T42.6X3	T42.6X4	T42.6X5	T42.6X6
Seed disinfectant or dressing	T6Ø.8X1	T6Ø.8X2	T6Ø.8X3	T6Ø.8X4	—	—
Seeds (poisonous)	T62.2X1	T62.2X2	T62.2X3	T62.2X4	—	—
Selegiline	T42.8X1	T42.8X2	T42.8X3	T42.8X4	T42.8X5	T42.8X6
Selenium NEC	T56.891	T56.892	T56.893	T56.894	—	—
disulfide or sulfide	T49.4X1	T49.4X2	T49.4X3	T49.4X4	T49.4X5	T49.4X6
fumes	T59.891	T59.892	T59.893	T59.894	—	—
sulfide	T49.4X1	T49.4X2	T49.4X3	T49.4X4	T49.4X5	T49.4X6
Selenomethionine (75Se)	T5Ø.8X1	T5Ø.8X2	T5Ø.8X3	T5Ø.8X4	T5Ø.8X5	T5Ø.8X6
Selsun	T49.4X1	T49.4X2	T49.4X3	T49.4X4	T49.4X5	T49.4X6
Semustine	T45.1X1	T45.1X2	T45.1X3	T45.1X4	T45.1X5	T45.1X6
Senega syrup	T48.4X1	T48.4X2	T48.4X3	T48.4X4	T48.4X5	T48.4X6
Senna	T47.2X1	T47.2X2	T47.2X3	T47.2X4	T47.2X5	T47.2X6
Sennoside A+B	T47.2X1	T47.2X2	T47.2X3	T47.2X4	T47.2X5	T47.2X6
Septisol	T49.2X1	T49.2X2	T49.2X3	T49.2X4	T49.2X5	T49.2X6
Seractide	T38.811	T38.812	T38.813	T38.814	T38.815	T38.816
Serax	T42.4X1	T42.4X2	T42.4X3	T42.4X4	T42.4X5	T42.4X6
Serenesil	T42.6X1	T42.6X2	T42.6X3	T42.6X4	T42.6X5	T42.6X6
Serenium (hydrochloride)	T37.91	T37.92	T37.93	T37.94	T37.95	T37.96
Serepax — *see* Oxazepam						
Serevent*	T48.6X1	T48.6X2	T48.6X3	T48.6X4	T48.6X5	T48.6X6
Sermorelin	T38.891	T38.892	T38.893	T38.894	T38.895	T38.896
Sernyl	T41.1X1	T41.1X2	T41.1X3	T41.1X4	T41.1X5	T41.1X6
Serotonin	T5Ø.991	T5Ø.992	T5Ø.993	T5Ø.994	T5Ø.995	T5Ø.996
Serpasil	T46.5X1	T46.5X2	T46.5X3	T46.5X4	T46.5X5	T46.5X6
Serrapeptase	T45.3X1	T45.3X2	T45.3X3	T45.3X4	T45.3X5	T45.3X6
Sertraline*	T43.221	T43.222	T43.223	T43.224	T43.225	T43.226
Serum						
anti-Rh	T5Ø.Z11	T5Ø.Z12	T5Ø.Z13	T5Ø.Z14	T5Ø.Z15	T5Ø.Z16
anti-snake-bite	T5Ø.Z11	T5Ø.Z12	T5Ø.Z13	T5Ø.Z14	T5Ø.Z15	T5Ø.Z16
antibotulinus	T5Ø.Z11	T5Ø.Z12	T5Ø.Z13	T5Ø.Z14	T5Ø.Z15	T5Ø.Z16
anticytotoxic	T5Ø.Z11	T5Ø.Z12	T5Ø.Z13	T5Ø.Z14	T5Ø.Z15	T5Ø.Z16
antidiphtheria	T5Ø.Z11	T5Ø.Z12	T5Ø.Z13	T5Ø.Z14	T5Ø.Z15	T5Ø.Z16
antimeningococcus	T5Ø.Z11	T5Ø.Z12	T5Ø.Z13	T5Ø.Z14	T5Ø.Z15	T5Ø.Z16
antitetanic	T5Ø.Z11	T5Ø.Z12	T5Ø.Z13	T5Ø.Z14	T5Ø.Z15	T5Ø.Z16
antitoxic	T5Ø.Z11	T5Ø.Z12	T5Ø.Z13	T5Ø.Z14	T5Ø.Z15	T5Ø.Z16
complement (inhibitor)	T45.8X1	T45.8X2	T45.8X3	T45.8X4	T45.8X5	T45.8X6
convalescent	T5Ø.Z11	T5Ø.Z12	T5Ø.Z13	T5Ø.Z14	T5Ø.Z15	T5Ø.Z16
hemolytic complement	T45.8X1	T45.8X2	T45.8X3	T45.8X4	T45.8X5	T45.8X6
immune (human)	T5Ø.Z11	T5Ø.Z12	T5Ø.Z13	T5Ø.Z14	T5Ø.Z15	T5Ø.Z16
protective NEC	T5Ø.Z11	T5Ø.Z12	T5Ø.Z13	T5Ø.Z14	T5Ø.Z15	T5Ø.Z16
Setastine	T45.ØX1	T45.ØX2	T45.ØX3	T45.ØX4	T45.ØX5	T45.ØX6
Setoperone	T43.591	T43.592	T43.593	T43.594	T43.595	T43.596
Sewer gas	T59.91	T59.92	T59.93	T59.94	—	—
Shampoo	T55.ØX1	T55.ØX2	T55.ØX3	T55.ØX4	—	—
Shellfish, noxious, nonbacterial	T61.781	T61.782	T61.783	T61.784	—	—
Sildenafil	T46.7X1	T46.7X2	T46.7X3	T46.7X4	T46.7X5	T46.7X6
Silibinin	T5Ø.991	T5Ø.992	T5Ø.993	T5Ø.994	T5Ø.995	T5Ø.996
Silicone NEC	T65.891	T65.892	T65.893	T65.894	—	—
medicinal	T49.3X1	T49.3X2	T49.3X3	T49.3X4	T49.3X5	T49.3X6
Silvadene	T49.ØX1	T49.ØX2	T49.ØX3	T49.ØX4	T49.ØX5	T49.ØX6
Silver	T49.ØX1	T49.ØX2	T49.ØX3	T49.ØX4	T49.ØX5	T49.ØX6
anti-infectives	T49.ØX1	T49.ØX2	T49.ØX3	T49.ØX4	T49.ØX5	T49.ØX6
arsphenamine	T37.8X1	T37.8X2	T37.8X3	T37.8X4	T37.8X5	T37.8X6
colloidal	T49.ØX1	T49.ØX2	T49.ØX3	T49.ØX4	T49.ØX5	T49.ØX6
nitrate	T49.ØX1	T49.ØX2	T49.ØX3	T49.ØX4	T49.ØX5	T49.ØX6
ophthalmic preparation	T49.5X1	T49.5X2	T49.5X3	T49.5X4	T49.5X5	T49.5X6
toughened (keratolytic)	T49.4X1	T49.4X2	T49.4X3	T49.4X4	T49.4X5	T49.4X6
nonmedicinal (dust)	T56.891	T56.892	T56.893	T56.894	—	—
protein	T49.5X1	T49.5X2	T49.5X3	T49.5X4	T49.5X5	T49.5X6
salvarsan	T37.8X1	T37.8X2	T37.8X3	T37.8X4	T37.8X5	T37.8X6
Silver — *continued*						
sulfadiazine	T49.4X1	T49.4X2	T49.4X3	T49.4X4	T49.4X5	T49.4X6
Silymarin	T5Ø.991	T5Ø.992	T5Ø.993	T5Ø.994	T5Ø.995	T5Ø.996
Simaldrate	T47.1X1	T47.1X2	T47.1X3	T47.1X4	T47.1X5	T47.1X6
Simazine	T6Ø.3X1	T6Ø.3X2	T6Ø.3X3	T6Ø.3X4	—	—
Simethicone	T47.1X1	T47.1X2	T47.1X3	T47.1X4	T47.1X5	T47.1X6
Simfibrate	T46.6X1	T46.6X2	T46.6X3	T46.6X4	T46.6X5	T46.6X6
Simvastatin	T46.6X1	T46.6X2	T46.6X3	T46.6X4	T46.6X5	T46.6X6
Sincalide	T5Ø.8X1	T5Ø.8X2	T5Ø.8X3	T5Ø.8X4	T5Ø.8X5	T5Ø.8X6
Sinequan	T43.Ø11	T43.Ø12	T43.Ø13	T43.Ø14	T43.Ø15	T43.Ø16
Singoserp	T46.5X1	T46.5X2	T46.5X3	T46.5X4	T46.5X5	T46.5X6
Singulair*	T48.6X1	T48.6X2	T48.6X3	T48.6X4	T48.6X5	T48.6X6
Sintrom	T45.511	T45.512	T45.513	T45.514	T45.515	T45.516
Sisomicin	T36.5X1	T36.5X2	T36.5X3	T36.5X4	T36.5X5	T36.5X6
Sitosterols	T46.6X1	T46.6X2	T46.6X3	T46.6X4	T46.6X5	T46.6X6
Skeletal muscle relaxants	T48.1X1	T48.1X2	T48.1X3	T48.1X4	T48.1X5	T48.1X6
Skin						
agents (external)	T49.91	T49.92	T49.93	T49.94	T49.95	T49.96
specified NEC	T49.8X1	T49.8X2	T49.8X3	T49.8X4	T49.8X5	T49.8X6
test antigen	T5Ø.8X1	T5Ø.8X2	T5Ø.8X3	T5Ø.8X4	T5Ø.8X5	T5Ø.8X6
Sleep-eze	T45.ØX1	T45.ØX2	T45.ØX3	T45.ØX4	T45.ØX5	T45.ØX6
Sleeping draught, pill	T42.71	T42.72	T42.73	T42.74	T42.75	T42.76
Smallpox vaccine	T5Ø.B11	T5Ø.B12	T5Ø.B13	T5Ø.B14	T5Ø.B15	T5Ø.B16
Smelter fumes NEC	T56.91	T56.92	T56.93	T56.94	—	—
Smog	T59.1X1	T59.1X2	T59.1X3	T59.1X4	—	—
Smoke NEC	T59.811	T59.812	T59.813	T59.814	—	—
Smooth muscle relaxant	T44.3X1	T44.3X2	T44.3X3	T44.3X4	T44.3X5	T44.3X6
Snail killer NEC	T6Ø.8X1	T6Ø.8X2	T6Ø.8X3	T6Ø.8X4	—	—
Snake venom or bite	T63.ØØ1	T63.ØØ2	T63.ØØ3	T63.ØØ4	—	—
hemocoagulase	T45.7X1	T45.7X2	T45.7X3	T45.7X4	T45.7X5	T45.7X6
Snuff	T65.211	T65.212	T65.213	T65.214	—	—
Soap (powder) (product)	T55.ØX1	T55.ØX2	T55.ØX3	T55.ØX4	—	—
enema	T47.4X1	T47.4X2	T47.4X3	T47.4X4	T47.4X5	T47.4X6
medicinal, soft	T49.2X1	T49.2X2	T49.2X3	T49.2X4	T49.2X5	T49.2X6
superfatted	T49.2X1	T49.2X2	T49.2X3	T49.2X4	T49.2X5	T49.2X6
Sobrerol	T48.4X1	T48.4X2	T48.4X3	T48.4X4	T48.4X5	T48.4X6
Soda (caustic)	T54.3X1	T54.3X2	T54.3X3	T54.3X4	—	—
bicarb	T47.1X1	T47.1X2	T47.1X3	T47.1X4	T47.1X5	T47.1X6
chlorinated — *see* Sodium, hypochlorite						
Sodium						
(L)-triiodothyronine	T38.1X1	T38.1X2	T38.1X3	T38.1X4	T38.1X5	T38.1X6
acetosulfone	T37.1X1	T37.1X2	T37.1X3	T37.1X4	T37.1X5	T37.1X6
acetrizoate	T5Ø.8X1	T5Ø.8X2	T5Ø.8X3	T5Ø.8X4	T5Ø.8X5	T5Ø.8X6
acid phosphate	T5Ø.3X1	T5Ø.3X2	T5Ø.3X3	T5Ø.3X4	T5Ø.3X5	T5Ø.3X6
alginate	T47.8X1	T47.8X2	T47.8X3	T47.8X4	T47.8X5	T47.8X6
amidotrizoate	T5Ø.8X1	T5Ø.8X2	T5Ø.8X3	T5Ø.8X4	T5Ø.8X5	T5Ø.8X6
aminohippurate*	T5Ø.8X1	T5Ø.8X2	T5Ø.8X3	T5Ø.8X4	T5Ø.8X5	T5Ø.8X6
aminopterin	T45.1X1	T45.1X2	T45.1X3	T45.1X4	T45.1X5	T45.1X6
amylosulfate	T47.8X1	T47.8X2	T47.8X3	T47.8X4	T47.8X5	T47.8X6
amytal	T42.3X1	T42.3X2	T42.3X3	T42.3X4	T42.3X5	T42.3X6
antimony gluconate	T37.3X1	T37.3X2	T37.3X3	T37.3X4	T37.3X5	T37.3X6
arsenate	T57.ØX1	T57.ØX2	T57.ØX3	T57.ØX4	—	—
aurothiomalate	T39.4X1	T39.4X2	T39.4X3	T39.4X4	T39.4X5	T39.4X6
aurothiosulfate	T39.4X1	T39.4X2	T39.4X3	T39.4X4	T39.4X5	T39.4X6
barbiturate	T42.3X1	T42.3X2	T42.3X3	T42.3X4	T42.3X5	T42.3X6
basic phosphate	T47.4X1	T47.4X2	T47.4X3	T47.4X4	T47.4X5	T47.4X6
bicarbonate	T47.1X1	T47.1X2	T47.1X3	T47.1X4	T47.1X5	T47.1X6
bichromate	T57.8X1	T57.8X2	T57.8X3	T57.8X4	—	—
biphosphate	T5Ø.3X1	T5Ø.3X2	T5Ø.3X3	T5Ø.3X4	T5Ø.3X5	T5Ø.3X6
bisulfate	T65.891	T65.892	T65.893	T65.894	—	—
borate						
cleanser	T57.8X1	T57.8X2	T57.8X3	T57.8X4	—	—
eye	T49.5X1	T49.5X2	T49.5X3	T49.5X4	T49.5X5	T49.5X6
therapeutic	T49.8X1	T49.8X2	T49.8X3	T49.8X4	T49.8X5	T49.8X6
bromide	T42.6X1	T42.6X2	T42.6X3	T42.6X4	T42.6X5	T42.6X6
cacodylate (nonmedicinal) NEC	T5Ø.8X1	T5Ø.8X2	T5Ø.8X3	T5Ø.8X4	T5Ø.8X5	T5Ø.8X6
anti-infective	T37.8X1	T37.8X2	T37.8X3	T37.8X4	T37.8X5	T37.8X6
herbicide	T6Ø.3X1	T6Ø.3X2	T6Ø.3X3	T6Ø.3X4	—	—
calcium edetate	T45.8X1	T45.8X2	T45.8X3	T45.8X4	T45.8X5	T45.8X6
carbonate NEC	T54.3X1	T54.3X2	T54.3X3	T54.3X4	—	—
chlorate NEC	T65.891	T65.892	T65.893	T65.894	—	—
herbicide	T54.91	T54.92	T54.93	T54.94	—	—
chloride	T5Ø.3X1	T5Ø.3X2	T5Ø.3X3	T5Ø.3X4	T5Ø.3X5	T5Ø.3X6
with glucose	T5Ø.3X1	T5Ø.3X2	T5Ø.3X3	T5Ø.3X4	T5Ø.3X5	T5Ø.3X6
chromate	T65.891	T65.892	T65.893	T65.894	—	—
citrate	T5Ø.991	T5Ø.992	T5Ø.993	T5Ø.994	T5Ø.995	T5Ø.996
cromoglicate	T48.6X1	T48.6X2	T48.6X3	T48.6X4	T48.6X5	T48.6X6
cyanide	T65.ØX1	T65.ØX2	T65.ØX3	T65.ØX4	—	—
cyclamate	T5Ø.3X1	T5Ø.3X2	T5Ø.3X3	T5Ø.3X4	T5Ø.3X5	T5Ø.3X6
dehydrocholate	T45.8X1	T45.8X2	T45.8X3	T45.8X4	T45.8X5	T45.8X6
diatrizoate	T5Ø.8X1	T5Ø.8X2	T5Ø.8X3	T5Ø.8X4	T5Ø.8X5	T5Ø.8X6

Substance	Poisoning, Accidental (unintentional)	Poisoning, Intentional Self-harm	Poisoning, Assault	Poisoning, Undetermined	Adverse Effect	Underdosing
Sodium — *continued*						
dibunate	T48.4X1	T48.4X2	T48.4X3	T48.4X4	T48.4X5	T48.4X6
dioctyl sulfosuccinate	T47.4X1	T47.4X2	T47.4X3	T47.4X4	T47.4X5	T47.4X6
dipantoyl ferrate	T45.8X1	T45.8X2	T45.8X3	T45.8X4	T45.8X5	T45.8X6
edetate	T45.8X1	T45.8X2	T45.8X3	T45.8X4	T45.8X5	T45.8X6
ethacrynate	T50.1X1	T50.1X2	T50.1X3	T50.1X4	T50.1X5	T50.1X6
etidronate*	T50.991	T50.992	T50.993	T50.994	T50.995	T50.996
feredetate	T45.8X1	T45.8X2	T45.8X3	T45.8X4	T45.8X5	T45.8X6
Fluoride — *see* Fluoride						
fluoroacetate (dust) (pesticide)	T60.4X1	T60.4X2	T60.4X3	T60.4X4	—	—
free salt	T50.3X1	T50.3X2	T50.3X3	T50.3X4	T50.3X5	T50.3X6
fusidate	T36.8X1	T36.8X2	T36.8X3	T36.8X4	T36.8X5	T36.8X6
glucaldrate	T47.1X1	T47.1X2	T47.1X3	T47.1X4	T47.1X5	T47.1X6
glucosulfone	T37.1X1	T37.1X2	T37.1X3	T37.1X4	T37.1X5	T37.1X6
glutamate	T45.8X1	T45.8X2	T45.8X3	T45.8X4	T45.8X5	T45.8X6
hydrogen carbonate	T50.3X1	T50.3X2	T50.3X3	T50.3X4	T50.3X5	T50.3X6
hydroxide	T54.3X1	T54.3X2	T54.3X3	T54.3X4	—	—
hypochlorite (bleach) NEC	T54.3X1	T54.3X2	T54.3X3	T54.3X4	—	—
disinfectant	T54.3X1	T54.3X2	T54.3X3	T54.3X4	—	—
medicinal (anti-infective) (external)	T49.0X1	T49.0X2	T49.0X3	T49.0X4	T49.0X5	T49.0X6
vapor	T54.3X1	T54.3X2	T54.3X3	T54.3X4	—	—
hyposulfite	T49.0X1	T49.0X2	T49.0X3	T49.0X4	T49.0X5	T49.0X6
indigotin disulfonate	T50.8X1	T50.8X2	T50.8X3	T50.8X4	T50.8X5	T50.8X6
iodide	T50.991	T50.992	T50.993	T50.994	T50.995	T50.996
I-131	T50.8X1	T50.8X2	T50.8X3	T50.8X4	T50.8X5	T50.8X6
therapeutic	T38.2X1	T38.2X2	T38.2X3	T38.2X4	T38.2X5	T38.2X6
iodohippurate (131I)	T50.8X1	T50.8X2	T50.8X3	T50.8X4	T50.8X5	T50.8X6
iopodate	T50.8X1	T50.8X2	T50.8X3	T50.8X4	T50.8X5	T50.8X6
iothalamate	T50.8X1	T50.8X2	T50.8X3	T50.8X4	T50.8X5	T50.8X6
iron edetate	T45.4X1	T45.4X2	T45.4X3	T45.4X4	T45.4X5	T45.4X6
L-triiodothyronine	T38.1X1	T38.1X2	T38.1X3	T38.1X4	T38.1X5	T38.1X6
lactate (compound solution)	T45.8X1	T45.8X2	T45.8X3	T45.8X4	T45.8X5	T45.8X6
lauryl (sulfate)	T49.2X1	T49.2X2	T49.2X3	T49.2X4	T49.2X5	T49.2X6
magnesium citrate	T50.991	T50.992	T50.993	T50.994	T50.995	T50.996
mersalate	T50.2X1	T50.2X2	T50.2X3	T50.2X4	T50.2X5	T50.2X6
metasilicate	T65.891	T65.892	T65.893	T65.894	—	—
metrizoate	T50.8X1	T50.8X2	T50.8X3	T50.8X4	T50.8X5	T50.8X6
monofluoroacetate (pesticide)	T60.1X1	T60.1X2	T60.1X3	T60.1X4	—	—
morrhuate	T46.8X1	T46.8X2	T46.8X3	T46.8X4	T46.8X5	T46.8X6
nafcillin	T36.0X1	T36.0X2	T36.0X3	T36.0X4	T36.0X5	T36.0X6
nitrate (oxidizing agent)	T65.891	T65.892	T65.893	T65.894	—	—
nitrite	T50.6X1	T50.6X2	T50.6X3	T50.6X4	T50.6X5	T50.6X6
nitroferricyanide	T46.5X1	T46.5X2	T46.5X3	T46.5X4	T46.5X5	T46.5X6
nitroprusside	T46.5X1	T46.5X2	T46.5X3	T46.5X4	T46.5X5	T46.5X6
oxalate	T65.891	T65.892	T65.893	T65.894	—	—
oxide/peroxide	T65.891	T65.892	T65.893	T65.894	—	—
oxybate	T41.291	T41.292	T41.293	T41.294	T41.295	T41.296
para-aminohippurate	T50.8X1	T50.8X2	T50.8X3	T50.8X4	T50.8X5	T50.8X6
perborate (nonmedicinal) NEC	T65.891	T65.892	T65.893	T65.894	—	—
medicinal	T49.0X1	T49.0X2	T49.0X3	T49.0X4	T49.0X5	T49.0X6
soap	T55.0X1	T55.0X2	T55.0X3	T55.0X4	—	—
percarbonate — *see* Sodium, perborate						
pertechnetate Tc99m	T50.8X1	T50.8X2	T50.8X3	T50.8X4	T50.8X5	T50.8X6
phosphate						
cellulose	T45.8X1	T45.8X2	T45.8X3	T45.8X4	T45.8X5	T45.8X6
dibasic	T47.2X1	T47.2X2	T47.2X3	T47.2X4	T47.2X5	T47.2X6
monobasic	T47.2X1	T47.2X2	T47.2X3	T47.2X4	T47.2X5	T47.2X6
phytate	T50.6X1	T50.6X2	T50.6X3	T50.6X4	T50.6X5	T50.6X6
picosulfate	T47.2X1	T47.2X2	T47.2X3	T47.2X4	T47.2X5	T47.2X6
polyhydroxyaluminium monocarbonate	T47.1X1	T47.1X2	T47.1X3	T47.1X4	T47.1X5	T47.1X6
polystyrene sulfonate	T50.3X1	T50.3X2	T50.3X3	T50.3X4	T50.3X5	T50.3X6
propionate	T49.0X1	T49.0X2	T49.0X3	T49.0X4	T49.0X5	T49.0X6
propyl hydroxybenzoate	T50.991	T50.992	T50.993	T50.994	T50.995	T50.996
psylliate	T46.8X1	T46.8X2	T46.8X3	T46.8X4	T46.8X5	T46.8X6
removing resins	T50.3X1	T50.3X2	T50.3X3	T50.3X4	T50.3X5	T50.3X6
salicylate	T39.091	T39.092	T39.093	T39.094	T39.095	T39.096
salt NEC	T50.3X1	T50.3X2	T50.3X3	T50.3X4	T50.3X5	T50.3X6
selenate	T60.2X1	T60.2X2	T60.2X3	T60.2X4	—	—
stibogluconate	T37.3X1	T37.3X2	T37.3X3	T37.3X4	T37.3X5	T37.3X6
sulfate	T47.4X1	T47.4X2	T47.4X3	T47.4X4	T47.4X5	T47.4X6
sulfoxone	T37.1X1	T37.1X2	T37.1X3	T37.1X4	T37.1X5	T37.1X6
tetradecyl sulfate	T46.8X1	T46.8X2	T46.8X3	T46.8X4	T46.8X5	T46.8X6
thiopental	T41.1X1	T41.1X2	T41.1X3	T41.1X4	T41.1X5	T41.1X6
thiosalicylate	T39.091	T39.092	T39.093	T39.094	T39.095	T39.096
thiosulfate	T50.6X1	T50.6X2	T50.6X3	T50.6X4	T50.6X5	T50.6X6
tolbutamide	T38.3X1	T38.3X2	T38.3X3	T38.3X4	T38.3X5	T38.3X6
Sodium — *continued*						
tyropanoate	T50.8X1	T50.8X2	T50.8X3	T50.8X4	T50.8X5	T50.8X6
valproate	T42.6X1	T42.6X2	T42.6X3	T42.6X4	T42.6X5	T42.6X6
versenate	T50.6X1	T50.6X2	T50.6X3	T50.6X4	T50.6X5	T50.6X6
Sodium-free salt	T50.901	T50.902	T50.903	T50.904	T50.905	T50.906
Sodium-removing resin	T50.3X1	T50.3X2	T50.3X3	T50.3X4	T50.3X5	T50.3X6
Soft soap	T55.0X1	T55.0X2	T55.0X3	T55.0X4	—	—
Solanine	T62.2X1	T62.2X2	T62.2X3	T62.2X4	—	—
berries	T62.1X1	T62.1X2	T62.1X3	T62.1X4	—	—
Solanum dulcamara	T62.2X1	T62.2X2	T62.2X3	T62.2X4	—	—
berries	T62.1X1	T62.1X2	T62.1X3	T62.1X4	—	—
Solapsone	T37.1X1	T37.1X2	T37.1X3	T37.1X4	T37.1X5	T37.1X6
Solaquin*	T49.8X1	T49.8X2	T49.8X3	T49.8X4	T49.8X5	T49.8X6
Solar lotion	T49.3X1	T49.3X2	T49.3X3	T49.3X4	T49.3X5	T49.3X6
Solasulfone	T37.1X1	T37.1X2	T37.1X3	T37.1X4	T37.1X5	T37.1X6
Soldering fluid	T65.891	T65.892	T65.893	T65.894	—	—
Solid substance	T65.91	T65.92	T65.93	T65.94	—	—
specified NEC	T65.891	T65.892	T65.893	T65.894	—	—
Solvent, industrial NEC	T52.91	T52.92	T52.93	T52.94	—	—
naphtha	T52.0X1	T52.0X2	T52.0X3	T52.0X4	—	—
petroleum	T52.0X1	T52.0X2	T52.0X3	T52.0X4	—	—
specified NEC	T52.8X1	T52.8X2	T52.8X3	T52.8X4	—	—
Soma	T42.8X1	T42.8X2	T42.8X3	T42.8X4	T42.8X5	T42.8X6
Somatorelin	T38.891	T38.892	T38.893	T38.894	T38.895	T38.896
Somatostatin	T38.991	T38.992	T38.993	T38.994	T38.995	T38.996
Somatotropin	T38.811	T38.812	T38.813	T38.814	T38.815	T38.816
Somatrem	T38.811	T38.812	T38.813	T38.814	T38.815	T38.816
Somatropin	T38.811	T38.812	T38.813	T38.814	T38.815	T38.816
Sominex	T45.0X1	T45.0X2	T45.0X3	T45.0X4	T45.0X5	T45.0X6
Somnos	T42.6X1	T42.6X2	T42.6X3	T42.6X4	T42.6X5	T42.6X6
Somonal	T42.3X1	T42.3X2	T42.3X3	T42.3X4	T42.3X5	T42.3X6
Soneryl	T42.3X1	T42.3X2	T42.3X3	T42.3X4	T42.3X5	T42.3X6
Soothing syrup	T50.901	T50.902	T50.903	T50.904	T50.905	T50.906
Sopor	T42.6X1	T42.6X2	T42.6X3	T42.6X4	T42.6X5	T42.6X6
Soporific	T42.71	T42.72	T42.73	T42.74	T42.75	T42.76
Soporific drug	T42.71	T42.72	T42.73	T42.74	T42.75	T42.76
specified type NEC	T42.6X1	T42.6X2	T42.6X3	T42.6X4	T42.6X5	T42.6X6
Sorbide nitrate	T46.3X1	T46.3X2	T46.3X3	T46.3X4	T46.3X5	T46.3X6
Sorbitol	T47.4X1	T47.4X2	T47.4X3	T47.4X4	T47.4X5	T47.4X6
Sotalol	T44.7X1	T44.7X2	T44.7X3	T44.7X4	T44.7X5	T44.7X6
Sotradecol	T46.8X1	T46.8X2	T46.8X3	T46.8X4	T46.8X5	T46.8X6
Soysterol	T46.6X1	T46.6X2	T46.6X3	T46.6X4	T46.6X5	T46.6X6
Spacoline	T44.3X1	T44.3X2	T44.3X3	T44.3X4	T44.3X5	T44.3X6
Spanish fly	T49.8X1	T49.8X2	T49.8X3	T49.8X4	T49.8X5	T49.8X6
Sparine	T43.3X1	T43.3X2	T43.3X3	T43.3X4	T43.3X5	T43.3X6
Sparteine	T48.0X1	T48.0X2	T48.0X3	T48.0X4	T48.0X5	T48.0X6
Spasmolytic						
anticholinergics	T44.3X1	T44.3X2	T44.3X3	T44.3X4	T44.3X5	T44.3X6
autonomic	T44.3X1	T44.3X2	T44.3X3	T44.3X4	T44.3X5	T44.3X6
bronchial NEC	T48.6X1	T48.6X2	T48.6X3	T48.6X4	T48.6X5	T48.6X6
quaternary ammonium	T44.3X1	T44.3X2	T44.3X3	T44.3X4	T44.3X5	T44.3X6
skeletal muscle NEC	T48.1X1	T48.1X2	T48.1X3	T48.1X4	T48.1X5	T48.1X6
Spectinomycin	T36.5X1	T36.5X2	T36.5X3	T36.5X4	T36.5X5	T36.5X6
Spectracef*	T36.1X1	T36.1X2	T36.1X3	T36.1X4	T36.1X5	T36.1X6
Speed	T43.651	T43.652	T43.653	T43.654	T43.655	T43.656
Spermicide	T49.8X1	T49.8X2	T49.8X3	T49.8X4	T49.8X5	T49.8X6
Spider (bite) (venom)	T63.391	T63.392	T63.393	T63.394	—	—
antivenin	T50.Z11	T50.Z12	T50.Z13	T50.Z14	T50.Z15	T50.Z16
Spigelia (root)	T37.4X1	T37.4X2	T37.4X3	T37.4X4	T37.4X5	T37.4X6
Spindle inactivator	T50.4X1	T50.4X2	T50.4X3	T50.4X4	T50.4X5	T50.4X6
Spiperone	T43.4X1	T43.4X2	T43.4X3	T43.4X4	T43.4X5	T43.4X6
Spiramycin	T36.3X1	T36.3X2	T36.3X3	T36.3X4	T36.3X5	T36.3X6
Spirapril	T46.4X1	T46.4X2	T46.4X3	T46.4X4	T46.4X5	T46.4X6
Spirilene	T43.591	T43.592	T43.593	T43.594	T43.595	T43.596
Spirit(s) (neutral) **NEC**	T51.0X1	T51.0X2	T51.0X3	T51.0X4	—	—
beverage	T51.0X1	T51.0X2	T51.0X3	T51.0X4	—	—
industrial	T51.0X1	T51.0X2	T51.0X3	T51.0X4	—	—
mineral	T52.0X1	T52.0X2	T52.0X3	T52.0X4	—	—
of salt — *see* Hydrochloric acid						
surgical	T51.0X1	T51.0X2	T51.0X3	T51.0X4	—	—
Spiriva*	T44.3X1	T44.3X2	T44.3X3	T44.3X4	T44.3X5	T44.3X6
Spironolactone	T50.0X1	T50.0X2	T50.0X3	T50.0X4	T50.0X5	T50.0X6
Spiroperidol	T43.4X1	T43.4X2	T43.4X3	T43.4X4	T43.4X5	T43.4X6
Sponge, absorbable (gelatin)	T45.7X1	T45.7X2	T45.7X3	T45.7X4	T45.7X5	T45.7X6
Sporostacin	T49.0X1	T49.0X2	T49.0X3	T49.0X4	T49.0X5	T49.0X6
Spray (aerosol)	T65.91	T65.92	T65.93	T65.94	—	—
cosmetic	T65.891	T65.892	T65.893	T65.894	—	—
medicinal NEC	T50.901	T50.902	T50.903	T50.904	T50.905	T50.906
pesticides — *see* Pesticide						
specified content — *see* specific substance						
Spurge flax	T62.2X1	T62.2X2	T62.2X3	T62.2X4	—	—

Substance	Poisoning, Accidental (unintentional)	Poisoning, Intentional Self-harm	Poisoning, Assault	Poisoning, Undetermined	Adverse Effect	Under-dosing
Spurges	T62.2X1	T62.2X2	T62.2X3	T62.2X4	—	—
Sputum viscosity-lowering drug	T48.4X1	T48.4X2	T48.4X3	T48.4X4	T48.4X5	T48.4X6
Squill	T46.ØX1	T46.ØX2	T46.ØX3	T46.ØX4	T46.ØX5	T46.ØX6
rat poison	T6Ø.4X1	T6Ø.4X2	T6Ø.4X3	T6Ø.4X4	—	—
Squirting cucumber (cathartic)	T47.2X1	T47.2X2	T47.2X3	T47.2X4	T47.2X5	T47.2X6
Stains	T65.6X1	T65.6X2	T65.6X3	T65.6X4	—	—
Stannous fluoride	T49.7X1	T49.7X2	T49.7X3	T49.7X4	T49.7X5	T49.7X6
Stanolone	T38.7X1	T38.7X2	T38.7X3	T38.7X4	T38.7X5	T38.7X6
Stanozolol	T38.7X1	T38.7X2	T38.7X3	T38.7X4	T38.7X5	T38.7X6
Staphisagria or stavesacre (pediculicide)	T49.ØX1	T49.ØX2	T49.ØX3	T49.ØX4	T49.ØX5	T49.ØX6
Starch	T5Ø.9Ø1	T5Ø.9Ø2	T5Ø.9Ø3	T5Ø.9Ø4	T5Ø.9Ø5	T5Ø.9Ø6
Stavzor*	T42.6X1	T42.6X2	T42.6X3	T42.6X4	T42.6X5	T42.6X6
Stelazine	T43.3X1	T43.3X2	T43.3X3	T43.3X4	T43.3X5	T43.3X6
Stemetil	T43.3X1	T43.3X2	T43.3X3	T43.3X4	T43.3X5	T43.3X6
Stepronin	T48.4X1	T48.4X2	T48.4X3	T48.4X4	T48.4X5	T48.4X6
Sterculia	T47.4X1	T47.4X2	T47.4X3	T47.4X4	T47.4X5	T47.4X6
Sternutator gas	T59.891	T59.892	T59.893	T59.894	—	—
Steroid	T38.ØX1	T38.ØX2	T38.ØX3	T38.ØX4	T38.ØX5	T38.ØX6
anabolic	T38.7X1	T38.7X2	T38.7X3	T38.7X4	T38.7X5	T38.7X6
androgenic	T38.7X1	T38.7X2	T38.7X3	T38.7X4	T38.7X5	T38.7X6
antineoplastic, hormone	T38.7X1	T38.7X2	T38.7X3	T38.7X4	T38.7X5	T38.7X6
estrogen	T38.5X1	T38.5X2	T38.5X3	T38.5X4	T38.5X5	T38.5X6
ENT agent	T49.6X1	T49.6X2	T49.6X3	T49.6X4	T49.6X5	T49.6X6
ophthalmic preparation	T49.5X1	T49.5X2	T49.5X3	T49.5X4	T49.5X5	T49.5X6
topical NEC	T49.ØX1	T49.ØX2	T49.ØX3	T49.ØX4	T49.ØX5	T49.ØX6
Stibine	T56.891	T56.892	T56.893	T56.894	—	—
Stibogluconate	T37.3X1	T37.3X2	T37.3X3	T37.3X4	T37.3X5	T37.3X6
Stibophen	T37.4X1	T37.4X2	T37.4X3	T37.4X4	T37.4X5	T37.4X6
Stilbamidine (isetionate)	T37.3X1	T37.3X2	T37.3X3	T37.3X4	T37.3X5	T37.3X6
Stilbestrol	T38.5X1	T38.5X2	T38.5X3	T38.5X4	T38.5X5	T38.5X6
Stilboestrol	T38.5X1	T38.5X2	T38.5X3	T38.5X4	T38.5X5	T38.5X6
Stimulant						
central nervous system — *see also* Psychostimulant	T43.6Ø1	T43.6Ø2	T43.6Ø3	T43.6Ø4	T43.6Ø5	T43.6Ø6
analeptics	T5Ø.7X1	T5Ø.7X2	T5Ø.7X3	T5Ø.7X4	T5Ø.7X5	T5Ø.7X6
opiate antagonist	T5Ø.7X1	T5Ø.7X2	T5Ø.7X3	T5Ø.7X4	T5Ø.7X5	T5Ø.7X6
psychotherapeutic NEC — *see also* Psychotherapeutic drug	T43.6Ø1	T43.6Ø2	T43.6Ø3	T43.6Ø4	T43.6Ø5	T43.6Ø6
specified NEC	T43.691	T43.692	T43.693	T43.694	T43.695	T43.696
respiratory	T48.9Ø1	T48.9Ø2	T48.9Ø3	T48.9Ø4	T48.9Ø5	T48.9Ø6
Stone-dissolving drug	T5Ø.9Ø1	T5Ø.9Ø2	T5Ø.9Ø3	T5Ø.9Ø4	T5Ø.9Ø5	T5Ø.9Ø6
Storage battery (cells) (acid)	T54.2X1	T54.2X2	T54.2X3	T54.2X4	—	—
Stovaine	T41.3X1	T41.3X2	T41.3X3	T41.3X4	T41.3X5	T41.3X6
infiltration (subcutaneous)	T41.3X1	T41.3X2	T41.3X3	T41.3X4	T41.3X5	T41.3X6
nerve block (peripheral) (plexus)	T41.3X1	T41.3X2	T41.3X3	T41.3X4	T41.3X5	T41.3X6
spinal	T41.3X1	T41.3X2	T41.3X3	T41.3X4	T41.3X5	T41.3X6
topical (surface)	T41.3X1	T41.3X2	T41.3X3	T41.3X4	T41.3X5	T41.3X6
Stovarsal	T37.8X1	T37.8X2	T37.8X3	T37.8X4	T37.8X5	T37.8X6
Stove gas — *see* Gas, stove						
Stoxil	T49.5X1	T49.5X2	T49.5X3	T49.5X4	T49.5X5	T49.5X6
Stramonium	T48.6X1	T48.6X2	T48.6X3	T48.6X4	T48.6X5	T48.6X6
natural state	T62.2X1	T62.2X2	T62.2X3	T62.2X4	—	—
Streptodornase	T45.3X1	T45.3X2	T45.3X3	T45.3X4	T45.3X5	T45.3X6
Streptoduocin	T36.5X1	T36.5X2	T36.5X3	T36.5X4	T36.5X5	T36.5X6
Streptokinase	T45.611	T45.612	T45.613	T45.614	T45.615	T45.616
Streptomycin (derivative)	T36.5X1	T36.5X2	T36.5X3	T36.5X4	T36.5X5	T36.5X6
Streptonivicin	T36.5X1	T36.5X2	T36.5X3	T36.5X4	T36.5X5	T36.5X6
Streptovarycin	T36.5X1	T36.5X2	T36.5X3	T36.5X4	T36.5X5	T36.5X6
Streptozocin	T45.1X1	T45.1X2	T45.1X3	T45.1X4	T45.1X5	T45.1X6
Streptozotocin	T45.1X1	T45.1X2	T45.1X3	T45.1X4	T45.1X5	T45.1X6
Stripper (paint) (solvent)	T52.8X1	T52.8X2	T52.8X3	T52.8X4	—	—
Strobane	T6Ø.1X1	T6Ø.1X2	T6Ø.1X3	T6Ø.1X4	—	—
Strofantina	T46.ØX1	T46.ØX2	T46.ØX3	T46.ØX4	T46.ØX5	T46.ØX6
Stromectol*	T37.4X1	T37.4X2	T37.4X3	T37.4X4	T37.4X5	T37.4X6
Strophanthin (g) (k)	T46.ØX1	T46.ØX2	T46.ØX3	T46.ØX4	T46.ØX5	T46.ØX6
Strophanthus	T46.ØX1	T46.ØX2	T46.ØX3	T46.ØX4	T46.ØX5	T46.ØX6
Strophantin	T46.ØX1	T46.ØX2	T46.ØX3	T46.ØX4	T46.ØX5	T46.ØX6
Strophantin-g	T46.ØX1	T46.ØX2	T46.ØX3	T46.ØX4	T46.ØX5	T46.ØX6
Strychnine (nonmedicinal) (pesticide) (salts)	T65.1X1	T65.1X2	T65.1X3	T65.1X4	—	—
medicinal	T48.291	T48.292	T48.293	T48.294	T48.295	T48.296
Strychnos (ignatii) — *see* Strychnine						
Styramate	T42.8X1	T42.8X2	T42.8X3	T42.8X4	T42.8X5	T42.8X6
Styrene	T65.891	T65.892	T65.893	T65.894	—	—
Succinimide, antiepileptic or anticonvulsant	T42.2X1	T42.2X2	T42.2X3	T42.2X4	T42.2X5	T42.2X6

Substance	Poisoning, Accidental (unintentional)	Poisoning, Intentional Self-harm	Poisoning, Assault	Poisoning, Undetermined	Adverse Effect	Under-dosing
Succinimide, antiepileptic or anticonvulsant — *continued*						
mercuric — *see* Mercury						
Succinylcholine	T48.1X1	T48.1X2	T48.1X3	T48.1X4	T48.1X5	T48.1X6
Succinylsulfathiazole	T37.ØX1	T37.ØX2	T37.ØX3	T37.ØX4	T37.ØX5	T37.ØX6
Sucralfate	T47.1X1	T47.1X2	T47.1X3	T47.1X4	T47.1X5	T47.1X6
Sucrose	T5Ø.3X1	T5Ø.3X2	T5Ø.3X3	T5Ø.3X4	T5Ø.3X5	T5Ø.3X6
Sufentanil	T4Ø.411	T4Ø.412	T4Ø.413	T4Ø.414	T4Ø.415	T4Ø.416
Sulbactam	T36.ØX1	T36.ØX2	T36.ØX3	T36.ØX4	T36.ØX5	T36.ØX6
Sulbenicillin	T36.ØX1	T36.ØX2	T36.ØX3	T36.ØX4	T36.ØX5	T36.ØX6
Sulbentine	T49.ØX1	T49.ØX2	T49.ØX3	T49.ØX4	T49.ØX5	T49.ØX6
Sulconazole*	T49.ØX1	T49.ØX2	T49.ØX3	T49.ØX4	T49.ØX5	T49.ØX6
Sulfacetamide	T49.ØX1	T49.ØX2	T49.ØX3	T49.ØX4	T49.ØX5	T49.ØX6
ophthalmic preparation	T49.5X1	T49.5X2	T49.5X3	T49.5X4	T49.5X5	T49.5X6
Sulfachlorpyridazine	T37.ØX1	T37.ØX2	T37.ØX3	T37.ØX4	T37.ØX5	T37.ØX6
Sulfacitine	T37.ØX1	T37.ØX2	T37.ØX3	T37.ØX4	T37.ØX5	T37.ØX6
Sulfadiasulfone sodium	T37.ØX1	T37.ØX2	T37.ØX3	T37.ØX4	T37.ØX5	T37.ØX6
Sulfadiazine	T37.ØX1	T37.ØX2	T37.ØX3	T37.ØX4	T37.ØX5	T37.ØX6
silver (topical)	T49.ØX1	T49.ØX2	T49.ØX3	T49.ØX4	T49.ØX5	T49.ØX6
Sulfadimethoxine	T37.ØX1	T37.ØX2	T37.ØX3	T37.ØX4	T37.ØX5	T37.ØX6
Sulfadimidine	T37.ØX1	T37.ØX2	T37.ØX3	T37.ØX4	T37.ØX5	T37.ØX6
Sulfadoxine	T37.ØX1	T37.ØX2	T37.ØX3	T37.ØX4	T37.ØX5	T37.ØX6
with pyrimethamine	T37.2X1	T37.2X2	T37.2X3	T37.2X4	T37.2X5	T37.2X6
Sulfaethidole	T37.ØX1	T37.ØX2	T37.ØX3	T37.ØX4	T37.ØX5	T37.ØX6
Sulfafurazole	T37.ØX1	T37.ØX2	T37.ØX3	T37.ØX4	T37.ØX5	T37.ØX6
Sulfaguanidine	T37.ØX1	T37.ØX2	T37.ØX3	T37.ØX4	T37.ØX5	T37.ØX6
Sulfalene	T37.ØX1	T37.ØX2	T37.ØX3	T37.ØX4	T37.ØX5	T37.ØX6
Sulfaloxate	T37.ØX1	T37.ØX2	T37.ØX3	T37.ØX4	T37.ØX5	T37.ØX6
Sulfaloxic acid	T37.ØX1	T37.ØX2	T37.ØX3	T37.ØX4	T37.ØX5	T37.ØX6
Sulfamazone	T39.2X1	T39.2X2	T39.2X3	T39.2X4	T39.2X5	T39.2X6
Sulfamerazine	T37.ØX1	T37.ØX2	T37.ØX3	T37.ØX4	T37.ØX5	T37.ØX6
Sulfameter	T37.ØX1	T37.ØX2	T37.ØX3	T37.ØX4	T37.ØX5	T37.ØX6
Sulfamethazine	T37.ØX1	T37.ØX2	T37.ØX3	T37.ØX4	T37.ØX5	T37.ØX6
Sulfamethizole	T37.ØX1	T37.ØX2	T37.ØX3	T37.ØX4	T37.ØX5	T37.ØX6
Sulfamethoxazole	T37.ØX1	T37.ØX2	T37.ØX3	T37.ØX4	T37.ØX5	T37.ØX6
with trimethoprim	T36.8X1	T36.8X2	T36.8X3	T36.8X4	T36.8X5	T36.8X6
Sulfamethoxydiazine	T37.ØX1	T37.ØX2	T37.ØX3	T37.ØX4	T37.ØX5	T37.ØX6
Sulfamethoxypyridazine	T37.ØX1	T37.ØX2	T37.ØX3	T37.ØX4	T37.ØX5	T37.ØX6
Sulfamethylthiazole	T37.ØX1	T37.ØX2	T37.ØX3	T37.ØX4	T37.ØX5	T37.ØX6
Sulfametoxydiazine	T37.ØX1	T37.ØX2	T37.ØX3	T37.ØX4	T37.ØX5	T37.ØX6
Sulfamidopyrine	T39.2X1	T39.2X2	T39.2X3	T39.2X4	T39.2X5	T39.2X6
Sulfamonomethoxine	T37.ØX1	T37.ØX2	T37.ØX3	T37.ØX4	T37.ØX5	T37.ØX6
Sulfamoxole	T37.ØX1	T37.ØX2	T37.ØX3	T37.ØX4	T37.ØX5	T37.ØX6
Sulfamylon	T49.ØX1	T49.ØX2	T49.ØX3	T49.ØX4	T49.ØX5	T49.ØX6
Sulfan blue (diagnostic dye)	T5Ø.8X1	T5Ø.8X2	T5Ø.8X3	T5Ø.8X4	T5Ø.8X5	T5Ø.8X6
Sulfanilamide	T37.ØX1	T37.ØX2	T37.ØX3	T37.ØX4	T37.ØX5	T37.ØX6
Sulfanilylguanidine	T37.ØX1	T37.ØX2	T37.ØX3	T37.ØX4	T37.ØX5	T37.ØX6
Sulfaperin	T37.ØX1	T37.ØX2	T37.ØX3	T37.ØX4	T37.ØX5	T37.ØX6
Sulfaphenazole	T37.ØX1	T37.ØX2	T37.ØX3	T37.ØX4	T37.ØX5	T37.ØX6
Sulfaphenylthiazole	T37.ØX1	T37.ØX2	T37.ØX3	T37.ØX4	T37.ØX5	T37.ØX6
Sulfaproxyline	T37.ØX1	T37.ØX2	T37.ØX3	T37.ØX4	T37.ØX5	T37.ØX6
Sulfapyridine	T37.ØX1	T37.ØX2	T37.ØX3	T37.ØX4	T37.ØX5	T37.ØX6
Sulfapyrimidine	T37.ØX1	T37.ØX2	T37.ØX3	T37.ØX4	T37.ØX5	T37.ØX6
Sulfarsphenamine	T37.8X1	T37.8X2	T37.8X3	T37.8X4	T37.8X5	T37.8X6
Sulfasalazine	T37.ØX1	T37.ØX2	T37.ØX3	T37.ØX4	T37.ØX5	T37.ØX6
Sulfasuxidine	T37.ØX1	T37.ØX2	T37.ØX3	T37.ØX4	T37.ØX5	T37.ØX6
Sulfasymazine	T37.ØX1	T37.ØX2	T37.ØX3	T37.ØX4	T37.ØX5	T37.ØX6
Sulfated amylopectin	T47.8X1	T47.8X2	T47.8X3	T47.8X4	T47.8X5	T47.8X6
Sulfathiazole	T37.ØX1	T37.ØX2	T37.ØX3	T37.ØX4	T37.ØX5	T37.ØX6
Sulfatostearate	T49.2X1	T49.2X2	T49.2X3	T49.2X4	T49.2X5	T49.2X6
Sulfatrim*	T36.8X1	T36.8X2	T36.8X3	T36.8X4	T36.8X5	T36.8X6
Sulfinpyrazone	T5Ø.4X1	T5Ø.4X2	T5Ø.4X3	T5Ø.4X4	T5Ø.4X5	T5Ø.4X6
Sulfiram	T49.ØX1	T49.ØX2	T49.ØX3	T49.ØX4	T49.ØX5	T49.ØX6
Sulfisomidine	T37.ØX1	T37.ØX2	T37.ØX3	T37.ØX4	T37.ØX5	T37.ØX6
Sulfisoxazole	T37.ØX1	T37.ØX2	T37.ØX3	T37.ØX4	T37.ØX5	T37.ØX6
ophthalmic preparation	T49.5X1	T49.5X2	T49.5X3	T49.5X4	T49.5X5	T49.5X6
Sulfobromophthalein (sodium)	T5Ø.8X1	T5Ø.8X2	T5Ø.8X3	T5Ø.8X4	T5Ø.8X5	T5Ø.8X6
Sulfobromphthalein	T5Ø.8X1	T5Ø.8X2	T5Ø.8X3	T5Ø.8X4	T5Ø.8X5	T5Ø.8X6
Sulfogaiacol	T48.4X1	T48.4X2	T48.4X3	T48.4X4	T48.4X5	T48.4X6
Sulfomyxin	T36.8X1	T36.8X2	T36.8X3	T36.8X4	T36.8X5	T36.8X6
Sulfonal	T42.6X1	T42.6X2	T42.6X3	T42.6X4	T42.6X5	T42.6X6
Sulfonamide NEC	T37.ØX1	T37.ØX2	T37.ØX3	T37.ØX4	T37.ØX5	T37.ØX6
eye	T49.5X1	T49.5X2	T49.5X3	T49.5X4	T49.5X5	T49.5X6
Sulfonazide	T37.1X1	T37.1X2	T37.1X3	T37.1X4	T37.1X5	T37.1X6
Sulfones	T37.1X1	T37.1X2	T37.1X3	T37.1X4	T37.1X5	T37.1X6
Sulfonethylmethane	T42.6X1	T42.6X2	T42.6X3	T42.6X4	T42.6X5	T42.6X6
Sulfonmethane	T42.6X1	T42.6X2	T42.6X3	T42.6X4	T42.6X5	T42.6X6
Sulfonphthal, sulfonphthol	T5Ø.8X1	T5Ø.8X2	T5Ø.8X3	T5Ø.8X4	T5Ø.8X5	T5Ø.8X6
Sulfonylurea derivatives, oral	T38.3X1	T38.3X2	T38.3X3	T38.3X4	T38.3X5	T38.3X6
Sulforidazine	T43.3X1	T43.3X2	T43.3X3	T43.3X4	T43.3X5	T43.3X6

Substance	Poisoning, Accidental (unintentional)	Poisoning, Intentional Self-harm	Poisoning, Assault	Poisoning, Undetermined	Adverse Effect	Under-dosing
Sulfoxone	T37.1X1	T37.1X2	T37.1X3	T37.1X4	T37.1X5	T37.1X6
Sulfur, sulfurated, sulfuric, sulfurous, sulfuryl (compounds NEC) (medicinal)	T49.4X1	T49.4X2	T49.4X3	T49.4X4	T49.4X5	T49.4X6
acid	T54.2X1	T54.2X2	T54.2X3	T54.2X4	—	—
dioxide (gas)	T59.1X1	T59.1X2	T59.1X3	T59.1X4	—	—
ether — *see* Ether(s)						
hydrogen	T59.6X1	T59.6X2	T59.6X3	T59.6X4	—	—
medicinal (keratolytic) (ointment) NEC	T49.4X1	T49.4X2	T49.4X3	T49.4X4	T49.4X5	T49.4X6
ointment	T49.0X1	T49.0X2	T49.0X3	T49.0X4	T49.0X5	T49.0X6
pesticide (vapor)	T60.91	T60.92	T60.93	T60.94	—	—
vapor NEC	T59.891	T59.892	T59.893	T59.894	—	—
Sulfuric acid	T54.2X1	T54.2X2	T54.2X3	T54.2X4	—	—
Sulglicotide	T47.1X1	T47.1X2	T47.1X3	T47.1X4	T47.1X5	T47.1X6
Sulindac	T39.391	T39.392	T39.393	T39.394	T39.395	T39.396
Sulisatin	T47.2X1	T47.2X2	T47.2X3	T47.2X4	T47.2X5	T47.2X6
Sulisobenzone	T49.3X1	T49.3X2	T49.3X3	T49.3X4	T49.3X5	T49.3X6
Sulkowitch's reagent	T50.8X1	T50.8X2	T50.8X3	T50.8X4	T50.8X5	T50.8X6
Sulmetozine	T44.3X1	T44.3X2	T44.3X3	T44.3X4	T44.3X5	T44.3X6
Suloctidil	T46.7X1	T46.7X2	T46.7X3	T46.7X4	T46.7X5	T46.7X6
Sulph- — *see also* Sulf-						
Sulphadiazine	T37.0X1	T37.0X2	T37.0X3	T37.0X4	T37.0X5	T37.0X6
Sulphadimethoxine	T37.0X1	T37.0X2	T37.0X3	T37.0X4	T37.0X5	T37.0X6
Sulphadimidine	T37.0X1	T37.0X2	T37.0X3	T37.0X4	T37.0X5	T37.0X6
Sulphadione	T37.1X1	T37.1X2	T37.1X3	T37.1X4	T37.1X5	T37.1X6
Sulphafurazole	T37.0X1	T37.0X2	T37.0X3	T37.0X4	T37.0X5	T37.0X6
Sulphamethizole	T37.0X1	T37.0X2	T37.0X3	T37.0X4	T37.0X5	T37.0X6
Sulphamethoxazole	T37.0X1	T37.0X2	T37.0X3	T37.0X4	T37.0X5	T37.0X6
Sulphan blue	T50.8X1	T50.8X2	T50.8X3	T50.8X4	T50.8X5	T50.8X6
Sulphaphenazole	T37.0X1	T37.0X2	T37.0X3	T37.0X4	T37.0X5	T37.0X6
Sulphapyridine	T37.0X1	T37.0X2	T37.0X3	T37.0X4	T37.0X5	T37.0X6
Sulphasalazine	T37.0X1	T37.0X2	T37.0X3	T37.0X4	T37.0X5	T37.0X6
Sulphinpyrazone	T50.4X1	T50.4X2	T50.4X3	T50.4X4	T50.4X5	T50.4X6
Sulpiride	T43.591	T43.592	T43.593	T43.594	T43.595	T43.596
Sulprostone	T48.0X1	T48.0X2	T48.0X3	T48.0X4	T48.0X5	T48.0X6
Sulpyrine	T39.2X1	T39.2X2	T39.2X3	T39.2X4	T39.2X5	T39.2X6
Sultamicillin	T36.0X1	T36.0X2	T36.0X3	T36.0X4	T36.0X5	T36.0X6
Sulthiame	T42.6X1	T42.6X2	T42.6X3	T42.6X4	T42.6X5	T42.6X6
Sultiame	T42.6X1	T42.6X2	T42.6X3	T42.6X4	T42.6X5	T42.6X6
Sultopride	T43.591	T43.592	T43.593	T43.594	T43.595	T43.596
Sumatriptan	T39.8X1	T39.8X2	T39.8X3	T39.8X4	T39.8X5	T39.8X6
Sumavel*	T39.8X1	T39.8X2	T39.8X3	T39.8X4	T39.8X5	T39.8X6
Sunflower seed oil	T46.6X1	T46.6X2	T46.6X3	T46.6X4	T46.6X5	T46.6X6
Superinone	T48.4X1	T48.4X2	T48.4X3	T48.4X4	T48.4X5	T48.4X6
Suprofen	T39.311	T39.312	T39.313	T39.314	T39.315	T39.316
Suramin (sodium)	T37.4X1	T37.4X2	T37.4X3	T37.4X4	T37.4X5	T37.4X6
Surfacaine	T41.3X1	T41.3X2	T41.3X3	T41.3X4	T41.3X5	T41.3X6
Surital	T41.1X1	T41.1X2	T41.1X3	T41.1X4	T41.1X5	T41.1X6
Sutilains	T45.3X1	T45.3X2	T45.3X3	T45.3X4	T45.3X5	T45.3X6
Suxamethonium (chloride)	T48.1X1	T48.1X2	T48.1X3	T48.1X4	T48.1X5	T48.1X6
Suxethonium (chloride)	T48.1X1	T48.1X2	T48.1X3	T48.1X4	T48.1X5	T48.1X6
Suxibuzone	T39.2X1	T39.2X2	T39.2X3	T39.2X4	T39.2X5	T39.2X6
Sweet niter spirit	T46.3X1	T46.3X2	T46.3X3	T46.3X4	T46.3X5	T46.3X6
Sweet oil (birch)	T49.3X1	T49.3X2	T49.3X3	T49.3X4	T49.3X5	T49.3X6
Sweetener	T50.901	T50.902	T50.903	T50.904	T50.905	T50.906
Sylvant*	T45.1X1	T45.1X2	T45.1X3	T45.1X4	T45.1X5	T45.1X6
Sym-dichloroethyl ether	T53.6X1	T53.6X2	T53.6X3	T53.6X4	—	—
Sympatholytic NEC	T44.8X1	T44.8X2	T44.8X3	T44.8X4	T44.8X5	T44.8X6
haloalkylamine	T44.8X1	T44.8X2	T44.8X3	T44.8X4	T44.8X5	T44.8X6
Sympathomimetic NEC	T44.901	T44.902	T44.903	T44.904	T44.905	T44.906
anti-common-cold	T48.5X1	T48.5X2	T48.5X3	T48.5X4	T48.5X5	T48.5X6
bronchodilator	T48.6X1	T48.6X2	T48.6X3	T48.6X4	T48.6X5	T48.6X6
specified NEC	T44.991	T44.992	T44.993	T44.994	T44.995	T44.996
Synagis	T50.B91	T50.B92	T50.B93	T50.B94	T50.B95	T50.B96
Synalar	T49.0X1	T49.0X2	T49.0X3	T49.0X4	T49.0X5	T49.0X6
Synthetic cannabinoids	T40.721	T40.722	T40.723	T40.724	T40.725	T40.726
Synthroid	T38.1X1	T38.1X2	T38.1X3	T38.1X4	T38.1X5	T38.1X6
Syntocinon	T48.0X1	T48.0X2	T48.0X3	T48.0X4	T48.0X5	T48.0X6
Syrosingopine	T46.5X1	T46.5X2	T46.5X3	T46.5X4	T46.5X5	T46.5X6
Systemic drug	T45.91	T45.92	T45.93	T45.94	T45.95	T45.96
specified NEC	T45.8X1	T45.8X2	T45.8X3	T45.8X4	T45.8X5	T45.8X6
Tablets — *see also* specified substance	T50.901	T50.902	T50.903	T50.904	T50.905	T50.906
Tace	T38.5X1	T38.5X2	T38.5X3	T38.5X4	T38.5X5	T38.5X6
Tacrine	T44.0X1	T44.0X2	T44.0X3	T44.0X4	T44.0X5	T44.0X6
Tadalafil	T46.7X1	T46.7X2	T46.7X3	T46.7X4	T46.7X5	T46.7X6
Talampicillin	T36.0X1	T36.0X2	T36.0X3	T36.0X4	T36.0X5	T36.0X6
Talbutal	T42.3X1	T42.3X2	T42.3X3	T42.3X4	T42.3X5	T42.3X6
Talc powder	T49.3X1	T49.3X2	T49.3X3	T49.3X4	T49.3X5	T49.3X6
Talcum	T49.3X1	T49.3X2	T49.3X3	T49.3X4	T49.3X5	T49.3X6
Taleranol	T38.6X1	T38.6X2	T38.6X3	T38.6X4	T38.6X5	T38.6X6

Substance	Poisoning, Accidental (unintentional)	Poisoning, Intentional Self-harm	Poisoning, Assault	Poisoning, Undetermined	Adverse Effect	Under-dosing
Taltz*	T39.391	T39.392	T39.393	T39.394	T39.395	T39.396
Tamoxifen	T38.6X1	T38.6X2	T38.6X3	T38.6X4	T38.6X5	T38.6X6
Tamsulosin	T44.6X1	T44.6X2	T44.6X3	T44.6X4	T44.6X5	T44.6X6
Tandearil, tanderil	T39.2X1	T39.2X2	T39.2X3	T39.2X4	T39.2X5	T39.2X6
Tannic acid	T49.2X1	T49.2X2	T49.2X3	T49.2X4	T49.2X5	T49.2X6
medicinal (astringent)	T49.2X1	T49.2X2	T49.2X3	T49.2X4	T49.2X5	T49.2X6
Tannin — *see* Tannic acid						
Tansy	T62.2X1	T62.2X2	T62.2X3	T62.2X4	—	—
TAO	T36.3X1	T36.3X2	T36.3X3	T36.3X4	T36.3X5	T36.3X6
Tapazole	T38.2X1	T38.2X2	T38.2X3	T38.2X4	T38.2X5	T38.2X6
Tar NEC	T52.0X1	T52.0X2	T52.0X3	T52.0X4	—	—
camphor	T60.1X1	T60.1X2	T60.1X3	T60.1X4	—	—
distillate	T49.1X1	T49.1X2	T49.1X3	T49.1X4	T49.1X5	T49.1X6
fumes	T59.891	T59.892	T59.893	T59.894	—	—
medicinal	T49.1X1	T49.1X2	T49.1X3	T49.1X4	T49.1X5	T49.1X6
ointment	T49.1X1	T49.1X2	T49.1X3	T49.1X4	T49.1X5	T49.1X6
Taractan	T43.591	T43.592	T43.593	T43.594	T43.595	T43.596
Tarantula (venomous)	T63.321	T63.322	T63.323	T63.324	—	—
Tartar emetic	T37.8X1	T37.8X2	T37.8X3	T37.8X4	T37.8X5	T37.8X6
Tartaric acid	T65.891	T65.892	T65.893	T65.894	—	—
Tartrate, laxative	T47.4X1	T47.4X2	T47.4X3	T47.4X4	T47.4X5	T47.4X6
Tartrated antimony (anti-infective)	T37.8X1	T37.8X2	T37.8X3	T37.8X4	T37.8X5	T37.8X6
Tauromustine	T45.1X1	T45.1X2	T45.1X3	T45.1X4	T45.1X5	T45.1X6
TCA — *see* Trichloroacetic acid						
TCDD	T53.7X1	T53.7X2	T53.7X3	T53.7X4	—	—
TDI (vapor)	T65.0X1	T65.0X2	T65.0X3	T65.0X4	—	—
Tear						
gas	T59.3X1	T59.3X2	T59.3X3	T59.3X4	—	—
solution	T49.5X1	T49.5X2	T49.5X3	T49.5X4	T49.5X5	T49.5X6
Tecentriq*	T45.1X1	T45.1X2	T45.1X3	T45.1X4	T45.1X5	T45.1X6
Teclothiazide	T50.2X1	T50.2X2	T50.2X3	T50.2X4	T50.2X5	T50.2X6
Teclozan	T37.3X1	T37.3X2	T37.3X3	T37.3X4	T37.3X5	T37.3X6
Tegafur	T45.1X1	T45.1X2	T45.1X3	T45.1X4	T45.1X5	T45.1X6
Tegretol	T42.1X1	T42.1X2	T42.1X3	T42.1X4	T42.1X5	T42.1X6
Teicoplanin	T36.8X1	T36.8X2	T36.8X3	T36.8X4	T36.8X5	T36.8X6
Telepaque	T50.8X1	T50.8X2	T50.8X3	T50.8X4	T50.8X5	T50.8X6
Tellurium	T56.891	T56.892	T56.893	T56.894	—	—
fumes	T56.891	T56.892	T56.893	T56.894	—	—
TEM	T45.1X1	T45.1X2	T45.1X3	T45.1X4	T45.1X5	T45.1X6
Temazepam	T42.4X1	T42.4X2	T42.4X3	T42.4X4	T42.4X5	T42.4X6
Temocillin	T36.0X1	T36.0X2	T36.0X3	T36.0X4	T36.0X5	T36.0X6
Tenamfetamine	T43.621	T43.622	T43.623	T43.624	T43.625	T43.626
Tenecteplase*	T45.611	T45.612	T45.613	T45.614	T45.615	T45.616
Teniposide	T45.1X1	T45.1X2	T45.1X3	T45.1X4	T45.1X5	T45.1X6
Tenitramine	T46.3X1	T46.3X2	T46.3X3	T46.3X4	T46.3X5	T46.3X6
Tenoglicin	T48.4X1	T48.4X2	T48.4X3	T48.4X4	T48.4X5	T48.4X6
Tenonitrozole	T37.3X1	T37.3X2	T37.3X3	T37.3X4	T37.3X5	T37.3X6
Tenormin*	T44.7X1	T44.7X2	T44.7X3	T44.7X4	T44.7X5	T44.7X6
Tenoxicam	T39.391	T39.392	T39.393	T39.394	T39.395	T39.396
TEPA	T45.1X1	T45.1X2	T45.1X3	T45.1X4	T45.1X5	T45.1X6
TEPP	T60.0X1	T60.0X2	T60.0X3	T60.0X4	—	—
Teprotide	T46.5X1	T46.5X2	T46.5X3	T46.5X4	T46.5X5	T46.5X6
Terazosin	T44.6X1	T44.6X2	T44.6X3	T44.6X4	T44.6X5	T44.6X6
Terbufos	T60.0X1	T60.0X2	T60.0X3	T60.0X4	—	—
Terbutaline	T48.6X1	T48.6X2	T48.6X3	T48.6X4	T48.6X5	T48.6X6
Terconazole	T49.0X1	T49.0X2	T49.0X3	T49.0X4	T49.0X5	T49.0X6
Terfenadine	T45.0X1	T45.0X2	T45.0X3	T45.0X4	T45.0X5	T45.0X6
Teriparatide (acetate)	T50.991	T50.992	T50.993	T50.994	T50.995	T50.996
Terizidone	T37.1X1	T37.1X2	T37.1X3	T37.1X4	T37.1X5	T37.1X6
Terlipressin	T38.891	T38.892	T38.893	T38.894	T38.895	T38.896
Terodiline	T46.3X1	T46.3X2	T46.3X3	T46.3X4	T46.3X5	T46.3X6
Teroxalene	T37.4X1	T37.4X2	T37.4X3	T37.4X4	T37.4X5	T37.4X6
Terpin (cis) **hydrate**	T48.4X1	T48.4X2	T48.4X3	T48.4X4	T48.4X5	T48.4X6
Terramycin	T36.4X1	T36.4X2	T36.4X3	T36.4X4	T36.4X5	T36.4X6
Tertatolol	T44.7X1	T44.7X2	T44.7X3	T44.7X4	T44.7X5	T44.7X6
Tessalon	T48.3X1	T48.3X2	T48.3X3	T48.3X4	T48.3X5	T48.3X6
Testolactone	T38.7X1	T38.7X2	T38.7X3	T38.7X4	T38.7X5	T38.7X6
Testosterone	T38.7X1	T38.7X2	T38.7X3	T38.7X4	T38.7X5	T38.7X6
Tetanus toxoid or vaccine	T50.A91	T50.A92	T50.A93	T50.A94	T50.A95	T50.A96
antitoxin	T50.Z11	T50.Z12	T50.Z13	T50.Z14	T50.Z15	T50.Z16
immune globulin (human)	T50.Z11	T50.Z12	T50.Z13	T50.Z14	T50.Z15	T50.Z16
toxoid	T50.A91	T50.A92	T50.A93	T50.A94	T50.A95	T50.A96
with diphtheria toxoid	T50.A21	T50.A22	T50.A23	T50.A24	T50.A25	T50.A26
with pertussis	T50.A11	T50.A12	T50.A13	T50.A14	T50.A15	T50.A16
Tetrabenazine	T43.591	T43.592	T43.593	T43.594	T43.595	T43.596
Tetracaine	T41.3X1	T41.3X2	T41.3X3	T41.3X4	T41.3X5	T41.3X6
nerve block (peripheral) (plexus)	T41.3X1	T41.3X2	T41.3X3	T41.3X4	T41.3X5	T41.3X6
regional	T41.3X1	T41.3X2	T41.3X3	T41.3X4	T41.3X5	T41.3X6
spinal	T41.3X1	T41.3X2	T41.3X3	T41.3X4	T41.3X5	T41.3X6
Tetrachlorethylene — *see* Tetrachloroethylene						

Substance	Poisoning, Accidental (unintentional)	Poisoning, Intentional Self-harm	Poisoning, Assault	Poisoning, Undetermined	Adverse Effect	Under-dosing
Tetrachlormethiazide	T50.2X1	T50.2X2	T50.2X3	T50.2X4	T50.2X5	T50.2X6
Tetrachloroethane	T53.6X1	T53.6X2	T53.6X3	T53.6X4	—	—
vapor	T53.6X1	T53.6X2	T53.6X3	T53.6X4	—	—
paint or varnish	T53.6X1	T53.6X2	T53.6X3	T53.6X4	—	—
Tetrachloroethylene	T53.3X1	T53.3X2	T53.3X3	T53.3X4	—	—
(liquid)						
medicinal	T37.4X1	T37.4X2	T37.4X3	T37.4X4	T37.4X5	T37.4X6
vapor	T53.3X1	T53.3X2	T53.3X3	T53.3X4	—	—
Tetrachloromethane — see Carbon tetrachloride						
Tetracosactide	T38.811	T38.812	T38.813	T38.814	T38.815	T38.816
Tetracosactrin	T38.811	T38.812	T38.813	T38.814	T38.815	T38.816
Tetracycline	T36.4X1	T36.4X2	T36.4X3	T36.4X4	T36.4X5	T36.4X6
ophthalmic preparation	T49.5X1	T49.5X2	T49.5X3	T49.5X4	T49.5X5	T49.5X6
topical NEC	T49.0X1	T49.0X2	T49.0X3	T49.0X4	T49.0X5	T49.0X6
Tetradifon	T60.8X1	T60.8X2	T60.8X3	T60.8X4	—	—
Tetradotoxin	T61.771	T61.772	T61.773	T61.774	—	—
Tetraethyl						
lead	T56.0X1	T56.0X2	T56.0X3	T56.0X4	—	—
pyrophosphate	T60.0X1	T60.0X2	T60.0X3	T60.0X4	—	—
Tetraethylammonium chloride	T44.2X1	T44.2X2	T44.2X3	T44.2X4	T44.2X5	T44.2X6
Tetraethylthiuram disulfide	T50.6X1	T50.6X2	T50.6X3	T50.6X4	T50.6X5	T50.6X6
Tetrahydroaminoacridine	T44.0X1	T44.0X2	T44.0X3	T44.0X4	T44.0X5	T44.0X6
Tetrahydrocannabinol	T40.711	T40.712	T40.713	T40.714	T40.715	T40.716
Tetrahydrofuran	T52.8X1	T52.8X2	T52.8X3	T52.8X4	—	—
Tetrahydrolipstatin*	T47.8X1	T47.8X2	T47.8X3	T47.8X4	T47.8X5	T47.8X6
Tetrahydronaphthalene	T52.8X1	T52.8X2	T52.8X3	T52.8X4	—	—
Tetrahydrozoline	T49.5X1	T49.5X2	T49.5X3	T49.5X4	T49.5X5	T49.5X6
Tetralin	T52.8X1	T52.8X2	T52.8X3	T52.8X4	—	—
Tetramethrin	T60.2X1	T60.2X2	T60.2X3	T60.2X4	—	—
Tetramethylthiuram (disulfide) NEC	T60.3X1	T60.3X2	T60.3X3	T60.3X4	—	—
medicinal	T49.0X1	T49.0X2	T49.0X3	T49.0X4	T49.0X5	T49.0X6
Tetramisole	T37.4X1	T37.4X2	T37.4X3	T37.4X4	T37.4X5	T37.4X6
Tetranicotinoyl fructose	T46.7X1	T46.7X2	T46.7X3	T46.7X4	T46.7X5	T46.7X6
Tetrazepam	T42.4X1	T42.4X2	T42.4X3	T42.4X4	T42.4X5	T42.4X6
Tetronal	T42.6X1	T42.6X2	T42.6X3	T42.6X4	T42.6X5	T42.6X6
Tetryl	T65.3X1	T65.3X2	T65.3X3	T65.3X4	—	—
Tetrylammonium chloride	T44.2X1	T44.2X2	T44.2X3	T44.2X4	T44.2X5	T44.2X6
Tetryzoline	T49.5X1	T49.5X2	T49.5X3	T49.5X4	T49.5X5	T49.5X6
Thalidomide	T45.1X1	T45.1X2	T45.1X3	T45.1X4	T45.1X5	T45.1X6
Thallium (compounds) (dust) NEC	T56.811	T56.812	T56.813	T56.814	—	—
pesticide	T60.4X1	T60.4X2	T60.4X3	T60.4X4	—	—
THC	T40.711	T40.712	T40.713	T40.714	T40.715	T40.716
Thebacon	T48.3X1	T48.3X2	T48.3X3	T48.3X4	T48.3X5	T48.3X6
Thebaine	T40.2X1	T40.2X2	T40.2X3	T40.2X4	T40.2X5	T40.2X6
Thenoic acid	T49.6X1	T49.6X2	T49.6X3	T49.6X4	T49.6X5	T49.6X6
Thenyldiamine	T45.0X1	T45.0X2	T45.0X3	T45.0X4	T45.0X5	T45.0X6
Theobromine (calcium salicylate)	T48.6X1	T48.6X2	T48.6X3	T48.6X4	T48.6X5	T48.6X6
sodium salicylate	T48.6X1	T48.6X2	T48.6X3	T48.6X4	T48.6X5	T48.6X6
Theolair*	T48.6X1	T48.6X2	T48.6X3	T48.6X4	T48.6X5	T48.6X6
Theophyllamine	T48.6X1	T48.6X2	T48.6X3	T48.6X4	T48.6X5	T48.6X6
Theophylline	T48.6X1	T48.6X2	T48.6X3	T48.6X4	T48.6X5	T48.6X6
aminobenzoic acid	T48.6X1	T48.6X2	T48.6X3	T48.6X4	T48.6X5	T48.6X6
ethylenediamine	T48.6X1	T48.6X2	T48.6X3	T48.6X4	T48.6X5	T48.6X6
piperazine	T48.6X1	T48.6X2	T48.6X3	T48.6X4	T48.6X5	T48.6X6
p-amino-benzoate						
Therevac*	T47.4X1	T47.4X2	T47.4X3	T47.4X4	T47.4X5	T47.4X6
Thiabendazole	T37.4X1	T37.4X2	T37.4X3	T37.4X4	T37.4X5	T37.4X6
Thialbarbital	T41.1X1	T41.1X2	T41.1X3	T41.1X4	T41.1X5	T41.1X6
Thiamazole	T38.2X1	T38.2X2	T38.2X3	T38.2X4	T38.2X5	T38.2X6
Thiambutosine	T37.1X1	T37.1X2	T37.1X3	T37.1X4	T37.1X5	T37.1X6
Thiamine	T45.2X1	T45.2X2	T45.2X3	T45.2X4	T45.2X5	T45.2X6
Thiamphenicol	T36.2X1	T36.2X2	T36.2X3	T36.2X4	T36.2X5	T36.2X6
Thiamylal	T41.1X1	T41.1X2	T41.1X3	T41.1X4	T41.1X5	T41.1X6
sodium	T41.1X1	T41.1X2	T41.1X3	T41.1X4	T41.1X5	T41.1X6
Thiazesim	T43.291	T43.292	T43.293	T43.294	T43.295	T43.296
Thiazides (diuretics)	T50.2X1	T50.2X2	T50.2X3	T50.2X4	T50.2X5	T50.2X6
Thiazinamium metilsulfate	T43.3X1	T43.3X2	T43.3X3	T43.3X4	T43.3X5	T43.3X6
Thiethylperazine	T43.3X1	T43.3X2	T43.3X3	T43.3X4	T43.3X5	T43.3X6
Thimerosal	T49.0X1	T49.0X2	T49.0X3	T49.0X4	T49.0X5	T49.0X6
ophthalmic preparation	T49.5X1	T49.5X2	T49.5X3	T49.5X4	T49.5X5	T49.5X6
Thioacetazone	T37.1X1	T37.1X2	T37.1X3	T37.1X4	T37.1X5	T37.1X6
with isoniazid	T37.1X1	T37.1X2	T37.1X3	T37.1X4	T37.1X5	T37.1X6
Thiobarbital sodium	T41.1X1	T41.1X2	T41.1X3	T41.1X4	T41.1X5	T41.1X6
Thiobarbiturate anesthetic	T41.1X1	T41.1X2	T41.1X3	T41.1X4	T41.1X5	T41.1X6
Thiobismol	T37.8X1	T37.8X2	T37.8X3	T37.8X4	T37.8X5	T37.8X6
Thiobutabarbital sodium	T41.1X1	T41.1X2	T41.1X3	T41.1X4	T41.1X5	T41.1X6
Thiocarbamate (insecticide)	T60.0X1	T60.0X2	T60.0X3	T60.0X4	—	—
Thiocarbamide	T38.2X1	T38.2X2	T38.2X3	T38.2X4	T38.2X5	T38.2X6
Thiocarbarsone	T37.8X1	T37.8X2	T37.8X3	T37.8X4	T37.8X5	T37.8X6
Thiocarlide	T37.1X1	T37.1X2	T37.1X3	T37.1X4	T37.1X5	T37.1X6
Thioctamide	T50.991	T50.992	T50.993	T50.994	T50.995	T50.996
Thioctic acid	T50.991	T50.992	T50.993	T50.994	T50.995	T50.996
Thiofos	T60.0X1	T60.0X2	T60.0X3	T60.0X4	—	—
Thioglycolate	T49.4X1	T49.4X2	T49.4X3	T49.4X4	T49.4X5	T49.4X6
Thioglycolic acid	T65.891	T65.892	T65.893	T65.894	—	—
Thioguanine	T45.1X1	T45.1X2	T45.1X3	T45.1X4	T45.1X5	T45.1X6
Thiomercaptomerin	T50.2X1	T50.2X2	T50.2X3	T50.2X4	T50.2X5	T50.2X6
Thiomerin	T50.2X1	T50.2X2	T50.2X3	T50.2X4	T50.2X5	T50.2X6
Thiomersal	T49.0X1	T49.0X2	T49.0X3	T49.0X4	T49.0X5	T49.0X6
Thionazin	T60.0X1	T60.0X2	T60.0X3	T60.0X4	—	—
Thiopental (sodium)	T41.1X1	T41.1X2	T41.1X3	T41.1X4	T41.1X5	T41.1X6
Thiopentone (sodium)	T41.1X1	T41.1X2	T41.1X3	T41.1X4	T41.1X5	T41.1X6
Thiopropazate	T43.3X1	T43.3X2	T43.3X3	T43.3X4	T43.3X5	T43.3X6
Thioproperazine	T43.3X1	T43.3X2	T43.3X3	T43.3X4	T43.3X5	T43.3X6
Thioridazine	T43.3X1	T43.3X2	T43.3X3	T43.3X4	T43.3X5	T43.3X6
Thiosinamine	T49.3X1	T49.3X2	T49.3X3	T49.3X4	T49.3X5	T49.3X6
Thiotepa	T45.1X1	T45.1X2	T45.1X3	T45.1X4	T45.1X5	T45.1X6
Thiothixene	T43.4X1	T43.4X2	T43.4X3	T43.4X4	T43.4X5	T43.4X6
Thiouracil (benzyl) (methyl) (propyl)	T38.2X1	T38.2X2	T38.2X3	T38.2X4	T38.2X5	T38.2X6
Thiourea	T38.2X1	T38.2X2	T38.2X3	T38.2X4	T38.2X5	T38.2X6
Thiphenamil	T44.3X1	T44.3X2	T44.3X3	T44.3X4	T44.3X5	T44.3X6
Thiram	T60.3X1	T60.3X2	T60.3X3	T60.3X4	—	—
medicinal	T49.2X1	T49.2X2	T49.2X3	T49.2X4	T49.2X5	T49.2X6
Thonzylamine (systemic)	T45.0X1	T45.0X2	T45.0X3	T45.0X4	T45.0X5	T45.0X6
mucosal decongestant	T48.5X1	T48.5X2	T48.5X3	T48.5X4	T48.5X5	T48.5X6
Thorazine	T43.3X1	T43.3X2	T43.3X3	T43.3X4	T43.3X5	T43.3X6
Thorium dioxide suspension	T50.8X1	T50.8X2	T50.8X3	T50.8X4	T50.8X5	T50.8X6
Thornapple	T62.2X1	T62.2X2	T62.2X3	T62.2X4	—	—
Throat drug NEC	T49.6X1	T49.6X2	T49.6X3	T49.6X4	T49.6X5	T49.6X6
Thrombate 111*	T45.511	T45.512	T45.513	T45.514	T45.515	T45.516
Thrombin	T45.7X1	T45.7X2	T45.7X3	T45.7X4	T45.7X5	T45.7X6
Thrombolysin	T45.611	T45.612	T45.613	T45.614	T45.615	T45.616
Thromboplastin	T45.7X1	T45.7X2	T45.7X3	T45.7X4	T45.7X5	T45.7X6
Thurfyl nicotinate	T46.7X1	T46.7X2	T46.7X3	T46.7X4	T46.7X5	T46.7X6
Thymol	T49.0X1	T49.0X2	T49.0X3	T49.0X4	T49.0X5	T49.0X6
Thymopentin	T37.5X1	T37.5X2	T37.5X3	T37.5X4	T37.5X5	T37.5X6
Thymoxamine	T46.7X1	T46.7X2	T46.7X3	T46.7X4	T46.7X5	T46.7X6
Thymus extract	T38.891	T38.892	T38.893	T38.894	T38.895	T38.896
Thyreotrophic hormone	T38.811	T38.812	T38.813	T38.814	T38.815	T38.816
Thyroglobulin	T38.1X1	T38.1X2	T38.1X3	T38.1X4	T38.1X5	T38.1X6
Thyroid (hormone)	T38.1X1	T38.1X2	T38.1X3	T38.1X4	T38.1X5	T38.1X6
Thyrolar	T38.1X1	T38.1X2	T38.1X3	T38.1X4	T38.1X5	T38.1X6
Thyrotrophin	T38.811	T38.812	T38.813	T38.814	T38.815	T38.816
Thyrotropic hormone	T38.811	T38.812	T38.813	T38.814	T38.815	T38.816
Thyroxine	T38.1X1	T38.1X2	T38.1X3	T38.1X4	T38.1X5	T38.1X6
Tiabendazole	T37.4X1	T37.4X2	T37.4X3	T37.4X4	T37.4X5	T37.4X6
Tiamizide	T50.2X1	T50.2X2	T50.2X3	T50.2X4	T50.2X5	T50.2X6
Tianeptine	T43.291	T43.292	T43.293	T43.294	T43.295	T43.296
Tiapamil	T46.1X1	T46.1X2	T46.1X3	T46.1X4	T46.1X5	T46.1X6
Tiapride	T43.591	T43.592	T43.593	T43.594	T43.595	T43.596
Tiaprofenic acid	T39.311	T39.312	T39.313	T39.314	T39.315	T39.316
Tiaramide	T39.8X1	T39.8X2	T39.8X3	T39.8X4	T39.8X5	T39.8X6
Ticagrelor*	T45.521	T45.522	T45.523	T45.524	T45.525	T45.526
Ticarcillin	T36.0X1	T36.0X2	T36.0X3	T36.0X4	T36.0X5	T36.0X6
Ticlatone	T49.0X1	T49.0X2	T49.0X3	T49.0X4	T49.0X5	T49.0X6
Ticlopidine	T45.521	T45.522	T45.523	T45.524	T45.525	T45.526
Ticrynafen	T50.1X1	T50.1X2	T50.1X3	T50.1X4	T50.1X5	T50.1X6
Tidiacic	T50.991	T50.992	T50.993	T50.994	T50.995	T50.996
Tiemonium	T44.3X1	T44.3X2	T44.3X3	T44.3X4	T44.3X5	T44.3X6
iodide	T44.3X1	T44.3X2	T44.3X3	T44.3X4	T44.3X5	T44.3X6
Tienilic acid	T50.1X1	T50.1X2	T50.1X3	T50.1X4	T50.1X5	T50.1X6
Tifenamil	T44.3X1	T44.3X2	T44.3X3	T44.3X4	T44.3X5	T44.3X6
Tigan	T45.0X1	T45.0X2	T45.0X3	T45.0X4	T45.0X5	T45.0X6
Tigloidine	T44.3X1	T44.3X2	T44.3X3	T44.3X4	T44.3X5	T44.3X6
Tilactase	T47.5X1	T47.5X2	T47.5X3	T47.5X4	T47.5X5	T47.5X6
Tiletamine	T41.291	T41.292	T41.293	T41.294	T41.295	T41.296
Tilidine	T40.491	T40.492	T40.493	T40.494	—	—
Timepidium bromide	T44.3X1	T44.3X2	T44.3X3	T44.3X4	T44.3X5	T44.3X6
Timiperone	T43.4X1	T43.4X2	T43.4X3	T43.4X4	T43.4X5	T43.4X6
Timolol	T44.7X1	T44.7X2	T44.7X3	T44.7X4	T44.7X5	T44.7X6
Tin (chloride) (dust) (oxide) NEC	T56.6X1	T56.6X2	T56.6X3	T56.6X4	—	—
anti-infectives	T37.8X1	T37.8X2	T37.8X3	T37.8X4	T37.8X5	T37.8X6
Tincture, iodine — see Iodine						
Tindal	T43.3X1	T43.3X2	T43.3X3	T43.3X4	T43.3X5	T43.3X6

Substance	Poisoning, Accidental (unintentional)	Poisoning, Intentional Self-harm	Poisoning, Assault	Poisoning, Undetermined	Adverse Effect	Under-dosing
Tinidazole	T37.3X1	T37.3X2	T37.3X3	T37.3X4	T37.3X5	T37.3X6
Tinoridine	T39.8X1	T39.8X2	T39.8X3	T39.8X4	T39.8X5	T39.8X6
Tiocarlide	T37.1X1	T37.1X2	T37.1X3	T37.1X4	T37.1X5	T37.1X6
Tioclomarol	T45.511	T45.512	T45.513	T45.514	T45.515	T45.516
Tioconazole	T49.0X1	T49.0X2	T49.0X3	T49.0X4	T49.0X5	T49.0X6
Tioguanine	T45.1X1	T45.1X2	T45.1X3	T45.1X4	T45.1X5	T45.1X6
Tiopronin	T50.991	T50.992	T50.993	T50.994	T50.995	T50.996
Tiotixene	T43.4X1	T43.4X2	T43.4X3	T43.4X4	T43.4X5	T43.4X6
Tioxolone	T49.4X1	T49.4X2	T49.4X3	T49.4X4	T49.4X5	T49.4X6
Tipepidine	T48.3X1	T48.3X2	T48.3X3	T48.3X4	T48.3X5	T48.3X6
Tiquizium bromide	T44.3X1	T44.3X2	T44.3X3	T44.3X4	T44.3X5	T44.3X6
Tiratricol	T38.1X1	T38.1X2	T38.1X3	T38.1X4	T38.1X5	T38.1X6
Tisopurine	T50.4X1	T50.4X2	T50.4X3	T50.4X4	T50.4X5	T50.4X6
Titanium (compounds) (vapor)	T56.891	T56.892	T56.893	T56.894	—	—
dioxide	T49.3X1	T49.3X2	T49.3X3	T49.3X4	T49.3X5	T49.3X6
ointment	T49.3X1	T49.3X2	T49.3X3	T49.3X4	T49.3X5	T49.3X6
oxide	T49.3X1	T49.3X2	T49.3X3	T49.3X4	T49.3X5	T49.3X6
tetrachloride	T56.891	T56.892	T56.893	T56.894	—	—
Titanocene	T56.891	T56.892	T56.893	T56.894	—	—
Titroid	T38.1X1	T38.1X2	T38.1X3	T38.1X4	T38.1X5	T38.1X6
Tizanidine	T42.8X1	T42.8X2	T42.8X3	T42.8X4	T42.8X5	T42.8X6
TMTD	T60.3X1	T60.3X2	T60.3X3	T60.3X4	—	—
TNT (fumes)	T65.3X1	T65.3X2	T65.3X3	T65.3X4	—	—
Toadstool	T62.0X1	T62.0X2	T62.0X3	T62.0X4	—	—
Tobacco NEC	T65.291	T65.292	T65.293	T65.294	—	—
cigarettes	T65.221	T65.222	T65.223	T65.224	—	—
Indian	T62.2X1	T62.2X2	T62.2X3	T62.2X4	—	—
smoke, second-hand	T65.221	T65.222	T65.223	T65.224	—	—
Tobraflex*	T49.5X1	T49.5X2	T49.5X3	T49.5X4	T49.5X5	T49.5X6
Tobramycin	T36.5X1	T36.5X2	T36.5X3	T36.5X4	T36.5X5	T36.5X6
Tocainide	T46.2X1	T46.2X2	T46.2X3	T46.2X4	T46.2X5	T46.2X6
Tocoferol	T45.2X1	T45.2X2	T45.2X3	T45.2X4	T45.2X5	T45.2X6
Tocopherol	T45.2X1	T45.2X2	T45.2X3	T45.2X4	T45.2X5	T45.2X6
acetate	T45.2X1	T45.2X2	T45.2X3	T45.2X4	T45.2X5	T45.2X6
Tocosamine	T48.0X1	T48.0X2	T48.0X3	T48.0X4	T48.0X5	T48.0X6
Todralazine	T46.5X1	T46.5X2	T46.5X3	T46.5X4	T46.5X5	T46.5X6
Tofisopam	T42.4X1	T42.4X2	T42.4X3	T42.4X4	T42.4X5	T42.4X6
Tofranil	T43.011	T43.012	T43.013	T43.014	T43.015	T43.016
Toilet deodorizer	T65.891	T65.892	T65.893	T65.894	—	—
Tolamolol	T44.7X1	T44.7X2	T44.7X3	T44.7X4	T44.7X5	T44.7X6
Tolazamide	T38.3X1	T38.3X2	T38.3X3	T38.3X4	T38.3X5	T38.3X6
Tolazoline	T46.7X1	T46.7X2	T46.7X3	T46.7X4	T46.7X5	T46.7X6
Tolbutamide (sodium)	T38.3X1	T38.3X2	T38.3X3	T38.3X4	T38.3X5	T38.3X6
Tolciclate	T49.0X1	T49.0X2	T49.0X3	T49.0X4	T49.0X5	T49.0X6
Tolmetin	T39.391	T39.392	T39.393	T39.394	T39.395	T39.396
Tolnaftate	T49.0X1	T49.0X2	T49.0X3	T49.0X4	T49.0X5	T49.0X6
Tolonidine	T46.5X1	T46.5X2	T46.5X3	T46.5X4	T46.5X5	T46.5X6
Toloxatone	T42.6X1	T42.6X2	T42.6X3	T42.6X4	T42.6X5	T42.6X6
Tolperisone	T44.3X1	T44.3X2	T44.3X3	T44.3X4	T44.3X5	T44.3X6
Tolserol	T42.8X1	T42.8X2	T42.8X3	T42.8X4	T42.8X5	T42.8X6
Toluene (liquid)	T52.2X1	T52.2X2	T52.2X3	T52.2X4	—	—
diisocyanate	T65.0X1	T65.0X2	T65.0X3	T65.0X4	—	—
Toluidine	T65.891	T65.892	T65.893	T65.894	—	—
vapor	T59.891	T59.892	T59.893	T59.894	—	—
Toluol (liquid)	T52.2X1	T52.2X2	T52.2X3	T52.2X4	—	—
vapor	T52.2X1	T52.2X2	T52.2X3	T52.2X4	—	—
Toluylenediamine	T65.3X1	T65.3X2	T65.3X3	T65.3X4	—	—
Tolylene-2,4-diisocyanate	T65.0X1	T65.0X2	T65.0X3	T65.0X4	—	—
Tonic NEC	T50.901	T50.902	T50.903	T50.904	T50.905	T50.906
Topical action drug NEC	T49.91	T49.92	T49.93	T49.94	T49.95	T49.96
ear, nose or throat	T49.6X1	T49.6X2	T49.6X3	T49.6X4	T49.6X5	T49.6X6
eye	T49.5X1	T49.5X2	T49.5X3	T49.5X4	T49.5X5	T49.5X6
skin	T49.91	T49.92	T49.93	T49.94	T49.95	T49.96
specified NEC	T49.8X1	T49.8X2	T49.8X3	T49.8X4	T49.8X5	T49.8X6
Toprol*	T44.7X1	T44.7X2	T44.7X3	T44.7X4	T44.7X5	T44.7X6
Toquizine	T44.3X1	T44.3X2	T44.3X3	T44.3X4	T44.3X5	T44.3X6
Toremifene	T38.6X1	T38.6X2	T38.6X3	T38.6X4	T38.6X5	T38.6X6
Tosylchloramide sodium	T49.8X1	T49.8X2	T49.8X3	T49.8X4	T49.8X5	T49.8X6
Toxaphene (dust) (spray)	T60.1X1	T60.1X2	T60.1X3	T60.1X4	—	—
Toxin, diphtheria (Schick Test)	T50.8X1	T50.8X2	T50.8X3	T50.8X4	T50.8X5	T50.8X6
Toxoid						
combined	T50.A21	T50.A22	T50.A23	T50.A24	T50.A25	T50.A26
diphtheria	T50.A91	T50.A92	T50.A93	T50.A94	T50.A95	T50.A96
tetanus	T50.A91	T50.A92	T50.A93	T50.A94	T50.A95	T50.A96
Trace element NEC	T45.8X1	T45.8X2	T45.8X3	T45.8X4	T45.8X5	T45.8X6
Tractor fuel NEC	T52.0X1	T52.0X2	T52.0X3	T52.0X4	—	—
Tragacanth	T50.991	T50.992	T50.993	T50.994	T50.995	T50.996
Tramadol	T40.421	T40.422	T40.423	T40.424	T40.425	T40.426
Tramazoline	T48.5X1	T48.5X2	T48.5X3	T48.5X4	T48.5X5	T48.5X6
Tranexamic acid	T45.621	T45.622	T45.623	T45.624	T45.625	T45.626
Tranilast	T45.0X1	T45.0X2	T45.0X3	T45.0X4	T45.0X5	T45.0X6

Substance	Poisoning, Accidental (unintentional)	Poisoning, Intentional Self-harm	Poisoning, Assault	Poisoning, Undetermined	Adverse Effect	Under-dosing
Tranquilizer NEC	T43.501	T43.502	T43.503	T43.504	T43.505	T43.506
with hypnotic or sedative	T42.6X1	T42.6X2	T42.6X3	T42.6X4	T42.6X5	T42.6X6
benzodiazepine NEC	T42.4X1	T42.4X2	T42.4X3	T42.4X4	T42.4X5	T42.4X6
butyrophenone NEC	T43.4X1	T43.4X2	T43.4X3	T43.4X4	T43.4X5	T43.4X6
carbamate	T43.591	T43.592	T43.593	T43.594	T43.595	T43.596
dimethylamine	T43.3X1	T43.3X2	T43.3X3	T43.3X4	T43.3X5	T43.3X6
ethylamine	T43.3X1	T43.3X2	T43.3X3	T43.3X4	T43.3X5	T43.3X6
hydroxyzine	T43.591	T43.592	T43.593	T43.594	T43.595	T43.596
major NEC	T43.501	T43.502	T43.503	T43.504	T43.505	T43.506
penothiazine NEC	T43.3X1	T43.3X2	T43.3X3	T43.3X4	T43.3X5	T43.3X6
phenothiazine-based	T43.3X1	T43.3X2	T43.3X3	T43.3X4	T43.3X5	T43.3X6
piperazine NEC	T43.3X1	T43.3X2	T43.3X3	T43.3X4	T43.3X5	T43.3X6
piperidine	T43.3X1	T43.3X2	T43.3X3	T43.3X4	T43.3X5	T43.3X6
propylamine	T43.3X1	T43.3X2	T43.3X3	T43.3X4	T43.3X5	T43.3X6
specified NEC	T43.591	T43.592	T43.593	T43.594	T43.595	T43.596
thioxanthene NEC	T43.591	T43.592	T43.593	T43.594	T43.595	T43.596
Tranxene	T42.4X1	T42.4X2	T42.4X3	T42.4X4	T42.4X5	T42.4X6
Tranylcypromine	T43.1X1	T43.1X2	T43.1X3	T43.1X4	T43.1X5	T43.1X6
Trapidil	T46.3X1	T46.3X2	T46.3X3	T46.3X4	T46.3X5	T46.3X6
Trasentine	T44.3X1	T44.3X2	T44.3X3	T44.3X4	T44.3X5	T44.3X6
Travert	T50.3X1	T50.3X2	T50.3X3	T50.3X4	T50.3X5	T50.3X6
Trazodone	T43.211	T43.212	T43.213	T43.214	T43.215	T43.216
Treanda*	T45.1X1	T45.1X2	T45.1X3	T45.1X4	T45.1X5	T45.1X6
Trecator	T37.1X1	T37.1X2	T37.1X3	T37.1X4	T37.1X5	T37.1X6
Treosulfan	T45.1X1	T45.1X2	T45.1X3	T45.1X4	T45.1X5	T45.1X6
Tretamine	T45.1X1	T45.1X2	T45.1X3	T45.1X4	T45.1X5	T45.1X6
Tretinoin	T49.0X1	T49.0X2	T49.0X3	T49.0X4	T49.0X5	T49.0X6
Tretoquinol	T48.6X1	T48.6X2	T48.6X3	T48.6X4	T48.6X5	T48.6X6
Triacetin	T49.0X1	T49.0X2	T49.0X3	T49.0X4	T49.0X5	T49.0X6
Triacetoxyanthracene	T49.4X1	T49.4X2	T49.4X3	T49.4X4	T49.4X5	T49.4X6
Triacetyloleandomycin	T36.3X1	T36.3X2	T36.3X3	T36.3X4	T36.3X5	T36.3X6
Triamcinolone	T38.0X1	T38.0X2	T38.0X3	T38.0X4	T38.0X5	T38.0X6
ENT agent	T49.6X1	T49.6X2	T49.6X3	T49.6X4	T49.6X5	T49.6X6
hexacetonide	T49.0X1	T49.0X2	T49.0X3	T49.0X4	T49.0X5	T49.0X6
ophthalmic preparation	T49.5X1	T49.5X2	T49.5X3	T49.5X4	T49.5X5	T49.5X6
topical NEC	T49.0X1	T49.0X2	T49.0X3	T49.0X4	T49.0X5	T49.0X6
Triampyzine	T44.3X1	T44.3X2	T44.3X3	T44.3X4	T44.3X5	T44.3X6
Triamterene	T50.2X1	T50.2X2	T50.2X3	T50.2X4	T50.2X5	T50.2X6
Triazine (herbicide)	T60.3X1	T60.3X2	T60.3X3	T60.3X4	—	—
Triaziquone	T45.1X1	T45.1X2	T45.1X3	T45.1X4	T45.1X5	T45.1X6
Triazolam	T42.4X1	T42.4X2	T42.4X3	T42.4X4	T42.4X5	T42.4X6
Triazole (herbicide)	T60.3X1	T60.3X2	T60.3X3	T60.3X4	—	—
Tribavirin*	T37.5X1	T37.5X2	T37.5X3	T37.5X4	T37.5X5	T37.5X6
Tribenoside	T46.991	T46.992	T46.993	T46.994	T46.995	T46.996
Tribromacetaldehyde	T42.6X1	T42.6X2	T42.6X3	T42.6X4	T42.6X5	T42.6X6
Tribromoethanol, rectal	T41.291	T41.292	T41.293	T41.294	T41.295	T41.296
Tribromomethane	T42.6X1	T42.6X2	T42.6X3	T42.6X4	T42.6X5	T42.6X6
Trichlorethane	T53.2X1	T53.2X2	T53.2X3	T53.2X4	—	—
Trichlorethylene	T53.2X1	T53.2X2	T53.2X3	T53.2X4	—	—
Trichlorfon	T60.0X1	T60.0X2	T60.0X3	T60.0X4	—	—
Trichlormethiazide	T50.2X1	T50.2X2	T50.2X3	T50.2X4	T50.2X5	T50.2X6
Trichlormethine	T45.1X1	T45.1X2	T45.1X3	T45.1X4	T45.1X5	T45.1X6
Trichloroacetic acid, Trichloracetic acid	T54.2X1	T54.2X2	T54.2X3	T54.2X4	—	—
medicinal	T49.4X1	T49.4X2	T49.4X3	T49.4X4	T49.4X5	T49.4X6
Trichloroethane	T53.2X1	T53.2X2	T53.2X3	T53.2X4	—	—
Trichloroethanol	T42.6X1	T42.6X2	T42.6X3	T42.6X4	T42.6X5	T42.6X6
Trichloroethyl phosphate	T42.6X1	T42.6X2	T42.6X3	T42.6X4	T42.6X5	T42.6X6
Trichloroethylene (liquid) (vapor)	T53.2X1	T53.2X2	T53.2X3	T53.2X4	—	—
anesthetic (gas)	T41.0X1	T41.0X2	T41.0X3	T41.0X4	T41.0X5	T41.0X6
vapor NEC	T53.2X1	T53.2X2	T53.2X3	T53.2X4	—	—
Trichlorofluoromethane NEC	T53.5X1	T53.5X2	T53.5X3	T53.5X4	—	—
Trichloronate	T60.0X1	T60.0X2	T60.0X3	T60.0X4	—	—
Trichloropropane	T53.6X1	T53.6X2	T53.6X3	T53.6X4	—	—
Trichlorotriethylamine	T45.1X1	T45.1X2	T45.1X3	T45.1X4	T45.1X5	T45.1X6
Trichomonacides NEC	T37.3X1	T37.3X2	T37.3X3	T37.3X4	T37.3X5	T37.3X6
Trichomycin	T36.7X1	T36.7X2	T36.7X3	T36.7X4	T36.7X5	T36.7X6
Triclobisonium chloride	T49.0X1	T49.0X2	T49.0X3	T49.0X4	T49.0X5	T49.0X6
Triclocarban	T49.0X1	T49.0X2	T49.0X3	T49.0X4	T49.0X5	T49.0X6
Triclofos	T42.6X1	T42.6X2	T42.6X3	T42.6X4	T42.6X5	T42.6X6
Triclosan	T49.0X1	T49.0X2	T49.0X3	T49.0X4	T49.0X5	T49.0X6
Tricosal*	T39.091	T39.092	T39.093	T39.094	T39.095	T39.096
Tricresyl phosphate	T65.891	T65.892	T65.893	T65.894	—	—
solvent	T52.91	T52.92	T52.93	T52.94	—	—
Tricyclamol chloride	T44.3X1	T44.3X2	T44.3X3	T44.3X4	T44.3X5	T44.3X6
Tridesilon	T49.0X1	T49.0X2	T49.0X3	T49.0X4	T49.0X5	T49.0X6
Tridihexethyl iodide	T44.3X1	T44.3X2	T44.3X3	T44.3X4	T44.3X5	T44.3X6
Tridione	T42.2X1	T42.2X2	T42.2X3	T42.2X4	T42.2X5	T42.2X6
Trientine	T45.8X1	T45.8X2	T45.8X3	T45.8X4	T45.8X5	T45.8X6
Triethanolamine NEC	T54.3X1	T54.3X2	T54.3X3	T54.3X4	—	—
detergent	T54.3X1	T54.3X2	T54.3X3	T54.3X4	—	—

*Optum Value-Add

☑ Additional Character May Be Required — Refer to the Tabular List for Character Selection

407

Table of Drugs and Chemicals

Tinidazole — Triethanolamine NEC

Substance	Poisoning, Accidental (unintentional)	Poisoning, Intentional Self-harm	Poisoning, Assault	Poisoning, Undetermined	Adverse Effect	Under-dosing
Triethanolamine — *continued*						
trinitrate (biphosphate)	T46.3X1	T46.3X2	T46.3X3	T46.3X4	T46.3X5	T46.3X6
Triethanomelamine	T45.1X1	T45.1X2	T45.1X3	T45.1X4	T45.1X5	T45.1X6
Triethylenemelamine	T45.1X1	T45.1X2	T45.1X3	T45.1X4	T45.1X5	T45.1X6
Triethylenephosphoramide	T45.1X1	T45.1X2	T45.1X3	T45.1X4	T45.1X5	T45.1X6
Triethylenethiophosphoramide	T45.1X1	T45.1X2	T45.1X3	T45.1X4	T45.1X5	T45.1X6
Trifluoperazine	T43.3X1	T43.3X2	T43.3X3	T43.3X4	T43.3X5	T43.3X6
Trifluoroethyl vinyl ether	T41.ØX1	T41.ØX2	T41.ØX3	T41.ØX4	T41.ØX5	T41.ØX6
Trifluperidol	T43.4X1	T43.4X2	T43.4X3	T43.4X4	T43.4X5	T43.4X6
Triflupromazine	T43.3X1	T43.3X2	T43.3X3	T43.3X4	T43.3X5	T43.3X6
Trifluridine	T37.5X1	T37.5X2	T37.5X3	T37.5X4	T37.5X5	T37.5X6
Triflusal	T45.521	T45.522	T45.523	T45.524	T45.525	T45.526
Trihexyphenidyl	T44.3X1	T44.3X2	T44.3X3	T44.3X4	T44.3X5	T44.3X6
Triiodothyronine	T38.1X1	T38.1X2	T38.1X3	T38.1X4	T38.1X5	T38.1X6
Trilene	T41.ØX1	T41.ØX2	T41.ØX3	T41.ØX4	T41.ØX5	T41.ØX6
Trilostane	T38.991	T38.992	T38.993	T38.994	T38.995	T38.996
Trimebutine	T44.3X1	T44.3X2	T44.3X3	T44.3X4	T44.3X5	T44.3X6
Trimecaine	T41.3X1	T41.3X2	T41.3X3	T41.3X4	T41.3X5	T41.3X6
Trimeprazine (tartrate)	T44.3X1	T44.3X2	T44.3X3	T44.3X4	T44.3X5	T44.3X6
Trimetaphan camsilate	T44.2X1	T44.2X2	T44.2X3	T44.2X4	T44.2X5	T44.2X6
Trimetazidine	T46.7X1	T46.7X2	T46.7X3	T46.7X4	T46.7X5	T46.7X6
Trimethadione	T42.2X1	T42.2X2	T42.2X3	T42.2X4	T42.2X5	T42.2X6
Trimethaphan	T44.2X1	T44.2X2	T44.2X3	T44.2X4	T44.2X5	T44.2X6
Trimethidinium	T44.2X1	T44.2X2	T44.2X3	T44.2X4	T44.2X5	T44.2X6
Trimethobenzamide	T45.ØX1	T45.ØX2	T45.ØX3	T45.ØX4	T45.ØX5	T45.ØX6
Trimethoprim	T37.8X1	T37.8X2	T37.8X3	T37.8X4	T37.8X5	T37.8X6
with sulfamethoxazole	T36.8X1	T36.8X2	T36.8X3	T36.8X4	T36.8X5	T36.8X6
Trimethylcarbinol	T51.3X1	T51.3X2	T51.3X3	T51.3X4	—	—
Trimethylpsoralen	T49.3X1	T49.3X2	T49.3X3	T49.3X4	T49.3X5	T49.3X6
Trimeton	T45.ØX1	T45.ØX2	T45.ØX3	T45.ØX4	T45.ØX5	T45.ØX6
Trimetrexate	T45.1X1	T45.1X2	T45.1X3	T45.1X4	T45.1X5	T45.1X6
Trimipramine	T43.Ø11	T43.Ø12	T43.Ø13	T43.Ø14	T43.Ø15	T43.Ø16
Trimox*	T36.ØX1	T36.ØX2	T36.ØX3	T36.ØX4	T36.ØX5	T36.ØX6
Trimustine	T45.1X1	T45.1X2	T45.1X3	T45.1X4	T45.1X5	T45.1X6
Trinitrine	T46.3X1	T46.3X2	T46.3X3	T46.3X4	T46.3X5	T46.3X6
Trinitrobenzol	T65.3X1	T65.3X2	T65.3X3	T65.3X4	—	—
Trinitrophenol	T65.3X1	T65.3X2	T65.3X3	T65.3X4	—	—
Trinitrotoluene (fumes)	T65.3X1	T65.3X2	T65.3X3	T65.3X4	—	—
Trional	T42.6X1	T42.6X2	T42.6X3	T42.6X4	T42.6X5	T42.6X6
Triorthocresyl phosphate	T65.891	T65.892	T65.893	T65.894	—	—
Trioxide of arsenic	T57.ØX1	T57.ØX2	T57.ØX3	T57.ØX4	—	—
Trioxysalen	T49.4X1	T49.4X2	T49.4X3	T49.4X4	T49.4X5	T49.4X6
Tripamide	T5Ø.2X1	T5Ø.2X2	T5Ø.2X3	T5Ø.2X4	T5Ø.2X5	T5Ø.2X6
Triparanol	T46.6X1	T46.6X2	T46.6X3	T46.6X4	T46.6X5	T46.6X6
Tripelennamine	T45.ØX1	T45.ØX2	T45.ØX3	T45.ØX4	T45.ØX5	T45.ØX6
Triperiden	T44.3X1	T44.3X2	T44.3X3	T44.3X4	T44.3X5	T44.3X6
Triperidol	T43.4X1	T43.4X2	T43.4X3	T43.4X4	T43.4X5	T43.4X6
Triphenylphosphate	T65.891	T65.892	T65.893	T65.894	—	—
Triple						
bromides	T42.6X1	T42.6X2	T42.6X3	T42.6X4	T42.6X5	T42.6X6
carbonate	T47.1X1	T47.1X2	T47.1X3	T47.1X4	T47.1X5	T47.1X6
vaccine						
DPT	T5Ø.A11	T5Ø.A12	T5Ø.A13	T5Ø.A14	T5Ø.A15	T5Ø.A16
including pertussis	T5Ø.A11	T5Ø.A12	T5Ø.A13	T5Ø.A14	T5Ø.A15	T5Ø.A16
MMR	T5Ø.B91	T5Ø.B92	T5Ø.B93	T5Ø.B94	T5Ø.B95	T5Ø.B96
Triprolidine	T45.ØX1	T45.ØX2	T45.ØX3	T45.ØX4	T45.ØX5	T45.ØX6
Trisodium hydrogen edetate	T5Ø.6X1	T5Ø.6X2	T5Ø.6X3	T5Ø.6X4	T5Ø.6X5	T5Ø.6X6
Trisoralen	T49.3X1	T49.3X2	T49.3X3	T49.3X4	T49.3X5	T49.3X6
Trisulfapyrimidines	T37.ØX1	T37.ØX2	T37.ØX3	T37.ØX4	T37.ØX5	T37.ØX6
Trithiozine	T44.3X1	T44.3X2	T44.3X3	T44.3X4	T44.3X5	T44.3X6
Tritiozine	T44.3X1	T44.3X2	T44.3X3	T44.3X4	T44.3X5	T44.3X6
Tritoqualine	T45.ØX1	T45.ØX2	T45.ØX3	T45.ØX4	T45.ØX5	T45.ØX6
Trizivir*	T37.5X1	T37.5X2	T37.5X3	T37.5X4	T37.5X5	T37.5X6
Trofosfamide	T45.1X1	T45.1X2	T45.1X3	T45.1X4	T45.1X5	T45.1X6
Troleandomycin	T36.3X1	T36.3X2	T36.3X3	T36.3X4	T36.3X5	T36.3X6
Trolnitrate (phosphate)	T46.3X1	T46.3X2	T46.3X3	T46.3X4	T46.3X5	T46.3X6
Tromantadine	T37.5X1	T37.5X2	T37.5X3	T37.5X4	T37.5X5	T37.5X6
Trometamol	T5Ø.2X1	T5Ø.2X2	T5Ø.2X3	T5Ø.2X4	T5Ø.2X5	T5Ø.2X6
Tromethamine	T5Ø.2X1	T5Ø.2X2	T5Ø.2X3	T5Ø.2X4	T5Ø.2X5	T5Ø.2X6
Tronothane	T41.3X1	T41.3X2	T41.3X3	T41.3X4	T41.3X5	T41.3X6
Tropacine	T44.3X1	T44.3X2	T44.3X3	T44.3X4	T44.3X5	T44.3X6
Tropatepine	T44.3X1	T44.3X2	T44.3X3	T44.3X4	T44.3X5	T44.3X6
Tropicamide	T44.3X1	T44.3X2	T44.3X3	T44.3X4	T44.3X5	T44.3X6
Trospium chloride	T44.3X1	T44.3X2	T44.3X3	T44.3X4	T44.3X5	T44.3X6
Troxerutin	T46.991	T46.992	T46.993	T46.994	T46.995	T46.996
Troxidone	T42.2X1	T42.2X2	T42.2X3	T42.2X4	T42.2X5	T42.2X6
Tryparsamide	T37.3X1	T37.3X2	T37.3X3	T37.3X4	T37.3X5	T37.3X6
Trypsin	T45.3X1	T45.3X2	T45.3X3	T45.3X4	T45.3X5	T45.3X6
Tryptizol	T43.Ø11	T43.Ø12	T43.Ø13	T43.Ø14	T43.Ø15	T43.Ø16
TSH	T38.811	T38.812	T38.813	T38.814	T38.815	T38.816
Tuaminoheptane	T48.5X1	T48.5X2	T48.5X3	T48.5X4	T48.5X5	T48.5X6

Substance	Poisoning, Accidental (unintentional)	Poisoning, Intentional Self-harm	Poisoning, Assault	Poisoning, Undetermined	Adverse Effect	Under-dosing
Tuberculin, purified protein derivative (PPD)	T5Ø.8X1	T5Ø.8X2	T5Ø.8X3	T5Ø.8X4	T5Ø.8X5	T5Ø.8X6
Tubocurare	T48.1X1	T48.1X2	T48.1X3	T48.1X4	T48.1X5	T48.1X6
Tubocurarine (chloride)	T48.1X1	T48.1X2	T48.1X3	T48.1X4	T48.1X5	T48.1X6
Tulobuterol	T48.6X1	T48.6X2	T48.6X3	T48.6X4	T48.6X5	T48.6X6
Turpentine (spirits of)	T52.8X1	T52.8X2	T52.8X3	T52.8X4	—	—
vapor	T52.8X1	T52.8X2	T52.8X3	T52.8X4	—	—
Twinrix*	T5Ø.B91	T5Ø.B92	T5Ø.B93	T5Ø.B94	T5Ø.B95	T5Ø.B96
Tybamate	T43.591	T43.592	T43.593	T43.594	T43.595	T43.596
Tygacil*	T36.4X1	T36.4X2	T36.4X3	T36.4X4	T36.4X5	T36.4X6
Tyloxapol	T48.4X1	T48.4X2	T48.4X3	T48.4X4	T48.4X5	T48.4X6
Tymazoline	T48.5X1	T48.5X2	T48.5X3	T48.5X4	T48.5X5	T48.5X6
Tymlos*	T5Ø.991	T5Ø.992	T5Ø.993	T5Ø.994	T5Ø.995	T5Ø.996
Typhoid-paratyphoid vaccine	T5Ø.A91	T5Ø.A92	T5Ø.A93	T5Ø.A94	T5Ø.A95	T5Ø.A96
Typhus vaccine	T5Ø.A91	T5Ø.A92	T5Ø.A93	T5Ø.A94	T5Ø.A95	T5Ø.A96
Tyropanoate	T5Ø.8X1	T5Ø.8X2	T5Ø.8X3	T5Ø.8X4	T5Ø.8X5	T5Ø.8X6
Tyrothricin	T49.6X1	T49.6X2	T49.6X3	T49.6X4	T49.6X5	T49.6X6
ENT agent	T49.6X1	T49.6X2	T49.6X3	T49.6X4	T49.6X5	T49.6X6
ophthalmic preparation	T49.5X1	T49.5X2	T49.5X3	T49.5X4	T49.5X5	T49.5X6
Ufenamate	T39.391	T39.392	T39.393	T39.394	T39.395	T39.396
Ultraviolet light protectant	T49.3X1	T49.3X2	T49.3X3	T49.3X4	T49.3X5	T49.3X6
Unasyn*	T36.ØX1	T36.ØX2	T36.ØX3	T36.ØX4	T36.ØX5	T36.ØX6
Undecenoic acid	T49.ØX1	T49.ØX2	T49.ØX3	T49.ØX4	T49.ØX5	T49.ØX6
Undecoylium	T49.ØX1	T49.ØX2	T49.ØX3	T49.ØX4	T49.ØX5	T49.ØX6
Undecylenic acid (derivatives)	T49.ØX1	T49.ØX2	T49.ØX3	T49.ØX4	T49.ØX5	T49.ØX6
Unithroid*	T38.1X1	T38.1X2	T38.1X3	T38.1X4	T38.1X5	T38.1X6
Unna's boot	T49.3X1	T49.3X2	T49.3X3	T49.3X4	T49.3X5	T49.3X6
Unsaturated fatty acid	T46.6X1	T46.6X2	T46.6X3	T46.6X4	T46.6X5	T46.6X6
Uracil mustard	T45.1X1	T45.1X2	T45.1X3	T45.1X4	T45.1X5	T45.1X6
Uramustine	T45.1X1	T45.1X2	T45.1X3	T45.1X4	T45.1X5	T45.1X6
Urapidil	T46.5X1	T46.5X2	T46.5X3	T46.5X4	T46.5X5	T46.5X6
Urari	T48.1X1	T48.1X2	T48.1X3	T48.1X4	T48.1X5	T48.1X6
Urate oxidase	T5Ø.4X1	T5Ø.4X2	T5Ø.4X3	T5Ø.4X4	T5Ø.4X5	T5Ø.4X6
Urea	T47.3X1	T47.3X2	T47.3X3	T47.3X4	T47.3X5	T47.3X6
peroxide	T49.ØX1	T49.ØX2	T49.ØX3	T49.ØX4	T49.ØX5	T49.ØX6
stibamine	T37.4X1	T37.4X2	T37.4X3	T37.4X4	T37.4X5	T37.4X6
topical	T49.8X1	T49.8X2	T49.8X3	T49.8X4	T49.8X5	T49.8X6
Ureaphil*	T48.ØX1	T48.ØX2	T48.ØX3	T48.ØX4	T48.ØX5	T48.ØX6
Urethane	T45.1X1	T45.1X2	T45.1X3	T45.1X4	T45.1X5	T45.1X6
Urginea (maritima) (scilla) — *see* Squill						
Uric acid metabolism drug NEC	T5Ø.4X1	T5Ø.4X2	T5Ø.4X3	T5Ø.4X4	T5Ø.4X5	T5Ø.4X6
Uricosuric agent	T5Ø.4X1	T5Ø.4X2	T5Ø.4X3	T5Ø.4X4	T5Ø.4X5	T5Ø.4X6
Urinary anti-infective	T37.8X1	T37.8X2	T37.8X3	T37.8X4	T37.8X5	T37.8X6
Urofollitropin	T38.811	T38.812	T38.813	T38.814	T38.815	T38.816
Urokinase	T45.611	T45.612	T45.613	T45.614	T45.615	T45.616
Urokon	T5Ø.8X1	T5Ø.8X2	T5Ø.8X3	T5Ø.8X4	T5Ø.8X5	T5Ø.8X6
Ursodeoxycholic acid	T5Ø.991	T5Ø.992	T5Ø.993	T5Ø.994	T5Ø.995	T5Ø.996
Ursodiol	T5Ø.991	T5Ø.992	T5Ø.993	T5Ø.994	T5Ø.995	T5Ø.996
Urtica	T62.2X1	T62.2X2	T62.2X3	T62.2X4	—	—
Utility gas — *see* Gas, utility						
Vaccine NEC	T5Ø.Z91	T5Ø.Z92	T5Ø.Z93	T5Ø.Z94	T5Ø.Z95	T5Ø.Z96
antineoplastic	T5Ø.Z91	T5Ø.Z92	T5Ø.Z93	T5Ø.Z94	T5Ø.Z95	T5Ø.Z96
bacterial NEC	T5Ø.A91	T5Ø.A92	T5Ø.A93	T5Ø.A94	T5Ø.A95	T5Ø.A96
mixed NEC	T5Ø.A21	T5Ø.A22	T5Ø.A23	T5Ø.A24	T5Ø.A25	T5Ø.A26
with						
other bacterial component	T5Ø.A21	T5Ø.A22	T5Ø.A23	T5Ø.A24	T5Ø.A25	T5Ø.A26
pertussis component	T5Ø.A11	T5Ø.A12	T5Ø.A13	T5Ø.A14	T5Ø.A15	T5Ø.A16
viral-rickettsial component	T5Ø.A21	T5Ø.A22	T5Ø.A23	T5Ø.A24	T5Ø.A25	T5Ø.A26
BCG	T5Ø.A91	T5Ø.A92	T5Ø.A93	T5Ø.A94	T5Ø.A95	T5Ø.A96
cholera	T5Ø.A91	T5Ø.A92	T5Ø.A93	T5Ø.A94	T5Ø.A95	T5Ø.A96
diphtheria	T5Ø.A91	T5Ø.A92	T5Ø.A93	T5Ø.A94	T5Ø.A95	T5Ø.A96
with tetanus	T5Ø.A21	T5Ø.A22	T5Ø.A23	T5Ø.A24	T5Ø.A25	T5Ø.A26
and pertussis	T5Ø.A11	T5Ø.A12	T5Ø.A13	T5Ø.A14	T5Ø.A15	T5Ø.A16
influenza	T5Ø.B91	T5Ø.B92	T5Ø.B93	T5Ø.B94	T5Ø.B95	T5Ø.B96
measles	T5Ø.B91	T5Ø.B92	T5Ø.B93	T5Ø.B94	T5Ø.B95	T5Ø.B96
with mumps and rubella	T5Ø.B91	T5Ø.B92	T5Ø.B93	T5Ø.B94	T5Ø.B95	T5Ø.B96
meningococcal	T5Ø.A91	T5Ø.A92	T5Ø.A93	T5Ø.A94	T5Ø.A95	T5Ø.A96
mumps	T5Ø.B91	T5Ø.B92	T5Ø.B93	T5Ø.B94	T5Ø.B95	T5Ø.B96
paratyphoid	T5Ø.A91	T5Ø.A92	T5Ø.A93	T5Ø.A94	T5Ø.A95	T5Ø.A96
pertussis	T5Ø.A11	T5Ø.A12	T5Ø.A13	T5Ø.A14	T5Ø.A15	T5Ø.A16
with diphtheria	T5Ø.A11	T5Ø.A12	T5Ø.A13	T5Ø.A14	T5Ø.A15	T5Ø.A16
and tetanus	T5Ø.A11	T5Ø.A12	T5Ø.A13	T5Ø.A14	T5Ø.A15	T5Ø.A16
with other component	T5Ø.A11	T5Ø.A12	T5Ø.A13	T5Ø.A14	T5Ø.A15	T5Ø.A16
plague	T5Ø.A91	T5Ø.A92	T5Ø.A93	T5Ø.A94	T5Ø.A95	T5Ø.A96
poliomyelitis	T5Ø.B91	T5Ø.B92	T5Ø.B93	T5Ø.B94	T5Ø.B95	T5Ø.B96
poliovirus	T5Ø.B91	T5Ø.B92	T5Ø.B93	T5Ø.B94	T5Ø.B95	T5Ø.B96

Substance	Poisoning, Accidental (unintentional)	Poisoning, Intentional Self-harm	Poisoning, Assault	Poisoning, Undetermined	Adverse Effect	Underdosing
Vaccine — continued						
rabies	T50.B91	T50.B92	T50.B93	T50.B94	T50.B95	T50.B96
respiratory syncytial virus	T50.B91	T50.B92	T50.B93	T50.B94	T50.B95	T50.B96
rickettsial NEC	T50.A91	T50.A92	T50.A93	T50.A94	T50.A95	T50.A96
with						
bacterial component	T50.A21	T50.A22	T50.A23	T50.A24	T50.A25	T50.A26
Rocky Mountain spotted fever	T50.A91	T50.A92	T50.A93	T50.A94	T50.A95	T50.A96
rubella	T50.B91	T50.B92	T50.B93	T50.B94	T50.B95	T50.B96
sabin oral	T50.B91	T50.B92	T50.B93	T50.B94	T50.B95	T50.B96
smallpox	T50.B11	T50.B12	T50.B13	T50.B14	T50.B15	T50.B16
TAB	T50.A91	T50.A92	T50.A93	T50.A94	T50.A95	T50.A96
tetanus	T50.A91	T50.A92	T50.A93	T50.A94	T50.A95	T50.A96
typhoid	T50.A91	T50.A92	T50.A93	T50.A94	T50.A95	T50.A96
typhus	T50.A91	T50.A92	T50.A93	T50.A94	T50.A95	T50.A96
viral NEC	T50.B91	T50.B92	T50.B93	T50.B94	T50.B95	T50.B96
yellow fever	T50.B91	T50.B92	T50.B93	T50.B94	T50.B95	T50.B96
Vaccinia immune globulin	T50.Z11	T50.Z12	T50.Z13	T50.Z14	T50.Z15	T50.Z16
Vaginal contraceptives	T49.8X1	T49.8X2	T49.8X3	T49.8X4	T49.8X5	T49.8X6
Valacyclovir*	T37.5X1	T37.5X2	T37.5X3	T37.5X4	T37.5X5	T37.5X6
Valerian						
root	T42.6X1	T42.6X2	T42.6X3	T42.6X4	T42.6X5	T42.6X6
tincture	T42.6X1	T42.6X2	T42.6X3	T42.6X4	T42.6X5	T42.6X6
Valethamate bromide	T44.3X1	T44.3X2	T44.3X3	T44.3X4	T44.3X5	T44.3X6
Valisone	T49.0X1	T49.0X2	T49.0X3	T49.0X4	T49.0X5	T49.0X6
Valium	T42.4X1	T42.4X2	T42.4X3	T42.4X4	T42.4X5	T42.4X6
Valmid	T42.6X1	T42.6X2	T42.6X3	T42.6X4	T42.6X5	T42.6X6
Valnoctamide	T42.6X1	T42.6X2	T42.6X3	T42.6X4	T42.6X5	T42.6X6
Valproate (sodium)	T42.6X1	T42.6X2	T42.6X3	T42.6X4	T42.6X5	T42.6X6
Valproic acid	T42.6X1	T42.6X2	T42.6X3	T42.6X4	T42.6X5	T42.6X6
Valpromide	T42.6X1	T42.6X2	T42.6X3	T42.6X4	T42.6X5	T42.6X6
Vanadium	T56.891	T56.892	T56.893	T56.894	—	—
Vancomycin	T36.8X1	T36.8X2	T36.8X3	T36.8X4	T36.8X5	T36.8X6
Vandazole*	T49.0X1	T49.0X2	T49.0X3	T49.0X4	T49.0X5	T49.0X6
Vapor — see also Gas	T59.91	T59.92	T59.93	T59.94	—	—
kiln (carbon monoxide)	T58.8X1	T58.8X2	T58.8X3	T58.8X4	—	—
lead — see lead						
specified source NEC	T59.891	T59.892	T59.893	T59.894	—	—
Vardenafil	T46.7X1	T46.7X2	T46.7X3	T46.7X4	T46.7X5	T46.7X6
Varicose reduction drug	T46.8X1	T46.8X2	T46.8X3	T46.8X4	T46.8X5	T46.8X6
Varnish	T65.4X1	T65.4X2	T65.4X3	T65.4X4	—	—
cleaner	T52.91	T52.92	T52.93	T52.94	—	—
Vaseline	T49.3X1	T49.3X2	T49.3X3	T49.3X4	T49.3X5	T49.3X6
Vasodilan	T46.7X1	T46.7X2	T46.7X3	T46.7X4	T46.7X5	T46.7X6
Vasodilator						
coronary NEC	T46.3X1	T46.3X2	T46.3X3	T46.3X4	T46.3X5	T46.3X6
peripheral NEC	T46.7X1	T46.7X2	T46.7X3	T46.7X4	T46.7X5	T46.7X6
Vasopressin	T38.891	T38.892	T38.893	T38.894	T38.895	T38.896
Vasopressor drugs	T38.891	T38.892	T38.893	T38.894	T38.895	T38.896
Vecuronium bromide	T48.1X1	T48.1X2	T48.1X3	T48.1X4	T48.1X5	T48.1X6
Vegetable extract, astringent	T49.2X1	T49.2X2	T49.2X3	T49.2X4	T49.2X5	T49.2X6
Venlafaxine	T43.211	T43.212	T43.213	T43.214	T43.215	T43.216
Venom, venomous (bite) (sting)	T63.91	T63.92	T63.93	T63.94	—	—
amphibian NEC	T63.831	T63.832	T63.833	T63.834	—	—
animal NEC	T63.891	T63.892	T63.893	T63.894	—	—
ant	T63.421	T63.422	T63.423	T63.424	—	—
arthropod NEC	T63.481	T63.482	T63.483	T63.484	—	—
bee	T63.441	T63.442	T63.443	T63.444	—	—
centipede	T63.411	T63.412	T63.413	T63.414	—	—
fish	T63.591	T63.592	T63.593	T63.594	—	—
frog	T63.811	T63.812	T63.813	T63.814	—	—
hornet	T63.451	T63.452	T63.453	T63.454	—	—
insect NEC	T63.481	T63.482	T63.483	T63.484	—	—
lizard	T63.121	T63.122	T63.123	T63.124	—	—
marine						
animals	T63.691	T63.692	T63.693	T63.694	—	—
bluebottle	T63.611	T63.612	T63.613	T63.614	—	—
jellyfish NEC	T63.621	T63.622	T63.623	T63.624	—	—
Portuguese Man-o-war	T63.611	T63.612	T63.613	T63.614	—	—
sea anemone	T63.631	T63.632	T63.633	T63.634	—	—
specified NEC	T63.691	T63.692	T63.693	T63.694	—	—
fish	T63.591	T63.592	T63.593	T63.594	—	—
plants	T63.711	T63.712	T63.713	T63.714	—	—
sting ray	T63.511	T63.512	T63.513	T63.514	—	—
millipede (tropical)	T63.411	T63.412	T63.413	T63.414	—	—
plant NEC	T63.791	T63.792	T63.793	T63.794	—	—
marine	T63.711	T63.712	T63.713	T63.714	—	—
reptile	T63.191	T63.192	T63.193	T63.194	—	—
gila monster	T63.111	T63.112	T63.113	T63.114	—	—
lizard NEC	T63.121	T63.122	T63.123	T63.124	—	—
scorpion	T63.2X1	T63.2X2	T63.2X3	T63.2X4	—	—
Venom, venomous — continued						
snake	T63.001	T63.002	T63.003	T63.004	—	—
African NEC	T63.081	T63.082	T63.083	T63.084	—	—
American (North) (South) NEC	T63.061	T63.062	T63.063	T63.064	—	—
Asian	T63.081	T63.082	T63.083	T63.084	—	—
Australian	T63.071	T63.072	T63.073	T63.074	—	—
cobra	T63.041	T63.042	T63.043	T63.044	—	—
coral snake	T63.021	T63.022	T63.023	T63.024	—	—
rattlesnake	T63.011	T63.012	T63.013	T63.014	—	—
specified NEC	T63.091	T63.092	T63.093	T63.094	—	—
taipan	T63.031	T63.032	T63.033	T63.034	—	—
specified NEC	T63.891	T63.892	T63.893	T63.894	—	—
spider	T63.301	T63.302	T63.303	T63.304	—	—
black widow	T63.311	T63.312	T63.313	T63.314	—	—
brown recluse	T63.331	T63.332	T63.333	T63.334	—	—
specified NEC	T63.391	T63.392	T63.393	T63.394	—	—
tarantula	T63.321	T63.322	T63.323	T63.324	—	—
sting ray	T63.511	T63.512	T63.513	T63.514	—	—
toad	T63.821	T63.822	T63.823	T63.824	—	—
wasp	T63.461	T63.462	T63.463	T63.464	—	—
Venous sclerosing drug NEC	T46.8X1	T46.8X2	T46.8X3	T46.8X4	T46.8X5	T46.8X6
Ventavis*	T46.7X1	T46.7X2	T46.7X3	T46.7X4	T46.7X5	T46.7X6
Ventolin — see Albuterol						
Veramon	T42.3X1	T42.3X2	T42.3X3	T42.3X4	T42.3X5	T42.3X6
Verapamil	T46.1X1	T46.1X2	T46.1X3	T46.1X4	T46.1X5	T46.1X6
Veratrine	T46.5X1	T46.5X2	T46.5X3	T46.5X4	T46.5X5	T46.5X6
Veratrum						
album	T62.2X1	T62.2X2	T62.2X3	T62.2X4	—	—
alkaloids	T46.5X1	T46.5X2	T46.5X3	T46.5X4	T46.5X5	T46.5X6
viride	T62.2X1	T62.2X2	T62.2X3	T62.2X4	—	—
Verdigris	T60.3X1	T60.3X2	T60.3X3	T60.3X4	—	—
Veronal	T42.3X1	T42.3X2	T42.3X3	T42.3X4	T42.3X5	T42.3X6
Veroxil	T37.4X1	T37.4X2	T37.4X3	T37.4X4	T37.4X5	T37.4X6
Versenate	T50.6X1	T50.6X2	T50.6X3	T50.6X4	T50.6X5	T50.6X6
Versidyne	T39.8X1	T39.8X2	T39.8X3	T39.8X4	T39.8X5	T39.8X6
Vetrabutine	T48.0X1	T48.0X2	T48.0X3	T48.0X4	T48.0X5	T48.0X6
Vexol*	T49.5X1	T49.5X2	T49.5X3	T49.5X4	T49.5X5	T49.5X6
Viagra*	T46.7X1	T46.7X2	T46.7X3	T46.7X4	T46.7X5	T46.7X6
Vibramycin*	T36.4X1	T36.4X2	T36.4X3	T36.4X4	T36.4X5	T36.4X6
Victrelis*	T37.5X1	T37.5X2	T37.5X3	T37.5X4	T37.5X5	T37.5X6
Vidarabine	T37.5X1	T37.5X2	T37.5X3	T37.5X4	T37.5X5	T37.5X6
Vienna						
green	T57.0X1	T57.0X2	T57.0X3	T57.0X4	—	—
insecticide	T60.2X1	T60.2X2	T60.2X3	T60.2X4	—	—
red	T57.0X1	T57.0X2	T57.0X3	T57.0X4	—	—
pharmaceutical dye	T50.991	T50.992	T50.993	T50.994	T50.995	T50.996
Vigabatrin	T42.6X1	T42.6X2	T42.6X3	T42.6X4	T42.6X5	T42.6X6
Viloxazine	T43.291	T43.292	T43.293	T43.294	T43.295	T43.296
Viminol	T39.8X1	T39.8X2	T39.8X3	T39.8X4	T39.8X5	T39.8X6
Vinbarbital, vinbarbitone	T42.3X1	T42.3X2	T42.3X3	T42.3X4	T42.3X5	T42.3X6
Vinblastine	T45.1X1	T45.1X2	T45.1X3	T45.1X4	T45.1X5	T45.1X6
Vinburnine	T46.7X1	T46.7X2	T46.7X3	T46.7X4	T46.7X5	T46.7X6
Vincamine	T45.1X1	T45.1X2	T45.1X3	T45.1X4	T45.1X5	T45.1X6
Vincristine	T45.1X1	T45.1X2	T45.1X3	T45.1X4	T45.1X5	T45.1X6
Vindesine	T45.1X1	T45.1X2	T45.1X3	T45.1X4	T45.1X5	T45.1X6
Vinesthene, vinethene	T41.0X1	T41.0X2	T41.0X3	T41.0X4	T41.0X5	T41.0X6
Vinorelbine tartrate	T45.1X1	T45.1X2	T45.1X3	T45.1X4	T45.1X5	T45.1X6
Vinpocetine	T46.7X1	T46.7X2	T46.7X3	T46.7X4	T46.7X5	T46.7X6
Vinyl						
acetate	T65.891	T65.892	T65.893	T65.894	—	—
bital	T42.3X1	T42.3X2	T42.3X3	T42.3X4	T42.3X5	T42.3X6
bromide	T65.891	T65.892	T65.893	T65.894	—	—
chloride	T59.891	T59.892	T59.893	T59.894	—	—
ether	T41.0X1	T41.0X2	T41.0X3	T41.0X4	T41.0X5	T41.0X6
Vinylbital	T42.3X1	T42.3X2	T42.3X3	T42.3X4	T42.3X5	T42.3X6
Vinylidene chloride	T65.891	T65.892	T65.893	T65.894	—	—
Vioform	T37.8X1	T37.8X2	T37.8X3	T37.8X4	T37.8X5	T37.8X6
topical	T49.0X1	T49.0X2	T49.0X3	T49.0X4	T49.0X5	T49.0X6
Viokase*	T47.5X1	T47.5X2	T47.5X3	T47.5X4	T47.5X5	T47.5X6
Viomycin	T36.8X1	T36.8X2	T36.8X3	T36.8X4	T36.8X5	T36.8X6
Viosterol	T45.2X1	T45.2X2	T45.2X3	T45.2X4	T45.2X5	T45.2X6
Viper (venom)	T63.091	T63.092	T63.093	T63.094	—	—
Viprynium	T37.4X1	T37.4X2	T37.4X3	T37.4X4	T37.4X5	T37.4X6
Viquidil	T46.7X1	T46.7X2	T46.7X3	T46.7X4	T46.7X5	T46.7X6
Viral vaccine NEC	T50.B91	T50.B92	T50.B93	T50.B94	T50.B95	T50.B96
Virginiamycin	T36.8X1	T36.8X2	T36.8X3	T36.8X4	T36.8X5	T36.8X6
Virugon	T37.5X1	T37.5X2	T37.5X3	T37.5X4	T37.5X5	T37.5X6
Viscous agent	T50.901	T50.902	T50.903	T50.904	T50.905	T50.906
Visine	T49.5X1	T49.5X2	T49.5X3	T49.5X4	T49.5X5	T49.5X6
Visnadine	T46.3X1	T46.3X2	T46.3X3	T46.3X4	T46.3X5	T46.3X6
Vitamin NEC	T45.2X1	T45.2X2	T45.2X3	T45.2X4	T45.2X5	T45.2X6

*Optum Value-Add

Vitamin NEC

Table of Drugs and Chemicals

Substance	Poisoning, Accidental (unintentional)	Poisoning, Intentional Self-harm	Poisoning, Assault	Poisoning, Undetermined	Adverse Effect	Under-dosing
Vitamin — continued						
A	T45.2X1	T45.2X2	T45.2X3	T45.2X4	T45.2X5	T45.2X6
B NEC	T45.2X1	T45.2X2	T45.2X3	T45.2X4	T45.2X5	T45.2X6
nicotinic acid	T46.7X1	T46.7X2	T46.7X3	T46.7X4	T46.7X5	T46.7X6
B1	T45.2X1	T45.2X2	T45.2X3	T45.2X4	T45.2X5	T45.2X6
B12	T45.2X1	T45.2X2	T45.2X3	T45.2X4	T45.2X5	T45.2X6
B15	T45.2X1	T45.2X2	T45.2X3	T45.2X4	T45.2X5	T45.2X6
B2	T45.2X1	T45.2X2	T45.2X3	T45.2X4	T45.2X5	T45.2X6
B6	T45.2X1	T45.2X2	T45.2X3	T45.2X4	T45.2X5	T45.2X6
C	T45.2X1	T45.2X2	T45.2X3	T45.2X4	T45.2X5	T45.2X6
D	T45.2X1	T45.2X2	T45.2X3	T45.2X4	T45.2X5	T45.2X6
D2	T45.2X1	T45.2X2	T45.2X3	T45.2X4	T45.2X5	T45.2X6
D3	T45.2X1	T45.2X2	T45.2X3	T45.2X4	T45.2X5	T45.2X6
E	T45.2X1	T45.2X2	T45.2X3	T45.2X4	T45.2X5	T45.2X6
E acetate	T45.2X1	T45.2X2	T45.2X3	T45.2X4	T45.2X5	T45.2X6
hematopoietic	T45.8X1	T45.8X2	T45.8X3	T45.8X4	T45.8X5	T45.8X6
K NEC	T45.7X1	T45.7X2	T45.7X3	T45.7X4	T45.7X5	T45.7X6
K1	T45.7X1	T45.7X2	T45.7X3	T45.7X4	T45.7X5	T45.7X6
K2	T45.7X1	T45.7X2	T45.7X3	T45.7X4	T45.7X5	T45.7X6
PP	T45.2X1	T45.2X2	T45.2X3	T45.2X4	T45.2X5	T45.2X6
ulceroprotectant	T47.1X1	T47.1X2	T47.1X3	T47.1X4	T47.1X5	T47.1X6
Vleminckx's solution	T49.4X1	T49.4X2	T49.4X3	T49.4X4	T49.4X5	T49.4X6
Voltaren — see Diclofenac sodium						
Voraxaze*	T50.6X1	T50.6X2	T50.6X3	T50.6X4	T50.6X5	T50.6X6
Warfarin	T45.511	T45.512	T45.513	T45.514	T45.515	T45.516
rodenticide	T60.4X1	T60.4X2	T60.4X3	T60.4X4	—	—
sodium	T45.511	T45.512	T45.513	T45.514	T45.515	T45.516
Wasp (sting)	T63.461	T63.462	T63.463	T63.464	—	—
Water						
balance drug	T50.3X1	T50.3X2	T50.3X3	T50.3X4	T50.3X5	T50.3X6
distilled	T50.3X1	T50.3X2	T50.3X3	T50.3X4	T50.3X5	T50.3X6
gas — see Gas, water						
incomplete combustion of — see Carbon, monoxide, fuel, utility						
hemlock	T62.2X1	T62.2X2	T62.2X3	T62.2X4	—	—
moccasin (venom)	T63.061	T63.062	T63.063	T63.064	—	—
purified	T50.3X1	T50.3X2	T50.3X3	T50.3X4	T50.3X5	T50.3X6
Wax (paraffin) (petroleum)	T52.0X1	T52.0X2	T52.0X3	T52.0X4	—	—
automobile	T65.891	T65.892	T65.893	T65.894	—	—
floor	T52.0X1	T52.0X2	T52.0X3	T52.0X4	—	—
Weed killers NEC	T60.3X1	T60.3X2	T60.3X3	T60.3X4	—	—
Wellbutrin*	T43.291	T43.292	T43.293	T43.294	T43.295	T43.296
Welldorm	T42.6X1	T42.6X2	T42.6X3	T42.6X4	T42.6X5	T42.6X6
Westcort*	T49.0X1	T49.0X2	T49.0X3	T49.0X4	T49.0X5	T49.0X6
White						
arsenic	T57.0X1	T57.0X2	T57.0X3	T57.0X4	—	—
hellebore	T62.2X1	T62.2X2	T62.2X3	T62.2X4	—	—
lotion (keratolytic)	T49.4X1	T49.4X2	T49.4X3	T49.4X4	T49.4X5	T49.4X6
spirit	T52.0X1	T52.0X2	T52.0X3	T52.0X4	—	—
Whitewash	T65.891	T65.892	T65.893	T65.894	—	—
Whole blood (human)	T45.8X1	T45.8X2	T45.8X3	T45.8X4	T45.8X5	T45.8X6
Wild						
black cherry	T62.2X1	T62.2X2	T62.2X3	T62.2X4	—	—
poisonous plants NEC	T62.2X1	T62.2X2	T62.2X3	T62.2X4	—	—
Window cleaning fluid	T65.891	T65.892	T65.893	T65.894	—	—
Wintergreen (oil)	T49.3X1	T49.3X2	T49.3X3	T49.3X4	T49.3X5	T49.3X6
Wisterine	T62.2X1	T62.2X2	T62.2X3	T62.2X4	—	—
Witch hazel	T49.2X1	T49.2X2	T49.2X3	T49.2X4	T49.2X5	T49.2X6
Wood alcohol or spirit	T51.1X1	T51.1X2	T51.1X3	T51.1X4	—	—
Wool fat (hydrous)	T49.3X1	T49.3X2	T49.3X3	T49.3X4	T49.3X5	T49.3X6
Woorali	T48.1X1	T48.1X2	T48.1X3	T48.1X4	T48.1X5	T48.1X6
Wormseed, American	T37.4X1	T37.4X2	T37.4X3	T37.4X4	T37.4X5	T37.4X6
Xamoterol	T44.5X1	T44.5X2	T44.5X3	T44.5X4	T44.5X5	T44.5X6
Xanax*	T42.4X1	T42.4X2	T42.4X3	T42.4X4	T42.4X5	T42.4X6
Xanthine diuretics	T50.2X1	T50.2X2	T50.2X3	T50.2X4	T50.2X5	T50.2X6
Xanthinol nicotinate	T46.7X1	T46.7X2	T46.7X3	T46.7X4	T46.7X5	T46.7X6
Xanthotoxin	T49.3X1	T49.3X2	T49.3X3	T49.3X4	T49.3X5	T49.3X6
Xantinol nicotinate	T46.7X1	T46.7X2	T46.7X3	T46.7X4	T46.7X5	T46.7X6
Xantocillin	T36.0X1	T36.0X2	T36.0X3	T36.0X4	T36.0X5	T36.0X6
Xenon (127Xe) (133Xe)	T50.8X1	T50.8X2	T50.8X3	T50.8X4	T50.8X5	T50.8X6
Xenysalate	T49.4X1	T49.4X2	T49.4X3	T49.4X4	T49.4X5	T49.4X6
Xibornol	T37.8X1	T37.8X2	T37.8X3	T37.8X4	T37.8X5	T37.8X6
Xigris	T45.511	T45.512	T45.513	T45.514	T45.515	T45.516
Xipamide	T50.2X1	T50.2X2	T50.2X3	T50.2X4	T50.2X5	T50.2X6
Xylazine	T65.841	T65.842	T65.843	T65.844	—	—
Xylene (vapor)	T52.2X1	T52.2X2	T52.2X3	T52.2X4	—	—
Xylocaine (infiltration) (topical)	T41.3X1	T41.3X2	T41.3X3	T41.3X4	T41.3X5	T41.3X6
nerve block (peripheral) (plexus)	T41.3X1	T41.3X2	T41.3X3	T41.3X4	T41.3X5	T41.3X6
spinal	T41.3X1	T41.3X2	T41.3X3	T41.3X4	T41.3X5	T41.3X6
Xylol (vapor)	T52.2X1	T52.2X2	T52.2X3	T52.2X4	—	—
Xylometazoline	T48.5X1	T48.5X2	T48.5X3	T48.5X4	T48.5X5	T48.5X6
Xylose*	T50.8X1	T50.8X2	T50.8X3	T50.8X4	T50.8X5	T50.8X6
Yaz*	T38.4X1	T38.4X2	T38.4X3	T38.4X4	T38.4X5	T38.4X6
Yeast	T45.2X1	T45.2X2	T45.2X3	T45.2X4	T45.2X5	T45.2X6
dried	T45.2X1	T45.2X2	T45.2X3	T45.2X4	T45.2X5	T45.2X6
Yellow						
fever vaccine	T50.B91	T50.B92	T50.B93	T50.B94	T50.B95	T50.B96
jasmine	T62.2X1	T62.2X2	T62.2X3	T62.2X4	—	—
phenolphthalein	T47.2X1	T47.2X2	T47.2X3	T47.2X4	T47.2X5	T47.2X6
Yervoy*	T45.1X1	T45.1X2	T45.1X3	T45.1X4	T45.1X5	T45.1X6
Yew	T62.2X1	T62.2X2	T62.2X3	T62.2X4	—	—
Yohimbic acid	T40.991	T40.992	T40.993	T40.994	T40.995	T40.996
Zactane	T39.8X1	T39.8X2	T39.8X3	T39.8X4	T39.8X5	T39.8X6
Zalcitabine	T37.5X1	T37.5X2	T37.5X3	T37.5X4	T37.5X5	T37.5X6
Zanaflex*	T48.1X1	T48.1X2	T48.1X3	T48.1X4	T48.1X5	T48.1X6
Zaroxolyn	T50.2X1	T50.2X2	T50.2X3	T50.2X4	T50.2X5	T50.2X6
Zephiran (topical)	T49.0X1	T49.0X2	T49.0X3	T49.0X4	T49.0X5	T49.0X6
ophthalmic preparation	T49.5X1	T49.5X2	T49.5X3	T49.5X4	T49.5X5	T49.5X6
Zeranol	T38.7X1	T38.7X2	T38.7X3	T38.7X4	T38.7X5	T38.7X6
Zerone	T51.1X1	T51.1X2	T51.1X3	T51.1X4	—	—
Zestril*	T46.4X1	T46.4X2	T46.4X3	T46.4X4	T46.4X5	T46.4X6
Zidovudine	T37.5X1	T37.5X2	T37.5X3	T37.5X4	T37.5X5	T37.5X6
Zilactin*	T41.3X1	T41.3X2	T41.3X3	T41.3X4	T41.3X5	T41.3X6
Zimeldine	T43.221	T43.222	T43.223	T43.224	T43.225	T43.226
Zinc (compounds) (fumes) (vapor)	T56.5X1	T56.5X2	T56.5X3	T56.5X4	—	—
NEC						
anti-infectives	T49.0X1	T49.0X2	T49.0X3	T49.0X4	T49.0X5	T49.0X6
antivaricose	T46.8X1	T46.8X2	T46.8X3	T46.8X4	T46.8X5	T46.8X6
bacitracin	T49.0X1	T49.0X2	T49.0X3	T49.0X4	T49.0X5	T49.0X6
chromate	T56.5X1	T56.5X2	T56.5X3	T56.5X4	—	—
gelatin	T49.3X1	T49.3X2	T49.3X3	T49.3X4	T49.3X5	T49.3X6
oxide	T49.3X1	T49.3X2	T49.3X3	T49.3X4	T49.3X5	T49.3X6
plaster	T49.3X1	T49.3X2	T49.3X3	T49.3X4	T49.3X5	T49.3X6
peroxide	T49.0X1	T49.0X2	T49.0X3	T49.0X4	T49.0X5	T49.0X6
pesticides	T56.5X1	T56.5X2	T56.5X3	T56.5X4	—	—
phosphide	T60.4X1	T60.4X2	T60.4X3	T60.4X4	—	—
pyrithionate	T49.4X1	T49.4X2	T49.4X3	T49.4X4	T49.4X5	T49.4X6
stearate	T49.3X1	T49.3X2	T49.3X3	T49.3X4	T49.3X5	T49.3X6
sulfate	T49.5X1	T49.5X2	T49.5X3	T49.5X4	T49.5X5	T49.5X6
ENT agent	T49.6X1	T49.6X2	T49.6X3	T49.6X4	T49.6X5	T49.6X6
ophthalmic solution	T49.5X1	T49.5X2	T49.5X3	T49.5X4	T49.5X5	T49.5X6
topical NEC	T49.0X1	T49.0X2	T49.0X3	T49.0X4	T49.0X5	T49.0X6
undecylenate	T49.0X1	T49.0X2	T49.0X3	T49.0X4	T49.0X5	T49.0X6
chloride (mouthwash)	T49.6X1	T49.6X2	T49.6X3	T49.6X4	T49.6X5	T49.6X6
Zineb	T60.0X1	T60.0X2	T60.0X3	T60.0X4	—	—
Zinostatin	T45.1X1	T45.1X2	T45.1X3	T45.1X4	T45.1X5	T45.1X6
Zipeprol	T48.3X1	T48.3X2	T48.3X3	T48.3X4	T48.3X5	T48.3X6
Zithromax*	T36.3X1	T36.3X2	T36.3X3	T36.3X4	T36.3X5	T36.3X6
Zocor*	T46.6X1	T46.6X2	T46.6X3	T46.6X4	T46.6X5	T46.6X6
Zofenopril	T46.4X1	T46.4X2	T46.4X3	T46.4X4	T46.4X5	T46.4X6
Zoloft*	T43.221	T43.222	T43.223	T43.224	T43.225	T43.226
Zolpidem	T42.6X1	T42.6X2	T42.6X3	T42.6X4	T42.6X5	T42.6X6
Zolpimist*	T42.6X1	T42.6X2	T42.6X3	T42.6X4	T42.6X5	T42.6X6
Zomepirac	T39.391	T39.392	T39.393	T39.394	T39.395	T39.396
Zopiclone	T42.6X1	T42.6X2	T42.6X3	T42.6X4	T42.6X5	T42.6X6
Zorubicin	T45.1X1	T45.1X2	T45.1X3	T45.1X4	T45.1X5	T45.1X6
Zotepine	T43.591	T43.592	T43.593	T43.594	T43.595	T43.596
Zovant	T45.511	T45.512	T45.513	T45.514	T45.515	T45.516
Zoxazolamine	T42.8X1	T42.8X2	T42.8X3	T42.8X4	T42.8X5	T42.8X6
Zuclopenthixol	T43.4X1	T43.4X2	T43.4X3	T43.4X4	T43.4X5	T43.4X6
Zyban*	T43.291	T43.292	T43.293	T43.294	T43.295	T43.296
Zyflo*	T48.6X1	T48.6X2	T48.6X3	T48.6X4	T48.6X5	T48.6X6
Zygadenus (venenosus)	T62.2X1	T62.2X2	T62.2X3	T62.2X4	—	—
Zyprexa	T43.591	T43.592	T43.593	T43.594	T43.595	T43.596
Zyzal*	T45.0X1	T45.0X2	T45.0X3	T45.0X4	T45.0X5	T45.0X6

☑ Additional Character May Be Required — Refer to the Tabular List for Character Selection   *Optum Value-Add

A

Abandonment (causing exposure to weather conditions) (with intent to injure or kill) NEC X58.- ☑

Abuse (adult) (child) (mental) (physical) (sexual) X58.- ☑

Accident (to) X58.- ☑
- aircraft (in transit) (powered) — *see also* Accident, transport, aircraft
  - due to, caused by cataclysm — *see* Forces of nature, by type
- animal-drawn vehicle — *see* Accident, transport, animal-drawn vehicle occupant
- animal-rider — *see* Accident, transport, animal-rider
- automobile — *see* Accident, transport, car occupant
- barefoot water skier V94.4- ☑
- boat, boating — *see also* Accident, watercraft
  - striking swimmer
    - powered V94.11- ☑
    - unpowered V94.12- ☑
- bus — *see* Accident, transport, bus occupant
- cable car, not on rails V98.0- ☑
  - on rails — *see* Accident, transport, streetcar occupant
- car — *see* Accident, transport, car occupant
- caused by, due to
  - animal NEC W64.- ☑
  - chain hoist W24.0- ☑
  - cold (excessive) — *see* Exposure, cold
  - corrosive liquid, substance — *see* Table of Drugs and Chemicals
  - cutting or piercing instrument — *see* Contact, with, by type of instrument
  - drive belt W24.0- ☑
  - electric
    - current — *see* Exposure, electric current
    - motor — *see also* Contact, with, by type of machine W31.3- ☑
      - current (of) W86.8- ☑
  - environmental factor NEC X58.- ☑
  - explosive material — *see* Explosion
  - fire, flames — *see* Exposure, fire
  - firearm missile — *see* Discharge, firearm by type
  - heat (excessive) — *see* Heat
  - hot — *see* Contact, with, hot
  - ignition — *see* Ignition
  - lifting device W24.0- ☑
  - lightning — *see* subcategory T75.0- ☑
    - causing fire — *see* Exposure, fire
  - machine, machinery — *see* Contact, with, by type of machine
  - natural factor NEC X58.- ☑
  - pulley (block) W24.0- ☑
  - radiation — *see* Radiation
  - steam X13.1- ☑
    - inhalation X13.0- ☑
    - pipe X16.- ☑
  - thunderbolt — *see* subcategory T75.0- ☑
    - causing fire — *see* Exposure, fire
  - transmission device W24.1- ☑
- coach — *see* Accident, transport, bus occupant
- coal car — *see* Accident, transport, industrial vehicle occupant
- diving — *see also* Fall, into, water
  - with
    - drowning or submersion — *see* Drowning
- forklift — *see* Accident, transport, industrial vehicle occupant
- heavy transport vehicle NOS — *see* Accident, transport, truck occupant
- ice yacht V98.2- ☑
- in
  - medical, surgical procedure
    - as, or due to misadventure — *see* Misadventure
    - causing an abnormal reaction or later complication without mention of misadventure — *see also* Complication of or following, by type of procedure Y84.9
- land yacht V98.1- ☑
- late effect of — *see* W00-X58 with 7th character S
- logging car — *see* Accident, transport, industrial vehicle occupant
- machine, machinery — *see also* Contact, with, by type of machine
  - on board watercraft V93.69- ☑
    - explosion — *see* Explosion, in, watercraft
    - fire — *see* Burn, on board watercraft
    - powered craft V93.63- ☑

Accident — *continued*
- machine, machinery — *see also* Contact, with, by type of machine — *continued*
  - on board watercraft — *continued*
    - powered craft — *continued*
      - ferry boat V93.61- ☑
      - fishing boat V93.62- ☑
      - jetskis V93.63- ☑
      - liner V93.61- ☑
      - merchant ship V93.60- ☑
      - passenger ship V93.61- ☑
      - sailboat V93.64- ☑
- mine tram — *see* Accident, transport, industrial vehicle occupant
- mobility scooter (motorized) — *see* Accident, transport, pedestrian, conveyance, specified type NEC
- motor scooter — *see* Accident, transport, motorcycle
- motor vehicle NOS (traffic) — *see also* Accident, transport V89.2- ☑
  - nontraffic V89.0- ☑
  - three-wheeled NOS — *see* Accident, transport, three-wheeled motor vehicle occupant
- motorcycle NOS — *see* Accident, transport, motorcycle
- nonmotor vehicle NOS (nontraffic) — *see also* Accident, transport V89.1- ☑
  - traffic NOS V89.3- ☑
- nontraffic (victim's mode of transport NOS) V88.9- ☑
  - collision (between) V88.7- ☑
    - bus and truck V88.5- ☑
    - car and
      - bus V88.3- ☑
      - pickup V88.2- ☑
      - three-wheeled motor vehicle V88.0- ☑
      - train V88.6- ☑
      - truck V88.4- ☑
      - two-wheeled motor vehicle V88.0- ☑
      - van V88.2- ☑
    - specified vehicle NEC and
      - three-wheeled motor vehicle V88.1- ☑
      - two-wheeled motor vehicle V88.1- ☑
    - known mode of transport — *see* Accident, transport, by type of vehicle
  - noncollision V88.8- ☑
- on board watercraft V93.89- ☑
  - powered craft V93.83- ☑
    - ferry boat V93.81- ☑
    - fishing boat V93.82- ☑
    - jetskis V93.83- ☑
    - liner V93.81- ☑
    - merchant ship V93.80- ☑
    - passenger ship V93.81- ☑
  - unpowered craft V93.88- ☑
    - canoe V93.85- ☑
    - inflatable V93.86- ☑
      - in tow
        - recreational V94.31- ☑
        - specified NEC V94.32- ☑
    - kayak V93.85- ☑
    - sailboat V93.84- ☑
    - surf-board V93.88- ☑
    - water skis V93.87- ☑
    - windsurfer V93.88- ☑
- parachutist V97.29- ☑
  - entangled in object V97.21- ☑
  - injured on landing V97.22- ☑
- pedal cycle — *see* Accident, transport, pedal cyclist
- pedestrian (on foot)
  - with
    - another pedestrian W51.- ☑
      - on pedestrian conveyance NEC V00.09- ☑
        - with fall W03.- ☑
          - due to ice or snow W00.0- ☑
    - rider of
      - hoverboard V00.038- ☑
      - Segway V00.038- ☑
      - standing
        - electric scooter V00.031- ☑
        - micro-mobility pedestrian conveyance NEC V00.038- ☑
      - roller skater (in-line) V00.01- ☑
      - skate boarder V00.02- ☑
      - transport vehicle — *see* Accident, transport
    - on pedestrian conveyance — *see* Accident, transport, pedestrian, conveyance
- pick-up truck or van — *see* Accident, transport, pickup truck occupant

Accident — *continued*
- quarry truck — *see* Accident, transport, industrial vehicle occupant
- railway vehicle (any) (in motion) — *see* Accident, transport, railway vehicle occupant
  - due to cataclysm — *see* Forces of nature, by type
- scooter (non-motorized) — *see* Accident, transport, pedestrian, conveyance, scooter
- sequelae of — *see* categories W00-X58 with 7th character S
- skateboard — *see* Accident, transport, pedestrian, conveyance, skateboard
- ski(ing) — *see* Accident, transport, pedestrian, conveyance
  - lift V98.3- ☑
- specified cause NEC X58.- ☑
- streetcar — *see* Accident, transport, streetcar occupant
- traffic (victim's mode of transport NOS) V87.9- ☑
  - collision (between) V87.7- ☑
    - bus and truck V87.5- ☑
    - car and
      - bus V87.3- ☑
      - pickup V87.2- ☑
      - three-wheeled motor vehicle V87.0- ☑
      - train V87.6- ☑
      - truck V87.4- ☑
      - two-wheeled motor vehicle V87.0- ☑
      - van V87.2- ☑
    - specified vehicle NEC V86.39- ☑
      - and
        - three-wheeled motor vehicle V87.1- ☑
        - two-wheeled motor vehicle V87.1- ☑
      - driver V86.09- ☑
      - passenger V86.19- ☑
      - person on outside V86.29- ☑
      - while boarding or alighting V86.49- ☑
    - known mode of transport — *see* Accident, transport, by type of vehicle
  - noncollision V87.8- ☑
- transport (involving injury to) V99.- ☑
  - 18 wheeler — *see* Accident, transport, truck occupant
  - agricultural vehicle occupant (nontraffic) V84.9- ☑
    - driver V84.5- ☑
    - hanger-on V84.7- ☑
    - passenger V84.6- ☑
    - traffic V84.3- ☑
      - driver V84.0- ☑
      - hanger-on V84.2- ☑
      - passenger V84.1- ☑
    - while boarding or alighting V84.4- ☑
  - aircraft NEC V97.89- ☑
    - military NEC V97.818- ☑
      - civilian injured by V97.811- ☑
      - with civilian aircraft V97.810- ☑
    - occupant injured (in)
      - nonpowered craft accident V96.9- ☑
        - balloon V96.00- ☑
          - collision V96.03- ☑
          - crash V96.01- ☑
          - explosion V96.05- ☑
          - fire V96.04- ☑
          - forced landing V96.02- ☑
          - specified type NEC V96.09- ☑
        - glider V96.20- ☑
          - collision V96.23- ☑
          - crash V96.21- ☑
          - explosion V96.25- ☑
          - fire V96.24- ☑
          - forced landing V96.22- ☑
          - specified type NEC V96.29- ☑
        - hang glider V96.10- ☑
          - collision V96.13- ☑
          - crash V96.11- ☑
          - explosion V96.15- ☑
          - fire V96.14- ☑
          - forced landing V96.12- ☑
          - specified type NEC V96.19- ☑
        - specified craft NEC V96.8- ☑
      - powered craft accident V95.9- ☑
        - fixed wing NEC
          - commercial V95.30- ☑
            - collision V95.33- ☑
            - crash V95.31- ☑
            - explosion V95.35- ☑
            - fire V95.34- ☑
            - forced landing V95.32- ☑

☑ Additional Character Required — Refer to the Tabular List for Character Selection

Accident — continued
- transport — *continued*
  - aircraft — *continued*
    - occupant injured — *continued*
      - powered craft accident — *continued*
        - fixed wing — *continued*
          - commercial — *continued*
            - specified type NEC V95.39- ☑
          - private V95.20- ☑
            - collision V95.23- ☑
            - crash V95.21- ☑
            - explosion V95.25- ☑
            - fire V95.24- ☑
            - forced landing V95.22- ☑
            - specified type NEC V95.29- ☑
        - glider V95.10- ☑
          - collision V95.13- ☑
          - crash V95.11- ☑
          - explosion V95.15- ☑
          - fire V95.14- ☑
          - forced landing V95.12- ☑
          - specified type NEC V95.19- ☑
        - helicopter V95.00- ☑
          - collision V95.03- ☑
          - crash V95.01- ☑
          - explosion V95.05- ☑
          - fire V95.04- ☑
          - forced landing V95.02- ☑
          - specified type NEC V95.09- ☑
        - spacecraft V95.40- ☑
          - collision V95.43- ☑
          - crash V95.41- ☑
          - explosion V95.45- ☑
          - fire V95.44- ☑
          - forced landing V95.42- ☑
          - specified type NEC V95.49- ☑
        - specified craft NEC V95.8- ☑
        - ultralight V95.10- ☑
          - collision V95.13- ☑
          - crash V95.11- ☑
          - explosion V95.15- ☑
          - fire V95.14- ☑
          - forced landing V95.12- ☑
          - specified type NEC V95.19- ☑
      - specified accident NEC V97.0- ☑
      - while boarding or alighting V97.1- ☑
    - person (injured by)
      - falling from, in or on aircraft V97.0- ☑
      - machinery on aircraft V97.89- ☑
      - on ground with aircraft involvement V97.39- ☑
      - rotating propeller V97.32- ☑
      - struck by object falling from aircraft V97.31- ☑
      - sucked into aircraft jet V97.33- ☑
      - while boarding or alighting aircraft V97.1- ☑
  - airport (battery-powered) passenger vehicle — *see* Accident, transport, industrial vehicle occupant
  - all-terrain vehicle occupant (nontraffic) V86.95- ☑
    - driver V86.55- ☑
    - dune buggy — *see* Accident, transport, dune buggy occupant
    - hanger-on V86.75- ☑
    - passenger V86.65- ☑
    - snowmobile — *see* Accident, transport, snowmobile occupant
    - specified type NEC V86.99- ☑
      - driver V86.59- ☑
      - passenger V86.69- ☑
      - person on outside V86.79- ☑
    - traffic V86.35- ☑
      - driver V86.05- ☑
      - hanger-on V86.25- ☑
      - passenger V86.15- ☑
      - while boarding or alighting V86.45- ☑
  - ambulance occupant (traffic) V86.31- ☑
    - driver V86.01- ☑
    - hanger-on V86.21- ☑
    - nontraffic V86.91- ☑
      - driver V86.51- ☑
      - hanger-on V86.71- ☑
      - passenger V86.61- ☑
    - passenger V86.11- ☑
    - while boarding or alighting V86.41- ☑
  - animal-drawn vehicle occupant (in) V80.929- ☑
    - collision (with)
      - animal V80.12- ☑

Accident — continued
- transport — *continued*
  - animal-drawn vehicle occupant — *continued*
    - collision — *continued*
      - animal — *continued*
        - being ridden V80.711- ☑
      - animal-drawn vehicle V80.721- ☑
      - bus V80.42- ☑
      - car V80.42- ☑
      - fixed or stationary object V80.82- ☑
      - military vehicle V80.920- ☑
      - nonmotor vehicle V80.791- ☑
      - pedal cycle V80.22- ☑
      - pedestrian V80.12- ☑
      - pickup V80.42- ☑
      - railway train or vehicle V80.62- ☑
      - specified motor vehicle NEC V80.52- ☑
      - streetcar V80.731- ☑
      - truck V80.42- ☑
      - two- or three-wheeled motor vehicle V80.32- ☑
      - van V80.42- ☑
    - noncollision V80.02- ☑
    - specified circumstance NEC V80.928- ☑
  - animal-rider V80.919- ☑
    - collision (with)
      - animal V80.11- ☑
        - being ridden V80.710- ☑
      - animal-drawn vehicle V80.720- ☑
      - bus V80.41- ☑
      - car V80.41- ☑
      - fixed or stationary object V80.81- ☑
      - military vehicle V80.910- ☑
      - nonmotor vehicle V80.790- ☑
      - pedal cycle V80.21- ☑
      - pedestrian V80.11- ☑
      - pickup V80.41- ☑
      - railway train or vehicle V80.61- ☑
      - specified motor vehicle NEC V80.51- ☑
      - streetcar V80.730- ☑
      - truck V80.41- ☑
      - two- or three-wheeled motor vehicle V80.31- ☑
      - van V80.41- ☑
    - noncollision V80.018- ☑
      - specified as horse rider V80.010- ☑
    - specified circumstance NEC V80.918- ☑
  - armored car — *see* Accident, transport, truck occupant
  - battery-powered truck (baggage) (mail) — *see* Accident, transport, industrial vehicle occupant
  - bus occupant V79.9- ☑
    - collision (with)
      - animal (traffic) V70.9- ☑
        - being ridden (traffic) V76.9- ☑
          - nontraffic V76.3- ☑
          - while boarding or alighting V76.4- ☑
        - nontraffic V70.3- ☑
        - while boarding or alighting V70.4- ☑
      - animal-drawn vehicle (traffic) V76.9- ☑
        - nontraffic V76.3- ☑
        - while boarding or alighting V76.4- ☑
      - bus (traffic) V74.9- ☑
        - nontraffic V74.3- ☑
        - while boarding or alighting V74.4- ☑
      - car (traffic) V73.9- ☑
        - nontraffic V73.3- ☑
        - while boarding or alighting V73.4- ☑
      - motor vehicle NOS (traffic) V79.60- ☑
        - nontraffic V79.20- ☑
        - specified type NEC (traffic) V79.69- ☑
          - nontraffic V79.29- ☑
      - pedal cycle (traffic) V71.9- ☑
        - nontraffic V71.3- ☑
        - while boarding or alighting V71.4- ☑
      - pickup truck (traffic) V73.9- ☑
        - nontraffic V73.3- ☑
        - while boarding or alighting V73.4- ☑
      - railway vehicle (traffic) V75.9- ☑
        - nontraffic V75.3- ☑
        - while boarding or alighting V75.4- ☑
      - specified vehicle NEC (traffic) V76.9- ☑
        - nontraffic V76.3- ☑
        - while boarding or alighting V76.4- ☑
      - stationary object (traffic) V77.9- ☑
        - nontraffic V77.3- ☑

Accident — continued
- transport — *continued*
  - bus occupant — *continued*
    - collision — *continued*
      - stationary object — *continued*
        - while boarding or alighting V77.4- ☑
      - streetcar (traffic) V76.9- ☑
        - nontraffic V76.3- ☑
        - while boarding or alighting V76.4- ☑
      - three wheeled motor vehicle (traffic) V72.9- ☑
        - nontraffic V72.3- ☑
        - while boarding or alighting V72.4- ☑
      - truck (traffic) V74.9- ☑
        - nontraffic V74.3- ☑
        - while boarding or alighting V74.4- ☑
      - two wheeled motor vehicle (traffic) V72.9- ☑
        - nontraffic V72.3- ☑
        - while boarding or alighting V72.4- ☑
      - van (traffic) V73.9- ☑
        - nontraffic V73.3- ☑
        - while boarding or alighting V73.4- ☑
    - driver
      - collision (with)
        - animal (traffic) V70.5- ☑
          - being ridden (traffic) V76.5- ☑
            - nontraffic V76.0- ☑
          - nontraffic V70.0- ☑
        - animal-drawn vehicle (traffic) V76.5- ☑
          - nontraffic V76.0- ☑
        - bus (traffic) V74.5- ☑
          - nontraffic V74.0- ☑
        - car (traffic) V73.5- ☑
          - nontraffic V73.0- ☑
        - motor vehicle NOS (traffic) V79.40- ☑
          - nontraffic V79.00- ☑
          - specified type NEC (traffic) V79.49- ☑
            - nontraffic V79.09- ☑
        - pedal cycle (traffic) V71.5- ☑
          - nontraffic V71.0- ☑
        - pickup truck (traffic) V73.5- ☑
          - nontraffic V73.0- ☑
        - railway vehicle (traffic) V75.5- ☑
          - nontraffic V75.0- ☑
        - specified vehicle NEC (traffic) V76.5- ☑
          - nontraffic V76.0- ☑
        - stationary object (traffic) V77.5- ☑
          - nontraffic V77.0- ☑
        - streetcar (traffic) V76.5- ☑
          - nontraffic V76.0- ☑
        - three wheeled motor vehicle (traffic) V72.5- ☑
          - nontraffic V72.0- ☑
        - truck (traffic) V74.5- ☑
          - nontraffic V74.0- ☑
        - two wheeled motor vehicle (traffic) V72.5- ☑
          - nontraffic V72.0- ☑
        - van (traffic) V73.5- ☑
          - nontraffic V73.0- ☑
      - noncollision accident (traffic) V78.5- ☑
        - nontraffic V78.0- ☑
    - hanger-on
      - collision (with)
        - animal (traffic) V70.7- ☑
          - being ridden (traffic) V76.7- ☑
            - nontraffic V76.2- ☑
          - nontraffic V70.2- ☑
        - animal-drawn vehicle (traffic) V76.7- ☑
          - nontraffic V76.2- ☑
        - bus (traffic) V74.7- ☑
          - nontraffic V74.2- ☑
        - car (traffic) V73.7- ☑
          - nontraffic V73.2- ☑
        - pedal cycle (traffic) V71.7- ☑
          - nontraffic V71.2- ☑
        - pickup truck (traffic) V73.7- ☑
          - nontraffic V73.2- ☑
        - railway vehicle (traffic) V75.7- ☑
          - nontraffic V75.2- ☑
        - specified vehicle NEC (traffic) V76.7- ☑
          - nontraffic V76.2- ☑
        - stationary object (traffic) V77.7- ☑
          - nontraffic V77.2- ☑
        - streetcar (traffic) V76.7- ☑
          - nontraffic V76.2- ☑

Accident — *continued*
  transport — *continued*
    bus occupant — *continued*
      hanger-on — *continued*
        collision — *continued*
          three wheeled motor vehicle (traffic) V72.7- ☑
            nontraffic V72.2- ☑
          truck (traffic) V74.7- ☑
            nontraffic V74.2- ☑
          two wheeled motor vehicle (traffic) V72.7- ☑
            nontraffic V72.2- ☑
          van (traffic) V73.7- ☑
            nontraffic V73.2- ☑
        noncollision accident (traffic) V78.7- ☑
          nontraffic V78.2- ☑
      noncollision accident (traffic) V78.9- ☑
        nontraffic V78.3- ☑
        while boarding or alighting V78.4- ☑
      nontraffic V79.3- ☑
      passenger
        collision (with)
          animal (traffic) V70.6- ☑
            being ridden (traffic) V76.6- ☑
              nontraffic V76.1- ☑
            nontraffic V70.1- ☑
          animal-drawn vehicle (traffic) V76.6- ☑
            nontraffic V76.1- ☑
          bus (traffic) V74.6- ☑
            nontraffic V74.1- ☑
          car (traffic) V73.6- ☑
            nontraffic V73.1- ☑
          motor vehicle NOS (traffic) V79.50- ☑
            nontraffic V79.10- ☑
            specified type NEC (traffic) V79.59- ☑
              nontraffic V79.19- ☑
          pedal cycle (traffic) V71.6- ☑
            nontraffic V71.1- ☑
          pickup truck (traffic) V73.6- ☑
            nontraffic V73.1- ☑
          railway vehicle (traffic) V75.6- ☑
            nontraffic V75.1- ☑
          specified vehicle NEC (traffic) V76.6- ☑
            nontraffic V76.1- ☑
          stationary object (traffic) V77.6- ☑
            nontraffic V77.1- ☑
          streetcar (traffic) V76.6- ☑
            nontraffic V76.1- ☑
          three wheeled motor vehicle (traffic) V72.6- ☑
            nontraffic V72.1- ☑
          truck (traffic) V74.6- ☑
            nontraffic V74.1- ☑
          two wheeled motor vehicle (traffic) V72.6- ☑
            nontraffic V72.1- ☑
          van (traffic) V73.6- ☑
            nontraffic V73.1- ☑
        noncollision accident (traffic) V78.6- ☑
          nontraffic V78.1- ☑
      specified type NEC V79.88- ☑
      military vehicle V79.81- ☑
    cable car, not on rails V98.0- ☑
      on rails — *see* Accident, transport, streetcar occupant
    car occupant V49.9- ☑
      ambulance occupant — *see* Accident, transport, ambulance occupant
      collision (with)
        animal (traffic) V40.9- ☑
          being ridden (traffic) V46.9- ☑
            nontraffic V46.3- ☑
            while boarding or alighting V46.4- ☑
          nontraffic V40.3- ☑
          while boarding or alighting V40.4- ☑
        animal-drawn vehicle (traffic) V46.9- ☑
          nontraffic V46.3- ☑
          while boarding or alighting V46.4- ☑
        bus (traffic) V44.9- ☑
          nontraffic V44.3- ☑
          while boarding or alighting V44.4- ☑
        car (traffic) V43.92- ☑
          nontraffic V43.32- ☑
          while boarding or alighting V43.42- ☑

Accident — *continued*
  transport — *continued*
    car occupant — *continued*
      collision — *continued*
        motor vehicle NOS (traffic) V49.60- ☑
          nontraffic V49.20- ☑
          specified type NEC (traffic) V49.69- ☑
            nontraffic V49.29- ☑
        pedal cycle (traffic) V41.9- ☑
          nontraffic V41.3- ☑
          while boarding or alighting V41.4- ☑
        pickup truck (traffic) V43.93- ☑
          nontraffic V43.33- ☑
          while boarding or alighting V43.43- ☑
        railway vehicle (traffic) V45.9- ☑
          nontraffic V45.3- ☑
          while boarding or alighting V45.4- ☑
        specified vehicle NEC (traffic) V46.9- ☑
          nontraffic V46.3- ☑
          while boarding or alighting V46.4- ☑
        sport utility vehicle (traffic) V43.91- ☑
          nontraffic V43.31- ☑
          while boarding or alighting V43.41- ☑
        stationary object (traffic) V47.9- ☑
          nontraffic V47.3- ☑
          while boarding or alighting V47.4- ☑
        streetcar (traffic) V46.9- ☑
          nontraffic V46.3- ☑
          while boarding or alighting V46.4- ☑
        three wheeled motor vehicle (traffic) V42.9- ☑
          nontraffic V42.3- ☑
          while boarding or alighting V42.4- ☑
        truck (traffic) V44.9- ☑
          nontraffic V44.3- ☑
          while boarding or alighting V44.4- ☑
        two wheeled motor vehicle (traffic) V42.9- ☑
          nontraffic V42.3- ☑
          while boarding or alighting V42.4- ☑
        van (traffic) V43.94- ☑
          nontraffic V43.34- ☑
          while boarding or alighting V43.44- ☑
      driver
        collision (with)
          animal (traffic) V40.5- ☑
            being ridden (traffic) V46.5- ☑
              nontraffic V46.0- ☑
            nontraffic V40.0- ☑
          animal-drawn vehicle (traffic) V46.5- ☑
            nontraffic V46.0- ☑
          bus (traffic) V44.5- ☑
            nontraffic V44.0- ☑
          car (traffic) V43.52- ☑
            nontraffic V43.02- ☑
          motor vehicle NOS (traffic) V49.40- ☑
            nontraffic V49.00- ☑
            specified type NEC (traffic) V49.49- ☑
              nontraffic V49.09- ☑
          pedal cycle (traffic) V41.5- ☑
            nontraffic V41.0- ☑
          pickup truck (traffic) V43.53- ☑
            nontraffic V43.03- ☑
          railway vehicle (traffic) V45.5- ☑
            nontraffic V45.0- ☑
          specified vehicle NEC (traffic) V46.5- ☑
            nontraffic V46.0- ☑
          sport utility vehicle (traffic) V43.51- ☑
            nontraffic V43.01- ☑
          stationary object (traffic) V47.5- ☑
            nontraffic V47.0- ☑
          streetcar (traffic) V46.5- ☑
            nontraffic V46.0- ☑
          three wheeled motor vehicle (traffic) V42.5- ☑
            nontraffic V42.0- ☑
          truck (traffic) V44.5- ☑
            nontraffic V44.0- ☑
          two wheeled motor vehicle (traffic) V42.5- ☑
            nontraffic V42.0- ☑
          van (traffic) V43.54- ☑
            nontraffic V43.04- ☑
        noncollision accident (traffic) V48.5- ☑
          nontraffic V48.0- ☑

Accident — *continued*
  transport — *continued*
    car occupant — *continued*
      hanger-on
        collision (with)
          animal (traffic) V40.7- ☑
            being ridden (traffic) V46.7- ☑
              nontraffic V46.2- ☑
            nontraffic V40.2- ☑
          animal-drawn vehicle (traffic) V46.7- ☑
            nontraffic V46.2- ☑
          bus (traffic) V44.7- ☑
            nontraffic V44.2- ☑
          car (traffic) V43.72- ☑
            nontraffic V43.22- ☑
          pedal cycle (traffic) V41.7- ☑
            nontraffic V41.2- ☑
          pickup truck (traffic) V43.73- ☑
            nontraffic V43.23- ☑
          railway vehicle (traffic) V45.7- ☑
            nontraffic V45.2- ☑
          specified vehicle NEC (traffic) V46.7- ☑
            nontraffic V46.2- ☑
          sport utility vehicle (traffic) V43.71- ☑
            nontraffic V43.21- ☑
          stationary object (traffic) V47.7- ☑
            nontraffic V47.2- ☑
          streetcar (traffic) V46.7- ☑
            nontraffic V46.2- ☑
          three wheeled motor vehicle (traffic) V42.7- ☑
            nontraffic V42.2- ☑
          truck (traffic) V44.7- ☑
            nontraffic V44.2- ☑
          two wheeled motor vehicle (traffic) V42.7- ☑
            nontraffic V42.2- ☑
          van (traffic) V43.74- ☑
            nontraffic V43.24- ☑
        noncollision accident (traffic) V48.7- ☑
          nontraffic V48.2- ☑
      noncollision accident (traffic) V48.9- ☑
        nontraffic V48.3- ☑
        while boarding or alighting V48.4- ☑
      nontraffic V49.3- ☑
      passenger
        collision (with)
          animal (traffic) V40.6- ☑
            being ridden (traffic) V46.6- ☑
              nontraffic V46.1- ☑
            nontraffic V40.1- ☑
          animal-drawn vehicle (traffic) V46.6- ☑
            nontraffic V46.1- ☑
          bus (traffic) V44.6- ☑
            nontraffic V44.1- ☑
          car (traffic) V43.62- ☑
            nontraffic V43.12- ☑
          motor vehicle NOS (traffic) V49.50- ☑
            nontraffic V49.10- ☑
            specified type NEC (traffic) V49.59- ☑
              nontraffic V49.19- ☑
          pedal cycle (traffic) V41.6- ☑
            nontraffic V41.1- ☑
          pickup truck (traffic) V43.63- ☑
            nontraffic V43.13- ☑
          railway vehicle (traffic) V45.6- ☑
            nontraffic V45.1- ☑
          specified vehicle NEC (traffic) V46.6- ☑
            nontraffic V46.1- ☑
          sport utility vehicle (traffic) V43.61- ☑
            nontraffic V43.11- ☑
          stationary object (traffic) V47.6- ☑
            nontraffic V47.1- ☑
          streetcar (traffic) V46.6- ☑
            nontraffic V46.1- ☑
          three wheeled motor vehicle (traffic) V42.6- ☑
            nontraffic V42.1- ☑
          truck (traffic) V44.6- ☑
            nontraffic V44.1- ☑
          two wheeled motor vehicle (traffic) V42.6- ☑
            nontraffic V42.1- ☑
          van (traffic) V43.64- ☑
            nontraffic V43.14- ☑

☑ Additional Character Required — Refer to the Tabular List for Character Selection

Accident
  Accident — *continued*
    transport — *continued*
      car occupant — *continued*
        passenger — *continued*
          noncollision accident (traffic) V48.6- ☑
            nontraffic V48.1- ☑
          specified type NEC V49.88- ☑
          military vehicle V49.81- ☑
      coal car — *see* Accident, transport, industrial vehicle occupant
      construction vehicle occupant (nontraffic) V85.9- ☑
        driver V85.5- ☑
        hanger-on V85.7- ☑
        passenger V85.6- ☑
        traffic V85.3- ☑
          driver V85.0- ☑
          hanger-on V85.2- ☑
          passenger V85.1- ☑
        while boarding or alighting V85.4- ☑
      dirt bike rider (nontraffic) V86.96- ☑
        driver V86.56- ☑
        hanger-on V86.76- ☑
        passenger V86.66- ☑
        traffic V86.36- ☑
          driver V86.06- ☑
          hanger-on V86.26- ☑
          passenger V86.16- ☑
        while boarding or alighting V86.46- ☑
      due to cataclysm — *see* Forces of nature, by type
      dune buggy occupant (nontraffic) V86.93- ☑
        driver V86.53- ☑
        hanger-on V86.73- ☑
        passenger V86.63- ☑
        traffic V86.33- ☑
          driver V86.03- ☑
          hanger-on V86.23- ☑
          passenger V86.13- ☑
        while boarding or alighting V86.43- ☑
      e-bicycle — *see* Accident, transport, electric (assisted) bicyclist
      e-bike — *see* Accident, transport, electric (assisted) bicyclist
      electric (assisted) bicyclist V29.91- ☑
        collision (with)
          animal (traffic) V20.91- ☑
            being ridden (traffic) V26.91- ☑
              nontraffic V26.21- ☑
              while boarding or alighting V26.31- ☑
            nontraffic V20.21- ☑
            while boarding or alighting V20.31- ☑
          animal-drawn vehicle (traffic) V26.91- ☑
            nontraffic V26.21- ☑
            while boarding or alighting V26.31- ☑
          bus (traffic) V24.91- ☑
            nontraffic V24.21- ☑
            while boarding or alighting V24.31- ☑
          car (traffic) V23.91- ☑
            nontraffic V23.21- ☑
            while boarding or alighting V23.31- ☑
          motor vehicle NOS (traffic) V29.601- ☑
            nontraffic V29.201- ☑
            specified type NEC (traffic) V29.691- ☑
              nontraffic V29.291- ☑
          pedal cycle (traffic) V21.91- ☑
            nontraffic V21.21- ☑
            while boarding or alighting V21.31- ☑
          pedestrian V20.91- ☑
            nontraffic V20.01- ☑
            while boarding or alighting V20.31- ☑
          pickup truck (traffic) V23.91- ☑
            nontraffic V23.21- ☑
            while boarding or alighting V23.31- ☑
          railway vehicle (traffic) V25.91- ☑
            nontraffic V25.21- ☑
            while boarding or alighting V25.31- ☑
          specified vehicle NEC (traffic) V26.91- ☑
            nontraffic V26.21- ☑
            while boarding or alighting V26.31- ☑
          stationary object (traffic) V27.91- ☑
            nontraffic V27.21- ☑
            while boarding or alighting V27.31- ☑
          streetcar (traffic) V26.91- ☑
            nontraffic V26.21- ☑
            while boarding or alighting V26.31- ☑
          three wheeled motor vehicle (traffic) V22.91- ☑

Accident — *continued*
  transport — *continued*
    electric bicyclist — *continued*
      collision — *continued*
        three wheeled motor vehicle — *continued*
          nontraffic V22.21- ☑
          while boarding or alighting V22.31- ☑
        truck (traffic) V24.91- ☑
          nontraffic V24.21- ☑
          while boarding or alighting V24.31- ☑
        two wheeled motor vehicle (traffic) V22.91- ☑
          nontraffic V22.21- ☑
          while boarding or alighting V22.31- ☑
        van (traffic) V23.91- ☑
          nontraffic V23.21- ☑
          while boarding or alighting V23.31- ☑
      driver
        collision (with)
          animal (traffic) V20.41- ☑
            being ridden (traffic) V26.41- ☑
              nontraffic V26.01- ☑
            nontraffic V20.01- ☑
          animal-drawn vehicle (traffic) V26.41- ☑
            nontraffic V26.01- ☑
          bus (traffic) V24.41- ☑
            nontraffic V24.01- ☑
          car (traffic) V23.41- ☑
            nontraffic V23.01- ☑
          motor vehicle NOS (traffic) V29.401- ☑
            nontraffic V29.001- ☑
            specified type NEC (traffic) V29.491- ☑
              nontraffic V29.091- ☑
          pedal cycle (traffic) V21.41- ☑
            nontraffic V21.01- ☑
          pedestrian
            nontraffic V20.01- ☑
            traffic V20.41- ☑
          pickup truck (traffic) V23.41- ☑
            nontraffic V23.01- ☑
          railway vehicle (traffic) V25.41- ☑
            nontraffic V25.01- ☑
          specified vehicle NEC (traffic) V26.41- ☑
            nontraffic V26.01- ☑
          stationary object (traffic) V27.41- ☑
            nontraffic V27.01- ☑
          streetcar (traffic) V26.41- ☑
            nontraffic V26.01- ☑
          three wheeled motor vehicle (traffic) V22.41- ☑
            nontraffic V22.01- ☑
          truck (traffic) V24.41- ☑
            nontraffic V24.01- ☑
          two wheeled motor vehicle (traffic) V22.41- ☑
            nontraffic V22.01- ☑
          van (traffic) V23.41- ☑
            nontraffic V23.01- ☑
        noncollision accident (traffic) V28.41- ☑
          nontraffic V28.01- ☑
      noncollision accident (traffic) V28.91- ☑
        nontraffic V28.21- ☑
        while boarding or alighting V28.31- ☑
      nontraffic V29.31- ☑
      passenger
        collision (with)
          animal (traffic) V20.51- ☑
            being ridden (traffic) V26.51- ☑
              nontraffic V26.11- ☑
            nontraffic V20.11- ☑
          animal-drawn vehicle (traffic) V26.51- ☑
            nontraffic V26.11- ☑
          bus (traffic) V24.51- ☑
            nontraffic V24.11- ☑
          car (traffic) V23.51- ☑
            nontraffic V23.11- ☑
          motor vehicle NOS (traffic) V29.501- ☑
            nontraffic V29.101- ☑
            specified type NEC (traffic) V29.591- ☑
              nontraffic V29.191- ☑
          pedal cycle (traffic) V21.51- ☑
            nontraffic V21.11- ☑
          pedestrian
            nontraffic V20.11- ☑
            traffic V20.51- ☑
          pickup truck (traffic) V23.51- ☑

Accident — *continued*
  transport — *continued*
    electric bicyclist — *continued*
      passenger — *continued*
        collision — *continued*
          pickup truck — *continued*
            nontraffic V23.11- ☑
          railway vehicle (traffic) V25.51- ☑
            nontraffic V25.11- ☑
          specified vehicle NEC (traffic) V26.51- ☑
            nontraffic V26.11- ☑
          stationary object (traffic) V27.51- ☑
            nontraffic V27.11- ☑
          streetcar (traffic) V26.51- ☑
            nontraffic V26.11- ☑
          three wheeled motor vehicle (traffic) V22.51- ☑
            nontraffic V22.11- ☑
          truck (traffic) V24.51- ☑
            nontraffic V24.11- ☑
          two wheeled motor vehicle (traffic) V22.51- ☑
            nontraffic V22.11- ☑
          van (traffic) V23.51- ☑
            nontraffic V23.11- ☑
        noncollision accident (traffic) V28.51- ☑
          nontraffic V28.11- ☑
      specified type NEC V29.881- ☑
      military vehicle V29.811- ☑
    forklift — *see* Accident, transport, industrial vehicle occupant
    go cart — *see* Accident, transport, all-terrain vehicle occupant
    golf cart — *see* Accident, transport, all-terrain vehicle occupant
    heavy transport vehicle occupant — *see* Accident, transport, truck occupant
    hoverboard V00.848- ☑
    ice yacht V98.2- ☑
    industrial vehicle occupant (nontraffic) V83.9- ☑
      driver V83.5- ☑
      hanger-on V83.7- ☑
      passenger V83.6- ☑
      traffic V83.3- ☑
        driver V83.0- ☑
        hanger-on V83.2- ☑
        passenger V83.1- ☑
      while boarding or alighting V83.4- ☑
    interurban electric car — *see* Accident, transport, streetcar
    land yacht V98.1- ☑
    logging car — *see* Accident, transport, industrial vehicle occupant
    military vehicle occupant (traffic) V86.34- ☑
      driver V86.04- ☑
      hanger-on V86.24- ☑
      nontraffic V86.94- ☑
        driver V86.54- ☑
        hanger-on V86.74- ☑
        passenger V86.64- ☑
      passenger V86.14- ☑
      while boarding or alighting V86.44- ☑
    mine tram — *see* Accident, transport, industrial vehicle occupant
    motor/cross bike rider — *see also* Accident, transport, dirt bike rider V86.96- ☑
    motor vehicle NEC occupant (traffic) V89.2- ☑
    motorcoach — *see* Accident, transport, bus occupant
    motorcycle V29.99- ☑
      collision (with)
        animal (traffic) V20.99- ☑
          being ridden (traffic) V26.99- ☑
            nontraffic V26.29- ☑
              while boarding or alighting V26.39- ☑
          nontraffic V20.29- ☑
          while boarding or alighting V20.39- ☑
        animal-drawn vehicle (traffic) V26.99- ☑
          nontraffic V26.29- ☑
          while boarding or alighting V26.39- ☑
        bus (traffic) V24.99- ☑
          nontraffic V24.29- ☑
          while boarding or alighting V24.39- ☑
        car (traffic) V23.99- ☑
          nontraffic V23.29- ☑
          while boarding or alighting V23.39- ☑
        motor vehicle NOS (traffic) V29.608- ☑

Accident — *continued*
  transport — *continued*
    motorcycle — *continued*
      collision — *continued*
        motor vehicle — *continued*
          nontraffic V29.208- ☑
          specified type NEC (traffic) V29.698- ☑
            nontraffic V29.298- ☑
        pedal cycle (traffic) V21.99- ☑
          nontraffic V21.29- ☑
          while boarding or alighting V21.39- ☑
        pickup truck (traffic) V23.99- ☑
          nontraffic V23.29- ☑
          while boarding or alighting V23.39- ☑
        railway vehicle (traffic) V25.99- ☑
          nontraffic V25.29- ☑
          while boarding or alighting V25.39- ☑
        specified vehicle NEC (traffic) V26.99- ☑
          nontraffic V26.29- ☑
          while boarding or alighting V26.39- ☑
        stationary object (traffic) V27.99- ☑
          nontraffic V27.29- ☑
          while boarding or alighting V27.39- ☑
        streetcar (traffic) V26.99- ☑
          nontraffic V26.29- ☑
          while boarding or alighting V26.39- ☑
        three wheeled motor vehicle (traffic) V22.99- ☑
          nontraffic V22.29- ☑
          while boarding or alighting V22.39- ☑
        truck (traffic) V24.99- ☑
          nontraffic V24.29- ☑
          while boarding or alighting V24.39- ☑
        two wheeled motor vehicle (traffic) V22.99- ☑
          nontraffic V22.29- ☑
          while boarding or alighting V22.39- ☑
        van (traffic) V23.99- ☑
          nontraffic V23.29- ☑
          while boarding or alighting V23.39- ☑
      driver
        collision (with)
          animal (traffic) V20.49- ☑
            being ridden (traffic) V26.49- ☑
              nontraffic V26.09- ☑
            nontraffic V20.09- ☑
          animal-drawn vehicle (traffic) V26.49- ☑
            nontraffic V26.09- ☑
          bus (traffic) V24.49- ☑
            nontraffic V24.09- ☑
          car (traffic) V23.49- ☑
            nontraffic V23.09- ☑
          motor vehicle NOS (traffic) V29.408- ☑
            nontraffic V29.008- ☑
            specified type NEC (traffic) V29.498- ☑
              nontraffic V29.098- ☑
          pedal cycle (traffic) V21.49- ☑
            nontraffic V21.09- ☑
          pedestrian
            nontraffic V20.09- ☑
            traffic V20.49- ☑
          pickup truck (traffic) V23.49- ☑
            nontraffic V23.09- ☑
          railway vehicle (traffic) V25.49- ☑
            nontraffic V25.09- ☑
          specified vehicle NEC (traffic) V26.49- ☑
            nontraffic V26.09- ☑
          stationary object (traffic) V27.49- ☑
            nontraffic V27.09- ☑
          streetcar (traffic) V26.49- ☑
            nontraffic V26.09- ☑
          three wheeled motor vehicle (traffic) V22.49- ☑
            nontraffic V22.09- ☑
          truck (traffic) V24.49- ☑
            nontraffic V24.09- ☑
          two wheeled motor vehicle (traffic) V22.49- ☑
            nontraffic V22.09- ☑
          van (traffic) V23.49- ☑
            nontraffic V23.09- ☑
        noncollision accident (traffic) V28.49- ☑
          nontraffic V28.09- ☑
      noncollision accident (traffic) V28.99- ☑
        nontraffic V28.29- ☑
        while boarding or alighting V28.39- ☑
      nontraffic V29.39- ☑
      passenger
        collision (with)
          animal (traffic) V20.59- ☑
            being ridden (traffic) V26.59- ☑
              nontraffic V26.19- ☑
            nontraffic V20.19- ☑
          animal-drawn vehicle (traffic) V26.59- ☑
            nontraffic V26.19- ☑
          bus (traffic) V24.59- ☑
            nontraffic V24.19- ☑
          car (traffic) V23.59- ☑
            nontraffic V23.19- ☑
          motor vehicle NOS (traffic) V29.508- ☑
            nontraffic V29.108- ☑
            specified type NEC (traffic) V29.598- ☑
              nontraffic V29.198- ☑
          pedal cycle (traffic) V21.59- ☑
            nontraffic V21.19- ☑
          pedestrian
            nontraffic V20.19- ☑
            traffic V20.59- ☑
          pickup truck (traffic) V23.59- ☑
            nontraffic V23.19- ☑
          railway vehicle (traffic) V25.59- ☑
            nontraffic V25.19- ☑
          specified vehicle NEC (traffic) V26.59- ☑
            nontraffic V26.19- ☑
          stationary object (traffic) V27.59- ☑
            nontraffic V27.19- ☑
          streetcar (traffic) V26.59- ☑
            nontraffic V26.19- ☑
          three wheeled motor vehicle (traffic) V22.59- ☑
            nontraffic V22.19- ☑
          truck (traffic) V24.59- ☑
            nontraffic V24.19- ☑
          two wheeled motor vehicle (traffic) V22.59- ☑
            nontraffic V22.19- ☑
          van (traffic) V23.59- ☑
            nontraffic V23.19- ☑
        noncollision accident (traffic) V28.59- ☑
          nontraffic V28.19- ☑
      specified type NEC V29.888- ☑
      military vehicle V29.818- ☑
    occupant (of)
      aircraft (powered) V95.9- ☑
        fixed wing
          commercial — *see* Accident, transport, aircraft, occupant, powered, fixed wing, commercial
          private — *see* Accident, transport, aircraft, occupant, powered, fixed wing, private
        nonpowered V96.9- ☑
        specified NEC V95.8- ☑
      airport battery-powered vehicle — *see* Accident, transport, industrial vehicle occupant
      all-terrain vehicle (ATV) — *see* Accident, transport, all-terrain vehicle occupant
      animal-drawn vehicle — *see* Accident, transport, animal-drawn vehicle occupant
      automobile — *see* Accident, transport, car occupant
      balloon V96.00- ☑
      battery-powered vehicle — *see* Accident, transport, industrial vehicle occupant
      bicycle — *see* Accident, transport, pedal cyclist
        motorized — *see* Accident, transport, motorcycle rider
      boat NEC — *see* Accident, watercraft
      bulldozer — *see* Accident, transport, construction vehicle occupant
      bus — *see* Accident, transport, bus occupant
      cable car (on rails) — *see also* Accident, transport, streetcar occupant
        not on rails V98.0- ☑
      car — *see also* Accident, transport, car occupant
        cable (on rails) — *see also* Accident, transport, streetcar occupant
          not on rails V98.0- ☑
      coach — *see* Accident, transport, bus occupant
      coal-car — *see* Accident, transport, industrial vehicle occupant
      digger — *see* Accident, transport, construction vehicle occupant
      dump truck — *see* Accident, transport, construction vehicle occupant
      earth-leveler — *see* Accident, transport, construction vehicle occupant
      farm machinery (self-propelled) — *see* Accident, transport, agricultural vehicle occupant
      forklift — *see* Accident, transport, industrial vehicle occupant
      glider (unpowered) V96.20- ☑
        hang V96.10- ☑
        powered (microlight) (ultralight) — *see* Accident, transport, aircraft, occupant, powered, glider
      glider (unpowered) NEC V96.20- ☑
      hang-glider V96.10- ☑
      harvester — *see* Accident, transport, agricultural vehicle occupant
      heavy (transport) vehicle — *see* Accident, transport, truck occupant
      helicopter — *see* Accident, transport, aircraft, occupant, helicopter
      ice-yacht V98.2- ☑
      kite (carrying person) V96.8- ☑
      land-yacht V98.1- ☑
      logging car — *see* Accident, transport, industrial vehicle occupant
      mechanical shovel — *see* Accident, transport, construction vehicle occupant
      microlight — *see* Accident, transport, aircraft, occupant, powered, glider
      minibus — *see* Accident, transport, pickup truck occupant
      minivan — *see* Accident, transport, pickup truck occupant
      moped — *see* Accident, transport, motorcycle
      motor scooter — *see* Accident, transport, motorcycle
      motorcycle (with sidecar) — *see* Accident, transport, motorcycle
      off-road motor-vehicle — *see also* Accident, transport, all-terrain vehicle occupant V86.99- ☑
      pedal cycle — *see also* Accident, transport, pedal cyclist
      pick-up (truck) — *see* Accident, transport, pickup truck occupant
      railway (train) (vehicle) (subterranean) (elevated) — *see* Accident, transport, railway vehicle occupant
      rickshaw — *see* Accident, transport, pedal cycle
        motorized — *see* Accident, transport, three-wheeled motor vehicle
        pedal driven — *see* Accident, transport, pedal cyclist
      road-roller — *see* Accident, transport, construction vehicle occupant
      ship NOS V94.9- ☑
      ski-lift (chair) (gondola) V98.3- ☑
      snowmobile — *see* Accident, transport, snowmobile occupant
      spacecraft, spaceship — *see* Accident, transport, aircraft, occupant, spacecraft
      sport utility vehicle — *see* Accident, transport, pickup truck occupant
      streetcar (interurban) (operating on public street or highway) — *see* Accident, transport, streetcar occupant
      SUV — *see* Accident, transport, pickup truck occupant
      teleferique V98.0- ☑
      three-wheeled vehicle (motorized) — *see also* Accident, transport, three-wheeled motor vehicle occupant
        nonmotorized — *see* Accident, transport, pedal cycle
      tractor (farm) (and trailer) — *see* Accident, transport, agricultural vehicle occupant
      train — *see* Accident, transport, railway vehicle occupant
      tram — *see* Accident, transport, streetcar occupant
        in mine or quarry — *see* Accident, transport, industrial vehicle occupant
      tricycle — *see* Accident, transport, pedal cycle

☑ **Additional Character Required** — Refer to the Tabular List for Character Selection

Accident — *continued*
   transport — *continued*
     occupant — *continued*
       tricycle — *see* Accident, transport, pedal cycle — *continued*
         motorized — *see* Accident, transport, three-wheeled motor vehicle
       trolley — *see* Accident, transport, streetcar occupant
       in mine or quarry — *see* Accident, transport, industrial vehicle occupant
       tub, in mine or quarry — *see* Accident, transport, industrial vehicle occupant
       ultralight — *see* Accident, transport, aircraft, occupant, powered, glider
       van — *see* Accident, transport, van occupant
       vehicle NEC V89.9- ☑
         heavy transport — *see* Accident, transport, truck occupant
         motor (traffic) NEC V89.2- ☑
         nontraffic NEC V89.0- ☑
       watercraft NOS V94.9- ☑
         causing drowning — *see* Drowning, resulting from accident to boat
     off-road motor-vehicle — *see also* Accident, transport, all-terrain vehicle occupant V86.99- ☑
     parachutist V97.29- ☑
       after accident to aircraft — *see* Accident, transport, aircraft
       entangled in object V97.21- ☑
       injured on landing V97.22- ☑
     pedal cyclist V19.9- ☑
       collision (with)
         animal (traffic) V10.9- ☑
           being ridden (traffic) V16.9- ☑
             nontraffic V16.2- ☑
             while boarding or alighting V16.3- ☑
           nontraffic V10.2- ☑
           while boarding or alighting V10.3- ☑
         animal-drawn vehicle (traffic) V16.9- ☑
           nontraffic V16.2- ☑
           while boarding or alighting V16.3- ☑
         bus (traffic) V14.9- ☑
           nontraffic V14.2- ☑
           while boarding or alighting V14.3- ☑
         car (traffic) V13.9- ☑
           nontraffic V13.2- ☑
           while boarding or alighting V13.3- ☑
         motor vehicle NOS (traffic) V19.60- ☑
           nontraffic V19.20- ☑
           specified type NEC (traffic) V19.69- ☑
             nontraffic V19.29- ☑
         pedal cycle (traffic) V11.9- ☑
           nontraffic V11.2- ☑
           while boarding or alighting V11.3- ☑
         pickup truck (traffic) V13.9- ☑
           nontraffic V13.2- ☑
           while boarding or alighting V13.3- ☑
         railway vehicle (traffic) V15.9- ☑
           nontraffic V15.2- ☑
           while boarding or alighting V15.3- ☑
         specified vehicle NEC (traffic) V16.9- ☑
           nontraffic V16.2- ☑
           while boarding or alighting V16.3- ☑
         stationary object (traffic) V17.9- ☑
           nontraffic V17.2- ☑
           while boarding or alighting V17.3- ☑
         streetcar (traffic) V16.9- ☑
           nontraffic V16.2- ☑
           while boarding or alighting V16.3- ☑
         three wheeled motor vehicle (traffic) V12.9- ☑
           nontraffic V12.2- ☑
           while boarding or alighting V12.3- ☑
         truck (traffic) V14.9- ☑
           nontraffic V14.2- ☑
           while boarding or alighting V14.3- ☑
         two wheeled motor vehicle (traffic) V12.9- ☑
           nontraffic V12.2- ☑
           while boarding or alighting V12.3- ☑
         van (traffic) V13.9- ☑
           nontraffic V13.2- ☑
           while boarding or alighting V13.3- ☑
       driver
         collision (with)
           animal (traffic) V10.4- ☑
             being ridden (traffic) V16.4- ☑

Accident — *continued*
   transport — *continued*
     pedal cyclist — *continued*
       driver — *continued*
         collision — *continued*
           animal — *continued*
             being ridden — *continued*
               nontraffic V16.0- ☑
             nontraffic V10.0- ☑
           animal-drawn vehicle (traffic) V16.4- ☑
             nontraffic V16.0- ☑
           bus (traffic) V14.4- ☑
             nontraffic V14.0- ☑
           car (traffic) V13.4- ☑
             nontraffic V13.0- ☑
           motor vehicle NOS (traffic) V19.40- ☑
             nontraffic V19.00- ☑
             specified type NEC (traffic) V19.49- ☑
               nontraffic V19.09- ☑
           pedal cycle (traffic) V11.4- ☑
             nontraffic V11.0- ☑
           pickup truck (traffic) V13.4- ☑
             nontraffic V13.0- ☑
           railway vehicle (traffic) V15.4- ☑
             nontraffic V15.0- ☑
           specified vehicle NEC (traffic) V16.4- ☑
             nontraffic V16.0- ☑
           stationary object (traffic) V17.4- ☑
             nontraffic V17.0- ☑
           streetcar (traffic) V16.4- ☑
             nontraffic V16.0- ☑
           three wheeled motor vehicle (traffic) V12.4- ☑
             nontraffic V12.0- ☑
           truck (traffic) V14.4- ☑
             nontraffic V14.0- ☑
           two wheeled motor vehicle (traffic) V12.4- ☑
             nontraffic V12.0- ☑
           van (traffic) V13.4- ☑
             nontraffic V13.0- ☑
         noncollision accident (traffic) V18.4- ☑
           nontraffic V18.0- ☑
       noncollision accident (traffic) V18.9- ☑
         nontraffic V18.2- ☑
         while boarding or alighting V18.3- ☑
       nontraffic V19.3- ☑
       passenger
         collision (with)
           animal (traffic) V10.5- ☑
             being ridden (traffic) V16.5- ☑
               nontraffic V16.1- ☑
             nontraffic V10.1- ☑
           animal-drawn vehicle (traffic) V16.5- ☑
             nontraffic V16.1- ☑
           bus (traffic) V14.5- ☑
             nontraffic V14.1- ☑
           car (traffic) V13.5- ☑
             nontraffic V13.1- ☑
           motor vehicle NOS (traffic) V19.50- ☑
             nontraffic V19.10- ☑
             specified type NEC (traffic) V19.59- ☑
               nontraffic V19.19- ☑
           pedal cycle (traffic) V11.5- ☑
             nontraffic V11.1- ☑
           pickup truck (traffic) V13.5- ☑
             nontraffic V13.1- ☑
           railway vehicle (traffic) V15.5- ☑
             nontraffic V15.1- ☑
           specified vehicle NEC (traffic) V16.5- ☑
             nontraffic V16.1- ☑
           stationary object (traffic) V17.5- ☑
             nontraffic V17.1- ☑
           streetcar (traffic) V16.5- ☑
             nontraffic V16.1- ☑
           three wheeled motor vehicle (traffic) V12.5- ☑
             nontraffic V12.1- ☑
           truck (traffic) V14.5- ☑
             nontraffic V14.1- ☑
           two wheeled motor vehicle (traffic) V12.5- ☑
             nontraffic V12.1- ☑
           van (traffic) V13.5- ☑
             nontraffic V13.1- ☑

Accident — *continued*
   transport — *continued*
     pedal cyclist — *continued*
       passenger — *continued*
         noncollision accident (traffic) V18.5- ☑
           nontraffic V18.1- ☑
       specified type NEC V19.88- ☑
       military vehicle V19.81- ☑
     pedestrian
       conveyance (occupant) V09.9- ☑
         baby stroller V00.828- ☑
           collision (with) V09.9- ☑
             animal being ridden or animal drawn vehicle V06.99- ☑
               nontraffic V06.09- ☑
               traffic V06.19- ☑
             bus or heavy transport V04.99- ☑
               nontraffic V04.09- ☑
               traffic V04.19- ☑
             car V03.99- ☑
               nontraffic V03.09- ☑
               traffic V03.19- ☑
             pedal cycle V01.99- ☑
               nontraffic V01.09- ☑
               traffic V01.19- ☑
             pick-up truck or van V03.99- ☑
               nontraffic V03.09- ☑
               traffic V03.19- ☑
             railway (train) (vehicle) V05.99- ☑
               nontraffic V05.09- ☑
               traffic V05.19- ☑
             stationary object V00.822- ☑
             streetcar V06.99- ☑
               nontraffic V06.09- ☑
               traffic V06.19- ☑
             two- or three-wheeled motor vehicle V02.99- ☑
               nontraffic V02.09- ☑
               traffic V02.19- ☑
             vehicle V09.9- ☑
               animal-drawn V06.99- ☑
                 nontraffic V06.09- ☑
                 traffic V06.19- ☑
               motor
                 nontraffic V09.00- ☑
                 traffic V09.20- ☑
           fall V00.821- ☑
           nontraffic V09.1- ☑
             involving motor vehicle NEC V09.00- ☑
           traffic V09.3- ☑
             involving motor vehicle NEC V09.20- ☑
         flat-bottomed NEC V00.388- ☑
           collision (with) V09.9- ☑
             animal being ridden or animal drawn vehicle V06.99- ☑
               nontraffic V06.09- ☑
               traffic V06.19- ☑
             bus or heavy transport V04.99- ☑
               nontraffic V04.09- ☑
               traffic V04.19- ☑
             car V03.99- ☑
               nontraffic V03.09- ☑
               traffic V03.19- ☑
             pedal cycle V01.99- ☑
               nontraffic V01.09- ☑
               traffic V01.19- ☑
             pick-up truck or van V03.99- ☑
               nontraffic V03.09- ☑
               traffic V03.19- ☑
             railway (train) (vehicle) V05.99- ☑
               nontraffic V05.09- ☑
               traffic V05.19- ☑
             stationary object V00.382- ☑
             streetcar V06.99- ☑
               nontraffic V06.09- ☑
               traffic V06.19- ☑
             two- or three-wheeled motor vehicle V02.99- ☑
               nontraffic V02.09- ☑
               traffic V02.19- ☑
             vehicle V09.9- ☑
               animal-drawn V06.99- ☑
                 nontraffic V06.09- ☑
                 traffic V06.19- ☑

Accident — continued
  transport — continued
    pedestrian — continued
      conveyance — continued
        flat-bottomed — continued
          collision — continued
            vehicle — continued
              motor
                nontraffic V09.00- ☑
                traffic V09.20- ☑
          fall V00.381- ☑
          nontraffic V09.1- ☑
            involving motor vehicle NEC V09.00- ☑
          snow
            board — see Accident, transport, pedestrian, conveyance, snow board
            ski — see Accident, transport, pedestrian, conveyance, skis (snow)
          traffic V09.3- ☑
            involving motor vehicle NEC V09.20- ☑
        gliding type NEC V00.288- ☑
          collision (with) V09.9- ☑
            animal being ridden or animal drawn vehicle V06.99- ☑
              nontraffic V06.09- ☑
              traffic V06.19- ☑
            bus or heavy transport V04.99- ☑
              nontraffic V04.09- ☑
              traffic V04.19- ☑
            car V03.99- ☑
              nontraffic V03.09- ☑
              traffic V03.19- ☑
            pedal cycle V01.99- ☑
              nontraffic V01.09- ☑
              traffic V01.19- ☑
            pick-up truck or van V03.99- ☑
              nontraffic V03.09- ☑
              traffic V03.19- ☑
            railway (train) (vehicle) V05.99- ☑
              nontraffic V05.09- ☑
              traffic V05.19- ☑
            stationary object V00.282- ☑
            streetcar V06.99- ☑
              nontraffic V06.09- ☑
              traffic V02.19- ☑
            two- or three-wheeled motor vehicle V02.99- ☑
              nontraffic V02.09- ☑
              traffic V02.19- ☑
            vehicle V09.9- ☑
              animal-drawn V06.99- ☑
                nontraffic V06.09- ☑
                traffic V06.19- ☑
              motor
                nontraffic V09.00- ☑
                traffic V09.20- ☑
          fall V00.281- ☑
          heelies — see Accident, transport, pedestrian, conveyance, heelies
          ice skate — see Accident, transport, pedestrian, conveyance, ice skate
          nontraffic V09.1- ☑
            involving motor vehicle NEC V09.00- ☑
          sled — see Accident, transport, pedestrian, conveyance, sled
          traffic V09.3- ☑
            involving motor vehicle NEC V09.20- ☑
          wheelies — see Accident, transport, pedestrian, conveyance, heelies
        heelies V00.158- ☑
          colliding with stationary object V00.152- ☑
          fall V00.151- ☑
        hoverboard
          collision with
            animal being ridden or animal drawn vehicle V06.938- ☑
              nontraffic V06.038- ☑
              traffic V06.138- ☑
            bus or heavy transport V04.938- ☑
              nontraffic V04.038- ☑
              traffic V04.138- ☑
            car V03.938- ☑
              nontraffic V03.038- ☑
              traffic V03.138- ☑

Accident — continued
  transport — continued
    pedestrian — continued
      conveyance — continued
        hoverboard — continued
          collision with — continued
            pedal cycle V01.938- ☑
              nontraffic V01.038- ☑
              traffic V01.138- ☑
            pick-up or van V03.938- ☑
              nontraffic V03.038- ☑
              traffic V03.138- ☑
            railway (train) (vehicle) V05.938- ☑
              nontraffic V05.038- ☑
              traffic V05.138- ☑
            streetcar V06.938- ☑
              nontraffic V06.038- ☑
              traffic V06.138- ☑
            three-wheeled motor vehicle V02.938- ☑
              nontraffic V02.038- ☑
              traffic V02.138- ☑
            two-wheeled motor vehicle V02.938- ☑
              nontraffic V02.038- ☑
              traffic V02.138- ☑
            vehicle, nonmotor, specified NEC V06.938- ☑
              nontraffic V06.038- ☑
              traffic V06.138- ☑
          fall V00.848- ☑
        ice skates V00.218- ☑
          collision (with) V09.9- ☑
            animal being ridden or animal drawn vehicle V06.99- ☑
              nontraffic V06.09- ☑
              traffic V06.19- ☑
            bus or heavy transport V04.99- ☑
              nontraffic V04.09- ☑
              traffic V04.19- ☑
            car V03.99- ☑
              nontraffic V03.09- ☑
              traffic V03.19- ☑
            pedal cycle V01.99- ☑
              nontraffic V01.09- ☑
              traffic V01.19- ☑
            pick-up truck or van V03.99- ☑
              nontraffic V03.09- ☑
              traffic V03.19- ☑
            railway (train) (vehicle) V05.99- ☑
              nontraffic V05.09- ☑
              traffic V05.19- ☑
            stationary object V00.212- ☑
            streetcar V06.99- ☑
              nontraffic V06.09- ☑
              traffic V06.19- ☑
            two- or three-wheeled motor vehicle V02.99- ☑
              nontraffic V02.09- ☑
              traffic V02.19- ☑
            vehicle V09.9- ☑
              animal-drawn V06.99- ☑
              nontraffic V06.09- ☑
              traffic V06.19- ☑
            motor
              nontraffic V09.00- ☑
              traffic V09.20- ☑
          fall V00.211- ☑
          nontraffic V09.1- ☑
            involving motor vehicle NEC V09.00- ☑
          traffic V09.3- ☑
            involving motor vehicle NEC V09.20- ☑
        motorized mobility scooter V00.838- ☑
          collision with stationary object V00.832- ☑
          fall from V00.831- ☑
          nontraffic V09.1- ☑
            involving motor vehicle V09.00- ☑
              military V09.01- ☑
              specified type NEC V09.09- ☑
        roller skates (non in-line) V00.128- ☑
          collision (with) V09.9- ☑
            animal being ridden or animal drawn vehicle V06.91- ☑
              nontraffic V06.01- ☑
              traffic V06.11- ☑

Accident — continued
  transport — continued
    pedestrian — continued
      conveyance — continued
        roller skates — continued
          collision — continued
            bus or heavy transport V04.91- ☑
              nontraffic V04.01- ☑
              traffic V04.11- ☑
            car V03.91- ☑
              nontraffic V03.01- ☑
              traffic V03.11- ☑
            pedal cycle V01.91- ☑
              nontraffic V01.01- ☑
              traffic V01.11- ☑
            pick-up truck or van V03.91- ☑
              nontraffic V03.01- ☑
              traffic V03.11- ☑
            railway (train) (vehicle) V05.91- ☑
              nontraffic V05.01- ☑
              traffic V05.11- ☑
            stationary object V00.122- ☑
            streetcar V06.91- ☑
              nontraffic V06.01- ☑
              traffic V06.11- ☑
            two- or three-wheeled motor vehicle V02.91- ☑
              nontraffic V02.01- ☑
              traffic V02.11- ☑
            vehicle V09.9- ☑
              animal-drawn V06.91- ☑
                nontraffic V06.01- ☑
                traffic V06.11- ☑
              motor
                nontraffic V09.00- ☑
                traffic V09.20- ☑
          fall V00.121- ☑
          in-line V00.118- ☑
            collision — see also Accident, transport, pedestrian, conveyance occupant, roller skates, collision with stationary object V00.112- ☑
            fall V00.111- ☑
          nontraffic V09.1- ☑
            involving motor vehicle NEC V09.00- ☑
          traffic V09.3- ☑
            involving motor vehicle NEC V09.20- ☑
        rolling shoes V00.158- ☑
          colliding with stationary object V00.152- ☑
          fall V00.151- ☑
        rolling type NEC V00.188- ☑
          collision (with) V09.9- ☑
            animal being ridden or animal drawn vehicle V06.99- ☑
              nontraffic V06.09- ☑
              traffic V06.19- ☑
            bus or heavy transport V04.99- ☑
              nontraffic V04.09- ☑
              traffic V04.19- ☑
            car V03.99- ☑
              nontraffic V03.09- ☑
              traffic V03.19- ☑
            pedal cycle V01.99- ☑
              nontraffic V01.09- ☑
              traffic V01.19- ☑
            pick-up truck or van V03.99- ☑
              nontraffic V03.09- ☑
              traffic V03.19- ☑
            railway (train) (vehicle) V05.99- ☑
              nontraffic V05.09- ☑
              traffic V05.19- ☑
            stationary object V00.182- ☑
            streetcar V06.99- ☑
              nontraffic V06.09- ☑
              traffic V06.19- ☑
            two- or three-wheeled motor vehicle V02.99- ☑
              nontraffic V02.09- ☑
              traffic V02.19- ☑
            vehicle V09.9- ☑
              animal-drawn V06.99- ☑
                nontraffic V06.09- ☑
                traffic V06.19- ☑

☑ Additional Character Required — Refer to the Tabular List for Character Selection

Accident

Accident — *continued*
- transport — *continued*
  - pedestrian — *continued*
    - conveyance — *continued*
      - rolling type — *continued*
        - collision — *continued*
          - vehicle — *continued*
            - motor
              - nontraffic V09.00- ☑
              - traffic V09.20- ☑
        - fall V00.181- ☑
        - in-line roller skate — *see* Accident, transport, pedestrian, conveyance, roller skate, in-line
        - nontraffic V09.1- ☑
          - involving motor vehicle NEC V09.00- ☑
        - roller skate — *see* Accident, transport, pedestrian, conveyance, roller skate
        - scooter (non-motorized) — *see* Accident, transport, pedestrian, conveyance, scooter
        - skateboard — *see* Accident, transport, pedestrian, conveyance, skateboard
        - traffic V09.3- ☑
          - involving motor vehicle NEC V09.20- ☑
      - scooter (non-motorized) V00.148- ☑
        - collision (with) V09.9- ☑
          - animal being ridden or animal drawn vehicle V06.99- ☑
            - nontraffic V06.09- ☑
            - traffic V06.19- ☑
          - bus or heavy transport V04.99- ☑
            - nontraffic V04.09- ☑
            - traffic V04.19- ☑
          - car V03.99- ☑
            - nontraffic V03.09- ☑
            - traffic V03.19- ☑
          - pedal cycle V01.99- ☑
            - nontraffic V01.09- ☑
            - traffic V01.19- ☑
          - pick-up truck or van V03.99- ☑
            - nontraffic V03.09- ☑
            - traffic V03.19- ☑
          - railway (train) (vehicle) V05.99- ☑
            - nontraffic V05.09- ☑
            - traffic V05.19- ☑
          - stationary object V00.142- ☑
          - streetcar V06.99- ☑
            - nontraffic V06.09- ☑
            - traffic V06.19- ☑
          - two- or three-wheeled motor vehicle V02.99- ☑
            - nontraffic V02.09- ☑
            - traffic V02.19- ☑
          - vehicle V09.9- ☑
            - animal-drawn V06.99- ☑
              - nontraffic V06.09- ☑
              - traffic V06.19- ☑
            - motor
              - nontraffic V09.00- ☑
              - traffic V09.20- ☑
        - fall V00.141- ☑
        - nontraffic V09.1- ☑
          - involving motor vehicle NEC V09.00- ☑
        - traffic V09.3- ☑
          - involving motor vehicle NEC V09.20- ☑
      - Segway
        - collision with
          - animal being ridden or animal drawn vehicle V06.938- ☑
            - nontraffic V06.038- ☑
            - traffic V06.138- ☑
          - bus or heavy transport V04.938- ☑
            - nontraffic V04.038- ☑
            - traffic V04.138- ☑
          - car V03.938- ☑
            - nontraffic V03.038- ☑
            - traffic V03.138- ☑
          - pedal cycle V01.938- ☑
            - nontraffic V01.038- ☑
            - traffic V01.138- ☑
          - pick-up or van V03.938- ☑
            - nontraffic V03.038- ☑
            - traffic V03.138- ☑
          - railway (train) (vehicle) V05.938- ☑
            - nontraffic V05.038- ☑

Accident — *continued*
- transport — *continued*
  - pedestrian — *continued*
    - conveyance — *continued*
      - Segway — *continued*
        - collision with — *continued*
          - railway — *continued*
            - traffic V05.138- ☑
          - streetcar V06.938- ☑
            - nontraffic V06.038- ☑
            - traffic V06.138- ☑
          - three-wheeled vehicle V02.938- ☑
            - nontraffic V02.038- ☑
            - traffic V02.138- ☑
          - two-wheeled vehicle V02.938- ☑
            - nontraffic V02.038- ☑
            - traffic V02.138- ☑
          - vehicle, nonmotor, specified NEC V06.938- ☑
            - nontraffic V06.038- ☑
            - traffic V06.138- ☑
        - fall V00.848- ☑
      - skateboard V00.138- ☑
        - collision (with) V09.9- ☑
          - animal being ridden or animal drawn vehicle V06.92- ☑
            - nontraffic V06.02- ☑
            - traffic V06.12- ☑
          - bus or heavy transport V04.92- ☑
            - nontraffic V04.02- ☑
            - traffic V04.12- ☑
          - car V03.92- ☑
            - nontraffic V03.02- ☑
            - traffic V03.12- ☑
          - pedal cycle V01.92- ☑
            - nontraffic V01.02- ☑
            - traffic V01.12- ☑
          - pick-up truck or van V03.92- ☑
            - nontraffic V03.02- ☑
            - traffic V03.12- ☑
          - railway (train) (vehicle) V05.92- ☑
            - nontraffic V05.02- ☑
            - traffic V05.12- ☑
          - stationary object V00.132- ☑
          - streetcar V06.92- ☑
            - nontraffic V06.02- ☑
            - traffic V06.12- ☑
          - two- or three-wheeled motor vehicle V02.92- ☑
            - nontraffic V02.02- ☑
            - traffic V02.12- ☑
          - vehicle V09.9- ☑
            - animal-drawn V06.92- ☑
              - nontraffic V06.02- ☑
              - traffic V06.12- ☑
            - motor
              - nontraffic V09.00- ☑
              - traffic V09.20- ☑
        - fall V00.131- ☑
        - nontraffic V09.1- ☑
          - involving motor vehicle NEC V09.00- ☑
        - traffic V09.3- ☑
          - involving motor vehicle NEC V09.20- ☑
      - skis (snow) V00.328- ☑
        - collision (with) V09.9- ☑
          - animal being ridden or animal drawn vehicle V06.99- ☑
            - nontraffic V06.09- ☑
            - traffic V06.19- ☑
          - bus or heavy transport V04.99- ☑
            - nontraffic V04.09- ☑
            - traffic V04.19- ☑
          - car V03.99- ☑
            - nontraffic V03.09- ☑
            - traffic V03.19- ☑
          - pedal cycle V01.99- ☑
            - nontraffic V01.09- ☑
            - traffic V01.19- ☑
          - pick-up truck or van V03.99- ☑
            - nontraffic V03.09- ☑
            - traffic V03.19- ☑
          - railway (train) (vehicle) V05.99- ☑
            - nontraffic V05.09- ☑
            - traffic V05.19- ☑
          - stationary object V00.322- ☑

Accident — *continued*
- transport — *continued*
  - pedestrian — *continued*
    - conveyance — *continued*
      - skis — *continued*
        - collision — *continued*
          - streetcar V06.99- ☑
            - nontraffic V06.09- ☑
            - traffic V06.19- ☑
          - two- or three-wheeled motor vehicle V02.99- ☑
            - nontraffic V02.09- ☑
            - traffic V02.19- ☑
          - vehicle V09.9- ☑
            - animal-drawn V06.99- ☑
              - nontraffic V06.09- ☑
              - traffic V06.19- ☑
            - motor
              - nontraffic V09.00- ☑
              - traffic V09.20- ☑
        - fall V00.321- ☑
        - nontraffic V09.1- ☑
          - involving motor vehicle NEC V09.00- ☑
        - traffic V09.3- ☑
          - involving motor vehicle NEC V09.20- ☑
      - sled V00.228- ☑
        - collision (with) V09.9- ☑
          - animal being ridden or animal drawn vehicle V06.99- ☑
            - nontraffic V06.09- ☑
            - traffic V06.19- ☑
          - bus or heavy transport V04.99- ☑
            - nontraffic V04.09- ☑
            - traffic V04.19- ☑
          - car V03.99- ☑
            - nontraffic V03.09- ☑
            - traffic V03.19- ☑
          - pedal cycle V01.99- ☑
            - nontraffic V01.09- ☑
            - traffic V01.19- ☑
          - pick-up truck or van V03.99- ☑
            - nontraffic V03.09- ☑
            - traffic V03.19- ☑
          - railway (train) (vehicle) V05.99- ☑
            - nontraffic V05.09- ☑
            - traffic V05.19- ☑
          - stationary object V00.222- ☑
          - streetcar V06.99- ☑
            - nontraffic V06.09- ☑
            - traffic V06.19- ☑
          - two- or three-wheeled motor vehicle V02.99- ☑
            - nontraffic V02.09- ☑
            - traffic V02.19- ☑
          - vehicle V09.9- ☑
            - animal-drawn V06.99- ☑
              - nontraffic V06.09- ☑
              - traffic V06.19- ☑
            - motor
              - nontraffic V09.00- ☑
              - traffic V09.20- ☑
        - fall V00.221- ☑
        - nontraffic V09.1- ☑
          - involving motor vehicle NEC V09.00- ☑
        - traffic V09.3- ☑
          - involving motor vehicle NEC V09.20- ☑
      - snow board V00.318- ☑
        - collision (with) V09.9- ☑
          - animal being ridden or animal drawn vehicle V06.99- ☑
            - nontraffic V06.09- ☑
            - traffic V06.19- ☑
          - bus or heavy transport V04.99- ☑
            - nontraffic V04.09- ☑
            - traffic V04.19- ☑
          - car V03.99- ☑
            - nontraffic V03.09- ☑
            - traffic V03.19- ☑
          - pedal cycle V01.99- ☑
            - nontraffic V01.09- ☑
            - traffic V01.19- ☑
          - pick-up truck or van V03.99- ☑
            - nontraffic V03.09- ☑
            - traffic V03.19- ☑
          - railway (train) (vehicle) V05.99- ☑

Accident — *continued*
  transport — *continued*
    pedestrian — *continued*
      conveyance — *continued*
        snow board — *continued*
          collision — *continued*
            railway — *continued*
              nontraffic V05.09- ☑
              traffic V05.19- ☑
            stationary object V00.312- ☑
            streetcar V06.99- ☑
              nontraffic V06.09- ☑
              traffic V06.19- ☑
            two- or three-wheeled motor vehicle V02.99- ☑
              nontraffic V02.09- ☑
              traffic V02.19- ☑
            vehicle V09.9- ☑
              animal-drawn V06.99- ☑
                nontraffic V06.09- ☑
                traffic V06.19- ☑
              motor
                nontraffic V09.00- ☑
                traffic V09.20- ☑
          fall V00.311- ☑
          nontraffic V09.1- ☑
            involving motor vehicle NEC V09.00- ☑
          traffic V09.3- ☑
            involving motor vehicle NEC V09.20- ☑
        specified type NEC V00.898- ☑
          collision (with) V09.9- ☑
            animal being ridden or animal drawn vehicle V06.99- ☑
              nontraffic V06.09- ☑
              traffic V06.19- ☑
            bus or heavy transport V04.99- ☑
              nontraffic V04.09- ☑
              traffic V04.19- ☑
            car V03.99- ☑
              nontraffic V03.09- ☑
              traffic V03.19- ☑
            pedal cycle V01.99- ☑
              nontraffic V01.09- ☑
              traffic V01.19- ☑
            pick-up truck or van V03.99- ☑
              nontraffic V03.09- ☑
              traffic V03.19- ☑
            railway (train) (vehicle) V05.99- ☑
              nontraffic V05.09- ☑
              traffic V05.19- ☑
            stationary object V00.892- ☑
            streetcar V06.99- ☑
              nontraffic V06.09- ☑
              traffic V06.19- ☑
            two- or three-wheeled motor vehicle V02.99- ☑
              nontraffic V02.09- ☑
              traffic V02.19- ☑
            vehicle V09.9- ☑
              animal-drawn V06.99- ☑
                nontraffic V06.09- ☑
                traffic V06.19- ☑
              motor
                nontraffic V09.00- ☑
                traffic V09.20- ☑
          fall V00.891- ☑
          nontraffic V09.1- ☑
            involving motor vehicle NEC V09.00- ☑
          traffic V09.3- ☑
            involving motor vehicle NEC V09.20- ☑
        standing
          electric scooter
            collision with
              animal being ridden or animal drawn vehicle V06.931- ☑
                nontraffic V06.031- ☑
                traffic V06.131- ☑
              bus or heavy transport V04.931- ☑
                nontraffic V04.031- ☑
                traffic V04.131- ☑
              car V03.931- ☑
                nontraffic V04.031- ☑
                traffic V04.131- ☑
              pedal cycle V01.931- ☑
                nontraffic V01.031- ☑

Accident — *continued*
  transport — *continued*
    pedestrian — *continued*
      conveyance — *continued*
        standing — *continued*
          electric scooter — *continued*
            collision with — *continued*
              pedal cycle — *continued*
                traffic V01.131- ☑
              pick-up or van V03.931- ☑
                nontraffic V03.031- ☑
                traffic V03.131- ☑
              railway (train) (vehicle) V05.931- ☑
                nontraffic V05.031- ☑
                traffic V05.131- ☑
              streetcar V06.931- ☑
                nontraffic V06.031- ☑
                traffic V06.131- ☑
              three-wheeled motor vehicle V02.931- ☑
                nontraffic V02.031- ☑
                traffic V02.131- ☑
              two-wheeled motor vehicle V02.931- ☑
                nontraffic V02.031- ☑
                traffic V02.131- ☑
              vehicle, nonmotor, specified NEC V06.931- ☑
                nontraffic V06.031- ☑
                traffic V06.131- ☑
            fall V00.841- ☑
          micro-mobility pedestrian conveyance
            collision with
              animal being ridden or animal drawn vehicle V06.938- ☑
                nontraffic V06.038- ☑
                traffic V06.138- ☑
              bus or heavy transport V04.938- ☑
                nontraffic V04.038- ☑
                traffic V04.138- ☑
              car V03.938- ☑
                nontraffic V03.038- ☑
                traffic V03.138- ☑
              pedal cycle V01.938- ☑
                nontraffic V01.038- ☑
                traffic V01.138- ☑
              pick-up or van V03.938- ☑
                nontraffic V03.038- ☑
                traffic V03.138- ☑
              railway (train) (vehicle) V05.938- ☑
                nontraffic V05.038- ☑
                traffic V05.138- ☑
              stationary object V00.842- ☑
              streetcar V06.938- ☑
                nontraffic V06.038- ☑
                traffic V06.138- ☑
              three-wheeled motor vehicle V02.938- ☑
                nontraffic V02.038- ☑
                traffic V02.138- ☑
              two-wheeled motor vehicle V02.938- ☑
                nontraffic V02.038- ☑
                traffic V02.138- ☑
              vehicle, nonmotor, specified NEC V06.938- ☑
                nontraffic V06.038- ☑
                traffic V06.138- ☑
            fall V00.848- ☑
          traffic V09.3- ☑
            involving motor vehicle V09.20- ☑
            military V09.21- ☑
            specified type NEC V09.29- ☑
        wheelchair (powered) V00.818- ☑
          collision (with) V09.9- ☑
            animal being ridden or animal drawn vehicle V06.99- ☑
              nontraffic V06.09- ☑
              traffic V06.19- ☑
            bus or heavy transport V04.99- ☑
              nontraffic V04.09- ☑
              traffic V04.19- ☑
            car V03.99- ☑
              nontraffic V03.09- ☑
              traffic V03.19- ☑
            pedal cycle V01.99- ☑

Accident — *continued*
  transport — *continued*
    pedestrian — *continued*
      conveyance — *continued*
        wheelchair — *continued*
          collision — *continued*
            pedal cycle — *continued*
              nontraffic V01.09- ☑
              traffic V01.19- ☑
            pick-up truck or van V03.99- ☑
              nontraffic V03.09- ☑
              traffic V03.19- ☑
            railway (train) (vehicle) V05.99- ☑
              nontraffic V05.09- ☑
              traffic V05.19- ☑
            stationary object V00.812- ☑
            streetcar V06.99- ☑
              nontraffic V06.09- ☑
              traffic V06.19- ☑
            two- or three-wheeled motor vehicle V02.99- ☑
              nontraffic V02.09- ☑
              traffic V02.19- ☑
            vehicle V09.9- ☑
              animal-drawn V06.99- ☑
                nontraffic V06.09- ☑
                traffic V06.19- ☑
              motor
                nontraffic V09.00- ☑
                traffic V09.20- ☑
          fall V00.811- ☑
          nontraffic V09.1- ☑
            involving motor vehicle NEC V09.00- ☑
          traffic V09.3- ☑
            involving motor vehicle NEC V09.20- ☑
        wheeled shoe V00.158- ☑
          colliding with stationary object V00.152- ☑
          fall V00.151- ☑
      on foot — *see also* Accident, pedestrian
        collision (with)
          animal being ridden or animal drawn vehicle V06.90- ☑
            nontraffic V06.00- ☑
            traffic V06.10- ☑
          bus or heavy transport V04.90- ☑
            nontraffic V04.00- ☑
            traffic V04.10- ☑
          car V03.90- ☑
            nontraffic V03.00- ☑
            traffic V03.10- ☑
          pedal cycle V01.90- ☑
            nontraffic V01.00- ☑
            traffic V01.10- ☑
          pick-up truck or van V03.90- ☑
            nontraffic V03.00- ☑
            traffic V03.10- ☑
          railway (train) (vehicle) V05.90- ☑
            nontraffic V05.00- ☑
            traffic V05.10- ☑
          streetcar V06.90- ☑
            nontraffic V06.00- ☑
            traffic V06.10- ☑
          two- or three-wheeled motor vehicle V02.90- ☑
            nontraffic V02.00- ☑
            traffic V02.10- ☑
          vehicle V09.9- ☑
            animal-drawn V06.90- ☑
              nontraffic V06.00- ☑
              traffic V06.10- ☑
            motor
        nontraffic V09.1- ☑
          involving motor vehicle V09.00- ☑
            military V09.01- ☑
            specified type NEC V09.09- ☑
        traffic V09.3- ☑
          involving motor vehicle V09.20- ☑
            military V09.21- ☑
            specified type NEC V09.29- ☑
      person NEC (unknown way or transportation) V99.- ☑
        collision (between)
          bus (with)
            heavy transport vehicle (traffic) V87.5- ☑
              nontraffic V88.5- ☑

Accident

Accident — *continued*
  transport — *continued*
    person — *continued*
      collision — *continued*
        car (with)
          bus (traffic) V87.3- ☑
            nontraffic V88.3- ☑
          heavy transport vehicle (traffic) V87.4- ☑
            nontraffic V88.4- ☑
          nontraffic V88.5- ☑
          pick-up truck or van (traffic) V87.2- ☑
            nontraffic V88.2- ☑
          train or railway vehicle (traffic) V87.6- ☑
            nontraffic V88.6- ☑
          two-or three-wheeled motor vehicle (traffic) V87.0- ☑
            nontraffic V88.0- ☑
        motor vehicle (traffic) NEC V87.7- ☑
          nontraffic V88.7- ☑
        two-or three-wheeled vehicle (with) (traffic)
          motor vehicle NEC V87.1- ☑
            nontraffic V88.1- ☑
        nonmotor vehicle (collision) (noncollision) (traffic) V87.9- ☑
          nontraffic V88.9- ☑
      pickup truck occupant V59.9- ☑
        collision (with)
          animal (traffic) V50.9- ☑
            being ridden (traffic) V56.9- ☑
              nontraffic V56.3- ☑
                while boarding or alighting V56.4- ☑
            nontraffic V50.3- ☑
            while boarding or alighting V50.4- ☑
          animal-drawn vehicle (traffic) V56.9- ☑
            nontraffic V56.3- ☑
            while boarding or alighting V56.4- ☑
          bus (traffic) V54.9- ☑
            nontraffic V54.3- ☑
            while boarding or alighting V54.4- ☑
          car (traffic) V53.9- ☑
            nontraffic V53.3- ☑
            while boarding or alighting V53.4- ☑
          motor vehicle NOS (traffic) V59.60- ☑
            nontraffic V59.20- ☑
            specified type NEC (traffic) V59.69- ☑
              nontraffic V59.29- ☑
          pedal cycle (traffic) V51.9- ☑
            nontraffic V51.3- ☑
            while boarding or alighting V51.4- ☑
          pickup truck (traffic) V53.9- ☑
            nontraffic V53.3- ☑
            while boarding or alighting V53.4- ☑
          railway vehicle (traffic) V55.9- ☑
            nontraffic V55.3- ☑
            while boarding or alighting V55.4- ☑
          specified vehicle NEC (traffic) V56.9- ☑
            nontraffic V56.3- ☑
            while boarding or alighting V56.4- ☑
          stationary object (traffic) V57.9- ☑
            nontraffic V57.3- ☑
            while boarding or alighting V57.4- ☑
          streetcar (traffic) V56.9- ☑
            nontraffic V56.3- ☑
            while boarding or alighting V56.4- ☑
          three wheeled motor vehicle (traffic) V52.9- ☑
            nontraffic V52.3- ☑
            while boarding or alighting V52.4- ☑
          truck (traffic) V54.9- ☑
            nontraffic V54.3- ☑
            while boarding or alighting V54.4- ☑
          two wheeled motor vehicle (traffic) V52.9- ☑
            nontraffic V52.3- ☑
            while boarding or alighting V52.4- ☑
          van (traffic) V53.9- ☑
            nontraffic V53.3- ☑
            while boarding or alighting V53.4- ☑
        driver
          collision (with)
            animal (traffic) V50.5- ☑
              being ridden (traffic) V56.5- ☑
                nontraffic V56.0- ☑
              nontraffic V50.0- ☑
            animal-drawn vehicle (traffic) V56.5- ☑
              nontraffic V56.0- ☑
            bus (traffic) V54.5- ☑

Accident — *continued*
  transport — *continued*
    pickup truck occupant — *continued*
      driver — *continued*
        collision — *continued*
          bus — *continued*
            nontraffic V54.0- ☑
          car (traffic) V53.5- ☑
            nontraffic V53.0- ☑
          motor vehicle NOS (traffic) V59.40- ☑
            nontraffic V59.00- ☑
            specified type NEC (traffic) V59.49- ☑
              nontraffic V59.09- ☑
          pedal cycle (traffic) V51.5- ☑
            nontraffic V51.0- ☑
          pickup truck (traffic) V53.5- ☑
            nontraffic V53.0- ☑
          railway vehicle (traffic) V55.5- ☑
            nontraffic V55.0- ☑
          specified vehicle NEC (traffic) V56.5- ☑
            nontraffic V56.0- ☑
          stationary object (traffic) V57.5- ☑
            nontraffic V57.0- ☑
          streetcar (traffic) V56.5- ☑
            nontraffic V56.0- ☑
          three wheeled motor vehicle (traffic) V52.5- ☑
            nontraffic V52.0- ☑
          truck (traffic) V54.5- ☑
            nontraffic V54.0- ☑
          two wheeled motor vehicle (traffic) V52.5- ☑
            nontraffic V52.0- ☑
          van (traffic) V53.5- ☑
            nontraffic V53.0- ☑
        noncollision accident (traffic) V58.5- ☑
          nontraffic V58.0- ☑
      hanger-on
        collision (with)
          animal (traffic) V50.7- ☑
            being ridden (traffic) V56.7- ☑
              nontraffic V56.2- ☑
            nontraffic V50.2- ☑
          animal-drawn vehicle (traffic) V56.7- ☑
            nontraffic V56.2- ☑
          bus (traffic) V54.7- ☑
            nontraffic V54.2- ☑
          car (traffic) V53.7- ☑
            nontraffic V53.2- ☑
          pedal cycle (traffic) V51.7- ☑
            nontraffic V51.2- ☑
          pickup truck (traffic) V53.7- ☑
            nontraffic V53.2- ☑
          railway vehicle (traffic) V55.7- ☑
            nontraffic V55.2- ☑
          specified vehicle NEC (traffic) V56.7- ☑
            nontraffic V56.2- ☑
          stationary object (traffic) V57.7- ☑
            nontraffic V57.2- ☑
          streetcar (traffic) V56.7- ☑
            nontraffic V56.2- ☑
          three wheeled motor vehicle (traffic) V52.7- ☑
            nontraffic V52.2- ☑
          truck (traffic) V54.7- ☑
            nontraffic V54.2- ☑
          two wheeled motor vehicle (traffic) V52.7- ☑
            nontraffic V52.2- ☑
          van (traffic) V53.7- ☑
            nontraffic V53.2- ☑
        noncollision accident (traffic) V58.7- ☑
          nontraffic V58.2- ☑
      noncollision accident (traffic) V58.9- ☑
        nontraffic V58.3- ☑
        while boarding or alighting V58.4- ☑
      nontraffic V59.3- ☑
      passenger
        collision (with)
          animal (traffic) V50.6- ☑
            being ridden (traffic) V56.6- ☑
              nontraffic V56.1- ☑
            nontraffic V50.1- ☑
          animal-drawn vehicle (traffic) V56.6- ☑
            nontraffic V56.1- ☑

Accident — *continued*
  transport — *continued*
    pickup truck occupant — *continued*
      passenger — *continued*
        collision — *continued*
          bus (traffic) V54.6- ☑
            nontraffic V54.1- ☑
          car (traffic) V53.6- ☑
            nontraffic V53.1- ☑
          motor vehicle NOS (traffic) V59.50- ☑
            nontraffic V59.10- ☑
            specified type NEC (traffic) V59.59- ☑
              nontraffic V59.19- ☑
          pedal cycle (traffic) V51.6- ☑
            nontraffic V51.1- ☑
          pickup truck (traffic) V53.6- ☑
            nontraffic V53.1- ☑
          railway vehicle (traffic) V55.6- ☑
            nontraffic V55.1- ☑
          specified vehicle NEC (traffic) V56.6- ☑
            nontraffic V56.1- ☑
          stationary object (traffic) V57.6- ☑
            nontraffic V57.1- ☑
          streetcar (traffic) V56.6- ☑
            nontraffic V56.1- ☑
          three wheeled motor vehicle (traffic) V52.6- ☑
            nontraffic V52.1- ☑
          truck (traffic) V54.6- ☑
            nontraffic V54.1- ☑
          two wheeled motor vehicle (traffic) V52.6- ☑
            nontraffic V52.1- ☑
          van (traffic) V53.6- ☑
            nontraffic V53.1- ☑
        noncollision accident (traffic) V58.6- ☑
          nontraffic V58.1- ☑
      specified type NEC V59.88- ☑
      military vehicle V59.81- ☑
    quarry truck — *see* Accident, transport, industrial vehicle occupant
    race car — *see* Accident, transport, motor vehicle NEC occupant
    railway vehicle occupant V81.9- ☑
      collision (with) V81.3- ☑
        motor vehicle (non-military) (traffic) V81.1- ☑
          military V81.83- ☑
          nontraffic V81.0- ☑
        rolling stock V81.2- ☑
        specified object NEC V81.3- ☑
      during derailment V81.7- ☑
        with antecedent collision — *see* Accident, transport, railway vehicle occupant, collision
      explosion V81.81- ☑
      fall (in railway vehicle) V81.5- ☑
        during derailment V81.7- ☑
          with antecedent collision — *see* Accident, transport, railway vehicle occupant, collision
        from railway vehicle V81.6- ☑
          during derailment V81.7- ☑
            with antecedent collision — *see* Accident, transport, railway vehicle occupant, collision
        while boarding or alighting V81.4- ☑
      fire V81.81- ☑
      object falling onto train V81.82- ☑
      specified type NEC V81.89- ☑
      while boarding or alighting V81.4- ☑
    Segway V00.848- ☑
    ski lift V98.3- ☑
    snowmobile occupant (nontraffic) V86.92- ☑
      driver V86.52- ☑
      hanger-on V86.72- ☑
      passenger V86.62- ☑
      traffic V86.32- ☑
        driver V86.02- ☑
        hanger-on V86.22- ☑
        passenger V86.12- ☑
      while boarding or alighting V86.42- ☑
    specified NEC V98.8- ☑
    sport utility vehicle occupant — *see also* Accident, transport, pickup truck occupant
    streetcar occupant V82.9- ☑
      collision (with) V82.3- ☑

Accident — *continued*
   transport — *continued*
      streetcar occupant — *continued*
         collision — *continued*
            motor vehicle (traffic) V82.1- ☑
               nontraffic V82.0- ☑
            rolling stock V82.2- ☑
         during derailment V82.7- ☑
            with antecedent collision — *see* Accident, transport, streetcar occupant, collision
         fall (in streetcar) V82.5- ☑
            during derailment V82.7- ☑
               with antecedent collision — *see* Accident, transport, streetcar occupant, collision
            from streetcar V82.6- ☑
               during derailment V82.7- ☑
                  with antecedent collision — *see* Accident, transport, streetcar occupant, collision
            while boarding or alighting V82.4- ☑
         while boarding or alighting V82.4- ☑
         specified type NEC V82.8- ☑
         while boarding or alighting V82.4- ☑
      three-wheeled motor vehicle occupant V39.9- ☑
         collision (with)
            animal (traffic) V30.9- ☑
               being ridden (traffic) V36.9- ☑
                  nontraffic V36.3- ☑
                     while boarding or alighting V36.4- ☑
               nontraffic V30.3- ☑
                  while boarding or alighting V30.4- ☑
            animal-drawn vehicle (traffic) V36.9- ☑
               nontraffic V36.3- ☑
               while boarding or alighting V36.4- ☑
            bus (traffic) V34.9- ☑
               nontraffic V34.3- ☑
               while boarding or alighting V34.4- ☑
            car (traffic) V33.9- ☑
               nontraffic V33.3- ☑
               while boarding or alighting V33.4- ☑
            motor vehicle NOS (traffic) V39.60- ☑
               nontraffic V39.20- ☑
               specified type NEC (traffic) V39.69- ☑
                  nontraffic V39.29- ☑
            pedal cycle (traffic) V31.9- ☑
               nontraffic V31.3- ☑
               while boarding or alighting V31.4- ☑
            pickup truck (traffic) V33.9- ☑
               nontraffic V33.3- ☑
               while boarding or alighting V33.4- ☑
            railway vehicle (traffic) V35.9- ☑
               nontraffic V35.3- ☑
               while boarding or alighting V35.4- ☑
            specified vehicle NEC (traffic) V36.9- ☑
               nontraffic V36.3- ☑
               while boarding or alighting V36.4- ☑
            stationary object (traffic) V37.9- ☑
               nontraffic V37.3- ☑
               while boarding or alighting V37.4- ☑
            streetcar (traffic) V36.9- ☑
               nontraffic V36.3- ☑
               while boarding or alighting V36.4- ☑
            three wheeled motor vehicle (traffic) V32.9- ☑
               nontraffic V32.3- ☑
               while boarding or alighting V32.4- ☑
            truck (traffic) V34.9- ☑
               nontraffic V34.3- ☑
               while boarding or alighting V34.4- ☑
            two wheeled motor vehicle (traffic) V32.9- ☑
               nontraffic V32.3- ☑
               while boarding or alighting V32.4- ☑
            van (traffic) V33.9- ☑
               nontraffic V33.3- ☑
               while boarding or alighting V33.4- ☑
         driver
            collision (with)
               animal (traffic) V30.5- ☑
                  being ridden (traffic) V36.5- ☑
                     nontraffic V36.0- ☑
                  nontraffic V30.0- ☑
               animal-drawn vehicle (traffic) V36.5- ☑
                 nontraffic V36.0- ☑
               bus (traffic) V34.5- ☑
                 nontraffic V34.0- ☑

Accident — *continued*
   transport — *continued*
      three-wheeled motor vehicle occupant — *continued*
         driver — *continued*
            collision — *continued*
               car (traffic) V33.5- ☑
                  nontraffic V33.0- ☑
               motor vehicle NOS (traffic) V39.40- ☑
                  nontraffic V39.00- ☑
                  specified type NEC (traffic) V39.49- ☑
                     nontraffic V39.09- ☑
               pedal cycle (traffic) V31.5- ☑
                  nontraffic V31.0- ☑
               pickup truck (traffic) V33.5- ☑
                  nontraffic V33.0- ☑
               railway vehicle (traffic) V35.5- ☑
                  nontraffic V35.0- ☑
               specified vehicle NEC (traffic) V36.5- ☑
                  nontraffic V36.0- ☑
               stationary object (traffic) V37.5- ☑
                  nontraffic V37.0- ☑
               streetcar (traffic) V36.5- ☑
                  nontraffic V36.0- ☑
               three wheeled motor vehicle (traffic) V32.5- ☑
                  nontraffic V32.0- ☑
               truck (traffic) V34.5- ☑
                  nontraffic V34.0- ☑
               two wheeled motor vehicle (traffic) V32.5- ☑
                  nontraffic V32.0- ☑
               van (traffic) V33.5- ☑
                  nontraffic V33.0- ☑
            noncollision accident (traffic) V38.5- ☑
               nontraffic V38.0- ☑
         hanger-on
            collision (with)
               animal (traffic) V30.7- ☑
                  being ridden (traffic) V36.7- ☑
                     nontraffic V36.2- ☑
                  nontraffic V30.2- ☑
               animal-drawn vehicle (traffic) V36.7- ☑
                 nontraffic V36.2- ☑
               bus (traffic) V34.7- ☑
                 nontraffic V34.2- ☑
               car (traffic) V33.7- ☑
                 nontraffic V33.2- ☑
               pedal cycle (traffic) V31.7- ☑
                 nontraffic V31.2- ☑
               pickup truck (traffic) V33.7- ☑
                 nontraffic V33.2- ☑
               railway vehicle (traffic) V35.7- ☑
                 nontraffic V35.2- ☑
               specified vehicle NEC (traffic) V36.7- ☑
                 nontraffic V36.2- ☑
               stationary object (traffic) V37.7- ☑
                 nontraffic V37.2- ☑
               streetcar (traffic) V36.7- ☑
                 nontraffic V36.2- ☑
               three wheeled motor vehicle (traffic) V32.7- ☑
                 nontraffic V32.2- ☑
               truck (traffic) V34.7- ☑
                 nontraffic V34.2- ☑
               two wheeled motor vehicle (traffic) V32.7- ☑
                 nontraffic V32.2- ☑
               van (traffic) V33.7- ☑
                 nontraffic V33.2- ☑
            noncollision accident (traffic) V38.7- ☑
               nontraffic V38.2- ☑
         noncollision accident (traffic) V38.9- ☑
            nontraffic V38.3- ☑
            while boarding or alighting V38.4- ☑
         nontraffic V39.3- ☑
         passenger
            collision (with)
               animal (traffic) V30.6- ☑
                  being ridden (traffic) V36.6- ☑
                     nontraffic V36.1- ☑
                  nontraffic V30.1- ☑
               animal-drawn vehicle (traffic) V36.6- ☑
                 nontraffic V36.1- ☑
               bus (traffic) V34.6- ☑

Accident — *continued*
   transport — *continued*
      three-wheeled motor vehicle occupant — *continued*
         passenger — *continued*
            collision — *continued*
               bus — *continued*
                  nontraffic V34.1- ☑
               car (traffic) V33.6- ☑
                 nontraffic V33.1- ☑
               motor vehicle NOS (traffic) V39.50- ☑
                 nontraffic V39.10- ☑
                 specified type NEC (traffic) V39.59- ☑
                   nontraffic V39.19- ☑
               pedal cycle (traffic) V31.6- ☑
                 nontraffic V31.1- ☑
               pickup truck (traffic) V33.6- ☑
                 nontraffic V33.1- ☑
               railway vehicle (traffic) V35.6- ☑
                 nontraffic V35.1- ☑
               specified vehicle NEC (traffic) V36.6- ☑
                 nontraffic V36.1- ☑
               stationary object (traffic) V37.6- ☑
                 nontraffic V37.1- ☑
               streetcar (traffic) V36.6- ☑
                 nontraffic V36.1- ☑
               three wheeled motor vehicle (traffic) V32.6- ☑
                 nontraffic V32.1- ☑
               truck (traffic) V34.6- ☑
                 nontraffic V34.1- ☑
               two wheeled motor vehicle (traffic) V32.6- ☑
                 nontraffic V32.1- ☑
               van (traffic) V33.6- ☑
                 nontraffic V33.1- ☑
            noncollision accident (traffic) V38.6- ☑
               nontraffic V38.1- ☑
         specified type NEC V39.89- ☑
         military vehicle V39.81- ☑
      tractor (farm) (and trailer) — *see* Accident, transport, agricultural vehicle occupant
      tram — *see* Accident, transport, streetcar
         in mine or quarry — *see* Accident, transport, industrial vehicle occupant
      trolley — *see* Accident, transport, streetcar
         in mine or quarry — *see* Accident, transport, industrial vehicle occupant
      truck (heavy) occupant V69.9- ☑
         collision (with)
            animal (traffic) V60.9- ☑
               being ridden (traffic) V66.9- ☑
                  nontraffic V66.3- ☑
                     while boarding or alighting V66.4- ☑
               nontraffic V60.3- ☑
                  while boarding or alighting V60.4- ☑
            animal-drawn vehicle (traffic) V66.9- ☑
               nontraffic V66.3- ☑
               while boarding or alighting V66.4- ☑
            bus (traffic) V64.9- ☑
               nontraffic V64.3- ☑
               while boarding or alighting V64.4- ☑
            car (traffic) V63.9- ☑
               nontraffic V63.3- ☑
               while boarding or alighting V63.4- ☑
            motor vehicle NOS (traffic) V69.60- ☑
               nontraffic V69.20- ☑
               specified type NEC (traffic) V69.69- ☑
                 nontraffic V69.29- ☑
            pedal cycle (traffic) V61.9- ☑
               nontraffic V61.3- ☑
               while boarding or alighting V61.4- ☑
            pickup truck (traffic) V63.9- ☑
               nontraffic V63.3- ☑
               while boarding or alighting V63.4- ☑
            railway vehicle (traffic) V65.9- ☑
               nontraffic V65.3- ☑
               while boarding or alighting V65.4- ☑
            specified vehicle NEC (traffic) V66.9- ☑
               nontraffic V66.3- ☑
               while boarding or alighting V66.4- ☑
            stationary object (traffic) V67.9- ☑
               nontraffic V67.3- ☑
               while boarding or alighting V67.4- ☑
            streetcar (traffic) V66.9- ☑
               nontraffic V66.3- ☑

☑ Additional Character Required — Refer to the Tabular List for Character Selection

Accident — *continued*
  transport — *continued*
    truck occupant — *continued*
      collision — *continued*
        streetcar — *continued*
          while boarding or alighting V66.4- ☑
        three wheeled motor vehicle (traffic) V62.9- ☑
          nontraffic V62.3- ☑
          while boarding or alighting V62.4- ☑
        truck (traffic) V64.9- ☑
          nontraffic V64.3- ☑
          while boarding or alighting V64.4- ☑
        two wheeled motor vehicle (traffic) V62.9- ☑
          nontraffic V62.3- ☑
          while boarding or alighting V62.4- ☑
        van (traffic) V63.9- ☑
          nontraffic V63.3- ☑
          while boarding or alighting V63.4- ☑
      driver
        collision (with)
          animal (traffic) V60.5- ☑
            being ridden (traffic) V66.5- ☑
              nontraffic V66.0- ☑
            nontraffic V60.0- ☑
          animal-drawn vehicle (traffic) V66.5- ☑
            nontraffic V66.0- ☑
          bus (traffic) V64.5- ☑
            nontraffic V64.0- ☑
          car (traffic) V63.5- ☑
            nontraffic V63.0- ☑
          motor vehicle NOS (traffic) V69.40- ☑
            nontraffic V69.00- ☑
            specified type NEC (traffic) V69.49- ☑
              nontraffic V69.09- ☑
          pedal cycle (traffic) V61.5- ☑
            nontraffic V61.0- ☑
          pickup truck (traffic) V63.5- ☑
            nontraffic V63.0- ☑
          railway vehicle (traffic) V65.5- ☑
            nontraffic V65.0- ☑
          specified vehicle NEC (traffic) V66.5- ☑
            nontraffic V66.0- ☑
          stationary object (traffic) V67.5- ☑
            nontraffic V67.0- ☑
          streetcar (traffic) V66.5- ☑
            nontraffic V66.0- ☑
          three wheeled motor vehicle (traffic)
            V62.5- ☑
            nontraffic V62.0- ☑
          truck (traffic) V64.5- ☑
            nontraffic V64.0- ☑
          two wheeled motor vehicle (traffic)
            V62.5- ☑
            nontraffic V62.0- ☑
          van (traffic) V63.5- ☑
            nontraffic V63.0- ☑
        noncollision accident (traffic) V68.5- ☑
          nontraffic V68.0- ☑
      dump — *see* Accident, transport, construction vehicle occupant
      hanger-on
        collision (with)
          animal (traffic) V60.7- ☑
            being ridden (traffic) V66.7- ☑
              nontraffic V66.2- ☑
            nontraffic V60.2- ☑
          animal-drawn vehicle (traffic) V66.7- ☑
            nontraffic V66.2- ☑
          bus (traffic) V64.7- ☑
            nontraffic V64.2- ☑
          car (traffic) V63.7- ☑
            nontraffic V63.2- ☑
          pedal cycle (traffic) V61.7- ☑
            nontraffic V61.2- ☑
          pickup truck (traffic) V63.7- ☑
            nontraffic V63.2- ☑
          railway vehicle (traffic) V65.7- ☑
            nontraffic V65.2- ☑
          specified vehicle NEC (traffic) V66.7- ☑
            nontraffic V66.2- ☑
          stationary object (traffic) V67.7- ☑
            nontraffic V67.2- ☑
          streetcar (traffic) V66.7- ☑
            nontraffic V66.2- ☑

Accident — *continued*
  transport — *continued*
    truck occupant — *continued*
      hanger-on — *continued*
        collision — *continued*
          three wheeled motor vehicle (traffic)
            V62.7- ☑
            nontraffic V62.2- ☑
          truck (traffic) V64.7- ☑
            nontraffic V64.2- ☑
          two wheeled motor vehicle (traffic)
            V62.7- ☑
            nontraffic V62.2- ☑
          van (traffic) V63.7- ☑
            nontraffic V63.2- ☑
        noncollision accident (traffic) V68.7- ☑
          nontraffic V68.2- ☑
      noncollision accident (traffic) V68.9- ☑
        nontraffic V68.3- ☑
        while boarding or alighting V68.4- ☑
      nontraffic V69.3- ☑
      passenger
        collision (with)
          animal (traffic) V60.6- ☑
            being ridden (traffic) V66.6- ☑
              nontraffic V66.1- ☑
            nontraffic V60.1- ☑
          animal-drawn vehicle (traffic) V66.6- ☑
            nontraffic V66.1- ☑
          bus (traffic) V64.6- ☑
            nontraffic V64.1- ☑
          car (traffic) V63.6- ☑
            nontraffic V63.1- ☑
          motor vehicle NOS (traffic) V69.50- ☑
            nontraffic V69.10- ☑
            specified type NEC (traffic) V69.59- ☑
              nontraffic V69.19- ☑
          pedal cycle (traffic) V61.6- ☑
            nontraffic V61.1- ☑
          pickup truck (traffic) V63.6- ☑
            nontraffic V63.1- ☑
          railway vehicle (traffic) V65.6- ☑
            nontraffic V65.1- ☑
          specified vehicle NEC (traffic) V66.6- ☑
            nontraffic V66.1- ☑
          stationary object (traffic) V67.6- ☑
            nontraffic V67.1- ☑
          streetcar (traffic) V66.6- ☑
            nontraffic V66.1- ☑
          three wheeled motor vehicle (traffic)
            V62.6- ☑
            nontraffic V62.1- ☑
          truck (traffic) V64.6- ☑
            nontraffic V64.1- ☑
          two wheeled motor vehicle (traffic)
            V62.6- ☑
            nontraffic V62.1- ☑
          van (traffic) V63.6- ☑
            nontraffic V63.1- ☑
        noncollision accident (traffic) V68.6- ☑
          nontraffic V68.1- ☑
      pickup — *see* Accident, transport, pickup truck occupant
      specified type NEC V69.88- ☑
      military vehicle V69.81- ☑
    van occupant V59.9- ☑
      collision (with)
        animal (traffic) V50.9- ☑
          being ridden (traffic) V56.9- ☑
            nontraffic V56.3- ☑
            while boarding or alighting V56.4- ☑
          nontraffic V50.3- ☑
          while boarding or alighting V50.4- ☑
        animal-drawn vehicle (traffic) V56.9- ☑
          nontraffic V56.3- ☑
          while boarding or alighting V56.4- ☑
        bus (traffic) V54.9- ☑
          nontraffic V54.3- ☑
          while boarding or alighting V54.4- ☑
        car (traffic) V53.9- ☑
          nontraffic V53.3- ☑
          while boarding or alighting V53.4- ☑
        motor vehicle NOS (traffic) V59.60- ☑
          nontraffic V59.20- ☑
          specified type NEC (traffic) V59.69- ☑

Accident — *continued*
  transport — *continued*
    van occupant — *continued*
      collision — *continued*
        motor vehicle — *continued*
          specified type — *continued*
            nontraffic V59.29- ☑
        pedal cycle (traffic) V51.9- ☑
          nontraffic V51.3- ☑
          while boarding or alighting V51.4- ☑
        pickup truck (traffic) V53.9- ☑
          nontraffic V53.3- ☑
          while boarding or alighting V53.4- ☑
        railway vehicle (traffic) V55.9- ☑
          nontraffic V55.3- ☑
          while boarding or alighting V55.4- ☑
        specified vehicle NEC (traffic) V56.9- ☑
          nontraffic V56.3- ☑
          while boarding or alighting V56.4- ☑
        stationary object (traffic) V57.9- ☑
          nontraffic V57.3- ☑
          while boarding or alighting V57.4- ☑
        streetcar (traffic) V56.9- ☑
          nontraffic V56.3- ☑
          while boarding or alighting V56.4- ☑
        three wheeled motor vehicle (traffic) V52.9- ☑
          nontraffic V52.3- ☑
          while boarding or alighting V52.4- ☑
        truck (traffic) V54.9- ☑
          nontraffic V54.3- ☑
          while boarding or alighting V54.4- ☑
        two wheeled motor vehicle (traffic) V52.9- ☑
          nontraffic V52.3- ☑
          while boarding or alighting V52.4- ☑
        van (traffic) V53.9- ☑
          nontraffic V53.3- ☑
          while boarding or alighting V53.4- ☑
      driver
        collision (with)
          animal (traffic) V50.5- ☑
            being ridden (traffic) V56.5- ☑
              nontraffic V56.0- ☑
            nontraffic V50.0- ☑
          animal-drawn vehicle (traffic) V56.5- ☑
            nontraffic V56.0- ☑
          bus (traffic) V54.5- ☑
            nontraffic V54.0- ☑
          car (traffic) V53.5- ☑
            nontraffic V53.0- ☑
          motor vehicle NOS (traffic) V59.40- ☑
            nontraffic V59.00- ☑
            specified type NEC (traffic) V59.49- ☑
              nontraffic V59.09- ☑
          pedal cycle (traffic) V51.5- ☑
            nontraffic V51.0- ☑
          pickup truck (traffic) V53.5- ☑
            nontraffic V53.0- ☑
          railway vehicle (traffic) V55.5- ☑
            nontraffic V55.0- ☑
          specified vehicle NEC (traffic) V56.5- ☑
            nontraffic V56.0- ☑
          stationary object (traffic) V57.5- ☑
            nontraffic V57.0- ☑
          streetcar (traffic) V56.5- ☑
            nontraffic V56.0- ☑
          three wheeled motor vehicle (traffic)
            V52.5- ☑
            nontraffic V52.0- ☑
          truck (traffic) V54.5- ☑
            nontraffic V54.0- ☑
          two wheeled motor vehicle (traffic)
            V52.5- ☑
            nontraffic V52.0- ☑
          van (traffic) V53.5- ☑
            nontraffic V53.0- ☑
        noncollision accident (traffic) V58.5- ☑
          nontraffic V58.0- ☑
      hanger-on
        collision (with)
          animal (traffic) V50.7- ☑
            being ridden (traffic) V56.7- ☑
              nontraffic V56.2- ☑
            nontraffic V50.2- ☑
          animal-drawn vehicle (traffic) V56.7- ☑
            nontraffic V56.2- ☑

Accident — *continued*
  transport — *continued*
    van occupant — *continued*
      hanger-on — *continued*
        collision — *continued*
          bus (traffic) V54.7- ☑
            nontraffic V54.2- ☑
          car (traffic) V53.7- ☑
            nontraffic V53.2- ☑
          pedal cycle (traffic) V51.7- ☑
            nontraffic V51.2- ☑
          pickup truck (traffic) V53.7- ☑
            nontraffic V53.2- ☑
          railway vehicle (traffic) V55.7- ☑
            nontraffic V55.2- ☑
          specified vehicle NEC (traffic) V56.7- ☑
            nontraffic V56.2- ☑
          stationary object (traffic) V57.7- ☑
            nontraffic V57.2- ☑
          streetcar (traffic) V56.7- ☑
            nontraffic V56.2- ☑
          three wheeled motor vehicle (traffic) V52.7- ☑
            nontraffic V52.2- ☑
          truck (traffic) V54.7- ☑
            nontraffic V54.2- ☑
          two wheeled motor vehicle (traffic) V52.7- ☑
            nontraffic V52.2- ☑
          van (traffic) V53.7- ☑
            nontraffic V53.2- ☑
        noncollision accident (traffic) V58.7- ☑
          nontraffic V58.2- ☑
      noncollision accident (traffic) V58.9- ☑
        nontraffic V58.3- ☑
      while boarding or alighting V58.4- ☑
      nontraffic V59.3- ☑
      passenger
        collision (with)
          animal (traffic) V50.6- ☑
            being ridden (traffic) V56.6- ☑
              nontraffic V56.1- ☑
            nontraffic V50.1- ☑
          animal-drawn vehicle (traffic) V56.6- ☑
            nontraffic V56.1- ☑
          bus (traffic) V54.6- ☑
            nontraffic V54.1- ☑
          car (traffic) V53.6- ☑
            nontraffic V53.1- ☑
          motor vehicle NOS (traffic) V59.50- ☑
            nontraffic V59.10- ☑
            specified type NEC (traffic) V59.59- ☑
              nontraffic V59.19- ☑
          pedal cycle (traffic) V51.6- ☑
            nontraffic V51.1- ☑
          pickup truck (traffic) V53.6- ☑
            nontraffic V53.1- ☑
          railway vehicle (traffic) V55.6- ☑
            nontraffic V55.1- ☑
          specified vehicle NEC (traffic) V56.6- ☑
            nontraffic V56.1- ☑
          stationary object (traffic) V57.6- ☑
            nontraffic V57.1- ☑
          streetcar (traffic) V56.6- ☑
            nontraffic V56.1- ☑
          three wheeled motor vehicle (traffic) V52.6- ☑
            nontraffic V52.1- ☑
          truck (traffic) V54.6- ☑
            nontraffic V54.1- ☑
          two wheeled motor vehicle (traffic) V52.6- ☑
            nontraffic V52.1- ☑
          van (traffic) V53.6- ☑
            nontraffic V53.1- ☑
        noncollision accident (traffic) V58.6- ☑
          nontraffic V58.1- ☑
      specified type NEC V59.88- ☑
      military vehicle V59.81- ☑
    watercraft occupant — *see* Accident, watercraft
    vehicle NEC V89.9- ☑
      animal-drawn NEC — *see* Accident, transport, animal-drawn vehicle occupant

Accident — *continued*
  vehicle — *continued*
    special
      agricultural — *see* Accident, transport, agricultural vehicle occupant
      construction — *see* Accident, transport, construction vehicle occupant
      industrial — *see* Accident, transport, industrial vehicle occupant
    three-wheeled NEC (motorized) — *see* Accident, transport, three-wheeled motor vehicle occupant
  watercraft V94.9- ☑
    causing
      drowning — *see* Drowning, due to, accident to, watercraft
      injury NEC V91.89- ☑
        crushed between craft and object V91.19- ☑
          powered craft V91.13- ☑
            ferry boat V91.11- ☑
            fishing boat V91.12- ☑
            jetskis V91.13- ☑
            liner V91.11- ☑
            merchant ship V91.10- ☑
            passenger ship V91.11- ☑
          unpowered craft V91.18- ☑
            canoe V91.15- ☑
            inflatable V91.16- ☑
            kayak V91.15- ☑
            sailboat V91.14- ☑
            surf-board V91.18- ☑
            windsurfer V91.18- ☑
        fall on board V91.29- ☑
          powered craft V91.23- ☑
            ferry boat V91.21- ☑
            fishing boat V91.22- ☑
            jetskis V91.23- ☑
            liner V91.21- ☑
            merchant ship V91.20- ☑
            passenger ship V91.21- ☑
          unpowered craft
            canoe V91.25- ☑
            inflatable V91.26- ☑
            kayak V91.25- ☑
            sailboat V91.24- ☑
        fire on board causing burn V91.09- ☑
          powered craft V91.03- ☑
            ferry boat V91.01- ☑
            fishing boat V91.02- ☑
            jetskis V91.03- ☑
            liner V91.01- ☑
            merchant ship V91.00- ☑
            passenger ship V91.01- ☑
          unpowered craft V91.08- ☑
            canoe V91.05- ☑
            inflatable V91.06- ☑
            kayak V91.05- ☑
            sailboat V91.04- ☑
            surf-board V91.08- ☑
            water skis V91.07- ☑
            windsurfer V91.08- ☑
        hit by falling object V91.39- ☑
          powered craft V91.33- ☑
            ferry boat V91.31- ☑
            fishing boat V91.32- ☑
            jetskis V91.33- ☑
            liner V91.31- ☑
            merchant ship V91.30- ☑
            passenger ship V91.31- ☑
          unpowered craft V91.38- ☑
            canoe V91.35- ☑
            inflatable V91.36- ☑
            kayak V91.35- ☑
            sailboat V91.34- ☑
            surf-board V91.38- ☑
            water skis V91.37- ☑
            windsurfer V91.38- ☑
        specified type NEC V91.89- ☑
          powered craft V91.83- ☑
            ferry boat V91.81- ☑
            fishing boat V91.82- ☑
            jetskis V91.83- ☑
            liner V91.81- ☑
            merchant ship V91.80- ☑
            passenger ship V91.81- ☑

Accident — *continued*
  watercraft — *continued*
    causing — *continued*
      injury — *continued*
        specified type — *continued*
          unpowered craft V91.88- ☑
            canoe V91.85- ☑
            inflatable V91.86- ☑
            kayak V91.85- ☑
            sailboat V91.84- ☑
            surf-board V91.88- ☑
            water skis V91.87- ☑
            windsurfer V91.88- ☑
    due to, caused by cataclysm — *see* Forces of nature, by type
    military NEC V94.818- ☑
      civilian in water injured by V94.811- ☑
      with civilian watercraft V94.810- ☑
    nonpowered, struck by
      nonpowered vessel V94.21- ☑
      powered vessel V94.22- ☑
    specified type NEC V94.89- ☑
    striking swimmer
      powered V94.11- ☑
      unpowered V94.12- ☑
Acid throwing (assault) Y08.89- ☑
Activity (involving) (of victim at time of event) Y93.9
  aerobic and step exercise (class) Y93.A3 (*following* Y93.7)
  alpine skiing Y93.23
  animal care NEC Y93.K9 (*following* Y93.7)
  arts and handcrafts NEC Y93.D9 (*following* Y93.7)
  athletics NEC Y93.79
  athletics played as a team or group NEC Y93.69
  athletics played individually NEC Y93.59
  badminton Y93.73
  baking Y93.G3 (*following* Y93.7)
  ballet Y93.41
  barbells Y93.B3 (*following* Y93.7)
  BASE (Building, Antenna, Span, Earth) jumping Y93.33
  baseball Y93.64
  basketball Y93.67
  bathing (personal) Y93.E1 (*following* Y93.7)
  beach volleyball Y93.68
  bike riding Y93.55
  blackout game Y93.85
  boogie boarding Y93.18
  bowling Y93.54
  boxing Y93.71
  brass instrument playing Y93.J4 (*following* Y93.7)
  building construction Y93.H3 (*following* Y93.7)
  bungee jumping Y93.34
  calisthenics Y93.A2 (*following* Y93.7)
  canoeing (in calm and turbulent water) Y93.16
  capture the flag Y93.6A
  cardiorespiratory exercise NEC Y93.A9 (*following* Y93.7)
  caregiving (providing) NEC Y93.F9 (*following* Y93.7)
    bathing Y93.F1 (*following* Y93.7)
    lifting Y93.F2 (*following* Y93.7)
  cellular
    communication device Y93.C2 (*following* Y93.7)
    telephone Y93.C2 (*following* Y93.7)
  challenge course Y93.A5 (*following* Y93.7)
  cheerleading Y93.45
  choking game Y93.85
  circuit training Y93.A4 (*following* Y93.7)
  cleaning
    floor Y93.E5 (*following* Y93.7)
  climbing NEC Y93.39
    mountain Y93.31
    rock Y93.31
    wall Y93.31
  clothing care and maintenance NEC Y93.E9 (*following* Y93.7)
  combatives Y93.75
  computer
    keyboarding Y93.C1 (*following* Y93.7)
    technology NEC Y93.C9 (*following* Y93.7)
  confidence course Y93.A5 (*following* Y93.7)
  construction (building) Y93.H3 (*following* Y93.7)
  cooking and baking Y93.G3 (*following* Y93.7)
  cool down exercises Y93.A2 (*following* Y93.7)
  cricket Y93.69
  crocheting Y93.D1 (*following* Y93.7)
  cross country skiing Y93.24
  dancing (all types) Y93.41
  digging
    dirt Y93.H1 (*following* Y93.7)
  dirt digging Y93.H1 (*following* Y93.7)

☑ Additional Character Required — Refer to the Tabular List for Character Selection

Activity

Activity — continued
- dishwashing Y93.G1 (*following* Y93.7)
- diving (platform) (springboard) Y93.12
  - underwater Y93.15
- dodge ball Y93.6A
- downhill skiing Y93.23
- drum playing Y93.J2 (*following* Y93.7)
- dumbbells Y93.B3 (*following* Y93.7)
- electronic
  - devices NEC Y93.C9 (*following* Y93.7)
    - hand held interactive Y93.C2 (*following* Y93.7)
  - game playing (using) (with)
    - interactive device Y93.C2 (*following* Y93.7)
    - keyboard or other stationary device Y93.C1 (*following* Y93.7)
- elliptical machine Y93.A1 (*following* Y93.7)
- exercise(s)
  - machines ((primarily) for)
    - cardiorespiratory conditioning Y93.A1 (*following* Y93.7)
    - muscle strengthening Y93.B1 (*following* Y93.7)
  - muscle strengthening (non-machine) NEC Y93.B9 (*following* Y93.7)
  - external motion NEC Y93.I9 (*following* Y93.7)
    - rollercoaster Y93.I1 (*following* Y93.7)
- fainting game Y93.85
- field hockey Y93.65
- figure skating (pairs) (singles) Y93.21
- flag football Y93.62
- floor mopping and cleaning Y93.E5 (*following* Y93.7)
- food preparation and clean up Y93.G1 (*following* Y93.7)
- football (American) NOS Y93.61
  - flag Y93.62
  - tackle Y93.61
  - touch Y93.62
- four square Y93.6A
- free weights Y93.B3 (*following* Y93.7)
- frisbee (ultimate) Y93.74
- furniture
  - building Y93.D3 (*following* Y93.7)
  - finishing Y93.D3 (*following* Y93.7)
  - repair Y93.D3 (*following* Y93.7)
- game playing (electronic)
  - using interactive device Y93.C2 (*following* Y93.7)
  - using keyboard or other stationary device Y93.C1 (*following* Y93.7)
- gardening Y93.H2 (*following* Y93.7)
- golf Y93.53
- grass drills Y93.A6 (*following* Y93.7)
- grilling and smoking food Y93.G2 (*following* Y93.7)
- grooming and shearing an animal Y93.K3 (*following* Y93.7)
- guerilla drills Y93.A6 (*following* Y93.7)
- gymnastics (rhythmic) Y93.43
- hand held interactive electronic device Y93.C2 (*following* Y93.7)
- handball Y93.73
- handcrafts NEC Y93.D9 (*following* Y93.7)
- hang gliding Y93.35
- hiking (on level or elevated terrain) Y93.01
- hockey (ice) Y93.22
  - field Y93.65
- horseback riding Y93.52
- household (interior) maintenance NEC Y93.E9 (*following* Y93.7)
- ice NEC Y93.29
  - dancing Y93.21
  - hockey Y93.22
  - skating Y93.21
- inline roller skating Y93.51
- ironing Y93.E4 (*following* Y93.7)
- judo Y93.75
- jumping jacks Y93.A2 (*following* Y93.7)
- jumping (off) NEC Y93.39
  - BASE (Building, Antenna, Span, Earth) Y93.33
  - bungee Y93.34
  - jacks Y93.A2 (*following* Y93.7)
  - rope Y93.56
- jumping rope Y93.56
- karate Y93.75
- kayaking (in calm and turbulent water) Y93.16
- keyboarding (computer) Y93.C1 (*following* Y93.7)
- kickball Y93.6A
- knitting Y93.D1 (*following* Y93.7)
- lacrosse Y93.65
- land maintenance NEC Y93.H9 (*following* Y93.7)
- landscaping Y93.H2 (*following* Y93.7)
- laundry Y93.E2 (*following* Y93.7)

Activity — continued
- machines (exercise)
  - primarily for cardiorespiratory conditioning Y93.A1 (*following* Y93.7)
  - primarily for muscle strengthening Y93.B1 (*following* Y93.7)
- maintenance
  - exterior building NEC Y93.H9 (*following* Y93.7)
  - household (interior) NEC Y93.E9 (*following* Y93.7)
  - land Y93.H9 (*following* Y93.7)
  - property Y93.H9 (*following* Y93.7)
- marching (on level or elevated terrain) Y93.01
- martial arts Y93.75
- microwave oven Y93.G3 (*following* Y93.7)
- milking an animal Y93.K2 (*following* Y93.7)
- mopping (floor) Y93.E5 (*following* Y93.7)
- mountain climbing Y93.31
- muscle strengthening
  - exercises (non-machine) NEC Y93.B9 (*following* Y93.7)
  - machines Y93.B1 (*following* Y93.7)
- musical keyboard (electronic) playing Y93.J1 (*following* Y93.7)
- nordic skiing Y93.24
- obstacle course Y93.A5 (*following* Y93.7)
- outdoor, specified NEC Y93.L9
- oven (microwave) Y93.G3 (*following* Y93.7)
- packing up and unpacking in moving to a new residence Y93.E6 (*following* Y93.7)
- parasailing Y93.19
- pass out game Y93.85
- percussion instrument playing NEC Y93.J2 (*following* Y93.7)
- personal
  - bathing and showering Y93.E1 (*following* Y93.7)
  - hygiene NEC Y93.E8 (*following* Y93.7)
  - showering Y93.E1 (*following* Y93.7)
- physical games generally associated with school recess, summer camp and children Y93.6A
- physical training NEC Y93.A9 (*following* Y93.7)
- piano playing Y93.J1 (*following* Y93.7)
- pickleball Y93.73
- pilates Y93.B4 (*following* Y93.7)
- platform diving Y93.12
- playing musical instrument
  - brass instrument Y93.J4 (*following* Y93.7)
  - drum Y93.J2 (*following* Y93.7)
  - musical keyboard (electronic) Y93.J1 (*following* Y93.7)
  - percussion instrument NEC Y93.J2 (*following* Y93.7)
  - piano Y93.J1 (*following* Y93.7)
  - string instrument Y93.J3 (*following* Y93.7)
  - winds instrument Y93.J4 (*following* Y93.7)
- property maintenance
  - exterior NEC Y93.H9 (*following* Y93.7)
  - interior NEC Y93.E9 (*following* Y93.7)
- protesting (political, social) Y93.89
- pruning (garden and lawn) Y93.H2 (*following* Y93.7)
- pull-ups Y93.B2 (*following* Y93.7)
- push-ups Y93.B2 (*following* Y93.7)
- racquetball Y93.73
- rafting (in calm and turbulent water) Y93.16
- raking (leaves) Y93.H1 (*following* Y93.7)
- rappelling Y93.32
- refereeing a sports activity Y93.81
- residential relocation Y93.E6 (*following* Y93.7)
- rhythmic gymnastics Y93.43
- rhythmic movement NEC Y93.49
- riding
  - horseback Y93.52
  - rollercoaster Y93.I1 (*following* Y93.7)
- rock climbing Y93.31
- roller skating (inline) Y93.51
- rollercoaster riding Y93.I1 (*following* Y93.7)
- rough housing and horseplay Y93.83
- rowing (in calm and turbulent water) Y93.16
- rugby Y93.63
- running Y93.02
- SCUBA diving Y93.15
- sewing Y93.D2 (*following* Y93.7)
- shoveling Y93.H1 (*following* Y93.7)
  - dirt Y93.H1 (*following* Y93.7)
  - snow Y93.H1 (*following* Y93.7)
- showering (personal) Y93.E1 (*following* Y93.7)
- sit-ups Y93.B2 (*following* Y93.7)
- skateboarding Y93.51
- skating (ice) Y93.21
  - roller Y93.51
- skiing (alpine) (downhill) Y93.23
  - cross country Y93.24
  - nordic Y93.24

Activity — continued
- skiing — continued
  - water Y93.17
- sledding (snow) Y93.23
- sleeping (sleep) Y93.84
- smoking and grilling food Y93.G2 (*following* Y93.7)
- snorkeling Y93.15
- snow NEC Y93.29
  - boarding Y93.23
  - shoveling Y93.H1 (*following* Y93.7)
  - sledding Y93.23
  - tubing Y93.23
- soccer Y93.66
- softball Y93.64
- specified NEC Y93.89
- spectator at an event Y93.82
- splitting wood Y93.L1
- sports NEC Y93.79
  - sports played as a team or group NEC Y93.69
  - sports played individually NEC Y93.59
- springboard diving Y93.12
- squash Y93.73
- stationary bike Y93.A1 (*following* Y93.7)
- step (stepping) exercise (class) Y93.A3 (*following* Y93.7)
- stepper machine Y93.A1 (*following* Y93.7)
- stove Y93.G3 (*following* Y93.7)
- string instrument playing Y93.J3 (*following* Y93.7)
- surfing Y93.18
  - wind Y93.18
- swimming Y93.11
- tackle football Y93.61
- tap dancing Y93.41
- tennis Y93.73
- tobogganing Y93.23
- touch football Y93.62
- track and field events (non-running) Y93.57
  - running Y93.02
- trampoline Y93.44
- treadmill Y93.A1 (*following* Y93.7)
- trimming shrubs Y93.H2 (*following* Y93.7)
- tubing (in calm and turbulent water) Y93.16
  - snow Y93.23
- ultimate frisbee Y93.74
- underwater diving Y93.15
- unpacking in moving to a new residence Y93.E6 (*following* Y93.7)
- use of stove, oven and microwave oven Y93.G3 (*following* Y93.7)
- vacuuming Y93.E3 (*following* Y93.7)
- volleyball (beach) (court) Y93.68
- wake boarding Y93.17
- walking (on level or elevated terrain) Y93.01
  - an animal Y93.K1 (*following* Y93.7)
- walking an animal Y93.K1 (*following* Y93.7)
- wall climbing Y93.31
- warm up and cool down exercises Y93.A2 (*following* Y93.7)
- water NEC Y93.19
  - aerobics Y93.14
  - craft NEC Y93.19
  - exercise Y93.14
  - polo Y93.13
  - skiing Y93.17
  - sliding Y93.18
  - survival training and testing Y93.19
- weeding (garden and lawn) Y93.H2 (*following* Y93.7)
- wind instrument playing Y93.J4 (*following* Y93.7)
- windsurfing Y93.18
- wrestling Y93.72
- yoga Y93.42

Adverse effect of drugs — *see* Table of Drugs and Chemicals
Aerosinusitis — *see* Air, pressure
After-effect, late — *see* Sequelae
Air
- blast in war operations — *see* War operations, air blast
- pressure
  - change, rapid
    - during
      - ascent W94.29-
        - while (in) (surfacing from)
          - aircraft W94.23-
          - deep water diving W94.21-
          - underground W94.22-
      - descent W94.39-
        - in
          - aircraft W94.31-
          - water W94.32-

Air — *continued*
- pressure — *continued*
  - high, prolonged W94.0- ☑
  - low, prolonged W94.12- ☑
    - due to residence or long visit at high altitude W94.11- ☑

Alpine sickness W94.11- ☑
Altitude sickness W94.11- ☑
Anaphylactic shock, anaphylaxis — *see* Table of Drugs and Chemicals
Andes disease W94.11- ☑
Arachnidism, arachnoidism X58.- ☑
Arson (with intent to injure or kill) X97.- ☑
Asphyxia, asphyxiation
- by
  - food (bone) (seed) — *see* categories T17 and T18.- ☑
  - gas — *see also* Table of Drugs and Chemicals
    - legal
      - execution — *see* Legal, intervention, gas
      - intervention — *see* Legal, intervention, gas
- from
  - fire — *see also* Exposure, fire
    - in war operations — *see* War operations, fire
  - ignition — *see* Ignition
  - vomitus T17.810- ☑
- in war operations — *see* War operations, restriction of airway

Aspiration
- food (any type) (into respiratory tract) (with asphyxia, obstruction respiratory tract, suffocation) — *see* categories T17 and T18.- ☑
- foreign body — *see* Foreign body, aspiration
- vomitus (with asphyxia, obstruction respiratory tract, suffocation) — *see* Index to Diseases and Injuries, Foreign body, respiratory tract

Assassination (attempt) — *see* Assault
Assault (homicidal) (by) (in) Y09
- arson X97.- ☑
- bite (of human being) Y04.1- ☑
- bodily force Y04.8- ☑
  - bite Y04.1- ☑
  - bumping into Y04.2- ☑
  - sexual (confirmed) T74.2- ☑
    - suspected T76.2- ☑
  - unarmed fight Y04.0- ☑
- bomb X96.9- ☑
  - antipersonnel X96.0- ☑
  - fertilizer X96.3- ☑
  - gasoline X96.1- ☑
  - letter X96.2- ☑
  - petrol X96.1- ☑
  - pipe X96.3- ☑
  - specified NEC X96.8- ☑
- brawl (hand) (fists) (foot) (unarmed) Y04.0- ☑
- burning, burns (by fire) NEC X97.- ☑
  - acid Y08.89- ☑
  - caustic, corrosive substance Y08.89- ☑
  - chemical from swallowing caustic, corrosive substance — *see* Table of Drugs and Chemicals
  - cigarette(s) X97.- ☑
  - hot object X98.9- ☑
    - fluid NEC X98.2- ☑
    - household appliance X98.3- ☑
    - specified NEC X98.8- ☑
    - steam X98.0- ☑
    - tap water X98.1- ☑
    - vapors X98.0- ☑
  - scalding — *see* Assault, burning
    - steam X98.0- ☑
  - vitriol Y08.89- ☑
- caustic, corrosive substance (gas) Y08.89- ☑
- crashing of
  - aircraft Y08.81- ☑
  - motor vehicle Y03.8- ☑
    - pushed in front of Y02.0- ☑
    - run over Y03.0- ☑
    - specified NEC Y03.8- ☑
- cutting or piercing instrument X99.9- ☑
  - dagger X99.2- ☑
  - glass X99.0- ☑
  - knife X99.1- ☑
  - specified NEC X99.8- ☑
  - sword X99.2- ☑
- dagger X99.2- ☑
- drowning (in) X92.9- ☑
  - bathtub X92.0- ☑

Assault — *continued*
- drowning — *continued*
  - natural water X92.3- ☑
  - specified NEC X92.8- ☑
  - swimming pool X92.1- ☑
    - following fall X92.2- ☑
- dynamite X96.8- ☑
- explosive(s) (material) X96.9- ☑
- fight (hand) (fists) (foot) (unarmed) Y04.0- ☑
  - with weapon — *see* Assault, by type of weapon
- fire X97.- ☑
- firearm X95.9- ☑
  - airgun X95.01- ☑
  - handgun X93.- ☑
  - hunting rifle X94.1- ☑
  - larger X94.9- ☑
    - specified NEC X94.8- ☑
  - machine gun X94.2- ☑
  - shotgun X94.0- ☑
  - specified NEC X95.8- ☑
- from high place Y01.- ☑
- gunshot (wound) NEC — *see* Assault, firearm, by type
- incendiary device X97.- ☑
- injury Y09
  - to child due to criminal abortion attempt NEC Y08.89- ☑
- knife X99.1- ☑
- late effect of — *see* categories X92-Y08 with 7th character S
- placing before moving object NEC Y02.8- ☑
  - motor vehicle Y02.0- ☑
- poisoning — *see* categories T36-T65 with 7th character S
- puncture, any part of body — *see* Assault, cutting or piercing instrument
- pushing
  - before moving object NEC Y02.8- ☑
    - motor vehicle Y02.0- ☑
    - subway train Y02.1- ☑
    - train Y02.1- ☑
  - from high place Y01.- ☑
- rape (confirmed) T74.2- ☑
  - suspected T76.2- ☑
- scalding — *see* Assault, burning
- sequelae of — *see* categories X92-Y08 with 7th character S
- sexual (by bodily force) T74.2- ☑
  - suspected T76.2- ☑
- shooting — *see* Assault, firearm
- specified means NEC Y08.89- ☑
- stab, any part of body — *see* Assault, cutting or piercing instrument
- steam X98.0- ☑
- striking against
  - other person Y04.2- ☑
  - sports equipment Y08.09- ☑
    - baseball bat Y08.02- ☑
    - hockey stick Y08.01- ☑
- struck by
  - sports equipment Y08.09- ☑
    - baseball bat Y08.02- ☑
    - hockey stick Y08.01- ☑
- submersion — *see* Assault, drowning
- violence Y09
- weapon Y09
  - blunt Y00.- ☑
  - cutting or piercing — *see* Assault, cutting or piercing instrument
  - firearm — *see* Assault, firearm
- wound Y09
  - cutting — *see* Assault, cutting or piercing instrument
  - gunshot — *see* Assault, firearm
  - knife X99.1- ☑
  - piercing — *see* Assault, cutting or piercing instrument
  - puncture — *see* Assault, cutting or piercing instrument
  - stab — *see* Assault, cutting or piercing instrument

Attack by mammals NEC W55.89- ☑
Avalanche — *see* Landslide
Aviator's disease — *see* Air, pressure

B

Barotitis, barodontalgia, barosinusitis, barotrauma (otitic) (sinus) — *see* Air, pressure
Battered (baby) (child) (person) (syndrome) X58.- ☑

Bayonet wound W26.1- ☑
- in
  - legal intervention — *see* Legal, intervention, sharp object, bayonet
  - war operations — *see* War operations, combat
- stated as undetermined whether accidental or intentional Y28.8- ☑
- suicide (attempt) X78.2- ☑

Bean in nose T17.1- ☑
Bed set on fire NEC — *see* Exposure, fire, uncontrolled, building, bed
Beheading (by guillotine)
- homicide X99.9- ☑
- legal execution — *see* Legal, intervention

Bending, injury in (prolonged) (static) X50.1- ☑
Bends — *see* Air, pressure, change
Bite, bitten by
- alligator W58.01- ☑
- arthropod (nonvenomous) NEC W57.- ☑
- bull W55.21- ☑
- cat W55.01- ☑
- cow W55.21- ☑
- crocodile W58.11- ☑
- dog W54.0- ☑
- goat W55.31- ☑
- hoof stock NEC W55.31- ☑
- horse W55.11- ☑
- human being (accidentally) W50.3- ☑
  - with intent to injure or kill Y04.1- ☑
  - as, or caused by, a crowd or human stampede (with fall) W52.- ☑
  - assault Y04.1- ☑
  - homicide (attempt) Y04.1- ☑
  - in
    - fight Y04.1- ☑
- insect (nonvenomous) W57.- ☑
- lizard (nonvenomous) W59.01- ☑
- mammal NEC W55.81- ☑
  - marine W56.31- ☑
- marine animal (nonvenomous) W56.81- ☑
- millipede W57.- ☑
- moray eel W56.51- ☑
- mouse W53.01- ☑
- person(s) (accidentally) W50.3- ☑
  - with intent to injure or kill Y04.1- ☑
  - as, or caused by, a crowd or human stampede (with fall) W52.- ☑
  - assault Y04.1- ☑
  - homicide (attempt) Y04.1- ☑
  - in
    - fight Y04.1- ☑
- pig W55.41- ☑
- raccoon W55.51- ☑
- rat W53.11- ☑
- reptile W59.81- ☑
  - lizard W59.01- ☑
  - snake W59.11- ☑
  - turtle W59.21- ☑
  - terrestrial W59.81- ☑
- rodent W53.81- ☑
  - mouse W53.01- ☑
  - rat W53.11- ☑
  - specified NEC W53.81- ☑
  - squirrel W53.21- ☑
- shark W56.41- ☑
- sheep W55.31- ☑
- snake (nonvenomous) W59.11- ☑
- spider (nonvenomous) W57.- ☑
- squirrel W53.21- ☑

Blast (air) in war operations — *see* War operations, blast
Blizzard X37.2- ☑
Blood alcohol level Y90.9
- less than 20mg/100ml Y90.0
- presence in blood, level not specified Y90.9
- 20-39mg/100ml Y90.1
- 40-59mg/100ml Y90.2
- 60-79mg/100ml Y90.3
- 80-99mg/100ml Y90.4
- 100-119mg/100ml Y90.5
- 120-199mg/100ml Y90.6
- 200-239mg/100ml Y90.7

Blow X58.- ☑
- by law-enforcing agent, police (on duty) — *see* Legal, intervention, manhandling
  - blunt object — *see* Legal, intervention, blunt object

Blowing up — *see* Explosion

☑ Additional Character Required — Refer to the Tabular List for Character Selection

Brawl (hand) (fists) (foot) Y04.0- ☑
Breakage (accidental) (part of)
    ladder (causing fall) W11.- ☑
    scaffolding (causing fall) W12.- ☑
Broken
    glass, contact with — *see* Contact, with, glass
    power line (causing electric shock) W85.- ☑
Bumping against, into (accidentally)
    object NEC W22.8- ☑
        caused by crowd or human stampede (with fall) W52.- ☑
        sports equipment W21.9- ☑
        with fall — *see* Fall, due to, bumping against, object
    person(s) W51.- ☑
        with fall W03.- ☑
            due to ice or snow W00.0- ☑
        assault Y04.2- ☑
        caused by, a crowd or human stampede (with fall) W52.- ☑
        homicide (attempt) Y04.2- ☑
    sports equipment W21.9- ☑
Burn, burned, burning (accidental) (by) (from) (on)
    acid NEC — *see* Table of Drugs and Chemicals
    bed linen — *see* Exposure, fire, uncontrolled, in building, bed
    blowtorch X08.8- ☑
        with ignition of clothing NEC X06.2- ☑
            nightwear X05.- ☑
    bonfire, campfire (controlled) — *see also* Exposure, fire, controlled, not in building)
        uncontrolled — *see* Exposure, fire, uncontrolled, not in building
    candle X08.8- ☑
        with ignition of clothing NEC X06.2- ☑
            nightwear X05.- ☑
    caustic liquid, substance (external) (internal) NEC — *see* Table of Drugs and Chemicals
    chemical (external) (internal) — *see also* Table of Drugs and Chemicals
        in war operations — *see* War operations. fire
    cigar(s) or cigarette(s) X08.8- ☑
        with ignition of clothing NEC X06.2- ☑
            nightwear X05.- ☑
    clothes, clothing NEC (from controlled fire) X06.2- ☑
        with conflagration — *see* Exposure, fire, uncontrolled, building
            not in building or structure — *see* Exposure, fire, uncontrolled, not in building
    cooker (hot) X15.8- ☑
        stated as undetermined whether accidental or intentional Y27.3- ☑
        suicide (attempt) X77.3- ☑
    electric blanket X16.- ☑
    engine (hot) X17.- ☑
    fire, flames — *see* Exposure, fire
    flare, Very pistol — *see* Discharge, firearm NEC
    heat
        from appliance (electrical) (household) X15.8- ☑
            cooker X15.8- ☑
            hotplate X15.2- ☑
            kettle X15.8- ☑
            light bulb X15.8- ☑
            saucepan X15.3- ☑
            skillet X15.3- ☑
            stated as undetermined whether accidental or intentional Y27.3- ☑
            stove X15.0- ☑
            suicide (attempt) X77.3- ☑
            toaster X15.1- ☑
        in local application or packing during medical or surgical procedure Y63.5
    heating
        appliance, radiator or pipe X16.- ☑
    homicide (attempt) — *see* Assault, burning
    hot
        air X14.1- ☑
        cooker X15.8- ☑
        drink X10.0- ☑
        engine X17.- ☑
        fat X10.2- ☑
        fluid NEC X12.- ☑
        food X10.1- ☑
        gases X14.1- ☑
        heating appliance X16.- ☑
        household appliance NEC X15.8- ☑
        kettle X15.8- ☑

Burn, burned, burning — *continued*
    hot — *continued*
        liquid NEC X12.- ☑
        machinery X17.- ☑
        metal (molten) (liquid) NEC X18.- ☑
        object (not producing fire or flames) NEC X19.- ☑
        oil (cooking) X10.2- ☑
        pipe(s) X16.- ☑
        radiator X16.- ☑
        saucepan (glass) (metal) X15.3- ☑
        stove (kitchen) X15.0- ☑
        substance NEC X19.- ☑
            caustic or corrosive NEC — *see* Table of Drugs and Chemicals
        toaster X15.1- ☑
        tool X17.- ☑
        vapor X13.1- ☑
        water (tap) — *see* Contact, with, hot, tap water
    hotplate X15.2- ☑
        suicide (attempt) X77.3- ☑
    ignition — *see* Ignition
    in war operations — *see* War operations, fire
    inflicted by other person X97.- ☑
        by hot objects, hot vapor, and steam — *see* Assault, burning, hot object
    internal, from swallowed caustic, corrosive liquid, substance — *see* Table of Drugs and Chemicals
    iron (hot) X15.8- ☑
        stated as undetermined whether accidental or intentional Y27.3- ☑
        suicide (attempt) X77.3- ☑
    kettle (hot) X15.8- ☑
        stated as undetermined whether accidental or intentional Y27.3- ☑
        suicide (attempt) X77.3- ☑
    lamp (flame) X08.8- ☑
        with ignition of clothing NEC X06.2- ☑
            nightwear X05.- ☑
    lighter (cigar) (cigarette) X08.8- ☑
        with ignition of clothing NEC X06.2- ☑
            nightwear X05.- ☑
    lightning — *see* subcategory T75.0- ☑
        causing fire — *see* Exposure, fire
    liquid (boiling) (hot) NEC X12.- ☑
        stated as undetermined whether accidental or intentional Y27.2- ☑
        suicide (attempt) X77.2- ☑
    local application of externally applied substance in medical or surgical care Y63.5
    machinery (hot) X17.- ☑
    matches X08.8- ☑
        with ignition of clothing NEC X06.2- ☑
            nightwear X05.- ☑
    mattress — *see* Exposure, fire, uncontrolled, building, bed
    medicament, externally applied Y63.5
    metal (hot) (liquid) (molten) NEC X18.- ☑
    nightwear (nightclothes, nightdress, gown, pajamas, robe) X05.- ☑
    object (hot) NEC X19.- ☑
    on board watercraft
        due to
            accident to watercraft V91.09- ☑
                powered craft V91.03- ☑
                    ferry boat V91.01- ☑
                    fishing boat V91.02- ☑
                    jetskis V91.03- ☑
                    liner V91.01- ☑
                    merchant ship V91.00- ☑
                    passenger ship V91.01- ☑
                unpowered craft V91.08- ☑
                    canoe V91.05- ☑
                    inflatable V91.06- ☑
                    kayak V91.05- ☑
                    sailboat V91.04- ☑
                    surf-board V91.08- ☑
                    water skis V91.07- ☑
                    windsurfer V91.08- ☑
            fire on board V93.09- ☑
                ferry boat V93.01- ☑
                fishing boat V93.02- ☑
                jetskis V93.03- ☑
                liner V93.01- ☑
                merchant ship V93.00- ☑
                passenger ship V93.01- ☑
                powered craft NEC V93.03- ☑

Burn, burned, burning — *continued*
    on board watercraft — *continued*
        due to — *continued*
            fire on board — *continued*
                sailboat V93.04- ☑
            specified heat source NEC on board V93.19- ☑
                ferry boat V93.11- ☑
                fishing boat V93.12- ☑
                jetskis V93.13- ☑
                liner V93.11- ☑
                merchant ship V93.10- ☑
                passenger ship V93.11- ☑
                powered craft NEC V93.13- ☑
                sailboat V93.14- ☑
    pipe (hot) X16.- ☑
    smoking X08.8- ☑
        with ignition of clothing NEC X06.2- ☑
            nightwear X05.- ☑
    powder — *see* Powder burn
    radiator (hot) X16.- ☑
    saucepan (hot) (glass) (metal) X15.3- ☑
        stated as undetermined whether accidental or intentional Y27.3- ☑
        suicide (attempt) X77.3- ☑
    self-inflicted X76.- ☑
        stated as undetermined whether accidental or intentional Y26.- ☑
    stated as undetermined whether accidental or intentional Y27.0- ☑
    steam X13.1- ☑
        pipe X16.- ☑
        stated as undetermined whether accidental or intentional Y27.8- ☑
        stated as undetermined whether accidental or intentional Y27.0- ☑
        suicide (attempt) X77.0- ☑
    stove (hot) (kitchen) X15.0- ☑
        stated as undetermined whether accidental or intentional Y27.3- ☑
        suicide (attempt) X77.3- ☑
    substance (hot) NEC X19.- ☑
        boiling X12.- ☑
        stated as undetermined whether accidental or intentional Y27.2- ☑
        suicide (attempt) X77.2- ☑
        molten (metal) X18.- ☑
    suicide (attempt) NEC X76.- ☑
        hot
            household appliance X77.3- ☑
            object X77.9- ☑
    therapeutic misadventure
        heat in local application or packing during medical or surgical procedure Y63.5
        overdose of radiation Y63.2
    toaster (hot) X15.1- ☑
        stated as undetermined whether accidental or intentional Y27.3- ☑
        suicide (attempt) X77.3- ☑
    tool (hot) X17.- ☑
    torch, welding X08.8- ☑
        with ignition of clothing NEC X06.2- ☑
            nightwear X05.- ☑
    trash fire (controlled) — *see* Exposure, fire, controlled, not in building
        uncontrolled — *see* Exposure, fire, uncontrolled, not in building
    vapor (hot) X13.1- ☑
        stated as undetermined whether accidental or intentional Y27.0- ☑
        suicide (attempt) X77.0- ☑
    Very pistol — *see* Discharge, firearm NEC
Butted by animal W55.82- ☑
    bull W55.22- ☑
    cow W55.22- ☑
    goat W55.32- ☑
    horse W55.12- ☑
    pig W55.42- ☑
    sheep W55.32- ☑

C

Caisson disease — *see* Air, pressure, change
Campfire (exposure to) (controlled) — *see also* Exposure, fire, controlled, not in building
    uncontrolled — *see* Exposure, fire, uncontrolled, not in building

Capital punishment (any means) — *see* Legal, intervention
Car sickness T75.3- ☑
Casualty (not due to war) NEC X58.- ☑
 war — *see* War operations
Cat
 bite W55.01- ☑
 scratch W55.03- ☑
Cataclysm, cataclysmic (any injury) NEC — *see* Forces of nature
Catching fire — *see* Exposure, fire
Caught
 between
  folding object W23.0- ☑
  objects (moving) W23.0- ☑
   and
    machinery — *see* Contact, with, by type of machine
    stationary W23.2- ☑
   stationary W23.1- ☑
    and moving W23.2- ☑
  sliding door and door frame W23.0- ☑
 by, in
  machinery (moving parts of) — *see* Contact, with, by type of machine
  washing-machine wringer W23.0- ☑
 under packing crate (due to losing grip) W23.1- ☑
Cave-in caused by cataclysmic earth surface movement or eruption — *see* Landslide
Change(s) in air pressure — *see* Air, pressure, change
Choked, choking (on) (any object except food or vomitus)
 food (bone) (seed) — *see* categories T17 and T18.- ☑
 vomitus T17.81- ☑
Civil insurrection — *see* War operations
Cloudburst (any injury) X37.8- ☑
Cold, exposure to (accidental) (excessive) (extreme) (natural) (place) NEC — *see* Exposure, cold
Collapse
 building W20.1- ☑
  burning (uncontrolled fire) X00.2- ☑
 dam or man-made structure (causing earth movement) X36.0- ☑
 machinery — *see* Contact, with, by type of machine
 structure W20.1- ☑
  burning (uncontrolled fire) X00.2- ☑
Collision (accidental) NEC — *see also* Accident, transport V89.9- ☑
 pedestrian W51.- ☑
  with fall W03.- ☑
   due to ice or snow W00.0- ☑
   involving pedestrian conveyance — *see* Accident, transport, pedestrian, conveyance
   and
    crowd or human stampede (with fall) W52.- ☑
    object W22.8- ☑
     with fall — *see* Fall, due to, bumping against, object
  person(s) — *see* Collision, pedestrian
 transport vehicle NEC V89.9- ☑
  and
   avalanche, fallen or not moving — *see* Accident, transport
    falling or moving — *see* Landslide
   landslide, fallen or not moving — *see* Accident, transport
    falling or moving — *see* Landslide
  due to cataclysm — *see* Forces of nature, by type
  intentional, purposeful suicide (attempt) — *see* Suicide, collision
Combustion, spontaneous — *see* Ignition
Complication (delayed) **of or following** (medical or surgical procedure) Y84.9
 with misadventure — *see* Misadventure
 amputation of limb(s) Y83.5
 anastomosis (arteriovenous) (blood vessel) (gastrojejunal) (tendon) (natural or artificial material) Y83.2
 aspiration (of fluid) Y84.4
  tissue Y84.8
 biopsy Y84.8
 blood
  sampling Y84.7
  transfusion
   procedure Y84.8
 bypass Y83.2
 catheterization (urinary) Y84.6
  cardiac Y84.0
 colostomy Y83.3
 cystostomy Y83.3

Complication (delayed) **of or following** — *continued*
 dialysis (kidney) Y84.1
 drug — *see* Table of Drugs and Chemicals
 due to misadventure — *see* Misadventure
 duodenostomy Y83.3
 electroshock therapy Y84.3
 external stoma, creation of Y83.3
 formation of external stoma Y83.3
 gastrostomy Y83.3
 graft Y83.2
 hypothermia (medically-induced) Y84.8
 implant, implantation (of)
  artificial
   internal device (cardiac pacemaker) (electrodes in brain) (heart valve prosthesis) (orthopedic) Y83.1
   material or tissue (for anastomosis or bypass) Y83.2
    with creation of external stoma Y83.3
  natural tissues (for anastomosis or bypass) Y83.2
   with creation of external stoma Y83.3
 infusion
  procedure Y84.8
 injection — *see* Table of Drugs and Chemicals
  procedure Y84.8
 insertion of gastric or duodenal sound Y84.5
 insulin-shock therapy Y84.3
 paracentesis (abdominal) (thoracic) (aspirative) Y84.4
 procedures other than surgical operation — *see* Complication of or following, by type of procedure
 radiological procedure or therapy Y84.2
 removal of organ (partial) (total) NEC Y83.6
 sampling
  blood Y84.7
  fluid NEC Y84.4
  tissue Y84.8
 shock therapy Y84.3
 surgical operation NEC — *see also* Complication of or following, by type of operation Y83.9
  reconstructive NEC Y83.4
   with
    anastomosis, bypass or graft Y83.2
    formation of external stoma Y83.3
  specified NEC Y83.8
 transfusion — *see also* Table of Drugs and Chemicals
  procedure Y84.8
 transplant, transplantation (heart) (kidney) (liver) (whole organ, any) Y83.0
  partial organ Y83.4
 ureterostomy Y83.3
 vaccination — *see also* Table of Drugs and Chemicals
  procedure Y84.8
Compression
 divers' squeeze — *see* Air, pressure, change
 trachea by
  food (lodged in esophagus) — *see* categories T17 and T18.- ☑
  vomitus (lodged in esophagus) T17.81- ☑
Conflagration — *see* Exposure, fire, uncontrolled
Constriction (external)
 hair W49.01- ☑
 jewelry W49.04- ☑
 ring W49.04- ☑
 rubber band W49.03- ☑
 specified item NEC W49.09- ☑
 string W49.02- ☑
 thread W49.02- ☑
Contact (accidental)
 with
  abrasive wheel (metalworking) W31.1- ☑
  alligator W58.09- ☑
   bite W58.01- ☑
   crushing W58.03- ☑
   strike W58.02- ☑
  amphibian W62.9- ☑
   frog W62.0- ☑
   toad W62.1- ☑
  animal (nonvenomous) NEC W64.- ☑
   marine W56.89- ☑
    bite W56.81- ☑
    dolphin — *see* Contact, with, dolphin
    fish NEC — *see* Contact, with, fish
    mammal — *see* Contact, with, mammal, marine
    orca — *see* Contact, with, orca
    sea lion — *see* Contact, with, sea lion
    shark — *see* Contact, with, shark
    strike W56.82- ☑
  animate mechanical force NEC W64.- ☑
  arrow W21.89- ☑

Contact — *continued*
 with — *continued*
  arrow — *continued*
   not thrown, projected or falling W45.8- ☑
  arthropods (nonvenomous) W57.- ☑
  axe W27.0- ☑
  band-saw (industrial) W31.2- ☑
  bayonet — *see* Bayonet wound
  bee(s) X58.- ☑
  bench-saw (industrial) W31.2- ☑
  bird W61.99- ☑
   bite W61.91- ☑
   chicken — *see* Contact, with, chicken
   duck — *see* Contact, with, duck
   goose — *see* Contact, with, goose
   macaw — *see* Contact, with, macaw
   parrot — *see* Contact, with, parrot
   psittacine — *see* Contact, with, psittacine
   strike W61.92- ☑
   turkey — *see* Contact, with, turkey
  blender W29.0- ☑
  boiling water X12.- ☑
   stated as undetermined whether accidental or intentional Y27.2- ☑
   suicide (attempt) X77.2- ☑
  bore, earth-drilling or mining (land) (seabed) W31.0- ☑
  buffalo — *see* Contact, with, hoof stock NEC
  bull W55.29- ☑
   bite W55.21- ☑
   gored W55.22- ☑
   strike W55.22- ☑
  bumper cars W31.81- ☑
  camel — *see* Contact, with, hoof stock NEC
  can
   lid W26.8- ☑
   opener W27.4- ☑
    powered W29.0- ☑
  cat W55.09- ☑
   bite W55.01- ☑
   scratch W55.03- ☑
  caterpillar (venomous) X58.- ☑
  centipede (venomous) X58.- ☑
  chain
   hoist W24.0- ☑
    agricultural operations W30.89- ☑
   saw W29.3- ☑
  chicken W61.39- ☑
   peck W61.33- ☑
   strike W61.32- ☑
  chisel W27.0- ☑
  circular saw W31.2- ☑
  cobra X58.- ☑
  combine (harvester) W30.0- ☑
  conveyer belt W24.1- ☑
  cooker (hot) X15.8- ☑
   stated as undetermined whether accidental or intentional Y27.3- ☑
   suicide (attempt) X77.3- ☑
  coral X58.- ☑
  cotton gin W31.82- ☑
  cow W55.29- ☑
   bite W55.21- ☑
   strike W55.22- ☑
  crane W24.0- ☑
   agricultural operations W30.89- ☑
  crocodile W58.19- ☑
   bite W58.11- ☑
   crushing W58.13- ☑
   strike W58.12- ☑
  dagger W26.1- ☑
   stated as undetermined whether accidental or intentional Y28.2- ☑
   suicide (attempt) X78.2- ☑
  dairy equipment W31.82- ☑
  dart W21.89- ☑
   not thrown, projected or falling W45.8- ☑
  deer — *see* Contact, with, hoof stock NEC
  derrick W24.0- ☑
   agricultural operations W30.89- ☑
    hay W30.2- ☑
  dog W54.8- ☑
   bite W54.0- ☑
   strike W54.1- ☑
  dolphin W56.09- ☑
   bite W56.01- ☑

☑ **Additional Character Required** — Refer to the Tabular List for Character Selection

Contact

Contact — *continued*
- with — *continued*
  - dolphin — *continued*
    - strike W56.02- ☑
  - donkey — *see* Contact, with, hoof stock NEC
  - drill (powered) W29.8-
    - earth (land) (seabed) W31.0- ☑
    - nonpowered W27.8- ☑
  - drive belt W24.0- ☑
    - agricultural operations W30.89- ☑
  - dry ice — *see* Exposure, cold, man-made
  - dryer (clothes) (powered) (spin) W29.2- ☑
  - duck W61.69- ☑
    - bite W61.61- ☑
    - strike W61.62- ☑
  - earth (-)
    - drilling machine (industrial) W31.0- ☑
    - scraping machine in stationary use W31.83- ☑
  - edge of stiff paper W26.2- ☑
  - electric
    - beater W29.0- ☑
    - blanket X16.- ☑
    - fan W29.2- ☑
      - commercial W31.82- ☑
    - knife W29.1- ☑
    - mixer W29.0- ☑
  - elevator (building) W24.0- ☑
    - agricultural operations W30.89- ☑
      - grain W30.3- ☑
  - engine(s), hot NEC X17.- ☑
  - excavating machine W31.0- ☑
  - farm machine W30.9- ☑
  - feces — *see* Contact, with, by type of animal
  - fer de lance X58.- ☑
  - fish W56.59- ☑
    - bite W56.51- ☑
    - shark — *see* Contact, with, shark
    - strike W56.52- ☑
  - fishing hook W45.3- ☑
  - flying horses W31.81- ☑
  - forging (metalworking) machine W31.1- ☑
  - fork W27.4- ☑
  - forklift (truck) W24.0- ☑
    - agricultural operations W30.89- ☑
  - frog W62.0- ☑
  - garden
    - cultivator (powered) W29.3- ☑
      - riding W30.89- ☑
    - fork W27.1- ☑
  - gas turbine W31.3- ☑
  - Gila monster X58.- ☑
  - giraffe — *see* Contact, with, hoof stock NEC
  - glass (sharp) (broken) W25.- ☑
    - assault X99.0- ☑
    - due to fall — *see* Fall, by type
    - stated as undetermined whether accidental or intentional Y28.0- ☑
    - suicide (attempt) X78.0- ☑
    - with subsequent fall W18.02- ☑
  - goat W55.39- ☑
    - bite W55.31- ☑
    - strike W55.32- ☑
  - goose W61.59- ☑
    - bite W61.51- ☑
    - strike W61.52- ☑
  - hand
    - saw W27.0- ☑
    - tool (not powered) NEC W27.8- ☑
      - powered W29.8- ☑
  - harvester W30.0- ☑
  - hay-derrick W30.2- ☑
  - heat NEC X19.- ☑
    - from appliance (electrical) (household) — *see* Contact, with, hot, household appliance heating appliance X16.- ☑
  - heating
    - appliance (hot) X16.- ☑
    - pad (electric) X16.- ☑
  - hedge-trimmer (powered) W29.3- ☑
  - hoe W27.1- ☑
  - hoist (chain) (shaft) NEC W24.0- ☑
    - agricultural W30.89- ☑
  - hoof stock NEC W55.39- ☑
    - bite W55.31- ☑
    - strike W55.32- ☑

Contact — *continued*
- with — *continued*
  - hornet(s) X58.- ☑
  - horse W55.19- ☑
    - bite W55.11- ☑
    - strike W55.12- ☑
  - hot
    - air X14.1- ☑
      - inhalation X14.0- ☑
    - cooker X15.8- ☑
    - cooking
      - pan X15.3- ☑
      - pot X15.3- ☑
    - drinks X10.0- ☑
    - engine X17.- ☑
    - fats X10.2- ☑
    - fluids NEC X12.- ☑
      - assault X98.2- ☑
      - suicide (attempt) X77.2- ☑
      - undetermined whether accidental or intentional Y27.2- ☑
    - food X10.1- ☑
    - gases X14.1- ☑
      - inhalation X14.0- ☑
    - heating appliance X16.- ☑
    - household appliance X15.8- ☑
      - assault X98.3- ☑
      - cooker X15.8- ☑
      - hotplate X15.2- ☑
      - kettle X15.8- ☑
      - light bulb X15.8- ☑
      - object NEC X19.- ☑
        - assault X98.8- ☑
        - stated as undetermined whether accidental or intentional Y27.9- ☑
        - suicide (attempt) X77.8- ☑
      - saucepan X15.3- ☑
      - skillet X15.3- ☑
      - stated as undetermined whether accidental or intentional Y27.3- ☑
      - stove X15.0- ☑
      - suicide (attempt) X77.3- ☑
      - toaster X15.1- ☑
    - kettle X15.8- ☑
    - light bulb X15.8- ☑
    - liquid NEC — *see also* Burn X12.- ☑
      - drinks X10.0- ☑
      - stated as undetermined whether accidental or intentional Y27.2- ☑
      - suicide (attempt) X77.2- ☑
      - tap water X11.8- ☑
        - stated as undetermined whether accidental or intentional Y27.1- ☑
        - suicide (attempt) X77.1- ☑
    - machinery X17.- ☑
    - metal (molten) (liquid) NEC X18.- ☑
    - object (not producing fire or flames) NEC X19.- ☑
    - oil (cooking) X10.2- ☑
    - pipe X16.- ☑
    - plate X15.2- ☑
    - radiator X16.- ☑
    - saucepan (glass) (metal) X15.3- ☑
    - skillet X15.3- ☑
    - stove (kitchen) X15.0- ☑
    - substance NEC X19.- ☑
    - tap-water X11.8- ☑
      - assault X98.1- ☑
      - heated on stove X12.- ☑
        - stated as undetermined whether accidental or intentional Y27.2- ☑
        - suicide (attempt) X77.2- ☑
      - in bathtub X11.0- ☑
      - running X11.1- ☑
      - stated as undetermined whether accidental or intentional Y27.1- ☑
      - suicide (attempt) X77.1- ☑
    - toaster X15.1- ☑
    - tool X17.- ☑
    - vapors X13.1- ☑
      - inhalation X13.0- ☑
    - water (tap) X11.8- ☑
      - boiling X12.- ☑
        - stated as undetermined whether accidental or intentional Y27.2- ☑
        - suicide (attempt) X77.2- ☑

Contact — *continued*
- with — *continued*
  - hot — *continued*
    - water — *continued*
      - heated on stove X12.- ☑
        - stated as undetermined whether accidental or intentional Y27.2- ☑
        - suicide (attempt) X77.2- ☑
      - in bathtub X11.0- ☑
      - running X11.1- ☑
        - stated as undetermined whether accidental or intentional Y27.1- ☑
        - suicide (attempt) X77.1- ☑
  - hotplate X15.2- ☑
  - ice-pick W27.4- ☑
  - insect (nonvenomous) NEC W57.- ☑
  - kettle (hot) X15.8- ☑
  - knife W26.0- ☑
    - assault X99.1- ☑
    - electric W29.1- ☑
    - stated as undetermined whether accidental or intentional Y28.1- ☑
    - suicide (attempt) X78.1- ☑
  - lathe (metalworking) W31.1- ☑
    - turnings W45.8- ☑
    - woodworking W31.2- ☑
  - lawnmower (powered) (ridden) W28.- ☑
    - causing electrocution W86.8- ☑
      - suicide (attempt) X83.1- ☑
    - unpowered W27.1- ☑
  - lift, lifting (devices) W24.0- ☑
    - agricultural operations W30.89- ☑
    - shaft W24.0- ☑
  - liquefied gas — *see* Exposure, cold, man-made
  - liquid air, hydrogen, nitrogen — *see* Exposure, cold, man-made
  - lizard (nonvenomous) W59.09- ☑
    - bite W59.01- ☑
    - strike W59.02- ☑
  - llama — *see* Contact, with, hoof stock NEC
  - macaw W61.19- ☑
    - bite W61.11- ☑
    - strike W61.12- ☑
  - machine, machinery W31.9- ☑
    - abrasive wheel W31.1- ☑
    - agricultural including animal-powered W30.9- ☑
      - combine harvester W30.0- ☑
      - grain storage elevator W30.3- ☑
      - hay derrick W30.2- ☑
      - power take-off device W30.1- ☑
      - reaper W30.0- ☑
      - specified NEC W30.89- ☑
      - thresher W30.0- ☑
      - transport vehicle, stationary W30.81- ☑
    - band saw W31.2- ☑
    - bench saw W31.2- ☑
    - circular saw W31.2- ☑
    - commercial NEC W31.82- ☑
    - drilling, metal (industrial) W31.1- ☑
    - earth-drilling W31.0- ☑
    - earthmoving or scraping W31.89- ☑
    - excavating W31.89- ☑
    - forging machine W31.1- ☑
    - gas turbine W31.3- ☑
    - hot X17.- ☑
    - internal combustion engine W31.3- ☑
    - land drill W31.0- ☑
    - lathe W31.1- ☑
    - lifting (devices) W24.0- ☑
    - metal drill W31.1- ☑
    - metalworking (industrial) W31.1- ☑
    - milling, metal W31.1- ☑
    - mining W31.0- ☑
    - molding W31.2- ☑
    - overhead plane W31.2- ☑
    - power press, metal W31.1- ☑
    - prime mover W31.3- ☑
    - printing W31.89- ☑
    - radial saw W31.2- ☑
    - recreational W31.81- ☑
    - roller-coaster W31.81- ☑
    - rolling mill, metal W31.1- ☑
    - sander W31.2- ☑
    - seabed drill W31.0- ☑

Contact — continued
　with — continued
　　machine, machinery — continued
　　　shaft
　　　　hoist W31.0- ☑
　　　　lift W31.0- ☑
　　　specified NEC W31.89- ☑
　　　spinning W31.89- ☑
　　　steam engine W31.3- ☑
　　　transmission W24.1- ☑
　　　undercutter W31.0- ☑
　　　water driven turbine W31.3- ☑
　　　weaving W31.89- ☑
　　　woodworking or forming (industrial) W31.2- ☑
　　mammal (feces) (urine) W55.89- ☑
　　　bull — see Contact, with, bull
　　　cat — see Contact, with, cat
　　　cow — see Contact, with, cow
　　　goat — see Contact, with, goat
　　　hoof stock — see Contact, with, hoof stock
　　　horse — see Contact, with, horse
　　　marine W56.39- ☑
　　　　dolphin — see Contact, with, dolphin
　　　　orca — see Contact, with, orca
　　　　sea lion — see Contact, with, sea lion
　　　　specified NEC W56.39- ☑
　　　　　bite W56.31- ☑
　　　　　strike W56.32- ☑
　　　pig — see Contact, with, pig
　　　raccoon — see Contact, with, raccoon
　　　rodent — see Contact, with, rodent
　　　sheep — see Contact, with, sheep
　　　specified NEC W55.89- ☑
　　　　bite W55.81- ☑
　　　　strike W55.82- ☑
　　marine
　　　animal W56.89- ☑
　　　　bite W56.81- ☑
　　　　dolphin — see Contact, with, dolphin
　　　　fish NEC — see Contact, with, fish
　　　　mammal — see Contact, with, mammal, marine
　　　　orca — see Contact, with, orca
　　　　sea lion — see Contact, with, sea lion
　　　　shark — see Contact, with, shark
　　　　strike W56.82- ☑
　　meat
　　　grinder (domestic) W29.0- ☑
　　　　industrial W31.82- ☑
　　　　nonpowered W27.4- ☑
　　　slicer (domestic) W29.0- ☑
　　　　industrial W31.82- ☑
　　merry go round W31.81- ☑
　　metal, hot (liquid) (molten) NEC X18.- ☑
　　millipede W57.- ☑
　　nail W45.0- ☑
　　　gun W29.4- ☑
　　needle (sewing) W27.3- ☑
　　　hypodermic W46.0- ☑
　　　　contaminated W46.1- ☑
　　object (blunt) NEC
　　　hot NEC X19.- ☑
　　　legal intervention — see Legal, intervention, blunt object
　　　sharp NEC W45.8- ☑
　　　　inflicted by other person NEC W45.8- ☑
　　　　stated as
　　　　　intentional homicide (attempt) — see Assault, cutting or piercing instrument
　　　　legal intervention — see Legal, intervention, sharp object
　　　　self-inflicted X78.9- ☑
　　orca W56.29- ☑
　　　bite W56.21- ☑
　　　strike W56.22- ☑
　　overhead plane W31.2- ☑
　　paper (as sharp object) W26.2- ☑
　　paper-cutter W27.5- ☑
　　parrot W61.09- ☑
　　　bite W61.01- ☑
　　　strike W61.02- ☑
　　pig W55.49- ☑
　　　bite W55.41- ☑
　　　strike W55.42- ☑
　　pipe, hot X16.- ☑
　　pitchfork W27.1- ☑

Contact — continued
　with — continued
　　plane (metal) (wood) W27.0- ☑
　　　overhead W31.2- ☑
　　plant thorns, spines, sharp leaves or other mechanisms W60.- ☑
　　powered
　　　garden cultivator W29.3- ☑
　　　household appliance, implement, or machine W29.8- ☑
　　　saw (industrial) W31.2- ☑
　　　　hand W29.8- ☑
　　printing machine W31.89- ☑
　　psittacine bird W61.29- ☑
　　　bite W61.21- ☑
　　　macaw — see Contact, with, macaw
　　　parrot — see Contact, with, parrot
　　　strike W61.22- ☑
　　pulley (block) (transmission) W24.0- ☑
　　　agricultural operations W30.89- ☑
　　raccoon W55.59- ☑
　　　bite W55.51- ☑
　　　strike W55.52- ☑
　　radial-saw (industrial) W31.2- ☑
　　radiator (hot) X16.- ☑
　　rake W27.1- ☑
　　rattlesnake X58.- ☑
　　reaper W30.0- ☑
　　reptile W59.89- ☑
　　　lizard — see Contact, with, lizard
　　　snake — see Contact, with, snake
　　　specified NEC W59.89- ☑
　　　　bite W59.81- ☑
　　　　crushing W59.83- ☑
　　　　strike W59.82- ☑
　　　turtle — see Contact, with, turtle
　　rivet gun (powered) W29.4- ☑
　　road scraper — see Accident, transport, construction vehicle
　　rodent (feces) (urine) W53.89- ☑
　　　bite W53.81- ☑
　　　mouse W53.09- ☑
　　　　bite W53.01- ☑
　　　rat W53.19- ☑
　　　　bite W53.11- ☑
　　　specified NEC W53.89- ☑
　　　　bite W53.81- ☑
　　　squirrel W53.29- ☑
　　　　bite W53.21- ☑
　　roller coaster W31.81- ☑
　　rope NEC W24.0- ☑
　　　agricultural operations W30.89- ☑
　　saliva — see Contact, with, by type of animal
　　sander W29.8- ☑
　　　industrial W31.2- ☑
　　saucepan (hot) (glass) (metal) X15.3- ☑
　　saw W27.0- ☑
　　　band (industrial) W31.2- ☑
　　　bench (industrial) W31.2- ☑
　　　chain W29.3- ☑
　　　hand W27.0- ☑
　　sawing machine, metal W31.1- ☑
　　scissors W27.2- ☑
　　scorpion X58.- ☑
　　screwdriver W27.0- ☑
　　　powered W29.8- ☑
　　sea
　　　anemone, cucumber or urchin (spine) X58.- ☑
　　　lion W56.19- ☑
　　　　bite W56.11- ☑
　　　　strike W56.12- ☑
　　serpent — see Contact, with, snake, by type
　　sewing-machine (electric) (powered) W29.2- ☑
　　　not powered W27.8- ☑
　　shaft (hoist) (lift) (transmission) NEC W24.0- ☑
　　　agricultural W30.89- ☑
　　shark W56.49- ☑
　　　bite W56.41- ☑
　　　strike W56.42- ☑
　　sharp object(s) W26.9- ☑
　　　specified NEC W26.8- ☑
　　shears (hand) W27.2- ☑
　　　powered (industrial) W31.1- ☑
　　　　domestic W29.2- ☑
　　sheep W55.39- ☑

Contact — continued
　with — continued
　　sheep — continued
　　　bite W55.31- ☑
　　　strike W55.32- ☑
　　shovel W27.8- ☑
　　　steam — see Accident, transport, construction vehicle
　　snake (nonvenomous) W59.19- ☑
　　　bite W59.11- ☑
　　　crushing W59.13- ☑
　　　strike W59.12- ☑
　　spade W27.1- ☑
　　spider (venomous) X58.- ☑
　　spin-drier W29.2- ☑
　　spinning machine W31.89- ☑
　　splinter W45.8- ☑
　　sports equipment W21.9- ☑
　　staple gun (powered) W29.8- ☑
　　steam X13.1- ☑
　　　engine W31.3- ☑
　　　inhalation X13.0- ☑
　　　pipe X16.- ☑
　　　shovel W31.89- ☑
　　stove (hot) (kitchen) X15.0- ☑
　　substance, hot NEC X19.- ☑
　　　molten (metal) X18.- ☑
　　sword W26.1- ☑
　　　assault X99.2- ☑
　　　stated as undetermined whether accidental or intentional Y28.2- ☑
　　　suicide (attempt) X78.2- ☑
　　tarantula X58.- ☑
　　thresher W30.0- ☑
　　tin can lid W26.8- ☑
　　toad W62.1- ☑
　　toaster (hot) X15.1- ☑
　　tool W27.8- ☑
　　　hand (not powered) W27.8- ☑
　　　　auger W27.0- ☑
　　　　axe W27.0- ☑
　　　　can opener W27.4- ☑
　　　　chisel W27.0- ☑
　　　　fork W27.4- ☑
　　　　garden W27.1- ☑
　　　　handsaw W27.0- ☑
　　　　hoe W27.1- ☑
　　　　ice-pick W27.4- ☑
　　　　kitchen utensil W27.4- ☑
　　　　manual
　　　　　lawn mower W27.1- ☑
　　　　　sewing machine W27.8- ☑
　　　　meat grinder W27.4- ☑
　　　　needle (sewing) W27.3- ☑
　　　　　hypodermic W46.0- ☑
　　　　　　contaminated W46.1- ☑
　　　　paper cutter W27.5- ☑
　　　　pitchfork W27.1- ☑
　　　　rake W27.1- ☑
　　　　scissors W27.2- ☑
　　　　screwdriver W27.0- ☑
　　　　specified NEC W27.8- ☑
　　　　workbench W27.0- ☑
　　　hot X17.- ☑
　　　powered W29.8- ☑
　　　　blender W29.0- ☑
　　　　　commercial W31.82- ☑
　　　　can opener W29.0- ☑
　　　　　commercial W31.82- ☑
　　　　chainsaw W29.3- ☑
　　　　clothes dryer W29.2- ☑
　　　　　commercial W31.82- ☑
　　　　dishwasher W29.2- ☑
　　　　　commercial W31.82- ☑
　　　　edger W29.3- ☑
　　　　electric fan W29.2- ☑
　　　　　commercial W31.82- ☑
　　　　electric knife W29.1- ☑
　　　　food processor W29.0- ☑
　　　　　commercial W31.82- ☑
　　　　garbage disposal W29.0- ☑
　　　　　commercial W31.82- ☑
　　　　garden tool W29.3- ☑
　　　　hedge trimmer W29.3- ☑
　　　　ice maker W29.0- ☑

☑ Additional Character Required — Refer to the Tabular List for Character Selection

Contact — continued
  with — continued
    tool — continued
      powered — continued
        ice maker — continued
          commercial W31.82- ☑
        kitchen appliance W29.0- ☑
          commercial W31.82- ☑
        lawn mower W28.- ☑
        meat grinder W29.0- ☑
          commercial W31.82- ☑
        mixer W29.0- ☑
          commercial W31.82- ☑
        rototiller W29.3- ☑
        sewing machine W29.2- ☑
          commercial W31.82- ☑
        washing machine W29.2- ☑
          commercial W31.82- ☑
      transmission device (belt, cable, chain, gear, pinion, shaft) W24.1- ☑
        agricultural operations W30.89- ☑
      turbine (gas) (water-driven) W31.3- ☑
      turkey W61.49- ☑
        peck W61.43- ☑
        strike W61.42- ☑
      turtle (nonvenomous) W59.29- ☑
        bite W59.21- ☑
        strike W59.22- ☑
      terrestrial W59.89- ☑
        bite W59.81- ☑
        crushing W59.83- ☑
        strike W59.82- ☑
      under-cutter W31.0- ☑
      urine — see Contact, with, by type of animal
      vehicle
        agricultural use (transport) — see Accident, transport, agricultural vehicle
          not on public highway W30.81- ☑
        industrial use (transport) — see Accident, transport, industrial vehicle
          not on public highway W31.83- ☑
        off-road use (transport) — see Accident, transport, all-terrain or off-road vehicle
          not on public highway W31.83- ☑
        special construction use (transport) — see Accident, transport, construction vehicle
          not on public highway W31.83- ☑
      venomous
        animal X58.- ☑
        arthropods X58.- ☑
        lizard X58.- ☑
        marine animal NEC X58.- ☑
        marine plant NEC X58.- ☑
        millipedes (tropical) X58.- ☑
        plant(s) X58.- ☑
        snake X58.- ☑
        spider X58.- ☑
        viper X58.- ☑
      washing-machine (powered) W29.2- ☑
      wasp X58.- ☑
      weaving-machine W31.89- ☑
      winch W24.0- ☑
        agricultural operations W30.89- ☑
      wire NEC W24.0- ☑
        agricultural operations W30.89- ☑
      wood slivers W45.8- ☑
      yellow jacket X58.- ☑
      zebra — see Contact, with, hoof stock NEC
  pressure X50.9- ☑
  stress X50.9- ☑
Coup de soleil X32.- ☑
Crash
  aircraft (in transit) (powered) V95.9- ☑
    balloon V96.01- ☑
    fixed wing NEC (private) V95.21- ☑
      commercial V95.31- ☑
    glider V96.21- ☑
      hang V96.11- ☑
      powered V95.11- ☑
    helicopter V95.01- ☑
    in war operations — see War operations, destruction of aircraft
    microlight V95.11- ☑
    nonpowered V96.9- ☑
      specified NEC V96.8- ☑
    powered NEC V95.8- ☑

Crash — continued
  aircraft — continued
    stated as
      homicide (attempt) Y08.81- ☑
      suicide (attempt) X83.0- ☑
    ultralight V95.11- ☑
  spacecraft V95.41- ☑
  transport vehicle NEC — see also Accident, transport V89.9- ☑
    homicide (attempt) Y03.8- ☑
    motor NEC (traffic) V89.2- ☑
      homicide (attempt) Y03.8- ☑
      suicide (attempt) — see Suicide, collision
Cruelty (mental) (physical) (sexual) X58.- ☑
Crushed (accidentally) X58.- ☑
  between objects (moving) (stationary and moving) W23.0- ☑
    stationary W23.1- ☑
  by
    alligator W58.03- ☑
    avalanche NEC — see Landslide
    cave-in W20.0- ☑
      caused by cataclysmic earth surface movement — see Landslide
    crocodile W58.13- ☑
    crowd or human stampede W52.- ☑
    falling
      aircraft V97.39- ☑
        in war operations — see War operations, destruction of aircraft
      earth, material W20.0- ☑
        caused by cataclysmic earth surface movement — see Landslide
      object NEC W20.8- ☑
    landslide NEC — see Landslide
    lizard (nonvenomous) W59.09- ☑
    machinery — see Contact, with, by type of machine
    reptile NEC W59.89- ☑
    snake (nonvenomous) W59.13- ☑
  in
    machinery — see Contact, with, by type of machine
Cut, cutting (any part of body) (accidental) — see also Contact, with, by object or machine
  during medical or surgical treatment as misadventure — see Index to Diseases and Injuries, Complications
  homicide (attempt) — see Assault, cutting or piercing instrument
  inflicted by other person — see Assault, cutting or piercing instrument
  legal
    execution — see Legal, intervention
    intervention — see Legal, intervention, sharp object
  machine NEC — see also Contact, with, by type of machine W31.9- ☑
  self-inflicted — see Suicide, cutting or piercing instrument
  suicide (attempt) — see Suicide, cutting or piercing instrument
Cyclone (any injury) X37.1- ☑

D

Decapitation (accidental circumstances) NEC X58.- ☑
  homicide X99.9- ☑
  legal execution — see Legal, intervention
Dehydration from lack of water X58.- ☑
Deprivation X58.- ☑
Derailment (accidental)
  railway (rolling stock) (train) (vehicle) (without antecedent collision) V81.7- ☑
    with antecedent collision — see Accident, transport, railway vehicle occupant
  streetcar (without antecedent collision) V82.7- ☑
    with antecedent collision — see Accident, transport, streetcar occupant
Descent
  parachute (voluntary) (without accident to aircraft) V97.29- ☑
    due to accident to aircraft — see Accident, transport, aircraft
Desertion X58.- ☑
Destitution X58.- ☑
Disability, late effect or sequela of injury — see Sequelae
Discharge (accidental)
  airgun W34.010- ☑
    assault X95.01- ☑

Discharge — continued
  airgun — continued
    homicide (attempt) X95.01- ☑
    stated as undetermined whether accidental or intentional Y24.0- ☑
    suicide (attempt) X74.01- ☑
  BB gun — see Discharge, airgun
  firearm (accidental) Y24.9- ☑
    accidental W34.00- ☑
    assault X95.9- ☑
    handgun (pistol) (revolver) Y22.- ☑
      accidental W32.0- ☑
      assault X93.- ☑
      homicide (attempt) X93.- ☑
      legal intervention — see Legal, intervention, firearm, handgun
      stated as undetermined whether accidental or intentional Y22.- ☑
      suicide (attempt) X72.- ☑
    homicide (attempt) X95.9- ☑
    hunting rifle Y23.1- ☑
      accidental W33.02- ☑
      assault X94.1- ☑
      homicide (attempt) X94.1- ☑
      legal intervention
        injuring
          bystander Y35.032- ☑
          law enforcement personnel Y35.031- ☑
          suspect Y35.033- ☑
          unspecified person Y35.039- ☑
      stated as undetermined whether accidental or intentional Y23.1- ☑
      suicide (attempt) X73.1- ☑
    larger Y23.9- ☑
      accidental W33.00- ☑
      assault X94.9- ☑
      homicide (attempt) X94.9- ☑
      hunting rifle — see Discharge, firearm, hunting rifle
      legal intervention — see Legal, intervention, firearm by type of firearm
      machine gun — see Discharge, firearm, machine gun
      shotgun — see Discharge, firearm, shotgun
      specified NEC Y23.8- ☑
        accidental W33.09- ☑
        assault X94.8- ☑
        homicide (attempt) X94.8- ☑
        legal intervention
          injuring
            bystander Y35.092- ☑
            law enforcement personnel Y35.091- ☑
            suspect Y35.093- ☑
            unspecified person Y35.099- ☑
        stated as undetermined whether accidental or intentional Y23.8- ☑
        suicide (attempt) X73.8- ☑
      stated as undetermined whether accidental or intentional Y23.9- ☑
      suicide (attempt) X73.9- ☑
    legal intervention
      injuring
        bystander Y35.002- ☑
        law enforcement personnel Y35.001- ☑
        suspect Y35.003- ☑
        unspecified person Y35.009- ☑
      using rubber bullet
        injuring
          bystander Y35.042- ☑
          law enforcement personnel Y35.041- ☑
          suspect Y35.043- ☑
          unspecified person Y35.049- ☑
    machine gun Y23.3- ☑
      accidental W33.03- ☑
      assault X94.2- ☑
      homicide (attempt) X94.2- ☑
      legal intervention — see Legal, intervention, firearm, machine gun
      stated as undetermined whether accidental or intentional Y23.3- ☑
      suicide (attempt) X73.2- ☑
    pellet gun — see Discharge, airgun
    shotgun Y23.0- ☑
      accidental W33.01- ☑
      assault X94.0- ☑
      homicide (attempt) X94.0- ☑

Discharge — *continued*
- firearm — *continued*
  - shotgun — *continued*
    - legal intervention — *see* Legal, intervention, firearm, specified NEC
    - stated as undetermined whether accidental or intentional Y23.0- ☑
    - suicide (attempt) X73.0- ☑
  - specified NEC W34.09- ☑
    - assault X95.8- ☑
    - homicide (attempt) X95.8- ☑
    - legal intervention — *see* Legal, intervention, firearm, specified NEC
    - stated as undetermined whether accidental or intentional Y24.8- ☑
    - suicide (attempt) X74.8- ☑
  - stated as undetermined whether accidental or intentional Y24.9- ☑
  - suicide (attempt) X74.9- ☑
  - Very pistol W34.09- ☑
    - assault X95.8- ☑
    - homicide (attempt) X95.8- ☑
    - stated as undetermined whether accidental or intentional Y24.8- ☑
    - suicide (attempt) X74.8- ☑
- firework(s) W39.- ☑
  - stated as undetermined whether accidental or intentional Y25.- ☑
- gas-operated gun NEC W34.018- ☑
  - airgun — *see* Discharge, airgun
  - assault X95.09- ☑
  - homicide (attempt) X95.09- ☑
  - paintball gun — *see* Discharge, paintball gun
  - stated as undetermined whether accidental or intentional Y24.8- ☑
  - suicide (attempt) X74.09- ☑
- gun NEC — *see also* Discharge, firearm NEC
  - air — *see* Discharge, airgun
  - BB — *see* Discharge, airgun
  - for single hand use — *see* Discharge, firearm, handgun
  - hand — *see* Discharge, firearm, handgun
  - machine — *see* Discharge, firearm, machine gun
  - other specified — *see* Discharge, firearm NEC
  - paintball — *see* Discharge, paintball gun
  - pellet — *see* Discharge, airgun
- handgun — *see* Discharge, firearm, handgun
- machine gun — *see* Discharge, firearm, machine gun
- paintball gun W34.011- ☑
  - assault X95.02- ☑
  - homicide (attempt) X95.02- ☑
  - stated as undetermined whether accidental or intentional Y24.8- ☑
  - suicide (attempt) X74.02- ☑
- pistol — *see* Discharge, firearm, handgun
  - flare — *see* Discharge, firearm, Very pistol
  - pellet — *see* Discharge, airgun
  - Very — *see* Discharge, firearm, Very pistol
- revolver — *see* Discharge, firearm, handgun
- rifle (hunting) — *see* Discharge, firearm, hunting rifle
- shotgun — *see* Discharge, firearm, shotgun
- spring-operated gun NEC W34.018- ☑
  - assault X95.09- ☑
  - homicide (attempt) X95.09- ☑
  - stated as undetermined whether accidental or intentional Y24.8- ☑
  - suicide (attempt) X74.09- ☑

Disease
- Andes W94.11- ☑
- aviator's — *see* Air, pressure
- range W94.11- ☑

Diver's disease, palsy, paralysis, squeeze — *see* Air, pressure

Diving (into water) — *see* Accident, diving

Dog bite W54.0- ☑

Dragged by transport vehicle NEC — *see also* Accident, transport V09.9- ☑

Drinking poison (accidental) — *see* Table of Drugs and Chemicals

Dropped (accidentally) **while being carried or supported by other person** W04.- ☑

Drowning (accidental) W74.- ☑
- assault X92.9- ☑
- due to
  - accident (to)
    - machinery — *see* Contact, with, by type of machine

Drowning — *continued*
- due to — *continued*
  - accident — *continued*
    - watercraft V90.89- ☑
      - burning V90.29- ☑
        - powered V90.23- ☑
          - fishing boat V90.22- ☑
          - jetskis V90.23- ☑
          - merchant ship V90.20- ☑
          - passenger ship V90.21- ☑
        - unpowered V90.28- ☑
          - canoe V90.25- ☑
          - inflatable V90.26- ☑
          - kayak V90.25- ☑
          - sailboat V90.24- ☑
          - water skis V90.27- ☑
      - crushed V90.39- ☑
        - powered V90.33- ☑
          - fishing boat V90.32- ☑
          - jetskis V90.33- ☑
          - merchant ship V90.30- ☑
          - passenger ship V90.31- ☑
        - unpowered V90.38- ☑
          - canoe V90.35- ☑
          - inflatable V90.36- ☑
          - kayak V90.35- ☑
          - sailboat V90.34- ☑
          - water skis V90.37- ☑
      - overturning V90.09- ☑
        - powered V90.03- ☑
          - fishing boat V90.02- ☑
          - jetskis V90.03- ☑
          - merchant ship V90.00- ☑
          - passenger ship V90.01- ☑
        - unpowered V90.08- ☑
          - canoe V90.05- ☑
          - inflatable V90.06- ☑
          - kayak V90.05- ☑
          - sailboat V90.04- ☑
      - sinking V90.19- ☑
        - powered V90.13- ☑
          - fishing boat V90.12- ☑
          - jetskis V90.13- ☑
          - merchant ship V90.10- ☑
          - passenger ship V90.11- ☑
        - unpowered V90.18- ☑
          - canoe V90.15- ☑
          - inflatable V90.16- ☑
          - kayak V90.15- ☑
          - sailboat V90.14- ☑
      - specified type NEC V90.89- ☑
        - powered V90.83- ☑
          - fishing boat V90.82- ☑
          - jetskis V90.83- ☑
          - merchant ship V90.80- ☑
          - passenger ship V90.81- ☑
        - unpowered V90.88- ☑
          - canoe V90.85- ☑
          - inflatable V90.86- ☑
          - kayak V90.85- ☑
          - sailboat V90.84- ☑
          - water skis V90.87- ☑
    - avalanche — *see* Landslide
    - cataclysmic
      - earth surface movement NEC — *see* Forces of nature, earth movement
      - storm — *see* Forces of nature, cataclysmic storm
    - cloudburst X37.8- ☑
    - cyclone X37.1- ☑
    - fall overboard (from) V92.09- ☑
      - powered craft V92.03- ☑
        - ferry boat V92.01- ☑
        - fishing boat V92.02- ☑
        - jetskis V92.03- ☑
        - liner V92.01- ☑
        - merchant ship V92.00- ☑
        - passenger ship V92.01- ☑
      - resulting from
        - accident to watercraft — *see* Drowning, due to, accident to, watercraft
        - being washed overboard (from) V92.29- ☑
          - powered craft V92.23- ☑
            - ferry boat V92.21- ☑
            - fishing boat V92.22- ☑
            - jetskis V92.23- ☑

Drowning — *continued*
- due to — *continued*
  - fall overboard — *continued*
    - resulting from — *continued*
      - being washed overboard — *continued*
        - powered craft — *continued*
          - liner V92.21- ☑
          - merchant ship V92.20- ☑
          - passenger ship V92.21- ☑
        - unpowered craft V92.28- ☑
          - canoe V92.25- ☑
          - inflatable V92.26- ☑
          - kayak V92.25- ☑
          - sailboat V92.24- ☑
          - surf-board V92.28- ☑
          - water skis V92.27- ☑
          - windsurfer V92.28- ☑
      - motion of watercraft V92.19- ☑
        - powered craft V92.13- ☑
          - ferry boat V92.11- ☑
          - fishing boat V92.12- ☑
          - jetskis V92.13- ☑
          - liner V92.11- ☑
          - merchant ship V92.10- ☑
          - passenger ship V92.11- ☑
        - unpowered craft
          - canoe V92.15- ☑
          - inflatable V92.16- ☑
          - kayak V92.15- ☑
          - sailboat V92.14- ☑
    - unpowered craft V92.08- ☑
      - canoe V92.05- ☑
      - inflatable V92.06- ☑
      - kayak V92.05- ☑
      - sailboat V92.04- ☑
      - surf-board V92.08- ☑
      - water skis V92.07- ☑
      - windsurfer V92.08- ☑
  - hurricane X37.0- ☑
  - jumping into water from watercraft (involved in accident) — *see also* Drowning, due to, accident to, watercraft
    - without accident to or on watercraft W16.711- ☑
  - tidal wave NEC — *see* Forces of nature, tidal wave
  - torrential rain X37.8- ☑
- following
  - fall
    - into
      - bathtub W16.211- ☑
      - bucket W16.221- ☑
      - fountain — *see* Drowning, following, fall, into, water, specified NEC
      - quarry — *see* Drowning, following, fall, into, water, specified NEC
      - reservoir — *see* Drowning, following, fall, into, water, specified NEC
      - swimming-pool W16.011- ☑
        - stated as undetermined whether accidental or intentional Y21.3- ☑
        - striking
          - bottom W16.021- ☑
          - wall W16.031- ☑
        - suicide (attempt) X71.2- ☑
      - water NOS W16.41- ☑
        - natural (lake) (open sea) (river) (stream) (pond) W16.111- ☑
          - striking
            - bottom W16.121- ☑
            - side W16.131- ☑
        - specified NEC W16.311- ☑
          - striking
            - bottom W16.321- ☑
            - wall W16.331- ☑
  - overboard NEC — *see* Drowning, due to, fall overboard
  - jump or dive
    - from boat W16.711- ☑
      - striking bottom W16.721- ☑
    - into
      - fountain — *see* Drowning, following, jump or dive, into, water, specified NEC
      - quarry — *see* Drowning, following, jump or dive, into, water, specified NEC
      - reservoir — *see* Drowning, following, jump or dive, into, water, specified NEC
      - swimming-pool W16.511- ☑

☑ **Additional Character Required** — Refer to the Tabular List for Character Selection

Drowning — *continued*
  following — *continued*
    jump or dive — *continued*
      into — *continued*
        swimming-pool — *continued*
          striking
            bottom W16.521- ☑
            wall W16.531- ☑
          suicide (attempt) X71.2- ☑
        water NOS W16.91- ☑
          natural (lake) (open sea) (river) (stream)
            (pond) W16.611- ☑
          specified NEC W16.811- ☑
            bottom W16.821- ☑
            striking
              bottom W16.821- ☑
              wall W16.831- ☑
          striking
            bottom W16.821- ☑
            wall W16.831- ☑
          striking bottom W16.621- ☑
  homicide (attempt) X92.9- ☑
  in
    bathtub (accidental) W65.- ☑
      assault X92.0- ☑
      following fall W16.211- ☑
      stated as undetermined whether accidental or
        intentional Y21.1- ☑
      stated as undetermined whether accidental or in-
        tentional Y21.0- ☑
      suicide (attempt) X71.0- ☑
    lake — *see* Drowning, in, natural water
    natural water (lake) (open sea) (river) (stream) (pond)
      W69.- ☑
      assault X92.3- ☑
      following
        dive or jump W16.611- ☑
          striking bottom W16.621- ☑
        fall W16.111- ☑
          striking
            bottom W16.121- ☑
            side W16.131- ☑
      stated as undetermined whether accidental or in-
        tentional Y21.4- ☑
      suicide (attempt) X71.3- ☑
    quarry — *see* Drowning, in, specified place NEC
    quenching tank — *see* Drowning, in, specified place
      NEC
    reservoir — *see* Drowning, in, specified place NEC
    river — *see* Drowning, in, natural water
    sea — *see* Drowning, in, natural water
    specified place NEC W73.- ☑
      assault X92.8- ☑
      following
        dive or jump W16.811- ☑
          striking
            bottom W16.821- ☑
            wall W16.831- ☑
        fall W16.311- ☑
          striking
            bottom W16.321- ☑
            wall W16.331- ☑
      stated as undetermined whether accidental or
        tentional Y21.8- ☑
      suicide (attempt) X71.8- ☑
    stream — *see* Drowning, in, natural water
    swimming-pool W67.- ☑
      assault X92.1- ☑
        following fall X92.2- ☑
      following
        dive or jump W16.511- ☑
          striking
            bottom W16.521- ☑
            wall W16.531- ☑
        fall W16.011- ☑
          striking
            bottom W16.021- ☑
            wall W16.031- ☑
      stated as undetermined whether accidental or in-
        tentional Y21.2- ☑
        following fall Y21.3- ☑
      suicide (attempt) X71.1- ☑
        following fall X71.2- ☑
    war operations — *see* War operations, restriction of
      airway

Drowning — *continued*
  resulting from accident to watercraft — *see* Drowning,
    due to, accident to, watercraft
  self-inflicted X71.9- ☑
  stated as undetermined whether accidental or intentional
    Y21.9- ☑
  suicide (attempt) X71.9- ☑

E

Earth falling (on) W20.0- ☑
  caused by cataclysmic earth surface movement or erup-
    tion — *see* Landslide
Earth (surface) **movement NEC** — *see* Forces of nature,
  earth movement
Earthquake (any injury) X34.- ☑
Effect(s) (adverse) **of**
  air pressure (any) — *see* Air, pressure
  cold, excessive (exposure to) — *see* Exposure, cold
  heat (excessive) — *see* Heat
  hot place (weather) — *see* Heat
  insolation X30.- ☑
  late — *see* Sequelae
  motion — *see* Motion
  nuclear explosion or weapon in war operations — *see*
    War operations, nuclear weapon
  radiation — *see* Radiation
  travel — *see* Travel
Electric shock (accidental) (by) (in) — *see* Exposure, electric
  current
Electrocution (accidental) — *see* Exposure, electric current
Endotracheal tube wrongly placed during anesthetic
  procedure
Entanglement
  in
    bed linen, causing suffocation T71.- ☑
    wheel of pedal cycle V19.88- ☑
Entry of foreign body or material — *see* Foreign body
Environmental pollution related condition — *see* category Z77
Execution, legal (any method) — *see* Legal, intervention
Exhaustion
  cold — *see* Exposure, cold
  due to excessive exertion — *see also* Overexertion
    X50.9- ☑
  heat — *see* Heat
Explosion (accidental) (of) (with secondary fire) W40.9- ☑
  acetylene W40.1- ☑
  aerosol can W36.1- ☑
  air tank (compressed) (in machinery) W36.2- ☑
  aircraft (in transit) (powered) NEC V95.9- ☑
    balloon V96.05- ☑
    fixed wing NEC (private) V95.25- ☑
      commercial V95.35- ☑
    glider V96.25- ☑
      hang V96.15- ☑
      powered V95.15- ☑
    helicopter V95.05- ☑
    in war operations — *see* War operations, destruction
      of aircraft
    microlight V95.15- ☑
    nonpowered V96.9- ☑
      specified NEC V96.8- ☑
    powered NEC V95.8- ☑
    stated as
      homicide (attempt) Y08.81- ☑
      suicide (attempt) X83.0- ☑
    ultralight V95.15- ☑
  anesthetic gas in operating room W40.1- ☑
  antipersonnel bomb W40.8- ☑
    assault X96.0- ☑
    homicide (attempt) X96.0- ☑
    suicide (attempt) X75.- ☑
  assault X96.9- ☑
  bicycle tire W37.0- ☑
  blasting (cap) (materials) W40.0- ☑
  boiler (machinery), not on transport vehicle W35.- ☑
    on watercraft — *see* Explosion, in, watercraft
  butane W40.1- ☑
  caused by other person X96.9- ☑
  coal gas W40.1- ☑
  detonator W40.0- ☑
  dump (munitions) W40.8- ☑
  dynamite W40.0- ☑
    in
      assault X96.8- ☑

Explosion — *continued*
  dynamite — *continued*
    in — *continued*
      homicide (attempt) X96.8- ☑
      legal intervention
        injuring
          bystander Y35.112- ☑
          law enforcement personnel Y35.111- ☑
          suspect Y35.113- ☑
          unspecified person Y35.119- ☑
      suicide (attempt) X75.- ☑
  explosive (material) W40.9- ☑
    gas W40.1- ☑
    in blasting operation W40.0- ☑
    specified NEC W40.8- ☑
      in
        assault X96.8- ☑
        homicide (attempt) X96.8- ☑
        legal intervention
          injuring
            bystander Y35.192- ☑
            law enforcement personnel Y35.191- ☑
            suspect Y35.193- ☑
            unspecified person Y35.199- ☑
        suicide (attempt) X75.- ☑
  factory (munitions) W40.8- ☑
  fertilizer bomb W40.8- ☑
    assault X96.3- ☑
    homicide (attempt) X96.3- ☑
    suicide (attempt) X75.- ☑
  fire-damp W40.1- ☑
  firearm (parts) NEC W34.19- ☑
    airgun W34.110- ☑
    BB gun W34.110- ☑
    gas, air or spring-operated gun NEC W34.118- ☑
    handgun W32.1- ☑
    hunting rifle W33.12- ☑
    larger firearm W33.10- ☑
      specified NEC W33.19- ☑
    machine gun W33.13- ☑
    paintball gun W34.111- ☑
    pellet gun W34.110- ☑
    shotgun W33.11- ☑
    Very pistol [flare] W34.19- ☑
  fireworks W39.- ☑
  gas (coal) (explosive) W40.1- ☑
    cylinder W36.9- ☑
      aerosol can W36.1- ☑
      air tank W36.2- ☑
      pressurized W36.3- ☑
      specified NEC W36.8- ☑
  gasoline (fumes) (tank) not in moving motor vehicle
    W40.1- ☑
    bomb W40.8- ☑
      assault X96.1- ☑
      homicide (attempt) X96.1- ☑
      suicide (attempt) X75.- ☑
    in motor vehicle — *see* Accident, transport, by type
      of vehicle
  grain store W40.8- ☑
  grenade W40.8- ☑
    in
      assault X96.8- ☑
      homicide (attempt) X96.8- ☑
      legal intervention
        injuring
          bystander Y35.192- ☑
          law enforcement personnel Y35.191- ☑
          suspect Y35.193- ☑
          unspecified person Y35.199- ☑
      suicide (attempt) X75.- ☑
  handgun (parts) — *see* Explosion, firearm, handgun
  homicide (attempt) X96.9- ☑
    antipersonnel bomb — *see* Explosion, antipersonnel
      bomb
    fertilizer bomb — *see* Explosion, fertilizer bomb
    gasoline bomb — *see* Explosion, gasoline bomb
    letter bomb — *see* Explosion, letter bomb
    pipe bomb — *see* Explosion, pipe bomb
    specified NEC X96.8- ☑
  hose, pressurized W37.8- ☑
  hot water heater, tank (in machinery) W35.- ☑
    on watercraft — *see* Explosion, in, watercraft
  in, on
    dump W40.8- ☑
    factory W40.8- ☑

Explosion — *continued*
  in, on — *continued*
    mine (of explosive gases) NEC W40.1- ☑
    watercraft V93.59- ☑
      powered craft V93.53- ☑
        ferry boat V93.51- ☑
        fishing boat V93.52- ☑
        jetskis V93.53- ☑
        liner V93.51- ☑
        merchant ship V93.50- ☑
        passenger ship V93.51- ☑
        sailboat V93.54- ☑
  letter bomb W40.8- ☑
    assault X96.2- ☑
    homicide (attempt) X96.2- ☑
    suicide (attempt) X75.- ☑
  machinery — *see also* Contact, with, by type of machine
    on board watercraft — *see* Explosion, in, watercraft
    pressure vessel — *see* Explosion, by type of vessel
  methane W40.1- ☑
  mine W40.1- ☑
  missile NEC W40.8- ☑
  mortar bomb W40.8- ☑
    in
      assault X96.8- ☑
      homicide (attempt) X96.8- ☑
      legal intervention
        injuring
          bystander Y35.192- ☑
          law enforcement personnel Y35.191- ☑
          suspect Y35.193- ☑
          unspecified person Y35.199- ☑
      suicide (attempt) X75.- ☑
  munitions (dump) (factory) W40.8- ☑
  pipe, pressurized W37.8- ☑
    bomb W40.8- ☑
      assault X96.4- ☑
      homicide (attempt) X96.4- ☑
      suicide (attempt) X75.- ☑
  pressure, pressurized
    cooker W38.- ☑
    gas tank (in machinery) W36.3- ☑
    hose W37.8- ☑
    pipe W37.8- ☑
    specified device NEC W38.- ☑
    tire W37.8- ☑
      bicycle W37.0- ☑
    vessel (in machinery) W38.- ☑
  propane W40.1- ☑
  self-inflicted X75.- ☑
  shell (artillery) NEC W40.8- ☑
    during war operations — *see* War operations, explosion
    in
      legal intervention
        injuring
          bystander Y35.122- ☑
          law enforcement personnel Y35.121- ☑
          suspect Y35.123- ☑
          unspecified person Y35.129- ☑
      war — *see* War operations, explosion
  spacecraft V95.45- ☑
  stated as undetermined whether accidental or intentional Y25.- ☑
  steam or water lines (in machinery) W37.8- ☑
  stove W40.9- ☑
  suicide (attempt) X75.- ☑
  tire, pressurized W37.8- ☑
    bicycle W37.0- ☑
  undetermined whether accidental or intentional Y25.- ☑
  vehicle tire NEC W37.8- ☑
    bicycle W37.0- ☑
  war operations — *see* War operations, explosion

Exposure (to) X58.- ☑
  air pressure change — *see* Air, pressure
  cold (accidental) (excessive) (extreme) (natural) (place) X31.- ☑
    assault Y08.89- ☑
    due to
      man-made conditions W93.8- ☑
        dry ice (contact) W93.01- ☑
          inhalation W93.02- ☑
        liquid air (contact) (hydrogen) (nitrogen) W93.11- ☑
          inhalation W93.12- ☑
        refrigeration unit (deep freeze) W93.2- ☑

Exposure — *continued*
  cold — *continued*
    due to — *continued*
      man-made conditions — *continued*
        suicide (attempt) X83.2- ☑
      weather (conditions) X31.- ☑
    homicide (attempt) Y08.89- ☑
    self-inflicted X83.2- ☑
  due to abandonment or neglect X58.- ☑
  electric current W86.8- ☑
    appliance (faulty) W86.8- ☑
      domestic W86.0- ☑
    caused by other person Y08.89- ☑
    conductor (faulty) W86.1- ☑
    control apparatus (faulty) W86.1- ☑
    electric power generating plant, distribution station W86.1- ☑
    electroshock gun — *see* Exposure, electric current, taser
    high-voltage cable W85.- ☑
    homicide (attempt) Y08.89- ☑
    legal execution — *see* Legal, intervention, specified means NEC
    lightning — *see* subcategory T75.0- ☑
    live rail W86.8- ☑
    misadventure in medical or surgical procedure in electroshock therapy Y63.4
    motor (electric) (faulty) W86.8- ☑
      domestic W86.0- ☑
    self-inflicted X83.1- ☑
    specified NEC W86.8- ☑
      domestic W86.0- ☑
    stun gun — *see* Exposure, electric current, taser
    suicide (attempt) X83.1- ☑
    taser W86.8- ☑
      assault Y08.89- ☑
      legal intervention — *see* category Y35.- ☑
      self-harm (intentional) X83.8- ☑
      undetermined intent Y33.- ☑
    third rail W86.8- ☑
    transformer (faulty) W86.1- ☑
    transmission lines W85.- ☑
  environmental tobacco smoke X58.- ☑
  excessive
    cold — *see* Exposure, cold
    heat (natural) NEC X30.- ☑
      man-made W92.- ☑
  factor(s) NOS X58.- ☑
    environmental NEC X58.- ☑
    man-made NEC W99.- ☑
      natural NEC — *see* Forces of nature
    specified NEC X58.- ☑
  fire, flames (accidental) X08.8- ☑
    assault X97.- ☑
    campfire — *see* Exposure, fire, controlled, not in building
    controlled (in)
      with ignition (of) clothing — *see also* Ignition, clothes X06.2- ☑
        nightwear X05.- ☑
      bonfire — *see* Exposure, fire, controlled, not in building
      brazier (in building or structure) — *see also* Exposure, fire, controlled, building
        not in building or structure — *see* Exposure, fire, controlled, not in building
      building or structure X02.0- ☑
        with
          fall from building X02.3- ☑
          injury due to building collapse X02.2- ☑
          jump from building X02.5- ☑
          smoke inhalation X02.1- ☑
          hit by object from building X02.4- ☑
          specified mode of injury NEC X02.8- ☑
      fireplace, furnace or stove — *see* Exposure, fire, controlled, building
      not in building or structure X03.0- ☑
        with
          fall X03.3- ☑
          smoke inhalation X03.1- ☑
          hit by object X03.4- ☑
          specified mode of injury NEC X03.8- ☑
      trash — *see* Exposure, fire, controlled, not in building
    fireplace — *see* Exposure, fire, controlled, building

Exposure — *continued*
  fire, flames — *continued*
    fittings or furniture (in building or structure) (uncontrolled) — *see* Exposure, fire, uncontrolled, building
    forest (uncontrolled) — *see* Exposure, fire, uncontrolled, not in building
    grass (uncontrolled) — *see* Exposure, fire, uncontrolled, not in building
    hay (uncontrolled) — *see* Exposure, fire, uncontrolled, not in building
    homicide (attempt) X97.- ☑
    ignition of highly flammable material X04.- ☑
    in, of, on, starting in
      machinery — *see* Contact, with, by type of machine
      motor vehicle (in motion) — *see also* Accident, transport, occupant by type of vehicle V87.8- ☑
        with collision — *see* Collision
      railway rolling stock, train, vehicle V81.81- ☑
        with collision — *see* Accident, transport, railway vehicle occupant
      streetcar (in motion) V82.8- ☑
        with collision — *see* Accident, transport, streetcar occupant
      transport vehicle NEC — *see also* Accident, transport
        with collision — *see* Collision
      war operations — *see also* War operations, fire from nuclear explosion — *see* War operations, nuclear weapons
      watercraft (in transit) (not in transit) V91.09- ☑
        localized — *see* Burn, on board watercraft, due to, fire on board
        powered craft V91.03- ☑
          ferry boat V91.01- ☑
          fishing boat V91.02- ☑
          jet skis V91.03- ☑
          liner V91.01- ☑
          merchant ship V91.00- ☑
          passenger ship V91.01- ☑
        unpowered craft V91.08- ☑
          canoe V91.05- ☑
          inflatable V91.06- ☑
          kayak V91.05- ☑
          sailboat V91.04- ☑
          surf-board V91.08- ☑
          waterskis V91.07- ☑
          windsurfer V91.08- ☑
    lumber (uncontrolled) — *see* Exposure, fire, uncontrolled, not in building
    mine (uncontrolled) — *see* Exposure, fire, uncontrolled, not in building
    prairie (uncontrolled) — *see* Exposure, fire, uncontrolled, not in building
    resulting from
      explosion — *see* Explosion
      lightning X08.8- ☑
    self-inflicted X76.- ☑
    specified NEC X08.8- ☑
    started by other person X97.- ☑
    stated as undetermined whether accidental or intentional Y26.- ☑
    stove — *see* Exposure, fire, controlled, building
    suicide (attempt) X76.- ☑
    tunnel (uncontrolled) — *see* Exposure, fire, uncontrolled, not in building
    uncontrolled
      in building or structure X00.0- ☑
        with
          fall from building X00.3- ☑
          injury due to building collapse X00.2- ☑
          jump from building X00.5- ☑
          smoke inhalation X00.1- ☑
        bed X08.00- ☑
          due to
            cigarette X08.01- ☑
            specified material NEC X08.09- ☑
        furniture NEC X08.20- ☑
          due to
            cigarette X08.21- ☑
            specified material NEC X08.29- ☑
        hit by object from building X00.4- ☑
        sofa X08.10- ☑
          due to
            cigarette X08.11- ☑

Exposure — *continued*
   fire, flames — *continued*
     uncontrolled — *continued*
       in building or structure — *continued*
         sofa — *continued*
           due to — *continued*
             specified material NEC X08.19- ☑
         specified mode of injury NEC X00.8- ☑
       not in building or structure (any) X01.0- ☑
         with
           fall X01.3- ☑
           smoke inhalation X01.1- ☑
         hit by object X01.4- ☑
         specified mode of injury NEC X01.8- ☑
       undetermined whether accidental or intentional Y26.- ☑
   forces of nature NEC — *see* Forces of nature
   G-forces (abnormal) W49.9- ☑
   gravitational forces (abnormal) W49.9- ☑
   heat (natural) NEC — *see* Heat
   high-pressure jet (hydraulic) (pneumatic) W49.9- ☑
   hydraulic jet W49.9- ☑
   inanimate mechanical force W49.9- ☑
   jet, high-pressure (hydraulic) (pneumatic) W49.9- ☑
   lightning — *see* subcategory T75.0- ☑
     causing fire — *see* Exposure, fire
   mechanical forces NEC W49.9- ☑
     animate NEC W64.- ☑
     inanimate NEC W49.9- ☑
   noise W42.9- ☑
     supersonic W42.0- ☑
   noxious substance — *see* Table of Drugs and Chemicals
   pneumatic jet W49.9- ☑
   prolonged in deep-freeze unit or refrigerator W93.2- ☑
   radiation — *see* Radiation
   smoke — *see also* Exposure, fire
     tobacco, second hand Z77.22
   specified factors NEC X58.- ☑
   sunlight X32.- ☑
     man-made (sun lamp) W89.8- ☑
       tanning bed W89.1- ☑
   supersonic waves W42.0- ☑
   transmission line(s), electric W85.- ☑
   vibration W49.9- ☑
   waves
     infrasound W49.9- ☑
     sound W42.9- ☑
     supersonic W42.0- ☑
   weather NEC — *see* Forces of nature
External cause status Y99.9
   child assisting in compensated work for family Y99.8
   civilian activity done for financial or other compensation Y99.0
   civilian activity done for income or pay Y99.0
   family member assisting in compensated work for other family member Y99.8
   hobby not done for income Y99.8
   leisure activity Y99.8
   military activity Y99.1
   off-duty activity of military personnel Y99.8
   recreation or sport not for income or while a student Y99.8
   specified NEC Y99.8
   student activity Y99.8
   volunteer activity Y99.2

F

Factors, supplemental
   alcohol
     blood level
       less than 20mg/100ml Y90.0
       presence in blood, level not specified Y90.9
       20-39mg/100ml Y90.1
       40-59mg/100ml Y90.2
       60-79mg/100ml Y90.3
       80-99mg/100ml Y90.4
       100-119mg/100ml Y90.5
       120-199mg/100ml Y90.6
       200-239mg/100ml Y90.7
       240mg/100ml or more Y90.8
     presence in blood, but level not specified Y90.9
   environmental-pollution-related condition- see Z57.- ☑
   nosocomial condition Y95
   work-related condition Y99.0
Failure
   in suture or ligature during surgical procedure Y65.2

Failure — *continued*
   mechanical, of instrument or apparatus (any) (during any medical or surgical procedure) Y65.8
   sterile precautions (during medical and surgical care) — *see* Misadventure, failure, sterile precautions, by type of procedure
   to
     introduce tube or instrument Y65.4
       endotracheal tube during anesthesia Y65.3
     make curve (transport vehicle) NEC — *see* Accident, transport
     remove tube or instrument Y65.4
Fall, falling (accidental) W19.- ☑
   building W20.1- ☑
     burning (uncontrolled fire) X00.3- ☑
   down
     embankment W17.81- ☑
     escalator W10.0- ☑
     hill W17.81- ☑
     ladder W11.- ☑
     ramp W10.2- ☑
     stairs, steps W10.9- ☑
   due to
     bumping against
       object W18.00- ☑
         sharp glass W18.02- ☑
         specified NEC W18.09- ☑
         sports equipment W18.01- ☑
       person W03.- ☑
         due to ice or snow W00.0- ☑
         on pedestrian conveyance — *see* Accident, transport, pedestrian, conveyance
     collision with another person W03.- ☑
       due to ice or snow W00.0- ☑
       involving pedestrian conveyance — *see* Accident, transport, pedestrian, conveyance
     grocery cart tipping over W17.82- ☑
     ice or snow W00.9- ☑
       from one level to another W00.2- ☑
       on stairs or steps W00.1- ☑
       involving pedestrian conveyance — *see* Accident, transport, pedestrian, conveyance
       on same level W00.0- ☑
     slipping (on moving sidewalk) W01.0- ☑
       with subsequent striking against object W01.10- ☑
         furniture W01.190- ☑
         sharp object W01.119- ☑
           glass W01.110- ☑
         power tool or machine W01.111- ☑
         specified NEC W01.118- ☑
         specified NEC W01.198- ☑
     striking against
       object W18.00- ☑
         sharp glass W18.02- ☑
         specified NEC W18.09- ☑
         sports equipment W18.01- ☑
       person W03.- ☑
         due to ice or snow W00.0- ☑
         on pedestrian conveyance — *see* Accident, transport, pedestrian, conveyance
   earth (with asphyxia or suffocation (by pressure)) — *see* Earth, falling
   from, off, out of
     aircraft NEC (with accident to aircraft NEC) V97.0- ☑
       while boarding or alighting V97.1- ☑
     balcony W13.0- ☑
     bed W06.- ☑
     boat, ship, watercraft NEC (with drowning or submersion) — *see* Drowning, due to, fall overboard
       with hitting bottom or object V94.0- ☑
     bridge W13.1- ☑
     building W13.9- ☑
       burning (uncontrolled fire) X00.3- ☑
     cavity W17.2- ☑
     chair W07.- ☑
     cherry picker W17.89- ☑
     cliff W15.- ☑
     dock W17.4- ☑
     embankment W17.81- ☑
     escalator W10.0- ☑
     flagpole W13.8- ☑
     furniture NEC W08.- ☑
     grocery cart W17.82- ☑
     haystack W17.89- ☑
     high place NEC W17.89- ☑

Fall, falling — *continued*
   from, off, out of — *continued*
     high place — *continued*
       stated as undetermined whether accidental or intentional Y30.- ☑
     hole W17.2- ☑
     incline W10.2- ☑
     ladder W11.- ☑
     lifting device W17.89- ☑
     machine, machinery — *see also* Contact, with, by type of machine
       not in operation W17.89- ☑
     manhole W17.1- ☑
     mobile elevated work platform [MEWP] W17.89- ☑
     motorized mobility scooter W05.2- ☑
     one level to another NEC W17.89- ☑
       intentional, purposeful, suicide (attempt) X80.- ☑
       stated as undetermined whether accidental or intentional Y30.- ☑
     pit W17.2- ☑
     playground equipment W09.8- ☑
       jungle gym W09.2- ☑
       slide W09.0- ☑
       swing W09.1- ☑
     quarry W17.89- ☑
     railing W13.9- ☑
     ramp W10.2- ☑
     roof W13.2- ☑
     scaffolding W12.- ☑
     scooter (nonmotorized) W05.1- ☑
       motorized mobility W05.2- ☑
     sky lift W17.89- ☑
     stairs, steps W10.9- ☑
       curb W10.1- ☑
       due to ice or snow W00.1- ☑
       escalator W10.0- ☑
       incline W10.2- ☑
       ramp W10.2- ☑
       sidewalk curb W10.1- ☑
       specified NEC W10.8- ☑
     standing
       electric scooter V00.841- ☑
       micro-mobility pedestrian conveyance V00.848- ☑
     stepladder W11.- ☑
     stool W08.- ☑
     storm drain W17.1- ☑
     streetcar NEC V82.6- ☑
       while boarding or alighting V82.4- ☑
       with antecedent collision — *see* Accident, transport, streetcar occupant
     structure NEC W13.8- ☑
       burning (uncontrolled fire) X00.3- ☑
     table W08.- ☑
     toilet W18.11- ☑
       with subsequent striking against object W18.12- ☑
     train NEC V81.6- ☑
       during derailment (without antecedent collision) V81.7- ☑
         with antecedent collision — *see* Accident, transport, railway vehicle occupant
       while boarding or alighting V81.4- ☑
     transport vehicle after collision — *see* Accident, transport, by type of vehicle, collision
     tree W14.- ☑
     vehicle (in motion) NEC — *see also* Accident, transport V89.9- ☑
       motor NEC — *see also* Accident, transport, occupant, by type of vehicle V87.8- ☑
       stationary W17.89- ☑
         while boarding or alighting — *see* Accident, transport, by type of vehicle, while boarding or alighting
     viaduct W13.8- ☑
     wall W13.8- ☑
     watercraft — *see also* Drowning, due to, fall overboard
       with hitting bottom or object V94.0- ☑
     well W17.0- ☑
     wheelchair, non-moving W05.0- ☑
       powered — *see* Accident, transport, pedestrian, conveyance occupant, specified type NEC
     window W13.4- ☑
   in, on
     aircraft NEC V97.0- ☑
       while boarding or alighting V97.1- ☑

Fall, falling — *continued*
  in, on — *continued*
    aircraft — *continued*
      with accident to aircraft V97.0- ☑
    bathtub (empty) W18.2- ☑
      filled W16.212- ☑
        causing drowning W16.211- ☑
    escalator W10.0- ☑
    incline W10.2- ☑
    ladder W11.- ☑
    machine, machinery — *see* Contact, with, by type of machine
    object, edged, pointed or sharp (with cut) — *see* Fall, by type
    playground equipment W09.8- ☑
      jungle gym W09.2- ☑
      slide W09.0- ☑
      swing W09.1- ☑
    ramp W10.2- ☑
    scaffolding W12.- ☑
    shower W18.2- ☑
      causing drowning W16.211- ☑
    staircase, stairs, steps W10.9- ☑
      curb W10.1- ☑
      due to ice or snow W00.1- ☑
      escalator W10.0- ☑
      incline W10.2- ☑
      specified NEC W10.8- ☑
    streetcar (without antecedent collision) V82.5- ☑
      with antecedent collision — *see* Accident, transport, streetcar occupant
      while boarding or alighting V82.4- ☑
    train (without antecedent collision) V81.5- ☑
      with antecedent collision — *see* Accident, transport, railway vehicle occupant
      during derailment (without antecedent collision) V81.7- ☑
        with antecedent collision — *see* Accident, transport, railway vehicle occupant
      while boarding or alighting V81.4- ☑
    transport vehicle after collision — *see* Accident, transport, by type of vehicle, collision
    watercraft V93.39- ☑
      due to
        accident to craft V91.29- ☑
          powered craft V91.23- ☑
            ferry boat V91.21- ☑
            fishing boat V91.22- ☑
            jetskis V91.23- ☑
            liner V91.21- ☑
            merchant ship V91.20- ☑
            passenger ship V91.21- ☑
          unpowered craft
            canoe V91.25- ☑
            inflatable V91.26- ☑
            kayak V91.25- ☑
            sailboat V91.24- ☑
        powered craft V93.33- ☑
          ferry boat V93.31- ☑
          fishing boat V93.32- ☑
          jetskis V93.33- ☑
          liner V93.31- ☑
          merchant ship V93.30- ☑
          passenger ship V93.31- ☑
        unpowered craft V93.38- ☑
          canoe V93.35- ☑
          inflatable V93.36- ☑
          kayak V93.35- ☑
          sailboat V93.34- ☑
          surf-board V93.38- ☑
          windsurfer V93.38- ☑
  into
    cavity W17.2- ☑
    dock W17.4- ☑
    fire — *see* Exposure, fire, by type
    haystack W17.89- ☑
    hole W17.2- ☑
    lake — *see* Fall, into, water
    manhole W17.1- ☑
    moving part of machinery — *see* Contact, with, by type of machine
    ocean — *see* Fall, into, water
    opening in surface NEC W17.89- ☑
    pit W17.2- ☑
    pond — *see* Fall, into, water
    quarry W17.89- ☑

Fall, falling — *continued*
  into — *continued*
    river — *see* Fall, into, water
    shaft W17.89- ☑
    storm drain W17.1- ☑
    stream — *see* Fall, into, water
    swimming pool — *see also* Fall, into, water, in, swimming pool
      empty W17.3- ☑
    tank W17.89- ☑
    water W16.42- ☑
      causing drowning W16.41- ☑
      from watercraft — *see* Drowning, due to, fall overboard
      hitting diving board W21.4- ☑
      in
        bathtub W16.212- ☑
          causing drowning W16.211- ☑
        bucket W16.222- ☑
          causing drowning W16.221- ☑
        natural body of water W16.112- ☑
          causing drowning W16.111- ☑
          striking
            bottom W16.122- ☑
              causing drowning W16.121- ☑
            side W16.132- ☑
              causing drowning W16.131- ☑
        specified water NEC W16.312- ☑
          causing drowning W16.311- ☑
          striking
            bottom W16.322- ☑
              causing drowning W16.321- ☑
            wall W16.332- ☑
              causing drowning W16.331- ☑
        swimming pool W16.012- ☑
          causing drowning W16.011- ☑
          striking
            bottom W16.022- ☑
              causing drowning W16.031- ☑
            wall W16.032- ☑
              causing drowning W16.021- ☑
        utility bucket W16.222- ☑
          causing drowning W16.221- ☑
    well W17.0- ☑
  involving
    bed W06.- ☑
    chair W07.- ☑
    furniture NEC W08.- ☑
    glass — *see* Fall, by type
    playground equipment W09.8- ☑
      jungle gym W09.2- ☑
      slide W09.0- ☑
      swing W09.1- ☑
    roller blades — *see* Accident, transport, pedestrian, conveyance
    skateboard(s) — *see* Accident, transport, pedestrian, conveyance
    skates (ice) (in line) (roller) — *see* Accident, transport, pedestrian, conveyance
    skis — *see* Accident, transport, pedestrian, conveyance
    table W08.- ☑
    wheelchair, non-moving W05.0- ☑
      powered — *see* Accident, transport, pedestrian, conveyance, specified type NEC
  object — *see* Struck by, object, falling
  off
    toilet W18.11- ☑
      with subsequent striking against object W18.12- ☑
  on same level W18.30- ☑
    due to
      specified NEC W18.39- ☑
      stepping on an object W18.31- ☑
  out of
    bed W06.- ☑
    building NEC W13.8- ☑
    chair W07.- ☑
    furniture NEC W08.- ☑
    wheelchair, non-moving W05.0- ☑
      powered — *see* Accident, transport, pedestrian, conveyance, specified type NEC
    window W13.4- ☑
  over
    animal W01.0- ☑
    cliff W15.- ☑

Fall, falling — *continued*
  over — *continued*
    embankment W17.81- ☑
    small object W01.0- ☑
    rock W20.8- ☑
    same level W18.30- ☑
      from
        being crushed, pushed, or stepped on by a crowd or human stampede W52.- ☑
        collision, pushing, shoving, by or with other person W03.- ☑
        slipping, stumbling, tripping W01.0- ☑
      involving ice or snow W00.0- ☑
        involving skates (ice) (roller), skateboard, skis — *see* Accident, transport, pedestrian, conveyance
    snowslide (avalanche) — *see* Landslide
    stone W20.8- ☑
    structure W20.1- ☑
      burning (uncontrolled fire) X00.3- ☑
    through
      bridge W13.1- ☑
      floor W13.3- ☑
      roof W13.2- ☑
      wall W13.8- ☑
      window W13.4- ☑
    timber W20.8- ☑
    tree (caused by lightning) W20.8- ☑
    while being carried or supported by other person(s) W04.- ☑
Fallen on by
  animal (not being ridden) NEC W55.89- ☑
Felo-de-se — *see* Suicide
Fight (hand) (fists) (foot) — *see* Assault, fight
Fire (accidental) — *see* Exposure, fire
Firearm discharge — *see* Discharge, firearm
Fireball effects from nuclear explosion in war operations — *see* War operations, nuclear weapons
Fireworks (explosion) W39.- ☑
Flash burns from explosion — *see* Explosion
Flood (any injury) (caused by) X38.- ☑
  collapse of man-made structure causing earth movement X36.0- ☑
  tidal wave — *see* Forces of nature, tidal wave
Food (any type) **in**
  air passages (with asphyxia, obstruction, or suffocation) — *see* categories T17 and T18.- ☑
  alimentary tract causing asphyxia (due to compression of trachea) — *see* categories T17 and T18.- ☑
Forces of nature X39.8- ☑
  avalanche X36.1- ☑
    causing transport accident — *see* Accident, transport, by type of vehicle
  blizzard X37.2- ☑
  cataclysmic storm X37.9- ☑
    with flood X38.- ☑
    blizzard X37.2- ☑
    cloudburst X37.8- ☑
    cyclone X37.1- ☑
    dust storm X37.3- ☑
    hurricane X37.0- ☑
    specified storm NEC X37.8- ☑
    storm surge X37.0- ☑
    tornado X37.1- ☑
    twister X37.1- ☑
    typhoon X37.0- ☑
  cloudburst X37.8- ☑
  cold (natural) X31.- ☑
  cyclone X37.1- ☑
  dam collapse causing earth movement X36.0- ☑
  dust storm X37.3- ☑
  earth movement X36.1- ☑
    caused by dam or structure collapse X36.0- ☑
    earthquake X34.- ☑
  earthquake X34.- ☑
  flood (caused by) X38.- ☑
    dam collapse X36.0- ☑
    tidal wave — *see* Forces of nature, tidal wave
  heat (natural) X30.- ☑
  hurricane X37.0- ☑
  landslide X36.1- ☑
    causing transport accident — *see* Accident, transport, by type of vehicle
  lightning — *see* subcategory T75.0- ☑
    causing fire — *see* Exposure, fire
  mudslide X36.1- ☑

☑ Additional Character Required — Refer to the Tabular List for Character Selection

Forces of nature — continued
mudslide — continued
  causing transport accident — see Accident, transport, by type of vehicle
radiation (natural) X39.08- ☑
  radon X39.01- ☑
radon X39.01- ☑
specified force NEC X39.8- ☑
storm surge X37.0- ☑
structure collapse causing earth movement X36.0- ☑
sunlight X32.- ☑
tidal wave X37.41- ☑
  due to
    earthquake X37.41- ☑
    landslide X37.43- ☑
    storm X37.42- ☑
    volcanic eruption X37.41- ☑
tornado X37.1- ☑
tsunami X37.41- ☑
twister X37.1- ☑
typhoon X37.0- ☑
volcanic eruption X35.- ☑

Foreign body
aspiration — see Index to Diseases and Injuries, Foreign body, respiratory tract
embedded in skin W45.- ☑
entering through
  natural orifice W44.9- ☑
    audio device W44.G1- ☑
    battery W44.A0- ☑
      button W44.A1- ☑
      cylindrical W44.A9- ☑
      other specified NEC W44.A9- ☑
    bezoar W44.F1- ☑
    bottle cap W44.E9- ☑
    can lid W44.E9- ☑
    combination metal and plastic
      jewelry W44.G3- ☑
      toy and toy part W44.G2- ☑
    dagger W44.H2- ☑
    dart W44.H1- ☑
    ear buds W44.G1- ☑
    food W44.F3- ☑
    glass W44.C0- ☑
      intact W44.C2- ☑
        bottle W44.C2- ☑
      shard W44.C1- ☑
      sharp W44.C1- ☑
    hearing aids W44.G1- ☑
    insect W44.F4- ☑
    knife W44.H2- ☑
    magnetic metal W44.D0- ☑
      bead W44.D1- ☑
      coin W44.D2- ☑
      jewelry W44.D4- ☑
      object specified NEC W44.D9- ☑
      toy W44.D3- ☑
    needle (hypodermic) (sewing) W44.H1- ☑
    non-magnetic metal W44.E0- ☑
      bead W44.E1- ☑
      coin W44.E2- ☑
      jewelry W44.E4- ☑
      object specified NEC W44.E9- ☑
      toy W44.E3- ☑
    objects of natural or organic material W44.F0- ☑
      specified NEC W44.F9- ☑
    other
      non-organic objects W44.G0- ☑
        specified NEC W44.G9- ☑
      sharp object unspecified W44.H0- ☑
    plastic
      bead W44.B1- ☑
      bottle W44.B5- ☑
      coin W44.B2- ☑
      jewelry W44.B4- ☑
      object W44.B0- ☑
        specified NEC W44.B9- ☑
      toy and toy part W44.B3- ☑
    pull tab W44.E9- ☑
    rubber band W44.F2- ☑
    safety pin W44.H1- ☑
    shard pottery W44.H9- ☑
    sharp object specified NEC W44.H9- ☑
    specified NEC W44.8- ☑
    sword W44.H2- ☑

Foreign body — continued
entering through — continued
  skin W45.8- ☑
    can lid W26.8- ☑
    fishing hook W45.3- ☑
    nail W45.0- ☑
    paper W26.2- ☑
    specified NEC W45.8- ☑
    splinter W45.8- ☑
Forest fire (exposure to) — see Exposure, fire, uncontrolled, not in building
Found injured X58.- ☑
  from exposure (to) — see Exposure
  on
    highway, road(way), street V89.9- ☑
    railway right of way V81.9- ☑
Fracture (circumstances unknown or unspecified) X58.- ☑
  due to specified cause NEC X58.- ☑
Freezing — see Exposure, cold
Frostbite X31.- ☑
  due to man-made conditions — see Exposure, cold, man-made
Frozen — see Exposure, cold

G
Gored by bull W55.22- ☑
Gunshot wound — see also Discharge, firearm, by type Y24.9- ☑

H
Hailstones, injured by X39.8- ☑
Hanged herself or himself T71.162- ☑
Hanging (accidental) — see also T71.16
  legal execution — see Legal, intervention, specified means NEC
Heat (effects of) (excessive) X30.- ☑
  due to
    man-made conditions W92.- ☑
      on board watercraft V93.29- ☑
        fishing boat V93.22- ☑
        merchant ship V93.20- ☑
        passenger ship V93.21- ☑
        sailboat V93.24- ☑
        specified powered craft NEC V93.23- ☑
    weather (conditions) X30.- ☑
  from
    electric heating apparatus causing burning X16.- ☑
    nuclear explosion in war operations — see War operations, nuclear weapons
    inappropriate in local application or packing in medical or surgical procedure Y63.5
Hemorrhage
  delayed following medical or surgical treatment without mention of misadventure — see Index to Diseases and Injuries, Complication(s)
  during medical or surgical treatment as misadventure — see Index to Diseases and Injuries, Complication(s)
High
  altitude (effects) — see Air, pressure, low
  level of radioactivity, effects — see Radiation
  pressure (effects) — see Air, pressure, high
  temperature, effects — see Heat
Hit, hitting (accidental) by — see Struck by
Hitting against — see Striking against
Homicide (attempt) (justifiable) — see Assault
Hot
  place, effects — see also Heat
  weather, effects X30.- ☑
House fire (uncontrolled) — see Exposure, fire, uncontrolled, building
Humidity, causing problem X39.8- ☑
Hunger X58.- ☑
Hurricane (any injury) X37.0- ☑
Hypobarism, hypobaropathy — see Air, pressure, low

I
Ictus
  caloris — see also Heat
  solaris X30.- ☑
Ignition (accidental) — see also Exposure, fire X08.8- ☑
  anesthetic gas in operating room W40.1- ☑
  apparel X06.2- ☑

Ignition — continued
apparel — continued
  from highly flammable material X04.- ☑
  nightwear X05.- ☑
bed linen (sheets) (spreads) (pillows) (mattress) — see Exposure, fire, uncontrolled, building, bed
benzine X04.- ☑
clothes, clothing NEC (from controlled fire) X06.2- ☑
  from
    highly flammable material X04.- ☑
ether X04.- ☑
  in operating room W40.1- ☑
explosive material — see Explosion
gasoline X04.- ☑
jewelry (plastic) (any) X06.0- ☑
kerosene X04.- ☑
material
  explosive — see Explosion
  highly flammable with secondary explosion X04.- ☑
nightwear X05.- ☑
paraffin X04.- ☑
petrol X04.- ☑
Immersion (accidental) — see also Drowning
  hand or foot due to cold (excessive) X31.- ☑
Implantation of quills of porcupine W55.89- ☑
Inanition (from) (hunger) X58.- ☑
  thirst X58.- ☑
Inappropriate operation performed
  correct operation on wrong side or body part (wrong side) (wrong site) Y65.53
  operation intended for another patient done on wrong patient Y65.52
  wrong operation performed on correct patient Y65.51
Inattention after, at birth (homicidal intent) (infanticidal intent) X58.- ☑
Incident, adverse
  device
    anesthesiology Y70.8
      accessory Y70.2
      diagnostic Y70.0
      miscellaneous Y70.8
      monitoring Y70.0
      prosthetic Y70.2
      rehabilitative Y70.1
      surgical Y70.3
      therapeutic Y70.1
    cardiovascular Y71.8
      accessory Y71.2
      diagnostic Y71.0
      miscellaneous Y71.8
      monitoring Y71.0
      prosthetic Y71.2
      rehabilitative Y71.1
      surgical Y71.3
      therapeutic Y71.1
    gastroenterology Y73.8
      accessory Y73.2
      diagnostic Y73.0
      miscellaneous Y73.8
      monitoring Y73.0
      prosthetic Y73.2
      rehabilitative Y73.1
      surgical Y73.3
      therapeutic Y73.1
    general
      hospital Y74.8
        accessory Y74.2
        diagnostic Y74.0
        miscellaneous Y74.8
        monitoring Y74.0
        prosthetic Y74.2
        rehabilitative Y74.1
        surgical Y74.3
        therapeutic Y74.1
      surgical Y81.8
        accessory Y81.2
        diagnostic Y81.0
        miscellaneous Y81.8
        monitoring Y81.0
        prosthetic Y81.2
        rehabilitative Y81.1
        surgical Y81.3
        therapeutic Y81.1
    gynecological Y76.8
      accessory Y76.2
      diagnostic Y76.0
      miscellaneous Y76.8
      monitoring Y76.0

Incident, adverse — *continued*
  device — *continued*
    gynecological — *continued*
      prosthetic Y76.2
      rehabilitative Y76.1
      surgical Y76.3
      therapeutic Y76.1
    medical Y82.9
      specified type NEC Y82.8
    neurological Y75.8
      accessory Y75.2
      diagnostic Y75.0
      miscellaneous Y75.8
      monitoring Y75.0
      prosthetic Y75.2
      rehabilitative Y75.1
      surgical Y75.3
      therapeutic Y75.1
    obstetrical Y76.8
      accessory Y76.2
      diagnostic Y76.0
      miscellaneous Y76.8
      monitoring Y76.0
      prosthetic Y76.2
      rehabilitative Y76.1
      surgical Y76.3
      therapeutic Y76.1
    ophthalmic Y77.8
      accessory Y77.2
      contact lens (rigid gas permeable) (soft (hydrophilic)) Y77.11
      diagnostic Y77.0
      miscellaneous Y77.8
      monitoring Y77.0
      prosthetic Y77.2
      rehabilitative Y77.19
      surgical Y77.3
      therapeutic Y77.19
    orthopedic Y79.8
      accessory Y79.2
      diagnostic Y79.0
      miscellaneous Y79.8
      monitoring Y79.0
      prosthetic Y79.2
      rehabilitative Y79.1
      surgical Y79.3
      therapeutic Y79.1
    otorhinolaryngological Y72.8
      accessory Y72.2
      diagnostic Y72.0
      miscellaneous Y72.8
      monitoring Y72.0
      prosthetic Y72.2
      rehabilitative Y72.1
      surgical Y72.3
      therapeutic Y72.1
    personal use Y74.8
      accessory Y74.2
      diagnostic Y74.0
      miscellaneous Y74.8
      monitoring Y74.0
      prosthetic Y74.2
      rehabilitative Y74.1
      surgical Y74.3
      therapeutic Y74.1
    physical medicine Y80.8
      accessory Y80.2
      diagnostic Y80.0
      miscellaneous Y80.8
      monitoring Y80.0
      prosthetic Y80.2
      rehabilitative Y80.1
      surgical Y80.3
      therapeutic Y80.1
    plastic surgical Y81.8
      accessory Y81.2
      diagnostic Y81.0
      miscellaneous Y81.8
      monitoring Y81.0
      prosthetic Y81.2
      rehabilitative Y81.1
      surgical Y81.3
      therapeutic Y81.1
    radiological Y78.8
      accessory Y78.2
      diagnostic Y78.0
      miscellaneous Y78.8
      monitoring Y78.0
      prosthetic Y78.2

Incident, adverse — *continued*
  device — *continued*
    radiological — *continued*
      rehabilitative Y78.1
      surgical Y78.3
      therapeutic Y78.1
    urology Y73.8
      accessory Y73.2
      diagnostic Y73.0
      miscellaneous Y73.8
      monitoring Y73.0
      prosthetic Y73.2
      rehabilitative Y73.1
      surgical Y73.3
      therapeutic Y73.1
Incineration (accidental) — *see* Exposure, fire
Infanticide — *see* Assault
Infrasound waves (causing injury) W49.9- ☑
Ingestion
  foreign body (causing injury) (with obstruction) — *see* Foreign body, alimentary canal
  poisonous
    plant(s) X58.- ☑
    substance NEC — *see* Table of Drugs and Chemicals
Inhalation
  excessively cold substance, man-made — *see* Exposure, cold, man-made
  food (any type) (into respiratory tract) (with asphyxia, obstruction respiratory tract, suffocation) — *see* categories T17 and T18.- ☑
  foreign body — *see* Foreign body, aspiration
  gastric contents (with asphyxia, obstruction respiratory passage, suffocation) T17.81- ☑
  hot air or gases X14.0- ☑
  liquid air, hydrogen, nitrogen W93.12- ☑
    suicide (attempt) X83.2- ☑
  steam X13.0- ☑
    assault X98.0- ☑
    stated as undetermined whether accidental or intentional Y27.0- ☑
    suicide (attempt) X77.0- ☑
  toxic gas — *see* Table of Drugs and Chemicals
  vomitus (with asphyxia, obstruction respiratory passage, suffocation) T17.81- ☑
Injury, injured (accidental(ly)) NOS X58.- ☑
  by, caused by, from
    assault — *see* Assault
    law-enforcing agent, police, in course of legal intervention — *see* Legal intervention
    suicide (attempt) X83.8- ☑
  due to, in
    civil insurrection — *see* War operations
    fight — *see also* Assault, fight Y04.0- ☑
    war operations — *see* War operations
  homicide — *see also* Assault Y09
  inflicted (by)
    in course of arrest (attempted), suppression of disturbance, maintenance of order, by law-enforcing agents — *see* Legal intervention
    other person
      stated as
        accidental X58.- ☑
        intentional, homicide (attempt) — *see* Assault
      undetermined whether accidental or intentional Y33.- ☑
  purposely (inflicted) by other person(s) — *see* Assault
  self-inflicted X83.8- ☑
    stated as accidental X58.- ☑
  specified cause NEC X58.- ☑
  undetermined whether accidental or intentional Y33.- ☑
Insolation, effects X30.- ☑
Insufficient nourishment X58.- ☑
Interruption of respiration (by)
  food (lodged in esophagus) — *see* categories T17 and T18.- ☑
  vomitus (lodged in esophagus) T17.81- ☑
Intervention, legal — *see* Legal intervention
Intoxication
  drug — *see* Table of Drugs and Chemicals
  poison — *see* Table of Drugs and Chemicals

J

Jammed (accidentally)
  between objects (moving) (stationary and moving) W23.0- ☑
    stationary W23.1- ☑

Jumped, jumping
  before moving object NEC X81.8- ☑
    motor vehicle X81.0- ☑
    subway train X81.1- ☑
    train X81.1- ☑
    undetermined whether accidental or intentional Y31.- ☑
  from
    boat (into water) voluntarily, without accident (to or on boat) W16.712- ☑
      striking bottom W16.722- ☑
        causing drowning W16.721- ☑
      with
        accident to or on boat — *see* Accident, watercraft
        drowning or submersion W16.711- ☑
          suicide (attempt) X71.3- ☑
    building — *see also* Jumped, from, high place W13.9- ☑
      burning (uncontrolled fire) X00.5- ☑
    high place NEC W17.89- ☑
      suicide (attempt) X80.- ☑
      undetermined whether accidental or intentional Y30.- ☑
    structure — *see also* Jumped, from, high place W13.9- ☑
      burning (uncontrolled fire) X00.5- ☑
  into water W16.92- ☑
    causing drowning W16.91- ☑
    from, off watercraft — *see* Jumped, from, boat
    in
      natural body W16.612- ☑
        causing drowning W16.611- ☑
        striking bottom W16.622- ☑
          causing drowning W16.621- ☑
      specified place NEC W16.812- ☑
        causing drowning W16.811- ☑
        striking
          bottom W16.822- ☑
            causing drowning W16.821- ☑
          wall W16.832- ☑
            causing drowning W16.831- ☑
      swimming pool W16.512- ☑
        causing drowning W16.511- ☑
        striking
          bottom W16.522- ☑
            causing drowning W16.521- ☑
          wall W16.532- ☑
            causing drowning W16.531- ☑
    suicide (attempt) X71.3- ☑

K

Kicked by
  animal NEC W55.82- ☑
  person(s) (accidentally) W50.1- ☑
    with intent to injure or kill Y04.0- ☑
    as, or caused by, a crowd or human stampede (with fall) W52.- ☑
    assault Y04.0- ☑
    homicide (attempt) Y04.0- ☑
    in
      fight Y04.0- ☑
      legal intervention
        injuring
          bystander Y35.812- ☑
          law enforcement personnel Y35.811- ☑
          suspect Y35.813- ☑
          unspecified person Y35.819- ☑
Kicking
  against
    object W22.8- ☑
      sports equipment W21.9- ☑
      stationary W22.09- ☑
        sports equipment W21.89- ☑
    person — *see* Striking against, person
  sports equipment W21.9- ☑
  carpet stretcher with knee X50.3- ☑
Killed, killing (accidentally) NOS — *see also* Injury X58.- ☑
  in
    action — *see* War operations
    brawl, fight (hand) (fists) (foot) Y04.0- ☑
      by weapon — *see also* Assault
        cutting, piercing — *see* Assault, cutting or piercing instrument

Killed, killing — *continued*
  in — *continued*
    brawl, fight — *continued*
      by weapon — *see also* Assault — *continued*
        firearm — *see* Discharge, firearm, by type, homicide
  self
    stated as
      accident NOS X58.- ☑
      suicide — *see* Suicide
      undetermined whether accidental or intentional Y33.- ☑
Kneeling (prolonged) (static) X50.1- ☑
Knocked down (accidentally) (by) NOS X58.- ☑
  animal (not being ridden) NEC — *see also* Struck by, by type of animal
  crowd or human stampede W52.- ☑
  person W51.- ☑
    in brawl, fight Y04.0- ☑
  transport vehicle NEC — *see also* Accident, transport V09.9- ☑

L

Laceration NEC — *see* Injury
Lack of
  care (helpless person) (infant) (newborn) X58.- ☑
  food except as result of abandonment or neglect X58.- ☑
    due to abandonment or neglect X58.- ☑
  water except as result of transport accident X58.- ☑
    due to transport accident — *see* Accident, transport, by type
  helpless person, infant, newborn X58.- ☑
Landslide (falling on transport vehicle) X36.1- ☑
  caused by collapse of man-made structure X36.0- ☑
Late effect — *see* Sequelae
Legal
  execution (any method) — *see* Legal, intervention
  intervention (by)
    baton — *see* Legal, intervention, blunt object, baton
    bayonet — *see* Legal, intervention, sharp object, bayonet
    blow — *see* Legal, intervention, manhandling
    blunt object
      baton
        injuring
          bystander Y35.312- ☑
          law enforcement personnel Y35.311- ☑
          suspect Y35.313- ☑
          unspecified person Y35.319- ☑
      injuring
        bystander Y35.302- ☑
        law enforcement personnel Y35.301- ☑
        suspect Y35.303- ☑
        unspecified person Y35.309- ☑
      specified NEC
        injuring
          bystander Y35.392- ☑
          law enforcement personnel Y35.391- ☑
          suspect Y35.393- ☑
          unspecified person Y35.399- ☑
      stave
        injuring
          bystander Y35.392- ☑
          law enforcement personnel Y35.391- ☑
          suspect Y35.393- ☑
          unspecified person Y35.399- ☑
    bomb — *see* Legal, intervention, explosive
    conducted energy device
      injuring
        bystander Y35.832- ☑
        law enforcement personnel Y35.831- ☑
        suspect Y35.833- ☑
        unspecified person Y35.839- ☑
    cutting or piercing instrument — *see* Legal, intervention, sharp object
    dynamite — *see* Legal, intervention, explosive, dynamite
    electroshock device (taser)
      injuring
        bystander Y35.832- ☑
        law enforcement personnel Y35.831- ☑
        suspect Y35.833- ☑
        unspecified person Y35.839- ☑

Legal — *continued*
  intervention — *continued*
    explosive(s)
      dynamite
        injuring
          bystander Y35.112- ☑
          law enforcement personnel Y35.111- ☑
          suspect Y35.113- ☑
          unspecified person Y35.119- ☑
      grenade
        injuring
          bystander Y35.192- ☑
          law enforcement personnel Y35.191- ☑
          suspect Y35.193- ☑
          unspecified person Y35.199- ☑
      injuring
        bystander Y35.102- ☑
        law enforcement personnel Y35.101- ☑
        suspect Y35.103- ☑
        unspecified person Y35.109- ☑
      mortar bomb
        injuring
          bystander Y35.192- ☑
          law enforcement personnel Y35.191- ☑
          suspect Y35.193- ☑
          unspecified person Y35.199- ☑
      shell
        injuring
          bystander Y35.122- ☑
          law enforcement personnel Y35.121- ☑
          suspect Y35.123- ☑
          unspecified person Y35.129- ☑
      specified NEC
        injuring
          bystander Y35.192- ☑
          law enforcement personnel Y35.191- ☑
          suspect Y35.193- ☑
          unspecified person Y35.199- ☑
    firearm(s) (discharge)
      handgun
        injuring
          bystander Y35.022- ☑
          law enforcement personnel Y35.021- ☑
          suspect Y35.023- ☑
          unspecified person Y35.029- ☑
      injuring
        bystander Y35.002- ☑
        law enforcement personnel Y35.001- ☑
        suspect Y35.003- ☑
        unspecified person Y35.009- ☑
      machine gun
        injuring
          bystander Y35.012- ☑
          law enforcement personnel Y35.011- ☑
          suspect Y35.013- ☑
          unspecified person Y35.019- ☑
      rifle pellet
        injuring
          bystander Y35.032- ☑
          law enforcement personnel Y35.031- ☑
          suspect Y35.033- ☑
          unspecified person Y35.039- ☑
      rubber bullet
        injuring
          bystander Y35.042- ☑
          law enforcement personnel Y35.041- ☑
          suspect Y35.043- ☑
          unspecified person Y35.049- ☑
      shotgun — *see* Legal, intervention, firearm, specified NEC
      specified NEC
        injuring
          bystander Y35.092- ☑
          law enforcement personnel Y35.091- ☑
          suspect Y35.093- ☑
          unspecified person Y35.099- ☑
    gas (asphyxiation) (poisoning)
      injuring
        bystander Y35.202- ☑
        law enforcement personnel Y35.201- ☑
        suspect Y35.203- ☑
        unspecified person Y35.209- ☑
      specified NEC
        injuring
          bystander Y35.292- ☑
          law enforcement personnel Y35.291- ☑

Legal — *continued*
  intervention — *continued*
    gas — *continued*
      specified — *continued*
        injuring — *continued*
          suspect Y35.293- ☑
          unspecified person Y35.299- ☑
      tear gas
        injuring
          bystander Y35.212- ☑
          law enforcement personnel Y35.211- ☑
          suspect Y35.213- ☑
          unspecified person Y35.219- ☑
    grenade — *see* Legal, intervention, explosive, grenade
    injuring
      bystander Y35.92- ☑
      law enforcement personnel Y35.91- ☑
      suspect Y35.93- ☑
      unspecified person Y35.99- ☑
    late effect (of) — *see with 7th character S* Y35.- ☑
    manhandling
      injuring
        bystander Y35.812- ☑
        law enforcement personnel Y35.811- ☑
        suspect Y35.813- ☑
        unspecified person Y35.819- ☑
    sequelae (of) — *see with 7th character S* Y35.- ☑
    sharp objects
      bayonet
        injuring
          bystander Y35.412- ☑
          law enforcement personnel Y35.411- ☑
          suspect Y35.413- ☑
          unspecified person Y35.419- ☑
      injuring
        bystander Y35.402- ☑
        law enforcement personnel Y35.401- ☑
        suspect Y35.403- ☑
        unspecified person Y35.409- ☑
      specified NEC
        injuring
          bystander Y35.492- ☑
          law enforcement personnel Y35.491- ☑
          suspect Y35.493- ☑
          unspecified person Y35.499- ☑
    specified means NEC
      injuring
        bystander Y35.892- ☑
        law enforcement personnel Y35.891- ☑
        suspect Y35.893- ☑
        unspecified person Y35.899- ☑
    stabbing — *see* Legal, intervention, sharp object
    stave — *see* Legal, intervention, blunt object, stave
    stun gun
      injuring
        bystander Y35.832- ☑
        law enforcement personnel Y35.831- ☑
        suspect Y35.833- ☑
        unspecified person Y35.839- ☑
    taser
      injuring
        bystander Y35.832- ☑
        law enforcement personnel Y35.831- ☑
        suspect Y35.833- ☑
        unspecified person Y35.839- ☑
    tear gas — *see* Legal, intervention, gas, tear gas
    truncheon — *see* Legal, intervention, blunt object, stave
Lifting — *see also* Overexertion
  heavy objects X50.0- ☑
  weights X50.0- ☑
Lightning (shock) (stroke) (struck by) — *see subcategory* T75.0- ☑
  causing fire — *see* Exposure, fire
Loss of control (transport vehicle) NEC — *see* Accident, transport
Lost at sea NOS — *see* Drowning, due to, fall overboard
Low
  pressure (effects) — *see* Air, pressure, low
  temperature (effects) — *see* Exposure, cold
Lying before train, vehicle or other moving object X81.8- ☑
  subway train X81.1- ☑
  train X81.1- ☑
  undetermined whether accidental or intentional Y31.- ☑
Lynching — *see* Assault

M

Malfunction (mechanism or component) (of)
   firearm W34.10- ☑
      airgun W34.110- ☑
      BB gun W34.110- ☑
      gas, air or spring-operated gun NEC W34.118- ☑
      handgun W32.1- ☑
      hunting rifle W33.12- ☑
      larger firearm W33.10- ☑
         specified NEC W33.19- ☑
      machine gun W33.13- ☑
      paintball gun W34.111- ☑
      pellet gun W34.110- ☑
      shotgun W33.11- ☑
      specified NEC W34.19- ☑
      Very pistol [flare] W34.19- ☑
   handgun — see Malfunction, firearm, handgun
Maltreatment — see Perpetrator
Mangled (accidentally) NOS X58.- ☑
Manhandling (in brawl, fight) Y04.0- ☑
   legal intervention — see Legal, intervention, manhandling
Manslaughter (nonaccidental) — see Assault
Mauled by animal NEC W55.89- ☑
Medical procedure, complication of (delayed or as an abnormal reaction without mention of misadventure) — see Complication of or following, by specified type of procedure
   due to or as a result of misadventure — see Misadventure
Melting (due to fire) — see also Exposure, fire
   apparel NEC X06.3- ☑
   clothes, clothing NEC X06.3- ☑
      nightwear X05.- ☑
   fittings or furniture (burning building) (uncontrolled fire) X00.8- ☑
   nightwear X05.- ☑
   plastic jewelry X06.1- ☑
Mental cruelty X58.- ☑
Military operations (injuries to military and civilians occurring during peacetime on military property and during routine military exercises and operations) (by) (from) (involving) Y37.90- ☑
   air blast Y37.20- ☑
   aircraft
      destruction — see Military operations, destruction of aircraft
      airway restriction — see Military operations, restriction of airways
      asphyxiation — see Military operations, restriction of airways
   biological weapons Y37.6X- ☑
   blast Y37.20- ☑
   blast fragments Y37.20- ☑
   blast overpressure
      high level (due to explosion) Y37.A2- ☑
      low level (due to explosion) Y37.A1- ☑
   blast wave Y37.20- ☑
   blast wind Y37.20- ☑
   bomb Y37.20- ☑
      dirty Y37.50- ☑
      gasoline Y37.31- ☑
      incendiary Y37.31- ☑
      petrol Y37.31- ☑
   bullet Y37.43- ☑
      incendiary Y37.32- ☑
      rubber Y37.41- ☑
   chemical weapons Y37.7X- ☑
   combat
      hand to hand (unarmed) combat Y37.44- ☑
      using blunt or piercing object Y37.45- ☑
   conflagration — see Military operations, fire
   conventional warfare NEC Y37.49- ☑
   depth-charge Y37.01- ☑
   destruction of aircraft Y37.10- ☑
      due to
         air to air missile Y37.11- ☑
         collision with other aircraft Y37.12- ☑
         detonation (accidental) of onboard munitions and explosives Y37.14- ☑
         enemy fire or explosives Y37.11- ☑
         explosive placed on aircraft Y37.11- ☑
         onboard fire Y37.13- ☑
         rocket propelled grenade [RPG] Y37.11- ☑
         small arms fire Y37.11- ☑

Military operations — continued
   destruction of aircraft — continued
      due to — continued
         surface to air missile Y37.11- ☑
         specified NEC Y37.19- ☑
   detonation (accidental) of
      onboard marine weapons Y37.05- ☑
      own munitions or munitions launch device Y37.24- ☑
   dirty bomb Y37.50- ☑
   explosion (of) Y37.20- ☑
      aerial bomb Y37.21- ☑
      bomb NOS — see also Military operations, bomb(s) Y37.20- ☑
      fragments Y37.20- ☑
      grenade Y37.29- ☑
      guided missile Y37.22- ☑
      improvised explosive device [IED] (person-borne) (roadside) (vehicle-borne) Y37.23- ☑
      land mine Y37.29- ☑
      marine mine (at sea) (in harbor) Y37.02- ☑
      marine weapon Y37.00- ☑
         specified NEC Y37.09- ☑
      own munitions or munitions launch device (accidental) Y37.24- ☑
      sea-based artillery shell Y37.03- ☑
      specified NEC Y37.29- ☑
      torpedo Y37.04- ☑
   fire Y37.30- ☑
      specified NEC Y37.39- ☑
   firearms
      discharge Y37.43- ☑
      pellets Y37.42- ☑
   flamethrower Y37.33- ☑
   fragments (from) (of)
      improvised explosive device [IED] (person-borne) (roadside) (vehicle-borne) Y37.26- ☑
      munitions Y37.25- ☑
      specified NEC Y37.29- ☑
      weapons Y37.27- ☑
   friendly fire Y37.92- ☑
   hand to hand (unarmed) combat Y37.44- ☑
   HLB overpressure Y37.A2- ☑
   hot substances — see Military operations, fire
   incendiary bullet Y37.32- ☑
   LLB overpressure Y37.A1- ☑
   nuclear weapon (effects of) Y37.50- ☑
      acute radiation exposure Y37.54- ☑
      blast pressure Y37.51- ☑
      direct blast Y37.51- ☑
      direct heat Y37.53- ☑
      fallout exposure Y37.54- ☑
      fireball Y37.53- ☑
      indirect blast (struck or crushed by blast debris) (being thrown by blast) Y37.52- ☑
      ionizing radiation (immediate exposure) Y37.54- ☑
      nuclear radiation Y37.54- ☑
      radiation
         ionizing (immediate exposure) Y37.54- ☑
         nuclear Y37.54- ☑
         thermal Y37.53- ☑
      secondary effects Y37.54- ☑
      specified NEC Y37.59- ☑
      thermal radiation Y37.53- ☑
   restriction of air (airway)
      intentional Y37.46- ☑
      unintentional Y37.47- ☑
   rubber bullets Y37.41- ☑
   shrapnel NOS Y37.29- ☑
   suffocation — see Military operations, restriction of airways
   unconventional warfare NEC Y37.7X- ☑
   underwater blast NOS Y37.00- ☑
   warfare
      conventional NEC Y37.49- ☑
      unconventional NEC Y37.7X- ☑
   weapon of mass destruction [WMD] Y37.91- ☑
   weapons
      biological weapons Y37.6X- ☑
      chemical Y37.7X- ☑
      nuclear (effects of) Y37.50- ☑
         acute radiation exposure Y37.54- ☑
         blast pressure Y37.51- ☑
         direct blast Y37.51- ☑
         direct heat Y37.53- ☑
         fallout exposure Y37.54- ☑
         fireball Y37.53- ☑

Military operations — continued
   weapons — continued
      nuclear — continued
         radiation
            ionizing (immediate exposure) Y37.54- ☑
            nuclear Y37.54- ☑
            thermal Y37.53- ☑
         secondary effects Y37.54- ☑
         specified NEC Y37.59- ☑
      of mass destruction [WMD] Y37.91- ☑
Misadventure(s) **to patient**(s) **during surgical or medical care** Y69
   contaminated medical or biological substance (blood, drug, fluid) Y64.9
      administered (by) NEC Y64.9
         immunization Y64.1
         infusion Y64.0
         injection Y64.1
         specified means NEC Y64.8
         transfusion Y64.0
         vaccination Y64.1
   excessive amount of blood or other fluid during transfusion or infusion Y63.0
   failure
      in dosage Y63.9
         electroshock therapy Y63.4
         inappropriate temperature (too hot or too cold) in local application and packing Y63.5
         infusion
            excessive amount of fluid Y63.0
            incorrect dilution of fluid Y63.1
         insulin-shock therapy Y63.4
         nonadministration of necessary drug or biological substance Y63.6
         overdose — see Table of Drugs and Chemicals
            radiation, in therapy Y63.2
         radiation
            overdose Y63.2
         specified procedure NEC Y63.8
         transfusion
            excessive amount of blood Y63.0
   mechanical, of instrument or apparatus (any) (during any procedure) Y65.8
   sterile precautions (during procedure) Y62.9
      aspiration of fluid or tissue (by puncture or catheterization, except heart) Y62.6
      biopsy (except needle aspiration) Y62.8
         needle (aspirating) Y62.6
      blood sampling Y62.6
      catheterization Y62.6
         heart Y62.5
      dialysis (kidney) Y62.2
      endoscopic examination Y62.4
      enema Y62.8
      immunization Y62.3
      infusion Y62.1
      injection Y62.3
      needle biopsy Y62.6
      paracentesis (abdominal) (thoracic) Y62.6
      perfusion Y62.2
      puncture (lumbar) Y62.6
      removal of catheter or packing Y62.8
      specified procedure NEC Y62.8
      surgical operation Y62.0
      transfusion Y62.1
      vaccination Y62.3
   suture or ligature during surgical procedure Y65.2
   to introduce or to remove tube or instrument — see Failure, to
   hemorrhage — see Index to Diseases and Injuries, Complication(s)
   inadvertent exposure of patient to radiation Y63.3
   inappropriate
      operation performed — see Inappropriate operation performed
      temperature (too hot or too cold) in local application or packing Y63.5
   infusion — see also Misadventure, by type, infusion Y69
      excessive amount of fluid Y63.0
      incorrect dilution of fluid Y63.1
      wrong fluid Y65.1
   mismatched blood in transfusion Y65.0
   nonadministration of necessary drug or biological substance Y63.6
   overdose — see Table of Drugs and Chemicals
      radiation (in therapy) Y63.2
   perforation — see Index to Diseases and Injuries, Complication(s)

☑ Additional Character Required — Refer to the Tabular List for Character Selection

Misadventure(s) to patient(s) during surgical or medical care — continued
- performance of inappropriate operation — see Inappropriate operation performed
- puncture — see Index to Diseases and Injuries, Complication(s)
- specified type NEC Y65.8
  - failure
    - suture or ligature during surgical operation Y65.2
    - to introduce or to remove tube or instrument — see Failure, to
  - infusion of wrong fluid Y65.1
  - performance of inappropriate operation — see Inappropriate operation performed
  - transfusion of mismatched blood Y65.0
  - wrong
    - fluid in infusion Y65.1
    - placement of endotracheal tube during anesthetic procedure Y65.3
- transfusion — see Misadventure, by type, transfusion
  - excessive amount of blood Y63.0
  - mismatched blood Y65.0
- wrong
  - drug given in error — see Table of Drugs and Chemicals
  - fluid in infusion Y65.1
  - placement of endotracheal tube during anesthetic procedure Y65.3

Mismatched blood in transfusion Y65.0
Motion sickness T75.3- ☑
Mountain sickness W94.11- ☑
Mudslide (of cataclysmic nature) — see Landslide
Murder (attempt) — see Assault

N

Nail
- contact with W45.0- ☑
  - gun W29.4- ☑
- embedded in skin W45.0- ☑

Neglect (criminal) (homicidal intent) X58.- ☑
Noise (causing injury) (pollution) W42.9- ☑
- supersonic W42.0- ☑

Nonadministration (of)
- drug or biological substance (necessary) Y63.6
- surgical and medical care Y66

Nosocomial condition Y95

O

Object
- falling
  - from, in, on, hitting
    - machinery — see Contact, with, by type of machine
  - set in motion by
    - accidental explosion or rupture of pressure vessel W38.- ☑
    - firearm — see Discharge, firearm, by type
    - machine(ry) — see Contact, with, by type of machine

Overdose (drug) — see Table of Drugs and Chemicals
- radiation Y63.2

Overexertion X50.9- ☑
- from
  - prolonged static or awkward postures X50.1- ☑
  - repetitive movements X50.3- ☑
  - specified strenuous movements or postures NEC X50.9- ☑
  - strenuous movement or load X50.0- ☑

Overexposure (accidental) (to)
- cold — see also Exposure, cold X31.- ☑
  - due to man-made conditions — see Exposure, cold, man-made
- heat — see also Heat X30.- ☑
- radiation — see Radiation
- radioactivity W88.0- ☑
- sun (sunburn) X32.- ☑
- weather NEC — see Forces of nature
- wind NEC — see Forces of nature

Overheated — see Heat
Overturning (accidental)
- machinery — see Contact, with, by type of machine
- transport vehicle NEC — see also Accident, transport V89.9- ☑
- watercraft (causing drowning, submersion) — see also Drowning, due to, accident to, watercraft, overturning

Overturning — continued
- watercraft — see also Drowning, due to, accident to, watercraft, overturning — continued
  - causing injury except drowning or submersion — see Accident, watercraft, causing, injury NEC

P

Parachute descent (voluntary) (without accident to aircraft) V97.29- ☑
- due to accident to aircraft — see Accident, transport, aircraft

Pecked by bird W61.99- ☑
Perforation during medical or surgical treatment as misadventure — see Index to Diseases and Injuries, Complication(s)

Perpetrator, perpetration, of assault, maltreatment and neglect (by) Y07.9
- acquaintance Y07.54
- aunt Y07.47
- boyfriend
  - current Y07.030
  - former Y07.031
- brother Y07.410
  - stepbrother Y07.435
- child (adopted) (biological) (foster) (in-law) (step) Y07.44
- coach Y07.53
- cousin
  - female Y07.491
  - male Y07.490
- daughter (adopted) (biological) (foster) (in-law) (step) Y07.44
- daycare provider Y07.519
  - at-home
    - adult care Y07.512
    - childcare Y07.510
  - care center
    - adult care Y07.513
    - childcare Y07.511
- family member NEC Y07.499
- father Y07.11
  - adoptive Y07.13
  - foster Y07.420
  - stepfather Y07.430
- foster father Y07.420
- foster mother Y07.421
- friend Y07.54
- girl friend
  - current Y07.040
  - former Y07.041
- grandchild (adopted) (biological) (foster) (in-law) (step) Y07.45
- granddaughter (adopted) (biological) (foster) (in-law) (step) Y07.45
- grandfather Y07.46
- grandmother Y07.46
- grandparent Y07.46
- grandson (adopted) (biological) (foster) (in-law) (step) Y07.45
- healthcare provider Y07.529
  - mental health Y07.521
  - specified NEC Y07.528
- husband
  - current Y07.010
  - former Y07.011
- instructor Y07.53
- mother Y07.12
  - adoptive Y07.14
  - foster Y07.421
  - stepmother Y07.433
- multiple perpetrators Y07.6
- non-binary
  - child (adopted) (biological) (foster) (in-law) (step) Y07.44
  - grandchild (adopted) (biological) (foster) (in-law) (step) Y07.45
  - grandparent Y07.46
  - parental sibling Y07.47
- nonfamily member Y07.50
  - specified NEC Y07.59
- nurse Y07.528
- occupational therapist Y07.528
- parental sibling Y07.47
- partner
  - female (dating) (intimate)
    - current Y07.040
    - former Y07.041

Perpetrator, perpetration, of assault, maltreatment and neglect — continued
- partner — continued
  - gender non-conforming
    - current Y07.050
    - former Y07.051
  - male (dating) (intimate)
    - current Y07.030
    - former Y07.031
  - non-binary
    - current Y07.050
    - former Y07.051
- of parent
  - female Y07.434
  - male Y07.432
- physical therapist Y07.528
- sister Y07.411
- son (adopted) (biological) (foster) (in-law) (step) Y07.44
- speech therapist Y07.528
- stepbrother Y07.435
- stepfather Y07.430
- stepmother Y07.433
- stepsister Y07.436
- teacher Y07.53
- uncle Y07.47
- wife
  - current Y07.020
  - former Y07.021

Piercing — see Contact, with, by type of object or machine
Pinched
- between objects (moving) (stationary and moving) W23.0- ☑
- stationary W23.1- ☑

Pinned under machine(ry) — see Contact, with, by type of machine

Place of occurrence Y92.9
- abandoned house Y92.89
- airplane Y92.813
- airport Y92.520
- ambulatory health services establishment NEC Y92.538
- ambulatory surgery center Y92.530
- amusement park Y92.831
- apartment (co-op) — see Place of occurrence, residence, apartment
- assembly hall Y92.29
- bank Y92.510
- bar Y92.59
- barn Y92.71
- baseball field Y92.320
- basketball court Y92.310
- beach Y92.832
- boarding house — see Place of occurrence, residence, boarding house
- boat Y92.814
- bowling alley Y92.39
- bridge Y92.89
- building under construction Y92.61
- bus Y92.811
  - station Y92.521
- cafe Y92.511
- campsite Y92.833
- campus — see Place of occurrence, school
- canal Y92.89
- car Y92.810
- casino Y92.59
- children's home — see Place of occurrence, residence, institutional, orphanage
- church Y92.22
- cinema Y92.26
- clubhouse Y92.29
- coal pit Y92.64
- college (community) Y92.214
- condominium — see Place of occurrence, residence, apartment
- construction area — see Place of occurrence, industrial and construction area
- convalescent home — see Place of occurrence, residence, institutional, nursing home
- court-house Y92.240
- cricket ground Y92.328
- cultural building Y92.258
  - art gallery Y92.250
  - museum Y92.251
  - music hall Y92.252
  - opera house Y92.253
  - specified NEC Y92.258
  - theater Y92.254
- dancehall Y92.252
- day nursery Y92.210

Place of occurrence — *continued*
- dentist office Y92.531
- derelict house Y92.89
- desert Y92.820
- dock NOS Y92.89
- dockyard Y92.62
- doctor's office Y92.531
- dormitory — *see* Place of occurrence, residence, institutional, school dormitory
- dry dock Y92.62
- factory (building) (premises) Y92.63
- farm (land under cultivation) (outbuildings) Y92.79
  - barn Y92.71
  - chicken coop Y92.72
  - field Y92.73
  - hen house Y92.72
  - house — *see* Place of occurrence, residence, house
  - orchard Y92.74
  - specified NEC Y92.79
- football field Y92.321
- forest Y92.821
- freeway Y92.411
- gallery Y92.250
- garage (commercial) Y92.59
  - boarding house Y92.044
  - military base Y92.135
  - mobile home Y92.025
  - nursing home Y92.124
  - orphanage Y92.114
  - private house Y92.015
  - reform school Y92.155
- gas station Y92.524
- gasworks Y92.69
- golf course Y92.39
- gravel pit Y92.64
- grocery Y92.512
- gymnasium Y92.39
- handball court Y92.318
- harbor Y92.89
- harness racing course Y92.39
- healthcare provider office Y92.531
- highway Y92.410
  - interstate Y92.411
- hill Y92.828
- hockey rink Y92.330
- home — *see* Place of occurrence, residence
- hospice — *see* Place of occurrence, residence, institutional, nursing home
- hospital Y92.239
  - cafeteria Y92.233
  - corridor Y92.232
  - operating room Y92.234
  - patient
    - bathroom Y92.231
    - room Y92.230
  - specified NEC Y92.238
- hotel Y92.59
- house — *see also* Place of occurrence, residence
  - abandoned Y92.89
  - under construction Y92.61
- industrial and construction area (yard) Y92.69
  - building under construction Y92.61
  - dock Y92.62
  - dry dock Y92.62
  - factory Y92.63
  - gasworks Y92.69
  - mine Y92.64
  - oil rig Y92.65
  - pit Y92.64
  - power station Y92.69
  - shipyard Y92.62
  - specified NEC Y92.69
  - tunnel under construction Y92.69
  - workshop Y92.69
- interstate Y92.411
- kindergarten Y92.211
- lacrosse field Y92.328
- lake Y92.838
  - wilderness Y92.828
- library Y92.241
- mall Y92.59
- market Y92.512
- marsh Y92.828
- military
  - base — *see* Place of occurrence, residence, institutional, military base
  - training ground Y92.84
- mine Y92.64
- mosque Y92.22

Place of occurrence — *continued*
- motel Y92.59
- motorway (interstate) Y92.411
- mountain Y92.828
- movie-house Y92.26
- museum Y92.251
- music-hall Y92.252
- not applicable Y92.9
- nuclear power station Y92.69
- nursing home — *see* Place of occurrence, residence, institutional, nursing home
- office building Y92.59
- offshore installation Y92.65
- oil rig Y92.65
- old people's home — *see* Place of occurrence, residence, institutional, specified NEC
- opera-house Y92.253
- orphanage — *see* Place of occurrence, residence, institutional, orphanage
- outpatient surgery center Y92.530
- park (public) Y92.830
  - amusement Y92.831
- parking garage Y92.89
  - lot Y92.481
- pavement Y92.480
- physician office Y92.531
- polo field Y92.328
- pond Y92.828
- post office Y92.242
- power station Y92.69
- prairie Y92.828
- prison — *see* Place of occurrence, residence, institutional, prison
- public
  - administration building Y92.248
    - city hall Y92.243
    - courthouse Y92.240
    - library Y92.241
    - post office Y92.242
    - specified NEC Y92.248
  - building NEC Y92.29
    - hall Y92.29
  - place NOS Y92.89
- race course Y92.39
- radio station Y92.59
- railway line (bridge) Y92.85
- ranch (outbuildings) — *see* Place of occurrence, farm
- recreation area Y92.838
  - amusement park Y92.831
  - beach Y92.832
  - campsite Y92.833
  - park (public) Y92.830
  - seashore Y92.832
  - specified NEC Y92.838
- reform school - — *see* Place of occurrence, residence, institutional, reform school
- religious institution Y92.22
- residence (non-institutional) (private) Y92.009
  - apartment Y92.039
    - bathroom Y92.031
    - bedroom Y92.032
    - kitchen Y92.030
    - specified NEC Y92.038
  - bathroom Y92.002
  - bedroom Y92.003
  - boarding house Y92.049
    - bathroom Y92.041
    - bedroom Y92.042
    - driveway Y92.043
    - garage Y92.044
    - garden Y92.046
    - kitchen Y92.040
    - specified NEC Y92.048
    - swimming pool Y92.045
    - yard Y92.046
  - dining room Y92.001
  - garden Y92.007
  - home Y92.009
  - house, single family Y92.019
    - bathroom Y92.012
    - bedroom Y92.013
    - dining room Y92.011
    - driveway Y92.014
    - garage Y92.015
    - garden Y92.017
    - kitchen Y92.010
    - specified NEC Y92.018
    - swimming pool Y92.016
    - yard Y92.017

Place of occurrence — *continued*
- residence — *continued*
  - institutional Y92.10
    - children's home — *see* Place of occurrence, residence, institutional, orphanage
    - hospice — *see* Place of occurrence, residence, institutional, nursing home
    - military base Y92.139
      - barracks Y92.133
      - garage Y92.135
      - garden Y92.137
      - kitchen Y92.130
      - mess hall Y92.131
      - specified NEC Y92.138
      - swimming pool Y92.136
      - yard Y92.137
    - nursing home Y92.129
      - bathroom Y92.121
      - bedroom Y92.122
      - driveway Y92.123
      - garage Y92.124
      - garden Y92.126
      - kitchen Y92.120
      - specified NEC Y92.128
      - swimming pool Y92.125
      - yard Y92.126
    - orphanage Y92.119
      - bathroom Y92.111
      - bedroom Y92.112
      - driveway Y92.113
      - garage Y92.114
      - garden Y92.116
      - kitchen Y92.110
      - specified NEC Y92.118
      - swimming pool Y92.115
      - yard Y92.116
    - prison Y92.149
      - bathroom Y92.142
      - cell Y92.143
      - courtyard Y92.147
      - dining room Y92.141
      - kitchen Y92.140
      - specified NEC Y92.148
      - swimming pool Y92.146
    - reform school Y92.159
      - bathroom Y92.152
      - bedroom Y92.153
      - dining room Y92.151
      - driveway Y92.154
      - garage Y92.155
      - garden Y92.157
      - kitchen Y92.150
      - specified NEC Y92.158
      - swimming pool Y92.156
      - yard Y92.157
    - school dormitory Y92.169
      - bathroom Y92.162
      - bedroom Y92.163
      - dining room Y92.161
      - kitchen Y92.160
      - specified NEC Y92.168
    - specified NEC Y92.199
      - bathroom Y92.192
      - bedroom Y92.193
      - dining room Y92.191
      - driveway Y92.194
      - garage Y92.195
      - garden Y92.197
      - kitchen Y92.190
      - specified NEC Y92.198
      - swimming pool Y92.196
      - yard Y92.197
  - kitchen Y92.000
  - mobile home Y92.029
    - bathroom Y92.022
    - bedroom Y92.023
    - dining room Y92.021
    - driveway Y92.024
    - garage Y92.025
    - garden Y92.027
    - kitchen Y92.020
    - specified NEC Y92.028
    - swimming pool Y92.026
    - yard Y92.027
  - specified place in residence NEC Y92.008
  - specified residence type NEC Y92.099
    - bathroom Y92.091
    - bedroom Y92.092
    - driveway Y92.093

Place of occurrence — *continued*
  residence — *continued*
    specified residence type — *continued*
      garage Y92.094
      garden Y92.096
      kitchen Y92.090
      specified NEC Y92.098
      swimming pool Y92.095
      yard Y92.096
  restaurant Y92.511
  riding school Y92.39
  river Y92.828
  road Y92.410
  rodeo ring Y92.39
  rugby field Y92.328
  same day surgery center Y92.530
  sand pit Y92.64
  school (private) (public) (state) Y92.219
    college Y92.214
    daycare center Y92.210
    elementary school Y92.211
    high school Y92.213
    kindergarten Y92.211
    middle school Y92.212
    specified NEC Y92.218
    trade school Y92.215
    university Y92.214
    vocational school Y92.215
  sea (shore) Y92.832
  senior citizen center Y92.29
  service area
    airport Y92.520
    bus station Y92.521
    gas station Y92.524
    highway rest stop Y92.523
    railway station Y92.522
  shipyard Y92.62
  shop (commercial) Y92.513
  sidewalk Y92.480
  silo Y92.79
  skating rink (roller) Y92.331
    ice Y92.330
  slaughter house Y92.86
  soccer field Y92.322
  specified place NEC Y92.89
  sports area Y92.39
    athletic
      court Y92.318
        basketball Y92.310
        specified NEC Y92.318
        squash Y92.311
        tennis Y92.312
      field Y92.328
        baseball Y92.320
        cricket ground Y92.328
        football Y92.321
        hockey Y92.328
        soccer Y92.322
        specified NEC Y92.328
    golf course Y92.39
    gymnasium Y92.39
    riding school Y92.39
    skating rink (roller) Y92.331
      ice Y92.330
    stadium Y92.39
    swimming pool Y92.34
  squash court Y92.311
  stadium Y92.39
  steeplechasing course Y92.39
  store Y92.512
  stream Y92.828
  street and highway Y92.410
    bike path Y92.482
    freeway Y92.411
    highway ramp Y92.415
    interstate highway Y92.411
    local residential or business street Y92.414
    motorway Y92.411
    parking lot Y92.481
    parkway Y92.412
    sidewalk Y92.480
    specified NEC Y92.488
    state road Y92.413
  subway car Y92.816
  supermarket Y92.512
  swamp Y92.828
  swimming pool (public) Y92.34
    private (at) Y92.095
      boarding house Y92.045

Place of occurrence — *continued*
  swimming pool — *continued*
    private — *continued*
      military base Y92.136
      mobile home Y92.026
      nursing home Y92.125
      orphanage Y92.115
      prison Y92.146
      reform school Y92.156
      single family residence Y92.016
  synagogue Y92.22
  tavern Y92.59
  television station Y92.59
  tennis court Y92.312
  theater Y92.254
  trade area Y92.59
    bank Y92.510
    cafe Y92.511
    casino Y92.59
    garage Y92.59
    hotel Y92.59
    market Y92.512
    office building Y92.59
    radio station Y92.59
    restaurant Y92.511
    shop Y92.513
    shopping mall Y92.59
    store Y92.512
    supermarket Y92.512
    television station Y92.59
    warehouse Y92.59
  trailer park, residential — *see* Place of occurrence, residence, mobile home
  trailer site NOS Y92.89
  train Y92.815
    station Y92.522
  truck Y92.812
  tunnel under construction Y92.69
  university Y92.214
  urgent (health) care center Y92.532
  vehicle (transport) Y92.818
    airplane Y92.813
    boat Y92.814
    bus Y92.811
    car Y92.810
    specified NEC Y92.818
    subway car Y92.816
    train Y92.815
    truck Y92.812
  warehouse Y92.59
  water reservoir Y92.89
  wilderness area Y92.828
    desert Y92.820
    forest Y92.821
    marsh Y92.828
    mountain Y92.828
    prairie Y92.828
    specified NEC Y92.828
    swamp Y92.828
  workshop Y92.69
  yard, private Y92.096
    boarding house Y92.046
    mobile home Y92.027
    single family house Y92.017
  youth center Y92.29
  zoo (zoological garden) Y92.834
Plumbism — *see* Table of Drugs and Chemicals, lead
Poisoning (accidental) (by) — *see also* Table of Drugs and Chemicals
  by plant, thorns, spines, sharp leaves or other mechanisms NEC X58.- ☑
  carbon monoxide
    generated by
      motor vehicle — *see* Accident, transport
      watercraft (in transit) (not in transit) V93.89- ☑
        ferry boat V93.81- ☑
        fishing boat V93.82- ☑
        jet skis V93.83- ☑
        liner V93.81- ☑
        merchant ship V93.80- ☑
        passenger ship V93.81- ☑
        powered craft NEC V93.83- ☑
  caused by injection of poisons into skin by plant thorns, spines, sharp leaves X58.- ☑
  marine or sea plants (venomous) X58.- ☑
  execution — *see* Legal, intervention, gas
  intervention
    by gas — *see* Legal, intervention, gas

Poisoning — *continued*
  execution — *see* Legal, intervention, gas — *continued*
  intervention — *continued*
    other specified means — *see* Legal, intervention, specified means NEC
  exhaust gas
    generated by
      motor vehicle — *see* Accident, transport
      watercraft (in transit) (not in transit) V93.89- ☑
        ferry boat V93.81- ☑
        fishing boat V93.82- ☑
        jet skis V93.83- ☑
        liner V93.81- ☑
        merchant ship V93.80- ☑
        passenger ship V93.81- ☑
        powered craft NEC V93.83- ☑
  fumes or smoke due to
    explosion — *see also* Explosion W40.9- ☑
    fire — *see* Exposure, fire
    ignition — *see* Ignition
  gas
    in legal intervention — *see* Legal, intervention, gas
    legal execution — *see* Legal, intervention, gas
  in war operations — *see* War operations
  legal
Powder burn (by) (from)
  airgun W34.110- ☑
  BB gun W34.110- ☑
  firearm NEC W34.19- ☑
  gas, air or spring-operated gun NEC W34.118- ☑
  handgun W32.1- ☑
  hunting rifle W33.12- ☑
  larger firearm W33.10- ☑
    specified NEC W33.19- ☑
  machine gun W33.13- ☑
  paintball gun W34.111- ☑
  pellet gun W34.110- ☑
  shotgun W33.11- ☑
  Very pistol [flare] W34.19- ☑
Premature cessation (of) **surgical and medical care** Y66
Privation (food) (water) X58.- ☑
Procedure (operation)
  correct, on wrong side or body part (wrong side) (wrong site) Y65.53
  intended for another patient done on wrong patient Y65.52
  performed on patient not scheduled for surgery Y65.52
  performed on wrong patient Y65.52
  wrong, performed on correct patient Y65.51
Prolonged
  sitting in transport vehicle — *see* Sitting
  stay in
    high altitude as cause of anoxia, barodontalgia, barotitis or hypoxia W94.11- ☑
    weightless environment X52.- ☑
Pulling, excessive — *see also* Overexertion X50.9- ☑
Puncture, puncturing — *see also* Contact, with, by type of object or machine
  by
    plant thorns, spines, sharp leaves or other mechanisms NEC W60.- ☑
  during medical or surgical treatment as misadventure — *see* Index to Diseases and Injuries, Complication(s)
Pushed, pushing (accidental) (injury in)
  by other person(s) (accidental) W51.- ☑
    as, or caused by, a crowd or human stampede (with fall) W52.- ☑
    before moving object NEC Y02.8- ☑
      motor vehicle Y02.0- ☑
      subway train Y02.1- ☑
      train Y02.1- ☑
    from
      high place NEC
        in accidental circumstances W17.89- ☑
        stated as
          intentional, homicide (attempt) Y01.- ☑
          undetermined whether accidental or intentional Y30.- ☑
      transport vehicle NEC — *see also* Accident, transport V89.9- ☑
        stated as
          intentional, homicide (attempt) Y08.89- ☑
  with fall W03.- ☑
    due to ice or snow W00.0- ☑
  overexertion X50.9- ☑

R

Radiation (exposure to)
  arc lamps W89.0- ☑
  atomic power plant (malfunction) NEC W88.1- ☑
  complication of or abnormal reaction to medical radiotherapy Y84.2
  electromagnetic, ionizing W88.0- ☑
  gamma rays W88.1- ☑
  in
    war operations (from or following nuclear explosion) — see War operations
  inadvertent exposure of patient (receiving test or therapy) Y63.3
  infrared (heaters and lamps) W90.1- ☑
    excessive heat from W92.- ☑
  ionized, ionizing (particles, artificially accelerated)
    radioisotopes W88.1- ☑
    specified NEC W88.8- ☑
    x-rays W88.0- ☑
  isotopes, radioactive — see Radiation, radioactive isotopes
  laser(s) W90.2- ☑
    in war operations — see War operations
    misadventure in medical care Y63.2
  light sources (man-made visible and ultraviolet) W89.9- ☑
    natural X32.- ☑
    specified NEC W89.8- ☑
    tanning bed W89.1- ☑
    welding light W89.0- ☑
  man-made visible light W89.9- ☑
    specified NEC W89.8- ☑
    tanning bed W89.1- ☑
    welding light W89.0- ☑
  microwave W90.8- ☑
  misadventure in medical or surgical procedure Y63.2
  natural NEC X39.08- ☑
    radon X39.01- ☑
  overdose (in medical or surgical procedure) Y63.2
  radar W90.0- ☑
  radioactive isotopes (any) W88.1- ☑
    atomic power plant malfunction W88.1- ☑
    misadventure in medical or surgical treatment Y63.2
  radiofrequency W90.0- ☑
  radium NEC W88.1- ☑
  sun X32.- ☑
  ultraviolet (light) (man-made) W89.9- ☑
    natural X32.- ☑
    specified NEC W89.8- ☑
    tanning bed W89.1- ☑
    welding light W89.0- ☑
  welding arc, torch, or light W89.0- ☑
    excessive heat from W92.- ☑
  x-rays (hard) (soft) W88.0- ☑
Range disease W94.11- ☑
Rape (attempted) (confirmed) T74.2- ☑
  suspected T76.2- ☑
Rat bite W53.11- ☑
Reaching (prolonged) (static) X50.1- ☑
Reaction, abnormal to medical procedure — see also Complication of or following, by type of procedure Y84.9
  biologicals — see Table of Drugs and Chemicals
  drugs — see Table of Drugs and Chemicals
  vaccine — see Table of Drugs and Chemicals
  with misadventure — see Misadventure
Recoil
  airgun W34.110- ☑
  BB gun W34.110- ☑
  firearm NEC W34.19- ☑
  gas, air or spring-operated gun NEC W34.118- ☑
  handgun W32.1- ☑
  hunting rifle W33.12- ☑
  larger firearm W33.10- ☑
    specified NEC W33.19- ☑
  machine gun W33.13- ☑
  paintball gun W34.111- ☑
  pellet W34.110- ☑
  shotgun W33.11- ☑
  Very pistol [flare] W34.19- ☑
Reduction in
  atmospheric pressure — see Air, pressure, change
Rock falling on or hitting (accidentally) (person) W20.8- ☑
  in cave-in W20.0- ☑

Run over (accidentally) (by)
  animal (not being ridden) NEC W55.89- ☑
  machinery — see Contact, with, by specified type of machine
  transport vehicle NEC — see also Accident, transport V09.9- ☑
    intentional homicide (attempt) Y03.0- ☑
    motor NEC V09.20- ☑
      intentional homicide (attempt) Y03.0- ☑
Running
  before moving object X81.8- ☑
  motor vehicle X81.0- ☑
Running off, away
  animal (being ridden) — see also Accident, transport V80.918- ☑
    not being ridden W55.89- ☑
  animal-drawn vehicle NEC — see also Accident, transport V80.928- ☑
  highway, road(way), street
    transport vehicle NEC — see also Accident, transport V89.9- ☑
Rupture pressurized devices — see Explosion, by type of device

S

Saturnism — see Table of Drugs and Chemicals, lead
Scald, scalding (accidental) (by) (from) (in) X19.- ☑
  air (hot) X14.1- ☑
  gases (hot) X14.1- ☑
  homicide (attempt) — see Assault, burning, hot object
  inflicted by other person
    stated as intentional, homicide (attempt) — see Assault, burning, hot object
  liquid (boiling) (hot) NEC X12.- ☑
    stated as undetermined whether accidental or intentional Y27.2- ☑
    suicide (attempt) X77.2- ☑
  local application of externally applied substance in medical or surgical care Y63.5
  metal (molten) (liquid) (hot) NEC X18.- ☑
  self-inflicted X77.9- ☑
  stated as undetermined whether accidental or intentional Y27.8- ☑
  steam X13.1- ☑
    assault X98.0- ☑
    stated as undetermined whether accidental or intentional Y27.0- ☑
    suicide (attempt) X77.0- ☑
  suicide (attempt) X77.9- ☑
  vapor (hot) X13.1- ☑
    assault X98.0- ☑
    stated as undetermined whether accidental or intentional Y27.0- ☑
    suicide (attempt) X77.0- ☑
Scratched by
  cat W55.03- ☑
  person(s) (accidentally) W50.4- ☑
    with intent to injure or kill Y04.0- ☑
    as, or caused by, a crowd or human stampede (with fall) W52.- ☑
    assault Y04.0- ☑
    homicide (attempt) Y04.0- ☑
    in
      fight Y04.0- ☑
      legal intervention
        injuring
          bystander Y35.892- ☑
          law enforcement personnel Y35.891- ☑
          suspect Y35.893- ☑
          unspecified person Y35.899- ☑
Seasickness T75.3- ☑
Self-harm NEC — see also External cause by type, undetermined whether accidental or intentional
  intentional — see Suicide
  poisoning NEC — see Table of Drugs and Chemicals, poisoning, accidental
Self-inflicted (injury) **NEC** — see also External cause by type, undetermined whether accidental or intentional
  intentional — see Suicide
  poisoning NEC — see Table of Drugs and Chemicals, poisoning, accidental
Sequelae (of)
  accident NEC — see W00-X58 with 7th character S
  assault (homicidal) (any means) — see X92-Y08 with 7th character S

Sequelae — continued
  homicide, attempt (any means) — see X92-Y08 with 7th character S
  injury undetermined whether accidentally or purposely inflicted — see Y21-Y33 with 7th character S
  intentional self-harm (classifiable to X71-X83) — see X71-X83 with 7th character S
  legal intervention — see with 7th character S Y35.- ☑
  motor vehicle accident — see V00-V99 with 7th character S
  suicide, attempt (any means) — see X71-X83 with 7th character S
  transport accident — see V00-V99 with 7th character S
  war operations — see War operations
Shock
  electric — see Exposure, electric current
  from electric appliance (any) (faulty) W86.8- ☑
    domestic W86.0- ☑
    suicide (attempt) X83.1- ☑
Shooting, shot (accidental(ly)) — see also Discharge, firearm, by type
  herself or himself — see Discharge, firearm by type, self-inflicted
  homicide (attempt) — see Discharge, firearm by type, homicide
  in war operations — see War operations
  inflicted by other person — see Discharge, firearm by type, homicide
    accidental — see Discharge, firearm, by type of firearm
  legal
    execution — see Legal, intervention, firearm
    intervention — see Legal, intervention, firearm
  self-inflicted — see Discharge, firearm by type, suicide
    accidental — see Discharge, firearm, by type of firearm
  suicide (attempt) — see Discharge, firearm by type, suicide
Shoving (accidentally) **by other person** — see Pushed, by other person
Sickness
  alpine W94.11- ☑
  motion — see Motion
  mountain W94.11- ☑
Sinking (accidental)
  watercraft (causing drowning, submersion) — see also Drowning, due to, accident to, watercraft, sinking
  causing injury except drowning or submersion — see Accident, watercraft, causing, injury NEC
Siriasis X32.- ☑
Sitting (prolonged) (static) X50.1- ☑
Slashed wrists — see Cut, self-inflicted
Slipping (accidental) (on same level) (with fall) W01.0- ☑
  on
    ice W00.0- ☑
      with skates — see Accident, transport, pedestrian, conveyance
    mud W01.0- ☑
    oil W01.0- ☑
    snow W00.0- ☑
      with skis — see Accident, transport, pedestrian, conveyance
    surface (slippery) (wet) NEC W01.0- ☑
  without fall W18.40- ☑
    due to
      specified NEC W18.49- ☑
      stepping from one level to another W18.43- ☑
      stepping into hole or opening W18.42- ☑
      stepping on object W18.41- ☑
Sliver, wood, contact with W45.8- ☑
Smoldering (due to fire) — see Exposure, fire
Sodomy (attempted) **by force** T74.2- ☑
Sound waves (causing injury) W42.9- ☑
  supersonic W42.0- ☑
Splinter, contact with W45.8- ☑
Stab, stabbing — see Cut
Standing (prolonged) (static) X50.1- ☑
Starvation X58.- ☑
Status of external cause Y99.9
  child assisting in compensated work for family Y99.8
  civilian activity done for financial or other compensation Y99.0
  civilian activity done for income or pay Y99.0
  family member assisting in compensated work for other family member Y99.8
  hobby not done for income Y99.8
  leisure activity Y99.8
  military activity Y99.1
  off-duty activity of military personnel Y99.8

Status of external cause — *continued*
  recreation or sport not for income or while a student Y99.8
  specified NEC Y99.8
  student activity Y99.8
  volunteer activity Y99.2

Stepped on
  by
    animal (not being ridden) NEC W55.89- ☑
    crowd or human stampede W52.- ☑
    person W50.0- ☑

Stepping on
  object W22.8- ☑
    sports equipment W21.9- ☑
    stationary W22.09- ☑
      sports equipment W21.89- ☑
    with fall W18.31- ☑
  person W51.- ☑
    by crowd or human stampede W52.- ☑
  sports equipment W21.9- ☑

Sting
  arthropod, nonvenomous W57.- ☑
  insect, nonvenomous W57.- ☑

Storm (cataclysmic) — *see* Forces of nature, cataclysmic storm

Straining, excessive — *see also* Overexertion X50.9- ☑

Strangling — *see* Strangulation

Strangulation (accidental) T71.- ☑

Strenuous movements — *see also* Overexertion X50.9- ☑

Striking against
  airbag (automobile) W22.10- ☑
    driver side W22.11- ☑
    front passenger side W22.12- ☑
    specified NEC W22.19- ☑
  bottom when
    diving or jumping into water (in) W16.822- ☑
      causing drowning W16.821- ☑
      from boat Y08.722- ☑
        causing drowning W16.721- ☑
      natural body W16.622- ☑
        causing drowning W16.821- ☑
      swimming pool W16.522- ☑
        causing drowning W16.521- ☑
    falling into water (in) W16.322- ☑
      causing drowning W16.321- ☑
      fountain — *see* Striking against, bottom when, falling into water, specified NEC
      natural body W16.122- ☑
        causing drowning W16.121- ☑
      reservoir — *see* Striking against, bottom when, falling into water, specified NEC
      specified NEC W16.322- ☑
        causing drowning W16.321- ☑
      swimming pool W16.022- ☑
        causing drowning W16.021- ☑
  diving board (swimming-pool) W21.4- ☑
  object W22.8- ☑
    caused by crowd or human stampede (with fall) W52.- ☑
    furniture W22.03- ☑
    lamppost W22.02- ☑
    sports equipment W21.9- ☑
    stationary W22.09- ☑
      sports equipment W21.89- ☑
    wall W22.01- ☑
    with
      drowning or submersion — *see* Drowning
      fall — *see* Fall, due to, bumping against, object
  person(s) W51.- ☑
    as, or caused by, a crowd or human stampede (with fall) W52.- ☑
    assault Y04.2- ☑
    homicide (attempt) Y04.2- ☑
    with fall W03.- ☑
      due to ice or snow W00.0- ☑
  sports equipment W21.9- ☑
  wall (when) W22.01- ☑
    diving or jumping into water (in) W16.832- ☑
      causing drowning W16.831- ☑
      swimming pool W16.532- ☑
        causing drowning W16.531- ☑
    falling into water (in) W16.332- ☑
      causing drowning W16.331- ☑
      fountain — *see* Striking against, wall when, falling into water, specified NEC
      natural body W16.132- ☑

Striking against — *continued*
  wall — *continued*
    falling into water — *continued*
      natural body — *continued*
        causing drowning W16.131- ☑
      reservoir — *see* Striking against, wall when, falling into water, specified NEC
      specified NEC W16.332- ☑
        causing drowning W16.331- ☑
      swimming pool W16.032- ☑
        causing drowning W16.031- ☑
    swimming pool (when) W22.042- ☑
      causing drowning W22.041- ☑
      diving or jumping into water W16.532- ☑
        causing drowning W16.531- ☑
      falling into water W16.032- ☑
        causing drowning W16.031- ☑

Struck (accidentally) **by**
  airbag (automobile) W22.10- ☑
    driver side W22.11- ☑
    front passenger side W22.12- ☑
    specified NEC W22.19- ☑
  alligator W58.02- ☑
  animal (not being ridden) NEC W55.89- ☑
  avalanche — *see* Landslide
  ball (hit) (thrown) W21.00- ☑
    assault Y08.09- ☑
    baseball W21.03- ☑
    basketball W21.05- ☑
    football W21.01- ☑
    golf ball W21.04- ☑
    soccer W21.02- ☑
    softball W21.07- ☑
    specified NEC W21.09- ☑
    volleyball W21.06- ☑
  bat or racquet
    baseball bat W21.11- ☑
      assault Y08.02- ☑
    golf club W21.13- ☑
      assault Y08.09- ☑
    specified NEC W21.19- ☑
      assault Y08.09- ☑
    tennis racquet W21.12- ☑
      assault Y08.09- ☑
  bullet — *see also* Discharge, firearm by type
    in war operations — *see* War operations
  crocodile W58.12- ☑
  dog W54.1- ☑
  flare, Very pistol — *see* Discharge, firearm NEC
  hailstones X39.8- ☑
  hockey (ice)
    field
      puck W21.221- ☑
      stick W21.211- ☑
    puck W21.220- ☑
    stick W21.210- ☑
      assault Y08.01- ☑
  landslide — *see* Landslide
  law-enforcement agent (on duty) — *see* Legal, intervention, manhandling
    with blunt object — *see* Legal, intervention, blunt object
  lightning T75.0- ☑
    causing fire — *see* Exposure, fire
  machine — *see* Contact, with, by type of machine
  mammal NEC W55.89- ☑
    marine W56.32- ☑
  marine animal W56.82- ☑
  missile
    firearm — *see* Discharge, firearm by type
    in war operations — *see* War operations, missile
  object W22.8- ☑
    blunt W22.8- ☑
      assault Y00.- ☑
      suicide (attempt) X79.- ☑
      undetermined whether accidental or intentional Y29.- ☑
    falling W20.8- ☑
      from, in, on
        building W20.1- ☑
          burning (uncontrolled fire) X00.4- ☑
        cataclysmic
          earth surface movement NEC — *see* Landslide
          storm — *see* Forces of nature, cataclysmic storm

Struck (accidentally) **by** — *continued*
  object — *continued*
    falling — *continued*
      from, in, on — *continued*
        cave-in W20.0- ☑
        earthquake X34.- ☑
        machine (in operation) — *see* Contact, with, by type of machine
        structure W20.1- ☑
          burning X00.4- ☑
        transport vehicle (in motion) — *see* Accident, transport, by type of vehicle
        watercraft V93.49- ☑
          due to
            accident to craft V91.39- ☑
              powered craft V91.33- ☑
                ferry boat V91.31- ☑
                fishing boat V91.32- ☑
                jetskis V91.33- ☑
                liner V91.31- ☑
                merchant ship V91.30- ☑
                passenger ship V91.31- ☑
            unpowered craft V91.38- ☑
              canoe V91.35- ☑
              inflatable V91.36- ☑
              kayak V91.35- ☑
              sailboat V91.34- ☑
              surf-board V91.38- ☑
              windsurfer V91.38- ☑
          powered craft V93.43- ☑
            ferry boat V93.41- ☑
            fishing boat V93.42- ☑
            jetskis V93.43- ☑
            liner V93.41- ☑
            merchant ship V93.40- ☑
            passenger ship V93.41- ☑
          unpowered craft V93.48- ☑
            sailboat V93.44- ☑
            surf-board V93.48- ☑
            windsurfer V93.48- ☑
    moving NEC W20.8- ☑
    projected W20.8- ☑
      assault Y00.- ☑
      in sports W21.9- ☑
        assault Y08.09- ☑
        ball W21.00- ☑
          baseball W21.03- ☑
          basketball W21.05- ☑
          football W21.01- ☑
          golf ball W21.04- ☑
          soccer W21.02- ☑
          softball W21.07- ☑
          specified NEC W21.09- ☑
          volleyball W21.06- ☑
        bat or racquet
          baseball bat W21.11- ☑
            assault Y08.02- ☑
          golf club W21.13- ☑
            assault Y08.09- ☑
          specified NEC W21.19- ☑
            assault Y08.09- ☑
          tennis racquet W21.12- ☑
            assault Y08.09- ☑
        hockey (ice)
          field
            puck W21.221- ☑
            stick W21.211- ☑
          puck W21.220- ☑
          stick W21.210- ☑
            assault Y08.01- ☑
        specified NEC W21.89- ☑
    set in motion by explosion — *see* Explosion
    thrown W20.8- ☑
      assault Y00.- ☑
      in sports W21.9- ☑
        assault Y08.09- ☑
        ball W21.00- ☑
          baseball W21.03- ☑
          basketball W21.05- ☑
          football W21.01- ☑
          golf ball W21.04- ☑
          soccer W21.02- ☑
          soft ball W21.07- ☑
          specified NEC W21.09- ☑
          volleyball W21.06- ☑

Struck (accidentally) **by** — *continued*
 object — *continued*
  thrown — *continued*
   in sports — *continued*
    bat or racquet
     baseball bat W21.11- ☑
      assault Y08.02- ☑
     golf club W21.13- ☑
      assault Y08.09- ☑
     specified NEC W21.19- ☑
      assault Y08.09- ☑
     tennis racquet W21.12- ☑
      assault Y08.09- ☑
    hockey (ice)
     field
      puck W21.221- ☑
      stick W21.211- ☑
     puck W21.220- ☑
     stick W21.210- ☑
      assault Y08.01- ☑
    specified NEC W21.89- ☑
 other person(s) W50.0- ☑
  with
   blunt object W22.8- ☑
    intentional, homicide (attempt) Y00.- ☑
    sports equipment W21.9- ☑
    undetermined whether accidental or intentional Y29.- ☑
   fall W03.- ☑
    due to ice or snow W00.0- ☑
   as, or caused by, a crowd or human stampede (with fall) W52.- ☑
   assault Y04.2- ☑
   homicide (attempt) Y04.2- ☑
   in legal intervention
    injuring
     bystander Y35.812- ☑
     law enforcement personnel Y35.811- ☑
     suspect Y35.813- ☑
     unspecified person Y35.819- ☑
   sports equipment W21.9- ☑
 police (on duty) — *see* Legal, intervention, manhandling
  with blunt object — *see* Legal, intervention, blunt object
 sports equipment W21.9- ☑
  assault Y08.09- ☑
  ball W21.00- ☑
   baseball W21.03- ☑
   basketball W21.05- ☑
   football W21.01- ☑
   golf ball W21.04- ☑
   soccer W21.02- ☑
   soft ball W21.07- ☑
   specified NEC W21.09- ☑
   volleyball W21.06- ☑
  bat or racquet
   baseball bat W21.11- ☑
    assault Y08.02- ☑
   golf club W21.13- ☑
    assault Y08.09- ☑
   specified NEC W21.19- ☑
   tennis racquet W21.12- ☑
    assault Y08.09- ☑
  cleats (shoe) W21.31- ☑
  foot wear NEC W21.39- ☑
  football helmet W21.81- ☑
  hockey (ice)
   field
    puck W21.221- ☑
    stick W21.211- ☑
   puck W21.220- ☑
   stick W21.210- ☑
    assault Y08.01- ☑
  skate blades W21.32- ☑
  specified NEC W21.89- ☑
   assault Y08.09- ☑
 thunderbolt — *see* subcategory T75.0- ☑
  causing fire — *see* Exposure, fire
 transport vehicle NEC — *see also* Accident, transport V09.9- ☑
  intentional, homicide (attempt) Y03.0- ☑
  motor NEC — *see also* Accident, transport V09.20- ☑
   homicide Y03.0- ☑
  vehicle (transport) NEC — *see* Accident, transport, by type of vehicle

Struck (accidentally) **by** — *continued*
 vehicle — *see* Accident, transport, by type of vehicle — *continued*
  stationary (falling from jack, hydraulic lift, ramp) W20.8- ☑
Stumbling
 over
  animal NEC W01.0- ☑
   with fall W18.09- ☑
  carpet, rug or (small) object W22.8- ☑
   with fall W18.09- ☑
  person W51.- ☑
   with fall W03.- ☑
    due to ice or snow W00.0- ☑
 without fall W18.40- ☑
  due to
   specified NEC W18.49- ☑
   stepping from one level to another W18.43- ☑
   stepping into hole or opening W18.42- ☑
   stepping on object W18.41- ☑
Submersion (accidental) — *see* Drowning
Suffocation (accidental) (by external means) (by pressure) (mechanical) — *see also* category T71.- ☑
 due to, by
  avalanche — *see* Landslide
  explosion — *see* Explosion
  fire — *see* Exposure, fire
  ignition — *see* Ignition
  landslide — *see* Landslide
 in
  burning building X00.8- ☑
  food, any type (aspiration) (ingestion) (inhalation) — *see* categories T17 and T18.- ☑
  machine(ry) — *see* Contact, with, by type of machine
  vomitus (aspiration) (inhalation) T17.81- ☑
Suicide, suicidal (attempted) (by) X83.8- ☑
 blunt object X79.- ☑
 burning, burns X76.- ☑
  hot object X77.9- ☑
   fluid NEC X77.2- ☑
   household appliance X77.3- ☑
   specified NEC X77.8- ☑
   steam X77.0- ☑
   tap water X77.1- ☑
   vapors X77.0- ☑
 caustic substance — *see* Table of Drugs and Chemicals
 cold, extreme X83.2- ☑
 collision of motor vehicle with
  motor vehicle X82.0- ☑
  specified NEC X82.8- ☑
  train X82.1- ☑
  tree X82.2- ☑
 crashing of aircraft X83.0- ☑
 cut (any part of body) X78.9- ☑
 cutting or piercing instrument X78.9- ☑
  dagger X78.2- ☑
  glass X78.0- ☑
  knife X78.1- ☑
  specified NEC X78.8- ☑
  sword X78.2- ☑
 drowning (in) X71.9- ☑
  bathtub X71.0- ☑
  natural water X71.3- ☑
  specified NEC X71.8- ☑
  swimming pool X71.1- ☑
   following fall X71.2- ☑
 electrocution X83.1- ☑
 explosive(s) (material) X75.- ☑
 fire, flames X76.- ☑
 firearm X74.9- ☑
  airgun X74.01- ☑
  handgun X72.- ☑
  hunting rifle X73.1- ☑
  larger X73.9- ☑
   specified NEC X73.8- ☑
  machine gun X73.2- ☑
  shotgun X73.0- ☑
  specified NEC X74.8- ☑
 hanging X83.8- ☑
 hot object — *see* Suicide, burning, hot object
 jumping
  before moving object X81.8- ☑
   motor vehicle X81.0- ☑
   subway train X81.1- ☑
   train X81.1- ☑
  from high place X80.- ☑

Suicide, suicidal — *continued*
 late effect of attempt — *see* X71-X83 with 7th character S
 lying before moving object, train, vehicle X81.8- ☑
 poisoning — *see* Table of Drugs and Chemicals
 puncture (any part of body) — *see* Suicide, cutting or piercing instrument
 scald — *see* Suicide, burning, hot object
 sequelae of attempt — *see* X71-X83 with 7th character S
 sharp object (any) — *see* Suicide, cutting or piercing instrument
 shooting — *see* Suicide, firearm
 specified means NEC X83.8- ☑
 stab (any part of body) — *see* Suicide, cutting or piercing instrument
 steam, hot vapors X77.0- ☑
 strangulation X83.8- ☑
 submersion — *see* Suicide, drowning
 suffocation X83.8- ☑
 wound NEC X83.8- ☑
Sunstroke X32.- ☑
Supersonic waves (causing injury) W42.0- ☑
Surgical procedure, complication of (delayed or as an abnormal reaction without mention of misadventure) — *see also* Complication of or following, by type of procedure
 due to or as a result of misadventure — *see* Misadventure
Swallowed, swallowing
 foreign body — *see* Foreign body, alimentary canal
 poison — *see* Table of Drugs and Chemicals
 substance
  caustic or corrosive — *see* Table of Drugs and Chemicals
  poisonous — *see* Table of Drugs and Chemicals

T

Tackle in sport W03.- ☑
Terrorism (involving) Y38.80- ☑
 biological weapons Y38.6X- ☑
 chemical weapons Y38.7X- ☑
 conflagration Y38.3X- ☑
 drowning and submersion Y38.89- ☑
 explosion Y38.2X- ☑
  destruction of aircraft Y38.1X- ☑
  marine weapons Y38.0X- ☑
 fire Y38.3X- ☑
 firearms Y38.4X- ☑
 hot substances Y38.3X- ☑
 lasers Y38.89- ☑
 nuclear weapons Y38.5X- ☑
 piercing or stabbing instruments Y38.89- ☑
 secondary effects Y38.9X- ☑
 specified method NEC Y38.89- ☑
 suicide bomber Y38.81- ☑
Thirst X58.- ☑
Threat to breathing
 aspiration — *see* Aspiration
 due to cave-in, falling earth or substance NEC T71.- ☑
Thrown (accidentally)
 against part (any) of or object in transport vehicle (in motion) NEC — *see also* Accident, transport
 from
  high place, homicide (attempt) Y01.- ☑
  machinery — *see* Contact, with, by type of machine
  transport vehicle NEC — *see also* Accident, transport V89.9- ☑
 off — *see* Thrown, from
Thunderbolt — *see* subcategory T75.0- ☑
 causing fire — *see* Exposure, fire
Tidal wave (any injury) **NEC** — *see* Forces of nature, tidal wave
Took
 overdose (drug) — *see* Table of Drugs and Chemicals
 poison — *see* Table of Drugs and Chemicals
Tornado (any injury) X37.1- ☑
Torrential rain (any injury) X37.8- ☑
Torture X58.- ☑
Trampled by animal NEC W55.89- ☑
Trapped (accidentally)
 between objects (moving) (stationary and moving) — *see* Caught
 by part (any) of
  electric (assisted) bicycle V29.881- ☑
  motorcycle V29.888- ☑
  pedal cycle V19.88- ☑

Trapped — *continued*
  by part of — *continued*
    transport vehicle NEC — *see also* Accident, transport V89.9- ☑

Travel (effects) (sickness) T75.3- ☑
Tree falling on or hitting (accidentally) (person) W20.8- ☑
Tripping
  over
    animal W01.0- ☑
      with fall W01.0- ☑
    carpet, rug or (small) object W22.8- ☑
      with fall W18.09- ☑
    person W51.- ☑
      with fall W03.- ☑
        due to ice or snow W00.0- ☑
  without fall W18.40- ☑
    due to
      specified NEC W18.49- ☑
      stepping from one level to another W18.43- ☑
      stepping into hole or opening W18.42- ☑
      stepping on object W18.41- ☑
Twisted by person(s) (accidentally) W50.2- ☑
  with intent to injure or kill Y04.0- ☑
  as, or caused by, a crowd or human stampede (with fall) W52.- ☑
  assault Y04.0- ☑
  homicide (attempt) Y04.0- ☑
  in
    fight Y04.0- ☑
    legal intervention — *see* Legal, intervention, manhandling
Twisting (prolonged) (static) X50.1- ☑

U

Underdosing of necessary drugs, medicaments or biological substances Y63.6
Undetermined intent (contact) (exposure)
  automobile collision Y32.- ☑
  blunt object Y29.- ☑
  drowning (submersion) (in) Y21.9- ☑
    bathtub Y21.0- ☑
      after fall Y21.1- ☑
    natural water (lake) (ocean) (pond) (river) (stream) Y21.4- ☑
    specified place NEC Y21.8- ☑
    swimming pool Y21.2- ☑
      after fall Y21.3- ☑
  explosive material Y25.- ☑
  fall, jump or push from high place Y30.- ☑
  falling, lying or running before moving object Y31.- ☑
  fire Y26.- ☑
  firearm discharge Y24.9- ☑
    airgun (BB) (pellet) Y24.0- ☑
    handgun (pistol) (revolver) Y22.- ☑
    hunting rifle Y23.1- ☑
    larger Y23.9- ☑
      hunting rifle Y23.1- ☑
      machine gun Y23.3- ☑
      military Y23.2- ☑
      shotgun Y23.0- ☑
      specified type NEC Y23.8- ☑
    machine gun Y23.3- ☑
    military Y23.2- ☑
    shotgun Y23.0- ☑
    specified type NEC Y24.8- ☑
    Very pistol Y24.8- ☑
  hot object Y27.9- ☑
    fluid NEC Y27.2- ☑
    household appliance Y27.3- ☑
    specified object NEC Y27.8- ☑
    steam Y27.0- ☑
    tap water Y27.1- ☑
    vapor Y27.0- ☑
  jump, fall or push from high place Y30.- ☑
  lying, falling or running before moving object Y31.- ☑
  motor vehicle crash Y32.- ☑
  push, fall or jump from high place Y30.- ☑
  running, falling or lying before moving object Y31.- ☑
  sharp object Y28.9- ☑
    dagger Y28.2- ☑
    glass Y28.0- ☑
    knife Y28.1- ☑
    specified object NEC Y28.8- ☑
    sword Y28.2- ☑

Undetermined intent — *continued*
  smoke Y26.- ☑
  specified event NEC Y33.- ☑
Use of hand as hammer X50.3- ☑

V

Vibration (causing injury) W49.9- ☑
Victim (of)
  avalanche — *see* Landslide
  earth movements NEC — *see* Forces of nature, earth movement
  earthquake X34.- ☑
  flood — *see* Flood
  landslide — *see* Landslide
  lightning — *see* subcategory T75.0- ☑
    causing fire — *see* Exposure, fire
  storm (cataclysmic) NEC — *see* Forces of nature, cataclysmic storm
  volcanic eruption X35.- ☑
Volcanic eruption (any injury) X35.- ☑
Vomitus, gastric contents in air passages (with asphyxia, obstruction or suffocation) T17.81- ☑

W

Walked into stationary object (any) W22.09- ☑
  furniture W22.03- ☑
  lamppost W22.02- ☑
  wall W22.01- ☑
War operations (injuries to military personnel and civilians during war, civil insurrection and peacekeeping missions) (by) (from) (involving) Y36.90- ☑
  after cessation of hostilities Y36.89- ☑
    explosion (of)
      bomb placed during war operations Y36.82- ☑
      mine placed during war operations Y36.81- ☑
    specified NEC Y36.88- ☑
  air blast Y36.20- ☑
  aircraft
    destruction — *see* War operations, destruction of aircraft
  airway restriction — *see* War operations, restriction of airways
  asphyxiation — *see* War operations, restriction of airways
  biological weapons Y36.6X- ☑
  blast Y36.20- ☑
  blast fragments Y36.20- ☑
  blast overpressure
    high level (due to explosion) Y36.A2- ☑
    low level (due to explosion) Y36.A1- ☑
  blast wave Y36.20- ☑
  blast wind Y36.20- ☑
  bomb Y36.20- ☑
    dirty Y36.50- ☑
    gasoline Y36.31- ☑
    incendiary Y36.31- ☑
    petrol Y36.31- ☑
  bullet Y36.43- ☑
    incendiary Y36.32- ☑
    rubber Y36.41- ☑
  chemical weapons Y36.7X- ☑
  combat
    hand to hand (unarmed) combat Y36.44- ☑
    using blunt or piercing object Y36.45- ☑
  conflagration — *see* War operations, fire
  conventional warfare NEC Y36.49- ☑
  depth-charge Y36.01- ☑
  destruction of aircraft Y36.10- ☑
    due to
      air to air missile Y36.11- ☑
      collision with other aircraft Y36.12- ☑
      detonation (accidental) of onboard munitions and explosives Y36.14- ☑
      enemy fire or explosives Y36.11- ☑
      explosive placed on aircraft Y36.11- ☑
      onboard fire Y36.13- ☑
      rocket propelled grenade [RPG] Y36.11- ☑
      small arms fire Y36.11- ☑
      surface to air missile Y36.11- ☑
    specified NEC Y36.19- ☑
  detonation (accidental) of
    onboard marine weapons Y36.05- ☑
    own munitions or munitions launch device Y36.24- ☑
  dirty bomb Y36.50- ☑
  explosion (of) Y36.20- ☑

War operations — *continued*
  explosion — *continued*
    aerial bomb Y36.21- ☑
    after cessation of hostilities
      bomb placed during war operations Y36.82- ☑
      mine placed during war operations Y36.81- ☑
    bomb NOS — *see also* War operations, bomb(s) Y36.20- ☑
    fragments Y36.20- ☑
    grenade Y36.29- ☑
    guided missile Y36.22- ☑
    improvised explosive device [IED] (person-borne) (roadside) (vehicle-borne) Y36.23- ☑
    land mine Y36.29- ☑
    marine mine (at sea) (in harbor) Y36.02- ☑
    marine weapon Y36.00- ☑
      specified NEC Y36.09- ☑
    own munitions or munitions launch device (accidental) Y36.24- ☑
    sea-based artillery shell Y36.03- ☑
    specified NEC Y36.29- ☑
    torpedo Y36.04- ☑
  fire Y36.30- ☑
    specified NEC Y36.39- ☑
  firearms
    discharge Y36.43- ☑
    pellets Y36.42- ☑
  flamethrower Y36.33- ☑
  fragments (from) (of)
    improvised explosive device [IED] (person-borne) (roadside) (vehicle-borne) Y36.26- ☑
    munitions Y36.25- ☑
    specified NEC Y36.29- ☑
    weapons Y36.27- ☑
  friendly fire Y36.92- ☑
  hand to hand (unarmed) combat Y36.44- ☑
  HLB overpressure Y36.A2- ☑
  hot substances — *see* War operations, fire
  incendiary bullet Y36.32- ☑
  LLB overpressure Y36.A1- ☑
  nuclear weapon (effects of) Y36.50- ☑
    acute radiation exposure Y36.54- ☑
    blast pressure Y36.51- ☑
    direct blast Y36.51- ☑
    direct heat Y36.53- ☑
    fallout exposure Y36.54- ☑
    fireball Y36.53- ☑
    indirect blast (struck or crushed by blast debris) (being thrown by blast) Y36.52- ☑
    ionizing radiation (immediate exposure) Y36.54- ☑
    nuclear radiation Y36.54- ☑
    radiation
      ionizing (immediate exposure) Y36.54- ☑
        nuclear Y36.54- ☑
        thermal Y36.53- ☑
    secondary effects Y36.54- ☑
    specified NEC Y36.59- ☑
    thermal radiation Y36.53- ☑
  restriction of air (airway)
    intentional Y36.46- ☑
    unintentional Y36.47- ☑
  rubber bullets Y36.41- ☑
  shrapnel NOS Y36.29- ☑
  suffocation — *see* War operations, restriction of airways
  unconventional warfare NEC Y36.7X- ☑
  underwater blast NOS Y36.00- ☑
  warfare
    conventional NEC Y36.49- ☑
    unconventional NEC Y36.7X- ☑
  weapon of mass destruction [WMD] Y36.91- ☑
  weapons
    biological weapons Y36.6X- ☑
    chemical Y36.7X- ☑
    nuclear (effects of) Y36.50- ☑
      acute radiation exposure Y36.54- ☑
      blast pressure Y36.51- ☑
      direct blast Y36.51- ☑
      direct heat Y36.53- ☑
      fallout exposure Y36.54- ☑
      fireball Y36.53- ☑
      radiation
        ionizing (immediate exposure) Y36.54- ☑
          nuclear Y36.54- ☑
          thermal Y36.53- ☑
      secondary effects Y36.54- ☑

War operations — *continued*
  weapons — *continued*
    nuclear — *continued*
      specified NEC Y36.59- ☑
      of mass destruction [WMD] Y36.91- ☑
Washed
  away by flood — *see* Flood
  off road by storm (transport vehicle) — *see* Forces of nature, cataclysmic storm

Weather exposure NEC — *see* Forces of nature
Weightlessness (causing injury) (effects of) (in spacecraft, real or simulated) X52.- ☑
Work related condition Y99.0
Wound (accidental) NEC — *see also* Injury X58.- ☑
  battle — *see also* War operations Y36.90- ☑
  gunshot — *see* Discharge, firearm by type

Wreck transport vehicle NEC — *see also* Accident, transport V89.9- ☑
Wrong
  device implanted into correct surgical site Y65.51
  fluid in infusion Y65.1
  patient, procedure performed on Y65.52
  procedure (operation) on correct patient Y65.51

ICD-10-CM Tabular List of Diseases and Injuries

Chapter 1. Certain Infectious and Parasitic Diseases (A00–B99), U07.1, U09.9

Chapter-specific Guidelines with Coding Examples
The chapter-specific guidelines from the ICD-10-CM Official Guidelines for Coding and Reporting have been provided below. Along with these guidelines are coding examples, contained in the shaded boxes, that have been developed to help illustrate the coding and/or sequencing guidance found in these guidelines.

a. **Human immunodeficiency virus (HIV) infections**
   1) **Code only confirmed cases**
      Code only confirmed cases of HIV infection/illness. This is an exception to the hospital inpatient guideline Section II, H.
      In this context, "confirmation" does not require documentation of positive serology or culture for HIV; the provider's diagnostic statement that the patient is HIV positive or has an HIV-related illness is sufficient.

      > Patient being seen for hypothyroidism with possible HIV infection
      >
      > **E03.9**   Hypothyroidism, unspecified
      >
      > *Explanation:* Only the hypothyroidism is coded in this scenario because it has not been confirmed that an HIV infection is present.

   2) **Selection and sequencing of HIV codes**
      (a) *HIV disease*
         If the term "AIDS" or "HIV disease" is documented or if the patient is treated for any HIV-related illness or is described as having any condition(s) resulting from the patient's HIV positive status; code B20, Human immunodeficiency virus [HIV], should be assigned.
      (b) **Patient admitted for HIV-related condition**
         If a patient is admitted for an HIV-related condition, the principal diagnosis should be B20, Human immunodeficiency virus [HIV] disease followed by additional diagnosis codes for all reported HIV-related conditions.
         An exception to this guideline is if the reason for admission is hemolytic-uremic syndrome associated with HIV disease. Assign code D59.31, Infection-associated hemolytic-uremic syndrome, followed by code B20, Human immunodeficiency virus [HIV] disease.

         > HIV with CMV
         >
         > **B20**   Human immunodeficiency virus [HIV] disease
         > **B25.9** Cytomegaloviral disease, unspecified
         >
         > *Explanation:* Cytomegaloviral infection is an HIV related condition, so the HIV diagnosis code is reported first, followed by the code for the CMV.

      (c) **Patient with HIV disease admitted for unrelated condition**
         If a patient with HIV disease is admitted for an unrelated condition (such as a traumatic injury), the code for the unrelated condition (e.g., the nature of injury code) should be the principal diagnosis. Code B20 would be reported as a secondary diagnosis. Codes for other documented conditions should also be reported as secondary diagnoses.

         > Sprain of the internal collateral ligament, right ankle; HIV
         >
         > **S93.491A** Sprain of other ligament of right ankle, initial encounter
         > **B20**   Human immunodeficiency virus [HIV] disease
         >
         > *Explanation:* The ankle sprain is not related to HIV, so it is the first-listed diagnosis code, and HIV is reported secondarily.

      (d) *Patient newly diagnosed with HIV disease*
         Whether the patient is newly diagnosed or has had previous admissions/encounters for HIV conditions is irrelevant to the sequencing decision.

         > Newly diagnosed multiple cutaneous Kaposi's sarcoma lesions in previously diagnosed HIV disease
         >
         > **B20**   Human immunodeficiency virus [HIV] disease
         > **C46.0** Kaposi's sarcoma of skin
         >
         > *Explanation:* Even though the HIV was diagnosed on a previous encounter, it is still sequenced first when coded with an HIV-related condition. Kaposi's sarcoma is an HIV-related condition.

      (e) **Asymptomatic human immunodeficiency virus**
         When "HIV positive," "HIV test positive," or similar terminology is documented, and there is no documentation of symptoms or HIV-related illness, code Z21, Asymptomatic human immunodeficiency virus [HIV] infection status, should be assigned.
      (f) *Inconclusive HIV serology*
         Patients with documentation of inconclusive HIV serology, may be assigned code R75, Inconclusive laboratory evidence of human immunodeficiency virus [HIV].
      (g) **Previously diagnosed HIV-related illness**
         Patients with documentation of a prior diagnosis of an HIV-related illness should be coded to B20. Once an HIV-related illness has developed, code B20 should always be assigned on every subsequent admission/encounter. Patients previously diagnosed with any HIV illness (B20) should never be assigned to R75, Inconclusive laboratory evidence of human immunodeficiency virus [HIV] or Z21, Asymptomatic human immunodeficiency virus [HIV] infection status.
      (h) **HIV Infection in pregnancy, childbirth and the puerperium**
         When a patient presents during pregnancy, childbirth or the puerperium with documented symptomatic HIV disease or an HIV related illness, assign a code from subcategory O98.7, Human immunodeficiency [HIV] disease complicating pregnancy, childbirth and the puerperium, followed by code B20 and additional code(s) for any HIV-related illness(es). Codes from Chapter 15 always take sequencing priority.

         When a patient presents during pregnancy, childbirth or the puerperium with documented asymptomatic HIV infection status or is HIV-positive, assign a code from subcategory O98.7 followed by code Z21.
      (i) *Encounters for HIV testing*
         If a patient without signs or symptoms is tested for HIV, assign code Z11.4, Encounter for screening for human immunodeficiency virus [HIV]. Use additional codes for any associated high-risk behavior, if applicable.

         If a patient with signs or symptoms of HIV presents for HIV testing, code the signs and symptoms. An additional counseling code Z71.7, Human immunodeficiency virus [HIV] counseling, may be assigned if counseling is provided during the encounter for the test. Code Z11.4, Encounter for screening for human immunodeficiency virus [HIV], should not be assigned if HIV signs or symptoms are present.

         When a patient presents for follow up regarding their HIV test results and the test result is negative, assign code Z71.7, Human immunodeficiency virus [HIV] counseling.

         If the results are positive, see previous guidelines and assign codes as appropriate.
      (j) *HIV disease or HIV positive status managed by antiretroviral medication*
         If a patient with documented HIV disease, HIV-related illness or AIDS is currently managed on antiretroviral medications, assign code B20, Human immunodeficiency virus [HIV] disease.

         If a patient with documented HIV positive status is currently managed on antiretroviral medication, assign code Z21, Asymptomatic human immunodeficiency virus [HIV] infection status, in the absence of any additional documentation of HIV disease, HIV-related illness or AIDS.

         Code Z79.899, Other long term (current) drug therapy, may be assigned as an additional code to identify the long-term (current) use of antiretroviral medications.
      (k) **Encounter for HIV prophylaxis measures**
         When a patient is seen for administration of pre-exposure prophylaxis medication for HIV, assign code Z29.81, Encounter for HIV pre-exposure prophylaxis. Pre-exposure prophylaxis (PrEP) is intended to prevent infection in people who are at risk for getting HIV through sex or injection drug use. Any risk factors for HIV should also be coded.

b. **Infectious agents as the cause of diseases classified to other chapters**
   Certain infections are classified in chapters other than Chapter 1 and no organism is identified as part of the infection code. In these instances, it is necessary to use an additional code from Chapter 1 to identify the organism.

A code from category B95, Streptococcus, Staphylococcus, and Enterococcus as the cause of diseases classified to other chapters, B96, Other bacterial agents as the cause of diseases classified to other chapters, or B97, Viral agents as the cause of diseases classified to other chapters, is to be used as an additional code to identify the organism. An instructional note will be found at the infection code advising that an additional organism code is required.

Acute *E. coli* cystitis

N30.00	Acute cystitis without hematuria
B96.20	Unspecified Escherichia coli [E.coli] as the cause of diseases classified elsewhere

Explanation: An instructional note under the category for the cystitis indicates to code also the specific organism.

c. **Infections resistant to antibiotics**

Many bacterial infections are resistant to current antibiotics. It is necessary to identify all infections documented as antibiotic resistant. Assign a code from category Z16, Resistance to antimicrobial drugs, following the infection code only if the infection code does not identify drug resistance.

Penicillin-resistant *Streptococcus pneumoniae* pneumonia

J13	Pneumonia due to Streptococcus pneumoniae
Z16.11	Resistance to penicillins

Explanation: Code Z16.11 is assigned as a secondary code to represent the penicillin resistance. This code includes resistance to amoxicillin and ampicillin.

d. **Sepsis, severe sepsis, and septic shock infections resistant to antibiotics**

1) **Coding of Sepsis and Severe Sepsis**

   (a) **Sepsis**

   For a diagnosis of sepsis, assign the appropriate code for the underlying systemic infection. If the type of infection or causal organism is not further specified, assign code A41.9, Sepsis, unspecified organism.

   A code from subcategory R65.2, Severe sepsis, should not be assigned unless severe sepsis or an associated acute organ dysfunction is documented.

   Gram-negative sepsis

A41.50	Gram-negative sepsis, unspecified

   Staphylococcal sepsis

A41.2	Sepsis due to unspecified staphylococcus

   Explanation: In both examples above the organism causing the sepsis is identified, therefore A41.9 Sepsis, unspecified organism, would not be appropriate as this code would not capture the highest degree of specificity found in the documentation. Do not use an additional code for severe sepsis unless an acute organ dysfunction was also documented as "associated with" or "due to" the sepsis or the sepsis was documented as "severe."

   (i) **Negative or inconclusive blood cultures and sepsis**

   Negative or inconclusive blood cultures do not preclude a diagnosis of sepsis in patients with clinical evidence of the condition; however, the provider should be queried.

   (ii) **Urosepsis**

   The term urosepsis is a nonspecific term. It is not to be considered synonymous with sepsis. It has no default code in the Alphabetic Index. Should a provider use this term, he/she must be queried for clarification.

   (iii) **Sepsis with organ dysfunction**

   If a patient has sepsis and associated acute organ dysfunction or multiple organ dysfunction (MOD), follow the instructions for coding severe sepsis.

   (iv) **Acute organ dysfunction that is not clearly associated with the sepsis**

   If a patient has sepsis and an acute organ dysfunction, but the medical record documentation indicates that the acute organ dysfunction is related to a medical condition other than the sepsis, do not assign a code from subcategory R65.2, Severe sepsis. An acute organ dysfunction must be associated with the sepsis in order to assign the severe sepsis code. If the documentation is not clear as to whether an acute organ dysfunction is related to the sepsis or another medical condition, query the provider.

Sepsis and acute respiratory failure due to COPD exacerbation

A41.9	Sepsis, unspecified organism
J44.1	Chronic obstructive pulmonary disease with (acute) exacerbation
J96.00	Acute respiratory failure, unspecified whether with hypoxia or hypercapnia

Explanation: Although acute organ dysfunction is present in the form of acute respiratory failure, severe sepsis (R65.2) is not coded in this example, as the acute respiratory failure is attributed to the COPD exacerbation rather than the sepsis. Sequencing of these codes would be determined by the reason for the encounter.

(b) **Severe sepsis**

The coding of severe sepsis requires a minimum of 2 codes: first a code for the underlying systemic infection, followed by a code from subcategory R65.2, Severe sepsis. If the causal organism is not documented, assign code A41.9, Sepsis, unspecified organism, for the infection. Additional code(s) for the associated acute organ dysfunction are also required.

Due to the complex nature of severe sepsis, some cases may require querying the provider prior to assignment of the codes.

2) **Septic shock**

Septic shock generally refers to circulatory failure associated with severe sepsis, and therefore, it represents a type of acute organ dysfunction.

For cases of septic shock, the code for the systemic infection should be sequenced first, followed by code R65.21, Severe sepsis with septic shock or code T81.12, Postprocedural septic shock. Any additional codes for the other acute organ dysfunctions should also be assigned. As noted in the sequencing instructions in the Tabular List, the code for septic shock cannot be assigned as a principal diagnosis.

Sepsis with septic shock

A41.9	Sepsis, unspecified organism
R65.21	Severe sepsis with septic shock

Explanation: Documentation of septic shock automatically implies severe sepsis as it is a form of acute organ dysfunction. Septic shock is not coded as the first-listed diagnosis; it is always preceded by the code for the systemic infection.

3) **Sequencing of severe sepsis**

If severe sepsis is present on admission, and meets the definition of principal diagnosis, the underlying systemic infection should be assigned as principal diagnosis followed by the appropriate code from subcategory R65.2 as required by the sequencing rules in the Tabular List. A code from subcategory R65.2 can never be assigned as a principal diagnosis.

When severe sepsis develops during an encounter (it was not present on admission), the underlying systemic infection and the appropriate code from subcategory R65.2 should be assigned as secondary diagnoses.

Severe sepsis may be present on admission, but the diagnosis may not be confirmed until sometime after admission. If the documentation is not clear whether severe sepsis was present on admission, the provider should be queried.

For infection-associated hemolytic-uremic syndrome with severe sepsis, see guideline I.C.1.d.9.

4) **Sepsis or severe sepsis with a localized infection**

If the reason for admission is sepsis or severe sepsis and a localized infection, such as pneumonia or cellulitis, a code(s) for the underlying systemic infection should be assigned first and the code for the localized infection should be assigned as a secondary diagnosis. If the patient has severe sepsis, a code from subcategory R65.2 should also be assigned as a secondary diagnosis. If the patient is admitted with a localized infection, such as pneumonia, and sepsis/severe sepsis doesn't develop until after admission, the localized infection should be assigned first, followed by the appropriate sepsis/severe sepsis codes.

For hemolytic-uremic syndrome associated with sepsis, see guideline I.C.1.d.9.

Patient presents with acute renal failure due to severe sepsis from *Pseudomonas pneumonia*

A41.52	Sepsis due to Pseudomonas
J15.1	Pneumonia due to Pseudomonas
R65.20	Severe sepsis without septic shock
N17.9	Acute kidney failure, unspecified

Explanation: If all conditions are present, the systemic infection (sepsis) is sequenced first followed by the codes for the localized infection (pneumonia), severe sepsis and any organ dysfunction.

5) Sepsis due to a postprocedural infection

(a) Documentation of causal relationship

As with all postprocedural complications, code assignment is based on the provider's documentation of the relationship between the infection and the procedure.

(b) Sepsis due to a postprocedural infection

For sepsis following a postprocedural wound (surgical site) infection, a code from T81.41 to T81.43, Infection following a procedure, T81.49, Infection following a procedure, other surgical site, or a code from O86.00 to O86.03, Infection of obstetric surgical wound, or code O86.09, Infection of obstetric surgical wound, other surgical site, that identifies the site of the infection should be sequenced first, if known. Assign an additional code for sepsis following a procedure (T81.44) or sepsis following an obstetrical procedure (O86.04). Use an additional code to identify the infectious agent. If the patient has severe sepsis, the appropriate code from subcategory R65.2 should also be assigned with the additional code(s) for any acute organ dysfunction.

For infections following infusion, transfusion, therapeutic injection, or immunization, a code from subcategory T80.2, Infections following infusion, transfusion, and therapeutic injection, or code T88.0-, Infection following immunization, should be coded first, followed by the code for the specific infection. If the patient has severe sepsis, the appropriate code from subcategory R65.2 should also be assigned, with the additional codes(s) for any acute organ dysfunction.

(c) Postprocedural infection and postprocedural septic shock

If a postprocedural infection has resulted in postprocedural septic shock, assign the codes indicated above for sepsis due to a postprocedural infection, followed by code T81.12-, Postprocedural septic shock. Do not assign code R65.21, Severe sepsis with septic shock. Additional code(s) should be assigned for any acute organ dysfunction.

6) Sepsis and severe sepsis associated with a noninfectious process (condition)

In some cases, a noninfectious process (condition) such as trauma, may lead to an infection which can result in sepsis or severe sepsis. If sepsis or severe sepsis is documented as associated with a noninfectious condition, such as a burn or serious injury, and this condition meets the definition for principal diagnosis, the code for the noninfectious condition should be sequenced first, followed by the code for the resulting infection. If severe sepsis is present, a code from subcategory R65.2 should also be assigned with any associated organ dysfunction(s) codes. It is not necessary to assign a code from subcategory R65.1, Systemic inflammatory response syndrome (SIRS) of non-infectious origin, for these cases.

If the infection meets the definition of principal diagnosis, it should be sequenced before the non-infectious condition. When both the associated non-infectious condition and the infection meet the definition of principal diagnosis, either may be assigned as principal diagnosis.

Only one code from category R65, Symptoms and signs specifically associated with systemic inflammation and infection, should be assigned. Therefore, when a non-infectious condition leads to an infection resulting in severe sepsis, assign the appropriate code from subcategory R65.2, Severe sepsis. Do not additionally assign a code from subcategory R65.1, Systemic inflammatory response syndrome (SIRS) of non-infectious origin.

See Section I.C.18. SIRS due to non-infectious process

7) Sepsis and septic shock complicating abortion, pregnancy, childbirth, and the puerperium

See Section I.C.15. Sepsis and septic shock complicating abortion, pregnancy, childbirth and the puerperium

8) Newborn sepsis

See Section I.C.16. f. Bacterial sepsis of Newborn

9) Hemolytic-uremic syndrome associated with sepsis

If the reason for admission is hemolytic-uremic syndrome that is associated with sepsis, assign code D59.31, Infection-associated hemolytic-uremic syndrome, as the principal diagnosis. Codes for the underlying systemic infection and any other conditions (such as severe sepsis) should be assigned as secondary diagnoses.

e. Methicillin resistant Staphylococcus aureus (MRSA) conditions

1) Selection and sequencing of MRSA codes

(a) Combination codes for MRSA infection

When a patient is diagnosed with an infection that is due to methicillin resistant *Staphylococcus aureus* (MRSA), and that infection has a combination code that includes the causal organism (e.g., sepsis, pneumonia) assign the appropriate combination code for the condition (e.g., code A41.02, Sepsis due to Methicillin resistant Staphylococcus aureus or code J15.212, Pneumonia due to Methicillin resistant Staphylococcus aureus). Do not assign code B95.62, Methicillin resistant Staphylococcus aureus infection as the cause of diseases classified elsewhere, as an additional code, because the combination code includes the type of infection and the MRSA organism. Do not assign a code from subcategory Z16.11, Resistance to penicillins, as an additional diagnosis.

See Section C.1. for instructions on coding and sequencing of sepsis and severe sepsis.

(b) Other codes for MRSA infection

When there is documentation of a current infection (e.g., wound infection, stitch abscess, urinary tract infection) due to MRSA, and that infection does not have a combination code that includes the causal organism, assign the appropriate code to identify the condition along with code B95.62, Methicillin resistant Staphylococcus aureus infection as the cause of diseases classified elsewhere for the MRSA infection. Do not assign a code from subcategory Z16.11, Resistance to penicillins.

(c) Methicillin susceptible Staphylococcus aureus (MSSA) and MRSA colonization

The condition or state of being colonized or carrying MSSA or MRSA is called colonization or carriage, while an individual person is described as being colonized or being a carrier.

Colonization means that MSSA or MSRA is present on or in the body without necessarily causing illness. A positive MRSA colonization test might be documented by the provider as "MRSA screen positive" or "MRSA nasal swab positive".

Assign code Z22.322, Carrier or suspected carrier of Methicillin resistant Staphylococcus aureus, for patients documented as having MRSA colonization. Assign code Z22.321, Carrier or suspected carrier of Methicillin susceptible Staphylococcus aureus, for patients documented as having MSSA colonization. Colonization is not necessarily indicative of a disease process or as the cause of a specific condition the patient may have unless documented as such by the provider.

(d) MRSA colonization and infection

If a patient is documented as having both MRSA colonization and infection during a hospital admission, code Z22.322, Carrier or suspected carrier of Methicillin resistant Staphylococcus aureus, and a code for the MRSA infection may both be assigned.

f. Zika virus infections

1) Code only confirmed cases

Code only a confirmed diagnosis of Zika virus (A92.5, Zika virus disease) as documented by the provider. This is an exception to the hospital inpatient guideline Section II, H. In this context, "confirmation" does not require documentation of the type of test performed; the provider's diagnostic statement that the condition is confirmed is sufficient. This code should be assigned regardless of the stated mode of transmission.

If the provider documents "suspected", "possible" or "probable" Zika, do not assign code A92.5. Assign a code(s) explaining the reason for encounter (such as fever, rash, or joint pain) or Z20.821, Contact with and (suspected) exposure to Zika virus.

g. Coronavirus infections

1) COVID-19 infection (infection due to SARS-CoV-2)

(a) Code only confirmed cases

Code only a confirmed diagnosis of the 2019 novel coronavirus disease (COVID-19) as documented by the provider. For a confirmed diagnosis, assign code U07.1, COVID-19. This is an exception to the hospital inpatient guideline Section II, H. In this context, "confirmation" does not require documentation of a positive test result for COVID-19; the provider's documentation that the individual has COVID-19 is sufficient.

If the provider documents "suspected," "possible," "probable," or "inconclusive" COVID-19, do not assign code U07.1. Instead, code the signs and symptoms reported. See guideline I.C.1.g.1.g.

> Patient presents with cough and a slight fever and fear they were exposed to the coronavirus. The provider documents cough, temperature of 99.4, lungs clear, rule out COVID-19.
>
> | | |
> |---|---|
> | R50.9 | Fever, unspecified |
> | R05.9 | Cough, unspecified |
> | Z20.822 | Contact with and (suspected) exposure to COVID-19 |
>
> *Explanation*: For patients who have been exposed or fear they have been exposed to coronavirus, report codes for signs and symptoms, followed by the Z code. Report U07.1 COVID-19, only when the diagnosis is confirmed through provider documentation.

(b) Sequencing of codes

When COVID-19 meets the definition of principal diagnosis, code U07.1, COVID-19, should be sequenced first, followed by the appropriate codes for associated manifestations, except when another guideline requires that certain codes be sequenced first, such as obstetrics, sepsis, or transplant complications.

For a COVID-19 infection that progresses to sepsis, see Section I.C.1.d. Sepsis, Severe Sepsis, and Septic Shock

See Section I.C.15.s. for COVID-19 infection in pregnancy, childbirth, and the puerperium

See Section I.C.16.h. for COVID-19 infection in newborn

For a COVID-19 infection in a lung transplant patient, see Section I.C.19.g.3.a. Transplant complications other than kidney.

(c) Acute respiratory manifestations of COVID-19

When the reason for the encounter/admission is a respiratory manifestation of COVID-19, assign code U07.1, COVID-19, as the principal/first-listed diagnosis and assign code(s) for the respiratory manifestation(s) as additional diagnoses.

The following conditions are examples of common respiratory manifestations of COVID-19.

(i) Pneumonia

For a patient with pneumonia confirmed as due to COVID-19, assign codes U07.1, COVID-19, and J12.82, Pneumonia due to coronavirus disease 2019.

(ii) Acute bronchitis

For a patient with acute bronchitis confirmed as due to COVID-19, assign codes U07.1, and J20.8, Acute bronchitis due to other specified organisms.

Bronchitis not otherwise specified (NOS) due to COVID-19 should be coded using code U07.1 and J40, Bronchitis, not specified as acute or chronic.

(iii) Lower respiratory infection

If the COVID-19 is documented as being associated with a lower respiratory infection, not otherwise specified (NOS), or an acute respiratory infection, NOS, codes U07.1 and J22, Unspecified acute lower respiratory infection, should be assigned.

If the COVID-19 is documented as being associated with a respiratory infection, NOS, codes U07.1 and J98.8, Other specified respiratory disorders, should be assigned.

(iv) Acute respiratory distress syndrome

For acute respiratory distress syndrome (ARDS) due to COVID-19, assign codes U07.1, and J80, Acute respiratory distress syndrome.

(v) Acute respiratory failure

For acute respiratory failure due to COVID-19, assign code U07.1, and code J96.0-, Acute respiratory failure.

(d) Non-respiratory manifestations of COVID-19

When the reason for the encounter/admission is a non-respiratory manifestation (e.g., viral enteritis) of COVID-19, assign code U07.1, COVID-19, as the principal/first-listed diagnosis and assign code(s) for the manifestation(s) as additional diagnoses.

(e) Exposure to COVID-19

For asymptomatic individuals with actual or suspected exposure to COVID-19, assign code Z20.822, Contact with and (suspected) exposure to COVID-19.

For symptomatic individuals with actual or suspected exposure to COVID-19 and the infection has been ruled out, or test results are inconclusive or unknown, assign code Z20.822, Contact with and (suspected) exposure to COVID-19. See guideline I.C.21.c.1, Contact/Exposure, for additional guidance regarding the use of category Z20 codes.

If COVID-19 is confirmed, see guideline I.C.1.g.1.a.

Patient was exposed to COVID-19 by a family member. They are asymptomatic and their test result is negative.

Z20.822   Contact with and (suspected) exposure to COVID-19

Explanation: Report Z20.822 for patients who have a negative test result but have known exposure to someone who has tested positive for COVID-19.

(f) Screening for COVID-19

For screening for COVID-19, including preoperative testing, assign code Z11.52, Encounter for screening for COVID-19.

(g) Signs and symptoms without definitive diagnosis of COVID-19

For patients presenting with any signs/symptoms associated with COVID-19 (such as fever, etc.) but a definitive diagnosis has not been established, assign the appropriate code(s) for each of the presenting signs and symptoms such as:

- R05.1, Acute cough, or R05.9, Cough, unspecified
- R06.02 Shortness of breath
- R50.9 Fever, unspecified

If a patient with signs/symptoms associated with COVID-19 also has an actual or suspected contact with or exposure to COVID-19, assign Z20.822, Contact with and (suspected) exposure to COVID19, as an additional code.

(h) Asymptomatic individuals who test positive for COVID-19

For asymptomatic individuals who test positive for COVID-19 and there is no provider documentation of a diagnosis of COVID-19, query the provider as to whether or not the individual has COVID-19. A false positive laboratory test is possible, and it is the provider's responsibility to confirm the diagnosis and document accordingly.

(i) Personal history of COVID-19

For patients with a history of COVID-19, assign code Z86.16, Personal history of COVID-19.

(j) Follow-up visits after COVID-19 infection has resolved

For individuals who previously had COVID-19, without residual symptom(s) or condition(s), and are being seen for follow-up evaluation, and COVID-19 test results are negative, assign codes Z09, Encounter for follow-up examination after completed treatment for conditions other than malignant neoplasm, and Z86.16, Personal history of COVID-19.

For follow-up visits for individuals with symptom(s) or condition(s) related to a previous COVID-19 infection, see guideline I.C.1.g.1.m.

See Section I.C.21.c.8, Factors influencing health states and contact with health services, Follow-up

(k) Encounter for antibody testing

For an encounter for antibody testing that is not being performed to confirm a current COVID-19 infection, nor is a follow-up test after resolution of COVID-19, assign Z01.84, Encounter for antibody response examination.

Follow the applicable guidelines above if the individual is being tested to confirm a current COVID-19 infection.

For follow-up testing after a COVID-19 infection, see guideline I.C.1.g.1.j.

(l) Multisystem inflammatory syndrome

For individuals with multisystem inflammatory syndrome (MIS) and COVID-19, assign code U07.1, COVID-19, as the principal/first-listed diagnosis and assign code M35.81, Multisystem inflammatory syndrome, as an additional diagnosis.

If an individual with a history of COVID-19 develops MIS, assign codes M35.81, Multisystem inflammatory syndrome, and U09.9, Post COVID-19 condition, unspecified.

If an individual with a known or suspected exposure to COVID-19, and no current COVID-19 infection or history of COVID-19, develops MIS, assign codes M35.81, Multisystem inflammatory syndrome, and Z20.822, Contact with and (suspected) exposure to COVID-19.

Additional codes should be assigned for any associated complications of MIS.

(m) Post COVID-19 condition

For sequela of COVID-19, or associated symptoms or conditions that develop following a previous COVID-19 infection, assign a code(s) for the specific symptom(s) or condition(s) related to the previous COVID-19 infection, if known, and code U09.9, Post COVID-19 condition, unspecified.

Code U09.9 should not be assigned for manifestations of an active (current) COVID-19 infection.

If a patient has a condition(s) associated with a previous COVID-19 infection and develops a new active (current) COVID-19 infection, code U09.9 may be assigned in conjunction with code U07.1, COVID-19, to identify that the patient also has a condition(s) associated with a previous COVID-19 infection. Code(s) for the specific condition(s) associated with the previous COVID-19 infection and code(s) for manifestation(s) of the new active (current) COVID-19 infection should also be assigned.

(n) Underimmunization for COVID-19 Status

Code Z28.310, Unvaccinated for COVID-19, may be assigned when the patient has not received a COVID-19 vaccine of any type. Code Z28.311, Partially vaccinated for COVID-19, may be assigned when the patient has been partially vaccinated for COVID-19 as per the recommendations of the Centers for Disease Control and Prevention (CDC) in place at the time of the encounter. For information, visit the CDC's website https://www.cdc.gov/covidschedule.

See Section I.B.14. for underimmunization documentation by clinicians other than patient's provider.

Chapter 1. Certain Infectious and Parasitic Diseases (A00-B99)

INCLUDES diseases generally recognized as communicable or transmissible
Use additional code to identify resistance to antimicrobial drugs (Z16.-)
EXCLUDES 1 certain localized infections - see body system-related chapters
EXCLUDES 2 carrier or suspected carrier of infectious disease (Z22.-)
infectious and parasitic diseases complicating pregnancy, childbirth and the puerperium (O98.-)
infectious and parasitic diseases specific to the perinatal period (P35-P39)
influenza and other acute respiratory infections (J00-J22)

This chapter contains the following blocks:
- A00-A09 Intestinal infectious diseases
- A15-A19 Tuberculosis
- A20-A28 Certain zoonotic bacterial diseases
- A30-A49 Other bacterial diseases
- A50-A64 Infections with a predominantly sexual mode of transmission
- A65-A69 Other spirochetal diseases
- A70-A74 Other diseases caused by chlamydiae
- A75-A79 Rickettsioses
- A80-A89 Viral and prion infections of the central nervous system
- A90-A99 Arthropod-borne viral fevers and viral hemorrhagic fevers
- B00-B09 Viral infections characterized by skin and mucous membrane lesions
- B10 Other human herpesviruses
- B15-B19 Viral hepatitis
- B20 Human immunodeficiency virus [HIV] disease
- B25-B34 Other viral diseases
- B35-B49 Mycoses
- B50-B64 Protozoal diseases
- B65-B83 Helminthiases
- B85-B89 Pediculosis, acariasis and other infestations
- B90-B94 Sequelae of infectious and parasitic diseases
- B95-B97 Bacterial and viral infectious agents
- B99 Other infectious diseases

Intestinal infectious diseases (A00-A09)

A00 Cholera
DEF: Acute infection of the bowel due to *Vibrio cholerae* that presents with profuse diarrhea, cramps, and vomiting, resulting in severe dehydration, electrolyte imbalance, and death. It is spread through ingestion of food or water contaminated with feces of infected persons.
- A00.0 Cholera due to Vibrio cholerae 01, biovar cholerae
  - Classical cholera
- A00.1 Cholera due to Vibrio cholerae 01, biovar eltor
  - Cholera eltor
- A00.9 Cholera, unspecified

A01 Typhoid and paratyphoid fevers
DEF: Paratyphoid fever: Prolonged febrile illness, caused by *Salmonella* serotypes other than *S. typhi*, especially *S. enterica* serotypes paratyphi A, B, and C.
DEF: Typhoid fever: Acute generalized illness caused by *Salmonella typhi*. Clinical features include fever, headache, abdominal pain, cough, toxemia, leukopenia, abnormal pulse, rose spots on the skin, bacteremia, hyperplasia of intestinal lymph nodes, mesenteric lymphadenopathy, and Peyer's patches in the intestines.
- A01.0 Typhoid fever
  - Infection due to Salmonella typhi
  - A01.00 Typhoid fever, unspecified
  - A01.01 Typhoid meningitis
  - A01.02 Typhoid fever with heart involvement
    - Typhoid endocarditis
    - Typhoid myocarditis
  - A01.03 Typhoid pneumonia
  - A01.04 Typhoid arthritis
  - A01.05 Typhoid osteomyelitis
  - A01.09 Typhoid fever with other complications
- A01.1 Paratyphoid fever A
- A01.2 Paratyphoid fever B
- A01.3 Paratyphoid fever C
- A01.4 Paratyphoid fever, unspecified
  - Infection due to Salmonella paratyphi NOS

A02 Other salmonella infections
INCLUDES infection or foodborne intoxication due to any Salmonella species other than S. typhi and S. paratyphi
- A02.0 Salmonella enteritis
  - Salmonellosis
  - **TIP:** Dehydration (E86.0) is a complication of salmonella enteritis and may be reported separately.
- A02.1 Salmonella sepsis
- A02.2 Localized salmonella infections
  - A02.20 Localized salmonella infection, unspecified
  - A02.21 Salmonella meningitis
  - A02.22 Salmonella pneumonia
  - A02.23 Salmonella arthritis
  - A02.24 Salmonella osteomyelitis
  - A02.25 Salmonella pyelonephritis
    - Salmonella tubulo-interstitial nephropathy
  - A02.29 Salmonella with other localized infection
- A02.8 Other specified salmonella infections
- A02.9 Salmonella infection, unspecified

A03 Shigellosis
DEF: Infection caused by the genus *Shigella*, of the family *Enterobacteriaceae* that is known to cause an acute dysenteric infection of the bowel with fever, drowsiness, anorexia, nausea, vomiting, bloody diarrhea, abdominal cramps, and distention.
- A03.0 Shigellosis due to Shigella dysenteriae
  - Group A shigellosis [Shiga-Kruse dysentery]
- A03.1 Shigellosis due to Shigella flexneri
  - Group B shigellosis
- A03.2 Shigellosis due to Shigella boydii
  - Group C shigellosis
- A03.3 Shigellosis due to Shigella sonnei
  - Group D shigellosis
- A03.8 Other shigellosis
- A03.9 Shigellosis, unspecified
  - Bacillary dysentery NOS

A04 Other bacterial intestinal infections
EXCLUDES 1 bacterial foodborne intoxications, NEC (A05.-)
tuberculous enteritis (A18.32)
DEF: *Escherichia coli*: Gram-negative, anaerobic bacteria of the family *Enterobacteriaceae* found in the large intestine of warm-blooded animals, generally as a nonpathologic entity aiding in digestion. They become pathogenic when an opportunity to grow somewhere outside this relationship presents itself, such as ingestion of fecal-contaminated food or water.
- A04.0 Enteropathogenic Escherichia coli infection
- A04.1 Enterotoxigenic Escherichia coli infection
- A04.2 Enteroinvasive Escherichia coli infection
- A04.3 Enterohemorrhagic Escherichia coli infection
  - **DEF:** *E. coli* infection penetrating the intestinal mucosa, producing microscopic ulceration and bleeding.
- A04.4 Other intestinal Escherichia coli infections
  - Escherichia coli enteritis NOS
- A04.5 Campylobacter enteritis
  - **TIP:** For Guillain-Barre syndrome occurring as a sequela of *Campylobacter enteritis*, assign code G61.0 as the first-listed diagnosis followed by B94.8 for the sequelae.
- A04.6 Enteritis due to Yersinia enterocolitica
  - **EXCLUDES 1** extraintestinal yersiniosis (A28.2)
- A04.7 Enterocolitis due to Clostridium difficile
  - Clostridioides difficile colitis
  - Foodborne intoxication by Clostridium difficile
  - Pseudomembraneous colitis
  - **AHA:** 2017,4Q,4
  - A04.71 Enterocolitis due to Clostridium difficile, recurrent
    - **AHA:** 2020,1Q,18
  - A04.72 Enterocolitis due to Clostridium difficile, not specified as recurrent
- A04.8 Other specified bacterial intestinal infections
- A04.9 Bacterial intestinal infection, unspecified
  - Bacterial enteritis NOS

A05 Other bacterial foodborne intoxications, not elsewhere classified
EXCLUDES 1 Clostridium difficile foodborne intoxication and infection (A04.7-)
Escherichia coli infection (A04.0-A04.4)
listeriosis (A32.-)
salmonella foodborne intoxication and infection (A02.-)
toxic effect of noxious foodstuffs (T61-T62)
- A05.0 Foodborne staphylococcal intoxication
  - **TIP:** Assign code A04.8 to report a staphylococcal infection when it is caused by the ingestion of contaminated food but not caused by *S. aureus* toxins.

A05.1 Botulism food poisoning
Botulism NOS
Classical foodborne intoxication due to Clostridium botulinum
EXCLUDES 1 infant botulism (A48.51)
wound botulism (A48.52)
DEF: Muscle-paralyzing neurotoxic disease caused by ingesting pre-formed toxin from the bacterium *Clostridium botulinum*. It causes vomiting and diarrhea, vision problems, slurred speech, difficulty swallowing, paralysis, and death.

A05.2 Foodborne Clostridium perfringens [Clostridium welchii] intoxication
Enteritis necroticans
Pig-bel

A05.3 Foodborne Vibrio parahaemolyticus intoxication
A05.4 Foodborne Bacillus cereus intoxication
A05.5 Foodborne Vibrio vulnificus intoxication
A05.8 Other specified bacterial foodborne intoxications
A05.9 Bacterial foodborne intoxication, unspecified

✓4th A06 Amebiasis
INCLUDES infection due to Entamoeba histolytica
EXCLUDES 1 other protozoal intestinal diseases (A07.-)
EXCLUDES 2 acanthamebiasis (B60.1-)
Naegleriasis (B60.2)
DEF: Infection with a single cell protozoan known as the amoeba. Transmission occurs through ingestion of feces, contaminated food or water, use of human feces as fertilizer, or person-to-person contact.

A06.0 Acute amebic dysentery
Acute amebiasis
Intestinal amebiasis NOS

A06.1 Chronic intestinal amebiasis
A06.2 Amebic nondysenteric colitis
A06.3 Ameboma of intestine
Ameboma NOS

A06.4 Amebic liver abscess COM
Hepatic amebiasis

A06.5 Amebic lung abscess HCC ESR COM
Amebic abscess of lung (and liver)

A06.6 Amebic brain abscess COM
Amebic abscess of brain (and liver) (and lung)

A06.7 Cutaneous amebiasis
✓5th A06.8 Amebic infection of other sites
A06.81 Amebic cystitis
A06.82 Other amebic genitourinary infections
Amebic balanitis
Amebic vesiculitis
Amebic vulvovaginitis

A06.89 Other amebic infections
Amebic appendicitis
Amebic splenic abscess

A06.9 Amebiasis, unspecified

✓4th A07 Other protozoal intestinal diseases
DEF: Protozoa: Group comprised of the simplest, single celled organisms, ranging in size from micro to macroscopic. They can live alone or in colonies, and do not show any differentiation in tissues. Most are motile and can live free in nature, but some are parasitic, causing disease in the variety of hosts they inhabit.

A07.0 Balantidiasis
Balantidial dysentery

A07.1 Giardiasis [lambliasis]
DEF: Infection caused by the flagellate protozoan *Giardia lamblia* causing gastrointestinal problems such as vomiting, chronic diarrhea, and weight loss. The most common parasite in the U.S., this is usually transmitted by ingesting contaminated water while in the cyst state, after which it latches onto the wall of the small intestine.

A07.2 Cryptosporidiosis HCC Rx ESR COM
DEF: Microscopic parasite found in water and one of the most common causes of waterborne gastrointestinal infectious disease in the United States. It is usually transmitted by ingesting contaminated drinking water or recreational water and causes profuse watery diarrhea, flatulence, abdominal pain, and cramping.

A07.3 Isosporiasis
Infection due to Isospora belli and Isospora hominis
Intestinal coccidiosis
Isosporosis

A07.4 Cyclosporiasis

A07.8 Other specified protozoal intestinal diseases
Intestinal microsporidiosis
Intestinal trichomoniasis
Sarcocystosis
Sarcosporidiosis

A07.9 Protozoal intestinal disease, unspecified
Flagellate diarrhea
Protozoal colitis
Protozoal diarrhea
Protozoal dysentery

✓4th A08 Viral and other specified intestinal infections
EXCLUDES 1 influenza with involvement of gastrointestinal tract (J09.X3, J10.2, J11.2)

A08.0 Rotaviral enteritis
✓5th A08.1 Acute gastroenteropathy due to Norwalk agent and other small round viruses
A08.11 Acute gastroenteropathy due to Norwalk agent
Acute gastroenteropathy due to Norovirus
Acute gastroenteropathy due to Norwalk-like agent
A08.19 Acute gastroenteropathy due to other small round viruses
Acute gastroenteropathy due to small round virus [SRV] NOS

A08.2 Adenoviral enteritis
✓5th A08.3 Other viral enteritis
A08.31 Calicivirus enteritis
A08.32 Astrovirus enteritis
A08.39 Other viral enteritis
Coxsackie virus enteritis
Echovirus enteritis
Enterovirus enteritis NEC
Torovirus enteritis

A08.4 Viral intestinal infection, unspecified
Viral enteritis NOS
Viral gastroenteritis NOS
Viral gastroenteropathy NOS
AHA: 2016,3Q,12

A08.8 Other specified intestinal infections

A09 Infectious gastroenteritis and colitis, unspecified
Infectious colitis NOS
Infectious enteritis NOS
Infectious gastroenteritis NOS
EXCLUDES 1 colitis NOS (K52.9)
diarrhea NOS (R19.7)
enteritis NOS (K52.9)
gastroenteritis NOS (K52.9)
noninfective gastroenteritis and colitis, unspecified (K52.9)
DEF: Colitis: Inflammation of mucous membranes of the colon.
DEF: Enteritis: Inflammation of mucous membranes of the small intestine.
DEF: Gastroenteritis: Inflammation of mucous membranes of the stomach and intestines.

Tuberculosis (A15-A19)

INCLUDES infections due to Mycobacterium tuberculosis and Mycobacterium bovis

▶Use additional code, if applicable, for associated cachexia (E88.A)◀

EXCLUDES 1
congenital tuberculosis (P37.0)
nonspecific reaction to test for tuberculosis without active tuberculosis (R76.1-)
pneumoconiosis associated with tuberculosis, any type in A15 (J65)
positive PPD (R76.11)
positive tuberculin skin test without active tuberculosis (R76.11)
sequelae of tuberculosis (B90.-)
silicotuberculosis (J65)

DEF: Bacterial infection that typically spreads by inhalation of an airborne agent that usually attacks the lungs, but may also affect other organs.

A15 Respiratory tuberculosis

A15.0 Tuberculosis of lung
Tuberculous bronchiectasis
Tuberculous fibrosis of lung
Tuberculous pneumonia
Tuberculous pneumothorax

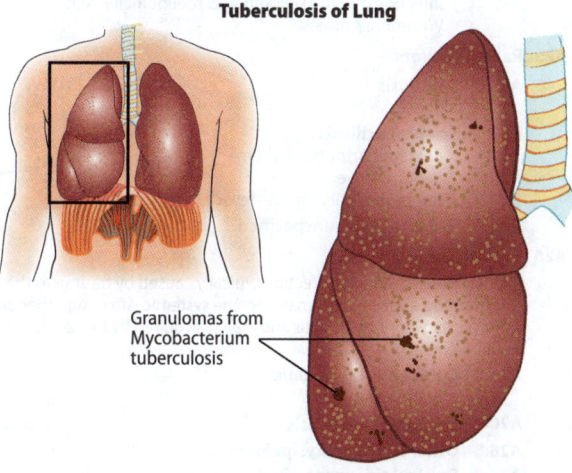
Tuberculosis of Lung
Granulomas from Mycobacterium tuberculosis

A15.4 Tuberculosis of intrathoracic lymph nodes
Tuberculosis of hilar lymph nodes
Tuberculosis of mediastinal lymph nodes
Tuberculosis of tracheobronchial lymph nodes
EXCLUDES 1 tuberculosis specified as primary (A15.7)

A15.5 Tuberculosis of larynx, trachea and bronchus
Tuberculosis of bronchus
Tuberculosis of glottis
Tuberculosis of larynx
Tuberculosis of trachea

A15.6 Tuberculous pleurisy
Tuberculosis of pleura Tuberculous empyema
EXCLUDES 1 primary respiratory tuberculosis (A15.7)

A15.7 Primary respiratory tuberculosis

A15.8 Other respiratory tuberculosis
Mediastinal tuberculosis
Nasopharyngeal tuberculosis
Tuberculosis of nose
Tuberculosis of sinus [any nasal]

A15.9 Respiratory tuberculosis unspecified

A17 Tuberculosis of nervous system

A17.0 Tuberculous meningitis
Tuberculosis of meninges (cerebral)(spinal)
Tuberculous leptomeningitis
EXCLUDES 1 tuberculous meningoencephalitis (A17.82)

A17.1 Meningeal tuberculoma
Tuberculoma of meninges (cerebral) (spinal)
EXCLUDES 2 tuberculoma of brain and spinal cord (A17.81)

A17.8 Other tuberculosis of nervous system

- **A17.81 Tuberculoma of brain and spinal cord**
  Tuberculous abscess of brain and spinal cord
- **A17.82 Tuberculous meningoencephalitis**
  Tuberculous myelitis
- **A17.83 Tuberculous neuritis**
  Tuberculous mononeuropathy

- **A17.89 Other tuberculosis of nervous system**
  Tuberculous polyneuropathy

A17.9 Tuberculosis of nervous system, unspecified

A18 Tuberculosis of other organs

A18.0 Tuberculosis of bones and joints

- **A18.01 Tuberculosis of spine**
  Pott's disease or curvature of spine
  Tuberculous arthritis
  Tuberculous osteomyelitis of spine
  Tuberculous spondylitis
- **A18.02 Tuberculous arthritis of other joints**
  Tuberculosis of hip (joint)
  Tuberculosis of knee (joint)
- **A18.03 Tuberculosis of other bones**
  Tuberculous mastoiditis
  Tuberculous osteomyelitis
- **A18.09 Other musculoskeletal tuberculosis**
  Tuberculous myositis
  Tuberculous synovitis
  Tuberculous tenosynovitis

A18.1 Tuberculosis of genitourinary system

- **A18.10 Tuberculosis of genitourinary system, unspecified**
- **A18.11 Tuberculosis of kidney and ureter**
- **A18.12 Tuberculosis of bladder**
- **A18.13 Tuberculosis of other urinary organs**
  Tuberculous urethritis
- **A18.14 Tuberculosis of prostate**
- **A18.15 Tuberculosis of other male genital organs**
- **A18.16 Tuberculosis of cervix**
- **A18.17 Tuberculous female pelvic inflammatory disease**
  Tuberculous endometritis
  Tuberculous oophoritis and salpingitis
- **A18.18 Tuberculosis of other female genital organs**
  Tuberculous ulceration of vulva

A18.2 Tuberculous peripheral lymphadenopathy
Tuberculous adenitis
EXCLUDES 2 tuberculosis of bronchial and mediastinal lymph nodes (A15.4)
tuberculosis of mesenteric and retroperitoneal lymph nodes (A18.39)
tuberculous tracheobronchial adenopathy (A15.4)

A18.3 Tuberculosis of intestines, peritoneum and mesenteric glands

- **A18.31 Tuberculous peritonitis**
  Tuberculous ascites
  DEF: Tuberculous inflammation of the membrane lining the abdomen.
- **A18.32 Tuberculous enteritis**
  Tuberculosis of anus and rectum
  Tuberculosis of intestine (large) (small)
- **A18.39 Retroperitoneal tuberculosis**
  Tuberculosis of mesenteric glands
  Tuberculosis of retroperitoneal (lymph glands)

A18.4 Tuberculosis of skin and subcutaneous tissue
Erythema induratum, tuberculous
Lupus exedens
Lupus vulgaris of eyelid
Lupus vulgaris NOS
Scrofuloderma
Tuberculosis of external ear
EXCLUDES 2 lupus erythematosus (L93.-)
systemic lupus erythematosus (M32.-)

A18.5 Tuberculosis of eye
EXCLUDES 2 lupus vulgaris of eyelid (A18.4)

- **A18.50 Tuberculosis of eye, unspecified**
- **A18.51 Tuberculous episcleritis**
- **A18.52 Tuberculous keratitis**
  Tuberculous interstitial keratitis
  Tuberculous keratoconjunctivitis (interstitial) (phlyctenular)
- **A18.53 Tuberculous chorioretinitis**
- **A18.54 Tuberculous iridocyclitis**
- **A18.59 Other tuberculosis of eye**
  Tuberculous conjunctivitis

A18.6 Tuberculosis of (inner) (middle) ear
Tuberculous otitis media
EXCLUDES 2 tuberculosis of external ear (A18.4)
tuberculous mastoiditis (A18.03)

A18.7 Tuberculosis of adrenal glands
Tuberculous Addison's disease

✓5th A18.8 Tuberculosis of other specified organs

- **A18.81** Tuberculosis of thyroid gland
- **A18.82** Tuberculosis of other endocrine glands
  - Tuberculosis of pituitary gland
  - Tuberculosis of thymus gland
- **A18.83** Tuberculosis of digestive tract organs, not elsewhere classified
  - *EXCLUDES 1* tuberculosis of intestine (A18.32)
- **A18.84** Tuberculosis of heart
  - Tuberculous cardiomyopathy
  - Tuberculous endocarditis
  - Tuberculous myocarditis
  - Tuberculous pericarditis
- **A18.85** Tuberculosis of spleen
- **A18.89** Tuberculosis of other sites
  - Tuberculosis of muscle
  - Tuberculous cerebral arteritis

✓4th A19 Miliary tuberculosis
INCLUDES
- disseminated tuberculosis
- generalized tuberculosis
- tuberculous polyserositis

- **A19.0** Acute miliary tuberculosis of a single specified site
- **A19.1** Acute miliary tuberculosis of multiple sites
- **A19.2** Acute miliary tuberculosis, unspecified
- **A19.8** Other miliary tuberculosis
- **A19.9** Miliary tuberculosis, unspecified

Certain zoonotic bacterial diseases (A20-A28)

✓4th A20 Plague
INCLUDES infection due to Yersinia pestis

- **A20.0** Bubonic plague
- **A20.1** Cellulocutaneous plague
- **A20.2** Pneumonic plague [ESR]
- **A20.3** Plague meningitis [COM]
- **A20.7** Septicemic plague [HCC][ESR][COM]
- **A20.8** Other forms of plague
  - Abortive plague
  - Asymptomatic plague
  - Pestis minor
- **A20.9** Plague, unspecified

✓4th A21 Tularemia
INCLUDES
- deer-fly fever
- infection due to Francisella tularensis
- rabbit fever

DEF: Febrile disease transmitted to humans by the bites of deer flies, fleas, and ticks, by inhaling aerosolized *F. tularensis*, or by ingesting contaminated food or water. Patients quickly develop fever, chills, weakness, headache, backache, and malaise.

- **A21.0** Ulceroglandular tularemia
- **A21.1** Oculoglandular tularemia
  - Ophthalmic tularemia
- **A21.2** Pulmonary tularemia [ESR]
- **A21.3** Gastrointestinal tularemia
  - Abdominal tularemia
- **A21.7** Generalized tularemia
- **A21.8** Other forms of tularemia
- **A21.9** Tularemia, unspecified

✓4th A22 Anthrax
INCLUDES infection due to Bacillus anthracis

- **A22.0** Cutaneous anthrax
  - Malignant carbuncle
  - Malignant pustule
- **A22.1** Pulmonary anthrax [ESR]
  - Inhalation anthrax
  - Ragpicker's disease
  - Woolsorter's disease
- **A22.2** Gastrointestinal anthrax
- **A22.7** Anthrax sepsis [HCC][ESR][COM]
- **A22.8** Other forms of anthrax
  - Anthrax meningitis
- **A22.9** Anthrax, unspecified

✓4th A23 Brucellosis
INCLUDES
- Malta fever
- Mediterranean fever
- undulant fever

- **A23.0** Brucellosis due to Brucella melitensis
- **A23.1** Brucellosis due to Brucella abortus
- **A23.2** Brucellosis due to Brucella suis
- **A23.3** Brucellosis due to Brucella canis
- **A23.8** Other brucellosis
- **A23.9** Brucellosis, unspecified

✓4th A24 Glanders and melioidosis

- **A24.0** Glanders
  - Infection due to Pseudomonas mallei
  - Malleus
- **A24.1** Acute and fulminating melioidosis
  - Melioidosis pneumonia
  - Melioidosis sepsis
- **A24.2** Subacute and chronic melioidosis
- **A24.3** Other melioidosis
- **A24.9** Melioidosis, unspecified
  - Infection due to Pseudomonas pseudomallei NOS
  - Whitmore's disease

✓4th A25 Rat-bite fevers

- **A25.0** Spirillosis
  - Sodoku
- **A25.1** Streptobacillosis
  - Epidemic arthritic erythema
  - Haverhill fever
  - Streptobacillary rat-bite fever
- **A25.9** Rat-bite fever, unspecified

✓4th A26 Erysipeloid
DEF: Acute cutaneous infection typically caused by trauma to the skin. Presenting as cellulitis, it may become systemic, affecting other organs. It is a gram-positive bacillus and mainly acquired by those who routinely handle meat.

- **A26.0** Cutaneous erysipeloid
  - Erythema migrans
- **A26.7** Erysipelothrix sepsis [HCC][ESR][COM]
- **A26.8** Other forms of erysipeloid
- **A26.9** Erysipeloid, unspecified

✓4th A27 Leptospirosis

- **A27.0** Leptospirosis icterohemorrhagica
  - Leptospiral or spirochetal jaundice (hemorrhagic)
  - Weil's disease
- **✓5th A27.8** Other forms of leptospirosis
  - **A27.81** Aseptic meningitis in leptospirosis [COM]
  - **A27.89** Other forms of leptospirosis
- **A27.9** Leptospirosis, unspecified

✓4th A28 Other zoonotic bacterial diseases, not elsewhere classified

- **A28.0** Pasteurellosis
- **A28.1** Cat-scratch disease
  - Cat-scratch fever
- **A28.2** Extraintestinal yersiniosis
  - *EXCLUDES 1* enteritis due to Yersinia enterocolitica (A04.6)
  - plague (A20.-)
- **A28.8** Other specified zoonotic bacterial diseases, not elsewhere classified
- **A28.9** Zoonotic bacterial disease, unspecified

Other bacterial diseases (A30-A49)
AHA: 2016,3Q,8-14

✓4th A30 Leprosy [Hansen's disease]
INCLUDES infection due to Mycobacterium leprae
EXCLUDES 1 sequelae of leprosy (B92)

- **A30.0** Indeterminate leprosy
  - I leprosy
- **A30.1** Tuberculoid leprosy
  - TT leprosy
- **A30.2** Borderline tuberculoid leprosy
  - BT leprosy
- **A30.3** Borderline leprosy
  - BB leprosy
- **A30.4** Borderline lepromatous leprosy
  - BL leprosy

HCC CMS-HCC   **Rx** Rx HCC   **ESR** ESRD HCC   **COM** Commercial HCC   **N** Newborn: 0   **P** Pediatric: 0-17   **M** Maternity: 9-64   **A** Adult: 15-124

A30.5 Lepromatous leprosy
  LL leprosy
A30.8 Other forms of leprosy
A30.9 Leprosy, unspecified

A31 Infection due to other mycobacteria
  EXCLUDES 2: leprosy (A30.-)
  tuberculosis (A15-A19)
  A31.0 Pulmonary mycobacterial infection [HCC] [Rx] [ESR] [COM]
    Infection due to Mycobacterium avium
    Infection due to Mycobacterium intracellulare [Battey bacillus]
    Infection due to Mycobacterium kansasii
  A31.1 Cutaneous mycobacterial infection
    Buruli ulcer
    Infection due to Mycobacterium marinum
    Infection due to Mycobacterium ulcerans
  A31.2 Disseminated mycobacterium avium-intracellulare complex (DMAC) [HCC] [Rx] [ESR] [COM]
    MAC sepsis
  A31.8 Other mycobacterial infections
  A31.9 Mycobacterial infection, unspecified
    Atypical mycobacterial infection NOS
    Mycobacteriosis NOS

A32 Listeriosis
  INCLUDES: listerial foodborne infection
  EXCLUDES 1: neonatal (disseminated) listeriosis (P37.2)
  A32.0 Cutaneous listeriosis
  A32.1 Listerial meningitis and meningoencephalitis
    A32.11 Listerial meningitis [COM]
    A32.12 Listerial meningoencephalitis [COM]
  A32.7 Listerial sepsis [HCC] [ESR] [COM]
  A32.8 Other forms of listeriosis
    A32.81 Oculoglandular listeriosis
    A32.82 Listerial endocarditis [COM]
    A32.89 Other forms of listeriosis
      Listerial cerebral arteritis
  A32.9 Listeriosis, unspecified

A33 Tetanus neonatorum [N]
A34 Obstetrical tetanus [COM] [M]
A35 Other tetanus [COM]
  Tetanus NOS
  EXCLUDES 1: obstetrical tetanus (A34)
  tetanus neonatorum (A33)
  DEF: Tetanus: Acute, often fatal, infectious disease caused by the anaerobic, spore-forming bacillus *Clostridium tetani*. The bacillus enters the body through a contaminated wound, burns, surgical wounds, or cutaneous ulcers. Symptoms include lockjaw, spasms, seizures, and paralysis.

A36 Diphtheria
  A36.0 Pharyngeal diphtheria
    Diphtheritic membranous angina
    Tonsillar diphtheria
  A36.1 Nasopharyngeal diphtheria
  A36.2 Laryngeal diphtheria
    Diphtheritic laryngotracheitis
  A36.3 Cutaneous diphtheria
    EXCLUDES 2: erythrasma (L08.1)
  A36.8 Other diphtheria
    A36.81 Diphtheritic cardiomyopathy [HCC] [Rx] [ESR] [COM]
      Diphtheritic myocarditis
    A36.82 Diphtheritic radiculomyelitis
    A36.83 Diphtheritic polyneuritis
    A36.84 Diphtheritic tubulo-interstitial nephropathy
    A36.85 Diphtheritic cystitis
    A36.86 Diphtheritic conjunctivitis
    A36.89 Other diphtheritic complications
      Diphtheritic peritonitis
  A36.9 Diphtheria, unspecified

A37 Whooping cough
  DEF: Acute, highly contagious respiratory tract infection caused by *Bordetella pertussis* and *B. bronchiseptica*. Whooping cough is known by its characteristic paroxysmal cough.
  A37.0 Whooping cough due to Bordetella pertussis
    A37.00 Whooping cough due to Bordetella pertussis without pneumonia
      Paroxysmal cough due to Bordetella pertussis without pneumonia
    A37.01 Whooping cough due to Bordetella pertussis with pneumonia
      Paroxysmal cough due to Bordetella pertussis with pneumonia
  A37.1 Whooping cough due to Bordetella parapertussis
    A37.10 Whooping cough due to Bordetella parapertussis without pneumonia
    A37.11 Whooping cough due to Bordetella parapertussis with pneumonia
  A37.8 Whooping cough due to other Bordetella species
    A37.80 Whooping cough due to other Bordetella species without pneumonia
    A37.81 Whooping cough due to other Bordetella species with pneumonia
  A37.9 Whooping cough, unspecified species
    A37.90 Whooping cough, unspecified species without pneumonia
    A37.91 Whooping cough, unspecified species with pneumonia

A38 Scarlet fever
  INCLUDES: scarlatina
  EXCLUDES 2: streptococcal sore throat (J02.0)
  DEF: Acute contagious disease caused by Group A bacteria, the same bacterium that causes strep throat. Individuals with strep throat can develop scarlet fever particularly if the infection is not treated with antibiotics. It is characterized by a red blush to the skin of the chest and abdomen and swelling of the nose, throat, and mouth.
  A38.0 Scarlet fever with otitis media
  A38.1 Scarlet fever with myocarditis [COM]
  A38.8 Scarlet fever with other complications
  A38.9 Scarlet fever, uncomplicated
    Scarlet fever, NOS

A39 Meningococcal infection
  DEF: Condition caused by *Neisseria meningitidis*, a bacteria that may invade the spinal cord, brain, heart, joints, optic nerve, or bloodstream.
  A39.0 Meningococcal meningitis [COM]
  A39.1 Waterhouse-Friderichsen syndrome [Rx] [ESR] [COM]
    Meningococcal hemorrhagic adrenalitis
    Meningococcic adrenal syndrome
  A39.2 Acute meningococcemia [HCC] [ESR] [COM]
  A39.3 Chronic meningococcemia [HCC] [ESR] [COM]
  A39.4 Meningococcemia, unspecified [HCC] [ESR] [COM]
  A39.5 Meningococcal heart disease
    A39.50 Meningococcal carditis, unspecified [COM]
    A39.51 Meningococcal endocarditis [COM]
    A39.52 Meningococcal myocarditis [COM]
    A39.53 Meningococcal pericarditis [COM]
  A39.8 Other meningococcal infections
    A39.81 Meningococcal encephalitis [COM]
    A39.82 Meningococcal retrobulbar neuritis
    A39.83 Meningococcal arthritis [HCC] [ESR] [COM]
    A39.84 Postmeningococcal arthritis [HCC] [ESR] [COM]
    A39.89 Other meningococcal infections
      Meningococcal conjunctivitis
  A39.9 Meningococcal infection, unspecified
    Meningococcal disease NOS

A40 Streptococcal sepsis ✓4th

Code first, if applicable, postprocedural sepsis (T81.44-)
sepsis due to central venous catheter (T80.211-)
streptococcal sepsis during labor (O75.3)
streptococcal sepsis following abortion or ectopic or molar pregnancy (O03.37, O03.87, O04.87, O07.37, O08.82)
streptococcal sepsis following immunization (T88.0-)
streptococcal sepsis following infusion, transfusion or therapeutic injection (T80.22-, T80.29-)

EXCLUDES 1
neonatal (P36.0-P36.1)
puerperal sepsis (O85)
sepsis due to Streptococcus, group D (A41.81)

AHA: 2020,2Q,8,28; 2019,4Q,65; 2018,4Q,89; 2018,1Q,16; 2016,1Q,32

- **A40.0** Sepsis due to streptococcus, group A `HCC` `ESR` `COM`
- **A40.1** Sepsis due to streptococcus, group B `HCC` `ESR` `COM`
  AHA: 2019,1Q,14
- **A40.3** Sepsis due to Streptococcus pneumoniae `HCC` `ESR` `COM`
  Pneumococcal sepsis
- **A40.8** Other streptococcal sepsis `HCC` `ESR` `COM`
- **A40.9** Streptococcal sepsis, unspecified `HCC` `ESR` `COM`

A41 Other sepsis ✓4th

Code first, if applicable, postprocedural sepsis (T81.44-)
sepsis due to central venous catheter (T80.211-)
sepsis during labor (O75.3)
sepsis following abortion, ectopic or molar pregnancy (O03.37, O03.87, O04.87, O07.37, O08.82)
sepsis following immunization (T88.0-)
sepsis following infusion, transfusion or therapeutic injection (T80.22-, T80.29-)

EXCLUDES 1
bacteremia NOS (R78.81)
neonatal (P36.-)
puerperal sepsis (O85)
streptococcal sepsis (A40.-)

EXCLUDES 2
sepsis (due to) (in) actinomycotic (A42.7)
sepsis (due to) (in) anthrax (A22.7)
sepsis (due to) (in) candidal (B37.7)
sepsis (due to) (in) Erysipelothrix (A26.7)
sepsis (due to) (in) extraintestinal yersiniosis (A28.2)
sepsis (due to) (in) gonococcal (A54.86)
sepsis (due to) (in) herpesviral (B00.7)
sepsis (due to) (in) listerial (A32.7)
sepsis (due to) (in) melioidosis (A24.1)
sepsis (due to) (in) meningococcal (A39.2-A39.4)
sepsis (due to) (in) plague (A20.7)
sepsis (due to) (in) tularemia (A21.7)
toxic shock syndrome (A48.3)

AHA: 2020,2Q,8,28; 2019,4Q,65; 2019,3Q,17; 2018,4Q,18; 2018,1Q,16; 2016,1Q,32; 2014,2Q,13

- **A41.0** Sepsis due to Staphylococcus aureus ✓5th
  - **A41.01** Sepsis due to Methicillin susceptible Staphylococcus aureus `HCC` `ESR` `COM`
    MSSA sepsis
    Staphylococcus aureus sepsis NOS
    AHA: 2020,2Q,17
  - **A41.02** Sepsis due to Methicillin resistant Staphylococcus aureus `HCC` `ESR` `COM`
- **A41.1** Sepsis due to other specified staphylococcus `HCC` `ESR` `COM`
  Coagulase negative staphylococcus sepsis
  AHA: 2024,1Q,19
- **A41.2** Sepsis due to unspecified staphylococcus `HCC` `ESR` `COM`
- **A41.3** Sepsis due to Hemophilus influenzae `HCC` `ESR` `COM`
- **A41.4** Sepsis due to anaerobes `HCC` `ESR` `COM`
  EXCLUDES 1 gas gangrene (A48.0)
- **A41.5** Sepsis due to other Gram-negative organisms ✓5th
  - **A41.50** Gram-negative sepsis, unspecified `HCC` `ESR` `COM`
    Gram-negative sepsis NOS
    AHA: 2020,2Q,28
  - **A41.51** Sepsis due to Escherichia coli [E. coli] `HCC` `ESR` `COM`
    AHA: 2020,2Q,17
  - **A41.52** Sepsis due to Pseudomonas `HCC` `ESR` `COM`
    Pseudomonas aeruginosa
  - **A41.53** Sepsis due to Serratia `HCC` `ESR` `COM`
  - **A41.54** Sepsis due to Acinetobacter baumannii `HCC` `ESR` `COM`
    AHA: 2023,4Q,4
  - **A41.59** Other Gram-negative sepsis `HCC` `ESR` `COM`

- **A41.8** Other specified sepsis ✓5th
  - **A41.81** Sepsis due to Enterococcus `HCC` `ESR` `COM`
    TIP: *E. faecium*, is a species of *Enterococcus* that is highly resistant to multiple antibiotics. Assign a code from category Z16 when resistance to antimicrobial drugs is documented.
  - **A41.89** Other specified sepsis `HCC` `ESR` `COM`
    AHA: 2020,2Q,8; 2017,1Q,51; 2016,3Q,8-14
- **A41.9** Sepsis, unspecified organism `HCC` `ESR` `COM`
  Septicemia NOS
  AHA: 2022,2Q,5; 2022,1Q,35; 2020,2Q,28

A42 Actinomycosis ✓4th

EXCLUDES 1 actinomycetoma (B47.1)

- **A42.0** Pulmonary actinomycosis `ESR`
- **A42.1** Abdominal actinomycosis
- **A42.2** Cervicofacial actinomycosis
- **A42.7** Actinomycotic sepsis `HCC` `ESR` `COM`
- **A42.8** Other forms of actinomycosis ✓5th
  - **A42.81** Actinomycotic meningitis `COM`
  - **A42.82** Actinomycotic encephalitis `COM`
  - **A42.89** Other forms of actinomycosis
- **A42.9** Actinomycosis, unspecified

A43 Nocardiosis ✓4th

DEF: Rare bacterial infection occurring most often in those with weakened immune systems. Can be acquired in soil, decaying plants, or standing water. It typically begins in the lungs and has a tendency to spread to other body systems.

- **A43.0** Pulmonary nocardiosis `ESR`
- **A43.1** Cutaneous nocardiosis
- **A43.8** Other forms of nocardiosis
- **A43.9** Nocardiosis, unspecified

A44 Bartonellosis ✓4th

- **A44.0** Systemic bartonellosis
  Oroya fever
- **A44.1** Cutaneous and mucocutaneous bartonellosis
  Verruga peruana
- **A44.8** Other forms of bartonellosis
- **A44.9** Bartonellosis, unspecified

A46 Erysipelas

EXCLUDES 1 postpartum or puerperal erysipelas (O86.89)

DEF: Skin infection affecting the upper dermis and superficial dermal lymphatics. Lesion edges are well-demarcated with distinct raised borders. It is often caused by group A *Streptococci*.

A48 Other bacterial diseases, not elsewhere classified ✓4th

EXCLUDES 1 actinomycetoma (B47.1)

- **A48.0** Gas gangrene `HCC` `ESR` `COM`
  Clostridial cellulitis
  Clostridial myonecrosis
  AHA: 2017,4Q,102
- **A48.1** Legionnaires' disease `HCC` `ESR` `COM`
  DEF: Severe and often fatal infection by *Legionella pneumophila*. Symptoms include high fever, gastrointestinal pain, headache, myalgia, dry cough, and pneumonia and it is usually transmitted through airborne water droplets via air conditioning systems or hot tubs.
- **A48.2** Nonpneumonic Legionnaires' disease [Pontiac fever]
- **A48.3** Toxic shock syndrome `HCC` `ESR` `COM`
  Use additional code to identify the organism (B95, B96)
  EXCLUDES 1
  endotoxic shock NOS (R57.8)
  sepsis NOS (A41.9)
  AHA: 2022,1Q,35
  DEF: Bacteria producing an endotoxin, such as *Staphylococci*, flood the body with the toxins producing a high fever, vomiting and diarrhea, decreasing blood pressure, a skin rash, and shock.
  Synonym(s): TSS.
- **A48.4** Brazilian purpuric fever
  Systemic Hemophilus aegyptius infection
- **A48.5** Other specified botulism ✓5th
  Non-foodborne intoxication due to toxins of Clostridium botulinum [C. botulinum]
  EXCLUDES 1 food poisoning due to toxins of Clostridium botulinum (A05.1)
  - **A48.51** Infant botulism `P`

	A48.52	**Wound** botulism
		Non-foodborne botulism NOS
		Use additional code for associated wound
	A48.8	Other specified bacterial diseases

✓4th **A49** **Bacterial** infection of unspecified site

EXCLUDES 1   bacterial agents as the cause of diseases classified elsewhere (B95-B96)
chlamydial infection NOS (A74.9)
meningococcal infection NOS (A39.9)
rickettsial infection NOS (A79.9)
spirochetal infection NOS (A69.9)

✓5th **A49.0** **Staphylococcal** infection, unspecified site

	A49.01	**Methicillin susceptible** Staphylococcus aureus infection, unspecified site
		Methicillin susceptible Staphylococcus aureus (MSSA) infection
		Staphylococcus aureus infection NOS
	A49.02	**Methicillin resistant** Staphylococcus aureus infection, unspecified site
		Methicillin resistant Staphylococcus aureus (MRSA) infection

A49.1	**Streptococcal** infection, unspecified site
A49.2	**Hemophilus influenzae** infection, unspecified site
A49.3	**Mycoplasma** infection, unspecified site
A49.8	Other bacterial infections of unspecified site
A49.9	Bacterial infection, unspecified
	EXCLUDES 1 bacteremia NOS (R78.81)

Infections with a predominantly sexual mode of transmission (A50-A64)

EXCLUDES 1   nonspecific and nongonococcal urethritis (N34.1)
Reiter's disease (M02.3-)
EXCLUDES 2   human immunodeficiency virus [HIV] disease (B20)
AHA: 2021,2Q,6

✓4th **A50** **Congenital** syphilis

✓5th **A50.0** **Early** congenital syphilis, **symptomatic**
Any congenital syphilitic condition specified as early or manifest less than two years after birth.

	A50.01	Early congenital syphilitic **oculopathy**
	A50.02	Early congenital syphilitic **osteochondropathy**
	A50.03	Early congenital syphilitic **pharyngitis**
		Early congenital syphilitic laryngitis
	A50.04	Early congenital syphilitic **pneumonia** COM
	A50.05	Early congenital syphilitic **rhinitis**
	A50.06	Early **cutaneous** congenital syphilis
	A50.07	Early **mucocutaneous** congenital syphilis
	A50.08	Early **visceral** congenital syphilis
	A50.09	Other early congenital syphilis, symptomatic

A50.1	**Early** congenital syphilis, **latent**
	Congenital syphilis without clinical manifestations, with positive serological reaction and negative spinal fluid test, less than two years after birth.
A50.2	**Early** congenital syphilis, **unspecified**
	Congenital syphilis NOS less than two years after birth.

✓5th **A50.3** **Late** congenital syphilitic **oculopathy**

EXCLUDES 1   Hutchinson's triad (A50.53)

	A50.30	Late congenital syphilitic oculopathy, unspecified
	A50.31	Late congenital syphilitic **interstitial keratitis**
	A50.32	Late congenital syphilitic **chorioretinitis**
	A50.39	Other late congenital syphilitic oculopathy

✓5th **A50.4** **Late** congenital **neurosyphilis [juvenile neurosyphilis]**

Use additional code to identify any associated mental disorder
EXCLUDES 1   Hutchinson's triad (A50.53)

	A50.40	Late congenital neurosyphilis, unspecified COM
		Juvenile neurosyphilis NOS
	A50.41	Late congenital syphilitic **meningitis** COM
	A50.42	Late congenital syphilitic **encephalitis** COM
	A50.43	Late congenital syphilitic **polyneuropathy** COM
	A50.44	Late congenital syphilitic **optic nerve atrophy** COM
	A50.45	**Juvenile general paresis** COM
		Dementia paralytica juvenilis
		Juvenile taboparetic neurosyphilis
	A50.49	Other late congenital neurosyphilis COM
		Juvenile tabes dorsalis

✓5th **A50.5** Other **late** congenital syphilis, **symptomatic**
Any congenital syphilitic condition specified as late or manifest two years or more after birth.

	A50.51	**Clutton's joints**
	A50.52	**Hutchinson's teeth**
	A50.53	**Hutchinson's triad**
	A50.54	Late congenital **cardiovascular syphilis** COM
	A50.55	Late congenital syphilitic **arthropathy** HCC ESR COM
	A50.56	Late congenital syphilitic **osteochondropathy**
	A50.57	**Syphilitic saddle nose**
	A50.59	Other late congenital syphilis, symptomatic

A50.6	**Late** congenital syphilis, **latent**
	Congenital syphilis without clinical manifestations, with positive serological reaction and negative spinal fluid test, two years or more after birth.
A50.7	**Late** congenital syphilis, **unspecified**
	Congenital syphilis NOS two years or more after birth.
A50.9	Congenital syphilis, unspecified

✓4th **A51** **Early** syphilis

DEF: Syphilis: Sexually transmitted disease caused by the *Treponema pallidum* spirochete. Syphilis usually exhibits cutaneous manifestations and may exist for years without symptoms.

A51.0	**Primary genital** syphilis
	Syphilitic chancre NOS
A51.1	**Primary anal** syphilis
A51.2	**Primary** syphilis of other sites

✓5th **A51.3** **Secondary** syphilis of **skin and mucous membranes**

DEF: Transitory or chronic cutaneous eruptions that present within two to 10 weeks following an initial syphilis infection that may include nontender lymphadenopathy along with alopecia and condylomata lata.

	A51.31	**Condyloma latum**
	A51.32	**Syphilitic alopecia**
	A51.39	Other secondary syphilis of skin
		Syphilitic leukoderma
		Syphilitic mucous patch
		EXCLUDES 1 late syphilitic leukoderma (A52.79)

✓5th **A51.4** Other **secondary** syphilis

	A51.41	Secondary syphilitic **meningitis** COM
	A51.42	Secondary syphilitic **female pelvic disease**
	A51.43	Secondary syphilitic **oculopathy**
		Secondary syphilitic chorioretinitis
		Secondary syphilitic iridocyclitis, iritis
		Secondary syphilitic uveitis
	A51.44	Secondary syphilitic **nephritis**
	A51.45	Secondary syphilitic **hepatitis**
	A51.46	Secondary syphilitic **osteopathy**
	A51.49	Other secondary syphilitic conditions
		Secondary syphilitic lymphadenopathy
		Secondary syphilitic myositis

A51.5	**Early** syphilis, **latent**
	Syphilis (acquired) without clinical manifestations, with positive serological reaction and negative spinal fluid test, less than two years after infection.
A51.9	Early syphilis, unspecified

✓4th **A52** **Late** syphilis

✓5th **A52.0** **Cardiovascular and cerebrovascular** syphilis

	A52.00	Cardiovascular syphilis, unspecified COM
	A52.01	Syphilitic **aneurysm of aorta** COM
	A52.02	Syphilitic **aortitis** COM
	A52.03	Syphilitic **endocarditis** COM
		Syphilitic aortic valve incompetence or stenosis
		Syphilitic mitral valve stenosis
		Syphilitic pulmonary valve regurgitation
	A52.04	Syphilitic cerebral **arteritis**
	A52.05	Other **cerebrovascular** syphilis COM
		Syphilitic cerebral aneurysm (ruptured) (non-ruptured)
		Syphilitic cerebral thrombosis
	A52.06	Other syphilitic **heart** involvement COM
		Syphilitic coronary artery disease
		Syphilitic myocarditis
		Syphilitic pericarditis
	A52.09	Other cardiovascular syphilis COM

✓5th **A52.1** **Symptomatic neurosyphilis**

	A52.10	Symptomatic neurosyphilis, unspecified COM

A52.11 Tabes dorsalis [COM]
  Locomotor ataxia (progressive)
  Tabetic neurosyphilis
A52.12 Other cerebrospinal syphilis [COM]
A52.13 Late syphilitic meningitis [COM]
A52.14 Late syphilitic encephalitis [COM]
A52.15 Late syphilitic neuropathy [COM]
  Late syphilitic acoustic neuritis
  Late syphilitic optic (nerve) atrophy
  Late syphilitic polyneuropathy
  Late syphilitic retrobulbar neuritis
A52.16 Charcôt's arthropathy (tabetic) [COM]
  DEF: Progressive neurologic arthropathy in which chronic degeneration of joints in the weight-bearing areas with peripheral hypertrophy occurs as a complication of a neuropathy disorder. Supporting structures relax from a loss of sensation resulting in chronic joint instability.
A52.17 General paresis [COM]
  Dementia paralytica
A52.19 Other symptomatic neurosyphilis [COM]
  Syphilitic parkinsonism
A52.2 Asymptomatic neurosyphilis [COM]
A52.3 Neurosyphilis, unspecified [COM]
  Gumma (syphilitic)
  Syphilis (late)
  Syphiloma
  AHA: 2021,2Q,6

✓5th **A52.7 Other symptomatic late syphilis**
  A52.71 Late syphilitic oculopathy
    Late syphilitic chorioretinitis
    Late syphilitic episcleritis
  A52.72 Syphilis of lung and bronchus
  A52.73 Symptomatic late syphilis of other respiratory organs
  A52.74 Syphilis of liver and other viscera
    Late syphilitic peritonitis
  A52.75 Syphilis of kidney and ureter
    Syphilitic glomerular disease
  A52.76 Other genitourinary symptomatic late syphilis
    Late syphilitic female pelvic inflammatory disease
  A52.77 Syphilis of bone and joint
  A52.78 Syphilis of other musculoskeletal tissue
    Late syphilitic bursitis
    Syphilis [stage unspecified] of bursa
    Syphilis [stage unspecified] of muscle
    Syphilis [stage unspecified] of synovium
    Syphilis [stage unspecified] of tendon
  A52.79 Other symptomatic late syphilis
    Late syphilitic leukoderma
    Syphilis of adrenal gland
    Syphilis of pituitary gland
    Syphilis of thyroid gland
    Syphilitic splenomegaly
    EXCLUDES 1 syphilitic leukoderma (secondary) (A51.39)

A52.8 Late syphilis, latent
  Syphilis (acquired) without clinical manifestations, with positive serological reaction and negative spinal fluid test, two years or more after infection
A52.9 Late syphilis, unspecified

✓4th **A53 Other and unspecified syphilis**
  A53.0 Latent syphilis, unspecified as early or late
    Latent syphilis NOS
    Positive serological reaction for syphilis
  A53.9 Syphilis, unspecified
    Infection due to Treponema pallidum NOS
    Syphilis (acquired) NOS
    EXCLUDES 1 syphilis NOS under two years of age (A50.2)

✓4th **A54 Gonococcal infection**
  DEF: Sexually transmitted bacterial infection caused by *Neisseria gonorrhoeae*. Women are often asymptomatic, while men tend to develop urinary symptoms quickly.

  ✓5th **A54.0 Gonococcal infection of lower genitourinary tract without periurethral or accessory gland abscess**
    EXCLUDES 1 gonococcal infection with genitourinary gland abscess (A54.1)
        gonococcal infection with periurethral abscess (A54.1)
    A54.00 Gonococcal infection of lower genitourinary tract, unspecified
    A54.01 Gonococcal cystitis and urethritis, unspecified
    A54.02 Gonococcal vulvovaginitis, unspecified
    A54.03 Gonococcal cervicitis, unspecified
    A54.09 Other gonococcal infection of lower genitourinary tract
  A54.1 Gonococcal infection of lower genitourinary tract with periurethral and accessory gland abscess
    Gonococcal Bartholin's gland abscess
  ✓5th **A54.2 Gonococcal pelviperitonitis and other gonococcal genitourinary infection**
    A54.21 Gonococcal infection of kidney and ureter
    A54.22 Gonococcal prostatitis
    A54.23 Gonococcal infection of other male genital organs
      Gonococcal epididymitis
      Gonococcal orchitis
    A54.24 Gonococcal female pelvic inflammatory disease
      Gonococcal pelviperitonitis
      EXCLUDES 1 gonococcal peritonitis (A54.85)
    A54.29 Other gonococcal genitourinary infections
  ✓5th **A54.3 Gonococcal infection of eye**
    A54.30 Gonococcal infection of eye, unspecified
    A54.31 Gonococcal conjunctivitis
      Ophthalmia neonatorum due to gonococcus
    A54.32 Gonococcal iridocyclitis
    A54.33 Gonococcal keratitis
    A54.39 Other gonococcal eye infection
      Gonococcal endophthalmia
  ✓5th **A54.4 Gonococcal infection of musculoskeletal system**
    A54.40 Gonococcal infection of musculoskeletal system, unspecified [HCC ESR COM]
    A54.41 Gonococcal spondylopathy [HCC ESR COM]
    A54.42 Gonococcal arthritis [HCC ESR COM]
      EXCLUDES 2 gonococcal infection of spine (A54.41)
    A54.43 Gonococcal osteomyelitis [HCC ESR COM]
      EXCLUDES 2 gonococcal infection of spine (A54.41)
    A54.49 Gonococcal infection of other musculoskeletal tissue [HCC ESR COM]
      Gonococcal bursitis
      Gonococcal myositis
      Gonococcal synovitis
      Gonococcal tenosynovitis
  A54.5 Gonococcal pharyngitis
  A54.6 Gonococcal infection of anus and rectum
  ✓5th **A54.8 Other gonococcal infections**
    A54.81 Gonococcal meningitis [COM]
    A54.82 Gonococcal brain abscess [COM]
    A54.83 Gonococcal heart infection [COM]
      Gonococcal endocarditis
      Gonococcal myocarditis
      Gonococcal pericarditis
    A54.84 Gonococcal pneumonia [ESR]
    A54.85 Gonococcal peritonitis [HCC ESR COM]
      EXCLUDES 1 gonococcal pelviperitonitis (A54.24)
    A54.86 Gonococcal sepsis [HCC ESR COM]
    A54.89 Other gonococcal infections
      Gonococcal keratoderma
      Gonococcal lymphadenitis
  A54.9 Gonococcal infection, unspecified

A55 Chlamydial lymphogranuloma (venereum)
  Climatic or tropical bubo
  Durand-Nicolas-Favre disease
  Esthiomene
  Lymphogranuloma inguinale

A56 Other sexually transmitted chlamydial diseases

INCLUDES sexually transmitted diseases due to Chlamydia trachomatis

EXCLUDES 1 neonatal chlamydial conjunctivitis (P39.1)
neonatal chlamydial pneumonia (P23.1)

EXCLUDES 2 chlamydial lymphogranuloma (A55)
conditions classified to A74.-

DEF: *Chlamydia trachomatis*: Bacterium that causes a common venereal disease. Symptoms of chlamydia are usually mild or absent, however, serious complications may cause irreversible damage, including cystitis, pelvic inflammatory disease, and infertility in women and discharge from the penis, prostatitis, and infertility in men. Genital chlamydial infection can cause arthritis, skin lesions, and inflammation of the eye and urethra.
Synonym(s): *Reiter's syndrome.*

- **A56.0** Chlamydial infection of lower genitourinary tract
  - **A56.00** Chlamydial infection of lower genitourinary tract, unspecified
  - **A56.01** Chlamydial cystitis and urethritis
  - **A56.02** Chlamydial vulvovaginitis
  - **A56.09** Other chlamydial infection of lower genitourinary tract
    Chlamydial cervicitis
- **A56.1** Chlamydial infection of pelviperitoneum and other genitourinary organs
  - **A56.11** Chlamydial female pelvic inflammatory disease
  - **A56.19** Other chlamydial genitourinary infection
    Chlamydial epididymitis
    Chlamydial orchitis
- **A56.2** Chlamydial infection of genitourinary tract, unspecified
- **A56.3** Chlamydial infection of anus and rectum
- **A56.4** Chlamydial infection of pharynx
- **A56.8** Sexually transmitted chlamydial infection of other sites

A57 Chancroid
Ulcus molle

DEF: Localized infection by *Haemophilus ducreyi*, causing genital ulcers and infecting the inguinal lymph nodes.

A58 Granuloma inguinale
Donovanosis

A59 Trichomoniasis

EXCLUDES 2 intestinal trichomoniasis (A07.8)

DEF: Infection with the parasitic, flagellated protozoa of the genus *Trichomonas*. This protozoon is found in the intestinal and genitourinary tracts of humans and in the mouth around tartar, cavities, and areas of periodontal disease.

- **A59.0** Urogenital trichomoniasis
  - **A59.00** Urogenital trichomoniasis, unspecified
    Fluor (vaginalis) due to Trichomonas
    Leukorrhea (vaginalis) due to Trichomonas
  - **A59.01** Trichomonal vulvovaginitis
  - **A59.02** Trichomonal prostatitis
  - **A59.03** Trichomonal cystitis and urethritis
  - **A59.09** Other urogenital trichomoniasis
    Trichomonas cervicitis
- **A59.8** Trichomoniasis of other sites
- **A59.9** Trichomoniasis, unspecified

A60 Anogenital herpesviral [herpes simplex] infections

- **A60.0** Herpesviral infection of genitalia and urogenital tract
  - **A60.00** Herpesviral infection of urogenital system, unspecified
  - **A60.01** Herpesviral infection of penis
  - **A60.02** Herpesviral infection of other male genital organs
  - **A60.03** Herpesviral cervicitis
  - **A60.04** Herpesviral vulvovaginitis
    Herpesviral [herpes simplex] ulceration
    Herpesviral [herpes simplex] vaginitis
    Herpesviral [herpes simplex] vulvitis
  - **A60.09** Herpesviral infection of other urogenital tract
    AHA: 2020,1Q,20
- **A60.1** Herpesviral infection of perianal skin and rectum
- **A60.9** Anogenital herpesviral infection, unspecified

A63 Other predominantly sexually transmitted diseases, not elsewhere classified

EXCLUDES 2 molluscum contagiosum (B08.1)
papilloma of cervix (D26.0)

- **A63.0** Anogenital (venereal) warts
  Anogenital warts due to (human) papillomavirus [HPV]
  Condyloma acuminatum
- **A63.8** Other specified predominantly sexually transmitted diseases

A64 Unspecified sexually transmitted disease

Other spirochetal diseases (A65-A69)

EXCLUDES 2 leptospirosis (A27.-)
syphilis (A50-A53)

A65 Nonvenereal syphilis
Bejel
Endemic syphilis
Njovera

A66 Yaws

INCLUDES bouba
frambesia (tropica)
pian

- **A66.0** Initial lesions of yaws
  Chancre of yaws
  Frambesia, initial or primary
  Initial frambesial ulcer
  Mother yaw
- **A66.1** Multiple papillomata and wet crab yaws
  Frambesioma
  Pianoma
  Plantar or palmar papilloma of yaws
- **A66.2** Other early skin lesions of yaws
  Cutaneous yaws, less than five years after infection
  Early yaws (cutaneous) (macular) (maculopapular) (micropapular) (papular)
  Frambeside of early yaws
- **A66.3** Hyperkeratosis of yaws
  Ghoul hand
  Hyperkeratosis, palmar or plantar (early) (late) due to yaws
  Worm-eaten soles
- **A66.4** Gummata and ulcers of yaws
  Gummatous frambeside
  Nodular late yaws (ulcerated)
- **A66.5** Gangosa
  Rhinopharyngitis mutilans
- **A66.6** Bone and joint lesions of yaws
  Yaws ganglion
  Yaws goundou
  Yaws gumma, bone
  Yaws gummatous osteitis or periostitis
  Yaws hydrarthrosis
  Yaws osteitis
  Yaws periostitis (hypertrophic)
- **A66.7** Other manifestations of yaws
  Juxta-articular nodules of yaws
  Mucosal yaws
- **A66.8** Latent yaws
  Yaws without clinical manifestations, with positive serology
- **A66.9** Yaws, unspecified

A67 Pinta [carate]

- **A67.0** Primary lesions of pinta
  Chancre (primary) of pinta
  Papule (primary) of pinta
- **A67.1** Intermediate lesions of pinta
  Erythematous plaques of pinta
  Hyperchromic lesions of pinta
  Hyperkeratosis of pinta
  Pintids
- **A67.2** Late lesions of pinta
  Achromic skin lesions of pinta
  Cicatricial skin lesions of pinta
  Dyschromic skin lesions of pinta
- **A67.3** Mixed lesions of pinta
  Achromic with hyperchromic skin lesions of pinta [carate]
- **A67.9** Pinta, unspecified

A68 Relapsing fevers

INCLUDES recurrent fever

EXCLUDES 2 Lyme disease (A69.2-)

- **A68.0** Louse-borne relapsing fever
  Relapsing fever due to Borrelia recurrentis
- **A68.1** Tick-borne relapsing fever
  Relapsing fever due to any Borrelia species other than Borrelia recurrentis
- **A68.9** Relapsing fever, unspecified

A69 Other spirochetal infections
A69.0 Necrotizing ulcerative stomatitis
Cancrum oris
Fusospirochetal gangrene
Noma
Stomatitis gangrenosa
A69.1 Other Vincent's infections
Fusospirochetal pharyngitis
Necrotizing ulcerative (acute) gingivitis
Necrotizing ulcerative (acute) gingivostomatitis
Spirochetal stomatitis
Trench mouth
Vincent's angina
Vincent's gingivitis
A69.2 Lyme disease
Erythema chronicum migrans due to Borrelia burgdorferi
DEF: Recurrent multisystem disorder through tick bites that begins with lesions of erythema chronicum migrans and is followed by arthritis of the large joints, myalgia, malaise, and neurological and cardiac manifestations.
A69.20 Lyme disease, unspecified
AHA: 2021,4Q,5
A69.21 Meningitis due to Lyme disease
A69.22 Other neurologic disorders in Lyme disease
Cranial neuritis
Meningoencephalitis
Polyneuropathy
A69.23 Arthritis due to Lyme disease
A69.29 Other conditions associated with Lyme disease
Myopericarditis due to Lyme disease
AHA: 2016,3Q,12
A69.8 Other specified spirochetal infections
A69.9 Spirochetal infection, unspecified

Other diseases caused by chlamydiae (A70-A74)
EXCLUDES 1: sexually transmitted chlamydial diseases (A55-A56)

A70 Chlamydia psittaci infections
Ornithosis
Parrot fever
Psittacosis

A71 Trachoma
EXCLUDES 1: sequelae of trachoma (B94.0)
A71.0 Initial stage of trachoma
Trachoma dubium
A71.1 Active stage of trachoma
Granular conjunctivitis (trachomatous)
Trachomatous follicular conjunctivitis
Trachomatous pannus
A71.9 Trachoma, unspecified

A74 Other diseases caused by chlamydiae
EXCLUDES 1: neonatal chlamydial conjunctivitis (P39.1)
neonatal chlamydial pneumonia (P23.1)
Reiter's disease (M02.3-)
sexually transmitted chlamydial diseases (A55-A56)
EXCLUDES 2: chlamydial pneumonia (J16.0)
A74.0 Chlamydial conjunctivitis
Paratrachoma
A74.8 Other chlamydial diseases
A74.81 Chlamydial peritonitis
A74.89 Other chlamydial diseases
A74.9 Chlamydial infection, unspecified
Chlamydiosis NOS

Rickettsioses (A75-A79)
DEF: Rickettsia: Condition caused by bacteria that live in lice/ticks transmitted to humans through bites.

A75 Typhus fever
EXCLUDES 1: rickettsiosis due to Ehrlichia sennetsu (A79.81)
A75.0 Epidemic louse-borne typhus fever due to Rickettsia prowazekii
Classical typhus (fever)
Epidemic (louse-borne) typhus
A75.1 Recrudescent typhus [Brill's disease]
Brill-Zinsser disease
A75.2 Typhus fever due to Rickettsia typhi
Murine (flea-borne) typhus
A75.3 Typhus fever due to Rickettsia tsutsugamushi
Scrub (mite-borne) typhus
Tsutsugamushi fever
Typhus fever due to Orientia Tsutsugamushi (scrub typhus)
A75.9 Typhus fever, unspecified
Typhus (fever) NOS

A77 Spotted fever [tick-borne rickettsioses]
A77.0 Spotted fever due to Rickettsia rickettsii
Rocky Mountain spotted fever
Sao Paulo fever
A77.1 Spotted fever due to Rickettsia conorii
African tick typhus
Boutonneuse fever
India tick typhus
Kenya tick typhus
Marseilles fever
Mediterranean tick fever
A77.2 Spotted fever due to Rickettsia siberica
North Asian tick fever
Siberian tick typhus
A77.3 Spotted fever due to Rickettsia australis
Queensland tick typhus
A77.4 Ehrlichiosis
EXCLUDES 1: anaplasmosis [A. phagocytophilum] (A79.82)
rickettsiosis due to Ehrlichia sennetsu (A79.81)
AHA: 2021,4Q,5
A77.40 Ehrlichiosis, unspecified
A77.41 Ehrlichiosis chaffeensis [E. chaffeensis]
A77.49 Other ehrlichiosis
Ehrlichiosis due to E. ewingii
Ehrlichiosis due to E. muris eauclairensis
A77.8 Other spotted fevers
Rickettsia 364D/R. philipii (Pacific Coast tick fever)
Spotted fever due to Rickettsia africae (African tick bite fever)
Spotted fever due to Rickettsia parkeri
A77.9 Spotted fever, unspecified
Tick-borne typhus NOS

A78 Q fever
Infection due to Coxiella burnetii
Nine Mile fever
Quadrilateral fever

A79 Other rickettsioses
A79.0 Trench fever
Quintan fever
Wolhynian fever
A79.1 Rickettsialpox due to Rickettsia akari
Kew Garden fever
Vesicular rickettsiosis
A79.8 Other specified rickettsioses
A79.81 Rickettsiosis due to Ehrlichia sennetsu
Rickettsiosis due to Neorickettsia sennetsu
A79.82 Anaplasmosis [A. phagocytophilum]
Transfusion transmitted A. phagocytophilum
AHA: 2021,4Q,4-5
A79.89 Other specified rickettsioses
A79.9 Rickettsiosis, unspecified
Rickettsial infection NOS

Viral and prion infections of the central nervous system (A80-A89)
EXCLUDES 1: postpolio syndrome (G14)
sequelae of poliomyelitis (B91)
sequelae of viral encephalitis (B94.1)

A80 Acute poliomyelitis
EXCLUDES 1: acute flaccid myelitis (G04.82)
A80.0 Acute paralytic poliomyelitis, vaccine-associated
A80.1 Acute paralytic poliomyelitis, wild virus, imported
A80.2 Acute paralytic poliomyelitis, wild virus, indigenous
A80.3 Acute paralytic poliomyelitis, other and unspecified
A80.30 Acute paralytic poliomyelitis, unspecified
A80.39 Other acute paralytic poliomyelitis
A80.4 Acute nonparalytic poliomyelitis
A80.9 Acute poliomyelitis, unspecified

A81 Atypical virus infections of central nervous system

INCLUDES diseases of the central nervous system caused by prions

Use additional code, if applicable, to identify:
  dementia with anxiety (F02.84, F02.A4, F02.B4, F02.C4)
  dementia with behavioral disturbance (F02.81-, F02.A1-, F02.B1-, F02.C1-)
  dementia with mood disturbance (F02.83, F02.A3, F02.B3, F02.C3)
  dementia with psychotic disturbance (F02.82, F02.A2, F02.B2, F02.C2)
  dementia without behavioral disturbance (F02.80, F02.A0, F02.B0, F02.C0)
  mild neurocognitive disorder due to known physiological condition (F06.7-)

A81.0 Creutzfeldt-Jakob disease
DEF: Communicable, rare spongiform encephalopathy occurring later in life with progressive destruction of the pyramidal and extrapyramidal systems eventually leading to death. Progressive dementia, wasting of muscles, tremor, and other symptoms are present.

- **A81.00** Creutzfeldt-Jakob disease, unspecified
  Jakob-Creutzfeldt disease, unspecified
- **A81.01** Variant Creutzfeldt-Jakob disease
  vCJD
- **A81.09** Other Creutzfeldt-Jakob disease
  CJD
  Familial Creutzfeldt-Jakob disease
  Iatrogenic Creutzfeldt-Jakob disease
  Sporadic Creutzfeldt-Jakob disease
  Subacute spongiform encephalopathy (with dementia)

A81.1 Subacute sclerosing panencephalitis
Dawson's inclusion body encephalitis
Van Bogaert's sclerosing leukoencephalopathy

A81.2 Progressive multifocal leukoencephalopathy
Multifocal leukoencephalopathy NOS

A81.8 Other atypical virus infections of central nervous system
- **A81.81** Kuru
- **A81.82** Gerstmann-Straussler-Scheinker syndrome
  GSS syndrome
- **A81.83** Fatal familial insomnia
  FFI
- **A81.89** Other atypical virus infections of central nervous system

A81.9 Atypical virus infection of central nervous system, unspecified
Prion diseases of the central nervous system NOS

A82 Rabies

- **A82.0** Sylvatic rabies
- **A82.1** Urban rabies
- **A82.9** Rabies, unspecified

A83 Mosquito-borne viral encephalitis

INCLUDES mosquito-borne viral meningoencephalitis

EXCLUDES 2 Venezuelan equine encephalitis (A92.2)
  West Nile fever (A92.3-)
  West Nile virus (A92.3-)

- **A83.0** Japanese encephalitis
- **A83.1** Western equine encephalitis
- **A83.2** Eastern equine encephalitis
- **A83.3** St Louis encephalitis
- **A83.4** Australian encephalitis
  Kunjin virus disease
- **A83.5** California encephalitis
  California meningoencephalitis
  La Crosse encephalitis
- **A83.6** Rocio virus disease
- **A83.8** Other mosquito-borne viral encephalitis
- **A83.9** Mosquito-borne viral encephalitis, unspecified

A84 Tick-borne viral encephalitis

INCLUDES tick-borne viral meningoencephalitis

- **A84.0** Far Eastern tick-borne encephalitis [Russian spring-summer encephalitis]
- **A84.1** Central European tick-borne encephalitis
- **A84.8** Other tick-borne viral encephalitis
  AHA: 2020,4Q,4-5
  - **A84.81** Powassan virus disease
  - **A84.89** Other tick-borne viral encephalitis
    Louping ill
    Code first, if applicable, transfusion related infection (T80.22-)
- **A84.9** Tick-borne viral encephalitis, unspecified

A85 Other viral encephalitis, not elsewhere classified

INCLUDES specified viral encephalomyelitis NEC
  specified viral meningoencephalitis NEC

EXCLUDES 1 encephalitis due to cytomegalovirus (B25.8)
  encephalitis due to herpesvirus [herpes simplex] (B00.4)
  encephalitis due to herpesvirus NEC (B10.0-)
  encephalitis due to measles virus (B05.0)
  encephalitis due to mumps virus (B26.2)
  encephalitis due to poliomyelitis virus (A80.-)
  encephalitis due to zoster (B02.0)
  lymphocytic choriomeningitis (A87.2)
  myalgic encephalomyelitis (G93.32)

- **A85.0** Enteroviral encephalitis
  Enteroviral encephalomyelitis
- **A85.1** Adenoviral encephalitis
  Adenoviral meningoencephalitis
- **A85.2** Arthropod-borne viral encephalitis, unspecified
  EXCLUDES 1 West nile virus with encephalitis (A92.31)
- **A85.8** Other specified viral encephalitis
  Encephalitis lethargica
  Von Economo-Cruchet disease

A86 Unspecified viral encephalitis
Viral encephalomyelitis NOS
Viral meningoencephalitis NOS

A87 Viral meningitis

EXCLUDES 1 meningitis due to herpesvirus [herpes simplex] (B00.3)
  meningitis due to measles virus (B05.1)
  meningitis due to mumps virus (B26.1)
  meningitis due to poliomyelitis virus (A80.-)
  meningitis due to zoster (B02.1)

DEF: Meningitis: Inflammation of the meningeal layers of the brain and spine.

- **A87.0** Enteroviral meningitis
  Coxsackievirus meningitis
  Echovirus meningitis
- **A87.1** Adenoviral meningitis
- **A87.2** Lymphocytic choriomeningitis
  Lymphocytic meningoencephalitis
- **A87.8** Other viral meningitis
- **A87.9** Viral meningitis, unspecified

A88 Other viral infections of central nervous system, not elsewhere classified

EXCLUDES 1 viral encephalitis NOS (A86)
  viral meningitis NOS (A87.9)

- **A88.0** Enteroviral exanthematous fever [Boston exanthem]
- **A88.1** Epidemic vertigo
- **A88.8** Other specified viral infections of central nervous system

A89 Unspecified viral infection of central nervous system

Arthropod-borne viral fevers and viral hemorrhagic fevers (A90-A99)

A90 Dengue fever [classical dengue]
EXCLUDES 1 dengue hemorrhagic fever (A91)
AHA: 2016,3Q,13

A91 Dengue hemorrhagic fever

A92 Other mosquito-borne viral fevers
EXCLUDES 1 Ross River disease (B33.1)

- **A92.0** Chikungunya virus disease
  Chikungunya (hemorrhagic) fever
- **A92.1** O'nyong-nyong fever
- **A92.2** Venezuelan equine fever
  Venezuelan equine encephalitis
  Venezuelan equine encephalomyelitis virus disease

Chapter 1. Certain Infectious and Parasitic Diseases

A92.3 West Nile virus infection
West Nile fever
AHA: 2016,3Q,12

- **A92.30** West Nile virus infection, unspecified
  West Nile fever NOS
  West Nile fever without complications
  West Nile virus NOS
- **A92.31** West Nile virus infection with encephalitis
  West Nile encephalitis
  West Nile encephalomyelitis
- **A92.32** West Nile virus infection with other neurologic manifestation
  Use additional code to specify the neurologic manifestation
- **A92.39** West Nile virus infection with other complications
  Use additional code to specify the other conditions

A92.4 Rift Valley fever

A92.5 Zika virus disease
Zika NOS
Zika virus fever
Zika virus infection
EXCLUDES 1: congenital Zika virus disease (P35.4)
AHA: 2016,4Q,4-7
DEF: Virus transmitted via a bite from an infected Aedes species mosquito. Common symptoms of the virus include fever, rash, joint pain, and conjunctivitis; they are usually mild in nature and may last from several days to a week. Most people who have the Zika virus do not require medical attention; however, in pregnant women, the Zika virus can cause a serious birth defect called microcephaly, as well as other severe fetal brain defects.
TIP: Assign code Z71.1, when a patient requests testing for Zika virus but in the absence of symptoms or recent exposure to the virus.
TIP: Code only confirmed diagnoses of Zika virus; documentation by the physician that the disease is confirmed is sufficient.

A92.8 Other specified mosquito-borne viral fevers

A92.9 Mosquito-borne viral fever, unspecified

A93 Other arthropod-borne viral fevers, not elsewhere classified

- **A93.0** Oropouche virus disease
  Oropouche fever
- **A93.1** Sandfly fever
  Pappataci fever
  Phlebotomus fever
- **A93.2** Colorado tick fever
- **A93.8** Other specified arthropod-borne viral fevers
  Piry virus disease
  Vesicular stomatitis virus disease [Indiana fever]

A94 Unspecified arthropod-borne viral fever
Arboviral fever NOS
Arbovirus infection NOS

A95 Yellow fever

- **A95.0** Sylvatic yellow fever
  Jungle yellow fever
- **A95.1** Urban yellow fever
- **A95.9** Yellow fever, unspecified

A96 Arenaviral hemorrhagic fever

- **A96.0** Junin hemorrhagic fever
  Argentinian hemorrhagic fever
- **A96.1** Machupo hemorrhagic fever
  Bolivian hemorrhagic fever
- **A96.2** Lassa fever
- **A96.8** Other arenaviral hemorrhagic fevers
- **A96.9** Arenaviral hemorrhagic fever, unspecified

A98 Other viral hemorrhagic fevers, not elsewhere classified
EXCLUDES 1: chikungunya hemorrhagic fever (A92.0)
dengue hemorrhagic fever (A91)

- **A98.0** Crimean-Congo hemorrhagic fever
  Central Asian hemorrhagic fever
- **A98.1** Omsk hemorrhagic fever
- **A98.2** Kyasanur Forest disease
- **A98.3** Marburg virus disease
- **A98.4** Ebola virus disease
- **A98.5** Hemorrhagic fever with renal syndrome
  Epidemic hemorrhagic fever
  Hantaan virus disease
  Hantavirus disease with renal manifestations
  Korean hemorrhagic fever
  Nephropathia epidemica
  Russian hemorrhagic fever
  Songo fever
  EXCLUDES 1: hantavirus (cardio)-pulmonary syndrome (B33.4)
- **A98.8** Other specified viral hemorrhagic fevers

A99 Unspecified viral hemorrhagic fever

Viral infections characterized by skin and mucous membrane lesions (B00-B09)

B00 Herpesviral [herpes simplex] infections
EXCLUDES 1: congenital herpesviral infections (P35.2)
EXCLUDES 2: anogenital herpesviral infection (A60.-)
gammaherpesviral mononucleosis (B27.0-)
herpangina (B08.5)

- **B00.0** Eczema herpeticum
  Kaposi's varicelliform eruption
- **B00.1** Herpesviral vesicular dermatitis
  Herpes simplex facialis
  Herpes simplex labialis
  Herpes simplex otitis externa
  Vesicular dermatitis of ear
  Vesicular dermatitis of lip
- **B00.2** Herpesviral gingivostomatitis and pharyngotonsillitis
  Herpesviral pharyngitis
- **B00.3** Herpesviral meningitis
- **B00.4** Herpesviral encephalitis
  Herpesviral meningoencephalitis
  Simian B disease
  EXCLUDES 1: herpesviral encephalitis due to herpesvirus 6 and 7 (B10.01, B10.09)
  non-simplex herpesviral encephalitis (B10.0-)
- **B00.5** Herpesviral ocular disease
  - **B00.50** Herpesviral ocular disease, unspecified
  - **B00.51** Herpesviral iridocyclitis
    Herpesviral iritis
    Herpesviral uveitis, anterior
  - **B00.52** Herpesviral keratitis
    Herpesviral keratoconjunctivitis
  - **B00.53** Herpesviral conjunctivitis
  - **B00.59** Other herpesviral disease of eye
    Herpesviral dermatitis of eyelid
- **B00.7** Disseminated herpesviral disease
  Herpesviral sepsis
- **B00.8** Other forms of herpesviral infections
  - **B00.81** Herpesviral hepatitis
  - **B00.82** Herpes simplex myelitis
  - **B00.89** Other herpesviral infection
    Herpesviral whitlow
- **B00.9** Herpesviral infection, unspecified
  Herpes simplex infection NOS

B01 Varicella [chickenpox]

- **B01.0** Varicella meningitis
- **B01.1** Varicella encephalitis, myelitis and encephalomyelitis
  Postchickenpox encephalitis, myelitis and encephalomyelitis
  - **B01.11** Varicella encephalitis and encephalomyelitis
    Postchickenpox encephalitis and encephalomyelitis
  - **B01.12** Varicella myelitis
    Postchickenpox myelitis
- **B01.2** Varicella pneumonia
- **B01.8** Varicella with other complications
  - **B01.81** Varicella keratitis
  - **B01.89** Other varicella complications
- **B01.9** Varicella without complication
  Varicella NOS

B02 Zoster [herpes zoster]
INCLUDES: shingles
zona

- **B02.0** Zoster encephalitis
  Zoster meningoencephalitis

| HCC CMS-HCC | Rx Rx HCC | ESR ESRD HCC | COM Commercial HCC | N Newborn: 0 | P Pediatric: 0-17 | M Maternity: 9-64 | A Adult: 15-124 |

Chapter 1. Certain Infectious and Parasitic Diseases

- **B02.1** Zoster meningitis [COM]
  - AHA: 2019,1Q,18
- ✓5th **B02.2** Zoster with other nervous system involvement
  - **B02.21** Postherpetic geniculate ganglionitis [Rx]
  - **B02.22** Postherpetic trigeminal neuralgia [Rx]
  - **B02.23** Postherpetic polyneuropathy [Rx]
  - **B02.24** Postherpetic myelitis [HCC Rx ESR COM]
    - Herpes zoster myelitis
  - **B02.29** Other postherpetic nervous system involvement [Rx]
    - Postherpetic radiculopathy
- ✓5th **B02.3** Zoster ocular disease
  - **B02.30** Zoster ocular disease, unspecified
  - **B02.31** Zoster conjunctivitis
  - **B02.32** Zoster iridocyclitis
  - **B02.33** Zoster keratitis
    - Herpes zoster keratoconjunctivitis
  - **B02.34** Zoster scleritis
  - **B02.39** Other herpes zoster eye disease
    - Zoster blepharitis
- **B02.7** Disseminated zoster
- **B02.8** Zoster with other complications
  - Herpes zoster otitis externa
- **B02.9** Zoster without complications
  - Zoster NOS

- **B03** Smallpox
  - NOTE: In 1980 the 33rd World Health Assembly declared that smallpox had been eradicated.
  - The classification is maintained for surveillance purposes.

- **B04** Monkeypox
  - Mpox
  - AHA: 2022,3Q,3-4

- ✓4th **B05** Measles
  - INCLUDES: morbilli
  - EXCLUDES 1: subacute sclerosing panencephalitis (A81.1)
  - **B05.0** Measles complicated by encephalitis [COM]
    - Postmeasles encephalitis
  - **B05.1** Measles complicated by meningitis [COM]
    - Postmeasles meningitis
  - **B05.2** Measles complicated by pneumonia
    - Postmeasles pneumonia
  - **B05.3** Measles complicated by otitis media
    - Postmeasles otitis media
  - **B05.4** Measles with intestinal complications
  - ✓5th **B05.8** Measles with other complications
    - **B05.81** Measles keratitis and keratoconjunctivitis
    - **B05.89** Other measles complications
  - **B05.9** Measles without complication
    - Measles NOS

- ✓4th **B06** Rubella [German measles]
  - EXCLUDES 1: congenital rubella (P35.0)
  - DEF: Highly contagious virus in which the symptoms are mild and short-lived in most people. Rubella during pregnancy, however, can result in abortion, stillbirth, or congenital defects.
  - ✓5th **B06.0** Rubella with neurological complications
    - **B06.00** Rubella with neurological complication, unspecified
    - **B06.01** Rubella encephalitis [COM]
      - Rubella meningoencephalitis
    - **B06.02** Rubella meningitis [COM]
    - **B06.09** Other neurological complications of rubella
  - ✓5th **B06.8** Rubella with other complications
    - **B06.81** Rubella pneumonia
    - **B06.82** Rubella arthritis [HCC ESR COM]
    - **B06.89** Other rubella complications
  - **B06.9** Rubella without complication
    - Rubella NOS

- ✓4th **B07** Viral warts
  - INCLUDES: verruca simplex
    - verruca vulgaris
    - viral warts due to human papillomavirus
  - EXCLUDES 2: anogenital (venereal) warts (A63.0)
    - papilloma of bladder (D41.4)
    - papilloma of cervix (D26.0)
    - papilloma larynx (D14.1)
  - **B07.0** Plantar wart
    - Verruca plantaris
  - **B07.8** Other viral warts
    - Common wart
    - Flat wart
    - Verruca plana
  - **B07.9** Viral wart, unspecified

- ✓4th **B08** Other viral infections characterized by skin and mucous membrane lesions, not elsewhere classified
  - EXCLUDES 1: vesicular stomatitis virus disease (A93.8)
  - ✓5th **B08.0** Other orthopoxvirus infections
    - EXCLUDES 2: monkeypox (B04)
    - ✓6th **B08.01** Cowpox and vaccinia not from vaccine
      - **B08.010** Cowpox
        - DEF: Disease contracted by milking infected cows. The vesicles usually appear on the fingers, hands, and adjacent areas and usually disappear without scarring. Other symptoms include local edema, lymphangitis, and regional lymphadenitis with or without fever.
      - **B08.011** Vaccinia not from vaccine
        - EXCLUDES 1: vaccinia (from vaccination) (generalized) (T88.1)
    - **B08.02** Orf virus disease
      - Contagious pustular dermatitis
      - Ecthyma contagiosum
    - **B08.03** Pseudocowpox [milker's node]
    - **B08.04** Paravaccinia, unspecified
    - **B08.09** Other orthopoxvirus infections
      - Orthopoxvirus infection NOS
  - **B08.1** Molluscum contagiosum
    - DEF: Benign poxvirus infection causing small bumps on the skin or conjunctiva, transmitted by close contact.
  - ✓5th **B08.2** Exanthema subitum [sixth disease]
    - Roseola infantum
    - **B08.20** Exanthema subitum [sixth disease], unspecified [P]
      - Roseola infantum, unspecified
    - **B08.21** Exanthema subitum [sixth disease] due to human herpesvirus 6 [P]
      - Roseola infantum due to human herpesvirus 6
    - **B08.22** Exanthema subitum [sixth disease] due to human herpesvirus 7 [P]
      - Roseola infantum due to human herpesvirus 7
  - **B08.3** Erythema infectiosum [fifth disease]
    - DEF: Infection with human parvovirus B19, mainly occurring in children. Symptoms include a low-grade fever, malaise, or a "cold" a few days before the appearance of a mild rash illness that presents as a "slapped-cheek" rash on the face and a lacy red rash on the trunk and limbs.
  - **B08.4** Enteroviral vesicular stomatitis with exanthem
    - Hand, foot and mouth disease
  - **B08.5** Enteroviral vesicular pharyngitis
    - Herpangina
    - DEF: Acute infectious Coxsackie virus infection causing throat lesions, fever, and vomiting that generally affects children in the summer.
  - ✓5th **B08.6** Parapoxvirus infections
    - **B08.60** Parapoxvirus infection, unspecified
    - **B08.61** Bovine stomatitis
    - **B08.62** Sealpox
    - **B08.69** Other parapoxvirus infections
  - ✓5th **B08.7** Yatapoxvirus infections
    - **B08.70** Yatapoxvirus infection, unspecified
    - **B08.71** Tanapox virus disease
    - **B08.72** Yaba pox virus disease
      - Yaba monkey tumor disease
    - **B08.79** Other yatapoxvirus infections

✓ Additional Character Required | ✓x7th Placeholder Alert | Manifestation | Unspecified Dx | Q QPP | UPD Unacceptable PDx

B08.8 Other specified viral infections characterized by skin and mucous membrane lesions
- Enteroviral lymphonodular pharyngitis
- Foot-and-mouth disease
- Poxvirus NEC

B09 Unspecified viral infection characterized by skin and mucous membrane lesions
- Viral enanthema NOS
- Viral exanthema NOS

Other human herpesviruses (B10)

B10 Other human herpesviruses
EXCLUDES 2:
- cytomegalovirus (B25.9)
- Epstein-Barr virus (B27.0-)
- herpes NOS (B00.9)
- herpes simplex (B00.-)
- herpes zoster (B02.-)
- human herpesvirus 1 and 2 (B00.-)
- human herpesvirus 3 (B01.-, B02.-)
- human herpesvirus 4 (B27.0-)
- human herpesvirus 5 (B25.-)
- human herpesvirus NOS (B00.-)
- varicella (B01.-)
- zoster (B02.-)

B10.0 Other human herpesvirus encephalitis
EXCLUDES 2:
- herpes encephalitis NOS (B00.4)
- herpes simplex encephalitis (B00.4)
- human herpesvirus encephalitis (B00.4)
- simian B herpes virus encephalitis (B00.4)

B10.01 Human herpesvirus 6 encephalitis [COM]
B10.09 Other human herpesvirus encephalitis [COM]
- Human herpesvirus 7 encephalitis
- AHA: 2024,2Q,21

B10.8 Other human herpesvirus infection
B10.81 Human herpesvirus 6 infection
B10.82 Human herpesvirus 7 infection
B10.89 Other human herpesvirus infection
- Human herpesvirus 8 infection
- Kaposi's sarcoma-associated herpesvirus infection

Viral hepatitis (B15-B19)

EXCLUDES 1: sequelae of viral hepatitis (B94.2)
EXCLUDES 2: cytomegaloviral hepatitis (B25.1)
herpesviral [herpes simplex] hepatitis (B00.81)

DEF: Hepatitis A: HAV infection that is self-limiting with flulike symptoms. Transmission is fecal-oral.
DEF: Hepatitis B: HBV infection that can be chronic and systemic. Transmission is bodily fluids.
DEF: Hepatitis C: HCV infection that can be chronic and systemic. Transmission is blood transfusion and unidentified agents.
DEF: Hepatitis D (delta): HDV that occurs only in the presence of hepatitis B virus. Transmission is contaminated blood in contact with mucous membranes.
DEF: Hepatitis E: HEV is an epidemic form. Transmission is fecal-oral, most often from contaminated water.

B15 Acute hepatitis A
B15.0 Hepatitis A with hepatic coma [COM]
B15.9 Hepatitis A without hepatic coma
- Hepatitis A (acute)(viral) NOS

B16 Acute hepatitis B
AHA: 2016,3Q,13
B16.0 Acute hepatitis B with delta-agent with hepatic coma [COM]
B16.1 Acute hepatitis B with delta-agent without hepatic coma
B16.2 Acute hepatitis B without delta-agent with hepatic coma [COM]
B16.9 Acute hepatitis B without delta-agent and without hepatic coma
- Hepatitis B (acute) (viral) NOS

B17 Other acute viral hepatitis
B17.0 Acute delta-(super) infection of hepatitis B carrier
B17.1 Acute hepatitis C
B17.10 Acute hepatitis C without hepatic coma [Rx]
- Acute hepatitis C NOS
B17.11 Acute hepatitis C with hepatic coma [Rx] [COM]
B17.2 Acute hepatitis E
B17.8 Other specified acute viral hepatitis
- Hepatitis non-A non-B (acute) (viral) NEC

B17.9 Acute viral hepatitis, unspecified
- Acute hepatitis NOS
- Acute infectious hepatitis NOS

B18 Chronic viral hepatitis
INCLUDES: carrier of viral hepatitis
▶Use additional code, if applicable, for ascites (R18.8)◀
AHA: 2017,1Q,41

B18.0 Chronic viral hepatitis B with delta-agent [HCC] [Rx] [ESR] [COM]
B18.1 Chronic viral hepatitis B without delta-agent [HCC] [Rx] [ESR] [COM]
- Carrier of viral hepatitis B
- Chronic (viral) hepatitis B
B18.2 Chronic viral hepatitis C [HCC] [Rx] [ESR] [COM]
- Carrier of viral hepatitis C
- AHA: 2018,1Q,4
B18.8 Other chronic viral hepatitis [HCC] [Rx] [ESR] [COM]
- Carrier of other viral hepatitis
B18.9 Chronic viral hepatitis, unspecified [HCC] [ESR] [COM]
- Carrier of unspecified viral hepatitis

B19 Unspecified viral hepatitis
B19.0 Unspecified viral hepatitis with hepatic coma [COM]
B19.1 Unspecified viral hepatitis B
B19.10 Unspecified viral hepatitis B without hepatic coma
- Unspecified viral hepatitis B NOS
B19.11 Unspecified viral hepatitis B with hepatic coma [COM]
B19.2 Unspecified viral hepatitis C
B19.20 Unspecified viral hepatitis C without hepatic coma [Rx]
- Viral hepatitis C NOS
B19.21 Unspecified viral hepatitis C with hepatic coma [Rx] [COM]
B19.9 Unspecified viral hepatitis without hepatic coma
- Viral hepatitis NOS

Human immunodeficiency virus [HIV] disease (B20)

B20 Human immunodeficiency virus [HIV] disease [HCC] [Rx] [ESR] [COM]
INCLUDES:
- acquired immune deficiency syndrome [AIDS]
- AIDS-related complex [ARC]
- HIV infection, symptomatic

Code first human immunodeficiency virus [HIV] disease complicating pregnancy, childbirth and the puerperium, if applicable (O98.7-)
Use additional code(s) to identify all manifestations of HIV infection
EXCLUDES 1:
- asymptomatic human immunodeficiency virus [HIV] infection status (Z21)
- exposure to HIV virus (Z20.6)
- inconclusive serologic evidence of HIV (R75)

AHA: 2022,1Q,36; 2021,2Q,6; 2021,1Q,52; 2020,4Q,97; 2020,2Q,12; 2019,1Q,8-11

Other viral diseases (B25-B34)

B25 Cytomegaloviral disease
EXCLUDES 1:
- congenital cytomegalovirus infection (P35.1)
- cytomegaloviral mononucleosis (B27.1-)

B25.0 Cytomegaloviral pneumonitis [HCC] [Rx] [ESR] [COM]
B25.1 Cytomegaloviral hepatitis [HCC] [Rx] [ESR] [COM]
B25.2 Cytomegaloviral pancreatitis [HCC] [Rx] [ESR] [COM]
B25.8 Other cytomegaloviral diseases [HCC] [Rx] [ESR] [COM]
- Cytomegaloviral encephalitis
B25.9 Cytomegaloviral disease, unspecified [HCC] [Rx] [ESR] [COM]

B26 Mumps
INCLUDES:
- epidemic parotitis
- infectious parotitis

B26.0 Mumps orchitis
B26.1 Mumps meningitis [COM]
B26.2 Mumps encephalitis [COM]
B26.3 Mumps pancreatitis [COM]
B26.8 Mumps with other complications
B26.81 Mumps hepatitis
B26.82 Mumps myocarditis [COM]
B26.83 Mumps nephritis
B26.84 Mumps polyneuropathy
B26.85 Mumps arthritis [HCC] [ESR] [COM]
B26.89 Other mumps complications

Chapter 1. Certain Infectious and Parasitic Diseases

B26.9 Mumps without complication
- Mumps NOS
- Mumps parotitis NOS

B27 Infectious mononucleosis
INCLUDES
- glandular fever
- monocytic angina
- Pfeiffer's disease

B27.0 Gammaherpesviral mononucleosis
- Mononucleosis due to Epstein-Barr virus
  - **B27.00** Gammaherpesviral mononucleosis without complication
  - **B27.01** Gammaherpesviral mononucleosis with polyneuropathy
  - **B27.02** Gammaherpesviral mononucleosis with meningitis [COM]
  - **B27.09** Gammaherpesviral mononucleosis with other complications
    - Hepatomegaly in gammaherpesviral mononucleosis
    - AHA: 2025,2Q,19; 2024,2Q,21

B27.1 Cytomegaloviral mononucleosis
  - **B27.10** Cytomegaloviral mononucleosis without complications
  - **B27.11** Cytomegaloviral mononucleosis with polyneuropathy
  - **B27.12** Cytomegaloviral mononucleosis with meningitis [COM]
  - **B27.19** Cytomegaloviral mononucleosis with other complication
    - Hepatomegaly in cytomegaloviral mononucleosis

B27.8 Other infectious mononucleosis
  - **B27.80** Other infectious mononucleosis without complication
  - **B27.81** Other infectious mononucleosis with polyneuropathy
  - **B27.82** Other infectious mononucleosis with meningitis [COM]
  - **B27.89** Other infectious mononucleosis with other complication
    - Hepatomegaly in other infectious mononucleosis

B27.9 Infectious mononucleosis, unspecified
  - **B27.90** Infectious mononucleosis, unspecified without complication
  - **B27.91** Infectious mononucleosis, unspecified with polyneuropathy
  - **B27.92** Infectious mononucleosis, unspecified with meningitis [COM]
  - **B27.99** Infectious mononucleosis, unspecified with other complication
    - Hepatomegaly in unspecified infectious mononucleosis

B30 Viral conjunctivitis
EXCLUDES 1
- herpesviral [herpes simplex] ocular disease (B00.5)
- ocular zoster (B02.3)

Viral Conjunctivitis

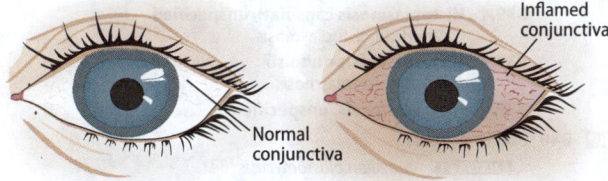

Normal conjunctiva / Inflamed conjunctiva

B30.0 Keratoconjunctivitis due to adenovirus
- Epidemic keratoconjunctivitis
- Shipyard eye

B30.1 Conjunctivitis due to adenovirus
- Acute adenoviral follicular conjunctivitis
- Swimming-pool conjunctivitis

B30.2 Viral pharyngoconjunctivitis

B30.3 Acute epidemic hemorrhagic conjunctivitis (enteroviral)
- Conjunctivitis due to coxsackievirus 24
- Conjunctivitis due to enterovirus 70
- Hemorrhagic conjunctivitis (acute)(epidemic)

B30.8 Other viral conjunctivitis
- Newcastle conjunctivitis

B30.9 Viral conjunctivitis, unspecified

B33 Other viral diseases, not elsewhere classified

B33.0 Epidemic myalgia
- Bornholm disease

B33.1 Ross River disease
- Epidemic polyarthritis and exanthema
- Ross River fever

B33.2 Viral carditis
- Coxsackie (virus) carditis
  - **B33.20** Viral carditis, unspecified [COM]
  - **B33.21** Viral endocarditis [COM]
  - **B33.22** Viral myocarditis [COM]
    - AHA: 2025,1Q,34
  - **B33.23** Viral pericarditis [COM]
  - **B33.24** Viral cardiomyopathy [HCC] [Rx] [ESR] [COM]

B33.3 Retrovirus infections, not elsewhere classified
- Retrovirus infection NOS

B33.4 Hantavirus (cardio)-pulmonary syndrome [HPS] [HCPS]
- Hantavirus disease with pulmonary manifestations
- Sin nombre virus disease
- Use additional code to identify any associated acute kidney failure (N17.9)
EXCLUDES 1
- hantavirus disease with renal manifestations (A98.5)
- hemorrhagic fever with renal manifestations (A98.5)

B33.8 Other specified viral diseases
EXCLUDES 1
- anogenital human papillomavirus infection (A63.0)
- viral warts due to human papillomavirus infection (B07)

B34 Viral infection of unspecified site
EXCLUDES 1
- anogenital human papillomavirus infection (A63.0)
- cytomegaloviral disease NOS (B25.9)
- herpesvirus [herpes simplex] infection NOS (B00.9)
- retrovirus infection NOS (B33.3)
- viral agents as the cause of diseases classified elsewhere (B97.-)
- viral warts due to human papillomavirus infection (B07)

B34.0 Adenovirus infection, unspecified

B34.1 Enterovirus infection, unspecified
- Coxsackievirus infection NOS
- Echovirus infection NOS

B34.2 Coronavirus infection, unspecified
EXCLUDES 1
- COVID-19 (U07.1)
- pneumonia due to SARS-associated coronavirus (J12.81)
- AHA: 2020,1Q,34-36

B34.3 Parvovirus infection, unspecified

B34.4 Papovavirus infection, unspecified

B34.8 Other viral infections of unspecified site

B34.9 Viral infection, unspecified
- Viremia NOS
- AHA: 2016,3Q,10

Mycoses (B35-B49)

EXCLUDES 2
- hypersensitivity pneumonitis due to organic dust (J67.-)
- mycosis fungoides (C84.0-)

B35 Dermatophytosis
INCLUDES
- favus
- infections due to species of Epidermophyton, Micro-sporum and Trichophyton
- tinea, any type except those in B36.-

DEF: Contagious superficial fungal infection of the skin that invades and grows in dead keratin.

B35.0 Tinea barbae and tinea capitis
- Beard ringworm
- Kerion
- Scalp ringworm
- Sycosis, mycotic

B35.1 Tinea unguium
- Dermatophytic onychia
- Dermatophytosis of nail
- Onychomycosis
- Ringworm of nails

B35.2 Tinea manuum
- Dermatophytosis of hand
- Hand ringworm

B35.3 Tinea pedis
- Athlete's foot
- Dermatophytosis of foot
- Foot ringworm

B35.4 Tinea corporis
- Ringworm of the body

B35.5 Tinea *imbricata*
Tokelau

B35.6 Tinea *cruris*
Dhobi itch
Groin ringworm
Jock itch

B35.8 Other dermatophytoses
Disseminated dermatophytosis
Granulomatous dermatophytosis

B35.9 Dermatophytosis, unspecified
Ringworm NOS

√4ᵗʰ **B36** Other superficial mycoses

B36.0 Pityriasis versicolor
Tinea flava
Tinea versicolor

B36.1 Tinea nigra
Keratomycosis nigricans palmaris
Microsporosis nigra
Pityriasis nigra

B36.2 White piedra
Tinea blanca

B36.3 Black piedra

B36.8 Other specified superficial mycoses

B36.9 Superficial mycosis, unspecified

√4ᵗʰ **B37** Candidiasis
INCLUDES: candidosis
moniliasis
EXCLUDES 1: neonatal candidiasis (P37.5)
DEF: *Candida:* Genus of yeast-like fungi that are commonly found in the mouth, skin, intestinal tract, and vagina. It may cause a white, cheesy discharge.

B37.0 Candidal *stomatitis*
Oral thrush

B37.1 *Pulmonary* candidiasis [HCC Rx ESR COM]
Candidal bronchitis
Candidal pneumonia

B37.2 Candidiasis of *skin and nail*
Candidal onychia
Candidal paronychia
EXCLUDES 2: diaper dermatitis (L22)

√5ᵗʰ **B37.3** Candidiasis of *vulva and vagina*
Candidal vulvovaginitis
Monilial vulvovaginitis
Vaginal thrush
AHA: 2022,4Q,4-5

B37.31 *Acute* candidiasis of vulva and vagina
Candidiasis of vulva and vagina NOS

B37.32 *Chronic* candidiasis of vulva and vagina
Recurrent candidiasis of vulva and vagina

√5ᵗʰ **B37.4** Candidiasis of other urogenital sites

B37.41 Candidal *cystitis and urethritis*

B37.42 Candidal *balanitis*

B37.49 Other urogenital candidiasis
Candidal pyelonephritis

B37.5 Candidal *meningitis* [COM]

B37.6 Candidal *endocarditis* [COM]

B37.7 Candidal *sepsis* [HCC Rx ESR COM]
Disseminated candidiasis
Systemic candidiasis
AHA: 2024,3Q,13; 2014,4Q,46

√5ᵗʰ **B37.8** Candidiasis of other sites

B37.81 Candidal *esophagitis* [HCC Rx ESR COM]

B37.82 Candidal *enteritis*
Candidal proctitis

B37.83 Candidal *cheilitis*

B37.84 Candidal *otitis externa*

B37.89 Other sites of candidiasis
Candidal osteomyelitis

B37.9 Candidiasis, unspecified
Thrush NOS

√4ᵗʰ **B38** Coccidioidomycosis

B38.0 *Acute pulmonary* coccidioidomycosis [ESR COM]

B38.1 *Chronic pulmonary* coccidioidomycosis [ESR COM]

B38.2 *Pulmonary* coccidioidomycosis, unspecified [ESR COM]

B38.3 *Cutaneous* coccidioidomycosis

B38.4 Coccidioidomycosis *meningitis* [COM]
DEF: *Coccidioides immitis* infection of the lining of the brain and/or spinal cord.

B38.7 *Disseminated* coccidioidomycosis
Generalized coccidioidomycosis

√5ᵗʰ **B38.8** Other forms of coccidioidomycosis

B38.81 *Prostatic* coccidioidomycosis

B38.89 Other forms of coccidioidomycosis

B38.9 Coccidioidomycosis, unspecified

√4ᵗʰ **B39** Histoplasmosis
Code first associated AIDS (B20)
Use additional code for any associated manifestations, such as:
endocarditis (I39)
meningitis (G02)
pericarditis (I32)
retinitis (H32)
DEF: Type of lung infection caused by breathing in fungal spores often found in the droppings of bats and birds or soil contaminated by their droppings.

B39.0 *Acute pulmonary* histoplasmosis capsulati [ESR COM]

B39.1 *Chronic pulmonary* histoplasmosis capsulati [ESR COM]

B39.2 Pulmonary histoplasmosis capsulati, unspecified [ESR COM]

B39.3 *Disseminated* histoplasmosis capsulati
Generalized histoplasmosis capsulati

B39.4 Histoplasmosis capsulati, unspecified
American histoplasmosis

B39.5 Histoplasmosis *duboisii*
African histoplasmosis

B39.9 Histoplasmosis, unspecified

√4ᵗʰ **B40** Blastomycosis
EXCLUDES 1: Brazilian blastomycosis (B41.-)
keloidal blastomycosis (B48.0)

B40.0 *Acute pulmonary* blastomycosis [ESR COM]

B40.1 *Chronic pulmonary* blastomycosis [ESR COM]

B40.2 *Pulmonary* blastomycosis, unspecified [ESR COM]

B40.3 *Cutaneous* blastomycosis

B40.7 *Disseminated* blastomycosis
Generalized blastomycosis

√5ᵗʰ **B40.8** Other forms of blastomycosis

B40.81 Blastomycotic *meningoencephalitis* [COM]
Meningomyelitis due to blastomycosis

B40.89 Other forms of blastomycosis

B40.9 Blastomycosis, unspecified

√4ᵗʰ **B41** Paracoccidioidomycosis
INCLUDES: Brazilian blastomycosis
Lutz' disease

B41.0 *Pulmonary* paracoccidioidomycosis [ESR COM]

- **B41.7** Disseminated paracoccidioidomycosis
  Generalized paracoccidioidomycosis
- **B41.8** Other forms of paracoccidioidomycosis
- **B41.9** Paracoccidioidomycosis, unspecified

B42 Sporotrichosis
- **B42.0** Pulmonary sporotrichosis
- **B42.1** Lymphocutaneous sporotrichosis
- **B42.7** Disseminated sporotrichosis
  Generalized sporotrichosis
- **B42.8** Other forms of sporotrichosis
  - **B42.81** Cerebral sporotrichosis
    Meningitis due to sporotrichosis
  - **B42.82** Sporotrichosis arthritis
  - **B42.89** Other forms of sporotrichosis
- **B42.9** Sporotrichosis, unspecified

B43 Chromomycosis and pheomycotic abscess
- **B43.0** Cutaneous chromomycosis
  Dermatitis verrucosa
- **B43.1** Pheomycotic brain abscess
  Cerebral chromomycosis
- **B43.2** Subcutaneous pheomycotic abscess and cyst
- **B43.8** Other forms of chromomycosis
- **B43.9** Chromomycosis, unspecified

B44 Aspergillosis
  INCLUDES aspergilloma
- **B44.0** Invasive pulmonary aspergillosis
- **B44.1** Other pulmonary aspergillosis
- **B44.2** Tonsillar aspergillosis
- **B44.7** Disseminated aspergillosis
  Generalized aspergillosis
- **B44.8** Other forms of aspergillosis
  - **B44.81** Allergic bronchopulmonary aspergillosis
  - **B44.89** Other forms of aspergillosis
- **B44.9** Aspergillosis, unspecified

B45 Cryptococcosis
- **B45.0** Pulmonary cryptococcosis
- **B45.1** Cerebral cryptococcosis
  Cryptococcal meningitis
  Cryptococcosis meningocerebralis
- **B45.2** Cutaneous cryptococcosis
- **B45.3** Osseous cryptococcosis
- **B45.7** Disseminated cryptococcosis
  Generalized cryptococcosis
- **B45.8** Other forms of cryptococcosis
- **B45.9** Cryptococcosis, unspecified

B46 Zygomycosis
- **B46.0** Pulmonary mucormycosis
- **B46.1** Rhinocerebral mucormycosis
- **B46.2** Gastrointestinal mucormycosis
- **B46.3** Cutaneous mucormycosis
  Subcutaneous mucormycosis
- **B46.4** Disseminated mucormycosis
  Generalized mucormycosis
- **B46.5** Mucormycosis, unspecified
- **B46.8** Other zygomycoses
  Entomophthoromycosis
- **B46.9** Zygomycosis, unspecified
  Phycomycosis NOS

B47 Mycetoma
- **B47.0** Eumycetoma
  Madura foot, mycotic
  Maduromycosis
- **B47.1** Actinomycetoma
- **B47.9** Mycetoma, unspecified
  Madura foot NOS

B48 Other mycoses, not elsewhere classified
- **B48.0** Lobomycosis
  Keloidal blastomycosis
  Lobo's disease
- **B48.1** Rhinosporidiosis
- **B48.2** Allescheriasis
  Infection due to Pseudallescheria boydii
  EXCLUDES 1 eumycetoma (B47.0)
- **B48.3** Geotrichosis
  Geotrichum stomatitis
- **B48.4** Penicillosis
  Talaromycosis
- **B48.8** Other specified mycoses
  Adiaspiromycosis
  Infection of tissue and organs by Alternaria
  Infection of tissue and organs by Drechslera
  Infection of tissue and organs by Fusarium
  Infection of tissue and organs by saprophytic fungi NEC
  AHA: 2014,4Q,46; 2014,2Q,13

B49 Unspecified mycosis
  Fungemia NOS

Protozoal diseases (B50-B64)
EXCLUDES 1 amebiasis (A06.-)
other protozoal intestinal diseases (A07.-)

B50 Plasmodium falciparum malaria
  INCLUDES mixed infections of Plasmodium falciparum with any other Plasmodium species
- **B50.0** Plasmodium falciparum malaria with cerebral complications
  Cerebral malaria NOS
- **B50.8** Other severe and complicated Plasmodium falciparum malaria
  Severe or complicated Plasmodium falciparum malaria NOS
- **B50.9** Plasmodium falciparum malaria, unspecified

B51 Plasmodium vivax malaria
  INCLUDES mixed infections of Plasmodium vivax with other Plasmodium species, except Plasmodium falciparum
  EXCLUDES 1 Plasmodium vivax with Plasmodium falciparum (B50.-)
- **B51.0** Plasmodium vivax malaria with rupture of spleen
- **B51.8** Plasmodium vivax malaria with other complications
- **B51.9** Plasmodium vivax malaria without complication
  Plasmodium vivax malaria NOS

B52 Plasmodium malariae malaria
  INCLUDES mixed infections of Plasmodium malariae with other Plasmodium species, except Plasmodium falciparum and Plasmodium vivax
  EXCLUDES 1 Plasmodium falciparum (B50.-)
  Plasmodium vivax (B51.-)
- **B52.0** Plasmodium malariae malaria with nephropathy
- **B52.8** Plasmodium malariae malaria with other complications
- **B52.9** Plasmodium malariae malaria without complication
  Plasmodium malariae malaria NOS

B53 Other specified malaria
- **B53.0** Plasmodium ovale malaria
  EXCLUDES 1 Plasmodium ovale with Plasmodium falciparum (B50.-)
  Plasmodium ovale with Plasmodium malariae (B52.-)
  Plasmodium ovale with Plasmodium vivax (B51.-)
- **B53.1** Malaria due to simian plasmodia
  EXCLUDES 1 malaria due to simian plasmodia with Plasmodium falciparum (B50.-)
  malaria due to simian plasmodia with Plasmodium malariae (B52.-)
  malaria due to simian plasmodia with Plasmodium ovale (B53.0)
  malaria due to simian plasmodia with Plasmodium vivax (B51.-)
- **B53.8** Other malaria, not elsewhere classified

B54 Unspecified malaria

B55 Leishmaniasis
- **B55.0** Visceral leishmaniasis
  Kala-azar
  Post-kala-azar dermal leishmaniasis
- **B55.1** Cutaneous leishmaniasis
- **B55.2** Mucocutaneous leishmaniasis
- **B55.9** Leishmaniasis, unspecified

B56 African trypanosomiasis
- **B56.0** Gambiense trypanosomiasis
  Infection due to Trypanosoma brucei gambiense
  West African sleeping sickness

B56.1 Rhodesiense trypanosomiasis
East African sleeping sickness
Infection due to Trypanosoma brucei rhodesiense

B56.9 African trypanosomiasis, unspecified
Sleeping sickness NOS

✓4th **B57 Chagas' disease**
INCLUDES American trypanosomiasis
infection due to Trypanosoma cruzi

B57.0 Acute Chagas' disease with heart involvement
Acute Chagas' disease with myocarditis

B57.1 Acute Chagas' disease without heart involvement
Acute Chagas' disease NOS

B57.2 Chagas' disease (chronic) with heart involvement
American trypanosomiasis NOS
Chagas' disease (chronic) NOS
Chagas' disease (chronic) with myocarditis
Trypanosomiasis NOS

✓5th **B57.3 Chagas' disease (chronic) with digestive system involvement**
  B57.30 Chagas' disease with digestive system involvement, unspecified
  B57.31 Megaesophagus in Chagas' disease
  B57.32 Megacolon in Chagas' disease
  B57.39 Other digestive system involvement in Chagas' disease

✓5th **B57.4 Chagas' disease (chronic) with nervous system involvement**
  B57.40 Chagas' disease with nervous system involvement, unspecified
  B57.41 Meningitis in Chagas' disease [COM]
  B57.42 Meningoencephalitis in Chagas' disease [COM]
  B57.49 Other nervous system involvement in Chagas' disease

B57.5 Chagas' disease (chronic) with other organ involvement

✓4th **B58 Toxoplasmosis**
INCLUDES infection due to Toxoplasma gondii
EXCLUDES 1 congenital toxoplasmosis (P37.1)

✓5th **B58.0 Toxoplasma oculopathy**
  B58.00 Toxoplasma oculopathy, unspecified
  B58.01 Toxoplasma chorioretinitis
  B58.09 Other toxoplasma oculopathy
    Toxoplasma uveitis

B58.1 Toxoplasma hepatitis

B58.2 Toxoplasma meningoencephalitis [HCC] [Rx] [ESR] [COM]

B58.3 Pulmonary toxoplasmosis [HCC] [Rx] [ESR] [COM]

✓5th **B58.8 Toxoplasmosis with other organ involvement**
  B58.81 Toxoplasma myocarditis [COM]
  B58.82 Toxoplasma myositis
  B58.83 Toxoplasma tubulo-interstitial nephropathy
    Toxoplasma pyelonephritis
  B58.89 Toxoplasmosis with other organ involvement

B58.9 Toxoplasmosis, unspecified

B59 Pneumocystosis [HCC] [Rx] [ESR] [COM]
Pneumonia due to Pneumocystis carinii
▶Pneumonia due to Pneumocystis jirovecii◀

✓4th **B60 Other protozoal diseases, not elsewhere classified**
EXCLUDES 1 cryptosporidiosis (A07.2)
intestinal microsporidiosis (A07.8)
isosporiasis (A07.3)

✓5th **B60.0 Babesiosis**
AHA: 2020,4Q,5-6
  B60.00 Babesiosis, unspecified
    Babesiosis due to unspecified Babesia species
    Piroplasmosis, unspecified
  B60.01 Babesiosis due to Babesia microti
    Infection due to B. microti
  B60.02 Babesiosis due to Babesia duncani
    Infection due to B. duncani and B. duncani-type species
  B60.03 Babesiosis due to Babesia divergens
    Babesiosis due to Babesia MO-1
    Infection due to B. divergens and B. divergens-like strains
  B60.09 Other babesiosis
    Babesiosis due to Babesia KO-1
    Babesiosis due to Babesia venatorum
    Infection due to other Babesia species
    Infection due to other protozoa of the order Piroplasmida
    Other piroplasmosis

✓5th **B60.1 Acanthamebiasis**
  B60.10 Acanthamebiasis, unspecified
  B60.11 Meningoencephalitis due to Acanthamoeba (culbertsoni) [COM]
  B60.12 Conjunctivitis due to Acanthamoeba
  B60.13 Keratoconjunctivitis due to Acanthamoeba
  B60.19 Other acanthamebic disease

B60.2 Naegleriasis
Primary amebic meningoencephalitis

B60.8 Other specified protozoal diseases
Microsporidiosis

B64 Unspecified protozoal disease

Helminthiases (B65-B83)

✓4th **B65 Schistosomiasis [bilharziasis]**
INCLUDES snail fever

B65.0 Schistosomiasis due to Schistosoma haematobium [urinary schistosomiasis]

B65.1 Schistosomiasis due to Schistosoma mansoni [intestinal schistosomiasis]

B65.2 Schistosomiasis due to Schistosoma japonicum
Asiatic schistosomiasis

B65.3 Cercarial dermatitis
Swimmer's itch

B65.8 Other schistosomiasis
Infection due to Schistosoma intercalatum
Infection due to Schistosoma mattheei
Infection due to Schistosoma mekongi

B65.9 Schistosomiasis, unspecified

✓4th **B66 Other fluke infections**
B66.0 Opisthorchiasis
Infection due to cat liver fluke
Infection due to Opisthorchis (felineus)(viverrini)

B66.1 Clonorchiasis
Chinese liver fluke disease
Infection due to Clonorchis sinensis
Oriental liver fluke disease

B66.2 Dicroceliasis
Infection due to Dicrocoelium dendriticum
Lancet fluke infection

B66.3 Fascioliasis
Infection due to Fasciola gigantica
Infection due to Fasciola hepatica
Infection due to Fasciola indica
Sheep liver fluke disease

B66.4 Paragonimiasis [ESR] [COM]
Infection due to Paragonimus species
Lung fluke disease
Pulmonary distomiasis

B66.5 Fasciolopsiasis
Infection due to Fasciolopsis buski
Intestinal distomiasis

B66.8 Other specified fluke infections
Echinostomiasis
Heterophyiasis
Metagonimiasis
Nanophyetiasis
Watsoniasis

B66.9 Fluke infection, unspecified

✓4th **B67 Echinococcosis**
INCLUDES hydatidosis

B67.0 Echinococcus granulosus infection of liver
B67.1 Echinococcus granulosus infection of lung [ESR] [COM]
B67.2 Echinococcus granulosus infection of bone

✓5th **B67.3 Echinococcus granulosus infection, other and multiple sites**
  B67.31 Echinococcus granulosus infection, thyroid gland
  B67.32 Echinococcus granulosus infection, multiple sites
  B67.39 Echinococcus granulosus infection, other sites

B67.4 Echinococcus granulosus infection, unspecified
Dog tapeworm (infection)

B67.5 Echinococcus multilocularis infection of liver

✓5th **B67.6 Echinococcus multilocularis infection, other and multiple sites**
  B67.61 Echinococcus multilocularis infection, multiple sites
  B67.69 Echinococcus multilocularis infection, other sites

B67.7 Echinococcus multilocularis infection, unspecified

B67.8 Echinococcosis, unspecified, of liver

B67.9 Echinococcosis, other and unspecified
B67.90 Echinococcosis, unspecified
Echinococcosis NOS
B67.99 Other echinococcosis

B68 Taeniasis
EXCLUDES 1 cysticercosis (B69.-)
B68.0 Taenia solium taeniasis
Pork tapeworm (infection)
B68.1 Taenia saginata taeniasis
Beef tapeworm (infection)
Infection due to adult tapeworm Taenia saginata
B68.9 Taeniasis, unspecified

B69 Cysticercosis
INCLUDES cysticerciasis infection due to larval form of Taenia solium
DEF: Condition that is developed when larvae or eggs of the tapeworm *Taenia solium* are ingested, most commonly in fecally contaminated water or undercooked pork.
B69.0 Cysticercosis of central nervous system
B69.1 Cysticercosis of eye
B69.8 Cysticercosis of other sites
B69.81 Myositis in cysticercosis
B69.89 Cysticercosis of other sites
B69.9 Cysticercosis, unspecified

B70 Diphyllobothriasis and sparganosis
B70.0 Diphyllobothriasis
Diphyllobothrium (adult) (latum) (pacificum) infection
Fish tapeworm (infection)
EXCLUDES 2 larval diphyllobothriasis (B70.1)
B70.1 Sparganosis
Infection due to Sparganum (mansoni) (proliferum)
Infection due to Spirometra larva
Larval diphyllobothriasis
Spirometrosis

B71 Other cestode infections
B71.0 Hymenolepiasis
Dwarf tapeworm infection
Rat tapeworm (infection)
B71.1 Dipylidiasis
B71.8 Other specified cestode infections
Coenurosis
B71.9 Cestode infection, unspecified
Tapeworm (infection) NOS

B72 Dracunculiasis
INCLUDES guinea worm infection
infection due to Dracunculus medinensis

B73 Onchocerciasis
INCLUDES onchocerca volvulus infection
onchocercosis
river blindness
B73.0 Onchocerciasis with eye disease
B73.00 Onchocerciasis with eye involvement, unspecified
B73.01 Onchocerciasis with endophthalmitis
B73.02 Onchocerciasis with glaucoma
B73.09 Onchocerciasis with other eye involvement
Infestation of eyelid due to onchocerciasis
B73.1 Onchocerciasis without eye disease

B74 Filariasis
EXCLUDES 2 onchocerciasis (B73)
tropical (pulmonary) eosinophilia NOS (J82.89)
B74.0 Filariasis due to Wuchereria bancrofti
Bancroftian elephantiasis
Bancroftian filariasis
B74.1 Filariasis due to Brugia malayi
B74.2 Filariasis due to Brugia timori
B74.3 Loiasis
Calabar swelling
Eyeworm disease of Africa
Loa loa infection
B74.4 Mansonelliasis
Infection due to Mansonella ozzardi
Infection due to Mansonella perstans
Infection due to Mansonella streptocerca
B74.8 Other filariases
Dirofilariasis
B74.9 Filariasis, unspecified

B75 Trichinellosis
INCLUDES infection due to Trichinella species
trichiniasis
DEF: Infection by *Trichinella spiralis*, the smallest of the parasitic nematodes, that is transmitted by eating undercooked pork or bear meat.
Synonym(s): Trichinosis.

B76 Hookworm diseases
INCLUDES uncinariasis
B76.0 Ancylostomiasis
Infection due to Ancylostoma species
B76.1 Necatoriasis
Infection due to Necator americanus
B76.8 Other hookworm diseases
B76.9 Hookworm disease, unspecified
Cutaneous larva migrans NOS

B77 Ascariasis
INCLUDES ascaridiasis
roundworm infection
B77.0 Ascariasis with intestinal complications
B77.8 Ascariasis with other complications
B77.81 Ascariasis pneumonia
B77.89 Ascariasis with other complications
B77.9 Ascariasis, unspecified

B78 Strongyloidiasis
EXCLUDES 1 trichostrongyliasis (B81.2)
B78.0 Intestinal strongyloidiasis
B78.1 Cutaneous strongyloidiasis
B78.7 Disseminated strongyloidiasis
B78.9 Strongyloidiasis, unspecified

B79 Trichuriasis
INCLUDES trichocephaliasis
whipworm (disease)(infection)

B80 Enterobiasis
INCLUDES oxyuriasis
pinworm infection
threadworm infection

B81 Other intestinal helminthiases, not elsewhere classified
EXCLUDES 1 angiostrongyliasis due to:
angiostrongylus cantonensis (B83.2)
parastrongylus cantonensis (B83.2)
B81.0 Anisakiasis
Infection due to Anisakis larva
B81.1 Intestinal capillariasis
Capillariasis NOS
Infection due to Capillaria philippinensis
EXCLUDES 2 hepatic capillariasis (B83.8)
B81.2 Trichostrongyliasis
B81.3 Intestinal angiostrongyliasis
Angiostrongyliasis due to:
Angiostrongylus costaricensis
Parastrongylus costaricensis
B81.4 Mixed intestinal helminthiases
Infection due to intestinal helminths classified to more than one of the categories B65.0-B81.3 and B81.8
Mixed helminthiasis NOS
B81.8 Other specified intestinal helminthiases
Infection due to Oesophagostomum species [esophagostomiasis]
Infection due to Ternidens diminutus [ternidensiasis]

B82 Unspecified intestinal parasitism
B82.0 Intestinal helminthiasis, unspecified
B82.9 Intestinal parasitism, unspecified

B83 Other helminthiases
EXCLUDES 1 capillariasis NOS (B81.1)
EXCLUDES 2 intestinal capillariasis (B81.1)
B83.0 Visceral larva migrans
Toxocariasis
B83.1 Gnathostomiasis
Wandering swelling
B83.2 Angiostrongyliasis due to Parastrongylus cantonensis
Eosinophilic meningoencephalitis due to Parastrongylus cantonensis
EXCLUDES 2 intestinal angiostrongyliasis (B81.3)
B83.3 Syngamiasis
Syngamosis

B83.4 Internal hirudiniasis
  EXCLUDES 2 external hirudiniasis (B88.3)

B83.8 Other specified helminthiases
  Acanthocephaliasis
  Gongylonemiasis
  Hepatic capillariasis
  Metastrongyliasis
  Thelaziasis

B83.9 Helminthiasis, unspecified
  Worms NOS
  EXCLUDES 1 intestinal helminthiasis NOS (B82.0)

Pediculosis, acariasis and other infestations (B85-B89)

B85 Pediculosis and phthiriasis

  B85.0 Pediculosis due to Pediculus humanus capitis
    Head-louse infestation

  B85.1 Pediculosis due to Pediculus humanus corporis
    Body-louse infestation

  B85.2 Pediculosis, unspecified

  B85.3 Phthiriasis
    Infestation by crab-louse
    Infestation by Phthirus pubis

  B85.4 Mixed pediculosis and phthiriasis
    Infestation classifiable to more than one of the categories B85.0-B85.3

B86 Scabies
  Sarcoptic itch
  DEF: Mite infestation that is caused by *Sarcoptes scabiei*. Scabies causes intense itching and sometimes secondary infection.

B87 Myiasis
  INCLUDES infestation by larva of flies

  B87.0 Cutaneous myiasis
    Creeping myiasis

  B87.1 Wound myiasis
    Traumatic myiasis

  B87.2 Ocular myiasis

  B87.3 Nasopharyngeal myiasis
    Laryngeal myiasis

  B87.4 Aural myiasis

  B87.8 Myiasis of other sites
    B87.81 Genitourinary myiasis
    B87.82 Intestinal myiasis
    B87.89 Myiasis of other sites

  B87.9 Myiasis, unspecified

B88 Other infestations

  B88.0 Other acariasis
    ~~Acarine dermatitis~~
    ~~Dermatitis due to Demodex species~~
    ~~Dermatitis due to Dermanyssus gallinae~~
    ~~Dermatitis due to Liponyssoides sanguineus~~
    ~~Trombiculosis~~
    EXCLUDES 2 scabies (B86)

  • **B88.01 Infestation by Demodex mites**
      Demodex brevis infestation
      Demodex folliculorum infestation
      Code also, if applicable, eyelid inflammation (H01.8-)

  • **B88.09 Other acariasis**
      Acarine dermatitis
      Dermatitis due to Dermanyssus gallinae
      Dermatitis due to Liponyssoides sanguineus
      Trombiculosis

  B88.1 Tungiasis [sandflea infestation]

  B88.2 Other arthropod infestations
    Scarabiasis

  B88.3 External hirudiniasis
    Leech infestation NOS
    EXCLUDES 2 internal hirudiniasis (B83.4)

  B88.8 Other specified infestations
    Ichthyoparasitism due to Vandellia cirrhosa
    Linguatulosis
    Porocephaliasis

  B88.9 Infestation, unspecified
    Infestation (skin) NOS
    Infestation by mites NOS
    Skin parasites NOS

B89 Unspecified parasitic disease

Sequelae of infectious and parasitic diseases (B90-B94)

NOTE Categories B90-B94 are to be used to indicate conditions in categories A00-B89 as the cause of sequelae, which are themselves classified elsewhere. The "sequelae" include conditions specified as such; they also include residuals of diseases classifiable to the above categories if there is evidence that the disease itself is no longer present. Codes from these categories are not to be used for chronic infections. Code chronic current infections to active infectious disease as appropriate.

Code first condition resulting from (sequela) the infectious or parasitic disease

B90 Sequelae of tuberculosis
  B90.0 Sequelae of central nervous system tuberculosis
  B90.1 Sequelae of genitourinary tuberculosis
  B90.2 Sequelae of tuberculosis of bones and joints
  B90.8 Sequelae of tuberculosis of other organs
    EXCLUDES 2 sequelae of respiratory tuberculosis (B90.9)
  B90.9 Sequelae of respiratory and unspecified tuberculosis
    Sequelae of tuberculosis NOS

B91 Sequelae of poliomyelitis
  EXCLUDES 1 postpolio syndrome (G14)

B92 Sequelae of leprosy

B94 Sequelae of other and unspecified infectious and parasitic diseases
  B94.0 Sequelae of trachoma
  B94.1 Sequelae of viral encephalitis
  B94.2 Sequelae of viral hepatitis
  B94.8 Sequelae of other specified infectious and parasitic diseases
    AHA: 2021,1Q,25-30,31-49; 2020,3Q,10-14; 2017,4Q,109
  B94.9 Sequelae of unspecified infectious and parasitic disease
    EXCLUDES 2 post COVID-19 condition (U09.9)

Bacterial and viral infectious agents (B95-B97)

NOTE These categories are provided for use as supplementary or additional codes to identify the infectious agent(s) in diseases classified elsewhere.

AHA: 2020,2Q,18; 2018,4Q,34; 2018,1Q,16

B95 Streptococcus, Staphylococcus, and Enterococcus as the cause of diseases classified elsewhere

  B95.0 Streptococcus, group A, as the cause of diseases classified elsewhere

  B95.1 Streptococcus, group B, as the cause of diseases classified elsewhere
    AHA: 2020,1Q,10; 2019,2Q,8-10

  B95.2 Enterococcus as the cause of diseases classified elsewhere

  B95.3 Streptococcus pneumoniae as the cause of diseases classified elsewhere

  B95.4 Other streptococcus as the cause of diseases classified elsewhere
    AHA: 2025,1Q,20

  B95.5 Unspecified streptococcus as the cause of diseases classified elsewhere

  B95.6 Staphylococcus aureus as the cause of diseases classified elsewhere

    B95.61 Methicillin susceptible Staphylococcus aureus infection as the cause of diseases classified elsewhere
      Methicillin susceptible Staphylococcus aureus (MSSA) infection as the cause of diseases classified elsewhere
      Staphylococcus aureus infection NOS as the cause of diseases classified elsewhere

    B95.62 Methicillin resistant Staphylococcus aureus infection as the cause of diseases classified elsewhere
      Methicillin resistant staphylococcus aureus (MRSA) infection as the cause of diseases classified elsewhere
      AHA: 2016,1Q,12

  B95.7 Other staphylococcus as the cause of diseases classified elsewhere

  B95.8 Unspecified staphylococcus as the cause of diseases classified elsewhere

B96 Other bacterial agents as the cause of diseases classified elsewhere

  B96.0 Mycoplasma pneumoniae [M. pneumoniae] as the cause of diseases classified elsewhere
    Pleuro-pneumonia-like-organism [PPLO]

- **B96.1** Klebsiella pneumoniae [K. pneumoniae] as the cause of diseases classified elsewhere [UPD]
- ✓5th **B96.2** Escherichia coli [E. coli] as the cause of diseases classified elsewhere
  - AHA: 2022,1Q,31
  - **B96.20** Unspecified Escherichia coli [E. coli] as the cause of diseases classified elsewhere [UPD]
    - Escherichia coli [E. coli] NOS
  - **B96.21** Shiga toxin-producing Escherichia coli [E. coli] [STEC] O157 as the cause of diseases classified elsewhere [UPD]
    - E. coli O157 with confirmation of Shiga toxin when H antigen is unknown, or is not H7
    - E. coli O157:H- (nonmotile) with confirmation of Shiga toxin
    - ▶O157:H7 Escherichia coli [E. coli] with or without confirmation of Shiga toxin-production◀
    - ▶Shiga toxin-producing Escherichia coli [E. coli] O157:H7 with or without confirmation of Shiga toxin-production◀
    - STEC O157:H7 with or without confirmation of Shiga toxin-production
  - **B96.22** Other specified Shiga toxin-producing Escherichia coli [E. coli] [STEC] as the cause of diseases classified elsewhere [UPD]
    - ▶Non-O157 Shiga toxin-producing Escherichia coli [E. coli]◀
    - ▶Non-O157 Shiga toxin-producing Escherichia coli [E. coli] with known O group◀
  - **B96.23** Unspecified Shiga toxin-producing Escherichia coli [E. coli] [STEC] as the cause of diseases classified elsewhere [UPD]
    - Shiga toxin-producing Escherichia coli [E. coli] with unspecified O group
    - STEC NOS
  - **B96.29** Other Escherichia coli [E. coli] as the cause of diseases classified elsewhere [UPD]
    - Non-Shiga toxin-producing E. coli
- **B96.3** Hemophilus influenzae [H. influenzae] as the cause of diseases classified elsewhere [UPD]
- **B96.4** Proteus (mirabilis) (morganii) as the cause of diseases classified elsewhere
- **B96.5** Pseudomonas (aeruginosa) (mallei) (pseudomallei) as the cause of diseases classified elsewhere [UPD]
  - AHA: 2015,1Q,18
- **B96.6** Bacteroides fragilis [B. fragilis] as the cause of diseases classified elsewhere [UPD]
- **B96.7** Clostridium perfringens [C. perfringens] as the cause of diseases classified elsewhere [UPD]
- ✓5th **B96.8** Other specified bacterial agents as the cause of diseases classified elsewhere
  - **B96.81** Helicobacter pylori [H. pylori] as the cause of diseases classified elsewhere [UPD]
  - **B96.82** Vibrio vulnificus as the cause of diseases classified elsewhere [UPD]
  - **B96.83** Acinetobacter baumannii as the cause of diseases classified elsewhere [UPD]
    - AHA: 2023,4Q,4
  - **B96.89** Other specified bacterial agents as the cause of diseases classified elsewhere [UPD]
- ✓4th **B97** Viral agents as the cause of diseases classified elsewhere
  - AHA: 2016,3Q,8-10,14
  - **B97.0** Adenovirus as the cause of diseases classified elsewhere [UPD]
  - ✓5th **B97.1** Enterovirus as the cause of diseases classified elsewhere
    - **B97.10** Unspecified enterovirus as the cause of diseases classified elsewhere [UPD]
    - **B97.11** Coxsackievirus as the cause of diseases classified elsewhere [UPD]
    - **B97.12** Echovirus as the cause of diseases classified elsewhere [UPD]
    - **B97.19** Other enterovirus as the cause of diseases classified elsewhere [UPD]
  - ✓5th **B97.2** Coronavirus as the cause of diseases classified elsewhere
    - **B97.21** SARS-associated coronavirus as the cause of diseases classified elsewhere [UPD]
      - EXCLUDES 1 pneumonia due to SARS-associated coronavirus (J12.81)
    - **B97.29** Other coronavirus as the cause of diseases classified elsewhere [UPD]
      - AHA: 2020,2Q,5; 2020,1Q,34-36
  - ✓5th **B97.3** Retrovirus as the cause of diseases classified elsewhere
    - EXCLUDES 1 human immunodeficiency virus [HIV] disease (B20)
    - **B97.30** Unspecified retrovirus as the cause of diseases classified elsewhere [UPD]
    - **B97.31** Lentivirus as the cause of diseases classified elsewhere [UPD]
    - **B97.32** Oncovirus as the cause of diseases classified elsewhere [UPD]
    - **B97.33** Human T-cell lymphotrophic virus, type I [HTLV-I] as the cause of diseases classified elsewhere [UPD]
    - **B97.34** Human T-cell lymphotrophic virus, type II [HTLV-II] as the cause of diseases classified elsewhere [UPD]
    - **B97.35** Human immunodeficiency virus, type 2 [HIV 2] as the cause of diseases classified elsewhere [HCC] [Rx] [ESR] [COM] [UPD]
    - **B97.39** Other retrovirus as the cause of diseases classified elsewhere [UPD]
  - **B97.4** Respiratory syncytial virus as the cause of diseases classified elsewhere [UPD]
    - RSV as the cause of diseases classified elsewhere
    - Code first related disorders, such as:
      - otitis media (H65.-)
      - upper respiratory infection (J06.9)
    - EXCLUDES 1 acute bronchiolitis due to respiratory syncytial virus (RSV) (J21.0)
      - acute bronchitis due to respiratory syncytial virus (RSV) (J20.5)
      - respiratory syncytial virus (RSV) pneumonia (J12.1)
  - **B97.5** Reovirus as the cause of diseases classified elsewhere [UPD]
  - **B97.6** Parvovirus as the cause of diseases classified elsewhere [UPD]
  - **B97.7** Papillomavirus as the cause of diseases classified elsewhere [UPD]
  - ✓5th **B97.8** Other viral agents as the cause of diseases classified elsewhere
    - **B97.81** Human metapneumovirus as the cause of diseases classified elsewhere [UPD]
    - **B97.89** Other viral agents as the cause of diseases classified elsewhere [UPD]

Other infectious diseases (B99)

- ✓4th **B99** Other and unspecified infectious diseases
  - **B99.8** Other infectious disease
  - **B99.9** Unspecified infectious disease

Chapter 2. Neoplasms (C00–D49)

Chapter-specific Guidelines with Coding Examples

The chapter-specific guidelines from the ICD-10-CM Official Guidelines for Coding and Reporting have been provided below. Along with these guidelines are coding examples, contained in the shaded boxes, that have been developed to help illustrate the coding and/or sequencing guidance found in these guidelines.

General guidelines

Chapter 2 of the ICD-10-CM contains the codes for most benign and all malignant neoplasms. Certain benign neoplasms, such as prostatic adenomas, may be found in the specific body system chapters. To properly code a neoplasm, it is necessary to determine from the record if the neoplasm is benign, in-situ, malignant, or of uncertain histologic behavior. If malignant, any secondary (metastatic) sites should also be determined.

Primary malignant neoplasms overlapping site boundaries

A primary malignant neoplasm that overlaps two or more contiguous (next to each other) sites should be classified to the subcategory/code .8 ('overlapping lesion'), unless the combination is specifically indexed elsewhere. For multiple neoplasms of the same site that are not contiguous such as tumors in different quadrants of the same breast, codes for each site should be assigned.

> A 62-year-old female with a malignant lesion of the upper lip that extends from the lipstick area to the labial frenulum
>
> **C00.8**   **Malignant neoplasm of overlapping sites of lip**
>
> *Explanation*: Because this is a single lesion that overlaps two contiguous sites, a single code for overlapping sites is assigned.

> A 74-year-old male is treated for two distinct malignant lesions, one in the mucosa of the upper lip and a second in the mucosa of the lower lip.
>
> **C00.3**   **Malignant neoplasm of upper lip, inner aspect**
>
> **C00.4**   **Malignant neoplasm of lower lip, inner aspect**
>
> *Explanation*: This patient has two distinct malignant lesions of the upper and lower lips. Because the lesions are not contiguous, two codes are reported.

Malignant neoplasm of ectopic tissue

Malignant neoplasms of ectopic tissue are to be coded to the site of origin mentioned, e.g., ectopic pancreatic malignant neoplasms involving the stomach are coded to malignant neoplasm of pancreas, unspecified (C25.9).

The neoplasm table in the Alphabetic Index should be referenced first. However, if the histological term is documented, that term should be referenced first, rather than going immediately to the Neoplasm Table, in order to determine which column in the Neoplasm Table is appropriate. For example, if the documentation indicates "adenoma," refer to the term in the Alphabetic Index to review the entries under this term and the instructional note to "see also neoplasm, by site, benign." The table provides the proper code based on the type of neoplasm and the site. It is important to select the proper column in the table that corresponds to the type of neoplasm. The Tabular List should then be referenced to verify that the correct code has been selected from the table and that a more specific site code does not exist.

See Section I.C.21. Factors influencing health status and contact with health services, Status, for information regarding Z15.0, codes for genetic susceptibility to cancer.

a. Admission/encounter for treatment of primary site

If the malignancy is chiefly responsible for occasioning the patient admission/encounter and treatment is directed at the primary site, designate the primary malignancy as the principal/first-listed diagnosis.

The only exception to this guideline is if the administration of chemotherapy, immunotherapy or external beam radiation therapy is chiefly responsible for occasioning the admission/encounter. In that case, assign the appropriate Z51.-- code as the first-listed or principal diagnosis, and the underlying diagnosis or problem for which the service is being performed as a secondary diagnosis.

b. Admission/encounter for treatment of secondary site

When a patient is admitted because of a primary neoplasm with metastasis and treatment is directed toward the secondary site only, the secondary neoplasm is designated as the principal diagnosis even though the primary malignancy is still present.

> Patient with primary prostate cancer with metastasis to lungs presents for wedge resection of mass in right lung
>
> **C78.01**   **Secondary malignant neoplasm of right lung**
>
> **C61**   **Malignant neoplasm of prostate**
>
> *Explanation*: Since the encounter is for treatment of the lung metastasis, the secondary lung metastasis is sequenced before the primary prostate cancer.

c. Coding and sequencing of complications

Coding and sequencing of complications associated with the malignancies or with the therapy thereof are subject to the following guidelines:

1) Anemia associated with malignancy

When admission/encounter is for management of an anemia associated with the malignancy, and the treatment is only for anemia, the appropriate code for the malignancy is sequenced as the principal or first-listed diagnosis followed by the appropriate code for the anemia (such as code D63.0, Anemia in neoplastic disease).

> Patient is seen for treatment of anemia in advanced primary liver cancer
>
> **C22.8**   **Malignant neoplasm of liver, primary, unspecified as to type**
>
> **D63.0**   **Anemia in neoplastic disease**
>
> *Explanation*: Even though the admission was solely to treat the anemia, this guideline indicates that the code for the malignancy is sequenced first.

2) Anemia associated with chemotherapy, immunotherapy and radiation therapy

When the admission/encounter is for management of an anemia associated with an adverse effect of the administration of chemotherapy or immunotherapy and the only treatment is for the anemia, the anemia code is sequenced first followed by the appropriate codes for the neoplasm and the adverse effect (T45.1X5, Adverse effect of antineoplastic and immunosuppressive drugs).

When the admission/encounter is for management of an anemia associated with an adverse effect of radiotherapy, the anemia code should be sequenced first, followed by the appropriate neoplasm code and code Y84.2, Radiological procedure and radiotherapy as the cause of abnormal reaction of the patient, or of later complication, without mention of misadventure at the time of the procedure.

> A 55-year-old male with a large malignant rectal tumor has been receiving external radiation therapy to shrink the tumor prior to planned surgery. He is referred today for a blood transfusion to treat anemia related to radiation therapy.
>
> **D64.89**   **Other specified anemias**
>
> **C20**   **Malignant neoplasm of rectum**
>
> **Y84.2**   **Radiological procedure and radiotherapy as the cause of abnormal reaction of the patient, or of later complication, without mention of misadventure at the time of the procedure**
>
> *Explanation*: The code for the anemia is sequenced first, followed by the code for the malignancy, and lastly the code for the abnormal reaction due to radiotherapy.

3) Management of dehydration due to the malignancy

When the admission/encounter is for management of dehydration due to the malignancy and only the dehydration is being treated (intravenous rehydration), the dehydration is sequenced first, followed by the code(s) for the malignancy.

4) Treatment of a complication resulting from a surgical procedure

When the admission/encounter is for treatment of a complication resulting from a surgical procedure, designate the complication as the principal or first-listed diagnosis if treatment is directed at resolving the complication.

Chapter 2. Neoplasms

d. **Primary malignancy previously excised**

When a primary malignancy has been previously excised or eradicated from its site and there is no further treatment directed to that site and there is no evidence of any existing primary malignancy at that site, a code from category Z85, Personal history of malignant neoplasm, should be used to indicate the former site of the malignancy. Any mention of extension, invasion, or metastasis to another site is coded as a secondary malignant neoplasm to that site. The secondary site may be the principal or first-listed diagnosis with the Z85 code used as a secondary code.

See section I.C.2.t. Secondary malignant neoplasm of lymphoid tissue.

> History of lung cancer, left upper lobectomy 18 months ago with no current treatment; MRI of the brain shows metastatic disease in the brain
>
> | | |
> |---|---|
> | C79.31 | Secondary malignant neoplasm of brain |
> | Z85.118 | Personal history of other malignant neoplasm of bronchus and lung |
>
> *Explanation*: The patient has undergone a diagnostic procedure that revealed metastatic lung cancer in the brain. The code for the secondary (metastatic) site is sequenced first, followed by a personal history code to identify the former site of the primary malignancy.

e. *Admissions/encounters involving antineoplastic chemotherapy, immunotherapy and radiation therapy*

1) **Episode of care involves surgical removal of neoplasm**

When an episode of care involves the surgical removal of a neoplasm, primary or secondary site, followed by adjunct chemotherapy or radiation treatment during the same episode of care, the code for the neoplasm should be assigned as principal or first-listed diagnosis.

2) *Patient admission/encounter chiefly for administration of antineoplastic chemotherapy, immunotherapy and radiation therapy*

If a patient admission/encounter is chiefly for the administration of chemotherapy, immunotherapy or external beam radiation therapy **for the treatment of a neoplasm,** assign code Z51.0, Encounter for antineoplastic radiation therapy, or Z51.11, Encounter for antineoplastic chemotherapy, or Z51.12, Encounter for antineoplastic immunotherapy as the first-listed or principal diagnosis. **If the reason for the encounter is more than one type of antineoplastic therapy, code Z51.0 and codes from subcategory Z51.1 may be assigned together, in which case one of these codes would be reported as a secondary diagnosis.**

The malignancy for which the therapy is being administered should be assigned as a secondary diagnosis.

If a patient admission/encounter is for the insertion or implantation of radioactive elements (e.g., brachytherapy) the appropriate code for the malignancy is sequenced as the principal or first-listed diagnosis. Code Z51.0 should not be assigned.

> Patient presents for second round of rituximab and fludarabine for his chronic B cell lymphocytic leukemia
>
> | | |
> |---|---|
> | Z51.11 | Encounter for antineoplastic chemotherapy |
> | Z51.12 | Encounter for antineoplastic immunotherapy |
> | C91.10 | Chronic lymphocytic leukemia of B-cell type not having achieved remission |
>
> *Explanation*: Rituximab is an antineoplastic immunotherapy while fludarabine is an antineoplastic chemotherapy. The two treatments are often used together. The encounter was solely for the purpose of administering this treatment and either can be sequenced first, before the neoplastic condition.

3) **Patient admitted for radiation therapy, chemotherapy or immunotherapy and develops complications**

When a patient is admitted for the purpose of external beam radiotherapy, immunotherapy or chemotherapy and develops complications such as uncontrolled nausea and vomiting or dehydration, the principal or first-listed diagnosis is Z51.0, Encounter for antineoplastic radiation therapy, or Z51.11, Encounter for antineoplastic chemotherapy, or Z51.12, Encounter for antineoplastic immunotherapy followed by any codes for the complications.

When a patient is admitted for the purpose of insertion or implantation of radioactive elements (e.g., brachytherapy) and develops complications such as uncontrolled nausea and vomiting or dehydration, the principal or first-listed diagnosis is the appropriate code for the malignancy followed by any codes for the complications.

f. **Admission/encounter to determine extent of malignancy**

When the reason for admission/encounter is to determine the extent of the malignancy, or for a procedure such as paracentesis or thoracentesis, the primary malignancy or appropriate metastatic site is designated as the principal or first-listed diagnosis, even though chemotherapy or radiotherapy is administered.

> Patient with left lung cancer with malignant pleural effusion being seen for paracentesis and initiation/administration of chemotherapy
>
> | | |
> |---|---|
> | C34.92 | Malignant neoplasm of unspecified part of left bronchus or lung |
> | J91.0 | Malignant pleural effusion |
> | Z51.11 | Encounter for antineoplastic chemotherapy |
>
> *Explanation*: The lung cancer is sequenced before the chemotherapy in this instance because the paracentesis for the malignant effusion is also being performed. An instructional note under the malignant effusion instructs that the lung cancer be sequenced first.

g. **Symptoms, signs, and abnormal findings listed in Chapter 18 associated with neoplasms**

Symptoms, signs, and ill-defined conditions listed in Chapter 18 characteristic of, or associated with, an existing primary or secondary site malignancy cannot be used to replace the malignancy as principal or first-listed diagnosis, regardless of the number of admissions or encounters for treatment and care of the neoplasm.

See Section I.C.21. Factors influencing health status and contact with health services, Encounter for prophylactic organ removal.

h. **Admission/encounter for pain control/management**

See Section I.C.6. for information on coding admission/encounter for pain control/management.

i. **Malignancy in two or more noncontiguous sites**

A patient may have more than one malignant tumor in the same organ. These tumors may represent different primaries or metastatic disease, depending on the site. Should the documentation be unclear, the provider should be queried as to the status of each tumor so that the correct codes can be assigned.

j. **Disseminated malignant neoplasm, unspecified**

Code C80.0, Disseminated malignant neoplasm, unspecified, is for use only in those cases where the patient has advanced metastatic disease and no known primary or secondary sites are specified. It should not be used in place of assigning codes for the primary site and all known secondary sites.

k. **Malignant neoplasm without specification of site**

Code C80.1, Malignant (primary) neoplasm, unspecified, equates to Cancer, unspecified. This code should only be used when no determination can be made as to the primary site of a malignancy. This code should rarely be used in the inpatient setting.

> Evaluation of painful hip leads to diagnosis of a metastatic bone lesion from an unknown primary neoplasm source
>
> | | |
> |---|---|
> | C79.51 | Secondary malignant neoplasm of bone |
> | C80.1 | Malignant (primary) neoplasm, unspecified |
>
> *Explanation*: If only the secondary site is known, use code C80.1 for the unknown primary site.

l. **Sequencing of neoplasm codes**

1) **Encounter for treatment of primary malignancy**

If the reason for the encounter is for treatment of a primary malignancy, assign the malignancy as the principal/first-listed diagnosis. The primary site is to be sequenced first, followed by any metastatic sites.

2) **Encounter for treatment of secondary malignancy**

When an encounter is for a primary malignancy with metastasis and treatment is directed toward the metastatic (secondary) site(s) only, the metastatic site(s) is designated as the principal/first-listed diagnosis. The primary malignancy is coded as an additional code.

Patient has primary colon cancer with metastasis to rib and is evaluated for possible excision of portion of rib bone	
C79.51	Secondary malignant neoplasm of bone
C18.9	Malignant neoplasm of colon, unspecified
Explanation: The treatment for this encounter is focused on the metastasis to the rib bone rather than the primary colon cancer, thus indicating that the bone metastasis is sequenced as the first-listed code.	

3) **Malignant neoplasm in a pregnant patient**

When a pregnant patient has a malignant neoplasm, a code from subcategory O9A.1-, Malignant neoplasm complicating pregnancy, childbirth, and the puerperium, should be sequenced first, followed by the appropriate code from Chapter 2 to indicate the type of neoplasm.

A 30-year-old pregnant female in first trimester evaluated for pituitary gland malignancy	
O9A.111	Malignant neoplasm complicating pregnancy, first trimester
C75.1	Malignant neoplasm of pituitary gland
Explanation: Codes from chapter 15 describing complications of pregnancy are sequenced as first-listed codes, further specified by codes from other chapters such as neoplastic, unless the pregnancy is documented as incidental to the condition. See also guideline 1.C.15.a.1.	

4) **Encounter for complication associated with a neoplasm**

When an encounter is for management of a complication associated with a neoplasm, such as dehydration, and the treatment is only for the complication, the complication is coded first, followed by the appropriate code(s) for the neoplasm.

The exception to this guideline is anemia. When the admission/encounter is for management of an anemia associated with the malignancy, and the treatment is only for anemia, the appropriate code for the malignancy is sequenced as the principal or first-listed diagnosis followed by code D63.0, Anemia in neoplastic disease.

Patient with pancreatic cancer is seen for initiation of TPN for cancer-related moderate protein-calorie malnutrition	
E44.0	Moderate protein-calorie malnutrition
C25.9	Malignant neoplasm of pancreas, unspecified
Explanation: The encounter is to initiate treatment for malnutrition, a common complication of many types of neoplasms, and is sequenced first.	

5) **Complication from surgical procedure for treatment of a neoplasm**

When an encounter is for treatment of a complication resulting from a surgical procedure performed for the treatment of the neoplasm, designate the complication as the principal/first-listed diagnosis. See the guideline regarding the coding of a current malignancy versus personal history to determine if the code for the neoplasm should also be assigned.

6) **Pathologic fracture due to a neoplasm**

When an encounter is for a pathological fracture due to a neoplasm, and the focus of treatment is the fracture, a code from subcategory M84.5, Pathological fracture in neoplastic disease, should be sequenced first, followed by the code for the neoplasm.

If the focus of treatment is the neoplasm with an associated pathological fracture, the neoplasm code should be sequenced first, followed by a code from M84.5 for the pathological fracture.

m. **Current malignancy versus personal history of malignancy**

When a primary malignancy has been excised but further treatment, such as an additional surgery for the malignancy, radiation therapy or chemotherapy is directed to that site, the primary malignancy code should be used until treatment is completed.

Female patient with ongoing chemotherapy after right mastectomy for breast cancer	
C50.911	Malignant neoplasm of unspecified site of right female breast
Z90.11	Acquired absence of right breast and nipple
Explanation: Even though the breast has been removed, the breast cancer is still being treated with chemotherapy and therefore is still coded as a current condition rather than personal history.	

When a primary malignancy has been previously excised or eradicated from its site, there is no further treatment (of the malignancy) directed to that site, and there is no evidence of any existing primary malignancy at that site, a code from category Z85, Personal history of malignant neoplasm, should be used to indicate the former site of the malignancy.

Codes from subcategories Z85.0 – Z85.85 should only be assigned for the former site of a primary malignancy, not the site of a secondary malignancy. Code Z85.89 may be assigned for the former site(s) of either a primary or secondary malignancy.

See Section I.C.21. Factors influencing health status and contact with health services, History (of)

n. **Leukemia, multiple myeloma, and malignant plasma cell neoplasms in remission versus personal history**

The categories for leukemia, and category C90, Multiple myeloma and malignant plasma cell neoplasms, have codes indicating whether or not the leukemia has achieved remission. There are also codes Z85.6, Personal history of leukemia, and Z85.79, Personal history of other malignant neoplasms of lymphoid, hematopoietic and related tissues. If the documentation is unclear as to whether the leukemia has achieved remission, the provider should be queried.

See Section I.C.21. Factors influencing health status and contact with health services, History (of)

o. **Aftercare following surgery for neoplasm**

See Section I.C.21. Factors influencing health status and contact with health services, Aftercare

p. **Follow-up care for completed treatment of a malignancy**

See Section I.C.21. Factors influencing health status and contact with health services, Follow-up

q. **Prophylactic organ removal for prevention of malignancy**

See Section I.C. 21, Factors influencing health status and contact with health services, Prophylactic organ removal

r. **Malignant neoplasm associated with transplanted organ**

A malignant neoplasm of a transplanted organ should be coded as a transplant complication. Assign first the appropriate code from category T86.-, Complications of transplanted organs and tissue, followed by code C80.2, Malignant neoplasm associated with transplanted organ. Use an additional code for the specific malignancy.

s. **Breast Implant Associated Anaplastic Large Cell Lymphoma**

Breast implant associated anaplastic large cell lymphoma (BIA-ALCL) is a type of lymphoma that can develop around breast implants. Assign code C84.7A, Anaplastic large cell lymphoma, ALK-negative, breast, for BIA-ALCL or C84.7B, Anaplastic large cell lymphoma, ALK-negative, in remission, for BIA-ALCL in remission. Do not assign a complication code from chapter 19.

t. **Secondary malignant neoplasm of lymphoid tissue**

When a malignant neoplasm of lymphoid tissue metastasizes beyond the lymph nodes, a code from categories C81-C85 with a final character identifying "extranodal and solid organ sites" should be assigned rather than a code for the secondary neoplasm of the affected solid organ. For example, for metastasis of diffuse large B-cell lymphoma to the lung, brain and left adrenal gland, assign code C83.398, Diffuse large B-cell lymphoma of other extranodal and solid organ sites.

Chapter 2. Neoplasms (C00-D49)

NOTE

Functional activity
All neoplasms are classified in this chapter, whether they are functionally active or not. An additional code from Chapter 4 may be used, to identify functional activity associated with any neoplasm.

Morphology [Histology]
Chapter 2 classifies neoplasms primarily by site (topography), with broad groupings for behavior, malignant, in situ, benign, etc. The Table of Neoplasms should be used to identify the correct topography code. In a few cases, such as for malignant melanoma and certain neuroendocrine tumors, the morphology (histologic type) is included in the category and codes.

Primary malignant neoplasms overlapping site boundaries
A primary malignant neoplasm that overlaps two or more contiguous (next to each other) sites should be classified to the subcategory/code .8 ("overlapping lesion"), unless the combination is specifically indexed elsewhere. For multiple neoplasms of the same site that are not contiguous, such as tumors in different quadrants of the same breast, codes for each site should be assigned.

Malignant neoplasm of ectopic tissue
Malignant neoplasms of ectopic tissue are to be coded to the site mentioned, e.g., ectopic pancreatic malignant neoplasms are coded to pancreas, unspecified (C25.9).

AHA: 2024,1Q,24; 2023,2Q,6; 2017,4Q,103; 2017,1Q,4,5-6,8

This chapter contains the following blocks:

C00-C14	Malignant neoplasms of lip, oral cavity and pharynx
C15-C26	Malignant neoplasms of digestive organs
C30-C39	Malignant neoplasms of respiratory and intrathoracic organs
C40-C41	Malignant neoplasms of bone and articular cartilage
C43-C44	Melanoma and other malignant neoplasms of skin
C45-C49	Malignant neoplasms of mesothelial and soft tissue
C50	Malignant neoplasms of breast
C51-C58	Malignant neoplasms of female genital organs
C60-C63	Malignant neoplasms of male genital organs
C64-C68	Malignant neoplasms of urinary tract
C69-C72	Malignant neoplasms of eye, brain and other parts of central nervous system
C73-C75	Malignant neoplasms of thyroid and other endocrine glands
C7A	Malignant neuroendocrine tumors
C7B	Secondary neuroendocrine tumors
C76-C80	Malignant neoplasms of ill-defined, other secondary and unspecified sites
C81-C96	Malignant neoplasms of lymphoid, hematopoietic and related tissue
D00-D09	In situ neoplasms
D10-D36	Benign neoplasms, except benign neuroendocrine tumors
D3A	Benign neuroendocrine tumors
D37-D48	Neoplasms of uncertain behavior, polycythemia vera and myelodysplastic syndromes
D49	Neoplasms of unspecified behavior

MALIGNANT NEOPLASMS (C00-C96)

Malignant neoplasms, stated or presumed to be primary (of specified sites), and certain specified histologies, except neuroendocrine, and of lymphoid, hematopoietic and related tissue (C00-C75)

AHA: 2022,1Q,16

TIP: Codes from this code block can be assigned for outpatient encounters based on the diagnosis listed in a pathology or cytology report when authenticated by a pathologist and available at the time of code assignment.

Malignant neoplasms of lip, oral cavity and pharynx (C00-C14)

C00 Malignant neoplasm of lip
   Use additional code to identify:
      alcohol abuse and dependence (F10.-)
      history of tobacco dependence (Z87.891)
      tobacco dependence (F17.-)
      tobacco use (Z72.0)
   EXCLUDES 1: malignant melanoma of lip (C43.0)
      Merkel cell carcinoma of lip (C4A.0)
      other and unspecified malignant neoplasm of skin of lip (C44.0-)

   C00.0 Malignant neoplasm of external upper lip
      Malignant neoplasm of lipstick area of upper lip
      Malignant neoplasm of upper lip NOS
      Malignant neoplasm of vermilion border of upper lip

   C00.1 Malignant neoplasm of external lower lip
      Malignant neoplasm of lipstick area of lower lip
      Malignant neoplasm of lower lip NOS
      Malignant neoplasm of vermilion border of lower lip

   C00.2 Malignant neoplasm of external lip, unspecified
      Malignant neoplasm of vermilion border of lip NOS

   C00.3 Malignant neoplasm of upper lip, inner aspect
      Malignant neoplasm of buccal aspect of upper lip
      Malignant neoplasm of frenulum of upper lip
      Malignant neoplasm of mucosa of upper lip
      Malignant neoplasm of oral aspect of upper lip

   C00.4 Malignant neoplasm of lower lip, inner aspect
      Malignant neoplasm of buccal aspect of lower lip
      Malignant neoplasm of frenulum of lower lip
      Malignant neoplasm of mucosa of lower lip
      Malignant neoplasm of oral aspect of lower lip

   C00.5 Malignant neoplasm of lip, unspecified, inner aspect
      Malignant neoplasm of buccal aspect of lip, unspecified
      Malignant neoplasm of frenulum of lip, unspecified
      Malignant neoplasm of mucosa of lip, unspecified
      Malignant neoplasm of oral aspect of lip, unspecified

   C00.6 Malignant neoplasm of commissure of lip, unspecified

   C00.8 Malignant neoplasm of overlapping sites of lip

   C00.9 Malignant neoplasm of lip, unspecified

C01 Malignant neoplasm of base of tongue
   Malignant neoplasm of dorsal surface of base of tongue
   Malignant neoplasm of fixed part of tongue NOS
   Malignant neoplasm of posterior third of tongue
   Use additional code to identify:
      alcohol abuse and dependence (F10.-)
      history of tobacco dependence (Z87.891)
      tobacco dependence (F17.-)
      tobacco use (Z72.0)

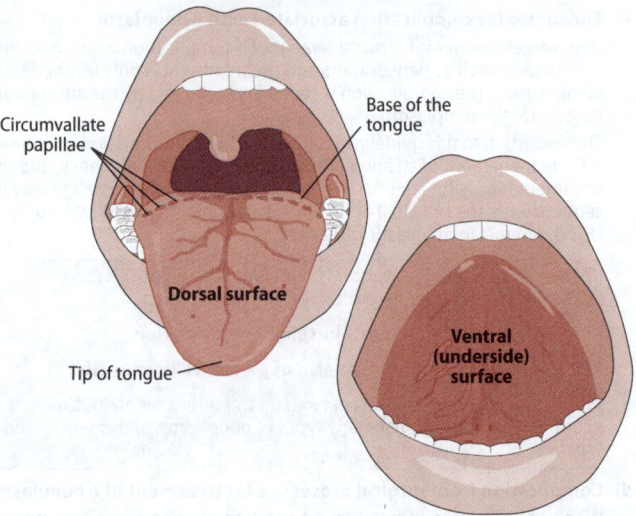

Malignant Neoplasm of Tongue

C02 Malignant neoplasm of other and unspecified parts of tongue
   Use additional code to identify:
      alcohol abuse and dependence (F10.-)
      history of tobacco dependence (Z87.891)
      tobacco dependence (F17.-)
      tobacco use (Z72.0)

   C02.0 Malignant neoplasm of dorsal surface of tongue
      Malignant neoplasm of anterior two-thirds of tongue, dorsal surface
      EXCLUDES 2: malignant neoplasm of dorsal surface of base of tongue (C01)

   C02.1 Malignant neoplasm of border of tongue
      Malignant neoplasm of tip of tongue

   C02.2 Malignant neoplasm of ventral surface of tongue
      Malignant neoplasm of anterior two-thirds of tongue, ventral surface
      Malignant neoplasm of frenulum linguae

   C02.3 Malignant neoplasm of anterior two-thirds of tongue, part unspecified
      Malignant neoplasm of middle third of tongue NOS
      Malignant neoplasm of mobile part of tongue NOS

   C02.4 Malignant neoplasm of lingual tonsil
      EXCLUDES 2: malignant neoplasm of tonsil NOS (C09.9)

Chapter 2. Neoplasms

C02.8 Malignant neoplasm of overlapping sites of tongue [HCC Rx ESR COM]
Malignant neoplasm of two or more contiguous sites of tongue

C02.9 Malignant neoplasm of tongue, unspecified [HCC Rx ESR COM]

✓4th C03 Malignant neoplasm of gum
INCLUDES malignant neoplasm of alveolar (ridge) mucosa
malignant neoplasm of gingiva
Use additional code to identify:
alcohol abuse and dependence (F10.-)
history of tobacco dependence (Z87.891)
tobacco dependence (F17.-)
tobacco use (Z72.0)
EXCLUDES 2 malignant odontogenic neoplasms (C41.0-C41.1)

C03.0 Malignant neoplasm of upper gum [HCC Rx ESR COM]
C03.1 Malignant neoplasm of lower gum [HCC Rx ESR COM]
C03.9 Malignant neoplasm of gum, unspecified [HCC Rx ESR COM]

✓4th C04 Malignant neoplasm of floor of mouth
Use additional code to identify:
alcohol abuse and dependence (F10.-)
history of tobacco dependence (Z87.891)
tobacco dependence (F17.-)
tobacco use (Z72.0)

C04.0 Malignant neoplasm of anterior floor of mouth [HCC Rx ESR COM]
Malignant neoplasm of anterior to the premolar-canine junction

C04.1 Malignant neoplasm of lateral floor of mouth [HCC Rx ESR COM]

C04.8 Malignant neoplasm of overlapping sites of floor of mouth [HCC Rx ESR COM]

C04.9 Malignant neoplasm of floor of mouth, unspecified [HCC Rx ESR COM]

✓4th C05 Malignant neoplasm of palate
Use additional code to identify:
alcohol abuse and dependence (F10.-)
history of tobacco dependence (Z87.891)
tobacco dependence (F17.-)
tobacco use (Z72.0)
EXCLUDES 1 Kaposi's sarcoma of palate (C46.2)

C05.0 Malignant neoplasm of hard palate [HCC Rx ESR COM]
C05.1 Malignant neoplasm of soft palate [HCC Rx ESR COM]
EXCLUDES 2 malignant neoplasm of nasopharyngeal surface of soft palate (C11.3)

C05.2 Malignant neoplasm of uvula [HCC Rx ESR COM]
C05.8 Malignant neoplasm of overlapping sites of palate [HCC Rx ESR COM]
C05.9 Malignant neoplasm of palate, unspecified [HCC Rx ESR COM]
Malignant neoplasm of roof of mouth

✓4th C06 Malignant neoplasm of other and unspecified parts of mouth
Use additional code to identify:
alcohol abuse and dependence (F10.-)
history of tobacco dependence (Z87.891)
tobacco dependence (F17.-)
tobacco use (Z72.0)

C06.0 Malignant neoplasm of cheek mucosa [HCC Rx ESR COM]
Malignant neoplasm of buccal mucosa NOS
Malignant neoplasm of internal cheek

C06.1 Malignant neoplasm of vestibule of mouth [HCC Rx ESR COM]
Malignant neoplasm of buccal sulcus (upper) (lower)
Malignant neoplasm of labial sulcus (upper) (lower)

C06.2 Malignant neoplasm of retromolar area [HCC Rx ESR COM]

✓5th C06.8 Malignant neoplasm of overlapping sites of other and unspecified parts of mouth
C06.80 Malignant neoplasm of overlapping sites of unspecified parts of mouth [HCC Rx ESR COM]
C06.89 Malignant neoplasm of overlapping sites of other parts of mouth [HCC Rx ESR COM]
"book leaf" neoplasm [ventral surface of tongue and floor of mouth]

C06.9 Malignant neoplasm of mouth, unspecified [HCC Rx ESR COM]
Malignant neoplasm of minor salivary gland, unspecified site
Malignant neoplasm of oral cavity NOS

C07 Malignant neoplasm of parotid gland [HCC Rx ESR COM]
Use additional code to identify:
alcohol abuse and dependence (F10.-)
exposure to environmental tobacco smoke (Z77.22)
exposure to tobacco smoke in the perinatal period (P96.81)
history of tobacco dependence (Z87.891)
occupational exposure to environmental tobacco smoke (Z57.31)
tobacco dependence (F17.-)
tobacco use (Z72.0)

✓4th C08 Malignant neoplasm of other and unspecified major salivary glands
INCLUDES malignant neoplasm of salivary ducts
Use additional code to identify:
alcohol abuse and dependence (F10.-)
exposure to environmental tobacco smoke (Z77.22)
exposure to tobacco smoke in the perinatal period (P96.81)
history of tobacco dependence (Z87.891)
occupational exposure to environmental tobacco smoke (Z57.31)
tobacco dependence (F17.-)
tobacco use (Z72.0)
EXCLUDES 1 malignant neoplasms of specified minor salivary glands which are classified according to their anatomical location
EXCLUDES 2 malignant neoplasms of minor salivary glands NOS (C06.9)
malignant neoplasm of parotid gland (C07)

C08.0 Malignant neoplasm of submandibular gland [HCC Rx ESR COM]
Malignant neoplasm of submaxillary gland

C08.1 Malignant neoplasm of sublingual gland [HCC Rx ESR COM]
C08.9 Malignant neoplasm of major salivary gland, unspecified [HCC Rx ESR COM]
Malignant neoplasm of salivary gland (major) NOS

✓4th C09 Malignant neoplasm of tonsil
Use additional code to identify:
alcohol abuse and dependence (F10.-)
exposure to environmental tobacco smoke (Z77.22)
exposure to tobacco smoke in the perinatal period (P96.81)
history of tobacco dependence (Z87.891)
occupational exposure to environmental tobacco smoke (Z57.31)
tobacco dependence (F17.-)
tobacco use (Z72.0)
EXCLUDES 2 malignant neoplasm of lingual tonsil (C02.4)
malignant neoplasm of pharyngeal tonsil (C11.1)

C09.0 Malignant neoplasm of tonsillar fossa [HCC ESR COM]
C09.1 Malignant neoplasm of tonsillar pillar (anterior) (posterior) [HCC ESR COM]
C09.8 Malignant neoplasm of overlapping sites of tonsil [HCC ESR COM]
C09.9 Malignant neoplasm of tonsil, unspecified [HCC ESR COM]
Malignant neoplasm of faucial tonsils
Malignant neoplasm of palatine tonsils
Malignant neoplasm of tonsil NOS

✓4th C10 Malignant neoplasm of oropharynx
Use additional code to identify:
alcohol abuse and dependence (F10.-)
exposure to environmental tobacco smoke (Z77.22)
exposure to tobacco smoke in the perinatal period (P96.81)
history of tobacco dependence (Z87.891)
occupational exposure to environmental tobacco smoke (Z57.31)
tobacco dependence (F17.-)
tobacco use (Z72.0)
EXCLUDES 2 malignant neoplasm of tonsil (C09.-)
DEF: Oropharynx: Middle portion of pharynx (throat); communicates with the oral cavity, nasopharynx and laryngopharynx.

C10.0 Malignant neoplasm of vallecula [HCC ESR COM]
C10.1 Malignant neoplasm of anterior surface of epiglottis [HCC ESR COM]
Malignant neoplasm of epiglottis, free border [margin]
Malignant neoplasm of glossoepiglottic fold(s)
EXCLUDES 2 malignant neoplasm of epiglottis (suprahyoid portion) NOS (C32.1)

C10.2 Malignant neoplasm of lateral wall of oropharynx [HCC ESR COM]
C10.3 Malignant neoplasm of posterior wall of oropharynx [HCC ESR COM]
C10.4 Malignant neoplasm of branchial cleft [HCC ESR COM]
Malignant neoplasm of branchial cyst [site of neoplasm]
C10.8 Malignant neoplasm of overlapping sites of oropharynx [HCC ESR COM]
Malignant neoplasm of junctional region of oropharynx

Chapter 2. Neoplasms

C10.9 Malignant neoplasm of oropharynx, unspecified `HCC` `ESR` `COM`

✓4th **C11** Malignant neoplasm of **nasopharynx**
Use additional code to identify:
exposure to environmental tobacco smoke (Z77.22)
exposure to tobacco smoke in the perinatal period (P96.81)
history of tobacco dependence (Z87.891)
occupational exposure to environmental tobacco smoke (Z57.31)
tobacco dependence (F17.-)
tobacco use (Z72.0)
DEF: Nasopharynx: Upper portion of pharynx (throat); communicates with the nasal cavities, oropharynx and tympanic cavities.

C11.0 Malignant neoplasm of **superior wall** of nasopharynx `HCC` `ESR` `COM`
Malignant neoplasm of roof of nasopharynx

C11.1 Malignant neoplasm of **posterior wall** of nasopharynx `HCC` `ESR` `COM`
Malignant neoplasm of adenoid
Malignant neoplasm of pharyngeal tonsil

C11.2 Malignant neoplasm of **lateral wall** of nasopharynx `HCC` `ESR` `COM`
Malignant neoplasm of fossa of Rosenmuller
Malignant neoplasm of opening of auditory tube
Malignant neoplasm of pharyngeal recess

C11.3 Malignant neoplasm of **anterior wall** of nasopharynx `HCC` `ESR` `COM`
Malignant neoplasm of floor of nasopharynx
Malignant neoplasm of nasopharyngeal (anterior) (posterior) surface of soft palate
Malignant neoplasm of posterior margin of nasal choana
Malignant neoplasm of posterior margin of nasal septum

C11.8 Malignant neoplasm of **overlapping sites** of nasopharynx `HCC` `ESR` `COM`

C11.9 Malignant neoplasm of nasopharynx, unspecified `HCC` `ESR` `COM`
Malignant neoplasm of nasopharyngeal wall NOS

C12 Malignant neoplasm of **pyriform sinus** `HCC` `ESR` `COM`
Malignant neoplasm of pyriform fossa
Use additional code to identify:
exposure to environmental tobacco smoke (Z77.22)
exposure to tobacco smoke in the perinatal period (P96.81)
history of tobacco dependence (Z87.891)
occupational exposure to environmental tobacco smoke (Z57.31)
tobacco dependence (F17.-)
tobacco use (Z72.0)

✓4th **C13** Malignant neoplasm of **hypopharynx**
Use additional code to identify:
exposure to environmental tobacco smoke (Z77.22)
exposure to tobacco smoke in the perinatal period (P96.81)
history of tobacco dependence (Z87.891)
occupational exposure to environmental tobacco smoke (Z57.31)
tobacco dependence (F17.-)
tobacco use (Z72.0)
EXCLUDES 2 malignant neoplasm of pyriform sinus (C12)
DEF: Hypopharynx: Lower portion of pharynx (throat); communicates with the oropharynx and the esophagus. **Synonym(s):** laryngopharynx.

C13.0 Malignant neoplasm of **postcricoid region** `HCC` `ESR` `COM`

C13.1 Malignant neoplasm of **aryepiglottic fold, hypopharyngeal aspect** `HCC` `ESR` `COM`
Malignant neoplasm of aryepiglottic fold NOS
Malignant neoplasm of aryepiglottic fold, marginal zone
Malignant neoplasm of interarytenoid fold NOS
Malignant neoplasm of interarytenoid fold, marginal zone
EXCLUDES 2 malignant neoplasm of aryepiglottic fold or interarytenoid fold, laryngeal aspect (C32.1)

C13.2 Malignant neoplasm of **posterior wall** of hypopharynx `HCC` `ESR` `COM`

C13.8 Malignant neoplasm of **overlapping sites** of hypopharynx `HCC` `ESR` `COM`

C13.9 Malignant neoplasm of hypopharynx, unspecified `HCC` `ESR` `COM`
Malignant neoplasm of hypopharyngeal wall NOS

✓4th **C14** Malignant neoplasm of **other and ill-defined sites in the lip, oral cavity and pharynx**
Use additional code to identify:
alcohol abuse and dependence (F10.-)
exposure to environmental tobacco smoke (Z77.22)
exposure to tobacco smoke in the perinatal period (P96.81)
history of tobacco dependence (Z87.891)
occupational exposure to environmental tobacco smoke (Z57.31)
tobacco dependence (F17.-)
tobacco use (Z72.0)
EXCLUDES 1 malignant neoplasm of oral cavity NOS (C06.9)

C14.0 Malignant neoplasm of pharynx, unspecified `HCC` `ESR` `COM`

C14.2 Malignant neoplasm of **Waldeyer's ring** `HCC` `ESR` `COM`
DEF: Waldeyer's ring: Ring of lymphoid tissue that is made up of the two palatine tonsils, the pharyngeal tonsil (adenoid), and the lingual tonsil. It functions as the defense against infection and assists with the development of the immune system.

C14.8 Malignant neoplasm of **overlapping sites** of lip, oral cavity and pharynx `HCC` `ESR` `COM`
Primary malignant neoplasm of two or more contiguous sites of lip, oral cavity and pharynx
EXCLUDES 1 "book leaf" neoplasm [ventral surface of tongue and floor of mouth] (C06.89)

Malignant neoplasms of digestive organs (C15-C26)

EXCLUDES 1 Kaposi's sarcoma of gastrointestinal sites (C46.4)
EXCLUDES 2 gastrointestinal stromal tumors (C49.A-)

✓4th **C15** Malignant neoplasm of **esophagus**
Use additional code to identify:
alcohol abuse and dependence (F10.-)
AHA: 2022,3Q,10

C15.3 Malignant neoplasm of **upper third** of esophagus `HCC` `ESR` `COM`

C15.4 Malignant neoplasm of **middle third** of esophagus `HCC` `ESR` `COM`

C15.5 Malignant neoplasm of **lower third** of esophagus `HCC` `ESR` `COM`
EXCLUDES 1 malignant neoplasm of cardio-esophageal junction (C16.0)

C15.8 Malignant neoplasm of **overlapping sites** of esophagus `HCC` `ESR` `COM`

C15.9 Malignant neoplasm of esophagus, unspecified `HCC` `ESR` `COM`

✓4th **C16** Malignant neoplasm of **stomach**
Use additional code to identify:
alcohol abuse and dependence (F10.-)
EXCLUDES 2 malignant carcinoid tumor of the stomach (C7A.092)

C16.0 Malignant neoplasm of **cardia** `HCC` `Rx` `ESR` `COM`
Malignant neoplasm of cardiac orifice
Malignant neoplasm of cardio-esophageal junction
Malignant neoplasm of esophagus and stomach
Malignant neoplasm of gastro-esophageal junction

C16.1 Malignant neoplasm of **fundus** of stomach `HCC` `Rx` `ESR` `COM`

C16.2 Malignant neoplasm of **body** of stomach `HCC` `Rx` `ESR` `COM`

C16.3 Malignant neoplasm of **pyloric** antrum `HCC` `Rx` `ESR` `COM`
Malignant neoplasm of gastric antrum

C16.4 Malignant neoplasm of **pylorus** `HCC` `Rx` `ESR` `COM`
Malignant neoplasm of prepylorus
Malignant neoplasm of pyloric canal

C16.5 Malignant neoplasm of **lesser curvature** of stomach, unspecified `HCC` `Rx` `ESR` `COM`
Malignant neoplasm of lesser curvature of stomach, not classifiable to C16.1-C16.4

C16.6 Malignant neoplasm of **greater curvature** of stomach, unspecified `HCC` `Rx` `ESR` `COM`
Malignant neoplasm of greater curvature of stomach, not classifiable to C16.0-C16.4

C16.8 Malignant neoplasm of **overlapping sites** of stomach `HCC` `Rx` `ESR` `COM`

C16.9 Malignant neoplasm of stomach, unspecified `HCC` `Rx` `ESR` `COM`
Gastric cancer NOS

✓4th **C17** Malignant neoplasm of **small intestine**
EXCLUDES 1 malignant carcinoid tumors of the small intestine (C7A.01)
AHA: 2016,1Q,19

C17.0 Malignant neoplasm of **duodenum** `HCC` `Rx` `ESR` `COM`

C17.1 Malignant neoplasm of **jejunum** `HCC` `Rx` `ESR` `COM`

`HCC` CMS-HCC `Rx` Rx HCC `ESR` ESRD HCC `COM` Commercial HCC **N** Newborn: 0 **P** Pediatric: 0-17 **M** Maternity: 9-64 **A** Adult: 15-124

Chapter 2. Neoplasms

C17.2 Malignant neoplasm of ileum
 EXCLUDES 1 malignant neoplasm of ileocecal valve (C18.0)

C17.3 Meckel's diverticulum, malignant
 EXCLUDES 1 Meckel's diverticulum, congenital (Q43.0)
 DEF: Congenital, abnormal remnant of embryonic digestive system development that leaves a sacculation or outpouching from the wall of the small intestine near the terminal part of the ileum made of acid-secreting tissue as in the stomach.

C17.8 Malignant neoplasm of overlapping sites of small intestine

C17.9 Malignant neoplasm of small intestine, unspecified

C18 Malignant neoplasm of colon
 EXCLUDES 1 malignant carcinoid tumors of the colon (C7A.02-)

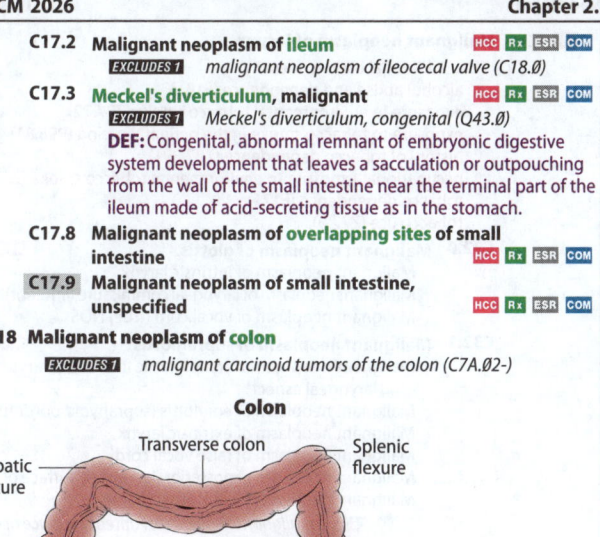

Colon

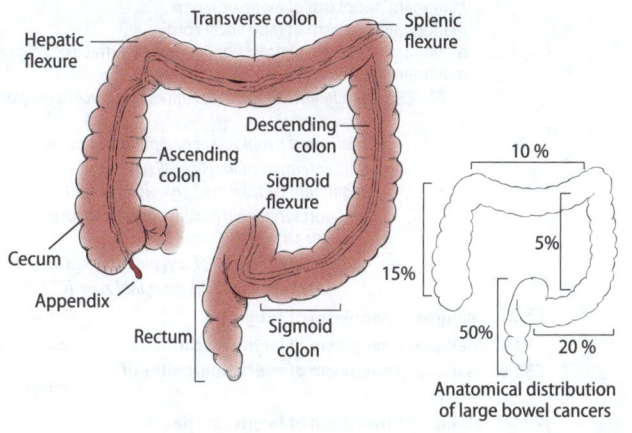

Anatomical distribution of large bowel cancers

C18.0 Malignant neoplasm of cecum
 Malignant neoplasm of ileocecal valve

C18.1 Malignant neoplasm of appendix

C18.2 Malignant neoplasm of ascending colon

C18.3 Malignant neoplasm of hepatic flexure

C18.4 Malignant neoplasm of transverse colon

C18.5 Malignant neoplasm of splenic flexure

C18.6 Malignant neoplasm of descending colon

C18.7 Malignant neoplasm of sigmoid colon
 Malignant neoplasm of sigmoid (flexure)
 EXCLUDES 1 malignant neoplasm of rectosigmoid junction (C19)

C18.8 Malignant neoplasm of overlapping sites of colon

C18.9 Malignant neoplasm of colon, unspecified
 Malignant neoplasm of large intestine NOS

C19 Malignant neoplasm of rectosigmoid junction
 Malignant neoplasm of colon with rectum
 Malignant neoplasm of rectosigmoid (colon)
 EXCLUDES 1 malignant carcinoid tumors of the colon (C7A.02-)

C20 Malignant neoplasm of rectum
 Malignant neoplasm of rectal ampulla
 EXCLUDES 1 malignant carcinoid tumor of the rectum (C7A.026)

C21 Malignant neoplasm of anus and anal canal
 EXCLUDES 2 malignant carcinoid tumors of the colon (C7A.02-)
 malignant melanoma of anal margin (C43.51)
 malignant melanoma of anal skin (C43.51)
 malignant melanoma of perianal skin (C43.51)
 other and unspecified malignant neoplasm of anal margin
  (C44.500, C44.510, C44.520, C44.590)
 other and unspecified malignant neoplasm of anal skin
  (C44.500, C44.510, C44.520, C44.590)
 other and unspecified malignant neoplasm of perianal skin
  (C44.500, C44.510, C44.520, C44.590)

C21.0 Malignant neoplasm of anus, unspecified

C21.1 Malignant neoplasm of anal canal
 Malignant neoplasm of anal sphincter

C21.2 Malignant neoplasm of cloacogenic zone

C21.8 Malignant neoplasm of overlapping sites of rectum, anus and anal canal
 Malignant neoplasm of anorectal junction
 Malignant neoplasm of anorectum
 Primary malignant neoplasm of two or more contiguous sites of rectum, anus and anal canal

C22 Malignant neoplasm of liver and intrahepatic bile ducts
 Use additional code to identify:
  alcohol abuse and dependence (F10.-)
  hepatitis B (B16.-, B18.0-B18.1)
  hepatitis C (B17.1-, B18.2)
 EXCLUDES 1 malignant neoplasm of biliary tract NOS (C24.9)
  secondary malignant neoplasm of liver and intrahepatic bile duct (C78.7)

C22.0 Liver cell carcinoma
 Hepatocellular carcinoma
 Hepatoma
 AHA: 2016,1Q,18

C22.1 Intrahepatic bile duct carcinoma
 Cholangiocarcinoma
 EXCLUDES 1 malignant neoplasm of hepatic duct (C24.0)
 AHA: 2023,1Q,24

C22.2 Hepatoblastoma

C22.3 Angiosarcoma of liver
 Kupffer cell sarcoma

C22.4 Other sarcomas of liver

C22.7 Other specified carcinomas of liver

C22.8 Malignant neoplasm of liver, primary, unspecified as to type

C22.9 Malignant neoplasm of liver, not specified as primary or secondary

C23 Malignant neoplasm of gallbladder

C24 Malignant neoplasm of other and unspecified parts of biliary tract
 EXCLUDES 1 malignant neoplasm of intrahepatic bile duct (C22.1)

C24.0 Malignant neoplasm of extrahepatic bile duct
 Malignant neoplasm of biliary duct or passage NOS
 Malignant neoplasm of common bile duct
 Malignant neoplasm of cystic duct
 Malignant neoplasm of hepatic duct

C24.1 Malignant neoplasm of ampulla of Vater
 DEF: Malignant neoplasm in the area of dilation at the juncture of the common bile and pancreatic ducts near the opening into the lumen of the duodenum.

C24.8 Malignant neoplasm of overlapping sites of biliary tract
 Malignant neoplasm involving both intrahepatic and extrahepatic bile ducts
 Primary malignant neoplasm of two or more contiguous sites of biliary tract

C24.9 Malignant neoplasm of biliary tract, unspecified

C25 Malignant neoplasm of pancreas
 Code also if applicable exocrine pancreatic insufficiency (K86.81)
 Use additional code to identify:
  alcohol abuse and dependence (F10.-)

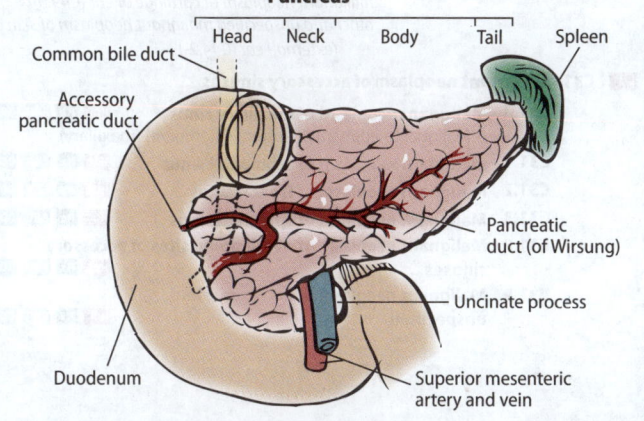

Pancreas

C25.0 Malignant neoplasm of head of pancreas

C25.1 Malignant neoplasm of body of pancreas

Chapter 2. Neoplasms

- **C25.2** Malignant neoplasm of tail of pancreas [HCC] [Rx] [ESR] [COM]
- **C25.3** Malignant neoplasm of pancreatic duct [HCC] [Rx] [ESR] [COM]
- **C25.4** Malignant neoplasm of endocrine pancreas [HCC] [Rx] [ESR] [COM]
  Malignant neoplasm of islets of Langerhans
  Use additional code to identify any functional activity
- **C25.7** Malignant neoplasm of other parts of pancreas [HCC] [Rx] [ESR] [COM]
  Malignant neoplasm of neck of pancreas
- **C25.8** Malignant neoplasm of overlapping sites of pancreas [HCC] [Rx] [COM]
- **C25.9** Malignant neoplasm of pancreas, unspecified [HCC] [Rx] [ESR] [COM]

✓4th **C26** Malignant neoplasm of other and ill-defined digestive organs
  EXCLUDES 1 malignant neoplasm of peritoneum and retroperitoneum (C48.-)
- **C26.0** Malignant neoplasm of intestinal tract, part unspecified [HCC] [ESR] [COM]
  Malignant neoplasm of intestine NOS
- **C26.1** Malignant neoplasm of spleen [HCC] [ESR] [COM]
  EXCLUDES 1 Hodgkin lymphoma (C81.-)
  non-Hodgkin lymphoma (C82-C85)
- **C26.9** Malignant neoplasm of ill-defined sites within the digestive system [HCC] [ESR] [COM]
  Malignant neoplasm of alimentary canal or tract NOS
  Malignant neoplasm of gastrointestinal tract NOS
  EXCLUDES 1 malignant neoplasm of abdominal NOS (C76.2)
  malignant neoplasm of intra-abdominal NOS (C76.2)

Malignant neoplasms of respiratory and intrathoracic organs (C30-C39)

INCLUDES malignant neoplasm of middle ear
EXCLUDES 1 mesothelioma (C45.-)

✓4th **C30** Malignant neoplasm of nasal cavity and middle ear
- **C30.0** Malignant neoplasm of nasal cavity [HCC] [Rx] [ESR] [COM]
  Malignant neoplasm of cartilage of nose
  Malignant neoplasm of internal nose
  Malignant neoplasm of nasal concha
  Malignant neoplasm of septum of nose
  Malignant neoplasm of vestibule of nose
  EXCLUDES 1 malignant neoplasm of nasal bone (C41.0)
  malignant melanoma of skin of nose (C43.31)
  malignant neoplasm of nose NOS (C76.0)
  malignant neoplasm of olfactory bulb (C72.2-)
  malignant neoplasm of posterior margin of nasal septum and choana (C11.2)
  malignant neoplasm of turbinates (C41.0)
  other and unspecified malignant neoplasm of skin of nose (C44.301, C44.311, C44.321, C44.391)
- **C30.1** Malignant neoplasm of middle ear [HCC] [Rx] [ESR] [COM]
  Malignant neoplasm of antrum tympanicum
  Malignant neoplasm of auditory tube
  Malignant neoplasm of eustachian tube
  Malignant neoplasm of inner ear
  Malignant neoplasm of mastoid air cells
  Malignant neoplasm of tympanic cavity
  EXCLUDES 1 malignant neoplasm of auricular canal (external) (C43.2-, C44.2-)
  malignant melanoma of skin of (external) ear (C43.2-)
  malignant neoplasm of bone of ear (meatus) (C41.0)
  malignant neoplasm of cartilage of ear (C49.0)
  other and unspecified malignant neoplasm of skin of (external) ear (C44.2-)

✓4th **C31** Malignant neoplasm of accessory sinuses
- **C31.0** Malignant neoplasm of maxillary sinus [HCC] [Rx] [ESR] [COM]
  Malignant neoplasm of antrum (Highmore) (maxillary)
- **C31.1** Malignant neoplasm of ethmoidal sinus [HCC] [Rx] [ESR] [COM]
- **C31.2** Malignant neoplasm of frontal sinus [HCC] [Rx] [ESR] [COM]
- **C31.3** Malignant neoplasm of sphenoid sinus [HCC] [Rx] [ESR] [COM]
- **C31.8** Malignant neoplasm of overlapping sites of accessory sinuses [HCC] [Rx] [COM]
- **C31.9** Malignant neoplasm of accessory sinus, unspecified [HCC] [Rx] [ESR] [COM]

✓4th **C32** Malignant neoplasm of larynx
  Use additional code to identify:
  alcohol abuse and dependence (F10.-)
  exposure to environmental tobacco smoke (Z77.22)
  exposure to tobacco smoke in the perinatal period (P96.81)
  history of tobacco dependence (Z87.891)
  occupational exposure to environmental tobacco smoke (Z57.31)
  tobacco dependence (F17.-)
  tobacco use (Z72.0)
- **C32.0** Malignant neoplasm of glottis [HCC] [ESR] [COM]
  Malignant neoplasm of intrinsic larynx
  Malignant neoplasm of laryngeal commissure (anterior)(posterior)
  Malignant neoplasm of vocal cord (true) NOS
- **C32.1** Malignant neoplasm of supraglottis [HCC] [ESR] [COM]
  Malignant neoplasm of aryepiglottic fold or interarytenoid fold, laryngeal aspect
  Malignant neoplasm of epiglottis (suprahyoid portion) NOS
  Malignant neoplasm of extrinsic larynx
  Malignant neoplasm of false vocal cord
  Malignant neoplasm of posterior (laryngeal) surface of epiglottis
  Malignant neoplasm of ventricular bands
  EXCLUDES 2 malignant neoplasm of anterior surface of epiglottis (C10.1)
  malignant neoplasm of aryepiglottic fold or interarytenoid fold NOS (C13.1)
  malignant neoplasm of aryepiglottic fold or interarytenoid fold, hypopharyngeal aspect (C13.1)
  malignant neoplasm of aryepiglottic fold or interarytenoid fold, marginal zone (C13.1)
- **C32.2** Malignant neoplasm of subglottis [HCC] [ESR] [COM]
- **C32.3** Malignant neoplasm of laryngeal cartilage [HCC] [ESR] [COM]
- **C32.8** Malignant neoplasm of overlapping sites of larynx [HCC] [ESR] [COM]
- **C32.9** Malignant neoplasm of larynx, unspecified [HCC] [ESR] [COM]

C33 Malignant neoplasm of trachea [HCC] [Rx] [ESR] [COM]
  Use additional code to identify:
  exposure to environmental tobacco smoke (Z77.22)
  exposure to tobacco smoke in the perinatal period (P96.81)
  history of tobacco dependence (Z87.891)
  occupational exposure to environmental tobacco smoke (Z57.31)
  tobacco dependence (F17.-)
  tobacco use (Z72.0)

✓4th **C34** Malignant neoplasm of bronchus and lung
  Use additional code to identify:
  exposure to environmental tobacco smoke (Z77.22)
  exposure to tobacco smoke in the perinatal period (P96.81)
  history of tobacco dependence (Z87.891)
  occupational exposure to environmental tobacco smoke (Z57.31)
  tobacco dependence (F17.-)
  tobacco use (Z72.0)
  EXCLUDES 1 Kaposi's sarcoma of lung (C46.5-)
  malignant carcinoid tumor of the bronchus and lung (C7A.090)
  AHA: 2023,1Q,20-21; 2022,4Q,22; 2019,1Q,16
  TIP: When documented, assign code I31.31 for associated malignant pericardial effusion. The neoplasm code should be sequenced first.

✓5th **C34.0** Malignant neoplasm of main bronchus
  Malignant neoplasm of carina
  Malignant neoplasm of hilus (of lung)
  - **C34.00** Malignant neoplasm of unspecified main bronchus [HCC] [Rx] [ESR] [COM] [Q]
  - **C34.01** Malignant neoplasm of right main bronchus [HCC] [Rx] [ESR] [COM] [Q]
  - **C34.02** Malignant neoplasm of left main bronchus [HCC] [Rx] [ESR] [COM] [Q]

✓5th **C34.1** Malignant neoplasm of upper lobe, bronchus or lung
  - **C34.10** Malignant neoplasm of upper lobe, unspecified bronchus or lung [HCC] [Rx] [ESR] [COM] [Q]
  - **C34.11** Malignant neoplasm of upper lobe, right bronchus or lung [HCC] [Rx] [ESR] [COM] [Q]
  - **C34.12** Malignant neoplasm of upper lobe, left bronchus or lung [HCC] [Rx] [ESR] [COM] [Q]
- **C34.2** Malignant neoplasm of middle lobe, bronchus or lung [HCC] [Rx] [ESR] [COM] [Q]

✓5th **C34.3** Malignant neoplasm of lower lobe, bronchus or lung
  - **C34.30** Malignant neoplasm of lower lobe, unspecified bronchus or lung [HCC] [Rx] [ESR] [COM] [Q]
  - **C34.31** Malignant neoplasm of lower lobe, right bronchus or lung [HCC] [Rx] [ESR] [COM] [Q]

Chapter 2. Neoplasms

- **C34.32** Malignant neoplasm of lower lobe, left bronchus or lung
- ✓5th **C34.8** Malignant neoplasm of overlapping sites of bronchus and lung
  - **C34.80** Malignant neoplasm of overlapping sites of unspecified bronchus and lung
  - **C34.81** Malignant neoplasm of overlapping sites of right bronchus and lung
  - **C34.82** Malignant neoplasm of overlapping sites of left bronchus and lung
- ✓5th **C34.9** Malignant neoplasm of unspecified part of bronchus or lung
  - **C34.90** Malignant neoplasm of unspecified part of unspecified bronchus or lung
    Lung cancer NOS
  - **C34.91** Malignant neoplasm of unspecified part of right bronchus or lung
  - **C34.92** Malignant neoplasm of unspecified part of left bronchus or lung

C37 Malignant neoplasm of thymus
  - EXCLUDES 1: malignant carcinoid tumor of the thymus (C7A.091)

✓4th **C38** Malignant neoplasm of heart, mediastinum and pleura
  - EXCLUDES 1: mesothelioma (C45.-)
  - **C38.0** Malignant neoplasm of heart
    Malignant neoplasm of pericardium
    - EXCLUDES 1: malignant neoplasm of great vessels (C49.3)
  - **C38.1** Malignant neoplasm of anterior mediastinum
  - **C38.2** Malignant neoplasm of posterior mediastinum
  - **C38.3** Malignant neoplasm of mediastinum, part unspecified
  - **C38.4** Malignant neoplasm of pleura
  - **C38.8** Malignant neoplasm of overlapping sites of heart, mediastinum and pleura

✓4th **C39** Malignant neoplasm of other and ill-defined sites in the respiratory system and intrathoracic organs
  Use additional code to identify:
    exposure to environmental tobacco smoke (Z77.22)
    exposure to tobacco smoke in the perinatal period (P96.81)
    history of tobacco dependence (Z87.891)
    occupational exposure to environmental tobacco smoke (Z57.31)
    tobacco dependence (F17.-)
    tobacco use (Z72.0)
  - EXCLUDES 1: intrathoracic malignant neoplasm NOS (C76.1)
    thoracic malignant neoplasm NOS (C76.1)
  - **C39.0** Malignant neoplasm of upper respiratory tract, part unspecified
  - **C39.9** Malignant neoplasm of lower respiratory tract, part unspecified
    Malignant neoplasm of respiratory tract NOS

Malignant neoplasms of bone and articular cartilage (C40-C41)

INCLUDES: malignant neoplasm of cartilage (articular) (joint)
  malignant neoplasm of periosteum
EXCLUDES 1: malignant neoplasm of bone marrow NOS (C96.9)
  malignant neoplasm of synovia (C49.-)

✓4th **C40** Malignant neoplasm of bone and articular cartilage of limbs
  Use additional code to identify major osseous defect, if applicable (M89.7-)
  - ✓5th **C40.0** Malignant neoplasm of scapula and long bones of upper limb
    - **C40.00** Malignant neoplasm of scapula and long bones of unspecified upper limb
    - **C40.01** Malignant neoplasm of scapula and long bones of right upper limb
    - **C40.02** Malignant neoplasm of scapula and long bones of left upper limb
  - ✓5th **C40.1** Malignant neoplasm of short bones of upper limb
    - **C40.10** Malignant neoplasm of short bones of unspecified upper limb
    - **C40.11** Malignant neoplasm of short bones of right upper limb
    - **C40.12** Malignant neoplasm of short bones of left upper limb
  - ✓5th **C40.2** Malignant neoplasm of long bones of lower limb
    - **C40.20** Malignant neoplasm of long bones of unspecified lower limb
    - **C40.21** Malignant neoplasm of long bones of right lower limb
    - **C40.22** Malignant neoplasm of long bones of left lower limb
  - ✓5th **C40.3** Malignant neoplasm of short bones of lower limb
    - **C40.30** Malignant neoplasm of short bones of unspecified lower limb
    - **C40.31** Malignant neoplasm of short bones of right lower limb
    - **C40.32** Malignant neoplasm of short bones of left lower limb
  - ✓5th **C40.8** Malignant neoplasm of overlapping sites of bone and articular cartilage of limb
    - **C40.80** Malignant neoplasm of overlapping sites of bone and articular cartilage of unspecified limb
    - **C40.81** Malignant neoplasm of overlapping sites of bone and articular cartilage of right limb
    - **C40.82** Malignant neoplasm of overlapping sites of bone and articular cartilage of left limb
  - ✓5th **C40.9** Malignant neoplasm of unspecified bones and articular cartilage of limb
    - **C40.90** Malignant neoplasm of unspecified bones and articular cartilage of unspecified limb
    - **C40.91** Malignant neoplasm of unspecified bones and articular cartilage of right limb
    - **C40.92** Malignant neoplasm of unspecified bones and articular cartilage of left limb

✓4th **C41** Malignant neoplasm of bone and articular cartilage of other and unspecified sites
  EXCLUDES 1: malignant neoplasm of bones of limbs (C40.-)
    malignant neoplasm of cartilage of ear (C49.0)
    malignant neoplasm of cartilage of eyelid (C49.0)
    malignant neoplasm of cartilage of larynx (C32.3)
    malignant neoplasm of cartilage of limbs (C40.-)
    malignant neoplasm of cartilage of nose (C30.0)
  - **C41.0** Malignant neoplasm of bones of skull and face
    Malignant neoplasm of maxilla (superior)
    Malignant neoplasm of orbital bone
    - EXCLUDES 2: carcinoma, any type except intraosseous or odontogenic of:
      malignant neoplasm of jaw bone (lower) (C41.1)
      maxillary sinus (C31.0)
      upper jaw (C03.0)
  - **C41.1** Malignant neoplasm of mandible
    Malignant neoplasm of inferior maxilla
    Malignant neoplasm of lower jaw bone
    - EXCLUDES 2: carcinoma, any type except intraosseous or odontogenic of:
      jaw NOS (C03.9)
      lower (C03.1)
      malignant neoplasm of upper jaw bone (C41.0)
  - **C41.2** Malignant neoplasm of vertebral column
    - EXCLUDES 1: malignant neoplasm of sacrum and coccyx (C41.4)
  - **C41.3** Malignant neoplasm of ribs, sternum and clavicle
  - **C41.4** Malignant neoplasm of pelvic bones, sacrum and coccyx
  - **C41.9** Malignant neoplasm of bone and articular cartilage, unspecified

Melanoma and other malignant neoplasms of skin (C43-C44)

✓4th **C43** Malignant melanoma of skin
  - EXCLUDES 1: melanoma in situ (D03.-)
  - EXCLUDES 2: malignant melanoma of skin of genital organs (C51-C52, C60.-, C63.-)
    Merkel cell carcinoma (C4A.-)
    sites other than skin - code to malignant neoplasm of the site
  - **C43.0** Malignant melanoma of lip
    - EXCLUDES 1: malignant neoplasm of vermilion border of lip (C00.0-C00.2)
  - ✓5th **C43.1** Malignant melanoma of eyelid, including canthus
    AHA: 2018,4Q,4
    - **C43.10** Malignant melanoma of unspecified eyelid, including canthus

---

✓ Additional Character Required   ✓x7th Placeholder Alert   Manifestation   Unspecified Dx   Q QPP   UPD Unacceptable PDx

Chapter 2. Neoplasms

- **C43.11** Malignant melanoma of right eyelid, including canthus ✓6th
  - **C43.111** Malignant melanoma of right upper eyelid, including canthus
  - **C43.112** Malignant melanoma of right lower eyelid, including canthus
- **C43.12** Malignant melanoma of left eyelid, including canthus ✓6th
  - **C43.121** Malignant melanoma of left upper eyelid, including canthus
  - **C43.122** Malignant melanoma of left lower eyelid, including canthus
- **C43.2** Malignant melanoma of ear and external auricular canal ✓5th
  - **C43.20** Malignant melanoma of unspecified ear and external auricular canal
  - **C43.21** Malignant melanoma of right ear and external auricular canal
  - **C43.22** Malignant melanoma of left ear and external auricular canal
- **C43.3** Malignant melanoma of other and unspecified parts of face ✓5th
  - **C43.30** Malignant melanoma of unspecified part of face
  - **C43.31** Malignant melanoma of nose
  - **C43.39** Malignant melanoma of other parts of face
- **C43.4** Malignant melanoma of scalp and neck
- **C43.5** Malignant melanoma of trunk ✓5th
  - EXCLUDES 2 — malignant neoplasm of anus NOS (C21.0)
    malignant neoplasm of scrotum (C63.2)
  - **C43.51** Malignant melanoma of anal skin
    Malignant melanoma of anal margin
    Malignant melanoma of perianal skin
  - **C43.52** Malignant melanoma of skin of breast
  - **C43.59** Malignant melanoma of other part of trunk
- **C43.6** Malignant melanoma of upper limb, including shoulder ✓5th
  - **C43.60** Malignant melanoma of unspecified upper limb, including shoulder
  - **C43.61** Malignant melanoma of right upper limb, including shoulder
  - **C43.62** Malignant melanoma of left upper limb, including shoulder
- **C43.7** Malignant melanoma of lower limb, including hip ✓5th
  - **C43.70** Malignant melanoma of unspecified lower limb, including hip
  - **C43.71** Malignant melanoma of right lower limb, including hip
  - **C43.72** Malignant melanoma of left lower limb, including hip
- **C43.8** Malignant melanoma of overlapping sites of skin
- **C43.9** Malignant melanoma of skin, unspecified
  Malignant melanoma of unspecified site of skin
  Melanoma (malignant) NOS

- **C4A** Merkel cell carcinoma ✓4th
  - DEF: Malignant cutaneous cancer predominantly found in elderly patients with sun exposure that usually presents as a flesh-colored or bluish-red lump typically seen on the neck, head, and face.
  - **C4A.0** Merkel cell carcinoma of lip
    - EXCLUDES 1 — malignant neoplasm of vermilion border of lip (C00.0-C00.2)
  - **C4A.1** Merkel cell carcinoma of eyelid, including canthus ✓5th
    AHA: 2018,4Q,4
    - **C4A.10** Merkel cell carcinoma of unspecified eyelid, including canthus
    - **C4A.11** Merkel cell carcinoma of right eyelid, including canthus ✓6th
      - **C4A.111** Merkel cell carcinoma of right upper eyelid, including canthus
      - **C4A.112** Merkel cell carcinoma of right lower eyelid, including canthus
    - **C4A.12** Merkel cell carcinoma of left eyelid, including canthus ✓6th
      - **C4A.121** Merkel cell carcinoma of left upper eyelid, including canthus
      - **C4A.122** Merkel cell carcinoma of left lower eyelid, including canthus
  - **C4A.2** Merkel cell carcinoma of ear and external auricular canal ✓5th
    - **C4A.20** Merkel cell carcinoma of unspecified ear and external auricular canal
    - **C4A.21** Merkel cell carcinoma of right ear and external auricular canal
    - **C4A.22** Merkel cell carcinoma of left ear and external auricular canal
  - **C4A.3** Merkel cell carcinoma of other and unspecified parts of face ✓5th
    - **C4A.30** Merkel cell carcinoma of unspecified part of face
    - **C4A.31** Merkel cell carcinoma of nose
    - **C4A.39** Merkel cell carcinoma of other parts of face
  - **C4A.4** Merkel cell carcinoma of scalp and neck
  - **C4A.5** Merkel cell carcinoma of trunk ✓5th
    - EXCLUDES 2 — malignant neoplasm of anus NOS (C21.0)
      malignant neoplasm of scrotum (C63.2)
    - **C4A.51** Merkel cell carcinoma of anal skin
      Merkel cell carcinoma of anal margin
      Merkel cell carcinoma of perianal skin
    - **C4A.52** Merkel cell carcinoma of skin of breast
    - **C4A.59** Merkel cell carcinoma of other part of trunk
  - **C4A.6** Merkel cell carcinoma of upper limb, including shoulder ✓5th
    - **C4A.60** Merkel cell carcinoma of unspecified upper limb, including shoulder
    - **C4A.61** Merkel cell carcinoma of right upper limb, including shoulder
    - **C4A.62** Merkel cell carcinoma of left upper limb, including shoulder
  - **C4A.7** Merkel cell carcinoma of lower limb, including hip ✓5th
    - **C4A.70** Merkel cell carcinoma of unspecified lower limb, including hip
    - **C4A.71** Merkel cell carcinoma of right lower limb, including hip
    - **C4A.72** Merkel cell carcinoma of left lower limb, including hip
  - **C4A.8** Merkel cell carcinoma of overlapping sites
  - **C4A.9** Merkel cell carcinoma, unspecified
    Merkel cell carcinoma NOS
    Merkel cell carcinoma of unspecified site

- **C44** Other and unspecified malignant neoplasm of skin ✓4th
  - INCLUDES — malignant neoplasm of sebaceous glands
    malignant neoplasm of sweat glands
  - EXCLUDES 1 — Kaposi's sarcoma of skin (C46.0)
    malignant melanoma of skin (C43.-)
    malignant neoplasm of skin of genital organs (C51-C52, C60.-, C63.2)
    Merkel cell carcinoma (C4A.-)
  - DEF: Basal cell carcinoma: Abnormal growth of skin cells that arises from the deepest layer of the epidermis and may present as an open sore, red patches, pink growth, or scar. Typically caused by sun exposure, it is one of the most common forms of skin cancer.
  - DEF: Squamous cell carcinoma: Uncontrolled growth of abnormal skin cells that arises from the outer layers of the skin (epidermis) and may present as an open sore. It is characterized by a firm, red nodule, elevated growth with a central depression, or a flat sore with a scaly crust.
  - **C44.0** Other and unspecified malignant neoplasm of skin of lip ✓5th
    - EXCLUDES 1 — malignant neoplasm of lip (C00.-)
    - **C44.00** Unspecified malignant neoplasm of skin of lip
    - **C44.01** Basal cell carcinoma of skin of lip
    - **C44.02** Squamous cell carcinoma of skin of lip
    - **C44.09** Other specified malignant neoplasm of skin of lip
  - **C44.1** Other and unspecified malignant neoplasm of skin of eyelid, including canthus ✓5th
    - EXCLUDES 1 — connective tissue of eyelid (C49.0)
    AHA: 2018,4Q,4
    - **C44.10** Unspecified malignant neoplasm of skin of eyelid, including canthus ✓6th
      - **C44.101** Unspecified malignant neoplasm of skin of unspecified eyelid, including canthus
      - **C44.102** Unspecified malignant neoplasm of skin of right eyelid, including canthus ✓7th

---

HCC CMS-HCC | Rx Rx HCC | ESR ESRD HCC | COM Commercial HCC | N Newborn: 0 | P Pediatric: 0-17 | M Maternity: 9-64 | A Adult: 15-124

- **C44.1021** Unspecified malignant neoplasm of skin of right upper eyelid, including canthus
- **C44.1022** Unspecified malignant neoplasm of skin of right lower eyelid, including canthus
- ✓7ᵗʰ **C44.109** Unspecified malignant neoplasm of skin of left eyelid, including canthus
  - **C44.1091** Unspecified malignant neoplasm of skin of left upper eyelid, including canthus
  - **C44.1092** Unspecified malignant neoplasm of skin of left lower eyelid, including canthus
- ✓6ᵗʰ **C44.11** Basal cell carcinoma of skin of eyelid, including canthus
  - **C44.111** Basal cell carcinoma of skin of unspecified eyelid, including canthus
  - ✓7ᵗʰ **C44.112** Basal cell carcinoma of skin of right eyelid, including canthus
    - **C44.1121** Basal cell carcinoma of skin of right upper eyelid, including canthus
    - **C44.1122** Basal cell carcinoma of skin of right lower eyelid, including canthus
  - ✓7ᵗʰ **C44.119** Basal cell carcinoma of skin of left eyelid, including canthus
    - **C44.1191** Basal cell carcinoma of skin of left upper eyelid, including canthus
    - **C44.1192** Basal cell carcinoma of skin of left lower eyelid, including canthus
- ✓6ᵗʰ **C44.12** Squamous cell carcinoma of skin of eyelid, including canthus
  - **C44.121** Squamous cell carcinoma of skin of unspecified eyelid, including canthus
  - ✓7ᵗʰ **C44.122** Squamous cell carcinoma of skin of right eyelid, including canthus
    - **C44.1221** Squamous cell carcinoma of skin of right upper eyelid, including canthus
    - **C44.1222** Squamous cell carcinoma of skin of right lower eyelid, including canthus
  - ✓7ᵗʰ **C44.129** Squamous cell carcinoma of skin of left eyelid, including canthus
    - **C44.1291** Squamous cell carcinoma of skin of left upper eyelid, including canthus
    - **C44.1292** Squamous cell carcinoma of skin of left lower eyelid, including canthus
- ✓6ᵗʰ **C44.13** Sebaceous cell carcinoma of skin of eyelid, including canthus
  - **C44.131** Sebaceous cell carcinoma of skin of unspecified eyelid, including canthus
  - ✓7ᵗʰ **C44.132** Sebaceous cell carcinoma of skin of right eyelid, including canthus
    - **C44.1321** Sebaceous cell carcinoma of skin of right upper eyelid, including canthus
    - **C44.1322** Sebaceous cell carcinoma of skin of right lower eyelid, including canthus
  - ✓7ᵗʰ **C44.139** Sebaceous cell carcinoma of skin of left eyelid, including canthus
    - **C44.1391** Sebaceous cell carcinoma of skin of left upper eyelid, including canthus
    - **C44.1392** Sebaceous cell carcinoma of skin of left lower eyelid, including canthus
- ✓6ᵗʰ **C44.19** Other specified malignant neoplasm of skin of eyelid, including canthus
  - **C44.191** Other specified malignant neoplasm of skin of unspecified eyelid, including canthus
  - ✓7ᵗʰ **C44.192** Other specified malignant neoplasm of skin of right eyelid, including canthus
    - **C44.1921** Other specified malignant neoplasm of skin of right upper eyelid, including canthus
    - **C44.1922** Other specified malignant neoplasm of skin of right lower eyelid, including canthus
  - ✓7ᵗʰ **C44.199** Other specified malignant neoplasm of skin of left eyelid, including canthus
    - **C44.1991** Other specified malignant neoplasm of skin of left upper eyelid, including canthus
    - **C44.1992** Other specified malignant neoplasm of skin of left lower eyelid, including canthus

- ✓5ᵗʰ **C44.2** Other and unspecified malignant neoplasm of skin of ear and external auricular canal
  - **EXCLUDES 1** connective tissue of ear (C49.0)
  - ✓6ᵗʰ **C44.20** Unspecified malignant neoplasm of skin of ear and external auricular canal
    - **C44.201** Unspecified malignant neoplasm of skin of unspecified ear and external auricular canal
    - **C44.202** Unspecified malignant neoplasm of skin of right ear and external auricular canal
    - **C44.209** Unspecified malignant neoplasm of skin of left ear and external auricular canal
  - ✓6ᵗʰ **C44.21** Basal cell carcinoma of skin of ear and external auricular canal
    - **C44.211** Basal cell carcinoma of skin of unspecified ear and external auricular canal
    - **C44.212** Basal cell carcinoma of skin of right ear and external auricular canal
    - **C44.219** Basal cell carcinoma of skin of left ear and external auricular canal
  - ✓6ᵗʰ **C44.22** Squamous cell carcinoma of skin of ear and external auricular canal
    - **C44.221** Squamous cell carcinoma of skin of unspecified ear and external auricular canal
    - **C44.222** Squamous cell carcinoma of skin of right ear and external auricular canal
    - **C44.229** Squamous cell carcinoma of skin of left ear and external auricular canal
  - ✓6ᵗʰ **C44.29** Other specified malignant neoplasm of skin of ear and external auricular canal
    - **C44.291** Other specified malignant neoplasm of skin of unspecified ear and external auricular canal
    - **C44.292** Other specified malignant neoplasm of skin of right ear and external auricular canal
    - **C44.299** Other specified malignant neoplasm of skin of left ear and external auricular canal

- ✓5ᵗʰ **C44.3** Other and unspecified malignant neoplasm of skin of other and unspecified parts of face
  - ✓6ᵗʰ **C44.30** Unspecified malignant neoplasm of skin of other and unspecified parts of face
    - **C44.300** Unspecified malignant neoplasm of skin of unspecified part of face
    - **C44.301** Unspecified malignant neoplasm of skin of nose
    - **C44.309** Unspecified malignant neoplasm of skin of other parts of face
  - ✓6ᵗʰ **C44.31** Basal cell carcinoma of skin of other and unspecified parts of face
    - **C44.310** Basal cell carcinoma of skin of unspecified parts of face
    - **C44.311** Basal cell carcinoma of skin of nose
    - **C44.319** Basal cell carcinoma of skin of other parts of face
  - ✓6ᵗʰ **C44.32** Squamous cell carcinoma of skin of other and unspecified parts of face
    - **C44.320** Squamous cell carcinoma of skin of unspecified parts of face
    - **C44.321** Squamous cell carcinoma of skin of nose
    - **C44.329** Squamous cell carcinoma of skin of other parts of face
  - ✓6ᵗʰ **C44.39** Other specified malignant neoplasm of skin of other and unspecified parts of face
    - **C44.390** Other specified malignant neoplasm of skin of unspecified parts of face
    - **C44.391** Other specified malignant neoplasm of skin of nose
    - **C44.399** Other specified malignant neoplasm of skin of other parts of face

Chapter 2. Neoplasms

- ✓5th **C44.4** Other and unspecified malignant neoplasm of skin of scalp and neck
  - **C44.40** Unspecified malignant neoplasm of skin of scalp and neck
  - **C44.41** Basal cell carcinoma of skin of scalp and neck
  - **C44.42** Squamous cell carcinoma of skin of scalp and neck
  - **C44.49** Other specified malignant neoplasm of skin of scalp and neck
- ✓5th **C44.5** Other and unspecified malignant neoplasm of skin of trunk
  - EXCLUDES 1 anus NOS (C21.0)
    scrotum (C63.2)
  - ✓6th **C44.50** Unspecified malignant neoplasm of skin of trunk
    - **C44.500** Unspecified malignant neoplasm of anal skin
      - Unspecified malignant neoplasm of anal margin
      - Unspecified malignant neoplasm of perianal skin
    - **C44.501** Unspecified malignant neoplasm of skin of breast
    - **C44.509** Unspecified malignant neoplasm of skin of other part of trunk
  - ✓6th **C44.51** Basal cell carcinoma of skin of trunk
    - **C44.510** Basal cell carcinoma of anal skin
      - Basal cell carcinoma of anal margin
      - Basal cell carcinoma of perianal skin
    - **C44.511** Basal cell carcinoma of skin of breast
    - **C44.519** Basal cell carcinoma of skin of other part of trunk
  - ✓6th **C44.52** Squamous cell carcinoma of skin of trunk
    - **C44.520** Squamous cell carcinoma of anal skin
      - Squamous cell carcinoma of anal margin
      - Squamous cell carcinoma of perianal skin
    - **C44.521** Squamous cell carcinoma of skin of breast
    - **C44.529** Squamous cell carcinoma of skin of other part of trunk
  - ✓6th **C44.59** Other specified malignant neoplasm of skin of trunk
    - **C44.590** Other specified malignant neoplasm of anal skin
      - Other specified malignant neoplasm of anal margin
      - Other specified malignant neoplasm of perianal skin
    - **C44.591** Other specified malignant neoplasm of skin of breast
    - **C44.599** Other specified malignant neoplasm of skin of other part of trunk
- ✓5th **C44.6** Other and unspecified malignant neoplasm of skin of upper limb, including shoulder
  - ✓6th **C44.60** Unspecified malignant neoplasm of skin of upper limb, including shoulder
    - **C44.601** Unspecified malignant neoplasm of skin of unspecified upper limb, including shoulder
    - **C44.602** Unspecified malignant neoplasm of skin of right upper limb, including shoulder
    - **C44.609** Unspecified malignant neoplasm of skin of left upper limb, including shoulder
  - ✓6th **C44.61** Basal cell carcinoma of skin of upper limb, including shoulder
    - **C44.611** Basal cell carcinoma of skin of unspecified upper limb, including shoulder
    - **C44.612** Basal cell carcinoma of skin of right upper limb, including shoulder
    - **C44.619** Basal cell carcinoma of skin of left upper limb, including shoulder
  - ✓6th **C44.62** Squamous cell carcinoma of skin of upper limb, including shoulder
    - **C44.621** Squamous cell carcinoma of skin of unspecified upper limb, including shoulder
    - **C44.622** Squamous cell carcinoma of skin of right upper limb, including shoulder
    - **C44.629** Squamous cell carcinoma of skin of left upper limb, including shoulder
  - ✓6th **C44.69** Other specified malignant neoplasm of skin of upper limb, including shoulder
    - **C44.691** Other specified malignant neoplasm of skin of unspecified upper limb, including shoulder
    - **C44.692** Other specified malignant neoplasm of skin of right upper limb, including shoulder
    - **C44.699** Other specified malignant neoplasm of skin of left upper limb, including shoulder
- ✓5th **C44.7** Other and unspecified malignant neoplasm of skin of lower limb, including hip
  - ✓6th **C44.70** Unspecified malignant neoplasm of skin of lower limb, including hip
    - **C44.701** Unspecified malignant neoplasm of skin of unspecified lower limb, including hip
    - **C44.702** Unspecified malignant neoplasm of skin of right lower limb, including hip
    - **C44.709** Unspecified malignant neoplasm of skin of left lower limb, including hip
  - ✓6th **C44.71** Basal cell carcinoma of skin of lower limb, including hip
    - **C44.711** Basal cell carcinoma of skin of unspecified lower limb, including hip
    - **C44.712** Basal cell carcinoma of skin of right lower limb, including hip
    - **C44.719** Basal cell carcinoma of skin of left lower limb, including hip
  - ✓6th **C44.72** Squamous cell carcinoma of skin of lower limb, including hip
    - **C44.721** Squamous cell carcinoma of skin of unspecified lower limb, including hip
    - **C44.722** Squamous cell carcinoma of skin of right lower limb, including hip
    - **C44.729** Squamous cell carcinoma of skin of left lower limb, including hip
  - ✓6th **C44.79** Other specified malignant neoplasm of skin of lower limb, including hip
    - **C44.791** Other specified malignant neoplasm of skin of unspecified lower limb, including hip
    - **C44.792** Other specified malignant neoplasm of skin of right lower limb, including hip
    - **C44.799** Other specified malignant neoplasm of skin of left lower limb, including hip
- ✓5th **C44.8** Other and unspecified malignant neoplasm of overlapping sites of skin
  - **C44.80** Unspecified malignant neoplasm of overlapping sites of skin
  - **C44.81** Basal cell carcinoma of overlapping sites of skin
  - **C44.82** Squamous cell carcinoma of overlapping sites of skin
  - **C44.89** Other specified malignant neoplasm of overlapping sites of skin
- ✓5th **C44.9** Other and unspecified malignant neoplasm of skin, unspecified
  - **C44.90** Unspecified malignant neoplasm of skin, unspecified
    - Malignant neoplasm of unspecified site of skin
  - **C44.91** Basal cell carcinoma of skin, unspecified
  - **C44.92** Squamous cell carcinoma of skin, unspecified
  - **C44.99** Other specified malignant neoplasm of skin, unspecified

Malignant neoplasms of mesothelial and soft tissue (C45-C49)

- ✓4th **C45** Mesothelioma
  - **DEF:** Rare type of cancer that forms in the thin layer of protective tissue that covers the majority of internal organs (mesothelium).
  - **C45.0** Mesothelioma of pleura HCC Rx ESR COM
    - EXCLUDES 1 other malignant neoplasm of pleura (C38.4)
    - **AHA:** 2017,2Q,11
    - **TIP:** For pleural mesothelioma that has metastasized to the chest wall, assign this code for the primary site along with C79.89 for metastatic cancer in the chest wall.
  - **C45.1** Mesothelioma of peritoneum HCC Rx ESR COM
    - Mesothelioma of cul-de-sac
    - Mesothelioma of mesentery
    - Mesothelioma of mesocolon
    - Mesothelioma of omentum
    - Mesothelioma of peritoneum (parietal) (pelvic)
    - EXCLUDES 1 other malignant neoplasm of soft tissue of peritoneum (C48.-)
  - **C45.2** Mesothelioma of pericardium HCC Rx ESR COM
    - EXCLUDES 1 other malignant neoplasm of pericardium (C38.0)
  - **C45.7** Mesothelioma of other sites HCC Rx ESR COM
  - **C45.9** Mesothelioma, unspecified HCC Rx ESR COM

C46 Kaposi's sarcoma
Code first any human immunodeficiency virus [HIV] disease (B20)
DEF: Malignant neoplasm that causes patches of abnormal tissue to grow under the skin, in the lining of the mouth, nose, and throat, in lymph nodes, or in other visceral organs. Kaposi's sarcoma is caused by human herpesvirus8 (HHV8).

- **C46.0** Kaposi's sarcoma of skin
- **C46.1** Kaposi's sarcoma of soft tissue
  - Kaposi's sarcoma of blood vessel
  - Kaposi's sarcoma of connective tissue
  - Kaposi's sarcoma of fascia
  - Kaposi's sarcoma of ligament
  - Kaposi's sarcoma of lymphatic(s) NEC
  - Kaposi's sarcoma of muscle
  - *EXCLUDES 2* Kaposi's sarcoma of lymph glands and nodes (C46.3)
- **C46.2** Kaposi's sarcoma of palate
- **C46.3** Kaposi's sarcoma of lymph nodes
- **C46.4** Kaposi's sarcoma of gastrointestinal sites
- **C46.5** Kaposi's sarcoma of lung
  - **AHA:** 2019,1Q,16
  - **TIP:** When documented, assign code I31.31 for associated malignant pericardial effusion. The neoplasm code should be sequenced first.
  - **C46.50** Kaposi's sarcoma of unspecified lung
  - **C46.51** Kaposi's sarcoma of right lung
  - **C46.52** Kaposi's sarcoma of left lung
- **C46.7** Kaposi's sarcoma of other sites
- **C46.9** Kaposi's sarcoma, unspecified
  - Kaposi's sarcoma of unspecified site

C47 Malignant neoplasm of peripheral nerves and autonomic nervous system
INCLUDES malignant neoplasm of sympathetic and parasympathetic nerves and ganglia
EXCLUDES 1 Kaposi's sarcoma of soft tissue (C46.1)

- **C47.0** Malignant neoplasm of peripheral nerves of head, face and neck
  - *EXCLUDES 1* malignant neoplasm of peripheral nerves of orbit (C69.6-)
- **C47.1** Malignant neoplasm of peripheral nerves of upper limb, including shoulder
  - **C47.10** Malignant neoplasm of peripheral nerves of unspecified upper limb, including shoulder
  - **C47.11** Malignant neoplasm of peripheral nerves of right upper limb, including shoulder
  - **C47.12** Malignant neoplasm of peripheral nerves of left upper limb, including shoulder
- **C47.2** Malignant neoplasm of peripheral nerves of lower limb, including hip
  - **C47.20** Malignant neoplasm of peripheral nerves of unspecified lower limb, including hip
  - **C47.21** Malignant neoplasm of peripheral nerves of right lower limb, including hip
  - **C47.22** Malignant neoplasm of peripheral nerves of left lower limb, including hip
- **C47.3** Malignant neoplasm of peripheral nerves of thorax
- **C47.4** Malignant neoplasm of peripheral nerves of abdomen
- **C47.5** Malignant neoplasm of peripheral nerves of pelvis
- **C47.6** Malignant neoplasm of peripheral nerves of trunk, unspecified
  - Malignant neoplasm of peripheral nerves of unspecified part of trunk
- **C47.8** Malignant neoplasm of overlapping sites of peripheral nerves and autonomic nervous system
- **C47.9** Malignant neoplasm of peripheral nerves and autonomic nervous system, unspecified
  - Malignant neoplasm of unspecified site of peripheral nerves and autonomic nervous system

C48 Malignant neoplasm of retroperitoneum and peritoneum
EXCLUDES 1 Kaposi's sarcoma of connective tissue (C46.1)
mesothelioma (C45.-)

- **C48.0** Malignant neoplasm of retroperitoneum
- **C48.1** Malignant neoplasm of specified parts of peritoneum
  - Malignant neoplasm of cul-de-sac
  - Malignant neoplasm of mesentery
  - Malignant neoplasm of mesocolon
  - Malignant neoplasm of omentum
  - Malignant neoplasm of parietal peritoneum
  - Malignant neoplasm of pelvic peritoneum
- **C48.2** Malignant neoplasm of peritoneum, unspecified
- **C48.8** Malignant neoplasm of overlapping sites of retroperitoneum and peritoneum

C49 Malignant neoplasm of other connective and soft tissue
INCLUDES
- malignant neoplasm of blood vessel
- malignant neoplasm of bursa
- malignant neoplasm of cartilage
- malignant neoplasm of fascia
- malignant neoplasm of fat
- malignant neoplasm of ligament, except uterine
- malignant neoplasm of lymphatic vessel
- malignant neoplasm of muscle
- malignant neoplasm of synovia
- malignant neoplasm of tendon (sheath)

EXCLUDES 1
- malignant neoplasm of cartilage (of):
- malignant neoplasm of connective tissue of breast (C50.-)
  - articular (C40-C41)
  - larynx (C32.3)
  - nose (C30.0)

EXCLUDES 2
- Kaposi's sarcoma of soft tissue (C46.1)
- malignant neoplasm of heart (C38.0)
- malignant neoplasm of peripheral nerves and autonomic nervous system (C47.-)
- malignant neoplasm of peritoneum (C48.2)
- malignant neoplasm of retroperitoneum (C48.0)
- malignant neoplasm of uterine ligament (C57.3)
- mesothelioma (C45.-)

- **C49.0** Malignant neoplasm of connective and soft tissue of head, face and neck
  - Malignant neoplasm of connective tissue of ear
  - Malignant neoplasm of connective tissue of eyelid
  - *EXCLUDES 1* connective tissue of orbit (C69.6-)
- **C49.1** Malignant neoplasm of connective and soft tissue of upper limb, including shoulder
  - **C49.10** Malignant neoplasm of connective and soft tissue of unspecified upper limb, including shoulder
  - **C49.11** Malignant neoplasm of connective and soft tissue of right upper limb, including shoulder
  - **C49.12** Malignant neoplasm of connective and soft tissue of left upper limb, including shoulder
- **C49.2** Malignant neoplasm of connective and soft tissue of lower limb, including hip
  - **C49.20** Malignant neoplasm of connective and soft tissue of unspecified lower limb, including hip
  - **C49.21** Malignant neoplasm of connective and soft tissue of right lower limb, including hip
  - **C49.22** Malignant neoplasm of connective and soft tissue of left lower limb, including hip
- **C49.3** Malignant neoplasm of connective and soft tissue of thorax
  - Malignant neoplasm of axilla
  - Malignant neoplasm of diaphragm
  - Malignant neoplasm of great vessels
  - *EXCLUDES 1* malignant neoplasm of breast (C50.-)
    - malignant neoplasm of heart (C38.0)
    - malignant neoplasm of mediastinum (C38.1-C38.3)
    - malignant neoplasm of thymus (C37)
  - **AHA:** 2015,3Q,19
- **C49.4** Malignant neoplasm of connective and soft tissue of abdomen
  - Malignant neoplasm of abdominal wall
  - Malignant neoplasm of hypochondrium
- **C49.5** Malignant neoplasm of connective and soft tissue of pelvis
  - Malignant neoplasm of buttock
  - Malignant neoplasm of groin
  - Malignant neoplasm of perineum

Chapter 2. Neoplasms

C49.6 Malignant neoplasm of connective and soft tissue of trunk, unspecified
Malignant neoplasm of back NOS

C49.8 Malignant neoplasm of overlapping sites of connective and soft tissue
Primary malignant neoplasm of two or more contiguous sites of connective and soft tissue

C49.9 Malignant neoplasm of connective and soft tissue, unspecified

✓5th **C49.A** Gastrointestinal stromal tumor
AHA: 2016,4Q,8
DEF: Uncommon malignant tumor found in the GI tract that originates from interstitial cells of the autonomic nervous system. Most occur in the stomach or small intestine but can originate anywhere in the GI tract.

- **C49.A0** Gastrointestinal stromal tumor, unspecified site
- **C49.A1** Gastrointestinal stromal tumor of esophagus
- **C49.A2** Gastrointestinal stromal tumor of stomach
- **C49.A3** Gastrointestinal stromal tumor of small intestine
- **C49.A4** Gastrointestinal stromal tumor of large intestine
- **C49.A5** Gastrointestinal stromal tumor of rectum
- **C49.A9** Gastrointestinal stromal tumor of other sites

Malignant neoplasms of breast (C50)

✓4th **C50** Malignant neoplasm of breast
INCLUDES: connective tissue of breast
Paget's disease of breast
Paget's disease of nipple
Use additional code to identify estrogen, and other hormones and factors receptor status (Z17.-)
EXCLUDES 1: skin of breast (C44.501, C44.511, C44.521, C44.591)
AHA: 2017,4Q,19

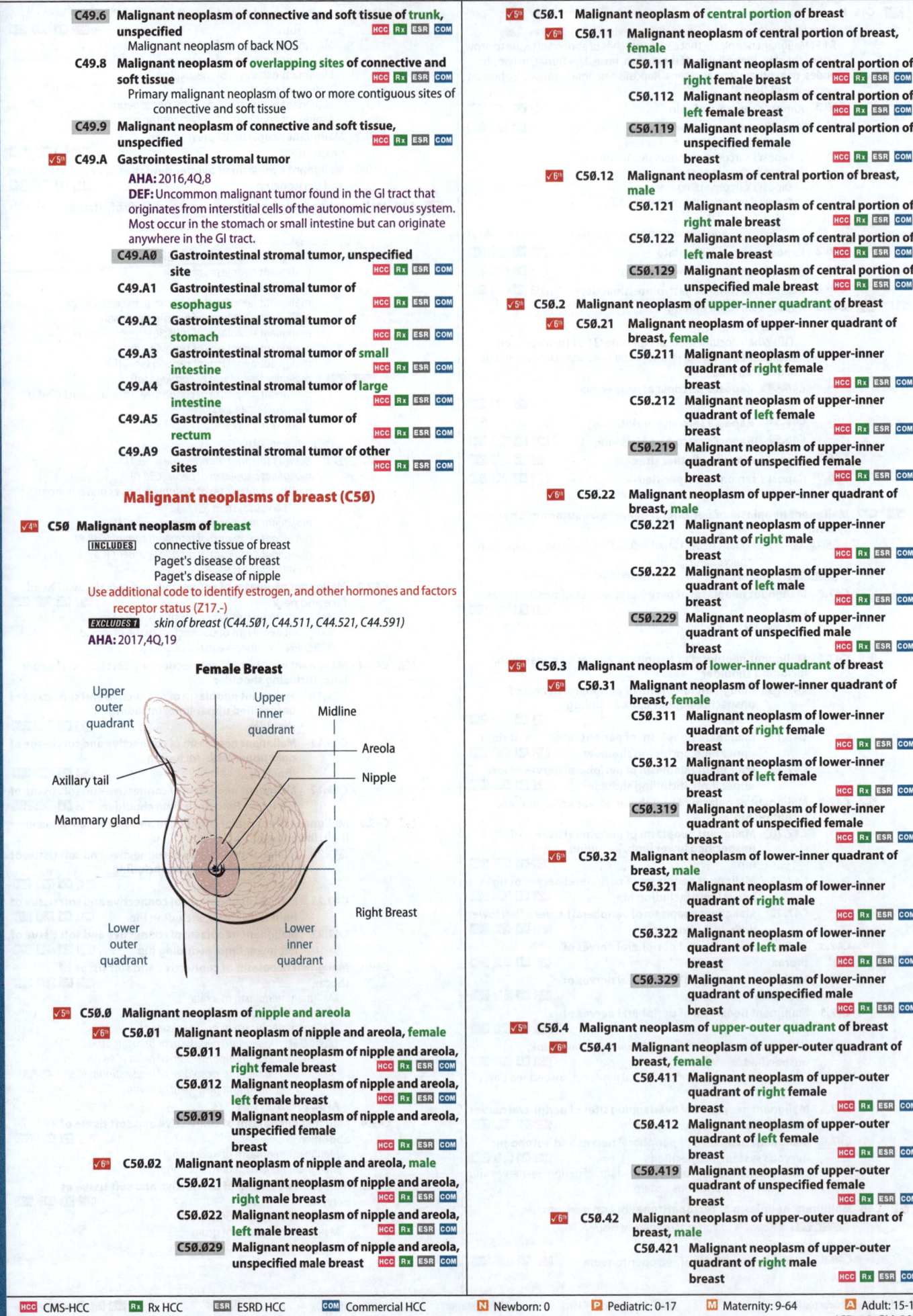

Female Breast — Upper outer quadrant, Upper inner quadrant, Midline, Areola, Nipple, Axillary tail, Mammary gland, Right Breast, Lower outer quadrant, Lower inner quadrant

✓5th **C50.0** Malignant neoplasm of nipple and areola
- ✓6th **C50.01** Malignant neoplasm of nipple and areola, female
  - **C50.011** Malignant neoplasm of nipple and areola, right female breast
  - **C50.012** Malignant neoplasm of nipple and areola, left female breast
  - **C50.019** Malignant neoplasm of nipple and areola, unspecified female breast
- ✓6th **C50.02** Malignant neoplasm of nipple and areola, male
  - **C50.021** Malignant neoplasm of nipple and areola, right male breast
  - **C50.022** Malignant neoplasm of nipple and areola, left male breast
  - **C50.029** Malignant neoplasm of nipple and areola, unspecified male breast

✓5th **C50.1** Malignant neoplasm of central portion of breast
- ✓6th **C50.11** Malignant neoplasm of central portion of breast, female
  - **C50.111** Malignant neoplasm of central portion of right female breast
  - **C50.112** Malignant neoplasm of central portion of left female breast
  - **C50.119** Malignant neoplasm of central portion of unspecified female breast
- ✓6th **C50.12** Malignant neoplasm of central portion of breast, male
  - **C50.121** Malignant neoplasm of central portion of right male breast
  - **C50.122** Malignant neoplasm of central portion of left male breast
  - **C50.129** Malignant neoplasm of central portion of unspecified male breast

✓5th **C50.2** Malignant neoplasm of upper-inner quadrant of breast
- ✓6th **C50.21** Malignant neoplasm of upper-inner quadrant of breast, female
  - **C50.211** Malignant neoplasm of upper-inner quadrant of right female breast
  - **C50.212** Malignant neoplasm of upper-inner quadrant of left female breast
  - **C50.219** Malignant neoplasm of upper-inner quadrant of unspecified female breast
- ✓6th **C50.22** Malignant neoplasm of upper-inner quadrant of breast, male
  - **C50.221** Malignant neoplasm of upper-inner quadrant of right male breast
  - **C50.222** Malignant neoplasm of upper-inner quadrant of left male breast
  - **C50.229** Malignant neoplasm of upper-inner quadrant of unspecified male breast

✓5th **C50.3** Malignant neoplasm of lower-inner quadrant of breast
- ✓6th **C50.31** Malignant neoplasm of lower-inner quadrant of breast, female
  - **C50.311** Malignant neoplasm of lower-inner quadrant of right female breast
  - **C50.312** Malignant neoplasm of lower-inner quadrant of left female breast
  - **C50.319** Malignant neoplasm of lower-inner quadrant of unspecified female breast
- ✓6th **C50.32** Malignant neoplasm of lower-inner quadrant of breast, male
  - **C50.321** Malignant neoplasm of lower-inner quadrant of right male breast
  - **C50.322** Malignant neoplasm of lower-inner quadrant of left male breast
  - **C50.329** Malignant neoplasm of lower-inner quadrant of unspecified male breast

✓5th **C50.4** Malignant neoplasm of upper-outer quadrant of breast
- ✓6th **C50.41** Malignant neoplasm of upper-outer quadrant of breast, female
  - **C50.411** Malignant neoplasm of upper-outer quadrant of right female breast
  - **C50.412** Malignant neoplasm of upper-outer quadrant of left female breast
  - **C50.419** Malignant neoplasm of upper-outer quadrant of unspecified female breast
- ✓6th **C50.42** Malignant neoplasm of upper-outer quadrant of breast, male
  - **C50.421** Malignant neoplasm of upper-outer quadrant of right male breast

---

HCC CMS-HCC | Rx Rx HCC | ESR ESRD HCC | COM Commercial HCC | N Newborn: 0 | P Pediatric: 0-17 | M Maternity: 9-64 | A Adult: 15-124

Chapter 2. Neoplasms

- **C50.422** Malignant neoplasm of upper-outer quadrant of left male breast `HCC` `Rx` `ESR` `COM`
- **C50.429** Malignant neoplasm of upper-outer quadrant of unspecified male breast `HCC` `Rx` `ESR` `COM`

√5th **C50.5** Malignant neoplasm of lower-outer quadrant of breast
- √6th **C50.51** Malignant neoplasm of lower-outer quadrant of breast, female
  - **C50.511** Malignant neoplasm of lower-outer quadrant of right female breast `HCC` `Rx` `ESR` `COM`
  - **C50.512** Malignant neoplasm of lower-outer quadrant of left female breast `HCC` `Rx` `ESR` `COM`
  - **C50.519** Malignant neoplasm of lower-outer quadrant of unspecified female breast `HCC` `Rx` `ESR` `COM`
- √6th **C50.52** Malignant neoplasm of lower-outer quadrant of breast, male
  - **C50.521** Malignant neoplasm of lower-outer quadrant of right male breast `HCC` `Rx` `ESR` `COM`
  - **C50.522** Malignant neoplasm of lower-outer quadrant of left male breast `HCC` `Rx` `ESR` `COM`
  - **C50.529** Malignant neoplasm of lower-outer quadrant of unspecified male breast `HCC` `Rx` `ESR` `COM`

√5th **C50.6** Malignant neoplasm of axillary tail of breast
- √6th **C50.61** Malignant neoplasm of axillary tail of breast, female
  - **C50.611** Malignant neoplasm of axillary tail of right female breast `HCC` `Rx` `ESR` `COM`
  - **C50.612** Malignant neoplasm of axillary tail of left female breast `HCC` `Rx` `ESR` `COM`
  - **C50.619** Malignant neoplasm of axillary tail of unspecified female breast `HCC` `Rx` `ESR` `COM`
- √6th **C50.62** Malignant neoplasm of axillary tail of breast, male
  - **C50.621** Malignant neoplasm of axillary tail of right male breast `HCC` `Rx` `ESR` `COM`
  - **C50.622** Malignant neoplasm of axillary tail of left male breast `HCC` `Rx` `ESR` `COM`
  - **C50.629** Malignant neoplasm of axillary tail of unspecified male breast `HCC` `Rx` `ESR` `COM`

√5th **C50.8** Malignant neoplasm of overlapping sites of breast
- √6th **C50.81** Malignant neoplasm of overlapping sites of breast, female
  - **C50.811** Malignant neoplasm of overlapping sites of right female breast `HCC` `Rx` `ESR` `COM`
  - **C50.812** Malignant neoplasm of overlapping sites of left female breast `HCC` `Rx` `ESR` `COM`
  - **C50.819** Malignant neoplasm of overlapping sites of unspecified female breast `HCC` `Rx` `ESR` `COM`
- √6th **C50.82** Malignant neoplasm of overlapping sites of breast, male
  - **C50.821** Malignant neoplasm of overlapping sites of right male breast `HCC` `Rx` `ESR` `COM`
  - **C50.822** Malignant neoplasm of overlapping sites of left male breast `HCC` `Rx` `ESR` `COM`
  - **C50.829** Malignant neoplasm of overlapping sites of unspecified male breast `HCC` `Rx` `ESR` `COM`

√5th **C50.9** Malignant neoplasm of breast of unspecified site
- √6th **C50.91** Malignant neoplasm of breast of unspecified site, female
  - **AHA:** 2022,3Q,10,14
  - **C50.911** Malignant neoplasm of unspecified site of right female breast `HCC` `Rx` `ESR` `COM`
  - **C50.912** Malignant neoplasm of unspecified site of left female breast `HCC` `Rx` `ESR` `COM`
  - **C50.919** Malignant neoplasm of unspecified site of unspecified female breast `HCC` `Rx` `ESR` `COM`
- √6th **C50.92** Malignant neoplasm of breast of unspecified site, male
  - **C50.921** Malignant neoplasm of unspecified site of right male breast `HCC` `Rx` `ESR` `COM`
  - **C50.922** Malignant neoplasm of unspecified site of left male breast `HCC` `Rx` `ESR` `COM`
  - **C50.929** Malignant neoplasm of unspecified site of unspecified male breast `HCC` `Rx` `ESR` `COM`

- √5th **C50.A** Malignant inflammatory neoplasm of breast
  - Inflammatory breast cancer (IBC)
  - **C50.A0** Malignant inflammatory neoplasm of unspecified breast
  - **C50.A1** Malignant inflammatory neoplasm of right breast
  - **C50.A2** Malignant inflammatory neoplasm of left breast

Malignant neoplasms of female genital organs (C51-C58)

INCLUDES malignant neoplasm of skin of female genital organs

√4th **C51** Malignant neoplasm of vulva
 EXCLUDES 1 carcinoma in situ of vulva (D07.1)
- **C51.0** Malignant neoplasm of labium majus `HCC` `ESR` `COM`
  Malignant neoplasm of Bartholin's [greater vestibular] gland
- **C51.1** Malignant neoplasm of labium minus `HCC` `ESR` `COM`
- **C51.2** Malignant neoplasm of clitoris `HCC` `ESR` `COM`
- **C51.8** Malignant neoplasm of overlapping sites of vulva
- **C51.9** Malignant neoplasm of vulva, unspecified `HCC` `ESR` `COM`
  Malignant neoplasm of external female genitalia NOS
  Malignant neoplasm of pudendum

C52 Malignant neoplasm of vagina `HCC` `ESR` `COM`
 EXCLUDES 1 carcinoma in situ of vagina (D07.2)

√4th **C53** Malignant neoplasm of cervix uteri
 EXCLUDES 1 carcinoma in situ of cervix uteri (D06.-)
 AHA: 2017,4Q,103
- **C53.0** Malignant neoplasm of endocervix `HCC` `ESR` `COM`
- **C53.1** Malignant neoplasm of exocervix `HCC` `ESR` `COM`
- **C53.8** Malignant neoplasm of overlapping sites of cervix uteri
- **C53.9** Malignant neoplasm of cervix uteri, unspecified `HCC` `ESR` `COM`

√4th **C54** Malignant neoplasm of corpus uteri
- **C54.0** Malignant neoplasm of isthmus uteri `HCC` `ESR` `COM`
  Malignant neoplasm of lower uterine segment
- **C54.1** Malignant neoplasm of endometrium `HCC` `ESR` `COM`
- **C54.2** Malignant neoplasm of myometrium `HCC` `ESR` `COM`
- **C54.3** Malignant neoplasm of fundus uteri `HCC` `ESR` `COM`
- **C54.8** Malignant neoplasm of overlapping sites of corpus uteri `HCC` `ESR` `COM`
  AHA: 2023,3Q,14
- **C54.9** Malignant neoplasm of corpus uteri, unspecified `HCC` `ESR` `COM`

C55 Malignant neoplasm of uterus, part unspecified `HCC` `ESR` `COM`

√4th **C56** Malignant neoplasm of ovary
 Use additional code to identify any functional activity
 AHA: 2025,2Q,16
- **C56.1** Malignant neoplasm of right ovary `HCC` `Rx` `ESR` `COM`
- **C56.2** Malignant neoplasm of left ovary `HCC` `Rx` `ESR` `COM`
- **C56.3** Malignant neoplasm of bilateral ovaries `HCC` `Rx` `ESR` `COM`
- **C56.9** Malignant neoplasm of unspecified ovary `HCC` `Rx` `ESR` `COM`

√4th **C57** Malignant neoplasm of other and unspecified female genital organs
- √5th **C57.0** Malignant neoplasm of fallopian tube
  Malignant neoplasm of oviduct
  Malignant neoplasm of uterine tube
  - **C57.00** Malignant neoplasm of unspecified fallopian tube `HCC` `ESR` `COM`
  - **C57.01** Malignant neoplasm of right fallopian tube `HCC` `Rx` `ESR` `COM`
  - **C57.02** Malignant neoplasm of left fallopian tube `HCC` `Rx` `ESR` `COM`
- √5th **C57.1** Malignant neoplasm of broad ligament
  - **C57.10** Malignant neoplasm of unspecified broad ligament `HCC` `Rx` `ESR` `COM`
  - **C57.11** Malignant neoplasm of right broad ligament `HCC` `Rx` `ESR` `COM`
  - **C57.12** Malignant neoplasm of left broad ligament `HCC` `Rx` `ESR` `COM`

Chapter 2. Neoplasms

- **C57.2** Malignant neoplasm of round ligament ✓5th
  - **C57.20** Malignant neoplasm of unspecified round ligament
  - **C57.21** Malignant neoplasm of right round ligament
  - **C57.22** Malignant neoplasm of left round ligament
- **C57.3** Malignant neoplasm of parametrium
  - Malignant neoplasm of uterine ligament NOS
- **C57.4** Malignant neoplasm of uterine adnexa, unspecified
- **C57.7** Malignant neoplasm of other specified female genital organs
  - Malignant neoplasm of wolffian body or duct
- **C57.8** Malignant neoplasm of overlapping sites of female genital organs
  - Primary malignant neoplasm of two or more contiguous sites of the female genital organs whose point of origin cannot be determined
  - Primary tubo-ovarian malignant neoplasm whose point of origin cannot be determined
  - Primary utero-ovarian malignant neoplasm whose point of origin cannot be determined
- **C57.9** Malignant neoplasm of female genital organ, unspecified
  - Malignant neoplasm of female genitourinary tract NOS
- **C58** Malignant neoplasm of placenta
  - **INCLUDES** choriocarcinoma NOS
    - chorionepithelioma NOS
  - **EXCLUDES 1** chorioadenoma (destruens) (D39.2)
    - hydatidiform mole NOS (O01.9)
    - invasive hydatidiform mole (D39.2)
    - male choriocarcinoma NOS (C62.9-)
    - malignant hydatidiform mole (D39.2)

Malignant neoplasms of male genital organs (C60-C63)

INCLUDES malignant neoplasm of skin of male genital organs

- ✓4th **C60** Malignant neoplasm of penis
  - **C60.0** Malignant neoplasm of prepuce
    - Malignant neoplasm of foreskin
  - **C60.1** Malignant neoplasm of glans penis
  - **C60.2** Malignant neoplasm of body of penis
    - Malignant neoplasm of corpus cavernosum
  - **C60.8** Malignant neoplasm of overlapping sites of penis
  - **C60.9** Malignant neoplasm of penis, unspecified
    - Malignant neoplasm of skin of penis NOS
- **C61** Malignant neoplasm of prostate
  - Use additional code, if applicable, to identify:
    - hormone sensitivity status (Z19.1-Z19.2)
    - rising PSA following treatment for malignant neoplasm of prostate (R97.21)
  - **EXCLUDES 1** malignant neoplasm of seminal vesicle (C63.7)
  - **AHA:** 2017,1Q,17
- ✓4th **C62** Malignant neoplasm of testis
  - Use additional code to identify any functional activity
  - ✓5th **C62.0** Malignant neoplasm of undescended testis
    - Malignant neoplasm of ectopic testis
    - Malignant neoplasm of retained testis
    - **C62.00** Malignant neoplasm of unspecified undescended testis
    - **C62.01** Malignant neoplasm of undescended right testis
    - **C62.02** Malignant neoplasm of undescended left testis
  - ✓5th **C62.1** Malignant neoplasm of descended testis
    - Malignant neoplasm of scrotal testis
    - **C62.10** Malignant neoplasm of unspecified descended testis
    - **C62.11** Malignant neoplasm of descended right testis
    - **C62.12** Malignant neoplasm of descended left testis
  - ✓5th **C62.9** Malignant neoplasm of testis, unspecified whether descended or undescended
    - **C62.90** Malignant neoplasm of unspecified testis, unspecified whether descended or undescended
      - Malignant neoplasm of testis NOS
    - **C62.91** Malignant neoplasm of right testis, unspecified whether descended or undescended
    - **C62.92** Malignant neoplasm of left testis, unspecified whether descended or undescended
- ✓4th **C63** Malignant neoplasm of other and unspecified male genital organs
  - ✓5th **C63.0** Malignant neoplasm of epididymis
    - **C63.00** Malignant neoplasm of unspecified epididymis
    - **C63.01** Malignant neoplasm of right epididymis
    - **C63.02** Malignant neoplasm of left epididymis
  - ✓5th **C63.1** Malignant neoplasm of spermatic cord
    - **C63.10** Malignant neoplasm of unspecified spermatic cord
    - **C63.11** Malignant neoplasm of right spermatic cord
    - **C63.12** Malignant neoplasm of left spermatic cord
  - **C63.2** Malignant neoplasm of scrotum
    - Malignant neoplasm of skin of scrotum
  - **C63.7** Malignant neoplasm of other specified male genital organs
    - Malignant neoplasm of seminal vesicle
    - Malignant neoplasm of tunica vaginalis
  - **C63.8** Malignant neoplasm of overlapping sites of male genital organs
    - Primary malignant neoplasm of two or more contiguous sites of male genital organs whose point of origin cannot be determined
  - **C63.9** Malignant neoplasm of male genital organ, unspecified
    - Malignant neoplasm of male genitourinary tract NOS

Malignant neoplasms of urinary tract (C64-C68)

- ✓4th **C64** Malignant neoplasm of kidney, except renal pelvis
  - **EXCLUDES 1** malignant carcinoid tumor of the kidney (C7A.093)
    - malignant neoplasm of renal calyces (C65.-)
    - malignant neoplasm of renal pelvis (C65.-)
  - **AHA:** 2025,2Q,11
  - **C64.1** Malignant neoplasm of right kidney, except renal pelvis
  - **C64.2** Malignant neoplasm of left kidney, except renal pelvis
  - **C64.9** Malignant neoplasm of unspecified kidney, except renal pelvis
- ✓4th **C65** Malignant neoplasm of renal pelvis
  - **INCLUDES** malignant neoplasm of pelviureteric junction
    - malignant neoplasm of renal calyces
  - **C65.1** Malignant neoplasm of right renal pelvis
  - **C65.2** Malignant neoplasm of left renal pelvis
  - **C65.9** Malignant neoplasm of unspecified renal pelvis
- ✓4th **C66** Malignant neoplasm of ureter
  - **EXCLUDES 1** malignant neoplasm of ureteric orifice of bladder (C67.6)
  - **C66.1** Malignant neoplasm of right ureter
  - **C66.2** Malignant neoplasm of left ureter
  - **C66.9** Malignant neoplasm of unspecified ureter
- ✓4th **C67** Malignant neoplasm of bladder
  - **AHA:** 2023,3Q,15
  - **C67.0** Malignant neoplasm of trigone of bladder
  - **C67.1** Malignant neoplasm of dome of bladder
  - **C67.2** Malignant neoplasm of lateral wall of bladder
  - **C67.3** Malignant neoplasm of anterior wall of bladder

C67.4	Malignant neoplasm of **posterior wall** of bladder	HCC Rx ESR COM
C67.5	Malignant neoplasm of **bladder neck**	HCC Rx ESR COM
	Malignant neoplasm of internal urethral orifice	
C67.6	Malignant neoplasm of **ureteric orifice**	HCC Rx ESR COM
C67.7	Malignant neoplasm of **urachus**	HCC Rx ESR COM
C67.8	Malignant neoplasm of **overlapping sites** of bladder	HCC Rx ESR COM
C67.9	Malignant neoplasm of bladder, unspecified	HCC Rx ESR COM
	AHA: 2016,1Q,19	

✓4th **C68** Malignant neoplasm of other and unspecified **urinary organs**

EXCLUDES 1   malignant neoplasm of female genitourinary tract NOS (C57.9)
malignant neoplasm of male genitourinary tract NOS (C63.9)

C68.0	Malignant neoplasm of **urethra**	HCC Rx ESR COM
	EXCLUDES 1 malignant neoplasm of urethral orifice of bladder (C67.5)	
C68.1	Malignant neoplasm of **paraurethral glands**	HCC Rx ESR COM
C68.8	Malignant neoplasm of **overlapping sites** of urinary organs	HCC Rx ESR COM
	Primary malignant neoplasm of two or more contiguous sites of urinary organs whose point of origin cannot be determined	
C68.9	Malignant neoplasm of urinary organ, unspecified	HCC Rx ESR COM
	Malignant neoplasm of urinary system NOS	

Malignant neoplasms of eye, brain and other parts of central nervous system (C69-C72)

✓4th **C69** Malignant neoplasm of **eye and adnexa**

EXCLUDES 1   malignant neoplasm of connective tissue of eyelid (C49.0)
malignant neoplasm of eyelid (skin) (C43.1-, C44.1-)
malignant neoplasm of optic nerve (C72.3-)

✓5th	**C69.0**	Malignant neoplasm of **conjunctiva**	
	C69.00	Malignant neoplasm of unspecified conjunctiva	HCC Rx ESR COM
	C69.01	Malignant neoplasm of **right** conjunctiva	HCC Rx ESR COM
	C69.02	Malignant neoplasm of **left** conjunctiva	HCC Rx ESR COM
✓5th	**C69.1**	Malignant neoplasm of **cornea**	
	C69.10	Malignant neoplasm of unspecified cornea	HCC Rx ESR COM
	C69.11	Malignant neoplasm of **right** cornea	HCC Rx ESR COM
	C69.12	Malignant neoplasm of **left** cornea	HCC Rx ESR COM
✓5th	**C69.2**	Malignant neoplasm of **retina**	
	EXCLUDES 1 dark area on retina (D49.81) neoplasm of unspecified behavior of retina and choroid (D49.81) retinal freckle (D49.81)		
	C69.20	Malignant neoplasm of unspecified retina	
	C69.21	Malignant neoplasm of **right** retina	HCC Rx ESR COM
	C69.22	Malignant neoplasm of **left** retina	HCC Rx ESR COM
✓5th	**C69.3**	Malignant neoplasm of **choroid**	
	C69.30	Malignant neoplasm of unspecified choroid	HCC Rx ESR COM
	C69.31	Malignant neoplasm of **right** choroid	HCC Rx ESR COM
	C69.32	Malignant neoplasm of **left** choroid	HCC Rx ESR COM
✓5th	**C69.4**	Malignant neoplasm of **ciliary body**	
	C69.40	Malignant neoplasm of unspecified ciliary body	HCC Rx ESR COM
	C69.41	Malignant neoplasm of **right** ciliary body	HCC Rx ESR COM
	C69.42	Malignant neoplasm of **left** ciliary body	HCC Rx ESR COM
✓5th	**C69.5**	Malignant neoplasm of **lacrimal gland and duct**	
	Malignant neoplasm of lacrimal sac Malignant neoplasm of nasolacrimal duct		
	C69.50	Malignant neoplasm of unspecified lacrimal gland and duct	HCC Rx ESR COM
	C69.51	Malignant neoplasm of **right** lacrimal gland and duct	HCC Rx ESR COM
	C69.52	Malignant neoplasm of **left** lacrimal gland and duct	HCC Rx ESR COM
✓5th	**C69.6**	Malignant neoplasm of **orbit**	
	Malignant neoplasm of connective tissue of orbit Malignant neoplasm of extraocular muscle Malignant neoplasm of peripheral nerves of orbit Malignant neoplasm of retrobulbar tissue Malignant neoplasm of retro-ocular tissue		
	EXCLUDES 1 malignant neoplasm of orbital bone (C41.0)		
	C69.60	Malignant neoplasm of unspecified orbit	HCC Rx ESR COM
	C69.61	Malignant neoplasm of **right** orbit	HCC Rx ESR COM
	C69.62	Malignant neoplasm of **left** orbit	HCC Rx ESR COM
✓5th	**C69.8**	Malignant neoplasm of **overlapping sites** of eye and adnexa	
	C69.80	Malignant neoplasm of overlapping sites of unspecified eye and adnexa	HCC Rx ESR COM
	C69.81	Malignant neoplasm of overlapping sites of **right** eye and adnexa	HCC Rx ESR COM
	C69.82	Malignant neoplasm of overlapping sites of **left** eye and adnexa	HCC Rx ESR COM
✓5th	**C69.9**	Malignant neoplasm of unspecified site of eye	
	Malignant neoplasm of eyeball		
	C69.90	Malignant neoplasm of unspecified site of unspecified eye	HCC Rx ESR COM
	C69.91	Malignant neoplasm of unspecified site of **right** eye	HCC Rx ESR COM
	C69.92	Malignant neoplasm of unspecified site of **left** eye	HCC Rx ESR COM

✓4th **C70** Malignant neoplasm of **meninges**

C70.0	Malignant neoplasm of **cerebral** meninges	HCC Rx ESR COM
C70.1	Malignant neoplasm of **spinal** meninges	HCC Rx ESR COM
C70.9	Malignant neoplasm of meninges, unspecified	HCC Rx ESR COM

✓4th **C71** Malignant neoplasm of **brain**

EXCLUDES 1   malignant neoplasm of cranial nerves (C72.2-C72.5)
retrobulbar malignant neoplasm (C69.6-)

Lobes of the Brain

C71.0	Malignant neoplasm of **cerebrum, except lobes and ventricles**	HCC Rx ESR COM
	Malignant neoplasm of supratentorial NOS	
C71.1	Malignant neoplasm of **frontal** lobe	HCC Rx ESR COM
C71.2	Malignant neoplasm of **temporal** lobe	HCC Rx ESR COM
C71.3	Malignant neoplasm of **parietal** lobe	HCC Rx ESR COM
C71.4	Malignant neoplasm of **occipital** lobe	HCC Rx ESR COM
C71.5	Malignant neoplasm of **cerebral** ventricle	HCC Rx ESR COM
	EXCLUDES 1 malignant neoplasm of fourth cerebral ventricle (C71.7)	
C71.6	Malignant neoplasm of **cerebellum**	HCC Rx ESR COM
C71.7	Malignant neoplasm of **brain stem**	HCC Rx ESR COM
	Infratentorial malignant neoplasm NOS Malignant neoplasm of fourth cerebral ventricle	
C71.8	Malignant neoplasm of **overlapping sites** of brain	HCC Rx ESR COM
C71.9	Malignant neoplasm of brain, unspecified	HCC Rx ESR COM
	AHA: 2014,3Q,3	

C72 Malignant neoplasm of spinal cord, cranial nerves and other parts of central nervous system

EXCLUDES 1: malignant neoplasm of meninges (C70.-)
malignant neoplasm of peripheral nerves and autonomic nervous system (C47.-)

- **C72.0** Malignant neoplasm of spinal cord
- **C72.1** Malignant neoplasm of cauda equina
- **C72.2** Malignant neoplasm of olfactory nerve
  - Malignant neoplasm of olfactory bulb
  - **C72.20** Malignant neoplasm of unspecified olfactory nerve
  - **C72.21** Malignant neoplasm of right olfactory nerve
  - **C72.22** Malignant neoplasm of left olfactory nerve
- **C72.3** Malignant neoplasm of optic nerve
  - **C72.30** Malignant neoplasm of unspecified optic nerve
  - **C72.31** Malignant neoplasm of right optic nerve
  - **C72.32** Malignant neoplasm of left optic nerve
- **C72.4** Malignant neoplasm of acoustic nerve
  - **C72.40** Malignant neoplasm of unspecified acoustic nerve
  - **C72.41** Malignant neoplasm of right acoustic nerve
  - **C72.42** Malignant neoplasm of left acoustic nerve
- **C72.5** Malignant neoplasm of other and unspecified cranial nerves
  - **C72.50** Malignant neoplasm of unspecified cranial nerve
    - Malignant neoplasm of cranial nerve NOS
  - **C72.59** Malignant neoplasm of other cranial nerves
- **C72.9** Malignant neoplasm of central nervous system, unspecified
  - Malignant neoplasm of nervous system NOS
  - Malignant neoplasm of unspecified site of central nervous system

Malignant neoplasms of thyroid and other endocrine glands (C73-C75)

- **C73** Malignant neoplasm of thyroid gland
  - Use additional code to identify any functional activity
- **C74** Malignant neoplasm of adrenal gland
  - TIP: If an adrenal gland tumor is described as functioning (producing too much of a hormone), additional codes should be assigned to report the functional activity.
  - **C74.0** Malignant neoplasm of cortex of adrenal gland
    - **C74.00** Malignant neoplasm of cortex of unspecified adrenal gland
    - **C74.01** Malignant neoplasm of cortex of right adrenal gland
    - **C74.02** Malignant neoplasm of cortex of left adrenal gland
  - **C74.1** Malignant neoplasm of medulla of adrenal gland
    - **C74.10** Malignant neoplasm of medulla of unspecified adrenal gland
    - **C74.11** Malignant neoplasm of medulla of right adrenal gland
    - **C74.12** Malignant neoplasm of medulla of left adrenal gland
  - **C74.9** Malignant neoplasm of unspecified part of adrenal gland
    - **C74.90** Malignant neoplasm of unspecified part of unspecified adrenal gland
    - **C74.91** Malignant neoplasm of unspecified part of right adrenal gland
    - **C74.92** Malignant neoplasm of unspecified part of left adrenal gland

C75 Malignant neoplasm of other endocrine glands and related structures

EXCLUDES 1: malignant carcinoid tumors (C7A.0-)
malignant neoplasm of adrenal gland (C74.-)
malignant neoplasm of endocrine pancreas (C25.4)
malignant neoplasm of islets of Langerhans (C25.4)
malignant neoplasm of ovary (C56.-)
malignant neoplasm of testis (C62.-)
malignant neoplasm of thymus (C37)
malignant neoplasm of thyroid gland (C73)
malignant neuroendocrine tumors (C7A.-)

- **C75.0** Malignant neoplasm of parathyroid gland
- **C75.1** Malignant neoplasm of pituitary gland
- **C75.2** Malignant neoplasm of craniopharyngeal duct
- **C75.3** Malignant neoplasm of pineal gland
- **C75.4** Malignant neoplasm of carotid body
- **C75.5** Malignant neoplasm of aortic body and other paraganglia
- **C75.8** Malignant neoplasm with pluriglandular involvement, unspecified
- **C75.9** Malignant neoplasm of endocrine gland, unspecified

Malignant neuroendocrine tumors (C7A)

- **C7A** Malignant neuroendocrine tumors
  - Code also any associated multiple endocrine neoplasia [MEN] syndromes (E31.2-)
  - Use additional code to identify any associated endocrine syndrome, such as:
    - carcinoid syndrome (E34.00)
  - EXCLUDES 2: malignant pancreatic islet cell tumors (C25.4)
    Merkel cell carcinoma (C4A.-)
  - AHA: 2019,3Q,7
  - DEF: Tumors comprised of cells that are capable of producing hormonal syndromes in which the normal hormonal balance required to support body system function is adversely affected.
  - **C7A.0** Malignant carcinoid tumors
    - AHA: 2019,3Q,7
    - DEF: Specific type of slow-growing neuroendocrine tumors. Carcinoid tumors occur most commonly in the hormone producing cells of the gastrointestinal tracts and can also occur in the pancreas, testes, ovaries, or lungs.
    - **C7A.00** Malignant carcinoid tumor of unspecified site
    - **C7A.01** Malignant carcinoid tumors of the small intestine
      - **C7A.010** Malignant carcinoid tumor of the duodenum
      - **C7A.011** Malignant carcinoid tumor of the jejunum
      - **C7A.012** Malignant carcinoid tumor of the ileum
      - **C7A.019** Malignant carcinoid tumor of the small intestine, unspecified portion
    - **C7A.02** Malignant carcinoid tumors of the appendix, large intestine, and rectum
      - **C7A.020** Malignant carcinoid tumor of the appendix
      - **C7A.021** Malignant carcinoid tumor of the cecum
      - **C7A.022** Malignant carcinoid tumor of the ascending colon
      - **C7A.023** Malignant carcinoid tumor of the transverse colon
      - **C7A.024** Malignant carcinoid tumor of the descending colon
      - **C7A.025** Malignant carcinoid tumor of the sigmoid colon
      - **C7A.026** Malignant carcinoid tumor of the rectum
      - **C7A.029** Malignant carcinoid tumor of the large intestine, unspecified portion
        - Malignant carcinoid tumor of the colon NOS

HCC CMS-HCC | Rx Rx HCC | ESR ESRD HCC | COM Commercial HCC | N Newborn: 0 | P Pediatric: 0-17 | M Maternity: 9-64 | A Adult: 15-124

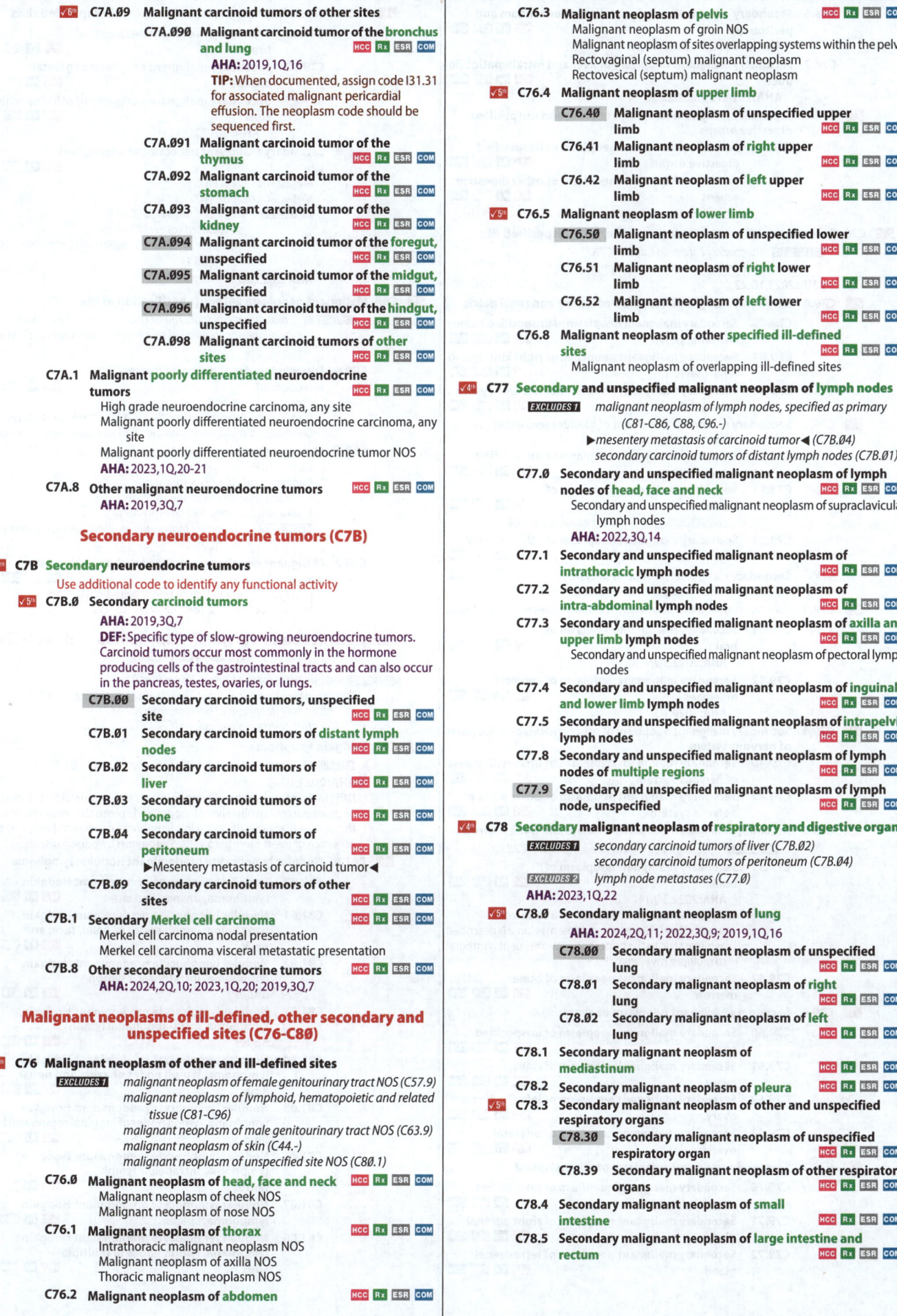

Chapter 2. Neoplasms

- **C78.6** Secondary malignant neoplasm of retroperitoneum and peritoneum [HCC Rx ESR COM]
  - **AHA:** 2025,2Q,16; 2017,2Q,12
- **C78.7** Secondary malignant neoplasm of liver and intrahepatic bile duct [HCC Rx ESR COM]
  - **AHA:** 2024,1Q,25; 2022,3Q,14
- **C78.8** Secondary malignant neoplasm of other and unspecified digestive organs
  - **C78.80** Secondary malignant neoplasm of unspecified digestive organ [HCC Rx ESR COM]
  - **C78.89** Secondary malignant neoplasm of other digestive organs [HCC Rx ESR COM]
    - Code also exocrine pancreatic insufficiency (K86.81)
- **C79** Secondary malignant neoplasm of other and unspecified sites
  - EXCLUDES 1: secondary carcinoid tumors (C7B.-)
    - secondary neuroendocrine tumors (C7B.-)
  - **AHA:** 2023,1Q,22
  - **C79.0** Secondary malignant neoplasm of kidney and renal pelvis
    - **C79.00** Secondary malignant neoplasm of unspecified kidney and renal pelvis [HCC Rx ESR COM]
    - **C79.01** Secondary malignant neoplasm of right kidney and renal pelvis [HCC Rx ESR COM]
    - **C79.02** Secondary malignant neoplasm of left kidney and renal pelvis [HCC Rx ESR COM]
  - **C79.1** Secondary malignant neoplasm of bladder and other and unspecified urinary organs
    - **C79.10** Secondary malignant neoplasm of unspecified urinary organs [HCC Rx ESR COM]
    - **C79.11** Secondary malignant neoplasm of bladder [HCC Rx ESR COM]
      - EXCLUDES 2: lymph node metastases (C77.0)
    - **C79.19** Secondary malignant neoplasm of other urinary organs [HCC Rx ESR COM]
  - **C79.2** Secondary malignant neoplasm of skin [HCC Rx ESR COM]
    - EXCLUDES 1: secondary Merkel cell carcinoma (C7B.1)
  - **C79.3** Secondary malignant neoplasm of brain and cerebral meninges
    - **C79.31** Secondary malignant neoplasm of brain [HCC Rx ESR COM]
      - **AHA:** 2022,3Q,9-10
    - **C79.32** Secondary malignant neoplasm of cerebral meninges [HCC Rx ESR COM]
      - **AHA:** 2020,1Q,13
  - **C79.4** Secondary malignant neoplasm of other and unspecified parts of nervous system
    - **C79.40** Secondary malignant neoplasm of unspecified part of nervous system [HCC Rx ESR COM]
    - **C79.49** Secondary malignant neoplasm of other parts of nervous system [HCC Rx ESR COM]
  - **C79.5** Secondary malignant neoplasm of bone and bone marrow
    - EXCLUDES 1: secondary carcinoid tumors of bone (C7B.03)
    - **C79.51** Secondary malignant neoplasm of bone [HCC Rx ESR COM]
      - **AHA:** 2022,3Q,14
      - **TIP:** Do not assign in addition to a code from subcategory C90.0 when multiple myeloma is described as metastatic to the bone; bone involvement is integral to multiple myeloma.
    - **C79.52** Secondary malignant neoplasm of bone marrow [HCC Rx ESR COM]
  - **C79.6** Secondary malignant neoplasm of ovary
    - **C79.60** Secondary malignant neoplasm of unspecified ovary [HCC Rx ESR COM]
    - **C79.61** Secondary malignant neoplasm of right ovary [HCC Rx ESR COM]
    - **C79.62** Secondary malignant neoplasm of left ovary [HCC Rx ESR COM]
    - **C79.63** Secondary malignant neoplasm of bilateral ovaries [HCC Rx ESR COM]
  - **C79.7** Secondary malignant neoplasm of adrenal gland
    - **C79.70** Secondary malignant neoplasm of unspecified adrenal gland [HCC Rx ESR COM]
    - **C79.71** Secondary malignant neoplasm of right adrenal gland [HCC Rx ESR COM]
    - **C79.72** Secondary malignant neoplasm of left adrenal gland [HCC Rx ESR COM]
  - **C79.8** Secondary malignant neoplasm of other specified sites
    - **C79.81** Secondary malignant neoplasm of breast [HCC Rx ESR COM]
    - **C79.82** Secondary malignant neoplasm of genital organs [HCC Rx ESR COM]
    - **C79.89** Secondary malignant neoplasm of other specified sites [HCC Rx ESR COM]
      - **AHA:** 2017,2Q,11
  - **C79.9** Secondary malignant neoplasm of unspecified site [HCC Rx ESR COM]
    - Metastatic cancer NOS
    - Metastatic disease NOS
    - EXCLUDES 1: carcinomatosis NOS (C80.0)
      - generalized cancer NOS (C80.0)
      - malignant (primary) neoplasm of unspecified site (C80.1)
    - **AHA:** 2023,2Q,5
- **C80** Malignant neoplasm without specification of site
  - EXCLUDES 1: malignant carcinoid tumor of unspecified site (C7A.00)
    - malignant neoplasm of specified multiple sites - code to each site
  - **C80.0** Disseminated malignant neoplasm, unspecified [HCC Rx ESR COM]
    - Carcinomatosis NOS
    - Generalized cancer, unspecified site (primary) (secondary)
    - Generalized malignancy, unspecified site (primary) (secondary)
  - **C80.1** Malignant (primary) neoplasm, unspecified [HCC ESR COM]
    - Cancer NOS
    - Cancer unspecified site (primary)
    - Carcinoma unspecified site (primary)
    - Malignancy unspecified site (primary)
    - EXCLUDES 1: secondary malignant neoplasm of unspecified site (C79.9)
  - **C80.2** Malignant neoplasm associated with transplanted organ [HCC Rx ESR COM UPD]
    - Code first complication of transplanted organ (T86.-)
    - Use additional code to identify the specific malignancy

Malignant neoplasms of lymphoid, hematopoietic and related tissue (C81-C96)

EXCLUDES 2: Kaposi's sarcoma of lymph nodes (C46.3)
- secondary and unspecified neoplasm of lymph nodes (C77.-)
- secondary neoplasm of bone marrow (C79.52)
- secondary neoplasm of spleen (C78.89)

- **C81** Hodgkin lymphoma
  - EXCLUDES 1: personal history of Hodgkin lymphoma (Z85.71)
  - **AHA:** 2023,1Q,22
  - **DEF:** Malignant disorder of lymphoid cells characterized by the presence of progressively swollen lymph nodes and spleen that may also involve the liver. A diagnosis of Hodgkin's lymphoma can be confirmed by the presence of Reed-Sternberg cells. **Synonym(s):** Hodgkin disease.
  - **C81.0** Nodular lymphocyte predominant Hodgkin lymphoma
    - **C81.00** Nodular lymphocyte predominant Hodgkin lymphoma, unspecified site [HCC Rx ESR COM]
    - **C81.01** Nodular lymphocyte predominant Hodgkin lymphoma, lymph nodes of head, face, and neck [HCC Rx ESR COM]
    - **C81.02** Nodular lymphocyte predominant Hodgkin lymphoma, intrathoracic lymph nodes [HCC Rx ESR COM]
    - **C81.03** Nodular lymphocyte predominant Hodgkin lymphoma, intra-abdominal lymph nodes [HCC Rx ESR COM]
    - **C81.04** Nodular lymphocyte predominant Hodgkin lymphoma, lymph nodes of axilla and upper limb [HCC Rx ESR COM]
    - **C81.05** Nodular lymphocyte predominant Hodgkin lymphoma, lymph nodes of inguinal region and lower limb [HCC Rx ESR COM]
    - **C81.06** Nodular lymphocyte predominant Hodgkin lymphoma, intrapelvic lymph nodes [HCC Rx ESR COM]
    - **C81.07** Nodular lymphocyte predominant Hodgkin lymphoma, spleen [HCC Rx ESR COM]
    - **C81.08** Nodular lymphocyte predominant Hodgkin lymphoma, lymph nodes of multiple sites [HCC Rx ESR COM]

C81.09 Nodular lymphocyte predominant Hodgkin lymphoma, extranodal and solid organ sites

C81.0A Nodular lymphocyte predominant Hodgkin lymphoma, in remission

C81.1 Nodular sclerosis Hodgkin lymphoma
Nodular sclerosis classical Hodgkin lymphoma

- **C81.10** Nodular sclerosis Hodgkin lymphoma, unspecified site
- **C81.11** Nodular sclerosis Hodgkin lymphoma, lymph nodes of head, face, and neck
- **C81.12** Nodular sclerosis Hodgkin lymphoma, intrathoracic lymph nodes
- **C81.13** Nodular sclerosis Hodgkin lymphoma, intra-abdominal lymph nodes
- **C81.14** Nodular sclerosis Hodgkin lymphoma, lymph nodes of axilla and upper limb
- **C81.15** Nodular sclerosis Hodgkin lymphoma, lymph nodes of inguinal region and lower limb
- **C81.16** Nodular sclerosis Hodgkin lymphoma, intrapelvic lymph nodes
- **C81.17** Nodular sclerosis Hodgkin lymphoma, spleen
- **C81.18** Nodular sclerosis Hodgkin lymphoma, lymph nodes of multiple sites
- **C81.19** Nodular sclerosis Hodgkin lymphoma, extranodal and solid organ sites
- **C81.1A** Nodular sclerosis Hodgkin lymphoma, in remission

C81.2 Mixed cellularity Hodgkin lymphoma
Mixed cellularity classical Hodgkin lymphoma

- **C81.20** Mixed cellularity Hodgkin lymphoma, unspecified site
- **C81.21** Mixed cellularity Hodgkin lymphoma, lymph nodes of head, face, and neck
- **C81.22** Mixed cellularity Hodgkin lymphoma, intrathoracic lymph nodes
- **C81.23** Mixed cellularity Hodgkin lymphoma, intra-abdominal lymph nodes
- **C81.24** Mixed cellularity Hodgkin lymphoma, lymph nodes of axilla and upper limb
- **C81.25** Mixed cellularity Hodgkin lymphoma, lymph nodes of inguinal region and lower limb
- **C81.26** Mixed cellularity Hodgkin lymphoma, intrapelvic lymph nodes
- **C81.27** Mixed cellularity Hodgkin lymphoma, spleen
- **C81.28** Mixed cellularity Hodgkin lymphoma, lymph nodes of multiple sites
- **C81.29** Mixed cellularity Hodgkin lymphoma, extranodal and solid organ sites
- **C81.2A** Mixed cellularity Hodgkin lymphoma, in remission

C81.3 Lymphocyte depleted Hodgkin lymphoma
Lymphocyte depleted classical Hodgkin lymphoma

- **C81.30** Lymphocyte depleted Hodgkin lymphoma, unspecified site
- **C81.31** Lymphocyte depleted Hodgkin lymphoma, lymph nodes of head, face, and neck
- **C81.32** Lymphocyte depleted Hodgkin lymphoma, intrathoracic lymph nodes
- **C81.33** Lymphocyte depleted Hodgkin lymphoma, intra-abdominal lymph nodes
- **C81.34** Lymphocyte depleted Hodgkin lymphoma, lymph nodes of axilla and upper limb
- **C81.35** Lymphocyte depleted Hodgkin lymphoma, lymph nodes of inguinal region and lower limb
- **C81.36** Lymphocyte depleted Hodgkin lymphoma, intrapelvic lymph nodes
- **C81.37** Lymphocyte depleted Hodgkin lymphoma, spleen
- **C81.38** Lymphocyte depleted Hodgkin lymphoma, lymph nodes of multiple sites
- **C81.39** Lymphocyte depleted Hodgkin lymphoma, extranodal and solid organ sites
- **C81.3A** Lymphocyte depleted Hodgkin lymphoma, in remission

C81.4 Lymphocyte-rich Hodgkin lymphoma
Lymphocyte-rich classical Hodgkin lymphoma

EXCLUDES 1 nodular lymphocyte predominant Hodgkin lymphoma (C81.0-)

- **C81.40** Lymphocyte-rich Hodgkin lymphoma, unspecified site
- **C81.41** Lymphocyte-rich Hodgkin lymphoma, lymph nodes of head, face, and neck
- **C81.42** Lymphocyte-rich Hodgkin lymphoma, intrathoracic lymph nodes
- **C81.43** Lymphocyte-rich Hodgkin lymphoma, intra-abdominal lymph nodes
- **C81.44** Lymphocyte-rich Hodgkin lymphoma, lymph nodes of axilla and upper limb
- **C81.45** Lymphocyte-rich Hodgkin lymphoma, lymph nodes of inguinal region and lower limb
- **C81.46** Lymphocyte-rich Hodgkin lymphoma, intrapelvic lymph nodes
- **C81.47** Lymphocyte-rich Hodgkin lymphoma, spleen
- **C81.48** Lymphocyte-rich Hodgkin lymphoma, lymph nodes of multiple sites
- **C81.49** Lymphocyte-rich Hodgkin lymphoma, extranodal and solid organ sites
- **C81.4A** Lymphocyte-rich Hodgkin lymphoma, in remission

C81.7 Other Hodgkin lymphoma
Classical Hodgkin lymphoma NOS
Other classical Hodgkin lymphoma

- **C81.70** Other Hodgkin lymphoma, unspecified site
- **C81.71** Other Hodgkin lymphoma, lymph nodes of head, face, and neck
- **C81.72** Other Hodgkin lymphoma, intrathoracic lymph nodes
- **C81.73** Other Hodgkin lymphoma, intra-abdominal lymph nodes
- **C81.74** Other Hodgkin lymphoma, lymph nodes of axilla and upper limb
- **C81.75** Other Hodgkin lymphoma, lymph nodes of inguinal region and lower limb
- **C81.76** Other Hodgkin lymphoma, intrapelvic lymph nodes
- **C81.77** Other Hodgkin lymphoma, spleen
- **C81.78** Other Hodgkin lymphoma, lymph nodes of multiple sites
- **C81.79** Other Hodgkin lymphoma, extranodal and solid organ sites
- **C81.7A** Other Hodgkin lymphoma, in remission

C81.9 Hodgkin lymphoma, unspecified

- **C81.90** Hodgkin lymphoma, unspecified, unspecified site
- **C81.91** Hodgkin lymphoma, unspecified, lymph nodes of head, face, and neck
- **C81.92** Hodgkin lymphoma, unspecified, intrathoracic lymph nodes
- **C81.93** Hodgkin lymphoma, unspecified, intra-abdominal lymph nodes
- **C81.94** Hodgkin lymphoma, unspecified, lymph nodes of axilla and upper limb
- **C81.95** Hodgkin lymphoma, unspecified, lymph nodes of inguinal region and lower limb
- **C81.96** Hodgkin lymphoma, unspecified, intrapelvic lymph nodes
- **C81.97** Hodgkin lymphoma, unspecified, spleen
- **C81.98** Hodgkin lymphoma, unspecified, lymph nodes of multiple sites
- **C81.99** Hodgkin lymphoma, unspecified, extranodal and solid organ sites
- **C81.9A** Hodgkin lymphoma, unspecified, in remission

C82 Follicular lymphoma

INCLUDES follicular lymphoma with or without diffuse areas
EXCLUDES 1 mature T/NK-cell lymphomas (C84.-)
personal history of non-Hodgkin lymphoma (Z85.72)

AHA: 2023,1Q,22

DEF: Most common subgroup of non-Hodgkin lymphomas (NHL), accounting for 20 to 30 percent of all NHLs. NHL is a B-cell lymphoma that is slow growing and characterized by the circular pattern of malignant cell growth with the cells clustered into identifiable nodules or follicles.

C82.0 Follicular lymphoma grade I
- **C82.00** Follicular lymphoma grade I, unspecified site
- **C82.01** Follicular lymphoma grade I, lymph nodes of head, face, and neck
- **C82.02** Follicular lymphoma grade I, intrathoracic lymph nodes
- **C82.03** Follicular lymphoma grade I, intra-abdominal lymph nodes
- **C82.04** Follicular lymphoma grade I, lymph nodes of axilla and upper limb
- **C82.05** Follicular lymphoma grade I, lymph nodes of inguinal region and lower limb
- **C82.06** Follicular lymphoma grade I, intrapelvic lymph nodes
- **C82.07** Follicular lymphoma grade I, spleen
- **C82.08** Follicular lymphoma grade I, lymph nodes of multiple sites
- **C82.09** Follicular lymphoma grade I, extranodal and solid organ sites
- **C82.0A** Follicular lymphoma grade I, in remission

C82.1 Follicular lymphoma grade II
- **C82.10** Follicular lymphoma grade II, unspecified site
- **C82.11** Follicular lymphoma grade II, lymph nodes of head, face, and neck
- **C82.12** Follicular lymphoma grade II, intrathoracic lymph nodes
- **C82.13** Follicular lymphoma grade II, intra-abdominal lymph nodes
- **C82.14** Follicular lymphoma grade II, lymph nodes of axilla and upper limb
- **C82.15** Follicular lymphoma grade II, lymph nodes of inguinal region and lower limb
- **C82.16** Follicular lymphoma grade II, intrapelvic lymph nodes
- **C82.17** Follicular lymphoma grade II, spleen
- **C82.18** Follicular lymphoma grade II, lymph nodes of multiple sites
- **C82.19** Follicular lymphoma grade II, extranodal and solid organ sites
- **C82.1A** Follicular lymphoma grade II, in remission

C82.2 Follicular lymphoma grade III, unspecified
- **C82.20** Follicular lymphoma grade III, unspecified, unspecified site
- **C82.21** Follicular lymphoma grade III, unspecified, lymph nodes of head, face, and neck
- **C82.22** Follicular lymphoma grade III, unspecified, intrathoracic lymph nodes
- **C82.23** Follicular lymphoma grade III, unspecified, intra-abdominal lymph nodes
- **C82.24** Follicular lymphoma grade III, unspecified, lymph nodes of axilla and upper limb
- **C82.25** Follicular lymphoma grade III, unspecified, lymph nodes of inguinal region and lower limb
- **C82.26** Follicular lymphoma grade III, unspecified, intrapelvic lymph nodes
- **C82.27** Follicular lymphoma grade III, unspecified, spleen
- **C82.28** Follicular lymphoma grade III, unspecified, lymph nodes of multiple sites
- **C82.29** Follicular lymphoma grade III, unspecified, extranodal and solid organ sites
- **C82.2A** Follicular lymphoma grade III, unspecified, in remission

C82.3 Follicular lymphoma grade IIIa
- **C82.30** Follicular lymphoma grade IIIa, unspecified site
- **C82.31** Follicular lymphoma grade IIIa, lymph nodes of head, face, and neck
- **C82.32** Follicular lymphoma grade IIIa, intrathoracic lymph nodes
- **C82.33** Follicular lymphoma grade IIIa, intra-abdominal lymph nodes
- **C82.34** Follicular lymphoma grade IIIa, lymph nodes of axilla and upper limb
- **C82.35** Follicular lymphoma grade IIIa, lymph nodes of inguinal region and lower limb
- **C82.36** Follicular lymphoma grade IIIa, intrapelvic lymph nodes
- **C82.37** Follicular lymphoma grade IIIa, spleen
- **C82.38** Follicular lymphoma grade IIIa, lymph nodes of multiple sites
- **C82.39** Follicular lymphoma grade IIIa, extranodal and solid organ sites
- **C82.3A** Follicular lymphoma grade IIIa, in remission

C82.4 Follicular lymphoma grade IIIb
- **C82.40** Follicular lymphoma grade IIIb, unspecified site
- **C82.41** Follicular lymphoma grade IIIb, lymph nodes of head, face, and neck
- **C82.42** Follicular lymphoma grade IIIb, intrathoracic lymph nodes
- **C82.43** Follicular lymphoma grade IIIb, intra-abdominal lymph nodes
- **C82.44** Follicular lymphoma grade IIIb, lymph nodes of axilla and upper limb
- **C82.45** Follicular lymphoma grade IIIb, lymph nodes of inguinal region and lower limb
- **C82.46** Follicular lymphoma grade IIIb, intrapelvic lymph nodes
- **C82.47** Follicular lymphoma grade IIIb, spleen
- **C82.48** Follicular lymphoma grade IIIb, lymph nodes of multiple sites
- **C82.49** Follicular lymphoma grade IIIb, extranodal and solid organ sites
- **C82.4A** Follicular lymphoma grade IIIb, in remission

C82.5 Diffuse follicle center lymphoma
- **C82.50** Diffuse follicle center lymphoma, unspecified site
- **C82.51** Diffuse follicle center lymphoma, lymph nodes of head, face, and neck
- **C82.52** Diffuse follicle center lymphoma, intrathoracic lymph nodes
- **C82.53** Diffuse follicle center lymphoma, intra-abdominal lymph nodes
- **C82.54** Diffuse follicle center lymphoma, lymph nodes of axilla and upper limb
- **C82.55** Diffuse follicle center lymphoma, lymph nodes of inguinal region and lower limb
- **C82.56** Diffuse follicle center lymphoma, intrapelvic lymph nodes
- **C82.57** Diffuse follicle center lymphoma, spleen
- **C82.58** Diffuse follicle center lymphoma, lymph nodes of multiple sites
- **C82.59** Diffuse follicle center lymphoma, extranodal and solid organ sites
- **C82.5A** Diffuse follicle center lymphoma, in remission

C82.6 Cutaneous follicle center lymphoma
- **C82.60** Cutaneous follicle center lymphoma, unspecified
- **C82.61** Cutaneous follicle center lymphoma, lymph nodes of head, face, and neck

Chapter 2. Neoplasms

- **C82.62** Cutaneous follicle center lymphoma, intrathoracic lymph nodes
- **C82.63** Cutaneous follicle center lymphoma, intra-abdominal lymph nodes
- **C82.64** Cutaneous follicle center lymphoma, lymph nodes of axilla and upper limb
- **C82.65** Cutaneous follicle center lymphoma, lymph nodes of inguinal region and lower limb
- **C82.66** Cutaneous follicle center lymphoma, intrapelvic lymph nodes
- **C82.67** Cutaneous follicle center lymphoma, spleen
- **C82.68** Cutaneous follicle center lymphoma, lymph nodes of multiple sites
- **C82.69** Cutaneous follicle center lymphoma, extranodal and solid organ sites
- **C82.6A** Cutaneous follicle center lymphoma, in remission

✓5th C82.8 Other types of follicular lymphoma
- **C82.80** Other types of follicular lymphoma, unspecified site
- **C82.81** Other types of follicular lymphoma, lymph nodes of head, face, and neck
- **C82.82** Other types of follicular lymphoma, intrathoracic lymph nodes
- **C82.83** Other types of follicular lymphoma, intra-abdominal lymph nodes
- **C82.84** Other types of follicular lymphoma, lymph nodes of axilla and upper limb
- **C82.85** Other types of follicular lymphoma, lymph nodes of inguinal region and lower limb
- **C82.86** Other types of follicular lymphoma, intrapelvic lymph nodes
- **C82.87** Other types of follicular lymphoma, spleen
- **C82.88** Other types of follicular lymphoma, lymph nodes of multiple sites
- **C82.89** Other types of follicular lymphoma, extranodal and solid organ sites
- **C82.8A** Other types of follicular lymphoma, in remission

✓5th C82.9 Follicular lymphoma, unspecified
- **C82.90** Follicular lymphoma, unspecified, unspecified site
- **C82.91** Follicular lymphoma, unspecified, lymph nodes of head, face, and neck
- **C82.92** Follicular lymphoma, unspecified, intrathoracic lymph nodes
- **C82.93** Follicular lymphoma, unspecified, intra-abdominal lymph nodes
- **C82.94** Follicular lymphoma, unspecified, lymph nodes of axilla and upper limb
- **C82.95** Follicular lymphoma, unspecified, lymph nodes of inguinal region and lower limb
- **C82.96** Follicular lymphoma, unspecified, intrapelvic lymph nodes
- **C82.97** Follicular lymphoma, unspecified, spleen
- **C82.98** Follicular lymphoma, unspecified, lymph nodes of multiple sites
- **C82.99** Follicular lymphoma, unspecified, extranodal and solid organ sites
- **C82.9A** Follicular lymphoma, unspecified, in remission

✓4th C83 Non-follicular lymphoma
EXCLUDES 1 personal history of non-Hodgkin lymphoma (Z85.72)
AHA: 2023,1Q,22

✓5th C83.0 Small cell B-cell lymphoma
Lymphoplasmacytic lymphoma
Nodal marginal zone lymphoma
Non-leukemic variant of B-CLL
Splenic marginal zone lymphoma
EXCLUDES 1 chronic lymphocytic leukemia (C91.1)
mature T/NK-cell lymphomas (C84.-)
Waldenstrom macroglobulinemia (C88.00)
AHA: 2023,1Q,18
DEF: Nonfollicular lymphoma that is rare, slow growing, and usually found in the older population.

- **C83.00** Small cell B-cell lymphoma, unspecified site
- **C83.01** Small cell B-cell lymphoma, lymph nodes of head, face, and neck
- **C83.02** Small cell B-cell lymphoma, intrathoracic lymph nodes
- **C83.03** Small cell B-cell lymphoma, intra-abdominal lymph nodes
- **C83.04** Small cell B-cell lymphoma, lymph nodes of axilla and upper limb
- **C83.05** Small cell B-cell lymphoma, lymph nodes of inguinal region and lower limb
- **C83.06** Small cell B-cell lymphoma, intrapelvic lymph nodes
- **C83.07** Small cell B-cell lymphoma, spleen
- **C83.08** Small cell B-cell lymphoma, lymph nodes of multiple sites
- **C83.09** Small cell B-cell lymphoma, extranodal and solid organ sites
- **C83.0A** Small cell B-cell lymphoma, in remission

✓5th C83.1 Mantle cell lymphoma
Centrocytic lymphoma
Malignant lymphomatous polyposis
DEF: Rare form of B-cell non-Hodgkin lymphoma named for the location of the tumor cell production, the mantle zone of the lymph nodes.

- **C83.10** Mantle cell lymphoma, unspecified site
- **C83.11** Mantle cell lymphoma, lymph nodes of head, face, and neck
- **C83.12** Mantle cell lymphoma, intrathoracic lymph nodes
- **C83.13** Mantle cell lymphoma, intra-abdominal lymph nodes
- **C83.14** Mantle cell lymphoma, lymph nodes of axilla and upper limb
- **C83.15** Mantle cell lymphoma, lymph nodes of inguinal region and lower limb
- **C83.16** Mantle cell lymphoma, intrapelvic lymph nodes
- **C83.17** Mantle cell lymphoma, spleen
- **C83.18** Mantle cell lymphoma, lymph nodes of multiple sites
- **C83.19** Mantle cell lymphoma, extranodal and solid organ sites
- **C83.1A** Mantle cell lymphoma, in remission
  Centrocytic lymphoma, in remission

✓5th C83.3 Diffuse large B-cell lymphoma
Anaplastic diffuse large B-cell lymphoma
CD30-positive diffuse large B-cell lymphoma
Centroblastic diffuse large B-cell lymphoma
Diffuse large B-cell lymphoma, subtype not specified
Immunoblastic diffuse large B-cell lymphoma
Plasmablastic diffuse large B-cell lymphoma
T-cell rich diffuse large B-cell lymphoma
EXCLUDES 1 mediastinal (thymic) large B-cell lymphoma (C85.2-)
mature T/NK-cell lymphomas (C84.-)
DEF: Nonfollicular lymphoma that is one of the more common types of lymphoma. This cancer is fast growing and affects any age but is found mostly in the older population.

- **C83.30** Diffuse large B-cell lymphoma, unspecified site

C83.31	Diffuse large B-cell lymphoma, lymph nodes of head, face, and neck	
C83.32	Diffuse large B-cell lymphoma, intrathoracic lymph nodes	
C83.33	Diffuse large B-cell lymphoma, intra-abdominal lymph nodes	
C83.34	Diffuse large B-cell lymphoma, lymph nodes of axilla and upper limb	
C83.35	Diffuse large B-cell lymphoma, lymph nodes of inguinal region and lower limb	
C83.36	Diffuse large B-cell lymphoma, intrapelvic lymph nodes	
C83.37	Diffuse large B-cell lymphoma, spleen	
C83.38	Diffuse large B-cell lymphoma, lymph nodes of multiple sites	

AHA: 2023, 1Q, 22

√6ᵗʰ **C83.39** Diffuse large B-cell lymphoma, extranodal and solid organ sites

AHA: 2024, 4Q, 4; 2023, 1Q, 22

- **C83.390** Primary central nervous system lymphoma
  - PCNSL of brain
  - PCNSL of meninges
  - PCNSL NOS
  - PCNSL of spinal cord
  - EXCLUDES 1: primary central nervous system lymphoma, Burkitt (C83.79)
    primary central nervous system lymphoma, lymphoblastic (C83.59)
    primary central nervous system lymphoma, other (C83.89)
    primary central nervous system lymphoma, peripheral T-cell (C84.49)
- **C83.398** Diffuse large B-cell lymphoma of other extranodal and solid organ sites
- **C83.3A** Diffuse large B-cell lymphoma, in remission

√5ᵗʰ **C83.5** Lymphoblastic (diffuse) lymphoma
- B-precursor lymphoma
- Lymphoblastic B-cell lymphoma
- Lymphoblastic lymphoma NOS
- Lymphoblastic T-cell lymphoma
- T-precursor lymphoma

DEF: Type of non-Hodgkin lymphoma considered lymphoma or leukemia—the determination is made based on the amount of bone marrow involvement. The cells are small to medium immature T-cells that often originate in the thymus where many of the T-cells are made.

- **C83.50** Lymphoblastic (diffuse) lymphoma, unspecified site
- **C83.51** Lymphoblastic (diffuse) lymphoma, lymph nodes of head, face, and neck
- **C83.52** Lymphoblastic (diffuse) lymphoma, intrathoracic lymph nodes
- **C83.53** Lymphoblastic (diffuse) lymphoma, intra-abdominal lymph nodes
- **C83.54** Lymphoblastic (diffuse) lymphoma, lymph nodes of axilla and upper limb
- **C83.55** Lymphoblastic (diffuse) lymphoma, lymph nodes of inguinal region and lower limb
- **C83.56** Lymphoblastic (diffuse) lymphoma, intrapelvic lymph nodes
- **C83.57** Lymphoblastic (diffuse) lymphoma, spleen
- **C83.58** Lymphoblastic (diffuse) lymphoma, lymph nodes of multiple sites
- **C83.59** Lymphoblastic (diffuse) lymphoma, extranodal and solid organ sites
- **C83.5A** Lymphoblastic (diffuse) lymphoma, in remission

√5ᵗʰ **C83.7** Burkitt lymphoma
- Atypical Burkitt lymphoma
- Burkitt-like lymphoma
- EXCLUDES 1: mature B-cell leukemia Burkitt type (C91.A-)

DEF: Malignancy of the lymphatic system, most often seen as a large bone-deteriorating lesion within the jaw or as an abdominal mass. It is a form of non-Hodgkin's lymphoma and is recognized as the fastest growing human tumor.

- **C83.70** Burkitt lymphoma, unspecified site
- **C83.71** Burkitt lymphoma, lymph nodes of head, face, and neck
- **C83.72** Burkitt lymphoma, intrathoracic lymph nodes
- **C83.73** Burkitt lymphoma, intra-abdominal lymph nodes
- **C83.74** Burkitt lymphoma, lymph nodes of axilla and upper limb
- **C83.75** Burkitt lymphoma, lymph nodes of inguinal region and lower limb
- **C83.76** Burkitt lymphoma, intrapelvic lymph nodes
- **C83.77** Burkitt lymphoma, spleen
- **C83.78** Burkitt lymphoma, lymph nodes of multiple sites
- **C83.79** Burkitt lymphoma, extranodal and solid organ sites
- **C83.7A** Burkitt lymphoma, in remission

√5ᵗʰ **C83.8** Other non-follicular lymphoma
- Intravascular large B-cell lymphoma
- Lymphoid granulomatosis
- Primary effusion B-cell lymphoma
- EXCLUDES 1: mediastinal (thymic) large B-cell lymphoma (C85.2-)
  T-cell rich B-cell lymphoma (C83.3-)

- **C83.80** Other non-follicular lymphoma, unspecified site
- **C83.81** Other non-follicular lymphoma, lymph nodes of head, face, and neck
- **C83.82** Other non-follicular lymphoma, intrathoracic lymph nodes
- **C83.83** Other non-follicular lymphoma, intra-abdominal lymph nodes
- **C83.84** Other non-follicular lymphoma, lymph nodes of axilla and upper limb
- **C83.85** Other non-follicular lymphoma, lymph nodes of inguinal region and lower limb
- **C83.86** Other non-follicular lymphoma, intrapelvic lymph nodes
- **C83.87** Other non-follicular lymphoma, spleen
- **C83.88** Other non-follicular lymphoma, lymph nodes of multiple sites
- **C83.89** Other non-follicular lymphoma, extranodal and solid organ sites
- **C83.8A** Other non-follicular lymphoma, in remission

√5ᵗʰ **C83.9** Non-follicular (diffuse) lymphoma, unspecified
- **C83.90** Non-follicular (diffuse) lymphoma, unspecified, unspecified site
- **C83.91** Non-follicular (diffuse) lymphoma, unspecified, lymph nodes of head, face, and neck
- **C83.92** Non-follicular (diffuse) lymphoma, unspecified, intrathoracic lymph nodes
- **C83.93** Non-follicular (diffuse) lymphoma, unspecified, intra-abdominal lymph nodes
- **C83.94** Non-follicular (diffuse) lymphoma, unspecified, lymph nodes of axilla and upper limb
- **C83.95** Non-follicular (diffuse) lymphoma, unspecified, lymph nodes of inguinal region and lower limb
- **C83.96** Non-follicular (diffuse) lymphoma, unspecified, intrapelvic lymph nodes
- **C83.97** Non-follicular (diffuse) lymphoma, unspecified, spleen
- **C83.98** Non-follicular (diffuse) lymphoma, unspecified, lymph nodes of multiple sites

	C83.99	Non-follicular (diffuse) lymphoma, unspecified, extranodal and solid organ sites HCC Rx ESR COM
	C83.9A	Non-follicular (diffuse) lymphoma, unspecified, in remission HCC Rx ESR COM

✓4th **C84 Mature T/NK-cell lymphomas**
  EXCLUDES 1 personal history of non-Hodgkin lymphoma (Z85.72)
  AHA: 2023,1Q,22

✓5th **C84.0 Mycosis fungoides**
  EXCLUDES 1 peripheral T-cell lymphoma, not elsewhere classified (C84.4-)
  DEF: Most common form of cutaneous T-cell lymphoma. A type of non-Hodgkin lymphoma in which white blood cells become cancerous and affect the skin and sometimes internal organs.
  Synonym(s): Alibert-Bazin syndrome.

- C84.00 Mycosis fungoides, unspecified site HCC Rx ESR COM
- C84.01 Mycosis fungoides, lymph nodes of head, face, and neck HCC Rx ESR COM
- C84.02 Mycosis fungoides, intrathoracic lymph nodes HCC Rx ESR COM
- C84.03 Mycosis fungoides, intra-abdominal lymph nodes HCC Rx ESR COM
- C84.04 Mycosis fungoides, lymph nodes of axilla and upper limb HCC Rx ESR COM
- C84.05 Mycosis fungoides, lymph nodes of inguinal region and lower limb HCC Rx ESR COM
- C84.06 Mycosis fungoides, intrapelvic lymph nodes HCC Rx ESR COM
- C84.07 Mycosis fungoides, spleen HCC Rx ESR COM
- C84.08 Mycosis fungoides, lymph nodes of multiple sites HCC Rx ESR COM
- C84.09 Mycosis fungoides, extranodal and solid organ sites HCC Rx ESR COM
- C84.0A Mycosis fungoides, in remission HCC Rx ESR COM

✓5th **C84.1 Sezary disease**
  DEF: Extension of mycosis fungoides that affects the blood and all of the skin, appearing as sunburn, rather than patches. It spreads to the lymph nodes and is often linked to a weakened immune system.

- C84.10 Sezary disease, unspecified site HCC Rx ESR COM
- C84.11 Sezary disease, lymph nodes of head, face, and neck HCC Rx ESR COM
- C84.12 Sezary disease, intrathoracic lymph nodes HCC Rx ESR COM
- C84.13 Sezary disease, intra-abdominal lymph nodes HCC Rx ESR COM
- C84.14 Sezary disease, lymph nodes of axilla and upper limb HCC Rx ESR COM
- C84.15 Sezary disease, lymph nodes of inguinal region and lower limb HCC Rx ESR COM
- C84.16 Sezary disease, intrapelvic lymph nodes HCC Rx ESR COM
- C84.17 Sezary disease, spleen HCC Rx ESR COM
- C84.18 Sezary disease, lymph nodes of multiple sites HCC Rx ESR COM
- C84.19 Sezary disease, extranodal and solid organ sites HCC Rx ESR COM
- C84.1A Sezary disease, in remission HCC Rx ESR COM

✓5th **C84.4 Peripheral T-cell lymphoma, not elsewhere classified**
  Lennert's lymphoma
  Lymphoepithelioid lymphoma
  Mature T-cell lymphoma, not elsewhere classified

- C84.40 Peripheral T-cell lymphoma, not elsewhere classified, unspecified site HCC Rx ESR COM
- C84.41 Peripheral T-cell lymphoma, not elsewhere classified, lymph nodes of head, face, and neck HCC Rx ESR COM
- C84.42 Peripheral T-cell lymphoma, not elsewhere classified, intrathoracic lymph nodes HCC Rx ESR COM
- C84.43 Peripheral T-cell lymphoma, not elsewhere classified, intra-abdominal lymph nodes HCC Rx ESR COM
- C84.44 Peripheral T-cell lymphoma, not elsewhere classified, lymph nodes of axilla and upper limb HCC Rx ESR COM
- C84.45 Peripheral T-cell lymphoma, not elsewhere classified, lymph nodes of inguinal region and lower limb HCC Rx ESR COM
- C84.46 Peripheral T-cell lymphoma, not elsewhere classified, intrapelvic lymph nodes HCC Rx ESR COM
- C84.47 Peripheral T-cell lymphoma, not elsewhere classified, spleen HCC Rx ESR COM
- C84.48 Peripheral T-cell lymphoma, not elsewhere classified, lymph nodes of multiple sites HCC Rx ESR COM
- C84.49 Peripheral T-cell lymphoma, not elsewhere classified, extranodal and solid organ sites HCC Rx ESR COM
- C84.4A Peripheral T-cell lymphoma, not elsewhere classified, in remission HCC Rx ESR COM

✓5th **C84.6 Anaplastic large cell lymphoma, ALK-positive**
  Anaplastic large cell lymphoma, CD30-positive

- C84.60 Anaplastic large cell lymphoma, ALK-positive, unspecified site HCC Rx ESR COM
- C84.61 Anaplastic large cell lymphoma, ALK-positive, lymph nodes of head, face, and neck HCC Rx ESR COM
- C84.62 Anaplastic large cell lymphoma, ALK-positive, intrathoracic lymph nodes HCC Rx ESR COM
- C84.63 Anaplastic large cell lymphoma, ALK-positive, intra-abdominal lymph nodes HCC Rx ESR COM
- C84.64 Anaplastic large cell lymphoma, ALK-positive, lymph nodes of axilla and upper limb HCC Rx ESR COM
- C84.65 Anaplastic large cell lymphoma, ALK-positive, lymph nodes of inguinal region and lower limb HCC Rx ESR COM
- C84.66 Anaplastic large cell lymphoma, ALK-positive, intrapelvic lymph nodes HCC Rx ESR COM
- C84.67 Anaplastic large cell lymphoma, ALK-positive, spleen HCC Rx ESR COM
- C84.68 Anaplastic large cell lymphoma, ALK-positive, lymph nodes of multiple sites HCC Rx ESR COM
- C84.69 Anaplastic large cell lymphoma, ALK-positive, extranodal and solid organ sites HCC Rx ESR COM
- C84.6A Anaplastic large cell lymphoma, ALK-positive, in remission HCC Rx ESR COM

✓5th **C84.7 Anaplastic large cell lymphoma, ALK-negative**
  EXCLUDES 1 primary cutaneous CD30-positive T-cell proliferations (C86.6-)

- C84.70 Anaplastic large cell lymphoma, ALK-negative, unspecified site HCC Rx ESR COM
- C84.71 Anaplastic large cell lymphoma, ALK-negative, lymph nodes of head, face, and neck HCC Rx ESR COM
- C84.72 Anaplastic large cell lymphoma, ALK-negative, intrathoracic lymph nodes HCC Rx ESR COM
- C84.73 Anaplastic large cell lymphoma, ALK-negative, intra-abdominal lymph nodes HCC Rx ESR COM
- C84.74 Anaplastic large cell lymphoma, ALK-negative, lymph nodes of axilla and upper limb HCC Rx ESR COM
- C84.75 Anaplastic large cell lymphoma, ALK-negative, lymph nodes of inguinal region and lower limb HCC Rx ESR COM
- C84.76 Anaplastic large cell lymphoma, ALK-negative, intrapelvic lymph nodes HCC Rx ESR COM
- C84.77 Anaplastic large cell lymphoma, ALK-negative, spleen HCC Rx ESR COM
- C84.78 Anaplastic large cell lymphoma, ALK-negative, lymph nodes of multiple sites HCC Rx ESR COM
- C84.79 Anaplastic large cell lymphoma, ALK-negative, extranodal and solid organ sites HCC Rx ESR COM
- C84.7A Anaplastic large cell lymphoma, ALK-negative, breast
  Breast implant associated anaplastic large cell lymphoma (BIA-ALCL)
  Use additional code to identify:
    breast implant status (Z98.82)
    personal history of breast implant removal (Z98.86)
  AHA: 2021,4Q,6
- C84.7B Anaplastic large cell lymphoma, ALK-negative, in remission HCC Rx ESR COM

✓5th **C84.A Cutaneous T-cell lymphoma, unspecified**
  AHA: 2021,2Q,6

- C84.A0 Cutaneous T-cell lymphoma, unspecified, unspecified site HCC Rx ESR COM
- C84.A1 Cutaneous T-cell lymphoma, unspecified lymph nodes of head, face, and neck HCC Rx ESR COM
- C84.A2 Cutaneous T-cell lymphoma, unspecified, intrathoracic lymph nodes HCC Rx ESR COM

Chapter 2. Neoplasms

- **C84.A3** Cutaneous T-cell lymphoma, unspecified, intra-abdominal lymph nodes
- **C84.A4** Cutaneous T-cell lymphoma, unspecified, lymph nodes of axilla and upper limb
- **C84.A5** Cutaneous T-cell lymphoma, unspecified, lymph nodes of inguinal region and lower limb
- **C84.A6** Cutaneous T-cell lymphoma, unspecified, intrapelvic lymph nodes
- **C84.A7** Cutaneous T-cell lymphoma, unspecified, spleen
- **C84.A8** Cutaneous T-cell lymphoma, unspecified, lymph nodes of multiple sites
- **C84.A9** Cutaneous T-cell lymphoma, unspecified, extranodal and solid organ sites
- **C84.AA** Cutaneous T-cell lymphoma, unspecified, in remission

C84.Z Other mature T/NK-cell lymphomas

NOTE If T-cell lineage or involvement is mentioned in conjunction with a specific lymphoma, code to the more specific description.

EXCLUDES 1
- angioimmunoblastic T-cell lymphoma (C86.50)
- blastic NK-cell lymphoma (C86.40)
- enteropathy-type T-cell lymphoma (C86.20)
- extranodal NK-cell lymphoma, nasal type (C86.00)
- hepatosplenic T-cell lymphoma (C86.10)
- primary cutaneous CD30-positive T-cell proliferations (C86.60)
- subcutaneous panniculitis-like T-cell lymphoma (C86.30)
- T-cell leukemia (C91.1-)

- **C84.Z0** Other mature T/NK-cell lymphomas, unspecified site
- **C84.Z1** Other mature T/NK-cell lymphomas, lymph nodes of head, face, and neck
- **C84.Z2** Other mature T/NK-cell lymphomas, intrathoracic lymph nodes
- **C84.Z3** Other mature T/NK-cell lymphomas, intra-abdominal lymph nodes
- **C84.Z4** Other mature T/NK-cell lymphomas, lymph nodes of axilla and upper limb
- **C84.Z5** Other mature T/NK-cell lymphomas, lymph nodes of inguinal region and lower limb
- **C84.Z6** Other mature T/NK-cell lymphomas, intrapelvic lymph nodes
- **C84.Z7** Other mature T/NK-cell lymphomas, spleen
- **C84.Z8** Other mature T/NK-cell lymphomas, lymph nodes of multiple sites
- **C84.Z9** Other mature T/NK-cell lymphomas, extranodal and solid organ sites
- **C84.ZA** Other mature T/NK-cell lymphomas, in remission

C84.9 Mature T/NK-cell lymphomas, unspecified

NK/T cell lymphoma NOS

EXCLUDES 1 mature T-cell lymphoma, not elsewhere classified (C84.4-)

- **C84.90** Mature T/NK-cell lymphomas, unspecified, unspecified site
- **C84.91** Mature T/NK-cell lymphomas, unspecified, lymph nodes of head, face, and neck
- **C84.92** Mature T/NK-cell lymphomas, unspecified, intrathoracic lymph nodes
- **C84.93** Mature T/NK-cell lymphomas, unspecified, intra-abdominal lymph nodes
- **C84.94** Mature T/NK-cell lymphomas, unspecified, lymph nodes of axilla and upper limb
- **C84.95** Mature T/NK-cell lymphomas, unspecified, lymph nodes of inguinal region and lower limb
- **C84.96** Mature T/NK-cell lymphomas, unspecified, intrapelvic lymph nodes
- **C84.97** Mature T/NK-cell lymphomas, unspecified, spleen
- **C84.98** Mature T/NK-cell lymphomas, unspecified, lymph nodes of multiple sites
- **C84.99** Mature T/NK-cell lymphomas, unspecified, extranodal and solid organ sites
- **C84.9A** Mature T/NK-cell lymphomas, unspecified, in remission

C85 Other specified and unspecified types of non-Hodgkin lymphoma

EXCLUDES 1 other specified types of T/NK-cell lymphoma (C86.-)
personal history of non-Hodgkin lymphoma (Z85.72)

AHA: 2023,1Q,22

C85.1 Unspecified B-cell lymphoma

NOTE If B-cell lineage or involvement is mentioned in conjunction with a specific lymphoma, code to the more specific description.

- **C85.10** Unspecified B-cell lymphoma, unspecified site
- **C85.11** Unspecified B-cell lymphoma, lymph nodes of head, face, and neck
- **C85.12** Unspecified B-cell lymphoma, intrathoracic lymph nodes
- **C85.13** Unspecified B-cell lymphoma, intra-abdominal lymph nodes
- **C85.14** Unspecified B-cell lymphoma, lymph nodes of axilla and upper limb
- **C85.15** Unspecified B-cell lymphoma, lymph nodes of inguinal region and lower limb
- **C85.16** Unspecified B-cell lymphoma, intrapelvic lymph nodes
- **C85.17** Unspecified B-cell lymphoma, spleen
- **C85.18** Unspecified B-cell lymphoma, lymph nodes of multiple sites
- **C85.19** Unspecified B-cell lymphoma, extranodal and solid organ sites
- **C85.1A** Unspecified B-cell lymphoma, in remission

C85.2 Mediastinal (thymic) large B-cell lymphoma

- **C85.20** Mediastinal (thymic) large B-cell lymphoma, unspecified site
- **C85.21** Mediastinal (thymic) large B-cell lymphoma, lymph nodes of head, face, and neck
- **C85.22** Mediastinal (thymic) large B-cell lymphoma, intrathoracic lymph nodes
- **C85.23** Mediastinal (thymic) large B-cell lymphoma, intra-abdominal lymph nodes
- **C85.24** Mediastinal (thymic) large B-cell lymphoma, lymph nodes of axilla and upper limb
- **C85.25** Mediastinal (thymic) large B-cell lymphoma, lymph nodes of inguinal region and lower limb
- **C85.26** Mediastinal (thymic) large B-cell lymphoma, intrapelvic lymph nodes
- **C85.27** Mediastinal (thymic) large B-cell lymphoma, spleen
- **C85.28** Mediastinal (thymic) large B-cell lymphoma, lymph nodes of multiple sites
- **C85.29** Mediastinal (thymic) large B-cell lymphoma, extranodal and solid organ sites
- **C85.2A** Mediastinal (thymic) large B-cell lymphoma, in remission

C85.8 Other specified types of non-Hodgkin lymphoma

- **C85.80** Other specified types of non-Hodgkin lymphoma, unspecified site
- **C85.81** Other specified types of non-Hodgkin lymphoma, lymph nodes of head, face, and neck
- **C85.82** Other specified types of non-Hodgkin lymphoma, intrathoracic lymph nodes
- **C85.83** Other specified types of non-Hodgkin lymphoma, intra-abdominal lymph nodes
- **C85.84** Other specified types of non-Hodgkin lymphoma, lymph nodes of axilla and upper limb
- **C85.85** Other specified types of non-Hodgkin lymphoma, lymph nodes of inguinal region and lower limb
- **C85.86** Other specified types of non-Hodgkin lymphoma, intrapelvic lymph nodes
- **C85.87** Other specified types of non-Hodgkin lymphoma, spleen

Chapter 2. Neoplasms

- **C85.88** Other specified types of non-Hodgkin lymphoma, lymph nodes of multiple sites
- **C85.89** Other specified types of non-Hodgkin lymphoma, extranodal and solid organ sites
- **C85.8A** Other specified types of non-Hodgkin lymphoma, in remission

C85.9 Non-Hodgkin lymphoma, unspecified
Lymphoma NOS
Malignant lymphoma NOS
Non-Hodgkin lymphoma NOS

- **C85.90** Non-Hodgkin lymphoma, unspecified, unspecified site
- **C85.91** Non-Hodgkin lymphoma, unspecified, lymph nodes of head, face, and neck
- **C85.92** Non-Hodgkin lymphoma, unspecified, intrathoracic lymph nodes
- **C85.93** Non-Hodgkin lymphoma, unspecified, intra-abdominal lymph nodes
- **C85.94** Non-Hodgkin lymphoma, unspecified, lymph nodes of axilla and upper limb
- **C85.95** Non-Hodgkin lymphoma, unspecified, lymph nodes of inguinal region and lower limb
- **C85.96** Non-Hodgkin lymphoma, unspecified, intrapelvic lymph nodes
- **C85.97** Non-Hodgkin lymphoma, unspecified, spleen
- **C85.98** Non-Hodgkin lymphoma, unspecified, lymph nodes of multiple sites
- **C85.99** Non-Hodgkin lymphoma, unspecified, extranodal and solid organ sites
- **C85.9A** Non-Hodgkin lymphoma, unspecified, in remission

C86 Other specified types of T/NK-cell lymphoma
EXCLUDES 1 anaplastic large cell lymphoma, ALK negative (C84.7-)
anaplastic large cell lymphoma, ALK positive (C84.6-)
mature T/NK-cell lymphomas (C84.-)
other specified types of non-Hodgkin lymphoma (C85.8-)

C86.0 Extranodal NK/T-cell lymphoma, nasal type
- **C86.00** Extranodal NK/T-cell lymphoma, nasal type not having achieved remission
  Extranodal NK/T-cell lymphoma, nasal type NOS
  Extranodal NK/T-cell lymphoma, nasal type with failed remission
- **C86.01** Extranodal NK/T-cell lymphoma, nasal type, in remission

C86.1 Hepatosplenic T-cell lymphoma
Alpha-beta and gamma delta types
- **C86.10** Hepatosplenic T-cell lymphoma not having achieved remission
  Hepatosplenic T-cell lymphoma NOS
  Hepatosplenic T-cell lymphoma with failed remission
- **C86.11** Hepatosplenic T-cell lymphoma, in remission

C86.2 Enteropathy-type (intestinal) T-cell lymphoma
Enteropathy associated T-cell lymphoma
- **C86.20** Enteropathy-type (intestinal) T-cell lymphoma not having achieved remission
  Enteropathy associated T-cell lymphoma NOS
  Enteropathy associated T-cell lymphoma not having achieved remission
  Enteropathy associated T-cell lymphoma with failed remission
  Enteropathy-type (intestinal) T-cell lymphoma NOS
  Enteropathy-type (intestinal) T-cell lymphoma with failed remission
- **C86.21** Enteropathy-type (intestinal) T-cell lymphoma, in remission
  Enteropathy associated T-cell lymphoma, in remission

C86.3 Subcutaneous panniculitis-like T-cell lymphoma
- **C86.30** Subcutaneous panniculitis-like T-cell lymphoma not having achieved remission
  Subcutaneous panniculitis-like T-cell lymphoma NOS
  Subcutaneous panniculitis-like T-cell lymphoma with failed remission
- **C86.31** Subcutaneous panniculitis-like T-cell lymphoma, in remission

C86.4 Blastic NK-cell lymphoma
Blastic plasmacytoid dendritic cell neoplasm (BPDCN)
- **C86.40** Blastic NK-cell lymphoma not having achieved remission
  Blastic NK-cell lymphoma NOS
  Blastic NK-cell lymphoma with failed remission
  Blastic plasmacytoid dendritic cell neoplasm (BPDCN) NOS
  Blastic plasmacytoid dendritic cell neoplasm (BPDCN) not having achieved remission
  Blastic plasmacytoid dendritic cell neoplasm (BPDCN) with failed remission
- **C86.41** Blastic NK-cell lymphoma, in remission
  Blastic plasmacytoid dendritic cell neoplasm (BPDCN), in remission

C86.5 Angioimmunoblastic T-cell lymphoma
Angioimmunoblastic lymphadenopathy with dysproteinemia (AILD)
- **C86.50** Angioimmunoblastic T-cell lymphoma not having achieved remission
  Angioimmunoblastic lymphadenopathy with dysproteinemia (AILD) NOS
  Angioimmunoblastic lymphadenopathy with dysproteinemia (AILD) not having achieved remission
  Angioimmunoblastic lymphadenopathy with dysproteinemia (AILD) with failed remission
  Angioimmunoblastic T-cell lymphoma NOS
  Angioimmunoblastic T-cell lymphoma with failed remission
- **C86.51** Angioimmunoblastic T-cell lymphoma, in remission
  Angioimmunoblastic lymphadenopathy with dysproteinemia (AILD), in remission

C86.6 Primary cutaneous CD30-positive T-cell proliferations
Lymphomatoid papulosis
Primary cutaneous anaplastic large cell lymphoma
Primary cutaneous CD30-positive large T-cell lymphoma
- **C86.60** Primary cutaneous CD30-positive T-cell proliferations not having achieved remission
  Lymphomatoid papulosis NOS
  Lymphomatoid papulosis not having achieved remission
  Lymphomatoid papulosis with failed remission
  Primary cutaneous anaplastic large cell lymphoma NOS
  Primary cutaneous anaplastic large cell lymphoma not having achieved remission
  Primary cutaneous anaplastic large cell lymphoma with failed remission
  Primary cutaneous CD30-positive large T-cell lymphoma NOS
  Primary cutaneous CD30-positive large T-cell lymphoma not having achieved remission
  Primary cutaneous CD30-positive large T-cell lymphoma with failed remission
  Primary cutaneous CD30-positive T-cell proliferations NOS
  Primary cutaneous CD30-positive T-cell proliferations with failed remission
- **C86.61** Primary cutaneous CD30-positive T-cell proliferations, in remission

C88 Malignant immunoproliferative diseases and certain other B-cell lymphomas
EXCLUDES 1 B-cell lymphoma, unspecified (C85.1-)
personal history of other malignant neoplasms of lymphoid, hematopoietic and related tissues (Z85.79)

C88.0 Waldenstrom macroglobulinemia
Lymphoplasmacytic lymphoma with IgM-production
Macroglobulinemia (idiopathic) (primary)
EXCLUDES 1 small cell B-cell lymphoma (C83.0)

C88.00 Waldenstrom macroglobulinemia not having achieved remission [HCC Rx ESR COM]
Lymphoplasmacytic lymphoma with IgM-production not having achieved remission
Lymphoplasmacytic lymphoma with IgM-production with failed remission
Lymphoplasmacytic lymphoma with IgM-production, NOS
Macroglobulinemia (idiopathic) (primary) NOS
Macroglobulinemia (idiopathic) (primary) not having achieved remission
Macroglobulinemia (idiopathic) (primary) with failed remission
Waldenstrom macroglobulinemia NOS
Waldenstrom macroglobulinemia with failed remission

C88.01 Waldenstrom macroglobulinemia, in remission [HCC Rx ESR COM]

C88.2 Heavy chain disease
Franklin disease
Gamma heavy chain disease
Mu heavy chain disease

C88.20 Heavy chain disease not having achieved remission [HCC Rx ESR COM]
Franklin disease NOS
Franklin disease not having achieved remission
Franklin disease with failed remission
Gamma heavy chain disease NOS
Gamma heavy chain disease not having achieved remission
Gamma heavy chain disease with failed remission
Heavy chain disease NOS
Heavy chain disease with failed remission
Mu heavy chain disease NOS
Mu heavy chain disease not having achieved remission
Mu heavy chain disease with failed remission

C88.21 Heavy chain disease, in remission [HCC Rx ESR COM]

C88.3 Immunoproliferative small intestinal disease
Alpha heavy chain disease
Mediterranean lymphoma

C88.30 Immunoproliferative small intestinal disease not having achieved remission [HCC Rx ESR COM]
Alpha heavy chain disease NOS
Alpha heavy chain disease not having achieved remission
Alpha heavy chain disease with failed remission
Immunoproliferative small intestinal disease NOS
Immunoproliferative small intestinal disease with failed remission
Mediterranean lymphoma NOS
Mediterranean lymphoma not having achieved remission
Mediterranean lymphoma with failed remission

C88.31 Immunoproliferative small intestinal disease, in remission [HCC Rx ESR COM]

C88.4 Extranodal marginal zone B-cell lymphoma of mucosa-associated lymphoid tissue [MALT-lymphoma]
Lymphoma of bronchial-associated lymphoid tissue [BALT-lymphoma]
Lymphoma of skin-associated lymphoid tissue [SALT-lymphoma]
EXCLUDES 1 high malignant (diffuse large B-cell) lymphoma (C83.3-)

C88.40 Extranodal marginal zone B-cell lymphoma of mucosa-associated lymphoid tissue [MALT-lymphoma] not having achieved remission [HCC Rx ESR COM]
Extranodal marginal zone B-cell lymphoma of mucosa-associated lymphoid tissue [MALT-lymphoma] NOS
Extranodal marginal zone B-cell lymphoma of mucosa-associated lymphoid tissue [MALT-lymphoma] with failed remission
Lymphoma of bronchial-associated lymphoid tissue [BALT-lymphoma] NOS
Lymphoma of bronchial-associated lymphoid tissue [BALT-lymphoma] not having achieved remission
Lymphoma of bronchial-associated lymphoid tissue [BALT-lymphoma] with failed remission
Lymphoma of skin-associated lymphoid tissue [SALT-lymphoma] NOS
Lymphoma of skin-associated lymphoid tissue [SALT-lymphoma] not having achieved remission
Lymphoma of skin-associated lymphoid tissue [SALT-lymphoma] with failed remission

C88.41 Extranodal marginal zone B-cell lymphoma of mucosa-associated lymphoid tissue [MALT-lymphoma], in remission [HCC Rx ESR COM]

C88.8 Other malignant immunoproliferative diseases

C88.80 Other malignant immunoproliferative diseases not having achieved remission [HCC Rx ESR COM]
Other malignant immunoproliferative diseases NOS
Other malignant immunoproliferative diseases with failed remission

C88.81 Other malignant immunoproliferative diseases, in remission [HCC Rx ESR COM]

C88.9 Malignant immunoproliferative disease, unspecified
Immunoproliferative disease NOS

C88.90 Malignant immunoproliferative disease, unspecified not having achieved remission [HCC Rx ESR COM]
Immunoproliferative disease NOS
Immunoproliferative disease NOS not having achieved remission
Immunoproliferative disease NOS with failed remission
Malignant immunoproliferative disease, unspecified NOS
Malignant immunoproliferative disease, unspecified with failed remission

C88.91 Malignant immunoproliferative disease, unspecified, in remission [HCC Rx ESR COM]

C90 Multiple myeloma and malignant plasma cell neoplasms
EXCLUDES 1 personal history of other malignant neoplasms of lymphoid, hematopoietic and related tissues (Z85.79)
AHA: 2019,2Q,30

C90.0 Multiple myeloma
Kahler's disease
Medullary plasmacytoma
Myelomatosis
Plasma cell myeloma
EXCLUDES 1 solitary myeloma (C90.3-)
solitary plasmactyoma (C90.3-)
AHA: 2021,3Q,5
TIP: Do not assign an additional code for bone metastasis (C79.51) when multiple myeloma is described as metastatic to the bone; bone involvement is integral to this disease process.
TIP: Smoldering multiple myeloma (SMM) is a plasma cell disorder that has not yet progressed to active multiple myeloma. Code D47.2 should be used when only SMM is documented.

C90.00 Multiple myeloma not having achieved remission [HCC Rx ESR COM]
Multiple myeloma NOS
Multiple myeloma with failed remission

C90.01 Multiple myeloma in remission [HCC Rx ESR COM]

C90.02 Multiple myeloma in relapse [HCC Rx ESR COM]

C90.1 Plasma cell leukemia
Plasmacytic leukemia
AHA: 2019,2Q,30

- **C90.10** Plasma cell leukemia not having achieved remission
  - Plasma cell leukemia NOS
  - Plasma cell leukemia with failed remission
- **C90.11** Plasma cell leukemia in remission
- **C90.12** Plasma cell leukemia in relapse

C90.2 Extramedullary plasmacytoma

- **C90.20** Extramedullary plasmacytoma not having achieved remission
  - Extramedullary plasmacytoma NOS
  - Extramedullary plasmacytoma with failed remission
- **C90.21** Extramedullary plasmacytoma in remission
- **C90.22** Extramedullary plasmacytoma in relapse

C90.3 Solitary plasmacytoma
Localized malignant plasma cell tumor NOS
Plasmacytoma NOS
Solitary myeloma

- **C90.30** Solitary plasmacytoma not having achieved remission
  - Solitary plasmacytoma NOS
  - Solitary plasmacytoma with failed remission
- **C90.31** Solitary plasmacytoma in remission
- **C90.32** Solitary plasmacytoma in relapse

C91 Lymphoid leukemia
EXCLUDES 1: personal history of leukemia (Z85.6)
AHA: 2020,1Q,13
DEF: Malignant proliferation of immature lymphocytes (white blood cells that make up lymphoid tissue), called lymphoblasts, that originate in the bone marrow. Can be acute (ALL) or chronic (CLL).

C91.0 Acute lymphoblastic leukemia [ALL]
NOTE: Codes in subcategory C91.0- should only be used for T-cell and B-cell precursor leukemia

- **C91.00** Acute lymphoblastic leukemia not having achieved remission
  - Acute lymphoblastic leukemia NOS
  - Acute lymphoblastic leukemia with failed remission
- **C91.01** Acute lymphoblastic leukemia, in remission
- **C91.02** Acute lymphoblastic leukemia, in relapse

C91.1 Chronic lymphocytic leukemia of B-cell type
Lymphoplasmacytic leukemia
Richter syndrome
EXCLUDES 1: lymphoplasmacytic lymphoma (C83.0-)
AHA: 2023,1Q,18

- **C91.10** Chronic lymphocytic leukemia of B-cell type not having achieved remission
  - Chronic lymphocytic leukemia of B-cell type NOS
  - Chronic lymphocytic leukemia of B-cell type with failed remission
- **C91.11** Chronic lymphocytic leukemia of B-cell type in remission
- **C91.12** Chronic lymphocytic leukemia of B-cell type in relapse

C91.3 Prolymphocytic leukemia of B-cell type

- **C91.30** Prolymphocytic leukemia of B-cell type not having achieved remission
  - Prolymphocytic leukemia of B-cell type NOS
  - Prolymphocytic leukemia of B-cell type with failed remission
- **C91.31** Prolymphocytic leukemia of B-cell type, in remission
- **C91.32** Prolymphocytic leukemia of B-cell type, in relapse

C91.4 Hairy cell leukemia
Leukemic reticuloendotheliosis
DEF: Rare type of leukemia that is slow growing and often also considered a type of lymphoma. The small B-cell lymphocytes appear with "hairy" projections under a microscope and are found mostly in the bone marrow, spleen, and blood.

- **C91.40** Hairy cell leukemia not having achieved remission
  - Hairy cell leukemia NOS
  - Hairy cell leukemia with failed remission
- **C91.41** Hairy cell leukemia, in remission
- **C91.42** Hairy cell leukemia, in relapse

C91.5 Adult T-cell lymphoma/leukemia (HTLV-1-associated)
Acute variant of adult T-cell lymphoma/leukemia (HTLV-1-associated)
Chronic variant of adult T-cell lymphoma/leukemia (HTLV-1-associated)
Lymphomatoid variant of adult T-cell lymphoma/leukemia (HTLV-1-associated)
Smouldering variant of adult T-cell lymphoma/leukemia (HTLV-1-associated)

- **C91.50** Adult T-cell lymphoma/leukemia (HTLV-1-associated) not having achieved remission
  - Adult T-cell lymphoma/leukemia (HTLV-1-associated) NOS
  - Adult T-cell lymphoma/leukemia (HTLV-1-associated) with failed remission
- **C91.51** Adult T-cell lymphoma/leukemia (HTLV-1-associated), in remission
- **C91.52** Adult T-cell lymphoma/leukemia (HTLV-1-associated), in relapse

C91.6 Prolymphocytic leukemia of T-cell type

- **C91.60** Prolymphocytic leukemia of T-cell type not having achieved remission
  - Prolymphocytic leukemia of T-cell type NOS
  - Prolymphocytic leukemia of T-cell type with failed remission
- **C91.61** Prolymphocytic leukemia of T-cell type, in remission
- **C91.62** Prolymphocytic leukemia of T-cell type, in relapse

C91.A Mature B-cell leukemia Burkitt-type
EXCLUDES 1: Burkitt lymphoma (C83.7-)

- **C91.A0** Mature B-cell leukemia Burkitt-type not having achieved remission
  - Mature B-cell leukemia Burkitt-type NOS
  - Mature B-cell leukemia Burkitt-type with failed remission
- **C91.A1** Mature B-cell leukemia Burkitt-type, in remission
- **C91.A2** Mature B-cell leukemia Burkitt-type, in relapse

C91.Z Other lymphoid leukemia
T-cell large granular lymphocytic leukemia (associated with rheumatoid arthritis)

- **C91.Z0** Other lymphoid leukemia not having achieved remission
  - Other lymphoid leukemia NOS
  - Other lymphoid leukemia with failed remission
- **C91.Z1** Other lymphoid leukemia, in remission
- **C91.Z2** Other lymphoid leukemia, in relapse

C91.9 Lymphoid leukemia, unspecified

- **C91.90** Lymphoid leukemia, unspecified not having achieved remission
  - Lymphoid leukemia NOS
  - Lymphoid leukemia with failed remission
- **C91.91** Lymphoid leukemia, unspecified, in remission
- **C91.92** Lymphoid leukemia, unspecified, in relapse

C92 Myeloid leukemia

INCLUDES
granulocytic leukemia
myelogenous leukemia

Code also, if applicable, pancytopenia (acquired) (D61.818)
EXCLUDES 1 personal history of leukemia (Z85.6)
AHA: 2020,1Q,13; 2019,1Q,16
DEF: Cancer that develops in immature myelocytes called myeloblasts. These are the cells that become white blood cells (except lymphocytes), red blood cells, or platelet-making cells. Can be acute (AML) or chronic (CML).
TIP: Pancytopenia, although common in some types of myeloid leukemias, is not always inherent. When it is documented, code D61.818 can be assigned in addition to a code from this category.

C92.0 Acute myeloblastic leukemia
Acute myeloblastic leukemia (with maturation)
Acute myeloblastic leukemia (without a FAB classification) NOS
Acute myeloblastic leukemia 1/ETO
Acute myeloblastic leukemia M0
Acute myeloblastic leukemia M1
Acute myeloblastic leukemia M2
Acute myeloblastic leukemia with t(8;21)
Acute myeloblastic leukemia, minimal differentiation
Refractory anemia with excess blasts in transformation [RAEBT]
EXCLUDES 1 acute exacerbation of chronic myeloid leukemia (C92.10)
refractory anemia with excess of blasts not in transformation (D46.2-)
AHA: 2018,4Q,87

- **C92.00** Acute myeloblastic leukemia, not having achieved remission
  Acute myeloblastic leukemia NOS
  Acute myeloblastic leukemia with failed remission
- **C92.01** Acute myeloblastic leukemia, in remission
  AHA: 2021,3Q,4
- **C92.02** Acute myeloblastic leukemia, in relapse
  AHA: 2023,1Q,23

C92.1 Chronic myeloid leukemia, BCR/ABL-positive
Chronic myelogenous leukemia with crisis of blast cells
Chronic myelogenous leukemia, Philadelphia chromosome (Ph1) positive
Chronic myelogenous leukemia, t(9;22) (q34;q11)
EXCLUDES 1 atypical chronic myeloid leukemia BCR/ABL-negative (C92.2-)
chronic myelomonocytic leukemia (C93.1-)
chronic myeloproliferative disease (D47.1)

- **C92.10** Chronic myeloid leukemia, BCR/ABL-positive, not having achieved remission
  Chronic myeloid leukemia, BCR/ABL-positive NOS
  Chronic myeloid leukemia, BCR/ABL-positive with failed remission
- **C92.11** Chronic myeloid leukemia, BCR/ABL-positive, in remission
- **C92.12** Chronic myeloid leukemia, BCR/ABL-positive, in relapse

C92.2 Atypical chronic myeloid leukemia, BCR/ABL-negative
- **C92.20** Atypical chronic myeloid leukemia, BCR/ABL-negative, not having achieved remission
  Atypical chronic myeloid leukemia, BCR/ABL-negative NOS
  Atypical chronic myeloid leukemia, BCR/ABL-negative with failed remission
- **C92.21** Atypical chronic myeloid leukemia, BCR/ABL-negative, in remission
- **C92.22** Atypical chronic myeloid leukemia, BCR/ABL-negative, in relapse

C92.3 Myeloid sarcoma
A malignant tumor of immature myeloid cells
Chloroma
Granulocytic sarcoma

- **C92.30** Myeloid sarcoma, not having achieved remission
  Myeloid sarcoma NOS
  Myeloid sarcoma with failed remission
- **C92.31** Myeloid sarcoma, in remission
- **C92.32** Myeloid sarcoma, in relapse

C92.4 Acute promyelocytic leukemia
AML M3
AML Me with t(15;17) and variants

- **C92.40** Acute promyelocytic leukemia, not having achieved remission
  Acute promyelocytic leukemia NOS
  Acute promyelocytic leukemia with failed remission
- **C92.41** Acute promyelocytic leukemia, in remission
- **C92.42** Acute promyelocytic leukemia, in relapse

C92.5 Acute myelomonocytic leukemia
AML M4
AML M4 Eo with inv(16) or t(16;16)

- **C92.50** Acute myelomonocytic leukemia, not having achieved remission
  Acute myelomonocytic leukemia NOS
  Acute myelomonocytic leukemia with failed remission
- **C92.51** Acute myelomonocytic leukemia, in remission
- **C92.52** Acute myelomonocytic leukemia, in relapse

C92.6 Acute myeloid leukemia with 11q23-abnormality
Acute myeloid leukemia with variation of MLL-gene

- **C92.60** Acute myeloid leukemia with 11q23-abnormality not having achieved remission
  Acute myeloid leukemia with 11q23-abnormality NOS
  Acute myeloid leukemia with 11q23-abnormality with failed remission
- **C92.61** Acute myeloid leukemia with 11q23-abnormality in remission
- **C92.62** Acute myeloid leukemia with 11q23-abnormality in relapse

C92.A Acute myeloid leukemia with multilineage dysplasia
Acute myeloid leukemia with dysplasia of remaining hematopoesis and/or myelodysplastic disease in its history

- **C92.A0** Acute myeloid leukemia with multilineage dysplasia, not having achieved remission
  Acute myeloid leukemia with multilineage dysplasia NOS
  Acute myeloid leukemia with multilineage dysplasia with failed remission
- **C92.A1** Acute myeloid leukemia with multilineage dysplasia, in remission
- **C92.A2** Acute myeloid leukemia with multilineage dysplasia, in relapse

C92.Z Other myeloid leukemia
- **C92.Z0** Other myeloid leukemia not having achieved remission
  Myeloid leukemia NEC
  Myeloid leukemia NEC with failed remission
- **C92.Z1** Other myeloid leukemia, in remission
- **C92.Z2** Other myeloid leukemia, in relapse

C92.9 Myeloid leukemia, unspecified
- **C92.90** Myeloid leukemia, unspecified, not having achieved remission
  Myeloid leukemia, unspecified NOS
  Myeloid leukemia, unspecified with failed remission
- **C92.91** Myeloid leukemia, unspecified in remission
- **C92.92** Myeloid leukemia, unspecified in relapse

C93 Monocytic leukemia

INCLUDES monocytoid leukemia
EXCLUDES 1 personal history of leukemia (Z85.6)
AHA: 2020,1Q,13

C93.0 Acute monoblastic/monocytic leukemia
AML M5
AML M5a
AML M5b

- **C93.00** Acute monoblastic/monocytic leukemia, not having achieved remission
  Acute monoblastic/monocytic leukemia NOS
  Acute monoblastic/monocytic leukemia with failed remission

Chapter 2. Neoplasms

- **C93.01** Acute monoblastic/monocytic leukemia, in remission
- **C93.02** Acute monoblastic/monocytic leukemia, in relapse

C93.1 Chronic myelomonocytic leukemia
Chronic monocytic leukemia
CMML with eosinophilia
CMML-1
CMML-2
Code also, if applicable, eosinophilia (D72.18)

- **C93.10** Chronic myelomonocytic leukemia not having achieved remission
  - Chronic myelomonocytic leukemia NOS
  - Chronic myelomonocytic leukemia with failed remission
- **C93.11** Chronic myelomonocytic leukemia, in remission
- **C93.12** Chronic myelomonocytic leukemia, in relapse

C93.3 Juvenile myelomonocytic leukemia

- **C93.30** Juvenile myelomonocytic leukemia, not having achieved remission
  - Juvenile myelomonocytic leukemia NOS
  - Juvenile myelomonocytic leukemia with failed remission
- **C93.31** Juvenile myelomonocytic leukemia, in remission
- **C93.32** Juvenile myelomonocytic leukemia, in relapse

C93.Z Other monocytic leukemia

- **C93.Z0** Other monocytic leukemia, not having achieved remission
  - Other monocytic leukemia NOS
- **C93.Z1** Other monocytic leukemia, in remission
- **C93.Z2** Other monocytic leukemia, in relapse

C93.9 Monocytic leukemia, unspecified

- **C93.90** Monocytic leukemia, unspecified, not having achieved remission
  - Monocytic leukemia, unspecified NOS
  - Monocytic leukemia, unspecified with failed remission
- **C93.91** Monocytic leukemia, unspecified in remission
- **C93.92** Monocytic leukemia, unspecified in relapse

C94 Other leukemias of specified cell type
EXCLUDES 1
- leukemic reticuloendotheliosis (C91.4-)
- myelodysplastic syndromes (D46.-)
- personal history of leukemia (Z85.6)
- plasma cell leukemia (C90.1-)

AHA: 2020,1Q,13

C94.0 Acute erythroid leukemia
Acute myeloid leukemia M6(a)(b)
Erythroleukemia
DEF: Erythroleukemia: Malignant blood dyscrasia (a myeloproliferative disorder).

- **C94.00** Acute erythroid leukemia, not having achieved remission
  - Acute erythroid leukemia NOS
  - Acute erythroid leukemia with failed remission
- **C94.01** Acute erythroid leukemia, in remission
- **C94.02** Acute erythroid leukemia, in relapse

C94.2 Acute megakaryoblastic leukemia
Acute megakaryocytic leukemia
Acute myeloid leukemia M7

- **C94.20** Acute megakaryoblastic leukemia not having achieved remission
  - Acute megakaryoblastic leukemia NOS
  - Acute megakaryoblastic leukemia with failed remission
- **C94.21** Acute megakaryoblastic leukemia, in remission
- **C94.22** Acute megakaryoblastic leukemia, in relapse

C94.3 Mast cell leukemia
AHA: 2017,4Q,5

- **C94.30** Mast cell leukemia not having achieved remission
  - Mast cell leukemia NOS
  - Mast cell leukemia with failed remission
- **C94.31** Mast cell leukemia, in remission
- **C94.32** Mast cell leukemia, in relapse

C94.4 Acute panmyelosis with myelofibrosis
Acute myelofibrosis
EXCLUDES 1
- myelofibrosis NOS (D75.81)
- secondary myelofibrosis NOS (D75.81)

- **C94.40** Acute panmyelosis with myelofibrosis not having achieved remission
  - Acute myelofibrosis NOS
  - Acute panmyelosis NOS
  - Acute panmyelosis with myelofibrosis with failed remission
- **C94.41** Acute panmyelosis with myelofibrosis, in remission
- **C94.42** Acute panmyelosis with myelofibrosis, in relapse

C94.6 Myelodysplastic disease, not elsewhere classified
Myelodysplastic/myeloproliferative neoplasm, unclassifiable
Myeloproliferative disease, not elsewhere classified

C94.8 Other specified leukemias
Acute basophilic leukemia
Aggressive NK-cell leukemia
Code also, if applicable, eosinophilia (D72.18)

- **C94.80** Other specified leukemias not having achieved remission
  - Other specified leukemia with failed remission
  - Other specified leukemias NOS
- **C94.81** Other specified leukemias, in remission
- **C94.82** Other specified leukemias, in relapse

C95 Leukemia of unspecified cell type
EXCLUDES 1 personal history of leukemia (Z85.6)
AHA: 2020,1Q,13

C95.0 Acute leukemia of unspecified cell type
Acute bilineal leukemia
Acute mixed lineage leukemia
Biphenotypic acute leukemia
Stem cell leukemia of unclear lineage
EXCLUDES 1 acute exacerbation of unspecified chronic leukemia (C95.10)

- **C95.00** Acute leukemia of unspecified cell type not having achieved remission
  - Acute leukemia NOS
  - Acute leukemia of unspecified cell type with failed remission
- **C95.01** Acute leukemia of unspecified cell type, in remission
- **C95.02** Acute leukemia of unspecified cell type, in relapse

C95.1 Chronic leukemia of unspecified cell type

- **C95.10** Chronic leukemia of unspecified cell type not having achieved remission
  - Chronic leukemia NOS
  - Chronic leukemia of unspecified cell type with failed remission
- **C95.11** Chronic leukemia of unspecified cell type, in remission
- **C95.12** Chronic leukemia of unspecified cell type, in relapse

C95.9 Leukemia, unspecified

- **C95.90** Leukemia, unspecified not having achieved remission
  - Leukemia NOS
  - Leukemia, unspecified with failed remission
- **C95.91** Leukemia, unspecified, in remission
- **C95.92** Leukemia, unspecified, in relapse

Chapter 2. Neoplasms

C96 Other and unspecified malignant neoplasms of lymphoid, hematopoietic and related tissue

EXCLUDES 1: personal history of other malignant neoplasms of lymphoid, hematopoietic and related tissues (Z85.79)

C96.0 Multifocal and multisystemic (disseminated) Langerhans-cell histiocytosis
Histiocytosis X, multisystemic
Letterer-Siwe disease

EXCLUDES 1: adult pulmonary Langerhans cell histiocytosis (J84.82)
multifocal and unisystemic Langerhans-cell histiocytosis (C96.5)
unifocal Langerhans-cell histiocytosis (C96.6)

C96.2 Malignant mast cell neoplasm

EXCLUDES 1: indolent mastocytosis (D47.02)
mast cell leukemia (C94.30)
mastocytosis (congenital) (cutaneous) (Q82.2)

AHA: 2017,4Q,5

DEF: Mast cell: Type of white blood cell found in the loose connective tissue of blood vessels and bronchioles responsible for acute hypersensitivity reactions, including anaphylactic shock. The IgE receptors on these cells bind with allergens causing cell degranulation and diffuse, widespread histamine release that results in airway constriction and vasodilation with decreased systemic blood pressure.

- **C96.20** Malignant mast cell neoplasm, unspecified
- **C96.21** Aggressive systemic mastocytosis
- **C96.22** Mast cell sarcoma
- **C96.29** Other malignant mast cell neoplasm

C96.4 Sarcoma of dendritic cells (accessory cells)
Follicular dendritic cell sarcoma
Interdigitating dendritic cell sarcoma
Langerhans cell sarcoma

C96.5 Multifocal and unisystemic Langerhans-cell histiocytosis
Hand-Schuller-Christian disease
Histiocytosis X, multifocal

EXCLUDES 1: multifocal and multisystemic (disseminated) Langerhans-cell histiocytosis (C96.0)
unifocal Langerhans-cell histiocytosis (C96.6)

C96.6 Unifocal Langerhans-cell histiocytosis
Eosinophilic granuloma
Histiocytosis X NOS
Histiocytosis X, unifocal
Langerhans-cell histiocytosis NOS

EXCLUDES 1: multifocal and multisysemic (disseminated) Langerhans-cell histiocytosis (C96.0)
multifocal and unisystemic Langerhans-cell histiocytosis (C96.5)

C96.A Histiocytic sarcoma
Malignant histiocytosis

C96.Z Other specified malignant neoplasms of lymphoid, hematopoietic and related tissue

C96.9 Malignant neoplasm of lymphoid, hematopoietic and related tissue, unspecified

In situ neoplasms (D00-D09)

INCLUDES: Bowen's disease
erythroplasia
grade III intraepithelial neoplasia
Queyrat's erythroplasia

AHA: 2023,3Q,15

D00 Carcinoma in situ of oral cavity, esophagus and stomach

EXCLUDES 1: melanoma in situ (D03.-)

D00.0 Carcinoma in situ of lip, oral cavity and pharynx

Use additional code to identify:
exposure to environmental tobacco smoke (Z77.22)
exposure to tobacco smoke in the perinatal period (P96.81)
history of tobacco dependence (Z87.891)
occupational exposure to environmental tobacco smoke (Z57.31)
tobacco dependence (F17.-)
tobacco use (Z72.0)

EXCLUDES 1: carcinoma in situ of aryepiglottic fold or interarytenoid fold, laryngeal aspect (D02.0)
carcinoma in situ of epiglottis NOS (D02.0)
carcinoma in situ of epiglottis suprahyoid portion (D02.0)
carcinoma in situ of skin of lip (D03.0, D04.0)

- **D00.00** Carcinoma in situ of oral cavity, unspecified site
- **D00.01** Carcinoma in situ of labial mucosa and vermilion border
- **D00.02** Carcinoma in situ of buccal mucosa
- **D00.03** Carcinoma in situ of gingiva and edentulous alveolar ridge
- **D00.04** Carcinoma in situ of soft palate
- **D00.05** Carcinoma in situ of hard palate
- **D00.06** Carcinoma in situ of floor of mouth
- **D00.07** Carcinoma in situ of tongue
- **D00.08** Carcinoma in situ of pharynx
  Carcinoma in situ of aryepiglottic fold NOS
  Carcinoma in situ of hypopharyngeal aspect of aryepiglottic fold
  Carcinoma in situ of marginal zone of aryepiglottic fold

D00.1 Carcinoma in situ of esophagus
D00.2 Carcinoma in situ of stomach

D01 Carcinoma in situ of other and unspecified digestive organs

EXCLUDES 1: melanoma in situ (D03.-)

D01.0 Carcinoma in situ of colon
EXCLUDES 1: carcinoma in situ of rectosigmoid junction (D01.1)

D01.1 Carcinoma in situ of rectosigmoid junction
D01.2 Carcinoma in situ of rectum
D01.3 Carcinoma in situ of anus and anal canal
Anal intraepithelial neoplasia III [AIN III]
Severe dysplasia of anus

EXCLUDES 1: anal intraepithelial neoplasia I and II [AIN I and AIN II] (K62.82)
carcinoma in situ of anal margin (D04.5)
carcinoma in situ of anal skin (D04.5)
carcinoma in situ of perianal skin (D04.5)

D01.4 Carcinoma in situ of other and unspecified parts of intestine
EXCLUDES 1: carcinoma in situ of ampulla of Vater (D01.5)

- **D01.40** Carcinoma in situ of unspecified part of intestine
- **D01.49** Carcinoma in situ of other parts of intestine

D01.5 Carcinoma in situ of liver, gallbladder and bile ducts
Carcinoma in situ of ampulla of Vater

D01.7 Carcinoma in situ of other specified digestive organs
Carcinoma in situ of pancreas

D01.9 Carcinoma in situ of digestive organ, unspecified

 CMS-HCC  Rx HCC ESRD HCC 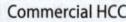 Commercial HCC 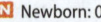 Newborn: 0 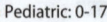 Pediatric: 0-17 Maternity: 9-64 Adult: 15-124

Chapter 2. Neoplasms

✓4th D02 Carcinoma in situ of middle ear and respiratory system
Use additional code to identify:
exposure to environmental tobacco smoke (Z77.22)
exposure to tobacco smoke in the perinatal period (P96.81)
history of tobacco dependence (Z87.891)
occupational exposure to environmental tobacco smoke (Z57.31)
tobacco dependence (F17.-)
tobacco use (Z72.0)
EXCLUDES 1   melanoma in situ (D03.-)

- **D02.0 Carcinoma in situ of larynx**
  Carcinoma in situ of aryepiglottic fold or interarytenoid fold, laryngeal aspect
  Carcinoma in situ of epiglottis (suprahyoid portion)
  EXCLUDES 1   carcinoma in situ of aryepiglottic fold or interarytenoid fold NOS (D00.08)
  carcinoma in situ of hypopharyngeal aspect (D00.08)
  carcinoma in situ of marginal zone (D00.08)
- **D02.1 Carcinoma in situ of trachea**
- **✓5th D02.2 Carcinoma in situ of bronchus and lung**
  - D02.20 Carcinoma in situ of unspecified bronchus and lung
  - D02.21 Carcinoma in situ of right bronchus and lung
  - D02.22 Carcinoma in situ of left bronchus and lung
- **D02.3 Carcinoma in situ of other parts of respiratory system**
  Carcinoma in situ of accessory sinuses
  Carcinoma in situ of middle ear
  Carcinoma in situ of nasal cavities
  EXCLUDES 1   carcinoma in situ of ear (external) (skin) (D04.2-)
  carcinoma in situ of nose NOS (D09.8)
  carcinoma in situ of skin of nose (D04.3)
- **D02.4 Carcinoma in situ of respiratory system, unspecified**

✓4th D03 Melanoma in situ
- **D03.0 Melanoma in situ of lip**
- **✓5th D03.1 Melanoma in situ of eyelid, including canthus**
  AHA: 2018,4Q,4
  - D03.10 Melanoma in situ of unspecified eyelid, including canthus
  - ✓6th D03.11 Melanoma in situ of right eyelid, including canthus
    - D03.111 Melanoma in situ of right upper eyelid, including canthus
    - D03.112 Melanoma in situ of right lower eyelid, including canthus
  - ✓6th D03.12 Melanoma in situ of left eyelid, including canthus
    - D03.121 Melanoma in situ of left upper eyelid, including canthus
    - D03.122 Melanoma in situ of left lower eyelid, including canthus
- **✓5th D03.2 Melanoma in situ of ear and external auricular canal**
  - D03.20 Melanoma in situ of unspecified ear and external auricular canal
  - D03.21 Melanoma in situ of right ear and external auricular canal
  - D03.22 Melanoma in situ of left ear and external auricular canal
- **✓5th D03.3 Melanoma in situ of other and unspecified parts of face**
  - D03.30 Melanoma in situ of unspecified part of face
  - D03.39 Melanoma in situ of other parts of face
- **D03.4 Melanoma in situ of scalp and neck**
- **✓5th D03.5 Melanoma in situ of trunk**
  - D03.51 Melanoma in situ of anal skin
    Melanoma in situ of anal margin
    Melanoma in situ of perianal skin
  - D03.52 Melanoma in situ of breast (skin) (soft tissue)
  - D03.59 Melanoma in situ of other part of trunk
- **✓5th D03.6 Melanoma in situ of upper limb, including shoulder**
  - D03.60 Melanoma in situ of unspecified upper limb, including shoulder
  - D03.61 Melanoma in situ of right upper limb, including shoulder
  - D03.62 Melanoma in situ of left upper limb, including shoulder
- **✓5th D03.7 Melanoma in situ of lower limb, including hip**
  - D03.70 Melanoma in situ of unspecified lower limb, including hip
  - D03.71 Melanoma in situ of right lower limb, including hip
  - D03.72 Melanoma in situ of left lower limb, including hip
- **D03.8 Melanoma in situ of other sites**
  Melanoma in situ of scrotum
  EXCLUDES 1   carcinoma in situ of scrotum (D07.61)
- **D03.9 Melanoma in situ, unspecified**

✓4th D04 Carcinoma in situ of skin
EXCLUDES 1   erythroplasia of Queyrat (penis) NOS (D07.4)
melanoma in situ (D03.-)
- **D04.0 Carcinoma in situ of skin of lip**
  EXCLUDES 2   carcinoma in situ of vermilion border of lip (D00.01)
- **✓5th D04.1 Carcinoma in situ of skin of eyelid, including canthus**
  AHA: 2018,4Q,4
  - D04.10 Carcinoma in situ of skin of unspecified eyelid, including canthus
  - ✓6th D04.11 Carcinoma in situ of skin of right eyelid, including canthus
    - D04.111 Carcinoma in situ of skin of right upper eyelid, including canthus
    - D04.112 Carcinoma in situ of skin of right lower eyelid, including canthus
  - ✓6th D04.12 Carcinoma in situ of skin of left eyelid, including canthus
    - D04.121 Carcinoma in situ of skin of left upper eyelid, including canthus
    - D04.122 Carcinoma in situ of skin of left lower eyelid, including canthus
- **✓5th D04.2 Carcinoma in situ of skin of ear and external auricular canal**
  - D04.20 Carcinoma in situ of skin of unspecified ear and external auricular canal
  - D04.21 Carcinoma in situ of skin of right ear and external auricular canal
  - D04.22 Carcinoma in situ of skin of left ear and external auricular canal
- **✓5th D04.3 Carcinoma in situ of skin of other and unspecified parts of face**
  - D04.30 Carcinoma in situ of skin of unspecified part of face
  - D04.39 Carcinoma in situ of skin of other parts of face
- **D04.4 Carcinoma in situ of skin of scalp and neck**
- **D04.5 Carcinoma in situ of skin of trunk**
  Carcinoma in situ of anal margin
  Carcinoma in situ of anal skin
  Carcinoma in situ of perianal skin
  Carcinoma in situ of skin of breast
  EXCLUDES 1   carcinoma in situ of anus NOS (D01.3)
  carcinoma in situ of scrotum (D07.61)
  carcinoma in situ of skin of genital organs (D07.-)
- **✓5th D04.6 Carcinoma in situ of skin of upper limb, including shoulder**
  - D04.60 Carcinoma in situ of skin of unspecified upper limb, including shoulder
  - D04.61 Carcinoma in situ of skin of right upper limb, including shoulder
  - D04.62 Carcinoma in situ of skin of left upper limb, including shoulder
- **✓5th D04.7 Carcinoma in situ of skin of lower limb, including hip**
  - D04.70 Carcinoma in situ of skin of unspecified lower limb, including hip
  - D04.71 Carcinoma in situ of skin of right lower limb, including hip
  - D04.72 Carcinoma in situ of skin of left lower limb, including hip
- **D04.8 Carcinoma in situ of skin of other sites**
- **D04.9 Carcinoma in situ of skin, unspecified**

✓4th D05 Carcinoma in situ of breast
EXCLUDES 1   carcinoma in situ of skin of breast (D04.5)
melanoma in situ of breast (skin) (D03.5)
Paget's disease of breast or nipple (C50.-)
EXCLUDES 2   malignant neoplasm of breast (C50.-)
- **✓5th D05.0 Lobular carcinoma in situ of breast**
  - D05.00 Lobular carcinoma in situ of unspecified breast
  - D05.01 Lobular carcinoma in situ of right breast
  - D05.02 Lobular carcinoma in situ of left breast

Chapter 2. Neoplasms

- ✓5th **D05.1** **Intraductal** carcinoma in situ of breast
  - **D05.10** Intraductal carcinoma in situ of unspecified breast
  - **D05.11** Intraductal carcinoma in situ of right breast
  - **D05.12** Intraductal carcinoma in situ of left breast
- ✓5th **D05.8** Other specified type of carcinoma in situ of breast
  - **D05.80** Other specified type of carcinoma in situ of unspecified breast
  - **D05.81** Other specified type of carcinoma in situ of right breast
  - **D05.82** Other specified type of carcinoma in situ of left breast
- ✓5th **D05.9** Unspecified type of carcinoma in situ of breast
  - **D05.90** Unspecified type of carcinoma in situ of unspecified breast
  - **D05.91** Unspecified type of carcinoma in situ of right breast
  - **D05.92** Unspecified type of carcinoma in situ of left breast
- ✓4th **D06** Carcinoma in situ of cervix uteri
  - INCLUDES
    - cervical adenocarcinoma in situ
    - cervical intraepithelial glandular neoplasia
    - cervical intraepithelial neoplasia III [CIN III]
    - severe dysplasia of cervix uteri
  - EXCLUDES 1
    - cervical intraepithelial neoplasia II [CIN II] (N87.1)
    - cytologic evidence of malignancy of cervix without histologic confirmation (R87.614)
    - high grade squamous intraepithelial lesion (HGSIL) of cervix (R87.613)
    - melanoma in situ of cervix (D03.5)
    - moderate cervical dysplasia (N87.1)
  - **D06.0** Carcinoma in situ of endocervix
  - **D06.1** Carcinoma in situ of exocervix
  - **D06.7** Carcinoma in situ of other parts of cervix
  - **D06.9** Carcinoma in situ of cervix, unspecified
- ✓4th **D07** Carcinoma in situ of other and unspecified genital organs
  - EXCLUDES 1 melanoma in situ of trunk (D03.5)
  - **D07.0** Carcinoma in situ of endometrium
  - **D07.1** Carcinoma in situ of vulva
    - Severe dysplasia of vulva
    - Vulvar intraepithelial neoplasia III [VIN III]
    - EXCLUDES 1
      - moderate dysplasia of vulva (N90.1)
      - vulvar intraepithelial neoplasia II [VIN II] (N90.1)
  - **D07.2** Carcinoma in situ of vagina
    - Severe dysplasia of vagina
    - Vaginal intraepithelial neoplasia III [VAIN III]
    - EXCLUDES 1
      - moderate dysplasia of vagina (N89.1)
      - vaginal intraepithelial neoplasia II [VIN II] (N89.1)
  - ✓5th **D07.3** Carcinoma in situ of other and unspecified female genital organs
    - **D07.30** Carcinoma in situ of unspecified female genital organs
    - **D07.39** Carcinoma in situ of other female genital organs
  - **D07.4** Carcinoma in situ of penis
    - Erythroplasia of Queyrat NOS
  - **D07.5** Carcinoma in situ of prostate
    - Prostatic intraepithelial neoplasia III (PIN III)
    - Severe dysplasia of prostate
    - EXCLUDES 1
      - dysplasia (mild) (moderate) of prostate (N42.3-)
      - prostatic intraepithelial neoplasia II [PIN II] (N42.3-)
  - ✓5th **D07.6** Carcinoma in situ of other and unspecified male genital organs
    - **D07.60** Carcinoma in situ of unspecified male genital organs
    - **D07.61** Carcinoma in situ of scrotum
    - **D07.69** Carcinoma in situ of other male genital organs
- ✓4th **D09** Carcinoma in situ of other and unspecified sites
  - EXCLUDES 1 melanoma in situ (D03.-)
  - **D09.0** Carcinoma in situ of bladder
  - ✓5th **D09.1** Carcinoma in situ of other and unspecified urinary organs
    - **D09.10** Carcinoma in situ of unspecified urinary organ
    - **D09.19** Carcinoma in situ of other urinary organs
  - ✓5th **D09.2** Carcinoma in situ of eye
    - EXCLUDES 1 carcinoma in situ of skin of eyelid (D04.1-)
    - **D09.20** Carcinoma in situ of unspecified eye
    - **D09.21** Carcinoma in situ of right eye
    - **D09.22** Carcinoma in situ of left eye
  - **D09.3** Carcinoma in situ of thyroid and other endocrine glands
    - EXCLUDES 1
      - carcinoma in situ of endocrine pancreas (D01.7)
      - carcinoma in situ of ovary (D07.39)
      - carcinoma in situ of testis (D07.69)
  - **D09.8** Carcinoma in situ of other specified sites
  - **D09.9** Carcinoma in situ, unspecified

Benign neoplasms, except benign neuroendocrine tumors (D10-D36)

- ✓4th **D10** Benign neoplasm of mouth and pharynx
  - **D10.0** Benign neoplasm of lip
    - Benign neoplasm of lip (frenulum) (inner aspect) (mucosa) (vermilion border)
    - EXCLUDES 1 benign neoplasm of skin of lip (D22.0, D23.0)
  - **D10.1** Benign neoplasm of tongue
    - Benign neoplasm of lingual tonsil
  - **D10.2** Benign neoplasm of floor of mouth
  - ✓5th **D10.3** Benign neoplasm of other and unspecified parts of mouth
    - **D10.30** Benign neoplasm of unspecified part of mouth
    - **D10.39** Benign neoplasm of other parts of mouth
      - Benign neoplasm of minor salivary gland NOS
      - EXCLUDES 1
        - benign odontogenic neoplasms (D16.4-D16.5)
        - benign neoplasm of mucosa of lip (D10.0)
        - benign neoplasm of nasopharyngeal surface of soft palate (D10.6)
  - **D10.4** Benign neoplasm of tonsil
    - Benign neoplasm of tonsil (faucial) (palatine)
    - EXCLUDES 1
      - benign neoplasm of lingual tonsil (D10.1)
      - benign neoplasm of pharyngeal tonsil (D10.6)
      - benign neoplasm of tonsillar fossa (D10.5)
      - benign neoplasm of tonsillar pillars (D10.5)
  - **D10.5** Benign neoplasm of other parts of oropharynx
    - Benign neoplasm of epiglottis, anterior aspect
    - Benign neoplasm of tonsillar fossa
    - Benign neoplasm of tonsillar pillars
    - Benign neoplasm of vallecula
    - EXCLUDES 1
      - benign neoplasm of epiglottis NOS (D14.1)
      - benign neoplasm of epiglottis, suprahyoid portion (D14.1)
    - **DEF:** Oropharynx: Middle portion of pharynx (throat); communicates with the oral cavity, nasopharynx and laryngopharynx.
  - **D10.6** Benign neoplasm of nasopharynx
    - Benign neoplasm of pharyngeal tonsil
    - Benign neoplasm of posterior margin of septum and choanae
    - **DEF:** Nasopharynx: Upper portion of pharynx (throat); communicates with the nasal cavities, oropharynx and tympanic cavities.
  - **D10.7** Benign neoplasm of hypopharynx
    - **DEF:** Hypopharynx: Lower portion of pharynx (throat); communicates with the oropharynx and the esophagus.
    - **Synonym(s):** laryngopharynx.
  - **D10.9** Benign neoplasm of pharynx, unspecified
- ✓4th **D11** Benign neoplasm of major salivary glands
  - EXCLUDES 1
    - benign neoplasms of specified minor salivary glands which are classified according to their anatomical location
    - benign neoplasms of minor salivary glands NOS (D10.39)
  - **D11.0** Benign neoplasm of parotid gland
  - **D11.7** Benign neoplasm of other major salivary glands
    - Benign neoplasm of sublingual salivary gland
    - Benign neoplasm of submandibular salivary gland
  - **D11.9** Benign neoplasm of major salivary gland, unspecified
- ✓4th **D12** Benign neoplasm of colon, rectum, anus and anal canal
  - EXCLUDES 2
    - benign carcinoid tumors of the large intestine, and rectum (D3A.02-)
    - polyp of colon NOS (K63.5)
  - **AHA:** 2018,2Q,14; 2017,1Q,15; 2015,2Q,14
  - **TIP:** Code K63.5 Polyp of colon, is assigned when documentation states hyperplastic colon polyps, regardless of the site in the colon. Slow-growing, hyperplastic polyps are not precancerous and are classified differently from benign or adenomatous polyps.
  - **D12.0** Benign neoplasm of cecum
    - Benign neoplasm of ileocecal valve
  - **D12.1** Benign neoplasm of appendix
    - EXCLUDES 1 benign carcinoid tumor of the appendix (D3A.020)
  - **D12.2** Benign neoplasm of ascending colon
  - **D12.3** Benign neoplasm of transverse colon
    - Benign neoplasm of hepatic flexure
    - Benign neoplasm of splenic flexure
    - **AHA:** 2017,1Q,16
  - **D12.4** Benign neoplasm of descending colon
  - **D12.5** Benign neoplasm of sigmoid colon

D12.6 Benign neoplasm of colon, unspecified
Adenomatosis of colon
Benign neoplasm of large intestine NOS
Polyposis (hereditary) of colon
EXCLUDES 1 ~~inflammatory polyp of colon (K51.4-)~~
EXCLUDES 2 ▶inflammatory polyp of colon (K51.4-)◀

D12.7 Benign neoplasm of rectosigmoid junction

D12.8 Benign neoplasm of rectum
EXCLUDES 1 benign carcinoid tumor of the rectum (D3A.026)
AHA: 2018,1Q,6

D12.9 Benign neoplasm of anus and anal canal
Benign neoplasm of anus NOS
EXCLUDES 1 benign neoplasm of anal margin (D22.5, D23.5)
benign neoplasm of anal skin (D22.5, D23.5)
benign neoplasm of perianal skin (D22.5, D23.5)

✓4th **D13 Benign neoplasm of other and ill-defined parts of digestive system**
EXCLUDES 1 benign stromal tumors of digestive system (D21.4)

D13.0 Benign neoplasm of esophagus

D13.1 Benign neoplasm of stomach
EXCLUDES 1 benign carcinoid tumor of the stomach (D3A.092)

D13.2 Benign neoplasm of duodenum
EXCLUDES 1 benign carcinoid tumor of the duodenum (D3A.010)

✓5th **D13.3 Benign neoplasm of other and unspecified parts of small intestine**
EXCLUDES 1 benign carcinoid tumors of the small intestine (D3A.01-)
benign neoplasm of ileocecal valve (D12.0)

    D13.30 Benign neoplasm of unspecified part of small intestine

    D13.39 Benign neoplasm of other parts of small intestine

D13.4 Benign neoplasm of liver
Benign neoplasm of intrahepatic bile ducts

D13.5 Benign neoplasm of extrahepatic bile ducts

D13.6 Benign neoplasm of pancreas
EXCLUDES 1 benign neoplasm of endocrine pancreas (D13.7)

D13.7 Benign neoplasm of endocrine pancreas
Benign neoplasm of islets of Langerhans
Islet cell tumor
Use additional code to identify any functional activity

✓5th **D13.9 Benign neoplasm of ill-defined sites within the digestive system**
AHA: 2023,4Q,4-5

    D13.91 Familial adenomatous polyposis
Code also associated conditions, such as:
benign neoplasm of colon (D12.6)
malignant neoplasm of colon (C18.-)

    D13.99 Benign neoplasm of ill-defined sites within the digestive system
Benign neoplasm of digestive system NOS
Benign neoplasm of intestine NOS
Benign neoplasm of spleen

✓4th **D14 Benign neoplasm of middle ear and respiratory system**

D14.0 Benign neoplasm of middle ear, nasal cavity and accessory sinuses
Benign neoplasm of cartilage of nose
EXCLUDES 1 benign neoplasm of auricular canal (external) (D22.2-, D23.2-)
benign neoplasm of bone of ear (D16.4)
benign neoplasm of bone of nose (D16.4)
benign neoplasm of cartilage of ear (D21.0)
benign neoplasm of ear (external)(skin) (D22.2-, D23.2-)
benign neoplasm of nose NOS (D36.7)
benign neoplasm of olfactory bulb (D33.3)
benign neoplasm of posterior margin of septum and choanae (D10.6)
benign neoplasm of skin of nose (D22.39, D23.39)
polyp of accessory sinus (J33.8)
polyp of ear (middle) (H74.4)
polyp of nasal (cavity) (J33.-)

D14.1 Benign neoplasm of larynx
Adenomatous polyp of larynx
Benign neoplasm of epiglottis (suprahyoid portion)
EXCLUDES 1 benign neoplasm of epiglottis, anterior aspect (D10.5)
polyp (nonadenomatous) of vocal cord or larynx (J38.1)

D14.2 Benign neoplasm of trachea

✓5th **D14.3 Benign neoplasm of bronchus and lung**
EXCLUDES 1 benign carcinoid tumor of the bronchus and lung (D3A.090)

    D14.30 Benign neoplasm of unspecified bronchus and lung

    D14.31 Benign neoplasm of right bronchus and lung

    D14.32 Benign neoplasm of left bronchus and lung

D14.4 Benign neoplasm of respiratory system, unspecified

✓4th **D15 Benign neoplasm of other and unspecified intrathoracic organs**
EXCLUDES 1 benign neoplasm of mesothelial tissue (D19.-)

D15.0 Benign neoplasm of thymus
EXCLUDES 1 benign carcinoid tumor of the thymus (D3A.091)

D15.1 Benign neoplasm of heart
EXCLUDES 1 benign neoplasm of great vessels (D21.3)

D15.2 Benign neoplasm of mediastinum
AHA: 2024,3Q,3

D15.7 Benign neoplasm of other specified intrathoracic organs

D15.9 Benign neoplasm of intrathoracic organ, unspecified

✓4th **D16 Benign neoplasm of bone and articular cartilage**
EXCLUDES 1 benign neoplasm of connective tissue of ear (D21.0)
benign neoplasm of connective tissue of eyelid (D21.0)
benign neoplasm of connective tissue of larynx (D14.1)
benign neoplasm of connective tissue of nose (D14.0)
benign neoplasm of synovia (D21.-)

✓5th **D16.0 Benign neoplasm of scapula and long bones of upper limb**

    D16.00 Benign neoplasm of scapula and long bones of unspecified upper limb

    D16.01 Benign neoplasm of scapula and long bones of right upper limb

    D16.02 Benign neoplasm of scapula and long bones of left upper limb

✓5th **D16.1 Benign neoplasm of short bones of upper limb**

    D16.10 Benign neoplasm of short bones of unspecified upper limb

    D16.11 Benign neoplasm of short bones of right upper limb

    D16.12 Benign neoplasm of short bones of left upper limb

✓5th **D16.2 Benign neoplasm of long bones of lower limb**

    D16.20 Benign neoplasm of long bones of unspecified lower limb

    D16.21 Benign neoplasm of long bones of right lower limb

    D16.22 Benign neoplasm of long bones of left lower limb

✓5th **D16.3 Benign neoplasm of short bones of lower limb**

    D16.30 Benign neoplasm of short bones of unspecified lower limb

    D16.31 Benign neoplasm of short bones of right lower limb

    D16.32 Benign neoplasm of short bones of left lower limb

D16.4 Benign neoplasm of bones of skull and face
Benign neoplasm of maxilla (superior)
Benign neoplasm of orbital bone
Keratocyst of maxilla
Keratocystic odontogenic tumor of maxilla
EXCLUDES 2 benign neoplasm of lower jaw bone (D16.5)

D16.5 Benign neoplasm of lower jaw bone
Keratocyst of mandible
Keratocystic odontogenic tumor of mandible

D16.6 Benign neoplasm of vertebral column
EXCLUDES 1 benign neoplasm of sacrum and coccyx (D16.8)

D16.7 Benign neoplasm of ribs, sternum and clavicle

D16.8 Benign neoplasm of pelvic bones, sacrum and coccyx

D16.9 Benign neoplasm of bone and articular cartilage, unspecified

✓4th **D17 Benign lipomatous neoplasm**

D17.0 Benign lipomatous neoplasm of skin and subcutaneous tissue of head, face and neck

D17.1 Benign lipomatous neoplasm of skin and subcutaneous tissue of trunk

✓5th **D17.2 Benign lipomatous neoplasm of skin and subcutaneous tissue of limb**

    D17.20 Benign lipomatous neoplasm of skin and subcutaneous tissue of unspecified limb

    D17.21 Benign lipomatous neoplasm of skin and subcutaneous tissue of right arm

    D17.22 Benign lipomatous neoplasm of skin and subcutaneous tissue of left arm

    D17.23 Benign lipomatous neoplasm of skin and subcutaneous tissue of right leg

    D17.24 Benign lipomatous neoplasm of skin and subcutaneous tissue of left leg

✓5th **D17.3 Benign lipomatous neoplasm of skin and subcutaneous tissue of other and unspecified sites**

    D17.30 Benign lipomatous neoplasm of skin and subcutaneous tissue of unspecified sites

    D17.39 Benign lipomatous neoplasm of skin and subcutaneous tissue of other sites

Chapter 2. Neoplasms

- **D17.4** Benign lipomatous neoplasm of intrathoracic organs
- **D17.5** Benign lipomatous neoplasm of intra-abdominal organs
  - EXCLUDES 1 benign lipomatous neoplasm of peritoneum and retroperitoneum (D17.79)
- **D17.6** Benign lipomatous neoplasm of spermatic cord
- ✓5th **D17.7** Benign lipomatous neoplasm of other sites
  - **D17.71** Benign lipomatous neoplasm of kidney
  - **D17.72** Benign lipomatous neoplasm of other genitourinary organ
  - **D17.79** Benign lipomatous neoplasm of other sites
    - Benign lipomatous neoplasm of peritoneum
    - Benign lipomatous neoplasm of retroperitoneum
- **D17.9** Benign lipomatous neoplasm, unspecified
  - Lipoma NOS
- ✓4th **D18** Hemangioma and lymphangioma, any site
  - EXCLUDES 1 benign neoplasm of glomus jugulare (D35.6)
    - blue or pigmented nevus (D22.-)
    - nevus NOS (D22.-)
    - vascular nevus (Q82.5)
  - ✓5th **D18.0** Hemangioma
    - Angioma NOS
    - Cavernous nevus
    - **DEF:** Common benign tumor usually occurring in infancy that is composed of newly formed blood vessels due to malformation of the angioblastic tissue.
    - **D18.00** Hemangioma unspecified site
    - **D18.01** Hemangioma of skin and subcutaneous tissue
    - **D18.02** Hemangioma of intracranial structures HCC Rx ESR COM
    - **D18.03** Hemangioma of intra-abdominal structures
    - **D18.09** Hemangioma of other sites
  - **D18.1** Lymphangioma, any site
    - AHA: 2018,3Q,31; 2018,2Q,13
- ✓4th **D19** Benign neoplasm of mesothelial tissue
  - **D19.0** Benign neoplasm of mesothelial tissue of pleura
  - **D19.1** Benign neoplasm of mesothelial tissue of peritoneum
  - **D19.7** Benign neoplasm of mesothelial tissue of other sites
  - **D19.9** Benign neoplasm of mesothelial tissue, unspecified
    - Benign mesothelioma NOS
- ✓4th **D20** Benign neoplasm of soft tissue of retroperitoneum and peritoneum
  - EXCLUDES 1 benign lipomatous neoplasm of peritoneum and retroperitoneum (D17.79)
    - benign neoplasm of mesothelial tissue (D19.-)
  - **D20.0** Benign neoplasm of soft tissue of retroperitoneum
  - **D20.1** Benign neoplasm of soft tissue of peritoneum
- ✓4th **D21** Other benign neoplasms of connective and other soft tissue
  - INCLUDES benign neoplasm of blood vessel
    - benign neoplasm of bursa
    - benign neoplasm of cartilage
    - benign neoplasm of fascia
    - benign neoplasm of fat
    - benign neoplasm of ligament, except uterine
    - benign neoplasm of lymphatic channel
    - benign neoplasm of muscle
    - benign neoplasm of synovia
    - benign neoplasm of tendon (sheath)
    - benign stromal tumors
  - EXCLUDES 1 benign neoplasm of articular cartilage (D16.-)
    - benign neoplasm of cartilage of larynx (D14.1)
    - benign neoplasm of cartilage of nose (D14.0)
    - benign neoplasm of connective tissue of breast (D24.-)
    - benign neoplasm of peripheral nerves and autonomic nervous system (D36.1-)
    - benign neoplasm of peritoneum (D20.1)
    - benign neoplasm of retroperitoneum (D20.0)
    - benign neoplasm of uterine ligament, any (D28.2)
    - benign neoplasm of vascular tissue (D18.-)
    - hemangioma (D18.0-)
    - lipomatous neoplasm (D17.-)
    - lymphangioma (D18.1)
    - uterine leiomyoma (D25.-)
  - **D21.0** Benign neoplasm of connective and other soft tissue of head, face and neck
    - Benign neoplasm of connective tissue of ear
    - Benign neoplasm of connective tissue of eyelid
    - EXCLUDES 1 benign neoplasm of connective tissue of orbit (D31.6-)
  - ✓5th **D21.1** Benign neoplasm of connective and other soft tissue of upper limb, including shoulder
    - **D21.10** Benign neoplasm of connective and other soft tissue of unspecified upper limb, including shoulder
    - **D21.11** Benign neoplasm of connective and other soft tissue of right upper limb, including shoulder
    - **D21.12** Benign neoplasm of connective and other soft tissue of left upper limb, including shoulder
  - ✓5th **D21.2** Benign neoplasm of connective and other soft tissue of lower limb, including hip
    - **D21.20** Benign neoplasm of connective and other soft tissue of unspecified lower limb, including hip
    - **D21.21** Benign neoplasm of connective and other soft tissue of right lower limb, including hip
    - **D21.22** Benign neoplasm of connective and other soft tissue of left lower limb, including hip
  - **D21.3** Benign neoplasm of connective and other soft tissue of thorax
    - Benign neoplasm of axilla
    - Benign neoplasm of diaphragm
    - Benign neoplasm of great vessels
    - EXCLUDES 1 benign neoplasm of heart (D15.1)
      - benign neoplasm of mediastinum (D15.2)
      - benign neoplasm of thymus (D15.0)
  - **D21.4** Benign neoplasm of connective and other soft tissue of abdomen
    - Benign stromal tumors of abdomen
  - **D21.5** Benign neoplasm of connective and other soft tissue of pelvis
    - EXCLUDES 1 benign neoplasm of any uterine ligament (D28.2)
      - uterine leiomyoma (D25.-)
  - **D21.6** Benign neoplasm of connective and other soft tissue of trunk, unspecified
    - Benign neoplasm of connective and other soft tissue of back NOS
  - **D21.9** Benign neoplasm of connective and other soft tissue, unspecified
- ✓4th **D22** Melanocytic nevi
  - INCLUDES atypical nevus
    - blue hairy pigmented nevus
    - nevus NOS
  - **D22.0** Melanocytic nevi of lip
  - ✓5th **D22.1** Melanocytic nevi of eyelid, including canthus
    - AHA: 2018,4Q,4
    - **D22.10** Melanocytic nevi of unspecified eyelid, including canthus
    - ✓6th **D22.11** Melanocytic nevi of right eyelid, including canthus
      - **D22.111** Melanocytic nevi of right upper eyelid, including canthus
      - **D22.112** Melanocytic nevi of right lower eyelid, including canthus
    - ✓6th **D22.12** Melanocytic nevi of left eyelid, including canthus
      - **D22.121** Melanocytic nevi of left upper eyelid, including canthus
      - **D22.122** Melanocytic nevi of left lower eyelid, including canthus
  - ✓5th **D22.2** Melanocytic nevi of ear and external auricular canal
    - **D22.20** Melanocytic nevi of unspecified ear and external auricular canal
    - **D22.21** Melanocytic nevi of right ear and external auricular canal
    - **D22.22** Melanocytic nevi of left ear and external auricular canal
  - ✓5th **D22.3** Melanocytic nevi of other and unspecified parts of face
    - **D22.30** Melanocytic nevi of unspecified part of face
    - **D22.39** Melanocytic nevi of other parts of face
  - **D22.4** Melanocytic nevi of scalp and neck
  - **D22.5** Melanocytic nevi of trunk
    - Melanocytic nevi of anal margin
    - Melanocytic nevi of anal skin
    - Melanocytic nevi of perianal skin
    - Melanocytic nevi of skin of breast
  - ✓5th **D22.6** Melanocytic nevi of upper limb, including shoulder
    - **D22.60** Melanocytic nevi of unspecified upper limb, including shoulder
    - **D22.61** Melanocytic nevi of right upper limb, including shoulder
    - **D22.62** Melanocytic nevi of left upper limb, including shoulder
  - ✓5th **D22.7** Melanocytic nevi of lower limb, including hip
    - **D22.70** Melanocytic nevi of unspecified lower limb, including hip

---

HCC CMS-HCC Rx Rx HCC ESR ESRD HCC COM Commercial HCC N Newborn: 0 P Pediatric: 0-17 M Maternity: 9-64 A Adult: 15-124

D22.71 Melanocytic nevi of right lower limb, including hip
D22.72 Melanocytic nevi of left lower limb, including hip
D22.9 Melanocytic nevi, unspecified

D23 Other benign neoplasms of skin
INCLUDES:
benign neoplasm of hair follicles
benign neoplasm of sebaceous glands
benign neoplasm of sweat glands
EXCLUDES 1: benign lipomatous neoplasms of skin (D17.0-D17.3)
EXCLUDES 2: melanocytic nevi (D22.-)

D23.0 Other benign neoplasm of skin of lip
  EXCLUDES 1: benign neoplasm of vermilion border of lip (D10.0)

D23.1 Other benign neoplasm of skin of eyelid, including canthus
  AHA: 2018,4Q,4
  D23.10 Other benign neoplasm of skin of unspecified eyelid, including canthus
  D23.11 Other benign neoplasm of skin of right eyelid, including canthus
    D23.111 Other benign neoplasm of skin of right upper eyelid, including canthus
    D23.112 Other benign neoplasm of skin of right lower eyelid, including canthus
  D23.12 Other benign neoplasm of skin of left eyelid, including canthus
    D23.121 Other benign neoplasm of skin of left upper eyelid, including canthus
    D23.122 Other benign neoplasm of skin of left lower eyelid, including canthus

D23.2 Other benign neoplasm of skin of ear and external auricular canal
  D23.20 Other benign neoplasm of skin of unspecified ear and external auricular canal
  D23.21 Other benign neoplasm of skin of right ear and external auricular canal
  D23.22 Other benign neoplasm of skin of left ear and external auricular canal

D23.3 Other benign neoplasm of skin of other and unspecified parts of face
  D23.30 Other benign neoplasm of skin of unspecified part of face
  D23.39 Other benign neoplasm of skin of other parts of face

D23.4 Other benign neoplasm of skin of scalp and neck

D23.5 Other benign neoplasm of skin of trunk
  Other benign neoplasm of anal margin
  Other benign neoplasm of anal skin
  Other benign neoplasm of perianal skin
  Other benign neoplasm of skin of breast
  EXCLUDES 1: benign neoplasm of anus NOS (D12.9)

D23.6 Other benign neoplasm of skin of upper limb, including shoulder
  D23.60 Other benign neoplasm of skin of unspecified upper limb, including shoulder
  D23.61 Other benign neoplasm of skin of right upper limb, including shoulder
  D23.62 Other benign neoplasm of skin of left upper limb, including shoulder

D23.7 Other benign neoplasm of skin of lower limb, including hip
  D23.70 Other benign neoplasm of skin of unspecified lower limb, including hip
  D23.71 Other benign neoplasm of skin of right lower limb, including hip
  D23.72 Other benign neoplasm of skin of left lower limb, including hip

D23.9 Other benign neoplasm of skin, unspecified

D24 Benign neoplasm of breast
INCLUDES:
benign neoplasm of connective tissue of breast
benign neoplasm of soft parts of breast
fibroadenoma of breast
EXCLUDES 2:
adenofibrosis of breast (N60.2)
benign cyst of breast (N60.-)
benign mammary dysplasia (N60.-)
benign neoplasm of skin of breast (D22.5, D23.5)
fibrocystic disease of breast (N60.-)

D24.1 Benign neoplasm of right breast
D24.2 Benign neoplasm of left breast
D24.9 Benign neoplasm of unspecified breast

D25 Leiomyoma of uterus
INCLUDES:
uterine fibroid
uterine fibromyoma
uterine myoma

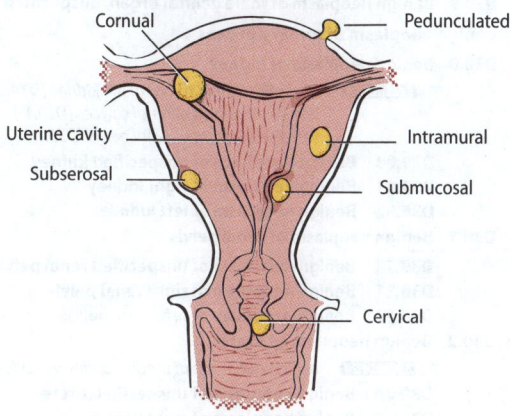
Uterine Leiomyomas (Fibroids)

D25.0 Submucous leiomyoma of uterus
D25.1 Intramural leiomyoma of uterus
  Interstitial leiomyoma of uterus
D25.2 Subserosal leiomyoma of uterus
  Subperitoneal leiomyoma of uterus
D25.9 Leiomyoma of uterus, unspecified

D26 Other benign neoplasms of uterus
D26.0 Other benign neoplasm of cervix uteri
D26.1 Other benign neoplasm of corpus uteri
D26.7 Other benign neoplasm of other parts of uterus
D26.9 Other benign neoplasm of uterus, unspecified

D27 Benign neoplasm of ovary
Use additional code to identify any functional activity
EXCLUDES 2:
corpus albicans cyst (N83.2-)
corpus luteum cyst (N83.1-)
endometrial cyst (N80.1-)
follicular (atretic) cyst (N83.0-)
graafian follicle cyst (N83.0-)
ovarian cyst NEC (N83.2-)
ovarian retention cyst (N83.2-)

D27.0 Benign neoplasm of right ovary
D27.1 Benign neoplasm of left ovary
D27.9 Benign neoplasm of unspecified ovary

D28 Benign neoplasm of other and unspecified female genital organs
INCLUDES:
adenomatous polyp
benign neoplasm of skin of female genital organs
benign teratoma
EXCLUDES 1:
epoophoron cyst (Q50.5)
fimbrial cyst (Q50.4)
Gartner's duct cyst (Q52.4)
parovarian cyst (Q50.5)

D28.0 Benign neoplasm of vulva
D28.1 Benign neoplasm of vagina
D28.2 Benign neoplasm of uterine tubes and ligaments
  Benign neoplasm of fallopian tube
  Benign neoplasm of uterine ligament (broad) (round)
D28.7 Benign neoplasm of other specified female genital organs
D28.9 Benign neoplasm of female genital organ, unspecified

D29 Benign neoplasm of male genital organs
INCLUDES: benign neoplasm of skin of male genital organs

D29.0 Benign neoplasm of penis
D29.1 Benign neoplasm of prostate
  EXCLUDES 1: enlarged prostate (N40.-)
D29.2 Benign neoplasm of testis
  Use additional code to identify any functional activity
  D29.20 Benign neoplasm of unspecified testis
  D29.21 Benign neoplasm of right testis
  D29.22 Benign neoplasm of left testis
D29.3 Benign neoplasm of epididymis
  D29.30 Benign neoplasm of unspecified epididymis
  D29.31 Benign neoplasm of right epididymis
  D29.32 Benign neoplasm of left epididymis

Chapter 2. Neoplasms

- **D29.4** Benign neoplasm of scrotum
  - Benign neoplasm of skin of scrotum
- **D29.8** Benign neoplasm of other specified male genital organs
  - Benign neoplasm of seminal vesicle
  - Benign neoplasm of spermatic cord
  - Benign neoplasm of tunica vaginalis
- **D29.9** Benign neoplasm of male genital organ, unspecified

- ✓4th **D30** Benign neoplasm of urinary organs
  - ✓5th **D30.0** Benign neoplasm of kidney
    - EXCLUDES 1: benign carcinoid tumor of the kidney (D3A.093)
      benign neoplasm of renal calyces (D30.1-)
      benign neoplasm of renal pelvis (D30.1-)
    - **D30.00** Benign neoplasm of unspecified kidney
    - **D30.01** Benign neoplasm of right kidney
    - **D30.02** Benign neoplasm of left kidney
  - ✓5th **D30.1** Benign neoplasm of renal pelvis
    - **D30.10** Benign neoplasm of unspecified renal pelvis
    - **D30.11** Benign neoplasm of right renal pelvis
    - **D30.12** Benign neoplasm of left renal pelvis
  - ✓5th **D30.2** Benign neoplasm of ureter
    - EXCLUDES 1: benign neoplasm of ureteric orifice of bladder (D30.3)
    - **D30.20** Benign neoplasm of unspecified ureter
    - **D30.21** Benign neoplasm of right ureter
    - **D30.22** Benign neoplasm of left ureter
  - **D30.3** Benign neoplasm of bladder
    - Benign neoplasm of ureteric orifice of bladder
    - Benign neoplasm of urethral orifice of bladder
  - **D30.4** Benign neoplasm of urethra
    - EXCLUDES 1: benign neoplasm of urethral orifice of bladder (D30.3)
  - **D30.8** Benign neoplasm of other specified urinary organs
    - Benign neoplasm of paraurethral glands
  - **D30.9** Benign neoplasm of urinary organ, unspecified
    - Benign neoplasm of urinary system NOS

- ✓4th **D31** Benign neoplasm of eye and adnexa
  - EXCLUDES 1: benign neoplasm of connective tissue of eyelid (D21.0)
    benign neoplasm of optic nerve (D33.3)
    benign neoplasm of skin of eyelid (D22.1-, D23.1-)
  - ✓5th **D31.0** Benign neoplasm of conjunctiva
    - **D31.00** Benign neoplasm of unspecified conjunctiva
    - **D31.01** Benign neoplasm of right conjunctiva
    - **D31.02** Benign neoplasm of left conjunctiva
  - ✓5th **D31.1** Benign neoplasm of cornea
    - **D31.10** Benign neoplasm of unspecified cornea
    - **D31.11** Benign neoplasm of right cornea
    - **D31.12** Benign neoplasm of left cornea
  - ✓5th **D31.2** Benign neoplasm of retina
    - EXCLUDES 1: dark area on retina (D49.81)
      hemangioma of retina (D49.81)
      neoplasm of unspecified behavior of retina and choroid (D49.81)
      retinal freckle (D49.81)
    - **D31.20** Benign neoplasm of unspecified retina
    - **D31.21** Benign neoplasm of right retina
    - **D31.22** Benign neoplasm of left retina
  - ✓5th **D31.3** Benign neoplasm of choroid
    - **D31.30** Benign neoplasm of unspecified choroid
    - **D31.31** Benign neoplasm of right choroid
    - **D31.32** Benign neoplasm of left choroid
  - ✓5th **D31.4** Benign neoplasm of ciliary body
    - **D31.40** Benign neoplasm of unspecified ciliary body
    - **D31.41** Benign neoplasm of right ciliary body
    - **D31.42** Benign neoplasm of left ciliary body
  - ✓5th **D31.5** Benign neoplasm of lacrimal gland and duct
    - Benign neoplasm of lacrimal sac
    - Benign neoplasm of nasolacrimal duct
    - **D31.50** Benign neoplasm of unspecified lacrimal gland and duct
    - **D31.51** Benign neoplasm of right lacrimal gland and duct
    - **D31.52** Benign neoplasm of left lacrimal gland and duct
  - ✓5th **D31.6** Benign neoplasm of unspecified site of orbit
    - Benign neoplasm of connective tissue of orbit
    - Benign neoplasm of extraocular muscle
    - Benign neoplasm of peripheral nerves of orbit
    - Benign neoplasm of retrobulbar tissue
    - Benign neoplasm of retro-ocular tissue
    - EXCLUDES 1: benign neoplasm of orbital bone (D16.4)
    - **D31.60** Benign neoplasm of unspecified site of unspecified orbit
    - **D31.61** Benign neoplasm of unspecified site of right orbit
    - **D31.62** Benign neoplasm of unspecified site of left orbit
  - ✓5th **D31.9** Benign neoplasm of unspecified part of eye
    - Benign neoplasm of eyeball
    - **D31.90** Benign neoplasm of unspecified part of unspecified eye
    - **D31.91** Benign neoplasm of unspecified part of right eye
    - **D31.92** Benign neoplasm of unspecified part of left eye

- ✓4th **D32** Benign neoplasm of meninges
  - **D32.0** Benign neoplasm of cerebral meninges HCC Rx ESR COM
  - **D32.1** Benign neoplasm of spinal meninges HCC Rx ESR COM
  - **D32.9** Benign neoplasm of meninges, unspecified HCC Rx ESR COM
    - Meningioma NOS

- ✓4th **D33** Benign neoplasm of brain and other parts of central nervous system
  - EXCLUDES 1: angioma (D18.0-)
    benign neoplasm of meninges (D32.-)
    benign neoplasm of peripheral nerves and autonomic nervous system (D36.1-)
    hemangioma (D18.0-)
    neurofibromatosis (Q85.0-)
    retro-ocular neoplasm (D31.6-)
  - **D33.0** Benign neoplasm of brain, supratentorial HCC Rx ESR COM
    - Benign neoplasm of cerebral ventricle
    - Benign neoplasm of cerebrum
    - Benign neoplasm of frontal lobe
    - Benign neoplasm of occipital lobe
    - Benign neoplasm of parietal lobe
    - Benign neoplasm of temporal lobe
    - EXCLUDES 1: benign neoplasm of fourth ventricle (D33.1)
  - **D33.1** Benign neoplasm of brain, infratentorial HCC Rx ESR COM
    - Benign neoplasm of brain stem
    - Benign neoplasm of cerebellum
    - Benign neoplasm of fourth ventricle
  - **D33.2** Benign neoplasm of brain, unspecified HCC Rx ESR COM
  - **D33.3** Benign neoplasm of cranial nerves HCC Rx ESR COM
    - Benign neoplasm of olfactory bulb
  - **D33.4** Benign neoplasm of spinal cord HCC Rx ESR COM
  - **D33.7** Benign neoplasm of other specified parts of central nervous system HCC Rx ESR COM
  - **D33.9** Benign neoplasm of central nervous system, unspecified HCC Rx ESR COM
    - Benign neoplasm of nervous system (central) NOS

- **D34** Benign neoplasm of thyroid gland
  - Use additional code to identify any functional activity

- ✓4th **D35** Benign neoplasm of other and unspecified endocrine glands
  - Use additional code to identify any functional activity
  - EXCLUDES 1: benign neoplasm of endocrine pancreas (D13.7)
    benign neoplasm of ovary (D27.-)
    benign neoplasm of testis (D29.2-)
    benign neoplasm of thymus (D15.0)
  - ✓5th **D35.0** Benign neoplasm of adrenal gland
    - **D35.00** Benign neoplasm of unspecified adrenal gland
    - **D35.01** Benign neoplasm of right adrenal gland
    - **D35.02** Benign neoplasm of left adrenal gland
  - **D35.1** Benign neoplasm of parathyroid gland
  - **D35.2** Benign neoplasm of pituitary gland HCC Rx ESR COM
    - AHA: 2014,3Q,22
  - **D35.3** Benign neoplasm of craniopharyngeal duct HCC Rx ESR COM
  - **D35.4** Benign neoplasm of pineal gland HCC Rx ESR COM
  - **D35.5** Benign neoplasm of carotid body
  - **D35.6** Benign neoplasm of aortic body and other paraganglia
    - Benign tumor of glomus jugulare
  - **D35.7** Benign neoplasm of other specified endocrine glands
  - **D35.9** Benign neoplasm of endocrine gland, unspecified
    - Benign neoplasm of unspecified endocrine gland

Chapter 2. Neoplasms

✓4th D36 Benign neoplasm of other and unspecified sites

- **D36.0** Benign neoplasm of lymph nodes
  - EXCLUDES 1: lymphangioma (D18.1)
- **✓5th D36.1** Benign neoplasm of peripheral nerves and autonomic nervous system
  - EXCLUDES 1: benign neoplasm of peripheral nerves of orbit (D31.6-)
    neurofibromatosis (Q85.0-)
  - **D36.10** Benign neoplasm of peripheral nerves and autonomic nervous system, unspecified
  - **D36.11** Benign neoplasm of peripheral nerves and autonomic nervous system of face, head, and neck
  - **D36.12** Benign neoplasm of peripheral nerves and autonomic nervous system, upper limb, including shoulder
  - **D36.13** Benign neoplasm of peripheral nerves and autonomic nervous system of lower limb, including hip
  - **D36.14** Benign neoplasm of peripheral nerves and autonomic nervous system of thorax
  - **D36.15** Benign neoplasm of peripheral nerves and autonomic nervous system of abdomen
  - **D36.16** Benign neoplasm of peripheral nerves and autonomic nervous system of pelvis
  - **D36.17** Benign neoplasm of peripheral nerves and autonomic nervous system of trunk, unspecified
- **D36.7** Benign neoplasm of other specified sites
  - Benign neoplasm of back NOS
  - Benign neoplasm of nose NOS
- **D36.9** Benign neoplasm, unspecified site

Benign neuroendocrine tumors (D3A)

✓4th D3A Benign neuroendocrine tumors

Code also any associated multiple endocrine neoplasia [MEN] syndromes (E31.2-)
Use additional code to identify any associated endocrine syndrome, such as:
carcinoid syndrome (E34.00)

EXCLUDES 2: benign pancreatic islet cell tumors (D13.7)

- **✓5th D3A.0 Benign carcinoid tumors**
  - **DEF:** Specific type of slow-growing neuroendocrine tumors. Carcinoid tumors occur most commonly in the hormone producing cells of the gastrointestinal tracts and can also occur in the pancreas, testes, ovaries, or lungs.
  - **D3A.00** Benign carcinoid tumor of unspecified site [HCC] [Rx]
    - Carcinoid tumor NOS
  - **✓6th D3A.01** Benign carcinoid tumors of the small intestine
    - **D3A.010** Benign carcinoid tumor of the duodenum [HCC] [Rx]
    - **D3A.011** Benign carcinoid tumor of the jejunum [HCC] [Rx]
    - **D3A.012** Benign carcinoid tumor of the ileum [HCC] [Rx]
    - **D3A.019** Benign carcinoid tumor of the small intestine, unspecified portion [HCC] [Rx]
  - **✓6th D3A.02** Benign carcinoid tumors of the appendix, large intestine, and rectum
    - **D3A.020** Benign carcinoid tumor of the appendix [HCC] [Rx]
    - **D3A.021** Benign carcinoid tumor of the cecum [HCC] [Rx]
    - **D3A.022** Benign carcinoid tumor of the ascending colon [HCC] [Rx]
    - **D3A.023** Benign carcinoid tumor of the transverse colon [HCC] [Rx]
    - **D3A.024** Benign carcinoid tumor of the descending colon [HCC] [Rx]
    - **D3A.025** Benign carcinoid tumor of the sigmoid colon [HCC] [Rx]
    - **D3A.026** Benign carcinoid tumor of the rectum [HCC] [Rx]
    - **D3A.029** Benign carcinoid tumor of the large intestine, unspecified portion [HCC] [Rx]
      - Benign carcinoid tumor of the colon NOS
  - **✓6th D3A.09** Benign carcinoid tumors of other sites
    - **D3A.090** Benign carcinoid tumor of the bronchus and lung [HCC] [Rx]
    - **D3A.091** Benign carcinoid tumor of the thymus [HCC] [Rx]
    - **D3A.092** Benign carcinoid tumor of the stomach [HCC] [Rx]
    - **D3A.093** Benign carcinoid tumor of the kidney [HCC] [Rx]
    - **D3A.094** Benign carcinoid tumor of the foregut, unspecified [HCC] [Rx]
    - **D3A.095** Benign carcinoid tumor of the midgut, unspecified [HCC] [Rx]
    - **D3A.096** Benign carcinoid tumor of the hindgut, unspecified [HCC] [Rx]
    - **D3A.098** Benign carcinoid tumors of other sites [HCC] [Rx]
  - **D3A.8** Other benign neuroendocrine tumors [HCC] [Rx]
    - Neuroendocrine tumor NOS

Neoplasms of uncertain behavior, polycythemia vera and myelodysplastic syndromes (D37-D48)

NOTE: Categories D37-D44, and D48 classify by site neoplasms of uncertain behavior, i.e., histologic confirmation whether the neoplasm is malignant or benign cannot be made.

EXCLUDES 1: neoplasms of unspecified behavior (D49.-)

✓4th D37 Neoplasm of uncertain behavior of oral cavity and digestive organs

EXCLUDES 1: stromal tumors of uncertain behavior of digestive system (D48.1-)

- **✓5th D37.0 Neoplasm of uncertain behavior of lip, oral cavity and pharynx**
  - EXCLUDES 1: neoplasm of uncertain behavior of aryepiglottic fold or interarytenoid fold, laryngeal aspect (D38.0)
    neoplasm of uncertain behavior of epiglottis NOS (D38.0)
    neoplasm of uncertain behavior of skin of lip (D48.5)
    neoplasm of uncertain behavior of suprahyoid portion of epiglottis (D38.0)
  - **D37.01** Neoplasm of uncertain behavior of lip
    - Neoplasm of uncertain behavior of vermilion border of lip
  - **D37.02** Neoplasm of uncertain behavior of tongue
  - **✓6th D37.03** Neoplasm of uncertain behavior of the major salivary glands
    - **D37.030** Neoplasm of uncertain behavior of the parotid salivary glands
    - **D37.031** Neoplasm of uncertain behavior of the sublingual salivary glands
    - **D37.032** Neoplasm of uncertain behavior of the submandibular salivary glands
    - **D37.039** Neoplasm of uncertain behavior of the major salivary glands, unspecified
  - **D37.04** Neoplasm of uncertain behavior of the minor salivary glands
    - Neoplasm of uncertain behavior of submucosal salivary glands of cheek
    - Neoplasm of uncertain behavior of submucosal salivary glands of hard palate
    - Neoplasm of uncertain behavior of submucosal salivary glands of lip
    - Neoplasm of uncertain behavior of submucosal salivary glands of soft palate
  - **D37.05** Neoplasm of uncertain behavior of pharynx
    - Neoplasm of uncertain behavior of aryepiglottic fold of pharynx NOS
    - Neoplasm of uncertain behavior of hypopharyngeal aspect of aryepiglottic fold of pharynx
    - Neoplasm of uncertain behavior of marginal zone of aryepiglottic fold of pharynx
  - **D37.09** Neoplasm of uncertain behavior of other specified sites of the oral cavity
- **D37.1** Neoplasm of uncertain behavior of stomach
- **D37.2** Neoplasm of uncertain behavior of small intestine
- **D37.3** Neoplasm of uncertain behavior of appendix
- **D37.4** Neoplasm of uncertain behavior of colon
- **D37.5** Neoplasm of uncertain behavior of rectum
  - Neoplasm of uncertain behavior of rectosigmoid junction
- **D37.6** Neoplasm of uncertain behavior of liver, gallbladder and bile ducts
  - Neoplasm of uncertain behavior of ampulla of Vater

D37.8 Neoplasm of uncertain behavior of other specified digestive organs
  Neoplasm of uncertain behavior of anal canal
  Neoplasm of uncertain behavior of anal sphincter
  Neoplasm of uncertain behavior of anus NOS
  Neoplasm of uncertain behavior of esophagus
  Neoplasm of uncertain behavior of intestine NOS
  Neoplasm of uncertain behavior of pancreas
  EXCLUDES 1   neoplasm of uncertain behavior of anal margin (D48.5)
      neoplasm of uncertain behavior of anal skin (D48.5)
      neoplasm of uncertain behavior of perianal skin (D48.5)

D37.9 Neoplasm of uncertain behavior of digestive organ, unspecified

D38 Neoplasm of uncertain behavior of middle ear and respiratory and intrathoracic organs
  EXCLUDES 1   neoplasm of uncertain behavior of heart (D48.7)

  D38.0 Neoplasm of uncertain behavior of larynx
    Neoplasm of uncertain behavior of aryepiglottic fold or interarytenoid fold, laryngeal aspect
    Neoplasm of uncertain behavior of epiglottis (suprahyoid portion)
    EXCLUDES 1   neoplasm of uncertain behavior of aryepiglottic fold or interarytenoid fold NOS (D37.05)
        neoplasm of uncertain behavior of hypopharyngeal aspect of aryepiglottic fold (D37.05)
        neoplasm of uncertain behavior of marginal zone of aryepiglottic fold (D37.05)

  D38.1 Neoplasm of uncertain behavior of trachea, bronchus and lung
  D38.2 Neoplasm of uncertain behavior of pleura
  D38.3 Neoplasm of uncertain behavior of mediastinum
  D38.4 Neoplasm of uncertain behavior of thymus
  D38.5 Neoplasm of uncertain behavior of other respiratory organs
    Neoplasm of uncertain behavior of accessory sinuses
    Neoplasm of uncertain behavior of cartilage of nose
    Neoplasm of uncertain behavior of middle ear
    Neoplasm of uncertain behavior of nasal cavities
    EXCLUDES 1   neoplasm of uncertain behavior of ear (external) (skin) (D48.5)
        neoplasm of uncertain behavior of nose NOS (D48.7)
        neoplasm of uncertain behavior of skin of nose (D48.5)

  D38.6 Neoplasm of uncertain behavior of respiratory organ, unspecified

D39 Neoplasm of uncertain behavior of female genital organs

  D39.0 Neoplasm of uncertain behavior of uterus
  D39.1 Neoplasm of uncertain behavior of ovary
    Use additional code to identify any functional activity
    D39.10 Neoplasm of uncertain behavior of unspecified ovary
    D39.11 Neoplasm of uncertain behavior of right ovary
    D39.12 Neoplasm of uncertain behavior of left ovary
  D39.2 Neoplasm of uncertain behavior of placenta
    Chorioadenoma destruens
    Invasive hydatidiform mole
    Malignant hydatidiform mole
    EXCLUDES 1   hydatidiform mole NOS (O01.9)
    AHA: 2023,3Q,14
  D39.8 Neoplasm of uncertain behavior of other specified female genital organs
    Neoplasm of uncertain behavior of skin of female genital organs
  D39.9 Neoplasm of uncertain behavior of female genital organ, unspecified

D40 Neoplasm of uncertain behavior of male genital organs

  D40.0 Neoplasm of uncertain behavior of prostate
  D40.1 Neoplasm of uncertain behavior of testis
    D40.10 Neoplasm of uncertain behavior of unspecified testis
    D40.11 Neoplasm of uncertain behavior of right testis
    D40.12 Neoplasm of uncertain behavior of left testis
  D40.8 Neoplasm of uncertain behavior of other specified male genital organs
    Neoplasm of uncertain behavior of skin of male genital organs
  D40.9 Neoplasm of uncertain behavior of male genital organ, unspecified

D41 Neoplasm of uncertain behavior of urinary organs

  D41.0 Neoplasm of uncertain behavior of kidney
    EXCLUDES 1   neoplasm of uncertain behavior of renal pelvis (D41.1-)
    D41.00 Neoplasm of uncertain behavior of unspecified kidney
    D41.01 Neoplasm of uncertain behavior of right kidney
    D41.02 Neoplasm of uncertain behavior of left kidney

  D41.1 Neoplasm of uncertain behavior of renal pelvis
    D41.10 Neoplasm of uncertain behavior of unspecified renal pelvis
    D41.11 Neoplasm of uncertain behavior of right renal pelvis
    D41.12 Neoplasm of uncertain behavior of left renal pelvis
  D41.2 Neoplasm of uncertain behavior of ureter
    D41.20 Neoplasm of uncertain behavior of unspecified ureter
    D41.21 Neoplasm of uncertain behavior of right ureter
    D41.22 Neoplasm of uncertain behavior of left ureter
  D41.3 Neoplasm of uncertain behavior of urethra
  D41.4 Neoplasm of uncertain behavior of bladder
  D41.8 Neoplasm of uncertain behavior of other specified urinary organs
  D41.9 Neoplasm of uncertain behavior of unspecified urinary organ

D42 Neoplasm of uncertain behavior of meninges
  D42.0 Neoplasm of uncertain behavior of cerebral meninges
  D42.1 Neoplasm of uncertain behavior of spinal meninges
  D42.9 Neoplasm of uncertain behavior of meninges, unspecified

D43 Neoplasm of uncertain behavior of brain and central nervous system
  EXCLUDES 1   neoplasm of uncertain behavior of peripheral nerves and autonomic nervous system (D48.2)

  D43.0 Neoplasm of uncertain behavior of brain, supratentorial
    Neoplasm of uncertain behavior of cerebral ventricle
    Neoplasm of uncertain behavior of cerebrum
    Neoplasm of uncertain behavior of frontal lobe
    Neoplasm of uncertain behavior of occipital lobe
    Neoplasm of uncertain behavior of parietal lobe
    Neoplasm of uncertain behavior of temporal lobe
    EXCLUDES 1   neoplasm of uncertain behavior of fourth ventricle (D43.1)
  D43.1 Neoplasm of uncertain behavior of brain, infratentorial
    Neoplasm of uncertain behavior of brain stem
    Neoplasm of uncertain behavior of cerebellum
    Neoplasm of uncertain behavior of fourth ventricle
    AHA: 2023,2Q,16
  D43.2 Neoplasm of uncertain behavior of brain, unspecified
  D43.3 Neoplasm of uncertain behavior of cranial nerves
  D43.4 Neoplasm of uncertain behavior of spinal cord
  D43.8 Neoplasm of uncertain behavior of other specified parts of central nervous system
  D43.9 Neoplasm of uncertain behavior of central nervous system, unspecified
    Neoplasm of uncertain behavior of nervous system (central) NOS

D44 Neoplasm of uncertain behavior of endocrine glands
  EXCLUDES 1   multiple endocrine adenomatosis (E31.2-)
      multiple endocrine neoplasia (E31.2-)
      neoplasm of uncertain behavior of endocrine pancreas (D37.8)
      neoplasm of uncertain behavior of ovary (D39.1-)
      neoplasm of uncertain behavior of testis (D40.1-)
      neoplasm of uncertain behavior of thymus (D38.4)

  D44.0 Neoplasm of uncertain behavior of thyroid gland
    AHA: 2024,3Q,3
  D44.1 Neoplasm of uncertain behavior of adrenal gland
    Use additional code to identify any functional activity
    D44.10 Neoplasm of uncertain behavior of unspecified adrenal gland
    D44.11 Neoplasm of uncertain behavior of right adrenal gland
    D44.12 Neoplasm of uncertain behavior of left adrenal gland
  D44.2 Neoplasm of uncertain behavior of parathyroid gland
  D44.3 Neoplasm of uncertain behavior of pituitary gland
    Use additional code to identify any functional activity
  D44.4 Neoplasm of uncertain behavior of craniopharyngeal duct
  D44.5 Neoplasm of uncertain behavior of pineal gland
  D44.6 Neoplasm of uncertain behavior of carotid body

Chapter 2. Neoplasms — D44.7–D47.9

D44.7 Neoplasm of uncertain behavior of aortic body and other paraganglia [HCC Rx ESR COM]
AHA: 2021,2Q,7; 2016,4Q,26

D44.9 Neoplasm of uncertain behavior of unspecified endocrine gland

D45 Polycythemia vera [HCC Rx ESR COM]
EXCLUDES 1 familial polycythemia (D75.0)
            secondary polycythemia (D75.1)
DEF: Abnormal proliferation of all bone marrow elements, increased red cell mass, and total blood volume. The etiology is unknown, but it is frequently associated with splenomegaly, leukocytosis, and thrombocythemia.

✓4th D46 Myelodysplastic syndromes
Use additional code for adverse effect, if applicable, to identify drug (T36-T50 with fifth or sixth character 5)
EXCLUDES 2 drug-induced aplastic anemia (D61.1)

D46.0 Refractory anemia without ring sideroblasts, so stated [HCC Rx ESR COM]
Refractory anemia without sideroblasts, without excess of blasts

D46.1 Refractory anemia with ring sideroblasts [HCC Rx ESR COM]
RARS

✓5th D46.2 Refractory anemia with excess of blasts [RAEB]

  D46.20 Refractory anemia with excess of blasts, unspecified [HCC Rx ESR COM]
  RAEB NOS

  D46.21 Refractory anemia with excess of blasts 1 [HCC Rx ESR COM]
  RAEB 1

  D46.22 Refractory anemia with excess of blasts 2
  RAEB 2

D46.A Refractory cytopenia with multilineage dysplasia [HCC Rx ESR COM]

D46.B Refractory cytopenia with multilineage dysplasia and ring sideroblasts [HCC Rx ESR COM]
RCMD RS

D46.C Myelodysplastic syndrome with isolated del(5q) chromosomal abnormality [HCC Rx ESR COM]
5q minus syndrome NOS
Myelodysplastic syndrome with 5q deletion

D46.4 Refractory anemia, unspecified [HCC Rx ESR COM]

D46.Z Other myelodysplastic syndromes [HCC Rx ESR COM]
EXCLUDES 1 chronic myelomonocytic leukemia (C93.1-)

D46.9 Myelodysplastic syndrome, unspecified [HCC Rx ESR COM]
Myelodysplasia NOS

✓4th D47 Other neoplasms of uncertain behavior of lymphoid, hematopoietic and related tissue

✓5th D47.0 Mast cell neoplasms of uncertain behavior
EXCLUDES 1 congenital cutaneous mastocytosis (Q82.2)
            histiocytic neoplasms of uncertain behavior (D47.Z9)
            malignant mast cell neoplasm (C96.2-)
AHA: 2017,4Q,5

  D47.01 Cutaneous mastocytosis [Rx]
  Diffuse cutaneous mastocytosis
  Maculopapular cutaneous mastocytosis
  Solitary mastocytoma
  Telangiectasia macularis eruptiva perstans
  Urticaria pigmentosa
  EXCLUDES 1 congenital (diffuse) (maculopapular) cutaneous mastocytosis (Q82.2)
              congenital urticaria pigmentosa (Q82.2)
              extracutaneous mastocytoma (D47.09)

  D47.02 Systemic mastocytosis [Rx]
  Indolent systemic mastocytosis
  Isolated bone marrow mastocytosis
  Smoldering systemic mastocytosis
  Systemic mastocytosis, with an associated hematological non-mast cell lineage disease (SM-AHNMD)
  Code also, if applicable, any associated hematological non-mast cell lineage disease, such as:
    acute myeloid leukemia (C92.6-, C92.A-)
    chronic myelomonocytic leukemia (C93.1-)
    essential thrombocytosis (D47.3)
    hypereosinophilic syndrome (D72.1)
    myelodysplastic syndrome (D46.9)
    myeloproliferative syndrome (D47.1)
    non-Hodgkin lymphoma (C82-C85)
    plasma cell myeloma (C90.0-)
    polycythemia vera (D45)
  EXCLUDES 1 aggressive systemic mastocytosis (C96.21)
              mast cell leukemia (C94.3-)

  D47.09 Other mast cell neoplasms of uncertain behavior [Rx]
  Extracutaneous mastocytoma
  Mast cell tumor NOS
  Mastocytoma NOS
  Mastocytosis NOS

D47.1 Chronic myeloproliferative disease [HCC Rx ESR COM]
Chronic neutrophilic leukemia
Myeloproliferative disease, unspecified
EXCLUDES 1 atypical chronic myeloid leukemia BCR/ABL-negative (C92.2-)
            chronic myeloid leukemia BCR/ABL-positive (C92.1-)
            myelofibrosis NOS (D75.81)
            myelophthisic anemia (D61.82)
            myelophthisis (D61.82)
            secondary myelofibrosis NOS (D75.81)

D47.2 Monoclonal gammopathy
Monoclonal gammopathy of undetermined significance [MGUS]
AHA: 2021,3Q,5
TIP: Smoldering multiple myeloma (SMM) is coded here.

D47.3 Essential (hemorrhagic) thrombocythemia [HCC Rx ESR COM]
Essential thrombocytosis
Idiopathic hemorrhagic thrombocythemia
Primary thrombocytosis
EXCLUDES 2 reactive thrombocytosis (D75.838)
            secondary thrombocytosis (D75.838)
            thrombocythemia NOS (D75.839)
            thrombocytosis NOS (D75.839)
DEF: Chronic myeloproliferative neoplasm involving production of excess blood platelets that may result in abnormal clotting or hemorrhaging.

D47.4 Osteomyelofibrosis [HCC Rx ESR COM]
Chronic idiopathic myelofibrosis
Myelofibrosis (idiopathic) (with myeloid metaplasia)
Myelosclerosis (megakaryocytic) with myeloid metaplasia
Secondary myelofibrosis in myeloproliferative disease
EXCLUDES 1 acute myelofibrosis (C94.4-)

✓5th D47.Z Other specified neoplasms of uncertain behavior of lymphoid, hematopoietic and related tissue
AHA: 2016,4Q,8

  D47.Z1 Post-transplant lymphoproliferative disorder (PTLD) [HCC ESR COM UPD]
  Code first complications of transplanted organs and tissue (T86.-)
  DEF: Excessive proliferation of B-cell lymphocytes following Epstein-Barr virus infection in organ transplant patients. It may progress to non-Hodgkin lymphoma.

  D47.Z2 Castleman disease [HCC Rx ESR COM]
  Code also, if applicable, human herpesvirus 8 infection (B10.89)
  EXCLUDES 2 Kaposi's sarcoma (C46.-)
  DEF: Rare disease of the lymph nodes and lymphoid tissues that closely mimics lymphoma.

  D47.Z9 Other specified neoplasms of uncertain behavior of lymphoid, hematopoietic and related tissue [HCC Rx ESR COM]
  Histiocytic tumors of uncertain behavior
  AHA: 2025,2Q,19

D47.9 Neoplasm of uncertain behavior of lymphoid, hematopoietic and related tissue, unspecified [HCC Rx ESR COM]
Lymphoproliferative disease NOS

✓ Additional Character Required   ✓x7th Placeholder Alert   Manifestation   Unspecified Dx   Q QPP   UPD Unacceptable PDx

Chapter 2. Neoplasms

D48 Neoplasm of uncertain behavior of other and unspecified sites
  EXCLUDES 1 neurofibromatosis (nonmalignant) (Q85.0-)

D48.0 Neoplasm of uncertain behavior of bone and articular cartilage
  EXCLUDES 1 neoplasm of uncertain behavior of cartilage of ear (D48.1-)
  neoplasm of uncertain behavior of cartilage of larynx (D38.0)
  neoplasm of uncertain behavior of cartilage of nose (D38.5)
  neoplasm of uncertain behavior of connective tissue of eyelid (D48.1-)
  neoplasm of uncertain behavior of synovia (D48.1-)

D48.1 Neoplasm of uncertain behavior of connective and other soft tissue
  Neoplasm of uncertain behavior of connective tissue of ear
  Neoplasm of uncertain behavior of connective tissue of eyelid
  Stromal tumors of uncertain behavior of digestive system
  EXCLUDES 1 neoplasm of uncertain behavior of articular cartilage (D48.0)
  neoplasm of uncertain behavior of cartilage of larynx (D38.0)
  neoplasm of uncertain behavior of cartilage of nose (D38.5)
  neoplasm of uncertain behavior of connective tissue of breast (D48.6-)
  AHA: 2023,4Q,5-6

  D48.11 Desmoid tumor
    ▶Aggressive fibromatosis◀
    D48.110 Desmoid tumor of head and neck
    D48.111 Desmoid tumor of chest wall
    D48.112 Desmoid tumor, intrathoracic
    D48.113 Desmoid tumor of abdominal wall
    D48.114 Desmoid tumor, intraabdominal
      Desmoid tumor of pelvic cavity
      Desmoid tumor, peritoneal, retroperitoneal
    D48.115 Desmoid tumor of upper extremity and shoulder girdle
    D48.116 Desmoid tumor of lower extremity and pelvic girdle
      Desmoid tumor of buttock
    D48.117 Desmoid tumor of back
    D48.118 Desmoid tumor of other site
    D48.119 Desmoid tumor of unspecified site

  D48.19 Other specified neoplasm of uncertain behavior of connective and other soft tissue

D48.2 Neoplasm of uncertain behavior of peripheral nerves and autonomic nervous system
  EXCLUDES 1 neoplasm of uncertain behavior of peripheral nerves of orbit (D48.7)

D48.3 Neoplasm of uncertain behavior of retroperitoneum

D48.4 Neoplasm of uncertain behavior of peritoneum

D48.5 Neoplasm of uncertain behavior of skin
  Neoplasm of uncertain behavior of anal margin
  Neoplasm of uncertain behavior of anal skin
  Neoplasm of uncertain behavior of perianal skin
  Neoplasm of uncertain behavior of skin of breast
  EXCLUDES 1 neoplasm of uncertain behavior of anus NOS (D37.8)
  neoplasm of uncertain behavior of skin of genital organs (D39.8, D40.8)
  neoplasm of uncertain behavior of vermilion border of lip (D37.0)

D48.6 Neoplasm of uncertain behavior of breast
  Cystosarcoma phyllodes
  Neoplasm of uncertain behavior of connective tissue of breast
  EXCLUDES 1 neoplasm of uncertain behavior of skin of breast (D48.5)

  D48.60 Neoplasm of uncertain behavior of unspecified breast
  D48.61 Neoplasm of uncertain behavior of right breast
  D48.62 Neoplasm of uncertain behavior of left breast

D48.7 Neoplasm of uncertain behavior of other specified sites
  Neoplasm of uncertain behavior of eye
  Neoplasm of uncertain behavior of heart
  Neoplasm of uncertain behavior of peripheral nerves of orbit
  EXCLUDES 1 neoplasm of uncertain behavior of connective tissue (D48.1-)
  neoplasm of uncertain behavior of skin of eyelid (D48.5)

D48.9 Neoplasm of uncertain behavior, unspecified

Neoplasms of unspecified behavior (D49)

D49 Neoplasms of unspecified behavior
  NOTE Category D49 classifies by site neoplasms of unspecified morphology and behavior. The term "mass", unless otherwise stated, is not to be regarded as a neoplastic growth.
  INCLUDES "growth" NOS
  neoplasm NOS
  new growth NOS
  tumor NOS
  EXCLUDES 1 neoplasms of uncertain behavior (D37-D44, D48)

D49.0 Neoplasm of unspecified behavior of digestive system
  EXCLUDES 1 neoplasm of unspecified behavior of margin of anus (D49.2)
  neoplasm of unspecified behavior of perianal skin (D49.2)
  neoplasm of unspecified behavior of skin of anus (D49.2)

D49.1 Neoplasm of unspecified behavior of respiratory system

D49.2 Neoplasm of unspecified behavior of bone, soft tissue, and skin
  EXCLUDES 1 neoplasm of unspecified behavior of anal canal (D49.0)
  neoplasm of unspecified behavior of anus NOS (D49.0)
  neoplasm of unspecified behavior of bone marrow (D49.89)
  neoplasm of unspecified behavior of cartilage of larynx (D49.1)
  neoplasm of unspecified behavior of cartilage of nose (D49.1)
  neoplasm of unspecified behavior of connective tissue of breast (D49.3)
  neoplasm of unspecified behavior of skin of genital organs (D49.59)
  neoplasm of unspecified behavior of vermilion border of lip (D49.0)

D49.3 Neoplasm of unspecified behavior of breast
  EXCLUDES 1 neoplasm of unspecified behavior of skin of breast (D49.2)

D49.4 Neoplasm of unspecified behavior of bladder

D49.5 Neoplasm of unspecified behavior of other genitourinary organs
  AHA: 2016,4Q,9

  D49.51 Neoplasm of unspecified behavior of kidney
    D49.511 Neoplasm of unspecified behavior of right kidney
    D49.512 Neoplasm of unspecified behavior of left kidney
    D49.519 Neoplasm of unspecified behavior of unspecified kidney
  D49.59 Neoplasm of unspecified behavior of other genitourinary organ

D49.6 Neoplasm of unspecified behavior of brain HCC Rx ESR COM
  EXCLUDES 1 neoplasm of unspecified behavior of cerebral meninges (D49.7)
  neoplasm of unspecified behavior of cranial nerves (D49.7)

D49.7 Neoplasm of unspecified behavior of endocrine glands and other parts of nervous system
  EXCLUDES 1 neoplasm of unspecified behavior of peripheral, sympathetic, and parasympathetic nerves and ganglia (D49.2)

D49.8 Neoplasm of unspecified behavior of other specified sites
  EXCLUDES 1 neoplasm of unspecified behavior of eyelid (skin) (D49.2)
  neoplasm of unspecified behavior of eyelid cartilage (D49.2)
  neoplasm of unspecified behavior of great vessels (D49.2)
  neoplasm of unspecified behavior of optic nerve (D49.7)

  D49.81 Neoplasm of unspecified behavior of retina and choroid
    Dark area on retina
    Retinal freckle
  D49.89 Neoplasm of unspecified behavior of other specified sites

D49.9 Neoplasm of unspecified behavior of unspecified site

HCC CMS-HCC Rx Rx HCC ESR ESRD HCC COM Commercial HCC N Newborn: 0 P Pediatric: 0-17 M Maternity: 9-64 A Adult: 15-124

Chapter 3. Disease of the Blood and Blood-Forming Organs and Certain Disorders Involving the Immune Mechanism (D50–D89)

Chapter-specific Guidelines with Coding Examples
Reserved for future guideline expansion.

Chapter 3. Diseases of the Blood and Blood-forming Organs and Certain Disorders Involving the Immune Mechanism (D50-D89)

EXCLUDES 2: autoimmune disease (systemic) NOS (M35.9)
certain conditions originating in the perinatal period (P00-P96)
complications of pregnancy, childbirth and the puerperium (O00-O9A)
congenital malformations, deformations and chromosomal abnormalities (Q00-Q99)
endocrine, nutritional and metabolic diseases (E00-E88)
human immunodeficiency virus [HIV] disease (B20)
injury, poisoning and certain other consequences of external causes (S00-T88)
neoplasms (C00-D49)
symptoms, signs and abnormal clinical and laboratory findings, not elsewhere classified (R00-R94)

This chapter contains the following blocks:
- D50-D53 Nutritional anemias
- D55-D59 Hemolytic anemias
- D60-D64 Aplastic and other anemias and other bone marrow failure syndromes
- D65-D69 Coagulation defects, purpura and other hemorrhagic conditions
- D70-D77 Other disorders of blood and blood-forming organs
- D78   Intraoperative and postprocedural complications of the spleen
- D80-D89 Certain disorders involving the immune mechanism

Nutritional anemias (D50-D53)

DEF: Nutritional anemia: The result of inadequate intake or absorption of a vitamin or mineral that impacts the production of red blood cells or causes them to develop abnormally affecting the size and shape.
TIP: Documentation must identify a link between anemia and the nutritional deficiency; low levels of a particular nutrient may occur concurrently with anemia but not cause the anemia.

✓4th D50 Iron deficiency anemia
INCLUDES: asiderotic anemia
hypochromic anemia

- **D50.0** Iron deficiency anemia **secondary to blood loss (chronic)**
  Posthemorrhagic anemia (chronic)
  EXCLUDES 1: acute posthemorrhagic anemia (D62)
  congenital anemia from fetal blood loss (P61.3)
  AHA: 2019,3Q,17

- **D50.1** **Sideropenic dysphagia**
  Kelly-Paterson syndrome
  Plummer-Vinson syndrome

- **D50.8** Other iron deficiency anemias
  Iron deficiency anemia due to inadequate dietary iron intake

- **D50.9** Iron deficiency anemia, unspecified

✓4th D51 Vitamin B12 deficiency anemia
EXCLUDES 1: vitamin B12 deficiency (E53.8)

- **D51.0** Vitamin B12 deficiency anemia due to **intrinsic factor deficiency**
  Addison anemia
  Biermer anemia
  Congenital intrinsic factor deficiency
  Pernicious (congenital) anemia
  DEF: Chronic progressive anemia due to vitamin B12 malabsorption, caused by lack of secretion of intrinsic factor, which is produced by the gastric mucosa of the stomach.

- **D51.1** Vitamin B12 deficiency anemia due to **selective vitamin B12 malabsorption with proteinuria**
  Imerslund (Gräsbeck) syndrome
  Megaloblastic hereditary anemia

- **D51.2** **Transcobalamin II deficiency**

- **D51.3** Other dietary vitamin B12 deficiency anemia
  Vegan anemia

- **D51.8** Other vitamin B12 deficiency anemias

- **D51.9** Vitamin B12 deficiency anemia, unspecified

✓4th D52 **Folate** deficiency anemia
EXCLUDES 1: folate deficiency without anemia (E53.8)
DEF: Deficiency in a B complex vitamin needed for the production of healthy red blood cells. Lack of folate, or folic acid, and other absorption conditions can cause anemia resulting in large, misshapen red blood cells called megaloblasts.

- **D52.0** **Dietary** folate deficiency anemia
  Nutritional megaloblastic anemia
  DEF: Result of a poor diet with inadequate intake of folate, which is needed to produce healthy red blood cells.

- **D52.1** **Drug-induced** folate deficiency anemia
  Use additional code for adverse effect, if applicable, to identify drug (T36-T50 with fifth or sixth character 5)

- **D52.8** Other folate deficiency anemias

- **D52.9** Folate deficiency anemia, unspecified
  Folic acid deficiency anemia NOS

✓4th D53 Other nutritional anemias
INCLUDES: megaloblastic anemia unresponsive to vitamin B12 or folate therapy

- **D53.0** **Protein** deficiency anemia
  Amino-acid deficiency anemia
  Orotaciduric anemia
  EXCLUDES 1: Lesch-Nyhan syndrome (E79.1)

- **D53.1** Other **megaloblastic** anemias, not elsewhere classified
  Megaloblastic anemia NOS
  EXCLUDES 1: Di Guglielmo's disease (C94.0)

- **D53.2** **Scorbutic** anemia
  EXCLUDES 1: scurvy (E54)

- **D53.8** Other specified nutritional anemias
  Anemia associated with deficiency of copper
  Anemia associated with deficiency of molybdenum
  Anemia associated with deficiency of zinc
  EXCLUDES 1: nutritional deficiencies without anemia, such as:
  copper deficiency NOS (E61.0)
  molybdenum deficiency NOS (E61.5)
  zinc deficiency NOS (E60)
  EXCLUDES 2: ▶nutritional deficiencies without anemia, such as:◄
  ▶copper deficiency NOS (E61.0)◄
  ▶molybdenum deficiency NOS (E61.5)◄
  ▶zinc deficiency NOS (E60)◄

- **D53.9** Nutritional anemia, unspecified
  Simple chronic anemia
  EXCLUDES 1: anemia NOS (D64.9)
  AHA: 2018,4Q,88

Hemolytic anemias (D55-D59)

✓4th D55 Anemia due to enzyme disorders
EXCLUDES 1: drug-induced enzyme deficiency anemia (D59.2)

- **D55.0** Anemia due to **glucose-6-phosphate dehydrogenase [G6PD] deficiency**
  Favism
  G6PD deficiency anemia
  EXCLUDES 1: glucose-6-phosphate dehydrogenase (G6PD) deficiency without anemia (D75.A)

- **D55.1** Anemia due to other disorders of **glutathione metabolism**
  Anemia (due to) enzyme deficiencies, except G6PD, related to the hexose monophosphate [HMP] shunt pathway
  Anemia (due to) hemolytic nonspherocytic (hereditary), type I

- ✓5th **D55.2** Anemia due to disorders of **glycolytic enzymes**
  EXCLUDES 1: disorders of glycolysis not associated with anemia (E74.81-)
  AHA: 2021,4Q,6-7
  - **D55.21** Anemia due to **pyruvate kinase deficiency**
    PK deficiency anemia
    Pyruvate kinase deficiency anemia
  - **D55.29** Anemia due to other disorders of glycolytic enzymes
    Hexokinase deficiency anemia
    Triose-phosphate isomerase deficiency anemia

- **D55.3** Anemia due to disorders of **nucleotide metabolism**
- **D55.8** Other anemias due to enzyme disorders
- **D55.9** Anemia due to enzyme disorder, unspecified

D56 Thalassemia

EXCLUDES 1 sickle-cell thalassemia (D57.4-)

DEF: Group of inherited disorders of hemoglobin metabolism causing mild to severe anemia. It is usually found in people of Mediterranean, African, Chinese, or Asian descent.

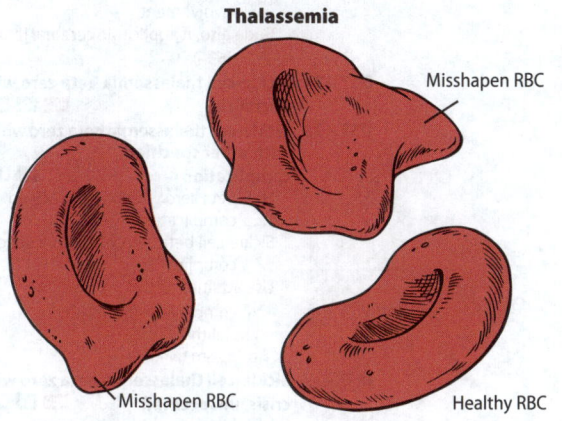
Thalassemia — Misshapen RBC, Healthy RBC

D56.0 Alpha thalassemia
Alpha thalassemia major
Hemoglobin H Constant Spring
Hemoglobin H disease
Hydrops fetalis due to alpha thalassemia
Severe alpha thalassemia
Triple gene defect alpha thalassemia

Use additional code, if applicable, for hydrops fetalis due to alpha thalassemia (P56.99)

EXCLUDES 1 alpha thalassemia trait or minor (D56.3)
asymptomatic alpha thalassemia (D56.3)
hydrops fetalis due to isoimmunization (P56.0)
hydrops fetalis not due to immune hemolysis (P83.2)

DEF: HBA1 and HBA2 genetic variant of chromosome 16 prevalent among those of African and Southeast Asian descent. Alpha thalassemia is associated with a wide spectrum of anemic presentation and includes hemoglobin H disease subtypes.

D56.1 Beta thalassemia
Beta thalassemia major
Cooley's anemia
Homozygous beta thalassemia
Severe beta thalassemia
Thalassemia intermedia
Thalassemia major

EXCLUDES 1 beta thalassemia minor (D56.3)
beta thalassemia trait (D56.3)
delta-beta thalassemia (D56.2)
hemoglobin E-beta thalassemia (D56.5)
sickle-cell beta thalassemia (D57.4-)

D56.2 Delta-beta thalassemia
Homozygous delta-beta thalassemia

EXCLUDES 1 delta-beta thalassemia minor (D56.3)
delta-beta thalassemia trait (D56.3)

D56.3 Thalassemia minor
Alpha thalassemia minor
Alpha thalassemia silent carrier
Alpha thalassemia trait
Beta thalassemia minor
Beta thalassemia trait
Delta-beta thalassemia minor
Delta-beta thalassemia trait
Thalassemia trait NOS

EXCLUDES 1 alpha thalassemia (D56.0)
beta thalassemia (D56.1)
delta-beta thalassemia (D56.2)
hemoglobin E-beta thalassemia (D56.5)
sickle-cell trait (D57.3)

DEF: Solitary abnormal gene that identifies a carrier of the disease, yet with an absence of symptoms or a clinically mild anemic presentation.

D56.4 Hereditary persistence of fetal hemoglobin [HPFH]

D56.5 Hemoglobin E-beta thalassemia
EXCLUDES 1 beta thalassemia (D56.1)
beta thalassemia minor (D56.3)
beta thalassemia trait (D56.3)
delta-beta thalassemia (D56.2)
delta-beta thalassemia trait (D56.3)
hemoglobin E disease (D58.2)
other hemoglobinopathies (D58.2)
sickle-cell beta thalassemia (D57.4-)

D56.8 Other thalassemias
Dominant thalassemia
Hemoglobin C thalassemia
Mixed thalassemia
Thalassemia with other hemoglobinopathy

EXCLUDES 1 hemoglobin C disease (D58.2)
hemoglobin E disease (D58.2)
other hemoglobinopathies (D58.2)
sickle-cell anemia (D57.-)
sickle-cell thalassemia (D57.4-)

D56.9 Thalassemia, unspecified
Mediterranean anemia (with other hemoglobinopathy)

D57 Sickle-cell disorders

Use additional code for any associated fever (R50.81)
EXCLUDES 1 other hemoglobinopathies (D58.-)
AHA: 2023,4Q,6-7; 2022,2Q,28

DEF: Severe, chronic inherited diseases caused by a genetic variation in hemoglobin protein of the red blood cell. The gene mutation causes the red blood cell to become hard, sticky, and crescent or sickle shaped, making it harder for red blood cells to travel through the bloodstream, disrupting blood flow and decreasing oxygen transport to tissues.

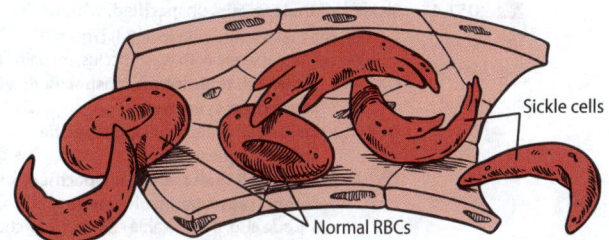
Sickle cell — Sickle cells, Normal RBCs

D57.0 Hb-SS disease with crisis
Hb-SS disease with (vaso-occlusive) pain
Sickle-cell disease with crisis
AHA: 2020,4Q,6-7

D57.00 Hb-SS disease with crisis, unspecified
Hb-SS disease with (painful) crisis NOS
Hb-SS disease with (vaso-occlusive) pain NOS

D57.01 Hb-SS disease with acute chest syndrome

D57.02 Hb-SS disease with splenic sequestration
AHA: 2025,1Q,24

D57.03 Hb-SS disease with cerebral vascular involvement
Code also, if applicable, cerebral infarction (I63.-)

D57.04 Hb-SS disease with dactylitis

D57.09 Hb-SS disease with crisis with other specified complication
Use additional code to identify complications, such as:
cholelithiasis (K80.-)
priapism (N48.32)

D57.1 Sickle-cell disease without crisis
Hb-SS disease without crisis
Sickle-cell anemia NOS
Sickle-cell disease NOS
Sickle-cell disorder NOS

D57.2 Sickle-cell/Hb-C disease
Hb-S/Hb-C disease
Hb-SC disease
AHA: 2020,4Q,6-7

D57.20 Sickle-cell/Hb-C disease without crisis

D57.21 Sickle-cell/Hb-C disease with crisis

D57.211 Sickle-cell/Hb-C disease with acute chest syndrome

D57.212 Sickle-cell/Hb-C disease with splenic sequestration `HCC` `ESR`

D57.213 Sickle-cell/Hb-C disease with cerebral vascular involvement `HCC` `ESR`
Code also, if applicable, cerebral infarction (I63.-)

D57.214 Sickle-cell/Hb-C disease with dactylitis `HCC` `ESR`

D57.218 Sickle-cell/Hb-C disease with crisis with other specified complication `HCC` `ESR`
Use additional code to identify complications, such as:
cholelithiasis (K80.-)
priapism (N48.32)

D57.219 Sickle-cell/Hb-C disease with crisis, unspecified `HCC` `ESR`
Sickle-cell/Hb-C disease with (vaso-occlusive) pain NOS
Sickle-cell/Hb-C disease with crisis NOS

D57.3 Sickle-cell trait `ESR`
Hb-S trait
Heterozygous hemoglobin S
DEF: Heterozygous genetic makeup characterized by one gene for normal hemoglobin and one for sickle-cell hemoglobin. The clinical disease is rarely present.

✓5th D57.4 Sickle-cell thalassemia
Sickle-cell beta thalassemia
Thalassemia Hb-S disease
AHA: 2020,4Q,6-7

D57.40 Sickle-cell thalassemia without crisis `HCC` `ESR`
Microdrepanocytosis
Sickle-cell thalassemia NOS

✓6th **D57.41** Sickle-cell thalassemia, unspecified, with crisis
Sickle-cell thalassemia with (painful) crisis NOS
Sickle-cell thalassemia with (vaso-occlusive) pain NOS

D57.411 Sickle-cell thalassemia, unspecified, with acute chest syndrome `HCC` `ESR`

D57.412 Sickle-cell thalassemia, unspecified, with splenic sequestration `HCC` `ESR`

D57.413 Sickle-cell thalassemia, unspecified, with cerebral vascular involvement `HCC` `ESR`
Code also, if applicable cerebral infarction (I63.-)

D57.414 Sickle-cell thalassemia, unspecified, with dactylitis `HCC` `ESR`

D57.418 Sickle-cell thalassemia, unspecified, with crisis with other specified complication `HCC` `ESR`
Use additional code to identify complications, such as:
cholelithiasis (K80.-)
priapism (N48.32)

D57.419 Sickle-cell thalassemia, unspecified, with crisis `HCC` `ESR`
Sickle-cell thalassemia with (painful) crisis NOS
Sickle-cell thalassemia with (vaso-occlusive) pain NOS

D57.42 Sickle-cell thalassemia beta zero without crisis `HCC` `Rx` `ESR` `COM`
HbS-beta zero without crisis
Sickle-cell beta zero without crisis

✓6th **D57.43** Sickle-cell thalassemia beta zero with crisis
HbS-beta zero with crisis
Sickle-cell beta zero with crisis

D57.431 Sickle-cell thalassemia beta zero with acute chest syndrome `HCC` `Rx` `ESR` `COM`
HbS-beta zero with acute chest syndrome
Sickle-cell beta zero with acute chest syndrome

D57.432 Sickle-cell thalassemia beta zero with splenic sequestration `HCC` `Rx` `ESR` `COM`
HbS-beta zero with splenic sequestration
Sickle-cell beta zero with splenic sequestration

D57.433 Sickle-cell thalassemia beta zero with cerebral vascular involvement `HCC` `Rx` `ESR` `COM`
HbS-beta zero with cerebral vascular involvement
Sickle-cell beta zero with cerebral vascular involvement
Code also, if applicable cerebral infarction (I63.-)

D57.434 Sickle-cell thalassemia beta zero with dactylitis `HCC` `Rx` `ESR` `COM`

D57.438 Sickle-cell thalassemia beta zero with crisis with other specified complication `HCC` `Rx` `ESR` `COM`
HbS-beta zero with other specified complication
Sickle-cell beta zero with other specified complication
Use additional code to identify complications, such as:
cholelithiasis (K80.-)
priapism (N48.32)

D57.439 Sickle-cell thalassemia beta zero with crisis, unspecified `HCC` `Rx` `ESR` `COM`
HbS-beta zero with other specified complication
Sickle-cell beta zero with crisis unspecified
Sickle-cell thalassemia beta zero with (painful) crisis NOS
Sickle-cell thalassemia beta zero with (vaso-occlusive) pain NOS

D57.44 Sickle-cell thalassemia beta plus without crisis `HCC` `ESR`
HbS-beta plus without crisis
Sickle-cell beta plus without crisis

✓6th **D57.45** Sickle-cell thalassemia beta plus with crisis
HbS-beta plus with crisis
Sickle-cell beta plus with crisis

D57.451 Sickle-cell thalassemia beta plus with acute chest syndrome `HCC` `ESR`
HbS-beta plus with acute chest syndrome
Sickle-cell beta plus with acute chest syndrome

D57.452 Sickle-cell thalassemia beta plus with splenic sequestration `HCC` `ESR`
HbS-beta plus with splenic sequestration
Sickle-cell beta plus with splenic sequestration

D57.453 Sickle-cell thalassemia beta plus with cerebral vascular involvement `HCC` `ESR`
HbS-beta plus with cerebral vascular involvement
Sickle-cell beta plus with cerebral vascular involvement
Code also, if applicable cerebral infarction (I63.-)

D57.454 Sickle-cell thalassemia beta plus with dactylitis `HCC` `ESR`

D57.458 Sickle-cell thalassemia beta plus with crisis with other specified complication `HCC` `ESR`
HbS-beta plus with crisis with other specified complication
Sickle-cell beta plus with crisis with other specified complication
Use additional code to identify complications, such as:
cholelithiasis (K80.-)
priapism (N48.32)

D57.459 Sickle-cell thalassemia beta plus with crisis, unspecified `HCC` `ESR`
HbS-beta plus with crisis with unspecified complication
Sickle-cell beta plus with crisis with unspecified complication
Sickle-cell thalassemia beta plus with (painful) crisis NOS
Sickle-cell thalassemia beta plus with (vaso-occlusive) pain NOS

`HCC` CMS-HCC `Rx` Rx HCC `ESR` ESRD HCC `COM` Commercial HCC   `N` Newborn: 0   `P` Pediatric: 0-17   `M` Maternity: 9-64   `A` Adult: 15-124

D57.8 Other sickle-cell disorders
Hb-SD disease
Hb-SE disease
AHA: 2020,4Q,6-7

- **D57.80** Other sickle-cell disorders without crisis [HCC] [ESR]
- **D57.81** Other sickle-cell disorders with crisis
  - **D57.811** Other sickle-cell disorders with acute chest syndrome [HCC] [ESR]
  - **D57.812** Other sickle-cell disorders with splenic sequestration [HCC] [ESR]
  - **D57.813** Other sickle-cell disorders with cerebral vascular involvement [HCC] [ESR]
    Code also, if applicable: cerebral infarction (I63.-)
  - **D57.814** Other sickle-cell disorders with dactylitis [HCC] [ESR]
  - **D57.818** Other sickle-cell disorders with crisis with other specified complication [HCC] [ESR]
    Use additional code to identify complications, such as:
       cholelithiasis (K80.-)
       priapism (N48.32)
  - **D57.819** Other sickle-cell disorders with crisis, unspecified [HCC] [ESR]
    Other sickle-cell disorders with (vaso-occlusive) pain NOS
    Other sickle-cell disorders with crisis NOS

D58 Other hereditary hemolytic anemias
EXCLUDES 1 hemolytic anemia of the newborn (P55.-)

D58.0 Hereditary spherocytosis [ESR]
Acholuric (familial) jaundice
Congenital (spherocytic) hemolytic icterus
Minkowski-Chauffard syndrome
DEF: Inherited condition caused by mutations to genes responsible for the production of proteins that form the membranes of red blood cells. The shape and flexibility of the red blood cell membrane is altered, diminishing the cell's ability to traverse the spleen, therefore becoming trapped and destroyed before the red blood cell has reached maturity.

D58.1 Hereditary elliptocytosis [ESR]
Elliptocytosis (congenital)
Ovalocytosis (congenital) (hereditary)

D58.2 Other hemoglobinopathies [ESR]
Abnormal hemoglobin NOS
Congenital Heinz body anemia
Hb-C disease
Hb-D disease
Hb-E disease
Hemoglobinopathy NOS
Unstable hemoglobin hemolytic disease
EXCLUDES 1 familial polycythemia (D75.0)
Hb-M disease (D74.0)
hemoglobin E-beta thalassemia (D56.5)
hereditary persistence of fetal hemoglobin [HPFH] (D56.4)
high-altitude polycythemia (D75.1)
methemoglobinemia (D74.-)
other hemoglobinopathies with thalassemia (D56.8)

D58.8 Other specified hereditary hemolytic anemias [ESR]
Stomatocytosis

D58.9 Hereditary hemolytic anemia, unspecified [ESR]

D59 Acquired hemolytic anemia
DEF: Non-hereditary anemia characterized by premature destruction of red blood cells caused by infectious organisms, poisons, and physical agents.

D59.0 Drug-induced autoimmune hemolytic anemia [Rx] [ESR] [COM]
Use additional code for adverse effect, if applicable, to identify drug (T36-T50 with fifth or sixth character 5)

D59.1 Other autoimmune hemolytic anemias
EXCLUDES 2 Evans syndrome (D69.41)
hemolytic disease of newborn (P55.-)
paroxysmal cold hemoglobinuria (D59.6)
AHA: 2020,4Q,7-8

- **D59.10** Autoimmune hemolytic anemia, unspecified [HCC] [Rx] [ESR] [COM]
- **D59.11** Warm autoimmune hemolytic anemia [HCC] [Rx] [ESR] [COM]
  Warm type (primary) (secondary) (symptomatic) autoimmune hemolytic anemia
  Warm type autoimmune hemolytic disease
- **D59.12** Cold autoimmune hemolytic anemia [HCC] [Rx] [ESR] [COM]
  Chronic cold hemagglutinin disease
  Cold agglutinin disease
  Cold agglutinin hemoglobinuria
  Cold type (primary) (secondary) (symptomatic) autoimmune hemolytic anemia
  Cold type autoimmune hemolytic disease
- **D59.13** Mixed type autoimmune hemolytic anemia [HCC] [Rx] [ESR] [COM]
  Mixed type autoimmune hemolytic disease
  Mixed type, cold and warm, (primary) (secondary) (symptomatic) autoimmune hemolytic anemia
- **D59.19** Other autoimmune hemolytic anemia [HCC] [Rx] [ESR] [COM]

D59.2 Drug-induced nonautoimmune hemolytic anemia [Rx] [ESR] [COM]
Drug-induced enzyme deficiency anemia
Use additional code for adverse effect, if applicable, to identify drug (T36-T50 with fifth or sixth character 5)

D59.3 Hemolytic-uremic syndrome
Code also, if applicable, any associated:
   acute kidney failure (N17.-)
   chronic kidney disease (N18.-)
AHA: 2022,4Q,5-6
DEF: Condition typically precipitated by infection causing low platelets and destruction of red blood cells resulting in hemolytic anemia. This cell damage and blockage of renal capillaries lead to kidney failure. Mainly affects children.

- **D59.30** Hemolytic-uremic syndrome, unspecified [HCC] [Rx] [ESR] [COM]
  Hemolytic-uremic syndrome NOS
- **D59.31** Infection-associated hemolytic-uremic syndrome [HCC] [Rx] [ESR] [COM]
  Shiga toxin-producing E. coli [STEC] related hemolytic uremic syndrome
  Typical hemolytic uremic syndrome
  Use additional code to identify associated infection, such as:
     E. coli infection (B96.2-)
     human immunodeficiency virus [HIV] disease (B20)
     pneumococcal meningitis (G00.1)
     pneumococcal pneumonia (J13)
     sepsis due to Streptococcus pneumoniae (A40.3)
     Shigella dysenteriae (A03.9)
     streptococcus pneumoniae as the cause of diseases classified elsewhere (B95.3)
- **D59.32** Hereditary hemolytic-uremic syndrome [HCC] [Rx] [ESR] [COM]
  Atypical hemolytic uremic syndrome with an identified genetic cause
  Code also, if applicable:
     defects in the complement system (D84.1)
     methylmalonic acidemia (E71.120)
- **D59.39** Other hemolytic-uremic syndrome [HCC] [Rx] [ESR] [COM]
  Atypical (nongenetic) hemolytic uremic syndrome
  Secondary hemolytic-uremic syndrome
  Code first, if applicable, any associated:
     complications of heart transplant (T86.2-)
     complications of kidney transplant (T86.1-)
     complications of liver transplant (T86.4-)
     COVID-19 (U07.1)
  Code also, if applicable, any associated condition, such as:
     hypertensive emergency (I16.1)
     malignant neoplasm (C00-C96)
     systemic lupus erythematosus (M32.-)
  Use additional code, if applicable, for adverse effect to identify drug (T36-T50 with fifth or sixth character 5)
  AHA: 2022,4Q,6

D59.4 Other nonautoimmune hemolytic anemias [HCC] [Rx] [ESR] [COM]
Mechanical hemolytic anemia
Microangiopathic hemolytic anemia
Toxic hemolytic anemia

Chapter 3. Diseases of the Blood and Blood-forming Organs

D59.5 **Paroxysmal nocturnal hemoglobinuria [Marchiafava-Micheli]** `HCC` `Rx` `ESR` `COM`
- EXCLUDES 1: hemoglobinuria NOS (R82.3)

D59.6 **Hemoglobinuria due to hemolysis from other external causes** `HCC` `Rx` `ESR` `COM`
- Hemoglobinuria from exertion
- March hemoglobinuria
- Paroxysmal cold hemoglobinuria
- Use additional code (Chapter 20) to identify external cause
- EXCLUDES 1: hemoglobinuria NOS (R82.3)

D59.8 **Other acquired hemolytic anemias** `HCC` `Rx` `ESR` `COM`

D59.9 **Acquired hemolytic anemia, unspecified** `HCC` `Rx` `ESR` `COM`
- Idiopathic hemolytic anemia, chronic

Aplastic and other anemias and other bone marrow failure syndromes (D60-D64)

D60 **Acquired pure red cell aplasia [erythroblastopenia]**
- INCLUDES: red cell aplasia (acquired) (adult) (with thymoma)
- EXCLUDES 1: congenital red cell aplasia (D61.01)
- DEF: Bone marrow failure characterized by underproduction of red blood cells while white blood cell and platelet production remains normal.

- **D60.0** **Chronic** acquired pure red cell aplasia `HCC` `Rx` `ESR` `COM`
- **D60.1** **Transient** acquired pure red cell aplasia `Rx` `ESR` `COM`
- **D60.8** **Other** acquired pure red cell aplasias `HCC` `Rx` `ESR` `COM`
- **D60.9** Acquired pure red cell aplasia, **unspecified** `HCC` `Rx` `ESR` `COM`

D61 **Other aplastic anemias and other bone marrow failure syndromes**
- EXCLUDES 2: neutropenia (D70.-)
- AHA: 2020,3Q,22; 2014,4Q,22
- DEF: Aplastic anemia: Bone marrow failure characterized by underproduction of red bloods cells, white blood cells and platelets.

- **D61.0** **Constitutional** aplastic anemia

  - **D61.01** **Constitutional (pure) red blood cell aplasia** `HCC` `Rx` `ESR` `COM`
    - Blackfan-Diamond syndrome
    - Congenital (pure) red cell aplasia
    - Familial hypoplastic anemia
    - Primary (pure) red cell aplasia
    - Red cell (pure) aplasia of infants
    - EXCLUDES 1: acquired red cell aplasia (D60.9)

  - **D61.02** **Shwachman-Diamond** syndrome `HCC` `Rx` `ESR` `COM`
    - Code also, if applicable, associated conditions such as:
      - acute myeloblastic leukemia (C92.0-)
      - exocrine pancreatic insufficiency (K86.81)
      - myelodysplastic syndrome (D46.-)
    - Use additional code, if applicable, for genetic susceptibility to other malignant neoplasm (Z15.09)
    - AHA: 2023,4Q,8

  - **D61.03** **Fanconi anemia** `HCC` `Rx` `ESR` `COM`
    - Fanconi pancytopenia
    - Fanconi's anemia
    - EXCLUDES 1: Fanconi syndrome (E72.0-)
    - AHA: 2024,4Q,5

  - **D61.09** **Other** constitutional aplastic anemia `HCC` `Rx` `ESR` `COM`
    - Pancytopenia with malformations

- **D61.1** **Drug-induced** aplastic anemia `Rx` `ESR` `COM`
  - Use additional code for adverse effect, if applicable, to identify drug (T36-T50 with fifth or sixth character 5)

- **D61.2** **Aplastic anemia due to other external agents** `HCC` `Rx` `ESR` `COM`
  - Code first, if applicable, toxic effects of substances chiefly nonmedicinal as to source (T51-T65)

- **D61.3** **Idiopathic** aplastic anemia `HCC` `Rx` `ESR` `COM`

- **D61.8** **Other specified aplastic anemias and other bone marrow failure syndromes**

  - **D61.81** **Pancytopenia**
    - EXCLUDES 1:
      - pancytopenia (due to) (with) aplastic anemia (D61.9)
      - pancytopenia (due to) (with) bone marrow infiltration (D61.82)
      - pancytopenia (due to) (with) congenital (pure) red cell aplasia (D61.01)
      - pancytopenia (due to) (with) hairy cell leukemia (C91.4-)
      - pancytopenia (due to) (with) human immunodeficiency virus disease (B20)
      - pancytopenia (due to) (with) leukoerythroblastic anemia (D61.82)
      - pancytopenia (due to) (with) myeloproliferative disease (D47.1)
    - EXCLUDES 2: pancytopenia (due to) (with) myelodysplastic syndromes (D46.-)
    - DEF: Shortage of all three blood cells: white, red, and platelets.

    - **D61.810** **Antineoplastic chemotherapy** induced **pancytopenia** `ESR`
      - EXCLUDES 2: aplastic anemia due to antineoplastic chemotherapy (D61.1)
      - AHA: 2020,3Q,22

    - **D61.811** **Other drug-induced** pancytopenia `ESR`
      - EXCLUDES 2: aplastic anemia due to drugs (D61.1)
      - AHA: 2023,3Q,4

    - **D61.818** **Other pancytopenia** `HCC` `ESR`
      - AHA: 2023,1Q,23; 2020,3Q,24; 2019,1Q,16
      - TIP: Assign this code in addition to myeloid leukemia codes (C92.-) when pancytopenia is documented. Although common in some types of myeloid leukemia, pancytopenia is not always inherent.

  - **D61.82** **Myelophthisis** `HCC` `Rx` `ESR` `COM`
    - Leukoerythroblastic anemia
    - Myelophthisic anemia
    - Panmyelophthisis
    - Code also the underlying disorder, such as:
      - malignant neoplasm of breast (C50.-)
      - tuberculosis (A15.-)
    - EXCLUDES 1:
      - idiopathic myelofibrosis (D47.1)
      - myelofibrosis NOS (D75.81)
      - myelofibrosis with myeloid metaplasia (D47.4)
      - primary myelofibrosis (D47.1)
      - secondary myelofibrosis (D75.81)
    - DEF: Condition that occurs when normal hematopoietic tissue in the bone marrow is replaced with abnormal tissue, such as fibrous tissue or tumors. Most commonly seen during the advanced stages of cancer.

  - **D61.89** **Other specified aplastic anemias and other bone marrow failure syndromes** `HCC` `Rx` `ESR` `COM`

- **D61.9** **Aplastic anemia, unspecified** `Rx` `ESR` `COM`
  - Hypoplastic anemia NOS
  - Medullary hypoplasia

D62 **Acute posthemorrhagic anemia**
- EXCLUDES 1:
  - anemia due to chronic blood loss (D50.0)
  - blood loss anemia NOS (D50.0)
  - congenital anemia from fetal blood loss (P61.3)
- AHA: 2023,1Q,15,16; 2019,3Q,11,17

D63 **Anemia in chronic diseases classified elsewhere**

- **D63.0** **Anemia in neoplastic disease**
  - Code first neoplasm (C00-D49)
  - EXCLUDES 1: aplastic anemia due to antineoplastic chemotherapy (D61.1)
  - EXCLUDES 2: anemia due to antineoplastic chemotherapy (D64.81)

- **D63.1** **Anemia in chronic kidney disease**
  - Erythropoietin resistant anemia (EPO resistant anemia)
  - Code first underlying chronic kidney disease (CKD) (N18.-)

D63.8 Anemia in other chronic diseases classified elsewhere
  Code first underlying disease, such as:
    diphyllobothriasis (B70.0)
    hookworm disease (B76.0-B76.9)
    hypothyroidism (E00.0-E03.9)
    malaria (B50.0-B54)
    symptomatic late syphilis (A52.79)
    tuberculosis (A18.89)

D64 Other anemias
  EXCLUDES 1 refractory anemia (D46.-)
    refractory anemia with excess blasts in transformation [RAEB T] (C92.0-)
  DEF: Sideroblastic anemia: Hereditary or secondary disorder in which the red blood cells cannot effectively use iron, a nutrient needed to make hemoglobin. Although the iron can enter the red blood cell it is not assimilated into the hemoglobin molecule and builds up ringed sideroblasts around the cell nucleus.

  D64.0 Hereditary sideroblastic anemia
    Sex-linked hypochromic sideroblastic anemia
  D64.1 Secondary sideroblastic anemia due to disease
    Code first underlying disease
  D64.2 Secondary sideroblastic anemia due to drugs and toxins
    Code first poisoning due to drug or toxin, if applicable (T36-T65 with fifth or sixth character 1-4)
    Use additional code for adverse effect, if applicable, to identify drug (T36-T50 with fifth or sixth character 5)
  D64.3 Other sideroblastic anemias
    Pyridoxine-responsive sideroblastic anemia NEC
    Sideroblastic anemia NOS
  D64.4 Congenital dyserythropoietic anemia
    Dyshematopoietic anemia (congenital)
    EXCLUDES 1 Blackfan-Diamond syndrome (D61.01)
      Di Guglielmo's disease (C94.0)
  D64.8 Other specified anemias
    D64.81 Anemia due to antineoplastic chemotherapy
      Antineoplastic chemotherapy induced anemia
      EXCLUDES 2 anemia in neoplastic disease (D63.0)
        aplastic anemia due to antineoplastic chemotherapy (D61.1)
      AHA: 2023,2Q,17; 2021,3Q,4; 2014,4Q,22
    D64.89 Other specified anemias
      Infantile pseudoleukemia
  D64.9 Anemia, unspecified
    AHA: 2020,3Q,24; 2018,4Q,88; 2017,1Q,7

Coagulation defects, purpura and other hemorrhagic conditions (D65-D69)

D65 Disseminated intravascular coagulation [defibrination syndrome]
  Afibrinogenemia, acquired
  Consumption coagulopathy
  COVID-19 associated diffuse or disseminated intravascular coagulopathy
  Diffuse or disseminated intravascular coagulation [DIC]
  Fibrinolytic hemorrhage, acquired
  Fibrinolytic purpura
  Purpura fulminans
  Code also, if applicable, associated condition
  EXCLUDES 1 disseminated intravascular coagulation (complicating):
    abortion or ectopic or molar pregnancy (O00-O07, O08.1)
    in newborn (P60)
    pregnancy, childbirth and the puerperium (O45.0, O46.0, O67.0, O72.3)
  AHA: 2021,1Q,39

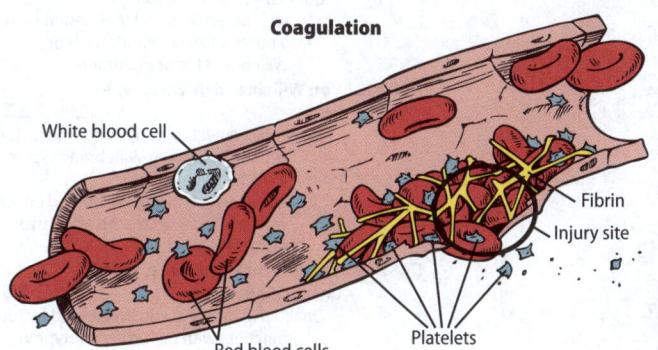

Coagulation
White blood cell
Fibrin
Injury site
Red blood cells
Platelets

D66 Hereditary factor VIII deficiency
  Classical hemophilia
  Deficiency factor VIII (with functional defect)
  Hemophilia A
  Hemophilia NOS
  EXCLUDES 1 factor VIII deficiency with vascular defect (D68.0-)
  AHA: 2022,4Q,9
  DEF: Hereditary, sex-linked lack of antihemophilic globulin (AHG) (factor VIII) that causes abnormal coagulation characterized by increased bleeding; large bruises of skin; bleeding in the mouth, nose, and gastrointestinal tract; and hemorrhages into joints, resulting in swelling and impaired function.
  TIP: Factor VIII deficiency may also be documented in patients with VWD. Only a code for the VWD should be reported; do not report code D66.

D67 Hereditary factor IX deficiency
  Christmas disease
  Factor IX deficiency (with functional defect)
  Hemophilia B
  Plasma thromboplastin component [PTC] deficiency

D68 Other coagulation defects
  EXCLUDES 1 abnormal coagulation profile NOS (R79.1)
  EXCLUDES 2 coagulation defects complicating abortion or ectopic or molar pregnancy (O00-O07, O08.1)
    coagulation defects complicating pregnancy, childbirth and the puerperium (O45.0, O46.0, O67.0, O72.3)
  AHA: 2016,1Q,14
  D68.0 Von Willebrand disease
    EXCLUDES 1 capillary fragility (hereditary) (D69.8)
      factor VIII deficiency NOS (D66)
      factor VIII deficiency with functional defect (D66)
    AHA: 2022,4Q,7-9
    DEF: Congenital, abnormal blood coagulation caused by deficient blood factor VII. Symptoms include excess or prolonged bleeding.
    TIP: Factor VIII deficiency may also be documented in patients with VWD. Only a code for the VWD should be reported; do not report code D66.
    D68.00 Von Willebrand disease, unspecified
    D68.01 Von Willebrand disease, type 1
      Partial quantitative deficiency of von Willebrand factor
      Type 1C von Willebrand disease
      AHA: 2022,4Q,9

D68.02 Von Willebrand disease, type 2
Qualitative defects of von Willebrand factor

D68.020 Von Willebrand disease, type 2A
Qualitative defects of von Willebrand factor with decreased platelet adhesion and selective deficiency of high-molecular-weight multimers

D68.021 Von Willebrand disease, type 2B
Qualitative defects of von Willebrand factor with high-molecular-weight von Willebrand factor loss
Qualitative defects of von Willebrand factor with hyper-adhesive forms
Qualitative defects of von Willebrand factor with increased affinity for platelet glycoprotein Ib

D68.022 Von Willebrand disease, type 2M
Qualitative defects of von Willebrand factor with defective platelet adhesion with a normal size distribution of von Willebrand factor multimers

D68.023 Von Willebrand disease, type 2N
Qualitative defects of von Willebrand factor with defective von Willebrand factor to factor VIII binding
Qualitative defects of von Willebrand factor with markedly decreased affinity for factor VIII

D68.029 Von Willebrand disease, type 2, unspecified
Qualitative defect in von Willebrand factor function, with no further subtyping

D68.03 Von Willebrand disease, type 3
(Near) complete absence of von Willebrand factor
Total quantitative deficiency of von Willebrand factor

D68.04 Acquired von Willebrand disease
Acquired von Willebrand syndrome

D68.09 Other von Willebrand disease
Platelet-type von Willebrand disease
Pseudo-von Willebrand disease
Code also, if applicable, qualitative platelet defects (D69.1)

D68.1 Hereditary factor XI deficiency
Hemophilia C
Plasma thromboplastin antecedent [PTA] deficiency
Rosenthal's disease

D68.2 Hereditary deficiency of other clotting factors
AC globulin deficiency
Congenital afibrinogenemia
Deficiency of factor I [fibrinogen]
Deficiency of factor II [prothrombin]
Deficiency of factor V [labile]
Deficiency of factor VII [stable]
Deficiency of factor X [Stuart-Prower]
Deficiency of factor XII [Hageman]
Deficiency of factor XIII [fibrin stabilizing]
Dysfibrinogenemia (congenital)
Hypoproconvertinemia
Owren's disease
Proaccelerin deficiency
AHA: 2025,2Q,3

D68.3 Hemorrhagic disorder due to circulating anticoagulants

D68.31 Hemorrhagic disorder due to intrinsic circulating anticoagulants, antibodies, or inhibitors

D68.311 Acquired hemophilia
Autoimmune hemophilia
Autoimmune inhibitors to clotting factors
Secondary hemophilia

D68.312 Antiphospholipid antibody with hemorrhagic disorder
Lupus anticoagulant (LAC) with hemorrhagic disorder
Systemic lupus erythematosus [SLE] inhibitor with hemorrhagic disorder

EXCLUDES 1 antiphospholipid antibody, finding without diagnosis (R76.0)
~~antiphospholipid antibody syndrome (D68.61)~~
~~antiphospholipid antibody with hypercoagulable state (D68.61)~~
~~lupus anticoagulant (LAC) with hypercoagulable state (D68.62)~~
~~systemic lupus erythematosus [SLE] inhibitor with hypercoagulable state (D68.62)~~
lupus anticoagulant (LAC) finding without diagnosis (R76.0)
systemic lupus erythematosus [SLE] inhibitor finding without diagnosis (R76.0)

EXCLUDES 2 ▶antiphospholipid antibody syndrome (D68.61)◀
▶antiphospholipid antibody with hypercoagulable state (D68.61)◀
▶lupus anticoagulant (LAC) with hypercoagulable state (D68.62)◀
▶systemic lupus erythematosus [SLE] inhibitor with hypercoagulable state (D68.62)◀

D68.318 Other hemorrhagic disorder due to intrinsic circulating anticoagulants, antibodies, or inhibitors
Antithromboplastinemia
Antithromboplastinogenemia
Hemorrhagic disorder due to intrinsic increase in anti-IXa
Hemorrhagic disorder due to intrinsic increase in antithrombin
Hemorrhagic disorder due to intrinsic increase in anti-VIIIa
Hemorrhagic disorder due to intrinsic increase in anti-XIa

D68.32 Hemorrhagic disorder due to extrinsic circulating anticoagulants
Drug-induced hemorrhagic disorder
Hemorrhagic disorder due to increase in anti-IIa
Hemorrhagic disorder due to increase in anti-Xa
Hyperheparinemia
Use additional code for adverse effect, if applicable, to identify drug (T45.515, T45.525)
AHA: 2021,1Q,4; 2016,1Q,14-15
TIP: Do not assign to identify routine therapeutic anticoagulation effects; assign only for documented adverse effects.

D68.4 Acquired coagulation factor deficiency
Deficiency of coagulation factor due to liver disease
Deficiency of coagulation factor due to vitamin K deficiency
EXCLUDES 1 vitamin K deficiency of newborn (P53)

D68.5 Primary thrombophilia
Primary hypercoagulable states
EXCLUDES 1
antiphospholipid syndrome (D68.61)
lupus anticoagulant (D68.62)
secondary activated protein C resistance (D68.69)
secondary antiphospholipid antibody syndrome (D68.69)
secondary lupus anticoagulant with hypercoagulable state (D68.69)
secondary systemic lupus erythematosus [SLE] inhibitor with hypercoagulable state (D68.69)
systemic lupus erythematosus [SLE] inhibitor finding without diagnosis (R76.0)
systemic lupus erythematosus [SLE] inhibitor with hemorrhagic disorder (D68.312)
thrombotic thrombocytopenic purpura (M31.19)

DEF: Thrombophilia: Increased tendency of the blood to clot, which can lead to thrombus or embolus formation.

D68.51 Activated protein C resistance
Factor V Leiden mutation
AHA: 2025,2Q,3

D68.52 Prothrombin gene mutation

D68.59 Other primary thrombophilia
Antithrombin III deficiency
Hypercoagulable state NOS
Primary hypercoagulable state NEC
Primary thrombophilia NEC
Protein C deficiency
Protein S deficiency
Thrombophilia NOS
AHA: 2021,2Q,8

D68.6 Other thrombophilia
Other hypercoagulable states
EXCLUDES 1
diffuse or disseminated intravascular coagulation [DIC] (D65)
heparin induced thrombocytopenia (HIT) (D75.82-)
hyperhomocysteinemia (E72.11)

D68.61 Antiphospholipid syndrome
Anticardiolipin syndrome
Antiphospholipid antibody syndrome
EXCLUDES 1
anti-phospholipid antibody, finding without diagnosis (R76.0)
~~anti-phospholipid antibody with hemorrhagic disorder (D68.312)~~
~~lupus anticoagulant syndrome (D68.62)~~
EXCLUDES 2
▶anti-phospholipid antibody with hemorrhagic disorder (D68.312)◀
▶lupus anticoagulant syndrome (D68.62)◀

D68.62 Lupus anticoagulant syndrome
Lupus anticoagulant
Presence of systemic lupus erythematosus [SLE] inhibitor
EXCLUDES 1
~~anticardiolipin syndrome (D68.61)~~
~~antiphospholipid syndrome (D68.61)~~
~~lupus anticoagulant (LAC) with hemorrhagic disorder (D68.312)~~
lupus anticoagulant (LAC) finding without diagnosis (R76.0)
EXCLUDES 2
▶anticardiolipin syndrome (D68.61)◀
▶antiphospholipid syndrome (D68.61)◀
▶lupus anticoagulant (LAC) with hemorrhagic disorder (D68.312)◀

D68.69 Other thrombophilia
COVID-19 associated hypercoagulability
Hypercoagulable states NEC
Secondary hypercoagulable state NOS
Code also, if applicable, associated condition
AHA: 2021,2Q,8

D68.8 Other specified coagulation defects
COVID-19 associated coagulopathy
Code also, if applicable, associated condition
EXCLUDES 1
hemorrhagic disease of newborn (P53)
AHA: 2021,1Q,39

D68.9 Coagulation defect, unspecified

D69 Purpura and other hemorrhagic conditions
EXCLUDES 1
benign hypergammaglobulinemic purpura (D89.0)
cryoglobulinemic purpura (D89.1)
essential (hemorrhagic) thrombocythemia (D47.3)
hemorrhagic thrombocythemia (D47.3)
purpura fulminans (D65)
thrombotic thrombocytopenic purpura (M31.19)
Waldenstrom hypergammaglobulinemic purpura (D89.0)

D69.0 Allergic purpura
Allergic vasculitis
Nonthrombocytopenic hemorrhagic purpura
Nonthrombocytopenic idiopathic purpura
Purpura anaphylactoid
Purpura Henoch(-Schonlein)
Purpura rheumatica
Vascular purpura
EXCLUDES 1
thrombocytopenic hemorrhagic purpura (D69.3)
AHA: 2020,3Q,26
DEF: Any hemorrhagic condition, thrombocytic or nonthrombocytopenic in origin, caused by a presumed allergic reaction.

D69.1 Qualitative platelet defects
Bernard-Soulier [giant platelet] syndrome
Glanzmann's disease
Grey platelet syndrome
Thromboasthenia (hemorrhagic) (hereditary)
Thrombocytopathy
EXCLUDES 1
hemolytic-uremic syndrome (D59.3-)
EXCLUDES 2
von Willebrand disease (D68.0-)

D69.2 Other nonthrombocytopenic purpura
Purpura NOS
Purpura simplex
Senile purpura

D69.3 Immune thrombocytopenic purpura
Hemorrhagic (thrombocytopenic) purpura
Idiopathic thrombocytopenic purpura
Tidal platelet dysgenesis
DEF: Tidal platelet dysgenesis: Fluctuation of platelet counts from normal to very low within periods of 20 to 40 days and may involve autoimmune platelet destruction.

D69.4 Other primary thrombocytopenia
EXCLUDES 1
transient neonatal thrombocytopenia (P61.0)
Wiskott-Aldrich syndrome (D82.0)

D69.41 Evans syndrome

D69.42 Congenital and hereditary thrombocytopenia purpura
Congenital thrombocytopenia
Hereditary thrombocytopenia
Code first congenital or hereditary disorder, such as:
thrombocytopenia with absent radius (TAR syndrome) (Q87.2)

D69.49 Other primary thrombocytopenia
Megakaryocytic hypoplasia
Primary thrombocytopenia NOS

D69.5 Secondary thrombocytopenia
EXCLUDES 1
heparin induced thrombocytopenia (HIT) (D75.82-)
transient thrombocytopenia of newborn (P61.0)

D69.51 Posttransfusion purpura
Posttransfusion purpura from whole blood (fresh) or blood products
PTP

D69.59 Other secondary thrombocytopenia
AHA: 2014,4Q,22

D69.6 Thrombocytopenia, unspecified
AHA: 2020,3Q,24

D69.8 Other specified hemorrhagic conditions
Capillary fragility (hereditary)
Vascular pseudohemophilia

D69.9 Hemorrhagic condition, unspecified

Other disorders of blood and blood-forming organs (D70-D77)

D70 Neutropenia
- **INCLUDES**
  - agranulocytosis
  - decreased absolute neutrophile count (ANC)
- Code also, if applicable, mucositis (J34.81, K12.3-, K92.81, N76.81)
- Use additional code for any associated:
  - fever (R50.81)
- **EXCLUDES 1**
  - neutropenic splenomegaly (D73.81)
  - transient neonatal neutropenia (P61.5)
- **DEF:** Abnormally low number of neutrophils. Neutrophils are phagocytic, meaning they surround and consume harmful pathogens, primarily bacteria. When neutrophil counts decrease the risk of infection increases.

- **D70.0 Congenital agranulocytosis**
  - Congenital neutropenia
  - Infantile genetic agranulocytosis
  - Kostmann's disease
- **D70.1 Agranulocytosis secondary to cancer chemotherapy**
  - Code also underlying neoplasm
  - Use additional code for adverse effect, if applicable, to identify drug (T45.1X5)
  - AHA: 2020,3Q,22; 2014,4Q,22
- **D70.2 Other drug-induced agranulocytosis**
  - Use additional code for adverse effect, if applicable, to identify drug (T36-T50 with fifth or sixth character 5)
- **D70.3 Neutropenia due to infection**
- **D70.4 Cyclic neutropenia**
  - Cyclic hematopoiesis
  - Periodic neutropenia
- **D70.8 Other neutropenia**
- **D70.9 Neutropenia, unspecified**
  - AHA: 2020,3Q,24

D71 Functional disorders of polymorphonuclear neutrophils
- ~~Cell membrane receptor complex [CR3] defect~~
- ~~Chronic (childhood) granulomatous disease~~
- ~~Congenital dysphagocytosis~~
- ~~Progressive septic granulomatosis~~

- **D71.1 Leukocyte adhesion deficiency**
  - LAD-I
  - LAD-II
  - LAD-III
  - Leukocyte adhesion deficiency type I
  - Leukocyte adhesion deficiency type II
  - Leukocyte adhesion deficiency type III
- **D71.8 Other functional disorders of polymorphonuclear neutrophils**
  - Cell membrane receptor complex [CR3] defect
  - Chronic (childhood) granulomatous disease
  - Congenital dysphagocytosis
  - Progressive septic granulomatosis
- **D71.9 Functional disorders of polymorphonuclear neutrophils, unspecified**

D72 Other disorders of white blood cells
- **EXCLUDES 1**
  - basophilia (D72.824)
  - immunity disorders (D80-D89)
  - neutropenia (D70)
  - preleukemia (syndrome) (D46.9)

- **D72.0 Genetic anomalies of leukocytes**
  - Alder (granulation) (granulocyte) anomaly
  - Alder syndrome
  - Hereditary leukocytic hypersegmentation
  - Hereditary leukocytic hyposegmentation
  - Hereditary leukomelanopathy
  - May-Hegglin (granulation) (granulocyte) anomaly
  - May-Hegglin syndrome
  - Pelger-Huet (granulation) (granulocyte) anomaly
  - Pelger-Huet syndrome
  - **EXCLUDES 1** Chediak (-Steinbrinck)-Higashi syndrome (E70.330)
- **D72.1 Eosinophilia**
  - **EXCLUDES 2**
    - Loffler's syndrome (J82.89)
    - pulmonary eosinophilia (J82.-)
  - AHA: 2020,4Q,8-10
  - **DEF:** Abnormally large accumulation or formation of eosinophils (nucleated, granular leukocytes) in the blood, characteristic of allergic states and infection.
  - **D72.10 Eosinophilia, unspecified**
  - **D72.11 Hypereosinophilic syndrome [HES]**
    - **D72.110 Idiopathic hypereosinophilic syndrome [IHES]**
    - **D72.111 Lymphocytic Variant Hypereosinophilic Syndrome [LHES]**
      - Lymphocyte variant hypereosinophilia
      - Code also, if applicable, any associated lymphocytic neoplastic disorder
    - **D72.118 Other hypereosinophilic syndrome**
      - Episodic angioedema with eosinophilia
      - Gleich's syndrome
    - **D72.119 Hypereosinophilic syndrome [HES], unspecified**
  - **D72.12 Drug rash with eosinophilia and systemic symptoms syndrome**
    - DRESS syndrome
    - Use additional code for adverse effect, if applicable, to identify drug (T36-T50 with fifth or sixth character 5)
  - **D72.18 Eosinophilia in diseases classified elsewhere**
    - Code first underlying disease, such as:
      - chronic myelomonocytic leukemia (C93.1-)
  - **D72.19 Other eosinophilia**
    - Familial eosinophilia
    - Hereditary eosinophilia
- **D72.8 Other specified disorders of white blood cells**
  - **EXCLUDES 1** leukemia (C91-C95)
  - **D72.81 Decreased white blood cell count**
    - **EXCLUDES 1** neutropenia (D70.-)
    - **D72.810 Lymphocytopenia**
      - Decreased lymphocytes
    - **D72.818 Other decreased white blood cell count**
      - Basophilic leukopenia
      - Eosinophilic leukopenia
      - Monocytopenia
      - Other decreased leukocytes
      - Plasmacytopenia
    - **D72.819 Decreased white blood cell count, unspecified**
      - Decreased leukocytes, unspecified
      - Leukocytopenia, unspecified
      - Leukopenia
      - **EXCLUDES 1** malignant leukopenia (D70.9)
  - **D72.82 Elevated white blood cell count**
    - **EXCLUDES 1** eosinophilia (D72.1)
    - **D72.820 Lymphocytosis (symptomatic)**
      - Elevated lymphocytes
    - **D72.821 Monocytosis (symptomatic)**
      - **EXCLUDES 1** infectious mononucleosis (B27.-)
    - **D72.822 Plasmacytosis**
    - **D72.823 Leukemoid reaction**
      - Basophilic leukemoid reaction
      - Leukemoid reaction NOS
      - Lymphocytic leukemoid reaction
      - Monocytic leukemoid reaction
      - Myelocytic leukemoid reaction
      - Neutrophilic leukemoid reaction
    - **D72.824 Basophilia**
      - **DEF:** Increase in the basophils of the blood, a type of white blood cell, often seen in conjunction with neoplastic disorders.
    - **D72.825 Bandemia**
      - Bandemia without diagnosis of specific infection
      - **EXCLUDES 1** confirmed infection - code to infection
        - leukemia (C91.-, C92.-, C93.-, C94.-, C95.-)
      - **DEF:** Increase in early neutrophil cells, called band cells, that may indicate infection.
    - **D72.828 Other elevated white blood cell count**
    - **D72.829 Elevated white blood cell count, unspecified**
      - Elevated leukocytes, unspecified
      - Leukocytosis, unspecified
  - **D72.89 Other specified disorders of white blood cells**
    - Abnormality of white blood cells NEC
- **D72.9 Disorder of white blood cells, unspecified**
  - Abnormal leukocyte differential NOS

D73 Diseases of spleen

D73.0 Hyposplenism
Atrophy of spleen
EXCLUDES 1 asplenia (congenital) (Q89.01)
postsurgical absence of spleen (Z90.81)
AHA: 2025,1Q,24

D73.1 Hypersplenism
EXCLUDES 1 neutropenic splenomegaly (D73.81)
primary splenic neutropenia (D73.81)
splenitis, splenomegaly in late syphilis (A52.79)
splenitis, splenomegaly in tuberculosis (A18.85)
splenomegaly congenital (Q89.0)
splenomegaly NOS (R16.1)

D73.2 Chronic congestive splenomegaly
D73.3 Abscess of spleen
D73.4 Cyst of spleen
D73.5 Infarction of spleen
Splenic rupture, nontraumatic
Torsion of spleen
EXCLUDES 1 rupture of spleen due to Plasmodium vivax malaria (B51.0)
traumatic rupture of spleen (S36.03-)

D73.8 Other diseases of spleen
D73.81 Neutropenic splenomegaly
Werner-Schultz disease
D73.89 Other diseases of spleen
Fibrosis of spleen NOS
Perisplenitis
Splenitis NOS

D73.9 Disease of spleen, unspecified

D74 Methemoglobinemia

D74.0 Congenital methemoglobinemia
Congenital NADH-methemoglobin reductase deficiency
Hemoglobin-M [Hb-M] disease
Methemoglobinemia, hereditary

D74.8 Other methemoglobinemias
Acquired methemoglobinemia (with sulfhemoglobinemia)
Toxic methemoglobinemia

D74.9 Methemoglobinemia, unspecified

D75 Other and unspecified diseases of blood and blood-forming organs
EXCLUDES 2 acute lymphadenitis (L04.-)
chronic lymphadenitis (I88.1)
enlarged lymph nodes (R59.-)
hypergammaglobulinemia NOS (D89.2)
lymphadenitis NOS (I88.9)
mesenteric lymphadenitis (acute) (chronic) (I88.0)

D75.0 Familial erythrocytosis
Benign polycythemia
Familial polycythemia
EXCLUDES 1 hereditary ovalocytosis (D58.1)

D75.1 Secondary polycythemia
Acquired polycythemia
Emotional polycythemia
Erythrocytosis NOS
Hypoxemic polycythemia
Nephrogenous polycythemia
Polycythemia due to erythropoietin
Polycythemia due to fall in plasma volume
Polycythemia due to high altitude
Polycythemia due to stress
Polycythemia NOS
Relative polycythemia
EXCLUDES 1 polycythemia neonatorum (P61.1)
polycythemia vera (D45)
DEF: Elevated number of red blood cells in circulating blood as a result of reduced oxygen supply to the tissues.

D75.8 Other specified diseases of blood and blood-forming organs
D75.81 Myelofibrosis
Myelofibrosis NOS
Secondary myelofibrosis NOS
Code first the underlying disorder, such as:
malignant neoplasm of breast (C50.-)
Use additional code for adverse effect, if applicable, to identify drug (T45.1X5)
Use additional code, if applicable, for associated therapy-related myelodysplastic syndrome (D46.-)
EXCLUDES 1 acute myelofibrosis (C94.4-)
idiopathic myelofibrosis (D47.1)
leukoerythroblastic anemia (D61.82)
myelofibrosis with myeloid metaplasia (D47.4)
myelophthisic anemia (D61.82)
myelophthisis (D61.82)
primary myelofibrosis (D47.1)

D75.82 Heparin induced thrombocytopenia (HIT)
Use additional code, if applicable, for adverse effect of heparin (T45.515-)
AHA: 2022,4Q,9-10
DEF: Immune-mediated reaction to heparin therapy causing an abrupt fall in platelet count and serious complications such as pulmonary embolism, stroke, AMI, or DVT.

D75.821 Non-immune heparin-induced thrombocytopenia
Non-immune HIT
Type 1 heparin-induced thrombocytopenia

D75.822 Immune-mediated heparin-induced thrombocytopenia
Immune-mediated HIT
Type 2 heparin-induced thrombocytopenia

D75.828 Other heparin-induced thrombocytopenia syndrome
Autoimmune heparin-induced thrombocytopenia syndrome
Delayed-onset heparin-induced thrombocytopenia
Persisting heparin-induced thrombocytopenia

D75.829 Heparin-induced thrombocytopenia, unspecified

D75.83 Thrombocytosis
EXCLUDES 2 essential thrombocythemia (D47.3)
AHA: 2021,4Q,7-8

D75.838 Other thrombocytosis
Reactive thrombocytosis
Secondary thrombocytosis
Code also underlying condition, if known and applicable

D75.839 Thrombocytosis, unspecified
Thrombocythemia NOS
Thrombocytosis NOS

D75.84 Other platelet-activating anti-PF4 disorders
Spontaneous heparin-induced thrombocytopenia syndrome (without heparin exposure)
Thrombosis with thrombocytopenia syndrome
Vaccine-induced thrombotic thrombocytopenia
Use additional code, if applicable, for adverse effect of other viral vaccine (T50.B95-)
AHA: 2022,4Q,9-10

D75.89 Other specified diseases of blood and blood-forming organs

D75.9 Disease of blood and blood-forming organs, unspecified

D75.A Glucose-6-phosphate dehydrogenase (G6PD) deficiency without anemia
EXCLUDES 1 glucose-6-phosphate dehydrogenase (G6PD) deficiency with anemia (D55.0)
AHA: 2019,4Q,4-5

D76 Other specified diseases with participation of lymphoreticular and reticulohistiocytic tissue

EXCLUDES 1
(Abt-) Letterer-Siwe disease (C96.0)
eosinophilic granuloma (C96.5)
Hand-Schuller-Christian disease (C96.5)
histiocytic medullary reticulosis (C96.9)
histiocytic sarcoma (C96.A)
histiocytosis X, multifocal (C96.5)
histiocytosis X, unifocal (C96.6)
Langerhans-cell histiocytosis NOS (C96.6)
Langerhans-cell histiocytosis, multifocal (C96.5)
Langerhans-cell histiocytosis, unifocal (C96.6)
leukemic reticuloendotheliosis (C91.4-)
lipomelanotic reticulosis (I89.8)
malignant histiocytosis (C96.A)
malignant reticulosis (C86.0)
nonlipid reticuloendotheliosis (C96.0)

D76.1 Hemophagocytic lymphohistiocytosis
Familial hemophagocytic reticulosis
Histiocytoses of mononuclear phagocytes

D76.2 Hemophagocytic syndrome, infection-associated
Use additional code to identify infectious agent or disease

D76.3 Other histiocytosis syndromes
Reticulohistiocytoma (giant-cell)
Sinus histiocytosis with massive lymphadenopathy
Xanthogranuloma

D77 Other disorders of blood and blood-forming organs in diseases classified elsewhere

Code first underlying disease, such as:
amyloidosis (E85.-)
congenital early syphilis (A50.0-)
echinococcosis (B67.0-B67.9)
malaria (B50.0-B54)
schistosomiasis [bilharziasis] (B65.0-B65.9)
vitamin C deficiency (E54)

EXCLUDES 1
rupture of spleen due to Plasmodium vivax malaria (B51.0)
splenitis, splenomegaly in late syphilis (A52.79)
splenitis, splenomegaly in tuberculosis (A18.85)

Intraoperative and postprocedural complications of the spleen (D78)

D78 Intraoperative and postprocedural complications of the spleen
AHA: 2016,4Q,9-10

D78.0 Intraoperative hemorrhage and hematoma of the spleen complicating a procedure
EXCLUDES 1 intraoperative hemorrhage and hematoma of the spleen due to accidental puncture or laceration during a procedure (D78.1-)

D78.01 Intraoperative hemorrhage and hematoma of the spleen complicating a procedure on the spleen
D78.02 Intraoperative hemorrhage and hematoma of the spleen complicating other procedure

D78.1 Accidental puncture and laceration of the spleen during a procedure
D78.11 Accidental puncture and laceration of the spleen during a procedure on the spleen
D78.12 Accidental puncture and laceration of the spleen during other procedure
AHA: 2022,1Q,22

D78.2 Postprocedural hemorrhage of the spleen following a procedure
D78.21 Postprocedural hemorrhage of the spleen following a procedure on the spleen
D78.22 Postprocedural hemorrhage of the spleen following other procedure

D78.3 Postprocedural hematoma and seroma of the spleen following a procedure
D78.31 Postprocedural hematoma of the spleen following a procedure on the spleen
D78.32 Postprocedural hematoma of the spleen following other procedure
D78.33 Postprocedural seroma of the spleen following a procedure on the spleen
D78.34 Postprocedural seroma of the spleen following other procedure

D78.8 Other intraoperative and postprocedural complications of the spleen
Use additional code, if applicable, to further specify disorder
D78.81 Other intraoperative complications of the spleen
D78.89 Other postprocedural complications of the spleen

Certain disorders involving the immune mechanism (D80-D89)

INCLUDES
defects in the complement system
immunodeficiency disorders, except human immunodeficiency virus [HIV] disease
sarcoidosis

EXCLUDES 1
autoimmune disease (systemic) NOS (M35.9)
functional disorders of polymorphonuclear neutrophils ▶(D71-)◀
human immunodeficiency virus [HIV] disease (B20)

D80 Immunodeficiency with predominantly antibody defects

D80.0 Hereditary hypogammaglobulinemia
Autosomal recessive agammaglobulinemia (Swiss type)
X-linked agammaglobulinemia [Bruton] (with growth hormone deficiency)

D80.1 Nonfamilial hypogammaglobulinemia
Agammaglobulinemia with immunoglobulin-bearing B-lymphocytes
Common variable agammaglobulinemia [CVAgamma]
Hypogammaglobulinemia NOS

D80.2 Selective deficiency of immunoglobulin A [IgA]

D80.3 Selective deficiency of immunoglobulin G [IgG] subclasses

D80.4 Selective deficiency of immunoglobulin M [IgM]

D80.5 Immunodeficiency with increased immunoglobulin M [IgM]

D80.6 Antibody deficiency with near-normal immunoglobulins or with hyperimmunoglobulinemia

D80.7 Transient hypogammaglobulinemia of infancy

D80.8 Other immunodeficiencies with predominantly antibody defects
Kappa light chain deficiency

D80.9 Immunodeficiency with predominantly antibody defects, unspecified

D81 Combined immunodeficiencies
EXCLUDES 1 autosomal recessive agammaglobulinemia (Swiss type) (D80.0)

D81.0 Severe combined immunodeficiency [SCID] with reticular dysgenesis

D81.1 Severe combined immunodeficiency [SCID] with low T- and B-cell numbers

D81.2 Severe combined immunodeficiency [SCID] with low or normal B-cell numbers

D81.3 Adenosine deaminase [ADA] deficiency
AHA: 2019,4Q,5-6

D81.30 Adenosine deaminase deficiency, unspecified
ADA deficiency NOS

D81.31 Severe combined immunodeficiency due to adenosine deaminase deficiency
ADA deficiency with SCID
Adenosine deaminase [ADA] deficiency with severe combined immunodeficiency

D81.32 Adenosine deaminase 2 deficiency
ADA2 deficiency
Adenosine deaminase deficiency type 2
Code also, if applicable, any associated manifestations, such as:
polyarteritis nodosa (M30.0)
stroke (I63.-)

D81.39 Other adenosine deaminase deficiency
Adenosine deaminase [ADA] deficiency type 1, NOS
Adenosine deaminase [ADA] deficiency type 1, without SCID
Adenosine deaminase [ADA] deficiency type 1, without severe combined immunodeficiency
Partial ADA deficiency (type 1)
Partial adenosine deaminase deficiency (type 1)

D81.4 Nezelof's syndrome

D81.5 Purine nucleoside phosphorylase [PNP] deficiency

D81.6 Major histocompatibility complex class I deficiency
Bare lymphocyte syndrome

D81.7 Major histocompatibility complex class II deficiency

Chapter 3. Diseases of the Blood and Blood-forming Organs

D81.8 Other combined immunodeficiencies
- **D81.81** Biotin-dependent carboxylase deficiency
  - Multiple carboxylase deficiency
  - EXCLUDES 1: biotin-dependent carboxylase deficiency due to dietary deficiency of biotin (E53.8)
  - **D81.810** Biotinidase deficiency
  - **D81.818** Other biotin-dependent carboxylase deficiency
    - Holocarboxylase synthetase deficiency
    - Other multiple carboxylase deficiency
  - **D81.819** Biotin-dependent carboxylase deficiency, unspecified
    - Multiple carboxylase deficiency, unspecified
- **D81.82** Activated Phosphoinositide 3-kinase Delta Syndrome [APDS]
  - p110d-activating mutation causing senescent T cells, lymphadenopathy, and immunodeficiency [PASLI] disease
  - Code also, if applicable, any associated manifestations, such as:
    - bronchiectasis (J47.-)
    - herpes virus infections (B00.-)
    - other acute respiratory tract infections (J00-J06; J20-J22)
    - other infections (A00-B99)
    - pneumonia (J12-J18)
  - AHA: 2022,4Q,11
- **D81.89** Other combined immunodeficiencies
- **D81.9** Combined immunodeficiency, unspecified
  - Severe combined immunodeficiency disorder [SCID] NOS

D82 Immunodeficiency associated with other major defects
- EXCLUDES 1: ataxia telangiectasia [Louis-Bar] (G11.3)
- **D82.0** Wiskott-Aldrich syndrome
  - Immunodeficiency with thrombocytopenia and eczema
- **D82.1** Di George's syndrome
  - Pharyngeal pouch syndrome
  - Thymic alymphoplasia
  - Thymic aplasia or hypoplasia with immunodeficiency
  - AHA: 2019,3Q,14
- **D82.2** Immunodeficiency with short-limbed stature
- **D82.3** Immunodeficiency following hereditary defective response to Epstein-Barr virus
  - X-linked lymphoproliferative disease
- **D82.4** Hyperimmunoglobulin E [IgE] syndrome
- **D82.8** Immunodeficiency associated with other specified major defects
- **D82.9** Immunodeficiency associated with major defect, unspecified

D83 Common variable immunodeficiency
- **D83.0** Common variable immunodeficiency with predominant abnormalities of B-cell numbers and function
- **D83.1** Common variable immunodeficiency with predominant immunoregulatory T-cell disorders
- **D83.2** Common variable immunodeficiency with autoantibodies to B- or T-cells
- **D83.8** Other common variable immunodeficiencies
- **D83.9** Common variable immunodeficiency, unspecified

D84 Other immunodeficiencies
- **D84.0** Lymphocyte function antigen-1 [LFA-1] defect
- **D84.1** Defects in the complement system
  - C1 esterase inhibitor [C1-INH] deficiency
- **D84.8** Other specified immunodeficiencies
  - AHA: 2020,4Q,10-12
  - **D84.81** Immunodeficiency due to conditions classified elsewhere
    - Code first underlying condition, such as:
      - chromosomal abnormalities (Q90-Q99)
      - diabetes mellitus (E08-E13)
      - malignant neoplasms (C00-C96)
    - EXCLUDES 1: certain disorders involving the immune mechanism (D80-D83, D84.0, D84.1, D84.9)
      - human immunodeficiency virus [HIV] disease (B20)
    - AHA: 2021,1Q,52
  - **D84.82** Immunodeficiency due to drugs and external causes
    - **D84.821** Immunodeficiency due to drugs
      - Immunodeficiency due to (current or past) medication
      - Use additional code for adverse effect if applicable, to identify adverse effect of drug (T36-T50 with fifth or six character 5)
      - Use additional code, if applicable, for associated long term (current) drug therapy drug or medication such as:
        - long term (current) drug therapy systemic steroids (Z79.52)
        - other long term (current) drug therapy (Z79.899)
    - **D84.822** Immunodeficiency due to external causes
      - Code also, if applicable, radiological procedure and radiotherapy (Y84.2)
      - Use additional code for external cause such as:
        - exposure to ionizing radiation (W88)
  - **D84.89** Other immunodeficiencies
- **D84.9** Immunodeficiency, unspecified
  - Immunocompromised NOS
  - Immunodeficient NOS
  - Immunosuppressed NOS
  - AHA: 2020,4Q,10

D86 Sarcoidosis
- DEF: Clustering of immune cells resulting in granuloma formation. Often affects the lungs and lymphatic system but can occur in other body sites.
- **D86.0** Sarcoidosis of lung
- **D86.1** Sarcoidosis of lymph nodes
- **D86.2** Sarcoidosis of lung with sarcoidosis of lymph nodes
- **D86.3** Sarcoidosis of skin
- **D86.8** Sarcoidosis of other sites
  - **D86.81** Sarcoid meningitis
  - **D86.82** Multiple cranial nerve palsies in sarcoidosis
  - **D86.83** Sarcoid iridocyclitis
  - **D86.84** Sarcoid pyelonephritis
    - Tubulo-interstitial nephropathy in sarcoidosis
  - **D86.85** Sarcoid myocarditis
  - **D86.86** Sarcoid arthropathy
    - Polyarthritis in sarcoidosis
  - **D86.87** Sarcoid myositis
  - **D86.89** Sarcoidosis of other sites
    - Hepatic granuloma
    - Uveoparotid fever [Heerfordt]
- **D86.9** Sarcoidosis, unspecified

D89 Other disorders involving the immune mechanism, not elsewhere classified
- EXCLUDES 1: hyperglobulinemia NOS (R77.1)
  - monoclonal gammopathy (of undetermined significance) (D47.2)
- EXCLUDES 2: transplant failure and rejection (T86.-)
- **D89.0** Polyclonal hypergammaglobulinemia
  - Benign hypergammaglobulinemic purpura
  - Polyclonal gammopathy NOS

Chapter 3. Diseases of the Blood and Blood-forming Organs

D89.1 Cryoglobulinemia `Rx` `ESR`
Cryoglobulinemic purpura
Cryoglobulinemic vasculitis
Essential cryoglobulinemia
Idiopathic cryoglobulinemia
Mixed cryoglobulinemia
Primary cryoglobulinemia
Secondary cryoglobulinemia

D89.2 Hypergammaglobulinemia, unspecified

D89.3 Immune reconstitution syndrome `Rx` `ESR` `COM`
Immune reconstitution inflammatory syndrome [IRIS]
Use additional code for adverse effect, if applicable, to identify drug (T36-T50 with fifth or sixth character 5)

✓5th D89.4 Mast cell activation syndrome and related disorders
EXCLUDES 1:
aggressive systemic mastocytosis (C96.21)
(indolent) systemic mastocytosis (D47.02)
(non-congenital) cutaneous mastocytosis (D47.01)
congenital cutaneous mastocytosis (Q82.2)
malignant mast cell neoplasm (C96.2-)
malignant mastocytoma (C96.29)
mast cell leukemia (C94.3-)
mast cell sarcoma (C96.22)
mastocytoma NOS (D47.09)
other mast cell neoplasms of uncertain behavior (D47.09)
systemic mastocytosis associated with a clonal hematologic non-mast cell lineage disease (SM-AHNMD) (D47.02)
AHA: 2016,4Q,11

- **D89.40** Mast cell activation, unspecified `Rx` `ESR` `COM`
  Mast cell activation disorder, unspecified
  Mast cell activation syndrome, NOS
- **D89.41** Monoclonal mast cell activation syndrome `Rx` `ESR` `COM`
- **D89.42** Idiopathic mast cell activation syndrome `Rx` `ESR` `COM`
- **D89.43** Secondary mast cell activation `Rx` `ESR` `COM`
  Secondary mast cell activation syndrome
  Code also underlying etiology, if known
- **D89.44** Hereditary alpha tryptasemia `Rx` `ESR` `COM`
  Use additional code, if applicable, for:
  allergy status, other than to drugs and biological substances (Z91.0-)
  personal history of anaphylaxis (Z87.892)
  AHA: 2021,4Q,8
- **D89.49** Other mast cell activation disorder `Rx` `ESR` `COM`
  Other mast cell activation syndrome

✓5th D89.8 Other specified disorders involving the immune mechanism, not elsewhere classified

- ✓6th **D89.81** Graft-versus-host disease
  Code first underlying cause, such as:
  complications of blood transfusion (T80.89)
  complications of transplanted organs and tissue (T86.-)
  Use additional code to identify associated manifestations, such as:
  desquamative dermatitis (L30.8)
  diarrhea (R19.7)
  elevated bilirubin (R17)
  hair loss (L65.9)
  AHA: 2023,3Q,19
  - **D89.810** Acute graft-versus-host disease `HCC` `Rx` `ESR` `COM` `UPD`
  - **D89.811** Chronic graft-versus-host disease `HCC` `Rx` `ESR` `COM` `UPD`
  - **D89.812** Acute on chronic graft-versus-host disease `HCC` `Rx` `ESR` `COM` `UPD`
  - **D89.813** Graft-versus-host disease, unspecified `HCC` `Rx` `ESR` `COM` `UPD`
- **D89.82** Autoimmune lymphoproliferative syndrome [ALPS] `ESR` `COM`
  DEF: Rare genetic alteration of the Fas protein that impairs normal cellular apoptosis (normal cell death), causing abnormal accumulation of lymphocytes in the lymph glands, liver, and spleen. Symptoms include neutropenia, anemia, and thrombocytopenia.
- ✓6th **D89.83** Cytokine release syndrome
  Code first underlying cause, such as:
  complications following infusion, transfusion and therapeutic injection (T80.89-)
  complications of transplanted organs and tissue (T86.-)
  Use additional code for adverse effect, if applicable, to identify immune checkpoint inhibitors and immunostimulant drugs (T45.AX5)
  Use additional code to identify associated manifestations
  AHA: 2020,4Q,12-15
  DEF: Form of systemic inflammatory response syndrome (SIRS) in which immune substances (cytokines) are released rapidly and in large amounts from the affected immune cells into the blood. The severity of associated symptoms or manifestations varies based on the underlying cause. This syndrome occurs as a complication of a disease, infection, or drug (often an adverse effect of immunotherapy in the form of treatment receiving monoclonal antibodies or Chimeric Antigen Receptor T [CAR-T] cells).
  - **D89.831** Cytokine release syndrome, grade 1 `UPD`
  - **D89.832** Cytokine release syndrome, grade 2 `UPD`
  - **D89.833** Cytokine release syndrome, grade 3 `UPD`
  - **D89.834** Cytokine release syndrome, grade 4 `UPD`
  - **D89.835** Cytokine release syndrome, grade 5 `UPD`
  - **D89.839** Cytokine release syndrome, grade unspecified `UPD`
- **D89.84** IgG4-related disease `HCC` `Rx` `ESR` `COM`
  Immunoglobulin G4-related disease
  AHA: 2023,4Q,9
- **D89.89** Other specified disorders involving the immune mechanism, not elsewhere classified `Rx` `ESR` `COM`
  EXCLUDES 1: human immunodeficiency virus disease (B20)
  AHA: 2017,4Q,109

D89.9 Disorder involving the immune mechanism, unspecified `Rx` `ESR` `COM`
Immune disease NOS
AHA: 2015,3Q,22

Chapter 4. Endocrine, Nutritional, and Metabolic Diseases (E00–E89)

Chapter-specific Guidelines with Coding Examples

The chapter-specific guidelines from the ICD-10-CM Official Guidelines for Coding and Reporting have been provided below. Along with these guidelines are coding examples, contained in the shaded boxes, that have been developed to help illustrate the coding and/or sequencing guidance found in these guidelines.

a. Diabetes mellitus

The diabetes mellitus codes are combination codes that include the type of diabetes mellitus, the body system affected, and the complications affecting that body system. As many codes within a particular category as are necessary to describe all of the complications of the disease may be used. They should be sequenced based on the reason for a particular encounter. Assign as many codes from categories E08–E13 as needed to identify all of the associated conditions that the patient has.

> Patient is seen for uncontrolled diabetes, type 2, with hyperglycemia diabetic nephropathy, and diabetic gastroparesis
>
> | | |
> |---|---|
> | E11.65 | Type 2 diabetes mellitus with hyperglycemia |
> | E11.21 | Type 2 diabetes mellitus with diabetic nephropathy |
> | E11.43 | Type 2 diabetes mellitus with diabetic autonomic (poly)neuropathy |
> | K31.84 | Gastroparesis |
>
> *Explanation*: Use as many codes to describe the diabetic complications as needed. Many are combination codes that describe more than one condition. Code first the reason for the encounter. The term "uncontrolled" can refer to either hyperglycemia or hypoglycemia. In this case, "uncontrolled" is described as "with hyperglycemia."

1) **Type of diabetes**

   The age of a patient is not the sole determining factor, though most type 1 diabetics develop the condition before reaching puberty. For this reason, type 1 diabetes mellitus is also referred to as juvenile diabetes.

   (a) Presymptomatic Type 1 diabetes mellitus

   Codes E10.A-, Type 1 diabetes mellitus, presymptomatic, are assigned for early-stage type 1 diabetes that predates the onset of symptoms.

   (b) Type 2 diabetes mellitus in remission

   Code E11.A, Type 2 diabetes mellitus without complications in remission, is assigned based on provider documentation that the diabetes mellitus is in remission. If the documentation is unclear as to whether the Type 2 diabetes mellitus has achieved remission, the provider should be queried. For example, the term "resolved" is not synonymous with remission.

2) **Type of diabetes mellitus not documented**

   If the type of diabetes mellitus is not documented in the medical record the default is E11.-, Type 2 diabetes mellitus.

> Office visit lists diabetic retinopathy with macular edema and hypertension on patient problem list
>
> | | |
> |---|---|
> | E11.311 | Type 2 diabetes mellitus with unspecified diabetic retinopathy with macular edema |
> | I10 | Essential (primary) hypertension |
>
> *Explanation*: Since the type of diabetes was not documented, default to category E11.

3) **Diabetes mellitus and the use of insulin, oral hypoglycemics, and injectable non-insulin drugs**

   If the documentation in a medical record does not indicate the type of diabetes but does indicate that the patient uses insulin, code E11-, Type 2 diabetes mellitus, should be assigned. Additional code(s) should be assigned from category Z79 to identify the long-term (current) use of insulin, oral hypoglycemic drugs, or injectable non-insulin antidiabetic, as follows:

   If the patient is treated with both oral hypoglycemic drugs and insulin, both code Z79.4, Long term (current) use of insulin, and code Z79.84, Long term (current) use of oral hypoglycemic drugs, should be assigned.

   If the patient is treated with both insulin and an injectable non-insulin antidiabetic drug, assign codes Z79.4, Long term (current) use of insulin, and Z79.85, Long-term (current) use of injectable non-insulin antidiabetic drugs.

   If the patient is treated with both oral hypoglycemic drugs and an injectable non-insulin antidiabetic drug, assign codes Z79.84, Long term (current) use of oral hypoglycemic drugs, and Z79.85, Long-term (current) use of injectable non-insulin antidiabetic drugs.

   Code Z79.4 should not be assigned if insulin is given temporarily to bring a type 2 patient's blood sugar under control during an encounter.

> Office visit lists chronic diabetes with daily insulin use on patient problem list
>
> | | |
> |---|---|
> | E11.9 | Type 2 diabetes mellitus without complications |
> | Z79.4 | Long term (current) use of insulin |
>
> *Explanation*: Do not assume that a patient on insulin must have type 1 diabetes. The default for diabetes without further specification defaults to type 2. Add the code for long term use of insulin.

4) **Diabetes mellitus in pregnancy and gestational diabetes**

   See Section I.C.15. Diabetes mellitus in pregnancy.
   See Section I.C.15. Gestational (pregnancy induced) diabetes

5) **Complications due to insulin pump malfunction**

   (a) Underdose of insulin due to insulin pump failure

   An underdose of insulin due to an insulin pump failure should be assigned to a code from subcategory T85.6, Mechanical complication of other specified internal and external prosthetic devices, implants and grafts, that specifies the type of pump malfunction, as the principal or first-listed code, followed by code T38.3X6-, Underdosing of insulin and oral hypoglycemic [antidiabetic] drugs. Additional codes for the type of diabetes mellitus and any associated complications due to the underdosing should also be assigned.

> A 24-year-old type 1 diabetic male treated in for hyperglycemia; insulin pump found to be malfunctioning and underdosing
>
> | | |
> |---|---|
> | T85.614A | Breakdown (mechanical) of insulin pump, initial encounter |
> | T38.3X6A | Underdosing of insulin and oral hypoglycemic [antidiabetic] drugs, initial encounter |
> | E10.65 | Type 1 diabetes mellitus with hyperglycemia |
>
> *Explanation*: The complication code for the mechanical breakdown of the pump is sequenced first, followed by the underdosing code and type of diabetes with complication. Code all other diabetic complication codes necessary to describe the patient's condition.

   (b) Overdose of insulin due to insulin pump failure

   The principal or first-listed code for an encounter due to an insulin pump malfunction resulting in an overdose of insulin, should also be T85.6-, Mechanical complication of other specified internal and external prosthetic devices, implants and grafts, followed by code T38.3X1-, Poisoning by insulin and oral hypoglycemic [antidiabetic] drugs, accidental (unintentional).

> A 24-year-old type 1 diabetic male found down with diabetic coma, brought into ED and treated for hypoglycemia; insulin pump found to be malfunctioning and overdosing
>
> | | |
> |---|---|
> | T85.614A | Breakdown (mechanical) of insulin pump, initial encounter |
> | T38.3X1A | Poisoning by insulin and oral hypoglycemic [antidiabetic] drugs, accidental (unintentional), initial encounter |
> | E10.641 | Type 1 diabetes mellitus with hypoglycemia with coma |
>
> *Explanation*: The complication code for the mechanical breakdown of the pump is sequenced first, followed by the poisoning code and type of diabetes with complication. All the characters in the combination code must be used to form a valid code and to fully describe the type of diabetes, the hypoglycemia, and the coma.

6) **Secondary diabetes mellitus**

   Codes under categories E08, Diabetes mellitus due to underlying condition, E09, Drug or chemical induced diabetes mellitus, and E13, Other specified diabetes mellitus, identify complications/manifestations associated with secondary diabetes mellitus. Secondary diabetes is always caused by another condition or event (e.g., cystic fibrosis, malignant neoplasm of pancreas, pancreatectomy, adverse effect of drug, or poisoning).

(a) Secondary diabetes mellitus and the use of insulin or oral hypoglycemic drugs

For patients with secondary diabetes mellitus who routinely use insulin, oral hypoglycemic drugs, or injectable non-insulin drugs, additional code(s) from category Z79 should be assigned to identify the long-term (current) use of insulin, oral hypoglycemic drugs, or non-injectable non-insulin drugs as follows:

If the patient is treated with both oral hypoglycemic drugs and insulin, both code Z79.4, Long term (current) use of insulin, and code Z79.84, Long term (current) use of oral hypoglycemic drugs, should be assigned.

If the patient is treated with both insulin and an injectable non-insulin antidiabetic drug, assign codes Z79.4, Long-term (current) use of insulin, and Z79.85, Long-term (current) use of injectable non-insulin antidiabetic drugs.

If the patient is treated with both oral hypoglycemic drugs and an injectable non-insulin antidiabetic drug, assign codes Z79.84, Long-term (current) use of oral hypoglycemic drugs, and Z79.85, Long-term (current) use of injectable non-insulin antidiabetic drugs.

Code Z79.4 should not be assigned if insulin is given temporarily to bring a secondary diabetic patient's blood sugar under control during an encounter.

Type 2 diabetic with no complications, normally only on oral metformin, is given insulin for three days to maintain glucose control while in the hospital recovering from surgery

E11.9 Type 2 diabetes mellitus without complications

Z79.84 Long term (current) use of oral hypoglycemic drugs

Explanation: Although the patient was given insulin for a short time during his hospital stay, the intent was only to maintain the patient's glucose levels while off his regular oral hypoglycemic medication, not for long term use. No code is needed for long term use of insulin, but a Z code for long term use of an oral hypoglycemic should be added to identify the chronic use of this drug.

Type 2 diabetic with diabetic polyneuropathy on insulin

E11.42 Type 2 diabetes mellitus with diabetic polyneuropathy

Z79.4 Long term (current) use of insulin

Explanation: Add a Z code for the long term use of insulin and the long term use of metformin because both are taken chronically.

(b) Assigning and sequencing secondary diabetes codes and its causes

The sequencing of the secondary diabetes codes in relationship to codes for the cause of the diabetes is based on the Tabular List instructions for categories E08, E09 and E13.

(i) Secondary diabetes mellitus due to pancreatectomy

For postpancreatectomy diabetes mellitus (lack of insulin due to the surgical removal of all or part of the pancreas), assign code E89.1, Postprocedural hypoinsulinemia. Assign a code from category E13 as the principal or first-listed diagnosis and a code from subcategory Z90.41, Acquired absence of pancreas, as an additional code.

(ii) Secondary diabetes due to drugs

Secondary diabetes may be caused by an adverse effect of correctly administered medications, poisoning or sequela of poisoning.

See section I.C.19.e. for coding of adverse effects and poisoning, and section I.C.20 for external cause code reporting.

Initial encounter for corticosteroid-induced diabetes mellitus

E09.9 Drug or chemical induced diabetes mellitus without complications

T38.0X5A Adverse effect of glucocorticoids and synthetic analogues, initial encounter

Explanation: If the diabetes is caused by an adverse effect of a drug, the diabetic condition is coded first. If it occurs from a poisoning or overdose, the poisoning code causing the diabetes is sequenced first.

b. Obesity

The obesity codes in category E66, Overweight and obesity, include codes related to the cause of obesity, such as drug-induced obesity (E66.1), and codes related to effects of obesity, such as code E66.2, Morbid (severe) obesity with alveolar hypoventilation. There are other codes related to obesity in other categories of the classification, such as E88.82, Obesity due to disruption of MC4R pathway; and codes in fifth character subcategory O99.21, Obesity complicating pregnancy, childbirth, and the puerperium.

1) Obesity class

The obesity class codes in subcategory E66.81, Obesity class, require a fifth character to convey the severity of obesity. The obesity class should be documented in the medical record by the provider for these codes to be assigned. The obesity class codes can be reported with other obesity codes in the classification found in Chapters 4 and 15 to fully describe the condition. However, if both class 3 obesity and morbid obesity are documented, only a code for class 3 obesity should be assigned as it is more specific.

Chapter 4. Endocrine, Nutritional and Metabolic Diseases (E00-E89)

NOTE All neoplasms, whether functionally active or not, are classified in Chapter 2. Appropriate codes in this chapter (i.e. E05.8, E07.0, E16-E31, E34.-) may be used as additional codes to indicate either functional activity by neoplasms and ectopic endocrine tissue or hyperfunction and hypofunction of endocrine glands associated with neoplasms and other conditions classified elsewhere.

EXCLUDES 1 transitory endocrine and metabolic disorders specific to newborn (P70-P74)

AHA: 2018,2Q,6

This chapter contains the following blocks:
- E00-E07 Disorders of thyroid gland
- E08-E13 Diabetes mellitus
- E15-E16 Other disorders of glucose regulation and pancreatic internal secretion
- E20-E35 Disorders of other endocrine glands
- E36 Intraoperative complications of endocrine system
- E40-E46 Malnutrition
- E50-E64 Other nutritional deficiencies
- E65-E68 Overweight, obesity and other hyperalimentation
- E70-E88 Metabolic disorders
- E89 Postprocedural endocrine and metabolic complications and disorders, not elsewhere classified

Disorders of thyroid gland (E00-E07)

E00 **Congenital iodine-deficiency syndrome**
Use additional code (F70-F79) to identify associated intellectual disabilities
EXCLUDES 1 subclinical iodine-deficiency hypothyroidism (E02)

- **E00.0** **Congenital iodine-deficiency syndrome, neurological type** Rx
  Endemic cretinism, neurological type
- **E00.1** **Congenital iodine-deficiency syndrome, myxedematous type** Rx
  Endemic cretinism, myxedematous type
  Endemic hypothyroid cretinism
- **E00.2** **Congenital iodine-deficiency syndrome, mixed type** Rx
  Endemic cretinism, mixed type
- **E00.9** **Congenital iodine-deficiency syndrome, unspecified** Rx
  Congenital iodine-deficiency hypothyroidism NOS
  Endemic cretinism NOS

E01 **Iodine-deficiency related thyroid disorders and allied conditions**
EXCLUDES 1 congenital iodine-deficiency syndrome (E00.-)
subclinical iodine-deficiency hypothyroidism (E02)

- **E01.0** **Iodine-deficiency related diffuse (endemic) goiter** Rx
- **E01.1** **Iodine-deficiency related multinodular (endemic) goiter** Rx
  Iodine-deficiency related nodular goiter
- **E01.2** **Iodine-deficiency related (endemic) goiter, unspecified** Rx
  Endemic goiter NOS
- **E01.8** **Other iodine-deficiency related thyroid disorders and allied conditions** Rx
  Acquired iodine-deficiency hypothyroidism NOS

E02 **Subclinical iodine-deficiency hypothyroidism** Rx
AHA: 2021,1Q,8

E03 **Other hypothyroidism**
EXCLUDES 1 iodine-deficiency related hypothyroidism (E00-E02)
postprocedural hypothyroidism (E89.0)
DEF: Hypothyroidism: Underproduction of thyroid hormone.

- **E03.0** **Congenital hypothyroidism with diffuse goiter** Rx
  Congenital goiter (nontoxic) NOS
  Congenital parenchymatous goiter (nontoxic)
  EXCLUDES 1 transitory congenital goiter with normal function (P72.0)
- **E03.1** **Congenital hypothyroidism without goiter** Rx
  Aplasia of thyroid (with myxedema)
  Congenital atrophy of thyroid
  Congenital hypothyroidism NOS
- **E03.2** **Hypothyroidism due to medicaments and other exogenous substances** Rx
  Code first poisoning due to drug or toxin, if applicable (T36-T65 with fifth or sixth character 1-4)
  Use additional code for adverse effect, if applicable, to identify drug (T36-T50 with fifth or sixth character 5)
- **E03.3** **Postinfectious hypothyroidism** Rx
- **E03.4** **Atrophy of thyroid (acquired)** Rx
  EXCLUDES 1 congenital atrophy of thyroid (E03.1)
- **E03.5** **Myxedema coma** HCC Rx ESR COM
- **E03.8** **Other specified hypothyroidism** Rx
  AHA: 2021,1Q,8
- **E03.9** **Hypothyroidism, unspecified** Rx
  Myxedema NOS
  AHA: 2024,1Q,14

E04 **Other nontoxic goiter**
EXCLUDES 1 congenital goiter (NOS) (diffuse) (parenchymatous) (E03.0)
iodine-deficiency related goiter (E00-E02)

- **E04.0** **Nontoxic diffuse goiter** Rx
  Diffuse (colloid) nontoxic goiter
  Simple nontoxic goiter
- **E04.1** **Nontoxic single thyroid nodule** Rx
  Colloid nodule (cystic) (thyroid)
  Nontoxic uninodular goiter
  Thyroid (cystic) nodule NOS
  DEF: Enlarged thyroid, commonly due to decreased thyroid production, with a single nodule. No clinical hypothyroidism.
- **E04.2** **Nontoxic multinodular goiter** Rx
  Cystic goiter NOS
  Multinodular (cystic) goiter NOS
  DEF: Enlarged thyroid, commonly due to decreased thyroid production with multiple nodules. No clinical hypothyroidism.
- **E04.8** **Other specified nontoxic goiter** Rx
- **E04.9** **Nontoxic goiter, unspecified** Rx
  Goiter NOS
  Nodular goiter (nontoxic) NOS

E05 **Thyrotoxicosis [hyperthyroidism]**
EXCLUDES 1 chronic thyroiditis with transient thyrotoxicosis (E06.2)
neonatal thyrotoxicosis (P72.1)
DEF: Excessive quantities of hormones from the thyroid gland caused by overproduction or loss of storage ability.

- **E05.0** **Thyrotoxicosis with diffuse goiter**
  Exophthalmic or toxic goiter NOS
  Graves' disease
  Toxic diffuse goiter
  DEF: Diffuse thyroid enlargement accompanied by hyperthyroidism, bulging eyes, and dermopathy.
  - **E05.00** **Thyrotoxicosis with diffuse goiter without thyrotoxic crisis or storm** Rx
  - **E05.01** **Thyrotoxicosis with diffuse goiter with thyrotoxic crisis or storm** Rx

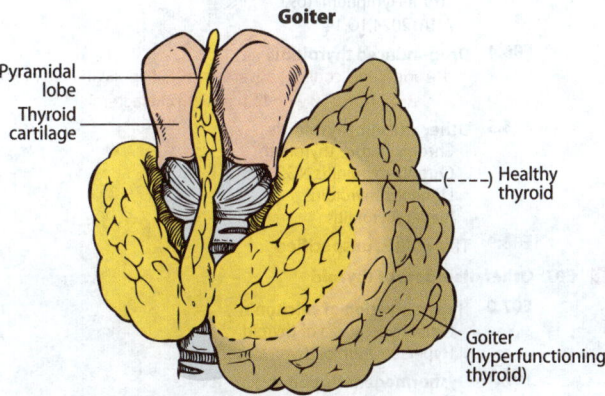

Goiter — Pyramidal lobe, Thyroid cartilage, Healthy thyroid, Goiter (hyperfunctioning thyroid)

- **E05.1** **Thyrotoxicosis with toxic single thyroid nodule**
  Thyrotoxicosis with toxic uninodular goiter
  DEF: Symptomatic hyperthyroidism with a single nodule on the enlarged thyroid gland. Onset of symptoms can be abrupt and include extreme nervousness, insomnia, weight loss, tremors, and psychosis or coma.
  - **E05.10** **Thyrotoxicosis with toxic single thyroid nodule without thyrotoxic crisis or storm** Rx
  - **E05.11** **Thyrotoxicosis with toxic single thyroid nodule with thyrotoxic crisis or storm** Rx
- **E05.2** **Thyrotoxicosis with toxic multinodular goiter**
  Toxic nodular goiter NOS
  - **E05.20** **Thyrotoxicosis with toxic multinodular goiter without thyrotoxic crisis or storm** Rx
  - **E05.21** **Thyrotoxicosis with toxic multinodular goiter with thyrotoxic crisis or storm** Rx
- **E05.3** **Thyrotoxicosis from ectopic thyroid tissue**
  - **E05.30** **Thyrotoxicosis from ectopic thyroid tissue without thyrotoxic crisis or storm** Rx

Chapter 4. Endocrine, Nutritional and Metabolic Diseases

E05.31 Thyrotoxicosis from ectopic thyroid tissue **with thyrotoxic crisis or storm** `Rx`

✓5th **E05.4 Thyrotoxicosis factitia**
- **E05.40** Thyrotoxicosis factitia **without thyrotoxic crisis or storm** `Rx`
- **E05.41** Thyrotoxicosis factitia **with thyrotoxic crisis or storm** `Rx`

✓5th **E05.8 Other thyrotoxicosis**
Overproduction of thyroid-stimulating hormone
- **E05.80** Other thyrotoxicosis **without thyrotoxic crisis or storm** `Rx`
- **E05.81** Other thyrotoxicosis **with thyrotoxic crisis or storm** `Rx`

✓5th **E05.9 Thyrotoxicosis, unspecified**
Hyperthyroidism NOS
- **E05.90** Thyrotoxicosis, unspecified **without thyrotoxic crisis or storm** `Rx`
- **E05.91** Thyrotoxicosis, unspecified **with thyrotoxic crisis or storm** `Rx`

✓4th **E06 Thyroiditis**
EXCLUDES 1 postpartum thyroiditis (O90.5)
DEF: Inflammation of the thyroid gland.

- **E06.0 Acute thyroiditis** `Rx`
  Abscess of thyroid
  Pyogenic thyroiditis
  Suppurative thyroiditis
  Use additional code (B95-B97) to identify infectious agent

- **E06.1 Subacute thyroiditis** `Rx`
  de Quervain thyroiditis
  Giant-cell thyroiditis
  Granulomatous thyroiditis
  Nonsuppurative thyroiditis
  Viral thyroiditis
  EXCLUDES 1 autoimmune thyroiditis (E06.3)

- **E06.2 Chronic thyroiditis with transient thyrotoxicosis** `Rx`
  EXCLUDES 1 autoimmune thyroiditis (E06.3)

- **E06.3 Autoimmune thyroiditis**
  Hashimoto's thyroiditis
  Hashitoxicosis (transient)
  Lymphadenoid goiter
  Lymphocytic thyroiditis
  Struma lymphomatosa
  AHA: 2024,1Q,14

- **E06.4 Drug-induced thyroiditis** `Rx`
  Use additional code for adverse effect, if applicable, to identify drug (T36-T50 with fifth or sixth character 5)

- **E06.5 Other chronic thyroiditis** `Rx`
  Chronic fibrous thyroiditis
  Chronic thyroiditis NOS
  Ligneous thyroiditis
  Riedel thyroiditis

- **E06.9 Thyroiditis, unspecified** `Rx`

✓4th **E07 Other disorders of thyroid**

- **E07.0 Hypersecretion of calcitonin** `Rx`
  C-cell hyperplasia of thyroid
  Hypersecretion of thyrocalcitonin

- **E07.1 Dyshormogenetic goiter** `Rx`
  Dyshormonogenetic goiter
  Familial dyshormogenetic goiter
  Familial dyshormogenetic goiter
  Pendred's syndrome
  EXCLUDES 1 transitory congenital goiter with normal function (P72.0)

✓5th **E07.8 Other specified disorders of thyroid**
- **E07.81 Sick-euthyroid syndrome**
  Euthyroid sick-syndrome
  DEF: Thyroid dysfunction caused by abnormal levels of thyroid hormones T3 and/or T4. This syndrome is often associated with starvation or critical illness.
- **E07.89 Other specified disorders of thyroid** `Rx`
  Abnormality of thyroid-binding globulin
  Hemorrhage of thyroid
  Infarction of thyroid

- **E07.9 Disorder of thyroid, unspecified** `Rx`

Diabetes mellitus (E08-E13)

AHA: 2020,1Q,12; 2018,2Q,6; 2017,4Q,100-101; 2016,2Q,36; 2016,1Q,11-13; 2013,4Q,114; 2013,3Q,20
TIP: There is no default code for diabetes mellitus documented only as uncontrolled. The provider must indicate whether the diabetic patient is hypoglycemic or hyperglycemic to determine the appropriate code.

✓4th **E08 Diabetes mellitus due to underlying condition**
Code first the underlying condition, such as:
  congenital rubella (P35.0)
  Cushing's syndrome (E24.-)
  cystic fibrosis (E84.-)
  malignant neoplasm (C00-C96)
  malnutrition (E40-E46)
  pancreatitis and other diseases of the pancreas (K85-K86.-)
Use additional code to identify control using:
  injectable non-insulin antidiabetic drugs (Z79.85)
  insulin (Z79.4)
  oral antidiabetic drugs (Z79.84)
  oral hypoglycemic drugs (Z79.84)
EXCLUDES 1 drug or chemical induced diabetes mellitus (E09.-)
  gestational diabetes (O24.4-)
  neonatal diabetes mellitus (P70.2)
  postpancreatectomy diabetes mellitus (E13.-)
  postprocedural diabetes mellitus (E13.-)
  secondary diabetes mellitus NEC (E13.-)
  type 1 diabetes mellitus (E10.-)
  type 2 diabetes mellitus (E11.-)

✓5th **E08.0 Diabetes mellitus due to underlying condition with hyperosmolarity**
DEF: Diabetic hyperosmolarity: Extremely high levels of glucose in the blood without ketones.
- **E08.00** *Diabetes mellitus due to underlying condition with hyperosmolarity without nonketotic hyperglycemic-hyperosmolar coma (NKHHC)* `HCC` `Rx` `ESR` `COM`
- **E08.01** *Diabetes mellitus due to underlying condition with hyperosmolarity with coma* `HCC` `Rx` `ESR` `COM`

✓5th **E08.1 Diabetes mellitus due to underlying condition with ketoacidosis**
DEF: Diabetic ketoacidosis: Potentially life-threatening complication due to a shortage of insulin in which the body switches to burning fatty acids and producing acidic ketone bodies.
- **E08.10** *Diabetes mellitus due to underlying condition with ketoacidosis without coma* `HCC` `Rx` `ESR` `COM`
- **E08.11** *Diabetes mellitus due to underlying condition with ketoacidosis with coma* `HCC` `Rx` `ESR` `COM`

✓5th **E08.2 Diabetes mellitus due to underlying condition with kidney complications**
AHA: 2019,3Q,3; 2018,4Q,88
- **E08.21** *Diabetes mellitus due to underlying condition with diabetic nephropathy* `HCC` `Rx` `ESR` `COM`
  Diabetes mellitus due to underlying condition with intercapillary glomerulosclerosis
  Diabetes mellitus due to underlying condition with intracapillary glomerulonephrosis
  Diabetes mellitus due to underlying condition with Kimmelstiel-Wilson disease
- **E08.22** *Diabetes mellitus due to underlying condition with diabetic chronic kidney disease* `HCC` `Rx` `ESR` `COM`
  Use additional code to identify stage of chronic kidney disease (N18.1-N18.6)
- **E08.29** *Diabetes mellitus due to underlying condition with other diabetic kidney complication* `HCC` `Rx` `ESR` `COM`
  Renal tubular degeneration in diabetes mellitus due to underlying condition

---

`HCC` CMS-HCC   `Rx` Rx HCC   `ESR` ESRD HCC   `COM` Commercial HCC   `N` Newborn: 0   `P` Pediatric: 0-17   `M` Maternity: 9-64   `A` Adult: 15-124

Chapter 4. Endocrine, Nutritional and Metabolic Diseases

E08.3 **Diabetes mellitus due to underlying condition with ophthalmic complications**
AHA: 2016,4Q,11-13

One of the following 7th characters is to be assigned to codes in subcategories E08.32, E08.33, E08.34, E08.35, and E08.37 to designate laterality of the disease:
1 right eye
2 left eye
3 bilateral
9 unspecified eye

- **E08.31** Diabetes mellitus due to underlying condition with unspecified diabetic retinopathy
  DEF: Diabetic retinopathy: Diabetic complication from damage to the retinal vessels resulting in vision problems that can progress to blindness.
  - **E08.311** Diabetes mellitus due to underlying condition with unspecified diabetic retinopathy with macular edema
  - **E08.319** Diabetes mellitus due to underlying condition with unspecified diabetic retinopathy without macular edema

- **E08.32** Diabetes mellitus due to underlying condition with mild nonproliferative diabetic retinopathy
  Diabetes mellitus due to underlying condition with nonproliferative diabetic retinopathy NOS
  - **E08.321** Diabetes mellitus due to underlying condition with mild nonproliferative diabetic retinopathy with macular edema
  - **E08.329** Diabetes mellitus due to underlying condition with mild nonproliferative diabetic retinopathy without macular edema

- **E08.33** Diabetes mellitus due to underlying condition with moderate nonproliferative diabetic retinopathy
  - **E08.331** Diabetes mellitus due to underlying condition with moderate nonproliferative diabetic retinopathy with macular edema
  - **E08.339** Diabetes mellitus due to underlying condition with moderate nonproliferative diabetic retinopathy without macular edema

- **E08.34** Diabetes mellitus due to underlying condition with severe nonproliferative diabetic retinopathy
  - **E08.341** Diabetes mellitus due to underlying condition with severe nonproliferative diabetic retinopathy with macular edema
  - **E08.349** Diabetes mellitus due to underlying condition with severe nonproliferative diabetic retinopathy without macular edema

- **E08.35** Diabetes mellitus due to underlying condition with proliferative diabetic retinopathy
  - **E08.351** Diabetes mellitus due to underlying condition with proliferative diabetic retinopathy with macular edema
  - **E08.352** Diabetes mellitus due to underlying condition with proliferative diabetic retinopathy with traction retinal detachment involving the macula
  - **E08.353** Diabetes mellitus due to underlying condition with proliferative diabetic retinopathy with traction retinal detachment not involving the macula
  - **E08.354** Diabetes mellitus due to underlying condition with proliferative diabetic retinopathy with combined traction retinal detachment and rhegmatogenous retinal detachment
  - **E08.355** Diabetes mellitus due to underlying condition with stable proliferative diabetic retinopathy
  - **E08.359** Diabetes mellitus due to underlying condition with proliferative diabetic retinopathy without macular edema

- **E08.36** Diabetes mellitus due to underlying condition with diabetic cataract
  AHA: 2019,2Q,30-31; 2016,4Q,142
- **E08.37** Diabetes mellitus due to underlying condition with diabetic macular edema, resolved following treatment
- **E08.39** Diabetes mellitus due to underlying condition with other diabetic ophthalmic complication
  Use additional code to identify manifestation, such as: diabetic glaucoma (H40-H42)
  AHA: 2023,3Q,19

E08.4 **Diabetes mellitus due to underlying condition with neurological complications**
- **E08.40** Diabetes mellitus due to underlying condition with diabetic neuropathy, unspecified
- **E08.41** Diabetes mellitus due to underlying condition with diabetic mononeuropathy
- **E08.42** Diabetes mellitus due to underlying condition with diabetic polyneuropathy
  Diabetes mellitus due to underlying condition with diabetic neuralgia
- **E08.43** Diabetes mellitus due to underlying condition with diabetic autonomic (poly)neuropathy
  Diabetes mellitus due to underlying condition with diabetic gastroparesis
  AHA: 2013,4Q,114
- **E08.44** Diabetes mellitus due to underlying condition with diabetic amyotrophy
- **E08.49** Diabetes mellitus due to underlying condition with other diabetic neurological complication

E08.5 **Diabetes mellitus due to underlying condition with circulatory complications**
- **E08.51** Diabetes mellitus due to underlying condition with diabetic peripheral angiopathy without gangrene
  AHA: 2018,3Q,3-4; 2018,2Q,7
- **E08.52** Diabetes mellitus due to underlying condition with diabetic peripheral angiopathy with gangrene
  Diabetes mellitus due to underlying condition with diabetic gangrene
  AHA: 2020,2Q,18; 2018,3Q,3; 2018,2Q,7; 2017,4Q,102
- **E08.59** Diabetes mellitus due to underlying condition with other circulatory complications

E08.6 **Diabetes mellitus due to underlying condition with other specified complications**
- **E08.61** Diabetes mellitus due to underlying condition with diabetic arthropathy
  - **E08.610** Diabetes mellitus due to underlying condition with diabetic neuropathic arthropathy
    Diabetes mellitus due to underlying condition with Charcôt's joints
    DEF: Charcot's joint: Progressive neurologic arthropathy in which chronic degeneration of joints in the weight-bearing areas with peripheral hypertrophy occurs as a complication of a neuropathy disorder. Supporting structures relax from a loss of sensation resulting in chronic joint instability.
  - **E08.618** Diabetes mellitus due to underlying condition with other diabetic arthropathy
    AHA: 2018,2Q,6
- **E08.62** Diabetes mellitus due to underlying condition with skin complications
  - **E08.620** Diabetes mellitus due to underlying condition with diabetic dermatitis
    Diabetes mellitus due to underlying condition with diabetic necrobiosis lipoidica

E08.621 *Diabetes mellitus due to underlying condition with foot ulcer* HCC Rx ESR COM
Use additional code to identify site of ulcer (L97.4-, L97.5-)
AHA: 2020,2Q,19
TIP: Do not assign a code for diabetic ulcer when the ulcer is closed/resolved or to report history of diabetic ulcers; Z86.31 Personal history of diabetic foot ulcer, may be assigned.

E08.622 *Diabetes mellitus due to underlying condition with other skin ulcer* HCC Rx ESR COM
Use additional code to identify site of ulcer (L97.1-L97.9, L98.41-L98.49)
AHA: 2021,1Q,7; 2017,4Q,17

E08.628 *Diabetes mellitus due to underlying condition with other skin complications* HCC Rx ESR COM

✓6th **E08.63** **Diabetes mellitus due to underlying condition with oral complications**

E08.630 *Diabetes mellitus due to underlying condition with periodontal disease* HCC Rx ESR COM

E08.638 *Diabetes mellitus due to underlying condition with other oral complications* HCC Rx ESR COM

✓6th **E08.64** **Diabetes mellitus due to underlying condition with hypoglycemia**
Use additional code for hypoglycemia level, if applicable (E16.A-)
AHA: 2017,1Q,42

E08.641 *Diabetes mellitus due to underlying condition with hypoglycemia with coma* HCC Rx ESR COM

E08.649 *Diabetes mellitus due to underlying condition with hypoglycemia without coma* HCC Rx ESR COM
AHA: 2016,3Q,42; 2015,3Q,21

E08.65 *Diabetes mellitus due to underlying condition with hyperglycemia* HCC Rx ESR COM
AHA: 2017,1Q,42; 2013,3Q,20

E08.69 *Diabetes mellitus due to underlying condition with other specified complication* HCC Rx ESR COM
Use additional code to identify complication
AHA: 2016,4Q,141; 2016,1Q,13

E08.8 *Diabetes mellitus due to underlying condition with unspecified complications* HCC Rx ESR COM

E08.9 *Diabetes mellitus due to underlying condition without complications* HCC Rx ESR COM
AHA: 2023,3Q,19; 2020,2Q,18

✓4th **E09** **Drug or chemical induced diabetes mellitus**
Code first poisoning due to drug or toxin, if applicable (T36-T65 with fifth or sixth character 1-4)
Use additional code for adverse effect, if applicable, to identify drug (T36-T50 with fifth or sixth character 5)
Use additional code to identify control using:
  injectable non-insulin antidiabetic drugs (Z79.85)
  insulin (Z79.4)
  oral antidiabetic drugs (Z79.84)
  oral hypoglycemic drugs (Z79.84)
EXCLUDES 1: diabetes mellitus due to underlying condition (E08.-)
  gestational diabetes (O24.4-)
  neonatal diabetes mellitus (P70.2)
  postpancreatectomy diabetes mellitus (E13.-)
  postprocedural diabetes mellitus (E13.-)
  secondary diabetes mellitus NEC (E13.-)
  type 1 diabetes mellitus (E10.-)
  type 2 diabetes mellitus (E11.-)

✓5th **E09.0** **Drug or chemical induced diabetes mellitus with hyperosmolarity**
DEF: Diabetic hyperosmolarity: Extremely high levels of glucose in the blood without ketones.

E09.00 **Drug or chemical induced diabetes mellitus with hyperosmolarity without nonketotic hyperglycemic-hyperosmolar coma (NKHHC)** Rx ESR COM

E09.01 **Drug or chemical induced diabetes mellitus with hyperosmolarity with coma** Rx ESR COM

✓5th **E09.1** **Drug or chemical induced diabetes mellitus with ketoacidosis**
DEF: Diabetic ketoacidosis: Potentially life-threatening complication due to a shortage of insulin in which the body switches to burning fatty acids and producing acidic ketone bodies.

E09.10 **Drug or chemical induced diabetes mellitus with ketoacidosis without coma** Rx ESR COM

E09.11 **Drug or chemical induced diabetes mellitus with ketoacidosis with coma** Rx ESR COM

✓5th **E09.2** **Drug or chemical induced diabetes mellitus with kidney complications**
AHA: 2019,3Q,3; 2018,4Q,88

E09.21 **Drug or chemical induced diabetes mellitus with diabetic nephropathy** Rx ESR COM
Drug or chemical induced diabetes mellitus with intercapillary glomerulosclerosis
Drug or chemical induced diabetes mellitus with intracapillary glomerulonephrosis
Drug or chemical induced diabetes mellitus with Kimmelstiel-Wilson disease

E09.22 **Drug or chemical induced diabetes mellitus with diabetic chronic kidney disease** Rx ESR COM
Use additional code to identify stage of chronic kidney disease (N18.1-N18.6)

E09.29 **Drug or chemical induced diabetes mellitus with other diabetic kidney complication** Rx ESR COM
Drug or chemical induced diabetes mellitus with renal tubular degeneration

✓5th **E09.3** **Drug or chemical induced diabetes mellitus with ophthalmic complications**
AHA: 2016,4Q,11-13

> One of the following 7th characters is to be assigned to codes in subcategories E09.32, E09.33, E09.34, E09.35, and E09.37 to designate laterality of the disease:
> 1 right eye
> 2 left eye
> 3 bilateral
> 9 unspecified eye

✓6th **E09.31** **Drug or chemical induced diabetes mellitus with unspecified diabetic retinopathy**
DEF: Diabetic retinopathy: Diabetic complication from damage to the retinal vessels resulting in vision problems that can progress to blindness.

E09.311 **Drug or chemical induced diabetes mellitus with unspecified diabetic retinopathy with macular edema** Rx ESR COM

E09.319 **Drug or chemical induced diabetes mellitus with unspecified diabetic retinopathy without macular edema** Rx ESR COM

✓6th **E09.32** **Drug or chemical induced diabetes mellitus with mild nonproliferative diabetic retinopathy**
Drug or chemical induced diabetes mellitus with nonproliferative diabetic retinopathy NOS

✓7th **E09.321** **Drug or chemical induced diabetes mellitus with mild nonproliferative diabetic retinopathy with macular edema** Rx ESR COM

✓7th **E09.329** **Drug or chemical induced diabetes mellitus with mild nonproliferative diabetic retinopathy without macular edema** Rx ESR COM

✓6th **E09.33** **Drug or chemical induced diabetes mellitus with moderate nonproliferative diabetic retinopathy**

✓7th **E09.331** **Drug or chemical induced diabetes mellitus with moderate nonproliferative diabetic retinopathy with macular edema** Rx ESR COM

✓7th **E09.339** **Drug or chemical induced diabetes mellitus with moderate nonproliferative diabetic retinopathy without macular edema** Rx ESR COM

✓6th **E09.34** **Drug or chemical induced diabetes mellitus with severe nonproliferative diabetic retinopathy**

✓7th **E09.341** **Drug or chemical induced diabetes mellitus with severe nonproliferative diabetic retinopathy with macular edema** Rx ESR COM

✓7th **E09.349** **Drug or chemical induced diabetes mellitus with severe nonproliferative diabetic retinopathy without macular edema** Rx ESR COM

E09.35 Drug or chemical induced diabetes mellitus with proliferative diabetic retinopathy

- **E09.351** Drug or chemical induced diabetes mellitus with proliferative diabetic retinopathy with macular edema
- **E09.352** Drug or chemical induced diabetes mellitus with proliferative diabetic retinopathy with traction retinal detachment involving the macula
- **E09.353** Drug or chemical induced diabetes mellitus with proliferative diabetic retinopathy with traction retinal detachment not involving the macula
- **E09.354** Drug or chemical induced diabetes mellitus with proliferative diabetic retinopathy with combined traction retinal detachment and rhegmatogenous retinal detachment
- **E09.355** Drug or chemical induced diabetes mellitus with stable proliferative diabetic retinopathy
- **E09.359** Drug or chemical induced diabetes mellitus with proliferative diabetic retinopathy without macular edema

E09.36 Drug or chemical induced diabetes mellitus with diabetic cataract
AHA: 2019,2Q,30-31; 2016,4Q,142

E09.37 Drug or chemical induced diabetes mellitus with diabetic macular edema, resolved following treatment

E09.39 Drug or chemical induced diabetes mellitus with other diabetic ophthalmic complication
Use additional code to identify manifestation, such as: diabetic glaucoma (H40-H42)
AHA: 2023,3Q,19

E09.4 Drug or chemical induced diabetes mellitus with neurological complications

- **E09.40** Drug or chemical induced diabetes mellitus with neurological complications with diabetic neuropathy, unspecified
- **E09.41** Drug or chemical induced diabetes mellitus with neurological complications with diabetic mononeuropathy
- **E09.42** Drug or chemical induced diabetes mellitus with neurological complications with diabetic polyneuropathy
  Drug or chemical induced diabetes mellitus with diabetic neuralgia
- **E09.43** Drug or chemical induced diabetes mellitus with neurological complications with diabetic autonomic (poly)neuropathy
  Drug or chemical induced diabetes mellitus with diabetic gastroparesis
  AHA: 2013,4Q,114
- **E09.44** Drug or chemical induced diabetes mellitus with neurological complications with diabetic amyotrophy
- **E09.49** Drug or chemical induced diabetes mellitus with neurological complications with other diabetic neurological complication

E09.5 Drug or chemical induced diabetes mellitus with circulatory complications

- **E09.51** Drug or chemical induced diabetes mellitus with diabetic peripheral angiopathy without gangrene
  AHA: 2018,3Q,3-4; 2018,2Q,7
- **E09.52** Drug or chemical induced diabetes mellitus with diabetic peripheral angiopathy with gangrene
  Drug or chemical induced diabetes mellitus with diabetic gangrene
  AHA: 2020,2Q,18; 2018,3Q,3; 2018,2Q,7; 2017,4Q,102
- **E09.59** Drug or chemical induced diabetes mellitus with other circulatory complications

E09.6 Drug or chemical induced diabetes mellitus with other specified complications

- **E09.61** Drug or chemical induced diabetes mellitus with diabetic arthropathy
  - **E09.610** Drug or chemical induced diabetes mellitus with diabetic neuropathic arthropathy
    Drug or chemical induced diabetes mellitus with Charcôt's joints
    DEF: Charcot's joint: Progressive neurologic arthropathy in which chronic degeneration of joints in the weight-bearing areas with peripheral hypertrophy occurs as a complication of a neuropathy disorder. Supporting structures relax from a loss of sensation resulting in chronic joint instability.
  - **E09.618** Drug or chemical induced diabetes mellitus with other diabetic arthropathy
    AHA: 2018,2Q,6

- **E09.62** Drug or chemical induced diabetes mellitus with skin complications
  - **E09.620** Drug or chemical induced diabetes mellitus with diabetic dermatitis
    Drug or chemical induced diabetes mellitus with diabetic necrobiosis lipoidica
  - **E09.621** Drug or chemical induced diabetes mellitus with foot ulcer
    Use additional code to identify site of ulcer (L97.4-, L97.5-)
    AHA: 2020,2Q,19
    TIP: Do not assign a code for diabetic ulcer when the ulcer is closed/resolved or to report history of diabetic ulcers; Z86.31 Personal history of diabetic foot ulcer, may be assigned.
  - **E09.622** Drug or chemical induced diabetes mellitus with other skin ulcer
    Use additional code to identify site of ulcer (L97.1-L97.9, L98.41-L98.49)
    AHA: 2021,1Q,7; 2017,4Q,17
  - **E09.628** Drug or chemical induced diabetes mellitus with other skin complications

- **E09.63** Drug or chemical induced diabetes mellitus with oral complications
  - **E09.630** Drug or chemical induced diabetes mellitus with periodontal disease
  - **E09.638** Drug or chemical induced diabetes mellitus with other oral complications

- **E09.64** Drug or chemical induced diabetes mellitus with hypoglycemia
  Use additional code for hypoglycemia level, if applicable (E16.A-)
  AHA: 2017,1Q,42
  - **E09.641** Drug or chemical induced diabetes mellitus with hypoglycemia with coma
  - **E09.649** Drug or chemical induced diabetes mellitus with hypoglycemia without coma
    AHA: 2016,3Q,42; 2015,3Q,21

- **E09.65** Drug or chemical induced diabetes mellitus with hyperglycemia
  AHA: 2017,1Q,42; 2013,3Q,20

- **E09.69** Drug or chemical induced diabetes mellitus with other specified complication
  Use additional code to identify complication
  AHA: 2016,4Q,141; 2016,1Q,13

E09.8 Drug or chemical induced diabetes mellitus with unspecified complications

E09.9 Drug or chemical induced diabetes mellitus without complications
AHA: 2023,3Q,19; 2020,2Q,18

Chapter 4. Endocrine, Nutritional and Metabolic Diseases

E10 Type 1 diabetes mellitus

INCLUDES
- brittle diabetes (mellitus)
- diabetes (mellitus) due to autoimmune process
- diabetes (mellitus) due to immune mediated pancreatic islet beta-cell destruction
- idiopathic diabetes (mellitus)
- juvenile onset diabetes (mellitus)
- ketosis-prone diabetes (mellitus)

EXCLUDES 1
- diabetes mellitus due to underlying condition (E08.-)
- drug or chemical induced diabetes mellitus (E09.-)
- gestational diabetes (O24.4-)
- hyperglycemia NOS (R73.9)
- neonatal diabetes mellitus (P70.2)
- postpancreatectomy diabetes mellitus (E13.-)
- postprocedural diabetes mellitus (E13.-)
- secondary diabetes mellitus NEC (E13.-)
- type 2 diabetes mellitus (E11.-)

AHA: 2023,2Q,10; 2020,3Q,30

E10.1 Type 1 diabetes mellitus with ketoacidosis
AHA: 2013,3Q,20
DEF: Diabetic ketoacidosis: Potentially life-threatening complication due to a shortage of insulin in which the body switches to burning fatty acids and producing acidic ketone bodies.

- **E10.10** Type 1 diabetes mellitus with ketoacidosis without coma
- **E10.11** Type 1 diabetes mellitus with ketoacidosis with coma

E10.2 Type 1 diabetes mellitus with kidney complications
AHA: 2019,3Q,3; 2018,4Q,88

- **E10.21** Type 1 diabetes mellitus with diabetic nephropathy
  - Type 1 diabetes mellitus with intercapillary glomerulosclerosis
  - Type 1 diabetes mellitus with intracapillary glomerulonephrosis
  - Type 1 diabetes mellitus with Kimmelstiel-Wilson disease
- **E10.22** Type 1 diabetes mellitus with diabetic chronic kidney disease
  - Use additional code to identify stage of chronic kidney disease (N18.1-N18.6)
  - AHA: 2024,3Q,12
- **E10.29** Type 1 diabetes mellitus with other diabetic kidney complication
  - Type 1 diabetes mellitus with renal tubular degeneration
  - AHA: 2016,1Q,13

E10.3 Type 1 diabetes mellitus with ophthalmic complications
AHA: 2016,4Q,11-13

> One of the following 7th characters is to be assigned to codes in subcategories E10.32, E10.33, E10.34, E10.35, and E10.37 to designate laterality of the disease:
> 1 right eye
> 2 left eye
> 3 bilateral
> 9 unspecified eye

- **E10.31** Type 1 diabetes mellitus with unspecified diabetic retinopathy
  - **DEF:** Diabetic retinopathy: Diabetic complication from damage to the retinal vessels resulting in vision problems that can progress to blindness.
  - **E10.311** Type 1 diabetes mellitus with unspecified diabetic retinopathy with macular edema
  - **E10.319** Type 1 diabetes mellitus with unspecified diabetic retinopathy without macular edema
- **E10.32** Type 1 diabetes mellitus with mild nonproliferative diabetic retinopathy
  - Type 1 diabetes mellitus with nonproliferative diabetic retinopathy NOS
  - **E10.321** Type 1 diabetes mellitus with mild nonproliferative diabetic retinopathy with macular edema
  - **E10.329** Type 1 diabetes mellitus with mild nonproliferative diabetic retinopathy without macular edema
- **E10.33** Type 1 diabetes mellitus with moderate nonproliferative diabetic retinopathy
  - **E10.331** Type 1 diabetes mellitus with moderate nonproliferative diabetic retinopathy with macular edema
  - **E10.339** Type 1 diabetes mellitus with moderate nonproliferative diabetic retinopathy without macular edema
- **E10.34** Type 1 diabetes mellitus with severe nonproliferative diabetic retinopathy
  - **E10.341** Type 1 diabetes mellitus with severe nonproliferative diabetic retinopathy with macular edema
  - **E10.349** Type 1 diabetes mellitus with severe nonproliferative diabetic retinopathy without macular edema
- **E10.35** Type 1 diabetes mellitus with proliferative diabetic retinopathy
  - **E10.351** Type 1 diabetes mellitus with proliferative diabetic retinopathy with macular edema
  - **E10.352** Type 1 diabetes mellitus with proliferative diabetic retinopathy with traction retinal detachment involving the macula
  - **E10.353** Type 1 diabetes mellitus with proliferative diabetic retinopathy with traction retinal detachment not involving the macula
  - **E10.354** Type 1 diabetes mellitus with proliferative diabetic retinopathy with combined traction retinal detachment and rhegmatogenous retinal detachment
  - **E10.355** Type 1 diabetes mellitus with stable proliferative diabetic retinopathy
  - **E10.359** Type 1 diabetes mellitus with proliferative diabetic retinopathy without macular edema
- **E10.36** Type 1 diabetes mellitus with diabetic cataract
  - AHA: 2019,2Q,30-31; 2016,4Q,142
- **E10.37** Type 1 diabetes mellitus with diabetic macular edema, resolved following treatment
- **E10.39** Type 1 diabetes mellitus with other diabetic ophthalmic complication
  - Use additional code to identify manifestation, such as: diabetic glaucoma (H40-H42)
  - AHA: 2023,3Q,19

E10.4 Type 1 diabetes mellitus with neurological complications
- **E10.40** Type 1 diabetes mellitus with diabetic neuropathy, unspecified
- **E10.41** Type 1 diabetes mellitus with diabetic mononeuropathy
- **E10.42** Type 1 diabetes mellitus with diabetic polyneuropathy
  - Type 1 diabetes mellitus with diabetic neuralgia
- **E10.43** Type 1 diabetes mellitus with diabetic autonomic (poly)neuropathy
  - Type 1 diabetes mellitus with diabetic gastroparesis
  - AHA: 2013,4Q,114
- **E10.44** Type 1 diabetes mellitus with diabetic amyotrophy
- **E10.49** Type 1 diabetes mellitus with other diabetic neurological complication

E10.5 Type 1 diabetes mellitus with circulatory complications
- **E10.51** Type 1 diabetes mellitus with diabetic peripheral angiopathy without gangrene
  - AHA: 2018,3Q,3-4; 2018,2Q,7
- **E10.52** Type 1 diabetes mellitus with diabetic peripheral angiopathy with gangrene
  - Type 1 diabetes mellitus with diabetic gangrene
  - AHA: 2020,2Q,18; 2018,3Q,3; 2018,2Q,7; 2017,4Q,102
- **E10.59** Type 1 diabetes mellitus with other circulatory complications

---

HCC CMS-HCC   Rx Rx HCC   ESR ESRD HCC   COM Commercial HCC   N Newborn: 0   P Pediatric: 0-17   M Maternity: 9-64   A Adult: 15-124

Chapter 4. Endocrine, Nutritional and Metabolic Diseases

E10.6 Type 1 diabetes mellitus with other specified complications
- **E10.61** Type 1 diabetes mellitus with diabetic arthropathy
  - **E10.610** Type 1 diabetes mellitus with diabetic neuropathic arthropathy `HCC` `Rx` `ESR` `COM` `Q`
    Type 1 diabetes mellitus with Charcôt's joints
    DEF: Charcot's joint: Progressive neurologic arthropathy in which chronic degeneration of joints in the weight-bearing areas with peripheral hypertrophy occurs as a complication of a neuropathy disorder. Supporting structures relax from a loss of sensation resulting in chronic joint instability.
  - **E10.618** Type 1 diabetes mellitus with other diabetic arthropathy `HCC` `Rx` `ESR` `COM` `Q`
    AHA: 2018,2Q,6
- **E10.62** Type 1 diabetes mellitus with skin complications
  - **E10.620** Type 1 diabetes mellitus with diabetic dermatitis `HCC` `Rx` `ESR` `COM` `Q`
    Type 1 diabetes mellitus with diabetic necrobiosis lipoidica
    AHA: 2024,3Q,12
  - **E10.621** Type 1 diabetes mellitus with foot ulcer `HCC` `Rx` `ESR` `COM` `Q`
    Use additional code to identify site of ulcer (L97.4-, L97.5-)
    AHA: 2020,2Q,19
    TIP: Do not assign a code for diabetic ulcer when the ulcer is closed/resolved or to report history of diabetic ulcers; Z86.31 Personal history of diabetic foot ulcer, may be assigned.
  - **E10.622** Type 1 diabetes mellitus with other skin ulcer `HCC` `Rx` `ESR` `COM` `Q`
    Use additional code to identify site of ulcer (L97.1-L97.9, L98.41-L98.49)
    AHA: 2021,1Q,7; 2017,4Q,17
  - **E10.628** Type 1 diabetes mellitus with other skin complications `HCC` `Rx` `ESR` `COM` `Q`
- **E10.63** Type 1 diabetes mellitus with oral complications
  - **E10.630** Type 1 diabetes mellitus with periodontal disease `HCC` `Rx` `ESR` `COM` `Q`
  - **E10.638** Type 1 diabetes mellitus with other oral complications `HCC` `Rx` `ESR` `COM` `Q`
- **E10.64** Type 1 diabetes mellitus with hypoglycemia
  Use additional code for hypoglycemia level, if applicable (E16.A-)
  AHA: 2017,1Q,42
  - **E10.641** Type 1 diabetes mellitus with hypoglycemia with coma `HCC` `Rx` `ESR` `COM` `Q`
  - **E10.649** Type 1 diabetes mellitus with hypoglycemia without coma `HCC` `Rx` `ESR` `COM` `Q`
    AHA: 2016,3Q,42; 2016,1Q,13; 2015,3Q,21
- **E10.65** Type 1 diabetes mellitus with hyperglycemia `HCC` `Rx` `ESR` `COM` `Q`
  AHA: 2022,1Q,28; 2017,1Q,42; 2013,3Q,20
- **E10.69** Type 1 diabetes mellitus with other specified complication `HCC` `Rx` `ESR` `COM` `Q`
  Use additional code to identify complication
  AHA: 2022,1Q,28; 2016,4Q,141; 2016,1Q,13

E10.8 Type 1 diabetes mellitus with unspecified complications `HCC` `Rx` `ESR` `COM` `Q`

E10.9 Type 1 diabetes mellitus without complications `HCC` `Rx` `ESR` `COM` `Q`
  AHA: 2023,3Q,19; 2020,2Q,18

E10.A Type 1 diabetes mellitus, presymptomatic
  Early-stage type 1 diabetes mellitus
  AHA: 2024,4Q,5
- **E10.A0** Type 1 diabetes mellitus, presymptomatic, unspecified
- **E10.A1** Type 1 diabetes mellitus, presymptomatic, Stage 1
  Multiple confirmed islet autoantibodies with normoglycemia
- **E10.A2** Type 1 diabetes mellitus, presymptomatic, Stage 2 `Q`
  Confirmed islet autoimmunity with dysglycemia

E11 Type 2 diabetes mellitus
  INCLUDES diabetes (mellitus) due to insulin secretory defect
  diabetes NOS
  insulin resistant diabetes (mellitus)
  Use additional code to identify control using:
    injectable non-insulin antidiabetic drugs (Z79.85)
    insulin (Z79.4)
    oral antidiabetic drugs (Z79.84)
    oral hypoglycemic drugs (Z79.84)
  EXCLUDES 1 diabetes mellitus due to underlying condition (E08.-)
    drug or chemical induced diabetes mellitus (E09.-)
    gestational diabetes (O24.4-)
    neonatal diabetes mellitus (P70.2)
    postpancreatectomy diabetes mellitus (E13.-)
    postprocedural diabetes mellitus (E13.-)
    secondary diabetes mellitus NEC (E13.-)
    type 1 diabetes mellitus (E10.-)
  AHA: 2020,3Q,30; 2020,1Q,12; 2016,2Q,10; 2013,1Q,26

E11.0 Type 2 diabetes mellitus with hyperosmolarity
  DEF: Diabetic hyperosmolarity: Extremely high levels of glucose in the blood without ketones.
- **E11.00** Type 2 diabetes mellitus with hyperosmolarity without nonketotic hyperglycemic-hyperosmolar coma (NKHHC) `HCC` `Rx` `ESR` `COM` `Q`
  AHA: 2022,1Q,28
- **E11.01** Type 2 diabetes mellitus with hyperosmolarity with coma `HCC` `Rx` `ESR` `COM` `Q`

E11.1 Type 2 diabetes mellitus with ketoacidosis
  AHA: 2017,4Q,6
  DEF: Diabetic ketoacidosis: Potentially life-threatening complication due to a shortage of insulin in which the body switches to burning fatty acids and producing acidic ketone bodies.
- **E11.10** Type 2 diabetes mellitus with ketoacidosis without coma `HCC` `Rx` `ESR` `COM`
- **E11.11** Type 2 diabetes mellitus with ketoacidosis with coma `HCC` `Rx` `ESR` `COM`

E11.2 Type 2 diabetes mellitus with kidney complications
  AHA: 2019,3Q,3; 2018,4Q,88
- **E11.21** Type 2 diabetes mellitus with diabetic nephropathy `HCC` `Rx` `ESR` `COM` `Q`
  Type 2 diabetes mellitus with intercapillary glomerulosclerosis
  Type 2 diabetes mellitus with intracapillary glomerulonephrosis
  Type 2 diabetes mellitus with Kimmelstiel-Wilson disease
- **E11.22** Type 2 diabetes mellitus with diabetic chronic kidney disease `HCC` `Rx` `ESR` `COM` `Q`
  Use additional code to identify stage of chronic kidney disease (N18.1-N18.6)
  AHA: 2024,3Q,12; 2022,3Q,15
- **E11.29** Type 2 diabetes mellitus with other diabetic kidney complication `HCC` `Rx` `ESR` `COM` `Q`
  Type 2 diabetes mellitus with renal tubular degeneration

E11.3 Type 2 diabetes mellitus with ophthalmic complications
  AHA: 2016,4Q,11-13

  One of the following 7th characters is to be assigned to codes in subcategories E11.32, E11.33, E11.34, E11.35, and E11.37 to designate laterality of the disease:
  1 right eye
  2 left eye
  3 bilateral
  9 unspecified eye

- **E11.31** Type 2 diabetes mellitus with unspecified diabetic retinopathy
  DEF: Diabetic retinopathy: Diabetic complication from damage to the retinal vessels resulting in vision problems that can progress to blindness.
  - **E11.311** Type 2 diabetes mellitus with unspecified diabetic retinopathy with macular edema `HCC` `Rx` `ESR` `COM` `Q`
  - **E11.319** Type 2 diabetes mellitus with unspecified diabetic retinopathy without macular edema `HCC` `Rx` `ESR` `COM` `Q`

E11.32 Type 2 diabetes mellitus with mild nonproliferative diabetic retinopathy
Type 2 diabetes mellitus with nonproliferative diabetic retinopathy NOS

- **E11.321** Type 2 diabetes mellitus with mild nonproliferative diabetic retinopathy with macular edema
- **E11.329** Type 2 diabetes mellitus with mild nonproliferative diabetic retinopathy without macular edema

E11.33 Type 2 diabetes mellitus with moderate nonproliferative diabetic retinopathy

- **E11.331** Type 2 diabetes mellitus with moderate nonproliferative diabetic retinopathy with macular edema
- **E11.339** Type 2 diabetes mellitus with moderate nonproliferative diabetic retinopathy without macular edema

E11.34 Type 2 diabetes mellitus with severe nonproliferative diabetic retinopathy

- **E11.341** Type 2 diabetes mellitus with severe nonproliferative diabetic retinopathy with macular edema
- **E11.349** Type 2 diabetes mellitus with severe nonproliferative diabetic retinopathy without macular edema

E11.35 Type 2 diabetes mellitus with proliferative diabetic retinopathy

- **E11.351** Type 2 diabetes mellitus with proliferative diabetic retinopathy with macular edema
- **E11.352** Type 2 diabetes mellitus with proliferative diabetic retinopathy with traction retinal detachment involving the macula
- **E11.353** Type 2 diabetes mellitus with proliferative diabetic retinopathy with traction retinal detachment not involving the macula
- **E11.354** Type 2 diabetes mellitus with proliferative diabetic retinopathy with combined traction retinal detachment and rhegmatogenous retinal detachment
- **E11.355** Type 2 diabetes mellitus with stable proliferative diabetic retinopathy
- **E11.359** Type 2 diabetes mellitus with proliferative diabetic retinopathy without macular edema

E11.36 Type 2 diabetes mellitus with diabetic cataract
AHA: 2019,2Q,30-31; 2016,4Q,142

E11.37 Type 2 diabetes mellitus with diabetic macular edema, resolved following treatment

E11.39 Type 2 diabetes mellitus with other diabetic ophthalmic complication
Use additional code to identify manifestation, such as: diabetic glaucoma (H40-H42)
AHA: 2023,3Q,19

E11.4 Type 2 diabetes mellitus with neurological complications
AHA: 2022,3Q,15

- **E11.40** Type 2 diabetes mellitus with diabetic neuropathy, unspecified
AHA: 2013,4Q,129
- **E11.41** Type 2 diabetes mellitus with diabetic mononeuropathy
- **E11.42** Type 2 diabetes mellitus with diabetic polyneuropathy
Type 2 diabetes mellitus with diabetic neuralgia
AHA: 2020,1Q,12
- **E11.43** Type 2 diabetes mellitus with diabetic autonomic (poly)neuropathy
Type 2 diabetes mellitus with diabetic gastroparesis
AHA: 2023,2Q,8; 2013,4Q,114
- **E11.44** Type 2 diabetes mellitus with diabetic amyotrophy

E11.49 Type 2 diabetes mellitus with other diabetic neurological complication

E11.5 Type 2 diabetes mellitus with circulatory complications

- **E11.51** Type 2 diabetes mellitus with diabetic peripheral angiopathy without gangrene
AHA: 2018,3Q,3-4; 2018,2Q,7
- **E11.52** Type 2 diabetes mellitus with diabetic peripheral angiopathy with gangrene
Type 2 diabetes mellitus with diabetic gangrene
AHA: 2020,2Q,18; 2018,3Q,3; 2018,2Q,7; 2017,4Q,102
- **E11.59** Type 2 diabetes mellitus with other circulatory complications

E11.6 Type 2 diabetes mellitus with other specified complications

- **E11.61** Type 2 diabetes mellitus with diabetic arthropathy
  - **E11.610** Type 2 diabetes mellitus with diabetic neuropathic arthropathy
    Type 2 diabetes mellitus with Charcôt's joints
    DEF: Charcot's joint: Progressive neurologic arthropathy in which chronic degeneration of joints in the weight-bearing areas with peripheral hypertrophy occurs as a complication of a neuropathy disorder. Supporting structures relax from a loss of sensation resulting in chronic joint instability.
  - **E11.618** Type 2 diabetes mellitus with other diabetic arthropathy
    AHA: 2018,2Q,6
- **E11.62** Type 2 diabetes mellitus with skin complications
  - **E11.620** Type 2 diabetes mellitus with diabetic dermatitis
    Type 2 diabetes mellitus with diabetic necrobiosis lipoidica
    AHA: 2024,3Q,12
  - **E11.621** Type 2 diabetes mellitus with foot ulcer
    Use additional code to identify site of ulcer (L97.4-, L97.5-)
    AHA: 2020,2Q,19; 2020,1Q,12
    TIP: Do not assign a code for diabetic ulcer when the ulcer is closed/resolved or to report history of diabetic ulcers; Z86.31 Personal history of diabetic foot ulcer, may be assigned.
  - **E11.622** Type 2 diabetes mellitus with other skin ulcer
    Use additional code to identify site of ulcer (L97.1-L97.9, L98.41-L98.49)
    AHA: 2021,1Q,7; 2017,4Q,17
  - **E11.628** Type 2 diabetes mellitus with other skin complications
- **E11.63** Type 2 diabetes mellitus with oral complications
  - **E11.630** Type 2 diabetes mellitus with periodontal disease
  - **E11.638** Type 2 diabetes mellitus with other oral complications
- **E11.64** Type 2 diabetes mellitus with hypoglycemia
  Use additional code for hypoglycemia level, if applicable (E16.A-)
  AHA: 2017,1Q,42
  - **E11.641** Type 2 diabetes mellitus with hypoglycemia with coma
  - **E11.649** Type 2 diabetes mellitus with hypoglycemia without coma
    AHA: 2016,3Q,42; 2015,3Q,21
- **E11.65** Type 2 diabetes mellitus with hyperglycemia
  AHA: 2023,2Q,10; 2022,1Q,28; 2017,1Q,42; 2013,3Q,20
- **E11.69** Type 2 diabetes mellitus with other specified complication
  Use additional code to identify complication
  AHA: 2020,1Q,12; 2016,4Q,141; 2016,1Q,13

E11.8 Type 2 diabetes mellitus with unspecified complications

E11.9 Type 2 diabetes mellitus without complications
EXCLUDES 1 ▶type 2 diabetes mellitus, without complications in remission (E11.A)◀
AHA: 2025,1Q,35; 2024,3Q,12; 2023,3Q,19; 2020,2Q,18

● **E11.A Type 2 diabetes mellitus without complications in remission**
EXCLUDES 1 type 2 diabetes mellitus, with complications (E11.0-E11.8)
type 2 diabetes mellitus, without complications not in remission (E11.9)

E13 Other specified diabetes mellitus
INCLUDES
 diabetes mellitus due to genetic defects of beta-cell function
 diabetes mellitus due to genetic defects in insulin action
 postpancreatectomy diabetes mellitus
 postprocedural diabetes mellitus
 secondary diabetes mellitus NEC

Use additional code to identify control using:
 injectable non-insulin antidiabetic drugs (Z79.85)
 insulin (Z79.4)
 oral antidiabetic drugs (Z79.84)
 oral hypoglycemic drugs (Z79.84)

EXCLUDES 1
 diabetes (mellitus) due to autoimmune process (E10.-)
 diabetes (mellitus) due to immune mediated pancreatic islet beta-cell destruction (E10.-)
 diabetes mellitus due to underlying condition (E08.-)
 drug or chemical induced diabetes mellitus (E09.-)
 gestational diabetes (O24.4-)
 neonatal diabetes mellitus (P70.2)
 type 1 diabetes mellitus (E10.-)

AHA: 2018,3Q,4; 2016,1Q,11-13
TIP: Use this category when the diabetes is documented as diabetes type 1.5. Synonymous terms used in the documentation may also include combined diabetes type 1 and type 2, latent autoimmune diabetes of adults (LADA), slow-progressing type 1 diabetes, or double diabetes.
TIP: When postprocedural or postpancreatectomy hypoinsulinemia (E89.1) is documented with postprocedural or postpancreatectomy diabetes mellitus (E13.-), code E89.1 should be sequenced first.

E13.0 Other specified diabetes mellitus with hyperosmolarity
DEF: Diabetic hyperosmolarity: Extremely high levels of glucose in the blood without ketones.

E13.00 Other specified diabetes mellitus with hyperosmolarity without nonketotic hyperglycemic-hyperosmolar coma (NKHHC)
E13.01 Other specified diabetes mellitus with hyperosmolarity with coma

E13.1 Other specified diabetes mellitus with ketoacidosis
AHA: 2016,2Q,10; 2013,1Q,26
DEF: Diabetic ketoacidosis: Potentially life-threatening complication due to a shortage of insulin in which the body switches to burning fatty acids and producing acidic ketone bodies.

E13.10 Other specified diabetes mellitus with ketoacidosis without coma
E13.11 Other specified diabetes mellitus with ketoacidosis with coma

E13.2 Other specified diabetes mellitus with kidney complications
AHA: 2019,3Q,3; 2018,4Q,88

E13.21 Other specified diabetes mellitus with diabetic nephropathy
 Other specified diabetes mellitus with intercapillary glomerulosclerosis
 Other specified diabetes mellitus with intracapillary glomerulonephrosis
 Other specified diabetes mellitus with Kimmelstiel-Wilson disease

E13.22 Other specified diabetes mellitus with diabetic chronic kidney disease
Use additional code to identify stage of chronic kidney disease (N18.1-N18.6)

E13.29 Other specified diabetes mellitus with other diabetic kidney complication
 Other specified diabetes mellitus with renal tubular degeneration

E13.3 Other specified diabetes mellitus with ophthalmic complications
AHA: 2016,4Q,11-13

One of the following 7th characters is to be assigned to codes in subcategories E13.32, E13.33, E13.34, E13.35, and E13.37 to designate laterality of the disease:
1 right eye
2 left eye
3 bilateral
9 unspecified eye

E13.31 Other specified diabetes mellitus with unspecified diabetic retinopathy
DEF: Diabetic retinopathy: Diabetic complication from damage to the retinal vessels resulting in vision problems that can progress to blindness.
 E13.311 Other specified diabetes mellitus with unspecified diabetic retinopathy with macular edema
 E13.319 Other specified diabetes mellitus with unspecified diabetic retinopathy without macular edema

E13.32 Other specified diabetes mellitus with mild nonproliferative diabetic retinopathy
 Other specified diabetes mellitus with nonproliferative diabetic retinopathy NOS
 E13.321 Other specified diabetes mellitus with mild nonproliferative diabetic retinopathy with macular edema
 E13.329 Other specified diabetes mellitus with mild nonproliferative diabetic retinopathy without macular edema

E13.33 Other specified diabetes mellitus with moderate nonproliferative diabetic retinopathy
 E13.331 Other specified diabetes mellitus with moderate nonproliferative diabetic retinopathy with macular edema
 E13.339 Other specified diabetes mellitus with moderate nonproliferative diabetic retinopathy without macular edema

E13.34 Other specified diabetes mellitus with severe nonproliferative diabetic retinopathy
 E13.341 Other specified diabetes mellitus with severe nonproliferative diabetic retinopathy with macular edema
 E13.349 Other specified diabetes mellitus with severe nonproliferative diabetic retinopathy without macular edema

E13.35 Other specified diabetes mellitus with proliferative diabetic retinopathy
 E13.351 Other specified diabetes mellitus with proliferative diabetic retinopathy with macular edema
 E13.352 Other specified diabetes mellitus with proliferative diabetic retinopathy with traction retinal detachment involving the macula
 E13.353 Other specified diabetes mellitus with proliferative diabetic retinopathy with traction retinal detachment not involving the macula
 E13.354 Other specified diabetes mellitus with proliferative diabetic retinopathy with combined traction retinal detachment and rhegmatogenous retinal detachment
 E13.355 Other specified diabetes mellitus with stable proliferative diabetic retinopathy
 E13.359 Other specified diabetes mellitus with proliferative diabetic retinopathy without macular edema

E13.36 Other specified diabetes mellitus with diabetic cataract
AHA: 2019,2Q,30-31; 2016,4Q,142

E13.37 Other specified diabetes mellitus with diabetic macular edema, resolved following treatment

E13.39 Other specified diabetes mellitus with other diabetic ophthalmic complication `HCC Rx ESR COM Q`
Use additional code to identify manifestation, such as: diabetic glaucoma (H40-H42)
AHA: 2023,3Q,19

✓5th **E13.4** Other specified diabetes mellitus with neurological complications

E13.40 Other specified diabetes mellitus with diabetic neuropathy, unspecified `HCC Rx ESR COM Q`

E13.41 Other specified diabetes mellitus with diabetic mononeuropathy `HCC Rx ESR COM Q`

E13.42 Other specified diabetes mellitus with diabetic polyneuropathy `HCC Rx ESR COM Q`
Other specified diabetes mellitus with diabetic neuralgia

E13.43 Other specified diabetes mellitus with diabetic autonomic (poly)neuropathy `HCC Rx ESR COM Q`
Other specified diabetes mellitus with diabetic gastroparesis
AHA: 2013,4Q,114

E13.44 Other specified diabetes mellitus with diabetic amyotrophy `HCC Rx ESR COM Q`

E13.49 Other specified diabetes mellitus with other diabetic neurological complication

✓5th **E13.5** Other specified diabetes mellitus with circulatory complications

E13.51 Other specified diabetes mellitus with diabetic peripheral angiopathy without gangrene `HCC Rx ESR COM Q`
AHA: 2018,3Q,3-4; 2018,2Q,7

E13.52 Other specified diabetes mellitus with diabetic peripheral angiopathy with gangrene `HCC Rx ESR COM Q`
Other specified diabetes mellitus with diabetic gangrene
AHA: 2020,2Q,18; 2018,3Q,3; 2018,2Q,7; 2017,4Q,102

E13.59 Other specified diabetes mellitus with other circulatory complications `HCC Rx ESR COM Q`

✓5th **E13.6** Other specified diabetes mellitus with other specified complications

✓6th **E13.61** Other specified diabetes mellitus with diabetic arthropathy

E13.610 Other specified diabetes mellitus with diabetic neuropathic arthropathy `HCC Rx ESR COM Q`
Other specified diabetes mellitus with Charcôt's joints
DEF: Charcot's joint: Progressive neurologic arthropathy in which chronic degeneration of joints in the weight-bearing areas with peripheral hypertrophy occurs as a complication of a neuropathy disorder. Supporting structures relax from a loss of sensation resulting in chronic joint instability.

E13.618 Other specified diabetes mellitus with other diabetic arthropathy `HCC Rx ESR COM Q`
AHA: 2018,2Q,6

✓6th **E13.62** Other specified diabetes mellitus with skin complications

E13.620 Other specified diabetes mellitus with diabetic dermatitis `HCC Rx ESR COM Q`
Other specified diabetes mellitus with diabetic necrobiosis lipoidica

E13.621 Other specified diabetes mellitus with foot ulcer `HCC Rx ESR COM Q`
Use additional code to identify site of ulcer (L97.4-, L97.5-)
AHA: 2020,2Q,19
TIP: Do not assign a code for diabetic ulcer when the ulcer is closed/resolved or to report history of diabetic ulcers; Z86.31 Personal history of diabetic foot ulcer, may be assigned.

E13.622 Other specified diabetes mellitus with other skin ulcer `HCC Rx ESR COM Q`
Use additional code to identify site of ulcer (L97.1-L97.9, L98.41-L98.49)
AHA: 2021,1Q,7; 2017,4Q,17

E13.628 Other specified diabetes mellitus with other skin complications `HCC Rx ESR COM Q`

✓6th **E13.63** Other specified diabetes mellitus with oral complications

E13.630 Other specified diabetes mellitus with periodontal disease `HCC Rx ESR COM Q`

E13.638 Other specified diabetes mellitus with other oral complications `HCC Rx ESR COM Q`

✓6th **E13.64** Other specified diabetes mellitus with hypoglycemia
Use additional code for hypoglycemia level, if applicable (E16.A-)
AHA: 2017,1Q,42

E13.641 Other specified diabetes mellitus with hypoglycemia with coma `HCC Rx ESR COM Q`

E13.649 Other specified diabetes mellitus with hypoglycemia without coma `HCC Rx ESR COM Q`
AHA: 2016,3Q,42; 2015,3Q,21

E13.65 Other specified diabetes mellitus with hyperglycemia `HCC Rx ESR COM Q`
AHA: 2017,1Q,42; 2013,3Q,20

E13.69 Other specified diabetes mellitus with other specified complication `HCC Rx ESR COM Q`
Use additional code to identify complication
AHA: 2016,4Q,141; 2016,1Q,13

E13.8 Other specified diabetes mellitus with unspecified complications `HCC Rx ESR COM Q`

E13.9 Other specified diabetes mellitus without complications `HCC Rx ESR COM Q`
AHA: 2023,3Q,19; 2020,2Q,18

Other disorders of glucose regulation and pancreatic internal secretion (E15-E16)

E15 Nondiabetic hypoglycemic coma `ESR COM`
INCLUDES drug-induced insulin coma in nondiabetic hyperinsulinism with hypoglycemic coma hypoglycemic coma NOS

✓4th **E16** Other disorders of pancreatic internal secretion

E16.0 Drug-induced hypoglycemia without coma
Use additional code for adverse effect, if applicable, to identify drug (T36-T50 with fifth or sixth character 5)
Use additional code for hypoglycemia level, if applicable (E16.A-)
EXCLUDES 1 diabetes with hypoglycemia without coma (E09.649)

E16.1 Other hypoglycemia
Functional hyperinsulinism
Functional nonhyperinsulinemic hypoglycemia
Hyperinsulinism NOS
Hyperplasia of pancreatic islet beta cells NOS
Use additional code for hypoglycemia level, if applicable (E16.A-)
EXCLUDES 1 diabetes with hypoglycemia (E08.649, E10.649, E11.649, E13.649)
hypoglycemia in infant of diabetic mother (P70.1)
neonatal hypoglycemia (P70.4)
AHA: 2024,2Q,10

E16.2 Hypoglycemia, unspecified
Use additional code for hypoglycemia level, if applicable (E16.A-)
EXCLUDES 1 diabetes with hypoglycemia (E08.649, E10.649, E11.649, E13.649)
AHA: 2024,4Q,7; 2016,3Q,42
TIP: Assign for nondiabetic hypoglycemic encephalopathy not further clarified in the documentation.

E16.3 Increased secretion of glucagon `Rx`
Hyperplasia of pancreatic endocrine cells with glucagon excess

E16.4 Increased secretion of gastrin `Rx`
Hypergastrinemia
Hyperplasia of pancreatic endocrine cells with gastrin excess
Zollinger-Ellison syndrome

Chapter 4. Endocrine, Nutritional and Metabolic Diseases

E16.8 Other specified disorders of pancreatic internal secretion Rx
  Increased secretion from endocrine pancreas of growth hormone-releasing hormone
  Increased secretion from endocrine pancreas of pancreatic polypeptide
  Increased secretion from endocrine pancreas of somatostatin
  Increased secretion from endocrine pancreas of vasoactive-intestinal polypeptide

E16.9 Disorder of pancreatic internal secretion, unspecified Rx
  Islet-cell hyperplasia NOS
  Pancreatic endocrine cell hyperplasia NOS

√5th **E16.A** Hypoglycemia level
  AHA: 2024,4Q,6-7
  E16.A1 Hypoglycemia level 1
    Decreased blood glucose level 1
  E16.A2 Hypoglycemia level 2
    Decreased blood glucose level 2
  E16.A3 Hypoglycemia level 3
    Decreased blood glucose level 3

Disorders of other endocrine glands (E20-E35)

EXCLUDES 1 galactorrhea (N64.3)
       gynecomastia (N62)

√4th **E20** Hypoparathyroidism
  EXCLUDES 1 Di George's syndrome (D82.1)
         postprocedural hypoparathyroidism (E89.2)
         tetany NOS (R29.0)
         transitory neonatal hypoparathyroidism (P71.4)

  E20.0 Idiopathic hypoparathyroidism Rx ESR COM
    DEF: Abnormally low secretion of parathyroid hormones, with unknown cause, which triggers decreased calcium and increased phosphorus in the blood that can result in cataracts, muscle cramps, tetany, tingling, or burning in the lips, fingers, and toes.

  E20.1 Pseudohypoparathyroidism

√5th **E20.8** Other hypoparathyroidism
  √6th **E20.81** Hypoparathyroidism due to impaired parathyroid hormone secretion
    AHA: 2023,4Q,9-11
    E20.810 Autosomal dominant hypocalcemia Rx ESR COM
      Autosomal dominant hypocalcemia type 1 (ADH1)
      Autosomal dominant hypocalcemia type 2 (ADH2)
      Code also, if applicable, any associated conditions, such as:
        calculus of kidney (N20.0)
        chronic kidney disease (N18.-)
        respiratory distress (J80, R06.-)
        seizure disorder (G40.-, R56.9)
    E20.811 Secondary hypoparathyroidism in diseases classified elsewhere Rx ESR COM
      Code first underlying condition, if known
    E20.812 Autoimmune hypoparathyroidism Rx ESR COM
      Code first, if applicable, underlying condition such as:
        autoimmune polyglandular failure (E31.0)
        Schmidt's syndrome (E31.0)
    E20.818 Other specified hypoparathyroidism due to impaired parathyroid hormone secretion Rx ESR COM
      Familial isolated hypoparathyroidism
    E20.819 Hypoparathyroidism due to impaired parathyroid hormone secretion, unspecified Rx ESR COM
  E20.89 Other specified hypoparathyroidism Rx ESR COM
    Familial hypoparathyroidism

  E20.9 Hypoparathyroidism, unspecified Rx ESR COM
    Parathyroid tetany

√4th **E21** Hyperparathyroidism and other disorders of parathyroid gland
  EXCLUDES 1 adult osteomalacia (M83.-)
         ectopic hyperparathyroidism (E34.2)
         hungry bone syndrome (E83.81)
         infantile and juvenile osteomalacia (E55.0)
  EXCLUDES 2 familial hypocalciuric hypercalcemia (E83.52)

  E21.0 Primary hyperparathyroidism Rx ESR COM
    Hyperplasia of parathyroid
    Osteitis fibrosa cystica generalisata [von Recklinghausen's disease of bone]
    DEF: Parathyroid dysfunction commonly caused by hyperplasia of two or more glands. Symptoms include hypercalcemia and increased parathyroid hormone levels.

  E21.1 Secondary hyperparathyroidism, not elsewhere classified Rx ESR COM
    EXCLUDES 1 secondary hyperparathyroidism of renal origin (N25.81)

  E21.2 Other hyperparathyroidism Rx ESR COM
    Tertiary hyperparathyroidism
    EXCLUDES 1 familial hypocalciuric hypercalcemia (E83.52)

  E21.3 Hyperparathyroidism, unspecified Rx ESR COM
  E21.4 Other specified disorders of parathyroid gland Rx ESR COM
  E21.5 Disorder of parathyroid gland, unspecified Rx ESR COM

√4th **E22** Hyperfunction of pituitary gland
  EXCLUDES 1 Cushing's syndrome (E24.-)
         Nelson's syndrome (E24.1)
         overproduction of ACTH not associated with Cushing's disease (E27.0)
         overproduction of pituitary ACTH (E24.0)
         overproduction of thyroid-stimulating hormone (E05.8-)

  E22.0 Acromegaly and pituitary gigantism HCC Rx ESR COM
    Overproduction of growth hormone
    EXCLUDES 1 constitutional gigantism (E34.4)
           constitutional tall stature (E34.4)
           increased secretion from endocrine pancreas of growth hormone-releasing hormone (E16.8)
    DEF: Acromegaly: Chronic condition caused by overproduction of the pituitary growth hormone resulting in enlarged skeletal parts and facial features.

  E22.1 Hyperprolactinemia Rx ESR COM
    Use additional code for adverse effect, if applicable, to identify drug (T36-T50 with fifth or sixth character 5)

  E22.2 Syndrome of inappropriate secretion of antidiuretic hormone Rx ESR COM

  E22.8 Other hyperfunction of pituitary gland Rx ESR COM
    Central precocious puberty

  E22.9 Hyperfunction of pituitary gland, unspecified Rx ESR COM

√4th **E23** Hypofunction and other disorders of the pituitary gland
  INCLUDES the listed conditions whether the disorder is in the pituitary or the hypothalamus
  EXCLUDES 1 postprocedural hypopituitarism (E89.3)
         short stature due to endocrine disorder (E34.3-)

  E23.0 Hypopituitarism Rx ESR COM
    Fertile eunuch syndrome
    Hypogonadotropic hypogonadism
    Idiopathic growth hormone deficiency
    Isolated deficiency of gonadotropin
    Isolated deficiency of growth hormone
    Isolated deficiency of pituitary hormone
    Kallmann's syndrome
    Lorain-Levi short stature
    Necrosis of pituitary gland (postpartum)
    Panhypopituitarism
    Pituitary cachexia
    Pituitary insufficiency NOS
    Pituitary short stature
    Sheehan's syndrome
    Simmonds' disease
    ▶Use additional code, if applicable, for associated cachexia (E88.A)◄
    AHA: 2024,1Q,15

  E23.1 Drug-induced hypopituitarism Rx ESR COM
    Use additional code for adverse effect, if applicable, to identify drug (T36-T50 with fifth or sixth character 5)

  E23.2 Diabetes insipidus Rx ESR COM
    EXCLUDES 1 nephrogenic diabetes insipidus (N25.1)

Chapter 4. Endocrine, Nutritional and Metabolic Diseases

E23.3 **Hypothalamic dysfunction, not elsewhere classified** `Rx` `ESR` `COM`
  EXCLUDES 1: Prader-Willi syndrome (Q87.11)
  Russell-Silver syndrome (Q87.19)
  AHA: 2024,1Q,15

E23.6 **Other disorders of pituitary gland** `Rx` `ESR` `COM`
  Abscess of pituitary
  Adiposogenital dystrophy

E23.7 **Disorder of pituitary gland, unspecified** `Rx` `ESR` `COM`

✓4th **E24** **Cushing's syndrome**
  EXCLUDES 1: congenital adrenal hyperplasia (E25.0)
  DEF: Abdominal striae, acne, hypertension, decreased carbohydrate tolerance, moon face, obesity, protein catabolism, and psychiatric disturbances resulting from increased adrenocortical secretion of cortisol caused by ACTH-dependent adrenocortical hyperplasia or tumor, or by steroid effects.

  E24.0 **Pituitary-dependent Cushing's disease** `HCC` `Rx` `ESR` `COM`
    Overproduction of pituitary ACTH
    Pituitary-dependent hypercorticalism

  E24.1 **Nelson's syndrome** `Rx` `ESR` `COM`

  E24.2 **Drug-induced Cushing's syndrome** `Rx` `ESR` `COM`
    Use additional code for adverse effect, if applicable, to identify drug (T36-T50 with fifth or sixth character 5)

  E24.3 **Ectopic ACTH syndrome** `Rx` `ESR` `COM`

  E24.4 **Alcohol-induced pseudo-Cushing's syndrome** `Rx` `ESR` `COM`

  E24.8 **Other Cushing's syndrome** `Rx` `ESR` `COM`

  E24.9 **Cushing's syndrome, unspecified** `Rx` `ESR` `COM`

✓4th **E25** **Adrenogenital disorders**
  INCLUDES: adrenogenital syndromes, virilizing or feminizing, whether acquired or due to adrenal hyperplasia consequent on inborn enzyme defects in hormone synthesis
  female adrenal pseudohermaphroditism
  female heterosexual precocious pseudopuberty
  male isosexual precocious pseudopuberty
  male macrogenitosomia praecox
  male sexual precocity with adrenal hyperplasia
  male virilization (female)
  EXCLUDES 1: chromosomal abnormalities (Q90-Q99)
  indeterminate sex and pseudohermaphroditism (Q56)

  E25.0 **Congenital adrenogenital disorders associated with enzyme deficiency** `Rx` `ESR` `COM`
    21-Hydroxylase deficiency
    Congenital adrenal hyperplasia
    Salt-losing congenital adrenal hyperplasia

  E25.8 **Other adrenogenital disorders** `Rx` `ESR` `COM`
    Idiopathic adrenogenital disorder
    Use additional code for adverse effect, if applicable, to identify drug (T36-T50 with fifth or sixth character 5)

  E25.9 **Adrenogenital disorder, unspecified** `Rx` `ESR` `COM`
    Adrenogenital syndrome NOS

✓4th **E26** **Hyperaldosteronism**

  ✓5th **E26.0** **Primary hyperaldosteronism**

    E26.01 **Conn's syndrome** `Rx` `ESR` `COM`
      Code also adrenal adenoma (D35.0-)

    E26.02 **Glucocorticoid-remediable aldosteronism** `Rx` `ESR` `COM`
      Familial aldosteronism type I
      DEF: Rare autosomal dominant familial form of primary aldosteronism in which the secretion of aldosterone is under the influence of adrenocorticotrophic hormone (ACTH) rather than the renin-angiotensin mechanism. Moderate hypersecretion of aldosterone and suppressed plasma renin activity that are rapidly reversed by administration of glucosteroids. Symptoms include hypertension and mild hypokalemia.

    E26.09 **Other primary hyperaldosteronism** `Rx` `ESR` `COM`
      Primary aldosteronism due to adrenal hyperplasia (bilateral)

  E26.1 **Secondary hyperaldosteronism** `Rx` `ESR` `COM`

  ✓5th **E26.8** **Other hyperaldosteronism**

    E26.81 **Bartter's syndrome** `Rx` `ESR` `COM`

    E26.89 **Other hyperaldosteronism** `Rx` `ESR` `COM`

  E26.9 **Hyperaldosteronism, unspecified** `Rx` `ESR` `COM`
    Aldosteronism NOS
    Hyperaldosteronism NOS

✓4th **E27** **Other disorders of adrenal gland**

  E27.0 **Other adrenocortical overactivity** `Rx` `ESR` `COM`
    Overproduction of ACTH, not associated with Cushing's disease
    Premature adrenarche
    EXCLUDES 1: Cushing's syndrome (E24.-)

  E27.1 **Primary adrenocortical insufficiency** `HCC` `Rx` `ESR` `COM`
    Addison's disease
    Autoimmune adrenalitis
    EXCLUDES 1: Addison only phenotype adrenoleukodystrophy (E71.528)
    amyloidosis (E85.-)
    tuberculous Addison's disease (A18.7)
    Waterhouse-Friderichsen syndrome (A39.1)

  E27.2 **Addisonian crisis** `Rx` `ESR` `COM`
    Adrenal crisis
    Adrenocortical crisis
    DEF: Life-threatening condition that occurs when there is not enough cortisol excreted from the adrenal glands. This condition may be due to injury to the adrenal glands or to the pituitary gland, which controls adrenal hormone secretion, or when a patient stops hydrocortisone treatment too quickly or too early.

  E27.3 **Drug-induced adrenocortical insufficiency** `Rx` `ESR` `COM`
    Use additional code for adverse effect, if applicable, to identify drug (T36-T50 with fifth or sixth character 5)

  ✓5th **E27.4** **Other and unspecified adrenocortical insufficiency**
    EXCLUDES 1: adrenoleukodystrophy [Addison-Schilder] (E71.528)
    Waterhouse-Friderichsen syndrome (A39.1)

    E27.40 **Unspecified adrenocortical insufficiency** `Rx` `ESR` `COM`
      Adrenocortical insufficiency NOS
      Hypoaldosteronism

    E27.49 **Other adrenocortical insufficiency** `Rx` `ESR` `COM`
      Adrenal hemorrhage
      Adrenal infarction
      AHA: 2024,1Q,15

  E27.5 **Adrenomedullary hyperfunction** `Rx` `ESR` `COM`
    Adrenomedullary hyperplasia
    Catecholamine hypersecretion
    ▶Code also, if applicable:◀
      ▶malignant pheochromocytoma (C74.1-)◀
      ▶pheochromocytoma (benign) (D35.0-)◀
      ▶secondary hypertension (I15.2)◀

  E27.8 **Other specified disorders of adrenal gland** `Rx` `ESR` `COM`
    Abnormality of cortisol-binding globulin

  E27.9 **Disorder of adrenal gland, unspecified** `Rx` `ESR` `COM`

✓4th **E28** **Ovarian dysfunction**
  EXCLUDES 1: isolated gonadotropin deficiency (E23.0)
  postprocedural ovarian failure (E89.4-)

  E28.0 **Estrogen excess**
    Use additional code for adverse effect, if applicable, to identify drug (T36-T50 with fifth or sixth character 5)

  E28.1 **Androgen excess**
    Hypersecretion of ovarian androgens
    Use additional code for adverse effect, if applicable, to identify drug (T36-T50 with fifth or sixth character 5)

  E28.2 **Polycystic ovarian syndrome**
    Sclerocystic ovary syndrome
    Stein-Leventhal syndrome
    AHA: 2022,2Q,16
    DEF: Common hormonal disorder among women of reproductive age that involves enlarged ovaries with numerous small cysts located along the outer ovarian edge.

  ✓5th **E28.3** **Primary ovarian failure**
    EXCLUDES 1: pure gonadal dysgenesis (Q99.1)
    Turner's syndrome (Q96.-)

    ✓6th **E28.31** **Premature menopause**

      E28.310 **Symptomatic premature menopause** `A`
        Symptoms such as flushing, sleeplessness, headache, lack of concentration, associated with premature menopause

      E28.319 **Asymptomatic premature menopause** `A`
        Premature menopause NOS

    E28.39 **Other primary ovarian failure**
      Decreased estrogen
      Resistant ovary syndrome

E28.8 Other ovarian dysfunction
Ovarian hyperfunction NOS
EXCLUDES 1: postprocedural ovarian failure (E89.4-)

E28.9 Ovarian dysfunction, unspecified

E29 Testicular dysfunction
EXCLUDES 1:
- androgen insensitivity syndrome (E34.5-)
- azoospermia or oligospermia NOS (N46.0-N46.1)
- isolated gonadotropin deficiency (E23.0)
- Klinefelter's syndrome (Q98.0-Q98.1, Q98.4)

E29.0 Testicular hyperfunction
Hypersecretion of testicular hormones

E29.1 Testicular hypofunction
5-delta-Reductase deficiency (with male pseudohermaphroditism)
Defective biosynthesis of testicular androgen NOS
Testicular hypogonadism NOS
Use additional code for adverse effect, if applicable, to identify drug (T36-T50 with fifth or sixth character 5)
EXCLUDES 1: postprocedural testicular hypofunction (E89.5)

E29.8 Other testicular dysfunction
E29.9 Testicular dysfunction, unspecified

E30 Disorders of puberty, not elsewhere classified

E30.0 Delayed puberty
Constitutional delay of puberty
Delayed sexual development

E30.1 Precocious puberty
Precocious menstruation
EXCLUDES 1:
- Albright (-McCune) (-Sternberg) syndrome (Q78.1)
- central precocious puberty (E22.8)
- congenital adrenal hyperplasia (E25.0)
- female heterosexual precocious pseudopuberty (E25.-)
- male isosexual precocious pseudopuberty (E25.-)

E30.8 Other disorders of puberty
Premature thelarche

E30.9 Disorder of puberty, unspecified

E31 Polyglandular dysfunction
EXCLUDES 1:
- ataxia telangiectasia [Louis-Bar] (G11.3)
- dystrophia myotonica [Steinert] (G71.11)
- pseudohypoparathyroidism (E20.1)

E31.0 Autoimmune polyglandular failure
Schmidt's syndrome

E31.1 Polyglandular hyperfunction
EXCLUDES 1:
- multiple endocrine adenomatosis (E31.2-)
- multiple endocrine neoplasia (E31.2-)

E31.2 Multiple endocrine neoplasia [MEN] syndromes
Multiple endocrine adenomatosis
Code also any associated malignancies and other conditions associated with the syndromes
DEF: Group of conditions in which several endocrine glands grow excessively (such as in adenomatous hyperplasia) and/or develop benign or malignant tumors. Tumors and hyperplasia associated with MEN often produce excess hormones, which impede normal physiology. There is no comprehensive cure known for MEN syndrome. Treatment is directed at the hyperplasia or tumors in each individual gland. Tumors are usually surgically removed and oral medications or hormonal injections are used to correct hormone imbalances.

E31.20 Multiple endocrine neoplasia [MEN] syndrome, unspecified
Multiple endocrine adenomatosis NOS
Multiple endocrine neoplasia [MEN] syndrome NOS

E31.21 Multiple endocrine neoplasia [MEN] type I
Wermer's syndrome

E31.22 Multiple endocrine neoplasia [MEN] type IIA
Sipple's syndrome

E31.23 Multiple endocrine neoplasia [MEN] type IIB

E31.8 Other polyglandular dysfunction
E31.9 Polyglandular dysfunction, unspecified

E32 Diseases of thymus
EXCLUDES 1:
- aplasia or hypoplasia of thymus with immunodeficiency (D82.1)
- myasthenia gravis (G70.0)

E32.0 Persistent hyperplasia of thymus
Hypertrophy of thymus

E32.1 Abscess of thymus

E32.8 Other diseases of thymus
EXCLUDES 1:
- aplasia or hypoplasia with immunodeficiency (D82.1)
- thymoma (D15.0)

E32.9 Disease of thymus, unspecified

E34 Other endocrine disorders
EXCLUDES 1: pseudohypoparathyroidism (E20.1)

E34.0 Carcinoid syndrome
Code also the underlying disorder, such as:
- primary neuroendocrine tumors (C7A.-)
- secondary neuroendocrine tumors (C7B.-)
AHA: 2024,4Q,8

E34.00 Carcinoid syndrome, unspecified
Carcinoid disease, unspecified

E34.01 Carcinoid heart syndrome
Carcinoid heart disease
Hedinger syndrome

E34.09 Other carcinoid syndrome
Carcinoid disease NEC
Carcinoid syndrome NEC
Other carcinoid disease

E34.1 Other hypersecretion of intestinal hormones
E34.2 Ectopic hormone secretion, not elsewhere classified
EXCLUDES 1: ectopic ACTH syndrome (E24.3)

E34.3 Short stature due to endocrine disorder
EXCLUDES 1:
- achondroplastic short stature (Q77.4)
- hypochondroplastic short stature (Q77.4)
- nutritional short stature (E45)
- pituitary short stature (E23.0)
- progeria (E34.8)
- renal short stature (N25.0)
- Russell-Silver syndrome (Q87.19)
- short stature (child) (R62.52)
- short stature in specific dysmorphic syndromes - code to syndrome - see Alphabetical Index
- short stature NOS (R62.52)
- short-limbed stature with immunodeficiency (D82.2)
AHA: 2022,4Q,11-13

E34.30 Short stature due to endocrine disorder, unspecified

E34.31 Constitutional short stature
Constitutional delay of growth, puberty, or maturation

E34.32 Genetic causes of short stature

E34.321 Primary insulin-like growth factor-1 (IGF-1) deficiency
Acid-labile subunit gene (IGFALS) defect
Growth hormone gene 1 (GH1) defect with growth hormone neutralizing antibodies
Growth hormone insensitivity syndrome (GHIS)
Insulin-like growth factor 1 gene (IGF1) defect
Laron type short stature
Severe primary insulin-like growth factor-1 deficiency (SPIGFD)
Signal transducer and activator of transcription 5B gene (STAT5b) defect

E34.322 Insulin-like growth factor-1 (IGF-1) resistance
Genetic syndrome with resistance to insulin-like growth factor-1
Insulin-like growth factor-1 receptor (IGF-1R) defect
Post-insulin-like growth factor-1 receptor signaling defect

E34.328 Other genetic causes of short stature
Short stature due to ACAN gene variant
Short stature due to aggrecan deficiency
Short stature due to NPR-2 gene variant

E34.329 Unspecified genetic causes of short stature

E34.39 Other short stature due to endocrine disorder

E34.4 Constitutional tall stature
Constitutional gigantism

Chapter 4. Endocrine, Nutritional and Metabolic Diseases

E34.5 **Androgen insensitivity syndrome**
DEF: X-linked recessive condition in which individuals that are chromosomally male fail to develop normal male external genitalia due to an abnormality on the X chromosome that prohibits the body, completely or in part, from recognizing the androgens produced. *Synonym(s):* AIS

- **E34.50** Androgen insensitivity syndrome, unspecified
  Androgen insensitivity NOS
- **E34.51** **Complete** androgen insensitivity syndrome
  Complete androgen insensitivity
  de Quervain syndrome
  Goldberg-Maxwell syndrome
- **E34.52** **Partial** androgen insensitivity syndrome
  Partial androgen insensitivity
  Reifenstein syndrome

E34.8 **Other specified endocrine disorders**
  Pineal gland dysfunction
  Progeria
  EXCLUDES 2 pseudohypoparathyroidism (E20.1)

E34.9 **Endocrine disorder, unspecified**
  Endocrine disturbance NOS
  Hormone disturbance NOS

E35 *Disorders of endocrine glands in diseases classified elsewhere*
  Code first underlying disease, such as:
    late congenital syphilis of thymus gland [Dubois disease] (A50.59)
  Use additional code, if applicable, to identify:
    sequelae of tuberculosis of other organs (B90.8)
  EXCLUDES 1
    Echinococcus granulosus infection of thyroid gland (B67.3)
    meningococcal hemorrhagic adrenalitis (A39.1)
    syphilis of endocrine gland (A52.79)
    tuberculosis of adrenal gland, except calcification (A18.7)
    tuberculosis of endocrine gland NEC (A18.82)
    tuberculosis of thyroid gland (A18.81)
    Waterhouse-Friderichsen syndrome (A39.1)

Intraoperative complications of endocrine system (E36)

E36 **Intraoperative complications of endocrine system**
  EXCLUDES 2 postprocedural endocrine and metabolic complications and disorders, not elsewhere classified (E89.-)

- **E36.0** **Intraoperative hemorrhage and hematoma** of an endocrine system organ or structure complicating a procedure
  EXCLUDES 1 intraoperative hemorrhage and hematoma of an endocrine system organ or structure due to accidental puncture or laceration during a procedure (E36.1-)
  - **E36.01** Intraoperative hemorrhage and hematoma of an endocrine system organ or structure complicating an endocrine system procedure
    AHA: 2020,1Q,19
  - **E36.02** Intraoperative hemorrhage and hematoma of an endocrine system organ or structure complicating other procedure

- **E36.1** **Accidental puncture and laceration** of an endocrine system organ or structure during a procedure
  - **E36.11** Accidental puncture and laceration of an endocrine system organ or structure during an endocrine system procedure
  - **E36.12** Accidental puncture and laceration of an endocrine system organ or structure during other procedure

- **E36.8** **Other intraoperative complications of endocrine system**
  Use additional code, if applicable, to further specify disorder

Malnutrition (E40-E46)

EXCLUDES 1 intestinal malabsorption (K90.-)
  sequelae of protein-calorie malnutrition (E64.0)
EXCLUDES 2 nutritional anemias (D50-D53)
  starvation (T73.0)
AHA: 2020,1Q,4-7; 2017,4Q,108; 2017,3Q,25
TIP: Assign additional code for BMI from category Z68, when documented. BMI can be based on documentation from clinicians who are not the patient's provider.
TIP: Malnutrition is not considered integral to cancer; assign the appropriate code in addition to the code for the specific type of cancer.

E40 **Kwashiorkor**
  Severe malnutrition with nutritional edema with dyspigmentation of skin and hair
  EXCLUDES 1 marasmic kwashiorkor (E42)

E41 **Nutritional marasmus**
  Severe malnutrition with marasmus
  EXCLUDES 1 marasmic kwashiorkor (E42)
  AHA: 2017,3Q,24
  DEF: Protein-calorie malabsorption or malnutrition in children characterized by tissue wasting, dehydration, and subcutaneous fat depletion. It may occur with infectious disease.

E42 **Marasmic kwashiorkor**
  Intermediate form severe protein-calorie malnutrition
  Severe protein-calorie malnutrition with signs of both kwashiorkor and marasmus

E43 **Unspecified severe protein-calorie malnutrition**
  Starvation edema
  AHA: 2022,1Q,13; 2020,1Q,5,6; 2017,4Q,108

E44 **Protein-calorie malnutrition of moderate and mild degree**
  AHA: 2020,1Q,5
- **E44.0** **Moderate** protein-calorie malnutrition
- **E44.1** **Mild** protein-calorie malnutrition

E45 **Retarded development following protein-calorie malnutrition**
  Nutritional short stature
  Nutritional stunting
  Physical retardation due to malnutrition

E46 **Unspecified protein-calorie malnutrition**
  Malnutrition NOS
  Protein-calorie imbalance NOS
  EXCLUDES 1 nutritional deficiency NOS (E63.9)
  AHA: 2018,4Q,82

Other nutritional deficiencies (E50-E64)

EXCLUDES 2 nutritional anemias (D50-D53)

E50 **Vitamin A deficiency**
  EXCLUDES 1 sequelae of vitamin A deficiency (E64.1)
- **E50.0** Vitamin A deficiency with conjunctival xerosis
- **E50.1** Vitamin A deficiency with Bitot's spot and conjunctival xerosis
  Bitot's spot in the young child
  DEF: Vitamin A deficiency with conjunctival dryness and superficial spots of keratinized epithelium.
- **E50.2** Vitamin A deficiency with corneal xerosis
- **E50.3** Vitamin A deficiency with corneal ulceration and xerosis
- **E50.4** Vitamin A deficiency with keratomalacia
  DEF: Vitamin A deficiency creating corneal dryness that progresses to corneal insensitivity, softness, and necrosis. It is usually bilateral.
- **E50.5** Vitamin A deficiency with night blindness
- **E50.6** Vitamin A deficiency with xerophthalmic scars of cornea
- **E50.7** Other ocular manifestations of vitamin A deficiency
  Xerophthalmia NOS
- **E50.8** Other manifestations of vitamin A deficiency
  Follicular keratosis
  Xeroderma
- **E50.9** Vitamin A deficiency, unspecified
  Hypovitaminosis A NOS

E51 **Thiamine deficiency**
  EXCLUDES 1 sequelae of thiamine deficiency (E64.8)
- **E51.1** **Beriberi**
  - **E51.11** **Dry** beriberi
    Beriberi NOS
    Beriberi with polyneuropathy
  - **E51.12** **Wet** beriberi
    Beriberi with cardiovascular manifestations
    Cardiovascular beriberi
    Shoshin disease
- **E51.2** **Wernicke's encephalopathy**
  DEF: Deficiency of vitamin B1 resulting in a triad of acute mental confusion, ataxia, and ophthalmoplegia. The vast majority of affected patients are alcoholics.
- **E51.8** Other manifestations of thiamine deficiency
- **E51.9** Thiamine deficiency, unspecified

E52 **Niacin deficiency [pellagra]**
  Niacin (-tryptophan) deficiency
  Nicotinamide deficiency
  Pellagra (alcoholic)
  EXCLUDES 1 sequelae of niacin deficiency (E64.8)

 CMS-HCC Rx HCC 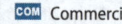 ESRD HCC 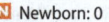 Commercial HCC **N** Newborn: 0 **P** Pediatric: 0-17 **M** Maternity: 9-64 **A** Adult: 15-124

Chapter 4. Endocrine, Nutritional and Metabolic Diseases

E53 Deficiency of other B group vitamins
- EXCLUDES 1: sequelae of vitamin B deficiency (E64.8)

E53.0 Riboflavin deficiency
- Ariboflavinosis
- Vitamin B2 deficiency

E53.1 Pyridoxine deficiency
- Vitamin B6 deficiency
- EXCLUDES 1: pyridoxine-responsive sideroblastic anemia (D64.3)

E53.8 Deficiency of other specified B group vitamins
- Biotin deficiency
- Cyanocobalamin deficiency
- Folate deficiency
- Folic acid deficiency
- Pantothenic acid deficiency
- Vitamin B12 deficiency
- EXCLUDES 1: folate deficiency anemia (D52.-)
- vitamin B12 deficiency anemia (D51.-)

E53.9 Vitamin B deficiency, unspecified

E54 Ascorbic acid deficiency
- Deficiency of vitamin C
- Scurvy
- EXCLUDES 1: scorbutic anemia (D53.2)
- sequelae of vitamin C deficiency (E64.2)
- DEF: Vitamin C deficiency causing swollen gums, myalgia, weight loss, and weakness.

E55 Vitamin D deficiency
- EXCLUDES 1: adult osteomalacia (M83.-)
- osteoporosis (M80.-)
- sequelae of rickets (E64.3)

E55.0 Rickets, active
- Infantile osteomalacia
- Juvenile osteomalacia
- EXCLUDES 1: celiac rickets (K90.0)
- Crohn's rickets (K50.-)
- hereditary vitamin D-dependent rickets (E83.32)
- inactive rickets (E64.3)
- renal rickets (N25.0)
- sequelae of rickets (E64.3)
- vitamin D-resistant rickets (E83.31)
- DEF: Rickets: Softening or weakening of the bones due to a lack of vitamin D, calcium, and phosphate.

E55.9 Vitamin D deficiency, unspecified
- Avitaminosis D

E56 Other vitamin deficiencies
- EXCLUDES 1: sequelae of other vitamin deficiencies (E64.8)

E56.0 Deficiency of vitamin E

E56.1 Deficiency of vitamin K
- EXCLUDES 1: deficiency of coagulation factor due to vitamin K deficiency (D68.4)
- vitamin K deficiency of newborn (P53)

E56.8 Deficiency of other vitamins

E56.9 Vitamin deficiency, unspecified

E58 Dietary calcium deficiency
- EXCLUDES 1: disorders of calcium metabolism (E83.5-)
- sequelae of calcium deficiency (E64.8)

E59 Dietary selenium deficiency
- Keshan disease
- EXCLUDES 1: sequelae of selenium deficiency (E64.8)

E60 Dietary zinc deficiency

E61 Deficiency of other nutrient elements
- Use additional code for adverse effect, if applicable, to identify drug (T36-T50 with fifth or sixth character 5)
- EXCLUDES 1: disorders of mineral metabolism (E83.-)
- iodine deficiency related thyroid disorders (E00-E02)
- sequelae of malnutrition and other nutritional deficiencies (E64.-)

E61.0 Copper deficiency

E61.1 Iron deficiency
- EXCLUDES 1: iron deficiency anemia (D50.-)

E61.2 Magnesium deficiency

E61.3 Manganese deficiency

E61.4 Chromium deficiency

E61.5 Molybdenum deficiency

E61.6 Vanadium deficiency

E61.7 Deficiency of multiple nutrient elements

E61.8 Deficiency of other specified nutrient elements

E61.9 Deficiency of nutrient element, unspecified

E63 Other nutritional deficiencies
- EXCLUDES 2: dehydration (E86.0)
- failure to thrive, adult (R62.7)
- failure to thrive, child (R62.51)
- feeding problems in newborn (P92.-)
- sequelae of malnutrition and other nutritional deficiencies (E64.-)

E63.0 Essential fatty acid [EFA] deficiency

E63.1 Imbalance of constituents of food intake

E63.8 Other specified nutritional deficiencies

E63.9 Nutritional deficiency, unspecified

E64 Sequelae of malnutrition and other nutritional deficiencies
- NOTE: This category is to be used to indicate conditions in categories E43, E44, E46, E50-E63 as the cause of sequelae, which are themselves classified elsewhere. The 'sequelae' include conditions specified as such; they also include the late effects of diseases classifiable to the above categories if the disease itself is no longer present
- Code first condition resulting from (sequela) of malnutrition and other nutritional deficiencies

E64.0 Sequelae of protein-calorie malnutrition
- EXCLUDES 2: retarded development following protein-calorie malnutrition (E45)

E64.1 Sequelae of vitamin A deficiency

E64.2 Sequelae of vitamin C deficiency

E64.3 Sequelae of rickets

E64.8 Sequelae of other nutritional deficiencies

E64.9 Sequelae of unspecified nutritional deficiency

Overweight, obesity and other hyperalimentation (E65-E68)

E65 Localized adiposity
- Fat pad

E66 Overweight and obesity
- Code first obesity complicating pregnancy, childbirth and the puerperium, if applicable (O99.21-)
- Use additional code to identify body mass index (BMI), if known, for adults (Z68.1-Z68.45) or pediatrics (Z68.5-)
- EXCLUDES 2: adiposogenital dystrophy (E23.6)
- lipomatosis dolorosa [Dercum] (E88.2)
- lipomatosis NOS (E88.2)
- Prader-Willi syndrome (Q87.11)
- AHA: 2025,1Q,4; 2022,3Q,6; 2018,4Q,77,79-80
- TIP: Do not assign a BMI code (Z68.-) when a pregnant patient is documented as being overweight or obese. Only a code from subcategory O99.21- and a code from this category should be assigned.

E66.0 Obesity due to excess calories

E66.01 Morbid (severe) obesity due to excess calories
- EXCLUDES 1: morbid (severe) obesity with alveolar hypoventilation (E66.2)
- AHA: 2025,1Q,17; 2022,3Q,6; 2022,2Q,9
- TIP: If both morbid obesity and class 3 obesity are documented, only the code for class 3 obesity (E66.813) should be assigned.

E66.09 Other obesity due to excess calories

E66.1 Drug-induced obesity
- Use additional code for adverse effect, if applicable, to identify drug (T36-T50 with fifth or sixth character 5)

E66.2 Morbid (severe) obesity with alveolar hypoventilation
- Obesity hypoventilation syndrome (OHS)
- Pickwickian syndrome

E66.3 Overweight
- AHA: 2018,4Q,78

E66.8 Other obesity
- AHA: 2024,4Q,8,11

E66.81 Obesity class
- AHA: 2025,1Q,17
- TIP: Assign a code for the specific class of obesity with any other obesity code within the classification (e.g., E66.1, E88.82, O99.21), except when both morbid obesity (E66.01) and class 3 obesity are documented. In this instance only the code for class 3 obesity should be assigned.

E66.811 Obesity, class 1

E66.812 Obesity, class 2

Chapter 4. Endocrine, Nutritional and Metabolic Diseases

E66.813 Obesity, class 3
E66.89 Other obesity not elsewhere classified
E66.9 Obesity, unspecified
  Obesity NOS
  AHA: 2021,2Q,10

E67 Other hyperalimentation
  EXCLUDES 1: hyperalimentation NOS (R63.2)
  sequelae of hyperalimentation (E68)
  E67.0 Hypervitaminosis A
  E67.1 Hypercarotenemia
    DEF: Elevated blood carotene level as a result of excessive carotenoid ingestion or an inability to convert carotenoids to vitamin A. Characteristics often include yellow discoloration of the skin, which may follow overeating of carotenoid-rich foods such as carrots, sweet potatoes, or squash.
  E67.2 Megavitamin-B6 syndrome
  E67.3 Hypervitaminosis D
  E67.8 Other specified hyperalimentation

E68 Sequelae of hyperalimentation
  Code first condition resulting from (sequela) of hyperalimentation

Metabolic disorders (E70-E88)

EXCLUDES 1: androgen insensitivity syndrome (E34.5-)
  congenital adrenal hyperplasia (E25.0)
  hemolytic anemias attributable to enzyme disorders (D55.-)
  Marfan syndrome (Q87.4-)
  5-alpha-reductase deficiency (E29.1)
EXCLUDES 2: Ehlers-Danlos syndromes (Q79.6-)
AHA: 2018,2Q,6

E70 Disorders of aromatic amino-acid metabolism
  E70.0 Classical phenylketonuria
  E70.1 Other hyperphenylalaninemias
  E70.2 Disorders of tyrosine metabolism
    EXCLUDES 1: transitory tyrosinemia of newborn (P74.5)
    E70.20 Disorder of tyrosine metabolism, unspecified
    E70.21 Tyrosinemia
      Hypertyrosinemia
    E70.29 Other disorders of tyrosine metabolism
      Alkaptonuria
      Ochronosis
  E70.3 Albinism
    DEF: Absence of pigment in skin, hair, and eyes. This genetic condition is often accompanied by astigmatism, photophobia, and nystagmus.
    E70.30 Albinism, unspecified
    E70.31 Ocular albinism
      E70.310 X-linked ocular albinism
      E70.311 Autosomal recessive ocular albinism
      E70.318 Other ocular albinism
      E70.319 Ocular albinism, unspecified
    E70.32 Oculocutaneous albinism
      EXCLUDES 1: Chediak-Higashi syndrome (E70.330)
      Hermansky-Pudlak syndrome (E70.331)
      E70.320 Tyrosinase negative oculocutaneous albinism
        Albinism I
        Oculocutaneous albinism ty-neg
      E70.321 Tyrosinase positive oculocutaneous albinism
        Albinism II
        Oculocutaneous albinism ty-pos
      E70.328 Other oculocutaneous albinism
        Cross syndrome
      E70.329 Oculocutaneous albinism, unspecified
    E70.33 Albinism with hematologic abnormality
      E70.330 Chediak-Higashi syndrome
      E70.331 Hermansky-Pudlak syndrome
      E70.338 Other albinism with hematologic abnormality
      E70.339 Albinism with hematologic abnormality, unspecified
    E70.39 Other specified albinism
      Piebaldism
  E70.4 Disorders of histidine metabolism
    E70.40 Disorders of histidine metabolism, unspecified
    E70.41 Histidinemia
    E70.49 Other disorders of histidine metabolism
  E70.5 Disorders of tryptophan metabolism
  E70.8 Other disorders of aromatic amino-acid metabolism
    AHA: 2020,4Q,15-16
    E70.81 Aromatic L-amino acid decarboxylase deficiency
      AADC deficiency
    E70.89 Other disorders of aromatic amino-acid metabolism
  E70.9 Disorder of aromatic amino-acid metabolism, unspecified

E71 Disorders of branched-chain amino-acid metabolism and fatty-acid metabolism
  E71.0 Maple-syrup-urine disease
  E71.1 Other disorders of branched-chain amino-acid metabolism
    E71.11 Branched-chain organic acidurias
      E71.110 Isovaleric acidemia
      E71.111 3-methylglutaconic aciduria
      E71.118 Other branched-chain organic acidurias
    E71.12 Disorders of propionate metabolism
      E71.120 Methylmalonic acidemia
      E71.121 Propionic acidemia
      E71.128 Other disorders of propionate metabolism
    E71.19 Other disorders of branched-chain amino-acid metabolism
      Hyperleucine-isoleucinemia
      Hypervalinemia
  E71.2 Disorder of branched-chain amino-acid metabolism, unspecified
  E71.3 Disorders of fatty-acid metabolism
    EXCLUDES 1: peroxisomal disorders (E71.5)
      Refsum's disease (G60.1)
      Schilder's disease (G37.0)
    EXCLUDES 2: carnitine deficiency due to inborn error of metabolism (E71.42)
    E71.30 Disorder of fatty-acid metabolism, unspecified
    E71.31 Disorders of fatty-acid oxidation
      E71.310 Long chain/very long chain acyl CoA dehydrogenase deficiency
        LCAD deficiency
        VLCAD deficiency
      E71.311 Medium chain acyl CoA dehydrogenase deficiency
        MCAD deficiency
      E71.312 Short chain acyl CoA dehydrogenase deficiency
        SCAD deficiency
      E71.313 Glutaric aciduria type II
        Glutaric aciduria type II A
        Glutaric aciduria type II B
        Glutaric aciduria type II C
        EXCLUDES 1: glutaric aciduria (type 1) NOS (E72.3)
      E71.314 Muscle carnitine palmitoyltransferase deficiency
      E71.318 Other disorders of fatty-acid oxidation
    E71.32 Disorders of ketone metabolism
    E71.39 Other disorders of fatty-acid metabolism

Chapter 4. Endocrine, Nutritional and Metabolic Diseases

E71.4 Disorders of carnitine metabolism
EXCLUDES 1: muscle carnitine palmitoyltransferase deficiency (E71.314)

- **E71.40** Disorder of carnitine metabolism, unspecified
- **E71.41** Primary carnitine deficiency
- **E71.42** Carnitine deficiency due to inborn errors of metabolism
  Code also associated inborn error or metabolism
- **E71.43** Iatrogenic carnitine deficiency
  - Carnitine deficiency due to hemodialysis
  - Carnitine deficiency due to Valproic acid therapy
- **E71.44** Other secondary carnitine deficiency
  - **E71.440** Ruvalcaba-Myhre-Smith syndrome
  - **E71.448** Other secondary carnitine deficiency

E71.5 Peroxisomal disorders
EXCLUDES 1: Schilder's disease (G37.0)

- **E71.50** Peroxisomal disorder, unspecified
- **E71.51** Disorders of peroxisome biogenesis
  - Group 1 peroxisomal disorders
  - **EXCLUDES 1:** Refsum's disease (G60.1)
  - **E71.510** Zellweger syndrome
  - **E71.511** Neonatal adrenoleukodystrophy
    - **EXCLUDES 1:** X-linked adrenoleukodystrophy (E71.42-)
  - **E71.518** Other disorders of peroxisome biogenesis
- **E71.52** X-linked adrenoleukodystrophy
  - **E71.520** Childhood cerebral X-linked adrenoleukodystrophy
  - **E71.521** Adolescent X-linked adrenoleukodystrophy
  - **E71.522** Adrenomyeloneuropathy
  - **E71.528** Other X-linked adrenoleukodystrophy
    - Addison only phenotype adrenoleukodystrophy
    - Addison-Schilder adrenoleukodystrophy
  - **E71.529** X-linked adrenoleukodystrophy, unspecified type
- **E71.53** Other group 2 peroxisomal disorders
- **E71.54** Other peroxisomal disorders
  - **E71.540** Rhizomelic chondrodysplasia punctata
    - **EXCLUDES 1:** chondrodysplasia punctata NOS (Q77.3)
  - **E71.541** Zellweger-like syndrome
  - **E71.542** Other group 3 peroxisomal disorders
  - **E71.548** Other peroxisomal disorders

E72 Other disorders of amino-acid metabolism
EXCLUDES 1: disorders of:
- gout (M1A.-, M10.-)
- aromatic amino-acid metabolism (E70.-)
- branched-chain amino-acid metabolism (E71.0-E71.2)
- fatty-acid metabolism (E71.3)
- purine and pyrimidine metabolism (E79.-)

E72.0 Disorders of amino-acid transport
EXCLUDES 1: disorders of tryptophan metabolism (E70.5)

- **E72.00** Disorders of amino-acid transport, unspecified
- **E72.01** Cystinuria
- **E72.02** Hartnup's disease
- **E72.03** Lowe's syndrome
  Use additional code for associated glaucoma (H42)
- **E72.04** Cystinosis
  - Fanconi (-de Toni) (-Debre) syndrome with cystinosis
  - **EXCLUDES 1:** Fanconi (-de Toni) (-Debre) syndrome without cystinosis (E72.09)
- **E72.09** Other disorders of amino-acid transport
  - Fanconi (-de Toni) (-Debre) syndrome, unspecified

E72.1 Disorders of sulfur-bearing amino-acid metabolism
EXCLUDES 1:
- cystinosis (E72.04)
- cystinuria (E72.01)
- transcobalamin II deficiency (D51.2)

- **E72.10** Disorders of sulfur-bearing amino-acid metabolism, unspecified
- **E72.11** Homocystinuria
  - Cystathionine synthase deficiency
  - **AHA:** 2021,4Q,28
- **E72.12** Methylenetetrahydrofolate reductase deficiency
- **E72.19** Other disorders of sulfur-bearing amino-acid metabolism
  - Cystathioninuria
  - Methioninemia
  - Sulfite oxidase deficiency

E72.2 Disorders of urea cycle metabolism
EXCLUDES 1: disorders of ornithine metabolism (E72.4)

- **E72.20** Disorder of urea cycle metabolism, unspecified
  - Hyperammonemia
  - **EXCLUDES 1:** hyperammonemia-hyperornithinemia-homocitrullinemia syndrome E72.4
  - transient hyperammonemia of newborn (P74.6)
- **E72.21** Argininemia
- **E72.22** Arginosuccinic aciduria
- **E72.23** Citrullinemia
- **E72.29** Other disorders of urea cycle metabolism

E72.3 Disorders of lysine and hydroxylysine metabolism
- Glutaric aciduria (type I)
- Glutaric aciduria NOS
- Hydroxylysinemia
- Hyperlysinemia
- **EXCLUDES 1:**
  - glutaric aciduria type II (E71.313)
  - Refsum's disease (G60.1)
  - Zellweger syndrome (E71.510)

E72.4 Disorders of ornithine metabolism
- Hyperammonemia-Hyperornithinemia-Homocitrullinemia syndrome
- Ornithine transcarbamylase deficiency
- Ornithinemia (types I, II)
- **EXCLUDES 1:** hereditary choroidal dystrophy (H31.2-)

E72.5 Disorders of glycine metabolism
- **E72.50** Disorder of glycine metabolism, unspecified
- **E72.51** Non-ketotic hyperglycinemia
- **E72.52** Trimethylaminuria
- **E72.53** Primary hyperoxaluria
  - Oxalosis
  - Oxaluria
  - **EXCLUDES 1:** ▶secondary hyperoxaluria (E72.54-)◀
  - **AHA:** 2018,4Q,29
  - **E72.530** Primary hyperoxaluria, type 1
  - **E72.538** Other specified primary hyperoxaluria
    - Primary hyperoxaluria, type 2
    - Primary hyperoxaluria, type 3
  - **E72.539** Primary hyperoxaluria, unspecified
- **E72.54** Secondary hyperoxaluria
  - **EXCLUDES 1:** primary hyperoxaluria (E72.53-)
  - **E72.540** Dietary hyperoxaluria
  - **E72.541** Enteric hyperoxaluria
  - **E72.548** Other secondary hyperoxaluria
  - **E72.549** Secondary hyperoxaluria, unspecified
- **E72.59** Other disorders of glycine metabolism
  - D-glycericacidemia
  - Hyperhydroxyprolinemia
  - Hyperprolinemia (types I, II)
  - Sarcosinemia

Chapter 4. Endocrine, Nutritional and Metabolic Diseases

E72.8 **Other specified disorders of amino-acid metabolism**
AHA: 2018,4Q,5

- **E72.81** **Disorders of gamma aminobutyric acid metabolism**
  - 4-hydroxybutyric aciduria
  - Disorders of GABA metabolism
  - GABA metabolic defect
  - GABA transaminase deficiency
  - GABA-T deficiency
  - Gamma-hydroxybutyric aciduria
  - SSADHD
  - Succinic semialdehyde dehydrogenase deficiency

- **E72.89** **Other specified disorders of amino-acid metabolism**
  - Disorders of beta-amino-acid metabolism
  - Disorders of gamma-glutamyl cycle

E72.9 **Disorder of amino-acid metabolism, unspecified**

E73 Lactose intolerance
DEF: Inability to break down sugar in dairy products due to a deficiency in the enzyme lactase.

- **E73.0** **Congenital** lactase deficiency
- **E73.1** **Secondary** lactase deficiency
- **E73.8** Other lactose intolerance
- **E73.9** Lactose intolerance, unspecified

E74 Other disorders of carbohydrate metabolism
EXCLUDES 1: diabetes mellitus (E08-E13)
hypoglycemia NOS (E16.2)
increased secretion of glucagon (E16.3)
mucopolysaccharidosis (E76.0-E76.3)

- **E74.0** **Glycogen storage** disease
  - **E74.00** Glycogen storage disease, unspecified
  - **E74.01** **von Gierke** disease
    - Type I glycogen storage disease
  - **E74.02** **Pompe** disease
    - Cardiac glycogenosis
    - Type II glycogen storage disease
  - **E74.03** **Cori** disease
    - Forbes disease
    - Type III glycogen storage disease
  - **E74.04** **McArdle** disease
    - Type V glycogen storage disease
  - **E74.05** **Lysosome-associated membrane protein 2 [LAMP2] deficiency**
    - Danon disease
    - Code also, if applicable, associated manifestations such as:
      - dilated cardiomyopathy (I42.0)
      - obstructive hypertrophic cardiomyopathy (I42.1)
    - AHA: 2023,4Q,11
  - **E74.09** Other glycogen storage disease
    - Andersen disease
    - Glycogen storage disease, types 0, IV, VI-XI
    - Hers disease
    - Liver phosphorylase deficiency
    - Muscle phosphofructokinase deficiency
    - Tauri disease

- **E74.1** **Disorders of fructose metabolism**
  - EXCLUDES 1: muscle phosphofructokinase deficiency (E74.09)
  - **E74.10** Disorder of fructose metabolism, unspecified
  - **E74.11** **Essential fructosuria**
    - Fructokinase deficiency
  - **E74.12** **Hereditary** fructose intolerance
    - Fructosemia
  - **E74.19** Other disorders of fructose metabolism
    - Fructose-1, 6-diphosphatase deficiency

- **E74.2** **Disorders of galactose metabolism**
  - **E74.20** Disorders of galactose metabolism, unspecified
  - **E74.21** **Galactosemia**
    - DEF: Any of three genetic disorders caused by a defective galactose metabolism. Symptoms include failure to thrive in infancy, jaundice, liver and spleen damage, cataracts, and mental retardation.
  - **E74.29** Other disorders of galactose metabolism
    - Galactokinase deficiency

- **E74.3** **Other disorders of intestinal carbohydrate absorption**
  - EXCLUDES 2: lactose intolerance (E73.-)
  - **E74.31** Sucrase-isomaltase deficiency
  - **E74.39** Other disorders of intestinal carbohydrate absorption
    - Disorder of intestinal carbohydrate absorption NOS
    - Glucose-galactose malabsorption
    - Sucrase deficiency

- **E74.4** **Disorders of pyruvate metabolism and gluconeogenesis**
  - Deficiency of phosphoenolpyruvate carboxykinase
  - Deficiency of pyruvate carboxylase
  - Deficiency of pyruvate dehydrogenase
  - EXCLUDES 1: disorders of pyruvate metabolism and gluconeogenesis with anemia (D55.-)
    Leigh's syndrome (G31.82)

- **E74.8** Other specified disorders of carbohydrate metabolism
  - AHA: 2020,4Q,16
  - **E74.81** Disorders of glucose transport, not elsewhere classified
    - **E74.810** Glucose transporter protein type 1 deficiency
      - De Vivo syndrome
      - Glucose transport defect, blood-brain barrier
      - Glut1 deficiency
      - GLUT1 deficiency syndrome 1, infantile onset
      - GLUT1 deficiency syndrome 2, childhood onset
    - **E74.818** Other disorders of glucose transport
      - (Familial) renal glycosuria
    - **E74.819** Disorders of glucose transport, unspecified
  - **E74.82** Disorders of citrate metabolism
    - AHA: 2024,4Q,10
    - **E74.820** SLC13A5 Citrate Transporter Disorder
    - **E74.829** Other disorders of citrate metabolism
  - **E74.89** Other specified disorders of carbohydrate metabolism
    - Essential pentosuria
    - AHA: 2023,3Q,3

- **E74.9** Disorder of carbohydrate metabolism, unspecified

E75 Disorders of sphingolipid metabolism and other lipid storage disorders
EXCLUDES 1: mucolipidosis, types I-III (E77.0-E77.1)
Refsum's disease (G60.1)

- **E75.0** **GM2 gangliosidosis**
  - **E75.00** GM2 gangliosidosis, unspecified
  - **E75.01** **Sandhoff** disease

HCC CMS-HCC | Rx Rx HCC | ESR ESRD HCC | COM Commercial HCC | N Newborn: 0 | P Pediatric: 0-17 | M Maternity: 9-64 | A Adult: 15-124

E75.02 Tay-Sachs disease
DEF: Genetic mutation of the HEXA gene that inhibits the breakdown of a toxic substance called ganglioside. The accumulation of ganglioside results in destruction of the neurons in the brain and spinal cord.

Tay-Sachs Disease

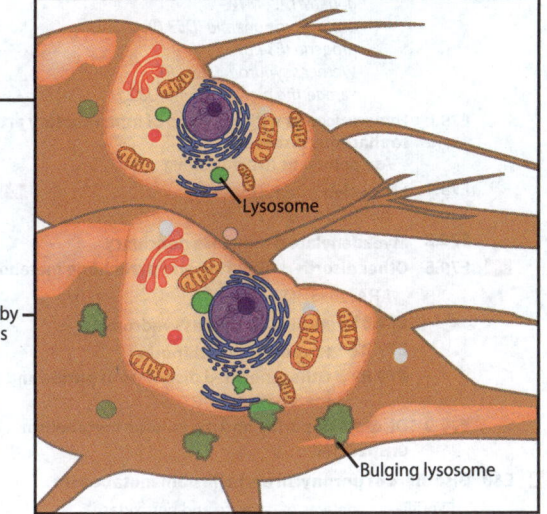

- **E75.09 Other GM2 gangliosidosis**
  - Adult GM2 gangliosidosis
  - Juvenile GM2 gangliosidosis
- **E75.1 Other and unspecified gangliosidosis**
  - **E75.10 Unspecified gangliosidosis**
    - Gangliosidosis NOS
  - **E75.11 Mucolipidosis IV**
  - **E75.19 Other gangliosidosis**
    - GM1 gangliosidosis
    - GM3 gangliosidosis
- **E75.2 Other sphingolipidosis**
  - EXCLUDES 1: adrenoleukodystrophy [Addison-Schilder] (E71.528)
  - **E75.21 Fabry (-Anderson) disease**
  - **E75.22 Gaucher disease**
  - **E75.23 Krabbe disease**
  - **E75.24 Niemann-Pick disease**
    - Acid sphingomyelinase deficiency (ASMD)
    - **E75.240 Niemann-Pick disease type A**
      - Acid sphingomyelinase deficiency type A (ASMD type A)
      - Infantile neurovisceral acid sphingomyelinase deficiency
    - **E75.241 Niemann-Pick disease type B**
      - Acid sphingomyelinase deficiency type B (ASMD type B)
      - Chronic visceral acid sphingomyelinase deficiency
    - **E75.242 Niemann-Pick disease type C**
    - **E75.243 Niemann-Pick disease type D**
    - **E75.244 Niemann-Pick disease type A/B**
      - Acid sphingomyelinase deficiency type A/B (ASMD type A/B)
      - Chronic neurovisceral acid sphingomyelinase deficiency
      - AHA: 2021,4Q,8-9
    - **E75.248 Other Niemann-Pick disease**
    - **E75.249 Niemann-Pick disease, unspecified**
      - Acid sphingomyelinase deficiency (ASMD) NOS
  - **E75.25 Metachromatic leukodystrophy**
  - **E75.26 Sulfatase deficiency**
    - Multiple sulfatase deficiency (MSD)
    - AHA: 2018,4Q,5-6
  - **E75.27 Pelizaeus-Merzbacher disease**
    - AHA: 2023,4Q,12-13
  - **E75.28 Canavan disease**
    - AHA: 2023,4Q,12-13
  - **E75.29 Other sphingolipidosis**
    - Farber's syndrome
    - Sulfatide lipidosis
- **E75.3 Sphingolipidosis, unspecified**
- **E75.4 Neuronal ceroid lipofuscinosis**
  - Batten disease
  - Bielschowsky-Jansky disease
  - Kufs disease
  - Spielmeyer-Vogt disease
- **E75.5 Other lipid storage disorders**
  - Cerebrotendinous cholesterosis [van Bogaert-Scherer-Epstein]
  - Wolman's disease
- **E75.6 Lipid storage disorder, unspecified**
- **E76 Disorders of glycosaminoglycan metabolism**
  - **E76.0 Mucopolysaccharidosis, type I**
    - **E76.01 Hurler's syndrome**
    - **E76.02 Hurler-Scheie syndrome**
    - **E76.03 Scheie's syndrome**
  - **E76.1 Mucopolysaccharidosis, type II**
    - Hunter's syndrome
  - **E76.2 Other mucopolysaccharidoses**
    - **E76.21 Morquio mucopolysaccharidoses**
      - **E76.210 Morquio A mucopolysaccharidoses**
        - Classic Morquio syndrome
        - Morquio syndrome A
        - Mucopolysaccharidosis, type IVA
      - **E76.211 Morquio B mucopolysaccharidoses**
        - Morquio syndrome B
        - Morquio-like mucopolysaccharidoses
        - Morquio-like syndrome
        - Mucopolysaccharidosis, type IVB
      - **E76.219 Morquio mucopolysaccharidoses, unspecified**
        - Morquio syndrome
        - Mucopolysaccharidosis, type IV
    - **E76.22 Sanfilippo mucopolysaccharidoses**
      - Mucopolysaccharidosis, type III (A) (B) (C) (D)
      - Sanfilippo A syndrome
      - Sanfilippo B syndrome
      - Sanfilippo C syndrome
      - Sanfilippo D syndrome
    - **E76.29 Other mucopolysaccharidoses**
      - beta-Glucuronidase deficiency
      - Maroteaux-Lamy (mild) (severe) syndrome
      - Mucopolysaccharidosis, types VI, VII
  - **E76.3 Mucopolysaccharidosis, unspecified**
  - **E76.8 Other disorders of glycosaminoglycan metabolism**
  - **E76.9 Glycosaminoglycan metabolism disorder, unspecified**
- **E77 Disorders of glycoprotein metabolism**
  - **E77.0 Defects in post-translational modification of lysosomal enzymes**
    - Mucolipidosis II [I-cell disease]
    - Mucolipidosis III [pseudo-Hurler polydystrophy]
  - **E77.1 Defects in glycoprotein degradation**
    - Aspartylglucosaminuria
    - Fucosidosis
    - Mannosidosis
    - Sialidosis [mucolipidosis I]
  - **E77.8 Other disorders of glycoprotein metabolism**
  - **E77.9 Disorder of glycoprotein metabolism, unspecified**

Additional Character Required | Placeholder Alert | Manifestation | Unspecified Dx | QPP | Unacceptable PDx

E78 Disorders of lipoprotein metabolism and other lipidemias
EXCLUDES 1 sphingolipidosis (E75.0-E75.3)

E78.0 Pure hypercholesterolemia
AHA: 2016,4Q,13-14

E78.00 Pure hypercholesterolemia, unspecified
(Pure) hypercholesterolemia NOS
Fredrickson's hyperlipoproteinemia, type IIa
Hyperbetalipoproteinemia
Low-density-lipoprotein-type [LDL] hyperlipoproteinemia
AHA: 2023,2Q,9; 2022,2Q,5-6

E78.01 Familial hypercholesterolemia
- E78.010 Homozygous familial hypercholesterolemia [HoFH]
- E78.011 Heterozygous familial hypercholesterolemia [HeFH]
- E78.019 Familial hypercholesterolemia, unspecified
  Familial hypercholesterolemia NOS

E78.1 Pure hyperglyceridemia
Elevated fasting triglycerides
Endogenous hyperglyceridemia
Fredrickson's hyperlipoproteinemia, type IV
Hyperlipidemia, group B
Hyperprebetalipoproteinemia
Very-low-density-lipoprotein-type [VLDL] hyperlipoproteinemia

E78.2 Mixed hyperlipidemia
Broad- or floating-betalipoproteinemia
Combined hyperlipidemia NOS
Elevated cholesterol with elevated triglycerides NEC
Fredrickson's hyperlipoproteinemia, type IIb or III
Hyperbetalipoproteinemia with prebetalipoproteinemia
Hypercholesteremia with endogenous hyperglyceridemia
Hyperlipidemia, group C
Tubo-eruptive xanthoma
Xanthoma tuberosum
EXCLUDES 1 cerebrotendinous cholesterosis [van Bogaert-Scherer-Epstein] (E75.5)
familial combined hyperlipidemia (E78.49)
AHA: 2023,2Q,9; 2022,2Q,6

E78.3 Hyperchylomicronemia
Chylomicron retention disease
Fredrickson's hyperlipoproteinemia, type I or V
Hyperlipidemia, group D
Mixed hyperglyceridemia

E78.4 Other hyperlipidemia
AHA: 2018,4Q,6

E78.41 Elevated Lipoprotein(a)
Elevated Lp(a)

E78.49 Other hyperlipidemia
Familial combined hyperlipidemia

E78.5 Hyperlipidemia, unspecified
AHA: 2022,2Q,5

E78.6 Lipoprotein deficiency
Abetalipoproteinemia
Depressed HDL cholesterol
High-density lipoprotein deficiency
Hypoalphalipoproteinemia
Hypobetalipoproteinemia (familial)
Lecithin cholesterol acyltransferase deficiency
Tangier disease

E78.7 Disorders of bile acid and cholesterol metabolism
EXCLUDES 1 Niemann-Pick disease type C (E75.242)

E78.70 Disorder of bile acid and cholesterol metabolism, unspecified

E78.71 Barth syndrome

E78.72 Smith-Lemli-Opitz syndrome

E78.79 Other disorders of bile acid and cholesterol metabolism
AHA: 2023,1Q,26

E78.8 Other disorders of lipoprotein metabolism
E78.81 Lipoid dermatoarthritis
E78.89 Other lipoprotein metabolism disorders

E78.9 Disorder of lipoprotein metabolism, unspecified

E79 Disorders of purine and pyrimidine metabolism
EXCLUDES 1
Ataxia-telangiectasia (Q87.19)
Bloom's syndrome (Q82.8)
calculus of kidney (N20.0)
Cockayne's syndrome (Q87.19)
combined immunodeficiency disorders (D81.-)
Fanconi's anemia (D61.09)
gout (M1A.-, M10.-)
orotaciduric anemia (D53.0)
progeria (E34.8)
Werner's syndrome (E34.8)
xeroderma pigmentosum (Q82.1)

E79.0 Hyperuricemia without signs of inflammatory arthritis and tophaceous disease
Asymptomatic hyperuricemia

E79.1 Lesch-Nyhan syndrome
HGPRT deficiency

E79.2 Myoadenylate deaminase deficiency

E79.8 Other disorders of purine and pyrimidine metabolism
AHA: 2023,4Q,12-13

E79.81 Aicardi-Goutieres syndrome
E79.82 Hereditary xanthinuria
E79.89 Other specified disorders of purine and pyrimidine metabolism

E79.9 Disorder of purine and pyrimidine metabolism, unspecified

E80 Disorders of porphyrin and bilirubin metabolism
INCLUDES defects of catalase and peroxidase

E80.0 Hereditary erythropoietic porphyria
Congenital erythropoietic porphyria
Erythropoietic protoporphyria

E80.1 Porphyria cutanea tarda

E80.2 Other and unspecified porphyria
E80.20 Unspecified porphyria
Porphyria NOS

E80.21 Acute intermittent (hepatic) porphyria

E80.29 Other porphyria
Hereditary coproporphyria

E80.3 Defects of catalase and peroxidase
Acatalasia [Takahara]

E80.4 Gilbert syndrome

E80.5 Crigler-Najjar syndrome

E80.6 Other disorders of bilirubin metabolism
Dubin-Johnson syndrome
Rotor's syndrome
AHA: 2022,3Q,7
TIP: Assign codes E80.6 and K76.89 to report benign recurrent intrahepatic cholestasis (BRIC) or progressive familial intrahepatic cholestasis (PFIC).

E80.7 Disorder of bilirubin metabolism, unspecified

E83 Disorders of mineral metabolism
EXCLUDES 1
dietary mineral deficiency (E58-E61)
parathyroid disorders (E20-E21)
vitamin D deficiency (E55.-)

E83.0 Disorders of copper metabolism
E83.00 Disorder of copper metabolism, unspecified

E83.01 Wilson's disease
Code also associated Kayser Fleischer ring (H18.04-)

E83.09 Other disorders of copper metabolism
Menkes' (kinky hair) (steely hair) disease

E83.1 Disorders of iron metabolism
EXCLUDES 1
iron deficiency anemia (D50.-)
sideroblastic anemia (D64.0-D64.3)

E83.10 Disorder of iron metabolism, unspecified

E83.11 Hemochromatosis
EXCLUDES 1
GALD (P78.84)
gestational alloimmune liver disease (P78.84)
neonatal hemochromatosis (P78.84)

E83.110 Hereditary hemochromatosis
Bronzed diabetes
Pigmentary cirrhosis (of liver)
Primary (hereditary) hemochromatosis

Chapter 4. Endocrine, Nutritional and Metabolic Diseases

- **E83.111** Hemochromatosis due to repeated red blood cell transfusions
  - Iron overload due to repeated red blood cell transfusions
  - Transfusion (red blood cell) associated hemochromatosis
- **E83.118** Other hemochromatosis [Rx]
- **E83.119** Hemochromatosis, unspecified [Rx]
- **E83.19** Other disorders of iron metabolism [Rx]
  - Use additional code, if applicable, for idiopathic pulmonary hemosiderosis (J84.03)

E83.2 Disorders of zinc metabolism
Acrodermatitis enteropathica

✓5th E83.3 Disorders of phosphorus metabolism and phosphatases
- EXCLUDES 1: adult osteomalacia (M83.-)
  - osteoporosis (M80.-)
- EXCLUDES 2: ▶disorders of pyrophosphate metabolism (E83.82-)◀
- **E83.30** Disorder of phosphorus metabolism, unspecified [Rx]
- **E83.31** Familial hypophosphatemia [HCC] [Rx]
  - Vitamin D-resistant osteomalacia
  - Vitamin D-resistant rickets
  - EXCLUDES 1: vitamin D-deficiency rickets (E55.0)
- **E83.32** Hereditary vitamin D-dependent rickets (type 1) (type 2) [Rx]
  - 25-hydroxyvitamin D 1-alpha-hydroxylase deficiency
  - Pseudovitamin D deficiency
  - Vitamin D receptor defect
- **E83.39** Other disorders of phosphorus metabolism [Rx]
  - Acid phosphatase deficiency
  - Hypophosphatasia

✓5th E83.4 Disorders of magnesium metabolism
- **E83.40** Disorders of magnesium metabolism, unspecified
- **E83.41** Hypermagnesemia
  - AHA: 2016,4Q,54
- **E83.42** Hypomagnesemia
- **E83.49** Other disorders of magnesium metabolism

✓5th E83.5 Disorders of calcium metabolism
- EXCLUDES 1:
  - autoimmune hypoparathyroidism (E20.812)
  - autosomal dominant hypocalcemia (E20.810)
  - chondrocalcinosis (M11.1-M11.2)
  - hungry bone syndrome (E83.81)
  - hyperparathyroidism (E21.0-E21.3)
  - secondary hypoparathyroidism in diseases classified elsewhere (E20.811)
- **E83.50** Unspecified disorder of calcium metabolism
- **E83.51** Hypocalcemia
- **E83.52** Hypercalcemia
  - Familial hypocalciuric hypercalcemia
- **E83.59** Other disorders of calcium metabolism

✓5th E83.8 Other disorders of mineral metabolism
- **E83.81** Hungry bone syndrome
- ● ✓6th **E83.82** Disorders of pyrophosphate metabolism
  - ● **E83.820** Generalized arterial calcification of infancy with unspecified genetic causality
    - Code also, if applicable, associated conditions such as:
      - heart failure (I50.-)
      - other secondary hypertension (I15.8)
  - ● **E83.821** ENPP1 deficiency causing generalized arterial calcification of infancy
    - Code also, if applicable, associated conditions such as:
      - heart failure (I50.-)
      - other secondary hypertension (I15.8)
  - ● **E83.822** ENPP1 deficiency causing autosomal recessive hypophosphatemic rickets type 2
  - ● **E83.823** ABCC6 deficiency causing generalized arterial calcification of infancy
    - Code also, if applicable, associated conditions such as:
      - heart failure (I50.-)
      - other secondary hypertension (I15.8)
  - ● **E83.824** ABCC6 deficiency causing pseudoxanthoma elasticum
  - ● **E83.825** CD73 deficiency causing arterial calcification
- **E83.89** Other disorders of mineral metabolism

E83.9 Disorder of mineral metabolism, unspecified

✓4th E84 Cystic fibrosis
- INCLUDES: mucoviscidosis
- Code also exocrine pancreatic insufficiency (K86.81)
- DEF: Genetic disorder affecting the respiratory, digestive, and reproductive systems in infants to young adults by disturbing exocrine gland function and causing chronic pulmonary disease with excess mucus production and pancreatic deficiency.
- **E84.0** Cystic fibrosis with pulmonary manifestations [HCC] [Rx] [ESR] [COM]
  - Use additional code to identify any infectious organism present, such as:
    - Pseudomonas (B96.5)
  - AHA: 2021,1Q,23
- ✓5th **E84.1** Cystic fibrosis with intestinal manifestations
  - **E84.11** Meconium ileus in cystic fibrosis [HCC] [Rx] [ESR] [COM] [N]
    - EXCLUDES 1: meconium ileus not due to cystic fibrosis (P76.0)
  - **E84.19** Cystic fibrosis with other intestinal manifestations [HCC] [Rx] [ESR] [COM]
    - Distal intestinal obstruction syndrome
- **E84.8** Cystic fibrosis with other manifestations [HCC] [Rx] [ESR] [COM]
- **E84.9** Cystic fibrosis, unspecified [HCC] [Rx] [ESR] [COM]

✓4th E85 Amyloidosis
- EXCLUDES 2: Alzheimer's disease (G30.0-)
- DEF: Conditions of diverse etiologies characterized by the accumulation of insoluble fibrillar proteins (amyloid) in various organs and tissues of the body, compromising vital functions.
- **E85.0** Non-neuropathic heredofamilial amyloidosis [HCC] [ESR] [COM]
  - Hereditary amyloid nephropathy
  - Code also associated disorders, such as:
    - autoinflammatory syndromes (M04.-)
  - EXCLUDES 2: transthyretin-related (ATTR) familial amyloid cardiomyopathy (E85.4)
- **E85.1** Neuropathic heredofamilial amyloidosis [HCC] [ESR] [COM]
  - Amyloid polyneuropathy (Portuguese)
  - Transthyretin-related (ATTR) familial amyloid polyneuropathy
  - AHA: 2012,4Q,99
- **E85.2** Heredofamilial amyloidosis, unspecified [HCC] [ESR] [COM]
- **E85.3** Secondary systemic amyloidosis [HCC] [ESR] [COM]
  - Hemodialysis-associated amyloidosis
- **E85.4** Organ-limited amyloidosis [HCC] [ESR] [COM]
  - Localized amyloidosis
  - Transthyretin-related (ATTR) familial amyloid cardiomyopathy
- ✓5th **E85.8** Other amyloidosis
  - AHA: 2017,4Q,7
  - **E85.81** Light chain (AL) amyloidosis [HCC] [ESR] [COM]
    - AHA: 2024,2Q,9
  - **E85.82** Wild-type transthyretin-related (ATTR) amyloidosis
    - Senile systemic amyloidosis (SSA)
  - **E85.89** Other amyloidosis [HCC] [ESR] [COM]
- **E85.9** Amyloidosis, unspecified [HCC] [ESR] [COM]

✓4th E86 Volume depletion
- Use additional code(s) for any associated disorders of electrolyte and acid-base balance (E87.-)
- EXCLUDES 1:
  - dehydration of newborn (P74.1)
  - postprocedural hypovolemic shock (T81.19)
  - traumatic hypovolemic shock (T79.4)
- EXCLUDES 2: hypovolemic shock NOS (R57.1)
- AHA: 2019,2Q,7; 2018,2Q,6
- **E86.0** Dehydration
  - AHA: 2019,2Q,7; 2019,1Q,12; 2014,1Q,7
  - TIP: Can be assigned in addition to hypernatremia (E87.0) or hyponatremia (E87.1), when documented.
- **E86.1** Hypovolemia
  - Depletion of volume of plasma
- **E86.9** Volume depletion, unspecified
  - DEF: Depletion of total body water (dehydration) and/or contraction of total intravascular plasma (hypovolemia).

Chapter 4. Endocrine, Nutritional and Metabolic Diseases

E87 Other disorders of fluid, electrolyte and acid-base balance

EXCLUDES 1:
- diabetes insipidus (E23.2)
- electrolyte imbalance associated with hyperemesis gravidarum (O21.1)
- electrolyte imbalance following ectopic or molar pregnancy (O08.5)
- familial periodic paralysis (G72.3)
- metabolic acidemia in newborn, unspecified (P19.9)

AHA: 2018,2Q,6

E87.0 Hyperosmolality and hypernatremia
Sodium [Na] excess
Sodium [Na] overload

EXCLUDES 2: diabetes with hyperosmolarity (E08, E09, E11, E13 with final characters .00 or .01)

AHA: 2022,1Q,28; 2014,1Q,7

TIP: Assign an additional code for dehydration (E86.0), when documented.

E87.1 Hypo-osmolality and hyponatremia
Sodium [Na] deficiency

EXCLUDES 1: syndrome of inappropriate secretion of antidiuretic hormone (E22.2)

AHA: 2014,1Q,7

TIP: Assign an additional code for dehydration (E86.0), when documented.

E87.2 Acidosis

EXCLUDES 1: diabetic acidosis - see categories E08-E10, E11, E13 with ketoacidosis

AHA: 2022,4Q,13-14; 2020,3Q,30

DEF: Reduction of alkaline in the blood and tissues caused by an increase in acid and decrease in bicarbonate.

E87.20 Acidosis, unspecified
Lactic acidosis NOS
Metabolic acidosis NOS
Code also, if applicable, respiratory failure with hypercapnia (J96. with 5th character 2)

E87.21 Acute metabolic acidosis
Acute lactic acidosis
AHA: 2024,4Q,16

E87.22 Chronic metabolic acidosis
Chronic lactic acidosis
Code first underlying etiology, if applicable
AHA: 2022,4Q,14

E87.29 Other acidosis
Respiratory acidosis NOS
EXCLUDES 2:
- acute respiratory acidosis (J96.02)
- chronic respiratory acidosis (J96.12)

E87.3 Alkalosis
Alkalosis NOS
Metabolic alkalosis
Respiratory alkalosis

E87.4 Mixed disorder of acid-base balance

E87.5 Hyperkalemia
Potassium [K] excess
Potassium [K] overload

E87.6 Hypokalemia
Potassium [K] deficiency

E87.7 Fluid overload
EXCLUDES 1:
- edema NOS (R60.9)
- fluid retention (R60.9)

E87.70 Fluid overload, unspecified
AHA: 2023,1Q,19

E87.71 Transfusion associated circulatory overload
Fluid overload due to transfusion (blood) (blood components)
TACO

E87.79 Other fluid overload

E87.8 Other disorders of electrolyte and fluid balance, not elsewhere classified
Electrolyte imbalance NOS
Hyperchloremia
Hypochloremia

E88 Other and unspecified metabolic disorders
Use additional codes for associated conditions
EXCLUDES 1: histiocytosis X (chronic) (C96.6)

E88.0 Disorders of plasma-protein metabolism, not elsewhere classified
EXCLUDES 1:
- monoclonal gammopathy (of undetermined significance) (D47.2)
- polyclonal hypergammaglobulinemia (D89.0)
- Waldenstrom macroglobulinemia (C88.00)

EXCLUDES 2: disorder of lipoprotein metabolism (E78.-)

E88.01 Alpha-1-antitrypsin deficiency
AAT deficiency

E88.02 Plasminogen deficiency
Dysplasminogenemia
Hypoplasminogenemia
Type 1 plasminogen deficiency
Type 2 plasminogen deficiency
Code also, if applicable, ligneous conjunctivitis ▶(H10.51-)◄
Use additional code for associated findings, such as:
- hydrocephalus (G91.4)
- otitis media (H67.-)
- respiratory disorder related to plasminogen deficiency (J99)

AHA: 2018,4Q,6-7

E88.09 Other disorders of plasma-protein metabolism, not elsewhere classified
Bisalbuminemia

E88.1 Lipodystrophy, not elsewhere classified
Lipodystrophy NOS
EXCLUDES 1: Whipple's disease (K90.81)

E88.10 Lipodystrophy, unspecified
Lipodystrophy NOS

E88.11 Partial lipodystrophy
Acquired partial lipodystrophy (APL)
Barraquer-Simons lipodystrophy
Familial partial lipodystrophy (FPLD)

E88.12 Generalized lipodystrophy
Acquired generalized lipodystrophy (AGL)
Berardinelli-Siep syndrome
Congenital generalized lipodystrophy (CGL)
Lawrence syndrome

E88.13 Localized lipodystrophy
Injection lipodystrophy
Insulin lipodystrophy

E88.14 HIV-associated lipodystrophy
Code first any human immunodeficiency virus [HIV] disease (B20)
Use additional code for adverse effect, if applicable, to identify drug (T37.5X5-)

E88.19 Other lipodystrophy, not elsewhere classified

E88.2 Lipomatosis, not elsewhere classified
Lipomatosis (Check) dolorosa [Dercum]
Lipomatosis NOS
AHA: 2025,1Q,26

E88.3 Tumor lysis syndrome
Tumor lysis syndrome (spontaneous)
Tumor lysis syndrome following antineoplastic drug chemotherapy
Use additional code for adverse effect, if applicable, to identify drug (T45.1X5)
AHA: 2020,1Q,37; 2019,2Q,24

DEF: Potentially fatal metabolic complication of tumor necrosis caused by spontaneous or treatment-related accumulation of byproducts from dying cancer cells. Symptoms include hyperkalemia, hyperphosphatemia, hypocalcemia, hyperuricemia, and hyperuricosuria.

E88.4 Mitochondrial metabolism disorders
EXCLUDES 1:
- disorders of pyruvate metabolism (E74.4)
- Kearns-Sayre syndrome (H49.81)
- Leber's disease (H47.22)
- Leigh's encephalopathy (G31.82)
- mitochondrial myopathy, NEC (G71.3)
- Reye's syndrome (G93.7)

E88.40 Mitochondrial metabolism disorder, unspecified

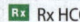

E88.41 **MELAS** syndrome
Mitochondrial myopathy, encephalopathy, lactic acidosis and stroke-like episodes

E88.42 **MERRF** syndrome
Myoclonic epilepsy associated with ragged-red fibers
Code also progressive myoclonic epilepsy (G40.3-)

E88.43 Disorders of mitochondrial tRNA synthetases
▶ARS2-related mitochondrial disorders◀
▶LBSL◀
▶Leukoencephalopathy with brainstem - spinal cord involvement - lactate elevation◀
▶Leukoencephalopathy with thalamus - brainstem involvement - high lactate◀
▶LTBL◀
▶Mitochondrial aminoacyl-tRNA synthetase disorders◀
▶Code also, if applicable, associated condition such as:◀
▶leukoencephalopathy (G93.49)◀
AHA: 2023,4Q,12-13

E88.49 Other mitochondrial metabolism disorders

✓5ᵗʰ **E88.8** Other specified metabolic disorders

✓6ᵗʰ **E88.81** Metabolic syndrome and other insulin resistance
Use additional codes for associated manifestations, such as:
obesity (E66.-)
AHA: 2023,4Q,13-14; 2022,3Q,6
DEF: Group of health risks that increase the likelihood of developing heart disease, stroke, and diabetes. These risks include certain parameters for blood pressure, cholesterol, and glucose levels.

E88.810 Metabolic syndrome
Dysmetabolic syndrome

E88.811 Insulin resistance syndrome, Type A

E88.818 Other insulin resistance
Insulin resistance syndrome, Type B

E88.819 Insulin resistance, unspecified

E88.82 Obesity due to disruption of MC4R pathway
Use additional code to identify body mass index (BMI), if known (Z68.-)
Use additional code, if applicable, to identify associated manifestations, such as polyphagia (R63.2)
AHA: 2024,4Q,10-11
TIP: Assign an additional code for the specific class of obesity (E66.811-E66.813), when documented.

E88.89 Other specified metabolic disorders
Launois-Bensaude adenolipomatosis
EXCLUDES 1 adult pulmonary Langerhans cell histiocytosis (J84.82)

E88.9 Metabolic disorder, unspecified

E88.A Wasting disease (syndrome) due to underlying condition
Cachexia due to underlying condition
Code first underlying condition
EXCLUDES 1 cachexia NOS (R64)
nutritional marasmus (E41)
EXCLUDES 2 failure to thrive (R62.51, R62.7)
AHA: 2023,4Q,14-15

Postprocedural endocrine and metabolic complications and disorders, not elsewhere classified (E89)

✓4ᵗʰ **E89** Postprocedural endocrine and metabolic complications and disorders, not elsewhere classified
EXCLUDES 2 intraoperative complications of endocrine system organ or structure (E36.0-, E36.1-, E36.8)

E89.0 Postprocedural hypothyroidism
Postirradiation hypothyroidism
Postsurgical hypothyroidism

E89.1 Postprocedural hypoinsulinemia
Postpancreatectomy hyperglycemia
Postsurgical hypoinsulinemia
Code first, if applicable, diabetes mellitus (postpancreatectomy) (postprocedural) (E13.-)
Use additional code, if applicable, to identify:
acquired absence of pancreas (Z90.41-)
insulin use (Z79.4)
EXCLUDES 1 transient postprocedural hyperglycemia (R73.9)
transient postprocedural hypoglycemia (E16.2)

E89.2 Postprocedural hypoparathyroidism
Parathyroprival tetany
AHA: 2023,3Q,13

E89.3 Postprocedural hypopituitarism
Postirradiation hypopituitarism

✓5ᵗʰ **E89.4** Postprocedural ovarian failure

E89.40 Asymptomatic postprocedural ovarian failure
Postprocedural ovarian failure NOS

E89.41 Symptomatic postprocedural ovarian failure
Symptoms such as flushing, sleeplessness, headache, lack of concentration, associated with postprocedural menopause

E89.5 Postprocedural testicular hypofunction

E89.6 Postprocedural adrenocortical (-medullary) hypofunction

✓5ᵗʰ **E89.8** Other postprocedural endocrine and metabolic complications and disorders
AHA: 2016,4Q,9-10

✓6ᵗʰ **E89.81** Postprocedural hemorrhage of an endocrine system organ or structure following a procedure

E89.810 Postprocedural hemorrhage of an endocrine system organ or structure following an endocrine system procedure

E89.811 Postprocedural hemorrhage of an endocrine system organ or structure following other procedure

✓6ᵗʰ **E89.82** Postprocedural hematoma and seroma of an endocrine system organ or structure

E89.820 Postprocedural hematoma of an endocrine system organ or structure following an endocrine system procedure

E89.821 Postprocedural hematoma of an endocrine system organ or structure following other procedure

E89.822 Postprocedural seroma of an endocrine system organ or structure following an endocrine system procedure

E89.823 Postprocedural seroma of an endocrine system organ or structure following other procedure

E89.89 Other postprocedural endocrine and metabolic complications and disorders
Use additional code, if applicable, to further specify disorder

Chapter 5. Mental, Behavioral and Neurodevelopmental Disorders (F01–F99)

Chapter-specific Guidelines with Coding Examples

The chapter-specific guidelines from the ICD-10-CM Official Guidelines for Coding and Reporting have been provided below. Along with these guidelines are coding examples, contained in the shaded boxes, that have been developed to help illustrate the coding and/or sequencing guidance found in these guidelines.

a. Pain disorders related to psychological factors

Assign code F45.41, for pain that is exclusively related to psychological disorders. As indicated by the Excludes 1 note under category G89, a code from category G89 should not be assigned with code F45.41.

> Chest pain determined to be persistent somatoform pain disorder
>
> **F45.41   Pain disorder exclusively related to psychological factors**
>
> *Explanation*: This pain was diagnosed as being exclusively psychological; therefore, no code from category G89 is added.

Code F45.42, Pain disorders with related psychological factors, should be used with a code from category G89, Pain, not elsewhere classified, if there is documentation of a psychological component for a patient with acute or chronic pain.
See Section I.C.6. Pain

b. Mental and behavioral disorders due to psychoactive substance use

1) In remission

Selection of codes describing "in remission" for categories F10-F19, Mental and behavioral disorders due to psychoactive substance use (categories F10-F19 with -.11, -.21, -.91) requires the provider's clinical judgment and are assigned only on the basis of provider documentation (as defined in the Official Guidelines for Coding and Reporting), unless otherwise instructed by the classification.

Mild substance use disorders in early or sustained remission are classified to the appropriate codes for substance abuse in remission, and moderate or severe substance use disorders in early or sustained remission are classified to the appropriate codes for substance dependence in remission.

> Physician documentation indicates the patient is seen to monitor progress on quitting cigarette smoking. The problem list indicates mild tobacco use disorder that is currently in remission.
>
> **F17.211   Nicotine dependence, cigarettes, in remission**
>
> *Explanation*: According to the index, Disorder, tobacco use, cigarettes (mild) (moderate) (severe), in remission (early) (sustained) is categorized to dependence (F17.211). Since the physician clearly documents mild cigarette use "disorder" and that the disorder is in remission, a code for nicotine dependence "in remission" is appropriate.

2) Psychoactive substance use, abuse and dependence

When the provider documentation refers to use, abuse and dependence of the same substance (e.g. alcohol, opioid, cannabis, etc.), only one code should be assigned to identify the pattern of use based on the following hierarchy:

- If both use and abuse are documented, assign only the code for abuse
- If both abuse and dependence are documented, assign only the code for dependence
- If use, abuse and dependence are all documented, assign only the code for dependence
- If both use and dependence are documented, assign only the code for dependence.

> History and physical notes cannabis dependence and ongoing cannabis abuse
>
> **F12.20   Cannabis dependence, uncomplicated**
>
> *Explanation*: In the hierarchy, the dependence code is used if both abuse and dependence are documented.

> Current problem list indicates daily opioid use with opioid abuse.
>
> **F11.10   Opioid abuse, uncomplicated**
>
> *Explanation*: In the hierarchy, the abuse code is used if both abuse and use are documented.

3) Psychoactive substance use, unspecified

As with all other unspecified diagnoses, the codes for unspecified psychoactive substance use (F10.9-, F11.9-, F12.9-, F13.9-, F14.9-, F15.9-, F16.9-, F18.9-, F19.9-) should only be assigned based on provider documentation and when they meet the definition of a reportable diagnosis (see Section III, Reporting Additional Diagnoses). These codes are to be used only when the psychoactive substance use is associated with a substance related disorder (chapter 5 disorders such as sexual dysfunction, sleep disorder, or a mental or behavioral disorder) or medical condition, and such a relationship is documented by the provider.

4) Medical conditions due to psychoactive substance use, abuse and dependence

Medical conditions due to substance use, abuse, and dependence are not classified as substance-induced disorders. Assign the diagnosis code for the medical condition as directed by the Alphabetical Index along with the appropriate psychoactive substance use, abuse or dependence code. For example, for alcoholic pancreatitis due to alcohol dependence, assign the appropriate code from subcategory K85.2, Alcohol induced acute pancreatitis, and the appropriate code from subcategory F10.2, such as code F10.20, Alcohol dependence, uncomplicated. It would not be appropriate to assign code F10.288, Alcohol dependence with other alcohol-induced disorder.

5) Blood alcohol level

A code from category Y90, Evidence of alcohol involvement determined by blood alcohol level, may be assigned when this information is documented and the patient's provider has documented a condition classifiable to category F10, Alcohol related disorders. The blood alcohol level does not need to be documented by the patient's provider in order for it to be coded.
See Section I.B.14. for blood alcohol level documentation by clinicians other than patient's provider.

c. Factitious disorder

Factitious disorder imposed on self or Munchausen's syndrome is a disorder in which a person falsely reports or causes his or her own physical or psychological signs or symptoms. For patients with documented factitious disorder on self or Munchausen's syndrome, assign the appropriate code from subcategory F68.1-, Factitious disorder imposed on self.

Munchausen's syndrome by proxy (MSBP) is a disorder in which a caregiver (perpetrator) falsely reports or causes an illness or injury in another person (victim) under his or her care, such as a child, an elderly adult, or a person who has a disability. The condition is also referred to as "factitious disorder imposed on another" or "factitious disorder by proxy." The perpetrator, not the victim, receives this diagnosis. Assign code F68.A, Factitious disorder imposed on another, to the perpetrator's record. For the victim of a patient suffering from MSBP, assign the appropriate code from categories T74, Adult and child abuse, neglect and other maltreatment, confirmed, or T76, Adult and child abuse, neglect and other maltreatment, suspected.
See Section I.C.19.f. Adult and child abuse, neglect and other maltreatment

d. Dementia

The ICD-10-CM classifies dementia (categories F01, F02, and F03) on the basis of the etiology and severity (unspecified, mild, moderate or severe). Selection of the appropriate severity level requires the provider's clinical judgment and codes should be assigned only on the basis of provider documentation (as defined in the Official Guidelines for Coding and Reporting), unless otherwise instructed by the classification. If the documentation does not provide information about the severity of the dementia, assign the appropriate code for unspecified severity.

If a patient is admitted to an inpatient acute care hospital or other inpatient facility setting with dementia at one severity level and it progresses to a higher severity level, assign one code for the highest severity level reported during the stay.

Chapter 5. Mental, Behavioral and Neurodevelopmental Disorders (F01-F99)

INCLUDES disorders of psychological development

EXCLUDES 2 symptoms, signs and abnormal clinical laboratory findings, not elsewhere classified (R00-R99)

This chapter contains the following blocks:
- F01-F09 Mental disorders due to known physiological conditions
- F10-F19 Mental and behavioral disorders due to psychoactive substance use
- F20-F29 Schizophrenia, schizotypal, delusional, and other non-mood psychotic disorders
- F30-F39 Mood [affective] disorders
- F40-F48 Anxiety, dissociative, stress-related, somatoform and other nonpsychotic mental disorders
- F50-F59 Behavioral syndromes associated with physiological disturbances and physical factors
- F60-F69 Disorders of adult personality and behavior
- F70-F79 Intellectual disabilities
- F80-F89 Pervasive and specific developmental disorders
- F90-F98 Behavioral and emotional disorders with onset usually occurring in childhood and adolescence
- F99 Unspecified mental disorder

Mental disorders due to known physiological conditions (F01-F09)

NOTE This block comprises a range of mental disorders grouped together on the basis of their having in common a demonstrable etiology in cerebral disease, brain injury, or other insult leading to cerebral dysfunction. The dysfunction may be primary, as in diseases, injuries, and insults that affect the brain directly and selectively; or secondary, as in systemic diseases and disorders that attack the brain only as one of the multiple organs or systems of the body that are involved.

✓4th F01 Vascular dementia

Vascular dementia as a result of infarction of the brain due to vascular disease, including hypertensive cerebrovascular disease.

INCLUDES arteriosclerotic dementia
major neurocognitive disorder due to vascular disease
multi-infarct dementia

Code first, if applicable, any causal condition
AHA: 2022,4Q,14-15

- ✓5th **F01.5** Vascular dementia, unspecified severity
  - **F01.50** Vascular dementia, unspecified severity, without behavioral disturbance, psychotic disturbance, mood disturbance, and anxiety HCC Rx ESR A
    Major neurocognitive disorder due to vascular disease NOS
    Vascular dementia NOS
    AHA: 2021,2Q,4
  - ✓6th **F01.51** Vascular dementia, unspecified severity, with behavioral disturbance
    - **F01.511** Vascular dementia, unspecified severity, with agitation HCC Rx ESR UPD A
      Major neurocognitive disorder due to vascular disease, unspecified severity, with aberrant motor behavior such as restlessness, rocking, pacing, or exit-seeking
      Major neurocognitive disorder due to vascular disease, unspecified severity, with verbal or physical behaviors such as profanity, shouting, threatening, anger, aggression, combativeness, or violence
      Vascular dementia, unspecified severity, with aberrant motor behavior such as restlessness, rocking, pacing, or exit-seeking
      Vascular dementia, unspecified severity, with verbal or physical behaviors such as profanity, shouting, threatening, anger, aggression, combativeness, or violence
    - **F01.518** Vascular dementia, unspecified severity, with other behavioral disturbance HCC Rx ESR UPD A
      Major neurocognitive disorder due to vascular disease, unspecified severity, with behavioral disturbances such as sleep disturbance, social disinhibition, or sexual disinhibition
      Vascular dementia, unspecified severity, with behavioral disturbances such as sleep disturbance, social disinhibition, or sexual disinhibition
      Use additional code, if applicable, to identify wandering in vascular dementia (Z91.83)
  - **F01.52** Vascular dementia, unspecified severity, with psychotic disturbance HCC Rx ESR UPD A
    Major neurocognitive disorder due to vascular disease, unspecified severity, with psychotic disturbance such as hallucinations, paranoia, suspiciousness, or delusional state
    Vascular dementia, unspecified severity, with psychotic disturbance such as hallucinations, paranoia, suspiciousness, or delusional state
  - **F01.53** Vascular dementia, unspecified severity, with mood disturbance HCC Rx ESR UPD A
    Major neurocognitive disorder due to vascular disease, unspecified severity, with mood disturbance such as depression, apathy, or anhedonia
    Vascular dementia, unspecified severity, with mood disturbance such as depression, apathy, or anhedonia
  - **F01.54** Vascular dementia, unspecified severity, with anxiety HCC Rx ESR UPD A
    Major neurocognitive disorder due to vascular disease, unspecified severity, with anxiety
- ✓5th **F01.A** Vascular dementia, mild
  EXCLUDES 1 mild neurocognitive disorder due to known physiological condition with or without behavioral disturbance (F06.7-)
  - **F01.A0** Vascular dementia, mild, without behavioral disturbance, psychotic disturbance, mood disturbance, and anxiety HCC Rx ESR UPD A
    Major neurocognitive disorder due to vascular disease, mild, NOS
    Vascular dementia, mild, NOS
  - ✓6th **F01.A1** Vascular dementia, mild, with behavioral disturbance
    - **F01.A11** Vascular dementia, mild, with agitation HCC Rx ESR UPD A
      Major neurocognitive disorder due to vascular disease, mild, with aberrant motor behavior such as restlessness, rocking, pacing, or exit-seeking
      Major neurocognitive disorder due to vascular disease, mild, with verbal or physical behaviors such as profanity, shouting, threatening, anger, aggression, combativeness, or violence
      Vascular dementia, mild, with aberrant motor behavior such as restlessness, rocking, pacing, or exit-seeking
      Vascular dementia, mild, with verbal or physical behaviors such as profanity, shouting, threatening, anger, aggression, combativeness, or violence
    - **F01.A18** Vascular dementia, mild, with other behavioral disturbance HCC Rx ESR UPD A
      Major neurocognitive disorder due to vascular disease, mild, with behavioral disturbances such as sleep disturbance, social disinhibition, or sexual disinhibition
      Vascular dementia, mild, with behavioral disturbances such as sleep disturbance, social disinhibition, or sexual disinhibition
      Use additional code, if applicable, to identify wandering in vascular dementia (Z91.83)

F01.A2 **Vascular dementia, mild, with psychotic disturbance** `HCC` `Rx` `ESR` `UPD` `A`
Major neurocognitive disorder due to vascular disease, mild, with psychotic disturbance such as hallucinations, paranoia, suspiciousness, or delusional state
Vascular dementia, mild, with psychotic disturbance such as hallucinations, paranoia, suspiciousness, or delusional state

F01.A3 **Vascular dementia, mild, with mood disturbance** `HCC` `Rx` `ESR` `UPD` `A`
Major neurocognitive disorder due to vascular disease, mild, with mood disturbance such as depression, apathy, or anhedonia
Vascular dementia, mild, with mood disturbance such as depression, apathy, or anhedonia

F01.A4 **Vascular dementia, mild, with anxiety** `HCC` `Rx` `ESR` `UPD` `A`
Major neurocognitive disorder due to vascular disease, mild, with anxiety

✓5th **F01.B** **Vascular dementia, moderate**

F01.B0 **Vascular dementia, moderate, without behavioral disturbance, psychotic disturbance, mood disturbance, and anxiety** `HCC` `Rx` `ESR` `UPD` `A`
Major neurocognitive disorder due to vascular disease, moderate, NOS
Vascular dementia, moderate, NOS

✓6th **F01.B1** **Vascular dementia, moderate, with behavioral disturbance**

F01.B11 **Vascular dementia, moderate, with agitation** `HCC` `Rx` `ESR` `UPD` `A`
Major neurocognitive disorder due to vascular disease, moderate, with aberrant motor behavior such as restlessness, rocking, pacing, or exit-seeking
Major neurocognitive disorder due to vascular disease, moderate, with verbal or physical behaviors such as profanity, shouting, threatening, anger, aggression, combativeness, or violence
Vascular dementia, moderate, with aberrant motor behavior such as restlessness, rocking, pacing, or exit-seeking
Vascular dementia, moderate, with verbal or physical behaviors such as profanity, shouting, threatening, anger, aggression, combativeness, or violence

F01.B18 **Vascular dementia, moderate, with other behavioral disturbance** `HCC` `Rx` `ESR` `UPD` `A`
Major neurocognitive disorder due to vascular disease, moderate, with behavioral disturbances such as sleep disturbance, social disinhibition, or sexual disinhibition
Vascular dementia, moderate, with behavioral disturbances such as sleep disturbance, social disinhibition, or sexual disinhibition
Use additional code, if applicable, to identify wandering in vascular dementia (Z91.83)

F01.B2 **Vascular dementia, moderate, with psychotic disturbance** `HCC` `Rx` `ESR` `UPD` `A`
Major neurocognitive disorder due to vascular disease, moderate, with psychotic disturbance such as hallucinations, paranoia, suspiciousness, or delusional state
Vascular dementia, moderate, with psychotic disturbance such as hallucinations, paranoia, suspiciousness, or delusional state

F01.B3 **Vascular dementia, moderate, with mood disturbance** `HCC` `Rx` `ESR` `UPD` `A`
Major neurocognitive disorder due to vascular disease, moderate, with mood disturbance such as depression, apathy, or anhedonia
Vascular dementia, moderate, with mood disturbance such as depression, apathy, or anhedonia

F01.B4 **Vascular dementia, moderate, with anxiety** `HCC` `Rx` `ESR` `UPD` `A`
Major neurocognitive disorder due to vascular disease, moderate, with anxiety

✓5th **F01.C** **Vascular dementia, severe**

F01.C0 **Vascular dementia, severe, without behavioral disturbance, psychotic disturbance, mood disturbance, and anxiety** `HCC` `Rx` `ESR` `UPD` `A`
Major neurocognitive disorder due to vascular disease, severe, NOS
Vascular dementia, severe, NOS

✓6th **F01.C1** **Vascular dementia, severe, with behavioral disturbance**

F01.C11 **Vascular dementia, severe, with agitation** `HCC` `Rx` `ESR` `UPD` `A`
Major neurocognitive disorder due to vascular disease, severe, with aberrant motor behavior such as restlessness, rocking, pacing, or exit-seeking
Major neurocognitive disorder due to vascular disease, severe, with verbal or physical behaviors such as profanity, shouting, threatening, anger, aggression, combativeness, or violence
Vascular dementia, severe, with aberrant motor behavior such as restlessness, rocking, pacing, or exit-seeking
Vascular dementia, severe, with verbal or physical behaviors such as profanity, shouting, threatening, anger, aggression, combativeness, or violence

F01.C18 **Vascular dementia, severe, with other behavioral disturbance** `HCC` `Rx` `ESR` `UPD` `A`
Major neurocognitive disorder due to vascular disease, severe, with behavioral disturbances such as sleep disturbance, social disinhibition, or sexual disinhibition
Vascular dementia, severe, with behavioral disturbances such as sleep disturbance, social disinhibition, or sexual disinhibition
Use additional code, if applicable, to identify wandering in vascular dementia (Z91.83)

F01.C2 **Vascular dementia, severe, with psychotic disturbance** `HCC` `Rx` `ESR` `UPD` `A`
Major neurocognitive disorder due to vascular disease, severe, with psychotic disturbance such as hallucinations, paranoia, suspiciousness, or delusional state
Vascular dementia, severe, with psychotic disturbance such as hallucinations, paranoia, suspiciousness, or delusional state

F01.C3 **Vascular dementia, severe, with mood disturbance** `HCC` `Rx` `ESR` `UPD` `A`
Major neurocognitive disorder due to vascular disease, severe, with mood disturbance such as depression, apathy, or anhedonia
Vascular dementia, severe, with mood disturbance such as depression, apathy, or anhedonia

F01.C4 **Vascular dementia, severe, with anxiety** `HCC` `Rx` `ESR` `UPD` `A`
Major neurocognitive disorder due to vascular disease, severe, with anxiety

F02 Dementia in other diseases classified elsewhere

INCLUDES major neurocognitive disorder in other diseases classified elsewhere

Code first the underlying physiological condition, such as:
- Alzheimer's (G30.-)
- cerebral lipidosis (E75.4)
- Creutzfeldt-Jakob disease (A81.0-)
- epilepsy and recurrent seizures (G40.-)
- frontotemporal dementia (G31.09)
- hepatolenticular degeneration (E83.01)
- human immunodeficiency virus [HIV] disease (B20)
- Huntington's disease (G10)
- hypercalcemia (E83.52)
- hypothyroidism, acquired (E00-E03.-)
- intoxications (T36-T65)
- Jakob-Creutzfeldt disease (A81.0-)
- multiple sclerosis ▶(G35-)◀
- neurocognitive disorder with Lewy bodies (G31.83)
- neurosyphilis (A52.17)
- niacin deficiency [pellagra] (E52)
- other frontotemporal neurocognitive disorder (G31.90)
- Parkinson's disease (G20.-)
- Pick's disease (G31.01)
- polyarteritis nodosa (M30.0)
- prion disease (A81.9)
- systemic lupus erythematosus (M32.-)
- traumatic brain injury (S06.-)
- trypanosomiasis (B56.-, B57.-)
- vitamin B deficiency (E53.8)

EXCLUDES 1 mild neurocognitive disorder due to known physiological condition with or without behavioral disturbance (F06.7-)

EXCLUDES 2 dementia in alcohol and psychoactive substance disorders (F10-F19, with .17, .27, .97)
vascular dementia (F01.5-, F01.A-, F01.B-, F01.C-)

AHA: 2022,4Q,14-15

F02.8 Dementia in other diseases classified elsewhere, unspecified severity

AHA: 2024,2Q,8; 2022,4Q,15; 2022,1Q,25; 2017,2Q,7; 2016,4Q,141; 2016,2Q,6

F02.80 Dementia in other diseases classified elsewhere, unspecified severity, *without* behavioral disturbance, psychotic disturbance, mood disturbance, and anxiety
Dementia in other diseases classified elsewhere NOS
Major neurocognitive disorder in other diseases classified elsewhere NOS

F02.81 Dementia in other diseases classified elsewhere, unspecified severity, with behavioral disturbance

F02.811 Dementia in other diseases classified elsewhere, unspecified severity, *with agitation*
Dementia in other diseases classified elsewhere, unspecified severity, with aberrant motor behavior such as restlessness, rocking, pacing, or exit-seeking
Dementia in other diseases classified elsewhere, unspecified severity, with verbal or physical behaviors such as profanity, shouting, threatening, anger, aggression, combativeness, or violence
Major neurocognitive disorder in other diseases classified elsewhere, unspecified severity, with aberrant motor behavior such as restlessness, rocking, pacing, or exit-seeking
Major neurocognitive disorder in other diseases classified elsewhere, unspecified severity, with verbal or physical behaviors such as profanity, shouting, threatening, anger, aggression, combativeness, or violence

F02.818 Dementia in other diseases classified elsewhere, unspecified severity, *with other behavioral disturbance*
Dementia in other diseases classified elsewhere with sleep disturbance, social disinhibition, or sexual disinhibition
Major neurocognitive disorder in other diseases classified elsewhere with sleep disturbance, social disinhibition, or sexual disinhibition
Use additional code, if applicable, to identify wandering in dementia in conditions classified elsewhere (Z91.83)

F02.82 Dementia in other diseases classified elsewhere, unspecified severity, *with psychotic disturbance*
Dementia in other diseases classified elsewhere, unspecified severity, with psychotic disturbance such as hallucinations, paranoia, suspiciousness, or delusional state
Major neurocognitive disorder in other diseases classified elsewhere, unspecified, with psychotic disturbance such as hallucinations, paranoia, suspiciousness, or delusional state

F02.83 Dementia in other diseases classified elsewhere, unspecified severity, *with mood disturbance*
Dementia in other diseases classified elsewhere, unspecified severity, with mood disturbance such as depression, apathy, or anhedonia
Major neurocognitive disorder in other diseases classified elsewhere unspecified severity,with mood disturbance such as with depression, apathy, or anhedonia

F02.84 Dementia in other diseases classified elsewhere, unspecified severity, *with anxiety*
Major neurocognitive disorder in other diseases classified elsewhere unspecified severity, with anxiety

F02.A Dementia in other diseases classified elsewhere, *mild*

EXCLUDES 1 mild neurocognitive disorder due to known physiological condition with or without behavioral disturbance (F06.7-)

F02.A0 Dementia in other diseases classified elsewhere, mild, *without* behavioral disturbance, psychotic disturbance, mood disturbance, and anxiety
Dementia in other diseases classified elsewhere, mild, NOS
Major neurocognitive disorder in other diseases classified elsewhere, mild, NOS

F02.A1 Dementia in other diseases classified elsewhere, mild, with behavioral disturbance

F02.A11 Dementia in other diseases classified elsewhere, mild, *with agitation*
Dementia in other diseases classified elsewhere, mild, with aberrant motor behavior such as restlessness, rocking, pacing, or exit-seeking
Dementia in other diseases classified elsewhere, mild, with verbal or physical behaviors such as profanity, shouting, threatening, anger, aggression, combativeness, or violence
Major neurocognitive disorder in other diseases classified elsewhere, mild, with aberrant motor behavior such as restlessness, rocking, pacing, or exit-seeking
Major neurocognitive disorder in other diseases classified elsewhere, mild, with verbal or physical behaviors such as profanity, shouting, threatening, anger, aggression, combativeness, or violence

F02.A18 Dementia in other diseases classified elsewhere, mild, with other behavioral disturbance [HCC] [Rx] [ESR] [UPD]

Dementia in other diseases classified elsewhere, mild, with behavioral disturbances such as sleep disturbance, social disinhibition, or sexual disinhibition

Major neurocognitive disorder in other diseases classified elsewhere, mild, with behavioral disturbances such as sleep disturbance, social disinhibition, or sexual disinhibition

Use additional code, if applicable, to identify wandering in dementia in conditions classified elsewhere (Z91.83)

F02.A2 Dementia in other diseases classified elsewhere, mild, with psychotic disturbance [HCC] [Rx] [ESR] [UPD]

Dementia in other diseases classified elsewhere, mild, with psychotic disturbance such as hallucinations, paranoia, suspiciousness, or delusional state

Major neurocognitive disorder in other diseases classified elsewhere, mild, with psychotic disturbance such as hallucinations, paranoia, suspiciousness, or delusional state

F02.A3 Dementia in other diseases classified elsewhere, mild, with mood disturbance [HCC] [Rx] [ESR] [UPD]

Dementia in other diseases classified elsewhere, mild, with mood disturbance such as depression, apathy, or anhedonia

Major neurocognitive disorder in other diseases classified elsewhere, mild, with mood disturbance such as depression, apathy, or anhedonia

F02.A4 Dementia in other diseases classified elsewhere, mild, with anxiety [HCC] [Rx] [ESR] [UPD]

Major neurocognitive disorder in other diseases classified elsewhere, mild, with anxiety

✓5th F02.B Dementia in other diseases classified elsewhere, moderate

F02.B0 Dementia in other diseases classified elsewhere, moderate, without behavioral disturbance, psychotic disturbance, mood disturbance, and anxiety [HCC] [Rx] [ESR] [UPD]

Dementia in other diseases classified elsewhere, moderate, NOS

Major neurocognitive disorder in other diseases classified elsewhere, moderate, NOS

✓6th F02.B1 Dementia in other diseases classified elsewhere, moderate, with behavioral disturbance

F02.B11 Dementia in other diseases classified elsewhere, moderate, with agitation [HCC] [Rx] [ESR] [UPD]

Dementia in other diseases classified elsewhere, moderate, with aberrant motor behavior such as restlessness, rocking, pacing, or exit-seeking

Dementia in other diseases classified elsewhere, moderate, with verbal or physical behaviors such as profanity, shouting, threatening, anger, aggression, combativeness, or violence

Major neurocognitive disorder in other diseases classified elsewhere, moderate, with aberrant motor behavior such as restlessness, rocking, pacing, or exit-seeking

Major neurocognitive disorder in other diseases classified elsewhere, moderate, with verbal or physical behaviors such as profanity, shouting, threatening, anger, aggression, combativeness, or violence

F02.B18 Dementia in other diseases classified elsewhere, moderate, with other behavioral disturbance [HCC] [Rx] [ESR] [UPD]

Dementia in other diseases classified elsewhere, moderate, with behavioral disturbances such as sleep disturbance, social disinhibition, or sexual disinhibition

Major neurocognitive disorder in other diseases classified elsewhere, moderate, with behavioral disturbance such as sleep disturbance, social disinhibition, or sexual disinhibition

Use additional code, if applicable, to identify wandering in dementia in conditions classified elsewhere (Z91.83)

F02.B2 Dementia in other diseases classified elsewhere, moderate, with psychotic disturbance [HCC] [Rx] [ESR] [UPD]

Dementia in other diseases classified elsewhere, moderate, with psychotic disturbance such as hallucinations, paranoia, suspiciousness, or delusional state

Major neurocognitive disorder in other diseases classified elsewhere, moderate, with psychotic disturbance such as hallucinations, paranoia, suspiciousness, or delusional state

F02.B3 Dementia in other diseases classified elsewhere, moderate, with mood disturbance [HCC] [Rx] [ESR] [UPD]

Dementia in other diseases classified elsewhere, moderate, with mood disturbance such as depression, apathy, or anhedonia

Major neurocognitive disorder in other diseases classified elsewhere, moderate, with mood disturbance such as depression, apathy, or anhedonia

F02.B4 Dementia in other diseases classified elsewhere, moderate, with anxiety [HCC] [Rx] [ESR] [UPD]

Major neurocognitive disorder in other diseases classified elsewhere, moderate, with anxiety

✓5th F02.C Dementia in other diseases classified elsewhere, severe

F02.C0 Dementia in other diseases classified elsewhere, severe, without behavioral disturbance, psychotic disturbance, mood disturbance, and anxiety [HCC] [Rx] [ESR] [UPD]

Dementia in other diseases classified elsewhere, severe, NOS

Major neurocognitive disorder in other diseases classified elsewhere, severe, NOS

✓6th F02.C1 Dementia in other diseases classified elsewhere, severe, with behavioral disturbance

F02.C11 Dementia in other diseases classified elsewhere, severe, with agitation [HCC] [Rx] [ESR] [UPD]

Dementia in other diseases classified elsewhere, severe, with aberrant motor behavior such as restlessness, rocking, pacing, or exit-seeking

Dementia in other diseases classified elsewhere, severe, with verbal or physical behaviors such as profanity, shouting, threatening, anger, aggression, combativeness, or violence

Major neurocognitive disorder in other diseases classified elsewhere, severe, with aberrant motor behavior such as restlessness, rocking, pacing, or exit-seeking

Major neurocognitive disorder in other diseases classified elsewhere, severe, with verbal or physical behaviors such as profanity, shouting, threatening, anger, aggression, combativeness, or violence

F02.C18 *Dementia in other diseases classified elsewhere, severe, with other behavioral disturbance* `HCC` `Rx` `ESR` `UPD`

Dementia in other diseases classified elsewhere, severe, with behavioral disturbances such as sleep disturbance, social disinhibition, or sexual disinhibition

Major neurocognitive disorder in other diseases classified elsewhere, severe, with behavioral disturbances such as sleep disturbance, social disinhibition, or sexual disinhibition

Use additional code, if applicable, to identify wandering in dementia in conditions classified elsewhere (Z91.83)

F02.C2 *Dementia in other diseases classified elsewhere, severe, with psychotic disturbance* `HCC` `Rx` `ESR` `UPD`

Dementia in other diseases classified elsewhere, severe, with psychotic disturbance such as hallucinations, paranoia, suspiciousness, or delusional state

Major neurocognitive disorder in other diseases classified elsewhere, severe, with psychotic disturbance such as hallucinations, paranoia, suspiciousness, or delusional state

F02.C3 *Dementia in other diseases classified elsewhere, severe, with mood disturbance* `HCC` `Rx` `ESR` `UPD`

Dementia in other diseases classified elsewhere, severe, with mood disturbance such as depression, apathy, or anhedonia

Major neurocognitive disorder in other diseases classified elsewhere, severe, with mood disturbance such as depression, apathy, or anhedonia

F02.C4 *Dementia in other diseases classified elsewhere, severe, with anxiety* `HCC` `Rx` `ESR` `UPD`

Major neurocognitive disorder in other diseases classified elsewhere, severe, with anxiety

✓4th **F03** **Unspecified dementia**

Major neurocognitive disorder NOS
Presenile dementia NOS
Presenile psychosis NOS
Primary degenerative dementia NOS
Senile dementia depressed or paranoid type
Senile dementia NOS
Senile psychosis NOS

EXCLUDES 2 dementia with delirium or acute confusional state (F05)
mild memory disturbance due to known physiological condition (F06.8)

AHA: 2022,4Q,14-15

✓5th **F03.9** **Unspecified dementia, unspecified severity**

F03.90 Unspecified dementia, unspecified severity, without behavioral disturbance, psychotic disturbance, mood disturbance, and anxiety `HCC` `Rx` `ESR` `UPD` `A`
Dementia NOS
AHA: 2024,2Q,8; 2021,2Q,4; 2012,4Q,92

✓6th **F03.91** Unspecified dementia, unspecified severity, with behavioral disturbance

F03.911 Unspecified dementia, unspecified severity, with agitation `HCC` `Rx` `ESR` `UPD` `A`
Unspecified dementia, unspecified severity, with aberrant motor behavior such as restlessness, rocking, pacing, or exit-seeking
Unspecified dementia, unspecified severity, with verbal or physical behaviors such as profanity, shouting, threatening, anger, aggression, combativeness, or violence

F03.918 Unspecified dementia, unspecified severity, with other behavioral disturbance `HCC` `Rx` `ESR` `UPD` `A`
Unspecified dementia, unspecified severity, with behavioral disturbances such as sleep disturbance, social disinhibition, or sexual disinhibition
Use additional code, if applicable, to identify wandering in unspecified dementia (Z91.83)

F03.92 Unspecified dementia, unspecified severity, with psychotic disturbance `HCC` `Rx` `ESR` `UPD` `A`
Unspecified dementia, unspecified severity, with psychotic disturbance such as hallucinations, paranoia, suspiciousness, or delusional state

F03.93 Unspecified dementia, unspecified severity, with mood disturbance `HCC` `Rx` `ESR` `UPD` `A`
Unspecified dementia, unspecified severity, with mood disturbance such as depression, apathy, or anhedonia

F03.94 Unspecified dementia, unspecified severity, with anxiety

✓5th **F03.A** Unspecified dementia, mild

EXCLUDES 1 mild neurocognitive disorder due to known physiological condition with or without behavioral disturbance (F06.7-)

F03.A0 Unspecified dementia, mild, without behavioral disturbance, psychotic disturbance, mood disturbance, and anxiety `HCC` `Rx` `ESR` `UPD` `A`
Dementia, mild, NOS

✓6th **F03.A1** Unspecified dementia, mild, with behavioral disturbance

F03.A11 Unspecified dementia, mild, with agitation `HCC` `Rx` `ESR` `UPD` `A`
Unspecified dementia, mild, with aberrant motor behavior such as restlessness, rocking, pacing, or exit-seeking
Unspecified dementia, mild, with verbal or physical behaviors such as profanity, shouting, threatening, anger, aggression, combativeness, or violence

F03.A18 Unspecified dementia, mild, with other behavioral disturbance `HCC` `Rx` `ESR` `UPD` `A`
Unspecified dementia, mild, with behavioral disturbances such as sleep disturbance, social disinhibition, or sexual disinhibition
Use additional code, if applicable, to identify wandering in unspecified dementia (Z91.83)

F03.A2 Unspecified dementia, mild, with psychotic disturbance `HCC` `Rx` `ESR` `UPD` `A`
Unspecified dementia, mild, with psychotic disturbance such as hallucinations, paranoia, suspiciousness, or delusional state

F03.A3 Unspecified dementia, mild, with mood disturbance `HCC` `Rx` `ESR` `UPD` `A`
Unspecified dementia, mild, with mood disturbance such as depression, apathy, or anhedonia

F03.A4 Unspecified dementia, mild, with anxiety

✓5th **F03.B** Unspecified dementia, moderate

F03.B0 Unspecified dementia, moderate, without behavioral disturbance, psychotic disturbance, mood disturbance, and anxiety `HCC` `Rx` `ESR` `UPD` `A`
Dementia, moderate, NOS

✓6th **F03.B1** Unspecified dementia, moderate, with behavioral disturbance

F03.B11 Unspecified dementia, moderate, with agitation `HCC` `Rx` `ESR` `UPD` `A`
Unspecified dementia, moderate, with aberrant motor behavior such as restlessness, rocking, pacing, or exit-seeking
Unspecified dementia, moderate, with verbal or physical behaviors such as profanity, shouting, threatening, anger, aggression, combativeness, or violence

F03.B18 Unspecified dementia, moderate, with other behavioral disturbance `HCC` `Rx` `ESR` `UPD` `A`
Unspecified dementia, moderate, with behavioral disturbances such as sleep disturbance, social disinhibition, or sexual disinhibition
Use additional code, if applicable, to identify wandering in unspecified dementia (Z91.83)

Chapter 5. Mental, Behavioral and Neurodevelopmental Disorders

F03.B2 **Unspecified dementia, moderate, with psychotic disturbance** `HCC` `Rx` `ESR` `UPD` `A`
  Unspecified dementia, moderate, with psychotic disturbance such as hallucinations, paranoia, suspiciousness, or delusional state

F03.B3 **Unspecified dementia, moderate, with mood disturbance** `HCC` `Rx` `ESR` `UPD` `A`
  Unspecified dementia, moderate, with mood disturbance such as depression, apathy, or anhedonia

F03.B4 **Unspecified dementia, moderate, with anxiety** `HCC` `Rx` `ESR` `UPD` `A`

✓5th **F03.C** **Unspecified dementia, severe**

  F03.C0 **Unspecified dementia, severe, without behavioral disturbance, psychotic disturbance, mood disturbance, and anxiety** `HCC` `Rx` `ESR` `UPD` `A`
    Dementia, severe, NOS

  ✓6th **F03.C1** **Unspecified dementia, severe, with behavioral disturbance**

    F03.C11 **Unspecified dementia, severe, with agitation** `HCC` `Rx` `ESR` `UPD` `A`
      Unspecified dementia, severe, with aberrant motor behavior such as restlessness, rocking, pacing, or exit-seeking
      Unspecified dementia, severe, with verbal or physical behaviors such as profanity, shouting, threatening, anger, aggression, combativeness, or violence

    F03.C18 **Unspecified dementia, severe, with other behavioral disturbance** `HCC` `Rx` `ESR` `UPD` `A`
      Unspecified dementia, severe, with behavioral disturbances such as sleep disturbance, social disinhibition, or sexual disinhibition
      Use additional code, if applicable, to identify wandering in unspecified dementia (Z91.83)

  F03.C2 **Unspecified dementia, severe, with psychotic disturbance** `HCC` `Rx` `ESR` `UPD` `A`
    Unspecified dementia, severe, with psychotic disturbance such as hallucinations, paranoia, suspiciousness, or delusional state

  F03.C3 **Unspecified dementia, severe, with mood disturbance** `HCC` `Rx` `ESR` `UPD` `A`
    Unspecified dementia, severe, with mood disturbance such as depression, apathy, or anhedonia
    AHA: 2023,4Q,14

  F03.C4 **Unspecified dementia, severe, with anxiety** `HCC` `Rx` `ESR` `UPD` `A`

F04 **Amnestic disorder due to known physiological condition** `Rx` `ESR`
  Korsakov's psychosis or syndrome, nonalcoholic
  Code first the underlying physiological condition
  EXCLUDES 1 amnesia NOS (R41.3)
              anterograde amnesia (R41.1)
              dissociative amnesia (F44.0)
              retrograde amnesia (R41.2)
  EXCLUDES 2 alcohol-induced or unspecified Korsakov's syndrome (F10.26, F10.96)
              Korsakov's syndrome induced by other psychoactive substances (F13.26, F13.96, F19.16, F19.26, F19.96)

F05 **Delirium due to known physiological condition** `UPD`
  Acute or subacute brain syndrome
  Acute or subacute confusional state (nonalcoholic)
  Acute or subacute infective psychosis
  Acute or subacute organic reaction
  Acute or subacute psycho-organic syndrome
  Delirium of mixed etiology
  Delirium superimposed on dementia
  Sundowning
  Code first the underlying physiological condition, such as: dementia (F03.9-)
  EXCLUDES 1 delirium NOS (R41.0)
  EXCLUDES 2 delirium tremens alcohol-induced or unspecified (F10.231, F10.921)
  AHA: 2019,2Q,34

✓4th **F06** **Other mental disorders due to known physiological condition**
  INCLUDES mental disorders due to endocrine disorder
            mental disorders due to exogenous hormone
            mental disorders due to exogenous toxic substance
            mental disorders due to primary cerebral disease
            mental disorders due to somatic illness
            mental disorders due to systemic disease affecting the brain
  Code first the underlying physiological condition
  EXCLUDES 1 unspecified dementia (F03.-)
  EXCLUDES 2 delirium due to known physiological condition (F05)
              dementia as classified in F01-F02
              other mental disorders associated with alcohol and other psychoactive substances (F10-F19)

  F06.0 **Psychotic disorder with hallucinations due to known physiological condition** `UPD`
    Organic hallucinatory state (nonalcoholic)
    EXCLUDES 2 hallucinations and perceptual disturbance induced by alcohol and other psychoactive substances (F10-F19 with .151, .251, .951)
                schizophrenia (F20.-)

  F06.1 **Catatonic disorder due to known physiological condition** `UPD`
    Catatonia associated with another mental disorder
    Catatonia NOS
    EXCLUDES 1 catatonic stupor (R40.1)
                stupor NOS (R40.1)
    EXCLUDES 2 catatonic schizophrenia (F20.2)
                dissociative stupor (F44.2)
    DEF: Catatonic: Abnormal neuropsychiatric state characterized by stupor, immobility or purposeless movements, or unresponsiveness in a person who otherwise appears awake.

  F06.2 **Psychotic disorder with delusions due to known physiological condition** `UPD`
    Paranoid and paranoid-hallucinatory organic states
    Schizophrenia-like psychosis in epilepsy
    EXCLUDES 2 alcohol and drug-induced psychotic disorder (F10-F19 with .150, .250, .950)
                brief psychotic disorder (F23)
                delusional disorder (F22)
                schizophrenia (F20.-)

  ✓5th **F06.3** **Mood disorder due to known physiological condition**
    EXCLUDES 2 mood disorders due to alcohol and other psychoactive substances (F10-F19 with .14, .24, .94)
                mood disorders, not due to known physiological condition or unspecified (F30-F39)

    F06.30 **Mood disorder due to known physiological condition, unspecified** `UPD`
    F06.31 **Mood disorder due to known physiological condition with depressive features** `UPD`
      Depressive disorder due to known physiological condition, with depressive features
    F06.32 **Mood disorder due to known physiological condition with major depressive-like episode** `UPD`
      Depressive disorder due to known physiological condition, with major depressive-like episode
    F06.33 **Mood disorder due to known physiological condition with manic features** `UPD`
      Bipolar and related disorder due to a known physiological condition, with manic features
      Bipolar and related disorder due to known physiological condition, with manic- or hypomanic-like episodes
    F06.34 **Mood disorder due to known physiological condition with mixed features** `UPD`
      Bipolar and related disorder due to known physiological condition, with mixed features
      Depressive disorder due to known physiological condition, with mixed features

  F06.4 **Anxiety disorder due to known physiological condition**
    EXCLUDES 2 anxiety disorders due to alcohol and other psychoactive substances (F10-F19 with .180, .280, .980)
                anxiety disorders, not due to known physiological condition or unspecified (F40.-, F41.-)

F06.7 Mild neurocognitive disorder due to known physiological condition
Mild neurocognitive impairment due to a known physiological condition

Code first the underlying physiological condition, such as:
- Alzheimer's disease (G30.-)
- human immunodeficiency virus [HIV] disease (B20)
- Huntington's disease (G10)
- neurocognitive disorder with Lewy bodies (G31.83)
- other frontotemporal neurocognitive disorder (G31.09)
- Parkinson's disease (G20.-)
- systemic lupus erythematosus (M32.-)
- traumatic brain injury (S06.-)
- vitamin B deficiency (E53.-)

EXCLUDES 1:
- age related cognitive decline (R41.81)
- altered mental status (R41.82)
- cerebral degeneration (G31.9)
- change in mental status (R41.82)
- cognitive deficits following (sequelae of) cerebral hemorrhage or infarction (I69.01-I69.11-, I69.21-I69.31-, I69.81-I69.91-)
- dementia (F01.-, F02.-, F03.-)
- mild cognitive impairment due to unknown or unspecified etiology (G31.84)
- neurologic neglect syndrome (R41.4)
- personality change, nonpsychotic (F68.8)

AHA: 2022,4Q,16

F06.70 Mild neurocognitive disorder due to known physiological condition without behavioral disturbance
Mild neurocognitive disorder due to known physiological condition, NOS

F06.71 Mild neurocognitive disorder due to known physiological condition with behavioral disturbance

F06.8 Other specified mental disorders due to known physiological condition
- Epileptic psychosis NOS
- Obsessive-compulsive and related disorder due to a known physiological condition
- Organic dissociative disorder
- Organic emotionally labile [asthenic] disorder

F07 Personality and behavioral disorders due to known physiological condition
Code first the underlying physiological condition

F07.0 Personality change due to known physiological condition
- Frontal lobe syndrome
- Limbic epilepsy personality syndrome
- Lobotomy syndrome
- Organic personality disorder
- Organic pseudopsychopathic personality
- Organic pseudoretarded personality
- Postleucotomy syndrome

EXCLUDES 1:
- mild cognitive impairment (G31.84)
- postconcussional syndrome (F07.81)
- postencephalitic syndrome (F07.89)
- signs and symptoms involving emotional state (R45.-)

EXCLUDES 2:
- specific personality disorder (F60.-)

F07.8 Other personality and behavioral disorders due to known physiological condition

F07.81 Postconcussional syndrome
Postcontusional syndrome (encephalopathy)
Post-traumatic brain syndrome, nonpsychotic

Use additional code to identify associated post-traumatic headache, if applicable (G44.3-)

EXCLUDES 1:
- current concussion (brain) (S06.0-)
- postencephalitic syndrome (F07.89)

DEF: Concussion symptoms that persist for weeks or months after a head injury. These symptoms may include headache, giddiness, fatigue, insomnia, mood fluctuation, and a subjective feeling of impaired intellectual function with extreme reaction to normal stressors.

F07.89 Other personality and behavioral disorders due to known physiological condition
Postencephalitic syndrome
Right hemispheric organic affective disorder

F07.9 Unspecified personality and behavioral disorder due to known physiological condition
Organic psychosyndrome

F09 Unspecified mental disorder due to known physiological condition
- Mental disorder NOS due to known physiological condition
- Organic brain syndrome NOS
- Organic mental disorder NOS
- Organic psychosis NOS
- Symptomatic psychosis NOS

Code first the underlying physiological condition

EXCLUDES 1:
- mild neurocognitive disorder due to known physiological condition (F06.7-)
- psychosis NOS (F29)

Mental and behavioral disorders due to psychoactive substance use (F10-F19)

AHA: 2022,4Q,16-17; 2022,1Q,34; 2020,1Q,9; 2018,4Q,69-70; 2017,4Q,8; 2017,2Q,27

TIP: Psychoactive substance withdrawal can occur in individuals who do not have a diagnosis of dependence but who use the substance regularly (i.e., use or abuse) and then reduce or cease the use.

F10 Alcohol related disorders
Use additional code for blood alcohol level, if applicable (Y90.-)

AHA: 2019,3Q,8

F10.1 Alcohol abuse
EXCLUDES 1:
- alcohol dependence (F10.2-)
- alcohol use, unspecified (F10.9-)

AHA: 2018,1Q,16; 2015,2Q,15

F10.10 Alcohol abuse, uncomplicated
Alcohol use disorder, mild

F10.11 Alcohol abuse, in remission
Alcohol use disorder, mild, in early remission
Alcohol use disorder, mild, in sustained remission

AHA: 2022,1Q,25

F10.12 Alcohol abuse with intoxication
- F10.120 Alcohol abuse with intoxication, uncomplicated
- F10.121 Alcohol abuse with intoxication delirium
- F10.129 Alcohol abuse with intoxication, unspecified

F10.13 Alcohol abuse, with withdrawal
AHA: 2020,4Q,16-17
- F10.130 Alcohol abuse with withdrawal, uncomplicated
- F10.131 Alcohol abuse with withdrawal delirium
- F10.132 Alcohol abuse with withdrawal with perceptual disturbance
- F10.139 Alcohol abuse with withdrawal, unspecified

F10.14 Alcohol abuse with alcohol-induced mood disorder
Alcohol use disorder, mild, with alcohol-induced bipolar or related disorder
Alcohol use disorder, mild, with alcohol-induced depressive disorder

F10.15 Alcohol abuse with alcohol-induced psychotic disorder
- F10.150 Alcohol abuse with alcohol-induced psychotic disorder with delusions
- F10.151 Alcohol abuse with alcohol-induced psychotic disorder with hallucinations
  DEF: Psychosis lasting less than six months with slight or no clouding of consciousness in which auditory hallucinations predominate.
- F10.159 Alcohol abuse with alcohol-induced psychotic disorder, unspecified

F10.18 Alcohol abuse with other alcohol-induced disorders
AHA: 2022,1Q,33
- F10.180 Alcohol abuse with alcohol-induced anxiety disorder
  AHA: 2022,1Q,25,33
- F10.181 Alcohol abuse with alcohol-induced sexual dysfunction
- F10.182 Alcohol abuse with alcohol-induced sleep disorder

	F10.188	Alcohol abuse with other alcohol-induced disorder [HCC] [ESR] [COM]
		AHA: 2022,1Q,25
	F10.19	Alcohol abuse with unspecified alcohol-induced disorder [ESR]

√5th **F10.2 Alcohol dependence**

EXCLUDES 1: alcohol abuse (F10.1-)
alcohol use, unspecified (F10.9-)

EXCLUDES 2: toxic effect of alcohol (T51.0-)

- **F10.20 Alcohol dependence, uncomplicated** [HCC] [ESR] [COM]
  Alcohol use disorder, moderate
  Alcohol use disorder, severe
  AHA: 2020,1Q,9

- **F10.21 Alcohol dependence, in remission** [HCC] [ESR] [COM]
  Alcohol use disorder, moderate, in early remission
  Alcohol use disorder, moderate, in sustained remission
  Alcohol use disorder, severe, in early remission
  Alcohol use disorder, severe, in sustained remission

√6th **F10.22 Alcohol dependence with intoxication**
  Acute drunkenness (in alcoholism)
  EXCLUDES 2: alcohol dependence with withdrawal (F10.23-)
  - F10.220 Alcohol dependence with intoxication, uncomplicated [HCC] [ESR] [COM]
  - F10.221 Alcohol dependence with intoxication delirium [HCC] [ESR] [COM]
  - F10.229 Alcohol dependence with intoxication, unspecified [HCC] [ESR] [COM]

√6th **F10.23 Alcohol dependence with withdrawal**
  EXCLUDES 2: alcohol dependence with intoxication (F10.22-)
  AHA: 2018,1Q,16; 2015,2Q,15
  - F10.230 Alcohol dependence with withdrawal, uncomplicated [HCC] [ESR] [COM]
  - F10.231 Alcohol dependence with withdrawal delirium [HCC] [ESR] [COM]
  - F10.232 Alcohol dependence with withdrawal with perceptual disturbance [HCC] [ESR] [COM]
  - F10.239 Alcohol dependence with withdrawal, unspecified [HCC] [ESR] [COM]

- **F10.24 Alcohol dependence with alcohol-induced mood disorder** [HCC] [ESR] [COM]
  Alcohol use disorder, moderate, with alcohol-induced bipolar or related disorder
  Alcohol use disorder, moderate, with alcohol-induced depressive disorder
  Alcohol use disorder, severe, with alcohol-induced bipolar or related disorder
  Alcohol use disorder, severe, with alcohol-induced depressive disorder

√6th **F10.25 Alcohol dependence with alcohol-induced psychotic disorder**
  - F10.250 Alcohol dependence with alcohol-induced psychotic disorder with delusions [HCC] [ESR] [COM]
  - F10.251 Alcohol dependence with alcohol-induced psychotic disorder with hallucinations [HCC] [ESR] [COM]
  - F10.259 Alcohol dependence with alcohol-induced psychotic disorder, unspecified [HCC] [ESR] [COM]

- **F10.26 Alcohol dependence with alcohol-induced persisting amnestic disorder** [HCC] [ESR] [COM]
  Alcohol use disorder, moderate, with alcohol-induced major neurocognitive disorder, amnestic-confabulatory type
  Alcohol use disorder, severe, with alcohol-induced major neurocognitive disorder, amnestic-confabulatory type
  DEF: Prominent and lasting reduced memory span and disordered time appreciation and confabulation that occurs in alcoholics as sequel to acute alcoholic psychosis.

- **F10.27 Alcohol dependence with alcohol-induced persisting dementia** [HCC] [ESR] [COM]
  Alcohol use disorder, moderate, with alcohol-induced major neurocognitive disorder, nonamnestic-confabulatory type
  Alcohol use disorder, severe, with alcohol-induced major neurocognitive disorder, nonamnestic-confabulatory type

√6th **F10.28 Alcohol dependence with other alcohol-induced disorders**
  - F10.280 Alcohol dependence with alcohol-induced anxiety disorder [HCC] [ESR] [COM]
  - F10.281 Alcohol dependence with alcohol-induced sexual dysfunction [HCC] [ESR] [COM]
  - F10.282 Alcohol dependence with alcohol-induced sleep disorder [HCC] [ESR] [COM]
  - F10.288 Alcohol dependence with other alcohol-induced disorder
    Alcohol use disorder, moderate, with alcohol-induced mild neurocognitive disorder
    Alcohol use disorder, severe, with alcohol-induced mild neurocognitive disorder
    AHA: 2020,1Q,9

- **F10.29 Alcohol dependence with unspecified alcohol-induced disorder** [HCC] [ESR] [COM]

√5th **F10.9 Alcohol use, unspecified**
  EXCLUDES 1: alcohol abuse (F10.1-)
  alcohol dependence (F10.2-)
  AHA: 2018,2Q,10-11
  TIP: Assign a substance use code only when the provider documents a relationship between the use and an associated physical, mental, or behavioral disorder. As with all diagnoses, substance use codes must meet the definition of a reportable diagnosis.

- **F10.90 Alcohol use, unspecified, uncomplicated**
- **F10.91 Alcohol use, unspecified, in remission**

√6th **F10.92 Alcohol use, unspecified with intoxication**
  - F10.920 Alcohol use, unspecified with intoxication, uncomplicated [ESR]
    AHA: 2018,2Q,10-11
  - F10.921 Alcohol use, unspecified with intoxication delirium [ESR]
  - F10.929 Alcohol use, unspecified with intoxication, unspecified [ESR]

√6th **F10.93 Alcohol use, unspecified with withdrawal**
  AHA: 2020,4Q,16-17
  - F10.930 Alcohol use, unspecified with withdrawal, uncomplicated [HCC] [ESR] [COM]
  - F10.931 Alcohol use, unspecified with withdrawal delirium [HCC] [ESR] [COM]
  - F10.932 Alcohol use, unspecified with withdrawal with perceptual disturbance [HCC] [ESR] [COM]
  - F10.939 Alcohol use, unspecified with withdrawal, unspecified [HCC] [ESR] [COM]

- **F10.94 Alcohol use, unspecified with alcohol-induced mood disorder** [HCC] [ESR] [COM]
  Alcohol induced bipolar or related disorder, without use disorder
  Alcohol induced depressive disorder, without use disorder

√6th **F10.95 Alcohol use, unspecified with alcohol-induced psychotic disorder**
  - F10.950 Alcohol use, unspecified with alcohol-induced psychotic disorder with delusions [HCC] [ESR] [COM]
  - F10.951 Alcohol use, unspecified with alcohol-induced psychotic disorder with hallucinations [HCC] [ESR] [COM]
  - F10.959 Alcohol use, unspecified with alcohol-induced psychotic disorder, unspecified [HCC] [ESR] [COM]
    Alcohol-induced psychotic disorder without use disorder

- **F10.96 Alcohol use, unspecified with alcohol-induced persisting amnestic disorder** [HCC] [ESR] [COM]
  Alcohol-induced major neurocognitive disorder, amnestic-confabulatory type, without use disorder

F10.97 Alcohol use, unspecified with alcohol-induced persisting dementia [HCC] [ESR] [COM]
  Alcohol-induced major neurocognitive disorder, nonamnestic-confabulatory type, without use disorder

√6ᵗʰ **F10.98** Alcohol use, unspecified with other alcohol-induced disorders
  F10.980 Alcohol use, unspecified with alcohol-induced anxiety disorder [HCC] [ESR] [COM]
    Alcohol induced anxiety disorder, without use disorder
  F10.981 Alcohol use, unspecified with alcohol-induced sexual dysfunction [HCC] [ESR] [COM]
    Alcohol induced sexual dysfunction, without use disorder
  F10.982 Alcohol use, unspecified with alcohol-induced sleep disorder [HCC] [ESR] [COM]
    Alcohol induced sleep disorder, without use disorder
  F10.988 Alcohol use, unspecified with other alcohol-induced disorder [HCC] [ESR] [COM]
    Alcohol induced mild neurocognitive disorder, without use disorder

F10.99 Alcohol use, unspecified with unspecified alcohol-induced disorder [ESR]

√4ᵗʰ **F11** Opioid related disorders

√5ᵗʰ **F11.1** Opioid abuse
  EXCLUDES 1 opioid dependence (F11.2-)
              opioid use, unspecified (F11.9-)
  F11.10 Opioid abuse, uncomplicated [HCC] [ESR]
    Opioid use disorder, mild
  F11.11 Opioid abuse, in remission [HCC] [ESR]
    Opioid use disorder, mild, in early remission
    Opioid use disorder, mild, in sustained remission

√6ᵗʰ **F11.12** Opioid abuse with intoxication
  F11.120 Opioid abuse with intoxication, uncomplicated [HCC] [ESR] [COM]
  F11.121 Opioid abuse with intoxication delirium [HCC] [ESR] [COM]
  F11.122 Opioid abuse with intoxication with perceptual disturbance [HCC] [ESR] [COM]
  F11.129 Opioid abuse with intoxication, unspecified [HCC] [ESR] [COM]

F11.13 Opioid abuse with withdrawal [HCC] [ESR] [COM]
  AHA: 2020,4Q,16-17

F11.14 Opioid abuse with opioid-induced mood disorder [HCC] [ESR] [COM]
  Opioid use disorder, mild, with opioid-induced depressive disorder

√6ᵗʰ **F11.15** Opioid abuse with opioid-induced psychotic disorder
  F11.150 Opioid abuse with opioid-induced psychotic disorder with delusions [HCC] [ESR] [COM]
  F11.151 Opioid abuse with opioid-induced psychotic disorder with hallucinations [HCC] [ESR] [COM]
  F11.159 Opioid abuse with opioid-induced psychotic disorder, unspecified [HCC] [ESR] [COM]

√6ᵗʰ **F11.18** Opioid abuse with other opioid-induced disorder
  F11.181 Opioid abuse with opioid-induced sexual dysfunction [HCC] [ESR] [COM]
  F11.182 Opioid abuse with opioid-induced sleep disorder [HCC] [ESR] [COM]
  F11.188 Opioid abuse with other opioid-induced disorder [HCC] [ESR] [COM]
    Opioid-associated amnestic syndrome with opioid abuse

F11.19 Opioid abuse with unspecified opioid-induced disorder [HCC] [ESR] [COM]

√5ᵗʰ **F11.2** Opioid dependence
  EXCLUDES 1 opioid abuse (F11.1-)
              opioid use, unspecified (F11.9-)
  EXCLUDES 2 opioid poisoning (T40.0-T40.2-)
  F11.20 Opioid dependence, uncomplicated [HCC] [ESR] [COM]
    Opioid use disorder, moderate
    Opioid use disorder, severe
  F11.21 Opioid dependence, in remission [HCC] [ESR] [COM]
    Opioid use disorder, moderate, in early remission
    Opioid use disorder, moderate, in sustained remission
    Opioid use disorder, severe, in early remission
    Opioid use disorder, severe, in sustained remission

√6ᵗʰ **F11.22** Opioid dependence with intoxication
  EXCLUDES 1 opioid dependence with withdrawal (F11.23)
  F11.220 Opioid dependence with intoxication, uncomplicated [HCC] [ESR] [COM]
  F11.221 Opioid dependence with intoxication delirium [HCC] [ESR] [COM]
  F11.222 Opioid dependence with intoxication with perceptual disturbance [HCC] [ESR] [COM]
  F11.229 Opioid dependence with intoxication, unspecified [HCC] [ESR] [COM]

F11.23 Opioid dependence with withdrawal [HCC] [ESR] [COM]
  EXCLUDES 1 opioid dependence with intoxication (F11.22-)

F11.24 Opioid dependence with opioid-induced mood disorder [HCC] [ESR] [COM]
  Opioid use disorder, moderate, with opioid induced depressive disorder

√6ᵗʰ **F11.25** Opioid dependence with opioid-induced psychotic disorder
  F11.250 Opioid dependence with opioid-induced psychotic disorder with delusions [HCC] [ESR] [COM]
  F11.251 Opioid dependence with opioid-induced psychotic disorder with hallucinations [HCC] [ESR] [COM]
  F11.259 Opioid dependence with opioid-induced psychotic disorder, unspecified [HCC] [ESR] [COM]

√6ᵗʰ **F11.28** Opioid dependence with other opioid-induced disorder
  F11.281 Opioid dependence with opioid-induced sexual dysfunction [HCC] [ESR] [COM]
  F11.282 Opioid dependence with opioid-induced sleep disorder [HCC] [ESR] [COM]
  F11.288 Opioid dependence with other opioid-induced disorder [HCC] [ESR] [COM]
    Opioid-associated amnestic syndrome with opioid dependence

F11.29 Opioid dependence with unspecified opioid-induced disorder [HCC] [ESR] [COM]

√5ᵗʰ **F11.9** Opioid use, unspecified
  EXCLUDES 1 opioid abuse (F11.1-)
              opioid dependence (F11.2-)
  TIP: Assign a substance use code only when the provider documents a relationship between the use and an associated physical, mental, or behavioral disorder. As with all diagnoses, substance use codes must meet the definition of a reportable diagnosis.
  F11.90 Opioid use, unspecified, uncomplicated
    AHA: 2018,2Q,10-11
  F11.91 Opioid use, unspecified, in remission

√6ᵗʰ **F11.92** Opioid use, unspecified with intoxication
  EXCLUDES 1 opioid use, unspecified with withdrawal (F11.93)
  F11.920 Opioid use, unspecified with intoxication, uncomplicated [HCC] [ESR] [COM]
  F11.921 Opioid use, unspecified with intoxication delirium [HCC] [ESR] [COM]
    Opioid-induced delirium
  F11.922 Opioid use, unspecified with intoxication with perceptual disturbance [HCC] [ESR] [COM]
  F11.929 Opioid use, unspecified with intoxication, unspecified [HCC] [ESR] [COM]

F11.93 Opioid use, unspecified with withdrawal
  EXCLUDES 1: opioid use, unspecified with intoxication (F11.92-)
F11.94 Opioid use, unspecified with opioid-induced mood disorder
  Opioid induced depressive disorder, without use disorder
F11.95 Opioid use, unspecified with opioid-induced psychotic disorder
  F11.950 Opioid use, unspecified with opioid-induced psychotic disorder with delusions
  F11.951 Opioid use, unspecified with opioid-induced psychotic disorder with hallucinations
  F11.959 Opioid use, unspecified with opioid-induced psychotic disorder, unspecified
F11.98 Opioid use, unspecified with other specified opioid-induced disorder
  F11.981 Opioid use, unspecified with opioid-induced sexual dysfunction
    Opioid induced sexual dysfunction, without use disorder
  F11.982 Opioid use, unspecified with opioid-induced sleep disorder
    Opioid induced sleep disorder, without use disorder
  F11.988 Opioid use, unspecified with other opioid-induced disorder
    Opioid induced anxiety disorder, without use disorder
    Opioid-associated amnestic syndrome without use disorder
F11.99 Opioid use, unspecified with unspecified opioid-induced disorder

F12 Cannabis related disorders
  INCLUDES: marijuana
  AHA: 2020,1Q,8

F12.1 Cannabis abuse
  EXCLUDES 1: cannabis dependence (F12.2-)
  cannabis use, unspecified (F12.9-)
  F12.10 Cannabis abuse, uncomplicated
    Cannabis use disorder, mild
  F12.11 Cannabis abuse, in remission
    Cannabis use disorder, mild, in early remission
    Cannabis use disorder, mild, in sustained remission
  F12.12 Cannabis abuse with intoxication
    F12.120 Cannabis abuse with intoxication, uncomplicated
    F12.121 Cannabis abuse with intoxication delirium
    F12.122 Cannabis abuse with intoxication with perceptual disturbance
    F12.129 Cannabis abuse with intoxication, unspecified
  F12.13 Cannabis abuse with withdrawal
    AHA: 2020,4Q,16-17
  F12.15 Cannabis abuse with psychotic disorder
    F12.150 Cannabis abuse with psychotic disorder with delusions
    F12.151 Cannabis abuse with psychotic disorder with hallucinations
    F12.159 Cannabis abuse with psychotic disorder, unspecified
  F12.18 Cannabis abuse with other cannabis-induced disorder
    F12.180 Cannabis abuse with cannabis-induced anxiety disorder
    F12.188 Cannabis abuse with other cannabis-induced disorder
      Cannabis use disorder, mild, with cannabis-induced sleep disorder
  F12.19 Cannabis abuse with unspecified cannabis-induced disorder

F12.2 Cannabis dependence
  EXCLUDES 1: cannabis abuse (F12.1-)
  cannabis use, unspecified (F12.9-)
  EXCLUDES 2: cannabis poisoning (T40.7-)
  F12.20 Cannabis dependence, uncomplicated
    Cannabis use disorder, moderate
    Cannabis use disorder, severe
  F12.21 Cannabis dependence, in remission
    Cannabis use disorder, moderate, in early remission
    Cannabis use disorder, moderate, in sustained remission
    Cannabis use disorder, severe, in early remission
    Cannabis use disorder, severe, in sustained remission
  F12.22 Cannabis dependence with intoxication
    F12.220 Cannabis dependence with intoxication, uncomplicated
    F12.221 Cannabis dependence with intoxication delirium
    F12.222 Cannabis dependence with intoxication with perceptual disturbance
    F12.229 Cannabis dependence with intoxication, unspecified
  F12.23 Cannabis dependence with withdrawal
    AHA: 2018,4Q,7
  F12.25 Cannabis dependence with psychotic disorder
    F12.250 Cannabis dependence with psychotic disorder with delusions
    F12.251 Cannabis dependence with psychotic disorder with hallucinations
    F12.259 Cannabis dependence with psychotic disorder, unspecified
  F12.28 Cannabis dependence with other cannabis-induced disorder
    F12.280 Cannabis dependence with cannabis-induced anxiety disorder
    F12.288 Cannabis dependence with other cannabis-induced disorder
      Cannabis use disorder, moderate, with cannabis-induced sleep disorder
      Cannabis use disorder, severe, with cannabis-induced sleep disorder
  F12.29 Cannabis dependence with unspecified cannabis-induced disorder

F12.9 Cannabis use, unspecified
  EXCLUDES 1: cannabis abuse (F12.1-)
  cannabis dependence (F12.2-)
  TIP: Assign a substance use code only when the provider documents a relationship between the use and an associated physical, mental, or behavioral disorder. As with all diagnoses, substance use codes must meet the definition of a reportable diagnosis.
  F12.90 Cannabis use, unspecified, uncomplicated
    AHA: 2023,3Q,18; 2018,2Q,10-11
  F12.91 Cannabis use, unspecified, in remission
  F12.92 Cannabis use, unspecified with intoxication
    F12.920 Cannabis use, unspecified with intoxication, uncomplicated
    F12.921 Cannabis use, unspecified with intoxication delirium
    F12.922 Cannabis use, unspecified with intoxication with perceptual disturbance
    F12.929 Cannabis use, unspecified with intoxication, unspecified
  F12.93 Cannabis use, unspecified with withdrawal
    AHA: 2018,4Q,7
  F12.95 Cannabis use, unspecified with psychotic disorder
    F12.950 Cannabis use, unspecified with psychotic disorder with delusions
    F12.951 Cannabis use, unspecified with psychotic disorder with hallucinations

F12.959 Cannabis use, unspecified with psychotic disorder, unspecified [HCC] [ESR] [COM]
  Cannabis induced psychotic disorder, without use disorder

✓6th **F12.98** Cannabis use, unspecified with other cannabis-induced disorder
  F12.980 Cannabis use, unspecified with anxiety disorder [HCC] [ESR] [COM]
    Cannabis induced anxiety disorder, without use disorder
  F12.988 Cannabis use, unspecified with other cannabis-induced disorder [HCC] [ESR] [COM]
    Cannabis induced sleep disorder, without use disorder

F12.99 Cannabis use, unspecified with unspecified cannabis-induced disorder [ESR] [COM]

✓4th **F13** Sedative, hypnotic, or anxiolytic related disorders
  ✓5th **F13.1** Sedative, hypnotic or anxiolytic-related abuse
    EXCLUDES 1 sedative, hypnotic or anxiolytic-related dependence (F13.2-)
      sedative, hypnotic, or anxiolytic use, unspecified (F13.9-)
    F13.10 Sedative, hypnotic or anxiolytic abuse, uncomplicated [HCC] [ESR]
      Sedative, hypnotic, or anxiolytic use disorder, mild
    F13.11 Sedative, hypnotic or anxiolytic abuse, in remission [HCC] [ESR]
      Sedative, hypnotic or anxiolytic use disorder, mild, in early remission
      Sedative, hypnotic or anxiolytic use disorder, mild, in sustained remission
    ✓6th **F13.12** Sedative, hypnotic or anxiolytic abuse with intoxication
      F13.120 Sedative, hypnotic or anxiolytic abuse with intoxication, uncomplicated [HCC] [ESR] [COM]
      F13.121 Sedative, hypnotic or anxiolytic abuse with intoxication delirium [HCC] [ESR] [COM]
      F13.129 Sedative, hypnotic or anxiolytic abuse with intoxication, unspecified [HCC] [ESR] [COM]
    ✓6th **F13.13** Sedative, hypnotic or anxiolytic abuse with withdrawal
      AHA: 2020,4Q,16-17
      F13.130 Sedative, hypnotic or anxiolytic abuse with withdrawal, uncomplicated [HCC] [ESR] [COM]
      F13.131 Sedative, hypnotic or anxiolytic abuse with withdrawal delirium [HCC] [ESR] [COM]
      F13.132 Sedative, hypnotic or anxiolytic abuse with withdrawal with perceptual disturbance [HCC] [ESR] [COM]
      F13.139 Sedative, hypnotic or anxiolytic abuse with withdrawal, unspecified [HCC] [ESR] [COM]
    F13.14 Sedative, hypnotic or anxiolytic abuse with sedative, hypnotic or anxiolytic-induced mood disorder [HCC] [ESR] [COM]
      Sedative, hypnotic, or anxiolytic use disorder, mild, with sedative, hypnotic, or anxiolytic-induced bipolar or related disorder
      Sedative, hypnotic, or anxiolytic use disorder, mild, with sedative, hypnotic, or anxiolytic-induced depressive disorder
    ✓6th **F13.15** Sedative, hypnotic or anxiolytic abuse with sedative, hypnotic or anxiolytic-induced psychotic disorder
      F13.150 Sedative, hypnotic or anxiolytic abuse with sedative, hypnotic or anxiolytic-induced psychotic disorder with delusions [HCC] [ESR] [COM]
      F13.151 Sedative, hypnotic or anxiolytic abuse with sedative, hypnotic or anxiolytic-induced psychotic disorder with hallucinations [HCC] [ESR] [COM]
      F13.159 Sedative, hypnotic or anxiolytic abuse with sedative, hypnotic or anxiolytic-induced psychotic disorder, unspecified [HCC] [ESR] [COM]
    ✓6th **F13.18** Sedative, hypnotic or anxiolytic abuse with other sedative, hypnotic or anxiolytic-induced disorders
      F13.180 Sedative, hypnotic or anxiolytic abuse with sedative, hypnotic or anxiolytic-induced anxiety disorder [HCC] [ESR] [COM]
      F13.181 Sedative, hypnotic or anxiolytic abuse with sedative, hypnotic or anxiolytic-induced sexual dysfunction [HCC] [ESR] [COM]
      F13.182 Sedative, hypnotic or anxiolytic abuse with sedative, hypnotic or anxiolytic-induced sleep disorder [HCC] [ESR] [COM]
      F13.188 Sedative, hypnotic or anxiolytic abuse with other sedative, hypnotic or anxiolytic-induced disorder [HCC] [ESR] [COM]
    F13.19 Sedative, hypnotic or anxiolytic abuse with unspecified sedative, hypnotic or anxiolytic-induced disorder [HCC] [ESR] [COM]
  ✓5th **F13.2** Sedative, hypnotic or anxiolytic-related dependence
    EXCLUDES 1 sedative, hypnotic or anxiolytic-related abuse (F13.1-)
      sedative, hypnotic, or anxiolytic use, unspecified (F13.9-)
    EXCLUDES 2 sedative, hypnotic, or anxiolytic poisoning (T42.-)
    F13.20 Sedative, hypnotic or anxiolytic dependence, uncomplicated [HCC] [ESR] [COM]
    F13.21 Sedative, hypnotic or anxiolytic dependence, in remission [HCC] [ESR] [COM]
      Sedative, hypnotic or anxiolytic use disorder, moderate, in early remission
      Sedative, hypnotic or anxiolytic use disorder, moderate, in sustained remission
      Sedative, hypnotic or anxiolytic use disorder, severe, in early remission
      Sedative, hypnotic or anxiolytic use disorder, severe, in sustained remission
    ✓6th **F13.22** Sedative, hypnotic or anxiolytic dependence with intoxication
      EXCLUDES 1 sedative, hypnotic or anxiolytic dependence with withdrawal (F13.23-)
      F13.220 Sedative, hypnotic or anxiolytic dependence with intoxication, uncomplicated [HCC] [ESR] [COM]
      F13.221 Sedative, hypnotic or anxiolytic dependence with intoxication delirium [HCC] [ESR] [COM]
      F13.229 Sedative, hypnotic or anxiolytic dependence with intoxication, unspecified [HCC] [ESR] [COM]
    ✓6th **F13.23** Sedative, hypnotic or anxiolytic dependence with withdrawal
      Sedative, hypnotic, or anxiolytic use disorder, moderate
      Sedative, hypnotic, or anxiolytic use disorder, severe
      EXCLUDES 1 sedative, hypnotic or anxiolytic dependence with intoxication (F13.22-)
      F13.230 Sedative, hypnotic or anxiolytic dependence with withdrawal, uncomplicated [HCC] [ESR] [COM]
      F13.231 Sedative, hypnotic or anxiolytic dependence with withdrawal delirium [HCC] [ESR] [COM]
      F13.232 Sedative, hypnotic or anxiolytic dependence with withdrawal with perceptual disturbance [HCC] [ESR] [COM]
        Sedative, hypnotic, or anxiolytic withdrawal with perceptual disturbances
      F13.239 Sedative, hypnotic or anxiolytic dependence with withdrawal, unspecified [HCC] [ESR] [COM]
        Sedative, hypnotic, or anxiolytic withdrawal without perceptual disturbances
    F13.24 Sedative, hypnotic or anxiolytic dependence with sedative, hypnotic or anxiolytic-induced mood disorder [HCC] [ESR] [COM]
      Sedative, hypnotic, or anxiolytic use disorder, moderate, with sedative, hypnotic, or anxiolytic-induced bipolar or related disorder
      Sedative, hypnotic, or anxiolytic use disorder, moderate, with sedative, hypnotic, or anxiolytic-induced depressive disorder
      Sedative, hypnotic, or anxiolytic use disorder, severe, with sedative, hypnotic, or anxiolytic-induced bipolar or related disorder
      Sedative, hypnotic, or anxiolytic use disorder, severe, with sedative, hypnotic, or anxiolytic-induced depressive disorder

[HCC] CMS-HCC   [Rx] Rx HCC   [ESR] ESRD HCC   [COM] Commercial HCC   N Newborn: 0   P Pediatric: 0-17   M Maternity: 9-64   A Adult: 15-124

F13.25 Sedative, hypnotic or anxiolytic dependence with sedative, hypnotic or anxiolytic-induced psychotic disorder

- **F13.250** Sedative, hypnotic or anxiolytic dependence with sedative, hypnotic or anxiolytic-induced psychotic disorder with **delusions** `HCC` `ESR` `COM`
- **F13.251** Sedative, hypnotic or anxiolytic dependence with sedative, hypnotic or anxiolytic-induced psychotic disorder with **hallucinations** `HCC` `ESR` `COM`
- **F13.259** Sedative, hypnotic or anxiolytic dependence with sedative, hypnotic or anxiolytic-induced psychotic disorder, unspecified

F13.26 Sedative, hypnotic or anxiolytic dependence with sedative, hypnotic or anxiolytic-induced **persisting amnestic disorder** `HCC` `ESR` `COM`

F13.27 Sedative, hypnotic or anxiolytic dependence with sedative, hypnotic or anxiolytic-induced **persisting dementia**

Sedative, hypnotic, or anxiolytic use disorder, moderate, with sedative, hypnotic, or anxiolytic induced major neurocognitive disorder

Sedative, hypnotic, or anxiolytic use disorder, severe, with sedative, hypnotic, or anxiolytic-induced major neurocognitive disorder

F13.28 Sedative, hypnotic or anxiolytic dependence with other sedative, hypnotic or anxiolytic-induced disorders

- **F13.280** Sedative, hypnotic or anxiolytic dependence with sedative, hypnotic or anxiolytic-induced **anxiety disorder** `HCC` `ESR` `COM`
- **F13.281** Sedative, hypnotic or anxiolytic dependence with sedative, hypnotic or anxiolytic-induced **sexual dysfunction** `HCC` `ESR` `COM`
- **F13.282** Sedative, hypnotic or anxiolytic dependence with sedative, hypnotic or anxiolytic-induced **sleep disorder** `HCC` `ESR` `COM`
- **F13.288** Sedative, hypnotic or anxiolytic dependence with other sedative, hypnotic or anxiolytic-induced disorder `HCC` `ESR` `COM`

    Sedative, hypnotic, or anxiolytic use disorder, moderate, with sedative, hypnotic, or anxiolytic-induced mild neurocognitive disorder

    Sedative, hypnotic, or anxiolytic use disorder, severe, with sedative, hypnotic, or anxiolytic-induced mild neurocognitive disorder

F13.29 Sedative, hypnotic or anxiolytic dependence with unspecified sedative, hypnotic or anxiolytic-induced disorder `HCC` `ESR` `COM`

F13.9 Sedative, hypnotic or anxiolytic-related use, unspecified

EXCLUDES 1 sedative, hypnotic or anxiolytic-related abuse (F13.1-)
sedative, hypnotic or anxiolytic-related dependence (F13.2-)

TIP: Assign a substance use code only when the provider documents a relationship between the use and an associated physical, mental, or behavioral disorder. As with all diagnoses, substance use codes must meet the definition of a reportable diagnosis.

- **F13.90** Sedative, hypnotic, or anxiolytic use, unspecified, **uncomplicated**
    AHA: 2018,2Q,10-11
- **F13.91** Sedative, hypnotic or anxiolytic use, unspecified, **in remission**
- **F13.92** Sedative, hypnotic or anxiolytic use, unspecified with **intoxication**
    EXCLUDES 1 sedative, hypnotic or anxiolytic use, unspecified with withdrawal (F13.93-)
    - **F13.920** Sedative, hypnotic or anxiolytic use, unspecified with intoxication, **uncomplicated** `HCC` `ESR` `COM`
    - **F13.921** Sedative, hypnotic or anxiolytic use, unspecified with intoxication **delirium** `HCC` `ESR` `COM`
        Sedative, hypnotic, or anxiolytic-induced delirium
    - **F13.929** Sedative, hypnotic or anxiolytic use, unspecified with intoxication, unspecified `HCC` `ESR` `COM`

- **F13.93** Sedative, hypnotic or anxiolytic use, unspecified with **withdrawal**
    EXCLUDES 1 sedative, hypnotic or anxiolytic use, unspecified with intoxication (F13.92-)
    - **F13.930** Sedative, hypnotic or anxiolytic use, unspecified with withdrawal, **uncomplicated** `HCC` `ESR` `COM`
    - **F13.931** Sedative, hypnotic or anxiolytic use, unspecified with withdrawal **delirium** `HCC` `ESR` `COM`
    - **F13.932** Sedative, hypnotic or anxiolytic use, unspecified with withdrawal with **perceptual disturbances** `HCC` `ESR` `COM`
    - **F13.939** Sedative, hypnotic or anxiolytic use, unspecified with withdrawal, unspecified `HCC` `ESR` `COM`

- **F13.94** Sedative, hypnotic or anxiolytic use, unspecified with sedative, hypnotic or anxiolytic-induced **mood disorder** `HCC` `ESR` `COM`
    Sedative, hypnotic, or anxiolytic-induced bipolar or related disorder, without use disorder
    Sedative, hypnotic, or anxiolytic-induced depressive disorder, without use disorder

- **F13.95** Sedative, hypnotic or anxiolytic use, unspecified with sedative, hypnotic or anxiolytic-induced **psychotic disorder**
    - **F13.950** Sedative, hypnotic or anxiolytic use, unspecified with sedative, hypnotic or anxiolytic-induced psychotic disorder with **delusions** `HCC` `ESR` `COM`
    - **F13.951** Sedative, hypnotic or anxiolytic use, unspecified with sedative, hypnotic or anxiolytic-induced psychotic disorder with **hallucinations** `HCC` `ESR` `COM`
    - **F13.959** Sedative, hypnotic or anxiolytic use, unspecified with sedative, hypnotic or anxiolytic-induced psychotic disorder, unspecified `HCC` `ESR` `COM`
        Sedative, hypnotic, or anxiolytic-induced psychotic disorder, without use disorder

- **F13.96** Sedative, hypnotic or anxiolytic use, unspecified with sedative, hypnotic or anxiolytic-induced **persisting amnestic disorder** `HCC` `ESR` `COM`

- **F13.97** Sedative, hypnotic or anxiolytic use, unspecified with sedative, hypnotic or anxiolytic-induced **persisting dementia** `HCC` `ESR` `COM`
    Sedative, hypnotic, or anxiolytic-induced major neurocognitive disorder, without use disorder

- **F13.98** Sedative, hypnotic or anxiolytic use, unspecified with other sedative, hypnotic or anxiolytic-induced disorders
    - **F13.980** Sedative, hypnotic or anxiolytic use, unspecified with sedative, hypnotic or anxiolytic-induced **anxiety disorder** `HCC` `ESR` `COM`
        Sedative, hypnotic, or anxiolytic-induced anxiety disorder, without use disorder
    - **F13.981** Sedative, hypnotic or anxiolytic use, unspecified with sedative, hypnotic or anxiolytic-induced **sexual dysfunction** `HCC` `ESR` `COM`
        Sedative, hypnotic, or anxiolytic-induced sexual dysfunction disorder, without use disorder
    - **F13.982** Sedative, hypnotic or anxiolytic use, unspecified with sedative, hypnotic or anxiolytic-induced **sleep disorder** `HCC` `ESR` `COM`
        Sedative, hypnotic, or anxiolytic-induced sleep disorder, without use disorder

F13.988 Sedative, hypnotic or anxiolytic use, unspecified with other sedative, hypnotic or anxiolytic-induced disorder [HCC] [ESR] [COM]
- Sedative, hypnotic, or anxiolytic-induced mild neurocognitive disorder

F13.99 Sedative, hypnotic or anxiolytic use, unspecified with unspecified sedative, hypnotic or anxiolytic-induced disorder [HCC] [ESR] [COM]

✓4ᵗʰ F14 Cocaine related disorders
EXCLUDES 2: other stimulant-related disorders (F15.-)

✓5ᵗʰ F14.1 Cocaine abuse
EXCLUDES 1: cocaine dependence (F14.2-)
cocaine use, unspecified (F14.9-)

- **F14.10** Cocaine abuse, uncomplicated [HCC] [ESR]
  - Cocaine use disorder, mild
- **F14.11** Cocaine abuse, in remission [HCC] [ESR]
  - Cocaine use disorder, mild, in early remission
  - Cocaine use disorder, mild, in sustained remission

✓6ᵗʰ F14.12 Cocaine abuse with intoxication
- **F14.120** Cocaine abuse with intoxication, uncomplicated [HCC] [ESR] [COM]
- **F14.121** Cocaine abuse with intoxication with delirium [HCC] [ESR] [COM]
- **F14.122** Cocaine abuse with intoxication with perceptual disturbance [HCC] [ESR] [COM]
- **F14.129** Cocaine abuse with intoxication, unspecified [HCC] [ESR] [COM]

- **F14.13** Cocaine abuse, unspecified with withdrawal [HCC] [ESR] [COM]
  - AHA: 2020,4Q,16-17

- **F14.14** Cocaine abuse with cocaine-induced mood disorder [HCC] [ESR] [COM]
  - Cocaine use disorder, mild, with cocaine-induced bipolar or related disorder
  - Cocaine use disorder, mild, with cocaine-induced depressive disorder

✓6ᵗʰ F14.15 Cocaine abuse with cocaine-induced psychotic disorder
- **F14.150** Cocaine abuse with cocaine-induced psychotic disorder with delusions [HCC] [ESR] [COM]
- **F14.151** Cocaine abuse with cocaine-induced psychotic disorder with hallucinations [HCC] [ESR] [COM]
- **F14.159** Cocaine abuse with cocaine-induced psychotic disorder, unspecified [HCC] [ESR] [COM]

✓6ᵗʰ F14.18 Cocaine abuse with other cocaine-induced disorder
- **F14.180** Cocaine abuse with cocaine-induced anxiety disorder [HCC] [ESR] [COM]
- **F14.181** Cocaine abuse with cocaine-induced sexual dysfunction [HCC] [ESR] [COM]
- **F14.182** Cocaine abuse with cocaine-induced sleep disorder [HCC] [ESR] [COM]
- **F14.188** Cocaine abuse with other cocaine-induced disorder [HCC] [ESR] [COM]
  - Cocaine use disorder, mild, with cocaine-induced obsessive compulsive or related disorder

- **F14.19** Cocaine abuse with unspecified cocaine-induced disorder [HCC] [ESR] [COM]

✓5ᵗʰ F14.2 Cocaine dependence
EXCLUDES 1: cocaine abuse (F14.1-)
cocaine use, unspecified (F14.9-)
EXCLUDES 2: cocaine poisoning (T40.5-)

- **F14.20** Cocaine dependence, uncomplicated [HCC] [ESR] [COM]
  - Cocaine use disorder, moderate
  - Cocaine use disorder, severe
- **F14.21** Cocaine dependence, in remission [HCC] [ESR] [COM]
  - Cocaine use disorder, moderate, in early remission
  - Cocaine use disorder, moderate, in sustained remission
  - Cocaine use disorder, severe, in early remission
  - Cocaine use disorder, severe, in sustained remission

✓6ᵗʰ F14.22 Cocaine dependence with intoxication
EXCLUDES 1: cocaine dependence with withdrawal (F14.23)

- **F14.220** Cocaine dependence with intoxication, uncomplicated [HCC] [ESR] [COM]
- **F14.221** Cocaine dependence with intoxication delirium [HCC] [ESR] [COM]
- **F14.222** Cocaine dependence with intoxication with perceptual disturbance [HCC] [ESR] [COM]
- **F14.229** Cocaine dependence with intoxication, unspecified [HCC] [ESR] [COM]

- **F14.23** Cocaine dependence with withdrawal [HCC] [ESR] [COM]
  - EXCLUDES 1: cocaine dependence with intoxication (F14.22-)

- **F14.24** Cocaine dependence with cocaine-induced mood disorder [HCC] [ESR] [COM]
  - Cocaine use disorder, moderate, with cocaine-induced bipolar or related disorder
  - Cocaine use disorder, moderate, with cocaine-induced depressive disorder
  - Cocaine use disorder, severe, with cocaine-induced bipolar or related disorder
  - Cocaine use disorder, severe, with cocaine-induced depressive disorder

✓6ᵗʰ F14.25 Cocaine dependence with cocaine-induced psychotic disorder
- **F14.250** Cocaine dependence with cocaine-induced psychotic disorder with delusions [HCC] [ESR] [COM]
- **F14.251** Cocaine dependence with cocaine-induced psychotic disorder with hallucinations [HCC] [ESR] [COM]
- **F14.259** Cocaine dependence with cocaine-induced psychotic disorder, unspecified [HCC] [ESR] [COM]

✓6ᵗʰ F14.28 Cocaine dependence with other cocaine-induced disorder
- **F14.280** Cocaine dependence with cocaine-induced anxiety disorder [HCC] [ESR] [COM]
- **F14.281** Cocaine dependence with cocaine-induced sexual dysfunction [HCC] [ESR] [COM]
- **F14.282** Cocaine dependence with cocaine-induced sleep disorder [HCC] [ESR] [COM]
- **F14.288** Cocaine dependence with other cocaine-induced disorder [HCC] [ESR] [COM]
  - Cocaine use disorder, moderate, with cocaine-induced obsessive compulsive or related disorder
  - Cocaine use disorder, severe, with cocaine-induced obsessive compulsive or related disorder

- **F14.29** Cocaine dependence with unspecified cocaine-induced disorder [HCC] [ESR] [COM]

✓5ᵗʰ F14.9 Cocaine use, unspecified
EXCLUDES 1: cocaine abuse (F14.1-)
cocaine dependence (F14.2-)

TIP: Assign a substance use code only when the provider documents a relationship between the use and an associated physical, mental, or behavioral disorder. As with all diagnoses, substance use codes must meet the definition of a reportable diagnosis.

- **F14.90** Cocaine use, unspecified, uncomplicated
  - AHA: 2018,2Q,10-11
- **F14.91** Cocaine use, unspecified, in remission

✓6ᵗʰ F14.92 Cocaine use, unspecified with intoxication
- **F14.920** Cocaine use, unspecified with intoxication, uncomplicated [HCC] [ESR] [COM]
- **F14.921** Cocaine use, unspecified with intoxication delirium [HCC] [ESR] [COM]
- **F14.922** Cocaine use, unspecified with intoxication with perceptual disturbance [HCC] [ESR] [COM]
- **F14.929** Cocaine use, unspecified with intoxication, unspecified [HCC] [ESR] [COM]

- **F14.93** Cocaine use, unspecified with withdrawal [HCC] [ESR] [COM]
  - AHA: 2020,4Q,16-17

- **F14.94** Cocaine use, unspecified with cocaine-induced mood disorder [HCC] [ESR] [COM]
  - Cocaine induced bipolar or related disorder, without use disorder
  - Cocaine induced depressive disorder, without use disorder

---

[HCC] CMS-HCC [Rx] Rx HCC [ESR] ESRD HCC [COM] Commercial HCC [N] Newborn: 0 [P] Pediatric: 0-17 [M] Maternity: 9-64 [A] Adult: 15-124

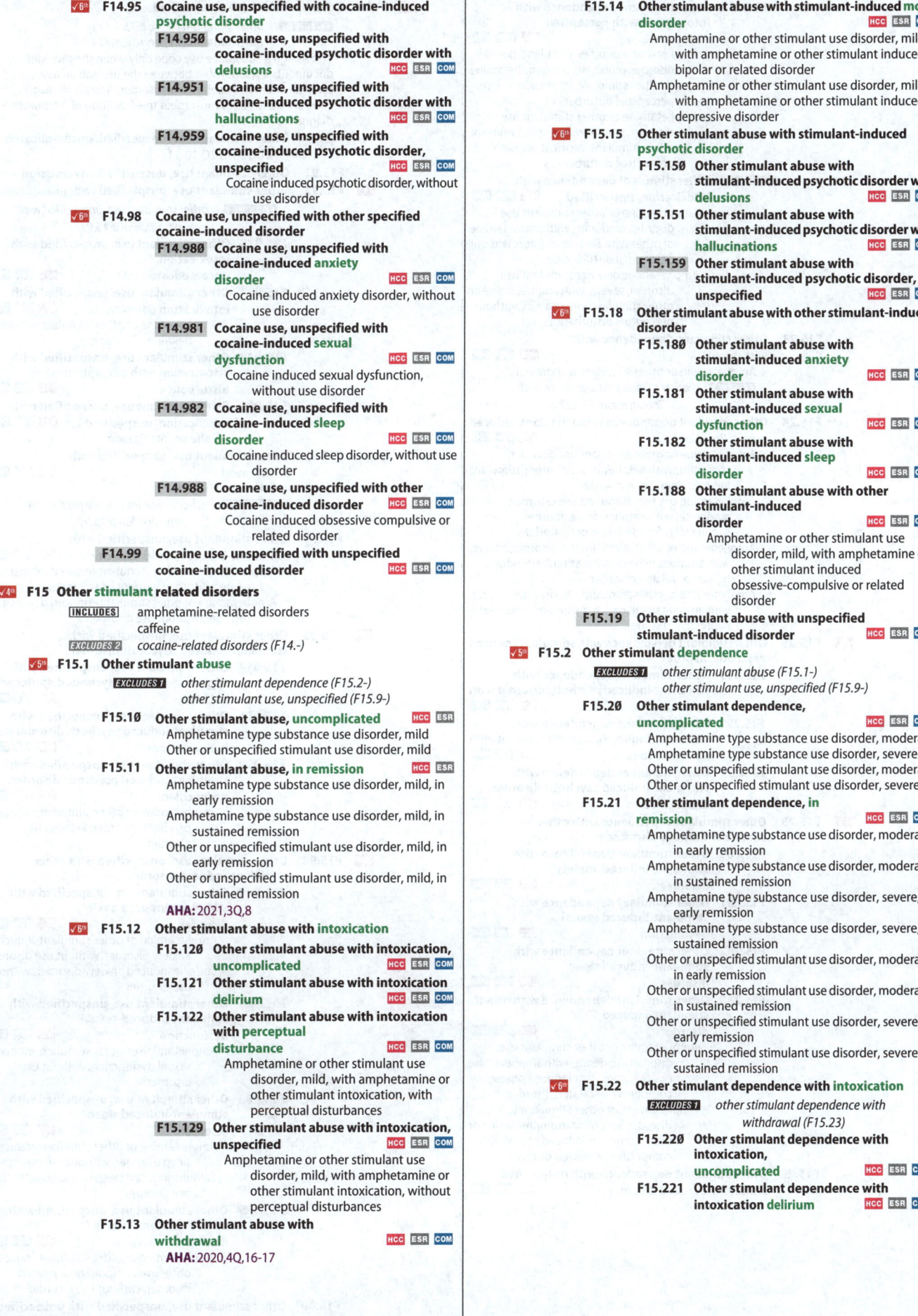

Chapter 5. Mental, Behavioral and Neurodevelopmental Disorders

F15.222 Other stimulant dependence with intoxication with perceptual disturbance `HCC` `ESR` `COM`
- Amphetamine or other stimulant use disorder, moderate, with amphetamine or other stimulant intoxication, with perceptual disturbances
- Amphetamine or other stimulant use disorder, severe, with amphetamine or other stimulant intoxication, with perceptual disturbances

F15.229 Other stimulant dependence with intoxication, unspecified `HCC` `ESR` `COM`
- Amphetamine or other stimulant use disorder, moderate, with amphetamine or other stimulant intoxication, without perceptual disturbances
- Amphetamine or other stimulant use disorder, severe, with amphetamine or other stimulant intoxication, without perceptual disturbances

F15.23 Other stimulant dependence with withdrawal `HCC` `ESR` `COM`
- Amphetamine or other stimulant withdrawal
- EXCLUDES 1: *other stimulant dependence with intoxication (F15.22-)*

F15.24 Other stimulant dependence with stimulant-induced mood disorder `HCC` `ESR` `COM`
- Amphetamine or other stimulant use disorder, moderate, with amphetamine or other stimulant induced depressive disorder
- Amphetamine or other stimulant use disorder, moderate, with amphetamine or other stimulant-induced bipolar or related disorder
- Amphetamine or other stimulant use disorder, severe, with amphetamine or other stimulant-induced bipolar or related disorder
- Amphetamine or other stimulant use disorder, severe, with amphetamine or other stimulant-induced depressive disorder

√6th **F15.25** Other stimulant dependence with stimulant-induced psychotic disorder
- **F15.250** Other stimulant dependence with stimulant-induced psychotic disorder with delusions `HCC` `ESR` `COM`
- **F15.251** Other stimulant dependence with stimulant-induced psychotic disorder with hallucinations `HCC` `ESR` `COM`
- **F15.259** Other stimulant dependence with stimulant-induced psychotic disorder, unspecified `HCC` `ESR` `COM`

√6th **F15.28** Other stimulant dependence with other stimulant-induced disorder
- **F15.280** Other stimulant dependence with stimulant-induced anxiety disorder `HCC` `ESR` `COM`
- **F15.281** Other stimulant dependence with stimulant-induced sexual dysfunction `HCC` `ESR` `COM`
- **F15.282** Other stimulant dependence with stimulant-induced sleep disorder `HCC` `ESR` `COM`
- **F15.288** Other stimulant dependence with other stimulant-induced disorder `HCC` `ESR` `COM`
  - Amphetamine or other stimulant use disorder, moderate, with amphetamine or other stimulant induced obsessive compulsive or related disorder
  - Amphetamine or other stimulant use disorder, severe, with amphetamine or other stimulant induced obsessive compulsive or related disorder

F15.29 Other stimulant dependence with unspecified stimulant-induced disorder `HCC` `ESR` `COM`

√5th **F15.9** Other stimulant use, unspecified
- EXCLUDES 1: *other stimulant abuse (F15.1-)*
  other stimulant dependence (F15.2-)
- **TIP:** Assign a substance use code only when the provider documents a relationship between the use and an associated physical, mental, or behavioral disorder. As with all diagnoses, substance use codes must meet the definition of a reportable diagnosis.

F15.90 Other stimulant use, unspecified, uncomplicated
- AHA: 2018,2Q,10-11

F15.91 Other stimulant use, unspecified, in remission

√6th **F15.92** Other stimulant use, unspecified with intoxication
- EXCLUDES 1: *other stimulant use, unspecified with withdrawal (F15.93)*
- **F15.920** Other stimulant use, unspecified with intoxication, uncomplicated `HCC` `ESR` `COM`
- **F15.921** Other stimulant use, unspecified with intoxication delirium `HCC` `ESR` `COM`
  - Amphetamine or other stimulant-induced delirium
- **F15.922** Other stimulant use, unspecified with intoxication with perceptual disturbance `HCC` `ESR` `COM`
- **F15.929** Other stimulant use, unspecified with intoxication, unspecified `HCC` `ESR` `COM`
  - Caffeine intoxication

F15.93 Other stimulant use, unspecified with withdrawal `HCC` `ESR` `COM`
- Caffeine withdrawal
- EXCLUDES 1: *other stimulant use, unspecified with intoxication (F15.92-)*

F15.94 Other stimulant use, unspecified with stimulant-induced mood disorder `HCC` `ESR` `COM`
- Amphetamine or other stimulant-induced bipolar or related disorder, without use disorder
- Amphetamine or other stimulant-induced depressive disorder, without use disorder

√6th **F15.95** Other stimulant use, unspecified with stimulant-induced psychotic disorder
- **F15.950** Other stimulant use, unspecified with stimulant-induced psychotic disorder with delusions `HCC` `ESR` `COM`
- **F15.951** Other stimulant use, unspecified with stimulant-induced psychotic disorder with hallucinations `HCC` `ESR` `COM`
- **F15.959** Other stimulant use, unspecified with stimulant-induced psychotic disorder, unspecified `HCC` `ESR` `COM`
  - Amphetamine or other stimulant-induced psychotic disorder, without use disorder

√6th **F15.98** Other stimulant use, unspecified with other stimulant-induced disorder
- **F15.980** Other stimulant use, unspecified with stimulant-induced anxiety disorder `HCC` `ESR` `COM`
  - Amphetamine or other stimulant-induced anxiety disorder, without use disorder
  - Caffeine induced anxiety disorder, without use disorder
- **F15.981** Other stimulant use, unspecified with stimulant-induced sexual dysfunction `HCC` `ESR` `COM`
  - Amphetamine or other stimulant-induced sexual dysfunction, without use disorder
- **F15.982** Other stimulant use, unspecified with stimulant-induced sleep disorder `HCC` `ESR` `COM`
  - Amphetamine or other stimulant-induced sleep disorder, without use disorder
  - Caffeine induced sleep disorder, without use disorder
- **F15.988** Other stimulant use, unspecified with other stimulant-induced disorder `HCC` `ESR` `COM`
  - Amphetamine or other stimulant-induced obsessive compulsive or related disorder, without use disorder

F15.99 Other stimulant use, unspecified with unspecified stimulant-induced disorder `HCC` `ESR` `COM`

`HCC` CMS-HCC   `Rx` Rx HCC   `ESR` ESRD HCC   `COM` Commercial HCC   **N** Newborn: 0   **P** Pediatric: 0-17   **M** Maternity: 9-64   **A** Adult: 15-124

F16 Hallucinogen related disorders

INCLUDES
- ecstasy
- PCP
- phencyclidine

AHA: 2018,4Q,31

F16.1 Hallucinogen abuse

EXCLUDES 1
- hallucinogen dependence (F16.2-)
- hallucinogen use, unspecified (F16.9-)

- **F16.10** Hallucinogen abuse, uncomplicated [HCC] [ESR]
  - Other hallucinogen use disorder, mild
  - Phencyclidine use disorder, mild

- **F16.11** Hallucinogen abuse, in remission [HCC] [ESR]
  - Other hallucinogen use disorder, mild, in early remission
  - Other hallucinogen use disorder, mild, in sustained remission
  - Phencyclidine use disorder, mild, in early remission
  - Phencyclidine use disorder, mild, in sustained remission

- **F16.12** Hallucinogen abuse with intoxication
  - **F16.120** Hallucinogen abuse with intoxication, uncomplicated [HCC] [ESR] [COM]
  - **F16.121** Hallucinogen abuse with intoxication with delirium [HCC] [ESR] [COM]
  - **F16.122** Hallucinogen abuse with intoxication with perceptual disturbance [HCC] [ESR] [COM]
  - **F16.129** Hallucinogen abuse with intoxication, unspecified [HCC] [ESR] [COM]

- **F16.14** Hallucinogen abuse with hallucinogen-induced mood disorder [HCC] [ESR] [COM]
  - Other hallucinogen use disorder, mild, with other hallucinogen induced bipolar or related disorder
  - Other hallucinogen use disorder, mild, with other hallucinogen induced depressive disorder
  - Phencyclidine use disorder, mild, with phencyclidine induced bipolar or related disorder
  - Phencyclidine use disorder, mild, with phencyclidine induced depressive disorder

- **F16.15** Hallucinogen abuse with hallucinogen-induced psychotic disorder
  - **F16.150** Hallucinogen abuse with hallucinogen-induced psychotic disorder with delusions [HCC] [ESR] [COM]
  - **F16.151** Hallucinogen abuse with hallucinogen-induced psychotic disorder with hallucinations [HCC] [ESR] [COM]
  - **F16.159** Hallucinogen abuse with hallucinogen-induced psychotic disorder, unspecified [HCC] [ESR] [COM]

- **F16.18** Hallucinogen abuse with other hallucinogen-induced disorder
  - **F16.180** Hallucinogen abuse with hallucinogen-induced anxiety disorder [HCC] [ESR] [COM]
  - **F16.183** Hallucinogen abuse with hallucinogen persisting perception disorder (flashbacks)
  - **F16.188** Hallucinogen abuse with other hallucinogen-induced disorder [HCC] [ESR] [COM]

- **F16.19** Hallucinogen abuse with unspecified hallucinogen-induced disorder [HCC] [ESR] [COM]

F16.2 Hallucinogen dependence

EXCLUDES 1
- hallucinogen abuse (F16.1-)
- hallucinogen use, unspecified (F16.9-)

- **F16.20** Hallucinogen dependence, uncomplicated [HCC] [ESR] [COM]
  - Other hallucinogen use disorder, moderate
  - Other hallucinogen use disorder, severe
  - Phencyclidine use disorder, moderate
  - Phencyclidine use disorder, severe

- **F16.21** Hallucinogen dependence, in remission [HCC] [ESR] [COM]
  - Other hallucinogen use disorder, moderate, in early remission
  - Other hallucinogen use disorder, moderate, in sustained remission
  - Other hallucinogen use disorder, severe, in early remission
  - Other hallucinogen use disorder, severe, in sustained remission
  - Phencyclidine use disorder, moderate, in early remission
  - Phencyclidine use disorder, moderate, in sustained remission
  - Phencyclidine use disorder, severe, in early remission
  - Phencyclidine use disorder, severe, in sustained remission

- **F16.22** Hallucinogen dependence with intoxication
  - **F16.220** Hallucinogen dependence with intoxication, uncomplicated [HCC] [ESR] [COM]
  - **F16.221** Hallucinogen dependence with intoxication with delirium [HCC] [ESR] [COM]
  - **F16.229** Hallucinogen dependence with intoxication, unspecified [HCC] [ESR] [COM]

- **F16.24** Hallucinogen dependence with hallucinogen-induced mood disorder [HCC] [ESR] [COM]
  - Other hallucinogen use disorder, moderate, with other hallucinogen induced bipolar or related disorder
  - Other hallucinogen use disorder, moderate, with other hallucinogen induced depressive disorder
  - Other hallucinogen use disorder, severe, with other hallucinogen-induced bipolar or related disorder
  - Other hallucinogen use disorder, severe, with other hallucinogen-induced depressive disorder
  - Phencyclidine use disorder, moderate, with phencyclidine induced bipolar or related disorder
  - Phencyclidine use disorder, moderate, with phencyclidine induced depressive disorder
  - Phencyclidine use disorder, severe, with phencyclidine induced bipolar or related disorder
  - Phencyclidine use disorder, severe, with phencyclidine-induced depressive disorder

- **F16.25** Hallucinogen dependence with hallucinogen-induced psychotic disorder
  - **F16.250** Hallucinogen dependence with hallucinogen-induced psychotic disorder with delusions [HCC] [ESR] [COM]
  - **F16.251** Hallucinogen dependence with hallucinogen-induced psychotic disorder with hallucinations [HCC] [ESR] [COM]
  - **F16.259** Hallucinogen dependence with hallucinogen-induced psychotic disorder, unspecified

- **F16.28** Hallucinogen dependence with other hallucinogen-induced disorder
  - **F16.280** Hallucinogen dependence with hallucinogen-induced anxiety disorder [HCC] [ESR] [COM]
  - **F16.283** Hallucinogen dependence with hallucinogen persisting perception disorder (flashbacks) [HCC] [ESR] [COM]
  - **F16.288** Hallucinogen dependence with other hallucinogen-induced disorder [HCC] [ESR] [COM]

- **F16.29** Hallucinogen dependence with unspecified hallucinogen-induced disorder [HCC] [ESR] [COM]

F16.9 Hallucinogen use, unspecified

EXCLUDES 1
- hallucinogen abuse (F16.1-)
- hallucinogen dependence (F16.2-)

TIP: Assign a substance use code only when the provider documents a relationship between the use and an associated physical, mental, or behavioral disorder. As with all diagnoses, substance use codes must meet the definition of a reportable diagnosis.

- **F16.90** Hallucinogen use, unspecified, uncomplicated
  - AHA: 2018,2Q,10-11
- **F16.91** Hallucinogen use, unspecified, in remission
- **F16.92** Hallucinogen use, unspecified with intoxication
  - **F16.920** Hallucinogen use, unspecified with intoxication, uncomplicated [HCC] [ESR] [COM]

F16.921 Hallucinogen use, unspecified with intoxication with delirium `HCC` `ESR` `COM`
 Other hallucinogen intoxication delirium
F16.929 Hallucinogen use, unspecified with intoxication, unspecified `HCC` `ESR` `COM`
F16.94 Hallucinogen use, unspecified with hallucinogen-induced mood disorder `HCC` `ESR` `COM`
 Other hallucinogen induced bipolar or related disorder, without use disorder
 Other hallucinogen induced depressive disorder, without use disorder
 Phencyclidine induced bipolar or related disorder, without use disorder
 Phencyclidine induced depressive disorder, without use disorder

✓6th **F16.95** Hallucinogen use, unspecified with hallucinogen-induced psychotic disorder
  F16.950 Hallucinogen use, unspecified with hallucinogen-induced psychotic disorder with delusions `HCC` `ESR` `COM`
  F16.951 Hallucinogen use, unspecified with hallucinogen-induced psychotic disorder with hallucinations `HCC` `ESR` `COM`
  F16.959 Hallucinogen use, unspecified with hallucinogen-induced psychotic disorder, unspecified `HCC` `ESR` `COM`
   Other hallucinogen induced psychotic disorder, without use disorder
   Phencyclidine induced psychotic disorder, without use disorder

✓6th **F16.98** Hallucinogen use, unspecified with other specified hallucinogen-induced disorder
  F16.980 Hallucinogen use, unspecified with hallucinogen-induced anxiety disorder `HCC` `ESR` `COM`
   Other hallucinogen-induced anxiety disorder, without use disorder
   Phencyclidine induced anxiety disorder, without use disorder
  F16.983 Hallucinogen use, unspecified with hallucinogen persisting perception disorder (flashbacks) `HCC` `ESR` `COM`
  F16.988 Hallucinogen use, unspecified with other hallucinogen-induced disorder `HCC` `ESR` `COM`
 F16.99 Hallucinogen use, unspecified with unspecified hallucinogen-induced disorder `HCC` `ESR` `COM`

✓4th **F17** Nicotine dependence
 EXCLUDES 1 history of tobacco dependence (Z87.891)
  tobacco use NOS (Z72.0)
 EXCLUDES 2 tobacco use (smoking) during pregnancy, childbirth and the puerperium (O99.33-)
  toxic effect of nicotine (T65.2-)
 AHA: 2013,4Q,108-109

✓5th **F17.2** Nicotine dependence
 ✓6th **F17.20** Nicotine dependence, unspecified
  F17.200 Nicotine dependence, unspecified, uncomplicated
   Tobacco use disorder, mild
   Tobacco use disorder, moderate
   Tobacco use disorder, severe
   AHA: 2016,1Q,36
   TIP: Assign when provider documentation indicates "smoker" without further specification.
  F17.201 Nicotine dependence, unspecified, in remission
   Tobacco use disorder, mild, in early remission
   Tobacco use disorder, mild, in sustained remission
   Tobacco use disorder, moderate, in early remission
   Tobacco use disorder, moderate, in sustained remission
   Tobacco use disorder, severe, in early remission
   Tobacco use disorder, severe, in sustained remission

  F17.203 Nicotine dependence unspecified, with withdrawal
   Tobacco withdrawal
  F17.208 Nicotine dependence, unspecified, with other nicotine-induced disorders
  F17.209 Nicotine dependence, unspecified, with unspecified nicotine-induced disorders
 ✓6th **F17.21** Nicotine dependence, cigarettes
  F17.210 Nicotine dependence, cigarettes, uncomplicated
   AHA: 2017,2Q,28-29
  F17.211 Nicotine dependence, cigarettes, in remission
   Tobacco use disorder, cigarettes, mild, in early remission
   Tobacco use disorder, cigarettes, mild, in sustained remission
   Tobacco use disorder, cigarettes, moderate, in early remission
   Tobacco use disorder, cigarettes, moderate, in sustained remission
   Tobacco use disorder, cigarettes, severe, in early remission
   Tobacco use disorder, cigarettes, severe, in sustained remission
  F17.213 Nicotine dependence, cigarettes, with withdrawal
  F17.218 Nicotine dependence, cigarettes, with other nicotine-induced disorders
  F17.219 Nicotine dependence, cigarettes, with unspecified nicotine-induced disorders
 ✓6th **F17.22** Nicotine dependence, chewing tobacco
  F17.220 Nicotine dependence, chewing tobacco, uncomplicated
  F17.221 Nicotine dependence, chewing tobacco, in remission
   Tobacco use disorder, chewing tobacco, mild, in early remission
   Tobacco use disorder, chewing tobacco, mild, in sustained remission
   Tobacco use disorder, chewing tobacco, moderate, in early remission
   Tobacco use disorder, chewing tobacco, moderate, in sustained remission
   Tobacco use disorder, chewing tobacco, severe, in early remission
   Tobacco use disorder, chewing tobacco, severe, in sustained remission
  F17.223 Nicotine dependence, chewing tobacco, with withdrawal
  F17.228 Nicotine dependence, chewing tobacco, with other nicotine-induced disorders
  F17.229 Nicotine dependence, chewing tobacco, with unspecified nicotine-induced disorders
 ✓6th **F17.29** Nicotine dependence, other tobacco product
  F17.290 Nicotine dependence, other tobacco product, uncomplicated
   AHA: 2017,2Q,28-29
  F17.291 Nicotine dependence, other tobacco product, in remission
   Tobacco use disorder, other tobacco product, mild, in early remission
   Tobacco use disorder, other tobacco product, mild, in sustained remission
   Tobacco use disorder, other tobacco product, moderate, in early remission
   Tobacco use disorder, other tobacco product, moderate, in sustained remission
   Tobacco use disorder, other tobacco product, severe, in early remission
   Tobacco use disorder, other tobacco product, severe, in sustained remission
  F17.293 Nicotine dependence, other tobacco product, with withdrawal
  F17.298 Nicotine dependence, other tobacco product, with other nicotine-induced disorders
  F17.299 Nicotine dependence, other tobacco product, with unspecified nicotine-induced disorders

F18 Inhalant related disorders
INCLUDES volatile solvents

F18.1 Inhalant abuse
EXCLUDES 1 inhalant dependence (F18.2-)
inhalant use, unspecified (F18.9-)

- **F18.10** Inhalant abuse, uncomplicated [HCC][ESR]
  Inhalant use disorder, mild
- **F18.11** Inhalant abuse, in remission [HCC][ESR]
  Inhalant use disorder, mild, in early remission
  Inhalant use disorder, mild, in sustained remission
- **F18.12** Inhalant abuse with intoxication
  - **F18.120** Inhalant abuse with intoxication, uncomplicated [HCC][ESR][COM]
  - **F18.121** Inhalant abuse with intoxication delirium [HCC][ESR][COM]
  - **F18.129** Inhalant abuse with intoxication, unspecified
- **F18.14** Inhalant abuse with inhalant-induced mood disorder [HCC][ESR][COM]
  Inhalant use disorder, mild, with inhalant induced depressive disorder
- **F18.15** Inhalant abuse with inhalant-induced psychotic disorder
  - **F18.150** Inhalant abuse with inhalant-induced psychotic disorder with delusions [HCC][ESR][COM]
  - **F18.151** Inhalant abuse with inhalant-induced psychotic disorder with hallucinations [HCC][ESR][COM]
  - **F18.159** Inhalant abuse with inhalant-induced psychotic disorder, unspecified [HCC][ESR][COM]
- **F18.17** Inhalant abuse with inhalant-induced dementia [HCC][ESR][COM]
  Inhalant use disorder, mild, with inhalant induced major neurocognitive disorder
- **F18.18** Inhalant abuse with other inhalant-induced disorders
  - **F18.180** Inhalant abuse with inhalant-induced anxiety disorder [HCC][ESR][COM]
  - **F18.188** Inhalant abuse with other inhalant-induced disorder
    Inhalant use disorder, mild, with inhalant induced mild neurocognitive disorder
- **F18.19** Inhalant abuse with unspecified inhalant-induced disorder [HCC][ESR][COM]

F18.2 Inhalant dependence
EXCLUDES 1 inhalant abuse (F18.1-)
inhalant use, unspecified (F18.9-)

- **F18.20** Inhalant dependence, uncomplicated [HCC][ESR]
  Inhalant use disorder, moderate
  Inhalant use disorder, severe
- **F18.21** Inhalant dependence, in remission [HCC][ESR]
  Inhalant use disorder, moderate, in early remission
  Inhalant use disorder, moderate, in sustained remission
  Inhalant use disorder, severe, in early remission
  Inhalant use disorder, severe, in sustained remission
- **F18.22** Inhalant dependence with intoxication
  - **F18.220** Inhalant dependence with intoxication, uncomplicated [HCC][ESR][COM]
  - **F18.221** Inhalant dependence with intoxication delirium [HCC][ESR][COM]
  - **F18.229** Inhalant dependence with intoxication, unspecified [HCC][ESR][COM]
- **F18.24** Inhalant dependence with inhalant-induced mood disorder [HCC][ESR][COM]
  Inhalant use disorder, moderate, with inhalant induced depressive disorder
  Inhalant use disorder, severe, with inhalant induced depressive disorder
- **F18.25** Inhalant dependence with inhalant-induced psychotic disorder
  - **F18.250** Inhalant dependence with inhalant-induced psychotic disorder with delusions [HCC][ESR][COM]
  - **F18.251** Inhalant dependence with inhalant-induced psychotic disorder with hallucinations [HCC][ESR][COM]
  - **F18.259** Inhalant dependence with inhalant-induced psychotic disorder, unspecified [HCC][ESR][COM]
- **F18.27** Inhalant dependence with inhalant-induced dementia [HCC][ESR][COM]
  Inhalant use disorder, moderate, with inhalant induced major neurocognitive disorder
  Inhalant use disorder, severe, with inhalant induced major neurocognitive disorder
- **F18.28** Inhalant dependence with other inhalant-induced disorders
  - **F18.280** Inhalant dependence with inhalant-induced anxiety disorder [HCC][ESR][COM]
  - **F18.288** Inhalant dependence with other inhalant-induced disorder
    Inhalant use disorder, moderate, with inhalant-induced mild neurocognitive disorder
    Inhalant use disorder, severe, with inhalant-induced mild neurocognitive disorder
- **F18.29** Inhalant dependence with unspecified inhalant-induced disorder [HCC][ESR][COM]

F18.9 Inhalant use, unspecified
EXCLUDES 1 inhalant abuse (F18.1-)
inhalant dependence (F18.2-)

TIP: Assign a substance use code only when the provider documents a relationship between the use and an associated physical, mental, or behavioral disorder. As with all diagnoses, substance use codes must meet the definition of a reportable diagnosis.

- **F18.90** Inhalant use, unspecified, uncomplicated
  AHA: 2018,2Q,10-11
- **F18.91** Inhalant use, unspecified, in remission
- **F18.92** Inhalant use, unspecified with intoxication
  - **F18.920** Inhalant use, unspecified with intoxication, uncomplicated [HCC][ESR][COM]
  - **F18.921** Inhalant use, unspecified with intoxication with delirium [HCC][ESR][COM]
  - **F18.929** Inhalant use, unspecified with intoxication, unspecified [HCC][ESR][COM]
- **F18.94** Inhalant use, unspecified with inhalant-induced mood disorder
  Inhalant induced depressive disorder
- **F18.95** Inhalant use, unspecified with inhalant-induced psychotic disorder
  - **F18.950** Inhalant use, unspecified with inhalant-induced psychotic disorder with delusions [HCC][ESR][COM]
  - **F18.951** Inhalant use, unspecified with inhalant-induced psychotic disorder with hallucinations [HCC][ESR][COM]
  - **F18.959** Inhalant use, unspecified with inhalant-induced psychotic disorder, unspecified [HCC][ESR][COM]
- **F18.97** Inhalant use, unspecified with inhalant-induced persisting dementia [HCC][ESR][COM]
  Inhalant-induced major neurocognitive disorder
- **F18.98** Inhalant use, unspecified with other inhalant-induced disorders
  - **F18.980** Inhalant use, unspecified with inhalant-induced anxiety disorder [HCC][ESR][COM]
  - **F18.988** Inhalant use, unspecified with other inhalant-induced disorder
    Inhalant-induced mild neurocognitive disorder
- **F18.99** Inhalant use, unspecified with unspecified inhalant-induced disorder [HCC][ESR][COM]

F19 Other psychoactive substance related disorders
INCLUDES polysubstance drug use (indiscriminate drug use)

F19.1 Other psychoactive substance abuse
EXCLUDES 1 other psychoactive substance dependence (F19.2-)
other psychoactive substance use, unspecified (F19.9-)

- **F19.10** Other psychoactive substance abuse, uncomplicated [HCC][ESR]
  Other (or unknown) substance use disorder, mild

F19.11 Other psychoactive substance abuse, in remission [HCC] [ESR]
  Other (or unknown) substance use disorder, mild, in early remission
  Other (or unknown) substance use disorder, mild, in sustained remission

✓6th **F19.12** Other psychoactive substance abuse with intoxication
  F19.120 Other psychoactive substance abuse with intoxication, uncomplicated [HCC] [ESR] [COM]
  F19.121 Other psychoactive substance abuse with intoxication delirium [HCC] [ESR] [COM]
  F19.122 Other psychoactive substance abuse with intoxication with perceptual disturbances [HCC] [ESR] [COM]
  F19.129 Other psychoactive substance abuse with intoxication, unspecified [HCC] [ESR] [COM]

✓6th **F19.13** Other psychoactive substance abuse with withdrawal
  AHA: 2020,4Q,16-17
  F19.130 Other psychoactive substance abuse with withdrawal, uncomplicated [HCC] [ESR] [COM]
  F19.131 Other psychoactive substance abuse with withdrawal delirium [HCC] [ESR] [COM]
  F19.132 Other psychoactive substance abuse with withdrawal with perceptual disturbance [HCC] [ESR] [COM]
  F19.139 Other psychoactive substance abuse with withdrawal, unspecified [HCC] [ESR] [COM]
    AHA: 2023,3Q,16

F19.14 Other psychoactive substance abuse with psychoactive substance-induced mood disorder [HCC] [ESR] [COM]
  Other (or unknown) substance use disorder, mild, with other (or unknown) substance-induced bipolar or related disorder
  Other (or unknown) substance use disorder, mild, with other (or unknown) substance-induced depressive disorder

✓6th **F19.15** Other psychoactive substance abuse with psychoactive substance-induced psychotic disorder
  F19.150 Other psychoactive substance abuse with psychoactive substance-induced psychotic disorder with delusions [HCC] [ESR] [COM]
  F19.151 Other psychoactive substance abuse with psychoactive substance-induced psychotic disorder with hallucinations [HCC] [ESR] [COM]
  F19.159 Other psychoactive substance abuse with psychoactive substance-induced psychotic disorder, unspecified [HCC] [ESR] [COM]

F19.16 Other psychoactive substance abuse with psychoactive substance-induced persisting amnestic disorder [HCC] [ESR] [COM]

F19.17 Other psychoactive substance abuse with psychoactive substance-induced persisting dementia [HCC] [ESR] [COM]
  Other (or unknown) substance use disorder, mild, with other (or unknown) substance-induced major neurocognitive disorder

✓6th **F19.18** Other psychoactive substance abuse with other psychoactive substance-induced disorders
  F19.180 Other psychoactive substance abuse with psychoactive substance-induced anxiety disorder [HCC] [ESR] [COM]
  F19.181 Other psychoactive substance abuse with psychoactive substance-induced sexual dysfunction [HCC] [ESR] [COM]
  F19.182 Other psychoactive substance abuse with psychoactive substance-induced sleep disorder [HCC] [ESR] [COM]
  F19.188 Other psychoactive substance abuse with other psychoactive substance-induced disorder [HCC] [ESR] [COM]
    Other (or unknown) substance use disorder, mild, with other (or unknown) substance induced mild neurocognitive disorder
    Other (or unknown) substance use disorder, mild, with other (or unknown) substance induced obsessive-compulsive or related disorder

F19.19 Other psychoactive substance abuse with unspecified psychoactive substance-induced disorder [HCC] [ESR] [COM]

✓5th **F19.2** Other psychoactive substance dependence
  EXCLUDES 1 other psychoactive substance abuse (F19.1-)
              other psychoactive substance use, unspecified (F19.9-)

  F19.20 Other psychoactive substance dependence, uncomplicated [HCC] [ESR] [COM]
    Other (or unknown) substance use disorder, moderate
    Other (or unknown) substance use disorder, severe

  F19.21 Other psychoactive substance dependence, in remission [HCC] [ESR] [COM]
    Other (or unknown) substance use disorder, moderate, in early remission
    Other (or unknown) substance use disorder, moderate, in sustained remission
    Other (or unknown) substance use disorder, severe, in early remission
    Other (or unknown) substance use disorder, severe, in sustained remission

  ✓6th **F19.22** Other psychoactive substance dependence with intoxication
    EXCLUDES 1 other psychoactive substance dependence with withdrawal (F19.23-)
    F19.220 Other psychoactive substance dependence with intoxication, uncomplicated [HCC] [ESR] [COM]
    F19.221 Other psychoactive substance dependence with intoxication delirium [HCC] [ESR] [COM]
    F19.222 Other psychoactive substance dependence with intoxication with perceptual disturbance [HCC] [ESR] [COM]
    F19.229 Other psychoactive substance dependence with intoxication, unspecified [HCC] [ESR] [COM]

  ✓6th **F19.23** Other psychoactive substance dependence with withdrawal
    EXCLUDES 1 other psychoactive substance dependence with intoxication (F19.22-)
    F19.230 Other psychoactive substance dependence with withdrawal, uncomplicated [HCC] [ESR] [COM]
    F19.231 Other psychoactive substance dependence with withdrawal delirium [HCC] [ESR] [COM]
    F19.232 Other psychoactive substance dependence with withdrawal with perceptual disturbance [HCC] [ESR] [COM]
    F19.239 Other psychoactive substance dependence with withdrawal, unspecified [HCC] [ESR] [COM]

  F19.24 Other psychoactive substance dependence with psychoactive substance-induced mood disorder [HCC] [ESR] [COM]
    Other (or unknown) substance use disorder, moderate, with other (or unknown) substance induced bipolar or related disorder
    Other (or unknown) substance use disorder, moderate, with other (or unknown) substance induced depressive disorder
    Other (or unknown) substance use disorder, severe, with other (or unknown) substance induced bipolar or related disorder
    Other (or unknown) substance use disorder, severe, with other (or unknown) substance induced depressive disorder

  ✓6th **F19.25** Other psychoactive substance dependence with psychoactive substance-induced psychotic disorder
    F19.250 Other psychoactive substance dependence with psychoactive substance-induced psychotic disorder with delusions [HCC] [ESR] [COM]

[HCC] CMS-HCC [Rx] Rx HCC [ESR] ESRD HCC [COM] Commercial HCC [N] Newborn: 0 [P] Pediatric: 0-17 [M] Maternity: 9-64 [A] Adult: 15-124

F19.251 Other psychoactive substance dependence with psychoactive substance-induced psychotic disorder with hallucinations

F19.259 Other psychoactive substance dependence with psychoactive substance-induced psychotic disorder, unspecified

F19.26 Other psychoactive substance dependence with psychoactive substance-induced persisting amnestic disorder

F19.27 Other psychoactive substance dependence with psychoactive substance-induced persisting dementia
- Other (or unknown) substance use disorder, moderate, with other (or unknown) substance induced major neurocognitive disorder
- Other (or unknown) substance use disorder, severe, with other (or unknown) substance induced major neurocognitive disorder

F19.28 Other psychoactive substance dependence with other psychoactive substance-induced disorders

F19.280 Other psychoactive substance dependence with psychoactive substance-induced anxiety disorder

F19.281 Other psychoactive substance dependence with psychoactive substance-induced sexual dysfunction

F19.282 Other psychoactive substance dependence with psychoactive substance-induced sleep disorder

F19.288 Other psychoactive substance dependence with other psychoactive substance-induced disorder
- Other (or unknown) substance use disorder, moderate, with other (or unknown) substance induced mild neurocognitive disorder
- Other (or unknown) substance use disorder, moderate, with other (or unknown) substance induced obsessive compulsive or related disorder
- Other (or unknown) substance use disorder, severe, with other (or unknown) substance induced mild neurocognitive disorder
- Other (or unknown) substance use disorder, severe, with other (or unknown) substance induced obsessive-compulsive or related disorder

F19.29 Other psychoactive substance dependence with unspecified psychoactive substance-induced disorder

F19.9 Other psychoactive substance use, unspecified
EXCLUDES 1: *other psychoactive substance abuse (F19.1-)*
other psychoactive substance dependence (F19.2-)
TIP: Assign a substance use code only when the provider documents a relationship between the use and an associated physical, mental, or behavioral disorder. As with all diagnoses, substance use codes must meet the definition of a reportable diagnosis.

F19.90 Other psychoactive substance use, unspecified, uncomplicated
AHA: 2018,2Q,10-11

F19.91 Other psychoactive substance use, unspecified, in remission

F19.92 Other psychoactive substance use, unspecified with intoxication
EXCLUDES 1: *other psychoactive substance use, unspecified with withdrawal (F19.93)*

F19.920 Other psychoactive substance use, unspecified with intoxication, uncomplicated

F19.921 Other psychoactive substance use, unspecified with intoxication with delirium
- Other (or unknown) substance-induced delirium

F19.922 Other psychoactive substance use, unspecified with intoxication with perceptual disturbance

F19.929 Other psychoactive substance use, unspecified with intoxication, unspecified

F19.93 Other psychoactive substance use, unspecified with withdrawal
EXCLUDES 1: *other psychoactive substance use, unspecified with intoxication (F19.92-)*

F19.930 Other psychoactive substance use, unspecified with withdrawal, uncomplicated

F19.931 Other psychoactive substance use, unspecified with withdrawal delirium

F19.932 Other psychoactive substance use, unspecified with withdrawal with perceptual disturbance

F19.939 Other psychoactive substance use, unspecified with withdrawal, unspecified

F19.94 Other psychoactive substance use, unspecified with psychoactive substance-induced mood disorder
- Other (or unknown) substance-induced bipolar or related disorder, without use disorder
- Other (or unknown) substance-induced depressive disorder, without use disorder

F19.95 Other psychoactive substance use, unspecified with psychoactive substance-induced psychotic disorder

F19.950 Other psychoactive substance use, unspecified with psychoactive substance-induced psychotic disorder with delusions

F19.951 Other psychoactive substance use, unspecified with psychoactive substance-induced psychotic disorder with hallucinations

F19.959 Other psychoactive substance use, unspecified with psychoactive substance-induced psychotic disorder, unspecified
- Other or unknown substance-induced psychotic disorder, without use disorder

F19.96 Other psychoactive substance use, unspecified with psychoactive substance-induced persisting amnestic disorder

F19.97 Other psychoactive substance use, unspecified with psychoactive substance-induced persisting dementia
- Other (or unknown) substance-induced major neurocognitive disorder, without use disorder

F19.98 Other psychoactive substance use, unspecified with other psychoactive substance-induced disorders

F19.980 Other psychoactive substance use, unspecified with psychoactive substance-induced anxiety disorder
- Other (or unknown) substance-induced anxiety disorder, without use disorder

F19.981 Other psychoactive substance use, unspecified with psychoactive substance-induced sexual dysfunction
- Other (or unknown) substance-induced sexual dysfunction, without use disorder

F19.982 Other psychoactive substance use, unspecified with psychoactive substance-induced sleep disorder
- Other (or unknown) substance-induced sleep disorder, without use disorder

F19.988 Other psychoactive substance use, unspecified with other psychoactive substance-induced disorder
- Other (or unknown) substance-induced mild neurocognitive disorder, without use disorder
- Other (or unknown) substance-induced obsessive-compulsive or related disorder, without use disorder

F19.99 Other psychoactive substance use, unspecified with unspecified psychoactive substance-induced disorder [HCC] [ESR] [COM]

Schizophrenia, schizotypal, delusional, and other non-mood psychotic disorders (F20-F29)

✓4th **F20 Schizophrenia**
Use additional code, if applicable, to identify:
other specified cognitive deficit (R41.84-)
EXCLUDES 1 brief psychotic disorder (F23)
cyclic schizophrenia (F25.0)
mood [affective] disorders with psychotic symptoms (F30.2, F31.2, F31.5, F31.64, F32.3, F33.3)
schizoaffective disorder (F25.-)
schizophrenic reaction NOS (F23)
EXCLUDES 2 schizophrenic reaction in:
alcoholism (F10.15-, F10.25-, F10.95-)
brain disease (F06.2)
epilepsy (F06.2)
psychoactive drug use (F11-F19 with .15. .25, .95)
schizotypal disorder (F21)
DEF: Group of disorders with disturbances in thought (delusions, hallucinations), mood (blunted, flattened, inappropriate affect), and sense of self. Schizophrenia also includes bizarre, purposeless behavior, repetitious activity, or inactivity.

F20.0 Paranoid schizophrenia [HCC] [Rx] [ESR] [COM]
Paraphrenic schizophrenia
EXCLUDES 1 involutional paranoid state (F22)
paranoia (F22)
DEF: Preoccupied with delusional suspicions and auditory hallucinations related to a single theme. This type of schizophrenia is usually hostile, grandiose, threatening, persecutory, and occasionally hypochondriacal.

F20.1 Disorganized schizophrenia [HCC] [Rx] [ESR] [COM]
Hebephrenia
Hebephrenic schizophrenia

F20.2 Catatonic schizophrenia [HCC] [Rx] [ESR] [COM]
Schizophrenic catalepsy
Schizophrenic catatonia
Schizophrenic flexibilitas cerea
EXCLUDES 1 catatonic stupor (R40.1)
DEF: Extreme changes in motor activity. One extreme is a decreased response or reaction to the environment and the other is spontaneous activity.

F20.3 Undifferentiated schizophrenia [HCC] [Rx] [ESR] [COM]
Atypical schizophrenia
EXCLUDES 1 acute schizophrenia-like psychotic disorder (F23)
EXCLUDES 2 post-schizophrenic depression (F32.89)

F20.5 Residual schizophrenia [HCC] [Rx] [ESR] [COM]
Restzustand (schizophrenic)
Schizophrenic residual state

✓5th **F20.8 Other schizophrenia**

F20.81 Schizophreniform disorder [HCC] [Rx] [ESR] [COM]
Schizophreniform psychosis NOS

F20.89 Other schizophrenia
Cenesthopathic schizophrenia
Simple schizophrenia

F20.9 Schizophrenia, unspecified [HCC] [Rx] [ESR] [COM]
AHA: 2019,2Q,32

F21 Schizotypal disorder [HCC] [Rx] [ESR] [COM]
Borderline schizophrenia
Latent schizophrenia
Latent schizophrenic reaction
Prepsychotic schizophrenia
Prodromal schizophrenia
Pseudoneurotic schizophrenia
Pseudopsychopathic schizophrenia
Schizotypal personality disorder
EXCLUDES 2 Asperger's syndrome (F84.5)
schizoid personality disorder (F60.1)
DEF: Disorder characterized by various oddities of thinking, perception, communication, and behavior that may be manifested as magical thinking, ideas of reference, paranoid ideation, recurrent illusions and derealization (depersonalization), or social isolation.

F22 Delusional disorders [HCC] [Rx] [ESR] [COM]
Delusional dysmorphophobia
Involutional paranoid state
Paranoia
Paranoia querulans
Paranoid psychosis
Paranoid state
Paraphrenia (late)
Sensitiver Beziehungswahn
EXCLUDES 1 mood [affective] disorders with psychotic symptoms (F30.2, F31.2, F31.5, F31.64, F32.3, F33.3)
paranoid schizophrenia (F20.0)
EXCLUDES 2 paranoid personality disorder (F60.0)
paranoid psychosis, psychogenic (F23)
paranoid reaction (F23)

F23 Brief psychotic disorder [HCC] [Rx] [ESR] [COM]
Paranoid reaction
Psychogenic paranoid psychosis
EXCLUDES 2 mood [affective] disorders with psychotic symptoms (F30.2, F31.2, F31.5, F31.64, F32.3, F33.3)
AHA: 2019,2Q,32

F24 Shared psychotic disorder [HCC] [Rx] [ESR] [COM]
Folie à deux
Induced paranoid disorder
Induced psychotic disorder

✓4th **F25 Schizoaffective disorders**
EXCLUDES 1 mood [affective] disorders with psychotic symptoms (F30.2, F31.2, F31.5, F31.64, F32.3, F33.3)
schizophrenia (F20.-)

F25.0 Schizoaffective disorder, bipolar type [HCC] [Rx] [ESR] [COM]
Cyclic schizophrenia
Schizoaffective disorder, manic type
Schizoaffective disorder, mixed type
Schizoaffective psychosis, bipolar type

F25.1 Schizoaffective disorder, depressive type [HCC] [Rx] [ESR] [COM]
Schizoaffective psychosis, depressive type

F25.8 Other schizoaffective disorders [HCC] [Rx] [ESR] [COM]

F25.9 Schizoaffective disorder, unspecified [HCC] [Rx] [ESR] [COM]
Schizoaffective psychosis NOS

F28 Other psychotic disorder not due to a substance or known physiological condition [HCC] [Rx] [ESR] [COM]
Chronic hallucinatory psychosis
Other specified schizophrenia spectrum and other psychotic disorder

F29 Unspecified psychosis not due to a substance or known physiological condition [HCC] [Rx] [ESR] [COM]
Psychosis NOS
Unspecified schizophrenia spectrum and other psychotic disorder
EXCLUDES 1 mental disorder NOS (F99)
unspecified mental disorder due to known physiological condition (F09)

Mood [affective] disorders (F30-F39)

✓4th **F30 Manic episode**
INCLUDES bipolar disorder, single manic episode
mixed affective episode
EXCLUDES 1 bipolar disorder (F31.-)
major depressive disorder, recurrent (F33.-)
major depressive disorder, single episode (F32.-)
DEF: Mania: Characterized by abnormal states of elation or excitement out of keeping with the individual's circumstances and varying from enhanced liveliness (hypomania) to violent, almost uncontrollable, excitement. Aggression and anger, flight of ideas, distractibility, impaired judgment, and grandiose ideas are common.

✓5th **F30.1 Manic episode without psychotic symptoms**

F30.10 Manic episode without psychotic symptoms, unspecified [HCC] [Rx] [ESR] [COM] [Q]

F30.11 Manic episode without psychotic symptoms, mild [HCC] [Rx] [ESR] [COM] [Q]

F30.12 Manic episode without psychotic symptoms, moderate [HCC] [Rx] [ESR] [COM] [Q]

F30.13 Manic episode, severe, without psychotic symptoms [HCC] [Rx] [ESR] [COM] [Q]

F30.2 Manic episode, severe with psychotic symptoms [HCC] [Rx] [ESR] [COM] [Q]
Mania with mood-congruent psychotic symptoms
Mania with mood-incongruent psychotic symptoms
Manic stupor

F30.3 Manic episode in partial remission [HCC] [Rx] [ESR] [COM] [Q]

[HCC] CMS-HCC   [Rx] Rx HCC   [ESR] ESRD HCC   [COM] Commercial HCC   [N] Newborn: 0   [P] Pediatric: 0-17   [M] Maternity: 9-64   [A] Adult: 15-124

Chapter 5. Mental, Behavioral and Neurodevelopmental Disorders

F30.4 Manic episode in full remission
F30.8 Other manic episodes
 Hypomania
F30.9 Manic episode, unspecified
 Mania NOS

F31 Bipolar disorder
INCLUDES
 bipolar I disorder
 bipolar type I disorder
 manic-depressive illness
 manic-depressive psychosis
 manic-depressive reaction
 seasonal bipolar disorder
EXCLUDES 1
 bipolar disorder, single manic episode (F30.-)
 major depressive disorder, recurrent (F33.-)
 major depressive disorder, single episode (F32.-)
EXCLUDES 2 cyclothymia (F34.0)
AHA: 2020,1Q,23

F31.0 Bipolar disorder, current episode hypomanic
F31.1 Bipolar disorder, current episode manic without psychotic features
 F31.10 Bipolar disorder, current episode manic without psychotic features, unspecified
 F31.11 Bipolar disorder, current episode manic without psychotic features, mild
 F31.12 Bipolar disorder, current episode manic without psychotic features, moderate
 F31.13 Bipolar disorder, current episode manic without psychotic features, severe
F31.2 Bipolar disorder, current episode manic severe with psychotic features
 Bipolar disorder, current episode manic with mood-congruent psychotic symptoms
 Bipolar disorder, current episode manic with mood-incongruent psychotic symptoms
 Bipolar I disorder, current or most recent episode manic with psychotic features
F31.3 Bipolar disorder, current episode depressed, mild or moderate severity
 F31.30 Bipolar disorder, current episode depressed, mild or moderate severity, unspecified
 F31.31 Bipolar disorder, current episode depressed, mild
 F31.32 Bipolar disorder, current episode depressed, moderate
F31.4 Bipolar disorder, current episode depressed, severe, without psychotic features
F31.5 Bipolar disorder, current episode depressed, severe, with psychotic features
 Bipolar disorder, current episode depressed with mood-congruent psychotic symptoms
 Bipolar disorder, current episode depressed with mood-incongruent psychotic symptoms
 Bipolar I disorder, current or most recent episode depressed, with psychotic features
F31.6 Bipolar disorder, current episode mixed
 F31.60 Bipolar disorder, current episode mixed, unspecified
 F31.61 Bipolar disorder, current episode mixed, mild
 F31.62 Bipolar disorder, current episode mixed, moderate
 F31.63 Bipolar disorder, current episode mixed, severe, without psychotic features
 F31.64 Bipolar disorder, current episode mixed, severe, with psychotic features
 Bipolar disorder, current episode mixed with mood-congruent psychotic symptoms
 Bipolar disorder, current episode mixed with mood-incongruent psychotic symptoms
F31.7 Bipolar disorder, currently in remission
 F31.70 Bipolar disorder, currently in remission, most recent episode unspecified
 F31.71 Bipolar disorder, in partial remission, most recent episode hypomanic
 F31.72 Bipolar disorder, in full remission, most recent episode hypomanic
 F31.73 Bipolar disorder, in partial remission, most recent episode manic
 F31.74 Bipolar disorder, in full remission, most recent episode manic
 F31.75 Bipolar disorder, in partial remission, most recent episode depressed
 F31.76 Bipolar disorder, in full remission, most recent episode depressed
 F31.77 Bipolar disorder, in partial remission, most recent episode mixed
 F31.78 Bipolar disorder, in full remission, most recent episode mixed
F31.8 Other bipolar disorders
 F31.81 Bipolar II disorder
 Bipolar disorder, type 2
 F31.89 Other bipolar disorder
 Recurrent manic episodes NOS
F31.9 Bipolar disorder, unspecified
 Manic depression
 AHA: 2020,1Q,23

F32 Depressive episode
INCLUDES
 single episode of agitated depression
 single episode of depressive reaction
 single episode of major depression
 single episode of psychogenic depression
 single episode of reactive depression
 single episode of vital depression
EXCLUDES 1
 bipolar disorder (F31.-)
 manic episode (F30.-)
 recurrent depressive disorder (F33.-)
EXCLUDES 2 adjustment disorder (F43.2)
AHA: 2020,1Q,23
DEF: Mood disorder that produces depression that may exhibit as sadness, low self-esteem, or guilt feelings. Other manifestations may be withdrawal from friends and family and interrupted sleep.

F32.0 Major depressive disorder, single episode, mild
F32.1 Major depressive disorder, single episode, moderate
F32.2 Major depressive disorder, single episode, severe without psychotic features
 AHA: 2024,4Q,14
F32.3 Major depressive disorder, single episode, severe with psychotic features
 Single episode of major depression with mood-congruent psychotic symptoms
 Single episode of major depression with mood-incongruent psychotic symptoms
 Single episode of major depression with psychotic symptoms
 Single episode of psychogenic depressive psychosis
 Single episode of psychotic depression
 Single episode of reactive depressive psychosis
F32.4 Major depressive disorder, single episode, in partial remission
F32.5 Major depressive disorder, single episode, in full remission
F32.8 Other depressive episodes
 AHA: 2016,4Q,14
 F32.81 Premenstrual dysphoric disorder
 EXCLUDES 1 premenstrual tension syndrome (N94.3)
 DEF: Severe manifestation of premenstrual syndrome (PMS) that can be disabling and destructive to day-to-day activities. It can exacerbate pre-existing emotional disorders, like depression and anxiety, and cause feelings of loss of control, fatigue, and irritability.
 F32.89 Other specified depressive episodes
 Atypical depression
 Post-schizophrenic depression
 Single episode of 'masked' depression NOS
F32.9 Major depressive disorder, single episode, unspecified
 Major depression NOS
 AHA: 2021,4Q,10; 2021,1Q,10; 2013,4Q,107
F32.A Depression, unspecified
 Depression NOS
 Depressive disorder NOS
 AHA: 2021,4Q,9-10

F33 Major depressive disorder, recurrent

INCLUDES
- recurrent episodes of depressive reaction
- recurrent episodes of endogenous depression
- recurrent episodes of major depression
- recurrent episodes of psychogenic depression
- recurrent episodes of reactive depression
- recurrent episodes of seasonal affective disorder
- recurrent episodes of seasonal depressive disorder
- recurrent episodes of vital depression

EXCLUDES 1
- bipolar disorder (F31.-)
- manic episode (F30.-)

AHA: 2020,1Q,23

DEF: Mood disorder that produces depression that may exhibit as sadness, low self-esteem, or guilt feelings. Other manifestations may be withdrawal from friends and family and interrupted sleep.

- **F33.0** Major depressive disorder, recurrent, mild
- **F33.1** Major depressive disorder, recurrent, moderate
- **F33.2** Major depressive disorder, recurrent, severe without psychotic features
- **F33.3** Major depressive disorder, recurrent, severe with psychotic symptoms
  - Endogenous depression with psychotic symptoms
  - Major depressive disorder, recurrent, with psychotic features
  - Recurrent severe episodes of major depression with mood-congruent psychotic symptoms
  - Recurrent severe episodes of major depression with mood-incongruent psychotic symptoms
  - Recurrent severe episodes of major depression with psychotic symptoms
  - Recurrent severe episodes of psychogenic depressive psychosis
  - Recurrent severe episodes of psychotic depression
  - Recurrent severe episodes of reactive depressive psychosis
- **F33.4** Major depressive disorder, recurrent, in remission
  - **F33.40** Major depressive disorder, recurrent, in remission, unspecified
  - **F33.41** Major depressive disorder, recurrent, in partial remission
  - **F33.42** Major depressive disorder, recurrent, in full remission
- **F33.8** Other recurrent depressive disorders
  - Recurrent brief depressive episodes
- **F33.9** Major depressive disorder, recurrent, unspecified
  - Monopolar depression NOS

F34 Persistent mood [affective] disorders

- **F34.0** Cyclothymic disorder
  - Affective personality disorder
  - Cycloid personality
  - Cyclothymia
  - Cyclothymic personality
  - **DEF:** Mood disorder characterized by fast and repeated alterations between hypomanic and depressed moods.
- **F34.1** Dysthymic disorder
  - Depressive neurosis
  - Depressive personality disorder
  - Dysthymia
  - Neurotic depression
  - Persistent anxiety depression
  - Persistent depressive disorder
  - **EXCLUDES 2**: anxiety depression (mild or not persistent) (F41.8)
  - **DEF:** Depression without psychosis. It is a less severe but persistent depression and is considered a mild to moderate chronic form of depression.
- **F34.8** Other persistent mood [affective] disorders
  - **AHA:** 2016,4Q,14
  - **F34.81** Disruptive mood dysregulation disorder
  - **F34.89** Other specified persistent mood disorders
- **F34.9** Persistent mood [affective] disorder, unspecified

F39 Unspecified mood [affective] disorder
Affective psychosis NOS

Anxiety, dissociative, stress-related, somatoform and other nonpsychotic mental disorders (F40-F48)

F40 Phobic anxiety disorders

DEF: Phobia: Broad-range anxiety with abnormally intense dread of certain objects or specific situations that would not normally have that effect.

- **F40.0** Agoraphobia
  - **DEF:** Profound anxiety or fear of leaving familiar settings like home, or being in unfamiliar locations or with strangers or crowds. Agoraphobia may or may not be preceded by recurrent panic attacks.
  - **F40.00** Agoraphobia, unspecified
  - **F40.01** Agoraphobia with panic disorder
    - Panic disorder with agoraphobia
    - **EXCLUDES 1** panic disorder without agoraphobia (F41.0)
  - **F40.02** Agoraphobia without panic disorder
- **F40.1** Social phobias
  - Anthropophobia
  - Social anxiety disorder
  - Social anxiety disorder of childhood
  - Social neurosis
  - **F40.10** Social phobia, unspecified
  - **F40.11** Social phobia, generalized
- **F40.2** Specific (isolated) phobias
  - **EXCLUDES 2** dysmorphophobia (nondelusional) (F45.22)
    - nosophobia (F45.22)
  - **F40.21** Animal type phobia
    - **F40.210** Arachnophobia
      - Fear of spiders
    - **F40.218** Other animal type phobia
  - **F40.22** Natural environment type phobia
    - **F40.220** Fear of thunderstorms
    - **F40.228** Other natural environment type phobia
  - **F40.23** Blood, injection, injury type phobia
    - **F40.230** Fear of blood
    - **F40.231** Fear of injections and transfusions
    - **F40.232** Fear of other medical care
    - **F40.233** Fear of injury
  - **F40.24** Situational type phobia
    - **F40.240** Claustrophobia
    - **F40.241** Acrophobia
    - **F40.242** Fear of bridges
    - **F40.243** Fear of flying
    - **F40.248** Other situational type phobia
  - **F40.29** Other specified phobia
    - **F40.290** Androphobia
      - Fear of men
    - **F40.291** Gynephobia
      - Fear of women
    - **F40.298** Other specified phobia
- **F40.8** Other phobic anxiety disorders
  - Phobic anxiety disorder of childhood
- **F40.9** Phobic anxiety disorder, unspecified
  - Phobia NOS
  - Phobic state NOS

F41 Other anxiety disorders

EXCLUDES 2 anxiety in:
- separation anxiety (F93.0)
- acute stress reaction (F43.0)
- neurasthenia (F48.8)
- psychophysiologic disorders (F45.-)
- transient adjustment reaction (F43.2)

- **F41.0** Panic disorder [episodic paroxysmal anxiety]
  - Panic attack
  - Panic state
  - **EXCLUDES 1** panic disorder with agoraphobia (F40.01)
  - **DEF:** Neurotic disorder characterized by recurrent panic or anxiety, apprehension, fear, or terror. Symptoms include shortness of breath, palpitations, dizziness, and shakiness; fear of dying may persist.

Chapter 5. Mental, Behavioral and Neurodevelopmental Disorders

F41.1 **Generalized anxiety disorder** [Rx]
  Anxiety neurosis
  Anxiety reaction
  Anxiety state
  Overanxious disorder
  EXCLUDES 2: neurasthenia (F48.8)

F41.3 **Other mixed anxiety disorders**

F41.8 **Other specified anxiety disorders**
  Anxiety depression (mild or not persistent)
  Anxiety hysteria
  Mixed anxiety and depressive disorder
  AHA: 2021,1Q,10

F41.9 **Anxiety disorder, unspecified**
  Anxiety NOS
  AHA: 2021,1Q,10

✓4th F42 Obsessive-compulsive disorder
  EXCLUDES 2: obsessive-compulsive personality (disorder) (F60.5)
  obsessive-compulsive symptoms occurring in depression ►(F32.-, F33.-)◄
  obsessive-compulsive symptoms occurring in schizophrenia (F20.-)
  AHA: 2016,4Q,14-15

  F42.2 **Mixed obsessional thoughts and acts** [Rx]
  F42.3 **Hoarding disorder** [Rx]
  F42.4 **Excoriation (skin-picking) disorder** [Rx]
    EXCLUDES 1: factitial dermatitis (L98.1)
    other specified behavioral and emotional disorders with onset usually occurring in early childhood and adolescence (F98.8)
  F42.8 **Other obsessive-compulsive disorder** [Rx]
    Anancastic neurosis
    Obsessive-compulsive neurosis
  F42.9 **Obsessive-compulsive disorder, unspecified** [Rx]

✓4th F43 Reaction to severe stress, and adjustment disorders
  F43.0 **Acute stress reaction**
    Acute crisis reaction
    Acute reaction to stress
    Combat and operational stress reaction
    Combat fatigue
    Crisis state
    Psychic shock

  ### ✓5th **F43.1** **Post-traumatic stress disorder (PTSD)**
    Traumatic neurosis
    DEF: Preoccupation with traumatic events beyond normal experience (i.e., rape, personal assault, etc.) that may also include recurring flashbacks of the trauma. Symptoms include difficulty remembering, sleeping, or concentrating, and guilt feelings for surviving.

    F43.10 **Post-traumatic stress disorder, unspecified** [Rx]
    F43.11 **Post-traumatic stress disorder, acute** [Rx]
    F43.12 **Post-traumatic stress disorder, chronic** [Rx]

  ### ✓5th **F43.2** **Adjustment disorders**
    Culture shock
    Grief reaction
    Hospitalism in children
    EXCLUDES 2: separation anxiety disorder of childhood (F93.0)

    F43.20 **Adjustment disorder, unspecified** [Rx]
    F43.21 **Adjustment disorder with depressed mood** [Rx]
      AHA: 2014,1Q,25
    F43.22 **Adjustment disorder with anxiety** [Rx]
    F43.23 **Adjustment disorder with mixed anxiety and depressed mood** [Rx]
    F43.24 **Adjustment disorder with disturbance of conduct** [Rx]
    F43.25 **Adjustment disorder with mixed disturbance of emotions and conduct** [Rx]
    F43.29 **Adjustment disorder with other symptoms** [Rx]

  ### ✓5th **F43.8** **Other reactions to severe stress**
    Other specified trauma and stressor-related disorder
    AHA: 2022,4Q,17
    F43.81 **Prolonged grief disorder**
      Complicated grief
      Complicated grief disorder
      Persistent complex bereavement disorder
    F43.89 **Other reactions to severe stress**

  F43.9 **Reaction to severe stress, unspecified**
    Trauma and stressor-related disorder, NOS
    Unspecified trauma and stressor-related disorder

✓4th F44 Dissociative and conversion disorders
  INCLUDES: conversion hysteria
  conversion reaction
  hysteria
  hysterical psychosis
  EXCLUDES 2: malingering [conscious simulation] (Z76.5)

  F44.0 **Dissociative amnesia** [HCC] [Rx] [ESR] [COM]
    EXCLUDES 1: amnesia NOS (R41.3)
    anterograde amnesia (R41.1)
    dissociative amnesia with dissociative fugue (F44.1)
    retrograde amnesia (R41.2)
    EXCLUDES 2: alcohol-or other psychoactive substance-induced amnestic disorder (F10, F13, F19 with .26, .96)
    amnestic disorder due to known physiological condition (F04)
    postictal amnesia in epilepsy (G40.-)

  F44.1 **Dissociative fugue** [HCC] [Rx] [ESR] [COM]
    Dissociative amnesia with dissociative fugue
    EXCLUDES 2: postictal fugue in epilepsy (G40.-)
    DEF: Dissociative hysteria identified by memory loss and flight from familiar surroundings to a completely separate environment. Episodes may last hours or days. Conscious activity is not associated with perception of surroundings and there is no later memory of the episode.

  F44.2 **Dissociative stupor** [Rx]
    EXCLUDES 1: catatonic stupor (R40.1)
    stupor NOS (R40.1)
    EXCLUDES 2: catatonic disorder due to known physiological condition (F06.1)
    depressive stupor (F32, F33)
    manic stupor (F30, F31)

  F44.4 **Conversion disorder with motor symptom or deficit** [Rx]
    Conversion disorder with abnormal movement
    Conversion disorder with speech symptoms
    Conversion disorder with swallowing symptoms
    Conversion disorder with weakness/paralysis
    Dissociative motor disorders
    Psychogenic aphonia
    Psychogenic dysphonia

  F44.5 **Conversion disorder with seizures or convulsions** [Rx]
    Conversion disorder with attacks or seizures
    Dissociative convulsions
    AHA: 2021,1Q,3; 2019,1Q,19

  F44.6 **Conversion disorder with sensory symptom or deficit** [Rx]
    Conversion disorder with anesthesia or sensory loss
    Conversion disorder with special sensory symptoms
    Dissociative anesthesia and sensory loss
    Psychogenic deafness

  F44.7 **Conversion disorder with mixed symptom presentation** [Rx]

  ### ✓5th **F44.8** **Other dissociative and conversion disorders**
    F44.81 **Dissociative identity disorder** [HCC] [Rx] [ESR] [COM]
      Multiple personality disorder
    F44.89 **Other dissociative and conversion disorders** [Rx]
      Ganser's syndrome
      Psychogenic confusion
      Psychogenic twilight state
      Trance and possession disorders

  F44.9 **Dissociative and conversion disorder, unspecified** [Rx]
    Dissociative disorder NOS

F45 Somatoform disorders

EXCLUDES 2: dissociative and conversion disorders (F44.-)
factitious disorders (F68.1-, F68.A)
hair-plucking (F63.3)
lalling (F80.0)
lisping (F80.0)
malingering [conscious simulation] (Z76.5)
nail-biting (F98.8)
psychological or behavioral factors associated with disorders or diseases classified elsewhere (F54)
sexual dysfunction, not due to a substance or known physiological condition (F52.-)
thumb-sucking (F98.8)
tic disorders (in childhood and adolescence) (F95.-)
Tourette's syndrome (F95.2)
trichotillomania (F63.3)

DEF: Types of disorders causing inconsistent physical symptoms that cannot be explained.

F45.0 Somatization disorder
Briquet's disorder
Multiple psychosomatic disorder

F45.1 Undifferentiated somatoform disorder
Somatic symptom disorder
Undifferentiated psychosomatic disorder

F45.2 Hypochondriacal disorders
EXCLUDES 2: delusional dysmorphophobia (F22)
fixed delusions about bodily functions or shape (F22)

- **F45.20** Hypochondriacal disorder, unspecified
- **F45.21** Hypochondriasis
  Hypochondriacal neurosis
  Illness anxiety disorder
- **F45.22** Body dysmorphic disorder
  Bigorexia
  Dysmorphophobia (nondelusional)
  Muscle dysmorphia
  Nosophobia
- **F45.29** Other hypochondriacal disorders

F45.4 Pain disorders related to psychological factors
EXCLUDES 1: pain NOS (R52)

- **F45.41** Pain disorder exclusively related to psychological factors
  Somatoform pain disorder (persistent)
- **F45.42** Pain disorder with related psychological factors
  Code also associated acute or chronic pain (G89.-)

F45.8 Other somatoform disorders
Psychogenic dysmenorrhea
Psychogenic dysphagia, including 'globus hystericus'
Psychogenic pruritus
Psychogenic torticollis
Somatoform autonomic dysfunction
Teeth grinding
EXCLUDES 1: sleep related teeth grinding (G47.63)

F45.9 Somatoform disorder, unspecified
Psychosomatic disorder NOS

F48 Other nonpsychotic mental disorders

F48.1 Depersonalization-derealization syndrome

F48.2 Pseudobulbar affect
Involuntary emotional expression disorder
Code first underlying cause, if known, such as:
amyotrophic lateral sclerosis (G12.21)
multiple sclerosis ▶(G35)◀
sequelae of cerebrovascular disease (I69.-)
sequelae of traumatic intracranial injury (S06.-)

F48.8 Other specified nonpsychotic mental disorders
Dhat syndrome
Neurasthenia
Occupational neurosis, including writer's cramp
Psychasthenia
Psychasthenic neurosis
Psychogenic syncope

F48.9 Nonpsychotic mental disorder, unspecified
Neurosis NOS

Behavioral syndromes associated with physiological disturbances and physical factors (F50-F59)

F50 Eating disorders

EXCLUDES 1: anorexia NOS (R63.0)
feeding problems of newborn (P92.-)
polyphagia (R63.2)

EXCLUDES 2: feeding difficulties (R63.3-)
feeding disorder in infancy or childhood (F98.2-)

AHA: 2022,1Q,13; 2018,4Q,82

TIP: Assign additional code for BMI from category Z68, when documented. BMI can be based on documentation from clinicians who are not the patient's provider.

F50.0 Anorexia nervosa
EXCLUDES 1: loss of appetite (R63.0)
psychogenic loss of appetite (F50.89)

AHA: 2024,4Q,12

DEF: Psychological eating disorder characterized by an intense fear of gaining weight and an unrealistic perception of body image that perpetuates the feeling of being fat or having too much fat. Avoidance of food and restrictive or unhealthy eating are common.

- **F50.00** Anorexia nervosa, unspecified
- **F50.01** Anorexia nervosa, restricting type
  - **F50.010** Anorexia nervosa, restricting type, mild
    Anorexia nervosa, restricting type, with a body mass index greater than or equal to 17 kg/m2
  - **F50.011** Anorexia nervosa, restricting type, moderate
    Anorexia nervosa, restricting type, with a body mass index of 16.0-16.99 kg/m2
  - **F50.012** Anorexia nervosa, restricting type, severe
    Anorexia nervosa, restricting type, with a body mass index of 15.0-15.99 kg/m2
    AHA: 2024,4Q,12
  - **F50.013** Anorexia nervosa, restricting type, extreme
    Anorexia nervosa, restricting type, with a body mass index of less than 15.0 kg/m2
  - **F50.014** Anorexia nervosa, restricting type, in remission
    Anorexia nervosa, restricting type, in full remission
    Anorexia nervosa, restricting type, in partial remission
  - **F50.019** Anorexia nervosa, restricting type, unspecified
- **F50.02** Anorexia nervosa, binge eating/purging type
  EXCLUDES 1: bulimia nervosa (F50.2-)
  - **F50.020** Anorexia nervosa, binge eating/purging type, mild
    Anorexia nervosa, binge eating/purging type, with a body mass index greater than or equal to 17 kg/m2
  - **F50.021** Anorexia nervosa, binge eating/purging type, moderate
    Anorexia nervosa, binge eating/purging type, with a body mass index of 16.0-16.99 kg/m2
  - **F50.022** Anorexia nervosa, binge eating/purging type, severe
    Anorexia nervosa, binge eating/purging type, with a body mass index of 15.0-15.99 kg/m2
  - **F50.023** Anorexia nervosa, binge eating/purging type, extreme
    Anorexia nervosa, binge eating/purging type, with a body mass index of less than 15.0 kg/m2
    AHA: 2024,4Q,13

Chapter 5. Mental, Behavioral and Neurodevelopmental Disorders

F50.024 Anorexia nervosa, binge eating/purging type, in remission `HCC` `Rx` `COM`
   Anorexia nervosa, binge eating/purging type, in full remission
   Anorexia nervosa, binge eating/purging type, in partial remission

F50.029 Anorexia nervosa, binge eating/purging type, unspecified `HCC` `Rx` `COM`

F50.2 Bulimia nervosa
   Bulimia NOS
   Hyperorexia nervosa
   EXCLUDES 1 anorexia nervosa, binge eating/purging type (F50.02-)
   AHA: 2024,4Q,12
   DEF: Episodic pattern of overeating (binge eating) followed by purging or extreme exercise accompanied by an awareness of the abnormal eating pattern with a fear of not being able to stop eating.

   F50.20 Bulimia nervosa, unspecified `HCC` `Rx` `COM`
   F50.21 Bulimia nervosa, mild `HCC` `Rx` `COM`
      Bulimia nervosa with 1-3 episodes of inappropriate compensatory behavior per week
   F50.22 Bulimia nervosa, moderate `HCC` `Rx` `COM`
      Bulimia nervosa with 4-7 episodes of inappropriate compensatory behavior per week
   F50.23 Bulimia nervosa, severe `HCC` `Rx` `COM`
      Bulimia nervosa with 8-13 episodes of inappropriate compensatory behavior per week
   F50.24 Bulimia nervosa, extreme `HCC` `Rx` `COM`
      Bulimia nervosa with 14 or more episodes of inappropriate compensatory behavior per week
   F50.25 Bulimia nervosa, in remission `HCC` `Rx` `COM`
      Bulimia nervosa, in full remission
      Bulimia nervosa, in partial remission

F50.8 Other eating disorders
   AHA: 2017,4Q,9; 2016,4Q,15-16

   F50.81 Binge eating disorder
      AHA: 2024,4Q,12
      F50.810 Binge eating disorder, mild `Rx`
         Binge eating disorder with 1-3 binge eating episodes per week
      F50.811 Binge eating disorder, moderate `Rx`
         Binge eating disorder with 4-7 binge eating episodes per week
      F50.812 Binge eating disorder, severe `Rx`
         Binge eating disorder with 8-13 binge eating episodes per week
      F50.813 Binge eating disorder, extreme `Rx`
         Binge eating disorder with 14 or more eating episodes per week
      F50.814 Binge eating disorder, in remission `Rx`
         Binge eating disorder, in full remission
         Binge eating disorder, in partial remission
      F50.819 Binge eating disorder, unspecified `Rx`

   F50.82 Avoidant/restrictive food intake disorder `Rx`
      Avoidant/restrictive food intake disorder, in remission
   F50.83 Pica in adults `Rx` `A`
      Pica in adults, in remission
      EXCLUDES 1 pica in infancy and childhood (F98.3)
      AHA: 2024,4Q,14
   F50.84 Rumination disorder in adults `Rx` `A`
      Rumination disorder in adults, in remission
      EXCLUDES 1 rumination disorder in infancy and childhood (F98.21)
      AHA: 2024,4Q,15
   F50.89 Other specified eating disorder `Rx`
      Psychogenic loss of appetite

F50.9 Eating disorder, unspecified `Rx`
   Atypical anorexia nervosa
   Atypical bulimia nervosa
   Feeding or eating disorder, unspecified
   Other specified feeding disorder

F51 Sleep disorders not due to a substance or known physiological condition
   EXCLUDES 2 organic sleep disorders (G47.-)

   F51.0 Insomnia not due to a substance or known physiological condition
      EXCLUDES 2 alcohol related insomnia (F10.182, F10.282, F10.982)
         drug-related insomnia (F11.182, F11.282, F11.982, F13.182, F13.282, F13.982, F14.182, F14.282, F14.982, F15.182, F15.282, F15.982, F19.182, F19.282, F19.982)
         insomnia due to known physiological condition (G47.0-)
         insomnia NOS (G47.0-)
         organic insomnia (G47.0-)
         sleep deprivation (Z72.820)

      F51.01 Primary insomnia
         Idiopathic insomnia
      F51.02 Adjustment insomnia
      F51.03 Paradoxical insomnia
      F51.04 Psychophysiologic insomnia
      F51.05 Insomnia due to other mental disorder
         Code also associated mental disorder
      F51.09 Other insomnia not due to a substance or known physiological condition

   F51.1 Hypersomnia not due to a substance or known physiological condition
      EXCLUDES 2 alcohol related hypersomnia (F10.182, F10.282, F10.982)
         drug-related hypersomnia (F11.182, F11.282, F11.982, F13.182, F13.282, F13.982, F14.182, F14.282, F14.982, F15.182, F15.282, F15.982, F19.182, F19.282, F19.982)
         hypersomnia due to known physiological condition (G47.10)
         hypersomnia NOS (G47.10)
         idiopathic hypersomnia (G47.11, G47.12)
         narcolepsy (G47.4-)

      F51.11 Primary hypersomnia
      F51.12 Insufficient sleep syndrome
         EXCLUDES 1 sleep deprivation (Z72.820)
      F51.13 Hypersomnia due to other mental disorder
         Code also associated mental disorder
      F51.19 Other hypersomnia not due to a substance or known physiological condition

   F51.3 Sleepwalking [somnambulism]
      Non-rapid eye movement sleep arousal disorders, sleepwalking type
   F51.4 Sleep terrors [night terrors]
      Non-rapid eye movement sleep arousal disorders, sleep terror type
   F51.5 Nightmare disorder
      Dream anxiety disorder
   F51.8 Other sleep disorders not due to a substance or known physiological condition
   F51.9 Sleep disorder not due to a substance or known physiological condition, unspecified
      Emotional sleep disorder NOS

F52 Sexual dysfunction not due to a substance or known physiological condition
   EXCLUDES 2 Dhat syndrome (F48.8)

   F52.0 Hypoactive sexual desire disorder
      Lack or loss of sexual desire
      Male hypoactive sexual desire disorder
      Sexual anhedonia
      EXCLUDES 1 decreased libido (R68.82)
   F52.1 Sexual aversion disorder
      Sexual aversion and lack of sexual enjoyment
   F52.2 Sexual arousal disorders
      Failure of genital response
      F52.21 Male erectile disorder
         Erectile disorder
         Psychogenic impotence
         EXCLUDES 1 impotence of organic origin (N52.-)
            impotence NOS (N52.-)
      F52.22 Female sexual arousal disorder
         Female sexual interest/arousal disorder
   F52.3 Orgasmic disorder
      Inhibited orgasm
      Psychogenic anorgasmy
      F52.31 Female orgasmic disorder

F52.32 **Male** orgasmic disorder
Delayed ejaculation

F52.4 **Premature ejaculation**

F52.5 **Vaginismus not due to a substance or known physiological condition**
Psychogenic vaginismus
EXCLUDES 2   vaginismus (due to a known physiological condition) (N94.2)
DEF: Psychogenic response resulting in painful contractions of the vaginal canal muscles. This condition can be severe enough to prevent sexual intercourse.

F52.6 **Dyspareunia not due to a substance or known physiological condition**
Genito-pelvic pain penetration disorder
Psychogenic dyspareunia
EXCLUDES 2   dyspareunia (due to a known physiological condition) (N94.1-)

F52.8 **Other sexual dysfunction not due to a substance or known physiological condition**
Excessive sexual drive
Nymphomania
Satyriasis

F52.9 **Unspecified sexual dysfunction not due to a substance or known physiological condition**
Sexual dysfunction NOS

√4th **F53** **Mental and behavioral disorders associated with the puerperium, not elsewhere classified**
EXCLUDES 1   mood disorders with psychotic features (F30.2, F31.2, F31.5, F31.64, F32.3, F33.3)
postpartum dysphoria (O90.6)
psychosis in schizophrenia, schizotypal, delusional, and other psychotic disorders (F20-F29)
AHA: 2018,4Q,8

F53.0 **Postpartum depression**   Rx M
Postnatal depression, NOS
Postpartum depression, NOS

F53.1 **Puerperal psychosis**   HCC Rx ESR COM M
Postpartum psychosis
Puerperal psychosis, NOS

F54 *Psychological and behavioral factors associated with disorders or diseases classified elsewhere*
Psychological factors affecting physical conditions
Code first the associated physical disorder, such as:
asthma (J45.-)
dermatitis (L23-L25)
gastric ulcer (K25.-)
mucous colitis (K58.-)
ulcerative colitis (K51.-)
urticaria (L50.-)
EXCLUDES 2   tension-type headache (G44.2)

√4th **F55** **Abuse of non-psychoactive substances**
EXCLUDES 2   abuse of psychoactive substances (F10-F19)

F55.0 **Abuse of** **antacids**

F55.1 **Abuse of** **herbal or folk remedies**
AHA: 2023,3Q,16

F55.2 **Abuse of** **laxatives**

F55.3 **Abuse of** **steroids or hormones**

F55.4 **Abuse of** **vitamins**

F55.8 **Abuse of other non-psychoactive substances**

F59 **Unspecified behavioral syndromes associated with physiological disturbances and physical factors**
Psychogenic physiological dysfunction NOS

Disorders of adult personality and behavior (F60-F69)

√4th **F60** **Specific personality disorders**

F60.0 **Paranoid** personality disorder   HCC Rx ESR COM
Expansive paranoid personality (disorder)
Fanatic personality (disorder)
Paranoid personality (disorder)
Querulant personality (disorder)
Sensitive paranoid personality (disorder)
EXCLUDES 2   paranoia (F22)
paranoia querulans (F22)
paranoid psychosis (F22)
paranoid schizophrenia (F20.0)
paranoid state (F22)

F60.1 **Schizoid** personality disorder   HCC Rx ESR COM
EXCLUDES 2   Asperger's syndrome (F84.5)
delusional disorder (F22)
schizoid disorder of childhood (F84.5)
schizophrenia (F20.-)
schizotypal disorder (F21)

F60.2 **Antisocial** personality disorder   HCC Rx ESR COM
Amoral personality (disorder)
Asocial personality (disorder)
Dissocial personality disorder
Psychopathic personality (disorder)
Sociopathic personality (disorder)
EXCLUDES 1   conduct disorders (F91.-)
EXCLUDES 2   borderline personality disorder (F60.3)

F60.3 **Borderline** personality disorder   HCC Rx ESR COM
Aggressive personality (disorder)
Emotionally unstable personality disorder
Explosive personality (disorder)
EXCLUDES 2   antisocial personality disorder (F60.2)

F60.4 **Histrionic** personality disorder   HCC Rx ESR COM
Hysterical personality (disorder)
Psychoinfantile personality (disorder)

F60.5 **Obsessive-compulsive** personality disorder   HCC Rx ESR COM
Anankastic personality (disorder)
Compulsive personality (disorder)
Obsessional personality (disorder)
EXCLUDES 2   obsessive-compulsive disorder (F42.-)

F60.6 **Avoidant** personality disorder   HCC Rx ESR COM
Anxious personality disorder

F60.7 **Dependent** personality disorder   HCC Rx ESR COM
Asthenic personality (disorder)
Inadequate personality (disorder)
Passive personality (disorder)
DEF: Lack of self-confidence, fear of abandonment, and an obsessive need to be taken care of.

√5th **F60.8** **Other specific personality disorders**

F60.81 **Narcissistic personality disorder**   HCC Rx ESR COM

F60.89 **Other specific personality disorders**   HCC Rx ESR COM
"Haltlose" type personality disorder
Eccentric personality disorder
Immature personality disorder
Passive-aggressive personality disorder
Psychoneurotic personality disorder
Self-defeating personality disorder

F60.9 **Personality disorder, unspecified**   HCC Rx ESR COM
Character disorder NOS
Character neurosis NOS
Pathological personality NOS

√4th **F63** **Impulse disorders**
EXCLUDES 2   habitual excessive use of alcohol or psychoactive substances (F10-F19)
impulse disorders involving sexual behavior (F65.-)

F63.0 **Pathological gambling**   Rx
Compulsive gambling
Gambling disorder
EXCLUDES 1   gambling and betting NOS (Z72.6)
EXCLUDES 2   excessive gambling by manic patients (F30, F31)
gambling in antisocial personality disorder (F60.2)

F63.1 **Pyromania**   Rx
Pathological fire-setting
EXCLUDES 2   fire-setting (by) (in):
adult with antisocial personality disorder (F60.2)
alcohol or psychoactive substance intoxication (F10-F19)
conduct disorders (F91.-)
mental disorders due to known physiological condition (F01-F09)
schizophrenia (F20.-)

Chapter 5. Mental, Behavioral and Neurodevelopmental Disorders

F63.2 **Kleptomania** [Rx]
Pathological stealing
EXCLUDES 1 — shoplifting as the reason for observation for suspected mental disorder (Z03.8)
EXCLUDES 2 — depressive disorder with stealing ▶(F31.-, F32.-, F33.-)◀
stealing due to underlying mental condition - code to mental condition
stealing in mental disorders due to known physiological condition (F01-F09)

F63.3 **Trichotillomania** [Rx]
Hair plucking
EXCLUDES 2 — other stereotyped movement disorder (F98.4)

F63.8 **Other impulse disorders**
- **F63.81** Intermittent explosive disorder [Rx]
- **F63.89** Other impulse disorders [Rx]

F63.9 **Impulse disorder, unspecified** [Rx]
Impulse control disorder NOS

F64 **Gender identity disorders**
AHA: 2016,4Q,16

F64.0 **Transsexualism**
Gender dysphoria in adolescents and adults
Gender identity disorder in adolescence and adulthood
Gender incongruence in adolescents and adults
Transgender
EXCLUDES 1 — gender identity disorder of childhood (F64.2)

F64.1 **Dual role transvestism**
Use additional code to identify sex reassignment status (Z87.890)
EXCLUDES 1 — gender identity disorder in childhood (F64.2)
EXCLUDES 2 — fetishistic transvestism (F65.1)

F64.2 **Gender identity disorder of childhood** [P]
Gender dysphoria in children
Gender incongruence of childhood
EXCLUDES 1 — gender identity disorder in adolescence and adulthood (F64.0)
EXCLUDES 2 — sexual maturation disorder (F66)

F64.8 **Other gender identity disorders**
Other specified gender dysphoria

F64.9 **Gender identity disorder, unspecified**
Gender dysphoria, unspecified
Gender incongruence, unspecified
Gender-role disorder NOS

F65 **Paraphilias**

F65.0 **Fetishism**
Fetishistic disorder

F65.1 **Transvestic fetishism**
Fetishistic transvestism
Transvestic disorder

F65.2 **Exhibitionism**
Exhibitionistic disorder

F65.3 **Voyeurism**
Voyeuristic disorder

F65.4 **Pedophilia**
Pedophilic disorder

F65.5 **Sadomasochism**
- **F65.50** Sadomasochism, unspecified
- **F65.51** Sexual masochism
  Sexual masochism disorder
- **F65.52** Sexual sadism
  Sexual sadism disorder

F65.8 **Other paraphilias**
- **F65.81** Frotteurism
  Frotteuristic disorder
- **F65.89** Other paraphilias
  Necrophilia
  Other specified paraphilic disorder

F65.9 **Paraphilia, unspecified**
Paraphilic disorder, unspecified
Sexual deviation NOS

F66 **Other sexual disorders**
Sexual maturation disorder
Sexual relationship disorder

F68 **Other disorders of adult personality and behavior**
AHA: 2018,4Q,9,65

F68.1 **Factitious disorder imposed on self**
Compensation neurosis
Elaboration of physical symptoms for psychological reasons
Hospital hopper syndrome
Münchausen's syndrome
Peregrinating patient
EXCLUDES 2 — factitial dermatitis (L98.1)
person feigning illness (with obvious motivation) (Z76.5)

- **F68.10** Factitious disorder imposed on self, unspecified [Rx]
- **F68.11** Factitious disorder imposed on self, with predominantly psychological signs and symptoms [Rx]
- **F68.12** Factitious disorder imposed on self, with predominantly physical signs and symptoms [Rx]
- **F68.13** Factitious disorder imposed on self, with combined psychological and physical signs and symptoms [Rx]

F68.A **Factitious disorder imposed on another** [Rx]
Factitious disorder by proxy
Münchausen's by proxy

F68.8 **Other specified disorders of adult personality and behavior**

F69 **Unspecified disorder of adult personality and behavior** [A]

Intellectual disabilities (F70-F79)

Code first any associated physical or developmental disorders
EXCLUDES 1 — borderline intellectual functioning, IQ above 70 to 84 (R41.83)

F70 **Mild intellectual disabilities** [Rx]
IQ level 50-55 to approximately 70
Mild mental subnormality

F71 **Moderate intellectual disabilities** [Rx]
IQ level 35-40 to 50-55
Moderate mental subnormality

F72 **Severe intellectual disabilities** [Rx]
IQ 20-25 to 35-40
Severe mental subnormality

F73 **Profound intellectual disabilities** [Rx]
IQ level below 20-25
Profound mental subnormality

F78 **Other intellectual disabilities** [Rx]

F78.A **Other genetic related intellectual disabilities**
AHA: 2021,4Q,10-11

- **F78.A1** **SYNGAP1-related intellectual disability** [Rx]
  Code also, if applicable, any associated:
  autism spectrum disorder (F84.0)
  autistic disorder (F84.0)
  encephalopathy (G93.4-)
  epilepsy and recurrent seizures (G40.-)
  other pervasive developmental disorders (F84.8)
  pervasive developmental disorder, NOS (F84.9)

- **F78.A9** **Other genetic related intellectual disability** [Rx]
  Code also, if applicable, any associated disorders

F79 **Unspecified intellectual disabilities** [Rx]
Mental deficiency NOS
Mental subnormality NOS

Pervasive and specific developmental disorders (F80-F89)

☑4th F80 Specific developmental disorders of speech and language

    F80.0 Phonological disorder
        Dyslalia
        Functional speech articulation disorder
        Lalling
        Lisping
        Phonological developmental disorder
        Speech articulation developmental disorder
        Speech-sound disorder
        EXCLUDES 1 speech articulation impairment due to aphasia NOS (R47.01)
                speech articulation impairment due to apraxia (R48.2)
        EXCLUDES 2 speech articulation impairment due to hearing loss (F80.4)
                speech articulation impairment due to intellectual disabilities (F70-F79)
                speech articulation impairment with expressive language developmental disorder (F80.1)
                speech articulation impairment with mixed receptive expressive language developmental disorder (F80.2)

    F80.1 Expressive language disorder
        Developmental dysphasia or aphasia, expressive type
        EXCLUDES 1 mixed receptive-expressive language disorder (F80.2)
                dysphasia and aphasia NOS (R47.-)
        EXCLUDES 2 acquired aphasia with epilepsy [Landau-Kleffner] (G40.80-)
                intellectual disabilities (F70-F79)
                pervasive developmental disorders (F84.-)
                selective mutism (F94.0)

    F80.2 Mixed receptive-expressive language disorder
        Developmental dysphasia or aphasia, receptive type
        Developmental Wernicke's aphasia
        EXCLUDES 1 central auditory processing disorder (H93.25)
                dysphasia or aphasia NOS (R47.-)
                expressive language disorder (F80.1)
                expressive type dysphasia or aphasia (F80.1)
                word deafness (H93.25)
        EXCLUDES 2 acquired aphasia with epilepsy [Landau-Kleffner] (G40.80-)
                intellectual disabilities (F70-F79)
                pervasive developmental disorders (F84.-)
                selective mutism (F94.0)

    F80.4 Speech and language development delay due to hearing loss
        Code also type of hearing loss (H90.-, H91.-)

    ☑5th F80.8 Other developmental disorders of speech and language
        AHA: 2017,1Q,27

        F80.81 Childhood onset fluency disorder
            Cluttering NOS
            Stuttering NOS
            EXCLUDES 1 adult onset fluency disorder (F98.5)
                fluency disorder (stuttering) following cerebrovascular disease (I69. with final characters -23)
                fluency disorder in conditions classified elsewhere (R47.82)

        F80.82 Social pragmatic communication disorder
            EXCLUDES 1 Asperger's syndrome (F84.5)
                autistic disorder (F84.0)
            AHA: 2016,4Q,16

        F80.89 Other developmental disorders of speech and language

    F80.9 Developmental disorder of speech and language, unspecified
        Communication disorder NOS
        Language disorder NOS

☑4th F81 Specific developmental disorders of scholastic skills

    F81.0 Specific reading disorder
        "Backward reading"
        Developmental dyslexia
        Specific learning disorder, with impairment in reading
        Specific reading retardation
        EXCLUDES 1 alexia NOS (R48.0)
                dyslexia NOS (R48.0)
        DEF: Serious impairment of reading skills unexplained in relation to general intelligence and teaching processes.

    F81.2 Mathematics disorder
        Developmental acalculia
        Developmental arithmetical disorder
        Developmental Gerstmann's syndrome
        Specific learning disorder, with impairment in mathematics
        EXCLUDES 1 acalculia NOS (R48.8)
        EXCLUDES 2 arithmetical difficulties associated with a reading disorder (F81.0)
                arithmetical difficulties associated with a spelling disorder (F81.81)
                arithmetical difficulties due to inadequate teaching (Z55.8)

    ☑5th F81.8 Other developmental disorders of scholastic skills

        F81.81 Disorder of written expression
            Specific learning disorder, with impairment in written expression
            Specific spelling disorder

        F81.89 Other developmental disorders of scholastic skills

    F81.9 Developmental disorder of scholastic skills, unspecified
        Knowledge acquisition disability NOS
        Learning disability NOS
        Learning disorder NOS

F82 Specific developmental disorder of motor function
    Clumsy child syndrome
    Developmental coordination disorder
    Developmental dyspraxia
    EXCLUDES 1 abnormalities of gait and mobility (R26.-)
        lack of coordination (R27.-)
    EXCLUDES 2 lack of coordination secondary to intellectual disabilities (F70-F79)

☑4th F84 Pervasive developmental disorders
Code also any associated medical condition and intellectual disabilities

    F84.0 Autistic disorder   [Rx] [COM]
        Autism spectrum disorder
        Infantile autism
        Infantile psychosis
        Kanner's syndrome
        EXCLUDES 1 Asperger's syndrome (F84.5)
        AHA: 2017,1Q,27
        TIP: When the encounter is focused on treatment of conditions related to autism spectrum disorder, first assign codes to identify the problem or manifestation receiving therapeutic services.

    F84.2 Rett's syndrome   [Rx] [COM]
        EXCLUDES 1 Asperger's syndrome (F84.5)
                autistic disorder (F84.0)
                other childhood disintegrative disorder (F84.3)

    F84.3 Other childhood disintegrative disorder   [Rx] [COM] [P]
        Dementia infantilis
        Disintegrative psychosis
        Heller's syndrome
        Symbiotic psychosis
        Use additional code to identify any associated neurological condition
        EXCLUDES 1 Asperger's syndrome (F84.5)
                autistic disorder (F84.0)
                Rett's syndrome (F84.2)

    F84.5 Asperger's syndrome   [Rx] [COM]
        Asperger's disorder
        Autistic psychopathy
        Schizoid disorder of childhood
        DEF: High-functioning form of autism. Children with this syndrome usually develop speech on schedule, are generally very intelligent, and communicate well, but have considerable social shortcomings. **Synonym(s):** AS.

    F84.8 Other pervasive developmental disorders   [Rx] [COM]
        Overactive disorder associated with intellectual disabilities and stereotyped movements

    F84.9 Pervasive developmental disorder, unspecified   [Rx] [COM]
        Atypical autism

F88 Other disorders of psychological development
    Developmental agnosia
    Global developmental delay
    Other specified neurodevelopmental disorder

F89 Unspecified disorder of psychological development
    Developmental disorder NOS
    Neurodevelopmental disorder NOS

Behavioral and emotional disorders with onset usually occurring in childhood and adolescence (F90-F98)

NOTE Codes within categories F90-F98 may be used regardless of the age of a patient. These disorders generally have onset within the childhood or adolescent years, but may continue throughout life or not be diagnosed until adulthood

F90 Attention-deficit hyperactivity disorders
INCLUDES attention deficit disorder with hyperactivity
attention deficit syndrome with hyperactivity
EXCLUDES 2 anxiety disorders (F40.-, F41.-)
mood [affective] disorders (F30-F39)
pervasive developmental disorders (F84.-)
schizophrenia (F20.-)

- **F90.0 Attention-deficit hyperactivity disorder, predominantly inattentive type**
  Attention-deficit/hyperactivity disorder, predominantly inattentive presentation
- **F90.1 Attention-deficit hyperactivity disorder, predominantly hyperactive type**
  Attention-deficit/hyperactivity disorder, predominantly hyperactive impulsive presentation
- **F90.2 Attention-deficit hyperactivity disorder, combined type**
  Attention-deficit/hyperactivity disorder, combined presentation
- **F90.8 Attention-deficit hyperactivity disorder, other type**
- **F90.9 Attention-deficit hyperactivity disorder, unspecified type**
  Attention-deficit hyperactivity disorder of childhood or adolescence NOS
  Attention-deficit hyperactivity disorder NOS

F91 Conduct disorders
EXCLUDES 1 antisocial behavior (Z72.81-)
antisocial personality disorder (F60.2)
EXCLUDES 2 conduct problems associated with attention-deficit hyperactivity disorder (F90.-)
mood [affective] disorders (F30-F39)
pervasive developmental disorders (F84.-)
schizophrenia (F20.-)

- **F91.0 Conduct disorder confined to family context**
- **F91.1 Conduct disorder, childhood-onset type**
  Conduct disorder, solitary aggressive type
  Unsocialized aggressive disorder
  Unsocialized conduct disorder
- **F91.2 Conduct disorder, adolescent-onset type**
  Conduct disorder, group type
  Socialized conduct disorder
- **F91.3 Oppositional defiant disorder**
- **F91.8 Other conduct disorders**
  Other specified conduct disorder
  Other specified disruptive disorder
- **F91.9 Conduct disorder, unspecified**
  Behavioral disorder NOS
  Conduct disorder NOS
  Disruptive behavior disorder NOS
  Disruptive disorder NOS

F93 Emotional disorders with onset specific to childhood
- **F93.0 Separation anxiety disorder of childhood**
  EXCLUDES 2 mood [affective] disorders (F30-F39)
  nonpsychotic mental disorders (F40-F48)
  phobic anxiety disorder of childhood (F40.8)
  social phobia (F40.1)
- **F93.8 Other childhood emotional disorders**
  Identity disorder
  EXCLUDES 2 gender identity disorder of childhood (F64.2)
- **F93.9 Childhood emotional disorder, unspecified**

F94 Disorders of social functioning with onset specific to childhood and adolescence
- **F94.0 Selective mutism**
  Elective mutism
  EXCLUDES 2 pervasive developmental disorders (F84.-)
  schizophrenia (F20.-)
  specific developmental disorders of speech and language (F80.-)
  transient mutism as part of separation anxiety in young children (F93.0)
- **F94.1 Reactive attachment disorder of childhood**
  Use additional code to identify any associated failure to thrive or growth retardation
  EXCLUDES 1 disinhibited attachment disorder of childhood (F94.2)
  normal variation in pattern of selective attachment
  EXCLUDES 2 Asperger's syndrome (F84.5)
  maltreatment syndromes (T74.-)
  sexual or physical abuse in childhood, resulting in psychosocial problems (Z62.81-)
- **F94.2 Disinhibited attachment disorder of childhood**
  Affectionless psychopathy
  Institutional syndrome
  EXCLUDES 1 reactive attachment disorder of childhood (F94.1)
  EXCLUDES 2 Asperger's syndrome (F84.5)
  attention-deficit hyperactivity disorders (F90.-)
  hospitalism in children (F43.2-)
- **F94.8 Other childhood disorders of social functioning**
- **F94.9 Childhood disorder of social functioning, unspecified**

F95 Tic disorder
- **F95.0 Transient tic disorder**
  Provisional tic disorder
- **F95.1 Chronic motor or vocal tic disorder**
- **F95.2 Tourette's disorder**
  Combined vocal and multiple motor tic disorder [de la Tourette]
  Tourette's syndrome
- **F95.8 Other tic disorders**
- **F95.9 Tic disorder, unspecified**
  Tic NOS

F98 Other behavioral and emotional disorders with onset usually occurring in childhood and adolescence
EXCLUDES 2 breath-holding spells (R06.89)
gender identity disorder of childhood (F64.2)
Kleine-Levin syndrome (G47.13)
obsessive-compulsive disorder (F42.-)
sleep disorders not due to a substance or known physiological condition (F51.-)

- **F98.0 Enuresis not due to a substance or known physiological condition**
  Enuresis (primary) (secondary) of nonorganic origin
  Functional enuresis
  Psychogenic enuresis
  Urinary incontinence of nonorganic origin
  EXCLUDES 1 enuresis NOS (R32)
- **F98.1 Encopresis not due to a substance or known physiological condition**
  Functional encopresis
  Incontinence of feces of nonorganic origin
  Psychogenic encopresis
  Use additional code to identify the cause of any coexisting constipation
  EXCLUDES 1 encopresis NOS (R15.-)
- **F98.2 Other feeding disorders of infancy and childhood**
  EXCLUDES 2 anorexia nervosa and other eating disorders (F50.-)
  feeding difficulties (R63.3-)
  feeding problems of newborn (P92.-)
  pica of infancy or childhood (F98.3)
  - **F98.21 Rumination disorder of infancy and childhood**
    Rumination disorder in infancy or childhood, in remission
    EXCLUDES 1 rumination disorder in adults (F50.84)
  - **F98.29 Other feeding disorders of infancy and early childhood**
- **F98.3 Pica of infancy and childhood**
  Pica in infancy or childhood, in remission
  EXCLUDES 1 pica in adults (F50.83)
- **F98.4 Stereotyped movement disorders**
  Stereotype/habit disorder
  EXCLUDES 1 abnormal involuntary movements (R25.-)
  EXCLUDES 2 compulsions in obsessive-compulsive disorder (F42.-)
  hair plucking (F63.3)
  movement disorders of organic origin (G20-G25)
  nail-biting (F98.8)
  nose-picking (F98.8)
  stereotypies that are part of a broader psychiatric condition (F01-F95)
  thumb-sucking (F98.8)
  tic disorders (F95.-)
  trichotillomania (F63.3)

F98.5 Adult onset fluency disorder
EXCLUDES 1   childhood onset fluency disorder (F80.81)
dysphasia (R47.02)
fluency disorder (stuttering) following cerebrovascular disease (I69. with final characters -23)
fluency disorder in conditions classified elsewhere (R47.82)
tic disorders (F95.-)

F98.8 Other specified behavioral and emotional disorders with onset usually occurring in childhood and adolescence
Excessive masturbation
Nail-biting
Nose-picking
Thumb-sucking

F98.9 Unspecified behavioral and emotional disorders with onset usually occurring in childhood and adolescence

Unspecified mental disorder (F99)

F99 Mental disorder, not otherwise specified
Mental illness NOS
EXCLUDES 1   unspecified mental disorder due to known physiological condition (F09)

Chapter 6. Diseases of the Nervous System (G00–G99)

Chapter-specific Guidelines with Coding Examples

The chapter-specific guidelines from the ICD-10-CM Official Guidelines for Coding and Reporting have been provided below. Along with these guidelines are coding examples, contained in the shaded boxes, that have been developed to help illustrate the coding and/or sequencing guidance found in these guidelines.

a. Dominant/nondominant side

Codes from category G81, Hemiplegia and hemiparesis, and subcategories G83.1, Monoplegia of lower limb, G83.2, Monoplegia of upper limb, and G83.3, Monoplegia, unspecified, identify whether the dominant or nondominant side is affected. Should the affected side be documented, but not specified as dominant or nondominant, and the classification system does not indicate a default, code selection is as follows:

- For ambidextrous patients, the default should be dominant.
- If the left side is affected, the default is non-dominant.
- If the right side is affected, the default is dominant.

> Hemiplegia affecting left side of ambidextrous patient
>
> **G81.92**   Hemiplegia, unspecified affecting left dominant side
>
> *Explanation*: Documentation states that the left side is affected and dominant is used for ambidextrous persons.

> Right spastic hemiplegia, unknown whether patient is right- or left-handed
>
> **G81.11**   Spastic hemiplegia affecting right dominant side
>
> *Explanation*: Since it is unknown whether the patient is right- or left-handed, if the right side is affected, the default is dominant.

b. Pain—Category G89

1) General coding information

Codes in category G89, Pain, not elsewhere classified, may be used in conjunction with codes from other categories and chapters to provide more detail about acute or chronic pain and neoplasm-related pain, unless otherwise indicated below.

If the pain is not specified as acute or chronic, post-thoracotomy, postprocedural, or neoplasm-related, do not assign codes from category G89.

A code from category G89 should not be assigned if the underlying (definitive) diagnosis is known, unless the reason for the encounter is pain control/ management and not management of the underlying condition.

When an admission or encounter is for a procedure aimed at treating the underlying condition (e.g., spinal fusion, kyphoplasty), a code for the underlying condition (e.g., vertebral fracture, spinal stenosis) should be assigned as the principal diagnosis. No code from category G89 should be assigned.

> Elderly patient with back pain is admitted for outpatient kyphoplasty for age-related osteopathic compression fracture at vertebra T3
>
> **M80.08XA**   Age-related osteoporosis with current pathological fracture, vertebra(e), initial encounter for fracture
>
> *Explanation*: No code is assigned for the pain as it is inherent in the underlying condition being treated.

(a) Category G89 codes as principal or first-listed diagnosis

Category G89 codes are acceptable as principal diagnosis or the first-listed code:

- When pain control or pain management is the reason for the admission/encounter (e.g., a patient with displaced intervertebral disc, nerve impingement and severe back pain presents for injection of steroid into the spinal canal). The underlying cause of the pain should be reported as an additional diagnosis, if known.

> Patient presents for steroid injection in the right elbow due to chronic pain associated with primary degenerative joint disease.
>
> **G89.29**   Other chronic pain
>
> **M19.021**   Primary osteoarthritis, right elbow
>
> *Explanation*: Since the encounter is for control of pain, not treating the underlying condition, the pain code is sequenced first followed by the underlying condition. The M25 pain code is not necessary as the underlying condition code represents the specific site.

- When a patient is admitted for the insertion of a neurostimulator for pain control, assign the appropriate pain code as the principal or first-listed diagnosis. When an admission or encounter is for a procedure aimed at treating the underlying condition and a neurostimulator is inserted for pain control during the same admission/encounter, a code for the underlying condition should be assigned as the principal diagnosis and the appropriate pain code should be assigned as a secondary diagnosis.

(b) Use of category G89 codes in conjunction with site specific pain codes

(i) Assigning category G89 and site-specific pain codes

Codes from category G89 may be used in conjunction with codes that identify the site of pain (including codes from chapter 18) if the category G89 code provides additional information. For example, if the code describes the site of the pain, but does not fully describe whether the pain is acute or chronic, then both codes should be assigned.

> Patient is seen to evaluate chronic right knee pain
>
> **M25.561**   Pain in right knee
>
> **G89.29**   Other chronic pain
>
> *Explanation*: No underlying condition has been determined yet so the pain would be the reason for the visit. The M25 pain code in this instance does not fully describe the condition as it does not represent that the pain is chronic. The G89 chronic pain code is assigned to provide specificity.

(ii) Sequencing of category G89 codes with site-specific pain codes

The sequencing of category G89 codes with site-specific pain codes (including chapter 18 codes), is dependent on the circumstances of the encounter/admission as follows:

- If the encounter is for pain control or pain management, assign the code from category G89 followed by the code identifying the specific site of pain (e.g., encounter for pain management for acute neck pain from trauma is assigned code G89.11, Acute pain due to trauma, followed by code M54.2, Cervicalgia, to identify the site of pain).

> Management of acute, traumatic left shoulder pain
>
> **G89.11**   Acute pain due to trauma
>
> **M25.512**   Pain in left shoulder
>
> *Explanation*: The reason for the encounter is to manage or control the pain, not to treat or evaluate an underlying condition. The G89 pain code is assigned as the first-listed diagnosis but in this instance does not fully describe the condition as it does not include the site and laterality. The M25 pain code is added to provide this information.

- If the encounter is for any other reason except pain control or pain management, and a related definitive diagnosis has not been established (confirmed) by the provider, assign the code for the specific site of pain first, followed by the appropriate code from category G89.

> Tests are performed to investigate the source of the patient's chronic epigastric abdominal pain
>
> **R10.13**   Epigastric pain
>
> **G89.29**   Other chronic pain
>
> *Explanation*: In this instance the patient's epigastric pain is not being treated; rather the source of the pain is being investigated. A code from chapter 18 for epigastric pain is sequenced before the additional specificity of the G89 code for the chronic pain.

2) Pain due to devices, implants and grafts

See Section I.C.19. Pain due to medical devices

3) Postoperative Pain

The provider's documentation should be used to guide the coding of postoperative pain, as well as *Section III. Reporting Additional Diagnoses* and *Section IV. Diagnostic Coding and Reporting in the Outpatient Setting*.

The default for post-thoracotomy and other postoperative pain not specified as acute or chronic is the code for the acute form.

Routine or expected postoperative pain immediately after surgery should not be coded.

> Pain pump dose is increased for the patient's unexpected, extreme pain post-thoracotomy
>
> **G89.12**   Acute post-thoracotomy pain
>
> *Explanation*: When acute or chronic is not documented, default to acute. The use of "unexpected, extreme" and the increase of medication dosage indicate that the pain was more than routine or expected.

(a) Postoperative pain not associated with specific postoperative complication

Postoperative pain not associated with a specific postoperative complication is assigned to the appropriate postoperative pain code in category G89.

(b) Postoperative pain associated with specific postoperative complication

Postoperative pain associated with a specific postoperative complication (such as painful wire sutures) is assigned to the appropriate code(s) found in Chapter 19, Injury, poisoning, and certain other consequences of external causes. If appropriate, use additional code(s) from category G89 to identify acute or chronic pain (G89.18 or G89.28).

4) Chronic pain

Chronic pain is classified to subcategory G89.2. There is no time frame defining when pain becomes chronic pain. The provider's documentation should be used to guide use of these codes.

5) Neoplasm related pain

Code G89.3 is assigned to pain documented as being related, associated or due to cancer, primary or secondary malignancy, or tumor. This code is assigned regardless of whether the pain is acute or chronic.

This code may be assigned as the principal or first-listed code when the stated reason for the admission/encounter is documented as pain control/pain management. The underlying neoplasm should be reported as an additional diagnosis.

> Patient referred today for pain management due to acute pain related to malignancy of the right breast.
>
> **G89.3**   Neoplasm related pain (acute)(chronic)
>
> **C50.911**   Malignant neoplasm of unspecified site of right female breast
>
> *Explanation*: Since the encounter was for pain medication management, the pain, rather than the neoplasm, was the reason for the encounter and is sequenced first. This "neoplasm-related pain" code includes both acute and chronic pain.

When the reason for the admission/encounter is management of the neoplasm and the pain associated with the neoplasm is also documented, code G89.3 may be assigned as an additional diagnosis. It is not necessary to assign an additional code for the site of the pain.

See Section I.C.2. for instructions on the sequencing of neoplasms for all other stated reasons or the admission/encounter (except for pain control/pain management).

> Patient with lung cancer presents with acute hip pain and is evaluated and found to have iliac bone metastasis
>
> **C79.51**   Secondary malignant neoplasm of bone
>
> **C34.90**   Malignant neoplasm of unspecified part of unspecified bronchus or lung
>
> **G89.3**   Neoplasm related pain (acute)(chronic)
>
> *Explanation*: The reason for the encounter was the evaluation and diagnosis of the bone metastasis, whose code would be assigned as first-listed, followed by codes for the primary neoplasm and the pain due to the iliac bone metastasis.

6) Chronic pain syndrome

Central pain syndrome (G89.0) and chronic pain syndrome (G89.4) are different than the term "chronic pain," and therefore codes should only be used when the provider has specifically documented this condition.

See Section I.C.5. Pain disorders related to psychological factors

Chapter 6. Diseases of the Nervous System (G00-G99)

EXCLUDES 2 certain conditions originating in the perinatal period (P04-P96)
certain infectious and parasitic diseases (A00-B99)
complications of pregnancy, childbirth and the puerperium (O00-O9A)
congenital malformations, deformations, and chromosomal abnormalities (Q00-Q99)
endocrine, nutritional and metabolic diseases (E00-E88)
injury, poisoning and certain other consequences of external causes (S00-T88)
neoplasms (C00-D49)
symptoms, signs and abnormal clinical and laboratory findings, not elsewhere classified (R00-R94)

This chapter contains the following blocks:
G00-G09 Inflammatory diseases of the central nervous system
G10-G14 Systemic atrophies primarily affecting the central nervous system
G20-G26 Extrapyramidal and movement disorders
G30-G32 Other degenerative diseases of the nervous system
G35-G37 Demyelinating diseases of the central nervous system
G40-G47 Episodic and paroxysmal disorders
G50-G59 Nerve, nerve root and plexus disorders
G60-G65 Polyneuropathies and other disorders of the peripheral nervous system
G70-G73 Diseases of myoneural junction and muscle
G80-G83 Cerebral palsy and other paralytic syndromes
G89-G99 Other disorders of the nervous system

Inflammatory diseases of the central nervous system (G00-G09)

√4th G00 Bacterial meningitis, not elsewhere classified
INCLUDES bacterial arachnoiditis
bacterial leptomeningitis
bacterial meningitis
bacterial pachymeningitis
EXCLUDES 1 bacterial meningoencephalitis (G04.2)
bacterial meningomyelitis (G04.2)
DEF: Inflammation of meningeal layers of the brain and spinal cord due to a bacterial infection.

G00.0 **Hemophilus** meningitis
Meningitis due to Hemophilus influenzae

G00.1 **Pneumococcal** meningitis
▶Meningitis due to Streptococcal pneumoniae◀

G00.2 **Streptococcal** meningitis
Use additional code to further identify organism (B95.0-B95.5)

G00.3 **Staphylococcal** meningitis
Use additional code to further identify organism (B95.61-B95.8)

G00.8 **Other bacterial** meningitis
Meningitis due to Escherichia coli
Meningitis due to Friedlander's bacillus
Meningitis due to Klebsiella
Use additional code to further identify organism (B96.-)

G00.9 Bacterial meningitis, unspecified
Meningitis due to gram-negative bacteria, unspecified
Purulent meningitis NOS
Pyogenic meningitis NOS
Suppurative meningitis NOS

G01 Meningitis in bacterial diseases classified elsewhere
Code first underlying disease
EXCLUDES 1 meningitis (in):
meningoencephalitis and meningomyelitis in bacterial diseases classified elsewhere (G05)
gonococcal (A54.81)
leptospirosis (A27.81)
listeriosis (A32.11)
Lyme disease (A69.21)
meningococcal (A39.0)
neurosyphilis (A52.13)
tuberculosis (A17.0)

G02 Meningitis in other infectious and parasitic diseases classified elsewhere
Code first underlying disease, such as:
African trypanosomiasis (B56.-)
poliovirus infection (A80.-)
EXCLUDES 1 candidal meningitis (B37.5)
coccidioidomycosis meningitis (B38.4)
cryptococcal meningitis (B45.1)
herpesviral [herpes simplex] meningitis (B00.3)
infectious mononucleosis complicated by meningitis (B27.- with fifth character 2)
measles complicated by meningitis (B05.1)
meningoencephalitis and meningomyelitis in other infectious and parasitic diseases classified elsewhere (G05)
mumps meningitis (B26.1)
rubella meningitis (B06.02)
varicella [chickenpox] meningitis (B01.0)
zoster meningitis (B02.1)

√4th G03 Meningitis due to other and unspecified causes
INCLUDES arachnoiditis NOS
leptomeningitis NOS
meningitis NOS
pachymeningitis NOS
EXCLUDES 1 meningoencephalitis (G04.-)
meningomyelitis (G04.-)

G03.0 **Nonpyogenic** meningitis
Aseptic meningitis
Nonbacterial meningitis
DEF: Type of meningitis where no bacterial, viral, or other infectious source exists that explains the meningitis symptomology.

G03.1 **Chronic** meningitis

G03.2 **Benign recurrent** meningitis [Mollaret]
DEF: Aseptic or noninfectious inflammation of the meninges with the presence of Mollaret cells in the spinal fluid. The patient experiences recurrent bouts of inflammation, lasting anywhere from two to five days.

G03.8 Meningitis due to other specified causes

G03.9 **Meningitis, unspecified**
Arachnoiditis (spinal) NOS

√4th G04 Encephalitis, myelitis and encephalomyelitis
INCLUDES acute ascending myelitis
meningoencephalitis
meningomyelitis
EXCLUDES 1 encephalopathy NOS (G93.40)
EXCLUDES 2 acute transverse myelitis (G37.3)
alcoholic encephalopathy (G31.2)
multiple sclerosis ▶(G35-)◀
myalgic encephalomyelitis (G93.32)
subacute necrotizing myelitis (G37.4)
toxic encephalitis (G92.8)
toxic encephalopathy (G92.8)
DEF: Encephalitis: Inflammation of the brain, often caused by viral or bacterial infection.
DEF: Encephalomyelitis: Inflammatory disease, often viral in nature, that affects the brain and spinal cord.
DEF: Myelitis: Inflammation of the spinal cord.

√5th G04.0 Acute disseminated encephalitis and encephalomyelitis (ADEM)
EXCLUDES 1 acute necrotizing hemorrhagic encephalopathy (G04.3-)
other noninfectious acute disseminated encephalomyelitis (noninfectious ADEM) (G04.81)

G04.00 Acute disseminated encephalitis and encephalomyelitis, unspecified

G04.01 **Postinfectious** acute disseminated encephalitis and encephalomyelitis (postinfectious ADEM)
EXCLUDES 1 post chickenpox encephalitis (B01.1)
post measles encephalitis (B05.0)
post measles myelitis (B05.1)

G04.02 **Postimmunization** acute disseminated encephalitis, myelitis and encephalomyelitis
Encephalitis, post immunization
Encephalomyelitis, post immunization
Use additional code to identify the vaccine (T50.A-, T50.B-, T50.Z-)

G04.1 Tropical spastic paraplegia

G04.2 Bacterial meningoencephalitis and meningomyelitis, not elsewhere classified

Chapter 6. Diseases of the Nervous System

G04.3 Acute necrotizing hemorrhagic encephalopathy
  EXCLUDES 1: acute disseminated encephalitis and encephalomyelitis (G04.0-)
  G04.30 Acute necrotizing hemorrhagic encephalopathy, unspecified
  G04.31 Postinfectious acute necrotizing hemorrhagic encephalopathy
  G04.32 Postimmunization acute necrotizing hemorrhagic encephalopathy
    Use additional code to identify the vaccine (T50.A-, T50.B-, T50.Z-)
  G04.39 Other acute necrotizing hemorrhagic encephalopathy
    Code also underlying etiology, if applicable

G04.8 Other encephalitis, myelitis and encephalomyelitis
  Code also any associated seizure (G40.-, R56.9)
  G04.81 Other encephalitis and encephalomyelitis
    Noninfectious acute disseminated encephalomyelitis (noninfectious ADEM)
  G04.82 Acute flaccid myelitis
    EXCLUDES 1: transverse myelitis (G37.3)
    AHA: 2021,4Q,11
  G04.89 Other myelitis
    AHA: 2020,1Q,14

G04.9 Encephalitis, myelitis and encephalomyelitis, unspecified
  G04.90 Encephalitis and encephalomyelitis, unspecified
    Ventriculitis (cerebral) NOS
  G04.91 Myelitis, unspecified

G05 Encephalitis, myelitis and encephalomyelitis in diseases classified elsewhere
  Code first underlying disease, such as:
    congenital toxoplasmosis encephalitis, myelitis and encephalomyelitis (P37.1)
    cytomegaloviral encephalitis, myelitis and encephalomyelitis (B25.8)
    encephalitis, myelitis and encephalomyelitis (in) systemic lupus erythematosus (M32.19)
    eosinophilic meningoencephalitis (B83.2)
    human immunodeficiency virus [HIV] disease (B20)
    poliovirus (A80.-)
    suppurative otitis media (H66.01-H66.4)
    systemic lupus erythematosus (M32.19)
    trichinellosis (B75)
  EXCLUDES 1: adenoviral encephalitis, myelitis and encephalomyelitis (A85.1)
    encephalitis, myelitis and encephalomyelitis (in) measles (B05.0)
    enteroviral encephalitis, myelitis and encephalomyelitis (A85.0)
    herpesviral [herpes simplex] encephalitis, myelitis and encephalomyelitis (B00.4)
    listerial encephalitis, myelitis and encephalomyelitis (A32.12)
    meningococcal encephalitis, myelitis and encephalomyelitis (A39.81)
    mumps encephalitis, myelitis and encephalomyelitis (B26.2)
    postchickenpox encephalitis, myelitis and encephalomyelitis (B01.1-)
    rubella encephalitis, myelitis and encephalomyelitis (B06.01)
    toxoplasmosis encephalitis, myelitis and encephalomyelitis (B58.2)
    zoster encephalitis, myelitis and encephalomyelitis (B02.0)
  G05.3 Encephalitis and encephalomyelitis in diseases classified elsewhere
    Meningoencephalitis in diseases classified elsewhere
    Code first underlying disease
  G05.4 Myelitis in diseases classified elsewhere
    Meningomyelitis in diseases classified elsewhere

G06 Intracranial and intraspinal abscess and granuloma
  Use additional code (B95-B97) to identify infectious agent
  DEF: Abscess: Circumscribed collection of pus resulting from bacteria, frequently associated with swelling and other signs of inflammation.
  DEF: Granuloma: Abnormal, dense collections of cells forming a mass or nodule of chronically inflamed tissue with granulations that is usually associated with an infective process.
  G06.0 Intracranial abscess and granuloma
    Brain [any part] abscess (embolic)
    Cerebellar abscess (embolic)
    Cerebral abscess (embolic)
    Intracranial epidural abscess or granuloma
    Intracranial extradural abscess or granuloma
    Intracranial subdural abscess or granuloma
    Otogenic abscess (embolic)
    EXCLUDES 1: tuberculous intracranial abscess and granuloma (A17.81)
  G06.1 Intraspinal abscess and granuloma
    Abscess (embolic) of spinal cord [any part]
    Intraspinal epidural abscess or granuloma
    Intraspinal extradural abscess or granuloma
    Intraspinal subdural abscess or granuloma
    EXCLUDES 1: tuberculous intraspinal abscess and granuloma (A17.81)
  G06.2 Extradural and subdural abscess, unspecified

G07 Intracranial and intraspinal abscess and granuloma in diseases classified elsewhere
  Code first underlying disease, such as:
    schistosomiasis granuloma of brain (B65.-)
  EXCLUDES 1: abscess of brain:
    tuberculoma of meninges (A17.1)
      amebic (A06.6)
      chromomycotic (B43.1)
      gonococcal (A54.82)
      tuberculous (A17.81)

G08 Intracranial and intraspinal phlebitis and thrombophlebitis
  Septic embolism of intracranial or intraspinal venous sinuses and veins
  Septic endophlebitis of intracranial or intraspinal venous sinuses and veins
  Septic phlebitis of intracranial or intraspinal venous sinuses and veins
  Septic thrombophlebitis of intracranial or intraspinal venous sinuses and veins
  Septic thrombosis of intracranial or intraspinal venous sinuses and veins
  EXCLUDES 1: intracranial phlebitis and thrombophlebitis complicating:
    nonpyogenic intracranial phlebitis and thrombophlebitis (I67.6)
      abortion, ectopic or molar pregnancy (O00-O07, O08.7)
      pregnancy, childbirth and the puerperium (O22.5, O87.3)
  EXCLUDES 2: intracranial phlebitis and thrombophlebitis complicating nonpyogenic intraspinal phlebitis and thrombophlebitis (G95.1)
  DEF: Inflammation and formation of a blood clot in a vein within the brain or spine, or their linings.

G09 Sequelae of inflammatory diseases of central nervous system
  NOTE: Category G09 is to be used to indicate conditions whose primary classification is to G00-G08 as the cause of sequelae, themselves classifiable elsewhere. The "sequelae" include conditions specified as residuals.
  Code first condition resulting from (sequela) of inflammatory diseases of central nervous system

Systemic atrophies primarily affecting the central nervous system (G10-G14)

G10 Huntington's disease
  Huntington's chorea
  Huntington's dementia
  Use additional code, if applicable, to identify:
    dementia with anxiety (F02.84, F02.A4, F02.B4, F02.C4)
    dementia with behavioral disturbance (F02.81-, F02.A1-, F02.B1-, F02.C1-)
    dementia with mood disturbance (F02.83, F02.A3, F02.B3, F02.C3)
    dementia with psychotic disturbance (F02.82, F02.A2, F02.B2, F02.C2)
    dementia without behavioral disturbance (F02.80, F02.A0, F02.B0, F02.C0)
    mild neurocognitive disorder due to known physiological condition (F06.7-)
  DEF: Genetic disease caused by degeneration of nerve cells in the brain, characterized by chronic progressive mental deterioration. Dementia and death occur within 15 to 20 years of onset.

G11 Hereditary ataxia

EXCLUDES 2: cerebral palsy (G80.-)
hereditary and idiopathic neuropathy (G60.-)
metabolic disorders (E70-E88)

DEF: Ataxia: Defect in muscular control or coordination due to a central nervous system disorder, particularly when voluntary muscular movements are attempted.

- **G11.0** Congenital nonpressive ataxia
- **G11.1** Early-onset cerebellar ataxia
  AHA: 2020,4Q,17-18
  - **G11.10** Early-onset cerebellar ataxia, unspecified
  - **G11.11** Friedreich ataxia
    Autosomal recessive Friedreich ataxia
    Friedreich ataxia with retained reflexes
  - **G11.19** Other early-onset cerebellar ataxia
    Early-onset cerebellar ataxia with essential tremor
    Early-onset cerebellar ataxia with myoclonus [Hunt's ataxia]
    Early-onset cerebellar ataxia with retained tendon reflexes
    X-linked recessive spinocerebellar ataxia
- **G11.2** Late-onset cerebellar ataxia
- **G11.3** Cerebellar ataxia with defective DNA repair
  Ataxia telangiectasia [Louis-Bar]
  EXCLUDES 2: Cockayne's syndrome (Q87.19)
  other disorders of purine and pyrimidine metabolism (E79.-)
  xeroderma pigmentosum (Q82.1)
- **G11.4** Hereditary spastic paraplegia
- **G11.5** Hypomyelination - hypogonadotropic hypogonadism - hypodontia
  4H syndrome
  Pol III-related leukodystrophy
  AHA: 2023,4Q,12-13
- **G11.6** Leukodystrophy with vanishing white matter disease
  AHA: 2023,4Q,12-13
- **G11.8** Other hereditary ataxias
- **G11.9** Hereditary ataxia, unspecified
  Hereditary cerebellar ataxia NOS
  Hereditary cerebellar degeneration
  Hereditary cerebellar disease
  Hereditary cerebellar syndrome

G12 Spinal muscular atrophy and related syndromes

- **G12.0** Infantile spinal muscular atrophy, type I [Werdnig-Hoffman]
- **G12.1** Other inherited spinal muscular atrophy
  Adult form spinal muscular atrophy
  Childhood form, type II spinal muscular atrophy
  Distal spinal muscular atrophy
  Juvenile form, type III spinal muscular atrophy [Kugelberg-Welander]
  Progressive bulbar palsy of childhood [Fazio-Londe]
  Scapuloperoneal form spinal muscular atrophy
- **G12.2** Motor neuron disease
  AHA: 2017,4Q,9-10
  - **G12.20** Motor neuron disease, unspecified
  - **G12.21** Amyotrophic lateral sclerosis
  - **G12.22** Progressive bulbar palsy
  - **G12.23** Primary lateral sclerosis
  - **G12.24** Familial motor neuron disease
  - **G12.25** Progressive spinal muscle atrophy
  - **G12.29** Other motor neuron disease
- **G12.8** Other spinal muscular atrophies and related syndromes
- **G12.9** Spinal muscular atrophy, unspecified

G13 Systemic atrophies primarily affecting central nervous system in diseases classified elsewhere

- **G13.0** Paraneoplastic neuromyopathy and neuropathy
  Carcinomatous neuromyopathy
  Sensorial paraneoplastic neuropathy [Denny Brown]
  Code first underlying neoplasm (C00-D49)
- **G13.1** Other systemic atrophy primarily affecting central nervous system in neoplastic disease
  Paraneoplastic limbic encephalopathy
  Code first underlying neoplasm (C00-D49)
- **G13.2** Systemic atrophy primarily affecting the central nervous system in myxedema
  Code first underlying disease, such as:
  hypothyroidism (E03.-)
  myxedematous congenital iodine deficiency (E00.1)
- **G13.8** Systemic atrophy primarily affecting central nervous system in other diseases classified elsewhere
  Code first underlying disease

G14 Postpolio syndrome

INCLUDES: postpolio myelitic syndrome
EXCLUDES 1: sequelae of poliomyelitis (B91)

Extrapyramidal and movement disorders (G20-G26)

G20 Parkinson's disease

Hemiparkinsonism
Idiopathic Parkinsonism or Parkinson's disease
Paralysis agitans
Primary Parkinsonism or Parkinson's disease
Use additional code, if applicable, to identify:
dementia with anxiety (F02.84, F02.A4, F02.B4, F02.C4)
dementia with behavioral disturbance (F02.81-, F02.A1-, F02.B1-, F02.C1-)
dementia with mood disturbance (F02.83, F02.A3, F02.B3, F02.C3)
dementia with psychotic disturbance (F02.82, F02.A2, F02.B2, F02.C2)
dementia without behavioral disturbance (F02.80, F02.A0, F02.B0, F02.C0)
mild neurocognitive disorder due to known physiological condition (F06.7-)
AHA: 2023,4Q,15-17; 2017,2Q,7; 2016,2Q,6
TIP: Repeated falls (R29.6) are not integral to Parkinson's disease and can be separately coded.

- **G20.A** Parkinson's disease without dyskinesia
  - **G20.A1** Parkinson's disease without dyskinesia, without mention of fluctuations
    Parkinson's disease NOS
    Parkinson's disease without dyskinesia, without mention of OFF episodes
  - **G20.A2** Parkinson's disease without dyskinesia, with fluctuations
    Parkinson's disease without dyskinesia, with OFF episodes
- **G20.B** Parkinson's disease with dyskinesia
  EXCLUDES 1: drug induced dystonia (G24.0-)
  - **G20.B1** Parkinson's disease with dyskinesia, without mention of fluctuations
    Parkinson's disease with dyskinesia, without mention of OFF episodes
  - **G20.B2** Parkinson's disease with dyskinesia, with fluctuations
    Parkinson's disease with dyskinesia, with OFF episodes
- **G20.C** Parkinsonism, unspecified
  Parkinsonism, NOS
  EXCLUDES 1: Parkinson's disease NOS (G20.A1)
  Parkinson's disease with dyskinesia (G20.B-)
  Parkinson's disease without dyskinesia (G20.A-)
  secondary parkinsonism (G21.-)

G21 Secondary parkinsonism

EXCLUDES 1: Huntington's disease (G10)
neurocognitive disorder with Lewy bodies (G31.83)
Shy-Drager syndrome (G90.3)
syphilitic Parkinsonism (A52.19)

- **G21.0** Malignant neuroleptic syndrome
  Use additional code for adverse effect, if applicable, to identify drug (T43.3X5, T43.4X5, T43.505, T43.595)
  EXCLUDES 1: neuroleptic induced parkinsonism (G21.11)
- **G21.1** Other drug-induced secondary parkinsonism
  - **G21.11** Neuroleptic induced parkinsonism
    Use additional code for adverse effect, if applicable, to identify drug (T43.3X5, T43.4X5, T43.505, T43.595)
    EXCLUDES 1: malignant neuroleptic syndrome (G21.0)

Chapter 6. Diseases of the Nervous System

G21.19 **Other drug induced secondary parkinsonism** `Rx` `ESR` `COM`
Other medication-induced parkinsonism
Use additional code for adverse effect, if applicable, to identify drug (T36-T50 with fifth or sixth character 5)

G21.2 **Secondary parkinsonism due to other external agents** `Rx` `ESR` `COM`
Code first (T51-T65) to identify external agent

G21.3 **Postencephalitic** parkinsonism `HCC` `Rx` `ESR` `COM`

G21.4 **Vascular** parkinsonism `HCC` `Rx` `ESR` `COM`

G21.8 Other secondary parkinsonism `HCC` `Rx` `ESR` `COM`

G21.9 Secondary parkinsonism, unspecified `HCC` `Rx` `ESR` `COM`

✓4th **G23** **Other degenerative diseases of basal ganglia**
EXCLUDES 2 multi-system degeneration of the autonomic nervous system (G90.3)

G23.0 **Hallervorden-Spatz disease** `HCC` `Rx` `ESR` `COM`
Pigmentary pallidal degeneration

G23.1 **Progressive supranuclear ophthalmoplegia [Steele-Richardson-Olszewski]** `HCC` `Rx` `ESR` `COM`
Progressive supranuclear palsy

G23.2 **Striatonigral degeneration** `HCC` `Rx` `ESR` `COM`

G23.3 **Hypomyelination with atrophy of the basal ganglia and cerebellum** `HCC` `Rx` `ESR` `COM`
H-ABC
▶TUBB4A-related neurologic disorders◀
AHA: 2023,4Q,12-13

G23.8 **Other specified degenerative diseases of basal ganglia** `HCC` `Rx` `ESR` `COM`
Calcification of basal ganglia

G23.9 Degenerative disease of basal ganglia, unspecified `HCC` `Rx` `ESR` `COM`

✓4th **G24** **Dystonia**
INCLUDES dyskinesia
EXCLUDES 2 athetoid cerebral palsy (G80.3)
DEF: Disorder of abnormal muscle tone, excessive or inadequate. Involuntary movements and prolonged muscle contractions result in tremors, abnormalities in posture, and twisting body motions that affect an isolated area or the whole body.

✓5th **G24.0** **Drug induced** dystonia
Use additional code for adverse effect, if applicable, to identify drug (T36-T50 with fifth or sixth character 5)

G24.01 **Drug induced subacute dyskinesia**
Drug induced blepharospasm
Drug induced orofacial dyskinesia
Neuroleptic induced tardive dyskinesia
Tardive dyskinesia

G24.02 **Drug induced acute dystonia**
Acute dystonic reaction to drugs
Neuroleptic induced acute dystonia

G24.09 Other drug induced dystonia

G24.1 **Genetic torsion** dystonia
(Schwalbe-) Ziehen-Oppenheim disease
Dystonia deformans progressiva
Dystonia musculorum deformans
Familial torsion dystonia
Idiopathic (torsion) dystonia NOS
Idiopathic familial dystonia

G24.2 **Idiopathic nonfamilial** dystonia

G24.3 **Spasmodic torticollis**
EXCLUDES 1 congenital torticollis (Q68.0)
hysterical torticollis (F44.4)
ocular torticollis (R29.891)
psychogenic torticollis (F45.8)
torticollis NOS (M43.6)
traumatic recurrent torticollis (S13.4)
DEF: Twisted, unnatural position of the neck due to contracted cervical muscles that pull the head to one side or cause involuntary shaking of the head.

G24.4 **Idiopathic orofacial** dystonia
Orofacial dyskinesia
EXCLUDES 1 drug induced orofacial dyskinesia (G24.01)

G24.5 **Blepharospasm**
EXCLUDES 1 drug induced blepharospasm (G24.01)
DEF: Involuntary contraction of the orbicularis oculi muscle, resulting in the eyelids being completely closed.

G24.8 Other dystonia
Acquired torsion dystonia NOS

G24.9 Dystonia, unspecified
Dyskinesia NOS

✓4th **G25** **Other extrapyramidal and movement disorders**
EXCLUDES 2 sleep related movement disorders (G47.6-)

G25.0 **Essential** tremor
Familial tremor
EXCLUDES 1 tremor NOS (R25.1)

G25.1 **Drug-induced** tremor
Use additional code for adverse effect, if applicable, to identify drug (T36-T50 with fifth or sixth character 5)

G25.2 Other specified forms of tremor
Intention tremor

G25.3 **Myoclonus**
Drug-induced myoclonus
Palatal myoclonus
Use additional code for adverse effect, if applicable, to identify drug (T36-T50 with fifth or sixth character 5)
EXCLUDES 1 facial myokymia (G51.4)
myoclonic epilepsy (G40.-)
DEF: Spasmodic, brief, involuntary muscle contractions that can be due to an undetermined etiology, drug-induced, or caused by a disease process.

G25.4 **Drug-induced chorea**
Use additional code for adverse effect, if applicable, to identify drug (T36-T50 with fifth or sixth character 5)

G25.5 Other chorea
Chorea NOS
EXCLUDES 1 chorea NOS with heart involvement (I02.0)
Huntington's chorea (G10)
rheumatic chorea (I02.-)
Sydenham's chorea (I02.-)

✓5th **G25.6** **Drug induced tics and other tics of organic origin**

G25.61 **Drug induced tics**
Use additional code for adverse effect, if applicable, to identify drug (T36-T50 with fifth or sixth character 5)

G25.69 Other tics of organic origin
EXCLUDES 1 habit spasm (F95.9)
tic NOS (F95.9)
Tourette's syndrome (F95.2)

✓5th **G25.7** **Other and unspecified drug induced movement disorders**
Use additional code for adverse effect, if applicable, to identify drug (T36-T50 with fifth or sixth character 5)

G25.70 Drug induced movement disorder, unspecified

G25.71 **Drug induced akathisia**
Drug induced acathisia
Neuroleptic induced acute akathisia
Tardive akathisia

G25.79 Other drug induced movement disorders

✓5th **G25.8** **Other specified extrapyramidal and movement disorders**

G25.81 **Restless legs syndrome**
DEF: Neurological disorder of unknown etiology creating an irresistible urge to move the legs, which may temporarily relieve the symptoms. This syndrome is accompanied by motor restlessness and sensations of pain, burning, prickling, or tingling.

G25.82 **Stiff-man syndrome**

G25.83 **Benign shuddering attacks**

G25.89 Other specified extrapyramidal and movement disorders

G25.9 Extrapyramidal and movement disorder, unspecified

G26 *Extrapyramidal and movement disorders in diseases classified elsewhere*
Code first underlying disease

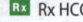 CMS-HCC Rx HCC 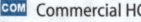 ESRD HCC 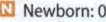 Commercial HCC Newborn: 0 Pediatric: 0-17 Maternity: 9-64 Adult: 15-124

Other degenerative diseases of the nervous system (G30-G32)

G30 Alzheimer's disease
  INCLUDES Alzheimer's dementia senile and presenile forms
  Use additional code, if applicable, to identify:
    delirium, if applicable (F05)
    dementia with anxiety (F02.84, F02.A4, F02.B4, F02.C4)
    dementia with behavioral disturbance (F02.81-, F02.A1-, F02.B1-, F02.C1-)
    dementia with mood disturbance (F02.83, F02.A3, F02.B3, F02.C3)
    dementia with psychotic disturbance (F02.82, F02.A2, F02.B2, F02.C2)
    dementia without behavioral disturbance (F02.80, F02.A0, F02.B0, F02.C0)
    mild neurocognitive disorder due to known physiological condition (F06.7-)
  EXCLUDES 1 senile degeneration of brain NEC (G31.1)
              senile dementia NOS (F03.-)
              senility NOS (R41.81)
  AHA: 2022,4Q,15; 2017,1Q,43
  TIP: A code from category F02 should always be assigned with a code from this category, even in the absence of documented dementia.
  TIP: Functional quadriplegia (R53.2) is not integral to Alzheimer's disease and can be coded in addition to codes from category G30.

  G30.0 Alzheimer's disease with early onset
  G30.1 Alzheimer's disease with late onset
  G30.8 Other Alzheimer's disease
  G30.9 Alzheimer's disease, unspecified
    AHA: 2016,2Q,6; 2012,4Q,95

G31 Other degenerative diseases of nervous system, not elsewhere classified
  Use additional code, if applicable, for codes G31.0-G31.83, G31.85-G31.9, to identify:
    dementia with anxiety (F02.84, F02.A4, F02.B4, F02.C4)
    dementia with behavioral disturbance (F02.81-, F02.A1-, F02.B1-, F02.C1-)
    dementia with mood disturbance (F02.83, F02.A3, F02.B3, F02.C3)
    dementia with psychotic disturbance (F02.82, F02.A2, F02.B2, F02.C2)
    dementia without behavioral disturbance (F02.80, F02.A0, F02.B0, F02.C0)
    mild neurocognitive disorder due to known physiological condition (F06.7-)
  EXCLUDES 2 Reye's syndrome (G93.7)

  G31.0 Frontotemporal dementia
    G31.01 Pick's disease
      Primary progressive aphasia
      Progressive isolated aphasia
      DEF: Progressive frontotemporal dementia with asymmetrical atrophy of the frontal and temporal regions of the cerebral cortex and abnormal rounded brain cells called Pick cells with the presence of abnormal staining of protein (called tau). Symptoms include prominent apathy, behavioral changes such as disinhibition and restlessness, echolalia, impairment of language, memory, and intellect, increased carelessness, poor personal hygiene, and decreased attention span.
    G31.09 Other frontotemporal neurocognitive disorder
      Frontal dementia
      Use additional code, if applicable, to identify mild neurocognitive disorders due to known physiological condition (F06.7-)

  G31.1 Senile degeneration of brain, not elsewhere classified
    EXCLUDES 1 Alzheimer's disease (G30.-)
                senility NOS (R41.81)

  G31.2 Degeneration of nervous system due to alcohol
    Alcoholic cerebellar ataxia
    Alcoholic cerebellar degeneration
    Alcoholic cerebral degeneration
    Alcoholic encephalopathy
    Dysfunction of the autonomic nervous system due to alcohol
    Code also associated alcoholism (F10.-)

  G31.8 Other specified degenerative diseases of nervous system
    G31.80 Leukodystrophy, unspecified
      AHA: 2023,4Q,12-13
    G31.81 Alpers disease
      Grey-matter degeneration
    G31.82 Leigh's disease
      Subacute necrotizing encephalopathy
    G31.83 Neurocognitive disorder with Lewy bodies
      Lewy body dementia
      Lewy body disease
      Use additional code, if applicable, to identify mild neurocognitive disorders due to known physiological condition (F06.7-)
      AHA: 2017,2Q,7; 2016,4Q,141
      DEF: Cerebral dementia with neurophysiologic changes, increased hippocampal volume, hypoperfusion in the occipital lobes, beta amyloid deposits with neurofibrillary tangles, and atrophy of the cortex and brainstem. Hallmark neuropsychological characteristics include fluctuating cognition with pronounced variation in attention and alertness, recurrent hallucinations, and Parkinsonism.
    G31.84 Mild cognitive impairment of uncertain or unknown etiology
      Mild cognitive disorder NOS
      Mild neurocognitive disorder of uncertain or unknown etiology
      Use additional code to identify presence of:
        alcohol abuse and dependence (F10.-)
        exposure to environmental tobacco smoke (Z77.22)
        history of tobacco dependence (Z87.891)
        hypertension (I10-I1A)
        occupational exposure to environmental tobacco smoke (Z57.31)
        tobacco dependence (F17.-)
        tobacco use (Z72.0)
      EXCLUDES 1 age related cognitive decline (R41.81)
                  altered mental status (R41.82)
                  cerebral degeneration (G31.9)
                  cerebrovascular diseases (I60-I69)
                  change in mental status (R41.82)
                  cognitive deficits following (sequelae of) cerebral hemorrhage or infarction (I69.01-, I69.11-, I69.21-, I69.31-, I69.81-, I69.91-)
                  cognitive impairment due to intracranial or head injury (S06.-)
                  dementia (F01.-, F02.-, F03.-)
                  mild neurocognitive disorder due to a known physiological condition (F06.7-)
                  neurologic neglect syndrome (R41.4)
                  personality change, nonpsychotic (F68.8)
      AHA: 2021,3Q,3
    G31.85 Corticobasal degeneration
    G31.86 Alexander disease
      AHA: 2023,4Q,12-13
    • **G31.87** Primary progressive apraxia of speech
    G31.89 Other specified degenerative diseases of nervous system
  G31.9 Degenerative disease of nervous system, unspecified
    AHA: 2021,3Q,3

G32 Other degenerative disorders of nervous system in diseases classified elsewhere
  G32.0 *Subacute combined degeneration of spinal cord in diseases classified elsewhere*
    Dana-Putnam syndrome
    Sclerosis of spinal cord (combined) (dorsolateral) (posterolateral)
    Code first underlying disease, such as:
      other dietary vitamin B12 deficiency anemia (D51.3)
      vitamin B12 deficiency (E53.8)
      vitamin B12 deficiency anemia due to intrinsic factor deficiency (D51.0)
      vitamin B12 deficiency anemia, unspecified (D51.8)
    EXCLUDES 1 syphilitic combined degeneration of spinal cord (A52.11)

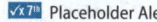

Chapter 6. Diseases of the Nervous System

G32.8 Other specified degenerative disorders of nervous system in diseases classified elsewhere
Code first underlying disease, such as:
amyloidosis cerebral degeneration (E85.-)
cerebral degeneration (due to) hypothyroidism (E00.0-E03.9)
cerebral degeneration (due to) neoplasm (C00-D49)
cerebral degeneration (due to) vitamin B deficiency, except thiamine (E52-E53.-)
EXCLUDES 1 superior hemorrhagic polioencephalitis [Wernicke's encephalopathy] (E51.2)

G32.81 Cerebellar ataxia in diseases classified elsewhere
Code first underlying disease, such as:
celiac disease (with gluten ataxia) (K90.0)
cerebellar ataxia (in) neoplastic disease (paraneoplastic cerebellar degeneration) (C00-D49)
non-celiac gluten ataxia (M35.9)
EXCLUDES 1 systemic atrophy primarily affecting the central nervous system in alcoholic cerebellar ataxia (G31.2)
systemic atrophy primarily affecting the central nervous system in myxedema (G13.2)

G32.89 Other specified degenerative disorders of nervous system in diseases classified elsewhere
Degenerative encephalopathy in diseases classified elsewhere

Demyelinating diseases of the central nervous system (G35-G37)

G35 Multiple sclerosis
~~Disseminated multiple sclerosis~~
~~Generalized multiple sclerosis~~
~~Multiple sclerosis of brain stem~~
~~Multiple sclerosis of cord~~
~~Multiple sclerosis NOS~~
AHA: 2021,1Q,7

- **G35.A** Relapsing-remitting multiple sclerosis
  EXCLUDES 1 demyelinating disease of central nervous system, unspecified (G37.9)
- **G35.B** Primary progressive multiple sclerosis
  - **G35.B0** Primary progressive multiple sclerosis, unspecified
  - **G35.B1** Active primary progressive multiple sclerosis
    Primary progressive multiple sclerosis with evidence of inflammatory disease activity
  - **G35.B2** Non-active primary progressive multiple sclerosis
    Primary progressive multiple sclerosis without evidence of inflammatory disease activity
- **G35.C** Secondary progressive multiple sclerosis
  - **G35.C0** Secondary progressive multiple sclerosis, unspecified
  - **G35.C1** Active secondary progressive multiple sclerosis
    Secondary progressive multiple sclerosis with evidence of inflammatory disease activity
  - **G35.C2** Non-active secondary progressive multiple sclerosis
    Secondary progressive multiple sclerosis without evidence of inflammatory disease activity
- **G35.D** Multiple sclerosis, unspecified
  Disseminated multiple sclerosis
  Generalized multiple sclerosis
  Multiple sclerosis of brain stem
  Multiple sclerosis of cord
  Multiple sclerosis NOS

G36 Other acute disseminated demyelination
EXCLUDES 1 postinfectious encephalitis and encephalomyelitis NOS (G04.01)
DEF: Demyelination: Abnormal loss of myelin, the protective white matter that insulates nerve endings and facilitates neuroreception and neurotransmission. When this substance is damaged, the nerve is short-circuited, resulting in impaired or loss of function.

G36.0 Neuromyelitis optica [Devic]
Demyelination in optic neuritis
EXCLUDES 1 optic neuritis NOS (H46)

G36.1 Acute and subacute hemorrhagic leukoencephalitis [Hurst]

G36.8 Other specified acute disseminated demyelination

G36.9 Acute disseminated demyelination, unspecified

G37 Other demyelinating diseases of central nervous system

G37.0 Diffuse sclerosis of central nervous system
Periaxial encephalitis
Schilder's disease
EXCLUDES 1 X linked adrenoleukodystrophy (E71.52-)

G37.1 Central demyelination of corpus callosum

G37.2 Central pontine myelinolysis
AHA: 2022,2Q,10

G37.3 Acute transverse myelitis in demyelinating disease of central nervous system
Acute transverse myelitis NOS
Acute transverse myelopathy
EXCLUDES 1 acute flaccid myelitis (G04.82)
multiple sclerosis ►(G35-)◄
neuromyelitis optica [Devic] (G36.0)

G37.4 Subacute necrotizing myelitis of central nervous system

G37.5 Concentric sclerosis [Balo] of central nervous system

G37.8 Other specified demyelinating diseases of central nervous system
AHA: 2023,4Q,18

  G37.81 Myelin oligodendrocyte glycoprotein antibody disease
  MOG antibody disease
  Code also associated manifestations, if known, such as:
  neuromyelitis optica (G36.0)
  noninfectious acute disseminated encephalomyelitis (G04.81)

  G37.89 Other specified demyelinating diseases of central nervous system

G37.9 Demyelinating disease of central nervous system, unspecified
►Clinically isolated syndromes◄

Episodic and paroxysmal disorders (G40-G47)

G40 Epilepsy and recurrent seizures
NOTE The following terms are to be considered equivalent to intractable: pharmacoresistant (pharmacologically resistant), treatment resistant, refractory (medically) and poorly controlled
EXCLUDES 1 conversion disorder with seizures (F44.5)
convulsions NOS (R56.9)
post traumatic seizures (R56.1)
seizure (convulsive) NOS (R56.9)
seizure of newborn (P90)
EXCLUDES 2 hippocampal sclerosis (G93.81)
mesial temporal sclerosis (G93.81)
temporal sclerosis (G93.81)
Todd's paralysis (G83.84)

G40.0 Localization-related (focal) (partial) idiopathic epilepsy and epileptic syndromes with seizures of localized onset
Benign childhood epilepsy with centrotemporal EEG spikes
Childhood epilepsy with occipital EEG paroxysms
EXCLUDES 1 adult onset localization-related epilepsy (G40.1-, G40.2-)

  G40.00 Localization-related (focal) (partial) idiopathic epilepsy and epileptic syndromes with seizures of localized onset, not intractable
  Localization-related (focal) (partial) idiopathic epilepsy and epileptic syndromes with seizures of localized onset without intractability

    G40.001 Localization-related (focal) (partial) idiopathic epilepsy and epileptic syndromes with seizures of localized onset, not intractable, with status epilepticus

    G40.009 Localization-related (focal) (partial) idiopathic epilepsy and epileptic syndromes with seizures of localized onset, not intractable, without status epilepticus
    Localization-related (focal) (partial) idiopathic epilepsy and epileptic syndromes with seizures of localized onset NOS

Chapter 6. Diseases of the Nervous System

- ✓6th **G40.01** Localization-related (focal) (partial) idiopathic epilepsy and epileptic syndromes with seizures of localized onset, **intractable**
  - **G40.011** Localization-related (focal) (partial) idiopathic epilepsy and epileptic syndromes with seizures of localized onset, intractable, **with status epilepticus** HCC Rx ESR COM
  - **G40.019** Localization-related (focal) (partial) idiopathic epilepsy and epileptic syndromes with seizures of localized onset, intractable, **without status epilepticus** HCC Rx ESR COM

- ✓5th **G40.1** Localization-related (focal) (partial) symptomatic epilepsy and epileptic syndromes with **simple partial seizures**
  - Attacks without alteration of consciousness
  - Epilepsia partialis continua [Kozhevnikof]
  - Simple partial seizures developing into secondarily generalized seizures
  - **AHA:** 2023,3Q,4
  - ✓6th **G40.10** Localization-related (focal) (partial) symptomatic epilepsy and epileptic syndromes with simple partial seizures, **not intractable**
    - Localization-related (focal) (partial) symptomatic epilepsy and epileptic syndromes with simple partial seizures without intractability
    - **G40.101** Localization-related (focal) (partial) symptomatic epilepsy and epileptic syndromes with simple partial seizures, not intractable, **with status epilepticus** HCC Rx ESR COM
    - **G40.109** Localization-related (focal) (partial) symptomatic epilepsy and epileptic syndromes with simple partial seizures, not intractable, **without status epilepticus** HCC Rx ESR COM
      - Localization-related (focal) (partial) symptomatic epilepsy and epileptic syndromes with simple partial seizures NOS
  - ✓6th **G40.11** Localization-related (focal) (partial) symptomatic epilepsy and epileptic syndromes with simple partial seizures, **intractable**
    - **G40.111** Localization-related (focal) (partial) symptomatic epilepsy and epileptic syndromes with simple partial seizures, intractable, **with status epilepticus** HCC Rx ESR COM
    - **G40.119** Localization-related (focal) (partial) symptomatic epilepsy and epileptic syndromes with simple partial seizures, intractable, **without status epilepticus** HCC Rx ESR COM

- ✓5th **G40.2** Localization-related (focal) (partial) symptomatic epilepsy and epileptic syndromes with **complex partial seizures**
  - Attacks with alteration of consciousness, often with automatisms
  - Complex partial seizures developing into secondarily generalized seizures
  - ✓6th **G40.20** Localization-related (focal) (partial) symptomatic epilepsy and epileptic syndromes with complex partial seizures, **not intractable**
    - Localization-related (focal) (partial) symptomatic epilepsy and epileptic syndromes with complex partial seizures without intractability
    - **G40.201** Localization-related (focal) (partial) symptomatic epilepsy and epileptic syndromes with complex partial seizures, not intractable, **with status epilepticus** HCC Rx ESR COM
    - **G40.209** Localization-related (focal) (partial) symptomatic epilepsy and epileptic syndromes with complex partial seizures, not intractable, **without status epilepticus** HCC Rx ESR COM
      - Localization-related (focal) (partial) symptomatic epilepsy and epileptic syndromes with complex partial seizures NOS

- ✓6th **G40.21** Localization-related (focal) (partial) symptomatic epilepsy and epileptic syndromes with complex partial seizures, **intractable**
  - **G40.211** Localization-related (focal) (partial) symptomatic epilepsy and epileptic syndromes with complex partial seizures, intractable, **with status epilepticus** HCC Rx ESR COM
  - **G40.219** Localization-related (focal) (partial) symptomatic epilepsy and epileptic syndromes with complex partial seizures, intractable, **without status epilepticus** HCC Rx ESR COM

- ✓5th **G40.3** **Generalized** idiopathic epilepsy and epileptic syndromes
  - Code also MERRF syndrome, if applicable (E88.42)
  - ✓6th **G40.30** Generalized idiopathic epilepsy and epileptic syndromes, **not intractable**
    - Generalized idiopathic epilepsy and epileptic syndromes without intractability
    - **G40.301** Generalized idiopathic epilepsy and epileptic syndromes, not intractable, **with status epilepticus** HCC Rx ESR COM
    - **G40.309** Generalized idiopathic epilepsy and epileptic syndromes, not intractable, **without status epilepticus** HCC Rx ESR COM
      - Generalized idiopathic epilepsy and epileptic syndromes NOS
  - ✓6th **G40.31** Generalized idiopathic epilepsy and epileptic syndromes, **intractable**
    - **G40.311** Generalized idiopathic epilepsy and epileptic syndromes, intractable, **with status epilepticus** HCC Rx ESR COM
    - **G40.319** Generalized idiopathic epilepsy and epileptic syndromes, intractable, **without status epilepticus** HCC Rx ESR COM

- ✓5th **G40.A** **Absence** epileptic syndrome
  - Absence epileptic syndrome, NOS
  - Childhood absence epilepsy [pyknolepsy]
  - Juvenile absence epilepsy
  - ✓6th **G40.A0** Absence epileptic syndrome, **not intractable**
    - **G40.A01** Absence epileptic syndrome, not intractable, **with status epilepticus** HCC Rx ESR COM
    - **G40.A09** Absence epileptic syndrome, not intractable, **without status epilepticus** HCC Rx ESR COM
  - ✓6th **G40.A1** Absence epileptic syndrome, **intractable**
    - **G40.A11** Absence epileptic syndrome, intractable, with status epilepticus HCC Rx ESR COM
    - **G40.A19** Absence epileptic syndrome, intractable, without status epilepticus HCC Rx ESR COM

- ✓5th **G40.B** **Juvenile myoclonic** epilepsy [impulsive petit mal]
  - ✓6th **G40.B0** Juvenile myoclonic epilepsy, **not intractable**
    - **G40.B01** Juvenile myoclonic epilepsy, not intractable, **with status epilepticus** HCC Rx ESR COM
    - **G40.B09** Juvenile myoclonic epilepsy, not intractable, **without status epilepticus** HCC Rx ESR COM
  - ✓6th **G40.B1** Juvenile myoclonic epilepsy, **intractable**
    - **G40.B11** Juvenile myoclonic epilepsy, intractable, with status epilepticus HCC Rx ESR COM
    - **G40.B19** Juvenile myoclonic epilepsy, intractable, without status epilepticus HCC Rx ESR COM

- ✓5th **G40.C** **Lafora progressive myoclonus** epilepsy
  - Lafora body disease
  - Code also, if applicable, associated conditions such as dementia (F02.8-)
  - **AHA:** 2023,4Q,18-19
  - ✓6th **G40.C0** Lafora progressive myoclonus epilepsy, **not intractable**
    - **G40.C01** Lafora progressive myoclonus epilepsy, not intractable, **with status epilepticus** HCC Rx ESR COM

✓ Additional Character Required ✓x7th Placeholder Alert Manifestation Unspecified Dx QPP UPD Unacceptable PDx

G40.C09 Lafora progressive myoclonus epilepsy, not intractable, without status epilepticus [HCC Rx ESR COM]
Lafora progressive myoclonus epilepsy NOS

✓6ᵗʰ **G40.C1** Lafora progressive myoclonus epilepsy, intractable

G40.C11 Lafora progressive myoclonus epilepsy, intractable, with status epilepticus [HCC Rx ESR COM]

G40.C19 Lafora progressive myoclonus epilepsy, intractable, without status epilepticus [HCC Rx ESR COM]

✓5ᵗʰ **G40.4** Other generalized epilepsy and epileptic syndromes
Epilepsy with grand mal seizures on awakening
Epilepsy with myoclonic absences
Epilepsy with myoclonic-astatic seizures
Grand mal seizure NOS
Nonspecific atonic epileptic seizures
Nonspecific clonic epileptic seizures
Nonspecific myoclonic epileptic seizures
Nonspecific tonic epileptic seizures
Nonspecific tonic-clonic epileptic seizures
Symptomatic early myoclonic encephalopathy

✓6ᵗʰ **G40.40** Other generalized epilepsy and epileptic syndromes, not intractable
Other generalized epilepsy and epileptic syndromes NOS
Other generalized epilepsy and epileptic syndromes without intractability

G40.401 Other generalized epilepsy and epileptic syndromes, not intractable, with status epilepticus [HCC Rx ESR COM]

G40.409 Other generalized epilepsy and epileptic syndromes, not intractable, without status epilepticus [HCC Rx ESR COM]

✓6ᵗʰ **G40.41** Other generalized epilepsy and epileptic syndromes, intractable

G40.411 Other generalized epilepsy and epileptic syndromes, intractable, with status epilepticus [HCC Rx ESR COM]

G40.419 Other generalized epilepsy and epileptic syndromes, intractable, without status epilepticus [HCC Rx ESR COM]

G40.42 Cyclin-Dependent Kinase-Like 5 Deficiency Disorder [HCC Rx ESR COM]
CDKL5
Use additional code, if known, to identify associated manifestations, such as:
cortical blindness (H47.61-)
global development delay (F88)
AHA: 2020,4Q,18-19

✓5ᵗʰ **G40.5** Epileptic seizures related to external causes
Epileptic seizures related to alcohol
Epileptic seizures related to drugs
Epileptic seizures related to hormonal changes
Epileptic seizures related to sleep deprivation
Epileptic seizures related to stress
Code also, if applicable, associated epilepsy and recurrent seizures (G40.-)
Use additional code for adverse effect, if applicable, to identify drug (T36-T50 with fifth or sixth character 5)

✓6ᵗʰ **G40.50** Epileptic seizures related to external causes, not intractable

G40.501 Epileptic seizures related to external causes, not intractable, with status epilepticus [HCC Rx ESR COM]

G40.509 Epileptic seizures related to external causes, not intractable, without status epilepticus [HCC Rx ESR COM]
Epileptic seizures related to external causes, NOS

✓5ᵗʰ **G40.8** Other epilepsy and recurrent seizures
Epilepsies and epileptic syndromes undetermined as to whether they are focal or generalized
Landau-Kleffner syndrome

✓6ᵗʰ **G40.80** Other epilepsy

G40.801 Other epilepsy, not intractable, with status epilepticus [HCC Rx ESR COM]
Other epilepsy without intractability with status epilepticus

G40.802 Other epilepsy, not intractable, without status epilepticus [HCC Rx ESR COM]
Other epilepsy NOS
Other epilepsy without intractability without status epilepticus

G40.803 Other epilepsy, intractable, with status epilepticus [HCC Rx ESR COM]

G40.804 Other epilepsy, intractable, without status epilepticus [HCC Rx ESR COM]

✓6ᵗʰ **G40.81** Lennox-Gastaut syndrome
DEF: Severe form of epilepsy with usual onset in early childhood. Seizures are frequent and difficult to treat, causing falls and intellectual impairment.

G40.811 Lennox-Gastaut syndrome, not intractable, with status epilepticus [HCC Rx ESR COM]

G40.812 Lennox-Gastaut syndrome, not intractable, without status epilepticus [HCC Rx ESR COM]

G40.813 Lennox-Gastaut syndrome, intractable, with status epilepticus [HCC Rx ESR COM]

G40.814 Lennox-Gastaut syndrome, intractable, without status epilepticus [HCC Rx ESR COM]

✓6ᵗʰ **G40.82** Epileptic spasms
Infantile spasms
Salaam attacks
West's syndrome

G40.821 Epileptic spasms, not intractable, with status epilepticus [HCC Rx ESR COM]

G40.822 Epileptic spasms, not intractable, without status epilepticus [HCC Rx ESR COM]

G40.823 Epileptic spasms, intractable, with status epilepticus [HCC Rx ESR COM]

G40.824 Epileptic spasms, intractable, without status epilepticus [HCC Rx ESR COM]

✓6ᵗʰ **G40.83** Dravet syndrome
Polymorphic epilepsy in infancy (PMEI)
Severe myoclonic epilepsy in infancy (SMEI)
AHA: 2020,4Q,19

G40.833 Dravet syndrome, intractable, with status epilepticus [HCC Rx ESR COM]

G40.834 Dravet syndrome, intractable, without status epilepticus [HCC Rx ESR COM]
Dravet syndrome NOS

✓6ᵗʰ **G40.84** KCNQ2-related epilepsy
AHA: 2024,4Q,15

G40.841 KCNQ2-related epilepsy, not intractable, with status epilepticus [HCC Rx ESR COM]

G40.842 KCNQ2-related epilepsy, not intractable, without status epilepticus [HCC Rx ESR COM]
KCNQ2-related epilepsy NOS

G40.843 KCNQ2-related epilepsy, intractable, with status epilepticus [HCC Rx ESR COM]

G40.844 KCNQ2-related epilepsy, intractable, without status epilepticus [HCC Rx ESR COM]

G40.89 Other seizures [HCC Rx ESR COM]
EXCLUDES 1 post traumatic seizures (R56.1)
recurrent seizures NOS (G40.909)
seizure NOS (R56.9)

✓5ᵗʰ **G40.9** Epilepsy, unspecified
AHA: 2019,1Q,19

✓6ᵗʰ **G40.90** Epilepsy, unspecified, not intractable
Epilepsy, unspecified, without intractability

G40.901 Epilepsy, unspecified, not intractable, with status epilepticus [HCC Rx ESR COM]

G40.909 Epilepsy, unspecified, not intractable, without status epilepticus [HCC Rx ESR COM]
Epilepsy NOS
Epileptic convulsions NOS
Epileptic fits NOS
Epileptic seizures NOS
Recurrent seizures NOS
Seizure disorder NOS
AHA: 2024,2Q,8; 2021,2Q,3; 2021,1Q,3

HCC CMS-HCC | Rx Rx HCC | ESR ESRD HCC | COM Commercial HCC | N Newborn: 0 | P Pediatric: 0-17 | M Maternity: 9-64 | A Adult: 15-124

G40.91 Epilepsy, unspecified, intractable
Intractable seizure disorder NOS
- G40.911 Epilepsy, unspecified, intractable, with status epilepticus
- G40.919 Epilepsy, unspecified, intractable, without status epilepticus

G43 Migraine

NOTE The following terms are to be considered equivalent to intractable: pharmacoresistant (pharmacologically resistant), treatment resistant, refractory (medically) and poorly controlled

Use additional code for adverse effect, if applicable, to identify drug (T36-T50 with fifth or sixth character 5)

EXCLUDES 1: headache NOS (R51.9)
lower half migraine (G44.00)
EXCLUDES 2: headache syndromes (G44.-)

DEF: Headaches that occur periodically on one or both sides of the head that may be associated with nausea and vomiting, sensitivity to light and sound, dizziness, distorted vision, and cognitive disturbances.

G43.0 Migraine without aura
Common migraine
EXCLUDES 1: chronic migraine without aura (G43.7-)

- G43.00 Migraine without aura, not intractable
  Migraine without aura without mention of refractory migraine
  - G43.001 Migraine without aura, not intractable, with status migrainosus
  - G43.009 Migraine without aura, not intractable, without status migrainosus
    Migraine without aura NOS
- G43.01 Migraine without aura, intractable
  Migraine without aura with refractory migraine
  - G43.011 Migraine without aura, intractable, with status migrainosus
  - G43.019 Migraine without aura, intractable, without status migrainosus

G43.1 Migraine with aura
Basilar migraine
Classical migraine
Migraine equivalents
Migraine preceded or accompanied by transient focal neurological phenomena
Migraine triggered seizures
Migraine with acute-onset aura
Migraine with aura without headache (migraine equivalents)
Migraine with prolonged aura
Migraine with typical aura
Retinal migraine
Code also any associated seizure (G40.-, R56.9)
EXCLUDES 1: chronic migraine with aura (G43.E-)
persistent migraine aura (G43.5-, G43.6-)

- G43.10 Migraine with aura, not intractable
  Migraine with aura without mention of refractory migraine
  - G43.101 Migraine with aura, not intractable, with status migrainosus
  - G43.109 Migraine with aura, not intractable, without status migrainosus
    Migraine with aura NOS
- G43.11 Migraine with aura, intractable
  Migraine with aura with refractory migraine
  - G43.111 Migraine with aura, intractable, with status migrainosus
  - G43.119 Migraine with aura, intractable, without status migrainosus

G43.4 Hemiplegic migraine
Familial migraine
Sporadic migraine
AHA: 2025,2Q,18

- G43.40 Hemiplegic migraine, not intractable
  Hemiplegic migraine without refractory migraine
  - G43.401 Hemiplegic migraine, not intractable, with status migrainosus
  - G43.409 Hemiplegic migraine, not intractable, without status migrainosus
    Hemiplegic migraine NOS
- G43.41 Hemiplegic migraine, intractable
  Hemiplegic migraine with refractory migraine
  - G43.411 Hemiplegic migraine, intractable, with status migrainosus
  - G43.419 Hemiplegic migraine, intractable, without status migrainosus

G43.5 Persistent migraine aura without cerebral infarction

- G43.50 Persistent migraine aura without cerebral infarction, not intractable
  Persistent migraine aura without cerebral infarction, without refractory migraine
  - G43.501 Persistent migraine aura without cerebral infarction, not intractable, with status migrainosus
  - G43.509 Persistent migraine aura without cerebral infarction, not intractable, without status migrainosus
    Persistent migraine aura NOS
- G43.51 Persistent migraine aura without cerebral infarction, intractable
  Persistent migraine aura without cerebral infarction, with refractory migraine
  - G43.511 Persistent migraine aura without cerebral infarction, intractable, with status migrainosus
  - G43.519 Persistent migraine aura without cerebral infarction, intractable, without status migrainosus

G43.6 Persistent migraine aura with cerebral infarction
Code also the type of cerebral infarction (I63.-)

- G43.60 Persistent migraine aura with cerebral infarction, not intractable
  Persistent migraine aura with cerebral infarction, without refractory migraine
  - G43.601 Persistent migraine aura with cerebral infarction, not intractable, with status migrainosus
  - G43.609 Persistent migraine aura with cerebral infarction, not intractable, without status migrainosus
- G43.61 Persistent migraine aura with cerebral infarction, intractable
  Persistent migraine aura with cerebral infarction, with refractory migraine
  - G43.611 Persistent migraine aura with cerebral infarction, intractable, with status migrainosus
  - G43.619 Persistent migraine aura with cerebral infarction, intractable, without status migrainosus

G43.7 Chronic migraine without aura
Transformed migraine
EXCLUDES 1: migraine without aura (G43.0-)

- G43.70 Chronic migraine without aura, not intractable
  Chronic migraine without aura, without refractory migraine
  - G43.701 Chronic migraine without aura, not intractable, with status migrainosus
  - G43.709 Chronic migraine without aura, not intractable, without status migrainosus
    Chronic migraine without aura NOS
- G43.71 Chronic migraine without aura, intractable
  Chronic migraine without aura, with refractory migraine
  - G43.711 Chronic migraine without aura, intractable, with status migrainosus
  - G43.719 Chronic migraine without aura, intractable, without status migrainosus

G43.A Cyclical vomiting
EXCLUDES 1: cyclical vomiting syndrome unrelated to migraine (R11.15)
AHA: 2019,4Q,15

- G43.A0 Cyclical vomiting, in migraine, not intractable
  Cyclical vomiting, without refractory migraine
- G43.A1 Cyclical vomiting, in migraine, intractable
  Cyclical vomiting, with refractory migraine

G43.B Ophthalmoplegic migraine

- **G43.B0** Ophthalmoplegic migraine, not intractable
  - Ophthalmoplegic migraine, without refractory migraine
- **G43.B1** Ophthalmoplegic migraine, intractable
  - Ophthalmoplegic migraine, with refractory migraine

G43.C Periodic headache syndromes in child or adult

- **G43.C0** Periodic headache syndromes in child or adult, not intractable
  - Periodic headache syndromes in child or adult, without refractory migraine
- **G43.C1** Periodic headache syndromes in child or adult, intractable
  - Periodic headache syndromes in child or adult, with refractory migraine

G43.D Abdominal migraine

- **G43.D0** Abdominal migraine, not intractable
  - Abdominal migraine, without refractory migraine
- **G43.D1** Abdominal migraine, intractable
  - Abdominal migraine, with refractory migraine

G43.8 Other migraine

- **G43.80** Other migraine, not intractable
  - Other migraine, without refractory migraine
  - **G43.801** Other migraine, not intractable, with status migrainosus
  - **G43.809** Other migraine, not intractable, without status migrainosus
- **G43.81** Other migraine, intractable
  - Other migraine, with refractory migraine
  - **G43.811** Other migraine, intractable, with status migrainosus
  - **G43.819** Other migraine, intractable, without status migrainosus
- **G43.82** Menstrual migraine, not intractable
  - Menstrual headache, not intractable
  - Menstrual migraine, without refractory migraine
  - Menstrually related migraine, not intractable
  - Pre-menstrual headache, not intractable
  - Pre-menstrual migraine, not intractable
  - Pure menstrual migraine, not intractable
  - Code also associated premenstrual tension syndrome (N94.3)
  - **G43.821** Menstrual migraine, not intractable, with status migrainosus
  - **G43.829** Menstrual migraine, not intractable, without status migrainosus
    - Menstrual migraine NOS
- **G43.83** Menstrual migraine, intractable
  - Menstrual headache, intractable
  - Menstrual migraine, with refractory migraine
  - Menstrually related migraine, intractable
  - Pre-menstrual headache, intractable
  - Pre-menstrual migraine, intractable
  - Pure menstrual migraine, intractable
  - Code also associated premenstrual tension syndrome (N94.3)
  - **G43.831** Menstrual migraine, intractable, with status migrainosus
  - **G43.839** Menstrual migraine, intractable, without status migrainosus

G43.9 Migraine, unspecified

- **G43.90** Migraine, unspecified, not intractable
  - Migraine, unspecified, without refractory migraine
  - **G43.901** Migraine, unspecified, not intractable, with status migrainosus
    - Status migrainosus NOS
  - **G43.909** Migraine, unspecified, not intractable, without status migrainosus
    - Migraine NOS
- **G43.91** Migraine, unspecified, intractable
  - Migraine, unspecified, with refractory migraine
  - **G43.911** Migraine, unspecified, intractable, with status migrainosus
  - **G43.919** Migraine, unspecified, intractable, without status migrainosus

G43.E Chronic migraine with aura

EXCLUDES 1: migraine with aura (G43.1-)
AHA: 2023,4Q,19-20

- **G43.E0** Chronic migraine with aura, not intractable
  - Chronic migraine with aura, without refractory migraine
  - **G43.E01** Chronic migraine with aura, not intractable, with status migrainosus
  - **G43.E09** Chronic migraine with aura, not intractable, without status migrainosus
    - Chronic migraine with aura NOS
- **G43.E1** Chronic migraine with aura, intractable
  - Chronic migraine with aura, with refractory migraine
  - **G43.E11** Chronic migraine with aura, intractable, with status migrainosus
  - **G43.E19** Chronic migraine with aura, intractable, without status migrainosus

G44 Other headache syndromes

EXCLUDES 1: headache NOS (R51.9)
EXCLUDES 2: atypical facial pain (G50.1)
headache due to lumbar puncture (G97.1)
migraines (G43.-)
trigeminal neuralgia (G50.0)

G44.0 Cluster headaches and other trigeminal autonomic cephalgias (TAC)

DEF: Cluster headache: Characteristic grouping or clustering of headaches that can last for a number of weeks or months and then completely disappear for months or years. They are typically not associated with gastrointestinal upset or light sensitivity as experienced in migraines.

- **G44.00** Cluster headache syndrome, unspecified
  - Ciliary neuralgia
  - Cluster headache NOS
  - Histamine cephalgia
  - Lower half migraine
  - Migrainous neuralgia
  - **G44.001** Cluster headache syndrome, unspecified, intractable
  - **G44.009** Cluster headache syndrome, unspecified, not intractable
    - Cluster headache syndrome NOS
- **G44.01** Episodic cluster headache
  - **G44.011** Episodic cluster headache, intractable
  - **G44.019** Episodic cluster headache, not intractable
    - Episodic cluster headache NOS
- **G44.02** Chronic cluster headache
  - **G44.021** Chronic cluster headache, intractable
  - **G44.029** Chronic cluster headache, not intractable
    - Chronic cluster headache NOS
- **G44.03** Episodic paroxysmal hemicrania
  - Paroxysmal hemicrania NOS
  - **G44.031** Episodic paroxysmal hemicrania, intractable
  - **G44.039** Episodic paroxysmal hemicrania, not intractable
    - Episodic paroxysmal hemicrania NOS
- **G44.04** Chronic paroxysmal hemicrania
  - **G44.041** Chronic paroxysmal hemicrania, intractable
  - **G44.049** Chronic paroxysmal hemicrania, not intractable
    - Chronic paroxysmal hemicrania NOS
- **G44.05** Short lasting unilateral neuralgiform headache with conjunctival injection and tearing (SUNCT)
  - **G44.051** Short lasting unilateral neuralgiform headache with conjunctival injection and tearing (SUNCT), intractable
  - **G44.059** Short lasting unilateral neuralgiform headache with conjunctival injection and tearing (SUNCT), not intractable
    - Short lasting unilateral neuralgiform headache with conjunctival injection and tearing (SUNCT) NOS
- **G44.09** Other trigeminal autonomic cephalgias (TAC)
  - **G44.091** Other trigeminal autonomic cephalgias (TAC), intractable
  - **G44.099** Other trigeminal autonomic cephalgias (TAC), not intractable

G44.1 **Vascular** headache, not elsewhere classified
  EXCLUDES 2: cluster headache (G44.0)
  complicated headache syndromes (G44.5-)
  drug-induced headache (G44.4-)
  migraine (G43.-)
  other specified headache syndromes (G44.8-)
  post-traumatic headache (G44.3-)
  tension-type headache (G44.2-)

G44.2 **Tension-type** headache
  G44.20 Tension-type headache, unspecified
    G44.201 Tension-type headache, unspecified, intractable
    G44.209 Tension-type headache, unspecified, not intractable
      Tension headache NOS
  G44.21 **Episodic** tension-type headache
    G44.211 Episodic tension-type headache, intractable
    G44.219 Episodic tension-type headache, not intractable
      Episodic tension-type headache NOS
  G44.22 **Chronic** tension-type headache
    G44.221 Chronic tension-type headache, intractable
    G44.229 Chronic tension-type headache, not intractable
      Chronic tension-type headache NOS

G44.3 **Post-traumatic** headache
  G44.30 Post-traumatic headache, unspecified
    G44.301 Post-traumatic headache, unspecified, intractable
    G44.309 Post-traumatic headache, unspecified, not intractable
      Post-traumatic headache NOS
  G44.31 **Acute** post-traumatic headache
    G44.311 Acute post-traumatic headache, intractable
    G44.319 Acute post-traumatic headache, not intractable
      Acute post-traumatic headache NOS
  G44.32 **Chronic** post-traumatic headache
    G44.321 Chronic post-traumatic headache, intractable
    G44.329 Chronic post-traumatic headache, not intractable
      Chronic post-traumatic headache NOS

G44.4 **Drug-induced** headache, not elsewhere classified
  Medication overuse headache
  Use additional code for adverse effect, if applicable, to identify drug (T36-T50 with fifth or sixth character 5)
  G44.40 Drug-induced headache, not elsewhere classified, not intractable
  G44.41 Drug-induced headache, not elsewhere classified, intractable

G44.5 **Complicated** headache syndromes
  G44.51 Hemicrania continua
    DEF: Persistent primary headache of unknown causation occurring on one side of the face and head. May last for more than three months, with daily and continuous pain of moderate intensity with severe exacerbations.
  G44.52 New daily persistent headache (NDPH)
  G44.53 Primary thunderclap headache
  G44.59 Other complicated headache syndrome

G44.8 Other specified headache syndromes
  EXCLUDES 2: headache with orthostatic or positional component, not elsewhere classifed (R51.0)
  G44.81 Hypnic headache
  G44.82 Headache associated with sexual activity
    Orgasmic headache
    Preorgasmic headache
  G44.83 Primary cough headache
  G44.84 Primary exertional headache
  G44.85 Primary stabbing headache
  G44.86 Cervicogenic headache
    Code also associated cervical spinal condition, if known
    AHA: 2021,4Q,11-12
  G44.89 Other headache syndrome

G45 Transient cerebral ischemic attacks and related syndromes
  EXCLUDES 1: neonatal cerebral ischemia (P91.0)
  transient retinal artery occlusion (H34.0-)
  AHA: 2023,1Q,37; 2018,2Q,9
  DEF: Transient cerebral ischemic attack: Intermittent or brief cerebral dysfunction from lack of oxygenation with no persistent neurological deficits associated with occlusive vascular disease. TIA may denote an impending cerebrovascular accident.
  G45.0 Vertebro-basilar artery syndrome
  G45.1 Carotid artery syndrome (hemispheric)
  G45.2 Multiple and bilateral precerebral artery syndromes
  G45.3 Amaurosis fugax
  G45.4 Transient global amnesia
    EXCLUDES 1: amnesia NOS (R41.3)
  G45.8 Other transient cerebral ischemic attacks and related syndromes
  G45.9 Transient cerebral ischemic attack, unspecified
    Spasm of cerebral artery
    TIA
    Transient cerebral ischemia NOS

G46 Vascular syndromes of brain in cerebrovascular diseases
  Code first underlying cerebrovascular disease (I60-I69)
  G46.0 Middle cerebral artery syndrome
  G46.1 Anterior cerebral artery syndrome
  G46.2 Posterior cerebral artery syndrome
  G46.3 Brain stem stroke syndrome
    Benedikt syndrome
    Claude syndrome
    Foville syndrome
    Millard-Gubler syndrome
    Wallenberg syndrome
    Weber syndrome
  G46.4 Cerebellar stroke syndrome
  G46.5 Pure motor lacunar syndrome
  G46.6 Pure sensory lacunar syndrome
  G46.7 Other lacunar syndromes
  G46.8 Other vascular syndromes of brain in cerebrovascular diseases

G47 Sleep disorders
  EXCLUDES 2: nightmares (F51.5)
  nonorganic sleep disorders (F51.-)
  sleep terrors (F51.4)
  sleepwalking (F51.3)
  G47.0 Insomnia
    EXCLUDES 2: alcohol related insomnia (F10.182, F10.282, F10.982)
    drug-related insomnia (F11.182, F11.282, F11.982, F13.182, F13.282, F13.982, F14.182, F14.282, F14.982, F15.182, F15.282, F15.982, F19.182, F19.282, F19.982)
    idiopathic insomnia (F51.01)
    insomnia due to a mental disorder (F51.05)
    insomnia not due to a substance or known physiological condition (F51.0-)
    nonorganic insomnia (F51.0-)
    primary insomnia (F51.01)
    sleep apnea (G47.3-)
    G47.00 Insomnia, unspecified
      Insomnia NOS
    G47.01 Insomnia due to medical condition
      Code also associated medical condition
    G47.09 Other insomnia
  G47.1 Hypersomnia
    EXCLUDES 2: alcohol-related hypersomnia (F10.182, F10.282, F10.982)
    drug-related hypersomnia (F11.182, F11.282, F11.982, F13.182, F13.282, F13.982, F14.182, F14.282, F14.982, F15.182, F15.282, F15.982, F19.182, F19.282, F19.982)
    hypersomnia due to a mental disorder (F51.13)
    hypersomnia not due to a substance or known physiological condition (F51.1-)
    primary hypersomnia (F51.11)
    sleep apnea (G47.3-)
    G47.10 Hypersomnia, unspecified
      Hypersomnia NOS
    G47.11 Idiopathic hypersomnia with long sleep time
      Idiopathic hypersomnia NOS
    G47.12 Idiopathic hypersomnia without long sleep time

Chapter 6. Diseases of the Nervous System

G47.13 **Recurrent** hypersomnia
  Kleine-Levin syndrome
  Menstrual related hypersomnia
G47.14 **Hypersomnia due to medical condition**
  Code also associated medical condition
G47.19 Other hypersomnia

√5th **G47.2** **Circadian rhythm sleep disorders**
  Disorders of the sleep wake schedule
  Inversion of nyctohemeral rhythm
  Inversion of sleep rhythm
  DEF: Circadian rhythm: Daily cycle (24-hour period) of physical, mental, and behavioral changes. It is largely influenced by environmental cues, such as changes in light or temperature.
  Synonym(s): *sleep/wake cycle.*

  G47.20 Circadian rhythm sleep disorder, unspecified type
    Sleep wake schedule disorder NOS
  G47.21 Circadian rhythm sleep disorder, **delayed sleep phase** type
    Delayed sleep phase syndrome
  G47.22 Circadian rhythm sleep disorder, **advanced sleep phase** type
  G47.23 Circadian rhythm sleep disorder, **irregular sleep wake** type
    Irregular sleep-wake pattern
  G47.24 Circadian rhythm sleep disorder, **free running** type
    Circadian rhythm sleep disorder, non-24-hour sleep-wake type
  G47.25 Circadian rhythm sleep disorder, **jet lag** type
  G47.26 Circadian rhythm sleep disorder, **shift work** type
  G47.27 *Circadian rhythm sleep disorder in conditions classified elsewhere*
    Code first underlying condition
  G47.29 Other circadian rhythm sleep disorder

√5th **G47.3** Sleep apnea
  Code also any associated underlying condition
  EXCLUDES 1   apnea NOS (R06.81)
    Cheyne-Stokes breathing (R06.3)
    pickwickian syndrome (E66.2)
    sleep apnea of newborn (P28.3-)

  G47.30 Sleep apnea, unspecified
    Sleep apnea NOS
  G47.31 **Primary central** sleep apnea
    Idiopathic central sleep apnea
  G47.32 **High altitude periodic breathing**
  G47.33 **Obstructive** sleep apnea **(adult) (pediatric)**
    Obstructive sleep apnea hypopnea
    EXCLUDES 1   *obstructive sleep apnea of newborn (P28.3-)*
  G47.34 Idiopathic sleep related nonobstructive alveolar hypoventilation
    Sleep related hypoxia
  G47.35 **Congenital central alveolar hypoventilation** syndrome
  G47.36 *Sleep related hypoventilation in conditions classified elsewhere*
    Sleep related hypoxemia in conditions classified elsewhere
    Code first underlying condition
  G47.37 *Central sleep apnea in conditions classified elsewhere*
    Code first underlying condition
  G47.39 Other sleep apnea

√5th **G47.4** Narcolepsy and cataplexy
  √6th **G47.41** Narcolepsy
    G47.411 Narcolepsy **with cataplexy**   Rx COM
    G47.419 Narcolepsy **without cataplexy**   Rx COM
      Narcolepsy NOS
  √6th **G47.42** Narcolepsy in conditions classified elsewhere
    Code first underlying condition
    G47.421 *Narcolepsy in conditions classified elsewhere with cataplexy*   Rx COM
    G47.429 *Narcolepsy in conditions classified elsewhere without cataplexy*   Rx COM

√5th **G47.5** Parasomnia
  EXCLUDES 1   alcohol induced parasomnia (F10.182, F10.282, F10.982)
    drug induced parasomnia (F11.182, F11.282, F11.982, F13.182, F13.282, F13.982, F14.182, F14.282, F14.982, F15.182, F15.282, F15.982, F19.182, F19.282, F19.982)
    parasomnia not due to a substance or known physiological condition (F51.8)

  G47.50 Parasomnia, unspecified
    Parasomnia NOS
  G47.51 Confusional arousals
  G47.52 REM sleep behavior disorder
  G47.53 Recurrent isolated sleep paralysis
  G47.54 *Parasomnia in conditions classified elsewhere*
    Code first underlying condition
  G47.59 Other parasomnia

√5th **G47.6** Sleep related movement disorders
  EXCLUDES 2   *restless legs syndrome (G25.81)*
  G47.61 **Periodic limb** movement disorder
  G47.62 Sleep related **leg cramps**
  G47.63 Sleep related **bruxism**
    EXCLUDES 1   *psychogenic bruxism (F45.8)*
  G47.69 Other sleep related movement disorders

G47.8 Other sleep disorders
  Other specified sleep-wake disorder
G47.9 Sleep disorder, unspecified
  Sleep disorder NOS
  Unspecified sleep-wake disorder

Nerve, nerve root and plexus disorders (G50-G59)

EXCLUDES 1   current traumatic nerve, nerve root and plexus disorders - see Injury, nerve by body region
  neuralgia NOS (M79.2)
  neuritis NOS (M79.2)
  peripheral neuritis in pregnancy (O26.82-)
  radiculitis NOS (M54.1-)

√4th **G50** Disorders of **trigeminal** nerve
  INCLUDES   disorders of 5th cranial nerve

  G50.0 **Trigeminal neuralgia**   Rx
    Syndrome of paroxysmal facial pain
    Tic douloureux
  G50.1 **Atypical facial pain**   Rx
  G50.8 Other disorders of trigeminal nerve   Rx
  G50.9 Disorder of trigeminal nerve, unspecified   Rx

√4th **G51** **Facial nerve** disorders
  INCLUDES   disorders of 7th cranial nerve

  G51.0 Bell's palsy
    Facial palsy
  G51.1 Geniculate ganglionitis
    EXCLUDES 1   *postherpetic geniculate ganglionitis (B02.21)*
  G51.2 Melkersson's syndrome
    Melkersson-Rosenthal syndrome
  √5th **G51.3** Clonic hemifacial spasm
    AHA: 2018,4Q,10
    G51.31 Clonic hemifacial spasm, **right**
    G51.32 Clonic hemifacial spasm, **left**
    G51.33 Clonic hemifacial spasm, **bilateral**
    G51.39 Clonic hemifacial spasm, unspecified
  G51.4 Facial myokymia
  G51.8 Other disorders of facial nerve
  G51.9 Disorder of facial nerve, unspecified

√4th **G52** Disorders of other **cranial nerves**
  EXCLUDES 2   *disorders of acoustic [8th] nerve (H93.3)*
    disorders of optic [2nd] nerve (H46, H47.0)
    paralytic strabismus due to nerve palsy (H49.0-H49.2)

  G52.0 Disorders of **olfactory** nerve
    Disorders of 1st cranial nerve
  G52.1 Disorders of **glossopharyngeal** nerve
    Disorders of 9th cranial nerve
    Glossopharyngeal neuralgia
  G52.2 Disorders of **vagus** nerve
    Disorders of pneumogastric [10th] nerve
  G52.3 Disorders of **hypoglossal** nerve
    Disorders of 12th cranial nerve

HCC CMS-HCC   Rx Rx HCC   ESR ESRD HCC   COM Commercial HCC   N Newborn: 0   P Pediatric: 0-17   M Maternity: 9-64   A Adult: 15-124

Chapter 6. Diseases of the Nervous System

G52.7 Disorders of multiple cranial nerves
Polyneuritis cranialis

G52.8 Disorders of other specified cranial nerves

G52.9 Cranial nerve disorder, unspecified

G53 *Cranial nerve disorders in diseases classified elsewhere*
Code first underlying disease, such as:
neoplasm (C00-D49)
EXCLUDES 1   *multiple cranial nerve palsy in sarcoidosis (D86.82)*
multiple cranial nerve palsy in syphilis (A52.15)
postherpetic geniculate ganglionitis (B02.21)
postherpetic trigeminal neuralgia (B02.22)

✓4th **G54** Nerve root and plexus disorders
EXCLUDES 1   *current traumatic nerve root and plexus disorders - see nerve injury by body region*
intervertebral disc disorders (M50-M51)
neuralgia or neuritis NOS (M79.2)
neuritis or radiculitis brachial NOS (M54.13)
neuritis or radiculitis lumbar NOS (M54.16)
neuritis or radiculitis lumbosacral NOS (M54.17)
neuritis or radiculitis thoracic NOS (M54.14)
radiculitis NOS (M54.10)
radiculopathy NOS (M54.10)
spondylosis (M47.-)

G54.0 Brachial plexus disorders
Thoracic outlet syndrome
AHA: 2023,2Q,8
DEF: Acquired disorder affecting the spinal nerves that send signals to the shoulder, arm, and hand, causing corresponding motor and sensory dysfunction. This disorder is characterized by regional paresthesia, pain, muscle weakness, and in severe cases paralysis.

G54.1 Lumbosacral plexus disorders

G54.2 Cervical root disorders, not elsewhere classified

G54.3 Thoracic root disorders, not elsewhere classified

G54.4 Lumbosacral root disorders, not elsewhere classified

G54.5 Neuralgic amyotrophy
Parsonage-Aldren-Turner syndrome
Shoulder-girdle neuritis
EXCLUDES 1   *neuralgic amyotrophy in diabetes mellitus (E08-E13 with .44)*

G54.6 Phantom limb syndrome with pain   HCC ESR COM

G54.7 Phantom limb syndrome without pain   HCC ESR COM
Phantom limb syndrome NOS

G54.8 Other nerve root and plexus disorders

G54.9 Nerve root and plexus disorder, unspecified

G55 *Nerve root and plexus compressions in diseases classified elsewhere*
Code first underlying disease, such as:
neoplasm (C00-D49)
EXCLUDES 1   *nerve root compression (due to) (in) ankylosing spondylitis (M45.-)*
nerve root compression (due to) (in) dorsopathies (M53.-, M54.-)
nerve root compression (due to) (in) intervertebral disc disorders (M50.1.-, M51.1.-)
nerve root compression (due to) (in) spondylopathies (M46.-, M48.-)
nerve root compression (due to) (in) spondylosis (M47.0-, M47.2-)

✓4th **G56** Mononeuropathies of upper limb
EXCLUDES 1   *current traumatic nerve disorder - see nerve injury by body region*
AHA: 2016,4Q,17-18

✓5th **G56.0** Carpal tunnel syndrome
DEF: Swelling and inflammation in the tendons or bursa surrounding the median nerve caused by repetitive activity. The resulting compression on the nerve causes pain, numbness, and tingling especially to the palm, index, middle finger, and thumb.
G56.00 Carpal tunnel syndrome, unspecified upper limb
G56.01 Carpal tunnel syndrome, right upper limb
G56.02 Carpal tunnel syndrome, left upper limb
G56.03 Carpal tunnel syndrome, bilateral upper limbs

✓5th **G56.1** Other lesions of median nerve
G56.10 Other lesions of median nerve, unspecified upper limb
G56.11 Other lesions of median nerve, right upper limb
G56.12 Other lesions of median nerve, left upper limb
G56.13 Other lesions of median nerve, bilateral upper limbs

✓5th **G56.2** Lesion of ulnar nerve
Tardy ulnar nerve palsy
G56.20 Lesion of ulnar nerve, unspecified upper limb
G56.21 Lesion of ulnar nerve, right upper limb
G56.22 Lesion of ulnar nerve, left upper limb
G56.23 Lesion of ulnar nerve, bilateral upper limbs

✓5th **G56.3** Lesion of radial nerve
G56.30 Lesion of radial nerve, unspecified upper limb
G56.31 Lesion of radial nerve, right upper limb
G56.32 Lesion of radial nerve, left upper limb
G56.33 Lesion of radial nerve, bilateral upper limbs

✓5th **G56.4** Causalgia of upper limb
Complex regional pain syndrome II of upper limb
EXCLUDES 1   *complex regional pain syndrome I of lower limb (G90.52-)*
complex regional pain syndrome I of upper limb (G90.51-)
complex regional pain syndrome II of lower limb (G57.7-)
reflex sympathetic dystrophy of lower limb (G90.52-)
reflex sympathetic dystrophy of upper limb (G90.51-)
G56.40 Causalgia of unspecified upper limb
G56.41 Causalgia of right upper limb
G56.42 Causalgia of left upper limb
G56.43 Causalgia of bilateral upper limbs

✓5th **G56.8** Other specified mononeuropathies of upper limb
Interdigital neuroma of upper limb
G56.80 Other specified mononeuropathies of unspecified upper limb
G56.81 Other specified mononeuropathies of right upper limb
G56.82 Other specified mononeuropathies of left upper limb
G56.83 Other specified mononeuropathies of bilateral upper limbs

✓5th **G56.9** Unspecified mononeuropathy of upper limb
G56.90 Unspecified mononeuropathy of unspecified upper limb
G56.91 Unspecified mononeuropathy of right upper limb
G56.92 Unspecified mononeuropathy of left upper limb
G56.93 Unspecified mononeuropathy of bilateral upper limbs

✓4th **G57** Mononeuropathies of lower limb
EXCLUDES 1   *current traumatic nerve disorder - see nerve injury by body region*
AHA: 2016,4Q,17-18

✓5th **G57.0** Lesion of sciatic nerve
EXCLUDES 1   *sciatica NOS (M54.3-)*
EXCLUDES 2   *sciatica attributed to intervertebral disc disorder (M51.1.-)*
G57.00 Lesion of sciatic nerve, unspecified lower limb
G57.01 Lesion of sciatic nerve, right lower limb
G57.02 Lesion of sciatic nerve, left lower limb
G57.03 Lesion of sciatic nerve, bilateral lower limbs

✓5th **G57.1** Meralgia paresthetica
Lateral cutaneous nerve of thigh syndrome
G57.10 Meralgia paresthetica, unspecified lower limb
G57.11 Meralgia paresthetica, right lower limb
G57.12 Meralgia paresthetica, left lower limb
G57.13 Meralgia paresthetica, bilateral lower limbs

✓5th **G57.2** Lesion of femoral nerve
G57.20 Lesion of femoral nerve, unspecified lower limb
G57.21 Lesion of femoral nerve, right lower limb
G57.22 Lesion of femoral nerve, left lower limb
G57.23 Lesion of femoral nerve, bilateral lower limbs

✓5th **G57.3** Lesion of lateral popliteal nerve
Peroneal nerve palsy
AHA: 2020,3Q,12
G57.30 Lesion of lateral popliteal nerve, unspecified lower limb
G57.31 Lesion of lateral popliteal nerve, right lower limb
G57.32 Lesion of lateral popliteal nerve, left lower limb
G57.33 Lesion of lateral popliteal nerve, bilateral lower limbs

✓5th **G57.4** Lesion of medial popliteal nerve
G57.40 Lesion of medial popliteal nerve, unspecified lower limb
G57.41 Lesion of medial popliteal nerve, right lower limb
G57.42 Lesion of medial popliteal nerve, left lower limb

G57.43 Lesion of medial popliteal nerve, bilateral lower limbs

√5th **G57.5 Tarsal tunnel syndrome**
- **G57.50** Tarsal tunnel syndrome, unspecified lower limb
- **G57.51** Tarsal tunnel syndrome, right lower limb
- **G57.52** Tarsal tunnel syndrome, left lower limb
- **G57.53** Tarsal tunnel syndrome, bilateral lower limbs

√5th **G57.6 Lesion of plantar nerve**
Morton's metatarsalgia
- **G57.60** Lesion of plantar nerve, unspecified lower limb
- **G57.61** Lesion of plantar nerve, right lower limb
- **G57.62** Lesion of plantar nerve, left lower limb
- **G57.63** Lesion of plantar nerve, bilateral lower limbs

√5th **G57.7 Causalgia of lower limb**
Complex regional pain syndrome II of lower limb
  EXCLUDES 1 complex regional pain syndrome I of lower limb (G90.52-)
  complex regional pain syndrome I of upper limb (G90.51-)
  complex regional pain syndrome II of upper limb (G56.4-)
  reflex sympathetic dystrophy of lower limb (G90.52-)
  reflex sympathetic dystrophy of upper limb (G90.51-)
- **G57.70** Causalgia of unspecified lower limb
- **G57.71** Causalgia of right lower limb
- **G57.72** Causalgia of left lower limb
- **G57.73** Causalgia of bilateral lower limbs

√5th **G57.8 Other specified mononeuropathies of lower limb**
Interdigital neuroma of lower limb
- **G57.80** Other specified mononeuropathies of unspecified lower limb
- **G57.81** Other specified mononeuropathies of right lower limb
- **G57.82** Other specified mononeuropathies of left lower limb
- **G57.83** Other specified mononeuropathies of bilateral lower limbs

√5th **G57.9 Unspecified mononeuropathy of lower limb**
- **G57.90** Unspecified mononeuropathy of unspecified lower limb
- **G57.91** Unspecified mononeuropathy of right lower limb
- **G57.92** Unspecified mononeuropathy of left lower limb
- **G57.93** Unspecified mononeuropathy of bilateral lower limbs

√4th **G58 Other mononeuropathies**
- **G58.0** Intercostal neuropathy
- **G58.7** Mononeuritis multiplex
- **G58.8** Other specified mononeuropathies
- **G58.9** Mononeuropathy, unspecified

G59 Mononeuropathy in diseases classified elsewhere
Code first underlying disease
  EXCLUDES 1 diabetic mononeuropathy (E08-E13 with .41)
  syphilitic nerve paralysis (A52.19)
  syphilitic neuritis (A52.15)
  tuberculous mononeuropathy (A17.83)

Polyneuropathies and other disorders of the peripheral nervous system (G60-G65)

EXCLUDES 1 neuralgia NOS (M79.2)
neuritis NOS (M79.2)
peripheral neuritis in pregnancy (O26.82-)
radiculitis NOS (M54.10)

√4th **G60 Hereditary and idiopathic neuropathy**
- **G60.0 Hereditary motor and sensory neuropathy**
  Charcôt-Marie-Tooth disease
  Dejerine-Sottas disease
  Hereditary motor and sensory neuropathy, types I-IV
  Hypertrophic neuropathy of infancy
  Peroneal muscular atrophy (axonal type) (hypertrophic type)
  Roussy-Levy syndrome
- **G60.1 Refsum's disease**
  Infantile Refsum disease
  DEF: Genetic disorder of the lipid metabolism characterized by retinitis pigmentosa, degenerative nerve disease, ataxia, and dry, rough, scaly skin.
- **G60.2** Neuropathy in association with hereditary ataxia
- **G60.3** Idiopathic progressive neuropathy
- **G60.8** Other hereditary and idiopathic neuropathies
  Dominantly inherited sensory neuropathy
  Morvan's disease
  Nelaton's syndrome
  Recessively inherited sensory neuropathy
- **G60.9** Hereditary and idiopathic neuropathy, unspecified

√4th **G61 Inflammatory polyneuropathy**
- **G61.0 Guillain-Barre syndrome** [Rx] [ESR] [COM]
  Acute (post-)infective polyneuritis
  Miller Fisher syndrome
  AHA: 2020,3Q,12; 2014,2Q,4
  DEF: Autoimmune disorder due to an immune response to foreign antigens with paraplegia of limbs, flaccid paralysis, ophthalmoplegia, ataxia, and areflexia. In most cases, this disorder is triggered by a mild viral infection, surgery, or following an immunization.
  TIP: Guillain-Barre syndrome can occur as a sequela of *Campylobacter* enteritis. Assign code B94.8 for the sequelae as an additional diagnosis.
- **G61.1 Serum neuropathy** [Rx] [ESR] [COM]
  Use additional code for adverse effect, if applicable, to identify serum (T50.-)
  √5th **G61.8 Other inflammatory polyneuropathies**
  - **G61.81 Chronic inflammatory demyelinating polyneuritis** [HCC] [Rx] [ESR] [COM]
  - **G61.82 Multifocal motor neuropathy** [HCC] [Rx] [ESR] [COM]
    MMN
    AHA: 2016,4Q,18
  - **G61.89** Other inflammatory polyneuropathies [Rx] [ESR] [COM]
- **G61.9** Inflammatory polyneuropathy, unspecified [Rx] [ESR] [COM]

√4th **G62 Other and unspecified polyneuropathies**
- **G62.0 Drug-induced polyneuropathy** [Rx] [ESR] [COM]
  Use additional code for adverse effect, if applicable, to identify drug (T36-T50 with fifth or sixth character 5)
- **G62.1 Alcoholic polyneuropathy** [Rx] [ESR] [COM]
  AHA: 2019,3Q,8
- **G62.2** Polyneuropathy due to other toxic agents [Rx] [ESR] [COM]
  Code first (T51-T65) to identify toxic agent
  √5th **G62.8 Other specified polyneuropathies**
  - **G62.81 Critical illness polyneuropathy** [Rx] [ESR] [COM]
    Acute motor neuropathy
  - **G62.82 Radiation-induced polyneuropathy** [Rx] [ESR] [COM]
    Use additional external cause code (W88-W90, X39.0-) to identify cause
  - **G62.89** Other specified polyneuropathies
    AHA: 2024,3Q,11; 2016,2Q,11
- **G62.9** Polyneuropathy, unspecified
  Neuropathy NOS

G63 Polyneuropathy in diseases classified elsewhere [Rx] [ESR] [COM]
Code first underlying disease, such as:
amyloidosis (E85.-)
endocrine disease, except diabetes (E00-E07, E15-E16, E20-E34)
metabolic diseases (E70-E88)
neoplasm (C00-D49)
nutritional deficiency (E40-E64)
  EXCLUDES 1 polyneuropathy (in):
  diabetes mellitus (E08-E13 with .42)
  diphtheria (A36.83)
  infectious mononucleosis complicated by polyneuropathy (B27.0-B27.9 with fifth character 1)
  Lyme disease (A69.22)
  mumps (B26.84)
  postherpetic (B02.23)
  rheumatoid arthritis (M05.5-)
  scleroderma (M34.83)
  systemic lupus erythematosus (M32.19)
AHA: 2024,3Q,11; 2023,3Q,19; 2021,1Q,7; 2012,4Q,99

G64 Other disorders of peripheral nervous system
Disorder of peripheral nervous system NOS

√4th **G65 Sequelae of inflammatory and toxic polyneuropathies**
Code first condition resulting from (sequela) of inflammatory and toxic polyneuropathies
- **G65.0** Sequelae of Guillain-Barre syndrome [Rx] [ESR] [COM]
- **G65.1** Sequelae of other inflammatory polyneuropathy [Rx] [ESR] [COM]
- **G65.2** Sequelae of toxic polyneuropathy [Rx] [ESR] [COM]

Diseases of myoneural junction and muscle (G70-G73)

- **G70** Myasthenia gravis and other myoneural disorders
  - EXCLUDES 1: botulism (A05.1, A48.51-A48.52)
  - transient neonatal myasthenia gravis (P94.0)
  - **G70.0** Myasthenia gravis
    - AHA: 2022,3Q,15
    - DEF: Autoimmune neuromuscular disorder caused by antibodies to the acetylcholine receptors at the neuromuscular junction, interfering with proper binding of the neurotransmitter from the neuron to the target muscle, causing muscle weakness, fatigue, and exhaustion, without pain or atrophy.
    - **G70.00** Myasthenia gravis without (acute) exacerbation
      - Myasthenia gravis NOS
    - **G70.01** Myasthenia gravis with (acute) exacerbation
      - Myasthenia gravis in crisis
  - **G70.1** Toxic myoneural disorders
    - Code first (T51-T65) to identify toxic agent
  - **G70.2** Congenital and developmental myasthenia
  - **G70.8** Other specified myoneural disorders
    - **G70.80** Lambert-Eaton syndrome, unspecified
      - Lambert-Eaton syndrome NOS
    - **G70.81** Lambert-Eaton syndrome in disease classified elsewhere
      - Code first underlying disease
      - EXCLUDES 1: Lambert-Eaton syndrome in neoplastic disease (G73.1)
    - **G70.89** Other specified myoneural disorders
  - **G70.9** Myoneural disorder, unspecified

- **G71** Primary disorders of muscles
  - EXCLUDES 2: arthrogryposis multiplex congenita (Q74.3)
  - metabolic disorders (E70-E88)
  - myositis (M60.-)
  - **G71.0** Muscular dystrophy
    - AHA: 2022,4Q,17-18; 2018,4Q,11-12
    - **G71.00** Muscular dystrophy, unspecified
    - **G71.01** Duchenne or Becker muscular dystrophy
      - Autosomal recessive, childhood type, muscular dystrophy resembling Duchenne or Becker muscular dystrophy
      - Benign [Becker] muscular dystrophy
      - Severe [Duchenne] muscular dystrophy
    - **G71.02** Facioscapulohumeral muscular dystrophy
      - Scapulohumeral muscular dystrophy
    - **G71.03** Limb girdle muscular dystrophies
      - **G71.031** Autosomal dominant limb girdle muscular dystrophy
        - LGMD D4 calpain-3-related
        - LGMD D5 collagen 6-related
        - Limb girdle muscular dystrophy type 1
      - **G71.032** Autosomal recessive limb girdle muscular dystrophy due to calpain-3 dysfunction
        - LGMD R1 calpain-3-related
        - Limb girdle muscular dystrophy type 2A
        - Primary calpainopathy
      - **G71.033** Limb girdle muscular dystrophy due to dysferlin dysfunction
        - Dysferlinopathy
        - LGMD R2 dysferlin-related
        - Limb girdle muscular dystrophy type 2B
        - Miyoshi Myopathy type 1
      - **G71.034** Limb girdle muscular dystrophy due to sarcoglycan dysfunction
        - **G71.0340** Limb girdle muscular dystrophy due to sarcoglycan dysfunction, unspecified
          - Sarcoglycanopathy, NOS
        - **G71.0341** Limb girdle muscular dystrophy due to alpha sarcoglycan dysfunction
          - Alpha sarcoglycanopathy
          - Limb girdle muscular dystrophy type 2D
          - Limb-girdle muscular dystrophy due to alpha-sarcoglycan deficiency
        - **G71.0342** Limb girdle muscular dystrophy due to beta sarcoglycan dysfunction
          - Beta sarcoglycanopathy
          - Limb girdle muscular dystrophy due to beta-sarcoglycan deficiency
          - Limb girdle muscular dystrophy type 2E
        - **G71.0349** Limb girdle muscular dystrophy due to other sarcoglycan dysfunction
          - Delta sarcoglycanopathy
          - Delta-sarcoglycan-related LGMD R6
          - Gamma sarcoglycanopathy
          - Gamma-sarcoglycan-related LGMD R5
          - Limb girdle muscular dystrophy type 2C
          - Limb girdle muscular dystrophy type 2F
      - **G71.035** Limb girdle muscular dystrophy due to anoctamin-5 dysfunction
        - Anoctamin-5-related LGMD R12
        - Anoctaminopathy
        - Autosomal recessive limb girdle muscular dystrophy type 2L
        - Miyoshi myopathy type 3
      - **G71.036** Limb girdle muscular dystrophy due to fukutin related protein dysfunction
        - LGMD R9 FKRP-related
        - Limb girdle muscular dystrophy due to FKRP deficiency
        - Limb girdle muscular dystrophy type 2I
      - **G71.038** Other limb girdle muscular dystrophy
        - ~~LGMD R9 FKRP-related~~
        - ~~Limb girdle muscular dystrophy due to fukutin related protein dysfunction~~
        - ~~Limb girdle muscular dystrophy type 2I~~
        - LGMD R22 collagen 6-related
        - Other autosomal recessive limb girdle muscular dystrophy
      - **G71.039** Limb girdle muscular dystrophy, unspecified
    - **G71.09** Other specified muscular dystrophies
      - Benign scapuloperoneal muscular dystrophy with early contractures [Emery-Dreifuss]
      - Congenital muscular dystrophy NOS
      - Congenital muscular dystrophy with specific morphological abnormalities of the muscle fiber
      - Distal muscular dystrophy
      - Ocular muscular dystrophy
      - Oculopharyngeal muscular dystrophy
      - Scapuloperoneal muscular dystrophy
  - **G71.1** Myotonic disorders
    - **G71.11** Myotonic muscular dystrophy
      - Dystrophia myotonica [Steinert]
      - Myotonia atrophica
      - Myotonic dystrophy
      - Proximal myotonic myopathy (PROMM)
      - Steinert disease
    - **G71.12** Myotonia congenita
      - Acetazolamide responsive myotonia congenita
      - Dominant myotonia congenita [Thomsen disease]
      - Myotonia levior
      - Recessive myotonia congenita [Becker disease]
    - **G71.13** Myotonic chondrodystrophy
      - Chondrodystrophic myotonia
      - Congenital myotonic chondrodystrophy
      - Schwartz-Jampel disease

Chapter 6. Diseases of the Nervous System

G71.14 **Drug induced** myotonia
Use additional code for adverse effect, if applicable, to identify drug (T36-T50 with fifth or sixth character 5)

G71.19 **Other specified myotonic disorders**
Myotonia fluctuans
Myotonia permanens
Neuromyotonia [Isaacs]
Paramyotonia congenita (of von Eulenburg)
Pseudomyotonia
Symptomatic myotonia

✓5th **G71.2** **Congenital myopathies**
EXCLUDES 2 arthrogryposis multiplex congenita (Q74.3)
AHA: 2020,4Q,19-21

G71.20 Congenital myopathy, unspecified [HCC ESR COM]

G71.21 **Nemaline** myopathy [HCC ESR COM]

✓6th **G71.22** **Centronuclear** myopathy

G71.220 **X-linked myotubular** myopathy [HCC ESR COM]
Myotubular (centronuclear) myopathy

G71.228 **Other centronuclear** myopathy [HCC ESR COM]
Autosomal centronuclear myopathy
Autosomal dominant centronuclear myopathy
Autosomal recessive centronuclear myopathy
Centronuclear myopathy, NOS

G71.29 **Other congenital myopathy** [HCC ESR COM]
Central core disease
Minicore disease
Multicore disease
Multiminicore disease

G71.3 **Mitochondrial myopathy**, not elsewhere classified
EXCLUDES 1 Kearns-Sayre syndrome (H49.81)
Leber's disease (H47.21)
Leigh's encephalopathy (G31.82)
mitochondrial metabolism disorders (E88.4.-)
Reye's syndrome (G93.7)

G71.8 Other primary disorders of muscles

G71.9 Primary disorder of muscle, unspecified
Hereditary myopathy NOS

✓4th **G72** **Other and unspecified myopathies**
EXCLUDES 1 arthrogryposis multiplex congenita (Q74.3)
dermatopolymyositis (M33.-)
ischemic infarction of muscle (M62.2-)
myositis (M60.-)
polymyositis (M33.2.-)

G72.0 **Drug-induced** myopathy
Use additional code for adverse effect, if applicable, to identify drug (T36-T50 with fifth or sixth character 5)

G72.1 **Alcoholic** myopathy
Use additional code to identify alcoholism (F10.-)

G72.2 Myopathy due to other toxic agents
Code first (T51-T65) to identify toxic agent

G72.3 **Periodic paralysis**
Familial periodic paralysis
Hyperkalemic periodic paralysis (familial)
Hypokalemic periodic paralysis (familial)
Myotonic periodic paralysis (familial)
Normokalemic paralysis (familial)
Potassium sensitive periodic paralysis
EXCLUDES 1 paramyotonia congenita (of von Eulenburg) (G71.19)

✓5th **G72.4** **Inflammatory and immune** myopathies, not elsewhere classified

G72.41 **Inclusion body myositis [IBM]** [HCC]

G72.49 Other inflammatory and immune myopathies, not elsewhere classified
Inflammatory myopathy NOS

✓5th **G72.8** Other specified myopathies

G72.81 **Critical illness** myopathy
Acute necrotizing myopathy
Acute quadriplegic myopathy
Intensive care (ICU) myopathy
Myopathy of critical illness
AHA: 2020,3Q,12

G72.89 Other specified myopathies

G72.9 **Myopathy, unspecified**

✓4th **G73** Disorders of myoneural junction and muscle in diseases classified elsewhere

G73.1 **Lambert-Eaton syndrome in neoplastic disease** [HCC Rx ESR COM UPD]
Code first underlying neoplasm (C00-D49)
EXCLUDES 1 Lambert-Eaton syndrome not associated with neoplasm (G70.80-G70.81)

G73.3 **Myasthenic syndromes in other diseases classified elsewhere** [HCC Rx ESR COM]
Code first underlying disease, such as:
neoplasm (C00-D49)
thyrotoxicosis (E05.-)

G73.7 **Myopathy in diseases classified elsewhere**
Code first underlying disease, such as:
glycogen storage disease (E74.0-)
hyperparathyroidism (E21.0, E21.3)
hypoparathyroidism (E20.-)
lipid storage disorders (E75.-)
EXCLUDES 1 myopathy in:
rheumatoid arthritis (M05.32)
sarcoidosis (D86.87)
scleroderma (M34.82)
Sjogren syndrome (M35.03)
systemic lupus erythematosus (M32.19)

Cerebral palsy and other paralytic syndromes (G80-G83)

✓4th **G80** **Cerebral palsy**
EXCLUDES 1 hereditary spastic paraplegia (G11.4)

G80.0 **Spastic quadriplegic** cerebral palsy [HCC ESR COM]
Congenital spastic paralysis (cerebral)

G80.1 **Spastic diplegic** cerebral palsy [HCC ESR COM]
Spastic cerebral palsy NOS

G80.2 **Spastic hemiplegic** cerebral palsy [HCC ESR COM]

G80.3 **Athetoid** cerebral palsy [HCC ESR COM]
Double athetosis (syndrome)
Dyskinetic cerebral palsy
Dystonic cerebral palsy
Vogt disease

G80.4 **Ataxic** cerebral palsy [HCC ESR COM]

G80.8 **Other cerebral palsy** [HCC ESR COM]
Mixed cerebral palsy syndromes

G80.9 **Cerebral palsy, unspecified** [HCC ESR COM]
Cerebral palsy NOS

✓4th **G81** **Hemiplegia and hemiparesis**
NOTE This category is to be used only when hemiplegia (complete)(incomplete) is reported without further specification, or is stated to be old or longstanding but of unspecified cause. The category is also for use in multiple coding to identify these types of hemiplegia resulting from any cause.
EXCLUDES 1 congenital cerebral palsy (G80.-)
hemiplegia and hemiparesis due to sequela of cerebrovascular disease (I69.05-, I69.15-, I69.25-, I69.35-, I69.85-, I69.95-)
AHA: 2015,1Q,25
TIP: If the documentation specifies the affected side but not whether it is the dominant or nondominant side, the default is as follows: for ambidextrous patients, the default is dominant; when the left side is affected, the default is nondominant; and when the right side is affected, the default is dominant.

✓5th **G81.0** **Flaccid** hemiplegia

G81.00 Flaccid hemiplegia affecting unspecified side [HCC ESR COM]

G81.01 Flaccid hemiplegia affecting **right dominant** side [HCC ESR COM]

G81.02 Flaccid hemiplegia affecting **left dominant** side [HCC ESR COM]

G81.03 Flaccid hemiplegia affecting **right nondominant** side [HCC ESR COM]

G81.04 Flaccid hemiplegia affecting **left nondominant** side [HCC ESR COM]

✓5th **G81.1** **Spastic** hemiplegia

G81.10 Spastic hemiplegia affecting unspecified side [HCC Rx ESR COM]

G81.11 Spastic hemiplegia affecting **right dominant** side [HCC Rx ESR COM]

G81.12 Spastic hemiplegia affecting **left dominant** side [HCC Rx ESR COM]

	G81.13	Spastic hemiplegia affecting right nondominant side
	G81.14	Spastic hemiplegia affecting left nondominant side
✓5th	**G81.9**	**Hemiplegia, unspecified**
		AHA: 2014,1Q,23
	G81.90	Hemiplegia, unspecified affecting unspecified side
	G81.91	Hemiplegia, unspecified affecting right dominant side
	G81.92	Hemiplegia, unspecified affecting left dominant side
	G81.93	Hemiplegia, unspecified affecting right nondominant side
	G81.94	Hemiplegia, unspecified affecting left nondominant side

✓4th **G82 Paraplegia (paraparesis) and quadriplegia (quadriparesis)**

NOTE This category is to be used only when the listed conditions are reported without further specification, or are stated to be old or longstanding but of unspecified cause. The category is also for use in multiple coding to identify these conditions resulting from any cause

EXCLUDES 1 congenital cerebral palsy (G80.-)
functional quadriplegia (R53.2)
hysterical paralysis (F44.4)

✓5th **G82.2 Paraplegia**
Paralysis of both lower limbs NOS
Paraparesis (lower) NOS
Paraplegia (lower) NOS
AHA: 2017,3Q,3

	G82.20	Paraplegia, unspecified
	G82.21	Paraplegia, complete
	G82.22	Paraplegia, incomplete

✓5th **G82.5 Quadriplegia**
AHA: 2024,2Q,23

	G82.50	Quadriplegia, unspecified
	G82.51	Quadriplegia, C1-C4 complete
	G82.52	Quadriplegia, C1-C4 incomplete
	G82.53	Quadriplegia, C5-C7 complete
	G82.54	Quadriplegia, C5-C7 incomplete

✓4th **G83 Other paralytic syndromes**

NOTE This category is to be used only when the listed conditions are reported without further specification, or are stated to be old or longstanding but of unspecified cause. The category is also for use in multiple coding to identify these conditions resulting from any cause.

INCLUDES paralysis (complete) (incomplete), except as in G80-G82

G83.0 Diplegia of upper limbs
Diplegia (upper)
Paralysis of both upper limbs

✓5th **G83.1 Monoplegia of lower limb**
Paralysis of lower limb
EXCLUDES 1 monoplegia of lower limbs due to sequela of cerebrovascular disease (I69.04-, I69.14-, I69.24-, I69.34-, I69.84-, I69.94-)

TIP: If the documentation specifies the affected side but not whether it is the dominant or nondominant side, the default is as follows: for ambidextrous patients, the default is dominant; when the left side is affected, the default is nondominant; and when the right side is affected, the default is dominant.

	G83.10	Monoplegia of lower limb affecting unspecified side
	G83.11	Monoplegia of lower limb affecting right dominant side
	G83.12	Monoplegia of lower limb affecting left dominant side
	G83.13	Monoplegia of lower limb affecting right nondominant side
	G83.14	Monoplegia of lower limb affecting left nondominant side

✓5th **G83.2 Monoplegia of upper limb**
Paralysis of upper limb
EXCLUDES 1 monoplegia of upper limbs due to sequela of cerebrovascular disease (I69.03-, I69.13-, I69.23-, I69.33-, I69.83-, I69.93-)

TIP: If the documentation specifies the affected side but not whether it is the dominant or nondominant side, the default is as follows: for ambidextrous patients, the default is dominant; when the left side is affected, the default is nondominant; and when the right side is affected, the default is dominant.

	G83.20	Monoplegia of upper limb affecting unspecified side
	G83.21	Monoplegia of upper limb affecting right dominant side
	G83.22	Monoplegia of upper limb affecting left dominant side
	G83.23	Monoplegia of upper limb affecting right nondominant side
	G83.24	Monoplegia of upper limb affecting left nondominant side

✓5th **G83.3 Monoplegia, unspecified**

TIP: If the documentation specifies the affected side but not whether it is the dominant or nondominant side, the default is as follows: for ambidextrous patients, the default is dominant; when the left side is affected, the default is nondominant; and when the right side is affected, the default is dominant.

	G83.30	Monoplegia, unspecified affecting unspecified side
	G83.31	Monoplegia, unspecified affecting right dominant side
	G83.32	Monoplegia, unspecified affecting left dominant side
	G83.33	Monoplegia, unspecified affecting right nondominant side
	G83.34	Monoplegia, unspecified affecting left nondominant side

G83.4 Cauda equina syndrome
Neurogenic bladder due to cauda equina syndrome
EXCLUDES 1 cord bladder NOS (G95.89)
neurogenic bladder NOS (N31.9)
AHA: 2024,1Q,17; 2020,3Q,24
DEF: Compression of the spinal nerve roots presenting with pain and tingling radiating down the buttocks, back of the thigh and calf, and into the foot in a sciatic manner with aching in the bladder, perineum, and sacrum. Loss of bowel and bladder control may also occur.

G83.5 Locked-in state
AHA: 2022,2Q,10

✓5th **G83.8 Other specified paralytic syndromes**
EXCLUDES 1 paralytic syndromes due to current spinal cord injury - code to spinal cord injury (S14, S24, S34)

	G83.81	Brown-Sequard syndrome
	G83.82	Anterior cord syndrome
	G83.83	Posterior cord syndrome
	G83.84	Todd's paralysis (postepileptic)
	G83.89	Other specified paralytic syndromes

G83.9 Paralytic syndrome, unspecified

Other disorders of the nervous system (G89-G99)

G89 Pain, not elsewhere classified ✓4th

Code also related psychological factors associated with pain (F45.42)

EXCLUDES 1: generalized pain NOS (R52)
pain disorders exclusively related to psychological factors (F45.41)
pain NOS (R52)

EXCLUDES 2: atypical face pain (G50.1)
headache syndromes (G44.-)
localized pain, unspecified type - code to pain by site, such as:
migraines (G43.-)
myalgia (M79.1-)
pain from prosthetic devices, implants, and grafts (T82.84, T83.84, T84.84, T85.84-)
phantom limb syndrome with pain (G54.6)
vulvar vestibulitis (N94.810)
vulvodynia (N94.81-)
  abdomen pain (R10.-)
  back pain (M54.9)
  breast pain (N64.4)
  chest pain (R07.1-R07.9)
  ear pain (H92.0-)
  eye pain (H57.1)
  headache (R51.9)
  joint pain (M25.5-)
  limb pain (M79.6-)
  lumbar region pain (M54.5-)
  painful urination (R30.9)
  pelvic and perineal pain ▶(R10.2-)◀
  renal colic (N23)
  shoulder pain (M25.51-)
  spine pain (M54.-)
  throat pain (R07.0)
  tongue pain (K14.6)
  tooth pain (K08.8)

G89.0 Central pain syndrome
Dejerine-Roussy syndrome
Myelopathic pain syndrome
Thalamic pain syndrome (hyperesthetic)

G89.1 Acute pain, not elsewhere classified ✓5th
  G89.11 Acute pain due to trauma
  G89.12 Acute post-thoracotomy pain
    Post-thoracotomy pain NOS
  G89.18 Other acute postprocedural pain
    Postoperative pain NOS
    Postprocedural pain NOS

G89.2 Chronic pain, not elsewhere classified ✓5th
  EXCLUDES 1: causalgia, lower limb (G57.7-)
  causalgia, upper limb (G56.4-)
  central pain syndrome (G89.0)
  chronic pain syndrome (G89.4)
  complex regional pain syndrome II, lower limb (G57.7-)
  complex regional pain syndrome II, upper limb (G56.4-)
  neoplasm related chronic pain (G89.3)
  reflex sympathetic dystrophy (G90.5-)
  G89.21 Chronic pain due to trauma
  G89.22 Chronic post-thoracotomy pain
  G89.28 Other chronic postprocedural pain
    Other chronic postoperative pain
  G89.29 Other chronic pain
    AHA: 2023,3Q,17

G89.3 Neoplasm related pain (acute) (chronic)
Cancer associated pain
Pain due to malignancy (primary) (secondary)
Tumor associated pain

G89.4 Chronic pain syndrome
Chronic pain associated with significant psychosocial dysfunction

G90 Disorders of autonomic nervous system ✓4th
  EXCLUDES 1: dysfunction of the autonomic nervous system due to alcohol (G31.2)

G90.0 Idiopathic peripheral autonomic neuropathy ✓5th
  G90.01 Carotid sinus syncope
    Carotid sinus syndrome
    DEF: Vagal activation caused by pressure on the carotid sinus baroreceptors. Sympathetic nerve impulses may cause sinus arrest or AV block.
  G90.09 Other idiopathic peripheral autonomic neuropathy
    Idiopathic peripheral autonomic neuropathy NOS

G90.1 Familial dysautonomia [Riley-Day] HCC Rx ESR COM

G90.2 Horner's syndrome
Bernard(-Horner) syndrome
Cervical sympathetic dystrophy or paralysis

G90.3 Multi-system degeneration of the autonomic nervous system HCC Rx ESR COM
Neurogenic orthostatic hypotension [Shy-Drager]
EXCLUDES 1: orthostatic hypotension NOS (I95.1)

G90.4 Autonomic dysreflexia
Use additional code to identify the cause, such as:
  fecal impaction (K56.41)
  pressure ulcer (pressure area) (L89.-)
  urinary tract infection (N39.0)

G90.5 Complex regional pain syndrome I (CRPS I) ✓5th
Reflex sympathetic dystrophy
EXCLUDES 1: causalgia of lower limb (G57.7-)
  causalgia of upper limb (G56.4-)
  complex regional pain syndrome II of lower limb (G57.7-)
  complex regional pain syndrome II of upper limb (G56.4-)
  G90.50 Complex regional pain syndrome I, unspecified
  G90.51 Complex regional pain syndrome I of upper limb ✓6th
    G90.511 Complex regional pain syndrome I of right upper limb
    G90.512 Complex regional pain syndrome I of left upper limb
    G90.513 Complex regional pain syndrome I of upper limb, bilateral
    G90.519 Complex regional pain syndrome I of unspecified upper limb
  G90.52 Complex regional pain syndrome I of lower limb ✓6th
    G90.521 Complex regional pain syndrome I of right lower limb
    G90.522 Complex regional pain syndrome I of left lower limb
    G90.523 Complex regional pain syndrome I of lower limb, bilateral
    G90.529 Complex regional pain syndrome I of unspecified lower limb
  G90.59 Complex regional pain syndrome I of other specified site

G90.8 Other disorders of autonomic nervous system ✓5th
AHA: 2023,2Q,8
  G90.81 Serotonin syndrome
    Serotonin toxicity
    Code first poisoning due to drug or toxin, such as:
      linezolid (T36.8X- with sixth character 1-4)
      monoamine oxidase inhibitors (T43.1X with sixth character 1-4)
      selective serotonin and norepinephrine reuptake inhibitors [SSNRI] (T43.21 with sixth character 1-4)
      selective serotonin reuptake inhibitors [SSRI] (T43.22 with sixth character 1-4)
    Use additional code for adverse effect, if applicable, to identify drug, such as:
    Use additional code, if applicable, to identify:
      disseminated intravascular coagulation (D65)
      hypertensive crisis (I16.-)
      linezolid (T36.8X5)
      metabolic acidosis (E87.2-)
      monoamine oxidase inhibitors (T43.1X5)
      selective serotonin and norepinephrine reuptake inhibitors [SSNRI] (T43.215)
      selective serotonin reuptake inhibitors [SSRI] (T43.225)
      shock, not elsewhere classified (R57.-)
      toxic encephalopathy (G92.-)
      ventricular tachycardia (I47.2-)
    AHA: 2024,4Q,16
  G90.89 Other disorders of autonomic nervous system

G90.9 Disorder of the autonomic nervous system, unspecified

G90.A Postural orthostatic tachycardia syndrome [POTS]
Chronic orthostatic intolerance
Postural tachycardia syndrome
AHA: 2022,4Q,19-20

Chapter 6. Diseases of the Nervous System

G90.B **LMNB1-related autosomal dominant leukodystrophy** `HCC` `ESR` `COM`
AHA: 2023,4Q,12-13

✓4th **G91** **Hydrocephalus**
INCLUDES: acquired hydrocephalus
EXCLUDES 1: Arnold-Chiari syndrome with hydrocephalus (Q07.-)
congenital hydrocephalus (Q03.-)
spina bifida with hydrocephalus (Q05.-)
DEF: Abnormal buildup of cerebrospinal fluid in the brain causing dilation of the ventricles.

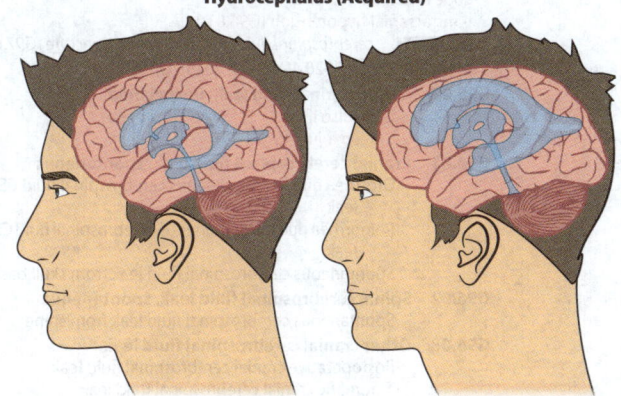

Hydrocephalus (Acquired)

Normal ventricles | Hydrocephalic ventricles

G91.0 **Communicating** hydrocephalus `HCC` `ESR` `COM`
Secondary normal pressure hydrocephalus

G91.1 **Obstructive** hydrocephalus `HCC` `ESR` `COM`
DEF: Obstruction of the cerebrospinal fluid passage from the brain into the spinal canal characterized by headaches, drowsiness, poor coordination, urinary incontinence, nausea, vomiting, and papilledema.

G91.2 **(Idiopathic) normal pressure** hydrocephalus `HCC` `ESR` `COM`
Normal pressure hydrocephalus NOS

G91.3 **Post-traumatic** hydrocephalus, unspecified `HCC` `ESR` `COM`

G91.4 *Hydrocephalus in diseases classified elsewhere* `HCC` `ESR` `COM`
Code first underlying condition, such as:
congenital syphilis (A50.4-)
neoplasm (C00-D49)
plasminogen deficiency (E88.02)
EXCLUDES 1: hydrocephalus due to congenital toxoplasmosis (P37.1)
AHA: 2014,3Q,3

G91.8 **Other** hydrocephalus `HCC` `ESR` `COM`
G91.9 **Hydrocephalus, unspecified** `HCC` `ESR` `COM`

✓4th **G92** **Toxic encephalopathy**
AHA: 2022,1Q,52; 2021,4Q,12-14; 2021,1Q,13; 2017,1Q,39-40
DEF: Brain tissue degeneration due to a toxic substance.

✓5th **G92.0** **Immune effector cell-associated neurotoxicity syndrome**
Code first underlying cause such as:
complications of immune effector cellular therapy (T80.82)
Code also, if applicable, associated signs and symptoms, such as:
cerebral edema (G93.6)
unspecified convulsions (R56.9)

G92.00 **Immune effector cell-associated neurotoxicity syndrome, grade unspecified** `UPD`
ICANS, grade unspecified

G92.01 **Immune effector cell-associated neurotoxicity syndrome, grade 1** `UPD`
ICANS, grade 1

G92.02 **Immune effector cell-associated neurotoxicity syndrome, grade 2** `UPD`
ICANS, grade 2

G92.03 **Immune effector cell-associated neurotoxicity syndrome, grade 3** `UPD`
ICANS, grade 3

G92.04 **Immune effector cell-associated neurotoxicity syndrome, grade 4** `UPD`
ICANS, grade 4

G92.05 **Immune effector cell-associated neurotoxicity syndrome, grade 5** `UPD`
ICANS, grade 5

G92.8 **Other toxic encephalopathy**
Toxic encephalitis
Toxic metabolic encephalopathy
Code first poisoning due to drug or toxin, if applicable, (T36-T65 with fifth or sixth character 1-4)
Use additional code for adverse effect, if applicable, to identify drug (T36-T50 with fifth or sixth character 5)
AHA: 2024,4Q,16; 2024,2Q,14; 2022,1Q,52

G92.9 **Unspecified toxic encephalopathy**
Code first poisoning due to drug or toxin, if applicable, (T36-T65 with fifth or sixth character 1-4)
Use additional code for adverse effect, if applicable, to identify drug (T36-T50 with fifth or sixth character 5)

✓4th **G93** **Other disorders of brain**

G93.0 **Cerebral cysts**
Arachnoid cyst
Porencephalic cyst, acquired
EXCLUDES 1: acquired periventricular cysts of newborn (P91.1)
congenital cerebral cysts (Q04.6)

G93.1 **Anoxic brain damage, not elsewhere classified** `HCC` `ESR` `COM`
EXCLUDES 1: cerebral anoxia due to anesthesia during labor and delivery (O74.3)
cerebral anoxia due to anesthesia during the puerperium (O89.2)
neonatal anoxia (P84)
DEF: Brain injury not resulting from birth trauma that is due to lack of oxygen. Brain cells, when deprived of oxygen, begin to expire after four minutes.

G93.2 **Benign intracranial hypertension**
Pseudotumor
EXCLUDES 1: hypertensive encephalopathy (I67.4)
obstructive hydrocephalus (G91.1)

✓5th **G93.3** **Postviral and related fatigue syndromes**
Use additional code, if applicable, for post COVID-19 condition, unspecified (U09.9)
EXCLUDES 1: chronic fatigue NOS (R53.82)
neurasthenia (F48.8)
AHA: 2022,4Q,20

G93.31 **Postviral fatigue** syndrome
G93.32 **Myalgic encephalomyelitis/chronic** fatigue syndrome
Chronic fatigue syndrome
ME/CFS
Myalgic encephalomyelitis

G93.39 **Other post infection and related fatigue syndromes**

✓5th **G93.4** **Other and unspecified encephalopathy**
EXCLUDES 2: alcoholic encephalopathy (G31.2)
encephalopathy in diseases classified elsewhere (G94)
hypertensive encephalopathy (I67.4)
toxic (metabolic) encephalopathy (G92.8)

G93.40 **Encephalopathy, unspecified**
AHA: 2017,2Q,8

G93.41 **Metabolic** encephalopathy
Septic encephalopathy
AHA: 2024,2Q,14; 2017,2Q,8; 2016,3Q,42; 2015,3Q,21
TIP: Assign separately when documented with diabetic hypoglycemia (E08.649, E09.649, E10.649, E11.649, E13.649).

G93.42 **Megalencephalic** leukoencephalopathy with subcortical cysts `HCC` `ESR` `COM`
AHA: 2023,4Q,12-13

G93.43 **Leukoencephalopathy with calcifications and cysts** `HCC` `ESR` `COM`
AHA: 2023,4Q,12-13

G93.44 **Adult-onset leukodystrophy** with axonal spheroids `HCC` `ESR` `COM` `A`
Adult-onset leukoencephalopathy with axonal spheroids and pigmented glia
AHA: 2023,4Q,12-13

Chapter 6. Diseases of the Nervous System

G93.45 **Developmental and epileptic encephalopathy** `HCC` `Rx` `ESR` `COM`
Early infantile epileptic encephalopathy
Code also, if applicable, associated disorders such as:
developmental disorder of speech and language (F80.-)
developmental disorders of scholastic skills (F81.-)
epilepsy, by specific type (G40.-)
intellectual disabilities (F70-F79)
other neurodevelopmental disorder (F88)
pervasive developmental disorders (F84.-)
AHA: 2024,4Q,17

G93.49 **Other encephalopathy**
Encephalopathy NEC
AHA: 2021,2Q,3; 2018,4Q,16; 2018,2Q,22,24; 2017,2Q,9

G93.5 **Compression of brain** `HCC` `ESR` `COM`
Arnold-Chiari type 1 compression of brain
Compression of brain (stem)
Herniation of brain (stem)
EXCLUDES 1 traumatic compression of brain (S06.A-)
AHA: 2020,2Q,31

G93.6 **Cerebral edema** `HCC` `Rx` `ESR` `COM`
EXCLUDES 1 cerebral edema due to birth injury (P11.0)
traumatic cerebral edema (S06.1-)
AHA: 2022,3Q,9-10

G93.7 **Reye's syndrome** `HCC` `Rx` `ESR` `COM` `P`
Code first poisoning due to salicylates, if applicable (T39.0-, with sixth character 1-4)
Use additional code for adverse effect due to salicylates, if applicable (T39.0-, with sixth character 5)
DEF: Rare childhood illness often developed after a viral upper respiratory infection. Symptoms include vomiting, elevated serum transaminase, brain swelling, disturbances of consciousness, seizures, and changes in liver and other viscera; it can be fatal.

✓5th **G93.8** **Other specified disorders of brain**

    G93.81 **Temporal sclerosis**
        Hippocampal sclerosis
        Mesial temporal sclerosis

    G93.82 **Brain death**

    G93.89 **Other specified disorders of brain**
        Postradiation encephalopathy
        AHA: 2024,2Q,15; 2020,2Q,24; 2019,3Q,8

G93.9 **Disorder of brain, unspecified**

G94 **Other disorders of brain in diseases classified elsewhere**
Code first underlying disease
EXCLUDES 1 encephalopathy in congenital syphilis (A50.49)
encephalopathy in influenza (J09.X9, J10.81, J11.81)
encephalopathy in syphilis (A52.19)
hydrocephalus in diseases classified elsewhere (G91.4)
AHA: 2018,2Q,22; 2017,2Q,8-9

✓4th **G95** **Other and unspecified diseases of spinal cord**
EXCLUDES 2 myelitis (G04.-)

   G95.0 **Syringomyelia and syringobulbia** `HCC` `Rx` `ESR` `COM`

✓5th **G95.1** **Vascular myelopathies**
EXCLUDES 2 intraspinal phlebitis and thrombophlebitis, except non-pyogenic (G08)

    G95.11 **Acute infarction of spinal cord (embolic) (nonembolic)** `HCC` `Rx` `ESR` `COM`
        Anoxia of spinal cord
        Arterial thrombosis of spinal cord

    G95.19 **Other vascular myelopathies** `HCC` `Rx` `ESR` `COM`
        Edema of spinal cord
        Hematomyelia
        Nonpyogenic intraspinal phlebitis and thrombophlebitis
        Subacute necrotic myelopathy
        AHA: 2024,3Q,5; 2023,3Q,21

✓5th **G95.2** **Other and unspecified cord compression**

    G95.20 **Unspecified cord compression** `HCC` `Rx` `ESR` `COM`
    G95.29 **Other cord compression** `HCC` `Rx` `ESR` `COM`

✓5th **G95.8** **Other specified diseases of spinal cord**
EXCLUDES 1 neurogenic bladder NOS (N31.9)
neurogenic bladder due to cauda equina syndrome (G83.4)
neuromuscular dysfunction of bladder without spinal cord lesion (N31.-)

    G95.81 **Conus medullaris syndrome** `HCC` `Rx` `ESR` `COM`

    G95.89 **Other specified diseases of spinal cord** `HCC` `Rx` `ESR` `COM`
        Cord bladder NOS
        Drug-induced myelopathy
        Radiation-induced myelopathy
        EXCLUDES 1 myelopathy NOS (G95.9)
        AHA: 2024,3Q,5

   G95.9 **Disease of spinal cord, unspecified** `HCC` `Rx` `ESR` `COM`
        Myelopathy NOS

✓4th **G96** **Other disorders of central nervous system**

✓5th **G96.0** **Cerebrospinal fluid leak**
Code also if applicable:
intracranial hypotension (G96.81-)
EXCLUDES 1 cerebrospinal fluid leak from spinal puncture (G97.0)
AHA: 2024,3Q,7; 2020,4Q,21-22; 2018,2Q,13

    G96.00 **Cerebrospinal fluid leak, unspecified**
        Code also if applicable:
        head injury (S00-S09)

    G96.01 **Cranial cerebrospinal fluid leak, spontaneous**
        Otorrhea due to spontaneous cerebrospinal fluid CSF leak
        Rhinorrhea due to spontaneous cerebrospinal fluid CSF leak
        Spontaneous cerebrospinal fluid leak from skull base

    G96.02 **Spinal cerebrospinal fluid leak, spontaneous**
        Spontaneous cerebrospinal fluid leak from spine

    G96.08 **Other cranial cerebrospinal fluid leak**
        Postoperative cranial cerebrospinal fluid leak
        Traumatic cranial cerebrospinal fluid leak
        Code also if applicable:
        head injury (S00 - S09)
        AHA: 2024,3Q,7

    G96.09 **Other spinal cerebrospinal fluid leak**
        Other spinal CSF leak
        Postoperative spinal cerebrospinal fluid leak
        Traumatic spinal cerebrospinal fluid leak
        Code also if applicable:
        head injury (S00 - S09)
        AHA: 2022,3Q,24

✓5th **G96.1** **Disorders of meninges, not elsewhere classified**

    G96.11 **Dural tear**
        Code also intracranial hypotension, if applicable (G96.81-)
        EXCLUDES 1 accidental puncture or laceration of dura during a procedure (G97.41)
        AHA: 2014,4Q,24

    G96.12 **Meningeal adhesions (cerebral) (spinal)**

✓6th **G96.19** **Other disorders of meninges, not elsewhere classified**
        AHA: 2020,4Q,22

        G96.191 **Perineural cyst**
            Cervical nerve root cyst
            Lumbar nerve root cyst
            Sacral nerve root cyst
            Tarlov cyst
            Thoracic nerve root cyst

        G96.198 **Other disorders of meninges, not elsewhere classified**

`HCC` CMS-HCC   `Rx` Rx HCC   `ESR` ESRD HCC   `COM` Commercial HCC   Newborn: 0    Pediatric: 0-17   Maternity: 9-64   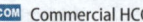 Adult: 15-124

Chapter 6. Diseases of the Nervous System

✓5ᵗʰ G96.8   Other specified disorders of central nervous system
　　AHA: 2020,4Q,21,23-24

　✓6ᵗʰ G96.81   Intracranial hypotension
　　Code also any associated diagnoses, such as:
　　　brachial amyotrophy (G54.5)
　　　cerebrospinal fluid leak from spine (G96.02)
　　　cranial nerve disorders in diseases classified elsewhere (G53)
　　　nerve root and compressions in diseases classified elsewhere (G55)
　　　nonpyogenic thrombosis of intracranial venous system (I67.6)
　　　nontraumatic intracerebral hemorrhage (I61.-)
　　　nontraumatic subdural hemorrhage (I62.0-)
　　　other and unspecified cord compression (G95.2-)
　　　other secondary parkinsonism (G21.8)
　　　reversible cerebrovascular vasoconstriction syndrome (I67.841)
　　　spinal cord herniation (G95.89)
　　　stroke (I63.-)
　　　syringomyelia (G95.0)
　　DEF: Central nervous system disorder resulting from a loss of cerebrospinal fluid (CSF) volume. More often associated with CSF leak at the level of the spine rather than the skull base, causes can be spontaneous, iatrogenic or traumatic spinal dura defects or holes, or overdrainage of CSF shunt devices. The most common symptom is headache.

　　　G96.810   Intracranial hypotension, unspecified
　　　G96.811   Intracranial hypotension, spontaneous
　　　　AHA: 2024,3Q,7
　　　G96.819   Other intracranial hypotension
　G96.89   Other specified disorders of central nervous system

G96.9   Disorder of central nervous system, unspecified

✓4ᵗʰ G97   Intraoperative and postprocedural complications and disorders of nervous system, not elsewhere classified
　EXCLUDES 2   intraoperative and postprocedural cerebrovascular infarction (I97.81-, I97.82-)
　AHA: 2016,4Q,9-10

　G97.0   Cerebrospinal fluid leak from spinal puncture
　　Code also any associated diagnoses or complications, such as:
　　　intracranial hypotension following a procedure (G97.83-G97.84)

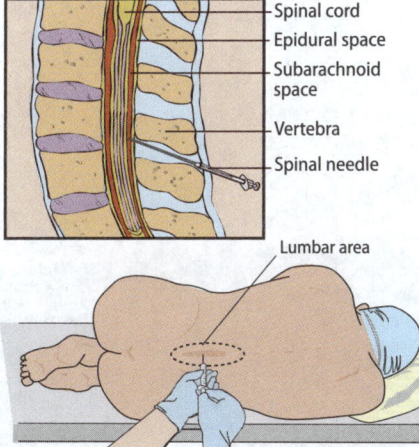
Spinal Puncture
- Spinal cord
- Epidural space
- Subarachnoid space
- Vertebra
- Spinal needle
- Lumbar area

　G97.1   Other reaction to spinal and lumbar puncture
　　Headache due to lumbar puncture
　　Other reaction to spinal dural puncture
　　Code also, if applicable, any associated headache with orthostatic component (R51.0)
　G97.2   Intracranial hypotension following ventricular shunting
　　Code also any associated diagnoses or complications

✓5ᵗʰ G97.3   Intraoperative hemorrhage and hematoma of a nervous system organ or structure complicating a procedure
　EXCLUDES 1   intraoperative hemorrhage and hematoma of a nervous system organ or structure due to accidental puncture and laceration during a procedure (G97.4-)

　G97.31   Intraoperative hemorrhage and hematoma of a nervous system organ or structure complicating a nervous system procedure
　G97.32   Intraoperative hemorrhage and hematoma of a nervous system organ or structure complicating other procedure

✓5ᵗʰ G97.4   Accidental puncture and laceration of a nervous system organ or structure during a procedure
　G97.41   Accidental puncture or laceration of dura during a procedure
　　Incidental (inadvertent) durotomy
　　Code also any associated diagnoses or complications
　　AHA: 2024,1Q,20-21; 2014,4Q,24
　G97.48   Accidental puncture and laceration of other nervous system organ or structure during a nervous system procedure
　G97.49   Accidental puncture and laceration of other nervous system organ or structure during other procedure

✓5ᵗʰ G97.5   Postprocedural hemorrhage of a nervous system organ or structure following a procedure
　G97.51   Postprocedural hemorrhage of a nervous system organ or structure following a nervous system procedure
　G97.52   Postprocedural hemorrhage of a nervous system organ or structure following other procedure

✓5ᵗʰ G97.6   Postprocedural hematoma and seroma of a nervous system organ or structure following a procedure
　G97.61   Postprocedural hematoma of a nervous system organ or structure following a nervous system procedure
　　AHA: 2025,2Q,26; 2024,3Q,5; 2020,3Q,24
　G97.62   Postprocedural hematoma of a nervous system organ or structure following other procedure
　　AHA: 2025,2Q,26
　G97.63   Postprocedural seroma of a nervous system organ or structure following a nervous system procedure
　G97.64   Postprocedural seroma of a nervous system organ or structure following other procedure

✓5ᵗʰ G97.8   Other intraoperative and postprocedural complications and disorders of nervous system
　Use additional code to further specify disorder
　AHA: 2020,4Q,23

　G97.81   Other intraoperative complications of nervous system
　G97.82   Other postprocedural complications and disorders of nervous system
　　AHA: 2022,1Q,34
　G97.83   Intracranial hypotension following lumbar cerebrospinal fluid shunting
　　Code also any associated diagnoses or complications
　G97.84   Intracranial hypotension following other procedure
　　Code also, if applicable:
　　　accidental puncture or laceration of dura during a procedure (G97.41)
　　　cerebrospinal fluid leak from spinal puncture (G97.0)

✓4ᵗʰ G98   Other disorders of nervous system not elsewhere classified
　INCLUDES   nervous system disorder NOS

　G98.0   Neurogenic arthritis, not elsewhere classified
　　Nonsyphilitic neurogenic arthropathy NEC
　　Nonsyphilitic neurogenic spondylopathy NEC
　　EXCLUDES 1   spondylopathy (in):
　　　syringomyelia and syringobulbia (G95.0)
　　　tabes dorsalis (A52.11)
　G98.8   Other disorders of nervous system
　　Nervous system disorder NOS

✓4ᵗʰ G99   Other disorders of nervous system in diseases classified elsewhere
　G99.0   Autonomic neuropathy in diseases classified elsewhere
　　Code first underlying disease, such as:
　　　amyloidosis (E85.-)
　　　gout (M1A.-, M10.-)
　　　hyperthyroidism (E05.-)
　　EXCLUDES 1   diabetic autonomic neuropathy (E08-E13 with .43)

G99.2 *Myelopathy in diseases classified elsewhere* `HCC` `Rx` `ESR` `COM`
Code first underlying disease, such as:
neoplasm (C00-D49)
EXCLUDES 1   myelopathy in:
intervertebral disease (M50.0-, M51.0-)
spondylosis (M47.0-, M47.1-)
AHA: 2018,3Q,18-19
TIP: Use this code in addition to a spondylolisthesis code (M43.1-) or a spinal stenosis code (M48.0-) when either of these disorders is documented as the cause of the myelopathy.

G99.8 *Other specified disorders of nervous system in diseases classified elsewhere*
Code first underlying disorder, such as:
amyloidosis (E85.-)
avitaminosis (E56.-)
EXCLUDES 1   nervous system involvement in:
cysticercosis (B69.0)
rubella (B06.0-)
syphilis (A52.1-)

Chapter 7. Diseases of the Eye and Adnexa (H00–H59)

Chapter-specific Guidelines with Coding Examples

The chapter-specific guidelines from the ICD-10-CM Official Guidelines for Coding and Reporting have been provided below. Along with these guidelines are coding examples, contained in the shaded boxes, that have been developed to help illustrate the coding and/or sequencing guidance found in these guidelines.

a. Glaucoma

1) Assigning glaucoma codes

Assign as many codes from category H40, Glaucoma, as needed to identify the type of glaucoma, the affected eye, and the glaucoma stage.

2) Bilateral glaucoma with same type and stage

When a patient has bilateral glaucoma and both eyes are documented as being the same type and stage, and there is a code for bilateral glaucoma, report only the code for the type of glaucoma, bilateral, with the seventh character for the stage.

> Bilateral mild stage primary open-angle glaucoma
>
> **H40.1131**   **Primary open-angle glaucoma, bilateral, mild stage**
>
> *Explanation*: In this scenario, the patient has the same type and stage of glaucoma in both eyes. As this type of glaucoma has a code for bilateral, assign only the code for the bilateral glaucoma with the seventh character for the stage.

When a patient has bilateral glaucoma and both eyes are documented as being the same type and stage, and the classification does not provide a code for bilateral glaucoma (i.e. subcategories H40.10 and H40.20) report only one code for the type of glaucoma with the appropriate seventh character for the stage.

> Bilateral open-angle glaucoma, severe stage; not specified as to type
>
> **H40.10X3**   **Unspecified open-angle glaucoma, severe stage**
>
> *Explanation*: In this scenario, the patient has glaucoma of the same type and stage of both eyes, but there is no code specifically for bilateral glaucoma. Only one code is assigned with the appropriate seventh character for the stage.

3) Bilateral glaucoma stage with different types or stages

When a patient has bilateral glaucoma and each eye is documented as having a different type or stage, and the classification distinguishes laterality, assign the appropriate code for each eye rather than the code for bilateral glaucoma.

> Bilateral chronic angle-closure glaucoma; right eye is documented as mild stage and left eye as moderate stage
>
> **H40.2211**   **Chronic angle-closure glaucoma, right eye, mild stage**
>
> **H40.2222**   **Chronic angle-closure glaucoma, left eye, moderate stage**
>
> *Explanation*: In this scenario the patient has the same type of glaucoma in both eyes, but each eye is at a different stage. Because the subcategory for this condition identifies laterality, one code is assigned for the right eye and one code is assigned for the left eye, each with the appropriate seventh character for the stage appended.

When a patient has bilateral glaucoma and each eye is documented as having a different type, and the classification does not distinguish laterality (i.e. subcategories H40.10 and H40.20), assign one code for each type of glaucoma with the appropriate seventh character for the stage.

> Documentation relates mild, unspecified primary angle-closure glaucoma of the left eye with mild unspecified open-angle glaucoma of the right eye
>
> **H40.20X1**   **Unspecified primary angle-closure glaucoma, mild stage**
>
> **H40.10X1**   **Unspecified open-angle glaucoma, mild stage**
>
> *Explanation*: In this scenario the patient has a different type of glaucoma in each eye and the classification does not distinguish laterality. A code for each type of glaucoma is assigned, each with the appropriate seventh character for the stage.

When a patient has bilateral glaucoma and each eye is documented as having the same type, but different stage, and the classification does not distinguish laterality (i.e. subcategories H40.10 and H40.20), assign a code for the type of glaucoma for each eye with the seventh character for the specific glaucoma stage documented for each eye.

> Bilateral open-angle glaucoma, not specified as to type; the right eye is documented to be in mild stage and the left eye as being in moderate stage
>
> **H40.10X1**   **Unspecified open-angle glaucoma, mild stage**
>
> **H40.10X2**   **Unspecified open-angle glaucoma, moderate stage**
>
> *Explanation*: In this scenario the patient has the same type of glaucoma in each eye but each eye is at a different stage, and the classification does not distinguish laterality at this subcategory level. Two codes are assigned; both codes represent the same type of glaucoma but each has a different seventh character identifying the appropriate stage for each eye.

4) Patient admitted with glaucoma and stage evolves during the admission

If a patient is admitted with glaucoma and the stage progresses during the admission, assign the code for highest stage documented.

5) Indeterminate stage glaucoma

Assignment of the seventh character "4" for "indeterminate stage" should be based on the clinical documentation. The seventh character "4" is used for glaucomas whose stage cannot be clinically determined. This seventh character should not be confused with the seventh character "0", unspecified, which should be assigned when there is no documentation regarding the stage of the glaucoma.

b. Blindness

If "blindness" or "low vision" of both eyes is documented but the visual impairment category is not documented, assign code H54.3, Unqualified visual loss, both eyes. If "blindness" or "low vision" in one eye is documented but the visual impairment category is not documented, assign a code from H54.6-, Unqualified visual loss, one eye. If "blindness" or "visual loss" is documented without any information about whether one or both eyes are affected, assign code H54.7, Unspecified visual loss.

> Patient assessment indicates moderately impaired/low vision in the left eye with no visual impairments in the right eye
>
> **H54.62**   **Unqualified visual loss, left eye, normal vision right eye**
>
> Report unqualified visual loss when the visual impairment category is not specified. In this case, only the left eye is impacted by visual loss with normal vision of the right eye documented.

Chapter 7. Diseases of the Eye and Adnexa (H00-H59)

NOTE Use an external cause code following the code for the eye condition, if applicable, to identify the cause of the eye condition

EXCLUDES 2
- certain conditions originating in the perinatal period (P04-P96)
- certain infectious and parasitic diseases (A00-B99)
- complications of pregnancy, childbirth and the puerperium (O00-O9A)
- congenital malformations, deformations, and chromosomal abnormalities (Q00-Q99)
- diabetes mellitus related eye conditions (E09.3-, E10.3-, E11.3-, E13.3-)
- endocrine, nutritional and metabolic diseases (E00-E88)
- injury (trauma) of eye and orbit (S05.-)
- injury, poisoning and certain other consequences of external causes (S00-T88)
- neoplasms (C00-D49)
- symptoms, signs and abnormal clinical and laboratory findings, not elsewhere classified (R00-R94)
- syphilis related eye disorders (A50.01, A50.3-, A51.43, A52.71)

This chapter contains the following blocks:
- H00-H05 Disorders of eyelid, lacrimal system and orbit
- H10-H11 Disorders of conjunctiva
- H15-H22 Disorders of sclera, cornea, iris and ciliary body
- H25-H28 Disorders of lens
- H30-H36 Disorders of choroid and retina
- H40-H42 Glaucoma
- H43-H44 Disorders of vitreous body and globe
- H46-H47 Disorders of optic nerve and visual pathways
- H49-H52 Disorders of ocular muscles, binocular movement, accommodation and refraction
- H53-H54 Visual disturbances and blindness
- H55-H57 Other disorders of eye and adnexa
- H59 Intraoperative and postprocedural complications and disorders of eye and adnexa, not elsewhere classified

Disorders of eyelid, lacrimal system and orbit (H00-H05)

EXCLUDES 2
- open wound of eyelid (S01.1-)
- superficial injury of eyelid (S00.1-, S00.2-)

H00 Hordeolum and chalazion

H00.0 Hordeolum (externum) (internum) of eyelid
DEF: Acute localized infection of the gland of Zeis (external hordeolum) or Molt or of the meibomian glands (internal hordeolum) of the orbit.

H00.01 Hordeolum externum
Hordeolum NOS
Stye
- H00.011 Hordeolum externum right upper eyelid
- H00.012 Hordeolum externum right lower eyelid
- H00.013 Hordeolum externum right eye, unspecified eyelid
- H00.014 Hordeolum externum left upper eyelid
- H00.015 Hordeolum externum left lower eyelid
- H00.016 Hordeolum externum left eye, unspecified eyelid
- H00.019 Hordeolum externum unspecified eye, unspecified eyelid

H00.02 Hordeolum internum
Infection of meibomian gland
- H00.021 Hordeolum internum right upper eyelid
- H00.022 Hordeolum internum right lower eyelid
- H00.023 Hordeolum internum right eye, unspecified eyelid
- H00.024 Hordeolum internum left upper eyelid
- H00.025 Hordeolum internum left lower eyelid
- H00.026 Hordeolum internum left eye, unspecified eyelid
- H00.029 Hordeolum internum unspecified eye, unspecified eyelid

H00.03 Abscess of eyelid
Furuncle of eyelid
- H00.031 Abscess of right upper eyelid
- H00.032 Abscess of right lower eyelid
- H00.033 Abscess of eyelid right eye, unspecified eyelid
- H00.034 Abscess of left upper eyelid
- H00.035 Abscess of left lower eyelid
- H00.036 Abscess of eyelid left eye, unspecified eyelid
- H00.039 Abscess of eyelid unspecified eye, unspecified eyelid

H00.1 Chalazion
Meibomian (gland) cyst
EXCLUDES 2 infected meibomian gland (H00.02-)
DEF: Noninfectious, obstructive mass in the oil gland of the eyelid that results in a small chronic lump or inflammation.
- H00.11 Chalazion right upper eyelid
- H00.12 Chalazion right lower eyelid
- H00.13 Chalazion right eye, unspecified eyelid
- H00.14 Chalazion left upper eyelid
- H00.15 Chalazion left lower eyelid
- H00.16 Chalazion left eye, unspecified eyelid
- H00.19 Chalazion unspecified eye, unspecified eyelid

H01 Other inflammation of eyelid

H01.0 Blepharitis
EXCLUDES 1 blepharoconjunctivitis (H10.5-)

H01.00 Unspecified blepharitis
AHA: 2018,4Q,13
- H01.001 Unspecified blepharitis right upper eyelid
- H01.002 Unspecified blepharitis right lower eyelid
- H01.003 Unspecified blepharitis right eye, unspecified eyelid
- H01.004 Unspecified blepharitis left upper eyelid
- H01.005 Unspecified blepharitis left lower eyelid
- H01.006 Unspecified blepharitis left eye, unspecified eyelid
- H01.009 Unspecified blepharitis unspecified eye, unspecified eyelid
- H01.00A Unspecified blepharitis right eye, upper and lower eyelids
- H01.00B Unspecified blepharitis left eye, upper and lower eyelids

H01.01 Ulcerative blepharitis
AHA: 2018,4Q,13
- H01.011 Ulcerative blepharitis right upper eyelid
- H01.012 Ulcerative blepharitis right lower eyelid
- H01.013 Ulcerative blepharitis right eye, unspecified eyelid
- H01.014 Ulcerative blepharitis left upper eyelid
- H01.015 Ulcerative blepharitis left lower eyelid
- H01.016 Ulcerative blepharitis left eye, unspecified eyelid
- H01.019 Ulcerative blepharitis unspecified eye, unspecified eyelid
- H01.01A Ulcerative blepharitis right eye, upper and lower eyelids
- H01.01B Ulcerative blepharitis left eye, upper and lower eyelids

H01.02 Squamous blepharitis
AHA: 2018,4Q,13
- H01.021 Squamous blepharitis right upper eyelid
- H01.022 Squamous blepharitis right lower eyelid
- H01.023 Squamous blepharitis right eye, unspecified eyelid
- H01.024 Squamous blepharitis left upper eyelid
- H01.025 Squamous blepharitis left lower eyelid
- H01.026 Squamous blepharitis left eye, unspecified eyelid
- H01.029 Squamous blepharitis unspecified eye, unspecified eyelid
- H01.02A Squamous blepharitis right eye, upper and lower eyelids
- H01.02B Squamous blepharitis left eye, upper and lower eyelids

H01.1 Noninfectious dermatoses of eyelid

H01.11 Allergic dermatitis of eyelid
Contact dermatitis of eyelid
- H01.111 Allergic dermatitis of right upper eyelid
- H01.112 Allergic dermatitis of right lower eyelid
- H01.113 Allergic dermatitis of right eye, unspecified eyelid
- H01.114 Allergic dermatitis of left upper eyelid
- H01.115 Allergic dermatitis of left lower eyelid
- H01.116 Allergic dermatitis of left eye, unspecified eyelid
- H01.119 Allergic dermatitis of unspecified eye, unspecified eyelid

H01.12 Discoid lupus erythematosus of eyelid
- H01.121 Discoid lupus erythematosus of right upper eyelid

Chapter 7. Diseases of the Eye and Adnexa

- H01.122 Discoid lupus erythematosus of right lower eyelid Rx
- H01.123 Discoid lupus erythematosus of right eye, unspecified eyelid Rx
- H01.124 Discoid lupus erythematosus of left upper eyelid
- H01.125 Discoid lupus erythematosus of left lower eyelid Rx
- H01.126 Discoid lupus erythematosus of left eye, unspecified eyelid Rx
- H01.129 Discoid lupus erythematosus of unspecified eye, unspecified eyelid Rx

✓6th H01.13 Eczematous dermatitis of eyelid
- H01.131 Eczematous dermatitis of right upper eyelid
- H01.132 Eczematous dermatitis of right lower eyelid
- H01.133 Eczematous dermatitis of right eye, unspecified eyelid
- H01.134 Eczematous dermatitis of left upper eyelid
- H01.135 Eczematous dermatitis of left lower eyelid
- H01.136 Eczematous dermatitis of left eye, unspecified eyelid
- H01.139 Eczematous dermatitis of unspecified eye, unspecified eyelid

✓6th H01.14 Xeroderma of eyelid
- H01.141 Xeroderma of right upper eyelid
- H01.142 Xeroderma of right lower eyelid
- H01.143 Xeroderma of right eye, unspecified eyelid
- H01.144 Xeroderma of left upper eyelid
- H01.145 Xeroderma of left lower eyelid
- H01.146 Xeroderma of left eye, unspecified eyelid
- H01.149 Xeroderma of unspecified eye, unspecified eyelid

▲ ✓5th H01.8 Other specified inflammations of eyelid
▶Code also, if applicable, infestation by Demodex mites (B88.01)◀
- • H01.81 Other specified inflammation of right upper eyelid
- • H01.82 Other specified inflammation of right lower eyelid
- • H01.83 Other specified inflammation of right eye, unspecified eyelid
- • H01.84 Other specified inflammation of left upper eyelid
- • H01.85 Other specified inflammation of left lower eyelid
- • H01.86 Other specified inflammation of left eye, unspecified eyelid
- • H01.89 Other specified inflammation of unspecified eye, unspecified eyelid
- • H01.8A Other specified inflammation of right eye, upper and lower eyelids
- • H01.8B Other specified inflammation of left eye, upper and lower eyelids

H01.9 Unspecified inflammation of eyelid
Inflammation of eyelid NOS

✓4th H02 Other disorders of eyelid
EXCLUDES 1 congenital malformations of eyelid (Q10.0-Q10.3)

Entropion and Ectropion

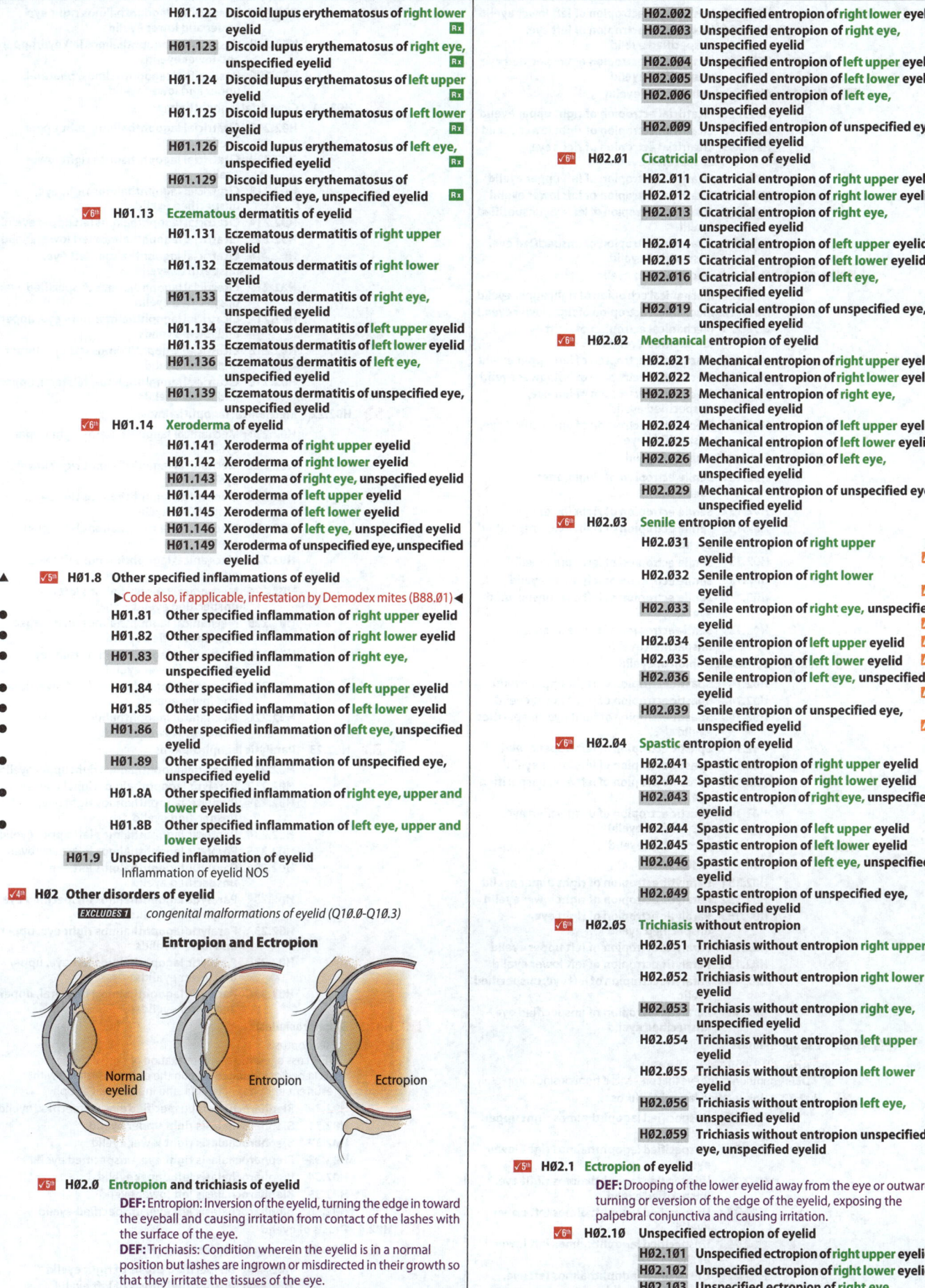

Normal eyelid | Entropion | Ectropion

✓5th H02.0 Entropion and trichiasis of eyelid
DEF: Entropion: Inversion of the eyelid, turning the edge in toward the eyeball and causing irritation from contact of the lashes with the surface of the eye.
DEF: Trichiasis: Condition wherein the eyelid is in a normal position but lashes are ingrown or misdirected in their growth so that they irritate the tissues of the eye.

✓6th H02.00 Unspecified entropion of eyelid
- H02.001 Unspecified entropion of right upper eyelid
- H02.002 Unspecified entropion of right lower eyelid
- H02.003 Unspecified entropion of right eye, unspecified eyelid
- H02.004 Unspecified entropion of left upper eyelid
- H02.005 Unspecified entropion of left lower eyelid
- H02.006 Unspecified entropion of left eye, unspecified eyelid
- H02.009 Unspecified entropion of unspecified eye, unspecified eyelid

✓6th H02.01 Cicatricial entropion of eyelid
- H02.011 Cicatricial entropion of right upper eyelid
- H02.012 Cicatricial entropion of right lower eyelid
- H02.013 Cicatricial entropion of right eye, unspecified eyelid
- H02.014 Cicatricial entropion of left upper eyelid
- H02.015 Cicatricial entropion of left lower eyelid
- H02.016 Cicatricial entropion of left eye, unspecified eyelid
- H02.019 Cicatricial entropion of unspecified eye, unspecified eyelid

✓6th H02.02 Mechanical entropion of eyelid
- H02.021 Mechanical entropion of right upper eyelid
- H02.022 Mechanical entropion of right lower eyelid
- H02.023 Mechanical entropion of right eye, unspecified eyelid
- H02.024 Mechanical entropion of left upper eyelid
- H02.025 Mechanical entropion of left lower eyelid
- H02.026 Mechanical entropion of left eye, unspecified eyelid
- H02.029 Mechanical entropion of unspecified eye, unspecified eyelid

✓6th H02.03 Senile entropion of eyelid
- H02.031 Senile entropion of right upper eyelid A
- H02.032 Senile entropion of right lower eyelid A
- H02.033 Senile entropion of right eye, unspecified eyelid A
- H02.034 Senile entropion of left upper eyelid A
- H02.035 Senile entropion of left lower eyelid A
- H02.036 Senile entropion of left eye, unspecified eyelid A
- H02.039 Senile entropion of unspecified eye, unspecified eyelid A

✓6th H02.04 Spastic entropion of eyelid
- H02.041 Spastic entropion of right upper eyelid
- H02.042 Spastic entropion of right lower eyelid
- H02.043 Spastic entropion of right eye, unspecified eyelid
- H02.044 Spastic entropion of left upper eyelid
- H02.045 Spastic entropion of left lower eyelid
- H02.046 Spastic entropion of left eye, unspecified eyelid
- H02.049 Spastic entropion of unspecified eye, unspecified eyelid

✓6th H02.05 Trichiasis without entropion
- H02.051 Trichiasis without entropion right upper eyelid
- H02.052 Trichiasis without entropion right lower eyelid
- H02.053 Trichiasis without entropion right eye, unspecified eyelid
- H02.054 Trichiasis without entropion left upper eyelid
- H02.055 Trichiasis without entropion left lower eyelid
- H02.056 Trichiasis without entropion left eye, unspecified eyelid
- H02.059 Trichiasis without entropion unspecified eye, unspecified eyelid

✓5th H02.1 Ectropion of eyelid
DEF: Drooping of the lower eyelid away from the eye or outward turning or eversion of the edge of the eyelid, exposing the palpebral conjunctiva and causing irritation.

✓6th H02.10 Unspecified ectropion of eyelid
- H02.101 Unspecified ectropion of right upper eyelid
- H02.102 Unspecified ectropion of right lower eyelid
- H02.103 Unspecified ectropion of right eye, unspecified eyelid
- H02.104 Unspecified ectropion of left upper eyelid

Chapter 7. Diseases of the Eye and Adnexa

- H02.105 Unspecified ectropion of left lower eyelid
- H02.106 Unspecified ectropion of left eye, unspecified eyelid
- H02.109 Unspecified ectropion of unspecified eye, unspecified eyelid

✓6th **H02.11** Cicatricial ectropion of eyelid
- H02.111 Cicatricial ectropion of right upper eyelid
- H02.112 Cicatricial ectropion of right lower eyelid
- H02.113 Cicatricial ectropion of right eye, unspecified eyelid
- H02.114 Cicatricial ectropion of left upper eyelid
- H02.115 Cicatricial ectropion of left lower eyelid
- H02.116 Cicatricial ectropion of left eye, unspecified eyelid
- H02.119 Cicatricial ectropion of unspecified eye, unspecified eyelid

✓6th **H02.12** Mechanical ectropion of eyelid
- H02.121 Mechanical ectropion of right upper eyelid
- H02.122 Mechanical ectropion of right lower eyelid
- H02.123 Mechanical ectropion of right eye, unspecified eyelid
- H02.124 Mechanical ectropion of left upper eyelid
- H02.125 Mechanical ectropion of left lower eyelid
- H02.126 Mechanical ectropion of left eye, unspecified eyelid
- H02.129 Mechanical ectropion of unspecified eye, unspecified eyelid

✓6th **H02.13** Senile ectropion of eyelid
- H02.131 Senile ectropion of right upper eyelid **A**
- H02.132 Senile ectropion of right lower eyelid **A**
- H02.133 Senile ectropion of right eye, unspecified eyelid **A**
- H02.134 Senile ectropion of left upper eyelid **A**
- H02.135 Senile ectropion of left lower eyelid **A**
- H02.136 Senile ectropion of left eye, unspecified eyelid **A**
- H02.139 Senile ectropion of unspecified eye, unspecified eyelid **A**

✓6th **H02.14** Spastic ectropion of eyelid
- H02.141 Spastic ectropion of right upper eyelid
- H02.142 Spastic ectropion of right lower eyelid
- H02.143 Spastic ectropion of right eye, unspecified eyelid
- H02.144 Spastic ectropion of left upper eyelid
- H02.145 Spastic ectropion of left lower eyelid
- H02.146 Spastic ectropion of left eye, unspecified eyelid
- H02.149 Spastic ectropion of unspecified eye, unspecified eyelid

✓6th **H02.15** Paralytic ectropion of eyelid
  AHA: 2018,4Q,13
- H02.151 Paralytic ectropion of right upper eyelid
- H02.152 Paralytic ectropion of right lower eyelid
- H02.153 Paralytic ectropion of right eye, unspecified eyelid
- H02.154 Paralytic ectropion of left upper eyelid
- H02.155 Paralytic ectropion of left lower eyelid
- H02.156 Paralytic ectropion of left eye, unspecified eyelid
- H02.159 Paralytic ectropion of unspecified eye, unspecified eyelid

✓5th **H02.2** Lagophthalmos
  AHA: 2018,4Q,14
  DEF: Condition of the eye that prevents it from closing completely.

✓6th **H02.20** Unspecified lagophthalmos
- H02.201 Unspecified lagophthalmos right upper eyelid
- H02.202 Unspecified lagophthalmos right lower eyelid
- H02.203 Unspecified lagophthalmos right eye, unspecified eyelid
- H02.204 Unspecified lagophthalmos left upper eyelid
- H02.205 Unspecified lagophthalmos left lower eyelid
- H02.206 Unspecified lagophthalmos left eye, unspecified eyelid
- H02.209 Unspecified lagophthalmos unspecified eye, unspecified eyelid
- H02.20A Unspecified lagophthalmos right eye, upper and lower eyelids
- H02.20B Unspecified lagophthalmos left eye, upper and lower eyelids
- H02.20C Unspecified lagophthalmos, bilateral, upper and lower eyelids

✓6th **H02.21** Cicatricial lagophthalmos
- H02.211 Cicatricial lagophthalmos right upper eyelid
- H02.212 Cicatricial lagophthalmos right lower eyelid
- H02.213 Cicatricial lagophthalmos right eye, unspecified eyelid
- H02.214 Cicatricial lagophthalmos left upper eyelid
- H02.215 Cicatricial lagophthalmos left lower eyelid
- H02.216 Cicatricial lagophthalmos left eye, unspecified eyelid
- H02.219 Cicatricial lagophthalmos unspecified eye, unspecified eyelid
- H02.21A Cicatricial lagophthalmos right eye, upper and lower eyelids
- H02.21B Cicatricial lagophthalmos left eye, upper and lower eyelids
- H02.21C Cicatricial lagophthalmos, bilateral, upper and lower eyelids

✓6th **H02.22** Mechanical lagophthalmos
- H02.221 Mechanical lagophthalmos right upper eyelid
- H02.222 Mechanical lagophthalmos right lower eyelid
- H02.223 Mechanical lagophthalmos right eye, unspecified eyelid
- H02.224 Mechanical lagophthalmos left upper eyelid
- H02.225 Mechanical lagophthalmos left lower eyelid
- H02.226 Mechanical lagophthalmos left eye, unspecified eyelid
- H02.229 Mechanical lagophthalmos unspecified eye, unspecified eyelid
- H02.22A Mechanical lagophthalmos right eye, upper and lower eyelids
- H02.22B Mechanical lagophthalmos left eye, upper and lower eyelids
- H02.22C Mechanical lagophthalmos, bilateral, upper and lower eyelids

✓6th **H02.23** Paralytic lagophthalmos
- H02.231 Paralytic lagophthalmos right upper eyelid
- H02.232 Paralytic lagophthalmos right lower eyelid
- H02.233 Paralytic lagophthalmos right eye, unspecified eyelid
- H02.234 Paralytic lagophthalmos left upper eyelid
- H02.235 Paralytic lagophthalmos left lower eyelid
- H02.236 Paralytic lagophthalmos left eye, unspecified eyelid
- H02.239 Paralytic lagophthalmos unspecified eye, unspecified eyelid
- H02.23A Paralytic lagophthalmos right eye, upper and lower eyelids
- H02.23B Paralytic lagophthalmos left eye, upper and lower eyelids
- H02.23C Paralytic lagophthalmos, bilateral, upper and lower eyelids

✓5th **H02.3** Blepharochalasis
  Pseudoptosis
  DEF: Loss of elasticity and relaxation of skin of the eyelid, thickened or indurated skin on the eyelid associated with recurrent episodes of edema, and intracellular atrophy.
- H02.30 Blepharochalasis unspecified eye, unspecified eyelid
- H02.31 Blepharochalasis right upper eyelid
- H02.32 Blepharochalasis right lower eyelid
- H02.33 Blepharochalasis right eye, unspecified eyelid
- H02.34 Blepharochalasis left upper eyelid
- H02.35 Blepharochalasis left lower eyelid
- H02.36 Blepharochalasis left eye, unspecified eyelid

✓5th **H02.4** Ptosis of eyelid
✓6th **H02.40** Unspecified ptosis of eyelid
- H02.401 Unspecified ptosis of right eyelid
- H02.402 Unspecified ptosis of left eyelid
- H02.403 Unspecified ptosis of bilateral eyelids
- H02.409 Unspecified ptosis of unspecified eyelid

H02.41 Mechanical ptosis of eyelid
- H02.411 Mechanical ptosis of right eyelid
- H02.412 Mechanical ptosis of left eyelid
- H02.413 Mechanical ptosis of bilateral eyelids
- H02.419 Mechanical ptosis of unspecified eyelid

H02.42 Myogenic ptosis of eyelid
- H02.421 Myogenic ptosis of right eyelid
- H02.422 Myogenic ptosis of left eyelid
- H02.423 Myogenic ptosis of bilateral eyelids
- H02.429 Myogenic ptosis of unspecified eyelid

H02.43 Paralytic ptosis of eyelid
Neurogenic ptosis of eyelid
- H02.431 Paralytic ptosis of right eyelid
- H02.432 Paralytic ptosis of left eyelid
- H02.433 Paralytic ptosis of bilateral eyelids
- H02.439 Paralytic ptosis unspecified eyelid

H02.5 Other disorders affecting eyelid function
EXCLUDES 2: blepharospasm (G24.5)
organic tic (G25.69)
psychogenic tic (F95.-)

H02.51 Abnormal innervation syndrome
- H02.511 Abnormal innervation syndrome right upper eyelid
- H02.512 Abnormal innervation syndrome right lower eyelid
- H02.513 Abnormal innervation syndrome right eye, unspecified eyelid
- H02.514 Abnormal innervation syndrome left upper eyelid
- H02.515 Abnormal innervation syndrome left lower eyelid
- H02.516 Abnormal innervation syndrome left eye, unspecified eyelid
- H02.519 Abnormal innervation syndrome unspecified eye, unspecified eyelid

H02.52 Blepharophimosis
Ankyloblepharon
- H02.521 Blepharophimosis right upper eyelid
- H02.522 Blepharophimosis right lower eyelid
- H02.523 Blepharophimosis right eye, unspecified eyelid
- H02.524 Blepharophimosis left upper eyelid
- H02.525 Blepharophimosis left lower eyelid
- H02.526 Blepharophimosis left eye, unspecified eyelid
- H02.529 Blepharophimosis unspecified eye, unspecified lid

H02.53 Eyelid retraction
Eyelid lag
- H02.531 Eyelid retraction right upper eyelid
- H02.532 Eyelid retraction right lower eyelid
- H02.533 Eyelid retraction right eye, unspecified eyelid
- H02.534 Eyelid retraction left upper eyelid
- H02.535 Eyelid retraction left lower eyelid
- H02.536 Eyelid retraction left eye, unspecified eyelid
- H02.539 Eyelid retraction unspecified eye, unspecified lid

H02.59 Other disorders affecting eyelid function
Deficient blink reflex
Sensory disorders

H02.6 Xanthelasma of eyelid
DEF: Condition in which there are small yellow tumors that occur on the eyelid, usually appearing near the nose.
- H02.60 Xanthelasma of unspecified eye, unspecified eyelid
- H02.61 Xanthelasma of right upper eyelid
- H02.62 Xanthelasma of right lower eyelid
- H02.63 Xanthelasma of right eye, unspecified eyelid
- H02.64 Xanthelasma of left upper eyelid
- H02.65 Xanthelasma of left lower eyelid
- H02.66 Xanthelasma of left eye, unspecified eyelid

H02.7 Other and unspecified degenerative disorders of eyelid and periocular area
- H02.70 Unspecified degenerative disorders of eyelid and periocular area

H02.71 Chloasma of eyelid and periocular area
Dyspigmentation of eyelid
Hyperpigmentation of eyelid
- H02.711 Chloasma of right upper eyelid and periocular area
- H02.712 Chloasma of right lower eyelid and periocular area
- H02.713 Chloasma of right eye, unspecified eyelid and periocular area
- H02.714 Chloasma of left upper eyelid and periocular area
- H02.715 Chloasma of left lower eyelid and periocular area
- H02.716 Chloasma of left eye, unspecified eyelid and periocular area
- H02.719 Chloasma of unspecified eye, unspecified eyelid and periocular area

H02.72 Madarosis of eyelid and periocular area
Hypotrichosis of eyelid
- H02.721 Madarosis of right upper eyelid and periocular area
- H02.722 Madarosis of right lower eyelid and periocular area
- H02.723 Madarosis of right eye, unspecified eyelid and periocular area
- H02.724 Madarosis of left upper eyelid and periocular area
- H02.725 Madarosis of left lower eyelid and periocular area
- H02.726 Madarosis of left eye, unspecified eyelid and periocular area
- H02.729 Madarosis of unspecified eye, unspecified eyelid and periocular area

H02.73 Vitiligo of eyelid and periocular area
Hypopigmentation of eyelid
- H02.731 Vitiligo of right upper eyelid and periocular area
- H02.732 Vitiligo of right lower eyelid and periocular area
- H02.733 Vitiligo of right eye, unspecified eyelid and periocular area
- H02.734 Vitiligo of left upper eyelid and periocular area
- H02.735 Vitiligo of left lower eyelid and periocular area
- H02.736 Vitiligo of left eye, unspecified eyelid and periocular area
- H02.739 Vitiligo of unspecified eye, unspecified eyelid and periocular area

H02.79 Other degenerative disorders of eyelid and periocular area

H02.8 Other specified disorders of eyelid

H02.81 Retained foreign body in eyelid
Use additional code to identify the type of retained foreign body (Z18.-)
EXCLUDES 1: laceration of eyelid with foreign body (S01.12-)
retained intraocular foreign body (H44.6-, H44.7-)
superficial foreign body of eyelid and periocular area (S00.25-)
- H02.811 Retained foreign body in right upper eyelid
- H02.812 Retained foreign body in right lower eyelid
- H02.813 Retained foreign body in right eye, unspecified eyelid
- H02.814 Retained foreign body in left upper eyelid
- H02.815 Retained foreign body in left lower eyelid
- H02.816 Retained foreign body in left eye, unspecified eyelid
- H02.819 Retained foreign body in unspecified eye, unspecified eyelid

H02.82 Cysts of eyelid
Sebaceous cyst of eyelid
- H02.821 Cysts of right upper eyelid
- H02.822 Cysts of right lower eyelid
- H02.823 Cysts of right eye, unspecified eyelid
- H02.824 Cysts of left upper eyelid
- H02.825 Cysts of left lower eyelid
- H02.826 Cysts of left eye, unspecified eyelid
- H02.829 Cysts of unspecified eye, unspecified eyelid

Chapter 7. Diseases of the Eye and Adnexa

H02.83 Dermatochalasis of eyelid
DEF: Acquired form of connective tissue disorder associated with decreased elastic tissue and abnormal elastin formation, resulting in loss of elasticity of the skin of the eyelid. It is generally associated with aging.
- H02.831 Dermatochalasis of right upper eyelid
- H02.832 Dermatochalasis of right lower eyelid
- H02.833 Dermatochalasis of right eye, unspecified eyelid
- H02.834 Dermatochalasis of left upper eyelid
- H02.835 Dermatochalasis of left lower eyelid
- H02.836 Dermatochalasis of left eye, unspecified eyelid
- H02.839 Dermatochalasis of unspecified eye, unspecified eyelid

H02.84 Edema of eyelid
Hyperemia of eyelid
- H02.841 Edema of right upper eyelid
- H02.842 Edema of right lower eyelid
- H02.843 Edema of right eye, unspecified eyelid
- H02.844 Edema of left upper eyelid
- H02.845 Edema of left lower eyelid
- H02.846 Edema of left eye, unspecified eyelid
- H02.849 Edema of unspecified eye, unspecified eyelid

H02.85 Elephantiasis of eyelid
- H02.851 Elephantiasis of right upper eyelid
- H02.852 Elephantiasis of right lower eyelid
- H02.853 Elephantiasis of right eye, unspecified eyelid
- H02.854 Elephantiasis of left upper eyelid
- H02.855 Elephantiasis of left lower eyelid
- H02.856 Elephantiasis of left eye, unspecified eyelid
- H02.859 Elephantiasis of unspecified eye, unspecified eyelid

H02.86 Hypertrichosis of eyelid
- H02.861 Hypertrichosis of right upper eyelid
- H02.862 Hypertrichosis of right lower eyelid
- H02.863 Hypertrichosis of right eye, unspecified eyelid
- H02.864 Hypertrichosis of left upper eyelid
- H02.865 Hypertrichosis of left lower eyelid
- H02.866 Hypertrichosis of left eye, unspecified eyelid
- H02.869 Hypertrichosis of unspecified eye, unspecified eyelid

H02.87 Vascular anomalies of eyelid
- H02.871 Vascular anomalies of right upper eyelid
- H02.872 Vascular anomalies of right lower eyelid
- H02.873 Vascular anomalies of right eye, unspecified eyelid
- H02.874 Vascular anomalies of left upper eyelid
- H02.875 Vascular anomalies of left lower eyelid
- H02.876 Vascular anomalies of left eye, unspecified eyelid
- H02.879 Vascular anomalies of unspecified eye, unspecified eyelid

H02.88 Meibomian gland dysfunction of eyelid
AHA: 2018,4Q,14-15
- H02.881 Meibomian gland dysfunction right upper eyelid
- H02.882 Meibomian gland dysfunction right lower eyelid
- H02.883 Meibomian gland dysfunction of right eye, unspecified eyelid
- H02.884 Meibomian gland dysfunction left upper eyelid
- H02.885 Meibomian gland dysfunction left lower eyelid
- H02.886 Meibomian gland dysfunction of left eye, unspecified eyelid
- H02.889 Meibomian gland dysfunction of unspecified eye, unspecified eyelid
- H02.88A Meibomian gland dysfunction right eye, upper and lower eyelids
- H02.88B Meibomian gland dysfunction left eye, upper and lower eyelids

H02.89 Other specified disorders of eyelid
Hemorrhage of eyelid

H02.9 Unspecified disorder of eyelid
Disorder of eyelid NOS

H04 Disorders of lacrimal system
EXCLUDES 1 congenital malformations of lacrimal system (Q10.4-Q10.6)

H04.0 Dacryoadenitis
DEF: Inflammation of the lacrimal gland.

H04.00 Unspecified dacryoadenitis
- H04.001 Unspecified dacryoadenitis, right lacrimal gland
- H04.002 Unspecified dacryoadenitis, left lacrimal gland
- H04.003 Unspecified dacryoadenitis, bilateral lacrimal glands
- H04.009 Unspecified dacryoadenitis, unspecified lacrimal gland

H04.01 Acute dacryoadenitis
- H04.011 Acute dacryoadenitis, right lacrimal gland
- H04.012 Acute dacryoadenitis, left lacrimal gland
- H04.013 Acute dacryoadenitis, bilateral lacrimal glands
- H04.019 Acute dacryoadenitis, unspecified lacrimal gland

H04.02 Chronic dacryoadenitis
- H04.021 Chronic dacryoadenitis, right lacrimal gland
- H04.022 Chronic dacryoadenitis, left lacrimal gland
- H04.023 Chronic dacryoadenitis, bilateral lacrimal glands
- H04.029 Chronic dacryoadenitis, unspecified lacrimal gland

H04.03 Chronic enlargement of lacrimal gland
- H04.031 Chronic enlargement of right lacrimal gland
- H04.032 Chronic enlargement of left lacrimal gland
- H04.033 Chronic enlargement of bilateral lacrimal glands
- H04.039 Chronic enlargement of unspecified lacrimal gland

H04.1 Other disorders of lacrimal gland

H04.11 Dacryops
- H04.111 Dacryops of right lacrimal gland
- H04.112 Dacryops of left lacrimal gland
- H04.113 Dacryops of bilateral lacrimal glands
- H04.119 Dacryops of unspecified lacrimal gland

H04.12 Dry eye syndrome
Tear film insufficiency, NOS
- H04.121 Dry eye syndrome of right lacrimal gland
- H04.122 Dry eye syndrome of left lacrimal gland
- H04.123 Dry eye syndrome of bilateral lacrimal glands
- H04.129 Dry eye syndrome of unspecified lacrimal gland

H04.13 Lacrimal cyst
Lacrimal cystic degeneration
- H04.131 Lacrimal cyst, right lacrimal gland
- H04.132 Lacrimal cyst, left lacrimal gland
- H04.133 Lacrimal cyst, bilateral lacrimal glands
- H04.139 Lacrimal cyst, unspecified lacrimal gland

H04.14 Primary lacrimal gland atrophy
- H04.141 Primary lacrimal gland atrophy, right lacrimal gland
- H04.142 Primary lacrimal gland atrophy, left lacrimal gland
- H04.143 Primary lacrimal gland atrophy, bilateral lacrimal glands
- H04.149 Primary lacrimal gland atrophy, unspecified lacrimal gland

H04.15 Secondary lacrimal gland atrophy
- H04.151 Secondary lacrimal gland atrophy, right lacrimal gland
- H04.152 Secondary lacrimal gland atrophy, left lacrimal gland
- H04.153 Secondary lacrimal gland atrophy, bilateral lacrimal glands
- H04.159 Secondary lacrimal gland atrophy, unspecified lacrimal gland

H04.16 Lacrimal gland dislocation
- H04.161 Lacrimal gland dislocation, right lacrimal gland

- H04.162 Lacrimal gland dislocation, left lacrimal gland
- H04.163 Lacrimal gland dislocation, bilateral lacrimal glands
- H04.169 Lacrimal gland dislocation, unspecified lacrimal gland
- H04.19 Other specified disorders of lacrimal gland

√5th **H04.2 Epiphora**

DEF: Excessive tearing or overflow of tears down the cheeks often due to a stricture in the lacrimal passages but can be caused by other conditions.

√6th **H04.20 Unspecified epiphora**
- H04.201 Unspecified epiphora, right side
- H04.202 Unspecified epiphora, left side
- H04.203 Unspecified epiphora, bilateral
- H04.209 Unspecified epiphora, unspecified side

√6th **H04.21 Epiphora due to excess lacrimation**
- H04.211 Epiphora due to excess lacrimation, right lacrimal gland
- H04.212 Epiphora due to excess lacrimation, left lacrimal gland
- H04.213 Epiphora due to excess lacrimation, bilateral lacrimal glands
- H04.219 Epiphora due to excess lacrimation, unspecified lacrimal gland

√6th **H04.22 Epiphora due to insufficient drainage**
- H04.221 Epiphora due to insufficient drainage, right side
- H04.222 Epiphora due to insufficient drainage, left side
- H04.223 Epiphora due to insufficient drainage, bilateral
- H04.229 Epiphora due to insufficient drainage, unspecified side

√5th **H04.3 Acute and unspecified inflammation of lacrimal passages**

EXCLUDES 1 neonatal dacryocystitis (P39.1)

√6th **H04.30 Unspecified dacryocystitis**
- H04.301 Unspecified dacryocystitis of right lacrimal passage
- H04.302 Unspecified dacryocystitis of left lacrimal passage
- H04.303 Unspecified dacryocystitis of bilateral lacrimal passages
- H04.309 Unspecified dacryocystitis of unspecified lacrimal passage

√6th **H04.31 Phlegmonous dacryocystitis**
- H04.311 Phlegmonous dacryocystitis of right lacrimal passage
- H04.312 Phlegmonous dacryocystitis of left lacrimal passage
- H04.313 Phlegmonous dacryocystitis of bilateral lacrimal passages
- H04.319 Phlegmonous dacryocystitis of unspecified lacrimal passage

√6th **H04.32 Acute dacryocystitis**

Acute dacryopericystitis
- H04.321 Acute dacryocystitis of right lacrimal passage
- H04.322 Acute dacryocystitis of left lacrimal passage
- H04.323 Acute dacryocystitis of bilateral lacrimal passages
- H04.329 Acute dacryocystitis of unspecified lacrimal passage

√6th **H04.33 Acute lacrimal canaliculitis**
- H04.331 Acute lacrimal canaliculitis of right lacrimal passage
- H04.332 Acute lacrimal canaliculitis of left lacrimal passage
- H04.333 Acute lacrimal canaliculitis of bilateral lacrimal passages
- H04.339 Acute lacrimal canaliculitis of unspecified lacrimal passage

√5th **H04.4 Chronic inflammation of lacrimal passages**

√6th **H04.41 Chronic dacryocystitis**
- H04.411 Chronic dacryocystitis of right lacrimal passage
- H04.412 Chronic dacryocystitis of left lacrimal passage
- H04.413 Chronic dacryocystitis of bilateral lacrimal passages
- H04.419 Chronic dacryocystitis of unspecified lacrimal passage

√6th **H04.42 Chronic lacrimal canaliculitis**
- H04.421 Chronic lacrimal canaliculitis of right lacrimal passage
- H04.422 Chronic lacrimal canaliculitis of left lacrimal passage
- H04.423 Chronic lacrimal canaliculitis of bilateral lacrimal passages
- H04.429 Chronic lacrimal canaliculitis of unspecified lacrimal passage

√6th **H04.43 Chronic lacrimal mucocele**
- H04.431 Chronic lacrimal mucocele of right lacrimal passage
- H04.432 Chronic lacrimal mucocele of left lacrimal passage
- H04.433 Chronic lacrimal mucocele of bilateral lacrimal passages
- H04.439 Chronic lacrimal mucocele of unspecified lacrimal passage

√5th **H04.5 Stenosis and insufficiency of lacrimal passages**

√6th **H04.51 Dacryolith**
- H04.511 Dacryolith of right lacrimal passage
- H04.512 Dacryolith of left lacrimal passage
- H04.513 Dacryolith of bilateral lacrimal passages
- H04.519 Dacryolith of unspecified lacrimal passage

√6th **H04.52 Eversion of lacrimal punctum**
- H04.521 Eversion of right lacrimal punctum
- H04.522 Eversion of left lacrimal punctum
- H04.523 Eversion of bilateral lacrimal punctum
- H04.529 Eversion of unspecified lacrimal punctum

√6th **H04.53 Neonatal obstruction of nasolacrimal duct**

EXCLUDES 1 congenital stenosis and stricture of lacrimal duct (Q10.5)
- H04.531 Neonatal obstruction of right nasolacrimal duct N
- H04.532 Neonatal obstruction of left nasolacrimal duct N
- H04.533 Neonatal obstruction of bilateral nasolacrimal duct N
- H04.539 Neonatal obstruction of unspecified nasolacrimal duct N

√6th **H04.54 Stenosis of lacrimal canaliculi**
- H04.541 Stenosis of right lacrimal canaliculi
- H04.542 Stenosis of left lacrimal canaliculi
- H04.543 Stenosis of bilateral lacrimal canaliculi
- H04.549 Stenosis of unspecified lacrimal canaliculi

√6th **H04.55 Acquired stenosis of nasolacrimal duct**
- H04.551 Acquired stenosis of right nasolacrimal duct
- H04.552 Acquired stenosis of left nasolacrimal duct
- H04.553 Acquired stenosis of bilateral nasolacrimal duct
- H04.559 Acquired stenosis of unspecified nasolacrimal duct

√6th **H04.56 Stenosis of lacrimal punctum**
- H04.561 Stenosis of right lacrimal punctum
- H04.562 Stenosis of left lacrimal punctum
- H04.563 Stenosis of bilateral lacrimal punctum
- H04.569 Stenosis of unspecified lacrimal punctum

√6th **H04.57 Stenosis of lacrimal sac**
- H04.571 Stenosis of right lacrimal sac
- H04.572 Stenosis of left lacrimal sac
- H04.573 Stenosis of bilateral lacrimal sac
- H04.579 Stenosis of unspecified lacrimal sac

√5th **H04.6 Other changes of lacrimal passages**

√6th **H04.61 Lacrimal fistula**
- H04.611 Lacrimal fistula right lacrimal passage
- H04.612 Lacrimal fistula left lacrimal passage
- H04.613 Lacrimal fistula bilateral lacrimal passages
- H04.619 Lacrimal fistula unspecified lacrimal passage

- H04.69 Other changes of lacrimal passages

Chapter 7. Diseases of the Eye and Adnexa

- ✓5th **H04.8** Other disorders of lacrimal system
  - ✓6th **H04.81** Granuloma of lacrimal passages
    - **H04.811** Granuloma of right lacrimal passage
    - **H04.812** Granuloma of left lacrimal passage
    - **H04.813** Granuloma of bilateral lacrimal passages
    - **H04.819** Granuloma of unspecified lacrimal passage
  - **H04.89** Other disorders of lacrimal system
- **H04.9** Disorder of lacrimal system, unspecified

- ✓4th **H05** Disorders of orbit
  - EXCLUDES 1 congenital malformation of orbit (Q10.7)
  - ✓5th **H05.0** Acute inflammation of orbit
    - **H05.00** Unspecified acute inflammation of orbit
    - ✓6th **H05.01** Cellulitis of orbit
      - Abscess of orbit
      - **H05.011** Cellulitis of right orbit
      - **H05.012** Cellulitis of left orbit
      - **H05.013** Cellulitis of bilateral orbits
      - **H05.019** Cellulitis of unspecified orbit
    - ✓6th **H05.02** Osteomyelitis of orbit
      - **H05.021** Osteomyelitis of right orbit
      - **H05.022** Osteomyelitis of left orbit
      - **H05.023** Osteomyelitis of bilateral orbits
      - **H05.029** Osteomyelitis of unspecified orbit
    - ✓6th **H05.03** Periostitis of orbit
      - **H05.031** Periostitis of right orbit
      - **H05.032** Periostitis of left orbit
      - **H05.033** Periostitis of bilateral orbits
      - **H05.039** Periostitis of unspecified orbit
    - ✓6th **H05.04** Tenonitis of orbit
      - **H05.041** Tenonitis of right orbit
      - **H05.042** Tenonitis of left orbit
      - **H05.043** Tenonitis of bilateral orbits
      - **H05.049** Tenonitis of unspecified orbit
  - ✓5th **H05.1** Chronic inflammatory disorders of orbit
    - **H05.10** Unspecified chronic inflammatory disorders of orbit
    - ✓6th **H05.11** Granuloma of orbit
      - Pseudotumor (inflammatory) of orbit
      - **H05.111** Granuloma of right orbit
      - **H05.112** Granuloma of left orbit
      - **H05.113** Granuloma of bilateral orbits
      - **H05.119** Granuloma of unspecified orbit
    - ✓6th **H05.12** Orbital myositis
      - **H05.121** Orbital myositis, right orbit
      - **H05.122** Orbital myositis, left orbit
      - **H05.123** Orbital myositis, bilateral
      - **H05.129** Orbital myositis, unspecified orbit
  - ✓5th **H05.2** Exophthalmic conditions
    - **H05.20** Unspecified exophthalmos
    - ✓6th **H05.21** Displacement (lateral) of globe
      - **H05.211** Displacement (lateral) of globe, right eye
      - **H05.212** Displacement (lateral) of globe, left eye
      - **H05.213** Displacement (lateral) of globe, bilateral
      - **H05.219** Displacement (lateral) of globe, unspecified eye
    - ✓6th **H05.22** Edema of orbit
      - Orbital congestion
      - **H05.221** Edema of right orbit
      - **H05.222** Edema of left orbit
      - **H05.223** Edema of bilateral orbit
      - **H05.229** Edema of unspecified orbit
    - ✓6th **H05.23** Hemorrhage of orbit
      - **H05.231** Hemorrhage of right orbit
      - **H05.232** Hemorrhage of left orbit
      - **H05.233** Hemorrhage of bilateral orbit
      - **H05.239** Hemorrhage of unspecified orbit
    - ✓6th **H05.24** Constant exophthalmos
      - **H05.241** Constant exophthalmos, right eye
      - **H05.242** Constant exophthalmos, left eye
      - **H05.243** Constant exophthalmos, bilateral
      - **H05.249** Constant exophthalmos, unspecified eye
    - ✓6th **H05.25** Intermittent exophthalmos
      - **H05.251** Intermittent exophthalmos, right eye
      - **H05.252** Intermittent exophthalmos, left eye
      - **H05.253** Intermittent exophthalmos, bilateral
      - **H05.259** Intermittent exophthalmos, unspecified eye
    - ✓6th **H05.26** Pulsating exophthalmos
      - **H05.261** Pulsating exophthalmos, right eye
      - **H05.262** Pulsating exophthalmos, left eye
      - **H05.263** Pulsating exophthalmos, bilateral
      - **H05.269** Pulsating exophthalmos, unspecified eye
  - ✓5th **H05.3** Deformity of orbit
    - EXCLUDES 1 congenital deformity of orbit (Q10.7)
      hypertelorism (Q75.2)
    - **H05.30** Unspecified deformity of orbit
    - ✓6th **H05.31** Atrophy of orbit
      - **H05.311** Atrophy of right orbit
      - **H05.312** Atrophy of left orbit
      - **H05.313** Atrophy of bilateral orbit
      - **H05.319** Atrophy of unspecified orbit
    - ✓6th **H05.32** Deformity of orbit due to bone disease
      - Code also associated bone disease
      - **H05.321** Deformity of right orbit due to bone disease
      - **H05.322** Deformity of left orbit due to bone disease
      - **H05.323** Deformity of bilateral orbits due to bone disease
      - **H05.329** Deformity of unspecified orbit due to bone disease
    - ✓6th **H05.33** Deformity of orbit due to trauma or surgery
      - **H05.331** Deformity of right orbit due to trauma or surgery
      - **H05.332** Deformity of left orbit due to trauma or surgery
      - **H05.333** Deformity of bilateral orbits due to trauma or surgery
      - **H05.339** Deformity of unspecified orbit due to trauma or surgery
    - ✓6th **H05.34** Enlargement of orbit
      - **H05.341** Enlargement of right orbit
      - **H05.342** Enlargement of left orbit
      - **H05.343** Enlargement of bilateral orbits
      - **H05.349** Enlargement of unspecified orbit
    - ✓6th **H05.35** Exostosis of orbit
      - **H05.351** Exostosis of right orbit
      - **H05.352** Exostosis of left orbit
      - **H05.353** Exostosis of bilateral orbits
      - **H05.359** Exostosis of unspecified orbit
  - ✓5th **H05.4** Enophthalmos
    - ✓6th **H05.40** Unspecified enophthalmos
      - **H05.401** Unspecified enophthalmos, right eye
      - **H05.402** Unspecified enophthalmos, left eye
      - **H05.403** Unspecified enophthalmos, bilateral
      - **H05.409** Unspecified enophthalmos, unspecified eye
    - ✓6th **H05.41** Enophthalmos due to atrophy of orbital tissue
      - **H05.411** Enophthalmos due to atrophy of orbital tissue, right eye
      - **H05.412** Enophthalmos due to atrophy of orbital tissue, left eye
      - **H05.413** Enophthalmos due to atrophy of orbital tissue, bilateral
      - **H05.419** Enophthalmos due to atrophy of orbital tissue, unspecified eye
    - ✓6th **H05.42** Enophthalmos due to trauma or surgery
      - **H05.421** Enophthalmos due to trauma or surgery, right eye
      - **H05.422** Enophthalmos due to trauma or surgery, left eye
      - **H05.423** Enophthalmos due to trauma or surgery, bilateral
      - **H05.429** Enophthalmos due to trauma or surgery, unspecified eye
  - ✓5th **H05.5** Retained (old) foreign body following penetrating wound of orbit
    - Retrobulbar foreign body
    - Use additional code to identify the type of retained foreign body (Z18.-)
    - EXCLUDES 1 current penetrating wound of orbit (S05.4-)
    - EXCLUDES 2 retained foreign body of eyelid (H02.81-)
      retained intraocular foreign body (H44.6-, H44.7-)
    - **H05.50** Retained (old) foreign body following penetrating wound of unspecified orbit

H05.51 Retained (old) foreign body following penetrating wound of **right** orbit
H05.52 Retained (old) foreign body following penetrating wound of **left** orbit
H05.53 Retained (old) foreign body following penetrating wound of **bilateral** orbits

√5th **H05.8** Other disorders of orbit
  √6th **H05.81** Cyst of orbit
    Encephalocele of orbit
    H05.811 Cyst of **right** orbit
    H05.812 Cyst of **left** orbit
    H05.813 Cyst of **bilateral** orbits
    H05.819 Cyst of unspecified orbit
  √6th **H05.82** Myopathy of extraocular muscles
    H05.821 Myopathy of extraocular muscles, **right** orbit
    H05.822 Myopathy of extraocular muscles, **left** orbit
    H05.823 Myopathy of extraocular muscles, **bilateral**
    H05.829 Myopathy of extraocular muscles, unspecified orbit
  • √6th **H05.83** **Thyroid orbitopathy**
    Graves' ophthalmopathy
    Graves' orbitopathy
    Thyroid eye disease
    Code also, if applicable, any associated conditions such as:
      autoimmune thyroiditis (E06.3)
      thyrotoxicosis with diffuse goiter (E05.0-)
  • **H05.831** Thyroid orbitopathy, **right** orbit
  • **H05.832** Thyroid orbitopathy, **left** orbit
  • **H05.833** Thyroid orbitopathy, **bilateral**
  • **H05.839** Thyroid orbitopathy, unspecified orbit
  H05.89 Other disorders of orbit
H05.9 Unspecified disorder of orbit

Disorders of conjunctiva (H10-H11)

√4th **H10** Conjunctivitis
  EXCLUDES 1 keratoconjunctivitis (H16.2-)
  √5th **H10.0** **Mucopurulent** conjunctivitis
    √6th **H10.01** Acute follicular conjunctivitis
      H10.011 Acute follicular conjunctivitis, **right** eye
      H10.012 Acute follicular conjunctivitis, **left** eye
      H10.013 Acute follicular conjunctivitis, **bilateral**
      H10.019 Acute follicular conjunctivitis, unspecified eye
    √6th **H10.02** Other mucopurulent conjunctivitis
      H10.021 Other mucopurulent conjunctivitis, **right** eye
      H10.022 Other mucopurulent conjunctivitis, **left** eye
      H10.023 Other mucopurulent conjunctivitis, **bilateral**
      H10.029 Other mucopurulent conjunctivitis, unspecified eye
  √5th **H10.1** **Acute atopic** conjunctivitis
    Acute papillary conjunctivitis
    H10.10 Acute atopic conjunctivitis, unspecified eye
    H10.11 Acute atopic conjunctivitis, **right** eye
    H10.12 Acute atopic conjunctivitis, **left** eye
    H10.13 Acute atopic conjunctivitis, **bilateral**
  √5th **H10.2** Other **acute** conjunctivitis
    √6th **H10.21** Acute **toxic** conjunctivitis
      Acute chemical conjunctivitis
      Code first (T51-T65) to identify chemical and intent
      EXCLUDES 1 burn and corrosion of eye and adnexa (T26.-)
      H10.211 Acute toxic conjunctivitis, **right** eye
      H10.212 Acute toxic conjunctivitis, **left** eye
      H10.213 Acute toxic conjunctivitis, **bilateral**
      H10.219 Acute toxic conjunctivitis, unspecified eye
    √6th **H10.22** **Pseudomembranous** conjunctivitis
      H10.221 Pseudomembranous conjunctivitis, **right** eye
      H10.222 Pseudomembranous conjunctivitis, **left** eye
      H10.223 Pseudomembranous conjunctivitis, **bilateral**
      H10.229 Pseudomembranous conjunctivitis, unspecified eye
    √6th **H10.23** **Serous** conjunctivitis, except viral
      EXCLUDES 1 viral conjunctivitis (B30.-)
      H10.231 Serous conjunctivitis, except viral, **right** eye
      H10.232 Serous conjunctivitis, except viral, **left** eye
      H10.233 Serous conjunctivitis, except viral, **bilateral**
      H10.239 Serous conjunctivitis, except viral, unspecified eye
  √5th **H10.3** Unspecified **acute** conjunctivitis
    EXCLUDES 1 ophthalmia neonatorum NOS (P39.1)
    H10.30 Unspecified acute conjunctivitis, unspecified eye
    H10.31 Unspecified acute conjunctivitis, **right** eye
    H10.32 Unspecified acute conjunctivitis, **left** eye
    H10.33 Unspecified acute conjunctivitis, **bilateral**
  √5th **H10.4** **Chronic** conjunctivitis
    √6th **H10.40** Unspecified chronic conjunctivitis
      H10.401 Unspecified chronic conjunctivitis, **right** eye
      H10.402 Unspecified chronic conjunctivitis, **left** eye
      H10.403 Unspecified chronic conjunctivitis, **bilateral**
      H10.409 Unspecified chronic conjunctivitis, unspecified eye
    √6th **H10.41** Chronic **giant papillary** conjunctivitis
      H10.411 Chronic giant papillary conjunctivitis, **right** eye
      H10.412 Chronic giant papillary conjunctivitis, **left** eye
      H10.413 Chronic giant papillary conjunctivitis, **bilateral**
      H10.419 Chronic giant papillary conjunctivitis, unspecified eye
    √6th **H10.42** **Simple** chronic conjunctivitis
      H10.421 Simple chronic conjunctivitis, **right** eye
      H10.422 Simple chronic conjunctivitis, **left** eye
      H10.423 Simple chronic conjunctivitis, **bilateral**
      H10.429 Simple chronic conjunctivitis, unspecified eye
    √6th **H10.43** Chronic **follicular** conjunctivitis
      H10.431 Chronic follicular conjunctivitis, **right** eye
      H10.432 Chronic follicular conjunctivitis, **left** eye
      H10.433 Chronic follicular conjunctivitis, **bilateral**
      H10.439 Chronic follicular conjunctivitis, unspecified eye
    H10.44 **Vernal** conjunctivitis
      EXCLUDES 1 vernal keratoconjunctivitis with limbar and corneal involvement (H16.26-)
    H10.45 Other chronic **allergic** conjunctivitis
  √5th **H10.5** Blepharoconjunctivitis
    √6th **H10.50** Unspecified blepharoconjunctivitis
      H10.501 Unspecified blepharoconjunctivitis, **right** eye
      H10.502 Unspecified blepharoconjunctivitis, **left** eye
      H10.503 Unspecified blepharoconjunctivitis, **bilateral**
      H10.509 Unspecified blepharoconjunctivitis, unspecified eye
    √6th **H10.51** **Ligneous** conjunctivitis
      Code also underlying condition if known, such as: plasminogen deficiency (E88.02)
      H10.511 Ligneous conjunctivitis, **right** eye
      H10.512 Ligneous conjunctivitis, **left** eye
      H10.513 Ligneous conjunctivitis, **bilateral**
      H10.519 Ligneous conjunctivitis, unspecified eye
    √6th **H10.52** **Angular** blepharoconjunctivitis
      H10.521 Angular blepharoconjunctivitis, **right** eye
      H10.522 Angular blepharoconjunctivitis, **left** eye
      H10.523 Angular blepharoconjunctivitis, **bilateral**
      H10.529 Angular blepharoconjunctivitis, unspecified eye
    √6th **H10.53** **Contact** blepharoconjunctivitis
      H10.531 Contact blepharoconjunctivitis, **right** eye
      H10.532 Contact blepharoconjunctivitis, **left** eye
      H10.533 Contact blepharoconjunctivitis, **bilateral**
      H10.539 Contact blepharoconjunctivitis, unspecified eye

Chapter 7. Diseases of the Eye and Adnexa

✓5th **H10.8** Other conjunctivitis
  ✓6th **H10.81** Pingueculitis
      EXCLUDES 1 pinguecula (H11.15-)
      H10.811 Pingueculitis, right eye
      H10.812 Pingueculitis, left eye
      H10.813 Pingueculitis, bilateral
      H10.819 Pingueculitis, unspecified eye
  ✓6th **H10.82** Rosacea conjunctivitis
      Code first underlying rosacea dermatitis (L71.-)
      AHA: 2018,4Q,15
      H10.821 Rosacea conjunctivitis, right eye
      H10.822 Rosacea conjunctivitis, left eye
      H10.823 Rosacea conjunctivitis, bilateral
      H10.829 Rosacea conjunctivitis, unspecified eye
  H10.89 Other conjunctivitis
H10.9 Unspecified conjunctivitis

✓4th **H11** Other disorders of conjunctiva
  EXCLUDES 1 keratoconjunctivitis (H16.2-)
  ✓5th **H11.0** Pterygium of eye
      EXCLUDES 1 pseudopterygium (H11.81-)
      DEF: Benign, wedge-shaped, conjunctival thickening that advances from the inner corner of the eye toward the cornea.

Pterygium

  ✓6th **H11.00** Unspecified pterygium of eye
      H11.001 Unspecified pterygium of right eye
      H11.002 Unspecified pterygium of left eye
      H11.003 Unspecified pterygium of eye, bilateral
      H11.009 Unspecified pterygium of unspecified eye
  ✓6th **H11.01** Amyloid pterygium
      H11.011 Amyloid pterygium of right eye
      H11.012 Amyloid pterygium of left eye
      H11.013 Amyloid pterygium of eye, bilateral
      H11.019 Amyloid pterygium of unspecified eye
  ✓6th **H11.02** Central pterygium of eye
      H11.021 Central pterygium of right eye
      H11.022 Central pterygium of left eye
      H11.023 Central pterygium of eye, bilateral
      H11.029 Central pterygium of unspecified eye
  ✓6th **H11.03** Double pterygium of eye
      H11.031 Double pterygium of right eye
      H11.032 Double pterygium of left eye
      H11.033 Double pterygium of eye, bilateral
      H11.039 Double pterygium of unspecified eye
  ✓6th **H11.04** Peripheral pterygium of eye, stationary
      H11.041 Peripheral pterygium, stationary, right eye
      H11.042 Peripheral pterygium, stationary, left eye
      H11.043 Peripheral pterygium, stationary, bilateral
      H11.049 Peripheral pterygium, stationary, unspecified eye
  ✓6th **H11.05** Peripheral pterygium of eye, progressive
      H11.051 Peripheral pterygium, progressive, right eye
      H11.052 Peripheral pterygium, progressive, left eye
      H11.053 Peripheral pterygium, progressive, bilateral
      H11.059 Peripheral pterygium, progressive, unspecified eye
  ✓6th **H11.06** Recurrent pterygium of eye
      H11.061 Recurrent pterygium of right eye
      H11.062 Recurrent pterygium of left eye
      H11.063 Recurrent pterygium of eye, bilateral
      H11.069 Recurrent pterygium of unspecified eye

✓5th **H11.1** Conjunctival degenerations and deposits
    EXCLUDES 2 pseudopterygium (H11.81)
    H11.10 Unspecified conjunctival degenerations
  ✓6th **H11.11** Conjunctival deposits
      H11.111 Conjunctival deposits, right eye
      H11.112 Conjunctival deposits, left eye
      H11.113 Conjunctival deposits, bilateral
      H11.119 Conjunctival deposits, unspecified eye
  ✓6th **H11.12** Conjunctival concretions
      H11.121 Conjunctival concretions, right eye
      H11.122 Conjunctival concretions, left eye
      H11.123 Conjunctival concretions, bilateral
      H11.129 Conjunctival concretions, unspecified eye
  ✓6th **H11.13** Conjunctival pigmentations
      Conjunctival argyrosis [argyria]
      H11.131 Conjunctival pigmentations, right eye
      H11.132 Conjunctival pigmentations, left eye
      H11.133 Conjunctival pigmentations, bilateral
      H11.139 Conjunctival pigmentations, unspecified eye
  ✓6th **H11.14** Conjunctival xerosis, unspecified
      EXCLUDES 1 xerosis of conjunctiva due to vitamin A deficiency (E50.0, E50.1)
      DEF: Abnormal dryness of the conjunctiva due to lack of sufficient tears or conjunctival secretions.
      H11.141 Conjunctival xerosis, unspecified, right eye
      H11.142 Conjunctival xerosis, unspecified, left eye
      H11.143 Conjunctival xerosis, unspecified, bilateral
      H11.149 Conjunctival xerosis, unspecified, unspecified eye
  ✓6th **H11.15** Pinguecula
      EXCLUDES 1 pingueculitis (H10.81-)
      DEF: Proliferation on the conjunctiva near the sclerocorneal junction, usually of the side of the nose and usually in older patients.

Pinguecula

      H11.151 Pinguecula, right eye
      H11.152 Pinguecula, left eye
      H11.153 Pinguecula, bilateral
      H11.159 Pinguecula, unspecified eye

✓5th **H11.2** Conjunctival scars
  ✓6th **H11.21** Conjunctival adhesions and strands (localized)
      H11.211 Conjunctival adhesions and strands (localized), right eye
      H11.212 Conjunctival adhesions and strands (localized), left eye
      H11.213 Conjunctival adhesions and strands (localized), bilateral
      H11.219 Conjunctival adhesions and strands (localized), unspecified eye
  ✓6th **H11.22** Conjunctival granuloma
      H11.221 Conjunctival granuloma, right eye
      H11.222 Conjunctival granuloma, left eye
      H11.223 Conjunctival granuloma, bilateral
      H11.229 Conjunctival granuloma, unspecified
  ✓6th **H11.23** Symblepharon
      H11.231 Symblepharon, right eye
      H11.232 Symblepharon, left eye
      H11.233 Symblepharon, bilateral
      H11.239 Symblepharon, unspecified eye
  ✓6th **H11.24** Scarring of conjunctiva
      H11.241 Scarring of conjunctiva, right eye
      H11.242 Scarring of conjunctiva, left eye
      H11.243 Scarring of conjunctiva, bilateral
      H11.249 Scarring of conjunctiva, unspecified eye

H11.3 Conjunctival hemorrhage
Subconjunctival hemorrhage
- H11.30 Conjunctival hemorrhage, unspecified eye
- H11.31 Conjunctival hemorrhage, right eye
- H11.32 Conjunctival hemorrhage, left eye
- H11.33 Conjunctival hemorrhage, bilateral

H11.4 Other conjunctival vascular disorders and cysts

H11.41 Vascular abnormalities of conjunctiva
Conjunctival aneurysm
- H11.411 Vascular abnormalities of conjunctiva, right eye
- H11.412 Vascular abnormalities of conjunctiva, left eye
- H11.413 Vascular abnormalities of conjunctiva, bilateral
- H11.419 Vascular abnormalities of conjunctiva, unspecified eye

H11.42 Conjunctival edema
- H11.421 Conjunctival edema, right eye
- H11.422 Conjunctival edema, left eye
- H11.423 Conjunctival edema, bilateral
- H11.429 Conjunctival edema, unspecified eye

H11.43 Conjunctival hyperemia
- H11.431 Conjunctival hyperemia, right eye
- H11.432 Conjunctival hyperemia, left eye
- H11.433 Conjunctival hyperemia, bilateral
- H11.439 Conjunctival hyperemia, unspecified eye

H11.44 Conjunctival cysts
- H11.441 Conjunctival cysts, right eye
- H11.442 Conjunctival cysts, left eye
- H11.443 Conjunctival cysts, bilateral
- H11.449 Conjunctival cysts, unspecified eye

H11.8 Other specified disorders of conjunctiva

H11.81 Pseudopterygium of conjunctiva
- H11.811 Pseudopterygium of conjunctiva, right eye
- H11.812 Pseudopterygium of conjunctiva, left eye
- H11.813 Pseudopterygium of conjunctiva, bilateral
- H11.819 Pseudopterygium of conjunctiva, unspecified eye

H11.82 Conjunctivochalasis
- H11.821 Conjunctivochalasis, right eye
- H11.822 Conjunctivochalasis, left eye
- H11.823 Conjunctivochalasis, bilateral
- H11.829 Conjunctivochalasis, unspecified eye

- H11.89 Other specified disorders of conjunctiva

H11.9 Unspecified disorder of conjunctiva

Disorders of sclera, cornea, iris and ciliary body (H15-H22)

H15 Disorders of sclera

H15.0 Scleritis

H15.00 Unspecified scleritis
- H15.001 Unspecified scleritis, right eye
- H15.002 Unspecified scleritis, left eye
- H15.003 Unspecified scleritis, bilateral
- H15.009 Unspecified scleritis, unspecified eye

H15.01 Anterior scleritis
- H15.011 Anterior scleritis, right eye
- H15.012 Anterior scleritis, left eye
- H15.013 Anterior scleritis, bilateral
- H15.019 Anterior scleritis, unspecified eye

H15.02 Brawny scleritis
- H15.021 Brawny scleritis, right eye
- H15.022 Brawny scleritis, left eye
- H15.023 Brawny scleritis, bilateral
- H15.029 Brawny scleritis, unspecified eye

H15.03 Posterior scleritis
Sclerotenonitis
- H15.031 Posterior scleritis, right eye
- H15.032 Posterior scleritis, left eye
- H15.033 Posterior scleritis, bilateral
- H15.039 Posterior scleritis, unspecified eye

H15.04 Scleritis with corneal involvement
- H15.041 Scleritis with corneal involvement, right eye
- H15.042 Scleritis with corneal involvement, left eye
- H15.043 Scleritis with corneal involvement, bilateral
- H15.049 Scleritis with corneal involvement, unspecified eye

H15.05 Scleromalacia perforans
- H15.051 Scleromalacia perforans, right eye
- H15.052 Scleromalacia perforans, left eye
- H15.053 Scleromalacia perforans, bilateral
- H15.059 Scleromalacia perforans, unspecified eye

H15.09 Other scleritis
Scleral abscess
- H15.091 Other scleritis, right eye
- H15.092 Other scleritis, left eye
- H15.093 Other scleritis, bilateral
- H15.099 Other scleritis, unspecified eye

H15.1 Episcleritis

H15.10 Unspecified episcleritis
- H15.101 Unspecified episcleritis, right eye
- H15.102 Unspecified episcleritis, left eye
- H15.103 Unspecified episcleritis, bilateral
- H15.109 Unspecified episcleritis, unspecified eye

H15.11 Episcleritis periodica fugax
- H15.111 Episcleritis periodica fugax, right eye
- H15.112 Episcleritis periodica fugax, left eye
- H15.113 Episcleritis periodica fugax, bilateral
- H15.119 Episcleritis periodica fugax, unspecified eye

H15.12 Nodular episcleritis
- H15.121 Nodular episcleritis, right eye
- H15.122 Nodular episcleritis, left eye
- H15.123 Nodular episcleritis, bilateral
- H15.129 Nodular episcleritis, unspecified eye

H15.8 Other disorders of sclera
EXCLUDES 2: blue sclera (Q13.5)
degenerative myopia (H44.2-)

H15.81 Equatorial staphyloma
- H15.811 Equatorial staphyloma, right eye
- H15.812 Equatorial staphyloma, left eye
- H15.813 Equatorial staphyloma, bilateral
- H15.819 Equatorial staphyloma, unspecified eye

H15.82 Localized anterior staphyloma
- H15.821 Localized anterior staphyloma, right eye
- H15.822 Localized anterior staphyloma, left eye
- H15.823 Localized anterior staphyloma, bilateral
- H15.829 Localized anterior staphyloma, unspecified eye

H15.83 Staphyloma posticum
- H15.831 Staphyloma posticum, right eye
- H15.832 Staphyloma posticum, left eye
- H15.833 Staphyloma posticum, bilateral
- H15.839 Staphyloma posticum, unspecified eye

H15.84 Scleral ectasia
- H15.841 Scleral ectasia, right eye
- H15.842 Scleral ectasia, left eye
- H15.843 Scleral ectasia, bilateral
- H15.849 Scleral ectasia, unspecified eye

H15.85 Ring staphyloma
- H15.851 Ring staphyloma, right eye
- H15.852 Ring staphyloma, left eye
- H15.853 Ring staphyloma, bilateral
- H15.859 Ring staphyloma, unspecified eye

- H15.89 Other disorders of sclera

H15.9 Unspecified disorder of sclera

H16 Keratitis
DEF: Condition in which the cornea becomes inflamed and irritated.

H16.0 Corneal ulcer

H16.00 Unspecified corneal ulcer
- H16.001 Unspecified corneal ulcer, right eye
- H16.002 Unspecified corneal ulcer, left eye
- H16.003 Unspecified corneal ulcer, bilateral
- H16.009 Unspecified corneal ulcer, unspecified eye

H16.01 Central corneal ulcer
- H16.011 Central corneal ulcer, right eye
- H16.012 Central corneal ulcer, left eye
- H16.013 Central corneal ulcer, bilateral

Chapter 7. Diseases of the Eye and Adnexa

H16.019 Central corneal ulcer, unspecified eye

H16.02 Ring corneal ulcer
- H16.021 Ring corneal ulcer, right eye
- H16.022 Ring corneal ulcer, left eye
- H16.023 Ring corneal ulcer, bilateral
- H16.029 Ring corneal ulcer, unspecified eye

H16.03 Corneal ulcer with hypopyon
- H16.031 Corneal ulcer with hypopyon, right eye
- H16.032 Corneal ulcer with hypopyon, left eye
- H16.033 Corneal ulcer with hypopyon, bilateral
- H16.039 Corneal ulcer with hypopyon, unspecified eye

H16.04 Marginal corneal ulcer
- H16.041 Marginal corneal ulcer, right eye
- H16.042 Marginal corneal ulcer, left eye
- H16.043 Marginal corneal ulcer, bilateral
- H16.049 Marginal corneal ulcer, unspecified eye

H16.05 Mooren's corneal ulcer
- H16.051 Mooren's corneal ulcer, right eye
- H16.052 Mooren's corneal ulcer, left eye
- H16.053 Mooren's corneal ulcer, bilateral
- H16.059 Mooren's corneal ulcer, unspecified eye

H16.06 Mycotic corneal ulcer
- H16.061 Mycotic corneal ulcer, right eye
- H16.062 Mycotic corneal ulcer, left eye
- H16.063 Mycotic corneal ulcer, bilateral
- H16.069 Mycotic corneal ulcer, unspecified eye

H16.07 Perforated corneal ulcer
- H16.071 Perforated corneal ulcer, right eye
- H16.072 Perforated corneal ulcer, left eye
- H16.073 Perforated corneal ulcer, bilateral
- H16.079 Perforated corneal ulcer, unspecified eye

H16.1 Other and unspecified superficial keratitis without conjunctivitis

H16.10 Unspecified superficial keratitis
- H16.101 Unspecified superficial keratitis, right eye
- H16.102 Unspecified superficial keratitis, left eye
- H16.103 Unspecified superficial keratitis, bilateral
- H16.109 Unspecified superficial keratitis, unspecified eye

H16.11 Macular keratitis
Areolar keratitis
Nummular keratitis
Stellate keratitis
Striate keratitis
- H16.111 Macular keratitis, right eye
- H16.112 Macular keratitis, left eye
- H16.113 Macular keratitis, bilateral
- H16.119 Macular keratitis, unspecified eye

H16.12 Filamentary keratitis
- H16.121 Filamentary keratitis, right eye
- H16.122 Filamentary keratitis, left eye
- H16.123 Filamentary keratitis, bilateral
- H16.129 Filamentary keratitis, unspecified eye

H16.13 Photokeratitis
Snow blindness
Welders keratitis
- H16.131 Photokeratitis, right eye
- H16.132 Photokeratitis, left eye
- H16.133 Photokeratitis, bilateral
- H16.139 Photokeratitis, unspecified eye

H16.14 Punctate keratitis
- H16.141 Punctate keratitis, right eye
- H16.142 Punctate keratitis, left eye
- H16.143 Punctate keratitis, bilateral
- H16.149 Punctate keratitis, unspecified eye

H16.2 Keratoconjunctivitis

H16.20 Unspecified keratoconjunctivitis
Superficial keratitis with conjunctivitis NOS
- H16.201 Unspecified keratoconjunctivitis, right eye
- H16.202 Unspecified keratoconjunctivitis, left eye
- H16.203 Unspecified keratoconjunctivitis, bilateral
- H16.209 Unspecified keratoconjunctivitis, unspecified eye

H16.21 Exposure keratoconjunctivitis
- H16.211 Exposure keratoconjunctivitis, right eye
- H16.212 Exposure keratoconjunctivitis, left eye
- H16.213 Exposure keratoconjunctivitis, bilateral
- H16.219 Exposure keratoconjunctivitis, unspecified eye

H16.22 Keratoconjunctivitis sicca, not specified as Sjögren's
EXCLUDES 1 Sjögren's syndrome (M35.01)
- H16.221 Keratoconjunctivitis sicca, not specified as Sjögren's, right eye
- H16.222 Keratoconjunctivitis sicca, not specified as Sjögren's, left eye
- H16.223 Keratoconjunctivitis sicca, not specified as Sjögren's, bilateral
  AHA: 2024,3Q,16
- H16.229 Keratoconjunctivitis sicca, not specified as Sjögren's, unspecified eye

H16.23 Neurotrophic keratoconjunctivitis
- H16.231 Neurotrophic keratoconjunctivitis, right eye
- H16.232 Neurotrophic keratoconjunctivitis, left eye
- H16.233 Neurotrophic keratoconjunctivitis, bilateral
- H16.239 Neurotrophic keratoconjunctivitis, unspecified eye

H16.24 Ophthalmia nodosa
- H16.241 Ophthalmia nodosa, right eye
- H16.242 Ophthalmia nodosa, left eye
- H16.243 Ophthalmia nodosa, bilateral
- H16.249 Ophthalmia nodosa, unspecified eye

H16.25 Phlyctenular keratoconjunctivitis
- H16.251 Phlyctenular keratoconjunctivitis, right eye
- H16.252 Phlyctenular keratoconjunctivitis, left eye
- H16.253 Phlyctenular keratoconjunctivitis, bilateral
- H16.259 Phlyctenular keratoconjunctivitis, unspecified eye

H16.26 Vernal keratoconjunctivitis, with limbar and corneal involvement
EXCLUDES 1 vernal conjunctivitis without limbar and corneal involvement (H10.44)
- H16.261 Vernal keratoconjunctivitis, with limbar and corneal involvement, right eye
- H16.262 Vernal keratoconjunctivitis, with limbar and corneal involvement, left eye
- H16.263 Vernal keratoconjunctivitis, with limbar and corneal involvement, bilateral
- H16.269 Vernal keratoconjunctivitis, with limbar and corneal involvement, unspecified eye

H16.29 Other keratoconjunctivitis
- H16.291 Other keratoconjunctivitis, right eye
- H16.292 Other keratoconjunctivitis, left eye
- H16.293 Other keratoconjunctivitis, bilateral
- H16.299 Other keratoconjunctivitis, unspecified eye

H16.3 Interstitial and deep keratitis

H16.30 Unspecified interstitial keratitis
- H16.301 Unspecified interstitial keratitis, right eye
- H16.302 Unspecified interstitial keratitis, left eye
- H16.303 Unspecified interstitial keratitis, bilateral
- H16.309 Unspecified interstitial keratitis, unspecified eye

H16.31 Corneal abscess
- H16.311 Corneal abscess, right eye
- H16.312 Corneal abscess, left eye
- H16.313 Corneal abscess, bilateral
- H16.319 Corneal abscess, unspecified eye

H16.32 Diffuse interstitial keratitis
Cogan's syndrome
- H16.321 Diffuse interstitial keratitis, right eye
- H16.322 Diffuse interstitial keratitis, left eye
- H16.323 Diffuse interstitial keratitis, bilateral
- H16.329 Diffuse interstitial keratitis, unspecified eye

H16.33 Sclerosing keratitis
- H16.331 Sclerosing keratitis, right eye
- H16.332 Sclerosing keratitis, left eye
- H16.333 Sclerosing keratitis, bilateral
- H16.339 Sclerosing keratitis, unspecified eye

H16.39 Other interstitial and deep keratitis
- H16.391 Other interstitial and deep keratitis, right eye

H16.4 Corneal neovascularization

- H16.392 Other interstitial and deep keratitis, left eye
- H16.393 Other interstitial and deep keratitis, bilateral
- H16.399 Other interstitial and deep keratitis, unspecified eye

H16.4 Corneal neovascularization

- **H16.40** Unspecified corneal neovascularization
  - H16.401 Unspecified corneal neovascularization, right eye
  - H16.402 Unspecified corneal neovascularization, left eye
  - H16.403 Unspecified corneal neovascularization, bilateral
  - H16.409 Unspecified corneal neovascularization, unspecified eye
- **H16.41** Ghost vessels (corneal)
  - H16.411 Ghost vessels (corneal), right eye
  - H16.412 Ghost vessels (corneal), left eye
  - H16.413 Ghost vessels (corneal), bilateral
  - H16.419 Ghost vessels (corneal), unspecified eye
- **H16.42** Pannus (corneal)
  - H16.421 Pannus (corneal), right eye
  - H16.422 Pannus (corneal), left eye
  - H16.423 Pannus (corneal), bilateral
  - H16.429 Pannus (corneal), unspecified eye
- **H16.43** Localized vascularization of cornea
  - H16.431 Localized vascularization of cornea, right eye
  - H16.432 Localized vascularization of cornea, left eye
  - H16.433 Localized vascularization of cornea, bilateral
  - H16.439 Localized vascularization of cornea, unspecified eye
- **H16.44** Deep vascularization of cornea
  - H16.441 Deep vascularization of cornea, right eye
  - H16.442 Deep vascularization of cornea, left eye
  - H16.443 Deep vascularization of cornea, bilateral
  - H16.449 Deep vascularization of cornea, unspecified eye

H16.8 Other keratitis
H16.9 Unspecified keratitis

H17 Corneal scars and opacities

H17.0 Adherent leukoma
- H17.00 Adherent leukoma, unspecified eye
- H17.01 Adherent leukoma, right eye
- H17.02 Adherent leukoma, left eye
- H17.03 Adherent leukoma, bilateral

H17.1 Central corneal opacity
- H17.10 Central corneal opacity, unspecified eye
- H17.11 Central corneal opacity, right eye
- H17.12 Central corneal opacity, left eye
- H17.13 Central corneal opacity, bilateral

H17.8 Other corneal scars and opacities
- **H17.81** Minor opacity of cornea
  - Corneal nebula
  - H17.811 Minor opacity of cornea, right eye
  - H17.812 Minor opacity of cornea, left eye
  - H17.813 Minor opacity of cornea, bilateral
  - H17.819 Minor opacity of cornea, unspecified eye
- **H17.82** Peripheral opacity of cornea
  - H17.821 Peripheral opacity of cornea, right eye
  - H17.822 Peripheral opacity of cornea, left eye
  - H17.823 Peripheral opacity of cornea, bilateral
  - H17.829 Peripheral opacity of cornea, unspecified eye
- **H17.89** Other corneal scars and opacities

H17.9 Unspecified corneal scar and opacity

H18 Other disorders of cornea

H18.0 Corneal pigmentations and deposits
- **H18.00** Unspecified corneal deposit
  - H18.001 Unspecified corneal deposit, right eye
  - H18.002 Unspecified corneal deposit, left eye
  - H18.003 Unspecified corneal deposit, bilateral
  - H18.009 Unspecified corneal deposit, unspecified eye
- **H18.01** Anterior corneal pigmentations
  - Staehli's line
  - H18.011 Anterior corneal pigmentations, right eye
  - H18.012 Anterior corneal pigmentations, left eye
  - H18.013 Anterior corneal pigmentations, bilateral
  - H18.019 Anterior corneal pigmentations, unspecified eye
- **H18.02** Argentous corneal deposits
  - H18.021 Argentous corneal deposits, right eye
  - H18.022 Argentous corneal deposits, left eye
  - H18.023 Argentous corneal deposits, bilateral
  - H18.029 Argentous corneal deposits, unspecified eye
- **H18.03** Corneal deposits in metabolic disorders
  - Code also associated metabolic disorder
  - H18.031 Corneal deposits in metabolic disorders, right eye
  - H18.032 Corneal deposits in metabolic disorders, left eye
  - H18.033 Corneal deposits in metabolic disorders, bilateral
  - H18.039 Corneal deposits in metabolic disorders, unspecified eye
- **H18.04** Kayser-Fleischer ring
  - Code also associated Wilson's disease (E83.01)
  - H18.041 Kayser-Fleischer ring, right eye
  - H18.042 Kayser-Fleischer ring, left eye
  - H18.043 Kayser-Fleischer ring, bilateral
  - H18.049 Kayser-Fleischer ring, unspecified eye
- **H18.05** Posterior corneal pigmentations
  - Krukenberg's spindle
  - H18.051 Posterior corneal pigmentations, right eye
  - H18.052 Posterior corneal pigmentations, left eye
  - H18.053 Posterior corneal pigmentations, bilateral
  - H18.059 Posterior corneal pigmentations, unspecified eye
- **H18.06** Stromal corneal pigmentations
  - Hematocornea
  - H18.061 Stromal corneal pigmentations, right eye
  - H18.062 Stromal corneal pigmentations, left eye
  - H18.063 Stromal corneal pigmentations, bilateral
  - H18.069 Stromal corneal pigmentations, unspecified eye

H18.1 Bullous keratopathy
DEF: Corneal swelling due to a damaged corneal endothelium. Bullous keratopathy is characterized by recurring, rupturing epithelial blisters causing glaucoma, iridocyclitis, and Fuchs' dystrophy.
- H18.10 Bullous keratopathy, unspecified eye
- H18.11 Bullous keratopathy, right eye
- H18.12 Bullous keratopathy, left eye
- H18.13 Bullous keratopathy, bilateral

H18.2 Other and unspecified corneal edema
- H18.20 Unspecified corneal edema
- **H18.21** Corneal edema secondary to contact lens
  - EXCLUDES 2: other corneal disorders due to contact lens (H18.82-)
  - H18.211 Corneal edema secondary to contact lens, right eye
  - H18.212 Corneal edema secondary to contact lens, left eye
  - H18.213 Corneal edema secondary to contact lens, bilateral
  - H18.219 Corneal edema secondary to contact lens, unspecified eye
- **H18.22** Idiopathic corneal edema
  - H18.221 Idiopathic corneal edema, right eye
  - H18.222 Idiopathic corneal edema, left eye
  - H18.223 Idiopathic corneal edema, bilateral
  - H18.229 Idiopathic corneal edema, unspecified eye
- **H18.23** Secondary corneal edema
  - H18.231 Secondary corneal edema, right eye
  - H18.232 Secondary corneal edema, left eye
  - H18.233 Secondary corneal edema, bilateral
  - H18.239 Secondary corneal edema, unspecified eye

H18.3 Changes of corneal membranes
- **H18.30** Unspecified corneal membrane change
- **H18.31** Folds and rupture in Bowman's membrane
  - H18.311 Folds and rupture in Bowman's membrane, right eye
  - H18.312 Folds and rupture in Bowman's membrane, left eye
  - H18.313 Folds and rupture in Bowman's membrane, bilateral
  - H18.319 Folds and rupture in Bowman's membrane, unspecified eye
- **H18.32** Folds in Descemet's membrane
  - H18.321 Folds in Descemet's membrane, right eye
  - H18.322 Folds in Descemet's membrane, left eye
  - H18.323 Folds in Descemet's membrane, bilateral
  - H18.329 Folds in Descemet's membrane, unspecified eye
- **H18.33** Rupture in Descemet's membrane
  - H18.331 Rupture in Descemet's membrane, right eye
  - H18.332 Rupture in Descemet's membrane, left eye
  - H18.333 Rupture in Descemet's membrane, bilateral
  - H18.339 Rupture in Descemet's membrane, unspecified eye

H18.4 Corneal degeneration
EXCLUDES 1: Mooren's ulcer (H16.0-)
recurrent erosion of cornea (H18.83-)
- **H18.40** Unspecified corneal degeneration
- **H18.41** Arcus senilis
  Senile corneal changes
  - H18.411 Arcus senilis, right eye
  - H18.412 Arcus senilis, left eye
  - H18.413 Arcus senilis, bilateral
  - H18.419 Arcus senilis, unspecified eye
- **H18.42** Band keratopathy
  - H18.421 Band keratopathy, right eye
  - H18.422 Band keratopathy, left eye
  - H18.423 Band keratopathy, bilateral
  - H18.429 Band keratopathy, unspecified eye
- **H18.43** Other calcerous corneal degeneration
- **H18.44** Keratomalacia
  EXCLUDES 1: keratomalacia due to vitamin A deficiency (E50.4)
  - H18.441 Keratomalacia, right eye
  - H18.442 Keratomalacia, left eye
  - H18.443 Keratomalacia, bilateral
  - H18.449 Keratomalacia, unspecified eye
- **H18.45** Nodular corneal degeneration
  - H18.451 Nodular corneal degeneration, right eye
  - H18.452 Nodular corneal degeneration, left eye
  - H18.453 Nodular corneal degeneration, bilateral
  - H18.459 Nodular corneal degeneration, unspecified eye
- **H18.46** Peripheral corneal degeneration
  - H18.461 Peripheral corneal degeneration, right eye
  - H18.462 Peripheral corneal degeneration, left eye
  - H18.463 Peripheral corneal degeneration, bilateral
  - H18.469 Peripheral corneal degeneration, unspecified eye
- **H18.49** Other corneal degeneration

H18.5 Hereditary corneal dystrophies
AHA: 2020,4Q,24
- **H18.50** Unspecified hereditary corneal dystrophies
  - H18.501 Unspecified hereditary corneal dystrophies, right eye
  - H18.502 Unspecified hereditary corneal dystrophies, left eye
  - H18.503 Unspecified hereditary corneal dystrophies, bilateral
  - H18.509 Unspecified hereditary corneal dystrophies, unspecified eye
- **H18.51** Endothelial corneal dystrophy
  Fuchs' dystrophy
  - H18.511 Endothelial corneal dystrophy, right eye
  - H18.512 Endothelial corneal dystrophy, left eye
  - H18.513 Endothelial corneal dystrophy, bilateral
  - H18.519 Endothelial corneal dystrophy, unspecified eye
- **H18.52** Epithelial (juvenile) corneal dystrophy
  - H18.521 Epithelial (juvenile) corneal dystrophy, right eye
  - H18.522 Epithelial (juvenile) corneal dystrophy, left eye
  - H18.523 Epithelial (juvenile) corneal dystrophy, bilateral
  - H18.529 Epithelial (juvenile) corneal dystrophy, unspecified eye
- **H18.53** Granular corneal dystrophy
  - H18.531 Granular corneal dystrophy, right eye
  - H18.532 Granular corneal dystrophy, left eye
  - H18.533 Granular corneal dystrophy, bilateral
  - H18.539 Granular corneal dystrophy, unspecified eye
- **H18.54** Lattice corneal dystrophy
  - H18.541 Lattice corneal dystrophy, right eye
  - H18.542 Lattice corneal dystrophy, left eye
  - H18.543 Lattice corneal dystrophy, bilateral
  - H18.549 Lattice corneal dystrophy, unspecified eye
- **H18.55** Macular corneal dystrophy
  - H18.551 Macular corneal dystrophy, right eye
  - H18.552 Macular corneal dystrophy, left eye
  - H18.553 Macular corneal dystrophy, bilateral
  - H18.559 Macular corneal dystrophy, unspecified eye
- **H18.59** Other hereditary corneal dystrophies
  - H18.591 Other hereditary corneal dystrophies, right eye
  - H18.592 Other hereditary corneal dystrophies, left eye
  - H18.593 Other hereditary corneal dystrophies, bilateral
  - H18.599 Other hereditary corneal dystrophies, unspecified eye

H18.6 Keratoconus
- **H18.60** Keratoconus, unspecified
  - H18.601 Keratoconus, unspecified, right eye
  - H18.602 Keratoconus, unspecified, left eye
  - H18.603 Keratoconus, unspecified, bilateral
  - H18.609 Keratoconus, unspecified, unspecified eye
- **H18.61** Keratoconus, stable
  - H18.611 Keratoconus, stable, right eye
  - H18.612 Keratoconus, stable, left eye
  - H18.613 Keratoconus, stable, bilateral
  - H18.619 Keratoconus, stable, unspecified eye
- **H18.62** Keratoconus, unstable
  Acute hydrops
  - H18.621 Keratoconus, unstable, right eye
  - H18.622 Keratoconus, unstable, left eye
  - H18.623 Keratoconus, unstable, bilateral
  - H18.629 Keratoconus, unstable, unspecified eye

H18.7 Other and unspecified corneal deformities
EXCLUDES 1: congenital malformations of cornea (Q13.3-Q13.4)
- **H18.70** Unspecified corneal deformity
- **H18.71** Corneal ectasia
  - H18.711 Corneal ectasia, right eye
  - H18.712 Corneal ectasia, left eye
  - H18.713 Corneal ectasia, bilateral
  - H18.719 Corneal ectasia, unspecified eye
- **H18.72** Corneal staphyloma
  - H18.721 Corneal staphyloma, right eye
  - H18.722 Corneal staphyloma, left eye
  - H18.723 Corneal staphyloma, bilateral
  - H18.729 Corneal staphyloma, unspecified eye
- **H18.73** Descemetocele
  - H18.731 Descemetocele, right eye
  - H18.732 Descemetocele, left eye
  - H18.733 Descemetocele, bilateral
  - H18.739 Descemetocele, unspecified eye
- **H18.79** Other corneal deformities
  - H18.791 Other corneal deformities, right eye
  - H18.792 Other corneal deformities, left eye
  - H18.793 Other corneal deformities, bilateral
  - H18.799 Other corneal deformities, unspecified eye

H18.8 Other specified disorders of cornea

H18.81 Anesthesia and hypoesthesia of cornea
- H18.811 Anesthesia and hypoesthesia of cornea, right eye
- H18.812 Anesthesia and hypoesthesia of cornea, left eye
- H18.813 Anesthesia and hypoesthesia of cornea, bilateral
- H18.819 Anesthesia and hypoesthesia of cornea, unspecified eye

H18.82 Corneal disorder due to contact lens
EXCLUDES 2: corneal edema due to contact lens (H18.21-)
- H18.821 Corneal disorder due to contact lens, right eye
- H18.822 Corneal disorder due to contact lens, left eye
- H18.823 Corneal disorder due to contact lens, bilateral
- H18.829 Corneal disorder due to contact lens, unspecified eye

H18.83 Recurrent erosion of cornea
- H18.831 Recurrent erosion of cornea, right eye
- H18.832 Recurrent erosion of cornea, left eye
- H18.833 Recurrent erosion of cornea, bilateral
- H18.839 Recurrent erosion of cornea, unspecified eye

H18.89 Other specified disorders of cornea
- H18.891 Other specified disorders of cornea, right eye
- H18.892 Other specified disorders of cornea, left eye
- H18.893 Other specified disorders of cornea, bilateral
- H18.899 Other specified disorders of cornea, unspecified eye

H18.9 Unspecified disorder of cornea

H20 Iridocyclitis

H20.0 Acute and subacute iridocyclitis
Acute anterior uveitis
Acute cyclitis
Acute iritis
Subacute anterior uveitis
Subacute cyclitis
Subacute iritis

EXCLUDES 1:
iridocyclitis, iritis, uveitis (due to) (in) diabetes mellitus (E08-E13 with .39)
iridocyclitis, iritis, uveitis (due to) (in) diphtheria (A36.89)
iridocyclitis, iritis, uveitis (due to) (in) gonococcal (A54.32)
iridocyclitis, iritis, uveitis (due to) (in) herpes (simplex) (B00.51)
iridocyclitis, iritis, uveitis (due to) (in) herpes zoster (B02.32)
iridocyclitis, iritis, uveitis (due to) (in) late congenital syphilis (A50.39)
iridocyclitis, iritis, uveitis (due to) (in) late syphilis (A52.71)
iridocyclitis, iritis, uveitis (due to) (in) sarcoidosis (D86.83)
iridocyclitis, iritis, uveitis (due to) (in) syphilis (A51.43)
iridocyclitis, iritis, uveitis (due to) (in) toxoplasmosis (B58.09)
iridocyclitis, iritis, uveitis (due to) (in) tuberculosis (A18.54)

- H20.00 Unspecified acute and subacute iridocyclitis

H20.01 Primary iridocyclitis
- H20.011 Primary iridocyclitis, right eye
- H20.012 Primary iridocyclitis, left eye
- H20.013 Primary iridocyclitis, bilateral
- H20.019 Primary iridocyclitis, unspecified eye

H20.02 Recurrent acute iridocyclitis
- H20.021 Recurrent acute iridocyclitis, right eye
- H20.022 Recurrent acute iridocyclitis, left eye
- H20.023 Recurrent acute iridocyclitis, bilateral
- H20.029 Recurrent acute iridocyclitis, unspecified eye

H20.03 Secondary infectious iridocyclitis
- H20.031 Secondary infectious iridocyclitis, right eye
- H20.032 Secondary infectious iridocyclitis, left eye
- H20.033 Secondary infectious iridocyclitis, bilateral
- H20.039 Secondary infectious iridocyclitis, unspecified eye

H20.04 Secondary noninfectious iridocyclitis
- H20.041 Secondary noninfectious iridocyclitis, right eye
- H20.042 Secondary noninfectious iridocyclitis, left eye
- H20.043 Secondary noninfectious iridocyclitis, bilateral
- H20.049 Secondary noninfectious iridocyclitis, unspecified eye

H20.05 Hypopyon
- H20.051 Hypopyon, right eye
- H20.052 Hypopyon, left eye
- H20.053 Hypopyon, bilateral
- H20.059 Hypopyon, unspecified eye

H20.1 Chronic iridocyclitis
Use additional code for any associated cataract (H26.21-)
EXCLUDES 2: posterior cyclitis (H30.2-)
- H20.10 Chronic iridocyclitis, unspecified eye
- H20.11 Chronic iridocyclitis, right eye
- H20.12 Chronic iridocyclitis, left eye
- H20.13 Chronic iridocyclitis, bilateral

H20.2 Lens-induced iridocyclitis
- H20.20 Lens-induced iridocyclitis, unspecified eye
- H20.21 Lens-induced iridocyclitis, right eye
- H20.22 Lens-induced iridocyclitis, left eye
- H20.23 Lens-induced iridocyclitis, bilateral

H20.8 Other iridocyclitis
EXCLUDES 2:
glaucomatocyclitis crises (H40.4-)
posterior cyclitis (H30.2-)
sympathetic uveitis (H44.13-)

H20.81 Fuchs' heterochromic cyclitis
- H20.811 Fuchs' heterochromic cyclitis, right eye
- H20.812 Fuchs' heterochromic cyclitis, left eye
- H20.813 Fuchs' heterochromic cyclitis, bilateral
- H20.819 Fuchs' heterochromic cyclitis, unspecified eye

H20.82 Vogt-Koyanagi syndrome
- H20.821 Vogt-Koyanagi syndrome, right eye
- H20.822 Vogt-Koyanagi syndrome, left eye
- H20.823 Vogt-Koyanagi syndrome, bilateral
- H20.829 Vogt-Koyanagi syndrome, unspecified eye

H20.9 Unspecified iridocyclitis
Uveitis NOS

H21 Other disorders of iris and ciliary body
EXCLUDES 2: sympathetic uveitis (H44.1-)

H21.0 Hyphema
EXCLUDES 1: traumatic hyphema (S05.1-)

Hyphema

Iris
Cornea
Hyphema

- H21.00 Hyphema, unspecified eye
- H21.01 Hyphema, right eye
- H21.02 Hyphema, left eye
- H21.03 Hyphema, bilateral

H21.1 Other vascular disorders of iris and ciliary body
Neovascularization of iris or ciliary body
Rubeosis iridis
Rubeosis of iris

H21.1X Other vascular disorders of iris and ciliary body
- H21.1X1 Other vascular disorders of iris and ciliary body, right eye
- H21.1X2 Other vascular disorders of iris and ciliary body, left eye
- H21.1X3 Other vascular disorders of iris and ciliary body, bilateral
- H21.1X9 Other vascular disorders of iris and ciliary body, unspecified eye

H21.2 Degeneration of iris and ciliary body

H21.21 Degeneration of chamber angle
- H21.211 Degeneration of chamber angle, right eye
- H21.212 Degeneration of chamber angle, left eye
- H21.213 Degeneration of chamber angle, bilateral
- H21.219 Degeneration of chamber angle, unspecified eye

H21.22 Degeneration of ciliary body
- H21.221 Degeneration of ciliary body, right eye
- H21.222 Degeneration of ciliary body, left eye
- H21.223 Degeneration of ciliary body, bilateral
- H21.229 Degeneration of ciliary body, unspecified eye

H21.23 Degeneration of iris (pigmentary)
Translucency of iris
- H21.231 Degeneration of iris (pigmentary), right eye
- H21.232 Degeneration of iris (pigmentary), left eye
- H21.233 Degeneration of iris (pigmentary), bilateral
- H21.239 Degeneration of iris (pigmentary), unspecified eye

H21.24 Degeneration of pupillary margin
- H21.241 Degeneration of pupillary margin, right eye
- H21.242 Degeneration of pupillary margin, left eye
- H21.243 Degeneration of pupillary margin, bilateral
- H21.249 Degeneration of pupillary margin, unspecified eye

H21.25 Iridoschisis
- H21.251 Iridoschisis, right eye
- H21.252 Iridoschisis, left eye
- H21.253 Iridoschisis, bilateral
- H21.259 Iridoschisis, unspecified eye

H21.26 Iris atrophy (essential) (progressive)
- H21.261 Iris atrophy (essential) (progressive), right eye
- H21.262 Iris atrophy (essential) (progressive), left eye
- H21.263 Iris atrophy (essential) (progressive), bilateral
- H21.269 Iris atrophy (essential) (progressive), unspecified eye

H21.27 Miotic pupillary cyst
- H21.271 Miotic pupillary cyst, right eye
- H21.272 Miotic pupillary cyst, left eye
- H21.273 Miotic pupillary cyst, bilateral
- H21.279 Miotic pupillary cyst, unspecified eye

H21.29 Other iris atrophy

H21.3 Cyst of iris, ciliary body and anterior chamber
EXCLUDES 2 miotic pupillary cyst (H21.27-)

H21.30 Idiopathic cysts of iris, ciliary body or anterior chamber
Cyst of iris, ciliary body or anterior chamber NOS
- H21.301 Idiopathic cysts of iris, ciliary body or anterior chamber, right eye
- H21.302 Idiopathic cysts of iris, ciliary body or anterior chamber, left eye
- H21.303 Idiopathic cysts of iris, ciliary body or anterior chamber, bilateral
- H21.309 Idiopathic cysts of iris, ciliary body or anterior chamber, unspecified eye

H21.31 Exudative cysts of iris or anterior chamber
- H21.311 Exudative cysts of iris or anterior chamber, right eye
- H21.312 Exudative cysts of iris or anterior chamber, left eye
- H21.313 Exudative cysts of iris or anterior chamber, bilateral
- H21.319 Exudative cysts of iris or anterior chamber, unspecified eye

H21.32 Implantation cysts of iris, ciliary body or anterior chamber
- H21.321 Implantation cysts of iris, ciliary body or anterior chamber, right eye
- H21.322 Implantation cysts of iris, ciliary body or anterior chamber, left eye
- H21.323 Implantation cysts of iris, ciliary body or anterior chamber, bilateral
- H21.329 Implantation cysts of iris, ciliary body or anterior chamber, unspecified eye

H21.33 Parasitic cyst of iris, ciliary body or anterior chamber
- H21.331 Parasitic cyst of iris, ciliary body or anterior chamber, right eye
- H21.332 Parasitic cyst of iris, ciliary body or anterior chamber, left eye
- H21.333 Parasitic cyst of iris, ciliary body or anterior chamber, bilateral
- H21.339 Parasitic cyst of iris, ciliary body or anterior chamber, unspecified eye

H21.34 Primary cyst of pars plana
- H21.341 Primary cyst of pars plana, right eye
- H21.342 Primary cyst of pars plana, left eye
- H21.343 Primary cyst of pars plana, bilateral
- H21.349 Primary cyst of pars plana, unspecified eye

H21.35 Exudative cyst of pars plana
DEF: Protein, fatty-filled bullous elevation of the nonpigmented outermost ciliary epithelium of pars plana, due to fluid leak from blood vessels.
- H21.351 Exudative cyst of pars plana, right eye
- H21.352 Exudative cyst of pars plana, left eye
- H21.353 Exudative cyst of pars plana, bilateral
- H21.359 Exudative cyst of pars plana, unspecified eye

H21.4 Pupillary membranes
Iris bombé
Pupillary occlusion
Pupillary seclusion
EXCLUDES 1 congenital pupillary membranes (Q13.8)
- H21.40 Pupillary membranes, unspecified eye
- H21.41 Pupillary membranes, right eye
- H21.42 Pupillary membranes, left eye
- H21.43 Pupillary membranes, bilateral

H21.5 Other and unspecified adhesions and disruptions of iris and ciliary body
EXCLUDES 1 corectopia (Q13.2)

H21.50 Unspecified adhesions of iris
Synechia (iris) NOS
- H21.501 Unspecified adhesions of iris, right eye
- H21.502 Unspecified adhesions of iris, left eye
- H21.503 Unspecified adhesions of iris, bilateral
- H21.509 Unspecified adhesions of iris and ciliary body, unspecified eye

H21.51 Anterior synechiae (iris)
- H21.511 Anterior synechiae (iris), right eye
- H21.512 Anterior synechiae (iris), left eye
- H21.513 Anterior synechiae (iris), bilateral
- H21.519 Anterior synechiae (iris), unspecified eye

H21.52 Goniosynechiae
- H21.521 Goniosynechiae, right eye
- H21.522 Goniosynechiae, left eye
- H21.523 Goniosynechiae, bilateral
- H21.529 Goniosynechiae, unspecified eye

H21.53 Iridodialysis
- H21.531 Iridodialysis, right eye
- H21.532 Iridodialysis, left eye
- H21.533 Iridodialysis, bilateral
- H21.539 Iridodialysis, unspecified eye

H21.54 Posterior synechiae (iris)
- H21.541 Posterior synechiae (iris), right eye
- H21.542 Posterior synechiae (iris), left eye
- H21.543 Posterior synechiae (iris), bilateral
- H21.549 Posterior synechiae (iris), unspecified eye

H21.55 Recession of chamber angle
- H21.551 Recession of chamber angle, right eye
- H21.552 Recession of chamber angle, left eye

H21.553 Recession of chamber angle, bilateral
H21.559 Recession of chamber angle, unspecified eye

H21.56 **Pupillary abnormalities**
 Deformed pupil
 Ectopic pupil
 Rupture of sphincter, pupil
 EXCLUDES 1   congenital deformity of pupil (Q13.2-)
 H21.561 Pupillary abnormality, right eye
 H21.562 Pupillary abnormality, left eye
 H21.563 Pupillary abnormality, bilateral
 H21.569 Pupillary abnormality, unspecified eye

H21.8 Other specified disorders of iris and ciliary body
 H21.81 Floppy iris syndrome
  Intraoperative floppy iris syndrome (IFIS)
  Use additional code for adverse effect, if applicable, to identify drug (T36-T50 with fifth or sixth character 5)
 H21.82 Plateau iris syndrome (post-iridectomy) (postprocedural)
 H21.89 Other specified disorders of iris and ciliary body

H21.9 Unspecified disorder of iris and ciliary body

H22 Disorders of iris and ciliary body in diseases classified elsewhere
 Code first underlying disease, such as:
  gout (M1A.-, M10.-)
  leprosy (A30.-)
  parasitic disease (B89)

Disorders of lens (H25-H28)

H25 Age-related cataract
 Senile cataract
 EXCLUDES 2   capsular glaucoma with pseudoexfoliation of lens (H40.1-)

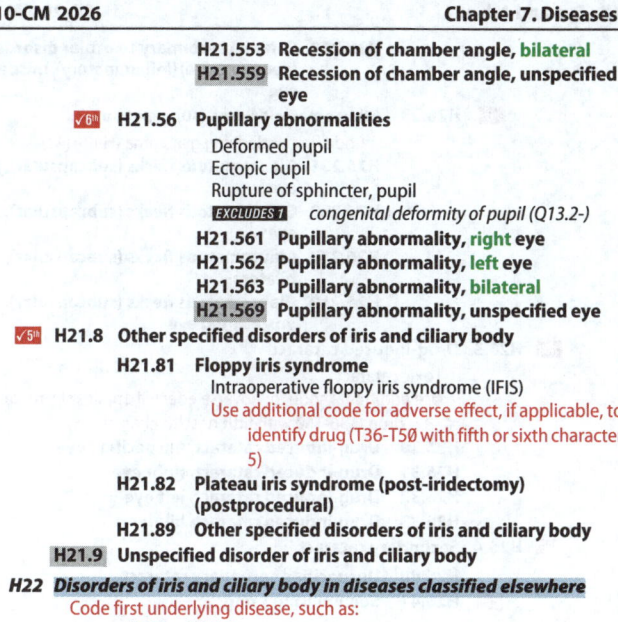

Cataracts

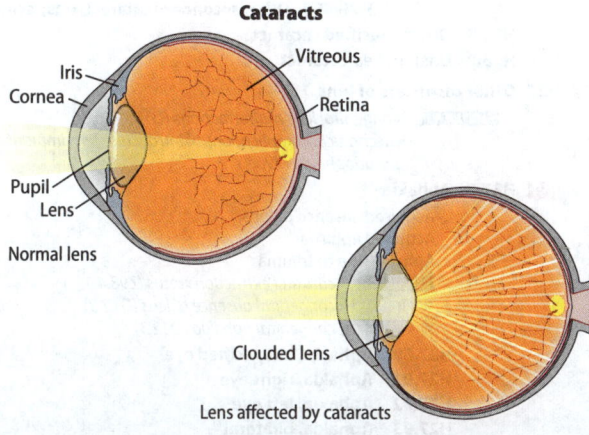

H25.0 **Age-related incipient cataract**
 H25.01 Cortical age-related cataract
  H25.011 Cortical age-related cataract, right eye
  H25.012 Cortical age-related cataract, left eye
  H25.013 Cortical age-related cataract, bilateral
  H25.019 Cortical age-related cataract, unspecified eye
 H25.03 Anterior subcapsular polar age-related cataract
  H25.031 Anterior subcapsular polar age-related cataract, right eye
  H25.032 Anterior subcapsular polar age-related cataract, left eye
  H25.033 Anterior subcapsular polar age-related cataract, bilateral
  H25.039 Anterior subcapsular polar age-related cataract, unspecified eye
 H25.04 Posterior subcapsular polar age-related cataract
  H25.041 Posterior subcapsular polar age-related cataract, right eye
  H25.042 Posterior subcapsular polar age-related cataract, left eye
  H25.043 Posterior subcapsular polar age-related cataract, bilateral
  H25.049 Posterior subcapsular polar age-related cataract, unspecified eye
 H25.09 Other age-related incipient cataract
  Coronary age-related cataract
  Punctate age-related cataract
  Water clefts
  H25.091 Other age-related incipient cataract, right eye
  H25.092 Other age-related incipient cataract, left eye
  H25.093 Other age-related incipient cataract, bilateral
  H25.099 Other age-related incipient cataract, unspecified eye

H25.1 Age-related nuclear cataract
 Cataracta brunescens
 Nuclear sclerosis cataract
 AHA: 2019,2Q,31; 2016,1Q,32
 H25.10 Age-related nuclear cataract, unspecified eye
 H25.11 Age-related nuclear cataract, right eye
 H25.12 Age-related nuclear cataract, left eye
 H25.13 Age-related nuclear cataract, bilateral

H25.2 Age-related cataract, morgagnian type
 Age-related hypermature cataract
 H25.20 Age-related cataract, morgagnian type, unspecified eye
 H25.21 Age-related cataract, morgagnian type, right eye
 H25.22 Age-related cataract, morgagnian type, left eye
 H25.23 Age-related cataract, morgagnian type, bilateral

H25.8 Other age-related cataract
 H25.81 Combined forms of age-related cataract
  AHA: 2019,2Q,30
  H25.811 Combined forms of age-related cataract, right eye
  H25.812 Combined forms of age-related cataract, left eye
  H25.813 Combined forms of age-related cataract, bilateral
  H25.819 Combined forms of age-related cataract, unspecified eye
 H25.89 Other age-related cataract

H25.9 Unspecified age-related cataract

H26 Other cataract
 EXCLUDES 1   congenital cataract (Q12.0)

H26.0 Infantile and juvenile cataract
 H26.00 Unspecified infantile and juvenile cataract
  H26.001 Unspecified infantile and juvenile cataract, right eye
  H26.002 Unspecified infantile and juvenile cataract, left eye
  H26.003 Unspecified infantile and juvenile cataract, bilateral
  H26.009 Unspecified infantile and juvenile cataract, unspecified eye
 H26.01 Infantile and juvenile cortical, lamellar, or zonular cataract
  H26.011 Infantile and juvenile cortical, lamellar, or zonular cataract, right eye
  H26.012 Infantile and juvenile cortical, lamellar, or zonular cataract, left eye
  H26.013 Infantile and juvenile cortical, lamellar, or zonular cataract, bilateral
  H26.019 Infantile and juvenile cortical, lamellar, or zonular cataract, unspecified eye
 H26.03 Infantile and juvenile nuclear cataract
  H26.031 Infantile and juvenile nuclear cataract, right eye
  H26.032 Infantile and juvenile nuclear cataract, left eye
  H26.033 Infantile and juvenile nuclear cataract, bilateral
  H26.039 Infantile and juvenile nuclear cataract, unspecified eye

Chapter 7. Diseases of the Eye and Adnexa

H26.04 **Anterior subcapsular polar** infantile and juvenile cataract
- H26.041 Anterior subcapsular polar infantile and juvenile cataract, **right** eye
- H26.042 Anterior subcapsular polar infantile and juvenile cataract, **left** eye
- H26.043 Anterior subcapsular polar infantile and juvenile cataract, **bilateral**
- H26.049 Anterior subcapsular polar infantile and juvenile cataract, **unspecified** eye

H26.05 **Posterior subcapsular polar** infantile and juvenile cataract
- H26.051 Posterior subcapsular polar infantile and juvenile cataract, **right** eye
- H26.052 Posterior subcapsular polar infantile and juvenile cataract, **left** eye
- H26.053 Posterior subcapsular polar infantile and juvenile cataract, **bilateral**
- H26.059 Posterior subcapsular polar infantile and juvenile cataract, **unspecified** eye

H26.06 **Combined forms** of infantile and juvenile cataract
- H26.061 Combined forms of infantile and juvenile cataract, **right** eye
- H26.062 Combined forms of infantile and juvenile cataract, **left** eye
- H26.063 Combined forms of infantile and juvenile cataract, **bilateral**
- H26.069 Combined forms of infantile and juvenile cataract, **unspecified** eye

H26.09 Other infantile and juvenile cataract

H26.1 **Traumatic** cataract
Use additional code (Chapter 20) to identify external cause

H26.10 Unspecified traumatic cataract
- H26.101 Unspecified traumatic cataract, **right** eye
- H26.102 Unspecified traumatic cataract, **left** eye
- H26.103 Unspecified traumatic cataract, **bilateral**
- H26.109 Unspecified traumatic cataract, **unspecified** eye

H26.11 **Localized** traumatic opacities
- H26.111 Localized traumatic opacities, **right** eye
- H26.112 Localized traumatic opacities, **left** eye
- H26.113 Localized traumatic opacities, **bilateral**
- H26.119 Localized traumatic opacities, **unspecified** eye

H26.12 **Partially resolved** traumatic cataract
- H26.121 Partially resolved traumatic cataract, **right** eye
- H26.122 Partially resolved traumatic cataract, **left** eye
- H26.123 Partially resolved traumatic cataract, **bilateral**
- H26.129 Partially resolved traumatic cataract, **unspecified** eye

H26.13 **Total** traumatic cataract
- H26.131 Total traumatic cataract, **right** eye
- H26.132 Total traumatic cataract, **left** eye
- H26.133 Total traumatic cataract, **bilateral**
- H26.139 Total traumatic cataract, **unspecified** eye

H26.2 **Complicated** cataract

H26.20 Unspecified complicated cataract
Cataracta complicata NOS

H26.21 Cataract **with neovascularization**
Code also, if applicable, associated condition, such as: chronic iridocyclitis (H20.1-)
- H26.211 Cataract with neovascularization, **right** eye
- H26.212 Cataract with neovascularization, **left** eye
- H26.213 Cataract with neovascularization, **bilateral**
- H26.219 Cataract with neovascularization, **unspecified** eye

H26.22 Cataract **secondary to ocular disorders** (degenerative) (inflammatory)
Code also associated ocular disorder
- H26.221 Cataract secondary to ocular disorders (degenerative) (inflammatory), **right** eye
- H26.222 Cataract secondary to ocular disorders (degenerative) (inflammatory), **left** eye
- H26.223 Cataract secondary to ocular disorders (degenerative) (inflammatory), **bilateral**
- H26.229 Cataract secondary to ocular disorders (degenerative) (inflammatory), unspecified eye

H26.23 **Glaucomatous flecks** (subcapsular)
Code first underlying glaucoma (H40-H42)
- H26.231 Glaucomatous flecks (subcapsular), **right** eye
- H26.232 Glaucomatous flecks (subcapsular), **left** eye
- H26.233 Glaucomatous flecks (subcapsular), **bilateral**
- H26.239 Glaucomatous flecks (subcapsular), **unspecified eye**

H26.3 **Drug-induced** cataract
Toxic cataract
Use additional code for adverse effect, if applicable, to identify drug (T36-T50 with fifth or sixth character 5)
- H26.30 Drug-induced cataract, unspecified eye
- H26.31 Drug-induced cataract, **right** eye
- H26.32 Drug-induced cataract, **left** eye
- H26.33 Drug-induced cataract, **bilateral**

H26.4 **Secondary** cataract

H26.40 Unspecified secondary cataract

H26.41 **Soemmering's ring**
- H26.411 Soemmering's ring, **right** eye
- H26.412 Soemmering's ring, **left** eye
- H26.413 Soemmering's ring, **bilateral**
- H26.419 Soemmering's ring, **unspecified** eye

H26.49 Other secondary cataract
AHA: 2018,2Q,14
- H26.491 Other secondary cataract, **right** eye
- H26.492 Other secondary cataract, **left** eye
- H26.493 Other secondary cataract, **bilateral**
- H26.499 Other secondary cataract, **unspecified** eye

H26.8 Other specified cataract

H26.9 Unspecified cataract

H27 Other disorders of lens
EXCLUDES 1 congenital lens malformations (Q12.-)
mechanical complications of intraocular lens implant (T85.2)
pseudophakia (Z96.1)

H27.0 **Aphakia**
Acquired absence of lens
Acquired aphakia
Aphakia due to trauma
EXCLUDES 1 cataract extraction status (Z98.4-)
congenital absence of lens (Q12.3)
congenital aphakia (Q12.3)
- H27.00 Aphakia, unspecified eye
- H27.01 Aphakia, **right** eye
- H27.02 Aphakia, **left** eye
- H27.03 Aphakia, **bilateral**

H27.1 **Dislocation of lens**

H27.10 Unspecified dislocation of lens

H27.11 **Subluxation of lens**
- H27.111 Subluxation of lens, **right** eye
- H27.112 Subluxation of lens, **left** eye
- H27.113 Subluxation of lens, **bilateral**
- H27.119 Subluxation of lens, **unspecified** eye

H27.12 **Anterior dislocation of lens**
- H27.121 Anterior dislocation of lens, **right** eye
- H27.122 Anterior dislocation of lens, **left** eye
- H27.123 Anterior dislocation of lens, **bilateral**
- H27.129 Anterior dislocation of lens, **unspecified** eye

H27.13 **Posterior dislocation of lens**
- H27.131 Posterior dislocation of lens, **right** eye
- H27.132 Posterior dislocation of lens, **left** eye
- H27.133 Posterior dislocation of lens, **bilateral**
- H27.139 Posterior dislocation of lens, **unspecified** eye

H27.8 Other specified disorders of lens

H27.9 Unspecified disorder of lens

H28 Cataract in diseases classified elsewhere
Code first underlying disease, such as:
   hypoparathyroidism (E20.-)
   myotonia (G71.1-)
   myxedema (E03.-)
   protein-calorie malnutrition (E40-E46)
   EXCLUDES 1 cataract in diabetes mellitus (E08.36, E09.36, E10.36, E11.36, E13.36)

Disorders of choroid and retina (H30-H36)

H30 Chorioretinal inflammation

H30.0 Focal chorioretinal inflammation
Focal chorioretinitis
Focal choroiditis
Focal retinitis
Focal retinochoroiditis

H30.00 Unspecified focal chorioretinal inflammation
Focal chorioretinitis NOS
Focal choroiditis NOS
Focal retinitis NOS
Focal retinochoroiditis NOS
- H30.001 Unspecified focal chorioretinal inflammation, right eye
- H30.002 Unspecified focal chorioretinal inflammation, left eye
- H30.003 Unspecified focal chorioretinal inflammation, bilateral
- H30.009 Unspecified focal chorioretinal inflammation, unspecified eye

H30.01 Focal chorioretinal inflammation, juxtapapillary
- H30.011 Focal chorioretinal inflammation, juxtapapillary, right eye
- H30.012 Focal chorioretinal inflammation, juxtapapillary, left eye
- H30.013 Focal chorioretinal inflammation, juxtapapillary, bilateral
- H30.019 Focal chorioretinal inflammation, juxtapapillary, unspecified eye

H30.02 Focal chorioretinal inflammation of posterior pole
- H30.021 Focal chorioretinal inflammation of posterior pole, right eye
- H30.022 Focal chorioretinal inflammation of posterior pole, left eye
- H30.023 Focal chorioretinal inflammation of posterior pole, bilateral
- H30.029 Focal chorioretinal inflammation of posterior pole, unspecified eye

H30.03 Focal chorioretinal inflammation, peripheral
- H30.031 Focal chorioretinal inflammation, peripheral, right eye
- H30.032 Focal chorioretinal inflammation, peripheral, left eye
- H30.033 Focal chorioretinal inflammation, peripheral, bilateral
- H30.039 Focal chorioretinal inflammation, peripheral, unspecified eye

H30.04 Focal chorioretinal inflammation, macular or paramacular
- H30.041 Focal chorioretinal inflammation, macular or paramacular, right eye
- H30.042 Focal chorioretinal inflammation, macular or paramacular, left eye
- H30.043 Focal chorioretinal inflammation, macular or paramacular, bilateral
- H30.049 Focal chorioretinal inflammation, macular or paramacular, unspecified eye

H30.1 Disseminated chorioretinal inflammation
Disseminated chorioretinitis
Disseminated choroiditis
Disseminated retinitis
Disseminated retinochoroiditis
EXCLUDES 2 exudative retinopathy (H35.02-)

H30.10 Unspecified disseminated chorioretinal inflammation
Disseminated chorioretinitis NOS
Disseminated choroiditis NOS
Disseminated retinitis NOS
Disseminated retinochoroiditis NOS
- H30.101 Unspecified disseminated chorioretinal inflammation, right eye
- H30.102 Unspecified disseminated chorioretinal inflammation, left eye
- H30.103 Unspecified disseminated chorioretinal inflammation, bilateral
- H30.109 Unspecified disseminated chorioretinal inflammation, unspecified eye

H30.11 Disseminated chorioretinal inflammation of posterior pole
- H30.111 Disseminated chorioretinal inflammation of posterior pole, right eye
- H30.112 Disseminated chorioretinal inflammation of posterior pole, left eye
- H30.113 Disseminated chorioretinal inflammation of posterior pole, bilateral
- H30.119 Disseminated chorioretinal inflammation of posterior pole, unspecified eye

H30.12 Disseminated chorioretinal inflammation, peripheral
- H30.121 Disseminated chorioretinal inflammation, peripheral right eye
- H30.122 Disseminated chorioretinal inflammation, peripheral, left eye
- H30.123 Disseminated chorioretinal inflammation, peripheral, bilateral
- H30.129 Disseminated chorioretinal inflammation, peripheral, unspecified eye

H30.13 Disseminated chorioretinal inflammation, generalized
- H30.131 Disseminated chorioretinal inflammation, generalized, right eye
- H30.132 Disseminated chorioretinal inflammation, generalized, left eye
- H30.133 Disseminated chorioretinal inflammation, generalized, bilateral
- H30.139 Disseminated chorioretinal inflammation, generalized, unspecified eye

H30.14 Acute posterior multifocal placoid pigment epitheliopathy
- H30.141 Acute posterior multifocal placoid pigment epitheliopathy, right eye
- H30.142 Acute posterior multifocal placoid pigment epitheliopathy, left eye
- H30.143 Acute posterior multifocal placoid pigment epitheliopathy, bilateral
- H30.149 Acute posterior multifocal placoid pigment epitheliopathy, unspecified eye

H30.2 Posterior cyclitis
Pars planitis
- H30.20 Posterior cyclitis, unspecified eye
- H30.21 Posterior cyclitis, right eye
- H30.22 Posterior cyclitis, left eye
- H30.23 Posterior cyclitis, bilateral

H30.8 Other chorioretinal inflammations

H30.81 Harada's disease
- H30.811 Harada's disease, right eye
- H30.812 Harada's disease, left eye
- H30.813 Harada's disease, bilateral
- H30.819 Harada's disease, unspecified eye

H30.89 Other chorioretinal inflammations
- H30.891 Other chorioretinal inflammations, right eye
- H30.892 Other chorioretinal inflammations, left eye
- H30.893 Other chorioretinal inflammations, bilateral
- H30.899 Other chorioretinal inflammations, unspecified eye

H30.9 Unspecified chorioretinal inflammation
Chorioretinitis NOS
Choroiditis NOS
Neuroretinitis NOS
Retinitis NOS
Retinochoroiditis NOS
- H30.90 Unspecified chorioretinal inflammation, unspecified eye
- H30.91 Unspecified chorioretinal inflammation, right eye
- H30.92 Unspecified chorioretinal inflammation, left eye
- H30.93 Unspecified chorioretinal inflammation, bilateral

H31 Other disorders of choroid

H31.0 Chorioretinal scars
EXCLUDES 2 postsurgical chorioretinal scars (H59.81-)

H31.00 Unspecified chorioretinal scars
- H31.001 Unspecified chorioretinal scars, right eye

- H31.002 Unspecified chorioretinal scars, left eye
- H31.003 Unspecified chorioretinal scars, bilateral
- H31.009 Unspecified chorioretinal scars, unspecified eye

✓6th H31.01 Macula scars of posterior pole (postinflammatory) (post-traumatic)
  EXCLUDES 1 postprocedural chorioretinal scar (H59.81-)
  - H31.011 Macula scars of posterior pole (postinflammatory) (post-traumatic), right eye
  - H31.012 Macula scars of posterior pole (postinflammatory) (post-traumatic), left eye
  - H31.013 Macula scars of posterior pole (postinflammatory) (post-traumatic), bilateral
  - H31.019 Macula scars of posterior pole (postinflammatory) (post-traumatic), unspecified eye

✓6th H31.02 Solar retinopathy
  - H31.021 Solar retinopathy, right eye
  - H31.022 Solar retinopathy, left eye
  - H31.023 Solar retinopathy, bilateral
  - H31.029 Solar retinopathy, unspecified eye

✓6th H31.09 Other chorioretinal scars
  - H31.091 Other chorioretinal scars, right eye
  - H31.092 Other chorioretinal scars, left eye
  - H31.093 Other chorioretinal scars, bilateral
  - H31.099 Other chorioretinal scars, unspecified eye

✓5th H31.1 Choroidal degeneration
  EXCLUDES 2 angioid streaks of macula (H35.33)

✓6th H31.10 Unspecified choroidal degeneration
  Choroidal sclerosis NOS
  - H31.101 Choroidal degeneration, unspecified, right eye
  - H31.102 Choroidal degeneration, unspecified, left eye
  - H31.103 Choroidal degeneration, unspecified, bilateral
  - H31.109 Choroidal degeneration, unspecified, unspecified eye

✓6th H31.11 Age-related choroidal atrophy
  - H31.111 Age-related choroidal atrophy, right eye [A]
  - H31.112 Age-related choroidal atrophy, left eye [A]
  - H31.113 Age-related choroidal atrophy, bilateral [A]
  - H31.119 Age-related choroidal atrophy, unspecified eye [A]

✓6th H31.12 Diffuse secondary atrophy of choroid
  - H31.121 Diffuse secondary atrophy of choroid, right eye
  - H31.122 Diffuse secondary atrophy of choroid, left eye
  - H31.123 Diffuse secondary atrophy of choroid, bilateral
  - H31.129 Diffuse secondary atrophy of choroid, unspecified eye

✓5th H31.2 Hereditary choroidal dystrophy
  EXCLUDES 2 hyperornithinemia (E72.4)
  ornithinemia (E72.4)
  - H31.20 Hereditary choroidal dystrophy, unspecified
  - H31.21 Choroideremia
  - H31.22 Choroidal dystrophy (central areolar) (generalized) (peripapillary)
  - H31.23 Gyrate atrophy, choroid
  - H31.29 Other hereditary choroidal dystrophy

✓5th H31.3 Choroidal hemorrhage and rupture

✓6th H31.30 Unspecified choroidal hemorrhage
  - H31.301 Unspecified choroidal hemorrhage, right eye
  - H31.302 Unspecified choroidal hemorrhage, left eye
  - H31.303 Unspecified choroidal hemorrhage, bilateral
  - H31.309 Unspecified choroidal hemorrhage, unspecified eye

✓6th H31.31 Expulsive choroidal hemorrhage
  - H31.311 Expulsive choroidal hemorrhage, right eye
  - H31.312 Expulsive choroidal hemorrhage, left eye
  - H31.313 Expulsive choroidal hemorrhage, bilateral
  - H31.319 Expulsive choroidal hemorrhage, unspecified eye

✓6th H31.32 Choroidal rupture
  - H31.321 Choroidal rupture, right eye
  - H31.322 Choroidal rupture, left eye
  - H31.323 Choroidal rupture, bilateral
  - H31.329 Choroidal rupture, unspecified eye

✓5th H31.4 Choroidal detachment

✓6th H31.40 Unspecified choroidal detachment
  - H31.401 Unspecified choroidal detachment, right eye
  - H31.402 Unspecified choroidal detachment, left eye
  - H31.403 Unspecified choroidal detachment, bilateral
  - H31.409 Unspecified choroidal detachment, unspecified eye

✓6th H31.41 Hemorrhagic choroidal detachment
  - H31.411 Hemorrhagic choroidal detachment, right eye
  - H31.412 Hemorrhagic choroidal detachment, left eye
  - H31.413 Hemorrhagic choroidal detachment, bilateral
  - H31.419 Hemorrhagic choroidal detachment, unspecified eye

✓6th H31.42 Serous choroidal detachment
  - H31.421 Serous choroidal detachment, right eye
  - H31.422 Serous choroidal detachment, left eye
  - H31.423 Serous choroidal detachment, bilateral
  - H31.429 Serous choroidal detachment, unspecified eye

- H31.8 Other specified disorders of choroid
- H31.9 Unspecified disorder of choroid

H32 Chorioretinal disorders in diseases classified elsewhere
Code first underlying disease, such as:
  congenital toxoplasmosis (P37.1)
  histoplasmosis (B39.-)
  leprosy (A30.-)
  EXCLUDES 1 chorioretinitis (in):
    toxoplasmosis (acquired) (B58.01)
    tuberculosis (A18.53)

✓4th H33 Retinal detachments and breaks
  EXCLUDES 1 detachment of retinal pigment epithelium (H35.72-, H35.73-)

✓5th H33.0 Retinal detachment with retinal break
  Rhegmatogenous retinal detachment
  EXCLUDES 1 serous retinal detachment (without retinal break) (H33.2-)

✓6th H33.00 Unspecified retinal detachment with retinal break
  - H33.001 Unspecified retinal detachment with retinal break, right eye
  - H33.002 Unspecified retinal detachment with retinal break, left eye
  - H33.003 Unspecified retinal detachment with retinal break, bilateral
  - H33.009 Unspecified retinal detachment with retinal break, unspecified eye

Chapter 7. Diseases of the Eye and Adnexa

- ✓6th **H33.01** Retinal detachment with single break
  - H33.011 Retinal detachment with single break, right eye
  - H33.012 Retinal detachment with single break, left eye
  - H33.013 Retinal detachment with single break, bilateral
  - H33.019 Retinal detachment with single break, unspecified eye
- ✓6th **H33.02** Retinal detachment with multiple breaks
  - H33.021 Retinal detachment with multiple breaks, right eye
  - H33.022 Retinal detachment with multiple breaks, left eye
  - H33.023 Retinal detachment with multiple breaks, bilateral
  - H33.029 Retinal detachment with multiple breaks, unspecified eye
- ✓6th **H33.03** Retinal detachment with giant retinal tear
  - H33.031 Retinal detachment with giant retinal tear, right eye
  - H33.032 Retinal detachment with giant retinal tear, left eye
  - H33.033 Retinal detachment with giant retinal tear, bilateral
  - H33.039 Retinal detachment with giant retinal tear, unspecified eye
- ✓6th **H33.04** Retinal detachment with retinal dialysis
  - H33.041 Retinal detachment with retinal dialysis, right eye
  - H33.042 Retinal detachment with retinal dialysis, left eye
  - H33.043 Retinal detachment with retinal dialysis, bilateral
  - H33.049 Retinal detachment with retinal dialysis, unspecified eye
- ✓6th **H33.05** Total retinal detachment
  - H33.051 Total retinal detachment, right eye
  - H33.052 Total retinal detachment, left eye
  - H33.053 Total retinal detachment, bilateral
  - H33.059 Total retinal detachment, unspecified eye
- ✓5th **H33.1** Retinoschisis and retinal cysts
  - EXCLUDES 1: congenital retinoschisis (Q14.1)
    microcystoid degeneration of retina (H35.42-)
  - ✓6th **H33.10** Unspecified retinoschisis
    - H33.101 Unspecified retinoschisis, right eye
    - H33.102 Unspecified retinoschisis, left eye
    - H33.103 Unspecified retinoschisis, bilateral
    - H33.109 Unspecified retinoschisis, unspecified eye
  - ✓6th **H33.11** Cyst of ora serrata
    - H33.111 Cyst of ora serrata, right eye
    - H33.112 Cyst of ora serrata, left eye
    - H33.113 Cyst of ora serrata, bilateral
    - H33.119 Cyst of ora serrata, unspecified eye
  - ✓6th **H33.12** Parasitic cyst of retina
    - H33.121 Parasitic cyst of retina, right eye
    - H33.122 Parasitic cyst of retina, left eye
    - H33.123 Parasitic cyst of retina, bilateral
    - H33.129 Parasitic cyst of retina, unspecified eye
  - ✓6th **H33.19** Other retinoschisis and retinal cysts
    Pseudocyst of retina
    - H33.191 Other retinoschisis and retinal cysts, right eye
    - H33.192 Other retinoschisis and retinal cysts, left eye
    - H33.193 Other retinoschisis and retinal cysts, bilateral
    - H33.199 Other retinoschisis and retinal cysts, unspecified eye
- ✓5th **H33.2** Serous retinal detachment
  Retinal detachment NOS
  Retinal detachment without retinal break
  - EXCLUDES 1: central serous chorioretinopathy (H35.71-)
  - H33.20 Serous retinal detachment, unspecified eye
  - H33.21 Serous retinal detachment, right eye
  - H33.22 Serous retinal detachment, left eye
  - H33.23 Serous retinal detachment, bilateral
- ✓5th **H33.3** Retinal breaks without detachment
  - EXCLUDES 1: chorioretinal scars after surgery for detachment (H59.81-)
    peripheral retinal degeneration without break (H35.4-)
  - EXCLUDES 2: ▶peripheral retinal degeneration without break (H35.4-)◀
  - ✓6th **H33.30** Unspecified retinal break
    - H33.301 Unspecified retinal break, right eye
    - H33.302 Unspecified retinal break, left eye
    - H33.303 Unspecified retinal break, bilateral
    - H33.309 Unspecified retinal break, unspecified eye
  - ✓6th **H33.31** Horseshoe tear of retina without detachment
    Operculum of retina without detachment
    - H33.311 Horseshoe tear of retina without detachment, right eye
    - H33.312 Horseshoe tear of retina without detachment, left eye
    - H33.313 Horseshoe tear of retina without detachment, bilateral
    - H33.319 Horseshoe tear of retina without detachment, unspecified eye
  - ✓6th **H33.32** Round hole of retina without detachment
    - H33.321 Round hole, right eye
    - H33.322 Round hole, left eye
    - H33.323 Round hole, bilateral
    - H33.329 Round hole, unspecified eye
  - ✓6th **H33.33** Multiple defects of retina without detachment
    - H33.331 Multiple defects of retina without detachment, right eye
    - H33.332 Multiple defects of retina without detachment, left eye
    - H33.333 Multiple defects of retina without detachment, bilateral
    - H33.339 Multiple defects of retina without detachment, unspecified eye
- ✓5th **H33.4** Traction detachment of retina
  Proliferative vitreo-retinopathy with retinal detachment
  - H33.40 Traction detachment of retina, unspecified eye
  - H33.41 Traction detachment of retina, right eye
  - H33.42 Traction detachment of retina, left eye
  - H33.43 Traction detachment of retina, bilateral
- **H33.8** Other retinal detachments
- ✓4th **H34** Retinal vascular occlusions
  - EXCLUDES 1: amaurosis fugax (G45.3)
  - ✓5th **H34.0** Transient retinal artery occlusion
    - H34.00 Transient retinal artery occlusion, unspecified eye
    - H34.01 Transient retinal artery occlusion, right eye
    - H34.02 Transient retinal artery occlusion, left eye
    - H34.03 Transient retinal artery occlusion, bilateral
  - ✓5th **H34.1** Central retinal artery occlusion
    - H34.10 Central retinal artery occlusion, unspecified eye
    - H34.11 Central retinal artery occlusion, right eye
    - H34.12 Central retinal artery occlusion, left eye
    - H34.13 Central retinal artery occlusion, bilateral
  - ✓5th **H34.2** Other retinal artery occlusions
    - ✓6th **H34.21** Partial retinal artery occlusion
      Hollenhorst's plaque
      Retinal microembolism
      - H34.211 Partial retinal artery occlusion, right eye
      - H34.212 Partial retinal artery occlusion, left eye
      - H34.213 Partial retinal artery occlusion, bilateral
      - H34.219 Partial retinal artery occlusion, unspecified eye
    - ✓6th **H34.23** Retinal artery branch occlusion
      - H34.231 Retinal artery branch occlusion, right eye
      - H34.232 Retinal artery branch occlusion, left eye
      - H34.233 Retinal artery branch occlusion, bilateral
      - H34.239 Retinal artery branch occlusion, unspecified eye

H34.8 Other retinal vascular occlusions
AHA: 2016,4Q,19

H34.81 Central retinal vein occlusion

One of the following 7th characters is to be assigned to codes in subcategory H34.81 to designate the severity of the occlusion:
- 0 with macular edema
- 1 with retinal neovascularization
- 2 stable/old central retinal vein occlusion

- **H34.811** Central retinal vein occlusion, **right eye** HCC
- **H34.812** Central retinal vein occlusion, **left eye** HCC
- **H34.813** Central retinal vein occlusion, **bilateral** HCC
- **H34.819** Central retinal vein occlusion, unspecified eye HCC

H34.82 Venous engorgement
Incipient retinal vein occlusion
Partial retinal vein occlusion
- **H34.821** Venous engorgement, **right** eye
- **H34.822** Venous engorgement, **left** eye
- **H34.823** Venous engorgement, **bilateral**
- **H34.829** Venous engorgement, unspecified eye

H34.83 Tributary (branch) retinal vein occlusion

One of the following 7th characters is to be assigned to codes in subcategory H34.83 to designate the severity of the occlusion:
- 0 with macular edema
- 1 with retinal neovascularization
- 2 stable/old tributary (branch) retinal vein occlusion

- **H34.831** Tributary (branch) retinal vein occlusion, **right** eye HCC
- **H34.832** Tributary (branch) retinal vein occlusion, **left** eye HCC
- **H34.833** Tributary (branch) retinal vein occlusion, **bilateral** HCC
- **H34.839** Tributary (branch) retinal vein occlusion, unspecified eye HCC

H34.9 Unspecified retinal vascular occlusion

H35 Other retinal disorders
EXCLUDES 2 diabetic retinal disorders (E08.311-E08.359, E09.311-E09.359, E10.311-E10.359, E11.311-E11.359, E13.311-E13.359)

H35.0 Background retinopathy and retinal vascular changes
Code also any associated hypertension (I10)

- **H35.00** Unspecified background retinopathy

- **H35.01** Changes in retinal vascular appearance
  Retinal vascular sheathing
  - **H35.011** Changes in retinal vascular appearance, **right** eye
  - **H35.012** Changes in retinal vascular appearance, **left** eye
  - **H35.013** Changes in retinal vascular appearance, **bilateral**
  - **H35.019** Changes in retinal vascular appearance, unspecified eye

- **H35.02** **Exudative** retinopathy
  Coats retinopathy
  - **H35.021** Exudative retinopathy, **right** eye
  - **H35.022** Exudative retinopathy, **left** eye
  - **H35.023** Exudative retinopathy, **bilateral**
  - **H35.029** Exudative retinopathy, unspecified eye

- **H35.03** **Hypertensive** retinopathy
  - **H35.031** Hypertensive retinopathy, **right** eye
  - **H35.032** Hypertensive retinopathy, **left** eye
  - **H35.033** Hypertensive retinopathy, **bilateral**
  - **H35.039** Hypertensive retinopathy, unspecified eye

- **H35.04** Retinal **micro-aneurysms,** unspecified
  - **H35.041** Retinal micro-aneurysms, unspecified, **right** eye
  - **H35.042** Retinal micro-aneurysms, unspecified, **left** eye
  - **H35.043** Retinal micro-aneurysms, unspecified, **bilateral**
  - **H35.049** Retinal micro-aneurysms, unspecified eye

- **H35.05** Retinal **neovascularization,** unspecified
  - **H35.051** Retinal neovascularization, unspecified, **right** eye
  - **H35.052** Retinal neovascularization, unspecified, **left** eye
  - **H35.053** Retinal neovascularization, unspecified, **bilateral**
  - **H35.059** Retinal neovascularization, unspecified, unspecified eye

- **H35.06** Retinal **vasculitis**
  Eales disease
  Retinal perivasculitis
  DEF: Sight-threatening intraocular inflammation of the retinal blood vessels that causes minimal, partial, or even complete blindness.
  - **H35.061** Retinal vasculitis, **right** eye
  - **H35.062** Retinal vasculitis, **left** eye
  - **H35.063** Retinal vasculitis, **bilateral**
  - **H35.069** Retinal vasculitis, unspecified eye

- **H35.07** Retinal **telangiectasis**
  - **H35.071** Retinal telangiectasis, **right** eye
  - **H35.072** Retinal telangiectasis, **left** eye
  - **H35.073** Retinal telangiectasis, **bilateral**
  - **H35.079** Retinal telangiectasis, unspecified eye

- **H35.09** Other intraretinal microvascular abnormalities
  Retinal varices

H35.1 Retinopathy of prematurity

- **H35.10** Retinopathy of prematurity, unspecified
  Retinopathy of prematurity NOS
  - **H35.101** Retinopathy of prematurity, unspecified, **right** eye
  - **H35.102** Retinopathy of prematurity, unspecified, **left** eye
  - **H35.103** Retinopathy of prematurity, unspecified, **bilateral**
  - **H35.109** Retinopathy of prematurity, unspecified, unspecified eye

- **H35.11** Retinopathy of prematurity, **stage 0**
  - **H35.111** Retinopathy of prematurity, stage 0, **right** eye
  - **H35.112** Retinopathy of prematurity, stage 0, **left** eye
  - **H35.113** Retinopathy of prematurity, stage 0, **bilateral**
  - **H35.119** Retinopathy of prematurity, stage 0, unspecified eye

- **H35.12** Retinopathy of prematurity, **stage 1**
  - **H35.121** Retinopathy of prematurity, stage 1, **right** eye
  - **H35.122** Retinopathy of prematurity, stage 1, **left** eye
  - **H35.123** Retinopathy of prematurity, stage 1, **bilateral**
  - **H35.129** Retinopathy of prematurity, stage 1, unspecified eye

- **H35.13** Retinopathy of prematurity, **stage 2**
  - **H35.131** Retinopathy of prematurity, stage 2, **right** eye
  - **H35.132** Retinopathy of prematurity, stage 2, **left** eye
  - **H35.133** Retinopathy of prematurity, stage 2, **bilateral**
  - **H35.139** Retinopathy of prematurity, stage 2, unspecified eye

- **H35.14** Retinopathy of prematurity, **stage 3**
  - **H35.141** Retinopathy of prematurity, stage 3, **right** eye
  - **H35.142** Retinopathy of prematurity, stage 3, **left** eye
  - **H35.143** Retinopathy of prematurity, stage 3, **bilateral**
  - **H35.149** Retinopathy of prematurity, stage 3, unspecified eye

- **H35.15** Retinopathy of prematurity, **stage 4**
  - **H35.151** Retinopathy of prematurity, stage 4, **right** eye
  - **H35.152** Retinopathy of prematurity, stage 4, **left** eye
  - **H35.153** Retinopathy of prematurity, stage 4, **bilateral**

	H35.159	Retinopathy of prematurity, stage 4, unspecified eye
✓6ᵗʰ H35.16		Retinopathy of prematurity, stage 5
	H35.161	Retinopathy of prematurity, stage 5, right eye
	H35.162	Retinopathy of prematurity, stage 5, left eye
	H35.163	Retinopathy of prematurity, stage 5, bilateral
	H35.169	Retinopathy of prematurity, stage 5, unspecified eye
✓6ᵗʰ H35.17		Retrolental fibroplasia
	H35.171	Retrolental fibroplasia, right eye
	H35.172	Retrolental fibroplasia, left eye
	H35.173	Retrolental fibroplasia, bilateral
	H35.179	Retrolental fibroplasia, unspecified eye

✓5ᵗʰ **H35.2** **Other non-diabetic proliferative retinopathy**
Proliferative vitreo-retinopathy
Thalassemia proliferative retinopathy
EXCLUDES 1 proliferative vitreo-retinopathy with retinal detachment (H33.4-)
EXCLUDES 2 proliferative sickle-cell retinopathy (H36.82-)

	H35.20	Other non-diabetic proliferative retinopathy, unspecified eye
	H35.21	Other non-diabetic proliferative retinopathy, right eye
	H35.22	Other non-diabetic proliferative retinopathy, left eye
	H35.23	Other non-diabetic proliferative retinopathy, bilateral

✓5ᵗʰ **H35.3** **Degeneration of macula and posterior pole**

H35.30 Unspecified macular degeneration
Age-related macular degeneration

✓6ᵗʰ **H35.31** **Nonexudative age-related macular degeneration**
Atrophic age-related macular degeneration
Dry age-related macular degeneration
AHA: 2016,4Q,20-21

One of the following 7th characters is to be assigned to each code in subcategory H35.31 to designate the stage of the disease:
0 stage unspecified
1 early dry stage
2 intermediate dry stage
3 advanced atrophic without subfoveal involvement/advanced dry stage
4 advanced atrophic with subfoveal involvement

✓7ᵗʰ H35.311	Nonexudative age-related macular degeneration, right eye
✓7ᵗʰ H35.312	Nonexudative age-related macular degeneration, left eye
✓7ᵗʰ H35.313	Nonexudative age-related macular degeneration, bilateral
✓7ᵗʰ H35.319	Nonexudative age-related macular degeneration, unspecified eye

✓6ᵗʰ **H35.32** **Exudative age-related macular degeneration**
Wet age-related macular degeneration
AHA: 2016,4Q,20-21

One of the following 7th characters is to be assigned to each code in subcategory H35.32 to designate the stage of the disease:
0 stage unspecified
1 with active choroidal neovascularization
2 with inactive choroidal neovascularization/with involuted or regressed neovascularization
3 with inactive scar

✓7ᵗʰ H35.321	Exudative age-related macular degeneration, right eye HCC ESR COM
✓7ᵗʰ H35.322	Exudative age-related macular degeneration, left eye HCC ESR COM
✓7ᵗʰ H35.323	Exudative age-related macular degeneration, bilateral HCC ESR COM
✓7ᵗʰ H35.329	Exudative age-related macular degeneration, unspecified eye HCC ESR COM

H35.33	**Angioid streaks** of macula
	DEF: Degeneration of the choroid, characterized by broad, irregular, dark brown streaks radiating from the optic disc; occurs with pseudoxanthoma elasticum or Paget's disease.

✓6ᵗʰ **H35.34** **Macular cyst, hole, or pseudohole**
H35.341	Macular cyst, hole, or pseudohole, right eye
H35.342	Macular cyst, hole, or pseudohole, left eye
H35.343	Macular cyst, hole, or pseudohole, bilateral
H35.349	Macular cyst, hole, or pseudohole, unspecified eye

✓6ᵗʰ **H35.35** **Cystoid macular degeneration**
EXCLUDES 1 cystoid macular edema following cataract surgery (H59.03-)
H35.351	Cystoid macular degeneration, right eye
H35.352	Cystoid macular degeneration, left eye
H35.353	Cystoid macular degeneration, bilateral
H35.359	Cystoid macular degeneration, unspecified eye

✓6ᵗʰ **H35.36** **Drusen (degenerative) of macula**
AHA: 2017,1Q,51; 2016,4Q,21
H35.361	Drusen (degenerative) of macula, right eye
H35.362	Drusen (degenerative) of macula, left eye
H35.363	Drusen (degenerative) of macula, bilateral
H35.369	Drusen (degenerative) of macula, unspecified eye

✓6ᵗʰ **H35.37** **Puckering of macula**
H35.371	Puckering of macula, right eye
H35.372	Puckering of macula, left eye
H35.373	Puckering of macula, bilateral
H35.379	Puckering of macula, unspecified eye

✓6ᵗʰ **H35.38** **Toxic maculopathy**
Code first poisoning due to drug or toxin, if applicable (T36-T65 with fifth or sixth character 1-4)
Use additional code for adverse effect, if applicable, to identify drug (T36-T50 with fifth or sixth character 5)
H35.381	Toxic maculopathy, right eye
H35.382	Toxic maculopathy, left eye
H35.383	Toxic maculopathy, bilateral
H35.389	Toxic maculopathy, unspecified eye

✓5ᵗʰ **H35.4** **Peripheral retinal degeneration**
EXCLUDES 1 hereditary retinal degeneration (dystrophy) (H35.5-)
  peripheral retinal degeneration with retinal break (H33.3-)
EXCLUDES 2 ▶peripheral retinal degeneration with retinal break (H33.3-)◄

H35.40 Unspecified peripheral retinal degeneration

✓6ᵗʰ **H35.41** **Lattice degeneration of retina**
Palisade degeneration of retina
DEF: Degeneration of the retina, often bilateral, that is usually benign. It is characterized by lines intersecting at irregular intervals in the peripheral retina. Retinal thinning and retinal holes may occur.
H35.411	Lattice degeneration of retina, right eye
H35.412	Lattice degeneration of retina, left eye
H35.413	Lattice degeneration of retina, bilateral
H35.419	Lattice degeneration of retina, unspecified eye

✓6ᵗʰ **H35.42** **Microcystoid degeneration of retina**
H35.421	Microcystoid degeneration of retina, right eye
H35.422	Microcystoid degeneration of retina, left eye
H35.423	Microcystoid degeneration of retina, bilateral
H35.429	Microcystoid degeneration of retina, unspecified eye

✓6ᵗʰ **H35.43** **Paving stone degeneration of retina**
H35.431	Paving stone degeneration of retina, right eye
H35.432	Paving stone degeneration of retina, left eye
H35.433	Paving stone degeneration of retina, bilateral
H35.439	Paving stone degeneration of retina, unspecified eye

Chapter 7. Diseases of the Eye and Adnexa

- **H35.44** **Age-related reticular** degeneration of retina
  - H35.441 Age-related reticular degeneration of retina, **right** eye
  - H35.442 Age-related reticular degeneration of retina, **left** eye
  - H35.443 Age-related reticular degeneration of retina, **bilateral**
  - H35.449 Age-related reticular degeneration of retina, unspecified eye
- **H35.45** **Secondary pigmentary** degeneration
  - H35.451 Secondary pigmentary degeneration, **right** eye
  - H35.452 Secondary pigmentary degeneration, **left** eye
  - H35.453 Secondary pigmentary degeneration, **bilateral**
  - H35.459 Secondary pigmentary degeneration, unspecified eye
- **H35.46** **Secondary vitreoretinal** degeneration
  - H35.461 Secondary vitreoretinal degeneration, **right** eye
  - H35.462 Secondary vitreoretinal degeneration, **left** eye
  - H35.463 Secondary vitreoretinal degeneration, **bilateral**
  - H35.469 Secondary vitreoretinal degeneration, unspecified eye
- **H35.5** Hereditary retinal dystrophy
  - EXCLUDES 1: dystrophies primarily involving Bruch's membrane (H31.1-)
  - H35.50 Unspecified hereditary retinal dystrophy
  - H35.51 **Vitreoretinal** dystrophy
  - H35.52 **Pigmentary** retinal dystrophy
    - Albipunctate retinal dystrophy
    - Retinitis pigmentosa
    - Tapetoretinal dystrophy
  - H35.53 Other dystrophies primarily involving the sensory retina
    - Stargardt's disease
  - H35.54 Dystrophies primarily involving the **retinal pigment epithelium**
    - Vitelliform retinal dystrophy
- **H35.6** Retinal hemorrhage
  - H35.60 Retinal hemorrhage, unspecified eye
  - H35.61 Retinal hemorrhage, **right** eye
  - H35.62 Retinal hemorrhage, **left** eye
  - H35.63 Retinal hemorrhage, **bilateral**
- **H35.7** Separation of retinal layers
  - EXCLUDES 1: retinal detachment (serous) (H33.2-)
    - rhegmatogenous retinal detachment (H33.0-)
  - H35.70 Unspecified separation of retinal layers
  - **H35.71** **Central serous** chorioretinopathy
    - H35.711 Central serous chorioretinopathy, **right** eye
    - H35.712 Central serous chorioretinopathy, **left** eye
    - H35.713 Central serous chorioretinopathy, **bilateral**
    - H35.719 Central serous chorioretinopathy, unspecified eye
  - **H35.72** **Serous** detachment of retinal pigment epithelium
    - H35.721 Serous detachment of retinal pigment epithelium, **right** eye
    - H35.722 Serous detachment of retinal pigment epithelium, **left** eye
    - H35.723 Serous detachment of retinal pigment epithelium, **bilateral**
    - H35.729 Serous detachment of retinal pigment epithelium, unspecified eye
  - **H35.73** **Hemorrhagic** detachment of retinal pigment epithelium
    - H35.731 Hemorrhagic detachment of retinal pigment epithelium, **right** eye
    - H35.732 Hemorrhagic detachment of retinal pigment epithelium, **left** eye
    - H35.733 Hemorrhagic detachment of retinal pigment epithelium, **bilateral**
    - H35.739 Hemorrhagic detachment of retinal pigment epithelium, unspecified eye

- **H35.8** Other specified retinal disorders
  - EXCLUDES 2: retinal hemorrhage (H35.6-)
  - H35.81 Retinal edema
    - Retinal cotton wool spots
  - H35.82 Retinal ischemia
  - H35.89 Other specified retinal disorders
- **H35.9** Unspecified retinal disorder

H36 Retinal disorders in diseases classified elsewhere
Code first underlying disease, such as:
  lipid storage disorders (E75.-)
  sickle-cell disorders (D57.-)
  EXCLUDES 1: arteriosclerotic retinopathy (H35.0-)
    diabetic retinopathy (E08.3-, E09.3-, E10.3-, E11.3-, E13.3-)
  AHA: 2023,4Q,20-21

- **H36.8** Other retinal disorders in diseases classified elsewhere
  - **H36.81** **Nonproliferative** sickle-cell retinopathy
    - H36.811 Nonproliferative sickle-cell retinopathy, **right** eye
    - H36.812 Nonproliferative sickle-cell retinopathy, **left** eye
    - H36.813 Nonproliferative sickle-cell retinopathy, **bilateral**
    - H36.819 Nonproliferative sickle-cell retinopathy, unspecified eye
  - **H36.82** **Proliferative** sickle-cell retinopathy
    - H36.821 Proliferative sickle-cell retinopathy, **right** eye
    - H36.822 Proliferative sickle-cell retinopathy, **left** eye
    - H36.823 Proliferative sickle-cell retinopathy, **bilateral**
    - H36.829 Proliferative sickle-cell retinopathy, unspecified eye
  - H36.89 Other retinal disorders in diseases classified elsewhere
    - Retinal dystrophy in lipid storage disorders

Glaucoma (H40-H42)

H40 Glaucoma
EXCLUDES 1: absolute glaucoma (H44.51-)
  congenital glaucoma (Q15.0)
  traumatic glaucoma due to birth injury (P15.3)

Open Angle/Angle Closure Glaucoma

- **H40.0** Glaucoma suspect
  - **H40.00** Preglaucoma, unspecified
    - H40.001 Preglaucoma, unspecified, **right** eye
    - H40.002 Preglaucoma, unspecified, **left** eye
    - H40.003 Preglaucoma, unspecified, **bilateral**
    - H40.009 Preglaucoma, unspecified, unspecified eye
  - **H40.01** **Open angle with borderline findings, low risk**
    - Open angle, low risk
    - H40.011 Open angle with borderline findings, low risk, **right** eye
    - H40.012 Open angle with borderline findings, low risk, **left** eye
    - H40.013 Open angle with borderline findings, low risk, **bilateral**
    - H40.019 Open angle with borderline findings, low risk, unspecified eye

Chapter 7. Diseases of the Eye and Adnexa

- ✓6th **H40.02** Open angle with borderline findings, high risk
  - Open angle, high risk
  - **H40.021** Open angle with borderline findings, high risk, right eye
  - **H40.022** Open angle with borderline findings, high risk, left eye
  - **H40.023** Open angle with borderline findings, high risk, bilateral
  - **H40.029** Open angle with borderline findings, high risk, unspecified eye
- ✓6th **H40.03** Anatomical narrow angle
  - Primary angle closure suspect
  - **H40.031** Anatomical narrow angle, right eye
  - **H40.032** Anatomical narrow angle, left eye
  - **H40.033** Anatomical narrow angle, bilateral
  - **H40.039** Anatomical narrow angle, unspecified eye
- ✓6th **H40.04** Steroid responder
  - **H40.041** Steroid responder, right eye
  - **H40.042** Steroid responder, left eye
  - **H40.043** Steroid responder, bilateral
  - **H40.049** Steroid responder, unspecified eye
- ✓6th **H40.05** Ocular hypertension
  - **H40.051** Ocular hypertension, right eye
  - **H40.052** Ocular hypertension, left eye
  - **H40.053** Ocular hypertension, bilateral
  - **H40.059** Ocular hypertension, unspecified eye
- ✓6th **H40.06** Primary angle closure without glaucoma damage
  - **H40.061** Primary angle closure without glaucoma damage, right eye
  - **H40.062** Primary angle closure without glaucoma damage, left eye
  - **H40.063** Primary angle closure without glaucoma damage, bilateral
  - **H40.069** Primary angle closure without glaucoma damage, unspecified eye
- ✓5th **H40.1** Open-angle glaucoma

  One of the following 7th characters is to be assigned to each code in subcategories H40.10, H40.11, H40.12, H40.13, and H40.14 to designate the stage of glaucoma.
  - 0 stage unspecified
  - 1 mild stage
  - 2 moderate stage
  - 3 severe stage
  - 4 indeterminate stage

  - ✓x 7th **H40.10** Unspecified open-angle glaucoma [Rx]
    - **TIP:** Only one code from this subcategory should be assigned when both left and right eyes are the same stage.
  - ✓6th **H40.11** Primary open-angle glaucoma
    - Chronic simple glaucoma
    - AHA: 2016,4Q,22
    - ✓7th **H40.111** Primary open-angle glaucoma, right eye [Rx] [Q]
    - ✓7th **H40.112** Primary open-angle glaucoma, left eye [Rx] [Q]
    - ✓7th **H40.113** Primary open-angle glaucoma, bilateral [Rx] [Q]
    - ✓7th **H40.119** Primary open-angle glaucoma, unspecified eye [Rx]
  - ✓6th **H40.12** Low-tension glaucoma
    - ✓7th **H40.121** Low-tension glaucoma, right eye [Rx] [Q]
    - ✓7th **H40.122** Low-tension glaucoma, left eye [Rx] [Q]
    - ✓7th **H40.123** Low-tension glaucoma, bilateral [Rx] [Q]
    - ✓7th **H40.129** Low-tension glaucoma, unspecified eye [Rx]
  - ✓6th **H40.13** Pigmentary glaucoma
    - ✓7th **H40.131** Pigmentary glaucoma, right eye [Rx]
    - ✓7th **H40.132** Pigmentary glaucoma, left eye [Rx]
    - ✓7th **H40.133** Pigmentary glaucoma, bilateral [Rx]
    - ✓7th **H40.139** Pigmentary glaucoma, unspecified eye [Rx]
  - ✓6th **H40.14** Capsular glaucoma with pseudoexfoliation of lens
    - ✓7th **H40.141** Capsular glaucoma with pseudoexfoliation of lens, right eye [Rx]
    - ✓7th **H40.142** Capsular glaucoma with pseudoexfoliation of lens, left eye [Rx]
    - ✓7th **H40.143** Capsular glaucoma with pseudoexfoliation of lens, bilateral [Rx]
    - ✓7th **H40.149** Capsular glaucoma with pseudoexfoliation of lens, unspecified eye [Rx]
  - ✓6th **H40.15** Residual stage of open-angle glaucoma
    - **H40.151** Residual stage of open-angle glaucoma, right eye [Rx] [Q]
    - **H40.152** Residual stage of open-angle glaucoma, left eye [Rx] [Q]
    - **H40.153** Residual stage of open-angle glaucoma, bilateral [Rx] [Q]
    - **H40.159** Residual stage of open-angle glaucoma, unspecified eye
- ✓5th **H40.2** Primary angle-closure glaucoma
  - EXCLUDES 1: aqueous misdirection (H40.83-)
  - malignant glaucoma (H40.83-)

  One of the following 7th characters is to be assigned to code H40.20 and H40.22 to designate the stage of glaucoma.
  - 0 stage unspecified
  - 1 mild stage
  - 2 moderate stage
  - 3 severe stage
  - 4 indeterminate stage

  - ✓x 7th **H40.20** Unspecified primary angle-closure glaucoma [Rx]
    - **TIP:** Only one code from this subcategory should be assigned when both left and right eyes are the same stage.
  - ✓6th **H40.21** Acute angle-closure glaucoma
    - Acute angle-closure glaucoma attack
    - Acute angle-closure glaucoma crisis
    - **H40.211** Acute angle-closure glaucoma, right eye
    - **H40.212** Acute angle-closure glaucoma, left eye
    - **H40.213** Acute angle-closure glaucoma, bilateral
    - **H40.219** Acute angle-closure glaucoma, unspecified eye
  - ✓6th **H40.22** Chronic angle-closure glaucoma
    - Chronic primary angle closure glaucoma
    - ✓7th **H40.221** Chronic angle-closure glaucoma, right eye [Rx]
    - ✓7th **H40.222** Chronic angle-closure glaucoma, left eye [Rx]
    - ✓7th **H40.223** Chronic angle-closure glaucoma, bilateral [Rx]
    - ✓7th **H40.229** Chronic angle-closure glaucoma, unspecified eye [Rx]
  - ✓6th **H40.23** Intermittent angle-closure glaucoma
    - **H40.231** Intermittent angle-closure glaucoma, right eye [Rx]
    - **H40.232** Intermittent angle-closure glaucoma, left eye [Rx]
    - **H40.233** Intermittent angle-closure glaucoma, bilateral [Rx]
    - **H40.239** Intermittent angle-closure glaucoma, unspecified eye [Rx]
  - ✓6th **H40.24** Residual stage of angle-closure glaucoma
    - **H40.241** Residual stage of angle-closure glaucoma, right eye [Rx]
    - **H40.242** Residual stage of angle-closure glaucoma, left eye [Rx]
    - **H40.243** Residual stage of angle-closure glaucoma, bilateral [Rx]
    - **H40.249** Residual stage of angle-closure glaucoma, unspecified eye
- ✓5th **H40.3** Glaucoma secondary to eye trauma
  - Code also underlying condition

  One of the following 7th characters is to be assigned to each code in subcategory H40.3 to designate the stage of glaucoma.
  - 0 stage unspecified
  - 1 mild stage
  - 2 moderate stage
  - 3 severe stage
  - 4 indeterminate stage

  - ✓x 7th **H40.30** Glaucoma secondary to eye trauma, unspecified eye [Rx]
  - ✓x 7th **H40.31** Glaucoma secondary to eye trauma, right eye [Rx]
  - ✓x 7th **H40.32** Glaucoma secondary to eye trauma, left eye [Rx]

Chapter 7. Diseases of the Eye and Adnexa

H40.33 Glaucoma secondary to eye trauma, **bilateral** ℞

H40.4 Glaucoma **secondary** to eye **inflammation**
Code also underlying condition

> One of the following 7th characters is to be assigned to each code in subcategory H40.4 to designate the stage of glaucoma.
> 0 stage unspecified
> 1 mild stage
> 2 moderate stage
> 3 severe stage
> 4 indeterminate stage

H40.40 Glaucoma secondary to eye inflammation, unspecified eye ℞
H40.41 Glaucoma secondary to eye inflammation, **right** eye ℞
H40.42 Glaucoma secondary to eye inflammation, **left** eye ℞
H40.43 Glaucoma secondary to eye inflammation, **bilateral** ℞

H40.5 Glaucoma **secondary** to other **eye disorders**
Code also underlying eye disorder

> One of the following 7th characters is to be assigned to each code in subcategory H40.5 to designate the stage of glaucoma.
> 0 stage unspecified
> 1 mild stage
> 2 moderate stage
> 3 severe stage
> 4 indeterminate stage

H40.50 Glaucoma secondary to other eye disorders, unspecified eye ℞
H40.51 Glaucoma secondary to other eye disorders, **right** eye ℞
H40.52 Glaucoma secondary to other eye disorders, **left** eye ℞
H40.53 Glaucoma secondary to other eye disorders, **bilateral** ℞

H40.6 Glaucoma **secondary** to **drugs**
Use additional code for adverse effect, if applicable, to identify drug (T36-T50 with fifth or sixth character 5)

> One of the following 7th characters is to be assigned to each code in subcategory H40.6 to designate the stage of glaucoma
> 0 stage unspecified
> 1 mild stage
> 2 moderate stage
> 3 severe stage
> 4 indeterminate stage

H40.60 Glaucoma secondary to drugs, unspecified eye ℞
H40.61 Glaucoma secondary to drugs, **right** eye ℞
H40.62 Glaucoma secondary to drugs, **left** eye ℞
H40.63 Glaucoma secondary to drugs, **bilateral** ℞

H40.8 Other glaucoma
  H40.81 Glaucoma with **increased episcleral venous pressure**
    H40.811 Glaucoma with increased episcleral venous pressure, **right** eye ℞
    H40.812 Glaucoma with increased episcleral venous pressure, **left** eye ℞
    H40.813 Glaucoma with increased episcleral venous pressure, **bilateral** ℞
    H40.819 Glaucoma with increased episcleral venous pressure, unspecified eye ℞
  H40.82 **Hypersecretion** glaucoma
    H40.821 Hypersecretion glaucoma, **right** eye ℞
    H40.822 Hypersecretion glaucoma, **left** eye ℞
    H40.823 Hypersecretion glaucoma, **bilateral** ℞
    H40.829 Hypersecretion glaucoma, unspecified eye ℞
  H40.83 **Aqueous misdirection**
    Malignant glaucoma
    H40.831 Aqueous misdirection, **right** eye ℞
    H40.832 Aqueous misdirection, **left** eye ℞
    H40.833 Aqueous misdirection, **bilateral** ℞
    H40.839 Aqueous misdirection, unspecified eye ℞
  H40.84 **Neovascular secondary angle closure** glaucoma
    Code first the underlying condition such as:
    central retinal vein occlusion (H34.81)
    diabetes mellitus (E08.39, E09.39, E10.39, E11.39, E13.39)
    retinal ischemia (H35.82)
    • **H40.841** Neovascular secondary angle closure glaucoma, **right** eye
    • **H40.842** Neovascular secondary angle closure glaucoma, **left** eye
    • **H40.843** Neovascular secondary angle closure glaucoma, **bilateral**
    • **H40.849** Neovascular secondary angle closure glaucoma, unspecified eye
  H40.89 Other specified glaucoma ℞

H40.9 Unspecified glaucoma ℞

H42 Glaucoma in diseases classified elsewhere ℞
Code first underlying condition, such as:
amyloidosis (E85.-)
aniridia (Q13.1)
glaucoma (in) diabetes mellitus (E08.39, E09.39, E10.39, E11.39, E13.39)
Lowe's syndrome (E72.03)
Rieger anomaly (Q13.81)
specified metabolic disorder (E70-E88)
EXCLUDES 1 glaucoma (in) onchocerciasis (B73.02)
glaucoma (in) syphilis (A52.71)
glaucoma (in) tuberculous (A18.59)
▶neovascular secondary angle closure glaucoma (H40.84-)◀

Disorders of vitreous body and globe (H43-H44)

H43 Disorders of vitreous body
  H43.0 Vitreous **prolapse**
    EXCLUDES 1 traumatic vitreous prolapse (S05.2-)
    vitreous syndrome following cataract surgery (H59.0-)
    H43.00 Vitreous prolapse, unspecified eye
    H43.01 Vitreous prolapse, **right** eye
    H43.02 Vitreous prolapse, **left** eye
    H43.03 Vitreous prolapse, **bilateral**
  H43.1 Vitreous **hemorrhage**
    H43.10 Vitreous hemorrhage, unspecified eye HCC ESR
    H43.11 Vitreous hemorrhage, **right** eye HCC ESR
    H43.12 Vitreous hemorrhage, **left** eye HCC ESR
    H43.13 Vitreous hemorrhage, **bilateral** HCC ESR
  H43.2 **Crystalline deposits** in vitreous body
    H43.20 Crystalline deposits in vitreous body, unspecified eye
    H43.21 Crystalline deposits in vitreous body, **right** eye
    H43.22 Crystalline deposits in vitreous body, **left** eye
    H43.23 Crystalline deposits in vitreous body, **bilateral**
  H43.3 Other vitreous opacities
    H43.31 Vitreous **membranes and strands**
      H43.311 Vitreous membranes and strands, **right** eye
      H43.312 Vitreous membranes and strands, **left** eye
      H43.313 Vitreous membranes and strands, **bilateral**
      H43.319 Vitreous membranes and strands, unspecified eye
    H43.39 Other vitreous opacities
      Vitreous floaters
      H43.391 Other vitreous opacities, **right** eye
      H43.392 Other vitreous opacities, **left** eye
      H43.393 Other vitreous opacities, **bilateral**
      H43.399 Other vitreous opacities, unspecified eye
  H43.8 Other disorders of vitreous body
    EXCLUDES 1 proliferative vitreo-retinopathy with retinal detachment (H33.4-)
    EXCLUDES 2 vitreous abscess (H44.02-)
    H43.81 Vitreous **degeneration**
      Vitreous detachment
      H43.811 Vitreous degeneration, **right** eye
      H43.812 Vitreous degeneration, **left** eye
      H43.813 Vitreous degeneration, **bilateral**
      H43.819 Vitreous degeneration, unspecified eye
    H43.82 Vitreomacular **adhesion**
      Vitreomacular traction
      H43.821 Vitreomacular adhesion, **right** eye A
      H43.822 Vitreomacular adhesion, **left** eye A

HCC CMS-HCC | ℞ Rx HCC | ESR ESRD HCC | COM Commercial HCC | N Newborn: 0 | P Pediatric: 0-17 | M Maternity: 9-64 | A Adult: 15-124

	H43.823	Vitreomacular adhesion, bilateral		H44.2B2	Degenerative myopia with macular hole, left eye
	H43.829	Vitreomacular adhesion, unspecified eye		H44.2B3	Degenerative myopia with macular hole, bilateral
H43.89		Other disorders of vitreous body		H44.2B9	Degenerative myopia with macular hole, unspecified eye
H43.9		Unspecified disorder of vitreous body			

H44 Disorders of globe

INCLUDES disorders affecting multiple structures of eye

H44.0 Purulent endophthalmitis
Use additional code to identify organism
EXCLUDES 1 bleb associated endophthalmitis (H59.4-)

- H44.00 Unspecified purulent endophthalmitis
  - H44.001 Unspecified purulent endophthalmitis, right eye
  - H44.002 Unspecified purulent endophthalmitis, left eye
  - H44.003 Unspecified purulent endophthalmitis, bilateral
  - H44.009 Unspecified purulent endophthalmitis, unspecified eye
- H44.01 Panophthalmitis (acute)
  - H44.011 Panophthalmitis (acute), right eye
  - H44.012 Panophthalmitis (acute), left eye
  - H44.013 Panophthalmitis (acute), bilateral
  - H44.019 Panophthalmitis (acute), unspecified eye
- H44.02 Vitreous abscess (chronic)
  - H44.021 Vitreous abscess (chronic), right eye
  - H44.022 Vitreous abscess (chronic), left eye
  - H44.023 Vitreous abscess (chronic), bilateral
  - H44.029 Vitreous abscess (chronic), unspecified eye

H44.1 Other endophthalmitis
EXCLUDES 1 bleb associated endophthalmitis (H59.4-)
EXCLUDES 2 ophthalmia nodosa (H16.2-)

- H44.11 Panuveitis
  DEF: Inflammation of all layers of the uvea of the eye, including the choroid, iris, and ciliary body. It also typically involves the lens, retina, optic nerve, and vitreous and causes reduced vision or blindness.
  - H44.111 Panuveitis, right eye
  - H44.112 Panuveitis, left eye
  - H44.113 Panuveitis, bilateral
  - H44.119 Panuveitis, unspecified eye
- H44.12 Parasitic endophthalmitis, unspecified
  - H44.121 Parasitic endophthalmitis, unspecified, right eye
  - H44.122 Parasitic endophthalmitis, unspecified, left eye
  - H44.123 Parasitic endophthalmitis, unspecified, bilateral
  - H44.129 Parasitic endophthalmitis, unspecified, unspecified eye
- H44.13 Sympathetic uveitis
  - H44.131 Sympathetic uveitis, right eye
  - H44.132 Sympathetic uveitis, left eye
  - H44.133 Sympathetic uveitis, bilateral
  - H44.139 Sympathetic uveitis, unspecified eye
- H44.19 Other endophthalmitis

H44.2 Degenerative myopia
Malignant myopia
AHA: 2017,4Q,10-11

- H44.20 Degenerative myopia, unspecified eye
- H44.21 Degenerative myopia, right eye
- H44.22 Degenerative myopia, left eye
- H44.23 Degenerative myopia, bilateral
- H44.2A Degenerative myopia with choroidal neovascularization
  Use additional code for any associated choroid disorders (H31.-)
  - H44.2A1 Degenerative myopia with choroidal neovascularization, right eye
  - H44.2A2 Degenerative myopia with choroidal neovascularization, left eye
  - H44.2A3 Degenerative myopia with choroidal neovascularization, bilateral
  - H44.2A9 Degenerative myopia with choroidal neovascularization, unspecified eye
- H44.2B Degenerative myopia with macular hole
  - H44.2B1 Degenerative myopia with macular hole, right eye
- H44.2C Degenerative myopia with retinal detachment
  Use additional code to identify the retinal detachment (H33.-)
  - H44.2C1 Degenerative myopia with retinal detachment, right eye
  - H44.2C2 Degenerative myopia with retinal detachment, left eye
  - H44.2C3 Degenerative myopia with retinal detachment, bilateral
  - H44.2C9 Degenerative myopia with retinal detachment, unspecified eye
- H44.2D Degenerative myopia with foveoschisis
  - H44.2D1 Degenerative myopia with foveoschisis, right eye
  - H44.2D2 Degenerative myopia with foveoschisis, left eye
  - H44.2D3 Degenerative myopia with foveoschisis, bilateral
  - H44.2D9 Degenerative myopia with foveoschisis, unspecified eye
- H44.2E Degenerative myopia with other maculopathy
  - H44.2E1 Degenerative myopia with other maculopathy, right eye
  - H44.2E2 Degenerative myopia with other maculopathy, left eye
  - H44.2E3 Degenerative myopia with other maculopathy, bilateral
  - H44.2E9 Degenerative myopia with other maculopathy, unspecified eye

H44.3 Other and unspecified degenerative disorders of globe
- H44.30 Unspecified degenerative disorder of globe
- H44.31 Chalcosis
  - H44.311 Chalcosis, right eye
  - H44.312 Chalcosis, left eye
  - H44.313 Chalcosis, bilateral
  - H44.319 Chalcosis, unspecified eye
- H44.32 Siderosis of eye
  DEF: Iron pigment deposits within tissue of the eyeball caused by high iron content of the blood. Symptoms include cataracts, rust-colored anterior subcapsular deposits, iris heterochromia, pupillary mydriasis, and depressed electroretinogram amplitudes.
  - H44.321 Siderosis of eye, right eye
  - H44.322 Siderosis of eye, left eye
  - H44.323 Siderosis of eye, bilateral
  - H44.329 Siderosis of eye, unspecified eye
- H44.39 Other degenerative disorders of globe
  - H44.391 Other degenerative disorders of globe, right eye
  - H44.392 Other degenerative disorders of globe, left eye
  - H44.393 Other degenerative disorders of globe, bilateral
  - H44.399 Other degenerative disorders of globe, unspecified eye

H44.4 Hypotony of eye
- H44.40 Unspecified hypotony of eye
- H44.41 Flat anterior chamber hypotony of eye
  - H44.411 Flat anterior chamber hypotony of right eye
  - H44.412 Flat anterior chamber hypotony of left eye
  - H44.413 Flat anterior chamber hypotony of eye, bilateral
  - H44.419 Flat anterior chamber hypotony of unspecified eye
- H44.42 Hypotony of eye due to ocular fistula
  - H44.421 Hypotony of right eye due to ocular fistula
  - H44.422 Hypotony of left eye due to ocular fistula
  - H44.423 Hypotony of eye due to ocular fistula, bilateral
  - H44.429 Hypotony of unspecified eye due to ocular fistula

H44.43 Hypotony of eye due to other ocular disorders
- **H44.431** Hypotony of eye due to other ocular disorders, right eye
- **H44.432** Hypotony of eye due to other ocular disorders, left eye
- **H44.433** Hypotony of eye due to other ocular disorders, bilateral
- **H44.439** Hypotony of eye due to other ocular disorders, unspecified eye

H44.44 Primary hypotony of eye
- **H44.441** Primary hypotony of right eye
- **H44.442** Primary hypotony of left eye
- **H44.443** Primary hypotony of eye, bilateral
- **H44.449** Primary hypotony of unspecified eye

H44.5 Degenerated conditions of globe
- **H44.50** Unspecified degenerated conditions of globe

H44.51 Absolute glaucoma
- **H44.511** Absolute glaucoma, right eye
- **H44.512** Absolute glaucoma, left eye
- **H44.513** Absolute glaucoma, bilateral
- **H44.519** Absolute glaucoma, unspecified eye

H44.52 Atrophy of globe
Phthisis bulbi
- **H44.521** Atrophy of globe, right eye
- **H44.522** Atrophy of globe, left eye
- **H44.523** Atrophy of globe, bilateral
- **H44.529** Atrophy of globe, unspecified eye

H44.53 Leucocoria
- **H44.531** Leucocoria, right eye
- **H44.532** Leucocoria, left eye
- **H44.533** Leucocoria, bilateral
- **H44.539** Leucocoria, unspecified eye

H44.6 Retained (old) intraocular foreign body, magnetic
Use additional code to identify magnetic foreign body (Z18.11)

EXCLUDES 1 current intraocular foreign body (S05.-)
EXCLUDES 2 retained foreign body in eyelid (H02.81-)
retained (old) foreign body following penetrating wound of orbit (H05.5-)
retained (old) intraocular foreign body, nonmagnetic (H44.7-)

H44.60 Unspecified retained (old) intraocular foreign body, magnetic
- **H44.601** Unspecified retained (old) intraocular foreign body, magnetic, right eye
- **H44.602** Unspecified retained (old) intraocular foreign body, magnetic, left eye
- **H44.603** Unspecified retained (old) intraocular foreign body, magnetic, bilateral
- **H44.609** Unspecified retained (old) intraocular foreign body, magnetic, unspecified eye

H44.61 Retained (old) magnetic foreign body in anterior chamber
- **H44.611** Retained (old) magnetic foreign body in anterior chamber, right eye
- **H44.612** Retained (old) magnetic foreign body in anterior chamber, left eye
- **H44.613** Retained (old) magnetic foreign body in anterior chamber, bilateral
- **H44.619** Retained (old) magnetic foreign body in anterior chamber, unspecified eye

H44.62 Retained (old) magnetic foreign body in iris or ciliary body
- **H44.621** Retained (old) magnetic foreign body in iris or ciliary body, right eye
- **H44.622** Retained (old) magnetic foreign body in iris or ciliary body, left eye
- **H44.623** Retained (old) magnetic foreign body in iris or ciliary body, bilateral
- **H44.629** Retained (old) magnetic foreign body in iris or ciliary body, unspecified eye

H44.63 Retained (old) magnetic foreign body in lens
- **H44.631** Retained (old) magnetic foreign body in lens, right eye
- **H44.632** Retained (old) magnetic foreign body in lens, left eye
- **H44.633** Retained (old) magnetic foreign body in lens, bilateral
- **H44.639** Retained (old) magnetic foreign body in lens, unspecified eye

H44.64 Retained (old) magnetic foreign body in posterior wall of globe
- **H44.641** Retained (old) magnetic foreign body in posterior wall of globe, right eye
- **H44.642** Retained (old) magnetic foreign body in posterior wall of globe, left eye
- **H44.643** Retained (old) magnetic foreign body in posterior wall of globe, bilateral
- **H44.649** Retained (old) magnetic foreign body in posterior wall of globe, unspecified eye

H44.65 Retained (old) magnetic foreign body in vitreous body
- **H44.651** Retained (old) magnetic foreign body in vitreous body, right eye
- **H44.652** Retained (old) magnetic foreign body in vitreous body, left eye
- **H44.653** Retained (old) magnetic foreign body in vitreous body, bilateral
- **H44.659** Retained (old) magnetic foreign body in vitreous body, unspecified eye

H44.69 Retained (old) intraocular foreign body, magnetic, in other or multiple sites
- **H44.691** Retained (old) intraocular foreign body, magnetic, in other or multiple sites, right eye
- **H44.692** Retained (old) intraocular foreign body, magnetic, in other or multiple sites, left eye
- **H44.693** Retained (old) intraocular foreign body, magnetic, in other or multiple sites, bilateral
- **H44.699** Retained (old) intraocular foreign body, magnetic, in other or multiple sites, unspecified eye

H44.7 Retained (old) intraocular foreign body, nonmagnetic
Use additional code to identify nonmagnetic foreign body (Z18.01-Z18.10, Z18.12, Z18.2-Z18.9)

EXCLUDES 1 current intraocular foreign body (S05.-)
EXCLUDES 2 retained foreign body in eyelid (H02.81-)
retained (old) foreign body following penetrating wound of orbit (H05.5-)
retained (old) intraocular foreign body, magnetic (H44.6-)

H44.70 Unspecified retained (old) intraocular foreign body, nonmagnetic
- **H44.701** Unspecified retained (old) intraocular foreign body, nonmagnetic, right eye
- **H44.702** Unspecified retained (old) intraocular foreign body, nonmagnetic, left eye
- **H44.703** Unspecified retained (old) intraocular foreign body, nonmagnetic, bilateral
- **H44.709** Unspecified retained (old) intraocular foreign body, nonmagnetic, unspecified eye
  Retained (old) intraocular foreign body NOS

H44.71 Retained (nonmagnetic) (old) foreign body in anterior chamber
- **H44.711** Retained (nonmagnetic) (old) foreign body in anterior chamber, right eye
- **H44.712** Retained (nonmagnetic) (old) foreign body in anterior chamber, left eye
- **H44.713** Retained (nonmagnetic) (old) foreign body in anterior chamber, bilateral
- **H44.719** Retained (nonmagnetic) (old) foreign body in anterior chamber, unspecified eye

H44.72 Retained (nonmagnetic) (old) foreign body in iris or ciliary body
- **H44.721** Retained (nonmagnetic) (old) foreign body in iris or ciliary body, right eye
- **H44.722** Retained (nonmagnetic) (old) foreign body in iris or ciliary body, left eye
- **H44.723** Retained (nonmagnetic) (old) foreign body in iris or ciliary body, bilateral
- **H44.729** Retained (nonmagnetic) (old) foreign body in iris or ciliary body, unspecified eye

H44.73 Retained (nonmagnetic) (old) foreign body in lens
- **H44.731** Retained (nonmagnetic) (old) foreign body in lens, right eye
- **H44.732** Retained (nonmagnetic) (old) foreign body in lens, left eye
- **H44.733** Retained (nonmagnetic) (old) foreign body in lens, bilateral

H44.739 Retained (nonmagnetic) (old) foreign body in lens, unspecified eye

✓6th **H44.74 Retained (nonmagnetic) (old) foreign body in posterior wall of globe**
- H44.741 Retained (nonmagnetic) (old) foreign body in posterior wall of globe, right eye
- H44.742 Retained (nonmagnetic) (old) foreign body in posterior wall of globe, left eye
- H44.743 Retained (nonmagnetic) (old) foreign body in posterior wall of globe, bilateral
- H44.749 Retained (nonmagnetic) (old) foreign body in posterior wall of globe, unspecified eye

✓6th **H44.75 Retained (nonmagnetic) (old) foreign body in vitreous body**
- H44.751 Retained (nonmagnetic) (old) foreign body in vitreous body, right eye
- H44.752 Retained (nonmagnetic) (old) foreign body in vitreous body, left eye
- H44.753 Retained (nonmagnetic) (old) foreign body in vitreous body, bilateral
- H44.759 Retained (nonmagnetic) (old) foreign body in vitreous body, unspecified eye

✓6th **H44.79 Retained (old) intraocular foreign body, nonmagnetic, in other or multiple sites**
- H44.791 Retained (old) intraocular foreign body, nonmagnetic, in other or multiple sites, right eye
- H44.792 Retained (old) intraocular foreign body, nonmagnetic, in other or multiple sites, left eye
- H44.793 Retained (old) intraocular foreign body, nonmagnetic, in other or multiple sites, bilateral
- H44.799 Retained (old) intraocular foreign body, nonmagnetic, in other or multiple sites, unspecified eye

✓5th **H44.8 Other disorders of globe**

✓6th **H44.81 Hemophthalmos**
   DEF: Pool of blood within the eyeball, not from a current injury.
- H44.811 Hemophthalmos, right eye
- H44.812 Hemophthalmos, left eye
- H44.813 Hemophthalmos, bilateral
- H44.819 Hemophthalmos, unspecified eye

✓6th **H44.82 Luxation of globe**
- H44.821 Luxation of globe, right eye
- H44.822 Luxation of globe, left eye
- H44.823 Luxation of globe, bilateral
- H44.829 Luxation of globe, unspecified eye

H44.89 Other disorders of globe
   AHA: 2022,1Q,33

H44.9 Unspecified disorder of globe

Disorders of optic nerve and visual pathways (H46-H47)

✓4th **H46 Optic neuritis**
   EXCLUDES 2: ischemic optic neuropathy (H47.01-)
   neuromyelitis optica [Devic] (G36.0)

✓5th **H46.0 Optic papillitis**
- H46.00 Optic papillitis, unspecified eye
- H46.01 Optic papillitis, right eye
- H46.02 Optic papillitis, left eye
- H46.03 Optic papillitis, bilateral

✓5th **H46.1 Retrobulbar neuritis**
   Retrobulbar neuritis NOS
   EXCLUDES 1: syphilitic retrobulbar neuritis (A52.15)
- H46.10 Retrobulbar neuritis, unspecified eye
- H46.11 Retrobulbar neuritis, right eye
- H46.12 Retrobulbar neuritis, left eye
- H46.13 Retrobulbar neuritis, bilateral

H46.2 Nutritional optic neuropathy

H46.3 Toxic optic neuropathy
   Code first (T51-T65) to identify cause

H46.8 Other optic neuritis

H46.9 Unspecified optic neuritis
   AHA: 2023,3Q,19

✓4th **H47 Other disorders of optic [2nd] nerve and visual pathways**

✓5th **H47.0 Disorders of optic nerve, not elsewhere classified**

✓6th **H47.01 Ischemic optic neuropathy**
- H47.011 Ischemic optic neuropathy, right eye
- H47.012 Ischemic optic neuropathy, left eye
- H47.013 Ischemic optic neuropathy, bilateral
- H47.019 Ischemic optic neuropathy, unspecified eye

✓6th **H47.02 Hemorrhage in optic nerve sheath**
- H47.021 Hemorrhage in optic nerve sheath, right eye
- H47.022 Hemorrhage in optic nerve sheath, left eye
- H47.023 Hemorrhage in optic nerve sheath, bilateral
- H47.029 Hemorrhage in optic nerve sheath, unspecified eye

✓6th **H47.03 Optic nerve hypoplasia**
- H47.031 Optic nerve hypoplasia, right eye
- H47.032 Optic nerve hypoplasia, left eye
- H47.033 Optic nerve hypoplasia, bilateral
- H47.039 Optic nerve hypoplasia, unspecified eye

✓6th **H47.09 Other disorders of optic nerve, not elsewhere classified**
   Compression of optic nerve
- H47.091 Other disorders of optic nerve, not elsewhere classified, right eye
- H47.092 Other disorders of optic nerve, not elsewhere classified, left eye
- H47.093 Other disorders of optic nerve, not elsewhere classified, bilateral
- H47.099 Other disorders of optic nerve, not elsewhere classified, unspecified eye

✓5th **H47.1 Papilledema**
   DEF: Swelling of the optic papilla, the raised area connected to the optic disk made up of nerves that enter the eyeball. It may be caused by increased intracranial pressure, decreased ocular pressure, or a retinal disorder.
- H47.10 Unspecified papilledema
- H47.11 Papilledema associated with increased intracranial pressure
- H47.12 Papilledema associated with decreased ocular pressure
- H47.13 Papilledema associated with retinal disorder

✓6th **H47.14 Foster-Kennedy syndrome**
- H47.141 Foster-Kennedy syndrome, right eye
- H47.142 Foster-Kennedy syndrome, left eye
- H47.143 Foster-Kennedy syndrome, bilateral
- H47.149 Foster-Kennedy syndrome, unspecified eye

✓5th **H47.2 Optic atrophy**
- H47.20 Unspecified optic atrophy

✓6th **H47.21 Primary optic atrophy**
- H47.211 Primary optic atrophy, right eye
- H47.212 Primary optic atrophy, left eye
- H47.213 Primary optic atrophy, bilateral
- H47.219 Primary optic atrophy, unspecified eye

H47.22 Hereditary optic atrophy
   Leber's optic atrophy

✓6th **H47.23 Glaucomatous optic atrophy**
- H47.231 Glaucomatous optic atrophy, right eye
- H47.232 Glaucomatous optic atrophy, left eye
- H47.233 Glaucomatous optic atrophy, bilateral
- H47.239 Glaucomatous optic atrophy, unspecified eye

✓6th **H47.29 Other optic atrophy**
   Temporal pallor of optic disc
- H47.291 Other optic atrophy, right eye
- H47.292 Other optic atrophy, left eye
- H47.293 Other optic atrophy, bilateral
- H47.299 Other optic atrophy, unspecified eye

✓5th **H47.3 Other disorders of optic disc**

✓6th **H47.31 Coloboma of optic disc**
- H47.311 Coloboma of optic disc, right eye
- H47.312 Coloboma of optic disc, left eye
- H47.313 Coloboma of optic disc, bilateral
- H47.319 Coloboma of optic disc, unspecified eye

Chapter 7. Diseases of the Eye and Adnexa

✓6th **H47.32** Drusen of optic disc
- H47.321 Drusen of optic disc, right eye
- H47.322 Drusen of optic disc, left eye
- H47.323 Drusen of optic disc, bilateral
- H47.329 Drusen of optic disc, unspecified eye

✓6th **H47.33** Pseudopapilledema of optic disc
- H47.331 Pseudopapilledema of optic disc, right eye
- H47.332 Pseudopapilledema of optic disc, left eye
- H47.333 Pseudopapilledema of optic disc, bilateral
- H47.339 Pseudopapilledema of optic disc, unspecified eye

✓6th **H47.39** Other disorders of optic disc
- H47.391 Other disorders of optic disc, right eye
- H47.392 Other disorders of optic disc, left eye
- H47.393 Other disorders of optic disc, bilateral
- H47.399 Other disorders of optic disc, unspecified eye

✓5th **H47.4** Disorders of optic chiasm
Code also underlying condition
- H47.41 Disorders of optic chiasm in (due to) inflammatory disorders
- H47.42 Disorders of optic chiasm in (due to) neoplasm
- H47.43 Disorders of optic chiasm in (due to) vascular disorders
- H47.49 Disorders of optic chiasm in (due to) other disorders

✓5th **H47.5** Disorders of other visual pathways
Disorders of optic tracts, geniculate nuclei and optic radiations
Code also underlying condition

✓6th **H47.51** Disorders of visual pathways in (due to) inflammatory disorders
- H47.511 Disorders of visual pathways in (due to) inflammatory disorders, right side
- H47.512 Disorders of visual pathways in (due to) inflammatory disorders, left side
- H47.519 Disorders of visual pathways in (due to) inflammatory disorders, unspecified side

✓6th **H47.52** Disorders of visual pathways in (due to) neoplasm
- H47.521 Disorders of visual pathways in (due to) neoplasm, right side
- H47.522 Disorders of visual pathways in (due to) neoplasm, left side
- H47.529 Disorders of visual pathways in (due to) neoplasm, unspecified side

✓6th **H47.53** Disorders of visual pathways in (due to) vascular disorders
- H47.531 Disorders of visual pathways in (due to) vascular disorders, right side
- H47.532 Disorders of visual pathways in (due to) vascular disorders, left side
- H47.539 Disorders of visual pathways in (due to) vascular disorders, unspecified side

✓5th **H47.6** Disorders of visual cortex
Code also underlying condition
EXCLUDES 1 injury to visual cortex S04.04-

✓6th **H47.61** Cortical blindness
- H47.611 Cortical blindness, right side of brain
- H47.612 Cortical blindness, left side of brain
- H47.619 Cortical blindness, unspecified side of brain

✓6th **H47.62** Disorders of visual cortex in (due to) inflammatory disorders
- H47.621 Disorders of visual cortex in (due to) inflammatory disorders, right side of brain
- H47.622 Disorders of visual cortex in (due to) inflammatory disorders, left side of brain
- H47.629 Disorders of visual cortex in (due to) inflammatory disorders, unspecified side of brain

✓6th **H47.63** Disorders of visual cortex in (due to) neoplasm
- H47.631 Disorders of visual cortex in (due to) neoplasm, right side of brain
- H47.632 Disorders of visual cortex in (due to) neoplasm, left side of brain
- H47.639 Disorders of visual cortex in (due to) neoplasm, unspecified side of brain

✓6th **H47.64** Disorders of visual cortex in (due to) vascular disorders
- H47.641 Disorders of visual cortex in (due to) vascular disorders, right side of brain
- H47.642 Disorders of visual cortex in (due to) vascular disorders, left side of brain
- H47.649 Disorders of visual cortex in (due to) vascular disorders, unspecified side of brain

H47.9 Unspecified disorder of visual pathways

Disorders of ocular muscles, binocular movement, accommodation and refraction (H49-H52)

EXCLUDES 2 nystagmus and other irregular eye movements (H55)

✓4th **H49** Paralytic strabismus
EXCLUDES 2 internal ophthalmoplegia (H52.51-)
internuclear ophthalmoplegia (H51.2-)
progressive supranuclear ophthalmoplegia (G23.1)
DEF: Strabismus: Misalignment of the eyes with the inability to move and focus in the same direction due to conditions affecting the muscles controlling them.

✓5th **H49.0** Third [oculomotor] nerve palsy
- H49.00 Third [oculomotor] nerve palsy, unspecified eye
- H49.01 Third [oculomotor] nerve palsy, right eye
- H49.02 Third [oculomotor] nerve palsy, left eye
- H49.03 Third [oculomotor] nerve palsy, bilateral

✓5th **H49.1** Fourth [trochlear] nerve palsy
- H49.10 Fourth [trochlear] nerve palsy, unspecified eye
- H49.11 Fourth [trochlear] nerve palsy, right eye
- H49.12 Fourth [trochlear] nerve palsy, left eye
- H49.13 Fourth [trochlear] nerve palsy, bilateral

✓5th **H49.2** Sixth [abducent] nerve palsy
- H49.20 Sixth [abducent] nerve palsy, unspecified eye
- H49.21 Sixth [abducent] nerve palsy, right eye
- H49.22 Sixth [abducent] nerve palsy, left eye
- H49.23 Sixth [abducent] nerve palsy, bilateral

✓5th **H49.3** Total (external) ophthalmoplegia
- H49.30 Total (external) ophthalmoplegia, unspecified eye
- H49.31 Total (external) ophthalmoplegia, right eye
- H49.32 Total (external) ophthalmoplegia, left eye
- H49.33 Total (external) ophthalmoplegia, bilateral

✓5th **H49.4** Progressive external ophthalmoplegia
EXCLUDES 1 Kearns-Sayre syndrome (H49.81-)
- H49.40 Progressive external ophthalmoplegia, unspecified eye
- H49.41 Progressive external ophthalmoplegia, right eye
- H49.42 Progressive external ophthalmoplegia, left eye
- H49.43 Progressive external ophthalmoplegia, bilateral

✓5th **H49.8** Other paralytic strabismus

✓6th **H49.81** Kearns-Sayre syndrome
Progressive external ophthalmoplegia with pigmentary retinopathy
Code also, if applicable, other manifestations, such as: heart block (I45.9)
- H49.811 Kearns-Sayre syndrome, right eye Rx ESR COM
- H49.812 Kearns-Sayre syndrome, left eye Rx ESR COM
- H49.813 Kearns-Sayre syndrome, bilateral Rx ESR COM
- H49.819 Kearns-Sayre syndrome, unspecified eye Rx ESR COM

✓6th **H49.88** Other paralytic strabismus
External ophthalmoplegia NOS
- H49.881 Other paralytic strabismus, right eye
- H49.882 Other paralytic strabismus, left eye
- H49.883 Other paralytic strabismus, bilateral
- H49.889 Other paralytic strabismus, unspecified eye

H49.9 Unspecified paralytic strabismus

✓4th **H50** Other strabismus
DEF: Strabismus: Misalignment of the eyes with the inability to move and focus in the same direction due to conditions affecting the muscles controlling them.

✓5th **H50.0** Esotropia
Convergent concomitant strabismus
EXCLUDES 1 intermittent esotropia (H50.31-, H50.32)
- H50.00 Unspecified esotropia

✓6th **H50.01** Monocular esotropia
- H50.011 Monocular esotropia, right eye

H50.012 Monocular esotropia, left eye
✓6ᵗʰ H50.02 Monocular esotropia with A pattern
H50.021 Monocular esotropia with A pattern, right eye
H50.022 Monocular esotropia with A pattern, left eye
✓6ᵗʰ H50.03 Monocular esotropia with V pattern
H50.031 Monocular esotropia with V pattern, right eye
H50.032 Monocular esotropia with V pattern, left eye
✓6ᵗʰ H50.04 Monocular esotropia with other noncomitancies
H50.041 Monocular esotropia with other noncomitancies, right eye
H50.042 Monocular esotropia with other noncomitancies, left eye
H50.05 Alternating esotropia
H50.06 Alternating esotropia with A pattern
H50.07 Alternating esotropia with V pattern
H50.08 Alternating esotropia with other noncomitancies

Eye Muscle Diseases

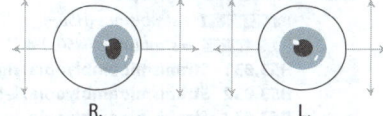
Monocular (one eye only) esotropia (inward)

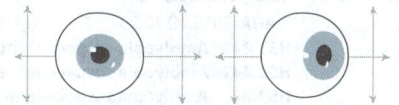
Monocular exotropia (outward)

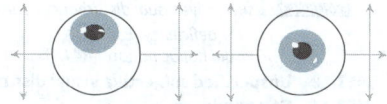
Monocular hypertropia (upward)

✓5ᵗʰ H50.1 Exotropia
Divergent concomitant strabismus
EXCLUDES 1 intermittent exotropia (H50.33-, H50.34)
H50.10 Unspecified exotropia
✓6ᵗʰ H50.11 Monocular exotropia
H50.111 Monocular exotropia, right eye
H50.112 Monocular exotropia, left eye
✓6ᵗʰ H50.12 Monocular exotropia with A pattern
H50.121 Monocular exotropia with A pattern, right eye
H50.122 Monocular exotropia with A pattern, left eye
✓6ᵗʰ H50.13 Monocular exotropia with V pattern
H50.131 Monocular exotropia with V pattern, right eye
H50.132 Monocular exotropia with V pattern, left eye
✓6ᵗʰ H50.14 Monocular exotropia with other noncomitancies
H50.141 Monocular exotropia with other noncomitancies, right eye
H50.142 Monocular exotropia with other noncomitancies, left eye
H50.15 Alternating exotropia
H50.16 Alternating exotropia with A pattern
H50.17 Alternating exotropia with V pattern
H50.18 Alternating exotropia with other noncomitancies
✓5ᵗʰ H50.2 Vertical strabismus
Hypertropia
H50.21 Vertical strabismus, right eye
H50.22 Vertical strabismus, left eye
✓5ᵗʰ H50.3 Intermittent heterotropia
H50.30 Unspecified intermittent heterotropia
✓6ᵗʰ H50.31 Intermittent monocular esotropia
H50.311 Intermittent monocular esotropia, right eye

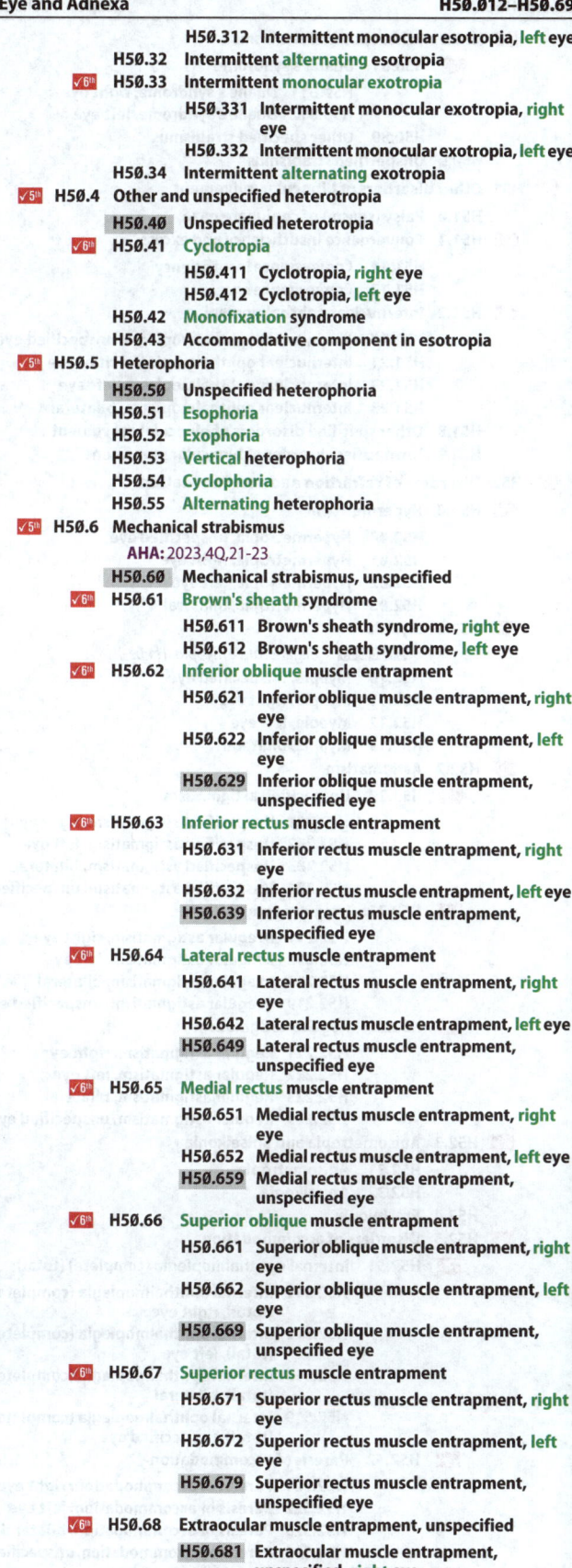

H50.8 Other specified strabismus
H50.81 Duane's syndrome
- H50.811 Duane's syndrome, right eye
- H50.812 Duane's syndrome, left eye
H50.89 Other specified strabismus
H50.9 Unspecified strabismus

H51 Other disorders of binocular movement
H51.0 Palsy (spasm) of conjugate gaze
H51.1 Convergence insufficiency and excess
- H51.11 Convergence insufficiency
- H51.12 Convergence excess
H51.2 Internuclear ophthalmoplegia
- H51.20 Internuclear ophthalmoplegia, unspecified eye
- H51.21 Internuclear ophthalmoplegia, right eye
- H51.22 Internuclear ophthalmoplegia, left eye
- H51.23 Internuclear ophthalmoplegia, bilateral
H51.8 Other specified disorders of binocular movement
H51.9 Unspecified disorder of binocular movement

H52 Disorders of refraction and accommodation
H52.0 Hypermetropia
- H52.00 Hypermetropia, unspecified eye
- H52.01 Hypermetropia, right eye
- H52.02 Hypermetropia, left eye
- H52.03 Hypermetropia, bilateral
H52.1 Myopia
EXCLUDES 1 degenerative myopia (H44.2-)
- H52.10 Myopia, unspecified eye
- H52.11 Myopia, right eye
- H52.12 Myopia, left eye
- H52.13 Myopia, bilateral
H52.2 Astigmatism
- H52.20 Unspecified astigmatism
  - H52.201 Unspecified astigmatism, right eye
  - H52.202 Unspecified astigmatism, left eye
  - H52.203 Unspecified astigmatism, bilateral
  - H52.209 Unspecified astigmatism, unspecified eye
- H52.21 Irregular astigmatism
  - H52.211 Irregular astigmatism, right eye
  - H52.212 Irregular astigmatism, left eye
  - H52.213 Irregular astigmatism, bilateral
  - H52.219 Irregular astigmatism, unspecified eye
- H52.22 Regular astigmatism
  - H52.221 Regular astigmatism, right eye
  - H52.222 Regular astigmatism, left eye
  - H52.223 Regular astigmatism, bilateral
  - H52.229 Regular astigmatism, unspecified eye
H52.3 Anisometropia and aniseikonia
- H52.31 Anisometropia
- H52.32 Aniseikonia
H52.4 Presbyopia
H52.5 Disorders of accommodation
- H52.51 Internal ophthalmoplegia (complete) (total)
  - H52.511 Internal ophthalmoplegia (complete) (total), right eye
  - H52.512 Internal ophthalmoplegia (complete) (total), left eye
  - H52.513 Internal ophthalmoplegia (complete) (total), bilateral
  - H52.519 Internal ophthalmoplegia (complete) (total), unspecified eye
- H52.52 Paresis of accommodation
  - H52.521 Paresis of accommodation, right eye
  - H52.522 Paresis of accommodation, left eye
  - H52.523 Paresis of accommodation, bilateral
  - H52.529 Paresis of accommodation, unspecified eye
- H52.53 Spasm of accommodation
  - H52.531 Spasm of accommodation, right eye
  - H52.532 Spasm of accommodation, left eye
  - H52.533 Spasm of accommodation, bilateral
  - H52.539 Spasm of accommodation, unspecified eye
H52.6 Other disorders of refraction
H52.7 Unspecified disorder of refraction

Visual disturbances and blindness (H53-H54)

H53 Visual disturbances
H53.0 Amblyopia ex anopsia
EXCLUDES 1 amblyopia due to vitamin A deficiency (E50.5)
- H53.00 Unspecified amblyopia
  - H53.001 Unspecified amblyopia, right eye
  - H53.002 Unspecified amblyopia, left eye
  - H53.003 Unspecified amblyopia, bilateral
  - H53.009 Unspecified amblyopia, unspecified eye
- H53.01 Deprivation amblyopia
  - H53.011 Deprivation amblyopia, right eye
  - H53.012 Deprivation amblyopia, left eye
  - H53.013 Deprivation amblyopia, bilateral
  - H53.019 Deprivation amblyopia, unspecified eye
- H53.02 Refractive amblyopia
  - H53.021 Refractive amblyopia, right eye
  - H53.022 Refractive amblyopia, left eye
  - H53.023 Refractive amblyopia, bilateral
  - H53.029 Refractive amblyopia, unspecified eye
- H53.03 Strabismic amblyopia
  EXCLUDES 1 strabismus (H50.-)
  EXCLUDES 2 ▶strabismus (H50.-)◄
  - H53.031 Strabismic amblyopia, right eye
  - H53.032 Strabismic amblyopia, left eye
  - H53.033 Strabismic amblyopia, bilateral
  - H53.039 Strabismic amblyopia, unspecified eye
- H53.04 Amblyopia suspect
  AHA: 2016,4Q,22-23
  - H53.041 Amblyopia suspect, right eye
  - H53.042 Amblyopia suspect, left eye
  - H53.043 Amblyopia suspect, bilateral
  - H53.049 Amblyopia suspect, unspecified eye
H53.1 Subjective visual disturbances
EXCLUDES 1 subjective visual disturbances due to vitamin A deficiency (E50.5)
visual hallucinations (R44.1)
- H53.10 Unspecified subjective visual disturbances
- H53.11 Day blindness
  Hemeralopia
- H53.12 Transient visual loss
  Scintillating scotoma
  EXCLUDES 1 amaurosis fugax (G45.3-)
  transient retinal artery occlusion (H34.0-)
  AHA: 2022,1Q,30
  - H53.121 Transient visual loss, right eye
  - H53.122 Transient visual loss, left eye
  - H53.123 Transient visual loss, bilateral
  - H53.129 Transient visual loss, unspecified eye
- H53.13 Sudden visual loss
  - H53.131 Sudden visual loss, right eye
  - H53.132 Sudden visual loss, left eye
  - H53.133 Sudden visual loss, bilateral
  - H53.139 Sudden visual loss, unspecified eye
- H53.14 Visual discomfort
  Asthenopia
  Photophobia
  - H53.141 Visual discomfort, right eye
  - H53.142 Visual discomfort, left eye
  - H53.143 Visual discomfort, bilateral
  - H53.149 Visual discomfort, unspecified
- H53.15 Visual distortions of shape and size
  Metamorphopsia
- H53.16 Psychophysical visual disturbances
- H53.19 Other subjective visual disturbances
  Visual halos
  AHA: 2022,1Q,30
H53.2 Diplopia
Double vision
H53.3 Other and unspecified disorders of binocular vision
- H53.30 Unspecified disorder of binocular vision
- H53.31 Abnormal retinal correspondence
- H53.32 Fusion with defective stereopsis
- H53.33 Simultaneous visual perception without fusion
- H53.34 Suppression of binocular vision

Chapter 7. Diseases of the Eye and Adnexa

H53.4 Visual field defects
- **H53.40** Unspecified visual field defects
- **H53.41** Scotoma involving central area
  - Central scotoma
  - AHA: 2022,1Q,30
  - **H53.411** Scotoma involving central area, right eye
  - **H53.412** Scotoma involving central area, left eye
  - **H53.413** Scotoma involving central area, bilateral
  - **H53.419** Scotoma involving central area, unspecified eye
- **H53.42** Scotoma of blind spot area
  - Enlarged blind spot
  - **H53.421** Scotoma of blind spot area, right eye
  - **H53.422** Scotoma of blind spot area, left eye
  - **H53.423** Scotoma of blind spot area, bilateral
  - **H53.429** Scotoma of blind spot area, unspecified eye
- **H53.43** Sector or arcuate defects
  - Arcuate scotoma
  - Bjerrum scotoma
  - **H53.431** Sector or arcuate defects, right eye
  - **H53.432** Sector or arcuate defects, left eye
  - **H53.433** Sector or arcuate defects, bilateral
  - **H53.439** Sector or arcuate defects, unspecified eye
- **H53.45** Other localized visual field defect
  - Peripheral visual field defect
  - Ring scotoma NOS
  - Scotoma NOS
  - **H53.451** Other localized visual field defect, right eye
  - **H53.452** Other localized visual field defect, left eye
  - **H53.453** Other localized visual field defect, bilateral
  - **H53.459** Other localized visual field defect, unspecified eye
- **H53.46** Homonymous bilateral field defects
  - Homonymous hemianopia
  - Homonymous hemianopsia
  - Quadrant anopia
  - Quadrant anopsia
  - **H53.461** Homonymous bilateral field defects, right side
  - **H53.462** Homonymous bilateral field defects, left side
  - **H53.469** Homonymous bilateral field defects, unspecified side
    - Homonymous bilateral field defects NOS
- **H53.47** Heteronymous bilateral field defects
  - Heteronymous hemianop(s)ia
- **H53.48** Generalized contraction of visual field
  - **H53.481** Generalized contraction of visual field, right eye
  - **H53.482** Generalized contraction of visual field, left eye
  - **H53.483** Generalized contraction of visual field, bilateral
  - **H53.489** Generalized contraction of visual field, unspecified eye

H53.5 Color vision deficiencies
- Color blindness
- EXCLUDES 2: day blindness (H53.11)
- **H53.50** Unspecified color vision deficiencies
  - Color blindness NOS
- **H53.51** Achromatopsia
  - DEF: Nonprogressive genetic visual disorder characterized by complete color blindness, decreased vision, and light sensitivity.
- **H53.52** Acquired color vision deficiency
- **H53.53** Deuteranomaly
  - Deuteranopia
  - DEF: Male-only genetic disorder causing difficulty in distinguishing green and red; no shortened spectrum.
- **H53.54** Protanomaly
  - Protanopia
- **H53.55** Tritanomaly
  - Tritanopia
- **H53.59** Other color vision deficiencies

H53.6 Night blindness
- EXCLUDES 1: night blindness due to vitamin A deficiency (E50.5)
- **H53.60** Unspecified night blindness
- **H53.61** Abnormal dark adaptation curve
- **H53.62** Acquired night blindness
- **H53.63** Congenital night blindness
- **H53.69** Other night blindness

H53.7 Vision sensitivity deficiencies
- **H53.71** Glare sensitivity
- **H53.72** Impaired contrast sensitivity

H53.8 Other visual disturbances

H53.9 Unspecified visual disturbance

H54 Blindness and low vision
- NOTE: For definition of visual impairment categories see table below
- Code first any associated underlying cause of the blindness
- EXCLUDES 1: amaurosis fugax (G45.3)
- AHA: 2017,4Q,11-12

- **H54.0** Blindness, both eyes
  - Visual impairment categories 3, 4, 5 in both eyes.
  - **H54.0X** Blindness, both eyes, different category levels
    - **H54.0X3** Blindness right eye, category 3
      - **H54.0X33** Blindness right eye category 3, blindness left eye category 3
      - **H54.0X34** Blindness right eye category 3, blindness left eye category 4
      - **H54.0X35** Blindness right eye category 3, blindness left eye category 5
    - **H54.0X4** Blindness right eye, category 4
      - **H54.0X43** Blindness right eye category 4, blindness left eye category 3
      - **H54.0X44** Blindness right eye category 4, blindness left eye category 4
      - **H54.0X45** Blindness right eye category 4, blindness left eye category 5
    - **H54.0X5** Blindness right eye, category 5
      - **H54.0X53** Blindness right eye category 5, blindness left eye category 3
      - **H54.0X54** Blindness right eye category 5, blindness left eye category 4
      - **H54.0X55** Blindness right eye category 5, blindness left eye category 5

- **H54.1** Blindness, one eye, low vision other eye
  - Visual impairment categories 3, 4, 5 in one eye, with categories 1 or 2 in the other eye.
  - **H54.10** Blindness, one eye, low vision other eye, unspecified eyes
  - **H54.11** Blindness, right eye, low vision left eye
    - **H54.113** Blindness right eye category 3, low vision left eye
      - **H54.1131** Blindness right eye category 3, low vision left eye category 1
      - **H54.1132** Blindness right eye category 3, low vision left eye category 2
    - **H54.114** Blindness right eye category 4, low vision left eye
      - **H54.1141** Blindness right eye category 4, low vision left eye category 1
      - **H54.1142** Blindness right eye category 4, low vision left eye category 2
    - **H54.115** Blindness right eye category 5, low vision left eye
      - **H54.1151** Blindness right eye category 5, low vision left eye category 1
      - **H54.1152** Blindness right eye category 5, low vision left eye category 2
  - **H54.12** Blindness, left eye, low vision right eye
    - **H54.121** Low vision right eye category 1, blindness left eye
      - **H54.1213** Low vision right eye category 1, blindness left eye category 3
      - **H54.1214** Low vision right eye category 1, blindness left eye category 4
      - **H54.1215** Low vision right eye category 1, blindness left eye category 5
    - **H54.122** Low vision right eye category 2, blindness left eye
      - **H54.1223** Low vision right eye category 2, blindness left eye category 3
      - **H54.1224** Low vision right eye category 2, blindness left eye category 4
      - **H54.1225** Low vision right eye category 2, blindness left eye category 5

H54.2–H57.10 Chapter 7. Diseases of the Eye and Adnexa

- **H54.2** Low vision, both eyes
  Visual impairment categories 1 or 2 in both eyes.
  - **H54.2X** Low vision, both eyes, different category levels
    - **H54.2X1** Low vision, right eye, category 1
      - H54.2X11 Low vision right eye category 1, low vision left eye category 1
      - H54.2X12 Low vision right eye category 1, low vision left eye category 2
    - **H54.2X2** Low vision, right eye, category 2
      - H54.2X21 Low vision right eye category 2, low vision left eye category 1
      - H54.2X22 Low vision right eye category 2, low vision left eye category 2
- **H54.3** Unqualified visual loss, both eyes
  Visual impairment category 9 in both eyes.
  TIP: Assign only when both eyes are documented as affected by blindness or low vision but the visual impairment category is not documented.
- **H54.4** Blindness, one eye
  Visual impairment categories 3, 4, 5 in one eye [normal vision in other eye]
  - H54.40 Blindness, one eye, unspecified eye
  - **H54.41** Blindness, right eye, normal vision left eye
    - **H54.413** Blindness, right eye, category 3
      - H54.413A Blindness right eye category 3, normal vision left eye
    - **H54.414** Blindness, right eye, category 4
      - H54.414A Blindness right eye category 4, normal vision left eye
    - **H54.415** Blindness, right eye, category 5
      - H54.415A Blindness right eye category 5, normal vision left eye
  - **H54.42** Blindness, left eye, normal vision right eye
    - **H54.42A** Blindness, left eye, category 3-5
      - H54.42A3 Blindness left eye category 3, normal vision right eye
      - H54.42A4 Blindness left eye category 4, normal vision right eye
      - H54.42A5 Blindness left eye category 5, normal vision right eye
- **H54.5** Low vision, one eye
  Visual impairment categories 1 or 2 in one eye [normal vision in other eye].
  - H54.50 Low vision, one eye, unspecified eye
  - **H54.51** Low vision, right eye, normal vision left eye
    - **H54.511** Low vision, right eye, category 1
      - H54.511A Low vision right eye category 1, normal vision left eye
    - **H54.512** Low vision, right eye, category 2
      - H54.512A Low vision right eye category 2, normal vision left eye
  - **H54.52** Low vision, left eye, normal vision right eye
    - **H54.52A** Low vision, left eye, category 1-2
      - H54.52A1 Low vision left eye category 1, normal vision right eye
      - H54.52A2 Low vision left eye category 2, normal vision right eye
- **H54.6** Unqualified visual loss, one eye
  Visual impairment category 9 in one eye [normal vision in other eye].
  TIP: Assign a code from this category only when one eye is documented as affected by blindness or low vision but the visual impairment category is not documented.
  - H54.60 Unqualified visual loss, one eye, unspecified
  - H54.61 Unqualified visual loss, right eye, normal vision left eye
  - H54.62 Unqualified visual loss, left eye, normal vision right eye
- **H54.7** Unspecified visual loss
  Visual impairment category 9 NOS
  TIP: Assign only when documentation specifies blindness, visual loss, or low vision but not whether one or both eyes are affected or the visual impairment category.
- **H54.8** Legal blindness, as defined in USA
  Blindness NOS according to USA definition
  EXCLUDES 1 legal blindness with specification of impairment level (H54.0-H54.7)
  NOTE The table below gives a classification of severity of visual impairment recommended by a WHO Study Group on the Prevention of Blindness, Geneva, 6-10 November 1972.

  If the extent of the visual field is taken into account, patients with a field no greater than 10 but greater than 5 around central fixation should be placed in category 3 and patients with a field no greater than 5 around central fixation should be placed in category 4, even if the central acuity is not impaired.

  The term "low vision" in category H54 comprises categories 1 and 2 of the table, the term "blindness" categories 3, 4 and 5, and the term "unqualified visual loss" category 9.

Category of visual impairment	Visual acuity with best possible correction	
	Maximum less than:	Minimum equal to or better than:
1	6/18 3/10 (0.3) 20/70	6/60 1/10 (0.1) 20/200
2	6/60 1/10 (0.1) 20/200	3/60 1/20 (0.05) 20/400
3	3/60 1/20 (0.05) 20/400	1/60 (finger counting at one meter) 1/50 (0.02) 5/300 (20/1200)
4	1/60 (finger counting at one meter) 1/50 (0.02) 5/300	Light perception
5	No light perception	
9	Undetermined or unspecified	

Other disorders of eye and adnexa (H55-H57)

- **H55** Nystagmus and other irregular eye movements
  - **H55.0** Nystagmus
    DEF: Rapid, rhythmic, involuntary movements of the eyeball in vertical, horizontal, rotational, or mixed directions.
    - H55.00 Unspecified nystagmus
    - H55.01 Congenital nystagmus
    - H55.02 Latent nystagmus
    - H55.03 Visual deprivation nystagmus
    - H55.04 Dissociated nystagmus
    - H55.09 Other forms of nystagmus
  - **H55.8** Other irregular eye movements
    AHA: 2020,4Q,25
    - H55.81 Deficient saccadic eye movements
    - H55.82 Deficient smooth pursuit eye movements
    - H55.89 Other irregular eye movements
- **H57** Other disorders of eye and adnexa
  - **H57.0** Anomalies of pupillary function
    - H57.00 Unspecified anomaly of pupillary function
    - H57.01 Argyll Robertson pupil, atypical
      EXCLUDES 1 syphilitic Argyll Robertson pupil (A52.19)
    - H57.02 Anisocoria
    - H57.03 Miosis
    - H57.04 Mydriasis
    - **H57.05** Tonic pupil
      - H57.051 Tonic pupil, right eye
      - H57.052 Tonic pupil, left eye
      - H57.053 Tonic pupil, bilateral
      - H57.059 Tonic pupil, unspecified eye
    - H57.09 Other anomalies of pupillary function
  - **H57.1** Ocular pain
    - H57.10 Ocular pain, unspecified eye

H57.11 Ocular pain, right eye
H57.12 Ocular pain, left eye
H57.13 Ocular pain, bilateral

H57.8 Other specified disorders of eye and adnexa
AHA: 2018,4Q,15-16

H57.81 Brow ptosis
H57.811 Brow ptosis, right
H57.812 Brow ptosis, left
H57.813 Brow ptosis, bilateral
H57.819 Brow ptosis, unspecified

H57.89 Other specified disorders of eye and adnexa

H57.8A Foreign body sensation eye (ocular)
AHA: 2023,4Q,23
H57.8A1 Foreign body sensation, right eye
H57.8A2 Foreign body sensation, left eye
H57.8A3 Foreign body sensation, bilateral eyes
H57.8A9 Foreign body sensation, unspecified eye

H57.9 Unspecified disorder of eye and adnexa

Intraoperative and postprocedural complications and disorders of eye and adnexa, not elsewhere classified (H59)

H59 Intraoperative and postprocedural complications and disorders of eye and adnexa, not elsewhere classified
EXCLUDES 1: mechanical complication of intraocular lens (T85.2)
mechanical complication of other ocular prosthetic devices, implants and grafts (T85.3)
pseudophakia (Z96.1)
secondary cataracts (H26.4-)

H59.0 Disorders of the eye following cataract surgery

H59.01 Keratopathy (bullous aphakic) following cataract surgery
Vitreal corneal syndrome
Vitreous (touch) syndrome
H59.011 Keratopathy (bullous aphakic) following cataract surgery, right eye
H59.012 Keratopathy (bullous aphakic) following cataract surgery, left eye
H59.013 Keratopathy (bullous aphakic) following cataract surgery, bilateral
H59.019 Keratopathy (bullous aphakic) following cataract surgery, unspecified eye

H59.02 Cataract (lens) fragments in eye following cataract surgery
H59.021 Cataract (lens) fragments in eye following cataract surgery, right eye
H59.022 Cataract (lens) fragments in eye following cataract surgery, left eye
H59.023 Cataract (lens) fragments in eye following cataract surgery, bilateral
H59.029 Cataract (lens) fragments in eye following cataract surgery, unspecified eye

H59.03 Cystoid macular edema following cataract surgery
H59.031 Cystoid macular edema following cataract surgery, right eye
H59.032 Cystoid macular edema following cataract surgery, left eye
H59.033 Cystoid macular edema following cataract surgery, bilateral
H59.039 Cystoid macular edema following cataract surgery, unspecified eye

H59.09 Other disorders of the eye following cataract surgery
H59.091 Other disorders of the right eye following cataract surgery
H59.092 Other disorders of the left eye following cataract surgery
H59.093 Other disorders of the eye following cataract surgery, bilateral
H59.099 Other disorders of unspecified eye following cataract surgery

H59.1 Intraoperative hemorrhage and hematoma of eye and adnexa complicating a procedure
EXCLUDES 1: intraoperative hemorrhage and hematoma of eye and adnexa due to accidental puncture or laceration during a procedure (H59.2-)

H59.11 Intraoperative hemorrhage and hematoma of eye and adnexa complicating an ophthalmic procedure
H59.111 Intraoperative hemorrhage and hematoma of right eye and adnexa complicating an ophthalmic procedure
H59.112 Intraoperative hemorrhage and hematoma of left eye and adnexa complicating an ophthalmic procedure
H59.113 Intraoperative hemorrhage and hematoma of eye and adnexa complicating an ophthalmic procedure, bilateral
H59.119 Intraoperative hemorrhage and hematoma of unspecified eye and adnexa complicating an ophthalmic procedure

H59.12 Intraoperative hemorrhage and hematoma of eye and adnexa complicating other procedure
H59.121 Intraoperative hemorrhage and hematoma of right eye and adnexa complicating other procedure
H59.122 Intraoperative hemorrhage and hematoma of left eye and adnexa complicating other procedure
H59.123 Intraoperative hemorrhage and hematoma of eye and adnexa complicating other procedure, bilateral
H59.129 Intraoperative hemorrhage and hematoma of unspecified eye and adnexa complicating other procedure

H59.2 Accidental puncture and laceration of eye and adnexa during a procedure

H59.21 Accidental puncture and laceration of eye and adnexa during an ophthalmic procedure
H59.211 Accidental puncture and laceration of right eye and adnexa during an ophthalmic procedure
H59.212 Accidental puncture and laceration of left eye and adnexa during an ophthalmic procedure
H59.213 Accidental puncture and laceration of eye and adnexa during an ophthalmic procedure, bilateral
H59.219 Accidental puncture and laceration of unspecified eye and adnexa during an ophthalmic procedure

H59.22 Accidental puncture and laceration of eye and adnexa during other procedure
H59.221 Accidental puncture and laceration of right eye and adnexa during other procedure
H59.222 Accidental puncture and laceration of left eye and adnexa during other procedure
H59.223 Accidental puncture and laceration of eye and adnexa during other procedure, bilateral
H59.229 Accidental puncture and laceration of unspecified eye and adnexa during other procedure

H59.3 Postprocedural hemorrhage, hematoma, and seroma of eye and adnexa following a procedure
AHA: 2016,4Q,9-10

H59.31 Postprocedural hemorrhage of eye and adnexa following an ophthalmic procedure
H59.311 Postprocedural hemorrhage of right eye and adnexa following an ophthalmic procedure
H59.312 Postprocedural hemorrhage of left eye and adnexa following an ophthalmic procedure
H59.313 Postprocedural hemorrhage of eye and adnexa following an ophthalmic procedure, bilateral
H59.319 Postprocedural hemorrhage of unspecified eye and adnexa following an ophthalmic procedure

H59.32 Postprocedural hemorrhage of eye and adnexa following other procedure
H59.321 Postprocedural hemorrhage of right eye and adnexa following other procedure
H59.322 Postprocedural hemorrhage of left eye and adnexa following other procedure
H59.323 Postprocedural hemorrhage of eye and adnexa following other procedure, bilateral
H59.329 Postprocedural hemorrhage of unspecified eye and adnexa following other procedure

H59.33 Postprocedural hematoma of eye and adnexa following an ophthalmic procedure
H59.331 Postprocedural hematoma of right eye and adnexa following an ophthalmic procedure
H59.332 Postprocedural hematoma of left eye and adnexa following an ophthalmic procedure

		H59.333	Postprocedural hematoma of eye and adnexa following an ophthalmic procedure, bilateral
		H59.339	Postprocedural hematoma of unspecified eye and adnexa following an ophthalmic procedure
	√6ᵗʰ H59.34		Postprocedural hematoma of eye and adnexa following other procedure
		H59.341	Postprocedural hematoma of right eye and adnexa following other procedure
		H59.342	Postprocedural hematoma of left eye and adnexa following other procedure
		H59.343	Postprocedural hematoma of eye and adnexa following other procedure, bilateral
		H59.349	Postprocedural hematoma of unspecified eye and adnexa following other procedure
	√6ᵗʰ H59.35		Postprocedural seroma of eye and adnexa following an ophthalmic procedure
		H59.351	Postprocedural seroma of right eye and adnexa following an ophthalmic procedure
		H59.352	Postprocedural seroma of left eye and adnexa following an ophthalmic procedure
		H59.353	Postprocedural seroma of eye and adnexa following an ophthalmic procedure, bilateral
		H59.359	Postprocedural seroma of unspecified eye and adnexa following an ophthalmic procedure
	√6ᵗʰ H59.36		Postprocedural seroma of eye and adnexa following other procedure
		H59.361	Postprocedural seroma of right eye and adnexa following other procedure
		H59.362	Postprocedural seroma of left eye and adnexa following other procedure
		H59.363	Postprocedural seroma of eye and adnexa following other procedure, bilateral
		H59.369	Postprocedural seroma of unspecified eye and adnexa following other procedure

√5ᵗʰ **H59.4 Inflammation (infection) of postprocedural bleb**
Postprocedural blebitis
EXCLUDES 1   filtering (vitreous) bleb after glaucoma surgery status (Z98.83)

	H59.40	Inflammation (infection) of postprocedural bleb, unspecified
	H59.41	Inflammation (infection) of postprocedural bleb, stage 1
	H59.42	Inflammation (infection) of postprocedural bleb, stage 2
	H59.43	Inflammation (infection) of postprocedural bleb, stage 3

Bleb endophthalmitis

√5ᵗʰ **H59.8 Other intraoperative and postprocedural complications and disorders of eye and adnexa, not elsewhere classified**

√6ᵗʰ **H59.81 Chorioretinal scars after surgery for detachment**

		H59.811	Chorioretinal scars after surgery for detachment, right eye
		H59.812	Chorioretinal scars after surgery for detachment, left eye
		H59.813	Chorioretinal scars after surgery for detachment, bilateral
		H59.819	Chorioretinal scars after surgery for detachment, unspecified eye
	H59.88		Other intraoperative complications of eye and adnexa, not elsewhere classified
	H59.89		Other postprocedural complications and disorders of eye and adnexa, not elsewhere classified

AHA: 2020,3Q,29

Chapter 8. Diseases of the Ear and Mastoid Process (H60–H95)

Chapter-specific Guidelines with Coding Examples
Reserved for future guideline expansion.

Chapter 8. Diseases of the Ear and Mastoid Process (H60-H95)

NOTE Use an external cause code following the code for the ear condition, if applicable, to identify the cause of the ear condition

EXCLUDES 2 certain conditions originating in the perinatal period (P04-P96)
certain infectious and parasitic diseases (A00-B99)
complications of pregnancy, childbirth and the puerperium (O00-O9A)
congenital malformations, deformations and chromosomal abnormalities (Q00-Q99)
endocrine, nutritional and metabolic diseases (E00-E88)
injury, poisoning and certain other consequences of external causes (S00-T88)
neoplasms (C00-D49)
symptoms, signs and abnormal clinical and laboratory findings, not elsewhere classified (R00-R94)

This chapter contains the following blocks:
H60-H62 Diseases of external ear
H65-H75 Diseases of middle ear and mastoid
H80-H83 Diseases of inner ear
H90-H94 Other disorders of ear
H95   Intraoperative and postprocedural complications and disorders of ear and mastoid process, not elsewhere classified

Diseases of external ear (H60-H62)

H60 Otitis externa

H60.0 Abscess of external ear
  Boil of external ear
  Carbuncle of auricle or external auditory canal
  Furuncle of external ear
  H60.00 Abscess of external ear, unspecified ear
  H60.01 Abscess of right external ear
  H60.02 Abscess of left external ear
  H60.03 Abscess of external ear, bilateral

H60.1 Cellulitis of external ear
  Cellulitis of auricle
  Cellulitis of external auditory canal
  H60.10 Cellulitis of external ear, unspecified ear
  H60.11 Cellulitis of right external ear
  H60.12 Cellulitis of left external ear
  H60.13 Cellulitis of external ear, bilateral

H60.2 Malignant otitis externa
  H60.20 Malignant otitis externa, unspecified ear
  H60.21 Malignant otitis externa, right ear
  H60.22 Malignant otitis externa, left ear
  H60.23 Malignant otitis externa, bilateral

H60.3 Other infective otitis externa
  H60.31 Diffuse otitis externa
    H60.311 Diffuse otitis externa, right ear
    H60.312 Diffuse otitis externa, left ear
    H60.313 Diffuse otitis externa, bilateral
    H60.319 Diffuse otitis externa, unspecified ear
  H60.32 Hemorrhagic otitis externa
    H60.321 Hemorrhagic otitis externa, right ear
    H60.322 Hemorrhagic otitis externa, left ear
    H60.323 Hemorrhagic otitis externa, bilateral
    H60.329 Hemorrhagic otitis externa, unspecified ear
  H60.33 Swimmer's ear
    DEF: Commonly occurs when water gets trapped in the ear after swimming.
    H60.331 Swimmer's ear, right ear
    H60.332 Swimmer's ear, left ear
    H60.333 Swimmer's ear, bilateral
    H60.339 Swimmer's ear, unspecified ear
  H60.39 Other infective otitis externa
    H60.391 Other infective otitis externa, right ear
    H60.392 Other infective otitis externa, left ear
    H60.393 Other infective otitis externa, bilateral
    H60.399 Other infective otitis externa, unspecified ear

H60.4 Cholesteatoma of external ear
  Keratosis obturans of external ear (canal)
  EXCLUDES 2 cholesteatoma of middle ear (H71.-)
  recurrent cholesteatoma of postmastoidectomy cavity (H95.0-)
  DEF: Cholesteatoma: Noncancerous cyst-like mass of cell debris, including cholesterol and epithelial cells resulting from trauma, repeated or improperly healed infections, and congenital enclosure of epidermal cells.
  H60.40 Cholesteatoma of external ear, unspecified ear
  H60.41 Cholesteatoma of right external ear
  H60.42 Cholesteatoma of left external ear
  H60.43 Cholesteatoma of external ear, bilateral

H60.5 Acute noninfective otitis externa
  H60.50 Unspecified acute noninfective otitis externa
    Acute otitis externa NOS
    H60.501 Unspecified acute noninfective otitis externa, right ear
    H60.502 Unspecified acute noninfective otitis externa, left ear
    H60.503 Unspecified acute noninfective otitis externa, bilateral
    H60.509 Unspecified acute noninfective otitis externa, unspecified ear
  H60.51 Acute actinic otitis externa
    H60.511 Acute actinic otitis externa, right ear
    H60.512 Acute actinic otitis externa, left ear
    H60.513 Acute actinic otitis externa, bilateral
    H60.519 Acute actinic otitis externa, unspecified ear
  H60.52 Acute chemical otitis externa
    H60.521 Acute chemical otitis externa, right ear
    H60.522 Acute chemical otitis externa, left ear
    H60.523 Acute chemical otitis externa, bilateral
    H60.529 Acute chemical otitis externa, unspecified ear
  H60.53 Acute contact otitis externa
    H60.531 Acute contact otitis externa, right ear
    H60.532 Acute contact otitis externa, left ear
    H60.533 Acute contact otitis externa, bilateral
    H60.539 Acute contact otitis externa, unspecified ear
  H60.54 Acute eczematoid otitis externa
    H60.541 Acute eczematoid otitis externa, right ear
    H60.542 Acute eczematoid otitis externa, left ear
    H60.543 Acute eczematoid otitis externa, bilateral
    H60.549 Acute eczematoid otitis externa, unspecified ear
  H60.55 Acute reactive otitis externa
    H60.551 Acute reactive otitis externa, right ear
    H60.552 Acute reactive otitis externa, left ear
    H60.553 Acute reactive otitis externa, bilateral
    H60.559 Acute reactive otitis externa, unspecified ear
  H60.59 Other noninfective acute otitis externa
    H60.591 Other noninfective acute otitis externa, right ear
    H60.592 Other noninfective acute otitis externa, left ear
    H60.593 Other noninfective acute otitis externa, bilateral
    H60.599 Other noninfective acute otitis externa, unspecified ear

H60.6 Unspecified chronic otitis externa
  H60.60 Unspecified chronic otitis externa, unspecified ear
  H60.61 Unspecified chronic otitis externa, right ear
  H60.62 Unspecified chronic otitis externa, left ear
  H60.63 Unspecified chronic otitis externa, bilateral

H60.8 Other otitis externa
  H60.8X Other otitis externa
    H60.8X1 Other otitis externa, right ear
    H60.8X2 Other otitis externa, left ear
    H60.8X3 Other otitis externa, bilateral
    H60.8X9 Other otitis externa, unspecified ear

H60.9 Unspecified otitis externa
  H60.90 Unspecified otitis externa, unspecified ear
  H60.91 Unspecified otitis externa, right ear

Chapter 8. Diseases of the Ear and Mastoid Process

H60.92 Unspecified otitis externa, left ear
H60.93 Unspecified otitis externa, bilateral

H61 Other disorders of external ear

H61.0 Chondritis and perichondritis of external ear
Chondrodermatitis nodularis chronica helicis
Perichondritis of auricle
Perichondritis of pinna

- **H61.00** Unspecified perichondritis of external ear
  - **H61.001** Unspecified perichondritis of right external ear
  - **H61.002** Unspecified perichondritis of left external ear
  - **H61.003** Unspecified perichondritis of external ear, bilateral
  - **H61.009** Unspecified perichondritis of external ear, unspecified ear

- **H61.01** Acute perichondritis of external ear
  - **H61.011** Acute perichondritis of right external ear
  - **H61.012** Acute perichondritis of left external ear
  - **H61.013** Acute perichondritis of external ear, bilateral
  - **H61.019** Acute perichondritis of external ear, unspecified ear

- **H61.02** Chronic perichondritis of external ear
  - **H61.021** Chronic perichondritis of right external ear
  - **H61.022** Chronic perichondritis of left external ear
  - **H61.023** Chronic perichondritis of external ear, bilateral
  - **H61.029** Chronic perichondritis of external ear, unspecified ear

- **H61.03** Chondritis of external ear
  Chondritis of auricle
  Chondritis of pinna
  AHA: 2015,1Q,18
  DEF: Infection that has progressed into the cartilage and presents as indurated and edematous skin over the pinna. Vascular compromise occurs with tissue necrosis and deformity.
  - **H61.031** Chondritis of right external ear
  - **H61.032** Chondritis of left external ear
  - **H61.033** Chondritis of external ear, bilateral
  - **H61.039** Chondritis of external ear, unspecified ear

H61.1 Noninfective disorders of pinna
EXCLUDES 2: cauliflower ear (M95.1-)
gouty tophi of ear (M1A.-)

- **H61.10** Unspecified noninfective disorders of pinna
  Disorder of pinna NOS
  - **H61.101** Unspecified noninfective disorders of pinna, right ear
  - **H61.102** Unspecified noninfective disorders of pinna, left ear
  - **H61.103** Unspecified noninfective disorders of pinna, bilateral
  - **H61.109** Unspecified noninfective disorders of pinna, unspecified ear

- **H61.11** Acquired deformity of pinna
  Acquired deformity of auricle
  EXCLUDES 2: cauliflower ear (M95.1-)
  - **H61.111** Acquired deformity of pinna, right ear
  - **H61.112** Acquired deformity of pinna, left ear
  - **H61.113** Acquired deformity of pinna, bilateral
  - **H61.119** Acquired deformity of pinna, unspecified ear

- **H61.12** Hematoma of pinna
  Hematoma of auricle
  - **H61.121** Hematoma of pinna, right ear
  - **H61.122** Hematoma of pinna, left ear
  - **H61.123** Hematoma of pinna, bilateral
  - **H61.129** Hematoma of pinna, unspecified ear

- **H61.19** Other noninfective disorders of pinna
  - **H61.191** Noninfective disorders of pinna, right ear
  - **H61.192** Noninfective disorders of pinna, left ear
  - **H61.193** Noninfective disorders of pinna, bilateral
  - **H61.199** Noninfective disorders of pinna, unspecified ear

H61.2 Impacted cerumen
Wax in ear
- **H61.20** Impacted cerumen, unspecified ear
- **H61.21** Impacted cerumen, right ear
- **H61.22** Impacted cerumen, left ear
- **H61.23** Impacted cerumen, bilateral

H61.3 Acquired stenosis of external ear canal
Collapse of external ear canal
EXCLUDES 1: postprocedural stenosis of external ear canal (H95.81-)

- **H61.30** Acquired stenosis of external ear canal, unspecified
  - **H61.301** Acquired stenosis of right external ear canal, unspecified
  - **H61.302** Acquired stenosis of left external ear canal, unspecified
  - **H61.303** Acquired stenosis of external ear canal, unspecified, bilateral
  - **H61.309** Acquired stenosis of external ear canal, unspecified, unspecified ear

- **H61.31** Acquired stenosis of external ear canal secondary to trauma
  - **H61.311** Acquired stenosis of right external ear canal secondary to trauma
  - **H61.312** Acquired stenosis of left external ear canal secondary to trauma
  - **H61.313** Acquired stenosis of external ear canal secondary to trauma, bilateral
  - **H61.319** Acquired stenosis of external ear canal secondary to trauma, unspecified ear

- **H61.32** Acquired stenosis of external ear canal secondary to inflammation and infection
  DEF: Narrowing of the external ear canal due to chronic inflammation or infection.
  - **H61.321** Acquired stenosis of right external ear canal secondary to inflammation and infection
  - **H61.322** Acquired stenosis of left external ear canal secondary to inflammation and infection
  - **H61.323** Acquired stenosis of external ear canal secondary to inflammation and infection, bilateral
  - **H61.329** Acquired stenosis of external ear canal secondary to inflammation and infection, unspecified ear

- **H61.39** Other acquired stenosis of external ear canal
  - **H61.391** Other acquired stenosis of right external ear canal
  - **H61.392** Other acquired stenosis of left external ear canal
  - **H61.393** Other acquired stenosis of external ear canal, bilateral
  - **H61.399** Other acquired stenosis of external ear canal, unspecified ear

H61.8 Other specified disorders of external ear

- **H61.81** Exostosis of external canal
  - **H61.811** Exostosis of right external canal
  - **H61.812** Exostosis of left external canal
  - **H61.813** Exostosis of external canal, bilateral
  - **H61.819** Exostosis of external canal, unspecified ear

- **H61.89** Other specified disorders of external ear
  - **H61.891** Other specified disorders of right external ear
  - **H61.892** Other specified disorders of left external ear
  - **H61.893** Other specified disorders of external ear, bilateral
  - **H61.899** Other specified disorders of external ear, unspecified ear

H61.9 Disorder of external ear, unspecified
- **H61.90** Disorder of external ear, unspecified, unspecified ear
- **H61.91** Disorder of right external ear, unspecified
- **H61.92** Disorder of left external ear, unspecified
- **H61.93** Disorder of external ear, unspecified, bilateral

H62 Disorders of external ear in diseases classified elsewhere

H62.4 Otitis externa in other diseases classified elsewhere
Code first underlying disease, such as:
erysipelas (A46)
impetigo (L01.0-)
EXCLUDES 1: otitis externa (in):
candidiasis (B37.84)
herpes viral [herpes simplex] (B00.1)
herpes zoster (B02.8)

- **H62.40** *Otitis externa in other diseases classified elsewhere, unspecified ear*

- **H62.41** Otitis externa in other diseases classified elsewhere, right ear
- **H62.42** Otitis externa in other diseases classified elsewhere, left ear
- **H62.43** Otitis externa in other diseases classified elsewhere, bilateral
- ✓5th **H62.8** Other disorders of external ear in diseases classified elsewhere
  - Code first underlying disease, such as:
  - gout (M1A.-, M10.-)
  - ✓6th **H62.8X** Other disorders of external ear in diseases classified elsewhere
    - **H62.8X1** Other disorders of right external ear in diseases classified elsewhere
    - **H62.8X2** Other disorders of left external ear in diseases classified elsewhere
    - **H62.8X3** Other disorders of external ear in diseases classified elsewhere, bilateral
    - **H62.8X9** Other disorders of external ear in diseases classified elsewhere, unspecified ear

Diseases of middle ear and mastoid (H65-H75)

- ✓4th **H65** Nonsuppurative otitis media
  - **INCLUDES** nonsuppurative otitis media with myringitis
  - Use additional code for any associated perforated tympanic membrane (H72.-)
  - Use additional code, if applicable, to identify:
    - exposure to environmental tobacco smoke (Z77.22)
    - exposure to tobacco smoke in the perinatal period (P96.81)
    - history of tobacco dependence (Z87.891)
    - infectious agent (B95-B97)
    - occupational exposure to environmental tobacco smoke (Z57.31)
    - tobacco dependence (F17.-)
    - tobacco use (Z72.0)
  - ✓5th **H65.0** Acute serous otitis media
    - Acute and subacute secretory otitis
    - **H65.00** Acute serous otitis media, unspecified ear
    - **H65.01** Acute serous otitis media, right ear
    - **H65.02** Acute serous otitis media, left ear
    - **H65.03** Acute serous otitis media, bilateral
    - **H65.04** Acute serous otitis media, recurrent, right ear
    - **H65.05** Acute serous otitis media, recurrent, left ear
    - **H65.06** Acute serous otitis media, recurrent, bilateral
    - **H65.07** Acute serous otitis media, recurrent, unspecified ear
  - ✓5th **H65.1** Other acute nonsuppurative otitis media
    - **EXCLUDES 1** otitic barotrauma (T70.0)
    - otitis media (acute) NOS (H66.9)
    - ✓6th **H65.11** Acute and subacute allergic otitis media (mucoid) (sanguinous) (serous)
      - **H65.111** Acute and subacute allergic otitis media (mucoid) (sanguinous) (serous), right ear
      - **H65.112** Acute and subacute allergic otitis media (mucoid) (sanguinous) (serous), left ear
      - **H65.113** Acute and subacute allergic otitis media (mucoid) (sanguinous) (serous), bilateral
      - **H65.114** Acute and subacute allergic otitis media (mucoid) (sanguinous) (serous), recurrent, right ear
      - **H65.115** Acute and subacute allergic otitis media (mucoid) (sanguinous) (serous), recurrent, left ear
      - **H65.116** Acute and subacute allergic otitis media (mucoid) (sanguinous) (serous), recurrent, bilateral
      - **H65.117** Acute and subacute allergic otitis media (mucoid) (sanguinous) (serous), recurrent, unspecified ear
      - **H65.119** Acute and subacute allergic otitis media (mucoid) (sanguinous) (serous), unspecified ear
    - ✓6th **H65.19** Other acute nonsuppurative otitis media
      - Acute and subacute mucoid otitis media
      - Acute and subacute nonsuppurative otitis media NOS
      - Acute and subacute sanguinous otitis media
      - Acute and subacute seromucinous otitis media
      - **H65.191** Other acute nonsuppurative otitis media, right ear
      - **H65.192** Other acute nonsuppurative otitis media, left ear
      - **H65.193** Other acute nonsuppurative otitis media, bilateral
      - **H65.194** Other acute nonsuppurative otitis media, recurrent, right ear
      - **H65.195** Other acute nonsuppurative otitis media, recurrent, left ear
      - **H65.196** Other acute nonsuppurative otitis media, recurrent, bilateral
      - **H65.197** Other acute nonsuppurative otitis media, recurrent, unspecified ear
      - **H65.199** Other acute nonsuppurative otitis media, unspecified ear
  - ✓5th **H65.2** Chronic serous otitis media
    - Chronic tubotympanic catarrh
    - **H65.20** Chronic serous otitis media, unspecified ear
    - **H65.21** Chronic serous otitis media, right ear
    - **H65.22** Chronic serous otitis media, left ear
    - **H65.23** Chronic serous otitis media, bilateral
  - ✓5th **H65.3** Chronic mucoid otitis media
    - Chronic mucinous otitis media
    - Chronic secretory otitis media
    - Chronic transudative otitis media
    - Glue ear
    - **EXCLUDES 1** adhesive middle ear disease (H74.1)
    - **H65.30** Chronic mucoid otitis media, unspecified ear
    - **H65.31** Chronic mucoid otitis media, right ear
    - **H65.32** Chronic mucoid otitis media, left ear
    - **H65.33** Chronic mucoid otitis media, bilateral
  - ✓5th **H65.4** Other chronic nonsuppurative otitis media
    - ✓6th **H65.41** Chronic allergic otitis media
      - **H65.411** Chronic allergic otitis media, right ear
      - **H65.412** Chronic allergic otitis media, left ear
      - **H65.413** Chronic allergic otitis media, bilateral
      - **H65.419** Chronic allergic otitis media, unspecified ear
    - ✓6th **H65.49** Other chronic nonsuppurative otitis media
      - Chronic exudative otitis media
      - Chronic nonsuppurative otitis media NOS
      - Chronic otitis media with effusion (nonpurulent)
      - Chronic seromucinous otitis media
      - **H65.491** Other chronic nonsuppurative otitis media, right ear
      - **H65.492** Other chronic nonsuppurative otitis media, left ear
      - **H65.493** Other chronic nonsuppurative otitis media, bilateral
      - **H65.499** Other chronic nonsuppurative otitis media, unspecified ear
  - ✓5th **H65.9** Unspecified nonsuppurative otitis media
    - Allergic otitis media NOS
    - Catarrhal otitis media NOS
    - Exudative otitis media NOS
    - Mucoid otitis media NOS
    - Otitis media with effusion (nonpurulent) NOS
    - Secretory otitis media NOS
    - Seromucinous otitis media NOS
    - Serous otitis media NOS
    - Transudative otitis media NOS
    - **H65.90** Unspecified nonsuppurative otitis media, unspecified ear
    - **H65.91** Unspecified nonsuppurative otitis media, right ear
    - **H65.92** Unspecified nonsuppurative otitis media, left ear
    - **H65.93** Unspecified nonsuppurative otitis media, bilateral
- ✓4th **H66** Suppurative and unspecified otitis media
  - **INCLUDES** suppurative and unspecified otitis media with myringitis
  - Use additional code to identify:
    - exposure to environmental tobacco smoke (Z77.22)
    - exposure to tobacco smoke in the perinatal period (P96.81)
    - history of tobacco dependence (Z87.891)
    - occupational exposure to environmental tobacco smoke (Z57.31)
    - tobacco dependence (F17.-)
    - tobacco use (Z72.0)
  - **AHA:** 2016,1Q,34
  - ✓5th **H66.0** Acute suppurative otitis media
    - ✓6th **H66.00** Acute suppurative otitis media without spontaneous rupture of ear drum
      - **H66.001** Acute suppurative otitis media without spontaneous rupture of ear drum, right ear
      - **H66.002** Acute suppurative otitis media without spontaneous rupture of ear drum, left ear

Chapter 8. Diseases of the Ear and Mastoid Process

- **H66.003** Acute suppurative otitis media without spontaneous rupture of ear drum, bilateral
- **H66.004** Acute suppurative otitis media without spontaneous rupture of ear drum, recurrent, right ear
- **H66.005** Acute suppurative otitis media without spontaneous rupture of ear drum, recurrent, left ear
- **H66.006** Acute suppurative otitis media without spontaneous rupture of ear drum, recurrent, bilateral
- **H66.007** Acute suppurative otitis media without spontaneous rupture of ear drum, recurrent, unspecified ear
- **H66.009** Acute suppurative otitis media without spontaneous rupture of ear drum, unspecified ear

✓6ᵗʰ **H66.01** Acute suppurative otitis media with spontaneous rupture of ear drum
  DEF: Sudden, severe inflammation of the middle ear, causing pressure that perforates the ear drum tissue.
- **H66.011** Acute suppurative otitis media with spontaneous rupture of ear drum, right ear
- **H66.012** Acute suppurative otitis media with spontaneous rupture of ear drum, left ear
- **H66.013** Acute suppurative otitis media with spontaneous rupture of ear drum, bilateral
- **H66.014** Acute suppurative otitis media with spontaneous rupture of ear drum, recurrent, right ear
- **H66.015** Acute suppurative otitis media with spontaneous rupture of ear drum, recurrent, left ear
- **H66.016** Acute suppurative otitis media with spontaneous rupture of ear drum, recurrent, bilateral
- **H66.017** Acute suppurative otitis media with spontaneous rupture of ear drum, recurrent, unspecified ear
- **H66.019** Acute suppurative otitis media with spontaneous rupture of ear drum, unspecified ear

✓5ᵗʰ **H66.1** Chronic tubotympanic suppurative otitis media
  Benign chronic suppurative otitis media
  Chronic tubotympanic disease
  Use additional code for any associated perforated tympanic membrane (H72.-)
- **H66.10** Chronic tubotympanic suppurative otitis media, unspecified
- **H66.11** Chronic tubotympanic suppurative otitis media, right ear
- **H66.12** Chronic tubotympanic suppurative otitis media, left ear
- **H66.13** Chronic tubotympanic suppurative otitis media, bilateral

✓5ᵗʰ **H66.2** Chronic atticoantral suppurative otitis media
  Chronic atticoantral disease
  Use additional code for any associated perforated tympanic membrane (H72.-)
- **H66.20** Chronic atticoantral suppurative otitis media, unspecified ear
- **H66.21** Chronic atticoantral suppurative otitis media, right ear
- **H66.22** Chronic atticoantral suppurative otitis media, left ear
- **H66.23** Chronic atticoantral suppurative otitis media, bilateral

✓5ᵗʰ **H66.3** Other chronic suppurative otitis media
  Chronic suppurative otitis media NOS
  Use additional code for any associated perforated tympanic membrane (H72.-)
  EXCLUDES 1 tuberculous otitis media (A18.6)

✓6ᵗʰ **H66.3X** Other chronic suppurative otitis media
- **H66.3X1** Other chronic suppurative otitis media, right ear
- **H66.3X2** Other chronic suppurative otitis media, left ear
- **H66.3X3** Other chronic suppurative otitis media, bilateral
- **H66.3X9** Other chronic suppurative otitis media, unspecified ear

✓5ᵗʰ **H66.4** Suppurative otitis media, unspecified
  Purulent otitis media NOS
  Use additional code for any associated perforated tympanic membrane (H72.-)
- **H66.40** Suppurative otitis media, unspecified, unspecified ear
- **H66.41** Suppurative otitis media, unspecified, right ear
- **H66.42** Suppurative otitis media, unspecified, left ear
- **H66.43** Suppurative otitis media, unspecified, bilateral

✓5ᵗʰ **H66.9** Otitis media, unspecified
  Acute otitis media NOS
  Chronic otitis media NOS
  Otitis media NOS
  Use additional code for any associated perforated tympanic membrane (H72.-)
- **H66.90** Otitis media, unspecified, unspecified ear
- **H66.91** Otitis media, unspecified, right ear
- **H66.92** Otitis media, unspecified, left ear
- **H66.93** Otitis media, unspecified, bilateral

✓4ᵗʰ **H67** Otitis media in diseases classified elsewhere
  Code first underlying disease, such as:
    plasminogen deficiency (E88.02)
    viral disease NEC (B00-B34)
  Use additional code for any associated perforated tympanic membrane (H72.-)
  EXCLUDES 1 otitis media in:
    influenza (J09.X9, J10.83, J11.83)
    measles (B05.3)
    scarlet fever (A38.0)
    tuberculosis (A18.6)
- **H67.1** Otitis media in diseases classified elsewhere, right ear
- **H67.2** Otitis media in diseases classified elsewhere, left ear
- **H67.3** Otitis media in diseases classified elsewhere, bilateral
- **H67.9** Otitis media in diseases classified elsewhere, unspecified ear

✓4ᵗʰ **H68** Eustachian salpingitis and obstruction
  DEF: Eustachian tube: Internal channel between the tympanic cavity and the nasopharynx that equalizes internal pressure to the outside pressure and drains mucous production from the middle ear.

✓5ᵗʰ **H68.0** Eustachian salpingitis
  ✓6ᵗʰ **H68.00** Unspecified Eustachian salpingitis
  - **H68.001** Unspecified Eustachian salpingitis, right ear
  - **H68.002** Unspecified Eustachian salpingitis, left ear
  - **H68.003** Unspecified Eustachian salpingitis, bilateral
  - **H68.009** Unspecified Eustachian salpingitis, unspecified ear

  ✓6ᵗʰ **H68.01** Acute Eustachian salpingitis
  - **H68.011** Acute Eustachian salpingitis, right ear
  - **H68.012** Acute Eustachian salpingitis, left ear
  - **H68.013** Acute Eustachian salpingitis, bilateral
  - **H68.019** Acute Eustachian salpingitis, unspecified ear

  ✓6ᵗʰ **H68.02** Chronic Eustachian salpingitis
  - **H68.021** Chronic Eustachian salpingitis, right ear
  - **H68.022** Chronic Eustachian salpingitis, left ear
  - **H68.023** Chronic Eustachian salpingitis, bilateral
  - **H68.029** Chronic Eustachian salpingitis, unspecified ear

✓5ᵗʰ **H68.1** Obstruction of Eustachian tube
  Stenosis of Eustachian tube
  Stricture of Eustachian tube
  ✓6ᵗʰ **H68.10** Unspecified obstruction of Eustachian tube
  - **H68.101** Unspecified obstruction of Eustachian tube, right ear
  - **H68.102** Unspecified obstruction of Eustachian tube, left ear
  - **H68.103** Unspecified obstruction of Eustachian tube, bilateral
  - **H68.109** Unspecified obstruction of Eustachian tube, unspecified ear

  ✓6ᵗʰ **H68.11** Osseous obstruction of Eustachian tube
  - **H68.111** Osseous obstruction of Eustachian tube, right ear
  - **H68.112** Osseous obstruction of Eustachian tube, left ear
  - **H68.113** Osseous obstruction of Eustachian tube, bilateral

Chapter 8. Diseases of the Ear and Mastoid Process

H68.119 Osseous obstruction of Eustachian tube, unspecified ear

✓6th H68.12 **Intrinsic cartilagenous** obstruction of Eustachian tube
- H68.121 Intrinsic cartilagenous obstruction of Eustachian tube, **right** ear
- H68.122 Intrinsic cartilagenous obstruction of Eustachian tube, **left** ear
- H68.123 Intrinsic cartilagenous obstruction of Eustachian tube, **bilateral**
- H68.129 Intrinsic cartilagenous obstruction of Eustachian tube, unspecified ear

✓6th H68.13 **Extrinsic cartilagenous** obstruction of Eustachian tube
Compression of Eustachian tube
- H68.131 Extrinsic cartilagenous obstruction of Eustachian tube, **right** ear
- H68.132 Extrinsic cartilagenous obstruction of Eustachian tube, **left** ear
- H68.133 Extrinsic cartilagenous obstruction of Eustachian tube, **bilateral**
- H68.139 Extrinsic cartilagenous obstruction of Eustachian tube, unspecified ear

✓4th **H69 Other and unspecified disorders of Eustachian tube**
DEF: Eustachian tube: Internal channel between the tympanic cavity and the nasopharynx that equalizes internal pressure to the outside pressure and drains mucous production from the middle ear.

✓5th H69.0 **Patulous** Eustachian tube
- H69.00 Patulous Eustachian tube, unspecified ear
- H69.01 Patulous Eustachian tube, **right** ear
- H69.02 Patulous Eustachian tube, **left** ear
- H69.03 Patulous Eustachian tube, **bilateral**

✓5th H69.8 Other specified disorders of Eustachian tube
- H69.80 Other specified disorders of Eustachian tube, unspecified ear
- H69.81 Other specified disorders of Eustachian tube, **right** ear
- H69.82 Other specified disorders of Eustachian tube, **left** ear
- H69.83 Other specified disorders of Eustachian tube, **bilateral**

✓5th H69.9 Unspecified Eustachian tube disorder
- H69.90 Unspecified Eustachian tube disorder, unspecified ear
- H69.91 Unspecified Eustachian tube disorder, **right** ear
- H69.92 Unspecified Eustachian tube disorder, **left** ear
- H69.93 Unspecified Eustachian tube disorder, **bilateral**

✓4th **H70 Mastoiditis and related conditions**

✓5th H70.0 **Acute** mastoiditis
Abscess of mastoid
Empyema of mastoid

✓6th H70.00 Acute mastoiditis **without complications**
- H70.001 Acute mastoiditis without complications, **right** ear
- H70.002 Acute mastoiditis without complications, **left** ear
- H70.003 Acute mastoiditis without complications, **bilateral**
- H70.009 Acute mastoiditis without complications, unspecified ear

✓6th H70.01 **Subperiosteal abscess** of mastoid
- H70.011 Subperiosteal abscess of mastoid, **right** ear
- H70.012 Subperiosteal abscess of mastoid, **left** ear
- H70.013 Subperiosteal abscess of mastoid, **bilateral**
- H70.019 Subperiosteal abscess of mastoid, unspecified ear

✓6th H70.09 Acute mastoiditis with other complications
- H70.091 Acute mastoiditis with other complications, **right** ear
- H70.092 Acute mastoiditis with other complications, **left** ear
- H70.093 Acute mastoiditis with other complications, **bilateral**
- H70.099 Acute mastoiditis with other complications, unspecified ear

✓5th H70.1 **Chronic** mastoiditis
Caries of mastoid
Fistula of mastoid
EXCLUDES 1 tuberculous mastoiditis (A18.03)
- H70.10 Chronic mastoiditis, unspecified ear
- H70.11 Chronic mastoiditis, **right** ear
- H70.12 Chronic mastoiditis, **left** ear
- H70.13 Chronic mastoiditis, **bilateral**

✓5th H70.2 **Petrositis**
Inflammation of petrous bone

✓6th H70.20 Unspecified petrositis
- H70.201 Unspecified petrositis, **right** ear
- H70.202 Unspecified petrositis, **left** ear
- H70.203 Unspecified petrositis, **bilateral**
- H70.209 Unspecified petrositis, unspecified ear

✓6th H70.21 **Acute** petrositis
DEF: Sudden, severe inflammation of the petrous temporal bone behind the ear, associated with a middle ear infection.
- H70.211 Acute petrositis, **right** ear
- H70.212 Acute petrositis, **left** ear
- H70.213 Acute petrositis, **bilateral**
- H70.219 Acute petrositis, unspecified ear

✓6th H70.22 **Chronic** petrositis
- H70.221 Chronic petrositis, **right** ear
- H70.222 Chronic petrositis, **left** ear
- H70.223 Chronic petrositis, **bilateral**
- H70.229 Chronic petrositis, unspecified ear

✓5th H70.8 Other mastoiditis and related conditions
EXCLUDES 1 preauricular sinus and cyst (Q18.1)
sinus, fistula, and cyst of branchial cleft (Q18.0)

✓6th H70.81 **Postauricular fistula**
- H70.811 Postauricular fistula, **right** ear
- H70.812 Postauricular fistula, **left** ear
- H70.813 Postauricular fistula, **bilateral**
- H70.819 Postauricular fistula, unspecified ear

✓6th H70.89 Other mastoiditis and related conditions
- H70.891 Other mastoiditis and related conditions, **right** ear
- H70.892 Other mastoiditis and related conditions, **left** ear
- H70.893 Other mastoiditis and related conditions, **bilateral**
- H70.899 Other mastoiditis and related conditions, unspecified ear

✓5th H70.9 Unspecified mastoiditis
- H70.90 Unspecified mastoiditis, unspecified ear
- H70.91 Unspecified mastoiditis, **right** ear
- H70.92 Unspecified mastoiditis, **left** ear
- H70.93 Unspecified mastoiditis, **bilateral**

✓4th **H71 Cholesteatoma of middle ear**
EXCLUDES 2 cholesteatoma of external ear (H60.4-)
recurrent cholesteatoma of postmastoidectomy cavity (H95.0-)
AHA: 2021,3Q,8
DEF: Cholesteatoma: Noncancerous cyst-like mass of cell debris, including cholesterol and epithelial cells resulting from trauma, repeated or improperly healed infections, and congenital enclosure of epidermal cells.

Cholesteatoma of Middle Ear

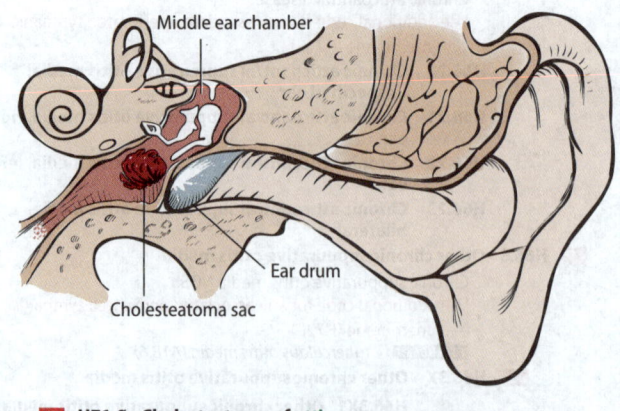

✓5th H71.0 Cholesteatoma of **attic**
- H71.00 Cholesteatoma of attic, unspecified ear
- H71.01 Cholesteatoma of attic, **right** ear
- H71.02 Cholesteatoma of attic, **left** ear
- H71.03 Cholesteatoma of attic, **bilateral**

✓5th H71.1 Cholesteatoma of **tympanum**
- H71.10 Cholesteatoma of tympanum, unspecified ear

- H71.11 Cholesteatoma of tympanum, right ear
- H71.12 Cholesteatoma of tympanum, left ear
- H71.13 Cholesteatoma of tympanum, bilateral

√5th **H71.2 Cholesteatoma of mastoid**
- H71.20 Cholesteatoma of mastoid, unspecified ear
- H71.21 Cholesteatoma of mastoid, right ear
- H71.22 Cholesteatoma of mastoid, left ear
- H71.23 Cholesteatoma of mastoid, bilateral

√5th **H71.3 Diffuse cholesteatosis**
AHA: 2021,3Q,8
- H71.30 Diffuse cholesteatosis, unspecified ear
- H71.31 Diffuse cholesteatosis, right ear
- H71.32 Diffuse cholesteatosis, left ear
- H71.33 Diffuse cholesteatosis, bilateral

√5th **H71.9 Unspecified cholesteatoma**
- H71.90 Unspecified cholesteatoma, unspecified ear
- H71.91 Unspecified cholesteatoma, right ear
- H71.92 Unspecified cholesteatoma, left ear
- H71.93 Unspecified cholesteatoma, bilateral

√4th **H72 Perforation of tympanic membrane**
INCLUDES persistent post-traumatic perforation of ear drum
postinflammatory perforation of ear drum
Code first any associated otitis media (H65.-, H66.1-, H66.2-, H66.3-, H66.4-, H66.9-, H67.-)
EXCLUDES 1 acute suppurative otitis media with rupture of the tympanic membrane (H66.01-)
traumatic rupture of ear drum (S09.2-)

√5th **H72.0 Central perforation of tympanic membrane**
- H72.00 Central perforation of tympanic membrane, unspecified ear
- H72.01 Central perforation of tympanic membrane, right ear
- H72.02 Central perforation of tympanic membrane, left ear
- H72.03 Central perforation of tympanic membrane, bilateral

√5th **H72.1 Attic perforation of tympanic membrane**
Perforation of pars flaccida
- H72.10 Attic perforation of tympanic membrane, unspecified ear
- H72.11 Attic perforation of tympanic membrane, right ear
- H72.12 Attic perforation of tympanic membrane, left ear
- H72.13 Attic perforation of tympanic membrane, bilateral

√5th **H72.2 Other marginal perforations of tympanic membrane**
√6th H72.2X Other marginal perforations of tympanic membrane
- H72.2X1 Other marginal perforations of tympanic membrane, right ear
- H72.2X2 Other marginal perforations of tympanic membrane, left ear
- H72.2X3 Other marginal perforations of tympanic membrane, bilateral
- H72.2X9 Other marginal perforations of tympanic membrane, unspecified ear

√5th **H72.8 Other perforations of tympanic membrane**
√6th H72.81 Multiple perforations of tympanic membrane
- H72.811 Multiple perforations of tympanic membrane, right ear
- H72.812 Multiple perforations of tympanic membrane, left ear
- H72.813 Multiple perforations of tympanic membrane, bilateral
- H72.819 Multiple perforations of tympanic membrane, unspecified ear

√6th H72.82 Total perforations of tympanic membrane
- H72.821 Total perforations of tympanic membrane, right ear
- H72.822 Total perforations of tympanic membrane, left ear
- H72.823 Total perforations of tympanic membrane, bilateral
- H72.829 Total perforations of tympanic membrane, unspecified ear

√5th **H72.9 Unspecified perforation of tympanic membrane**
- H72.90 Unspecified perforation of tympanic membrane, unspecified ear
- H72.91 Unspecified perforation of tympanic membrane, right ear
- H72.92 Unspecified perforation of tympanic membrane, left ear
- H72.93 Unspecified perforation of tympanic membrane, bilateral

√4th **H73 Other disorders of tympanic membrane**

√5th **H73.0 Acute myringitis**
EXCLUDES 1 acute myringitis with otitis media (H65, H66)
√6th H73.00 Unspecified acute myringitis
Acute tympanitis NOS
- H73.001 Acute myringitis, right ear
- H73.002 Acute myringitis, left ear
- H73.003 Acute myringitis, bilateral
- H73.009 Acute myringitis, unspecified ear

√6th H73.01 Bullous myringitis
DEF: Bacterial or viral otitis media that is characterized by the appearance of serous or hemorrhagic blebs on the ear drum and sudden onset of severe pain in ear.
- H73.011 Bullous myringitis, right ear
- H73.012 Bullous myringitis, left ear
- H73.013 Bullous myringitis, bilateral
- H73.019 Bullous myringitis, unspecified ear

√6th H73.09 Other acute myringitis
- H73.091 Other acute myringitis, right ear
- H73.092 Other acute myringitis, left ear
- H73.093 Other acute myringitis, bilateral
- H73.099 Other acute myringitis, unspecified ear

√5th **H73.1 Chronic myringitis**
Chronic tympanitis
EXCLUDES 1 chronic myringitis with otitis media (H65, H66)
- H73.10 Chronic myringitis, unspecified ear
- H73.11 Chronic myringitis, right ear
- H73.12 Chronic myringitis, left ear
- H73.13 Chronic myringitis, bilateral

√5th **H73.2 Unspecified myringitis**
- H73.20 Unspecified myringitis, unspecified ear
- H73.21 Unspecified myringitis, right ear
- H73.22 Unspecified myringitis, left ear
- H73.23 Unspecified myringitis, bilateral

√5th **H73.8 Other specified disorders of tympanic membrane**
√6th H73.81 Atrophic flaccid tympanic membrane
- H73.811 Atrophic flaccid tympanic membrane, right ear
- H73.812 Atrophic flaccid tympanic membrane, left ear
- H73.813 Atrophic flaccid tympanic membrane, bilateral
- H73.819 Atrophic flaccid tympanic membrane, unspecified ear

√6th H73.82 Atrophic nonflaccid tympanic membrane
- H73.821 Atrophic nonflaccid tympanic membrane, right ear
- H73.822 Atrophic nonflaccid tympanic membrane, left ear
- H73.823 Atrophic nonflaccid tympanic membrane, bilateral
- H73.829 Atrophic nonflaccid tympanic membrane, unspecified ear

√6th H73.89 Other specified disorders of tympanic membrane
- H73.891 Other specified disorders of tympanic membrane, right ear
- H73.892 Other specified disorders of tympanic membrane, left ear
- H73.893 Other specified disorders of tympanic membrane, bilateral
- H73.899 Other specified disorders of tympanic membrane, unspecified ear

√5th **H73.9 Unspecified disorder of tympanic membrane**
- H73.90 Unspecified disorder of tympanic membrane, unspecified ear
- H73.91 Unspecified disorder of tympanic membrane, right ear
- H73.92 Unspecified disorder of tympanic membrane, left ear
- H73.93 Unspecified disorder of tympanic membrane, bilateral

Chapter 8. Diseases of the Ear and Mastoid Process

- ✓4th **H74** Other disorders of middle ear mastoid
  - EXCLUDES 2 mastoiditis (H70.-)
  - ✓5th **H74.0** Tympanosclerosis
    - **DEF:** Calcification of tissue in the ear drum, middle ear bones, and middle ear canal.
    - H74.01 Tympanosclerosis, right ear
    - H74.02 Tympanosclerosis, left ear
    - H74.03 Tympanosclerosis, bilateral
    - H74.09 Tympanosclerosis, unspecified ear
  - ✓5th **H74.1** Adhesive middle ear disease
    - Adhesive otitis
    - EXCLUDES 1 glue ear (H65.3-)
    - H74.11 Adhesive right middle ear disease
    - H74.12 Adhesive left middle ear disease
    - H74.13 Adhesive middle ear disease, bilateral
    - H74.19 Adhesive middle ear disease, unspecified ear
  - ✓5th **H74.2** Discontinuity and dislocation of ear ossicles
    - H74.20 Discontinuity and dislocation of ear ossicles, unspecified ear
    - H74.21 Discontinuity and dislocation of right ear ossicles
    - H74.22 Discontinuity and dislocation of left ear ossicles
    - H74.23 Discontinuity and dislocation of ear ossicles, bilateral
  - ✓5th **H74.3** Other acquired abnormalities of ear ossicles
    - ✓6th **H74.31** Ankylosis of ear ossicles
      - H74.311 Ankylosis of ear ossicles, right ear
      - H74.312 Ankylosis of ear ossicles, left ear
      - H74.313 Ankylosis of ear ossicles, bilateral
      - H74.319 Ankylosis of ear ossicles, unspecified ear
    - ✓6th **H74.32** Partial loss of ear ossicles
      - H74.321 Partial loss of ear ossicles, right ear
      - H74.322 Partial loss of ear ossicles, left ear
      - H74.323 Partial loss of ear ossicles, bilateral
      - H74.329 Partial loss of ear ossicles, unspecified ear
    - ✓6th **H74.39** Other acquired abnormalities of ear ossicles
      - H74.391 Other acquired abnormalities of right ear ossicles
      - H74.392 Other acquired abnormalities of left ear ossicles
      - H74.393 Other acquired abnormalities of ear ossicles, bilateral
      - H74.399 Other acquired abnormalities of ear ossicles, unspecified ear
  - ✓5th **H74.4** Polyp of middle ear
    - H74.40 Polyp of middle ear, unspecified ear
    - H74.41 Polyp of right middle ear
    - H74.42 Polyp of left middle ear
    - H74.43 Polyp of middle ear, bilateral
  - ✓5th **H74.8** Other specified disorders of middle ear and mastoid
    - ✓6th **H74.8X** Other specified disorders of middle ear and mastoid
      - H74.8X1 Other specified disorders of right middle ear and mastoid
      - H74.8X2 Other specified disorders of left middle ear and mastoid
      - H74.8X3 Other specified disorders of middle ear and mastoid, bilateral
      - H74.8X9 Other specified disorders of middle ear and mastoid, unspecified ear
  - ✓5th **H74.9** Unspecified disorder of middle ear and mastoid
    - H74.90 Unspecified disorder of middle ear and mastoid, unspecified ear
    - H74.91 Unspecified disorder of right middle ear and mastoid
    - H74.92 Unspecified disorder of left middle ear and mastoid
    - H74.93 Unspecified disorder of middle ear and mastoid, bilateral
- ✓4th **H75** Other disorders of middle ear and mastoid in diseases classified elsewhere
  - Code first underlying disease
  - ✓5th **H75.0** Mastoiditis in infectious and parasitic diseases classified elsewhere
    - EXCLUDES 1 mastoiditis (in):
      - syphilis (A52.77)
      - tuberculosis (A18.03)
    - H75.00 *Mastoiditis in infectious and parasitic diseases classified elsewhere, unspecified ear*
    - H75.01 *Mastoiditis in infectious and parasitic diseases classified elsewhere, right ear*
    - H75.02 *Mastoiditis in infectious and parasitic diseases classified elsewhere, left ear*
    - H75.03 *Mastoiditis in infectious and parasitic diseases classified elsewhere, bilateral*
  - ✓5th **H75.8** Other specified disorders of middle ear and mastoid in diseases classified elsewhere
    - H75.80 *Other specified disorders of middle ear and mastoid in diseases classified elsewhere, unspecified ear*
    - H75.81 *Other specified disorders of right middle ear and mastoid in diseases classified elsewhere*
    - H75.82 *Other specified disorders of left middle ear and mastoid in diseases classified elsewhere*
    - H75.83 *Other specified disorders of middle ear and mastoid in diseases classified elsewhere, bilateral*

Diseases of inner ear (H80-H83)

- ✓4th **H80** Otosclerosis
  - INCLUDES otospongiosis
  - ✓5th **H80.0** Otosclerosis involving oval window, nonobliterative
    - H80.00 Otosclerosis involving oval window, nonobliterative, unspecified ear
    - H80.01 Otosclerosis involving oval window, nonobliterative, right ear
    - H80.02 Otosclerosis involving oval window, nonobliterative, left ear
    - H80.03 Otosclerosis involving oval window, nonobliterative, bilateral
  - ✓5th **H80.1** Otosclerosis involving oval window, obliterative
    - H80.10 Otosclerosis involving oval window, obliterative, unspecified ear
    - H80.11 Otosclerosis involving oval window, obliterative, right ear
    - H80.12 Otosclerosis involving oval window, obliterative, left ear
    - H80.13 Otosclerosis involving oval window, obliterative, bilateral
  - ✓5th **H80.2** Cochlear otosclerosis
    - Otosclerosis involving otic capsule
    - Otosclerosis involving round window
    - H80.20 Cochlear otosclerosis, unspecified ear
    - H80.21 Cochlear otosclerosis, right ear
    - H80.22 Cochlear otosclerosis, left ear
    - H80.23 Cochlear otosclerosis, bilateral
  - ✓5th **H80.8** Other otosclerosis
    - H80.80 Other otosclerosis, unspecified ear
    - H80.81 Other otosclerosis, right ear
    - H80.82 Other otosclerosis, left ear
    - H80.83 Other otosclerosis, bilateral
  - ✓5th **H80.9** Unspecified otosclerosis
    - H80.90 Unspecified otosclerosis, unspecified ear
    - H80.91 Unspecified otosclerosis, right ear
    - H80.92 Unspecified otosclerosis, left ear
    - H80.93 Unspecified otosclerosis, bilateral
- ✓4th **H81** Disorders of vestibular function
  - EXCLUDES 1 epidemic vertigo (A88.1)
    - vertigo NOS (R42)
  - ✓5th **H81.0** Meniere's disease
    - Labyrinthine hydrops
    - Meniere's syndrome or vertigo
    - **DEF:** Distended membranous labyrinth of the middle ear from fluctuating pressure of fluid (hydrops) that causes vertigo, tinnitus, pressure, and hearing loss that may last on and off for several hours. Episodes may occur in clusters or may subside for weeks, months, or even years.
    - H81.01 Meniere's disease, right ear
    - H81.02 Meniere's disease, left ear
    - H81.03 Meniere's disease, bilateral
    - H81.09 Meniere's disease, unspecified ear
  - ✓5th **H81.1** Benign paroxysmal vertigo
    - H81.10 Benign paroxysmal vertigo, unspecified ear
    - H81.11 Benign paroxysmal vertigo, right ear
    - H81.12 Benign paroxysmal vertigo, left ear
    - H81.13 Benign paroxysmal vertigo, bilateral

Chapter 8. Diseases of the Ear and Mastoid Process

H81.2 **Vestibular neuronitis**
 DEF: Transient benign vertigo caused by inflammation of the vestibular nerve. It is characterized by response to caloric stimulation on one side and nystagmus with rhythmic movement of the eyes. Normal auditory function is present.
- H81.20 Vestibular neuronitis, unspecified ear
- H81.21 Vestibular neuronitis, right ear
- H81.22 Vestibular neuronitis, left ear
- H81.23 Vestibular neuronitis, bilateral

H81.3 **Other peripheral vertigo**
 H81.31 Aural vertigo
- H81.311 Aural vertigo, right ear
- H81.312 Aural vertigo, left ear
- H81.313 Aural vertigo, bilateral
- H81.319 Aural vertigo, unspecified ear

 H81.39 Other peripheral vertigo
 Lermoyez' syndrome
 Otogenic vertigo
 Peripheral vertigo NOS
- H81.391 Other peripheral vertigo, right ear
- H81.392 Other peripheral vertigo, left ear
- H81.393 Other peripheral vertigo, bilateral
- H81.399 Other peripheral vertigo, unspecified ear

H81.4 **Vertigo of central origin**
 Central positional nystagmus

H81.8 **Other disorders of vestibular function**
 H81.8X Other disorders of vestibular function
- H81.8X1 Other disorders of vestibular function, right ear
- H81.8X2 Other disorders of vestibular function, left ear
- H81.8X3 Other disorders of vestibular function, bilateral
- H81.8X9 Other disorders of vestibular function, unspecified ear
 AHA: 2022,2Q,12

H81.9 **Unspecified disorder of vestibular function**
 Vertiginous syndrome NOS
- H81.90 Unspecified disorder of vestibular function, unspecified ear
- H81.91 Unspecified disorder of vestibular function, right ear
- H81.92 Unspecified disorder of vestibular function, left ear
- H81.93 Unspecified disorder of vestibular function, bilateral

H82 **Vertiginous syndromes in diseases classified elsewhere**
 Code first underlying disease
 EXCLUDES 1 epidemic vertigo (A88.1)
- H82.1 *Vertiginous syndromes in diseases classified elsewhere, right ear*
- H82.2 *Vertiginous syndromes in diseases classified elsewhere, left ear*
- H82.3 *Vertiginous syndromes in diseases classified elsewhere, bilateral*
- H82.9 *Vertiginous syndromes in diseases classified elsewhere, unspecified ear*

H83 **Other diseases of inner ear**
 H83.0 Labyrinthitis
 DEF: Inflammation of the inner ear, or labyrinth, characterized by pus, vertigo, dizziness, nausea, and hearing loss.
- H83.01 Labyrinthitis, right ear
- H83.02 Labyrinthitis, left ear
- H83.03 Labyrinthitis, bilateral
- H83.09 Labyrinthitis, unspecified ear

 H83.1 Labyrinthine fistula
- H83.11 Labyrinthine fistula, right ear
- H83.12 Labyrinthine fistula, left ear
- H83.13 Labyrinthine fistula, bilateral
- H83.19 Labyrinthine fistula, unspecified ear

 H83.2 Labyrinthine dysfunction
 Labyrinthine hypersensitivity
 Labyrinthine hypofunction
 Labyrinthine loss of function
 DEF: Decreased function of the labyrinth sensors.
 H83.2X Labyrinthine dysfunction
- H83.2X1 Labyrinthine dysfunction, right ear
- H83.2X2 Labyrinthine dysfunction, left ear
- H83.2X3 Labyrinthine dysfunction, bilateral
- H83.2X9 Labyrinthine dysfunction, unspecified ear

 H83.3 Noise effects on inner ear
 Acoustic trauma of inner ear
 Noise-induced hearing loss of inner ear
 H83.3X Noise effects on inner ear
- H83.3X1 Noise effects on right inner ear
- H83.3X2 Noise effects on left inner ear
- H83.3X3 Noise effects on inner ear, bilateral
- H83.3X9 Noise effects on inner ear, unspecified ear

 H83.8 Other specified diseases of inner ear
 H83.8X Other specified diseases of inner ear
- H83.8X1 Other specified diseases of right inner ear
- H83.8X2 Other specified diseases of left inner ear
- H83.8X3 Other specified diseases of inner ear, bilateral
- H83.8X9 Other specified diseases of inner ear, unspecified ear

 H83.9 Unspecified disease of inner ear
- H83.90 Unspecified disease of inner ear, unspecified ear
- H83.91 Unspecified disease of right inner ear
- H83.92 Unspecified disease of left inner ear
- H83.93 Unspecified disease of inner ear, bilateral

Other disorders of ear (H90-H94)

H90 **Conductive and sensorineural hearing loss**
 EXCLUDES 1 deaf nonspeaking NEC (H91.3)
 deafness NOS (H91.9-)
 hearing loss NOS (H91.9-)
 noise-induced hearing loss (H83.3-)
 ototoxic hearing loss (H91.0-)
 sudden (idiopathic) hearing loss (H91.2-)
 AHA: 2015,2Q,7
 DEF: Conductive hearing loss: Hearing loss due to the inability of soundwaves to move from the outer (external) ear to the inner ear.
 DEF: Sensorineural hearing loss: Hearing loss that occurs from damage to the hair cells of the inner ear or problems with the nerve pathways from the inner ear to the brain.

 H90.0 Conductive hearing loss, bilateral
 H90.1 Conductive hearing loss, unilateral with unrestricted hearing on the contralateral side
- H90.11 Conductive hearing loss, unilateral, right ear, with unrestricted hearing on the contralateral side
- H90.12 Conductive hearing loss, unilateral, left ear, with unrestricted hearing on the contralateral side

 H90.2 Conductive hearing loss, unspecified
 Conductive deafness NOS

 H90.3 Sensorineural hearing loss, bilateral
 H90.4 Sensorineural hearing loss, unilateral with unrestricted hearing on the contralateral side
- H90.41 Sensorineural hearing loss, unilateral, right ear, with unrestricted hearing on the contralateral side
- H90.42 Sensorineural hearing loss, unilateral, left ear, with unrestricted hearing on the contralateral side

 H90.5 Unspecified sensorineural hearing loss
 Central hearing loss NOS
 Congenital deafness NOS
 Neural hearing loss NOS
 Perceptive hearing loss NOS
 Sensorineural deafness NOS
 Sensory hearing loss NOS
 EXCLUDES 1 abnormal auditory perception (H93.2-)
 psychogenic deafness (F44.6)

 H90.6 Mixed conductive and sensorineural hearing loss, bilateral
 AHA: 2015,2Q,7

 H90.7 Mixed conductive and sensorineural hearing loss, unilateral with unrestricted hearing on the contralateral side
- H90.71 Mixed conductive and sensorineural hearing loss, unilateral, right ear, with unrestricted hearing on the contralateral side
- H90.72 Mixed conductive and sensorineural hearing loss, unilateral, left ear, with unrestricted hearing on the contralateral side

 H90.8 Mixed conductive and sensorineural hearing loss, unspecified

Chapter 8. Diseases of the Ear and Mastoid Process

- ✓5th **H90.A** Conductive and sensorineural hearing loss with restricted hearing on the contralateral side
  AHA: 2016,4Q,23-25
  - ✓6th **H90.A1** Conductive hearing loss, unilateral, with restricted hearing on the contralateral side
    - **H90.A11** Conductive hearing loss, unilateral, right ear with restricted hearing on the contralateral side
    - **H90.A12** Conductive hearing loss, unilateral, left ear with restricted hearing on the contralateral side
  - ✓6th **H90.A2** Sensorineural hearing loss, unilateral, with restricted hearing on the contralateral side
    - **H90.A21** Sensorineural hearing loss, unilateral, right ear, with restricted hearing on the contralateral side
    - **H90.A22** Sensorineural hearing loss, unilateral, left ear, with restricted hearing on the contralateral side
  - ✓6th **H90.A3** Mixed conductive and sensorineural hearing loss, unilateral with restricted hearing on the contralateral side
    - **H90.A31** Mixed conductive and sensorineural hearing loss, unilateral, right ear with restricted hearing on the contralateral side
    - **H90.A32** Mixed conductive and sensorineural hearing, unilateral, left ear with restricted hearing on the contralateral side

- ✓4th **H91** Other and unspecified hearing loss
  EXCLUDES 1 abnormal auditory perception (H93.2-)
  hearing loss as classified in H90.-
  impacted cerumen (H61.2-)
  noise-induced hearing loss (H83.3-)
  psychogenic deafness (F44.6)
  transient ischemic deafness (H93.01-)
  - ✓5th **H91.0** Ototoxic hearing loss
    Code first poisoning due to drug or toxin, if applicable (T36-T65 with fifth or sixth character 1-4)
    Use additional code for adverse effect, if applicable, to identify drug (T36-T50 with fifth or sixth character 5)
    - **H91.01** Ototoxic hearing loss, right ear
    - **H91.02** Ototoxic hearing loss, left ear
    - **H91.03** Ototoxic hearing loss, bilateral
    - **H91.09** Ototoxic hearing loss, unspecified ear
  - ✓5th **H91.1** Presbycusis
    Presbyacusia
    - **H91.10** Presbycusis, unspecified ear
    - **H91.11** Presbycusis, right ear
    - **H91.12** Presbycusis, left ear
    - **H91.13** Presbycusis, bilateral
  - ✓5th **H91.2** Sudden idiopathic hearing loss
    Sudden hearing loss NOS
    - **H91.20** Sudden idiopathic hearing loss, unspecified ear
    - **H91.21** Sudden idiopathic hearing loss, right ear
    - **H91.22** Sudden idiopathic hearing loss, left ear
    - **H91.23** Sudden idiopathic hearing loss, bilateral
  - **H91.3** Deaf nonspeaking, not elsewhere classified
  - ✓5th **H91.8** Other specified hearing loss
    - ✓6th **H91.8X** Other specified hearing loss
      - **H91.8X1** Other specified hearing loss, right ear
      - **H91.8X2** Other specified hearing loss, left ear
      - **H91.8X3** Other specified hearing loss, bilateral
      - **H91.8X9** Other specified hearing loss, unspecified ear
  - ✓5th **H91.9** Unspecified hearing loss
    Deafness NOS
    High frequency deafness
    Low frequency deafness
    - **H91.90** Unspecified hearing loss, unspecified ear
    - **H91.91** Unspecified hearing loss, right ear
    - **H91.92** Unspecified hearing loss, left ear
    - **H91.93** Unspecified hearing loss, bilateral

- ✓4th **H92** Otalgia and effusion of ear
  - ✓5th **H92.0** Otalgia
    - **H92.01** Otalgia, right ear
    - **H92.02** Otalgia, left ear
    - **H92.03** Otalgia, bilateral
    - **H92.09** Otalgia, unspecified ear
  - ✓5th **H92.1** Otorrhea
    EXCLUDES 1 leakage of cerebrospinal fluid through ear (G96.0)
    - **H92.10** Otorrhea, unspecified ear
    - **H92.11** Otorrhea, right ear
    - **H92.12** Otorrhea, left ear
    - **H92.13** Otorrhea, bilateral
  - ✓5th **H92.2** Otorrhagia
    EXCLUDES 1 traumatic otorrhagia - code to injury
    - **H92.20** Otorrhagia, unspecified ear
    - **H92.21** Otorrhagia, right ear
    - **H92.22** Otorrhagia, left ear
    - **H92.23** Otorrhagia, bilateral

- ✓4th **H93** Other disorders of ear, not elsewhere classified
  - ✓5th **H93.0** Degenerative and vascular disorders of ear
    EXCLUDES 1 presbycusis (H91.1)
    - ✓6th **H93.01** Transient ischemic deafness
      - **H93.011** Transient ischemic deafness, right ear
      - **H93.012** Transient ischemic deafness, left ear
      - **H93.013** Transient ischemic deafness, bilateral
      - **H93.019** Transient ischemic deafness, unspecified ear
    - ✓6th **H93.09** Unspecified degenerative and vascular disorders of ear
      - **H93.091** Unspecified degenerative and vascular disorders of right ear
      - **H93.092** Unspecified degenerative and vascular disorders of left ear
      - **H93.093** Unspecified degenerative and vascular disorders of ear, bilateral
      - **H93.099** Unspecified degenerative and vascular disorders of unspecified ear
  - ✓5th **H93.1** Tinnitus
    - **H93.11** Tinnitus, right ear
    - **H93.12** Tinnitus, left ear
    - **H93.13** Tinnitus, bilateral
    - **H93.19** Tinnitus, unspecified ear
  - ✓5th **H93.A** Pulsatile tinnitus
    AHA: 2023,2Q,18; 2016,4Q,25-26
    - **H93.A1** Pulsatile tinnitus, right ear
    - **H93.A2** Pulsatile tinnitus, left ear
    - **H93.A3** Pulsatile tinnitus, bilateral
    - **H93.A9** Pulsatile tinnitus, unspecified ear
  - ✓5th **H93.2** Other abnormal auditory perceptions
    EXCLUDES 2 auditory hallucinations (R44.0)
    - ✓6th **H93.21** Auditory recruitment
      - **H93.211** Auditory recruitment, right ear
      - **H93.212** Auditory recruitment, left ear
      - **H93.213** Auditory recruitment, bilateral
      - **H93.219** Auditory recruitment, unspecified ear
    - ✓6th **H93.22** Diplacusis
      - **H93.221** Diplacusis, right ear
      - **H93.222** Diplacusis, left ear
      - **H93.223** Diplacusis, bilateral
      - **H93.229** Diplacusis, unspecified ear
    - ✓6th **H93.23** Hyperacusis
      DEF: Exceptionally acute sense of hearing caused by such conditions as Bell's palsy. This term may also refer to painful sensitivity to sounds.
      - **H93.231** Hyperacusis, right ear
      - **H93.232** Hyperacusis, left ear
      - **H93.233** Hyperacusis, bilateral
      - **H93.239** Hyperacusis, unspecified ear
    - ✓6th **H93.24** Temporary auditory threshold shift
      - **H93.241** Temporary auditory threshold shift, right ear
      - **H93.242** Temporary auditory threshold shift, left ear
      - **H93.243** Temporary auditory threshold shift, bilateral
      - **H93.249** Temporary auditory threshold shift, unspecified ear
    - **H93.25** Central auditory processing disorder
      Congenital auditory imperception
      Word deafness
      EXCLUDES 1 mixed receptive-expressive language disorder (F80.2)

Chapter 8. Diseases of the Ear and Mastoid Process

- **H93.29** Other abnormal auditory perceptions
  - H93.291 Other abnormal auditory perceptions, right ear
  - H93.292 Other abnormal auditory perceptions, left ear
  - H93.293 Other abnormal auditory perceptions, bilateral
  - H93.299 Other abnormal auditory perceptions, unspecified ear
- **H93.3** Disorders of acoustic nerve
  - Disorder of 8th cranial nerve
  - **EXCLUDES 1** acoustic neuroma (D33.3)
  - syphilitic acoustic neuritis (A52.15)
  - **H93.3X** Disorders of acoustic nerve
    - H93.3X1 Disorders of right acoustic nerve
    - H93.3X2 Disorders of left acoustic nerve
    - H93.3X3 Disorders of bilateral acoustic nerves
    - H93.3X9 Disorders of unspecified acoustic nerve
- **H93.8** Other specified disorders of ear
  - **H93.8X** Other specified disorders of ear
    - H93.8X1 Other specified disorders of right ear
    - H93.8X2 Other specified disorders of left ear
    - H93.8X3 Other specified disorders of ear, bilateral
    - H93.8X9 Other specified disorders of ear, unspecified ear
- **H93.9** Unspecified disorder of ear
  - H93.90 Unspecified disorder of ear, unspecified ear
  - H93.91 Unspecified disorder of right ear
  - H93.92 Unspecified disorder of left ear
  - H93.93 Unspecified disorder of ear, bilateral

- **H94** Other disorders of ear in diseases classified elsewhere
  - **H94.0** Acoustic neuritis in infectious and parasitic diseases classified elsewhere
    - Code first underlying disease, such as:
    - parasitic disease (B65-B89)
    - **EXCLUDES 1** acoustic neuritis (in):
      - herpes zoster (B02.29)
      - syphilis (A52.15)
    - H94.00 Acoustic neuritis in infectious and parasitic diseases classified elsewhere, unspecified ear
    - H94.01 Acoustic neuritis in infectious and parasitic diseases classified elsewhere, right ear
    - H94.02 Acoustic neuritis in infectious and parasitic diseases classified elsewhere, left ear
    - H94.03 Acoustic neuritis in infectious and parasitic diseases classified elsewhere, bilateral
  - **H94.8** Other specified disorders of ear in diseases classified elsewhere
    - Code first underlying disease, such as:
    - congenital syphilis (A50.0)
    - **EXCLUDES 1** aural myiasis (B87.4)
    - syphilitic labyrinthitis (A52.79)
    - H94.80 Other specified disorders of ear in diseases classified elsewhere, unspecified ear
    - H94.81 Other specified disorders of right ear in diseases classified elsewhere
    - H94.82 Other specified disorders of left ear in diseases classified elsewhere
    - H94.83 Other specified disorders of ear in diseases classified elsewhere, bilateral

Intraoperative and postprocedural complications and disorders of ear and mastoid process, not elsewhere classified (H95)

- **H95** Intraoperative and postprocedural complications and disorders of ear and mastoid process, not elsewhere classified
  - AHA: 2016,4Q,9-10
  - **H95.0** Recurrent cholesteatoma of postmastoidectomy cavity
    - H95.00 Recurrent cholesteatoma of postmastoidectomy cavity, unspecified ear
    - H95.01 Recurrent cholesteatoma of postmastoidectomy cavity, right ear
    - H95.02 Recurrent cholesteatoma of postmastoidectomy cavity, left ear
    - H95.03 Recurrent cholesteatoma of postmastoidectomy cavity, bilateral ears
  - **H95.1** Other disorders of ear and mastoid process following mastoidectomy
    - **H95.11** Chronic inflammation of postmastoidectomy cavity
      - H95.111 Chronic inflammation of postmastoidectomy cavity, right ear
      - H95.112 Chronic inflammation of postmastoidectomy cavity, left ear
      - H95.113 Chronic inflammation of postmastoidectomy cavity, bilateral ears
      - H95.119 Chronic inflammation of postmastoidectomy cavity, unspecified ear
    - **H95.12** Granulation of postmastoidectomy cavity
      - H95.121 Granulation of postmastoidectomy cavity, right ear
      - H95.122 Granulation of postmastoidectomy cavity, left ear
      - H95.123 Granulation of postmastoidectomy cavity, bilateral ears
      - H95.129 Granulation of postmastoidectomy cavity, unspecified ear
    - **H95.13** Mucosal cyst of postmastoidectomy cavity
      - H95.131 Mucosal cyst of postmastoidectomy cavity, right ear
      - H95.132 Mucosal cyst of postmastoidectomy cavity, left ear
      - H95.133 Mucosal cyst of postmastoidectomy cavity, bilateral ears
      - H95.139 Mucosal cyst of postmastoidectomy cavity, unspecified ear
    - **H95.19** Other disorders following mastoidectomy
      - H95.191 Other disorders following mastoidectomy, right ear
      - H95.192 Other disorders following mastoidectomy, left ear
      - H95.193 Other disorders following mastoidectomy, bilateral ears
      - H95.199 Other disorders following mastoidectomy, unspecified ear
  - **H95.2** Intraoperative hemorrhage and hematoma of ear and mastoid process complicating a procedure
    - **EXCLUDES 1** intraoperative hemorrhage and hematoma of ear and mastoid process due to accidental puncture or laceration during a procedure (H95.3-)
    - H95.21 Intraoperative hemorrhage and hematoma of ear and mastoid process complicating a procedure on the ear and mastoid process
    - H95.22 Intraoperative hemorrhage and hematoma of ear and mastoid process complicating other procedure
  - **H95.3** Accidental puncture and laceration of ear and mastoid process during a procedure
    - H95.31 Accidental puncture and laceration of the ear and mastoid process during a procedure on the ear and mastoid process
    - H95.32 Accidental puncture and laceration of the ear and mastoid process during other procedure
  - **H95.4** Postprocedural hemorrhage of ear and mastoid process following a procedure
    - H95.41 Postprocedural hemorrhage of ear and mastoid process following a procedure on the ear and mastoid process
    - H95.42 Postprocedural hemorrhage of ear and mastoid process following other procedure
  - **H95.5** Postprocedural hematoma and seroma of ear and mastoid process following a procedure
    - H95.51 Postprocedural hematoma of ear and mastoid process following a procedure on the ear and mastoid process
    - H95.52 Postprocedural hematoma of ear and mastoid process following other procedure
    - H95.53 Postprocedural seroma of ear and mastoid process following a procedure on the ear and mastoid process
    - H95.54 Postprocedural seroma of ear and mastoid process following other procedure
  - **H95.8** Other intraoperative and postprocedural complications and disorders of the ear and mastoid process, not elsewhere classified
    - **EXCLUDES 2** postprocedural complications and disorders following mastoidectomy (H95.0-, H95.1-)
    - **H95.81** Postprocedural stenosis of external ear canal
      - H95.811 Postprocedural stenosis of right external ear canal

---

Additional Character Required | Placeholder Alert | Manifestation | Unspecified Dx | QPP | UPD Unacceptable PDx

- **H95.812** Postprocedural stenosis of left external ear canal
- **H95.813** Postprocedural stenosis of external ear canal, bilateral
- **H95.819** Postprocedural stenosis of unspecified external ear canal
- **H95.88** Other intraoperative complications and disorders of the ear and mastoid process, not elsewhere classified
  Use additional code, if applicable, to further specify disorder
- **H95.89** Other postprocedural complications and disorders of the ear and mastoid process, not elsewhere classified
  Use additional code, if applicable, to further specify disorder

Chapter 9. Diseases of the Circulatory System (I00–I99)

Chapter-specific Guidelines with Coding Examples
The chapter-specific guidelines from the ICD-10-CM Official Guidelines for Coding and Reporting have been provided below. Along with these guidelines are coding examples, contained in the shaded boxes, that have been developed to help illustrate the coding and/or sequencing guidance found in these guidelines.

a. Hypertension
The classification presumes a causal relationship between hypertension and heart involvement and between hypertension and kidney involvement, as the two conditions are linked by the term "with" in the Alphabetic Index. These conditions should be coded as related even in the absence of provider documentation explicitly linking them, unless the documentation clearly states the conditions are unrelated.

For hypertension and conditions not specifically linked by relational terms such as "with," "associated with" or "due to" in the classification, provider documentation must link the conditions in order to code them as related.

1) **Hypertension with heart disease**

   Hypertension with heart conditions classified to I50.-, Heart failure, I51.4, Myocarditis, unspecified, I51.89, Other ill-defined heart diseases, and I51.9, Heart disease, unspecified, is assigned to a code from category I11, Hypertensive heart disease. Use additional code(s) from category I50, Heart failure, or I51, Complications and ill-defined descriptions of heart disease, to identify the heart condition.

   Hypertension with heart conditions classified to I51.5, Myocardial degeneration, or I51.7, Cardiomegaly, is assigned to a code from category I11, Hypertensive heart disease. No additional code is assigned to identify the specific heart condition.

   The same heart conditions (I50.-, I51.4-I51.7, I51.89, I51.9) with hypertension are coded separately if the provider has documented they are unrelated to the hypertension. **The applicable hypertension code I10, Essential (primary) hypertension, or a code from category I15, Secondary hypertension, should be assigned. Sequence according to the circumstances of the admission/encounter.**

2) **Hypertensive chronic kidney disease**

   Assign codes from category I12, Hypertensive chronic kidney disease, when both hypertension and a condition classifiable to category N18, Chronic kidney disease (CKD), are present. CKD should not be coded as hypertensive if the provider indicates the CKD is not related to the hypertension.

   The appropriate code from category N18 should be used as a secondary code with a code from category I12 to identify the stage of chronic kidney disease.
   See Section I.C.14. Chronic kidney disease.

   If a patient has hypertensive chronic kidney disease and acute renal failure, the acute renal failure should also be coded. Sequence according to the circumstances of the admission/encounter.

3) **Hypertensive heart and chronic kidney disease**

   The codes in category I13, Hypertensive heart and chronic kidney disease, are combination codes that include hypertension, heart disease and chronic kidney disease. Assign codes from combination category I13, Hypertensive heart and chronic kidney disease, when there is hypertension with both heart and chronic kidney disease. If heart failure is present, assign an additional code from category I50 to identify the type of heart failure.

   The appropriate code from category N18, Chronic kidney disease, should be used as a secondary code with a code from category I13 to identify the stage of chronic kidney disease.
   See Section I.C.14. Chronic kidney disease.

   The Includes note at I13 specifies that the conditions included at I11 and I12 are included together in I13. If a patient has hypertension, heart disease and chronic kidney disease, then a code from I13 should be used, not codes from I11 or I12.

   For patients with both acute renal failure and chronic kidney disease, the acute renal failure should also be coded. Sequence according to the circumstances of the admission/encounter.

Hypertensive heart and kidney disease with congestive heart failure and stage 2 chronic kidney disease	
I13.0	Hypertensive heart and chronic kidney disease with heart failure and stage 1 through stage 4 chronic kidney disease, or unspecified chronic kidney disease
I50.9	Heart failure, unspecified
N18.2	Chronic kidney disease, stage 2 (mild)

   Explanation: Combination codes in category I13 are used to report conditions classifiable to *both* categories I11 and I12. Do not report conditions classifiable to I11 and I12 separately. Use additional codes to report type of heart failure and stage of CKD.

4) **Hypertensive cerebrovascular disease**

   For hypertensive cerebrovascular disease, first assign the appropriate code from categories I60-I69, followed by the appropriate hypertension code.

5) **Hypertensive retinopathy**

   Subcategory H35.0, Background retinopathy and retinal vascular changes, should be used along with a code from categories I10-I15, in the Hypertensive diseases section, to include the systemic hypertension. The sequencing is based on the reason for the encounter.

6) **Hypertension, secondary**

   Secondary hypertension is due to an underlying condition. Two codes are required: one to identify the underlying etiology and one from category I15 to identify the hypertension. Sequencing of codes is determined by the reason for admission/encounter.

Renovascular hypertension due to renal artery atherosclerosis	
I15.0	Renovascular hypertension
I70.1	Atherosclerosis of renal artery

   Explanation: Secondary hypertension requires two codes: a code to identify the etiology and the appropriate I15 code.

7) **Hypertension, transient**

   Assign code R03.0, Elevated blood pressure reading without diagnosis of hypertension, unless patient has an established diagnosis of hypertension. Assign code O13.-, Gestational [pregnancy-induced] hypertension without significant proteinuria, or O14.-, Pre-eclampsia, for transient hypertension of pregnancy.

8) **Hypertension, controlled**

   This diagnostic statement usually refers to an existing state of hypertension under control by therapy. Assign the appropriate code from categories I10-I15, Hypertensive diseases.

9) **Hypertension, uncontrolled**

   Uncontrolled hypertension may refer to untreated hypertension or hyper- tension not responding to current therapeutic regimen. In either case, assign the appropriate code from categories I10-I15, Hypertensive diseases.

10) **Hypertensive crisis**

    Assign a code from category I16, Hypertensive crisis, for documented hypertensive urgency, hypertensive emergency or unspecified hypertensive crisis. Code also any identified hypertensive disease (I10-I15). The sequencing is based on the reason for the encounter.

11) **Pulmonary hypertension**

    Pulmonary hypertension is classified to category I27, Other pulmonary heart diseases. For secondary pulmonary hypertension (I27.1, I27.2-), code also any associated conditions or adverse effects of drugs or toxins. The sequencing is based on the reason for the encounter, except for adverse effects of drugs (See Section I.C.19.e.).

12) **Hypertension, Resistant**

    Resistant hypertension refers to blood pressure of a patient with hypertension that remains above goal in spite of the use of antihypertensive medications. Assign code I1A.0, Resistant hypertension, as an additional code when apparent treatment resistant hypertension, treatment resistant hypertension, or true resistant hypertension is documented by the provider. A code for the specific type of existing hypertension is sequenced first, if known.

b. Atherosclerotic coronary artery disease and angina
ICD-10-CM has combination codes for atherosclerotic heart disease with angina pectoris. The subcategories for these codes are I25.11, Atherosclerotic heart disease of native coronary artery with angina pectoris and I25.7, Atherosclerosis of coronary artery bypass graft(s) and coronary artery of transplanted heart with angina pectoris.

When using one of these combination codes it is not necessary to use an additional code for angina pectoris. A causal relationship can be assumed in a patient with both atherosclerosis and angina pectoris, unless the documentation indicates the angina is due to something other than the atherosclerosis.

If a patient with coronary artery disease is admitted due to an acute myocardial infarction (AMI), the AMI should be sequenced before the coronary artery disease.

See Section I.C.9. Acute myocardial infarction (AMI)

> Patient is being seen for spastic angina pectoris. She also has a documented history of progressive coronary artery disease of the native vessels.
>
> | I25.111 | Atherosclerotic heart disease of native coronary artery with angina pectoris with documented spasm |
> |---|---|
>
> *Explanation*: Report the combination code for atherosclerotic heart disease (coronary artery disease) with angina pectoris. A causal relationship is assumed in a patient with both atherosclerosis and angina pectoris, unless the documentation indicates the angina is due to something other than the atherosclerosis. When using one of these combination codes, it is not necessary to use an additional code for angina pectoris.

c. **Intraoperative and postprocedural cerebrovascular accident**

Medical record documentation should clearly specify the cause- and- effect relationship between the medical intervention and the cerebrovascular accident in order to assign a code for intraoperative or postprocedural cerebrovascular accident.

Proper code assignment depends on whether it was an infarction or hemorrhage and whether it occurred intraoperatively or postoperatively. If it was a cerebral hemorrhage, code assignment depends on the type of procedure performed.

> Embolic cerebral infarction of the right middle cerebral artery that occurred during hip replacement surgery. The surgeon documented as due to the surgery.
>
> | I97.811 | Intraoperative cerebrovascular infarction during other surgery |
> |---|---|
> | I63.411 | Cerebral infarction due to embolism of right middle cerebral artery |
>
> *Explanation*: Code assignment for intraoperative or postprocedural cerebrovascular accident is based on the provider's documentation of a cause-and-effect relationship between the condition and the procedure. Proper code assignment also depends on whether the cerebrovascular accident was an infarction or hemorrhage, occurred intraoperatively or postoperatively, and the type of procedure performed.

d. **Sequelae of cerebrovascular disease**

1) **Category I69, Sequelae of cerebrovascular disease**

   Category I69 is used to indicate conditions classifiable to categories I60-I67 as the causes of sequela (neurologic deficits), themselves classified elsewhere. These "late effects" include neurologic deficits that persist after initial onset of conditions classifiable to categories I60-I67. The neurologic deficits caused by cerebrovascular disease may be present from the onset or may arise at any time after the onset of the condition classifiable to categories I60-I67.

   Codes from category I69, Sequelae of cerebrovascular disease, that specify hemiplegia, hemiparesis and monoplegia identify whether the dominant or nondominant side is affected. Should the affected side be documented, but not specified as dominant or nondominant, and the classification system does not indicate a default, code selection is as follows:
   - For ambidextrous patients, the default should be dominant.
   - If the left side is affected, the default is non-dominant.
   - If the right side is affected, the default is dominant.

2) **Codes from category I69 with codes from I60–I67**

   Codes from category I69 may be assigned on a health care record with codes from I60-I67, if the patient has a current cerebrovascular disease and deficits from an old cerebrovascular disease.

3) **Codes from category I69 and personal history of transient ischemic attack (TIA) and cerebral infarction (Z86.73)**

   Codes from category I69 should not be assigned if the patient does not have neurologic deficits.

   See Section I.C.21. 4. History (of) for use of personal history codes

e. **Acute myocardial infarction (AMI)**

1) **Type 1 ST elevation myocardial infarction (STEMI) and non-ST elevation myocardial infarction (NSTEMI)**

   The ICD-10-CM codes for type 1 acute myocardial infarction (AMI) identify the site, such as anterolateral wall or true posterior wall.

Subcategories I21.0-I21.2 and code I21.3 are used for type 1 ST elevation myocardial infarction (STEMI). Code I21.4, Non-ST elevation (NSTEMI) myocardial infarction, is used for type 1 non-ST elevation myocardial infarction (NSTEMI) and nontransmural MIs.

If a type 1 NSTEMI evolves to STEMI, assign the STEMI code. If a type 1 STEMI converts to NSTEMI due to thrombolytic therapy, it is still coded as STEMI.

For encounters occurring while the myocardial infarction is equal to, or less than, four weeks old, including transfers to another acute setting or a postacute setting, and the myocardial infarction meets the definition for "other diagnoses" (see Section III, Reporting Additional Diagnoses), codes from category I21 may continue to be reported. For encounters after the 4-week time frame and the patient is still receiving care related to the myocardial infarction, the appropriate aftercare code should be assigned, rather than a code from category I21. For old or healed myocardial infarctions not requiring further care, code I25.2, Old myocardial infarction, may be assigned.

2) **Acute myocardial infarction, unspecified**

   Code I21.9, Acute myocardial infarction, unspecified, is the default for unspecified acute myocardial infarction or unspecified type. If only type 1 STEMI or transmural MI without the site is documented, assign code I21.3, ST elevation (STEMI) myocardial infarction of unspecified site.

3) **AMI documented as nontransmural or subendocardial but site provided**

   If an AMI is documented as nontransmural or subendocardial, but the site is provided, it is still coded as a subendocardial AMI.

   See Section I.C.21.3.for information on coding status post administration of tPA in a different facility within the last 24 hours.

4) **Subsequent acute myocardial infarction**

   A code from category I22, Subsequent ST elevation (STEMI) and non-ST elevation (NSTEMI) myocardial infarction, is to be used when a patient who has suffered a type 1 or unspecified AMI has a new AMI within the 4-week time frame of the initial AMI. A code from category I22 must be used in conjunction with a code from category I21. The sequencing of the I22 and I21 codes depends on the circumstances of the encounter.

   Do not assign code I22 for subsequent myocardial infarctions other than type 1 or unspecified. For subsequent type 2 AMI assign only code I21.A1. For subsequent type 4 or type 5 AMI, assign only code I21.A9.

   If a subsequent myocardial infarction of one type occurs within 4 weeks of a myocardial infarction of a different type, assign the appropriate codes from category I21 to identify each type. Do not assign a code from I22. Codes from category I22 should only be assigned if both the initial and subsequent myocardial infarctions are type 1 or unspecified.

   > Patient suffered an acute NSTEMI 14 days ago and is now seen for an inferior STEMI.
   >
   > | I22.1 | Subsequent ST elevation (STEMI) myocardial infarction of inferior wall |
   > |---|---|
   > | I21.4 | Non-ST elevation (NSTEMI) myocardial infarction |
   >
   > *Explanation*: Both MIs were type 1, and the current MI occurred within the four-week time frame; therefore a code for the current/subsequent STEMI (I22.1) is reported as well as a code for the previous NSTEMI (I21.4).

5) **Other types of myocardial infarction**

   The ICD-10-CM provides codes for different types of myocardial infarction. Type 1 myocardial infarctions are assigned to codes I21.0-I21.4.

   Type 2 myocardial infarction (myocardial infarction due to demand ischemia or secondary to ischemic imbalance) is assigned to code I21.A1, Myocardial infarction type 2 with the underlying cause coded first, if applicable. Do not assign code I24.89, Other forms of acute ischemic heart disease, for the demand ischemia. If a type 2 AMI is described as NSTEMI or STEMI, only assign code I21.A1. Codes I21.01-I21.4 should only be assigned for type 1 AMIs.

   Acute myocardial infarctions type 3, 4a, 4b, 4c and 5 are assigned to code I21.A9, Other myocardial infarction type.

   The "Code also" and "Code first" notes should be followed related to complications, and for coding of postprocedural myocardial infarctions during or following cardiac surgery.

6) **Myocardial infarction with coronary microvascular dysfunction**

   Coronary microvascular dysfunction (CMD) is a condition that impacts the microvasculature by restricting microvascular flow and increasing microvascular resistance. Code I21.B, Myocardial infarction with coronary microvascular dysfunction, is assigned for myocardial infarction with coronary microvascular disease, myocardial infarction with coronary microvascular dysfunction, and myocardial infarction with non-obstructive coronary arteries (MINOCA) with microvascular disease.

Chapter 9. Diseases of the Circulatory System (I00-I99)

EXCLUDES 2 certain conditions originating in the perinatal period (P04-P96)
certain infectious and parasitic diseases (A00-B99)
complications of pregnancy, childbirth and the puerperium (O00-O9A)
congenital malformations, deformations, and chromosomal abnormalities (Q00-Q99)
endocrine, nutritional and metabolic diseases (E00-E88)
injury, poisoning and certain other consequences of external causes (S00-T88)
neoplasms (C00-D49)
symptoms, signs and abnormal clinical and laboratory findings, not elsewhere classified (R00-R94)
systemic connective tissue disorders (M30-M36)
transient cerebral ischemic attacks and related syndromes (G45.-)

This chapter contains the following blocks:
- I00-I02 Acute rheumatic fever
- I05-I09 Chronic rheumatic heart diseases
- I10-I1A Hypertensive diseases
- I20-I25 Ischemic heart diseases
- I26-I28 Pulmonary heart disease and diseases of pulmonary circulation
- I30-I5A Other forms of heart disease
- I60-I69 Cerebrovascular diseases
- I70-I79 Diseases of arteries, arterioles and capillaries
- I80-I89 Diseases of veins, lymphatic vessels and lymph nodes, not elsewhere classified
- I95-I99 Other and unspecified disorders of the circulatory system

Acute rheumatic fever (I00-I02)

DEF: Rheumatic fever: Inflammatory disease that can follow a throat infection by group A *streptococci*. Complications can involve the joints (arthritis), subcutaneous tissue (nodules), skin (erythema marginatum), heart (carditis), or brain (chorea).

I00 Rheumatic fever without heart involvement
INCLUDES arthritis, rheumatic, acute or subacute
EXCLUDES 1 rheumatic fever with heart involvement (I01.0-I01.9)

I01 Rheumatic fever with heart involvement
EXCLUDES 1 chronic diseases of rheumatic origin (I05-I09) unless rheumatic fever is also present or there is evidence of reactivation or activity of the rheumatic process

I01.0 Acute rheumatic pericarditis
Any condition in I00 with pericarditis
Rheumatic pericarditis (acute)
EXCLUDES 1 acute pericarditis not specified as rheumatic (I30.-)

I01.1 Acute rheumatic endocarditis
Acute rheumatic valvulitis
Any condition in I00 with endocarditis or valvulitis

I01.2 Acute rheumatic myocarditis
Any condition in I00 with myocarditis

I01.8 Other acute rheumatic heart disease
Acute rheumatic pancarditis
Any condition in I00 with other or multiple types of heart involvement

I01.9 Acute rheumatic heart disease, unspecified
Any condition in I00 with unspecified type of heart involvement
Rheumatic carditis, acute
Rheumatic heart disease, active or acute

I02 Rheumatic chorea
INCLUDES Sydenham's chorea
EXCLUDES 1 chorea NOS (G25.5)
Huntington's chorea (G10)

I02.0 Rheumatic chorea with heart involvement
Chorea NOS with heart involvement
Rheumatic chorea with heart involvement of any type classifiable under I01.-

I02.9 Rheumatic chorea without heart involvement
Rheumatic chorea NOS

Chronic rheumatic heart diseases (I05-I09)

I05 Rheumatic mitral valve diseases
INCLUDES conditions classifiable to both I05.0 and I05.2-I05.9, whether specified as rheumatic or not
EXCLUDES 1 mitral valve disease specified as nonrheumatic (I34.-)
mitral valve disease with aortic and/or tricuspid valve involvement (I08.-)

I05.0 Rheumatic mitral stenosis
Mitral (valve) obstruction (rheumatic)

I05.1 Rheumatic mitral insufficiency
Rheumatic mitral incompetence
Rheumatic mitral regurgitation
EXCLUDES 1 mitral insufficiency not specified as rheumatic (I34.0)

I05.2 Rheumatic mitral stenosis with insufficiency
Rheumatic mitral stenosis with incompetence or regurgitation

I05.8 Other rheumatic mitral valve diseases
Rheumatic mitral (valve) failure

I05.9 Rheumatic mitral valve disease, unspecified
Rheumatic mitral (valve) disorder (chronic) NOS

I06 Rheumatic aortic valve diseases
EXCLUDES 1 aortic valve disease not specified as rheumatic (I35.-)
aortic valve disease with mitral and/or tricuspid valve involvement (I08.-)

I06.0 Rheumatic aortic stenosis
Rheumatic aortic (valve) obstruction

I06.1 Rheumatic aortic insufficiency
Rheumatic aortic incompetence
Rheumatic aortic regurgitation

I06.2 Rheumatic aortic stenosis with insufficiency
Rheumatic aortic stenosis with incompetence or regurgitation

I06.8 Other rheumatic aortic valve diseases

I06.9 Rheumatic aortic valve disease, unspecified
Rheumatic aortic (valve) disease NOS

I07 Rheumatic tricuspid valve diseases
INCLUDES rheumatic tricuspid valve diseases specified as rheumatic or unspecified
EXCLUDES 1 tricuspid valve disease specified as nonrheumatic (I36.-)
tricuspid valve disease with aortic and/or mitral valve involvement (I08.-)

I07.0 Rheumatic tricuspid stenosis
Tricuspid (valve) stenosis (rheumatic)

I07.1 Rheumatic tricuspid insufficiency
Tricuspid (valve) insufficiency (rheumatic)

I07.2 Rheumatic tricuspid stenosis and insufficiency

I07.8 Other rheumatic tricuspid valve diseases

I07.9 Rheumatic tricuspid valve disease, unspecified
Rheumatic tricuspid valve disorder NOS

I08 Multiple valve diseases
INCLUDES multiple valve diseases specified as rheumatic or unspecified
EXCLUDES 1 endocarditis, valve unspecified (I38)
rheumatic valve disease NOS (I09.1)
EXCLUDES 2 multiple valve disease specified as nonrheumatic (I34.-, I35.-, I36.-, I37.-, I38., Q22.-, Q23.-,Q24.8-)

I08.0 Rheumatic disorders of both mitral and aortic valves
Involvement of both mitral and aortic valves specified as rheumatic or unspecified
AHA: 2025,1Q,19; 2019,2Q,5

I08.1 Rheumatic disorders of both mitral and tricuspid valves

I08.2 Rheumatic disorders of both aortic and tricuspid valves

I08.3 Combined rheumatic disorders of mitral, aortic and tricuspid valves

I08.8 Other rheumatic multiple valve diseases

I08.9 Rheumatic multiple valve disease, unspecified

I09 Other rheumatic heart diseases

I09.0 Rheumatic myocarditis
EXCLUDES 1 myocarditis not specified as rheumatic (I51.4)

I09.1 Rheumatic diseases of endocardium, valve unspecified
Rheumatic endocarditis (chronic)
Rheumatic valvulitis (chronic)
EXCLUDES 1 endocarditis, valve unspecified (I38)

I09.2 Chronic rheumatic pericarditis
Adherent pericardium, rheumatic
Chronic rheumatic mediastinopericarditis
Chronic rheumatic myopericarditis
EXCLUDES 1 chronic pericarditis not specified as rheumatic (I31.-)

I09.8 Other specified rheumatic heart diseases

  I09.81 Rheumatic heart failure   HCC Rx ESR COM
  Use additional code to identify type of heart failure (I50.-)

  I09.89 Other specified rheumatic heart diseases
  Rheumatic disease of pulmonary valve

I09.9 Rheumatic heart disease, unspecified
Rheumatic carditis
EXCLUDES 1 rheumatoid carditis (M05.31)

Hypertensive diseases (I10-I1A)

Use additional code to identify:
  exposure to environmental tobacco smoke (Z77.22)
  history of tobacco dependence (Z87.891)
  occupational exposure to environmental tobacco smoke (Z57.31)
  tobacco dependence (F17.-)
  tobacco use (Z72.0)

EXCLUDES 1 neonatal hypertension (P29.2)
  primary pulmonary hypertension (I27.0)

EXCLUDES 2 hypertensive disease complicating pregnancy, childbirth and the puerperium (O10-O11, O13-O16)

I10 Essential (primary) hypertension
INCLUDES high blood pressure
  hypertension (arterial) (benign) (essential) (malignant) (primary) (systemic)

EXCLUDES 1 hypertensive disease complicating pregnancy, childbirth and the puerperium (O10-O11, O13-O16)

EXCLUDES 2 essential (primary) hypertension involving vessels of brain (I60-I69)
  essential (primary) hypertension involving vessels of eye (H35.0-)

AHA: 2023,4Q,24; 2022,1Q,36; 2020,1Q,12; 2018,2Q,9; 2016,4Q,27

I11 Hypertensive heart disease
INCLUDES any condition in I50.- or I51.4-I51.7, I51.89, I51.9 due to hypertension

AHA: 2018,2Q,9

TIP: Do not assign a code from this category when provider documentation indicates the heart disease is attributable to another cause.

I11.0 Hypertensive heart disease with heart failure
  Hypertensive heart failure
  Use additional code to identify type of heart failure (I50.-)
  AHA: 2017,1Q,47

I11.9 Hypertensive heart disease without heart failure
  Hypertensive heart disease NOS

I12 Hypertensive chronic kidney disease
INCLUDES any condition in N18 and N26 — due to hypertension
  arteriosclerosis of kidney
  arteriosclerotic nephritis (chronic) (interstitial)
  hypertensive nephropathy
  nephrosclerosis

EXCLUDES 1 hypertension due to kidney disease (I15.0, I15.1)
  renovascular hypertension (I15.0)
  secondary hypertension (I15.-)

EXCLUDES 2 acute kidney failure (N17.-)

AHA: 2019,3Q,3; 2018,4Q,88; 2016,3Q,22

TIP: Do not assign a code from this category when provider documentation indicates the chronic kidney disease (CKD) is attributable to another cause.

I12.0 Hypertensive chronic kidney disease with stage 5 chronic kidney disease or end stage renal disease
  Use additional code to identify the stage of chronic kidney disease (N18.5, N18.6)

I12.9 Hypertensive chronic kidney disease with stage 1 through stage 4 chronic kidney disease, or unspecified chronic kidney disease
  Hypertensive chronic kidney disease NOS
  Hypertensive renal disease NOS
  Use additional code to identify the stage of chronic kidney disease (N18.1-N18.4, N18.9)

I13 Hypertensive heart and chronic kidney disease
INCLUDES any condition in I11.- with any condition in I12.-
  cardiorenal disease
  cardiovascular renal disease

TIP: Do not assign a code from this category when provider documentation indicates the heart and/or chronic kidney disease is attributable to another cause.

I13.0 Hypertensive heart and chronic kidney disease with heart failure and stage 1 through stage 4 chronic kidney disease, or unspecified chronic kidney disease
  Use additional code to identify stage of chronic kidney disease (N18.1-N18.4, N18.9)
  Use additional code to identify type of heart failure (I50.-)

I13.1 Hypertensive heart and chronic kidney disease without heart failure

I13.10 Hypertensive heart and chronic kidney disease without heart failure, with stage 1 through stage 4 chronic kidney disease, or unspecified chronic kidney disease
  Hypertensive heart disease and hypertensive chronic kidney disease NOS
  Use additional code to identify the stage of chronic kidney disease (N18.1-N18.4, N18.9)

I13.11 Hypertensive heart and chronic kidney disease without heart failure, with stage 5 chronic kidney disease, or end stage renal disease
  Use additional code to identify the stage of chronic kidney disease (N18.5, N18.6)

I13.2 Hypertensive heart and chronic kidney disease with heart failure and with stage 5 chronic kidney disease, or end stage renal disease
  Use additional code to identify the stage of chronic kidney disease (N18.5, N18.6)
  Use additional code to identify type of heart failure (I50.-)

I15 Secondary hypertension
Code also underlying condition

EXCLUDES 1 postprocedural hypertension (I97.3)

EXCLUDES 2 secondary hypertension involving vessels of brain (I60-I69)
  secondary hypertension involving vessels of eye (H35.0-)

I15.0 Renovascular hypertension

I15.1 Hypertension secondary to other renal disorders
  AHA: 2016,3Q,22

I15.2 Hypertension secondary to endocrine disorders
  AHA: 2023,2Q,16

I15.8 Other secondary hypertension

I15.9 Secondary hypertension, unspecified

I16 Hypertensive crisis
Code also any identified hypertensive disease (I10-I15, I1A)
AHA: 2016,4Q,26-28

I16.0 Hypertensive urgency

I16.1 Hypertensive emergency
  Use additional code, if applicable, to identify specific organ dysfunction, such as:
    acute kidney injury (N17.-)
    acute myocardial infarction (I21.-)
    acute pulmonary edema (left and/or right ventricular failure) (J81.0, I50.-)
    aortic dissection (I71.0-)
    cerebral hemorrhage (I60.-, I61.-, I62.-)
    cerebral infarction (I63.-)
    eclampsia (O15.-)
    hypertensive encephalopathy (I67.4)
    seizure (R56.9)
  AHA: 2023,4Q,24

I16.9 Hypertensive crisis, unspecified

I1A Other hypertension
AHA: 2023,4Q,23-25

I1A.0 Resistant hypertension
  Apparent treatment resistant hypertension
  Treatment resistant hypertension
  True resistant hypertension
  Code first specific type of existing hypertension, if known, such as:
    essential hypertension (I10)
    secondary hypertension (I15.-)

Ischemic heart diseases (I20-I25)

Code also the presence of hypertension (I10-I1A)

I20 **Angina pectoris**
Use additional code to identify:
exposure to environmental tobacco smoke (Z77.22)
history of tobacco dependence (Z87.891)
occupational exposure to environmental tobacco smoke (Z57.31)
tobacco dependence (F17.-)
tobacco use (Z72.0)

EXCLUDES 1 angina pectoris with atherosclerotic heart disease of native coronary arteries (I25.1-)
atherosclerosis of coronary artery bypass graft(s) and coronary artery of transplanted heart with angina pectoris (I25.7-)
postinfarction angina (I23.7)

DEF: Chest pain due to reduced blood flow resulting in a lack of oxygen to the heart muscles.

- **I20.0** **Unstable** angina
  Accelerated angina
  Crescendo angina
  De novo effort angina
  Intermediate coronary syndrome
  Preinfarction syndrome
  Worsening effort angina

- **I20.1** Angina pectoris with **documented spasm**
  Angiospastic angina
  Prinzmetal angina
  Spasm-induced angina
  Variant angina

- **I20.2** **Refractory** angina pectoris
  AHA: 2022,4Q,20-21

- **I20.8** Other forms of angina pectoris
  Use additional code(s) for symptoms associated with angina equivalent
  AHA: 2023,4Q,25-26

  - **I20.81** Angina pectoris with coronary microvascular dysfunction
    Angina pectoris with coronary microvascular disease

  - **I20.89** Other forms of angina pectoris
    Angina of effort
    Angina equivalent
    Coronary slow flow syndrome
    Stable angina
    Stenocardia

- **I20.9** Angina pectoris, unspecified
  Angina NOS
  Anginal syndrome
  Cardiac angina
  Ischemic chest pain

I21 **Acute myocardial infarction**
INCLUDES cardiac infarction
coronary (artery) embolism
coronary (artery) occlusion
coronary (artery) rupture
coronary (artery) thrombosis
infarction of heart, myocardium, or ventricle
myocardial infarction specified as acute or with a stated duration of 4 weeks (28 days) or less from onset

Use additional code, if applicable, to identify:
exposure to environmental tobacco smoke (Z77.22)
history of tobacco dependence (Z87.891)
occupational exposure to environmental tobacco smoke (Z57.31)
status post administration of tPA (rtPA) in a different facility within the last 24 hours prior to admission to current facility (Z92.82)
tobacco dependence (F17.-)
tobacco use (Z72.0)

EXCLUDES 2 old myocardial infarction (I25.2)
postmyocardial infarction syndrome (I24.1)
subsequent type 1 myocardial infarction (I22.-)

AHA: 2019,2Q,5; 2018,4Q,68; 2018,3Q,5; 2017,4Q,12-14; 2017,1Q,44-45; 2016,4Q,140; 2015,2Q,16; 2013,1Q,25; 2012,4Q,96,102-103

TIP: When chronic total occlusion and myocardial infarction are documented as being in different vessels, assign code I25.82 Chronic total occlusion of coronary artery, in addition to the myocardial infarction code.

- **I21.0** ST elevation (STEMI) myocardial infarction of **anterior wall**
  Type 1 ST elevation myocardial infarction of anterior wall
  DEF: ST elevation myocardial infarction: Complete obstruction of one or more coronary arteries causing decreased blood flow (ischemia) and necrosis of myocardial muscle cells.

  - **I21.01** ST elevation (STEMI) myocardial infarction involving **left main** coronary artery

  - **I21.02** ST elevation (STEMI) myocardial infarction involving **left anterior descending** coronary artery
    ST elevation (STEMI) myocardial infarction involving diagonal coronary artery
    AHA: 2013,1Q,25

  - **I21.09** ST elevation (STEMI) myocardial infarction involving **other** coronary artery of anterior wall
    Acute transmural myocardial infarction of anterior wall
    Anteroapical transmural (Q wave) infarction (acute)
    Anterolateral transmural (Q wave) infarction (acute)
    Anteroseptal transmural (Q wave) infarction (acute)
    Transmural (Q wave) infarction (acute) (of) anterior (wall) NOS
    AHA: 2012,4Q,102-103

- **I21.1** ST elevation (STEMI) myocardial infarction of **inferior wall**
  Type 1 ST elevation myocardial infarction of inferior wall
  DEF: ST elevation myocardial infarction: Complete obstruction of one or more coronary arteries causing decreased blood flow (ischemia) and necrosis of myocardial muscle cells.

  - **I21.11** ST elevation (STEMI) myocardial infarction involving **right** coronary artery
    Inferoposterior transmural (Q wave) infarction (acute)

  - **I21.19** ST elevation (STEMI) myocardial infarction involving **other** coronary artery of inferior wall
    Acute transmural myocardial infarction of inferior wall
    Inferolateral transmural (Q wave) infarction (acute)
    Transmural (Q wave) infarction (acute) (of) diaphragmatic wall
    Transmural (Q wave) infarction (acute) (of) inferior (wall) NOS
    EXCLUDES 2 ST elevation (STEMI) myocardial infarction involving left circumflex coronary artery (I21.21)
    AHA: 2012,4Q,96

- **I21.2** ST elevation (STEMI) myocardial infarction of other sites
  Type 1 ST elevation myocardial infarction of other sites
  DEF: ST elevation myocardial infarction: Complete obstruction of one or more coronary arteries causing decreased blood flow (ischemia) and necrosis of myocardial muscle cells.

  - **I21.21** ST elevation (STEMI) myocardial infarction involving **left circumflex** coronary artery
    ST elevation (STEMI) myocardial infarction involving oblique marginal coronary artery

Chapter 9. Diseases of the Circulatory System

I21.29 ST elevation (STEMI) myocardial infarction involving other sites `HCC` `Rx` `ESR` `COM`
  Acute transmural myocardial infarction of other sites
  Apical-lateral transmural (Q wave) infarction (acute)
  Basal-lateral transmural (Q wave) infarction (acute)
  High lateral transmural (Q wave) infarction (acute)
  Lateral (wall) NOS transmural (Q wave) infarction (acute)
  Posterior (true) transmural (Q wave) infarction (acute)
  Posterobasal transmural (Q wave) infarction (acute)
  Posterolateral transmural (Q wave) infarction (acute)
  Posteroseptal transmural (Q wave) infarction (acute)
  Septal transmural (Q wave) infarction (acute) NOS

I21.3 ST elevation (STEMI) myocardial infarction of unspecified site `HCC` `Rx` `ESR` `COM`
  Acute transmural myocardial infarction of unspecified site
  Transmural (Q wave) myocardial infarction NOS
  Type 1 ST elevation myocardial infarction of unspecified site
  DEF: ST elevation myocardial infarction: Complete obstruction of one or more coronary arteries causing decreased blood flow (ischemia) and necrosis of myocardial muscle cells.

I21.4 Non-ST elevation (NSTEMI) myocardial infarction `HCC` `Rx` `ESR` `COM`
  Acute subendocardial myocardial infarction
  Non-Q wave myocardial infarction NOS
  Nontransmural myocardial infarction NOS
  Type 1 non-ST elevation myocardial infarction
  AHA: 2025,2Q,26; 2025,1Q,20; 2024,1Q,28; 2023,2Q,29; 2021,3Q,6; 2019,2Q,33; 2017,1Q,44-45
  DEF: Partial obstruction of one or more coronary arteries that causes decreased blood flow (ischemia) and may cause partial thickness necrosis of myocardial muscle cells.

I21.9 Acute myocardial infarction, unspecified `HCC` `Rx` `ESR` `COM`
  Myocardial infarction (acute) NOS

√5th I21.A Other type of myocardial infarction
  AHA: 2019,2Q,5

  I21.A1 Myocardial infarction type 2 `HCC` `Rx` `ESR` `COM`
    Myocardial infarction due to demand ischemia
    Myocardial infarction secondary to ischemic imbalance
    Code first, if applicable, the underlying cause, such as:
      anemia (D50.0-D64.9)
      chronic obstructive pulmonary disease (J44.-)
      paroxysmal tachycardia (I47.0-I47.9)
      shock (R57.0-R57.9)
    AHA: 2019,4Q,53; 2017,4Q,13-14
    DEF: Often referred to as due to demand ischemia, myocardial infarction (MI) type 2 refers to an MI due to ischemia and necrosis resulting from an oxygen imbalance to the heart. This mismatch between oxygen decreased supply and increased demand is caused by conditions other than coronary artery disease such as vasospasm, embolism, anemia, hypertension, hypotension, or arrhythmias.

  I21.A9 Other myocardial infarction type `HCC` `Rx` `ESR` `COM`
    Myocardial infarction associated with revascularization procedure
    Myocardial infarction type 3
    Myocardial infarction type 4a
    Myocardial infarction type 4b
    Myocardial infarction type 4c
    Myocardial infarction type 5
    Code first, if applicable, postprocedural myocardial infarction following cardiac surgery (I97.190), or postprocedural myocardial infarction during cardiac surgery (I97.790)
    Code also complication, if known and applicable, such as:
      (acute) stent occlusion (T82.897-)
      (acute) stent stenosis (T82.855-)
      (acute) stent thrombosis (T82.867-)
      cardiac arrest due to underlying cardiac condition (I46.2)
      complication of percutaneous coronary intervention (PCI) (I97.89)
      occlusion of coronary artery bypass graft (T82.218-)
    AHA: 2021,3Q,6; 2019,2Q,33

I21.B Myocardial infarction with coronary microvascular dysfunction `HCC` `Rx` `ESR` `COM`
  Myocardial infarction with coronary microvascular disease
  Myocardial infarction with nonobstructive coronary arteries [MINOCA] with microvascular disease
  AHA: 2023,4Q,25-26

√4th I22 Subsequent ST elevation (STEMI) and non-ST elevation (NSTEMI) myocardial infarction
  INCLUDES acute myocardial infarction occurring within four weeks (28 days) of a previous acute myocardial infarction, regardless of site
    cardiac infarction
    coronary (artery) embolism
    coronary (artery) occlusion
    coronary (artery) rupture
    coronary (artery) thrombosis
    infarction of heart, myocardium, or ventricle
    recurrent myocardial infarction
    reinfarction of myocardium
    rupture of heart, myocardium, or ventricle
    subsequent type 1 myocardial infarction
  Use additional code, if applicable, to identify:
    exposure to environmental tobacco smoke (Z77.22)
    history of tobacco dependence (Z87.891)
    occupational exposure to environmental tobacco smoke (Z57.31)
    status post administration of tPA (rtPA) in a different facility within the last 24 hours prior to admission to current facility (Z92.82)
    tobacco dependence (F17.-)
    tobacco use (Z72.0)
  EXCLUDES 1 subsequent myocardial infarction, type 2 (I21.A1)
    subsequent myocardial infarction of other type (type 3) (type 4) (type 5) (I21.A9)
  AHA: 2018,4Q,68; 2018,3Q,5; 2017,4Q,12-13; 2017,2Q,11; 2013,1Q,25; 2012,4Q,97,102-103
  DEF: Non-ST elevation myocardial infarction: Partial obstruction of one or more coronary arteries that causes decreased blood flow (ischemia) and may cause partial thickness necrosis of myocardial muscle cells.
  DEF: ST elevation myocardial infarction: Complete obstruction of one or more coronary arteries causing decreased blood flow (ischemia) and necrosis of myocardial muscle cells.
  TIP: When chronic total occlusion and myocardial infarction are documented as being in different vessels, assign code I25.82 Chronic total occlusion of coronary artery, in addition to the myocardial infarction code.

  I22.0 Subsequent ST elevation (STEMI) myocardial infarction of anterior wall `HCC` `Rx` `ESR` `COM`
    Subsequent acute transmural myocardial infarction of anterior wall
    Subsequent anteroapical transmural (Q wave) infarction (acute)
    Subsequent anterolateral transmural (Q wave) infarction (acute)
    Subsequent anteroseptal transmural (Q wave) infarction (acute)
    Subsequent transmural (Q wave) infarction (acute)(of) anterior (wall) NOS

  I22.1 Subsequent ST elevation (STEMI) myocardial infarction of inferior wall `HCC` `Rx` `ESR` `COM`
    Subsequent acute transmural myocardial infarction of inferior wall
    Subsequent inferolateral transmural (Q wave) infarction (acute)
    Subsequent inferoposterior transmural (Q wave) infarction (acute)
    Subsequent transmural (Q wave) infarction (acute)(of) diaphragmatic wall
    Subsequent transmural (Q wave) infarction (acute)(of) inferior (wall) NOS
    AHA: 2012,4Q,102

  I22.2 Subsequent non-ST elevation (NSTEMI) myocardial infarction `HCC` `Rx` `ESR` `COM`
    Subsequent acute subendocardial myocardial infarction
    Subsequent non-Q wave myocardial infarction NOS
    Subsequent nontransmural myocardial infarction NOS

 CMS-HCC   Rx HCC   `ESR` ESRD HCC   `COM` Commercial HCC   `N` Newborn: 0   `P` Pediatric: 0-17   `M` Maternity: 9-64   `A` Adult: 15-124

Chapter 9. Diseases of the Circulatory System

I22.8 **Subsequent ST elevation (STEMI) myocardial infarction of other sites** `HCC` `Rx` `ESR` `COM`
- Subsequent acute transmural myocardial infarction of other sites
- Subsequent apical-lateral transmural (Q wave) myocardial infarction (acute)
- Subsequent basal-lateral transmural (Q wave) myocardial infarction (acute)
- Subsequent high lateral transmural (Q wave) myocardial infarction (acute)
- Subsequent posterior (true) transmural (Q wave) myocardial infarction (acute)
- Subsequent posterobasal transmural (Q wave) myocardial infarction (acute)
- Subsequent posterolateral transmural (Q wave) myocardial infarction (acute)
- Subsequent posteroseptal transmural (Q wave) myocardial infarction (acute)
- Subsequent septal NOS transmural (Q wave) myocardial infarction (acute)
- Subsequent transmural (Q wave) myocardial infarction (acute)(of) lateral (wall) NOS

I22.9 **Subsequent ST elevation (STEMI) myocardial infarction of unspecified site** `HCC` `Rx` `ESR` `COM`
- Subsequent acute myocardial infarction of unspecified site
- Subsequent myocardial infarction (acute) NOS

✓4th **I23** **Certain current complications following ST elevation (STEMI) and non-ST elevation (NSTEMI) myocardial infarction (within the 28 day period)**
AHA: 2017,2Q,11
DEF: Non-ST elevation myocardial infarction: Partial obstruction of one or more coronary arteries that causes decreased blood flow (ischemia) and may cause partial thickness necrosis of myocardial muscle cells.
DEF: ST elevation myocardial infarction: Complete obstruction of one or more coronary arteries causing decreased blood flow (ischemia) and necrosis of myocardial muscle cells.

I23.0 **Hemopericardium** as current complication following acute myocardial infarction `HCC` `Rx` `ESR` `COM` `A`
  EXCLUDES 1 hemopericardium not specified as current complication following acute myocardial infarction (I31.2)

I23.1 **Atrial septal defect** as current complication following acute myocardial infarction `HCC` `Rx` `ESR` `COM` `A`
  EXCLUDES 1 acquired atrial septal defect not specified as current complication following acute myocardial infarction (I51.0)

I23.2 **Ventricular septal defect** as current complication following acute myocardial infarction `HCC` `Rx` `ESR` `COM` `A`
  EXCLUDES 1 acquired ventricular septal defect not specified as current complication following acute myocardial infarction (I51.0)

I23.3 **Rupture of cardiac wall** without hemopericardium as current complication following acute myocardial infarction `HCC` `Rx` `ESR` `COM` `A`

I23.4 **Rupture of chordae tendineae** as current complication following acute myocardial infarction `HCC` `Rx` `ESR` `COM` `A`
  EXCLUDES 1 rupture of chordae tendineae not specified as current complication following acute myocardial infarction (I51.1)

I23.5 **Rupture of papillary muscle** as current complication following acute myocardial infarction `HCC` `Rx` `ESR` `COM` `A`
  EXCLUDES 1 rupture of papillary muscle not specified as current complication following acute myocardial infarction (I51.2)

I23.6 **Thrombosis of atrium, auricular appendage, and ventricle** as current complications following acute myocardial infarction `HCC` `Rx` `ESR` `COM` `A`
  EXCLUDES 1 thrombosis of atrium, auricular appendage, and ventricle not specified as current complication following acute myocardial infarction (I51.3)

I23.7 **Postinfarction angina** `HCC` `Rx` `ESR` `COM` `A`
AHA: 2015,2Q,16
TIP: When postinfarction angina occurs with atherosclerotic coronary artery disease, code both I23.7 and I25.118 for atherosclerotic disease with other forms of angina pectoris.

I23.8 **Other current complications following acute myocardial infarction** `HCC` `Rx` `ESR` `COM` `A`

✓4th **I24** **Other acute ischemic heart diseases**
  EXCLUDES 1 angina pectoris (I20.-)
             transient myocardial ischemia in newborn (P29.4)
  EXCLUDES 2 non-ischemic myocardial injury (I5A)

I24.0 **Acute coronary thrombosis not resulting in myocardial infarction** `HCC` `Rx` `ESR` `COM`
- Acute coronary (artery) (vein) embolism not resulting in myocardial infarction
- Acute coronary (artery) (vein) occlusion not resulting in myocardial infarction
- Acute coronary (artery) (vein) thromboembolism not resulting in myocardial infarction
  EXCLUDES 1 atherosclerotic heart disease (I25.1-)
AHA: 2013,1Q,24

I24.1 **Dressler's syndrome** `HCC` `Rx` `ESR` `COM`
- Postmyocardial infarction syndrome
  EXCLUDES 1 postinfarction angina (I23.7)
DEF: Fever, leukocytosis, chest pain, evidence of pericarditis, pleurisy, and pneumonia occurring days or weeks after a myocardial infarction.

✓5th **I24.8** **Other forms of acute ischemic heart disease**
  EXCLUDES 1 myocardial infarction due to demand ischemia (I21.A1)
AHA: 2023,4Q,25-26; 2019,4Q,53; 2017,4Q,13

I24.81 **Acute coronary microvascular dysfunction** `HCC` `Rx` `ESR` `COM`
- Acute (presentation of) coronary microvascular disease

I24.89 **Other forms of acute ischemic heart disease** `HCC` `Rx` `ESR` `COM`

I24.9 **Acute ischemic heart disease, unspecified** `HCC` `Rx` `ESR` `COM`
  EXCLUDES 1 ischemic heart disease (chronic) NOS (I25.9)

✓4th **I25** **Chronic ischemic heart disease**
Use additional code to identify:
  chronic total occlusion of coronary artery (I25.82)
  exposure to environmental tobacco smoke (Z77.22)
  history of tobacco dependence (Z87.891)
  occupational exposure to environmental tobacco smoke (Z57.31)
  tobacco dependence (F17.-)
  tobacco use (Z72.0)
  EXCLUDES 2 non-ischemic myocardial injury (I5A)
AHA: 2025,1Q,20; 2022,4Q,20-21

✓5th **I25.1** **Atherosclerotic heart disease of native coronary artery**
- Atherosclerotic cardiovascular disease
- Coronary (artery) atheroma
- Coronary (artery) atherosclerosis
- Coronary (artery) disease
- Coronary (artery) sclerosis
Use additional code, if applicable, to identify:
  coronary atherosclerosis due to calcified coronary lesion (I25.84)
  coronary atherosclerosis due to lipid rich plaque (I25.83)
  EXCLUDES 2 atheroembolism (I75.-)
             atherosclerosis of coronary artery bypass graft(s) and transplanted heart (I25.7-)

I25.10 **Atherosclerotic heart disease of native coronary artery without angina pectoris** `Rx` `A`
- Atherosclerotic heart disease NOS
AHA: 2024,1Q,28; 2021,3Q,6-7; 2015,2Q,16; 2012,4Q,92

✓6th **I25.11** **Atherosclerotic heart disease of native coronary artery with angina pectoris**
AHA: 2024,1Q,28

I25.110 **Atherosclerotic heart disease of native coronary artery with unstable angina pectoris** `HCC` `Rx` `ESR` `COM` `A`
  EXCLUDES 1 unstable angina without atherosclerotic heart disease (I20.0)

I25.111 Atherosclerotic heart disease of native coronary artery with angina pectoris with **documented spasm** `Rx` `ESR` `A`
EXCLUDES 1 — angina pectoris with documented spasm without atherosclerotic heart disease (I20.1)

I25.112 Atherosclerotic heart disease of native coronary artery with **refractory** angina pectoris `Rx` `ESR` `A`

I25.118 Atherosclerotic heart disease of native coronary artery with other forms of angina pectoris `Rx` `ESR` `A`
EXCLUDES 1 — other forms of angina pectoris without atherosclerotic heart disease (I20.8-)
AHA: 2015,2Q,16
TIP: When postinfarction angina occurs with atherosclerotic coronary artery disease, code both I23.7 and I25.118 for atherosclerotic disease with other forms of angina pectoris.

I25.119 Atherosclerotic heart disease of native coronary artery with unspecified angina pectoris `Rx` `ESR` `A`
Atherosclerotic heart disease with angina NOS
Atherosclerotic heart disease with ischemic chest pain
EXCLUDES 1 — unspecified angina pectoris without atherosclerotic heart disease (I20.9)

I25.2 Old myocardial infarction `Rx`
Healed myocardial infarction
Past myocardial infarction diagnosed by ECG or other investigation, but currently presenting no symptoms

I25.3 Aneurysm of heart `Rx`
Mural aneurysm
Ventricular aneurysm

✓5th **I25.4** Coronary artery aneurysm and dissection

I25.41 Coronary artery aneurysm `Rx`
Coronary arteriovenous fistula, acquired
EXCLUDES 1 — congenital coronary (artery) aneurysm (Q24.5)

I25.42 Coronary artery dissection `Rx`
DEF: Tear in the intimal arterial wall of a coronary artery resulting in the sudden intrusion of blood within the layers of the wall.

I25.5 Ischemic cardiomyopathy `Rx`
EXCLUDES 2 — coronary atherosclerosis (I25.1-, I25.7-)
AHA: 2022,3Q,17

I25.6 Silent myocardial ischemia `Rx`

✓5th **I25.7** Atherosclerosis of coronary artery **bypass graft(s)** and coronary artery of **transplanted heart** with angina pectoris
Use additional code, if applicable, to identify:
coronary atherosclerosis due to calcified coronary lesion (I25.84)
coronary atherosclerosis due to lipid rich plaque (I25.83)
EXCLUDES 1 — atherosclerosis of bypass graft(s) of transplanted heart without angina pectoris (I25.812)
atherosclerosis of coronary artery bypass graft(s) without angina pectoris (I25.810)
atherosclerosis of native coronary artery of transplanted heart without angina pectoris (I25.811)

✓6th **I25.70** Atherosclerosis of coronary artery **bypass graft(s)**, unspecified, with angina pectoris

I25.700 Atherosclerosis of coronary artery bypass graft(s), unspecified, with **unstable** angina pectoris `HCC` `Rx` `ESR` `COM` `A`
EXCLUDES 1 — unstable angina pectoris without atherosclerosis of coronary artery bypass graft (I20.0)

I25.701 Atherosclerosis of coronary artery bypass graft(s), unspecified, with angina pectoris with **documented spasm** `Rx` `ESR` `A`
EXCLUDES 1 — angina pectoris with documented spasm without atherosclerosis of coronary artery bypass graft (I20.1)

I25.702 Atherosclerosis of coronary artery bypass graft(s), unspecified, with **refractory** angina pectoris `Rx` `ESR` `A`
AHA: 2022,4Q,21

I25.708 Atherosclerosis of coronary artery bypass graft(s), unspecified, with other forms of angina pectoris `Rx` `ESR` `A`
EXCLUDES 1 — other forms of angina pectoris without atherosclerosis of coronary artery bypass graft (I20.8-)

I25.709 Atherosclerosis of coronary artery bypass graft(s), unspecified, with unspecified angina pectoris `Rx` `ESR` `A`
EXCLUDES 1 — unspecified angina pectoris without atherosclerosis of coronary artery bypass graft (I20.9)

✓6th **I25.71** Atherosclerosis of **autologous vein** coronary artery bypass graft(s) with angina pectoris

I25.710 Atherosclerosis of autologous vein coronary artery bypass graft(s) with **unstable** angina pectoris `HCC` `Rx` `ESR` `COM` `A`
EXCLUDES 1 — unstable angina without atherosclerosis of autologous vein coronary artery bypass graft(s) (I20.0)
EXCLUDES 2 — embolism or thrombus of coronary artery bypass graft(s) (T82.8-)

I25.711 Atherosclerosis of autologous vein coronary artery bypass graft(s) with angina pectoris with **documented spasm** `Rx` `ESR` `A`
EXCLUDES 1 — angina pectoris with documented spasm without atherosclerosis of autologous vein coronary artery bypass graft(s) (I20.1)

I25.712 Atherosclerosis of autologous vein coronary artery bypass graft(s) with **refractory** angina pectoris `Rx` `ESR` `A`

I25.718 Atherosclerosis of autologous vein coronary artery bypass graft(s) with other forms of angina pectoris `Rx` `ESR` `A`
EXCLUDES 1 — other forms of angina pectoris without atherosclerosis of autologous vein coronary artery bypass graft(s) (I20.8-)

I25.719 Atherosclerosis of autologous vein coronary artery bypass graft(s) with unspecified angina pectoris `Rx` `ESR` `A`
EXCLUDES 1 — unspecified angina pectoris without atherosclerosis of autologous vein coronary artery bypass graft(s) (I20.9)

`HCC` CMS-HCC `Rx` Rx HCC `ESR` ESRD HCC  Commercial HCC `N` Newborn: 0 `P` Pediatric: 0-17 `M` Maternity: 9-64 `A` Adult: 15-124

I25.72 Atherosclerosis of autologous artery coronary artery bypass graft(s) with angina pectoris
Atherosclerosis of internal mammary artery graft with angina pectoris

- **I25.720** Atherosclerosis of autologous artery coronary artery bypass graft(s) with unstable angina pectoris `HCC` `Rx` `ESR` `COM` `A`
  - EXCLUDES 1: unstable angina without atherosclerosis of autologous artery coronary artery bypass graft(s) (I20.0)
- **I25.721** Atherosclerosis of autologous artery coronary artery bypass graft(s) with angina pectoris with documented spasm `Rx` `ESR` `A`
  - EXCLUDES 1: angina pectoris with documented spasm without atherosclerosis of autologous artery coronary artery bypass graft(s) (I20.1)
- **I25.722** Atherosclerosis of autologous artery coronary artery bypass graft(s) with refractory angina pectoris `Rx` `ESR` `A`
- **I25.728** Atherosclerosis of autologous artery coronary artery bypass graft(s) with other forms of angina pectoris `Rx` `ESR` `A`
  - EXCLUDES 1: other forms of angina pectoris without atherosclerosis of autologous artery coronary artery bypass graft(s) (I20.8-)
- **I25.729** Atherosclerosis of autologous artery coronary artery bypass graft(s) with unspecified angina pectoris `Rx` `ESR` `A`
  - EXCLUDES 1: unspecified angina pectoris without atherosclerosis of autologous artery coronary artery bypass graft(s) (I20.9)

I25.73 Atherosclerosis of nonautologous biological coronary artery bypass graft(s) with angina pectoris

- **I25.730** Atherosclerosis of nonautologous biological coronary artery bypass graft(s) with unstable angina pectoris `HCC` `Rx` `ESR` `COM` `A`
  - EXCLUDES 1: unstable angina without atherosclerosis of nonautologous biological coronary artery bypass graft(s) (I20.0)
- **I25.731** Atherosclerosis of nonautologous biological coronary artery bypass graft(s) with angina pectoris with documented spasm `Rx` `ESR` `A`
  - EXCLUDES 1: angina pectoris with documented spasm without atherosclerosis of nonautologous biological coronary artery bypass graft(s) (I20.1)
- **I25.732** Atherosclerosis of nonautologous biological coronary artery bypass graft(s) with refractory angina pectoris `Rx` `ESR` `A`
- **I25.738** Atherosclerosis of nonautologous biological coronary artery bypass graft(s) with other forms of angina pectoris `Rx` `ESR` `A`
  - EXCLUDES 1: other forms of angina pectoris without atherosclerosis of nonautologous biological coronary artery bypass graft(s) (I20.8-)
- **I25.739** Atherosclerosis of nonautologous biological coronary artery bypass graft(s) with unspecified angina pectoris `Rx` `ESR` `A`
  - EXCLUDES 1: unspecified angina pectoris without atherosclerosis of nonautologous biological coronary artery bypass graft(s) (I20.9)

I25.75 Atherosclerosis of native coronary artery of transplanted heart with angina pectoris
EXCLUDES 1: atherosclerosis of native coronary artery of transplanted heart without angina pectoris (I25.811)

- **I25.750** Atherosclerosis of native coronary artery of transplanted heart with unstable angina `HCC` `Rx` `ESR` `COM` `A`
- **I25.751** Atherosclerosis of native coronary artery of transplanted heart with angina pectoris with documented spasm `Rx` `ESR` `A`
- **I25.752** Atherosclerosis of native coronary artery of transplanted heart with refractory angina pectoris `Rx` `ESR` `A`
- **I25.758** Atherosclerosis of native coronary artery of transplanted heart with other forms of angina pectoris `Rx` `ESR` `A`
- **I25.759** Atherosclerosis of native coronary artery of transplanted heart with unspecified angina pectoris `Rx` `ESR`

I25.76 Atherosclerosis of bypass graft of coronary artery of transplanted heart with angina pectoris
EXCLUDES 1: atherosclerosis of bypass graft of coronary artery of transplanted heart without angina pectoris (I25.812)

- **I25.760** Atherosclerosis of bypass graft of coronary artery of transplanted heart with unstable angina `HCC` `Rx` `ESR` `COM` `A`
- **I25.761** Atherosclerosis of bypass graft of coronary artery of transplanted heart with angina pectoris with documented spasm `Rx` `ESR` `A`
- **I25.762** Atherosclerosis of bypass graft of coronary artery of transplanted heart with refractory angina pectoris `Rx` `ESR` `A`
- **I25.768** Atherosclerosis of bypass graft of coronary artery of transplanted heart with other forms of angina pectoris `Rx` `ESR` `A`
- **I25.769** Atherosclerosis of bypass graft of coronary artery of transplanted heart with unspecified angina pectoris `Rx` `ESR` `A`

I25.79 Atherosclerosis of other coronary artery bypass graft(s) with angina pectoris

- **I25.790** Atherosclerosis of other coronary artery bypass graft(s) with unstable angina pectoris `HCC` `Rx` `ESR` `COM` `A`
  - EXCLUDES 1: unstable angina without atherosclerosis of other coronary artery bypass graft(s) (I20.0)
- **I25.791** Atherosclerosis of other coronary artery bypass graft(s) with angina pectoris with documented spasm `Rx` `ESR` `A`
  - EXCLUDES 1: angina pectoris with documented spasm without atherosclerosis of other coronary artery bypass graft(s) (I20.1)
- **I25.792** Atherosclerosis of other coronary artery bypass graft(s) with refractory angina pectoris `Rx` `ESR` `A`
- **I25.798** Atherosclerosis of other coronary artery bypass graft(s) with other forms of angina pectoris `Rx` `ESR` `A`
  - EXCLUDES 1: other forms of angina pectoris without atherosclerosis of other coronary artery bypass graft(s) (I20.8-)

I25.799 Atherosclerosis of other coronary artery bypass graft(s) with unspecified angina pectoris Rx ESR A
EXCLUDES 1: unspecified angina pectoris without atherosclerosis of other coronary artery bypass graft(s) (I20.9)

I25.8 Other forms of chronic ischemic heart disease

I25.81 Atherosclerosis of other coronary vessels without angina pectoris
Use additional code, if applicable, to identify:
coronary atherosclerosis due to calcified coronary lesion (I25.84)
coronary atherosclerosis due to lipid rich plaque (I25.83)
EXCLUDES 2: atherosclerotic heart disease of native coronary artery without angina pectoris (I25.10)

I25.810 Atherosclerosis of coronary artery bypass graft(s) without angina pectoris Rx A
Atherosclerosis of coronary artery bypass graft NOS
EXCLUDES 1: atherosclerosis of coronary bypass graft(s) with angina pectoris (I25.70-I25.73-, I25.79-)

I25.811 Atherosclerosis of native coronary artery of transplanted heart without angina pectoris Rx
Atherosclerosis of native coronary artery of transplanted heart NOS
EXCLUDES 1: atherosclerosis of native coronary artery of transplanted heart with angina pectoris (I25.75-)

I25.812 Atherosclerosis of bypass graft of coronary artery of transplanted heart without angina pectoris Rx A
Atherosclerosis of bypass graft of transplanted heart NOS
EXCLUDES 1: atherosclerosis of bypass graft of transplanted heart with angina pectoris (I25.76)

I25.82 Chronic total occlusion of coronary artery Rx UPD
Complete occlusion of coronary artery
Total occlusion of coronary artery
Code first coronary atherosclerosis (I25.1-, I25.7-, I25.81-)
EXCLUDES 1: acute coronary occlusion with myocardial infarction (I21.0-I21.B, I22.-)
acute coronary occlusion without myocardial infarction (I24.0)
AHA: 2018,3Q,5
DEF: Complete blockage of the coronary artery due to plaque accumulation over an extended period of time, resulting in substantial reduction of blood flow. Symptoms include angina or chest pain.
TIP: Report this code in addition to a code from category I21 or I22 when the chronic total occlusion and the myocardial infarction are documented as being in different vessels.

I25.83 Coronary atherosclerosis due to lipid rich plaque Rx UPD A
Code first coronary atherosclerosis (I25.1-, I25.7-, I25.81-)

I25.84 Coronary atherosclerosis due to calcified coronary lesion Rx UPD
Coronary atherosclerosis due to severely calcified coronary lesion
Code first coronary atherosclerosis (I25.1-, I25.7-, I25.81-)

I25.85 Chronic coronary microvascular dysfunction Rx
Chronic (presentation of) coronary microvascular disease
Coronary microvascular dysfunction NOS
AHA: 2023,4Q,25-26

I25.89 Other forms of chronic ischemic heart disease Rx

I25.9 Chronic ischemic heart disease, unspecified Rx
Ischemic heart disease (chronic) NOS

Pulmonary heart disease and diseases of pulmonary circulation (I26-I28)

I26 Pulmonary embolism
INCLUDES: pulmonary (acute)(artery)(vein) infarction
pulmonary (acute) (artery)(vein) thromboembolism
pulmonary (acute)(artery)(vein) thrombosis
EXCLUDES 1: cor pulmonale without embolism (I27.81)
EXCLUDES 2: chronic pulmonary embolism (I27.82)
personal history of pulmonary embolism (Z86.711)
pulmonary embolism complicating abortion, ectopic or molar pregnancy (O00-O07, O08.2)
pulmonary embolism complicating pregnancy, childbirth and the puerperium (O88.-)
pulmonary embolism due to complications of surgical and medical care (T80.0, T81.7-, T82.8-)
pulmonary embolism due to trauma (T79.0, T79.1)
septic (non-pulmonary) arterial embolism (I76)
AHA: 2022,3Q,8

I26.0 Pulmonary embolism with acute cor pulmonale
DEF: Cor pulmonale: Heart-lung disease appearing in identifiable forms as chronic or acute. The chronic form of this heart-lung disease is marked by dilation, hypertrophy and failure of the right ventricle due to a disease that has affected the function of the lungs, excluding congenital or left heart diseases and is also called chronic cardiopulmonary disease. The acute form is an overload of the right ventricle from a rapid onset of pulmonary hypertension, usually arising from a pulmonary embolism.

I26.01 Septic pulmonary embolism with acute cor pulmonale HCC Rx ESR COM UPD
Code first underlying infection

I26.02 Saddle embolus of pulmonary artery with acute cor pulmonale HCC Rx ESR COM

I26.03 Cement embolism of pulmonary artery with acute cor pulmonale HCC Rx ESR COM UPD
Code first complication of other artery following a procedure (T81.718)
AHA: 2024,4Q,17

I26.04 Fat embolism of pulmonary artery with acute cor pulmonale HCC Rx ESR COM
Code first, if applicable:
complication of other artery following a procedure (T81.718)
traumatic fat embolism (T79.1)
AHA: 2024,4Q,17

I26.09 Other pulmonary embolism with acute cor pulmonale HCC Rx ESR COM
Acute cor pulmonale NOS
Other thrombotic pulmonary embolism with acute cor pulmonale
AHA: 2014,4Q,21

I26.9 Pulmonary embolism without acute cor pulmonale

I26.90 Septic pulmonary embolism without acute cor pulmonale HCC Rx ESR COM UPD
Code first underlying infection

I26.92 Saddle embolus of pulmonary artery without acute cor pulmonale HCC Rx ESR COM

I26.93 Single subsegmental thrombotic pulmonary embolism without acute cor pulmonale HCC Rx ESR COM
Subsegmental pulmonary embolism NOS
AHA: 2021,2Q,9; 2019,4Q,6-7

I26.94 Multiple subsegmental thrombotic pulmonary emboli without acute cor pulmonale HCC Rx ESR COM
AHA: 2022,2Q,13; 2021,2Q,9; 2019,4Q,6-7

I26.95 Cement embolism of pulmonary artery without acute cor pulmonale HCC Rx ESR COM UPD
Code first complication of other artery following a procedure (T81.718)
AHA: 2024,4Q,17,19

I26.96 Fat embolism of pulmonary artery without acute cor pulmonale HCC Rx ESR COM
Code first, if applicable:
complication of other artery following a procedure (T81.718)
traumatic fat embolism (T79.1)
AHA: 2024,4Q,17,19

I26.99 Other pulmonary embolism without acute cor pulmonale
  Acute pulmonary embolism NOS
  Other thrombotic pulmonary embolism without acute cor pulmonale
  Pulmonary embolism NOS
  AHA: 2022,2Q,13; 2020,3Q,10-11; 2019,2Q,22

I27 Other pulmonary heart diseases

I27.0 Primary pulmonary hypertension
  Heritable pulmonary arterial hypertension
  Idiopathic pulmonary arterial hypertension
  Primary group 1 pulmonary hypertension
  Primary pulmonary arterial hypertension
  EXCLUDES 1 persistent pulmonary hypertension of newborn (P29.30)
    pulmonary hypertension NOS (I27.20)
    secondary pulmonary arterial hypertension (I27.21)
    secondary pulmonary hypertension (I27.29)
  DEF: Condition that occurs when pressure within the pulmonary artery is elevated and vascular resistance is observed in the lungs.

I27.1 Kyphoscoliotic heart disease

I27.2 Other secondary pulmonary hypertension
  Code also associated underlying condition
  EXCLUDES 1 Eisenmenger's syndrome (I27.83)
  AHA: 2017,4Q,14-15; 2014,4Q,21
  DEF: Condition that occurs when pressure within the pulmonary artery is elevated and vascular resistance is observed in the lungs.

  I27.20 Pulmonary hypertension, unspecified
    Pulmonary hypertension NOS

  I27.21 Secondary pulmonary arterial hypertension
    (Associated) (drug-induced) (toxin-induced) (secondary) group 1 pulmonary hypertension
    (Associated) (drug-induced) (toxin-induced) pulmonary arterial hypertension NOS
    Code also associated conditions if applicable, or adverse effects of drugs or toxins, such as:
      adverse effect of appetite depressants (T50.5X5)
      congenital heart disease (Q20-Q28)
      human immunodeficiency virus [HIV] disease (B20)
      polymyositis (M33.2-)
      portal hypertension (K76.6)
      rheumatoid arthritis (M05.-)
      schistosomiasis (B65.-)
      Sjogren syndrome (M35.0-)
      systemic sclerosis (M34.-)

  I27.22 Pulmonary hypertension due to left heart disease
    Group 2 pulmonary hypertension
    Code also associated left heart disease, if known, such as:
      multiple valve disease (I08.-)
      rheumatic aortic valve diseases (I06.-)
      rheumatic mitral valve diseases (I05.-)

  I27.23 Pulmonary hypertension due to lung diseases and hypoxia
    Group 3 pulmonary hypertension
    Code also associated lung disease, if known, such as:
      bronchiectasis (J47.-)
      cystic fibrosis with pulmonary manifestations (E84.0)
      interstitial lung disease (J84.-)
      pleural effusion (J90)
      sleep apnea (G47.3-)

  I27.24 Chronic thromboembolic pulmonary hypertension
    Group 4 pulmonary hypertension
    Code also associated pulmonary embolism, if applicable (I26.-, I27.82)

  I27.29 Other secondary pulmonary hypertension
    Group 5 pulmonary hypertension
    Pulmonary hypertension due to hematologic disorders
    Pulmonary hypertension due to metabolic disorders
    Pulmonary hypertension due to other systemic disorders
    Pulmonary hypertension with unclear multifactorial mechanisms
    Code also other associated disorders, if known, such as:
      chronic myeloid leukemia (C92.10-C92.22)
      essential thrombocythemia (D47.3)
      Gaucher disease (E75.22)
      hypertensive chronic kidney disease with end stage renal disease (I12.0, I13.11, I13.2)
      hyperthyroidism (E05.-)
      hypothyroidism (E00-E03)
      polycythemia vera (D45)
      sarcoidosis (D86.-)
    AHA: 2016,2Q,8

I27.8 Other specified pulmonary heart diseases

  I27.81 Cor pulmonale (chronic)
    Cor pulmonale NOS
    Code also, if applicable, right heart failure (I50.81-)
    EXCLUDES 1 acute cor pulmonale (I26.0-)
    AHA: 2014,4Q,21
    DEF: Heart-lung disease appearing in identifiable forms as chronic or acute. The chronic form of this heart-lung disease is marked by dilation, hypertrophy and failure of the right ventricle due to a disease that has affected the function of the lungs, excluding congenital or left heart diseases and is also called chronic cardiopulmonary disease. The acute form is an overload of the right ventricle from a rapid onset of pulmonary hypertension, usually arising from a pulmonary embolism.

  I27.82 Chronic pulmonary embolism
    Use additional code, if applicable, for associated long-term (current) use of anticoagulants (Z79.01)
    EXCLUDES 1 personal history of pulmonary embolism (Z86.711)
    AHA: 2021,2Q,9
    DEF: Long-standing condition commonly associated with pulmonary hypertension in which small blood clots travel to the lungs repeatedly over many weeks, months, or years, requiring continuation of established anticoagulant or thrombolytic therapy.

  I27.83 Eisenmenger's syndrome
    (Irreversible) Eisenmenger's disease
    Eisenmenger's complex
    Pulmonary hypertension with right to left shunt related to congenital heart disease
    Code also underlying heart defect, if known, such as:
      atrial septal defect (Q21.1-)
      Eisenmenger's defect (Q21.8)
      patent ductus arteriosus (Q25.0)
      ventricular septal defect (Q21.0)
    DEF: Pulmonary hypertension with congenital communication between two circulations resulting in a right to left shunt. This causes reduced oxygen saturation in the arterial blood, leading to cyanosis and organ damage. Once it develops, this life-threating condition is irreversible.

  I27.84 Fontan related circulation
    I27.840 Fontan-associated liver disease [FALD]
    I27.841 Fontan-associated lymphatic dysfunction
      Code also associated conditions such as:
        chylothorax (J94.0)
        Fontan associated protein-losing enteropathy (K90.89)
        plastic (obstructive) bronchitis (J44.89)
    I27.848 Other Fontan-associated condition
      Use additional code to specify the Fontan associated condition
    I27.849 Fontan related circulation, unspecified

  I27.89 Other specified pulmonary heart diseases

I27.9 Pulmonary heart disease, unspecified
  Chronic cardiopulmonary disease

Chapter 9. Diseases of the Circulatory System

✓4th I28 Other diseases of pulmonary vessels

I28.0 Arteriovenous fistula of pulmonary vessels `HCC` `Rx` `ESR` `COM`
  EXCLUDES 1   congenital arteriovenous fistula (Q25.72)

I28.1 Aneurysm of pulmonary artery `HCC` `Rx` `ESR` `COM`
  EXCLUDES 1   congenital aneurysm (Q25.79)
           congenital arteriovenous aneurysm (Q25.72)

I28.8 Other diseases of pulmonary vessels `HCC` `Rx` `ESR` `COM`
  Pulmonary arteritis
  Pulmonary endarteritis
  Rupture of pulmonary vessels
  Stenosis of pulmonary vessels
  Stricture of pulmonary vessels

I28.9 Disease of pulmonary vessels, unspecified `HCC` `Rx` `ESR` `COM`

Other forms of heart disease (I30-I5A)

✓4th I30 Acute pericarditis
  INCLUDES   acute mediastinopericarditis
           acute myopericarditis
           acute pericardial effusion
           acute pleuropericarditis
           acute pneumopericarditis
  EXCLUDES 1   Dressler's syndrome (I24.1)
           rheumatic pericarditis (acute) (I01.0)
           viral pericarditis due to Coxsackie virus (B33.23)
  DEF: Pericarditis: Inflammation affecting the pericardium, the fibroserous membrane that surrounds the heart.

I30.0 Acute nonspecific idiopathic pericarditis `COM`

I30.1 Infective pericarditis `COM`
  Pneumococcal pericarditis
  Pneumopyopericardium
  Purulent pericarditis
  Pyopericarditis
  Pyopericardium
  Pyopneumopericardium
  Staphylococcal pericarditis
  Streptococcal pericarditis
  Suppurative pericarditis
  Viral pericarditis
  Use additional code (B95-B97) to identify infectious agent

I30.8 Other forms of acute pericarditis `COM`

I30.9 Acute pericarditis, unspecified `COM`

✓4th I31 Other diseases of pericardium
  EXCLUDES 1   diseases of pericardium specified as rheumatic (I09.2)
           postcardiotomy syndrome (I97.0)
           traumatic injury to pericardium (S26.-)

I31.0 Chronic adhesive pericarditis `COM`
  Accretio cordis
  Adherent pericardium
  Adhesive mediastinopericarditis

I31.1 Chronic constrictive pericarditis `COM`
  Concretio cordis
  Pericardial calcification

I31.2 Hemopericardium, not elsewhere classified `COM`
  EXCLUDES 1   hemopericardium as current complication following
              acute myocardial infarction (I23.0)
           malignant pericardial effusion (I31.31)
  DEF: Presence of blood in the pericardial sac (pericardium). It can lead to potentially fatal cardiac tamponade if enough blood enters the pericardial cavity.

✓5th I31.3 Pericardial effusion (noninflammatory)
  EXCLUDES 1   acute pericardial effusion (I30.9)
  AHA: 2022,4Q,22; 2019,1Q,16

  I31.31 Malignant pericardial effusion in diseases classified elsewhere `HCC` `COM`
    Code first underlying neoplasm (C00-D49)
    AHA: 2022,4Q,22

  I31.39 Other pericardial effusion (noninflammatory) `COM`
    Chylopericardium

I31.4 Cardiac tamponade `COM` `UPD`
  Code first underlying cause
  DEF: Life-threatening condition in which fluid or blood accumulates in the space between the muscle of the heart (myocardium) and the outer sac that covers the heart (pericardium), resulting in compression of the heart.

Cardiac Tamponade

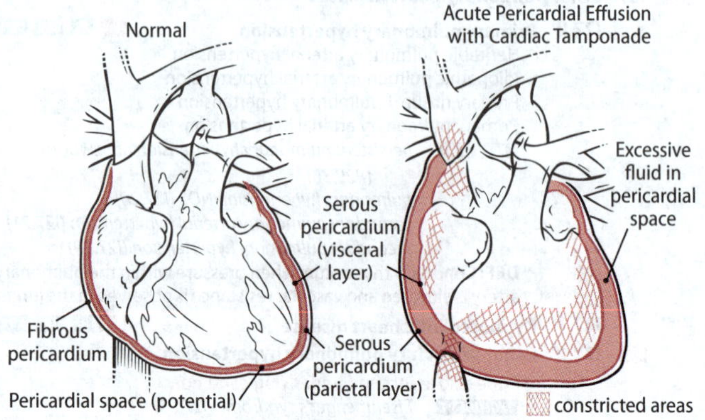

Normal — Acute Pericardial Effusion with Cardiac Tamponade
Serous pericardium (visceral layer)
Excessive fluid in pericardial space
Fibrous pericardium
Serous pericardium (parietal layer)
Pericardial space (potential)
constricted areas

I31.8 Other specified diseases of pericardium `COM`
  Epicardial plaques
  Focal pericardial adhesions

I31.9 Disease of pericardium, unspecified `COM`
  Pericarditis (chronic) NOS

I32 Pericarditis in diseases classified elsewhere `COM`
  Code first underlying disease
  EXCLUDES 1   pericarditis (in):
           coxsackie (virus) (B33.23)
           gonococcal (A54.83)
           meningococcal (A39.53)
           rheumatoid (arthritis) (M05.31)
           syphilitic (A52.06)
           systemic lupus erythematosus (M32.12)
           tuberculosis (A18.84)
  DEF: Pericarditis: Inflammation affecting the pericardium, the fibroserous membrane that surrounds the heart.

✓4th I33 Acute and subacute endocarditis
  EXCLUDES 1   acute rheumatic endocarditis (I01.1)
           endocarditis NOS (I38)
  DEF: Endocarditis: Inflammatory disease of the interior lining of the heart chamber and heart valves.

I33.0 Acute and subacute infective endocarditis `COM`
  Bacterial endocarditis (acute) (subacute)
  Endocarditis lenta (acute) (subacute)
  Infective endocarditis (acute) (subacute) NOS
  Malignant endocarditis (acute) (subacute)
  Purulent endocarditis (acute) (subacute)
  Septic endocarditis (acute) (subacute)
  Ulcerative endocarditis (acute) (subacute)
  Vegetative endocarditis (acute) (subacute)
  Use additional code (B95-B97) to identify infectious agent
  AHA: 2025,1Q,19,20

I33.9 Acute and subacute endocarditis, unspecified `COM`
  Acute endocarditis NOS
  Acute myoendocarditis NOS
  Acute periendocarditis NOS
  Subacute endocarditis NOS
  Subacute myoendocarditis NOS
  Subacute periendocarditis NOS

Chapter 9. Diseases of the Circulatory System

I34 Nonrheumatic mitral valve disorders
   EXCLUDES 1:
      mitral valve disease (I05.9)
      mitral valve disorder specified as congenital (Q23.2, Q23.9)
      mitral valve disorder specified as rheumatic (I05.-)
      mitral valve disorder of unspecified cause with diseases of aortic and/or tricuspid valve(s) (I08.-)
      mitral valve disorder of unspecified cause with mitral stenosis or obstruction (I05.0)
      mitral valve failure (I05.8)
      mitral valve stenosis (I05.0)

- **I34.0** Nonrheumatic mitral (valve) insufficiency
  Nonrheumatic mitral (valve) incompetence NOS
  Nonrheumatic mitral (valve) regurgitation NOS
  Code also, if applicable:
     nonrheumatic mitral (valve) annulus calcification (I34.81)
  AHA: 2025,1Q,19

- **I34.1** Nonrheumatic mitral (valve) prolapse
  Floppy nonrheumatic mitral valve syndrome
  EXCLUDES 1: Marfan's syndrome (Q87.4-)

- **I34.2** Nonrheumatic mitral (valve) stenosis
  Code also, if applicable:
     nonrheumatic mitral (valve) annulus calcification (I34.81)

- **I34.8** Other nonrheumatic mitral valve disorders
  AHA: 2022,4Q,23
  - **I34.81** Nonrheumatic mitral (valve) annulus calcification
    Mitral (valve) annulus calcification NOS
    Nonrheumatic mitral (valve) annular calcification
    Code also, if applicable:
       nonrheumatic mitral (valve) insufficiency (I34.0)
       nonrheumatic mitral (valve) stenosis (I34.2)
  - **I34.89** Other nonrheumatic mitral valve disorders

- **I34.9** Nonrheumatic mitral valve disorder, unspecified

I35 Nonrheumatic aortic valve disorders
   Code also, if applicable, bicuspid aortic valve (Q23.81)
   EXCLUDES 2:
      aortic valve disorder of unspecified cause but with diseases of mitral and/or tricuspid valve(s) (I08.-)
      aortic valve disorder specified as congenital (Q23.0, Q23.1)
      aortic valve disorder specified as rheumatic (I06.-)
      hypertrophic subaortic stenosis (I42.1)

- **I35.0** Nonrheumatic aortic (valve) stenosis
  AHA: 2024,4Q,26
- **I35.1** Nonrheumatic aortic (valve) insufficiency
  Nonrheumatic aortic (valve) incompetence NOS
  Nonrheumatic aortic (valve) regurgitation NOS
- **I35.2** Nonrheumatic aortic (valve) stenosis with insufficiency
- **I35.8** Other nonrheumatic aortic valve disorders
- **I35.9** Nonrheumatic aortic valve disorder, unspecified

I36 Nonrheumatic tricuspid valve disorders
   EXCLUDES 1:
      tricuspid valve disorders of unspecified cause (I07.-)
      tricuspid valve disorders specified as congenital (Q22.4, Q22.8, Q22.9)
      tricuspid valve disorders specified as rheumatic (I07.-)
      tricuspid valve disorders with aortic and/or mitral valve involvement (I08.-)

- **I36.0** Nonrheumatic tricuspid (valve) stenosis
- **I36.1** Nonrheumatic tricuspid (valve) insufficiency
  Nonrheumatic tricuspid (valve) incompetence
  Nonrheumatic tricuspid (valve) regurgitation
- **I36.2** Nonrheumatic tricuspid (valve) stenosis with insufficiency
- **I36.8** Other nonrheumatic tricuspid valve disorders
- **I36.9** Nonrheumatic tricuspid valve disorder, unspecified

I37 Nonrheumatic pulmonary valve disorders
   EXCLUDES 1:
      pulmonary valve disorder specified as congenital (Q22.1, Q22.2, Q22.3)
      pulmonary valve disorder specified as rheumatic (I09.89)

- **I37.0** Nonrheumatic pulmonary valve stenosis
- **I37.1** Nonrheumatic pulmonary valve insufficiency
  Nonrheumatic pulmonary valve incompetence
  Nonrheumatic pulmonary valve regurgitation
- **I37.2** Nonrheumatic pulmonary valve stenosis with insufficiency
- **I37.8** Other nonrheumatic pulmonary valve disorders
- **I37.9** Nonrheumatic pulmonary valve disorder, unspecified

I38 Endocarditis, valve unspecified
   INCLUDES:
      endocarditis (chronic) NOS
      valvular incompetence NOS
      valvular insufficiency NOS
      valvular regurgitation NOS
      valvular stenosis NOS
      valvulitis (chronic) NOS
   EXCLUDES 1:
      congenital insufficiency of cardiac valve NOS (Q24.8)
      congenital stenosis of cardiac valve NOS (Q24.8)
      endocardial fibroelastosis (I42.4)
      endocarditis specified as rheumatic (I09.1)
DEF: Endocarditis: Inflammatory disease of the interior lining of the heart chamber and heart valves.

I39 *Endocarditis and heart valve disorders in diseases classified elsewhere*
Code first underlying disease, such as:
   Q fever (A78)
   EXCLUDES 1: endocardial involvement in:
      candidiasis (B37.6)
      gonococcal infection (A54.83)
      Libman-Sacks disease (M32.11)
      listerosis (A32.82)
      meningococcal infection (A39.51)
      rheumatoid arthritis (M05.31)
      syphilis (A52.03)
      tuberculosis (A18.84)
      typhoid fever (A01.02)
DEF: Endocarditis: Inflammatory disease of the interior lining of the heart chamber and heart valves.

I40 Acute myocarditis
   INCLUDES: subacute myocarditis
   EXCLUDES 1: acute rheumatic myocarditis (I01.2)
DEF: Myocarditis: Inflammation of the middle layer of the heart, which is composed of muscle tissue.

- **I40.0** Infective myocarditis
  Septic myocarditis
  Use additional code (B95-B97) to identify infectious agent
- **I40.1** Isolated myocarditis
  Fiedler's myocarditis
  Giant cell myocarditis
  Idiopathic myocarditis
- **I40.8** Other acute myocarditis
- **I40.9** Acute myocarditis, unspecified

I41 *Myocarditis in diseases classified elsewhere*
Code first underlying disease, such as:
   typhus (A75.0-A75.9)
   EXCLUDES 1: myocarditis (in):
      acute (B57.0)
      Chagas' disease (chronic) (B57.2)
      coxsackie (virus) infection (B33.22)
      diphtheritic (A36.81)
      gonococcal (A54.83)
      influenzal (J09.X9, J10.82, J11.82)
      meningococcal (A39.52)
      mumps (B26.82)
      rheumatoid arthritis (M05.31)
      sarcoid (D86.85)
      syphilis (A52.06)
      toxoplasmosis (B58.81)
      tuberculous (A18.84)
DEF: Myocarditis: Inflammation of the middle layer of the heart, which is composed of muscle tissue.

I42 Cardiomyopathy
   INCLUDES: myocardiopathy
Code first pre-existing cardiomyopathy complicating pregnancy and puerperium (O99.4)
   EXCLUDES 2:
      ischemic cardiomyopathy (I25.5)
      peripartum cardiomyopathy (O90.3)
      ventricular hypertrophy (I51.7)

- **I42.0** Dilated cardiomyopathy
  Congestive cardiomyopathy
- **I42.1** Obstructive hypertrophic cardiomyopathy
  Hypertrophic subaortic stenosis (idiopathic)
  DEF: Cardiomyopathy marked by left ventricle hypertrophy and an enlarged septum that result in obstructed blood flow, arrhythmias, mitral regurgitation, and sudden cardiac death.
  TIP: When this condition is described as inherited, assign code Q24.8.

I42.2 Other **hypertrophic** cardiomyopathy [HCC Rx ESR COM]
Nonobstructive hypertrophic cardiomyopathy

I42.3 **Endomyocardial (eosinophilic)** disease [HCC Rx ESR COM]
Endomyocardial (tropical) fibrosis
Löffler's endocarditis

I42.4 **Endocardial fibroelastosis** [HCC Rx ESR COM]
Congenital cardiomyopathy
Elastomyofibrosis

I42.5 Other **restrictive** cardiomyopathy [HCC Rx ESR COM]
Constrictive cardiomyopathy NOS

I42.6 **Alcoholic** cardiomyopathy [HCC Rx ESR COM]
Code also presence of alcoholism (F10.-)

I42.7 **Cardiomyopathy due to drug and external agent** [Rx COM]
Code first poisoning due to drug or toxin, if applicable (T36-T65 with fifth or sixth character 1-4)
Use additional code for adverse effect, if applicable, to identify drug (T36-T50 with fifth or sixth character 5)
AHA: 2021,3Q,8

I42.8 Other cardiomyopathies [HCC Rx ESR COM]

I42.9 Cardiomyopathy, unspecified [HCC Rx ESR COM]
Cardiomyopathy (primary) (secondary) NOS

I43 **Cardiomyopathy in diseases classified elsewhere** [HCC Rx ESR COM]
Code first underlying disease, such as:
amyloidosis (E85.-)
glycogen storage disease (E74.0-)
gout (M10.0-)
thyrotoxicosis (E05.0-E05.9-)
EXCLUDES 1   cardiomyopathy (in):
coxsackie (virus) (B33.24)
diphtheria (A36.81)
sarcoidosis (D86.85)
tuberculosis (A18.84)
AHA: 2024,2Q,9

I44 **Atrioventricular and left bundle-branch block** ✓4th

I44.0 Atrioventricular block, **first degree**

I44.1 Atrioventricular block, **second degree**
Atrioventricular block, type I and II
Möbitz block, type I and II
Second degree block, type I and II
Wenckebach's block

I44.2 Atrioventricular block, **complete** [HCC ESR COM]
Complete heart block NOS
Third degree block
AHA: 2025,2Q,4; 2019,2Q,4

✓5th **I44.3** Other and unspecified **atrioventricular** block
Atrioventricular block NOS
I44.30 Unspecified atrioventricular block
I44.39 Other atrioventricular block

I44.4 **Left anterior fascicular** block

I44.5 **Left posterior fascicular** block

✓5th **I44.6** Other and unspecified fascicular block
I44.60 Unspecified fascicular block
Left bundle-branch hemiblock NOS
I44.69 Other fascicular block

I44.7 Left bundle-branch block, unspecified

Conduction Disorders

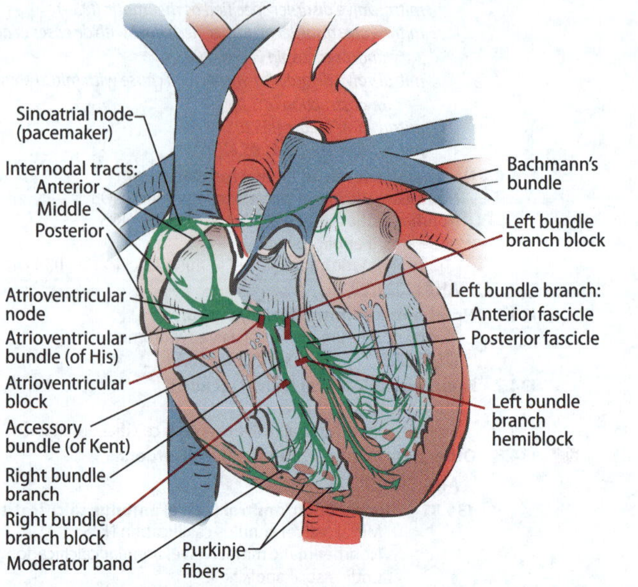

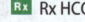

I45 Other conduction disorders ✓4th

I45.0 **Right fascicular** block

✓5th **I45.1** Other and unspecified right bundle-branch block
I45.10 Unspecified right bundle-branch block
Right bundle-branch block NOS
I45.19 Other right bundle-branch block

I45.2 **Bifascicular** block

I45.3 **Trifascicular** block

I45.4 Nonspecific intraventricular block
Bundle-branch block NOS

I45.5 Other specified heart block
Sinoatrial block
Sinoauricular block
EXCLUDES 1   heart block NOS (I45.9)

I45.6 Pre-excitation syndrome
Accelerated atrioventricular conduction
Accessory atrioventricular conduction
Anomalous atrioventricular excitation
Lown-Ganong-Levine syndrome
Pre-excitation atrioventricular conduction
Wolff-Parkinson-White syndrome

✓5th **I45.8** Other specified conduction disorders
I45.81 Long QT syndrome
DEF: Condition characterized by recurrent syncope, malignant arrhythmias, and sudden death. This syndrome has a characteristic prolonged Q-T interval on an electrocardiogram.
I45.89 Other specified conduction disorders
Atrioventricular [AV] dissociation
Interference dissociation
Isorhythmic dissociation
Nonparoxysmal AV nodal tachycardia
AHA: 2013,2Q,31

I45.9 Conduction disorder, unspecified
Heart block NOS
Stokes-Adams syndrome

✓4th **I46** Cardiac arrest
EXCLUDES 2   cardiogenic shock (R57.0)
AHA: 2019,2Q,4-5

I46.2 Cardiac arrest **due to underlying cardiac condition** [HCC ESR COM UPD]
Code first underlying cardiac condition
AHA: 2024,1Q,27

I46.8 Cardiac arrest due to other underlying condition [HCC ESR COM UPD]
Code first underlying condition

I46.9 Cardiac arrest, cause unspecified [HCC ESR COM]
AHA: 2020,3Q,26

Chapter 9. Diseases of the Circulatory System

I47 Paroxysmal tachycardia
Code first tachycardia complicating:
  abortion or ectopic or molar pregnancy (O00-O07, O08.8)
  obstetric surgery and procedures (O75.4)
  EXCLUDES 1 tachycardia NOS (R00.0)
    sinoauricular tachycardia NOS (R00.0)
    sinus [sinusal] tachycardia NOS (R00.0)

- **I47.0 Re-entry ventricular arrhythmia**
- **I47.1 Supraventricular tachycardia**
  AHA: 2023,4Q,26-27
  - **I47.10 Supraventricular tachycardia, unspecified**
  - **I47.11 Inappropriate sinus tachycardia, so stated**
    IST
  - **I47.19 Other supraventricular tachycardia**
    Atrial (paroxysmal) tachycardia
    Atrioventricular [AV] (paroxysmal) tachycardia
    Atrioventricular re-entrant (nodal) tachycardia [AVNRT] [AVRT]
    Junctional (paroxysmal) tachycardia
    Nodal (paroxysmal) tachycardia
- **I47.2 Ventricular tachycardia**
  AHA: 2022,4Q,23-24; 2021,3Q,11; 2013,3Q,23
  - **I47.20 Ventricular tachycardia, unspecified**
  - **I47.21 Torsades de pointes**
    Code also, if applicable, long QT syndrome (I45.81)
    Use additional code for adverse effect, if applicable, to identify drug (T36-T50 with fifth or sixth character 5)
    AHA: 2022,4Q,24
    DEF: Torsades de pointes (TdP): Accelerated heart rhythm, anywhere between 150 and 300 beats per minute, that initiates in the lower chambers of the heart (ventricles). Most commonly occurs in the setting of inherited or medication-induced long QT syndrome.
  - **I47.29 Other ventricular tachycardia**
- **I47.9 Paroxysmal tachycardia, unspecified**
  Bouveret (-Hoffman) syndrome

I48 Atrial fibrillation and flutter

- **I48.0 Paroxysmal atrial fibrillation**
  AHA: 2021,2Q,8; 2018,3Q,6
- **I48.1 Persistent atrial fibrillation**
  EXCLUDES 1 permanent atrial fibrillation (I48.21)
  AHA: 2021,2Q,8; 2019,4Q,7; 2019,2Q,3; 2018,3Q,6
  - **I48.11 Longstanding persistent atrial fibrillation**
  - **I48.19 Other persistent atrial fibrillation**
    Chronic persistent atrial fibrillation
    Persistent atrial fibrillation, NOS
    AHA: 2019,4Q,7
- **I48.2 Chronic atrial fibrillation**
  AHA: 2021,2Q,8; 2019,4Q,7; 2019,2Q,3; 2018,3Q,6
  - **I48.20 Chronic atrial fibrillation, unspecified**
    EXCLUDES 1 chronic persistent atrial fibrillation (I48.19)
  - **I48.21 Permanent atrial fibrillation**
- **I48.3 Typical atrial flutter**
  Type I atrial flutter
- **I48.4 Atypical atrial flutter**
  Type II atrial flutter
- **I48.9 Unspecified atrial fibrillation and atrial flutter**
  - **I48.91 Unspecified atrial fibrillation**
  - **I48.92 Unspecified atrial flutter**

I49 Other cardiac arrhythmias
Code first cardiac arrhythmia complicating:
  abortion or ectopic or molar pregnancy (O00-O07, O08.8)
  obstetric surgery and procedures (O75.4)
  EXCLUDES 2 bradycardia NOS (R00.1)
    neonatal dysrhythmia (P29.1-)
    sinoatrial bradycardia (R00.1)
    sinus bradycardia (R00.1)
    vagal bradycardia (R00.1)

- **I49.0 Ventricular fibrillation and flutter**
  - **I49.01 Ventricular fibrillation**
    AHA: 2022,2Q,14
  - **I49.02 Ventricular flutter**
- **I49.1 Atrial premature depolarization**
  Atrial premature beats
- **I49.2 Junctional premature depolarization**
- **I49.3 Ventricular premature depolarization**
  AHA: 2020,2Q,23
- **I49.4 Other and unspecified premature depolarization**
  - **I49.40 Unspecified premature depolarization**
    Premature beats NOS
  - **I49.49 Other premature depolarization**
    Ectopic beats
    Extrasystoles
    Extrasystolic arrhythmias
    Premature contractions
- **I49.5 Sick sinus syndrome**
  Tachycardia-bradycardia syndrome
  AHA: 2019,1Q,33
  TIP: The presence of a pacemaker controls but does not cure sick sinus syndrome and therefore is considered a reportable chronic condition. When a pacemaker is evaluated by a provider, this code and code Z95.0 Presence of cardiac pacemaker, should be reported, even in the absence of any notable changes or management.
- **I49.8 Other specified cardiac arrhythmias**
  Brugada syndrome
  Coronary sinus rhythm disorder
  Ectopic rhythm disorder
  Nodal rhythm disorder
  AHA: 2025,2Q,4
- **I49.9 Cardiac arrhythmia, unspecified**
  Arrhythmia (cardiac) NOS

I50 Heart failure
Code first:
  heart failure complicating abortion or ectopic or molar pregnancy (O00-O07, O08.8)
  heart failure due to hypertension (I11.0)
  heart failure due to hypertension with chronic kidney disease (I13.-)
  heart failure following surgery (I97.13-)
  obstetric surgery and procedures (O75.4)
  rheumatic heart failure (I09.81)
  EXCLUDES 2 cardiac arrest (I46.-)
    neonatal cardiac failure (P29.0)
  AHA: 2018,4Q,67; 2018,2Q,9; 2017,1Q,47; 2014,1Q,25; 2013,2Q,33

- **I50.1 Left ventricular failure, unspecified**
  Cardiac asthma
  Edema of lung with heart disease NOS
  Edema of lung with heart failure
  Left heart failure
  Pulmonary edema with heart disease NOS
  Pulmonary edema with heart failure
  EXCLUDES 1 edema of lung without heart disease or heart failure (J81.-)
    pulmonary edema without heart disease or failure (J81.-)
- **I50.2 Systolic (congestive) heart failure**
  Heart failure with reduced ejection fraction [HFrEF]
  Systolic left ventricular heart failure
  Code also end stage heart failure, if applicable (I50.84)
  EXCLUDES 1 combined systolic (congestive) and diastolic (congestive) heart failure (I50.4-)
  AHA: 2020,3Q,32; 2017,1Q,46; 2016,1Q,10
  - **I50.20 Unspecified systolic (congestive) heart failure**
  - **I50.21 Acute systolic (congestive) heart failure**
  - **I50.22 Chronic systolic (congestive) heart failure**

Chapter 9. Diseases of the Circulatory System

I50.23 Acute on chronic systolic (congestive) heart failure [HCC Rx ESR COM]

√5th I50.3 Diastolic (congestive) heart failure
Diastolic left ventricular heart failure
Heart failure with normal ejection fraction
Heart failure with preserved ejection fraction [HFpEF]
Code also end stage heart failure, if applicable (I50.84)
EXCLUDES 1 combined systolic (congestive) and diastolic (congestive) heart failure (I50.4-)
AHA: 2024,2Q,9; 2020,3Q,32; 2017,1Q,46; 2016,1Q,10

- **I50.30** Unspecified diastolic (congestive) heart failure [HCC Rx ESR COM]
- **I50.31** Acute diastolic (congestive) heart failure [HCC Rx ESR COM]
  AHA: 2025,2Q,5
- **I50.32** Chronic diastolic (congestive) heart failure [HCC Rx ESR COM]
  AHA: 2023,3Q,14
  DEF: HFimpEF: Heart failure with improved ejection fraction
  DEF: HFrecEF: Heart failure with recovered ejection fraction
- **I50.33** Acute on chronic diastolic (congestive) heart failure [HCC Rx ESR COM]

√5th I50.4 Combined systolic (congestive) and diastolic (congestive) heart failure
Combined systolic and diastolic left ventricular heart failure
Heart failure with reduced ejection fraction and diastolic dysfunction
Code also end stage heart failure, if applicable (I50.84)
AHA: 2017,1Q,46; 2016,1Q,10

- **I50.40** Unspecified combined systolic (congestive) and diastolic (congestive) heart failure [HCC Rx ESR COM]
- **I50.41** Acute combined systolic (congestive) and diastolic (congestive) heart failure [HCC Rx ESR COM]
- **I50.42** Chronic combined systolic (congestive) and diastolic (congestive) heart failure [HCC Rx ESR COM]
- **I50.43** Acute on chronic combined systolic (congestive) and diastolic (congestive) heart failure [HCC Rx ESR COM]

√5th I50.8 Other heart failure
AHA: 2022,3Q,16; 2017,4Q,15-16

- **√6th I50.81** Right heart failure
  Right ventricular failure
  AHA: 2023,3Q,14
  - **I50.810** Right heart failure, unspecified [HCC Rx ESR COM]
    Right heart failure without mention of left heart failure
    Right ventricular failure NOS
  - **I50.811** Acute right heart failure [HCC Rx ESR COM]
    Acute (isolated) right ventricular failure
    Acute isolated right heart failure
  - **I50.812** Chronic right heart failure [HCC Rx ESR COM]
    Chronic (isolated) right ventricular failure
    Chronic isolated right heart failure
  - **I50.813** Acute on chronic right heart failure [HCC Rx ESR COM]
    Acute decompensation of chronic (isolated) right ventricular failure
    Acute exacerbation of chronic (isolated) right ventricular failure
    Acute on chronic (isolated) right ventricular failure
    Acute on chronic isolated right heart failure
  - **I50.814** Right heart failure due to left heart failure [HCC Rx ESR COM]
    Right ventricular failure secondary to left ventricular failure
    Code also the type of left ventricular failure, if known (I50.2-I50.43)
    EXCLUDES 1 right heart failure with but not due to left heart failure (I50.82)
- **I50.82** Biventricular heart failure [HCC Rx ESR COM]
  Code also the type of left ventricular failure as systolic, diastolic, or combined, if known (I50.2-I50.43)
- **I50.83** High output heart failure [HCC Rx ESR COM]
  DEF: Occurs when the high demand for blood exceeds the capacity of a normally functioning heart to meet the demand.
- **I50.84** End stage heart failure [HCC Rx ESR COM]
  Stage D heart failure
  Code also the type of heart failure as systolic, diastolic, or combined, if known (I50.2-I50.43)
- **I50.89** Other heart failure [HCC Rx ESR COM]

I50.9 Heart failure, unspecified [HCC Rx ESR COM]
Cardiac, heart or myocardial failure NOS
Congestive heart disease
Congestive heart failure NOS
EXCLUDES 2 fluid overload unrelated to congestive heart failure (E87.70)
AHA: 2017,4Q,15-16; 2017,1Q,45-46; 2014,4Q,21; 2012,4Q,92

√4th I51 Complications and ill-defined descriptions of heart disease
EXCLUDES 1 any condition in I51.4-I51.9 due to hypertension (I11.-)
any condition in I51.4-I51.9 due to hypertension and chronic kidney disease (I13.-)
heart disease specified as rheumatic (I00-I09)
EXCLUDES 2 ▶heart disease specified as rheumatic (I00-I09)◀

- **I51.0** Cardiac septal defect, acquired [A]
  Acquired septal atrial defect (old)
  Acquired septal auricular defect (old)
  Acquired septal ventricular defect (old)
  EXCLUDES 1 cardiac septal defect as current complication following acute myocardial infarction (I23.1, I23.2)
  DEF: Abnormal communication between opposite heart chambers due to a defect of the septum. It is not present at birth.
- **I51.1** Rupture of chordae tendineae, not elsewhere classified [HCC Rx ESR COM]
  EXCLUDES 1 rupture of chordae tendineae as current complication following acute myocardial infarction (I23.4)
- **I51.2** Rupture of papillary muscle, not elsewhere classified [HCC Rx ESR COM]
  EXCLUDES 1 rupture of papillary muscle as current complication following acute myocardial infarction (I23.5)
- **I51.3** Intracardiac thrombosis, not elsewhere classified
  Apical thrombosis (old)
  Atrial thrombosis (old)
  Auricular thrombosis (old)
  Mural thrombosis (old)
  Ventricular thrombosis (old)
  EXCLUDES 1 intracardiac thrombosis as current complication following acute myocardial infarction (I23.6)
  AHA: 2013,1Q,24
- **I51.4** Myocarditis, unspecified [HCC Rx ESR COM]
  Chronic (interstitial) myocarditis
  Myocardial fibrosis
  Myocarditis NOS
  EXCLUDES 1 acute or subacute myocarditis (I40.-)
  AHA: 2018,4Q,67; 2018,2Q,9
- **I51.5** Myocardial degeneration [HCC Rx ESR COM]
  Fatty degeneration of heart or myocardium
  Myocardial disease
  Senile degeneration of heart or myocardium
  EXCLUDES 1 ▶myocardial degeneration due to hypertension (I11.-)◀
  ▶myocardial degeneration due to hypertension and chronic kidney disease (I13.-)◀
  AHA: 2018,4Q,67; 2018,2Q,9
- **I51.7** Cardiomegaly
  Cardiac dilatation
  Cardiac hypertrophy
  Ventricular dilatation
  EXCLUDES 1 ▶cardiomegaly due to hypertension (I11.-)◀
  ▶cardiomegaly due to hypertension and chronic kidney disease (I13.-)◀
  AHA: 2018,4Q,67; 2018,2Q,9

I51.8 Other ill-defined heart diseases
AHA: 2018,2Q,9

I51.81 Takotsubo syndrome
Reversible left ventricular dysfunction following sudden emotional stress
Stress induced cardiomyopathy
Takotsubo cardiomyopathy
Transient left ventricular apical ballooning syndrome
DEF: Complex of symptoms mimicking myocardial infarct in absence of heart disease, with the majority of cases occurring in postmenopausal women. Heart muscles are temporarily weakened, and a sudden, massive surge of adrenalin stuns the heart, greatly reducing the ability to pump blood.

I51.89 Other ill-defined heart diseases
Carditis (acute)(chronic)
Pancarditis (acute)(chronic)
AHA: 2019,2Q,5; 2018,4Q,67

I51.9 Heart disease, unspecified
AHA: 2018,4Q,67; 2018,2Q,9

I52 Other heart disorders in diseases classified elsewhere
Code first underlying disease, such as:
congenital syphilis (A50.5)
mucopolysaccharidosis (E76.3)
schistosomiasis (B65.0-B65.9)
EXCLUDES 1 heart disease (in):
gonococcal infection (A54.83)
meningococcal infection (A39.50)
rheumatoid arthritis (M05.31)
syphilis (A52.06)

I5A Non-ischemic myocardial injury (non-traumatic)
Acute (non-ischemic) myocardial injury
Chronic (non-ischemic) myocardial injury
Unspecified (non-ischemic) myocardial injury
Code first the underlying cause, if known and applicable, such as:
acute kidney failure (N17.-)
acute myocarditis (I40.-)
cardiomyopathy (I42.-)
chronic kidney disease (CKD) (N18.-)
heart failure (I50.-)
hypertensive urgency (I16.0)
nonrheumatic aortic valve disorders (I35.-)
paroxysmal tachycardia (I47.-)
pulmonary embolism (I26.-)
pulmonary hypertension (I27.0, I27.2-)
sepsis (A41.-)
takotsubo syndrome (I51.81)
EXCLUDES 1 acute myocardial infarction (I21.-)
injury of heart (S26.-)
EXCLUDES 2 other acute ischemic heart diseases (I24.-)
AHA: 2021,4Q,14-15

Cerebrovascular diseases (I60-I69)

Use additional code to identify presence of:
alcohol abuse and dependence (F10.-)
exposure to environmental tobacco smoke (Z77.22)
history of tobacco dependence (Z87.891)
hypertension (I10-I1A)
occupational exposure to environmental tobacco smoke (Z57.31)
tobacco dependence (F17.-)
tobacco use (Z72.0)
EXCLUDES 1 traumatic intracranial hemorrhage (S06.-)
AHA: 2014,3Q,5; 2012,4Q,91-92

I60 Nontraumatic subarachnoid hemorrhage
Use additional code, if known, to indicate National Institutes of Health Stroke Scale (NIHSS) score (R29.7-)
EXCLUDES 1 syphilitic ruptured cerebral aneurysm (A52.05)
EXCLUDES 2 sequelae of subarachnoid hemorrhage (I69.0-)

I60.0 Nontraumatic subarachnoid hemorrhage from carotid siphon and bifurcation
- **I60.00** Nontraumatic subarachnoid hemorrhage from unspecified carotid siphon and bifurcation
- **I60.01** Nontraumatic subarachnoid hemorrhage from right carotid siphon and bifurcation
- **I60.02** Nontraumatic subarachnoid hemorrhage from left carotid siphon and bifurcation

I60.1 Nontraumatic subarachnoid hemorrhage from middle cerebral artery
- **I60.10** Nontraumatic subarachnoid hemorrhage from unspecified middle cerebral artery
- **I60.11** Nontraumatic subarachnoid hemorrhage from right middle cerebral artery
- **I60.12** Nontraumatic subarachnoid hemorrhage from left middle cerebral artery

I60.2 Nontraumatic subarachnoid hemorrhage from anterior communicating artery

I60.3 Nontraumatic subarachnoid hemorrhage from posterior communicating artery
- **I60.30** Nontraumatic subarachnoid hemorrhage from unspecified posterior communicating artery
- **I60.31** Nontraumatic subarachnoid hemorrhage from right posterior communicating artery
- **I60.32** Nontraumatic subarachnoid hemorrhage from left posterior communicating artery

I60.4 Nontraumatic subarachnoid hemorrhage from basilar artery

I60.5 Nontraumatic subarachnoid hemorrhage from vertebral artery
- **I60.50** Nontraumatic subarachnoid hemorrhage from unspecified vertebral artery
- **I60.51** Nontraumatic subarachnoid hemorrhage from right vertebral artery
- **I60.52** Nontraumatic subarachnoid hemorrhage from left vertebral artery

I60.6 Nontraumatic subarachnoid hemorrhage from other intracranial arteries

I60.7 Nontraumatic subarachnoid hemorrhage from unspecified intracranial artery
Ruptured (congenital) berry aneurysm
Ruptured (congenital) cerebral aneurysm
Subarachnoid hemorrhage (nontraumatic) from cerebral artery NOS
Subarachnoid hemorrhage (nontraumatic) from communicating artery NOS
EXCLUDES 1 berry aneurysm, nonruptured (I67.1)

I60.8 Other nontraumatic subarachnoid hemorrhage
Meningeal hemorrhage
Rupture of cerebral arteriovenous malformation

I60.9 Nontraumatic subarachnoid hemorrhage, unspecified

I61 Nontraumatic intracerebral hemorrhage
Use additional code, if known, to indicate National Institutes of Health Stroke Scale (NIHSS) score (R29.7-)
EXCLUDES 2 sequelae of intracerebral hemorrhage (I69.1-)
AHA: 2022,3Q,9-10; 2017,2Q,9-10

I61.0 Nontraumatic intracerebral hemorrhage in hemisphere, subcortical
Deep intracerebral hemorrhage (nontraumatic)
AHA: 2016,4Q,27

I61.1 Nontraumatic intracerebral hemorrhage in hemisphere, cortical
Cerebral lobe hemorrhage (nontraumatic)
Superficial intracerebral hemorrhage (nontraumatic)

I61.2 Nontraumatic intracerebral hemorrhage in hemisphere, unspecified

I61.3 Nontraumatic intracerebral hemorrhage in brain stem
AHA: 2023,4Q,42

I61.4 Nontraumatic intracerebral hemorrhage in cerebellum

I61.5 Nontraumatic intracerebral hemorrhage, intraventricular

I61.6 Nontraumatic intracerebral hemorrhage, multiple localized

I61.8 Other nontraumatic intracerebral hemorrhage
AHA: 2024,2Q,25

I61.9 Nontraumatic intracerebral hemorrhage, unspecified

I62 Other and unspecified nontraumatic intracranial hemorrhage
Use additional code, if known, to indicate National Institutes of Health Stroke Scale (NIHSS) score (R29.7-)
EXCLUDES 2 sequelae of intracranial hemorrhage (I69.2)

I62.0 Nontraumatic subdural hemorrhage
- **I62.00** Nontraumatic subdural hemorrhage, unspecified
- **I62.01** Nontraumatic acute subdural hemorrhage

I62.02 Nontraumatic subacute subdural hemorrhage `HCC` `ESR` `COM`

I62.03 Nontraumatic chronic subdural hemorrhage `HCC` `ESR` `COM`

I62.1 Nontraumatic extradural hemorrhage `HCC` `ESR` `COM`
Nontraumatic epidural hemorrhage
AHA: 2023,3Q,21

I62.9 Nontraumatic intracranial hemorrhage, unspecified `HCC` `ESR` `COM`

√4th **I63** Cerebral infarction
INCLUDES occlusion and stenosis of cerebral and precerebral arteries, resulting in cerebral infarction
Use additional code, if applicable, to identify status post administration of tPA (rtPA) in a different facility within the last 24 hours prior to admission to current facility (Z92.82)
Use additional code, if known, to indicate National Institutes of Health Stroke Scale (NIHSS) score (R29.7-)
EXCLUDES 1 neonatal cerebral infarction (P91.82-)
EXCLUDES 2 chronic, without residual deficits (sequelae) (Z86.73)
sequelae of cerebral infarction (I69.3-)
AHA: 2024,1Q,26; 2017,2Q,9-10; 2016,4Q,28,61-62; 2015,1Q,25; 2014,1Q,23
TIP: Weakness on one side of the body documented as secondary to stroke is synonymous with hemiparesis/hemiplegia (G81.-). Weakness of one limb documented as secondary to stroke is synonymous with monoplegia (G83.1-, G83.2-, G83.3-).

√5th **I63.0** Cerebral infarction due to thrombosis of precerebral arteries

I63.00 Cerebral infarction due to thrombosis of unspecified precerebral artery `HCC` `ESR` `COM`

√6th **I63.01** Cerebral infarction due to thrombosis of vertebral artery

I63.011 Cerebral infarction due to thrombosis of right vertebral artery `HCC` `ESR` `COM`

I63.012 Cerebral infarction due to thrombosis of left vertebral artery `HCC` `ESR` `COM`

I63.013 Cerebral infarction due to thrombosis of bilateral vertebral arteries `HCC` `ESR` `COM`

I63.019 Cerebral infarction due to thrombosis of unspecified vertebral artery `HCC` `ESR` `COM`

I63.02 Cerebral infarction due to thrombosis of basilar artery `HCC` `ESR` `COM`

√6th **I63.03** Cerebral infarction due to thrombosis of carotid artery

I63.031 Cerebral infarction due to thrombosis of right carotid artery `HCC` `ESR` `COM`

I63.032 Cerebral infarction due to thrombosis of left carotid artery `HCC` `ESR` `COM`

I63.033 Cerebral infarction due to thrombosis of bilateral carotid arteries `HCC` `ESR` `COM`

I63.039 Cerebral infarction due to thrombosis of unspecified carotid artery `HCC` `ESR` `COM`

I63.09 Cerebral infarction due to thrombosis of other precerebral artery `HCC` `ESR` `COM`

√5th **I63.1** Cerebral infarction due to embolism of precerebral arteries

I63.10 Cerebral infarction due to embolism of unspecified precerebral artery `HCC` `ESR` `COM`

√6th **I63.11** Cerebral infarction due to embolism of vertebral artery

I63.111 Cerebral infarction due to embolism of right vertebral artery `HCC` `ESR` `COM`

I63.112 Cerebral infarction due to embolism of left vertebral artery `HCC` `ESR` `COM`

I63.113 Cerebral infarction due to embolism of bilateral vertebral arteries `HCC` `ESR` `COM`

I63.119 Cerebral infarction due to embolism of unspecified vertebral artery `HCC` `ESR` `COM`

I63.12 Cerebral infarction due to embolism of basilar artery `HCC` `ESR` `COM`

√6th **I63.13** Cerebral infarction due to embolism of carotid artery

I63.131 Cerebral infarction due to embolism of right carotid artery `HCC` `ESR` `COM`

I63.132 Cerebral infarction due to embolism of left carotid artery `HCC` `ESR` `COM`

I63.133 Cerebral infarction due to embolism of bilateral carotid arteries `HCC` `ESR` `COM`

I63.139 Cerebral infarction due to embolism of unspecified carotid artery `HCC` `ESR` `COM`

I63.19 Cerebral infarction due to embolism of other precerebral artery `HCC` `ESR` `COM`

√5th **I63.2** Cerebral infarction due to unspecified occlusion or stenosis of precerebral arteries
AHA: 2020,3Q,27-28

I63.20 Cerebral infarction due to unspecified occlusion or stenosis of unspecified precerebral arteries `HCC` `ESR` `COM`

√6th **I63.21** Cerebral infarction due to unspecified occlusion or stenosis of vertebral arteries

I63.211 Cerebral infarction due to unspecified occlusion or stenosis of right vertebral artery `HCC` `ESR` `COM`

I63.212 Cerebral infarction due to unspecified occlusion or stenosis of left vertebral artery `HCC` `ESR` `COM`

I63.213 Cerebral infarction due to unspecified occlusion or stenosis of bilateral vertebral arteries `HCC` `ESR` `COM`

I63.219 Cerebral infarction due to unspecified occlusion or stenosis of unspecified vertebral artery `HCC` `ESR` `COM`

I63.22 Cerebral infarction due to unspecified occlusion or stenosis of basilar artery `HCC` `ESR` `COM`

√6th **I63.23** Cerebral infarction due to unspecified occlusion or stenosis of carotid arteries

I63.231 Cerebral infarction due to unspecified occlusion or stenosis of right carotid arteries `HCC` `ESR` `COM`

I63.232 Cerebral infarction due to unspecified occlusion or stenosis of left carotid arteries `HCC` `ESR` `COM`

I63.233 Cerebral infarction due to unspecified occlusion or stenosis of bilateral carotid arteries `HCC` `ESR` `COM`

I63.239 Cerebral infarction due to unspecified occlusion or stenosis of unspecified carotid artery `HCC` `ESR` `COM`

I63.29 Cerebral infarction due to unspecified occlusion or stenosis of other precerebral arteries `HCC` `ESR` `COM`

√5th **I63.3** Cerebral infarction due to thrombosis of cerebral arteries

I63.30 Cerebral infarction due to thrombosis of unspecified cerebral artery `HCC` `ESR` `COM`

√6th **I63.31** Cerebral infarction due to thrombosis of middle cerebral artery

I63.311 Cerebral infarction due to thrombosis of right middle cerebral artery `HCC` `ESR` `COM`

I63.312 Cerebral infarction due to thrombosis of left middle cerebral artery `HCC` `ESR` `COM`

I63.313 Cerebral infarction due to thrombosis of bilateral middle cerebral arteries `HCC` `ESR` `COM`

I63.319 Cerebral infarction due to thrombosis of unspecified middle cerebral artery `HCC` `ESR` `COM`

√6th **I63.32** Cerebral infarction due to thrombosis of anterior cerebral artery

I63.321 Cerebral infarction due to thrombosis of right anterior cerebral artery `HCC` `ESR` `COM`

I63.322 Cerebral infarction due to thrombosis of left anterior cerebral artery `HCC` `ESR` `COM`

I63.323 Cerebral infarction due to thrombosis of bilateral anterior cerebral arteries `HCC` `ESR` `COM`

I63.329 Cerebral infarction due to thrombosis of unspecified anterior cerebral artery `HCC` `ESR` `COM`

√6th **I63.33** Cerebral infarction due to thrombosis of posterior cerebral artery

I63.331 Cerebral infarction due to thrombosis of right posterior cerebral artery `HCC` `ESR` `COM`

I63.332 Cerebral infarction due to thrombosis of left posterior cerebral artery `HCC` `ESR` `COM`

I63.333 Cerebral infarction due to thrombosis of bilateral posterior cerebral arteries `HCC` `ESR` `COM`

Chapter 9. Diseases of the Circulatory System

- **I63.339** Cerebral infarction due to thrombosis of unspecified posterior cerebral artery `HCC` `ESR` `COM`
- √6th **I63.34** Cerebral infarction due to thrombosis of cerebellar artery
  - **I63.341** Cerebral infarction due to thrombosis of right cerebellar artery `HCC` `ESR` `COM`
  - **I63.342** Cerebral infarction due to thrombosis of left cerebellar artery `HCC` `ESR` `COM`
  - **I63.343** Cerebral infarction due to thrombosis of bilateral cerebellar arteries `HCC` `ESR` `COM`
  - **I63.349** Cerebral infarction due to thrombosis of unspecified cerebellar artery `HCC` `ESR` `COM`
- **I63.39** Cerebral infarction due to thrombosis of other cerebral artery `HCC` `ESR` `COM`
- √5th **I63.4** Cerebral infarction due to embolism of cerebral arteries
  - **I63.40** Cerebral infarction due to embolism of unspecified cerebral artery
  - √6th **I63.41** Cerebral infarction due to embolism of middle cerebral artery
    - **I63.411** Cerebral infarction due to embolism of right middle cerebral artery `HCC` `ESR` `COM`
    - **I63.412** Cerebral infarction due to embolism of left middle cerebral artery `HCC` `ESR` `COM`
    - **I63.413** Cerebral infarction due to embolism of bilateral middle cerebral arteries
    - **I63.419** Cerebral infarction due to embolism of unspecified middle cerebral artery `HCC` `ESR` `COM`
  - √6th **I63.42** Cerebral infarction due to embolism of anterior cerebral artery
    - **I63.421** Cerebral infarction due to embolism of right anterior cerebral artery `HCC` `ESR` `COM`
    - **I63.422** Cerebral infarction due to embolism of left anterior cerebral artery `HCC` `ESR` `COM`
    - **I63.423** Cerebral infarction due to embolism of bilateral anterior cerebral arteries `HCC` `ESR` `COM`
    - **I63.429** Cerebral infarction due to embolism of unspecified anterior cerebral artery `HCC` `ESR` `COM`
  - √6th **I63.43** Cerebral infarction due to embolism of posterior cerebral artery
    - **I63.431** Cerebral infarction due to embolism of right posterior cerebral artery `HCC` `ESR` `COM`
    - **I63.432** Cerebral infarction due to embolism of left posterior cerebral artery `HCC` `ESR` `COM`
    - **I63.433** Cerebral infarction due to embolism of bilateral posterior cerebral arteries `HCC` `ESR` `COM`
    - **I63.439** Cerebral infarction due to embolism of unspecified posterior cerebral artery `HCC` `ESR` `COM`
  - √6th **I63.44** Cerebral infarction due to embolism of cerebellar artery
    - **I63.441** Cerebral infarction due to embolism of right cerebellar artery `HCC` `ESR` `COM`
    - **I63.442** Cerebral infarction due to embolism of left cerebellar artery `HCC` `ESR` `COM`
    - **I63.443** Cerebral infarction due to embolism of bilateral cerebellar arteries `HCC` `ESR` `COM`
    - **I63.449** Cerebral infarction due to embolism of unspecified cerebellar artery `HCC` `ESR` `COM`
  - **I63.49** Cerebral infarction due to embolism of other cerebral artery `HCC` `ESR` `COM`
- √5th **I63.5** Cerebral infarction due to unspecified occlusion or stenosis of cerebral arteries
  - **I63.50** Cerebral infarction due to unspecified occlusion or stenosis of unspecified cerebral artery `HCC` `ESR` `COM`
  - √6th **I63.51** Cerebral infarction due to unspecified occlusion or stenosis of middle cerebral artery
    - **I63.511** Cerebral infarction due to unspecified occlusion or stenosis of right middle cerebral artery `HCC` `ESR` `COM`
    - **I63.512** Cerebral infarction due to unspecified occlusion or stenosis of left middle cerebral artery `HCC` `ESR` `COM`
    - **I63.513** Cerebral infarction due to unspecified occlusion or stenosis of bilateral middle cerebral arteries `HCC` `ESR` `COM`
    - **I63.519** Cerebral infarction due to unspecified occlusion or stenosis of unspecified middle cerebral artery `HCC` `ESR` `COM`
  - √6th **I63.52** Cerebral infarction due to unspecified occlusion or stenosis of anterior cerebral artery
    - **I63.521** Cerebral infarction due to unspecified occlusion or stenosis of right anterior cerebral artery `HCC` `ESR` `COM`
    - **I63.522** Cerebral infarction due to unspecified occlusion or stenosis of left anterior cerebral artery `HCC` `ESR` `COM`
    - **I63.523** Cerebral infarction due to unspecified occlusion or stenosis of bilateral anterior cerebral arteries `HCC` `ESR` `COM`
    - **I63.529** Cerebral infarction due to unspecified occlusion or stenosis of unspecified anterior cerebral artery `HCC` `ESR` `COM`
  - √6th **I63.53** Cerebral infarction due to unspecified occlusion or stenosis of posterior cerebral artery
    - **I63.531** Cerebral infarction due to unspecified occlusion or stenosis of right posterior cerebral artery `HCC` `ESR` `COM`
    - **I63.532** Cerebral infarction due to unspecified occlusion or stenosis of left posterior cerebral artery `HCC` `ESR` `COM`
    - **I63.533** Cerebral infarction due to unspecified occlusion or stenosis of bilateral posterior cerebral arteries `HCC` `ESR` `COM`
    - **I63.539** Cerebral infarction due to unspecified occlusion or stenosis of unspecified posterior cerebral artery `HCC` `ESR` `COM`
  - √6th **I63.54** Cerebral infarction due to unspecified occlusion or stenosis of cerebellar artery
    - **I63.541** Cerebral infarction due to unspecified occlusion or stenosis of right cerebellar artery `HCC` `ESR` `COM`
    - **I63.542** Cerebral infarction due to unspecified occlusion or stenosis of left cerebellar artery `HCC` `ESR` `COM`
    - **I63.543** Cerebral infarction due to unspecified occlusion or stenosis of bilateral cerebellar arteries `HCC` `ESR` `COM`
    - **I63.549** Cerebral infarction due to unspecified occlusion or stenosis of unspecified cerebellar artery `HCC` `ESR` `COM`
  - **I63.59** Cerebral infarction due to unspecified occlusion or stenosis of other cerebral artery `HCC` `ESR` `COM`
- **I63.6** Cerebral infarction due to cerebral venous thrombosis, nonpyogenic `HCC` `ESR` `COM`
- √5th **I63.8** Other cerebral infarction
  - **AHA:** 2018,4Q,16
  - **I63.81** Other cerebral infarction due to occlusion or stenosis of small artery `HCC` `ESR` `COM`
    Lacunar infarction
    AHA: 2020,3Q,27
  - **I63.89** Other cerebral infarction `HCC` `ESR` `COM`
    AHA: 2024,1Q,32; 2022,1Q,25
- **I63.9** Cerebral infarction, unspecified `HCC` `ESR` `COM`
  Stroke NOS
  EXCLUDES 2 transient cerebral ischemic attacks and related syndromes (G45.-)
  AHA: 2020,2Q,29
  TIP: When provider documentation does not identify the location of an infarction, imaging reports can be used to pinpoint the location and lead to a more specific infarction code.

Chapter 9. Diseases of the Circulatory System

I65 **Occlusion and stenosis of precerebral arteries, not resulting in cerebral infarction**
- INCLUDES
  - embolism of precerebral artery
  - narrowing of precerebral artery
  - obstruction (complete) (partial) of precerebral artery
  - thrombosis of precerebral artery
- EXCLUDES 1
  - insufficiency, NOS, of precerebral artery (G45.-)
  - insufficiency of precerebral arteries causing cerebral infarction (I63.0-I63.2)
- AHA: 2018,2Q,9

I65.0 Occlusion and stenosis of vertebral artery
- I65.01 Occlusion and stenosis of right vertebral artery
- I65.02 Occlusion and stenosis of left vertebral artery
- I65.03 Occlusion and stenosis of bilateral vertebral arteries
- I65.09 Occlusion and stenosis of unspecified vertebral artery

I65.1 Occlusion and stenosis of basilar artery

I65.2 Occlusion and stenosis of carotid artery
- AHA: 2021,1Q,4; 2020,3Q,28
- I65.21 Occlusion and stenosis of right carotid artery
- I65.22 Occlusion and stenosis of left carotid artery
- I65.23 Occlusion and stenosis of bilateral carotid arteries
- I65.29 Occlusion and stenosis of unspecified carotid artery

I65.8 Occlusion and stenosis of other precerebral arteries

I65.9 Occlusion and stenosis of unspecified precerebral artery
- Occlusion and stenosis of precerebral artery NOS

I66 **Occlusion and stenosis of cerebral arteries, not resulting in cerebral infarction**
- INCLUDES
  - embolism of cerebral artery
  - narrowing of cerebral artery
  - obstruction (complete) (partial) of cerebral artery
  - thrombosis of cerebral artery
- EXCLUDES 1
  - occlusion and stenosis of cerebral artery causing cerebral infarction (I63.3-I63.5)

I66.0 Occlusion and stenosis of middle cerebral artery
- I66.01 Occlusion and stenosis of right middle cerebral artery
- I66.02 Occlusion and stenosis of left middle cerebral artery
- I66.03 Occlusion and stenosis of bilateral middle cerebral arteries
- I66.09 Occlusion and stenosis of unspecified middle cerebral artery

I66.1 Occlusion and stenosis of anterior cerebral artery
- I66.11 Occlusion and stenosis of right anterior cerebral artery
- I66.12 Occlusion and stenosis of left anterior cerebral artery
- I66.13 Occlusion and stenosis of bilateral anterior cerebral arteries
- I66.19 Occlusion and stenosis of unspecified anterior cerebral artery

I66.2 Occlusion and stenosis of posterior cerebral artery
- I66.21 Occlusion and stenosis of right posterior cerebral artery
- I66.22 Occlusion and stenosis of left posterior cerebral artery
- I66.23 Occlusion and stenosis of bilateral posterior cerebral arteries
- I66.29 Occlusion and stenosis of unspecified posterior cerebral artery

I66.3 Occlusion and stenosis of cerebellar arteries

I66.8 Occlusion and stenosis of other cerebral arteries
- Occlusion and stenosis of perforating arteries

I66.9 Occlusion and stenosis of unspecified cerebral artery

I67 **Other cerebrovascular diseases**
- EXCLUDES 1
  - occlusion and stenosis of cerebral artery causing cerebral infarction (I63.3-I63.5-)
  - occlusion and stenosis of precerebral artery causing cerebral infarction (I63.2-)
- EXCLUDES 2
  - sequelae of the listed conditions (I69.8)

I67.0 Dissection of cerebral arteries, nonruptured
- EXCLUDES 1 ruptured cerebral arteries (I60.7)
- AHA: 2021,3Q,5
- DEF: Dissecting aneurysm: Tear within an arterial wall that allows blood to accumulate between the outer and middle layers, creating a false lumen.

I67.1 Cerebral aneurysm, nonruptured
- Cerebral aneurysm NOS
- Cerebral arteriovenous fistula, acquired
- Internal carotid artery aneurysm, intracranial portion
- Internal carotid artery aneurysm, NOS
- EXCLUDES 1
  - congenital cerebral aneurysm, nonruptured (Q28.-)
  - ruptured cerebral aneurysm (I60.7)
- AHA: 2021,3Q,5
- TIP: A diagnosis of dissecting aneurysm should be coded to the dissection code, I67.0. The bulging/aneurysm, although present, occurred secondary to the dissection. The dissection represents the most significant problem.

Berry Aneurysm

Berry aneurysms form at the site of a weakness in an arterial wall, often at a junction

Berry aneurysm

- Anterior communicating artery 40%
- Anterior cerebral artery
- Internal carotid 20%
- Middle cerebral artery 34%
- Posterior cerebral artery 4%
- Posterior communicating artery
- Basilar artery

Common sites of berry aneurysms in the circle of Willis arteries

I67.2 Cerebral atherosclerosis
- Atheroma of cerebral and precerebral arteries

I67.3 Progressive vascular leukoencephalopathy
- Binswanger's disease

I67.4 Hypertensive encephalopathy
- Code also, if applicable, associated hypertensive conditions such as:
  - essential (primary) hypertension (I10)
  - hypertensive chronic kidney disease (I12.-)
  - hypertensive heart and chronic kidney disease (I13.-)
  - hypertensive heart disease (I11.-)
- EXCLUDES 2 insufficiency, NOS, of precerebral arteries (G45.2)
- AHA: 2023,4Q,24

I67.5 Moyamoya disease
- DEF: Cerebrovascular ischemia. Vessels occlude and rupture, causing tiny hemorrhages at the base of brain. It affects predominantly Japanese people.

I67.6 Nonpyogenic thrombosis of intracranial venous system
- Nonpyogenic thrombosis of cerebral vein
- Nonpyogenic thrombosis of intracranial venous sinus
- EXCLUDES 1 nonpyogenic thrombosis of intracranial venous system causing infarction (I63.6)

I67.7 Cerebral arteritis, not elsewhere classified
- Granulomatous angiitis of the nervous system
- EXCLUDES 1 allergic granulomatous angiitis (M30.1)

I67.8 Other specified cerebrovascular diseases
- I67.81 Acute cerebrovascular insufficiency
  - Acute cerebrovascular insufficiency unspecified as to location or reversibility
- I67.82 Cerebral ischemia
  - Chronic cerebral ischemia
- I67.83 Posterior reversible encephalopathy syndrome
  - PRES

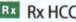

Chapter 9. Diseases of the Circulatory System

✓6th I67.84 Cerebral vasospasm and vasoconstriction
- **I67.841 Reversible cerebrovascular vasoconstriction syndrome**
  - Call-Fleming syndrome
  - Code first underlying condition, if applicable, such as eclampsia (O15.00-O15.9)
- **I67.848 Other cerebrovascular vasospasm and vasoconstriction**

✓6th I67.85 Hereditary cerebrovascular diseases
AHA: 2018,4Q,17
- **I67.850 Cerebral autosomal dominant arteriopathy with subcortical infarcts and leukoencephalopathy**
  - CADASIL
  - Code also any associated diagnoses, such as:
    - epilepsy (G40.-)
    - stroke (I63.-)
    - vascular dementia (F01.-)
- **I67.858 Other hereditary cerebrovascular disease**

I67.89 Other cerebrovascular disease
AHA: 2023,2Q,18

I67.9 Cerebrovascular disease, unspecified

✓4th I68 Cerebrovascular disorders in diseases classified elsewhere

I68.0 Cerebral amyloid angiopathy
Code first underlying amyloidosis (E85.-)

I68.2 Cerebral arteritis in other diseases classified elsewhere
Code first underlying disease
EXCLUDES 1: cerebral arteritis (in):
- listerosis (A32.89)
- syphilis (A52.04)
- systemic lupus erythematosus (M32.19)
- tuberculosis (A18.89)

I68.8 Other cerebrovascular disorders in diseases classified elsewhere
Code first underlying disease
EXCLUDES 1: syphilitic cerebral aneurysm (A52.05)

✓4th I69 Sequelae of cerebrovascular disease

NOTE: Category I69 is to be used to indicate conditions in I60-I67 as the cause of sequelae. The "sequelae" include conditions specified as such or as residuals which may occur at any time after the onset of the causal condition

EXCLUDES 1:
- personal history of cerebral infarction without residual deficit (Z86.73)
- personal history of prolonged reversible ischemic neurologic deficit (PRIND) (Z86.73)
- personal history of reversible ischemic neurologcial deficit (RIND) (Z86.73)
- sequelae of traumatic intracranial injury (S06.-)

AHA: 2023,1Q,37; 2020,2Q,29; 2017,1Q,47; 2016,4Q,28; 2015,1Q,25; 2012,4Q,106

TIP: For codes describing hemiplegia, hemiparesis, and monoplegia; if the documentation identifies the affected side but not whether it is the dominant or nondominant side, the default is as follows: for ambidextrous patients, the default is dominant; when the left side is affected, the default is nondominant; and when the right side is affected, the default is dominant.

TIP: Weakness on one side of the body (unilateral weakness) documented as secondary to old cerebrovascular disease is synonymous with hemiparesis/hemiplegia. Weakness of one limb documented as secondary to old cerebrovascular disease is synonymous with monoplegia.

✓5th I69.0 Sequelae of nontraumatic subarachnoid hemorrhage

- **I69.00 Unspecified sequelae of nontraumatic subarachnoid hemorrhage**

- **✓6th I69.01 Cognitive deficits following nontraumatic subarachnoid hemorrhage**
  - **I69.010 Attention and concentration deficit following nontraumatic subarachnoid hemorrhage**
  - **I69.011 Memory deficit following nontraumatic subarachnoid hemorrhage**
  - **I69.012 Visuospatial deficit and spatial neglect following nontraumatic subarachnoid hemorrhage**
  - **I69.013 Psychomotor deficit following nontraumatic subarachnoid hemorrhage**
  - **I69.014 Frontal lobe and executive function deficit following nontraumatic subarachnoid hemorrhage**
  - **I69.015 Cognitive social or emotional deficit following nontraumatic subarachnoid hemorrhage**
  - **I69.018 Other symptoms and signs involving cognitive functions following nontraumatic subarachnoid hemorrhage**
  - **I69.019 Unspecified symptoms and signs involving cognitive functions following nontraumatic subarachnoid hemorrhage**

- **✓6th I69.02 Speech and language deficits following nontraumatic subarachnoid hemorrhage**
  - **I69.020 Aphasia following nontraumatic subarachnoid hemorrhage**
  - **I69.021 Dysphasia following nontraumatic subarachnoid hemorrhage**
  - **I69.022 Dysarthria following nontraumatic subarachnoid hemorrhage**
  - **I69.023 Fluency disorder following nontraumatic subarachnoid hemorrhage**
    - Stuttering following nontraumatic subarachnoid hemorrhage
  - **I69.028 Other speech and language deficits following nontraumatic subarachnoid hemorrhage**

- **✓6th I69.03 Monoplegia of upper limb following nontraumatic subarachnoid hemorrhage**
  AHA: 2017,1Q,47
  - **I69.031 Monoplegia of upper limb following nontraumatic subarachnoid hemorrhage affecting right dominant side** HCC ESR COM
  - **I69.032 Monoplegia of upper limb following nontraumatic subarachnoid hemorrhage affecting left dominant side** HCC ESR COM
  - **I69.033 Monoplegia of upper limb following nontraumatic subarachnoid hemorrhage affecting right non-dominant side** HCC ESR COM
  - **I69.034 Monoplegia of upper limb following nontraumatic subarachnoid hemorrhage affecting left non-dominant side** HCC ESR COM
  - **I69.039 Monoplegia of upper limb following nontraumatic subarachnoid hemorrhage affecting unspecified side** HCC ESR COM

- **✓6th I69.04 Monoplegia of lower limb following nontraumatic subarachnoid hemorrhage**
  AHA: 2017,1Q,47
  - **I69.041 Monoplegia of lower limb following nontraumatic subarachnoid hemorrhage affecting right dominant side** HCC ESR COM
  - **I69.042 Monoplegia of lower limb following nontraumatic subarachnoid hemorrhage affecting left dominant side** HCC ESR COM
  - **I69.043 Monoplegia of lower limb following nontraumatic subarachnoid hemorrhage affecting right non-dominant side** HCC ESR COM
  - **I69.044 Monoplegia of lower limb following nontraumatic subarachnoid hemorrhage affecting left non-dominant side** HCC ESR COM
  - **I69.049 Monoplegia of lower limb following nontraumatic subarachnoid hemorrhage affecting unspecified side** HCC ESR COM

- **✓6th I69.05 Hemiplegia and hemiparesis following nontraumatic subarachnoid hemorrhage**
  AHA: 2015,1Q,25
  - **I69.051 Hemiplegia and hemiparesis following nontraumatic subarachnoid hemorrhage affecting right dominant side** HCC ESR COM
  - **I69.052 Hemiplegia and hemiparesis following nontraumatic subarachnoid hemorrhage affecting left dominant side** HCC ESR COM
  - **I69.053 Hemiplegia and hemiparesis following nontraumatic subarachnoid hemorrhage affecting right non-dominant side**

✓ Additional Character Required | ✓x7th Placeholder Alert | Manifestation | Unspecified Dx | Q QPP | UPD Unacceptable PDx

I69.Ø54 Hemiplegia and hemiparesis following nontraumatic subarachnoid hemorrhage affecting left non-dominant side [HCC] [ESR] [COM]

I69.Ø59 Hemiplegia and hemiparesis following nontraumatic subarachnoid hemorrhage affecting unspecified side [HCC] [ESR] [COM]

√6th **I69.Ø6** Other paralytic syndrome following nontraumatic subarachnoid hemorrhage

Use additional code to identify type of paralytic syndrome, such as:
locked-in state (G83.5)
quadriplegia (G82.5-)

EXCLUDES 1 hemiplegia/hemiparesis following nontraumatic subarachnoid hemorrhage (I69.Ø5-)
monoplegia of lower limb following nontraumatic subarachnoid hemorrhage (I69.Ø4-)
monoplegia of upper limb following nontraumatic subarachnoid hemorrhage (I69.Ø3-)

I69.Ø61 Other paralytic syndrome following nontraumatic subarachnoid hemorrhage affecting right dominant side [HCC] [ESR] [COM]

I69.Ø62 Other paralytic syndrome following nontraumatic subarachnoid hemorrhage affecting left dominant side [HCC] [ESR] [COM]

I69.Ø63 Other paralytic syndrome following nontraumatic subarachnoid hemorrhage affecting right non-dominant side [HCC] [ESR] [COM]

I69.Ø64 Other paralytic syndrome following nontraumatic subarachnoid hemorrhage affecting left non-dominant side [HCC] [ESR] [COM]

I69.Ø65 Other paralytic syndrome following nontraumatic subarachnoid hemorrhage, bilateral [HCC] [ESR] [COM]

I69.Ø69 Other paralytic syndrome following nontraumatic subarachnoid hemorrhage affecting unspecified side [HCC] [ESR] [COM]

√6th **I69.Ø9** Other sequelae of nontraumatic subarachnoid hemorrhage

I69.Ø9Ø Apraxia following nontraumatic subarachnoid hemorrhage

I69.Ø91 Dysphagia following nontraumatic subarachnoid hemorrhage
Use additional code to identify the type of dysphagia, if known (R13.11-R13.19)

I69.Ø92 Facial weakness following nontraumatic subarachnoid hemorrhage
Facial droop following nontraumatic subarachnoid hemorrhage

I69.Ø93 Ataxia following nontraumatic subarachnoid hemorrhage

I69.Ø98 Other sequelae following nontraumatic subarachnoid hemorrhage
Alterations of sensation following nontraumatic subarachnoid hemorrhage
Disturbance of vision following nontraumatic subarachnoid hemorrhage
Use additional code to identify the sequelae

√5th **I69.1** Sequelae of nontraumatic intracerebral hemorrhage

I69.1Ø Unspecified sequelae of nontraumatic intracerebral hemorrhage

√6th **I69.11** Cognitive deficits following nontraumatic intracerebral hemorrhage

I69.11Ø Attention and concentration deficit following nontraumatic intracerebral hemorrhage

I69.111 Memory deficit following nontraumatic intracerebral hemorrhage

I69.112 Visuospatial deficit and spatial neglect following nontraumatic intracerebral hemorrhage

I69.113 Psychomotor deficit following nontraumatic intracerebral hemorrhage

I69.114 Frontal lobe and executive function deficit following nontraumatic intracerebral hemorrhage

I69.115 Cognitive social or emotional deficit following nontraumatic intracerebral hemorrhage

I69.118 Other symptoms and signs involving cognitive functions following nontraumatic intracerebral hemorrhage

I69.119 Unspecified symptoms and signs involving cognitive functions following nontraumatic intracerebral hemorrhage

√6th **I69.12** Speech and language deficits following nontraumatic intracerebral hemorrhage

I69.12Ø Aphasia following nontraumatic intracerebral hemorrhage

I69.121 Dysphasia following nontraumatic intracerebral hemorrhage

I69.122 Dysarthria following nontraumatic intracerebral hemorrhage

I69.123 Fluency disorder following nontraumatic intracerebral hemorrhage
Stuttering following nontraumatic intracerebral hemorrhage

I69.128 Other speech and language deficits following nontraumatic intracerebral hemorrhage

√6th **I69.13** Monoplegia of upper limb following nontraumatic intracerebral hemorrhage
AHA: 2017,1Q,47

I69.131 Monoplegia of upper limb following nontraumatic intracerebral hemorrhage affecting right dominant side [HCC] [ESR] [COM]

I69.132 Monoplegia of upper limb following nontraumatic intracerebral hemorrhage affecting left dominant side [HCC] [ESR] [COM]

I69.133 Monoplegia of upper limb following nontraumatic intracerebral hemorrhage affecting right non-dominant side [HCC] [ESR] [COM]

I69.134 Monoplegia of upper limb following nontraumatic intracerebral hemorrhage affecting left non-dominant side [HCC] [ESR] [COM]

I69.139 Monoplegia of upper limb following nontraumatic intracerebral hemorrhage affecting unspecified side [HCC] [ESR] [COM]

√6th **I69.14** Monoplegia of lower limb following nontraumatic intracerebral hemorrhage
AHA: 2017,1Q,47

I69.141 Monoplegia of lower limb following nontraumatic intracerebral hemorrhage affecting right dominant side [HCC] [ESR] [COM]

I69.142 Monoplegia of lower limb following nontraumatic intracerebral hemorrhage affecting left dominant side [HCC] [ESR] [COM]

I69.143 Monoplegia of lower limb following nontraumatic intracerebral hemorrhage affecting right non-dominant side [HCC] [ESR] [COM]

I69.144 Monoplegia of lower limb following nontraumatic intracerebral hemorrhage affecting left non-dominant side [HCC] [ESR] [COM]

I69.149 Monoplegia of lower limb following nontraumatic intracerebral hemorrhage affecting unspecified side [HCC] [ESR] [COM]

√6th **I69.15** Hemiplegia and hemiparesis following nontraumatic intracerebral hemorrhage
AHA: 2015,1Q,25

I69.151 Hemiplegia and hemiparesis following nontraumatic intracerebral hemorrhage affecting right dominant side [HCC] [ESR] [COM]

I69.152 Hemiplegia and hemiparesis following nontraumatic intracerebral hemorrhage affecting left dominant side [HCC] [ESR] [COM]

[HCC] CMS-HCC   [Rx] Rx HCC   [ESR] ESRD HCC   [COM] Commercial HCC   [N] Newborn: 0   [P] Pediatric: 0-17   [M] Maternity: 9-64   [A] Adult: 15-124

- **I69.153** Hemiplegia and hemiparesis following nontraumatic intracerebral hemorrhage affecting **right non-dominant** side [HCC] [ESR] [COM]
- **I69.154** Hemiplegia and hemiparesis following nontraumatic intracerebral hemorrhage affecting **left non-dominant** side [HCC] [ESR] [COM]
- **I69.159** Hemiplegia and hemiparesis following nontraumatic intracerebral hemorrhage affecting unspecified side [HCC] [ESR] [COM]

✓6ᵗʰ **I69.16** Other **paralytic syndrome** following nontraumatic intracerebral hemorrhage

Use additional code to identify type of paralytic syndrome, such as:
locked-in state (G83.5)
quadriplegia (G82.5-)

EXCLUDES 1 hemiplegia/hemiparesis following nontraumatic intracerebral hemorrhage (I69.15-)
monoplegia of lower limb following nontraumatic intracerebral hemorrhage (I69.14-)
monoplegia of upper limb following nontraumatic intracerebral hemorrhage (I69.13-)

- **I69.161** Other paralytic syndrome following nontraumatic intracerebral hemorrhage affecting **right dominant** side [HCC] [ESR] [COM]
- **I69.162** Other paralytic syndrome following nontraumatic intracerebral hemorrhage affecting **left dominant** side [HCC] [ESR] [COM]
- **I69.163** Other paralytic syndrome following nontraumatic intracerebral hemorrhage affecting **right non-dominant** side
- **I69.164** Other paralytic syndrome following nontraumatic intracerebral hemorrhage affecting **left non-dominant** side [HCC] [ESR] [COM]
- **I69.165** Other paralytic syndrome following nontraumatic intracerebral hemorrhage, **bilateral** [HCC] [ESR] [COM]
- **I69.169** Other paralytic syndrome following nontraumatic intracerebral hemorrhage affecting unspecified side [HCC] [ESR] [COM]

✓6ᵗʰ **I69.19** Other sequelae of nontraumatic intracerebral hemorrhage
- **I69.190** **Apraxia** following nontraumatic intracerebral hemorrhage
- **I69.191** **Dysphagia** following nontraumatic intracerebral hemorrhage
  Use additional code to identify the type of dysphagia, if known (R13.11-R13.19)
- **I69.192** **Facial weakness** following nontraumatic intracerebral hemorrhage
  Facial droop following nontraumatic intracerebral hemorrhage
- **I69.193** **Ataxia** following nontraumatic intracerebral hemorrhage
- **I69.198** Other sequelae of nontraumatic intracerebral hemorrhage
  Alteration of sensations following nontraumatic intracerebral hemorrhage
  Disturbance of vision following nontraumatic intracerebral hemorrhage
  Use additional code to identify the sequelae

✓5ᵗʰ **I69.2** Sequelae of other nontraumatic **intracranial** hemorrhage

- **I69.20** Unspecified sequelae of other nontraumatic intracranial hemorrhage

✓6ᵗʰ **I69.21** **Cognitive deficits** following other nontraumatic intracranial hemorrhage
- **I69.210** **Attention and concentration** deficit following other nontraumatic intracranial hemorrhage
- **I69.211** **Memory** deficit following other nontraumatic intracranial hemorrhage
- **I69.212** **Visuospatial** deficit and **spatial neglect** following other nontraumatic intracranial hemorrhage
- **I69.213** **Psychomotor** deficit following other nontraumatic intracranial hemorrhage
- **I69.214** **Frontal lobe and executive function** deficit following other nontraumatic intracranial hemorrhage
- **I69.215** **Cognitive social or emotional** deficit following other nontraumatic intracranial hemorrhage
- **I69.218** Other symptoms and signs involving cognitive functions following other nontraumatic intracranial hemorrhage
- **I69.219** Unspecified symptoms and signs involving cognitive functions following other nontraumatic intracranial hemorrhage

✓6ᵗʰ **I69.22** **Speech and language deficits** following other nontraumatic intracranial hemorrhage
- **I69.220** **Aphasia** following other nontraumatic intracranial hemorrhage
- **I69.221** **Dysphasia** following other nontraumatic intracranial hemorrhage
- **I69.222** **Dysarthria** following other nontraumatic intracranial hemorrhage
- **I69.223** **Fluency** disorder following other nontraumatic intracranial hemorrhage
  Stuttering following other nontraumatic intracranial hemorrhage
- **I69.228** Other speech and language deficits following other nontraumatic intracranial hemorrhage

✓6ᵗʰ **I69.23** **Monoplegia of upper limb** following other nontraumatic intracranial hemorrhage
  AHA: 2017,1Q,47
- **I69.231** Monoplegia of upper limb following other nontraumatic intracranial hemorrhage affecting **right dominant** side [HCC] [ESR] [COM]
- **I69.232** Monoplegia of upper limb following other nontraumatic intracranial hemorrhage affecting **left dominant** side [HCC] [ESR] [COM]
- **I69.233** Monoplegia of upper limb following other nontraumatic intracranial hemorrhage affecting **right non-dominant** side [HCC] [ESR] [COM]
- **I69.234** Monoplegia of upper limb following other nontraumatic intracranial hemorrhage affecting **left non-dominant** side [HCC] [ESR] [COM]
- **I69.239** Monoplegia of upper limb following other nontraumatic intracranial hemorrhage affecting unspecified side [HCC] [ESR] [COM]

✓6ᵗʰ **I69.24** **Monoplegia of lower limb** following other nontraumatic intracranial hemorrhage
  AHA: 2017,1Q,47
- **I69.241** Monoplegia of lower limb following other nontraumatic intracranial hemorrhage affecting **right dominant** side [HCC] [ESR] [COM]
- **I69.242** Monoplegia of lower limb following other nontraumatic intracranial hemorrhage affecting **left dominant** side [HCC] [ESR] [COM]
- **I69.243** Monoplegia of lower limb following other nontraumatic intracranial hemorrhage affecting **right non-dominant** side [HCC] [ESR] [COM]
- **I69.244** Monoplegia of lower limb following other nontraumatic intracranial hemorrhage affecting **left non-dominant** side [HCC] [ESR] [COM]
- **I69.249** Monoplegia of lower limb following other nontraumatic intracranial hemorrhage affecting unspecified side [HCC] [ESR] [COM]

✓6ᵗʰ **I69.25** **Hemiplegia and hemiparesis** following other nontraumatic intracranial hemorrhage
  AHA: 2015,1Q,25
- **I69.251** Hemiplegia and hemiparesis following other nontraumatic intracranial hemorrhage affecting **right dominant** side [HCC] [ESR] [COM]

Chapter 9. Diseases of the Circulatory System

I69.252 Hemiplegia and hemiparesis following other nontraumatic intracranial hemorrhage affecting **left dominant** side HCC ESR COM

I69.253 Hemiplegia and hemiparesis following other nontraumatic intracranial hemorrhage affecting **right non-dominant** side HCC ESR COM

I69.254 Hemiplegia and hemiparesis following other nontraumatic intracranial hemorrhage affecting **left non-dominant** side HCC ESR COM

I69.259 Hemiplegia and hemiparesis following other nontraumatic intracranial hemorrhage affecting unspecified side HCC ESR COM

✓6th **I69.26** Other **paralytic syndrome** following other nontraumatic intracranial hemorrhage
Use additional code to identify type of paralytic syndrome, such as:
locked-in state (G83.5)
quadriplegia (G82.5-)
EXCLUDES 1 hemiplegia/hemiparesis following other nontraumatic intracranial hemorrhage (I69.25-)
monoplegia of lower limb following other nontraumatic intracranial hemorrhage (I69.24-)
monoplegia of upper limb following other nontraumatic intracranial hemorrhage (I69.23-)

I69.261 Other paralytic syndrome following other nontraumatic intracranial hemorrhage affecting **right dominant** side HCC ESR COM

I69.262 Other paralytic syndrome following other nontraumatic intracranial hemorrhage affecting **left dominant** side HCC ESR COM

I69.263 Other paralytic syndrome following other nontraumatic intracranial hemorrhage affecting **right non-dominant** side HCC ESR COM

I69.264 Other paralytic syndrome following other nontraumatic intracranial hemorrhage affecting **left non-dominant** side HCC ESR COM

I69.265 Other paralytic syndrome following other nontraumatic intracranial hemorrhage, **bilateral** HCC ESR COM

I69.269 Other paralytic syndrome following other nontraumatic intracranial hemorrhage affecting unspecified side HCC ESR COM

✓6th **I69.29** Other sequelae of other nontraumatic intracranial hemorrhage

I69.290 **Apraxia** following other nontraumatic intracranial hemorrhage

I69.291 **Dysphagia** following other nontraumatic intracranial hemorrhage
Use additional code to identify the type of dysphagia, if known (R13.11-R13.19)

I69.292 **Facial weakness** following other nontraumatic intracranial hemorrhage
Facial droop following other nontraumatic intracranial hemorrhage

I69.293 **Ataxia** following other nontraumatic intracranial hemorrhage

I69.298 Other sequelae of other nontraumatic intracranial hemorrhage
Alteration of sensation following other nontraumatic intracranial hemorrhage
Disturbance of vision following other nontraumatic intracranial hemorrhage
Use additional code to identify the sequelae

✓5th **I69.3** Sequelae of **cerebral infarction**
Sequelae of stroke NOS
AHA: 2013,4Q,127-128; 2012,4Q,92,94

I69.30 Unspecified sequelae of cerebral infarction

✓6th **I69.31** **Cognitive** deficits following cerebral infarction

I69.310 **Attention and concentration** deficit following cerebral infarction

I69.311 **Memory** deficit following cerebral infarction

I69.312 **Visuospatial** deficit and **spatial neglect** following cerebral infarction

I69.313 **Psychomotor** deficit following cerebral infarction

I69.314 **Frontal lobe and executive function** deficit following cerebral infarction

I69.315 **Cognitive social or emotional** deficit following cerebral infarction

I69.318 Other symptoms and signs involving cognitive functions following cerebral infarction

I69.319 Unspecified symptoms and signs involving cognitive functions following cerebral infarction

✓6th **I69.32** **Speech and language deficits** following cerebral infarction

I69.320 **Aphasia** following cerebral infarction

I69.321 **Dysphasia** following cerebral infarction
AHA: 2012,4Q,91

I69.322 **Dysarthria** following cerebral infarction
EXCLUDES 2 transient ischemic attack (TIA) (G45.9)

I69.323 **Fluency disorder** following cerebral infarction
Stuttering following cerebral infarction

I69.328 Other speech and language deficits following cerebral infarction

✓6th **I69.33** **Monoplegia of upper limb** following cerebral infarction
AHA: 2017,1Q,47

I69.331 Monoplegia of upper limb following cerebral infarction affecting **right dominant** side HCC ESR COM

I69.332 Monoplegia of upper limb following cerebral infarction affecting **left dominant** side HCC ESR COM

I69.333 Monoplegia of upper limb following cerebral infarction affecting **right non-dominant** side HCC ESR COM

I69.334 Monoplegia of upper limb following cerebral infarction affecting **left non-dominant** side HCC ESR COM

I69.339 Monoplegia of upper limb following cerebral infarction affecting unspecified side HCC ESR COM

✓6th **I69.34** **Monoplegia of lower limb** following cerebral infarction
AHA: 2017,1Q,47

I69.341 Monoplegia of lower limb following cerebral infarction affecting **right dominant** side HCC ESR COM

I69.342 Monoplegia of lower limb following cerebral infarction affecting **left dominant** side HCC ESR COM

I69.343 Monoplegia of lower limb following cerebral infarction affecting **right non-dominant** side HCC ESR COM

I69.344 Monoplegia of lower limb following cerebral infarction affecting **left non-dominant** side HCC ESR COM

I69.349 Monoplegia of lower limb following cerebral infarction affecting unspecified side HCC ESR COM

✓6th **I69.35** **Hemiplegia and hemiparesis** following cerebral infarction
AHA: 2015,1Q,25

I69.351 Hemiplegia and hemiparesis following cerebral infarction affecting **right dominant** side HCC ESR COM
EXCLUDES 2 transient ischemic attack (TIA) (G45.9)

I69.352 Hemiplegia and hemiparesis following cerebral infarction affecting **left dominant** side HCC ESR COM

I69.353 Hemiplegia and hemiparesis following cerebral infarction affecting **right non-dominant** side HCC ESR COM

I69.354 Hemiplegia and hemiparesis following cerebral infarction affecting left non-dominant side [HCC] [ESR] [COM]
AHA: 2012,4Q,91

I69.359 Hemiplegia and hemiparesis following cerebral infarction affecting unspecified side [HCC] [ESR] [COM]

I69.36 Other paralytic syndrome following cerebral infarction
Use additional code to identify type of paralytic syndrome, such as:
locked-in state (G83.5)
quadriplegia (G82.5-)
EXCLUDES 1 hemiplegia/hemiparesis following cerebral infarction (I69.35-)
monoplegia of lower limb following cerebral infarction (I69.34-)
monoplegia of upper limb following cerebral infarction (I69.33-)

I69.361 Other paralytic syndrome following cerebral infarction affecting right dominant side

I69.362 Other paralytic syndrome following cerebral infarction affecting left dominant side [HCC] [ESR] [COM]

I69.363 Other paralytic syndrome following cerebral infarction affecting right non-dominant side [HCC] [ESR] [COM]

I69.364 Other paralytic syndrome following cerebral infarction affecting left non-dominant side [HCC] [ESR] [COM]

I69.365 Other paralytic syndrome following cerebral infarction, bilateral [HCC] [ESR] [COM]

I69.369 Other paralytic syndrome following cerebral infarction affecting unspecified side [HCC] [ESR] [COM]

I69.39 Other sequelae of cerebral infarction

I69.390 Apraxia following cerebral infarction

I69.391 Dysphagia following cerebral infarction
Use additional code to identify the type of dysphagia, if known (R13.11-R13.19)

I69.392 Facial weakness following cerebral infarction
Facial droop following cerebral infarction
AHA: 2024,2Q,13

I69.393 Ataxia following cerebral infarction

I69.398 Other sequelae of cerebral infarction
Alteration of sensation following cerebral infarction
Disturbance of vision following cerebral infarction
Use additional code to identify the sequelae
AHA: 2024,2Q,13; 2020,2Q,29

I69.8 Sequelae of other cerebrovascular diseases
EXCLUDES 1 sequelae of traumatic intracranial injury (S06.-)

I69.80 Unspecified sequelae of other cerebrovascular disease

I69.81 Cognitive deficits following other cerebrovascular disease

I69.810 Attention and concentration deficit following other cerebrovascular disease

I69.811 Memory deficit following other cerebrovascular disease

I69.812 Visuospatial deficit and spatial neglect following other cerebrovascular disease

I69.813 Psychomotor deficit following other cerebrovascular disease

I69.814 Frontal lobe and executive function deficit following other cerebrovascular disease

I69.815 Cognitive social or emotional deficit following other cerebrovascular disease

I69.818 Other symptoms and signs involving cognitive functions following other cerebrovascular disease

I69.819 Unspecified symptoms and signs involving cognitive functions following other cerebrovascular disease

I69.82 Speech and language deficits following other cerebrovascular disease

I69.820 Aphasia following other cerebrovascular disease

I69.821 Dysphasia following other cerebrovascular disease

I69.822 Dysarthria following other cerebrovascular disease

I69.823 Fluency disorder following other cerebrovascular disease
Stuttering following other cerebrovascular disease

I69.828 Other speech and language deficits following other cerebrovascular disease
AHA: 2019,3Q,8

I69.83 Monoplegia of upper limb following other cerebrovascular disease
AHA: 2017,1Q,47

I69.831 Monoplegia of upper limb following other cerebrovascular disease affecting right dominant side [HCC] [ESR] [COM]

I69.832 Monoplegia of upper limb following other cerebrovascular disease affecting left dominant side [HCC] [ESR] [COM]

I69.833 Monoplegia of upper limb following other cerebrovascular disease affecting right non-dominant side [HCC] [ESR] [COM]

I69.834 Monoplegia of upper limb following other cerebrovascular disease affecting left non-dominant side [HCC] [ESR] [COM]

I69.839 Monoplegia of upper limb following other cerebrovascular disease affecting unspecified side [HCC] [ESR] [COM]

I69.84 Monoplegia of lower limb following other cerebrovascular disease
AHA: 2017,1Q,47

I69.841 Monoplegia of lower limb following other cerebrovascular disease affecting right dominant side [HCC] [ESR] [COM]

I69.842 Monoplegia of lower limb following other cerebrovascular disease affecting left dominant side [HCC] [ESR] [COM]

I69.843 Monoplegia of lower limb following other cerebrovascular disease affecting right non-dominant side [HCC] [ESR] [COM]

I69.844 Monoplegia of lower limb following other cerebrovascular disease affecting left non-dominant side [HCC] [ESR] [COM]

I69.849 Monoplegia of lower limb following other cerebrovascular disease affecting unspecified side [HCC] [ESR] [COM]

I69.85 Hemiplegia and hemiparesis following other cerebrovascular disease
AHA: 2015,1Q,25

I69.851 Hemiplegia and hemiparesis following other cerebrovascular disease affecting right dominant side [HCC] [ESR] [COM]

I69.852 Hemiplegia and hemiparesis following other cerebrovascular disease affecting left dominant side [HCC] [ESR] [COM]

I69.853 Hemiplegia and hemiparesis following other cerebrovascular disease affecting right non-dominant side [HCC] [ESR] [COM]

I69.854 Hemiplegia and hemiparesis following other cerebrovascular disease affecting left non-dominant side [HCC] [ESR] [COM]

I69.859 Hemiplegia and hemiparesis following other cerebrovascular disease affecting unspecified side [HCC] [ESR] [COM]

I69.86 Other paralytic syndrome following other cerebrovascular disease
Use additional code to identify type of paralytic syndrome, such as:
locked-in state (G83.5)
quadriplegia (G82.5-)
EXCLUDES 1 hemiplegia/hemiparesis following other cerebrovascular disease (I69.85-)
monoplegia of lower limb following other cerebrovascular disease (I69.84-)
monoplegia of upper limb following other cerebrovascular disease (I69.83-)

I69.861 Other paralytic syndrome following other cerebrovascular disease affecting right dominant side [HCC] [ESR] [COM]

I69.862 Other paralytic syndrome following other cerebrovascular disease affecting **left dominant** side HCC ESR COM

I69.863 Other paralytic syndrome following other cerebrovascular disease affecting **right non-dominant** side HCC ESR COM

I69.864 Other paralytic syndrome following other cerebrovascular disease affecting **left non-dominant** side HCC ESR COM

I69.865 Other paralytic syndrome following other cerebrovascular disease, **bilateral** HCC ESR COM

I69.869 Other paralytic syndrome following other cerebrovascular disease affecting unspecified side HCC ESR COM

√6ᵗʰ **I69.89** Other sequelae of other cerebrovascular disease

I69.890 **Apraxia** following other cerebrovascular disease

I69.891 **Dysphagia** following other cerebrovascular disease

Use additional code to identify the type of dysphagia, if known (R13.11-R13.19)

I69.892 **Facial weakness** following other cerebrovascular disease

Facial droop following other cerebrovascular disease

I69.893 **Ataxia** following other cerebrovascular disease

I69.898 Other sequelae of other cerebrovascular disease

Alteration of sensation following other cerebrovascular disease

Disturbance of vision following other cerebrovascular disease

Use additional code to identify the sequelae

√5ᵗʰ **I69.9** Sequelae of unspecified **cerebrovascular diseases**

EXCLUDES 1 sequelae of stroke (I69.3)
sequelae of traumatic intracranial injury (S06.-)

I69.90 Unspecified sequelae of unspecified cerebrovascular disease

√6ᵗʰ **I69.91** **Cognitive deficits** following unspecified cerebrovascular disease

I69.910 **Attention and concentration** deficit following unspecified cerebrovascular disease

I69.911 **Memory** deficit following unspecified cerebrovascular disease

I69.912 **Visuospatial** deficit and **spatial neglect** following unspecified cerebrovascular disease

I69.913 **Psychomotor** deficit following unspecified cerebrovascular disease

I69.914 **Frontal lobe and executive function** deficit following unspecified cerebrovascular disease

I69.915 **Cognitive social or emotional** deficit following unspecified cerebrovascular disease

I69.918 Other symptoms and signs involving cognitive functions following unspecified cerebrovascular disease

I69.919 Unspecified symptoms and signs involving cognitive functions following unspecified cerebrovascular disease

√6ᵗʰ **I69.92** **Speech and language deficits** following unspecified cerebrovascular disease

I69.920 **Aphasia** following unspecified cerebrovascular disease

I69.921 **Dysphasia** following unspecified cerebrovascular disease

I69.922 **Dysarthria** following unspecified cerebrovascular disease

I69.923 **Fluency disorder** following unspecified cerebrovascular disease

Stuttering following unspecified cerebrovascular disease

I69.928 Other speech and language deficits following unspecified cerebrovascular disease

√6ᵗʰ **I69.93** **Monoplegia of upper limb** following unspecified cerebrovascular disease

AHA: 2017,1Q,47

I69.931 Monoplegia of upper limb following unspecified cerebrovascular disease affecting **right dominant** side HCC ESR COM

I69.932 Monoplegia of upper limb following unspecified cerebrovascular disease affecting **left dominant** side HCC ESR COM

I69.933 Monoplegia of upper limb following unspecified cerebrovascular disease affecting **right non-dominant** side HCC ESR COM

I69.934 Monoplegia of upper limb following unspecified cerebrovascular disease affecting **left non-dominant** side HCC ESR COM

I69.939 Monoplegia of upper limb following unspecified cerebrovascular disease affecting unspecified side HCC ESR COM

√6ᵗʰ **I69.94** **Monoplegia of lower limb** following unspecified cerebrovascular disease

AHA: 2017,1Q,47

I69.941 Monoplegia of lower limb following unspecified cerebrovascular disease affecting **right dominant** side HCC ESR COM

I69.942 Monoplegia of lower limb following unspecified cerebrovascular disease affecting **left dominant** side HCC ESR COM

I69.943 Monoplegia of lower limb following unspecified cerebrovascular disease affecting **right non-dominant** side HCC ESR COM

I69.944 Monoplegia of lower limb following unspecified cerebrovascular disease affecting **left non-dominant** side HCC ESR COM

I69.949 Monoplegia of lower limb following unspecified cerebrovascular disease affecting unspecified side HCC ESR COM

√6ᵗʰ **I69.95** **Hemiplegia and hemiparesis** following unspecified cerebrovascular disease

AHA: 2015,1Q,25

I69.951 Hemiplegia and hemiparesis following unspecified cerebrovascular disease affecting **right dominant** side HCC ESR COM

I69.952 Hemiplegia and hemiparesis following unspecified cerebrovascular disease affecting **left dominant** side HCC ESR COM

I69.953 Hemiplegia and hemiparesis following unspecified cerebrovascular disease affecting **right non-dominant** side HCC ESR COM

I69.954 Hemiplegia and hemiparesis following unspecified cerebrovascular disease affecting **left non-dominant** side HCC ESR COM

I69.959 Hemiplegia and hemiparesis following unspecified cerebrovascular disease affecting unspecified side HCC ESR COM

HCC CMS-HCC | Rx Rx HCC | ESR ESRD HCC | COM Commercial HCC | N Newborn: 0 | P Pediatric: 0-17 | M Maternity: 9-64 | A Adult: 15-124

Chapter 9. Diseases of the Circulatory System

I69.96 Other paralytic syndrome following unspecified cerebrovascular disease
Use additional code to identify type of paralytic syndrome, such as:
locked-in state (G83.5)
quadriplegia (G82.5-)
EXCLUDES 1: hemiplegia/hemiparesis following unspecified cerebrovascular disease (I69.95-)
monoplegia of lower limb following unspecified cerebrovascular disease (I69.94-)
monoplegia of upper limb following unspecified cerebrovascular disease (I69.93-)

- **I69.961** Other paralytic syndrome following unspecified cerebrovascular disease affecting right dominant side
- **I69.962** Other paralytic syndrome following unspecified cerebrovascular disease affecting left dominant side
- **I69.963** Other paralytic syndrome following unspecified cerebrovascular disease affecting right non-dominant side
- **I69.964** Other paralytic syndrome following unspecified cerebrovascular disease affecting left non-dominant side
- **I69.965** Other paralytic syndrome following unspecified cerebrovascular disease, bilateral
- **I69.969** Other paralytic syndrome following unspecified cerebrovascular disease affecting unspecified side

I69.99 Other sequelae of unspecified cerebrovascular disease

- **I69.990** Apraxia following unspecified cerebrovascular disease
- **I69.991** Dysphagia following unspecified cerebrovascular disease
  Use additional code to identify the type of dysphagia, if known (R13.11-R13.19)
- **I69.992** Facial weakness following unspecified cerebrovascular disease
  Facial droop following unspecified cerebrovascular disease
- **I69.993** Ataxia following unspecified cerebrovascular disease
- **I69.998** Other sequelae following unspecified cerebrovascular disease
  Alteration in sensation following unspecified cerebrovascular disease
  Disturbance of vision following unspecified cerebrovascular disease
  Use additional code to identify the sequelae

Diseases of arteries, arterioles and capillaries (I70-I79)

I70 Atherosclerosis
INCLUDES:
arterial degeneration
arteriolosclerosis
arteriosclerosis
arteriosclerotic vascular disease
arteriovascular degeneration
atheroma
endarteritis deformans or obliterans
senile arteritis
senile endarteritis
vascular degeneration
Use additional code to identify:
exposure to environmental tobacco smoke (Z77.22)
history of tobacco dependence (Z87.891)
occupational exposure to environmental tobacco smoke (Z57.31)
tobacco dependence (F17.-)
tobacco use (Z72.0)
EXCLUDES 2: arteriosclerotic cardiovascular disease (I25.1-)
arteriosclerotic heart disease (I25.1-)
atheroembolism (I75.-)
cerebral atherosclerosis (I67.2)
coronary atherosclerosis (I25.1-)
mesenteric atherosclerosis (K55.1)
precerebral atherosclerosis (I67.2)
primary pulmonary atherosclerosis (I27.0)

I70.0 Atherosclerosis of aorta

I70.1 Atherosclerosis of renal artery
Goldblatt's kidney
EXCLUDES 2: atherosclerosis of renal arterioles (I12.-)

I70.2 Atherosclerosis of native arteries of the extremities
Monckeberg's (medial) sclerosis
Use additional code, if applicable, to identify chronic total occlusion of artery of extremity (I70.92)
EXCLUDES 2: atherosclerosis of bypass graft of extremities (I70.30-I70.79)
AHA: 2020,4Q,98; 2018,3Q,4; 2018,2Q,7

- **I70.20** Unspecified atherosclerosis of native arteries of extremities
  - **I70.201** Unspecified atherosclerosis of native arteries of extremities, right leg
  - **I70.202** Unspecified atherosclerosis of native arteries of extremities, left leg
  - **I70.203** Unspecified atherosclerosis of native arteries of extremities, bilateral legs
  - **I70.208** Unspecified atherosclerosis of native arteries of extremities, other extremity
  - **I70.209** Unspecified atherosclerosis of native arteries of extremities, unspecified extremity

- **I70.21** Atherosclerosis of native arteries of extremities with intermittent claudication
  - **I70.211** Atherosclerosis of native arteries of extremities with intermittent claudication, right leg
  - **I70.212** Atherosclerosis of native arteries of extremities with intermittent claudication, left leg
  - **I70.213** Atherosclerosis of native arteries of extremities with intermittent claudication, bilateral legs
  - **I70.218** Atherosclerosis of native arteries of extremities with intermittent claudication, other extremity
  - **I70.219** Atherosclerosis of native arteries of extremities with intermittent claudication, unspecified extremity

I70.22 Atherosclerosis of native arteries of extremities with rest pain
INCLUDES: any condition classifiable to I70.21-
chronic limb-threatening ischemia of native arteries of extremities with rest pain
chronic limb-threatening ischemia NOS of native arteries of extremities
critical limb ischemia of native arteries of extremities with rest pain
critical limb ischemia NOS of native arteries of extremities

- **I70.221** Atherosclerosis of native arteries of extremities with rest pain, right leg
- **I70.222** Atherosclerosis of native arteries of extremities with rest pain, left leg
- **I70.223** Atherosclerosis of native arteries of extremities with rest pain, bilateral legs
- **I70.228** Atherosclerosis of native arteries of extremities with rest pain, other extremity
- **I70.229** Atherosclerosis of native arteries of extremities with rest pain, unspecified extremity

I70.23 Atherosclerosis of native arteries of right leg with ulceration
INCLUDES: any condition classifiable to I70.211 and I70.221
chronic limb-threatening ischemia of native arteries of right leg with ulceration
critical limb ischemia of native arteries of right leg with ulceration

Use additional code to identify severity of ulcer (L97.-)

- **I70.231** Atherosclerosis of native arteries of right leg with ulceration of thigh
- **I70.232** Atherosclerosis of native arteries of right leg with ulceration of calf
- **I70.233** Atherosclerosis of native arteries of right leg with ulceration of ankle
- **I70.234** Atherosclerosis of native arteries of right leg with ulceration of heel and midfoot
  Atherosclerosis of native arteries of right leg with ulceration of plantar surface of midfoot
- **I70.235** Atherosclerosis of native arteries of right leg with ulceration of other part of foot
  Atherosclerosis of native arteries of right leg extremities with ulceration of toe
- **I70.238** Atherosclerosis of native arteries of right leg with ulceration of other part of lower leg
- **I70.239** Atherosclerosis of native arteries of right leg with ulceration of unspecified site

I70.24 Atherosclerosis of native arteries of left leg with ulceration
INCLUDES: any condition classifiable to I70.212 and I70.222
chronic limb-threatening ischemia of native arteries of left leg with ulceration
critical limb ischemia of native arteries of left leg with ulceration

Use additional code to identify severity of ulcer (L97.-)

- **I70.241** Atherosclerosis of native arteries of left leg with ulceration of thigh
- **I70.242** Atherosclerosis of native arteries of left leg with ulceration of calf
- **I70.243** Atherosclerosis of native arteries of left leg with ulceration of ankle
- **I70.244** Atherosclerosis of native arteries of left leg with ulceration of heel and midfoot
  Atherosclerosis of native arteries of left leg with ulceration of plantar surface of midfoot
- **I70.245** Atherosclerosis of native arteries of left leg with ulceration of other part of foot
  Atherosclerosis of native arteries of left leg extremities with ulceration of toe
- **I70.248** Atherosclerosis of native arteries of left leg with ulceration of other part of lower leg
- **I70.249** Atherosclerosis of native arteries of left leg with ulceration of unspecified site

I70.25 Atherosclerosis of native arteries of other extremities with ulceration
INCLUDES: any condition classifiable to I70.218 and I70.228

Use additional code to identify the severity of the ulcer (L98.49-)

I70.26 Atherosclerosis of native arteries of extremities with gangrene
INCLUDES: any condition classifiable to I70.21-, I70.22-, I70.23-, I70.24-, and I70.25-
chronic limb-threatening ischemia of native arteries of extremities with gangrene
critical limb ischemia of native arteries of extremities with gangrene

Use additional code to identify the severity of any ulcer (L97.-, L98.49-), if applicable

- **I70.261** Atherosclerosis of native arteries of extremities with gangrene, right leg
- **I70.262** Atherosclerosis of native arteries of extremities with gangrene, left leg
- **I70.263** Atherosclerosis of native arteries of extremities with gangrene, bilateral legs
- **I70.268** Atherosclerosis of native arteries of extremities with gangrene, other extremity
- **I70.269** Atherosclerosis of native arteries of extremities with gangrene, unspecified extremity

I70.29 Other atherosclerosis of native arteries of extremities
- **I70.291** Other atherosclerosis of native arteries of extremities, right leg
- **I70.292** Other atherosclerosis of native arteries of extremities, left leg
- **I70.293** Other atherosclerosis of native arteries of extremities, bilateral legs
- **I70.298** Other atherosclerosis of native arteries of extremities, other extremity
- **I70.299** Other atherosclerosis of native arteries of extremities, unspecified extremity

I70.3 Atherosclerosis of unspecified type of bypass graft(s) of the extremities
Use additional code, if applicable, to identify chronic total occlusion of artery of extremity (I70.92)

EXCLUDES 1: embolism or thrombus of bypass graft(s) of extremities (T82.8-)

AHA: 2020,4Q,98

I70.30 Unspecified atherosclerosis of unspecified type of bypass graft(s) of the extremities
- **I70.301** Unspecified atherosclerosis of unspecified type of bypass graft(s) of the extremities, right leg
- **I70.302** Unspecified atherosclerosis of unspecified type of bypass graft(s) of the extremities, left leg

I70.303 Unspecified atherosclerosis of unspecified type of bypass graft(s) of the extremities, bilateral legs `ESR` `A`

I70.308 Unspecified atherosclerosis of unspecified type of bypass graft(s) of the extremities, other extremity `ESR` `A`

I70.309 Unspecified atherosclerosis of unspecified type of bypass graft(s) of the extremities, unspecified extremity `ESR` `A`

✓6th **I70.31** Atherosclerosis of unspecified type of bypass graft(s) of the extremities with intermittent claudication

I70.311 Atherosclerosis of unspecified type of bypass graft(s) of the extremities with intermittent claudication, right leg `ESR` `A`

I70.312 Atherosclerosis of unspecified type of bypass graft(s) of the extremities with intermittent claudication, left leg `ESR` `A`

I70.313 Atherosclerosis of unspecified type of bypass graft(s) of the extremities with intermittent claudication, bilateral legs `ESR` `A`

I70.318 Atherosclerosis of unspecified type of bypass graft(s) of the extremities with intermittent claudication, other extremity `ESR` `A`

I70.319 Atherosclerosis of unspecified type of bypass graft(s) of the extremities with intermittent claudication, unspecified extremity `ESR` `A`

✓6th **I70.32** Atherosclerosis of unspecified type of bypass graft(s) of the extremities with rest pain

INCLUDES any condition classifiable to I70.31-
chronic limb-threatening ischemia NOS of unspecified type of bypass graft(s) of the extremities
chronic limb-threatening ischemia of unspecified type of bypass graft(s) of the extremities with rest pain
critical limb ischemia NOS of unspecified type of bypass graft(s) of the extremities
critical limb ischemia of unspecified type of bypass graft(s) of the extremities with rest pain

I70.321 Atherosclerosis of unspecified type of bypass graft(s) of the extremities with rest pain, right leg `HCC` `ESR` `A`

I70.322 Atherosclerosis of unspecified type of bypass graft(s) of the extremities with rest pain, left leg `HCC` `ESR` `A`

I70.323 Atherosclerosis of unspecified type of bypass graft(s) of the extremities with rest pain, bilateral legs `HCC` `ESR` `A`

I70.328 Atherosclerosis of unspecified type of bypass graft(s) of the extremities with rest pain, other extremity `HCC` `ESR` `A`

I70.329 Atherosclerosis of unspecified type of bypass graft(s) of the extremities with rest pain, unspecified extremity `HCC` `ESR` `A`

✓6th **I70.33** Atherosclerosis of unspecified type of bypass graft(s) of the right leg with ulceration

INCLUDES any condition classifiable to I70.311 and I70.321
chronic limb-threatening ischemia of unspecified type of bypass graft(s) of the right leg with ulceration
critical limb ischemia of unspecified type of bypass graft(s) of the right leg with ulceration

Use additional code to identify severity of ulcer (L97.-)

I70.331 Atherosclerosis of unspecified type of bypass graft(s) of the right leg with ulceration of thigh `HCC` `Rx` `ESR` `COM` `A`

I70.332 Atherosclerosis of unspecified type of bypass graft(s) of the right leg with ulceration of calf `HCC` `Rx` `ESR` `COM` `A`

I70.333 Atherosclerosis of unspecified type of bypass graft(s) of the right leg with ulceration of ankle `HCC` `Rx` `ESR` `COM` `A`

I70.334 Atherosclerosis of unspecified type of bypass graft(s) of the right leg with ulceration of heel and midfoot `HCC` `Rx` `ESR` `COM` `A`

Atherosclerosis of unspecified type of bypass graft(s) of right leg with ulceration of plantar surface of midfoot

I70.335 Atherosclerosis of unspecified type of bypass graft(s) of the right leg with ulceration of other part of foot `HCC` `Rx` `ESR` `COM` `A`

Atherosclerosis of unspecified type of bypass graft(s) of the right leg with ulceration of toe

I70.338 Atherosclerosis of unspecified type of bypass graft(s) of the right leg with ulceration of other part of lower leg `HCC` `Rx` `ESR` `COM` `A`

I70.339 Atherosclerosis of unspecified type of bypass graft(s) of the right leg with ulceration of unspecified site `HCC` `Rx` `ESR` `COM` `A`

✓6th **I70.34** Atherosclerosis of unspecified type of bypass graft(s) of the left leg with ulceration

INCLUDES any condition classifiable to I70.312 and I70.322
chronic limb-threatening ischemia of unspecified type of bypass graft(s) of the left leg with ulceration
critical limb ischemia of unspecified type of bypass graft(s) of the left leg with ulceration

Use additional code to identify severity of ulcer (L97.-)

I70.341 Atherosclerosis of unspecified type of bypass graft(s) of the left leg with ulceration of thigh `HCC` `Rx` `ESR` `COM` `A`

I70.342 Atherosclerosis of unspecified type of bypass graft(s) of the left leg with ulceration of calf `HCC` `Rx` `ESR` `COM` `A`

I70.343 Atherosclerosis of unspecified type of bypass graft(s) of the left leg with ulceration of ankle `HCC` `Rx` `ESR` `COM` `A`

I70.344 Atherosclerosis of unspecified type of bypass graft(s) of the left leg with ulceration of heel and midfoot `HCC` `Rx` `ESR` `COM` `A`

Atherosclerosis of unspecified type of bypass graft(s) of left leg with ulceration of plantar surface of midfoot

I70.345 Atherosclerosis of unspecified type of bypass graft(s) of the left leg with ulceration of other part of foot `HCC` `Rx` `ESR` `COM` `A`

Atherosclerosis of unspecified type of bypass graft(s) of the left leg with ulceration of toe

I70.348 Atherosclerosis of unspecified type of bypass graft(s) of the left leg with ulceration of other part of lower leg `HCC` `Rx` `ESR` `COM` `A`

I70.349 Atherosclerosis of unspecified type of bypass graft(s) of the left leg with ulceration of unspecified site `HCC` `Rx` `ESR` `COM` `A`

I70.35 Atherosclerosis of unspecified type of bypass graft(s) of other extremity with ulceration `HCC` `Rx` `ESR` `COM` `A`

INCLUDES any condition classifiable to I70.318 and I70.328

Use additional code to identify severity of ulcer (L98.49-)

I70.36 Atherosclerosis of unspecified type of bypass graft(s) of the extremities with gangrene

INCLUDES any condition classifiable to I70.31-, I70.32-, I70.33-, I70.34-, I70.35
chronic limb-threatening ischemia of unspecified type of bypass graft(s) of the extremities with gangrene
critical limb ischemia of unspecified type of bypass graft(s) of the extremities with gangrene

Use additional code to identify the severity of any ulcer (L97.-, L98.49-), if applicable

- **I70.361** Atherosclerosis of unspecified type of bypass graft(s) of the extremities with gangrene, right leg
- **I70.362** Atherosclerosis of unspecified type of bypass graft(s) of the extremities with gangrene, left leg
- **I70.363** Atherosclerosis of unspecified type of bypass graft(s) of the extremities with gangrene, bilateral legs
- **I70.368** Atherosclerosis of unspecified type of bypass graft(s) of the extremities with gangrene, other extremity
- **I70.369** Atherosclerosis of unspecified type of bypass graft(s) of the extremities with gangrene, unspecified extremity

I70.39 Other atherosclerosis of unspecified type of bypass graft(s) of the extremities

- **I70.391** Other atherosclerosis of unspecified type of bypass graft(s) of the extremities, right leg
- **I70.392** Other atherosclerosis of unspecified type of bypass graft(s) of the extremities, left leg
- **I70.393** Other atherosclerosis of unspecified type of bypass graft(s) of the extremities, bilateral legs
- **I70.398** Other atherosclerosis of unspecified type of bypass graft(s) of the extremities, other extremity
- **I70.399** Other atherosclerosis of unspecified type of bypass graft(s) of the extremities, unspecified extremity

I70.4 Atherosclerosis of autologous vein bypass graft(s) of the extremities

Use additional code, if applicable, to identify chronic total occlusion of artery of extremity (I70.92)
AHA: 2020,4Q,98

I70.40 Unspecified atherosclerosis of autologous vein bypass graft(s) of the extremities

- **I70.401** Unspecified atherosclerosis of autologous vein bypass graft(s) of the extremities, right leg
- **I70.402** Unspecified atherosclerosis of autologous vein bypass graft(s) of the extremities, left leg
- **I70.403** Unspecified atherosclerosis of autologous vein bypass graft(s) of the extremities, bilateral legs
- **I70.408** Unspecified atherosclerosis of autologous vein bypass graft(s) of the extremities, other extremity
- **I70.409** Unspecified atherosclerosis of autologous vein bypass graft(s) of the extremities, unspecified extremity

I70.41 Atherosclerosis of autologous vein bypass graft(s) of the extremities with intermittent claudication

- **I70.411** Atherosclerosis of autologous vein bypass graft(s) of the extremities with intermittent claudication, right leg
- **I70.412** Atherosclerosis of autologous vein bypass graft(s) of the extremities with intermittent claudication, left leg
- **I70.413** Atherosclerosis of autologous vein bypass graft(s) of the extremities with intermittent claudication, bilateral legs
- **I70.418** Atherosclerosis of autologous vein bypass graft(s) of the extremities with intermittent claudication, other extremity
- **I70.419** Atherosclerosis of autologous vein bypass graft(s) of the extremities with intermittent claudication, unspecified extremity

I70.42 Atherosclerosis of autologous vein bypass graft(s) of the extremities with rest pain

INCLUDES any condition classifiable to I70.41-
chronic limb-threatening ischemia of autologous vein bypass graft(s) of the extremities with rest pain
chronic limb-threatening ischemia NOS of autologous vein bypass graft(s) of the extremities
critical limb ischemia of autologous vein bypass graft(s) of the extremities with rest pain
critical limb ischemia NOS of autologous vein bypass graft(s) of the extremities

- **I70.421** Atherosclerosis of autologous vein bypass graft(s) of the extremities with rest pain, right leg
- **I70.422** Atherosclerosis of autologous vein bypass graft(s) of the extremities with rest pain, left leg
- **I70.423** Atherosclerosis of autologous vein bypass graft(s) of the extremities with rest pain, bilateral legs
- **I70.428** Atherosclerosis of autologous vein bypass graft(s) of the extremities with rest pain, other extremity
- **I70.429** Atherosclerosis of autologous vein bypass graft(s) of the extremities with rest pain, unspecified extremity

I70.43 Atherosclerosis of autologous vein bypass graft(s) of the right leg with ulceration

INCLUDES any condition classifiable to I70.411 and I70.421
chronic limb-threatening ischemia of autologous vein bypass graft(s) of the right leg with ulceration
critical limb ischemia of autologous vein bypass graft(s) of the right leg with ulceration

Use additional code to identify severity of ulcer (L97.-)

- **I70.431** Atherosclerosis of autologous vein bypass graft(s) of the right leg with ulceration of thigh
- **I70.432** Atherosclerosis of autologous vein bypass graft(s) of the right leg with ulceration of calf
- **I70.433** Atherosclerosis of autologous vein bypass graft(s) of the right leg with ulceration of ankle
- **I70.434** Atherosclerosis of autologous vein bypass graft(s) of the right leg with ulceration of heel and midfoot
  Atherosclerosis of autologous vein bypass graft(s) of right leg with ulceration of plantar surface of midfoot
- **I70.435** Atherosclerosis of autologous vein bypass graft(s) of the right leg with ulceration of other part of foot
  Atherosclerosis of autologous vein bypass graft(s) of right leg with ulceration of toe
- **I70.438** Atherosclerosis of autologous vein bypass graft(s) of the right leg with ulceration of other part of lower leg
- **I70.439** Atherosclerosis of autologous vein bypass graft(s) of the right leg with ulceration of unspecified site

I70.44–I70.528

- **I70.44** ✓6th Atherosclerosis of autologous vein bypass graft(s) of the **left leg** with **ulceration**
  - INCLUDES: any condition classifiable to I70.412 and I70.422
    chronic limb-threatening ischemia of autologous vein bypass graft(s) of the left leg with ulceration
    critical limb ischemia of autologous vein bypass graft(s) of the left leg with ulceration
  - Use additional code to identify severity of ulcer (L97.-)
  - **I70.441** Atherosclerosis of autologous vein bypass graft(s) of the left leg with ulceration of **thigh** HCC Rx ESR COM
  - **I70.442** Atherosclerosis of autologous vein bypass graft(s) of the left leg with ulceration of **calf** HCC Rx ESR COM
  - **I70.443** Atherosclerosis of autologous vein bypass graft(s) of the left leg with ulceration of **ankle** HCC Rx ESR COM
  - **I70.444** Atherosclerosis of autologous vein bypass graft(s) of the left leg with ulceration of **heel and midfoot** HCC Rx ESR COM
    Atherosclerosis of autologous vein bypass graft(s) of left leg with ulceration of plantar surface of midfoot
  - **I70.445** Atherosclerosis of autologous vein bypass graft(s) of the left leg with ulceration of **other part of foot** HCC Rx ESR COM
    Atherosclerosis of autologous vein bypass graft(s) of left leg with ulceration of toe
  - **I70.448** Atherosclerosis of autologous vein bypass graft(s) of the left leg with ulceration of other part of lower leg HCC Rx ESR COM
  - **I70.449** Atherosclerosis of autologous vein bypass graft(s) of the left leg with ulceration of unspecified site HCC Rx ESR COM
- **I70.45** Atherosclerosis of autologous vein bypass graft(s) of other extremity with **ulceration** HCC Rx ESR COM
  - INCLUDES: any condition classifiable to I70.418, I70.428, and I70.438
  - Use additional code to identify severity of ulcer (L98.49)
- **I70.46** ✓6th Atherosclerosis of autologous vein bypass graft(s) of the extremities with **gangrene**
  - INCLUDES: any condition classifiable to I70.41-, I70.42-, and I70.43-, I70.44-, I70.45
    chronic limb-threatening ischemia of autologous vein bypass graft(s) of the extremities with gangrene
    critical limb ischemia of autologous vein bypass graft(s) of the extremities with gangrene
  - Use additional code to identify the severity of any ulcer (L97.-, L98.49-), if applicable
  - **I70.461** Atherosclerosis of autologous vein bypass graft(s) of the extremities with gangrene, **right leg** HCC ESR COM
  - **I70.462** Atherosclerosis of autologous vein bypass graft(s) of the extremities with gangrene, **left leg** HCC ESR COM
  - **I70.463** Atherosclerosis of autologous vein bypass graft(s) of the extremities with gangrene, **bilateral legs** HCC ESR COM
  - **I70.468** Atherosclerosis of autologous vein bypass graft(s) of the extremities with gangrene, other extremity HCC ESR COM
  - **I70.469** Atherosclerosis of autologous vein bypass graft(s) of the extremities with gangrene, unspecified extremity HCC ESR COM
- **I70.49** ✓6th Other atherosclerosis of autologous vein bypass graft(s) of the extremities
  - **I70.491** Other atherosclerosis of autologous vein bypass graft(s) of the extremities, **right leg** ESR
  - **I70.492** Other atherosclerosis of autologous vein bypass graft(s) of the extremities, **left leg** ESR
  - **I70.493** Other atherosclerosis of autologous vein bypass graft(s) of the extremities, **bilateral legs** ESR
  - **I70.498** Other atherosclerosis of autologous vein bypass graft(s) of the extremities, other extremity ESR
  - **I70.499** Other atherosclerosis of autologous vein bypass graft(s) of the extremities, unspecified extremity ESR
- **I70.5** ✓5th Atherosclerosis of **nonautologous biological bypass graft(s)** of the **extremities**
  - Use additional code, if applicable, to identify chronic total occlusion of artery of extremity (I70.92)
  - AHA: 2020,4Q,98
  - **I70.50** ✓6th Unspecified atherosclerosis of nonautologous biological bypass graft(s) of the extremities
    - **I70.501** Unspecified atherosclerosis of nonautologous biological bypass graft(s) of the extremities, **right leg** ESR
    - **I70.502** Unspecified atherosclerosis of nonautologous biological bypass graft(s) of the extremities, **left leg** ESR
    - **I70.503** Unspecified atherosclerosis of nonautologous biological bypass graft(s) of the extremities, **bilateral legs**
    - **I70.508** Unspecified atherosclerosis of nonautologous biological bypass graft(s) of the extremities, other extremity ESR
    - **I70.509** Unspecified atherosclerosis of nonautologous biological bypass graft(s) of the extremities, unspecified extremity ESR
  - **I70.51** ✓6th Atherosclerosis of nonautologous biological bypass graft(s) of the extremities **intermittent claudication**
    - **I70.511** Atherosclerosis of nonautologous biological bypass graft(s) of the extremities with intermittent claudication, **right leg** ESR
    - **I70.512** Atherosclerosis of nonautologous biological bypass graft(s) of the extremities with intermittent claudication, **left leg** ESR
    - **I70.513** Atherosclerosis of nonautologous biological bypass graft(s) of the extremities with intermittent claudication, **bilateral legs** ESR
    - **I70.518** Atherosclerosis of nonautologous biological bypass graft(s) of the extremities with intermittent claudication, other extremity ESR
    - **I70.519** Atherosclerosis of nonautologous biological bypass graft(s) of the extremities with intermittent claudication, unspecified extremity ESR
  - **I70.52** ✓6th Atherosclerosis of nonautologous biological bypass graft(s) of the extremities with **rest pain**
    - INCLUDES: any condition classifiable to I70.51-
      chronic limb-threatening ischemia of nonautologous biological bypass graft(s) of the extremities with rest pain
      chronic limb-threatening ischemia NOS of nonautologous biological bypass graft(s) of the extremities
      critical limb ischemia of nonautologous biological bypass graft(s) of the extremities with rest pain
      critical limb ischemia NOS of nonautologous biological bypass graft(s) of the extremities
    - **I70.521** Atherosclerosis of nonautologous biological bypass graft(s) of the extremities with rest pain, **right leg** HCC ESR
    - **I70.522** Atherosclerosis of nonautologous biological bypass graft(s) of the extremities with rest pain, **left leg** HCC ESR
    - **I70.523** Atherosclerosis of nonautologous biological bypass graft(s) of the extremities with rest pain, **bilateral legs** HCC ESR
    - **I70.528** Atherosclerosis of nonautologous biological bypass graft(s) of the extremities with rest pain, other extremity HCC ESR

I70.529 Atherosclerosis of nonautologous biological bypass graft(s) of the extremities with rest pain, unspecified extremity `HCC` `ESR` `A`

✓6ᵗʰ **I70.53** Atherosclerosis of nonautologous biological bypass graft(s) of the right leg with ulceration

INCLUDES
any condition classifiable to I70.511 and I70.521
chronic limb-threatening ischemia of nonautologous biological bypass graft(s) of the right leg with ulceration
critical limb ischemia of nonautologous biological bypass graft(s) of the right leg with ulceration

Use additional code to identify severity of ulcer (L97.-)

I70.531 Atherosclerosis of nonautologous biological bypass graft(s) of the right leg with ulceration of thigh `HCC` `Rx` `ESR` `COM` `A`

I70.532 Atherosclerosis of nonautologous biological bypass graft(s) of the right leg with ulceration of calf `HCC` `Rx` `ESR` `COM` `A`

I70.533 Atherosclerosis of nonautologous biological bypass graft(s) of the right leg with ulceration of ankle `HCC` `Rx` `ESR` `COM` `A`

I70.534 Atherosclerosis of nonautologous biological bypass graft(s) of the right leg with ulceration of heel and midfoot `HCC` `Rx` `ESR` `COM` `A`
Atherosclerosis of nonautologous biological bypass graft(s) of right leg with ulceration of plantar surface of midfoot

I70.535 Atherosclerosis of nonautologous biological bypass graft(s) of the right leg with ulceration of other part of foot `HCC` `Rx` `ESR` `COM` `A`
Atherosclerosis of nonautologous biological bypass graft(s) of the right leg with ulceration of toe

I70.538 Atherosclerosis of nonautologous biological bypass graft(s) of the right leg with ulceration of other part of lower leg `HCC` `Rx` `ESR` `COM` `A`

I70.539 Atherosclerosis of nonautologous biological bypass graft(s) of the right leg with ulceration of unspecified site `HCC` `Rx` `ESR` `COM` `A`

✓6ᵗʰ **I70.54** Atherosclerosis of nonautologous biological bypass graft(s) of the left leg with ulceration

INCLUDES
any condition classifiable to I70.512 and I70.522
chronic limb-threatening ischemia of nonautologous biological bypass graft(s) of the left leg with ulceration
critical limb ischemia of nonautologous biological bypass graft(s) of the left leg with ulceration

Use additional code to identify severity of ulcer (L97.-)

I70.541 Atherosclerosis of nonautologous biological bypass graft(s) of the left leg with ulceration of thigh `HCC` `Rx` `ESR` `COM` `A`

I70.542 Atherosclerosis of nonautologous biological bypass graft(s) of the left leg with ulceration of calf `HCC` `Rx` `ESR` `COM` `A`

I70.543 Atherosclerosis of nonautologous biological bypass graft(s) of the left leg with ulceration of ankle `HCC` `Rx` `ESR` `COM` `A`

I70.544 Atherosclerosis of nonautologous biological bypass graft(s) of the left leg with ulceration of heel and midfoot `HCC` `Rx` `ESR` `COM` `A`
Atherosclerosis of nonautologous biological bypass graft(s) of left leg with ulceration of plantar surface of midfoot

I70.545 Atherosclerosis of nonautologous biological bypass graft(s) of the left leg with ulceration of other part of foot `HCC` `Rx` `ESR` `COM` `A`
Atherosclerosis of nonautologous biological bypass graft(s) of the left leg with ulceration of toe

I70.548 Atherosclerosis of nonautologous biological bypass graft(s) of the left leg with ulceration of other part of lower leg `HCC` `Rx` `ESR` `COM` `A`

I70.549 Atherosclerosis of nonautologous biological bypass graft(s) of the left leg with ulceration of unspecified site `HCC` `Rx` `ESR` `COM` `A`

I70.55 Atherosclerosis of nonautologous biological bypass graft(s) of other extremity with ulceration `HCC` `ESR` `COM` `A`

INCLUDES
any condition classifiable to I70.518, I70.528, and I70.538

Use additional code to identify severity of ulcer (L98.49)

✓6ᵗʰ **I70.56** Atherosclerosis of nonautologous biological bypass graft(s) of the extremities with gangrene

INCLUDES
any condition classifiable to I70.51-, I70.52-, and I70.53-, I70.54-, I70.55
chronic limb-threatening ischemia of nonautologous biological bypass graft(s) of the extremities with gangrene
critical limb ischemia of nonautologous biological bypass graft(s) of the extremities with gangrene

Use additional code to identify the severity of any ulcer (L97.-, L98.49-), if applicable

I70.561 Atherosclerosis of nonautologous biological bypass graft(s) of the extremities with gangrene, right leg `HCC` `ESR` `COM` `A`

I70.562 Atherosclerosis of nonautologous biological bypass graft(s) of the extremities with gangrene, left leg `HCC` `ESR` `COM` `A`

I70.563 Atherosclerosis of nonautologous biological bypass graft(s) of the extremities with gangrene, bilateral legs `HCC` `ESR` `COM` `A`

I70.568 Atherosclerosis of nonautologous biological bypass graft(s) of the extremities with gangrene, other extremity `HCC` `ESR` `COM` `A`

I70.569 Atherosclerosis of nonautologous biological bypass graft(s) of the extremities with gangrene, unspecified extremity `HCC` `ESR` `COM` `A`

✓6ᵗʰ **I70.59** Other atherosclerosis of nonautologous biological bypass graft(s) of the extremities

I70.591 Other atherosclerosis of nonautologous biological bypass graft(s) of the extremities, right leg `ESR`

I70.592 Other atherosclerosis of nonautologous biological bypass graft(s) of the extremities, left leg `ESR`

I70.593 Other atherosclerosis of nonautologous biological bypass graft(s) of the extremities, bilateral legs `ESR`

I70.598 Other atherosclerosis of nonautologous biological bypass graft(s) of the extremities, other extremity `ESR`

I70.599 Other atherosclerosis of nonautologous biological bypass graft(s) of the extremities, unspecified extremity `ESR` `A`

✓5ᵗʰ **I70.6** Atherosclerosis of nonbiological bypass graft(s) of the extremities
Use additional code, if applicable, to identify chronic total occlusion of artery of extremity (I70.92)
AHA: 2020,4Q,98

✓6ᵗʰ **I70.60** Unspecified atherosclerosis of nonbiological bypass graft(s) of the extremities

I70.601 Unspecified atherosclerosis of nonbiological bypass graft(s) of the extremities, right leg `ESR` `A`

- **I70.602** Unspecified atherosclerosis of nonbiological bypass graft(s) of the extremities, **left leg**
- **I70.603** Unspecified atherosclerosis of nonbiological bypass graft(s) of the extremities, **bilateral legs**
- **I70.608** Unspecified atherosclerosis of nonbiological bypass graft(s) of the extremities, **other extremity**
- **I70.609** Unspecified atherosclerosis of nonbiological bypass graft(s) of the extremities, **unspecified extremity**

√6th **I70.61** Atherosclerosis of nonbiological bypass graft(s) of the extremities with **intermittent claudication**
- **I70.611** Atherosclerosis of nonbiological bypass graft(s) of the extremities with intermittent claudication, **right leg**
- **I70.612** Atherosclerosis of nonbiological bypass graft(s) of the extremities with intermittent claudication, **left leg**
- **I70.613** Atherosclerosis of nonbiological bypass graft(s) of the extremities with intermittent claudication, **bilateral legs**
- **I70.618** Atherosclerosis of nonbiological bypass graft(s) of the extremities with intermittent claudication, **other extremity**
- **I70.619** Atherosclerosis of nonbiological bypass graft(s) of the extremities with intermittent claudication, **unspecified extremity**

√6th **I70.62** Atherosclerosis of nonbiological bypass graft(s) of the extremities with **rest pain**

INCLUDES
- any condition classifiable to I70.61-
- chronic limb-threatening ischemia of nonbiological bypass graft(s) of the extremities with rest pain
- chronic limb-threatening ischemia NOS of nonbiological bypass graft(s) of the extremities
- critical limb ischemia of nonbiological bypass graft(s) of the extremities with rest pain
- critical limb ischemia NOS of nonbiological bypass graft(s) of the extremities

- **I70.621** Atherosclerosis of nonbiological bypass graft(s) of the extremities with rest pain, **right leg**
- **I70.622** Atherosclerosis of nonbiological bypass graft(s) of the extremities with rest pain, **left leg**
- **I70.623** Atherosclerosis of nonbiological bypass graft(s) of the extremities with rest pain, **bilateral legs**
- **I70.628** Atherosclerosis of nonbiological bypass graft(s) of the extremities with rest pain, **other extremity**
- **I70.629** Atherosclerosis of nonbiological bypass graft(s) of the extremities with rest pain, **unspecified extremity**

√6th **I70.63** Atherosclerosis of nonbiological bypass graft(s) of the **right leg** with **ulceration**

INCLUDES
- any condition classifiable to I70.611 and I70.621
- chronic limb-threatening ischemia of nonbiological bypass graft(s) of the right leg with ulceration
- critical limb ischemia of nonbiological bypass graft(s) of the right leg with ulceration

Use additional code to identify severity of ulcer (L97.-)

- **I70.631** Atherosclerosis of nonbiological bypass graft(s) of the right leg with ulceration of **thigh**
- **I70.632** Atherosclerosis of nonbiological bypass graft(s) of the right leg with ulceration of **calf**
- **I70.633** Atherosclerosis of nonbiological bypass graft(s) of the right leg with ulceration of **ankle**
- **I70.634** Atherosclerosis of nonbiological bypass graft(s) of the right leg with ulceration of **heel and midfoot**
  - Atherosclerosis of nonbiological bypass graft(s) of right leg with ulceration of plantar surface of midfoot
- **I70.635** Atherosclerosis of nonbiological bypass graft(s) of the right leg with ulceration of **other part of foot**
  - Atherosclerosis of nonbiological bypass graft(s) of the right leg with ulceration of toe
- **I70.638** Atherosclerosis of nonbiological bypass graft(s) of the right leg with ulceration of **other part of lower leg**
- **I70.639** Atherosclerosis of nonbiological bypass graft(s) of the right leg with ulceration of **unspecified site**

√6th **I70.64** Atherosclerosis of nonbiological bypass graft(s) of the **left leg** with **ulceration**

INCLUDES
- any condition classifiable to I70.612 and I70.622
- chronic limb-threatening ischemia of nonbiological bypass graft(s) of the left leg with ulceration
- critical limb ischemia of nonbiological bypass graft(s) of the left leg with ulceration

Use additional code to identify severity of ulcer (L97.-)

- **I70.641** Atherosclerosis of nonbiological bypass graft(s) of the left leg with ulceration of **thigh**
- **I70.642** Atherosclerosis of nonbiological bypass graft(s) of the left leg with ulceration of **calf**
- **I70.643** Atherosclerosis of nonbiological bypass graft(s) of the left leg with ulceration of **ankle**
- **I70.644** Atherosclerosis of nonbiological bypass graft(s) of the left leg with ulceration of **heel and midfoot**
  - Atherosclerosis of nonbiological bypass graft(s) of left leg with ulceration of plantar surface of midfoot
- **I70.645** Atherosclerosis of nonbiological bypass graft(s) of the left leg with ulceration of **other part of foot**
  - Atherosclerosis of nonbiological bypass graft(s) of the left leg with ulceration of toe
- **I70.648** Atherosclerosis of nonbiological bypass graft(s) of the left leg with ulceration of **other part of lower leg**
- **I70.649** Atherosclerosis of nonbiological bypass graft(s) of the left leg with ulceration of **unspecified site**

I70.65 Atherosclerosis of nonbiological bypass graft(s) of other extremity with **ulceration**

INCLUDES any condition classifiable to I70.618 and I70.628

Use additional code to identify severity of ulcer (L98.49)

√6th **I70.66** Atherosclerosis of nonbiological bypass graft(s) of the extremities with **gangrene**

INCLUDES
- any condition classifiable to I70.61-, I70.62-, I70.63-, I70.64-, I70.65
- chronic limb-threatening ischemia of nonbiological bypass graft(s) of the extremities with gangrene
- critical limb ischemia of nonbiological bypass graft(s) of the extremities with gangrene

Use additional code to identify the severity of any ulcer (L97.-, L98.49-), if applicable

- **I70.661** Atherosclerosis of nonbiological bypass graft(s) of the extremities with gangrene, **right leg**

I70.662	Atherosclerosis of nonbiological bypass graft(s) of the extremities with gangrene, left leg
I70.663	Atherosclerosis of nonbiological bypass graft(s) of the extremities with gangrene, bilateral legs
I70.668	Atherosclerosis of nonbiological bypass graft(s) of the extremities with gangrene, other extremity
I70.669	Atherosclerosis of nonbiological bypass graft(s) of the extremities with gangrene, unspecified extremity

I70.69 Other atherosclerosis of nonbiological bypass graft(s) of the extremities

I70.691	Other atherosclerosis of nonbiological bypass graft(s) of the extremities, right leg
I70.692	Other atherosclerosis of nonbiological bypass graft(s) of the extremities, left leg
I70.693	Other atherosclerosis of nonbiological bypass graft(s) of the extremities, bilateral legs
I70.698	Other atherosclerosis of nonbiological bypass graft(s) of the extremities, other extremity
I70.699	Other atherosclerosis of nonbiological bypass graft(s) of the extremities, unspecified extremity

I70.7 Atherosclerosis of other type of bypass graft(s) of the extremities

Use additional code, if applicable, to identify chronic total occlusion of artery of extremity (I70.92)

AHA: 2020,4Q,98

I70.70 Unspecified atherosclerosis of other type of bypass graft(s) of the extremities

I70.701	Unspecified atherosclerosis of other type of bypass graft(s) of the extremities, right leg
I70.702	Unspecified atherosclerosis of other type of bypass graft(s) of the extremities, left leg
I70.703	Unspecified atherosclerosis of other type of bypass graft(s) of the extremities, bilateral legs
I70.708	Unspecified atherosclerosis of other type of bypass graft(s) of the extremities, other extremity
I70.709	Unspecified atherosclerosis of other type of bypass graft(s) of the extremities, unspecified extremity

I70.71 Atherosclerosis of other type of bypass graft(s) of the extremities with intermittent claudication

I70.711	Atherosclerosis of other type of bypass graft(s) of the extremities with intermittent claudication, right leg
I70.712	Atherosclerosis of other type of bypass graft(s) of the extremities with intermittent claudication, left leg
I70.713	Atherosclerosis of other type of bypass graft(s) of the extremities with intermittent claudication, bilateral legs
I70.718	Atherosclerosis of other type of bypass graft(s) of the extremities with intermittent claudication, other extremity
I70.719	Atherosclerosis of other type of bypass graft(s) of the extremities with intermittent claudication, unspecified extremity

I70.72 Atherosclerosis of other type of bypass graft(s) of the extremities with rest pain

INCLUDES
any condition classifiable to I70.71-
chronic limb-threatening ischemia NOS of other type of bypass graft(s) of the extremities
chronic limb-threatening ischemia of other type of bypass graft(s) of the extremities with rest pain
critical limb ischemia NOS of other type of bypass graft(s) of the extremities
critical limb ischemia of other type of bypass graft(s) of the extremities with rest pain

I70.721	Atherosclerosis of other type of bypass graft(s) of the extremities with rest pain, right leg
I70.722	Atherosclerosis of other type of bypass graft(s) of the extremities with rest pain, left leg
I70.723	Atherosclerosis of other type of bypass graft(s) of the extremities with rest pain, bilateral legs
I70.728	Atherosclerosis of other type of bypass graft(s) of the extremities with rest pain, other extremity
I70.729	Atherosclerosis of other type of bypass graft(s) of the extremities with rest pain, unspecified extremity

I70.73 Atherosclerosis of other type of bypass graft(s) of the right leg with ulceration

INCLUDES
any condition classifiable to I70.711 and I70.721
chronic limb-threatening ischemia of other type of bypass graft(s) of the right leg with ulceration
critical limb ischemia of other type of bypass graft(s) of the right leg with ulceration

Use additional code to identify severity of ulcer (L97.-)

I70.731	Atherosclerosis of other type of bypass graft(s) of the right leg with ulceration of thigh
I70.732	Atherosclerosis of other type of bypass graft(s) of the right leg with ulceration of calf
I70.733	Atherosclerosis of other type of bypass graft(s) of the right leg with ulceration of ankle
I70.734	Atherosclerosis of other type of bypass graft(s) of the right leg with ulceration of heel and midfoot
	Atherosclerosis of other type of bypass graft(s) of right leg with ulceration of plantar surface of midfoot
I70.735	Atherosclerosis of other type of bypass graft(s) of the right leg with ulceration of other part of foot
	Atherosclerosis of other type of bypass graft(s) of right leg with ulceration of toe
I70.738	Atherosclerosis of other type of bypass graft(s) of the right leg with ulceration of other part of lower leg
I70.739	Atherosclerosis of other type of bypass graft(s) of the right leg with ulceration of unspecified site

Chapter 9. Diseases of the Circulatory System

I70.74 Atherosclerosis of other type of bypass graft(s) of the left leg with ulceration
- **INCLUDES** any condition classifiable to I70.712 and I70.722
- chronic limb-threatening ischemia of other type of bypass graft(s) of the left leg with ulceration
- critical limb ischemia of other type of bypass graft(s) of the left leg with ulceration
- *Use additional code to identify severity of ulcer (L97.-)*

  I70.741 Atherosclerosis of other type of bypass graft(s) of the left leg with ulceration of thigh
  I70.742 Atherosclerosis of other type of bypass graft(s) of the left leg with ulceration of calf
  I70.743 Atherosclerosis of other type of bypass graft(s) of the left leg with ulceration of ankle
  I70.744 Atherosclerosis of other type of bypass graft(s) of the left leg with ulceration of heel and midfoot
  - Atherosclerosis of other type of bypass graft(s) of left leg with ulceration of plantar surface of midfoot

  I70.745 Atherosclerosis of other type of bypass graft(s) of the left leg with ulceration of other part of foot
  - Atherosclerosis of other type of bypass graft(s) of left leg with ulceration of toe

  I70.748 Atherosclerosis of other type of bypass graft(s) of the left leg with ulceration of other part of lower leg
  I70.749 Atherosclerosis of other type of bypass graft(s) of the left leg with ulceration of unspecified site

I70.75 Atherosclerosis of other type of bypass graft(s) of other extremity with ulceration
- **INCLUDES** any condition classifiable to I70.718 and I70.728
- *Use additional code to identify severity of ulcer (L98.49)*

I70.76 Atherosclerosis of other type of bypass graft(s) of the extremities with gangrene
- **INCLUDES** any condition classifiable to I70.71-, I70.72-, I70.73-, I70.74-, I70.75
- chronic limb-threatening ischemia of other type of bypass graft(s) of the extremities with gangrene
- critical limb ischemia of other type of bypass graft(s) of the extremities with gangrene
- *Use additional code to identify the severity of any ulcer (L97.-, L98.49-), if applicable*

  I70.761 Atherosclerosis of other type of bypass graft(s) of the extremities with gangrene, right leg
  I70.762 Atherosclerosis of other type of bypass graft(s) of the extremities with gangrene, left leg
  I70.763 Atherosclerosis of other type of bypass graft(s) of the extremities with gangrene, bilateral legs
  I70.768 Atherosclerosis of other type of bypass graft(s) of the extremities with gangrene, other extremity
  I70.769 Atherosclerosis of other type of bypass graft(s) of the extremities with gangrene, unspecified extremity

I70.79 Other atherosclerosis of other type of bypass graft(s) of the extremities
  I70.791 Other atherosclerosis of other type of bypass graft(s) of the extremities, right leg
  I70.792 Other atherosclerosis of other type of bypass graft(s) of the extremities, left leg
  I70.793 Other atherosclerosis of other type of bypass graft(s) of the extremities, bilateral legs
  I70.798 Other atherosclerosis of other type of bypass graft(s) of the extremities, other extremity
  I70.799 Other atherosclerosis of other type of bypass graft(s) of the extremities, unspecified extremity

I70.8 Atherosclerosis of other arteries
- **TIP:** Arteriosclerosis of the iliac arteries is coded here.

I70.9 Other and unspecified atherosclerosis
- **EXCLUDES 2** ▶disorders of pyrophosphate metabolism (E83.82-)◀

  I70.90 Unspecified atherosclerosis
  I70.91 Generalized atherosclerosis
  I70.92 Chronic total occlusion of artery of the extremities
  - Complete occlusion of artery of the extremities
  - Total occlusion of artery of the extremities
  - *Code first atherosclerosis of arteries of the extremities (I70.2-, I70.3-, I70.4-, I70.5-, I70.6-, I70.7-)*

I71 Aortic aneurysm and dissection
Code first, if applicable:
- syphilitic aortic aneurysm (A52.01)
- traumatic aortic aneurysm (S25.09, S35.09)

AHA: 2022,4Q,24-26
TIP: A diagnosis of dissecting aneurysm should be coded to subcategory I71.0 only. The bulging/aneurysm, although present, occurred secondary to the dissection. The dissection represents the most significant problem.

I71.0 Dissection of aorta
  I71.00 Dissection of unspecified site of aorta
  I71.01 Dissection of thoracic aorta
  - **AHA:** 2024,2Q,17
    I71.010 Dissection of ascending aorta
    I71.011 Dissection of aortic arch
    I71.012 Dissection of descending thoracic aorta
    I71.019 Dissection of thoracic aorta, unspecified
  I71.02 Dissection of abdominal aorta
  I71.03 Dissection of thoracoabdominal aorta

I71.1 Thoracic aortic aneurysm, ruptured
  I71.10 Thoracic aortic aneurysm, ruptured, unspecified
  I71.11 Aneurysm of the ascending aorta, ruptured
  I71.12 Aneurysm of the aortic arch, ruptured
  I71.13 Aneurysm of the descending thoracic aorta, ruptured

I71.2 Thoracic aortic aneurysm, without rupture
  I71.20 Thoracic aortic aneurysm, without rupture, unspecified
  I71.21 Aneurysm of the ascending aorta, without rupture
  I71.22 Aneurysm of the aortic arch, without rupture
  I71.23 Aneurysm of the descending thoracic aorta, without rupture

I71.3 Abdominal aortic aneurysm, ruptured
  I71.30 Abdominal aortic aneurysm, ruptured, unspecified
  I71.31 Pararenal abdominal aortic aneurysm, ruptured
  I71.32 Juxtarenal abdominal aortic aneurysm, ruptured
  I71.33 Infrarenal abdominal aortic aneurysm, ruptured

I71.4 Abdominal aortic aneurysm, without rupture
  I71.40 Abdominal aortic aneurysm, without rupture, unspecified
  I71.41 Pararenal abdominal aortic aneurysm, without rupture
  - **AHA:** 2024,2Q,16
  I71.42 Juxtarenal abdominal aortic aneurysm, without rupture
  I71.43 Infrarenal abdominal aortic aneurysm, without rupture

Chapter 9. Diseases of the Circulatory System

I71.5 **Thoracoabdominal** aortic aneurysm, **ruptured**
- **I71.50** Thoracoabdominal aortic aneurysm, ruptured, unspecified `HCC` `ESR` `COM`
- **I71.51** **Supraceliac** aneurysm of the thoracoabdominal aorta, ruptured `HCC` `ESR` `COM`
- **I71.52** **Paravisceral** aneurysm of the thoracoabdominal aorta, ruptured `HCC` `ESR` `COM`

I71.6 **Thoracoabdominal** aortic aneurysm, **without rupture**
- **I71.60** Thoracoabdominal aortic aneurysm, without rupture, unspecified `ESR`
- **I71.61** **Supraceliac** aneurysm of the thoracoabdominal aorta, without rupture `ESR`
- **I71.62** **Paravisceral** aneurysm of the thoracoabdominal aorta, without rupture `ESR`

I71.8 Aortic aneurysm of unspecified site, **ruptured** `HCC` `ESR` `COM`
Rupture of aorta NOS

I71.9 Aortic aneurysm of unspecified site, **without rupture** `ESR`
Aneurysm of aorta
Dilatation of aorta
Hyaline necrosis of aorta

I72 Other aneurysm
- **INCLUDES** aneurysm (cirsoid) (false) (ruptured)
- **EXCLUDES 2**
  - acquired aneurysm (I77.0)
  - aneurysm (of) aorta (I71.-)
  - aneurysm (of) arteriovenous NOS (Q27.3-)
  - carotid artery dissection (I77.71)
  - cerebral (nonruptured) aneurysm (I67.1)
  - coronary aneurysm (I25.4)
  - coronary artery dissection (I25.42)
  - dissection of artery NEC (I77.79)
  - dissection of precerebral artery, congenital (nonruptured) (Q28.1)
  - heart aneurysm (I25.3)
  - iliac artery dissection (I77.72)
  - precerebral artery, congential (nonruptured) (Q28.1)
  - pulmonary artery aneurysm (I28.1)
  - renal artery dissection (I77.73)
  - retinal aneurysm (H35.0)
  - ruptured cerebral aneurysm (I60.7)
  - varicose aneurysm (I77.0)
  - vertebral artery dissection (I77.74)

AHA: 2016,4Q,28-29

- **I72.0** Aneurysm of **carotid** artery `ESR`
  Aneurysm of common carotid artery
  Aneurysm of external carotid artery
  Aneurysm of internal carotid artery, extracranial portion
  - **EXCLUDES 1** aneurysm of internal carotid artery, intracranial portion (I67.1)
    aneurysm of internal carotid artery NOS (I67.1)
- **I72.1** Aneurysm of artery of **upper extremity** `ESR`
- **I72.2** Aneurysm of **renal** artery `ESR`
- **I72.3** Aneurysm of **iliac** artery `ESR`
- **I72.4** Aneurysm of artery of **lower extremity** `ESR`
  AHA: 2019,2Q,21
- **I72.5** Aneurysm of other precerebral arteries `ESR`
  Aneurysm of basilar artery (trunk)
  - **EXCLUDES 2**
    - aneurysm of carotid artery (I72.0)
    - aneurysm of vertebral artery (I72.6)
    - dissection of carotid artery (I77.71)
    - dissection of other precerebral arteries (I77.75)
    - dissection of vertebral artery (I77.74)
- **I72.6** Aneurysm of **vertebral** artery `ESR`
  - **EXCLUDES 2** dissection of vertebral artery (I77.74)
- **I72.8** Aneurysm of other specified arteries `ESR`

I72.9 Aneurysm of unspecified site `ESR`

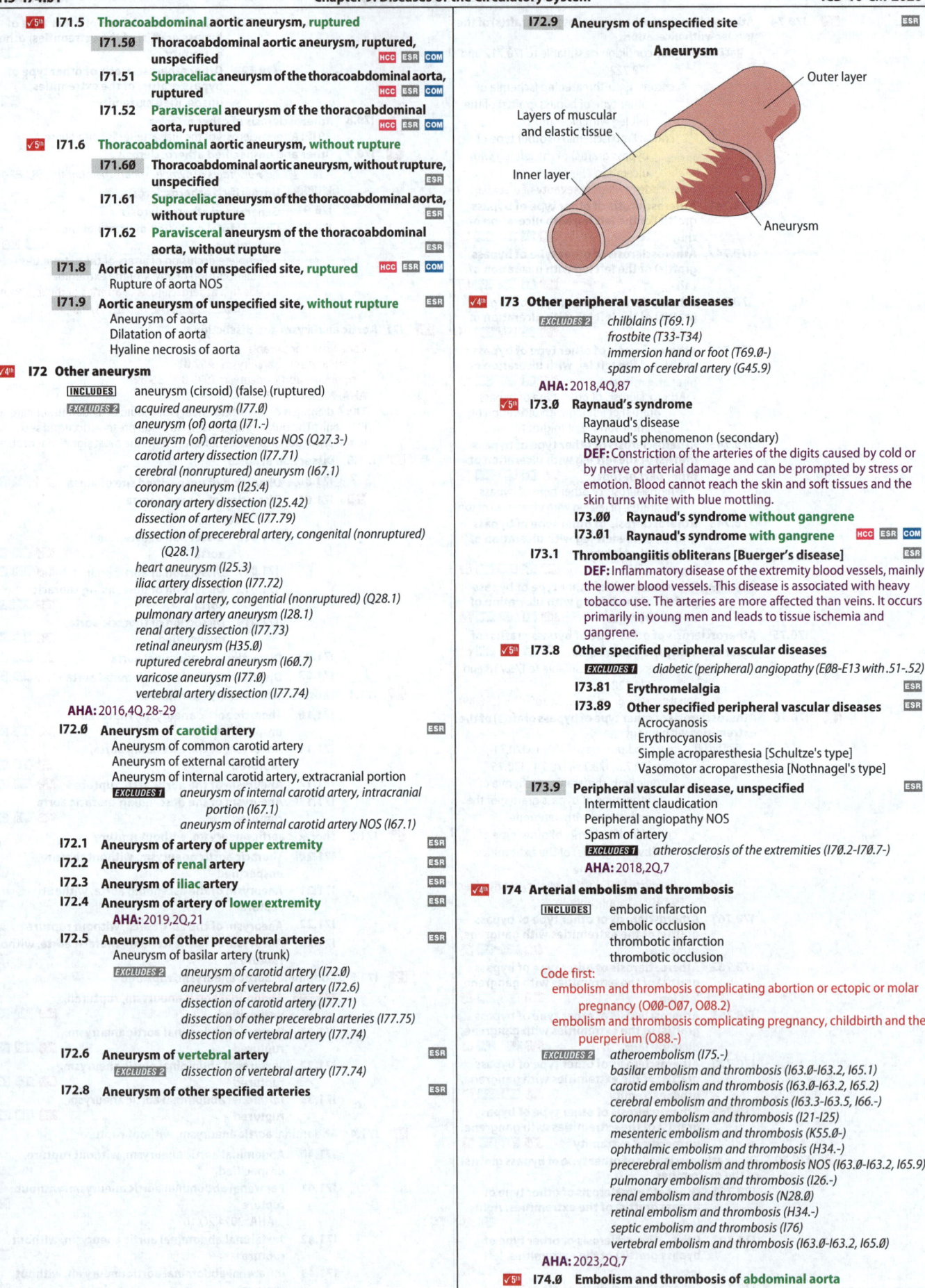
Aneurysm — Outer layer, Layers of muscular and elastic tissue, Inner layer, Aneurysm

I73 Other peripheral vascular diseases
- **EXCLUDES 2**
  - chilblains (T69.1)
  - frostbite (T33-T34)
  - immersion hand or foot (T69.0-)
  - spasm of cerebral artery (G45.9)

AHA: 2018,4Q,87

- **I73.0** Raynaud's syndrome
  Raynaud's disease
  Raynaud's phenomenon (secondary)
  DEF: Constriction of the arteries of the digits caused by cold or by nerve or arterial damage and can be prompted by stress or emotion. Blood cannot reach the skin and soft tissues and the skin turns white with blue mottling.
  - **I73.00** Raynaud's syndrome **without gangrene**
  - **I73.01** Raynaud's syndrome **with gangrene** `HCC` `ESR` `COM`
- **I73.1** Thromboangiitis obliterans [Buerger's disease] `ESR`
  DEF: Inflammatory disease of the extremity blood vessels, mainly the lower blood vessels. This disease is associated with heavy tobacco use. The arteries are more affected than veins. It occurs primarily in young men and leads to tissue ischemia and gangrene.
- **I73.8** Other specified peripheral vascular diseases
  - **EXCLUDES 1** diabetic (peripheral) angiopathy (E08-E13 with .51-.52)
  - **I73.81** Erythromelalgia
  - **I73.89** Other specified peripheral vascular diseases `ESR`
    Acrocyanosis
    Erythrocyanosis
    Simple acroparesthesia [Schultze's type]
    Vasomotor acroparesthesia [Nothnagel's type]
- **I73.9** Peripheral vascular disease, unspecified `ESR`
  Intermittent claudication
  Peripheral angiopathy NOS
  Spasm of artery
  - **EXCLUDES 1** atherosclerosis of the extremities (I70.2-I70.7-)
  AHA: 2018,2Q,7

I74 Arterial embolism and thrombosis
- **INCLUDES**
  - embolic infarction
  - embolic occlusion
  - thrombotic infarction
  - thrombotic occlusion
- **Code first:**
  - embolism and thrombosis complicating abortion or ectopic or molar pregnancy (O00-O07, O08.2)
  - embolism and thrombosis complicating pregnancy, childbirth and the puerperium (O88.-)
- **EXCLUDES 2**
  - atheroembolism (I75.-)
  - basilar embolism and thrombosis (I63.0-I63.2, I65.1)
  - carotid embolism and thrombosis (I63.0-I63.2, I65.2)
  - cerebral embolism and thrombosis (I63.3-I63.5, I66.-)
  - coronary embolism and thrombosis (I21-I25)
  - mesenteric embolism and thrombosis (K55.0-)
  - ophthalmic embolism and thrombosis (H34.-)
  - precerebral embolism and thrombosis NOS (I63.0-I63.2, I65.9)
  - pulmonary embolism and thrombosis (I26.-)
  - renal embolism and thrombosis (N28.0)
  - retinal embolism and thrombosis (H34.-)
  - septic embolism and thrombosis (I76)
  - vertebral embolism and thrombosis (I63.0-I63.2, I65.0)

AHA: 2023,2Q,7

- **I74.0** Embolism and thrombosis of **abdominal aorta**
  - **I74.01** **Saddle** embolus of abdominal aorta `HCC` `ESR` `COM`

`HCC` CMS-HCC `Rx` Rx HCC `ESR` ESRD HCC `COM` Commercial HCC **N** Newborn: 0 **P** Pediatric: 0-17 **M** Maternity: 9-64 **A** Adult: 15-124

Chapter 9. Diseases of the Circulatory System

I74.09 Other arterial embolism and thrombosis of abdominal aorta [HCC] [ESR] [COM]
- Aortic bifurcation syndrome
- Aortoiliac obstruction
- Leriche's syndrome

✓5th **I74.1** Embolism and thrombosis of other and unspecified parts of aorta
- **I74.10** Embolism and thrombosis of unspecified parts of aorta [HCC] [ESR] [COM]
- **I74.11** Embolism and thrombosis of thoracic aorta [HCC] [ESR] [COM]
- **I74.19** Embolism and thrombosis of other parts of aorta [HCC] [ESR] [COM]

I74.2 Embolism and thrombosis of arteries of the upper extremities [HCC] [ESR] [COM]

I74.3 Embolism and thrombosis of arteries of the lower extremities [HCC] [ESR] [COM]

I74.4 Embolism and thrombosis of arteries of extremities, unspecified [HCC] [ESR] [COM]
- Peripheral arterial embolism NOS

I74.5 Embolism and thrombosis of iliac artery [HCC] [ESR] [COM]

I74.8 Embolism and thrombosis of other arteries [HCC] [ESR] [COM]

I74.9 Embolism and thrombosis of unspecified artery [HCC] [ESR] [COM]

✓4th **I75** Atheroembolism
- INCLUDES: atherothrombotic microembolism, cholesterol embolism

✓5th **I75.0** Atheroembolism of extremities
- ✓6th **I75.01** Atheroembolism of upper extremity
  - **I75.011** Atheroembolism of right upper extremity [HCC] [ESR] [COM]
  - **I75.012** Atheroembolism of left upper extremity [HCC] [ESR] [COM]
  - **I75.013** Atheroembolism of bilateral upper extremities [HCC] [ESR] [COM]
  - **I75.019** Atheroembolism of unspecified upper extremity [HCC] [ESR] [COM]
- ✓6th **I75.02** Atheroembolism of lower extremity
  - **I75.021** Atheroembolism of right lower extremity [HCC] [ESR] [COM]
  - **I75.022** Atheroembolism of left lower extremity [HCC] [ESR] [COM]
  - **I75.023** Atheroembolism of bilateral lower extremities [HCC] [ESR] [COM]
  - **I75.029** Atheroembolism of unspecified lower extremity [HCC] [ESR] [COM]

✓5th **I75.8** Atheroembolism of other sites
- **I75.81** Atheroembolism of kidney [HCC] [ESR] [COM]
  - Use additional code for any associated acute kidney failure and chronic kidney disease (N17.-, N18.-)
- **I75.89** Atheroembolism of other site [HCC] [ESR] [COM]

I76 Septic arterial embolism [HCC] [ESR] [COM] [UPD]
- Code first underlying infection, such as:
  - infective endocarditis (I33.0)
  - lung abscess (J85.-)
- Use additional code to identify the site of the embolism (I74.-)
- EXCLUDES 2: septic pulmonary embolism (I26.01, I26.90)

✓4th **I77** Other disorders of arteries and arterioles
- EXCLUDES 2: collagen (vascular) diseases (M30-M36)
  - hypersensitivity angiitis (M31.0)
  - pulmonary artery (I28.-)

I77.0 Arteriovenous fistula, acquired [ESR]
- Aneurysmal varix
- Arteriovenous aneurysm, acquired
- EXCLUDES 1: arteriovenous aneurysm NOS (Q27.3-)
  - presence of arteriovenous shunt (fistula) for dialysis (Z99.2)
  - traumatic - see injury of blood vessel by body region
- EXCLUDES 2: cerebral (I67.1)
  - coronary (I25.4)
- DEF: Communication between an artery and vein caused by trauma or invasive procedures.

I77.1 Stricture of artery [ESR]
- Narrowing of artery
- AHA: 2021,3Q,12

I77.2 Rupture of artery [ESR]
- Erosion of artery
- Fistula of artery
- Ulcer of artery
- EXCLUDES 1: traumatic rupture of artery - see injury of blood vessel by body region

I77.3 Arterial fibromuscular dysplasia [ESR]
- Fibromuscular hyperplasia (of) carotid artery
- Fibromuscular hyperplasia (of) renal artery

I77.4 Celiac artery compression syndrome [ESR]
- AHA: 2021,3Q,12

I77.5 Necrosis of artery [ESR]

I77.6 Arteritis, unspecified [ESR]
- Aortitis NOS
- Endarteritis NOS
- EXCLUDES 1: arteritis or endarteritis:
  - aortic arch (M31.4)
  - cerebral NEC (I67.7)
  - coronary (I25.89)
  - deformans (I70.-)
  - giant cell (M31.5, M31.6)
  - obliterans (I70.-)
  - senile (I70.-)

✓5th **I77.7** Other arterial dissection
- EXCLUDES 2: dissection of aorta (I71.0-)
  - dissection of coronary artery (I25.42)
- AHA: 2016,4Q,28-29
- **I77.70** Dissection of unspecified artery [ESR] [COM]
- **I77.71** Dissection of carotid artery [ESR] [COM]
- **I77.72** Dissection of iliac artery [ESR] [COM]
- **I77.73** Dissection of renal artery [ESR] [COM]
- **I77.74** Dissection of vertebral artery [ESR] [COM]
  - EXCLUDES 2: aneurysm of vertebral artery (I72.6)
  - AHA: 2024,1Q,26
- **I77.75** Dissection of other precerebral arteries [ESR] [COM]
  - Dissection of basilar artery (trunk)
  - EXCLUDES 2: aneurysm of carotid artery (I72.0)
    - aneurysm of other precerebral arteries (I72.5)
    - aneurysm of vertebral artery (I72.6)
    - dissection of carotid artery (I77.71)
    - dissection of vertebral artery (I77.74)
- **I77.76** Dissection of artery of upper extremity [ESR] [COM]
- **I77.77** Dissection of artery of lower extremity [ESR] [COM]
- **I77.79** Dissection of other specified artery [ESR] [COM]

✓5th **I77.8** Other specified disorders of arteries and arterioles
- ✓6th **I77.81** Aortic ectasia
  - Ectasis aorta
  - EXCLUDES 1: aortic aneurysm and dissection (I71.-)
  - **I77.810** Thoracic aortic ectasia [ESR]
  - **I77.811** Abdominal aortic ectasia [ESR]
  - **I77.812** Thoracoabdominal aortic ectasia [ESR]
  - **I77.819** Aortic ectasia, unspecified site [ESR]
- **I77.82** Antineutrophilic cytoplasmic antibody [ANCA] vasculitis [HCC] [Rx] [ESR] [COM]
  - ANCA associated vasculitis
  - ANCA positive vasculitis
  - EXCLUDES 2: eosinophilic granulomatosis with polyangiitis (M30.1)
    - granulomatosis with polyangiitis (M31.3-)
    - microscopic polyangiitis (M31.7)
  - AHA: 2022,4Q,26-27
- **I77.89** Other specified disorders of arteries and arterioles [ESR]
  - AHA: 2021,1Q,23

I77.9 Disorder of arteries and arterioles, unspecified [ESR]
- AHA: 2021,1Q,4; 2018,2Q,7

✓4th **I78** Diseases of capillaries

I78.0 Hereditary hemorrhagic telangiectasia [ESR]
- Rendu-Osler-Weber disease

Chapter 9. Diseases of the Circulatory System

I78.1 Nevus, non-neoplastic
Araneus nevus
Senile nevus
Spider nevus
Stellar nevus
EXCLUDES 1 nevus NOS (D22.-)
vascular NOS (Q82.5)
EXCLUDES 2 blue nevus (D22.-)
flammeus nevus (Q82.5)
hairy nevus (D22.-)
melanocytic nevus (D22.-)
pigmented nevus (D22.-)
portwine nevus (Q82.5)
sanguineous nevus (Q82.5)
strawberry nevus (Q82.5)
verrucous nevus (Q82.5)
AHA: 2019,1Q,21

I78.8 Other diseases of capillaries
I78.9 Disease of capillaries, unspecified

✓4th **I79** Disorders of arteries, arterioles and capillaries in diseases classified elsewhere

I79.0 Aneurysm of aorta in diseases classified elsewhere [ESR]
Code first underlying disease
EXCLUDES 1 syphilitic aneurysm (A52.01)

I79.1 Aortitis in diseases classified elsewhere [ESR]
Code first underlying disease
EXCLUDES 1 syphilitic aortitis (A52.02)

I79.8 Other disorders of arteries, arterioles and capillaries in diseases classified elsewhere [ESR]
Code first underlying disease, such as:
amyloidosis (E85.-)
EXCLUDES 1 diabetic (peripheral) angiopathy (E08-E13 with .51-.52)
syphilitic endarteritis (A52.09)
tuberculous endarteritis (A18.89)

Diseases of veins, lymphatic vessels and lymph nodes, not elsewhere classified (I80-I89)

✓4th **I80** Phlebitis and thrombophlebitis
INCLUDES endophlebitis
inflammation, vein
periphlebitis
suppurative phlebitis
▶Code first, if applicable:◀
phlebitis and thrombophlebitis complicating abortion, ectopic or molar pregnancy (O00-O07, O08.7)
phlebitis and thrombophlebitis complicating pregnancy, childbirth and the puerperium (O22.-, O87.-)
EXCLUDES 1 venous embolism and thrombosis of lower extremities (I82.4-, I82.5-, I82.81-)

✓5th **I80.0** Phlebitis and thrombophlebitis of superficial vessels of lower extremities
Phlebitis and thrombophlebitis of femoropopliteal vein

I80.00 Phlebitis and thrombophlebitis of superficial vessels of unspecified lower extremity
I80.01 Phlebitis and thrombophlebitis of superficial vessels of right lower extremity
I80.02 Phlebitis and thrombophlebitis of superficial vessels of left lower extremity
I80.03 Phlebitis and thrombophlebitis of superficial vessels of lower extremities, bilateral

✓5th **I80.1** Phlebitis and thrombophlebitis of femoral vein
Phlebitis and thrombophlebitis of common femoral vein
Phlebitis and thrombophlebitis of deep femoral vein

I80.10 Phlebitis and thrombophlebitis of unspecified femoral vein [HCC Rx ESR COM]
I80.11 Phlebitis and thrombophlebitis of right femoral vein [HCC Rx ESR COM]
I80.12 Phlebitis and thrombophlebitis of left femoral vein [HCC Rx ESR COM]
I80.13 Phlebitis and thrombophlebitis of femoral vein, bilateral [HCC Rx ESR COM]

✓5th **I80.2** Phlebitis and thrombophlebitis of other and unspecified deep vessels of lower extremities

✓6th **I80.20** Phlebitis and thrombophlebitis of unspecified deep vessels of lower extremities
I80.201 Phlebitis and thrombophlebitis of unspecified deep vessels of right lower extremity [HCC Rx ESR COM]
I80.202 Phlebitis and thrombophlebitis of unspecified deep vessels of left lower extremity [HCC Rx ESR COM]
I80.203 Phlebitis and thrombophlebitis of unspecified deep vessels of lower extremities, bilateral [HCC Rx ESR COM]
I80.209 Phlebitis and thrombophlebitis of unspecified deep vessels of unspecified lower extremity [HCC Rx ESR COM]

✓6th **I80.21** Phlebitis and thrombophlebitis of iliac vein
Phlebitis and thrombophlebitis of common iliac vein
Phlebitis and thrombophlebitis of external iliac vein
Phlebitis and thrombophlebitis of internal iliac vein
I80.211 Phlebitis and thrombophlebitis of right iliac vein [HCC Rx ESR COM]
I80.212 Phlebitis and thrombophlebitis of left iliac vein [HCC Rx ESR COM]
I80.213 Phlebitis and thrombophlebitis of iliac vein, bilateral [HCC Rx ESR COM]
I80.219 Phlebitis and thrombophlebitis of unspecified iliac vein [HCC Rx ESR COM]

✓6th **I80.22** Phlebitis and thrombophlebitis of popliteal vein
I80.221 Phlebitis and thrombophlebitis of right popliteal vein [HCC Rx ESR COM]
I80.222 Phlebitis and thrombophlebitis of left popliteal vein [HCC Rx ESR COM]
I80.223 Phlebitis and thrombophlebitis of popliteal vein, bilateral [HCC Rx ESR COM]
I80.229 Phlebitis and thrombophlebitis of unspecified popliteal vein [HCC Rx ESR COM]

✓6th **I80.23** Phlebitis and thrombophlebitis of tibial vein
Phlebitis and thrombophlebitis of anterior tibial vein
Phlebitis and thrombophlebitis of posterior tibial vein
I80.231 Phlebitis and thrombophlebitis of right tibial vein [HCC Rx ESR COM]
I80.232 Phlebitis and thrombophlebitis of left tibial vein [HCC Rx ESR COM]
I80.233 Phlebitis and thrombophlebitis of tibial vein, bilateral [HCC Rx ESR COM]
I80.239 Phlebitis and thrombophlebitis of unspecified tibial vein [HCC Rx ESR COM]

✓6th **I80.24** Phlebitis and thrombophlebitis of peroneal vein
AHA: 2019,4Q,8
I80.241 Phlebitis and thrombophlebitis of right peroneal vein [HCC Rx ESR COM]
I80.242 Phlebitis and thrombophlebitis of left peroneal vein [HCC Rx ESR COM]
I80.243 Phlebitis and thrombophlebitis of peroneal vein, bilateral [HCC Rx ESR COM]
I80.249 Phlebitis and thrombophlebitis of unspecified peroneal vein [HCC Rx ESR COM]

✓6th **I80.25** Phlebitis and thrombophlebitis of calf muscular vein
Phlebitis and thrombophlebitis of calf muscular vein, NOS
Phlebitis and thrombophlebitis of gastrocnemial vein
Phlebitis and thrombophlebitis of soleal vein
AHA: 2019,4Q,8
I80.251 Phlebitis and thrombophlebitis of right calf muscular vein [HCC Rx ESR COM]
I80.252 Phlebitis and thrombophlebitis of left calf muscular vein [HCC Rx ESR COM]
I80.253 Phlebitis and thrombophlebitis of calf muscular vein, bilateral [HCC Rx ESR COM]
I80.259 Phlebitis and thrombophlebitis of unspecified calf muscular vein [HCC Rx ESR COM]

✓6th **I80.29** Phlebitis and thrombophlebitis of other deep vessels of lower extremities
I80.291 Phlebitis and thrombophlebitis of other deep vessels of right lower extremity [HCC Rx ESR COM]
I80.292 Phlebitis and thrombophlebitis of other deep vessels of left lower extremity [HCC Rx ESR COM]
I80.293 Phlebitis and thrombophlebitis of other deep vessels of lower extremity, bilateral [HCC Rx ESR COM]

[HCC] CMS-HCC [Rx] Rx HCC [ESR] ESRD HCC [COM] Commercial HCC [N] Newborn: 0 [P] Pediatric: 0-17 [M] Maternity: 9-64 [A] Adult: 15-124

- **I80.299** Phlebitis and thrombophlebitis of other deep vessels of unspecified lower extremity [HCC Rx ESR COM]
- **I80.3** Phlebitis and thrombophlebitis of lower extremities, unspecified
- **I80.8** Phlebitis and thrombophlebitis of other sites
- **I80.9** Phlebitis and thrombophlebitis of unspecified site

I81 Portal vein thrombosis
Portal (vein) obstruction

EXCLUDES 2: hepatic vein thrombosis (I82.0)
phlebitis of portal vein (K75.1)

AHA: 2019,4Q,68

✓4th I82 Other venous embolism and thrombosis
Code first venous embolism and thrombosis complicating:
abortion, ectopic or molar pregnancy (O00-O07, O08.7)
pregnancy, childbirth and the puerperium (O22.-, O87.-)

EXCLUDES 2: venous embolism and thrombosis (of):
cerebral (I63.6, I67.6)
coronary (I21-I25)
intracranial and intraspinal, septic or NOS (G08)
intracranial, nonpyogenic (I67.6)
intraspinal, nonpyogenic (G95.1)
mesenteric (K55.0-)
portal (I81)
pulmonary (I26.-)

- **I82.0** Budd-Chiari syndrome [HCC Rx ESR COM]
  Hepatic vein thrombosis
  DEF: Thrombosis or other obstruction of the hepatic veins. Symptoms include an enlarged liver, extensive collateral vessels, intractable ascites, and severe portal hypertension.
- **I82.1** Thrombophlebitis migrans
- ✓5th **I82.2** Embolism and thrombosis of vena cava and other thoracic veins
  - ✓6th **I82.21** Embolism and thrombosis of superior vena cava
    - **I82.210** Acute embolism and thrombosis of superior vena cava [HCC Rx ESR COM]
      Embolism and thrombosis of superior vena cava NOS
    - **I82.211** Chronic embolism and thrombosis of superior vena cava [HCC Rx ESR COM]
  - ✓6th **I82.22** Embolism and thrombosis of inferior vena cava
    - **I82.220** Acute embolism and thrombosis of inferior vena cava [HCC Rx ESR COM]
      Embolism and thrombosis of inferior vena cava NOS
    - **I82.221** Chronic embolism and thrombosis of inferior vena cava [HCC Rx ESR COM]
  - ✓6th **I82.29** Embolism and thrombosis of other thoracic veins
    Embolism and thrombosis of brachiocephalic (innominate) vein
    - **I82.290** Acute embolism and thrombosis of other thoracic veins [HCC Rx ESR COM]
    - **I82.291** Chronic embolism and thrombosis of other thoracic veins [HCC Rx ESR COM]
- **I82.3** Embolism and thrombosis of renal vein [HCC Rx ESR COM]
- ✓5th **I82.4** Acute embolism and thrombosis of deep veins of lower extremity
  - ✓6th **I82.40** Acute embolism and thrombosis of unspecified deep veins of lower extremity
    Deep vein thrombosis NOS
    DVT NOS
    EXCLUDES 1: acute embolism and thrombosis of unspecified deep veins of distal lower extremity (I82.4Z-)
    acute embolism and thrombosis of unspecified deep veins of proximal lower extremity (I82.4Y-)
    - **I82.401** Acute embolism and thrombosis of unspecified deep veins of right lower extremity [HCC Rx ESR COM]
    - **I82.402** Acute embolism and thrombosis of unspecified deep veins of left lower extremity [HCC Rx ESR COM]
    - **I82.403** Acute embolism and thrombosis of unspecified deep veins of lower extremity, bilateral [HCC Rx ESR COM]
    - **I82.409** Acute embolism and thrombosis of unspecified deep veins of unspecified lower extremity [HCC Rx ESR COM]
  - ✓6th **I82.41** Acute embolism and thrombosis of femoral vein
    Acute embolism and thrombosis of common femoral vein
    Acute embolism and thrombosis of deep femoral vein
    AHA: 2023,3Q,12
    - **I82.411** Acute embolism and thrombosis of right femoral vein [HCC Rx ESR COM]
    - **I82.412** Acute embolism and thrombosis of left femoral vein [HCC Rx ESR COM]
    - **I82.413** Acute embolism and thrombosis of femoral vein, bilateral
    - **I82.419** Acute embolism and thrombosis of unspecified femoral vein [HCC Rx ESR COM]
  - ✓6th **I82.42** Acute embolism and thrombosis of iliac vein
    Acute embolism and thrombosis of common iliac vein
    Acute embolism and thrombosis of external iliac vein
    Acute embolism and thrombosis of internal iliac vein
    - **I82.421** Acute embolism and thrombosis of right iliac vein [HCC Rx ESR COM]
    - **I82.422** Acute embolism and thrombosis of left iliac vein [HCC Rx ESR COM]
    - **I82.423** Acute embolism and thrombosis of iliac vein, bilateral
    - **I82.429** Acute embolism and thrombosis of unspecified iliac vein [HCC Rx ESR COM]
  - ✓6th **I82.43** Acute embolism and thrombosis of popliteal vein
    - **I82.431** Acute embolism and thrombosis of right popliteal vein [HCC Rx ESR COM]
    - **I82.432** Acute embolism and thrombosis of left popliteal vein
    - **I82.433** Acute embolism and thrombosis of popliteal vein, bilateral [HCC Rx ESR COM]
    - **I82.439** Acute embolism and thrombosis of unspecified popliteal vein [HCC Rx ESR COM]
  - ✓6th **I82.44** Acute embolism and thrombosis of tibial vein
    Acute embolism and thrombosis of anterior tibial vein
    Acute embolism and thrombosis of posterior tibial vein
    - **I82.441** Acute embolism and thrombosis of right tibial vein [HCC Rx ESR COM]
    - **I82.442** Acute embolism and thrombosis of left tibial vein [HCC Rx ESR COM]
    - **I82.443** Acute embolism and thrombosis of tibial vein, bilateral [HCC Rx ESR COM]
    - **I82.449** Acute embolism and thrombosis of unspecified tibial vein
  - ✓6th **I82.45** Acute embolism and thrombosis of peroneal vein
    AHA: 2019,4Q,8-10
    - **I82.451** Acute embolism and thrombosis of right peroneal vein [HCC Rx ESR COM]
    - **I82.452** Acute embolism and thrombosis of left peroneal vein [HCC Rx ESR COM]
    - **I82.453** Acute embolism and thrombosis of peroneal vein, bilateral
    - **I82.459** Acute embolism and thrombosis of unspecified peroneal vein [HCC Rx ESR COM]
  - ✓6th **I82.46** Acute embolism and thrombosis of calf muscular vein
    Acute embolism and thrombosis of calf muscular vein, NOS
    Acute embolism and thrombosis of gastrocnemial vein
    Acute embolism and thrombosis of soleal vein
    AHA: 2019,4Q,8-10
    - **I82.461** Acute embolism and thrombosis of right calf muscular vein [HCC Rx ESR COM]
    - **I82.462** Acute embolism and thrombosis of left calf muscular vein [HCC Rx ESR COM]
    - **I82.463** Acute embolism and thrombosis of calf muscular vein, bilateral [HCC Rx ESR COM]
    - **I82.469** Acute embolism and thrombosis of unspecified calf muscular vein [HCC Rx ESR COM]
  - ✓6th **I82.49** Acute embolism and thrombosis of other specified deep vein of lower extremity
    - **I82.491** Acute embolism and thrombosis of other specified deep vein of right lower extremity [HCC Rx ESR COM]

Chapter 9. Diseases of the Circulatory System

- **I82.492** Acute embolism and thrombosis of other specified deep vein of **left** lower extremity `HCC` `Rx` `ESR` `COM`
- **I82.493** Acute embolism and thrombosis of other specified deep vein of lower extremity, **bilateral** `HCC` `Rx` `ESR` `COM`
- **I82.499** Acute embolism and thrombosis of other specified deep vein of unspecified lower extremity `HCC` `Rx` `ESR` `COM`

✓6ᵗʰ I82.4Y Acute embolism and thrombosis of unspecified deep veins of **proximal** lower extremity
Acute embolism and thrombosis of deep vein of thigh NOS
Acute embolism and thrombosis of deep vein of upper leg NOS
- **I82.4Y1** Acute embolism and thrombosis of unspecified deep veins of **right** proximal lower extremity `HCC` `Rx` `ESR` `COM`
- **I82.4Y2** Acute embolism and thrombosis of unspecified deep veins of **left** proximal lower extremity `HCC` `Rx` `ESR` `COM`
- **I82.4Y3** Acute embolism and thrombosis of unspecified deep veins of proximal lower extremity, **bilateral** `HCC` `Rx` `ESR` `COM`
- **I82.4Y9** Acute embolism and thrombosis of unspecified deep veins of unspecified proximal lower extremity `HCC` `Rx` `ESR` `COM`

✓6ᵗʰ I82.4Z Acute embolism and thrombosis of unspecified deep veins of **distal** lower extremity
Acute embolism and thrombosis of deep vein of calf NOS
Acute embolism and thrombosis of deep vein of lower leg NOS
- **I82.4Z1** Acute embolism and thrombosis of unspecified deep veins of **right** distal lower extremity `HCC` `Rx` `ESR` `COM`
- **I82.4Z2** Acute embolism and thrombosis of unspecified deep veins of **left** distal lower extremity `HCC` `Rx` `ESR` `COM`
- **I82.4Z3** Acute embolism and thrombosis of unspecified deep veins of distal lower extremity, **bilateral** `HCC` `Rx` `ESR` `COM`
- **I82.4Z9** Acute embolism and thrombosis of unspecified deep veins of unspecified distal lower extremity `HCC` `Rx` `ESR` `COM`

✓5ᵗʰ I82.5 **Chronic** embolism and thrombosis of **deep veins of lower extremity**
Use additional code, if applicable, for associated long-term (current) use of anticoagulants (Z79.01)
EXCLUDES 1 personal history of venous embolism and thrombosis (Z86.718)
AHA: 2020,2Q,20

✓6ᵗʰ I82.50 Chronic embolism and thrombosis of unspecified deep veins of lower extremity
EXCLUDES 1 chronic embolism and thrombosis of unspecified deep veins of distal lower extremity (I82.5Z-)
chronic embolism and thrombosis of unspecified deep veins of proximal lower extremity (I82.5Y-)
- **I82.501** Chronic embolism and thrombosis of unspecified deep veins of **right** lower extremity `HCC` `Rx` `ESR` `COM`
- **I82.502** Chronic embolism and thrombosis of unspecified deep veins of **left** lower extremity `HCC` `Rx` `ESR` `COM`
- **I82.503** Chronic embolism and thrombosis of unspecified deep veins of lower extremity, **bilateral** `HCC` `Rx` `ESR` `COM`
- **I82.509** Chronic embolism and thrombosis of unspecified deep veins of unspecified lower extremity `HCC` `Rx` `ESR` `COM`

✓6ᵗʰ I82.51 Chronic embolism and thrombosis of **femoral vein**
Chronic embolism and thrombosis of common femoral vein
Chronic embolism and thrombosis of deep femoral vein
- **I82.511** Chronic embolism and thrombosis of **right** femoral vein `HCC` `Rx` `ESR` `COM`
- **I82.512** Chronic embolism and thrombosis of **left** femoral vein `HCC` `Rx` `ESR` `COM`
- **I82.513** Chronic embolism and thrombosis of femoral vein, **bilateral** `HCC` `Rx` `ESR` `COM`
- **I82.519** Chronic embolism and thrombosis of unspecified femoral vein `HCC` `Rx` `ESR` `COM`

✓6ᵗʰ I82.52 Chronic embolism and thrombosis of **iliac vein**
Chronic embolism and thrombosis of common iliac vein
Chronic embolism and thrombosis of external iliac vein
Chronic embolism and thrombosis of internal iliac vein
- **I82.521** Chronic embolism and thrombosis of **right** iliac vein `HCC` `Rx` `ESR` `COM`
- **I82.522** Chronic embolism and thrombosis of **left** iliac vein `HCC` `Rx` `ESR` `COM`
- **I82.523** Chronic embolism and thrombosis of iliac vein, **bilateral** `HCC` `Rx` `ESR` `COM`
- **I82.529** Chronic embolism and thrombosis of unspecified iliac vein `HCC` `Rx` `ESR` `COM`

✓6ᵗʰ I82.53 Chronic embolism and thrombosis of **popliteal vein**
- **I82.531** Chronic embolism and thrombosis of **right** popliteal vein `HCC` `Rx` `ESR` `COM`
- **I82.532** Chronic embolism and thrombosis of **left** popliteal vein `HCC` `Rx` `ESR` `COM`
- **I82.533** Chronic embolism and thrombosis of popliteal vein, **bilateral** `HCC` `Rx` `ESR` `COM`
- **I82.539** Chronic embolism and thrombosis of unspecified popliteal vein `HCC` `Rx` `ESR` `COM`

✓6ᵗʰ I82.54 Chronic embolism and thrombosis of **tibial vein**
Chronic embolism and thrombosis of anterior tibial vein
Chronic embolism and thrombosis of posterior tibial vein
- **I82.541** Chronic embolism and thrombosis of **right** tibial vein `HCC` `Rx` `ESR` `COM`
- **I82.542** Chronic embolism and thrombosis of **left** tibial vein `HCC` `Rx` `ESR` `COM`
- **I82.543** Chronic embolism and thrombosis of tibial vein, **bilateral** `HCC` `Rx` `ESR` `COM`
- **I82.549** Chronic embolism and thrombosis of unspecified tibial vein `HCC` `Rx` `ESR` `COM`

✓6ᵗʰ I82.55 Chronic embolism and thrombosis of **peroneal vein**
AHA: 2019,4Q,8-10
- **I82.551** Chronic embolism and thrombosis of **right** peroneal vein `HCC` `Rx` `ESR` `COM`
- **I82.552** Chronic embolism and thrombosis of **left** peroneal vein `HCC` `Rx` `ESR` `COM`
- **I82.553** Chronic embolism and thrombosis of peroneal vein, **bilateral** `HCC` `Rx` `ESR` `COM`
- **I82.559** Chronic embolism and thrombosis of unspecified peroneal vein `HCC` `Rx` `ESR` `COM`

✓6ᵗʰ I82.56 Chronic embolism and thrombosis of **calf muscular vein**
Chronic embolism and thrombosis of calf muscular vein NOS
Chronic embolism and thrombosis of gastrocnemial vein
Chronic embolism and thrombosis of soleal vein
AHA: 2019,4Q,8-10
- **I82.561** Chronic embolism and thrombosis of **right** calf muscular vein `HCC` `Rx` `ESR` `COM`
- **I82.562** Chronic embolism and thrombosis of **left** calf muscular vein `HCC` `Rx` `ESR` `COM`
- **I82.563** Chronic embolism and thrombosis of calf muscular vein, **bilateral** `HCC` `Rx` `ESR` `COM`
- **I82.569** Chronic embolism and thrombosis of unspecified calf muscular vein `HCC` `Rx` `ESR` `COM`

✓6ᵗʰ I82.59 Chronic embolism and thrombosis of other specified deep vein of lower extremity
- **I82.591** Chronic embolism and thrombosis of other specified deep vein of **right** lower extremity `HCC` `Rx` `ESR` `COM`
- **I82.592** Chronic embolism and thrombosis of other specified deep vein of **left** lower extremity `HCC` `Rx` `ESR` `COM`
- **I82.593** Chronic embolism and thrombosis of other specified deep vein of lower extremity, **bilateral** `HCC` `Rx` `ESR` `COM`

I82.599 Chronic embolism and thrombosis of other specified deep vein of unspecified lower extremity

✓6th **I82.5Y** Chronic embolism and thrombosis of unspecified deep veins of proximal lower extremity
Chronic embolism and thrombosis of deep veins of thigh NOS
Chronic embolism and thrombosis of deep veins of upper leg NOS

I82.5Y1 Chronic embolism and thrombosis of unspecified deep veins of right proximal lower extremity

I82.5Y2 Chronic embolism and thrombosis of unspecified deep veins of left proximal lower extremity

I82.5Y3 Chronic embolism and thrombosis of unspecified deep veins of proximal lower extremity, bilateral

I82.5Y9 Chronic embolism and thrombosis of unspecified deep veins of unspecified proximal lower extremity

✓6th **I82.5Z** Chronic embolism and thrombosis of unspecified deep veins of distal lower extremity
Chronic embolism and thrombosis of deep veins of calf NOS
Chronic embolism and thrombosis of deep veins of lower leg NOS

I82.5Z1 Chronic embolism and thrombosis of unspecified deep veins of right distal lower extremity

I82.5Z2 Chronic embolism and thrombosis of unspecified deep veins of left distal lower extremity

I82.5Z3 Chronic embolism and thrombosis of unspecified deep veins of distal lower extremity, bilateral

I82.5Z9 Chronic embolism and thrombosis of unspecified deep veins of unspecified distal lower extremity

✓5th **I82.6** Acute embolism and thrombosis of veins of upper extremity

✓6th **I82.60** Acute embolism and thrombosis of unspecified veins of upper extremity

I82.601 Acute embolism and thrombosis of unspecified veins of right upper extremity

I82.602 Acute embolism and thrombosis of unspecified veins of left upper extremity

I82.603 Acute embolism and thrombosis of unspecified veins of upper extremity, bilateral

I82.609 Acute embolism and thrombosis of unspecified veins of unspecified upper extremity

✓6th **I82.61** Acute embolism and thrombosis of superficial veins of upper extremity
Acute embolism and thrombosis of antecubital vein
Acute embolism and thrombosis of basilic vein
Acute embolism and thrombosis of cephalic vein

I82.611 Acute embolism and thrombosis of superficial veins of right upper extremity

I82.612 Acute embolism and thrombosis of superficial veins of left upper extremity

I82.613 Acute embolism and thrombosis of superficial veins of upper extremity, bilateral

I82.619 Acute embolism and thrombosis of superficial veins of unspecified upper extremity

✓6th **I82.62** Acute embolism and thrombosis of deep veins of upper extremity
Acute embolism and thrombosis of brachial vein
Acute embolism and thrombosis of radial vein
Acute embolism and thrombosis of ulnar vein

I82.621 Acute embolism and thrombosis of deep veins of right upper extremity

I82.622 Acute embolism and thrombosis of deep veins of left upper extremity

I82.623 Acute embolism and thrombosis of deep veins of upper extremity, bilateral

I82.629 Acute embolism and thrombosis of deep veins of unspecified upper extremity

✓5th **I82.7** Chronic embolism and thrombosis of veins of upper extremity
Use additional code, if applicable, for associated long-term (current) use of anticoagulants (Z79.01)
EXCLUDES 1 personal history of venous embolism and thrombosis (Z86.718)

✓6th **I82.70** Chronic embolism and thrombosis of unspecified veins of upper extremity

I82.701 Chronic embolism and thrombosis of unspecified veins of right upper extremity

I82.702 Chronic embolism and thrombosis of unspecified veins of left upper extremity

I82.703 Chronic embolism and thrombosis of unspecified veins of upper extremity, bilateral

I82.709 Chronic embolism and thrombosis of unspecified veins of unspecified upper extremity

✓6th **I82.71** Chronic embolism and thrombosis of superficial veins of upper extremity
Chronic embolism and thrombosis of antecubital vein
Chronic embolism and thrombosis of basilic vein
Chronic embolism and thrombosis of cephalic vein

I82.711 Chronic embolism and thrombosis of superficial veins of right upper extremity

I82.712 Chronic embolism and thrombosis of superficial veins of left upper extremity

I82.713 Chronic embolism and thrombosis of superficial veins of upper extremity, bilateral

I82.719 Chronic embolism and thrombosis of superficial veins of unspecified upper extremity

✓6th **I82.72** Chronic embolism and thrombosis of deep veins of upper extremity
Chronic embolism and thrombosis of brachial vein
Chronic embolism and thrombosis of radial vein
Chronic embolism and thrombosis of ulnar vein

I82.721 Chronic embolism and thrombosis of deep veins of right upper extremity

I82.722 Chronic embolism and thrombosis of deep veins of left upper extremity

I82.723 Chronic embolism and thrombosis of deep veins of upper extremity, bilateral

I82.729 Chronic embolism and thrombosis of deep veins of unspecified upper extremity

✓5th **I82.A** Embolism and thrombosis of axillary vein

✓6th **I82.A1** Acute embolism and thrombosis of axillary vein

I82.A11 Acute embolism and thrombosis of right axillary vein

I82.A12 Acute embolism and thrombosis of left axillary vein

I82.A13 Acute embolism and thrombosis of axillary vein, bilateral

I82.A19 Acute embolism and thrombosis of unspecified axillary vein

✓6th **I82.A2** Chronic embolism and thrombosis of axillary vein

I82.A21 Chronic embolism and thrombosis of right axillary vein

I82.A22 Chronic embolism and thrombosis of left axillary vein

I82.A23 Chronic embolism and thrombosis of axillary vein, bilateral

I82.A29 Chronic embolism and thrombosis of unspecified axillary vein

✓5th **I82.B** Embolism and thrombosis of subclavian vein

✓6th **I82.B1** Acute embolism and thrombosis of subclavian vein

I82.B11 Acute embolism and thrombosis of right subclavian vein

I82.B12 Acute embolism and thrombosis of left subclavian vein

Chapter 9. Diseases of the Circulatory System

- **I82.B13** Acute embolism and thrombosis of subclavian vein, bilateral `HCC` `Rx` `ESR` `COM`
- **I82.B19** Acute embolism and thrombosis of unspecified subclavian vein `HCC` `Rx` `ESR` `COM`
- √6th **I82.B2** Chronic embolism and thrombosis of subclavian vein
  - **I82.B21** Chronic embolism and thrombosis of right subclavian vein `HCC` `Rx` `ESR` `COM`
  - **I82.B22** Chronic embolism and thrombosis of left subclavian vein `HCC` `Rx` `ESR` `COM`
  - **I82.B23** Chronic embolism and thrombosis of subclavian vein, bilateral `HCC` `Rx` `ESR` `COM`
  - **I82.B29** Chronic embolism and thrombosis of unspecified subclavian vein `HCC` `Rx` `ESR` `COM`
- √5th **I82.C** Embolism and thrombosis of internal jugular vein
  - √6th **I82.C1** Acute embolism and thrombosis of internal jugular vein
    - **I82.C11** Acute embolism and thrombosis of right internal jugular vein `HCC` `Rx` `ESR` `COM`
    - **I82.C12** Acute embolism and thrombosis of left internal jugular vein `HCC` `Rx` `ESR` `COM`
    - **I82.C13** Acute embolism and thrombosis of internal jugular vein, bilateral `HCC` `Rx` `ESR` `COM`
    - **I82.C19** Acute embolism and thrombosis of unspecified internal jugular vein `HCC` `Rx` `ESR` `COM`
  - √6th **I82.C2** Chronic embolism and thrombosis of internal jugular vein
    - **I82.C21** Chronic embolism and thrombosis of right internal jugular vein `HCC` `Rx` `ESR` `COM`
    - **I82.C22** Chronic embolism and thrombosis of left internal jugular vein `HCC` `Rx` `ESR` `COM`
    - **I82.C23** Chronic embolism and thrombosis of internal jugular vein, bilateral `HCC` `Rx` `ESR` `COM`
    - **I82.C29** Chronic embolism and thrombosis of unspecified internal jugular vein `HCC` `Rx` `ESR` `COM`
- √5th **I82.8** Embolism and thrombosis of other specified veins
  - *Use additional code, if applicable, for associated long-term (current) use of anticoagulants (Z79.01)*
  - √6th **I82.81** Embolism and thrombosis of superficial veins of lower extremities
    - Embolism and thrombosis of saphenous vein (greater) (lesser)
    - **I82.811** Embolism and thrombosis of superficial veins of right lower extremity
    - **I82.812** Embolism and thrombosis of superficial veins of left lower extremity
    - **I82.813** Embolism and thrombosis of superficial veins of lower extremities, bilateral
    - **I82.819** Embolism and thrombosis of superficial veins of unspecified lower extremity
  - √6th **I82.89** Embolism and thrombosis of other specified veins
    - **I82.890** Acute embolism and thrombosis of other specified veins
    - **I82.891** Chronic embolism and thrombosis of other specified veins
- √5th **I82.9** Embolism and thrombosis of unspecified vein
  - **I82.90** Acute embolism and thrombosis of unspecified vein
    - Embolism of vein NOS
    - Thrombosis (vein) NOS
  - **I82.91** Chronic embolism and thrombosis of unspecified vein
- √4th **I83** Varicose veins of lower extremities
  - EXCLUDES 2 *varicose veins complicating pregnancy (O22.0-)*
    varicose veins complicating the puerperium (O87.4)
  - √5th **I83.0** Varicose veins of lower extremities with ulcer
    - *Use additional code to identify severity of ulcer (L97.-)*
    - √6th **I83.00** Varicose veins of unspecified lower extremity with ulcer
      - **I83.001** Varicose veins of unspecified lower extremity with ulcer of thigh `HCC` `ESR` `COM` `A`
      - **I83.002** Varicose veins of unspecified lower extremity with ulcer of calf `HCC` `ESR` `COM` `A`
      - **I83.003** Varicose veins of unspecified lower extremity with ulcer of ankle `HCC` `ESR` `COM` `A`
      - **I83.004** Varicose veins of unspecified lower extremity with ulcer of heel and midfoot `HCC` `ESR` `COM` `A`
        - Varicose veins of unspecified lower extremity with ulcer of plantar surface of midfoot
      - **I83.005** Varicose veins of unspecified lower extremity with ulcer other part of foot `HCC` `ESR` `COM` `A`
        - Varicose veins of unspecified lower extremity with ulcer of toe
      - **I83.008** Varicose veins of unspecified lower extremity with ulcer other part of lower leg `HCC` `ESR` `COM` `A`
      - **I83.009** Varicose veins of unspecified lower extremity with ulcer of unspecified site `HCC` `ESR` `COM` `A`
    - √6th **I83.01** Varicose veins of right lower extremity with ulcer
      - **I83.011** Varicose veins of right lower extremity with ulcer of thigh `HCC` `ESR` `COM` `A`
      - **I83.012** Varicose veins of right lower extremity with ulcer of calf `HCC` `ESR` `COM` `A`
      - **I83.013** Varicose veins of right lower extremity with ulcer of ankle `HCC` `ESR` `COM` `A`
      - **I83.014** Varicose veins of right lower extremity with ulcer of heel and midfoot `HCC` `ESR` `COM` `A`
        - Varicose veins of right lower extremity with ulcer of plantar surface of midfoot
      - **I83.015** Varicose veins of right lower extremity with ulcer other part of foot `HCC` `ESR` `COM` `A`
        - Varicose veins of right lower extremity with ulcer of toe
      - **I83.018** Varicose veins of right lower extremity with ulcer other part of lower leg `HCC` `ESR` `COM` `A`
      - **I83.019** Varicose veins of right lower extremity with ulcer of unspecified site `HCC` `ESR` `COM` `A`
    - √6th **I83.02** Varicose veins of left lower extremity with ulcer
      - **I83.021** Varicose veins of left lower extremity with ulcer of thigh `HCC` `ESR` `COM` `A`
      - **I83.022** Varicose veins of left lower extremity with ulcer of calf `HCC` `ESR` `COM` `A`
      - **I83.023** Varicose veins of left lower extremity with ulcer of ankle `HCC` `ESR` `COM` `A`
      - **I83.024** Varicose veins of left lower extremity with ulcer of heel and midfoot `HCC` `ESR` `COM` `A`
        - Varicose veins of left lower extremity with ulcer of plantar surface of midfoot
      - **I83.025** Varicose veins of left lower extremity with ulcer other part of foot `HCC` `ESR` `COM` `A`
        - Varicose veins of left lower extremity with ulcer of toe
      - **I83.028** Varicose veins of left lower extremity with ulcer other part of lower leg `HCC` `ESR` `COM` `A`
      - **I83.029** Varicose veins of left lower extremity with ulcer of unspecified site `HCC` `ESR` `COM` `A`
  - √5th **I83.1** Varicose veins of lower extremities with inflammation
    - **I83.10** Varicose veins of unspecified lower extremity with inflammation `A`
    - **I83.11** Varicose veins of right lower extremity with inflammation `A`
    - **I83.12** Varicose veins of left lower extremity with inflammation `A`

I83.2 Varicose veins of lower extremities with both ulcer and inflammation
Use additional code to identify severity of ulcer (L97.-)

I83.20 Varicose veins of unspecified lower extremity with both ulcer and inflammation
- **I83.201** Varicose veins of unspecified lower extremity with both ulcer of thigh and inflammation
- **I83.202** Varicose veins of unspecified lower extremity with both ulcer of calf and inflammation
- **I83.203** Varicose veins of unspecified lower extremity with both ulcer of ankle and inflammation
- **I83.204** Varicose veins of unspecified lower extremity with both ulcer of heel and midfoot and inflammation
  - Varicose veins of unspecified lower extremity with both ulcer of plantar surface of midfoot and inflammation
- **I83.205** Varicose veins of unspecified lower extremity with both ulcer other part of foot and inflammation
  - Varicose veins of unspecified lower extremity with both ulcer of toe and inflammation
- **I83.208** Varicose veins of unspecified lower extremity with both ulcer of other part of lower extremity and inflammation
- **I83.209** Varicose veins of unspecified lower extremity with both ulcer of unspecified site and inflammation

I83.21 Varicose veins of right lower extremity with both ulcer and inflammation
- **I83.211** Varicose veins of right lower extremity with both ulcer of thigh and inflammation
- **I83.212** Varicose veins of right lower extremity with both ulcer of calf and inflammation
- **I83.213** Varicose veins of right lower extremity with both ulcer of ankle and inflammation
- **I83.214** Varicose veins of right lower extremity with both ulcer of heel and midfoot and inflammation
  - Varicose veins of right lower extremity with both ulcer of plantar surface of midfoot and inflammation
- **I83.215** Varicose veins of right lower extremity with both ulcer other part of foot and inflammation
  - Varicose veins of right lower extremity with both ulcer of toe and inflammation
- **I83.218** Varicose veins of right lower extremity with both ulcer of other part of lower extremity and inflammation
- **I83.219** Varicose veins of right lower extremity with both ulcer of unspecified site and inflammation

I83.22 Varicose veins of left lower extremity with both ulcer and inflammation
- **I83.221** Varicose veins of left lower extremity with both ulcer of thigh and inflammation
- **I83.222** Varicose veins of left lower extremity with both ulcer of calf and inflammation
- **I83.223** Varicose veins of left lower extremity with both ulcer of ankle and inflammation
- **I83.224** Varicose veins of left lower extremity with both ulcer of heel and midfoot and inflammation
  - Varicose veins of left lower extremity with both ulcer of plantar surface of midfoot and inflammation
- **I83.225** Varicose veins of left lower extremity with both ulcer other part of foot and inflammation
  - Varicose veins of left lower extremity with both ulcer of toe and inflammation
- **I83.228** Varicose veins of left lower extremity with both ulcer of other part of lower extremity and inflammation
- **I83.229** Varicose veins of left lower extremity with both ulcer of unspecified site and inflammation

I83.8 Varicose veins of lower extremities with other complications

I83.81 Varicose veins of lower extremities with pain
- **I83.811** Varicose veins of right lower extremity with pain
- **I83.812** Varicose veins of left lower extremity with pain
- **I83.813** Varicose veins of bilateral lower extremities with pain
- **I83.819** Varicose veins of unspecified lower extremity with pain

I83.89 Varicose veins of lower extremities with other complications
Varicose veins of lower extremities with edema
Varicose veins of lower extremities with swelling
- **I83.891** Varicose veins of right lower extremity with other complications
- **I83.892** Varicose veins of left lower extremity with other complications
- **I83.893** Varicose veins of bilateral lower extremities with other complications
- **I83.899** Varicose veins of unspecified lower extremity with other complications

I83.9 Asymptomatic varicose veins of lower extremities
Phlebectasia of lower extremities
Varicose veins of lower extremities
Varix of lower extremities

- **I83.90** Asymptomatic varicose veins of unspecified lower extremity
  - Varicose veins NOS
- **I83.91** Asymptomatic varicose veins of right lower extremity
- **I83.92** Asymptomatic varicose veins of left lower extremity
- **I83.93** Asymptomatic varicose veins of bilateral lower extremities

I85 Esophageal varices
Use additional code to identify:
alcohol abuse and dependence (F10.-)

I85.0 Esophageal varices
Idiopathic esophageal varices
Primary esophageal varices
- **I85.00** Esophageal varices without bleeding
  - Esophageal varices NOS
- **I85.01** Esophageal varices with bleeding

I85.1 Secondary esophageal varices
Esophageal varices secondary to alcoholic liver disease
Esophageal varices secondary to cirrhosis of liver
Esophageal varices secondary to schistosomiasis
Esophageal varices secondary to toxic liver disease
Code first underlying disease
- **I85.10** Secondary esophageal varices without bleeding
- **I85.11** Secondary esophageal varices with bleeding

I86 Varicose veins of other sites
EXCLUDES 1 varicose veins of unspecified site (I83.9-)
EXCLUDES 2 retinal varices (H35.0-)

- **I86.0** Sublingual varices
  - DEF: Distended, tortuous veins beneath the tongue.
- **I86.1** Scrotal varices
  - Varicocele
- **I86.2** Pelvic varices
- **I86.3** Vulval varices
  - EXCLUDES 1 vulval varices complicating childbirth and the puerperium (O87.8)
  - vulval varices complicating pregnancy (O22.1-)
- **I86.4** Gastric varices

Chapter 9. Diseases of the Circulatory System

I86.8 **Varicose veins of other specified sites**
Varicose ulcer of nasal septum

✓4th I87 Other disorders of veins

✓5th I87.0 Postthrombotic syndrome
Chronic venous hypertension due to deep vein thrombosis
Postphlebitic syndrome
EXCLUDES 1 chronic venous hypertension without deep vein thrombosis (I87.3-)

✓6th I87.00 Postthrombotic syndrome without complications
Asymptomatic postthrombotic syndrome

- **I87.001** Postthrombotic syndrome without complications of right lower extremity
- **I87.002** Postthrombotic syndrome without complications of left lower extremity
- **I87.003** Postthrombotic syndrome without complications of bilateral lower extremity
- **I87.009** Postthrombotic syndrome without complications of unspecified extremity
  Postthrombotic syndrome NOS

✓6th I87.01 Postthrombotic syndrome with ulcer
Use additional code to specify site and severity of ulcer (L97.-)

- **I87.011** Postthrombotic syndrome with ulcer of right lower extremity [HCC] [ESR] [COM]
- **I87.012** Postthrombotic syndrome with ulcer of left lower extremity [HCC] [ESR] [COM]
- **I87.013** Postthrombotic syndrome with ulcer of bilateral lower extremity [HCC] [ESR] [COM]
- **I87.019** Postthrombotic syndrome with ulcer of unspecified lower extremity [HCC] [ESR] [COM]

✓6th I87.02 Postthrombotic syndrome with inflammation

- **I87.021** Postthrombotic syndrome with inflammation of right lower extremity
- **I87.022** Postthrombotic syndrome with inflammation of left lower extremity
- **I87.023** Postthrombotic syndrome with inflammation of bilateral lower extremity
- **I87.029** Postthrombotic syndrome with inflammation of unspecified lower extremity

✓6th I87.03 Postthrombotic syndrome with ulcer and inflammation
Use additional code to specify site and severity of ulcer (L97.-)

- **I87.031** Postthrombotic syndrome with ulcer and inflammation of right lower extremity [HCC] [ESR] [COM]
- **I87.032** Postthrombotic syndrome with ulcer and inflammation of left lower extremity [HCC] [ESR] [COM]
- **I87.033** Postthrombotic syndrome with ulcer and inflammation of bilateral lower extremity [HCC] [ESR] [COM]
- **I87.039** Postthrombotic syndrome with ulcer and inflammation of unspecified lower extremity [HCC] [ESR] [COM]

✓6th I87.09 Postthrombotic syndrome with other complications

- **I87.091** Postthrombotic syndrome with other complications of right lower extremity
- **I87.092** Postthrombotic syndrome with other complications of left lower extremity
- **I87.093** Postthrombotic syndrome with other complications of bilateral lower extremity
- **I87.099** Postthrombotic syndrome with other complications of unspecified lower extremity

I87.1 Compression of vein
Stricture of vein
Vena cava syndrome (inferior) (superior)
EXCLUDES 2 compression of pulmonary vein (I28.8)
AHA: 2023,2Q,8

I87.2 Venous insufficiency (chronic) (peripheral)
Stasis dermatitis
Code also, if applicable, associated hypertensive conditions such as:
essential (primary) hypertension (I10)
hypertensive chronic kidney disease (I12.-)
hypertensive heart and chronic kidney disease (I13.-)
hypertensive heart disease (I11.-)
Use additional code, if applicable, to specify site and severity of ulcer (L97.-)
EXCLUDES 1 stasis dermatitis with varicose veins of lower extremities (I83.1-, I83.2-)
AHA: 2025,1Q,35; 2024,1Q,16
DEF: Insufficient drainage of venous blood in any part of the body that results in edema or dermatosis.

✓5th I87.3 Chronic venous hypertension (idiopathic)
Stasis edema
EXCLUDES 1 chronic venous hypertension due to deep vein thrombosis (I87.0-)
varicose veins of lower extremities (I83.-)

✓6th I87.30 Chronic venous hypertension (idiopathic) without complications
Asymptomatic chronic venous hypertension (idiopathic)

- **I87.301** Chronic venous hypertension (idiopathic) without complications of right lower extremity
- **I87.302** Chronic venous hypertension (idiopathic) without complications of left lower extremity
- **I87.303** Chronic venous hypertension (idiopathic) without complications of bilateral lower extremity
- **I87.309** Chronic venous hypertension (idiopathic) without complications of unspecified lower extremity
  Chronic venous hypertension NOS

✓6th I87.31 Chronic venous hypertension (idiopathic) with ulcer
Use additional code to specify site and severity of ulcer (L97.-)

- **I87.311** Chronic venous hypertension (idiopathic) with ulcer of right lower extremity [HCC] [ESR] [COM]
- **I87.312** Chronic venous hypertension (idiopathic) with ulcer of left lower extremity [HCC] [ESR] [COM]
- **I87.313** Chronic venous hypertension (idiopathic) with ulcer of bilateral lower extremity [HCC] [ESR] [COM]
- **I87.319** Chronic venous hypertension (idiopathic) with ulcer of unspecified lower extremity [HCC] [ESR] [COM]

✓6th I87.32 Chronic venous hypertension (idiopathic) with inflammation

- **I87.321** Chronic venous hypertension (idiopathic) with inflammation of right lower extremity
- **I87.322** Chronic venous hypertension (idiopathic) with inflammation of left lower extremity
- **I87.323** Chronic venous hypertension (idiopathic) with inflammation of bilateral lower extremity
- **I87.329** Chronic venous hypertension (idiopathic) with inflammation of unspecified lower extremity

✓6th I87.33 Chronic venous hypertension (idiopathic) with ulcer and inflammation
Use additional code to specify site and severity of ulcer (L97.-)

- **I87.331** Chronic venous hypertension (idiopathic) with ulcer and inflammation of right lower extremity [HCC] [ESR] [COM]
- **I87.332** Chronic venous hypertension (idiopathic) with ulcer and inflammation of left lower extremity [HCC] [ESR] [COM]
- **I87.333** Chronic venous hypertension (idiopathic) with ulcer and inflammation of bilateral lower extremity [HCC] [ESR] [COM]
- **I87.339** Chronic venous hypertension (idiopathic) with ulcer and inflammation of unspecified lower extremity [HCC] [ESR] [COM]

[HCC] CMS-HCC [Rx] Rx HCC [ESR] ESRD HCC [COM] Commercial HCC N Newborn: 0 P Pediatric: 0-17 M Maternity: 9-64 A Adult: 15-124

Chapter 9. Diseases of the Circulatory System

- √6th **I87.39 Chronic venous hypertension (idiopathic) with other complications**
  - **I87.391** Chronic venous hypertension (idiopathic) with other complications of right lower extremity
  - **I87.392** Chronic venous hypertension (idiopathic) with other complications of left lower extremity
  - **I87.393** Chronic venous hypertension (idiopathic) with other complications of bilateral lower extremity
  - **I87.399** Chronic venous hypertension (idiopathic) with other complications of unspecified lower extremity
- **I87.8 Other specified disorders of veins**
  - Phlebosclerosis
  - Venofibrosis
- **I87.9 Disorder of vein, unspecified**

√4th **I88 Nonspecific lymphadenitis**
  - EXCLUDES 1: acute lymphadenitis, except mesenteric (L04.-)
    - enlarged lymph nodes NOS (R59.-)
    - human immunodeficiency virus [HIV] disease resulting in generalized lymphadenopathy (B20)
- **I88.0 Nonspecific mesenteric lymphadenitis**
  - Mesenteric lymphadenitis (acute)(chronic)
- **I88.1 Chronic lymphadenitis, except mesenteric**
  - Adenitis
  - Lymphadenitis
- **I88.8 Other nonspecific lymphadenitis**
- **I88.9 Nonspecific lymphadenitis, unspecified**
  - Lymphadenitis NOS

√4th **I89 Other noninfective disorders of lymphatic vessels and lymph nodes**
  - EXCLUDES 1: chylocele, tunica vaginalis (nonfilarial) NOS (N50.89)
    - enlarged lymph nodes NOS (R59.-)
    - filarial chylocele (B74.-)
    - hereditary lymphedema (Q82.0)
- **I89.0 Lymphedema, not elsewhere classified**
  - Elephantiasis (nonfilarial) NOS
  - Lymphangiectasis
  - Obliteration, lymphatic vessel
  - Praecox lymphedema
  - Secondary lymphedema
  - EXCLUDES 1: postmastectomy lymphedema (I97.2)
  - AHA: 2024,1Q,16
- **I89.1 Lymphangitis**
  - Chronic lymphangitis
  - Lymphangitis NOS
  - Subacute lymphangitis
  - EXCLUDES 1: acute lymphangitis (L03.-)
- **I89.8 Other specified noninfective disorders of lymphatic vessels and lymph nodes**
  - Chylocele (nonfilarial)
  - Chylous ascites
  - Chylous cyst
  - Lipomelanotic reticulosis
  - Lymph node or vessel fistula
  - Lymph node or vessel infarction
  - Lymph node or vessel rupture
- **I89.9 Noninfective disorder of lymphatic vessels and lymph nodes, unspecified**
  - Disease of lymphatic vessels NOS

Other and unspecified disorders of the circulatory system (I95-I99)

√4th **I95 Hypotension**
  - EXCLUDES 1: cardiovascular collapse (R57.9)
    - maternal hypotension syndrome (O26.5-)
    - nonspecific low blood pressure reading NOS (R03.1)
- **I95.0 Idiopathic hypotension**
- **I95.1 Orthostatic hypotension**
  - Hypotension, postural
  - EXCLUDES 1: neurogenic orthostatic hypotension [Shy-Drager] (G90.3)
    - orthostatic hypotension due to drugs (I95.2)
  - AHA: 2023,2Q,8
- **I95.2 Hypotension due to drugs**
  - Orthostatic hypotension due to drugs
  - Use additional code for adverse effect, if applicable, to identify drug (T36-T50 with fifth or sixth character 5)
- **I95.3 Hypotension of hemodialysis**
  - Intra-dialytic hypotension
- √5th **I95.8 Other hypotension**
  - **I95.81** Postprocedural hypotension
  - **I95.89** Other hypotension
    - Chronic hypotension
- **I95.9 Hypotension, unspecified**

I96 Gangrene, not elsewhere classified HCC ESR COM
  - Gangrenous cellulitis
  - EXCLUDES 1: gangrene in atherosclerosis of native arteries of the extremities (I70.26)
    - gangrene of certain specified sites - see Alphabetical Index
    - gangrene in hernia (K40.1, K40.4, K41.1, K41.4, K42.1, K43.1-, K44.1, K45.1, K46.1)
    - gangrene in other peripheral vascular diseases (I73.-)
    - gas gangrene (A48.0)
    - pyoderma gangrenosum (L88)
  - EXCLUDES 2: gangrene in diabetes mellitus (E08-E13 with .52)
  - AHA: 2022,3Q,13; 2018,4Q,87; 2018,3Q,3; 2017,3Q,6; 2013,2Q,34

√4th **I97 Intraoperative and postprocedural complications and disorders of circulatory system, not elsewhere classified**
  - EXCLUDES 2: postprocedural shock (T81.1-)
  - AHA: 2021,1Q,13; 2019,2Q,21
- **I97.0 Postcardiotomy syndrome**
- √5th **I97.1 Other postprocedural cardiac functional disturbances**
  - EXCLUDES 2: acute pulmonary insufficiency following thoracic surgery (J95.1)
    - intraoperative cardiac functional disturbances (I97.7-)
  - √6th **I97.11 Postprocedural cardiac insufficiency**
    - **I97.110** Postprocedural cardiac insufficiency following cardiac surgery
    - **I97.111** Postprocedural cardiac insufficiency following other surgery
  - √6th **I97.12 Postprocedural cardiac arrest**
    - **I97.120** Postprocedural cardiac arrest following cardiac surgery
    - **I97.121** Postprocedural cardiac arrest following other surgery
  - √6th **I97.13 Postprocedural heart failure**
    - Use additional code to identify the heart failure (I50.-)
    - **I97.130** Postprocedural heart failure following cardiac surgery
    - **I97.131** Postprocedural heart failure following other surgery
  - √6th **I97.19 Other postprocedural cardiac functional disturbances**
    - Use additional code, if applicable, to further specify disorder
    - **I97.190** Other postprocedural cardiac functional disturbances following cardiac surgery
      - Use additional code, if applicable, for type 4 or type 5 myocardial infarction, to further specify disorder
      - AHA: 2019,2Q,33
    - **I97.191** Other postprocedural cardiac functional disturbances following other surgery
- **I97.2 Postmastectomy lymphedema syndrome** A
  - Elephantiasis due to mastectomy
  - Obliteration of lymphatic vessels
- **I97.3 Postprocedural hypertension**
- √5th **I97.4 Intraoperative hemorrhage and hematoma of a circulatory system organ or structure complicating a procedure**
  - EXCLUDES 1: intraoperative hemorrhage and hematoma of a circulatory system organ or structure due to accidental puncture and laceration during a procedure (I97.5-)
  - EXCLUDES 2: intraoperative cerebrovascular hemorrhage complicating a procedure (G97.3-)
  - √6th **I97.41 Intraoperative hemorrhage and hematoma of a circulatory system organ or structure complicating a circulatory system procedure**
    - **I97.410** Intraoperative hemorrhage and hematoma of a circulatory system organ or structure complicating a cardiac catheterization
    - **I97.411** Intraoperative hemorrhage and hematoma of a circulatory system organ or structure complicating a cardiac bypass

- **I97.418** Intraoperative hemorrhage and hematoma of a circulatory system organ or structure complicating other circulatory system procedure
- **I97.42** Intraoperative hemorrhage and hematoma of a circulatory system organ or structure complicating other procedure
  - AHA: 2020,1Q,19
- √5th **I97.5** Accidental puncture and laceration of a circulatory system organ or structure during a procedure
  - EXCLUDES 2: accidental puncture and laceration of brain during a procedure (G97.4-)
  - **I97.51** Accidental puncture and laceration of a circulatory system organ or structure during a circulatory system procedure
    - AHA: 2019,2Q,24
  - **I97.52** Accidental puncture and laceration of a circulatory system organ or structure during other procedure
- √5th **I97.6** Postprocedural hemorrhage, hematoma and seroma of a circulatory system organ or structure following a procedure
  - EXCLUDES 2: postprocedural cerebrovascular hemorrhage complicating a procedure (G97.5-)
  - AHA: 2016,4Q,9-10
  - √6th **I97.61** Postprocedural hemorrhage of a circulatory system organ or structure following a circulatory system procedure
    - **I97.610** Postprocedural hemorrhage of a circulatory system organ or structure following a cardiac catheterization
    - **I97.611** Postprocedural hemorrhage of a circulatory system organ or structure following cardiac bypass
    - **I97.618** Postprocedural hemorrhage of a circulatory system organ or structure following other circulatory system procedure
  - √6th **I97.62** Postprocedural hemorrhage, hematoma and seroma of a circulatory system organ or structure following other procedure
    - **I97.620** Postprocedural hemorrhage of a circulatory system organ or structure following other procedure
    - **I97.621** Postprocedural hematoma of a circulatory system organ or structure following other procedure
    - **I97.622** Postprocedural seroma of a circulatory system organ or structure following other procedure
  - √6th **I97.63** Postprocedural hematoma of a circulatory system organ or structure following a circulatory system procedure
    - **I97.630** Postprocedural hematoma of a circulatory system organ or structure following a cardiac catheterization
    - **I97.631** Postprocedural hematoma of a circulatory system organ or structure following cardiac bypass
    - **I97.638** Postprocedural hematoma of a circulatory system organ or structure following other circulatory system procedure
  - √6th **I97.64** Postprocedural seroma of a circulatory system organ or structure following a circulatory system procedure
    - **I97.640** Postprocedural seroma of a circulatory system organ or structure following a cardiac catheterization
    - **I97.641** Postprocedural seroma of a circulatory system organ or structure following cardiac bypass
    - **I97.648** Postprocedural seroma of a circulatory system organ or structure following other circulatory system procedure
- √5th **I97.7** Intraoperative cardiac functional disturbances
  - EXCLUDES 2: acute pulmonary insufficiency following thoracic surgery (J95.1)
  - postprocedural cardiac functional disturbances (I97.1-)
  - √6th **I97.71** Intraoperative cardiac arrest
    - **I97.710** Intraoperative cardiac arrest during cardiac surgery
    - **I97.711** Intraoperative cardiac arrest during other surgery
  - √6th **I97.79** Other intraoperative cardiac functional disturbances
    - Use additional code, if applicable, to further specify disorder
    - **I97.790** Other intraoperative cardiac functional disturbances during cardiac surgery
    - **I97.791** Other intraoperative cardiac functional disturbances during other surgery
- √5th **I97.8** Other intraoperative and postprocedural complications and disorders of the circulatory system, not elsewhere classified
  - Use additional code, if applicable, to further specify disorder
  - √6th **I97.81** Intraoperative cerebrovascular infarction
    - **I97.810** Intraoperative cerebrovascular infarction during cardiac surgery ESR
    - **I97.811** Intraoperative cerebrovascular infarction during other surgery ESR
  - √6th **I97.82** Postprocedural cerebrovascular infarction
    - **I97.820** Postprocedural cerebrovascular infarction following cardiac surgery ESR
    - **I97.821** Postprocedural cerebrovascular infarction following other surgery ESR
  - **I97.88** Other intraoperative complications of the circulatory system, not elsewhere classified
  - **I97.89** Other postprocedural complications and disorders of the circulatory system, not elsewhere classified
    - AHA: 2025,2Q,5; 2024,1Q,26; 2021,3Q,33; 2020,3Q,3-8; 2019,2Q,33
- √4th **I99** Other and unspecified disorders of circulatory system
  - **I99.8** Other disorder of circulatory system
    - AHA: 2020,4Q,98
  - **I99.9** Unspecified disorder of circulatory system

Chapter 10. Diseases of the Respiratory System (J00–J99), U07.0

Chapter-specific Guidelines with Coding Examples
The chapter-specific guidelines from the ICD-10-CM Official Guidelines for Coding and Reporting have been provided below. Along with these guidelines are coding examples, contained in the shICD-10-CM 2026aded boxes, that have been developed to help illustrate the coding and/or sequencing guidance found in these guidelines.

a. Chronic obstructive pulmonary disease [COPD] and asthma

1) Acute exacerbation of chronic obstructive bronchitis and asthma
The codes in categories J44 and J45 distinguish between uncomplicated cases and those in acute exacerbation. An acute exacerbation is a worsening or a decompensation of a chronic condition. An acute exacerbation is not equivalent to an infection superimposed on a chronic condition, though an exacerbation may be triggered by an infection.

> Acute streptococcal bronchitis with acute exacerbation of COPD
>
> | | |
> |---|---|
> | J20.2 | Acute bronchitis due to streptococcus |
> | J44.0 | Chronic obstructive pulmonary disease with (acute) lower respiratory infection |
> | J44.1 | Chronic obstructive pulmonary disease with (acute) exacerbation |
>
> *Explanation*: ICD-10-CM uses combination codes to create organism-specific classifications for acute bronchitis. Category J44 codes include combination codes with severity components, which differentiate between COPD with acute lower respiratory infection (acute bronchitis), COPD with acute exacerbation, and COPD without mention of a complication (unspecified).
>
> An acute exacerbation is a worsening or a decompensation of a chronic condition. An acute exacerbation is not equivalent to an infection superimposed on a chronic condition, though an exacerbation may be triggered by an infection, as in this example.

> Exacerbation of moderate persistent asthma with status asthmaticus
>
> | | |
> |---|---|
> | J45.42 | Moderate persistent asthma with status asthmaticus |
>
> *Explanation*: Category J45 Asthma includes severity-specific subcategories and fifth-character codes to distinguish between uncomplicated cases, those in acute exacerbation, and those with status asthmaticus.

b. Acute respiratory failure

1) Acute respiratory failure as principal diagnosis
A code from subcategory J96.0, Acute respiratory failure, or subcategory J96.2, Acute and chronic respiratory failure, may be assigned as a principal diagnosis when it is the condition established after study to be chiefly responsible for occasioning the admission to the hospital, and the selection is supported by the Alphabetic Index and Tabular List. However, chapter-specific coding guidelines (such as obstetrics, poisoning, HIV, newborn) that provide sequencing direction take precedence.

> Acute hypoxic respiratory failure due to exacerbation of chronic obstructive bronchitis
>
> | | |
> |---|---|
> | J96.01 | Acute respiratory failure with hypoxia |
> | J44.1 | Chronic obstructive pulmonary disease with (acute) exacerbation |
>
> *Explanation*: Category J96 classifies respiratory failure with combination codes that designate the severity and the presence of hypoxia and hypercapnia. Code J96.01 is sequenced as the first-listed diagnosis, as the reason for the encounter. Respiratory failure may be assigned as a principal diagnosis when it is the condition established after study to be chiefly responsible for occasioning the encounter and the selection is supported by the Alphabetic Index and Tabular List.

2) Acute respiratory failure as secondary diagnosis
Respiratory failure may be listed as a secondary diagnosis if it occurs after admission, or if it is present on admission, but does not meet the definition of principal diagnosis.

> Acute respiratory failure due to accidental oxycodone overdose
>
> | | |
> |---|---|
> | T40.2X1A | Poisoning by other opioids, accidental (unintentional), initial encounter |
> | J96.00 | Acute respiratory failure, unspecified whether with hypoxia or hypercapnia |
>
> *Explanation*: Respiratory failure may be assigned as a principal diagnosis when it is the condition established after study to be chiefly responsible for occasioning the encounter, and the selection is supported by the Alphabetic Index and Tabular List. However, chapter-specific coding guidelines, such as poisoning, that provide sequencing direction take precedence. When coding a poisoning or reaction to the improper use of a medication (e.g., overdose, wrong substance given or taken in error, wrong route of administration), first assign the appropriate code from categories T36–T50. Use additional code(s) for all manifestations of the poisoning. In this instance, the respiratory failure is a manifestation of the poisoning and is sequenced as a secondary diagnosis.

3) Sequencing of acute respiratory failure and another acute condition
When a patient is admitted with respiratory failure and another acute condition, (e.g., myocardial infarction, cerebrovascular accident, aspiration pneumonia), the principal diagnosis will not be the same in every situation. This applies whether the other acute condition is a respiratory or nonrespiratory condition. Selection of the principal diagnosis will be dependent on the circumstances of admission. If both the respiratory failure and the other acute condition are equally responsible for occasioning the admission to the hospital, and there are no chapter-specific sequencing rules, the guideline regarding two or more diagnoses that equally meet the definition for principal diagnosis (*Section II, C.*) may be applied in these situations.

If the documentation is not clear as to whether acute respiratory failure and another condition are equally responsible for occasioning the admission, query the provider for clarification.

> Patient presents with acute pneumococcal pneumonia and acute respiratory failure
>
> | | |
> |---|---|
> | J96.00 | Acute respiratory failure, unspecified whether with hypoxia or hypercapnia |
> | J13 | Pneumonia due to Streptococcus pneumoniae |
>
> *Explanation*: When a patient is seen for respiratory failure and another acute condition, such as a bacterial pneumonia, the principal or first-listed diagnosis is not the same in every situation. This applies whether the other acute condition is a respiratory or nonrespiratory condition. The principal diagnosis depends on the problem chiefly responsible for the encounter.

c. Influenza due to certain identified influenza viruses
Code only confirmed cases of influenza due to certain identified influenza viruses (category J09), and due to other identified influenza virus (category J10). This is an exception to the hospital inpatient guideline Section II, H. (Uncertain Diagnosis).

In this context, "confirmation" does not require documentation of positive laboratory testing specific for avian or other novel influenza A or other identified influenza virus. However, coding should be based on the provider's diagnostic statement that the patient has avian influenza, or other novel influenza A, for category J09, or has another particular identified strain of influenza, such as H1N1 or H3N2, but not identified as novel or variant, for category J10.

If the provider records "suspected" or "possible" or "probable" avian influenza, or novel influenza, or other identified influenza, then the appropriate influenza code from category J11, Influenza due to unidentified influenza virus, should be assigned. A code from category J09, Influenza due to certain identified influenza viruses, should not be assigned nor should a code from category J10, Influenza due to other identified influenza virus.

Influenza due to avian influenza virus with pneumonia

J09.X1   Influenza due to identified novel influenza A virus with pneumonia

Explanation: Codes in category J09 Influenza due to certain identified influenza viruses should be assigned only for confirmed cases. "Confirmation" does not require positive laboratory testing of a specific influenza virus but does need to be based on the provider's diagnostic statement, which should not include terms such as "possible," "probable," or "suspected."

d. Ventilator associated pneumonia

1) Documentation of ventilator associated pneumonia

As with all procedural or postprocedural complications, code assignment is based on the provider's documentation of the relationship between the condition and the procedure.

Code J95.851, Ventilator associated pneumonia, should be assigned only when the provider has documented ventilator associated pneumonia (VAP). An additional code to identify the organism (e.g., Pseudomonas aeruginosa, code B96.5) should also be assigned. Do not assign an additional code from categories J12-J18 to identify the type of pneumonia.

Code J95.851 should not be assigned for cases where the patient has pneumonia and is on a mechanical ventilator and the provider has not specifically stated that the pneumonia is ventilator-associated pneumonia. If the documentation is unclear as to whether the patient has a pneumonia that is a complication attributable to the mechanical ventilator, query the provider.

2) Ventilator associated pneumonia develops after admission

A patient may be admitted with one type of pneumonia (e.g., code J13, Pneumonia due to Streptococcus pneumonia) and subsequently develop VAP. In this instance, the principal diagnosis would be the appropriate code from categories J12-J18 for the pneumonia diagnosed at the time of admission. Code J95.851, Ventilator associated pneumonia, would be assigned as an additional diagnosis when the provider has also documented the presence of ventilator associated pneumonia.

e. Vaping-related disorders

For patients presenting with condition(s) related to vaping, assign code U07.0, Vaping-related disorder, as the principal diagnosis. For lung injury due to vaping, assign only code U07.0. Assign additional codes for other manifestations, such as acute respiratory failure (subcategory J96.0-) or pneumonitis (code J68.0).

Associated respiratory signs and symptoms due to vaping, such as cough, shortness of breath, etc., are not coded separately, when a definitive diagnosis has been established. However, it would be appropriate to code separately any gastrointestinal symptoms, such as diarrhea and abdominal pain.

See Section I.C.1.g.1.c.i. for Pneumonia confirmed as due to COVID-19

Chapter 10. Diseases of the Respiratory System (J00-J99)

NOTE When a respiratory condition is described as occurring in more than one site and is not specifically indexed, it should be classified to the lower anatomic site (e.g., tracheobronchitis to bronchitis in J40).

Use additional code, where applicable, to identify:
- exposure to environmental tobacco smoke (Z77.22)
- exposure to tobacco smoke in the perinatal period (P96.81)
- history of tobacco dependence (Z87.891)
- occupational exposure to environmental tobacco smoke (Z57.31)
- tobacco dependence (F17.-)
- tobacco use (Z72.0)

EXCLUDES 2
- certain conditions originating in the perinatal period (P04-P96)
- certain infectious and parasitic diseases (A00-B99)
- complications of pregnancy, childbirth and the puerperium (O00-O9A)
- congenital malformations, deformations and chromosomal abnormalities (Q00-Q99)
- endocrine, nutritional and metabolic diseases (E00-E88)
- injury, poisoning and certain other consequences of external causes (S00-T88)
- neoplasms (C00-D49)
- smoke inhalation (T59.81-)
- symptoms, signs and abnormal clinical and laboratory findings, not elsewhere classified (R00-R94)

This chapter contains the following blocks:
- J00-J06 Acute upper respiratory infections
- J09-J18 Influenza and pneumonia
- J20-J22 Other acute lower respiratory infections
- J30-J39 Other diseases of upper respiratory tract
- J40-J4A Chronic lower respiratory diseases
- J60-J70 Lung diseases due to external agents
- J80-J84 Other respiratory diseases principally affecting the interstitium
- J85-J86 Suppurative and necrotic conditions of the lower respiratory tract
- J90-J94 Other diseases of the pleura
- J95 Intraoperative and postprocedural complications and disorders of respiratory system, not elsewhere classified
- J96-J99 Other diseases of the respiratory system

Acute upper respiratory infections (J00-J06)

EXCLUDES 1 chronic obstructive pulmonary disease with acute lower respiratory infection (J44.0)

J00 Acute nasopharyngitis [common cold]
Acute rhinitis
Coryza (acute)
Infective nasopharyngitis NOS
Infective rhinitis
Nasal catarrh, acute
Nasopharyngitis NOS

EXCLUDES 1
- acute pharyngitis (J02.-)
- acute sore throat NOS (J02.9)
- influenza virus with other respiratory manifestations (J09.X2, J10.1, J11.1)
- pharyngitis NOS (J02.9)
- rhinitis NOS (J31.0)
- sore throat NOS (J02.9)

EXCLUDES 2
- allergic rhinitis (J30.1-J30.9)
- chronic pharyngitis (J31.2)
- chronic rhinitis (J31.0)
- chronic sore throat (J31.2)
- nasopharyngitis, chronic (J31.1)
- vasomotor rhinitis (J30.0)

J01 Acute sinusitis
INCLUDES
- acute abscess of sinus
- acute empyema of sinus
- acute infection of sinus
- acute inflammation of sinus
- acute suppuration of sinus

Use additional code (B95-B97) to identify infectious agent

EXCLUDES 1 sinusitis NOS (J32.9)
EXCLUDES 2 chronic sinusitis (J32.0-J32.8)

J01.0 Acute maxillary sinusitis
Acute antritis
- J01.00 Acute maxillary sinusitis, unspecified
- J01.01 Acute recurrent maxillary sinusitis

J01.1 Acute frontal sinusitis
- J01.10 Acute frontal sinusitis, unspecified
- J01.11 Acute recurrent frontal sinusitis

J01.2 Acute ethmoidal sinusitis
- J01.20 Acute ethmoidal sinusitis, unspecified
- J01.21 Acute recurrent ethmoidal sinusitis

J01.3 Acute sphenoidal sinusitis
- J01.30 Acute sphenoidal sinusitis, unspecified
- J01.31 Acute recurrent sphenoidal sinusitis

J01.4 Acute pansinusitis
- J01.40 Acute pansinusitis, unspecified
- J01.41 Acute recurrent pansinusitis

J01.8 Other acute sinusitis
- J01.80 Other acute sinusitis
  Acute sinusitis involving more than one sinus but not pansinusitis
- J01.81 Other acute recurrent sinusitis
  Acute recurrent sinusitis involving more than one sinus but not pansinusitis

J01.9 Acute sinusitis, unspecified
- J01.90 Acute sinusitis, unspecified
- J01.91 Acute recurrent sinusitis, unspecified

J02 Acute pharyngitis
INCLUDES acute sore throat
EXCLUDES 1
- acute laryngopharyngitis (J06.0)
- peritonsillar abscess (J36)
- pharyngeal abscess (J39.1)
- retropharyngeal abscess (J39.0)

EXCLUDES 2 chronic pharyngitis (J31.2)

J02.0 Streptococcal pharyngitis
Septic pharyngitis
Streptococcal sore throat
EXCLUDES 2 scarlet fever (A38.-)

J02.8 Acute pharyngitis due to other specified organisms
Use additional code (B95-B97) to identify infectious agent
EXCLUDES 1
- acute pharyngitis due to coxsackie virus (B08.5)
- acute pharyngitis due to gonococcus (A54.5)
- acute pharyngitis due to herpes [simplex] virus (B00.2)
- acute pharyngitis due to infectious mononucleosis (B27.-)
- enteroviral vesicular pharyngitis (B08.5)

J02.9 Acute pharyngitis, unspecified
Gangrenous pharyngitis (acute)
Infective pharyngitis (acute) NOS
Pharyngitis (acute) NOS
Sore throat (acute) NOS
Suppurative pharyngitis (acute)
Ulcerative pharyngitis (acute)
EXCLUDES 1 influenza virus with other respiratory manifestations (J09.X2, J10.1, J11.1)

J03 Acute tonsillitis
EXCLUDES 1
- acute sore throat (J02.-)
- hypertrophy of tonsils (J35.1)
- peritonsillar abscess (J36)
- sore throat NOS (J02.9)
- streptococcal sore throat (J02.0)

EXCLUDES 2 chronic tonsillitis (J35.0)

J03.0 Streptococcal tonsillitis
- J03.00 Acute streptococcal tonsillitis, unspecified
- J03.01 Acute recurrent streptococcal tonsillitis

J03.8 Acute tonsillitis due to other specified organisms
Use additional code (B95-B97) to identify infectious agent
EXCLUDES 1
- diphtheritic tonsillitis (A36.0)
- herpesviral pharyngotonsillitis (B00.2)
- streptococcal tonsillitis (J03.0)
- tuberculous tonsillitis (A15.8)
- Vincent's tonsillitis (A69.1)

- J03.80 Acute tonsillitis due to other specified organisms
- J03.81 Acute recurrent tonsillitis due to other specified organisms

J03.9 Acute tonsillitis, unspecified
Follicular tonsillitis (acute)
Gangrenous tonsillitis (acute)
Infective tonsillitis (acute)
Tonsillitis (acute) NOS
Ulcerative tonsillitis (acute)
EXCLUDES 1 influenza virus with other respiratory manifestations (J09.X2, J10.1, J11.1)

- J03.90 Acute tonsillitis, unspecified
- J03.91 Acute recurrent tonsillitis, unspecified

Chapter 10. Diseases of the Respiratory System

J04 Acute laryngitis and tracheitis ✓4th

Code also influenza, if present, such as:
influenza due to identified novel influenza A virus with other respiratory manifestations (J09.X2)
influenza due to other identified influenza virus with other respiratory manifestations (J10.1)
influenza due to unidentified influenza virus with other respiratory manifestations (J11.1)
Use additional code (B95-B97) to identify infectious agent
EXCLUDES 1 acute obstructive laryngitis [croup] and epiglottitis (J05.-)
EXCLUDES 2 laryngismus (stridulus) (J38.5)

J04.0 Acute laryngitis
Edematous laryngitis (acute)
Laryngitis (acute) NOS
Subglottic laryngitis (acute)
Suppurative laryngitis (acute)
Ulcerative laryngitis (acute)
EXCLUDES 1 acute obstructive laryngitis (J05.0)
EXCLUDES 2 chronic laryngitis (J37.0)

J04.1 Acute tracheitis ✓5th
Acute viral tracheitis
Catarrhal tracheitis (acute)
Tracheitis (acute) NOS
EXCLUDES 2 chronic tracheitis (J42)

- **J04.10** Acute tracheitis without obstruction
- **J04.11** Acute tracheitis with obstruction

J04.2 Acute laryngotracheitis
Laryngotracheitis NOS
Tracheitis (acute) with laryngitis (acute)
EXCLUDES 1 acute obstructive laryngotracheitis (J05.0)
EXCLUDES 2 chronic laryngotracheitis (J37.1)

J04.3 Supraglottitis, unspecified ✓5th

- **J04.30** Supraglottitis, unspecified, without obstruction
- **J04.31** Supraglottitis, unspecified, with obstruction

J05 Acute obstructive laryngitis [croup] and epiglottitis ✓4th

Code also, influenza, if present, such as:
influenza due to identified novel influenza A virus with other respiratory manifestations (J09.X2)
influenza due to other identified influenza virus with other respiratory manifestations (J10.1)
influenza due to unidentified influenza virus with other respiratory manifestations (J11.1)
Use additional code (B95-B97) to identify infectious agent

J05.0 Acute obstructive laryngitis [croup]
Obstructive laryngitis (acute) NOS
Obstructive laryngotracheitis NOS
DEF: Acute laryngeal obstruction due to allergies, foreign bodies, or in the majority of cases a viral infection. Symptoms include a harsh, barking cough, hoarseness, and a persistent, high-pitched respiratory sound (stridor).

J05.1 Acute epiglottitis ✓5th
EXCLUDES 2 epiglottitis, chronic (J37.0)

- **J05.10** Acute epiglottitis without obstruction
  Epiglottitis NOS
- **J05.11** Acute epiglottitis with obstruction

J06 Acute upper respiratory infections of multiple and unspecified sites ✓4th

EXCLUDES 1 acute respiratory infection NOS (J22)
influenza virus with other respiratory manifestations (J09.X2, J10.1, J11.1)
streptococcal pharyngitis (J02.0)

J06.0 Acute laryngopharyngitis

J06.9 Acute upper respiratory infection, unspecified
Upper respiratory disease, acute
Upper respiratory infection NOS
Use additional code (B95-B97) to identify infectious agent, if known, such as:
respiratory syncytial virus (RSV) (B97.4)
AHA: 2020,1Q,22

Influenza and pneumonia (J09-J18)

Use additional code, if applicable, to identify resistance to antimicrobial drugs (Z16.-)
EXCLUDES 2 allergic or eosinophilic pneumonia (J82)
aspiration pneumonia NOS (J69.0)
meconium pneumonia (P24.01)
neonatal aspiration pneumonia (P24.-)
pneumonia due to solids and liquids (J69.-)
congenital pneumonia (P23.9)
lipid pneumonia (J69.1)
rheumatic pneumonia (I00)
ventilator associated pneumonia (J95.851)
AHA: 2017,4Q,96

J09 Influenza due to certain identified influenza viruses ✓4th

EXCLUDES 1 influenza A/H1N1 (J10.-)
influenza due to other identified influenza virus (J10.-)
influenza due to unidentified influenza virus (J11.-)
seasonal influenza due to other identified influenza virus (J10.-)
seasonal influenza due to unidentified influenza virus (J11.-)

J09.X Influenza due to identified novel influenza A virus ✓5th
Avian influenza
Bird influenza
Influenza A/H5N1
Influenza of other animal origin, not bird or swine
Swine influenza virus (viruses that normally cause infections in pigs)
AHA: 2016,3Q,10

- **J09.X1 Influenza due to identified novel influenza A virus with pneumonia**
  Code also, if applicable, associated:
  lung abscess (J85.1)
  other specified type of pneumonia

- **J09.X2 Influenza due to identified novel influenza A virus with other respiratory manifestations**
  Influenza due to identified novel influenza A virus NOS
  Influenza due to identified novel influenza A virus with laryngitis
  Influenza due to identified novel influenza A virus with pharyngitis
  Influenza due to identified novel influenza A virus with upper respiratory symptoms
  Use additional code, if applicable, for associated:
  pleural effusion (J91.8)
  sinusitis (J01.-)

- **J09.X3 Influenza due to identified novel influenza A virus with gastrointestinal manifestations**
  Influenza due to identified novel influenza A virus gastroenteritis
  EXCLUDES 1 'intestinal flu' [viral gastroenteritis] (A08.-)

- **J09.X9 Influenza due to identified novel influenza A virus with other manifestations**
  Influenza due to identified novel influenza A virus with encephalopathy
  Influenza due to identified novel influenza A virus with myocarditis
  Influenza due to identified novel influenza A virus with otitis media
  Use additional code to identify manifestation

J10 Influenza due to other identified influenza virus ✓4th

INCLUDES influenza A (non-novel)
influenza B
influenza C
EXCLUDES 1 influenza due to avian influenza virus (J09.X-)
influenza due to swine flu (J09.X-)
influenza due to unidentifed influenza virus (J11.-)

J10.0 Influenza due to other identified influenza virus with pneumonia ✓5th
Code also associated lung abscess, if applicable (J85.1)

- **J10.00** Influenza due to other identified influenza virus with unspecified type of pneumonia
- **J10.01** Influenza due to other identified influenza virus with the same other identified influenza virus pneumonia
- **J10.08** Influenza due to other identified influenza virus with other specified pneumonia
  Code also other specified type of pneumonia

Chapter 10. Diseases of the Respiratory System

J10.1 Influenza due to other identified influenza virus with **other respiratory manifestations**
Influenza due to other identified influenza virus NOS
Influenza due to other identified influenza virus with laryngitis
Influenza due to other identified influenza virus with pharyngitis
Influenza due to other identified influenza virus with upper respiratory symptoms
Use additional code for associated pleural effusion, if applicable (J91.8)
Use additional code for associated sinusitis, if applicable (J01.-)
AHA: 2016,3Q,10-11

J10.2 Influenza due to other identified influenza virus with **gastrointestinal manifestations**
Influenza due to other identified influenza virus gastroenteritis
EXCLUDES 1 "intestinal flu" [viral gastroenteritis] (A08.-)

√5th **J10.8** Influenza due to other identified influenza virus with other manifestations

- **J10.81** Influenza due to other identified influenza virus with **encephalopathy**
- **J10.82** Influenza due to other identified influenza virus with **myocarditis**
- **J10.83** Influenza due to other identified influenza virus with **otitis media**
  Use additional code for any associated perforated tympanic membrane (H72.-)
- **J10.89** Influenza due to other identified influenza virus with other manifestations
  Use additional codes to identify the manifestations

√4th **J11** Influenza due to **unidentified** influenza virus

√5th **J11.0** Influenza due to unidentified influenza virus with **pneumonia**
Code also associated lung abscess, if applicable (J85.1)
AHA: 2016,3Q,11

- **J11.00** Influenza due to unidentified influenza virus with unspecified type of pneumonia
  Influenza with pneumonia NOS
- **J11.08** Influenza due to unidentified influenza virus with **specified** pneumonia
  Code also other specified type of pneumonia

J11.1 Influenza due to unidentified influenza virus with **other respiratory manifestations**
Influenza NOS
Influenza with upper respiratory symptoms NOS
Influenzal laryngitis NOS
Influenzal pharyngitis NOS
Use additional code for associated pleural effusion, if applicable (J91.8)
Use additional code for associated sinusitis, if applicable (J01.-)

J11.2 Influenza due to unidentified influenza virus with **gastrointestinal manifestations**
Influenza gastroenteritis NOS
EXCLUDES 1 "intestinal flu" [viral gastroenteritis] (A08.-)

√5th **J11.8** Influenza due to unidentified influenza virus with other manifestations

- **J11.81** Influenza due to unidentified influenza virus with **encephalopathy**
  Influenzal encephalopathy NOS
- **J11.82** Influenza due to unidentified influenza virus with **myocarditis**
  Influenzal myocarditis NOS
- **J11.83** Influenza due to unidentified influenza virus with **otitis media**
  Influenzal otitis media NOS
  Use additional code for any associated perforated tympanic membrane (H72.-)
- **J11.89** Influenza due to unidentified influenza virus with other manifestations
  Use additional codes to identify the manifestations

√4th **J12** Viral pneumonia, not elsewhere classified
INCLUDES bronchopneumonia due to viruses other than influenza viruses
Code first associated influenza, if applicable (J09.X1, J10.0-, J11.0-)
Code also associated abscess, if applicable (J85.1)
EXCLUDES 2 aspiration pneumonia due to anesthesia during labor and delivery (O74.0)
aspiration pneumonia due to anesthesia during pregnancy (O29)
aspiration pneumonia due to anesthesia during puerperium (O89.0)
aspiration pneumonia due to solids and liquids (J69.-)
aspiration pneumonia NOS (J69.0)
congenital pneumonia (P23.0)
congenital rubella pneumonitis (P35.0)
interstitial pneumonia NOS (J84.9)
lipid pneumonia (J69.1)
neonatal aspiration pneumonia (P24.-)
AHA: 2020,2Q,28; 2019,1Q,35; 2018,3Q,24; 2016,3Q,15; 2013,4Q,118

J12.0 **Adenoviral** pneumonia

J12.1 **Respiratory syncytial** virus pneumonia
RSV pneumonia

J12.2 **Parainfluenza** virus pneumonia

J12.3 **Human metapneumovirus** pneumonia

√5th **J12.8** Other viral pneumonia

- **J12.81** Pneumonia due to **SARS-associated coronavirus**
  Severe acute respiratory syndrome NOS
  DEF: Inflammation of the lungs with consolidation, caused by the severe adult respiratory syndrome (SARS)-associated coronavirus or SARS-CoV. This pneumonia should not be confused with that caused by SARS-CoV-2 (COVID-19).
- **J12.82** Pneumonia due to **coronavirus disease 2019** UPD
  Pneumonia due to 2019 novel coronavirus (SARS-CoV-2)
  Pneumonia due to COVID-19
  Code first COVID-19 (U07.1)
  AHA: 2021,1Q,25-30,31-49
- **J12.89** Other viral pneumonia
  AHA: 2021,1Q,33-34; 2020,2Q,8,11; 2020,1Q,34-36

J12.9 Viral pneumonia, unspecified

J13 Pneumonia due to **Streptococcus pneumoniae** ESR
Bronchopneumonia due to S. pneumoniae
Code first, if applicable, associated influenza (J09.X1, J10.0-, J11.0-)
Code also, if applicable, any associated condition such as:
abscess (J85.1)
aspiration pneumonia (J69.-)
EXCLUDES 1 congenital pneumonia due to S. pneumoniae (P23.6)
lobar pneumonia, unspecified organism (J18.1)
pneumonia due to other streptococci (J15.3-J15.4)
AHA: 2020,2Q,28; 2019,1Q,35; 2018,3Q,24; 2016,3Q,15; 2013,4Q,118

J14 Pneumonia due to **Hemophilus influenzae** ESR
Bronchopneumonia due to H. influenzae
Code first, if applicable, associated influenza (J09.X1, J10.0-, J11.0-)
Code also, if applicable, any associated condition such as:
abscess (J85.1)
aspiration pneumonia (J69.-)
EXCLUDES 1 congenital pneumonia due to H. influenzae (P23.6)
AHA: 2020,2Q,28; 2019,1Q,35; 2018,3Q,24; 2016,3Q,15; 2013,4Q,118

√4th **J15** **Bacterial** pneumonia, not elsewhere classified
INCLUDES Bronchopneumonia due to bacteria other than S. pneumoniae and H. influenzae
Code first, if applicable, associated influenza (J09.X1, J10.0-, J11.0-)
Code also, if applicable, any associated condition such as:
abscess (J85.1)
aspiration pneumonia (J69.-)
EXCLUDES 1 chlamydial pneumonia (J16.0)
congenital pneumonia (P23.-)
Legionnaires' disease (A48.1)
spirochetal pneumonia (A69.8)
AHA: 2020,2Q,28; 2019,1Q,35; 2018,3Q,24; 2016,3Q,15; 2013,4Q,118

J15.0 Pneumonia due to **Klebsiella pneumoniae** HCC ESR COM

J15.1 Pneumonia due to **Pseudomonas** HCC ESR COM

√5th **J15.2** Pneumonia due to **staphylococcus**

- **J15.20** Pneumonia due to staphylococcus, unspecified HCC ESR COM

J15.21 Pneumonia due to Staphylococcus aureus

- **J15.21** Pneumonia due to Staphylococcus aureus
  - **J15.211** Pneumonia due to methicillin susceptible Staphylococcus aureus [HCC] [ESR] [COM]
    - MSSA pneumonia
    - Pneumonia due to Staphylococcus aureus NOS
  - **J15.212** Pneumonia due to methicillin resistant Staphylococcus aureus [HCC] [ESR] [COM]
  - **J15.29** Pneumonia due to other staphylococcus [HCC] [ESR] [COM]
- **J15.3** Pneumonia due to streptococcus, group B [ESR]
- **J15.4** Pneumonia due to other streptococci [ESR]
  - EXCLUDES 1: pneumonia due to streptococcus, group B (J15.3)
    pneumonia due to Streptococcus pneumoniae (J13)
- **J15.5** Pneumonia due to Escherichia coli [HCC] [ESR] [COM]
- **J15.6** Pneumonia due to other Gram-negative bacteria
  - AHA: 2023,4Q,27; 2020,2Q,28
  - **J15.61** Pneumonia due to Acinetobacter baumannii [HCC] [ESR] [COM]
  - **J15.69** Pneumonia due to other Gram-negative bacteria [HCC] [ESR] [COM]
    - Pneumonia due to other aerobic Gram-negative bacteria
    - Pneumonia due to Serratia marcescens
- **J15.7** Pneumonia due to Mycoplasma pneumoniae
- **J15.8** Pneumonia due to other specified bacteria [HCC] [ESR] [COM]
- **J15.9** Unspecified bacterial pneumonia
  - Pneumonia due to gram-positive bacteria

J16 Pneumonia due to other infectious organisms, not elsewhere classified

Code first, if applicable, associated influenza (J09.X1, J10.0-, J11.0-)
Code also, if applicable, any associated condition such as:
- abscess (J85.1)
- aspiration pneumonia (J69.-)

EXCLUDES 1:
- congenital pneumonia (P23.-)
- ornithosis (A70)
- pneumocystosis (B59)
- pneumonia NOS (J18.9)

AHA: 2020,2Q,28; 2019,1Q,35; 2018,3Q,24; 2016,3Q,15; 2013,4Q,118

- **J16.0** Chlamydial pneumonia
- **J16.8** Pneumonia due to other specified infectious organisms

J17 Pneumonia in diseases classified elsewhere

Code first underlying disease, such as:
- Q fever (A78)
- rheumatic fever (I00)
- schistosomiasis (B65.0-B65.9)

Code also, if applicable, any associated condition such as:
- abscess (J85.1)
- aspiration pneumonia (J69.-)

EXCLUDES 1:
- candidial pneumonia (B37.1)
- chlamydial pneumonia (J16.0)
- gonorrheal pneumonia (A54.84)
- histoplasmosis pneumonia (B39.0-B39.2)
- measles pneumonia (B05.2)
- nocardiosis pneumonia (A43.0)
- pneumocystosis (B59)
- pneumonia due to Pneumocystis carinii (B59)
- ▶pneumonia due to Pneumocystis jirovecii◀ (B59)
- pneumonia in actinomycosis (A42.0)
- pneumonia in anthrax (A22.1)
- pneumonia in ascariasis (B77.81)
- pneumonia in aspergillosis (B44.0-B44.1)
- pneumonia in coccidioidomycosis (B38.0-B38.2)
- pneumonia in cytomegalovirus disease (B25.0)
- pneumonia in toxoplasmosis (B58.3)
- rubella pneumonia (B06.81)
- salmonella pneumonia (A02.22)
- spirochetal infection NEC with pneumonia (A69.8)
- tularemia pneumonia (A21.2)
- typhoid fever with pneumonia (A01.03)
- varicella pneumonia (B01.2)
- whooping cough with pneumonia (A37 with fifth character 1)

AHA: 2020,2Q,28; 2019,1Q,35; 2016,3Q,15; 2013,4Q,118

J18 Pneumonia, unspecified organism

Code first, if applicable, associated influenza (J09.X1, J10.0-, J11.0-)
Code also, if applicable, any associated condition such as:
- aspiration pneumonia (J69.-)

EXCLUDES 1:
- congenital pneumonia (P23.0)
- drug-induced interstitial lung disorder (J70.2-J70.4)
- interstitial pneumonia NOS (J84.9)
- neonatal aspiration pneumonia (P24.-)
- pneumonitis due to fumes and vapors (J68.0)
- usual interstitial pneumonia (J84.178)

EXCLUDES 2:
- abscess of lung with pneumonia (J85.1)
- aspiration pneumonia due to anesthesia during labor and delivery (O74.0)
- aspiration pneumonia due to anesthesia during pregnancy (O29)
- aspiration pneumonia due to anesthesia during puerperium (O89.0)
- aspiration pneumonia due to solids and liquids (J69.-)
- aspiration pneumonia NOS (J69.0)
- lipid pneumonia (J69.1)
- pneumonitis due to external agents (J67-J70)

AHA: 2020,2Q,28; 2019,1Q,35; 2016,3Q,15; 2013,4Q,118

- **J18.0** Bronchopneumonia, unspecified organism
  - EXCLUDES 1:
    - hypostatic bronchopneumonia (J18.2)
    - lipid pneumonia (J69.1)
  - EXCLUDES 2:
    - acute bronchiolitis (J21.-)
    - chronic bronchiolitis (J44.89)
    - other specified chronic obstructive pulmonary disease (J44.89)
- **J18.1** Lobar pneumonia, unspecified organism [ESR]
  - AHA: 2019,3Q,37; 2018,3Q,24
  - **DEF:** Lobar pneumonia is characterized by consolidated inflammation confined or localized to only one or a few lobes of the lung. The consolidation affects primarily the alveolar air spaces, unlike bronchopneumonia, which arises from the bronchi or bronchioles and affects a wide area without any localization.
  - **TIP:** Documentation of right upper lobe, left upper lobe, right lower lobe, left lower lobe, or right middle lobe pneumonia alone is not synonymous with "lobar pneumonia," nor should a diagnosis of lobar pneumonia be assumed based on an imaging report that identifies pneumonia in a specific lobe. Assign J18.1 only when the provider specifically documents "lobar pneumonia" without specifying a causal organism.
- **J18.2** Hypostatic pneumonia, unspecified organism [COM]
  - Hypostatic bronchopneumonia
  - Passive pneumonia
- **J18.8** Other pneumonia, unspecified organism
- **J18.9** Pneumonia, unspecified organism
  - AHA: 2020,2Q,28; 2019,3Q,15; 2019,2Q,28; 2014,3Q,4; 2013,4Q,119; 2012,4Q,94

Other acute lower respiratory infections (J20-J22)

EXCLUDES 2 chronic obstructive pulmonary disease with acute lower respiratory infection (J44.0)

J20 Acute bronchitis
INCLUDES
- acute and subacute bronchitis (with) bronchospasm
- acute and subacute bronchitis (with) tracheitis
- acute and subacute bronchitis (with) tracheobronchitis, acute
- acute and subacute fibrinous bronchitis
- acute and subacute membranous bronchitis
- acute and subacute purulent bronchitis
- acute and subacute septic bronchitis

EXCLUDES 1
- bronchitis NOS (J40)
- tracheobronchitis NOS (J40)

EXCLUDES 2
- acute bronchitis with bronchiectasis (J47.0)
- acute bronchitis with chronic obstructive asthma (J44.0)
- acute bronchitis with chronic obstructive pulmonary disease (J44.0)
- allergic bronchitis NOS ▶(J45.909)◄
- bronchitis due to chemicals, fumes and vapors (J68.0)
- chronic bronchitis NOS (J42)
- chronic mucopurulent bronchitis (J41.1)
- chronic obstructive bronchitis (J44.-)
- chronic obstructive tracheobronchitis (J44.-)
- chronic simple bronchitis (J41.0)
- chronic tracheobronchitis (J42)

AHA: 2019,1Q,35; 2016,3Q,10,16

DEF: Acute inflammation of the main branches of the bronchial tree due to infectious or irritant agents. Symptoms include cough with a varied production of sputum, fever, substernal soreness, and lung rales. Bronchitis usually lasts three to 10 days.

- **J20.0** Acute bronchitis due to **Mycoplasma pneumoniae**
- **J20.1** Acute bronchitis due to **Hemophilus influenzae**
- **J20.2** Acute bronchitis due to **streptococcus**
- **J20.3** Acute bronchitis due to **coxsackievirus**
- **J20.4** Acute bronchitis due to **parainfluenza virus**
- **J20.5** Acute bronchitis due to **respiratory syncytial virus**
  Acute bronchitis due to RSV
- **J20.6** Acute bronchitis due to **rhinovirus**
- **J20.7** Acute bronchitis due to **echovirus**
- **J20.8** Acute bronchitis due to other specified organisms
  AHA: 2020,1Q,34-36
- **J20.9** Acute bronchitis, unspecified

J21 Acute bronchiolitis
INCLUDES acute bronchiolitis with bronchospasm
EXCLUDES 2 respiratory bronchiolitis interstitial lung disease (J84.115)

- **J21.0** Acute bronchiolitis due to **respiratory syncytial virus**
  Acute bronchiolitis due to RSV
- **J21.1** Acute bronchiolitis due to **human metapneumovirus**
- **J21.8** Acute bronchiolitis due to other specified organisms
- **J21.9** Acute bronchiolitis, unspecified
  Bronchiolitis (acute)
  EXCLUDES 1 chronic bronchiolitis (J44.89)

J22 Unspecified acute lower respiratory infection
Acute (lower) respiratory (tract) infection NOS
EXCLUDES 1 upper respiratory infection (acute) (J06.9)
AHA: 2020,1Q,22,34-36

Other diseases of upper respiratory tract (J30-J39)

J30 Vasomotor and allergic rhinitis
INCLUDES spasmodic rhinorrhea
EXCLUDES 1
- allergic rhinitis with asthma (bronchial) (J45.909)
- rhinitis NOS (J31.0)

- **J30.0** **Vasomotor** rhinitis
  DEF: Noninfectious and nonallergic type of rhinitis for which the cause is often unknown. Symptoms often mimic those of allergic rhinitis with a diagnosis of vasomotor rhinitis typically made after ruling out allergens as the cause.
- **J30.1** **Allergic** rhinitis **due to pollen**
  Allergy NOS due to pollen
  Hay fever
  Pollinosis
- **J30.2** Other **seasonal allergic** rhinitis
- **J30.5** Allergic rhinitis **due to food**
- **J30.8** Other allergic rhinitis
  - **J30.81** Allergic rhinitis due to **animal** (cat) (dog) **hair and dander**
  - **J30.89** Other allergic rhinitis
    Perennial allergic rhinitis
- **J30.9** Allergic rhinitis, unspecified

J31 Chronic rhinitis, nasopharyngitis and pharyngitis

- **J31.0** Chronic rhinitis
  - Atrophic rhinitis (chronic)
  - Granulomatous rhinitis (chronic)
  - Hypertrophic rhinitis (chronic)
  - Obstructive rhinitis (chronic)
  - Ozena
  - Purulent rhinitis (chronic)
  - Rhinitis (chronic) NOS
  - Ulcerative rhinitis (chronic)

  EXCLUDES 1
  - allergic rhinitis (J30.1-J30.9)
  - vasomotor rhinitis (J30.0)

  DEF: Persistent inflammation of the mucous membranes of the nose, characterized by a postnasal drip.

- **J31.1** Chronic nasopharyngitis
  EXCLUDES 2 acute nasopharyngitis (J00)
  DEF: Persistent inflammation of the mucous membranes extending from the nares to the pharynx. It is characterized by constant irritation in the nasopharynx and postnasal drip.

- **J31.2** Chronic pharyngitis
  - Atrophic pharyngitis (chronic)
  - Chronic sore throat
  - Granular pharyngitis (chronic)
  - Hypertrophic pharyngitis (chronic)

  EXCLUDES 2 acute pharyngitis (J02.9)

J32 Chronic sinusitis
INCLUDES
- sinus abscess
- sinus empyema
- sinus infection
- sinus suppuration

Use additional code to identify:
infectious agent (B95-B97)

EXCLUDES 2 acute sinusitis (J01.-)

- **J32.0** Chronic **maxillary** sinusitis
  - Antritis (chronic)
  - Maxillary sinusitis NOS
- **J32.1** Chronic **frontal** sinusitis
  - Frontal sinusitis NOS
- **J32.2** Chronic **ethmoidal** sinusitis
  - Ethmoidal sinusitis NOS
  - EXCLUDES 1 Woakes' ethmoiditis (J33.1)
- **J32.3** Chronic **sphenoidal** sinusitis
  - Sphenoidal sinusitis NOS
- **J32.4** Chronic **pansinusitis**
  - Pansinusitis NOS
- **J32.8** Other chronic sinusitis
  - Sinusitis (chronic) involving more than one sinus but not pansinusitis
- **J32.9** Chronic sinusitis, unspecified
  - Sinusitis (chronic) NOS

J33 Nasal polyp
EXCLUDES 1 adenomatous polyps (D14.0)

- **J33.0** Polyp of nasal cavity
  - Choanal polyp
  - Nasopharyngeal polyp
- **J33.1** Polypoid sinus degeneration
  - Woakes' syndrome or ethmoiditis
- **J33.8** Other polyp of sinus
  - Accessory polyp of sinus
  - Ethmoidal polyp of sinus
  - Maxillary polyp of sinus
  - Sphenoidal polyp of sinus
- **J33.9** Nasal polyp, unspecified

J34 Other and unspecified disorders of nose and nasal sinuses
EXCLUDES 2 varicose ulcer of nasal septum (I86.8)

- **J34.0** Abscess, furuncle and carbuncle of nose
  - Cellulitis of nose
  - Necrosis of nose
  - Ulceration of nose
- **J34.1** Cyst and mucocele of nose and nasal sinus

J34.2 Deviated nasal septum
Deflection or deviation of septum (nasal) (acquired)
> EXCLUDES 1 congenital deviated nasal septum (Q67.4)

DEF: Condition in which the nasal septum, a thin wall composed of cartilage and bone that separates the two nostrils, is crooked or displaced from the midline.

J34.3 Hypertrophy of nasal turbinates
DEF: Overgrowth of bones within the nasal turbinate, which are ridges of bone and soft tissue that project from the sidewalls of the nasal passages. Hypertrophy can cause obstruction of the nasal passages.

✓5th J34.8 Other specified disorders of nose and nasal sinuses

J34.81 Nasal mucositis (ulcerative)
Code also type of associated therapy, such as:
  antineoplastic and immunosuppressive drugs (T45.1X-)
  radiological procedure and radiotherapy (Y84.2)
> EXCLUDES 2 gastrointestinal mucositis (ulcerative) (K92.81)
> mucositis (ulcerative) of vagina and vulva (N76.81)
> oral mucositis (ulcerative) (K12.3-)

✓6th J34.82 Nasal valve collapse
Nasal valve compromise
Nasal valve stenosis
Code first underlying cause, such as:
  deviated nasal septum (J34.2)
AHA: 2024,4Q,20

✓7th J34.820 Internal nasal valve collapse

J34.8200 Internal nasal valve collapse, unspecified

J34.8201 Internal nasal valve collapse, static
Narrowing of the septum, head of the inferior turbinate and the upper lateral cartilage

J34.8202 Internal nasal valve collapse, dynamic
Collapse or falling of the upper, middle sidewall of the nose on inspiration

✓7th J34.821 External nasal valve collapse

J34.8210 External nasal valve collapse, unspecified

J34.8211 External nasal valve collapse, static
Fixed narrowing of the caudal septum, lower lateral cartilage, alar rim and nasal sill

J34.8212 External nasal valve collapse, dynamic
Collapse or falling of the lower sidewall or nostril of the nose on inspiration

J34.829 Nasal valve collapse, unspecified
Nasal valve collapse, NOS

J34.89 Other specified disorders of nose and nasal sinuses
Perforation of nasal septum NOS
Rhinolith

J34.9 Unspecified disorder of nose and nasal sinuses

✓4th J35 Chronic diseases of tonsils and adenoids

✓5th J35.0 Chronic tonsillitis and adenoiditis
> EXCLUDES 2 acute tonsillitis (J03.-)

J35.01 Chronic tonsillitis
J35.02 Chronic adenoiditis
J35.03 Chronic tonsillitis and adenoiditis

J35.1 Hypertrophy of tonsils
Enlargement of tonsils
> EXCLUDES 1 hypertrophy of tonsils with tonsillitis (J35.0-)

J35.2 Hypertrophy of adenoids
Enlargement of adenoids
> EXCLUDES 1 hypertrophy of adenoids with adenoiditis (J35.0-)

J35.3 Hypertrophy of tonsils with hypertrophy of adenoids
> EXCLUDES 1 hypertrophy of tonsils and adenoids with tonsillitis and adenoiditis (J35.03)

J35.8 Other chronic diseases of tonsils and adenoids
Adenoid vegetations
Amygdalolith
Calculus, tonsil
Cicatrix of tonsil (and adenoid)
Tonsillar tag
Ulcer of tonsil

J35.9 Chronic disease of tonsils and adenoids, unspecified
Disease (chronic) of tonsils and adenoids NOS

J36 Peritonsillar abscess
> INCLUDES abscess of tonsil
> peritonsillar cellulitis
> quinsy

Use additional code (B95-B97) to identify infectious agent
> EXCLUDES 1 acute tonsillitis (J03.-)
> chronic tonsillitis (J35.0)
> retropharyngeal abscess (J39.0)
> tonsillitis NOS (J03.9-)

✓4th J37 Chronic laryngitis and laryngotracheitis
Use additional code to identify:
  exposure to environmental tobacco smoke (Z77.22)
  exposure to tobacco smoke in the perinatal period (P96.81)
  history of tobacco dependence (Z87.891)
  infectious agent (B95-B97)
  occupational exposure to environmental tobacco smoke (Z57.31)
  tobacco dependence (F17.-)
  tobacco use (Z72.0)

J37.0 Chronic laryngitis
Catarrhal laryngitis
Hypertrophic laryngitis
Sicca laryngitis
> EXCLUDES 2 acute laryngitis (J04.0)
> obstructive (acute) laryngitis (J05.0)

J37.1 Chronic laryngotracheitis
Laryngitis, chronic, with tracheitis (chronic)
Tracheitis, chronic, with laryngitis
> EXCLUDES 1 chronic tracheitis (J42)
> EXCLUDES 2 acute laryngotracheitis (J04.2)
> acute tracheitis (J04.1)

✓4th J38 Diseases of vocal cords and larynx, not elsewhere classified
> EXCLUDES 1 congenital laryngeal stridor (P28.89)
> obstructive laryngitis (acute) (J05.0)
> postprocedural subglottic stenosis (J95.5)
> stridor (R06.1)
> ulcerative laryngitis (J04.0)

✓5th J38.0 Paralysis of vocal cords and larynx
Laryngoplegia
Paralysis of glottis

J38.00 Paralysis of vocal cords and larynx, unspecified
J38.01 Paralysis of vocal cords and larynx, unilateral
AHA: 2025,1Q,27
J38.02 Paralysis of vocal cords and larynx, bilateral

J38.1 Polyp of vocal cord and larynx
> EXCLUDES 1 adenomatous polyps (D14.1)

J38.2 Nodules of vocal cords
Chorditis (fibrinous)(nodosa)(tuberosa)
Singer's nodes
Teacher's nodes

J38.3 Other diseases of vocal cords
Abscess of vocal cords
Cellulitis of vocal cords
Granuloma of vocal cords
Leukokeratosis of vocal cords
Leukoplakia of vocal cords

J38.4 Edema of larynx
Edema (of) glottis
Subglottic edema
Supraglottic edema
> EXCLUDES 1 acute obstructive laryngitis [croup] (J05.0)
> edematous laryngitis (J04.0)

J38.5 Laryngeal spasm
Laryngismus (stridulus)

J38.6 Stenosis of larynx

J38.7 Other diseases of larynx
Abscess of larynx
Cellulitis of larynx
Disease of larynx NOS
Necrosis of larynx
Pachyderma of larynx
Perichondritis of larynx
Ulcer of larynx

✓4th J39 Other diseases of upper respiratory tract
EXCLUDES 1   acute respiratory infection NOS (J22)
              acute upper respiratory infection (J06.9)
              upper respiratory inflammation due to chemicals, gases, fumes or vapors (J68.2)

J39.0 Retropharyngeal and parapharyngeal abscess
Peripharyngeal abscess
EXCLUDES 1   peritonsillar abscess (J36)
DEF: Purulent infection behind the pharynx and the front of the precerebral fascia, characterized by neck stiffness, cervical lymphadenopathy, sore throat, fever, and stridor.

J39.1 Other abscess of pharynx
Cellulitis of pharynx
Nasopharyngeal abscess

J39.2 Other diseases of pharynx
Cyst of pharynx
Edema of pharynx
EXCLUDES 2   chronic pharyngitis (J31.2)
              ulcerative pharyngitis (J02.9)

J39.3 Upper respiratory tract hypersensitivity reaction, site unspecified
EXCLUDES 1   hypersensitivity reaction of upper respiratory tract, such as:
              extrinsic allergic alveolitis (J67.9)
              pneumoconiosis (J60-J67.9)

J39.8 Other specified diseases of upper respiratory tract
AHA: 2023,1Q,30

J39.9 Disease of upper respiratory tract, unspecified

Chronic lower respiratory diseases (J40-J4A)

EXCLUDES 1   bronchitis due to chemicals, gases, fumes and vapors (J68.0)
EXCLUDES 2   cystic fibrosis (E84.-)

J40 Bronchitis, not specified as acute or chronic
Bronchitis NOS
Bronchitis with tracheitis NOS
Catarrhal bronchitis
Tracheobronchitis NOS
Use additional code to identify:
    exposure to environmental tobacco smoke (Z77.22)
    exposure to tobacco smoke in the perinatal period (P96.81)
    history of tobacco dependence (Z87.891)
    occupational exposure to environmental tobacco smoke (Z57.31)
    tobacco dependence (F17.-)
    tobacco use (Z72.0)
EXCLUDES 1   acute bronchitis (J20.-)
              allergic bronchitis NOS ▶(J45.909)◀
              asthmatic bronchitis NOS (J45.9-)
              bronchitis due to chemicals, gases, fumes and vapors (J68.0)
AHA: 2020,1Q,34-36

✓4th J41 Simple and mucopurulent chronic bronchitis
Use additional code to identify:
    exposure to environmental tobacco smoke (Z77.22)
    exposure to tobacco smoke in the perinatal period (P96.81)
    history of tobacco dependence (Z87.891)
    occupational exposure to environmental tobacco smoke (Z57.31)
    tobacco dependence (F17.-)
    tobacco use (Z72.0)
EXCLUDES 2   chronic bronchitis NOS (J42)
              chronic obstructive pulmonary disease (J44.-)

J41.0 Simple chronic bronchitis HCC Rx ESR COM
J41.1 Mucopurulent chronic bronchitis HCC Rx ESR COM
J41.8 Mixed simple and mucopurulent chronic bronchitis HCC Rx ESR COM

J42 Unspecified chronic bronchitis HCC Rx ESR COM
Chronic bronchitis NOS
Chronic tracheitis
Chronic tracheobronchitis
Use additional code to identify:
    exposure to environmental tobacco smoke (Z77.22)
    exposure to tobacco smoke in the perinatal period (P96.81)
    history of tobacco dependence (Z87.891)
    occupational exposure to environmental tobacco smoke (Z57.31)
    tobacco dependence (F17.-)
    tobacco use (Z72.0)
EXCLUDES 1   bronchiolitis obliterans and bronchiolitis obliterans syndrome (J44.81)
              chronic asthmatic bronchitis (J44.-)
              chronic bronchitis with airways obstruction (J44.-)
              chronic emphysematous bronchitis (J44.-)
              chronic obstructive pulmonary disease NOS (J44.9)
              simple and mucopurulent chronic bronchitis (J41.-)

✓4th J43 Emphysema
EXCLUDES 1   compensatory emphysema (J98.3)
              emphysema due to inhalation of chemicals, gases, fumes or vapors (J68.4)
              interstitial emphysema (J98.2)
              mediastinal emphysema (J98.2)
              neonatal interstitial emphysema (P25.0)
              surgical (subcutaneous) emphysema (T81.82)
EXCLUDES 2   ▶emphysema due to inhalation of chemicals, gases, fumes or vapors (J68.4)◀
              emphysema with chronic (obstructive) bronchitis (J44.-)
              emphysematous (obstructive) bronchitis (J44.-)
              traumatic subcutaneous emphysema (T79.7)
DEF: Pathological condition in which there is destructive enlargement of the air sacs in the lungs resulting in damage and lack of elasticity to the alveolar walls, commonly seen in long-term smokers.

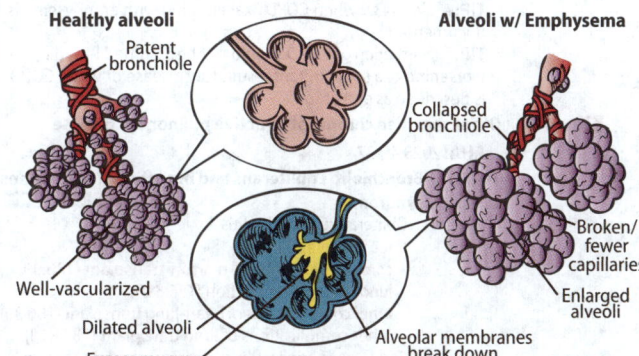

Emphysema

J43.0 Unilateral pulmonary emphysema [MacLeod's syndrome] HCC Rx ESR COM
Swyer-James syndrome
Unilateral emphysema
Unilateral hyperlucent lung
Unilateral pulmonary artery functional hypoplasia
Unilateral transparency of lung

J43.1 Panlobular emphysema HCC Rx ESR COM
Panacinar emphysema

J43.2 Centrilobular emphysema HCC Rx ESR COM

J43.8 Other emphysema HCC Rx ESR COM

J43.9 Emphysema, unspecified HCC Rx ESR COM
Bullous emphysema (lung)(pulmonary)
Emphysema (lung)(pulmonary) NOS
Emphysematous bleb
Vesicular emphysema (lung)(pulmonary)
AHA: 2024,2Q,4; 2019,1Q,34-36; 2017,4Q,97-98

J44 Other chronic obstructive pulmonary disease ✓4th

INCLUDES
asthma with chronic obstructive pulmonary disease
chronic asthmatic (obstructive) bronchitis
chronic bronchitis with airway obstruction
chronic bronchitis with emphysema
chronic emphysematous bronchitis
chronic obstructive asthma
chronic obstructive bronchitis
chronic obstructive tracheobronchitis

Code also type of asthma, if applicable (J45.-)

EXCLUDES 1
chronic bronchitis NOS (J42)
chronic simple and mucopurulent bronchitis (J41.-)
chronic tracheitis (J42)
chronic tracheobronchitis (J42)

EXCLUDES 2
bronchiectasis (J47.-)
▶chronic bronchitis NOS (J42)◀
▶chronic simple and mucopurulent bronchitis (J41.-)◀
▶chronic tracheitis (J42)◀
▶chronic tracheobronchitis (J42)◀
emphysema without chronic bronchitis (J43.-)

AHA: 2024,2Q,3–5; 2019,1Q,34-36; 2017,4Q,97-98; 2017,1Q,25-26; 2016,3Q,15-16; 2013,4Q,109

J44.0 Chronic obstructive pulmonary disease with (acute) lower respiratory infection [HCC Rx ESR COM]
Code also to identify the infection
AHA: 2019,1Q,35; 2017,4Q,96; 2017,1Q,24-25
TIP: Do not assign when only aspiration pneumonia is present. Aspiration pneumonia is not classified as a respiratory infection.

J44.1 Chronic obstructive pulmonary disease with (acute) exacerbation [HCC Rx ESR COM]
Decompensated COPD
Decompensated COPD with (acute) exacerbation

EXCLUDES 2
chronic obstructive pulmonary disease [COPD] with acute bronchitis (J44.0)
lung diseases due to external agents (J60-J70)

AHA: 2019,1Q,34; 2017,4Q,96; 2017,1Q,26; 2016,1Q,36
TIP: Assign J43.9 when COPD exacerbation with emphysema is documented.
TIP: Exacerbation of COPD should not be assumed based upon worsening of a concomitant respiratory disease or when COPD is described as end-stage.

J44.8 Other specified chronic obstructive pulmonary disease ✓5th
AHA: 2023,4Q,27

J44.81 Bronchiolitis obliterans and bronchiolitis obliterans syndrome [HCC Rx ESR COM]
Obliterative bronchiolitis
Code first, if applicable:
complication of bone marrow transplant (T86.09)
lung transplant rejection (T86.810)
other complications of heart-lung transplant (T86.39)
other complications of lung transplant (T86.818)
Code also, if applicable, associated conditions, such as:
chronic graft-versus-host disease (D89.811)
chronic lung allograft dysfunction (J4A.-)
chronic respiratory conditions due to chemicals, gases, fumes and vapors (J68.4)
complication of stem cell transplant (T86.5)
heart-lung transplant rejection (T86.31)

J44.89 Other specified chronic obstructive pulmonary disease [HCC Rx ESR COM]
Chronic asthmatic (obstructive) bronchitis
Chronic emphysematous bronchitis

J44.9 Chronic obstructive pulmonary disease, unspecified [HCC Rx ESR COM]
Chronic obstructive airway disease NOS
Chronic obstructive lung disease NOS

EXCLUDES 2 lung diseases due to external agents (J60-J70)
AHA: 2019,1Q,36; 2017,4Q,96-97; 2016,1Q,36; 2014,4Q,21; 2013,4Q,109

J4A Chronic lung allograft dysfunction ✓4th
Code first, if applicable:
heart-lung transplant rejection (T86.31)
lung transplant rejection (T86.810)
other complications of heart-lung transplant (T86.39)
other complications of lung transplant (T86.818)
Code also, if applicable, bronchiolitis obliterans syndrome (J44.81)
AHA: 2023,4Q,28

J4A.0 Restrictive allograft syndrome [HCC Rx ESR COM]
Code also, if applicable, for mixed chronic lung allograft dysfunction, bronchiolitis obliterans syndrome (J44.81)

J4A.8 Other chronic lung allograft dysfunction [HCC Rx ESR COM]

J4A.9 Chronic lung allograft dysfunction, unspecified [HCC Rx ESR COM]

J45 Asthma ✓4th

INCLUDES
allergic (predominantly) asthma
allergic bronchitis NOS
allergic rhinitis with asthma
atopic asthma
extrinsic allergic asthma
hay fever with asthma
idiosyncratic asthma
intrinsic nonallergic asthma
nonallergic asthma

Use additional code to identify:
eosinophilic asthma (J82.83)
exposure to environmental tobacco smoke (Z77.22)
exposure to tobacco smoke in the perinatal period (P96.81)
history of tobacco dependence (Z87.891)
occupational exposure to environmental tobacco smoke (Z57.31)
tobacco dependence (F17.-)
tobacco use (Z72.0)

EXCLUDES 1
detergent asthma (J69.8)
miner's asthma (J60)
wheezing NOS (R06.2)
wood asthma (J67.8)

EXCLUDES 2
asthma with chronic obstructive pulmonary disease (J44.89)
chronic asthmatic (obstructive) bronchitis (J44.89)
chronic obstructive asthma (J44.89)
other specified chronic obstructive pulmonary disease (J44.89)

AHA: 2024,2Q,3; 2023,1Q,17; 2019,1Q,36; 2017,1Q,25-26; 2012,4Q,99
DEF: Status asthmaticus: Severe, intractable episode of asthma that is unresponsive to normal therapeutic measures.

J45.2 Mild intermittent asthma ✓5th

J45.20 Mild intermittent asthma, uncomplicated [Rx COM]
Mild intermittent asthma NOS

J45.21 Mild intermittent asthma with (acute) exacerbation [Rx COM]

J45.22 Mild intermittent asthma with status asthmaticus [Rx COM]

J45.3 Mild persistent asthma ✓5th

J45.30 Mild persistent asthma, uncomplicated [Rx COM]
Mild persistent asthma NOS

J45.31 Mild persistent asthma with (acute) exacerbation [Rx COM]
AHA: 2016,1Q,35

J45.32 Mild persistent asthma with status asthmaticus [Rx COM]

J45.4 Moderate persistent asthma ✓5th

J45.40 Moderate persistent asthma, uncomplicated [Rx COM]
Moderate persistent asthma NOS

J45.41 Moderate persistent asthma with (acute) exacerbation [Rx COM]
AHA: 2017,1Q,26

J45.42 Moderate persistent asthma with status asthmaticus [Rx COM]

J45.5 Severe persistent asthma ✓5th

J45.50 Severe persistent asthma, uncomplicated [HCC Rx COM]
Severe persistent asthma NOS

J45.51 Severe persistent asthma with (acute) exacerbation [HCC Rx COM]

J45.52 Severe persistent asthma with status asthmaticus [HCC Rx COM]

Chapter 10. Diseases of the Respiratory System

J45.9 Other and unspecified asthma

J45.90 Unspecified asthma
Asthmatic bronchitis NOS
Childhood asthma NOS
Late onset asthma
AHA: 2017,4Q,96; 2017,1Q,25

- **J45.901** Unspecified asthma with (acute) exacerbation
- **J45.902** Unspecified asthma with status asthmaticus
- **J45.909** Unspecified asthma, uncomplicated
  Asthma NOS
  EXCLUDES 2: lung diseases due to external agents (J60-J70)
  AHA: 2017,1Q,25

J45.99 Other asthma
- **J45.990** Exercise induced bronchospasm
- **J45.991** Cough variant asthma
- **J45.998** Other asthma

J47 Bronchiectasis
INCLUDES: bronchiolectasis
Use additional code to identify:
  exposure to environmental tobacco smoke (Z77.22)
  exposure to tobacco smoke in the perinatal period (P96.81)
  history of tobacco dependence (Z87.891)
  occupational exposure to environmental tobacco smoke (Z57.31)
  tobacco dependence (F17.-)
  tobacco use (Z72.0)
EXCLUDES 1: congenital bronchiectasis (Q33.4)
  tuberculous bronchiectasis (current disease) (A15.0)
DEF: Dilation of the bronchi with mucus production and persistent cough due to infection or chronic conditions that causes diminished lung capacity and frequent infections of the lung.

- **J47.0 Bronchiectasis with acute lower respiratory infection**
  Bronchiectasis with acute bronchitis
  Code also to identify infection, if applicable
- **J47.1 Bronchiectasis with (acute) exacerbation**
  AHA: 2021,1Q,23
- **J47.9 Bronchiectasis, uncomplicated**
  Bronchiectasis NOS
  AHA: 2024,2Q,5

Lung diseases due to external agents (J60-J70)

EXCLUDES 2: asthma (J45.-)
  malignant neoplasm of bronchus and lung (C34.-)
DEF: Pneumoconiosis: Condition caused by inhaling inorganic dust particles, typically associated with occupations that require regular exposure to mineral dusts. A form of interstitial lung disease that contributes to the inflammation of the air sacs, causing the lung tissue to harden.

J60 Coalworker's pneumoconiosis
Anthracosilicosis
Anthracosis
Black lung disease
Coalworker's lung
EXCLUDES 1: coalworker pneumoconiosis with tuberculosis, any type in A15 (J65)

J61 Pneumoconiosis due to asbestos and other mineral fibers
Asbestosis
EXCLUDES 1: pleural plaque with asbestosis (J92.0)
  pneumoconiosis with tuberculosis, any type in A15 (J65)

J62 Pneumoconiosis due to dust containing silica
INCLUDES: silicotic fibrosis (massive) of lung
EXCLUDES 1: pneumoconiosis with tuberculosis, any type in A15 (J65)

- **J62.0 Pneumoconiosis due to talc dust**
- **J62.8 Pneumoconiosis due to other dust containing silica**
  Silicosis NOS

J63 Pneumoconiosis due to other inorganic dusts
EXCLUDES 1: pneumoconiosis with tuberculosis, any type in A15 (J65)

- **J63.0 Aluminosis (of lung)**
- **J63.1 Bauxite fibrosis (of lung)**
- **J63.2 Berylliosis**
- **J63.3 Graphite fibrosis (of lung)**
- **J63.4 Siderosis**
  AHA: 2019,3Q,8
- **J63.5 Stannosis**
- **J63.6 Pneumoconiosis due to other specified inorganic dusts**

J64 Unspecified pneumoconiosis
EXCLUDES 1: pneumonoconiosis with tuberculosis, any type in A15 (J65)

J65 Pneumoconiosis associated with tuberculosis
Any condition in J60-J64 with tuberculosis, any type in A15
Silicotuberculosis
► Use additional code, if applicable, for associated cachexia (E88.A) ◄

J66 Airway disease due to specific organic dust
EXCLUDES 2: allergic alveolitis (J67.-)
  asbestosis (J61)
  bagassosis (J67.1)
  farmer's lung (J67.0)
  hypersensitivity pneumonitis due to organic dust (J67.-)
  reactive airways dysfunction syndrome (J68.3)

- **J66.0 Byssinosis**
  Airway disease due to cotton dust
- **J66.1 Flax-dressers' disease**
- **J66.2 Cannabinosis**
- **J66.8 Airway disease due to other specific organic dusts**

J67 Hypersensitivity pneumonitis due to organic dust
INCLUDES: allergic alveolitis and pneumonitis due to inhaled organic dust and particles of fungal, actinomycetic or other origin
EXCLUDES 1: pneumonitis due to inhalation of chemicals, gases, fumes or vapors (J68.0)

- **J67.0 Farmer's lung**
  Harvester's lung
  Haymaker's lung
  Moldy hay disease
- **J67.1 Bagassosis**
  Bagasse disease
  Bagasse pneumonitis
- **J67.2 Bird fancier's lung**
  Budgerigar fancier's disease or lung
  Pigeon fancier's disease or lung
- **J67.3 Suberosis**
  Corkhandler's disease or lung
  Corkworker's disease or lung
- **J67.4 Maltworker's lung**
  Alveolitis due to Aspergillus clavatus
- **J67.5 Mushroom-worker's lung**
- **J67.6 Maple-bark-stripper's lung**
  Alveolitis due to Cryptostroma corticale
  Cryptostromosis
- **J67.7 Air conditioner and humidifier lung**
  Allergic alveolitis due to fungal, thermophilic actinomycetes and other organisms growing in ventilation [air conditioning] systems
- **J67.8 Hypersensitivity pneumonitis due to other organic dusts**
  Cheese-washer's lung
  Coffee-worker's lung
  Fish-meal worker's lung
  Furrier's lung
  Sequoiosis
- **J67.9 Hypersensitivity pneumonitis due to unspecified organic dust**
  Allergic alveolitis (extrinsic) NOS
  Hypersensitivity pneumonitis NOS

J68 Respiratory conditions due to inhalation of chemicals, gases, fumes and vapors
Code first (T51-T65) to identify cause
Use additional code to identify associated respiratory conditions, such as: acute respiratory failure (J96.0-)

- **J68.0 Bronchitis and pneumonitis due to chemicals, gases, fumes and vapors**
  Chemical bronchitis (acute)
  AHA: 2019,2Q,31

J68.1 **Pulmonary edema** due to chemicals, gases, fumes and vapors [HCC] [ESR] [COM]
    Chemical pulmonary edema (acute) (chronic)
    EXCLUDES 1 pulmonary edema (acute) (chronic) NOS (J81.-)

J68.2 **Upper respiratory inflammation** due to chemicals, gases, fumes and vapors, not elsewhere classified [HCC] [ESR] [COM]

J68.3 Other **acute and subacute respiratory conditions** due to chemicals, gases, fumes and vapors [HCC] [ESR] [COM]
    Reactive airways dysfunction syndrome

J68.4 **Chronic respiratory conditions** due to chemicals, gases, fumes and vapors [HCC] [ESR] [COM]
    obliterative bronchiolitis (J44.81)
    Code also, if applicable, chronic conditions, such as:
      emphysema (J43.-)
      pulmonary fibrosis (J84.10)
    EXCLUDES 1 chronic pulmonary edema due to chemicals, gases, fumes and vapors (J68.1)

J68.8 Other respiratory conditions due to chemicals, gases, fumes and vapors [HCC] [ESR] [COM]

J68.9 Unspecified respiratory condition due to chemicals, gases, fumes and vapors [HCC] [ESR] [COM]

✓4th **J69** Pneumonitis due to solids and liquids
    Codes also, if applicable, other types of pneumonias
    EXCLUDES 1 neonatal aspiration syndromes (P24.-)
      postprocedural pneumonitis (J95.4)
    AHA: 2017,1Q,24
    DEF: Pneumonitis: Noninfectious inflammation of the walls of the alveoli in the lung tissue due to inhalation of food, vomit, oils, essences, or other solids or liquids.

J69.0 Pneumonitis due to **inhalation of food and vomit** [HCC] [ESR] [COM]
    Aspiration pneumonia (due to) food (regurgitated)
    Aspiration pneumonia (due to) gastric secretions
    Aspiration pneumonia (due to) milk
    Aspiration pneumonia (due to) vomit
    Aspiration pneumonia NOS
    Code also any associated foreign body in respiratory tract (T17.-)
    EXCLUDES 1 chemical pneumonitis due to anesthesia (J95.4)
      obstetric aspiration pneumonitis (O74.0)
    AHA: 2020,2Q,11,28; 2019,3Q,17; 2019,2Q,6,31

J69.1 Pneumonitis due to **inhalation of oils and essences** [HCC] [ESR] [COM]
    Exogenous lipoid pneumonia
    Lipid pneumonia NOS
    Code first (T51-T65) to identify substance
    EXCLUDES 1 endogenous lipoid pneumonia (J84.89)

J69.8 Pneumonitis due to inhalation of other solids and liquids [HCC] [ESR] [COM]
    Pneumonitis due to aspiration of blood
    Pneumonitis due to aspiration of detergent
    Code first (T51-T65) to identify substance

✓4th **J70** Respiratory conditions due to other external agents

J70.0 **Acute** pulmonary manifestations due to **radiation** [ESR] [COM]
    Radiation pneumonitis
    Use additional code (W88-W90, X39.0-) to identify the external cause

J70.1 **Chronic** and other pulmonary manifestations due to **radiation** [ESR] [COM]
    Fibrosis of lung following radiation
    Use additional code (W88-W90, X39.0-) to identify the external cause

J70.2 **Acute drug-induced interstitial** lung disorders [ESR]
    Use additional code for adverse effect, if applicable, to identify drug (T36-T50 with fifth or sixth character 5)
    EXCLUDES 1 interstitial pneumonia NOS (J84.9)
      lymphoid interstitial pneumonia (J84.2)
    AHA: 2019,2Q,28

J70.3 **Chronic drug-induced interstitial** lung disorders [ESR]
    Use additional code for adverse effect, if applicable, to identify drug (T36-T50 with fifth or sixth character 5)
    EXCLUDES 1 interstitial pneumonia NOS (J84.9)
      lymphoid interstitial pneumonia (J84.2)

J70.4 Drug-induced interstitial lung disorders, unspecified [ESR]
    Use additional code for adverse effect, if applicable, to identify drug (T36-T50 with fifth or sixth character 5)
    EXCLUDES 1 interstitial pneumonia NOS (J84.9)
      lymphoid interstitial pneumonia (J84.2)
    AHA: 2019,2Q,28

J70.5 Respiratory conditions due to **smoke inhalation** [ESR]
    Code first smoke inhalation (T59.81-)
    EXCLUDES 2 smoke inhalation due to chemicals, gases, fumes and vapors (J68.9)
    AHA: 2013,4Q,121

J70.8 Respiratory conditions due to other specified external agents [ESR]
    Code first (T51-T65) to identify the external agent

J70.9 Respiratory conditions due to unspecified external agent [ESR]
    Code first (T51-T65) to identify the external agent

Other respiratory diseases principally affecting the interstitium (J80-J84)

J80 Acute respiratory distress syndrome [HCC] [ESR] [COM]
    Acute respiratory distress syndrome in adult or child
    Adult hyaline membrane disease
    EXCLUDES 1 respiratory distress syndrome in newborn (perinatal) (P22.0)
    AHA: 2021,1Q,23; 2020,4Q,96; 2020,1Q,34-36; 2017,1Q,26
    DEF: Lung inflammation or injury resulting in a build-up of fluid in the air sacs, preventing the passage of oxygen from the air into the bloodstream.

✓4th **J81** Pulmonary edema
    Use additional code to identify:
      exposure to environmental tobacco smoke (Z77.22)
      history of tobacco dependence (Z87.891)
      occupational exposure to environmental tobacco smoke (Z57.31)
      tobacco dependence (F17.-)
      tobacco use (Z72.0)
    EXCLUDES 1 chemical (acute) pulmonary edema (J68.1)
      hypostatic pneumonia (J18.2)
      passive pneumonia (J18.2)
      pulmonary edema due to external agents (J60-J70)
      pulmonary edema with heart disease NOS (I50.1)
      pulmonary edema with heart failure (I50.1)
    DEF: Accumulation of fluid in the air sacs of the lungs, making it difficult to breathe.

J81.0 **Acute** pulmonary edema [HCC] [ESR] [COM]
    Acute edema of lung
    AHA: 2023,1Q,25; 2020,3Q,27

J81.1 **Chronic** pulmonary edema [COM]
    Pulmonary congestion (chronic) (passive)
    Pulmonary edema NOS

✓4th **J82** Pulmonary eosinophilia, not elsewhere classified
    EXCLUDES 2 pulmonary eosinophilia due to aspergillosis (B44.-)
      pulmonary eosinophilia due to drugs (J70.2-J70.4)
      pulmonary eosinophilia due to specified parasitic infection (B50-B83)
      pulmonary eosinophilia due to systemic connective tissue disorders (M30-M36)
      pulmonary infiltrate NOS (R91.8)
    DEF: Infiltration of eosinophils (white blood cells of the immune system) into the parenchyma of the lungs, resulting in cough, fever, and dyspnea.

✓5th **J82.8** Pulmonary eosinophilia, not elsewhere classified
    AHA: 2020,4Q,25-27

    J82.81 **Chronic** eosinophilic pneumonia [HCC] [Rx] [ESR] [COM]
      Eosinophilic pneumonia, NOS

    J82.82 **Acute** eosinophilic pneumonia

    J82.83 **Eosinophilic** asthma [Rx] [COM]
      Code first asthma, by type, such as:
        mild intermittent asthma (J45.2-)
        mild persistent asthma (J45.3-)
        moderate persistent asthma (J45.4-)
        severe persistent asthma (J45.5-)

    J82.89 Other pulmonary eosinophilia, not elsewhere classified [ESR] [COM]
      Allergic pneumonia
      Loffler's pneumonia
      Tropical (pulmonary) eosinophilia NOS

J84 Other interstitial pulmonary diseases

Code also, if applicable, associated condition

EXCLUDES 1 drug-induced interstitial lung disorders (J70.2-J70.4)
interstitial emphysema (J98.2)

EXCLUDES 2 lung diseases due to external agents (J60-J70)

DEF: Interstitial: Within the small spaces or gaps occurring in tissue or organs.

J84.0 Alveolar and parieto-alveolar conditions

J84.01 Alveolar proteinosis
DEF: Reduced ventilation due to proteinaceous deposits on alveoli. Symptoms include dyspnea, cough, chest pain, weakness, weight loss, and hemoptysis.

J84.02 Pulmonary alveolar microlithiasis

J84.03 Idiopathic pulmonary hemosiderosis
Essential brown induration of lung
Code first underlying disease, such as:
  disorders of iron metabolism (E83.1-)
EXCLUDES 1 acute idiopathic pulmonary hemorrhage in infants [AIPHI] (R04.81)
DEF: Fibrosis of the alveolar walls marked by abnormal accumulation of iron as hemosiderin in the lungs. It primarily affects children and symptoms include anemia, fluid in the lungs, and blood in the sputum. Etiology is unknown.

J84.09 Other alveolar and parieto-alveolar conditions

J84.1 Other interstitial pulmonary diseases with fibrosis

▶Code also, if applicable, pulmonary fibrosis (chronic) due to inhalation of chemicals, gases, fumes or vapors (J68.4)◀

EXCLUDES 1 pulmonary fibrosis (chronic) due to inhalation of chemicals, gases, fumes or vapors (J68.4)
pulmonary fibrosis (chronic) following radiation (J70.1)

J84.10 Pulmonary fibrosis, unspecified
Capillary fibrosis of lung
Cirrhosis of lung (chronic) NOS
Fibrosis of lung (atrophic) (chronic) (confluent) (massive) (perialveolar) (peribronchial) NOS
Induration of lung (chronic) NOS
Postinflammatory pulmonary fibrosis
AHA: 2024,2Q,20

J84.11 Idiopathic interstitial pneumonia
EXCLUDES 1 lymphoid interstitial pneumonia (J84.2)
pneumocystis pneumonia (B59)

J84.111 Idiopathic interstitial pneumonia, not otherwise specified

J84.112 Idiopathic pulmonary fibrosis
Cryptogenic fibrosing alveolitis
Idiopathic fibrosing alveolitis

J84.113 Idiopathic non-specific interstitial pneumonitis
EXCLUDES 1 non-specific interstitial pneumonia NOS, or due to known underlying cause (J84.89)

J84.114 Acute interstitial pneumonitis
Hamman-Rich syndrome
EXCLUDES 1 pneumocystis pneumonia (B59)

J84.115 Respiratory bronchiolitis interstitial lung disease

J84.116 Cryptogenic organizing pneumonia
EXCLUDES 1 organizing pneumonia NOS, or due to known underlying cause (J84.89)

J84.117 Desquamative interstitial pneumonia

J84.17 Other interstitial pulmonary diseases with fibrosis in diseases classified elsewhere
AHA: 2020,4Q,27-28

J84.170 Interstitial lung disease with progressive fibrotic phenotype in diseases classified elsewhere
Progressive fibrotic interstitial lung disease
Code first underlying disease, such as:
  lung diseases due to external agents (J60-J70)
  rheumatoid arthritis (M05.00-M06.9)
  sarcoidosis (D86.-)
  systemic connective tissue disorders (M30-M36)

J84.178 Other interstitial pulmonary diseases with fibrosis in diseases classified elsewhere
Interstitial pneumonia (nonspecific) (usual) due to collagen vascular disease
Interstitial pneumonia (nonspecific) (usual) in diseases classified elsewhere
Organizing pneumonia due to collagen vascular disease
Organizing pneumonia in diseases classified elsewhere
Code first underlying disease, such as:
  progressive systemic sclerosis (M34.0)
  rheumatoid arthritis (M05.00-M06.9)
  systemic lupus erythematosis (M32.0-M32.9)

J84.2 Lymphoid interstitial pneumonia
Lymphoid interstitial pneumonitis

J84.8 Other specified interstitial pulmonary diseases
EXCLUDES 1 exogenous lipoid pneumonia (J69.1)
unspecified lipoid pneumonia (J69.1)

J84.81 Lymphangioleiomyomatosis
Lymphangiomyomatosis

J84.82 Adult pulmonary Langerhans cell histiocytosis
Adult PLCH

J84.83 Surfactant mutations of the lung
DEF: Genetic disorder resulting in insufficient secretion of a complex mixture of phospholipids and proteins that reduce surface tension in the alveoli following the onset of breathing to facilitate lung expansion in the newborn. It is the leading indication for pediatric lung transplantation.

J84.84 Other interstitial lung diseases of childhood

J84.841 Neuroendocrine cell hyperplasia of infancy

J84.842 Pulmonary interstitial glycogenosis

J84.843 Alveolar capillary dysplasia with vein misalignment

J84.848 Other interstitial lung diseases of childhood

J84.89 Other specified interstitial pulmonary diseases
Endogenous lipoid pneumonia
Interstitial pneumonitis
Non-specific interstitial pneumonitis NOS
Organizing pneumonia NOS
Code first, if applicable:
  poisoning due to drug or toxin (T51-T65 with fifth or sixth character to indicate intent), for toxic pneumonopathy
  underlying cause of pneumonopathy, if known
Use additional code, for adverse effect, to identify drug (T36-T50 with fifth or sixth character 5), if drug-induced
EXCLUDES 1 cryptogenic organizing pneumonia (J84.116)
idiopathic non-specific interstitial pneumonitis (J84.113)
lipoid pneumonia, exogenous or unspecified (J69.1)
lymphoid interstitial pneumonia (J84.2)
AHA: 2021,4Q,106; 2021,1Q,48; 2019,2Q,28

J84.9 Interstitial pulmonary disease, unspecified
Interstitial pneumonia NOS

Suppurative and necrotic conditions of the lower respiratory tract (J85-J86)

✓4ᵗʰ J85 Abscess of lung and mediastinum
Use additional code (B95-B97) to identify infectious agent
- **J85.0** Gangrene and necrosis of lung HCC ESR COM
- **J85.1** Abscess of lung with pneumonia HCC ESR COM
  Code also the type of pneumonia
- **J85.2** Abscess of lung without pneumonia HCC ESR COM
  Abscess of lung NOS
- **J85.3** Abscess of mediastinum HCC ESR COM

✓4ᵗʰ J86 Pyothorax
Use additional code (B95-B97) to identify infectious agent
EXCLUDES 1 abscess of lung (J85.-)
  pyothorax due to tuberculosis (A15.6)
DEF: Collection of pus in the pleural space that is commonly caused by an infection that spreads from the lung, such as bacterial pneumonia or a lung abscess.

- **J86.0** Pyothorax with fistula HCC ESR COM
  Any condition classifiable to J86.9 with fistula
  Bronchocutaneous fistula
  Bronchopleural fistula
  Hepatopleural fistula
  Mediastinal fistula
  Pleural fistula
  Thoracic fistula
  Code also, if applicable, disruption of internal operation (surgical) wound (T81.32-)
  AHA: 2024,3Q,4
  DEF: Purulent infection of the respiratory cavity, with communication from a cavity to another structure.

- **J86.9** Pyothorax without fistula HCC ESR COM
  Abscess of pleura
  Abscess of thorax
  Empyema (chest) (lung) (pleura)
  Fibrinopurulent pleurisy
  Purulent pleurisy
  Pyopneumothorax
  Septic pleurisy
  Seropurulent pleurisy
  Suppurative pleurisy

Other diseases of the pleura (J90-J94)

J90 Pleural effusion, not elsewhere classified
Encysted pleurisy
Pleural effusion NOS
Pleurisy with effusion (exudative) (serous)
EXCLUDES 1 chylous (pleural) effusion (J94.0)
  malignant pleural effusion (J91.0)
  pleurisy NOS (R09.1)
  tuberculous pleural effusion (A15.6)
DEF: Collection of lymph and other fluid within the pleural space.

✓4ᵗʰ J91 Pleural effusion in conditions classified elsewhere
EXCLUDES 2 pleural effusion in heart failure (I50.-)
  pleural effusion in systemic lupus erythematosus (M32.13)
DEF: Collection of lymph and other fluid within the pleural space.

- **J91.0** Malignant pleural effusion HCC
  Code first underlying neoplasm (C00-D49)
  AHA: 2024,2Q,11; 2022,3Q,14

- **J91.8** Pleural effusion in other conditions classified elsewhere
  Code first underlying disease, such as:
    filariasis (B74.0-B74.9)
    influenza (J09.X2, J10.1, J11.1)
  AHA: 2024,3Q,4; 2015,2Q,15
  TIP: Assign this code as a secondary diagnosis to congestive heart failure (I50.-) only if pleural effusion is specifically evaluated or treated.

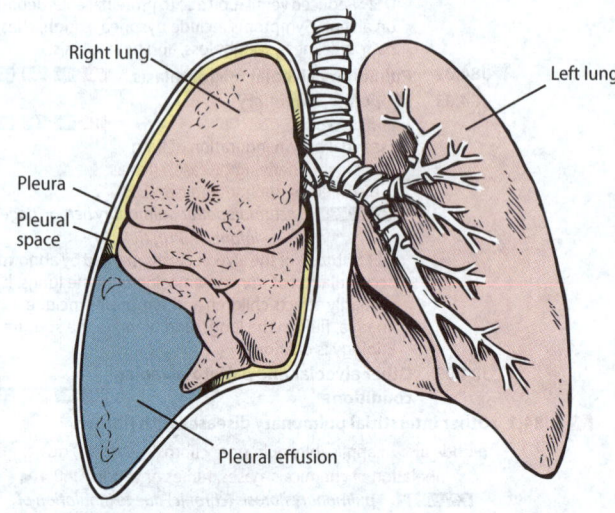
Pleural Effusion

✓4ᵗʰ J92 Pleural plaque
INCLUDES pleural thickening
DEF: Areas of fibrous thickening that form on the parietal or visceral pleura, the membranes that line the ribs and lungs.

- **J92.0** Pleural plaque with presence of asbestos
- **J92.9** Pleural plaque without asbestos
  Pleural plaque NOS

✓4ᵗʰ J93 Pneumothorax and air leak
EXCLUDES 1 congenital or perinatal pneumothorax (P25.1)
  postprocedural air leak (J95.812)
  postprocedural pneumothorax (J95.811)
  pyopneumothorax (J86.-)
  traumatic pneumothorax (S27.0)
  tuberculous (current disease) pneumothorax (A15.-)
DEF: Pneumothorax: Lung displacement due to abnormal leakage of air or gas that is trapped in the pleural space formed by the membrane that encloses the lungs and lines the thoracic cavity.

- **J93.0** Spontaneous tension pneumothorax
  DEF: Leaking air from the lung into the lining, causing collapse.

- **✓5ᵗʰ J93.1** Other spontaneous pneumothorax
  - **J93.11** Primary spontaneous pneumothorax
  - **J93.12** Secondary spontaneous pneumothorax UPD
    Code first underlying condition, such as:
      catamenial pneumothorax due to endometriosis (N80.B-)
      cystic fibrosis (E84.-)
      eosinophilic pneumonia (J82.81-J82.82)
      lymphangioleiomyomatosis (J84.81)
      malignant neoplasm of bronchus and lung (C34.-)
      Marfan syndrome (Q87.4-)
      pneumonia due to Pneumocystis carinii (B59)
      secondary malignant neoplasm of lung (C78.0-)
      spontaneous rupture of the esophagus (K22.3)

- **✓5ᵗʰ J93.8** Other pneumothorax and air leak
  - **J93.81** Chronic pneumothorax
  - **J93.82** Other air leak
    Persistent air leak
  - **J93.83** Other pneumothorax
    Acute pneumothorax
    Spontaneous pneumothorax NOS
    AHA: 2020,3Q,9-10

- **J93.9** Pneumothorax, unspecified
  Pneumothorax NOS

Chapter 10. Diseases of the Respiratory System

J94 Other pleural conditions ✓4th
- EXCLUDES 1: pleurisy NOS (R09.1)
  - traumatic hemopneumothorax (S27.2)
  - traumatic hemothorax (S27.1)
  - tuberculous pleural conditions (current disease) (A15.-)

J94.0 Chylous effusion
- Chyliform effusion
- DEF: Fluid within the pleural space due to the leaking of lymph contents into the space, usually as a result of thoracic duct damage or injury or mediastinal lymphoma.

J94.1 Fibrothorax
- DEF: Fibrosis within the pleural lining of the lungs commonly seen as a stiff layer surrounding the lung typically attributed to traumatic hemothorax or pleural effusion.

J94.2 Hemothorax
- Hemopneumothorax

J94.8 Other specified pleural conditions
- Hydropneumothorax
- Hydrothorax
- AHA: 2024,3Q,4; 2021,1Q,48

J94.9 Pleural condition, unspecified

Intraoperative and postprocedural complications and disorders of respiratory system, not elsewhere classified (J95)

J95 Intraoperative and postprocedural complications and disorders of respiratory system, not elsewhere classified ✓4th
- EXCLUDES 2: aspiration pneumonia (J69.-)
  - emphysema (subcutaneous) resulting from a procedure (T81.82)
  - hypostatic pneumonia (J18.2)
  - pulmonary manifestations due to radiation (J70.0-J70.1)

J95.0 Tracheostomy complications ✓5th
- DEF: Tracheostomy: Formation of a tracheal opening on the neck surface with tube insertion to allow for respiration in cases of obstruction or decreased patency. A tracheostomy may be planned or performed on an emergency basis for temporary or long-term use.

- **J95.00** Unspecified tracheostomy complication HCC ESR COM
- **J95.01** Hemorrhage from tracheostomy stoma HCC ESR COM
- **J95.02** Infection of tracheostomy stoma HCC ESR COM
  - Use additional code to identify type of infection, such as:
    - cellulitis of neck (L03.221)
    - sepsis (A40, A41.-)
- **J95.03** Malfunction of tracheostomy stoma HCC ESR COM
  - Mechanical complication of tracheostomy stoma
  - Obstruction of tracheostomy airway
  - Tracheal stenosis due to tracheostomy
- **J95.04** Tracheo-esophageal fistula following tracheostomy HCC ESR COM
- **J95.09** Other tracheostomy complication HCC ESR COM

J95.1 Acute pulmonary insufficiency following thoracic surgery ESR
- EXCLUDES 2: functional disturbances following cardiac surgery (I97.0, I97.1-)

J95.2 Acute pulmonary insufficiency following nonthoracic surgery ESR
- EXCLUDES 2: functional disturbances following cardiac surgery (I97.0, I97.1-)

J95.3 Chronic pulmonary insufficiency following surgery ESR
- EXCLUDES 2: functional disturbances following cardiac surgery (I97.0, I97.1-)

J95.4 Chemical pneumonitis due to anesthesia
- Mendelson's syndrome
- Postprocedural aspiration pneumonia
- Use additional code for adverse effect, if applicable, to identify drug (T41.- with fifth or sixth character 5)
- EXCLUDES 1: aspiration pneumonitis due to anesthesia complicating labor and delivery (O74.0)
  - aspiration pneumonitis due to anesthesia complicating pregnancy (O29)
  - aspiration pneumonitis due to anesthesia complicating the puerperium (O89.01)

J95.5 Postprocedural subglottic stenosis

J95.6 Intraoperative hemorrhage and hematoma of a respiratory system organ or structure complicating a procedure ✓5th
- EXCLUDES 1: intraoperative hemorrhage and hematoma of a respiratory system organ or structure due to accidental puncture and laceration during procedure (J95.7-)

- **J95.61** Intraoperative hemorrhage and hematoma of a respiratory system organ or structure complicating a respiratory system procedure
- **J95.62** Intraoperative hemorrhage and hematoma of a respiratory system organ or structure complicating other procedure

J95.7 Accidental puncture and laceration of a respiratory system organ or structure during a procedure ✓5th
- EXCLUDES 2: postprocedural pneumothorax (J95.811)

- **J95.71** Accidental puncture and laceration of a respiratory system organ or structure during a respiratory system procedure
- **J95.72** Accidental puncture and laceration of a respiratory system organ or structure during other procedure

J95.8 Other intraoperative and postprocedural complications and disorders of respiratory system, not elsewhere classified ✓5th
- AHA: 2016,4Q,9-10

- **J95.81 Postprocedural pneumothorax and air leak** ✓6th
  - **J95.811** Postprocedural pneumothorax
    - AHA: 2021,1Q,48
  - **J95.812** Postprocedural air leak

- **J95.82 Postprocedural respiratory failure** ✓6th
  - EXCLUDES 1: respiratory failure in other conditions (J96.-)
  - **J95.821** Acute postprocedural respiratory failure ESR
    - Postprocedural respiratory failure NOS
    - AHA: 2024,4Q,19
  - **J95.822** Acute and chronic postprocedural respiratory failure ESR

- **J95.83 Postprocedural hemorrhage of a respiratory system organ or structure following a procedure** ✓6th
  - AHA: 2023,2Q,28
  - **J95.830** Postprocedural hemorrhage of a respiratory system organ or structure following a respiratory system procedure
  - **J95.831** Postprocedural hemorrhage of a respiratory system organ or structure following other procedure

- **J95.84 Transfusion-related acute lung injury (TRALI)**
  - DEF: Relatively rare, but serious, pulmonary complication of blood transfusion, with acute respiratory distress, noncardiogenic pulmonary edema, cyanosis, hypoxemia, hypotension, fever, and chills.

- **J95.85 Complication of respirator [ventilator]** ✓6th
  - **J95.850** Mechanical complication of respirator HCC ESR COM
    - EXCLUDES 1: encounter for respirator [ventilator] dependence during power failure (Z99.12)
  - **J95.851** Ventilator associated pneumonia HCC ESR
    - Ventilator associated pneumonitis
    - Use additional code to identify the organism, if known (B95.-, B96.-, B97.-)
    - EXCLUDES 1: ventilator lung in newborn (P27.8)
    - AHA: 2020,2Q,17; 2017,1Q,25
  - **J95.859** Other complication of respirator [ventilator] HCC ESR COM
    - AHA: 2021,1Q,48

- **J95.86 Postprocedural hematoma and seroma of a respiratory system organ or structure following a procedure** ✓6th
  - **J95.860** Postprocedural hematoma of a respiratory system organ or structure following a respiratory system procedure
  - **J95.861** Postprocedural hematoma of a respiratory system organ or structure following other procedure
  - **J95.862** Postprocedural seroma of a respiratory system organ or structure following a respiratory system procedure

---

✓ Additional Character Required | ✓7th Placeholder Alert | Manifestation | Unspecified Dx | Q QPP | UPD Unacceptable PDx

J95.863 Postprocedural seroma of a respiratory system organ or structure following other procedure

J95.87 Transfusion-associated dyspnea (TAD)
- EXCLUDES 1: transfusion associated circulatory overload (TACO) (E87.71)
- transfusion-related acute lung injury (TRALI) (J95.84)
- AHA: 2022,4Q,27

J95.88 Other intraoperative complications of respiratory system, not elsewhere classified

J95.89 Other postprocedural complications and disorders of respiratory system, not elsewhere classified
- Use additional code to identify disorder, such as:
  - aspiration pneumonia (J69.-)
  - bacterial or viral pneumonia (J12-J18)
- EXCLUDES 2: acute pulmonary insufficiency following thoracic surgery (J95.1)
- postprocedural subglottic stenosis (J95.5)

Other diseases of the respiratory system (J96-J99)

J96 Respiratory failure, not elsewhere classified
- EXCLUDES 1: acute respiratory distress syndrome (J80)
  - cardiorespiratory failure (R09.2)
  - newborn respiratory distress syndrome (P22.0)
  - postprocedural respiratory failure (J95.82-)
  - respiratory arrest (R09.2)
  - respiratory arrest of newborn (P28.81)
  - respiratory failure of newborn (P28.5)
- AHA: 2021,1Q,27,44-45; 2020,4Q,96

J96.0 Acute respiratory failure
- **J96.00** Acute respiratory failure, unspecified whether with hypoxia or hypercapnia
  - AHA: 2016,3Q,14; 2013,4Q,121
- **J96.01** Acute respiratory failure with hypoxia
  - AHA: 2024,2Q,11; 2020,3Q,12
- **J96.02** Acute respiratory failure with hypercapnia
  - Acute respiratory acidosis

J96.1 Chronic respiratory failure
- **J96.10** Chronic respiratory failure, unspecified whether with hypoxia or hypercapnia
  - AHA: 2016,1Q,38; 2015,1Q,21
- **J96.11** Chronic respiratory failure with hypoxia
  - AHA: 2013,4Q,129
- **J96.12** Chronic respiratory failure with hypercapnia
  - Chronic respiratory acidosis

J96.2 Acute and chronic respiratory failure
- Acute on chronic respiratory failure
- **J96.20** Acute and chronic respiratory failure, unspecified whether with hypoxia or hypercapnia
- **J96.21** Acute and chronic respiratory failure with hypoxia
- **J96.22** Acute and chronic respiratory failure with hypercapnia

J96.9 Respiratory failure, unspecified
- **J96.90** Respiratory failure, unspecified, unspecified whether with hypoxia or hypercapnia
- **J96.91** Respiratory failure, unspecified with hypoxia
- **J96.92** Respiratory failure, unspecified with hypercapnia

J98 Other respiratory disorders
- Use additional code to identify:
  - exposure to environmental tobacco smoke (Z77.22)
  - exposure to tobacco smoke in the perinatal period (P96.81)
  - history of tobacco dependence (Z87.891)
  - occupational exposure to environmental tobacco smoke (Z57.31)
  - tobacco dependence (F17.-)
  - tobacco use (Z72.0)
- EXCLUDES 1: newborn apnea (P28.4-)
  - newborn sleep apnea (P28.3-)
- EXCLUDES 2: apnea NOS (R06.81)
  - sleep apnea (G47.3-)

J98.0 Diseases of bronchus, not elsewhere classified
- **J98.01** Acute bronchospasm
  - EXCLUDES 1: acute bronchiolitis with bronchospasm (J21.-)
    - acute bronchitis with bronchospasm (J20.-)
    - asthma (J45.-)
    - exercise induced bronchospasm (J45.990)
- **J98.09** Other diseases of bronchus, not elsewhere classified
  - Broncholithiasis
  - Calcification of bronchus
  - Stenosis of bronchus
  - Tracheobronchial collapse
  - Tracheobronchial dyskinesia
  - Ulcer of bronchus
  - AHA: 2022,3Q,8

J98.1 Pulmonary collapse
- EXCLUDES 1: therapeutic collapse of lung status (Z98.3)
- **J98.11** Atelectasis
  - EXCLUDES 1: newborn atelectasis
    - tuberculous atelectasis (current disease) (A15)
  - DEF: Collapse of lung tissue affecting part or all of one lung, preventing normal oxygen absorption to healthy tissues.
- **J98.19** Other pulmonary collapse

J98.2 Interstitial emphysema
- Mediastinal emphysema
- EXCLUDES 1: emphysema NOS (J43.9)
  - emphysema in newborn (P25.0)
  - surgical emphysema (subcutaneous) (T81.82)
  - traumatic subcutaneous emphysema (T79.7)

J98.3 Compensatory emphysema
- DEF: Distention of all or part of the lung caused by disease processes or surgical intervention that decreased volume in another part of the lung, causing an overcompensation reaction. Compensatory emphysema occurs in association with pneumonias, pleural effusions, atelectasis, empyema, and pneumothorax.

J98.4 Other disorders of lung
- Calcification of lung
- Cystic lung disease (acquired)
- Lung disease NOS
- Pulmolithiasis
- EXCLUDES 1: acute interstitial pneumonitis (J84.114)
  - pulmonary insufficiency following surgery (J95.1-J95.2)
- AHA: 2024,2Q,20

J98.5 Diseases of mediastinum, not elsewhere classified
- EXCLUDES 2: abscess of mediastinum (J85.3)
- AHA: 2016,4Q,29
- **J98.51** Mediastinitis
  - Code first underlying condition, if applicable, such as postoperative mediastinitis (T81.-)
- **J98.59** Other diseases of mediastinum, not elsewhere classified
  - Fibrosis of mediastinum
  - Hernia of mediastinum
  - Retraction of mediastinum

J98.6 Disorders of diaphragm
- Diaphragmatitis
- Paralysis of diaphragm
- Relaxation of diaphragm
- EXCLUDES 1: congenital malformation of diaphragm NEC (Q79.1)
  - congenital diaphragmatic hernia (Q79.0)
- EXCLUDES 2: diaphragmatic hernia (K44.-)

J98.8 Other specified respiratory disorders
- AHA: 2025,2Q,7; 2020,1Q,34-36

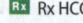 CMS-HCC  Rx HCC 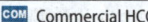 ESRD HCC 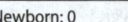 Commercial HCC 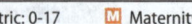 Newborn: 0 · Pediatric: 0-17 · Maternity: 9-64 · Adult: 15-124

J98.9 Respiratory disorder, unspecified
Respiratory disease (chronic) NOS

J99 Respiratory disorders in diseases classified elsewhere HCC Rx ESR COM
Code first underlying disease, such as:
amyloidosis (E85.-)
ankylosing spondylitis (M45.-)
congenital syphilis (A50.-)
cryoglobulinemia (D89.1)
early congenital syphilis (A50.0-)
plasminogen deficiency (E88.02)
schistosomiasis (B65.0-B65.9)

EXCLUDES 1 respiratory disorders in:
amebiasis (A06.5)
blastomycosis (B40.0-B40.2)
candidiasis (B37.1)
coccidioidomycosis (B38.0-B38.2)
cystic fibrosis with pulmonary manifestations (E84.0)
dermatomyositis (M33.01, M33.11)
histoplasmosis (B39.0-B39.2)
late syphilis (A52.72, A52.73)
polymyositis (M33.21)
Sjogren syndrome (M35.02)
systemic lupus erythematosus (M32.13)
systemic sclerosis (M34.81)
Wegener's granulomatosis (M31.30-M31.31)

Chapter 11. Diseases of the Digestive System (K00–K95)

Chapter-specific Guidelines with Coding Examples
Reserved for future guideline expansion.

Chapter 11. Diseases of the Digestive System (K00-K95)

EXCLUDES 2
certain conditions originating in the perinatal period (P04-P96)
certain infectious and parasitic diseases (A00-B99)
complications of pregnancy, childbirth and the puerperium (O00-O9A)
congenital malformations, deformations and chromosomal abnormalities (Q00-Q99)
endocrine, nutritional and metabolic diseases (E00-E88)
injury, poisoning and certain other consequences of external causes (S00-T88)
neoplasms (C00-D49)
symptoms, signs and abnormal clinical and laboratory findings, not elsewhere classified (R00-R94)

This chapter contains the following blocks:
- K00-K14 Diseases of oral cavity and salivary glands
- K20-K31 Diseases of esophagus, stomach and duodenum
- K35-K38 Diseases of appendix
- K40-K46 Hernia
- K50-K52 Noninfective enteritis and colitis
- K55-K64 Other diseases of intestines
- K65-K68 Diseases of peritoneum and retroperitoneum
- K70-K77 Diseases of liver
- K80-K87 Disorders of gallbladder, biliary tract and pancreas
- K90-K95 Other diseases of the digestive system

Diseases of oral cavity and salivary glands (K00-K14)

K00 Disorders of tooth development and eruption
EXCLUDES 2 embedded and impacted teeth (K01.-)

K00.0 Anodontia
Hypodontia
Oligodontia
EXCLUDES 1 acquired absence of teeth (K08.1-)
DEF: Partial or complete absence of teeth due to a congenital defect involving the tooth bud.

K00.1 Supernumerary teeth
Distomolar
Fourth molar
Mesiodens
Paramolar
Supplementary teeth
EXCLUDES 2 supernumerary roots (K00.2)

K00.2 Abnormalities of size and form of teeth
Concrescence of teeth
Dens evaginatus
Dens in dente
Dens invaginatus
Enamel pearls
Fusion of teeth
Gemination of teeth
Macrodontia
Microdontia
Peg-shaped [conical] teeth
Supernumerary roots
Taurodontism
Tuberculum paramolare
EXCLUDES 1 abnormalities of teeth due to congenital syphilis (A50.5)
tuberculum Carabelli, which is regarded as a normal variation and should not be coded

K00.3 Mottled teeth
Dental fluorosis
Mottling of enamel
Nonfluoride enamel opacities
EXCLUDES 2 deposits [accretions] on teeth (K03.6)

K00.4 Disturbances in tooth formation
Aplasia and hypoplasia of cementum
Dilaceration of tooth
Enamel hypoplasia (neonatal) (postnatal) (prenatal)
Regional odontodysplasia
Turner's tooth
EXCLUDES 1 Hutchinson's teeth and mulberry molars in congenital syphilis (A50.5)
EXCLUDES 2 mottled teeth (K00.3)

K00.5 Hereditary disturbances in tooth structure, not elsewhere classified
Amelogenesis imperfecta
Dentinal dysplasia
Dentinogenesis imperfecta
Odontogenesis imperfecta
Shell teeth

K00.6 Disturbances in tooth eruption
Dentia praecox
Natal tooth
Neonatal tooth
Premature eruption of tooth
Premature shedding of primary [deciduous] tooth
Prenatal teeth
Retained [persistent] primary tooth
EXCLUDES 2 embedded and impacted teeth (K01.-)

K00.7 Teething syndrome

K00.8 Other disorders of tooth development
Color changes during tooth formation
Intrinsic staining of teeth NOS
EXCLUDES 2 posteruptive color changes (K03.7)

K00.9 Disorder of tooth development, unspecified
Disorder of odontogenesis NOS

K01 Embedded and impacted teeth
EXCLUDES 1 abnormal position of fully erupted teeth (M26.3-)

K01.0 Embedded teeth

K01.1 Impacted teeth

K02 Dental caries
INCLUDES
caries of dentine
dental cavities
early childhood caries
pre-eruptive caries
recurrent caries (dentino enamel junction) (enamel) (to the pulp)
tooth decay

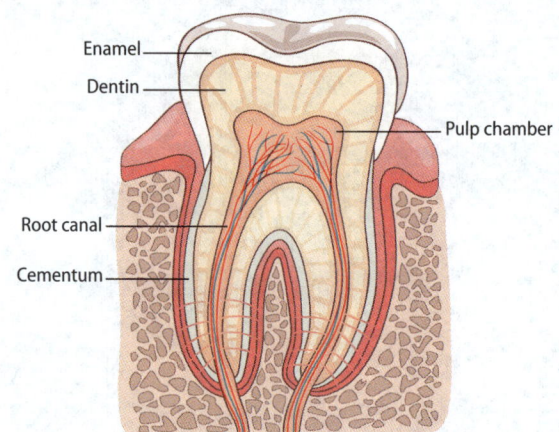

Tooth Anatomy

K02.3 Arrested dental caries
Arrested coronal and root caries

K02.5 Dental caries on pit and fissure surface
Dental caries on chewing surface of tooth

K02.51 Dental caries on pit and fissure surface limited to enamel
White spot lesions [initial caries] on pit and fissure surface of tooth

K02.52 Dental caries on pit and fissure surface penetrating into dentin
Primary dental caries, cervical origin

K02.53 Dental caries on pit and fissure surface penetrating into pulp

K02.6 Dental caries on smooth surface

K02.61 Dental caries on smooth surface limited to enamel
White spot lesions [initial caries] on smooth surface of tooth

K02.62 Dental caries on smooth surface penetrating into dentin

K02.63 Dental caries on smooth surface penetrating into pulp

K02.7 Dental root caries

K02.9 Dental caries, unspecified

Chapter 11. Diseases of the Digestive System

✓4th K03 Other diseases of hard tissues of teeth
EXCLUDES 2: bruxism (F45.8)
dental caries (K02.-)
teeth-grinding NOS (F45.8)

K03.0 Excessive attrition of teeth
Approximal wear of teeth
Occlusal wear of teeth
DEF: Attrition: In dentistry, wearing away or erosion of tooth surface from abrasive food or grinding teeth.

K03.1 Abrasion of teeth
Dentifrice abrasion of teeth
Habitual abrasion of teeth
Occupational abrasion of teeth
Ritual abrasion of teeth
Traditional abrasion of teeth
Wedge defect NOS

K03.2 Erosion of teeth
Erosion of teeth due to diet
Erosion of teeth due to drugs and medicaments
Erosion of teeth due to persistent vomiting
Erosion of teeth NOS
Idiopathic erosion of teeth
Occupational erosion of teeth

K03.3 Pathological resorption of teeth
Internal granuloma of pulp
Resorption of teeth (external)

K03.4 Hypercementosis
Cementation hyperplasia

K03.5 Ankylosis of teeth

K03.6 Deposits [accretions] on teeth
Betel deposits [accretions] on teeth
Black deposits [accretions] on teeth
Extrinsic staining of teeth NOS
Green deposits [accretions] on teeth
Materia alba deposits [accretions] on teeth
Orange deposits [accretions] on teeth
Staining of teeth NOS
Subgingival dental calculus
Supragingival dental calculus
Tobacco deposits [accretions] on teeth

K03.7 Posteruptive color changes of dental hard tissues
EXCLUDES 2: deposits [accretions] on teeth (K03.6)

✓5th K03.8 Other specified diseases of hard tissues of teeth
K03.81 Cracked tooth
EXCLUDES 1: asymptomatic craze lines in enamel - omit code
broken or fractured tooth due to trauma (S02.5)
K03.89 Other specified diseases of hard tissues of teeth

K03.9 Disease of hard tissues of teeth, unspecified

✓4th K04 Diseases of pulp and periapical tissues
AHA: 2016,4Q,29-30

✓5th K04.0 Pulpitis
Acute pulpitis
Chronic (hyperplastic) (ulcerative) pulpitis
K04.01 Reversible pulpitis
K04.02 Irreversible pulpitis

K04.1 Necrosis of pulp
Pulpal gangrene

K04.2 Pulp degeneration
Denticles
Pulpal calcifications
Pulpal stones

K04.3 Abnormal hard tissue formation in pulp
Secondary or irregular dentine

K04.4 Acute apical periodontitis of pulpal origin
Acute apical periodontitis NOS
EXCLUDES 1: acute periodontitis (K05.2-)
DEF: Severe inflammation of the area surrounding the tip of a tooth's root that is often secondary to infection or trauma.

K04.5 Chronic apical periodontitis
Apical or periapical granuloma
Apical periodontitis NOS
EXCLUDES 1: chronic apical periodontitis (K05.3-)

K04.6 Periapical abscess with sinus
Dental abscess with sinus
Dentoalveolar abscess with sinus

K04.7 Periapical abscess without sinus
Dental abscess without sinus
Dentoalveolar abscess without sinus

K04.8 Radicular cyst
Apical (periodontal) cyst
Periapical cyst
Residual radicular cyst
EXCLUDES 2: lateral periodontal cyst (K09.0)
DEF: Most common odontogenic cyst in tissue around the tooth apex due to chronic inflammation of dental pulp.

✓5th K04.9 Other and unspecified diseases of pulp and periapical tissues
K04.90 Unspecified diseases of pulp and periapical tissues
K04.99 Other diseases of pulp and periapical tissues

✓4th K05 Gingivitis and periodontal diseases
Use additional code to identify:
alcohol abuse and dependence (F10.-)
exposure to environmental tobacco smoke (Z77.22)
exposure to tobacco smoke in the perinatal period (P96.81)
history of tobacco dependence (Z87.891)
occupational exposure to environmental tobacco smoke (Z57.31)
tobacco dependence (F17.-)
tobacco use (Z72.0)
AHA: 2016,4Q,29-30

✓5th K05.0 Acute gingivitis
EXCLUDES 1: acute necrotizing ulcerative gingivitis (A69.1)
herpesviral [herpes simplex] gingivostomatitis (B00.2)
K05.00 Acute gingivitis, plaque induced
Acute gingivitis NOS
Plaque induced gingival disease
K05.01 Acute gingivitis, non-plaque induced

✓5th K05.1 Chronic gingivitis
Desquamative gingivitis (chronic)
Gingivitis (chronic) NOS
Hyperplastic gingivitis (chronic)
Pregnancy associated gingivitis
Simple marginal gingivitis (chronic)
Ulcerative gingivitis (chronic)
Code first, if applicable, diseases of the digestive system complicating pregnancy (O99.61-)
K05.10 Chronic gingivitis, plaque induced
Chronic gingivitis NOS
Gingivitis NOS
K05.11 Chronic gingivitis, non-plaque induced

✓5th K05.2 Aggressive periodontitis
Acute pericoronitis
EXCLUDES 1: acute apical periodontitis (K04.4)
periapical abscess (K04.7)
periapical abscess with sinus (K04.6)
K05.20 Aggressive periodontitis, unspecified
✓6th K05.21 Aggressive periodontitis, localized
Periodontal abscess
K05.211 Aggressive periodontitis, localized, slight
K05.212 Aggressive periodontitis, localized, moderate
K05.213 Aggressive periodontitis, localized, severe
K05.219 Aggressive periodontitis, localized, unspecified severity
✓6th K05.22 Aggressive periodontitis, generalized
K05.221 Aggressive periodontitis, generalized, slight
K05.222 Aggressive periodontitis, generalized, moderate
K05.223 Aggressive periodontitis, generalized, severe
K05.229 Aggressive periodontitis, generalized, unspecified severity

✓5th K05.3 Chronic periodontitis
Chronic pericoronitis
Complex periodontitis
Periodontitis NOS
Simplex periodontitis
EXCLUDES 1: chronic apical periodontitis (K04.5)
K05.30 Chronic periodontitis, unspecified
✓6th K05.31 Chronic periodontitis, localized
K05.311 Chronic periodontitis, localized, slight
K05.312 Chronic periodontitis, localized, moderate
K05.313 Chronic periodontitis, localized, severe
K05.319 Chronic periodontitis, localized, unspecified severity

Chapter 11. Diseases of the Digestive System

- ✓6th **K05.32** Chronic periodontitis, generalized
  - **K05.321** Chronic periodontitis, generalized, slight
  - **K05.322** Chronic periodontitis, generalized, moderate
  - **K05.323** Chronic periodontitis, generalized, severe
  - **K05.329** Chronic periodontitis, generalized, unspecified severity
- **K05.4** Periodontosis
  - Juvenile periodontosis
- **K05.5** Other periodontal diseases
  - Combined periodontic-endodontic lesion
  - Narrow gingival width (of periodontal soft tissue)
  - EXCLUDES 2 leukoplakia of gingiva (K13.21)
- **K05.6** Periodontal disease, unspecified

✓4th **K06** Other disorders of gingiva and edentulous alveolar ridge
- EXCLUDES 2
  - acute gingivitis (K05.0)
  - atrophy of edentulous alveolar ridge (K08.2)
  - chronic gingivitis (K05.1)
  - gingivitis NOS (K05.1)
- AHA: 2016,4Q,29-30

✓5th **K06.0** Gingival recession
- Gingival recession (postinfective) (postprocedural)
- AHA: 2017,4Q,16
  - ✓6th **K06.01** Gingival recession, localized
    - **K06.010** Localized gingival recession, unspecified
      - Localized gingival recession, NOS
    - **K06.011** Localized gingival recession, minimal
    - **K06.012** Localized gingival recession, moderate
    - **K06.013** Localized gingival recession, severe
  - ✓6th **K06.02** Gingival recession, generalized
    - **K06.020** Generalized gingival recession, unspecified
      - Generalized gingival recession, NOS
    - **K06.021** Generalized gingival recession, minimal
    - **K06.022** Generalized gingival recession, moderate
    - **K06.023** Generalized gingival recession, severe
- **K06.1** Gingival enlargement
  - Gingival fibromatosis
- **K06.2** Gingival and edentulous alveolar ridge lesions associated with trauma
  - Irritative hyperplasia of edentulous ridge [denture hyperplasia]
  - Use additional code (Chapter 20) to identify external cause or denture status (Z97.2)
- **K06.3** Horizontal alveolar bone loss
- **K06.8** Other specified disorders of gingiva and edentulous alveolar ridge
  - Fibrous epulis
  - Flabby alveolar ridge
  - Giant cell epulis
  - Peripheral giant cell granuloma of gingiva
  - Pyogenic granuloma of gingiva
  - Vertical ridge deficiency
  - EXCLUDES 2 gingival cyst (K09.0)
- **K06.9** Disorder of gingiva and edentulous alveolar ridge, unspecified

✓4th **K08** Other disorders of teeth and supporting structures
- EXCLUDES 2
  - dentofacial anomalies [including malocclusion] (M26.-)
  - disorders of jaw (M27.-)
- AHA: 2016,4Q,29-30
- **K08.0** Exfoliation of teeth due to systemic causes
  - Code also underlying systemic condition
- ✓5th **K08.1** Complete loss of teeth
  - Acquired loss of teeth, complete
  - EXCLUDES 1
    - congenital absence of teeth (K00.0)
    - exfoliation of teeth due to systemic causes (K08.0)
    - partial loss of teeth (K08.4-)
  - ✓6th **K08.10** Complete loss of teeth, unspecified cause
    - **K08.101** Complete loss of teeth, unspecified cause, class I
    - **K08.102** Complete loss of teeth, unspecified cause, class II
    - **K08.103** Complete loss of teeth, unspecified cause, class III
    - **K08.104** Complete loss of teeth, unspecified cause, class IV
    - **K08.109** Complete loss of teeth, unspecified cause, unspecified class
      - Edentulism NOS
  - ✓6th **K08.11** Complete loss of teeth due to trauma
    - **K08.111** Complete loss of teeth due to trauma, class I
    - **K08.112** Complete loss of teeth due to trauma, class II
    - **K08.113** Complete loss of teeth due to trauma, class III
    - **K08.114** Complete loss of teeth due to trauma, class IV
    - **K08.119** Complete loss of teeth due to trauma, unspecified class
  - ✓6th **K08.12** Complete loss of teeth due to periodontal diseases
    - **K08.121** Complete loss of teeth due to periodontal diseases, class I
    - **K08.122** Complete loss of teeth due to periodontal diseases, class II
    - **K08.123** Complete loss of teeth due to periodontal diseases, class III
    - **K08.124** Complete loss of teeth due to periodontal diseases, class IV
    - **K08.129** Complete loss of teeth due to periodontal diseases, unspecified class
  - ✓6th **K08.13** Complete loss of teeth due to caries
    - **K08.131** Complete loss of teeth due to caries, class I
    - **K08.132** Complete loss of teeth due to caries, class II
    - **K08.133** Complete loss of teeth due to caries, class III
    - **K08.134** Complete loss of teeth due to caries, class IV
    - **K08.139** Complete loss of teeth due to caries, unspecified class
  - ✓6th **K08.19** Complete loss of teeth due to other specified cause
    - **K08.191** Complete loss of teeth due to other specified cause, class I
    - **K08.192** Complete loss of teeth due to other specified cause, class II
    - **K08.193** Complete loss of teeth due to other specified cause, class III
    - **K08.194** Complete loss of teeth due to other specified cause, class IV
    - **K08.199** Complete loss of teeth due to other specified cause, unspecified class
- ✓5th **K08.2** Atrophy of edentulous alveolar ridge
  - **K08.20** Unspecified atrophy of edentulous alveolar ridge
    - Atrophy of the mandible NOS
    - Atrophy of the maxilla NOS
  - **K08.21** Minimal atrophy of the mandible
    - Minimal atrophy of the edentulous mandible
  - **K08.22** Moderate atrophy of the mandible
    - Moderate atrophy of the edentulous mandible
  - **K08.23** Severe atrophy of the mandible
    - Severe atrophy of the edentulous mandible
  - **K08.24** Minimal atrophy of maxilla
    - Minimal atrophy of the edentulous maxilla
  - **K08.25** Moderate atrophy of the maxilla
    - Moderate atrophy of the edentulous maxilla
  - **K08.26** Severe atrophy of the maxilla
    - Severe atrophy of the edentulous maxilla
- **K08.3** Retained dental root
- ✓5th **K08.4** Partial loss of teeth
  - Acquired loss of teeth, partial
  - EXCLUDES 1
    - complete loss of teeth (K08.1-)
    - congenital absence of teeth (K00.0)
  - EXCLUDES 2 exfoliation of teeth due to systemic causes (K08.0)
  - ✓6th **K08.40** Partial loss of teeth, unspecified cause
    - **K08.401** Partial loss of teeth, unspecified cause, class I
    - **K08.402** Partial loss of teeth, unspecified cause, class II
    - **K08.403** Partial loss of teeth, unspecified cause, class III
    - **K08.404** Partial loss of teeth, unspecified cause, class IV
    - **K08.409** Partial loss of teeth, unspecified cause, unspecified class
      - Tooth extraction status NOS
  - ✓6th **K08.41** Partial loss of teeth due to trauma
    - **K08.411** Partial loss of teeth due to trauma, class I

Chapter 11. Diseases of the Digestive System

- K08.412 Partial loss of teeth due to trauma, class II
- K08.413 Partial loss of teeth due to trauma, class III
- K08.414 Partial loss of teeth due to trauma, class IV
- K08.419 Partial loss of teeth due to trauma, unspecified class

✓6th K08.42 Partial loss of teeth due to periodontal diseases
- K08.421 Partial loss of teeth due to periodontal diseases, class I
- K08.422 Partial loss of teeth due to periodontal diseases, class II
- K08.423 Partial loss of teeth due to periodontal diseases, class III
- K08.424 Partial loss of teeth due to periodontal diseases, class IV
- K08.429 Partial loss of teeth due to periodontal diseases, unspecified class

✓6th K08.43 Partial loss of teeth due to caries
- K08.431 Partial loss of teeth due to caries, class I
- K08.432 Partial loss of teeth due to caries, class II
- K08.433 Partial loss of teeth due to caries, class III
- K08.434 Partial loss of teeth due to caries, class IV
- K08.439 Partial loss of teeth due to caries, unspecified class

✓6th K08.49 Partial loss of teeth due to other specified cause
- K08.491 Partial loss of teeth due to other specified cause, class I
- K08.492 Partial loss of teeth due to other specified cause, class II
- K08.493 Partial loss of teeth due to other specified cause, class III
- K08.494 Partial loss of teeth due to other specified cause, class IV
- K08.499 Partial loss of teeth due to other specified cause, unspecified class

✓5th K08.5 Unsatisfactory restoration of tooth
Defective bridge, crown, filling
Defective dental restoration
EXCLUDES 1 dental restoration status (Z98.811)
EXCLUDES 2 endosseous dental implant failure (M27.6-)
unsatisfactory endodontic treatment (M27.5-)

- K08.50 Unsatisfactory restoration of tooth, unspecified
  Defective dental restoration NOS
- K08.51 Open restoration margins of tooth
  Dental restoration failure of marginal integrity
  Open margin on tooth restoration
  Poor gingival margin to tooth restoration
- K08.52 Unrepairable overhanging of dental restorative materials
  Overhanging of tooth restoration

✓6th K08.53 Fractured dental restorative material
EXCLUDES 1 cracked tooth (K03.81)
traumatic fracture of tooth (S02.5)
- K08.530 Fractured dental restorative material without loss of material
- K08.531 Fractured dental restorative material with loss of material
- K08.539 Fractured dental restorative material, unspecified

- K08.54 Contour of existing restoration of tooth biologically incompatible with oral health
  Dental restoration failure of periodontal anatomical integrity
  Unacceptable contours of existing restoration of tooth
  Unacceptable morphology of existing restoration of tooth
- K08.55 Allergy to existing dental restorative material
  Use additional code to identify the specific type of allergy
- K08.56 Poor aesthetic of existing restoration of tooth
  Dental restoration aesthetically inadequate or displeasing
- K08.59 Other unsatisfactory restoration of tooth
  Other defective dental restoration

✓5th K08.8 Other specified disorders of teeth and supporting structures
- K08.81 Primary occlusal trauma
- K08.82 Secondary occlusal trauma
- K08.89 Other specified disorders of teeth and supporting structures
  Enlargement of alveolar ridge NOS
  Insufficient anatomic crown height
  Insufficient clinical crown length
  Irregular alveolar process
  Toothache NOS
- K08.9 Disorder of teeth and supporting structures, unspecified

✓4th K09 Cysts of oral region, not elsewhere classified
INCLUDES lesions showing histological features both of aneurysmal cyst and of another fibro-osseous lesion
EXCLUDES 2 cysts of jaw (M27.0-, M27.4-)
radicular cyst (K04.8)

- K09.0 Developmental odontogenic cysts
  Dentigerous cyst
  Eruption cyst
  Follicular cyst
  Gingival cyst
  Lateral periodontal cyst
  Primordial cyst
  EXCLUDES 2 keratocysts (D16.4, D16.5)
  odontogenic keratocystic tumors (D16.4, D16.5)
- K09.1 Developmental (nonodontogenic) cysts of oral region
  Cyst (of) incisive canal
  Cyst (of) palatine of papilla
  Globulomaxillary cyst
  Median palatal cyst
  Nasoalveolar cyst
  Nasolabial cyst
  Nasopalatine duct cyst
- K09.8 Other cysts of oral region, not elsewhere classified
  Dermoid cyst
  Epidermoid cyst
  Epstein's pearl
  Lymphoepithelial cyst
- K09.9 Cyst of oral region, unspecified

✓4th K11 Diseases of salivary glands
Use additional code to identify:
alcohol abuse and dependence (F10.-)
exposure to environmental tobacco smoke (Z77.22)
exposure to tobacco smoke in the perinatal period (P96.81)
history of tobacco dependence (Z87.891)
occupational exposure to environmental tobacco smoke (Z57.31)
tobacco dependence (F17.-)
tobacco use (Z72.0)

- K11.0 Atrophy of salivary gland
- K11.1 Hypertrophy of salivary gland
  DEF: Overgrowth of or enlarged salivary gland tissue caused by infection, salivary duct blockage, autoimmune diseases, and benign and malignant tumors.

✓5th K11.2 Sialoadenitis
Parotitis
EXCLUDES 1 epidemic parotitis (B26.-)
mumps (B26.-)
uveoparotid fever [Heerfordt] (D86.89)
DEF: Inflammation of the salivary gland.
- K11.20 Sialoadenitis, unspecified
- K11.21 Acute sialoadenitis
  EXCLUDES 1 acute recurrent sialoadenitis (K11.22)
- K11.22 Acute recurrent sialoadenitis
- K11.23 Chronic sialoadenitis

- K11.3 Abscess of salivary gland
- K11.4 Fistula of salivary gland
  EXCLUDES 1 congenital fistula of salivary gland (Q38.4)
- K11.5 Sialolithiasis
  Calculus of salivary gland or duct
  Stone of salivary gland or duct
- K11.6 Mucocele of salivary gland
  Mucous extravasation cyst of salivary gland
  Mucous retention cyst of salivary gland
  Ranula
- K11.7 Disturbances of salivary secretion
  Hypoptyalism
  Ptyalism
  Xerostomia
  EXCLUDES 2 dry mouth NOS (R68.2)

K11.8 Other diseases of salivary glands
Benign lymphoepithelial lesion of salivary gland
Mikulicz' disease
Necrotizing sialometaplasia
Sialectasia
Stenosis of salivary duct
Stricture of salivary duct
- EXCLUDES 1: Sjogren syndrome (M35.0-)

K11.9 Disease of salivary gland, unspecified
Sialoadenopathy NOS

K12 Stomatitis and related lesions
Use additional code to identify:
- alcohol abuse and dependence (F10.-)
- exposure to environmental tobacco smoke (Z77.22)
- exposure to tobacco smoke in the perinatal period (P96.81)
- history of tobacco dependence (Z87.891)
- occupational exposure to environmental tobacco smoke (Z57.31)
- tobacco dependence (F17.-)
- tobacco use (Z72.0)
- EXCLUDES 1:
  - cancrum oris (A69.0)
  - cheilitis (K13.0)
  - gangrenous stomatitis (A69.0)
  - herpesviral [herpes simplex] gingivostomatitis (B00.2)
  - noma (A69.0)

K12.0 Recurrent oral aphthae
Aphthous stomatitis (major) (minor)
Bednar's aphthae
Periadenitis mucosa necrotica recurrens
Recurrent aphthous ulcer
Stomatitis herpetiformis

DEF: Disorder of unknown etiology with small oval or round painful ulcers of the mouth marked by a grayish exudate and a red halo effect.

K12.1 Other forms of stomatitis
Denture stomatitis
Stomatitis NOS
Ulcerative stomatitis
Vesicular stomatitis
- EXCLUDES 1:
  - acute necrotizing ulcerative stomatitis (A69.1)
  - Vincent's stomatitis (A69.1)

K12.2 Cellulitis and abscess of mouth
Cellulitis of mouth (floor)
Submandibular abscess
- EXCLUDES 2:
  - abscess of salivary gland (K11.3)
  - abscess of tongue (K14.0)
  - periapical abscess (K04.6-K04.7)
  - periodontal abscess (K05.21)
  - peritonsillar abscess (J36)

K12.3 Oral mucositis (ulcerative)
Mucositis (oral) (oropharyneal)
- EXCLUDES 2:
  - gastrointestinal mucositis (ulcerative) (K92.81)
  - mucositis (ulcerative) of vagina and vulva (N76.81)
  - nasal mucositis (ulcerative) (J34.81)

K12.30 Oral mucositis (ulcerative), unspecified

K12.31 Oral mucositis (ulcerative) due to **antineoplastic therapy**
Use additional code for adverse effect, if applicable, to identify antineoplastic and immunosuppressive drugs (T45.1X5)
Use additional code for other antineoplastic therapy, such as:
radiological procedure and radiotherapy (Y84.2)

K12.32 Oral mucositis (ulcerative) due to other drugs
Use additional code for adverse effect, if applicable, to identify drug (T36-T50 with fifth or sixth character 5)

K12.33 Oral mucositis (ulcerative) due to **radiation**
Use additional external cause code (W88-W90, X39.0-) to identify cause

K12.39 Other oral mucositis (ulcerative)
Viral oral mucositis (ulcerative)

K13 Other diseases of lip and oral mucosa
INCLUDES epithelial disturbances of tongue
Use additional code to identify:
- alcohol abuse and dependence (F10.-)
- exposure to environmental tobacco smoke (Z77.22)
- exposure to tobacco smoke in the perinatal period (P96.81)
- history of tobacco dependence (Z87.891)
- occupational exposure to environmental tobacco smoke (Z57.31)
- tobacco dependence (F17.-)
- tobacco use (Z72.0)
- EXCLUDES 2:
  - certain disorders of gingiva and edentulous alveolar ridge (K05-K06)
  - cysts of oral region (K09.-)
  - diseases of tongue (K14.-)
  - stomatitis and related lesions (K12.-)

K13.0 Diseases of lips
Abscess of lips
Angular cheilitis
Cellulitis of lips
Cheilitis NOS
Cheilodynia
Cheilosis
Exfoliative cheilitis
Fistula of lips
Glandular cheilitis
Hypertrophy of lips
Perlèche NEC
- EXCLUDES 1:
  - ariboflavinosis (E53.0)
  - cheilitis due to radiation-related disorders (L55-L59)
  - congenital fistula of lips (Q38.0)
  - congenital hypertrophy of lips (Q18.6)
  - perlèche due to candidiasis (B37.83)
  - perlèche due to riboflavin deficiency (E53.0)

K13.1 Cheek and lip biting

K13.2 Leukoplakia and other disturbances of oral epithelium, including tongue
- EXCLUDES 1:
  - carcinoma in situ of oral epithelium (D00.0-)
  - hairy leukoplakia (K13.3)

DEF: Leukoplakia: Thickened white patches or lesions appearing on a mucous membrane, such as oral mucosa or tongue.

K13.21 Leukoplakia of **oral mucosa, including tongue**
Leukokeratosis of oral mucosa
Leukoplakia of gingiva, lips, tongue
- EXCLUDES 1:
  - hairy leukoplakia (K13.3)
  - leukokeratosis nicotina palati (K13.24)

K13.22 **Minimal keratinized residual ridge mucosa**
Minimal keratinization of alveolar ridge mucosa

K13.23 **Excessive keratinized residual ridge mucosa**
Excessive keratinization of alveolar ridge mucosa

K13.24 **Leukokeratosis nicotina palati**
Smoker's palate

K13.29 Other disturbances of oral epithelium, including tongue
Erythroplakia of mouth or tongue
Focal epithelial hyperplasia of mouth or tongue
Leukoedema of mouth or tongue
Other oral epithelium disturbances

K13.3 Hairy leukoplakia

K13.4 Granuloma and granuloma-like lesions of oral mucosa
Eosinophilic granuloma
Granuloma pyogenicum
Verrucous xanthoma

K13.5 Oral submucous fibrosis
Submucous fibrosis of tongue

K13.6 Irritative hyperplasia of oral mucosa
- EXCLUDES 2: irritative hyperplasia of edentulous ridge [denture hyperplasia] (K06.2)

K13.7 Other and unspecified lesions of oral mucosa

K13.70 Unspecified lesions of oral mucosa

K13.79 Other lesions of oral mucosa
Focal oral mucinosis
AHA: 2022,2Q,7

K14 Diseases of tongue
Use additional code to identify:
  alcohol abuse and dependence (F10.-)
  exposure to environmental tobacco smoke (Z77.22)
  history of tobacco dependence (Z87.891)
  occupational exposure to environmental tobacco smoke (Z57.31)
  tobacco dependence (F17.-)
  tobacco use (Z72.0)
  EXCLUDES 2   erythroplakia (K13.29)
              focal epithelial hyperplasia (K13.29)
              hairy leukoplakia (K13.3)
              leukoedema of tongue (K13.29)
              leukoplakia of tongue (K13.21)
              macroglossia (congenital) (Q38.2)
              submucous fibrosis of tongue (K13.5)

K14.0 Glossitis
Abscess of tongue
Ulceration (traumatic) of tongue
EXCLUDES 1   atrophic glossitis (K14.4)
DEF: Inflammation and swelling of the tongue that may be associated with infection, adverse drug reactions, smoking, or injury.

K14.1 Geographic tongue
Benign migratory glossitis
Glossitis areata exfoliativa

K14.2 Median rhomboid glossitis

K14.3 Hypertrophy of tongue papillae
Black hairy tongue
Coated tongue
Hypertrophy of foliate papillae
Lingua villosa nigra

K14.4 Atrophy of tongue papillae
Atrophic glossitis

K14.5 Plicated tongue
Fissured tongue
Furrowed tongue
Scrotal tongue
EXCLUDES 1   fissured tongue, congenital (Q38.3)

K14.6 Glossodynia
Glossopyrosis
Painful tongue

K14.8 Other diseases of tongue
Atrophy of tongue
Crenated tongue
Enlargement of tongue
Glossocele
Glossoptosis
Hypertrophy of tongue

K14.9 Disease of tongue, unspecified
Glossopathy NOS

Diseases of esophagus, stomach and duodenum (K20-K31)
EXCLUDES 2   hiatus hernia (K44.-)

K20 Esophagitis
Use additional code to identify:
  alcohol abuse and dependence (F10.-)
EXCLUDES 1   erosion of esophagus (K22.1-)
            esophagitis with gastro-esophageal reflux disease (K21.0-)
            reflux esophagitis (K21.0-)
            ulcerative esophagitis (K22.1-)
EXCLUDES 2   eosinophilic gastritis or gastroenteritis (K52.81)
AHA: 2023,1Q,20

K20.0 Eosinophilic esophagitis
AHA: 2020,4Q,9

K20.8 Other esophagitis
AHA: 2020,4Q,28-29

K20.80 Other esophagitis without bleeding
Abscess of esophagus
Other esophagitis NOS

K20.81 Other esophagitis with bleeding

K20.9 Esophagitis, unspecified
AHA: 2020,4Q,28-29

K20.90 Esophagitis, unspecified without bleeding
Esophagitis NOS

K20.91 Esophagitis, unspecified with bleeding

K21 Gastro-esophageal reflux disease
EXCLUDES 1   newborn esophageal reflux (P78.83)

K21.0 Gastro-esophageal reflux disease with esophagitis
AHA: 2020,4Q,28-29

K21.00 Gastro-esophageal reflux disease with esophagitis, without bleeding
Reflux esophagitis

K21.01 Gastro-esophageal reflux disease with esophagitis, with bleeding

K21.9 Gastro-esophageal reflux disease without esophagitis
Esophageal reflux NOS
AHA: 2016,1Q,18

K22 Other diseases of esophagus
EXCLUDES 2   esophageal varices (I85.-)

K22.0 Achalasia of cardia
Achalasia NOS
Cardiospasm
EXCLUDES 1   congenital cardiospasm (Q39.5)
DEF: Esophageal motility disorder that is caused by absence of the esophageal peristalsis and impaired relaxation of the lower esophageal sphincter. It is characterized by dysphagia, regurgitation, and heartburn.

K22.1 Ulcer of esophagus
Barrett's ulcer
Erosion of esophagus
Fungal ulcer of esophagus
Peptic ulcer of esophagus
Ulcer of esophagus due to ingestion of chemicals
Ulcer of esophagus due to ingestion of drugs and medicaments
Ulcerative esophagitis
Code first poisoning due to drug or toxin, if applicable (T36-T65 with fifth or sixth character 1-4)
Use additional code for adverse effect, if applicable, to identify drug (T36-T50 with fifth or sixth character 5)
EXCLUDES 1   Barrett's esophagus (K22.7-)
AHA: 2018,3Q,22; 2017,3Q,27
TIP: Assign a code for "with bleeding" when an esophageal ulcer and bleeding (hematemesis) are documented. The ICD-10-CM classification assumes the two are related without the provider linking the two conditions. Evidence of bleeding during a procedure is not required.

K22.10 Ulcer of esophagus without bleeding
Ulcer of esophagus NOS

K22.11 Ulcer of esophagus with bleeding
EXCLUDES 2   bleeding esophageal varices (I85.01, I85.11)
AHA: 2023,1Q,20
TIP: For bleeding esophageal ulcers resulting from anticoagulant therapy, assign this code, code D68.32 Hemorrhagic disorder due to extrinsic circulating anticoagulant, and adverse effect code T45.515- with the appropriate seventh character.

K22.2 Esophageal obstruction
Compression of esophagus
Constriction of esophagus
Stenosis of esophagus
Stricture of esophagus
EXCLUDES 1   congenital stenosis or stricture of esophagus (Q39.3)

K22.3 Perforation of esophagus
Rupture of esophagus
EXCLUDES 1   traumatic perforation of (thoracic) esophagus (S27.8-)

K22.4 Dyskinesia of esophagus
Corkscrew esophagus
Diffuse esophageal spasm
Spasm of esophagus
EXCLUDES 1   cardiospasm (K22.0)
AHA: 2025,2Q,17

K22.5 Diverticulum of esophagus, acquired
Esophageal pouch, acquired
EXCLUDES 1   diverticulum of esophagus (congenital) (Q39.6)

K22.6 Gastro-esophageal laceration-hemorrhage syndrome
Mallory-Weiss syndrome

K22.7 Barrett's esophagus
Barrett's disease
Barrett's syndrome
EXCLUDES 1: Barrett's ulcer (K22.1)
malignant neoplasm of esophagus (C15.-)
DEF: Metaplastic disorder in which specialized columnar epithelial cells replace the normal squamous epithelial cells. Secondary to chronic gastroesophageal reflux damage to the mucosa, this disorder increases the risk of developing adenocarcinoma.

- **K22.70** Barrett's esophagus without dysplasia
  Barrett's esophagus NOS
- **K22.71** Barrett's esophagus with dysplasia
  - **K22.710** Barrett's esophagus with low grade dysplasia
  - **K22.711** Barrett's esophagus with high grade dysplasia
  - **K22.719** Barrett's esophagus with dysplasia, unspecified

K22.8 Other specified diseases of esophagus
EXCLUDES 2: esophageal varices (I85.-)
Paterson-Kelly syndrome (D50.1)
AHA: 2021,4Q,15; 2020,1Q,16

- **K22.81** Esophageal polyp
  EXCLUDES 1: benign neoplasm of esophagus (D13.0)
- **K22.82** Esophagogastric junction polyp
  EXCLUDES 1: benign neoplasm of stomach (D13.1)
- **K22.89** Other specified disease of esophagus
  Hemorrhage of esophagus NOS
  AHA: 2024,2Q,26

K22.9 Disease of esophagus, unspecified

K23 Disorders of esophagus in diseases classified elsewhere
Code first underlying disease, such as:
congenital syphilis (A50.5)
EXCLUDES 1: late syphilis (A52.79)
megaesophagus due to Chagas' disease (B57.31)
tuberculosis (A18.83)

K25 Gastric ulcer
INCLUDES: erosion (acute) of stomach
pylorus ulcer (peptic)
stomach ulcer (peptic)
Use additional code to identify:
alcohol abuse and dependence (F10.-)
EXCLUDES 1: acute gastritis (K29.0-)
peptic ulcer NOS (K27.-)
AHA: 2021,1Q,9,11; 2017,3Q,27
TIP: Assign a code for "with hemorrhage" when a gastric ulcer and GI bleeding are documented. The ICD-10-CM classification assumes the two are related without the provider linking the two conditions. Evidence of bleeding during a procedure is not required.
TIP: For bleeding ulcers resulting from anticoagulant therapy, assign the appropriate "with hemorrhage" ulcer code from this category, code D68.32 Hemorrhagic disorder due to extrinsic circulating anticoagulant, and adverse effect code T45.515- with the appropriate seventh character.

- **K25.0** Acute gastric ulcer with hemorrhage
  AHA: 2023,1Q,16
- **K25.1** Acute gastric ulcer with perforation
- **K25.2** Acute gastric ulcer with both hemorrhage and perforation
- **K25.3** Acute gastric ulcer without hemorrhage or perforation
- **K25.4** Chronic or unspecified gastric ulcer with hemorrhage
- **K25.5** Chronic or unspecified gastric ulcer with perforation
- **K25.6** Chronic or unspecified gastric ulcer with both hemorrhage and perforation
- **K25.7** Chronic gastric ulcer without hemorrhage or perforation
- **K25.9** Gastric ulcer, unspecified as acute or chronic, without hemorrhage or perforation

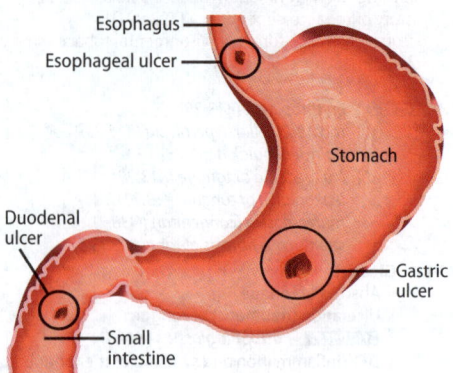

Gastrointestinal Ulcers

K26 Duodenal ulcer
INCLUDES: duodenum ulcer (peptic)
erosion (acute) of duodenum
postpyloric ulcer (peptic)
Use additional code to identify:
alcohol abuse and dependence (F10.-)
EXCLUDES 1: peptic ulcer NOS (K27.-)
AHA: 2023,2Q,11; 2017,3Q,27
TIP: Assign a code for "with hemorrhage" when a duodenal ulcer and GI bleeding are documented. The ICD-10-CM classification assumes the two are related without the provider linking the two conditions. Evidence of bleeding during a procedure is not required.
TIP: For bleeding ulcers resulting from anticoagulant therapy, assign the appropriate "with hemorrhage" ulcer code from this category, code D68.32 Hemorrhagic disorder due to extrinsic circulating anticoagulant, and adverse effect code T45.515- with the appropriate seventh character.

- **K26.0** Acute duodenal ulcer with hemorrhage
- **K26.1** Acute duodenal ulcer with perforation
- **K26.2** Acute duodenal ulcer with both hemorrhage and perforation
- **K26.3** Acute duodenal ulcer without hemorrhage or perforation
- **K26.4** Chronic or unspecified duodenal ulcer with hemorrhage
  AHA: 2016,1Q,14
- **K26.5** Chronic or unspecified duodenal ulcer with perforation
- **K26.6** Chronic or unspecified duodenal ulcer with both hemorrhage and perforation
- **K26.7** Chronic duodenal ulcer without hemorrhage or perforation
- **K26.9** Duodenal ulcer, unspecified as acute or chronic, without hemorrhage or perforation

K27 Peptic ulcer, site unspecified
INCLUDES: gastroduodenal ulcer NOS
peptic ulcer NOS
Use additional code to identify:
alcohol abuse and dependence (F10.-)
EXCLUDES 1: peptic ulcer of newborn (P78.82)
AHA: 2017,3Q,27
TIP: Assign a code for "with hemorrhage" when a peptic ulcer and GI bleeding are documented. The ICD-10-CM classification assumes the two are related without the provider linking the two conditions. Evidence of bleeding during a procedure is not required.
TIP: For bleeding ulcers resulting from anticoagulant therapy, assign the appropriate "with hemorrhage" ulcer code from this category, code D68.32 Hemorrhagic disorder due to extrinsic circulating anticoagulant, and adverse effect code T45.515- with the appropriate seventh character.

- **K27.0** Acute peptic ulcer, site unspecified, with hemorrhage
- **K27.1** Acute peptic ulcer, site unspecified, with perforation
- **K27.2** Acute peptic ulcer, site unspecified, with both hemorrhage and perforation
- **K27.3** Acute peptic ulcer, site unspecified, without hemorrhage or perforation
- **K27.4** Chronic or unspecified peptic ulcer, site unspecified, with hemorrhage
- **K27.5** Chronic or unspecified peptic ulcer, site unspecified, with perforation
- **K27.6** Chronic or unspecified peptic ulcer, site unspecified, with both hemorrhage and perforation

K27.7 Chronic peptic ulcer, site unspecified, without hemorrhage or perforation
K27.9 Peptic ulcer, site unspecified, unspecified as acute or chronic, without hemorrhage or perforation

K28 Gastrojejunal ulcer
  INCLUDES anastomotic ulcer (peptic) or erosion
  gastrocolic ulcer (peptic) or erosion
  gastrointestinal ulcer (peptic) or erosion
  gastrojejunal ulcer (peptic) or erosion
  jejunal ulcer (peptic) or erosion
  marginal ulcer (peptic) or erosion
  stomal ulcer (peptic) or erosion
  Use additional code to identify:
    alcohol abuse and dependence (F10.-)
  EXCLUDES 1 primary ulcer of small intestine (K63.3)
  AHA: 2017,3Q,27
  TIP: Assign a code for "with hemorrhage" when a gastrojejunal ulcer and GI bleeding are documented. The ICD-10-CM classification assumes the two are related without the provider linking the two conditions. Evidence of bleeding during a procedure is not required.
  TIP: For bleeding ulcers resulting from anticoagulant therapy, assign the appropriate "with hemorrhage" ulcer code from this category, code D68.32 Hemorrhagic disorder due to extrinsic circulating anticoagulant, and adverse effect code T45.515- with the appropriate seventh character.

K28.0 Acute gastrojejunal ulcer with hemorrhage
K28.1 Acute gastrojejunal ulcer with perforation
K28.2 Acute gastrojejunal ulcer with both hemorrhage and perforation
K28.3 Acute gastrojejunal ulcer without hemorrhage or perforation
K28.4 Chronic or unspecified gastrojejunal ulcer with hemorrhage
  AHA: 2023,3Q,10
K28.5 Chronic or unspecified gastrojejunal ulcer with perforation
K28.6 Chronic or unspecified gastrojejunal ulcer with both hemorrhage and perforation
K28.7 Chronic gastrojejunal ulcer without hemorrhage or perforation
K28.9 Gastrojejunal ulcer, unspecified as acute or chronic, without hemorrhage or perforation

K29 Gastritis and duodenitis
  EXCLUDES 1 eosinophilic gastritis or gastroenteritis (K52.81)
  Zollinger-Ellison syndrome (E16.4)
  AHA: 2018,3Q,22
  TIP: Assign a code for "with bleeding" when gastritis or duodenitis and GI bleeding are documented. The ICD-10-CM classification assumes the two are related without the provider linking the two conditions. Evidence of bleeding during a procedure is not required.
  TIP: For bleeding ulcers resulting from anticoagulant therapy, assign the appropriate "with hemorrhage" ulcer code from this category, code D68.32 Hemorrhagic disorder due to extrinsic circulating anticoagulant, and adverse effect code T45.515- with the appropriate seventh character.

K29.0 Acute gastritis
  Use additional code to identify:
    alcohol abuse and dependence (F10.-)
  EXCLUDES 1 erosion (acute) of stomach (K25.-)
  K29.00 Acute gastritis without bleeding
  K29.01 Acute gastritis with bleeding
K29.2 Alcoholic gastritis
  Use additional code to identify:
    alcohol abuse and dependence (F10.-)
  K29.20 Alcoholic gastritis without bleeding
  K29.21 Alcoholic gastritis with bleeding
K29.3 Chronic superficial gastritis
  K29.30 Chronic superficial gastritis without bleeding
  K29.31 Chronic superficial gastritis with bleeding
K29.4 Chronic atrophic gastritis
  Gastric atrophy
  K29.40 Chronic atrophic gastritis without bleeding
  K29.41 Chronic atrophic gastritis with bleeding
K29.5 Unspecified chronic gastritis
  Chronic antral gastritis
  Chronic fundal gastritis
  K29.50 Unspecified chronic gastritis without bleeding
  K29.51 Unspecified chronic gastritis with bleeding
K29.6 Other gastritis
  Giant hypertrophic gastritis
  Granulomatous gastritis
  Menetrier's disease
  K29.60 Other gastritis without bleeding
  K29.61 Other gastritis with bleeding
K29.7 Gastritis, unspecified
  K29.70 Gastritis, unspecified, without bleeding
  K29.71 Gastritis, unspecified, with bleeding
K29.8 Duodenitis
  K29.80 Duodenitis without bleeding
    AHA: 2025,2Q,5
  K29.81 Duodenitis with bleeding
K29.9 Gastroduodenitis, unspecified
  K29.90 Gastroduodenitis, unspecified, without bleeding
  K29.91 Gastroduodenitis, unspecified, with bleeding

K30 Functional dyspepsia
  Indigestion
  EXCLUDES 1 dyspepsia NOS (R10.13)
  heartburn (R12)
  nervous dyspepsia (F45.8)
  neurotic dyspepsia (F45.8)
  psychogenic dyspepsia (F45.8)

K31 Other diseases of stomach and duodenum
  INCLUDES functional disorders of stomach
  EXCLUDES 2 diabetic gastroparesis (E08.43, E09.43, E10.43, E11.43, E13.43)
  diverticulum of duodenum (K57.00-K57.13)

K31.0 Acute dilatation of stomach
  Acute distention of stomach
K31.1 Adult hypertrophic pyloric stenosis
  Pyloric stenosis NOS
  EXCLUDES 1 congenital or infantile pyloric stenosis (Q40.0)
  AHA: 2023,3Q,11
K31.2 Hourglass stricture and stenosis of stomach
  EXCLUDES 1 congenital hourglass stomach (Q40.2)
  hourglass contraction of stomach (K31.89)
K31.3 Pylorospasm, not elsewhere classified
  EXCLUDES 1 congenital or infantile pylorospasm (Q40.0)
  neurotic pylorospasm (F45.8)
  psychogenic pylorospasm (F45.8)
K31.4 Gastric diverticulum
  EXCLUDES 1 congenital diverticulum of stomach (Q40.2)
K31.5 Obstruction of duodenum
  Constriction of duodenum
  Duodenal ileus (chronic)
  Stenosis of duodenum
  Stricture of duodenum
  Volvulus of duodenum
  EXCLUDES 1 congenital stenosis of duodenum (Q41.0)
K31.6 Fistula of stomach and duodenum
  Gastrocolic fistula
  Gastrojejunocolic fistula
  Code also, if applicable, disruption of internal operation (surgical) wound (T81.32-)
K31.7 Polyp of stomach and duodenum
  EXCLUDES 1 adenomatous polyp of stomach (D13.1)
  AHA: 2020,1Q,16
K31.8 Other specified diseases of stomach and duodenum
  K31.81 Angiodysplasia of stomach and duodenum
    TIP: Assign a code for "with bleeding" when angiodysplasia of the stomach or the duodenum and GI bleeding are documented. The ICD-10-CM classification assumes the two are related without the provider linking the two conditions. Evidence of bleeding during a procedure is not required.
    K31.811 Angiodysplasia of stomach and duodenum with bleeding
      AHA: 2023,1Q,16
    K31.819 Angiodysplasia of stomach and duodenum without bleeding
      Angiodysplasia of stomach and duodenum NOS
  K31.82 Dieulafoy lesion (hemorrhagic) of stomach and duodenum
    EXCLUDES 2 Dieulafoy lesion of intestine (K63.81)
    DEF: Abnormally large submucosal artery protruding through a defect in the stomach mucosa or intestines that can cause massive and life-threatening hemorrhaging.
  K31.83 Achlorhydria
    DEF: Absence of hydrochloric acid in gastric secretions due to gastric mucosa atrophy. Achlorhydria is unresponsive to histamines.

K31.84 **Gastroparesis**
Gastroparalysis
Code first underlying disease, if known, such as:
anorexia nervosa (F50.0-)
diabetes mellitus (E08.43, E09.43, E10.43, E11.43, E13.43)
scleroderma (M34.-)
AHA: 2013,4Q,114

K31.89 **Other diseases of stomach and duodenum**
AHA: 2024,2Q,26; 2020,1Q,15; 2017,1Q,28

K31.9 **Disease of stomach and duodenum, unspecified**

√5th **K31.A** **Gastric intestinal metaplasia**
AHA: 2021,4Q,15-16

K31.A0 **Gastric intestinal metaplasia, unspecified**
Gastric intestinal metaplasia indefinite for dysplasia
Gastric intestinal metaplasia NOS

√6th **K31.A1** **Gastric intestinal metaplasia without dysplasia**

K31.A11 Gastric intestinal metaplasia without dysplasia, involving the antrum

K31.A12 Gastric intestinal metaplasia without dysplasia, involving the body (corpus)

K31.A13 Gastric intestinal metaplasia without dysplasia, involving the fundus

K31.A14 Gastric intestinal metaplasia without dysplasia, involving the cardia

K31.A15 Gastric intestinal metaplasia without dysplasia, involving multiple sites

K31.A19 Gastric intestinal metaplasia without dysplasia, unspecified site

√6th **K31.A2** **Gastric intestinal metaplasia with dysplasia**

K31.A21 Gastric intestinal metaplasia with low grade dysplasia

K31.A22 Gastric intestinal metaplasia with high grade dysplasia

K31.A29 Gastric intestinal metaplasia with dysplasia, unspecified

Diseases of appendix (K35-K38)

√4th **K35** **Acute appendicitis**
AHA: 2018,4Q,17-18

√5th **K35.2** **Acute appendicitis with generalized peritonitis**
AHA: 2023,4Q,28-29

√6th **K35.20** **Acute appendicitis with generalized peritonitis, without abscess**

K35.200 Acute appendicitis with generalized peritonitis, without perforation or abscess
(Acute) appendicitis with generalized peritonitis without rupture or perforation of appendix NOS

K35.201 Acute appendicitis with generalized peritonitis, with perforation, without abscess
Appendicitis (acute) with generalized (diffuse) peritonitis following rupture or perforation of appendix NOS

K35.209 Acute appendicitis with generalized peritonitis, without abscess, unspecified as to perforation
(Acute) appendicitis with generalized peritonitis NOS

√6th **K35.21** **Acute appendicitis with generalized peritonitis, with abscess**

K35.210 Acute appendicitis with generalized peritonitis, without perforation, with abscess
(Acute) appendicitis with generalized peritonitis without rupture or perforation of appendix, with abscess

K35.211 Acute appendicitis with generalized peritonitis, with perforation and abscess
Appendicitis (acute) with generalized (diffuse) peritonitis following rupture or perforation of appendix, with abscess

K35.219 Acute appendicitis with generalized peritonitis, with abscess, unspecified as to perforation
(Acute) appendicitis with generalized peritonitis and abscess NOS

√5th **K35.3** **Acute appendicitis with localized peritonitis**

K35.30 Acute appendicitis with localized peritonitis, without perforation or gangrene
Acute appendicitis with localized peritonitis NOS

K35.31 Acute appendicitis with localized peritonitis and gangrene, without perforation

K35.32 Acute appendicitis with perforation, localized peritonitis, and gangrene, without abscess
(Acute) appendicitis with perforation NOS
Perforated appendix NOS
Ruptured appendix (with localized peritonitis) NOS
AHA: 2020,1Q,16

K35.33 Acute appendicitis with perforation, localized peritonitis, and gangrene, with abscess
(Acute) appendicitis with (peritoneal) abscess NOS
Ruptured appendix with localized peritonitis and abscess

√5th **K35.8** **Other and unspecified acute appendicitis**

K35.80 Unspecified acute appendicitis
Acute appendicitis NOS
Acute appendicitis without (localized) (generalized) peritonitis

√6th **K35.89** **Other acute appendicitis**
AHA: 2020,1Q,16

K35.890 Other acute appendicitis without perforation or gangrene

K35.891 Other acute appendicitis without perforation, with gangrene
(Acute) appendicitis with gangrene NOS

K36 **Other appendicitis**
Chronic appendicitis
Recurrent appendicitis

K37 **Unspecified appendicitis**
EXCLUDES 1   unspecified appendicitis with peritonitis (K35.2-, K35.3-)

√4th **K38** **Other diseases of appendix**

K38.0 Hyperplasia of appendix

K38.1 Appendicular concretions
Fecalith of appendix
Stercolith of appendix

K38.2 Diverticulum of appendix

K38.3 Fistula of appendix

K38.8 Other specified diseases of appendix
Intussusception of appendix

K38.9 Disease of appendix, unspecified

Hernia (K40-K46)

NOTE Hernia with both gangrene and obstruction is classified to hernia with gangrene.

INCLUDES acquired hernia
congenital [except diaphragmatic or hiatus] hernia
recurrent hernia

AHA: 2021,3Q,30-31

TIP: Do not assign a code for bilateral hernia when the right and left sides have differing pathology. For example, two codes would be assigned for bilateral femoral hernia in which the left side is incarcerated (with obstruction) but the right side is not incarcerated; the code for bilateral would not apply in this case.

√4th **K40** **Inguinal hernia**
INCLUDES   bubonocele
direct inguinal hernia
double inguinal hernia
indirect inguinal hernia
inguinal hernia NOS
oblique inguinal hernia
scrotal hernia
DEF: Within the groin region.

√5th **K40.0** **Bilateral inguinal hernia, with obstruction, without gangrene**
Incarcerated inguinal hernia (bilateral) without gangrene
Inguinal hernia (bilateral) causing obstruction without gangrene
Irreducible inguinal hernia (bilateral) without gangrene
Strangulated inguinal hernia (bilateral) without gangrene

K40.00 Bilateral inguinal hernia, with obstruction, without gangrene, not specified as recurrent
Bilateral inguinal hernia, with obstruction, without gangrene NOS

K40.01 Bilateral inguinal hernia, with obstruction, without gangrene, recurrent

Chapter 11. Diseases of the Digestive System

√5th K40.1 Bilateral inguinal hernia, with gangrene
  - K40.10 Bilateral inguinal hernia, with gangrene, not specified as recurrent
    - Bilateral inguinal hernia, with gangrene NOS
  - K40.11 Bilateral inguinal hernia, with gangrene, recurrent

√5th K40.2 Bilateral inguinal hernia, without obstruction or gangrene
  - K40.20 Bilateral inguinal hernia, without obstruction or gangrene, not specified as recurrent
    - Bilateral inguinal hernia NOS
  - K40.21 Bilateral inguinal hernia, without obstruction or gangrene, recurrent

√5th K40.3 Unilateral inguinal hernia, with obstruction, without gangrene
  - Incarcerated inguinal hernia (unilateral) without gangrene
  - Inguinal hernia (unilateral) causing obstruction without gangrene
  - Irreducible inguinal hernia (unilateral) without gangrene
  - Strangulated inguinal hernia (unilateral) without gangrene
  - K40.30 Unilateral inguinal hernia, with obstruction, without gangrene, not specified as recurrent
    - Inguinal hernia, with obstruction NOS
    - Unilateral inguinal hernia, with obstruction, without gangrene NOS
  - K40.31 Unilateral inguinal hernia, with obstruction, without gangrene, recurrent

√5th K40.4 Unilateral inguinal hernia, with gangrene
  - K40.40 Unilateral inguinal hernia, with gangrene, not specified as recurrent
    - Inguinal hernia with gangrene NOS
    - Unilateral inguinal hernia with gangrene NOS
  - K40.41 Unilateral inguinal hernia, with gangrene, recurrent

√5th K40.9 Unilateral inguinal hernia, without obstruction or gangrene
  - K40.90 Unilateral inguinal hernia, without obstruction or gangrene, not specified as recurrent
    - Inguinal hernia NOS
    - Unilateral inguinal hernia NOS
  - K40.91 Unilateral inguinal hernia, without obstruction or gangrene, recurrent

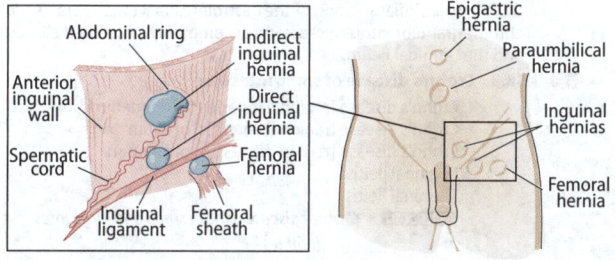

Hernia Sites

√4th K41 Femoral hernia

  √5th K41.0 Bilateral femoral hernia, with obstruction, without gangrene
  - Femoral hernia (bilateral) causing obstruction, without gangrene
  - Incarcerated femoral hernia (bilateral), without gangrene
  - Irreducible femoral hernia (bilateral), without gangrene
  - Strangulated femoral hernia (bilateral), without gangrene
  - K41.00 Bilateral femoral hernia, with obstruction, without gangrene, not specified as recurrent
    - Bilateral femoral hernia, with obstruction, without gangrene NOS
  - K41.01 Bilateral femoral hernia, with obstruction, without gangrene, recurrent

  √5th K41.1 Bilateral femoral hernia, with gangrene
  - K41.10 Bilateral femoral hernia, with gangrene, not specified as recurrent
    - Bilateral femoral hernia, with gangrene NOS
  - K41.11 Bilateral femoral hernia, with gangrene, recurrent

  √5th K41.2 Bilateral femoral hernia, without obstruction or gangrene
  - K41.20 Bilateral femoral hernia, without obstruction or gangrene, not specified as recurrent
    - Bilateral femoral hernia NOS
  - K41.21 Bilateral femoral hernia, without obstruction or gangrene, recurrent

√5th K41.3 Unilateral femoral hernia, with obstruction, without gangrene
  - Femoral hernia (unilateral) causing obstruction, without gangrene
  - Incarcerated femoral hernia (unilateral), without gangrene
  - Irreducible femoral hernia (unilateral), without gangrene
  - Strangulated femoral hernia (unilateral), without gangrene
  - K41.30 Unilateral femoral hernia, with obstruction, without gangrene, not specified as recurrent
    - Femoral hernia, with obstruction NOS
    - Unilateral femoral hernia, with obstruction NOS
  - K41.31 Unilateral femoral hernia, with obstruction, without gangrene, recurrent

√5th K41.4 Unilateral femoral hernia, with gangrene
  - K41.40 Unilateral femoral hernia, with gangrene, not specified as recurrent
    - Femoral hernia, with gangrene NOS
    - Unilateral femoral hernia, with gangrene NOS
  - K41.41 Unilateral femoral hernia, with gangrene, recurrent

√5th K41.9 Unilateral femoral hernia, without obstruction or gangrene
  - K41.90 Unilateral femoral hernia, without obstruction or gangrene, not specified as recurrent
    - Femoral hernia NOS
    - Unilateral femoral hernia NOS
  - K41.91 Unilateral femoral hernia, without obstruction or gangrene, recurrent

√4th K42 Umbilical hernia
  - INCLUDES paraumbilical hernia
  - EXCLUDES 1 omphalocele (Q79.2)

  K42.0 Umbilical hernia with obstruction, without gangrene
  - Incarcerated umbilical hernia, without gangrene
  - Irreducible umbilical hernia, without gangrene
  - Strangulated umbilical hernia, without gangrene
  - Umbilical hernia causing obstruction, without gangrene

  K42.1 Umbilical hernia with gangrene
  - Gangrenous umbilical hernia

  K42.9 Umbilical hernia without obstruction or gangrene
  - Umbilical hernia NOS

√4th K43 Ventral hernia
  DEF: Condition in which a loop of bowel protrudes through a weakness in the abdominal wall muscles that may occur as a birth defect, past surgical site (incisional), or form at a stomal site (parastomal).

  K43.0 Incisional hernia with obstruction, without gangrene
  - Incarcerated incisional hernia, without gangrene
  - Incisional hernia causing obstruction, without gangrene
  - Irreducible incisional hernia, without gangrene
  - Strangulated incisional hernia, without gangrene

  K43.1 Incisional hernia with gangrene
  - Gangrenous incisional hernia
  - **AHA:** 2020,2Q,22

  K43.2 Incisional hernia without obstruction or gangrene
  - Incisional hernia NOS

  K43.3 Parastomal hernia with obstruction, without gangrene
  - Incarcerated parastomal hernia, without gangrene
  - Irreducible parastomal hernia, without gangrene
  - Parastomal hernia causing obstruction, without gangrene
  - Strangulated parastomal hernia, without gangrene

  K43.4 Parastomal hernia with gangrene
  - Gangrenous parastomal hernia

  K43.5 Parastomal hernia without obstruction or gangrene
  - Parastomal hernia NOS

Chapter 11. Diseases of the Digestive System

K43.6 Other and unspecified ventral hernia with obstruction, without gangrene
Epigastric hernia causing obstruction, without gangrene
Hypogastric hernia causing obstruction, without gangrene
Incarcerated epigastric hernia without gangrene
Incarcerated hypogastric hernia without gangrene
Incarcerated midline hernia without gangrene
Incarcerated spigelian hernia without gangrene
Incarcerated subxiphoid hernia without gangrene
Irreducible epigastric hernia without gangrene
Irreducible hypogastric hernia without gangrene
Irreducible midline hernia without gangrene
Irreducible spigelian hernia without gangrene
Irreducible subxiphoid hernia without gangrene
Midline hernia causing obstruction, without gangrene
Spigelian hernia causing obstruction, without gangrene
Strangulated epigastric hernia without gangrene
Strangulated hypogastric hernia without gangrene
Strangulated midline hernia without gangrene
Strangulated spigelian hernia without gangrene
Strangulated subxiphoid hernia without gangrene
Subxiphoid hernia causing obstruction, without gangrene

K43.7 Other and unspecified ventral hernia with gangrene
Any condition listed under K43.6 specified as gangrenous

K43.9 Ventral hernia without obstruction or gangrene
Epigastric hernia
Ventral hernia NOS

✓4th K44 Diaphragmatic hernia
INCLUDES hiatus hernia (esophageal) (sliding)
paraesophageal hernia
EXCLUDES 1 congenital diaphragmatic hernia (Q79.0)
congenital hiatus hernia (Q40.1)

DEF: Protrusion of an abdominal organ, usually the stomach, through the esophageal opening within the diaphragm and occurring in two types: the sliding hiatal hernia and the paraesophageal hernia.

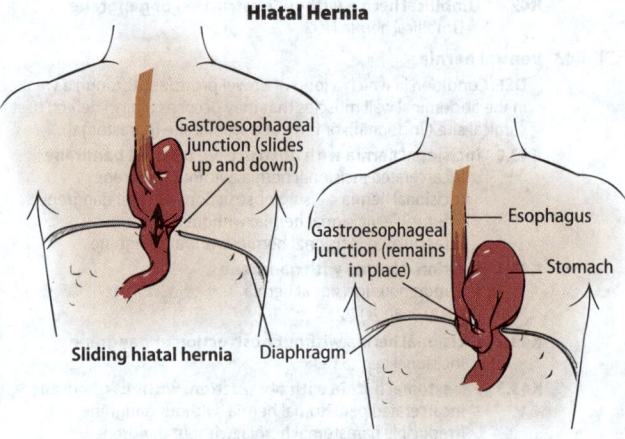

Hiatal Hernia

K44.0 Diaphragmatic hernia with obstruction, without gangrene
Diaphragmatic hernia causing obstruction
Incarcerated diaphragmatic hernia
Irreducible diaphragmatic hernia
Strangulated diaphragmatic hernia
AHA: 2022,2Q,13

K44.1 Diaphragmatic hernia with gangrene
Gangrenous diaphragmatic hernia

K44.9 Diaphragmatic hernia without obstruction or gangrene
Diaphragmatic hernia NOS

✓4th K45 Other abdominal hernia
INCLUDES abdominal hernia, specified site NEC
lumbar hernia
obturator hernia
pudendal hernia
retroperitoneal hernia
sciatic hernia

K45.0 Other specified abdominal hernia with obstruction, without gangrene
Other specified abdominal hernia causing obstruction
Other specified incarcerated abdominal hernia
Other specified irreducible abdominal hernia
Other specified strangulated abdominal hernia

K45.1 Other specified abdominal hernia with gangrene
Any condition listed under K45 specified as gangrenous
AHA: 2024,2Q,22

K45.8 Other specified abdominal hernia without obstruction or gangrene

✓4th K46 Unspecified abdominal hernia
INCLUDES enterocele
epiplocele
hernia NOS
interstitial hernia
intestinal hernia
intra-abdominal hernia
EXCLUDES 1 vaginal enterocele (N81.5)

K46.0 Unspecified abdominal hernia with obstruction, without gangrene
Unspecified abdominal hernia causing obstruction
Unspecified incarcerated abdominal hernia
Unspecified irreducible abdominal hernia
Unspecified strangulated abdominal hernia

K46.1 Unspecified abdominal hernia with gangrene
Any condition listed under K46 specified as gangrenous

K46.9 Unspecified abdominal hernia without obstruction or gangrene
Abdominal hernia NOS

Noninfective enteritis and colitis (K50-K52)

INCLUDES noninfective inflammatory bowel disease
EXCLUDES 1 irritable bowel syndrome (K58.-)
megacolon (K59.3-)

✓4th K50 Crohn's disease [regional enteritis]
INCLUDES granulomatous enteritis
Use additional code to identify any associated fistulas, if applicable:
Use additional code to identify manifestations, such as:
anal fistula (K60.3-)
anorectal fistula (K60.5-)
pyoderma gangrenosum (L88)
rectal fistula (K60.4-)
EXCLUDES 1 ulcerative colitis (K51.-)
AHA: 2019,3Q,5; 2012,4Q,104

DEF: Chronic inflammation of the gastrointestinal tract characterized by chronic granulomatous disease, most commonly affecting the intestines and the terminal ileum.

✓5th K50.0 Crohn's disease of small intestine
Crohn's disease [regional enteritis] of duodenum
Crohn's disease [regional enteritis] of ileum
Crohn's disease [regional enteritis] of jejunum
Regional ileitis
Terminal ileitis
EXCLUDES 1 Crohn's disease of both small and large intestine (K50.8-)

K50.00 Crohn's disease of small intestine without complications

✓6th K50.01 Crohn's disease of small intestine with complications
K50.011 Crohn's disease of small intestine with rectal bleeding
K50.012 Crohn's disease of small intestine with intestinal obstruction
K50.013 Crohn's disease of small intestine with fistula
K50.014 Crohn's disease of small intestine with abscess
AHA: 2012,4Q,104
K50.018 Crohn's disease of small intestine with other complication
K50.019 Crohn's disease of small intestine with unspecified complications

✓5th K50.1 Crohn's disease of large intestine
Crohn's disease [regional enteritis] of colon
Crohn's disease [regional enteritis] of large bowel
Crohn's disease [regional enteritis] of rectum
Granulomatous colitis
Regional colitis
EXCLUDES 1 Crohn's disease of both small and large intestine (K50.8)

K50.10 Crohn's disease of large intestine without complications

✓6th K50.11 Crohn's disease of large intestine with complications
K50.111 Crohn's disease of large intestine with rectal bleeding

K50.112 Crohn's disease of large intestine with intestinal obstruction
K50.113 Crohn's disease of large intestine with fistula
K50.114 Crohn's disease of large intestine with abscess
K50.118 Crohn's disease of large intestine with other complication
K50.119 Crohn's disease of large intestine with unspecified complications

√5ᵗʰ **K50.8 Crohn's disease of both small and large intestine**
K50.80 Crohn's disease of both small and large intestine without complications
√6ᵗʰ K50.81 Crohn's disease of both small and large intestine with complications
K50.811 Crohn's disease of both small and large intestine with rectal bleeding
K50.812 Crohn's disease of both small and large intestine with intestinal obstruction
K50.813 Crohn's disease of both small and large intestine with fistula
K50.814 Crohn's disease of both small and large intestine with abscess
K50.818 Crohn's disease of both small and large intestine with other complication
K50.819 Crohn's disease of both small and large intestine with unspecified complications

√5ᵗʰ **K50.9 Crohn's disease, unspecified**
K50.90 Crohn's disease, unspecified, without complications
 Crohn's disease NOS
 Regional enteritis NOS
√6ᵗʰ K50.91 Crohn's disease, unspecified, with complications
K50.911 Crohn's disease, unspecified, with rectal bleeding
K50.912 Crohn's disease, unspecified, with intestinal obstruction
K50.913 Crohn's disease, unspecified, with fistula
K50.914 Crohn's disease, unspecified, with abscess
K50.918 Crohn's disease, unspecified, with other complication
K50.919 Crohn's disease, unspecified, with unspecified complications

√4ᵗʰ **K51 Ulcerative colitis**
Use additional code to identify any associated fistulas, if applicable:
Use additional code to identify manifestations, such as:
 anal fistula (K60.3-)
 anorectal fistula (K60.5-)
 pyoderma gangrenosum (L88)
 rectal fistula (K60.4-)
EXCLUDES 1 Crohn's disease [regional enteritis] (K50.-)

√5ᵗʰ **K51.0 Ulcerative (chronic) pancolitis**
 Backwash ileitis
K51.00 Ulcerative (chronic) pancolitis without complications
 Ulcerative (chronic) pancolitis NOS
√6ᵗʰ K51.01 Ulcerative (chronic) pancolitis with complications
K51.011 Ulcerative (chronic) pancolitis with rectal bleeding
K51.012 Ulcerative (chronic) pancolitis with intestinal obstruction
K51.013 Ulcerative (chronic) pancolitis with fistula
K51.014 Ulcerative (chronic) pancolitis with abscess
K51.018 Ulcerative (chronic) pancolitis with other complication
K51.019 Ulcerative (chronic) pancolitis with unspecified complications

√5ᵗʰ **K51.2 Ulcerative (chronic) proctitis**
K51.20 Ulcerative (chronic) proctitis without complications
 Ulcerative (chronic) proctitis NOS
√6ᵗʰ K51.21 Ulcerative (chronic) proctitis with complications
K51.211 Ulcerative (chronic) proctitis with rectal bleeding
K51.212 Ulcerative (chronic) proctitis with intestinal obstruction
K51.213 Ulcerative (chronic) proctitis with fistula
K51.214 Ulcerative (chronic) proctitis with abscess
K51.218 Ulcerative (chronic) proctitis with other complication
K51.219 Ulcerative (chronic) proctitis with unspecified complications

√5ᵗʰ **K51.3 Ulcerative (chronic) rectosigmoiditis**
K51.30 Ulcerative (chronic) rectosigmoiditis without complications
 Ulcerative (chronic) rectosigmoiditis NOS
√6ᵗʰ K51.31 Ulcerative (chronic) rectosigmoiditis with complications
K51.311 Ulcerative (chronic) rectosigmoiditis with rectal bleeding
K51.312 Ulcerative (chronic) rectosigmoiditis with intestinal obstruction
K51.313 Ulcerative (chronic) rectosigmoiditis with fistula
K51.314 Ulcerative (chronic) rectosigmoiditis with abscess
K51.318 Ulcerative (chronic) rectosigmoiditis with other complication
K51.319 Ulcerative (chronic) rectosigmoiditis with unspecified complications

√5ᵗʰ **K51.4 Inflammatory polyps of colon**
EXCLUDES 2 adenomatous polyp of colon (D12.6)
 polyposis of colon (D12.6)
 polyps of colon NOS (K63.5)
K51.40 Inflammatory polyps of colon without complications
 Inflammatory polyps of colon NOS
√6ᵗʰ K51.41 Inflammatory polyps of colon with complications
K51.411 Inflammatory polyps of colon with rectal bleeding
K51.412 Inflammatory polyps of colon with intestinal obstruction
K51.413 Inflammatory polyps of colon with fistula
K51.414 Inflammatory polyps of colon with abscess
K51.418 Inflammatory polyps of colon with other complication
K51.419 Inflammatory polyps of colon with unspecified complications

√5ᵗʰ **K51.5 Left sided colitis**
 Left hemicolitis
K51.50 Left sided colitis without complications
 Left sided colitis NOS
√6ᵗʰ K51.51 Left sided colitis with complications
K51.511 Left sided colitis with rectal bleeding
K51.512 Left sided colitis with intestinal obstruction
K51.513 Left sided colitis with fistula
K51.514 Left sided colitis with abscess
K51.518 Left sided colitis with other complication
K51.519 Left sided colitis with unspecified complications

K51.8 Other ulcerative colitis

- **K51.80** Other ulcerative colitis without complications [HCC Rx ESR COM]
- **K51.81** Other ulcerative colitis with complications
  - **K51.811** Other ulcerative colitis with rectal bleeding [HCC Rx ESR COM]
  - **K51.812** Other ulcerative colitis with intestinal obstruction [HCC Rx ESR COM]
  - **K51.813** Other ulcerative colitis with fistula [HCC Rx ESR COM]
  - **K51.814** Other ulcerative colitis with abscess [HCC Rx ESR COM]
  - **K51.818** Other ulcerative colitis with other complication [HCC Rx ESR COM]
  - **K51.819** Other ulcerative colitis with unspecified complications [HCC Rx ESR COM]

K51.9 Ulcerative colitis, unspecified

- **K51.90** Ulcerative colitis, unspecified, without complications [HCC Rx ESR COM]
- **K51.91** Ulcerative colitis, unspecified, with complications
  - **K51.911** Ulcerative colitis, unspecified with rectal bleeding [HCC Rx ESR COM]
  - **K51.912** Ulcerative colitis, unspecified with intestinal obstruction [HCC Rx ESR COM]
  - **K51.913** Ulcerative colitis, unspecified with fistula [HCC Rx ESR COM]
  - **K51.914** Ulcerative colitis, unspecified with abscess [HCC Rx ESR COM]
  - **K51.918** Ulcerative colitis, unspecified with other complication [HCC Rx ESR COM]
  - **K51.919** Ulcerative colitis, unspecified with unspecified complications [HCC Rx ESR COM]

K52 Other and unspecified noninfective gastroenteritis and colitis

AHA: 2016,4Q,30-31

- **K52.0** Gastroenteritis and colitis due to radiation
- **K52.1** Toxic gastroenteritis and colitis
  - Drug-induced gastroenteritis and colitis
  - Code first (T51-T65) to identify toxic agent
  - Use additional code for adverse effect, if applicable, to identify drug (T36-T50 with fifth or sixth character 5)
  - **AHA:** 2019,1Q,17
- **K52.2** Allergic and dietetic gastroenteritis and colitis
  - Food hypersensitivity gastroenteritis or colitis
  - Use additional code to identify type of food allergy (Z91.01-, Z91.02-)
  - EXCLUDES 2: allergic eosinophilic colitis (K52.82)
    - allergic eosinophilic esophagitis (K20.0)
    - allergic eosinophilic gastritis (K52.81)
    - allergic eosinophilic gastroenteritis (K52.81)
  - **DEF:** True immunoglobulin E (IgE)-mediated allergic reaction of the lining of the stomach, intestines, or colon to food proteins. It causes nausea, vomiting, diarrhea, and abdominal cramping.
  - **K52.21** Food protein-induced enterocolitis syndrome
    - FPIES
    - Use additional code for hypovolemic shock, if present (R57.1)
  - **K52.22** Food protein-induced enteropathy
  - **K52.29** Other allergic and dietetic gastroenteritis and colitis
    - Allergic proctocolitis
    - Food hypersensitivity gastroenteritis or colitis
    - Food protein-induced proctocolitis
    - Food-induced eosinophilic proctocolitis
    - Immediate gastrointestinal hypersensitivity
    - Milk protein-induced proctocolitis
- **K52.3** Indeterminate colitis
  - Colonic inflammatory bowel disease unclassified (IBDU)
  - EXCLUDES 1: unspecified colitis (K52.9)
- **K52.8** Other specified noninfective gastroenteritis and colitis
  - **K52.81** Eosinophilic gastritis or gastroenteritis
    - Eosinophilic enteritis
    - EXCLUDES 2: eosinophilic esophagitis (K20.0)
    - **DEF:** Disorder involving the accumulation of eosinophil in the lining of the stomach or multiple levels of the gastrointestinal tract, but without a known cause such as connective tissue disease, drug reaction, malignancy, or parasitic infection.
  - **K52.82** Eosinophilic colitis
    - EXCLUDES 2: allergic proctocolitis (K52.29)
      - food protein-induced enterocolitis syndrome (FPIES) (K52.21)
      - food protein-induced proctocolitis (K52.29)
      - food-induced eosinophilic proctocolitis (K52.29)
      - milk protein-induced proctocolitis (K52.29)
    - **DEF:** Disorder involving the accumulation of eosinophil in the tissues lining the colon, but without a known cause such as connective tissue disease, drug reaction, malignancy, or parasitic infection. The resultant inflammation may cause extreme abdominal pain, diarrhea, or bloody stool.
  - **K52.83** Microscopic colitis
    - **K52.831** Collagenous colitis [Rx]
    - **K52.832** Lymphocytic colitis [Rx]
    - **K52.838** Other microscopic colitis [Rx]
    - **K52.839** Microscopic colitis, unspecified [Rx]
  - **K52.89** Other specified noninfective gastroenteritis and colitis
    - **AHA:** 2019,1Q,20
- **K52.9** Noninfective gastroenteritis and colitis, unspecified
  - Colitis NOS
  - Enteritis NOS
  - Gastroenteritis NOS
  - Ileitis NOS
  - Jejunitis NOS
  - Sigmoiditis NOS
  - EXCLUDES 1: diarrhea NOS (R19.7)
    - functional diarrhea (K59.1)
    - infectious gastroenteritis and colitis NOS (A09)
    - neonatal diarrhea (noninfective) (P78.3)
    - psychogenic diarrhea (F45.8)
  - **AHA:** 2021,3Q,3

Other diseases of intestines (K55-K64)

K55 Vascular disorders of intestine

- EXCLUDES 1: necrotizing enterocolitis of newborn (P77.-)
- EXCLUDES 2: angioectasia (angiodysplasia) duodenum (K31.81-)
- **AHA:** 2016,4Q,32

- **K55.0** Acute vascular disorders of intestine
  - Infarction of appendices epiploicae
  - Mesenteric (artery) (vein) embolism
  - Mesenteric (artery) (vein) infarction
  - Mesenteric (artery) (vein) thrombosis
  - **AHA:** 2019,4Q,68
  - **K55.01** Acute (reversible) ischemia of small intestine
    - **K55.011** Focal (segmental) acute (reversible) ischemia of small intestine [ESR COM]
    - **K55.012** Diffuse acute (reversible) ischemia of small intestine [ESR COM]
    - **K55.019** Acute (reversible) ischemia of small intestine, extent unspecified [ESR COM]
  - **K55.02** Acute infarction of small intestine
    - Gangrene of small intestine
    - Necrosis of small intestine
    - **K55.021** Focal (segmental) acute infarction of small intestine [ESR COM]
    - **K55.022** Diffuse acute infarction of small intestine [ESR COM]
    - **K55.029** Acute infarction of small intestine, extent unspecified [ESR COM]
  - **K55.03** Acute (reversible) ischemia of large intestine
    - Acute fulminant ischemic colitis
    - Subacute ischemic colitis
    - **K55.031** Focal (segmental) acute (reversible) ischemia of large intestine [ESR COM]
    - **K55.032** Diffuse acute (reversible) ischemia of large intestine [ESR COM]
    - **K55.039** Acute (reversible) ischemia of large intestine, extent unspecified [ESR COM]
    - **AHA:** 2019,4Q,68
  - **K55.04** Acute infarction of large intestine
    - Gangrene of large intestine
    - Necrosis of large intestine
    - **K55.041** Focal (segmental) acute infarction of large intestine [ESR COM]

Chapter 11. Diseases of the Digestive System

K55.042 Diffuse acute infarction of large intestine
K55.049 Acute infarction of large intestine, extent unspecified

K55.05 Acute (reversible) ischemia of intestine, part unspecified
- **K55.051** Focal (segmental) acute (reversible) ischemia of intestine, part unspecified
- **K55.052** Diffuse acute (reversible) ischemia of intestine, part unspecified
- **K55.059** Acute (reversible) ischemia of intestine, part and extent unspecified

K55.06 Acute infarction of intestine, part unspecified
- Acute intestinal infarction
- Gangrene of intestine
- Necrosis of intestine
- **K55.061** Focal (segmental) acute infarction of intestine, part unspecified
- **K55.062** Diffuse acute infarction of intestine, part unspecified
- **K55.069** Acute infarction of intestine, part and extent unspecified

K55.1 Chronic vascular disorders of intestine
- Chronic ischemic colitis
- Chronic ischemic enteritis
- Chronic ischemic enterocolitis
- Ischemic stricture of intestine
- Mesenteric atherosclerosis
- Mesenteric vascular insufficiency

K55.2 Angiodysplasia of colon
  AHA: 2018,3Q,21
  TIP: Assign a code for "with hemorrhage" when angiodysplasia and GI bleeding are documented. The ICD-10-CM classification assumes the two are related without the provider linking the two conditions. Evidence of bleeding during a procedure is not required.
- **K55.20** Angiodysplasia of colon without hemorrhage
- **K55.21** Angiodysplasia of colon with hemorrhage
  DEF: Small vascular abnormalities due to fragile blood vessels in the colon, resulting in blood loss from the gastrointestinal (GI) tract.

K55.3 Necrotizing enterocolitis
  EXCLUDES 1: necrotizing enterocolitis of newborn (P77.-)
  EXCLUDES 2: necrotizing enterocolitis due to Clostridium difficile (A04.7-)
- **K55.30** Necrotizing enterocolitis, unspecified
  - Necrotizing enterocolitis, NOS
- **K55.31** Stage 1 necrotizing enterocolitis
  - Necrotizing enterocolitis without pneumatosis, without perforation
- **K55.32** Stage 2 necrotizing enterocolitis
  - Necrotizing enterocolitis with pneumatosis, without perforation
- **K55.33** Stage 3 necrotizing enterocolitis
  - Necrotizing enterocolitis with perforation
  - Necrotizing enterocolitis with pneumatosis and perforation

K55.8 Other vascular disorders of intestine

K55.9 Vascular disorder of intestine, unspecified
- Ischemic colitis
- Ischemic enteritis
- Ischemic enterocolitis

K56 Paralytic ileus and intestinal obstruction without hernia
  EXCLUDES 1:
  - congenital stricture or stenosis of intestine (Q41-Q42)
  - cystic fibrosis with meconium ileus (E84.11)
  - ischemic stricture of intestine (K55.1)
  - meconium ileus NOS (P76.0)
  - neonatal intestinal obstructions classifiable to P76.-
  - obstruction of duodenum (K31.5)
  - postprocedural intestinal obstruction (K91.3-)
  EXCLUDES 2: stenosis of anus or rectum (K62.4)

K56.0 Paralytic ileus
- Paralysis of bowel
- Paralysis of colon
- Paralysis of intestine
  EXCLUDES 1:
  - gallstone ileus (K56.3)
  - ileus NOS (K56.7)
  - obstructive ileus NOS (K56.69-)
  DEF: Intestinal obstruction due to paralysis of bowel motility or peristalsis.

K56.1 Intussusception
- Intussusception or invagination of bowel
- Intussusception or invagination of colon
- Intussusception or invagination of intestine
- Intussusception or invagination of rectum
  EXCLUDES 2: intussusception of appendix (K38.8)
  AHA: 2023,3Q,11
  DEF: Intestinal obstruction due to prolapse of a bowel section into an adjacent section. It occurs primarily in children and symptoms include acute abdominal pain, vomiting, and passage of blood and mucus from the rectum.

K56.2 Volvulus
- Strangulation of colon or intestine
- Torsion of colon or intestine
- Twist of colon or intestine
  EXCLUDES 2: volvulus of duodenum (K31.5)
  AHA: 2024,2Q,22
  DEF: Twisting, knotting, or entanglement of the bowel on itself that may quickly compromise oxygen supply to the intestinal tissues. A volvulus usually occurs at the sigmoid and ileocecal areas of the intestines.

Volvulus

Knotted intestine (volvulus)

K56.3 Gallstone ileus
- Obstruction of intestine by gallstone

K56.4 Other impaction of intestine
- **K56.41** Fecal impaction
  EXCLUDES 1: constipation (K59.0-)
  EXCLUDES 2: incomplete defecation (R15.0)
  AHA: 2024,2Q,6
- **K56.49** Other impaction of intestine

K56.5 Intestinal adhesions [bands] with obstruction (postinfection)
- Abdominal hernia due to adhesions with obstruction
- Peritoneal adhesions [bands] with intestinal obstruction (postinfection)
  AHA: 2017,4Q,16-17
- **K56.50** Intestinal adhesions [bands], unspecified as to partial versus complete obstruction
  - Intestinal adhesions with obstruction NOS
- **K56.51** Intestinal adhesions [bands], with partial obstruction
  - Intestinal adhesions with incomplete obstruction

	K56.52	Intestinal adhesions [bands] with complete obstruction [HCC][ESR][COM]
✓5th K56.6		Other and unspecified intestinal obstruction
		AHA: 2017,4Q,16-17; 2017,2Q,12
✓6th	K56.60	Unspecified intestinal obstruction
	K56.600	Partial intestinal obstruction, unspecified as to cause [HCC][ESR][COM]
		Incomplete intestinal obstruction, NOS
	K56.601	Complete intestinal obstruction, unspecified as to cause [HCC][ESR][COM]
	K56.609	Unspecified intestinal obstruction, unspecified as to partial versus complete obstruction [HCC][ESR][COM]
		Intestinal obstruction NOS
✓6th	K56.69	Other intestinal obstruction
		Enterostenosis NOS
		Obstructive ileus NOS
		Occlusion of colon or intestine NOS
		Stenosis of colon or intestine NOS
		Stricture of colon or intestine NOS
	K56.690	Other partial intestinal obstruction [HCC][ESR][COM]
		Other incomplete intestinal obstruction
	K56.691	Other complete intestinal obstruction [HCC][ESR][COM]
	K56.699	Other intestinal obstruction unspecified as to partial versus complete obstruction [HCC][ESR][COM]
		Other intestinal obstruction, NEC
		AHA: 2023,3Q,10
	K56.7	Ileus, unspecified [HCC][ESR][COM]
		EXCLUDES 1 obstructive ileus (K56.69-)
		EXCLUDES 2 intestinal obstruction with hernia (K40-K46)
		AHA: 2017,1Q,40

✓4th **K57 Diverticular disease of intestine**
Code also if applicable peritonitis K65.-
EXCLUDES 1 congenital diverticulum of intestine (Q43.8)
Meckel's diverticulum (Q43.0)
EXCLUDES 2 diverticulum of appendix (K38.2)
AHA: 2022,1Q,26-27; 2021,1Q,9,11; 2018,3Q,21
TIP: Assign a code for "with bleeding" when diverticular disease of the intestine and GI bleeding are documented. The ICD-10-CM classification assumes the two are related without the provider linking the two conditions. Evidence of bleeding during a procedure is not required.

✓5th K57.0		Diverticulitis of small intestine with perforation and abscess
	EXCLUDES 1	diverticulitis of both small and large intestine with perforation and abscess (K57.4-)
	K57.00	Diverticulitis of small intestine with perforation and abscess without bleeding
	K57.01	Diverticulitis of small intestine with perforation and abscess with bleeding
✓5th K57.1		Diverticular disease of small intestine without perforation or abscess
	EXCLUDES 1	diverticular disease of both small and large intestine without perforation or abscess (K57.5-)
	K57.10	Diverticulosis of small intestine without perforation or abscess without bleeding
		Diverticular disease of small intestine NOS
	K57.11	Diverticulosis of small intestine without perforation or abscess with bleeding
	K57.12	Diverticulitis of small intestine without perforation or abscess without bleeding
	K57.13	Diverticulitis of small intestine without perforation or abscess with bleeding
✓5th K57.2		Diverticulitis of large intestine with perforation and abscess
	EXCLUDES 1	diverticulitis of both small and large intestine with perforation and abscess (K57.4-)
	K57.20	Diverticulitis of large intestine with perforation and abscess without bleeding
		AHA: 2025,2Q,6
	K57.21	Diverticulitis of large intestine with perforation and abscess with bleeding

✓5th K57.3		Diverticular disease of large intestine without perforation or abscess
	EXCLUDES 1	diverticular disease of both small and large intestine without perforation or abscess (K57.5-)
	K57.30	Diverticulosis of large intestine without perforation or abscess without bleeding
		Diverticular disease of colon NOS
	K57.31	Diverticulosis of large intestine without perforation or abscess with bleeding
	K57.32	Diverticulitis of large intestine without perforation or abscess without bleeding
	K57.33	Diverticulitis of large intestine without perforation or abscess with bleeding
✓5th K57.4		Diverticulitis of both small and large intestine with perforation and abscess
	K57.40	Diverticulitis of both small and large intestine with perforation and abscess without bleeding
	K57.41	Diverticulitis of both small and large intestine with perforation and abscess with bleeding
✓5th K57.5		Diverticular disease of both small and large intestine without perforation or abscess
	K57.50	Diverticulosis of both small and large intestine without perforation or abscess without bleeding
		Diverticular disease of both small and large intestine NOS
	K57.51	Diverticulosis of both small and large intestine without perforation or abscess with bleeding
	K57.52	Diverticulitis of both small and large intestine without perforation or abscess without bleeding
	K57.53	Diverticulitis of both small and large intestine without perforation or abscess with bleeding
✓5th K57.8		Diverticulitis of intestine, part unspecified, with perforation and abscess
	K57.80	Diverticulitis of intestine, part unspecified, with perforation and abscess without bleeding
	K57.81	Diverticulitis of intestine, part unspecified, with perforation and abscess with bleeding
✓5th K57.9		Diverticular disease of intestine, part unspecified, without perforation or abscess
	K57.90	Diverticulosis of intestine, part unspecified, without perforation or abscess without bleeding
		Diverticular disease of intestine NOS
	K57.91	Diverticulosis of intestine, part unspecified, without perforation or abscess with bleeding
	K57.92	Diverticulitis of intestine, part unspecified, without perforation or abscess without bleeding
	K57.93	Diverticulitis of intestine, part unspecified, without perforation or abscess with bleeding

✓4th **K58 Irritable bowel syndrome**
INCLUDES irritable colon
spastic colon
AHA: 2016,4Q,32-33

	K58.0	Irritable bowel syndrome with diarrhea
	K58.1	Irritable bowel syndrome with constipation
	K58.2	Mixed irritable bowel syndrome
	K58.8	Other irritable bowel syndrome
	K58.9	Irritable bowel syndrome, unspecified
		Irritable bowel syndrome NOS

✓4th **K59 Other functional intestinal disorders**
EXCLUDES 1 change in bowel habit NOS (R19.4)
intestinal malabsorption (K90.-)
psychogenic intestinal disorders (F45.8)
EXCLUDES 2 functional disorders of stomach (K31.-)

✓5th K59.0		Constipation
	EXCLUDES 1	fecal impaction (K56.41)
	EXCLUDES 2	incomplete defecation (R15.0)
	AHA: 2024,2Q,6; 2016,4Q,33	
	K59.00	Constipation, unspecified
	K59.01	Slow transit constipation
		DEF: Delay in the transit of fecal material through the colon secondary to smooth muscle dysfunction or decreased peristaltic contractions along the colon.
	K59.02	Outlet dysfunction constipation
		AHA: 2023,1Q,24
		TIP: Report this code for documented pelvic floor dyssynergia, outlet type constipation, or anismus.

K59.03 **Drug induced** constipation
Use additional code for adverse effect, if applicable, to identify drug (T36-T50 with fifth or sixth character 5)

K59.04 **Chronic idiopathic** constipation
Functional constipation

K59.09 **Other** constipation
Chronic constipation

K59.1 **Functional diarrhea**
EXCLUDES 1: diarrhea NOS (R19.7)
irritable bowel syndrome with diarrhea (K58.0)

K59.2 **Neurogenic bowel, not elsewhere classified**
DEF: Disorder of bowel due to a spinal cord lesion because of injury or as a complication of conditions such as multiple sclerosis (MS) or spina bifida. Loss of bowel control is the primary symptom, manifested as constipation or bowel incontinence.

✓5th **K59.3** **Megacolon, not elsewhere classified**
Dilatation of colon
Code first, if applicable (T51-T65) to identify toxic agent
EXCLUDES 1: congenital megacolon (aganglionic) (Q43.1)
megacolon (due to) (in) Chagas' disease (B57.32)
megacolon (due to) (in) Clostridium difficile (A04.7-)
megacolon (due to) (in) Hirschsprung's disease (Q43.1)
AHA: 2016,4Q,33-34

  K59.31 **Toxic megacolon** HCC ESR COM
  K59.39 **Other megacolon**
  Megacolon NOS

K59.4 **Anal spasm**
Proctalgia fugax

✓5th **K59.8** **Other specified functional intestinal disorders**
AHA: 2020,4Q,29-30

  K59.81 **Ogilvie syndrome**
  Acute colonic pseudo-obstruction (ACPO)
  K59.89 **Other specified functional intestinal disorders**
  Atony of colon
  Pseudo-obstruction (acute) (chronic) of intestine

K59.9 **Functional intestinal disorder, unspecified**

✓4th **K60** **Fissure and fistula of anal and rectal regions**
EXCLUDES 1: fissure and fistula of anal and rectal regions with abscess or cellulitis (K61.-)
EXCLUDES 2: abscess or cellulitis of anal and rectal regions (K61.-)
anal sphincter tear (healed) (nontraumatic) (old) (K62.81)
AHA: 2024,4Q,21

K60.0 **Acute** anal fissure
K60.1 **Chronic** anal fissure
K60.2 Anal fissure, unspecified

✓5th **K60.3** Anal fistula
Code first, if applicable:
Crohn's disease (K50.-)
ulcerative colitis (K51.-)
EXCLUDES 1: congenital fistula (Q43.6)

  K60.30 **Anal fistula, unspecified**
  Anal fistula NOS

  ✓6th **K60.31** **Anal fistula, simple**
  Low intersphincteric anal fistula
  Superficial anal fistula
    K60.311 **Anal fistula, simple, initial**
    Anal fistula, simple, new
    K60.312 **Anal fistula, simple, persistent**
    Anal fistula, simple, chronic
    K60.313 **Anal fistula, simple, recurrent**
    Anal fistula simple, occurring following complete healing
    K60.319 **Anal fistula, simple, unspecified**

  ✓6th **K60.32** **Anal fistula, complex**
  Extrasphincteric anal fistula
  High intersphincteric anal fistula
  Suprasphincteric anal fistula
  Transsphincteric anal fistula
  Code also, if applicable:
  perianal abscess (K61.0)
  rectovaginal fistula (N82.3)
  stenosis of anus and rectum (K62.4)
    K60.321 **Anal fistula, complex, initial**
    Anal fistula, complex, new
    K60.322 **Anal fistula, complex, persistent**
    Anal fistula, complex, chronic
    K60.323 **Anal fistula, complex, recurrent**
    Anal fistula complex, occurring following complete healing
    K60.329 **Anal fistula, complex, unspecified**

✓5th **K60.4** **Rectal fistula**
Fistula of rectum to skin
Code first, if applicable:
Crohn's disease (K50.-)
ulcerative colitis (K51.-)
EXCLUDES 1: congenital fistula (Q43.6)
rectovaginal fistula (N82.3)
vesicorectal fistual (N32.1)

  K60.40 **Rectal fistula, unspecified**
  Rectal fistula NOS

  ✓6th **K60.41** **Rectal fistula, simple**
  Low intersphincteric rectal fistula
  Superficial rectal fistula
    K60.411 **Rectal fistula, simple, initial**
    Rectal, fistula, simple, new
    K60.412 **Rectal fistula, simple, persistent**
    Rectal fistula, simple, chronic
    K60.413 **Rectal fistula, simple, recurrent**
    Rectal fistula simple, occurring following complete healing
    K60.419 **Rectal fistula, simple, unspecified**

  ✓6th **K60.42** **Rectal fistula, complex**
  Extrasphincteric rectal fistula
  High intersphincteric rectal fistula
  Suprasphincteric rectal fistula
  Transsphincteric rectal fistula
  Code also, if applicable:
  perianal abscess (K61.0)
  rectovaginal fistula (N82.3)
  stenosis of anus and rectum (K62.4)
    K60.421 **Rectal fistula, complex, initial**
    Rectal fistula, complex, new
    K60.422 **Rectal fistula, complex, persistent**
    Rectal fistula, complex, chronic
    K60.423 **Rectal fistula, complex, recurrent**
    Rectal fistula complex occurring following complete healing
    K60.429 **Rectal fistula, complex, unspecified**

✓5th **K60.5** **Anorectal fistula**
Code first, if applicable:
Crohn's disease (K50.-)
ulcerative colitis (K51.-)
EXCLUDES 1: congenital fistula (Q43.6)

  K60.50 **Anorectal fistula, unspecified**
  Anorectal fistula NOS

  ✓6th **K60.51** **Anorectal fistula, simple**
  Low intersphincteric anorectal fistula
  Superficial anorectal fistula
    K60.511 **Anorectal fistula, simple, initial**
    Anorectal fistula, simple, new
    K60.512 **Anorectal fistula, simple, persistent**
    Anorectal fistula, simple, chronic
    K60.513 **Anorectal fistula, simple, recurrent**
    Anorectal fistula simple, occurring following complete healing
    K60.519 **Anorectal fistula, simple, unspecified**

  ✓6th **K60.52** **Anorectal fistula, complex**
  Extrasphincteric anorectal fistula
  High intersphincteric anorectal fistula
  Suprasphincteric anorectal fistula
  Transsphincteric anorectal fistula
  Code also, if applicable:
  perianal abscess (K61.0)
  rectovaginal fistula (N82.3)
  stenosis of anus and rectum (K62.4)
    K60.521 **Anorectal fistula, complex, initial**
    Anorectal fistula, complex, new
    K60.522 **Anorectal fistula, complex, persistent**
    Anorectal fistula, complex, chronic
    K60.523 **Anorectal fistula, complex, recurrent**
    Anorectal fistula complex, occurring following complete healing
    K60.529 **Anorectal fistula, complex, unspecified**

K61 Abscess of anal and rectal regions
INCLUDES: abscess of anal and rectal regions
cellulitis of anal and rectal regions

K61.0 Anal abscess
Perianal abscess
EXCLUDES 2: intrasphincteric abscess (K61.4)

K61.1 Rectal abscess
Perirectal abscess
EXCLUDES 1: ischiorectal abscess (K61.39)
AHA: 2012,4Q,104

K61.2 Anorectal abscess

K61.3 Ischiorectal abscess
AHA: 2018,4Q,19

K61.31 Horseshoe abscess
K61.39 Other ischiorectal abscess
Abscess of ischiorectal fossa
Ischiorectal abscess, NOS

K61.4 Intrasphincteric abscess
Intersphincteric abscess

K61.5 Supralevator abscess
AHA: 2018,4Q,19

K62 Other diseases of anus and rectum
INCLUDES: anal canal
EXCLUDES 2: colostomy and enterostomy malfunction (K94.0-, K94.1-)
fecal incontinence (R15.-)
hemorrhoids (K64.-)

K62.0 Anal polyp
K62.1 Rectal polyp
EXCLUDES 1: adenomatous polyp (D12.8)
AHA: 2018,1Q,6

K62.2 Anal prolapse
Prolapse of anal canal

K62.3 Rectal prolapse
Prolapse of rectal mucosa

K62.4 Stenosis of anus and rectum
Stricture of anus (sphincter)
AHA: 2019,2Q,13

K62.5 Hemorrhage of anus and rectum
EXCLUDES 1: gastrointestinal bleeding NOS (K92.2)
melena (K92.1)
neonatal rectal hemorrhage (P54.2)
AHA: 2019,1Q,21

K62.6 Ulcer of anus and rectum
Solitary ulcer of anus and rectum
Stercoral ulcer of anus and rectum
EXCLUDES 1: fissure and fistula of anus and rectum (K60.-)
ulcerative colitis (K51.-)

K62.7 Radiation proctitis
Use additional code to identify the type of radiation (W88.-) or radiation therapy (Y84.2)
AHA: 2019,1Q,21

K62.8 Other specified diseases of anus and rectum
EXCLUDES 2: ulcerative proctitis (K51.2)

K62.81 Anal sphincter tear (healed) (nontraumatic) (old)
Tear of anus, nontraumatic
Use additional code for any associated fecal incontinence (R15.-)
EXCLUDES 2: anal fissure (K60.-)
anal sphincter tear (healed) (old) complicating delivery (O34.7-)
traumatic tear of anal sphincter (S31.831)

K62.82 Dysplasia of anus
Anal intraepithelial neoplasia I and II (AIN I and II) (histologically confirmed)
Dysplasia of anus NOS
Mild and moderate dysplasia of anus (histologically confirmed)
EXCLUDES 1: abnormal results from anal cytologic examination without histologic confirmation (R85.61-)
anal intraepithelial neoplasia III (D01.3)
carcinoma in situ of anus (D01.3)
HGSIL of anus (R85.613)
severe dysplasia of anus (D01.3)

K62.89 Other specified diseases of anus and rectum
Proctitis NOS
Use additional code for any associated fecal incontinence (R15.-)

K62.9 Disease of anus and rectum, unspecified

K63 Other diseases of intestine

K63.0 Abscess of intestine
EXCLUDES 1: abscess of intestine with Crohn's disease (K50.014, K50.114, K50.814, K50.914)
abscess of intestine with diverticular disease (K57.0, K57.2, K57.4, K57.8)
abscess of intestine with ulcerative colitis (K51.014, K51.214, K51.314, K51.414, K51.514, K51.814, K51.914)
EXCLUDES 2: abscess of anal and rectal regions (K61.-)
abscess of appendix (K35.3-)

K63.1 Perforation of intestine (nontraumatic)
Perforation (nontraumatic) of rectum
EXCLUDES 1: perforation (nontraumatic) of duodenum (K26.-)
perforation (nontraumatic) of intestine with diverticular disease (K57.0, K57.2, K57.4, K57.8)
EXCLUDES 2: perforation (nontraumatic) of appendix (K35.2-, K35.3-)
AHA: 2025,2Q,8; 2020,2Q,22

K63.2 Fistula of intestine
Code also, if applicable, disruption of internal operation (surgical) wound (T81.32-)
EXCLUDES 1: fistula of duodenum (K31.6)
fistula of intestine with Crohn's disease (K50.013, K50.113, K50.813, K50.913)
fistula of intestine with ulcerative colitis (K51.013, K51.213, K51.313, K51.413, K51.513, K51.813, K51.913)
EXCLUDES 2: fistula of anal and rectal regions (K60.-)
fistula of appendix (K38.3)
intestinal-genital fistula, female (N82.2-N82.4)
vesicointestinal fistula (N32.1)
AHA: 2017,3Q,4

K63.3 Ulcer of intestine
Primary ulcer of small intestine
EXCLUDES 1: duodenal ulcer (K26.-)
gastrointestinal ulcer (K28.-)
gastrojejunal ulcer (K28.-)
jejunal ulcer (K28.-)
peptic ulcer, site unspecified (K27.-)
ulcer of anus or rectum (K62.6)
ulcer of intestine with perforation (K63.1)
ulcerative colitis (K51.-)

K63.4 Enteroptosis
K63.5 Polyp of colon
EXCLUDES 2: adenomatous polyp of colon (D12.-)
inflammatory polyp of colon (K51.4-)
polyposis of colon (D12.6)
AHA: 2019,1Q,33; 2018,2Q,14; 2017,1Q,15; 2015,2Q,14
TIP: Assign this code when documentation states hyperplastic colon polyp regardless of the site in the colon. Slow-growing, hyperplastic polyps are not precancerous and are classified differently from benign or adenomatous polyps.

K63.8 Other specified diseases of intestine

K63.81 Dieulafoy lesion of intestine
EXCLUDES 1: Dieulafoy lesion of stomach and duodenum (K31.82)
DEF: Abnormally large submucosal artery protruding through a defect in the stomach mucosa or intestines that can cause massive and life-threatening hemorrhaging.

K63.82 Intestinal microbial overgrowth
AHA: 2023,4Q,29-30

K63.821 Small intestinal bacterial overgrowth
K63.8211 Small intestinal bacterial overgrowth, hydrogen-subtype
K63.8212 Small intestinal bacterial overgrowth, hydrogen sulfide-subtype
K63.8219 Small intestinal bacterial overgrowth, unspecified

K63.822 Small intestinal fungal overgrowth
K63.829 Intestinal methanogen overgrowth, unspecified

K63.89 Other specified diseases of intestine
AHA: 2013,2Q,31

K63.9 Disease of intestine, unspecified

K64 Hemorrhoids and perianal venous thrombosis
INCLUDES piles
EXCLUDES 1 hemorrhoids complicating childbirth and the puerperium (O87.2)
hemorrhoids complicating pregnancy (O22.4)

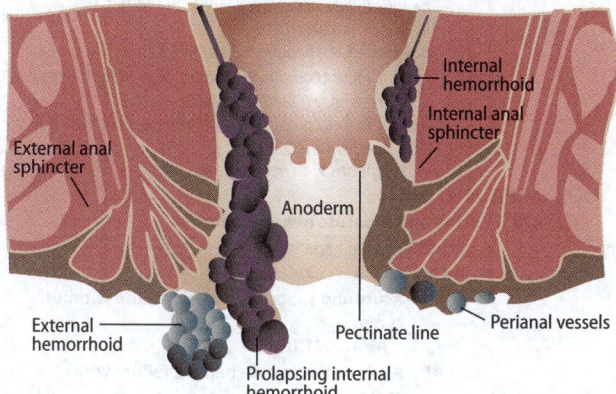
Hemorrhoids

K64.0 First degree hemorrhoids
Grade/stage I hemorrhoids
Hemorrhoids (bleeding) without prolapse outside of anal canal

K64.1 Second degree hemorrhoids
Grade/stage II hemorrhoids
Hemorrhoids (bleeding) that prolapse with straining, but retract spontaneously

K64.2 Third degree hemorrhoids
Grade/stage III hemorrhoids
Hemorrhoids (bleeding) that prolapse with straining and require manual replacement back inside anal canal

K64.3 Fourth degree hemorrhoids
Grade/stage IV hemorrhoids
Hemorrhoids (bleeding) with prolapsed tissue that cannot be manually replaced

K64.4 Residual hemorrhoidal skin tags
External hemorrhoids, NOS
Skin tags of anus

K64.5 Perianal venous thrombosis
External hemorrhoids with thrombosis
Perianal hematoma
Thrombosed hemorrhoids NOS

K64.8 Other hemorrhoids
Internal hemorrhoids, without mention of degree
Prolapsed hemorrhoids, degree not specified

K64.9 Unspecified hemorrhoids
Hemorrhoids (bleeding) NOS
Hemorrhoids (bleeding) without mention of degree

Diseases of peritoneum and retroperitoneum (K65-K68)

K65 Peritonitis
Code also if applicable diverticular disease of intestine (K57.-)
Use additional code (B95-B97), to identify infectious agent, if known
EXCLUDES 1 acute appendicitis with generalized peritonitis (K35.2-)
aseptic peritonitis (T81.6)
benign paroxysmal peritonitis (E85.0)
chemical peritonitis (T81.6)
gonococcal peritonitis (A54.85)
neonatal peritonitis (P78.0-P78.1)
pelvic peritonitis, female (N73.3-N73.5)
periodic familial peritonitis (E85.0)
peritonitis due to talc or other foreign substance (T81.6)
peritonitis in chlamydia (A74.81)
peritonitis in diphtheria (A36.89)
peritonitis in syphilis (late) (A52.74)
peritonitis in tuberculosis (A18.31)
peritonitis with or following abortion or ectopic or molar pregnancy (O00-O07, O08.0)
peritonitis with or following appendicitis (K35.-)
puerperal peritonitis (O85)
retroperitoneal infections (K68.-)

K65.0 Generalized (acute) peritonitis
Pelvic peritonitis (acute), male
Subphrenic peritonitis (acute)
Suppurative peritonitis (acute)

K65.1 Peritoneal abscess
Abdominopelvic abscess
Abscess (of) omentum
Abscess (of) peritoneum
Mesenteric abscess
Retrocecal abscess
Subdiaphragmatic abscess
Subhepatic abscess
Subphrenic abscess
AHA: 2024,1Q,20; 2022,1Q,26; 2019,1Q,15

K65.2 Spontaneous bacterial peritonitis
EXCLUDES 1 bacterial peritonitis NOS (K65.9)

K65.3 Choleperitonitis
Peritonitis due to bile
DEF: Inflammation of the peritoneum due to leakage of bile into the peritoneal cavity resulting from rupture of the bile passages or gallbladder.

K65.4 Sclerosing mesenteritis
(Idiopathic) sclerosing mesenteric fibrosis
Fat necrosis of peritoneum
Mesenteric lipodystrophy
Mesenteric panniculitis
Retractile mesenteritis

K65.8 Other peritonitis
Chronic proliferative peritonitis
Peritonitis due to urine

K65.9 Peritonitis, unspecified
Bacterial peritonitis NOS
AHA: 2022,1Q,27; 2013,2Q,31

K66 Other disorders of peritoneum
EXCLUDES 2 ascites (R18.-)
peritoneal effusion (chronic) (R18.8)

K66.0 Peritoneal adhesions (postprocedural) (postinfection)
Adhesions (of) abdominal (wall)
Adhesions (of) diaphragm
Adhesions (of) intestine
Adhesions (of) male pelvis
Adhesions (of) omentum
Adhesions (of) stomach
Adhesive bands
Mesenteric adhesions
EXCLUDES 1 peritoneal adhesions with intestinal obstruction (K56.5-)
EXCLUDES 2 female pelvic adhesions [bands] (N73.6)
female pelvic postprocedural adhesions (N99.4)

K66.1 Hemoperitoneum
Peritoneal hematoma
Peritoneal hemorrhage
EXCLUDES 1 traumatic hemoperitoneum (S36.8-)
EXCLUDES 2 retroperitoneal hematoma (K68.3)
retroperitoneal hemorrhage (K68.3)
AHA: 2022,1Q,22-23

K66.8 Other specified disorders of peritoneum
K66.9 Disorder of peritoneum, unspecified

K67 Disorders of peritoneum in infectious diseases classified elsewhere
Code first underlying disease, such as:
congenital syphilis (A50.0)
helminthiasis (B65.0-B83.9)
EXCLUDES 1 peritonitis in chlamydia (A74.81)
peritonitis in diphtheria (A36.89)
peritonitis in gonococcal (A54.85)
peritonitis in syphilis (late) (A52.74)
peritonitis in tuberculosis (A18.31)

K68 Disorders of retroperitoneum

K68.1 Retroperitoneal abscess
K68.11 Postprocedural retroperitoneal abscess
EXCLUDES 2 infection following procedure (T81.4-)
K68.12 Psoas muscle abscess
K68.19 Other retroperitoneal abscess
AHA: 2025,2Q,6; 2023,2Q,27; 2019,1Q,15
TIP: This code should be used for a diagnosis of internal presacral abscess. If an intra-abdominal abscess is also present, code K65.1 can also be assigned; sequencing depends on the circumstances of admission.

K68.2 Retroperitoneal fibrosis
Code also, if applicable, associated obstruction of ureter (N13.5)
AHA: 2023,4Q,30-31

K68.3 Retroperitoneal hematoma
Retroperitoneal hemorrhage
AHA: 2023,4Q,30-31

K68.9 Other disorders of retroperitoneum

Diseases of liver (K70-K77)

EXCLUDES 1: jaundice NOS (R17)
EXCLUDES 2: hemochromatosis (E83.11-)
Reye's syndrome (G93.7)
viral hepatitis (B15-B19)
Wilson's disease (E83.01)

✓4th K70 Alcoholic liver disease
Use additional code to identify:
alcohol abuse and dependence (F10.-)

K70.0 Alcoholic fatty liver [A]

✓5th K70.1 Alcoholic hepatitis
- **K70.10** Alcoholic hepatitis without ascites [HCC] [COM] [A]
- **K70.11** Alcoholic hepatitis with ascites [HCC] [COM] [A]

K70.2 Alcoholic fibrosis and sclerosis of liver [A]

✓5th K70.3 Alcoholic cirrhosis of liver
Alcoholic cirrhosis NOS
- **K70.30** Alcoholic cirrhosis of liver without ascites [HCC] [ESR] [COM] [A]
- **K70.31** Alcoholic cirrhosis of liver with ascites [HCC] [ESR] [COM] [A]
AHA: 2018,1Q,4

✓5th K70.4 Alcoholic hepatic failure
Acute alcoholic hepatic failure
Alcoholic hepatic failure NOS
Chronic alcoholic hepatic failure
Subacute alcoholic hepatic failure
- **K70.40** Alcoholic hepatic failure without coma [HCC] [ESR] [COM] [A]
- **K70.41** Alcoholic hepatic failure with coma [HCC] [ESR] [COM] [A]

K70.9 Alcoholic liver disease, unspecified [ESR] [A]

✓4th K71 Toxic liver disease
INCLUDES: drug-induced idiosyncratic (unpredictable) liver disease
drug-induced toxic (predictable) liver disease
Code first poisoning due to drug or toxin, if applicable (T36-T65 with fifth or sixth character 1-4)
Use additional code for adverse effect, if applicable, to identify drug (T36-T50 with fifth or sixth character 5)
EXCLUDES 2: alcoholic liver disease (K70.-)
Budd-Chiari syndrome (I82.0)

K71.0 Toxic liver disease with cholestasis
"Pure" cholestasis
Cholestasis with hepatocyte injury

✓5th K71.1 Toxic liver disease with hepatic necrosis
Hepatic failure (acute) (chronic) due to drugs
- **K71.10** Toxic liver disease with hepatic necrosis, without coma [COM]
- **K71.11** Toxic liver disease with hepatic necrosis, with coma [ESR] [COM]

K71.2 Toxic liver disease with acute hepatitis

K71.3 Toxic liver disease with chronic persistent hepatitis [HCC] [COM]

K71.4 Toxic liver disease with chronic lobular hepatitis [HCC] [COM]

✓5th K71.5 Toxic liver disease with chronic active hepatitis
Toxic liver disease with lupoid hepatitis
- **K71.50** Toxic liver disease with chronic active hepatitis without ascites [HCC] [COM]
- **K71.51** Toxic liver disease with chronic active hepatitis with ascites [HCC] [COM]
AHA: 2018,1Q,4

K71.6 Toxic liver disease with hepatitis, not elsewhere classified

K71.7 Toxic liver disease with fibrosis and cirrhosis of liver [HCC] [COM]

K71.8 Toxic liver disease with other disorders of liver
Toxic liver disease with focal nodular hyperplasia
Toxic liver disease with hepatic granulomas
Toxic liver disease with peliosis hepatis
Toxic liver disease with veno-occlusive disease of liver
AHA: 2024,1Q,25; 2015,2Q,17

K71.9 Toxic liver disease, unspecified

✓4th K72 Hepatic failure, not elsewhere classified
INCLUDES: fulminant hepatitis NEC, with hepatic failure
liver (cell) necrosis with hepatic failure
malignant hepatitis NEC, with hepatic failure
yellow liver atrophy or dystrophy
► Use additional code, if applicable, for ascites (R18.8) ◄
EXCLUDES 1: alcoholic hepatic failure (K70.4)
hepatic failure with toxic liver disease (K71.1-)
icterus of newborn (P55-P59)
postprocedural hepatic failure (K91.82)
EXCLUDES 2: hepatic failure complicating abortion or ectopic or molar pregnancy (O00-O07, O08.8)
hepatic failure complicating pregnancy, childbirth and the puerperium (O26.6-)
viral hepatitis with hepatic coma (B15-B19)
AHA: 2017,1Q,41

✓5th K72.0 Acute and subacute hepatic failure
Acute non-viral hepatitis NOS
AHA: 2015,2Q,17; 2014,2Q,13
- **K72.00** Acute and subacute hepatic failure without coma [COM]
AHA: 2021,1Q,13
- **K72.01** Acute and subacute hepatic failure with coma [ESR] [COM]

✓5th K72.1 Chronic hepatic failure
End stage liver disease
- **K72.10** Chronic hepatic failure without coma [HCC] [ESR] [COM]
AHA: 2021,1Q,13
- **K72.11** Chronic hepatic failure with coma [HCC] [ESR] [COM]

✓5th K72.9 Hepatic failure, unspecified
- **K72.90** Hepatic failure, unspecified without coma [HCC] [ESR] [COM]
AHA: 2022,1Q,52; 2018,4Q,20; 2016,2Q,35
- **K72.91** Hepatic failure, unspecified with coma [HCC] [ESR] [COM]
Hepatic coma NOS

✓4th K73 Chronic hepatitis, not elsewhere classified
► Use additional code, if applicable, for ascites (R18.8) ◄
EXCLUDES 1: alcoholic hepatitis (chronic) (K70.1-)
drug-induced hepatitis (chronic) (K71.-)
granulomatous hepatitis (chronic) NEC (K75.3)
reactive, nonspecific hepatitis (chronic) (K75.2)
viral hepatitis (chronic) (B15-B19)

K73.0 Chronic persistent hepatitis, not elsewhere classified [HCC] [ESR] [COM]

K73.1 Chronic lobular hepatitis, not elsewhere classified [HCC] [ESR] [COM]

K73.2 Chronic active hepatitis, not elsewhere classified [HCC] [ESR] [COM]

K73.8 Other chronic hepatitis, not elsewhere classified [HCC] [ESR] [COM]

K73.9 Chronic hepatitis, unspecified [HCC] [ESR] [COM]

✓4th K74 Fibrosis and cirrhosis of liver
Code also, if applicable, viral hepatitis (acute) (chronic) (B15-B19)
EXCLUDES 1: alcoholic cirrhosis (of liver) (K70.3)
alcoholic fibrosis of liver (K70.2)
cardiac sclerosis of liver (K76.1)
cirrhosis (of liver) with toxic liver disease (K71.7)
congenital cirrhosis (of liver) (P78.81)
pigmentary cirrhosis (of liver) (E83.110)

✓5th K74.0 Hepatic fibrosis
Code first underlying liver disease, such as:
nonalcoholic steatohepatitis (NASH) (K75.81)
AHA: 2020,4Q,30-31
- **K74.00** Hepatic fibrosis, unspecified
- **K74.01** Hepatic fibrosis, early fibrosis
Hepatic fibrosis, stage F1 or stage F2
- **K74.02** Hepatic fibrosis, advanced fibrosis
Hepatic fibrosis, stage F3
EXCLUDES 1: cirrhosis of liver (K74.6-)
hepatic fibrosis, stage F4 (K74.6-)

K74.1 Hepatic sclerosis

K74.2 Hepatic fibrosis with hepatic sclerosis

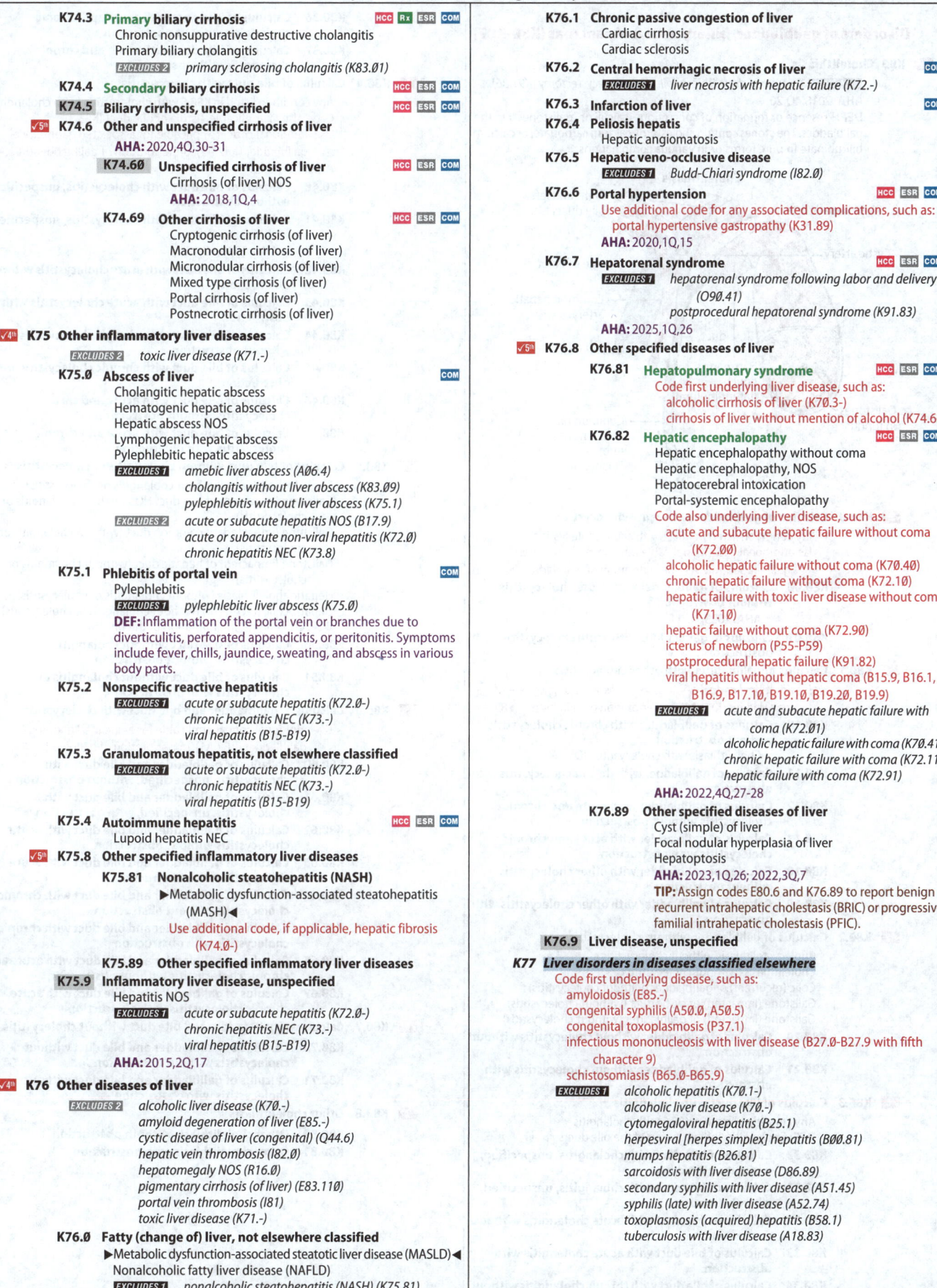

Disorders of gallbladder, biliary tract and pancreas (K80-K87)

√4th K80 Cholelithiasis
EXCLUDES 1 *retained cholelithiasis following cholecystectomy (K91.86)*
AHA: 2018,4Q,20
DEF: Presence or formation of concretions (calculi or "gallstones") in the gallbladder. The stones contain cholesterol, calcium carbonate, or calcium bilirubinate in pure forms or in various combinations.

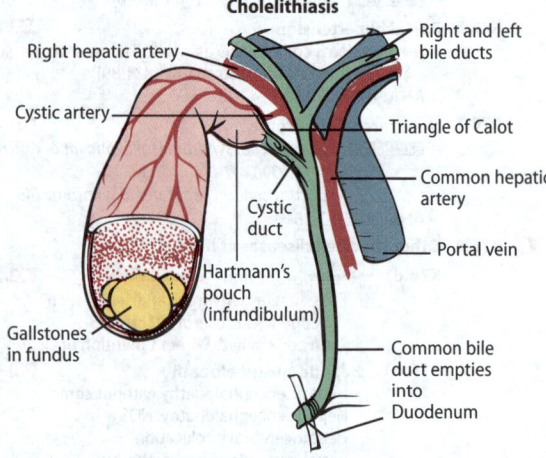

Cholelithiasis

√5th K80.0 Calculus of gallbladder with acute cholecystitis
Any condition listed in K80.2 with acute cholecystitis
Use additional code if applicable for associated gangrene of gallbladder (K82.A1), or perforation of gallbladder (K82.A2)

K80.00 Calculus of gallbladder with acute cholecystitis without obstruction
AHA: 2023,2Q,11

K80.01 Calculus of gallbladder with acute cholecystitis with obstruction

√5th K80.1 Calculus of gallbladder with other cholecystitis
Use additional code if applicable for associated gangrene of gallbladder (K82.A1), or perforation of gallbladder (K82.A2)

K80.10 Calculus of gallbladder with chronic cholecystitis without obstruction
Cholelithiasis with cholecystitis NOS

K80.11 Calculus of gallbladder with chronic cholecystitis with obstruction

K80.12 Calculus of gallbladder with acute and chronic cholecystitis without obstruction

K80.13 Calculus of gallbladder with acute and chronic cholecystitis with obstruction

K80.18 Calculus of gallbladder with other cholecystitis without obstruction

K80.19 Calculus of gallbladder with other cholecystitis with obstruction

√5th K80.2 Calculus of gallbladder without cholecystitis
Cholecystolithiasis without cholecystitis
Cholelithiasis (without cholecystitis)
Colic (recurrent) of gallbladder (without cholecystitis)
Gallstone (impacted) of cystic duct (without cholecystitis)
Gallstone (impacted) of gallbladder (without cholecystitis)

K80.20 Calculus of gallbladder without cholecystitis without obstruction

K80.21 Calculus of gallbladder without cholecystitis with obstruction

√5th K80.3 Calculus of bile duct with cholangitis
Any condition listed in K80.5 with cholangitis
DEF: Cholangitis: Inflammation of the bile ducts.

K80.30 Calculus of bile duct with cholangitis, unspecified, without obstruction

K80.31 Calculus of bile duct with cholangitis, unspecified, with obstruction

K80.32 Calculus of bile duct with acute cholangitis without obstruction

K80.33 Calculus of bile duct with acute cholangitis with obstruction

K80.34 Calculus of bile duct with chronic cholangitis without obstruction

K80.35 Calculus of bile duct with chronic cholangitis with obstruction

K80.36 Calculus of bile duct with acute and chronic cholangitis without obstruction

K80.37 Calculus of bile duct with acute and chronic cholangitis with obstruction

√5th K80.4 Calculus of bile duct with cholecystitis
Any condition listed in K80.5 with cholecystitis (with cholangitis)
Code also, if applicable, fistula of bile duct (K83.3)
Use additional code if applicable for associated gangrene of gallbladder (K82.A1), or perforation of gallbladder (K82.A2)
AHA: 2019,1Q,17

K80.40 Calculus of bile duct with cholecystitis, unspecified, without obstruction

K80.41 Calculus of bile duct with cholecystitis, unspecified, with obstruction
AHA: 2019,1Q,17

K80.42 Calculus of bile duct with acute cholecystitis without obstruction

K80.43 Calculus of bile duct with acute cholecystitis with obstruction

K80.44 Calculus of bile duct with chronic cholecystitis without obstruction

K80.45 Calculus of bile duct with chronic cholecystitis with obstruction

K80.46 Calculus of bile duct with acute and chronic cholecystitis without obstruction

K80.47 Calculus of bile duct with acute and chronic cholecystitis with obstruction

√5th K80.5 Calculus of bile duct without cholangitis or cholecystitis
Choledocholithiasis (without cholangitis or cholecystitis)
Gallstone (impacted) of bile duct NOS (without cholangitis or cholecystitis)
Gallstone (impacted) of common duct (without cholangitis or cholecystitis)
Gallstone (impacted) of hepatic duct (without cholangitis or cholecystitis)
Hepatic cholelithiasis (without cholangitis or cholecystitis)
Hepatic colic (recurrent) (without cholangitis or cholecystitis)
DEF: Cholangitis: Inflammation of the bile ducts.

K80.50 Calculus of bile duct without cholangitis or cholecystitis without obstruction

K80.51 Calculus of bile duct without cholangitis or cholecystitis with obstruction

√5th K80.6 Calculus of gallbladder and bile duct with cholecystitis
Use additional code if applicable for associated gangrene of gallbladder (K82.A1), or perforation of gallbladder (K82.A2)

K80.60 Calculus of gallbladder and bile duct with cholecystitis, unspecified, without obstruction

K80.61 Calculus of gallbladder and bile duct with cholecystitis, unspecified, with obstruction

K80.62 Calculus of gallbladder and bile duct with acute cholecystitis without obstruction

K80.63 Calculus of gallbladder and bile duct with acute cholecystitis with obstruction

K80.64 Calculus of gallbladder and bile duct with chronic cholecystitis without obstruction

K80.65 Calculus of gallbladder and bile duct with chronic cholecystitis with obstruction

K80.66 Calculus of gallbladder and bile duct with acute and chronic cholecystitis without obstruction

K80.67 Calculus of gallbladder and bile duct with acute and chronic cholecystitis with obstruction

√5th K80.7 Calculus of gallbladder and bile duct without cholecystitis

K80.70 Calculus of gallbladder and bile duct without cholecystitis without obstruction

K80.71 Calculus of gallbladder and bile duct without cholecystitis with obstruction

√5th K80.8 Other cholelithiasis

K80.80 Other cholelithiasis without obstruction

K80.81 Other cholelithiasis with obstruction

Chapter 11. Diseases of the Digestive System

✓4th K81 Cholecystitis
Use additional code if applicable for associated gangrene of gallbladder (K82.A1), or perforation of gallbladder (K82.A2)
EXCLUDES 1 cholecystitis with cholelithiasis (K80.-)
AHA: 2018,4Q,20

- **K81.0 Acute cholecystitis**
  - Abscess of gallbladder
  - Angiocholecystitis
  - Emphysematous (acute) cholecystitis
  - Empyema of gallbladder
  - Gangrene of gallbladder
  - Gangrenous cholecystitis
  - Suppurative cholecystitis
- **K81.1 Chronic cholecystitis**
- **K81.2 Acute cholecystitis with chronic cholecystitis**
- **K81.9 Cholecystitis, unspecified**

✓4th K82 Other diseases of gallbladder
EXCLUDES 1 nonvisualization of gallbladder (R93.2)
postcholecystectomy syndrome (K91.5)

- **K82.0 Obstruction of gallbladder**
  - Occlusion of cystic duct or gallbladder without cholelithiasis
  - Stenosis of cystic duct or gallbladder without cholelithiasis
  - Stricture of cystic duct or gallbladder without cholelithiasis
  - EXCLUDES 1 obstruction of gallbladder with cholelithiasis (K80.-)
- **K82.1 Hydrops of gallbladder**
  - Mucocele of gallbladder
- **K82.2 Perforation of gallbladder**
  - Rupture of cystic duct or gallbladder
  - EXCLUDES 1 perforation of gallbladder in cholecystitis (K82.A2)
- **K82.3 Fistula of gallbladder**
  - Cholecystocolic fistula
  - Cholecystoduodenal fistula
  - Code also, if applicable, disruption of internal operation (surgical) wound (T81.32-)
- **K82.4 Cholesterolosis of gallbladder**
  - Strawberry gallbladder
  - EXCLUDES 1 cholesterolosis of gallbladder with cholecystitis (K81.-)
    cholesterolosis of gallbladder with cholelithiasis (K80.-)
- **K82.8 Other specified diseases of gallbladder**
  - Adhesions of cystic duct or gallbladder
  - Atrophy of cystic duct or gallbladder
  - Cyst of cystic duct or gallbladder
  - Dyskinesia of cystic duct or gallbladder
  - Hypertrophy of cystic duct or gallbladder
  - Nonfunctioning of cystic duct or gallbladder
  - Ulcer of cystic duct or gallbladder
- **K82.9 Disease of gallbladder, unspecified**
- **✓5th K82.A Disorders of gallbladder in diseases classified elsewhere**
  - Code first the type of cholecystitis (K81.-), or cholelithiasis with cholecystitis (K80.00-K80.19, K80.40-K80.47, K80.60-K80.67)
  - AHA: 2018,4Q,19-20
  - **K82.A1 Gangrene of gallbladder in cholecystitis**
  - **K82.A2 Perforation of gallbladder in cholecystitis**

✓4th K83 Other diseases of biliary tract
EXCLUDES 1 postcholecystectomy syndrome (K91.5)
EXCLUDES 2 conditions involving the cystic duct (K81-K82)
conditions involving the gallbladder (K81-K82)

- **✓5th K83.0 Cholangitis**
  - EXCLUDES 1 cholangitic liver abscess (K75.0)
    cholangitis with choledocholithiasis (K80.3-, K80.4-)
  - EXCLUDES 2 chronic nonsuppurative destructive cholangitis (K74.3)
    primary biliary cholangitis (K74.3)
    primary biliary cirrhosis (K74.3)
  - AHA: 2018,4Q,20
  - **K83.01 Primary sclerosing cholangitis** HCC
  - **K83.09 Other cholangitis** HCC
    - Ascending cholangitis
    - Cholangitis NOS
    - Primary cholangitis
    - Recurrent cholangitis
    - Sclerosing cholangitis
    - Secondary cholangitis
    - Stenosing cholangitis
    - Suppurative cholangitis
- **K83.1 Obstruction of bile duct** HCC
  - Occlusion of bile duct without cholelithiasis
  - Stenosis of bile duct without cholelithiasis
  - Stricture of bile duct without cholelithiasis
  - EXCLUDES 1 congenital obstruction of bile duct (Q44.3)
    obstruction of bile duct with cholelithiasis (K80.-)
  - AHA: 2023,1Q,26; 2016,1Q,18
- **K83.2 Perforation of bile duct**
  - Rupture of bile duct
- **K83.3 Fistula of bile duct**
  - Choledochoduodenal fistula
  - AHA: 2019,1Q,17
- **K83.4 Spasm of sphincter of Oddi**
- **K83.5 Biliary cyst**
- **K83.8 Other specified diseases of biliary tract**
  - Adhesions of biliary tract
  - Atrophy of biliary tract
  - Hypertrophy of biliary tract
  - Ulcer of biliary tract
- **K83.9 Disease of biliary tract, unspecified**

✓4th K85 Acute pancreatitis
INCLUDES acute (recurrent) pancreatitis
subacute pancreatitis
AHA: 2016,4Q,34

- **✓5th K85.0 Idiopathic acute pancreatitis**
  - **K85.00 Idiopathic acute pancreatitis without necrosis or infection** COM
  - **K85.01 Idiopathic acute pancreatitis with uninfected necrosis** COM
  - **K85.02 Idiopathic acute pancreatitis with infected necrosis** COM
- **✓5th K85.1 Biliary acute pancreatitis**
  - Gallstone pancreatitis
  - AHA: 2023,2Q,11
  - **K85.10 Biliary acute pancreatitis without necrosis or infection** COM
  - **K85.11 Biliary acute pancreatitis with uninfected necrosis** COM
  - **K85.12 Biliary acute pancreatitis with infected necrosis** COM
- **✓5th K85.2 Alcohol induced acute pancreatitis**
  - EXCLUDES 2 alcohol induced chronic pancreatitis (K86.0)
  - **K85.20 Alcohol induced acute pancreatitis without necrosis or infection** COM
    - AHA: 2020,1Q,9
  - **K85.21 Alcohol induced acute pancreatitis with uninfected necrosis** COM
  - **K85.22 Alcohol induced acute pancreatitis with infected necrosis** COM
- **✓5th K85.3 Drug induced acute pancreatitis**
  - Use additional code for adverse effect, if applicable, to identify drug (T36-T50 with fifth or sixth character 5)
  - Use additional code to identify drug abuse and dependence (F11.-F17.-)
  - **K85.30 Drug induced acute pancreatitis without necrosis or infection** COM
  - **K85.31 Drug induced acute pancreatitis with uninfected necrosis** COM
  - **K85.32 Drug induced acute pancreatitis with infected necrosis** COM
- **✓5th K85.8 Other acute pancreatitis**
  - **K85.80 Other acute pancreatitis without necrosis or infection** COM
  - **K85.81 Other acute pancreatitis with uninfected necrosis** COM
  - **K85.82 Other acute pancreatitis with infected necrosis** COM
- **✓5th K85.9 Acute pancreatitis, unspecified**
  - Pancreatitis NOS
  - **K85.90 Acute pancreatitis without necrosis or infection, unspecified** COM
  - **K85.91 Acute pancreatitis with uninfected necrosis, unspecified** COM
  - **K85.92 Acute pancreatitis with infected necrosis, unspecified** COM

Chapter 11. Diseases of the Digestive System

K86 Other diseases of pancreas
EXCLUDES 2: fibrocystic disease of pancreas (E84.-)
islet cell tumor (of pancreas) (D13.7)
pancreatic steatorrhea (K90.3)

- **K86.0 Alcohol-induced chronic pancreatitis** `HCC` `Rx` `ESR` `COM`
  Code also exocrine pancreatic insufficiency (K86.81)
  Use additional code to identify:
  alcohol abuse and dependence (F10.-)
  EXCLUDES 2: alcohol induced acute pancreatitis (K85.2-)

- **K86.1 Other chronic pancreatitis** `HCC` `Rx` `ESR` `COM`
  Chronic pancreatitis NOS
  Infectious chronic pancreatitis
  Recurrent chronic pancreatitis
  Relapsing chronic pancreatitis
  Code also exocrine pancreatic insufficiency (K86.81)

- **K86.2 Cyst of pancreas** `Rx`
- **K86.3 Pseudocyst of pancreas** `Rx`
- **K86.8 Other specified diseases of pancreas**
  AHA: 2016,4Q,34-35
  - **K86.81 Exocrine pancreatic insufficiency** `Rx`
  - **K86.89 Other specified diseases of pancreas** `Rx`
    Aseptic pancreatic necrosis, unrelated to acute pancreatitis
    Atrophy of pancreas
    Calculus of pancreas
    Cirrhosis of pancreas
    Fibrosis of pancreas
    Pancreatic fat necrosis, unrelated to acute pancreatitis
    Pancreatic infantilism
    Pancreatic necrosis NOS, unrelated to acute pancreatitis
    AHA: 2024,3Q,4
- **K86.9 Disease of pancreas, unspecified** `Rx`

K87 Disorders of gallbladder, biliary tract and pancreas in diseases classified elsewhere `Rx`
Code first underlying disease
EXCLUDES 1: cytomegaloviral pancreatitis (B25.2)
mumps pancreatitis (B26.3)
syphilitic gallbladder (A52.74)
syphilitic pancreas (A52.74)
tuberculosis of gallbladder (A18.83)
tuberculosis of pancreas (A18.83)

Other diseases of the digestive system (K90-K95)

K90 Intestinal malabsorption
EXCLUDES 1: intestinal malabsorption following gastrointestinal surgery (K91.2)
AHA: 2017,4Q,108

- **K90.0 Celiac disease** `Rx`
  Celiac disease with steatorrhea
  Celiac gluten-sensitive enteropathy
  Nontropical sprue
  Code also exocrine pancreatic insufficiency (K86.81)
  Use additional code for associated disorders including:
  dermatitis herpetiformis (L13.0)
  gluten ataxia (G32.81)
  DEF: Malabsorption syndrome due to gluten consumption. Symptoms include fetid, bulky, frothy, oily stools; a distended abdomen; gas; asthenia; electrolyte depletion; and vitamin B, D, and K deficiency.

- **K90.1 Tropical sprue** `Rx`
  Sprue NOS
  Tropical steatorrhea

- **K90.2 Blind loop syndrome, not elsewhere classified** `Rx`
  Blind loop syndrome NOS
  EXCLUDES 1: congenital blind loop syndrome (Q43.8)
  postsurgical blind loop syndrome (K91.2)

- **K90.3 Pancreatic steatorrhea** `Rx`

- **K90.4 Other malabsorption due to intolerance**
  EXCLUDES 2: celiac gluten-sensitive enteropathy (K90.0)
  lactose intolerance (E73.-)
  AHA: 2016,4Q,35-36
  - **K90.41 Non-celiac gluten sensitivity**
    Gluten sensitivity NOS
    Non-celiac gluten sensitive enteropathy

  - **K90.49 Malabsorption due to intolerance, not elsewhere classified** `Rx`
    Malabsorption due to intolerance to carbohydrate
    Malabsorption due to intolerance to fat
    Malabsorption due to intolerance to protein
    Malabsorption due to intolerance to starch

- **K90.8 Other intestinal malabsorption**
  AHA: 2023,4Q,31-33
  - **K90.81 Whipple's disease** `Rx`
  - **K90.82 Short bowel syndrome**
    Short gut syndrome
    EXCLUDES 1: ▶postsurgical malabsorption, not elsewhere classified (K91.2)◀
    - **K90.821 Short bowel syndrome with colon in continuity** `Rx`
      Short bowel syndrome with colonic continuity
    - **K90.822 Short bowel syndrome without colon in continuity** `Rx`
      Short bowel syndrome without colonic continuity
      ▶Use additional code, if applicable, for colostomy status (Z93.3)◀
    - **K90.829 Short bowel syndrome, unspecified** `Rx`
  - **K90.83 Intestinal failure** `Rx`
  - **K90.89 Other intestinal malabsorption** `Rx`
- **K90.9 Intestinal malabsorption, unspecified** `Rx`

K91 Intraoperative and postprocedural complications and disorders of digestive system, not elsewhere classified
EXCLUDES 2: complications of artificial opening of digestive system (K94.-)
complications of bariatric procedures (K95.-)
gastrojejunal ulcer (K28.-)
postprocedural (radiation) retroperitoneal abscess (K68.11)
radiation colitis (K52.0)
radiation gastroenteritis (K52.0)
radiation proctitis (K62.7)
AHA: 2016,4Q,9-10

- **K91.0 Vomiting following gastrointestinal surgery**
- **K91.1 Postgastric surgery syndromes**
  Dumping syndrome
  Postgastrectomy syndrome
  Postvagotomy syndrome
- **K91.2 Postsurgical malabsorption, not elsewhere classified** `Rx`
  Postsurgical blind loop syndrome
  EXCLUDES 1: malabsorption osteomalacia in adults (M83.2)
  malabsorption osteoporosis, postsurgical (M80.8-, M81.8)
- **K91.3 Postprocedural intestinal obstruction**
  AHA: 2017,4Q,16-17; 2017,1Q,40
  - **K91.30 Postprocedural intestinal obstruction, unspecified as to partial versus complete**
    Postprocedural intestinal obstruction NOS
  - **K91.31 Postprocedural partial intestinal obstruction**
    Postprocedural incomplete intestinal obstruction
  - **K91.32 Postprocedural complete intestinal obstruction**
- **K91.5 Postcholecystectomy syndrome**
- **K91.6 Intraoperative hemorrhage and hematoma of a digestive system organ or structure complicating a procedure**
  EXCLUDES 1: intraoperative hemorrhage and hematoma of a digestive system organ or structure due to accidental puncture and laceration during a procedure (K91.7-)
  - **K91.61 Intraoperative hemorrhage and hematoma of a digestive system organ or structure complicating a digestive system procedure**
    AHA: 2020,1Q,19
  - **K91.62 Intraoperative hemorrhage and hematoma of a digestive system organ or structure complicating other procedure**
- **K91.7 Accidental puncture and laceration of a digestive system organ or structure during a procedure**
  AHA: 2022,1Q,51
  - **K91.71 Accidental puncture and laceration of a digestive system organ or structure during a digestive system procedure**
    AHA: 2021,2Q,11

K91.72 Accidental puncture and laceration of a digestive system organ or structure during other procedure
AHA: 2019,2Q,23

✓5th K91.8 Other intraoperative and postprocedural complications and disorders of digestive system

K91.81 Other intraoperative complications of digestive system

K91.82 Postprocedural hepatic failure

K91.83 Postprocedural hepatorenal syndrome

✓6th K91.84 Postprocedural hemorrhage of a digestive system organ or structure following a procedure

K91.840 Postprocedural hemorrhage of a digestive system organ or structure following a digestive system procedure
AHA: 2016,1Q,15

K91.841 Postprocedural hemorrhage of a digestive system organ or structure following other procedure

✓6th K91.85 Complications of intestinal pouch

K91.850 Pouchitis HCC ESR COM
Inflammation of internal ileoanal pouch
DEF: Inflammatory complication of an existing surgically created ileoanal pouch, resulting in multiple GI complaints, including diarrhea, abdominal pain, rectal bleeding, fecal urgency, or incontinence.

K91.858 Other complications of intestinal pouch HCC ESR COM
AHA: 2019,2Q,13

K91.86 Retained cholelithiasis following cholecystectomy

✓6th K91.87 Postprocedural hematoma and seroma of a digestive system organ or structure following a procedure

K91.870 Postprocedural hematoma of a digestive system organ or structure following a digestive system procedure
AHA: 2022,1Q,24

K91.871 Postprocedural hematoma of a digestive system organ or structure following other procedure

K91.872 Postprocedural seroma of a digestive system organ or structure following a digestive system procedure

K91.873 Postprocedural seroma of a digestive system organ or structure following other procedure

K91.89 Other postprocedural complications and disorders of digestive system
Use additional code, if applicable, to further specify disorder
EXCLUDES 2 postprocedural retroperitoneal abscess (K68.11)
AHA: 2020,2Q,22; 2017,1Q,40

✓4th K92 Other diseases of digestive system
EXCLUDES 1 neonatal gastrointestinal hemorrhage (P54.0-P54.3)

K92.0 Hematemesis

K92.1 Melena
EXCLUDES 1 occult blood in feces (R19.5)

K92.2 Gastrointestinal hemorrhage, unspecified
Gastric hemorrhage NOS
Intestinal hemorrhage NOS
EXCLUDES 1 acute hemorrhagic gastritis (K29.01)
angiodysplasia of stomach with hemorrhage (K31.811)
diverticular disease with hemorrhage (K57.-)
gastritis and duodenitis with hemorrhage (K29.-)
hemorrhage of anus and rectum (K62.5)
peptic ulcer with hemorrhage (K25-K28)
AHA: 2021,1Q,11

✓5th K92.8 Other specified diseases of the digestive system

K92.81 Gastrointestinal mucositis (ulcerative)
Code also type of associated therapy, such as:
antineoplastic and immunosuppressive drugs (T45.1X-)
radiological procedure and radiotherapy (Y84.2)
EXCLUDES 2 mucositis (ulcerative) of vagina and vulva (N76.81)
nasal mucositis (ulcerative) (J34.81)
oral mucositis (ulcerative) (K12.3-)

K92.89 Other specified diseases of the digestive system

K92.9 Disease of digestive system, unspecified

✓4th K94 Complications of artificial openings of the digestive system

✓5th K94.0 Colostomy complications

K94.00 Colostomy complication, unspecified HCC ESR COM

K94.01 Colostomy hemorrhage HCC ESR COM

K94.02 Colostomy infection HCC ESR COM
Use additional code to specify type of infection, such as:
cellulitis of abdominal wall (L03.311)
sepsis (A40.-, A41.-)

K94.03 Colostomy malfunction HCC ESR COM
Mechanical complication of colostomy

K94.09 Other complications of colostomy HCC ESR COM

✓5th K94.1 Enterostomy complications

K94.10 Enterostomy complication, unspecified HCC ESR COM

K94.11 Enterostomy hemorrhage HCC ESR COM

K94.12 Enterostomy infection HCC ESR COM
Use additional code to specify type of infection, such as:
cellulitis of abdominal wall (L03.311)
sepsis (A40.-, A41.-)

K94.13 Enterostomy malfunction HCC ESR COM
Mechanical complication of enterostomy

K94.19 Other complications of enterostomy HCC ESR COM

✓5th K94.2 Gastrostomy complications

K94.20 Gastrostomy complication, unspecified HCC ESR COM

K94.21 Gastrostomy hemorrhage HCC ESR COM

K94.22 Gastrostomy infection HCC ESR COM
Use additional code to specify type of infection, such as:
cellulitis of abdominal wall (L03.311)
sepsis (A40.-, A41.-)

K94.23 Gastrostomy malfunction HCC ESR COM
Mechanical complication of gastrostomy
AHA: 2019,1Q,26

K94.29 Other complications of gastrostomy HCC ESR COM

✓5th K94.3 Esophagostomy complications

K94.30 Esophagostomy complications, unspecified HCC ESR COM

K94.31 Esophagostomy hemorrhage HCC ESR COM

K94.32 Esophagostomy infection HCC ESR COM
Use additional code to identify the infection

K94.33 Esophagostomy malfunction HCC ESR COM
Mechanical complication of esophagostomy

K94.39 Other complications of esophagostomy HCC ESR COM

✓4th K95 Complications of bariatric procedures

✓5th K95.0 Complications of gastric band procedure

K95.01 Infection due to gastric band procedure
Use additional code to specify type of infection or organism, such as:
bacterial and viral infectious agents (B95.-, B96.-)
cellulitis of abdominal wall (L03.311)
sepsis (A40.-, A41.-)

K95.09 Other complications of gastric band procedure
Use additional code, if applicable, to further specify complication

✓5th K95.8 Complications of other bariatric procedure
EXCLUDES 1 complications of gastric band surgery (K95.0-)

K95.81 Infection due to other bariatric procedure
Use additional code to specify type of infection or organism, such as:
bacterial and viral infectious agents (B95.-, B96.-)
cellulitis of abdominal wall (L03.311)
sepsis (A40.-, A41.-)

K95.89 Other complications of other bariatric procedure
Use additional code, if applicable, to further specify complication

Chapter 12. Diseases of the Skin and Subcutaneous Tissue (L00–L99)

Chapter-specific Guidelines with Coding Examples

The chapter-specific guidelines from the ICD-10-CM Official Guidelines for Coding and Reporting have been provided below. Along with these guidelines are coding examples, contained in the shaded boxes, that have been developed to help illustrate the coding and/or sequencing guidance found in these guidelines.

a. Pressure ulcer stage codes

1) Pressure ulcer stages

Codes in category L89, Pressure ulcer, identify the site and stage of the pressure ulcer.

The ICD-10-CM classifies pressure ulcer stages based on severity, which is designated by stages 1-4, deep tissue pressure injury, unspecified stage, and unstageable.

Assign as many codes from category L89 as needed to identify all the pressure ulcers the patient has, if applicable.

See Section I.B.14. for pressure ulcer stage documentation by clinicians other than patient's provider.

> Stage 3 pressure ulcer left ankle, 6 x 7 cm that invades the fascia; stage 2 pressure ulcer of left hip
>
> **L89.523** Pressure ulcer of left ankle, stage 3
>
> **L89.222** Pressure ulcer of left hip, stage 2
>
> *Explanation:* Patient has a left ankle pressure ulcer documented as stage 3 and a left hip pressure ulcer documented as stage 2. Combination codes from category L89 Pressure ulcer, identify the site of the pressure ulcer as well as the stage. Assign as many codes from category L89 as needed to identify all the pressure ulcers the patient has.

2) Unstageable pressure ulcers

Assignment of the code for unstageable pressure ulcer (L89.--0) should be based on the clinical documentation. These codes are used for pressure ulcers whose stage cannot be clinically determined (e.g., the ulcer is covered by eschar or has been treated with a skin or muscle graft). This code should not be confused with the codes for unspecified stage (L89.--9). When there is no documentation regarding the stage of the pressure ulcer, assign the appropriate code for unspecified stage (L89.--9).

> Pressure ulcer of the right lower back documented as unstageable due to the presence of thick eschar covering the ulcer
>
> **L89.130** Pressure ulcer of right lower back, unstageable
>
> *Explanation:* Codes for unstageable pressure ulcers are assigned when the stage cannot be clinically determined (e.g., the ulcer is covered by eschar or has been treated with a skin or muscle graft).

If during an encounter, the stage of an unstageable pressure ulcer is revealed after debridement, assign only the code for the stage revealed following debridement.

3) Documented pressure ulcer stage

Assignment of the pressure ulcer stage code should be guided by clinical documentation of the stage or documentation of the terms found in the Alphabetic Index. For clinical terms describing the stage that are not found in the Alphabetic Index, and there is no documentation of the stage, the provider should be queried.

> Left heel pressure ulcer with partial thickness skin loss involving the dermis
>
> **L89.622** Pressure ulcer of left heel, stage 2
>
> *Explanation:* Code assignment for the pressure ulcer stage should be guided by either the clinical documentation of the stage or the documentation of terms found in the Alphabetic Index. The clinical documentation describing the left heel pressure ulcer "partial thickness skin loss involving the dermis" matches the ICD-10-CM index parenthetical description for stage 2 "(abrasion, blister, partial thickness skin loss involving epidermis and/or dermis)."

4) Patients admitted with pressure ulcers documented as healed

No code is assigned if the documentation states that the pressure ulcer is completely healed at the time of admission.

> Patient receiving follow-up examination of a completely healed pressure ulcer of the foot
>
> **Z09** Encounter for follow-up examination after completed treatment for conditions other than malignant neoplasm
>
> **Z87.2** Personal history of diseases of the skin and subcutaneous tissue
>
> *Explanation:* Assign only codes for the reason for the encounter and the personal history of the pressure ulcer. Personal history code Z87.2 includes conditions classifiable to L00–L99 such as pressure ulcer. No code is assigned for a pressure ulcer documented as completely healed.

5) Pressure ulcers documented as healing

Pressure ulcers described as healing should be assigned the appropriate pressure ulcer stage code based on the documentation in the medical record. If the documentation does not provide information about the stage of the healing pressure ulcer, assign the appropriate code for unspecified stage.

If the documentation is unclear as to whether the patient has a current (new) pressure ulcer or if the patient is being treated for a healing pressure ulcer, query the provider.

For ulcers that were present on admission but healed at the time of discharge, assign the code for the site and stage of the pressure ulcer at the time of admission.

6) Patient admitted with pressure ulcer evolving into another stage during the admission

If a patient is admitted to an inpatient hospital with a pressure ulcer at one stage and it progresses to a higher stage, two separate codes should be assigned: one code for the site and stage of the ulcer on admission and a second code for the same ulcer site and the highest stage reported during the stay.

7) Pressure-induced deep tissue damage

For pressure-induced deep tissue damage or deep tissue pressure injury, assign only the appropriate code for pressure-induced deep tissue damage (L89.--6).

b. Non-pressure chronic ulcers

1) Patients admitted with non-pressure ulcers documented as healed

No code is assigned if the documentation states that the non-pressure ulcer is completely healed at the time of admission.

2) Non-pressure ulcers documented as healing

Non-pressure ulcers described as healing should be assigned the appropriate non-pressure ulcer code based on the documentation in the medical record. If the documentation does not provide information about the severity of the healing non-pressure ulcer, assign the appropriate code for unspecified severity.

If the documentation is unclear as to whether the patient has a current (new) non-pressure ulcer or if the patient is being treated for a healing non-pressure ulcer, query the provider.

For ulcers that were present on admission but healed at the time of discharge, assign the code for the site and severity of the non-pressure ulcer at the time of admission.

3) Patient admitted with non-pressure ulcer that progresses to another severity level during the admission

If a patient is admitted to an inpatient hospital with a non-pressure ulcer at one severity level and it progresses to a higher severity level, two separate codes should be assigned: one code for the site and severity level of the ulcer on admission and a second code for the same ulcer site and the highest severity level reported during the stay.

See Section I.B.14. for pressure ulcer stage documentation by clinicians other than patient's provider.

Chapter 12. Diseases of the Skin and Subcutaneous Tissue (L00-L99)

EXCLUDES 2   certain conditions originating in the perinatal period (P04-P96)
certain infectious and parasitic diseases (A00-B99)
complications of pregnancy, childbirth and the puerperium (O00-O9A)
congenital malformations, deformations, and chromosomal abnormalities (Q00-Q99)
endocrine, nutritional and metabolic diseases (E00-E88)
lipomelanotic reticulosis (I89.8)
neoplasms (C00-D49)
symptoms, signs and abnormal clinical and laboratory findings, not elsewhere classified (R00-R94)
systemic connective tissue disorders (M30-M36)
viral warts (B07.-)

AHA: 2022,2Q,7

This chapter contains the following blocks:

L00-L08	Infections of the skin and subcutaneous tissue
L10-L14	Bullous disorders
L20-L30	Dermatitis and eczema
L40-L45	Papulosquamous disorders
L49-L54	Urticaria and erythema
L55-L59	Radiation-related disorders of the skin and subcutaneous tissue
L60-L75	Disorders of skin appendages
L76	Intraoperative and postprocedural complications of skin and subcutaneous tissue
L80-L99	Other disorders of the skin and subcutaneous tissue

Infections of the skin and subcutaneous tissue (L00-L08)

Use additional code (B95-B97) to identify infectious agent

EXCLUDES 2   hordeolum (H00.0)
infective dermatitis (L30.3)
local infections of skin classified in Chapter 1
lupus panniculitis (L93.2)
panniculitis NOS (M79.3)
panniculitis of neck and back (M54.0-)
perlèche NOS (K13.0)
perlèche due to candidiasis (B37.0)
perlèche due to riboflavin deficiency (E53.0)
pyogenic granuloma (L98.0)
relapsing panniculitis [Weber-Christian] (M35.6)
viral warts (B07.-)
zoster (B02.-)

L00   **Staphylococcal scalded skin syndrome**   COM
Ritter's disease
Use additional code to identify percentage of skin exfoliation (L49.-)
EXCLUDES 1   bullous impetigo (L01.03)
pemphigus neonatorum (L01.03)
toxic epidermal necrolysis [Lyell] (L51.2)
DEF: Infectious skin disease of children younger than 5 years marked by eruptions ranging from a few localized blisters to widespread, easily ruptured, fine vesicles and bullae affecting almost the entire body. It results in exfoliation of large planes of skin and leaves raw areas.

✓4ᵗʰ **L01**   **Impetigo**
EXCLUDES 1   impetigo herpetiformis (L40.1)
DEF: Acute, superficial, highly contagious skin infection commonly occurring in children. Skin lesions usually appear on the face and consist of vesicles and bullae that burst and form yellow crusts.

✓5ᵗʰ **L01.0**   **Impetigo**
Impetigo contagiosa
Impetigo vulgaris
L01.00   **Impetigo, unspecified**
Impetigo NOS
L01.01   **Non-bullous impetigo**
L01.02   **Bockhart's impetigo**
Impetigo follicularis
Perifolliculitis NOS
Superficial pustular perifolliculitis
DEF: Superficial inflammation of the hair follicles commonly caused by *Staphylococcus aureus* that manifests as rounded, sphere-shaped, pustular eruptions in the areas of the scalp, beard, underarms, extremities, and buttocks.
L01.03   **Bullous impetigo**
Impetigo neonatorum
Pemphigus neonatorum
L01.09   **Other impetigo**
Ulcerative impetigo
L01.1   **Impetiginization of other dermatoses**

✓4ᵗʰ **L02**   **Cutaneous abscess, furuncle and carbuncle**
Use additional code to identify organism (B95-B96)
EXCLUDES 2   abscess of anus and rectal regions (K61.-)
abscess of female genital organs (external) (N76.4)
abscess of male genital organs (external) (N48.2, N49.-)
DEF: Carbuncle: Infection of the skin that arises from a collection of interconnected infected boils or furuncles, usually from hair follicles infected by *Staphylococcus*. This condition can produce pus and form drainage cavities.
DEF: Furuncle: Inflamed, painful abscess, cyst, or nodule on the skin caused by bacteria, often *Staphylococcus,* entering along the hair follicle.

✓5ᵗʰ **L02.0**   **Cutaneous abscess, furuncle and carbuncle of face**
EXCLUDES 2   abscess of ear, external (H60.0)
abscess of eyelid (H00.0)
abscess of head [any part, except face] (L02.8)
abscess of lacrimal gland (H04.0)
abscess of lacrimal passages (H04.3)
abscess of mouth (K12.2)
abscess of nose (J34.0)
abscess of orbit (H05.0)
submandibular abscess (K12.2)
L02.01   **Cutaneous abscess** of face
L02.02   **Furuncle** of face
Boil of face
Folliculitis of face
L02.03   **Carbuncle** of face

✓5ᵗʰ **L02.1**   **Cutaneous abscess, furuncle and carbuncle of neck**
L02.11   **Cutaneous abscess** of neck
L02.12   **Furuncle** of neck
Boil of neck
Folliculitis of neck
L02.13   **Carbuncle** of neck

✓5ᵗʰ **L02.2**   **Cutaneous abscess, furuncle and carbuncle of trunk**
EXCLUDES 1   non-newborn omphalitis (L08.82)
omphalitis of newborn (P38.-)
EXCLUDES 2   abscess of breast (N61.1)
abscess of buttocks (L02.3)
abscess of female external genital organs (N76.4)
abscess of hip (L02.4)
abscess of male external genital organs (N48.2, N49.-)
✓6ᵗʰ **L02.21**   **Cutaneous abscess** of trunk
L02.211   **Cutaneous abscess of** abdominal wall
L02.212   **Cutaneous abscess of** back [any part, except buttock and flank]
L02.213   **Cutaneous abscess of** chest wall
L02.214   **Cutaneous abscess of** groin
L02.215   **Cutaneous abscess of** perineum
L02.216   **Cutaneous abscess of** umbilicus
L02.217   **Cutaneous abscess of** flank
L02.219   Cutaneous abscess of trunk, unspecified
✓6ᵗʰ **L02.22**   **Furuncle** of trunk
Boil of trunk
Folliculitis of trunk
L02.221   **Furuncle of** abdominal wall
L02.222   **Furuncle of** back [any part, except buttock and flank]
L02.223   **Furuncle of** chest wall
L02.224   **Furuncle of** groin
L02.225   **Furuncle of** perineum
L02.226   **Furuncle of** umbilicus
L02.227   **Furuncle of** flank
L02.229   **Furuncle of trunk, unspecified**
✓6ᵗʰ **L02.23**   **Carbuncle** of trunk
L02.231   **Carbuncle of** abdominal wall
L02.232   **Carbuncle of** back [any part, except buttock]
L02.233   **Carbuncle of** chest wall
L02.234   **Carbuncle of** groin
L02.235   **Carbuncle of** perineum
L02.236   **Carbuncle of** umbilicus
L02.239   **Carbuncle of trunk, unspecified**

✓5ᵗʰ **L02.3**   **Cutaneous abscess, furuncle and carbuncle of** buttock
EXCLUDES 1   pilonidal cyst with abscess (L05.01)
L02.31   **Cutaneous abscess** of buttock
Cutaneous abscess of gluteal region

Chapter 12. Diseases of the Skin and Subcutaneous Tissue

- **L02.32** **Furuncle** of buttock
  - Boil of buttock
  - Folliculitis of buttock
  - Furuncle of gluteal region
- **L02.33** **Carbuncle** of buttock
  - Carbuncle of gluteal region
- ✓5th **L02.4** **Cutaneous abscess, furuncle and carbuncle of** limb
  - EXCLUDES 2: cutaneous abscess, furuncle and carbuncle of foot (L02.6-)
  - cutaneous abscess, furuncle and carbuncle of groin (L02.214, L02.224, L02.234)
  - cutaneous abscess, furuncle and carbuncle of hand (L02.5-)
  - ✓6th **L02.41** **Cutaneous abscess** of limb
    - **L02.411** Cutaneous abscess of right axilla
    - **L02.412** Cutaneous abscess of left axilla
    - **L02.413** Cutaneous abscess of right upper limb
    - **L02.414** Cutaneous abscess of left upper limb
    - **L02.415** Cutaneous abscess of right lower limb
    - **L02.416** Cutaneous abscess of left lower limb
    - **L02.419** Cutaneous abscess of limb, unspecified
  - ✓6th **L02.42** **Furuncle** of limb
    - Boil of limb
    - Folliculitis of limb
    - **L02.421** Furuncle of right axilla
    - **L02.422** Furuncle of left axilla
    - **L02.423** Furuncle of right upper limb
    - **L02.424** Furuncle of left upper limb
    - **L02.425** Furuncle of right lower limb
    - **L02.426** Furuncle of left lower limb
    - **L02.429** Furuncle of limb, unspecified
  - ✓6th **L02.43** **Carbuncle** of limb
    - **L02.431** Carbuncle of right axilla
    - **L02.432** Carbuncle of left axilla
    - **L02.433** Carbuncle of right upper limb
    - **L02.434** Carbuncle of left upper limb
    - **L02.435** Carbuncle of right lower limb
    - **L02.436** Carbuncle of left lower limb
    - **L02.439** Carbuncle of limb, unspecified
- ✓5th **L02.5** **Cutaneous abscess, furuncle and carbuncle of** hand
  - ✓6th **L02.51** **Cutaneous abscess** of hand
    - **L02.511** Cutaneous abscess of right hand
    - **L02.512** Cutaneous abscess of left hand
    - **L02.519** Cutaneous abscess of unspecified hand
  - ✓6th **L02.52** **Furuncle** hand
    - Boil of hand
    - Folliculitis of hand
    - **L02.521** Furuncle right hand
    - **L02.522** Furuncle left hand
    - **L02.529** Furuncle unspecified hand
  - ✓6th **L02.53** **Carbuncle** of hand
    - **L02.531** Carbuncle of right hand
    - **L02.532** Carbuncle of left hand
    - **L02.539** Carbuncle of unspecified hand
- ✓5th **L02.6** **Cutaneous abscess, furuncle and carbuncle of** foot
  - ✓6th **L02.61** **Cutaneous abscess** of foot
    - **L02.611** Cutaneous abscess of right foot
    - **L02.612** Cutaneous abscess of left foot
    - **L02.619** Cutaneous abscess of unspecified foot
  - ✓6th **L02.62** **Furuncle** of foot
    - Boil of foot
    - Folliculitis of foot
    - **L02.621** Furuncle of right foot
    - **L02.622** Furuncle of left foot
    - **L02.629** Furuncle of unspecified foot
  - ✓6th **L02.63** **Carbuncle** of foot
    - **L02.631** Carbuncle of right foot
    - **L02.632** Carbuncle of left foot
    - **L02.639** Carbuncle of unspecified foot
- ✓5th **L02.8** **Cutaneous abscess, furuncle and carbuncle of other sites**
  - ✓6th **L02.81** **Cutaneous abscess** of other sites
    - **L02.811** Cutaneous abscess of head [any part, except face]
    - **L02.818** Cutaneous abscess of other sites
  - ✓6th **L02.82** **Furuncle** of other sites
    - Boil of other sites
    - Folliculitis of other sites
    - **L02.821** Furuncle of head [any part, except face]
    - **L02.828** Furuncle of other sites
  - ✓6th **L02.83** **Carbuncle** of other sites
    - **L02.831** Carbuncle of head [any part, except face]
    - **L02.838** Carbuncle of other sites
- ✓5th **L02.9** **Cutaneous abscess, furuncle and carbuncle, unspecified**
  - **L02.91** **Cutaneous abscess**, unspecified
  - **L02.92** **Furuncle**, unspecified
    - Boil NOS
    - Furunculosis NOS
  - **L02.93** **Carbuncle**, unspecified
- ✓4th **L03** **Cellulitis and acute lymphangitis**
  - EXCLUDES 2: cellulitis of anal and rectal region (K61.-)
  - cellulitis of external auditory canal (H60.1)
  - cellulitis of eyelid (H00.0)
  - cellulitis of female external genital organs (N76.4)
  - cellulitis of lacrimal apparatus (H04.3)
  - cellulitis of male external genital organs (N48.2, N49.-)
  - cellulitis of mouth (K12.2)
  - cellulitis of nose (J34.0)
  - eosinophilic cellulitis [Wells] (L98.3)
  - febrile neutrophilic dermatosis [Sweet] (L98.2)
  - lymphangitis (chronic) (subacute) (I89.1)
  - **AHA:** 2017,4Q,100
  - **DEF:** Cellulitis: Infection of the skin and subcutaneous tissues, most often caused by *Staphylococcus* or *Streptococcus* bacteria secondary to a cutaneous lesion. Progression of the inflammation may lead to abscess and tissue death, or even systemic infection-like bacteremia.
  - **DEF:** Lymphangitis: Inflammation of the lymph channels most often caused by *Streptococcus*.
  - ✓5th **L03.0** **Cellulitis and acute lymphangitis of** finger and toe
    - Infection of nail
    - Onychia
    - Paronychia
    - Perionychia
    - ✓6th **L03.01** **Cellulitis** of finger
      - Felon
      - Whitlow
      - EXCLUDES 1: herpetic whitlow (B00.89)
      - **DEF:** Felon: Superficial bacterial skin infection at the tip of the finger.
      - **L03.011** Cellulitis of right finger
      - **L03.012** Cellulitis of left finger
      - **L03.019** Cellulitis of unspecified finger
    - ✓6th **L03.02** **Acute lymphangitis** of finger
      - Hangnail with lymphangitis of finger
      - **L03.021** Acute lymphangitis of right finger
      - **L03.022** Acute lymphangitis of left finger
      - **L03.029** Acute lymphangitis of unspecified finger
    - ✓6th **L03.03** **Cellulitis** of toe
      - **L03.031** Cellulitis of right toe
      - **L03.032** Cellulitis of left toe
      - **L03.039** Cellulitis of unspecified toe
    - ✓6th **L03.04** **Acute lymphangitis** of toe
      - Hangnail with lymphangitis of toe
      - **L03.041** Acute lymphangitis of right toe
      - **L03.042** Acute lymphangitis of left toe
      - **L03.049** Acute lymphangitis of unspecified toe
  - ✓5th **L03.1** **Cellulitis and acute lymphangitis of other parts of limb**
    - ✓6th **L03.11** **Cellulitis** of other parts of limb
      - EXCLUDES 2: cellulitis of fingers (L03.01-)
      - cellulitis of toes (L03.03-)
      - groin (L03.314)
      - **L03.111** Cellulitis of right axilla
      - **L03.112** Cellulitis of left axilla
      - **L03.113** Cellulitis of right upper limb
      - **L03.114** Cellulitis of left upper limb
      - **L03.115** Cellulitis of right lower limb
      - **L03.116** Cellulitis of left lower limb
      - **L03.119** Cellulitis of unspecified part of limb
    - ✓6th **L03.12** **Acute lymphangitis** of other parts of limb
      - EXCLUDES 2: acute lymphangitis of fingers (L03.2-)
      - acute lymphangitis of groin (L03.324)
      - acute lymphangitis of toes (L03.04-)
      - **L03.121** Acute lymphangitis of right axilla

Chapter 12. Diseases of the Skin and Subcutaneous Tissue

- L03.122 Acute lymphangitis of **left axilla**
- L03.123 Acute lymphangitis of **right upper** limb
- L03.124 Acute lymphangitis of **left upper** limb
- L03.125 Acute lymphangitis of **right lower** limb
- L03.126 Acute lymphangitis of **left lower** limb
- L03.129 Acute lymphangitis of unspecified part of limb

L03.2 Cellulitis and acute lymphangitis of **face and neck**

L03.21 Cellulitis and acute lymphangitis of **face**

- **L03.211 Cellulitis** of face
  - EXCLUDES 2:
    - abscess of orbit (H05.01-)
    - cellulitis of ear (H60.1-)
    - cellulitis of eyelid (H00.0-)
    - cellulitis of head (L03.81)
    - cellulitis of lacrimal apparatus (H04.3)
    - cellulitis of lip (K13.0)
    - cellulitis of mouth (K12.2)
    - cellulitis of nose (internal) (J34.0)
    - cellulitis of orbit (H05.01-)
    - cellulitis of scalp (L03.81)
  - AHA: 2013,4Q,123
- **L03.212 Acute lymphangitis** of face
- **L03.213 Periorbital cellulitis**
  - Preseptal cellulitis
  - AHA: 2016,4Q,36

L03.22 Cellulitis and acute lymphangitis of **neck**

- **L03.221 Cellulitis** of neck
- **L03.222 Acute lymphangitis** of neck

L03.3 Cellulitis and acute lymphangitis of **trunk**

L03.31 **Cellulitis** of trunk

EXCLUDES 2:
- cellulitis of anal and rectal regions (K61.-)
- cellulitis of breast NOS (N61.0)
- cellulitis of female external genital organs (N76.4)
- cellulitis of male external genital organs (N48.2, N49.-)
- omphalitis of newborn (P38.-)
- puerperal cellulitis of breast (O91.2)

- **L03.311 Cellulitis of abdominal wall**
  - EXCLUDES 2: cellulitis of umbilicus (L03.316)
  - cellulitis of groin (L03.314)
- L03.312 Cellulitis of **back** [any part except buttock]
- L03.313 Cellulitis of **chest wall**
- L03.314 Cellulitis of **groin**
- L03.315 Cellulitis of **perineum**
- L03.316 Cellulitis of **umbilicus**
- L03.317 Cellulitis of **buttock**
- L03.319 Cellulitis of trunk, unspecified
- L03.31A Cellulitis of **flank**

L03.32 **Acute lymphangitis** of trunk

- L03.321 Acute lymphangitis of **abdominal wall**
- L03.322 Acute lymphangitis of **back** [any part except buttock]
- L03.323 Acute lymphangitis of **chest wall**
- L03.324 Acute lymphangitis of **groin**
- L03.325 Acute lymphangitis of **perineum**
- L03.326 Acute lymphangitis of **umbilicus**
- L03.327 Acute lymphangitis of **buttock**
- L03.329 Acute lymphangitis of trunk, unspecified
- L03.32A Acute lymphangitis of **flank**

L03.8 Cellulitis and acute lymphangitis of other sites

L03.81 **Cellulitis** of other sites

- **L03.811 Cellulitis of head** [any part, except face]
  - Cellulitis of scalp
  - EXCLUDES 2: cellulitis of face (L03.211)
- L03.818 Cellulitis of other sites

L03.89 **Acute lymphangitis** of other sites

- **L03.891 Acute lymphangitis of head** [any part, except face]
- L03.898 Acute lymphangitis of other sites

L03.9 Cellulitis and acute lymphangitis, unspecified

- **L03.90 Cellulitis**, unspecified
- **L03.91 Acute lymphangitis**, unspecified
  - EXCLUDES 1: lymphangitis NOS (I89.1)

L04 Acute lymphadenitis

INCLUDES:
- abscess (acute) of lymph nodes, except mesenteric
- acute lymphadenitis, except mesenteric

EXCLUDES 1:
- chronic or subacute lymphadenitis, except mesenteric (I88.1)
- enlarged lymph nodes (R59.-)
- human immunodeficiency virus [HIV] disease resulting in generalized lymphadenopathy (B20)
- lymphadenitis NOS (I88.9)
- nonspecific mesenteric lymphadenitis (I88.0)

DEF: Inflammation or enlargement of the lymph nodes.

- L04.0 Acute lymphadenitis of **face, head and neck**
- L04.1 Acute lymphadenitis of **trunk**
- L04.2 Acute lymphadenitis of **upper limb**
  - Acute lymphadenitis of axilla
  - Acute lymphadenitis of shoulder
- L04.3 Acute lymphadenitis of **lower limb**
  - Acute lymphadenitis of hip
  - EXCLUDES 2: acute lymphadenitis of groin (L04.1)
- L04.8 Acute lymphadenitis of other sites
- L04.9 Acute lymphadenitis, unspecified

L05 Pilonidal cyst and sinus

DEF: Pilonidal cyst: Sac or sinus cavity of trapped epithelial tissues in the sacrococcygeal region, usually associated with ingrown hair.

DEF: Pilonidal sinus: Fistula, tract, or channel that extends from an infected area of ingrown hair to another site within the skin or out to the skin surface.

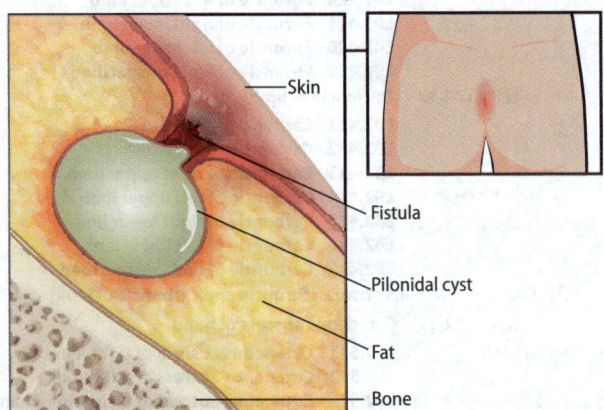

Pilonidal Cyst — Skin, Fistula, Pilonidal cyst, Fat, Bone

L05.0 Pilonidal cyst and sinus **with abscess**

- **L05.01 Pilonidal cyst with abscess**
  - Pilonidal abscess
  - Pilonidal dimple with abscess
  - Postanal dimple with abscess
  - EXCLUDES 2: congenital sacral dimple (Q82.6)
  - parasacral dimple (Q82.6)
- **L05.02 Pilonidal sinus with abscess**
  - Coccygeal fistula with abscess
  - Coccygeal sinus with abscess
  - Pilonidal fistula with abscess

L05.9 Pilonidal cyst and sinus **without abscess**

- **L05.91 Pilonidal cyst without abscess**
  - Pilonidal cyst NOS
  - Pilonidal dimple
  - Postanal dimple
  - EXCLUDES 2: congenital sacral dimple (Q82.6)
  - parasacral dimple (Q82.6)
- **L05.92 Pilonidal sinus without abscess**
  - Coccygeal fistula
  - Coccygeal sinus without abscess
  - Pilonidal fistula

L08 Other local infections of skin and subcutaneous tissue

L08.0 Pyoderma

- Dermatitis gangrenosa
- Purulent dermatitis
- Septic dermatitis
- Suppurative dermatitis

EXCLUDES 1:
- pyoderma gangrenosum (L88)
- pyoderma vegetans (L08.81)

DEF: Any superficial skin disease commonly characterized by the discharging of pus not attributed to another condition.

L08.1 Erythrasma
DEF: Chronic, superficial skin infection of brown scaly patches, commonly found in skin folds most prevalent in the overweight or diabetic population.

L08.8 Other specified local infections of the skin and subcutaneous tissue
- **L08.81** Pyoderma vegetans
  - EXCLUDES 1: pyoderma gangrenosum (L88)
  - pyoderma NOS (L08.0)
- **L08.82** Omphalitis not of newborn
  - EXCLUDES 1: omphalitis of newborn (P38.-)
- **L08.89** Other specified local infections of the skin and subcutaneous tissue

L08.9 Local infection of the skin and subcutaneous tissue, unspecified

Bullous disorders (L10-L14)

EXCLUDES 1: benign familial pemphigus [Hailey-Hailey] (Q82.8)
staphylococcal scalded skin syndrome (L00)
toxic epidermal necrolysis [Lyell] (L51.2)

L10 Pemphigus
  EXCLUDES 1: pemphigus neonatorum (L01.03)
- **L10.0** Pemphigus vulgaris
- **L10.1** Pemphigus vegetans
- **L10.2** Pemphigus foliaceous
- **L10.3** Brazilian pemphigus [fogo selvagem]
- **L10.4** Pemphigus erythematosus
  Senear-Usher syndrome
- **L10.5** Drug-induced pemphigus
  Use additional code for adverse effect, if applicable, to identify drug (T36-T50 with fifth or sixth character 5)
- **L10.8** Other pemphigus
  - **L10.81** Paraneoplastic pemphigus
  - **L10.89** Other pemphigus
- **L10.9** Pemphigus, unspecified

L11 Other acantholytic disorders
- **L11.0** Acquired keratosis follicularis
  EXCLUDES 1: keratosis follicularis (congenital) [Darier-White] (Q82.8)
  AHA: 2021,3Q,10
- **L11.1** Transient acantholytic dermatosis [Grover]
- **L11.8** Other specified acantholytic disorders
- **L11.9** Acantholytic disorder, unspecified

L12 Pemphigoid
  EXCLUDES 1: herpes gestationis (O26.4-)
  impetigo herpetiformis (L40.1)
- **L12.0** Bullous pemphigoid
- **L12.1** Cicatricial pemphigoid
  Benign mucous membrane pemphigoid
  DEF: Chronic autoimmune disease characterized by subepidermal blistering lesions of the mucosa, including the conjunctiva. It is seen predominantly in the elderly and produces adhesions and scarring.
- **L12.2** Chronic bullous disease of childhood
  Juvenile dermatitis herpetiformis
- **L12.3** Acquired epidermolysis bullosa
  EXCLUDES 1: epidermolysis bullosa (congenital) (Q81.-)
  - **L12.30** Acquired epidermolysis bullosa, unspecified
  - **L12.31** Epidermolysis bullosa due to drug
    Use additional code for adverse effect, if applicable, to identify drug (T36-T50 with fifth or sixth character 5)
  - **L12.35** Other acquired epidermolysis bullosa
- **L12.8** Other pemphigoid
- **L12.9** Pemphigoid, unspecified

L13 Other bullous disorders
- **L13.0** Dermatitis herpetiformis
  Duhring's disease
  Hydroa herpetiformis
  EXCLUDES 1: juvenile dermatitis herpetiformis (L12.2)
  senile dermatitis herpetiformis (L12.0)
  DEF: Skin disease to which people are genetically predisposed resulting from an immunological response to gluten. Dermatitis herpetiformis is an extremely pruritic eruption of various lesions that frequently heal, leaving hyperpigmentation or hypopigmentation and occasionally scarring. It is usually associated with asymptomatic gluten-sensitive enteropathy.
- **L13.1** Subcorneal pustular dermatitis
  Sneddon-Wilkinson disease
- **L13.8** Other specified bullous disorders
- **L13.9** Bullous disorder, unspecified

L14 Bullous disorders in diseases classified elsewhere
  Code first underlying disease

Dermatitis and eczema (L20-L30)

NOTE: In this block the terms dermatitis and eczema are used synonymously and interchangeably.

EXCLUDES 2: chronic (childhood) granulomatous disease ▶(D71-)◄
dermatitis gangrenosa (L08.0)
dermatitis herpetiformis (L13.0)
dry skin dermatitis (L85.3)
factitial dermatitis (L98.1)
perioral dermatitis (L71.0)
radiation-related disorders of the skin and subcutaneous tissue (L55-L59)
stasis dermatitis (I87.2)

L20 Atopic dermatitis
- **L20.0** Besnier's prurigo
- **L20.8** Other atopic dermatitis
  EXCLUDES 2: circumscribed neurodermatitis (L28.0)
  - **L20.81** Atopic neurodermatitis
    Diffuse neurodermatitis
  - **L20.82** Flexural eczema
  - **L20.83** Infantile (acute) (chronic) eczema
  - **L20.84** Intrinsic (allergic) eczema
  - **L20.89** Other atopic dermatitis
- **L20.9** Atopic dermatitis, unspecified

L21 Seborrheic dermatitis
  EXCLUDES 2: infective dermatitis (L30.3)
  seborrheic keratosis (L82.-)
- **L21.0** Seborrhea capitis
  Cradle cap
  AHA: 2018,1Q,6
  TIP: Assign for dandruff in an adult patient.
- **L21.1** Seborrheic infantile dermatitis
- **L21.8** Other seborrheic dermatitis
- **L21.9** Seborrheic dermatitis, unspecified
  Seborrhea NOS

L22 Diaper dermatitis
  Diaper erythema
  Diaper rash
  Psoriasiform diaper rash
  AHA: 2021,4Q,18

L23 Allergic contact dermatitis
  EXCLUDES 1: allergy NOS (T78.40)
  contact dermatitis NOS (L25.9)
  dermatitis NOS (L30.9)
  EXCLUDES 2: dermatitis due to substances taken internally (L27.-)
  dermatitis of eyelid (H01.1-)
  diaper dermatitis (L22)
  eczema of external ear (H60.5-)
  irritant contact dermatitis (L24.-)
  perioral dermatitis (L71.0)
  radiation-related disorders of the skin and subcutaneous tissue (L55-L59)
- **L23.0** Allergic contact dermatitis due to metals
  Allergic contact dermatitis due to chromium
  Allergic contact dermatitis due to nickel
- **L23.1** Allergic contact dermatitis due to adhesives
- **L23.2** Allergic contact dermatitis due to cosmetics

Chapter 12. Diseases of the Skin and Subcutaneous Tissue

L23.3 **Allergic contact dermatitis due to drugs in contact with skin**
Use additional code for adverse effect, if applicable, to identify drug (T36-T50 with fifth or sixth character 5)
EXCLUDES 2 — dermatitis due to ingested drugs and medicaments (L27.0-L27.1)

L23.4 **Allergic contact dermatitis due to dyes**

L23.5 **Allergic contact dermatitis due to other chemical products**
Allergic contact dermatitis due to cement
Allergic contact dermatitis due to insecticide
Allergic contact dermatitis due to plastic
Allergic contact dermatitis due to rubber

L23.6 **Allergic contact dermatitis due to food in contact with the skin**
EXCLUDES 2 — dermatitis due to ingested food (L27.2)

L23.7 **Allergic contact dermatitis due to plants, except food**
EXCLUDES 2 — allergy NOS due to pollen (J30.1)

✓5th **L23.8** **Allergic contact dermatitis due to other agents**
  L23.81 Allergic contact dermatitis due to animal (cat) (dog) dander
    Allergic contact dermatitis due to animal (cat) (dog) hair
  L23.89 Allergic contact dermatitis due to other agents

L23.9 **Allergic contact dermatitis, unspecified cause**
Allergic contact eczema NOS

✓4th **L24** **Irritant contact dermatitis**
  EXCLUDES 1 — allergy NOS (T78.40)
    contact dermatitis NOS (L25.9)
    dermatitis NOS (L30.9)
  EXCLUDES 2 — allergic contact dermatitis (L23.-)
    dermatitis due to substances taken internally (L27.-)
    dermatitis of eyelid (H01.1-)
    diaper dermatitis (L22)
    eczema of external ear (H60.5-)
    perioral dermatitis (L71.0)
    radiation-related disorders of the skin and subcutaneous tissue (L55-L59)

L24.0 **Irritant contact dermatitis due to detergents**

L24.1 **Irritant contact dermatitis due to oils and greases**

L24.2 **Irritant contact dermatitis due to solvents**
Irritant contact dermatitis due to chlorocompound
Irritant contact dermatitis due to cyclohexane
Irritant contact dermatitis due to ester
Irritant contact dermatitis due to glycol
Irritant contact dermatitis due to hydrocarbon
Irritant contact dermatitis due to ketone

L24.3 **Irritant contact dermatitis due to cosmetics**

L24.4 **Irritant contact dermatitis due to drugs in contact with skin**
Use additional code for adverse effect, if applicable, to identify drug (T36-T50 with fifth or sixth character 5)

L24.5 **Irritant contact dermatitis due to other chemical products**
Irritant contact dermatitis due to cement
Irritant contact dermatitis due to insecticide
Irritant contact dermatitis due to plastic
Irritant contact dermatitis due to rubber

L24.6 **Irritant contact dermatitis due to food in contact with skin**
EXCLUDES 2 — dermatitis due to ingested food (L27.2)

L24.7 **Irritant contact dermatitis due to plants, except food**
EXCLUDES 2 — allergy NOS to pollen (J30.1)

✓5th **L24.8** **Irritant contact dermatitis due to other agents**
  L24.81 Irritant contact dermatitis due to metals
    Irritant contact dermatitis due to chromium
    Irritant contact dermatitis due to nickel
  L24.89 Irritant contact dermatitis due to other agents
    Irritant contact dermatitis due to dyes

L24.9 **Irritant contact dermatitis, unspecified cause**
Irritant contact eczema NOS

✓5th **L24.A** **Irritant contact dermatitis due to friction or contact with body fluids**
  EXCLUDES 1 — irritant contact dermatitis related to stoma or fistula (L24.B-)
  EXCLUDES 2 — erythema intertrigo (L30.4)
  AHA: 2021,4Q,16-18
  L24.A0 Irritant contact dermatitis due to friction or contact with body fluids, unspecified
  L24.A1 Irritant contact dermatitis due to saliva
  L24.A2 Irritant contact dermatitis due to fecal, urinary or dual incontinence
    EXCLUDES 1 — diaper dermatitis (L22)

L24.A9 **Irritant contact dermatitis due friction or contact with other specified body fluids**
Irritant contact dermatitis related to endotracheal tube
Wound fluids, exudate

✓5th **L24.B** **Irritant contact dermatitis related to stoma or fistula**
Use additional code to identify any artificial opening status (Z93.-), if applicable, for contact dermatitis related to stoma secretions
AHA: 2021,4Q,16-18
  L24.B0 Irritant contact dermatitis related to unspecified stoma or fistula
    Irritant contact dermatitis related to fistula NOS
    Irritant contact dermatitis related to stoma NOS
  L24.B1 Irritant contact dermatitis related to digestive stoma or fistula
    Irritant contact dermatitis related to gastrostomy
    Irritant contact dermatitis related to jejunostomy
    Irritant contact dermatitis related to saliva or spit fistula
  L24.B2 Irritant contact dermatitis related to respiratory stoma or fistula
    Irritant contact dermatitis related to tracheostomy
  L24.B3 Irritant contact dermatitis related to fecal or urinary stoma or fistula
    Irritant contact dermatitis related to colostomy
    Irritant contact dermatitis related to enterocutaneous fistula
    Irritant contact dermatitis related to ileostomy

✓4th **L25** **Unspecified contact dermatitis**
  EXCLUDES 1 — allergic contact dermatitis (L23.-)
    allergy NOS (T78.40)
    dermatitis NOS (L30.9)
    irritant contact dermatitis (L24.-)
  EXCLUDES 2 — dermatitis due to ingested substances (L27.-)
    dermatitis of eyelid (H01.1-)
    eczema of external ear (H60.5-)
    perioral dermatitis (L71.0)
    radiation-related disorders of the skin and subcutaneous tissue (L55-L59)

L25.0 **Unspecified contact dermatitis due to cosmetics**

L25.1 **Unspecified contact dermatitis due to drugs in contact with skin**
Use additional code for adverse effect, if applicable, to identify drug (T36-T50 with fifth or sixth character 5)
EXCLUDES 2 — dermatitis due to ingested drugs and medicaments (L27.0-L27.1)

L25.2 **Unspecified contact dermatitis due to dyes**

L25.3 **Unspecified contact dermatitis due to other chemical products**
Unspecified contact dermatitis due to cement
Unspecified contact dermatitis due to insecticide

L25.4 **Unspecified contact dermatitis due to food in contact with skin**
EXCLUDES 2 — dermatitis due to ingested food (L27.2)

L25.5 **Unspecified contact dermatitis due to plants, except food**
EXCLUDES 1 — nettle rash (L50.9)
EXCLUDES 2 — allergy NOS due to pollen (J30.1)

L25.8 **Unspecified contact dermatitis due to other agents**

L25.9 **Unspecified contact dermatitis, unspecified cause**
Contact dermatitis (occupational) NOS
Contact eczema (occupational) NOS

L26 **Exfoliative dermatitis**
Hebra's pityriasis
EXCLUDES 1 — Ritter's disease (L00)

✓4th **L27** **Dermatitis due to substances taken internally**
  EXCLUDES 1 — allergy NOS (T78.40)
  EXCLUDES 2 — adverse food reaction, except dermatitis (T78.0-T78.1)
    contact dermatitis (L23-L25)
    drug photoallergic response (L56.1)
    drug phototoxic response (L56.0)
    urticaria (L50.-)

L27.0 **Generalized skin eruption due to drugs and medicaments taken internally**
Use additional code for adverse effect, if applicable, to identify drug (T36-T50 with fifth or sixth character 5)

L27.1 **Localized skin eruption due to drugs and medicaments taken internally**
Use additional code for adverse effect, if applicable, to identify drug (T36-T50 with fifth or sixth character 5)

Chapter 12. Diseases of the Skin and Subcutaneous Tissue

- **L27.2** Dermatitis due to ingested food
  - *EXCLUDES 2* dermatitis due to food in contact with skin (L23.6, L24.6, L25.4)
- **L27.8** Dermatitis due to other substances taken internally
- **L27.9** Dermatitis due to unspecified substance taken internally

✓4th L28 Lichen simplex chronicus and prurigo
- **L28.0** Lichen simplex chronicus
  - Circumscribed neurodermatitis
  - Lichen NOS
- **L28.1** Prurigo nodularis
- **L28.2** Other prurigo
  - Prurigo Hebra
  - Prurigo mitis
  - Prurigo NOS
  - Urticaria papulosa

✓4th L29 Pruritus
- *EXCLUDES 1* neurotic excoriation (L98.1)
  - psychogenic pruritus (F45.8)
- **L29.0** Pruritus ani
- **L29.1** Pruritus scroti
- **L29.2** Pruritus vulvae
- **L29.3** Anogenital pruritus, unspecified
- ✓5th **L29.8** Other pruritus
  - **L29.81** Cholestatic pruritus
    - Code also, if applicable, type of liver disease
    - Use additional code for adverse effect, if applicable, to identify drug (T36-T50 with fifth or sixth character 5)
    - AHA: 2024,4Q,22
  - **L29.89** Other pruritus
- **L29.9** Pruritus, unspecified
  - Itch NOS

✓4th L30 Other and unspecified dermatitis
- *EXCLUDES 2* contact dermatitis (L23-L25)
  - dry skin dermatitis (L85.3)
  - small plaque parapsoriasis (L41.3)
  - stasis dermatitis (I87.2)
- **L30.0** Nummular dermatitis
- **L30.1** Dyshidrosis [pompholyx]
- **L30.2** Cutaneous autosensitization
  - Candidid [levurid]
  - Dermatophytid
  - Eczematid
- **L30.3** Infective dermatitis
  - Infectious eczematoid dermatitis
- **L30.4** Erythema intertrigo
- **L30.5** Pityriasis alba
  - AHA: 2018,1Q,6
- **L30.8** Other specified dermatitis
- **L30.9** Dermatitis, unspecified
  - Eczema NOS

Papulosquamous disorders (L40-L45)

✓4th L40 Psoriasis
DEF: Chronic autoimmune condition that speeds up skin cell growth, causing excessive immature skin cells to form raised, rounded erythematous lesions covered by dry, silvery scaling patches. Most commonly found on the scalp, elbows, knees, hands, feet, and genitals, it can also affect the joints with stiffness and swelling.
- **L40.0** Psoriasis vulgaris [Rx]
  - Nummular psoriasis
  - Plaque psoriasis
- **L40.1** Generalized pustular psoriasis [Rx]
  - Impetigo herpetiformis
  - Von Zumbusch's disease
- **L40.2** Acrodermatitis continua [Rx]
- **L40.3** Pustulosis palmaris et plantaris [Rx]
- **L40.4** Guttate psoriasis [Rx]
- ✓5th **L40.5** Arthropathic psoriasis
  - **L40.50** Arthropathic psoriasis, unspecified [HCC] [Rx] [ESR] [COM]
  - **L40.51** Distal interphalangeal psoriatic arthropathy [HCC] [Rx] [ESR] [COM]
  - **L40.52** Psoriatic arthritis mutilans [HCC] [Rx] [ESR] [COM]
  - **L40.53** Psoriatic spondylitis [HCC] [Rx] [ESR] [COM]
  - **L40.54** Psoriatic juvenile arthropathy [HCC] [Rx] [ESR] [COM]
  - **L40.59** Other psoriatic arthropathy [HCC] [Rx] [ESR] [COM]
- **L40.8** Other psoriasis [Rx]
  - Flexural psoriasis
- **L40.9** Psoriasis, unspecified [Rx]

✓4th L41 Parapsoriasis
- *EXCLUDES 1* poikiloderma vasculare atrophicans (L94.5)
- **L41.0** Pityriasis lichenoides et varioliformis acuta [Rx]
  - Mucha-Habermann disease
- **L41.1** Pityriasis lichenoides chronica [Rx]
- **L41.3** Small plaque parapsoriasis [Rx]
- **L41.4** Large plaque parapsoriasis [Rx]
- **L41.5** Retiform parapsoriasis [Rx]
- **L41.8** Other parapsoriasis [Rx]
- **L41.9** Parapsoriasis, unspecified [Rx]

L42 Pityriasis rosea

✓4th L43 Lichen planus
- *EXCLUDES 1* lichen planopilaris (L66.1-)
- **L43.0** Hypertrophic lichen planus
- **L43.1** Bullous lichen planus
- **L43.2** Lichenoid drug reaction
  - Use additional code for adverse effect, if applicable, to identify drug (T36-T50 with fifth or sixth character 5)
- **L43.3** Subacute (active) lichen planus
  - Lichen planus tropicus
- **L43.8** Other lichen planus
- **L43.9** Lichen planus, unspecified

✓4th L44 Other papulosquamous disorders
- **L44.0** Pityriasis rubra pilaris
- **L44.1** Lichen nitidus
  - **DEF:** Chronic, inflammatory, asymptomatic skin disorder, characterized by numerous glistening, flat-topped, discrete, skin-colored micropapules, most often on the penis, lower abdomen, inner thighs, wrists, forearms, breasts, and buttocks.
- **L44.2** Lichen striatus
- **L44.3** Lichen ruber moniliformis
- **L44.4** Infantile papular acrodermatitis [Gianotti-Crosti] [P]
- **L44.8** Other specified papulosquamous disorders
- **L44.9** Papulosquamous disorder, unspecified

L45 Papulosquamous disorders in diseases classified elsewhere
Code first underlying disease

Urticaria and erythema (L49-L54)
- *EXCLUDES 1* Lyme disease (A69.2-)
  - rosacea (L71.-)

✓4th L49 Exfoliation due to erythematous conditions according to extent of body surface involved
Code first erythematous condition causing exfoliation, such as:
- (Staphylococcal) scalded skin syndrome (L00)
- Ritter's disease (L00)
- Stevens-Johnson syndrome (L51.1)
- Stevens-Johnson syndrome-toxic epidermal necrolysis overlap syndrome (L51.3)
- toxic epidermal necrolysis (L51.2)

DEF: Exfoliation: Falling or sloughing off skin in layers.
- **L49.0** Exfoliation due to erythematous condition involving less than 10 percent of body surface [UPD]
  - Exfoliation due to erythematous condition NOS
- **L49.1** Exfoliation due to erythematous condition involving 10-19 percent of body surface [COM] [UPD]
- **L49.2** Exfoliation due to erythematous condition involving 20-29 percent of body surface [COM] [UPD]
- **L49.3** Exfoliation due to erythematous condition involving 30-39 percent of body surface [COM] [UPD]
- **L49.4** Exfoliation due to erythematous condition involving 40-49 percent of body surface [COM] [UPD]
- **L49.5** Exfoliation due to erythematous condition involving 50-59 percent of body surface [COM] [UPD]
- **L49.6** Exfoliation due to erythematous condition involving 60-69 percent of body surface [COM] [UPD]
- **L49.7** Exfoliation due to erythematous condition involving 70-79 percent of body surface [COM] [UPD]
- **L49.8** Exfoliation due to erythematous condition involving 80-89 percent of body surface [COM] [UPD]
- **L49.9** Exfoliation due to erythematous condition involving 90 or more percent of body surface [COM] [UPD]

✓ Additional Character Required | ✓x7th Placeholder Alert | Manifestation | Unspecified Dx | Q QPP | UPD Unacceptable PDx

Chapter 12. Diseases of the Skin and Subcutaneous Tissue

L50 Urticaria
EXCLUDES 1
- allergic contact dermatitis (L23.-)
- angioneurotic edema (T78.3)
- giant urticaria (T78.3)
- hereditary angio-edema (D84.1)
- Quincke's edema (T78.3)
- serum urticaria (T80.6-)
- solar urticaria (L56.3)
- urticaria neonatorum (P83.8)
- urticaria papulosa (L28.2)
- urticaria pigmentosa (D47.01)

DEF: Eruption of itching edema of the skin. **Synonym(s):** hives.

- **L50.0** Allergic urticaria
- **L50.1** Idiopathic urticaria
- **L50.2** Urticaria due to cold and heat
  - **EXCLUDES 2** familial cold urticaria (M04.2)
- **L50.3** Dermatographic urticaria
- **L50.4** Vibratory urticaria
- **L50.5** Cholinergic urticaria
- **L50.6** Contact urticaria
- **L50.8** Other urticaria
  - Chronic urticaria
  - Recurrent periodic urticaria
- **L50.9** Urticaria, unspecified

L51 Erythema multiforme
Use additional code for adverse effect, if applicable, to identify drug (T36-T50 with fifth or sixth character 5)
Use additional code to identify associated manifestations, such as:
Use additional code to identify percentage of skin exfoliation (L49.-)
- arthropathy associated with dermatological disorders (M14.8-)
- conjunctival edema (H11.42)
- conjunctivitis (H10.22-)
- corneal scars and opacities (H17.-)
- corneal ulcer (H16.0-)
- edema of eyelid (H02.84-)
- inflammation of eyelid ▶(H01.8-)◀
- keratoconjunctivitis sicca (H16.22-)
- mechanical lagophthalmos (H02.22-)
- stomatitis (K12.-)
- symblepharon (H11.23-)

EXCLUDES 1
- staphylococcal scalded skin syndrome (L00)
- Ritter's disease (L00)

DEF: Acute complex of symptoms with a varied pattern of skin eruptions, such as macular, bullous, papular, nodose, or vesicular lesions on the neck, face, and legs. Erythema (redness of skin and mucous membranes) multiforme (multiple forms) is a hypersensitivity (allergic) reaction that can occur at any age but primarily affects children or young adults.

- **L51.0** Nonbullous erythema multiforme
- **L51.1** Stevens-Johnson syndrome
- **L51.2** Toxic epidermal necrolysis [Lyell]
- **L51.3** Stevens-Johnson syndrome-toxic epidermal necrolysis overlap syndrome
  - SJS-TEN overlap syndrome
- **L51.8** Other erythema multiforme
- **L51.9** Erythema multiforme, unspecified
  - Erythema iris
  - Erythema multiforme major NOS
  - Erythema multiforme minor NOS
  - Herpes iris

L52 Erythema nodosum
EXCLUDES 1 tuberculous erythema nodosum (A18.4)

DEF: Form of panniculitis (inflammation of the fat layer beneath the skin) most often occurring in women. Commonly seen as a hypersensitivity reaction to infections, drugs, sarcoidosis, and specific enteropathies. The acute stage is associated with fever, malaise, and arthralgia. The lesions are pink to blue in color as tender nodules and are found on the front of the legs below the knees.

L53 Other erythematous conditions
EXCLUDES 1
- erythema ab igne (L59.0)
- erythema due to external agents in contact with skin (L23-L25)
- erythema intertrigo (L30.4)

- **L53.0** Toxic erythema
  - Code first poisoning due to drug or toxin, if applicable (T36-T65 with fifth or sixth character 1-4)
  - Use additional code for adverse effect, if applicable, to identify drug (T36-T50 with fifth or sixth character 5)
  - **EXCLUDES 2** neonatal erythema toxicum (P83.1)
- **L53.1** Erythema annulare centrifugum
- **L53.2** Erythema marginatum
- **L53.3** Other chronic figurate erythema
- **L53.8** Other specified erythematous conditions
- **L53.9** Erythematous condition, unspecified
  - Erythema NOS
  - Erythroderma NOS

L54 Erythema in diseases classified elsewhere
Code first underlying disease

Radiation-related disorders of the skin and subcutaneous tissue (L55-L59)

L55 Sunburn
- **L55.0** Sunburn of first degree
- **L55.1** Sunburn of second degree
- **L55.2** Sunburn of third degree
- **L55.9** Sunburn, unspecified

L56 Other acute skin changes due to ultraviolet radiation
Use additional code to identify the source of the ultraviolet radiation (W89, X32)

- **L56.0** Drug phototoxic response
  - Use additional code for adverse effect, if applicable, to identify drug (T36-T50 with fifth or sixth character 5)
- **L56.1** Drug photoallergic response
  - Use additional code for adverse effect, if applicable, to identify drug (T36-T50 with fifth or sixth character 5)
- **L56.2** Photocontact dermatitis [berloque dermatitis]
- **L56.3** Solar urticaria
- **L56.4** Polymorphous light eruption
- **L56.5** Disseminated superficial actinic porokeratosis (DSAP)
  - **DEF:** Autosomal dominant skin condition occurring in sun-exposed areas of the skin (particularly the arms and legs), characterized by superficial annular, keratotic, brownish-red spots or thickenings with depressed centers and sharp, ridged borders. It may evolve into squamous cell carcinoma.
- **L56.8** Other specified acute skin changes due to ultraviolet radiation
- **L56.9** Acute skin change due to ultraviolet radiation, unspecified

L57 Skin changes due to chronic exposure to nonionizing radiation
Use additional code to identify the source of the ultraviolet radiation (W89), or other nonionizing radiation (W90)

- **L57.0** Actinic keratosis
  - Keratosis NOS
  - Senile keratosis
  - Solar keratosis
- **L57.1** Actinic reticuloid
- **L57.2** Cutis rhomboidalis nuchae
- **L57.3** Poikiloderma of Civatte
- **L57.4** Cutis laxa senilis
  - Elastosis senilis
- **L57.5** Actinic granuloma
- **L57.8** Other skin changes due to chronic exposure to nonionizing radiation
  - Farmer's skin
  - Sailor's skin
  - Solar dermatitis
- **L57.9** Skin changes due to chronic exposure to nonionizing radiation, unspecified

L58 Radiodermatitis
Use additional code to identify the source of the radiation (W88, W90)

- **L58.0** Acute radiodermatitis
- **L58.1** Chronic radiodermatitis
- **L58.9** Radiodermatitis, unspecified

L59 Other disorders of skin and subcutaneous tissue related to radiation
- **L59.0** Erythema ab igne [dermatitis ab igne]
- **L59.8** Other specified disorders of the skin and subcutaneous tissue related to radiation
  - AHA: 2017,1Q,33
- **L59.9** Disorder of the skin and subcutaneous tissue related to radiation, unspecified

Disorders of skin appendages (L60-L75)

EXCLUDES 1   congenital malformations of integument (Q84.-)

✓4th L60 Nail disorders
    EXCLUDES 2   clubbing of nails (R68.3)
                     onychia and paronychia (L03.0-)

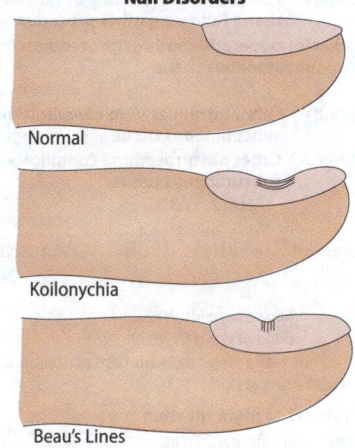

Nail Disorders — Normal, Koilonychia, Beau's Lines

- L60.0 Ingrowing nail
- L60.1 Onycholysis
- L60.2 Onychogryphosis
- L60.3 Nail dystrophy
- L60.4 Beau's lines
- L60.5 Yellow nail syndrome
- L60.8 Other nail disorders
- L60.9 Nail disorder, unspecified

L62 Nail disorders in diseases classified elsewhere
Code first underlying disease, such as:
   pachydermoperiostosis (M89.4-)

✓4th L63 Alopecia areata
- L63.0 Alopecia (capitis) totalis
- L63.1 Alopecia universalis
- L63.2 Ophiasis
- L63.8 Other alopecia areata
- L63.9 Alopecia areata, unspecified

✓4th L64 Androgenic alopecia
    INCLUDES   male-pattern baldness
- L64.0 Drug-induced androgenic alopecia
    Use additional code for adverse effect, if applicable, to identify drug (T36-T50 with fifth or sixth character 5)
- L64.8 Other androgenic alopecia
- L64.9 Androgenic alopecia, unspecified

✓4th L65 Other nonscarring hair loss
Use additional code for adverse effect, if applicable, to identify drug (T36-T50 with fifth or sixth character 5)
    EXCLUDES 1   trichotillomania (F63.3)
- L65.0 Telogen effluvium
    DEF: Form of nonscarring alopecia characterized by shedding of hair from premature telogen development in follicles due to stress, including shock, childbirth, surgery, drugs, or weight loss.
- L65.1 Anagen effluvium
- L65.2 Alopecia mucinosa
- L65.8 Other specified nonscarring hair loss
- L65.9 Nonscarring hair loss, unspecified
    Alopecia NOS

✓4th L66 Cicatricial alopecia [scarring hair loss]
- L66.0 Pseudopelade
- ✓5th L66.1 Lichen planopilaris
    AHA: 2024,4Q,23
    - L66.10 Lichen planopilaris, unspecified
    - L66.11 Classic lichen planopilaris
        Follicular lichen planus
    - L66.12 Frontal fibrosing alopecia
        FFA
    - L66.19 Other lichen planopilaris
        Lassueur Graham-Little Piccardi syndrome
- L66.2 Folliculitis decalvans
- L66.3 Perifolliculitis capitis abscedens
- L66.4 Folliculitis ulerythematosa reticulata
- ✓5th L66.8 Other cicatricial alopecia
    AHA: 2024,4Q,23; 2015,1Q,19
    - L66.81 Central centrifugal cicatricial alopecia
        CCCA
    - L66.89 Other cicatricial alopecia
- L66.9 Cicatricial alopecia, unspecified

✓4th L67 Hair color and hair shaft abnormalities
    EXCLUDES 1   monilethrix (Q84.1)
                     pili annulati (Q84.1)
                     telogen effluvium (L65.0)
- L67.0 Trichorrhexis nodosa
- L67.1 Variations in hair color
    Canities
    Greyness, hair (premature)
    Heterochromia of hair
    Poliosis circumscripta, acquired
    Poliosis NOS
- L67.8 Other hair color and hair shaft abnormalities
    Fragilitas crinium
- L67.9 Hair color and hair shaft abnormality, unspecified

✓4th L68 Hypertrichosis
    INCLUDES   excess hair
    EXCLUDES 1   congenital hypertrichosis (Q84.2)
                     persistent lanugo (Q84.2)
- L68.0 Hirsutism
- L68.1 Acquired hypertrichosis lanuginosa
- L68.2 Localized hypertrichosis
- L68.3 Polytrichia
- L68.8 Other hypertrichosis
- L68.9 Hypertrichosis, unspecified

✓4th L70 Acne
    EXCLUDES 2   acne keloid (L73.0)
- L70.0 Acne vulgaris
- L70.1 Acne conglobata
- L70.2 Acne varioliformis
    Acne necrotica miliaris
    DEF: Rare form of acne characterized by development of persistent brown papulopustules followed by scar formation. This type of acne usually presents on the brow and temporoparietal part of the scalp.
- L70.3 Acne tropica
- L70.4 Infantile acne
- L70.5 Acné excoriée
    Acné excoriée des jeunes filles
    Picker's acne
- L70.8 Other acne
- L70.9 Acne, unspecified

✓4th L71 Rosacea
Use additional code for adverse effect, if applicable, to identify drug (T36-T50 with fifth or sixth character 5)
- L71.0 Perioral dermatitis
- L71.1 Rhinophyma
- L71.8 Other rosacea
    AHA: 2018,4Q,15
- L71.9 Rosacea, unspecified

✓4th L72 Follicular cysts of skin and subcutaneous tissue
- L72.0 Epidermal cyst
- ✓5th L72.1 Pilar and trichodermal cyst
    - L72.11 Pilar cyst
    - L72.12 Trichodermal cyst
        Trichilemmal (proliferating) cyst
- L72.2 Steatocystoma multiplex
- L72.3 Sebaceous cyst
    EXCLUDES 2   pilar cyst (L72.11)
                     trichilemmal (proliferating) cyst (L72.12)
- L72.8 Other follicular cysts of the skin and subcutaneous tissue
- L72.9 Follicular cyst of the skin and subcutaneous tissue, unspecified

✓4th L73 Other follicular disorders
- L73.0 Acne keloid
- L73.1 Pseudofolliculitis barbae

Chapter 12. Diseases of the Skin and Subcutaneous Tissue

- **L73.2** Hidradenitis suppurativa
- **L73.8** Other specified follicular disorders
  - Sycosis barbae
- **L73.9** Follicular disorder, unspecified

☑4th **L74** Eccrine sweat disorders
- EXCLUDES 2: generalized hyperhidrosis (R61)
- **DEF:** Eccrine sweat glands: Glands found in the dermal and hypodermal layer of the skin throughout the body, particularly on the forehead, scalp, axillae, palms, and soles. These glands produce watery and neutral or slightly acidic sweat.
- **L74.0** Miliaria rubra
- **L74.1** Miliaria crystallina
- **L74.2** Miliaria profunda
  - Miliaria tropicalis
- **L74.3** Miliaria, unspecified
- **L74.4** Anhidrosis
  - Hypohidrosis
  - **DEF:** Inability to sweat normally. When the body can't cool itself through perspiration it can lead to heatstroke, a life-threatening condition.
- ☑5th **L74.5** Focal hyperhidrosis
  - ☑6th **L74.51** Primary focal hyperhidrosis
    - **L74.510** Primary focal hyperhidrosis, axilla
    - **L74.511** Primary focal hyperhidrosis, face
    - **L74.512** Primary focal hyperhidrosis, palms
    - **L74.513** Primary focal hyperhidrosis, soles
    - **L74.519** Primary focal hyperhidrosis, unspecified
  - **L74.52** Secondary focal hyperhidrosis
    - Frey's syndrome
- **L74.8** Other eccrine sweat disorders
- **L74.9** Eccrine sweat disorder, unspecified
  - Sweat gland disorder NOS

☑4th **L75** Apocrine sweat disorders
- EXCLUDES 1: dyshidrosis (L30.1)
  - hidradenitis suppurativa (L73.2)
- **DEF:** Apocrine sweat glands: Found in the axilla, areola, and circumanal region, these glands begin to function in puberty and produce viscid milky secretions in response to external stimuli.
- **L75.0** Bromhidrosis
- **L75.1** Chromhidrosis
- **L75.2** Apocrine miliaria
  - Fox-Fordyce disease
  - **DEF:** Chronic, usually pruritic disease evidenced by small follicular papular eruptions, especially in the axillary and pubic areas. Apocrine miliaria develops from the closure and rupture of the affected apocrine glands' intraepidermal portion of the ducts.
- **L75.8** Other apocrine sweat disorders
- **L75.9** Apocrine sweat disorder, unspecified

Intraoperative and postprocedural complications of skin and subcutaneous tissue (L76)

☑4th **L76** Intraoperative and postprocedural complications of skin and subcutaneous tissue
- AHA: 2016,4Q,9-10
- ☑5th **L76.0** Intraoperative hemorrhage and hematoma of skin and subcutaneous tissue complicating a procedure
  - EXCLUDES 1: intraoperative hemorrhage and hematoma of skin and subcutaneous tissue due to accidental puncture and laceration during a procedure (L76.1-)
  - **L76.01** Intraoperative hemorrhage and hematoma of skin and subcutaneous tissue complicating a dermatologic procedure
  - **L76.02** Intraoperative hemorrhage and hematoma of skin and subcutaneous tissue complicating other procedure
- ☑5th **L76.1** Accidental puncture and laceration of skin and subcutaneous tissue during a procedure
  - **L76.11** Accidental puncture and laceration of skin and subcutaneous tissue during a dermatologic procedure
  - **L76.12** Accidental puncture and laceration of skin and subcutaneous tissue during other procedure
- ☑5th **L76.2** Postprocedural hemorrhage of skin and subcutaneous tissue following a procedure
  - **L76.21** Postprocedural hemorrhage of skin and subcutaneous tissue following a dermatologic procedure
  - **L76.22** Postprocedural hemorrhage of skin and subcutaneous tissue following other procedure
- ☑5th **L76.3** Postprocedural hematoma and seroma of skin and subcutaneous tissue following a procedure
  - **L76.31** Postprocedural hematoma of skin and subcutaneous tissue following a dermatologic procedure
  - **L76.32** Postprocedural hematoma of skin and subcutaneous tissue following other procedure
  - **L76.33** Postprocedural seroma of skin and subcutaneous tissue following a dermatologic procedure
  - **L76.34** Postprocedural seroma of skin and subcutaneous tissue following other procedure
- ☑5th **L76.8** Other intraoperative and postprocedural complications of skin and subcutaneous tissue
  - Use additional code, if applicable, to further specify disorder
  - **L76.81** Other intraoperative complications of skin and subcutaneous tissue
  - **L76.82** Other postprocedural complications of skin and subcutaneous tissue
    - AHA: 2017,3Q,6

Other disorders of the skin and subcutaneous tissue (L80-L99)

L80 Vitiligo
- EXCLUDES 2: vitiligo of eyelids (H02.73-)
  - vitiligo of vulva (N90.89)
- **DEF:** Persistent, progressive development of nonpigmented white patches on otherwise normal skin.

☑4th **L81** Other disorders of pigmentation
- EXCLUDES 1: birthmark NOS (Q82.5)
  - Peutz-Jeghers syndrome (Q85.89)
- EXCLUDES 2: nevus - see Alphabetical Index
- **L81.0** Postinflammatory hyperpigmentation
- **L81.1** Chloasma
- **L81.2** Freckles
- **L81.3** Cafe au lait spots
- **L81.4** Other melanin hyperpigmentation
  - Lentigo
- **L81.5** Leukoderma, not elsewhere classified
- **L81.6** Other disorders of diminished melanin formation
- **L81.7** Pigmented purpuric dermatosis
  - Angioma serpiginosum
- **L81.8** Other specified disorders of pigmentation
  - Iron pigmentation
  - Tattoo pigmentation
- **L81.9** Disorder of pigmentation, unspecified

☑4th **L82** Seborrheic keratosis
- INCLUDES: basal cell papilloma
  - dermatosis papulosa nigra
  - Leser-Trélat disease
- EXCLUDES 2: seborrheic dermatitis (L21.-)
- **DEF:** Common, benign, noninvasive, lightly pigmented, warty growth composed of basaloid cells that usually appear at middle age as soft, easily crumbling plaques on the face, trunk, and extremities.
- **L82.0** Inflamed seborrheic keratosis
  - AHA: 2023,2Q,12; 2021,3Q,10
- **L82.1** Other seborrheic keratosis
  - Seborrheic keratosis NOS

L83 Acanthosis nigricans
- Confluent and reticulated papillomatosis
- **DEF:** Diffuse, velvety hyperplasia of the spinous skin layer of the axilla and other body folds marked by gray, brown, or black pigmentation. In adult form, it is often associated with malignant acanthosis nigricans in a benign, nevoid form relatively generalized.

L84 Corns and callosities
- Callus
- Clavus

☑4th **L85** Other epidermal thickening
- EXCLUDES 2: hypertrophic disorders of the skin (L91.-)
- **L85.0** Acquired ichthyosis
  - EXCLUDES 1: congenital ichthyosis (Q80.-)
- **L85.1** Acquired keratosis [keratoderma] palmaris et plantaris
  - EXCLUDES 1: inherited keratosis palmaris et plantaris (Q82.8)
- **L85.2** Keratosis punctata (palmaris et plantaris)
- **L85.3** Xerosis cutis
  - Dry skin dermatitis
- **L85.8** Other specified epidermal thickening
  - Cutaneous horn
- **L85.9** Epidermal thickening, unspecified

L86 Keratoderma in diseases classified elsewhere

Code first underlying disease, such as:
Reiter's disease (M02.3-)

EXCLUDES 1
- gonococcal keratoderma (A54.89)
- gonococcal keratosis (A54.89)
- keratoderma due to vitamin A deficiency (E50.8)
- keratosis due to vitamin A deficiency (E50.8)
- xeroderma due to vitamin A deficiency (E50.8)

✓4th L87 Transepidermal elimination disorders

EXCLUDES 1 granuloma annulare (perforating) (L92.0)

L87.0 Keratosis follicularis et parafollicularis in cutem penetrans
- Hyperkeratosis follicularis penetrans
- Kyrle disease

L87.1 Reactive perforating collagenosis

L87.2 Elastosis perforans serpiginosa

L87.8 Other transepidermal elimination disorders

L87.9 Transepidermal elimination disorder, unspecified

L88 Pyoderma gangrenosum   HCC Rx COM
Phagedenic pyoderma

EXCLUDES 1 dermatitis gangrenosa (L08.0)

DEF: Persistent debilitating skin disease characterized by irregular, boggy, blue-red ulcerations, with central healing and undermined edges.

✓4th L89 Pressure ulcer

INCLUDES
- bed sore
- decubitus ulcer
- plaster ulcer
- pressure area
- pressure sore

Code first any associated gangrene (I96)

EXCLUDES 2
- decubitus (trophic) ulcer of cervix (uteri) (N86)
- diabetic ulcers (E08.621, E08.622, E09.621, E09.622, E10.621, E10.622, E11.621, E11.622, E13.621, E13.622)
- non-pressure chronic ulcer of skin (L97.-)
- skin infections (L00-L08)
- varicose ulcer (I83.0, I83.2)

AHA: 2022,2Q,8; 2021,1Q,24; 2019,4Q,10-11,54; 2018,4Q,69; 2018,3Q,3; 2018,2Q,21; 2017,4Q,109; 2017,1Q,49; 2016,4Q,143

TIP: The stage of a diagnosed pressure ulcer can be based on documentation from clinicians who are not the patient's provider.

Four Stages of Pressure Ulcer

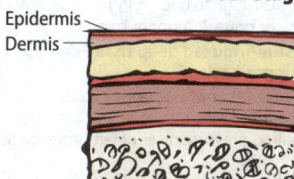

Stage 1
Persistent focal edema

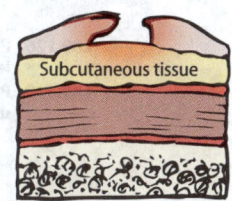

Stage 2
Abrasion, blister, partial thickness skin loss involving epidermis and/or dermis

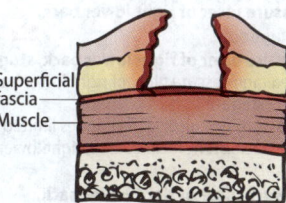

Stage 3
Full thickness skin loss involving damage or necrosis of subcutaneous tissue

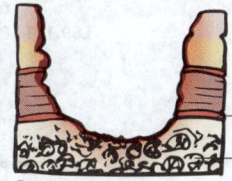

Stage 4
Necrosis of soft tissues through to underlying muscle, tendon, or bone

✓5th L89.0 Pressure ulcer of elbow

✓6th L89.00 Pressure ulcer of unspecified elbow

L89.000 Pressure ulcer of unspecified elbow, unstageable   HCC ESR

L89.001 Pressure ulcer of unspecified elbow, stage 1
- Healing pressure ulcer of unspecified elbow, stage 1
- Pressure pre-ulcer skin changes limited to persistent focal edema, unspecified elbow

L89.002 Pressure ulcer of unspecified elbow, stage 2   HCC ESR
- Healing pressure ulcer of unspecified elbow, stage 2
- Pressure ulcer with abrasion, blister, partial thickness skin loss involving epidermis and/or dermis, unspecified elbow

L89.003 Pressure ulcer of unspecified elbow, stage 3   HCC ESR
- Healing pressure ulcer of unspecified elbow, stage 3
- Pressure ulcer with full thickness skin loss involving damage or necrosis of subcutaneous tissue, unspecified elbow

L89.004 Pressure ulcer of unspecified elbow, stage 4   HCC ESR
- Healing pressure ulcer of unspecified elbow, stage 4
- Pressure ulcer with necrosis of soft tissues through to underlying muscle, tendon, or bone, unspecified elbow

L89.006 Pressure-induced deep tissue damage of unspecified elbow

L89.009 Pressure ulcer of unspecified elbow, unspecified stage
- Healing pressure ulcer of elbow NOS
- Healing pressure ulcer of unspecified elbow, unspecified stage

✓6th L89.01 Pressure ulcer of right elbow

L89.010 Pressure ulcer of right elbow, unstageable   HCC ESR

L89.011 Pressure ulcer of right elbow, stage 1
- Healing pressure ulcer of right elbow, stage 1
- Pressure pre-ulcer skin changes limited to persistent focal edema, right elbow

L89.012 Pressure ulcer of right elbow, stage 2   HCC ESR
- Healing pressure ulcer of right elbow, stage 2
- Pressure ulcer with abrasion, blister, partial thickness skin loss involving epidermis and/or dermis, right elbow

L89.013 Pressure ulcer of right elbow, stage 3   HCC ESR
- Healing pressure ulcer of right elbow, stage 3
- Pressure ulcer with full thickness skin loss involving damage or necrosis of subcutaneous tissue, right elbow

L89.014 Pressure ulcer of right elbow, stage 4   HCC ESR
- Healing pressure ulcer of right elbow, stage 4
- Pressure ulcer with necrosis of soft tissues through to underlying muscle, tendon, or bone, right elbow

L89.016 Pressure-induced deep tissue damage of right elbow

L89.019 Pressure ulcer of right elbow, unspecified stage
- Healing pressure ulcer of right elbow NOS

✓6th L89.02 Pressure ulcer of left elbow

L89.020 Pressure ulcer of left elbow, unstageable   HCC ESR

L89.021 Pressure ulcer of left elbow, stage 1
- Healing pressure ulcer of left elbow, stage 1
- Pressure pre-ulcer skin changes limited to persistent focal edema, left elbow

L89.022 Pressure ulcer of left elbow, stage 2   HCC ESR
- Healing pressure ulcer of left elbow, stage 2
- Pressure ulcer with abrasion, blister, partial thickness skin loss involving epidermis and/or dermis, left elbow

L89.023 Pressure ulcer of left elbow, stage 3   HCC ESR
- Healing pressure ulcer of left elbow, stage 3
- Pressure ulcer with full thickness skin loss involving damage or necrosis of subcutaneous tissue, left elbow

L89.024 **Pressure ulcer of left elbow, stage 4** `HCC` `ESR`
  Healing pressure ulcer of left elbow, stage 4
  Pressure ulcer with necrosis of soft tissues through to underlying muscle, tendon, or bone, left elbow

L89.026 **Pressure-induced deep tissue damage of left elbow**

L89.029 **Pressure ulcer of left elbow, unspecified stage**
  Healing pressure ulcer of left elbow NOS

L89.1 Pressure ulcer of back

L89.10 Pressure ulcer of unspecified part of back

L89.100 **Pressure ulcer of unspecified part of back, unstageable** `HCC` `ESR`

L89.101 **Pressure ulcer of unspecified part of back, stage 1**
  Healing pressure ulcer of unspecified part of back, stage 1
  Pressure pre-ulcer skin changes limited to persistent focal edema, unspecified part of back

L89.102 **Pressure ulcer of unspecified part of back, stage 2** `HCC` `ESR`
  Healing pressure ulcer of unspecified part of back, stage 2
  Pressure ulcer with abrasion, blister, partial thickness skin loss involving epidermis and/or dermis, unspecified part of back

L89.103 **Pressure ulcer of unspecified part of back, stage 3** `HCC` `ESR`
  Healing pressure ulcer of unspecified part of back, stage 3
  Pressure ulcer with full thickness skin loss involving damage or necrosis of subcutaneous tissue, unspecified part of back

L89.104 **Pressure ulcer of unspecified part of back, stage 4** `HCC` `ESR`
  Healing pressure ulcer of unspecified part of back, stage 4
  Pressure ulcer with necrosis of soft tissues through to underlying muscle, tendon, or bone, unspecified part of back

L89.106 **Pressure-induced deep tissue damage of unspecified part of back**

L89.109 **Pressure ulcer of unspecified part of back, unspecified stage**
  Healing pressure ulcer of unspecified part of back NOS
  Healing pressure ulcer of unspecified part of back, unspecified stage

L89.11 Pressure ulcer of right upper back
  Pressure ulcer of right shoulder blade

L89.110 **Pressure ulcer of right upper back, unstageable** `HCC` `ESR`

L89.111 **Pressure ulcer of right upper back, stage 1**
  Healing pressure ulcer of right upper back, stage 1
  Pressure pre-ulcer skin changes limited to persistent focal edema, right upper back

L89.112 **Pressure ulcer of right upper back, stage 2** `HCC` `ESR`
  Healing pressure ulcer of right upper back, stage 2
  Pressure ulcer with abrasion, blister, partial thickness skin loss involving epidermis and/or dermis, right upper back

L89.113 **Pressure ulcer of right upper back, stage 3** `HCC` `ESR`
  Healing pressure ulcer of right upper back, stage 3
  Pressure ulcer with full thickness skin loss involving damage or necrosis of subcutaneous tissue, right upper back

L89.114 **Pressure ulcer of right upper back, stage 4** `HCC` `ESR`
  Healing pressure ulcer of right upper back, stage 4
  Pressure ulcer with necrosis of soft tissues through to underlying muscle, tendon, or bone, right upper back

L89.116 **Pressure-induced deep tissue damage of right upper back**

L89.119 **Pressure ulcer of right upper back, unspecified stage**
  Healing pressure ulcer of right upper back NOS
  Healing pressure ulcer of right upper back, unspecified stage

L89.12 Pressure ulcer of left upper back
  Pressure ulcer of left shoulder blade

L89.120 **Pressure ulcer of left upper back, unstageable** `HCC` `ESR`

L89.121 **Pressure ulcer of left upper back, stage 1**
  Healing pressure ulcer of left upper back, stage 1
  Pressure pre-ulcer skin changes limited to persistent focal edema, left upper back

L89.122 **Pressure ulcer of left upper back, stage 2** `HCC` `ESR`
  Healing pressure ulcer of left upper back, stage 2
  Pressure ulcer with abrasion, blister, partial thickness skin loss involving epidermis and/or dermis, left upper back

L89.123 **Pressure ulcer of left upper back, stage 3** `HCC` `ESR`
  Healing pressure ulcer of left upper back, stage 3
  Pressure ulcer with full thickness skin loss involving damage or necrosis of subcutaneous tissue, left upper back

L89.124 **Pressure ulcer of left upper back, stage 4** `HCC` `ESR`
  Healing pressure ulcer of left upper back, stage 4
  Pressure ulcer with necrosis of soft tissues through to underlying muscle, tendon, or bone, left upper back

L89.126 **Pressure-induced deep tissue damage of left upper back**

L89.129 **Pressure ulcer of left upper back, unspecified stage**
  Healing pressure ulcer of left upper back NOS
  Healing pressure ulcer of left upper back, unspecified stage

L89.13 Pressure ulcer of right lower back

L89.130 **Pressure ulcer of right lower back, unstageable** `HCC` `ESR`

L89.131 **Pressure ulcer of right lower back, stage 1**
  Healing pressure ulcer of right lower back, stage 1
  Pressure pre-ulcer skin changes limited to persistent focal edema, right lower back

L89.132 **Pressure ulcer of right lower back, stage 2** `HCC` `ESR`
  Healing pressure ulcer of right lower back, stage 2
  Pressure ulcer with abrasion, blister, partial thickness skin loss involving epidermis and/or dermis, right lower back

L89.133 **Pressure ulcer of right lower back, stage 3** `HCC` `ESR`
  Healing pressure ulcer of right lower back, stage 3
  Pressure ulcer with full thickness skin loss involving damage or necrosis of subcutaneous tissue, right lower back

L89.134 **Pressure ulcer of right lower back, stage 4**
 Healing pressure ulcer of right lower back, stage 4
 Pressure ulcer with necrosis of soft tissues through to underlying muscle, tendon, or bone, right lower back

L89.136 **Pressure-induced deep tissue damage of right lower back**

L89.139 **Pressure ulcer of right lower back, unspecified stage**
 Healing pressure ulcer of right lower back NOS
 Healing pressure ulcer of right lower back, unspecified stage

L89.14 **Pressure ulcer of left lower back**

L89.140 **Pressure ulcer of left lower back, unstageable**

L89.141 **Pressure ulcer of left lower back, stage 1**
 Healing pressure ulcer of left lower back, stage 1
 Pressure pre-ulcer skin changes limited to persistent focal edema, left lower back

L89.142 **Pressure ulcer of left lower back, stage 2**
 Healing pressure ulcer of left lower back, stage 2
 Pressure ulcer with abrasion, blister, partial thickness skin loss involving epidermis and/or dermis, left lower back

L89.143 **Pressure ulcer of left lower back, stage 3**
 Healing pressure ulcer of left lower back, stage 3
 Pressure ulcer with full thickness skin loss involving damage or necrosis of subcutaneous tissue, left lower back

L89.144 **Pressure ulcer of left lower back, stage 4**
 Healing pressure ulcer of left lower back, stage 4
 Pressure ulcer with necrosis of soft tissues through to underlying muscle, tendon, or bone, left lower back

L89.146 **Pressure-induced deep tissue damage of left lower back**

L89.149 **Pressure ulcer of left lower back, unspecified stage**
 Healing pressure ulcer of left lower back NOS
 Healing pressure ulcer of left lower back, unspecified stage

L89.15 **Pressure ulcer of sacral region**
 Pressure ulcer of coccyx
 Pressure ulcer of tailbone
 AHA: 2021,3Q,10

L89.150 **Pressure ulcer of sacral region, unstageable**

L89.151 **Pressure ulcer of sacral region, stage 1**
 Healing pressure ulcer of sacral region, stage 1
 Pressure pre-ulcer skin changes limited to persistent focal edema, sacral region

L89.152 **Pressure ulcer of sacral region, stage 2**
 Healing pressure ulcer of sacral region, stage 2
 Pressure ulcer with abrasion, blister, partial thickness skin loss involving epidermis and/or dermis, sacral region

L89.153 **Pressure ulcer of sacral region, stage 3**
 Healing pressure ulcer of sacral region, stage 3
 Pressure ulcer with full thickness skin loss involving damage or necrosis of subcutaneous tissue, sacral region

L89.154 **Pressure ulcer of sacral region, stage 4**
 Healing pressure ulcer of sacral region, stage 4
 Pressure ulcer with necrosis of soft tissues through to underlying muscle, tendon, or bone, sacral region
 AHA: 2022,2Q,8

L89.156 **Pressure-induced deep tissue damage of sacral region**

L89.159 **Pressure ulcer of sacral region, unspecified stage**
 Healing pressure ulcer of sacral region NOS
 Healing pressure ulcer of sacral region, unspecified stage

L89.2 **Pressure ulcer of hip**

L89.20 **Pressure ulcer of unspecified hip**

L89.200 **Pressure ulcer of unspecified hip, unstageable**

L89.201 **Pressure ulcer of unspecified hip, stage 1**
 Healing pressure ulcer of unspecified hip back, stage 1
 Pressure pre-ulcer skin changes limited to persistent focal edema, unspecified hip

L89.202 **Pressure ulcer of unspecified hip, stage 2**
 Healing pressure ulcer of unspecified hip, stage 2
 Pressure ulcer with abrasion, blister, partial thickness skin loss involving epidermis and/or dermis, unspecified hip

L89.203 **Pressure ulcer of unspecified hip, stage 3**
 Healing pressure ulcer of unspecified hip, stage 3
 Pressure ulcer with full thickness skin loss involving damage or necrosis of subcutaneous tissue, unspecified hip

L89.204 **Pressure ulcer of unspecified hip, stage 4**
 Healing pressure ulcer of unspecified hip, stage 4
 Pressure ulcer with necrosis of soft tissues through to underlying muscle, tendon, or bone, unspecified hip

L89.206 **Pressure-induced deep tissue damage of unspecified hip**

L89.209 **Pressure ulcer of unspecified hip, unspecified stage**
 Healing pressure ulcer of unspecified hip NOS
 Healing pressure ulcer of unspecified hip, unspecified stage

L89.21 **Pressure ulcer of right hip**

L89.210 **Pressure ulcer of right hip, unstageable**

L89.211 **Pressure ulcer of right hip, stage 1**
 Healing pressure ulcer of right hip back, stage 1
 Pressure pre-ulcer skin changes limited to persistent focal edema, right hip

L89.212 **Pressure ulcer of right hip, stage 2**
 Healing pressure ulcer of right hip, stage 2
 Pressure ulcer with abrasion, blister, partial thickness skin loss involving epidermis and/or dermis, right hip

L89.213 **Pressure ulcer of right hip, stage 3**
 Healing pressure ulcer of right hip, stage 3
 Pressure ulcer with full thickness skin loss involving damage or necrosis of subcutaneous tissue, right hip

L89.214 **Pressure ulcer of right hip, stage 4**
 Healing pressure ulcer of right hip, stage 4
 Pressure ulcer with necrosis of soft tissues through to underlying muscle, tendon, or bone, right hip

L89.216 **Pressure-induced deep tissue damage of right hip**

- **L89.219** Pressure ulcer of right hip, unspecified stage
  - Healing pressure ulcer of right hip NOS
  - Healing pressure ulcer of right hip, unspecified stage

- **L89.22** Pressure ulcer of left hip
  - **L89.220** Pressure ulcer of left hip, unstageable [HCC] [ESR]
  - **L89.221** Pressure ulcer of left hip, stage 1
    - Healing pressure ulcer of left hip back, stage 1
    - Pressure pre-ulcer skin changes limited to persistent focal edema, left hip
  - **L89.222** Pressure ulcer of left hip, stage 2 [HCC] [ESR]
    - Healing pressure ulcer of left hip, stage 2
    - Pressure ulcer with abrasion, blister, partial thickness skin loss involving epidermis and/or dermis, left hip
  - **L89.223** Pressure ulcer of left hip, stage 3 [HCC] [ESR]
    - Healing pressure ulcer of left hip, stage 3
    - Pressure ulcer with full thickness skin loss involving damage or necrosis of subcutaneous tissue, left hip
  - **L89.224** Pressure ulcer of left hip, stage 4 [HCC] [ESR]
    - Healing pressure ulcer of left hip, stage 4
    - Pressure ulcer with necrosis of soft tissues through to underlying muscle, tendon, or bone, left hip
  - **L89.226** Pressure-induced deep tissue damage of left hip
  - **L89.229** Pressure ulcer of left hip, unspecified stage
    - Healing pressure ulcer of left hip NOS
    - Healing pressure ulcer of left hip, unspecified stage

- **L89.3** Pressure ulcer of buttock
  - AHA: 2021,3Q,10
  - **L89.30** Pressure ulcer of unspecified buttock
    - **L89.300** Pressure ulcer of unspecified buttock, unstageable [HCC] [ESR]
    - **L89.301** Pressure ulcer of unspecified buttock, stage 1
      - Healing pressure ulcer of unspecified buttock, stage 1
      - Pressure pre-ulcer skin changes limited to persistent focal edema, unspecified buttock
    - **L89.302** Pressure ulcer of unspecified buttock, stage 2 [HCC] [ESR]
      - Healing pressure ulcer of unspecified buttock, stage 2
      - Pressure ulcer with abrasion, blister, partial thickness skin loss involving epidermis and/or dermis, unspecified buttock
    - **L89.303** Pressure ulcer of unspecified buttock, stage 3 [HCC] [ESR]
      - Healing pressure ulcer of unspecified buttock, stage 3
      - Pressure ulcer with full thickness skin loss involving damage or necrosis of subcutaneous tissue, unspecified buttock
    - **L89.304** Pressure ulcer of unspecified buttock, stage 4 [HCC] [ESR]
      - Healing pressure ulcer of unspecified buttock, stage 4
      - Pressure ulcer with necrosis of soft tissues through to underlying muscle, tendon, or bone, unspecified buttock
    - **L89.306** Pressure-induced deep tissue damage of unspecified buttock
    - **L89.309** Pressure ulcer of unspecified buttock, unspecified stage
      - Healing pressure ulcer of unspecified buttock NOS
      - Healing pressure ulcer of unspecified buttock, unspecified stage
  - **L89.31** Pressure ulcer of right buttock
    - **L89.310** Pressure ulcer of right buttock, unstageable [HCC] [ESR]
    - **L89.311** Pressure ulcer of right buttock, stage 1
      - Healing pressure ulcer of right buttock, stage 1
      - Pressure pre-ulcer skin changes limited to persistent focal edema, right buttock
    - **L89.312** Pressure ulcer of right buttock, stage 2 [HCC] [ESR]
      - Healing pressure ulcer of right buttock, stage 2
      - Pressure ulcer with abrasion, blister, partial thickness skin loss involving epidermis and/or dermis, right buttock
    - **L89.313** Pressure ulcer of right buttock, stage 3 [HCC] [ESR]
      - Healing pressure ulcer of right buttock, stage 3
      - Pressure ulcer with full thickness skin loss involving damage or necrosis of subcutaneous tissue, right buttock
    - **L89.314** Pressure ulcer of right buttock, stage 4 [HCC] [ESR]
      - Healing pressure ulcer of right buttock, stage 4
      - Pressure ulcer with necrosis of soft tissues through to underlying muscle, tendon, or bone, right buttock
    - **L89.316** Pressure-induced deep tissue damage of right buttock
    - **L89.319** Pressure ulcer of right buttock, unspecified stage
      - Healing pressure ulcer of right buttock NOS
      - Healing pressure ulcer of right buttock, unspecified stage
  - **L89.32** Pressure ulcer of left buttock
    - **L89.320** Pressure ulcer of left buttock, unstageable [HCC] [ESR]
    - **L89.321** Pressure ulcer of left buttock, stage 1
      - Healing pressure ulcer of left buttock, stage 1
      - Pressure pre-ulcer skin changes limited to persistent focal edema, left buttock
    - **L89.322** Pressure ulcer of left buttock, stage 2 [HCC] [ESR]
      - Healing pressure ulcer of left buttock, stage 2
      - Pressure ulcer with abrasion, blister, partial thickness skin loss involving epidermis and/or dermis, left buttock
    - **L89.323** Pressure ulcer of left buttock, stage 3 [HCC] [ESR]
      - Healing pressure ulcer of left buttock, stage 3
      - Pressure ulcer with full thickness skin loss involving damage or necrosis of subcutaneous tissue, left buttock
    - **L89.324** Pressure ulcer of left buttock, stage 4 [HCC] [ESR]
      - Healing pressure ulcer of left buttock, stage 4
      - Pressure ulcer with necrosis of soft tissues through to underlying muscle, tendon, or bone, left buttock
    - **L89.326** Pressure-induced deep tissue damage of left buttock
    - **L89.329** Pressure ulcer of left buttock, unspecified stage
      - Healing pressure ulcer of left buttock NOS
      - Healing pressure ulcer of left buttock, unspecified stage

- **L89.4** Pressure ulcer of contiguous site of back, buttock and hip
  - **L89.40** Pressure ulcer of contiguous site of back, buttock and hip, unspecified stage
    - Healing pressure ulcer of contiguous site of back, buttock and hip NOS
    - Healing pressure ulcer of contiguous site of back, buttock and hip, unspecified stage

L89.41 **Pressure ulcer of contiguous site of back, buttock and hip, stage 1**
Healing pressure ulcer of contiguous site of back, buttock and hip, stage 1
Pressure pre-ulcer skin changes limited to persistent focal edema, contiguous site of back, buttock and hip

L89.42 **Pressure ulcer of contiguous site of back, buttock and hip, stage 2** HCC ESR
Healing pressure ulcer of contiguous site of back, buttock and hip, stage 2
Pressure ulcer with abrasion, blister, partial thickness skin loss involving epidermis and/or dermis, contiguous site of back, buttock and hip

L89.43 **Pressure ulcer of contiguous site of back, buttock and hip, stage 3** HCC ESR
Healing pressure ulcer of contiguous site of back, buttock and hip, stage 3
Pressure ulcer with full thickness skin loss involving damage or necrosis of subcutaneous tissue, contiguous site of back, buttock and hip

L89.44 **Pressure ulcer of contiguous site of back, buttock and hip, stage 4** HCC ESR
Healing pressure ulcer of contiguous site of back, buttock and hip, stage 4
Pressure ulcer with necrosis of soft tissues through to underlying muscle, tendon, or bone, contiguous site of back, buttock and hip

L89.45 **Pressure ulcer of contiguous site of back, buttock and hip, unstageable** HCC ESR

L89.46 **Pressure-induced deep tissue damage of contiguous site of back, buttock and hip**

✓5th **L89.5** **Pressure ulcer of ankle**

✓6th **L89.50** **Pressure ulcer of unspecified ankle**

L89.500 **Pressure ulcer of unspecified ankle, unstageable** HCC ESR

L89.501 **Pressure ulcer of unspecified ankle, stage 1**
Healing pressure ulcer of unspecified ankle, stage 1
Pressure pre-ulcer skin changes limited to persistent focal edema, unspecified ankle

L89.502 **Pressure ulcer of unspecified ankle, stage 2** HCC ESR
Healing pressure ulcer of unspecified ankle, stage 2
Pressure ulcer with abrasion, blister, partial thickness skin loss involving epidermis and/or dermis, unspecified ankle

L89.503 **Pressure ulcer of unspecified ankle, stage 3** HCC ESR
Healing pressure ulcer of unspecified ankle, stage 3
Pressure ulcer with full thickness skin loss involving damage or necrosis of subcutaneous tissue, unspecified ankle

L89.504 **Pressure ulcer of unspecified ankle, stage 4** HCC ESR
Healing pressure ulcer of unspecified ankle, stage 4
Pressure ulcer with necrosis of soft tissues through to underlying muscle, tendon, or bone, unspecified ankle

L89.506 **Pressure-induced deep tissue damage of unspecified ankle**

L89.509 **Pressure ulcer of unspecified ankle, unspecified stage**
Healing pressure ulcer of unspecified ankle NOS
Healing pressure ulcer of unspecified ankle, unspecified stage

✓6th **L89.51** **Pressure ulcer of right ankle**

L89.510 **Pressure ulcer of right ankle, unstageable** HCC ESR

L89.511 **Pressure ulcer of right ankle, stage 1**
Healing pressure ulcer of right ankle, stage 1
Pressure pre-ulcer skin changes limited to persistent focal edema, right ankle

L89.512 **Pressure ulcer of right ankle, stage 2** HCC ESR
Healing pressure ulcer of right ankle, stage 2
Pressure ulcer with abrasion, blister, partial thickness skin loss involving epidermis and/or dermis, right ankle

L89.513 **Pressure ulcer of right ankle, stage 3** HCC ESR
Healing pressure ulcer of right ankle, stage 3
Pressure ulcer with full thickness skin loss involving damage or necrosis of subcutaneous tissue, right ankle

L89.514 **Pressure ulcer of right ankle, stage 4** HCC ESR
Healing pressure ulcer of right ankle, stage 4
Pressure ulcer with necrosis of soft tissues through to underlying muscle, tendon, or bone, right ankle

L89.516 **Pressure-induced deep tissue damage of right ankle**

L89.519 **Pressure ulcer of right ankle, unspecified stage**
Healing pressure ulcer of right ankle NOS
Healing pressure ulcer of right ankle, unspecified stage

✓6th **L89.52** **Pressure ulcer of left ankle**

L89.520 **Pressure ulcer of left ankle, unstageable** HCC ESR

L89.521 **Pressure ulcer of left ankle, stage 1**
Healing pressure ulcer of left ankle, stage 1
Pressure pre-ulcer skin changes limited to persistent focal edema, left ankle

L89.522 **Pressure ulcer of left ankle, stage 2** HCC ESR
Healing pressure ulcer of left ankle, stage 2
Pressure ulcer with abrasion, blister, partial thickness skin loss involving epidermis and/or dermis, left ankle

L89.523 **Pressure ulcer of left ankle, stage 3** HCC ESR
Healing pressure ulcer of left ankle, stage 3
Pressure ulcer with full thickness skin loss involving damage or necrosis of subcutaneous tissue, left ankle

L89.524 **Pressure ulcer of left ankle, stage 4** HCC ESR
Healing pressure ulcer of left ankle, stage 4
Pressure ulcer with necrosis of soft tissues through to underlying muscle, tendon, or bone, left ankle

L89.526 **Pressure-induced deep tissue damage of left ankle**

L89.529 **Pressure ulcer of left ankle, unspecified stage**
Healing pressure ulcer of left ankle NOS
Healing pressure ulcer of left ankle, unspecified stage

✓5th **L89.6** **Pressure ulcer of heel**

✓6th **L89.60** **Pressure ulcer of unspecified heel**

L89.600 **Pressure ulcer of unspecified heel, unstageable** HCC ESR

L89.601 **Pressure ulcer of unspecified heel, stage 1**
Healing pressure ulcer of unspecified heel, stage 1
Pressure pre-ulcer skin changes limited to persistent focal edema, unspecified heel

L89.602 **Pressure ulcer of unspecified heel, stage 2** HCC ESR
Healing pressure ulcer of unspecified heel, stage 2
Pressure ulcer with abrasion, blister, partial thickness skin loss involving epidermis and/or dermis, unspecified heel

L89.603 **Pressure ulcer of unspecified heel, stage 3** HCC ESR
Healing pressure ulcer of unspecified heel, stage 3
Pressure ulcer with full thickness skin loss involving damage or necrosis of subcutaneous tissue, unspecified heel

- **L89.604** Pressure ulcer of unspecified heel, stage 4
  - Healing pressure ulcer of unspecified heel, stage 4
  - Pressure ulcer with necrosis of soft tissues through to underlying muscle, tendon, or bone, unspecified heel
- **L89.606** Pressure-induced deep tissue damage of unspecified heel
- **L89.609** Pressure ulcer of unspecified heel, unspecified stage
  - Healing pressure ulcer of unspecified heel NOS
  - Healing pressure ulcer of unspecified heel, unspecified stage

L89.61 Pressure ulcer of right heel
- **L89.610** Pressure ulcer of right heel, unstageable
- **L89.611** Pressure ulcer of right heel, stage 1
  - Healing pressure ulcer of right heel, stage 1
  - Pressure pre-ulcer skin changes limited to persistent focal edema, right heel
- **L89.612** Pressure ulcer of right heel, stage 2
  - Healing pressure ulcer of right heel, stage 2
  - Pressure ulcer with abrasion, blister, partial thickness skin loss involving epidermis and/or dermis, right heel
- **L89.613** Pressure ulcer of right heel, stage 3
  - Healing pressure ulcer of right heel, stage 3
  - Pressure ulcer with full thickness skin loss involving damage or necrosis of subcutaneous tissue, right heel
- **L89.614** Pressure ulcer of right heel, stage 4
  - Healing pressure ulcer of right heel, stage 4
  - Pressure ulcer with necrosis of soft tissues through to underlying muscle, tendon, or bone, right heel
- **L89.616** Pressure-induced deep tissue damage of right heel
- **L89.619** Pressure ulcer of right heel, unspecified stage
  - Healing pressure ulcer of right heel NOS
  - Healing pressure ulcer of right heel, unspecified stage

L89.62 Pressure ulcer of left heel
- **L89.620** Pressure ulcer of left heel, unstageable
- **L89.621** Pressure ulcer of left heel, stage 1
  - Healing pressure ulcer of left heel, stage 1
  - Pressure pre-ulcer skin changes limited to persistent focal edema, left heel
- **L89.622** Pressure ulcer of left heel, stage 2
  - Healing pressure ulcer of left heel, stage 2
  - Pressure ulcer with abrasion, blister, partial thickness skin loss involving epidermis and/or dermis, left heel
- **L89.623** Pressure ulcer of left heel, stage 3
  - Healing pressure ulcer of left heel, stage 3
  - Pressure ulcer with full thickness skin loss involving damage or necrosis of subcutaneous tissue, left heel
- **L89.624** Pressure ulcer of left heel, stage 4
  - Healing pressure ulcer of left heel, stage 4
  - Pressure ulcer with necrosis of soft tissues through to underlying muscle, tendon, or bone, left heel
- **L89.626** Pressure-induced deep tissue damage of left heel
- **L89.629** Pressure ulcer of left heel, unspecified stage
  - Healing pressure ulcer of left heel NOS
  - Healing pressure ulcer of left heel, unspecified stage

L89.8 Pressure ulcer of other site

L89.81 Pressure ulcer of head
Pressure ulcer of face
- **L89.810** Pressure ulcer of head, unstageable
- **L89.811** Pressure ulcer of head, stage 1
  - Healing pressure ulcer of head, stage 1
  - Pressure pre-ulcer skin changes limited to persistent focal edema, head
- **L89.812** Pressure ulcer of head, stage 2
  - Healing pressure ulcer of head, stage 2
  - Pressure ulcer with abrasion, blister, partial thickness skin loss involving epidermis and/or dermis, head
- **L89.813** Pressure ulcer of head, stage 3
  - Healing pressure ulcer of head, stage 3
  - Pressure ulcer with full thickness skin loss involving damage or necrosis of subcutaneous tissue, head
- **L89.814** Pressure ulcer of head, stage 4
  - Healing pressure ulcer of head, stage 4
  - Pressure ulcer with necrosis of soft tissues through to underlying muscle, tendon, or bone, head
- **L89.816** Pressure-induced deep tissue damage of head
- **L89.819** Pressure ulcer of head, unspecified stage
  - Healing pressure ulcer of head NOS
  - Healing pressure ulcer of head, unspecified stage

L89.89 Pressure ulcer of other site
- **L89.890** Pressure ulcer of other site, unstageable
- **L89.891** Pressure ulcer of other site, stage 1
  - Healing pressure ulcer of other site, stage 1
  - Pressure pre-ulcer skin changes limited to persistent focal edema, other site
- **L89.892** Pressure ulcer of other site, stage 2
  - Healing pressure ulcer of other site, stage 2
  - Pressure ulcer with abrasion, blister, partial thickness skin loss involving epidermis and/or dermis, other site
- **L89.893** Pressure ulcer of other site, stage 3
  - Healing pressure ulcer of other site, stage 3
  - Pressure ulcer with full thickness skin loss involving damage or necrosis of subcutaneous tissue, other site
- **L89.894** Pressure ulcer of other site, stage 4
  - Healing pressure ulcer of other site, stage 4
  - Pressure ulcer with necrosis of soft tissues through to underlying muscle, tendon, or bone, other site
- **L89.896** Pressure-induced deep tissue damage of other site
- **L89.899** Pressure ulcer of other site, unspecified stage
  - Healing pressure ulcer of other site NOS
  - Healing pressure ulcer of other site, unspecified stage

L89.9 Pressure ulcer of unspecified site
- **L89.90** Pressure ulcer of unspecified site, unspecified stage
  - Healing pressure ulcer of unspecified site NOS
  - Healing pressure ulcer of unspecified site, unspecified stage
- **L89.91** Pressure ulcer of unspecified site, stage 1
  - Healing pressure ulcer of unspecified site, stage 1
  - Pressure pre-ulcer skin changes limited to persistent focal edema, unspecified site
- **L89.92** Pressure ulcer of unspecified site, stage 2
  - Healing pressure ulcer of unspecified site, stage 2
  - Pressure ulcer with abrasion, blister, partial thickness skin loss involving epidermis and/or dermis, unspecified site
- **L89.93** Pressure ulcer of unspecified site, stage 3
  - Healing pressure ulcer of unspecified site, stage 3
  - Pressure ulcer with full thickness skin loss involving damage or necrosis of subcutaneous tissue, unspecified site

Chapter 12. Diseases of the Skin and Subcutaneous Tissue

L89.94 Pressure ulcer of unspecified site, stage 4
 Healing pressure ulcer of unspecified site, stage 4
 Pressure ulcer with necrosis of soft tissues through to underlying muscle, tendon, or bone, unspecified site

L89.95 Pressure ulcer of unspecified site, unstageable

L89.96 Pressure-induced deep tissue damage of unspecified site

L90 Atrophic disorders of skin

L90.0 Lichen sclerosus et atrophicus
 EXCLUDES 2: lichen sclerosus of external female genital organs (N90.4)
 lichen sclerosus of external male genital organs (N48.0)

L90.1 Anetoderma of Schweninger-Buzzi

L90.2 Anetoderma of Jadassohn-Pellizzari

L90.3 Atrophoderma of Pasini and Pierini

L90.4 Acrodermatitis chronica atrophicans

L90.5 Scar conditions and fibrosis of skin
 Adherent scar (skin)
 Cicatrix
 Disfigurement of skin due to scar
 Fibrosis of skin NOS
 Scar NOS
 EXCLUDES 2: hypertrophic scar (L91.0)
 keloid scar (L91.0)
 AHA: 2016,2Q,5; 2015,1Q,19

L90.6 Striae atrophicae

L90.8 Other atrophic disorders of skin

L90.9 Atrophic disorder of skin, unspecified

L91 Hypertrophic disorders of skin

L91.0 Hypertrophic scar
 Keloid
 Keloid scar
 EXCLUDES 2: acne keloid (L73.0)
 scar NOS (L90.5)
 DEF: Overgrowth of scar tissue due to excess amounts of collagen during connective tissue repair, occurring mainly on the upper trunk and face.

L91.8 Other hypertrophic disorders of the skin

L91.9 Hypertrophic disorder of the skin, unspecified

L92 Granulomatous disorders of skin and subcutaneous tissue

 EXCLUDES 2: actinic granuloma (L57.5)

L92.0 Granuloma annulare
 Perforating granuloma annulare

L92.1 Necrobiosis lipoidica, not elsewhere classified
 EXCLUDES 1: necrobiosis lipoidica associated with diabetes mellitus (E08-E13 with .620)

L92.2 Granuloma faciale [eosinophilic granuloma of skin]

L92.3 Foreign body granuloma of the skin and subcutaneous tissue
 Use additional code to identify the type of retained foreign body (Z18.-)

L92.8 Other granulomatous disorders of the skin and subcutaneous tissue

L92.9 Granulomatous disorder of the skin and subcutaneous tissue, unspecified
 EXCLUDES 2: umbilical granuloma (P83.81)
 AHA: 2017,4Q,21-22

L93 Lupus erythematosus

Use additional code for adverse effect, if applicable, to identify drug (T36-T50 with fifth or sixth character 5)
 EXCLUDES 1: lupus exedens (A18.4)
 lupus vulgaris (A18.4)
 scleroderma (M34.-)
 systemic lupus erythematosus (M32.-)
 DEF: Inflammatory, autoimmune skin condition in which the body's autoimmune system attacks healthy tissue of the integumentary system.

L93.0 Discoid lupus erythematosus
 Lupus erythematosus NOS

L93.1 Subacute cutaneous lupus erythematosus

L93.2 Other local lupus erythematosus
 Lupus erythematosus profundus
 Lupus panniculitis

L94 Other localized connective tissue disorders

 EXCLUDES 1: systemic connective tissue disorders (M30-M36)

L94.0 Localized scleroderma [morphea]
 Circumscribed scleroderma

L94.1 Linear scleroderma
 En coup de sabre lesion

L94.2 Calcinosis cutis

L94.3 Sclerodactyly

L94.4 Gottron's papules

L94.5 Poikiloderma vasculare atrophicans

L94.6 Ainhum

L94.8 Other specified localized connective tissue disorders

L94.9 Localized connective tissue disorder, unspecified

L95 Vasculitis limited to skin, not elsewhere classified

 EXCLUDES 1: angioma serpiginosum (L81.7)
 Henoch(-Schonlein) purpura (D69.0)
 hypersensitivity angiitis (M31.0)
 lupus panniculitis (L93.2)
 panniculitis of neck and back (M54.0-)
 panniculitis NOS (M79.3)
 polyarteritis nodosa (M30.0)
 relapsing panniculitis (M35.6)
 rheumatoid vasculitis (M05.2)
 serum sickness (T80.6-)
 urticaria (L50.-)
 Wegener's granulomatosis (M31.3-)

L95.0 Livedoid vasculitis
 Atrophie blanche (en plaque)

L95.1 Erythema elevatum diutinum

L95.8 Other vasculitis limited to the skin

L95.9 Vasculitis limited to the skin, unspecified

L97 Non-pressure chronic ulcer of lower limb, not elsewhere classified

 INCLUDES: chronic ulcer of skin of lower limb NOS
 non-healing ulcer of skin
 non-infected sinus of skin
 trophic ulcer NOS
 tropical ulcer NOS
 ulcer of skin of lower limb NOS

Code first any associated underlying condition, such as:
 any associated gangrene (I96)
 atherosclerosis of the lower extremities (I70.23-, I70.24-, I70.33-, I70.34-, I70.43-, I70.44-, I70.53-, I70.54-, I70.63-, I70.64-, I70.73-, I70.74-)
 chronic venous hypertension (I87.31-, I87.33-)
 diabetic ulcers (E08.621, E08.622, E09.621, E09.622, E10.621, E10.622, E11.621, E11.622, E13.621, E13.622)
 postphlebitic syndrome (I87.01-, I87.03-)
 postthrombotic syndrome (I87.01-, I87.03-)
 varicose ulcer (I83.0-, I83.2-)
 EXCLUDES 2: pressure ulcer (pressure area) (L89.-)
 skin infections (L00-L08)
 specific infections classified to A00-B99
 AHA: 2021,1Q,7; 2020,2Q,19; 2018,4Q,69; 2017,4Q,17
 TIP: The depth and/or severity of a diagnosed nonpressure ulcer can be determined based on medical record documentation from clinicians who are not the patient's provider.

L97.1 Non-pressure chronic ulcer of thigh

 L97.10 Non-pressure chronic ulcer of unspecified thigh

  L97.101 Non-pressure chronic ulcer of unspecified thigh limited to breakdown of skin

  L97.102 Non-pressure chronic ulcer of unspecified thigh with fat layer exposed

  L97.103 Non-pressure chronic ulcer of unspecified thigh with necrosis of muscle

  L97.104 Non-pressure chronic ulcer of unspecified thigh with necrosis of bone

  L97.105 Non-pressure chronic ulcer of unspecified thigh with muscle involvement without evidence of necrosis

  L97.106 Non-pressure chronic ulcer of unspecified thigh with bone involvement without evidence of necrosis

  L97.108 Non-pressure chronic ulcer of unspecified thigh with other specified severity

L97.109 Non-pressure chronic ulcer of unspecified thigh with unspecified severity `HCC` `Rx` `ESR` `COM`

√6th **L97.11** Non-pressure chronic ulcer of right thigh
- **L97.111** Non-pressure chronic ulcer of right thigh limited to breakdown of skin `HCC` `Rx` `ESR` `COM`
- **L97.112** Non-pressure chronic ulcer of right thigh with fat layer exposed `HCC` `Rx` `ESR` `COM`
- **L97.113** Non-pressure chronic ulcer of right thigh with necrosis of muscle `HCC` `Rx` `ESR` `COM`
- **L97.114** Non-pressure chronic ulcer of right thigh with necrosis of bone `HCC` `Rx` `ESR` `COM`
- **L97.115** Non-pressure chronic ulcer of right thigh with muscle involvement without evidence of necrosis `HCC` `Rx` `ESR` `COM`
- **L97.116** Non-pressure chronic ulcer of right thigh with bone involvement without evidence of necrosis `HCC` `Rx` `ESR` `COM`
- **L97.118** Non-pressure chronic ulcer of right thigh with other specified severity `HCC` `Rx` `ESR` `COM`
- **L97.119** Non-pressure chronic ulcer of right thigh with unspecified severity `HCC` `Rx` `ESR` `COM`

√6th **L97.12** Non-pressure chronic ulcer of left thigh
- **L97.121** Non-pressure chronic ulcer of left thigh limited to breakdown of skin `HCC` `Rx` `ESR` `COM`
- **L97.122** Non-pressure chronic ulcer of left thigh with fat layer exposed `HCC` `Rx` `ESR` `COM`
- **L97.123** Non-pressure chronic ulcer of left thigh with necrosis of muscle `HCC` `Rx` `ESR` `COM`
- **L97.124** Non-pressure chronic ulcer of left thigh with necrosis of bone `HCC` `Rx` `ESR` `COM`
- **L97.125** Non-pressure chronic ulcer of left thigh with muscle involvement without evidence of necrosis `HCC` `Rx` `ESR` `COM`
- **L97.126** Non-pressure chronic ulcer of left thigh with bone involvement without evidence of necrosis `HCC` `Rx` `ESR` `COM`
- **L97.128** Non-pressure chronic ulcer of left thigh with other specified severity `HCC` `Rx` `ESR` `COM`
- **L97.129** Non-pressure chronic ulcer of left thigh with unspecified severity `HCC` `Rx` `ESR` `COM`

√5th **L97.2** Non-pressure chronic ulcer of calf
▶Non-pressure chronic ulcer of shin◀
AHA: 2024,1Q,16

√6th **L97.20** Non-pressure chronic ulcer of unspecified calf
- **L97.201** Non-pressure chronic ulcer of unspecified calf limited to breakdown of skin `HCC` `Rx` `ESR` `COM`
- **L97.202** Non-pressure chronic ulcer of unspecified calf with fat layer exposed `HCC` `Rx` `ESR` `COM`
- **L97.203** Non-pressure chronic ulcer of unspecified calf with necrosis of muscle `HCC` `Rx` `ESR` `COM`
- **L97.204** Non-pressure chronic ulcer of unspecified calf with necrosis of bone `HCC` `Rx` `ESR` `COM`
- **L97.205** Non-pressure chronic ulcer of unspecified calf with muscle involvement without evidence of necrosis `HCC` `Rx` `ESR` `COM`
- **L97.206** Non-pressure chronic ulcer of unspecified calf with bone involvement without evidence of necrosis `HCC` `Rx` `ESR` `COM`
- **L97.208** Non-pressure chronic ulcer of unspecified calf with other specified severity `HCC` `Rx` `ESR` `COM`
- **L97.209** Non-pressure chronic ulcer of unspecified calf with unspecified severity `HCC` `Rx` `ESR` `COM`

√6th **L97.21** Non-pressure chronic ulcer of right calf
- **L97.211** Non-pressure chronic ulcer of right calf limited to breakdown of skin `HCC` `Rx` `ESR` `COM`
- **L97.212** Non-pressure chronic ulcer of right calf with fat layer exposed `HCC` `Rx` `ESR` `COM`
- **L97.213** Non-pressure chronic ulcer of right calf with necrosis of muscle `HCC` `Rx` `ESR` `COM`
- **L97.214** Non-pressure chronic ulcer of right calf with necrosis of bone `HCC` `Rx` `ESR` `COM`
- **L97.215** Non-pressure chronic ulcer of right calf with muscle involvement without evidence of necrosis `HCC` `Rx` `ESR` `COM`
- **L97.216** Non-pressure chronic ulcer of right calf with bone involvement without evidence of necrosis `HCC` `Rx` `ESR` `COM`
- **L97.218** Non-pressure chronic ulcer of right calf with other specified severity `HCC` `Rx` `ESR` `COM`
- **L97.219** Non-pressure chronic ulcer of right calf with unspecified severity `HCC` `Rx` `ESR` `COM`

√6th **L97.22** Non-pressure chronic ulcer of left calf
- **L97.221** Non-pressure chronic ulcer of left calf limited to breakdown of skin `HCC` `Rx` `ESR` `COM`
- **L97.222** Non-pressure chronic ulcer of left calf with fat layer exposed `HCC` `Rx` `ESR` `COM`
- **L97.223** Non-pressure chronic ulcer of left calf with necrosis of muscle `HCC` `Rx` `ESR` `COM`
- **L97.224** Non-pressure chronic ulcer of left calf with necrosis of bone `HCC` `Rx` `ESR` `COM`
- **L97.225** Non-pressure chronic ulcer of left calf with muscle involvement without evidence of necrosis `HCC` `Rx` `ESR` `COM`
- **L97.226** Non-pressure chronic ulcer of left calf with bone involvement without evidence of necrosis `HCC` `Rx` `ESR` `COM`
- **L97.228** Non-pressure chronic ulcer of left calf with other specified severity `HCC` `Rx` `ESR` `COM`
- **L97.229** Non-pressure chronic ulcer of left calf with unspecified severity `HCC` `Rx` `ESR` `COM`

√5th **L97.3** Non-pressure chronic ulcer of ankle

√6th **L97.30** Non-pressure chronic ulcer of unspecified ankle
- **L97.301** Non-pressure chronic ulcer of unspecified ankle limited to breakdown of skin `HCC` `Rx` `ESR` `COM`
- **L97.302** Non-pressure chronic ulcer of unspecified ankle with fat layer exposed `HCC` `Rx` `ESR` `COM`
- **L97.303** Non-pressure chronic ulcer of unspecified ankle with necrosis of muscle `HCC` `Rx` `ESR` `COM`
- **L97.304** Non-pressure chronic ulcer of unspecified ankle with necrosis of bone `HCC` `Rx` `ESR` `COM`
- **L97.305** Non-pressure chronic ulcer of unspecified ankle with muscle involvement without evidence of necrosis `HCC` `Rx` `ESR` `COM`
- **L97.306** Non-pressure chronic ulcer of unspecified ankle with bone involvement without evidence of necrosis `HCC` `Rx` `ESR` `COM`
- **L97.308** Non-pressure chronic ulcer of unspecified ankle with other specified severity `HCC` `Rx` `ESR` `COM`
- **L97.309** Non-pressure chronic ulcer of unspecified ankle with unspecified severity `HCC` `Rx` `ESR` `COM`

√6th **L97.31** Non-pressure chronic ulcer of right ankle
- **L97.311** Non-pressure chronic ulcer of right ankle limited to breakdown of skin `HCC` `Rx` `ESR` `COM`
- **L97.312** Non-pressure chronic ulcer of right ankle with fat layer exposed `HCC` `Rx` `ESR` `COM`
- **L97.313** Non-pressure chronic ulcer of right ankle with necrosis of muscle `HCC` `Rx` `ESR` `COM`
- **L97.314** Non-pressure chronic ulcer of right ankle with necrosis of bone `HCC` `Rx` `ESR` `COM`
- **L97.315** Non-pressure chronic ulcer of right ankle with muscle involvement without evidence of necrosis `HCC` `Rx` `ESR` `COM`
- **L97.316** Non-pressure chronic ulcer of right ankle with bone involvement without evidence of necrosis `HCC` `Rx` `ESR` `COM`

Chapter 12. Diseases of the Skin and Subcutaneous Tissue

- L97.318 Non-pressure chronic ulcer of right ankle with other specified severity
- L97.319 Non-pressure chronic ulcer of right ankle with unspecified severity
- L97.32 Non-pressure chronic ulcer of left ankle
  - L97.321 Non-pressure chronic ulcer of left ankle limited to breakdown of skin
  - L97.322 Non-pressure chronic ulcer of left ankle with fat layer exposed
  - L97.323 Non-pressure chronic ulcer of left ankle with necrosis of muscle
  - L97.324 Non-pressure chronic ulcer of left ankle with necrosis of bone
  - L97.325 Non-pressure chronic ulcer of left ankle with muscle involvement without evidence of necrosis
  - L97.326 Non-pressure chronic ulcer of left ankle with bone involvement without evidence of necrosis
  - L97.328 Non-pressure chronic ulcer of left ankle with other specified severity
  - L97.329 Non-pressure chronic ulcer of left ankle with unspecified severity
- L97.4 Non-pressure chronic ulcer of heel and midfoot
  Non-pressure chronic ulcer of plantar surface of midfoot
  - L97.40 Non-pressure chronic ulcer of unspecified heel and midfoot
    - L97.401 Non-pressure chronic ulcer of unspecified heel and midfoot limited to breakdown of skin
    - L97.402 Non-pressure chronic ulcer of unspecified heel and midfoot with fat layer exposed
    - L97.403 Non-pressure chronic ulcer of unspecified heel and midfoot with necrosis of muscle
    - L97.404 Non-pressure chronic ulcer of unspecified heel and midfoot with necrosis of bone
    - L97.405 Non-pressure chronic ulcer of unspecified heel and midfoot with muscle involvement without evidence of necrosis
    - L97.406 Non-pressure chronic ulcer of unspecified heel and midfoot with bone involvement without evidence of necrosis
    - L97.408 Non-pressure chronic ulcer of unspecified heel and midfoot with other specified severity
    - L97.409 Non-pressure chronic ulcer of unspecified heel and midfoot with unspecified severity
  - L97.41 Non-pressure chronic ulcer of right heel and midfoot
    - L97.411 Non-pressure chronic ulcer of right heel and midfoot limited to breakdown of skin
    - L97.412 Non-pressure chronic ulcer of right heel and midfoot with fat layer exposed
      - AHA: 2020,2Q,19
    - L97.413 Non-pressure chronic ulcer of right heel and midfoot with necrosis of muscle
    - L97.414 Non-pressure chronic ulcer of right heel and midfoot with necrosis of bone
    - L97.415 Non-pressure chronic ulcer of right heel and midfoot with muscle involvement without evidence of necrosis
    - L97.416 Non-pressure chronic ulcer of right heel and midfoot with bone involvement without evidence of necrosis
  - L97.418 Non-pressure chronic ulcer of right heel and midfoot with other specified severity
  - L97.419 Non-pressure chronic ulcer of right heel and midfoot with unspecified severity
  - L97.42 Non-pressure chronic ulcer of left heel and midfoot
    - L97.421 Non-pressure chronic ulcer of left heel and midfoot limited to breakdown of skin
      - AHA: 2016,1Q,12
    - L97.422 Non-pressure chronic ulcer of left heel and midfoot with fat layer exposed
      - AHA: 2020,2Q,19
    - L97.423 Non-pressure chronic ulcer of left heel and midfoot with necrosis of muscle
    - L97.424 Non-pressure chronic ulcer of left heel and midfoot with necrosis of bone
    - L97.425 Non-pressure chronic ulcer of left heel and midfoot with muscle involvement without evidence of necrosis
    - L97.426 Non-pressure chronic ulcer of left heel and midfoot with bone involvement without evidence of necrosis
    - L97.428 Non-pressure chronic ulcer of left heel and midfoot with other specified severity
    - L97.429 Non-pressure chronic ulcer of left heel and midfoot with unspecified severity
- L97.5 Non-pressure chronic ulcer of other part of foot
  Non-pressure chronic ulcer of toe
  - L97.50 Non-pressure chronic ulcer of other part of unspecified foot
    - L97.501 Non-pressure chronic ulcer of other part of unspecified foot limited to breakdown of skin
    - L97.502 Non-pressure chronic ulcer of other part of unspecified foot with fat layer exposed
    - L97.503 Non-pressure chronic ulcer of other part of unspecified foot with necrosis of muscle
    - L97.504 Non-pressure chronic ulcer of other part of unspecified foot with necrosis of bone
    - L97.505 Non-pressure chronic ulcer of other part of unspecified foot with muscle involvement without evidence of necrosis
    - L97.506 Non-pressure chronic ulcer of other part of unspecified foot with bone involvement without evidence of necrosis
    - L97.508 Non-pressure chronic ulcer of other part of unspecified foot with other specified severity
    - L97.509 Non-pressure chronic ulcer of other part of unspecified foot with unspecified severity
  - L97.51 Non-pressure chronic ulcer of other part of right foot
    - AHA: 2020,1Q,12
    - L97.511 Non-pressure chronic ulcer of other part of right foot limited to breakdown of skin
    - L97.512 Non-pressure chronic ulcer of other part of right foot with fat layer exposed
      - AHA: 2020,2Q,19
    - L97.513 Non-pressure chronic ulcer of other part of right foot with necrosis of muscle
    - L97.514 Non-pressure chronic ulcer of other part of right foot with necrosis of bone

---

✓ Additional Character Required ✓x7th Placeholder Alert Manifestation Unspecified Dx Q QPP UPD Unacceptable PDx

		L97.515	Non-pressure chronic ulcer of other part of right foot with muscle involvement without evidence of necrosis `HCC` `Rx` `ESR` `COM`
		L97.516	Non-pressure chronic ulcer of other part of right foot with bone involvement without evidence of necrosis `HCC` `Rx` `ESR` `COM`
		L97.518	Non-pressure chronic ulcer of other part of right foot with other specified severity `HCC` `Rx` `ESR` `COM`
		L97.519	Non-pressure chronic ulcer of other part of right foot with unspecified severity `HCC` `Rx` `ESR` `COM`
	✓6th L97.52		Non-pressure chronic ulcer of other part of left foot
			AHA: 2020,1Q,12
		L97.521	Non-pressure chronic ulcer of other part of left foot limited to breakdown of skin `HCC` `Rx` `ESR` `COM`
		L97.522	Non-pressure chronic ulcer of other part of left foot with fat layer exposed `HCC` `Rx` `ESR` `COM`
			AHA: 2020,2Q,19
		L97.523	Non-pressure chronic ulcer of other part of left foot with necrosis of muscle `HCC` `Rx` `ESR` `COM`
		L97.524	Non-pressure chronic ulcer of other part of left foot with necrosis of bone `HCC` `Rx` `ESR` `COM`
		L97.525	Non-pressure chronic ulcer of other part of left foot with muscle involvement without evidence of necrosis `HCC` `Rx` `ESR` `COM`
		L97.526	Non-pressure chronic ulcer of other part of left foot with bone involvement without evidence of necrosis `HCC` `Rx` `ESR` `COM`
		L97.528	Non-pressure chronic ulcer of other part of left foot with other specified severity `HCC` `Rx` `ESR` `COM`
		L97.529	Non-pressure chronic ulcer of other part of left foot with unspecified severity `HCC` `Rx` `ESR` `COM`
✓5th L97.8			Non-pressure chronic ulcer of other part of lower leg
	✓6th L97.80		Non-pressure chronic ulcer of other part of unspecified lower leg
		L97.801	Non-pressure chronic ulcer of other part of unspecified lower leg limited to breakdown of skin `HCC` `Rx` `ESR` `COM`
		L97.802	Non-pressure chronic ulcer of other part of unspecified lower leg with fat layer exposed `HCC` `Rx` `ESR` `COM`
		L97.803	Non-pressure chronic ulcer of other part of unspecified lower leg with necrosis of muscle `HCC` `Rx` `ESR` `COM`
		L97.804	Non-pressure chronic ulcer of other part of unspecified lower leg with necrosis of bone `HCC` `Rx` `ESR` `COM`
		L97.805	Non-pressure chronic ulcer of other part of unspecified lower leg with muscle involvement without evidence of necrosis `HCC` `Rx` `ESR` `COM`
		L97.806	Non-pressure chronic ulcer of other part of unspecified lower leg with bone involvement without evidence of necrosis `HCC` `Rx` `ESR` `COM`
		L97.808	Non-pressure chronic ulcer of other part of unspecified lower leg with other specified severity `HCC` `Rx` `ESR` `COM`
		L97.809	Non-pressure chronic ulcer of other part of unspecified lower leg with unspecified severity `HCC` `Rx` `ESR` `COM`
	✓6th L97.81		Non-pressure chronic ulcer of other part of right lower leg
		L97.811	Non-pressure chronic ulcer of other part of right lower leg limited to breakdown of skin `HCC` `Rx` `ESR` `COM`
		L97.812	Non-pressure chronic ulcer of other part of right lower leg with fat layer exposed `HCC` `Rx` `ESR` `COM`
		L97.813	Non-pressure chronic ulcer of other part of right lower leg with necrosis of muscle `HCC` `Rx` `ESR` `COM`
		L97.814	Non-pressure chronic ulcer of other part of right lower leg with necrosis of bone `HCC` `Rx` `ESR` `COM`
		L97.815	Non-pressure chronic ulcer of other part of right lower leg with muscle involvement without evidence of necrosis `HCC` `Rx` `ESR` `COM`
		L97.816	Non-pressure chronic ulcer of other part of right lower leg with bone involvement without evidence of necrosis `HCC` `Rx` `ESR` `COM`
		L97.818	Non-pressure chronic ulcer of other part of right lower leg with other specified severity `HCC` `Rx` `ESR` `COM`
		L97.819	Non-pressure chronic ulcer of other part of right lower leg with unspecified severity `HCC` `Rx` `ESR` `COM`
	✓6th L97.82		Non-pressure chronic ulcer of other part of left lower leg
		L97.821	Non-pressure chronic ulcer of other part of left lower leg limited to breakdown of skin `HCC` `Rx` `ESR` `COM`
		L97.822	Non-pressure chronic ulcer of other part of left lower leg with fat layer exposed `HCC` `Rx` `ESR` `COM`
		L97.823	Non-pressure chronic ulcer of other part of left lower leg with necrosis of muscle `HCC` `Rx` `ESR` `COM`
		L97.824	Non-pressure chronic ulcer of other part of left lower leg with necrosis of bone `HCC` `Rx` `ESR` `COM`
		L97.825	Non-pressure chronic ulcer of other part of left lower leg with muscle involvement without evidence of necrosis `HCC` `Rx` `ESR` `COM`
		L97.826	Non-pressure chronic ulcer of other part of left lower leg with bone involvement without evidence of necrosis `HCC` `Rx` `ESR` `COM`
		L97.828	Non-pressure chronic ulcer of other part of left lower leg with other specified severity `HCC` `Rx` `ESR` `COM`
		L97.829	Non-pressure chronic ulcer of other part of left lower leg with unspecified severity `HCC` `Rx` `ESR` `COM`
✓5th L97.9			Non-pressure chronic ulcer of unspecified part of lower leg
			AHA: 2025,1Q,35
	✓6th L97.90		Non-pressure chronic ulcer of unspecified part of unspecified lower leg
		L97.901	Non-pressure chronic ulcer of unspecified part of unspecified lower leg limited to breakdown of skin `HCC` `Rx` `ESR` `COM`
		L97.902	Non-pressure chronic ulcer of unspecified part of unspecified lower leg with fat layer exposed `HCC` `Rx` `ESR` `COM`
		L97.903	Non-pressure chronic ulcer of unspecified part of unspecified lower leg with necrosis of muscle `HCC` `Rx` `ESR` `COM`
		L97.904	Non-pressure chronic ulcer of unspecified part of unspecified lower leg with necrosis of bone `HCC` `Rx` `ESR` `COM`
		L97.905	Non-pressure chronic ulcer of unspecified part of unspecified lower leg with muscle involvement without evidence of necrosis `HCC` `Rx` `ESR` `COM`
		L97.906	Non-pressure chronic ulcer of unspecified part of unspecified lower leg with bone involvement without evidence of necrosis `HCC` `Rx` `ESR` `COM`
		L97.908	Non-pressure chronic ulcer of unspecified part of unspecified lower leg with other specified severity `HCC` `Rx` `ESR` `COM`
		L97.909	Non-pressure chronic ulcer of unspecified part of unspecified lower leg with unspecified severity `HCC` `Rx` `ESR` `COM`
	✓6th L97.91		Non-pressure chronic ulcer of unspecified part of right lower leg
		L97.911	Non-pressure chronic ulcer of unspecified part of right lower leg limited to breakdown of skin `HCC` `Rx` `ESR` `COM`

`HCC` CMS-HCC `Rx` Rx HCC `ESR` ESRD HCC `COM` Commercial HCC `N` Newborn: 0 `P` Pediatric: 0-17 `M` Maternity: 9-64 `A` Adult: 15-124

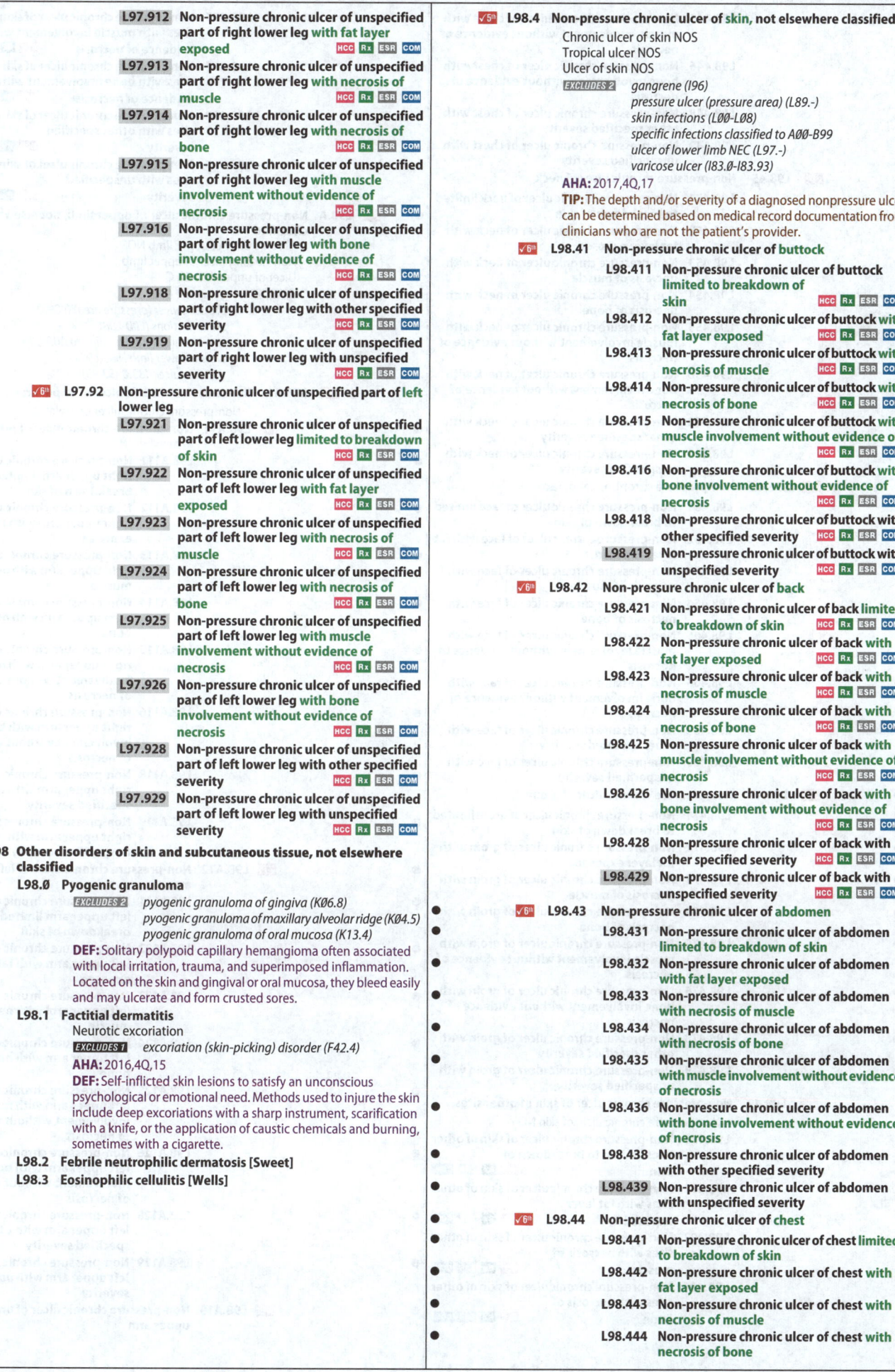

Chapter 12. Diseases of the Skin and Subcutaneous Tissue

- L98.445 Non-pressure chronic ulcer of chest with muscle involvement without evidence of necrosis
- L98.446 Non-pressure chronic ulcer of chest with bone involvement without evidence of necrosis
- L98.448 Non-pressure chronic ulcer of chest with other specified severity
- L98.449 Non-pressure chronic ulcer of chest with unspecified severity
- √6ᵗʰ L98.45 Non-pressure chronic ulcer of neck
  - L98.451 Non-pressure chronic ulcer of neck limited to breakdown of skin
  - L98.452 Non-pressure chronic ulcer of neck with fat layer exposed
  - L98.453 Non-pressure chronic ulcer of neck with necrosis of muscle
  - L98.454 Non-pressure chronic ulcer of neck with necrosis of bone
  - L98.455 Non-pressure chronic ulcer of neck with muscle involvement without evidence of necrosis
  - L98.456 Non-pressure chronic ulcer of neck with bone involvement without evidence of necrosis
  - L98.458 Non-pressure chronic ulcer of neck with other specified severity
  - L98.459 Non-pressure chronic ulcer of neck with unspecified severity
- √6ᵗʰ L98.46 Non-pressure chronic ulcer of face
  - L98.461 Non-pressure chronic ulcer of face limited to breakdown of skin
  - L98.462 Non-pressure chronic ulcer of face with fat layer exposed
  - L98.463 Non-pressure chronic ulcer of face with necrosis of muscle
  - L98.464 Non-pressure chronic ulcer of face with necrosis of bone
  - L98.465 Non-pressure chronic ulcer of face with muscle involvement without evidence of necrosis
  - L98.466 Non-pressure chronic ulcer of face with bone involvement without evidence of necrosis
  - L98.468 Non-pressure chronic ulcer of face with other specified severity
  - L98.469 Non-pressure chronic ulcer of face with unspecified severity
- √6ᵗʰ L98.47 Non-pressure chronic ulcer of groin
  - L98.471 Non-pressure chronic ulcer of groin limited to breakdown of skin
  - L98.472 Non-pressure chronic ulcer of groin with fat layer exposed
  - L98.473 Non-pressure chronic ulcer of groin with necrosis of muscle
  - L98.474 Non-pressure chronic ulcer of groin with necrosis of bone
  - L98.475 Non-pressure chronic ulcer of groin with muscle involvement without evidence of necrosis
  - L98.476 Non-pressure chronic ulcer of groin with bone involvement without evidence of necrosis
  - L98.478 Non-pressure chronic ulcer of groin with other specified severity
  - L98.479 Non-pressure chronic ulcer of groin with unspecified severity
- √6ᵗʰ L98.49 Non-pressure chronic ulcer of skin of other sites
  - Non-pressure chronic ulcer of skin NOS
  - L98.491 Non-pressure chronic ulcer of skin of other sites limited to breakdown of skin HCC Rx ESR COM
  - L98.492 Non-pressure chronic ulcer of skin of other sites with fat layer exposed HCC Rx ESR COM
  - L98.493 Non-pressure chronic ulcer of skin of other sites with necrosis of muscle HCC Rx ESR COM
  - L98.494 Non-pressure chronic ulcer of skin of other sites with necrosis of bone HCC Rx ESR COM
  - L98.495 Non-pressure chronic ulcer of skin of other sites with muscle involvement without evidence of necrosis HCC Rx ESR COM
  - L98.496 Non-pressure chronic ulcer of skin of other sites with bone involvement without evidence of necrosis HCC Rx ESR COM
  - L98.498 Non-pressure chronic ulcer of skin of other sites with other specified severity HCC Rx ESR COM
  - L98.499 Non-pressure chronic ulcer of skin of other sites with unspecified severity HCC Rx ESR COM
- √5ᵗʰ L98.A Non-pressure chronic ulcer of upper limb, not elsewhere classified
  - Chronic ulcer of upper limb NOS
  - Non-healing ulcer of upper limb
  - Ulcer of upper limb NEC
  - EXCLUDES 2 gangrene (I96)
    pressure ulcer (pressure area) (L89.-)
    skin infections (L00-L08)
    specific infections classified to A00-B99
    ulcer of lower limb NEC (L97.-)
    varicose ulcer (I83.0-I83.93)
  - √6ᵗʰ L98.A1 Non-pressure chronic ulcer of upper arm
    - Non-pressure chronic ulcer of axilla
    - √7ᵗʰ L98.A11 Non-pressure chronic ulcer of right upper arm
      - L98.A111 Non-pressure chronic ulcer of right upper arm limited to breakdown of skin
      - L98.A112 Non-pressure chronic ulcer of right upper arm with fat layer exposed
      - L98.A113 Non-pressure chronic ulcer of right upper arm with necrosis of muscle
      - L98.A114 Non-pressure chronic ulcer of right upper arm with necrosis of bone
      - L98.A115 Non-pressure chronic ulcer of right upper arm with muscle involvement without evidence of necrosis
      - L98.A116 Non-pressure chronic ulcer of right upper arm with bone involvement without evidence of necrosis
      - L98.A118 Non-pressure chronic ulcer of right upper arm with other specified severity
      - L98.A119 Non-pressure chronic ulcer of right upper arm with unspecified severity
    - √7ᵗʰ L98.A12 Non-pressure chronic ulcer of left upper arm
      - L98.A121 Non-pressure chronic ulcer of left upper arm limited to breakdown of skin
      - L98.A122 Non-pressure chronic ulcer of left upper arm with fat layer exposed
      - L98.A123 Non-pressure chronic ulcer of left upper arm with necrosis of muscle
      - L98.A124 Non-pressure chronic ulcer of left upper arm with necrosis of bone
      - L98.A125 Non-pressure chronic ulcer of left upper arm with muscle involvement without evidence of necrosis
      - L98.A126 Non-pressure chronic ulcer of left upper arm with bone involvement without evidence of necrosis
      - L98.A128 Non-pressure chronic ulcer of left upper arm with other specified severity
      - L98.A129 Non-pressure chronic ulcer of left upper arm with unspecified severity
    - √7ᵗʰ L98.A19 Non-pressure chronic ulcer of unspecified upper arm

---

HCC CMS-HCC   Rx Rx HCC   ESR ESRD HCC   COM Commercial HCC   N Newborn: 0   P Pediatric: 0-17   M Maternity: 9-64   A Adult: 15-124

- L98.A191 Non-pressure chronic ulcer of unspecified upper arm limited to breakdown of skin
- L98.A192 Non-pressure chronic ulcer of unspecified upper arm with fat layer exposed
- L98.A193 Non-pressure chronic ulcer of unspecified upper arm with necrosis of muscle
- L98.A194 Non-pressure chronic ulcer of unspecified upper arm with necrosis of bone
- L98.A195 Non-pressure chronic ulcer of unspecified upper arm with muscle involvement without evidence of necrosis
- L98.A196 Non-pressure chronic ulcer of unspecified upper arm with bone involvement without evidence of necrosis
- L98.A198 Non-pressure chronic ulcer of unspecified upper arm with other specified severity
- L98.A199 Non-pressure chronic ulcer of unspecified upper arm with unspecified severity
- ✓6th L98.A2 Non-pressure chronic ulcer of forearm
  - ✓7th L98.A21 Non-pressure chronic ulcer of right forearm
    - L98.A211 Non-pressure chronic ulcer of right forearm limited to breakdown of skin
    - L98.A212 Non-pressure chronic ulcer of right forearm with fat layer exposed
    - L98.A213 Non-pressure chronic ulcer of right forearm with necrosis of muscle
    - L98.A214 Non-pressure chronic ulcer of right forearm with necrosis of bone
    - L98.A215 Non-pressure chronic ulcer of right forearm with muscle involvement without evidence of necrosis
    - L98.A216 Non-pressure chronic ulcer of right forearm with bone involvement without evidence of necrosis
    - L98.A218 Non-pressure chronic ulcer of right forearm with other specified severity
    - L98.A219 Non-pressure chronic ulcer of right forearm with unspecified severity
  - ✓7th L98.A22 Non-pressure chronic ulcer of left forearm
    - L98.A221 Non-pressure chronic ulcer of left forearm limited to breakdown of skin
    - L98.A222 Non-pressure chronic ulcer of left forearm with fat layer exposed
    - L98.A223 Non-pressure chronic ulcer of left forearm with necrosis of muscle
    - L98.A224 Non-pressure chronic ulcer of left forearm with necrosis of bone
    - L98.A225 Non-pressure chronic ulcer of left forearm with muscle involvement without evidence of necrosis
    - L98.A226 Non-pressure chronic ulcer of left forearm with bone involvement without evidence of necrosis
    - L98.A228 Non-pressure chronic ulcer of left forearm with other specified severity
    - L98.A229 Non-pressure chronic ulcer of left forearm with unspecified severity
  - ✓7th L98.A29 Non-pressure chronic ulcer of unspecified forearm
    - L98.A291 Non-pressure chronic ulcer of unspecified forearm limited to breakdown of skin
    - L98.A292 Non-pressure chronic ulcer of unspecified forearm with fat layer exposed
    - L98.A293 Non-pressure chronic ulcer of unspecified forearm with necrosis of muscle
    - L98.A294 Non-pressure chronic ulcer of unspecified forearm with necrosis of bone
    - L98.A295 Non-pressure chronic ulcer of unspecified forearm with muscle involvement without evidence of necrosis
    - L98.A296 Non-pressure chronic ulcer of unspecified forearm with bone involvement without evidence of necrosis
    - L98.A298 Non-pressure chronic ulcer of unspecified forearm with other specified severity
    - L98.A299 Non-pressure chronic ulcer of unspecified forearm with unspecified severity
- ✓6th L98.A3 Non-pressure chronic ulcer of hand
  - ✓7th L98.A31 Non-pressure chronic ulcer of right hand
    - L98.A311 Non-pressure chronic ulcer of right hand limited to breakdown of skin
    - L98.A312 Non-pressure chronic ulcer of right hand with fat layer exposed
    - L98.A313 Non-pressure chronic ulcer of right hand with necrosis of muscle
    - L98.A314 Non-pressure chronic ulcer of right hand with necrosis of bone
    - L98.A315 Non-pressure chronic ulcer of right hand with muscle involvement without evidence of necrosis
    - L98.A316 Non-pressure chronic ulcer of right hand with bone involvement without evidence of necrosis
    - L98.A318 Non-pressure chronic ulcer of right hand with other specified severity
    - L98.A319 Non-pressure chronic ulcer of right hand with unspecified severity
  - ✓7th L98.A32 Non-pressure chronic ulcer of left hand
    - L98.A321 Non-pressure chronic ulcer of left hand limited to breakdown of skin
    - L98.A322 Non-pressure chronic ulcer of left hand with fat layer exposed
    - L98.A323 Non-pressure chronic ulcer of left hand with necrosis of muscle
    - L98.A324 Non-pressure chronic ulcer of left hand with necrosis of bone
    - L98.A325 Non-pressure chronic ulcer of left hand with muscle involvement without evidence of necrosis
    - L98.A326 Non-pressure chronic ulcer of left hand with bone involvement without evidence of necrosis
    - L98.A328 Non-pressure chronic ulcer of left hand with other specified severity
    - L98.A329 Non-pressure chronic ulcer of left hand with unspecified severity
  - ✓7th L98.A39 Non-pressure chronic ulcer of unspecified hand
    - L98.A391 Non-pressure chronic ulcer of unspecified hand limited to breakdown of skin

- L98.A392 Non-pressure chronic ulcer of unspecified hand with fat layer exposed
- L98.A393 Non-pressure chronic ulcer of unspecified hand with necrosis of muscle
- L98.A394 Non-pressure chronic ulcer of unspecified hand with necrosis of bone
- L98.A395 Non-pressure chronic ulcer of unspecified hand with muscle involvement without evidence of necrosis
- L98.A396 Non-pressure chronic ulcer of unspecified hand with bone involvement without evidence of necrosis
- L98.A398 Non-pressure chronic ulcer of unspecified hand with other specified severity
- L98.A399 Non-pressure chronic ulcer of unspecified hand with unspecified severity

L98.5 Mucinosis of the skin
Focal mucinosis
Lichen myxedematosus
Reticular erythematous mucinosis

EXCLUDES 1 focal oral mucinosis (K13.79)
myxedema (E03.9)

L98.6 Other infiltrative disorders of the skin and subcutaneous tissue
EXCLUDES 1 hyalinosis cutis et mucosae (E78.89)

L98.7 Excessive and redundant skin and subcutaneous tissue
Loose or sagging skin following dietary weight loss
Loose or sagging skin, following bariatric surgery weight loss
Loose or sagging skin, NOS

EXCLUDES 2 acquired excess or redundant skin of eyelid (H02.3-)
congenital excess or redundant skin of eyelid (Q10.3)
skin changes due to chronic exposure to nonionizing radiation (L57.-)

AHA: 2022,3Q,11; 2016,4Q,36

L98.8 Other specified disorders of the skin and subcutaneous tissue
AHA: 2013,2Q,32

L98.9 Disorder of the skin and subcutaneous tissue, unspecified

L99 Other disorders of skin and subcutaneous tissue in diseases classified elsewhere
Code first underlying disease, such as:
amyloidosis (E85.-)

EXCLUDES 1 skin disorders in diabetes (E08-E13 with .62-)
skin disorders in gonorrhea (A54.89)
skin disorders in syphilis (A51.31, A52.79)

AHA: 2021,1Q,39

Chapter 13. Diseases of the Musculoskeletal System and Connective Tissue (M00–M99)

Chapter-specific Guidelines with Coding Examples

The chapter-specific guidelines from the ICD-10-CM Official Guidelines for Coding and Reporting have been provided below. Along with these guidelines are coding examples, contained in the shaded boxes, that have been developed to help illustrate the coding and/or sequencing guidance found in these guidelines.

a. Site and laterality

Most of the codes within Chapter 13 have site and laterality designations. The site represents the bone, joint or the muscle involved.

1) Bone versus joint

For certain conditions, the bone may be affected at the upper or lower end, (e.g., avascular necrosis of bone, M87, Osteoporosis, M80, M81). Though the portion of the bone affected may be at the joint, the site designation will be the bone, not the joint.

> Idiopathic avascular necrosis of the femoral head of the left hip joint
>
> **M87.052   Idiopathic aseptic necrosis of left femur**
>
> *Explanation:* For certain conditions such as avascular necrosis, the bone may be affected at the joint, but the site designation is the bone, not the joint.

2) Multiple sites

Codes describing specified sites are assigned individually by site when documented. When the specified site(s) are not documented, assign the appropriate code for "multiple sites."

b. Acute traumatic versus chronic or recurrent musculoskeletal conditions

Many musculoskeletal conditions are a result of previous injury or trauma to a site, or are recurrent conditions. Bone, joint or muscle conditions that are the result of a healed injury are usually found in chapter 13. Recurrent bone, joint or muscle conditions are also usually found in chapter 13. Any current, acute injury should be coded to the appropriate injury code from chapter 19. Chronic or recurrent conditions should generally be coded with a code from chapter 13. If it is difficult to determine from the documentation in the record which code is best to describe a condition, query the provider.

> Acute traumatic bucket handle tear of right medial meniscus
>
> **S83.211A   Bucket-handle tear of medial meniscus, current injury, right knee, initial encounter**
>
> *Explanation:* Any current, acute injury is not coded in chapter 13. It should instead be coded to the appropriate injury code from chapter 19.

> Old bucket handle tear of right medial meniscus
>
> **M23.203   Derangement of unspecified medial meniscus due to old tear or injury, right knee**
>
> *Explanation:* Chronic or recurrent conditions should generally be coded with a code from chapter 13.

c. Coding of Pathologic Fractures

7th character A is for use as long as the patient is receiving active treatment for the fracture. Examples of active treatment are: surgical treatment, emergency department encounter, evaluation and continuing treatment by the same or a different physician. While the patient may be seen by a new or different provider over the course of treatment for a pathological fracture, assignment of the 7th character is based on whether the patient is undergoing active treatment and not whether the provider is seeing the patient for the first time.

> Pathologic fracture of left foot, unknown cause, currently under active treatment by a follow-up provider
>
> **M84.475A   Pathological fracture, left foot, initial encounter for fracture**
>
> *Explanation:* Seventh character A is for use as long as the patient is receiving active treatment for a pathologic fracture. Examples of active treatment are surgical treatment, emergency department encounter, evaluation, and continuing treatment by the same or a different physician.
>
> The seventh character is based on whether the patient is undergoing active treatment and not whether the provider is seeing the patient for the first time.

7th character D is to be used for encounters after the patient has completed active treatment for the fracture and is receiving routine care for the fracture during the healing or recovery phase. The other 7th characters, listed under each subcategory in the Tabular List, are to be used for subsequent encounters for treatment of problems associated with the healing, such as malunions, nonunions, and sequelae.

Care for complications of surgical treatment for fracture repairs during the healing or recovery phase should be coded with the appropriate complication codes.

See Section I.C.19. Coding of traumatic fractures.

d. Osteoporosis

Osteoporosis is a systemic condition, meaning that all bones of the musculoskeletal system are affected. Therefore, site is not a component of the codes under category M81, Osteoporosis without current pathological fracture. The site codes under category M80, Osteoporosis with current pathological fracture, identify the site of the fracture, not the osteoporosis.

1) Osteoporosis without pathological fracture

Category M81, Osteoporosis without current pathological fracture, is for use for patients with osteoporosis who do not currently have a pathologic fracture due to the osteoporosis, even if they have had a fracture in the past. For patients with a history of osteoporosis fractures, status code Z87.310, Personal history of (healed) osteoporosis fracture, should follow the code from M81.

> Age-related osteoporosis with healed osteoporotic fracture of the lumbar vertebra
>
> **M81.0   Age-related osteoporosis without current pathological fracture**
>
> **Z87.310   Personal history of (healed) osteoporosis fracture**
>
> *Explanation:* Category M81 is used for patients with osteoporosis who do not currently have a pathologic fracture due to the osteoporosis. To report a previous (healed) fracture, status code Z87.310 Personal history of (healed) osteoporosis fracture, should follow the code from M81.

2) Osteoporosis with current pathological fracture

Category M80, Osteoporosis with current pathological fracture, is for patients who have a current pathologic fracture at the time of an encounter. The codes under M80 identify the site of the fracture. A code from category M80, not a traumatic fracture code, should be used for any patient with known osteoporosis who suffers a fracture, even if the patient had a minor fall or trauma, if that fall or trauma would not usually break a normal, healthy bone.

> Disuse osteoporosis with current fracture of right shoulder sustained lifting a grocery bag, initial encounter
>
> **M80.811A   Other osteoporosis with current pathological fracture, right shoulder, initial encounter for fracture**
>
> *Explanation:* A code from category M80, not a traumatic fracture code, should be used for any patient with known osteoporosis who suffers a fracture, even if the patient had a minor fall or trauma, if that fall or trauma would not usually break a normal, healthy bone.

e. Multisystem inflammatory syndrome

See Section I.C.1.g.1.l. for Multisystem Inflammatory Syndrome

Muscle/Tendon Table

ICD-10-CM categorizes certain muscles and tendons in the upper and lower extremities by their action (e.g., extension, flexion), their anatomical location (e.g., posterior, anterior), and/or whether they are intrinsic or extrinsic to a certain anatomical area. The Muscle/Tendon Table is provided at the beginning of chapters 13 and 19 as a resource to help users when code selection depends on one or more of these characteristics. A **TIP** has been placed at those categories and/or subcategories that relate to this table. Please note that this table is not all-inclusive, and proper code assignment should be based on the provider's documentation.

Body Region	Muscle	Extensor Tendon	Flexor Tendon	Other Tendon
Shoulder				
	Deltoid	Posterior deltoid	Anterior deltoid	
	Rotator cuff			
	Infraspinatus			Infraspinatus
	Subscapularis			Subscapularis
	Supraspinatus			Supraspinatus
	Teres minor			Teres minor
	Teres major	Teres major		
Upper arm				
	Anterior muscles			
	Biceps brachii — long head		Biceps brachii — long head	
	Biceps brachii — short head		Biceps brachii — short head	
	Brachialis		Brachialis	
	Coracobrachialis		Coracobrachialis	
	Posterior muscles			
	Triceps brachii	Triceps brachii		
Forearm				
	Anterior muscles			
	Flexors			
	Deep			
	Flexor digitorum profundus		Flexor digitorum profundus	
	Flexor pollicis longus		Flexor pollicis longus	
	Intermediate			
	Flexor digitorum superficialis		Flexor digitorum superficialis	
	Superficial			
	Flexor carpi radialis		Flexor carpi radialis	
	Flexor carpi ulnaris		Flexor carpi ulnaris	
	Palmaris longus		Palmaris longus	
	Pronators			
	Pronator quadratus			Pronator quadratus
	Pronator teres			Pronator teres
	Posterior muscles			
	Extensors			
	Deep			
	Abductor pollicis longus			Abductor pollicis longus
	Extensor indicis	Extensor indicis		
	Extensor pollicis brevis	Extensor pollicis brevis		
	Extensor pollicis longus	Extensor pollicis longus		
	Superficial			
	Brachioradialis			Brachioradialis
	Extensor carpi radialis brevis	Extensor carpi radialis brevis		
	Extensor carpi radialis longus	Extensor carpi radialis longus		
	Extensor carpi ulnaris	Extensor carpi ulnaris		
	Extensor digiti minimi	Extensor digiti minimi		
	Extensor digitorum	Extensor digitorum		
	Anconeus	Anconeus		
	Supinator			Supinator

Body Region	Muscle	Extensor Tendon	Flexor Tendon	Other Tendon
Hand				
Extrinsic — attach to a site in the forearm as well as a site in the hand with action related to hand movement at the wrist				
	Extensor carpi radialis brevis	Extensor carpi radialis brevis		
	Extensor carpi radialis longus	Extensor carpi radialis longus		
	Extensor carpi ulnaris	Extensor carpi ulnaris		
	Flexor carpi radialis		Flexor carpi radialis	
	Flexor carpi ulnaris		Flexor carpi ulnaris	
	Flexor digitorum superficialis		Flexor digitorum superficialis	
	Palmaris longus		Palmaris longus	
Extrinsic — attach to a site in the forearm as well as a site in the hand with action in the hand related to finger movement				
	Adductor pollicis longus			Adductor pollicis longus
	Extensor digiti minimi	Extensor digiti minimi		
	Extensor digitorum	Extensor digitorum		
	Extensor indicis	Extensor indicis		
	Flexor digitorum profundus		Flexor digitorum profundus	
	Flexor digitorum superficialis		Flexor digitorum superficialis	
Extrinsic — attach to a site in the forearm as well as a site in the hand with action in the hand related to thumb movement				
	Extensor pollicis brevis	Extensor pollicis brevis		
	Extensor pollicis longus	Extensor pollicis longus		
	Flexor pollicis longus		Flexor pollicis longus	
Intrinsic — found within the hand only				
	Adductor pollicis			Adductor pollicis
	Dorsal interossei	Dorsal interossei	Dorsal interossei	
	Lumbricals	Lumbricals	Lumbricals	
	Palmaris brevis			Palmaris brevis
	Palmar interossei	Palmar interossei	Palmar interossei	
	Hypothenar muscles			
	Abductor digiti minimi			Abductor digiti minimi
	Flexor digiti minimi brevis		Flexor digiti minimi brevis	
	Opponens digiti minimi		Opponens digiti minimi	
	Thenar muscles			
	Abductor pollicis brevis			Abductor pollicis brevis
	Flexor pollicis brevis		Flexor pollicis brevis	
	Opponens pollicis		Opponens pollicis	
Thigh				
	Anterior muscles			
	Iliopsoas		Iliopsoas	
	Pectineus		Pectineus	
	Quadriceps	Quadriceps		
	Rectus femoris	Rectus femoris — Extends knee	Rectus femoris — Flexes hip	
	Vastus intermedius	Vastus intermedius		
	Vastus lateralis	Vastus lateralis		
	Vastus medialis	Vastus medialis		
	Sartorius		Sartorius	
	Medial muscles			
	Adductor brevis			Adductor brevis
	Adductor longus			Adductor longus
	Adductor magnus			Adductor magnus
	Gracilis			Gracilis
	Obturator externus			Obturator externus
	Posterior muscles			
	Hamstring	Hamstring — Extends hip	Hamstring — Flexes knee	
	Biceps femoris	Biceps femoris	Biceps femoris	
	Semimembranosus	Semimembranosus	Semimembranosus	
	Semitendinosus	Semitendinosus	Semitendinosus	

Body Region	Muscle	Extensor Tendon	Flexor Tendon	Other Tendon
Lower leg				
	Anterior muscles			
	Extensor digitorum longus	Extensor digitorum longus		
	Extensor hallucis longus	Extensor hallucis longus		
	Fibularis (peroneus) tertius	Fibularis (peroneus) tertius		
	Tibialis anterior	Tibialis anterior		Tibialis anterior
	Lateral muscles			
	Fibularis (peroneus) brevis		Fibularis (peroneus) brevis	
	Fibularis (peroneus) longus		Fibularis (peroneus) longus	
	Posterior muscles			
	Deep			
	Flexor digitorum longus		Flexor digitorum longus	
	Flexor hallucis longus		Flexor hallucis longus	
	Popliteus		Popliteus	
	Tibialis posterior		Tibialis posterior	
	Superficial			
	Gastrocnemius		Gastrocnemius	
	Plantaris		Plantaris	
	Soleus		Soleus	
				Calcaneal (Achilles)
Ankle/Foot				
Extrinsic — attach to a site in the lower leg as well as a site in the foot with action related to foot movement at the ankle				
	Plantaris		Plantaris	
	Soleus		Soleus	
	Tibialis anterior	Tibialis anterior		
	Tibialis posterior		Tibialis posterior	
Extrinsic — attach to a site in the lower leg as well as a site in the foot with action in the foot related to toe movement				
	Extensor digitorum longus	Extensor digitorum longus		
	Extensor hallucis longus	Extensor hallucis longus		
	Flexor digitorum longus		Flexor digitorum longus	
	Flexor hallucis longus		Flexor hallucis longus	
Intrinsic — found within the ankle/foot only				
	Dorsal muscles			
	Extensor digitorum brevis	Extensor digitorum brevis		
	Extensor hallucis brevis	Extensor hallucis brevis		
	Plantar muscles			
	Abductor digiti minimi		Abductor digiti minimi	
	Abductor hallucis		Abductor hallucis	
	Dorsal interossei	Dorsal interossei	Dorsal interossei	
	Flexor digiti minimi brevis		Flexor digiti minimi brevis	
	Flexor digitorum brevis		Flexor digitorum brevis	
	Flexor hallucis brevis		Flexor hallucis brevis	
	Lumbricals	Lumbricals	Lumbricals	
	Quadratus plantae		Quadratus plantae	
	Plantar interossei	Plantar interossei	Plantar interossei	

Chapter 13. Diseases of the Musculoskeletal System and Connective Tissue (M00-M99)

NOTE Use an external cause code following the code for the musculoskeletal condition, if applicable, to identify the cause of the musculoskeletal condition

EXCLUDES 2
- arthropathic psoriasis (L40.5-)
- certain conditions originating in the perinatal period (P04-P96)
- certain infectious and parasitic diseases (A00-B99)
- compartment syndrome (traumatic) (T79.A-)
- complications of pregnancy, childbirth and the puerperium (O00-O9A)
- congenital malformations, deformations, and chromosomal abnormalities (Q00-Q99)
- endocrine, nutritional and metabolic diseases (E00-E88)
- injury, poisoning and certain other consequences of external causes (S00-T88)
- neoplasms (C00-D49)
- symptoms, signs and abnormal clinical and laboratory findings, not elsewhere classified (R00-R94)

This chapter contains the following blocks:
- M00-M02 Infectious arthropathies
- M04 Autoinflammatory syndromes
- M05-M14 Inflammatory polyarthropathies
- M15-M19 Osteoarthritis
- M20-M25 Other joint disorders
- M26-M27 Dentofacial anomalies [including malocclusion] and other disorders of jaw
- M30-M36 Systemic connective tissue disorders
- M40-M43 Deforming dorsopathies
- M45-M49 Spondylopathies
- M50-M54 Other dorsopathies
- M60-M63 Disorders of muscles
- M65-M67 Disorders of synovium and tendon
- M70-M79 Other soft tissue disorders
- M80-M85 Disorders of bone density and structure
- M86-M90 Other osteopathies
- M91-M94 Chondropathies
- M95 Other disorders of the musculoskeletal system and connective tissue
- M96 Intraoperative and postprocedural complications and disorders of musculoskeletal system, not elsewhere classified
- M97 Periprosthetic fracture around internal prosthetic joint
- M99 Biomechanical lesions, not elsewhere classified

ARTHROPATHIES (M00-M25)

INCLUDES disorders affecting predominantly peripheral (limb) joints

Infectious arthropathies (M00-M02)

NOTE This block comprises arthropathies due to microbiological agents. Distinction is made between the following types of etiological relationship:

a) direct infection of joint, where organisms invade synovial tissue and microbial antigen is present in the joint;

b) indirect infection, which may be of two types: a reactive arthropathy, where microbial infection of the body is established but neither organisms nor antigens can be identified in the joint, and a postinfective arthropathy, where microbial antigen is present but recovery of an organism is inconstant and evidence of local multiplication is lacking.

AHA: 2019,3Q,16

✓4th M00 Pyogenic arthritis

EXCLUDES 2 infection and inflammatory reaction due to internal joint prosthesis (T84.5-)

AHA: 2022,1Q,31

DEF: Pyogenic: Relating to or involving pus production, often referred to as suppurative or purulent.

✓5th M00.0 Staphylococcal arthritis and polyarthritis
Use additional code (B95.61-B95.8) to identify bacterial agent

- M00.00 Staphylococcal arthritis, unspecified joint
- ✓6th M00.01 Staphylococcal arthritis, shoulder
  - M00.011 Staphylococcal arthritis, right shoulder
  - M00.012 Staphylococcal arthritis, left shoulder
  - M00.019 Staphylococcal arthritis, unspecified shoulder
- ✓6th M00.02 Staphylococcal arthritis, elbow
  - M00.021 Staphylococcal arthritis, right elbow
  - M00.022 Staphylococcal arthritis, left elbow
  - M00.029 Staphylococcal arthritis, unspecified elbow
- ✓6th M00.03 Staphylococcal arthritis, wrist
  Staphylococcal arthritis of carpal bones
  - M00.031 Staphylococcal arthritis, right wrist
  - M00.032 Staphylococcal arthritis, left wrist
  - M00.039 Staphylococcal arthritis, unspecified wrist
- ✓6th M00.04 Staphylococcal arthritis, hand
  Staphylococcal arthritis of metacarpus and phalanges
  - M00.041 Staphylococcal arthritis, right hand
  - M00.042 Staphylococcal arthritis, left hand
  - M00.049 Staphylococcal arthritis, unspecified hand
- ✓6th M00.05 Staphylococcal arthritis, hip
  - M00.051 Staphylococcal arthritis, right hip
  - M00.052 Staphylococcal arthritis, left hip
  - M00.059 Staphylococcal arthritis, unspecified hip
- ✓6th M00.06 Staphylococcal arthritis, knee
  - M00.061 Staphylococcal arthritis, right knee
  - M00.062 Staphylococcal arthritis, left knee
  - M00.069 Staphylococcal arthritis, unspecified knee
- ✓6th M00.07 Staphylococcal arthritis, ankle and foot
  Staphylococcal arthritis, tarsus, metatarsus and phalanges
  - M00.071 Staphylococcal arthritis, right ankle and foot
  - M00.072 Staphylococcal arthritis, left ankle and foot
  - M00.079 Staphylococcal arthritis, unspecified ankle and foot
- M00.08 Staphylococcal arthritis, vertebrae
- M00.09 Staphylococcal polyarthritis

✓5th M00.1 Pneumococcal arthritis and polyarthritis
- M00.10 Pneumococcal arthritis, unspecified joint
- ✓6th M00.11 Pneumococcal arthritis, shoulder
  - M00.111 Pneumococcal arthritis, right shoulder
  - M00.112 Pneumococcal arthritis, left shoulder
  - M00.119 Pneumococcal arthritis, unspecified shoulder
- ✓6th M00.12 Pneumococcal arthritis, elbow
  - M00.121 Pneumococcal arthritis, right elbow
  - M00.122 Pneumococcal arthritis, left elbow
  - M00.129 Pneumococcal arthritis, unspecified elbow
- ✓6th M00.13 Pneumococcal arthritis, wrist
  Pneumococcal arthritis of carpal bones
  - M00.131 Pneumococcal arthritis, right wrist
  - M00.132 Pneumococcal arthritis, left wrist
  - M00.139 Pneumococcal arthritis, unspecified wrist
- ✓6th M00.14 Pneumococcal arthritis, hand
  Pneumococcal arthritis of metacarpus and phalanges
  - M00.141 Pneumococcal arthritis, right hand
  - M00.142 Pneumococcal arthritis, left hand
  - M00.149 Pneumococcal arthritis, unspecified hand

M00.15 Pneumococcal arthritis, hip
- M00.151 Pneumococcal arthritis, right hip
- M00.152 Pneumococcal arthritis, left hip
- M00.159 Pneumococcal arthritis, unspecified hip

M00.16 Pneumococcal arthritis, knee
- M00.161 Pneumococcal arthritis, right knee
- M00.162 Pneumococcal arthritis, left knee
- M00.169 Pneumococcal arthritis, unspecified knee

M00.17 Pneumococcal arthritis, ankle and foot
Pneumococcal arthritis, tarsus, metatarsus and phalanges
- M00.171 Pneumococcal arthritis, right ankle and foot
- M00.172 Pneumococcal arthritis, left ankle and foot
- M00.179 Pneumococcal arthritis, unspecified ankle and foot

- M00.18 Pneumococcal arthritis, vertebrae
- M00.19 Pneumococcal polyarthritis

M00.2 Other streptococcal arthritis and polyarthritis
Use additional code (B95.0-B95.2, B95.4-B95.5) to identify bacterial agent

- M00.20 Other streptococcal arthritis, unspecified joint

M00.21 Other streptococcal arthritis, shoulder
- M00.211 Other streptococcal arthritis, right shoulder
- M00.212 Other streptococcal arthritis, left shoulder
- M00.219 Other streptococcal arthritis, unspecified shoulder

M00.22 Other streptococcal arthritis, elbow
- M00.221 Other streptococcal arthritis, right elbow
- M00.222 Other streptococcal arthritis, left elbow
- M00.229 Other streptococcal arthritis, unspecified elbow

M00.23 Other streptococcal arthritis, wrist
Other streptococcal arthritis of carpal bones
- M00.231 Other streptococcal arthritis, right wrist
- M00.232 Other streptococcal arthritis, left wrist
- M00.239 Other streptococcal arthritis, unspecified wrist

M00.24 Other streptococcal arthritis, hand
Other streptococcal arthritis metacarpus and phalanges
- M00.241 Other streptococcal arthritis, right hand
- M00.242 Other streptococcal arthritis, left hand
- M00.249 Other streptococcal arthritis, unspecified hand

M00.25 Other streptococcal arthritis, hip
- M00.251 Other streptococcal arthritis, right hip
- M00.252 Other streptococcal arthritis, left hip
- M00.259 Other streptococcal arthritis, unspecified hip

M00.26 Other streptococcal arthritis, knee
- M00.261 Other streptococcal arthritis, right knee
- M00.262 Other streptococcal arthritis, left knee
- M00.269 Other streptococcal arthritis, unspecified knee

M00.27 Other streptococcal arthritis, ankle and foot
Other streptococcal arthritis, tarsus, metatarsus and phalanges
- M00.271 Other streptococcal arthritis, right ankle and foot
- M00.272 Other streptococcal arthritis, left ankle and foot
- M00.279 Other streptococcal arthritis, unspecified ankle and foot

- M00.28 Other streptococcal arthritis, vertebrae
- M00.29 Other streptococcal polyarthritis

M00.8 Arthritis and polyarthritis due to other bacteria
Use additional code (B96) to identify bacteria

- M00.80 Arthritis due to other bacteria, unspecified joint

M00.81 Arthritis due to other bacteria, shoulder
- M00.811 Arthritis due to other bacteria, right shoulder
- M00.812 Arthritis due to other bacteria, left shoulder
- M00.819 Arthritis due to other bacteria, unspecified shoulder

M00.82 Arthritis due to other bacteria, elbow
- M00.821 Arthritis due to other bacteria, right elbow
- M00.822 Arthritis due to other bacteria, left elbow
- M00.829 Arthritis due to other bacteria, unspecified elbow

M00.83 Arthritis due to other bacteria, wrist
Arthritis due to other bacteria, carpal bones
- M00.831 Arthritis due to other bacteria, right wrist
- M00.832 Arthritis due to other bacteria, left wrist
- M00.839 Arthritis due to other bacteria, unspecified wrist

M00.84 Arthritis due to other bacteria, hand
Arthritis due to other bacteria, metacarpus and phalanges
- M00.841 Arthritis due to other bacteria, right hand
- M00.842 Arthritis due to other bacteria, left hand
- M00.849 Arthritis due to other bacteria, unspecified hand

M00.85 Arthritis due to other bacteria, hip
- M00.851 Arthritis due to other bacteria, right hip
- M00.852 Arthritis due to other bacteria, left hip
- M00.859 Arthritis due to other bacteria, unspecified hip

M00.86 Arthritis due to other bacteria, knee
AHA: 2019,3Q,16
- M00.861 Arthritis due to other bacteria, right knee
- M00.862 Arthritis due to other bacteria, left knee
- M00.869 Arthritis due to other bacteria, unspecified knee

M00.87 Arthritis due to other bacteria, ankle and foot
Arthritis due to other bacteria, tarsus, metatarsus, and phalanges
- M00.871 Arthritis due to other bacteria, right ankle and foot
- M00.872 Arthritis due to other bacteria, left ankle and foot
- M00.879 Arthritis due to other bacteria, unspecified ankle and foot

- M00.88 Arthritis due to other bacteria, vertebrae
- M00.89 Polyarthritis due to other bacteria

M00.9 Pyogenic arthritis, unspecified
Infective arthritis NOS

Chapter 13. Diseases of the Musculoskeletal System and Connective Tissue

M01 Direct infections of joint in infectious and parasitic diseases classified elsewhere

Code first underlying disease, such as:
- leprosy [Hansen's disease] (A30.-)
- mycoses (B35-B49)
- O'nyong-nyong fever (A92.1)
- paratyphoid fever (A01.1-A01.4)

EXCLUDES 1
- arthropathy in Lyme disease (A69.23)
- gonococcal arthritis (A54.42)
- meningococcal arthritis (A39.83)
- mumps arthritis (B26.85)
- postinfective arthropathy (M02.-)
- postmeningococcal arthritis (A39.84)
- reactive arthritis (M02.3)
- rubella arthritis (B06.82)
- sarcoidosis arthritis (D86.86)
- tuberculosis arthritis (A18.01-A18.02)
- typhoid fever arthritis (A01.04)

M01.X Direct infection of joint in infectious and parasitic diseases classified elsewhere

- **M01.X0** Direct infection of unspecified joint in infectious and parasitic diseases classified elsewhere
- **M01.X1** Direct infection of shoulder joint in infectious and parasitic diseases classified elsewhere
  - **M01.X11** Direct infection of right shoulder in infectious and parasitic diseases classified elsewhere
  - **M01.X12** Direct infection of left shoulder in infectious and parasitic diseases classified elsewhere
  - **M01.X19** Direct infection of unspecified shoulder in infectious and parasitic diseases classified elsewhere
- **M01.X2** Direct infection of elbow in infectious and parasitic diseases classified elsewhere
  - **M01.X21** Direct infection of right elbow in infectious and parasitic diseases classified elsewhere
  - **M01.X22** Direct infection of left elbow in infectious and parasitic diseases classified elsewhere
  - **M01.X29** Direct infection of unspecified elbow in infectious and parasitic diseases classified elsewhere
- **M01.X3** Direct infection of wrist in infectious and parasitic diseases classified elsewhere
  - Direct infection of carpal bones in infectious and parasitic diseases classified elsewhere
  - **M01.X31** Direct infection of right wrist in infectious and parasitic diseases classified elsewhere
  - **M01.X32** Direct infection of left wrist in infectious and parasitic diseases classified elsewhere
  - **M01.X39** Direct infection of unspecified wrist in infectious and parasitic diseases classified elsewhere
- **M01.X4** Direct infection of hand in infectious and parasitic diseases classified elsewhere
  - Direct infection of metacarpus and phalanges in infectious and parasitic diseases classified elsewhere
  - **M01.X41** Direct infection of right hand in infectious and parasitic diseases classified elsewhere
  - **M01.X42** Direct infection of left hand in infectious and parasitic diseases classified elsewhere
  - **M01.X49** Direct infection of unspecified hand in infectious and parasitic diseases classified elsewhere
- **M01.X5** Direct infection of hip in infectious and parasitic diseases classified elsewhere
  - **M01.X51** Direct infection of right hip in infectious and parasitic diseases classified elsewhere
  - **M01.X52** Direct infection of left hip in infectious and parasitic diseases classified elsewhere
  - **M01.X59** Direct infection of unspecified hip in infectious and parasitic diseases classified elsewhere
- **M01.X6** Direct infection of knee in infectious and parasitic diseases classified elsewhere
  - **M01.X61** Direct infection of right knee in infectious and parasitic diseases classified elsewhere
  - **M01.X62** Direct infection of left knee in infectious and parasitic diseases classified elsewhere
  - **M01.X69** Direct infection of unspecified knee in infectious and parasitic diseases classified elsewhere
- **M01.X7** Direct infection of ankle and foot in infectious and parasitic diseases classified elsewhere
  - Direct infection of tarsus, metatarsus and phalanges in infectious and parasitic diseases classified elsewhere
  - **M01.X71** Direct infection of right ankle and foot in infectious and parasitic diseases classified elsewhere
  - **M01.X72** Direct infection of left ankle and foot in infectious and parasitic diseases classified elsewhere
  - **M01.X79** Direct infection of unspecified ankle and foot in infectious and parasitic diseases classified elsewhere
- **M01.X8** Direct infection of vertebrae in infectious and parasitic diseases classified elsewhere
- **M01.X9** Direct infection of multiple joints in infectious and parasitic diseases classified elsewhere

M02 Postinfective and reactive arthropathies

Code first underlying disease, such as:
- congenital syphilis [Clutton's joints] (A50.5)
- enteritis due to Yersinia enterocolitica (A04.6)
- infective endocarditis (I33.0)
- viral hepatitis (B15-B19)

EXCLUDES 1
- Behcet's disease (M35.2)
- direct infections of joint in infectious and parasitic diseases classified elsewhere (M01.-)
- mumps arthritis (B26.85)
- postmeningococcal arthritis (A39.84)
- rheumatic fever (I00)
- rubella arthritis (B06.82)
- syphilis arthritis (late) (A52.77)
- tabetic arthropathy [Charcôt's] (A52.16)

M02.0 Arthropathy following intestinal bypass

- **M02.00** Arthropathy following intestinal bypass, unspecified site
- **M02.01** Arthropathy following intestinal bypass, shoulder
  - **M02.011** Arthropathy following intestinal bypass, right shoulder
  - **M02.012** Arthropathy following intestinal bypass, left shoulder
  - **M02.019** Arthropathy following intestinal bypass, unspecified shoulder
- **M02.02** Arthropathy following intestinal bypass, elbow
  - **M02.021** Arthropathy following intestinal bypass, right elbow
  - **M02.022** Arthropathy following intestinal bypass, left elbow
  - **M02.029** Arthropathy following intestinal bypass, unspecified elbow
- **M02.03** Arthropathy following intestinal bypass, wrist
  - Arthropathy following intestinal bypass, carpal bones
  - **M02.031** Arthropathy following intestinal bypass, right wrist
  - **M02.032** Arthropathy following intestinal bypass, left wrist
  - **M02.039** Arthropathy following intestinal bypass, unspecified wrist
- **M02.04** Arthropathy following intestinal bypass, hand
  - Arthropathy following intestinal bypass, metacarpals and phalanges
  - **M02.041** Arthropathy following intestinal bypass, right hand
  - **M02.042** Arthropathy following intestinal bypass, left hand
  - **M02.049** Arthropathy following intestinal bypass, unspecified hand
- **M02.05** Arthropathy following intestinal bypass, hip
  - **M02.051** Arthropathy following intestinal bypass, right hip

Chapter 13. Diseases of the Musculoskeletal System and Connective Tissue

- M02.052 Arthropathy following intestinal bypass, left hip
- M02.059 Arthropathy following intestinal bypass, unspecified hip
- ✓6th **M02.06** Arthropathy following intestinal bypass, knee
  - M02.061 Arthropathy following intestinal bypass, right knee
  - M02.062 Arthropathy following intestinal bypass, left knee
  - M02.069 Arthropathy following intestinal bypass, unspecified knee
- ✓6th **M02.07** Arthropathy following intestinal bypass, ankle and foot
  - Arthropathy following intestinal bypass, tarsus, metatarsus and phalanges
  - M02.071 Arthropathy following intestinal bypass, right ankle and foot
  - M02.072 Arthropathy following intestinal bypass, left ankle and foot
  - M02.079 Arthropathy following intestinal bypass, unspecified ankle and foot
- **M02.08** Arthropathy following intestinal bypass, vertebrae
- **M02.09** Arthropathy following intestinal bypass, multiple sites

✓5th M02.1 Postdysenteric arthropathy
- M02.10 Postdysenteric arthropathy, unspecified site [HCC] [ESR] [COM]
- ✓6th **M02.11** Postdysenteric arthropathy, shoulder
  - M02.111 Postdysenteric arthropathy, right shoulder [HCC] [ESR] [COM]
  - M02.112 Postdysenteric arthropathy, left shoulder [HCC] [ESR] [COM]
  - M02.119 Postdysenteric arthropathy, unspecified shoulder [HCC] [ESR] [COM]
- ✓6th **M02.12** Postdysenteric arthropathy, elbow
  - M02.121 Postdysenteric arthropathy, right elbow [HCC] [ESR] [COM]
  - M02.122 Postdysenteric arthropathy, left elbow [HCC] [ESR] [COM]
  - M02.129 Postdysenteric arthropathy, unspecified elbow
- ✓6th **M02.13** Postdysenteric arthropathy, wrist
  - Postdysenteric arthropathy, carpal bones
  - M02.131 Postdysenteric arthropathy, right wrist [HCC] [ESR] [COM]
  - M02.132 Postdysenteric arthropathy, left wrist [HCC] [ESR] [COM]
  - M02.139 Postdysenteric arthropathy, unspecified wrist [HCC] [ESR] [COM]
- ✓6th **M02.14** Postdysenteric arthropathy, hand
  - Postdysenteric arthropathy, metacarpus and phalanges
  - M02.141 Postdysenteric arthropathy, right hand [HCC] [ESR] [COM]
  - M02.142 Postdysenteric arthropathy, left hand [HCC] [ESR] [COM]
  - M02.149 Postdysenteric arthropathy, unspecified hand [HCC] [ESR] [COM]
- ✓6th **M02.15** Postdysenteric arthropathy, hip
  - M02.151 Postdysenteric arthropathy, right hip [HCC] [ESR] [COM]
  - M02.152 Postdysenteric arthropathy, left hip [HCC] [ESR] [COM]
  - M02.159 Postdysenteric arthropathy, unspecified hip [HCC] [ESR] [COM]
- ✓6th **M02.16** Postdysenteric arthropathy, knee
  - M02.161 Postdysenteric arthropathy, right knee [HCC] [ESR] [COM]
  - M02.162 Postdysenteric arthropathy, left knee [HCC] [ESR] [COM]
  - M02.169 Postdysenteric arthropathy, unspecified knee [HCC] [ESR] [COM]
- ✓6th **M02.17** Postdysenteric arthropathy, ankle and foot
  - Postdysenteric arthropathy, tarsus, metatarsus and phalanges
  - M02.171 Postdysenteric arthropathy, right ankle and foot [HCC] [ESR] [COM]
  - M02.172 Postdysenteric arthropathy, left ankle and foot [HCC] [ESR] [COM]
  - M02.179 Postdysenteric arthropathy, unspecified ankle and foot [HCC] [ESR] [COM]
- M02.18 Postdysenteric arthropathy, vertebrae [HCC] [ESR] [COM]
- M02.19 Postdysenteric arthropathy, multiple sites [HCC] [ESR] [COM]

✓5th M02.2 Postimmunization arthropathy
- M02.20 Postimmunization arthropathy, unspecified site
- ✓6th **M02.21** Postimmunization arthropathy, shoulder
  - M02.211 Postimmunization arthropathy, right shoulder
  - M02.212 Postimmunization arthropathy, left shoulder
  - M02.219 Postimmunization arthropathy, unspecified shoulder
- ✓6th **M02.22** Postimmunization arthropathy, elbow
  - M02.221 Postimmunization arthropathy, right elbow
  - M02.222 Postimmunization arthropathy, left elbow
  - M02.229 Postimmunization arthropathy, unspecified elbow
- ✓6th **M02.23** Postimmunization arthropathy, wrist
  - Postimmunization arthropathy, carpal bones
  - M02.231 Postimmunization arthropathy, right wrist
  - M02.232 Postimmunization arthropathy, left wrist
  - M02.239 Postimmunization arthropathy, unspecified wrist
- ✓6th **M02.24** Postimmunization arthropathy, hand
  - Postimmunization arthropathy, metacarpus and phalanges
  - M02.241 Postimmunization arthropathy, right hand
  - M02.242 Postimmunization arthropathy, left hand
  - M02.249 Postimmunization arthropathy, unspecified hand
- ✓6th **M02.25** Postimmunization arthropathy, hip
  - M02.251 Postimmunization arthropathy, right hip
  - M02.252 Postimmunization arthropathy, left hip
  - M02.259 Postimmunization arthropathy, unspecified hip
- ✓6th **M02.26** Postimmunization arthropathy, knee
  - M02.261 Postimmunization arthropathy, right knee
  - M02.262 Postimmunization arthropathy, left knee
  - M02.269 Postimmunization arthropathy, unspecified knee
- ✓6th **M02.27** Postimmunization arthropathy, ankle and foot
  - Postimmunization arthropathy, tarsus, metatarsus and phalanges
  - M02.271 Postimmunization arthropathy, right ankle and foot
  - M02.272 Postimmunization arthropathy, left ankle and foot
  - M02.279 Postimmunization arthropathy, unspecified ankle and foot
- M02.28 Postimmunization arthropathy, vertebrae
- M02.29 Postimmunization arthropathy, multiple sites

✓5th M02.3 Reiter's disease
Reactive arthritis
DEF: Arthritis, iridocyclitis, and urethritis, sometimes with diarrhea. While symptoms may recur, arthritis is constant.
- M02.30 Reiter's disease, unspecified site [HCC] [Rx] [ESR] [COM]
- ✓6th **M02.31** Reiter's disease, shoulder
  - M02.311 Reiter's disease, right shoulder [HCC] [Rx] [ESR] [COM]
  - M02.312 Reiter's disease, left shoulder [HCC] [Rx] [ESR] [COM]
  - M02.319 Reiter's disease, unspecified shoulder [HCC] [Rx] [ESR] [COM]
- ✓6th **M02.32** Reiter's disease, elbow
  - M02.321 Reiter's disease, right elbow [HCC] [Rx] [ESR] [COM]
  - M02.322 Reiter's disease, left elbow [HCC] [Rx] [ESR] [COM]
  - M02.329 Reiter's disease, unspecified elbow [HCC] [Rx] [ESR] [COM]
- ✓6th **M02.33** Reiter's disease, wrist
  - Reiter's disease, carpal bones
  - M02.331 Reiter's disease, right wrist [HCC] [Rx] [ESR] [COM]

[HCC] CMS-HCC [Rx] Rx HCC [ESR] ESRD HCC [COM] Commercial HCC N Newborn: 0 P Pediatric: 0-17 M Maternity: 9-64 A Adult: 15-124

Chapter 13. Diseases of the Musculoskeletal System and Connective Tissue

- M02.332 Reiter's disease, left wrist
- M02.339 Reiter's disease, unspecified wrist
- ✓6th **M02.34** Reiter's disease, hand
  - Reiter's disease, metacarpus and phalanges
  - M02.341 Reiter's disease, right hand
  - M02.342 Reiter's disease, left hand
  - M02.349 Reiter's disease, unspecified hand
- ✓6th **M02.35** Reiter's disease, hip
  - M02.351 Reiter's disease, right hip
  - M02.352 Reiter's disease, left hip
  - M02.359 Reiter's disease, unspecified hip
- ✓6th **M02.36** Reiter's disease, knee
  - M02.361 Reiter's disease, right knee
  - M02.362 Reiter's disease, left knee
  - M02.369 Reiter's disease, unspecified knee
- ✓6th **M02.37** Reiter's disease, ankle and foot
  - Reiter's disease, tarsus, metatarsus and phalanges
  - M02.371 Reiter's disease, right ankle and foot
  - M02.372 Reiter's disease, left ankle and foot
  - M02.379 Reiter's disease, unspecified ankle and foot
- **M02.38** Reiter's disease, vertebrae
- **M02.39** Reiter's disease, multiple sites
- ✓5th **M02.8** Other reactive arthropathies
  - M02.80 Other reactive arthropathies, unspecified site
  - ✓6th **M02.81** Other reactive arthropathies, shoulder
    - M02.811 Other reactive arthropathies, right shoulder
    - M02.812 Other reactive arthropathies, left shoulder
    - M02.819 Other reactive arthropathies, unspecified shoulder
  - ✓6th **M02.82** Other reactive arthropathies, elbow
    - M02.821 Other reactive arthropathies, right elbow
    - M02.822 Other reactive arthropathies, left elbow
    - M02.829 Other reactive arthropathies, unspecified elbow
  - ✓6th **M02.83** Other reactive arthropathies, wrist
    - Other reactive arthropathies, carpal bones
    - M02.831 Other reactive arthropathies, right wrist
    - M02.832 Other reactive arthropathies, left wrist
    - M02.839 Other reactive arthropathies, unspecified wrist
  - ✓6th **M02.84** Other reactive arthropathies, hand
    - Other reactive arthropathies, metacarpus and phalanges
    - M02.841 Other reactive arthropathies, right hand
    - M02.842 Other reactive arthropathies, left hand
    - M02.849 Other reactive arthropathies, unspecified hand
  - ✓6th **M02.85** Other reactive arthropathies, hip
    - M02.851 Other reactive arthropathies, right hip
    - M02.852 Other reactive arthropathies, left hip
    - M02.859 Other reactive arthropathies, unspecified hip
  - ✓6th **M02.86** Other reactive arthropathies, knee
    - M02.861 Other reactive arthropathies, right knee
    - M02.862 Other reactive arthropathies, left knee
    - M02.869 Other reactive arthropathies, unspecified knee
  - ✓6th **M02.87** Other reactive arthropathies, ankle and foot
    - Other reactive arthropathies, tarsus, metatarsus and phalanges
    - M02.871 Other reactive arthropathies, right ankle and foot
    - M02.872 Other reactive arthropathies, left ankle and foot
    - M02.879 Other reactive arthropathies, unspecified ankle and foot
  - **M02.88** Other reactive arthropathies, vertebrae
  - **M02.89** Other reactive arthropathies, multiple sites
- **M02.9** Reactive arthropathy, unspecified

Autoinflammatory syndromes (M04)

✓4th **M04** Autoinflammatory syndromes
  EXCLUDES 2 Crohn's disease (K50.-)
  AHA: 2016,4Q,37

- **M04.1** Periodic fever syndromes
  - Familial Mediterranean fever
  - Hyperimmunoglobin D syndrome
  - Mevalonate kinase deficiency
  - Tumor necrosis factor receptor associated periodic syndrome [TRAPS]
- **M04.2** Cryopyrin-associated periodic syndromes
  - Chronic infantile neurological, cutaneous and articular syndrome [CINCA]
  - Familial cold autoinflammatory syndrome
  - Familial cold urticaria
  - Muckle-Wells syndrome
  - Neonatal onset multisystemic inflammatory disorder [NOMID]
- **M04.8** Other autoinflammatory syndromes
  - Blau syndrome
  - Deficiency of interleukin 1 receptor antagonist [DIRA]
  - Majeed syndrome
  - Periodic fever, aphthous stomatitis, pharyngitis, and adenopathy syndrome [PFAPA]
  - Pyogenic arthritis, pyoderma gangrenosum, and acne syndrome [PAPA]
- **M04.9** Autoinflammatory syndrome, unspecified

Inflammatory polyarthropathies (M05-M14)

✓4th **M05** Rheumatoid arthritis with rheumatoid factor
  EXCLUDES 1 juvenile rheumatoid arthritis (M08.-)
  rheumatic fever (I00)
  rheumatoid arthritis of spine (M45.-)
  AHA: 2020,4Q,31-32
  DEF: Rheumatoid arthritis: Autoimmune systemic disease that causes chronic inflammation of the joints and other areas of the body, manifested by inflammatory changes in articular structures and synovial membranes, atrophy, and loss in bone density.

- ✓5th **M05.0** Felty's syndrome
  - Rheumatoid arthritis with splenoadenomegaly and leukopenia
  - M05.00 Felty's syndrome, unspecified site
  - ✓6th **M05.01** Felty's syndrome, shoulder
    - M05.011 Felty's syndrome, right shoulder
    - M05.012 Felty's syndrome, left shoulder
    - M05.019 Felty's syndrome, unspecified shoulder
  - ✓6th **M05.02** Felty's syndrome, elbow
    - M05.021 Felty's syndrome, right elbow
    - M05.022 Felty's syndrome, left elbow
    - M05.029 Felty's syndrome, unspecified elbow

M05.03–M05.242 Chapter 13. Diseases of the Musculoskeletal System and Connective Tissue

- ✓6th **M05.03** Felty's syndrome, wrist
  - Felty's syndrome, carpal bones
  - **M05.031** Felty's syndrome, right wrist `HCC` `Rx` `ESR` `COM`
  - **M05.032** Felty's syndrome, left wrist `HCC` `Rx` `ESR` `COM`
  - **M05.039** Felty's syndrome, unspecified wrist `HCC` `Rx` `ESR` `COM`
- ✓6th **M05.04** Felty's syndrome, hand
  - Felty's syndrome, metacarpus and phalanges
  - **M05.041** Felty's syndrome, right hand `HCC` `Rx` `ESR` `COM`
  - **M05.042** Felty's syndrome, left hand `HCC` `Rx` `ESR` `COM`
  - **M05.049** Felty's syndrome, unspecified hand `HCC` `Rx` `ESR` `COM`
- ✓6th **M05.05** Felty's syndrome, hip
  - **M05.051** Felty's syndrome, right hip `HCC` `Rx` `ESR` `COM`
  - **M05.052** Felty's syndrome, left hip `HCC` `Rx` `ESR` `COM`
  - **M05.059** Felty's syndrome, unspecified hip `HCC` `Rx` `ESR` `COM`
- ✓6th **M05.06** Felty's syndrome, knee
  - **M05.061** Felty's syndrome, right knee `HCC` `Rx` `ESR` `COM`
  - **M05.062** Felty's syndrome, left knee `HCC` `Rx` `ESR` `COM`
  - **M05.069** Felty's syndrome, unspecified knee `HCC` `Rx` `ESR` `COM`
- ✓6th **M05.07** Felty's syndrome, ankle and foot
  - Felty's syndrome, tarsus, metatarsus and phalanges
  - **M05.071** Felty's syndrome, right ankle and foot `HCC` `Rx` `ESR` `COM`
  - **M05.072** Felty's syndrome, left ankle and foot `HCC` `Rx` `ESR` `COM`
  - **M05.079** Felty's syndrome, unspecified ankle and foot `HCC` `Rx` `ESR` `COM`
  - **M05.09** Felty's syndrome, multiple sites `HCC` `Rx` `ESR` `COM`
- ✓5th **M05.1** Rheumatoid lung disease with rheumatoid arthritis
  - **M05.10** Rheumatoid lung disease with rheumatoid arthritis of unspecified site `HCC` `Rx` `ESR` `COM`
  - ✓6th **M05.11** Rheumatoid lung disease with rheumatoid arthritis of shoulder
    - **M05.111** Rheumatoid lung disease with rheumatoid arthritis of right shoulder `HCC` `Rx` `ESR` `COM`
    - **M05.112** Rheumatoid lung disease with rheumatoid arthritis of left shoulder `HCC` `Rx` `ESR` `COM`
    - **M05.119** Rheumatoid lung disease with rheumatoid arthritis of unspecified shoulder `HCC` `Rx` `ESR` `COM`
  - ✓6th **M05.12** Rheumatoid lung disease with rheumatoid arthritis of elbow
    - **M05.121** Rheumatoid lung disease with rheumatoid arthritis of right elbow `HCC` `Rx` `ESR` `COM`
    - **M05.122** Rheumatoid lung disease with rheumatoid arthritis of left elbow `HCC` `Rx` `ESR` `COM`
    - **M05.129** Rheumatoid lung disease with rheumatoid arthritis of unspecified elbow `HCC` `Rx` `ESR` `COM`
  - ✓6th **M05.13** Rheumatoid lung disease with rheumatoid arthritis of wrist
    - Rheumatoid lung disease with rheumatoid arthritis, carpal bones
    - **M05.131** Rheumatoid lung disease with rheumatoid arthritis of right wrist `HCC` `Rx` `ESR` `COM`
    - **M05.132** Rheumatoid lung disease with rheumatoid arthritis of left wrist `HCC` `Rx` `ESR` `COM`
    - **M05.139** Rheumatoid lung disease with rheumatoid arthritis of unspecified wrist `HCC` `Rx` `ESR` `COM`
  - ✓6th **M05.14** Rheumatoid lung disease with rheumatoid arthritis of hand
    - Rheumatoid lung disease with rheumatoid arthritis, metacarpus and phalanges
    - **M05.141** Rheumatoid lung disease with rheumatoid arthritis of right hand `HCC` `Rx` `ESR` `COM`
    - **M05.142** Rheumatoid lung disease with rheumatoid arthritis of left hand `HCC` `Rx` `ESR` `COM`
    - **M05.149** Rheumatoid lung disease with rheumatoid arthritis of unspecified hand `HCC` `Rx` `ESR` `COM`
  - ✓6th **M05.15** Rheumatoid lung disease with rheumatoid arthritis of hip
    - **M05.151** Rheumatoid lung disease with rheumatoid arthritis of right hip `HCC` `Rx` `ESR` `COM`
    - **M05.152** Rheumatoid lung disease with rheumatoid arthritis of left hip `HCC` `Rx` `ESR` `COM`
    - **M05.159** Rheumatoid lung disease with rheumatoid arthritis of unspecified hip `HCC` `Rx` `ESR` `COM`
  - ✓6th **M05.16** Rheumatoid lung disease with rheumatoid arthritis of knee
    - **M05.161** Rheumatoid lung disease with rheumatoid arthritis of right knee `HCC` `Rx` `ESR` `COM`
    - **M05.162** Rheumatoid lung disease with rheumatoid arthritis of left knee `HCC` `Rx` `ESR` `COM`
    - **M05.169** Rheumatoid lung disease with rheumatoid arthritis of unspecified knee `HCC` `Rx` `ESR` `COM`
  - ✓6th **M05.17** Rheumatoid lung disease with rheumatoid arthritis of ankle and foot
    - Rheumatoid lung disease with rheumatoid arthritis, tarsus, metatarsus and phalanges
    - **M05.171** Rheumatoid lung disease with rheumatoid arthritis of right ankle and foot `HCC` `Rx` `ESR` `COM`
    - **M05.172** Rheumatoid lung disease with rheumatoid arthritis of left ankle and foot `HCC` `Rx` `ESR` `COM`
    - **M05.179** Rheumatoid lung disease with rheumatoid arthritis of unspecified ankle and foot `HCC` `Rx` `ESR` `COM`
  - **M05.19** Rheumatoid lung disease with rheumatoid arthritis of multiple sites `HCC` `Rx` `ESR` `COM`
- ✓5th **M05.2** Rheumatoid vasculitis with rheumatoid arthritis
  - **M05.20** Rheumatoid vasculitis with rheumatoid arthritis of unspecified site `HCC` `Rx` `ESR` `COM`
  - ✓6th **M05.21** Rheumatoid vasculitis with rheumatoid arthritis of shoulder
    - **M05.211** Rheumatoid vasculitis with rheumatoid arthritis of right shoulder `HCC` `Rx` `ESR` `COM`
    - **M05.212** Rheumatoid vasculitis with rheumatoid arthritis of left shoulder `HCC` `Rx` `ESR` `COM`
    - **M05.219** Rheumatoid vasculitis with rheumatoid arthritis of unspecified shoulder `HCC` `Rx` `ESR` `COM`
  - ✓6th **M05.22** Rheumatoid vasculitis with rheumatoid arthritis of elbow
    - **M05.221** Rheumatoid vasculitis with rheumatoid arthritis of right elbow `HCC` `Rx` `ESR` `COM`
    - **M05.222** Rheumatoid vasculitis with rheumatoid arthritis of left elbow `HCC` `Rx` `ESR` `COM`
    - **M05.229** Rheumatoid vasculitis with rheumatoid arthritis of unspecified elbow `HCC` `Rx` `ESR` `COM`
  - ✓6th **M05.23** Rheumatoid vasculitis with rheumatoid arthritis of wrist
    - Rheumatoid vasculitis with rheumatoid arthritis, carpal bones
    - **M05.231** Rheumatoid vasculitis with rheumatoid arthritis of right wrist `HCC` `Rx` `ESR` `COM`
    - **M05.232** Rheumatoid vasculitis with rheumatoid arthritis of left wrist `HCC` `Rx` `ESR` `COM`
    - **M05.239** Rheumatoid vasculitis with rheumatoid arthritis of unspecified wrist `HCC` `Rx` `ESR` `COM`
  - ✓6th **M05.24** Rheumatoid vasculitis with rheumatoid arthritis of hand
    - Rheumatoid vasculitis with rheumatoid arthritis, metacarpus and phalanges
    - **M05.241** Rheumatoid vasculitis with rheumatoid arthritis of right hand `HCC` `Rx` `ESR` `COM`
    - **M05.242** Rheumatoid vasculitis with rheumatoid arthritis of left hand `HCC` `Rx` `ESR` `COM`

`HCC` CMS-HCC   `Rx` Rx HCC   `ESR` ESRD HCC   `COM` Commercial HCC   `N` Newborn: 0   `P` Pediatric: 0–17   `M` Maternity: 9–64   `A` Adult: 15–124

Chapter 13. Diseases of the Musculoskeletal System and Connective Tissue

M05.249 Rheumatoid vasculitis with rheumatoid arthritis of unspecified hand

✓6th M05.25 Rheumatoid vasculitis with rheumatoid arthritis of hip
- M05.251 Rheumatoid vasculitis with rheumatoid arthritis of right hip
- M05.252 Rheumatoid vasculitis with rheumatoid arthritis of left hip
- M05.259 Rheumatoid vasculitis with rheumatoid arthritis of unspecified hip

✓6th M05.26 Rheumatoid vasculitis with rheumatoid arthritis of knee
- M05.261 Rheumatoid vasculitis with rheumatoid arthritis of right knee
- M05.262 Rheumatoid vasculitis with rheumatoid arthritis of left knee
- M05.269 Rheumatoid vasculitis with rheumatoid arthritis of unspecified knee

✓6th M05.27 Rheumatoid vasculitis with rheumatoid arthritis of ankle and foot
  Rheumatoid vasculitis with rheumatoid arthritis, tarsus, metatarsus and phalanges
- M05.271 Rheumatoid vasculitis with rheumatoid arthritis of right ankle and foot
- M05.272 Rheumatoid vasculitis with rheumatoid arthritis of left ankle and foot
- M05.279 Rheumatoid vasculitis with rheumatoid arthritis of unspecified ankle and foot

M05.29 Rheumatoid vasculitis with rheumatoid arthritis of multiple sites

✓5th M05.3 Rheumatoid heart disease with rheumatoid arthritis
  Rheumatoid carditis
  Rheumatoid endocarditis
  Rheumatoid myocarditis
  Rheumatoid pericarditis

M05.30 Rheumatoid heart disease with rheumatoid arthritis of unspecified site

✓6th M05.31 Rheumatoid heart disease with rheumatoid arthritis of shoulder
- M05.311 Rheumatoid heart disease with rheumatoid arthritis of right shoulder
- M05.312 Rheumatoid heart disease with rheumatoid arthritis of left shoulder
- M05.319 Rheumatoid heart disease with rheumatoid arthritis of unspecified shoulder

✓6th M05.32 Rheumatoid heart disease with rheumatoid arthritis of elbow
- M05.321 Rheumatoid heart disease with rheumatoid arthritis of right elbow
- M05.322 Rheumatoid heart disease with rheumatoid arthritis of left elbow
- M05.329 Rheumatoid heart disease with rheumatoid arthritis of unspecified elbow

✓6th M05.33 Rheumatoid heart disease with rheumatoid arthritis of wrist
  Rheumatoid heart disease with rheumatoid arthritis, carpal bones
- M05.331 Rheumatoid heart disease with rheumatoid arthritis of right wrist
- M05.332 Rheumatoid heart disease with rheumatoid arthritis of left wrist
- M05.339 Rheumatoid heart disease with rheumatoid arthritis of unspecified wrist

✓6th M05.34 Rheumatoid heart disease with rheumatoid arthritis of hand
  Rheumatoid heart disease with rheumatoid arthritis, metacarpus and phalanges
- M05.341 Rheumatoid heart disease with rheumatoid arthritis of right hand
- M05.342 Rheumatoid heart disease with rheumatoid arthritis of left hand
- M05.349 Rheumatoid heart disease with rheumatoid arthritis of unspecified hand

✓6th M05.35 Rheumatoid heart disease with rheumatoid arthritis of hip
- M05.351 Rheumatoid heart disease with rheumatoid arthritis of right hip
- M05.352 Rheumatoid heart disease with rheumatoid arthritis of left hip
- M05.359 Rheumatoid heart disease with rheumatoid arthritis of unspecified hip

✓6th M05.36 Rheumatoid heart disease with rheumatoid arthritis of knee
- M05.361 Rheumatoid heart disease with rheumatoid arthritis of right knee
- M05.362 Rheumatoid heart disease with rheumatoid arthritis of left knee
- M05.369 Rheumatoid heart disease with rheumatoid arthritis of unspecified knee

✓6th M05.37 Rheumatoid heart disease with rheumatoid arthritis of ankle and foot
  Rheumatoid heart disease with rheumatoid arthritis, tarsus, metatarsus and phalanges
- M05.371 Rheumatoid heart disease with rheumatoid arthritis of right ankle and foot
- M05.372 Rheumatoid heart disease with rheumatoid arthritis of left ankle and foot
- M05.379 Rheumatoid heart disease with rheumatoid arthritis of unspecified ankle and foot

M05.39 Rheumatoid heart disease with rheumatoid arthritis of multiple sites

✓5th M05.4 Rheumatoid myopathy with rheumatoid arthritis

M05.40 Rheumatoid myopathy with rheumatoid arthritis of unspecified site

✓6th M05.41 Rheumatoid myopathy with rheumatoid arthritis of shoulder
- M05.411 Rheumatoid myopathy with rheumatoid arthritis of right shoulder
- M05.412 Rheumatoid myopathy with rheumatoid arthritis of left shoulder
- M05.419 Rheumatoid myopathy with rheumatoid arthritis of unspecified shoulder

✓6th M05.42 Rheumatoid myopathy with rheumatoid arthritis of elbow
- M05.421 Rheumatoid myopathy with rheumatoid arthritis of right elbow
- M05.422 Rheumatoid myopathy with rheumatoid arthritis of left elbow
- M05.429 Rheumatoid myopathy with rheumatoid arthritis of unspecified elbow

✓6th M05.43 Rheumatoid myopathy with rheumatoid arthritis of wrist
  Rheumatoid myopathy with rheumatoid arthritis, carpal bones
- M05.431 Rheumatoid myopathy with rheumatoid arthritis of right wrist
- M05.432 Rheumatoid myopathy with rheumatoid arthritis of left wrist

---

✓ Additional Character Required ✓7th Placeholder Alert Manifestation Unspecified Dx Q QPP UPD Unacceptable PDx

- **M05.439** Rheumatoid myopathy with rheumatoid arthritis of unspecified wrist
- ✓6th **M05.44** Rheumatoid myopathy with rheumatoid arthritis of hand
  - Rheumatoid myopathy with rheumatoid arthritis, metacarpus and phalanges
  - **M05.441** Rheumatoid myopathy with rheumatoid arthritis of right hand
  - **M05.442** Rheumatoid myopathy with rheumatoid arthritis of left hand
  - **M05.449** Rheumatoid myopathy with rheumatoid arthritis of unspecified hand
- ✓6th **M05.45** Rheumatoid myopathy with rheumatoid arthritis of hip
  - **M05.451** Rheumatoid myopathy with rheumatoid arthritis of right hip
  - **M05.452** Rheumatoid myopathy with rheumatoid arthritis of left hip
  - **M05.459** Rheumatoid myopathy with rheumatoid arthritis of unspecified hip
- ✓6th **M05.46** Rheumatoid myopathy with rheumatoid arthritis of knee
  - **M05.461** Rheumatoid myopathy with rheumatoid arthritis of right knee
  - **M05.462** Rheumatoid myopathy with rheumatoid arthritis of left knee
  - **M05.469** Rheumatoid myopathy with rheumatoid arthritis of unspecified knee
- ✓6th **M05.47** Rheumatoid myopathy with rheumatoid arthritis of ankle and foot
  - Rheumatoid myopathy with rheumatoid arthritis, tarsus, metatarsus and phalanges
  - **M05.471** Rheumatoid myopathy with rheumatoid arthritis of right ankle and foot
  - **M05.472** Rheumatoid myopathy with rheumatoid arthritis of left ankle and foot
  - **M05.479** Rheumatoid myopathy with rheumatoid arthritis of unspecified ankle and foot
- **M05.49** Rheumatoid myopathy with rheumatoid arthritis of multiple sites
- ✓5th **M05.5** Rheumatoid polyneuropathy with rheumatoid arthritis
  - **M05.50** Rheumatoid polyneuropathy with rheumatoid arthritis of unspecified site
  - ✓6th **M05.51** Rheumatoid polyneuropathy with rheumatoid arthritis of shoulder
    - **M05.511** Rheumatoid polyneuropathy with rheumatoid arthritis of right shoulder
    - **M05.512** Rheumatoid polyneuropathy with rheumatoid arthritis of left shoulder
    - **M05.519** Rheumatoid polyneuropathy with rheumatoid arthritis of unspecified shoulder
  - ✓6th **M05.52** Rheumatoid polyneuropathy with rheumatoid arthritis of elbow
    - **M05.521** Rheumatoid polyneuropathy with rheumatoid arthritis of right elbow
    - **M05.522** Rheumatoid polyneuropathy with rheumatoid arthritis of left elbow
    - **M05.529** Rheumatoid polyneuropathy with rheumatoid arthritis of unspecified elbow
  - ✓6th **M05.53** Rheumatoid polyneuropathy with rheumatoid arthritis of wrist
    - Rheumatoid polyneuropathy with rheumatoid arthritis, carpal bones
    - **M05.531** Rheumatoid polyneuropathy with rheumatoid arthritis of right wrist
    - **M05.532** Rheumatoid polyneuropathy with rheumatoid arthritis of left wrist
    - **M05.539** Rheumatoid polyneuropathy with rheumatoid arthritis of unspecified wrist
  - ✓6th **M05.54** Rheumatoid polyneuropathy with rheumatoid arthritis of hand
    - Rheumatoid polyneuropathy with rheumatoid arthritis, metacarpus and phalanges
    - **M05.541** Rheumatoid polyneuropathy with rheumatoid arthritis of right hand
    - **M05.542** Rheumatoid polyneuropathy with rheumatoid arthritis of left hand
    - **M05.549** Rheumatoid polyneuropathy with rheumatoid arthritis of unspecified hand
  - ✓6th **M05.55** Rheumatoid polyneuropathy with rheumatoid arthritis of hip
    - **M05.551** Rheumatoid polyneuropathy with rheumatoid arthritis of right hip
    - **M05.552** Rheumatoid polyneuropathy with rheumatoid arthritis of left hip
    - **M05.559** Rheumatoid polyneuropathy with rheumatoid arthritis of unspecified hip
  - ✓6th **M05.56** Rheumatoid polyneuropathy with rheumatoid arthritis of knee
    - **M05.561** Rheumatoid polyneuropathy with rheumatoid arthritis of right knee
    - **M05.562** Rheumatoid polyneuropathy with rheumatoid arthritis of left knee
    - **M05.569** Rheumatoid polyneuropathy with rheumatoid arthritis of unspecified knee
  - ✓6th **M05.57** Rheumatoid polyneuropathy with rheumatoid arthritis of ankle and foot
    - Rheumatoid polyneuropathy with rheumatoid arthritis, tarsus, metatarsus and phalanges
    - **M05.571** Rheumatoid polyneuropathy with rheumatoid arthritis of right ankle and foot
    - **M05.572** Rheumatoid polyneuropathy with rheumatoid arthritis of left ankle and foot
    - **M05.579** Rheumatoid polyneuropathy with rheumatoid arthritis of unspecified ankle and foot
  - **M05.59** Rheumatoid polyneuropathy with rheumatoid arthritis of multiple sites
- ✓5th **M05.6** Rheumatoid arthritis with involvement of other organs and systems
  - **M05.60** Rheumatoid arthritis of unspecified site with involvement of other organs and systems
  - ✓6th **M05.61** Rheumatoid arthritis of shoulder with involvement of other organs and systems
    - **M05.611** Rheumatoid arthritis of right shoulder with involvement of other organs and systems
    - **M05.612** Rheumatoid arthritis of left shoulder with involvement of other organs and systems
    - **M05.619** Rheumatoid arthritis of unspecified shoulder with involvement of other organs and systems
  - ✓6th **M05.62** Rheumatoid arthritis of elbow with involvement of other organs and systems
    - **M05.621** Rheumatoid arthritis of right elbow with involvement of other organs and systems
    - **M05.622** Rheumatoid arthritis of left elbow with involvement of other organs and systems

Chapter 13. Diseases of the Musculoskeletal System and Connective Tissue

- M05.629 Rheumatoid arthritis of unspecified elbow with involvement of other organs and systems [HCC] [Rx] [ESR] [COM]
- ✓6th **M05.63** Rheumatoid arthritis of **wrist** with involvement of other organs and systems
  - Rheumatoid arthritis of carpal bones with involvement of other organs and systems
  - M05.631 Rheumatoid arthritis of **right** wrist with involvement of other organs and systems
  - M05.632 Rheumatoid arthritis of **left** wrist with involvement of other organs and systems [HCC] [Rx] [ESR] [COM]
  - M05.639 Rheumatoid arthritis of unspecified wrist with involvement of other organs and systems
- ✓6th **M05.64** Rheumatoid arthritis of **hand** with involvement of other organs and systems
  - Rheumatoid arthritis of metacarpus and phalanges with involvement of other organs and systems
  - M05.641 Rheumatoid arthritis of **right** hand with involvement of other organs and systems [HCC] [Rx] [ESR] [COM]
  - M05.642 Rheumatoid arthritis of **left** hand with involvement of other organs and systems
  - M05.649 Rheumatoid arthritis of unspecified hand with involvement of other organs and systems [HCC] [Rx] [ESR] [COM]
- ✓6th **M05.65** Rheumatoid arthritis of **hip** with involvement of other organs and systems
  - M05.651 Rheumatoid arthritis of **right** hip with involvement of other organs and systems [HCC] [Rx] [ESR] [COM]
  - M05.652 Rheumatoid arthritis of **left** hip with involvement of other organs and systems [HCC] [Rx] [ESR] [COM]
  - M05.659 Rheumatoid arthritis of unspecified hip with involvement of other organs and systems [HCC] [Rx] [ESR] [COM]
- ✓6th **M05.66** Rheumatoid arthritis of **knee** with involvement of other organs and systems
  - M05.661 Rheumatoid arthritis of **right** knee with involvement of other organs and systems [HCC] [Rx] [ESR] [COM]
  - M05.662 Rheumatoid arthritis of **left** knee with involvement of other organs and systems [HCC] [Rx] [ESR] [COM]
  - M05.669 Rheumatoid arthritis of unspecified knee with involvement of other organs and systems [HCC] [Rx] [ESR] [COM]
- ✓6th **M05.67** Rheumatoid arthritis of **ankle and foot** with involvement of other organs and systems
  - Rheumatoid arthritis of tarsus, metatarsus and phalanges with involvement of other organs and systems
  - M05.671 Rheumatoid arthritis of **right** ankle and foot with involvement of other organs and systems [HCC] [Rx] [ESR] [COM]
  - M05.672 Rheumatoid arthritis of **left** ankle and foot with involvement of other organs and systems [HCC] [Rx] [ESR] [COM]
  - M05.679 Rheumatoid arthritis of unspecified ankle and foot with involvement of other organs and systems [HCC] [Rx] [ESR] [COM]
- M05.69 Rheumatoid arthritis of **multiple sites** with involvement of other organs and systems [HCC] [Rx] [ESR] [COM]
- ✓5th **M05.7** Rheumatoid arthritis **with rheumatoid factor without organ or systems involvement**
  - M05.70 Rheumatoid arthritis with rheumatoid factor of unspecified site without organ or systems involvement [HCC] [Rx] [ESR] [COM]
  - ✓6th **M05.71** Rheumatoid arthritis with rheumatoid factor of **shoulder** without organ or systems involvement
    - M05.711 Rheumatoid arthritis with rheumatoid factor of **right** shoulder without organ or systems involvement [HCC] [Rx] [ESR] [COM]
    - M05.712 Rheumatoid arthritis with rheumatoid factor of **left** shoulder without organ or systems involvement [HCC] [Rx] [ESR] [COM]
    - M05.719 Rheumatoid arthritis with rheumatoid factor of unspecified shoulder without organ or systems involvement [HCC] [Rx] [ESR] [COM]
  - ✓6th **M05.72** Rheumatoid arthritis with rheumatoid factor of **elbow** without organ or systems involvement
    - M05.721 Rheumatoid arthritis with rheumatoid factor of **right** elbow without organ or systems involvement [HCC] [Rx] [ESR] [COM]
    - M05.722 Rheumatoid arthritis with rheumatoid factor of **left** elbow without organ or systems involvement [HCC] [Rx] [ESR] [COM]
    - M05.729 Rheumatoid arthritis with rheumatoid factor of unspecified elbow without organ or systems involvement [HCC] [Rx] [ESR] [COM]
  - ✓6th **M05.73** Rheumatoid arthritis with rheumatoid factor of **wrist** without organ or systems involvement
    - M05.731 Rheumatoid arthritis with rheumatoid factor of **right** wrist without organ or systems involvement [HCC] [Rx] [ESR] [COM]
    - M05.732 Rheumatoid arthritis with rheumatoid factor of **left** wrist without organ or systems involvement [HCC] [Rx] [ESR] [COM]
    - M05.739 Rheumatoid arthritis with rheumatoid factor of unspecified wrist without organ or systems involvement [HCC] [Rx] [ESR] [COM]
  - ✓6th **M05.74** Rheumatoid arthritis with rheumatoid factor of **hand** without organ or systems involvement
    - M05.741 Rheumatoid arthritis with rheumatoid factor of **right** hand without organ or systems involvement [HCC] [Rx] [ESR] [COM]
    - M05.742 Rheumatoid arthritis with rheumatoid factor of **left** hand without organ or systems involvement [HCC] [Rx] [ESR] [COM]
    - M05.749 Rheumatoid arthritis with rheumatoid factor of unspecified hand without organ or systems involvement [HCC] [Rx] [ESR] [COM]
  - ✓6th **M05.75** Rheumatoid arthritis with rheumatoid factor of **hip** without organ or systems involvement
    - M05.751 Rheumatoid arthritis with rheumatoid factor of **right** hip without organ or systems involvement [HCC] [Rx] [ESR] [COM]
    - M05.752 Rheumatoid arthritis with rheumatoid factor of **left** hip without organ or systems involvement [HCC] [Rx] [ESR] [COM]
    - M05.759 Rheumatoid arthritis with rheumatoid factor of unspecified hip without organ or systems involvement [HCC] [Rx] [ESR] [COM]
  - ✓6th **M05.76** Rheumatoid arthritis with rheumatoid factor of **knee** without organ or systems involvement
    - M05.761 Rheumatoid arthritis with rheumatoid factor of **right** knee without organ or systems involvement [HCC] [Rx] [ESR] [COM]
    - M05.762 Rheumatoid arthritis with rheumatoid factor of **left** knee without organ or systems involvement [HCC] [Rx] [ESR] [COM]
    - M05.769 Rheumatoid arthritis with rheumatoid factor of unspecified knee without organ or systems involvement [HCC] [Rx] [ESR] [COM]
  - ✓6th **M05.77** Rheumatoid arthritis with rheumatoid factor of **ankle and foot** without organ or systems involvement
    - M05.771 Rheumatoid arthritis with rheumatoid factor of **right** ankle and foot without organ or systems involvement [HCC] [Rx] [ESR] [COM]
    - M05.772 Rheumatoid arthritis with rheumatoid factor of **left** ankle and foot without organ or systems involvement [HCC] [Rx] [ESR] [COM]
    - M05.779 Rheumatoid arthritis with rheumatoid factor of unspecified ankle and foot without organ or systems involvement [HCC] [Rx] [ESR] [COM]
  - M05.79 Rheumatoid arthritis with rheumatoid factor of **multiple sites** without organ or systems involvement [HCC] [Rx] [ESR] [COM]
  - M05.7A Rheumatoid arthritis with rheumatoid factor of other specified site without organ or systems involvement
- ✓5th **M05.8** Other rheumatoid arthritis **with rheumatoid factor**
  - M05.80 Other rheumatoid arthritis with rheumatoid factor of unspecified site [HCC] [Rx] [ESR] [COM]

M05.81–M06.09 Chapter 13. Diseases of the Musculoskeletal System and Connective Tissue

- ✓6th **M05.81** Other rheumatoid arthritis with rheumatoid factor of shoulder
  - **M05.811** Other rheumatoid arthritis with rheumatoid factor of right shoulder `HCC` `Rx` `ESR` `COM`
  - **M05.812** Other rheumatoid arthritis with rheumatoid factor of left shoulder `HCC` `Rx` `ESR` `COM`
  - **M05.819** Other rheumatoid arthritis with rheumatoid factor of unspecified shoulder `HCC` `Rx` `ESR` `COM`
- ✓6th **M05.82** Other rheumatoid arthritis with rheumatoid factor of elbow
  - **M05.821** Other rheumatoid arthritis with rheumatoid factor of right elbow `HCC` `Rx` `ESR` `COM`
  - **M05.822** Other rheumatoid arthritis with rheumatoid factor of left elbow `HCC` `Rx` `ESR` `COM`
  - **M05.829** Other rheumatoid arthritis with rheumatoid factor of unspecified elbow `HCC` `Rx` `ESR` `COM`
- ✓6th **M05.83** Other rheumatoid arthritis with rheumatoid factor of wrist
  - **M05.831** Other rheumatoid arthritis with rheumatoid factor of right wrist `HCC` `Rx` `ESR` `COM`
  - **M05.832** Other rheumatoid arthritis with rheumatoid factor of left wrist `HCC` `Rx` `ESR` `COM`
  - **M05.839** Other rheumatoid arthritis with rheumatoid factor of unspecified wrist `HCC` `Rx` `ESR` `COM`
- ✓6th **M05.84** Other rheumatoid arthritis with rheumatoid factor of hand
  - **M05.841** Other rheumatoid arthritis with rheumatoid factor of right hand `HCC` `Rx` `ESR` `COM`
  - **M05.842** Other rheumatoid arthritis with rheumatoid factor of left hand `HCC` `Rx` `ESR` `COM`
  - **M05.849** Other rheumatoid arthritis with rheumatoid factor of unspecified hand `HCC` `Rx` `ESR` `COM`
- ✓6th **M05.85** Other rheumatoid arthritis with rheumatoid factor of hip
  - **M05.851** Other rheumatoid arthritis with rheumatoid factor of right hip `HCC` `Rx` `ESR` `COM`
  - **M05.852** Other rheumatoid arthritis with rheumatoid factor of left hip `HCC` `Rx` `ESR` `COM`
  - **M05.859** Other rheumatoid arthritis with rheumatoid factor of unspecified hip `HCC` `Rx` `ESR` `COM`
- ✓6th **M05.86** Other rheumatoid arthritis with rheumatoid factor of knee
  - **M05.861** Other rheumatoid arthritis with rheumatoid factor of right knee `HCC` `Rx` `ESR` `COM`
  - **M05.862** Other rheumatoid arthritis with rheumatoid factor of left knee `HCC` `Rx` `ESR` `COM`
  - **M05.869** Other rheumatoid arthritis with rheumatoid factor of unspecified knee `HCC` `Rx` `ESR` `COM`
- ✓6th **M05.87** Other rheumatoid arthritis with rheumatoid factor of ankle and foot
  - **M05.871** Other rheumatoid arthritis with rheumatoid factor of right ankle and foot `HCC` `Rx` `ESR` `COM`
  - **M05.872** Other rheumatoid arthritis with rheumatoid factor of left ankle and foot `HCC` `Rx` `ESR` `COM`
  - **M05.879** Other rheumatoid arthritis with rheumatoid factor of unspecified ankle and foot `HCC` `Rx` `ESR` `COM`
- **M05.89** Other rheumatoid arthritis with rheumatoid factor of multiple sites `HCC` `Rx` `ESR` `COM`
- **M05.8A** Other rheumatoid arthritis with rheumatoid factor of other specified site `HCC` `Rx` `ESR` `COM`

- **M05.9** Rheumatoid arthritis with rheumatoid factor, unspecified `HCC` `Rx` `ESR` `COM`
- • **M05.A** Abnormal rheumatoid factor and anti-citrullinated protein antibody with rheumatoid arthritis
  Code first rheumatoid arthritis with rheumatoid factor by site, if known (M05.00-M05.8A)

✓4th **M06** Other rheumatoid arthritis
  AHA: 2020,4Q,31-32
  DEF: Rheumatoid arthritis: Autoimmune systemic disease that causes chronic inflammation of the joints and other areas of the body, manifested by inflammatory changes in articular structures and synovial membranes, atrophy, and loss in bone density.

- ✓5th **M06.0** Rheumatoid arthritis without rheumatoid factor
  - **M06.00** Rheumatoid arthritis without rheumatoid factor, unspecified site `HCC` `Rx` `ESR` `COM`
  - ✓6th **M06.01** Rheumatoid arthritis without rheumatoid factor, shoulder
    - **M06.011** Rheumatoid arthritis without rheumatoid factor, right shoulder `HCC` `Rx` `ESR` `COM`
    - **M06.012** Rheumatoid arthritis without rheumatoid factor, left shoulder `HCC` `Rx` `ESR` `COM`
    - **M06.019** Rheumatoid arthritis without rheumatoid factor, unspecified shoulder `HCC` `Rx` `ESR` `COM`
  - ✓6th **M06.02** Rheumatoid arthritis without rheumatoid factor, elbow
    - **M06.021** Rheumatoid arthritis without rheumatoid factor, right elbow `HCC` `Rx` `ESR` `COM`
    - **M06.022** Rheumatoid arthritis without rheumatoid factor, left elbow `HCC` `Rx` `ESR` `COM`
    - **M06.029** Rheumatoid arthritis without rheumatoid factor, unspecified elbow `HCC` `Rx` `ESR` `COM`
  - ✓6th **M06.03** Rheumatoid arthritis without rheumatoid factor, wrist
    - **M06.031** Rheumatoid arthritis without rheumatoid factor, right wrist `HCC` `Rx` `ESR` `COM`
    - **M06.032** Rheumatoid arthritis without rheumatoid factor, left wrist `HCC` `Rx` `ESR` `COM`
    - **M06.039** Rheumatoid arthritis without rheumatoid factor, unspecified wrist `HCC` `Rx` `ESR` `COM`
  - ✓6th **M06.04** Rheumatoid arthritis without rheumatoid factor, hand
    - **M06.041** Rheumatoid arthritis without rheumatoid factor, right hand `HCC` `Rx` `ESR` `COM`
    - **M06.042** Rheumatoid arthritis without rheumatoid factor, left hand `HCC` `Rx` `ESR` `COM`
    - **M06.049** Rheumatoid arthritis without rheumatoid factor, unspecified hand `HCC` `Rx` `ESR` `COM`
  - ✓6th **M06.05** Rheumatoid arthritis without rheumatoid factor, hip
    - **M06.051** Rheumatoid arthritis without rheumatoid factor, right hip `HCC` `Rx` `ESR` `COM`
    - **M06.052** Rheumatoid arthritis without rheumatoid factor, left hip `HCC` `Rx` `ESR` `COM`
    - **M06.059** Rheumatoid arthritis without rheumatoid factor, unspecified hip `HCC` `Rx` `ESR` `COM`
  - ✓6th **M06.06** Rheumatoid arthritis without rheumatoid factor, knee
    - **M06.061** Rheumatoid arthritis without rheumatoid factor, right knee `HCC` `Rx` `ESR` `COM`
    - **M06.062** Rheumatoid arthritis without rheumatoid factor, left knee `HCC` `Rx` `ESR` `COM`
    - **M06.069** Rheumatoid arthritis without rheumatoid factor, unspecified knee `HCC` `Rx` `ESR` `COM`
  - ✓6th **M06.07** Rheumatoid arthritis without rheumatoid factor, ankle and foot
    - **M06.071** Rheumatoid arthritis without rheumatoid factor, right ankle and foot `HCC` `Rx` `ESR` `COM`
    - **M06.072** Rheumatoid arthritis without rheumatoid factor, left ankle and foot `HCC` `Rx` `ESR` `COM`
    - **M06.079** Rheumatoid arthritis without rheumatoid factor, unspecified ankle and foot `HCC` `Rx` `ESR` `COM`
  - **M06.08** Rheumatoid arthritis without rheumatoid factor, vertebrae `HCC` `Rx` `ESR` `COM`
  - **M06.09** Rheumatoid arthritis without rheumatoid factor, multiple sites `HCC` `Rx` `ESR` `COM`

`HCC` CMS-HCC `Rx` Rx HCC `ESR` ESRD HCC `COM` Commercial HCC **N** Newborn: 0 **P** Pediatric: 0-17 **M** Maternity: 9-64 **A** Adult: 15-124

	M06.0A	Rheumatoid arthritis without rheumatoid factor, other specified site [HCC] [Rx] [ESR] [COM]

	M06.1	Adult-onset Still's disease [HCC] [Rx] [ESR] [COM] [A]

EXCLUDES 1 Still's disease NOS (M08.2-)

DEF: Type of systemic arthritis characterized by a transient rash and spiking fevers. This condition may resolve or develop into a chronic condition and may affect internal organs, as well as joints.
Synonym(s): AOSD

√5th **M06.2 Rheumatoid bursitis**

- M06.20 Rheumatoid bursitis, unspecified site [HCC] [Rx] [ESR] [COM]
- √6th M06.21 Rheumatoid bursitis, shoulder
  - M06.211 Rheumatoid bursitis, right shoulder [HCC] [Rx] [ESR] [COM]
  - M06.212 Rheumatoid bursitis, left shoulder [HCC] [Rx] [ESR] [COM]
  - M06.219 Rheumatoid bursitis, unspecified shoulder [HCC] [Rx] [ESR] [COM]
- √6th M06.22 Rheumatoid bursitis, elbow
  - M06.221 Rheumatoid bursitis, right elbow [HCC] [Rx] [ESR] [COM]
  - M06.222 Rheumatoid bursitis, left elbow [HCC] [Rx] [ESR] [COM]
  - M06.229 Rheumatoid bursitis, unspecified elbow [HCC] [Rx] [ESR] [COM]
- √6th M06.23 Rheumatoid bursitis, wrist
  - M06.231 Rheumatoid bursitis, right wrist [HCC] [Rx] [ESR] [COM]
  - M06.232 Rheumatoid bursitis, left wrist [HCC] [Rx] [ESR] [COM]
  - M06.239 Rheumatoid bursitis, unspecified wrist [HCC] [Rx] [ESR] [COM]
- √6th M06.24 Rheumatoid bursitis, hand
  - M06.241 Rheumatoid bursitis, right hand [HCC] [Rx] [ESR] [COM]
  - M06.242 Rheumatoid bursitis, left hand [HCC] [Rx] [ESR] [COM]
  - M06.249 Rheumatoid bursitis, unspecified hand [HCC] [Rx] [ESR] [COM]
- √6th M06.25 Rheumatoid bursitis, hip
  - M06.251 Rheumatoid bursitis, right hip [HCC] [Rx] [ESR] [COM]
  - M06.252 Rheumatoid bursitis, left hip [HCC] [Rx] [ESR] [COM]
  - M06.259 Rheumatoid bursitis, unspecified hip [HCC] [Rx] [ESR] [COM]
- √6th M06.26 Rheumatoid bursitis, knee
  - M06.261 Rheumatoid bursitis, right knee [HCC] [Rx] [ESR] [COM]
  - M06.262 Rheumatoid bursitis, left knee [HCC] [Rx] [ESR] [COM]
  - M06.269 Rheumatoid bursitis, unspecified knee [HCC] [Rx] [ESR] [COM]
- √6th M06.27 Rheumatoid bursitis, ankle and foot
  - M06.271 Rheumatoid bursitis, right ankle and foot [HCC] [Rx] [ESR] [COM]
  - M06.272 Rheumatoid bursitis, left ankle and foot [HCC] [Rx] [ESR] [COM]
  - M06.279 Rheumatoid bursitis, unspecified ankle and foot [HCC] [Rx] [ESR] [COM]
- M06.28 Rheumatoid bursitis, vertebrae [HCC] [Rx] [ESR] [COM]
- M06.29 Rheumatoid bursitis, multiple sites [HCC] [Rx] [ESR] [COM]

√5th **M06.3 Rheumatoid nodule**

- M06.30 Rheumatoid nodule, unspecified site [HCC] [Rx] [ESR] [COM]
- √6th M06.31 Rheumatoid nodule, shoulder
  - M06.311 Rheumatoid nodule, right shoulder [HCC] [Rx] [ESR] [COM]
  - M06.312 Rheumatoid nodule, left shoulder [HCC] [Rx] [ESR] [COM]
  - M06.319 Rheumatoid nodule, unspecified shoulder [HCC] [Rx] [ESR] [COM]
- √6th M06.32 Rheumatoid nodule, elbow
  - M06.321 Rheumatoid nodule, right elbow [HCC] [Rx] [ESR] [COM]
  - M06.322 Rheumatoid nodule, left elbow [HCC] [Rx] [ESR] [COM]
  - M06.329 Rheumatoid nodule, unspecified elbow [HCC] [Rx] [ESR] [COM]
- √6th M06.33 Rheumatoid nodule, wrist
  - M06.331 Rheumatoid nodule, right wrist [HCC] [Rx] [ESR] [COM]
  - M06.332 Rheumatoid nodule, left wrist [HCC] [Rx] [ESR] [COM]
  - M06.339 Rheumatoid nodule, unspecified wrist [HCC] [Rx] [ESR] [COM]
- √6th M06.34 Rheumatoid nodule, hand
  - M06.341 Rheumatoid nodule, right hand [HCC] [Rx] [ESR] [COM]
  - M06.342 Rheumatoid nodule, left hand [HCC] [Rx] [ESR] [COM]
  - M06.349 Rheumatoid nodule, unspecified hand [HCC] [Rx] [ESR] [COM]
- √6th M06.35 Rheumatoid nodule, hip
  - M06.351 Rheumatoid nodule, right hip [HCC] [Rx] [ESR] [COM]
  - M06.352 Rheumatoid nodule, left hip [HCC] [Rx] [ESR] [COM]
  - M06.359 Rheumatoid nodule, unspecified hip [HCC] [Rx] [ESR] [COM]
- √6th M06.36 Rheumatoid nodule, knee
  - M06.361 Rheumatoid nodule, right knee [HCC] [Rx] [ESR] [COM]
  - M06.362 Rheumatoid nodule, left knee [HCC] [Rx] [ESR] [COM]
  - M06.369 Rheumatoid nodule, unspecified knee [HCC] [Rx] [ESR] [COM]
- √6th M06.37 Rheumatoid nodule, ankle and foot
  - M06.371 Rheumatoid nodule, right ankle and foot [HCC] [Rx] [ESR] [COM]
  - M06.372 Rheumatoid nodule, left ankle and foot [HCC] [Rx] [ESR] [COM]
  - M06.379 Rheumatoid nodule, unspecified ankle and foot [HCC] [Rx] [ESR] [COM]
- M06.38 Rheumatoid nodule, vertebrae [HCC] [Rx] [ESR] [COM]
- M06.39 Rheumatoid nodule, multiple sites [HCC] [Rx] [ESR] [COM]

M06.4 Inflammatory polyarthropathy

EXCLUDES 1 polyarthritis NOS (M13.0)
AHA: 2025,2Q,9-10; 2024,1Q,17

√5th **M06.8 Other specified rheumatoid arthritis**

- M06.80 Other specified rheumatoid arthritis, unspecified site [HCC] [Rx] [ESR] [COM]
- √6th M06.81 Other specified rheumatoid arthritis, shoulder
  - M06.811 Other specified rheumatoid arthritis, right shoulder [HCC] [Rx] [ESR] [COM]
  - M06.812 Other specified rheumatoid arthritis, left shoulder [HCC] [Rx] [ESR] [COM]
  - M06.819 Other specified rheumatoid arthritis, unspecified shoulder [HCC] [Rx] [ESR] [COM]
- √6th M06.82 Other specified rheumatoid arthritis, elbow
  - M06.821 Other specified rheumatoid arthritis, right elbow [HCC] [Rx] [ESR] [COM]
  - M06.822 Other specified rheumatoid arthritis, left elbow [HCC] [Rx] [ESR] [COM]
  - M06.829 Other specified rheumatoid arthritis, unspecified elbow [HCC] [Rx] [ESR] [COM]
- √6th M06.83 Other specified rheumatoid arthritis, wrist
  - M06.831 Other specified rheumatoid arthritis, right wrist [HCC] [Rx] [ESR] [COM]
  - M06.832 Other specified rheumatoid arthritis, left wrist [HCC] [Rx] [ESR] [COM]
  - M06.839 Other specified rheumatoid arthritis, unspecified wrist [HCC] [Rx] [ESR] [COM]
- √6th M06.84 Other specified rheumatoid arthritis, hand
  - M06.841 Other specified rheumatoid arthritis, right hand [HCC] [Rx] [ESR] [COM]
  - M06.842 Other specified rheumatoid arthritis, left hand [HCC] [Rx] [ESR] [COM]
  - M06.849 Other specified rheumatoid arthritis, unspecified hand [HCC] [Rx] [ESR] [COM]

- ✓6th **M06.85** Other specified rheumatoid arthritis, hip
  - **M06.851** Other specified rheumatoid arthritis, right hip `HCC` `Rx` `ESR` `COM`
  - **M06.852** Other specified rheumatoid arthritis, left hip `HCC` `Rx` `ESR` `COM`
  - **M06.859** Other specified rheumatoid arthritis, unspecified hip `HCC` `Rx` `ESR` `COM`
- ✓6th **M06.86** Other specified rheumatoid arthritis, knee
  - **M06.861** Other specified rheumatoid arthritis, right knee `HCC` `Rx` `ESR` `COM`
  - **M06.862** Other specified rheumatoid arthritis, left knee `HCC` `Rx` `ESR` `COM`
  - **M06.869** Other specified rheumatoid arthritis, unspecified knee `HCC` `Rx` `ESR` `COM`
- ✓6th **M06.87** Other specified rheumatoid arthritis, ankle and foot
  - **M06.871** Other specified rheumatoid arthritis, right ankle and foot `HCC` `Rx` `ESR` `COM`
  - **M06.872** Other specified rheumatoid arthritis, left ankle and foot `HCC` `Rx` `ESR` `COM`
  - **M06.879** Other specified rheumatoid arthritis, unspecified ankle and foot
- **M06.88** Other specified rheumatoid arthritis, vertebrae `HCC` `Rx` `ESR` `COM`
- **M06.89** Other specified rheumatoid arthritis, multiple sites `HCC` `Rx` `ESR` `COM`
- **M06.8A** Other specified rheumatoid arthritis, other specified site `HCC` `Rx` `ESR` `COM`
- **M06.9** Rheumatoid arthritis, unspecified `HCC` `Rx` `ESR` `COM`
  - **AHA:** 2024,1Q,17

✓4th M07 Enteropathic arthropathies

Code also associated enteropathy, such as:
  regional enteritis [Crohn's disease] (K50.-)
  ulcerative colitis (K51.-)

EXCLUDES 1 psoriatic arthropathies (L40.5-)

- ✓5th **M07.6** Enteropathic arthropathies
  - **M07.60** Enteropathic arthropathies, unspecified site
  - ✓6th **M07.61** Enteropathic arthropathies, shoulder
    - **M07.611** Enteropathic arthropathies, right shoulder
    - **M07.612** Enteropathic arthropathies, left shoulder
    - **M07.619** Enteropathic arthropathies, unspecified shoulder
  - ✓6th **M07.62** Enteropathic arthropathies, elbow
    - **M07.621** Enteropathic arthropathies, right elbow
    - **M07.622** Enteropathic arthropathies, left elbow
    - **M07.629** Enteropathic arthropathies, unspecified elbow
  - ✓6th **M07.63** Enteropathic arthropathies, wrist
    - **M07.631** Enteropathic arthropathies, right wrist
    - **M07.632** Enteropathic arthropathies, left wrist
    - **M07.639** Enteropathic arthropathies, unspecified wrist
  - ✓6th **M07.64** Enteropathic arthropathies, hand
    - **M07.641** Enteropathic arthropathies, right hand
    - **M07.642** Enteropathic arthropathies, left hand
    - **M07.649** Enteropathic arthropathies, unspecified hand
  - ✓6th **M07.65** Enteropathic arthropathies, hip
    - **M07.651** Enteropathic arthropathies, right hip
    - **M07.652** Enteropathic arthropathies, left hip
    - **M07.659** Enteropathic arthropathies, unspecified hip
  - ✓6th **M07.66** Enteropathic arthropathies, knee
    - **M07.661** Enteropathic arthropathies, right knee
    - **M07.662** Enteropathic arthropathies, left knee
    - **M07.669** Enteropathic arthropathies, unspecified knee
  - ✓6th **M07.67** Enteropathic arthropathies, ankle and foot
    - **M07.671** Enteropathic arthropathies, right ankle and foot
    - **M07.672** Enteropathic arthropathies, left ankle and foot
    - **M07.679** Enteropathic arthropathies, unspecified ankle and foot
  - **M07.68** Enteropathic arthropathies, vertebrae
  - **M07.69** Enteropathic arthropathies, multiple sites

✓4th M08 Juvenile arthritis

Code also any associated underlying condition, such as:
  regional enteritis [Crohn's disease] (K50.-)
  ulcerative colitis (K51.-)

EXCLUDES 1 arthropathy in Whipple's disease (M14.8)
  Felty's syndrome (M05.0)
  juvenile dermatomyositis (M33.0-)
  psoriatic juvenile arthropathy (L40.54)

AHA: 2020,4Q,31-32

- ✓5th **M08.0** Unspecified juvenile rheumatoid arthritis
  Juvenile rheumatoid arthritis with or without rheumatoid factor
  - **M08.00** Unspecified juvenile rheumatoid arthritis of unspecified site `HCC` `Rx` `ESR` `COM`
  - ✓6th **M08.01** Unspecified juvenile rheumatoid arthritis, shoulder
    - **M08.011** Unspecified juvenile rheumatoid arthritis, right shoulder `HCC` `Rx` `ESR` `COM`
    - **M08.012** Unspecified juvenile rheumatoid arthritis, left shoulder `HCC` `Rx` `ESR` `COM`
    - **M08.019** Unspecified juvenile rheumatoid arthritis, unspecified shoulder `HCC` `Rx` `ESR` `COM`
  - ✓6th **M08.02** Unspecified juvenile rheumatoid arthritis of elbow
    - **M08.021** Unspecified juvenile rheumatoid arthritis, right elbow `HCC` `Rx` `ESR` `COM`
    - **M08.022** Unspecified juvenile rheumatoid arthritis, left elbow `HCC` `Rx` `ESR` `COM`
    - **M08.029** Unspecified juvenile rheumatoid arthritis, unspecified elbow `HCC` `Rx` `ESR` `COM`
  - ✓6th **M08.03** Unspecified juvenile rheumatoid arthritis, wrist
    - **M08.031** Unspecified juvenile rheumatoid arthritis, right wrist `HCC` `Rx` `ESR` `COM`
    - **M08.032** Unspecified juvenile rheumatoid arthritis, left wrist `HCC` `Rx` `ESR` `COM`
    - **M08.039** Unspecified juvenile rheumatoid arthritis, unspecified wrist `HCC` `Rx` `ESR` `COM`
  - ✓6th **M08.04** Unspecified juvenile rheumatoid arthritis, hand
    - **M08.041** Unspecified juvenile rheumatoid arthritis, right hand `HCC` `Rx` `ESR` `COM`
    - **M08.042** Unspecified juvenile rheumatoid arthritis, left hand `HCC` `Rx` `ESR` `COM`
    - **M08.049** Unspecified juvenile rheumatoid arthritis, unspecified hand `HCC` `Rx` `ESR` `COM`
  - ✓6th **M08.05** Unspecified juvenile rheumatoid arthritis, hip
    - **M08.051** Unspecified juvenile rheumatoid arthritis, right hip `HCC` `Rx` `ESR` `COM`
    - **M08.052** Unspecified juvenile rheumatoid arthritis, left hip `HCC` `Rx` `ESR` `COM`
    - **M08.059** Unspecified juvenile rheumatoid arthritis, unspecified hip `HCC` `Rx` `ESR` `COM`
  - ✓6th **M08.06** Unspecified juvenile rheumatoid arthritis, knee
    - **M08.061** Unspecified juvenile rheumatoid arthritis, right knee `HCC` `Rx` `ESR` `COM`
    - **M08.062** Unspecified juvenile rheumatoid arthritis, left knee `HCC` `Rx` `ESR` `COM`
    - **M08.069** Unspecified juvenile rheumatoid arthritis, unspecified knee `HCC` `Rx` `ESR` `COM`
  - ✓6th **M08.07** Unspecified juvenile rheumatoid arthritis, ankle and foot
    - **M08.071** Unspecified juvenile rheumatoid arthritis, right ankle and foot `HCC` `Rx` `ESR` `COM`
    - **M08.072** Unspecified juvenile rheumatoid arthritis, left ankle and foot `HCC` `Rx` `ESR` `COM`
    - **M08.079** Unspecified juvenile rheumatoid arthritis, unspecified ankle and foot `HCC` `Rx` `ESR` `COM`
  - **M08.08** Unspecified juvenile rheumatoid arthritis, vertebrae `HCC` `Rx` `ESR` `COM`
  - **M08.09** Unspecified juvenile rheumatoid arthritis, multiple sites `HCC` `Rx` `ESR` `COM`
  - **M08.0A** Unspecified juvenile rheumatoid arthritis, other specified site `HCC` `Rx` `ESR` `COM`
- **M08.1** Juvenile ankylosing spondylitis `HCC` `Rx` `ESR` `COM`
  EXCLUDES 1 ankylosing spondylitis in adults (M45.0-)

Chapter 13. Diseases of the Musculoskeletal System and Connective Tissue

√5th **M08.2 Juvenile rheumatoid arthritis with systemic onset**
Still's disease NOS
EXCLUDES 1 adult-onset Still's disease (M06.1-)
DEF: Systemic juvenile rheumatoid arthritis characterized by a transient rash and spiking fevers that may affect internal organs, as well as joints.

- M08.20 Juvenile rheumatoid arthritis with systemic onset, unspecified site
- √6th M08.21 Juvenile rheumatoid arthritis with systemic onset, shoulder
  - M08.211 Juvenile rheumatoid arthritis with systemic onset, right shoulder
  - M08.212 Juvenile rheumatoid arthritis with systemic onset, left shoulder
  - M08.219 Juvenile rheumatoid arthritis with systemic onset, unspecified shoulder
- √6th M08.22 Juvenile rheumatoid arthritis with systemic onset, elbow
  - M08.221 Juvenile rheumatoid arthritis with systemic onset, right elbow
  - M08.222 Juvenile rheumatoid arthritis with systemic onset, left elbow
  - M08.229 Juvenile rheumatoid arthritis with systemic onset, unspecified elbow
- √6th M08.23 Juvenile rheumatoid arthritis with systemic onset, wrist
  - M08.231 Juvenile rheumatoid arthritis with systemic onset, right wrist
  - M08.232 Juvenile rheumatoid arthritis with systemic onset, left wrist
  - M08.239 Juvenile rheumatoid arthritis with systemic onset, unspecified wrist
- √6th M08.24 Juvenile rheumatoid arthritis with systemic onset, hand
  - M08.241 Juvenile rheumatoid arthritis with systemic onset, right hand
  - M08.242 Juvenile rheumatoid arthritis with systemic onset, left hand
  - M08.249 Juvenile rheumatoid arthritis with systemic onset, unspecified hand
- √6th M08.25 Juvenile rheumatoid arthritis with systemic onset, hip
  - M08.251 Juvenile rheumatoid arthritis with systemic onset, right hip
  - M08.252 Juvenile rheumatoid arthritis with systemic onset, left hip
  - M08.259 Juvenile rheumatoid arthritis with systemic onset, unspecified hip
- √6th M08.26 Juvenile rheumatoid arthritis with systemic onset, knee
  - M08.261 Juvenile rheumatoid arthritis with systemic onset, right knee
  - M08.262 Juvenile rheumatoid arthritis with systemic onset, left knee
  - M08.269 Juvenile rheumatoid arthritis with systemic onset, unspecified knee
- √6th M08.27 Juvenile rheumatoid arthritis with systemic onset, ankle and foot
  - M08.271 Juvenile rheumatoid arthritis with systemic onset, right ankle and foot
  - M08.272 Juvenile rheumatoid arthritis with systemic onset, left ankle and foot
  - M08.279 Juvenile rheumatoid arthritis with systemic onset, unspecified ankle and foot
- M08.28 Juvenile rheumatoid arthritis with systemic onset, vertebrae
- M08.29 Juvenile rheumatoid arthritis with systemic onset, multiple sites
- M08.2A Juvenile rheumatoid arthritis with systemic onset, other specified site

M08.3 Juvenile rheumatoid polyarthritis (seronegative)

√5th **M08.4 Pauciarticular juvenile rheumatoid arthritis**
- M08.40 Pauciarticular juvenile rheumatoid arthritis, unspecified site
- √6th M08.41 Pauciarticular juvenile rheumatoid arthritis, shoulder
  - M08.411 Pauciarticular juvenile rheumatoid arthritis, right shoulder
  - M08.412 Pauciarticular juvenile rheumatoid arthritis, left shoulder
  - M08.419 Pauciarticular juvenile rheumatoid arthritis, unspecified shoulder
- √6th M08.42 Pauciarticular juvenile rheumatoid arthritis, elbow
  - M08.421 Pauciarticular juvenile rheumatoid arthritis, right elbow
  - M08.422 Pauciarticular juvenile rheumatoid arthritis, left elbow
  - M08.429 Pauciarticular juvenile rheumatoid arthritis, unspecified elbow
- √6th M08.43 Pauciarticular juvenile rheumatoid arthritis, wrist
  - M08.431 Pauciarticular juvenile rheumatoid arthritis, right wrist
  - M08.432 Pauciarticular juvenile rheumatoid arthritis, left wrist
  - M08.439 Pauciarticular juvenile rheumatoid arthritis, unspecified wrist
- √6th M08.44 Pauciarticular juvenile rheumatoid arthritis, hand
  - M08.441 Pauciarticular juvenile rheumatoid arthritis, right hand
  - M08.442 Pauciarticular juvenile rheumatoid arthritis, left hand
  - M08.449 Pauciarticular juvenile rheumatoid arthritis, unspecified hand
- √6th M08.45 Pauciarticular juvenile rheumatoid arthritis, hip
  - M08.451 Pauciarticular juvenile rheumatoid arthritis, right hip
  - M08.452 Pauciarticular juvenile rheumatoid arthritis, left hip
  - M08.459 Pauciarticular juvenile rheumatoid arthritis, unspecified hip
- √6th M08.46 Pauciarticular juvenile rheumatoid arthritis, knee
  - M08.461 Pauciarticular juvenile rheumatoid arthritis, right knee
  - M08.462 Pauciarticular juvenile rheumatoid arthritis, left knee
  - M08.469 Pauciarticular juvenile rheumatoid arthritis, unspecified knee
- √6th M08.47 Pauciarticular juvenile rheumatoid arthritis, ankle and foot
  - M08.471 Pauciarticular juvenile rheumatoid arthritis, right ankle and foot
  - M08.472 Pauciarticular juvenile rheumatoid arthritis, left ankle and foot
  - M08.479 Pauciarticular juvenile rheumatoid arthritis, unspecified ankle and foot
- M08.48 Pauciarticular juvenile rheumatoid arthritis, vertebrae
- M08.4A Pauciarticular juvenile rheumatoid arthritis, other specified site

Additional Character Required | √x7th Placeholder Alert | Manifestation | Unspecified Dx | Q QPP | UPD Unacceptable PDx

M08.8 Other juvenile arthritis

- **M08.80** Other juvenile arthritis, unspecified site
- **M08.81** Other juvenile arthritis, shoulder
  - **M08.811** Other juvenile arthritis, right shoulder
  - **M08.812** Other juvenile arthritis, left shoulder
  - **M08.819** Other juvenile arthritis, unspecified shoulder
- **M08.82** Other juvenile arthritis, elbow
  - **M08.821** Other juvenile arthritis, right elbow
  - **M08.822** Other juvenile arthritis, left elbow
  - **M08.829** Other juvenile arthritis, unspecified elbow
- **M08.83** Other juvenile arthritis, wrist
  - **M08.831** Other juvenile arthritis, right wrist
  - **M08.832** Other juvenile arthritis, left wrist
  - **M08.839** Other juvenile arthritis, unspecified wrist
- **M08.84** Other juvenile arthritis, hand
  - **M08.841** Other juvenile arthritis, right hand
  - **M08.842** Other juvenile arthritis, left hand
  - **M08.849** Other juvenile arthritis, unspecified hand
- **M08.85** Other juvenile arthritis, hip
  - **M08.851** Other juvenile arthritis, right hip
  - **M08.852** Other juvenile arthritis, left hip
  - **M08.859** Other juvenile arthritis, unspecified hip
- **M08.86** Other juvenile arthritis, knee
  - **M08.861** Other juvenile arthritis, right knee
  - **M08.862** Other juvenile arthritis, left knee
  - **M08.869** Other juvenile arthritis, unspecified knee
- **M08.87** Other juvenile arthritis, ankle and foot
  - **M08.871** Other juvenile arthritis, right ankle and foot
  - **M08.872** Other juvenile arthritis, left ankle and foot
  - **M08.879** Other juvenile arthritis, unspecified ankle and foot
- **M08.88** Other juvenile arthritis, other specified site
  - Other juvenile arthritis, vertebrae
- **M08.89** Other juvenile arthritis, multiple sites

M08.9 Juvenile arthritis, unspecified

EXCLUDES 1 juvenile rheumatoid arthritis, unspecified (M08.0-)

- **M08.90** Juvenile arthritis, unspecified, unspecified site
- **M08.91** Juvenile arthritis, unspecified, shoulder
  - **M08.911** Juvenile arthritis, unspecified, right shoulder
  - **M08.912** Juvenile arthritis, unspecified, left shoulder
  - **M08.919** Juvenile arthritis, unspecified, unspecified shoulder
- **M08.92** Juvenile arthritis, unspecified, elbow
  - **M08.921** Juvenile arthritis, unspecified, right elbow
  - **M08.922** Juvenile arthritis, unspecified, left elbow
  - **M08.929** Juvenile arthritis, unspecified, unspecified elbow
- **M08.93** Juvenile arthritis, unspecified, wrist
  - **M08.931** Juvenile arthritis, unspecified, right wrist
  - **M08.932** Juvenile arthritis, unspecified, left wrist
  - **M08.939** Juvenile arthritis, unspecified, unspecified wrist
- **M08.94** Juvenile arthritis, unspecified, hand
  - **M08.941** Juvenile arthritis, unspecified, right hand
  - **M08.942** Juvenile arthritis, unspecified, left hand
  - **M08.949** Juvenile arthritis, unspecified, unspecified hand
- **M08.95** Juvenile arthritis, unspecified, hip
  - **M08.951** Juvenile arthritis, unspecified, right hip
  - **M08.952** Juvenile arthritis, unspecified, left hip
  - **M08.959** Juvenile arthritis, unspecified, unspecified hip
- **M08.96** Juvenile arthritis, unspecified, knee
  - **M08.961** Juvenile arthritis, unspecified, right knee
  - **M08.962** Juvenile arthritis, unspecified, left knee
  - **M08.969** Juvenile arthritis, unspecified, unspecified knee
- **M08.97** Juvenile arthritis, unspecified, ankle and foot
  - **M08.971** Juvenile arthritis, unspecified, right ankle and foot
  - **M08.972** Juvenile arthritis, unspecified, left ankle and foot
  - **M08.979** Juvenile arthritis, unspecified, unspecified ankle and foot
- **M08.98** Juvenile arthritis, unspecified, vertebrae
- **M08.99** Juvenile arthritis, unspecified, multiple sites
- **M08.9A** Juvenile arthritis, unspecified, other specified site

M1A Chronic gout

Use additional code to identify:
  autonomic neuropathy in diseases classified elsewhere (G99.0)
  calculus of urinary tract in diseases classified elsewhere (N22)
  cardiomyopathy in diseases classified elsewhere (I43)
  disorders of external ear in diseases classified elsewhere (H61.1-, H62.8-)
  disorders of iris and ciliary body in diseases classified elsewhere (H22)
  glomerular disorders in diseases classified elsewhere (N08)

EXCLUDES 1 gout NOS (M10.-)
EXCLUDES 2 acute gout (M10.-)

The appropriate 7th character is to be added to each code from category M1A.
0 without tophus (tophi)
1 with tophus (tophi)

M1A.0 Idiopathic chronic gout
Chronic gouty bursitis
Primary chronic gout

- **M1A.00** Idiopathic chronic gout, unspecified site
- **M1A.01** Idiopathic chronic gout, shoulder
  - **M1A.011** Idiopathic chronic gout, right shoulder
  - **M1A.012** Idiopathic chronic gout, left shoulder
  - **M1A.019** Idiopathic chronic gout, unspecified shoulder
- **M1A.02** Idiopathic chronic gout, elbow
  - **M1A.021** Idiopathic chronic gout, right elbow
  - **M1A.022** Idiopathic chronic gout, left elbow
  - **M1A.029** Idiopathic chronic gout, unspecified elbow
- **M1A.03** Idiopathic chronic gout, wrist
  - **M1A.031** Idiopathic chronic gout, right wrist
  - **M1A.032** Idiopathic chronic gout, left wrist
  - **M1A.039** Idiopathic chronic gout, unspecified wrist
- **M1A.04** Idiopathic chronic gout, hand
  - **M1A.041** Idiopathic chronic gout, right hand

Chapter 13. Diseases of the Musculoskeletal System and Connective Tissue

- √7th M1A.042 Idiopathic chronic gout, left hand
- √7th M1A.049 Idiopathic chronic gout, unspecified hand
- √6th M1A.05 Idiopathic chronic gout, hip
  - √7th M1A.051 Idiopathic chronic gout, right hip
  - √7th M1A.052 Idiopathic chronic gout, left hip
  - √7th M1A.059 Idiopathic chronic gout, unspecified hip
- √6th M1A.06 Idiopathic chronic gout, knee
  - √7th M1A.061 Idiopathic chronic gout, right knee
  - √7th M1A.062 Idiopathic chronic gout, left knee
  - √7th M1A.069 Idiopathic chronic gout, unspecified knee
- √6th M1A.07 Idiopathic chronic gout, ankle and foot
  - √7th M1A.071 Idiopathic chronic gout, right ankle and foot
  - √7th M1A.072 Idiopathic chronic gout, left ankle and foot
  - √7th M1A.079 Idiopathic chronic gout, unspecified ankle and foot
- √x7th M1A.08 Idiopathic chronic gout, vertebrae
- √x7th M1A.09 Idiopathic chronic gout, multiple sites
- √5th **M1A.1** **Lead-induced** chronic gout
  Code first toxic effects of lead and its compounds (T56.0-)
  - √x7th M1A.10 Lead-induced chronic gout, unspecified site
  - √6th M1A.11 Lead-induced chronic gout, shoulder
    - √7th M1A.111 Lead-induced chronic gout, right shoulder
    - √7th M1A.112 Lead-induced chronic gout, left shoulder
    - √7th M1A.119 Lead-induced chronic gout, unspecified shoulder
  - √6th M1A.12 Lead-induced chronic gout, elbow
    - √7th M1A.121 Lead-induced chronic gout, right elbow
    - √7th M1A.122 Lead-induced chronic gout, left elbow
    - √7th M1A.129 Lead-induced chronic gout, unspecified elbow
  - √6th M1A.13 Lead-induced chronic gout, wrist
    - √7th M1A.131 Lead-induced chronic gout, right wrist
    - √7th M1A.132 Lead-induced chronic gout, left wrist
    - √7th M1A.139 Lead-induced chronic gout, unspecified wrist
  - √6th M1A.14 Lead-induced chronic gout, hand
    - √7th M1A.141 Lead-induced chronic gout, right hand
    - √7th M1A.142 Lead-induced chronic gout, left hand
    - √7th M1A.149 Lead-induced chronic gout, unspecified hand
  - √6th M1A.15 Lead-induced chronic gout, hip
    - √7th M1A.151 Lead-induced chronic gout, right hip
    - √7th M1A.152 Lead-induced chronic gout, left hip
    - √7th M1A.159 Lead-induced chronic gout, unspecified hip
  - √6th M1A.16 Lead-induced chronic gout, knee
    - √7th M1A.161 Lead-induced chronic gout, right knee
    - √7th M1A.162 Lead-induced chronic gout, left knee
    - √7th M1A.169 Lead-induced chronic gout, unspecified knee
  - √6th M1A.17 Lead-induced chronic gout, ankle and foot
    - √7th M1A.171 Lead-induced chronic gout, right ankle and foot
    - √7th M1A.172 Lead-induced chronic gout, left ankle and foot
    - √7th M1A.179 Lead-induced chronic gout, unspecified ankle and foot
  - √x7th M1A.18 Lead-induced chronic gout, vertebrae
  - √x7th M1A.19 Lead-induced chronic gout, multiple sites
- √5th **M1A.2** **Drug-induced** chronic gout
  Use additional code for adverse effect, if applicable, to identify drug (T36-T50 with fifth or sixth character 5)
  - √x7th M1A.20 Drug-induced chronic gout, unspecified site
  - √6th M1A.21 Drug-induced chronic gout, shoulder
    - √7th M1A.211 Drug-induced chronic gout, right shoulder
    - √7th M1A.212 Drug-induced chronic gout, left shoulder
    - √7th M1A.219 Drug-induced chronic gout, unspecified shoulder
  - √6th M1A.22 Drug-induced chronic gout, elbow
    - √7th M1A.221 Drug-induced chronic gout, right elbow
- √7th M1A.222 Drug-induced chronic gout, left elbow
- √7th M1A.229 Drug-induced chronic gout, unspecified elbow
- √6th M1A.23 Drug-induced chronic gout, wrist
  - √7th M1A.231 Drug-induced chronic gout, right wrist
  - √7th M1A.232 Drug-induced chronic gout, left wrist
  - √7th M1A.239 Drug-induced chronic gout, unspecified wrist
- √6th M1A.24 Drug-induced chronic gout, hand
  - √7th M1A.241 Drug-induced chronic gout, right hand
  - √7th M1A.242 Drug-induced chronic gout, left hand
  - √7th M1A.249 Drug-induced chronic gout, unspecified hand
- √6th M1A.25 Drug-induced chronic gout, hip
  - √7th M1A.251 Drug-induced chronic gout, right hip
  - √7th M1A.252 Drug-induced chronic gout, left hip
  - √7th M1A.259 Drug-induced chronic gout, unspecified hip
- √6th M1A.26 Drug-induced chronic gout, knee
  - √7th M1A.261 Drug-induced chronic gout, right knee
  - √7th M1A.262 Drug-induced chronic gout, left knee
  - √7th M1A.269 Drug-induced chronic gout, unspecified knee
- √6th M1A.27 Drug-induced chronic gout, ankle and foot
  - √7th M1A.271 Drug-induced chronic gout, right ankle and foot
  - √7th M1A.272 Drug-induced chronic gout, left ankle and foot
  - √7th M1A.279 Drug-induced chronic gout, unspecified ankle and foot
- √x7th M1A.28 Drug-induced chronic gout, vertebrae
- √x7th M1A.29 Drug-induced chronic gout, multiple sites
- √5th **M1A.3** Chronic gout **due to renal impairment**
  Code first associated renal disease
  - √x7th M1A.30 Chronic gout due to renal impairment, unspecified site
  - √6th M1A.31 Chronic gout due to renal impairment, shoulder
    - √7th M1A.311 Chronic gout due to renal impairment, right shoulder
    - √7th M1A.312 Chronic gout due to renal impairment, left shoulder
    - √7th M1A.319 Chronic gout due to renal impairment, unspecified shoulder
  - √6th M1A.32 Chronic gout due to renal impairment, elbow
    - √7th M1A.321 Chronic gout due to renal impairment, right elbow
    - √7th M1A.322 Chronic gout due to renal impairment, left elbow
    - √7th M1A.329 Chronic gout due to renal impairment, unspecified elbow
  - √6th M1A.33 Chronic gout due to renal impairment, wrist
    - √7th M1A.331 Chronic gout due to renal impairment, right wrist
    - √7th M1A.332 Chronic gout due to renal impairment, left wrist
    - √7th M1A.339 Chronic gout due to renal impairment, unspecified wrist
  - √6th M1A.34 Chronic gout due to renal impairment, hand
    - √7th M1A.341 Chronic gout due to renal impairment, right hand
    - √7th M1A.342 Chronic gout due to renal impairment, left hand
    - √7th M1A.349 Chronic gout due to renal impairment, unspecified hand
  - √6th M1A.35 Chronic gout due to renal impairment, hip
    - √7th M1A.351 Chronic gout due to renal impairment, right hip
    - √7th M1A.352 Chronic gout due to renal impairment, left hip
    - √7th M1A.359 Chronic gout due to renal impairment, unspecified hip
  - √6th M1A.36 Chronic gout due to renal impairment, knee
    - √7th M1A.361 Chronic gout due to renal impairment, right knee
    - √7th M1A.362 Chronic gout due to renal impairment, left knee

	✓7th	M1A.369	Chronic gout due to renal impairment, unspecified knee
	✓6th	M1A.37	Chronic gout due to renal impairment, ankle and foot
		✓7th M1A.371	Chronic gout due to renal impairment, right ankle and foot
		✓7th M1A.372	Chronic gout due to renal impairment, left ankle and foot
		✓7th M1A.379	Chronic gout due to renal impairment, unspecified ankle and foot
	✓x7th	M1A.38	Chronic gout due to renal impairment, vertebrae
	✓x7th	M1A.39	Chronic gout due to renal impairment, multiple sites

✓5th M1A.4 Other secondary chronic gout

Code first associated condition

- ✓x7th **M1A.40** Other secondary chronic gout, unspecified site
- ✓6th **M1A.41** Other secondary chronic gout, shoulder
  - ✓7th M1A.411 Other secondary chronic gout, right shoulder
  - ✓7th M1A.412 Other secondary chronic gout, left shoulder
  - ✓7th M1A.419 Other secondary chronic gout, unspecified shoulder
- ✓6th **M1A.42** Other secondary chronic gout, elbow
  - ✓7th M1A.421 Other secondary chronic gout, right elbow
  - ✓7th M1A.422 Other secondary chronic gout, left elbow
  - ✓7th M1A.429 Other secondary chronic gout, unspecified elbow
- ✓6th **M1A.43** Other secondary chronic gout, wrist
  - ✓7th M1A.431 Other secondary chronic gout, right wrist
  - ✓7th M1A.432 Other secondary chronic gout, left wrist
  - ✓7th M1A.439 Other secondary chronic gout, unspecified wrist
- ✓6th **M1A.44** Other secondary chronic gout, hand
  - ✓7th M1A.441 Other secondary chronic gout, right hand
  - ✓7th M1A.442 Other secondary chronic gout, left hand
  - ✓7th M1A.449 Other secondary chronic gout, unspecified hand
- ✓6th **M1A.45** Other secondary chronic gout, hip
  - ✓7th M1A.451 Other secondary chronic gout, right hip
  - ✓7th M1A.452 Other secondary chronic gout, left hip
  - ✓7th M1A.459 Other secondary chronic gout, unspecified hip
- ✓6th **M1A.46** Other secondary chronic gout, knee
  - ✓7th M1A.461 Other secondary chronic gout, right knee
  - ✓7th M1A.462 Other secondary chronic gout, left knee
  - ✓7th M1A.469 Other secondary chronic gout, unspecified knee
- ✓6th **M1A.47** Other secondary chronic gout, ankle and foot
  - ✓7th M1A.471 Other secondary chronic gout, right ankle and foot
  - ✓7th M1A.472 Other secondary chronic gout, left ankle and foot
  - ✓7th M1A.479 Other secondary chronic gout, unspecified ankle and foot
- ✓x7th **M1A.48** Other secondary chronic gout, vertebrae
- ✓x7th **M1A.49** Other secondary chronic gout, multiple sites

✓x7th **M1A.9 Chronic gout, unspecified**

✓4th M10 Gout

Acute gout
Gout attack
Gout flare
Podagra

Use additional code to identify:
 autonomic neuropathy in diseases classified elsewhere (G99.0)
 calculus of urinary tract in diseases classified elsewhere (N22)
 cardiomyopathy in diseases classified elsewhere (I43)
 disorders of external ear in diseases classified elsewhere (H61.1-, H62.8-)
 disorders of iris and ciliary body in diseases classified elsewhere (H22)
 glomerular disorders in diseases classified elsewhere (N08)

EXCLUDES 2 chronic gout (M1A.-)

DEF: Purine and pyrimidine metabolic disorders, manifested by hyperuricemia and recurrent acute inflammatory arthritis. Monosodium urate or monohydrate crystals may be deposited in and around the joints, leading to joint destruction and severe crippling.

✓5th M10.0 Idiopathic gout

Gouty bursitis
Primary gout

- **M10.00** Idiopathic gout, unspecified site
- ✓6th **M10.01** Idiopathic gout, shoulder
  - M10.011 Idiopathic gout, right shoulder
  - M10.012 Idiopathic gout, left shoulder
  - M10.019 Idiopathic gout, unspecified shoulder
- ✓6th **M10.02** Idiopathic gout, elbow
  - M10.021 Idiopathic gout, right elbow
  - M10.022 Idiopathic gout, left elbow
  - M10.029 Idiopathic gout, unspecified elbow
- ✓6th **M10.03** Idiopathic gout, wrist
  - M10.031 Idiopathic gout, right wrist
  - M10.032 Idiopathic gout, left wrist
  - M10.039 Idiopathic gout, unspecified wrist
- ✓6th **M10.04** Idiopathic gout, hand
  - M10.041 Idiopathic gout, right hand
  - M10.042 Idiopathic gout, left hand
  - M10.049 Idiopathic gout, unspecified hand
- ✓6th **M10.05** Idiopathic gout, hip
  - M10.051 Idiopathic gout, right hip
  - M10.052 Idiopathic gout, left hip
  - M10.059 Idiopathic gout, unspecified hip
- ✓6th **M10.06** Idiopathic gout, knee
  - M10.061 Idiopathic gout, right knee
  - M10.062 Idiopathic gout, left knee
  - M10.069 Idiopathic gout, unspecified knee
- ✓6th **M10.07** Idiopathic gout, ankle and foot
  - M10.071 Idiopathic gout, right ankle and foot
  - M10.072 Idiopathic gout, left ankle and foot
  - M10.079 Idiopathic gout, unspecified ankle and foot
- **M10.08** Idiopathic gout, vertebrae
- **M10.09** Idiopathic gout, multiple sites

✓5th M10.1 Lead-induced gout

Code first toxic effects of lead and its compounds (T56.0-)

- **M10.10** Lead-induced gout, unspecified site
- ✓6th **M10.11** Lead-induced gout, shoulder
  - M10.111 Lead-induced gout, right shoulder
  - M10.112 Lead-induced gout, left shoulder
  - M10.119 Lead-induced gout, unspecified shoulder
- ✓6th **M10.12** Lead-induced gout, elbow
  - M10.121 Lead-induced gout, right elbow
  - M10.122 Lead-induced gout, left elbow
  - M10.129 Lead-induced gout, unspecified elbow
- ✓6th **M10.13** Lead-induced gout, wrist
  - M10.131 Lead-induced gout, right wrist
  - M10.132 Lead-induced gout, left wrist
  - M10.139 Lead-induced gout, unspecified wrist
- ✓6th **M10.14** Lead-induced gout, hand
  - M10.141 Lead-induced gout, right hand
  - M10.142 Lead-induced gout, left hand
  - M10.149 Lead-induced gout, unspecified hand
- ✓6th **M10.15** Lead-induced gout, hip
  - M10.151 Lead-induced gout, right hip
  - M10.152 Lead-induced gout, left hip
  - M10.159 Lead-induced gout, unspecified hip
- ✓6th **M10.16** Lead-induced gout, knee
  - M10.161 Lead-induced gout, right knee
  - M10.162 Lead-induced gout, left knee

	M10.169	Lead-induced gout, unspecified knee
✓6ᵗʰ M10.17		Lead-induced gout, ankle and foot
	M10.171	Lead-induced gout, right ankle and foot
	M10.172	Lead-induced gout, left ankle and foot
	M10.179	Lead-induced gout, unspecified ankle and foot
M10.18		Lead-induced gout, vertebrae
M10.19		Lead-induced gout, multiple sites

✓5ᵗʰ **M10.2 Drug-induced** gout

Use additional code for adverse effect, if applicable, to identify drug (T36-T50 with fifth or sixth character 5)

	M10.20	Drug-induced gout, unspecified site
✓6ᵗʰ M10.21		Drug-induced gout, shoulder
	M10.211	Drug-induced gout, right shoulder
	M10.212	Drug-induced gout, left shoulder
	M10.219	Drug-induced gout, unspecified shoulder
✓6ᵗʰ M10.22		Drug-induced gout, elbow
	M10.221	Drug-induced gout, right elbow
	M10.222	Drug-induced gout, left elbow
	M10.229	Drug-induced gout, unspecified elbow
✓6ᵗʰ M10.23		Drug-induced gout, wrist
	M10.231	Drug-induced gout, right wrist
	M10.232	Drug-induced gout, left wrist
	M10.239	Drug-induced gout, unspecified wrist
✓6ᵗʰ M10.24		Drug-induced gout, hand
	M10.241	Drug-induced gout, right hand
	M10.242	Drug-induced gout, left hand
	M10.249	Drug-induced gout, unspecified hand
✓6ᵗʰ M10.25		Drug-induced gout, hip
	M10.251	Drug-induced gout, right hip
	M10.252	Drug-induced gout, left hip
	M10.259	Drug-induced gout, unspecified hip
✓6ᵗʰ M10.26		Drug-induced gout, knee
	M10.261	Drug-induced gout, right knee
	M10.262	Drug-induced gout, left knee
	M10.269	Drug-induced gout, unspecified knee
✓6ᵗʰ M10.27		Drug-induced gout, ankle and foot
	M10.271	Drug-induced gout, right ankle and foot
	M10.272	Drug-induced gout, left ankle and foot
	M10.279	Drug-induced gout, unspecified ankle and foot
M10.28		Drug-induced gout, vertebrae
M10.29		Drug-induced gout, multiple sites

✓5ᵗʰ **M10.3 Gout due to renal impairment**

Code first associated renal disease

	M10.30	Gout due to renal impairment, unspecified site
✓6ᵗʰ M10.31		Gout due to renal impairment, shoulder
	M10.311	Gout due to renal impairment, right shoulder
	M10.312	Gout due to renal impairment, left shoulder
	M10.319	Gout due to renal impairment, unspecified shoulder
✓6ᵗʰ M10.32		Gout due to renal impairment, elbow
	M10.321	Gout due to renal impairment, right elbow
	M10.322	Gout due to renal impairment, left elbow
	M10.329	Gout due to renal impairment, unspecified elbow
✓6ᵗʰ M10.33		Gout due to renal impairment, wrist
	M10.331	Gout due to renal impairment, right wrist
	M10.332	Gout due to renal impairment, left wrist
	M10.339	Gout due to renal impairment, unspecified wrist
✓6ᵗʰ M10.34		Gout due to renal impairment, hand
	M10.341	Gout due to renal impairment, right hand
	M10.342	Gout due to renal impairment, left hand
	M10.349	Gout due to renal impairment, unspecified hand
✓6ᵗʰ M10.35		Gout due to renal impairment, hip
	M10.351	Gout due to renal impairment, right hip
	M10.352	Gout due to renal impairment, left hip
	M10.359	Gout due to renal impairment, unspecified hip
✓6ᵗʰ M10.36		Gout due to renal impairment, knee
	M10.361	Gout due to renal impairment, right knee
	M10.362	Gout due to renal impairment, left knee
	M10.369	Gout due to renal impairment, unspecified knee
✓6ᵗʰ M10.37		Gout due to renal impairment, ankle and foot
	M10.371	Gout due to renal impairment, right ankle and foot
	M10.372	Gout due to renal impairment, left ankle and foot
	M10.379	Gout due to renal impairment, unspecified ankle and foot
M10.38		Gout due to renal impairment, vertebrae
M10.39		Gout due to renal impairment, multiple sites

✓5ᵗʰ **M10.4 Other secondary gout**

Code first associated condition

	M10.40	Other secondary gout, unspecified site
✓6ᵗʰ M10.41		Other secondary gout, shoulder
	M10.411	Other secondary gout, right shoulder
	M10.412	Other secondary gout, left shoulder
	M10.419	Other secondary gout, unspecified shoulder
✓6ᵗʰ M10.42		Other secondary gout, elbow
	M10.421	Other secondary gout, right elbow
	M10.422	Other secondary gout, left elbow
	M10.429	Other secondary gout, unspecified elbow
✓6ᵗʰ M10.43		Other secondary gout, wrist
	M10.431	Other secondary gout, right wrist
	M10.432	Other secondary gout, left wrist
	M10.439	Other secondary gout, unspecified wrist
✓6ᵗʰ M10.44		Other secondary gout, hand
	M10.441	Other secondary gout, right hand
	M10.442	Other secondary gout, left hand
	M10.449	Other secondary gout, unspecified hand
✓6ᵗʰ M10.45		Other secondary gout, hip
	M10.451	Other secondary gout, right hip
	M10.452	Other secondary gout, left hip
	M10.459	Other secondary gout, unspecified hip
✓6ᵗʰ M10.46		Other secondary gout, knee
	M10.461	Other secondary gout, right knee
	M10.462	Other secondary gout, left knee
	M10.469	Other secondary gout, unspecified knee
✓6ᵗʰ M10.47		Other secondary gout, ankle and foot
	M10.471	Other secondary gout, right ankle and foot
	M10.472	Other secondary gout, left ankle and foot
	M10.479	Other secondary gout, unspecified ankle and foot
M10.48		Other secondary gout, vertebrae
M10.49		Other secondary gout, multiple sites

M10.9 Gout, unspecified
Gout NOS

✓4ᵗʰ **M11 Other crystal arthropathies**

✓5ᵗʰ **M11.0 Hydroxyapatite deposition disease**

DEF: Disease caused by deposits of calcium phosphate crystals in the soft tissues close to the joint (especially tendons) or in the joints. These calcifications can be mono or polyarticular and can cause destruction of the joint involved.

	M11.00	Hydroxyapatite deposition disease, unspecified site
✓6ᵗʰ M11.01		Hydroxyapatite deposition disease, shoulder
	M11.011	Hydroxyapatite deposition disease, right shoulder
	M11.012	Hydroxyapatite deposition disease, left shoulder
	M11.019	Hydroxyapatite deposition disease, unspecified shoulder
✓6ᵗʰ M11.02		Hydroxyapatite deposition disease, elbow
	M11.021	Hydroxyapatite deposition disease, right elbow
	M11.022	Hydroxyapatite deposition disease, left elbow
	M11.029	Hydroxyapatite deposition disease, unspecified elbow
✓6ᵗʰ M11.03		Hydroxyapatite deposition disease, wrist
	M11.031	Hydroxyapatite deposition disease, right wrist
	M11.032	Hydroxyapatite deposition disease, left wrist
	M11.039	Hydroxyapatite deposition disease, unspecified wrist

Chapter 13. Diseases of the Musculoskeletal System and Connective Tissue

- ✓6th **M11.04** Hydroxyapatite deposition disease, hand
  - M11.041 Hydroxyapatite deposition disease, right hand
  - M11.042 Hydroxyapatite deposition disease, left hand
  - M11.049 Hydroxyapatite deposition disease, unspecified hand
- ✓6th **M11.05** Hydroxyapatite deposition disease, hip
  - M11.051 Hydroxyapatite deposition disease, right hip
  - M11.052 Hydroxyapatite deposition disease, left hip
  - M11.059 Hydroxyapatite deposition disease, unspecified hip
- ✓6th **M11.06** Hydroxyapatite deposition disease, knee
  - M11.061 Hydroxyapatite deposition disease, right knee
  - M11.062 Hydroxyapatite deposition disease, left knee
  - M11.069 Hydroxyapatite deposition disease, unspecified knee
- ✓6th **M11.07** Hydroxyapatite deposition disease, ankle and foot
  - M11.071 Hydroxyapatite deposition disease, right ankle and foot
  - M11.072 Hydroxyapatite deposition disease, left ankle and foot
  - M11.079 Hydroxyapatite deposition disease, unspecified ankle and foot
- **M11.08** Hydroxyapatite deposition disease, vertebrae
- **M11.09** Hydroxyapatite deposition disease, multiple sites

✓5th **M11.1** Familial chondrocalcinosis
- **M11.10** Familial chondrocalcinosis, unspecified site
- ✓6th **M11.11** Familial chondrocalcinosis, shoulder
  - M11.111 Familial chondrocalcinosis, right shoulder
  - M11.112 Familial chondrocalcinosis, left shoulder
  - M11.119 Familial chondrocalcinosis, unspecified shoulder
- ✓6th **M11.12** Familial chondrocalcinosis, elbow
  - M11.121 Familial chondrocalcinosis, right elbow
  - M11.122 Familial chondrocalcinosis, left elbow
  - M11.129 Familial chondrocalcinosis, unspecified elbow
- ✓6th **M11.13** Familial chondrocalcinosis, wrist
  - M11.131 Familial chondrocalcinosis, right wrist
  - M11.132 Familial chondrocalcinosis, left wrist
  - M11.139 Familial chondrocalcinosis, unspecified wrist
- ✓6th **M11.14** Familial chondrocalcinosis, hand
  - M11.141 Familial chondrocalcinosis, right hand
  - M11.142 Familial chondrocalcinosis, left hand
  - M11.149 Familial chondrocalcinosis, unspecified hand
- ✓6th **M11.15** Familial chondrocalcinosis, hip
  - M11.151 Familial chondrocalcinosis, right hip
  - M11.152 Familial chondrocalcinosis, left hip
  - M11.159 Familial chondrocalcinosis, unspecified hip
- ✓6th **M11.16** Familial chondrocalcinosis, knee
  - M11.161 Familial chondrocalcinosis, right knee
  - M11.162 Familial chondrocalcinosis, left knee
  - M11.169 Familial chondrocalcinosis, unspecified knee
- ✓6th **M11.17** Familial chondrocalcinosis, ankle and foot
  - M11.171 Familial chondrocalcinosis, right ankle and foot
  - M11.172 Familial chondrocalcinosis, left ankle and foot
  - M11.179 Familial chondrocalcinosis, unspecified ankle and foot
- **M11.18** Familial chondrocalcinosis, vertebrae
- **M11.19** Familial chondrocalcinosis, multiple sites

✓5th **M11.2** Other chondrocalcinosis
  Chondrocalcinosis NOS
  AHA: 2018,3Q,20
  TIP: Pseudogout is captured with codes in this subcategory.
- **M11.20** Other chondrocalcinosis, unspecified site
- ✓6th **M11.21** Other chondrocalcinosis, shoulder
  - M11.211 Other chondrocalcinosis, right shoulder
  - M11.212 Other chondrocalcinosis, left shoulder
  - M11.219 Other chondrocalcinosis, unspecified shoulder
- ✓6th **M11.22** Other chondrocalcinosis, elbow
  - M11.221 Other chondrocalcinosis, right elbow
  - M11.222 Other chondrocalcinosis, left elbow
  - M11.229 Other chondrocalcinosis, unspecified elbow
- ✓6th **M11.23** Other chondrocalcinosis, wrist
  - M11.231 Other chondrocalcinosis, right wrist
  - M11.232 Other chondrocalcinosis, left wrist
  - M11.239 Other chondrocalcinosis, unspecified wrist
- ✓6th **M11.24** Other chondrocalcinosis, hand
  - M11.241 Other chondrocalcinosis, right hand
  - M11.242 Other chondrocalcinosis, left hand
  - M11.249 Other chondrocalcinosis, unspecified hand
- ✓6th **M11.25** Other chondrocalcinosis, hip
  - M11.251 Other chondrocalcinosis, right hip
  - M11.252 Other chondrocalcinosis, left hip
  - M11.259 Other chondrocalcinosis, unspecified hip
- ✓6th **M11.26** Other chondrocalcinosis, knee
  - M11.261 Other chondrocalcinosis, right knee
  - M11.262 Other chondrocalcinosis, left knee
  - M11.269 Other chondrocalcinosis, unspecified knee
- ✓6th **M11.27** Other chondrocalcinosis, ankle and foot
  - M11.271 Other chondrocalcinosis, right ankle and foot
  - M11.272 Other chondrocalcinosis, left ankle and foot
  - M11.279 Other chondrocalcinosis, unspecified ankle and foot
- **M11.28** Other chondrocalcinosis, vertebrae
- **M11.29** Other chondrocalcinosis, multiple sites

✓5th **M11.8** Other specified crystal arthropathies
- **M11.80** Other specified crystal arthropathies, unspecified site
- ✓6th **M11.81** Other specified crystal arthropathies, shoulder
  - M11.811 Other specified crystal arthropathies, right shoulder
  - M11.812 Other specified crystal arthropathies, left shoulder
  - M11.819 Other specified crystal arthropathies, unspecified shoulder
- ✓6th **M11.82** Other specified crystal arthropathies, elbow
  - M11.821 Other specified crystal arthropathies, right elbow
  - M11.822 Other specified crystal arthropathies, left elbow
  - M11.829 Other specified crystal arthropathies, unspecified elbow
- ✓6th **M11.83** Other specified crystal arthropathies, wrist
  - M11.831 Other specified crystal arthropathies, right wrist
  - M11.832 Other specified crystal arthropathies, left wrist
  - M11.839 Other specified crystal arthropathies, unspecified wrist
- ✓6th **M11.84** Other specified crystal arthropathies, hand
  - M11.841 Other specified crystal arthropathies, right hand
  - M11.842 Other specified crystal arthropathies, left hand
  - M11.849 Other specified crystal arthropathies, unspecified hand
- ✓6th **M11.85** Other specified crystal arthropathies, hip
  - M11.851 Other specified crystal arthropathies, right hip
  - M11.852 Other specified crystal arthropathies, left hip
  - M11.859 Other specified crystal arthropathies, unspecified hip
- ✓6th **M11.86** Other specified crystal arthropathies, knee
  - M11.861 Other specified crystal arthropathies, right knee
  - M11.862 Other specified crystal arthropathies, left knee
  - M11.869 Other specified crystal arthropathies, unspecified knee

Chapter 13. Diseases of the Musculoskeletal System and Connective Tissue

- ✓6th **M11.87** Other specified crystal arthropathies, ankle and foot
  - **M11.871** Other specified crystal arthropathies, right ankle and foot
  - **M11.872** Other specified crystal arthropathies, left ankle and foot
  - **M11.879** Other specified crystal arthropathies, unspecified ankle and foot
- **M11.88** Other specified crystal arthropathies, vertebrae
- **M11.89** Other specified crystal arthropathies, multiple sites
- **M11.9** Crystal arthropathy, unspecified

✓4th **M12** Other and unspecified arthropathy
  - **EXCLUDES 1** arthrosis (M15-M19)
    cricoarytenoid arthropathy (J38.7)
  - ✓5th **M12.0** Chronic postrheumatic arthropathy [Jaccoud]
    - **M12.00** Chronic postrheumatic arthropathy [Jaccoud], unspecified site HCC Rx ESR COM
    - ✓6th **M12.01** Chronic postrheumatic arthropathy [Jaccoud], shoulder
      - **M12.011** Chronic postrheumatic arthropathy [Jaccoud], right shoulder HCC Rx ESR COM
      - **M12.012** Chronic postrheumatic arthropathy [Jaccoud], left shoulder HCC Rx ESR COM
      - **M12.019** Chronic postrheumatic arthropathy [Jaccoud], unspecified shoulder HCC Rx ESR COM
    - ✓6th **M12.02** Chronic postrheumatic arthropathy [Jaccoud], elbow
      - **M12.021** Chronic postrheumatic arthropathy [Jaccoud], right elbow HCC Rx ESR COM
      - **M12.022** Chronic postrheumatic arthropathy [Jaccoud], left elbow HCC Rx ESR COM
      - **M12.029** Chronic postrheumatic arthropathy [Jaccoud], unspecified elbow HCC Rx ESR COM
    - ✓6th **M12.03** Chronic postrheumatic arthropathy [Jaccoud], wrist
      - **M12.031** Chronic postrheumatic arthropathy [Jaccoud], right wrist HCC Rx ESR COM
      - **M12.032** Chronic postrheumatic arthropathy [Jaccoud], left wrist HCC Rx ESR COM
      - **M12.039** Chronic postrheumatic arthropathy [Jaccoud], unspecified wrist HCC Rx ESR COM
    - ✓6th **M12.04** Chronic postrheumatic arthropathy [Jaccoud], hand
      - **M12.041** Chronic postrheumatic arthropathy [Jaccoud], right hand HCC Rx ESR COM
      - **M12.042** Chronic postrheumatic arthropathy [Jaccoud], left hand HCC Rx ESR COM
      - **M12.049** Chronic postrheumatic arthropathy [Jaccoud], unspecified hand HCC Rx ESR COM
    - ✓6th **M12.05** Chronic postrheumatic arthropathy [Jaccoud], hip
      - **M12.051** Chronic postrheumatic arthropathy [Jaccoud], right hip HCC Rx ESR COM
      - **M12.052** Chronic postrheumatic arthropathy [Jaccoud], left hip HCC Rx ESR COM
      - **M12.059** Chronic postrheumatic arthropathy [Jaccoud], unspecified hip HCC Rx ESR COM
    - ✓6th **M12.06** Chronic postrheumatic arthropathy [Jaccoud], knee
      - **M12.061** Chronic postrheumatic arthropathy [Jaccoud], right knee HCC Rx ESR COM
      - **M12.062** Chronic postrheumatic arthropathy [Jaccoud], left knee HCC Rx ESR COM
      - **M12.069** Chronic postrheumatic arthropathy [Jaccoud], unspecified knee HCC Rx ESR COM
    - ✓6th **M12.07** Chronic postrheumatic arthropathy [Jaccoud], ankle and foot
      - **M12.071** Chronic postrheumatic arthropathy [Jaccoud], right ankle and foot HCC Rx ESR COM
      - **M12.072** Chronic postrheumatic arthropathy [Jaccoud], left ankle and foot HCC Rx ESR COM
      - **M12.079** Chronic postrheumatic arthropathy [Jaccoud], unspecified ankle and foot HCC Rx ESR COM
    - **M12.08** Chronic postrheumatic arthropathy [Jaccoud], other specified site HCC Rx ESR COM
      Chronic postrheumatic arthropathy [Jaccoud], vertebrae
    - **M12.09** Chronic postrheumatic arthropathy [Jaccoud], multiple sites HCC Rx ESR COM
  - ✓5th **M12.1** Kaschin-Beck disease
    Osteochondroarthrosis deformans endemica
    - **M12.10** Kaschin-Beck disease, unspecified site
    - ✓6th **M12.11** Kaschin-Beck disease, shoulder
      - **M12.111** Kaschin-Beck disease, right shoulder
      - **M12.112** Kaschin-Beck disease, left shoulder
      - **M12.119** Kaschin-Beck disease, unspecified shoulder
    - ✓6th **M12.12** Kaschin-Beck disease, elbow
      - **M12.121** Kaschin-Beck disease, right elbow
      - **M12.122** Kaschin-Beck disease, left elbow
      - **M12.129** Kaschin-Beck disease, unspecified elbow
    - ✓6th **M12.13** Kaschin-Beck disease, wrist
      - **M12.131** Kaschin-Beck disease, right wrist
      - **M12.132** Kaschin-Beck disease, left wrist
      - **M12.139** Kaschin-Beck disease, unspecified wrist
    - ✓6th **M12.14** Kaschin-Beck disease, hand
      - **M12.141** Kaschin-Beck disease, right hand
      - **M12.142** Kaschin-Beck disease, left hand
      - **M12.149** Kaschin-Beck disease, unspecified hand
    - ✓6th **M12.15** Kaschin-Beck disease, hip
      - **M12.151** Kaschin-Beck disease, right hip
      - **M12.152** Kaschin-Beck disease, left hip
      - **M12.159** Kaschin-Beck disease, unspecified hip
    - ✓6th **M12.16** Kaschin-Beck disease, knee
      - **M12.161** Kaschin-Beck disease, right knee
      - **M12.162** Kaschin-Beck disease, left knee
      - **M12.169** Kaschin-Beck disease, unspecified knee
    - ✓6th **M12.17** Kaschin-Beck disease, ankle and foot
      - **M12.171** Kaschin-Beck disease, right ankle and foot
      - **M12.172** Kaschin-Beck disease, left ankle and foot
      - **M12.179** Kaschin-Beck disease, unspecified ankle and foot
    - **M12.18** Kaschin-Beck disease, vertebrae
    - **M12.19** Kaschin-Beck disease, multiple sites
  - ✓5th **M12.2** Villonodular synovitis (pigmented)
    - **M12.20** Villonodular synovitis (pigmented), unspecified site
    - ✓6th **M12.21** Villonodular synovitis (pigmented), shoulder
      - **M12.211** Villonodular synovitis (pigmented), right shoulder
      - **M12.212** Villonodular synovitis (pigmented), left shoulder
      - **M12.219** Villonodular synovitis (pigmented), unspecified shoulder
    - ✓6th **M12.22** Villonodular synovitis (pigmented), elbow
      - **M12.221** Villonodular synovitis (pigmented), right elbow
      - **M12.222** Villonodular synovitis (pigmented), left elbow
      - **M12.229** Villonodular synovitis (pigmented), unspecified elbow
    - ✓6th **M12.23** Villonodular synovitis (pigmented), wrist
      - **M12.231** Villonodular synovitis (pigmented), right wrist
      - **M12.232** Villonodular synovitis (pigmented), left wrist
      - **M12.239** Villonodular synovitis (pigmented), unspecified wrist
    - ✓6th **M12.24** Villonodular synovitis (pigmented), hand
      - **M12.241** Villonodular synovitis (pigmented), right hand
      - **M12.242** Villonodular synovitis (pigmented), left hand
      - **M12.249** Villonodular synovitis (pigmented), unspecified hand
    - ✓6th **M12.25** Villonodular synovitis (pigmented), hip
      - **M12.251** Villonodular synovitis (pigmented), right hip
      - **M12.252** Villonodular synovitis (pigmented), left hip
      - **M12.259** Villonodular synovitis (pigmented), unspecified hip

---

✓ Additional Character Required ✓x7th Placeholder Alert Manifestation Unspecified Dx QPP UPD Unacceptable PDx

Chapter 13. Diseases of the Musculoskeletal System and Connective Tissue

M12.26 Villonodular synovitis (pigmented), knee
- **M12.261** Villonodular synovitis (pigmented), right knee
- **M12.262** Villonodular synovitis (pigmented), left knee
- **M12.269** Villonodular synovitis (pigmented), unspecified knee

M12.27 Villonodular synovitis (pigmented), ankle and foot
- **M12.271** Villonodular synovitis (pigmented), right ankle and foot
- **M12.272** Villonodular synovitis (pigmented), left ankle and foot
- **M12.279** Villonodular synovitis (pigmented), unspecified ankle and foot

M12.28 Villonodular synovitis (pigmented), other specified site
  Villonodular synovitis (pigmented), vertebrae

M12.29 Villonodular synovitis (pigmented), multiple sites

M12.3 Palindromic rheumatism
  DEF: Sudden and recurring attacks of moderate to severe joint pain and swelling generally occurring in the hands or feet of unknown etiology. After the attack subsides, the joints appear normal again.

- **M12.30** Palindromic rheumatism, unspecified site
- **M12.31** Palindromic rheumatism, shoulder
  - **M12.311** Palindromic rheumatism, right shoulder
  - **M12.312** Palindromic rheumatism, left shoulder
  - **M12.319** Palindromic rheumatism, unspecified shoulder
- **M12.32** Palindromic rheumatism, elbow
  - **M12.321** Palindromic rheumatism, right elbow
  - **M12.322** Palindromic rheumatism, left elbow
  - **M12.329** Palindromic rheumatism, unspecified elbow
- **M12.33** Palindromic rheumatism, wrist
  - **M12.331** Palindromic rheumatism, right wrist
  - **M12.332** Palindromic rheumatism, left wrist
  - **M12.339** Palindromic rheumatism, unspecified wrist
- **M12.34** Palindromic rheumatism, hand
  - **M12.341** Palindromic rheumatism, right hand
  - **M12.342** Palindromic rheumatism, left hand
  - **M12.349** Palindromic rheumatism, unspecified hand
- **M12.35** Palindromic rheumatism, hip
  - **M12.351** Palindromic rheumatism, right hip
  - **M12.352** Palindromic rheumatism, left hip
  - **M12.359** Palindromic rheumatism, unspecified hip
- **M12.36** Palindromic rheumatism, knee
  - **M12.361** Palindromic rheumatism, right knee
  - **M12.362** Palindromic rheumatism, left knee
  - **M12.369** Palindromic rheumatism, unspecified knee
- **M12.37** Palindromic rheumatism, ankle and foot
  - **M12.371** Palindromic rheumatism, right ankle and foot
  - **M12.372** Palindromic rheumatism, left ankle and foot
  - **M12.379** Palindromic rheumatism, unspecified ankle and foot
- **M12.38** Palindromic rheumatism, other specified site
  Palindromic rheumatism, vertebrae
- **M12.39** Palindromic rheumatism, multiple sites

M12.4 Intermittent hydrarthrosis
- **M12.40** Intermittent hydrarthrosis, unspecified site
- **M12.41** Intermittent hydrarthrosis, shoulder
  - **M12.411** Intermittent hydrarthrosis, right shoulder
  - **M12.412** Intermittent hydrarthrosis, left shoulder
  - **M12.419** Intermittent hydrarthrosis, unspecified shoulder
- **M12.42** Intermittent hydrarthrosis, elbow
  - **M12.421** Intermittent hydrarthrosis, right elbow
  - **M12.422** Intermittent hydrarthrosis, left elbow
  - **M12.429** Intermittent hydrarthrosis, unspecified elbow
- **M12.43** Intermittent hydrarthrosis, wrist
  - **M12.431** Intermittent hydrarthrosis, right wrist
  - **M12.432** Intermittent hydrarthrosis, left wrist
  - **M12.439** Intermittent hydrarthrosis, unspecified wrist
- **M12.44** Intermittent hydrarthrosis, hand
  - **M12.441** Intermittent hydrarthrosis, right hand
  - **M12.442** Intermittent hydrarthrosis, left hand
  - **M12.449** Intermittent hydrarthrosis, unspecified hand
- **M12.45** Intermittent hydrarthrosis, hip
  - **M12.451** Intermittent hydrarthrosis, right hip
  - **M12.452** Intermittent hydrarthrosis, left hip
  - **M12.459** Intermittent hydrarthrosis, unspecified hip
- **M12.46** Intermittent hydrarthrosis, knee
  - **M12.461** Intermittent hydrarthrosis, right knee
  - **M12.462** Intermittent hydrarthrosis, left knee
  - **M12.469** Intermittent hydrarthrosis, unspecified knee
- **M12.47** Intermittent hydrarthrosis, ankle and foot
  - **M12.471** Intermittent hydrarthrosis, right ankle and foot
  - **M12.472** Intermittent hydrarthrosis, left ankle and foot
  - **M12.479** Intermittent hydrarthrosis, unspecified ankle and foot
- **M12.48** Intermittent hydrarthrosis, other site
- **M12.49** Intermittent hydrarthrosis, multiple sites

M12.5 Traumatic arthropathy
  EXCLUDES 1 current injury—see Alphabetic Index
  post-traumatic osteoarthritis of first carpometacarpal joint (M18.2-M18.3)
  post-traumatic osteoarthritis of hip (M16.4-M16.5)
  post-traumatic osteoarthritis of knee (M17.2-M17.3)
  post-traumatic osteoarthritis NOS (M19.1-)
  post-traumatic osteoarthritis of other single joints (M19.1-)
  AHA: 2015,1Q,17

- **M12.50** Traumatic arthropathy, unspecified site
- **M12.51** Traumatic arthropathy, shoulder
  - **M12.511** Traumatic arthropathy, right shoulder
  - **M12.512** Traumatic arthropathy, left shoulder
  - **M12.519** Traumatic arthropathy, unspecified shoulder
- **M12.52** Traumatic arthropathy, elbow
  - **M12.521** Traumatic arthropathy, right elbow
  - **M12.522** Traumatic arthropathy, left elbow
  - **M12.529** Traumatic arthropathy, unspecified elbow
- **M12.53** Traumatic arthropathy, wrist
  - **M12.531** Traumatic arthropathy, right wrist
  - **M12.532** Traumatic arthropathy, left wrist
  - **M12.539** Traumatic arthropathy, unspecified wrist
- **M12.54** Traumatic arthropathy, hand
  - **M12.541** Traumatic arthropathy, right hand
  - **M12.542** Traumatic arthropathy, left hand
  - **M12.549** Traumatic arthropathy, unspecified hand
- **M12.55** Traumatic arthropathy, hip
  - **M12.551** Traumatic arthropathy, right hip
  - **M12.552** Traumatic arthropathy, left hip
  - **M12.559** Traumatic arthropathy, unspecified hip
- **M12.56** Traumatic arthropathy, knee
  - **M12.561** Traumatic arthropathy, right knee
  - **M12.562** Traumatic arthropathy, left knee
  - **M12.569** Traumatic arthropathy, unspecified knee
- **M12.57** Traumatic arthropathy, ankle and foot
  - **M12.571** Traumatic arthropathy, right ankle and foot
  - **M12.572** Traumatic arthropathy, left ankle and foot
  - **M12.579** Traumatic arthropathy, unspecified ankle and foot
- **M12.58** Traumatic arthropathy, other specified site
  Traumatic arthropathy, vertebrae
- **M12.59** Traumatic arthropathy, multiple sites

M12.8 Other specific arthropathies, not elsewhere classified
  Transient arthropathy
- **M12.80** Other specific arthropathies, not elsewhere classified, unspecified site
- **M12.81** Other specific arthropathies, not elsewhere classified, shoulder
  - **M12.811** Other specific arthropathies, not elsewhere classified, right shoulder

Chapter 13. Diseases of the Musculoskeletal System and Connective Tissue

- M12.812 Other specific arthropathies, not elsewhere classified, left shoulder
- M12.819 Other specific arthropathies, not elsewhere classified, unspecified shoulder

M12.82 Other specific arthropathies, not elsewhere classified, elbow
- M12.821 Other specific arthropathies, not elsewhere classified, right elbow
- M12.822 Other specific arthropathies, not elsewhere classified, left elbow
- M12.829 Other specific arthropathies, not elsewhere classified, unspecified elbow

M12.83 Other specific arthropathies, not elsewhere classified, wrist
- M12.831 Other specific arthropathies, not elsewhere classified, right wrist
- M12.832 Other specific arthropathies, not elsewhere classified, left wrist
- M12.839 Other specific arthropathies, not elsewhere classified, unspecified wrist

M12.84 Other specific arthropathies, not elsewhere classified, hand
- M12.841 Other specific arthropathies, not elsewhere classified, right hand
- M12.842 Other specific arthropathies, not elsewhere classified, left hand
- M12.849 Other specific arthropathies, not elsewhere classified, unspecified hand

M12.85 Other specific arthropathies, not elsewhere classified, hip
- M12.851 Other specific arthropathies, not elsewhere classified, right hip
- M12.852 Other specific arthropathies, not elsewhere classified, left hip
- M12.859 Other specific arthropathies, not elsewhere classified, unspecified hip

M12.86 Other specific arthropathies, not elsewhere classified, knee
- M12.861 Other specific arthropathies, not elsewhere classified, right knee
- M12.862 Other specific arthropathies, not elsewhere classified, left knee
- M12.869 Other specific arthropathies, not elsewhere classified, unspecified knee

M12.87 Other specific arthropathies, not elsewhere classified, ankle and foot
- M12.871 Other specific arthropathies, not elsewhere classified, right ankle and foot
- M12.872 Other specific arthropathies, not elsewhere classified, left ankle and foot
- M12.879 Other specific arthropathies, not elsewhere classified, unspecified ankle and foot

M12.88 Other specific arthropathies, not elsewhere classified, other specified site
   Other specific arthropathies, not elsewhere classified, vertebrae

M12.89 Other specific arthropathies, not elsewhere classified, multiple sites

M12.9 Arthropathy, unspecified

M13 Other arthritis
EXCLUDES 1 arthrosis (M15-M19)
   osteoarthritis (M15-M19)

M13.0 Polyarthritis, unspecified

M13.1 Monoarthritis, not elsewhere classified
- **M13.10** Monoarthritis, not elsewhere classified, unspecified site
- **M13.11** Monoarthritis, not elsewhere classified, shoulder
  - M13.111 Monoarthritis, not elsewhere classified, right shoulder
  - M13.112 Monoarthritis, not elsewhere classified, left shoulder
  - M13.119 Monoarthritis, not elsewhere classified, unspecified shoulder
- **M13.12** Monoarthritis, not elsewhere classified, elbow
  - M13.121 Monoarthritis, not elsewhere classified, right elbow
  - M13.122 Monoarthritis, not elsewhere classified, left elbow
  - M13.129 Monoarthritis, not elsewhere classified, unspecified elbow
- **M13.13** Monoarthritis, not elsewhere classified, wrist
  - M13.131 Monoarthritis, not elsewhere classified, right wrist
  - M13.132 Monoarthritis, not elsewhere classified, left wrist
  - M13.139 Monoarthritis, not elsewhere classified, unspecified wrist
- **M13.14** Monoarthritis, not elsewhere classified, hand
  - M13.141 Monoarthritis, not elsewhere classified, right hand
  - M13.142 Monoarthritis, not elsewhere classified, left hand
  - M13.149 Monoarthritis, not elsewhere classified, unspecified hand
- **M13.15** Monoarthritis, not elsewhere classified, hip
  - M13.151 Monoarthritis, not elsewhere classified, right hip
  - M13.152 Monoarthritis, not elsewhere classified, left hip
  - M13.159 Monoarthritis, not elsewhere classified, unspecified hip
- **M13.16** Monoarthritis, not elsewhere classified, knee
  - M13.161 Monoarthritis, not elsewhere classified, right knee
  - M13.162 Monoarthritis, not elsewhere classified, left knee
  - M13.169 Monoarthritis, not elsewhere classified, unspecified knee
- **M13.17** Monoarthritis, not elsewhere classified, ankle and foot
  - M13.171 Monoarthritis, not elsewhere classified, right ankle and foot
  - M13.172 Monoarthritis, not elsewhere classified, left ankle and foot
  - M13.179 Monoarthritis, not elsewhere classified, unspecified ankle and foot

M13.8 Other specified arthritis
   Allergic arthritis
   EXCLUDES 1 osteoarthritis (M15-M19)
- **M13.80** Other specified arthritis, unspecified site
   AHA: 2025,2Q,9
- **M13.81** Other specified arthritis, shoulder
  - M13.811 Other specified arthritis, right shoulder
  - M13.812 Other specified arthritis, left shoulder
  - M13.819 Other specified arthritis, unspecified shoulder
- **M13.82** Other specified arthritis, elbow
  - M13.821 Other specified arthritis, right elbow
  - M13.822 Other specified arthritis, left elbow
  - M13.829 Other specified arthritis, unspecified elbow
- **M13.83** Other specified arthritis, wrist
  - M13.831 Other specified arthritis, right wrist
  - M13.832 Other specified arthritis, left wrist
  - M13.839 Other specified arthritis, unspecified wrist
- **M13.84** Other specified arthritis, hand
  - M13.841 Other specified arthritis, right hand
  - M13.842 Other specified arthritis, left hand
  - M13.849 Other specified arthritis, unspecified hand
- **M13.85** Other specified arthritis, hip
  - M13.851 Other specified arthritis, right hip
  - M13.852 Other specified arthritis, left hip
  - M13.859 Other specified arthritis, unspecified hip
- **M13.86** Other specified arthritis, knee
  - M13.861 Other specified arthritis, right knee
  - M13.862 Other specified arthritis, left knee
  - M13.869 Other specified arthritis, unspecified knee
- **M13.87** Other specified arthritis, ankle and foot
  - M13.871 Other specified arthritis, right ankle and foot
  - M13.872 Other specified arthritis, left ankle and foot
  - M13.879 Other specified arthritis, unspecified ankle and foot
- **M13.88** Other specified arthritis, other site
- **M13.89** Other specified arthritis, multiple sites
   AHA: 2025,2Q,10

✓ Additional Character Required ✓x7ᵗʰ Placeholder Alert Manifestation Unspecified Dx QPP UPD Unacceptable PDx

M14 Arthropathies in other diseases classified elsewhere

EXCLUDES 1
arthropathy in:
enteropathic arthropathies (M07.-)
juvenile psoriatic arthropathy (L40.54)
lipoid dermatoarthritis (E78.81)
diabetes mellitus (E08-E13 with .61-)
hematological disorders (M36.2-M36.3)
hypersensitivity reactions (M36.4)
neoplastic disease (M36.1)
neurosyphillis (A52.16)
sarcoidosis (D86.86)

M14.6 Charcot's joint
Neuropathic arthropathy

EXCLUDES 1 Charcôt's joint in diabetes mellitus (E08-E13 with .610)
Charcôt's joint in tabes dorsalis (A52.16)

DEF: Progressive neurologic arthropathy in which chronic degeneration of joints in the weight-bearing areas with peripheral hypertrophy occurs as a complication of a neuropathy disorder. Supporting structures relax from a loss of sensation resulting in chronic joint instability.

- **M14.60** Charcot's joint, unspecified site
- **M14.61** Charcôt's joint, shoulder
  - M14.611 Charcôt's joint, right shoulder
  - M14.612 Charcôt's joint, left shoulder
  - M14.619 Charcot's joint, unspecified shoulder
- **M14.62** Charcôt's joint, elbow
  - M14.621 Charcôt's joint, right elbow
  - M14.622 Charcôt's joint, left elbow
  - M14.629 Charcot's joint, unspecified elbow
- **M14.63** Charcôt's joint, wrist
  - M14.631 Charcôt's joint, right wrist
  - M14.632 Charcôt's joint, left wrist
  - M14.639 Charcot's joint, unspecified wrist
- **M14.64** Charcôt's joint, hand
  - M14.641 Charcôt's joint, right hand
  - M14.642 Charcôt's joint, left hand
  - M14.649 Charcot's joint, unspecified hand
- **M14.65** Charcôt's joint, hip
  - M14.651 Charcôt's joint, right hip
  - M14.652 Charcôt's joint, left hip
  - M14.659 Charcot's joint, unspecified hip
- **M14.66** Charcôt's joint, knee
  - M14.661 Charcôt's joint, right knee
  - M14.662 Charcôt's joint, left knee
  - M14.669 Charcot's joint, unspecified knee
- **M14.67** Charcôt's joint, ankle and foot
  - M14.671 Charcôt's joint, right ankle and foot
  - M14.672 Charcôt's joint, left ankle and foot
  - M14.679 Charcot's joint, unspecified ankle and foot
- **M14.68** Charcôt's joint, vertebrae
- **M14.69** Charcôt's joint, multiple sites

M14.8 Arthropathies in other specified diseases classified elsewhere
Code first underlying disease, such as:
amyloidosis (E85.-)
erythema multiforme (L51.-)
erythema nodosum (L52)
hemochromatosis (E83.11-)
hyperparathyroidism (E21.-)
hypothyroidism (E00-E03)
sickle-cell disorders (D57.-)
thyrotoxicosis [hyperthyroidism] (E05.-)
Whipple's disease (K90.81)

- **M14.80** Arthropathies in other specified diseases classified elsewhere, unspecified site
- **M14.81** Arthropathies in other specified diseases classified elsewhere, shoulder
  - M14.811 Arthropathies in other specified diseases classified elsewhere, right shoulder
  - M14.812 Arthropathies in other specified diseases classified elsewhere, left shoulder
  - M14.819 Arthropathies in other specified diseases classified elsewhere, unspecified shoulder
- **M14.82** Arthropathies in other specified diseases classified elsewhere, elbow
  - M14.821 Arthropathies in other specified diseases classified elsewhere, right elbow
  - M14.822 Arthropathies in other specified diseases classified elsewhere, left elbow
  - M14.829 Arthropathies in other specified diseases classified elsewhere, unspecified elbow
- **M14.83** Arthropathies in other specified diseases classified elsewhere, wrist
  - M14.831 Arthropathies in other specified diseases classified elsewhere, right wrist
  - M14.832 Arthropathies in other specified diseases classified elsewhere, left wrist
  - M14.839 Arthropathies in other specified diseases classified elsewhere, unspecified wrist
- **M14.84** Arthropathies in other specified diseases classified elsewhere, hand
  - M14.841 Arthropathies in other specified diseases classified elsewhere, right hand
  - M14.842 Arthropathies in other specified diseases classified elsewhere, left hand
  - M14.849 Arthropathies in other specified diseases classified elsewhere, unspecified hand
- **M14.85** Arthropathies in other specified diseases classified elsewhere, hip
  - M14.851 Arthropathies in other specified diseases classified elsewhere, right hip
  - M14.852 Arthropathies in other specified diseases classified elsewhere, left hip
  - M14.859 Arthropathies in other specified diseases classified elsewhere, unspecified hip
- **M14.86** Arthropathies in other specified diseases classified elsewhere, knee
  - M14.861 Arthropathies in other specified diseases classified elsewhere, right knee
  - M14.862 Arthropathies in other specified diseases classified elsewhere, left knee
  - M14.869 Arthropathies in other specified diseases classified elsewhere, unspecified knee
- **M14.87** Arthropathies in other specified diseases classified elsewhere, ankle and foot
  - M14.871 Arthropathies in other specified diseases classified elsewhere, right ankle and foot
  - M14.872 Arthropathies in other specified diseases classified elsewhere, left ankle and foot
  - M14.879 Arthropathies in other specified diseases classified elsewhere, unspecified ankle and foot
- **M14.88** Arthropathies in other specified diseases classified elsewhere, vertebrae
- **M14.89** Arthropathies in other specified diseases classified elsewhere, multiple sites

Osteoarthritis (M15-M19)

EXCLUDES 2 osteoarthritis of spine (M47.-)
AHA: 2020,2Q,14; 2016,4Q,147
TIP: Assign a primary osteoarthritis code when the site of the osteoarthritis is documented but the type of osteoarthritis — primary, secondary, generalized, or post-traumatic — is not documented. Primary is considered the default.

M15 Polyosteoarthritis

INCLUDES arthritis of multiple sites
EXCLUDES 1 bilateral involvement of single joint (M16-M19)

- **M15.0** Primary generalized (osteo)arthritis
- **M15.1** Heberden's nodes (with arthropathy)
  Interphalangeal distal osteoarthritis
- **M15.2** Bouchard's nodes (with arthropathy)
  Juxtaphalangeal distal osteoarthritis
- **M15.3** Secondary multiple arthritis
  Post-traumatic polyosteoarthritis
- **M15.4** Erosive (osteo)arthritis
- **M15.8** Other polyosteoarthritis
- **M15.9** Polyosteoarthritis, unspecified
  Generalized osteoarthritis NOS

M16 Osteoarthritis of hip
AHA: 2016,4Q,146

- **M16.0** Bilateral primary osteoarthritis of hip
  AHA: 2018,2Q,15
- **M16.1** Unilateral primary osteoarthritis of hip
  Primary osteoarthritis of hip NOS
  AHA: 2018,2Q,15
  - M16.10 Unilateral primary osteoarthritis, unspecified hip
  - M16.11 Unilateral primary osteoarthritis, right hip
  - M16.12 Unilateral primary osteoarthritis, left hip
- **M16.2** Bilateral osteoarthritis resulting from hip dysplasia

Chapter 13. Diseases of the Musculoskeletal System and Connective Tissue

M16.3 Unilateral osteoarthritis resulting from hip dysplasia
Dysplastic osteoarthritis of hip NOS
- **M16.30** Unilateral osteoarthritis resulting from hip dysplasia, unspecified hip
- **M16.31** Unilateral osteoarthritis resulting from hip dysplasia, right hip
- **M16.32** Unilateral osteoarthritis resulting from hip dysplasia, left hip

M16.4 Bilateral post-traumatic osteoarthritis of hip

M16.5 Unilateral post-traumatic osteoarthritis of hip
Post-traumatic osteoarthritis of hip NOS
- **M16.50** Unilateral post-traumatic osteoarthritis, unspecified hip
- **M16.51** Unilateral post-traumatic osteoarthritis, right hip
- **M16.52** Unilateral post-traumatic osteoarthritis, left hip

M16.6 Other bilateral secondary osteoarthritis of hip

M16.7 Other unilateral secondary osteoarthritis of hip
Secondary osteoarthritis of hip NOS

M16.9 Osteoarthritis of hip, unspecified

M17 Osteoarthritis of knee
AHA: 2016,4Q,146-147

M17.0 Bilateral primary osteoarthritis of knee
AHA: 2018,2Q,15

M17.1 Unilateral primary osteoarthritis of knee
Primary osteoarthritis of knee NOS
AHA: 2018,2Q,15
- **M17.10** Unilateral primary osteoarthritis, unspecified knee
- **M17.11** Unilateral primary osteoarthritis, right knee
- **M17.12** Unilateral primary osteoarthritis, left knee

M17.2 Bilateral post-traumatic osteoarthritis of knee

M17.3 Unilateral post-traumatic osteoarthritis of knee
Post-traumatic osteoarthritis of knee NOS
- **M17.30** Unilateral post-traumatic osteoarthritis, unspecified knee
- **M17.31** Unilateral post-traumatic osteoarthritis, right knee
- **M17.32** Unilateral post-traumatic osteoarthritis, left knee

M17.4 Other bilateral secondary osteoarthritis of knee

M17.5 Other unilateral secondary osteoarthritis of knee
Secondary osteoarthritis of knee NOS

M17.9 Osteoarthritis of knee, unspecified

M18 Osteoarthritis of first carpometacarpal joint

M18.0 Bilateral primary osteoarthritis of first carpometacarpal joints

M18.1 Unilateral primary osteoarthritis of first carpometacarpal joint
Primary osteoarthritis of first carpometacarpal joint NOS
- **M18.10** Unilateral primary osteoarthritis of first carpometacarpal joint, unspecified hand
- **M18.11** Unilateral primary osteoarthritis of first carpometacarpal joint, right hand
- **M18.12** Unilateral primary osteoarthritis of first carpometacarpal joint, left hand

M18.2 Bilateral post-traumatic osteoarthritis of first carpometacarpal joints

M18.3 Unilateral post-traumatic osteoarthritis of first carpometacarpal joint
Post-traumatic osteoarthritis of first carpometacarpal joint NOS
- **M18.30** Unilateral post-traumatic osteoarthritis of first carpometacarpal joint, unspecified hand
- **M18.31** Unilateral post-traumatic osteoarthritis of first carpometacarpal joint, right hand
- **M18.32** Unilateral post-traumatic osteoarthritis of first carpometacarpal joint, left hand

M18.4 Other bilateral secondary osteoarthritis of first carpometacarpal joints

M18.5 Other unilateral secondary osteoarthritis of first carpometacarpal joint
Secondary osteoarthritis of first carpometacarpal joint NOS
- **M18.50** Other unilateral secondary osteoarthritis of first carpometacarpal joint, unspecified hand
- **M18.51** Other unilateral secondary osteoarthritis of first carpometacarpal joint, right hand
- **M18.52** Other unilateral secondary osteoarthritis of first carpometacarpal joint, left hand

M18.9 Osteoarthritis of first carpometacarpal joint, unspecified

M19 Other and unspecified osteoarthritis
EXCLUDES 1 polyarthritis (M15.-)
EXCLUDES 2 arthrosis of spine (M47.-)
hallux rigidus (M20.2)
osteoarthritis of spine (M47.-)
AHA: 2020,4Q,31-32

M19.0 Primary osteoarthritis of other joints
AHA: 2018,2Q,15; 2016,4Q,145
- **M19.01** Primary osteoarthritis, shoulder
  - **M19.011** Primary osteoarthritis, right shoulder
  - **M19.012** Primary osteoarthritis, left shoulder
  - **M19.019** Primary osteoarthritis, unspecified shoulder
- **M19.02** Primary osteoarthritis, elbow
  - **M19.021** Primary osteoarthritis, right elbow
  - **M19.022** Primary osteoarthritis, left elbow
  - **M19.029** Primary osteoarthritis, unspecified elbow
- **M19.03** Primary osteoarthritis, wrist
  - **M19.031** Primary osteoarthritis, right wrist
  - **M19.032** Primary osteoarthritis, left wrist
  - **M19.039** Primary osteoarthritis, unspecified wrist
- **M19.04** Primary osteoarthritis, hand
  - **EXCLUDES 2** primary osteoarthritis of first carpometacarpal joint (M18.0-, M18.1-)
  - **M19.041** Primary osteoarthritis, right hand
  - **M19.042** Primary osteoarthritis, left hand
  - **M19.049** Primary osteoarthritis, unspecified hand
- **M19.07** Primary osteoarthritis ankle and foot
  - **M19.071** Primary osteoarthritis, right ankle and foot
  - **M19.072** Primary osteoarthritis, left ankle and foot
  - **M19.079** Primary osteoarthritis, unspecified ankle and foot
- **M19.09** Primary osteoarthritis, other specified site

M19.1 Post-traumatic osteoarthritis of other joints
- **M19.11** Post-traumatic osteoarthritis, shoulder
  - **M19.111** Post-traumatic osteoarthritis, right shoulder
  - **M19.112** Post-traumatic osteoarthritis, left shoulder
  - **M19.119** Post-traumatic osteoarthritis, unspecified shoulder
- **M19.12** Post-traumatic osteoarthritis, elbow
  - **M19.121** Post-traumatic osteoarthritis, right elbow
  - **M19.122** Post-traumatic osteoarthritis, left elbow
  - **M19.129** Post-traumatic osteoarthritis, unspecified elbow
- **M19.13** Post-traumatic osteoarthritis, wrist
  - **M19.131** Post-traumatic osteoarthritis, right wrist
  - **M19.132** Post-traumatic osteoarthritis, left wrist
  - **M19.139** Post-traumatic osteoarthritis, unspecified wrist
- **M19.14** Post-traumatic osteoarthritis, hand
  - **EXCLUDES 2** post-traumatic osteoarthritis of first carpometacarpal joint (M18.2-, M18.3-)
  - **M19.141** Post-traumatic osteoarthritis, right hand
  - **M19.142** Post-traumatic osteoarthritis, left hand
  - **M19.149** Post-traumatic osteoarthritis, unspecified hand
- **M19.17** Post-traumatic osteoarthritis, ankle and foot
  - **M19.171** Post-traumatic osteoarthritis, right ankle and foot
  - **M19.172** Post-traumatic osteoarthritis, left ankle and foot
  - **M19.179** Post-traumatic osteoarthritis, unspecified ankle and foot
- **M19.19** Post-traumatic osteoarthritis, other specified site

M19.2 Secondary osteoarthritis of other joints
- **M19.21** Secondary osteoarthritis, shoulder
  - **M19.211** Secondary osteoarthritis, right shoulder
  - **M19.212** Secondary osteoarthritis, left shoulder
  - **M19.219** Secondary osteoarthritis, unspecified shoulder
- **M19.22** Secondary osteoarthritis, elbow
  - **M19.221** Secondary osteoarthritis, right elbow
  - **M19.222** Secondary osteoarthritis, left elbow

Chapter 13. Diseases of the Musculoskeletal System and Connective Tissue

M19.229 Secondary osteoarthritis, unspecified elbow
✓6th M19.23 Secondary osteoarthritis, wrist
    M19.231 Secondary osteoarthritis, right wrist
    M19.232 Secondary osteoarthritis, left wrist
    M19.239 Secondary osteoarthritis, unspecified wrist
✓6th M19.24 Secondary osteoarthritis, hand
    M19.241 Secondary osteoarthritis, right hand
    M19.242 Secondary osteoarthritis, left hand
    M19.249 Secondary osteoarthritis, unspecified hand
✓6th M19.27 Secondary osteoarthritis, ankle and foot
    M19.271 Secondary osteoarthritis, right ankle and foot
    M19.272 Secondary osteoarthritis, left ankle and foot
    M19.279 Secondary osteoarthritis, unspecified ankle and foot
M19.29 Secondary osteoarthritis, other specified site

✓5th **M19.9 Osteoarthritis, unspecified site**
    TIP: Assign M19.90 when neither the site nor the type of osteoarthritis — primary, secondary, or post-traumatic — is documented.
    M19.90 Unspecified osteoarthritis, unspecified site
        Arthritis NOS
        Arthrosis NOS
        Osteoarthritis NOS
        AHA: 2016,4Q,145-147
    M19.91 Primary osteoarthritis, unspecified site
        Primary osteoarthritis NOS
    M19.92 Post-traumatic osteoarthritis, unspecified site
        Post-traumatic osteoarthritis NOS
    M19.93 Secondary osteoarthritis, unspecified site
        Secondary osteoarthritis NOS

Other joint disorders (M20-M25)

EXCLUDES 2 joints of the spine (M40-M54)

✓4th **M20 Acquired deformities of fingers and toes**
    EXCLUDES 1 acquired absence of fingers and toes (Z89.-)
        congenital absence of fingers and toes (Q71.3-, Q72.3-)
        congenital deformities and malformations of fingers and toes (Q66.-, Q68-Q70, Q74.-)

✓5th **M20.0 Deformity of finger(s)**
    EXCLUDES 1 clubbing of fingers (R68.3)
        palmar fascial fibromatosis [Dupuytren] (M72.0)
        trigger finger (M65.3)
✓6th M20.00 Unspecified deformity of finger(s)
    M20.001 Unspecified deformity of right finger(s)
    M20.002 Unspecified deformity of left finger(s)
    M20.009 Unspecified deformity of unspecified finger(s)
✓6th M20.01 Mallet finger
    M20.011 Mallet finger of right finger(s)
    M20.012 Mallet finger of left finger(s)
    M20.019 Mallet finger of unspecified finger(s)
✓6th M20.02 Boutonnière deformity
    DEF: Deformity of the finger caused by flexion of the proximal interphalangeal joint and hyperextension of the distal joint. The deformity results from rheumatoid arthritis, osteoarthritis, or injury.
    M20.021 Boutonnière deformity of right finger(s)
    M20.022 Boutonnière deformity of left finger(s)
    M20.029 Boutonniere deformity of unspecified finger(s)
✓6th M20.03 Swan-neck deformity
    DEF: Flexed distal and hyperextended proximal interphalangeal joint most commonly caused by rheumatoid arthritis.
    M20.031 Swan-neck deformity of right finger(s)
    M20.032 Swan-neck deformity of left finger(s)
    M20.039 Swan-neck deformity of unspecified finger(s)
✓6th M20.09 Other deformity of finger(s)
    M20.091 Other deformity of right finger(s)
    M20.092 Other deformity of left finger(s)
    M20.099 Other deformity of finger(s), unspecified finger(s)

✓5th **M20.1 Hallux valgus (acquired)**
    EXCLUDES 2 bunion (M21.6-)
    AHA: 2016,4Q,38
    DEF: Deformity in which the great toe deviates toward the other toes and may even be positioned over or under the second toe.

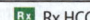

Hallux Valgus — Hallux valgus; Medial eminence of metatarsal bone; Right foot

    M20.10 Hallux valgus (acquired), unspecified foot
    M20.11 Hallux valgus (acquired), right foot
    M20.12 Hallux valgus (acquired), left foot
✓5th **M20.2 Hallux rigidus**
    M20.20 Hallux rigidus, unspecified foot
    M20.21 Hallux rigidus, right foot
    M20.22 Hallux rigidus, left foot
✓5th **M20.3 Hallux varus (acquired)**
    DEF: Deformity in which the great toe deviates away from the other toes.
    M20.30 Hallux varus (acquired), unspecified foot
    M20.31 Hallux varus (acquired), right foot
    M20.32 Hallux varus (acquired), left foot
✓5th **M20.4 Other hammer toe(s) (acquired)**
    M20.40 Other hammer toe(s) (acquired), unspecified foot
    M20.41 Other hammer toe(s) (acquired), right foot
    M20.42 Other hammer toe(s) (acquired), left foot
✓5th M20.5 Other deformities of toe(s) (acquired)
    ✓6th M20.5X Other deformities of toe(s) (acquired)
        M20.5X1 Other deformities of toe(s) (acquired), right foot
        M20.5X2 Other deformities of toe(s) (acquired), left foot
        M20.5X9 Other deformities of toe(s) (acquired), unspecified foot
✓5th **M20.6 Acquired deformities of toe(s), unspecified**
    M20.60 Acquired deformities of toe(s), unspecified, unspecified foot
    M20.61 Acquired deformities of toe(s), unspecified, right foot
    M20.62 Acquired deformities of toe(s), unspecified, left foot

✓4th **M21 Other acquired deformities of limbs**
    EXCLUDES 1 acquired absence of limb (Z89.-)
        congenital absence of limbs (Q71-Q73)
        congenital deformities and malformations of limbs (Q65-Q66, Q68-Q74)
    EXCLUDES 2 acquired deformities of fingers or toes (M20.-)
        coxa plana (M91.2)

✓5th **M21.0 Valgus deformity, not elsewhere classified**
    EXCLUDES 1 metatarsus valgus (Q66.6)
        talipes calcaneovalgus (Q66.4-)
    M21.00 Valgus deformity, not elsewhere classified, unspecified site
    ✓6th M21.02 Valgus deformity, not elsewhere classified, elbow
        Cubitus valgus
        M21.021 Valgus deformity, not elsewhere classified, right elbow
        M21.022 Valgus deformity, not elsewhere classified, left elbow

M21.029 Valgus deformity, not elsewhere classified, unspecified elbow

M21.05 Valgus deformity, not elsewhere classified, hip
M21.051 Valgus deformity, not elsewhere classified, right hip
M21.052 Valgus deformity, not elsewhere classified, left hip
M21.059 Valgus deformity, not elsewhere classified, unspecified hip

M21.06 Valgus deformity, not elsewhere classified, knee
Genu valgum
Knock knee
DEF: Genu valga/valgum: Condition in which the thighs slant inward, causing the knees to be angled abnormally close together, leaving the space between the ankles wider than normal.

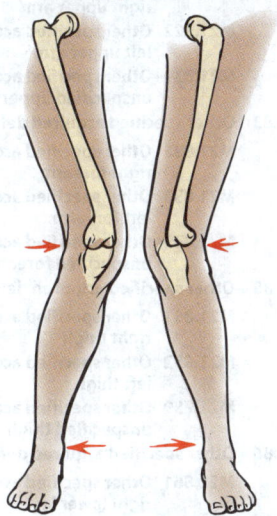
Genu Valga (knock-knee)

M21.16 Varus deformity, not elsewhere classified, knee
Bow leg
Genu varum
DEF: Genu varus/varum: Condition in which the thighs and/or legs are bowed in an outward curve with an abnormally increased space between the knees.

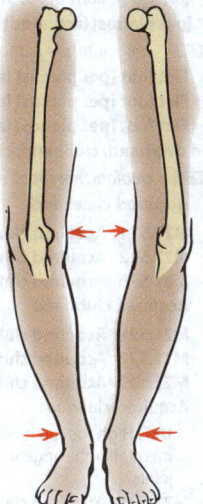
Genu Varus (bowleg)

M21.061 Valgus deformity, not elsewhere classified, right knee
M21.062 Valgus deformity, not elsewhere classified, left knee
M21.069 Valgus deformity, not elsewhere classified, unspecified knee

M21.07 Valgus deformity, not elsewhere classified, ankle
M21.071 Valgus deformity, not elsewhere classified, right ankle
M21.072 Valgus deformity, not elsewhere classified, left ankle
M21.079 Valgus deformity, not elsewhere classified, unspecified ankle

M21.1 Varus deformity, not elsewhere classified
EXCLUDES 1 metatarsus varus (Q66.22-)
tibia vara (M92.51-)

M21.10 Varus deformity, not elsewhere classified, unspecified site

M21.12 Varus deformity, not elsewhere classified, elbow
Cubitus varus, elbow
M21.121 Varus deformity, not elsewhere classified, right elbow
M21.122 Varus deformity, not elsewhere classified, left elbow
M21.129 Varus deformity, not elsewhere classified, unspecified elbow

M21.15 Varus deformity, not elsewhere classified, hip
M21.151 Varus deformity, not elsewhere classified, right hip
M21.152 Varus deformity, not elsewhere classified, left hip
M21.159 Varus deformity, not elsewhere classified, unspecified hip

M21.161 Varus deformity, not elsewhere classified, right knee
M21.162 Varus deformity, not elsewhere classified, left knee
M21.169 Varus deformity, not elsewhere classified, unspecified knee

M21.17 Varus deformity, not elsewhere classified, ankle
M21.171 Varus deformity, not elsewhere classified, right ankle
M21.172 Varus deformity, not elsewhere classified, left ankle
M21.179 Varus deformity, not elsewhere classified, unspecified ankle

M21.2 Flexion deformity
M21.20 Flexion deformity, unspecified site
M21.21 Flexion deformity, shoulder
M21.211 Flexion deformity, right shoulder
M21.212 Flexion deformity, left shoulder
M21.219 Flexion deformity, unspecified shoulder

M21.22 Flexion deformity, elbow
M21.221 Flexion deformity, right elbow
M21.222 Flexion deformity, left elbow
M21.229 Flexion deformity, unspecified elbow

M21.23 Flexion deformity, wrist
M21.231 Flexion deformity, right wrist
M21.232 Flexion deformity, left wrist
M21.239 Flexion deformity, unspecified wrist

M21.24 Flexion deformity, finger joints
M21.241 Flexion deformity, right finger joints
M21.242 Flexion deformity, left finger joints
M21.249 Flexion deformity, unspecified finger joints

M21.25 Flexion deformity, hip
M21.251 Flexion deformity, right hip
M21.252 Flexion deformity, left hip
M21.259 Flexion deformity, unspecified hip

M21.26 Flexion deformity, knee
M21.261 Flexion deformity, right knee
M21.262 Flexion deformity, left knee
M21.269 Flexion deformity, unspecified knee

M21.27 Flexion deformity, ankle and toes
M21.271 Flexion deformity, right ankle and toes
M21.272 Flexion deformity, left ankle and toes
M21.279 Flexion deformity, unspecified ankle and toes

M21.3 Wrist or foot drop (acquired)

M21.33 Wrist drop (acquired)
- M21.331 Wrist drop, right wrist
- M21.332 Wrist drop, left wrist
- M21.339 Wrist drop, unspecified wrist

M21.37 Foot drop (acquired)
- M21.371 Foot drop, right foot
- M21.372 Foot drop, left foot
- M21.379 Foot drop, unspecified foot

M21.4 Flat foot [pes planus] (acquired)
EXCLUDES 1 congenital pes planus (Q66.5-)
- M21.40 Flat foot [pes planus] (acquired), unspecified foot
- M21.41 Flat foot [pes planus] (acquired), right foot
- M21.42 Flat foot [pes planus] (acquired), left foot

M21.5 Acquired clawhand, clubhand, clawfoot and clubfoot
EXCLUDES 1 clubfoot, not specified as acquired (Q66.89)

M21.51 Acquired clawhand
- M21.511 Acquired clawhand, right hand
- M21.512 Acquired clawhand, left hand
- M21.519 Acquired clawhand, unspecified hand

M21.52 Acquired clubhand
- M21.521 Acquired clubhand, right hand
- M21.522 Acquired clubhand, left hand
- M21.529 Acquired clubhand, unspecified hand

M21.53 Acquired clawfoot
DEF: High foot arch with hyperextended toes at the metatarsophalangeal joint and flexed toes at the distal joints.
- M21.531 Acquired clawfoot, right foot
- M21.532 Acquired clawfoot, left foot
- M21.539 Acquired clawfoot, unspecified foot

M21.54 Acquired clubfoot
DEF: Acquired anomaly of the foot with the heel elevated and rotated outward and the toes pointing inward.
- M21.541 Acquired clubfoot, right foot
- M21.542 Acquired clubfoot, left foot
- M21.549 Acquired clubfoot, unspecified foot

M21.6 Other acquired deformities of foot
EXCLUDES 2 deformities of toe (acquired) (M20.1-M20.6-)
AHA: 2016,4Q,38

M21.61 Bunion
- M21.611 Bunion of right foot
- M21.612 Bunion of left foot
- M21.619 Bunion of unspecified foot

M21.62 Bunionette
- M21.621 Bunionette of right foot
- M21.622 Bunionette of left foot
- M21.629 Bunionette of unspecified foot

M21.6X Other acquired deformities of foot
AHA: 2023,3Q,20
- M21.6X1 Other acquired deformities of right foot
- M21.6X2 Other acquired deformities of left foot
- M21.6X9 Other acquired deformities of unspecified foot

M21.7 Unequal limb length (acquired)
NOTE: The site used should correspond to the shorter limb
- M21.70 Unequal limb length (acquired), unspecified site

M21.72 Unequal limb length (acquired), humerus
- M21.721 Unequal limb length (acquired), right humerus
- M21.722 Unequal limb length (acquired), left humerus
- M21.729 Unequal limb length (acquired), unspecified humerus

M21.73 Unequal limb length (acquired), ulna and radius
- M21.731 Unequal limb length (acquired), right ulna
- M21.732 Unequal limb length (acquired), left ulna
- M21.733 Unequal limb length (acquired), right radius
- M21.734 Unequal limb length (acquired), left radius
- M21.739 Unequal limb length (acquired), unspecified ulna and radius

M21.75 Unequal limb length (acquired), femur
- M21.751 Unequal limb length (acquired), right femur
- M21.752 Unequal limb length (acquired), left femur
- M21.759 Unequal limb length (acquired), unspecified femur

M21.76 Unequal limb length (acquired), tibia and fibula
- M21.761 Unequal limb length (acquired), right tibia
- M21.762 Unequal limb length (acquired), left tibia
- M21.763 Unequal limb length (acquired), right fibula
- M21.764 Unequal limb length (acquired), left fibula
- M21.769 Unequal limb length (acquired), unspecified tibia and fibula

M21.8 Other specified acquired deformities of limbs
EXCLUDES 2 coxa plana (M91.2)
- M21.80 Other specified acquired deformities of unspecified limb

M21.82 Other specified acquired deformities of upper arm
- M21.821 Other specified acquired deformities of right upper arm
- M21.822 Other specified acquired deformities of left upper arm
- M21.829 Other specified acquired deformities of unspecified upper arm

M21.83 Other specified acquired deformities of forearm
- M21.831 Other specified acquired deformities of right forearm
- M21.832 Other specified acquired deformities of left forearm
- M21.839 Other specified acquired deformities of unspecified forearm

M21.85 Other specified acquired deformities of thigh
- M21.851 Other specified acquired deformities of right thigh
- M21.852 Other specified acquired deformities of left thigh
- M21.859 Other specified acquired deformities of unspecified thigh

M21.86 Other specified acquired deformities of lower leg
- M21.861 Other specified acquired deformities of right lower leg
- M21.862 Other specified acquired deformities of left lower leg
- M21.869 Other specified acquired deformities of unspecified lower leg

M21.9 Unspecified acquired deformity of limb and hand
- M21.90 Unspecified acquired deformity of unspecified limb

M21.92 Unspecified acquired deformity of upper arm
- M21.921 Unspecified acquired deformity of right upper arm
- M21.922 Unspecified acquired deformity of left upper arm
- M21.929 Unspecified acquired deformity of unspecified upper arm

M21.93 Unspecified acquired deformity of forearm
- M21.931 Unspecified acquired deformity of right forearm
- M21.932 Unspecified acquired deformity of left forearm
- M21.939 Unspecified acquired deformity of unspecified forearm

M21.94 Unspecified acquired deformity of hand
- M21.941 Unspecified acquired deformity of hand, right hand
- M21.942 Unspecified acquired deformity of hand, left hand
- M21.949 Unspecified acquired deformity of hand, unspecified hand

M21.95 Unspecified acquired deformity of thigh
- M21.951 Unspecified acquired deformity of right thigh
- M21.952 Unspecified acquired deformity of left thigh
- M21.959 Unspecified acquired deformity of unspecified thigh

M21.96 Unspecified acquired deformity of lower leg
- M21.961 Unspecified acquired deformity of right lower leg
- M21.962 Unspecified acquired deformity of left lower leg

M21.969 Unspecified acquired deformity of unspecified lower leg

M22 Disorder of patella
EXCLUDES 2 traumatic dislocation of patella (S83.0-)

M22.0 Recurrent dislocation of patella
- M22.00 Recurrent dislocation of patella, unspecified knee
- M22.01 Recurrent dislocation of patella, right knee
- M22.02 Recurrent dislocation of patella, left knee

M22.1 Recurrent subluxation of patella
Incomplete dislocation of patella
- M22.10 Recurrent subluxation of patella, unspecified knee
- M22.11 Recurrent subluxation of patella, right knee
- M22.12 Recurrent subluxation of patella, left knee

M22.2 Patellofemoral disorders
- M22.2X Patellofemoral disorders
  - M22.2X1 Patellofemoral disorders, right knee
  - M22.2X2 Patellofemoral disorders, left knee
  - M22.2X9 Patellofemoral disorders, unspecified knee

M22.3 Other derangements of patella
- M22.3X Other derangements of patella
  - M22.3X1 Other derangements of patella, right knee
  - M22.3X2 Other derangements of patella, left knee
  - M22.3X9 Other derangements of patella, unspecified knee

M22.4 Chondromalacia patellae
- M22.40 Chondromalacia patellae, unspecified knee
- M22.41 Chondromalacia patellae, right knee
- M22.42 Chondromalacia patellae, left knee

M22.8 Other disorders of patella
- M22.8X Other disorders of patella
  - M22.8X1 Other disorders of patella, right knee
  - M22.8X2 Other disorders of patella, left knee
  - M22.8X9 Other disorders of patella, unspecified knee

M22.9 Unspecified disorder of patella
- M22.90 Unspecified disorder of patella, unspecified knee
- M22.91 Unspecified disorder of patella, right knee
- M22.92 Unspecified disorder of patella, left knee

M23 Internal derangement of knee
EXCLUDES 1
- ankylosis (M24.66)
- deformity of knee (M21.-)
- osteochondritis dissecans (M93.2)

EXCLUDES 2
- current injury - see injury of knee and lower leg (S80-S89)
- recurrent dislocation or subluxation of joints (M24.4)
- recurrent dislocation or subluxation of patella (M22.0-M22.1)

M23.0 Cystic meniscus
- M23.00 Cystic meniscus, unspecified meniscus
  - Cystic meniscus, unspecified lateral meniscus
  - Cystic meniscus, unspecified medial meniscus
  - M23.000 Cystic meniscus, unspecified lateral meniscus, right knee
  - M23.001 Cystic meniscus, unspecified lateral meniscus, left knee
  - M23.002 Cystic meniscus, unspecified lateral meniscus, unspecified knee
  - M23.003 Cystic meniscus, unspecified medial meniscus, right knee
  - M23.004 Cystic meniscus, unspecified medial meniscus, left knee
  - M23.005 Cystic meniscus, unspecified medial meniscus, unspecified knee
  - M23.006 Cystic meniscus, unspecified meniscus, right knee
  - M23.007 Cystic meniscus, unspecified meniscus, left knee
  - M23.009 Cystic meniscus, unspecified meniscus, unspecified knee
- M23.01 Cystic meniscus, anterior horn of medial meniscus
  - M23.011 Cystic meniscus, anterior horn of medial meniscus, right knee
  - M23.012 Cystic meniscus, anterior horn of medial meniscus, left knee
  - M23.019 Cystic meniscus, anterior horn of medial meniscus, unspecified knee
- M23.02 Cystic meniscus, posterior horn of medial meniscus
  - M23.021 Cystic meniscus, posterior horn of medial meniscus, right knee
  - M23.022 Cystic meniscus, posterior horn of medial meniscus, left knee
  - M23.029 Cystic meniscus, posterior horn of medial meniscus, unspecified knee
- M23.03 Cystic meniscus, other medial meniscus
  - M23.031 Cystic meniscus, other medial meniscus, right knee
  - M23.032 Cystic meniscus, other medial meniscus, left knee
  - M23.039 Cystic meniscus, other medial meniscus, unspecified knee
- M23.04 Cystic meniscus, anterior horn of lateral meniscus
  - M23.041 Cystic meniscus, anterior horn of lateral meniscus, right knee
  - M23.042 Cystic meniscus, anterior horn of lateral meniscus, left knee
  - M23.049 Cystic meniscus, anterior horn of lateral meniscus, unspecified knee
- M23.05 Cystic meniscus, posterior horn of lateral meniscus
  - M23.051 Cystic meniscus, posterior horn of lateral meniscus, right knee
  - M23.052 Cystic meniscus, posterior horn of lateral meniscus, left knee
  - M23.059 Cystic meniscus, posterior horn of lateral meniscus, unspecified knee
- M23.06 Cystic meniscus, other lateral meniscus
  - M23.061 Cystic meniscus, other lateral meniscus, right knee
  - M23.062 Cystic meniscus, other lateral meniscus, left knee
  - M23.069 Cystic meniscus, other lateral meniscus, unspecified knee

M23.2 Derangement of meniscus due to old tear or injury
Old bucket-handle tear
AHA: 2019,2Q,26

Derangement of Meniscus

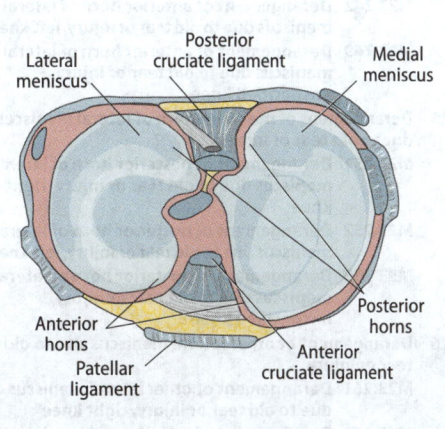
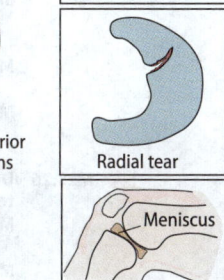

Overhead view of right knee

- M23.20 Derangement of unspecified meniscus due to old tear or injury
  - Derangement of unspecified lateral meniscus due to old tear or injury
  - Derangement of unspecified medial meniscus due to old tear or injury
  - M23.200 Derangement of unspecified lateral meniscus due to old tear or injury, right knee
  - M23.201 Derangement of unspecified lateral meniscus due to old tear or injury, left knee
  - M23.202 Derangement of unspecified lateral meniscus due to old tear or injury, unspecified knee
  - M23.203 Derangement of unspecified medial meniscus due to old tear or injury, right knee
  - M23.204 Derangement of unspecified medial meniscus due to old tear or injury, left knee

Chapter 13. Diseases of the Musculoskeletal System and Connective Tissue

- **M23.205** Derangement of unspecified medial meniscus due to old tear or injury, unspecified knee
- **M23.206** Derangement of unspecified meniscus due to old tear or injury, right knee
- **M23.207** Derangement of unspecified meniscus due to old tear or injury, left knee
- **M23.209** Derangement of unspecified meniscus due to old tear or injury, unspecified knee

✓6ᵗʰ **M23.21** Derangement of anterior horn of medial meniscus due to old tear or injury
- **M23.211** Derangement of anterior horn of medial meniscus due to old tear or injury, right knee
- **M23.212** Derangement of anterior horn of medial meniscus due to old tear or injury, left knee
- **M23.219** Derangement of anterior horn of medial meniscus due to old tear or injury, unspecified knee

✓6ᵗʰ **M23.22** Derangement of posterior horn of medial meniscus due to old tear or injury
- **M23.221** Derangement of posterior horn of medial meniscus due to old tear or injury, right knee
- **M23.222** Derangement of posterior horn of medial meniscus due to old tear or injury, left knee
- **M23.229** Derangement of posterior horn of medial meniscus due to old tear or injury, unspecified knee

✓6ᵗʰ **M23.23** Derangement of other medial meniscus due to old tear or injury
- **M23.231** Derangement of other medial meniscus due to old tear or injury, right knee
- **M23.232** Derangement of other medial meniscus due to old tear or injury, left knee
- **M23.239** Derangement of other medial meniscus due to old tear or injury, unspecified knee

✓6ᵗʰ **M23.24** Derangement of anterior horn of lateral meniscus due to old tear or injury
- **M23.241** Derangement of anterior horn of lateral meniscus due to old tear or injury, right knee
- **M23.242** Derangement of anterior horn of lateral meniscus due to old tear or injury, left knee
- **M23.249** Derangement of anterior horn of lateral meniscus due to old tear or injury, unspecified knee

✓6ᵗʰ **M23.25** Derangement of posterior horn of lateral meniscus due to old tear or injury
- **M23.251** Derangement of posterior horn of lateral meniscus due to old tear or injury, right knee
- **M23.252** Derangement of posterior horn of lateral meniscus due to old tear or injury, left knee
- **M23.259** Derangement of posterior horn of lateral meniscus due to old tear or injury, unspecified knee

✓6ᵗʰ **M23.26** Derangement of other lateral meniscus due to old tear or injury
- **M23.261** Derangement of other lateral meniscus due to old tear or injury, right knee
- **M23.262** Derangement of other lateral meniscus due to old tear or injury, left knee
- **M23.269** Derangement of other lateral meniscus due to old tear or injury, unspecified knee

✓5ᵗʰ **M23.3** Other meniscus derangements
Degenerate meniscus
Detached meniscus
Retained meniscus

✓6ᵗʰ **M23.30** Other meniscus derangements, unspecified meniscus
Other meniscus derangements, unspecified lateral meniscus
Other meniscus derangements, unspecified medial meniscus
- **M23.300** Other meniscus derangements, unspecified lateral meniscus, right knee
- **M23.301** Other meniscus derangements, unspecified lateral meniscus, left knee
- **M23.302** Other meniscus derangements, unspecified lateral meniscus, unspecified knee
- **M23.303** Other meniscus derangements, unspecified medial meniscus, right knee
- **M23.304** Other meniscus derangements, unspecified medial meniscus, left knee
- **M23.305** Other meniscus derangements, unspecified medial meniscus, unspecified knee
- **M23.306** Other meniscus derangements, unspecified meniscus, right knee
- **M23.307** Other meniscus derangements, unspecified meniscus, left knee
- **M23.309** Other meniscus derangements, unspecified meniscus, unspecified knee

✓6ᵗʰ **M23.31** Other meniscus derangements, anterior horn of medial meniscus
- **M23.311** Other meniscus derangements, anterior horn of medial meniscus, right knee
- **M23.312** Other meniscus derangements, anterior horn of medial meniscus, left knee
- **M23.319** Other meniscus derangements, anterior horn of medial meniscus, unspecified knee

✓6ᵗʰ **M23.32** Other meniscus derangements, posterior horn of medial meniscus
- **M23.321** Other meniscus derangements, posterior horn of medial meniscus, right knee
- **M23.322** Other meniscus derangements, posterior horn of medial meniscus, left knee
- **M23.329** Other meniscus derangements, posterior horn of medial meniscus, unspecified knee

✓6ᵗʰ **M23.33** Other meniscus derangements, other medial meniscus
- **M23.331** Other meniscus derangements, other medial meniscus, right knee
- **M23.332** Other meniscus derangements, other medial meniscus, left knee
- **M23.339** Other meniscus derangements, other medial meniscus, unspecified knee

✓6ᵗʰ **M23.34** Other meniscus derangements, anterior horn of lateral meniscus
- **M23.341** Other meniscus derangements, anterior horn of lateral meniscus, right knee
- **M23.342** Other meniscus derangements, anterior horn of lateral meniscus, left knee
- **M23.349** Other meniscus derangements, anterior horn of lateral meniscus, unspecified knee

✓6ᵗʰ **M23.35** Other meniscus derangements, posterior horn of lateral meniscus
- **M23.351** Other meniscus derangements, posterior horn of lateral meniscus, right knee
- **M23.352** Other meniscus derangements, posterior horn of lateral meniscus, left knee
- **M23.359** Other meniscus derangements, posterior horn of lateral meniscus, unspecified knee

✓6ᵗʰ **M23.36** Other meniscus derangements, other lateral meniscus
- **M23.361** Other meniscus derangements, other lateral meniscus, right knee
- **M23.362** Other meniscus derangements, other lateral meniscus, left knee
- **M23.369** Other meniscus derangements, other lateral meniscus, unspecified knee

✓5ᵗʰ **M23.4** Loose body in knee
- **M23.40** Loose body in knee, unspecified knee
- **M23.41** Loose body in knee, right knee
- **M23.42** Loose body in knee, left knee

✓5ᵗʰ **M23.5** Chronic instability of knee
- **M23.50** Chronic instability of knee, unspecified knee
- **M23.51** Chronic instability of knee, right knee
- **M23.52** Chronic instability of knee, left knee

✓5ᵗʰ **M23.6** Other spontaneous disruption of ligament(s) of knee

✓6ᵗʰ **M23.60** Other spontaneous disruption of unspecified ligament of knee
- **M23.601** Other spontaneous disruption of unspecified ligament of right knee
- **M23.602** Other spontaneous disruption of unspecified ligament of left knee
- **M23.609** Other spontaneous disruption of unspecified ligament of unspecified knee

✓6ᵗʰ **M23.61** Other spontaneous disruption of anterior cruciate ligament of knee
- **M23.611** Other spontaneous disruption of anterior cruciate ligament of right knee
- **M23.612** Other spontaneous disruption of anterior cruciate ligament of left knee

Chapter 13. Diseases of the Musculoskeletal System and Connective Tissue

- M23.619 Other spontaneous disruption of anterior cruciate ligament of unspecified knee
- ✓6th **M23.62** Other spontaneous disruption of posterior cruciate ligament of knee
  - M23.621 Other spontaneous disruption of posterior cruciate ligament of right knee
  - M23.622 Other spontaneous disruption of posterior cruciate ligament of left knee
  - M23.629 Other spontaneous disruption of posterior cruciate ligament of unspecified knee
- ✓6th **M23.63** Other spontaneous disruption of medial collateral ligament of knee
  - M23.631 Other spontaneous disruption of medial collateral ligament of right knee
  - M23.632 Other spontaneous disruption of medial collateral ligament of left knee
  - M23.639 Other spontaneous disruption of medial collateral ligament of unspecified knee
- ✓6th **M23.64** Other spontaneous disruption of lateral collateral ligament of knee
  - M23.641 Other spontaneous disruption of lateral collateral ligament of right knee
  - M23.642 Other spontaneous disruption of lateral collateral ligament of left knee
  - M23.649 Other spontaneous disruption of lateral collateral ligament of unspecified knee
- ✓6th **M23.67** Other spontaneous disruption of capsular ligament of knee
  - M23.671 Other spontaneous disruption of capsular ligament of right knee
  - M23.672 Other spontaneous disruption of capsular ligament of left knee
  - M23.679 Other spontaneous disruption of capsular ligament of unspecified knee
- ✓5th **M23.8** Other internal derangements of knee
  - Laxity of ligament of knee
  - Snapping knee
  - ✓6th **M23.8X** Other internal derangements of knee
    - M23.8X1 Other internal derangements of right knee
    - M23.8X2 Other internal derangements of left knee
    - M23.8X9 Other internal derangements of unspecified knee
- ✓5th **M23.9** Unspecified internal derangement of knee
  - M23.90 Unspecified internal derangement of unspecified knee
  - M23.91 Unspecified internal derangement of right knee
  - M23.92 Unspecified internal derangement of left knee

- ✓4th **M24** Other specific joint derangements
  - EXCLUDES 1: current injury - see injury of joint by body region
  - EXCLUDES 2: ganglion (M67.4)
    - snapping knee (M23.8-)
    - temporomandibular joint disorders (M26.6-)
  - AHA: 2020,4Q,31-32
  - ✓5th **M24.0** Loose body in joint
    - EXCLUDES 2: loose body in knee (M23.4)
    - M24.00 Loose body in unspecified joint
    - ✓6th **M24.01** Loose body in shoulder
      - M24.011 Loose body in right shoulder
      - M24.012 Loose body in left shoulder
      - M24.019 Loose body in unspecified shoulder
    - ✓6th **M24.02** Loose body in elbow
      - M24.021 Loose body in right elbow
      - M24.022 Loose body in left elbow
      - M24.029 Loose body in unspecified elbow
    - ✓6th **M24.03** Loose body in wrist
      - M24.031 Loose body in right wrist
      - M24.032 Loose body in left wrist
      - M24.039 Loose body in unspecified wrist
    - ✓6th **M24.04** Loose body in finger joints
      - M24.041 Loose body in right finger joint(s)
      - M24.042 Loose body in left finger joint(s)
      - M24.049 Loose body in unspecified finger joint(s)
    - ✓6th **M24.05** Loose body in hip
      - M24.051 Loose body in right hip
      - M24.052 Loose body in left hip
      - M24.059 Loose body in unspecified hip
    - ✓6th **M24.07** Loose body in ankle and toe joints
      - M24.071 Loose body in right ankle
      - M24.072 Loose body in left ankle
      - M24.073 Loose body in unspecified ankle
      - M24.074 Loose body in right toe joint(s)
      - M24.075 Loose body in left toe joint(s)
      - M24.076 Loose body in unspecified toe joint(s)
    - M24.08 Loose body, other site
  - ✓5th **M24.1** Other articular cartilage disorders
    - EXCLUDES 2: chondrocalcinosis (M11.1-, M11.2-)
      - internal derangement of knee (M23.-)
      - metastatic calcification (E83.59)
      - ochronosis (E70.29)
    - M24.10 Other articular cartilage disorders, unspecified site
    - ✓6th **M24.11** Other articular cartilage disorders, shoulder
      - M24.111 Other articular cartilage disorders, right shoulder
      - M24.112 Other articular cartilage disorders, left shoulder
      - M24.119 Other articular cartilage disorders, unspecified shoulder
    - ✓6th **M24.12** Other articular cartilage disorders, elbow
      - M24.121 Other articular cartilage disorders, right elbow
      - M24.122 Other articular cartilage disorders, left elbow
      - M24.129 Other articular cartilage disorders, unspecified elbow
    - ✓6th **M24.13** Other articular cartilage disorders, wrist
      - M24.131 Other articular cartilage disorders, right wrist
      - M24.132 Other articular cartilage disorders, left wrist
      - M24.139 Other articular cartilage disorders, unspecified wrist
    - ✓6th **M24.14** Other articular cartilage disorders, hand
      - M24.141 Other articular cartilage disorders, right hand
      - M24.142 Other articular cartilage disorders, left hand
      - M24.149 Other articular cartilage disorders, unspecified hand
    - ✓6th **M24.15** Other articular cartilage disorders, hip
      - M24.151 Other articular cartilage disorders, right hip
      - M24.152 Other articular cartilage disorders, left hip
      - M24.159 Other articular cartilage disorders, unspecified hip
    - ✓6th **M24.17** Other articular cartilage disorders, ankle and foot
      - M24.171 Other articular cartilage disorders, right ankle
      - M24.172 Other articular cartilage disorders, left ankle
      - M24.173 Other articular cartilage disorders, unspecified ankle
      - M24.174 Other articular cartilage disorders, right foot
      - M24.175 Other articular cartilage disorders, left foot
      - M24.176 Other articular cartilage disorders, unspecified foot
    - M24.19 Other articular cartilage disorders, other specified site
  - ✓5th **M24.2** Disorder of ligament
    - Instability secondary to old ligament injury
    - Ligamentous laxity NOS
    - EXCLUDES 1: familial ligamentous laxity (M35.7)
    - EXCLUDES 2: internal derangement of knee (M23.5-M23.8X9)
    - M24.20 Disorder of ligament, unspecified site
    - ✓6th **M24.21** Disorder of ligament, shoulder
      - M24.211 Disorder of ligament, right shoulder
      - M24.212 Disorder of ligament, left shoulder
      - M24.219 Disorder of ligament, unspecified shoulder
    - ✓6th **M24.22** Disorder of ligament, elbow
      - M24.221 Disorder of ligament, right elbow
      - M24.222 Disorder of ligament, left elbow
      - M24.229 Disorder of ligament, unspecified elbow
    - ✓6th **M24.23** Disorder of ligament, wrist
      - M24.231 Disorder of ligament, right wrist
      - M24.232 Disorder of ligament, left wrist
      - M24.239 Disorder of ligament, unspecified wrist

✓ Additional Character Required ✓x7th Placeholder Alert Manifestation Unspecified Dx Q QPP UPD Unacceptable PDx

M24.24 Disorder of ligament, hand
- M24.241 Disorder of ligament, right hand
- M24.242 Disorder of ligament, left hand
- M24.249 Disorder of ligament, unspecified hand

M24.25 Disorder of ligament, hip
- M24.251 Disorder of ligament, right hip
- M24.252 Disorder of ligament, left hip
- M24.259 Disorder of ligament, unspecified hip

M24.27 Disorder of ligament, ankle and foot
- M24.271 Disorder of ligament, right ankle
- M24.272 Disorder of ligament, left ankle
- M24.273 Disorder of ligament, unspecified ankle
- M24.274 Disorder of ligament, right foot
- M24.275 Disorder of ligament, left foot
- M24.276 Disorder of ligament, unspecified foot

M24.28 Disorder of ligament, vertebrae
AHA: 2023,2Q,13

M24.29 Disorder of ligament, other specified site

M24.3 Pathological dislocation of joint, not elsewhere classified
EXCLUDES 1: congenital dislocation or displacement of joint - see congenital malformations and deformations of the musculoskeletal system (Q65-Q79)
current injury - see injury of joints and ligaments by body region
recurrent dislocation of joint (M24.4-)

M24.30 Pathological dislocation of unspecified joint, not elsewhere classified

M24.31 Pathological dislocation of shoulder, not elsewhere classified
- M24.311 Pathological dislocation of right shoulder, not elsewhere classified
- M24.312 Pathological dislocation of left shoulder, not elsewhere classified
- M24.319 Pathological dislocation of unspecified shoulder, not elsewhere classified

M24.32 Pathological dislocation of elbow, not elsewhere classified
- M24.321 Pathological dislocation of right elbow, not elsewhere classified
- M24.322 Pathological dislocation of left elbow, not elsewhere classified
- M24.329 Pathological dislocation of unspecified elbow, not elsewhere classified

M24.33 Pathological dislocation of wrist, not elsewhere classified
- M24.331 Pathological dislocation of right wrist, not elsewhere classified
- M24.332 Pathological dislocation of left wrist, not elsewhere classified
- M24.339 Pathological dislocation of unspecified wrist, not elsewhere classified

M24.34 Pathological dislocation of hand, not elsewhere classified
- M24.341 Pathological dislocation of right hand, not elsewhere classified
- M24.342 Pathological dislocation of left hand, not elsewhere classified
- M24.349 Pathological dislocation of unspecified hand, not elsewhere classified

M24.35 Pathological dislocation of hip, not elsewhere classified
AHA: 2022,1Q,32
- M24.351 Pathological dislocation of right hip, not elsewhere classified
- M24.352 Pathological dislocation of left hip, not elsewhere classified
- M24.359 Pathological dislocation of unspecified hip, not elsewhere classified

M24.36 Pathological dislocation of knee, not elsewhere classified
- M24.361 Pathological dislocation of right knee, not elsewhere classified
- M24.362 Pathological dislocation of left knee, not elsewhere classified
- M24.369 Pathological dislocation of unspecified knee, not elsewhere classified

M24.37 Pathological dislocation of ankle and foot, not elsewhere classified
- M24.371 Pathological dislocation of right ankle, not elsewhere classified
- M24.372 Pathological dislocation of left ankle, not elsewhere classified
- M24.373 Pathological dislocation of unspecified ankle, not elsewhere classified
- M24.374 Pathological dislocation of right foot, not elsewhere classified
- M24.375 Pathological dislocation of left foot, not elsewhere classified
- M24.376 Pathological dislocation of unspecified foot, not elsewhere classified

M24.39 Pathological dislocation of other specified joint, not elsewhere classified

M24.4 Recurrent dislocation of joint
Recurrent subluxation of joint
EXCLUDES 2: recurrent dislocation of patella (M22.0-M22.1)
recurrent vertebral dislocation (M43.3-, M43.4, M43.5-)

M24.40 Recurrent dislocation, unspecified joint

M24.41 Recurrent dislocation, shoulder
- M24.411 Recurrent dislocation, right shoulder
- M24.412 Recurrent dislocation, left shoulder
- M24.419 Recurrent dislocation, unspecified shoulder

M24.42 Recurrent dislocation, elbow
- M24.421 Recurrent dislocation, right elbow
- M24.422 Recurrent dislocation, left elbow
- M24.429 Recurrent dislocation, unspecified elbow

M24.43 Recurrent dislocation, wrist
- M24.431 Recurrent dislocation, right wrist
- M24.432 Recurrent dislocation, left wrist
- M24.439 Recurrent dislocation, unspecified wrist

M24.44 Recurrent dislocation, hand and finger(s)
- M24.441 Recurrent dislocation, right hand
- M24.442 Recurrent dislocation, left hand
- M24.443 Recurrent dislocation, unspecified hand
- M24.444 Recurrent dislocation, right finger
- M24.445 Recurrent dislocation, left finger
- M24.446 Recurrent dislocation, unspecified finger

M24.45 Recurrent dislocation, hip
- M24.451 Recurrent dislocation, right hip
- M24.452 Recurrent dislocation, left hip
- M24.459 Recurrent dislocation, unspecified hip

M24.46 Recurrent dislocation, knee
- M24.461 Recurrent dislocation, right knee
- M24.462 Recurrent dislocation, left knee
- M24.469 Recurrent dislocation, unspecified knee

M24.47 Recurrent dislocation, ankle, foot and toes
- M24.471 Recurrent dislocation, right ankle
- M24.472 Recurrent dislocation, left ankle
- M24.473 Recurrent dislocation, unspecified ankle
- M24.474 Recurrent dislocation, right foot
- M24.475 Recurrent dislocation, left foot
- M24.476 Recurrent dislocation, unspecified foot
- M24.477 Recurrent dislocation, right toe(s)
- M24.478 Recurrent dislocation, left toe(s)
- M24.479 Recurrent dislocation, unspecified toe(s)

M24.49 Recurrent dislocation, other specified joint

M24.5 Contracture of joint
EXCLUDES 1: contracture of muscle without contracture of joint (M62.4-)
contracture of tendon (sheath) without contracture of joint (M62.4-)
Dupuytren's contracture (M72.0)
EXCLUDES 2: acquired deformities of limbs (M20-M21)
AHA: 2016,2Q,6

M24.50 Contracture, unspecified joint

M24.51 Contracture, shoulder
- M24.511 Contracture, right shoulder
- M24.512 Contracture, left shoulder
- M24.519 Contracture, unspecified shoulder

M24.52 Contracture, elbow
- M24.521 Contracture, right elbow
- M24.522 Contracture, left elbow
- M24.529 Contracture, unspecified elbow

M24.53 Contracture, wrist
- M24.531 Contracture, right wrist
- M24.532 Contracture, left wrist
- M24.539 Contracture, unspecified wrist

- **M24.54** Contracture, hand
  - M24.541 Contracture, right hand
  - M24.542 Contracture, left hand
  - M24.549 Contracture, unspecified hand
- **M24.55** Contracture, hip
  - M24.551 Contracture, right hip
  - M24.552 Contracture, left hip
  - M24.559 Contracture, unspecified hip
- **M24.56** Contracture, knee
  - M24.561 Contracture, right knee
  - M24.562 Contracture, left knee
  - M24.569 Contracture, unspecified knee
- **M24.57** Contracture, ankle and foot
  - M24.571 Contracture, right ankle
  - M24.572 Contracture, left ankle
  - M24.573 Contracture, unspecified ankle
  - M24.574 Contracture, right foot
  - M24.575 Contracture, left foot
  - M24.576 Contracture, unspecified foot
- M24.59 Contracture, other specified joint

M24.6 Ankylosis of joint
- EXCLUDES 1: stiffness of joint without ankylosis (M25.6-)
- EXCLUDES 2: spine (M43.2-)
- AHA: 2025,1Q,25
- DEF: Ankylosis: Abnormal union or fusion of bones in a joint, which is normally moveable.
  - M24.60 Ankylosis, unspecified joint
  - **M24.61** Ankylosis, shoulder
    - M24.611 Ankylosis, right shoulder
    - M24.612 Ankylosis, left shoulder
    - M24.619 Ankylosis, unspecified shoulder
  - **M24.62** Ankylosis, elbow
    - M24.621 Ankylosis, right elbow
    - M24.622 Ankylosis, left elbow
    - M24.629 Ankylosis, unspecified elbow
  - **M24.63** Ankylosis, wrist
    - M24.631 Ankylosis, right wrist
    - M24.632 Ankylosis, left wrist
    - M24.639 Ankylosis, unspecified wrist
  - **M24.64** Ankylosis, hand
    - M24.641 Ankylosis, right hand
    - M24.642 Ankylosis, left hand
    - M24.649 Ankylosis, unspecified hand
  - **M24.65** Ankylosis, hip
    - M24.651 Ankylosis, right hip
    - M24.652 Ankylosis, left hip
    - M24.659 Ankylosis, unspecified hip
  - **M24.66** Ankylosis, knee
    - M24.661 Ankylosis, right knee
    - M24.662 Ankylosis, left knee
    - M24.669 Ankylosis, unspecified knee
  - **M24.67** Ankylosis, ankle and foot
    - M24.671 Ankylosis, right ankle
    - M24.672 Ankylosis, left ankle
    - M24.673 Ankylosis, unspecified ankle
    - M24.674 Ankylosis, right foot
    - M24.675 Ankylosis, left foot
    - M24.676 Ankylosis, unspecified foot
  - M24.69 Ankylosis, other specified joint

M24.7 Protrusio acetabuli
- DEF: Intrapelvic protrusion of the acetabulum characterized by the sinking of the floor of the acetabulum, causing the femoral head to protrude. It limits hip movement and is of unknown etiology. Synonym(s): Otto's pelvis.

M24.8 Other specific joint derangements, not elsewhere classified
- EXCLUDES 2: iliotibial band syndrome (M76.3)
  - M24.80 Other specific joint derangements of unspecified joint, not elsewhere classified
  - **M24.81** Other specific joint derangements of shoulder, not elsewhere classified
    - M24.811 Other specific joint derangements of right shoulder, not elsewhere classified
    - M24.812 Other specific joint derangements of left shoulder, not elsewhere classified
    - M24.819 Other specific joint derangements of unspecified shoulder, not elsewhere classified
  - **M24.82** Other specific joint derangements of elbow, not elsewhere classified
    - M24.821 Other specific joint derangements of right elbow, not elsewhere classified
    - M24.822 Other specific joint derangements of left elbow, not elsewhere classified
    - M24.829 Other specific joint derangements of unspecified elbow, not elsewhere classified
  - **M24.83** Other specific joint derangements of wrist, not elsewhere classified
    - M24.831 Other specific joint derangements of right wrist, not elsewhere classified
    - M24.832 Other specific joint derangements of left wrist, not elsewhere classified
    - M24.839 Other specific joint derangements of unspecified wrist, not elsewhere classified
  - **M24.84** Other specific joint derangements of hand, not elsewhere classified
    - M24.841 Other specific joint derangements of right hand, not elsewhere classified
    - M24.842 Other specific joint derangements of left hand, not elsewhere classified
    - M24.849 Other specific joint derangements of unspecified hand, not elsewhere classified
  - **M24.85** Other specific joint derangements of hip, not elsewhere classified
    - Irritable hip
    - M24.851 Other specific joint derangements of right hip, not elsewhere classified
    - M24.852 Other specific joint derangements of left hip, not elsewhere classified
    - M24.859 Other specific joint derangements of unspecified hip, not elsewhere classified
  - **M24.87** Other specific joint derangements of ankle and foot, not elsewhere classified
    - M24.871 Other specific joint derangements of right ankle, not elsewhere classified
    - M24.872 Other specific joint derangements of left ankle, not elsewhere classified
    - M24.873 Other specific joint derangements of unspecified ankle, not elsewhere classified
    - M24.874 Other specific joint derangements of right foot, not elsewhere classified
    - M24.875 Other specific joint derangements left foot, not elsewhere classified
    - M24.876 Other specific joint derangements of unspecified foot, not elsewhere classified
  - M24.89 Other specific joint derangement of other specified joint, not elsewhere classified

M24.9 Joint derangement, unspecified

M25 Other joint disorder, not elsewhere classified
- EXCLUDES 2:
  - abnormality of gait and mobility (R26.-)
  - acquired deformities of limb (M20-M21)
  - calcification of bursa (M71.4-)
  - calcification of shoulder (joint) (M75.3)
  - calcification of tendon (M65.2-)
  - difficulty in walking (R26.2)
  - temporomandibular joint disorder (M26.6-)
- AHA: 2020,4Q,31-32

M25.0 Hemarthrosis
- EXCLUDES 1: current injury - see injury of joint by body region
  hemophilic arthropathy (M36.2)
  - M25.00 Hemarthrosis, unspecified joint
  - **M25.01** Hemarthrosis, shoulder
    - M25.011 Hemarthrosis, right shoulder
    - M25.012 Hemarthrosis, left shoulder
    - M25.019 Hemarthrosis, unspecified shoulder
  - **M25.02** Hemarthrosis, elbow
    - M25.021 Hemarthrosis, right elbow
    - M25.022 Hemarthrosis, left elbow
    - M25.029 Hemarthrosis, unspecified elbow
  - **M25.03** Hemarthrosis, wrist
    - M25.031 Hemarthrosis, right wrist
    - M25.032 Hemarthrosis, left wrist
    - M25.039 Hemarthrosis, unspecified wrist
  - **M25.04** Hemarthrosis, hand
    - M25.041 Hemarthrosis, right hand
    - M25.042 Hemarthrosis, left hand
    - M25.049 Hemarthrosis, unspecified hand

M25.05 Hemarthrosis, hip
- M25.051 Hemarthrosis, right hip
- M25.052 Hemarthrosis, left hip
- M25.059 Hemarthrosis, unspecified hip

M25.06 Hemarthrosis, knee
- M25.061 Hemarthrosis, right knee
- M25.062 Hemarthrosis, left knee
- M25.069 Hemarthrosis, unspecified knee

M25.07 Hemarthrosis, ankle and foot
- M25.071 Hemarthrosis, right ankle
- M25.072 Hemarthrosis, left ankle
- M25.073 Hemarthrosis, unspecified ankle
- M25.074 Hemarthrosis, right foot
- M25.075 Hemarthrosis, left foot
- M25.076 Hemarthrosis, unspecified foot

M25.08 Hemarthrosis, other specified site
Hemarthrosis, vertebrae

M25.1 Fistula of joint
- M25.10 Fistula, unspecified joint

M25.11 Fistula, shoulder
- M25.111 Fistula, right shoulder
- M25.112 Fistula, left shoulder
- M25.119 Fistula, unspecified shoulder

M25.12 Fistula, elbow
- M25.121 Fistula, right elbow
- M25.122 Fistula, left elbow
- M25.129 Fistula, unspecified elbow

M25.13 Fistula, wrist
- M25.131 Fistula, right wrist
- M25.132 Fistula, left wrist
- M25.139 Fistula, unspecified wrist

M25.14 Fistula, hand
- M25.141 Fistula, right hand
- M25.142 Fistula, left hand
- M25.149 Fistula, unspecified hand

M25.15 Fistula, hip
- M25.151 Fistula, right hip
- M25.152 Fistula, left hip
- M25.159 Fistula, unspecified hip

M25.16 Fistula, knee
- M25.161 Fistula, right knee
- M25.162 Fistula, left knee
- M25.169 Fistula, unspecified knee

M25.17 Fistula, ankle and foot
- M25.171 Fistula, right ankle
- M25.172 Fistula, left ankle
- M25.173 Fistula, unspecified ankle
- M25.174 Fistula, right foot
- M25.175 Fistula, left foot
- M25.176 Fistula, unspecified foot

M25.18 Fistula, other specified site
Fistula, vertebrae

M25.2 Flail joint
DEF: Hinged joint that exhibits an abnormal or excessive degree of range and mobility.
- M25.20 Flail joint, unspecified joint

M25.21 Flail joint, shoulder
- M25.211 Flail joint, right shoulder
- M25.212 Flail joint, left shoulder
- M25.219 Flail joint, unspecified shoulder

M25.22 Flail joint, elbow
- M25.221 Flail joint, right elbow
- M25.222 Flail joint, left elbow
- M25.229 Flail joint, unspecified elbow

M25.23 Flail joint, wrist
- M25.231 Flail joint, right wrist
- M25.232 Flail joint, left wrist
- M25.239 Flail joint, unspecified wrist

M25.24 Flail joint, hand
- M25.241 Flail joint, right hand
- M25.242 Flail joint, left hand
- M25.249 Flail joint, unspecified hand

M25.25 Flail joint, hip
- M25.251 Flail joint, right hip
- M25.252 Flail joint, left hip
- M25.259 Flail joint, unspecified hip

M25.26 Flail joint, knee
- M25.261 Flail joint, right knee
- M25.262 Flail joint, left knee
- M25.269 Flail joint, unspecified knee

M25.27 Flail joint, ankle and foot
- M25.271 Flail joint, right ankle and foot
- M25.272 Flail joint, left ankle and foot
- M25.279 Flail joint, unspecified ankle and foot

M25.28 Flail joint, other site

M25.3 Other instability of joint
EXCLUDES 1 instability of joint secondary to old ligament injury (M24.2-)
instability of joint secondary to removal of joint prosthesis (M96.8-)
EXCLUDES 2 spinal instabilities (M53.2-)

- M25.30 Other instability, unspecified joint

M25.31 Other instability, shoulder
- M25.311 Other instability, right shoulder
- M25.312 Other instability, left shoulder
- M25.319 Other instability, unspecified shoulder

M25.32 Other instability, elbow
- M25.321 Other instability, right elbow
- M25.322 Other instability, left elbow
- M25.329 Other instability, unspecified elbow

M25.33 Other instability, wrist
- M25.331 Other instability, right wrist
- M25.332 Other instability, left wrist
- M25.339 Other instability, unspecified wrist

M25.34 Other instability, hand
- M25.341 Other instability, right hand
- M25.342 Other instability, left hand
- M25.349 Other instability, unspecified hand

M25.35 Other instability, hip
- M25.351 Other instability, right hip
- M25.352 Other instability, left hip
- M25.359 Other instability, unspecified hip

M25.36 Other instability, knee
- M25.361 Other instability, right knee
- M25.362 Other instability, left knee
- M25.369 Other instability, unspecified knee

M25.37 Other instability, ankle and foot
- M25.371 Other instability, right ankle
- M25.372 Other instability, left ankle
- M25.373 Other instability, unspecified ankle
- M25.374 Other instability, right foot
- M25.375 Other instability, left foot
- M25.376 Other instability, unspecified foot

M25.39 Other instability, other specified joint

M25.4 Effusion of joint
EXCLUDES 1 hydrarthrosis in yaws (A66.6)
intermittent hydrarthrosis (M12.4-)
other infective (teno)synovitis (M65.1-)

- M25.40 Effusion, unspecified joint

M25.41 Effusion, shoulder
- M25.411 Effusion, right shoulder
- M25.412 Effusion, left shoulder
- M25.419 Effusion, unspecified shoulder

M25.42 Effusion, elbow
- M25.421 Effusion, right elbow
- M25.422 Effusion, left elbow
- M25.429 Effusion, unspecified elbow

M25.43 Effusion, wrist
- M25.431 Effusion, right wrist
- M25.432 Effusion, left wrist
- M25.439 Effusion, unspecified wrist

M25.44 Effusion, hand
- M25.441 Effusion, right hand
- M25.442 Effusion, left hand
- M25.449 Effusion, unspecified hand

M25.45 Effusion, hip
- M25.451 Effusion, right hip
- M25.452 Effusion, left hip
- M25.459 Effusion, unspecified hip

- **M25.46** Effusion, knee
  - M25.461 Effusion, right knee
  - M25.462 Effusion, left knee
  - M25.469 Effusion, unspecified knee
- **M25.47** Effusion, ankle and foot
  - M25.471 Effusion, right ankle
  - M25.472 Effusion, left ankle
  - M25.473 Effusion, unspecified ankle
  - M25.474 Effusion, right foot
  - M25.475 Effusion, left foot
  - M25.476 Effusion, unspecified foot
- **M25.48** Effusion, other site
- **M25.5** Pain in joint
  - EXCLUDES 2: pain in fingers (M79.64-)
  - pain in foot (M79.67-)
  - pain in hand (M79.64-)
  - pain in limb (M79.6-)
  - pain in toes (M79.67-)
  - **M25.50** Pain in unspecified joint
  - **M25.51** Pain in shoulder
    - M25.511 Pain in right shoulder
    - M25.512 Pain in left shoulder
    - M25.519 Pain in unspecified shoulder
  - **M25.52** Pain in elbow
    - M25.521 Pain in right elbow
    - M25.522 Pain in left elbow
    - M25.529 Pain in unspecified elbow
  - **M25.53** Pain in wrist
    - M25.531 Pain in right wrist
    - M25.532 Pain in left wrist
    - M25.539 Pain in unspecified wrist
  - **M25.54** Pain in joints of hand
    - AHA: 2016,4Q,38
    - M25.541 Pain in joints of right hand
    - M25.542 Pain in joints of left hand
    - M25.549 Pain in joints of unspecified hand
      - Pain in joints of hand NOS
  - **M25.55** Pain in hip
    - M25.551 Pain in right hip
    - M25.552 Pain in left hip
    - M25.559 Pain in unspecified hip
  - **M25.56** Pain in knee
    - M25.561 Pain in right knee
    - M25.562 Pain in left knee
    - M25.569 Pain in unspecified knee
  - **M25.57** Pain in ankle and joints of foot
    - M25.571 Pain in right ankle and joints of right foot
    - M25.572 Pain in left ankle and joints of left foot
    - M25.579 Pain in unspecified ankle and joints of unspecified foot
  - **M25.59** Pain in other specified joint
- **M25.6** Stiffness of joint, not elsewhere classified
  - EXCLUDES 1: ankylosis of joint (M24.6-)
  - contracture of joint (M24.5-)
  - **M25.60** Stiffness of unspecified joint, not elsewhere classified
  - **M25.61** Stiffness of shoulder, not elsewhere classified
    - M25.611 Stiffness of right shoulder, not elsewhere classified
    - M25.612 Stiffness of left shoulder, not elsewhere classified
    - M25.619 Stiffness of unspecified shoulder, not elsewhere classified
  - **M25.62** Stiffness of elbow, not elsewhere classified
    - M25.621 Stiffness of right elbow, not elsewhere classified
    - M25.622 Stiffness of left elbow, not elsewhere classified
    - M25.629 Stiffness of unspecified elbow, not elsewhere classified
  - **M25.63** Stiffness of wrist, not elsewhere classified
    - M25.631 Stiffness of right wrist, not elsewhere classified
    - M25.632 Stiffness of left wrist, not elsewhere classified
    - M25.639 Stiffness of unspecified wrist, not elsewhere classified
  - **M25.64** Stiffness of hand, not elsewhere classified
    - M25.641 Stiffness of right hand, not elsewhere classified
    - M25.642 Stiffness of left hand, not elsewhere classified
    - M25.649 Stiffness of unspecified hand, not elsewhere classified
  - **M25.65** Stiffness of hip, not elsewhere classified
    - M25.651 Stiffness of right hip, not elsewhere classified
    - M25.652 Stiffness of left hip, not elsewhere classified
    - M25.659 Stiffness of unspecified hip, not elsewhere classified
  - **M25.66** Stiffness of knee, not elsewhere classified
    - M25.661 Stiffness of right knee, not elsewhere classified
    - M25.662 Stiffness of left knee, not elsewhere classified
    - M25.669 Stiffness of unspecified knee, not elsewhere classified
  - **M25.67** Stiffness of ankle and foot, not elsewhere classified
    - M25.671 Stiffness of right ankle, not elsewhere classified
    - M25.672 Stiffness of left ankle, not elsewhere classified
    - M25.673 Stiffness of unspecified ankle, not elsewhere classified
    - M25.674 Stiffness of right foot, not elsewhere classified
    - M25.675 Stiffness of left foot, not elsewhere classified
    - M25.676 Stiffness of unspecified foot, not elsewhere classified
  - **M25.69** Stiffness of other specified joint, not elsewhere classified
- **M25.7** Osteophyte
  - **M25.70** Osteophyte, unspecified joint
  - **M25.71** Osteophyte, shoulder
    - M25.711 Osteophyte, right shoulder
    - M25.712 Osteophyte, left shoulder
    - M25.719 Osteophyte, unspecified shoulder
  - **M25.72** Osteophyte, elbow
    - M25.721 Osteophyte, right elbow
    - M25.722 Osteophyte, left elbow
    - M25.729 Osteophyte, unspecified elbow
  - **M25.73** Osteophyte, wrist
    - M25.731 Osteophyte, right wrist
    - M25.732 Osteophyte, left wrist
    - M25.739 Osteophyte, unspecified wrist
  - **M25.74** Osteophyte, hand
    - M25.741 Osteophyte, right hand
    - M25.742 Osteophyte, left hand
    - M25.749 Osteophyte, unspecified hand
  - **M25.75** Osteophyte, hip
    - M25.751 Osteophyte, right hip
    - M25.752 Osteophyte, left hip
    - M25.759 Osteophyte, unspecified hip
  - **M25.76** Osteophyte, knee
    - M25.761 Osteophyte, right knee
    - M25.762 Osteophyte, left knee
    - M25.769 Osteophyte, unspecified knee
  - **M25.77** Osteophyte, ankle and foot
    - M25.771 Osteophyte, right ankle
    - M25.772 Osteophyte, left ankle
    - M25.773 Osteophyte, unspecified ankle
    - M25.774 Osteophyte, right foot
    - M25.775 Osteophyte, left foot
    - M25.776 Osteophyte, unspecified foot
  - **M25.78** Osteophyte, vertebrae
- **M25.8** Other specified joint disorders
  - **M25.80** Other specified joint disorders, unspecified joint
  - **M25.81** Other specified joint disorders, shoulder
    - AHA: 2022,3Q,18
    - M25.811 Other specified joint disorders, right shoulder
    - M25.812 Other specified joint disorders, left shoulder

M25.819–M26.59 — Chapter 13. Diseases of the Musculoskeletal System and Connective Tissue — ICD-10-CM 2026

- M25.819 Other specified joint disorders, unspecified shoulder
- ✓6th M25.82 Other specified joint disorders, elbow
  - M25.821 Other specified joint disorders, right elbow
  - M25.822 Other specified joint disorders, left elbow
  - M25.829 Other specified joint disorders, unspecified elbow
- ✓6th M25.83 Other specified joint disorders, wrist
  - M25.831 Other specified joint disorders, right wrist
  - M25.832 Other specified joint disorders, left wrist
  - M25.839 Other specified joint disorders, unspecified wrist
- ✓6th M25.84 Other specified joint disorders, hand
  - M25.841 Other specified joint disorders, right hand
  - M25.842 Other specified joint disorders, left hand
  - M25.849 Other specified joint disorders, unspecified hand
- ✓6th M25.85 Other specified joint disorders, hip
  - AHA: 2014,4Q,25
  - M25.851 Other specified joint disorders, right hip
  - M25.852 Other specified joint disorders, left hip
  - M25.859 Other specified joint disorders, unspecified hip
- ✓6th M25.86 Other specified joint disorders, knee
  - M25.861 Other specified joint disorders, right knee
  - M25.862 Other specified joint disorders, left knee
  - M25.869 Other specified joint disorders, unspecified knee
- ✓6th M25.87 Other specified joint disorders, ankle and foot
  - M25.871 Other specified joint disorders, right ankle and foot
  - M25.872 Other specified joint disorders, left ankle and foot
  - M25.879 Other specified joint disorders, unspecified ankle and foot
- M25.9 Joint disorder, unspecified

Dentofacial anomalies [including malocclusion] and other disorders of jaw (M26-M27)

EXCLUDES 1 hemifacial atrophy or hypertrophy (Q67.4)
unilateral condylar hyperplasia or hypoplasia (M27.8)

- ✓4th M26 Dentofacial anomalies [including malocclusion]
  - ✓5th M26.0 Major anomalies of jaw size
    - EXCLUDES 1 acromegaly (E22.0)
    - Robin's syndrome (Q87.0)
    - M26.00 Unspecified anomaly of jaw size
    - M26.01 Maxillary hyperplasia
    - M26.02 Maxillary hypoplasia
      - AHA: 2014,3Q,23
    - M26.03 Mandibular hyperplasia
    - M26.04 Mandibular hypoplasia
    - M26.05 Macrogenia
    - M26.06 Microgenia
    - M26.07 Excessive tuberosity of jaw
      - Entire maxillary tuberosity
    - M26.09 Other specified anomalies of jaw size
  - ✓5th M26.1 Anomalies of jaw-cranial base relationship
    - M26.10 Unspecified anomaly of jaw-cranial base relationship
    - M26.11 Maxillary asymmetry
    - M26.12 Other jaw asymmetry
    - M26.19 Other specified anomalies of jaw-cranial base relationship
      - AHA: 2020,1Q,21
  - ✓5th M26.2 Anomalies of dental arch relationship
    - M26.20 Unspecified anomaly of dental arch relationship
    - ✓6th M26.21 Malocclusion, Angle's class
      - M26.211 Malocclusion, Angle's class I
        - Neutro-occlusion
      - M26.212 Malocclusion, Angle's class II
        - Disto-occlusion Division I
        - Disto-occlusion Division II
      - M26.213 Malocclusion, Angle's class III
        - Mesio-occlusion
      - M26.219 Malocclusion, Angle's class, unspecified
    - ✓6th M26.22 Open occlusal relationship
      - M26.220 Open anterior occlusal relationship
        - Anterior open bite
      - M26.221 Open posterior occlusal relationship
        - Posterior open bite
    - M26.23 Excessive horizontal overlap
      - Excessive horizontal overjet
    - M26.24 Reverse articulation
      - Crossbite (anterior) (posterior)
    - M26.25 Anomalies of interarch distance
    - M26.29 Other anomalies of dental arch relationship
      - Midline deviation of dental arch
      - Overbite (excessive) deep
      - Overbite (excessive) horizontal
      - Overbite (excessive) vertical
      - Posterior lingual occlusion of mandibular teeth
  - ✓5th M26.3 Anomalies of tooth position of fully erupted tooth or teeth
    - EXCLUDES 2 embedded and impacted teeth (K01.-)
    - M26.30 Unspecified anomaly of tooth position of fully erupted tooth or teeth
      - Abnormal spacing of fully erupted tooth or teeth NOS
      - Displacement of fully erupted tooth or teeth NOS
      - Transposition of fully erupted tooth or teeth NOS
    - M26.31 Crowding of fully erupted teeth
    - M26.32 Excessive spacing of fully erupted teeth
      - Diastema of fully erupted tooth or teeth NOS
    - M26.33 Horizontal displacement of fully erupted tooth or teeth
      - Tipped tooth or teeth
      - Tipping of fully erupted tooth
    - M26.34 Vertical displacement of fully erupted tooth or teeth
      - Extruded tooth
      - Infraeruption of tooth or teeth
      - Supraeruption of tooth or teeth
    - M26.35 Rotation of fully erupted tooth or teeth
    - M26.36 Insufficient interocclusal distance of fully erupted teeth (ridge)
      - Lack of adequate intermaxillary vertical dimension of fully erupted teeth
    - M26.37 Excessive interocclusal distance of fully erupted teeth
      - Excessive intermaxillary vertical dimension of fully erupted teeth
      - Loss of occlusal vertical dimension of fully erupted teeth
    - M26.39 Other anomalies of tooth position of fully erupted tooth or teeth
  - M26.4 Malocclusion, unspecified
  - ✓5th M26.5 Dentofacial functional abnormalities
    - EXCLUDES 1 bruxism (F45.8)
    - teeth-grinding NOS (F45.8)
    - M26.50 Dentofacial functional abnormalities, unspecified
    - M26.51 Abnormal jaw closure
    - M26.52 Limited mandibular range of motion
    - M26.53 Deviation in opening and closing of the mandible
    - M26.54 Insufficient anterior guidance
      - Insufficient anterior occlusal guidance
    - M26.55 Centric occlusion maximum intercuspation discrepancy
      - EXCLUDES 1 centric occlusion NOS (M26.59)
    - M26.56 Non-working side interference
      - Balancing side interference
    - M26.57 Lack of posterior occlusal support
    - M26.59 Other dentofacial functional abnormalities
      - Centric occlusion (of teeth) NOS
      - Malocclusion due to abnormal swallowing
      - Malocclusion due to mouth breathing
      - Malocclusion due to tongue, lip or finger habits

HCC CMS-HCC | Rx HCC | ESRD HCC | COM Commercial HCC | N Newborn: 0 | P Pediatric: 0-17 | M Maternity: 9-64 | A Adult: 15-124

M26.6 Temporomandibular joint disorders

EXCLUDES 2: current temporomandibular joint dislocation (S03.0)
current temporomandibular joint sprain (S03.4)

AHA: 2016,4Q,38-39

Temporomandibular Joint

Cutaway view of temporomandibular joint (TMJ) — Cutaway detail, Upper joint space, Articular disc (meniscus), Lower joint space, Condyle, Mandible

- **M26.60** Temporomandibular joint disorder, unspecified
  - **M26.601** Right temporomandibular joint disorder, unspecified
  - **M26.602** Left temporomandibular joint disorder, unspecified
  - **M26.603** Bilateral temporomandibular joint disorder, unspecified
  - **M26.609** Unspecified temporomandibular joint disorder, unspecified side
    - Temporomandibular joint disorder NOS
- **M26.61** Adhesions and ankylosis of temporomandibular joint
  - **M26.611** Adhesions and ankylosis of right temporomandibular joint
  - **M26.612** Adhesions and ankylosis of left temporomandibular joint
  - **M26.613** Adhesions and ankylosis of bilateral temporomandibular joint
  - **M26.619** Adhesions and ankylosis of temporomandibular joint, unspecified side
- **M26.62** Arthralgia of temporomandibular joint
  - **M26.621** Arthralgia of right temporomandibular joint
  - **M26.622** Arthralgia of left temporomandibular joint
  - **M26.623** Arthralgia of bilateral temporomandibular joint
  - **M26.629** Arthralgia of temporomandibular joint, unspecified side
- **M26.63** Articular disc disorder of temporomandibular joint
  - **M26.631** Articular disc disorder of right temporomandibular joint
  - **M26.632** Articular disc disorder of left temporomandibular joint
  - **M26.633** Articular disc disorder of bilateral temporomandibular joint
  - **M26.639** Articular disc disorder of temporomandibular joint, unspecified side
- **M26.64** Arthritis of temporomandibular joint
  - AHA: 2020,4Q,32
  - **M26.641** Arthritis of right temporomandibular joint
  - **M26.642** Arthritis of left temporomandibular joint
  - **M26.643** Arthritis of bilateral temporomandibular joint
  - **M26.649** Arthritis of unspecified temporomandibular joint
- **M26.65** Arthropathy of temporomandibular joint
  - AHA: 2020,4Q,32
  - **M26.651** Arthropathy of right temporomandibular joint
  - **M26.652** Arthropathy of left temporomandibular joint
  - **M26.653** Arthropathy of bilateral temporomandibular joint
  - **M26.659** Arthropathy of unspecified temporomandibular joint
- **M26.69** Other specified disorders of temporomandibular joint

M26.7 Dental alveolar anomalies
- **M26.70** Unspecified alveolar anomaly
- **M26.71** Alveolar maxillary hyperplasia
- **M26.72** Alveolar mandibular hyperplasia
- **M26.73** Alveolar maxillary hypoplasia
- **M26.74** Alveolar mandibular hypoplasia
- **M26.79** Other specified alveolar anomalies

M26.8 Other dentofacial anomalies
- **M26.81** Anterior soft tissue impingement
  - Anterior soft tissue impingement on teeth
- **M26.82** Posterior soft tissue impingement
  - Posterior soft tissue impingement on teeth
- **M26.89** Other dentofacial anomalies

M26.9 Dentofacial anomaly, unspecified

M27 Other diseases of jaws

M27.0 Developmental disorders of jaws
Latent bone cyst of jaw
Stafne's cyst
Torus mandibularis
Torus palatinus

M27.1 Giant cell granuloma, central
Giant cell granuloma NOS
EXCLUDES 1: peripheral giant cell granuloma (K06.8)

M27.2 Inflammatory conditions of jaws
Osteitis of jaw(s)
Osteomyelitis (neonatal) jaw(s)
Osteoradionecrosis jaw(s)
Periostitis jaw(s)
Sequestrum of jaw bone
Use additional code (W88-W90, X39.0) to identify radiation, if radiation-induced
EXCLUDES 2: osteonecrosis of jaw due to drug (M87.180)

M27.3 Alveolitis of jaws
Alveolar osteitis
Dry socket

M27.4 Other and unspecified cysts of jaw
EXCLUDES 1: cysts of oral region (K09.-)
latent bone cyst of jaw (M27.0)
Stafne's cyst (M27.0)

- **M27.40** Unspecified cyst of jaw
  - Cyst of jaw NOS
- **M27.49** Other cysts of jaw
  - Aneurysmal cyst of jaw
  - Hemorrhagic cyst of jaw
  - Traumatic cyst of jaw

M27.5 Periradicular pathology associated with previous endodontic treatment
- **M27.51** Perforation of root canal space due to endodontic treatment
- **M27.52** Endodontic overfill
- **M27.53** Endodontic underfill
- **M27.59** Other periradicular pathology associated with previous endodontic treatment

M27.6 Endosseous dental implant failure
- **M27.61** Osseointegration failure of dental implant
  - Hemorrhagic complications of dental implant placement
  - Iatrogenic osseointegration failure of dental implant
  - Osseointegration failure of dental implant due to complications of systemic disease
  - Osseointegration failure of dental implant due to poor bone quality
  - Pre-integration failure of dental implant NOS
  - Pre-osseointegration failure of dental implant
- **M27.62** Post-osseointegration biological failure of dental implant
  - Failure of dental implant due to lack of attached gingiva
  - Failure of dental implant due to occlusal trauma (caused by poor prosthetic design)
  - Failure of dental implant due to parafunctional habits
  - Failure of dental implant due to periodontal infection (peri-implantitis)
  - Failure of dental implant due to poor oral hygiene
  - Iatrogenic post-osseointegration failure of dental implant
  - Post-osseointegration failure of dental implant due to complications of systemic disease

Chapter 13. Diseases of the Musculoskeletal System and Connective Tissue

M27.63 Post-osseointegration mechanical failure of dental implant
  Failure of dental prosthesis causing loss of dental implant
  Fracture of dental implant
  EXCLUDES 2 cracked tooth (K03.81)
    fractured dental restorative material with loss of material (K08.531)
    fractured dental restorative material without loss of material (K08.530)
    fractured tooth (S02.5)

M27.69 Other endosseous dental implant failure
  Dental implant failure NOS

M27.8 Other specified diseases of jaws
  Cherubism
  Exostosis
  Fibrous dysplasia
  Unilateral condylar hyperplasia
  Unilateral condylar hypoplasia
  EXCLUDES 1 jaw pain (R68.84)

M27.9 Disease of jaws, unspecified

Systemic connective tissue disorders (M30-M36)

INCLUDES
  autoimmune disease NOS
  collagen (vascular) disease NOS
  systemic autoimmune disease
  systemic collagen (vascular) disease
EXCLUDES 1 autoimmune disease, single organ or single cell-type -code to relevant condition category

✓4th M30 Polyarteritis nodosa and related conditions
  EXCLUDES 1 microscopic polyarteritis (M31.7)

  M30.0 Polyarteritis nodosa [HCC Rx ESR COM]

  M30.1 Polyarteritis with lung involvement [Churg-Strauss] [HCC Rx ESR COM]
    Allergic granulomatous angiitis
    Eosinophilic granulomatosis with polyangiitis [EGPA]
    AHA: 2021,1Q,23

  M30.2 Juvenile polyarteritis [HCC Rx ESR COM]

  M30.3 Mucocutaneous lymph node syndrome [Kawasaki] [HCC Rx ESR COM]

  M30.8 Other conditions related to polyarteritis nodosa [HCC Rx ESR COM]
    Polyangiitis overlap syndrome

✓4th M31 Other necrotizing vasculopathies

  M31.0 Hypersensitivity angiitis [HCC Rx ESR COM]
    Goodpasture's syndrome

  ✓5th M31.1 Thrombotic microangiopathy
    AHA: 2021,4Q,19

    M31.10 Thrombotic microangiopathy, unspecified [HCC Rx ESR COM]

    M31.11 Hematopoietic stem cell transplantation-associated thrombotic microangiopathy [HSCT-TMA] [HCC Rx ESR COM]
      Transplant-associated thrombotic microangiopathy [TA-TMA]
      Code first if applicable:
        complications of bone marrow transplant (T86.0-)
        complications of stem cell transplant (T86.5)
      Use additional code to identify specific organ dysfunction, such as:
        acute kidney failure (N17.-)
        acute respiratory distress syndrome (J80)
        capillary leak syndrome (I78.8)
        diffuse alveolar hemorrhage (R04.89)
        encephalopathy (metabolic) (septic) (G93.41)
        fluid overload, unspecified (E87.70)
        graft versus host disease (D89.81-)
        hemolytic uremic syndrome (D59.3-)
        hepatic failure (K72.-)
        hepatic veno-occlusive disease (K76.5)
        idiopathic interstitial pneumonia (J84.11-)
        sinusoidal obstruction syndrome (K76.5)

    M31.19 Other thrombotic microangiopathy [HCC Rx ESR COM]
      Thrombotic thrombocytopenic purpura

  M31.2 Lethal midline granuloma [HCC Rx ESR COM]

  ✓5th M31.3 Wegener's granulomatosis
    Granulomatosis with polyangiitis
    Necrotizing respiratory granulomatosis
    AHA: 2021,1Q,23

    M31.30 Wegener's granulomatosis without renal involvement [HCC Rx ESR COM]
      Wegener's granulomatosis NOS
      AHA: 2021,2Q,10

    M31.31 Wegener's granulomatosis with renal involvement [HCC Rx ESR COM]

  M31.4 Aortic arch syndrome [Takayasu] [HCC Rx ESR COM]

  M31.5 Giant cell arteritis with polymyalgia rheumatica [HCC Rx ESR COM]

  M31.6 Other giant cell arteritis [HCC Rx ESR COM]

  M31.7 Microscopic polyangiitis
    Microscopic polyarteritis
    EXCLUDES 1 polyarteritis nodosa (M30.0)
    AHA: 2021,1Q,23

  M31.8 Other specified necrotizing vasculopathies [HCC ESR]
    Hypocomplementemic vasculitis
    Septic vasculitis

  M31.9 Necrotizing vasculopathy, unspecified [HCC ESR]

✓4th M32 Systemic lupus erythematosus (SLE)
  EXCLUDES 1 lupus erythematosus (discoid) (NOS) (L93.0)
  AHA: 2020,4Q,11; 2018,3Q,14
  TIP: There is no default code for "lupus NOS." Query the provider for the specific type of lupus in order to assign the appropriate code.

  M32.0 Drug-induced systemic lupus erythematosus [Rx ESR COM]
    Use additional code for adverse effect, if applicable, to identify drug (T36-T50 with fifth or sixth character 5)

  ✓5th M32.1 Systemic lupus erythematosus with organ or system involvement

    M32.10 Systemic lupus erythematosus, organ or system involvement unspecified [HCC Rx ESR COM]

    M32.11 Endocarditis in systemic lupus erythematosus [HCC Rx ESR COM]
      Libman-Sacks disease

    M32.12 Pericarditis in systemic lupus erythematosus [HCC Rx ESR COM]
      Lupus pericarditis

    M32.13 Lung involvement in systemic lupus erythematosus [HCC Rx ESR COM]
      Pleural effusion due to systemic lupus erythematosus

    M32.14 Glomerular disease in systemic lupus erythematosus [HCC Rx ESR COM]
      Lupus renal disease NOS
      AHA: 2013,4Q,125

    M32.15 Tubulo-interstitial nephropathy in systemic lupus erythematosus [HCC Rx ESR COM]

    M32.19 Other organ or system involvement in systemic lupus erythematosus [HCC Rx ESR COM]
      Use additional code(s) to identify organ or system involvement, such as encephalitis (G05.3)

  M32.8 Other forms of systemic lupus erythematosus [HCC Rx ESR COM]

  M32.9 Systemic lupus erythematosus, unspecified [HCC Rx ESR COM]
    SLE NOS
    Systemic lupus erythematosus NOS
    Systemic lupus erythematosus without organ involvement

✓4th M33 Dermatopolymyositis
  AHA: 2017,4Q,18

  ✓5th M33.0 Juvenile dermatomyositis

    M33.00 Juvenile dermatomyositis, organ involvement unspecified [HCC Rx ESR COM]

    M33.01 Juvenile dermatomyositis with respiratory involvement [HCC Rx ESR COM]

    M33.02 Juvenile dermatomyositis with myopathy [HCC Rx ESR COM]

    M33.03 Juvenile dermatomyositis without myopathy [HCC Rx ESR COM]

    M33.09 Juvenile dermatomyositis with other organ involvement [HCC Rx ESR COM]

  ✓5th M33.1 Other dermatomyositis
    Adult dermatomyositis

    M33.10 Other dermatomyositis, organ involvement unspecified [HCC Rx ESR COM]

[HCC] CMS-HCC [Rx] Rx HCC [ESR] ESRD HCC [COM] Commercial HCC [N] Newborn: 0 [P] Pediatric: 0-17 [M] Maternity: 9-64 [A] Adult: 15-124

	M33.11	Other dermatomyositis with respiratory involvement	HCC Rx ESR COM
	M33.12	Other dermatomyositis with myopathy	HCC Rx ESR COM
	M33.13	Other dermatomyositis without myopathy	
		Dermatomyositis NOS	
	M33.19	Other dermatomyositis with other organ involvement	HCC Rx ESR COM

✓5ᵗʰ **M33.2 Polymyositis**
- M33.20 Polymyositis, organ involvement unspecified — HCC Rx ESR COM
- M33.21 Polymyositis with respiratory involvement — HCC Rx ESR COM
- M33.22 Polymyositis with myopathy — HCC Rx ESR COM
- M33.29 Polymyositis with other organ involvement — HCC Rx ESR COM

✓5ᵗʰ **M33.9 Dermatopolymyositis, unspecified**
- M33.90 Dermatopolymyositis, unspecified, organ involvement unspecified — HCC Rx ESR COM
- M33.91 Dermatopolymyositis, unspecified with respiratory involvement — HCC Rx ESR COM
- M33.92 Dermatopolymyositis, unspecified with myopathy — HCC Rx ESR COM
- M33.93 Dermatopolymyositis, unspecified without myopathy — HCC Rx ESR COM
- M33.99 Dermatopolymyositis, unspecified with other organ involvement — HCC Rx ESR COM

✓4ᵗʰ **M34 Systemic sclerosis [scleroderma]**
  EXCLUDES 1 circumscribed scleroderma (L94.0)
              neonatal scleroderma (P83.88)

- **M34.0 Progressive systemic sclerosis** — HCC Rx ESR COM
- **M34.1 CR(E)ST syndrome** — HCC Rx ESR COM
  Combination of calcinosis, Raynaud's phenomenon, esophageal dysfunction, sclerodactyly, telangiectasia
- **M34.2 Systemic sclerosis induced by drug and chemical** — Rx ESR COM
  Code first poisoning due to drug or toxin, if applicable (T36-T65 with fifth or sixth character 1-4)
  Use additional code for adverse effect, if applicable, to identify drug (T36-T50 with fifth or sixth character 5)

✓5ᵗʰ **M34.8 Other forms of systemic sclerosis**
- M34.81 Systemic sclerosis with lung involvement — HCC Rx ESR COM
  Code also if applicable:
    other interstitial pulmonary diseases (J84.89)
    secondary pulmonary arterial hypertension (I27.21)
- M34.82 Systemic sclerosis with myopathy — HCC Rx ESR COM
- M34.83 Systemic sclerosis with polyneuropathy — HCC Rx ESR COM
- M34.89 Other systemic sclerosis — HCC Rx ESR COM

M34.9 Systemic sclerosis, unspecified — HCC Rx ESR COM

✓4ᵗʰ **M35 Other systemic involvement of connective tissue**
  EXCLUDES 1 reactive perforating collagenosis (L87.1)

✓5ᵗʰ **M35.0 Sjogren syndrome**
  Sicca syndrome
  Use additional code to identify associated manifestations
  EXCLUDES 1 dry mouth, unspecified (R68.2)
  AHA: 2024,3Q,16; 2021,4Q,20
  DEF: Autoimmune disease associated with keratoconjunctivitis, laryngopharyngitis, rhinitis, dry mouth, enlarged parotid gland, and chronic polyarthritis.

- M35.00 Sjogren syndrome, unspecified — Rx ESR COM
- M35.01 Sjogren syndrome with keratoconjunctivitis — Rx ESR COM
- M35.02 Sjogren syndrome with lung involvement — HCC Rx ESR COM
- M35.03 Sjogren syndrome with myopathy — Rx ESR COM
- M35.04 Sjogren syndrome with tubulo-interstitial nephropathy — Rx ESR COM
  Renal tubular acidosis in sicca syndrome
- M35.05 Sjogren syndrome with inflammatory arthritis — Rx ESR COM
- M35.06 Sjogren syndrome with peripheral nervous system involvement — Rx ESR COM
- M35.07 Sjogren syndrome with central nervous system involvement — Rx ESR COM
- M35.08 Sjogren syndrome with gastrointestinal involvement — Rx ESR COM
- M35.0A Sjogren syndrome with glomerular disease — Rx ESR COM
- M35.0B Sjogren syndrome with vasculitis — Rx ESR COM
- M35.0C Sjogren syndrome with dental involvement — Rx ESR COM
- M35.09 Sjogren syndrome with other organ involvement — Rx ESR COM

M35.1 Other overlap syndromes — Rx ESR COM
  Mixed connective tissue disease
  EXCLUDES 1 polyangiitis overlap syndrome (M30.8)

M35.2 Behcet's disease — HCC Rx ESR COM

M35.3 Polymyalgia rheumatica — ESR COM
  EXCLUDES 1 polymyalgia rheumatica with giant cell arteritis (M31.5)

M35.4 Diffuse (eosinophilic) fasciitis

M35.5 Multifocal fibrosclerosis — Rx ESR COM

M35.6 Relapsing panniculitis [Weber-Christian]
  EXCLUDES 1 lupus panniculitis (L93.2)
              panniculitis NOS (M79.3-)

M35.7 Hypermobility syndrome
  Familial ligamentous laxity
  EXCLUDES 1 ligamentous laxity, NOS (M24.2-)
  EXCLUDES 2 Ehlers-Danlos syndromes (Q79.6-)

✓5ᵗʰ **M35.8 Other specified systemic involvement of connective tissue**
  AHA: 2021,1Q,36; 2020,3Q,13-14

- M35.81 Multisystem inflammatory syndrome — HCC ESR COM
  MIS-A
  MIS-C
  Multisystem inflammatory syndrome in adults
  Multisystem inflammatory syndrome in children
  Pediatric inflammatory multisystem syndrome
  PIMS
  Code first, if applicable, COVID-19 (U07.1)
  Code also any associated complications such as:
    acute hepatic failure (K72.0-)
    acute kidney failure (N17.-)
    acute myocarditis (I40.-)
    acute respiratory distress syndrome (J80)
    cardiac arrhythmia (I47-I49.-)
    pneumonia due to COVID-19 (J12.82)
    severe sepsis (R65.2-)
    viral cardiomyopathy (B33.24)
    viral pericarditis (B33.23)
  Use additional code, if applicable, for:
    exposure to COVID-19 or SARS-CoV-2 infection (Z20.822)
    personal history of COVID-19 (Z86.16)
    post COVID-19 condition (U09.9)
  AHA: 2021,4Q,102; 2021,1Q,29,36,41
  DEF: Hyperinflammatory condition that seems to be largely associated with past or present coronavirus disease 2019 (COVID-19) infection. Predominantly occurring in children, with less frequent occurrences in adults, symptoms often include fever, laboratory evidence of inflammation, and evidence of clinically severe illness requiring hospitalization with multisystem (two or more) organ involvement. **Synonym(s):** MIS, MIS-C.

- M35.89 Other specified systemic involvement of connective tissue — Rx ESR COM

M35.9 Systemic involvement of connective tissue, unspecified — Rx ESR COM
  Autoimmune disease (systemic) NOS
  Collagen (vascular) disease NOS

✓4ᵗʰ **M36 Systemic disorders of connective tissue in diseases classified elsewhere**
  EXCLUDES 2 arthropathies in diseases classified elsewhere (M14.-)

- **M36.0 Dermato(poly)myositis in neoplastic disease** — HCC Rx ESR COM
  Code first underlying neoplasm (C00-D49)
- **M36.1 Arthropathy in neoplastic disease**
  Code first underlying neoplasm, such as:
    leukemia (C91-C95)
    malignant histiocytosis (C96.A)
    multiple myeloma (C90.0)

M36.2 Hemophilic arthropathy
Hemarthrosis in hemophilic arthropathy
Code first underlying disease, such as:
- factor IX deficiency (D67)
- factor VIII deficiency (D66)
- hemophilia (classical) (D66)
- hemophilia B (D67)
- hemophilia C (D68.1)
- with vascular defect (D68.0-)

M36.3 Arthropathy in other blood disorders
▶Code first underlying disease, such as:◀
- ▶disease of blood and blood-forming organs, unspecified (D75.9)◀
- ▶other hemoglobinopathies (D58.2)◀
- ▶thalassemia (D56.-)◀

M36.4 Arthropathy in hypersensitivity reactions classified elsewhere
Code first underlying disease, such as:
- Henoch (-Schonlein) purpura (D69.0)
- serum sickness (T80.6-)

M36.8 Systemic disorders of connective tissue in other diseases classified elsewhere   Rx ESR COM
Code first underlying disease, such as:
- alkaptonuria (E70.29)
- hypogammaglobulinemia (D80.-)
- ochronosis (E70.29)

DORSOPATHIES (M40-M54)

Deforming dorsopathies (M40-M43)

✓4th M40 Kyphosis and lordosis
Code first underlying disease
EXCLUDES 1 congenital kyphosis and lordosis (Q76.4)
kyphoscoliosis (M41.-)
postprocedural kyphosis and lordosis (M96.-)

Kyphosis and Lordosis

Kyphosis: Excessive convexity in the thoracic region

Lordosis: Excessive concavity in the lumbar region

✓5th M40.0 Postural kyphosis
EXCLUDES 1 osteochondrosis of spine (M42.-)
- M40.00 Postural kyphosis, site unspecified
- M40.03 Postural kyphosis, cervicothoracic region
- M40.04 Postural kyphosis, thoracic region
- M40.05 Postural kyphosis, thoracolumbar region

✓5th M40.1 Other secondary kyphosis
- M40.10 Other secondary kyphosis, site unspecified UPD
- M40.12 Other secondary kyphosis, cervical region UPD
- M40.13 Other secondary kyphosis, cervicothoracic region UPD
- M40.14 Other secondary kyphosis, thoracic region UPD
- M40.15 Other secondary kyphosis, thoracolumbar region UPD

✓5th M40.2 Other and unspecified kyphosis
✓6th M40.20 Unspecified kyphosis
- M40.202 Unspecified kyphosis, cervical region
- M40.203 Unspecified kyphosis, cervicothoracic region
- M40.204 Unspecified kyphosis, thoracic region
- M40.205 Unspecified kyphosis, thoracolumbar region
- M40.209 Unspecified kyphosis, site unspecified

✓6th M40.29 Other kyphosis
- M40.292 Other kyphosis, cervical region
- M40.293 Other kyphosis, cervicothoracic region
- M40.294 Other kyphosis, thoracic region
- M40.295 Other kyphosis, thoracolumbar region
- M40.299 Other kyphosis, site unspecified

✓5th M40.3 Flatback syndrome
- M40.30 Flatback syndrome, site unspecified
- M40.35 Flatback syndrome, thoracolumbar region
- M40.36 Flatback syndrome, lumbar region
- M40.37 Flatback syndrome, lumbosacral region

✓5th M40.4 Postural lordosis
Acquired lordosis
- M40.40 Postural lordosis, site unspecified
- M40.45 Postural lordosis, thoracolumbar region
- M40.46 Postural lordosis, lumbar region
- M40.47 Postural lordosis, lumbosacral region

✓5th M40.5 Lordosis, unspecified
- M40.50 Lordosis, unspecified, site unspecified
- M40.55 Lordosis, unspecified, thoracolumbar region
- M40.56 Lordosis, unspecified, lumbar region
- M40.57 Lordosis, unspecified, lumbosacral region

✓4th M41 Scoliosis
INCLUDES kyphoscoliosis
EXCLUDES 1 congenital scoliosis due to bony malformation (Q76.3)
congenital scoliosis NOS (Q67.5)
kyphoscoliotic heart disease (I27.1)
postural congenital scoliosis (Q67.5)
EXCLUDES 2 postprocedural scoliosis (M96.89)
postradiation scoliosis (M96.5)
AHA: 2022,1Q,30

Scoliosis

Lateral curvature of spine

✓5th M41.0 Infantile idiopathic scoliosis
AHA: 2014,4Q,26
- M41.00 Infantile idiopathic scoliosis, site unspecified
- M41.02 Infantile idiopathic scoliosis, cervical region
- M41.03 Infantile idiopathic scoliosis, cervicothoracic region
- M41.04 Infantile idiopathic scoliosis, thoracic region
- M41.05 Infantile idiopathic scoliosis, thoracolumbar region
- M41.06 Infantile idiopathic scoliosis, lumbar region
- M41.07 Infantile idiopathic scoliosis, lumbosacral region
- M41.08 Infantile idiopathic scoliosis, sacral and sacrococcygeal region

✓5th M41.1 Juvenile and adolescent idiopathic scoliosis
✓6th M41.11 Juvenile idiopathic scoliosis
AHA: 2014,4Q,28
- M41.112 Juvenile idiopathic scoliosis, cervical region
- M41.113 Juvenile idiopathic scoliosis, cervicothoracic region
- M41.114 Juvenile idiopathic scoliosis, thoracic region
- M41.115 Juvenile idiopathic scoliosis, thoracolumbar region
- M41.116 Juvenile idiopathic scoliosis, lumbar region

- **M41.117** Juvenile idiopathic scoliosis, lumbosacral region
- **M41.119** Juvenile idiopathic scoliosis, site unspecified

√6th **M41.12** Adolescent idiopathic scoliosis
  AHA: 2024,1Q,23
- **M41.122** Adolescent idiopathic scoliosis, cervical region
- **M41.123** Adolescent idiopathic scoliosis, cervicothoracic region
- **M41.124** Adolescent idiopathic scoliosis, thoracic region
  AHA: 2024,3Q,13
- **M41.125** Adolescent idiopathic scoliosis, thoracolumbar region
- **M41.126** Adolescent idiopathic scoliosis, lumbar region
- **M41.127** Adolescent idiopathic scoliosis, lumbosacral region
- **M41.129** Adolescent idiopathic scoliosis, site unspecified

√5th **M41.2** Other idiopathic scoliosis
- **M41.20** Other idiopathic scoliosis, site unspecified
- **M41.22** Other idiopathic scoliosis, cervical region
- **M41.23** Other idiopathic scoliosis, cervicothoracic region
- **M41.24** Other idiopathic scoliosis, thoracic region
- **M41.25** Other idiopathic scoliosis, thoracolumbar region
- **M41.26** Other idiopathic scoliosis, lumbar region
- **M41.27** Other idiopathic scoliosis, lumbosacral region

√5th **M41.3** Thoracogenic scoliosis
- **M41.30** Thoracogenic scoliosis, site unspecified
- **M41.34** Thoracogenic scoliosis, thoracic region
- **M41.35** Thoracogenic scoliosis, thoracolumbar region

√5th **M41.4** Neuromuscular scoliosis
  Scoliosis secondary to cerebral palsy, Friedreich's ataxia, poliomyelitis and other neuromuscular disorders
  Code also underlying condition
  AHA: 2014,4Q,27
- **M41.40** Neuromuscular scoliosis, site unspecified
- **M41.41** Neuromuscular scoliosis, occipito-atlanto-axial region
- **M41.42** Neuromuscular scoliosis, cervical region
- **M41.43** Neuromuscular scoliosis, cervicothoracic region
- **M41.44** Neuromuscular scoliosis, thoracic region
- **M41.45** Neuromuscular scoliosis, thoracolumbar region
- **M41.46** Neuromuscular scoliosis, lumbar region
- **M41.47** Neuromuscular scoliosis, lumbosacral region

√5th **M41.5** Other secondary scoliosis
  Code first underlying disease
  AHA: 2019,1Q,19
- **M41.50** Other secondary scoliosis, site unspecified UPD
- **M41.52** Other secondary scoliosis, cervical region UPD
- **M41.53** Other secondary scoliosis, cervicothoracic region UPD
- **M41.54** Other secondary scoliosis, thoracic region UPD
- **M41.55** Other secondary scoliosis, thoracolumbar region UPD
- **M41.56** Other secondary scoliosis, lumbar region UPD
- **M41.57** Other secondary scoliosis, lumbosacral region UPD

√5th **M41.8** Other forms of scoliosis
  AHA: 2022,1Q,30
- **M41.80** Other forms of scoliosis, site unspecified
- **M41.82** Other forms of scoliosis, cervical region
- **M41.83** Other forms of scoliosis, cervicothoracic region
- **M41.84** Other forms of scoliosis, thoracic region
- **M41.85** Other forms of scoliosis, thoracolumbar region
- **M41.86** Other forms of scoliosis, lumbar region
- **M41.87** Other forms of scoliosis, lumbosacral region

M41.9 Scoliosis, unspecified
  AHA: 2022,1Q,30

√4th **M42** Spinal osteochondrosis

√5th **M42.0** Juvenile osteochondrosis of spine
  Calve's disease
  Scheuermann's disease
  EXCLUDES 1 postural kyphosis (M40.0)
- **M42.00** Juvenile osteochondrosis of spine, site unspecified COM
- **M42.01** Juvenile osteochondrosis of spine, occipito-atlanto-axial region COM
- **M42.02** Juvenile osteochondrosis of spine, cervical region COM
- **M42.03** Juvenile osteochondrosis of spine, cervicothoracic region COM
- **M42.04** Juvenile osteochondrosis of spine, thoracic region COM
- **M42.05** Juvenile osteochondrosis of spine, thoracolumbar region COM
- **M42.06** Juvenile osteochondrosis of spine, lumbar region COM
- **M42.07** Juvenile osteochondrosis of spine, lumbosacral region COM
- **M42.08** Juvenile osteochondrosis of spine, sacral and sacrococcygeal region COM
- **M42.09** Juvenile osteochondrosis of spine, multiple sites in spine COM

√5th **M42.1** Adult osteochondrosis of spine
- **M42.10** Adult osteochondrosis of spine, site unspecified A
- **M42.11** Adult osteochondrosis of spine, occipito-atlanto-axial region A
- **M42.12** Adult osteochondrosis of spine, cervical region A
- **M42.13** Adult osteochondrosis of spine, cervicothoracic region A
- **M42.14** Adult osteochondrosis of spine, thoracic region A
- **M42.15** Adult osteochondrosis of spine, thoracolumbar region A
- **M42.16** Adult osteochondrosis of spine, lumbar region A
- **M42.17** Adult osteochondrosis of spine, lumbosacral region A
- **M42.18** Adult osteochondrosis of spine, sacral and sacrococcygeal region A
- **M42.19** Adult osteochondrosis of spine, multiple sites in spine A

M42.9 Spinal osteochondrosis, unspecified

√4th **M43** Other deforming dorsopathies
  EXCLUDES 1 congenital spondylolysis and spondylolisthesis (Q76.2)
  hemivertebra (Q76.3-Q76.4)
  Klippel-Feil syndrome (Q76.1)
  lumbarization and sacralization (Q76.4)
  platyspondylisis (Q76.4)
  spina bifida occulta (Q76.0)
  spinal curvature in osteoporosis (M80.-)
  spinal curvature in Paget's disease of bone [osteitis deformans] (M88.-)

√5th **M43.0** Spondylolysis
  EXCLUDES 1 congenital spondylolysis (Q76.2)
  spondylolisthesis (M43.1)
  AHA: 2023,3Q,20
- **M43.00** Spondylolysis, site unspecified
- **M43.01** Spondylolysis, occipito-atlanto-axial region
- **M43.02** Spondylolysis, cervical region
- **M43.03** Spondylolysis, cervicothoracic region
- **M43.04** Spondylolysis, thoracic region
- **M43.05** Spondylolysis, thoracolumbar region
- **M43.06** Spondylolysis, lumbar region
- **M43.07** Spondylolysis, lumbosacral region
- **M43.08** Spondylolysis, sacral and sacrococcygeal region
- **M43.09** Spondylolysis, multiple sites in spine

√5th **M43.1** Spondylolisthesis
  EXCLUDES 1 acute traumatic of lumbosacral region (S33.1)
  acute traumatic of sites other than lumbosacral - code to Fracture, vertebra, by region
  congenital spondylolisthesis (Q76.2)
  AHA: 2023,3Q,20; 2020,2Q,21; 2018,3Q,18
  DEF: anterolisthesis: Forward displacement of one vertebra slipping over another. This condition can cause compression of the nerve roots exiting the spine.
  DEF: retrolisthesis: Backward displacement of one vertebra slipping over another. This condition can cause compression of the nerve roots exiting the spine.
  TIP: Code also any associated radiculopathy (M54.1-) and/or myelopathy (G99.2).
- **M43.10** Spondylolisthesis, site unspecified
- **M43.11** Spondylolisthesis, occipito-atlanto-axial region
- **M43.12** Spondylolisthesis, cervical region

Chapter 13. Diseases of the Musculoskeletal System and Connective Tissue

- M43.13 Spondylolisthesis, cervicothoracic region
- M43.14 Spondylolisthesis, thoracic region
- M43.15 Spondylolisthesis, thoracolumbar region
- M43.16 Spondylolisthesis, lumbar region
  AHA: 2024,1Q,17
- M43.17 Spondylolisthesis, lumbosacral region
- M43.18 Spondylolisthesis, sacral and sacrococcygeal region
- M43.19 Spondylolisthesis, multiple sites in spine

M43.2 Fusion of spine
Ankylosis of spinal joint
  EXCLUDES 1 ankylosing spondylitis (M45.0-)
  congenital fusion of spine (Q76.4)
  EXCLUDES 2 arthrodesis status (Z98.1)
  pseudoarthrosis after fusion or arthrodesis (M96.0)

- M43.20 Fusion of spine, site unspecified
- M43.21 Fusion of spine, occipito-atlanto-axial region
- M43.22 Fusion of spine, cervical region
- M43.23 Fusion of spine, cervicothoracic region
- M43.24 Fusion of spine, thoracic region
- M43.25 Fusion of spine, thoracolumbar region
- M43.26 Fusion of spine, lumbar region
- M43.27 Fusion of spine, lumbosacral region
- M43.28 Fusion of spine, sacral and sacrococcygeal region

- M43.3 Recurrent atlantoaxial dislocation with myelopathy
- M43.4 Other recurrent atlantoaxial dislocation

M43.5 Other recurrent vertebral dislocation
  EXCLUDES 1 biomechanical lesions NEC (M99.-)

- M43.5X Other recurrent vertebral dislocation
  - M43.5X2 Other recurrent vertebral dislocation, cervical region
  - M43.5X3 Other recurrent vertebral dislocation, cervicothoracic region
  - M43.5X4 Other recurrent vertebral dislocation, thoracic region
  - M43.5X5 Other recurrent vertebral dislocation, thoracolumbar region
  - M43.5X6 Other recurrent vertebral dislocation, lumbar region
  - M43.5X7 Other recurrent vertebral dislocation, lumbosacral region
  - M43.5X8 Other recurrent vertebral dislocation, sacral and sacrococcygeal region
  - M43.5X9 Other recurrent vertebral dislocation, site unspecified

M43.6 Torticollis
  EXCLUDES 1 congenital (sternomastoid) torticollis (Q68.0)
  current injury - see Injury, of spine, by body region
  ocular torticollis (R29.891)
  psychogenic torticollis (F45.8)
  spasmodic torticollis (G24.3)
  torticollis due to birth injury (P15.2)
  DEF: Twisted, unnatural position of the neck due to contracted cervical muscles that pull the head to one side.

M43.8 Other specified deforming dorsopathies
  EXCLUDES 2 kyphosis and lordosis (M40.-)
  scoliosis (M41.-)

- M43.8X Other specified deforming dorsopathies
  - M43.8X1 Other specified deforming dorsopathies, occipito-atlanto-axial region
  - M43.8X2 Other specified deforming dorsopathies, cervical region
  - M43.8X3 Other specified deforming dorsopathies, cervicothoracic region
  - M43.8X4 Other specified deforming dorsopathies, thoracic region
  - M43.8X5 Other specified deforming dorsopathies, thoracolumbar region
  - M43.8X6 Other specified deforming dorsopathies, lumbar region
  - M43.8X7 Other specified deforming dorsopathies, lumbosacral region
  - M43.8X8 Other specified deforming dorsopathies, sacral and sacrococcygeal region
  - M43.8X9 Other specified deforming dorsopathies, site unspecified

- M43.9 Deforming dorsopathy, unspecified
  Curvature of spine NOS

Spondylopathies (M45-M49)

M45 Ankylosing spondylitis
Rheumatoid arthritis of spine
  EXCLUDES 1 arthropathy in Reiter's disease (M02.3-)
  juvenile (ankylosing) spondylitis (M08.1)
  EXCLUDES 2 Behcet's disease (M35.2)

- M45.0 Ankylosing spondylitis of multiple sites in spine
- M45.1 Ankylosing spondylitis of occipito-atlanto-axial region
- M45.2 Ankylosing spondylitis of cervical region
- M45.3 Ankylosing spondylitis of cervicothoracic region
- M45.4 Ankylosing spondylitis of thoracic region
- M45.5 Ankylosing spondylitis of thoracolumbar region
- M45.6 Ankylosing spondylitis lumbar region
- M45.7 Ankylosing spondylitis of lumbosacral region
- M45.8 Ankylosing spondylitis sacral and sacrococcygeal region
- M45.9 Ankylosing spondylitis of unspecified sites in spine

M45.A Non-radiographic axial spondyloarthritis
  AHA: 2021,4Q,21-22
- M45.A0 Non-radiographic axial spondyloarthritis of unspecified sites in spine
- M45.A1 Non-radiographic axial spondyloarthritis of occipito-atlanto-axial region
- M45.A2 Non-radiographic axial spondyloarthritis of cervical region
- M45.A3 Non-radiographic axial spondyloarthritis of cervicothoracic region
- M45.A4 Non-radiographic axial spondyloarthritis of thoracic region
- M45.A5 Non-radiographic axial spondyloarthritis of thoracolumbar region
- M45.A6 Non-radiographic axial spondyloarthritis of lumbar region
- M45.A7 Non-radiographic axial spondyloarthritis of lumbosacral region
- M45.A8 Non-radiographic axial spondyloarthritis of sacral and sacrococcygeal region
- M45.AB Non-radiographic axial spondyloarthritis of multiple sites in spine

M46 Other inflammatory spondylopathies

M46.0 Spinal enthesopathy
Disorder of ligamentous or muscular attachments of spine
- M46.00 Spinal enthesopathy, site unspecified
- M46.01 Spinal enthesopathy, occipito-atlanto-axial region
- M46.02 Spinal enthesopathy, cervical region
- M46.03 Spinal enthesopathy, cervicothoracic region
- M46.04 Spinal enthesopathy, thoracic region
- M46.05 Spinal enthesopathy, thoracolumbar region
- M46.06 Spinal enthesopathy, lumbar region
- M46.07 Spinal enthesopathy, lumbosacral region
- M46.08 Spinal enthesopathy, sacral and sacrococcygeal region
- M46.09 Spinal enthesopathy, multiple sites in spine

- M46.1 Sacroiliitis, not elsewhere classified
  AHA: 2020,2Q,14
  DEF: Inflammation of the sacroiliac joint (situated at the juncture of the sacrum and hip). Symptoms include pain in the buttocks or lower back that can extend down one or both legs.

M46.2 Osteomyelitis of vertebra
- M46.20 Osteomyelitis of vertebra, site unspecified
- M46.21 Osteomyelitis of vertebra, occipito-atlanto-axial region
- M46.22 Osteomyelitis of vertebra, cervical region
- M46.23 Osteomyelitis of vertebra, cervicothoracic region

Chapter 13. Diseases of the Musculoskeletal System and Connective Tissue

- **M46.24** Osteomyelitis of vertebra, thoracic region [HCC] [ESR] [COM]
- **M46.25** Osteomyelitis of vertebra, thoracolumbar region [HCC] [ESR] [COM]
- **M46.26** Osteomyelitis of vertebra, lumbar region [HCC] [ESR] [COM]
- **M46.27** Osteomyelitis of vertebra, lumbosacral region [HCC] [ESR] [COM]
- **M46.28** Osteomyelitis of vertebra, sacral and sacrococcygeal region [HCC] [ESR] [COM]

✓5th M46.3 Infection of intervertebral disc (pyogenic)
Use additional code (B95-B97) to identify infectious agent
- **M46.30** Infection of intervertebral disc (pyogenic), site unspecified [HCC] [ESR] [COM]
- **M46.31** Infection of intervertebral disc (pyogenic), occipito-atlanto-axial region [HCC] [ESR] [COM]
- **M46.32** Infection of intervertebral disc (pyogenic), cervical region [HCC] [ESR] [COM]
- **M46.33** Infection of intervertebral disc (pyogenic), cervicothoracic region [HCC] [ESR] [COM]
- **M46.34** Infection of intervertebral disc (pyogenic), thoracic region [HCC] [ESR] [COM]
- **M46.35** Infection of intervertebral disc (pyogenic), thoracolumbar region [HCC] [ESR] [COM]
- **M46.36** Infection of intervertebral disc (pyogenic), lumbar region [HCC] [ESR] [COM]
- **M46.37** Infection of intervertebral disc (pyogenic), lumbosacral region [HCC] [ESR] [COM]
- **M46.38** Infection of intervertebral disc (pyogenic), sacral and sacrococcygeal region [HCC] [ESR] [COM]
- **M46.39** Infection of intervertebral disc (pyogenic), multiple sites in spine [HCC] [ESR] [COM]

✓5th M46.4 Discitis, unspecified
- **M46.40** Discitis, unspecified, site unspecified
- **M46.41** Discitis, unspecified, occipito-atlanto-axial region
- **M46.42** Discitis, unspecified, cervical region
- **M46.43** Discitis, unspecified, cervicothoracic region
- **M46.44** Discitis, unspecified, thoracic region
- **M46.45** Discitis, unspecified, thoracolumbar region
- **M46.46** Discitis, unspecified, lumbar region
- **M46.47** Discitis, unspecified, lumbosacral region
- **M46.48** Discitis, unspecified, sacral and sacrococcygeal region
- **M46.49** Discitis, unspecified, multiple sites in spine

✓5th M46.5 Other infective spondylopathies
- **M46.50** Other infective spondylopathies, site unspecified [ESR]
- **M46.51** Other infective spondylopathies, occipito-atlanto-axial region [ESR]
- **M46.52** Other infective spondylopathies, cervical region [ESR]
- **M46.53** Other infective spondylopathies, cervicothoracic region [ESR]
- **M46.54** Other infective spondylopathies, thoracic region [ESR]
- **M46.55** Other infective spondylopathies, thoracolumbar region [ESR]
- **M46.56** Other infective spondylopathies, lumbar region [ESR]
- **M46.57** Other infective spondylopathies, lumbosacral region [ESR]
- **M46.58** Other infective spondylopathies, sacral and sacrococcygeal region [ESR]
- **M46.59** Other infective spondylopathies, multiple sites in spine [ESR]

✓5th M46.8 Other specified inflammatory spondylopathies
- **M46.80** Other specified inflammatory spondylopathies, site unspecified [ESR]
- **M46.81** Other specified inflammatory spondylopathies, occipito-atlanto-axial region [ESR]
- **M46.82** Other specified inflammatory spondylopathies, cervical region [ESR]
- **M46.83** Other specified inflammatory spondylopathies, cervicothoracic region [ESR]
- **M46.84** Other specified inflammatory spondylopathies, thoracic region [ESR]
- **M46.85** Other specified inflammatory spondylopathies, thoracolumbar region [ESR]
- **M46.86** Other specified inflammatory spondylopathies, lumbar region [ESR]
- **M46.87** Other specified inflammatory spondylopathies, lumbosacral region [ESR]
- **M46.88** Other specified inflammatory spondylopathies, sacral and sacrococcygeal region [ESR]
- **M46.89** Other specified inflammatory spondylopathies, multiple sites in spine

✓5th M46.9 Unspecified inflammatory spondylopathy
- **M46.90** Unspecified inflammatory spondylopathy, site unspecified [ESR]
- **M46.91** Unspecified inflammatory spondylopathy, occipito-atlanto-axial region [ESR]
- **M46.92** Unspecified inflammatory spondylopathy, cervical region [ESR]
  AHA: 2019,3Q,10
- **M46.93** Unspecified inflammatory spondylopathy, cervicothoracic region [ESR]
- **M46.94** Unspecified inflammatory spondylopathy, thoracic region [ESR]
- **M46.95** Unspecified inflammatory spondylopathy, thoracolumbar region [ESR]
- **M46.96** Unspecified inflammatory spondylopathy, lumbar region [ESR]
- **M46.97** Unspecified inflammatory spondylopathy, lumbosacral region [ESR]
- **M46.98** Unspecified inflammatory spondylopathy, sacral and sacrococcygeal region [ESR]
- **M46.99** Unspecified inflammatory spondylopathy, multiple sites in spine [ESR]

✓4th M47 Spondylosis
INCLUDES arthrosis or osteoarthritis of spine
degeneration of facet joints
AHA: 2020,1Q,17; 2019,3Q,10-11; 2016,4Q,147

✓5th M47.0 Anterior spinal and vertebral artery compression syndromes
✓6th M47.01 Anterior spinal artery compression syndromes
- **M47.011** Anterior spinal artery compression syndromes, occipito-atlanto-axial region
- **M47.012** Anterior spinal artery compression syndromes, cervical region
  AHA: 2023,1Q,37
- **M47.013** Anterior spinal artery compression syndromes, cervicothoracic region
- **M47.014** Anterior spinal artery compression syndromes, thoracic region
- **M47.015** Anterior spinal artery compression syndromes, thoracolumbar region
- **M47.016** Anterior spinal artery compression syndromes, lumbar region
- **M47.019** Anterior spinal artery compression syndromes, site unspecified

✓6th M47.02 Vertebral artery compression syndromes
- **M47.021** Vertebral artery compression syndromes, occipito-atlanto-axial region
- **M47.022** Vertebral artery compression syndromes, cervical region
  AHA: 2023,1Q,37
- **M47.029** Vertebral artery compression syndromes, site unspecified

✓5th M47.1 Other spondylosis with myelopathy
Spondylogenic compression of spinal cord
EXCLUDES 1 vertebral subluxation (M43.3-M43.5X9)
AHA: 2020,1Q,17
- **M47.10** Other spondylosis with myelopathy, site unspecified
- **M47.11** Other spondylosis with myelopathy, occipito-atlanto-axial region
- **M47.12** Other spondylosis with myelopathy, cervical region
- **M47.13** Other spondylosis with myelopathy, cervicothoracic region
- **M47.14** Other spondylosis with myelopathy, thoracic region
- **M47.15** Other spondylosis with myelopathy, thoracolumbar region
- **M47.16** Other spondylosis with myelopathy, lumbar region

✓5th M47.2 Other spondylosis with radiculopathy
AHA: 2020,1Q,17
- **M47.20** Other spondylosis with radiculopathy, site unspecified

- **M47.21** Other spondylosis with radiculopathy, occipito-atlanto-axial region
- **M47.22** Other spondylosis with radiculopathy, cervical region
- **M47.23** Other spondylosis with radiculopathy, cervicothoracic region
- **M47.24** Other spondylosis with radiculopathy, thoracic region
- **M47.25** Other spondylosis with radiculopathy, thoracolumbar region
- **M47.26** Other spondylosis with radiculopathy, lumbar region
- **M47.27** Other spondylosis with radiculopathy, lumbosacral region
- **M47.28** Other spondylosis with radiculopathy, sacral and sacrococcygeal region

✓5th **M47.8** Other spondylosis
  - ✓6th **M47.81** Spondylosis without myelopathy or radiculopathy
    - **AHA:** 2019,3Q,10-11; 2018,2Q,14
    - **M47.811** Spondylosis without myelopathy or radiculopathy, occipito-atlanto-axial region
    - **M47.812** Spondylosis without myelopathy or radiculopathy, cervical region
    - **M47.813** Spondylosis without myelopathy or radiculopathy, cervicothoracic region
    - **M47.814** Spondylosis without myelopathy or radiculopathy, thoracic region
    - **M47.815** Spondylosis without myelopathy or radiculopathy, thoracolumbar region
    - **M47.816** Spondylosis without myelopathy or radiculopathy, lumbar region
    - **M47.817** Spondylosis without myelopathy or radiculopathy, lumbosacral region
    - **M47.818** Spondylosis without myelopathy or radiculopathy, sacral and sacrococcygeal region
    - **M47.819** Spondylosis without myelopathy or radiculopathy, site unspecified
  - ✓6th **M47.89** Other spondylosis
    - **M47.891** Other spondylosis, occipito-atlanto-axial region
    - **M47.892** Other spondylosis, cervical region
    - **M47.893** Other spondylosis, cervicothoracic region
    - **M47.894** Other spondylosis, thoracic region
    - **M47.895** Other spondylosis, thoracolumbar region
    - **M47.896** Other spondylosis, lumbar region
    - **M47.897** Other spondylosis, lumbosacral region
    - **M47.898** Other spondylosis, sacral and sacrococcygeal region
    - **M47.899** Other spondylosis, site unspecified
- **M47.9** Spondylosis, unspecified

✓4th **M48** Other spondylopathies
  - ✓5th **M48.0** Spinal stenosis
    - Caudal stenosis
    - **AHA:** 2020,1Q,17; 2018,3Q,18-19
    - **TIP:** Code also any associated radiculopathy (M54.1-) and/or myelopathy (G99.2).
    - **M48.00** Spinal stenosis, site unspecified
    - **M48.01** Spinal stenosis, occipito-atlanto-axial region
    - **M48.02** Spinal stenosis, cervical region
    - **M48.03** Spinal stenosis, cervicothoracic region
    - **M48.04** Spinal stenosis, thoracic region
    - **M48.05** Spinal stenosis, thoracolumbar region
    - ✓6th **M48.06** Spinal stenosis, lumbar region
      - **AHA:** 2018,3Q,19; 2017,4Q,18-19
      - **M48.061** Spinal stenosis, lumbar region without neurogenic claudication
        - Spinal stenosis, lumbar region NOS
      - **M48.062** Spinal stenosis, lumbar region with neurogenic claudication
    - **M48.07** Spinal stenosis, lumbosacral region
    - **M48.08** Spinal stenosis, sacral and sacrococcygeal region
  - ✓5th **M48.1** Ankylosing hyperostosis [Forestier]
    - Diffuse idiopathic skeletal hyperostosis [DISH]
    - **M48.10** Ankylosing hyperostosis [Forestier], site unspecified
    - **M48.11** Ankylosing hyperostosis [Forestier], occipito-atlanto-axial region
    - **M48.12** Ankylosing hyperostosis [Forestier], cervical region
    - **M48.13** Ankylosing hyperostosis [Forestier], cervicothoracic region
    - **M48.14** Ankylosing hyperostosis [Forestier], thoracic region
    - **M48.15** Ankylosing hyperostosis [Forestier], thoracolumbar region
    - **M48.16** Ankylosing hyperostosis [Forestier], lumbar region
    - **M48.17** Ankylosing hyperostosis [Forestier], lumbosacral region
    - **M48.18** Ankylosing hyperostosis [Forestier], sacral and sacrococcygeal region
    - **M48.19** Ankylosing hyperostosis [Forestier], multiple sites in spine
  - ✓5th **M48.2** Kissing spine
    - **M48.20** Kissing spine, site unspecified
    - **M48.21** Kissing spine, occipito-atlanto-axial region
    - **M48.22** Kissing spine, cervical region
    - **M48.23** Kissing spine, cervicothoracic region
    - **M48.24** Kissing spine, thoracic region
    - **M48.25** Kissing spine, thoracolumbar region
    - **M48.26** Kissing spine, lumbar region
    - **M48.27** Kissing spine, lumbosacral region
  - ✓5th **M48.3** Traumatic spondylopathy
    - **M48.30** Traumatic spondylopathy, site unspecified
    - **M48.31** Traumatic spondylopathy, occipito-atlanto-axial region
    - **M48.32** Traumatic spondylopathy, cervical region
    - **M48.33** Traumatic spondylopathy, cervicothoracic region
    - **M48.34** Traumatic spondylopathy, thoracic region
    - **M48.35** Traumatic spondylopathy, thoracolumbar region
    - **M48.36** Traumatic spondylopathy, lumbar region
    - **M48.37** Traumatic spondylopathy, lumbosacral region
    - **M48.38** Traumatic spondylopathy, sacral and sacrococcygeal region
  - ✓5th **M48.4** Fatigue fracture of vertebra
    - Stress fracture of vertebra
    - **EXCLUDES 1** pathological fracture NOS (M84.4-)
      pathological fracture of vertebra due to neoplasm (M84.58)
      pathological fracture of vertebra due to osteoporosis (M80.-)
      pathological fracture of vertebra due to other diagnosis (M84.68)
      traumatic fracture of vertebrae (S12.0-S12.3-, S22.0-, S32.0-)

    The appropriate 7th character is to be added to each code from subcategory M48.4.
    - A initial encounter for fracture
    - D subsequent encounter for fracture with routine healing
    - G subsequent encounter for fracture with delayed healing
    - S sequela of fracture

    - ✓x7th **M48.40** Fatigue fracture of vertebra, site unspecified
    - ✓x7th **M48.41** Fatigue fracture of vertebra, occipito-atlanto-axial region
    - ✓x7th **M48.42** Fatigue fracture of vertebra, cervical region
    - ✓x7th **M48.43** Fatigue fracture of vertebra, cervicothoracic region
    - ✓x7th **M48.44** Fatigue fracture of vertebra, thoracic region
    - ✓x7th **M48.45** Fatigue fracture of vertebra, thoracolumbar region
    - ✓x7th **M48.46** Fatigue fracture of vertebra, lumbar region
    - ✓x7th **M48.47** Fatigue fracture of vertebra, lumbosacral region
    - ✓x7th **M48.48** Fatigue fracture of vertebra, sacral and sacrococcygeal region

M48.5 Collapsed vertebra, not elsewhere classified
Collapsed vertebra NOS
Compression fracture of vertebra NOS
Wedging of vertebra NOS
EXCLUDES 1
current injury - see Injury of spine, by body region
fatigue fracture of vertebra (M48.4)
pathological fracture NOS (M84.4-)
pathological fracture of vertebra due to neoplasm (M84.58)
pathological fracture of vertebra due to osteoporosis (M80.-)
pathological fracture of vertebra due to other diagnosis (M84.68)
stress fracture of vertebra (M48.4-)
traumatic fracture of vertebra (S12.-, S22.-, S32.-)

> The appropriate 7th character is to be added to each code from subcategory M48.5.
> A   initial encounter for fracture
> D   subsequent encounter for fracture with routine healing
> G   subsequent encounter for fracture with delayed healing
> S   sequela of fracture

- M48.50 Collapsed vertebra, not elsewhere classified, site unspecified
- M48.51 Collapsed vertebra, not elsewhere classified, occipito-atlanto-axial region
- M48.52 Collapsed vertebra, not elsewhere classified, cervical region
- M48.53 Collapsed vertebra, not elsewhere classified, cervicothoracic region
- M48.54 Collapsed vertebra, not elsewhere classified, thoracic region
- M48.55 Collapsed vertebra, not elsewhere classified, thoracolumbar region
- M48.56 Collapsed vertebra, not elsewhere classified, lumbar region
- M48.57 Collapsed vertebra, not elsewhere classified, lumbosacral region
- M48.58 Collapsed vertebra, not elsewhere classified, sacral and sacrococcygeal region

M48.8 Other specified spondylopathies
Ossification of posterior longitudinal ligament

M48.8X Other specified spondylopathies
- M48.8X1 Other specified spondylopathies, occipito-atlanto-axial region
- M48.8X2 Other specified spondylopathies, cervical region
- M48.8X3 Other specified spondylopathies, cervicothoracic region
- M48.8X4 Other specified spondylopathies, thoracic region
- M48.8X5 Other specified spondylopathies, thoracolumbar region
- M48.8X6 Other specified spondylopathies, lumbar region
- M48.8X7 Other specified spondylopathies, lumbosacral region
- M48.8X8 Other specified spondylopathies, sacral and sacrococcygeal region
- M48.8X9 Other specified spondylopathies, site unspecified

M48.9 Spondylopathy, unspecified

M49 Spondylopathies in diseases classified elsewhere
INCLUDES
curvature of spine in diseases classified elsewhere
deformity of spine in diseases classified elsewhere
kyphosis in diseases classified elsewhere
scoliosis in diseases classified elsewhere
spondylopathy in diseases classified elsewhere

Code first underlying disease, such as:
brucellosis (A23.-)
Charcôt-Marie-Tooth disease (G60.0)
enterobacterial infections (A01-A04)
osteitis fibrosa cystica (E21.0)

EXCLUDES 1
curvature of spine in tuberculosis [Pott's] (A18.01)
enteropathic arthropathies (M07.-)
gonococcal spondylitis (A54.41)
neuropathic [tabes dorsalis] spondylitis (A52.11)
neuropathic spondylopathy in syringomyelia (G95.0)
neuropathic spondylopathy in tabes dorsalis (A52.11)
nonsyphilitic neuropathic spondylopathy NEC (G98.0)
spondylitis in syphilis (acquired) (A52.77)
tuberculous spondylitis (A18.01)
typhoid fever spondylitis (A01.05)

M49.8 Spondylopathy in diseases classified elsewhere
- M49.80 Spondylopathy in diseases classified elsewhere, site unspecified
- M49.81 Spondylopathy in diseases classified elsewhere, occipito-atlanto-axial region
- M49.82 Spondylopathy in diseases classified elsewhere, cervical region
- M49.83 Spondylopathy in diseases classified elsewhere, cervicothoracic region
- M49.84 Spondylopathy in diseases classified elsewhere, thoracic region
- M49.85 Spondylopathy in diseases classified elsewhere, thoracolumbar region
- M49.86 Spondylopathy in diseases classified elsewhere, lumbar region
- M49.87 Spondylopathy in diseases classified elsewhere, lumbosacral region
- M49.88 Spondylopathy in diseases classified elsewhere, sacral and sacrococcygeal region
- M49.89 Spondylopathy in diseases classified elsewhere, multiple sites in spine

Other dorsopathies (M50-M54)

EXCLUDES 1
current injury - see injury of spine by body region
discitis NOS (M46.4-)

M50 Cervical disc disorders
INCLUDES
cervicothoracic disc disorders
cervicothoracic disc disorders with cervicalgia
AHA: 2016,4Q,39-40; 2016,1Q,17

M50.0 Cervical disc disorder with myelopathy
AHA: 2018,3Q,19
- M50.00 Cervical disc disorder with myelopathy, unspecified cervical region
- M50.01 Cervical disc disorder with myelopathy, high cervical region
  C2-C3 disc disorder with myelopathy
  C3-C4 disc disorder with myelopathy
- M50.02 Cervical disc disorder with myelopathy, mid-cervical region
  - M50.020 Cervical disc disorder with myelopathy, mid-cervical region, unspecified level
  - M50.021 Cervical disc disorder at C4-C5 level with myelopathy
    C4-C5 disc disorder with myelopathy
  - M50.022 Cervical disc disorder at C5-C6 level with myelopathy
    C5-C6 disc disorder with myelopathy
  - M50.023 Cervical disc disorder at C6-C7 level with myelopathy
    C6-C7 disc disorder with myelopathy
- M50.03 Cervical disc disorder with myelopathy, cervicothoracic region
  C7-T1 disc disorder with myelopathy

M50.1 Cervical disc disorder with radiculopathy
EXCLUDES 2 brachial radiculitis NOS (M54.13)
AHA: 2018,3Q,19
- M50.10 Cervical disc disorder with radiculopathy, unspecified cervical region

Chapter 13. Diseases of the Musculoskeletal System and Connective Tissue

- **M50.11** Cervical disc disorder with radiculopathy, **high cervical** region
  - C2-C3 disc disorder with radiculopathy
  - C3 radiculopathy due to disc disorder
  - C3-C4 disc disorder with radiculopathy
  - C4 radiculopathy due to disc disorder
- ✓6th **M50.12** Cervical disc disorder with radiculopathy, **mid-cervical** region
  - **M50.120** Mid-cervical disc disorder, unspecified level
  - **M50.121** Cervical disc disorder at **C4-C5 level** with radiculopathy
    - C4-C5 disc disorder with radiculopathy
    - C5 radiculopathy due to disc disorder
  - **M50.122** Cervical disc disorder at **C5-C6 level** with radiculopathy
    - C5-C6 disc disorder with radiculopathy
    - C6 radiculopathy due to disc disorder
  - **M50.123** Cervical disc disorder at **C6-C7 level** with radiculopathy
    - C6-C7 disc disorder with radiculopathy
    - C7 radiculopathy due to disc disorder
- **M50.13** Cervical disc disorder with radiculopathy, **cervicothoracic** region
  - C7-T1 disc disorder with radiculopathy
  - C8 radiculopathy due to disc disorder
- ✓5th **M50.2** Other cervical disc **displacement**
  - **M50.20** Other cervical disc displacement, unspecified cervical region
  - **M50.21** Other cervical disc displacement, **high cervical** region
    - Other C2-C3 cervical disc displacement
    - Other C3-C4 cervical disc displacement
  - ✓6th **M50.22** Other cervical disc displacement, **mid-cervical** region
    - **M50.220** Other cervical disc displacement, mid-cervical region, unspecified level
    - **M50.221** Other cervical disc displacement at **C4-C5 level**
      - Other C4-C5 cervical disc displacement
    - **M50.222** Other cervical disc displacement at **C5-C6 level**
      - Other C5-C6 cervical disc displacement
    - **M50.223** Other cervical disc displacement at **C6-C7 level**
      - Other C6-C7 cervical disc displacement
  - **M50.23** Other cervical disc displacement, **cervicothoracic** region
    - Other C7-T1 cervical disc displacement
- ✓5th **M50.3** Other cervical disc **degeneration**
  - **M50.30** Other cervical disc degeneration, unspecified cervical region
  - **M50.31** Other cervical disc degeneration, **high cervical** region
    - Other C2-C3 cervical disc degeneration
    - Other C3-C4 cervical disc degeneration
  - ✓6th **M50.32** Other cervical disc degeneration, **mid-cervical** region
    - **M50.320** Other cervical disc degeneration, mid-cervical region, unspecified level
    - **M50.321** Other cervical disc degeneration at **C4-C5 level**
      - Other C4-C5 cervical disc degeneration
    - **M50.322** Other cervical disc degeneration at **C5-C6 level**
      - Other C5-C6 cervical disc degeneration
    - **M50.323** Other cervical disc degeneration at **C6-C7 level**
      - Other C6-C7 cervical disc degeneration
  - **M50.33** Other cervical disc degeneration, **cervicothoracic** region
    - Other C7-T1 cervical disc degeneration
- ✓5th **M50.8** Other cervical disc disorders
  - **M50.80** Other cervical disc disorders, unspecified cervical region
  - **M50.81** Other cervical disc disorders, **high cervical** region
    - Other C2-C3 cervical disc disorders
    - Other C3-C4 cervical disc disorders
  - ✓6th **M50.82** Other cervical disc disorders, **mid-cervical** region
    - **M50.820** Other cervical disc disorders, mid-cervical region, unspecified level
    - **M50.821** Other cervical disc disorders at **C4-C5 level**
      - Other C4-C5 cervical disc disorders
    - **M50.822** Other cervical disc disorders at **C5-C6 level**
      - Other C5-C6 cervical disc disorders
    - **M50.823** Other cervical disc disorders at **C6-C7 level**
      - Other C6-C7 cervical disc disorders
  - **M50.83** Other cervical disc disorders, **cervicothoracic** region
    - Other C7-T1 cervical disc disorders
- ✓5th **M50.9** Cervical disc disorder, unspecified
  - **M50.90** Cervical disc disorder, unspecified, unspecified cervical region
  - **M50.91** Cervical disc disorder, unspecified, **high cervical** region
    - C2-C3 cervical disc disorder, unspecified
    - C3-C4 cervical disc disorder, unspecified
  - ✓6th **M50.92** Cervical disc disorder, unspecified, **mid-cervical** region
    - **M50.920** Unspecified cervical disc disorder, mid-cervical region, unspecified level
    - **M50.921** Unspecified cervical disc disorder at **C4-C5 level**
      - Unspecified C4-C5 cervical disc disorder
    - **M50.922** Unspecified cervical disc disorder at **C5-C6 level**
      - Unspecified C5-C6 cervical disc disorder
    - **M50.923** Unspecified cervical disc disorder at **C6-C7 level**
      - Unspecified C6-C7 cervical disc disorder
  - **M50.93** Cervical disc disorder, unspecified, **cervicothoracic** region
    - C7-T1 cervical disc disorder, unspecified

- ✓4th **M51** Thoracic, thoracolumbar, and lumbosacral intervertebral disc disorders
  - EXCLUDES 2 cervical and cervicothoracic disc disorders (M50.-)
  - sacral and sacrococcygeal disorders (M53.3)
  - ✓5th **M51.0** Thoracic, thoracolumbar and lumbosacral intervertebral disc disorders **with myelopathy**
    - **M51.04** Intervertebral disc disorders with myelopathy, **thoracic** region
    - **M51.05** Intervertebral disc disorders with myelopathy, **thoracolumbar** region
    - **M51.06** Intervertebral disc disorders with myelopathy, **lumbar** region
  - ✓5th **M51.1** Thoracic, thoracolumbar and lumbosacral intervertebral disc disorders **with radiculopathy**
    - Sciatica due to intervertebral disc disorder
    - EXCLUDES 1 lumbar radiculitis NOS (M54.16)
    - sciatica NOS (M54.3)
    - AHA: 2018,3Q,18
    - **M51.14** Intervertebral disc disorders with radiculopathy, **thoracic** region
    - **M51.15** Intervertebral disc disorders with radiculopathy, **thoracolumbar** region
    - **M51.16** Intervertebral disc disorders with radiculopathy, **lumbar** region
    - **M51.17** Intervertebral disc disorders with radiculopathy, **lumbosacral** region
  - ✓5th **M51.2** Other thoracic, thoracolumbar and lumbosacral intervertebral disc **displacement**
    - Lumbago due to displacement of intervertebral disc
    - AHA: 2022,1Q,26

Displacement Intervertebral Disc

Normal Top View — Nucleus pulposus, Lamina, Ligamentum flavum, Disc annulus

Herniated Top View — Nucleus pulposus, Herniates through annulus, Spinal cord, Spinal nerve

- **M51.24** Other intervertebral disc displacement, **thoracic** region
- **M51.25** Other intervertebral disc displacement, **thoracolumbar** region
- **M51.26** Other intervertebral disc displacement, **lumbar** region

 CMS-HCC Rx HCC 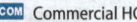 ESRD HCC 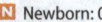 Commercial HCC 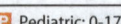 N Newborn: 0 • P Pediatric: 0-17 • M Maternity: 9-64 • A Adult: 15-124

Chapter 13. Diseases of the Musculoskeletal System and Connective Tissue

M51.27 Other intervertebral disc displacement, **lumbosacral** region

✓5th **M51.3 Other thoracic, thoracolumbar and lumbosacral intervertebral disc degeneration**
AHA: 2022,1Q,26; 2018,2Q,15; 2013,3Q,22

- M51.34 Other intervertebral disc degeneration, **thoracic** region
- M51.35 Other intervertebral disc degeneration, **thoracolumbar** region

✓6th M51.36 Other intervertebral disc degeneration, **lumbar** region
AHA: 2024,4Q,24

- M51.360 Other intervertebral disc degeneration, lumbar region **with discogenic back pain only**
  Other intervertebral disc degeneration, lumbar region with axial back pain only
- M51.361 Other intervertebral disc degeneration, lumbar region **with lower extremity pain only**
  Other intervertebral disc degeneration, lumbar region with leg pain only
  Other intervertebral disc degeneration, lumbar region with referred sclerotomal pain only
- M51.362 Other intervertebral disc degeneration, lumbar region **with discogenic back pain and lower extremity pain**
  Other intervertebral disc degeneration, lumbar region with axial back pain and referred sclerotomal pain
  Other intervertebral disc degeneration, lumbar region with discogenic back pain and leg pain
- M51.369 Other intervertebral disc degeneration, lumbar region **without mention of lumbar back pain or lower extremity pain**
  Other intervertebral disc degeneration, lumbar region without mention of lumbar back pain or leg pain
  Other intervertebral disc degeneration, lumbar region, NOS

✓6th M51.37 Other intervertebral disc degeneration, **lumbosacral** region
AHA: 2024,4Q,24

- M51.370 Other intervertebral disc degeneration, lumbosacral region **with discogenic back pain only**
  Other intervertebral disc degeneration, lumbosacral region with axial back pain only
- M51.371 Other intervertebral disc degeneration, lumbosacral region **with lower extremity pain only**
  Other intervertebral disc degeneration, lumbosacral region with leg pain only
  Other intervertebral disc degeneration, lumbosacral region with referred sclerotomal pain only
- M51.372 Other intervertebral disc degeneration, lumbosacral region **with discogenic back pain and lower extremity pain**
  Other intervertebral disc degeneration, lumbosacral region with axial back pain and referred sclerotomal pain
  Other intervertebral disc degeneration, lumbosacral region with discogenic back pain and leg pain
- M51.379 Other intervertebral disc degeneration, lumbosacral region **without mention of lumbar back pain or lower extremity pain**
  Other intervertebral disc degeneration, lumbosacral region without mention of lumbar back pain or leg pain
  Other intervertebral disc degeneration, lumbosacral region, NOS

✓5th **M51.4 Schmorl's nodes**
DEF: Irregular bone defect in the margin of the vertebral body that causes herniation into the end plate of the vertebral body.

- M51.44 Schmorl's nodes, **thoracic** region
- M51.45 Schmorl's nodes, **thoracolumbar** region
- M51.46 Schmorl's nodes, **lumbar** region
- M51.47 Schmorl's nodes, **lumbosacral** region

✓5th **M51.8 Other thoracic, thoracolumbar and lumbosacral intervertebral disc disorders**

- M51.84 Other intervertebral disc disorders, **thoracic** region
- M51.85 Other intervertebral disc disorders, **thoracolumbar** region
- M51.86 Other intervertebral disc disorders, **lumbar** region
- M51.87 Other intervertebral disc disorders, **lumbosacral** region

M51.9 Unspecified thoracic, thoracolumbar and lumbosacral intervertebral disc disorder

✓5th **M51.A Other lumbar and lumbosacral annulus fibrosus disc defects**
AHA: 2022,4Q,28-29

- M51.A0 Intervertebral annulus fibrosus defect, **lumbar** region, unspecified size
  Code first, if applicable, lumbar disc herniation (M51.06, M51.16, M51.26)
- M51.A1 Intervertebral annulus fibrosus defect, **small, lumbar** region
  Code first, if applicable, lumbar disc herniation (M51.06, M51.16, M51.26)
- M51.A2 Intervertebral annulus fibrosus defect, **large, lumbar** region
  Code first, if applicable, lumbar disc herniation (M51.06, M51.16, M51.26)
- M51.A3 Intervertebral annulus fibrosus defect, **lumbosacral** region, unspecified size
  Code first, if applicable, lumbosacral disc herniation (M51.17, M51.27)
- M51.A4 Intervertebral annulus fibrosus defect, **small, lumbosacral** region
  Code first, if applicable, lumbosacral disc herniation (M51.17, M51.27)
- M51.A5 Intervertebral annulus fibrosus defect, **large, lumbosacral** region
  Code first, if applicable, lumbosacral disc herniation (M51.17, M51.27)

✓4th **M53 Other and unspecified dorsopathies, not elsewhere classified**

M53.0 Cervicocranial syndrome
  Posterior cervical sympathetic syndrome

M53.1 Cervicobrachial syndrome
  EXCLUDES 2 cervical disc disorder (M50.-)
             thoracic outlet syndrome (G54.0)

✓5th M53.2 Spinal instabilities
  ✓6th M53.2X Spinal **instabilities**
  - M53.2X1 Spinal instabilities, **occipito-atlanto-axial** region
  - M53.2X2 Spinal instabilities, **cervical** region
  - M53.2X3 Spinal instabilities, **cervicothoracic** region
  - M53.2X4 Spinal instabilities, **thoracic** region
  - M53.2X5 Spinal instabilities, **thoracolumbar** region
  - M53.2X6 Spinal instabilities, **lumbar** region
  - M53.2X7 Spinal instabilities, **lumbosacral** region
  - M53.2X8 Spinal instabilities, **sacral and sacrococcygeal** region
  - M53.2X9 Spinal instabilities, site unspecified

M53.3 Sacrococcygeal disorders, not elsewhere classified
  Coccygodynia

✓5th **M53.8 Other specified dorsopathies**
- M53.80 Other specified dorsopathies, site unspecified
- M53.81 Other specified dorsopathies, **occipito-atlanto-axial** region
- M53.82 Other specified dorsopathies, **cervical** region
- M53.83 Other specified dorsopathies, **cervicothoracic** region
- M53.84 Other specified dorsopathies, **thoracic** region
- M53.85 Other specified dorsopathies, **thoracolumbar** region
- M53.86 Other specified dorsopathies, **lumbar** region
- M53.87 Other specified dorsopathies, **lumbosacral** region
- M53.88 Other specified dorsopathies, **sacral and sacrococcygeal** region

M53.9 Dorsopathy, unspecified

✓4th **M54 Dorsalgia**
  EXCLUDES 1 psychogenic dorsalgia (F45.41)

✓5th M54.0 Panniculitis affecting regions of neck and back
  EXCLUDES 1 lupus panniculitis (L93.2)
             panniculitis NOS (M79.3)
             relapsing [Weber-Christian] panniculitis (M35.6)

- M54.00 Panniculitis affecting regions of neck and back, site unspecified

M54.01	Panniculitis affecting regions of neck and back, **occipito-atlanto-axial** region
M54.02	Panniculitis affecting regions of neck and back, **cervical** region
M54.03	Panniculitis affecting regions of neck and back, **cervicothoracic** region
M54.04	Panniculitis affecting regions of neck and back, **thoracic** region
M54.05	Panniculitis affecting regions of neck and back, **thoracolumbar** region
M54.06	Panniculitis affecting regions of neck and back, **lumbar** region
M54.07	Panniculitis affecting regions of neck and back, **lumbosacral** region
M54.08	Panniculitis affecting regions of neck and back, **sacral and sacrococcygeal** region
M54.09	Panniculitis affecting regions, neck and back, **multiple sites** in spine

√5th **M54.1 Radiculopathy**
Brachial neuritis or radiculitis NOS
Lumbar neuritis or radiculitis NOS
Lumbosacral neuritis or radiculitis NOS
Radiculitis NOS
Thoracic neuritis or radiculitis NOS
EXCLUDES 1 neuralgia and neuritis NOS (M79.2)
radiculopathy with cervical disc disorder (M50.1)
radiculopathy with lumbar and other intervertebral disc disorder (M51.1-)
radiculopathy with spondylosis (M47.2-)
AHA: 2018,3Q,18
TIP: A code from this subcategory can be used in addition to a spondylolisthesis code (M43.1-) or a spinal stenosis code (M48.0-) when either condition is documented as the cause of the radiculopathy.

M54.10	Radiculopathy, site unspecified
M54.11	Radiculopathy, **occipito-atlanto-axial** region
M54.12	Radiculopathy, **cervical** region
M54.13	Radiculopathy, **cervicothoracic** region
M54.14	Radiculopathy, **thoracic** region
M54.15	Radiculopathy, **thoracolumbar** region
M54.16	Radiculopathy, **lumbar** region
M54.17	Radiculopathy, **lumbosacral** region
M54.18	Radiculopathy, **sacral and sacrococcygeal** region

M54.2 Cervicalgia
EXCLUDES 1 cervicalgia due to intervertebral cervical disc disorder (M50.-)

√5th **M54.3 Sciatica**
EXCLUDES 1 intervertebral disc degeneration, lumbar region with lower extremity pain only (M51.361)
intervertebral disc degeneration, lumbosacral region with lower extremity pain only (M51.371)
lesion of sciatic nerve (G57.0)
sciatica due to intervertebral disc disorder (M51.1-)
sciatica with lumbago (M54.4-)

M54.30	Sciatica, unspecified side
M54.31	Sciatica, **right** side
M54.32	Sciatica, **left** side

√5th **M54.4 Lumbago with sciatica**
EXCLUDES 1 intervertebral disc degeneration, lumbar region with discogenic back pain and lower extremity pain (M51.362)
intervertebral disc degeneration, lumbosacral region with discogenic back pain and lower extremity pain (M51.372)
lumbago with sciatica due to intervertebral disc disorder (M51.1-)
AHA: 2016,2Q,7

M54.40	Lumbago with sciatica, unspecified side
M54.41	Lumbago with sciatica, **right** side
M54.42	Lumbago with sciatica, **left** side

√5th **M54.5 Low back pain**
EXCLUDES 1 intervertebral disc degeneration, lumbar region with discogenic back pain only (M51.360)
intervertebral disc degeneration, lumbosacral region with discogenic back pain only (M51.370)
low back strain (S39.012)
lumbago due to intervertebral disc displacement (M51.2-)
lumbago with sciatica (M54.4-)
AHA: 2021,4Q,22

M54.50	Low back pain, unspecified
	Loin pain
	Lumbago NOS
M54.51	**Vertebrogenic** low back pain
	Low back vertebral endplate pain
M54.59	Other low back pain

M54.6 Pain in thoracic spine
EXCLUDES 1 pain in thoracic spine due to intervertebral disc disorder (M51.-)

√5th **M54.8 Other dorsalgia**
EXCLUDES 1 dorsalgia in thoracic region (M54.6)
low back pain (M54.5-)

M54.81	Occipital neuralgia
M54.89	Other dorsalgia

M54.9 Dorsalgia, unspecified
Back pain NOS
Backache NOS

SOFT TISSUE DISORDERS (M60-M79)

Disorders of muscles (M60-M63)

EXCLUDES 1 dermatopolymyositis (M33.-)
myopathy in amyloidosis (E85.-)
myopathy in polyarteritis nodosa (M30.0)
myopathy in rheumatoid arthritis (M05.32)
myopathy in scleroderma (M34.-)
myopathy in Sjögren's syndrome (M35.03)
myopathy in systemic lupus erythematosus (M32.-)
EXCLUDES 2 muscular dystrophies and myopathies (G71-G72)

√4th **M60 Myositis**
EXCLUDES 2 inclusion body myositis [IBM] (G72.41)

√5th **M60.0 Infective myositis**
Tropical pyomyositis
Use additional code (B95-B97) to identify infectious agent

√6th **M60.00 Infective myositis, unspecified site**

M60.000	Infective myositis, unspecified **right** arm
	Infective myositis, right upper limb NOS
M60.001	Infective myositis, unspecified **left** arm
	Infective myositis, left upper limb NOS
M60.002	Infective myositis, unspecified **arm**
	Infective myositis, upper limb NOS
M60.003	Infective myositis, unspecified **right leg**
	Infective myositis, right lower limb NOS
M60.004	Infective myositis, unspecified **left leg**
	Infective myositis, left lower limb NOS
M60.005	Infective myositis, unspecified **leg**
	Infective myositis, lower limb NOS
M60.009	Infective myositis, unspecified site

√6th **M60.01 Infective myositis, shoulder**

M60.011	Infective myositis, **right** shoulder
M60.012	Infective myositis, **left** shoulder
M60.019	Infective myositis, unspecified shoulder

√6th **M60.02 Infective myositis, upper arm**

M60.021	Infective myositis, **right** upper arm
M60.022	Infective myositis, **left** upper arm
M60.029	Infective myositis, unspecified upper arm

√6th **M60.03 Infective myositis, forearm**

M60.031	Infective myositis, **right** forearm
M60.032	Infective myositis, **left** forearm
M60.039	Infective myositis, unspecified forearm

√6th **M60.04 Infective myositis, hand and fingers**

M60.041	Infective myositis, **right** hand
M60.042	Infective myositis, **left** hand
M60.043	Infective myositis, unspecified hand
M60.044	Infective myositis, **right** finger(s)
M60.045	Infective myositis, **left** finger(s)
M60.046	Infective myositis, unspecified finger(s)

Chapter 13. Diseases of the Musculoskeletal System and Connective Tissue

- ☑6th **M60.05** Infective myositis, thigh
  - M60.051 Infective myositis, right thigh
  - M60.052 Infective myositis, left thigh
  - M60.059 Infective myositis, unspecified thigh
- ☑6th **M60.06** Infective myositis, lower leg
  - M60.061 Infective myositis, right lower leg
  - M60.062 Infective myositis, left lower leg
  - M60.069 Infective myositis, unspecified lower leg
- ☑6th **M60.07** Infective myositis, ankle, foot and toes
  - M60.070 Infective myositis, right ankle
  - M60.071 Infective myositis, left ankle
  - M60.072 Infective myositis, unspecified ankle
  - M60.073 Infective myositis, right foot
  - M60.074 Infective myositis, left foot
  - M60.075 Infective myositis, unspecified foot
  - M60.076 Infective myositis, right toe(s)
  - M60.077 Infective myositis, left toe(s)
  - M60.078 Infective myositis, unspecified toe(s)
- **M60.08** Infective myositis, other site
- **M60.09** Infective myositis, multiple sites
- ☑5th **M60.1** Interstitial myositis
  - M60.10 Interstitial myositis of unspecified site
  - ☑6th **M60.11** Interstitial myositis, shoulder
    - M60.111 Interstitial myositis, right shoulder
    - M60.112 Interstitial myositis, left shoulder
    - M60.119 Interstitial myositis, unspecified shoulder
  - ☑6th **M60.12** Interstitial myositis, upper arm
    - M60.121 Interstitial myositis, right upper arm
    - M60.122 Interstitial myositis, left upper arm
    - M60.129 Interstitial myositis, unspecified upper arm
  - ☑6th **M60.13** Interstitial myositis, forearm
    - M60.131 Interstitial myositis, right forearm
    - M60.132 Interstitial myositis, left forearm
    - M60.139 Interstitial myositis, unspecified forearm
  - ☑6th **M60.14** Interstitial myositis, hand
    - M60.141 Interstitial myositis, right hand
    - M60.142 Interstitial myositis, left hand
    - M60.149 Interstitial myositis, unspecified hand
  - ☑6th **M60.15** Interstitial myositis, thigh
    - M60.151 Interstitial myositis, right thigh
    - M60.152 Interstitial myositis, left thigh
    - M60.159 Interstitial myositis, unspecified thigh
  - ☑6th **M60.16** Interstitial myositis, lower leg
    - M60.161 Interstitial myositis, right lower leg
    - M60.162 Interstitial myositis, left lower leg
    - M60.169 Interstitial myositis, unspecified lower leg
  - ☑6th **M60.17** Interstitial myositis, ankle and foot
    - M60.171 Interstitial myositis, right ankle and foot
    - M60.172 Interstitial myositis, left ankle and foot
    - M60.179 Interstitial myositis, unspecified ankle and foot
  - **M60.18** Interstitial myositis, other site
  - **M60.19** Interstitial myositis, multiple sites
- ☑5th **M60.2** Foreign body granuloma of soft tissue, not elsewhere classified
  Use additional code to identify the type of retained foreign body (Z18.-)
  EXCLUDES 1 foreign body granuloma of skin and subcutaneous tissue (L92.3)
  - M60.20 Foreign body granuloma of soft tissue, not elsewhere classified, unspecified site
  - ☑6th **M60.21** Foreign body granuloma of soft tissue, not elsewhere classified, shoulder
    - M60.211 Foreign body granuloma of soft tissue, not elsewhere classified, right shoulder
    - M60.212 Foreign body granuloma of soft tissue, not elsewhere classified, left shoulder
    - M60.219 Foreign body granuloma of soft tissue, not elsewhere classified, unspecified shoulder
  - ☑6th **M60.22** Foreign body granuloma of soft tissue, not elsewhere classified, upper arm
    - M60.221 Foreign body granuloma of soft tissue, not elsewhere classified, right upper arm
    - M60.222 Foreign body granuloma of soft tissue, not elsewhere classified, left upper arm
    - M60.229 Foreign body granuloma of soft tissue, not elsewhere classified, unspecified upper arm
  - ☑6th **M60.23** Foreign body granuloma of soft tissue, not elsewhere classified, forearm
    - M60.231 Foreign body granuloma of soft tissue, not elsewhere classified, right forearm
    - M60.232 Foreign body granuloma of soft tissue, not elsewhere classified, left forearm
    - M60.239 Foreign body granuloma of soft tissue, not elsewhere classified, unspecified forearm
  - ☑6th **M60.24** Foreign body granuloma of soft tissue, not elsewhere classified, hand
    - M60.241 Foreign body granuloma of soft tissue, not elsewhere classified, right hand
    - M60.242 Foreign body granuloma of soft tissue, not elsewhere classified, left hand
    - M60.249 Foreign body granuloma of soft tissue, not elsewhere classified, unspecified hand
  - ☑6th **M60.25** Foreign body granuloma of soft tissue, not elsewhere classified, thigh
    - M60.251 Foreign body granuloma of soft tissue, not elsewhere classified, right thigh
    - M60.252 Foreign body granuloma of soft tissue, not elsewhere classified, left thigh
    - M60.259 Foreign body granuloma of soft tissue, not elsewhere classified, unspecified thigh
  - ☑6th **M60.26** Foreign body granuloma of soft tissue, not elsewhere classified, lower leg
    - M60.261 Foreign body granuloma of soft tissue, not elsewhere classified, right lower leg
    - M60.262 Foreign body granuloma of soft tissue, not elsewhere classified, left lower leg
    - M60.269 Foreign body granuloma of soft tissue, not elsewhere classified, unspecified lower leg
  - ☑6th **M60.27** Foreign body granuloma of soft tissue, not elsewhere classified, ankle and foot
    - M60.271 Foreign body granuloma of soft tissue, not elsewhere classified, right ankle and foot
    - M60.272 Foreign body granuloma of soft tissue, not elsewhere classified, left ankle and foot
    - M60.279 Foreign body granuloma of soft tissue, not elsewhere classified, unspecified ankle and foot
  - **M60.28** Foreign body granuloma of soft tissue, not elsewhere classified, other site
- ☑5th **M60.8** Other myositis
  - M60.80 Other myositis, unspecified site
  - ☑6th **M60.81** Other myositis shoulder
    - M60.811 Other myositis, right shoulder
    - M60.812 Other myositis, left shoulder
    - M60.819 Other myositis, unspecified shoulder
  - ☑6th **M60.82** Other myositis, upper arm
    - M60.821 Other myositis, right upper arm
    - M60.822 Other myositis, left upper arm
    - M60.829 Other myositis, unspecified upper arm
  - ☑6th **M60.83** Other myositis, forearm
    - M60.831 Other myositis, right forearm
    - M60.832 Other myositis, left forearm
    - M60.839 Other myositis, unspecified forearm
  - ☑6th **M60.84** Other myositis, hand
    - M60.841 Other myositis, right hand
    - M60.842 Other myositis, left hand
    - M60.849 Other myositis, unspecified hand
  - ☑6th **M60.85** Other myositis, thigh
    - M60.851 Other myositis, right thigh
    - M60.852 Other myositis, left thigh
    - M60.859 Other myositis, unspecified thigh
  - ☑6th **M60.86** Other myositis, lower leg
    - M60.861 Other myositis, right lower leg
    - M60.862 Other myositis, left lower leg
    - M60.869 Other myositis, unspecified lower leg
  - ☑6th **M60.87** Other myositis, ankle and foot
    - M60.871 Other myositis, right ankle and foot
    - M60.872 Other myositis, left ankle and foot
    - M60.879 Other myositis, unspecified ankle and foot
  - **M60.88** Other myositis, other site
  - **M60.89** Other myositis, multiple sites
- **M60.9** Myositis, unspecified

M61 Calcification and ossification of muscle

M61.0 Myositis ossificans traumatica
- M61.00 Myositis ossificans traumatica, unspecified site
- M61.01 Myositis ossificans traumatica, shoulder
  - M61.011 Myositis ossificans traumatica, right shoulder
  - M61.012 Myositis ossificans traumatica, left shoulder
  - M61.019 Myositis ossificans traumatica, unspecified shoulder
- M61.02 Myositis ossificans traumatica, upper arm
  - M61.021 Myositis ossificans traumatica, right upper arm
  - M61.022 Myositis ossificans traumatica, left upper arm
  - M61.029 Myositis ossificans traumatica, unspecified upper arm
- M61.03 Myositis ossificans traumatica, forearm
  - M61.031 Myositis ossificans traumatica, right forearm
  - M61.032 Myositis ossificans traumatica, left forearm
  - M61.039 Myositis ossificans traumatica, unspecified forearm
- M61.04 Myositis ossificans traumatica, hand
  - M61.041 Myositis ossificans traumatica, right hand
  - M61.042 Myositis ossificans traumatica, left hand
  - M61.049 Myositis ossificans traumatica, unspecified hand
- M61.05 Myositis ossificans traumatica, thigh
  - M61.051 Myositis ossificans traumatica, right thigh
  - M61.052 Myositis ossificans traumatica, left thigh
  - M61.059 Myositis ossificans traumatica, unspecified thigh
- M61.06 Myositis ossificans traumatica, lower leg
  - M61.061 Myositis ossificans traumatica, right lower leg
  - M61.062 Myositis ossificans traumatica, left lower leg
  - M61.069 Myositis ossificans traumatica, unspecified lower leg
- M61.07 Myositis ossificans traumatica, ankle and foot
  - M61.071 Myositis ossificans traumatica, right ankle and foot
  - M61.072 Myositis ossificans traumatica, left ankle and foot
  - M61.079 Myositis ossificans traumatica, unspecified ankle and foot
- M61.08 Myositis ossificans traumatica, other site
- M61.09 Myositis ossificans traumatica, multiple sites

M61.1 Myositis ossificans progressiva
Fibrodysplasia ossificans progressiva
- M61.10 Myositis ossificans progressiva, unspecified site
- M61.11 Myositis ossificans progressiva, shoulder
  - M61.111 Myositis ossificans progressiva, right shoulder
  - M61.112 Myositis ossificans progressiva, left shoulder
  - M61.119 Myositis ossificans progressiva, unspecified shoulder
- M61.12 Myositis ossificans progressiva, upper arm
  - M61.121 Myositis ossificans progressiva, right upper arm
  - M61.122 Myositis ossificans progressiva, left upper arm
  - M61.129 Myositis ossificans progressiva, unspecified upper arm
- M61.13 Myositis ossificans progressiva, forearm
  - M61.131 Myositis ossificans progressiva, right forearm
  - M61.132 Myositis ossificans progressiva, left forearm
  - M61.139 Myositis ossificans progressiva, unspecified forearm
- M61.14 Myositis ossificans progressiva, hand and finger(s)
  - M61.141 Myositis ossificans progressiva, right hand
  - M61.142 Myositis ossificans progressiva, left hand
  - M61.143 Myositis ossificans progressiva, unspecified hand
  - M61.144 Myositis ossificans progressiva, right finger(s)
  - M61.145 Myositis ossificans progressiva, left finger(s)
  - M61.146 Myositis ossificans progressiva, unspecified finger(s)
- M61.15 Myositis ossificans progressiva, thigh
  - M61.151 Myositis ossificans progressiva, right thigh
  - M61.152 Myositis ossificans progressiva, left thigh
  - M61.159 Myositis ossificans progressiva, unspecified thigh
- M61.16 Myositis ossificans progressiva, lower leg
  - M61.161 Myositis ossificans progressiva, right lower leg
  - M61.162 Myositis ossificans progressiva, left lower leg
  - M61.169 Myositis ossificans progressiva, unspecified lower leg
- M61.17 Myositis ossificans progressiva, ankle, foot and toe(s)
  - M61.171 Myositis ossificans progressiva, right ankle
  - M61.172 Myositis ossificans progressiva, left ankle
  - M61.173 Myositis ossificans progressiva, unspecified ankle
  - M61.174 Myositis ossificans progressiva, right foot
  - M61.175 Myositis ossificans progressiva, left foot
  - M61.176 Myositis ossificans progressiva, unspecified foot
  - M61.177 Myositis ossificans progressiva, right toe(s)
  - M61.178 Myositis ossificans progressiva, left toe(s)
  - M61.179 Myositis ossificans progressiva, unspecified toe(s)
- M61.18 Myositis ossificans progressiva, other site
- M61.19 Myositis ossificans progressiva, multiple sites

M61.2 Paralytic calcification and ossification of muscle
Myositis ossificans associated with quadriplegia or paraplegia
- M61.20 Paralytic calcification and ossification of muscle, unspecified site
- M61.21 Paralytic calcification and ossification of muscle, shoulder
  - M61.211 Paralytic calcification and ossification of muscle, right shoulder
  - M61.212 Paralytic calcification and ossification of muscle, left shoulder
  - M61.219 Paralytic calcification and ossification of muscle, unspecified shoulder
- M61.22 Paralytic calcification and ossification of muscle, upper arm
  - M61.221 Paralytic calcification and ossification of muscle, right upper arm
  - M61.222 Paralytic calcification and ossification of muscle, left upper arm
  - M61.229 Paralytic calcification and ossification of muscle, unspecified upper arm
- M61.23 Paralytic calcification and ossification of muscle, forearm
  - M61.231 Paralytic calcification and ossification of muscle, right forearm
  - M61.232 Paralytic calcification and ossification of muscle, left forearm
  - M61.239 Paralytic calcification and ossification of muscle, unspecified forearm
- M61.24 Paralytic calcification and ossification of muscle, hand
  - M61.241 Paralytic calcification and ossification of muscle, right hand
  - M61.242 Paralytic calcification and ossification of muscle, left hand
  - M61.249 Paralytic calcification and ossification of muscle, unspecified hand
- M61.25 Paralytic calcification and ossification of muscle, thigh
  - M61.251 Paralytic calcification and ossification of muscle, right thigh
  - M61.252 Paralytic calcification and ossification of muscle, left thigh
  - M61.259 Paralytic calcification and ossification of muscle, unspecified thigh
- M61.26 Paralytic calcification and ossification of muscle, lower leg
  - M61.261 Paralytic calcification and ossification of muscle, right lower leg

- **M61.262** Paralytic calcification and ossification of muscle, left lower leg
- **M61.269** Paralytic calcification and ossification of muscle, unspecified lower leg
- ✓6th **M61.27** Paralytic calcification and ossification of muscle, ankle and foot
  - **M61.271** Paralytic calcification and ossification of muscle, right ankle and foot
  - **M61.272** Paralytic calcification and ossification of muscle, left ankle and foot
  - **M61.279** Paralytic calcification and ossification of muscle, unspecified ankle and foot
- **M61.28** Paralytic calcification and ossification of muscle, other site
- **M61.29** Paralytic calcification and ossification of muscle, multiple sites
- ✓5th **M61.3** Calcification and ossification of muscles associated with burns
  - *Myositis ossificans associated with burns*
  - **M61.30** Calcification and ossification of muscles associated with burns, unspecified site
  - ✓6th **M61.31** Calcification and ossification of muscles associated with burns, shoulder
    - **M61.311** Calcification and ossification of muscles associated with burns, right shoulder
    - **M61.312** Calcification and ossification of muscles associated with burns, left shoulder
    - **M61.319** Calcification and ossification of muscles associated with burns, unspecified shoulder
  - ✓6th **M61.32** Calcification and ossification of muscles associated with burns, upper arm
    - **M61.321** Calcification and ossification of muscles associated with burns, right upper arm
    - **M61.322** Calcification and ossification of muscles associated with burns, left upper arm
    - **M61.329** Calcification and ossification of muscles associated with burns, unspecified upper arm
  - ✓6th **M61.33** Calcification and ossification of muscles associated with burns, forearm
    - **M61.331** Calcification and ossification of muscles associated with burns, right forearm
    - **M61.332** Calcification and ossification of muscles associated with burns, left forearm
    - **M61.339** Calcification and ossification of muscles associated with burns, unspecified forearm
  - ✓6th **M61.34** Calcification and ossification of muscles associated with burns, hand
    - **M61.341** Calcification and ossification of muscles associated with burns, right hand
    - **M61.342** Calcification and ossification of muscles associated with burns, left hand
    - **M61.349** Calcification and ossification of muscles associated with burns, unspecified hand
  - ✓6th **M61.35** Calcification and ossification of muscles associated with burns, thigh
    - **M61.351** Calcification and ossification of muscles associated with burns, right thigh
    - **M61.352** Calcification and ossification of muscles associated with burns, left thigh
    - **M61.359** Calcification and ossification of muscles associated with burns, unspecified thigh
  - ✓6th **M61.36** Calcification and ossification of muscles associated with burns, lower leg
    - **M61.361** Calcification and ossification of muscles associated with burns, right lower leg
    - **M61.362** Calcification and ossification of muscles associated with burns, left lower leg
    - **M61.369** Calcification and ossification of muscles associated with burns, unspecified lower leg
  - ✓6th **M61.37** Calcification and ossification of muscles associated with burns, ankle and foot
    - **M61.371** Calcification and ossification of muscles associated with burns, right ankle and foot
    - **M61.372** Calcification and ossification of muscles associated with burns, left ankle and foot
    - **M61.379** Calcification and ossification of muscles associated with burns, unspecified ankle and foot
  - **M61.38** Calcification and ossification of muscles associated with burns, other site
- **M61.39** Calcification and ossification of muscles associated with burns, multiple sites
- ✓5th **M61.4** Other calcification of muscle
  - EXCLUDES 1 *calcific tendinitis NOS (M65.2-)*
  - *calcific tendinitis of shoulder (M75.3)*
  - **M61.40** Other calcification of muscle, unspecified site
  - ✓6th **M61.41** Other calcification of muscle, shoulder
    - **M61.411** Other calcification of muscle, right shoulder
    - **M61.412** Other calcification of muscle, left shoulder
    - **M61.419** Other calcification of muscle, unspecified shoulder
  - ✓6th **M61.42** Other calcification of muscle, upper arm
    - **M61.421** Other calcification of muscle, right upper arm
    - **M61.422** Other calcification of muscle, left upper arm
    - **M61.429** Other calcification of muscle, unspecified upper arm
  - ✓6th **M61.43** Other calcification of muscle, forearm
    - **M61.431** Other calcification of muscle, right forearm
    - **M61.432** Other calcification of muscle, left forearm
    - **M61.439** Other calcification of muscle, unspecified forearm
  - ✓6th **M61.44** Other calcification of muscle, hand
    - **M61.441** Other calcification of muscle, right hand
    - **M61.442** Other calcification of muscle, left hand
    - **M61.449** Other calcification of muscle, unspecified hand
  - ✓6th **M61.45** Other calcification of muscle, thigh
    - **M61.451** Other calcification of muscle, right thigh
    - **M61.452** Other calcification of muscle, left thigh
    - **M61.459** Other calcification of muscle, unspecified thigh
  - ✓6th **M61.46** Other calcification of muscle, lower leg
    - **M61.461** Other calcification of muscle, right lower leg
    - **M61.462** Other calcification of muscle, left lower leg
    - **M61.469** Other calcification of muscle, unspecified lower leg
  - ✓6th **M61.47** Other calcification of muscle, ankle and foot
    - **M61.471** Other calcification of muscle, right ankle and foot
    - **M61.472** Other calcification of muscle, left ankle and foot
    - **M61.479** Other calcification of muscle, unspecified ankle and foot
  - **M61.48** Other calcification of muscle, other site
  - **M61.49** Other calcification of muscle, multiple sites
- ✓5th **M61.5** Other ossification of muscle
  - **M61.50** Other ossification of muscle, unspecified site
  - ✓6th **M61.51** Other ossification of muscle, shoulder
    - **M61.511** Other ossification of muscle, right shoulder
    - **M61.512** Other ossification of muscle, left shoulder
    - **M61.519** Other ossification of muscle, unspecified shoulder
  - ✓6th **M61.52** Other ossification of muscle, upper arm
    - **M61.521** Other ossification of muscle, right upper arm
    - **M61.522** Other ossification of muscle, left upper arm
    - **M61.529** Other ossification of muscle, unspecified upper arm
  - ✓6th **M61.53** Other ossification of muscle, forearm
    - **M61.531** Other ossification of muscle, right forearm
    - **M61.532** Other ossification of muscle, left forearm
    - **M61.539** Other ossification of muscle, unspecified forearm
  - ✓6th **M61.54** Other ossification of muscle, hand
    - **M61.541** Other ossification of muscle, right hand
    - **M61.542** Other ossification of muscle, left hand
    - **M61.549** Other ossification of muscle, unspecified hand
  - ✓6th **M61.55** Other ossification of muscle, thigh
    - **M61.551** Other ossification of muscle, right thigh
    - **M61.552** Other ossification of muscle, left thigh
      - **AHA:** 2024,3Q,14
    - **M61.559** Other ossification of muscle, unspecified thigh

- **M61.56** Other ossification of muscle, lower leg
  - **M61.561** Other ossification of muscle, right lower leg
  - **M61.562** Other ossification of muscle, left lower leg
  - **M61.569** Other ossification of muscle, unspecified lower leg
- **M61.57** Other ossification of muscle, ankle and foot
  - **M61.571** Other ossification of muscle, right ankle and foot
  - **M61.572** Other ossification of muscle, left ankle and foot
  - **M61.579** Other ossification of muscle, unspecified ankle and foot
- **M61.58** Other ossification of muscle, other site
- **M61.59** Other ossification of muscle, multiple sites
- **M61.9** Calcification and ossification of muscle, unspecified

M62 Other disorders of muscle
EXCLUDES 1
- alcoholic myopathy (G72.1)
- cramp and spasm (R25.2)
- drug-induced myopathy (G72.0)
- myalgia (M79.1-)
- stiff-man syndrome (G25.82)

EXCLUDES 2
- nontraumatic hematoma of muscle (M79.81)

- **M62.0** Separation of muscle (nontraumatic)
  - Diastasis of muscle
  - EXCLUDES 1
    - diastasis recti complicating pregnancy, labor and delivery (O71.8)
    - traumatic separation of muscle - see strain of muscle by body region
  - **M62.00** Separation of muscle (nontraumatic), unspecified site
  - **M62.01** Separation of muscle (nontraumatic), shoulder
    - **M62.011** Separation of muscle (nontraumatic), right shoulder
    - **M62.012** Separation of muscle (nontraumatic), left shoulder
    - **M62.019** Separation of muscle (nontraumatic), unspecified shoulder
  - **M62.02** Separation of muscle (nontraumatic), upper arm
    - **M62.021** Separation of muscle (nontraumatic), right upper arm
    - **M62.022** Separation of muscle (nontraumatic), left upper arm
    - **M62.029** Separation of muscle (nontraumatic), unspecified upper arm
  - **M62.03** Separation of muscle (nontraumatic), forearm
    - **M62.031** Separation of muscle (nontraumatic), right forearm
    - **M62.032** Separation of muscle (nontraumatic), left forearm
    - **M62.039** Separation of muscle (nontraumatic), unspecified forearm
  - **M62.04** Separation of muscle (nontraumatic), hand
    - **M62.041** Separation of muscle (nontraumatic), right hand
    - **M62.042** Separation of muscle (nontraumatic), left hand
    - **M62.049** Separation of muscle (nontraumatic), unspecified hand
  - **M62.05** Separation of muscle (nontraumatic), thigh
    - **M62.051** Separation of muscle (nontraumatic), right thigh
    - **M62.052** Separation of muscle (nontraumatic), left thigh
    - **M62.059** Separation of muscle (nontraumatic), unspecified thigh
  - **M62.06** Separation of muscle (nontraumatic), lower leg
    - **M62.061** Separation of muscle (nontraumatic), right lower leg
    - **M62.062** Separation of muscle (nontraumatic), left lower leg
    - **M62.069** Separation of muscle (nontraumatic), unspecified lower leg
  - **M62.07** Separation of muscle (nontraumatic), ankle and foot
    - **M62.071** Separation of muscle (nontraumatic), right ankle and foot
    - **M62.072** Separation of muscle (nontraumatic), left ankle and foot
    - **M62.079** Separation of muscle (nontraumatic), unspecified ankle and foot
  - **M62.08** Separation of muscle (nontraumatic), other site
- **M62.1** Other rupture of muscle (nontraumatic)
  - EXCLUDES 1
    - traumatic rupture of muscle - see strain of muscle by body region
  - EXCLUDES 2
    - rupture of tendon (M66.-)
  - **M62.10** Other rupture of muscle (nontraumatic), unspecified site
  - **M62.11** Other rupture of muscle (nontraumatic), shoulder
    - **M62.111** Other rupture of muscle (nontraumatic), right shoulder
    - **M62.112** Other rupture of muscle (nontraumatic), left shoulder
    - **M62.119** Other rupture of muscle (nontraumatic), unspecified shoulder
  - **M62.12** Other rupture of muscle (nontraumatic), upper arm
    - **M62.121** Other rupture of muscle (nontraumatic), right upper arm
    - **M62.122** Other rupture of muscle (nontraumatic), left upper arm
    - **M62.129** Other rupture of muscle (nontraumatic), unspecified upper arm
  - **M62.13** Other rupture of muscle (nontraumatic), forearm
    - **M62.131** Other rupture of muscle (nontraumatic), right forearm
    - **M62.132** Other rupture of muscle (nontraumatic), left forearm
    - **M62.139** Other rupture of muscle (nontraumatic), unspecified forearm
  - **M62.14** Other rupture of muscle (nontraumatic), hand
    - **M62.141** Other rupture of muscle (nontraumatic), right hand
    - **M62.142** Other rupture of muscle (nontraumatic), left hand
    - **M62.149** Other rupture of muscle (nontraumatic), unspecified hand
  - **M62.15** Other rupture of muscle (nontraumatic), thigh
    - **M62.151** Other rupture of muscle (nontraumatic), right thigh
    - **M62.152** Other rupture of muscle (nontraumatic), left thigh
    - **M62.159** Other rupture of muscle (nontraumatic), unspecified thigh
  - **M62.16** Other rupture of muscle (nontraumatic), lower leg
    - **M62.161** Other rupture of muscle (nontraumatic), right lower leg
    - **M62.162** Other rupture of muscle (nontraumatic), left lower leg
    - **M62.169** Other rupture of muscle (nontraumatic), unspecified lower leg
  - **M62.17** Other rupture of muscle (nontraumatic), ankle and foot
    - **M62.171** Other rupture of muscle (nontraumatic), right ankle and foot
    - **M62.172** Other rupture of muscle (nontraumatic), left ankle and foot
    - **M62.179** Other rupture of muscle (nontraumatic), unspecified ankle and foot
  - **M62.18** Other rupture of muscle (nontraumatic), other site
- **M62.2** Nontraumatic ischemic infarction of muscle
  - EXCLUDES 1
    - compartment syndrome (traumatic) (T79.A-)
    - nontraumatic compartment syndrome (M79.A-)
    - rhabdomyolysis (M62.82)
    - traumatic ischemia of muscle (T79.6)
    - Volkmann's ischemic contracture (T79.6)
  - **M62.20** Nontraumatic ischemic infarction of muscle, unspecified site
  - **M62.21** Nontraumatic ischemic infarction of muscle, shoulder
    - **M62.211** Nontraumatic ischemic infarction of muscle, right shoulder
    - **M62.212** Nontraumatic ischemic infarction of muscle, left shoulder
    - **M62.219** Nontraumatic ischemic infarction of muscle, unspecified shoulder
  - **M62.22** Nontraumatic ischemic infarction of muscle, upper arm
    - **M62.221** Nontraumatic ischemic infarction of muscle, right upper arm

	M62.222	Nontraumatic ischemic infarction of muscle, left upper arm
	M62.229	Nontraumatic ischemic infarction of muscle, unspecified upper arm
M62.23		Nontraumatic ischemic infarction of muscle, forearm
	M62.231	Nontraumatic ischemic infarction of muscle, right forearm
	M62.232	Nontraumatic ischemic infarction of muscle, left forearm
	M62.239	Nontraumatic ischemic infarction of muscle, unspecified forearm
M62.24		Nontraumatic ischemic infarction of muscle, hand
	M62.241	Nontraumatic ischemic infarction of muscle, right hand
	M62.242	Nontraumatic ischemic infarction of muscle, left hand
	M62.249	Nontraumatic ischemic infarction of muscle, unspecified hand
M62.25		Nontraumatic ischemic infarction of muscle, thigh
	M62.251	Nontraumatic ischemic infarction of muscle, right thigh
	M62.252	Nontraumatic ischemic infarction of muscle, left thigh
	M62.259	Nontraumatic ischemic infarction of muscle, unspecified thigh
M62.26		Nontraumatic ischemic infarction of muscle, lower leg
	M62.261	Nontraumatic ischemic infarction of muscle, right lower leg
	M62.262	Nontraumatic ischemic infarction of muscle, left lower leg
	M62.269	Nontraumatic ischemic infarction of muscle, unspecified lower leg
M62.27		Nontraumatic ischemic infarction of muscle, ankle and foot
	M62.271	Nontraumatic ischemic infarction of muscle, right ankle and foot
	M62.272	Nontraumatic ischemic infarction of muscle, left ankle and foot
	M62.279	Nontraumatic ischemic infarction of muscle, unspecified ankle and foot
M62.28		Nontraumatic ischemic infarction of muscle, other site
M62.3		Immobility syndrome (paraplegic)
M62.4		**Contracture of muscle**
		Contracture of tendon (sheath)
		EXCLUDES 1 contracture of joint (M24.5-)
	M62.40	Contracture of muscle, unspecified site
M62.41		Contracture of muscle, shoulder
	M62.411	Contracture of muscle, right shoulder
	M62.412	Contracture of muscle, left shoulder
	M62.419	Contracture of muscle, unspecified shoulder
M62.42		Contracture of muscle, upper arm
	M62.421	Contracture of muscle, right upper arm
	M62.422	Contracture of muscle, left upper arm
	M62.429	Contracture of muscle, unspecified upper arm
M62.43		Contracture of muscle, forearm
	M62.431	Contracture of muscle, right forearm
	M62.432	Contracture of muscle, left forearm
	M62.439	Contracture of muscle, unspecified forearm
M62.44		Contracture of muscle, hand
	M62.441	Contracture of muscle, right hand
	M62.442	Contracture of muscle, left hand
	M62.449	Contracture of muscle, unspecified hand
M62.45		Contracture of muscle, thigh
	M62.451	Contracture of muscle, right thigh
	M62.452	Contracture of muscle, left thigh
	M62.459	Contracture of muscle, unspecified thigh
M62.46		Contracture of muscle, lower leg
		AHA: 2023,2Q,14
	M62.461	Contracture of muscle, right lower leg
	M62.462	Contracture of muscle, left lower leg
	M62.469	Contracture of muscle, unspecified lower leg
M62.47		Contracture of muscle, ankle and foot
	M62.471	Contracture of muscle, right ankle and foot
	M62.472	Contracture of muscle, left ankle and foot
	M62.479	Contracture of muscle, unspecified ankle and foot
	M62.48	Contracture of muscle, other site
	M62.49	Contracture of muscle, multiple sites
M62.5		**Muscle wasting and atrophy, not elsewhere classified**
		Disuse atrophy NEC
		EXCLUDES 1 neuralgic amyotrophy (G54.5)
		progressive muscular atrophy (G12.21)
		sarcopenia (M62.84)
		EXCLUDES 2 pelvic muscle wasting (N81.84)
	M62.50	Muscle wasting and atrophy, not elsewhere classified, unspecified site
M62.51		Muscle wasting and atrophy, not elsewhere classified, shoulder
	M62.511	Muscle wasting and atrophy, not elsewhere classified, right shoulder
	M62.512	Muscle wasting and atrophy, not elsewhere classified, left shoulder
	M62.519	Muscle wasting and atrophy, not elsewhere classified, unspecified shoulder
M62.52		Muscle wasting and atrophy, not elsewhere classified, upper arm
	M62.521	Muscle wasting and atrophy, not elsewhere classified, right upper arm
	M62.522	Muscle wasting and atrophy, not elsewhere classified, left upper arm
	M62.529	Muscle wasting and atrophy, not elsewhere classified, unspecified upper arm
M62.53		Muscle wasting and atrophy, not elsewhere classified, forearm
	M62.531	Muscle wasting and atrophy, not elsewhere classified, right forearm
	M62.532	Muscle wasting and atrophy, not elsewhere classified, left forearm
	M62.539	Muscle wasting and atrophy, not elsewhere classified, unspecified forearm
M62.54		Muscle wasting and atrophy, not elsewhere classified, hand
	M62.541	Muscle wasting and atrophy, not elsewhere classified, right hand
	M62.542	Muscle wasting and atrophy, not elsewhere classified, left hand
	M62.549	Muscle wasting and atrophy, not elsewhere classified, unspecified hand
M62.55		Muscle wasting and atrophy, not elsewhere classified, thigh
	M62.551	Muscle wasting and atrophy, not elsewhere classified, right thigh
	M62.552	Muscle wasting and atrophy, not elsewhere classified, left thigh
	M62.559	Muscle wasting and atrophy, not elsewhere classified, unspecified thigh
M62.56		Muscle wasting and atrophy, not elsewhere classified, lower leg
	M62.561	Muscle wasting and atrophy, not elsewhere classified, right lower leg
	M62.562	Muscle wasting and atrophy, not elsewhere classified, left lower leg
	M62.569	Muscle wasting and atrophy, not elsewhere classified, unspecified lower leg
M62.57		Muscle wasting and atrophy, not elsewhere classified, ankle and foot
	M62.571	Muscle wasting and atrophy, not elsewhere classified, right ankle and foot
	M62.572	Muscle wasting and atrophy, not elsewhere classified, left ankle and foot
	M62.579	Muscle wasting and atrophy, not elsewhere classified, unspecified ankle and foot
	M62.58	Muscle wasting and atrophy, not elsewhere classified, other site
	M62.59	Muscle wasting and atrophy, not elsewhere classified, multiple sites
M62.5A		Muscle wasting and atrophy, not elsewhere classified, back
		AHA: 2022,4Q,29
	M62.5A0	Muscle wasting and atrophy, not elsewhere classified, back, cervical
	M62.5A1	Muscle wasting and atrophy, not elsewhere classified, back, thoracic
	M62.5A2	Muscle wasting and atrophy, not elsewhere classified, back, lumbosacral
	M62.5A9	Muscle wasting and atrophy, not elsewhere classified, back, unspecified level

M62.8 Other specified disorders of muscle
EXCLUDES 2: nontraumatic hematoma of muscle (M79.81)

M62.81 Muscle weakness (generalized)
EXCLUDES 1: muscle weakness in sarcopenia (M62.84)

M62.82 Rhabdomyolysis
EXCLUDES 1: traumatic rhabdomyolysis (T79.6)
AHA: 2024,4Q,16; 2019,2Q,12
DEF: Rapid disintegration or destruction of skeletal muscle caused by direct or indirect injury, resulting in the excretion of muscle protein myoglobin into the urine.

M62.83 Muscle spasm
- M62.830 Muscle spasm of back
- M62.831 Muscle spasm of calf
  - Charley-horse
- M62.838 Other muscle spasm

M62.84 Sarcopenia
Age-related sarcopenia
Code first underlying disease, if applicable, such as:
- disorders of myoneural junction and muscle disease in diseases classified elsewhere (G73.-)
- other and unspecified myopathies (G72.-)
- primary disorders of muscles (G71.-)

AHA: 2016,4Q,41

M62.85 Dysfunction of the multifidus muscles, lumbar region
AHA: 2024,4Q,25

M62.89 Other specified disorders of muscle
Muscle (sheath) hernia

M62.9 Disorder of muscle, unspecified

M63 Disorders of muscle in diseases classified elsewhere
Code first underlying disease, such as:
- leprosy (A30.-)
- neoplasm (C49.-, C79.89, D21.-, D48.1-)
- schistosomiasis (B65.-)
- trichinellosis (B75)

EXCLUDES 1:
- myopathy in cysticercosis (B69.81)
- myopathy in endocrine diseases (G73.7)
- myopathy in metabolic diseases (G73.7)
- myopathy in sarcoidosis (D86.87)
- myopathy in secondary syphilis (A51.49)
- myopathy in syphilis (late) (A52.78)
- myopathy in toxoplasmosis (B58.82)
- myopathy in tuberculosis (A18.09)

M63.8 Disorders of muscle in diseases classified elsewhere

M63.80 *Disorders of muscle in diseases classified elsewhere, unspecified site*

M63.81 Disorders of muscle in diseases classified elsewhere, shoulder
- M63.811 *Disorders of muscle in diseases classified elsewhere, right shoulder*
- M63.812 *Disorders of muscle in diseases classified elsewhere, left shoulder*
- M63.819 *Disorders of muscle in diseases classified elsewhere, unspecified shoulder*

M63.82 Disorders of muscle in diseases classified elsewhere, upper arm
- M63.821 *Disorders of muscle in diseases classified elsewhere, right upper arm*
- M63.822 *Disorders of muscle in diseases classified elsewhere, left upper arm*
- M63.829 *Disorders of muscle in diseases classified elsewhere, unspecified upper arm*

M63.83 Disorders of muscle in diseases classified elsewhere, forearm
- M63.831 *Disorders of muscle in diseases classified elsewhere, right forearm*
- M63.832 *Disorders of muscle in diseases classified elsewhere, left forearm*
- M63.839 *Disorders of muscle in diseases classified elsewhere, unspecified forearm*

M63.84 Disorders of muscle in diseases classified elsewhere, hand
- M63.841 *Disorders of muscle in diseases classified elsewhere, right hand*
- M63.842 *Disorders of muscle in diseases classified elsewhere, left hand*
- M63.849 *Disorders of muscle in diseases classified elsewhere, unspecified hand*

M63.85 Disorders of muscle in diseases classified elsewhere, thigh
- M63.851 *Disorders of muscle in diseases classified elsewhere, right thigh*
- M63.852 *Disorders of muscle in diseases classified elsewhere, left thigh*
- M63.859 *Disorders of muscle in diseases classified elsewhere, unspecified thigh*

M63.86 Disorders of muscle in diseases classified elsewhere, lower leg
- M63.861 *Disorders of muscle in diseases classified elsewhere, right lower leg*
- M63.862 *Disorders of muscle in diseases classified elsewhere, left lower leg*
- M63.869 *Disorders of muscle in diseases classified elsewhere, unspecified lower leg*

M63.87 Disorders of muscle in diseases classified elsewhere, ankle and foot
- M63.871 *Disorders of muscle in diseases classified elsewhere, right ankle and foot*
- M63.872 *Disorders of muscle in diseases classified elsewhere, left ankle and foot*
- M63.879 *Disorders of muscle in diseases classified elsewhere, unspecified ankle and foot*

M63.88 *Disorders of muscle in diseases classified elsewhere, other site*

M63.89 *Disorders of muscle in diseases classified elsewhere, multiple sites*

Disorders of synovium and tendon (M65-M67)

M65 Synovitis and tenosynovitis
EXCLUDES 1:
- chronic crepitant synovitis of hand and wrist (M70.0-)
- current injury - see injury of ligament or tendon by body region
- soft tissue disorders related to use, overuse and pressure (M70.-)

M65.0 Abscess of tendon sheath
Use additional code (B95-B96) to identify bacterial agent.

M65.00 Abscess of tendon sheath, unspecified site

M65.01 Abscess of tendon sheath, shoulder
- M65.011 Abscess of tendon sheath, right shoulder
- M65.012 Abscess of tendon sheath, left shoulder
- M65.019 Abscess of tendon sheath, unspecified shoulder

M65.02 Abscess of tendon sheath, upper arm
- M65.021 Abscess of tendon sheath, right upper arm
- M65.022 Abscess of tendon sheath, left upper arm
- M65.029 Abscess of tendon sheath, unspecified upper arm

M65.03 Abscess of tendon sheath, forearm
- M65.031 Abscess of tendon sheath, right forearm
- M65.032 Abscess of tendon sheath, left forearm
- M65.039 Abscess of tendon sheath, unspecified forearm

M65.04 Abscess of tendon sheath, hand
- M65.041 Abscess of tendon sheath, right hand
- M65.042 Abscess of tendon sheath, left hand
- M65.049 Abscess of tendon sheath, unspecified hand

M65.05 Abscess of tendon sheath, thigh
- M65.051 Abscess of tendon sheath, right thigh
- M65.052 Abscess of tendon sheath, left thigh
- M65.059 Abscess of tendon sheath, unspecified thigh

M65.06 Abscess of tendon sheath, lower leg
- M65.061 Abscess of tendon sheath, right lower leg
- M65.062 Abscess of tendon sheath, left lower leg
- M65.069 Abscess of tendon sheath, unspecified lower leg

M65.07 Abscess of tendon sheath, ankle and foot
- M65.071 Abscess of tendon sheath, right ankle and foot
- M65.072 Abscess of tendon sheath, left ankle and foot
- M65.079 Abscess of tendon sheath, unspecified ankle and foot

M65.08 Abscess of tendon sheath, other site

M65.1 Other infective (teno)synovitis
M65.10 Other infective (teno)synovitis, unspecified site

	M65.11	Other infective (teno)synovitis, shoulder
		M65.111 Other infective (teno)synovitis, right shoulder
		M65.112 Other infective (teno)synovitis, left shoulder
		M65.119 Other infective (teno)synovitis, unspecified shoulder
✓6th	M65.12	Other infective (teno)synovitis, elbow
		M65.121 Other infective (teno)synovitis, right elbow
		M65.122 Other infective (teno)synovitis, left elbow
		M65.129 Other infective (teno)synovitis, unspecified elbow
✓6th	M65.13	Other infective (teno)synovitis, wrist
		M65.131 Other infective (teno)synovitis, right wrist
		M65.132 Other infective (teno)synovitis, left wrist
		M65.139 Other infective (teno)synovitis, unspecified wrist
✓6th	M65.14	Other infective (teno)synovitis, hand
		M65.141 Other infective (teno)synovitis, right hand
		M65.142 Other infective (teno)synovitis, left hand
		M65.149 Other infective (teno)synovitis, unspecified hand
✓6th	M65.15	Other infective (teno)synovitis, hip
		M65.151 Other infective (teno)synovitis, right hip
		M65.152 Other infective (teno)synovitis, left hip
		M65.159 Other infective (teno)synovitis, unspecified hip
✓6th	M65.16	Other infective (teno)synovitis, knee
		M65.161 Other infective (teno)synovitis, right knee
		M65.162 Other infective (teno)synovitis, left knee
		M65.169 Other infective (teno)synovitis, unspecified knee
✓6th	M65.17	Other infective (teno)synovitis, ankle and foot
		M65.171 Other infective (teno)synovitis, right ankle and foot
		M65.172 Other infective (teno)synovitis, left ankle and foot
		M65.179 Other infective (teno)synovitis, unspecified ankle and foot
	M65.18	Other infective (teno)synovitis, other site
	M65.19	Other infective (teno)synovitis, multiple sites
✓5th	M65.2	Calcific tendinitis
		EXCLUDES 1 tendinitis as classified in M75-M77
		calcified tendinitis of shoulder (M75.3)
		M65.20 Calcific tendinitis, unspecified site
✓6th	M65.22	Calcific tendinitis, upper arm
		M65.221 Calcific tendinitis, right upper arm
		M65.222 Calcific tendinitis, left upper arm
		M65.229 Calcific tendinitis, unspecified upper arm
✓6th	M65.23	Calcific tendinitis, forearm
		M65.231 Calcific tendinitis, right forearm
		M65.232 Calcific tendinitis, left forearm
		M65.239 Calcific tendinitis, unspecified forearm
✓6th	M65.24	Calcific tendinitis, hand
		M65.241 Calcific tendinitis, right hand
		M65.242 Calcific tendinitis, left hand
		M65.249 Calcific tendinitis, unspecified hand
✓6th	M65.25	Calcific tendinitis, thigh
		M65.251 Calcific tendinitis, right thigh
		M65.252 Calcific tendinitis, left thigh
		M65.259 Calcific tendinitis, unspecified thigh
✓6th	M65.26	Calcific tendinitis, lower leg
		M65.261 Calcific tendinitis, right lower leg
		M65.262 Calcific tendinitis, left lower leg
		M65.269 Calcific tendinitis, unspecified lower leg
✓6th	M65.27	Calcific tendinitis, ankle and foot
		M65.271 Calcific tendinitis, right ankle and foot
		M65.272 Calcific tendinitis, left ankle and foot
		M65.279 Calcific tendinitis, unspecified ankle and foot
	M65.28	Calcific tendinitis, other site
	M65.29	Calcific tendinitis, multiple sites
✓5th	M65.3	Trigger finger
		Nodular tendinous disease
		M65.30 Trigger finger, unspecified finger
✓6th	M65.31	Trigger thumb
		M65.311 Trigger thumb, right thumb
		M65.312 Trigger thumb, left thumb
		M65.319 Trigger thumb, unspecified thumb
✓6th	M65.32	Trigger finger, index finger
		M65.321 Trigger finger, right index finger
		M65.322 Trigger finger, left index finger
		M65.329 Trigger finger, unspecified index finger
✓6th	M65.33	Trigger finger, middle finger
		M65.331 Trigger finger, right middle finger
		M65.332 Trigger finger, left middle finger
		M65.339 Trigger finger, unspecified middle finger
✓6th	M65.34	Trigger finger, ring finger
		M65.341 Trigger finger, right ring finger
		M65.342 Trigger finger, left ring finger
		M65.349 Trigger finger, unspecified ring finger
✓6th	M65.35	Trigger finger, little finger
		M65.351 Trigger finger, right little finger
		M65.352 Trigger finger, left little finger
		M65.359 Trigger finger, unspecified little finger
	M65.4	Radial styloid tenosynovitis [de Quervain]
✓6th	M65.8	Other synovitis and tenosynovitis
		M65.80 Other synovitis and tenosynovitis, unspecified site
✓6th	M65.81	Other synovitis and tenosynovitis, shoulder
		M65.811 Other synovitis and tenosynovitis, right shoulder
		M65.812 Other synovitis and tenosynovitis, left shoulder
		M65.819 Other synovitis and tenosynovitis, unspecified shoulder
✓6th	M65.82	Other synovitis and tenosynovitis, upper arm
		M65.821 Other synovitis and tenosynovitis, right upper arm
		M65.822 Other synovitis and tenosynovitis, left upper arm
		M65.829 Other synovitis and tenosynovitis, unspecified upper arm
✓6th	M65.83	Other synovitis and tenosynovitis, forearm
		M65.831 Other synovitis and tenosynovitis, right forearm
		M65.832 Other synovitis and tenosynovitis, left forearm
		M65.839 Other synovitis and tenosynovitis, unspecified forearm
✓6th	M65.84	Other synovitis and tenosynovitis, hand
		M65.841 Other synovitis and tenosynovitis, right hand
		M65.842 Other synovitis and tenosynovitis, left hand
		M65.849 Other synovitis and tenosynovitis, unspecified hand
✓6th	M65.85	Other synovitis and tenosynovitis, thigh
		M65.851 Other synovitis and tenosynovitis, right thigh
		M65.852 Other synovitis and tenosynovitis, left thigh
		M65.859 Other synovitis and tenosynovitis, unspecified thigh
✓6th	M65.86	Other synovitis and tenosynovitis, lower leg
		M65.861 Other synovitis and tenosynovitis, right lower leg
		M65.862 Other synovitis and tenosynovitis, left lower leg
		M65.869 Other synovitis and tenosynovitis, unspecified lower leg
✓6th	M65.87	Other synovitis and tenosynovitis, ankle and foot
		M65.871 Other synovitis and tenosynovitis, right ankle and foot
		M65.872 Other synovitis and tenosynovitis, left ankle and foot
		M65.879 Other synovitis and tenosynovitis, unspecified ankle and foot
	M65.88	Other synovitis and tenosynovitis, other site
	M65.89	Other synovitis and tenosynovitis, multiple sites
✓5th	M65.9	Synovitis and tenosynovitis, unspecified
		AHA: 2024,4Q,25
		M65.90 Unspecified synovitis and tenosynovitis, unspecified site

	M65.91	Unspecified synovitis and tenosynovitis, shoulder
	M65.911	Unspecified synovitis and tenosynovitis, right shoulder
	M65.912	Unspecified synovitis and tenosynovitis, left shoulder
	M65.919	Unspecified synovitis and tenosynovitis, unspecified shoulder
✓6th M65.92		Unspecified synovitis and tenosynovitis, upper arm
	M65.921	Unspecified synovitis and tenosynovitis, right upper arm
	M65.922	Unspecified synovitis and tenosynovitis, left upper arm
	M65.929	Unspecified synovitis and tenosynovitis, unspecified upper arm
✓6th M65.93		Unspecified synovitis and tenosynovitis, forearm
	M65.931	Unspecified synovitis and tenosynovitis, right forearm
	M65.932	Unspecified synovitis and tenosynovitis, left forearm
	M65.939	Unspecified synovitis and tenosynovitis, unspecified forearm
✓6th M65.94		Unspecified synovitis and tenosynovitis, hand
	M65.941	Unspecified synovitis and tenosynovitis, right hand
	M65.942	Unspecified synovitis and tenosynovitis, left hand
	M65.949	Unspecified synovitis and tenosynovitis, unspecified hand
✓6th M65.95		Unspecified synovitis and tenosynovitis, thigh
	M65.951	Unspecified synovitis and tenosynovitis, right thigh
	M65.952	Unspecified synovitis and tenosynovitis, left thigh
	M65.959	Unspecified synovitis and tenosynovitis, unspecified thigh
✓6th M65.96		Unspecified synovitis and tenosynovitis, lower leg
	M65.961	Unspecified synovitis and tenosynovitis, right lower leg
	M65.962	Unspecified synovitis and tenosynovitis, left lower leg
	M65.969	Unspecified synovitis and tenosynovitis, unspecified lower leg
✓6th M65.97		Unspecified synovitis and tenosynovitis, ankle and foot
	M65.971	Unspecified synovitis and tenosynovitis, right ankle and foot
	M65.972	Unspecified synovitis and tenosynovitis, left ankle and foot
	M65.979	Unspecified synovitis and tenosynovitis, unspecified ankle and foot
	M65.98	Unspecified synovitis and tenosynovitis, other site
	M65.99	Unspecified synovitis and tenosynovitis, multiple sites

✓4th **M66 Spontaneous rupture of synovium and tendon**

INCLUDES rupture that occurs when a normal force is applied to tissues that are inferred to have less than normal strength

EXCLUDES 2 rotator cuff syndrome (M75.1-)
rupture where an abnormal force is applied to normal tissue - see injury of tendon by body region

	M66.0	Rupture of popliteal cyst
✓5th M66.1		Rupture of synovium

Rupture of synovial cyst
EXCLUDES 2 rupture of popliteal cyst (M66.0)

	M66.10	Rupture of synovium, unspecified joint
✓6th M66.11		Rupture of synovium, shoulder
	M66.111	Rupture of synovium, right shoulder
	M66.112	Rupture of synovium, left shoulder
	M66.119	Rupture of synovium, unspecified shoulder
✓6th M66.12		Rupture of synovium, elbow
	M66.121	Rupture of synovium, right elbow
	M66.122	Rupture of synovium, left elbow
	M66.129	Rupture of synovium, unspecified elbow
✓6th M66.13		Rupture of synovium, wrist
	M66.131	Rupture of synovium, right wrist
	M66.132	Rupture of synovium, left wrist
	M66.139	Rupture of synovium, unspecified wrist
✓6th M66.14		Rupture of synovium, hand and fingers
	M66.141	Rupture of synovium, right hand
	M66.142	Rupture of synovium, left hand
	M66.143	Rupture of synovium, unspecified hand
	M66.144	Rupture of synovium, right finger(s)
	M66.145	Rupture of synovium, left finger(s)
	M66.146	Rupture of synovium, unspecified finger(s)
✓6th M66.15		Rupture of synovium, hip
	M66.151	Rupture of synovium, right hip
	M66.152	Rupture of synovium, left hip
	M66.159	Rupture of synovium, unspecified hip
✓6th M66.17		Rupture of synovium, ankle, foot and toes
	M66.171	Rupture of synovium, right ankle
	M66.172	Rupture of synovium, left ankle
	M66.173	Rupture of synovium, unspecified ankle
	M66.174	Rupture of synovium, right foot
	M66.175	Rupture of synovium, left foot
	M66.176	Rupture of synovium, unspecified foot
	M66.177	Rupture of synovium, right toe(s)
	M66.178	Rupture of synovium, left toe(s)
	M66.179	Rupture of synovium, unspecified toe(s)
	M66.18	Rupture of synovium, other site
✓5th M66.2		**Spontaneous rupture of extensor tendons**

TIP: Refer to the Muscle/Tendon table at the beginning of this chapter.

	M66.20	Spontaneous rupture of extensor tendons, unspecified site
✓6th M66.21		Spontaneous rupture of extensor tendons, shoulder
	M66.211	Spontaneous rupture of extensor tendons, right shoulder
	M66.212	Spontaneous rupture of extensor tendons, left shoulder
	M66.219	Spontaneous rupture of extensor tendons, unspecified shoulder
✓6th M66.22		Spontaneous rupture of extensor tendons, upper arm
	M66.221	Spontaneous rupture of extensor tendons, right upper arm
	M66.222	Spontaneous rupture of extensor tendons, left upper arm
	M66.229	Spontaneous rupture of extensor tendons, unspecified upper arm
✓6th M66.23		Spontaneous rupture of extensor tendons, forearm
	M66.231	Spontaneous rupture of extensor tendons, right forearm
	M66.232	Spontaneous rupture of extensor tendons, left forearm
	M66.239	Spontaneous rupture of extensor tendons, unspecified forearm
✓6th M66.24		Spontaneous rupture of extensor tendons, hand
	M66.241	Spontaneous rupture of extensor tendons, right hand
	M66.242	Spontaneous rupture of extensor tendons, left hand
	M66.249	Spontaneous rupture of extensor tendons, unspecified hand
✓6th M66.25		Spontaneous rupture of extensor tendons, thigh
	M66.251	Spontaneous rupture of extensor tendons, right thigh
	M66.252	Spontaneous rupture of extensor tendons, left thigh
	M66.259	Spontaneous rupture of extensor tendons, unspecified thigh
✓6th M66.26		Spontaneous rupture of extensor tendons, lower leg
	M66.261	Spontaneous rupture of extensor tendons, right lower leg
	M66.262	Spontaneous rupture of extensor tendons, left lower leg
	M66.269	Spontaneous rupture of extensor tendons, unspecified lower leg
✓6th M66.27		Spontaneous rupture of extensor tendons, ankle and foot
	M66.271	Spontaneous rupture of extensor tendons, right ankle and foot
	M66.272	Spontaneous rupture of extensor tendons, left ankle and foot
	M66.279	Spontaneous rupture of extensor tendons, unspecified ankle and foot
	M66.28	Spontaneous rupture of extensor tendons, other site
	M66.29	Spontaneous rupture of extensor tendons, multiple sites

Chapter 13. Diseases of the Musculoskeletal System and Connective Tissue

✓5th **M66.3 Spontaneous rupture of flexor tendons**
   TIP: Refer to the Muscle/Tendon table at the beginning of this chapter.
   - M66.30 Spontaneous rupture of flexor tendons, unspecified site
   - ✓6th M66.31 Spontaneous rupture of flexor tendons, shoulder
      - M66.311 Spontaneous rupture of flexor tendons, right shoulder
      - M66.312 Spontaneous rupture of flexor tendons, left shoulder
      - M66.319 Spontaneous rupture of flexor tendons, unspecified shoulder
   - ✓6th M66.32 Spontaneous rupture of flexor tendons, upper arm
      - M66.321 Spontaneous rupture of flexor tendons, right upper arm
      - M66.322 Spontaneous rupture of flexor tendons, left upper arm
      - M66.329 Spontaneous rupture of flexor tendons, unspecified upper arm
   - ✓6th M66.33 Spontaneous rupture of flexor tendons, forearm
      - M66.331 Spontaneous rupture of flexor tendons, right forearm
      - M66.332 Spontaneous rupture of flexor tendons, left forearm
      - M66.339 Spontaneous rupture of flexor tendons, unspecified forearm
   - ✓6th M66.34 Spontaneous rupture of flexor tendons, hand
      - M66.341 Spontaneous rupture of flexor tendons, right hand
      - M66.342 Spontaneous rupture of flexor tendons, left hand
      - M66.349 Spontaneous rupture of flexor tendons, unspecified hand
   - ✓6th M66.35 Spontaneous rupture of flexor tendons, thigh
      - M66.351 Spontaneous rupture of flexor tendons, right thigh
      - M66.352 Spontaneous rupture of flexor tendons, left thigh
      - M66.359 Spontaneous rupture of flexor tendons, unspecified thigh
   - ✓6th M66.36 Spontaneous rupture of flexor tendons, lower leg
      - M66.361 Spontaneous rupture of flexor tendons, right lower leg
      - M66.362 Spontaneous rupture of flexor tendons, left lower leg
      - M66.369 Spontaneous rupture of flexor tendons, unspecified lower leg
   - ✓6th M66.37 Spontaneous rupture of flexor tendons, ankle and foot
      - M66.371 Spontaneous rupture of flexor tendons, right ankle and foot
      - M66.372 Spontaneous rupture of flexor tendons, left ankle and foot
      - M66.379 Spontaneous rupture of flexor tendons, unspecified ankle and foot
   - M66.38 Spontaneous rupture of flexor tendons, other site
   - M66.39 Spontaneous rupture of flexor tendons, multiple sites

✓5th **M66.8 Spontaneous rupture of other tendons**
   TIP: Refer to the Muscle/Tendon table at the beginning of this chapter.
   - M66.80 Spontaneous rupture of other tendons, unspecified site
   - ✓6th M66.81 Spontaneous rupture of other tendons, shoulder
      - M66.811 Spontaneous rupture of other tendons, right shoulder
      - M66.812 Spontaneous rupture of other tendons, left shoulder
      - M66.819 Spontaneous rupture of other tendons, unspecified shoulder
   - ✓6th M66.82 Spontaneous rupture of other tendons, upper arm
      - M66.821 Spontaneous rupture of other tendons, right upper arm
      - M66.822 Spontaneous rupture of other tendons, left upper arm
      - M66.829 Spontaneous rupture of other tendons, unspecified upper arm
   - ✓6th M66.83 Spontaneous rupture of other tendons, forearm
      - M66.831 Spontaneous rupture of other tendons, right forearm
      - M66.832 Spontaneous rupture of other tendons, left forearm
      - M66.839 Spontaneous rupture of other tendons, unspecified forearm
   - ✓6th M66.84 Spontaneous rupture of other tendons, hand
      - M66.841 Spontaneous rupture of other tendons, right hand
      - M66.842 Spontaneous rupture of other tendons, left hand
      - M66.849 Spontaneous rupture of other tendons, unspecified hand
   - ✓6th M66.85 Spontaneous rupture of other tendons, thigh
      - M66.851 Spontaneous rupture of other tendons, right thigh
      - M66.852 Spontaneous rupture of other tendons, left thigh
      - M66.859 Spontaneous rupture of other tendons, unspecified thigh
   - ✓6th M66.86 Spontaneous rupture of other tendons, lower leg
      - M66.861 Spontaneous rupture of other tendons, right lower leg
      - M66.862 Spontaneous rupture of other tendons, left lower leg
      - M66.869 Spontaneous rupture of other tendons, unspecified lower leg
   - ✓6th M66.87 Spontaneous rupture of other tendons, ankle and foot
      - M66.871 Spontaneous rupture of other tendons, right ankle and foot
      - M66.872 Spontaneous rupture of other tendons, left ankle and foot
      - M66.879 Spontaneous rupture of other tendons, unspecified ankle and foot
   - M66.88 Spontaneous rupture of other tendons, other sites
   - M66.89 Spontaneous rupture of other tendons, multiple sites

M66.9 Spontaneous rupture of unspecified tendon
   Rupture at musculotendinous junction, nontraumatic

✓4th **M67 Other disorders of synovium and tendon**
   EXCLUDES 1: palmar fascial fibromatosis [Dupuytren] (M72.0)
   tendinitis NOS (M77.9-)
   xanthomatosis localized to tendons (E78.2)

   ✓5th **M67.0 Short Achilles tendon (acquired)**
      - M67.00 Short Achilles tendon (acquired), unspecified ankle
      - M67.01 Short Achilles tendon (acquired), right ankle
      - M67.02 Short Achilles tendon (acquired), left ankle

   ✓5th **M67.2 Synovial hypertrophy, not elsewhere classified**
      EXCLUDES 1: villonodular synovitis (pigmented) (M12.2-)
      - M67.20 Synovial hypertrophy, not elsewhere classified, unspecified site
      - ✓6th M67.21 Synovial hypertrophy, not elsewhere classified, shoulder
         - M67.211 Synovial hypertrophy, not elsewhere classified, right shoulder
         - M67.212 Synovial hypertrophy, not elsewhere classified, left shoulder
         - M67.219 Synovial hypertrophy, not elsewhere classified, unspecified shoulder
      - ✓6th M67.22 Synovial hypertrophy, not elsewhere classified, upper arm
         - M67.221 Synovial hypertrophy, not elsewhere classified, right upper arm
         - M67.222 Synovial hypertrophy, not elsewhere classified, left upper arm
         - M67.229 Synovial hypertrophy, not elsewhere classified, unspecified upper arm
      - ✓6th M67.23 Synovial hypertrophy, not elsewhere classified, forearm
         - M67.231 Synovial hypertrophy, not elsewhere classified, right forearm
         - M67.232 Synovial hypertrophy, not elsewhere classified, left forearm
         - M67.239 Synovial hypertrophy, not elsewhere classified, unspecified forearm
      - ✓6th M67.24 Synovial hypertrophy, not elsewhere classified, hand
         - M67.241 Synovial hypertrophy, not elsewhere classified, right hand
         - M67.242 Synovial hypertrophy, not elsewhere classified, left hand
         - M67.249 Synovial hypertrophy, not elsewhere classified, unspecified hand

M67.25–M67.829 Chapter 13. Diseases of the Musculoskeletal System and Connective Tissue

- ✓6th **M67.25** Synovial hypertrophy, not elsewhere classified, thigh
  - M67.251 Synovial hypertrophy, not elsewhere classified, right thigh
  - M67.252 Synovial hypertrophy, not elsewhere classified, left thigh
  - M67.259 Synovial hypertrophy, not elsewhere classified, unspecified thigh
- ✓6th **M67.26** Synovial hypertrophy, not elsewhere classified, lower leg
  - M67.261 Synovial hypertrophy, not elsewhere classified, right lower leg
  - M67.262 Synovial hypertrophy, not elsewhere classified, left lower leg
  - M67.269 Synovial hypertrophy, not elsewhere classified, unspecified lower leg
- ✓6th **M67.27** Synovial hypertrophy, not elsewhere classified, ankle and foot
  - M67.271 Synovial hypertrophy, not elsewhere classified, right ankle and foot
  - M67.272 Synovial hypertrophy, not elsewhere classified, left ankle and foot
  - M67.279 Synovial hypertrophy, not elsewhere classified, unspecified ankle and foot
- **M67.28** Synovial hypertrophy, not elsewhere classified, other site
- **M67.29** Synovial hypertrophy, not elsewhere classified, multiple sites
- ✓5th **M67.3** Transient synovitis
  - Toxic synovitis
  - EXCLUDES 1   palindromic rheumatism (M12.3-)
  - **M67.30** Transient synovitis, unspecified site
  - ✓6th **M67.31** Transient synovitis, shoulder
    - M67.311 Transient synovitis, right shoulder
    - M67.312 Transient synovitis, left shoulder
    - M67.319 Transient synovitis, unspecified shoulder
  - ✓6th **M67.32** Transient synovitis, elbow
    - M67.321 Transient synovitis, right elbow
    - M67.322 Transient synovitis, left elbow
    - M67.329 Transient synovitis, unspecified elbow
  - ✓6th **M67.33** Transient synovitis, wrist
    - M67.331 Transient synovitis, right wrist
    - M67.332 Transient synovitis, left wrist
    - M67.339 Transient synovitis, unspecified wrist
  - ✓6th **M67.34** Transient synovitis, hand
    - M67.341 Transient synovitis, right hand
    - M67.342 Transient synovitis, left hand
    - M67.349 Transient synovitis, unspecified hand
  - ✓6th **M67.35** Transient synovitis, hip
    - M67.351 Transient synovitis, right hip
    - M67.352 Transient synovitis, left hip
    - M67.359 Transient synovitis, unspecified hip
  - ✓6th **M67.36** Transient synovitis, knee
    - M67.361 Transient synovitis, right knee
    - M67.362 Transient synovitis, left knee
    - M67.369 Transient synovitis, unspecified knee
  - ✓6th **M67.37** Transient synovitis, ankle and foot
    - M67.371 Transient synovitis, right ankle and foot
    - M67.372 Transient synovitis, left ankle and foot
    - M67.379 Transient synovitis, unspecified ankle and foot
  - **M67.38** Transient synovitis, other site
  - **M67.39** Transient synovitis, multiple sites
- ✓5th **M67.4** Ganglion
  - Ganglion of joint or tendon (sheath)
  - EXCLUDES 1   ganglion in yaws (A66.6)
  - EXCLUDES 2   cyst of bursa (M71.2-M71.3)
  -             cyst of synovium (M71.2-M71.3)
  - **DEF:** Fluid-filled, benign cyst appearing on a tendon sheath or aponeurosis, frequently connecting to an underlying joint.
  - **M67.40** Ganglion, unspecified site
  - ✓6th **M67.41** Ganglion, shoulder
    - M67.411 Ganglion, right shoulder
    - M67.412 Ganglion, left shoulder
    - M67.419 Ganglion, unspecified shoulder
  - ✓6th **M67.42** Ganglion, elbow
    - M67.421 Ganglion, right elbow
    - M67.422 Ganglion, left elbow
    - M67.429 Ganglion, unspecified elbow
  - ✓6th **M67.43** Ganglion, wrist

Ganglion of Wrist

- M67.431 Ganglion, right wrist
- M67.432 Ganglion, left wrist
- M67.439 Ganglion, unspecified wrist
- ✓6th **M67.44** Ganglion, hand
  - M67.441 Ganglion, right hand
  - M67.442 Ganglion, left hand
  - M67.449 Ganglion, unspecified hand
- ✓6th **M67.45** Ganglion, hip
  - M67.451 Ganglion, right hip
  - M67.452 Ganglion, left hip
  - M67.459 Ganglion, unspecified hip
- ✓6th **M67.46** Ganglion, knee
  - M67.461 Ganglion, right knee
  - M67.462 Ganglion, left knee
  - M67.469 Ganglion, unspecified knee
- ✓6th **M67.47** Ganglion, ankle and foot
  - M67.471 Ganglion, right ankle and foot
  - M67.472 Ganglion, left ankle and foot
  - M67.479 Ganglion, unspecified ankle and foot
- **M67.48** Ganglion, other site
- **M67.49** Ganglion, multiple sites
- ✓5th **M67.5** Plica syndrome
  - Plica knee
  - **M67.50** Plica syndrome, unspecified knee
  - **M67.51** Plica syndrome, right knee
  - **M67.52** Plica syndrome, left knee
- ✓5th **M67.8** Other specified disorders of synovium and tendon
  - **M67.80** Other specified disorders of synovium and tendon, unspecified site
  - ✓6th **M67.81** Other specified disorders of synovium and tendon, shoulder
    - M67.811 Other specified disorders of synovium, right shoulder
    - M67.812 Other specified disorders of synovium, left shoulder
    - M67.813 Other specified disorders of tendon, right shoulder
    - M67.814 Other specified disorders of tendon, left shoulder
    - M67.819 Other specified disorders of synovium and tendon, unspecified shoulder
  - ✓6th **M67.82** Other specified disorders of synovium and tendon, elbow
    - M67.821 Other specified disorders of synovium, right elbow
    - M67.822 Other specified disorders of synovium, left elbow
    - M67.823 Other specified disorders of tendon, right elbow
    - M67.824 Other specified disorders of tendon, left elbow
    - M67.829 Other specified disorders of synovium and tendon, unspecified elbow

	✓6th	**M67.83**	Other specified disorders of synovium and tendon, wrist
		M67.831	Other specified disorders of synovium, right wrist
		M67.832	Other specified disorders of synovium, left wrist
		M67.833	Other specified disorders of tendon, right wrist
		M67.834	Other specified disorders of tendon, left wrist
		M67.839	Other specified disorders of synovium and tendon, unspecified wrist
	✓6th	**M67.84**	Other specified disorders of synovium and tendon, hand
		M67.841	Other specified disorders of synovium, right hand
		M67.842	Other specified disorders of synovium, left hand
		M67.843	Other specified disorders of tendon, right hand
		M67.844	Other specified disorders of tendon, left hand
		M67.849	Other specified disorders of synovium and tendon, unspecified hand
	✓6th	**M67.85**	Other specified disorders of synovium and tendon, hip
		M67.851	Other specified disorders of synovium, right hip
		M67.852	Other specified disorders of synovium, left hip
		M67.853	Other specified disorders of tendon, right hip
		M67.854	Other specified disorders of tendon, left hip
		M67.859	Other specified disorders of synovium and tendon, unspecified hip
	✓6th	**M67.86**	Other specified disorders of synovium and tendon, knee
		M67.861	Other specified disorders of synovium, right knee
		M67.862	Other specified disorders of synovium, left knee
		M67.863	Other specified disorders of tendon, right knee
		M67.864	Other specified disorders of tendon, left knee
		M67.869	Other specified disorders of synovium and tendon, unspecified knee
	✓6th	**M67.87**	Other specified disorders of synovium and tendon, ankle and foot
		M67.871	Other specified disorders of synovium, right ankle and foot
		M67.872	Other specified disorders of synovium, left ankle and foot
		M67.873	Other specified disorders of tendon, right ankle and foot
		M67.874	Other specified disorders of tendon, left ankle and foot
		M67.879	Other specified disorders of synovium and tendon, unspecified ankle and foot
		M67.88	Other specified disorders of synovium and tendon, other site
		M67.89	Other specified disorders of synovium and tendon, multiple sites
✓5th	**M67.9**		Unspecified disorder of synovium and tendon
		M67.90	Unspecified disorder of synovium and tendon, unspecified site
	✓6th	**M67.91**	Unspecified disorder of synovium and tendon, shoulder
		M67.911	Unspecified disorder of synovium and tendon, right shoulder
		M67.912	Unspecified disorder of synovium and tendon, left shoulder
		M67.919	Unspecified disorder of synovium and tendon, unspecified shoulder
	✓6th	**M67.92**	Unspecified disorder of synovium and tendon, upper arm
		M67.921	Unspecified disorder of synovium and tendon, right upper arm
		M67.922	Unspecified disorder of synovium and tendon, left upper arm
		M67.929	Unspecified disorder of synovium and tendon, unspecified upper arm
	✓6th	**M67.93**	Unspecified disorder of synovium and tendon, forearm
		M67.931	Unspecified disorder of synovium and tendon, right forearm
		M67.932	Unspecified disorder of synovium and tendon, left forearm
		M67.939	Unspecified disorder of synovium and tendon, unspecified forearm
	✓6th	**M67.94**	Unspecified disorder of synovium and tendon, hand
		M67.941	Unspecified disorder of synovium and tendon, right hand
		M67.942	Unspecified disorder of synovium and tendon, left hand
		M67.949	Unspecified disorder of synovium and tendon, unspecified hand
	✓6th	**M67.95**	Unspecified disorder of synovium and tendon, thigh
		M67.951	Unspecified disorder of synovium and tendon, right thigh
		M67.952	Unspecified disorder of synovium and tendon, left thigh
		M67.959	Unspecified disorder of synovium and tendon, unspecified thigh
	✓6th	**M67.96**	Unspecified disorder of synovium and tendon, lower leg
		M67.961	Unspecified disorder of synovium and tendon, right lower leg
		M67.962	Unspecified disorder of synovium and tendon, left lower leg
		M67.969	Unspecified disorder of synovium and tendon, unspecified lower leg
	✓6th	**M67.97**	Unspecified disorder of synovium and tendon, ankle and foot
		M67.971	Unspecified disorder of synovium and tendon, right ankle and foot
		M67.972	Unspecified disorder of synovium and tendon, left ankle and foot
		M67.979	Unspecified disorder of synovium and tendon, unspecified ankle and foot
		M67.98	Unspecified disorder of synovium and tendon, other site
		M67.99	Unspecified disorder of synovium and tendon, multiple sites

Other soft tissue disorders (M70-M79)

✓4th **M70** Soft tissue disorders related to use, overuse and pressure

    INCLUDES soft tissue disorders of occupational origin

    Use additional external cause code to identify activity causing disorder (Y93.-)

    EXCLUDES 1 bursitis NOS (M71.9-)
    EXCLUDES 2 bursitis of shoulder (M75.5)
                    enthesopathies (M76-M77)
                    pressure ulcer (pressure area) (L89.-)

	✓5th	**M70.0**		Crepitant synovitis (acute) (chronic) of hand and wrist
		✓6th	**M70.03**	Crepitant synovitis (acute) (chronic), wrist
			M70.031	Crepitant synovitis (acute) (chronic), right wrist
			M70.032	Crepitant synovitis (acute) (chronic), left wrist
			M70.039	Crepitant synovitis (acute) (chronic), unspecified wrist
		✓6th	**M70.04**	Crepitant synovitis (acute) (chronic), hand
			M70.041	Crepitant synovitis (acute) (chronic), right hand
			M70.042	Crepitant synovitis (acute) (chronic), left hand
			M70.049	Crepitant synovitis (acute) (chronic), unspecified hand
	✓5th	**M70.1**		Bursitis of hand
			M70.10	Bursitis, unspecified hand
			M70.11	Bursitis, right hand
			M70.12	Bursitis, left hand
	✓5th	**M70.2**		Olecranon bursitis
			M70.20	Olecranon bursitis, unspecified elbow
			M70.21	Olecranon bursitis, right elbow
			M70.22	Olecranon bursitis, left elbow
	✓5th	**M70.3**		Other bursitis of elbow
			M70.30	Other bursitis of elbow, unspecified elbow
			M70.31	Other bursitis of elbow, right elbow
			M70.32	Other bursitis of elbow, left elbow

✅ Additional Character Required   ✓x7th Placeholder Alert   Manifestation   Unspecified Dx   Q QPP   UPD Unacceptable PDx

M70.4 Prepatellar bursitis
- M70.40 Prepatellar bursitis, unspecified knee
- M70.41 Prepatellar bursitis, right knee
- M70.42 Prepatellar bursitis, left knee

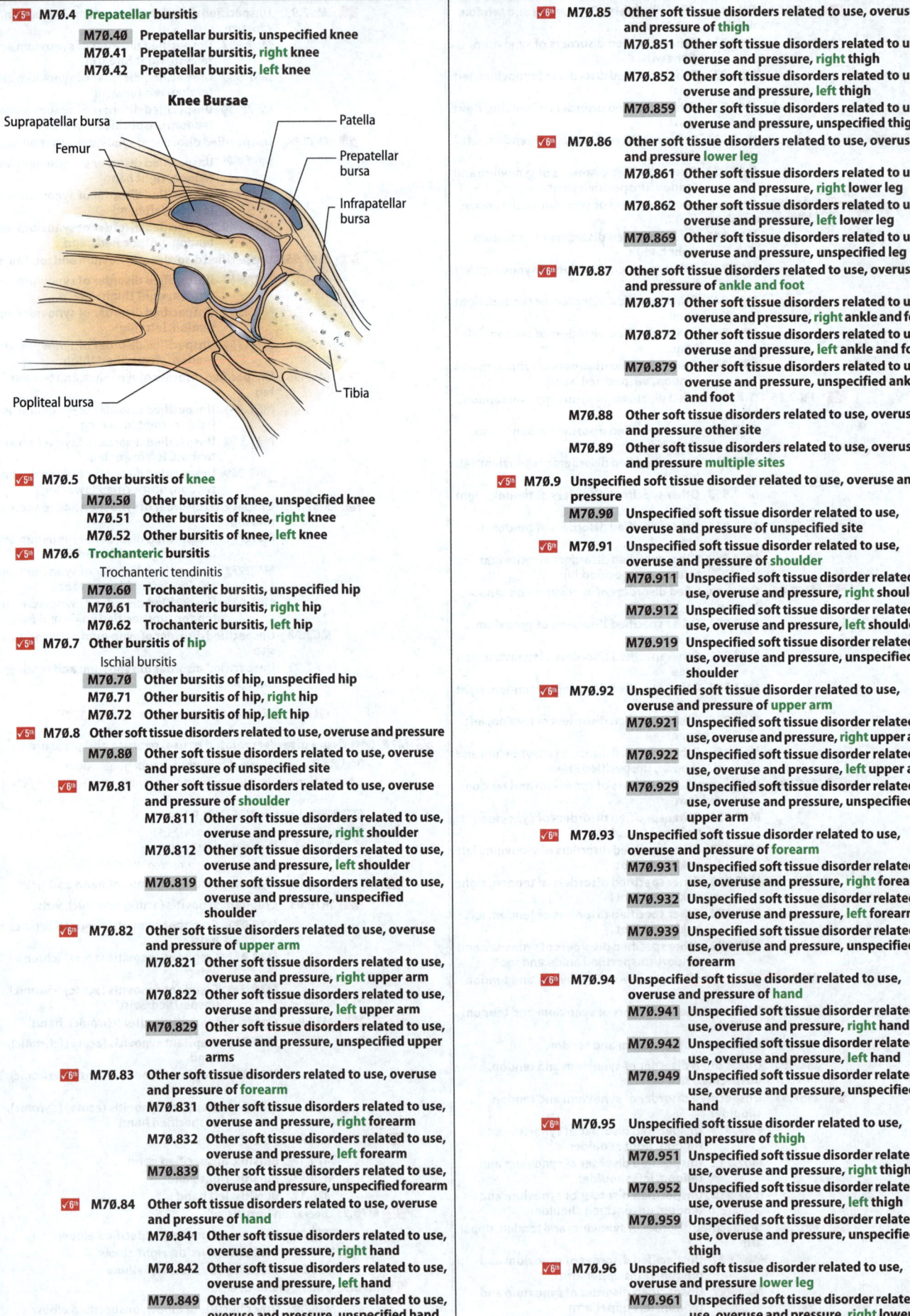

Knee Bursae

M70.5 Other bursitis of knee
- M70.50 Other bursitis of knee, unspecified knee
- M70.51 Other bursitis of knee, right knee
- M70.52 Other bursitis of knee, left knee

M70.6 Trochanteric bursitis
Trochanteric tendinitis
- M70.60 Trochanteric bursitis, unspecified hip
- M70.61 Trochanteric bursitis, right hip
- M70.62 Trochanteric bursitis, left hip

M70.7 Other bursitis of hip
Ischial bursitis
- M70.70 Other bursitis of hip, unspecified hip
- M70.71 Other bursitis of hip, right hip
- M70.72 Other bursitis of hip, left hip

M70.8 Other soft tissue disorders related to use, overuse and pressure
- M70.80 Other soft tissue disorders related to use, overuse and pressure of unspecified site
- M70.81 Other soft tissue disorders related to use, overuse and pressure of shoulder
  - M70.811 Other soft tissue disorders related to use, overuse and pressure, right shoulder
  - M70.812 Other soft tissue disorders related to use, overuse and pressure, left shoulder
  - M70.819 Other soft tissue disorders related to use, overuse and pressure, unspecified shoulder
- M70.82 Other soft tissue disorders related to use, overuse and pressure of upper arm
  - M70.821 Other soft tissue disorders related to use, overuse and pressure, right upper arm
  - M70.822 Other soft tissue disorders related to use, overuse and pressure, left upper arm
  - M70.829 Other soft tissue disorders related to use, overuse and pressure, unspecified upper arms
- M70.83 Other soft tissue disorders related to use, overuse and pressure of forearm
  - M70.831 Other soft tissue disorders related to use, overuse and pressure, right forearm
  - M70.832 Other soft tissue disorders related to use, overuse and pressure, left forearm
  - M70.839 Other soft tissue disorders related to use, overuse and pressure, unspecified forearm
- M70.84 Other soft tissue disorders related to use, overuse and pressure of hand
  - M70.841 Other soft tissue disorders related to use, overuse and pressure, right hand
  - M70.842 Other soft tissue disorders related to use, overuse and pressure, left hand
  - M70.849 Other soft tissue disorders related to use, overuse and pressure, unspecified hand
- M70.85 Other soft tissue disorders related to use, overuse and pressure of thigh
  - M70.851 Other soft tissue disorders related to use, overuse and pressure, right thigh
  - M70.852 Other soft tissue disorders related to use, overuse and pressure, left thigh
  - M70.859 Other soft tissue disorders related to use, overuse and pressure, unspecified thigh
- M70.86 Other soft tissue disorders related to use, overuse and pressure lower leg
  - M70.861 Other soft tissue disorders related to use, overuse and pressure, right lower leg
  - M70.862 Other soft tissue disorders related to use, overuse and pressure, left lower leg
  - M70.869 Other soft tissue disorders related to use, overuse and pressure, unspecified leg
- M70.87 Other soft tissue disorders related to use, overuse and pressure of ankle and foot
  - M70.871 Other soft tissue disorders related to use, overuse and pressure, right ankle and foot
  - M70.872 Other soft tissue disorders related to use, overuse and pressure, left ankle and foot
  - M70.879 Other soft tissue disorders related to use, overuse and pressure, unspecified ankle and foot
- M70.88 Other soft tissue disorders related to use, overuse and pressure other site
- M70.89 Other soft tissue disorders related to use, overuse and pressure multiple sites

M70.9 Unspecified soft tissue disorder related to use, overuse and pressure
- M70.90 Unspecified soft tissue disorder related to use, overuse and pressure of unspecified site
- M70.91 Unspecified soft tissue disorder related to use, overuse and pressure of shoulder
  - M70.911 Unspecified soft tissue disorder related to use, overuse and pressure, right shoulder
  - M70.912 Unspecified soft tissue disorder related to use, overuse and pressure, left shoulder
  - M70.919 Unspecified soft tissue disorder related to use, overuse and pressure, unspecified shoulder
- M70.92 Unspecified soft tissue disorder related to use, overuse and pressure of upper arm
  - M70.921 Unspecified soft tissue disorder related to use, overuse and pressure, right upper arm
  - M70.922 Unspecified soft tissue disorder related to use, overuse and pressure, left upper arm
  - M70.929 Unspecified soft tissue disorder related to use, overuse and pressure, unspecified upper arm
- M70.93 Unspecified soft tissue disorder related to use, overuse and pressure of forearm
  - M70.931 Unspecified soft tissue disorder related to use, overuse and pressure, right forearm
  - M70.932 Unspecified soft tissue disorder related to use, overuse and pressure, left forearm
  - M70.939 Unspecified soft tissue disorder related to use, overuse and pressure, unspecified forearm
- M70.94 Unspecified soft tissue disorder related to use, overuse and pressure of hand
  - M70.941 Unspecified soft tissue disorder related to use, overuse and pressure, right hand
  - M70.942 Unspecified soft tissue disorder related to use, overuse and pressure, left hand
  - M70.949 Unspecified soft tissue disorder related to use, overuse and pressure, unspecified hand
- M70.95 Unspecified soft tissue disorder related to use, overuse and pressure of thigh
  - M70.951 Unspecified soft tissue disorder related to use, overuse and pressure, right thigh
  - M70.952 Unspecified soft tissue disorder related to use, overuse and pressure, left thigh
  - M70.959 Unspecified soft tissue disorder related to use, overuse and pressure, unspecified thigh
- M70.96 Unspecified soft tissue disorder related to use, overuse and pressure lower leg
  - M70.961 Unspecified soft tissue disorder related to use, overuse and pressure, right lower leg
  - M70.962 Unspecified soft tissue disorder related to use, overuse and pressure, left lower leg

M70.969 Unspecified soft tissue disorder related to use, overuse and pressure, unspecified lower leg

M70.97 Unspecified soft tissue disorder related to use, overuse and pressure of ankle and foot
    M70.971 Unspecified soft tissue disorder related to use, overuse and pressure, right ankle and foot
    M70.972 Unspecified soft tissue disorder related to use, overuse and pressure, left ankle and foot
    M70.979 Unspecified soft tissue disorder related to use, overuse and pressure, unspecified ankle and foot

M70.98 Unspecified soft tissue disorder related to use, overuse and pressure other

M70.99 Unspecified soft tissue disorder related to use, overuse and pressure multiple sites

M71 Other bursopathies

EXCLUDES 1: bunion (M20.1)
bursitis related to use, overuse or pressure (M70.-)
enthesopathies (M76-M77)

M71.0 Abscess of bursa
Use additional code (B95.-, B96.-) to identify causative organism

  M71.00 Abscess of bursa, unspecified site
  M71.01 Abscess of bursa, shoulder
    M71.011 Abscess of bursa, right shoulder
    M71.012 Abscess of bursa, left shoulder
    M71.019 Abscess of bursa, unspecified shoulder
  M71.02 Abscess of bursa, elbow
    M71.021 Abscess of bursa, right elbow
    M71.022 Abscess of bursa, left elbow
    M71.029 Abscess of bursa, unspecified elbow
  M71.03 Abscess of bursa, wrist
    M71.031 Abscess of bursa, right wrist
    M71.032 Abscess of bursa, left wrist
    M71.039 Abscess of bursa, unspecified wrist
  M71.04 Abscess of bursa, hand
    M71.041 Abscess of bursa, right hand
    M71.042 Abscess of bursa, left hand
    M71.049 Abscess of bursa, unspecified hand
  M71.05 Abscess of bursa, hip
    M71.051 Abscess of bursa, right hip
    M71.052 Abscess of bursa, left hip
    M71.059 Abscess of bursa, unspecified hip
  M71.06 Abscess of bursa, knee
    M71.061 Abscess of bursa, right knee
    M71.062 Abscess of bursa, left knee
    M71.069 Abscess of bursa, unspecified knee
  M71.07 Abscess of bursa, ankle and foot
    M71.071 Abscess of bursa, right ankle and foot
    M71.072 Abscess of bursa, left ankle and foot
    M71.079 Abscess of bursa, unspecified ankle and foot
  M71.08 Abscess of bursa, other site
  M71.09 Abscess of bursa, multiple sites

M71.1 Other infective bursitis
Use additional code (B95.-, B96.-) to identify causative organism

  M71.10 Other infective bursitis, unspecified site
  M71.11 Other infective bursitis, shoulder
    M71.111 Other infective bursitis, right shoulder
    M71.112 Other infective bursitis, left shoulder
    M71.119 Other infective bursitis, unspecified shoulder
  M71.12 Other infective bursitis, elbow
    M71.121 Other infective bursitis, right elbow
    M71.122 Other infective bursitis, left elbow
    M71.129 Other infective bursitis, unspecified elbow
  M71.13 Other infective bursitis, wrist
    M71.131 Other infective bursitis, right wrist
    M71.132 Other infective bursitis, left wrist
    M71.139 Other infective bursitis, unspecified wrist
  M71.14 Other infective bursitis, hand
    M71.141 Other infective bursitis, right hand
    M71.142 Other infective bursitis, left hand
    M71.149 Other infective bursitis, unspecified hand
  M71.15 Other infective bursitis, hip
    M71.151 Other infective bursitis, right hip
    M71.152 Other infective bursitis, left hip
    M71.159 Other infective bursitis, unspecified hip
  M71.16 Other infective bursitis, knee
    M71.161 Other infective bursitis, right knee
    M71.162 Other infective bursitis, left knee
    M71.169 Other infective bursitis, unspecified knee
  M71.17 Other infective bursitis, ankle and foot
    M71.171 Other infective bursitis, right ankle and foot
    M71.172 Other infective bursitis, left ankle and foot
    M71.179 Other infective bursitis, unspecified ankle and foot
  M71.18 Other infective bursitis, other site
  M71.19 Other infective bursitis, multiple sites

M71.2 Synovial cyst of popliteal space [Baker]
EXCLUDES 1: synovial cyst of popliteal space with rupture (M66.0)
DEF: Sac filled with clear synovial fluid in adults, usually secondary to disease inside the joint, located on the back of the knee in the popliteal fossa area. In children, the cyst usually represents a ganglion of one of the tendons in the knee.

Baker's Cyst

Baker's cyst connected to knee joint synovial cavity

  M71.20 Synovial cyst of popliteal space [Baker], unspecified knee
  M71.21 Synovial cyst of popliteal space [Baker], right knee
  M71.22 Synovial cyst of popliteal space [Baker], left knee

M71.3 Other bursal cyst
Synovial cyst NOS
EXCLUDES 1: synovial cyst with rupture (M66.1-)

  M71.30 Other bursal cyst, unspecified site
  M71.31 Other bursal cyst, shoulder
    M71.311 Other bursal cyst, right shoulder
    M71.312 Other bursal cyst, left shoulder
    M71.319 Other bursal cyst, unspecified shoulder
  M71.32 Other bursal cyst, elbow
    M71.321 Other bursal cyst, right elbow
    M71.322 Other bursal cyst, left elbow
    M71.329 Other bursal cyst, unspecified elbow
  M71.33 Other bursal cyst, wrist
    M71.331 Other bursal cyst, right wrist
    M71.332 Other bursal cyst, left wrist
    M71.339 Other bursal cyst, unspecified wrist
  M71.34 Other bursal cyst, hand
    M71.341 Other bursal cyst, right hand
    M71.342 Other bursal cyst, left hand
    M71.349 Other bursal cyst, unspecified hand
  M71.35 Other bursal cyst, hip
    M71.351 Other bursal cyst, right hip
    M71.352 Other bursal cyst, left hip
    M71.359 Other bursal cyst, unspecified hip
  M71.37 Other bursal cyst, ankle and foot
    M71.371 Other bursal cyst, right ankle and foot
    M71.372 Other bursal cyst, left ankle and foot

Chapter 13. Diseases of the Musculoskeletal System and Connective Tissue

M71.379 Other bursal cyst, unspecified ankle and foot
M71.38 Other bursal cyst, other site
M71.39 Other bursal cyst, multiple sites

✓5th **M71.4 Calcium deposit in bursa**
   EXCLUDES 2   calcium deposit in bursa of shoulder (M75.3)
   M71.40 Calcium deposit in bursa, unspecified site
   ✓6th M71.42 Calcium deposit in bursa, elbow
      M71.421 Calcium deposit in bursa, right elbow
      M71.422 Calcium deposit in bursa, left elbow
      M71.429 Calcium deposit in bursa, unspecified elbow
   ✓6th M71.43 Calcium deposit in bursa, wrist
      M71.431 Calcium deposit in bursa, right wrist
      M71.432 Calcium deposit in bursa, left wrist
      M71.439 Calcium deposit in bursa, unspecified wrist
   ✓6th M71.44 Calcium deposit in bursa, hand
      M71.441 Calcium deposit in bursa, right hand
      M71.442 Calcium deposit in bursa, left hand
      M71.449 Calcium deposit in bursa, unspecified hand
   ✓6th M71.45 Calcium deposit in bursa, hip
      M71.451 Calcium deposit in bursa, right hip
      M71.452 Calcium deposit in bursa, left hip
      M71.459 Calcium deposit in bursa, unspecified hip
   ✓6th M71.46 Calcium deposit in bursa, knee
      M71.461 Calcium deposit in bursa, right knee
      M71.462 Calcium deposit in bursa, left knee
      M71.469 Calcium deposit in bursa, unspecified knee
   ✓6th M71.47 Calcium deposit in bursa, ankle and foot
      M71.471 Calcium deposit in bursa, right ankle and foot
      M71.472 Calcium deposit in bursa, left ankle and foot
      M71.479 Calcium deposit in bursa, unspecified ankle and foot
   M71.48 Calcium deposit in bursa, other site
   M71.49 Calcium deposit in bursa, multiple sites

✓5th **M71.5 Other bursitis, not elsewhere classified**
   EXCLUDES 1   bursitis NOS (M71.9-)
   EXCLUDES 2   bursitis of shoulder (M75.5)
                bursitis of tibial collateral [Pellegrini-Stieda] (M76.4-)
   M71.50 Other bursitis, not elsewhere classified, unspecified site
   ✓6th M71.52 Other bursitis, not elsewhere classified, elbow
      M71.521 Other bursitis, not elsewhere classified, right elbow
      M71.522 Other bursitis, not elsewhere classified, left elbow
      M71.529 Other bursitis, not elsewhere classified, unspecified elbow
   ✓6th M71.53 Other bursitis, not elsewhere classified, wrist
      M71.531 Other bursitis, not elsewhere classified, right wrist
      M71.532 Other bursitis, not elsewhere classified, left wrist
      M71.539 Other bursitis, not elsewhere classified, unspecified wrist
   ✓6th M71.54 Other bursitis, not elsewhere classified, hand
      M71.541 Other bursitis, not elsewhere classified, right hand
      M71.542 Other bursitis, not elsewhere classified, left hand
      M71.549 Other bursitis, not elsewhere classified, unspecified hand
   ✓6th M71.55 Other bursitis, not elsewhere classified, hip
      M71.551 Other bursitis, not elsewhere classified, right hip
      M71.552 Other bursitis, not elsewhere classified, left hip
      M71.559 Other bursitis, not elsewhere classified, unspecified hip
   ✓6th M71.56 Other bursitis, not elsewhere classified, knee
      M71.561 Other bursitis, not elsewhere classified, right knee
      M71.562 Other bursitis, not elsewhere classified, left knee
      M71.569 Other bursitis, not elsewhere classified, unspecified knee
   ✓6th M71.57 Other bursitis, not elsewhere classified, ankle and foot
      M71.571 Other bursitis, not elsewhere classified, right ankle and foot
      M71.572 Other bursitis, not elsewhere classified, left ankle and foot
      M71.579 Other bursitis, not elsewhere classified, unspecified ankle and foot
   M71.58 Other bursitis, not elsewhere classified, other site

✓5th **M71.8 Other specified bursopathies**
   M71.80 Other specified bursopathies, unspecified site
   ✓6th M71.81 Other specified bursopathies, shoulder
      M71.811 Other specified bursopathies, right shoulder
      M71.812 Other specified bursopathies, left shoulder
      M71.819 Other specified bursopathies, unspecified shoulder
   ✓6th M71.82 Other specified bursopathies, elbow
      M71.821 Other specified bursopathies, right elbow
      M71.822 Other specified bursopathies, left elbow
      M71.829 Other specified bursopathies, unspecified elbow
   ✓6th M71.83 Other specified bursopathies, wrist
      M71.831 Other specified bursopathies, right wrist
      M71.832 Other specified bursopathies, left wrist
      M71.839 Other specified bursopathies, unspecified wrist
   ✓6th M71.84 Other specified bursopathies, hand
      M71.841 Other specified bursopathies, right hand
      M71.842 Other specified bursopathies, left hand
      M71.849 Other specified bursopathies, unspecified hand
   ✓6th M71.85 Other specified bursopathies, hip
      M71.851 Other specified bursopathies, right hip
      M71.852 Other specified bursopathies, left hip
      M71.859 Other specified bursopathies, unspecified hip
   ✓6th M71.86 Other specified bursopathies, knee
      M71.861 Other specified bursopathies, right knee
      M71.862 Other specified bursopathies, left knee
      M71.869 Other specified bursopathies, unspecified knee
   ✓6th M71.87 Other specified bursopathies, ankle and foot
      M71.871 Other specified bursopathies, right ankle and foot
      M71.872 Other specified bursopathies, left ankle and foot
      M71.879 Other specified bursopathies, unspecified ankle and foot
   M71.88 Other specified bursopathies, other site
   M71.89 Other specified bursopathies, multiple sites

M71.9 Bursopathy, unspecified
   Bursitis NOS

✓4th **M72 Fibroblastic disorders**
   EXCLUDES 2   retroperitoneal fibromatosis (D48.3)
   M72.0 Palmar fascial fibromatosis [Dupuytren] A
      DEF: Dupuytren's contracture: Flexion deformity of a finger, due to shortened, thickened fibrosing of palmar fascia. The cause is unknown, but it is associated with long-standing epilepsy.
   M72.1 Knuckle pads
   M72.2 Plantar fascial fibromatosis
      Plantar fasciitis
      DEF: Rapid-growing and multiplanar nodular swellings and pain in the foot that is not associated with contractures.
   M72.4 Pseudosarcomatous fibromatosis
      Nodular fasciitis
   M72.6 Necrotizing fasciitis HCC ESR COM
      Use additional code (B95.-, B96.-) to identify causative organism

---

HCC CMS-HCC   Rx Rx HCC   ESR ESRD HCC   COM Commercial HCC   N Newborn: 0   P Pediatric: 0-17   M Maternity: 9-64   A Adult: 15-124

M72.8 Other fibroblastic disorders
Abscess of fascia
Fasciitis NEC
Other infective fasciitis
Use additional code to (B95.-, B96.-) identify causative organism
EXCLUDES 1: diffuse (eosinophilic) fasciitis (M35.4)
necrotizing fasciitis (M72.6)
nodular fasciitis (M72.4)
perirenal fasciitis NOS (N13.5)
perirenal fasciitis with infection (N13.6)
plantar fasciitis (M72.2)
AHA: 2025,1Q,31

M72.9 Fibroblastic disorder, unspecified
Fasciitis NOS
Fibromatosis NOS

M75 Shoulder lesions
EXCLUDES 2: shoulder-hand syndrome (M89.0-)

M75.0 Adhesive capsulitis of shoulder
Frozen shoulder
Periarthritis of shoulder
AHA: 2015,2Q,23
- M75.00 Adhesive capsulitis of unspecified shoulder
- M75.01 Adhesive capsulitis of right shoulder
- M75.02 Adhesive capsulitis of left shoulder

M75.1 Rotator cuff tear or rupture, not specified as traumatic
Rotator cuff syndrome
Supraspinatus syndrome
Supraspinatus tear or rupture, not specified as traumatic
EXCLUDES 1: tear of rotator cuff, traumatic (S46.01-)

- **M75.10** Unspecified rotator cuff tear or rupture, not specified as traumatic
  - M75.100 Unspecified rotator cuff tear or rupture of unspecified shoulder, not specified as traumatic
  - M75.101 Unspecified rotator cuff tear or rupture of right shoulder, not specified as traumatic
  - M75.102 Unspecified rotator cuff tear or rupture of left shoulder, not specified as traumatic

- **M75.11** Incomplete rotator cuff tear or rupture not specified as traumatic
  - M75.110 Incomplete rotator cuff tear or rupture of unspecified shoulder, not specified as traumatic
  - M75.111 Incomplete rotator cuff tear or rupture of right shoulder, not specified as traumatic
  - M75.112 Incomplete rotator cuff tear or rupture of left shoulder, not specified as traumatic

- **M75.12** Complete rotator cuff tear or rupture not specified as traumatic
  - M75.120 Complete rotator cuff tear or rupture of unspecified shoulder, not specified as traumatic
  - M75.121 Complete rotator cuff tear or rupture of right shoulder, not specified as traumatic
  - M75.122 Complete rotator cuff tear or rupture of left shoulder, not specified as traumatic

M75.2 Bicipital tendinitis
- M75.20 Bicipital tendinitis, unspecified shoulder
- M75.21 Bicipital tendinitis, right shoulder
- M75.22 Bicipital tendinitis, left shoulder

M75.3 Calcific tendinitis of shoulder
Calcified bursa of shoulder
- M75.30 Calcific tendinitis of unspecified shoulder
- M75.31 Calcific tendinitis of right shoulder
- M75.32 Calcific tendinitis of left shoulder

M75.4 Impingement syndrome of shoulder
AHA: 2022,3Q,18
- M75.40 Impingement syndrome of unspecified shoulder
- M75.41 Impingement syndrome of right shoulder
- M75.42 Impingement syndrome of left shoulder

M75.5 Bursitis of shoulder
- M75.50 Bursitis of unspecified shoulder
- M75.51 Bursitis of right shoulder
- M75.52 Bursitis of left shoulder

M75.8 Other shoulder lesions
- M75.80 Other shoulder lesions, unspecified shoulder
- M75.81 Other shoulder lesions, right shoulder
- M75.82 Other shoulder lesions, left shoulder

M75.9 Shoulder lesion, unspecified
- M75.90 Shoulder lesion, unspecified, unspecified shoulder
- M75.91 Shoulder lesion, unspecified, right shoulder
- M75.92 Shoulder lesion, unspecified, left shoulder

M76 Enthesopathies, lower limb, excluding foot
EXCLUDES 2: bursitis due to use, overuse and pressure (M70.-)
enthesopathies of ankle and foot (M77.5-)

M76.0 Gluteal tendinitis
- M76.00 Gluteal tendinitis, unspecified hip
- M76.01 Gluteal tendinitis, right hip
- M76.02 Gluteal tendinitis, left hip

M76.1 Psoas tendinitis
- M76.10 Psoas tendinitis, unspecified hip
- M76.11 Psoas tendinitis, right hip
- M76.12 Psoas tendinitis, left hip

M76.2 Iliac crest spur
- M76.20 Iliac crest spur, unspecified hip
- M76.21 Iliac crest spur, right hip
- M76.22 Iliac crest spur, left hip

M76.3 Iliotibial band syndrome
- M76.30 Iliotibial band syndrome, unspecified leg
- M76.31 Iliotibial band syndrome, right leg
- M76.32 Iliotibial band syndrome, left leg

M76.4 Tibial collateral bursitis [Pellegrini-Stieda]
- M76.40 Tibial collateral bursitis [Pellegrini-Stieda], unspecified leg
- M76.41 Tibial collateral bursitis [Pellegrini-Stieda], right leg
- M76.42 Tibial collateral bursitis [Pellegrini-Stieda], left leg

M76.5 Patellar tendinitis
- M76.50 Patellar tendinitis, unspecified knee
- M76.51 Patellar tendinitis, right knee
- M76.52 Patellar tendinitis, left knee

M76.6 Achilles tendinitis
Achilles bursitis
- M76.60 Achilles tendinitis, unspecified leg
- M76.61 Achilles tendinitis, right leg
- M76.62 Achilles tendinitis, left leg

M76.7 Peroneal tendinitis
- M76.70 Peroneal tendinitis, unspecified leg
- M76.71 Peroneal tendinitis, right leg
- M76.72 Peroneal tendinitis, left leg

M76.8 Other specified enthesopathies of lower limb, excluding foot
- **M76.81** Anterior tibial syndrome
  - M76.811 Anterior tibial syndrome, right leg
  - M76.812 Anterior tibial syndrome, left leg
  - M76.819 Anterior tibial syndrome, unspecified leg
- **M76.82** Posterior tibial tendinitis
  - M76.821 Posterior tibial tendinitis, right leg
  - M76.822 Posterior tibial tendinitis, left leg
  - M76.829 Posterior tibial tendinitis, unspecified leg
- **M76.89** Other specified enthesopathies of lower limb, excluding foot
  - M76.891 Other specified enthesopathies of right lower limb, excluding foot
  - M76.892 Other specified enthesopathies of left lower limb, excluding foot
  - M76.899 Other specified enthesopathies of unspecified lower limb, excluding foot

M76.9 Unspecified enthesopathy, lower limb, excluding foot

M77 Other enthesopathies
EXCLUDES 1: bursitis NOS (M71.9-)
EXCLUDES 2: bursitis due to use, overuse and pressure (M70.-)
osteophyte (M25.7)
spinal enthesopathy (M46.0-)

M77.0 Medial epicondylitis
- M77.00 Medial epicondylitis, unspecified elbow
- M77.01 Medial epicondylitis, right elbow
- M77.02 Medial epicondylitis, left elbow

M77.1 Lateral epicondylitis
Tennis elbow
- M77.10 Lateral epicondylitis, unspecified elbow
- M77.11 Lateral epicondylitis, right elbow
- M77.12 Lateral epicondylitis, left elbow

Chapter 13. Diseases of the Musculoskeletal System and Connective Tissue

M77.2 Periarthritis of wrist
- M77.20 Periarthritis, unspecified wrist
- M77.21 Periarthritis, right wrist
- M77.22 Periarthritis, left wrist

M77.3 Calcaneal spur
DEF: Overgrowth of calcaneus bone on the underside of the heel that causes pain on walking. Calcaneal spur is due to a chronic avulsion injury of the plantar fascia from the calcaneus.
- M77.30 Calcaneal spur, unspecified foot
- M77.31 Calcaneal spur, right foot
- M77.32 Calcaneal spur, left foot

M77.4 Metatarsalgia
EXCLUDES 1   Morton's metatarsalgia (G57.6)
- M77.40 Metatarsalgia, unspecified foot
- M77.41 Metatarsalgia, right foot
- M77.42 Metatarsalgia, left foot

M77.5 Other enthesopathy of foot and ankle
- M77.50 Other enthesopathy of unspecified foot and ankle
- M77.51 Other enthesopathy of right foot and ankle
- M77.52 Other enthesopathy of left foot and ankle

M77.8 Other enthesopathies, not elsewhere classified

M77.9 Enthesopathy, unspecified
Bone spur NOS
Capsulitis NOS
Periarthritis NOS
Tendinitis NOS

M79 Other and unspecified soft tissue disorders, not elsewhere classified
EXCLUDES 1   psychogenic rheumatism (F45.8)
soft tissue pain, psychogenic (F45.41)

M79.0 Rheumatism, unspecified
EXCLUDES 1   fibromyalgia (M79.7)
palindromic rheumatism (M12.3-)

M79.1 Myalgia
Myofascial pain syndrome
EXCLUDES 1   fibromyalgia (M79.7)
myositis (M60.-)
AHA: 2018,4Q,21
- M79.10 Myalgia, unspecified site
- M79.11 Myalgia of mastication muscle
- M79.12 Myalgia of auxiliary muscles, head and neck
- M79.18 Myalgia, other site

M79.2 Neuralgia and neuritis, unspecified
EXCLUDES 1   brachial radiculitis NOS (M54.1)
lumbosacral radiculitis NOS (M54.1)
mononeuropathies (G56-G58)
radiculitis NOS (M54.1)
sciatica (M54.3-M54.4)
TIP: Assign for documented neuropathic pain.

M79.3 Panniculitis, unspecified
EXCLUDES 1   lupus panniculitis (L93.2)
neck and back panniculitis (M54.0-)
relapsing [Weber-Christian] panniculitis (M35.6)
AHA: 2024,1Q,16

M79.4 Hypertrophy of (infrapatellar) fat pad

M79.5 Residual foreign body in soft tissue
EXCLUDES 1   foreign body granuloma of skin and subcutaneous tissue (L92.5)
foreign body granuloma of soft tissue (M60.2-)
AHA: 2023,2Q,27

M79.6 Pain in limb, hand, foot, fingers and toes
EXCLUDES 2   pain in joint (M25.5-)
- **M79.60** Pain in limb, unspecified
  - M79.601 Pain in right arm
    Pain in right upper limb NOS
  - M79.602 Pain in left arm
    Pain in left upper limb NOS
  - M79.603 Pain in arm, unspecified
    Pain in upper limb NOS
  - M79.604 Pain in right leg
    Pain in right lower limb NOS
  - M79.605 Pain in left leg
    Pain in left lower limb NOS
  - M79.606 Pain in leg, unspecified
    Pain in lower limb NOS
  - M79.609 Pain in unspecified limb
    Pain in limb NOS

- **M79.62** Pain in upper arm
  Pain in axillary region
  - M79.621 Pain in right upper arm
  - M79.622 Pain in left upper arm
  - M79.629 Pain in unspecified upper arm
- **M79.63** Pain in forearm
  - M79.631 Pain in right forearm
  - M79.632 Pain in left forearm
  - M79.639 Pain in unspecified forearm
- **M79.64** Pain in hand and fingers
  - M79.641 Pain in right hand
  - M79.642 Pain in left hand
  - M79.643 Pain in unspecified hand
  - M79.644 Pain in right finger(s)
  - M79.645 Pain in left finger(s)
  - M79.646 Pain in unspecified finger(s)
- **M79.65** Pain in thigh
  - M79.651 Pain in right thigh
  - M79.652 Pain in left thigh
  - M79.659 Pain in unspecified thigh
- **M79.66** Pain in lower leg
  - M79.661 Pain in right lower leg
  - M79.662 Pain in left lower leg
  - M79.669 Pain in unspecified lower leg
- **M79.67** Pain in foot and toes
  - M79.671 Pain in right foot
  - M79.672 Pain in left foot
  - M79.673 Pain in unspecified foot
  - M79.674 Pain in right toe(s)
  - M79.675 Pain in left toe(s)
  - M79.676 Pain in unspecified toe(s)

M79.7 Fibromyalgia
Fibromyositis
Fibrositis
Myofibrositis

M79.A Nontraumatic compartment syndrome
Code first, if applicable, associated postprocedural complication
EXCLUDES 1   compartment syndrome NOS (T79.A-)
fibromyalgia (M79.7)
nontraumatic ischemic infarction of muscle (M62.2-)
traumatic compartment syndrome (T79.A-)
- **M79.A1** Nontraumatic compartment syndrome of upper extremity
  Nontraumatic compartment syndrome of shoulder, arm, forearm, wrist, hand, and fingers
  - M79.A11 Nontraumatic compartment syndrome of right upper extremity
  - M79.A12 Nontraumatic compartment syndrome of left upper extremity
  - M79.A19 Nontraumatic compartment syndrome of unspecified upper extremity
- **M79.A2** Nontraumatic compartment syndrome of lower extremity
  Nontraumatic compartment syndrome of hip, buttock, thigh, leg, foot, and toes
  - M79.A21 Nontraumatic compartment syndrome of right lower extremity
  - M79.A22 Nontraumatic compartment syndrome of left lower extremity
  - M79.A29 Nontraumatic compartment syndrome of unspecified lower extremity
- **M79.A3** Nontraumatic compartment syndrome of abdomen
- **M79.A9** Nontraumatic compartment syndrome of other sites

M79.8 Other specified soft tissue disorders
- **M79.81** Nontraumatic hematoma of soft tissue
  Nontraumatic hematoma of muscle
  Nontraumatic seroma of muscle and soft tissue
- **M79.89** Other specified soft tissue disorders
  Polyalgia

M79.9 Soft tissue disorder, unspecified

OSTEOPATHIES AND CHONDROPATHIES (M80-M94)

Disorders of bone density and structure (M80-M85)

M80 Osteoporosis with current pathological fracture
- **INCLUDES** osteoporosis with current fragility fracture
- Use additional code to identify major osseous defect, if applicable (M89.7-)
- **EXCLUDES 1**
  - collapsed vertebra NOS (M48.5)
  - pathological fracture NOS (M84.4)
  - wedging of vertebra NOS (M48.5)
- **EXCLUDES 2** personal history of (healed) osteoporosis fracture (Z87.310)
- **AHA:** 2018,2Q,12
- **TIP:** The site codes in this category identify the site of the fracture, not the site of the osteoporosis.

> The appropriate 7th character is to be added to each code from category M80:
> - A   initial encounter for fracture
> - D   subsequent encounter for fracture with routine healing
> - G   subsequent encounter for fracture with delayed healing
> - K   subsequent encounter for fracture with nonunion
> - P   subsequent encounter for fracture with malunion
> - S   sequela

- **M80.0** Age-related osteoporosis with current pathological fracture
  - Involutional osteoporosis with current pathological fracture
  - Osteoporosis NOS with current pathological fracture
  - Postmenopausal osteoporosis with current pathological fracture
  - Senile osteoporosis with current pathological fracture
  - **M80.00** Age-related osteoporosis with current pathological fracture, unspecified site
  - **M80.01** Age-related osteoporosis with current pathological fracture, shoulder
    - **M80.011** Age-related osteoporosis with current pathological fracture, right shoulder
    - **M80.012** Age-related osteoporosis with current pathological fracture, left shoulder
    - **M80.019** Age-related osteoporosis with current pathological fracture, unspecified shoulder
  - **M80.02** Age-related osteoporosis with current pathological fracture, humerus
    - **M80.021** Age-related osteoporosis with current pathological fracture, right humerus
    - **M80.022** Age-related osteoporosis with current pathological fracture, left humerus
    - **M80.029** Age-related osteoporosis with current pathological fracture, unspecified humerus
  - **M80.03** Age-related osteoporosis with current pathological fracture, forearm
    - Age-related osteoporosis with current pathological fracture of wrist
    - **M80.031** Age-related osteoporosis with current pathological fracture, right forearm
    - **M80.032** Age-related osteoporosis with current pathological fracture, left forearm
    - **M80.039** Age-related osteoporosis with current pathological fracture, unspecified forearm
  - **M80.04** Age-related osteoporosis with current pathological fracture, hand
    - **M80.041** Age-related osteoporosis with current pathological fracture, right hand
    - **M80.042** Age-related osteoporosis with current pathological fracture, left hand
    - **M80.049** Age-related osteoporosis with current pathological fracture, unspecified hand
  - **M80.05** Age-related osteoporosis with current pathological fracture, femur
    - Age-related osteoporosis with current pathological fracture of hip
    - **M80.051** Age-related osteoporosis with current pathological fracture, right femur
    - **M80.052** Age-related osteoporosis with current pathological fracture, left femur
    - **M80.059** Age-related osteoporosis with current pathological fracture, unspecified femur
  - **M80.06** Age-related osteoporosis with current pathological fracture, lower leg
    - **M80.061** Age-related osteoporosis with current pathological fracture, right lower leg
    - **M80.062** Age-related osteoporosis with current pathological fracture, left lower leg
    - **M80.069** Age-related osteoporosis with current pathological fracture, unspecified lower leg
  - **M80.07** Age-related osteoporosis with current pathological fracture, ankle and foot
    - **M80.071** Age-related osteoporosis with current pathological fracture, right ankle and foot
    - **M80.072** Age-related osteoporosis with current pathological fracture, left ankle and foot
    - **M80.079** Age-related osteoporosis with current pathological fracture, unspecified ankle and foot
  - **M80.08** Age-related osteoporosis with current pathological fracture, vertebra(e)
  - **M80.0A** Age-related osteoporosis with current pathological fracture, other site
    - **AHA:** 2020,4Q,32-33
  - **M80.0B** Age-related osteoporosis with current pathological fracture, pelvis
    - **AHA:** 2023,4Q,33-34
    - **M80.0B1** Age-related osteoporosis with current pathological fracture, right pelvis
    - **M80.0B2** Age-related osteoporosis with current pathological fracture, left pelvis
    - **M80.0B9** Age-related osteoporosis with current pathological fracture, unspecified pelvis

- **M80.8** Other osteoporosis with current pathological fracture
  - Drug-induced osteoporosis with current pathological fracture
  - Idiopathic osteoporosis with current pathological fracture
  - Osteoporosis of disuse with current pathological fracture
  - Postoophorectomy osteoporosis with current pathological fracture
  - Postsurgical malabsorption osteoporosis with current pathological fracture
  - Post-traumatic osteoporosis with current pathological fracture
  - Use additional code for adverse effect, if applicable, to identify drug (T36-T50 with fifth or sixth character 5)
  - **M80.80** Other osteoporosis with current pathological fracture, unspecified site
  - **M80.81** Other osteoporosis with pathological fracture, shoulder
    - **M80.811** Other osteoporosis with current pathological fracture, right shoulder
    - **M80.812** Other osteoporosis with current pathological fracture, left shoulder
    - **M80.819** Other osteoporosis with current pathological fracture, unspecified shoulder
  - **M80.82** Other osteoporosis with current pathological fracture, humerus
    - **M80.821** Other osteoporosis with current pathological fracture, right humerus

Chapter 13. Diseases of the Musculoskeletal System and Connective Tissue

- ✓7ᵗʰ **M80.822** Other osteoporosis with current pathological fracture, left humerus [Rx] [Q]
- ✓7ᵗʰ **M80.829** Other osteoporosis with current pathological fracture, unspecified humerus [Rx] [Q]
- ✓6ᵗʰ **M80.83** Other osteoporosis with current pathological fracture, forearm
  Other osteoporosis with current pathological fracture of wrist
  - ✓7ᵗʰ **M80.831** Other osteoporosis with current pathological fracture, right forearm [Rx] [Q]
  - ✓7ᵗʰ **M80.832** Other osteoporosis with current pathological fracture, left forearm [Rx] [Q]
  - ✓7ᵗʰ **M80.839** Other osteoporosis with current pathological fracture, unspecified forearm [Rx] [Q]
- ✓6ᵗʰ **M80.84** Other osteoporosis with current pathological fracture, hand
  - ✓7ᵗʰ **M80.841** Other osteoporosis with current pathological fracture, right hand [Rx] [Q]
  - ✓7ᵗʰ **M80.842** Other osteoporosis with current pathological fracture, left hand [Rx] [Q]
  - ✓7ᵗʰ **M80.849** Other osteoporosis with current pathological fracture, unspecified hand [Rx] [Q]
- ✓6ᵗʰ **M80.85** Other osteoporosis with current pathological fracture, femur
  Other osteoporosis with current pathological fracture of hip
  - ✓7ᵗʰ **M80.851** Other osteoporosis with current pathological fracture, right femur [HCC] [Rx] [ESR] [COM] [Q]
  - ✓7ᵗʰ **M80.852** Other osteoporosis with current pathological fracture, left femur [HCC] [Rx] [ESR] [COM] [Q]
  - ✓7ᵗʰ **M80.859** Other osteoporosis with current pathological fracture, unspecified femur [HCC] [Rx] [ESR] [COM] [Q]
- ✓6ᵗʰ **M80.86** Other osteoporosis with current pathological fracture, lower leg
  - ✓7ᵗʰ **M80.861** Other osteoporosis with current pathological fracture, right lower leg [Rx] [Q]
  - ✓7ᵗʰ **M80.862** Other osteoporosis with current pathological fracture, left lower leg [Rx] [Q]
  - ✓7ᵗʰ **M80.869** Other osteoporosis with current pathological fracture, unspecified lower leg [Rx] [Q]
- ✓6ᵗʰ **M80.87** Other osteoporosis with current pathological fracture, ankle and foot
  - ✓7ᵗʰ **M80.871** Other osteoporosis with current pathological fracture, right ankle and foot [Rx] [Q]
  - ✓7ᵗʰ **M80.872** Other osteoporosis with current pathological fracture, left ankle and foot [Rx] [Q]
  - ✓7ᵗʰ **M80.879** Other osteoporosis with current pathological fracture, unspecified ankle and foot [Rx] [Q]
- ✓x 7ᵗʰ **M80.88** Other osteoporosis with current pathological fracture, vertebra(e) [HCC] [Rx] [ESR] [COM]
- ✓x 7ᵗʰ **M80.8A** Other osteoporosis with current pathological fracture, other site [Rx] [Q]
  AHA: 2020,4Q,32
- ✓6ᵗʰ **M80.8B** Other osteoporosis with current pathological fracture, pelvis
  AHA: 2023,4Q,33-34
  - ✓7ᵗʰ **M80.8B1** Other osteoporosis with current pathological fracture, right pelvis [Rx] [Q]
  - ✓7ᵗʰ **M80.8B2** Other osteoporosis with current pathological fracture, left pelvis [Rx] [Q]
  - ✓7ᵗʰ **M80.8B9** Other osteoporosis with current pathological fracture, unspecified pelvis [Rx] [Q]

- ✓4ᵗʰ **M81** Osteoporosis without current pathological fracture
  Use additional code to identify:
   major osseous defect, if applicable (M89.7-)
   personal history of (healed) osteoporosis fracture, if applicable (Z87.310)
  EXCLUDES 1 osteoporosis with current pathological fracture (M80.-)
   Sudeck's atrophy (M89.0)
  - **M81.0** Age-related osteoporosis without current pathological fracture [Rx] [Q] [A]
    Involutional osteoporosis without current pathological fracture
    Osteoporosis NOS
    Postmenopausal osteoporosis without current pathological fracture
    Senile osteoporosis without current pathological fracture
  - **M81.6** Localized osteoporosis [Lequesne] [Rx] [Q]
    EXCLUDES 1 Sudeck's atrophy (M89.0)
  - **M81.8** Other osteoporosis without current pathological fracture [Rx] [Q]
    Drug-induced osteoporosis without current pathological fracture
    Idiopathic osteoporosis without current pathological fracture
    Osteoporosis of disuse without current pathological fracture
    Postoophorectomy osteoporosis without current pathological fracture
    Postsurgical malabsorption osteoporosis without current pathological fracture
    Post-traumatic osteoporosis without current pathological fracture
    Use additional code for adverse effect, if applicable, to identify drug (T36-T50 with fifth or sixth character 5)

- ✓4ᵗʰ **M83** Adult osteomalacia
  EXCLUDES 1 infantile and juvenile osteomalacia (E55.0)
   renal osteodystrophy (N25.0)
   rickets (active) (E55.0)
   rickets (active) sequelae (E64.3)
   vitamin D-resistant osteomalacia (E83.31)
   vitamin D-resistant rickets (active) (E83.31)
  - **M83.0** Puerperal osteomalacia [Rx] [M]
  - **M83.1** Senile osteomalacia [Rx] [A]
  - **M83.2** Adult osteomalacia due to malabsorption [Rx] [A]
    Postsurgical malabsorption osteomalacia in adults
  - **M83.3** Adult osteomalacia due to malnutrition [Rx] [A]
  - **M83.4** Aluminum bone disease [Rx]
  - **M83.5** Other drug-induced osteomalacia in adults [Rx] [A]
    Use additional code for adverse effect, if applicable, to identify drug (T36-T50 with fifth or sixth character 5)
  - **M83.8** Other adult osteomalacia [Rx] [A]
  - **M83.9** Adult osteomalacia, unspecified [Rx] [A]

- ✓4ᵗʰ **M84** Disorder of continuity of bone
  EXCLUDES 2 traumatic fracture of bone-see fracture, by site
  - ✓5ᵗʰ **M84.3** Stress fracture
    Fatigue fracture
    March fracture
    Stress fracture NOS
    Stress reaction
    Use additional external cause code(s) to identify the cause of the stress fracture
    EXCLUDES 1 pathological fracture due to osteoporosis (M80.-)
     pathological fracture NOS (M84.4.-)
     traumatic fracture (S12.-, S22.-, S32.-, S42.-, S52.-, S62.-, S72.-, S82.-, S92.-)
    EXCLUDES 2 personal history of (healed) stress (fatigue) fracture (Z87.312)
     stress fracture of vertebra (M48.4-)

    > The appropriate 7th character is to be added to each code from subcategory M84.3.
    > A initial encounter for fracture
    > D subsequent encounter for fracture with routine healing
    > G subsequent encounter for fracture with delayed healing
    > K subsequent encounter for fracture with nonunion
    > P subsequent encounter for fracture with malunion
    > S sequela

    - ✓x 7ᵗʰ **M84.30** Stress fracture, unspecified site
    - ✓6ᵗʰ **M84.31** Stress fracture, shoulder
      - ✓7ᵗʰ **M84.311** Stress fracture, right shoulder [Q]
      - ✓7ᵗʰ **M84.312** Stress fracture, left shoulder [Q]
      - ✓7ᵗʰ **M84.319** Stress fracture, unspecified shoulder [Q]
    - ✓6ᵗʰ **M84.32** Stress fracture, humerus
      - ✓7ᵗʰ **M84.321** Stress fracture, right humerus [Q]

[HCC] CMS-HCC [Rx] Rx HCC [ESR] ESRD HCC [COM] Commercial HCC [N] Newborn: 0 [P] Pediatric: 0-17 [M] Maternity: 9-64 [A] Adult: 15-124

Chapter 13. Diseases of the Musculoskeletal System and Connective Tissue

M84.322–M84.519

- 7ᵗʰ **M84.322** Stress fracture, left humerus Q
- 7ᵗʰ **M84.329** Stress fracture, unspecified humerus Q
- 6ᵗʰ **M84.33** Stress fracture, ulna and radius
  - 7ᵗʰ **M84.331** Stress fracture, right ulna Q
  - 7ᵗʰ **M84.332** Stress fracture, left ulna Q
  - 7ᵗʰ **M84.333** Stress fracture, right radius Q
  - 7ᵗʰ **M84.334** Stress fracture, left radius Q
  - 7ᵗʰ **M84.339** Stress fracture, unspecified ulna and radius Q
- 6ᵗʰ **M84.34** Stress fracture, hand and fingers
  - 7ᵗʰ **M84.341** Stress fracture, right hand Q
  - 7ᵗʰ **M84.342** Stress fracture, left hand Q
  - 7ᵗʰ **M84.343** Stress fracture, unspecified hand Q
  - 7ᵗʰ **M84.344** Stress fracture, right finger(s)
  - 7ᵗʰ **M84.345** Stress fracture, left finger(s)
  - 7ᵗʰ **M84.346** Stress fracture, unspecified finger(s)
- 6ᵗʰ **M84.35** Stress fracture, pelvis and femur
  Stress fracture, hip
  - 7ᵗʰ **M84.350** Stress fracture, pelvis Q
  - 7ᵗʰ **M84.351** Stress fracture, right femur Q
  - 7ᵗʰ **M84.352** Stress fracture, left femur Q
  - 7ᵗʰ **M84.353** Stress fracture, unspecified femur Q
  - 7ᵗʰ **M84.359** Stress fracture, hip, unspecified Q
- 6ᵗʰ **M84.36** Stress fracture, tibia and fibula
  - 7ᵗʰ **M84.361** Stress fracture, right tibia Q
  - 7ᵗʰ **M84.362** Stress fracture, left tibia Q
  - 7ᵗʰ **M84.363** Stress fracture, right fibula Q
  - 7ᵗʰ **M84.364** Stress fracture, left fibula Q
  - 7ᵗʰ **M84.369** Stress fracture, unspecified tibia and fibula Q
- 6ᵗʰ **M84.37** Stress fracture, ankle, foot and toes
  - 7ᵗʰ **M84.371** Stress fracture, right ankle Q
  - 7ᵗʰ **M84.372** Stress fracture, left ankle Q
  - 7ᵗʰ **M84.373** Stress fracture, unspecified ankle Q
  - 7ᵗʰ **M84.374** Stress fracture, right foot Q
  - 7ᵗʰ **M84.375** Stress fracture, left foot Q
  - 7ᵗʰ **M84.376** Stress fracture, unspecified foot Q
  - 7ᵗʰ **M84.377** Stress fracture, right toe(s)
  - 7ᵗʰ **M84.378** Stress fracture, left toe(s)
  - 7ᵗʰ **M84.379** Stress fracture, unspecified toe(s)
- √x7ᵗʰ **M84.38** Stress fracture, other site Q
  - EXCLUDES 2: stress fracture of vertebra (M48.4-)
- 5ᵗʰ **M84.4** Pathological fracture, not elsewhere classified
  Chronic fracture
  Pathological fracture NOS
  EXCLUDES 1: collapsed vertebra NEC (M48.5)
  pathological fracture in neoplastic disease (M84.5-)
  pathological fracture in osteoporosis (M80.-)
  pathological fracture in other disease (M84.6-)
  stress fracture (M84.3-)
  traumatic fracture (S12.-, S22.-, S32.-, S42.-, S52.-, S62.-, S72.-, S82.-, S92.-)
  EXCLUDES 2: personal history of (healed) pathological fracture (Z87.311)

  The appropriate 7th character is to be added to each code from subcategory M84.4.
  - A initial encounter for fracture
  - D subsequent encounter for fracture with routine healing
  - G subsequent encounter for fracture with delayed healing
  - K subsequent encounter for fracture with nonunion
  - P subsequent encounter for fracture with malunion
  - S sequela

- √x7ᵗʰ **M84.40** Pathological fracture, unspecified site Rx
- 6ᵗʰ **M84.41** Pathological fracture, shoulder
  - 7ᵗʰ **M84.411** Pathological fracture, right shoulder Rx
  - 7ᵗʰ **M84.412** Pathological fracture, left shoulder Rx
  - 7ᵗʰ **M84.419** Pathological fracture, unspecified shoulder Rx
- 6ᵗʰ **M84.42** Pathological fracture, humerus
  - 7ᵗʰ **M84.421** Pathological fracture, right humerus Rx
  - 7ᵗʰ **M84.422** Pathological fracture, left humerus Rx
  - 7ᵗʰ **M84.429** Pathological fracture, unspecified humerus Rx
- 6ᵗʰ **M84.43** Pathological fracture, ulna and radius
  - 7ᵗʰ **M84.431** Pathological fracture, right ulna Rx
  - 7ᵗʰ **M84.432** Pathological fracture, left ulna Rx
  - 7ᵗʰ **M84.433** Pathological fracture, right radius Rx
  - 7ᵗʰ **M84.434** Pathological fracture, left radius Rx
  - 7ᵗʰ **M84.439** Pathological fracture, unspecified ulna and radius Rx
- 6ᵗʰ **M84.44** Pathological fracture, hand and fingers
  - 7ᵗʰ **M84.441** Pathological fracture, right hand Rx
  - 7ᵗʰ **M84.442** Pathological fracture, left hand Rx
  - 7ᵗʰ **M84.443** Pathological fracture, unspecified hand Rx
  - 7ᵗʰ **M84.444** Pathological fracture, right finger(s)
  - 7ᵗʰ **M84.445** Pathological fracture, left finger(s)
  - 7ᵗʰ **M84.446** Pathological fracture, unspecified finger(s) Rx
- 6ᵗʰ **M84.45** Pathological fracture, femur and pelvis
  AHA: 2016,4Q,43
  - 7ᵗʰ **M84.451** Pathological fracture, right femur HCC Rx ESR COM
  - 7ᵗʰ **M84.452** Pathological fracture, left femur HCC Rx ESR COM
  - 7ᵗʰ **M84.453** Pathological fracture, unspecified femur HCC Rx ESR COM
  - 7ᵗʰ **M84.454** Pathological fracture, pelvis Rx
  - 7ᵗʰ **M84.459** Pathological fracture, hip, unspecified HCC Rx ESR COM
- 6ᵗʰ **M84.46** Pathological fracture, tibia and fibula
  - 7ᵗʰ **M84.461** Pathological fracture, right tibia Rx
  - 7ᵗʰ **M84.462** Pathological fracture, left tibia Rx
  - 7ᵗʰ **M84.463** Pathological fracture, right fibula Rx
  - 7ᵗʰ **M84.464** Pathological fracture, left fibula Rx
  - 7ᵗʰ **M84.469** Pathological fracture, unspecified tibia and fibula Rx
- 6ᵗʰ **M84.47** Pathological fracture, ankle, foot and toes
  - 7ᵗʰ **M84.471** Pathological fracture, right ankle Rx
  - 7ᵗʰ **M84.472** Pathological fracture, left ankle Rx
  - 7ᵗʰ **M84.473** Pathological fracture, unspecified ankle Rx
  - 7ᵗʰ **M84.474** Pathological fracture, right foot Rx
  - 7ᵗʰ **M84.475** Pathological fracture, left foot Rx
  - 7ᵗʰ **M84.476** Pathological fracture, unspecified foot Rx
  - 7ᵗʰ **M84.477** Pathological fracture, right toe(s) Rx
  - 7ᵗʰ **M84.478** Pathological fracture, left toe(s) Rx
  - 7ᵗʰ **M84.479** Pathological fracture, unspecified toe(s) Rx
- √x7ᵗʰ **M84.48** Pathological fracture, other site Rx
- 5ᵗʰ **M84.5** Pathological fracture in neoplastic disease
  Code also underlying neoplasm

  The appropriate 7th character is to be added to each code from subcategory M84.5.
  - A initial encounter for fracture
  - D subsequent encounter for fracture with routine healing
  - G subsequent encounter for fracture with delayed healing
  - K subsequent encounter for fracture with nonunion
  - P subsequent encounter for fracture with malunion
  - S sequela

- √x7ᵗʰ **M84.50** Pathological fracture in neoplastic disease, unspecified site Rx
- 6ᵗʰ **M84.51** Pathological fracture in neoplastic disease, shoulder
  - 7ᵗʰ **M84.511** Pathological fracture in neoplastic disease, right shoulder Rx
  - 7ᵗʰ **M84.512** Pathological fracture in neoplastic disease, left shoulder Rx
  - 7ᵗʰ **M84.519** Pathological fracture in neoplastic disease, unspecified shoulder Rx

✓ Additional Character Required | √x7ᵗʰ Placeholder Alert | Manifestation | Unspecified Dx | Q QPP | UPD Unacceptable PDx

M84.52 Pathological fracture in neoplastic disease, humerus
- M84.521 Pathological fracture in neoplastic disease, right humerus
- M84.522 Pathological fracture in neoplastic disease, left humerus
- M84.529 Pathological fracture in neoplastic disease, unspecified humerus

M84.53 Pathological fracture in neoplastic disease, ulna and radius
- M84.531 Pathological fracture in neoplastic disease, right ulna
- M84.532 Pathological fracture in neoplastic disease, left ulna
- M84.533 Pathological fracture in neoplastic disease, right radius
- M84.534 Pathological fracture in neoplastic disease, left radius
- M84.539 Pathological fracture in neoplastic disease, unspecified ulna and radius

M84.54 Pathological fracture in neoplastic disease, hand
- M84.541 Pathological fracture in neoplastic disease, right hand
- M84.542 Pathological fracture in neoplastic disease, left hand
- M84.549 Pathological fracture in neoplastic disease, unspecified hand

M84.55 Pathological fracture in neoplastic disease, pelvis and femur
- M84.550 Pathological fracture in neoplastic disease, pelvis
- M84.551 Pathological fracture in neoplastic disease, right femur
- M84.552 Pathological fracture in neoplastic disease, left femur
- M84.553 Pathological fracture in neoplastic disease, unspecified femur
- M84.559 Pathological fracture in neoplastic disease, hip, unspecified

M84.56 Pathological fracture in neoplastic disease, tibia and fibula
- M84.561 Pathological fracture in neoplastic disease, right tibia
- M84.562 Pathological fracture in neoplastic disease, left tibia
- M84.563 Pathological fracture in neoplastic disease, right fibula
- M84.564 Pathological fracture in neoplastic disease, left fibula
- M84.569 Pathological fracture in neoplastic disease, unspecified tibia and fibula

M84.57 Pathological fracture in neoplastic disease, ankle and foot
- M84.571 Pathological fracture in neoplastic disease, right ankle
- M84.572 Pathological fracture in neoplastic disease, left ankle
- M84.573 Pathological fracture in neoplastic disease, unspecified ankle
- M84.574 Pathological fracture in neoplastic disease, right foot
- M84.575 Pathological fracture in neoplastic disease, left foot
- M84.576 Pathological fracture in neoplastic disease, unspecified foot

M84.58 Pathological fracture in neoplastic disease, other specified site
Pathological fracture in neoplastic disease, vertebrae

M84.6 Pathological fracture in other disease
Code also underlying condition

EXCLUDES 1 pathological fracture in osteoporosis (M80.-)

The appropriate 7th character is to be added to each code from subcategory M84.6.
- A initial encounter for fracture
- D subsequent encounter for fracture with routine healing
- G subsequent encounter for fracture with delayed healing
- K subsequent encounter for fracture with nonunion
- P subsequent encounter for fracture with malunion
- S sequela

M84.60 Pathological fracture in other disease, unspecified site

M84.61 Pathological fracture in other disease, shoulder
- M84.611 Pathological fracture in other disease, right shoulder
- M84.612 Pathological fracture in other disease, left shoulder
- M84.619 Pathological fracture in other disease, unspecified shoulder

M84.62 Pathological fracture in other disease, humerus
- M84.621 Pathological fracture in other disease, right humerus
- M84.622 Pathological fracture in other disease, left humerus
- M84.629 Pathological fracture in other disease, unspecified humerus

M84.63 Pathological fracture in other disease, ulna and radius
- M84.631 Pathological fracture in other disease, right ulna
- M84.632 Pathological fracture in other disease, left ulna
- M84.633 Pathological fracture in other disease, right radius
- M84.634 Pathological fracture in other disease, left radius
- M84.639 Pathological fracture in other disease, unspecified ulna and radius

M84.64 Pathological fracture in other disease, hand
- M84.641 Pathological fracture in other disease, right hand
- M84.642 Pathological fracture in other disease, left hand
- M84.649 Pathological fracture in other disease, unspecified hand

M84.65 Pathological fracture in other disease, pelvis and femur
- M84.650 Pathological fracture in other disease, pelvis
- M84.651 Pathological fracture in other disease, right femur
- M84.652 Pathological fracture in other disease, left femur
- M84.653 Pathological fracture in other disease, unspecified femur
- M84.659 Pathological fracture in other disease, hip, unspecified

M84.66 Pathological fracture in other disease, tibia and fibula
- M84.661 Pathological fracture in other disease, right tibia
- M84.662 Pathological fracture in other disease, left tibia
- M84.663 Pathological fracture in other disease, right fibula
- M84.664 Pathological fracture in other disease, left fibula
- M84.669 Pathological fracture in other disease, unspecified tibia and fibula

M84.67 Pathological fracture in other disease, ankle and foot
- M84.671 Pathological fracture in other disease, right ankle
- M84.672 Pathological fracture in other disease, left ankle
- M84.673 Pathological fracture in other disease, unspecified ankle
- M84.674 Pathological fracture in other disease, right foot

Chapter 13. Diseases of the Musculoskeletal System and Connective Tissue

- ✓7th **M84.675** Pathological fracture in other disease, **left foot** Rx
- ✓7th **M84.676** Pathological fracture in other disease, **unspecified foot** Rx
- ✓x7th **M84.68** Pathological fracture in other disease, other site Rx
- ✓5th **M84.7** Nontraumatic fracture, not elsewhere classified
  - ✓6th **M84.75** **Atypical** femoral fracture
    - **AHA:** 2016,4Q,41-42

    > The appropriate 7th character is to be added to each code from M84.75.
    > A initial encounter for fracture
    > D subsequent encounter for fracture with routine healing
    > G subsequent encounter for fracture with delayed healing
    > K subsequent encounter for fracture with nonunion
    > P subsequent encounter for fracture with malunion
    > S sequela

    - ✓7th **M84.750** Atypical femoral fracture, unspecified Q
    - ✓7th **M84.751** **Incomplete** atypical femoral fracture, **right** leg Q
    - ✓7th **M84.752** **Incomplete** atypical femoral fracture, **left** leg Q
    - ✓7th **M84.753** **Incomplete** atypical femoral fracture, **unspecified** leg Q
    - ✓7th **M84.754** **Complete transverse** atypical femoral fracture, **right** leg HCC ESR COM Q
    - ✓7th **M84.755** **Complete transverse** atypical femoral fracture, **left** leg HCC ESR COM Q
    - ✓7th **M84.756** **Complete transverse** atypical femoral fracture, **unspecified** leg HCC ESR COM Q
    - ✓7th **M84.757** **Complete oblique** atypical femoral fracture, **right** leg HCC ESR COM Q
    - ✓7th **M84.758** **Complete oblique** atypical femoral fracture, **left** leg HCC ESR COM Q
    - ✓7th **M84.759** **Complete oblique** atypical femoral fracture, **unspecified** leg HCC ESR COM Q
- ✓5th **M84.8** Other disorders of continuity of bone
  - **M84.80** Other disorders of continuity of bone, unspecified site
  - ✓6th **M84.81** Other disorders of continuity of bone, **shoulder**
    - **M84.811** Other disorders of continuity of bone, **right** shoulder
    - **M84.812** Other disorders of continuity of bone, **left** shoulder
    - **M84.819** Other disorders of continuity of bone, unspecified shoulder
  - ✓6th **M84.82** Other disorders of continuity of bone, **humerus**
    - **M84.821** Other disorders of continuity of bone, **right** humerus
    - **M84.822** Other disorders of continuity of bone, **left** humerus
    - **M84.829** Other disorders of continuity of bone, unspecified humerus
  - ✓6th **M84.83** Other disorders of continuity of bone, **ulna and radius**
    - **M84.831** Other disorders of continuity of bone, **right ulna**
    - **M84.832** Other disorders of continuity of bone, **left ulna**
    - **M84.833** Other disorders of continuity of bone, **right radius**
    - **M84.834** Other disorders of continuity of bone, **left radius**
    - **M84.839** Other disorders of continuity of bone, unspecified ulna and radius
  - ✓6th **M84.84** Other disorders of continuity of bone, **hand**
    - **M84.841** Other disorders of continuity of bone, **right** hand
    - **M84.842** Other disorders of continuity of bone, **left** hand
    - **M84.849** Other disorders of continuity of bone, unspecified hand
  - ✓6th **M84.85** Other disorders of continuity of bone, **pelvic region and thigh**
    - **M84.851** Other disorders of continuity of bone, **right** pelvic region and thigh
    - **M84.852** Other disorders of continuity of bone, **left** pelvic region and thigh
    - **M84.859** Other disorders of continuity of bone, unspecified pelvic region and thigh
  - ✓6th **M84.86** Other disorders of continuity of bone, **tibia and fibula**
    - **M84.861** Other disorders of continuity of bone, **right tibia**
    - **M84.862** Other disorders of continuity of bone, **left tibia**
    - **M84.863** Other disorders of continuity of bone, **right fibula**
    - **M84.864** Other disorders of continuity of bone, **left fibula**
    - **M84.869** Other disorders of continuity of bone, unspecified tibia and fibula
  - ✓6th **M84.87** Other disorders of continuity of bone, **ankle and foot**
    - **M84.871** Other disorders of continuity of bone, **right** ankle and foot
    - **M84.872** Other disorders of continuity of bone, **left** ankle and foot
    - **M84.879** Other disorders of continuity of bone, unspecified ankle and foot
  - **M84.88** Other disorders of continuity of bone, other site
- **M84.9** Disorder of continuity of bone, unspecified
- ✓4th **M85** Other disorders of bone density and structure
  - EXCLUDES 1 osteogenesis imperfecta (Q78.0)
  - osteopetrosis (Q78.2)
  - osteopoikilosis (Q78.8)
  - polyostotic fibrous dysplasia (Q78.1)
  - ✓5th **M85.0** Fibrous dysplasia (monostotic)
    - EXCLUDES 2 fibrous dysplasia of jaw (M27.8)
    - **M85.00** Fibrous dysplasia (monostotic), unspecified site
    - ✓6th **M85.01** Fibrous dysplasia (monostotic), **shoulder**
      - **M85.011** Fibrous dysplasia (monostotic), **right** shoulder
      - **M85.012** Fibrous dysplasia (monostotic), **left** shoulder
      - **M85.019** Fibrous dysplasia (monostotic), unspecified shoulder
    - ✓6th **M85.02** Fibrous dysplasia (monostotic), **upper arm**
      - **M85.021** Fibrous dysplasia (monostotic), **right** upper arm
      - **M85.022** Fibrous dysplasia (monostotic), **left** upper arm
      - **M85.029** Fibrous dysplasia (monostotic), unspecified upper arm
    - ✓6th **M85.03** Fibrous dysplasia (monostotic), **forearm**
      - **M85.031** Fibrous dysplasia (monostotic), **right** forearm
      - **M85.032** Fibrous dysplasia (monostotic), **left** forearm
      - **M85.039** Fibrous dysplasia (monostotic), unspecified forearm
    - ✓6th **M85.04** Fibrous dysplasia (monostotic), **hand**
      - **M85.041** Fibrous dysplasia (monostotic), **right** hand
      - **M85.042** Fibrous dysplasia (monostotic), **left** hand
      - **M85.049** Fibrous dysplasia (monostotic), unspecified hand
    - ✓6th **M85.05** Fibrous dysplasia (monostotic), **thigh**
      - **M85.051** Fibrous dysplasia (monostotic), **right** thigh
      - **M85.052** Fibrous dysplasia (monostotic), **left** thigh
      - **M85.059** Fibrous dysplasia (monostotic), unspecified thigh
    - ✓6th **M85.06** Fibrous dysplasia (monostotic), **lower leg**
      - **M85.061** Fibrous dysplasia (monostotic), **right** lower leg
      - **M85.062** Fibrous dysplasia (monostotic), **left** lower leg
      - **M85.069** Fibrous dysplasia (monostotic), unspecified lower leg
    - ✓6th **M85.07** Fibrous dysplasia (monostotic), **ankle and foot**
      - **M85.071** Fibrous dysplasia (monostotic), **right** ankle and foot
      - **M85.072** Fibrous dysplasia (monostotic), **left** ankle and foot
      - **M85.079** Fibrous dysplasia (monostotic), unspecified ankle and foot
    - **M85.08** Fibrous dysplasia (monostotic), other site
    - **M85.09** Fibrous dysplasia (monostotic), **multiple sites**

✓ Additional Character Required | ✓x7th Placeholder Alert | Manifestation | Unspecified Dx | Q QPP | UPD Unacceptable PDx

Chapter 13. Diseases of the Musculoskeletal System and Connective Tissue

- ✓5th **M85.1** Skeletal fluorosis
  - **M85.10** Skeletal fluorosis, unspecified site
  - ✓6th **M85.11** Skeletal fluorosis, shoulder
    - **M85.111** Skeletal fluorosis, right shoulder
    - **M85.112** Skeletal fluorosis, left shoulder
    - **M85.119** Skeletal fluorosis, unspecified shoulder
  - ✓6th **M85.12** Skeletal fluorosis, upper arm
    - **M85.121** Skeletal fluorosis, right upper arm
    - **M85.122** Skeletal fluorosis, left upper arm
    - **M85.129** Skeletal fluorosis, unspecified upper arm
  - ✓6th **M85.13** Skeletal fluorosis, forearm
    - **M85.131** Skeletal fluorosis, right forearm
    - **M85.132** Skeletal fluorosis, left forearm
    - **M85.139** Skeletal fluorosis, unspecified forearm
  - ✓6th **M85.14** Skeletal fluorosis, hand
    - **M85.141** Skeletal fluorosis, right hand
    - **M85.142** Skeletal fluorosis, left hand
    - **M85.149** Skeletal fluorosis, unspecified hand
  - ✓6th **M85.15** Skeletal fluorosis, thigh
    - **M85.151** Skeletal fluorosis, right thigh
    - **M85.152** Skeletal fluorosis, left thigh
    - **M85.159** Skeletal fluorosis, unspecified thigh
  - ✓6th **M85.16** Skeletal fluorosis, lower leg
    - **M85.161** Skeletal fluorosis, right lower leg
    - **M85.162** Skeletal fluorosis, left lower leg
    - **M85.169** Skeletal fluorosis, unspecified lower leg
  - ✓6th **M85.17** Skeletal fluorosis, ankle and foot
    - **M85.171** Skeletal fluorosis, right ankle and foot
    - **M85.172** Skeletal fluorosis, left ankle and foot
    - **M85.179** Skeletal fluorosis, unspecified ankle and foot
  - **M85.18** Skeletal fluorosis, other site
  - **M85.19** Skeletal fluorosis, multiple sites
- **M85.2** Hyperostosis of skull
  - **DEF:** Abnormal bone growth on the inner aspect of the cranial bones.
- ✓5th **M85.3** Osteitis condensans
  - **M85.30** Osteitis condensans, unspecified site
  - ✓6th **M85.31** Osteitis condensans, shoulder
    - **M85.311** Osteitis condensans, right shoulder
    - **M85.312** Osteitis condensans, left shoulder
    - **M85.319** Osteitis condensans, unspecified shoulder
  - ✓6th **M85.32** Osteitis condensans, upper arm
    - **M85.321** Osteitis condensans, right upper arm
    - **M85.322** Osteitis condensans, left upper arm
    - **M85.329** Osteitis condensans, unspecified upper arm
  - ✓6th **M85.33** Osteitis condensans, forearm
    - **M85.331** Osteitis condensans, right forearm
    - **M85.332** Osteitis condensans, left forearm
    - **M85.339** Osteitis condensans, unspecified forearm
  - ✓6th **M85.34** Osteitis condensans, hand
    - **M85.341** Osteitis condensans, right hand
    - **M85.342** Osteitis condensans, left hand
    - **M85.349** Osteitis condensans, unspecified hand
  - ✓6th **M85.35** Osteitis condensans, thigh
    - **M85.351** Osteitis condensans, right thigh
    - **M85.352** Osteitis condensans, left thigh
    - **M85.359** Osteitis condensans, unspecified thigh
  - ✓6th **M85.36** Osteitis condensans, lower leg
    - **M85.361** Osteitis condensans, right lower leg
    - **M85.362** Osteitis condensans, left lower leg
    - **M85.369** Osteitis condensans, unspecified lower leg
  - ✓6th **M85.37** Osteitis condensans, ankle and foot
    - **M85.371** Osteitis condensans, right ankle and foot
    - **M85.372** Osteitis condensans, left ankle and foot
    - **M85.379** Osteitis condensans, unspecified ankle and foot
  - **M85.38** Osteitis condensans, other site
  - **M85.39** Osteitis condensans, multiple sites
- ✓5th **M85.4** Solitary bone cyst
  - *EXCLUDES 2* solitary cyst of jaw (M27.4)
  - **M85.40** Solitary bone cyst, unspecified site
  - ✓6th **M85.41** Solitary bone cyst, shoulder
    - **M85.411** Solitary bone cyst, right shoulder
    - **M85.412** Solitary bone cyst, left shoulder
    - **M85.419** Solitary bone cyst, unspecified shoulder
  - ✓6th **M85.42** Solitary bone cyst, humerus
    - **M85.421** Solitary bone cyst, right humerus
    - **M85.422** Solitary bone cyst, left humerus
    - **M85.429** Solitary bone cyst, unspecified humerus
  - ✓6th **M85.43** Solitary bone cyst, ulna and radius
    - **M85.431** Solitary bone cyst, right ulna and radius
    - **M85.432** Solitary bone cyst, left ulna and radius
    - **M85.439** Solitary bone cyst, unspecified ulna and radius
  - ✓6th **M85.44** Solitary bone cyst, hand
    - **M85.441** Solitary bone cyst, right hand
    - **M85.442** Solitary bone cyst, left hand
    - **M85.449** Solitary bone cyst, unspecified hand
  - ✓6th **M85.45** Solitary bone cyst, pelvis
    - **M85.451** Solitary bone cyst, right pelvis
    - **M85.452** Solitary bone cyst, left pelvis
    - **M85.459** Solitary bone cyst, unspecified pelvis
  - ✓6th **M85.46** Solitary bone cyst, tibia and fibula
    - **M85.461** Solitary bone cyst, right tibia and fibula
    - **M85.462** Solitary bone cyst, left tibia and fibula
    - **M85.469** Solitary bone cyst, unspecified tibia and fibula
  - ✓6th **M85.47** Solitary bone cyst, ankle and foot
    - **M85.471** Solitary bone cyst, right ankle and foot
    - **M85.472** Solitary bone cyst, left ankle and foot
    - **M85.479** Solitary bone cyst, unspecified ankle and foot
  - **M85.48** Solitary bone cyst, other site
- ✓5th **M85.5** Aneurysmal bone cyst
  - *EXCLUDES 2* aneurysmal cyst of jaw (M27.4)
  - **DEF:** Solitary bone lesion that bulges into the periosteum and is marked by a calcified rim.
  - **M85.50** Aneurysmal bone cyst, unspecified site
  - ✓6th **M85.51** Aneurysmal bone cyst, shoulder
    - **M85.511** Aneurysmal bone cyst, right shoulder
    - **M85.512** Aneurysmal bone cyst, left shoulder
    - **M85.519** Aneurysmal bone cyst, unspecified shoulder
  - ✓6th **M85.52** Aneurysmal bone cyst, upper arm
    - **M85.521** Aneurysmal bone cyst, right upper arm
    - **M85.522** Aneurysmal bone cyst, left upper arm
    - **M85.529** Aneurysmal bone cyst, unspecified upper arm
  - ✓6th **M85.53** Aneurysmal bone cyst, forearm
    - **M85.531** Aneurysmal bone cyst, right forearm
    - **M85.532** Aneurysmal bone cyst, left forearm
    - **M85.539** Aneurysmal bone cyst, unspecified forearm
  - ✓6th **M85.54** Aneurysmal bone cyst, hand
    - **M85.541** Aneurysmal bone cyst, right hand
    - **M85.542** Aneurysmal bone cyst, left hand
    - **M85.549** Aneurysmal bone cyst, unspecified hand
  - ✓6th **M85.55** Aneurysmal bone cyst, thigh
    - **M85.551** Aneurysmal bone cyst, right thigh
    - **M85.552** Aneurysmal bone cyst, left thigh
    - **M85.559** Aneurysmal bone cyst, unspecified thigh
  - ✓6th **M85.56** Aneurysmal bone cyst, lower leg
    - **M85.561** Aneurysmal bone cyst, right lower leg
    - **M85.562** Aneurysmal bone cyst, left lower leg
    - **M85.569** Aneurysmal bone cyst, unspecified lower leg
  - ✓6th **M85.57** Aneurysmal bone cyst, ankle and foot
    - **M85.571** Aneurysmal bone cyst, right ankle and foot
    - **M85.572** Aneurysmal bone cyst, left ankle and foot
    - **M85.579** Aneurysmal bone cyst, unspecified ankle and foot
  - **M85.58** Aneurysmal bone cyst, other site
  - **M85.59** Aneurysmal bone cyst, multiple sites
- ✓5th **M85.6** Other cyst of bone
  - *EXCLUDES 1* cyst of jaw NEC (M27.4)
  - osteitis fibrosa cystica generalisata [von Recklinghausen's disease of bone] (E21.0)
  - **M85.60** Other cyst of bone, unspecified site
  - ✓6th **M85.61** Other cyst of bone, shoulder
    - **M85.611** Other cyst of bone, right shoulder

	M85.612	Other cyst of bone, left shoulder
	M85.619	Other cyst of bone, unspecified shoulder
✓6th M85.62		Other cyst of bone, upper arm
	M85.621	Other cyst of bone, right upper arm
	M85.622	Other cyst of bone, left upper arm
	M85.629	Other cyst of bone, unspecified upper arm
✓6th M85.63		Other cyst of bone, forearm
	M85.631	Other cyst of bone, right forearm
	M85.632	Other cyst of bone, left forearm
	M85.639	Other cyst of bone, unspecified forearm
✓6th M85.64		Other cyst of bone, hand
	M85.641	Other cyst of bone, right hand
	M85.642	Other cyst of bone, left hand
	M85.649	Other cyst of bone, unspecified hand
✓6th M85.65		Other cyst of bone, thigh
	M85.651	Other cyst of bone, right thigh
	M85.652	Other cyst of bone, left thigh
	M85.659	Other cyst of bone, unspecified thigh
✓6th M85.66		Other cyst of bone, lower leg
	M85.661	Other cyst of bone, right lower leg
	M85.662	Other cyst of bone, left lower leg
	M85.669	Other cyst of bone, unspecified lower leg
✓6th M85.67		Other cyst of bone, ankle and foot
	M85.671	Other cyst of bone, right ankle and foot
	M85.672	Other cyst of bone, left ankle and foot
	M85.679	Other cyst of bone, unspecified ankle and foot
	M85.68	Other cyst of bone, other site
	M85.69	Other cyst of bone, multiple sites

✓5th **M85.8** Other specified disorders of bone density and structure
Hyperostosis of bones, except skull
Osteosclerosis, acquired
 EXCLUDES 1 diffuse idiopathic skeletal hyperostosis [DISH] (M48.1)
  osteosclerosis congenita (Q77.4)
  osteosclerosis fragilitas (generalista) (Q78.2)
  osteosclerosis myelofibrosis (D75.81)

	M85.80	Other specified disorders of bone density and structure, unspecified site
✓6th M85.81		Other specified disorders of bone density and structure, shoulder
	M85.811	Other specified disorders of bone density and structure, right shoulder
	M85.812	Other specified disorders of bone density and structure, left shoulder
	M85.819	Other specified disorders of bone density and structure, unspecified shoulder
✓6th M85.82		Other specified disorders of bone density and structure, upper arm
	M85.821	Other specified disorders of bone density and structure, right upper arm
	M85.822	Other specified disorders of bone density and structure, left upper arm
	M85.829	Other specified disorders of bone density and structure, unspecified upper arm
✓6th M85.83		Other specified disorders of bone density and structure, forearm
	M85.831	Other specified disorders of bone density and structure, right forearm
	M85.832	Other specified disorders of bone density and structure, left forearm
	M85.839	Other specified disorders of bone density and structure, unspecified forearm
✓6th M85.84		Other specified disorders of bone density and structure, hand
	M85.841	Other specified disorders of bone density and structure, right hand
	M85.842	Other specified disorders of bone density and structure, left hand
	M85.849	Other specified disorders of bone density and structure, unspecified hand
✓6th M85.85		Other specified disorders of bone density and structure, thigh
	M85.851	Other specified disorders of bone density and structure, right thigh
	M85.852	Other specified disorders of bone density and structure, left thigh
	M85.859	Other specified disorders of bone density and structure, unspecified thigh
✓6th M85.86		Other specified disorders of bone density and structure, lower leg
	M85.861	Other specified disorders of bone density and structure, right lower leg
	M85.862	Other specified disorders of bone density and structure, left lower leg
	M85.869	Other specified disorders of bone density and structure, unspecified lower leg
✓6th M85.87		Other specified disorders of bone density and structure, ankle and foot
	M85.871	Other specified disorders of bone density and structure, right ankle and foot
	M85.872	Other specified disorders of bone density and structure, left ankle and foot
	M85.879	Other specified disorders of bone density and structure, unspecified ankle and foot
	M85.88	Other specified disorders of bone density and structure, other site
	M85.89	Other specified disorders of bone density and structure, multiple sites
M85.9		Disorder of bone density and structure, unspecified

AHA: 2021,3Q,11

Other osteopathies (M86-M90)

 EXCLUDES 1 postprocedural osteopathies (M96.-)

✓4th **M86** Osteomyelitis
Use additional code (B95-B97) to identify infectious agent
Use additional code to identify major osseous defect, if applicable (M89.7-)
 EXCLUDES 1 osteomyelitis due to:
  echinococcus (B67.2)
  gonococcus (A54.43)
  salmonella (A02.24)
 EXCLUDES 2 osteomyelitis of:
  orbit (H05.0-)
  petrous bone (H70.2-)
  vertebra (M46.2-)

AHA: 2025,2Q,13

✓5th **M86.0** Acute hematogenous osteomyelitis

	M86.00	Acute hematogenous osteomyelitis, unspecified site
✓6th M86.01		Acute hematogenous osteomyelitis, shoulder
	M86.011	Acute hematogenous osteomyelitis, right shoulder
	M86.012	Acute hematogenous osteomyelitis, left shoulder
	M86.019	Acute hematogenous osteomyelitis, unspecified shoulder
✓6th M86.02		Acute hematogenous osteomyelitis, humerus
	M86.021	Acute hematogenous osteomyelitis, right humerus
	M86.022	Acute hematogenous osteomyelitis, left humerus
	M86.029	Acute hematogenous osteomyelitis, unspecified humerus
✓6th M86.03		Acute hematogenous osteomyelitis, radius and ulna
	M86.031	Acute hematogenous osteomyelitis, right radius and ulna
	M86.032	Acute hematogenous osteomyelitis, left radius and ulna
	M86.039	Acute hematogenous osteomyelitis, unspecified radius and ulna
✓6th M86.04		Acute hematogenous osteomyelitis, hand
	M86.041	Acute hematogenous osteomyelitis, right hand
	M86.042	Acute hematogenous osteomyelitis, left hand
	M86.049	Acute hematogenous osteomyelitis, unspecified hand
✓6th M86.05		Acute hematogenous osteomyelitis, femur
	M86.051	Acute hematogenous osteomyelitis, right femur
	M86.052	Acute hematogenous osteomyelitis, left femur
	M86.059	Acute hematogenous osteomyelitis, unspecified femur

M86.06 Acute hematogenous osteomyelitis, tibia and fibula
- **M86.061** Acute hematogenous osteomyelitis, right tibia and fibula [HCC] [ESR] [COM]
- **M86.062** Acute hematogenous osteomyelitis, left tibia and fibula [HCC] [ESR] [COM]
- **M86.069** Acute hematogenous osteomyelitis, unspecified tibia and fibula [HCC] [ESR] [COM]

M86.07 Acute hematogenous osteomyelitis, ankle and foot
- **M86.071** Acute hematogenous osteomyelitis, right ankle and foot [HCC] [ESR] [COM]
- **M86.072** Acute hematogenous osteomyelitis, left ankle and foot [HCC] [ESR] [COM]
- **M86.079** Acute hematogenous osteomyelitis, unspecified ankle and foot [HCC] [ESR] [COM]

M86.08 Acute hematogenous osteomyelitis, other sites

M86.09 Acute hematogenous osteomyelitis, multiple sites [HCC] [ESR] [COM]

M86.1 Other acute osteomyelitis
M86.10 Other acute osteomyelitis, unspecified site [HCC] [ESR] [COM]

M86.11 Other acute osteomyelitis, shoulder
- **M86.111** Other acute osteomyelitis, right shoulder [HCC] [ESR] [COM]
- **M86.112** Other acute osteomyelitis, left shoulder [HCC] [ESR] [COM]
- **M86.119** Other acute osteomyelitis, unspecified shoulder [HCC] [ESR] [COM]

M86.12 Other acute osteomyelitis, humerus
- **M86.121** Other acute osteomyelitis, right humerus [HCC] [ESR] [COM]
- **M86.122** Other acute osteomyelitis, left humerus [HCC] [ESR] [COM]
- **M86.129** Other acute osteomyelitis, unspecified humerus [HCC] [ESR] [COM]

M86.13 Other acute osteomyelitis, radius and ulna
- **M86.131** Other acute osteomyelitis, right radius and ulna [HCC] [ESR] [COM]
- **M86.132** Other acute osteomyelitis, left radius and ulna [HCC] [ESR] [COM]
- **M86.139** Other acute osteomyelitis, unspecified radius and ulna [HCC] [ESR] [COM]

M86.14 Other acute osteomyelitis, hand
- **M86.141** Other acute osteomyelitis, right hand [HCC] [ESR] [COM]
- **M86.142** Other acute osteomyelitis, left hand [HCC] [ESR] [COM]
- **M86.149** Other acute osteomyelitis, unspecified hand [HCC] [ESR] [COM]

M86.15 Other acute osteomyelitis, femur
- **M86.151** Other acute osteomyelitis, right femur [HCC] [ESR] [COM]
- **M86.152** Other acute osteomyelitis, left femur [HCC] [ESR] [COM]
- **M86.159** Other acute osteomyelitis, unspecified femur [HCC] [ESR] [COM]

M86.16 Other acute osteomyelitis, tibia and fibula
- **M86.161** Other acute osteomyelitis, right tibia and fibula [HCC] [ESR] [COM]
- **M86.162** Other acute osteomyelitis, left tibia and fibula [HCC] [ESR] [COM]
- **M86.169** Other acute osteomyelitis, unspecified tibia and fibula [HCC] [ESR] [COM]

M86.17 Other acute osteomyelitis, ankle and foot
AHA: 2020,1Q,12
- **M86.171** Other acute osteomyelitis, right ankle and foot [HCC] [ESR] [COM]
- **M86.172** Other acute osteomyelitis, left ankle and foot [HCC] [ESR] [COM]
- **M86.179** Other acute osteomyelitis, unspecified ankle and foot [HCC] [ESR] [COM]

M86.18 Other acute osteomyelitis, other site [HCC] [ESR] [COM]

M86.19 Other acute osteomyelitis, multiple sites [HCC] [ESR] [COM]

M86.2 Subacute osteomyelitis
M86.20 Subacute osteomyelitis, unspecified site [HCC] [ESR] [COM]

M86.21 Subacute osteomyelitis, shoulder
- **M86.211** Subacute osteomyelitis, right shoulder [HCC] [ESR] [COM]
- **M86.212** Subacute osteomyelitis, left shoulder [HCC] [ESR] [COM]
- **M86.219** Subacute osteomyelitis, unspecified shoulder [HCC] [ESR] [COM]

M86.22 Subacute osteomyelitis, humerus
- **M86.221** Subacute osteomyelitis, right humerus [HCC] [ESR] [COM]
- **M86.222** Subacute osteomyelitis, left humerus [HCC] [ESR] [COM]
- **M86.229** Subacute osteomyelitis, unspecified humerus [HCC] [ESR] [COM]

M86.23 Subacute osteomyelitis, radius and ulna
- **M86.231** Subacute osteomyelitis, right radius and ulna [HCC] [ESR] [COM]
- **M86.232** Subacute osteomyelitis, left radius and ulna [HCC] [ESR] [COM]
- **M86.239** Subacute osteomyelitis, unspecified radius and ulna [HCC] [ESR] [COM]

M86.24 Subacute osteomyelitis, hand
- **M86.241** Subacute osteomyelitis, right hand [HCC] [ESR] [COM]
- **M86.242** Subacute osteomyelitis, left hand [HCC] [ESR] [COM]
- **M86.249** Subacute osteomyelitis, unspecified hand [HCC] [ESR] [COM]

M86.25 Subacute osteomyelitis, femur
- **M86.251** Subacute osteomyelitis, right femur [HCC] [ESR] [COM]
- **M86.252** Subacute osteomyelitis, left femur [HCC] [ESR] [COM]
- **M86.259** Subacute osteomyelitis, unspecified femur [HCC] [ESR] [COM]

M86.26 Subacute osteomyelitis, tibia and fibula
- **M86.261** Subacute osteomyelitis, right tibia and fibula [HCC] [ESR] [COM]
- **M86.262** Subacute osteomyelitis, left tibia and fibula [HCC] [ESR] [COM]
- **M86.269** Subacute osteomyelitis, unspecified tibia and fibula [HCC] [ESR] [COM]

M86.27 Subacute osteomyelitis, ankle and foot
- **M86.271** Subacute osteomyelitis, right ankle and foot [HCC] [ESR] [COM]
- **M86.272** Subacute osteomyelitis, left ankle and foot [HCC] [ESR] [COM]
- **M86.279** Subacute osteomyelitis, unspecified ankle and foot [HCC] [ESR] [COM]

M86.28 Subacute osteomyelitis, other site

M86.29 Subacute osteomyelitis, multiple sites [HCC] [ESR] [COM]

M86.3 Chronic multifocal osteomyelitis
M86.30 Chronic multifocal osteomyelitis, unspecified site [HCC] [ESR] [COM]

M86.31 Chronic multifocal osteomyelitis, shoulder
- **M86.311** Chronic multifocal osteomyelitis, right shoulder [HCC] [ESR] [COM]
- **M86.312** Chronic multifocal osteomyelitis, left shoulder [HCC] [ESR] [COM]
- **M86.319** Chronic multifocal osteomyelitis, unspecified shoulder [HCC] [ESR] [COM]

M86.32 Chronic multifocal osteomyelitis, humerus
- **M86.321** Chronic multifocal osteomyelitis, right humerus [HCC] [ESR] [COM]
- **M86.322** Chronic multifocal osteomyelitis, left humerus [HCC] [ESR] [COM]
- **M86.329** Chronic multifocal osteomyelitis, unspecified humerus [HCC] [ESR] [COM]

M86.33 Chronic multifocal osteomyelitis, radius and ulna
- **M86.331** Chronic multifocal osteomyelitis, right radius and ulna [HCC] [ESR] [COM]

		M86.332	Chronic multifocal osteomyelitis, left radius and ulna [HCC] [ESR] [COM]
		M86.339	Chronic multifocal osteomyelitis, unspecified radius and ulna [HCC] [ESR] [COM]
✓6th	M86.34		Chronic multifocal osteomyelitis, hand
		M86.341	Chronic multifocal osteomyelitis, right hand [HCC] [ESR] [COM]
		M86.342	Chronic multifocal osteomyelitis, left hand [HCC] [ESR] [COM]
		M86.349	Chronic multifocal osteomyelitis, unspecified hand
✓6th	M86.35		Chronic multifocal osteomyelitis, femur
		M86.351	Chronic multifocal osteomyelitis, right femur [HCC] [ESR] [COM]
		M86.352	Chronic multifocal osteomyelitis, left femur [HCC] [ESR] [COM]
		M86.359	Chronic multifocal osteomyelitis, unspecified femur
✓6th	M86.36		Chronic multifocal osteomyelitis, tibia and fibula
		M86.361	Chronic multifocal osteomyelitis, right tibia and fibula
		M86.362	Chronic multifocal osteomyelitis, left tibia and fibula
		M86.369	Chronic multifocal osteomyelitis, unspecified tibia and fibula
✓6th	M86.37		Chronic multifocal osteomyelitis, ankle and foot
		M86.371	Chronic multifocal osteomyelitis, right ankle and foot [HCC] [ESR] [COM]
		M86.372	Chronic multifocal osteomyelitis, left ankle and foot
		M86.379	Chronic multifocal osteomyelitis, unspecified ankle and foot [HCC] [ESR] [COM]
	M86.38		Chronic multifocal osteomyelitis, other site [HCC] [ESR] [COM]
	M86.39		Chronic multifocal osteomyelitis, multiple sites [HCC] [ESR] [COM]
✓5th	M86.4		Chronic osteomyelitis with draining sinus
		M86.40	Chronic osteomyelitis with draining sinus, unspecified site [HCC] [ESR] [COM]
✓6th	M86.41		Chronic osteomyelitis with draining sinus, shoulder
		M86.411	Chronic osteomyelitis with draining sinus, right shoulder [HCC] [ESR] [COM]
		M86.412	Chronic osteomyelitis with draining sinus, left shoulder [HCC] [ESR] [COM]
		M86.419	Chronic osteomyelitis with draining sinus, unspecified shoulder [HCC] [ESR] [COM]
✓6th	M86.42		Chronic osteomyelitis with draining sinus, humerus
		M86.421	Chronic osteomyelitis with draining sinus, right humerus
		M86.422	Chronic osteomyelitis with draining sinus, left humerus [HCC] [ESR] [COM]
		M86.429	Chronic osteomyelitis with draining sinus, unspecified humerus [HCC] [ESR] [COM]
✓6th	M86.43		Chronic osteomyelitis with draining sinus, radius and ulna
		M86.431	Chronic osteomyelitis with draining sinus, right radius and ulna [HCC] [ESR] [COM]
		M86.432	Chronic osteomyelitis with draining sinus, left radius and ulna [HCC] [ESR] [COM]
		M86.439	Chronic osteomyelitis with draining sinus, unspecified radius and ulna [HCC] [ESR] [COM]
✓6th	M86.44		Chronic osteomyelitis with draining sinus, hand
		M86.441	Chronic osteomyelitis with draining sinus, right hand [HCC] [ESR] [COM]
		M86.442	Chronic osteomyelitis with draining sinus, left hand [HCC] [ESR] [COM]
		M86.449	Chronic osteomyelitis with draining sinus, unspecified hand [HCC] [ESR] [COM]
✓6th	M86.45		Chronic osteomyelitis with draining sinus, femur
		M86.451	Chronic osteomyelitis with draining sinus, right femur
		M86.452	Chronic osteomyelitis with draining sinus, left femur [HCC] [ESR] [COM]
		M86.459	Chronic osteomyelitis with draining sinus, unspecified femur [HCC] [ESR] [COM]
✓6th	M86.46		Chronic osteomyelitis with draining sinus, tibia and fibula
		M86.461	Chronic osteomyelitis with draining sinus, right tibia and fibula [HCC] [ESR] [COM]
		M86.462	Chronic osteomyelitis with draining sinus, left tibia and fibula [HCC] [ESR] [COM]
		M86.469	Chronic osteomyelitis with draining sinus, unspecified tibia and fibula [HCC] [ESR] [COM]
✓6th	M86.47		Chronic osteomyelitis with draining sinus, ankle and foot
		M86.471	Chronic osteomyelitis with draining sinus, right ankle and foot [HCC] [ESR] [COM]
		M86.472	Chronic osteomyelitis with draining sinus, left ankle and foot [HCC] [ESR] [COM]
		M86.479	Chronic osteomyelitis with draining sinus, unspecified ankle and foot [HCC] [ESR] [COM]
	M86.48		Chronic osteomyelitis with draining sinus, other site [HCC] [ESR] [COM]
	M86.49		Chronic osteomyelitis with draining sinus, multiple sites [HCC] [ESR] [COM]
✓5th	M86.5		Other chronic hematogenous osteomyelitis
		M86.50	Other chronic hematogenous osteomyelitis, unspecified site [HCC] [ESR] [COM]
✓6th	M86.51		Other chronic hematogenous osteomyelitis, shoulder
		M86.511	Other chronic hematogenous osteomyelitis, right shoulder
		M86.512	Other chronic hematogenous osteomyelitis, left shoulder [HCC] [ESR] [COM]
		M86.519	Other chronic hematogenous osteomyelitis, unspecified shoulder
✓6th	M86.52		Other chronic hematogenous osteomyelitis, humerus
		M86.521	Other chronic hematogenous osteomyelitis, right humerus
		M86.522	Other chronic hematogenous osteomyelitis, left humerus [HCC] [ESR] [COM]
		M86.529	Other chronic hematogenous osteomyelitis, unspecified humerus [HCC] [ESR] [COM]
✓6th	M86.53		Other chronic hematogenous osteomyelitis, radius and ulna
		M86.531	Other chronic hematogenous osteomyelitis, right radius and ulna [HCC] [ESR] [COM]
		M86.532	Other chronic hematogenous osteomyelitis, left radius and ulna [HCC] [ESR] [COM]
		M86.539	Other chronic hematogenous osteomyelitis, unspecified radius and ulna [HCC] [ESR] [COM]
✓6th	M86.54		Other chronic hematogenous osteomyelitis, hand
		M86.541	Other chronic hematogenous osteomyelitis, right hand [HCC] [ESR] [COM]
		M86.542	Other chronic hematogenous osteomyelitis, left hand [HCC] [ESR] [COM]
		M86.549	Other chronic hematogenous osteomyelitis, unspecified hand [HCC] [ESR] [COM]
✓6th	M86.55		Other chronic hematogenous osteomyelitis, femur
		M86.551	Other chronic hematogenous osteomyelitis, right femur [HCC] [ESR] [COM]
		M86.552	Other chronic hematogenous osteomyelitis, left femur
		M86.559	Other chronic hematogenous osteomyelitis, unspecified femur [HCC] [ESR] [COM]
✓6th	M86.56		Other chronic hematogenous osteomyelitis, tibia and fibula
		M86.561	Other chronic hematogenous osteomyelitis, right tibia and fibula [HCC] [ESR] [COM]
		M86.562	Other chronic hematogenous osteomyelitis, left tibia and fibula [HCC] [ESR] [COM]

Chapter 13. Diseases of the Musculoskeletal System and Connective Tissue

- M86.569 Other chronic hematogenous osteomyelitis, unspecified tibia and fibula
- ✓6th M86.57 Other chronic hematogenous osteomyelitis, ankle and foot
  - M86.571 Other chronic hematogenous osteomyelitis, right ankle and foot
  - M86.572 Other chronic hematogenous osteomyelitis, left ankle and foot
  - M86.579 Other chronic hematogenous osteomyelitis, unspecified ankle and foot
- M86.58 Other chronic hematogenous osteomyelitis, other site
- M86.59 Other chronic hematogenous osteomyelitis, multiple sites
- ✓5th M86.6 Other chronic osteomyelitis
  - M86.60 Other chronic osteomyelitis, unspecified site
  - ✓6th M86.61 Other chronic osteomyelitis, shoulder
    - M86.611 Other chronic osteomyelitis, right shoulder
    - M86.612 Other chronic osteomyelitis, left shoulder
    - M86.619 Other chronic osteomyelitis, unspecified shoulder
  - ✓6th M86.62 Other chronic osteomyelitis, humerus
    - M86.621 Other chronic osteomyelitis, right humerus
    - M86.622 Other chronic osteomyelitis, left humerus
    - M86.629 Other chronic osteomyelitis, unspecified humerus
  - ✓6th M86.63 Other chronic osteomyelitis, radius and ulna
    - M86.631 Other chronic osteomyelitis, right radius and ulna
    - M86.632 Other chronic osteomyelitis, left radius and ulna
    - M86.639 Other chronic osteomyelitis, unspecified radius and ulna
  - ✓6th M86.64 Other chronic osteomyelitis, hand
    - M86.641 Other chronic osteomyelitis, right hand
    - M86.642 Other chronic osteomyelitis, left hand
    - M86.649 Other chronic osteomyelitis, unspecified hand
  - ✓6th M86.65 Other chronic osteomyelitis, thigh
    - M86.651 Other chronic osteomyelitis, right thigh
    - M86.652 Other chronic osteomyelitis, left thigh
    - M86.659 Other chronic osteomyelitis, unspecified thigh
  - ✓6th M86.66 Other chronic osteomyelitis, tibia and fibula
    - M86.661 Other chronic osteomyelitis, right tibia and fibula
    - M86.662 Other chronic osteomyelitis, left tibia and fibula
    - M86.669 Other chronic osteomyelitis, unspecified tibia and fibula
  - ✓6th M86.67 Other chronic osteomyelitis, ankle and foot
    - M86.671 Other chronic osteomyelitis, right ankle and foot
      - AHA: 2016,1Q,13
    - M86.672 Other chronic osteomyelitis, left ankle and foot
    - M86.679 Other chronic osteomyelitis, unspecified ankle and foot
  - M86.68 Other chronic osteomyelitis, other site
  - M86.69 Other chronic osteomyelitis, multiple sites
- ✓5th M86.8 Other osteomyelitis
  - Brodie's abscess
  - AHA: 2022,1Q,31
  - ✓6th M86.8X Other osteomyelitis
    - M86.8X0 Other osteomyelitis, multiple sites
    - M86.8X1 Other osteomyelitis, shoulder
    - M86.8X2 Other osteomyelitis, upper arm
    - M86.8X3 Other osteomyelitis, forearm
    - M86.8X4 Other osteomyelitis, hand
    - M86.8X5 Other osteomyelitis, thigh
    - M86.8X6 Other osteomyelitis, lower leg
    - M86.8X7 Other osteomyelitis, ankle and foot
    - M86.8X8 Other osteomyelitis, other site
    - M86.8X9 Other osteomyelitis, unspecified sites
- M86.9 Osteomyelitis, unspecified
  - Infection of bone NOS
  - Periostitis without osteomyelitis
- ✓4th M87 Osteonecrosis
  - INCLUDES avascular necrosis of bone
  - Use additional code to identify major osseous defect, if applicable (M89.7-)
  - EXCLUDES 1 juvenile osteonecrosis (M91-M92)
  - osteochondropathies (M90-M93)
  - ✓5th M87.0 Idiopathic aseptic necrosis of bone
    - M87.00 Idiopathic aseptic necrosis of unspecified bone
    - ✓6th M87.01 Idiopathic aseptic necrosis of shoulder
      - Idiopathic aseptic necrosis of clavicle and scapula
      - M87.011 Idiopathic aseptic necrosis of right shoulder
      - M87.012 Idiopathic aseptic necrosis of left shoulder
      - M87.019 Idiopathic aseptic necrosis of unspecified shoulder
    - ✓6th M87.02 Idiopathic aseptic necrosis of humerus
      - M87.021 Idiopathic aseptic necrosis of right humerus
      - M87.022 Idiopathic aseptic necrosis of left humerus
      - M87.029 Idiopathic aseptic necrosis of unspecified humerus
    - ✓6th M87.03 Idiopathic aseptic necrosis of radius, ulna and carpus
      - M87.031 Idiopathic aseptic necrosis of right radius
      - M87.032 Idiopathic aseptic necrosis of left radius
      - M87.033 Idiopathic aseptic necrosis of unspecified radius
      - M87.034 Idiopathic aseptic necrosis of right ulna
      - M87.035 Idiopathic aseptic necrosis of left ulna
      - M87.036 Idiopathic aseptic necrosis of unspecified ulna
      - M87.037 Idiopathic aseptic necrosis of right carpus
      - M87.038 Idiopathic aseptic necrosis of left carpus
      - M87.039 Idiopathic aseptic necrosis of unspecified carpus
    - ✓6th M87.04 Idiopathic aseptic necrosis of hand and fingers
      - Idiopathic aseptic necrosis of metacarpals and phalanges of hands
      - M87.041 Idiopathic aseptic necrosis of right hand
      - M87.042 Idiopathic aseptic necrosis of left hand
      - M87.043 Idiopathic aseptic necrosis of unspecified hand

M87.044	Idiopathic aseptic necrosis of right finger(s) HCC Rx ESR COM
M87.045	Idiopathic aseptic necrosis of left finger(s) HCC Rx ESR COM
M87.046	Idiopathic aseptic necrosis of unspecified finger(s) HCC Rx ESR COM

√6th **M87.05** Idiopathic aseptic necrosis of pelvis and femur
- M87.050 Idiopathic aseptic necrosis of pelvis HCC Rx ESR COM
- M87.051 Idiopathic aseptic necrosis of right femur HCC Rx ESR COM
- M87.052 Idiopathic aseptic necrosis of left femur HCC Rx ESR COM
- M87.059 Idiopathic aseptic necrosis of unspecified femur HCC Rx ESR COM

√6th **M87.06** Idiopathic aseptic necrosis of tibia and fibula
- M87.061 Idiopathic aseptic necrosis of right tibia HCC Rx ESR COM
- M87.062 Idiopathic aseptic necrosis of left tibia HCC Rx ESR COM
- M87.063 Idiopathic aseptic necrosis of unspecified tibia HCC Rx ESR COM
- M87.064 Idiopathic aseptic necrosis of right fibula HCC Rx ESR COM
- M87.065 Idiopathic aseptic necrosis of left fibula HCC Rx ESR COM
- M87.066 Idiopathic aseptic necrosis of unspecified fibula HCC Rx ESR COM

√6th **M87.07** Idiopathic aseptic necrosis of ankle, foot and toes
  Idiopathic aseptic necrosis of metatarsus, tarsus, and phalanges of toes
- M87.071 Idiopathic aseptic necrosis of right ankle HCC Rx ESR COM
- M87.072 Idiopathic aseptic necrosis of left ankle HCC Rx ESR COM
- M87.073 Idiopathic aseptic necrosis of unspecified ankle HCC Rx ESR COM
- M87.074 Idiopathic aseptic necrosis of right foot HCC Rx ESR COM
- M87.075 Idiopathic aseptic necrosis of left foot HCC Rx ESR COM
- M87.076 Idiopathic aseptic necrosis of unspecified foot HCC Rx ESR COM
- M87.077 Idiopathic aseptic necrosis of right toe(s) HCC Rx ESR COM
- M87.078 Idiopathic aseptic necrosis of left toe(s) HCC Rx ESR COM
- M87.079 Idiopathic aseptic necrosis of unspecified toe(s) HCC Rx ESR COM

M87.08 Idiopathic aseptic necrosis of bone, other site
M87.09 Idiopathic aseptic necrosis of bone, multiple sites HCC Rx ESR COM

√5th **M87.1** Osteonecrosis due to drugs
  Use additional code for adverse effect, if applicable, to identify drug (T36-T50 with fifth or sixth character 5)
- M87.10 Osteonecrosis due to drugs, unspecified bone Rx ESR COM

√6th **M87.11** Osteonecrosis due to drugs, shoulder
- M87.111 Osteonecrosis due to drugs, right shoulder Rx ESR COM
- M87.112 Osteonecrosis due to drugs, left shoulder Rx ESR COM
- M87.119 Osteonecrosis due to drugs, unspecified shoulder Rx ESR COM

√6th **M87.12** Osteonecrosis due to drugs, humerus
- M87.121 Osteonecrosis due to drugs, right humerus Rx ESR COM
- M87.122 Osteonecrosis due to drugs, left humerus Rx ESR COM
- M87.129 Osteonecrosis due to drugs, unspecified humerus Rx ESR COM

√6th **M87.13** Osteonecrosis due to drugs of radius, ulna and carpus
- M87.131 Osteonecrosis due to drugs of right radius Rx ESR COM
- M87.132 Osteonecrosis due to drugs of left radius Rx ESR COM
- M87.133 Osteonecrosis due to drugs of unspecified radius Rx ESR COM
- M87.134 Osteonecrosis due to drugs of right ulna Rx ESR COM
- M87.135 Osteonecrosis due to drugs of left ulna Rx ESR COM
- M87.136 Osteonecrosis due to drugs of unspecified ulna Rx ESR COM
- M87.137 Osteonecrosis due to drugs of right carpus Rx ESR COM
- M87.138 Osteonecrosis due to drugs of left carpus Rx ESR COM
- M87.139 Osteonecrosis due to drugs of unspecified carpus Rx ESR COM

√6th **M87.14** Osteonecrosis due to drugs, hand and fingers
- M87.141 Osteonecrosis due to drugs, right hand Rx ESR COM
- M87.142 Osteonecrosis due to drugs, left hand Rx ESR COM
- M87.143 Osteonecrosis due to drugs, unspecified hand Rx ESR COM
- M87.144 Osteonecrosis due to drugs, right finger(s) Rx ESR COM
- M87.145 Osteonecrosis due to drugs, left finger(s) Rx ESR COM
- M87.146 Osteonecrosis due to drugs, unspecified finger(s) Rx ESR COM

√6th **M87.15** Osteonecrosis due to drugs, pelvis and femur
- M87.150 Osteonecrosis due to drugs, pelvis Rx ESR COM
- M87.151 Osteonecrosis due to drugs, right femur Rx ESR COM
- M87.152 Osteonecrosis due to drugs, left femur Rx ESR COM
- M87.159 Osteonecrosis due to drugs, unspecified femur Rx ESR COM

√6th **M87.16** Osteonecrosis due to drugs, tibia and fibula
- M87.161 Osteonecrosis due to drugs, right tibia Rx ESR COM
- M87.162 Osteonecrosis due to drugs, left tibia Rx ESR COM
- M87.163 Osteonecrosis due to drugs, unspecified tibia Rx ESR COM
- M87.164 Osteonecrosis due to drugs, right fibula Rx ESR COM
- M87.165 Osteonecrosis due to drugs, left fibula Rx ESR COM
- M87.166 Osteonecrosis due to drugs, unspecified fibula Rx ESR COM

√6th **M87.17** Osteonecrosis due to drugs, ankle, foot and toes
- M87.171 Osteonecrosis due to drugs, right ankle Rx ESR COM
- M87.172 Osteonecrosis due to drugs, left ankle Rx ESR COM
- M87.173 Osteonecrosis due to drugs, unspecified ankle Rx ESR COM
- M87.174 Osteonecrosis due to drugs, right foot Rx ESR COM
- M87.175 Osteonecrosis due to drugs, left foot Rx ESR COM
- M87.176 Osteonecrosis due to drugs, unspecified foot Rx ESR COM
- M87.177 Osteonecrosis due to drugs, right toe(s) Rx ESR COM
- M87.178 Osteonecrosis due to drugs, left toe(s) Rx ESR COM
- M87.179 Osteonecrosis due to drugs, unspecified toe(s) Rx ESR COM

√6th **M87.18** Osteonecrosis due to drugs, other site
- M87.180 Osteonecrosis due to drugs, jaw Rx ESR COM
- M87.188 Osteonecrosis due to drugs, other site Rx ESR COM

M87.19 Osteonecrosis due to drugs, multiple sites Rx ESR COM

M87.2 Osteonecrosis due to previous trauma

- **M87.20** Osteonecrosis due to previous trauma, unspecified bone
- **M87.21** Osteonecrosis due to previous trauma, shoulder
  - **M87.211** Osteonecrosis due to previous trauma, right shoulder
  - **M87.212** Osteonecrosis due to previous trauma, left shoulder
  - **M87.219** Osteonecrosis due to previous trauma, unspecified shoulder
- **M87.22** Osteonecrosis due to previous trauma, humerus
  - **M87.221** Osteonecrosis due to previous trauma, right humerus
  - **M87.222** Osteonecrosis due to previous trauma, left humerus
  - **M87.229** Osteonecrosis due to previous trauma, unspecified humerus
- **M87.23** Osteonecrosis due to previous trauma of radius, ulna and carpus
  - **M87.231** Osteonecrosis due to previous trauma of right radius
  - **M87.232** Osteonecrosis due to previous trauma of left radius
  - **M87.233** Osteonecrosis due to previous trauma of unspecified radius
  - **M87.234** Osteonecrosis due to previous trauma of right ulna
  - **M87.235** Osteonecrosis due to previous trauma of left ulna
  - **M87.236** Osteonecrosis due to previous trauma of unspecified ulna
  - **M87.237** Osteonecrosis due to previous trauma of right carpus
  - **M87.238** Osteonecrosis due to previous trauma of left carpus
  - **M87.239** Osteonecrosis due to previous trauma of unspecified carpus
- **M87.24** Osteonecrosis due to previous trauma, hand and fingers
  - **M87.241** Osteonecrosis due to previous trauma, right hand
  - **M87.242** Osteonecrosis due to previous trauma, left hand
  - **M87.243** Osteonecrosis due to previous trauma, unspecified hand
  - **M87.244** Osteonecrosis due to previous trauma, right finger(s)
  - **M87.245** Osteonecrosis due to previous trauma, left finger(s)
  - **M87.246** Osteonecrosis due to previous trauma, unspecified finger(s)
- **M87.25** Osteonecrosis due to previous trauma, pelvis and femur
  - **M87.250** Osteonecrosis due to previous trauma, pelvis
  - **M87.251** Osteonecrosis due to previous trauma, right femur
  - **M87.252** Osteonecrosis due to previous trauma, left femur
  - **M87.256** Osteonecrosis due to previous trauma, unspecified femur
- **M87.26** Osteonecrosis due to previous trauma, tibia and fibula
  - **M87.261** Osteonecrosis due to previous trauma, right tibia
  - **M87.262** Osteonecrosis due to previous trauma, left tibia
  - **M87.263** Osteonecrosis due to previous trauma, unspecified tibia
  - **M87.264** Osteonecrosis due to previous trauma, right fibula
  - **M87.265** Osteonecrosis due to previous trauma, left fibula
  - **M87.266** Osteonecrosis due to previous trauma, unspecified fibula
- **M87.27** Osteonecrosis due to previous trauma, ankle, foot and toes
  - **M87.271** Osteonecrosis due to previous trauma, right ankle
  - **M87.272** Osteonecrosis due to previous trauma, left ankle
  - **M87.273** Osteonecrosis due to previous trauma, unspecified ankle
  - **M87.274** Osteonecrosis due to previous trauma, right foot
  - **M87.275** Osteonecrosis due to previous trauma, left foot
  - **M87.276** Osteonecrosis due to previous trauma, unspecified foot
  - **M87.277** Osteonecrosis due to previous trauma, right toe(s)
  - **M87.278** Osteonecrosis due to previous trauma, left toe(s)
  - **M87.279** Osteonecrosis due to previous trauma, unspecified toe(s)
- **M87.28** Osteonecrosis due to previous trauma, other site
- **M87.29** Osteonecrosis due to previous trauma, multiple sites

M87.3 Other secondary osteonecrosis

- **M87.30** Other secondary osteonecrosis, unspecified bone
- **M87.31** Other secondary osteonecrosis, shoulder
  - **M87.311** Other secondary osteonecrosis, right shoulder
  - **M87.312** Other secondary osteonecrosis, left shoulder
  - **M87.319** Other secondary osteonecrosis, unspecified shoulder
- **M87.32** Other secondary osteonecrosis, humerus
  - **M87.321** Other secondary osteonecrosis, right humerus
  - **M87.322** Other secondary osteonecrosis, left humerus
  - **M87.329** Other secondary osteonecrosis, unspecified humerus
- **M87.33** Other secondary osteonecrosis of radius, ulna and carpus
  - **M87.331** Other secondary osteonecrosis of right radius
  - **M87.332** Other secondary osteonecrosis of left radius
  - **M87.333** Other secondary osteonecrosis of unspecified radius
  - **M87.334** Other secondary osteonecrosis of right ulna
  - **M87.335** Other secondary osteonecrosis of left ulna
  - **M87.336** Other secondary osteonecrosis of unspecified ulna
  - **M87.337** Other secondary osteonecrosis of right carpus
  - **M87.338** Other secondary osteonecrosis of left carpus
  - **M87.339** Other secondary osteonecrosis of unspecified carpus
- **M87.34** Other secondary osteonecrosis, hand and fingers
  - **M87.341** Other secondary osteonecrosis, right hand
  - **M87.342** Other secondary osteonecrosis, left hand
  - **M87.343** Other secondary osteonecrosis, unspecified hand
  - **M87.344** Other secondary osteonecrosis, right finger(s)
  - **M87.345** Other secondary osteonecrosis, left finger(s)
  - **M87.346** Other secondary osteonecrosis, unspecified finger(s)
- **M87.35** Other secondary osteonecrosis, pelvis and femur
  - **M87.350** Other secondary osteonecrosis, pelvis
  - **M87.351** Other secondary osteonecrosis, right femur
  - **M87.352** Other secondary osteonecrosis, left femur

Chapter 13. Diseases of the Musculoskeletal System and Connective Tissue

- M87.353 Other secondary osteonecrosis, unspecified femur [HCC] [Rx] [ESR] [COM]
- ✓6th **M87.36** Other secondary osteonecrosis, **tibia and fibula**
  - M87.361 Other secondary osteonecrosis, **right tibia** [HCC] [Rx] [ESR] [COM]
  - M87.362 Other secondary osteonecrosis, **left tibia** [HCC] [Rx] [ESR] [COM]
  - M87.363 Other secondary osteonecrosis, unspecified tibia [HCC] [Rx] [ESR] [COM]
  - M87.364 Other secondary osteonecrosis, **right fibula** [HCC] [Rx] [ESR] [COM]
  - M87.365 Other secondary osteonecrosis, **left fibula** [HCC] [Rx] [ESR] [COM]
  - M87.366 Other secondary osteonecrosis, unspecified fibula [HCC] [Rx] [ESR] [COM]
- ✓6th **M87.37** Other secondary osteonecrosis, **ankle and foot**
  - M87.371 Other secondary osteonecrosis, **right ankle** [HCC] [Rx] [ESR] [COM]
  - M87.372 Other secondary osteonecrosis, **left ankle** [HCC] [Rx] [ESR] [COM]
  - M87.373 Other secondary osteonecrosis, unspecified ankle [HCC] [Rx] [ESR] [COM]
  - M87.374 Other secondary osteonecrosis, **right foot** [HCC] [Rx] [ESR] [COM]
  - M87.375 Other secondary osteonecrosis, **left foot** [HCC] [Rx] [ESR] [COM]
  - M87.376 Other secondary osteonecrosis, unspecified foot [HCC] [Rx] [ESR] [COM]
  - M87.377 Other secondary osteonecrosis, **right toe(s)** [HCC] [Rx] [ESR] [COM]
  - M87.378 Other secondary osteonecrosis, **left toe(s)** [HCC] [Rx] [ESR] [COM]
  - M87.379 Other secondary osteonecrosis, unspecified toe(s) [HCC] [Rx] [ESR] [COM]
- M87.38 Other secondary osteonecrosis, other site
- M87.39 Other secondary osteonecrosis, **multiple sites** [HCC] [Rx] [ESR] [COM]
- ✓5th **M87.8** Other osteonecrosis
  - M87.80 Other osteonecrosis, unspecified bone [HCC] [Rx] [ESR] [COM]
  - ✓6th **M87.81** Other osteonecrosis, **shoulder**
    - M87.811 Other osteonecrosis, **right shoulder** [HCC] [Rx] [ESR] [COM]
    - M87.812 Other osteonecrosis, **left shoulder** [HCC] [Rx] [ESR] [COM]
    - M87.819 Other osteonecrosis, unspecified shoulder [HCC] [Rx] [ESR] [COM]
  - ✓6th **M87.82** Other osteonecrosis, **humerus**
    - M87.821 Other osteonecrosis, **right humerus** [HCC] [Rx] [ESR] [COM]
    - M87.822 Other osteonecrosis, **left humerus** [HCC] [Rx] [ESR] [COM]
    - M87.829 Other osteonecrosis, unspecified humerus [HCC] [Rx] [ESR] [COM]
  - ✓6th **M87.83** Other osteonecrosis of **radius, ulna and carpus**
    - M87.831 Other osteonecrosis of **right radius** [HCC] [Rx] [ESR] [COM]
    - M87.832 Other osteonecrosis of **left radius** [HCC] [Rx] [ESR] [COM]
    - M87.833 Other osteonecrosis of unspecified radius [HCC] [Rx] [ESR] [COM]
    - M87.834 Other osteonecrosis of **right ulna** [HCC] [Rx] [ESR] [COM]
    - M87.835 Other osteonecrosis of **left ulna** [HCC] [Rx] [ESR] [COM]
    - M87.836 Other osteonecrosis of unspecified ulna [HCC] [Rx] [ESR] [COM]
    - M87.837 Other osteonecrosis of **right carpus** [HCC] [Rx] [ESR] [COM]
    - M87.838 Other osteonecrosis of **left carpus** [HCC] [Rx] [ESR] [COM]
    - M87.839 Other osteonecrosis of unspecified carpus [HCC] [Rx] [ESR] [COM]
  - ✓6th **M87.84** Other osteonecrosis, **hand and fingers**
    - M87.841 Other osteonecrosis, **right hand** [HCC] [Rx] [ESR] [COM]
    - M87.842 Other osteonecrosis, **left hand** [HCC] [Rx] [ESR] [COM]
    - M87.843 Other osteonecrosis, unspecified hand [HCC] [Rx] [ESR] [COM]
    - M87.844 Other osteonecrosis, **right finger(s)** [HCC] [Rx] [ESR] [COM]
    - M87.845 Other osteonecrosis, **left finger(s)** [HCC] [Rx] [ESR] [COM]
    - M87.849 Other osteonecrosis, unspecified finger(s) [HCC] [Rx] [ESR] [COM]
  - ✓6th **M87.85** Other osteonecrosis, **pelvis and femur**
    - M87.850 Other osteonecrosis, **pelvis** [HCC] [Rx] [ESR] [COM]
    - M87.851 Other osteonecrosis, **right femur** [HCC] [Rx] [ESR] [COM]
    - M87.852 Other osteonecrosis, **left femur** [HCC] [Rx] [ESR] [COM]
    - M87.859 Other osteonecrosis, unspecified femur [HCC] [Rx] [ESR] [COM]
  - ✓6th **M87.86** Other osteonecrosis, **tibia and fibula**
    - M87.861 Other osteonecrosis, **right tibia** [HCC] [Rx] [ESR] [COM]
    - M87.862 Other osteonecrosis, **left tibia** [HCC] [Rx] [ESR] [COM]
    - M87.863 Other osteonecrosis, unspecified tibia [HCC] [Rx] [ESR] [COM]
    - M87.864 Other osteonecrosis, **right fibula** [HCC] [Rx] [ESR] [COM]
    - M87.865 Other osteonecrosis, **left fibula** [HCC] [Rx] [ESR] [COM]
    - M87.869 Other osteonecrosis, unspecified fibula [HCC] [Rx] [ESR] [COM]
  - ✓6th **M87.87** Other osteonecrosis, **ankle, foot and toes**
    - M87.871 Other osteonecrosis, **right ankle** [HCC] [Rx] [ESR] [COM]
    - M87.872 Other osteonecrosis, **left ankle** [HCC] [Rx] [ESR] [COM]
    - M87.873 Other osteonecrosis, unspecified ankle [HCC] [Rx] [ESR] [COM]
    - M87.874 Other osteonecrosis, **right foot** [HCC] [Rx] [ESR] [COM]
    - M87.875 Other osteonecrosis, **left foot** [HCC] [Rx] [ESR] [COM]
    - M87.876 Other osteonecrosis, unspecified foot [HCC] [Rx] [ESR] [COM]
    - M87.877 Other osteonecrosis, **right toe(s)** [HCC] [Rx] [ESR] [COM]
    - M87.878 Other osteonecrosis, **left toe(s)** [HCC] [Rx] [ESR] [COM]
    - M87.879 Other osteonecrosis, unspecified toe(s) [HCC] [Rx] [ESR] [COM]
  - M87.88 Other osteonecrosis, other site [HCC] [Rx] [ESR] [COM]
  - M87.89 Other osteonecrosis, **multiple sites** [HCC] [Rx] [ESR] [COM]
- M87.9 Osteonecrosis, unspecified [HCC] [Rx] [ESR] [COM]
  Necrosis of bone NOS

✓4th **M88** Osteitis deformans [Paget's disease of bone]

EXCLUDES 1 osteitis deformans in neoplastic disease (M90.6)
DEF: Bone disease characterized by numerous cycles of bone resorption by the body. Resorption is followed by accelerated repair attempts, causing bone deformities and bowing, with associated fractures and pain.

- M88.0 Osteitis deformans of **skull**
- M88.1 Osteitis deformans of **vertebrae**
- ✓5th **M88.8** Osteitis deformans of other bones
  - ✓6th **M88.81** Osteitis deformans of **shoulder**
    - M88.811 Osteitis deformans of **right** shoulder
    - M88.812 Osteitis deformans of **left** shoulder
    - M88.819 Osteitis deformans of unspecified shoulder
  - ✓6th **M88.82** Osteitis deformans of **upper arm**
    - M88.821 Osteitis deformans of **right** upper arm
    - M88.822 Osteitis deformans of **left** upper arm
    - M88.829 Osteitis deformans of unspecified upper arm
  - ✓6th **M88.83** Osteitis deformans of **forearm**
    - M88.831 Osteitis deformans of **right** forearm
    - M88.832 Osteitis deformans of **left** forearm
    - M88.839 Osteitis deformans of unspecified forearm

- ✓6th **M88.84** Osteitis deformans of hand
  - M88.841 Osteitis deformans of right hand
  - M88.842 Osteitis deformans of left hand
  - M88.849 Osteitis deformans of unspecified hand
- ✓6th **M88.85** Osteitis deformans of thigh
  - M88.851 Osteitis deformans of right thigh
  - M88.852 Osteitis deformans of left thigh
  - M88.859 Osteitis deformans of unspecified thigh
- ✓6th **M88.86** Osteitis deformans of lower leg
  - M88.861 Osteitis deformans of right lower leg
  - M88.862 Osteitis deformans of left lower leg
  - M88.869 Osteitis deformans of unspecified lower leg
- ✓6th **M88.87** Osteitis deformans of ankle and foot
  - M88.871 Osteitis deformans of right ankle and foot
  - M88.872 Osteitis deformans of left ankle and foot
  - M88.879 Osteitis deformans of unspecified ankle and foot
- **M88.88** Osteitis deformans of other bones
  - EXCLUDES 2 osteitis deformans of skull (M88.0)
    osteitis deformans of vertebrae (M88.1)
- **M88.89** Osteitis deformans of multiple sites
- **M88.9** Osteitis deformans of unspecified bone

✓4th **M89** Other disorders of bone

- ✓5th **M89.0** Algoneurodystrophy
  - Shoulder-hand syndrome
  - Sudeck's atrophy
  - EXCLUDES 1 causalgia, lower limb (G57.7-)
    causalgia, upper limb (G56.4-)
    complex regional pain syndrome II, lower limb (G57.7-)
    complex regional pain syndrome II, upper limb (G56.4-)
    reflex sympathetic dystrophy (G90.5-)
  - **M89.00** Algoneurodystrophy, unspecified site
  - ✓6th **M89.01** Algoneurodystrophy, shoulder
    - M89.011 Algoneurodystrophy, right shoulder
    - M89.012 Algoneurodystrophy, left shoulder
    - M89.019 Algoneurodystrophy, unspecified shoulder
  - ✓6th **M89.02** Algoneurodystrophy, upper arm
    - M89.021 Algoneurodystrophy, right upper arm
    - M89.022 Algoneurodystrophy, left upper arm
    - M89.029 Algoneurodystrophy, unspecified upper arm
  - ✓6th **M89.03** Algoneurodystrophy, forearm
    - M89.031 Algoneurodystrophy, right forearm
    - M89.032 Algoneurodystrophy, left forearm
    - M89.039 Algoneurodystrophy, unspecified forearm
  - ✓6th **M89.04** Algoneurodystrophy, hand
    - M89.041 Algoneurodystrophy, right hand
    - M89.042 Algoneurodystrophy, left hand
    - M89.049 Algoneurodystrophy, unspecified hand
  - ✓6th **M89.05** Algoneurodystrophy, thigh
    - M89.051 Algoneurodystrophy, right thigh
    - M89.052 Algoneurodystrophy, left thigh
    - M89.059 Algoneurodystrophy, unspecified thigh
  - ✓6th **M89.06** Algoneurodystrophy, lower leg
    - M89.061 Algoneurodystrophy, right lower leg
    - M89.062 Algoneurodystrophy, left lower leg
    - M89.069 Algoneurodystrophy, unspecified lower leg
  - ✓6th **M89.07** Algoneurodystrophy, ankle and foot
    - M89.071 Algoneurodystrophy, right ankle and foot
    - M89.072 Algoneurodystrophy, left ankle and foot
    - M89.079 Algoneurodystrophy, unspecified ankle and foot
  - **M89.08** Algoneurodystrophy, other site
  - **M89.09** Algoneurodystrophy, multiple sites
- ✓5th **M89.1** Physeal arrest
  - Arrest of growth plate
  - Epiphyseal arrest
  - Growth plate arrest
  - ✓6th **M89.12** Physeal arrest, humerus
    - M89.121 Complete physeal arrest, right proximal humerus
    - M89.122 Complete physeal arrest, left proximal humerus
    - M89.123 Partial physeal arrest, right proximal humerus
    - M89.124 Partial physeal arrest, left proximal humerus
    - M89.125 Complete physeal arrest, right distal humerus
    - M89.126 Complete physeal arrest, left distal humerus
    - M89.127 Partial physeal arrest, right distal humerus
    - M89.128 Partial physeal arrest, left distal humerus
    - M89.129 Physeal arrest, humerus, unspecified
  - ✓6th **M89.13** Physeal arrest, forearm
    - M89.131 Complete physeal arrest, right distal radius
    - M89.132 Complete physeal arrest, left distal radius
    - M89.133 Partial physeal arrest, right distal radius
    - M89.134 Partial physeal arrest, left distal radius
    - M89.138 Other physeal arrest of forearm
    - M89.139 Physeal arrest, forearm, unspecified
  - ✓6th **M89.15** Physeal arrest, femur
    - M89.151 Complete physeal arrest, right proximal femur
    - M89.152 Complete physeal arrest, left proximal femur
    - M89.153 Partial physeal arrest, right proximal femur
    - M89.154 Partial physeal arrest, left proximal femur
    - M89.155 Complete physeal arrest, right distal femur
    - M89.156 Complete physeal arrest, left distal femur
    - M89.157 Partial physeal arrest, right distal femur
    - M89.158 Partial physeal arrest, left distal femur
    - M89.159 Physeal arrest, femur, unspecified
  - ✓6th **M89.16** Physeal arrest, lower leg
    - M89.160 Complete physeal arrest, right proximal tibia
    - M89.161 Complete physeal arrest, left proximal tibia
    - M89.162 Partial physeal arrest, right proximal tibia
    - M89.163 Partial physeal arrest, left proximal tibia
    - M89.164 Complete physeal arrest, right distal tibia
    - M89.165 Complete physeal arrest, left distal tibia
    - M89.166 Partial physeal arrest, right distal tibia
    - M89.167 Partial physeal arrest, left distal tibia
    - M89.168 Other physeal arrest of lower leg
    - M89.169 Physeal arrest, lower leg, unspecified
  - **M89.18** Physeal arrest, other site
- ✓5th **M89.2** Other disorders of bone development and growth
  - **M89.20** Other disorders of bone development and growth, unspecified site
  - ✓6th **M89.21** Other disorders of bone development and growth, shoulder
    - M89.211 Other disorders of bone development and growth, right shoulder
    - M89.212 Other disorders of bone development and growth, left shoulder
    - M89.219 Other disorders of bone development and growth, unspecified shoulder
  - ✓6th **M89.22** Other disorders of bone development and growth, humerus
    - M89.221 Other disorders of bone development and growth, right humerus
    - M89.222 Other disorders of bone development and growth, left humerus
    - M89.229 Other disorders of bone development and growth, unspecified humerus
  - ✓6th **M89.23** Other disorders of bone development and growth, ulna and radius
    - M89.231 Other disorders of bone development and growth, right ulna
    - M89.232 Other disorders of bone development and growth, left ulna
    - M89.233 Other disorders of bone development and growth, right radius
    - M89.234 Other disorders of bone development and growth, left radius
    - M89.239 Other disorders of bone development and growth, unspecified ulna and radius
  - ✓6th **M89.24** Other disorders of bone development and growth, hand
    - M89.241 Other disorders of bone development and growth, right hand
    - M89.242 Other disorders of bone development and growth, left hand
    - M89.249 Other disorders of bone development and growth, unspecified hand

Chapter 13. Diseases of the Musculoskeletal System and Connective Tissue

- ✓6th **M89.25** Other disorders of bone development and growth, femur
  - M89.251 Other disorders of bone development and growth, right femur
  - M89.252 Other disorders of bone development and growth, left femur
  - M89.259 Other disorders of bone development and growth, unspecified femur
- ✓6th **M89.26** Other disorders of bone development and growth, tibia and fibula
  - M89.261 Other disorders of bone development and growth, right tibia
  - M89.262 Other disorders of bone development and growth, left tibia
  - M89.263 Other disorders of bone development and growth, right fibula
  - M89.264 Other disorders of bone development and growth, left fibula
  - M89.269 Other disorders of bone development and growth, unspecified lower leg
- ✓6th **M89.27** Other disorders of bone development and growth, ankle and foot
  - M89.271 Other disorders of bone development and growth, right ankle and foot
  - M89.272 Other disorders of bone development and growth, left ankle and foot
  - M89.279 Other disorders of bone development and growth, unspecified ankle and foot
- **M89.28** Other disorders of bone development and growth, other site
- **M89.29** Other disorders of bone development and growth, multiple sites
- ✓5th **M89.3** Hypertrophy of bone
  - **M89.30** Hypertrophy of bone, unspecified site
  - ✓6th **M89.31** Hypertrophy of bone, shoulder
    - M89.311 Hypertrophy of bone, right shoulder
    - M89.312 Hypertrophy of bone, left shoulder
    - M89.319 Hypertrophy of bone, unspecified shoulder
  - ✓6th **M89.32** Hypertrophy of bone, humerus
    - M89.321 Hypertrophy of bone, right humerus
    - M89.322 Hypertrophy of bone, left humerus
    - M89.329 Hypertrophy of bone, unspecified humerus
  - ✓6th **M89.33** Hypertrophy of bone, ulna and radius
    - M89.331 Hypertrophy of bone, right ulna
    - M89.332 Hypertrophy of bone, left ulna
    - M89.333 Hypertrophy of bone, right radius
    - M89.334 Hypertrophy of bone, left radius
    - M89.339 Hypertrophy of bone, unspecified ulna and radius
  - ✓6th **M89.34** Hypertrophy of bone, hand
    - M89.341 Hypertrophy of bone, right hand
    - M89.342 Hypertrophy of bone, left hand
    - M89.349 Hypertrophy of bone, unspecified hand
  - ✓6th **M89.35** Hypertrophy of bone, femur
    - M89.351 Hypertrophy of bone, right femur
    - M89.352 Hypertrophy of bone, left femur
    - M89.359 Hypertrophy of bone, unspecified femur
  - ✓6th **M89.36** Hypertrophy of bone, tibia and fibula
    - M89.361 Hypertrophy of bone, right tibia
    - M89.362 Hypertrophy of bone, left tibia
    - M89.363 Hypertrophy of bone, right fibula
    - M89.364 Hypertrophy of bone, left fibula
    - M89.369 Hypertrophy of bone, unspecified tibia and fibula
  - ✓6th **M89.37** Hypertrophy of bone, ankle and foot
    - M89.371 Hypertrophy of bone, right ankle and foot
    - M89.372 Hypertrophy of bone, left ankle and foot
    - M89.379 Hypertrophy of bone, unspecified ankle and foot
  - **M89.38** Hypertrophy of bone, other site
  - **M89.39** Hypertrophy of bone, multiple sites
- ✓5th **M89.4** Other hypertrophic osteoarthropathy
  - Marie-Bamberger disease
  - Pachydermoperiostosis
  - **M89.40** Other hypertrophic osteoarthropathy, unspecified site
  - ✓6th **M89.41** Other hypertrophic osteoarthropathy, shoulder
    - M89.411 Other hypertrophic osteoarthropathy, right shoulder
    - M89.412 Other hypertrophic osteoarthropathy, left shoulder
    - M89.419 Other hypertrophic osteoarthropathy, unspecified shoulder
  - ✓6th **M89.42** Other hypertrophic osteoarthropathy, upper arm
    - M89.421 Other hypertrophic osteoarthropathy, right upper arm
    - M89.422 Other hypertrophic osteoarthropathy, left upper arm
    - M89.429 Other hypertrophic osteoarthropathy, unspecified upper arm
  - ✓6th **M89.43** Other hypertrophic osteoarthropathy, forearm
    - M89.431 Other hypertrophic osteoarthropathy, right forearm
    - M89.432 Other hypertrophic osteoarthropathy, left forearm
    - M89.439 Other hypertrophic osteoarthropathy, unspecified forearm
  - ✓6th **M89.44** Other hypertrophic osteoarthropathy, hand
    - M89.441 Other hypertrophic osteoarthropathy, right hand
    - M89.442 Other hypertrophic osteoarthropathy, left hand
    - M89.449 Other hypertrophic osteoarthropathy, unspecified hand
  - ✓6th **M89.45** Other hypertrophic osteoarthropathy, thigh
    - M89.451 Other hypertrophic osteoarthropathy, right thigh
    - M89.452 Other hypertrophic osteoarthropathy, left thigh
    - M89.459 Other hypertrophic osteoarthropathy, unspecified thigh
  - ✓6th **M89.46** Other hypertrophic osteoarthropathy, lower leg
    - M89.461 Other hypertrophic osteoarthropathy, right lower leg
    - M89.462 Other hypertrophic osteoarthropathy, left lower leg
    - M89.469 Other hypertrophic osteoarthropathy, unspecified lower leg
  - ✓6th **M89.47** Other hypertrophic osteoarthropathy, ankle and foot
    - M89.471 Other hypertrophic osteoarthropathy, right ankle and foot
    - M89.472 Other hypertrophic osteoarthropathy, left ankle and foot
    - M89.479 Other hypertrophic osteoarthropathy, unspecified ankle and foot
  - **M89.48** Other hypertrophic osteoarthropathy, other site
  - **M89.49** Other hypertrophic osteoarthropathy, multiple sites
- ✓5th **M89.5** Osteolysis
  - Use additional code to identify major osseous defect, if applicable (M89.7-)
  - EXCLUDES 2: periprosthetic osteolysis of internal prosthetic joint (T84.05-)
  - **M89.50** Osteolysis, unspecified site
  - ✓6th **M89.51** Osteolysis, shoulder
    - M89.511 Osteolysis, right shoulder
    - M89.512 Osteolysis, left shoulder
    - M89.519 Osteolysis, unspecified shoulder
  - ✓6th **M89.52** Osteolysis, upper arm
    - M89.521 Osteolysis, right upper arm
    - M89.522 Osteolysis, left upper arm
    - M89.529 Osteolysis, unspecified upper arm
  - ✓6th **M89.53** Osteolysis, forearm
    - M89.531 Osteolysis, right forearm
    - M89.532 Osteolysis, left forearm
    - M89.539 Osteolysis, unspecified forearm
  - ✓6th **M89.54** Osteolysis, hand
    - M89.541 Osteolysis, right hand
    - M89.542 Osteolysis, left hand
    - M89.549 Osteolysis, unspecified hand
  - ✓6th **M89.55** Osteolysis, thigh
    - M89.551 Osteolysis, right thigh
    - M89.552 Osteolysis, left thigh
    - M89.559 Osteolysis, unspecified thigh
  - ✓6th **M89.56** Osteolysis, lower leg
    - M89.561 Osteolysis, right lower leg
    - M89.562 Osteolysis, left lower leg
    - M89.569 Osteolysis, unspecified lower leg

Chapter 13. Diseases of the Musculoskeletal System and Connective Tissue

M89.57 Osteolysis, ankle and foot
- M89.571 Osteolysis, right ankle and foot
- M89.572 Osteolysis, left ankle and foot
- M89.579 Osteolysis, unspecified ankle and foot

M89.58 Osteolysis, other site

M89.59 Osteolysis, multiple sites

M89.6 Osteopathy after poliomyelitis
Use additional code (B91) to identify previous poliomyelitis
EXCLUDES 1 postpolio syndrome (G14)

- **M89.60** Osteopathy after poliomyelitis, unspecified site
- **M89.61** Osteopathy after poliomyelitis, shoulder
  - M89.611 Osteopathy after poliomyelitis, right shoulder
  - M89.612 Osteopathy after poliomyelitis, left shoulder
  - M89.619 Osteopathy after poliomyelitis, unspecified shoulder
- **M89.62** Osteopathy after poliomyelitis, upper arm
  - M89.621 Osteopathy after poliomyelitis, right upper arm
  - M89.622 Osteopathy after poliomyelitis, left upper arm
  - M89.629 Osteopathy after poliomyelitis, unspecified upper arm
- **M89.63** Osteopathy after poliomyelitis, forearm
  - M89.631 Osteopathy after poliomyelitis, right forearm
  - M89.632 Osteopathy after poliomyelitis, left forearm
  - M89.639 Osteopathy after poliomyelitis, unspecified forearm
- **M89.64** Osteopathy after poliomyelitis, hand
  - M89.641 Osteopathy after poliomyelitis, right hand
  - M89.642 Osteopathy after poliomyelitis, left hand
  - M89.649 Osteopathy after poliomyelitis, unspecified hand
- **M89.65** Osteopathy after poliomyelitis, thigh
  - M89.651 Osteopathy after poliomyelitis, right thigh
  - M89.652 Osteopathy after poliomyelitis, left thigh
  - M89.659 Osteopathy after poliomyelitis, unspecified thigh
- **M89.66** Osteopathy after poliomyelitis, lower leg
  - M89.661 Osteopathy after poliomyelitis, right lower leg
  - M89.662 Osteopathy after poliomyelitis, left lower leg
  - M89.669 Osteopathy after poliomyelitis, unspecified lower leg
- **M89.67** Osteopathy after poliomyelitis, ankle and foot
  - M89.671 Osteopathy after poliomyelitis, right ankle and foot
  - M89.672 Osteopathy after poliomyelitis, left ankle and foot
  - M89.679 Osteopathy after poliomyelitis, unspecified ankle and foot
- **M89.68** Osteopathy after poliomyelitis, other site
- **M89.69** Osteopathy after poliomyelitis, multiple sites

M89.7 Major osseous defect
Code first underlying disease, if known, such as:
aseptic necrosis of bone (M87.-)
malignant neoplasm of bone (C40.-)
osteolysis (M89.5-)
osteomyelitis (M86.-)
osteonecrosis (M87.-)
osteoporosis (M80.-, M81.-)
periprosthetic osteolysis (T84.05-)

- **M89.70** Major osseous defect, unspecified site
- **M89.71** Major osseous defect, shoulder region
  Major osseous defect clavicle or scapula
  - M89.711 Major osseous defect, right shoulder region
  - M89.712 Major osseous defect, left shoulder region
  - M89.719 Major osseous defect, unspecified shoulder region
- **M89.72** Major osseous defect, humerus
  - M89.721 Major osseous defect, right humerus
  - M89.722 Major osseous defect, left humerus
  - M89.729 Major osseous defect, unspecified humerus
- **M89.73** Major osseous defect, forearm
  Major osseous defect of radius and ulna
  - M89.731 Major osseous defect, right forearm
  - M89.732 Major osseous defect, left forearm
  - M89.739 Major osseous defect, unspecified forearm
- **M89.74** Major osseous defect, hand
  Major osseous defect of carpus, fingers, metacarpus
  - M89.741 Major osseous defect, right hand
  - M89.742 Major osseous defect, left hand
  - M89.749 Major osseous defect, unspecified hand
- **M89.75** Major osseous defect, pelvic region and thigh
  Major osseous defect of femur and pelvis
  - M89.751 Major osseous defect, right pelvic region and thigh
  - M89.752 Major osseous defect, left pelvic region and thigh
  - M89.759 Major osseous defect, unspecified pelvic region and thigh
- **M89.76** Major osseous defect, lower leg
  Major osseous defect of fibula and tibia
  - M89.761 Major osseous defect, right lower leg
  - M89.762 Major osseous defect, left lower leg
  - M89.769 Major osseous defect, unspecified lower leg
- **M89.77** Major osseous defect, ankle and foot
  Major osseous defect of metatarsus, tarsus, toes
  - M89.771 Major osseous defect, right ankle and foot
  - M89.772 Major osseous defect, left ankle and foot
  - M89.779 Major osseous defect, unspecified ankle and foot
- **M89.78** Major osseous defect, other site
- **M89.79** Major osseous defect, multiple sites

M89.8 Other specified disorders of bone
Infantile cortical hyperostoses
Post-traumatic subperiosteal ossification
AHA: 2022,2Q,10

- **M89.8X** Other specified disorders of bone
  - M89.8X0 Other specified disorders of bone, multiple sites
  - M89.8X1 Other specified disorders of bone, shoulder
  - M89.8X2 Other specified disorders of bone, upper arm
  - M89.8X3 Other specified disorders of bone, forearm
    AHA: 2019,3Q,9
  - M89.8X4 Other specified disorders of bone, hand
  - M89.8X5 Other specified disorders of bone, thigh
  - M89.8X6 Other specified disorders of bone, lower leg
  - M89.8X7 Other specified disorders of bone, ankle and foot
  - M89.8X8 Other specified disorders of bone, other site
    AHA: 2025,2Q,13; 2023,2Q,18
  - M89.8X9 Other specified disorders of bone, unspecified site

M89.9 Disorder of bone, unspecified

M90 Osteopathies in diseases classified elsewhere

EXCLUDES 1 osteochondritis, osteomyelitis, and osteopathy (in):
- cryptococcosis (B45.3)
- diabetes mellitus (E08-E13 with .69-)
- gonococcal (A54.43)
- neurogenic syphilis (A52.11)
- renal osteodystrophy (N25.0)
- salmonellosis (A02.24)
- secondary syphilis (A51.46)
- syphilis (late) (A52.77)

M90.5 Osteonecrosis in diseases classified elsewhere
Code first underlying disease, such as:
- caisson disease (T70.3)
- hemoglobinopathy (D50-D64)

- M90.50 Osteonecrosis in diseases classified elsewhere, unspecified site
- M90.51 Osteonecrosis in diseases classified elsewhere, shoulder
  - M90.511 Osteonecrosis in diseases classified elsewhere, right shoulder
  - M90.512 Osteonecrosis in diseases classified elsewhere, left shoulder
  - M90.519 Osteonecrosis in diseases classified elsewhere, unspecified shoulder
- M90.52 Osteonecrosis in diseases classified elsewhere, upper arm
  - M90.521 Osteonecrosis in diseases classified elsewhere, right upper arm
  - M90.522 Osteonecrosis in diseases classified elsewhere, left upper arm
  - M90.529 Osteonecrosis in diseases classified elsewhere, unspecified upper arm
- M90.53 Osteonecrosis in diseases classified elsewhere, forearm
  - M90.531 Osteonecrosis in diseases classified elsewhere, right forearm
  - M90.532 Osteonecrosis in diseases classified elsewhere, left forearm
  - M90.539 Osteonecrosis in diseases classified elsewhere, unspecified forearm
- M90.54 Osteonecrosis in diseases classified elsewhere, hand
  - M90.541 Osteonecrosis in diseases classified elsewhere, right hand
  - M90.542 Osteonecrosis in diseases classified elsewhere, left hand
  - M90.549 Osteonecrosis in diseases classified elsewhere, unspecified hand
- M90.55 Osteonecrosis in diseases classified elsewhere, thigh
  - M90.551 Osteonecrosis in diseases classified elsewhere, right thigh
  - M90.552 Osteonecrosis in diseases classified elsewhere, left thigh
  - M90.559 Osteonecrosis in diseases classified elsewhere, unspecified thigh
- M90.56 Osteonecrosis in diseases classified elsewhere, lower leg
  - M90.561 Osteonecrosis in diseases classified elsewhere, right lower leg
  - M90.562 Osteonecrosis in diseases classified elsewhere, left lower leg
  - M90.569 Osteonecrosis in diseases classified elsewhere, unspecified lower leg
- M90.57 Osteonecrosis in diseases classified elsewhere, ankle and foot
  - M90.571 Osteonecrosis in diseases classified elsewhere, right ankle and foot
  - M90.572 Osteonecrosis in diseases classified elsewhere, left ankle and foot
  - M90.579 Osteonecrosis in diseases classified elsewhere, unspecified ankle and foot
- M90.58 Osteonecrosis in diseases classified elsewhere, other site
- M90.59 Osteonecrosis in diseases classified elsewhere, multiple sites

M90.6 Osteitis deformans in neoplastic diseases
Osteitis deformans in malignant neoplasm of bone
Code first the neoplasm (C40.-, C41.-)
EXCLUDES 1 osteitis deformans [Paget's disease of bone] (M88.-)

- M90.60 Osteitis deformans in neoplastic diseases, unspecified site
- M90.61 Osteitis deformans in neoplastic diseases, shoulder
  - M90.611 Osteitis deformans in neoplastic diseases, right shoulder
  - M90.612 Osteitis deformans in neoplastic diseases, left shoulder
  - M90.619 Osteitis deformans in neoplastic diseases, unspecified shoulder
- M90.62 Osteitis deformans in neoplastic diseases, upper arm
  - M90.621 Osteitis deformans in neoplastic diseases, right upper arm
  - M90.622 Osteitis deformans in neoplastic diseases, left upper arm
  - M90.629 Osteitis deformans in neoplastic diseases, unspecified upper arm
- M90.63 Osteitis deformans in neoplastic diseases, forearm
  - M90.631 Osteitis deformans in neoplastic diseases, right forearm
  - M90.632 Osteitis deformans in neoplastic diseases, left forearm
  - M90.639 Osteitis deformans in neoplastic diseases, unspecified forearm
- M90.64 Osteitis deformans in neoplastic diseases, hand
  - M90.641 Osteitis deformans in neoplastic diseases, right hand
  - M90.642 Osteitis deformans in neoplastic diseases, left hand
  - M90.649 Osteitis deformans in neoplastic diseases, unspecified hand
- M90.65 Osteitis deformans in neoplastic diseases, thigh
  - M90.651 Osteitis deformans in neoplastic diseases, right thigh
  - M90.652 Osteitis deformans in neoplastic diseases, left thigh
  - M90.659 Osteitis deformans in neoplastic diseases, unspecified thigh
- M90.66 Osteitis deformans in neoplastic diseases, lower leg
  - M90.661 Osteitis deformans in neoplastic diseases, right lower leg
  - M90.662 Osteitis deformans in neoplastic diseases, left lower leg
  - M90.669 Osteitis deformans in neoplastic diseases, unspecified lower leg
- M90.67 Osteitis deformans in neoplastic diseases, ankle and foot
  - M90.671 Osteitis deformans in neoplastic diseases, right ankle and foot
  - M90.672 Osteitis deformans in neoplastic diseases, left ankle and foot
  - M90.679 Osteitis deformans in neoplastic diseases, unspecified ankle and foot
- M90.68 Osteitis deformans in neoplastic diseases, other site
- M90.69 Osteitis deformans in neoplastic diseases, multiple sites

M90.8 Osteopathy in diseases classified elsewhere
Code first underlying disease, such as:
- rickets (E55.0)
- vitamin-D-resistant rickets (E83.31)

- M90.80 Osteopathy in diseases classified elsewhere, unspecified site
- M90.81 Osteopathy in diseases classified elsewhere, shoulder
  - M90.811 Osteopathy in diseases classified elsewhere, right shoulder
  - M90.812 Osteopathy in diseases classified elsewhere, left shoulder
  - M90.819 Osteopathy in diseases classified elsewhere, unspecified shoulder

Chapter 13. Diseases of the Musculoskeletal System and Connective Tissue

- ✓6th **M90.82** Osteopathy in diseases classified elsewhere, **upper arm**
  - M90.821 Osteopathy in diseases classified elsewhere, **right** upper arm
  - M90.822 Osteopathy in diseases classified elsewhere, **left** upper arm
  - M90.829 Osteopathy in diseases classified elsewhere, **unspecified** upper arm
- ✓6th **M90.83** Osteopathy in diseases classified elsewhere, **forearm**
  - M90.831 Osteopathy in diseases classified elsewhere, **right** forearm
  - M90.832 Osteopathy in diseases classified elsewhere, **left** forearm
  - M90.839 Osteopathy in diseases classified elsewhere, **unspecified** forearm
- ✓6th **M90.84** Osteopathy in diseases classified elsewhere, **hand**
  - M90.841 Osteopathy in diseases classified elsewhere, **right** hand
  - M90.842 Osteopathy in diseases classified elsewhere, **left** hand
  - M90.849 Osteopathy in diseases classified elsewhere, **unspecified** hand
- ✓6th **M90.85** Osteopathy in diseases classified elsewhere, **thigh**
  - M90.851 Osteopathy in diseases classified elsewhere, **right** thigh
  - M90.852 Osteopathy in diseases classified elsewhere, **left** thigh
  - M90.859 Osteopathy in diseases classified elsewhere, **unspecified** thigh
- ✓6th **M90.86** Osteopathy in diseases classified elsewhere, **lower leg**
  - M90.861 Osteopathy in diseases classified elsewhere, **right** lower leg
  - M90.862 Osteopathy in diseases classified elsewhere, **left** lower leg
  - M90.869 Osteopathy in diseases classified elsewhere, **unspecified** lower leg
- ✓6th **M90.87** Osteopathy in diseases classified elsewhere, **ankle and foot**
  - M90.871 Osteopathy in diseases classified elsewhere, **right** ankle and foot
  - M90.872 Osteopathy in diseases classified elsewhere, **left** ankle and foot
  - M90.879 Osteopathy in diseases classified elsewhere, **unspecified** ankle and foot
- **M90.88** Osteopathy in diseases classified elsewhere, other site
- **M90.89** Osteopathy in diseases classified elsewhere, **multiple sites**

Chondropathies (M91-M94)

EXCLUDES 1: postprocedural chondropathies (M96.-)

- ✓4th **M91 Juvenile osteochondrosis of hip and pelvis**
  - EXCLUDES 1: slipped upper femoral epiphysis (nontraumatic) (M93.0-)
  - **M91.0** Juvenile osteochondrosis of **pelvis** [COM]
    - Osteochondrosis (juvenile) of acetabulum
    - Osteochondrosis (juvenile) of iliac crest [Buchanan]
    - Osteochondrosis (juvenile) of ischiopubic synchondrosis [van Neck]
    - Osteochondrosis (juvenile) of symphysis pubis [Pierson]
  - ✓5th **M91.1** Juvenile osteochondrosis of **head of femur** [Legg-Calve-Perthes]
    - M91.10 Juvenile osteochondrosis of head of femur [Legg-Calve-Perthes], unspecified leg
    - M91.11 Juvenile osteochondrosis of head of femur [Legg-Calve-Perthes], **right** leg
    - M91.12 Juvenile osteochondrosis of head of femur [Legg-Calve-Perthes], **left** leg
  - ✓5th **M91.2 Coxa plana**
    - Hip deformity due to previous juvenile osteochondrosis
    - M91.20 Coxa plana, unspecified hip
    - M91.21 Coxa plana, **right** hip
    - M91.22 Coxa plana, **left** hip
  - ✓5th **M91.3 Pseudocoxalgia**
    - M91.30 Pseudocoxalgia, unspecified hip
    - M91.31 Pseudocoxalgia, **right** hip
    - M91.32 Pseudocoxalgia, **left** hip
  - ✓5th **M91.4 Coxa magna**
    - M91.40 Coxa magna, unspecified hip
    - M91.41 Coxa magna, **right** hip
    - M91.42 Coxa magna, **left** hip
  - ✓5th **M91.8** Other juvenile osteochondrosis of hip and pelvis
    - Juvenile osteochondrosis after reduction of congenital dislocation of hip
    - M91.80 Other juvenile osteochondrosis of hip and pelvis, unspecified leg
    - M91.81 Other juvenile osteochondrosis of hip and pelvis, **right** leg
    - M91.82 Other juvenile osteochondrosis of hip and pelvis, **left** leg
  - ✓5th **M91.9** Juvenile osteochondrosis of hip and pelvis, unspecified
    - M91.90 Juvenile osteochondrosis of hip and pelvis, unspecified, unspecified leg
    - M91.91 Juvenile osteochondrosis of hip and pelvis, unspecified, **right** leg
    - M91.92 Juvenile osteochondrosis of hip and pelvis, unspecified, **left** leg
- ✓4th **M92 Other juvenile osteochondrosis**
  - ✓5th **M92.0** Juvenile osteochondrosis of **humerus**
    - Osteochondrosis (juvenile) of capitulum of humerus [Panner]
    - Osteochondrosis (juvenile) of head of humerus [Haas]
    - M92.00 Juvenile osteochondrosis of humerus, unspecified arm
    - M92.01 Juvenile osteochondrosis of humerus, **right** arm
    - M92.02 Juvenile osteochondrosis of humerus, **left** arm
  - ✓5th **M92.1** Juvenile osteochondrosis of **radius and ulna**
    - Osteochondrosis (juvenile) of lower ulna [Burns]
    - Osteochondrosis (juvenile) of radial head [Brailsford]
    - M92.10 Juvenile osteochondrosis of radius and ulna, unspecified arm
    - M92.11 Juvenile osteochondrosis of radius and ulna, **right** arm
    - M92.12 Juvenile osteochondrosis of radius and ulna, **left** arm
  - ✓5th **M92.2** Juvenile osteochondrosis, **hand**
    - ✓6th M92.20 Unspecified juvenile osteochondrosis, **hand**
      - M92.201 Unspecified juvenile osteochondrosis, **right** hand
      - M92.202 Unspecified juvenile osteochondrosis, **left** hand
      - M92.209 Unspecified juvenile osteochondrosis, unspecified hand
    - ✓6th M92.21 Osteochondrosis (juvenile) of **carpal lunate** [Kienbock]
      - M92.211 Osteochondrosis (juvenile) of carpal lunate [Kienbock], **right** hand
      - M92.212 Osteochondrosis (juvenile) of carpal lunate [Kienbock], **left** hand
      - M92.219 Osteochondrosis (juvenile) of carpal lunate [Kienbock], unspecified hand
    - ✓6th M92.22 Osteochondrosis (juvenile) of **metacarpal heads** [Mauclaire]
      - M92.221 Osteochondrosis (juvenile) of metacarpal heads [Mauclaire], **right** hand
      - M92.222 Osteochondrosis (juvenile) of metacarpal heads [Mauclaire], **left** hand
      - M92.229 Osteochondrosis (juvenile) of metacarpal heads [Mauclaire], unspecified hand
    - ✓6th M92.29 Other juvenile osteochondrosis, **hand**
      - M92.291 Other juvenile osteochondrosis, **right** hand
      - M92.292 Other juvenile osteochondrosis, **left** hand
      - M92.299 Other juvenile osteochondrosis, unspecified hand
  - ✓5th **M92.3** Other juvenile osteochondrosis, **upper limb**
    - M92.30 Other juvenile osteochondrosis, unspecified upper limb
    - M92.31 Other juvenile osteochondrosis, **right** upper limb
    - M92.32 Other juvenile osteochondrosis, **left** upper limb
  - ✓5th **M92.4** Juvenile osteochondrosis of **patella**
    - Osteochondrosis (juvenile) of primary patellar center [Kohler]
    - Osteochondrosis (juvenile) of secondary patellar centre [Sinding Larsen]
    - M92.40 Juvenile osteochondrosis of patella, unspecified knee
    - M92.41 Juvenile osteochondrosis of patella, **right** knee
    - M92.42 Juvenile osteochondrosis of patella, **left** knee

Chapter 13. Diseases of the Musculoskeletal System and Connective Tissue

- ✓5th **M92.5** Juvenile osteochondrosis of **tibia and fibula**
  - AHA: 2020,4Q,33-34
  - ✓6th **M92.50** Unspecified juvenile osteochondrosis of tibia and fibula
    - **M92.501** Unspecified juvenile osteochondrosis, **right** leg
    - **M92.502** Unspecified juvenile osteochondrosis, **left** leg
    - **M92.503** Unspecified juvenile osteochondrosis, **bilateral** leg
    - **M92.509** Unspecified juvenile osteochondrosis, unspecified leg
  - ✓6th **M92.51** Juvenile osteochondrosis of **proximal tibia**
    - Blount disease
    - Tibia vara
    - **M92.511** Juvenile osteochondrosis of proximal tibia, **right** leg
    - **M92.512** Juvenile osteochondrosis of proximal tibia, **left** leg
    - **M92.513** Juvenile osteochondrosis of proximal tibia, **bilateral**
    - **M92.519** Juvenile osteochondrosis of proximal tibia, unspecified leg
  - ✓6th **M92.52** Juvenile osteochondrosis of **tibia tubercle**
    - Osgood-Schlatter disease
    - **M92.521** Juvenile osteochondrosis of tibia tubercle, **right** leg
    - **M92.522** Juvenile osteochondrosis of tibia tubercle, **left** leg
    - **M92.523** Juvenile osteochondrosis of tibia tubercle, **bilateral**
    - **M92.529** Juvenile osteochondrosis of tibia tubercle, unspecified leg
  - ✓6th **M92.59** Other juvenile osteochondrosis of tibia and fibula
    - **M92.591** Other juvenile osteochondrosis of tibia and fibula, **right** leg
    - **M92.592** Other juvenile osteochondrosis of tibia and fibula, **left** leg
    - **M92.593** Other juvenile osteochondrosis of tibia and fibula, **bilateral**
    - **M92.599** Other juvenile osteochondrosis of tibia and fibula, unspecified leg
- ✓5th **M92.6** Juvenile osteochondrosis of **tarsus**
  - Osteochondrosis (juvenile) of calcaneum [Sever]
  - Osteochondrosis (juvenile) of os tibiale externum [Haglund]
  - Osteochondrosis (juvenile) of talus [Diaz]
  - Osteochondrosis (juvenile) of tarsal navicular [Kohler]
  - **M92.60** Juvenile osteochondrosis of tarsus, unspecified ankle
  - **M92.61** Juvenile osteochondrosis of tarsus, **right** ankle
  - **M92.62** Juvenile osteochondrosis of tarsus, **left** ankle
- ✓5th **M92.7** Juvenile osteochondrosis of **metatarsus**
  - Osteochondrosis (juvenile) of fifth metatarsus [Iselin]
  - Osteochondrosis (juvenile) of second metatarsus [Freiberg]
  - **M92.70** Juvenile osteochondrosis of metatarsus, unspecified foot
  - **M92.71** Juvenile osteochondrosis of metatarsus, **right** foot
  - **M92.72** Juvenile osteochondrosis of metatarsus, **left** foot
- **M92.8** Other specified juvenile osteochondrosis
  - DEF: Calcaneal apophysitis: Inflammation of the calcaneus at the point of Achilles tendon insertion usually occurring in boys ages 8 to 14. Pain, tenderness, and localized swelling are present.
- **M92.9** Juvenile osteochondrosis, unspecified
  - Juvenile apophysitis NOS
  - Juvenile epiphysitis NOS
  - Juvenile osteochondritis NOS
  - Juvenile osteochondrosis NOS
- ✓4th **M93** Other osteochondropathies
  - EXCLUDES 2 osteochondrosis of spine (M42.-)
  - ✓5th **M93.0** Slipped upper femoral epiphysis (nontraumatic)
    - Slipped capital femoral epiphysis (SCFE)
    - Slipped upper femoral epiphysis (SUFE)
    - Use additional code for associated chondrolysis (M94.3)
    - AHA: 2022,4Q,30-31
    - ✓6th **M93.00** Unspecified slipped upper femoral epiphysis (nontraumatic)
      - **M93.001** Unspecified slipped upper femoral epiphysis (nontraumatic), **right** hip
      - **M93.002** Unspecified slipped upper femoral epiphysis (nontraumatic), **left** hip
      - **M93.003** Unspecified slipped upper femoral epiphysis (nontraumatic), unspecified hip
      - **M93.004** Unspecified slipped upper femoral epiphysis (nontraumatic), **bilateral** hips
    - ✓6th **M93.01** Acute slipped upper femoral epiphysis, **stable** (nontraumatic)
      - **M93.011** Acute slipped upper femoral epiphysis, stable (nontraumatic), **right** hip
      - **M93.012** Acute slipped upper femoral epiphysis, stable (nontraumatic), **left** hip
      - **M93.013** Acute slipped upper femoral epiphysis, stable (nontraumatic), unspecified hip
      - **M93.014** Acute slipped upper femoral epiphysis, stable (nontraumatic), **bilateral** hips
    - ✓6th **M93.02** **Chronic** slipped upper femoral epiphysis, stable (nontraumatic)
      - **M93.021** Chronic slipped upper femoral epiphysis, stable (nontraumatic), **right** hip
      - **M93.022** Chronic slipped upper femoral epiphysis, stable (nontraumatic), **left** hip
      - **M93.023** Chronic slipped upper femoral epiphysis, stable (nontraumatic), unspecified hip
      - **M93.024** Chronic slipped upper femoral epiphysis, stable (nontraumatic), **bilateral** hips
    - ✓6th **M93.03** **Acute on chronic** slipped upper femoral epiphysis, **stable** (nontraumatic)
      - **M93.031** Acute on chronic slipped upper femoral epiphysis, stable (nontraumatic), **right** hip
      - **M93.032** Acute on chronic slipped upper femoral epiphysis, stable (nontraumatic), **left** hip
      - **M93.033** Acute on chronic slipped upper femoral epiphysis, stable (nontraumatic), unspecified hip
      - **M93.034** Acute on chronic slipped upper femoral epiphysis, stable (nontraumatic), **bilateral** hips
    - ✓6th **M93.04** **Acute** slipped upper femoral epiphysis, **unstable** (nontraumatic)
      - **M93.041** Acute slipped upper femoral epiphysis, unstable (nontraumatic), **right** hip
      - **M93.042** Acute slipped upper femoral epiphysis, unstable (nontraumatic), **left** hip
      - **M93.043** Acute slipped upper femoral epiphysis, unstable (nontraumatic), unspecified hip
      - **M93.044** Acute slipped upper femoral epiphysis, unstable (nontraumatic), **bilateral** hips
    - ✓6th **M93.05** **Acute on chronic** slipped upper femoral epiphysis, **unstable** (nontraumatic)
      - **M93.051** Acute on chronic slipped upper femoral epiphysis, unstable (nontraumatic), **right** hip
      - **M93.052** Acute on chronic slipped upper femoral epiphysis, unstable (nontraumatic), **left** hip
      - **M93.053** Acute on chronic slipped upper femoral epiphysis, unstable (nontraumatic), unspecified hip
      - **M93.054** Acute on chronic slipped upper femoral epiphysis, unstable (nontraumatic), **bilateral** hips
    - ✓6th **M93.06** **Acute** slipped upper femoral epiphysis, unspecified stability (nontraumatic)
      - **M93.061** Acute slipped upper femoral epiphysis, unspecified stability (nontraumatic), **right** hip
      - **M93.062** Acute slipped upper femoral epiphysis, unspecified stability (nontraumatic), **left** hip
      - **M93.063** Acute slipped upper femoral epiphysis, unspecified stability (nontraumatic), unspecified hip

	M93.064	Acute slipped upper femoral epiphysis, unspecified stability (nontraumatic), bilateral hips COM
✓6ᵗʰ M93.07		**Acute on chronic** slipped upper femoral epiphysis, unspecified stability (nontraumatic)
	M93.071	Acute on chronic slipped upper femoral epiphysis, unspecified stability (nontraumatic), **right** hip COM
	M93.072	Acute on chronic slipped upper femoral epiphysis, unspecified stability (nontraumatic), **left** hip COM
	M93.073	Acute on chronic slipped upper femoral epiphysis, unspecified stability (nontraumatic), unspecified hip COM
	M93.074	Acute on chronic slipped upper femoral epiphysis, unspecified stability (nontraumatic), **bilateral** hips COM
M93.1		Kienbock's disease of adults A
		Adult osteochondrosis of carpal lunates
✓5ᵗʰ M93.2		Osteochondritis dissecans
		DEF: Avascular necrosis caused by lack of blood flow to the bone and cartilage of a joint causing the bone to die. This can result in splinters or pieces of cartilage breaking off in the joint.
	M93.20	Osteochondritis dissecans of unspecified site
✓6ᵗʰ M93.21		Osteochondritis dissecans of **shoulder**
	M93.211	Osteochondritis dissecans, **right** shoulder
	M93.212	Osteochondritis dissecans, **left** shoulder
	M93.219	Osteochondritis dissecans, unspecified shoulder
✓6ᵗʰ M93.22		Osteochondritis dissecans of **elbow**
	M93.221	Osteochondritis dissecans, **right** elbow
	M93.222	Osteochondritis dissecans, **left** elbow
	M93.229	Osteochondritis dissecans, unspecified elbow
✓6ᵗʰ M93.23		Osteochondritis dissecans of **wrist**
	M93.231	Osteochondritis dissecans, **right** wrist
	M93.232	Osteochondritis dissecans, **left** wrist
	M93.239	Osteochondritis dissecans, unspecified wrist
✓6ᵗʰ M93.24		Osteochondritis dissecans of joints of **hand**
	M93.241	Osteochondritis dissecans, joints of **right** hand
	M93.242	Osteochondritis dissecans, joints of **left** hand
	M93.249	Osteochondritis dissecans, joints of unspecified hand
✓6ᵗʰ M93.25		Osteochondritis dissecans of **hip**
	M93.251	Osteochondritis dissecans, **right** hip
	M93.252	Osteochondritis dissecans, **left** hip
	M93.259	Osteochondritis dissecans, unspecified hip
✓6ᵗʰ M93.26		Osteochondritis dissecans **knee**
	M93.261	Osteochondritis dissecans, **right** knee
	M93.262	Osteochondritis dissecans, **left** knee
	M93.269	Osteochondritis dissecans, unspecified knee
✓6ᵗʰ M93.27		Osteochondritis dissecans of **ankle and joints of foot**
	M93.271	Osteochondritis dissecans, **right** ankle and joints of **right** foot
	M93.272	Osteochondritis dissecans, **left** ankle and joints of **left** foot
	M93.279	Osteochondritis dissecans, unspecified ankle and joints of foot
	M93.28	Osteochondritis dissecans other site
	M93.29	Osteochondritis dissecans **multiple sites**
✓5ᵗʰ M93.8		Other specified osteochondropathies
	M93.80	Other specified osteochondropathies of unspecified site
✓6ᵗʰ M93.81		Other specified osteochondropathies of **shoulder**
	M93.811	Other specified osteochondropathies, **right** shoulder
	M93.812	Other specified osteochondropathies, **left** shoulder
	M93.819	Other specified osteochondropathies, unspecified shoulder
✓6ᵗʰ M93.82		Other specified osteochondropathies of **upper arm**
	M93.821	Other specified osteochondropathies, **right** upper arm
	M93.822	Other specified osteochondropathies, **left** upper arm
	M93.829	Other specified osteochondropathies, unspecified upper arm
✓6ᵗʰ M93.83		Other specified osteochondropathies of **forearm**
	M93.831	Other specified osteochondropathies, **right** forearm
	M93.832	Other specified osteochondropathies, **left** forearm
	M93.839	Other specified osteochondropathies, unspecified forearm
✓6ᵗʰ M93.84		Other specified osteochondropathies of **hand**
	M93.841	Other specified osteochondropathies, **right** hand
	M93.842	Other specified osteochondropathies, **left** hand
	M93.849	Other specified osteochondropathies, unspecified hand
✓6ᵗʰ M93.85		Other specified osteochondropathies of **thigh**
	M93.851	Other specified osteochondropathies, **right** thigh
	M93.852	Other specified osteochondropathies, **left** thigh
	M93.859	Other specified osteochondropathies, unspecified thigh
✓6ᵗʰ M93.86		Other specified osteochondropathies **lower leg**
	M93.861	Other specified osteochondropathies, **right** lower leg
	M93.862	Other specified osteochondropathies, **left** lower leg
	M93.869	Other specified osteochondropathies, unspecified lower leg
✓6ᵗʰ M93.87		Other specified osteochondropathies of **ankle and foot**
	M93.871	Other specified osteochondropathies, **right** ankle and foot
	M93.872	Other specified osteochondropathies, **left** ankle and foot
	M93.879	Other specified osteochondropathies, unspecified ankle and foot
	M93.88	Other specified osteochondropathies other
	M93.89	Other specified osteochondropathies **multiple sites**
✓5ᵗʰ M93.9		Osteochondropathy, unspecified
		Apophysitis NOS
		Epiphysitis NOS
		Osteochondritis NOS
		Osteochondrosis NOS
	M93.90	Osteochondropathy, unspecified of unspecified site
✓6ᵗʰ M93.91		Osteochondropathy, unspecified of **shoulder**
	M93.911	Osteochondropathy, unspecified, **right** shoulder
	M93.912	Osteochondropathy, unspecified, **left** shoulder
	M93.919	Osteochondropathy, unspecified, unspecified shoulder
✓6ᵗʰ M93.92		Osteochondropathy, unspecified of **upper arm**
	M93.921	Osteochondropathy, unspecified, **right** upper arm
	M93.922	Osteochondropathy, unspecified, **left** upper arm
	M93.929	Osteochondropathy, unspecified, unspecified upper arm
✓6ᵗʰ M93.93		Osteochondropathy, unspecified of **forearm**
	M93.931	Osteochondropathy, unspecified, **right** forearm
	M93.932	Osteochondropathy, unspecified, **left** forearm
	M93.939	Osteochondropathy, unspecified, unspecified forearm
✓6ᵗʰ M93.94		Osteochondropathy, unspecified of **hand**
	M93.941	Osteochondropathy, unspecified, **right** hand
	M93.942	Osteochondropathy, unspecified, **left** hand
	M93.949	Osteochondropathy, unspecified, unspecified hand
✓6ᵗʰ M93.95		Osteochondropathy, unspecified of **thigh**
	M93.951	Osteochondropathy, unspecified, **right** thigh
	M93.952	Osteochondropathy, unspecified, **left** thigh
	M93.959	Osteochondropathy, unspecified, unspecified thigh

Chapter 13. Diseases of the Musculoskeletal System and Connective Tissue

- **M93.96** Osteochondropathy, unspecified lower leg
  - M93.961 Osteochondropathy, unspecified, right lower leg
  - M93.962 Osteochondropathy, unspecified, left lower leg
  - M93.969 Osteochondropathy, unspecified, unspecified lower leg
- **M93.97** Osteochondropathy, unspecified of ankle and foot
  - M93.971 Osteochondropathy, unspecified, right ankle and foot
  - M93.972 Osteochondropathy, unspecified, left ankle and foot
  - M93.979 Osteochondropathy, unspecified, unspecified ankle and foot
- M93.98 Osteochondropathy, unspecified other
- M93.99 Osteochondropathy, unspecified multiple sites

M94 Other disorders of cartilage

- **M94.0** Chondrocostal junction syndrome [Tietze]
  Costochondritis
- **M94.1** Relapsing polychondritis
- **M94.2** Chondromalacia
  - EXCLUDES 1: chondromalacia patellae (M22.4)
  - M94.20 Chondromalacia, unspecified site
  - **M94.21** Chondromalacia, shoulder
    - M94.211 Chondromalacia, right shoulder
    - M94.212 Chondromalacia, left shoulder
    - M94.219 Chondromalacia, unspecified shoulder
  - **M94.22** Chondromalacia, elbow
    - M94.221 Chondromalacia, right elbow
    - M94.222 Chondromalacia, left elbow
    - M94.229 Chondromalacia, unspecified elbow
  - **M94.23** Chondromalacia, wrist
    - M94.231 Chondromalacia, right wrist
    - M94.232 Chondromalacia, left wrist
    - M94.239 Chondromalacia, unspecified wrist
  - **M94.24** Chondromalacia, joints of hand
    - M94.241 Chondromalacia, joints of right hand
    - M94.242 Chondromalacia, joints of left hand
    - M94.249 Chondromalacia, joints of unspecified hand
  - **M94.25** Chondromalacia, hip
    - M94.251 Chondromalacia, right hip
    - M94.252 Chondromalacia, left hip
    - M94.259 Chondromalacia, unspecified hip
  - **M94.26** Chondromalacia, knee
    - M94.261 Chondromalacia, right knee
    - M94.262 Chondromalacia, left knee
    - M94.269 Chondromalacia, unspecified knee
  - **M94.27** Chondromalacia, ankle and joints of foot
    - M94.271 Chondromalacia, right ankle and joints of right foot
    - M94.272 Chondromalacia, left ankle and joints of left foot
    - M94.279 Chondromalacia, unspecified ankle and joints of foot
  - M94.28 Chondromalacia, other site
  - M94.29 Chondromalacia, multiple sites
- **M94.3** Chondrolysis
  Code first any associated slipped upper femoral epiphysis (nontraumatic) (M93.0-)
  - **M94.35** Chondrolysis, hip
    - M94.351 Chondrolysis, right hip
    - M94.352 Chondrolysis, left hip
    - M94.359 Chondrolysis, unspecified hip
- **M94.8** Other specified disorders of cartilage
  - **M94.8X** Other specified disorders of cartilage
    - M94.8X0 Other specified disorders of cartilage, multiple sites
    - M94.8X1 Other specified disorders of cartilage, shoulder
    - M94.8X2 Other specified disorders of cartilage, upper arm
    - M94.8X3 Other specified disorders of cartilage, forearm
    - M94.8X4 Other specified disorders of cartilage, hand
    - M94.8X5 Other specified disorders of cartilage, thigh
    - M94.8X6 Other specified disorders of cartilage, lower leg
    - M94.8X7 Other specified disorders of cartilage, ankle and foot
    - M94.8X8 Other specified disorders of cartilage, other site
    - M94.8X9 Other specified disorders of cartilage, unspecified sites
- M94.9 Disorder of cartilage, unspecified

Other disorders of the musculoskeletal system and connective tissue (M95)

M95 Other acquired deformities of musculoskeletal system and connective tissue

EXCLUDES 2:
- acquired absence of limbs and organs (Z89-Z90)
- acquired deformities of limbs (M20-M21)
- congenital malformations and deformations of the musculoskeletal system (Q65-Q79)
- deforming dorsopathies (M40-M43)
- dentofacial anomalies [including malocclusion] (M26.-)
- postprocedural musculoskeletal disorders (M96.-)

- **M95.0** Acquired deformity of nose
  - EXCLUDES 2: deviated nasal septum (J34.2)
- **M95.1** Cauliflower ear
  - EXCLUDES 2: other acquired deformities of ear (H61.1)
  - DEF: Acquired deformity of the external ear due to injury or subsequent perichondritis.
  - M95.10 Cauliflower ear, unspecified ear
  - M95.11 Cauliflower ear, right ear
  - M95.12 Cauliflower ear, left ear
- **M95.2** Other acquired deformity of head
  AHA: 2023,1Q,30; 2022,1Q,34
- **M95.3** Acquired deformity of neck
- **M95.4** Acquired deformity of chest and rib
  AHA: 2022,2Q,14; 2014,4Q,26-27
- **M95.5** Acquired deformity of pelvis
  - EXCLUDES 1: maternal care for known or suspected disproportion (O33.-)
- M95.8 Other specified acquired deformities of musculoskeletal system
- M95.9 Acquired deformity of musculoskeletal system, unspecified

Intraoperative and postprocedural complications and disorders of musculoskeletal system, not elsewhere classified (M96)

M96 Intraoperative and postprocedural complications and disorders of musculoskeletal system, not elsewhere classified

EXCLUDES 2:
- arthropathy following intestinal bypass (M02.0-)
- complications of internal orthopedic prosthetic devices, implants and grafts (T84.-)
- disorders associated with osteoporosis (M80)
- periprosthetic fracture around internal prosthetic joint (M97.-)
- presence of functional implants and other devices (Z96-Z97)

- **M96.0** Pseudarthrosis after fusion or arthrodesis
- **M96.1** Postlaminectomy syndrome, not elsewhere classified
  AHA: 2024,1Q,17
- **M96.2** Postradiation kyphosis
- **M96.3** Postlaminectomy kyphosis
- **M96.4** Postsurgical lordosis
- **M96.5** Postradiation scoliosis
- **M96.6** Fracture of bone following insertion of orthopedic implant, joint prosthesis, or bone plate
  Intraoperative fracture of bone during insertion of orthopedic implant, joint prosthesis, or bone plate
  - EXCLUDES 2: complication of internal orthopedic devices, implants or grafts (T84.-)
  - **M96.62** Fracture of humerus following insertion of orthopedic implant, joint prosthesis, or bone plate
    - M96.621 Fracture of humerus following insertion of orthopedic implant, joint prosthesis, or bone plate, right arm
    - M96.622 Fracture of humerus following insertion of orthopedic implant, joint prosthesis, or bone plate, left arm
    - M96.629 Fracture of humerus following insertion of orthopedic implant, joint prosthesis, or bone plate, unspecified arm

M96.63 Fracture of radius or ulna following insertion of orthopedic implant, joint prosthesis, or bone plate
- **M96.631** Fracture of radius or ulna following insertion of orthopedic implant, joint prosthesis, or bone plate, right arm
- **M96.632** Fracture of radius or ulna following insertion of orthopedic implant, joint prosthesis, or bone plate, left arm
- **M96.639** Fracture of radius or ulna following insertion of orthopedic implant, joint prosthesis, or bone plate, unspecified arm

M96.65 Fracture of pelvis following insertion of orthopedic implant, joint prosthesis, or bone plate

M96.66 Fracture of femur following insertion of orthopedic implant, joint prosthesis, or bone plate
- **M96.661** Fracture of femur following insertion of orthopedic implant, joint prosthesis, or bone plate, right leg
- **M96.662** Fracture of femur following insertion of orthopedic implant, joint prosthesis, or bone plate, left leg
- **M96.669** Fracture of femur following insertion of orthopedic implant, joint prosthesis, or bone plate, unspecified leg

M96.67 Fracture of tibia or fibula following insertion of orthopedic implant, joint prosthesis, or bone plate
- **M96.671** Fracture of tibia or fibula following insertion of orthopedic implant, joint prosthesis, or bone plate, right leg
- **M96.672** Fracture of tibia or fibula following insertion of orthopedic implant, joint prosthesis, or bone plate, left leg
- **M96.679** Fracture of tibia or fibula following insertion of orthopedic implant, joint prosthesis, or bone plate, unspecified leg

M96.69 Fracture of other bone following insertion of orthopedic implant, joint prosthesis, or bone plate

M96.8 Other intraoperative and postprocedural complications and disorders of musculoskeletal system, not elsewhere classified
AHA: 2016,4Q,9-10

M96.81 Intraoperative hemorrhage and hematoma of a musculoskeletal structure complicating a procedure
EXCLUDES 1 intraoperative hemorrhage and hematoma of a musculoskeletal structure due to accidental puncture and laceration during a procedure (M96.82-)
- **M96.810** Intraoperative hemorrhage and hematoma of a musculoskeletal structure complicating a musculoskeletal system procedure
- **M96.811** Intraoperative hemorrhage and hematoma of a musculoskeletal structure complicating other procedure

M96.82 Accidental puncture and laceration of a musculoskeletal structure during a procedure
- **M96.820** Accidental puncture and laceration of a musculoskeletal structure during a musculoskeletal system procedure
- **M96.821** Accidental puncture and laceration of a musculoskeletal structure during other procedure

M96.83 Postprocedural hemorrhage of a musculoskeletal structure following a procedure
- **M96.830** Postprocedural hemorrhage of a musculoskeletal structure following a musculoskeletal system procedure
- **M96.831** Postprocedural hemorrhage of a musculoskeletal structure following other procedure

M96.84 Postprocedural hematoma and seroma of a musculoskeletal structure following a procedure
- **M96.840** Postprocedural hematoma of a musculoskeletal structure following a musculoskeletal system procedure
- **M96.841** Postprocedural hematoma of a musculoskeletal structure following other procedure
AHA: 2016,4Q,10

- **M96.842** Postprocedural seroma of a musculoskeletal structure following a musculoskeletal system procedure
- **M96.843** Postprocedural seroma of a musculoskeletal structure following other procedure
AHA: 2023,2Q,13; 2018,3Q,6

M96.89 Other intraoperative and postprocedural complications and disorders of the musculoskeletal system
Instability of joint secondary to removal of joint prosthesis
Use additional code, if applicable, to further specify disorder
AHA: 2024,1Q,17,23; 2023,2Q,14; 2022,2Q,14; 2021,1Q,5

M96.A Fracture of ribs, sternum and thorax associated with compression of the chest and cardiopulmonary resuscitation
AHA: 2022,4Q,31-33
- **M96.A1** Fracture of sternum associated with chest compression and cardiopulmonary resuscitation
  Fracture of xiphoid process associated with chest compression and cardiopulmonary resuscitation
- **M96.A2** Fracture of one rib associated with chest compression and cardiopulmonary resuscitation
- **M96.A3** Multiple fractures of ribs associated with chest compression and cardiopulmonary resuscitation
AHA: 2022,4Q,32
- **M96.A4** Flail chest associated with chest compression and cardiopulmonary resuscitation
- **M96.A9** Other fracture associated with chest compression and cardiopulmonary resuscitation

Periprosthetic fractures around internal prosthetic joint (M97)

M97 Periprosthetic fracture around internal prosthetic joint
Code first, if known, the specific type and cause of fracture, such as traumatic or pathological
EXCLUDES 2 fracture of bone following insertion of orthopedic implant, joint prosthesis or bone plate (M96.6-)
breakage (fracture) of prosthetic joint (T84.01-)
AHA: 2016,4Q,42-43

The appropriate 7th character is to be added to each code from category M97.
A initial encounter
D subsequent encounter
S sequela

M97.0 Periprosthetic fracture around internal prosthetic hip joint
AHA: 2018,1Q,21; 2016,4Q,42
- **M97.01** Periprosthetic fracture around internal prosthetic right hip joint
- **M97.02** Periprosthetic fracture around internal prosthetic left hip joint

M97.1 Periprosthetic fracture around internal prosthetic knee joint
- **M97.11** Periprosthetic fracture around internal prosthetic right knee joint
- **M97.12** Periprosthetic fracture around internal prosthetic left knee joint

M97.2 Periprosthetic fracture around internal prosthetic ankle joint
- **M97.21** Periprosthetic fracture around internal prosthetic right ankle joint
- **M97.22** Periprosthetic fracture around internal prosthetic left ankle joint

M97.3 Periprosthetic fracture around internal prosthetic shoulder joint
- **M97.31** Periprosthetic fracture around internal prosthetic right shoulder joint
- **M97.32** Periprosthetic fracture around internal prosthetic left shoulder joint

M97.4 Periprosthetic fracture around internal prosthetic elbow joint
- **M97.41** Periprosthetic fracture around internal prosthetic right elbow joint
- **M97.42** Periprosthetic fracture around internal prosthetic left elbow joint

√x7th **M97.8** Periprosthetic fracture around other internal prosthetic joint
- Periprosthetic fracture around internal prosthetic finger joint
- Periprosthetic fracture around internal prosthetic spinal joint
- Periprosthetic fracture around internal prosthetic toe joint
- Periprosthetic fracture around internal prosthetic wrist joint

Use additional code to identify the joint (Z96.6-)

√x7th **M97.9** Periprosthetic fracture around unspecified internal prosthetic joint

Biomechanical lesions, not elsewhere classified (M99)

√4th **M99** Biomechanical lesions, not elsewhere classified

NOTE This category should not be used if the condition can be classified elsewhere.

DEF: Biomechanical lesion: Term used by osteopathic and chiropractic physicians to describe musculoskeletal conditions treated that are not more appropriately classified elsewhere.

√5th **M99.0** Segmental and somatic dysfunction
- M99.00 Segmental and somatic dysfunction of head region
- M99.01 Segmental and somatic dysfunction of cervical region
- M99.02 Segmental and somatic dysfunction of thoracic region
- M99.03 Segmental and somatic dysfunction of lumbar region
- M99.04 Segmental and somatic dysfunction of sacral region
- M99.05 Segmental and somatic dysfunction of pelvic region
- M99.06 Segmental and somatic dysfunction of lower extremity
- M99.07 Segmental and somatic dysfunction of upper extremity
- M99.08 Segmental and somatic dysfunction of rib cage
- M99.09 Segmental and somatic dysfunction of abdomen and other regions

√5th **M99.1** Subluxation complex (vertebral)
- M99.10 Subluxation complex (vertebral) of head region
- M99.11 Subluxation complex (vertebral) of cervical region
- M99.12 Subluxation complex (vertebral) of thoracic region
- M99.13 Subluxation complex (vertebral) of lumbar region
- M99.14 Subluxation complex (vertebral) of sacral region
- M99.15 Subluxation complex (vertebral) of pelvic region
- M99.16 Subluxation complex (vertebral) of lower extremity
- M99.17 Subluxation complex (vertebral) of upper extremity
- M99.18 Subluxation complex (vertebral) of rib cage
- M99.19 Subluxation complex (vertebral) of abdomen and other regions

√5th **M99.2** Subluxation stenosis of neural canal
- M99.20 Subluxation stenosis of neural canal of head region
- M99.21 Subluxation stenosis of neural canal of cervical region
- M99.22 Subluxation stenosis of neural canal of thoracic region
- M99.23 Subluxation stenosis of neural canal of lumbar region
- M99.24 Subluxation stenosis of neural canal of sacral region
- M99.25 Subluxation stenosis of neural canal of pelvic region
- M99.26 Subluxation stenosis of neural canal of lower extremity
- M99.27 Subluxation stenosis of neural canal of upper extremity
- M99.28 Subluxation stenosis of neural canal of rib cage
- M99.29 Subluxation stenosis of neural canal of abdomen and other regions

√5th **M99.3** Osseous stenosis of neural canal
- M99.30 Osseous stenosis of neural canal of head region
- M99.31 Osseous stenosis of neural canal of cervical region
- M99.32 Osseous stenosis of neural canal of thoracic region
- M99.33 Osseous stenosis of neural canal of lumbar region
- M99.34 Osseous stenosis of neural canal of sacral region
- M99.35 Osseous stenosis of neural canal of pelvic region
- M99.36 Osseous stenosis of neural canal of lower extremity
- M99.37 Osseous stenosis of neural canal of upper extremity
- M99.38 Osseous stenosis of neural canal of rib cage
- M99.39 Osseous stenosis of neural canal of abdomen and other regions

√5th **M99.4** Connective tissue stenosis of neural canal
- M99.40 Connective tissue stenosis of neural canal of head region
- M99.41 Connective tissue stenosis of neural canal of cervical region
- M99.42 Connective tissue stenosis of neural canal of thoracic region
- M99.43 Connective tissue stenosis of neural canal of lumbar region
- M99.44 Connective tissue stenosis of neural canal of sacral region
- M99.45 Connective tissue stenosis of neural canal of pelvic region
- M99.46 Connective tissue stenosis of neural canal of lower extremity
- M99.47 Connective tissue stenosis of neural canal of upper extremity
- M99.48 Connective tissue stenosis of neural canal of rib cage
- M99.49 Connective tissue stenosis of neural canal of abdomen and other regions

√5th **M99.5** Intervertebral disc stenosis of neural canal
- M99.50 Intervertebral disc stenosis of neural canal of head region
- M99.51 Intervertebral disc stenosis of neural canal of cervical region
- M99.52 Intervertebral disc stenosis of neural canal of thoracic region
- M99.53 Intervertebral disc stenosis of neural canal of lumbar region
- M99.54 Intervertebral disc stenosis of neural canal of sacral region
- M99.55 Intervertebral disc stenosis of neural canal of pelvic region
- M99.56 Intervertebral disc stenosis of neural canal of lower extremity
- M99.57 Intervertebral disc stenosis of neural canal of upper extremity
- M99.58 Intervertebral disc stenosis of neural canal of rib cage
- M99.59 Intervertebral disc stenosis of neural canal of abdomen and other regions

√5th **M99.6** Osseous and subluxation stenosis of intervertebral foramina
- M99.60 Osseous and subluxation stenosis of intervertebral foramina of head region
- M99.61 Osseous and subluxation stenosis of intervertebral foramina of cervical region
- M99.62 Osseous and subluxation stenosis of intervertebral foramina of thoracic region
- M99.63 Osseous and subluxation stenosis of intervertebral foramina of lumbar region
- M99.64 Osseous and subluxation stenosis of intervertebral foramina of sacral region
- M99.65 Osseous and subluxation stenosis of intervertebral foramina of pelvic region
- M99.66 Osseous and subluxation stenosis of intervertebral foramina of lower extremity
- M99.67 Osseous and subluxation stenosis of intervertebral foramina of upper extremity
- M99.68 Osseous and subluxation stenosis of intervertebral foramina of rib cage
- M99.69 Osseous and subluxation stenosis of intervertebral foramina of abdomen and other regions

√5th **M99.7** Connective tissue and disc stenosis of intervertebral foramina
- M99.70 Connective tissue and disc stenosis of intervertebral foramina of head region
- M99.71 Connective tissue and disc stenosis of intervertebral foramina of cervical region
- M99.72 Connective tissue and disc stenosis of intervertebral foramina of thoracic region
- M99.73 Connective tissue and disc stenosis of intervertebral foramina of lumbar region
- M99.74 Connective tissue and disc stenosis of intervertebral foramina of sacral region
- M99.75 Connective tissue and disc stenosis of intervertebral foramina of pelvic region
- M99.76 Connective tissue and disc stenosis of intervertebral foramina of lower extremity
- M99.77 Connective tissue and disc stenosis of intervertebral foramina of upper extremity
- M99.78 Connective tissue and disc stenosis of intervertebral foramina of rib cage
- M99.79 Connective tissue and disc stenosis of intervertebral foramina of abdomen and other regions

√5th **M99.8** Other biomechanical lesions
- M99.80 Other biomechanical lesions of head region
- M99.81 Other biomechanical lesions of cervical region
- M99.82 Other biomechanical lesions of thoracic region
- M99.83 Other biomechanical lesions of lumbar region
- M99.84 Other biomechanical lesions of sacral region

M99.85 Other biomechanical lesions of pelvic region
M99.86 Other biomechanical lesions of lower extremity
M99.87 Other biomechanical lesions of upper extremity
M99.88 Other biomechanical lesions of rib cage
M99.89 Other biomechanical lesions of abdomen and other regions
M99.9 Biomechanical lesion, unspecified

Chapter 14. Diseases of Genitourinary System (N00–N99)

Chapter-specific Guidelines with Coding Examples

The chapter-specific guidelines from the ICD-10-CM Official Guidelines for Coding and Reporting have been provided below. Along with these guidelines are coding examples, contained in the shaded boxes, that have been developed to help illustrate the coding and/or sequencing guidance found in these guidelines.

a. Chronic kidney disease

1) Stages of chronic kidney disease (CKD)

The ICD-10-CM classifies CKD based on severity. The severity of CKD is designated by stages 1-5. Stage 2, code N18.2, equates to mild CKD; stage 3, codes N18.30-N18.32, equate to moderate CKD; and stage 4, code N18.4, equates to severe CKD. Code N18.6, End stage renal disease (ESRD), is assigned when the provider has documented end-stage renal disease (ESRD).

If both a stage of CKD and ESRD are documented, assign code N18.6 only.

> Stage 5 chronic kidney disease with ESRD requiring chronic dialysis
>
> **N18.6**   End stage renal disease
>
> **Z99.2**   Dependence on renal dialysis
>
> *Explanation:* The diagnostic statement indicates the patient has chronic kidney disease, documented both as stage 5 and as ESRD requiring chronic dialysis. Code N18.6 End stage renal disease (ESRD), is assigned when the provider has documented end-stage-renal disease (ESRD). If both a stage of CKD and ESRD are documented, assign code N18.6 only.

2) Chronic kidney disease and kidney transplant status

Patients who have undergone kidney transplant may still have some form of chronic kidney disease (CKD) because the kidney transplant may not fully restore kidney function. Therefore, the presence of CKD alone does not constitute a transplant complication. Assign the appropriate N18 code for the patient's stage of CKD and code Z94.0, Kidney transplant status. If a transplant complication such as failure or rejection or other transplant complication is documented, see section I.C.19.g for information on coding complications of a kidney transplant. If the documentation is unclear as to whether the patient has a complication of the transplant, query the provider.

> Patient with residual chronic kidney disease stage 1 after kidney transplant
>
> **N18.1**   Chronic kidney disease, stage 1
>
> **Z94.0**   Kidney transplant status
>
> *Explanation:* Patients who have undergone kidney transplant may still have some form of chronic kidney disease (CKD) because the kidney transplant may not fully restore kidney function. The presence of CKD alone does not constitute a transplant complication. Assign the appropriate N18 code for the patient's stage of CKD and code Z94.0 Kidney transplant status.

3) Chronic kidney disease with other conditions

Patients with CKD may also suffer from other serious conditions, most commonly diabetes mellitus and hypertension. The sequencing of the CKD code in relationship to codes for other contributing conditions is based on the conventions in the Tabular List.

See I.C.9. Hypertensive chronic kidney disease.
See I.C.19. Chronic kidney disease and kidney transplant complications.

> Type 1 diabetic chronic kidney disease, stage 2
>
> **E10.22**   Type 1 diabetes mellitus with diabetic chronic kidney disease
>
> **N18.2**   Chronic kidney disease, stage 2 (mild)
>
> *Explanation:* Patients with CKD may also suffer from other serious conditions such as diabetes mellitus. The sequencing of the CKD code in relationship to codes for other contributing conditions is based on the conventions in the Tabular List. Diabetic CKD code E10.22 includes an instructional note to "Use additional code to identify stage of chronic kidney disease (N18.1–N18.6)," thus providing sequencing direction.

Chapter 14. Diseases of the Genitourinary System (N00-N99)

EXCLUDES 2
certain conditions originating in the perinatal period (P04-P96)
certain infectious and parasitic diseases (A00-B99)
complications of pregnancy, childbirth and the puerperium (O00-O9A)
congenital malformations, deformations and chromosomal abnormalities (Q00-Q99)
endocrine, nutritional and metabolic diseases (E00-E88)
injury, poisoning and certain other consequences of external causes (S00-T88)
neoplasms (C00-D49)
symptoms, signs and abnormal clinical and laboratory findings, not elsewhere classified (R00-R94)

This chapter contains the following blocks:
N00-N08 Glomerular diseases
N10-N16 Renal tubulo-interstitial diseases
N17-N19 Acute kidney failure and chronic kidney disease
N20-N23 Urolithiasis
N25-N29 Other disorders of kidney and ureter
N30-N39 Other diseases of the urinary system
N40-N53 Diseases of male genital organs
N60-N65 Disorders of breast
N70-N77 Inflammatory diseases of female pelvic organs
N80-N98 Noninflammatory disorders of female genital tract
N99 Intraoperative and postprocedural complications and disorders of genitourinary system, not elsewhere classified

Glomerular diseases (N00-N08)

Code also any associated kidney failure (N17-N19).
EXCLUDES 1 hypertensive chronic kidney disease (I12.-)
AHA: 2020,4Q,34-35
DEF: Glomeruli: Clusters of microscopic blood vessels located within the kidneys containing small pores through which waste products are filtered from the blood and urine is formed.
DEF: Glomerulonephritis: Disease of the kidney with diffuse inflammation of the capillary loops of the glomeruli.

N00 Acute nephritic syndrome
INCLUDES
acute glomerular disease
acute glomerulonephritis
acute nephritis
EXCLUDES 1 acute tubulo-interstitial nephritis (N10)
nephritic syndrome NOS (N05.-)
AHA: 2021,1Q,23

N00.0 Acute nephritic syndrome with minor glomerular abnormality
Acute nephritic syndrome with minimal change lesion

N00.1 Acute nephritic syndrome with focal and segmental glomerular lesions
Acute nephritic syndrome with focal and segmental hyalinosis
Acute nephritic syndrome with focal and segmental sclerosis
Acute nephritic syndrome with focal glomerulonephritis

N00.2 Acute nephritic syndrome with diffuse membranous glomerulonephritis

N00.3 Acute nephritic syndrome with diffuse mesangial proliferative glomerulonephritis

N00.4 Acute nephritic syndrome with diffuse endocapillary proliferative glomerulonephritis

N00.5 Acute nephritic syndrome with diffuse mesangiocapillary glomerulonephritis
Acute nephritic syndrome with membranoproliferative glomerulonephritis, types 1 and 3, or NOS
EXCLUDES 1 acute nephritic syndrome with C3 glomerulonephritis (N00.A)
acute nephritic syndrome with C3 glomerulopathy (N00.A)

N00.6 Acute nephritic syndrome with dense deposit disease
Acute nephritic syndrome with C3 glomerulopathy with dense deposit disease
Acute nephritic syndrome with membranoproliferative glomerulonephritis, type 2

N00.7 Acute nephritic syndrome with diffuse crescentic glomerulonephritis
Acute nephritic syndrome with extracapillary glomerulonephritis

N00.8 Acute nephritic syndrome with other morphologic changes
Acute nephritic syndrome with proliferative glomerulonephritis NOS

N00.9 Acute nephritic syndrome with unspecified morphologic changes

N00.A Acute nephritic syndrome with C3 glomerulonephritis
Acute nephritic syndrome with C3 glomerulopathy, NOS
EXCLUDES 1 acute nephritic syndrome (with C3 glomerulopathy) with dense deposit disease (N00.6)

N00.B Acute nephritic syndrome with immune complex membranoproliferative glomerulonephritis

N00.B1 Acute nephritic syndrome with idiopathic immune complex membranoproliferative glomerulonephritis (IC-MPGN)

N00.B2 Acute nephritic syndrome with secondary immune complex membranoproliferative glomerulonephritis (IC-MPGN)

N01 Rapidly progressive nephritic syndrome
INCLUDES
rapidly progressive glomerular disease
rapidly progressive glomerulonephritis
rapidly progressive nephritis
EXCLUDES 1 nephritic syndrome NOS (N05.-)
AHA: 2021,1Q,23

N01.0 Rapidly progressive nephritic syndrome with minor glomerular abnormality
Rapidly progressive nephritic syndrome with minimal change lesion

N01.1 Rapidly progressive nephritic syndrome with focal and segmental glomerular lesions
Rapidly progressive nephritic syndrome with focal and segmental hyalinosis
Rapidly progressive nephritic syndrome with focal and segmental sclerosis
Rapidly progressive nephritic syndrome with focal glomerulonephritis

N01.2 Rapidly progressive nephritic syndrome with diffuse membranous glomerulonephritis

N01.3 Rapidly progressive nephritic syndrome with diffuse mesangial proliferative glomerulonephritis

N01.4 Rapidly progressive nephritic syndrome with diffuse endocapillary proliferative glomerulonephritis

N01.5 Rapidly progressive nephritic syndrome with diffuse mesangiocapillary glomerulonephritis
Rapidly progressive nephritic syndrome with membranoproliferative glomerulonephritis, types 1 and 3, or NOS
EXCLUDES 1 rapidly progressive nephritic syndrome with C3 glomerulonephritis (N01.A)
rapidly progressive nephritic syndrome with C3 glomerulopathy (N01.A)

N01.6 Rapidly progressive nephritic syndrome with dense deposit disease
Rapidly progressive nephritic syndrome with C3 glomerulopathy with dense deposit disease
Rapidly progressive nephritic syndrome with membranoproliferative glomerulonephritis, type 2

N01.7 Rapidly progressive nephritic syndrome with diffuse crescentic glomerulonephritis
Rapidly progressive nephritic syndrome with extracapillary glomerulonephritis

N01.8 Rapidly progressive nephritic syndrome with other morphologic changes
Rapidly progressive nephritic syndrome with proliferative glomerulonephritis NOS

N01.9 Rapidly progressive nephritic syndrome with unspecified morphologic changes

N01.A Rapidly progressive nephritic syndrome with C3 glomerulonephritis
Rapidly progressive nephritic syndrome with C3 glomerulopathy, NOS
EXCLUDES 1 rapidly progressive nephritic syndrome (with C3 glomerulopathy) with dense deposit disease (N01.6)

N02 Recurrent and persistent hematuria
EXCLUDES 1 acute cystitis with hematuria (N30.01)
hematuria NOS (R31.9)
hematuria not associated with specified morphologic lesions (R31.-)

N02.0 Recurrent and persistent hematuria with minor glomerular abnormality
Recurrent and persistent hematuria with minimal change lesion

N02.1 Recurrent and persistent hematuria with focal and segmental glomerular lesions
Recurrent and persistent hematuria with focal and segmental hyalinosis
Recurrent and persistent hematuria with focal and segmental sclerosis
Recurrent and persistent hematuria with focal glomerulonephritis

N02.2 Recurrent and persistent hematuria with diffuse membranous glomerulonephritis

N02.3 **Recurrent and persistent hematuria with diffuse mesangial proliferative glomerulonephritis**

N02.4 **Recurrent and persistent hematuria with diffuse endocapillary proliferative glomerulonephritis**

N02.5 **Recurrent and persistent hematuria with diffuse mesangiocapillary glomerulonephritis**
Recurrent and persistent hematuria with membranoproliferative glomerulonephritis, types 1 and 3, or NOS
EXCLUDES 1 *recurrent and persistent hematuria with C3 glomerulonephritis (N02.A)*
recurrent and persistent hematuria with C3 glomerulopathy (N02.A)

N02.6 **Recurrent and persistent hematuria with dense deposit disease**
Recurrent and persistent hematuria with C3 glomerulopathy with dense deposit disease
Recurrent and persistent hematuria with membranoproliferative glomerulonephritis, type 2

N02.7 **Recurrent and persistent hematuria with diffuse crescentic glomerulonephritis**
Recurrent and persistent hematuria with extracapillary glomerulonephritis

N02.8 **Recurrent and persistent hematuria with other morphologic changes**
Recurrent and persistent hematuria with proliferative glomerulonephritis NOS

N02.9 **Recurrent and persistent hematuria with unspecified morphologic changes**
AHA: 2017,2Q,5

N02.A **Recurrent and persistent hematuria with C3 glomerulonephritis**
Recurrent and persistent hematuria with C3 glomerulopathy
EXCLUDES 1 *recurrent and persistent hematuria (with C3 glomerulopathy) with dense deposit disease (N02.6)*

N02.B **Recurrent and persistent immunoglobulin A nephropathy**
AHA: 2023,4Q,34-35

N02.B1 **Recurrent and persistent immunoglobulin A nephropathy with glomerular lesion**

N02.B2 **Recurrent and persistent immunoglobulin A nephropathy with focal and segmental glomerular lesion**
Recurrent and persistent immunoglobulin A nephropathy with focal and segmental hyalinosis or sclerosis

N02.B3 **Recurrent and persistent immunoglobulin A nephropathy with diffuse membranoproliferative glomerulonephritis**

N02.B4 **Recurrent and persistent immunoglobulin A nephropathy with diffuse membranous glomerulonephritis**

N02.B5 **Recurrent and persistent immunoglobulin A nephropathy with diffuse mesangial proliferative glomerulonephritis**

N02.B6 **Recurrent and persistent immunoglobulin A nephropathy with diffuse mesangiocapillary glomerulonephritis**

N02.B9 **Other recurrent and persistent immunoglobulin A nephropathy**

N03 **Chronic nephritic syndrome**
INCLUDES chronic glomerular disease
chronic glomerulonephritis
chronic nephritis
EXCLUDES 1 *chronic tubulo-interstitial nephritis (N11.-)*
diffuse sclerosing glomerulonephritis (N05.8-)
nephritic syndrome NOS (N05.-)
AHA: 2021,1Q,23
DEF: Slow, progressive type of nephritis characterized by inflammation of the capillary loops in the glomeruli of the kidney, which leads to renal failure.

N03.0 **Chronic nephritic syndrome with minor glomerular abnormality**
Chronic nephritic syndrome with minimal change lesion

N03.1 **Chronic nephritic syndrome with focal and segmental glomerular lesions**
Chronic nephritic syndrome with focal and segmental hyalinosis
Chronic nephritic syndrome with focal and segmental sclerosis
Chronic nephritic syndrome with focal glomerulonephritis

N03.2 **Chronic nephritic syndrome with diffuse membranous glomerulonephritis**

N03.3 **Chronic nephritic syndrome with diffuse mesangial proliferative glomerulonephritis**

N03.4 **Chronic nephritic syndrome with diffuse endocapillary proliferative glomerulonephritis**

N03.5 **Chronic nephritic syndrome with diffuse mesangiocapillary glomerulonephritis**
Chronic nephritic syndrome with membranoproliferative glomerulonephritis, types 1 and 3, or NOS
EXCLUDES 1 *chronic nephritic syndrome with C3 glomerulonephritis (N03.A)*
chronic nephritic syndrome with C3 glomerulopathy (N03.A)

N03.6 **Chronic nephritic syndrome with dense deposit disease**
Chronic nephritic syndrome with C3 glomerulopathy with dense deposit disease
Chronic nephritic syndrome with membranoproliferative glomerulonephritis, type 2

N03.7 **Chronic nephritic syndrome with diffuse crescentic glomerulonephritis**
Chronic nephritic syndrome with extracapillary glomerulonephritis

N03.8 **Chronic nephritic syndrome with other morphologic changes**
Chronic nephritic syndrome with proliferative glomerulonephritis NOS

N03.9 **Chronic nephritic syndrome with unspecified morphologic changes**

N03.A **Chronic nephritic syndrome with C3 glomerulonephritis**
Chronic nephritic syndrome with C3 glomerulopathy
EXCLUDES 1 *chronic nephritic syndrome (with C3 glomerulopathy) with dense deposit disease (N03.6)*

N04 **Nephrotic syndrome**
INCLUDES congenital nephrotic syndrome
lipoid nephrosis

N04.0 **Nephrotic syndrome with minor glomerular abnormality**
Nephrotic syndrome with minimal change lesion
AHA: 2024,3Q,14-15

N04.1 **Nephrotic syndrome with focal and segmental glomerular lesions**
Nephrotic syndrome with focal and segmental hyalinosis
Nephrotic syndrome with focal and segmental sclerosis
Nephrotic syndrome with focal glomerulonephritis

N04.2 **Nephrotic syndrome with diffuse membranous glomerulonephritis**
AHA: 2023,4Q,35-36

N04.20 **Nephrotic syndrome with diffuse membranous glomerulonephritis, unspecified**
Membranous nephropathy NOS with nephrotic syndrome

N04.21 **Primary membranous nephropathy with nephrotic syndrome**
Idiopathic membranous nephropathy with nephrotic syndrome

N04.22 **Secondary membranous nephropathy with nephrotic syndrome**
Code first, if applicable, other disease or disorder or poisoning causing membranous nephropathy
Use additional code, if applicable, for adverse effect of drug causing membranous nephropathy

N04.29 **Other nephrotic syndrome with diffuse membranous glomerulonephritis**

N04.3 **Nephrotic syndrome with diffuse mesangial proliferative glomerulonephritis**

N04.4 **Nephrotic syndrome with diffuse endocapillary proliferative glomerulonephritis**

N04.5 **Nephrotic syndrome with diffuse mesangiocapillary glomerulonephritis**
Nephrotic syndrome with membranoproliferative glomerulonephritis, types 1 and 3, or NOS
EXCLUDES 1 *nephrotic syndrome with C3 glomerulonephritis (N04.A)*
nephrotic syndrome with C3 glomerulopathy (N04.A)

N04.6 **Nephrotic syndrome with dense deposit disease**
Nephrotic syndrome with C3 glomerulopathy with dense deposit disease
Nephrotic syndrome with membranoproliferative glomerulonephritis, type 2

N04.7 **Nephrotic syndrome with diffuse crescentic glomerulonephritis**
Nephrotic syndrome with extracapillary glomerulonephritis

N04.8 **Nephrotic syndrome with other morphologic changes**
Nephrotic syndrome with proliferative glomerulonephritis NOS

N04.9 **Nephrotic syndrome with unspecified morphologic changes**

N04.A **Nephrotic syndrome with C3 glomerulonephritis**
Nephrotic syndrome with C3 glomerulopathy
EXCLUDES 1 *nephrotic syndrome (with C3 glomerulopathy) with dense deposit disease (N04.6)*

- ✓5th **N04.B** Nephrotic syndrome with immune complex membranoproliferative glomerulonephritis (IC-MPGN)
- **N04.B1** Nephrotic syndrome with idiopathic immune complex membranoproliferative glomerulonephritis (IC-MPGN)
- **N04.B2** Nephrotic syndrome with secondary immune complex membranoproliferative glomerulonephritis (IC-MPGN)

✓4th **N05** Unspecified nephritic syndrome
  - INCLUDES: glomerular disease NOS
    - glomerulonephritis NOS
    - nephritis NOS
    - nephropathy NOS and renal disease NOS with morphological lesion specified in .0-.8
  - EXCLUDES 1: nephropathy NOS with no stated morphological lesion (N28.9)
    - renal disease NOS with no stated morphological lesion (N28.9)
    - tubulo-interstitial nephritis NOS (N12)

- **N05.0** Unspecified nephritic syndrome with minor glomerular abnormality
  - Unspecified nephritic syndrome with minimal change lesion
- **N05.1** Unspecified nephritic syndrome with focal and segmental glomerular lesions
  - Unspecified nephritic syndrome with focal and segmental hyalinosis
  - Unspecified nephritic syndrome with focal and segmental sclerosis
  - Unspecified nephritic syndrome with focal glomerulonephritis
- **N05.2** Unspecified nephritic syndrome with diffuse membranous glomerulonephritis
- **N05.3** Unspecified nephritic syndrome with diffuse mesangial proliferative glomerulonephritis
- **N05.4** Unspecified nephritic syndrome with diffuse endocapillary proliferative glomerulonephritis
- **N05.5** Unspecified nephritic syndrome with diffuse mesangiocapillary glomerulonephritis
  - Unspecified nephritic syndrome with membranoproliferative glomerulonephritis, types 1 and 3, or NOS
  - EXCLUDES 1: unspecified nephritic syndrome with C3 glomerulonephritis (N05.A)
    - unspecified nephritic syndrome with C3 glomerulopathy (N05.A)
- **N05.6** Unspecified nephritic syndrome with dense deposit disease
  - Unspecified nephritic syndrome with C3 glomerulopathy with dense deposit disease
  - Unspecified nephritic syndrome with membranoproliferative glomerulonephritis, type 2
- **N05.7** Unspecified nephritic syndrome with diffuse crescentic glomerulonephritis
  - Unspecified nephritic syndrome with extracapillary glomerulonephritis
- **N05.8** Unspecified nephritic syndrome with other morphologic changes
  - Unspecified nephritic syndrome with proliferative glomerulonephritis NOS
- **N05.9** Unspecified nephritic syndrome with unspecified morphologic changes
- **N05.A** Unspecified nephritic syndrome with C3 glomerulonephritis
  - Unspecified nephritic syndrome with C3 glomerulopathy
  - EXCLUDES 1: unspecified nephritic syndrome (with C3 glomerulopathy) with dense deposit disease (N05.6)

✓4th **N06** Isolated proteinuria with specified morphological lesion
  - EXCLUDES 1: proteinuria not associated with specific morphologic lesions (R80.0)

- **N06.0** Isolated proteinuria with minor glomerular abnormality
  - Isolated proteinuria with minimal change lesion
- **N06.1** Isolated proteinuria with focal and segmental glomerular lesions
  - Isolated proteinuria with focal and segmental hyalinosis
  - Isolated proteinuria with focal and segmental sclerosis
  - Isolated proteinuria with focal glomerulonephritis
- ✓5th **N06.2** Isolated proteinuria with diffuse membranous glomerulonephritis
  - AHA: 2023,4Q,35-36
  - **N06.20** Isolated proteinuria with diffuse membranous glomerulonephritis, unspecified
    - Membranous nephropathy, NOS
    - EXCLUDES 1: membranous nephropathy NOS with nephrotic syndrome (N04.20)
  - **N06.21** Primary membranous nephropathy with isolated proteinuria
    - Idiopathic membranous nephropathy (with isolated proteinuria)
    - Primary membranous nephropathy, NOS
    - EXCLUDES 1: primary membranous nephropathy with nephrotic syndrome (N04.21)
  - **N06.22** Secondary membranous nephropathy with isolated proteinuria
    - Secondary membranous nephropathy, NOS
    - Code first, if applicable, other disease or disorder or poisoning causing membranous nephropathy
    - Use additional code, if applicable, for adverse effect of drug causing membranous nephropathy
    - EXCLUDES 1: secondary membranous nephropathy with nephrotic syndrome (N04.22)
  - **N06.29** Other isolated proteinuria with diffuse membranous glomerulonephritis
- **N06.3** Isolated proteinuria with diffuse mesangial proliferative glomerulonephritis
- **N06.4** Isolated proteinuria with diffuse endocapillary proliferative glomerulonephritis
- **N06.5** Isolated proteinuria with diffuse mesangiocapillary glomerulonephritis
  - Isolated proteinuria with membranoproliferative glomerulonephritis, types 1 and 3, or NOS
  - EXCLUDES 1: isolated proteinuria with C3 glomerulonephritis (N06.A)
    - isolated proteinuria with C3 glomerulopathy (N06.A)
- **N06.6** Isolated proteinuria with dense deposit disease
  - Isolated proteinuria with C3 glomerulopathy with dense deposit disease
  - Isolated proteinuria with membranoproliferative glomerulonephritis, type 2
- **N06.7** Isolated proteinuria with diffuse crescentic glomerulonephritis
  - Isolated proteinuria with extracapillary glomerulonephritis
- **N06.8** Isolated proteinuria with other morphologic lesion
  - Isolated proteinuria with proliferative glomerulonephritis NOS
- **N06.9** Isolated proteinuria with unspecified morphologic lesion
- **N06.A** Isolated proteinuria with C3 glomerulonephritis
  - Isolated proteinuria with C3 glomerulopathy
  - EXCLUDES 1: isolated proteinuria (with C3 glomerulopathy) with dense deposit disease (N06.6)

✓4th **N07** Hereditary nephropathy, not elsewhere classified
  - EXCLUDES 2: Alport's syndrome (Q87.81-)
    - hereditary amyloid nephropathy (E85.-)
    - nail patella syndrome (Q87.2)
    - non-neuropathic heredofamilial amyloidosis (E85.-)

- **N07.0** Hereditary nephropathy, not elsewhere classified with minor glomerular abnormality
  - Hereditary nephropathy, not elsewhere classified with minimal change lesion
- **N07.1** Hereditary nephropathy, not elsewhere classified with focal and segmental glomerular lesions
  - Hereditary nephropathy, not elsewhere classified with focal and segmental hyalinosis
  - Hereditary nephropathy, not elsewhere classified with focal and segmental sclerosis
  - Hereditary nephropathy, not elsewhere classified with focal glomerulonephritis
- **N07.2** Hereditary nephropathy, not elsewhere classified with diffuse membranous glomerulonephritis
- **N07.3** Hereditary nephropathy, not elsewhere classified with diffuse mesangial proliferative glomerulonephritis
- **N07.4** Hereditary nephropathy, not elsewhere classified with diffuse endocapillary proliferative glomerulonephritis
- **N07.5** Hereditary nephropathy, not elsewhere classified with diffuse mesangiocapillary glomerulonephritis
  - Hereditary nephropathy, not elsewhere classified with membranoproliferative glomerulonephritis, types 1 and 3, or NOS
  - EXCLUDES 1: hereditary nephropathy, not elsewhere classified with C3 glomerulonephritis (N07.A)
    - hereditary nephropathy, not elsewhere classified with C3 glomerulopathy (N07.A)
- **N07.6** Hereditary nephropathy, not elsewhere classified with dense deposit disease
  - Hereditary nephropathy, not elsewhere classified with C3 glomerulopathy with dense deposit disease
  - Hereditary nephropathy, not elsewhere classified with membranoproliferative glomerulonephritis, type 2

N07.7 Hereditary nephropathy, not elsewhere classified with diffuse crescentic glomerulonephritis
Hereditary nephropathy, not elsewhere classified with extracapillary glomerulonephritis

N07.8 Hereditary nephropathy, not elsewhere classified with other morphologic lesions
Hereditary nephropathy, not elsewhere classified with proliferative glomerulonephritis NOS

N07.9 Hereditary nephropathy, not elsewhere classified with unspecified morphologic lesions

N07.A Hereditary nephropathy, not elsewhere classified with C3 glomerulonephritis
Hereditary nephropathy, not elsewhere classified with C3 glomerulopathy
EXCLUDES 1 — *hereditary nephropathy, not elsewhere classified (with C3 glomerulopathy) with dense deposit disease (N07.6)*

• **N07.B Hereditary nephropathy, not elsewhere classified with APOL1-mediated kidney disease [AMKD]**
AMKD (with glomerulonephritis)
AMKD (with glomerulosclerosis)

N08 Glomerular disorders in diseases classified elsewhere
Glomerulonephritis
Nephritis
Nephropathy
Code first underlying disease, such as:
  amyloidosis (E85.-)
  congenital syphilis (A50.5)
  cryoglobulinemia (D89.1)
  disseminated intravascular coagulation (D65)
  gout (M1A.-, M10.-)
  microscopic polyangiitis (M31.7)
  multiple myeloma (C90.0-)
  sepsis (A40.0-A41.9)
  sickle-cell disease (D57.0-D57.8)
EXCLUDES 1 — *glomerulonephritis, nephritis and nephropathy (in):*
  pyelonephritis in diseases classified elsewhere (N16)
  renal tubulo-interstitial disorders classified elsewhere (N16)
    antiglomerular basement membrane disease (M31.0)
    diabetes (E08-E13 with .21)
    gonococcal (A54.21)
    Goodpasture's syndrome (M31.0)
    hemolytic-uremic syndrome (D59.3-)
    lupus (M32.14)
    mumps (B26.83)
    syphilis (A52.75)
    systemic lupus erythematosus (M32.14)
    Wegener's granulomatosis (M31.31)

Renal tubulo-interstitial diseases (N10-N16)

INCLUDES pyelonephritis
EXCLUDES 1 *pyeloureteritis cystica (N28.85)*

N10 Acute pyelonephritis
Acute infectious interstitial nephritis
Acute pyelitis
Acute tubulo-interstitial nephritis
Hemoglobin nephrosis
Myoglobin nephrosis
Use additional code (B95-B97), to identify infectious agent
AHA: 2020,3Q,25; 2019,3Q,13

✓4th **N11 Chronic tubulo-interstitial nephritis**
INCLUDES chronic infectious interstitial nephritis
  chronic pyelitis
  chronic pyelonephritis
Use additional code (B95-B97), to identify infectious agent

N11.0 Nonobstructive reflux-associated chronic pyelonephritis
Pyelonephritis (chronic) associated with (vesicoureteral) reflux
EXCLUDES 1 *vesicoureteral reflux NOS (N13.70)*

N11.1 Chronic obstructive pyelonephritis
Pyelonephritis (chronic) associated with anomaly of pelviureteric junction
Pyelonephritis (chronic) associated with anomaly of pyeloureteric junction
Pyelonephritis (chronic) associated with crossing of vessel
Pyelonephritis (chronic) associated with kinking of ureter
Pyelonephritis (chronic) associated with obstruction of ureter
Pyelonephritis (chronic) associated with stricture of pelviureteric junction
Pyelonephritis (chronic) associated with stricture of ureter
EXCLUDES 1 *calculous pyelonephritis (N20.9)*
  obstructive uropathy (N13.-)

N11.8 Other chronic tubulo-interstitial nephritis
Nonobstructive chronic pyelonephritis NOS

N11.9 Chronic tubulo-interstitial nephritis, unspecified
Chronic interstitial nephritis NOS
Chronic pyelitis NOS
Chronic pyelonephritis NOS

N12 Tubulo-interstitial nephritis, not specified as acute or chronic
Interstitial nephritis NOS
Pyelitis NOS
Pyelonephritis NOS
EXCLUDES 1 *calculous pyelonephritis (N20.9)*

✓4th **N13 Obstructive and reflux uropathy**
EXCLUDES 2 *calculus of kidney and ureter without hydronephrosis (N20.-)*
  congenital obstructive defects of renal pelvis and ureter (Q62.0-Q62.3)
  hydronephrosis with ureteropelvic junction obstruction (Q62.11)
  obstructive pyelonephritis (N11.1)
DEF: Hydronephrosis: Distension of the kidney caused by an accumulation of urine that cannot flow out due to an obstruction that may be caused by conditions such as kidney stones or vesicoureteral reflux.

N13.0 Hydronephrosis with ureteropelvic junction obstruction
Hydronephrosis due to acquired occlusion of ureteropelvic junction
EXCLUDES 2 *hydronephrosis with ureteropelvic junction obstruction due to calculus (N13.2)*
AHA: 2016,4Q,43

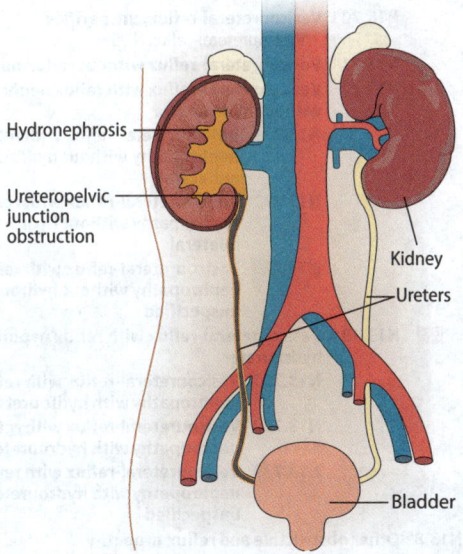

Hydronephrosis/UPJ Obstruction

N13.1 Hydronephrosis with ureteral stricture, not elsewhere classified
EXCLUDES 1 *hydronephrosis with ureteral stricture with infection (N13.6)*

N13.2 Hydronephrosis with renal and ureteral calculous obstruction
EXCLUDES 1 *hydronephrosis with renal and ureteral calculous obstruction with infection (N13.6)*

✓5th **N13.3 Other and unspecified hydronephrosis**
EXCLUDES 1 *hydronephrosis with infection (N13.6)*
  N13.30 Unspecified hydronephrosis
  N13.39 Other hydronephrosis

Chapter 14. Diseases of the Genitourinary System

N13.4 Hydroureter
   EXCLUDES 1
   congenital hydroureter (Q62.3-)
   hydroureter with infection (N13.6)
   vesicoureteral-reflux with hydroureter (N13.73-)
   DEF: Abnormal enlargement or distension of the ureter with water or urine caused by an obstruction.

N13.5 Crossing vessel and stricture of ureter without hydronephrosis
   Kinking and stricture of ureter without hydronephrosis
   EXCLUDES 1
   crossing vessel and stricture of ureter without hydronephrosis with infection (N13.6)

N13.6 Pyonephrosis
   Conditions in N13.0-N13.5 with infection
   Obstructive uropathy with infection
   Use additional code (B95-B97), to identify infectious agent
   AHA: 2018,2Q,21

√5th **N13.7 Vesicoureteral-reflux**
   EXCLUDES 1
   reflux-associated pyelonephritis (N11.0)
   DEF: Urine passage from the bladder flows backward up into the ureter and kidneys that can lead to bacterial infection and an increase in hydrostatic pressure, causing kidney damage.

Vesicoureteral Reflux

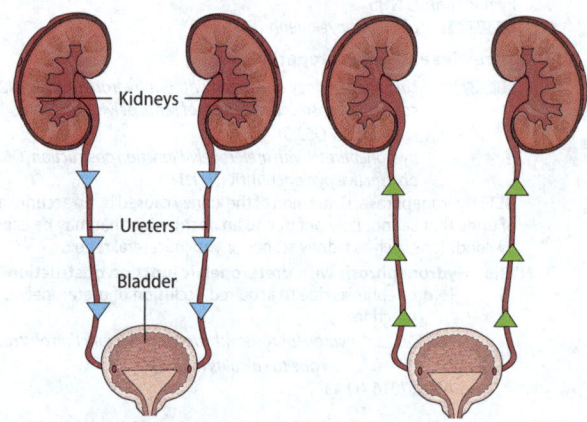

Normal flow of urine — Urine flowing the wrong way (VUR)

   N13.70 Vesicoureteral-reflux, unspecified
      Vesicoureteral-reflux NOS
   N13.71 Vesicoureteral-reflux without reflux nephropathy
√6th **N13.72 Vesicoureteral-reflux with reflux nephropathy without hydroureter**
      N13.721 Vesicoureteral-reflux with reflux nephropathy without hydroureter, unilateral
      N13.722 Vesicoureteral-reflux with reflux nephropathy without hydroureter, bilateral
      N13.729 Vesicoureteral-reflux with reflux nephropathy without hydroureter, unspecified
√6th **N13.73 Vesicoureteral-reflux with reflux nephropathy with hydroureter**
      N13.731 Vesicoureteral-reflux with reflux nephropathy with hydroureter, unilateral
      N13.732 Vesicoureteral-reflux with reflux nephropathy with hydroureter, bilateral
      N13.739 Vesicoureteral-reflux with reflux nephropathy with hydroureter, unspecified

N13.8 Other obstructive and reflux uropathy
   Urinary tract obstruction due to specified cause
   Code first, if applicable, any causal condition, such as:
      enlarged prostate (N40.1)

N13.9 Obstructive and reflux uropathy, unspecified
   Urinary tract obstruction NOS

√4th **N14 Drug- and heavy-metal-induced tubulo-interstitial and tubular conditions**
   Code first poisoning due to drug or toxin, if applicable (T36-T65 with fifth or sixth character 1-4)
   Use additional code for adverse effect, if applicable, to identify drug (T36-T50 with fifth or sixth character 5)

   N14.0 Analgesic nephropathy

√5th **N14.1 Nephropathy induced by other drugs, medicaments and biological substances**
   AHA: 2022,4Q,33; 2021,3Q,9-10
      N14.11 Contrast-induced nephropathy
         Contrast medium, radiography nephropathy
         EXCLUDES 2 acute kidney failure (N17.-)
      N14.19 Nephropathy induced by other drugs, medicaments and biological substances

   N14.2 Nephropathy induced by unspecified drug, medicament or biological substance
   N14.3 Nephropathy induced by heavy metals
   N14.4 Toxic nephropathy, not elsewhere classified

√4th **N15 Other renal tubulo-interstitial diseases**
   N15.0 Balkan nephropathy
      Balkan endemic nephropathy
   N15.1 Renal and perinephric abscess
   N15.8 Other specified renal tubulo-interstitial diseases
   N15.9 Renal tubulo-interstitial disease, unspecified
      Infection of kidney NOS
      EXCLUDES 1 urinary tract infection NOS (N39.0)

N16 Renal tubulo-interstitial disorders in diseases classified elsewhere
   Pyelonephritis
   Tubulo-interstitial nephritis
   Code first underlying disease, such as:
      brucellosis (A23.0-A23.9)
      cryoglobulinemia (D89.1)
      glycogen storage disease (E74.0-)
      leukemia (C91-C95)
      lymphoma (C81.0-C85.9, C96.0-C96.9)
      multiple myeloma (C90.0-)
      sepsis (A40.0-A41.9)
      Wilson's disease (E83.01)
   EXCLUDES 1
      diphtheritic pyelonephritis and tubulo-interstitial nephritis (A36.84)
      pyelonephritis and tubulo-interstitial nephritis in candidiasis (B37.49)
      pyelonephritis and tubulo-interstitial nephritis in cystinosis (E72.04)
      pyelonephritis and tubulo-interstitial nephritis in salmonella infection (A02.25)
      pyelonephritis and tubulo-interstitial nephritis in sarcoidosis (D86.84)
      pyelonephritis and tubulo-interstitial nephritis in Sjogren syndrome (M35.04)
      pyelonephritis and tubulo-interstitial nephritis in systemic lupus erythematosus (M32.15)
      pyelonephritis and tubulo-interstitial nephritis in toxoplasmosis (B58.83)
      renal tubular degeneration in diabetes (E08-E13 with .29)
      syphilitic pyelonephritis and tubulo-interstitial nephritis (A52.75)

Acute kidney failure and chronic kidney disease (N17-N19)

EXCLUDES 2
   congenital renal failure (P96.0)
   drug- and heavy-metal-induced tubulo-interstitial and tubular conditions (N14.-)
   extrarenal uremia (R39.2)
   hemolytic-uremic syndrome (D59.3-)
   hepatorenal syndrome (K76.7)
   postpartum hepatorenal syndrome (O90.41)
   posttraumatic renal failure (T79.5)
   prerenal uremia (R39.2)
   renal failure complicating abortion or ectopic or molar pregnancy (O00-O07, O08.4)
   renal failure following labor and delivery (O90.41)
   renal failure postprocedural (N99.0)

√4th **N17 Acute kidney failure**
   Code also associated underlying condition
   EXCLUDES 1 posttraumatic renal failure (T79.5)
   AHA: 2020,3Q,22; 2019,2Q,7; 2019,1Q,12; 2013,4Q,124

   N17.0 Acute kidney failure with tubular necrosis
      Acute tubular necrosis
      Renal tubular necrosis
      Tubular necrosis NOS
      AHA: 2024,3Q,15; 2022,4Q,33; 2021,3Q,10

   N17.1 Acute kidney failure with acute cortical necrosis
      Acute cortical necrosis
      Cortical necrosis NOS
      Renal cortical necrosis

Chapter 14. Diseases of the Genitourinary System

N17.2 Acute kidney failure with medullary necrosis `ESR`
  Acute medullary [papillary] necrosis
  Medullary [papillary] necrosis NOS
  Renal medullary [papillary] necrosis

N17.8 Other acute kidney failure `ESR`
  AHA: 2025,1Q,26

N17.9 Acute kidney failure, unspecified `ESR`
  Acute kidney injury (nontraumatic)
  EXCLUDES 2 traumatic kidney injury (S37.0-)

✓4th N18 Chronic kidney disease (CKD)
  Code first any associated:
    diabetic chronic kidney disease (E08.22, E09.22, E10.22, E11.22, E13.22)
    hypertensive chronic kidney disease (I12.-, I13.-)
  ▶Use additional code, if applicable, to identify:◀
    ▶associated cachexia (E88.A)◀
    ▶kidney transplant status (Z94.0)◀
  AHA: 2025,2Q,8; 2023,1Q,17; 2022,4Q,14; 2019,3Q,3; 2018,4Q,88; 2013,1Q,24
  TIP: CKD/ESRD occurring in an individual with a history of kidney transplant should not be assumed to be a transplant complication unless specifically indicated as such by provider documentation.

  N18.1 Chronic kidney disease, stage 1
  N18.2 Chronic kidney disease, stage 2 (mild)
  ✓5th N18.3 Chronic kidney disease, stage 3 (moderate)
    AHA: 2020,4Q,35
    N18.30 Chronic kidney disease, stage 3 unspecified `HCC` `ESR`
    N18.31 Chronic kidney disease, stage 3a `HCC` `ESR`
    N18.32 Chronic kidney disease, stage 3b `HCC` `ESR`
  N18.4 Chronic kidney disease, stage 4 (severe) `HCC` `Rx` `ESR` `COM`
  N18.5 Chronic kidney disease, stage 5 `HCC` `Rx` `ESR` `COM`
    EXCLUDES 1 chronic kidney disease, stage 5 requiring chronic dialysis (N18.6)
    DEF: End-stage renal disease (ESRD) with a GFR value of 15 ml/min or less not yet requiring chronic dialysis.
    TIP: When both ESRD and CKD 5 are documented, code only for ESRD.
  N18.6 End stage renal disease `HCC` `Rx` `ESR` `COM`
    Chronic kidney disease requiring chronic dialysis
    Use additional code to identify dialysis status (Z99.2)
    AHA: 2023,1Q,19; 2022,3Q,15; 2016,3Q,22; 2016,1Q,12; 2013,4Q,124-125
    TIP: When both ESRD and CKD 5 are documented, code only for ESRD.
  N18.9 Chronic kidney disease, unspecified
    Chronic renal disease
    Chronic renal failure NOS
    Chronic renal insufficiency
    Chronic uremia NOS
    Diffuse sclerosing glomerulonephritis NOS

N19 Unspecified kidney failure
  Uremia NOS
  EXCLUDES 1 acute kidney failure (N17.-)
    chronic kidney disease (N18.-)
    chronic uremia (N18.9)
    extrarenal uremia (R39.2)
    prerenal uremia (R39.2)
    renal insufficiency (acute) (N28.9)
    uremia of newborn (P96.0)

Urolithiasis (N20-N23)

AHA: 2017,1Q,5; 2015,2Q,8
TIP: Codes from this code block can be assigned based on the diagnosis listed in a radiology report when authenticated by a radiologist and available at the time of code assignment.

✓4th N20 Calculus of kidney and ureter
  Calculous pyelonephritis
  EXCLUDES 1 nephrocalcinosis (E83.59)
    that with hydronephrosis (N13.2)
  AHA: 2019,3Q,13

  N20.0 Calculus of kidney
    Nephrolithiasis NOS
    Renal calculus
    Renal stone
    Staghorn calculus
    Stone in kidney
    AHA: 2019,3Q,13

  N20.1 Calculus of ureter
    Calculus of the ureteropelvic junction
    Ureteric stone
    AHA: 2016,3Q,22
  N20.2 Calculus of kidney with calculus of ureter
  N20.9 Urinary calculus, unspecified

✓4th N21 Calculus of lower urinary tract
  INCLUDES calculus of lower urinary tract with cystitis and urethritis
  N21.0 Calculus in bladder
    Calculus in diverticulum of bladder
    Urinary bladder stone
    EXCLUDES 2 staghorn calculus (N20.0)
  N21.1 Calculus in urethra
    EXCLUDES 2 calculus of prostate (N42.0)
  N21.8 Other lower urinary tract calculus
  N21.9 Calculus of lower urinary tract, unspecified
    EXCLUDES 2 calculus of urinary tract NOS (N20.9)

N22 Calculus of urinary tract in diseases classified elsewhere
  Code first underlying disease, such as:
    gout (M1A.-, M10.-)
    schistosomiasis (B65.0-B65.9)

N23 Unspecified renal colic

Other disorders of kidney and ureter (N25-N29)

EXCLUDES 2 disorders of kidney and ureter with urolithiasis (N20-N23)

✓4th N25 Disorders resulting from impaired renal tubular function
  N25.0 Renal osteodystrophy `Rx`
    Azotemic osteodystrophy
    Phosphate-losing tubular disorders
    Renal rickets
    Renal short stature
    EXCLUDES 2 metabolic disorders classifiable to E70-E88
    DEF: Various bone diseases occurring when kidney function is impaired or fails. Abnormal levels of phosphorous and calcium can lead to osteomalacia, osteoporosis, or osteosclerosis.
  N25.1 Nephrogenic diabetes insipidus `Rx` `ESR` `COM`
    EXCLUDES 1 diabetes insipidus NOS (E23.2)
    DEF: Type of diabetes due to the inability of renal tubules to reabsorb water back into the body. It is not responsive to vasopressin (antidiuretic hormone) and it is characterized by excessive thirst and excessive urine production. It may develop into chronic renal insufficiency.
  ✓5th N25.8 Other disorders resulting from impaired renal tubular function
    N25.81 Secondary hyperparathyroidism of renal origin `Rx` `ESR` `COM`
      EXCLUDES 1 secondary hyperparathyroidism, non-renal (E21.1)
      EXCLUDES 2 metabolic disorders classifiable to E70-E88
      DEF: Parathyroid dysfunction caused by chronic renal failure. Phosphate clearance and vitamin D production is impaired resulting in lowered calcium blood levels and an excessive production of parathyroid hormone.
    N25.89 Other disorders resulting from impaired renal tubular function
      Hypokalemic nephropathy
      Lightwood-Albright syndrome
      Renal tubular acidosis NOS
  N25.9 Disorder resulting from impaired renal tubular function, unspecified

✓4th N26 Unspecified contracted kidney
  EXCLUDES 1 contracted kidney due to hypertension (I12.-)
    diffuse sclerosing glomerulonephritis (N05.8.-)
    hypertensive nephrosclerosis (arteriolar) (arteriosclerotic) (I12.-)
    small kidney of unknown cause (N27.-)
  N26.1 Atrophy of kidney (terminal)
  N26.2 Page kidney `Rx`
  N26.9 Renal sclerosis, unspecified

✓4th N27 Small kidney of unknown cause
  INCLUDES oligonephronia
  N27.0 Small kidney, unilateral
  N27.1 Small kidney, bilateral
  N27.9 Small kidney, unspecified

☑ Additional Character Required 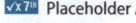 Placeholder Alert Manifestation Unspecified Dx QPP UPD Unacceptable PDx

Chapter 14. Diseases of the Genitourinary System

✓4th N28 Other disorders of kidney and ureter, not elsewhere classified

- **N28.0 Ischemia and infarction of kidney** [ESR] [COM]
  - Renal artery embolism
  - Renal artery obstruction
  - Renal artery occlusion
  - Renal artery thrombosis
  - Renal infarct
  - EXCLUDES 1 atherosclerosis of renal artery (extrarenal part) (I70.1)
    - congenital stenosis of renal artery (Q27.1)
    - Goldblatt's kidney (I70.1)

- **N28.1 Cyst of kidney, acquired**
  - Cyst (multiple) (solitary) of kidney (acquired)
  - EXCLUDES 1 cystic kidney disease (congenital) (Q61.-)

- ✓5th **N28.8 Other specified disorders of kidney and ureter**
  - EXCLUDES 1 hydroureter (N13.4)
    - ureteric stricture with hydronephrosis (N13.1)
    - ureteric stricture without hydronephrosis (N13.5)
  - **N28.81 Hypertrophy of kidney**
  - **N28.82 Megaloureter**
  - **N28.83 Nephroptosis**
  - **N28.84 Pyelitis cystica**
  - **N28.85 Pyeloureteritis cystica**
  - **N28.86 Ureteritis cystica**
  - **N28.89 Other specified disorders of kidney and ureter**
    - AHA: 2025,2Q,8; 2023,3Q,5

- **N28.9 Disorder of kidney and ureter, unspecified**
  - Nephropathy NOS
  - Renal disease (acute) NOS
  - Renal insufficiency (acute)
  - EXCLUDES 1 chronic renal insufficiency (N18.9)
    - unspecified nephritic syndrome (N05.-)
  - AHA: 2016,1Q,13

N29 Other disorders of kidney and ureter in diseases classified elsewhere
- Code first underlying disease, such as:
  - amyloidosis (E85.-)
  - nephrocalcinosis (E83.59)
  - schistosomiasis (B65.0-B65.9)
- EXCLUDES 1 disorders of kidney and ureter in:
  - cystinosis (E72.0)
  - gonorrhea (A54.21)
  - syphilis (A52.75)
  - tuberculosis (A18.11)

Other diseases of the urinary system (N30-N39)

EXCLUDES 2 urinary infection (complicating):
- abortion or ectopic or molar pregnancy (O00-O07, O08.8)
- pregnancy, childbirth and the puerperium (O23.-, O75.3, O86.2-)

✓4th N30 Cystitis
- Use additional code to identify infectious agent (B95-B97)
- EXCLUDES 1 prostatocystitis (N41.3)
- AHA: 2017,1Q,6
- DEF: Inflammation of the urinary bladder. Symptoms include dysuria, frequency of urination, urgency, and hematuria.

- ✓5th **N30.0 Acute cystitis**
  - EXCLUDES 1 irradiation cystitis (N30.4-)
    - trigonitis (N30.3-)
  - **N30.00 Acute cystitis without hematuria**
  - **N30.01 Acute cystitis with hematuria**

- ✓5th **N30.1 Interstitial cystitis (chronic)**
  - **N30.10 Interstitial cystitis (chronic) without hematuria**
  - **N30.11 Interstitial cystitis (chronic) with hematuria**

- ✓5th **N30.2 Other chronic cystitis**
  - **N30.20 Other chronic cystitis without hematuria**
  - **N30.21 Other chronic cystitis with hematuria**

- ✓5th **N30.3 Trigonitis**
  - Urethrotrigonitis
  - **N30.30 Trigonitis without hematuria**
  - **N30.31 Trigonitis with hematuria**

- ✓5th **N30.4 Irradiation cystitis**
  - **N30.40 Irradiation cystitis without hematuria**
  - **N30.41 Irradiation cystitis with hematuria**

- ✓5th **N30.8 Other cystitis**
  - Abscess of bladder
  - **N30.80 Other cystitis without hematuria**
  - **N30.81 Other cystitis with hematuria**

- ✓5th **N30.9 Cystitis, unspecified**
  - **N30.90 Cystitis, unspecified without hematuria**
  - **N30.91 Cystitis, unspecified with hematuria**

✓4th N31 Neuromuscular dysfunction of bladder, not elsewhere classified
- Use additional code to identify any associated urinary incontinence (N39.3-N39.4-)
- EXCLUDES 1 cord bladder NOS (G95.89)
  - neurogenic bladder due to cauda equina syndrome (G83.4)
  - neuromuscular dysfunction due to spinal cord lesion (G95.89)

- **N31.0 Uninhibited neuropathic bladder, not elsewhere classified**
- **N31.1 Reflex neuropathic bladder, not elsewhere classified**
- **N31.2 Flaccid neuropathic bladder, not elsewhere classified**
  - Atonic (motor) (sensory) neuropathic bladder
  - Autonomous neuropathic bladder
  - Nonreflex neuropathic bladder
- **N31.8 Other neuromuscular dysfunction of bladder**
- **N31.9 Neuromuscular dysfunction of bladder, unspecified**
  - Neurogenic bladder dysfunction NOS

✓4th N32 Other disorders of bladder
- EXCLUDES 2 calculus of bladder (N21.0)
  - cystocele (N81.1-)
  - hernia or prolapse of bladder, female (N81.1-)

- **N32.0 Bladder-neck obstruction**
  - Bladder-neck stenosis (acquired)
  - EXCLUDES 1 congenital bladder-neck obstruction (Q64.3-)
  - DEF: Bladder outlet and vesicourethral obstruction that occurs as a consequence of benign prostatic hypertrophy or prostatic cancer. It may also occur in either sex due to strictures, radiation, cystoscopy, catheterization, injury, infection, blood clots, bladder cancer, impaction, or other disease that compresses the bladder neck.

- **N32.1 Vesicointestinal fistula**
  - Vesicorectal fistula
  - AHA: 2025,2Q,6

- **N32.2 Vesical fistula, not elsewhere classified**
  - EXCLUDES 1 fistula between bladder and female genital tract (N82.0-N82.1)

- **N32.3 Diverticulum of bladder**
  - EXCLUDES 1 congenital diverticulum of bladder (Q64.6)
    - diverticulitis of bladder (N30.8-)

- ✓5th **N32.8 Other specified disorders of bladder**
  - **N32.81 Overactive bladder**
    - Detrusor muscle hyperactivity
    - EXCLUDES 1 frequent urination due to specified bladder condition — code to condition
    - DEF: Sudden involuntary contractions of the muscular wall of the bladder that results in a sudden, strong urge to urinate.
  - **N32.89 Other specified disorders of bladder**
    - Bladder hemorrhage
    - Bladder hypertrophy
    - Calcified bladder
    - Contracted bladder

- **N32.9 Bladder disorder, unspecified**

N33 Bladder disorders in diseases classified elsewhere
- Code first underlying disease, such as:
  - schistosomiasis (B65.0-B65.9)
- EXCLUDES 1 bladder disorder in syphilis (A52.76)
  - bladder disorder in tuberculosis (A18.12)
  - candidal cystitis (B37.41)
  - chlamydial cystitis (A56.01)
  - cystitis in gonorrhea (A54.01)
  - cystitis in neurogenic bladder (N31.-)
  - diphtheritic cystitis (A36.85)
  - neurogenic bladder (N31.-)
  - syphilitic cystitis (A52.76)
  - trichomonal cystitis (A59.03)

✓4th N34 Urethritis and urethral syndrome
- Use additional code (B95-B97), to identify infectious agent
- EXCLUDES 2 Reiter's disease (M02.3-)
  - urethritis in diseases with a predominantly sexual mode of transmission (A50-A64)
  - urethrotrigonitis (N30.3-)
- AHA: 2017,1Q,6

- **N34.0 Urethral abscess**
  - Abscess (of) Cowper's gland
  - Abscess (of) Littre's gland
  - Abscess (of) urethral (gland)
  - Periurethral abscess
  - EXCLUDES 1 urethral caruncle (N36.2)

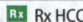

N34.1 Nonspecific urethritis
  Nongonococcal urethritis
  Nonvenereal urethritis

N34.2 Other urethritis
  Meatitis, urethral
  Postmenopausal urethritis
  Ulcer of urethra (meatus)
  Urethritis NOS

N34.3 Urethral syndrome, unspecified

✓4th **N35 Urethral stricture**
  EXCLUDES 1 congenital urethral stricture (Q64.3-)
              postprocedural urethral stricture (N99.1-)
  AHA: 2018,4Q,21-22

✓5th **N35.0 Post-traumatic urethral stricture**
  Urethral stricture due to injury
  EXCLUDES 1 postprocedural urethral stricture (N99.1-)

  ✓6th **N35.01 Post-traumatic urethral stricture, male**
    N35.010 Post-traumatic urethral stricture, male, meatal
    N35.011 Post-traumatic bulbous urethral stricture
    N35.012 Post-traumatic membranous urethral stricture
    N35.013 Post-traumatic anterior urethral stricture
    N35.014 Post-traumatic urethral stricture, male, unspecified
    N35.016 Post-traumatic urethral stricture, male, overlapping sites

  ✓6th **N35.02 Post-traumatic urethral stricture, female**
    N35.021 Urethral stricture due to childbirth
    N35.028 Other post-traumatic urethral stricture, female

✓5th **N35.1 Postinfective urethral stricture, not elsewhere classified**
  EXCLUDES 1 gonococcal urethral stricture (A54.01)
              syphilitic urethral stricture (A52.76)
              urethral stricture associated with schistosomiasis (B65.-, N29)

  ✓6th **N35.11 Postinfective urethral stricture, not elsewhere classified, male**
    N35.111 Postinfective urethral stricture, not elsewhere classified, male, meatal
    N35.112 Postinfective bulbous urethral stricture, not elsewhere classified, male
    N35.113 Postinfective membranous urethral stricture, not elsewhere classified, male
    N35.114 Postinfective anterior urethral stricture, not elsewhere classified, male
    N35.116 Postinfective urethral stricture, not elsewhere classified, male, overlapping sites
    N35.119 Postinfective urethral stricture, not elsewhere classified, male, unspecified

  N35.12 Postinfective urethral stricture, not elsewhere classified, female

✓5th **N35.8 Other urethral stricture**
  EXCLUDES 1 postprocedural urethral stricture (N99.1-)

  ✓6th **N35.81 Other urethral stricture, male**
    N35.811 Other urethral stricture, male, meatal
    N35.812 Other bulbous urethral stricture, male
    N35.813 Other membranous urethral stricture, male
    N35.814 Other anterior urethral stricture, male
    N35.816 Other urethral stricture, male, overlapping sites
    N35.819 Other urethral stricture, male, unspecified site

  N35.82 Other urethral stricture, female

✓5th **N35.9 Urethral stricture, unspecified**
  ✓6th **N35.91 Urethral stricture, unspecified, male**
    N35.911 Unspecified urethral stricture, male, meatal
    N35.912 Unspecified bulbous urethral stricture, male
    N35.913 Unspecified membranous urethral stricture, male
    N35.914 Unspecified anterior urethral stricture, male
    N35.916 Unspecified urethral stricture, male, overlapping sites
    N35.919 Unspecified urethral stricture, male, unspecified site
             Pinhole meatus NOS
             Urethral stricture NOS

  N35.92 Unspecified urethral stricture, female

✓4th **N36 Other disorders of urethra**

  N36.0 Urethral fistula
    Urethroperineal fistula
    Urethrorectal fistula
    Urinary fistula NOS
    EXCLUDES 1 urethroscrotal fistula (N50.89)
                urethrovaginal fistula (N82.1)
                urethrovesicovaginal fistula (N82.1)

  N36.1 Urethral diverticulum
  N36.2 Urethral caruncle

  ✓5th **N36.4 Urethral functional and muscular disorders**
    Use additional code to identify associated urinary stress incontinence (N39.3)
    N36.41 Hypermobility of urethra
    N36.42 Intrinsic sphincter deficiency (ISD)
    N36.43 Combined hypermobility of urethra and intrinsic sphincter deficiency
    N36.44 Muscular disorders of urethra
            Bladder sphincter dyssynergy

  N36.5 Urethral false passage
  N36.8 Other specified disorders of urethra
    EXCLUDES 1 congenital urethrocele (Q64.7)
                female urethrocele (N81.0)
    AHA: 2022,2Q,7

  N36.9 Urethral disorder, unspecified

N37 Urethral disorders in diseases classified elsewhere
  Code first underlying disease
  EXCLUDES 1 urethritis (in):
                candidal infection (B37.41)
                chlamydial (A56.01)
                gonorrhea (A54.01)
                syphilis (A52.76)
                trichomonal infection (A59.03)
                tuberculosis (A18.13)

✓4th **N39 Other disorders of urinary system**
  EXCLUDES 2 hematuria NOS (R31.-)
              proteinuria NOS (R80.-)
              recurrent or persistent hematuria (N02.-)
              recurrent or persistent hematuria with specified morphological lesion (N02.-)

  N39.0 Urinary tract infection, site not specified
    Use additional code (B95-B97), to identify infectious agent
    EXCLUDES 1 candidiasis of urinary tract (B37.4-)
                neonatal urinary tract infection (P39.3)
                pyuria (R82.81)
                urinary tract infection of specified site, such as:
                  cystitis (N30.-)
                  pyonephrosis (N13.6)
                  urethritis (N34.-)
    AHA: 2019,3Q,17; 2018,2Q,21,22; 2018,1Q,16; 2017,1Q,6; 2012,4Q,94

  N39.3 Stress incontinence (female) (male)
    Code also any associated overactive bladder (N32.81)
    EXCLUDES 1 mixed incontinence (N39.46)

  ✓5th **N39.4 Other specified urinary incontinence**
    Code also any associated overactive bladder (N32.81)
    EXCLUDES 1 enuresis NOS (R32)
                functional urinary incontinence (R39.81)
                urinary incontinence associated with cognitive impairment (R39.81)
                urinary incontinence of nonorganic origin (F98.0)
                urinary incontinence NOS (R32)

    N39.41 Urge incontinence
            EXCLUDES 1 mixed incontinence (N39.46)
    N39.42 Incontinence without sensory awareness
            Insensible (urinary) incontinence
    N39.43 Post-void dribbling
    N39.44 Nocturnal enuresis
            EXCLUDES 2 nocturnal polyuria (R35.81)
    N39.45 Continuous leakage
    N39.46 Mixed incontinence
            Urge and stress incontinence

✓6th **N39.49** **Other specified urinary incontinence**
   AHA: 2016,4Q,44
   N39.490 **Overflow incontinence**
   N39.491 **Coital incontinence**
   N39.492 **Postural (urinary) incontinence**
   N39.498 **Other specified urinary incontinence**
      Reflex incontinence
      Total incontinence
N39.8 **Other specified disorders of urinary system**
N39.9 **Disorder of urinary system, unspecified**

Diseases of male genital organs (N40-N53)

✓4th **N40** **Benign prostatic hyperplasia**
   INCLUDES adenofibromatous hypertrophy of prostate
      benign hypertrophy of the prostate
      benign prostatic hypertrophy
      BPH
      enlarged prostate
      nodular prostate
      polyp of prostate
   EXCLUDES 1 benign neoplasms of prostate (adenoma, benign) (fibroadenoma) (fibroma) (myoma) (D29.1)
   EXCLUDES 2 malignant neoplasm of prostate (C61)
   DEF: Enlargement of the prostate gland due to an abnormal proliferation of fibrostromal tissue in the paraurethral glands. This condition causes impingement of the urethra resulting in obstructed urinary flow.

   N40.0 **Benign prostatic hyperplasia without lower urinary tract symptoms**
      Enlarged prostate NOS
      Enlarged prostate without LUTS

   N40.1 **Benign prostatic hyperplasia with lower urinary tract symptoms**
      Enlarged prostate with LUTS
      Use additional code for associated symptoms, when specified:
         incomplete bladder emptying (R39.14)
         nocturia (R35.1)
         straining on urination (R39.16)
         urinary frequency (R35.0)
         urinary hesitancy (R39.11)
         urinary incontinence (N39.4-)
         urinary obstruction (N13.8)
         urinary retention (R33.8)
         urinary urgency (R39.15)
         weak urinary stream (R39.12)
      AHA: 2018,4Q,55

   N40.2 **Nodular prostate without lower urinary tract symptoms**
      Nodular prostate without LUTS

   N40.3 **Nodular prostate with lower urinary tract symptoms**
      Use additional code for associated symptoms, when specified:
         incomplete bladder emptying (R39.14)
         nocturia (R35.1)
         straining on urination (R39.16)
         urinary frequency (R35.0)
         urinary hesitancy (R39.11)
         urinary incontinence (N39.4-)
         urinary obstruction (N13.8)
         urinary retention (R33.8)
         urinary urgency (R39.15)
         weak urinary stream (R39.12)

✓4th **N41** **Inflammatory diseases of prostate**
   Use additional code (B95-B97), to identify infectious agent
   N41.0 **Acute prostatitis**
      AHA: 2024,1Q,16
   N41.1 **Chronic prostatitis**
   N41.2 **Abscess of prostate**
   N41.3 **Prostatocystitis**
      AHA: 2024,1Q,16
   N41.4 **Granulomatous prostatitis**
   N41.8 **Other inflammatory diseases of prostate**
   N41.9 **Inflammatory disease of prostate, unspecified**
      Prostatitis NOS

✓4th **N42** **Other and unspecified disorders of prostate**
   N42.0 **Calculus of prostate**
      Prostatic stone
      DEF: Formation of a small, solid stone often composed of calcium carbonate or calcium phosphate in the prostate gland.

   N42.1 **Congestion and hemorrhage of prostate**
      EXCLUDES 1 enlarged prostate (N40.-)
         hematuria (R31.-)
         hyperplasia of prostate (N40.-)
         inflammatory diseases of prostate (N41.-)

   ✓5th **N42.3** **Dysplasia of prostate**
      AHA: 2016,4Q,44
      N42.30 **Unspecified dysplasia of prostate**
      N42.31 **Prostatic intraepithelial neoplasia**
         PIN
         Prostatic intraepithelial neoplasia I (PIN I)
         Prostatic intraepithelial neoplasia II (PIN II)
         EXCLUDES 1 prostatic intraepithelial neoplasia III (PIN III) (D07.5)
         DEF: Abnormality of shape and size of the intraepithelial tissues of the prostate. It is a premalignant condition characterized by stalks and absence of a basilar cell layer.
      N42.32 **Atypical small acinar proliferation of prostate**
      N42.39 **Other dysplasia of prostate**

   ✓5th **N42.8** **Other specified disorders of prostate**
      N42.81 **Prostatodynia syndrome**
         Painful prostate syndrome
      N42.82 **Prostatosis syndrome**
      N42.83 **Cyst of prostate**
      N42.89 **Other specified disorders of prostate**
   N42.9 **Disorder of prostate, unspecified**

✓4th **N43** **Hydrocele and spermatocele**
   INCLUDES hydrocele of spermatic cord, testis or tunica vaginalis
   EXCLUDES 1 congenital hydrocele (P83.5)
   DEF: Hydrocele: Serous fluid that collects in the tunica vaginalis of the scrotum along the spermatic cord in males.

   N43.0 **Encysted hydrocele**
   N43.1 **Infected hydrocele**
      Use additional code (B95-B97), to identify infectious agent
   N43.2 **Other hydrocele**

Hydrocele

Testicle
Scrotum

Normal | Noncommunicating hydrocele | Communicating hydrocele | Hydrocele of the cord

   N43.3 **Hydrocele, unspecified**
   ✓5th **N43.4** **Spermatocele of epididymis**
      Spermatic cyst
      DEF: Spermatocele: Noncancerous accumulation of fluid and dead sperm cells normally located at the head of the epididymis that exhibits itself as a hard, smooth scrotal mass and do not normally require treatment unless they become enlarged or cause pain.
      N43.40 **Spermatocele of epididymis, unspecified**
      N43.41 **Spermatocele of epididymis, single**
      N43.42 **Spermatocele of epididymis, multiple**

✓4th **N44** **Noninflammatory disorders of testis**
   ✓5th **N44.0** **Torsion of testis**
      N44.00 **Torsion of testis, unspecified**
      N44.01 **Extravaginal torsion of spermatic cord**
         DEF: Torsion of the spermatic cord just below the tunica vaginalis attachments.
      N44.02 **Intravaginal torsion of spermatic cord**
         Torsion of spermatic cord NOS
      N44.03 **Torsion of appendix testis**
      N44.04 **Torsion of appendix epididymis**
   N44.1 **Cyst of tunica albuginea testis**
   N44.2 **Benign cyst of testis**
   N44.8 **Other noninflammatory disorders of the testis**

N45 Orchitis and epididymitis
Use additional code (B95-B97), to identify infectious agent
- **N45.1** Epididymitis
- **N45.2** Orchitis
- **N45.3** Epididymo-orchitis
- **N45.4** Abscess of epididymis or testis

N46 Male infertility
EXCLUDES 1 vasectomy status (Z98.52)

N46.0 Azoospermia
Absolute male infertility
Male infertility due to germinal (cell) aplasia
Male infertility due to spermatogenic arrest (complete)
DEF: Failure of the development of sperm or the absence of sperm in semen.

- **N46.01** Organic azoospermia
  Azoospermia NOS
- **N46.02** Azoospermia due to extratesticular causes
  Code also associated cause
  - **N46.021** Azoospermia due to drug therapy
  - **N46.022** Azoospermia due to infection
  - **N46.023** Azoospermia due to obstruction of efferent ducts
  - **N46.024** Azoospermia due to radiation
  - **N46.025** Azoospermia due to systemic disease
  - **N46.029** Azoospermia due to other extratesticular causes

N46.1 Oligospermia
Male infertility due to germinal cell desquamation
Male infertility due to hypospermatogenesis
Male infertility due to incomplete spermatogenic arrest
DEF: Insufficient production of sperm in semen.

- **N46.11** Organic oligospermia
  Oligospermia NOS
- **N46.12** Oligospermia due to extratesticular causes
  Code also associated cause
  - **N46.121** Oligospermia due to drug therapy
  - **N46.122** Oligospermia due to infection
  - **N46.123** Oligospermia due to obstruction of efferent ducts
  - **N46.124** Oligospermia due to radiation
  - **N46.125** Oligospermia due to systemic disease
  - **N46.129** Oligospermia due to other extratesticular causes

N46.8 Other male infertility
N46.9 Male infertility, unspecified

N47 Disorders of prepuce
- **N47.0** Adherent prepuce, newborn
- **N47.1** Phimosis
  DEF: Condition in which the foreskin is contracted and cannot be drawn back behind the glans penis.
- **N47.2** Paraphimosis
- **N47.3** Deficient foreskin
- **N47.4** Benign cyst of prepuce
- **N47.5** Adhesions of prepuce and glans penis
- **N47.6** Balanoposthitis
  Use additional code (B95-B97), to identify infectious agent
  EXCLUDES 1 balanitis (N48.1)
- **N47.7** Other inflammatory diseases of prepuce
  Use additional code (B95-B97), to identify infectious agent
- **N47.8** Other disorders of prepuce

N48 Other disorders of penis
N48.0 Leukoplakia of penis
Balanitis xerotica obliterans
Kraurosis of penis
Lichen sclerosus of external male genital organs
EXCLUDES 1 carcinoma in situ of penis (D07.4)

N48.1 Balanitis
Use additional code (B95-B97), to identify infectious agent
EXCLUDES 1 amebic balanitis (A06.8)
balanitis xerotica obliterans (N48.0)
candidal balanitis (B37.42)
gonococcal balanitis (A54.23)
herpesviral [herpes simplex] balanitis (A60.01)
DEF: Inflammation of the glans penis, most often affecting uncircumcised males.

N48.2 Other inflammatory disorders of penis
Use additional code (B95-B97), to identify infectious agent
EXCLUDES 1 balanitis (N48.1)
balanitis xerotica obliterans (N48.0)
balanoposthitis (N47.6)
- **N48.21** Abscess of corpus cavernosum and penis
- **N48.22** Cellulitis of corpus cavernosum and penis
- **N48.29** Other inflammatory disorders of penis

N48.3 Priapism
Painful erection
Code first underlying cause
- **N48.30** Priapism, unspecified
- **N48.31** Priapism due to trauma
- **N48.32** Priapism due to disease classified elsewhere
- **N48.33** Priapism, drug-induced
- **N48.39** Other priapism

N48.5 Ulcer of penis
N48.6 Induration penis plastica
Peyronie's disease
Plastic induration of penis

N48.8 Other specified disorders of penis
- **N48.81** Thrombosis of superficial vein of penis
- **N48.82** Acquired torsion of penis
  Acquired torsion of penis NOS
  EXCLUDES 1 congenital torsion of penis (Q55.63)
- **N48.83** Acquired buried penis
  EXCLUDES 1 congenital hidden penis (Q55.64)
- **N48.89** Other specified disorders of penis

N48.9 Disorder of penis, unspecified

N49 Inflammatory disorders of male genital organs, not elsewhere classified
Use additional code (B95-B97), to identify infectious agent
EXCLUDES 1 inflammation of penis (N48.1, N48.2-)
orchitis and epididymitis (N45.-)

- **N49.0** Inflammatory disorders of seminal vesicle
  Vesiculitis NOS
- **N49.1** Inflammatory disorders of spermatic cord, tunica vaginalis and vas deferens
  Vasitis
- **N49.2** Inflammatory disorders of scrotum
- **N49.3** Fournier gangrene
  AHA: 2020,2Q,18
- **N49.8** Inflammatory disorders of other specified male genital organs
  Inflammation of multiple sites in male genital organs
- **N49.9** Inflammatory disorder of unspecified male genital organ
  Abscess of unspecified male genital organ
  Boil of unspecified male genital organ
  Carbuncle of unspecified male genital organ
  Cellulitis of unspecified male genital organ

N50 Other and unspecified disorders of male genital organs
EXCLUDES 2 torsion of testis (N44.0-)

- **N50.0** Atrophy of testis
- **N50.1** Vascular disorders of male genital organs
  Hematocele, NOS, of male genital organs
  Hemorrhage of male genital organs
  Thrombosis of male genital organs
- **N50.3** Cyst of epididymis
- **N50.8** Other specified disorders of male genital organs
  AHA: 2016,4Q,45
  - **N50.81** Testicular pain
    - **N50.811** Right testicular pain
    - **N50.812** Left testicular pain
    - **N50.819** Testicular pain, unspecified
  - **N50.82** Scrotal pain

N50.89 Other specified disorders of the male genital organs
Atrophy of scrotum, seminal vesicle, spermatic cord, tunica vaginalis and vas deferens
Chylocele, tunica vaginalis (nonfilarial) NOS
Edema of scrotum, seminal vesicle, spermatic cord, tunica vaginalis and vas deferens
Hypertrophy of scrotum, seminal vesicle, spermatic cord, tunica vaginalis and vas deferens
Stricture of spermatic cord, tunica vaginalis, and vas deferens
Ulcer of scrotum, seminal vesicle, spermatic cord, testis, tunica vaginalis and vas deferens
Urethroscrotal fistula

N50.9 Disorder of male genital organs, unspecified

N51 Disorders of male genital organs in diseases classified elsewhere
Code first underlying disease, such as:
filariasis (B74.0-B74.9)
EXCLUDES 1: amebic balanitis (A06.8)
candidal balanitis (B37.42)
gonococcal balanitis (A54.23)
gonococcal prostatitis (A54.22)
herpesviral [herpes simplex] balanitis (A60.01)
trichomonal prostatitis (A59.02)
tuberculous prostatitis (A18.14)

N52 Male erectile dysfunction
EXCLUDES 1: psychogenic impotence (F52.21)

- **N52.0** Vasculogenic erectile dysfunction
  - **N52.01** Erectile dysfunction due to arterial insufficiency
  - **N52.02** Corporo-venous occlusive erectile dysfunction
  - **N52.03** Combined arterial insufficiency and corporo-venous occlusive erectile dysfunction
- **N52.1** Erectile dysfunction due to diseases classified elsewhere
  Code first underlying disease
- **N52.2** Drug-induced erectile dysfunction
- **N52.3** Postprocedural erectile dysfunction
  AHA: 2016,4Q,45
  - **N52.31** Erectile dysfunction following radical prostatectomy
  - **N52.32** Erectile dysfunction following radical cystectomy
  - **N52.33** Erectile dysfunction following urethral surgery
  - **N52.34** Erectile dysfunction following simple prostatectomy
  - **N52.35** Erectile dysfunction following radiation therapy
  - **N52.36** Erectile dysfunction following interstitial seed therapy
  - **N52.37** Erectile dysfunction following prostate ablative therapy
    Erectile dysfunction following cryotherapy
    Erectile dysfunction following other prostate ablative therapies
    Erectile dysfunction following ultrasound ablative therapies
  - **N52.39** Other and unspecified postprocedural erectile dysfunction
- **N52.8** Other male erectile dysfunction
- **N52.9** Male erectile dysfunction, unspecified
  Impotence NOS

N53 Other male sexual dysfunction
EXCLUDES 1: psychogenic sexual dysfunction (F52.-)

- **N53.1** Ejaculatory dysfunction
  EXCLUDES 1: premature ejaculation (F52.4)
  - **N53.11** Retarded ejaculation
  - **N53.12** Painful ejaculation
  - **N53.13** Anejaculatory orgasm
  - **N53.14** Retrograde ejaculation
    DEF: Form of male sexual dysfunction in which the semen enters the bladder instead of going out through the urethra during ejaculation.
  - **N53.19** Other ejaculatory dysfunction
    Ejaculatory dysfunction NOS
- **N53.8** Other male sexual dysfunction
- **N53.9** Unspecified male sexual dysfunction

Disorders of breast (N60-N65)

EXCLUDES 1: disorders of breast associated with childbirth (O91-O92)

N60 Benign mammary dysplasia
INCLUDES: fibrocystic mastopathy

- **N60.0** Solitary cyst of breast
  Cyst of breast
  - **N60.01** Solitary cyst of right breast
  - **N60.02** Solitary cyst of left breast
  - **N60.09** Solitary cyst of unspecified breast
- **N60.1** Diffuse cystic mastopathy
  Cystic breast
  Fibrocystic disease of breast
  EXCLUDES 1: diffuse cystic mastopathy with epithelial proliferation (N60.3-)
  - **N60.11** Diffuse cystic mastopathy of right breast
  - **N60.12** Diffuse cystic mastopathy of left breast
  - **N60.19** Diffuse cystic mastopathy of unspecified breast
- **N60.2** Fibroadenosis of breast
  Adenofibrosis of breast
  EXCLUDES 2: fibroadenoma of breast (D24.-)
  - **N60.21** Fibroadenosis of right breast
  - **N60.22** Fibroadenosis of left breast
  - **N60.29** Fibroadenosis of unspecified breast
- **N60.3** Fibrosclerosis of breast
  Cystic mastopathy with epithelial proliferation
  - **N60.31** Fibrosclerosis of right breast
  - **N60.32** Fibrosclerosis of left breast
  - **N60.39** Fibrosclerosis of unspecified breast
- **N60.4** Mammary duct ectasia
  - **N60.41** Mammary duct ectasia of right breast
  - **N60.42** Mammary duct ectasia of left breast
  - **N60.49** Mammary duct ectasia of unspecified breast
- **N60.8** Other benign mammary dysplasias
  - **N60.81** Other benign mammary dysplasias of right breast
  - **N60.82** Other benign mammary dysplasias of left breast
  - **N60.89** Other benign mammary dysplasias of unspecified breast
- **N60.9** Unspecified benign mammary dysplasia
  - **N60.91** Unspecified benign mammary dysplasia of right breast
  - **N60.92** Unspecified benign mammary dysplasia of left breast
  - **N60.99** Unspecified benign mammary dysplasia of unspecified breast

N61 Inflammatory disorders of breast
EXCLUDES 1: inflammatory carcinoma of breast ▶(C50.A-)◀
inflammatory disorder of breast associated with childbirth (O91.-)
neonatal infective mastitis (P39.0)
thrombophlebitis of breast [Mondor's disease] (I80.8)

- **N61.0** Mastitis without abscess
  Cellulitis (acute) (nonpuerperal) (subacute) of breast NOS
  Cellulitis (acute) (nonpuerperal) (subacute) of nipple NOS
  Infective mastitis (acute) (nonpuerperal) (subacute)
  Mastitis (acute) (nonpuerperal) (subacute) NOS
- **N61.1** Abscess of the breast and nipple
  Abscess (acute) (chronic) (nonpuerperal) of areola
  Abscess (acute) (chronic) (nonpuerperal) of breast
  Carbuncle of breast
  Mastitis with abscess
- **N61.2** Granulomatous mastitis
  AHA: 2020,4Q,35
  - **N61.20** Granulomatous mastitis, unspecified breast
  - **N61.21** Granulomatous mastitis, right breast
  - **N61.22** Granulomatous mastitis, left breast
  - **N61.23** Granulomatous mastitis, bilateral breast

N62 Hypertrophy of breast
Gynecomastia
Hypertrophy of breast NOS
Massive pubertal hypertrophy of breast
EXCLUDES 1: breast engorgement of newborn (P83.4)
disproportion of reconstructed breast (N65.1)
AHA: 2023,3Q,22

Chapter 14. Diseases of the Genitourinary System

N63 Unspecified lump in breast
Nodule(s) NOS in breast
AHA: 2022,3Q,8; 2019,4Q,12; 2017,4Q,19

- **N63.0** Unspecified lump in unspecified breast
- **N63.1** Unspecified lump in the right breast
  - **N63.10** Unspecified lump in the right breast, unspecified quadrant
  - **N63.11** Unspecified lump in the right breast, upper outer quadrant
  - **N63.12** Unspecified lump in the right breast, upper inner quadrant
  - **N63.13** Unspecified lump in the right breast, lower outer quadrant
  - **N63.14** Unspecified lump in the right breast, lower inner quadrant
  - **N63.15** Unspecified lump in the right breast, overlapping quadrants
- **N63.2** Unspecified lump in the left breast
  - **N63.20** Unspecified lump in the left breast, unspecified quadrant
  - **N63.21** Unspecified lump in the left breast, upper outer quadrant
  - **N63.22** Unspecified lump in the left breast, upper inner quadrant
  - **N63.23** Unspecified lump in the left breast, lower outer quadrant
  - **N63.24** Unspecified lump in the left breast, lower inner quadrant
  - **N63.25** Unspecified lump in the left breast, overlapping quadrants
- **N63.3** Unspecified lump in axillary tail
  - **N63.31** Unspecified lump in axillary tail of the right breast
  - **N63.32** Unspecified lump in axillary tail of the left breast
- **N63.4** Unspecified lump in breast, subareolar
  - **N63.41** Unspecified lump in right breast, subareolar
  - **N63.42** Unspecified lump in left breast, subareolar

N64 Other disorders of breast
EXCLUDES 2: mechanical complication of breast prosthesis and implant (T85.4-)

- **N64.0** Fissure and fistula of nipple
- **N64.1** Fat necrosis of breast
  - Fat necrosis (segmental) of breast
  - Code first breast necrosis due to breast graft (T85.898)
- **N64.2** Atrophy of breast
- **N64.3** Galactorrhea not associated with childbirth
- **N64.4** Mastodynia
- **N64.5** Other signs and symptoms in breast
  - EXCLUDES 2: abnormal findings on diagnostic imaging of breast (R92.-)
  - **N64.51** Induration of breast
  - **N64.52** Nipple discharge
    - EXCLUDES 1: abnormal findings in nipple discharge (R89.-)
  - **N64.53** Retraction of nipple
  - **N64.59** Other signs and symptoms in breast
- **N64.8** Other specified disorders of breast
  - **N64.81** Ptosis of breast
    - EXCLUDES 1: ptosis of native breast in relation to reconstructed breast (N65.1)
  - **N64.82** Hypoplasia of breast
    - Micromastia
    - EXCLUDES 1: congenital absence of breast (Q83.0)
    - hypoplasia of native breast in relation to reconstructed breast (N65.1)
  - **N64.89** Other specified disorders of breast
    - Galactocele
    - Subinvolution of breast (postlactational)
    - AHA: 2019,1Q,32; 2018,1Q,3
- **N64.9** Disorder of breast, unspecified

N65 Deformity and disproportion of reconstructed breast

- **N65.0** Deformity of reconstructed breast
  - Contour irregularity in reconstructed breast
  - Excess tissue in reconstructed breast
  - Misshapen reconstructed breast
- **N65.1** Disproportion of reconstructed breast
  - Breast asymmetry between native breast and reconstructed breast
  - Disproportion between native breast and reconstructed breast

Inflammatory diseases of female pelvic organs (N70-N77)

EXCLUDES 1: inflammatory diseases of female pelvic organs complicating:
abortion or ectopic or molar pregnancy (O00-O07, O08.0)
pregnancy, childbirth and the puerperium (O23.-, O75.3, O85, O86.-)

N70 Salpingitis and oophoritis
INCLUDES:
- abscess (of) fallopian tube
- abscess (of) ovary
- pyosalpinx
- salpingo-oophoritis
- tubo-ovarian abscess
- tubo-ovarian inflammatory disease

Use additional code (B95-B97), to identify infectious agent
EXCLUDES 1: gonococcal infection (A54.24)
tuberculous infection (A18.17)

- **N70.0** Acute salpingitis and oophoritis
  - **N70.01** Acute salpingitis
  - **N70.02** Acute oophoritis
  - **N70.03** Acute salpingitis and oophoritis
- **N70.1** Chronic salpingitis and oophoritis
  - Hydrosalpinx
  - **N70.11** Chronic salpingitis
  - **N70.12** Chronic oophoritis
  - **N70.13** Chronic salpingitis and oophoritis
- **N70.9** Salpingitis and oophoritis, unspecified
  - **N70.91** Salpingitis, unspecified
  - **N70.92** Oophoritis, unspecified
  - **N70.93** Salpingitis and oophoritis, unspecified

N71 Inflammatory disease of uterus, except cervix
INCLUDES:
- endo (myo) metritis
- metritis
- myometritis
- pyometra
- uterine abscess

Use additional code (B95-B97), to identify infectious agent
EXCLUDES 1: hyperplastic endometritis (N85.0-)
infection of uterus following delivery (O85, O86.-)

- **N71.0** Acute inflammatory disease of uterus
- **N71.1** Chronic inflammatory disease of uterus
- **N71.9** Inflammatory disease of uterus, unspecified

N72 Inflammatory disease of cervix uteri
INCLUDES:
- cervicitis (with or without erosion or ectropion)
- endocervicitis (with or without erosion or ectropion)
- exocervicitis (with or without erosion or ectropion)

Use additional code (B95-B97), to identify infectious agent
EXCLUDES 1: erosion and ectropion of cervix without cervicitis (N86)

N73 Other female pelvic inflammatory diseases
Use additional code (B95-B97), to identify infectious agent

- **N73.0** Acute parametritis and pelvic cellulitis
  - Abscess of broad ligament
  - Abscess of parametrium
  - Pelvic cellulitis, female
  - DEF: Parametritis: Inflammation of the parametrium.
- **N73.1** Chronic parametritis and pelvic cellulitis
  - Any condition in N73.0 specified as chronic
  - EXCLUDES 1: tuberculous parametritis and pelvic cellulitis (A18.17)
- **N73.2** Unspecified parametritis and pelvic cellulitis
  - Any condition in N73.0 unspecified whether acute or chronic
- **N73.3** Female acute pelvic peritonitis
- **N73.4** Female chronic pelvic peritonitis
  - EXCLUDES 1: tuberculous pelvic (female) peritonitis (A18.17)
- **N73.5** Female pelvic peritonitis, unspecified
- **N73.6** Female pelvic peritoneal adhesions (postinfective)
  - EXCLUDES 2: postprocedural pelvic peritoneal adhesions (N99.4)
  - AHA: 2014,1Q,6
- **N73.8** Other specified female pelvic inflammatory diseases
- **N73.9** Female pelvic inflammatory disease, unspecified
  - Female pelvic infection or inflammation NOS

N74 Female pelvic inflammatory disorders in diseases classified elsewhere
Code first underlying disease
EXCLUDES 1: chlamydial cervicitis (A56.02)
chlamydial pelvic inflammatory disease (A56.11)
gonococcal cervicitis (A54.03)
gonococcal pelvic inflammatory disease (A54.24)
herpesviral [herpes simplex] cervicitis (A60.03)
herpesviral [herpes simplex] pelvic inflammatory disease (A60.09)
syphilitic cervicitis (A52.76)
syphilitic pelvic inflammatory disease (A52.76)
trichomonal cervicitis (A59.09)
tuberculous cervicitis (A18.16)
tuberculous pelvic inflammatory disease (A18.17)

N75 Diseases of Bartholin's gland
DEF: Bartholin's gland: Mucous-producing gland found in the vestibular bulbs on either side of the vaginal orifice and connected to the mucosal membrane at the opening by a duct.

N75.0 Cyst of Bartholin's gland
N75.1 Abscess of Bartholin's gland
AHA: 2025,1Q,22
N75.8 Other diseases of Bartholin's gland
Bartholinitis
N75.9 Disease of Bartholin's gland, unspecified

N76 Other inflammation of vagina and vulva
Use additional code (B95-B97), to identify infectious agent
EXCLUDES 2: senile (atrophic) vaginitis (N95.2)
vulvar vestibulitis (N94.810)

N76.0 Acute vaginitis
Acute vulvovaginitis
Vaginitis NOS
Vulvovaginitis NOS
N76.1 Subacute and chronic vaginitis
Chronic vulvovaginitis
Subacute vulvovaginitis
N76.2 Acute vulvitis
Vulvitis NOS
N76.3 Subacute and chronic vulvitis
N76.4 Abscess of vulva
Furuncle of vulva
N76.5 Ulceration of vagina
N76.6 Ulceration of vulva
N76.8 Other specified inflammation of vagina and vulva
N76.81 Mucositis (ulcerative) of vagina and vulva
Code also type of associated therapy, such as:
antineoplastic and immunosuppressive drugs (T45.1X-)
radiological procedure and radiotherapy (Y84.2)
EXCLUDES 2: gastrointestinal mucositis (ulcerative) (K92.81)
nasal mucositis (ulcerative) (J34.81)
oral mucositis (ulcerative) (K12.3-)
N76.82 Fournier disease of vagina and vulva HCC ESR COM
Fournier gangrene of vagina and vulva
Code also, if applicable, diabetes mellitus (E08-E13 with .9)
EXCLUDES 1: gangrene in diabetes mellitus (E08-E13 with .52)
AHA: 2022,4Q,34
N76.89 Other specified inflammation of vagina and vulva

N77 Vulvovaginal ulceration and inflammation in diseases classified elsewhere
N77.0 Ulceration of vulva in diseases classified elsewhere
Code first underlying disease, such as:
Behcet's disease (M35.2)
EXCLUDES 1: ulceration of vulva in gonococcal infection (A54.02)
ulceration of vulva in herpesviral [herpes simplex] infection (A60.04)
ulceration of vulva in syphilis (A51.0)
ulceration of vulva in tuberculosis (A18.18)

N77.1 Vaginitis, vulvitis and vulvovaginitis in diseases classified elsewhere
Code first underlying disease, such as:
pinworm (B80)
EXCLUDES 1: candidal vulvovaginitis (B37.3-)
chlamydial vulvovaginitis (A56.02)
gonococcal vulvovaginitis (A54.02)
herpesviral [herpes simplex] vulvovaginitis (A60.04)
trichomonal vulvovaginitis (A59.01)
tuberculous vulvovaginitis (A18.18)
vulvovaginitis in early syphilis (A51.0)
vulvovaginitis in late syphilis (A52.76)

Noninflammatory disorders of female genital tract (N80-N98)

N80 Endometriosis
AHA: 2022,4Q,34-36
DEF: Aberrant uterine mucosal tissue appearing in areas of the pelvic cavity outside of its normal location, lining the uterus, and inflaming surrounding tissues often resulting in infertility or spontaneous abortion.

N80.0 Endometriosis of uterus
Endometriosis of the cervix
EXCLUDES 1: stromal endometriosis (D39.0)
N80.00 Endometriosis of the uterus, unspecified
N80.01 Superficial endometriosis of the uterus
N80.02 Deep endometriosis of the uterus
Deep retrocervical endometriosis
N80.03 Adenomyosis of the uterus
Adenomyosis NOS

N80.1 Endometriosis of ovary
N80.10 Endometriosis of ovary, unspecified depth
N80.101 Endometriosis of right ovary, unspecified depth
N80.102 Endometriosis of left ovary, unspecified depth
N80.103 Endometriosis of bilateral ovaries, unspecified depth
N80.109 Endometriosis of ovary, unspecified side, unspecified depth
Endometriosis of ovary NOS
N80.11 Superficial endometriosis of the ovary
N80.111 Superficial endometriosis of right ovary
AHA: 2022,4Q,35
N80.112 Superficial endometriosis of left ovary
N80.113 Superficial endometriosis of bilateral ovaries
N80.119 Superficial endometriosis of ovary, unspecified ovary
N80.12 Deep endometriosis of ovary
Deep ovarian endometriosis
Endometrioma
N80.121 Deep endometriosis of right ovary
N80.122 Deep endometriosis of left ovary
N80.123 Deep endometriosis of bilateral ovaries
N80.129 Deep endometriosis of ovary, unspecified ovary

N80.2 Endometriosis of fallopian tube
N80.20 Endometriosis of fallopian tube, unspecified depth
N80.201 Endometriosis of right fallopian tube, unspecified depth
N80.202 Endometriosis of left fallopian tube, unspecified depth
N80.203 Endometriosis of bilateral fallopian tubes, unspecified depth
N80.209 Endometriosis of unspecified fallopian tube, unspecified depth
Endometriosis fallopian tube NOS
N80.21 Superficial endometriosis of fallopian tube
N80.211 Superficial endometriosis of right fallopian tube
N80.212 Superficial endometriosis of left fallopian tube
N80.213 Superficial endometriosis of bilateral fallopian tubes
N80.219 Superficial endometriosis of unspecified fallopian tube
N80.22 Deep endometriosis of the fallopian tube
Deep endometriosis involving muscular wall of fallopian tube
N80.221 Deep endometriosis of right fallopian tube

- **N80.222** Deep endometriosis of left fallopian tube
- **N80.223** Deep endometriosis of bilateral fallopian tubes
- **N80.229** Deep endometriosis of unspecified fallopian tube

N80.3 Endometriosis of pelvic peritoneum

- **N80.30** Endometriosis of pelvic peritoneum, unspecified
  - Endometriosis of the retroperitoneum NOS
- **N80.31** Endometriosis of the anterior cul-de-sac
  - **N80.311** Superficial endometriosis of the anterior cul-de-sac
  - **N80.312** Deep endometriosis of the anterior cul-de-sac
  - **N80.319** Endometriosis of the anterior cul-de-sac, unspecified depth
    - Endometriosis of the anterior cul-de-sac NOS
- **N80.32** Endometriosis of the posterior cul-de-sac
  - **N80.321** Superficial endometriosis of the posterior cul-de-sac
  - **N80.322** Deep endometriosis of the posterior cul-de-sac
  - **N80.329** Endometriosis of the posterior cul-de-sac, unspecified depth
    - Endometriosis of the posterior cul-de-sac NOS
- **N80.33** Superficial endometriosis of the pelvic sidewall
  - **N80.331** Superficial endometriosis of the right pelvic sidewall
  - **N80.332** Superficial endometriosis of the left pelvic sidewall
  - **N80.333** Superficial endometriosis of bilateral pelvic sidewall
  - **N80.339** Superficial endometriosis of pelvic sidewall, unspecified side
- **N80.34** Deep endometriosis of the pelvic sidewall
  - **N80.341** Deep endometriosis of the right pelvic sidewall
  - **N80.342** Deep endometriosis of the left pelvic sidewall
  - **N80.343** Deep endometriosis of the bilateral pelvic sidewall
  - **N80.349** Deep endometriosis of the pelvic sidewall, unspecified side
    - AHA: 2022,4Q,36
- **N80.35** Endometriosis of the pelvic sidewall, unspecified depth
  - **N80.351** Endometriosis of the right pelvic sidewall, unspecified depth
  - **N80.352** Endometriosis of the left pelvic sidewall, unspecified depth
  - **N80.353** Endometriosis of bilateral pelvic sidewall, unspecified depth
  - **N80.359** Endometriosis of pelvic sidewall, unspecified side, unspecified depth
    - Endometriosis of the pelvic sidewall NOS
- **N80.36** Superficial endometriosis of the pelvic brim
  - **N80.361** Superficial endometriosis of the right pelvic brim
  - **N80.362** Superficial endometriosis of the left pelvic brim
  - **N80.363** Superficial endometriosis of bilateral pelvic brim
  - **N80.369** Superficial endometriosis of the pelvic brim, unspecified side
- **N80.37** Deep endometriosis of the pelvic brim
  - **N80.371** Deep endometriosis of the right pelvic brim
  - **N80.372** Deep endometriosis of the left pelvic brim
  - **N80.373** Deep endometriosis of bilateral pelvic brim
  - **N80.379** Deep endometriosis of the pelvic brim, unspecified side
- **N80.38** Endometriosis of the pelvic brim, unspecified depth
  - **N80.381** Endometriosis of the right pelvic brim, unspecified depth
  - **N80.382** Endometriosis of the left pelvic brim, unspecified depth
  - **N80.383** Endometriosis of bilateral pelvic brim, unspecified depth
  - **N80.389** Endometriosis of the pelvic brim, unspecified side, unspecified depth
    - Endometriosis of the pelvic brim NOS
- **N80.3A** Superficial endometriosis of the uterosacral ligament(s)
  - **N80.3A1** Superficial endometriosis of the right uterosacral ligament
  - **N80.3A2** Superficial endometriosis of the left uterosacral ligament
  - **N80.3A3** Superficial endometriosis of the bilateral uterosacral ligament(s)
  - **N80.3A9** Superficial endometriosis of the uterosacral ligament(s), unspecified side
- **N80.3B** Deep endometriosis of the uterosacral ligament(s)
  - **N80.3B1** Deep endometriosis of the right uterosacral ligament
  - **N80.3B2** Deep endometriosis of the left uterosacral ligament
  - **N80.3B3** Deep endometriosis of bilateral uterosacral ligament(s)
  - **N80.3B9** Deep endometriosis of the uterosacral ligament(s), unspecified side
- **N80.3C** Endometriosis of the uterosacral ligament(s), unspecified depth
  - **N80.3C1** Endometriosis of the right uterosacral ligament, unspecified depth
  - **N80.3C2** Endometriosis of the left uterosacral ligament, unspecified depth
  - **N80.3C3** Endometriosis of bilateral uterosacral ligament(s), unspecified depth
  - **N80.3C9** Endometriosis of the uterosacral ligament(s), unspecified side, unspecified depth
    - Endometriosis of the uterosacral ligament(s) NOS
- **N80.39** Endometriosis of other pelvic peritoneum
  - **N80.391** Superficial endometriosis of the pelvic peritoneum, other specified sites
  - **N80.392** Deep endometriosis of the pelvic peritoneum, other specified sites
  - **N80.399** Endometriosis of the pelvic peritoneum, other specified sites, unspecified depth

N80.4 Endometriosis of rectovaginal septum and vagina

- **N80.40** Endometriosis of rectovaginal septum, unspecified involvement of vagina
  - Endometriosis of the rectovaginal septum, NOS
- **N80.41** Endometriosis of rectovaginal septum without involvement of vagina
- **N80.42** Endometriosis of rectovaginal septum with involvement of vagina

N80.5 Endometriosis of intestine

- **N80.50** Endometriosis of intestine, unspecified
- **N80.51** Endometriosis of the rectum
  - **N80.511** Superficial endometriosis of the rectum
  - **N80.512** Deep endometriosis of the rectum
    - Deep endometriosis of the rectum, multifocal
  - **N80.519** Endometriosis of the rectum, unspecified depth
    - Endometriosis of the rectum NOS
- **N80.52** Endometriosis of the sigmoid colon
  - **N80.521** Superficial endometriosis of the sigmoid colon
  - **N80.522** Deep endometriosis of the sigmoid colon
  - **N80.529** Endometriosis of the sigmoid colon, unspecified depth
    - Endometriosis of the sigmoid colon NOS
- **N80.53** Endometriosis of the cecum
  - **N80.531** Superficial endometriosis of the cecum
  - **N80.532** Deep endometriosis of the cecum
  - **N80.539** Endometriosis of the cecum, unspecified depth
    - Endometriosis of the cecum NOS
- **N80.54** Endometriosis of the appendix
  - **N80.541** Superficial endometriosis of the appendix
  - **N80.542** Deep endometriosis of the appendix
  - **N80.549** Endometriosis of the appendix, unspecified depth
    - Endometriosis of the appendix NOS

Chapter 14. Diseases of the Genitourinary System

N80.55 **Endometriosis of other parts of the colon**
  Endometriosis of descending colon
  Endometriosis of transverse colon
  N80.551 Superficial endometriosis of other parts of the colon
  N80.552 Deep endometriosis of other parts of the colon
  N80.559 Endometriosis of other parts of the colon, unspecified depth
    Endometriosis of colon NOS
N80.56 **Endometriosis of the small intestine**
  N80.561 Superficial endometriosis of the small intestine
  N80.562 Deep endometriosis of the small intestine
    Deep endometriosis of the small intestine, multifocal
  N80.569 Endometriosis of the small intestine, unspecified depth
    Endometriosis of the small intestine NOS
N80.6 Endometriosis in cutaneous scar
N80.A Endometriosis of bladder and ureters
  N80.A0 Endometriosis of bladder, unspecified depth
    Endometriosis of bladder NOS
  N80.A1 Superficial endometriosis of bladder
  N80.A2 Deep endometriosis of bladder
  N80.A4 Superficial endometriosis of ureter
    Extrinsic endometriosis of ureter
    Code also, if applicable, obstructive and reflux uropathy (N13.-)
    N80.A41 Superficial endometriosis of right ureter
    N80.A42 Superficial endometriosis of left ureter
    N80.A43 Superficial endometriosis of bilateral ureters
    N80.A49 Superficial endometriosis of unspecified ureter
  N80.A5 Deep endometriosis of ureter
    Intrinsic endometriosis of ureter
    Code also, if applicable, obstructive and reflux uropathy (N13.-)
    N80.A51 Deep endometriosis of right ureter
    N80.A52 Deep endometriosis of left ureter
    N80.A53 Deep endometriosis of bilateral ureters
    N80.A59 Deep endometriosis of unspecified ureter
  N80.A6 Endometriosis of ureter, unspecified depth
    Code also, if applicable, obstructive and reflux uropathy (N13.-)
    N80.A61 Endometriosis of right ureter, unspecified depth
    N80.A62 Endometriosis of left ureter, unspecified depth
    N80.A63 Endometriosis of bilateral ureters, unspecified depth
    N80.A69 Endometriosis of unspecified ureter, unspecified depth
N80.B Endometriosis of cardiothoracic space
  Endometriosis of thorax
  Code also, if applicable:
    catamenial hemothorax (J94.2)
    catamenial pneumothorax (J93.12)
  N80.B1 Endometriosis of pleura
  N80.B2 Endometriosis of lung
  N80.B3 Endometriosis of diaphragm
    N80.B31 Superficial endometriosis of diaphragm
    N80.B32 Deep endometriosis of diaphragm
    N80.B39 Endometriosis of diaphragm, unspecified depth
      Endometriosis of the diaphragm NOS
  N80.B4 Endometriosis of the pericardial space
  N80.B5 Endometriosis of the mediastinal space
  N80.B6 Endometriosis of cardiothoracic space
N80.C Endometriosis of the abdomen
  N80.C0 Endometriosis of the abdomen, unspecified
    Endometriosis of the abdomen NOS
  N80.C1 Endometriosis of the anterior abdominal wall
    N80.C10 Endometriosis of the anterior abdominal wall, subcutaneous tissue
    N80.C11 Endometriosis of the anterior abdominal wall, fascia and muscular layers
    N80.C19 Endometriosis of the anterior abdominal wall, unspecified depth
      Endometriosis of the anterior abdominal wall NOS
  N80.C2 Endometriosis of the umbilicus
  N80.C3 Endometriosis of the inguinal canal
  N80.C4 Endometriosis of extra-pelvic abdominal peritoneum
  N80.C9 Endometriosis of other site of abdomen
N80.D Endometriosis of the pelvic nerves
  Endometriosis of the nerves of the retroperitoneum
  N80.D0 Endometriosis of the pelvic nerves, unspecified
    Endometriosis of nerve of the retroperitoneum, NOS
  N80.D1 Endometriosis of the sacral splanchnic nerves
    Endometriosis of the pelvic splanchnic nerves
  N80.D2 Endometriosis of the sacral nerve roots
  N80.D3 Endometriosis of the obturator nerve
  N80.D4 Endometriosis of the sciatic nerve
  N80.D5 Endometriosis of the pudendal nerve
  N80.D6 Endometriosis of the femoral nerve
  N80.D9 Endometriosis of other pelvic nerve
    Endometriosis of the other nerves of the retroperitoneum
N80.8 Other endometriosis
  Endometriosis of other site
N80.9 Endometriosis, unspecified
N81 **Female genital prolapse**
  EXCLUDES 1 genital prolapse complicating pregnancy, labor or delivery (O34.5-)
    prolapse and hernia of ovary and fallopian tube (N83.4-)
    prolapse of vaginal vault after hysterectomy (N99.3)

Types of Pelvic Organ Prolapse

Urethrocele — Bladder, Uterus, Rectum, Urethra, Vaginal canal, Urethrocele
Cystocele — Bladder, Uterus, Rectum, Urethra, Vaginal canal, Cystocele
Rectocele — Bladder, Uterus, Rectum, Urethra, Vaginal canal, Rectocele
Enterocele — Bladder, Uterus, Enterocele, Urethra, Vaginal canal, Terminal ileum

  N81.0 Urethrocele
    EXCLUDES 1 urethrocele with cystocele (N81.1-)
      urethrocele with prolapse of uterus (N81.2-N81.4)
  N81.1 Cystocele
    Cystocele with urethrocele
    Cystourethrocele
    EXCLUDES 1 cystocele with prolapse of uterus (N81.2-N81.4)
    N81.10 Cystocele, unspecified
      Prolapse of (anterior) vaginal wall NOS
    N81.11 Cystocele, midline
    N81.12 Cystocele, lateral
      Paravaginal cystocele
      DEF: Detachment of the lateral support connections of the vagina at the arcus tendineus fasciae pelvis (ATFP) that results in bladder drop. The bladder herniates into the vagina laterally.
  N81.2 Incomplete uterovaginal prolapse
    First degree uterine prolapse
    Prolapse of cervix NOS
    Second degree uterine prolapse
    EXCLUDES 1 cervical stump prolapse (N81.85)
  N81.3 Complete uterovaginal prolapse
    Procidentia (uteri) NOS
    Third degree uterine prolapse

N81.4 Uterovaginal prolapse, unspecified
  Prolapse of uterus NOS
N81.5 Vaginal enterocele
  EXCLUDES 1: enterocele with prolapse of uterus (N81.2-N81.4)
N81.6 Rectocele
  Prolapse of posterior vaginal wall
  Use additional code for any associated fecal incontinence, if applicable (R15.-)
  EXCLUDES 1: rectocele with prolapse of uterus (N81.2-N81.4)
  EXCLUDES 2: perineocele (N81.81)
  rectal prolapse (K62.3)
N81.8 Other female genital prolapse
  N81.81 Perineocele
  N81.82 Incompetence or weakening of pubocervical tissue
  N81.83 Incompetence or weakening of rectovaginal tissue
  N81.84 Pelvic muscle wasting
    Disuse atrophy of pelvic muscles and anal sphincter
  N81.85 Cervical stump prolapse
  N81.89 Other female genital prolapse
    Deficient perineum
    Old laceration of muscles of pelvic floor
N81.9 Female genital prolapse, unspecified

N82 Fistulae involving female genital tract
  EXCLUDES 1: vesicointestinal fistulae (N32.1)
  N82.0 Vesicovaginal fistula
  N82.1 Other female urinary-genital tract fistulae
    Cervicovesical fistula
    Ureterovaginal fistula
    Urethrovaginal fistula
    Uteroureteric fistula
    Uterovesical fistula
    AHA: 2017,3Q,3
  N82.2 Fistula of vagina to small intestine
  N82.3 Fistula of vagina to large intestine
    Rectovaginal fistula
  N82.4 Other female intestinal-genital tract fistulae
    Intestinouterine fistula
  N82.5 Female genital tract-skin fistulae
    Uterus to abdominal wall fistula
    Vaginoperineal fistula
  N82.8 Other female genital tract fistulae
  N82.9 Female genital tract fistula, unspecified

N83 Noninflammatory disorders of ovary, fallopian tube and broad ligament
  EXCLUDES 2: hydrosalpinx (N70.1-)
  AHA: 2016,4Q,46
  N83.0 Follicular cyst of ovary
    Cyst of graafian follicle
    Hemorrhagic follicular cyst (of ovary)
    N83.00 Follicular cyst of ovary, unspecified side
    N83.01 Follicular cyst of right ovary
    N83.02 Follicular cyst of left ovary
  N83.1 Corpus luteum cyst
    Hemorrhagic corpus luteum cyst
    AHA: 2022,1Q,23
    N83.10 Corpus luteum cyst of ovary, unspecified side
    N83.11 Corpus luteum cyst of right ovary
    N83.12 Corpus luteum cyst of left ovary
  N83.2 Other and unspecified ovarian cysts
    EXCLUDES 1: developmental ovarian cyst (Q50.1)
      neoplastic ovarian cyst (D27.-)
      polycystic ovarian syndrome (E28.2)
      Stein-Leventhal syndrome (E28.2)
    AHA: 2022,1Q,23
    N83.20 Unspecified ovarian cysts
      N83.201 Unspecified ovarian cyst, right side
      N83.202 Unspecified ovarian cyst, left side
      N83.209 Unspecified ovarian cyst, unspecified side
        Ovarian cyst, NOS
    N83.29 Other ovarian cysts
      Retention cyst of ovary
      Simple cyst of ovary
      N83.291 Other ovarian cyst, right side
      N83.292 Other ovarian cyst, left side
      N83.299 Other ovarian cyst, unspecified side
  N83.3 Acquired atrophy of ovary and fallopian tube
    N83.31 Acquired atrophy of ovary
      N83.311 Acquired atrophy of right ovary
      N83.312 Acquired atrophy of left ovary
      N83.319 Acquired atrophy of ovary, unspecified side
        Acquired atrophy of ovary, NOS
    N83.32 Acquired atrophy of fallopian tube
      N83.321 Acquired atrophy of right fallopian tube
      N83.322 Acquired atrophy of left fallopian tube
      N83.329 Acquired atrophy of fallopian tube, unspecified side
        Acquired atrophy of fallopian tube, NOS
    N83.33 Acquired atrophy of ovary and fallopian tube
      N83.331 Acquired atrophy of right ovary and fallopian tube
      N83.332 Acquired atrophy of left ovary and fallopian tube
      N83.339 Acquired atrophy of ovary and fallopian tube, unspecified side
        Acquired atrophy of ovary and fallopian tube, NOS
  N83.4 Prolapse and hernia of ovary and fallopian tube
    N83.40 Prolapse and hernia of ovary and fallopian tube, unspecified side
      Prolapse and hernia of ovary and fallopian tube, NOS
    N83.41 Prolapse and hernia of right ovary and fallopian tube
    N83.42 Prolapse and hernia of left ovary and fallopian tube
  N83.5 Torsion of ovary, ovarian pedicle and fallopian tube
    Torsion of accessory tube
    N83.51 Torsion of ovary and ovarian pedicle
      N83.511 Torsion of right ovary and ovarian pedicle
      N83.512 Torsion of left ovary and ovarian pedicle
      N83.519 Torsion of ovary and ovarian pedicle, unspecified side
        Torsion of ovary and ovarian pedicle, NOS
    N83.52 Torsion of fallopian tube
      Torsion of hydatid of Morgagni
      N83.521 Torsion of right fallopian tube
      N83.522 Torsion of left fallopian tube
      N83.529 Torsion of fallopian tube, unspecified side
        Torsion of fallopian tube, NOS
    N83.53 Torsion of ovary, ovarian pedicle and fallopian tube
  N83.6 Hematosalpinx
    EXCLUDES 1: hematosalpinx (with) (in):
      hematocolpos (N89.7)
      hematometra (N85.7)
      tubal pregnancy (O00.1-)
  N83.7 Hematoma of broad ligament
  N83.8 Other noninflammatory disorders of ovary, fallopian tube and broad ligament
    Broad ligament laceration syndrome [Allen-Masters]
  N83.9 Noninflammatory disorder of ovary, fallopian tube and broad ligament, unspecified

N84 Polyp of female genital tract
  EXCLUDES 1: adenomatous polyp (D28.-)
    placental polyp (O90.89)
  N84.0 Polyp of corpus uteri
    Polyp of endometrium
    Polyp of uterus NOS
    EXCLUDES 1: polypoid endometrial hyperplasia (N85.0-)
  N84.1 Polyp of cervix uteri
    Mucous polyp of cervix
  N84.2 Polyp of vagina
  N84.3 Polyp of vulva
    Polyp of labia
  N84.8 Polyp of other parts of female genital tract
  N84.9 Polyp of female genital tract, unspecified

Chapter 14. Diseases of the Genitourinary System

N85 Other noninflammatory disorders of uterus, except cervix
  EXCLUDES 1
    endometriosis (N80.-)
    inflammatory diseases of uterus (N71.-)
    noninflammatory disorders of cervix, except malposition (N86-N88)
    polyp of corpus uteri (N84.0)
    uterine prolapse (N81.-)

  N85.0 Endometrial hyperplasia
    N85.00 Endometrial hyperplasia, unspecified
      Hyperplasia (adenomatous) (cystic) (glandular) of endometrium
      Hyperplastic endometritis
    N85.01 Benign endometrial hyperplasia
      Endometrial hyperplasia (complex) (simple) without atypia
    N85.02 Endometrial intraepithelial neoplasia [EIN]
      Endometrial hyperplasia with atypia
      EXCLUDES 1 malignant neoplasm of endometrium (with endometrial intraepithelial neoplasia [EIN]) (C54.1)

  N85.2 Hypertrophy of uterus
    Bulky or enlarged uterus
    EXCLUDES 1 puerperal hypertrophy of uterus (O90.89)

  N85.3 Subinvolution of uterus
    EXCLUDES 1 puerperal subinvolution of uterus (O90.89)

  N85.4 Malposition of uterus
    Anteversion of uterus
    Retroflexion of uterus
    Retroversion of uterus
    EXCLUDES 1 malposition of uterus complicating pregnancy, labor or delivery (O34.5-, O65.5)

  N85.5 Inversion of uterus
    EXCLUDES 1 current obstetric trauma (O71.2)
      postpartum inversion of uterus (O71.2)
    DEF: Abnormality in which the uterus turns inside out.

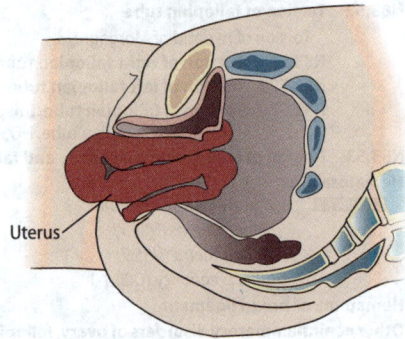

Inversion of Uterus

  N85.6 Intrauterine synechiae
  N85.7 Hematometra
    Hematosalpinx with hematometra
    EXCLUDES 1 hematometra with hematocolpos (N89.7)
    DEF: Accumulation of blood within the uterus.
  N85.8 Other specified noninflammatory disorders of uterus
    Atrophy of uterus, acquired
    Fibrosis of uterus NOS
  N85.9 Noninflammatory disorder of uterus, unspecified
    Disorder of uterus NOS
  N85.A Isthmocele
    Isthmocele (non-pregnant state)
    Code also any associated conditions such as:
      abnormal uterine and vaginal bleeding, unspecified (N93.9)
      female infertility of uterine origin (N97.2)
      pelvic and perineal pain ▶(R10.2-)◀
    EXCLUDES 1 maternal care for cesarean scar defect (isthmocele) (O34.22)
    AHA: 2022,4Q,36-37

N86 Erosion and ectropion of cervix uteri
  Decubitus (trophic) ulcer of cervix
  Eversion of cervix
  EXCLUDES 1 erosion and ectropion of cervix with cervicitis (N72)

N87 Dysplasia of cervix uteri
  EXCLUDES 1
    abnormal results from cervical cytologic examination without histologic confirmation (R87.61-)
    carcinoma in situ of cervix uteri (D06.-)
    cervical intraepithelial neoplasia III [CIN III] (D06.-)
    HGSIL of cervix (R87.613)
    severe dysplasia of cervix uteri (D06.-)

  N87.0 Mild cervical dysplasia
    Cervical intraepithelial neoplasia I [CIN I]
  N87.1 Moderate cervical dysplasia
    Cervical intraepithelial neoplasia II [CIN II]
  N87.9 Dysplasia of cervix uteri, unspecified
    Anaplasia of cervix
    Cervical atypism
    Cervical dysplasia NOS

N88 Other noninflammatory disorders of cervix uteri
  EXCLUDES 2 inflammatory disease of cervix (N72)
    polyp of cervix (N84.1)

  N88.0 Leukoplakia of cervix uteri
  N88.1 Old laceration of cervix uteri
    Adhesions of cervix
    EXCLUDES 1 current obstetric trauma (O71.3)
  N88.2 Stricture and stenosis of cervix uteri
    EXCLUDES 1 stricture and stenosis of cervix uteri complicating labor (O65.5)
  N88.3 Incompetence of cervix uteri
    Investigation and management of (suspected) cervical incompetence in a nonpregnant woman
    EXCLUDES 1 cervical incompetence complicating pregnancy (O34.3-)
    DEF: Inadequate functioning of the cervix marked by abnormal widening during pregnancy and causing premature birth or miscarriage.
  N88.4 Hypertrophic elongation of cervix uteri
  N88.8 Other specified noninflammatory disorders of cervix uteri
    EXCLUDES 1 current obstetric trauma (O71.3)
  N88.9 Noninflammatory disorder of cervix uteri, unspecified

N89 Other noninflammatory disorders of vagina
  EXCLUDES 1
    abnormal results from vaginal cytologic examination without histologic confirmation (R87.62-)
    carcinoma in situ of vagina (D07.2)
    HGSIL of vagina (R87.623)
    inflammation of vagina (N76.-)
    senile (atrophic) vaginitis (N95.2)
    severe dysplasia of vagina (D07.2)
    trichomonal leukorrhea (A59.00)
    vaginal intraepithelial neoplasia [VAIN], grade III (D07.2)

  N89.0 Mild vaginal dysplasia
    Vaginal intraepithelial neoplasia [VAIN], grade I
  N89.1 Moderate vaginal dysplasia
    Vaginal intraepithelial neoplasia [VAIN], grade II
  N89.3 Dysplasia of vagina, unspecified
  N89.4 Leukoplakia of vagina
  N89.5 Stricture and atresia of vagina
    Vaginal adhesions
    Vaginal stenosis
    EXCLUDES 1 congenital atresia or stricture (Q52.4)
      postprocedural adhesions of vagina (N99.2)
  N89.6 Tight hymenal ring
    Rigid hymen
    Tight introitus
    EXCLUDES 1 imperforate hymen (Q52.3)
  N89.7 Hematocolpos
    Hematocolpos with hematometra or hematosalpinx
    AHA: 2016,4Q,58
  N89.8 Other specified noninflammatory disorders of vagina
    Leukorrhea NOS
    Old vaginal laceration
    Pessary ulcer of vagina
    EXCLUDES 1 current obstetric trauma (O70.-, O71.4, O71.7-O71.8)
      old laceration involving muscles of pelvic floor (N81.8)
  N89.9 Noninflammatory disorder of vagina, unspecified

N90 Other noninflammatory disorders of vulva and perineum

EXCLUDES 1
- anogenital (venereal) warts (A63.0)
- carcinoma in situ of vulva (D07.1)
- condyloma acuminatum (A63.0)
- current obstetric trauma (O70.-, O71.7-O71.8)
- inflammation of vulva (N76.-)
- severe dysplasia of vulva (D07.1)
- vulvar intraepithelial neoplasm III [VIN III] (D07.1)

N90.0 Mild vulvar dysplasia
Vulvar intraepithelial neoplasia [VIN], grade I

N90.1 Moderate vulvar dysplasia
Vulvar intraepithelial neoplasia [VIN], grade II

N90.3 Dysplasia of vulva, unspecified

N90.4 Leukoplakia of vulva
- Dystrophy of vulva
- Kraurosis of vulva
- Lichen sclerosus of external female genital organs

N90.5 Atrophy of vulva
Stenosis of vulva

N90.6 Hypertrophy of vulva
AHA: 2016,4Q,46

- **N90.60** Unspecified hypertrophy of vulva
  Unspecified hypertrophy of labia
- **N90.61** Childhood asymmetric labium majus enlargement
  CALME
- **N90.69** Other specified hypertrophy of vulva
  Other specified hypertrophy of labia

N90.7 Vulvar cyst

N90.8 Other specified noninflammatory disorders of vulva and perineum

- **N90.81** Female genital mutilation status
  Female genital cutting status
  - **N90.810** Female genital mutilation status, unspecified
    - Female genital cutting status, unspecified
    - Female genital mutilation status NOS
  - **N90.811** Female genital mutilation Type I status
    - Clitorectomy status
    - Female genital cutting Type I status
  - **N90.812** Female genital mutilation Type II status
    - Clitorectomy with excision of labia minora status
    - Female genital cutting Type II status
  - **N90.813** Female genital mutilation Type III status
    - Female genital cutting Type III status
    - Infibulation status
  - **N90.818** Other female genital mutilation status
    - Female genital cutting Type IV status
    - Female genital mutilation Type IV status
    - Other female genital cutting status
- **N90.89** Other specified noninflammatory disorders of vulva and perineum
  - Adhesions of vulva
  - Hypertrophy of clitoris

N90.9 Noninflammatory disorder of vulva and perineum, unspecified

N91 Absent, scanty and rare menstruation

EXCLUDES 1 ovarian dysfunction (E28.-)

N91.0 Primary amenorrhea
N91.1 Secondary amenorrhea
N91.2 Amenorrhea, unspecified
N91.3 Primary oligomenorrhea
N91.4 Secondary oligomenorrhea
N91.5 Oligomenorrhea, unspecified
Hypomenorrhea NOS

N92 Excessive, frequent and irregular menstruation

EXCLUDES 1
- postmenopausal bleeding (N95.0)
- precocious puberty (menstruation) (E30.1)

N92.0 Excessive and frequent menstruation with regular cycle
- Heavy periods NOS
- Menorrhagia NOS
- Polymenorrhea

N92.1 Excessive and frequent menstruation with irregular cycle
- Irregular intermenstrual bleeding
- Irregular, shortened intervals between menstrual bleeding
- Menometrorrhagia
- Metrorrhagia

N92.2 Excessive menstruation at puberty
- Excessive bleeding associated with onset of menstrual periods
- Pubertal menorrhagia
- Puberty bleeding

N92.3 Ovulation bleeding
Regular intermenstrual bleeding

N92.4 Excessive bleeding in the premenopausal period
- Climacteric menorrhagia or metrorrhagia
- Menopausal menorrhagia or metrorrhagia
- Perimenopausal bleeding
- Perimenopausal menorrhagia or metrorrhagia
- Preclimacteric menorrhagia or metrorrhagia
- Premenopausal menorrhagia or metrorrhagia

N92.5 Other specified irregular menstruation

N92.6 Irregular menstruation, unspecified
- Irregular bleeding NOS
- Irregular periods NOS

EXCLUDES 1 irregular menstruation with:
- lengthened intervals or scanty bleeding (N91.3-N91.5)
- shortened intervals or excessive bleeding (N92.1)

N93 Other abnormal uterine and vaginal bleeding

EXCLUDES 1
- neonatal vaginal hemorrhage (P54.6)
- precocious puberty (menstruation) (E30.1)
- pseudomenses (P54.6)

N93.0 Postcoital and contact bleeding
N93.1 Pre-pubertal vaginal bleeding
AHA: 2016,4Q,47

N93.8 Other specified abnormal uterine and vaginal bleeding
Dysfunctional or functional uterine or vaginal bleeding NOS

N93.9 Abnormal uterine and vaginal bleeding, unspecified

N94 Pain and other conditions associated with female genital organs and menstrual cycle

N94.0 Mittelschmerz
DEF: One-sided, lower abdominal pain occurring between menstrual periods that is associated with ovulation.

N94.1 Dyspareunia
EXCLUDES 1 psychogenic dyspareunia (F52.6)
AHA: 2016,4Q,47

- **N94.10** Unspecified dyspareunia
- **N94.11** Superficial (introital) dyspareunia
- **N94.12** Deep dyspareunia
- **N94.19** Other specified dyspareunia

N94.2 Vaginismus
EXCLUDES 1 psychogenic vaginismus (F52.5)
DEF: Spontaneous contractions of the muscles surrounding the vagina, causing it to constrict or close.

N94.3 Premenstrual tension syndrome
Code also associated menstrual migraine (G43.82-, G43.83-)
EXCLUDES 1 premenstrual dysphoric disorder (F32.81)

N94.4 Primary dysmenorrhea
N94.5 Secondary dysmenorrhea
N94.6 Dysmenorrhea, unspecified
EXCLUDES 1 psychogenic dysmenorrhea (F45.8)

N94.8 Other specified conditions associated with female genital organs and menstrual cycle

- **N94.81** Vulvodynia
  - **N94.810** Vulvar vestibulitis
  - **N94.818** Other vulvodynia
  - **N94.819** Vulvodynia, unspecified
    Vulvodynia NOS
- **N94.89** Other specified conditions associated with female genital organs and menstrual cycle
  DEF: Hydrocele: Serous fluid that collects in the canal of Nuck in females.

N94.9 Unspecified condition associated with female genital organs and menstrual cycle

N95 Menopausal and other perimenopausal disorders

Menopausal and other perimenopausal disorders due to naturally occurring (age-related) menopause and perimenopause

EXCLUDES 1
excessive bleeding in the premenopausal period (N92.4)
menopausal and perimenopausal disorders due to artificial or premature menopause (E89.4-, E28.31-)
premature menopause (E28.31-)

EXCLUDES 2
postmenopausal osteoporosis (M81.0-)
postmenopausal osteoporosis with current pathological fracture (M80.0-)
postmenopausal urethritis (N34.2)

- **N95.0** Postmenopausal bleeding
- **N95.1** Menopausal and female climacteric states
  Symptoms such as flushing, sleeplessness, headache, lack of concentration, associated with natural (age-related) menopause
  Use additional code for associated symptoms
  EXCLUDES 1
  asymptomatic menopausal state (Z78.0)
  symptoms associated with artificial menopause (E89.41)
  symptoms associated with premature menopause (E28.310)
- **N95.2** Postmenopausal atrophic vaginitis
  Senile (atrophic) vaginitis
- **N95.8** Other specified menopausal and perimenopausal disorders
- **N95.9** Unspecified menopausal and perimenopausal disorder

N96 Recurrent pregnancy loss

Investigation or care in a nonpregnant woman with history of recurrent pregnancy loss

EXCLUDES 1
recurrent pregnancy loss with current pregnancy (O26.2-)

N97 Female infertility

INCLUDES
inability to achieve a pregnancy
sterility, female NOS

EXCLUDES 2
female infertility associated with:
hypopituitarism (E23.0)
incompetence of cervix uteri (N88.3)
Stein-Leventhal syndrome (E28.2)

DEF: Infertility: Inability to conceive for at least one year with regular intercourse.
DEF: Primary infertility: Infertility occurring in patients who have never conceived.
DEF: Secondary infertility: Infertility occurring in patients who have previously conceived.

- **N97.0** Female infertility associated with anovulation
  AHA: 2022,2Q,16
- **N97.1** Female infertility of tubal origin
  Female infertility associated with congenital anomaly of tube
  Female infertility due to tubal block
  Female infertility due to tubal occlusion
  Female infertility due to tubal stenosis
- **N97.2** Female infertility of uterine origin
  Female infertility associated with congenital anomaly of uterus
  Female infertility due to nonimplantation of ovum
- **N97.8** Female infertility of other origin
  AHA: 2022,2Q,15
- **N97.9** Female infertility, unspecified

N98 Complications associated with artificial fertilization

- **N98.0** Infection associated with artificial insemination
- **N98.1** Hyperstimulation of ovaries
  Hyperstimulation of ovaries associated with induced ovulation
  Hyperstimulation of ovaries NOS
- **N98.2** Complications of attempted introduction of fertilized ovum following in vitro fertilization
- **N98.3** Complications of attempted introduction of embryo in embryo transfer
- **N98.8** Other complications associated with artificial fertilization
- **N98.9** Complication associated with artificial fertilization, unspecified

Intraoperative and postprocedural complications and disorders of genitourinary system, not elsewhere classified (N99)

N99 Intraoperative and postprocedural complications and disorders of genitourinary system, not elsewhere classified

EXCLUDES 2
irradiation cystitis (N30.4-)
postoophorectomy osteoporosis with current pathological fracture (M80.8-)
postoophorectomy osteoporosis without current pathological fracture (M81.8)

- **N99.0** Postprocedural (acute) (chronic) kidney failure
  Use additional code to type of kidney disease
- **N99.1** Postprocedural urethral stricture
  Postcatheterization urethral stricture
  - **N99.11** Postprocedural urethral stricture, male
    AHA: 2016,4Q,47-48
    - **N99.110** Postprocedural urethral stricture, male, meatal
    - **N99.111** Postprocedural bulbous urethral stricture, male
    - **N99.112** Postprocedural membranous urethral stricture, male
    - **N99.113** Postprocedural anterior bulbous urethral stricture, male
    - **N99.114** Postprocedural urethral stricture, male, unspecified
    - **N99.115** Postprocedural fossa navicularis urethral stricture
    - **N99.116** Postprocedural urethral stricture, male, overlapping sites
  - **N99.12** Postprocedural urethral stricture, female
- **N99.2** Postprocedural adhesions of vagina
- **N99.3** Prolapse of vaginal vault after hysterectomy
- **N99.4** Postprocedural pelvic peritoneal adhesions
  EXCLUDES 2
  pelvic peritoneal adhesions NOS (N73.6)
  postinfective pelvic peritoneal adhesions (N73.6)
- **N99.5** Complications of stoma of urinary tract
  EXCLUDES 2
  mechanical complication of urinary catheter (T83.0-)
  AHA: 2016,4Q,48
  - **N99.51** Complication of cystostomy
    - **N99.510** Cystostomy hemorrhage
    - **N99.511** Cystostomy infection
    - **N99.512** Cystostomy malfunction
    - **N99.518** Other cystostomy complication
  - **N99.52** Complication of incontinent external stoma of urinary tract
    - **N99.520** Hemorrhage of incontinent external stoma of urinary tract
    - **N99.521** Infection of incontinent external stoma of urinary tract
    - **N99.522** Malfunction of incontinent external stoma of urinary tract
    - **N99.523** Herniation of incontinent stoma of urinary tract
    - **N99.524** Stenosis of incontinent stoma of urinary tract
    - **N99.528** Other complication of incontinent external stoma of urinary tract
  - **N99.53** Complication of continent stoma of urinary tract
    - **N99.530** Hemorrhage of continent stoma of urinary tract
    - **N99.531** Infection of continent stoma of urinary tract
    - **N99.532** Malfunction of continent stoma of urinary tract
    - **N99.533** Herniation of continent stoma of urinary tract
    - **N99.534** Stenosis of continent stoma of urinary tract
    - **N99.538** Other complication of continent stoma of urinary tract

- **N99.6** **Intraoperative hemorrhage and hematoma** of a genitourinary system organ or structure complicating a procedure
  - EXCLUDES 1: intraoperative hemorrhage and hematoma of a genitourinary system organ or structure due to accidental puncture or laceration during a procedure (N99.7-)
  - **N99.61** Intraoperative hemorrhage and hematoma of a genitourinary system organ or structure complicating a genitourinary system procedure
  - **N99.62** Intraoperative hemorrhage and hematoma of a genitourinary system organ or structure complicating other procedure
- **N99.7** **Accidental puncture and laceration** of a genitourinary system organ or structure during a procedure
  - **N99.71** Accidental puncture and laceration of a genitourinary system organ or structure during a genitourinary system procedure
  - **N99.72** Accidental puncture and laceration of a genitourinary system organ or structure during other procedure
- **N99.8** Other intraoperative and postprocedural complications and disorders of genitourinary system
  - AHA: 2016,4Q,9-10
  - **N99.81** Other intraoperative complications of genitourinary system
  - **N99.82** Postprocedural hemorrhage of a genitourinary system organ or structure following a procedure
    - **N99.820** Postprocedural hemorrhage of a genitourinary system organ or structure following a genitourinary system procedure
      - AHA: 2025,2Q,20-21
    - **N99.821** Postprocedural hemorrhage of a genitourinary system organ or structure following other procedure
  - **N99.83** Residual ovary syndrome
  - **N99.84** Postprocedural hematoma and seroma of a genitourinary system organ or structure following a procedure
    - **N99.840** Postprocedural hematoma of a genitourinary system organ or structure following a genitourinary system procedure
    - **N99.841** Postprocedural hematoma of a genitourinary system organ or structure following other procedure
    - **N99.842** Postprocedural seroma of a genitourinary system organ or structure following a genitourinary system procedure
    - **N99.843** Postprocedural seroma of a genitourinary system organ or structure following other procedure
  - **N99.85** Post endometrial ablation syndrome
    - AHA: 2019,4Q,12
  - **N99.89** Other postprocedural complications and disorders of genitourinary system

Chapter 15. Pregnancy, Childbirth, and the Puerperium (O00–O9A)

Chapter-specific Guidelines with Coding Examples

The chapter-specific guidelines from the ICD-10-CM Official Guidelines for Coding and Reporting have been provided below. Along with these guidelines are coding examples, contained in the shaded boxes, that have been developed to help illustrate the coding and/or sequencing guidance found in these guidelines.

a. General rules for obstetric cases

1) Codes from Chapter 15 and sequencing priority

Obstetric cases require codes from chapter 15, codes in the range O00-O9A, Pregnancy, Childbirth, and the Puerperium. Chapter 15 codes have sequencing priority over codes from other chapters. Additional codes from other chapters may be used in conjunction with chapter 15 codes to further specify conditions. Should the provider document that the pregnancy is incidental to the encounter, then code Z33.1, Pregnant state, incidental, should be used in place of any chapter 15 codes. It is the provider's responsibility to state that the condition being treated is not affecting the pregnancy.

> Bladder abscess in pregnant patient at 25 weeks' gestation
>
> **O23.12** Infections of bladder in pregnancy, second trimester
>
> **N30.80** Other cystitis without hematuria
>
> **Z3A.25** 25 weeks gestation of pregnancy
>
> *Explanation:* The documentation does not indicate that the pregnancy is incidental or in any way unaffected by the bladder abscess; therefore, an obstetrics code should be sequenced first. An additional code was provided to identify the specific bladder condition as this information is not called out specifically in the obstetrics code.

2) Chapter 15 codes used only on the maternal record

Chapter 15 codes are to be used only on the maternal record, never on the record of the newborn.

3) Final character for trimester

The majority of codes in Chapter 15 have a final character indicating the trimester of pregnancy. The timeframes for the trimesters are indicated at the beginning of the chapter. If trimester is not a component of a code, it is because the condition always occurs in a specific trimester, or the concept of trimester of pregnancy is not applicable. Certain codes have characters for only certain trimesters because the condition does not occur in all trimesters, but it may occur in more than just one. Assignment of the final character for trimester should be based on the provider's documentation of the trimester (or number of weeks) for the current admission/encounter. This applies to the assignment of trimester for pre-existing conditions as well as those that develop during or are due to the pregnancy. The provider's documentation of the number of weeks may be used to assign the appropriate code identifying the trimester.

> Pregnant patient at 21 weeks' gestation admitted with excessive vomiting
>
> **O21.2** Late vomiting of pregnancy
>
> **Z3A.21** 21 weeks gestation of pregnancy
>
> *Explanation:* Category O21 classifies vomiting in pregnancy. Although code selection is based on whether the vomiting is before or after 20 completed weeks, these codes are not further classified by trimester. If vomiting only in the second trimester was documented, the provider should be queried for the specific week of gestation, as this will affect code selection.

Whenever delivery occurs during the current admission, and there is an "in childbirth" option for the obstetric complication being coded, the "in childbirth" code should be assigned. When the classification does not provide an obstetric code with an "in childbirth" option, it is appropriate to assign a code describing the current trimester.

4) Selection of trimester for inpatient admissions that encompass more than one trimester

In instances when a patient is admitted to a hospital for complications of pregnancy during one trimester and remains in the hospital into a subsequent trimester, the trimester character for the antepartum complication code should be assigned on the basis of the trimester when the complication developed, not the trimester of the discharge. If the condition developed prior to the current admission/encounter or represents a pre-existing condition, the trimester character for the trimester at the time of the admission/encounter should be assigned.

5) Unspecified trimester

Each category that includes codes for trimester has a code for "unspecified trimester." The "unspecified trimester" code should rarely be used, such as when the documentation in the record is insufficient to determine the trimester and it is not possible to obtain clarification.

6) 7th character for fetus identification

Where applicable, a 7th character is to be assigned for certain categories (O31, O32, O33.3 - O33.6, O35, O36, O40, O41, O60.1, O60.2, O64, and O69) to identify the fetus for which the complication code applies.

Assign 7th character "0":

- For single gestations.
- When the documentation in the record is insufficient to determine the fetus affected and it is not possible to obtain clarification.
- When it is not possible to clinically determine which fetus is affected.

> Maternal patient with twin gestations is seen after ultrasound identifies fetus B to be in breech presentation
>
> **O32.1XX2** Maternal care for breech presentation, fetus 2
>
> *Explanation:* The documentation indicates that although there are two fetuses, only one fetus is determined to be in breech presentation. Whether fetus 2 or fetus B is used, the coder can assign the seventh character of 2 to identify the second fetus as the one in breech.

7) Completed weeks of gestation

In ICD-10-CM, "completed" weeks of gestation refers to full weeks. For example, if the provider documents gestation at 39 weeks and 6 days, the code for 39 weeks of gestation should be assigned, as the patient has not yet reached 40 completed weeks.

b. Selection of OB principal or first-listed diagnosis

1) Routine outpatient prenatal visits

For routine outpatient prenatal visits when no complications are present, a code from category Z34, Encounter for supervision of normal pregnancy, should be used as the first-listed diagnosis. These codes should not be used in conjunction with chapter 15 codes.

2) Supervision of high-risk pregnancy

Codes from category O09, Supervision of high-risk pregnancy, are intended for use only during the prenatal period. For complications during the labor or delivery episode as a result of a high-risk pregnancy, assign the applicable complication codes from Chapter 15. If there are no complications during the labor or delivery episode, assign code O80, Encounter for full-term uncomplicated delivery.

For routine prenatal outpatient visits for patients with high-risk pregnancies, a code from category O09, Supervision of high-risk pregnancy, should be used as the first-listed diagnosis. Secondary chapter 15 codes may be used in conjunction with these codes if appropriate.

> 36-year-old seen in labor with second child at 39 weeks' gestation, delivered a healthy baby, delivery complicated by tear of fourchette that was repaired
>
> **O70.0** First degree perineal laceration during delivery
>
> **Z3A.39** 39 weeks gestation of pregnancy
>
> **Z37.0** Single live birth
>
> Explanation: Although this patient is over 35 and having her second child (elderly multigravida), do not append a code from subcategory O09.52-. A code describing the tear of the fourchette, which complicated the delivery, should be used in addition to the applicable Z codes.

3) Episodes when no delivery occurs

In episodes when no delivery occurs, the principal diagnosis should correspond to the principal complication of the pregnancy which necessitated the encounter. Should more than one complication exist, all of which are treated or monitored, any of the complication codes may be sequenced first.

4) When a delivery occurs

When an obstetric patient is admitted and delivers during that admission, the condition that prompted the admission should be sequenced as the principal diagnosis. If multiple conditions prompted the admission, sequence the one most related to the delivery as the principal diagnosis. A code for any complication of the delivery should be assigned as an additional diagnosis. In cases of cesarean delivery, if the patient was admitted with a condition that resulted in the performance of a cesarean procedure, that condition should be selected as the principal diagnosis. If the reason for the admission was unrelated to the condition resulting in the cesarean delivery, the condition related to the reason for the admission should be selected as the principal diagnosis.

> Maternal patient with diet-controlled gestational diabetes was seen at 38 weeks' gestation in obstructed labor due to footling presentation; cesarean performed for the malpresentation
>
> | | |
> |---|---|
> | O64.8XX0 | Obstructed labor due to other malposition and malpresentation, not applicable or unspecified |
> | O24.420 | Gestational diabetes mellitus in childbirth, diet controlled |
> | Z3A.38 | 38 weeks gestation of pregnancy |
> | Z37.0 | Single live birth |
>
> *Explanation:* The obstructed labor necessitated the cesarean procedure.

5) **Outcome of delivery**

A code from category Z37, Outcome of delivery, should be included on every maternal record when a delivery has occurred. These codes are not to be used on subsequent records or on the newborn record.

c. **Pre-existing conditions versus conditions due to the pregnancy**

Certain categories in Chapter 15 distinguish between conditions of the mother that existed prior to pregnancy (pre-existing) and those that are a direct result of pregnancy. When assigning codes from Chapter 15, it is important to assess if a condition was pre-existing prior to pregnancy or developed during or due to the pregnancy in order to assign the correct code.

Categories that do not distinguish between pre-existing and pregnancy-related conditions may be used for either. It is acceptable to use codes specifically for the puerperium with codes complicating pregnancy and childbirth if a condition arises postpartum during the delivery encounter.

> Type 2 diabetic patient presents at 19 weeks gestation for glucose check. Patient has been taking oral metformin for several years and currently is experiencing no diabetic complications.
>
> | | |
> |---|---|
> | O24.112 | Pre-existing type 2 diabetes mellitus, in pregnancy, second trimester |
> | E11.9 | Type 2 diabetes mellitus without complications |
> | Z79.84 | Long term (current) use of oral hypoglycemic drugs |
>
> *Explanation:* The documentation states that the patient has been on a diabetic medication (oral metformin) for several years, indicating the patient was diabetic prior to becoming pregnant. Reporting pre-existing Type 2 diabetes in a pregnant patient requires two codes to capture the condition, a code from category O24 and a code from category E11. A note at E11 indicates that the code for long-term use of oral hypoglycemic drugs should also be reported.

d. **Pre-existing hypertension in pregnancy**

Category O10, Pre-existing hypertension complicating pregnancy, childbirth and the puerperium, includes codes for hypertensive heart and hypertensive chronic kidney disease. When assigning one of the O10 codes that includes hypertensive heart disease or hypertensive chronic kidney disease, it is necessary to add a secondary code from the appropriate hypertension category to specify the type of heart failure or chronic kidney disease.

See Section I.C.9. Hypertension.

e. **Fetal conditions affecting the management of the mother**

1) **Codes from categories O35 and O36**

Codes from categories O35, Maternal care for known or suspected fetal abnormality and damage, and O36, Maternal care for other fetal problems, are assigned only when the fetal condition is actually responsible for modifying the management of the mother, i.e., by requiring diagnostic studies, additional observation, special care, or termination of pregnancy. The fact that the fetal condition exists does not justify assigning a code from this series to the mother's record.

> A patient with twin gestation is seen for spotting 15 weeks into her pregnancy; the doctors also suspect fetal hydrocephalus. Patient is instructed to return in one week for additional diagnostic testing, sooner if the problem worsens.
>
> | | |
> |---|---|
> | O35.00X0 | Maternal care for (suspected) central nervous system malformation or damage in fetus, unspecified, not applicable or unspecified |
> | O26.852 | Spotting complicating pregnancy, second trimester |
> | Z3A.15 | 15 weeks gestation of pregnancy |
>
> *Explanation:* Whether the fetal hydrocephalus was suspected or confirmed, an additional code is warranted for this condition since documentation indicates the patient is to return sooner than her routine visit for further testing.

2) **In utero surgery**

In cases when surgery is performed on the fetus, a diagnosis code from category O35, Maternal care for known or suspected fetal abnormality and damage, should be assigned identifying the fetal condition. Assign the appropriate procedure code for the procedure performed.

No code from Chapter 16, the perinatal codes, should be used on the mother's record to identify fetal conditions. Surgery performed in utero on a fetus is still to be coded as an obstetric encounter.

f. **HIV infection in pregnancy, childbirth and the puerperium**

During pregnancy, childbirth or the puerperium, a patient admitted because of an HIV-related illness should receive a principal diagnosis from subcategory O98.7-, Human immunodeficiency [HIV] disease complicating pregnancy, childbirth and the puerperium, followed by the code(s) for the HIV-related illness(es).

Patients with asymptomatic HIV infection status admitted during pregnancy, childbirth, or the puerperium should receive codes of O98.7- and Z21, Asymptomatic human immunodeficiency virus [HIV] infection status.

> A previously asymptomatic HIV patient who is 13 weeks pregnant is evaluated for HIV-related candidal bronchitis
>
> | | |
> |---|---|
> | O98.711 | Human immunodeficiency virus [HIV] disease complicating pregnancy, first trimester |
> | B20 | Human immunodeficiency virus [HIV] disease |
> | B37.1 | Pulmonary candidiasis |
> | Z3A.13 | 13 weeks gestation of pregnancy |
>
> *Explanation:* Because candidal bronchitis is an AIDS-related condition, this patient is now considered to have HIV disease. An obstetrics code indicating that HIV is complicating the pregnancy is coded first, followed by B20 for HIV disease as well as a code for the candidal bronchitis.

g. **Diabetes mellitus in pregnancy**

Diabetes mellitus is a significant complicating factor in pregnancy. Pregnant patients who are diabetic should be assigned a code from category O24, Diabetes mellitus in pregnancy, childbirth, and the puerperium, first, followed by the appropriate diabetes code(s) (E08-E13) from Chapter 4.

h. **Long term use of insulin and oral hypoglycemics**

See section I.C.4.a.3 for information on the long term-use of insulin and oral hypoglycemics.

i. **Gestational (pregnancy induced) diabetes**

Gestational (pregnancy induced) diabetes can occur during the second and third trimester of pregnancy in patients who were not diabetic prior to pregnancy. Gestational diabetes can cause complications in the pregnancy similar to those of pre-existing diabetes mellitus. It also puts the patient at greater risk of developing diabetes after the pregnancy.

Codes for gestational diabetes are in subcategory O24.4, Gestational diabetes mellitus. No other code from category O24, Diabetes mellitus in pregnancy, childbirth, and the puerperium, should be used with a code from O24.4.

The codes under subcategory O24.4 include diet controlled, insulin controlled, and controlled by oral hypoglycemic drugs. If a patient with gestational diabetes is treated with both diet and insulin, only the code for insulin-controlled is required. If a patient with gestational diabetes is treated with both diet and oral hypoglycemic medications, only the code for "controlled by oral hypoglycemic drugs" is required. Codes Z79.4, Long-term (current) use of insulin, Z79.84, Long-term (current) use of oral hypoglycemic drugs, and Z79.85, Long-term (current) use of injectable non-insulin antidiabetic drugs, should not be assigned with codes from subcategory O24.4.

An abnormal glucose tolerance in pregnancy is assigned a code from subcategory O99.81, Abnormal glucose complicating pregnancy, childbirth, and the puerperium.

j. **Sepsis and septic shock complicating abortion, pregnancy, childbirth and the puerperium**

When assigning a chapter 15 code for sepsis complicating abortion, pregnancy, childbirth, and the puerperium, a code for the specific type of infection should be assigned as an additional diagnosis. If severe sepsis is present, a code from subcategory R65.2, Severe sepsis, and code(s) for associated organ dysfunction(s) should also be assigned as additional diagnoses.

> Patient is seen several days after a miscarriage with sepsis; cultures return MSSA
>
> **O03.87** Sepsis following complete or unspecified spontaneous abortion
>
> **B95.61** Methicillin susceptible Staphylococcus aureus infection as the cause of diseases classified elsewhere
>
> *Explanation:* The type of infection that caused this patient to become septic was methicillin susceptible *Staphylococcus aureus* (MSSA), which as a secondary code helps capture all aspects related to this patient's septic condition.

k. **Puerperal sepsis**

Code O85, Puerperal sepsis, should be assigned with a secondary code to identify the causal organism (e.g., for a bacterial infection, assign a code from category B95-B96, Bacterial infections in conditions classified elsewhere). A code from category A40, Streptococcal sepsis, or A41, Other sepsis, should not be used for puerperal sepsis. If applicable, use additional codes to identify severe sepsis (R65.2-) and any associated acute organ dysfunction.

Code O85 should not be assigned for sepsis following an obstetrical procedure (See Section I.C.1.d.5.b., Sepsis due to a postprocedural infection).

l. **Alcohol, tobacco and drug use during pregnancy, childbirth and the puerperium**

1) **Alcohol use during pregnancy, childbirth and the puerperium**

Codes under subcategory O99.31, Alcohol use complicating pregnancy, childbirth, and the puerperium, should be assigned for any pregnancy case when a patient uses alcohol during the pregnancy or postpartum. A secondary code from category F10, Alcohol related disorders, should also be assigned to identify manifestations of the alcohol use.

2) **Tobacco use during pregnancy, childbirth and the puerperium**

Codes under subcategory O99.33, Smoking (tobacco) complicating pregnancy, childbirth, and the puerperium, should be assigned for any pregnancy case when a patient uses any type of tobacco product during the pregnancy or postpartum.

A secondary code from category F17, Nicotine dependence, should also be assigned to identify the type of nicotine dependence.

3) **Drug use during pregnancy, childbirth and the puerperium**

Codes under subcategory O99.32, Drug use complicating pregnancy, childbirth, and the puerperium, should be assigned for any pregnancy case when a patient uses drugs during the pregnancy or postpartum. This can involve illegal drugs, or inappropriate use or abuse of prescription drugs. Secondary code(s) from categories F11-F16 and F18-F19 should also be assigned to identify manifestations of the drug use.

m. **Poisoning, toxic effects, adverse effects and underdosing in a pregnant patient**

A code from subcategory O9A.2, Injury, poisoning and certain other consequences of external causes complicating pregnancy, childbirth, and the puerperium, should be sequenced first, followed by the appropriate injury, poisoning, toxic effect, adverse effect or underdosing code, and then the additional code(s) that specifies the condition caused by the poisoning, toxic effect, adverse effect or underdosing.

See Section I.C.19. Adverse effects, poisoning, underdosing and toxic effects.

> Patient treated for accidental carbon monoxide poisoning from a gas heating implement; the patient is 18 weeks' pregnant
>
> **O9A.212** Injury, poisoning and certain other consequences of external causes complicating pregnancy, second trimester
>
> **T58.11XA** Toxic effect of carbon monoxide from utility gas, accidental (unintentional), initial encounter
>
> **Z3A.18** 18 weeks gestation of pregnancy
>
> *Explanation:* Although the carbon monoxide poisoning is the reason for the encounter, a code from the obstetrics chapter must be sequenced first. Chapter 15 codes have sequencing priority over codes from other chapters.

n. **Normal delivery, code O80**

1) **Encounter for full term uncomplicated delivery**

Code O80 should be assigned when a patient is admitted for a full-term normal delivery and delivers a single, healthy infant without any complications antepartum, during the delivery, or postpartum during the delivery episode. Code O80 is always a principal diagnosis. It is not to be used if any other code from chapter 15 is needed to describe a current complication of the antenatal, delivery, or postnatal period. Additional codes from other chapters may be used with code O80 if they are not related to or are in any way complicating the pregnancy.

2) **Uncomplicated delivery with resolved antepartum complication**

Code O80 may be used if the patient had a complication at some point during the pregnancy, but the complication is not present at the time of the admission for delivery.

> Patient presents in labor at 39 weeks' gestation and delivers a healthy newborn; patient had abnormal glucose levels in her first trimester, which have since resolved
>
> **O80** Encounter for full-term uncomplicated delivery
>
> **Z37.0** Single live birth
>
> *Explanation:* The abnormal glucose levels during the first trimester cannot be coded if they are not affecting the patient's current trimester. Without additional complications associated with the pregnancy, fetus, or mother, code O80 is appropriate.

3) **Outcome of delivery for O80**

Z37.0, Single live birth, is the only outcome of delivery code appropriate for use with O80.

o. **The peripartum and postpartum periods**

1) **Peripartum and postpartum periods**

The postpartum period begins immediately after delivery and continues for six weeks following delivery. The peripartum period is defined as the last month of pregnancy to five months postpartum.

2) **Peripartum and postpartum complication**

A postpartum complication is any complication occurring within the six-week period.

3) **Pregnancy-related complications after 6-week period**

Chapter 15 codes may also be used to describe pregnancy-related complications after the peripartum or postpartum period if the provider documents that a condition is pregnancy related.

> Patient referred for varicose veins. She had a baby boy three months ago; the varicose veins started to appear one month ago. The doctor attributes the patient's pregnancy as the cause of the varicose veins, which continue to be painful and bother the patient. She is seeking surgical relief.
>
> **O87.4** Varicose veins of the lower extremity in the puerperium
>
> *Explanation:* Although the varicose veins occurred several months after the delivery of the newborn, the doctor attributed the varicose veins to pregnancy and therefore a code from chapter 15 is appropriate.

4) **Admission for routine postpartum care following delivery outside hospital**

When the mother delivers outside the hospital prior to admission and is admitted for routine postpartum care and no complications are noted, code Z39.0, Encounter for care and examination of mother immediately after delivery, should be assigned as the principal diagnosis.

5) Pregnancy associated cardiomyopathy

Pregnancy associated cardiomyopathy, code O90.3, is unique in that it may be diagnosed in the third trimester of pregnancy but may continue to progress months after delivery. For this reason, it is referred to as peripartum cardiomyopathy. Code O90.3 is only for use when the cardiomyopathy develops as a result of pregnancy in a patient who did not have pre-existing heart disease.

p. Code O94, Sequelae of complication of pregnancy, childbirth, and the puerperium

1) Code O94

Code O94, Sequelae of complication of pregnancy, childbirth, and the puerperium, is for use in those cases when an initial complication of a pregnancy develops a sequela or sequelae requiring care or treatment at a future date.

2) After the initial postpartum period

This code may be used at any time after the initial postpartum period.

3) Sequencing of code O94

This code, like all sequela codes, is to be sequenced following the code describing the sequelae of the complication.

q. Termination of pregnancy and spontaneous abortions

1) Abortion with liveborn fetus

When an attempted termination of pregnancy results in a liveborn fetus, assign code Z33.2, Encounter for elective termination of pregnancy and a code from category Z37, Outcome of Delivery.

2) Retained products of conception following an abortion

Subsequent encounters for retained products of conception following a spontaneous abortion or elective termination of pregnancy, without complications are assigned O03.4, Incomplete spontaneous abortion without complication, or code O07.4, Failed attempted termination of pregnancy without complication. This advice is appropriate even when the patient was discharged previously with a discharge diagnosis of complete abortion. If the patient has a specific complication associated with the spontaneous abortion or elective termination of pregnancy in addition to retained products of conception, assign the appropriate complication code (e.g., O03.-, O04.-, O07.-) instead of code O03.4 or O07.4.

> Patient was seen two days ago for complete spontaneous abortion but returns today for urinary tract infection (UTI) with ultrasound showing retained products of conception
>
> **O03.38**   **Urinary tract infection following incomplete spontaneous abortion**
>
> *Explanation:* Although the diagnosis from the patient's previous stay indicated that the patient had a complete abortion, it is now determined that there were actually retained products of conception (POC). An abortion with retained POC is considered incomplete and in this case resulted in the patient developing a UTI.

3) Complications leading to abortion

Codes from Chapter 15 may be used as additional codes to identify any documented complications of the pregnancy in conjunction with codes in categories in O04, O07 and O08.

4) Hemorrhage following elective abortion

For hemorrhage post elective abortion, assign code O04.6, Delayed or excessive hemorrhage following (induced) termination of pregnancy. Do not assign code O72.1, Other immediate postpartum hemorrhage, as this code should not be assigned for post abortion conditions.

r. Abuse in a pregnant patient

For suspected or confirmed cases of abuse of a pregnant patient, a code(s) from subcategories O9A.3, Physical abuse complicating pregnancy, childbirth, and the puerperium, O9A.4, Sexual abuse complicating pregnancy, childbirth, and the puerperium, and O9A.5, Psychological abuse complicating pregnancy, childbirth, and the puerperium, should be sequenced first, followed by the appropriate codes (if applicable) to identify any associated current injury due to physical abuse, sexual abuse, and the perpetrator of abuse.

See Section I.C.19. Adult and child abuse, neglect and other maltreatment.

s. COVID-19 infection in pregnancy, childbirth, and the puerperium

During pregnancy, childbirth or the puerperium, when COVID-19 is the reason for admission/encounter, code O98.5-, Other viral diseases complicating pregnancy, childbirth and the puerperium, should be sequenced as the principal/first-listed diagnosis, and code U07.1, COVID-19, and the appropriate codes for associated manifestation(s) should be assigned as additional diagnoses. Codes from Chapter 15 always take sequencing priority.

If the reason for admission/encounter is unrelated to COVID-19 but the patient **has been diagnosed with** COVID-19 during the admission/encounter, the appropriate code for the reason for admission/encounter should be sequenced as the principal/first-listed diagnosis, and codes O98.5- and U07.1, as well as the appropriate codes for associated COVID-19 manifestations, should be assigned as additional diagnoses.

Chapter 15. Pregnancy, Childbirth and the Puerperium (O00-O9A)

NOTE CODES FROM THIS CHAPTER ARE FOR USE ONLY ON MATERNAL RECORDS, NEVER ON NEWBORN RECORDS

Codes from this chapter are for use for conditions related to or aggravated by the pregnancy, childbirth, or by the puerperium (maternal causes or obstetric causes)

NOTE Trimesters are counted from the first day of the last menstrual period. They are defined as follows:
1st trimester- less than 14 weeks 0 days
2nd trimester- 14 weeks 0 days to less than 28 weeks 0 days
3rd trimester- 28 weeks 0 days until delivery

Use additional code, if applicable, from category Z3A, Weeks of gestation, to identify the specific week of the pregnancy, if known.

EXCLUDES 1 supervision of normal pregnancy (Z34.-)
EXCLUDES 2 mental and behavioral disorders associated with the puerperium (F53.-)
obstetrical tetanus (A34)
postpartum necrosis of pituitary gland (E23.0)
puerperal osteomalacia (M83.0)

AHA: 2016,1Q,3-5; 2014,3Q,17

This chapter contains the following blocks:
- O00-O08 Pregnancy with abortive outcome
- O09 Supervision of high risk pregnancy
- O10-O16 Edema, proteinuria and hypertensive disorders in pregnancy, childbirth and the puerperium
- O20-O29 Other maternal disorders predominantly related to pregnancy
- O30-O48 Maternal care related to the fetus and amniotic cavity and possible delivery problems
- O60-O77 Complications of labor and delivery
- O80-O82 Encounter for delivery
- O85-O92 Complications predominantly related to the puerperium
- O94-O9A Other obstetric conditions, not elsewhere classified

Pregnancy with abortive outcome (O00-O08)

EXCLUDES 1 continuing pregnancy in multiple gestation after abortion of one fetus or more (O31.1-, O31.3-)

TIP: Do not assign a code from category Z3A with codes in this code block.

✓4th O00 Ectopic pregnancy
INCLUDES ruptured ectopic pregnancy
Use additional code from category O08 to identify any associated complication
AHA: 2016,4Q,48-50; 2014,3Q,17
DEF: Implantation of a fertilized egg outside the uterus, usually in the fallopian tube or abdomen that requires emergency treatment.

✓5th O00.0 Abdominal pregnancy
EXCLUDES 1 maternal care for viable fetus in abdominal pregnancy (O36.7-)

- O00.00 **Abdominal pregnancy without intrauterine pregnancy**
  Abdominal pregnancy NOS
- O00.01 **Abdominal pregnancy with intrauterine pregnancy**

✓5th O00.1 Tubal pregnancy
Fallopian pregnancy
Rupture of (fallopian) tube due to pregnancy
Tubal abortion
AHA: 2017,4Q,20

✓6th O00.10 Tubal pregnancy without intrauterine pregnancy
Tubal pregnancy NOS
- O00.101 **Right tubal pregnancy without intrauterine pregnancy**
- O00.102 **Left tubal pregnancy without intrauterine pregnancy**
- O00.109 Unspecified tubal pregnancy without intrauterine pregnancy

✓6th O00.11 Tubal pregnancy with intrauterine pregnancy
- O00.111 **Right tubal pregnancy with intrauterine pregnancy**
- O00.112 **Left tubal pregnancy with intrauterine pregnancy**
- O00.119 Unspecified tubal pregnancy with intrauterine pregnancy

✓5th O00.2 Ovarian pregnancy
AHA: 2017,4Q,20

✓6th O00.20 Ovarian pregnancy without intrauterine pregnancy
Ovarian pregnancy NOS
- O00.201 **Right ovarian pregnancy without intrauterine pregnancy**
- O00.202 **Left ovarian pregnancy without intrauterine pregnancy**
- O00.209 Unspecified ovarian pregnancy without intrauterine pregnancy

✓6th O00.21 Ovarian pregnancy with intrauterine pregnancy
- O00.211 **Right ovarian pregnancy with intrauterine pregnancy**
- O00.212 **Left ovarian pregnancy with intrauterine pregnancy**
- O00.219 Unspecified ovarian pregnancy with intrauterine pregnancy

✓5th O00.8 Other ectopic pregnancy
Cervical pregnancy
Cornual pregnancy
Intraligamentous pregnancy
Mural pregnancy

- O00.80 **Other ectopic pregnancy without intrauterine pregnancy**
  Other ectopic pregnancy NOS
- O00.81 **Other ectopic pregnancy with intrauterine pregnancy**

✓5th O00.9 Ectopic pregnancy, unspecified
- O00.90 **Unspecified ectopic pregnancy without intrauterine pregnancy**
  Ectopic pregnancy NOS
- O00.91 **Unspecified ectopic pregnancy with intrauterine pregnancy**

✓4th O01 Hydatidiform mole
Use additional code from category O08 to identify any associated complication
EXCLUDES 1 chorioadenoma (destruens) (D39.2)
malignant hydatidiform mole (D39.2)
AHA: 2014,3Q,17
DEF: Abnormal product of pregnancy, marked by a mass of cysts resembling a bunch of grapes due to chorionic villi proliferation and dissolution. It must be surgically removed.

- O01.0 **Classical hydatidiform mole**
  Complete hydatidiform mole
- O01.1 **Incomplete and partial hydatidiform mole**
- O01.9 **Hydatidiform mole, unspecified**
  Trophoblastic disease NOS
  Vesicular mole NOS

✓4th O02 Other abnormal products of conception
Use additional code from category O08 to identify any associated complication
EXCLUDES 1 papyraceous fetus (O31.0-)
AHA: 2014,3Q,17

- O02.0 **Blighted ovum and nonhydatidiform mole**
  Carneous mole
  Fleshy mole
  Intrauterine mole NOS
  Molar pregnancy NEC
  Pathological ovum
- O02.1 **Missed abortion**
  Early fetal death, before completion of 20 weeks of gestation, with retention of dead fetus
  EXCLUDES 1 failed induced abortion (O07.-)
  fetal death (intrauterine) (late) (O36.4)
  missed abortion with blighted ovum (O02.0)
  missed abortion with hydatidiform mole (O01.-)
  missed abortion with nonhydatidiform (O02.0)
  missed abortion with other abnormal products of conception (O02.8-)
  missed delivery (O36.4)
  stillbirth (P95)
  AHA: 2025,1Q,18; 2022,2Q,3; 2019,3Q,11

Chapter 15. Pregnancy, Childbirth and the Puerperium

O02.8 **Other specified abnormal products of conception**
  EXCLUDES 1: abnormal products of conception with blighted ovum (O02.0)
  abnormal products of conception with hydatidiform mole (O01.-)
  abnormal products of conception with nonhydatidiform mole (O02.0)

- **O02.81** **Inappropriate change in quantitative human chorionic gonadotropin (hCG) in early pregnancy**
  Biochemical pregnancy
  Chemical pregnancy
  Inappropriate level of quantitative human chorionic gonadotropin (hCG) for gestational age in early pregnancy
- **O02.89** **Other abnormal products of conception**

O02.9 **Abnormal product of conception, unspecified**

O03 Spontaneous abortion

  NOTE: Incomplete abortion includes retained products of conception following spontaneous abortion
  INCLUDES: miscarriage
  AHA: 2025,1Q,18; 2023,1Q,17

- **O03.0** **Genital tract and pelvic infection following incomplete spontaneous abortion**
  Endometritis following incomplete spontaneous abortion
  Oophoritis following incomplete spontaneous abortion
  Parametritis following incomplete spontaneous abortion
  Pelvic peritonitis following incomplete spontaneous abortion
  Salpingitis following incomplete spontaneous abortion
  Salpingo-oophoritis following incomplete spontaneous abortion
  EXCLUDES 1: sepsis following incomplete spontaneous abortion (O03.37)
  urinary tract infection following incomplete spontaneous abortion (O03.38)

- **O03.1** **Delayed or excessive hemorrhage following incomplete spontaneous abortion**
  Afibrinogenemia following incomplete spontaneous abortion
  Defibrination syndrome following incomplete spontaneous abortion
  Hemolysis following incomplete spontaneous abortion
  Intravascular coagulation following incomplete spontaneous abortion
  AHA: 2022,1Q,19

- **O03.2** **Embolism following incomplete spontaneous abortion**
  Air embolism following incomplete spontaneous abortion
  Amniotic fluid embolism following incomplete spontaneous abortion
  Blood-clot embolism following incomplete spontaneous abortion
  Embolism NOS following incomplete spontaneous abortion
  Fat embolism following incomplete spontaneous abortion
  Pulmonary embolism following incomplete spontaneous abortion
  Pyemic embolism following incomplete spontaneous abortion
  Septic or septicopyemic embolism following incomplete spontaneous abortion
  Soap embolism following incomplete spontaneous abortion

- **O03.3** **Other and unspecified complications following incomplete spontaneous abortion**
  - **O03.30** **Unspecified complication following incomplete spontaneous abortion**
  - **O03.31** **Shock following incomplete spontaneous abortion**
    Circulatory collapse following incomplete spontaneous abortion
    Shock (postprocedural) following incomplete spontaneous abortion
    EXCLUDES 1: shock due to infection following incomplete spontaneous abortion (O03.37)
  - **O03.32** **Renal failure following incomplete spontaneous abortion**
    Kidney failure (acute) following incomplete spontaneous abortion
    Oliguria following incomplete spontaneous abortion
    Renal shutdown following incomplete spontaneous abortion
    Renal tubular necrosis following incomplete spontaneous abortion
    Uremia following incomplete spontaneous abortion
  - **O03.33** **Metabolic disorder following incomplete spontaneous abortion**
  - **O03.34** **Damage to pelvic organs following incomplete spontaneous abortion**
    Laceration, perforation, tear or chemical damage of bladder following incomplete spontaneous abortion
    Laceration, perforation, tear or chemical damage of bowel following incomplete spontaneous abortion
    Laceration, perforation, tear or chemical damage of broad ligament following incomplete spontaneous abortion
    Laceration, perforation, tear or chemical damage of cervix following incomplete spontaneous abortion
    Laceration, perforation, tear or chemical damage of periurethral tissue following incomplete spontaneous abortion
    Laceration, perforation, tear or chemical damage of uterus following incomplete spontaneous abortion
    Laceration, perforation, tear or chemical damage of vagina following incomplete spontaneous abortion
  - **O03.35** **Other venous complications following incomplete spontaneous abortion**
  - **O03.36** **Cardiac arrest following incomplete spontaneous abortion**
  - **O03.37** **Sepsis following incomplete spontaneous abortion**
    Use additional code to identify infectious agent (B95-B97)
    Use additional code to identify severe sepsis, if applicable (R65.2-)
    EXCLUDES 1: septic or septicopyemic embolism following incomplete spontaneous abortion (O03.2)
  - **O03.38** **Urinary tract infection following incomplete spontaneous abortion**
    Cystitis following incomplete spontaneous abortion
  - **O03.39** **Incomplete spontaneous abortion with other complications**

- **O03.4** **Incomplete spontaneous abortion without complication**

- **O03.5** **Genital tract and pelvic infection following complete or unspecified spontaneous abortion**
  Endometritis following complete or unspecified spontaneous abortion
  Oophoritis following complete or unspecified spontaneous abortion
  Parametritis following complete or unspecified spontaneous abortion
  Pelvic peritonitis following complete or unspecified spontaneous abortion
  Salpingitis following complete or unspecified spontaneous abortion
  Salpingo-oophoritis following complete or unspecified spontaneous abortion
  EXCLUDES 1: sepsis following complete or unspecified spontaneous abortion (O03.87)
  urinary tract infection following complete or unspecified spontaneous abortion (O03.88)

- **O03.6** **Delayed or excessive hemorrhage following complete or unspecified spontaneous abortion**
  Afibrinogenemia following complete or unspecified spontaneous abortion
  Defibrination syndrome following complete or unspecified spontaneous abortion
  Hemolysis following complete or unspecified spontaneous abortion
  Intravascular coagulation following complete or unspecified spontaneous abortion
  AHA: 2022,1Q,19

O03.7 **Embolism** following **complete or unspecified** spontaneous abortion
- Air embolism following complete or unspecified spontaneous abortion
- Amniotic fluid embolism following complete or unspecified spontaneous abortion
- Blood-clot embolism following complete or unspecified spontaneous abortion
- Embolism NOS following complete or unspecified spontaneous abortion
- Fat embolism following complete or unspecified spontaneous abortion
- Pulmonary embolism following complete or unspecified spontaneous abortion
- Pyemic embolism following complete or unspecified spontaneous abortion
- Septic or septicopyemic embolism following complete or unspecified spontaneous abortion
- Soap embolism following complete or unspecified spontaneous abortion

O03.8 Other and unspecified complications following complete or unspecified spontaneous abortion

    O03.80 Unspecified complication following **complete or unspecified** spontaneous abortion

    O03.81 **Shock** following **complete or unspecified** spontaneous abortion
- Circulatory collapse following complete or unspecified spontaneous abortion
- Shock (postprocedural) following complete or unspecified spontaneous abortion

        EXCLUDES 1: shock due to infection following complete or unspecified spontaneous abortion (O03.87)

    O03.82 **Renal failure** following **complete or unspecified** spontaneous abortion
- Kidney failure (acute) following complete or unspecified spontaneous abortion
- Oliguria following complete or unspecified spontaneous abortion
- Renal shutdown following complete or unspecified spontaneous abortion
- Renal tubular necrosis following complete or unspecified spontaneous abortion
- Uremia following complete or unspecified spontaneous abortion

    O03.83 **Metabolic** disorder following **complete or unspecified** spontaneous abortion

    O03.84 **Damage to pelvic organs** following **complete or unspecified** spontaneous abortion
- Laceration, perforation, tear or chemical damage of bladder following complete or unspecified spontaneous abortion
- Laceration, perforation, tear or chemical damage of bowel following complete or unspecified spontaneous abortion
- Laceration, perforation, tear or chemical damage of broad ligament following complete or unspecified spontaneous abortion
- Laceration, perforation, tear or chemical damage of cervix following complete or unspecified spontaneous abortion
- Laceration, perforation, tear or chemical damage of periurethral tissue following complete or unspecified spontaneous abortion
- Laceration, perforation, tear or chemical damage of uterus following complete or unspecified spontaneous abortion
- Laceration, perforation, tear or chemical damage of vagina following complete or unspecified spontaneous abortion

    O03.85 Other **venous** complications following **complete or unspecified** spontaneous abortion

    O03.86 **Cardiac arrest** following **complete or unspecified** spontaneous abortion

    O03.87 **Sepsis** following **complete or unspecified** spontaneous abortion

        Use additional code to identify infectious agent (B95-B97)
        Use additional code to identify severe sepsis, if applicable (R65.2-)

        EXCLUDES 1: septic or septicopyemic embolism following complete or unspecified spontaneous abortion (O03.7)

    O03.88 **Urinary tract infection** following **complete or unspecified** spontaneous abortion
- Cystitis following complete or unspecified spontaneous abortion

    O03.89 **Complete or unspecified** spontaneous abortion with **other complications**

O03.9 **Complete or unspecified** spontaneous abortion **without complication**
- Miscarriage NOS
- Spontaneous abortion NOS

O04 **Complications** following (induced) **termination of pregnancy**

    INCLUDES: complications following (induced) termination of pregnancy
    EXCLUDES 2: encounter for elective termination of pregnancy (Z33.2)
        failed attempted termination of pregnancy (O07.-)

O04.5 **Genital tract and pelvic infection** following (induced) **termination of pregnancy**
- Endometritis following (induced) termination of pregnancy
- Oophoritis following (induced) termination of pregnancy
- Parametritis following (induced) termination of pregnancy
- Pelvic peritonitis following (induced) termination of pregnancy
- Salpingitis following (induced) termination of pregnancy
- Salpingo-oophoritis following (induced) termination of pregnancy

    EXCLUDES 1: sepsis following (induced) termination of pregnancy (O04.87)
        urinary tract infection following (induced) termination of pregnancy (O04.88)

O04.6 **Delayed or excessive hemorrhage** following (induced) **termination of pregnancy**
- Afibrinogenemia following (induced) termination of pregnancy
- Defibrination syndrome following (induced) termination of pregnancy
- Hemolysis following (induced) termination of pregnancy
- Intravascular coagulation following (induced) termination of pregnancy

    AHA: 2025,1Q,18; 2023,2Q,15; 2019,3Q,11

O04.7 **Embolism** following (induced) **termination of pregnancy**
- Air embolism following (induced) termination of pregnancy
- Amniotic fluid embolism following (induced) termination of pregnancy
- Blood-clot embolism following (induced) termination of pregnancy
- Embolism NOS following (induced) termination of pregnancy
- Fat embolism following (induced) termination of pregnancy
- Pulmonary embolism following (induced) termination of pregnancy
- Pyemic embolism following (induced) termination of pregnancy
- Septic or septicopyemic embolism following (induced) termination of pregnancy
- Soap embolism following (induced) termination of pregnancy

O04.8 (Induced) termination of pregnancy with other and unspecified complications

    O04.80 (Induced) termination of pregnancy with unspecified complications

    O04.81 **Shock** following (induced) **termination of pregnancy**
- Circulatory collapse following (induced) termination of pregnancy
- Shock (postprocedural) following (induced) termination of pregnancy

        EXCLUDES 1: shock due to infection following (induced) termination of pregnancy (O04.87)

    O04.82 **Renal failure** following (induced) **termination of pregnancy**
- Kidney failure (acute) following (induced) termination of pregnancy
- Oliguria following (induced) termination of pregnancy
- Renal shutdown following (induced) termination of pregnancy
- Renal tubular necrosis following (induced) termination of pregnancy
- Uremia following (induced) termination of pregnancy

    O04.83 **Metabolic disorder** following (induced) **termination of pregnancy**

O04.84 Damage to pelvic organs following (induced) termination of pregnancy M
　Laceration, perforation, tear or chemical damage of bladder following (induced) termination of pregnancy
　Laceration, perforation, tear or chemical damage of bowel following (induced) termination of pregnancy
　Laceration, perforation, tear or chemical damage of broad ligament following (induced) termination of pregnancy
　Laceration, perforation, tear or chemical damage of cervix following (induced) termination of pregnancy
　Laceration, perforation, tear or chemical damage of periurethral tissue following (induced) termination of pregnancy
　Laceration, perforation, tear or chemical damage of uterus following (induced) termination of pregnancy
　Laceration, perforation, tear or chemical damage of vagina following (induced) termination of pregnancy

O04.85 Other venous complications following (induced) termination of pregnancy M

O04.86 Cardiac arrest following (induced) termination of pregnancy M

O04.87 Sepsis following (induced) termination of pregnancy M
　Use additional code to identify infectious agent (B95-B97)
　Use additional code to identify severe sepsis, if applicable (R65.2-)
　　EXCLUDES 1　septic or septicopyemic embolism following (induced) termination of pregnancy (O04.7)

O04.88 Urinary tract infection following (induced) termination of pregnancy M
　Cystitis following (induced) termination of pregnancy

O04.89 (Induced) termination of pregnancy with other complications M

✓4th **O07 Failed attempted termination of pregnancy**
　INCLUDES　failure of attempted induction of termination of pregnancy
　　incomplete elective abortion
　EXCLUDES 1　incomplete spontaneous abortion (O03.0-)

O07.0 Genital tract and pelvic infection following failed attempted termination of pregnancy M
　Endometritis following failed attempted termination of pregnancy
　Oophoritis following failed attempted termination of pregnancy
　Parametritis following failed attempted termination of pregnancy
　Pelvic peritonitis following failed attempted termination of pregnancy
　Salpingitis following failed attempted termination of pregnancy
　Salpingo-oophoritis following failed attempted termination of pregnancy
　　EXCLUDES 1　sepsis following failed attempted termination of pregnancy (O07.37)
　　urinary tract infection following failed attempted termination of pregnancy (O07.38)

O07.1 Delayed or excessive hemorrhage following failed attempted termination of pregnancy M
　Afibrinogenemia following failed attempted termination of pregnancy
　Defibrination syndrome following failed attempted termination of pregnancy
　Hemolysis following failed attempted termination of pregnancy
　Intravascular coagulation following failed attempted termination of pregnancy

O07.2 Embolism following failed attempted termination of pregnancy M
　Air embolism following failed attempted termination of pregnancy
　Amniotic fluid embolism following failed attempted termination of pregnancy
　Blood-clot embolism following failed attempted termination of pregnancy
　Embolism NOS following failed attempted termination of pregnancy
　Fat embolism following failed attempted termination of pregnancy
　Pulmonary embolism following failed attempted termination of pregnancy
　Pyemic embolism following failed attempted termination of pregnancy
　Septic or septicopyemic embolism following failed attempted termination of pregnancy
　Soap embolism following failed attempted termination of pregnancy

✓5th **O07.3 Failed attempted termination of pregnancy with other and unspecified complications**
　O07.30 Failed attempted termination of pregnancy with unspecified complications M
　O07.31 Shock following failed attempted termination of pregnancy M
　　Circulatory collapse following failed attempted termination of pregnancy
　　Shock (postprocedural) following failed attempted termination of pregnancy
　　　EXCLUDES 1　shock due to infection following failed attempted termination of pregnancy (O07.37)
　O07.32 Renal failure following failed attempted termination of pregnancy M
　　Kidney failure (acute) following failed attempted termination of pregnancy
　　Oliguria following failed attempted termination of pregnancy
　　Renal shutdown following failed attempted termination of pregnancy
　　Renal tubular necrosis following failed attempted termination of pregnancy
　　Uremia following failed attempted termination of pregnancy
　O07.33 Metabolic disorder following failed attempted termination of pregnancy M
　O07.34 Damage to pelvic organs following failed attempted termination of pregnancy M
　　Laceration, perforation, tear or chemical damage of bladder following failed attempted termination of pregnancy
　　Laceration, perforation, tear or chemical damage of bowel following failed attempted termination of pregnancy
　　Laceration, perforation, tear or chemical damage of broad ligament following failed attempted termination of pregnancy
　　Laceration, perforation, tear or chemical damage of cervix following failed attempted termination of pregnancy
　　Laceration, perforation, tear or chemical damage of periurethral tissue following failed attempted termination of pregnancy
　　Laceration, perforation, tear or chemical damage of uterus following failed attempted termination of pregnancy
　　Laceration, perforation, tear or chemical damage of vagina following failed attempted termination of pregnancy
　O07.35 Other venous complications following failed attempted termination of pregnancy M
　O07.36 Cardiac arrest following failed attempted termination of pregnancy M
　O07.37 Sepsis following failed attempted termination of pregnancy M
　　Use additional code (B95-B97), to identify infectious agent
　　Use additional code (R65.2-) to identify severe sepsis, if applicable
　　　EXCLUDES 1　septic or septicopyemic embolism following failed attempted termination of pregnancy (O07.2)

HCC CMS-HCC　　Rx Rx HCC　　ESRD ESRD HCC　　COM Commercial HCC　　N Newborn: 0　　P Pediatric: 0-17　　M Maternity: 9-64　　A Adult: 15-124

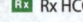

Chapter 15. Pregnancy, Childbirth and the Puerperium

O07.38 **Urinary tract infection** following failed attempted termination of pregnancy [M]
 Cystitis following failed attempted termination of pregnancy

O07.39 Failed attempted termination of pregnancy with other complications [M]

O07.4 Failed attempted termination of pregnancy without complication [M]

☑4th **O08** **Complications following ectopic and molar pregnancy**
 This category is for use with categories O00-O02 to identify any associated complications
 AHA: 2025,1Q,18

O08.0 **Genital tract and pelvic infection** following ectopic and molar pregnancy [COM] [M]
 Endometritis following ectopic and molar pregnancy
 Oophoritis following ectopic and molar pregnancy
 Parametritis following ectopic and molar pregnancy
 Pelvic peritonitis following ectopic and molar pregnancy
 Salpingitis following ectopic and molar pregnancy
 Salpingo-oophoritis following ectopic and molar pregnancy
 EXCLUDES 1 sepsis following ectopic and molar pregnancy (O08.82)
 urinary tract infection (O08.83)

O08.1 **Delayed or excessive hemorrhage** following ectopic and molar pregnancy [COM] [M]
 Afibrinogenemia following ectopic and molar pregnancy
 Defibrination syndrome following ectopic and molar pregnancy
 Hemolysis following ectopic and molar pregnancy
 Intravascular coagulation following ectopic and molar pregnancy
 EXCLUDES 1 delayed or excessive hemorrhage due to incomplete abortion (O03.1)

O08.2 **Embolism** following ectopic and molar pregnancy [COM] [M]
 Air embolism following ectopic and molar pregnancy
 Amniotic fluid embolism following ectopic and molar pregnancy
 Blood-clot embolism following ectopic and molar pregnancy
 Embolism NOS following ectopic and molar pregnancy
 Fat embolism following ectopic and molar pregnancy
 Pulmonary embolism following ectopic and molar pregnancy
 Pyemic embolism following ectopic and molar pregnancy
 Septic or septicopyemic embolism following ectopic and molar pregnancy
 Soap embolism following ectopic and molar pregnancy

O08.3 **Shock** following ectopic and molar pregnancy [COM] [M]
 Circulatory collapse following ectopic and molar pregnancy
 Shock (postprocedural) following ectopic and molar pregnancy
 EXCLUDES 1 shock due to infection following ectopic and molar pregnancy (O08.82)

O08.4 **Renal failure** following ectopic and molar pregnancy [COM] [M]
 Kidney failure (acute) following ectopic and molar pregnancy
 Oliguria following ectopic and molar pregnancy
 Renal shutdown following ectopic and molar pregnancy
 Renal tubular necrosis following ectopic and molar pregnancy
 Uremia following ectopic and molar pregnancy

O08.5 **Metabolic disorders** following an ectopic and molar pregnancy [COM] [M]

O08.6 **Damage to pelvic organs and tissues** following an ectopic and molar pregnancy [COM] [M]
 Laceration, perforation, tear or chemical damage of bladder following an ectopic and molar pregnancy
 Laceration, perforation, tear or chemical damage of bowel following an ectopic and molar pregnancy
 Laceration, perforation, tear or chemical damage of broad ligament following an ectopic and molar pregnancy
 Laceration, perforation, tear or chemical damage of cervix following an ectopic and molar pregnancy
 Laceration, perforation, tear or chemical damage of periurethral tissue following an ectopic and molar pregnancy
 Laceration, perforation, tear or chemical damage of uterus following an ectopic and molar pregnancy
 Laceration, perforation, tear or chemical damage of vagina following an ectopic and molar pregnancy

O08.7 Other venous complications following an ectopic and molar pregnancy [COM] [M]

☑5th **O08.8** Other complications following an ectopic and molar pregnancy
 O08.81 **Cardiac arrest** following an ectopic and molar pregnancy [COM] [M]

O08.82 **Sepsis** following ectopic and molar pregnancy [COM] [M]
 Use additional code (B95-B97), to identify infectious agent
 Use additional code (R65.2-) to identify severe sepsis, if applicable
 EXCLUDES 1 septic or septicopyemic embolism following ectopic and molar pregnancy (O08.2)

O08.83 **Urinary tract infection** following an ectopic and molar pregnancy [COM] [M]
 Cystitis following an ectopic and molar pregnancy

O08.89 Other complications following an ectopic and molar pregnancy [COM] [M]

O08.9 Unspecified complication following an ectopic and molar pregnancy [COM] [M]

Supervision of high risk pregnancy (O09)

☑4th **O09** **Supervision of high risk pregnancy**
 AHA: 2019,3Q,5; 2016,4Q,48-50,150

☑5th **O09.0** Supervision of pregnancy with **history of infertility**
 O09.00 Supervision of pregnancy with history of infertility, unspecified trimester [COM] [M]
 O09.01 Supervision of pregnancy with history of infertility, **first trimester** [COM] [M]
 O09.02 Supervision of pregnancy with history of infertility, **second trimester** [COM] [M]
 O09.03 Supervision of pregnancy with history of infertility, **third trimester** [COM] [M]

☑5th **O09.1** Supervision of pregnancy with **history of ectopic** pregnancy
 O09.10 Supervision of pregnancy with history of ectopic pregnancy, unspecified trimester [COM] [M]
 O09.11 Supervision of pregnancy with history of ectopic pregnancy, **first trimester** [COM] [M]
 O09.12 Supervision of pregnancy with history of ectopic pregnancy, **second trimester** [COM] [M]
 O09.13 Supervision of pregnancy with history of ectopic pregnancy, **third trimester** [COM] [M]

☑5th **O09.A** Supervision of pregnancy with **history of molar** pregnancy
 DEF: Molar pregnancy: Trophoblastic neoplasm that mimics pregnancy by proliferating from a pathologic ovum and resulting only in a mass of cysts resembling grapes, 80 percent of which are benign, but require surgical removal.
 O09.A0 Supervision of pregnancy with history of molar pregnancy, unspecified trimester [COM] [M]
 O09.A1 Supervision of pregnancy with history of molar pregnancy, **first trimester** [COM] [M]
 O09.A2 Supervision of pregnancy with history of molar pregnancy, **second trimester** [COM] [M]
 O09.A3 Supervision of pregnancy with history of molar pregnancy, **third trimester** [COM] [M]

☑5th **O09.2** Supervision of pregnancy with other poor reproductive or obstetric history
 EXCLUDES 2 pregnancy care for patient with history of recurrent pregnancy loss (O26.2-)

☑6th **O09.21** Supervision of pregnancy with history of **pre-term labor**
 O09.211 Supervision of pregnancy with history of pre-term labor, **first trimester** [COM] [M]
 O09.212 Supervision of pregnancy with history of pre-term labor, **second trimester** [COM] [M]
 O09.213 Supervision of pregnancy with history of pre-term labor, **third trimester** [COM] [M]
 O09.219 Supervision of pregnancy with history of pre-term labor, unspecified trimester [COM] [M]

☑6th **O09.29** Supervision of pregnancy with other poor reproductive or obstetric history
 Supervision of pregnancy with history of neonatal death
 Supervision of pregnancy with history of stillbirth
 O09.291 Supervision of pregnancy with other poor reproductive or obstetric history, **first trimester** [COM] [M]
 O09.292 Supervision of pregnancy with other poor reproductive or obstetric history, **second trimester** [COM] [M]
 O09.293 Supervision of pregnancy with other poor reproductive or obstetric history, **third trimester** [COM] [M]

Chapter 15. Pregnancy, Childbirth and the Puerperium

- **O09.299** Supervision of pregnancy with other poor reproductive or obstetric history, unspecified trimester [COM] [M]
- ✓5th **O09.3** Supervision of pregnancy with insufficient antenatal care
  - Supervision of concealed pregnancy
  - Supervision of hidden pregnancy
  - **O09.30** Supervision of pregnancy with insufficient antenatal care, unspecified trimester [COM] [M]
  - **O09.31** Supervision of pregnancy with insufficient antenatal care, first trimester [COM] [M]
  - **O09.32** Supervision of pregnancy with insufficient antenatal care, second trimester [COM] [M]
  - **O09.33** Supervision of pregnancy with insufficient antenatal care, third trimester [COM] [M]
- ✓5th **O09.4** Supervision of pregnancy with grand multiparity
  - **O09.40** Supervision of pregnancy with grand multiparity, unspecified trimester [COM] [M]
  - **O09.41** Supervision of pregnancy with grand multiparity, first trimester [COM] [M]
  - **O09.42** Supervision of pregnancy with grand multiparity, second trimester [COM] [M]
  - **O09.43** Supervision of pregnancy with grand multiparity, third trimester [COM] [M]
- ✓5th **O09.5** Supervision of elderly primigravida and multigravida
  - Pregnancy for a female 35 years and older at expected date of delivery
  - ✓6th **O09.51** Supervision of elderly primigravida
    - **O09.511** Supervision of elderly primigravida, first trimester [COM] [M]
    - **O09.512** Supervision of elderly primigravida, second trimester [COM] [M]
    - **O09.513** Supervision of elderly primigravida, third trimester [COM] [M]
    - **O09.519** Supervision of elderly primigravida, unspecified trimester [COM] [M]
  - ✓6th **O09.52** Supervision of elderly multigravida
    - **O09.521** Supervision of elderly multigravida, first trimester [COM] [M]
    - **O09.522** Supervision of elderly multigravida, second trimester [COM] [M]
    - **O09.523** Supervision of elderly multigravida, third trimester [COM] [M]
    - **O09.529** Supervision of elderly multigravida, unspecified trimester [COM] [M]
- ✓5th **O09.6** Supervision of young primigravida and multigravida
  - Supervision of pregnancy for a female less than 16 years old at expected date of delivery
  - ✓6th **O09.61** Supervision of young primigravida
    - **O09.611** Supervision of young primigravida, first trimester [COM] [M]
    - **O09.612** Supervision of young primigravida, second trimester [COM] [M]
    - **O09.613** Supervision of young primigravida, third trimester [COM] [M]
    - **O09.619** Supervision of young primigravida, unspecified trimester [COM] [M]
  - ✓6th **O09.62** Supervision of young multigravida
    - **O09.621** Supervision of young multigravida, first trimester [COM] [M]
    - **O09.622** Supervision of young multigravida, second trimester [COM] [M]
    - **O09.623** Supervision of young multigravida, third trimester [COM] [M]
    - **O09.629** Supervision of young multigravida, unspecified trimester [COM] [M]
- ✓5th **O09.7** Supervision of high risk pregnancy due to social problems
  - **O09.70** Supervision of high risk pregnancy due to social problems, unspecified trimester [COM] [M]
  - **O09.71** Supervision of high risk pregnancy due to social problems, first trimester [COM] [M]
  - **O09.72** Supervision of high risk pregnancy due to social problems, second trimester [COM] [M]
  - **O09.73** Supervision of high risk pregnancy due to social problems, third trimester [COM] [M]
- ✓5th **O09.8** Supervision of other high risk pregnancies
  - ✓6th **O09.81** Supervision of pregnancy resulting from assisted reproductive technology
    - Supervision of pregnancy resulting from in-vitro fertilization
    - EXCLUDES 2 gestational carrier status (Z33.3)
    - **O09.811** Supervision of pregnancy resulting from assisted reproductive technology, first trimester [COM] [M]
    - **O09.812** Supervision of pregnancy resulting from assisted reproductive technology, second trimester [COM] [M]
    - **O09.813** Supervision of pregnancy resulting from assisted reproductive technology, third trimester [COM] [M]
    - **O09.819** Supervision of pregnancy resulting from assisted reproductive technology, unspecified trimester [COM] [M]
  - ✓6th **O09.82** Supervision of pregnancy with history of in utero procedure during previous pregnancy
    - **O09.821** Supervision of pregnancy with history of in utero procedure during previous pregnancy, first trimester [COM] [M]
    - **O09.822** Supervision of pregnancy with history of in utero procedure during previous pregnancy, second trimester [COM] [M]
    - **O09.823** Supervision of pregnancy with history of in utero procedure during previous pregnancy, third trimester [COM] [M]
    - **O09.829** Supervision of pregnancy with history of in utero procedure during previous pregnancy, unspecified trimester [COM] [M]
      - EXCLUDES 1 supervision of pregnancy affected by in utero procedure during current pregnancy (O35.7)
  - ✓6th **O09.89** Supervision of other high risk pregnancies
    - **O09.891** Supervision of other high risk pregnancies, first trimester [COM] [M]
    - **O09.892** Supervision of other high risk pregnancies, second trimester [COM] [M]
    - **O09.893** Supervision of other high risk pregnancies, third trimester [COM] [M]
    - **O09.899** Supervision of other high risk pregnancies, unspecified trimester [COM] [M]
- ✓5th **O09.9** Supervision of high risk pregnancy, unspecified
  - **O09.90** Supervision of high risk pregnancy, unspecified, unspecified trimester [COM] [M]
  - **O09.91** Supervision of high risk pregnancy, unspecified, first trimester [COM] [M]
  - **O09.92** Supervision of high risk pregnancy, unspecified, second trimester [COM] [M]
  - **O09.93** Supervision of high risk pregnancy, unspecified, third trimester [COM] [M]

Edema, proteinuria and hypertensive disorders in pregnancy, childbirth and the puerperium (O10-O16)

AHA: 2016,4Q,50

- ✓4th **O10** Pre-existing hypertension complicating pregnancy, childbirth and the puerperium
  - INCLUDES pre-existing hypertension with pre-existing proteinuria complicating pregnancy, childbirth and the puerperium
  - EXCLUDES 2 pre-existing hypertension with superimposed pre-eclampsia complicating pregnancy, childbirth and the puerperium (O11.-)
  - **AHA:** 2025,2Q,17
  - ✓5th **O10.0** Pre-existing essential hypertension complicating pregnancy, childbirth and the puerperium
    - Any condition in I10 specified as a reason for obstetric care during pregnancy, childbirth or the puerperium
    - ✓6th **O10.01** Pre-existing essential hypertension complicating pregnancy
      - **O10.011** Pre-existing essential hypertension complicating pregnancy, first trimester [COM] [M]
      - **O10.012** Pre-existing essential hypertension complicating pregnancy, second trimester [COM] [M]

Chapter 15. Pregnancy, Childbirth and the Puerperium

- O10.013 Pre-existing essential hypertension complicating pregnancy, third trimester [COM] [M]
- O10.019 Pre-existing essential hypertension complicating pregnancy, unspecified trimester [COM] [M]
- O10.02 Pre-existing essential hypertension complicating childbirth [COM] [M]
- O10.03 Pre-existing essential hypertension complicating the puerperium [COM] [M]
- ✓5th O10.1 Pre-existing hypertensive heart disease complicating pregnancy, childbirth and the puerperium
  - Any condition in I11 specified as a reason for obstetric care during pregnancy, childbirth or the puerperium
  - Use additional code from I11 to identify the type of hypertensive heart disease
  - ✓6th O10.11 Pre-existing hypertensive heart disease complicating pregnancy
    - O10.111 Pre-existing hypertensive heart disease complicating pregnancy, first trimester [COM] [M]
    - O10.112 Pre-existing hypertensive heart disease complicating pregnancy, second trimester [COM] [M]
    - O10.113 Pre-existing hypertensive heart disease complicating pregnancy, third trimester [COM] [M]
    - O10.119 Pre-existing hypertensive heart disease complicating pregnancy, unspecified trimester [COM] [M]
  - O10.12 Pre-existing hypertensive heart disease complicating childbirth [COM] [M]
  - O10.13 Pre-existing hypertensive heart disease complicating the puerperium [COM] [M]
- ✓5th O10.2 Pre-existing hypertensive chronic kidney disease complicating pregnancy, childbirth and the puerperium
  - Any condition in I12 specified as a reason for obstetric care during pregnancy, childbirth or the puerperium
  - Use additional code from I12 to identify the type of hypertensive chronic kidney disease
  - ✓6th O10.21 Pre-existing hypertensive chronic kidney disease complicating pregnancy
    - O10.211 Pre-existing hypertensive chronic kidney disease complicating pregnancy, first trimester [COM] [M]
    - O10.212 Pre-existing hypertensive chronic kidney disease complicating pregnancy, second trimester [COM] [M]
    - O10.213 Pre-existing hypertensive chronic kidney disease complicating pregnancy, third trimester [COM] [M]
    - O10.219 Pre-existing hypertensive chronic kidney disease complicating pregnancy, unspecified trimester [COM] [M]
  - O10.22 Pre-existing hypertensive chronic kidney disease complicating childbirth [COM] [M]
  - O10.23 Pre-existing hypertensive chronic kidney disease complicating the puerperium [COM] [M]
- ✓5th O10.3 Pre-existing hypertensive heart and chronic kidney disease complicating pregnancy, childbirth and the puerperium
  - Any condition in I13 specified as a reason for obstetric care during pregnancy, childbirth or the puerperium
  - Use additional code from I13 to identify the type of hypertensive heart and chronic kidney disease
  - ✓6th O10.31 Pre-existing hypertensive heart and chronic kidney disease complicating pregnancy
    - O10.311 Pre-existing hypertensive heart and chronic kidney disease complicating pregnancy, first trimester [COM] [M]
    - O10.312 Pre-existing hypertensive heart and chronic kidney disease complicating pregnancy, second trimester [COM] [M]
    - O10.313 Pre-existing hypertensive heart and chronic kidney disease complicating pregnancy, third trimester [COM] [M]
    - O10.319 Pre-existing hypertensive heart and chronic kidney disease complicating pregnancy, unspecified trimester [COM] [M]
  - O10.32 Pre-existing hypertensive heart and chronic kidney disease complicating childbirth [COM] [M]
  - O10.33 Pre-existing hypertensive heart and chronic kidney disease complicating the puerperium [COM] [M]
- ✓5th O10.4 Pre-existing secondary hypertension complicating pregnancy, childbirth and the puerperium
  - Any condition in I15 specified as a reason for obstetric care during pregnancy, childbirth or the puerperium
  - Use additional code from I15 to identify the type of secondary hypertension
  - ✓6th O10.41 Pre-existing secondary hypertension complicating pregnancy
    - O10.411 Pre-existing secondary hypertension complicating pregnancy, first trimester [COM] [M]
    - O10.412 Pre-existing secondary hypertension complicating pregnancy, second trimester [COM] [M]
    - O10.413 Pre-existing secondary hypertension complicating pregnancy, third trimester [COM] [M]
    - O10.419 Pre-existing secondary hypertension complicating pregnancy, unspecified trimester [COM] [M]
  - O10.42 Pre-existing secondary hypertension complicating childbirth [COM] [M]
  - O10.43 Pre-existing secondary hypertension complicating the puerperium [COM] [M]
- ✓5th O10.9 Unspecified pre-existing hypertension complicating pregnancy, childbirth and the puerperium
  - ✓6th O10.91 Unspecified pre-existing hypertension complicating pregnancy
    - **AHA:** 2025,2Q,17
    - O10.911 Unspecified pre-existing hypertension complicating pregnancy, first trimester [COM] [M]
    - O10.912 Unspecified pre-existing hypertension complicating pregnancy, second trimester [COM] [M]
    - O10.913 Unspecified pre-existing hypertension complicating pregnancy, third trimester [COM] [M]
    - O10.919 Unspecified pre-existing hypertension complicating pregnancy, unspecified trimester [COM] [M]
  - O10.92 Unspecified pre-existing hypertension complicating childbirth [COM] [M]
  - O10.93 Unspecified pre-existing hypertension complicating the puerperium [COM] [M]
- ✓4th O11 Pre-existing hypertension with pre-eclampsia
  - INCLUDES conditions in O10 complicated by pre-eclampsia
  - pre-eclampsia superimposed pre-existing in hypertension
  - Use additional code from O10 to identify the type of hypertension
  - **DEF:** Complication of pregnancy manifesting in the development of borderline hypertension, protein in the urine, and unresponsive swelling between the 20th week of pregnancy and the end of the first week following birth in mild to moderate cases. Severe preeclampsia presents with hypertension, associated with marked swelling, proteinuria, abdominal pain, and/or visual changes.
  - O11.1 Pre-existing hypertension with pre-eclampsia, first trimester [COM] [M]
  - O11.2 Pre-existing hypertension with pre-eclampsia, second trimester [COM] [M]
  - O11.3 Pre-existing hypertension with pre-eclampsia, third trimester [COM] [M]
  - O11.4 Pre-existing hypertension with pre-eclampsia, complicating childbirth [COM] [M]
  - O11.5 Pre-existing hypertension with pre-eclampsia, complicating the puerperium [COM] [M]
  - O11.9 Pre-existing hypertension with pre-eclampsia, unspecified trimester [COM] [M]
- ✓4th O12 Gestational [pregnancy-induced] edema and proteinuria without hypertension
  - ✓5th O12.0 Gestational edema
    - O12.00 Gestational edema, unspecified trimester [COM] [M]
    - O12.01 Gestational edema, first trimester [COM] [M]
    - O12.02 Gestational edema, second trimester [COM] [M]
    - O12.03 Gestational edema, third trimester [COM] [M]
    - O12.04 Gestational edema, complicating childbirth [COM] [M]
    - O12.05 Gestational edema, complicating the puerperium [COM] [M]

☑ Additional Character Required ✓x7th Placeholder Alert Manifestation Unspecified Dx Q QPP UPD Unacceptable PDx

O12.1 Gestational proteinuria
- **O12.10** Gestational proteinuria, unspecified trimester
- **O12.11** Gestational proteinuria, first trimester
- **O12.12** Gestational proteinuria, second trimester
- **O12.13** Gestational proteinuria, third trimester
- **O12.14** Gestational proteinuria, complicating childbirth
- **O12.15** Gestational proteinuria, complicating the puerperium

O12.2 Gestational edema with proteinuria
- **O12.20** Gestational edema with proteinuria, unspecified trimester
- **O12.21** Gestational edema with proteinuria, first trimester
- **O12.22** Gestational edema with proteinuria, second trimester
- **O12.23** Gestational edema with proteinuria, third trimester
- **O12.24** Gestational edema with proteinuria, complicating childbirth
- **O12.25** Gestational edema with proteinuria, complicating the puerperium

O13 Gestational [pregnancy-induced] hypertension without significant proteinuria
INCLUDES gestational hypertension NOS
transient hypertension of pregnancy
AHA: 2016,1Q,5

- **O13.1** Gestational [pregnancy-induced] hypertension without significant proteinuria, first trimester
- **O13.2** Gestational [pregnancy-induced] hypertension without significant proteinuria, second trimester
- **O13.3** Gestational [pregnancy-induced] hypertension without significant proteinuria, third trimester
- **O13.4** Gestational [pregnancy-induced] hypertension without significant proteinuria, complicating childbirth
- **O13.5** Gestational [pregnancy-induced] hypertension without significant proteinuria, complicating the puerperium
- **O13.9** Gestational [pregnancy-induced] hypertension without significant proteinuria, unspecified trimester

O14 Pre-eclampsia
EXCLUDES 1 pre-existing hypertension with pre-eclampsia (O11)
DEF: Complication of pregnancy manifesting in the development of borderline hypertension, protein in the urine, and unresponsive swelling between the 20th week of pregnancy and the end of the first week following birth in mild to moderate cases. Severe preeclampsia presents with hypertension, associated with marked swelling, proteinuria, abdominal pain, and/or visual changes.

O14.0 Mild to moderate pre-eclampsia
AHA: 2019,3Q,12; 2019,2Q,8
- **O14.00** Mild to moderate pre-eclampsia, unspecified trimester
- **O14.02** Mild to moderate pre-eclampsia, second trimester
- **O14.03** Mild to moderate pre-eclampsia, third trimester
- **O14.04** Mild to moderate pre-eclampsia, complicating childbirth
  AHA: 2019,2Q,8
- **O14.05** Mild to moderate pre-eclampsia, complicating the puerperium

O14.1 Severe pre-eclampsia
EXCLUDES 1 HELLP syndrome (O14.2-)
AHA: 2019,3Q,12
- **O14.10** Severe pre-eclampsia, unspecified trimester
- **O14.12** Severe pre-eclampsia, second trimester
- **O14.13** Severe pre-eclampsia, third trimester
- **O14.14** Severe pre-eclampsia complicating childbirth
- **O14.15** Severe pre-eclampsia, complicating the puerperium

O14.2 HELLP syndrome
Severe pre-eclampsia with hemolysis, elevated liver enzymes and low platelet count (HELLP)
AHA: 2019,3Q,12
- **O14.20** HELLP syndrome (HELLP), unspecified trimester
- **O14.22** HELLP syndrome (HELLP), second trimester
- **O14.23** HELLP syndrome (HELLP), third trimester
- **O14.24** HELLP syndrome, complicating childbirth
- **O14.25** HELLP syndrome, complicating the puerperium

O14.9 Unspecified pre-eclampsia
- **O14.90** Unspecified pre-eclampsia, unspecified trimester
- **O14.92** Unspecified pre-eclampsia, second trimester
- **O14.93** Unspecified pre-eclampsia, third trimester
- **O14.94** Unspecified pre-eclampsia, complicating childbirth
- **O14.95** Unspecified pre-eclampsia, complicating the puerperium

O15 Eclampsia
INCLUDES convulsions following conditions in O10-O14 and O16
DEF: Tetany and toxemia producing seizure activity or coma in a pregnant patient who most often has presented with prior preeclampsia (i.e., hypertension, albuminuria, and edema).

O15.0 Eclampsia complicating pregnancy
- **O15.00** Eclampsia complicating pregnancy, unspecified trimester
- **O15.02** Eclampsia complicating pregnancy, second trimester
- **O15.03** Eclampsia complicating pregnancy, third trimester
- **O15.1** Eclampsia complicating labor
- **O15.2** Eclampsia complicating the puerperium
- **O15.9** Eclampsia, unspecified as to time period
  Eclampsia NOS

O16 Unspecified maternal hypertension
- **O16.1** Unspecified maternal hypertension, first trimester
- **O16.2** Unspecified maternal hypertension, second trimester
- **O16.3** Unspecified maternal hypertension, third trimester
- **O16.4** Unspecified maternal hypertension, complicating childbirth
- **O16.5** Unspecified maternal hypertension, complicating the puerperium
- **O16.9** Unspecified maternal hypertension, unspecified trimester

Other maternal disorders predominantly related to pregnancy (O20-O29)

EXCLUDES 2 maternal care related to the fetus and amniotic cavity and possible delivery problems (O30-O48)
maternal diseases classifiable elsewhere but complicating pregnancy, labor and delivery, and the puerperium (O98-O99)

O20 Hemorrhage in early pregnancy
INCLUDES hemorrhage before completion of 20 weeks gestation
EXCLUDES 1 pregnancy with abortive outcome (O00-O08)

- **O20.0** Threatened abortion
  Hemorrhage specified as due to threatened abortion
  DEF: Bloody discharge during pregnancy. The cervix may be dilated and pregnancy threatened, but the pregnancy is not terminated.
- **O20.8** Other hemorrhage in early pregnancy
  AHA: 2023,3Q,18
- **O20.9** Hemorrhage in early pregnancy, unspecified

O21 Excessive vomiting in pregnancy
- **O21.0** Mild hyperemesis gravidarum
  Hyperemesis gravidarum, mild or unspecified, starting before the end of the 20th week of gestation

Chapter 15. Pregnancy, Childbirth and the Puerperium

O21.1 **Hyperemesis gravidarum with metabolic disturbance** [COM] [M]
- Hyperemesis gravidarum, starting before the end of the 20th week of gestation, with metabolic disturbance such as carbohydrate depletion
- Hyperemesis gravidarum, starting before the end of the 20th week of gestation, with metabolic disturbance such as dehydration
- Hyperemesis gravidarum, starting before the end of the 20th week of gestation, with metabolic disturbance such as electrolyte imbalance

O21.2 **Late vomiting of pregnancy** [COM] [M]
- Excessive vomiting starting after 20 completed weeks of gestation

O21.8 **Other vomiting complicating pregnancy** [COM] [M]
- Vomiting due to diseases classified elsewhere, complicating pregnancy
- Use additional code, to identify cause

O21.9 **Vomiting of pregnancy, unspecified** [COM] [M]

O22 **Venous complications and hemorrhoids in pregnancy**
- EXCLUDES 1: venous complications of:
  - abortion NOS (O03.9)
  - ectopic or molar pregnancy (O08.7)
  - failed attempted abortion (O07.35)
  - induced abortion (O04.85)
  - spontaneous abortion (O03.89)
- EXCLUDES 2: obstetric pulmonary embolism (O88.-)
  - venous complications and hemorrhoids of childbirth and the puerperium (O87.-)

O22.0 **Varicose veins of lower extremity in pregnancy**
- Varicose veins NOS in pregnancy
- DEF: Distended, tortuous veins of the lower extremities associated with pregnancy.
  - **O22.00** Varicose veins of lower extremity in pregnancy, unspecified trimester [COM] [M]
  - **O22.01** Varicose veins of lower extremity in pregnancy, first trimester [COM] [M]
  - **O22.02** Varicose veins of lower extremity in pregnancy, second trimester [COM] [M]
  - **O22.03** Varicose veins of lower extremity in pregnancy, third trimester [COM] [M]

O22.1 **Genital varices in pregnancy**
- Perineal varices in pregnancy
- Vaginal varices in pregnancy
- Vulval varices in pregnancy
  - **O22.10** Genital varices in pregnancy, unspecified trimester [COM] [M]
  - **O22.11** Genital varices in pregnancy, first trimester [COM] [M]
  - **O22.12** Genital varices in pregnancy, second trimester [COM] [M]
  - **O22.13** Genital varices in pregnancy, third trimester [COM] [M]

O22.2 **Superficial thrombophlebitis in pregnancy**
- Phlebitis in pregnancy NOS
- Thrombophlebitis of legs in pregnancy
- Thrombosis in pregnancy NOS
- Use additional code to identify the superficial thrombophlebitis (I80.0-)
  - **O22.20** Superficial thrombophlebitis in pregnancy, unspecified trimester [COM] [M]
  - **O22.21** Superficial thrombophlebitis in pregnancy, first trimester [COM] [M]
  - **O22.22** Superficial thrombophlebitis in pregnancy, second trimester [COM] [M]
  - **O22.23** Superficial thrombophlebitis in pregnancy, third trimester [COM] [M]

O22.3 **Deep phlebothrombosis in pregnancy**
- Deep vein thrombosis, antepartum
- Use additional code to identify the deep vein thrombosis (I82.4-, I82.5-, I82.62-, I82.72-)
- Use additional code, if applicable, for associated long-term (current) use of anticoagulants (Z79.01)
  - **O22.30** Deep phlebothrombosis in pregnancy, unspecified trimester [COM] [M]
  - **O22.31** Deep phlebothrombosis in pregnancy, first trimester [COM] [M]
  - **O22.32** Deep phlebothrombosis in pregnancy, second trimester [COM] [M]
  - **O22.33** Deep phlebothrombosis in pregnancy, third trimester [COM] [M]

O22.4 **Hemorrhoids in pregnancy**
- **O22.40** Hemorrhoids in pregnancy, unspecified trimester [COM] [M]
- **O22.41** Hemorrhoids in pregnancy, first trimester [COM] [M]
- **O22.42** Hemorrhoids in pregnancy, second trimester [COM] [M]
- **O22.43** Hemorrhoids in pregnancy, third trimester [COM] [M]

O22.5 **Cerebral venous thrombosis in pregnancy**
- Cerebrovenous sinus thrombosis in pregnancy
  - **O22.50** Cerebral venous thrombosis in pregnancy, unspecified trimester [COM] [M]
  - **O22.51** Cerebral venous thrombosis in pregnancy, first trimester [COM] [M]
  - **O22.52** Cerebral venous thrombosis in pregnancy, second trimester [COM] [M]
  - **O22.53** Cerebral venous thrombosis in pregnancy, third trimester [COM] [M]

O22.8 **Other venous complications in pregnancy**
- **O22.8X** Other venous complications in pregnancy
  - **O22.8X1** Other venous complications in pregnancy, first trimester [COM] [M]
  - **O22.8X2** Other venous complications in pregnancy, second trimester [COM] [M]
  - **O22.8X3** Other venous complications in pregnancy, third trimester [COM] [M]
  - **O22.8X9** Other venous complications in pregnancy, unspecified trimester [COM] [M]

O22.9 **Venous complication in pregnancy, unspecified**
- Gestational phlebitis NOS
- Gestational phlebopathy NOS
- Gestational thrombosis NOS
  - **O22.90** Venous complication in pregnancy, unspecified, unspecified trimester [COM] [M]
  - **O22.91** Venous complication in pregnancy, unspecified, first trimester [COM] [M]
  - **O22.92** Venous complication in pregnancy, unspecified, second trimester [COM] [M]
  - **O22.93** Venous complication in pregnancy, unspecified, third trimester [COM] [M]

O23 **Infections of genitourinary tract in pregnancy**
- Use additional code to identify organism (B95.-, B96.-)
- EXCLUDES 2: gonococcal infections complicating pregnancy, childbirth and the puerperium (O98.2)
  - infections with a predominantly sexual mode of transmission NOS complicating pregnancy, childbirth and the puerperium (O98.3)
  - syphilis complicating pregnancy, childbirth and the puerperium (O98.1)
  - tuberculosis of genitourinary system complicating pregnancy, childbirth and the puerperium (O98.0)
  - venereal disease NOS complicating pregnancy, childbirth and the puerperium (O98.3)
- AHA: 2018,2Q,20

O23.0 **Infections of kidney in pregnancy**
- Pyelonephritis in pregnancy
  - **O23.00** Infections of kidney in pregnancy, unspecified trimester [COM] [M]
  - **O23.01** Infections of kidney in pregnancy, first trimester [COM] [M]
  - **O23.02** Infections of kidney in pregnancy, second trimester [COM] [M]
  - **O23.03** Infections of kidney in pregnancy, third trimester [COM] [M]

O23.1 **Infections of bladder in pregnancy**
- **O23.10** Infections of bladder in pregnancy, unspecified trimester [COM] [M]
- **O23.11** Infections of bladder in pregnancy, first trimester [COM] [M]
- **O23.12** Infections of bladder in pregnancy, second trimester [COM] [M]
- **O23.13** Infections of bladder in pregnancy, third trimester [COM] [M]

O23.2 **Infections of urethra in pregnancy**
- **O23.20** Infections of urethra in pregnancy, unspecified trimester [COM] [M]

Chapter 15. Pregnancy, Childbirth and the Puerperium

- **O23.21** Infections of urethra in pregnancy, first trimester
- **O23.22** Infections of urethra in pregnancy, second trimester
- **O23.23** Infections of urethra in pregnancy, third trimester
- **O23.3** Infections of other parts of urinary tract in pregnancy
  - **O23.30** Infections of other parts of urinary tract in pregnancy, unspecified trimester
  - **O23.31** Infections of other parts of urinary tract in pregnancy, first trimester
  - **O23.32** Infections of other parts of urinary tract in pregnancy, second trimester
  - **O23.33** Infections of other parts of urinary tract in pregnancy, third trimester
- **O23.4** Unspecified infection of urinary tract in pregnancy
  - **O23.40** Unspecified infection of urinary tract in pregnancy, unspecified trimester
  - **O23.41** Unspecified infection of urinary tract in pregnancy, first trimester
  - **O23.42** Unspecified infection of urinary tract in pregnancy, second trimester
  - **O23.43** Unspecified infection of urinary tract in pregnancy, third trimester
- **O23.5** Infections of the genital tract in pregnancy
  - **O23.51** Infection of cervix in pregnancy
    - **O23.511** Infections of cervix in pregnancy, first trimester
    - **O23.512** Infections of cervix in pregnancy, second trimester
    - **O23.513** Infections of cervix in pregnancy, third trimester
    - **O23.519** Infections of cervix in pregnancy, unspecified trimester
  - **O23.52** Salpingo-oophoritis in pregnancy
    - Oophoritis in pregnancy
    - Salpingitis in pregnancy
    - **O23.521** Salpingo-oophoritis in pregnancy, first trimester
    - **O23.522** Salpingo-oophoritis in pregnancy, second trimester
    - **O23.523** Salpingo-oophoritis in pregnancy, third trimester
    - **O23.529** Salpingo-oophoritis in pregnancy, unspecified trimester
  - **O23.59** Infection of other part of genital tract in pregnancy
    - **AHA:** 2025,1Q,22; 2022,1Q,20
    - **O23.591** Infection of other part of genital tract in pregnancy, first trimester
    - **O23.592** Infection of other part of genital tract in pregnancy, second trimester
    - **O23.593** Infection of other part of genital tract in pregnancy, third trimester
    - **O23.599** Infection of other part of genital tract in pregnancy, unspecified trimester
- **O23.9** Unspecified genitourinary tract infection in pregnancy
  - Genitourinary tract infection in pregnancy NOS
  - **AHA:** 2025,1Q,22
  - **O23.90** Unspecified genitourinary tract infection in pregnancy, unspecified trimester
  - **O23.91** Unspecified genitourinary tract infection in pregnancy, first trimester
  - **O23.92** Unspecified genitourinary tract infection in pregnancy, second trimester
  - **O23.93** Unspecified genitourinary tract infection in pregnancy, third trimester

- **O24** Diabetes mellitus in pregnancy, childbirth and the puerperium
  - **O24.0** Pre-existing type 1 diabetes mellitus, in pregnancy, childbirth and the puerperium
    - Juvenile onset diabetes mellitus, in pregnancy, childbirth and the puerperium
    - Ketosis-prone diabetes mellitus in pregnancy, childbirth and the puerperium
    - Use additional code from category E10 to further identify any manifestations
    - **O24.01** Pre-existing type 1 diabetes mellitus, in pregnancy
      - **O24.011** Pre-existing type 1 diabetes mellitus, in pregnancy, first trimester
      - **O24.012** Pre-existing type 1 diabetes mellitus, in pregnancy, second trimester
      - **O24.013** Pre-existing type 1 diabetes mellitus, in pregnancy, third trimester
      - **O24.019** Pre-existing type 1 diabetes mellitus, in pregnancy, unspecified trimester
    - **O24.02** Pre-existing type 1 diabetes mellitus, in childbirth
    - **O24.03** Pre-existing type 1 diabetes mellitus, in the puerperium
  - **O24.1** Pre-existing type 2 diabetes mellitus, in pregnancy, childbirth and the puerperium
    - Insulin-resistant diabetes mellitus in pregnancy, childbirth and the puerperium
    - Use additional code (for):
      - from category E11 to further identify any manifestations
      - injectable non-insulin antidiabetic drugs (Z79.85)
      - long-term (current) use of insulin (Z79.4)
    - **O24.11** Pre-existing type 2 diabetes mellitus, in pregnancy
      - **O24.111** Pre-existing type 2 diabetes mellitus, in pregnancy, first trimester
      - **O24.112** Pre-existing type 2 diabetes mellitus, in pregnancy, second trimester
      - **O24.113** Pre-existing type 2 diabetes mellitus, in pregnancy, third trimester
      - **O24.119** Pre-existing type 2 diabetes mellitus, in pregnancy, unspecified trimester
    - **O24.12** Pre-existing type 2 diabetes mellitus, in childbirth
    - **O24.13** Pre-existing type 2 diabetes mellitus, in the puerperium
  - **O24.3** Unspecified pre-existing diabetes mellitus in pregnancy, childbirth and the puerperium
    - Use additional code (for):
      - from category E11 to further identify any manifestation
      - injectable non-insulin antidiabetic drugs (Z79.85)
      - long-term (current) use of insulin (Z79.4)
    - **O24.31** Unspecified pre-existing diabetes mellitus in pregnancy
      - **O24.311** Unspecified pre-existing diabetes mellitus in pregnancy, first trimester
      - **O24.312** Unspecified pre-existing diabetes mellitus in pregnancy, second trimester
      - **O24.313** Unspecified pre-existing diabetes mellitus in pregnancy, third trimester
      - **O24.319** Unspecified pre-existing diabetes mellitus in pregnancy, unspecified trimester
    - **O24.32** Unspecified pre-existing diabetes mellitus in childbirth
    - **O24.33** Unspecified pre-existing diabetes mellitus in the puerperium
  - **O24.4** Gestational diabetes mellitus
    - Diabetes mellitus arising in pregnancy
    - Gestational diabetes mellitus NOS
    - **AHA:** 2020,3Q,30; 2016,4Q,50; 2015,4Q,34
    - **O24.41** Gestational diabetes mellitus in pregnancy
      - **O24.410** Gestational diabetes mellitus in pregnancy, diet controlled
      - **O24.414** Gestational diabetes mellitus in pregnancy, insulin controlled

Chapter 15. Pregnancy, Childbirth and the Puerperium

- **O24.415** Gestational diabetes mellitus in pregnancy, controlled by oral hypoglycemic drugs
  - Gestational diabetes mellitus in pregnancy, controlled by oral antidiabetic drugs
- **O24.419** Gestational diabetes mellitus in pregnancy, unspecified control
- ✓6th **O24.42** Gestational diabetes mellitus in childbirth
  - AHA: 2016, 1Q, 5
  - **O24.420** Gestational diabetes mellitus in childbirth, diet controlled
  - **O24.424** Gestational diabetes mellitus in childbirth, insulin controlled
  - **O24.425** Gestational diabetes mellitus in childbirth, controlled by oral hypoglycemic drugs
    - Gestational diabetes mellitus in childbirth, controlled by oral antidiabetic drugs
  - **O24.429** Gestational diabetes mellitus in childbirth, unspecified control
- ✓6th **O24.43** Gestational diabetes mellitus in the puerperium
  - **O24.430** Gestational diabetes mellitus in the puerperium, diet controlled
  - **O24.434** Gestational diabetes mellitus in the puerperium, insulin controlled
  - **O24.435** Gestational diabetes mellitus in puerperium, controlled by oral hypoglycemic drugs
    - Gestational diabetes mellitus in puerperium, controlled by oral antidiabetic drugs
  - **O24.439** Gestational diabetes mellitus in the puerperium, unspecified control
- ✓5th **O24.8** Other pre-existing diabetes mellitus in pregnancy, childbirth, and the puerperium
  - Use additional code (for):
    - from categories E08, E09 and E13 to further identify any manifestation
    - injectable non-insulin antidiabetic drugs (Z79.85)
    - long-term (current) use of insulin (Z79.4)
  - ✓6th **O24.81** Other pre-existing diabetes mellitus in pregnancy
    - **O24.811** Other pre-existing diabetes mellitus in pregnancy, first trimester
    - **O24.812** Other pre-existing diabetes mellitus in pregnancy, second trimester
    - **O24.813** Other pre-existing diabetes mellitus in pregnancy, third trimester
    - **O24.819** Other pre-existing diabetes mellitus in pregnancy, unspecified trimester
  - **O24.82** Other pre-existing diabetes mellitus in childbirth
  - **O24.83** Other pre-existing diabetes mellitus in the puerperium
- ✓5th **O24.9** Unspecified diabetes mellitus in pregnancy, childbirth and the puerperium
  - Use additional code (for):
    - from categories E08, E09 and E13 to further identify any manifestation
    - injectable non-insulin antidiabetic drugs (Z79.85)
    - long-term (current) use of insulin (Z79.4)
  - ✓6th **O24.91** Unspecified diabetes mellitus in pregnancy
    - **O24.911** Unspecified diabetes mellitus in pregnancy, first trimester
    - **O24.912** Unspecified diabetes mellitus in pregnancy, second trimester
    - **O24.913** Unspecified diabetes mellitus in pregnancy, third trimester
    - **O24.919** Unspecified diabetes mellitus in pregnancy, unspecified trimester
  - **O24.92** Unspecified diabetes mellitus in childbirth
  - **O24.93** Unspecified diabetes mellitus in the puerperium
- ✓4th **O25** Malnutrition in pregnancy, childbirth and the puerperium
  - ✓5th **O25.1** Malnutrition in pregnancy
    - **O25.10** Malnutrition in pregnancy, unspecified trimester
    - **O25.11** Malnutrition in pregnancy, first trimester
    - **O25.12** Malnutrition in pregnancy, second trimester
    - **O25.13** Malnutrition in pregnancy, third trimester
  - **O25.2** Malnutrition in childbirth
  - **O25.3** Malnutrition in the puerperium
- ✓4th **O26** Maternal care for other conditions predominantly related to pregnancy
  - ✓5th **O26.0** Excessive weight gain in pregnancy
    - EXCLUDES 2 gestational edema (O12.0, O12.2)
    - **O26.00** Excessive weight gain in pregnancy, unspecified trimester
    - **O26.01** Excessive weight gain in pregnancy, first trimester
    - **O26.02** Excessive weight gain in pregnancy, second trimester
    - **O26.03** Excessive weight gain in pregnancy, third trimester
  - ✓5th **O26.1** Low weight gain in pregnancy
    - **O26.10** Low weight gain in pregnancy, unspecified trimester
    - **O26.11** Low weight gain in pregnancy, first trimester
    - **O26.12** Low weight gain in pregnancy, second trimester
    - **O26.13** Low weight gain in pregnancy, third trimester
  - ✓5th **O26.2** Pregnancy care for patient with recurrent pregnancy loss
    - **O26.20** Pregnancy care for patient with recurrent pregnancy loss, unspecified trimester
    - **O26.21** Pregnancy care for patient with recurrent pregnancy loss, first trimester
    - **O26.22** Pregnancy care for patient with recurrent pregnancy loss, second trimester
    - **O26.23** Pregnancy care for patient with recurrent pregnancy loss, third trimester
  - ✓5th **O26.3** Retained intrauterine contraceptive device in pregnancy
    - **O26.30** Retained intrauterine contraceptive device in pregnancy, unspecified trimester
    - **O26.31** Retained intrauterine contraceptive device in pregnancy, first trimester
    - **O26.32** Retained intrauterine contraceptive device in pregnancy, second trimester
    - **O26.33** Retained intrauterine contraceptive device in pregnancy, third trimester
  - ✓5th **O26.4** Herpes gestationis
    - DEF: Rare skin disorder of unknown origin that appears on the abdomen in the second and third trimester as intensely itchy blisters that spread to other sites.
    - **O26.40** Herpes gestationis, unspecified trimester
    - **O26.41** Herpes gestationis, first trimester
    - **O26.42** Herpes gestationis, second trimester
    - **O26.43** Herpes gestationis, third trimester
  - ✓5th **O26.5** Maternal hypotension syndrome
    - Supine hypotensive syndrome
    - **O26.50** Maternal hypotension syndrome, unspecified trimester
    - **O26.51** Maternal hypotension syndrome, first trimester
    - **O26.52** Maternal hypotension syndrome, second trimester
    - **O26.53** Maternal hypotension syndrome, third trimester
  - ✓5th **O26.6** Liver and biliary tract disorders in pregnancy, childbirth and the puerperium
    - Use additional code to identify the specific disorder
    - EXCLUDES 2 hepatorenal syndrome following labor and delivery (O90.41)
    - ✓6th **O26.61** Liver and biliary tract disorders in pregnancy
      - **O26.611** Liver and biliary tract disorders in pregnancy, first trimester
      - **O26.612** Liver and biliary tract disorders in pregnancy, second trimester
      - **O26.613** Liver and biliary tract disorders in pregnancy, third trimester

---

✓ Additional Character Required   ✓x7th Placeholder Alert   Manifestation   Unspecified Dx   Q QPP   UPD Unacceptable PDx

- **O26.619** Liver and biliary tract disorders in pregnancy, unspecified trimester [COM] [M]
- **O26.62** Liver and biliary tract disorders in **childbirth** [COM] [M]
  - AHA: 2023,1Q,26
- **O26.63** Liver and biliary tract disorders in the **puerperium** [COM] [M]
- ✓6th **O26.64** Intrahepatic cholestasis of **pregnancy**
  - ▶Use additional code for hepatic obstruction (K76.89)◀
  - AHA: 2023,4Q,36-37
  - **O26.641** Intrahepatic cholestasis of pregnancy, **first trimester** [COM] [M]
  - **O26.642** Intrahepatic cholestasis of pregnancy, **second trimester** [COM] [M]
  - **O26.643** Intrahepatic cholestasis of pregnancy, **third trimester** [COM] [M]
  - **O26.649** Intrahepatic cholestasis of pregnancy, unspecified trimester [COM] [M]
- ✓5th **O26.7** Subluxation of symphysis (pubis) in pregnancy, childbirth and the puerperium
  - EXCLUDES 1 traumatic separation of symphysis (pubis) during childbirth (O71.6)
  - ✓6th **O26.71** Subluxation of symphysis (pubis) in **pregnancy**
    - **O26.711** Subluxation of symphysis (pubis) in pregnancy, **first trimester** [COM] [M]
    - **O26.712** Subluxation of symphysis (pubis) in pregnancy, **second trimester** [COM] [M]
    - **O26.713** Subluxation of symphysis (pubis) in pregnancy, **third trimester** [COM] [M]
    - **O26.719** Subluxation of symphysis (pubis) in pregnancy, unspecified trimester [COM] [M]
  - **O26.72** Subluxation of symphysis (pubis) in **childbirth** [COM] [M]
  - **O26.73** Subluxation of symphysis (pubis) in the **puerperium** [COM] [M]
- ✓5th **O26.8** Other specified pregnancy related conditions
  - ✓6th **O26.81** Pregnancy related exhaustion and fatigue
    - **O26.811** Pregnancy related exhaustion and fatigue, **first trimester** [COM] [M]
    - **O26.812** Pregnancy related exhaustion and fatigue, **second trimester** [COM] [M]
    - **O26.813** Pregnancy related exhaustion and fatigue, **third trimester** [COM] [M]
    - **O26.819** Pregnancy related exhaustion and fatigue, unspecified trimester [COM] [M]
  - ✓6th **O26.82** Pregnancy related peripheral neuritis
    - **O26.821** Pregnancy related peripheral neuritis, **first trimester** [COM] [M]
    - **O26.822** Pregnancy related peripheral neuritis, **second trimester** [COM] [M]
    - **O26.823** Pregnancy related peripheral neuritis, **third trimester** [COM] [M]
    - **O26.829** Pregnancy related peripheral neuritis, unspecified trimester [COM] [M]
  - ✓6th **O26.83** Pregnancy related renal disease
    - Use additional code to identify the specific disorder
    - **O26.831** Pregnancy related renal disease, **first trimester** [COM] [M]
    - **O26.832** Pregnancy related renal disease, **second trimester** [COM] [M]
    - **O26.833** Pregnancy related renal disease, **third trimester** [COM] [M]
    - **O26.839** Pregnancy related renal disease, unspecified trimester [COM] [M]
  - ✓6th **O26.84** Uterine size-date discrepancy complicating pregnancy
    - EXCLUDES 1 encounter for suspected problem with fetal growth ruled out (Z03.74)
    - **O26.841** Uterine size-date discrepancy, **first trimester** [COM] [M]
    - **O26.842** Uterine size-date discrepancy, **second trimester** [COM] [M]
    - **O26.843** Uterine size-date discrepancy, **third trimester** [COM] [M]
    - **O26.849** Uterine size-date discrepancy, unspecified trimester [COM] [M]
  - ✓6th **O26.85** Spotting complicating pregnancy
    - **O26.851** Spotting complicating pregnancy, **first trimester** [COM] [M]
    - **O26.852** Spotting complicating pregnancy, **second trimester** [COM] [M]
    - **O26.853** Spotting complicating pregnancy, **third trimester** [COM] [M]
    - **O26.859** Spotting complicating pregnancy, unspecified trimester [COM] [M]
  - **O26.86** Pruritic urticarial papules and plaques of pregnancy (PUPPP) [COM] [M]
    - Polymorphic eruption of pregnancy
  - ✓6th **O26.87** Cervical shortening
    - EXCLUDES 1 encounter for suspected cervical shortening ruled out (Z03.75)
    - DEF: Cervix that has shortened to less than 25 mm before the 24th week of pregnancy. A shortened cervix is a warning sign for impending premature delivery and is treated by cervical cerclage placement or progesterone.
    - **O26.872** Cervical shortening, **second trimester** [COM] [M]
    - **O26.873** Cervical shortening, **third trimester** [COM] [M]
    - **O26.879** Cervical shortening, unspecified trimester [COM] [M]
  - ✓6th **O26.89** Other specified pregnancy related conditions
    - Use additional code, if applicable, to identify specific condition such as insulin resistance (E88.81-)
    - AHA: 2015,3Q,40
    - **O26.891** Other specified pregnancy related conditions, **first trimester** [COM] [M]
    - **O26.892** Other specified pregnancy related conditions, **second trimester** [COM] [M]
    - **O26.893** Other specified pregnancy related conditions, **third trimester** [COM] [M]
    - **O26.899** Other specified pregnancy related conditions, unspecified trimester [COM] [M]
- ✓5th **O26.9** Pregnancy related conditions, unspecified
  - **O26.90** Pregnancy related conditions, unspecified, unspecified trimester [COM] [M]
  - **O26.91** Pregnancy related conditions, unspecified, **first trimester** [COM] [M]
  - **O26.92** Pregnancy related conditions, unspecified, **second trimester** [COM] [M]
  - **O26.93** Pregnancy related conditions, unspecified, **third trimester** [COM] [M]

✓4th **O28** Abnormal findings on antenatal screening of mother
  - EXCLUDES 1 diagnostic findings classified elsewhere - see Alphabetical Index
  - **O28.0** Abnormal **hematological** finding on antenatal screening of mother [M]
  - **O28.1** Abnormal **biochemical** finding on antenatal screening of mother [M]
  - **O28.2** Abnormal **cytological** finding on antenatal screening of mother [M]
  - **O28.3** Abnormal **ultrasonic** finding on antenatal screening of mother [M]
  - **O28.4** Abnormal **radiological** finding on antenatal screening of mother [M]
  - **O28.5** Abnormal **chromosomal and genetic** finding on antenatal screening of mother [M]
  - **O28.8** Other abnormal findings on antenatal screening of mother [M]
  - **O28.9** Unspecified abnormal findings on antenatal screening of mother [M]

Chapter 15. Pregnancy, Childbirth and the Puerperium

O29 Complications of anesthesia during pregnancy
INCLUDES maternal complications arising from the administration of a general, regional or local anesthetic, analgesic or other sedation during pregnancy

Use additional code, if necessary, to identify the complication

EXCLUDES 2 complications of anesthesia during labor and delivery (O74.-)
complications of anesthesia during the puerperium (O89.-)

O29.0 Pulmonary complications of anesthesia during pregnancy

O29.01 Aspiration pneumonitis due to anesthesia during pregnancy
Inhalation of stomach contents or secretions NOS due to anesthesia during pregnancy
Mendelson's syndrome due to anesthesia during pregnancy

- O29.011 Aspiration pneumonitis due to anesthesia during pregnancy, first trimester
- O29.012 Aspiration pneumonitis due to anesthesia during pregnancy, second trimester
- O29.013 Aspiration pneumonitis due to anesthesia during pregnancy, third trimester
- O29.019 Aspiration pneumonitis due to anesthesia during pregnancy, unspecified trimester

O29.02 Pressure collapse of lung due to anesthesia during pregnancy
- O29.021 Pressure collapse of lung due to anesthesia during pregnancy, first trimester
- O29.022 Pressure collapse of lung due to anesthesia during pregnancy, second trimester
- O29.023 Pressure collapse of lung due to anesthesia during pregnancy, third trimester
- O29.029 Pressure collapse of lung due to anesthesia during pregnancy, unspecified trimester

O29.09 Other pulmonary complications of anesthesia during pregnancy
- O29.091 Other pulmonary complications of anesthesia during pregnancy, first trimester
- O29.092 Other pulmonary complications of anesthesia during pregnancy, second trimester
- O29.093 Other pulmonary complications of anesthesia during pregnancy, third trimester
- O29.099 Other pulmonary complications of anesthesia during pregnancy, unspecified trimester

O29.1 Cardiac complications of anesthesia during pregnancy

O29.11 Cardiac arrest due to anesthesia during pregnancy
- O29.111 Cardiac arrest due to anesthesia during pregnancy, first trimester
- O29.112 Cardiac arrest due to anesthesia during pregnancy, second trimester
- O29.113 Cardiac arrest due to anesthesia during pregnancy, third trimester
- O29.119 Cardiac arrest due to anesthesia during pregnancy, unspecified trimester

O29.12 Cardiac failure due to anesthesia during pregnancy
- O29.121 Cardiac failure due to anesthesia during pregnancy, first trimester
- O29.122 Cardiac failure due to anesthesia during pregnancy, second trimester
- O29.123 Cardiac failure due to anesthesia during pregnancy, third trimester
- O29.129 Cardiac failure due to anesthesia during pregnancy, unspecified trimester

O29.19 Other cardiac complications of anesthesia during pregnancy
- O29.191 Other cardiac complications of anesthesia during pregnancy, first trimester
- O29.192 Other cardiac complications of anesthesia during pregnancy, second trimester
- O29.193 Other cardiac complications of anesthesia during pregnancy, third trimester
- O29.199 Other cardiac complications of anesthesia during pregnancy, unspecified trimester

O29.2 Central nervous system complications of anesthesia during pregnancy

O29.21 Cerebral anoxia due to anesthesia during pregnancy
- O29.211 Cerebral anoxia due to anesthesia during pregnancy, first trimester
- O29.212 Cerebral anoxia due to anesthesia during pregnancy, second trimester
- O29.213 Cerebral anoxia due to anesthesia during pregnancy, third trimester
- O29.219 Cerebral anoxia due to anesthesia during pregnancy, unspecified trimester

O29.29 Other central nervous system complications of anesthesia during pregnancy
- O29.291 Other central nervous system complications of anesthesia during pregnancy, first trimester
- O29.292 Other central nervous system complications of anesthesia during pregnancy, second trimester
- O29.293 Other central nervous system complications of anesthesia during pregnancy, third trimester
- O29.299 Other central nervous system complications of anesthesia during pregnancy, unspecified trimester

O29.3 Toxic reaction to local anesthesia during pregnancy

O29.3X Toxic reaction to local anesthesia during pregnancy
- O29.3X1 Toxic reaction to local anesthesia during pregnancy, first trimester
- O29.3X2 Toxic reaction to local anesthesia during pregnancy, second trimester
- O29.3X3 Toxic reaction to local anesthesia during pregnancy, third trimester
- O29.3X9 Toxic reaction to local anesthesia during pregnancy, unspecified trimester

O29.4 Spinal and epidural anesthesia induced headache during pregnancy
- O29.40 Spinal and epidural anesthesia induced headache during pregnancy, unspecified trimester
- O29.41 Spinal and epidural anesthesia induced headache during pregnancy, first trimester
- O29.42 Spinal and epidural anesthesia induced headache during pregnancy, second trimester
- O29.43 Spinal and epidural anesthesia induced headache during pregnancy, third trimester

O29.5 Other complications of spinal and epidural anesthesia during pregnancy

O29.5X Other complications of spinal and epidural anesthesia during pregnancy
- O29.5X1 Other complications of spinal and epidural anesthesia during pregnancy, first trimester
- O29.5X2 Other complications of spinal and epidural anesthesia during pregnancy, second trimester
- O29.5X3 Other complications of spinal and epidural anesthesia during pregnancy, third trimester
- O29.5X9 Other complications of spinal and epidural anesthesia during pregnancy, unspecified trimester

O29.6 Failed or difficult intubation for anesthesia during pregnancy
- O29.60 Failed or difficult intubation for anesthesia during pregnancy, unspecified trimester
- O29.61 Failed or difficult intubation for anesthesia during pregnancy, first trimester
- O29.62 Failed or difficult intubation for anesthesia during pregnancy, second trimester
- O29.63 Failed or difficult intubation for anesthesia during pregnancy, third trimester

O29.8 Other complications of anesthesia during pregnancy
O29.8X Other complications of anesthesia during pregnancy
- O29.8X1 Other complications of anesthesia during pregnancy, first trimester
- O29.8X2 Other complications of anesthesia during pregnancy, second trimester
- O29.8X3 Other complications of anesthesia during pregnancy, third trimester
- O29.8X9 Other complications of anesthesia during pregnancy, unspecified trimester

O29.9 Unspecified complication of anesthesia during pregnancy
- O29.90 Unspecified complication of anesthesia during pregnancy, unspecified trimester
- O29.91 Unspecified complication of anesthesia during pregnancy, first trimester
- O29.92 Unspecified complication of anesthesia during pregnancy, second trimester
- O29.93 Unspecified complication of anesthesia during pregnancy, third trimester

Maternal care related to the fetus and amniotic cavity and possible delivery problems (O30-O48)

O30 Multiple gestation
Code also any complications specific to multiple gestation
AHA: 2016,4Q,51

O30.0 Twin pregnancy
O30.00 Twin pregnancy, unspecified number of placenta and unspecified number of amniotic sacs
- O30.001 Twin pregnancy, unspecified number of placenta and unspecified number of amniotic sacs, first trimester
- O30.002 Twin pregnancy, unspecified number of placenta and unspecified number of amniotic sacs, second trimester
- O30.003 Twin pregnancy, unspecified number of placenta and unspecified number of amniotic sacs, third trimester
- O30.009 Twin pregnancy, unspecified number of placenta and unspecified number of amniotic sacs, unspecified trimester

O30.01 Twin pregnancy, monochorionic/monoamniotic
Twin pregnancy, one placenta, one amniotic sac
EXCLUDES 1 conjoined twins (O30.02-)
- O30.011 Twin pregnancy, monochorionic/monoamniotic, first trimester
- O30.012 Twin pregnancy, monochorionic/monoamniotic, second trimester
- O30.013 Twin pregnancy, monochorionic/monoamniotic, third trimester
- O30.019 Twin pregnancy, monochorionic/monoamniotic, unspecified trimester

O30.02 Conjoined twin pregnancy
- O30.021 Conjoined twin pregnancy, first trimester
- O30.022 Conjoined twin pregnancy, second trimester
- O30.023 Conjoined twin pregnancy, third trimester
- O30.029 Conjoined twin pregnancy, unspecified trimester

O30.03 Twin pregnancy, monochorionic/diamniotic
Twin pregnancy, one placenta, two amniotic sacs
- O30.031 Twin pregnancy, monochorionic/diamniotic, first trimester
- O30.032 Twin pregnancy, monochorionic/diamniotic, second trimester
- O30.033 Twin pregnancy, monochorionic/diamniotic, third trimester
- O30.039 Twin pregnancy, monochorionic/diamniotic, unspecified trimester

O30.04 Twin pregnancy, dichorionic/diamniotic
Twin pregnancy, two placentae, two amniotic sacs
- O30.041 Twin pregnancy, dichorionic/diamniotic, first trimester
- O30.042 Twin pregnancy, dichorionic/diamniotic, second trimester
- O30.043 Twin pregnancy, dichorionic/diamniotic, third trimester
- O30.049 Twin pregnancy, dichorionic/diamniotic, unspecified trimester

O30.09 Twin pregnancy, unable to determine number of placenta and number of amniotic sacs
- O30.091 Twin pregnancy, unable to determine number of placenta and number of amniotic sacs, first trimester
- O30.092 Twin pregnancy, unable to determine number of placenta and number of amniotic sacs, second trimester
- O30.093 Twin pregnancy, unable to determine number of placenta and number of amniotic sacs, third trimester
- O30.099 Twin pregnancy, unable to determine number of placenta and number of amniotic sacs, unspecified trimester

O30.1 Triplet pregnancy
O30.10 Triplet pregnancy, unspecified number of placenta and unspecified number of amniotic sacs
AHA: 2016,2Q,8
- O30.101 Triplet pregnancy, unspecified number of placenta and unspecified number of amniotic sacs, first trimester
- O30.102 Triplet pregnancy, unspecified number of placenta and unspecified number of amniotic sacs, second trimester
- O30.103 Triplet pregnancy, unspecified number of placenta and unspecified number of amniotic sacs, third trimester
- O30.109 Triplet pregnancy, unspecified number of placenta and unspecified number of amniotic sacs, unspecified trimester

O30.11 Triplet pregnancy with two or more monochorionic fetuses
- O30.111 Triplet pregnancy with two or more monochorionic fetuses, first trimester
- O30.112 Triplet pregnancy with two or more monochorionic fetuses, second trimester
- O30.113 Triplet pregnancy with two or more monochorionic fetuses, third trimester
- O30.119 Triplet pregnancy with two or more monochorionic fetuses, unspecified trimester

O30.12 Triplet pregnancy with two or more monoamniotic fetuses
- O30.121 Triplet pregnancy with two or more monoamniotic fetuses, first trimester
- O30.122 Triplet pregnancy with two or more monoamniotic fetuses, second trimester
- O30.123 Triplet pregnancy with two or more monoamniotic fetuses, third trimester
- O30.129 Triplet pregnancy with two or more monoamniotic fetuses, unspecified trimester

O30.13 Triplet pregnancy, trichorionic/triamniotic
AHA: 2018,4Q,22
- O30.131 Triplet pregnancy, trichorionic/triamniotic, first trimester
- O30.132 Triplet pregnancy, trichorionic/triamniotic, second trimester
- O30.133 Triplet pregnancy, trichorionic/triamniotic, third trimester

Chapter 15. Pregnancy, Childbirth and the Puerperium

- **O30.139** Triplet pregnancy, trichorionic/triamniotic, unspecified trimester
- ✓6th **O30.19** Triplet pregnancy, unable to determine number of placenta and number of amniotic sacs
  - **O30.191** Triplet pregnancy, unable to determine number of placenta and number of amniotic sacs, first trimester
  - **O30.192** Triplet pregnancy, unable to determine number of placenta and number of amniotic sacs, second trimester
  - **O30.193** Triplet pregnancy, unable to determine number of placenta and number of amniotic sacs, third trimester
  - **O30.199** Triplet pregnancy, unable to determine number of placenta and number of amniotic sacs, unspecified trimester
- ✓5th **O30.2** Quadruplet pregnancy
  - ✓6th **O30.20** Quadruplet pregnancy, unspecified number of placenta and unspecified number of amniotic sacs
    - **O30.201** Quadruplet pregnancy, unspecified number of placenta and unspecified number of amniotic sacs, first trimester
    - **O30.202** Quadruplet pregnancy, unspecified number of placenta and unspecified number of amniotic sacs, second trimester
    - **O30.203** Quadruplet pregnancy, unspecified number of placenta and unspecified number of amniotic sacs, third trimester
    - **O30.209** Quadruplet pregnancy, unspecified number of placenta and unspecified number of amniotic sacs, unspecified trimester
  - ✓6th **O30.21** Quadruplet pregnancy with two or more monochorionic fetuses
    - **O30.211** Quadruplet pregnancy with two or more monochorionic fetuses, first trimester
    - **O30.212** Quadruplet pregnancy with two or more monochorionic fetuses, second trimester
    - **O30.213** Quadruplet pregnancy with two or more monochorionic fetuses, third trimester
    - **O30.219** Quadruplet pregnancy with two or more monochorionic fetuses, unspecified trimester
  - ✓6th **O30.22** Quadruplet pregnancy with two or more monoamniotic fetuses
    - **O30.221** Quadruplet pregnancy with two or more monoamniotic fetuses, first trimester
    - **O30.222** Quadruplet pregnancy with two or more monoamniotic fetuses, second trimester
    - **O30.223** Quadruplet pregnancy with two or more monoamniotic fetuses, third trimester
    - **O30.229** Quadruplet pregnancy with two or more monoamniotic fetuses, unspecified trimester
  - ✓6th **O30.23** Quadruplet pregnancy, quadrachorionic/quadra-amniotic
    - **AHA:** 2018,4Q,22
    - **O30.231** Quadruplet pregnancy, quadrachorionic/quadra-amniotic, first trimester
    - **O30.232** Quadruplet pregnancy, quadrachorionic/quadra-amniotic, second trimester
    - **O30.233** Quadruplet pregnancy, quadrachorionic/quadra-amniotic, third trimester
    - **O30.239** Quadruplet pregnancy, quadrachorionic/quadra-amniotic, unspecified trimester
- ✓6th **O30.29** Quadruplet pregnancy, unable to determine number of placenta and number of amniotic sacs
  - **O30.291** Quadruplet pregnancy, unable to determine number of placenta and number of amniotic sacs, first trimester
  - **O30.292** Quadruplet pregnancy, unable to determine number of placenta and number of amniotic sacs, second trimester
  - **O30.293** Quadruplet pregnancy, unable to determine number of placenta and number of amniotic sacs, third trimester
  - **O30.299** Quadruplet pregnancy, unable to determine number of placenta and number of amniotic sacs, unspecified trimester
- ✓5th **O30.8** Other specified multiple gestation

  Multiple gestation pregnancy greater then quadruplets
  - ✓6th **O30.80** Other specified multiple gestation, unspecified number of placenta and unspecified number of amniotic sacs
    - **O30.801** Other specified multiple gestation, unspecified number of placenta and unspecified number of amniotic sacs, first trimester
    - **O30.802** Other specified multiple gestation, unspecified number of placenta and unspecified number of amniotic sacs, second trimester
    - **O30.803** Other specified multiple gestation, unspecified number of placenta and unspecified number of amniotic sacs, third trimester
    - **O30.809** Other specified multiple gestation, unspecified number of placenta and unspecified number of amniotic sacs, unspecified trimester
  - ✓6th **O30.81** Other specified multiple gestation with two or more monochorionic fetuses
    - **O30.811** Other specified multiple gestation with two or more monochorionic fetuses, first trimester
    - **O30.812** Other specified multiple gestation with two or more monochorionic fetuses, second trimester
    - **O30.813** Other specified multiple gestation with two or more monochorionic fetuses, third trimester
    - **O30.819** Other specified multiple gestation with two or more monochorionic fetuses, unspecified trimester
  - ✓6th **O30.82** Other specified multiple gestation with two or more monoamniotic fetuses
    - **O30.821** Other specified multiple gestation with two or more monoamniotic fetuses, first trimester
    - **O30.822** Other specified multiple gestation with two or more monoamniotic fetuses, second trimester
    - **O30.823** Other specified multiple gestation with two or more monoamniotic fetuses, third trimester
    - **O30.829** Other specified multiple gestation with two or more monoamniotic fetuses, unspecified trimester
  - ✓6th **O30.83** Other specified multiple gestation, number of chorions and amnions are both equal to the number of fetuses

    Heptachorionic, hepta-amniotic pregnancy (septuplets)
    Hexachorionic, hexa-amniotic pregnancy (sextuplets)
    Pentachorionic, penta-amniotic pregnancy (quintuplets)
    AHA: 2018,4Q,22
    - **O30.831** Other specified multiple gestation, number of chorions and amnions are both equal to the number of fetuses, first trimester
    - **O30.832** Other specified multiple gestation, number of chorions and amnions are both equal to the number of fetuses, second trimester

O30.833–O32.0 Chapter 15. Pregnancy, Childbirth and the Puerperium

O30.833 Other specified multiple gestation, number of chorions and amnions are both equal to the number of fetuses, *third trimester* COM M

O30.839 Other specified multiple gestation, number of chorions and amnions are both equal to the number of fetuses, *unspecified trimester* COM M

✓6ᵗʰ **O30.89** Other specified multiple gestation, *unable to determine number* of placenta and number of amniotic sacs

O30.891 Other specified multiple gestation, unable to determine number of placenta and number of amniotic sacs, *first trimester* COM M

O30.892 Other specified multiple gestation, unable to determine number of placenta and number of amniotic sacs, *second trimester* COM M

O30.893 Other specified multiple gestation, unable to determine number of placenta and number of amniotic sacs, *third trimester* COM M

O30.899 Other specified multiple gestation, unable to determine number of placenta and number of amniotic sacs, *unspecified trimester* COM M

✓5ᵗʰ **O30.9** Multiple gestation, unspecified
Multiple pregnancy NOS

O30.90 Multiple gestation, unspecified, unspecified trimester COM M

O30.91 Multiple gestation, unspecified, *first trimester* COM M

O30.92 Multiple gestation, unspecified, *second trimester* COM M

O30.93 Multiple gestation, unspecified, *third trimester* COM M

✓4ᵗʰ **O31** Complications specific to multiple gestation
EXCLUDES 2 delayed delivery of second twin, triplet, etc. (O63.2)
malpresentation of one fetus or more (O32.9)
placental transfusion syndromes (O43.0-)
AHA: 2012,4Q,107

One of the following 7th characters is to be assigned to each code under category O31. 7th character Ø is for single gestations and multiple gestations where the fetus is unspecified. 7th characters 1 through 9 are for cases of multiple gestations to identify the fetus for which the code applies. The appropriate code from category O30, Multiple gestation, must also be assigned when assigning a code from category O31 that has a 7th character of 1 through 9.
Ø not applicable or unspecified
1 fetus 1
2 fetus 2
3 fetus 3
4 fetus 4
5 fetus 5
9 other fetus

✓5ᵗʰ **O31.0** Papyraceous fetus
Fetus compressus
DEF: Fetus that has died, but remains in utero for weeks before delivery, becoming compacted and mummified in appearance, with skin resembling parchment. Occurs most commonly in multigestational pregnancies. *Synonym(s):* paper doll fetus.

✓x7ᵗʰ **O31.00** Papyraceous fetus, unspecified trimester COM M
✓x7ᵗʰ **O31.01** Papyraceous fetus, *first trimester* COM M
✓x7ᵗʰ **O31.02** Papyraceous fetus, *second trimester* COM M
✓x7ᵗʰ **O31.03** Papyraceous fetus, *third trimester* COM M

✓5ᵗʰ **O31.1** Continuing pregnancy *after spontaneous abortion* of one fetus or more

✓x7ᵗʰ **O31.10** Continuing pregnancy after spontaneous abortion of one fetus or more, unspecified trimester COM M
✓x7ᵗʰ **O31.11** Continuing pregnancy after spontaneous abortion of one fetus or more, *first trimester* COM M
✓x7ᵗʰ **O31.12** Continuing pregnancy after spontaneous abortion of one fetus or more, *second trimester* COM M
✓x7ᵗʰ **O31.13** Continuing pregnancy after spontaneous abortion of one fetus or more, *third trimester* COM M

✓5ᵗʰ **O31.2** Continuing pregnancy *after intrauterine death* of one fetus or more

✓x7ᵗʰ **O31.20** Continuing pregnancy after intrauterine death of one fetus or more, unspecified trimester COM M
✓x7ᵗʰ **O31.21** Continuing pregnancy after intrauterine death of one fetus or more, *first trimester* COM M
✓x7ᵗʰ **O31.22** Continuing pregnancy after intrauterine death of one fetus or more, *second trimester* COM M
✓x7ᵗʰ **O31.23** Continuing pregnancy after intrauterine death of one fetus or more, *third trimester* COM M

✓5ᵗʰ **O31.3** Continuing pregnancy after *elective fetal reduction* of one fetus or more
Continuing pregnancy after selective termination of one fetus or more

✓x7ᵗʰ **O31.30** Continuing pregnancy after elective fetal reduction of one fetus or more, unspecified trimester COM M
✓x7ᵗʰ **O31.31** Continuing pregnancy after elective fetal reduction of one fetus or more, *first trimester* COM M
✓x7ᵗʰ **O31.32** Continuing pregnancy after elective fetal reduction of one fetus or more, *second trimester* COM M
✓x7ᵗʰ **O31.33** Continuing pregnancy after elective fetal reduction of one fetus or more, *third trimester* COM M

✓5ᵗʰ **O31.8** Other complications specific to multiple gestation COM

✓6ᵗʰ **O31.8X** Other complications specific to multiple gestation

✓7ᵗʰ **O31.8X1** Other complications specific to multiple gestation, *first trimester* M
✓7ᵗʰ **O31.8X2** Other complications specific to multiple gestation, *second trimester* M
✓7ᵗʰ **O31.8X3** Other complications specific to multiple gestation, *third trimester* M
✓7ᵗʰ **O31.8X9** Other complications specific to multiple gestation, unspecified trimester M

✓4ᵗʰ **O32** Maternal care for malpresentation of fetus
INCLUDES the listed conditions as a reason for observation, hospitalization or other obstetric care of the mother, or for cesarean delivery before onset of labor
EXCLUDES 1 malpresentation of fetus with obstructed labor (O64.-)
AHA: 2012,4Q,107

One of the following 7th characters is to be assigned to each code under category O32. 7th character Ø is for single gestations and multiple gestations where the fetus is unspecified. 7th characters 1 through 9 are for cases of multiple gestations to identify the fetus for which the code applies. The appropriate code from category O30, Multiple gestation, must also be assigned when assigning a code from category O32 that has a 7th character of 1 through 9.
Ø not applicable or unspecified
1 fetus 1
2 fetus 2
3 fetus 3
4 fetus 4
5 fetus 5
9 other fetus

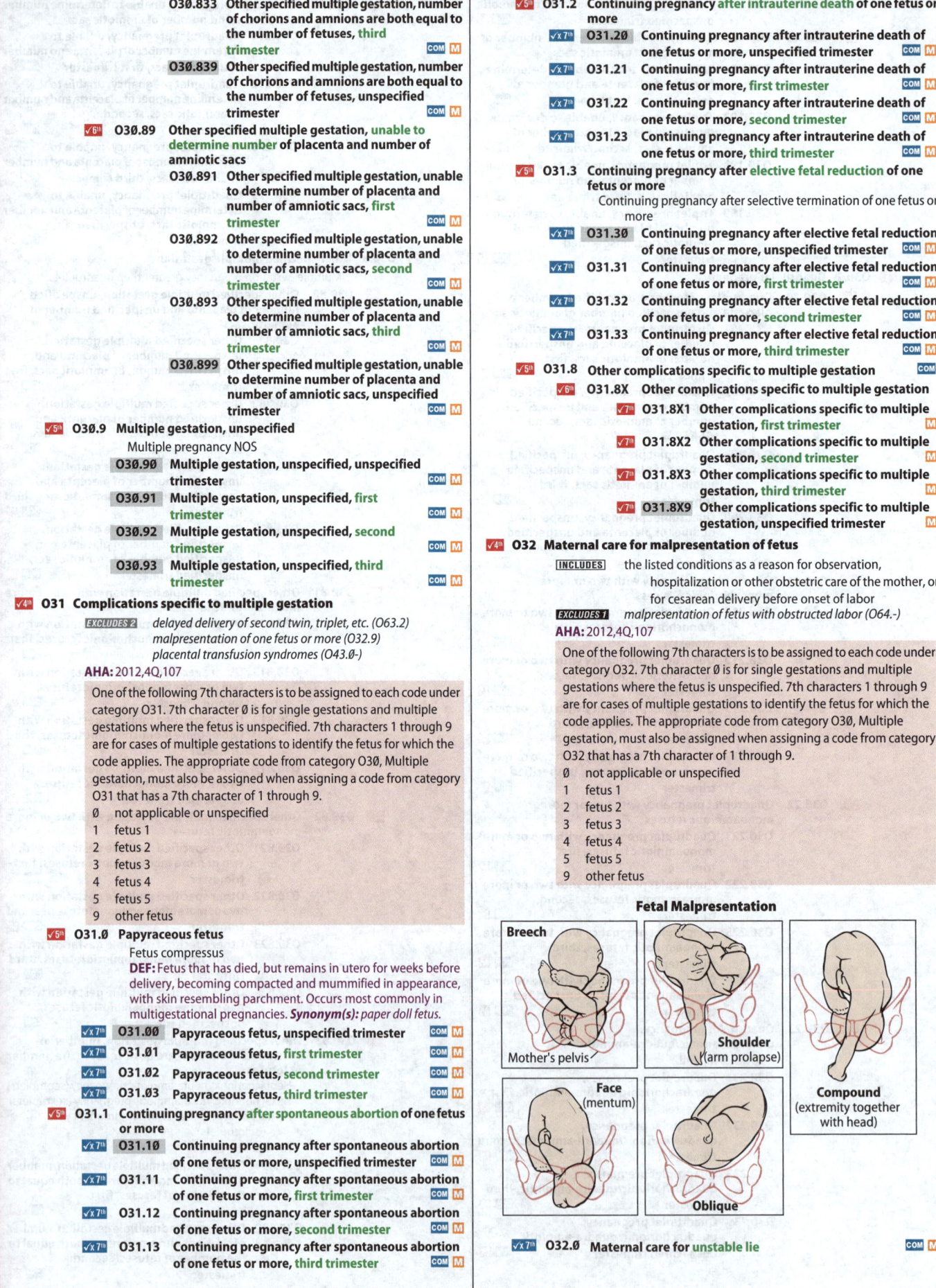

Fetal Malpresentation
Breech — Mother's pelvis
Shoulder (arm prolapse)
Compound (extremity together with head)
Face (mentum)
Oblique

✓x7ᵗʰ **O32.0** Maternal care for *unstable lie* COM M

O32.1 Maternal care for breech presentation
Maternal care for buttocks presentation
Maternal care for complete breech
Maternal care for frank breech

EXCLUDES 1 footling presentation (O32.8)
incomplete breech (O32.8)

DEF: Fetus presentation in a longitudinal lie with the buttocks or feet closest to birth canal that may require external cephalic version or cesarean delivery.

O32.2 Maternal care for transverse and oblique lie
Maternal care for oblique presentation
Maternal care for transverse presentation

O32.3 Maternal care for face, brow and chin presentation

O32.4 Maternal care for high head at term
Maternal care for failure of head to enter pelvic brim

O32.6 Maternal care for compound presentation

O32.8 Maternal care for other malpresentation of fetus
Maternal care for footling presentation
Maternal care for incomplete breech

O32.9 Maternal care for malpresentation of fetus, unspecified

O33 Maternal care for disproportion
INCLUDES the listed conditions as a reason for observation, hospitalization or other obstetric care of the mother, or for cesarean delivery before onset of labor

EXCLUDES 1 disproportion with obstructed labor (O65-O66)

O33.0 Maternal care for disproportion due to deformity of maternal pelvic bones
Maternal care for disproportion due to pelvic deformity causing disproportion NOS

O33.1 Maternal care for disproportion due to generally contracted pelvis
Maternal care for disproportion due to contracted pelvis NOS causing disproportion

O33.2 Maternal care for disproportion due to inlet contraction of pelvis
Maternal care for disproportion due to inlet contraction (pelvis) causing disproportion

O33.3 Maternal care for disproportion due to outlet contraction of pelvis
Maternal care for disproportion due to mid-cavity contraction (pelvis)
Maternal care for disproportion due to outlet contraction (pelvis)

One of the following 7th characters is to be assigned to code O33.3. 7th character 0 is for single gestations and multiple gestations where the fetus is unspecified. 7th characters 1 through 9 are for cases of multiple gestations to identify the fetus for which the code applies. The appropriate code from category O30, Multiple gestation, must also be assigned when assigning code O33.3 with a 7th character of 1 through 9.
- 0 not applicable or unspecified
- 1 fetus 1
- 2 fetus 2
- 3 fetus 3
- 4 fetus 4
- 5 fetus 5
- 9 other fetus

O33.4 Maternal care for disproportion of mixed maternal and fetal origin

One of the following 7th characters is to be assigned to code O33.4. 7th character 0 is for single gestations and multiple gestations where the fetus is unspecified. 7th characters 1 through 9 are for cases of multiple gestations to identify the fetus for which the code applies. The appropriate code from category O30, Multiple gestation, must also be assigned when assigning code O33.4 with a 7th character of 1 through 9.
- 0 not applicable or unspecified
- 1 fetus 1
- 2 fetus 2
- 3 fetus 3
- 4 fetus 4
- 5 fetus 5
- 9 other fetus

O33.5 Maternal care for disproportion due to unusually large fetus
Maternal care for disproportion due to disproportion of fetal origin with normally formed fetus
Maternal care for disproportion due to fetal disproportion NOS

One of the following 7th characters is to be assigned to code O33.5. 7th character 0 is for single gestations and multiple gestations where the fetus is unspecified. 7th characters 1 through 9 are for cases of multiple gestations to identify the fetus for which the code applies. The appropriate code from category O30, Multiple gestation, must also be assigned when assigning code O33.5 with a 7th character of 1 through 9.
- 0 not applicable or unspecified
- 1 fetus 1
- 2 fetus 2
- 3 fetus 3
- 4 fetus 4
- 5 fetus 5
- 9 other fetus

O33.6 Maternal care for disproportion due to hydrocephalic fetus

One of the following 7th characters is to be assigned to code O33.6. 7th character 0 is for single gestations and multiple gestations where the fetus is unspecified. 7th characters 1 through 9 are for cases of multiple gestations to identify the fetus for which the code applies. The appropriate code from category O30, Multiple gestation, must also be assigned when assigning code O33.6 with a 7th character of 1 through 9.
- 0 not applicable or unspecified
- 1 fetus 1
- 2 fetus 2
- 3 fetus 3
- 4 fetus 4
- 5 fetus 5
- 9 other fetus

O33.7 Maternal care for disproportion due to other fetal deformities
Maternal care for disproportion due to fetal ascites
Maternal care for disproportion due to fetal hydrops
Maternal care for disproportion due to fetal meningomyelocele
Maternal care for disproportion due to fetal sacral teratoma
Maternal care for disproportion due to fetal tumor

EXCLUDES 1 obstructed labor due to other fetal deformities (O66.3)
AHA: 2016,4Q,51

One of the following 7th characters is to be assigned to code O33.7. 7th character 0 is for single gestations and multiple gestations where the fetus is unspecified. 7th characters 1 through 9 are for cases of multiple gestations to identify the fetus for which the code applies. The appropriate code from category O30, Multiple gestation, must also be assigned when assigning code O33.7 with a 7th character of 1 through 9.
- 0 not applicable or unspecified
- 1 fetus 1
- 2 fetus 2
- 3 fetus 3
- 4 fetus 4
- 5 fetus 5
- 9 other fetus

O33.8 Maternal care for disproportion of other origin

O33.9 Maternal care for disproportion, unspecified
Maternal care for disproportion due to cephalopelvic disproportion NOS
Maternal care for disproportion due to fetopelvic disproportion NOS

O34 Maternal care for abnormality of pelvic organs
INCLUDES the listed conditions as a reason for hospitalization or other obstetric care of the mother, or for cesarean delivery before onset of labor

Code first any associated obstructed labor (O65.5)
Use additional code for specific condition

O34.0 Maternal care for congenital malformation of uterus
Maternal care for double uterus
Maternal care for uterus bicornis

O34.00 Maternal care for unspecified congenital malformation of uterus, unspecified trimester

	O34.01	Maternal care for unspecified congenital malformation of uterus, first trimester
	O34.02	Maternal care for unspecified congenital malformation of uterus, second trimester
	O34.03	Maternal care for unspecified congenital malformation of uterus, third trimester
√5th O34.1		Maternal care for benign tumor of corpus uteri
	EXCLUDES 2	maternal care for benign tumor of cervix (O34.4-) maternal care for malignant neoplasm of uterus (O9A.1-)
	O34.10	Maternal care for benign tumor of corpus uteri, unspecified trimester
	O34.11	Maternal care for benign tumor of corpus uteri, first trimester
	O34.12	Maternal care for benign tumor of corpus uteri, second trimester
	O34.13	Maternal care for benign tumor of corpus uteri, third trimester
√5th O34.2		Maternal care due to uterine scar from previous surgery
	AHA: 2020,4Q,36; 2016,4Q,76	
√6th O34.21		Maternal care for scar from previous cesarean delivery
	AHA: 2018,3Q,23; 2016,4Q,51-52	
	O34.211	Maternal care for low transverse scar from previous cesarean delivery
	O34.212	Maternal care for vertical scar from previous cesarean delivery
		Maternal care for classical scar from previous cesarean delivery
	O34.218	Maternal care for other type scar from previous cesarean delivery
		Mid-transverse T incision
	O34.219	Maternal care for unspecified type scar from previous cesarean delivery
	O34.22	Maternal care for cesarean scar defect (isthmocele)
	O34.29	Maternal care due to uterine scar from other previous surgery
		Maternal care due to uterine scar from other transmural uterine incision
√5th O34.3		Maternal care for cervical incompetence
		Maternal care for cerclage with or without cervical incompetence Maternal care for Shirodkar suture with or without cervical incompetence
		DEF: Inadequate functioning of the cervix marked by abnormal widening during pregnancy and causing premature birth or miscarriage.
	O34.30	Maternal care for cervical incompetence, unspecified trimester
	O34.31	Maternal care for cervical incompetence, first trimester
	O34.32	Maternal care for cervical incompetence, second trimester
	O34.33	Maternal care for cervical incompetence, third trimester
√5th O34.4		Maternal care for other abnormalities of cervix
	O34.40	Maternal care for other abnormalities of cervix, unspecified trimester
	O34.41	Maternal care for other abnormalities of cervix, first trimester
	O34.42	Maternal care for other abnormalities of cervix, second trimester
	O34.43	Maternal care for other abnormalities of cervix, third trimester
√5th O34.5		Maternal care for other abnormalities of gravid uterus
√6th O34.51		Maternal care for incarceration of gravid uterus
	O34.511	Maternal care for incarceration of gravid uterus, first trimester
	O34.512	Maternal care for incarceration of gravid uterus, second trimester
	O34.513	Maternal care for incarceration of gravid uterus, third trimester
	O34.519	Maternal care for incarceration of gravid uterus, unspecified trimester
√6th O34.52		Maternal care for prolapse of gravid uterus
	O34.521	Maternal care for prolapse of gravid uterus, first trimester
	O34.522	Maternal care for prolapse of gravid uterus, second trimester
	O34.523	Maternal care for prolapse of gravid uterus, third trimester
	O34.529	Maternal care for prolapse of gravid uterus, unspecified trimester
√6th O34.53		Maternal care for retroversion of gravid uterus
	O34.531	Maternal care for retroversion of gravid uterus, first trimester
	O34.532	Maternal care for retroversion of gravid uterus, second trimester
	O34.533	Maternal care for retroversion of gravid uterus, third trimester
	O34.539	Maternal care for retroversion of gravid uterus, unspecified trimester
√6th O34.59		Maternal care for other abnormalities of gravid uterus
	O34.591	Maternal care for other abnormalities of gravid uterus, first trimester
	O34.592	Maternal care for other abnormalities of gravid uterus, second trimester
	O34.593	Maternal care for other abnormalities of gravid uterus, third trimester
	O34.599	Maternal care for other abnormalities of gravid uterus, unspecified trimester
√5th O34.6		Maternal care for abnormality of vagina
	EXCLUDES 2	maternal care for vaginal varices in pregnancy (O22.1-)
	O34.60	Maternal care for abnormality of vagina, unspecified trimester
	O34.61	Maternal care for abnormality of vagina, first trimester
	O34.62	Maternal care for abnormality of vagina, second trimester
	O34.63	Maternal care for abnormality of vagina, third trimester
√5th O34.7		Maternal care for abnormality of vulva and perineum
	EXCLUDES 2	maternal care for perineal and vulval varices in pregnancy (O22.1-)
	O34.70	Maternal care for abnormality of vulva and perineum, unspecified trimester
	O34.71	Maternal care for abnormality of vulva and perineum, first trimester
	O34.72	Maternal care for abnormality of vulva and perineum, second trimester
	O34.73	Maternal care for abnormality of vulva and perineum, third trimester
√5th O34.8		Maternal care for other abnormalities of pelvic organs
	O34.80	Maternal care for other abnormalities of pelvic organs, unspecified trimester
	O34.81	Maternal care for other abnormalities of pelvic organs, first trimester
	O34.82	Maternal care for other abnormalities of pelvic organs, second trimester
	O34.83	Maternal care for other abnormalities of pelvic organs, third trimester
√5th O34.9		Maternal care for abnormality of pelvic organ, unspecified
	O34.90	Maternal care for abnormality of pelvic organ, unspecified, unspecified trimester
	O34.91	Maternal care for abnormality of pelvic organ, unspecified, first trimester
	O34.92	Maternal care for abnormality of pelvic organ, unspecified, second trimester
	O34.93	Maternal care for abnormality of pelvic organ, unspecified, third trimester

Chapter 15. Pregnancy, Childbirth and the Puerperium

O35 **Maternal care for known or suspected fetal abnormality and damage** ✓4th

> INCLUDES the listed conditions in the fetus as a reason for hospitalization or other obstetric care to the mother, or for termination of pregnancy
>
> Code also any associated maternal condition
>
> EXCLUDES 1 encounter for suspected maternal and fetal conditions ruled out (Z03.7-)
>
> AHA: 2022,4Q,37

> One of the following 7th characters is to be assigned to each code under category O35. 7th character 0 is for single gestations and multiple gestations where the fetus is unspecified. 7th characters 1 through 9 are for cases of multiple gestations to identify the fetus for which the code applies. The appropriate code from category O30, Multiple gestation, must also be assigned when assigning a code from category O35 that has a 7th character of 1 through 9.
> - 0 not applicable or unspecified
> - 1 fetus 1
> - 2 fetus 2
> - 3 fetus 3
> - 4 fetus 4
> - 5 fetus 5
> - 9 other fetus

- ✓5th **O35.0** Maternal care for (suspected) central nervous system malformation in fetus
  - EXCLUDES 2 chromosomal abnormality in fetus (O35.1-)
  - ✓x7th **O35.00** Maternal care for (suspected) central nervous system malformation or damage in fetus, unspecified
  - ✓x7th **O35.01** Maternal care for (suspected) central nervous system malformation or damage in fetus, agenesis of the corpus callosum
  - ✓x7th **O35.02** Maternal care for (suspected) central nervous system malformation or damage in fetus, anencephaly
  - ✓x7th **O35.03** Maternal care for (suspected) central nervous system malformation or damage in fetus, choroid plexus cysts
  - ✓x7th **O35.04** Maternal care for (suspected) central nervous system malformation or damage in fetus, encephalocele
  - ✓x7th **O35.05** Maternal care for (suspected) central nervous system malformation or damage in fetus, holoprosencephaly
    - AHA: 2024,3Q,9
  - ✓x7th **O35.06** Maternal care for (suspected) central nervous system malformation or damage in fetus, hydrocephaly
    - Maternal care for fetal hydrocephalus
  - ✓x7th **O35.07** Maternal care for (suspected) central nervous system malformation or damage in fetus, microcephaly
  - ✓x7th **O35.08** Maternal care for (suspected) central nervous system malformation or damage in fetus, spina bifida
  - ✓x7th **O35.09** Maternal care for (suspected) other central nervous system malformation or damage in fetus

- ✓5th **O35.1** Maternal care for (suspected) chromosomal abnormality in fetus
  - AHA: 2023,2Q,15
  - ✓x7th **O35.10** Maternal care for (suspected) chromosomal abnormality in fetus, unspecified
  - ✓x7th **O35.11** Maternal care for (suspected) chromosomal abnormality in fetus, Trisomy 13
  - ✓x7th **O35.12** Maternal care for (suspected) chromosomal abnormality in fetus, Trisomy 18
  - ✓x7th **O35.13** Maternal care for (suspected) chromosomal abnormality in fetus, Trisomy 21
  - ✓x7th **O35.14** Maternal care for (suspected) chromosomal abnormality in fetus, Turner Syndrome
  - ✓x7th **O35.15** Maternal care for (suspected) chromosomal abnormality in fetus, sex chromosome abnormality
  - ✓x7th **O35.19** Maternal care for (suspected) chromosomal abnormality in fetus, other chromosomal abnormality

- ✓x7th **O35.A** Maternal care for other (suspected) fetal abnormality and damage, fetal facial anomalies
- ✓x7th **O35.B** Maternal care for other (suspected) fetal abnormality and damage, fetal cardiac anomalies
- ✓x7th **O35.C** Maternal care for other (suspected) fetal abnormality and damage, fetal pulmonary anomalies
- ✓x7th **O35.D** Maternal care for other (suspected) fetal abnormality and damage, fetal gastrointestinal anomalies
- ✓x7th **O35.E** Maternal care for other (suspected) fetal abnormality and damage, fetal genitourinary anomalies
- ✓x7th **O35.F** Maternal care for other (suspected) fetal abnormality and damage, fetal musculoskeletal anomalies of trunk
  - EXCLUDES 2 maternal care for other (suspected) fetal abnormality and damage, fetal lower extremities anomalies (O35.H)
  - maternal care for other (suspected) fetal abnormality and damage, fetal upper extremities anomalies (O35.G)
- ✓x7th **O35.G** Maternal care for other (suspected) fetal abnormality and damage, fetal upper extremities anomalies
- ✓x7th **O35.H** Maternal care for other (suspected) fetal abnormality and damage, fetal lower extremities anomalies
- ✓x7th **O35.2** Maternal care for (suspected) hereditary disease in fetus
  - EXCLUDES 2 chromosomal abnormality in fetus (O35.1-)
- ✓x7th **O35.3** Maternal care for (suspected) damage to fetus from viral disease in mother
  - Maternal care for damage to fetus from maternal cytomegalovirus infection
  - Maternal care for damage to fetus from maternal rubella
- ✓x7th **O35.4** Maternal care for (suspected) damage to fetus from alcohol
- ✓x7th **O35.5** Maternal care for (suspected) damage to fetus by drugs
  - Maternal care for damage to fetus from drug addiction
- ✓x7th **O35.6** Maternal care for (suspected) damage to fetus by radiation
- ✓x7th **O35.7** Maternal care for (suspected) damage to fetus by other medical procedures
  - Maternal care for damage to fetus by amniocentesis
  - Maternal care for damage to fetus by biopsy procedures
  - Maternal care for damage to fetus by hematological investigation
  - Maternal care for damage to fetus by intrauterine contraceptive device
  - Maternal care for damage to fetus by intrauterine surgery
- ✓x7th **O35.8** Maternal care for other (suspected) fetal abnormality and damage
  - Maternal care for damage to fetus from maternal listeriosis
  - Maternal care for damage to fetus from maternal toxoplasmosis
- ✓x7th **O35.9** Maternal care for (suspected) fetal abnormality and damage, unspecified

O36 **Maternal care for other fetal problems** ✓4th

> INCLUDES the listed conditions in the fetus as a reason for hospitalization or other obstetric care of the mother, or for termination of pregnancy
>
> EXCLUDES 1 encounter for suspected maternal and fetal conditions ruled out (Z03.7-)
> placental transfusion syndromes (O43.0-)
>
> EXCLUDES 2 labor and delivery complicated by fetal stress (O77.-)
>
> AHA: 2015,3Q,40

> One of the following 7th characters is to be assigned to each code under category O36. 7th character 0 is for single gestations and multiple gestations where the fetus is unspecified. 7th characters 1 through 9 are for cases of multiple gestations to identify the fetus for which the code applies. The appropriate code from category O30, Multiple gestation, must also be assigned when assigning a code from category O36 that has a 7th character of 1 through 9.
> - 0 not applicable or unspecified
> - 1 fetus 1
> - 2 fetus 2
> - 3 fetus 3
> - 4 fetus 4
> - 5 fetus 5
> - 9 other fetus

- ✓5th **O36.0** Maternal care for rhesus isoimmunization
  - Maternal care for Rh incompatibility (with hydrops fetalis)
  - ✓6th **O36.01** Maternal care for anti-D [Rh] antibodies
    - AHA: 2014,4Q,17
    - ✓7th **O36.011** Maternal care for anti-D [Rh] antibodies, first trimester

---

Additional Character Required | ✓x7th Placeholder Alert | Manifestation | Unspecified Dx | QPP | UPD Unacceptable PDx

- **O36.012** Maternal care for anti-D [Rh] antibodies, second trimester
- **O36.013** Maternal care for anti-D [Rh] antibodies, third trimester
- **O36.019** Maternal care for anti-D [Rh] antibodies, unspecified trimester
- **O36.09** Maternal care for other rhesus isoimmunization
  - **O36.091** Maternal care for other rhesus isoimmunization, first trimester
  - **O36.092** Maternal care for other rhesus isoimmunization, second trimester
  - **O36.093** Maternal care for other rhesus isoimmunization, third trimester
  - **O36.099** Maternal care for other rhesus isoimmunization, unspecified trimester
- **O36.1** Maternal care for other isoimmunization
  Maternal care for ABO isoimmunization
  - **O36.11** Maternal care for Anti-A sensitization
    Maternal care for isoimmunization NOS (with hydrops fetalis)
    - **O36.111** Maternal care for Anti-A sensitization, first trimester
    - **O36.112** Maternal care for Anti-A sensitization, second trimester
    - **O36.113** Maternal care for Anti-A sensitization, third trimester
    - **O36.119** Maternal care for Anti-A sensitization, unspecified trimester
  - **O36.19** Maternal care for other isoimmunization
    Maternal care for Anti-B sensitization
    - **O36.191** Maternal care for other isoimmunization, first trimester
    - **O36.192** Maternal care for other isoimmunization, second trimester
    - **O36.193** Maternal care for other isoimmunization, third trimester
    - **O36.199** Maternal care for other isoimmunization, unspecified trimester
- **O36.2** Maternal care for hydrops fetalis
  Maternal care for hydrops fetalis NOS
  Maternal care for hydrops fetalis not associated with isoimmunization
  EXCLUDES 1: hydrops fetalis associated with ABO isoimmunization (O36.1-)
  hydrops fetalis associated with rhesus isoimmunization (O36.0-)
  DEF: Hydrops fetalis: Abnormal fluid buildup in at least two of the following fetal organ spaces: the skin (edema), abdomen (ascites), around the heart (pericardia effusion), and around the lung (pleural effusion). Fluid accumulation may also occur in the mother as polyhydramnios and edema of the placenta.
  - **O36.20** Maternal care for hydrops fetalis, unspecified trimester
  - **O36.21** Maternal care for hydrops fetalis, first trimester
  - **O36.22** Maternal care for hydrops fetalis, second trimester
  - **O36.23** Maternal care for hydrops fetalis, third trimester
- **O36.4** Maternal care for intrauterine death
  Maternal care for intrauterine fetal death after completion of 20 weeks of gestation
  Maternal care for intrauterine fetal death NOS
  Maternal care for late fetal death
  Maternal care for missed delivery
  EXCLUDES 1: missed abortion (O02.1)
  stillbirth (P95)
  AHA: 2022,2Q,3
- **O36.5** Maternal care for known or suspected poor fetal growth
  - **O36.51** Maternal care for known or suspected placental insufficiency
    - **O36.511** Maternal care for known or suspected placental insufficiency, first trimester
    - **O36.512** Maternal care for known or suspected placental insufficiency, second trimester
    - **O36.513** Maternal care for known or suspected placental insufficiency, third trimester
    - **O36.519** Maternal care for known or suspected placental insufficiency, unspecified trimester
  - **O36.59** Maternal care for other known or suspected poor fetal growth
    Maternal care for known or suspected light-for-dates NOS
    Maternal care for known or suspected small-for-dates NOS
    - **O36.591** Maternal care for other known or suspected poor fetal growth, first trimester
    - **O36.592** Maternal care for other known or suspected poor fetal growth, second trimester
    - **O36.593** Maternal care for other known or suspected poor fetal growth, third trimester
      AHA: 2024,3Q,10
    - **O36.599** Maternal care for other known or suspected poor fetal growth, unspecified trimester
- **O36.6** Maternal care for excessive fetal growth
  Maternal care for known or suspected large-for-dates
  - **O36.60** Maternal care for excessive fetal growth, unspecified trimester
  - **O36.61** Maternal care for excessive fetal growth, first trimester
  - **O36.62** Maternal care for excessive fetal growth, second trimester
  - **O36.63** Maternal care for excessive fetal growth, third trimester
- **O36.7** Maternal care for viable fetus in abdominal pregnancy
  - **O36.70** Maternal care for viable fetus in abdominal pregnancy, unspecified trimester
  - **O36.71** Maternal care for viable fetus in abdominal pregnancy, first trimester
  - **O36.72** Maternal care for viable fetus in abdominal pregnancy, second trimester
  - **O36.73** Maternal care for viable fetus in abdominal pregnancy, third trimester
- **O36.8** Maternal care for other specified fetal problems
  - **O36.80** Pregnancy with inconclusive fetal viability
    Encounter to determine fetal viability of pregnancy
    AHA: 2019,2Q,29
  - **O36.81** Decreased fetal movements
    - **O36.812** Decreased fetal movements, second trimester
    - **O36.813** Decreased fetal movements, third trimester
    - **O36.819** Decreased fetal movements, unspecified trimester
  - **O36.82** Fetal anemia and thrombocytopenia
    - **O36.821** Fetal anemia and thrombocytopenia, first trimester
    - **O36.822** Fetal anemia and thrombocytopenia, second trimester
    - **O36.823** Fetal anemia and thrombocytopenia, third trimester
    - **O36.829** Fetal anemia and thrombocytopenia, unspecified trimester

O36.83 Maternal care for abnormalities of the fetal heart rate or rhythm
- Maternal care for depressed fetal heart rate tones
- Maternal care for fetal bradycardia
- Maternal care for fetal heart rate abnormal variability
- Maternal care for fetal heart rate decelerations
- Maternal care for fetal heart rate irregularity
- Maternal care for fetal tachycardia
- Maternal care for non-reassuring fetal heart rate or rhythm

AHA: 2017,4Q,20

TIP: Assign for documented fetal tachycardia, bradycardia, decelerations, or loss of variability detected during antenatal testing.

- **O36.831** Maternal care for abnormalities of the fetal heart rate or rhythm, **first trimester**
- **O36.832** Maternal care for abnormalities of the fetal heart rate or rhythm, **second trimester**
- **O36.833** Maternal care for abnormalities of the fetal heart rate or rhythm, **third trimester**
- **O36.839** Maternal care for abnormalities of the fetal heart rate or rhythm, **unspecified trimester**

O36.89 Maternal care for other specified fetal problems
- **O36.891** Maternal care for other specified fetal problems, **first trimester**
- **O36.892** Maternal care for other specified fetal problems, **second trimester**
- **O36.893** Maternal care for other specified fetal problems, **third trimester**
- **O36.899** Maternal care for other specified fetal problems, **unspecified trimester**

O36.9 Maternal care for fetal problem, unspecified
- **O36.90** Maternal care for fetal problem, unspecified, **unspecified trimester**
- **O36.91** Maternal care for fetal problem, unspecified, **first trimester**
- **O36.92** Maternal care for fetal problem, unspecified, **second trimester**
- **O36.93** Maternal care for fetal problem, unspecified, **third trimester**

O40 Polyhydramnios
INCLUDES hydramnios
EXCLUDES 1 encounter for suspected maternal and fetal conditions ruled out (Z03.7-)

AHA: 2016,1Q,4
DEF: Excess amniotic fluid surrounding the fetus, typically defined as a total fluid volume of greater than 24 cm.

One of the following 7th characters is to be assigned to each code under category O40. 7th character 0 is for single gestations and multiple gestations where the fetus is unspecified. 7th characters 1 through 9 are for cases of multiple gestations to identify the fetus for which the code applies. The appropriate code from category O30, Multiple gestation, must also be assigned when assigning a code from category O40 that has a 7th character of 1 through 9.
- 0 not applicable or unspecified
- 1 fetus 1
- 2 fetus 2
- 3 fetus 3
- 4 fetus 4
- 5 fetus 5
- 9 other fetus

- **O40.1** Polyhydramnios, **first trimester**
- **O40.2** Polyhydramnios, **second trimester**
- **O40.3** Polyhydramnios, **third trimester**
- **O40.9** Polyhydramnios, **unspecified trimester**

O41 Other disorders of amniotic fluid and membranes
EXCLUDES 1 encounter for suspected maternal and fetal conditions ruled out (Z03.7-)

One of the following 7th characters is to be assigned to each code under category O41. 7th character 0 is for single gestations and multiple gestations where the fetus is unspecified. 7th characters 1 through 9 are for cases of multiple gestations to identify the fetus for which the code applies. The appropriate code from category O30, Multiple gestation, must also be assigned when assigning a code from category O41 that has a 7th character of 1 through 9.
- 0 not applicable or unspecified
- 1 fetus 1
- 2 fetus 2
- 3 fetus 3
- 4 fetus 4
- 5 fetus 5
- 9 other fetus

O41.0 Oligohydramnios
Oligohydramnios without rupture of membranes
DEF: Low amniotic fluid, occurring most frequently in the last trimester.
- **O41.00** Oligohydramnios, unspecified trimester
- **O41.01** Oligohydramnios, **first trimester**
- **O41.02** Oligohydramnios, **second trimester**
- **O41.03** Oligohydramnios, **third trimester**

O41.1 Infection of amniotic sac and membranes
- **O41.10** Infection of amniotic sac and membranes, unspecified
  - **O41.101** Infection of amniotic sac and membranes, unspecified, **first trimester**
  - **O41.102** Infection of amniotic sac and membranes, unspecified, **second trimester**
  - **O41.103** Infection of amniotic sac and membranes, unspecified, **third trimester**
  - **O41.109** Infection of amniotic sac and membranes, unspecified, **unspecified trimester**
- **O41.12** Chorioamnionitis
  AHA: 2019,2Q,34
  - **O41.121** Chorioamnionitis, **first trimester**
  - **O41.122** Chorioamnionitis, **second trimester**
  - **O41.123** Chorioamnionitis, **third trimester**
  - **O41.129** Chorioamnionitis, **unspecified trimester**
- **O41.14** Placentitis
  - **O41.141** Placentitis, **first trimester**
  - **O41.142** Placentitis, **second trimester**
  - **O41.143** Placentitis, **third trimester**
  - **O41.149** Placentitis, **unspecified trimester**

O41.8 Other specified disorders of amniotic fluid and membranes
- **O41.8X** Other specified disorders of amniotic fluid and membranes
  AHA: 2024,1Q,13
  - **O41.8X1** Other specified disorders of amniotic fluid and membranes, **first trimester**
  - **O41.8X2** Other specified disorders of amniotic fluid and membranes, **second trimester**
  - **O41.8X3** Other specified disorders of amniotic fluid and membranes, **third trimester**
  - **O41.8X9** Other specified disorders of amniotic fluid and membranes, **unspecified trimester**

O41.9 Disorder of amniotic fluid and membranes, unspecified
- **O41.90** Disorder of amniotic fluid and membranes, unspecified, **unspecified trimester**
- **O41.91** Disorder of amniotic fluid and membranes, unspecified, **first trimester**
- **O41.92** Disorder of amniotic fluid and membranes, unspecified, **second trimester**
- **O41.93** Disorder of amniotic fluid and membranes, unspecified, **third trimester**

O42 Premature rupture of membranes
AHA: 2023,3Q,17; 2016,1Q,3

O42.0 Premature rupture of membranes, onset of labor within 24 hours of rupture

- **O42.00** Premature rupture of membranes, onset of labor within 24 hours of rupture, unspecified weeks of gestation
- **O42.01** Preterm premature rupture of membranes, onset of labor within 24 hours of rupture
  Premature rupture of membranes before 37 completed weeks of gestation
  - **O42.011** Preterm premature rupture of membranes, onset of labor within 24 hours of rupture, first trimester
  - **O42.012** Preterm premature rupture of membranes, onset of labor within 24 hours of rupture, second trimester
  - **O42.013** Preterm premature rupture of membranes, onset of labor within 24 hours of rupture, third trimester
  - **O42.019** Preterm premature rupture of membranes, onset of labor within 24 hours of rupture, unspecified trimester
- **O42.02** Full-term premature rupture of membranes, onset of labor within 24 hours of rupture
  Premature rupture of membranes at or after 37 completed weeks of gestation, onset of labor within 24 hours of rupture

O42.1 Premature rupture of membranes, onset of labor more than 24 hours following rupture
AHA: 2016,1Q,5

- **O42.10** Premature rupture of membranes, onset of labor more than 24 hours following rupture, unspecified weeks of gestation
- **O42.11** Preterm premature rupture of membranes, onset of labor more than 24 hours following rupture
  Premature rupture of membranes before 37 completed weeks of gestation
  - **O42.111** Preterm premature rupture of membranes, onset of labor more than 24 hours following rupture, first trimester
  - **O42.112** Preterm premature rupture of membranes, onset of labor more than 24 hours following rupture, second trimester
  - **O42.113** Preterm premature rupture of membranes, onset of labor more than 24 hours following rupture, third trimester
  - **O42.119** Preterm premature rupture of membranes, onset of labor more than 24 hours following rupture, unspecified trimester
- **O42.12** Full-term premature rupture of membranes, onset of labor more than 24 hours following rupture
  Premature rupture of membranes at or after 37 completed weeks of gestation, onset of labor more than 24 hours following rupture

O42.9 Premature rupture of membranes, unspecified as to length of time between rupture and onset of labor

- **O42.90** Premature rupture of membranes, unspecified as to length of time between rupture and onset of labor, unspecified weeks of gestation
- **O42.91** Preterm premature rupture of membranes, unspecified as to length of time between rupture and onset of labor
  Premature rupture of membranes before 37 completed weeks of gestation
  - **O42.911** Preterm premature rupture of membranes, unspecified as to length of time between rupture and onset of labor, first trimester
  - **O42.912** Preterm premature rupture of membranes, unspecified as to length of time between rupture and onset of labor, second trimester
  - **O42.913** Preterm premature rupture of membranes, unspecified as to length of time between rupture and onset of labor, third trimester
  - **O42.919** Preterm premature rupture of membranes, unspecified as to length of time between rupture and onset of labor, unspecified trimester
- **O42.92** Full-term premature rupture of membranes, unspecified as to length of time between rupture and onset of labor
  Premature rupture of membranes at or after 37 completed weeks of gestation, unspecified as to length of time between rupture and onset of labor

O43 Placental disorders

EXCLUDES 2: maternal care for poor fetal growth due to placental insufficiency (O36.5-)
placenta previa (O44.-)
placental polyp (O90.89)
placentitis (O41.14-)
premature separation of placenta [abruptio placentae] (O45.-)

O43.0 Placental transfusion syndromes

- **O43.01** Fetomaternal placental transfusion syndrome
  Maternofetal placental transfusion syndrome
  - **O43.011** Fetomaternal placental transfusion syndrome, first trimester
  - **O43.012** Fetomaternal placental transfusion syndrome, second trimester
  - **O43.013** Fetomaternal placental transfusion syndrome, third trimester
  - **O43.019** Fetomaternal placental transfusion syndrome, unspecified trimester
- **O43.02** Fetus-to-fetus placental transfusion syndrome
  DEF: Condition in which an imbalance in amniotic fluid occurs due to uneven blood flow between twins sharing a placenta.

  Twin to Twin Transfusion Syndrome (TTTS)
  Healthy twins — Twins with TTTS

  - **O43.021** Fetus-to-fetus placental transfusion syndrome, first trimester
  - **O43.022** Fetus-to-fetus placental transfusion syndrome, second trimester
  - **O43.023** Fetus-to-fetus placental transfusion syndrome, third trimester
  - **O43.029** Fetus-to-fetus placental transfusion syndrome, unspecified trimester

O43.1 Malformation of placenta

- **O43.10** Malformation of placenta, unspecified
  Abnormal placenta NOS
  - **O43.101** Malformation of placenta, unspecified, first trimester
  - **O43.102** Malformation of placenta, unspecified, second trimester
  - **O43.103** Malformation of placenta, unspecified, third trimester
  - **O43.109** Malformation of placenta, unspecified trimester
- **O43.11** Circumvallate placenta
  - **O43.111** Circumvallate placenta, first trimester
  - **O43.112** Circumvallate placenta, second trimester
  - **O43.113** Circumvallate placenta, third trimester
  - **O43.119** Circumvallate placenta, unspecified trimester

Chapter 15. Pregnancy, Childbirth and the Puerperium

- **O43.12** Velamentous insertion of umbilical cord
  - **O43.121** Velamentous insertion of umbilical cord, first trimester
  - **O43.122** Velamentous insertion of umbilical cord, second trimester
  - **O43.123** Velamentous insertion of umbilical cord, third trimester
  - **O43.129** Velamentous insertion of umbilical cord, unspecified trimester
- **O43.19** Other malformation of placenta
  - **O43.191** Other malformation of placenta, first trimester
  - **O43.192** Other malformation of placenta, second trimester
  - **O43.193** Other malformation of placenta, third trimester
  - **O43.199** Other malformation of placenta, unspecified trimester

O43.2 Morbidly adherent placenta
  Code also associated third stage postpartum hemorrhage, if applicable (O72.0)
  EXCLUDES 1 retained placenta (O73.-)

- **O43.21** Placenta accreta
  DEF: Condition where the placenta adheres too deeply to the uterine wall; often associated with placenta previa.
  - **O43.211** Placenta accreta, first trimester
  - **O43.212** Placenta accreta, second trimester
  - **O43.213** Placenta accreta, third trimester
  - **O43.219** Placenta accreta, unspecified trimester
- **O43.22** Placenta increta
  AHA: 2022,1Q,20
  DEF: Condition where the placenta adheres too deeply to the uterine wall and penetrates the muscle; often associated with placenta previa.
  - **O43.221** Placenta increta, first trimester
  - **O43.222** Placenta increta, second trimester
  - **O43.223** Placenta increta, third trimester
  - **O43.229** Placenta increta, unspecified trimester
- **O43.23** Placenta percreta
  DEF: Condition where the placenta attaches through the uterine muscle and may invade other organs, resulting in antenatal complications, premature delivery, retention of all or a portion of the placenta, or postpartum bleeding.
  - **O43.231** Placenta percreta, first trimester
  - **O43.232** Placenta percreta, second trimester
  - **O43.233** Placenta percreta, third trimester
  - **O43.239** Placenta percreta, unspecified trimester

O43.8 Other placental disorders
- **O43.81** Placental infarction
  - **O43.811** Placental infarction, first trimester
  - **O43.812** Placental infarction, second trimester
  - **O43.813** Placental infarction, third trimester
  - **O43.819** Placental infarction, unspecified trimester
- **O43.89** Other placental disorders
  Placental dysfunction
  - **O43.891** Other placental disorders, first trimester
  - **O43.892** Other placental disorders, second trimester
  - **O43.893** Other placental disorders, third trimester
  - **O43.899** Other placental disorders, unspecified trimester

O43.9 Unspecified placental disorder
- **O43.90** Unspecified placental disorder, unspecified trimester
- **O43.91** Unspecified placental disorder, first trimester
- **O43.92** Unspecified placental disorder, second trimester
- **O43.93** Unspecified placental disorder, third trimester

O44 Placenta previa
AHA: 2016,4Q,52-53
DEF: Placenta implanted in the lower segment of the uterus, which commonly causes hemorrhage in the last trimester of pregnancy.

O44.0 Complete placenta previa NOS or without hemorrhage
  Placenta previa NOS
- **O44.00** Complete placenta previa NOS or without hemorrhage, unspecified trimester
- **O44.01** Complete placenta previa NOS or without hemorrhage, first trimester
- **O44.02** Complete placenta previa NOS or without hemorrhage, second trimester
- **O44.03** Complete placenta previa NOS or without hemorrhage, third trimester

O44.1 Complete placenta previa with hemorrhage
  EXCLUDES 1 labor and delivery complicated by hemorrhage from vasa previa (O69.4)
- **O44.10** Complete placenta previa with hemorrhage, unspecified trimester
- **O44.11** Complete placenta previa with hemorrhage, first trimester
- **O44.12** Complete placenta previa with hemorrhage, second trimester
- **O44.13** Complete placenta previa with hemorrhage, third trimester

O44.2 Partial placenta previa without hemorrhage
  Marginal placenta previa, NOS or without hemorrhage
- **O44.20** Partial placenta previa NOS or without hemorrhage, unspecified trimester
- **O44.21** Partial placenta previa NOS or without hemorrhage, first trimester
- **O44.22** Partial placenta previa NOS or without hemorrhage, second trimester
- **O44.23** Partial placenta previa NOS or without hemorrhage, third trimester

O44.3 Partial placenta previa with hemorrhage
  Marginal placenta previa with hemorrhage
- **O44.30** Partial placenta previa with hemorrhage, unspecified trimester
- **O44.31** Partial placenta previa with hemorrhage, first trimester
- **O44.32** Partial placenta previa with hemorrhage, second trimester
- **O44.33** Partial placenta previa with hemorrhage, third trimester

O44.4 Low lying placenta NOS or without hemorrhage
  Low implantation of placenta NOS or without hemorrhage
- **O44.40** Low lying placenta NOS or without hemorrhage, unspecified trimester
- **O44.41** Low lying placenta NOS or without hemorrhage, first trimester
- **O44.42** Low lying placenta NOS or without hemorrhage, second trimester
- **O44.43** Low lying placenta NOS or without hemorrhage, third trimester

O44.5 Low lying placenta with hemorrhage
  Low implantation of placenta with hemorrhage
- **O44.50** Low lying placenta with hemorrhage, unspecified trimester
- **O44.51** Low lying placenta with hemorrhage, first trimester
- **O44.52** Low lying placenta with hemorrhage, second trimester
- **O44.53** Low lying placenta with hemorrhage, third trimester

O45 Premature separation of placenta [abruptio placentae]

O45.0 Premature separation of placenta with coagulation defect

O45.00 Premature separation of placenta with coagulation defect, unspecified
- **O45.001** Premature separation of placenta with coagulation defect, unspecified, first trimester
- **O45.002** Premature separation of placenta with coagulation defect, unspecified, second trimester
- **O45.003** Premature separation of placenta with coagulation defect, unspecified, third trimester
- **O45.009** Premature separation of placenta with coagulation defect, unspecified, unspecified trimester

O45.01 Premature separation of placenta with afibrinogenemia
Premature separation of placenta with hypofibrinogenemia
- **O45.011** Premature separation of placenta with afibrinogenemia, first trimester
- **O45.012** Premature separation of placenta with afibrinogenemia, second trimester
- **O45.013** Premature separation of placenta with afibrinogenemia, third trimester
- **O45.019** Premature separation of placenta with afibrinogenemia, unspecified trimester

O45.02 Premature separation of placenta with disseminated intravascular coagulation
- **O45.021** Premature separation of placenta with disseminated intravascular coagulation, first trimester
- **O45.022** Premature separation of placenta with disseminated intravascular coagulation, second trimester
- **O45.023** Premature separation of placenta with disseminated intravascular coagulation, third trimester
- **O45.029** Premature separation of placenta with disseminated intravascular coagulation, unspecified trimester

O45.09 Premature separation of placenta with other coagulation defect
- **O45.091** Premature separation of placenta with other coagulation defect, first trimester
- **O45.092** Premature separation of placenta with other coagulation defect, second trimester
- **O45.093** Premature separation of placenta with other coagulation defect, third trimester
- **O45.099** Premature separation of placenta with other coagulation defect, unspecified trimester

O45.8 Other premature separation of placenta

O45.8X Other premature separation of placenta
- **O45.8X1** Other premature separation of placenta, first trimester
- **O45.8X2** Other premature separation of placenta, second trimester
- **O45.8X3** Other premature separation of placenta, third trimester
- **O45.8X9** Other premature separation of placenta, unspecified trimester

O45.9 Premature separation of placenta, unspecified
Abruptio placentae NOS
- **O45.90** Premature separation of placenta, unspecified, unspecified trimester
- **O45.91** Premature separation of placenta, unspecified, first trimester
- **O45.92** Premature separation of placenta, unspecified, second trimester
- **O45.93** Premature separation of placenta, unspecified, third trimester

O46 Antepartum hemorrhage, not elsewhere classified

EXCLUDES 1 hemorrhage in early pregnancy (O20.-)
intrapartum hemorrhage NEC (O67.-)
placenta previa (O44.-)
premature separation of placenta [abruptio placentae] (O45.-)

DEF: Uterine hemorrhage prior to delivery that is not related to placenta previa or abruptio placentae.

O46.0 Antepartum hemorrhage with coagulation defect

O46.00 Antepartum hemorrhage with coagulation defect, unspecified
- **O46.001** Antepartum hemorrhage with coagulation defect, unspecified, first trimester
- **O46.002** Antepartum hemorrhage with coagulation defect, unspecified, second trimester
- **O46.003** Antepartum hemorrhage with coagulation defect, unspecified, third trimester
- **O46.009** Antepartum hemorrhage with coagulation defect, unspecified, unspecified trimester

O46.01 Antepartum hemorrhage with afibrinogenemia
Antepartum hemorrhage with hypofibrinogenemia
- **O46.011** Antepartum hemorrhage with afibrinogenemia, first trimester
- **O46.012** Antepartum hemorrhage with afibrinogenemia, second trimester
- **O46.013** Antepartum hemorrhage with afibrinogenemia, third trimester
- **O46.019** Antepartum hemorrhage with afibrinogenemia, unspecified trimester

O46.02 Antepartum hemorrhage with disseminated intravascular coagulation
- **O46.021** Antepartum hemorrhage with disseminated intravascular coagulation, first trimester
- **O46.022** Antepartum hemorrhage with disseminated intravascular coagulation, second trimester
- **O46.023** Antepartum hemorrhage with disseminated intravascular coagulation, third trimester
- **O46.029** Antepartum hemorrhage with disseminated intravascular coagulation, unspecified trimester

O46.09 Antepartum hemorrhage with other coagulation defect
- **O46.091** Antepartum hemorrhage with other coagulation defect, first trimester
- **O46.092** Antepartum hemorrhage with other coagulation defect, second trimester
- **O46.093** Antepartum hemorrhage with other coagulation defect, third trimester
- **O46.099** Antepartum hemorrhage with other coagulation defect, unspecified trimester

O46.8 Other antepartum hemorrhage

O46.8X Other antepartum hemorrhage
- **O46.8X1** Other antepartum hemorrhage, first trimester
- **O46.8X2** Other antepartum hemorrhage, second trimester
- **O46.8X3** Other antepartum hemorrhage, third trimester
- **O46.8X9** Other antepartum hemorrhage, unspecified trimester

O46.9 Antepartum hemorrhage, unspecified
- **O46.90** Antepartum hemorrhage, unspecified, unspecified trimester
- **O46.91** Antepartum hemorrhage, unspecified, first trimester
- **O46.92** Antepartum hemorrhage, unspecified, second trimester

Chapter 15. Pregnancy, Childbirth and the Puerperium

O46.93 Antepartum hemorrhage, unspecified, third trimester

O47 False labor
- INCLUDES: Braxton Hicks contractions; threatened labor
- EXCLUDES 1: preterm labor (O60.-)
- AHA: 2021,1Q,10

O47.0 False labor before 37 completed weeks of gestation
- **O47.00** False labor before 37 completed weeks of gestation, unspecified trimester
- **O47.02** False labor before 37 completed weeks of gestation, second trimester
- **O47.03** False labor before 37 completed weeks of gestation, third trimester

O47.1 False labor at or after 37 completed weeks of gestation

O47.9 False labor, unspecified

O48 Late pregnancy
- AHA: 2022,2Q,3

O48.0 Post-term pregnancy
- Pregnancy over 40 completed weeks to 42 completed weeks gestation

O48.1 Prolonged pregnancy
- Pregnancy which has advanced beyond 42 completed weeks gestation
- AHA: 2016,1Q,5

Complications of labor and delivery (O60-O77)

O60 Preterm labor
- INCLUDES: onset (spontaneous) of labor before 37 completed weeks of gestation
- EXCLUDES 1: false labor (O47.0-); threatened labor NOS (O47.0-)

O60.0 Preterm labor without delivery
- **O60.00** Preterm labor without delivery, unspecified trimester
- **O60.02** Preterm labor without delivery, second trimester
- **O60.03** Preterm labor without delivery, third trimester

O60.1 Preterm labor with preterm delivery
- AHA: 2016,2Q,10

One of the following 7th characters is to be assigned to each code under subcategory O60.1. 7th character 0 is for single gestations and multiple gestations where the fetus is unspecified. 7th characters 1 through 9 are for cases of multiple gestations to identify the fetus for which the code applies. The appropriate code from category O30, Multiple gestation, must also be assigned when assigning a code from subcategory O60.1 that has a 7th character of 1 through 9.
- 0 not applicable or unspecified
- 1 fetus 1
- 2 fetus 2
- 3 fetus 3
- 4 fetus 4
- 5 fetus 5
- 9 other fetus

- **O60.10** Preterm labor with preterm delivery, unspecified trimester
  - Preterm labor with delivery NOS
- **O60.12** Preterm labor second trimester with preterm delivery second trimester
- **O60.13** Preterm labor second trimester with preterm delivery third trimester
- **O60.14** Preterm labor third trimester with preterm delivery third trimester

O60.2 Term delivery with preterm labor

One of the following 7th characters is to be assigned to each code under subcategory O60.2. 7th character 0 is for single gestations and multiple gestations where the fetus is unspecified. 7th characters 1 through 9 are for cases of multiple gestations to identify the fetus for which the code applies. The appropriate code from category O30, Multiple gestation, must also be assigned when assigning a code from subcategory O60.2 that has a 7th character of 1 through 9.
- 0 not applicable or unspecified
- 1 fetus 1
- 2 fetus 2
- 3 fetus 3
- 4 fetus 4
- 5 fetus 5
- 9 other fetus

- **O60.20** Term delivery with preterm labor, unspecified trimester
- **O60.22** Term delivery with preterm labor, second trimester
- **O60.23** Term delivery with preterm labor, third trimester

O61 Failed induction of labor

O61.0 Failed medical induction of labor
- Failed induction (of labor) by oxytocin
- Failed induction (of labor) by prostaglandins

O61.1 Failed instrumental induction of labor
- Failed mechanical induction (of labor)
- Failed surgical induction (of labor)

O61.8 Other failed induction of labor

O61.9 Failed induction of labor, unspecified

O62 Abnormalities of forces of labor
- DEF: Uterine inertia: Weak or poorly coordinated contractions of the uterus during labor.

O62.0 Primary inadequate contractions
- Failure of cervical dilatation
- Primary hypotonic uterine dysfunction
- Uterine inertia during latent phase of labor
- AHA: 2024,1Q,13

O62.1 Secondary uterine inertia
- Arrested active phase of labor
- Secondary hypotonic uterine dysfunction

O62.2 Other uterine inertia
- Atony of uterus NOS
- Atony of uterus without hemorrhage
- Desultory labor
- Hypotonic uterine dysfunction NOS
- Irregular labor
- Poor contractions
- Slow slope active phase of labor
- Uterine inertia NOS
- EXCLUDES 1: atony of uterus with hemorrhage (postpartum) (O72.1); postpartum atony of uterus without hemorrhage (O75.89)
- DEF: Uterine atony: Failure of the uterine muscles to contract after the fetus and placenta are delivered.

O62.3 Precipitate labor
- DEF: Rapid labor with delivery occurring in three hours or less from the onset of contractions.

O62.4 Hypertonic, incoordinate, and prolonged uterine contractions
- Cervical spasm
- Contraction ring dystocia
- Dyscoordinate labor
- Hour-glass contraction of uterus
- Hypertonic uterine dysfunction
- Incoordinate uterine action
- Tetanic contractions
- Uterine dystocia NOS
- Uterine spasm
- EXCLUDES 1: dystocia (fetal) (maternal) NOS (O66.9)

O62.8 Other abnormalities of forces of labor

O62.9 Abnormality of forces of labor, unspecified

O63 Long labor

O63.0 Prolonged first stage (of labor)

O63.1 Prolonged second stage (of labor)

O63.2 Delayed delivery of second twin, triplet, etc.

Chapter 15. Pregnancy, Childbirth and the Puerperium

O63.9 Long labor, unspecified
Prolonged labor NOS

O64 Obstructed labor due to malposition and malpresentation of fetus

One of the following 7th characters is to be assigned to each code under category O64. 7th character 0 is for single gestations and multiple gestations where the fetus is unspecified. 7th characters 1 through 9 are for cases of multiple gestations to identify the fetus for which the code applies. The appropriate code from category O30, Multiple gestation, must also be assigned when assigning a code from category O64 that has a 7th character of 1 through 9.

  0 not applicable or unspecified
  1 fetus 1
  2 fetus 2
  3 fetus 3
  4 fetus 4
  5 fetus 5
  9 other fetus

Fetal Malposition

- Breech
- Mother's pelvis
- Shoulder (arm prolapse)
- Face (mentum)
- Compound (extremity together with head)
- Oblique

O64.0 Obstructed labor due to incomplete rotation of fetal head
Deep transverse arrest
Obstructed labor due to persistent occipitoiliac (position)
Obstructed labor due to persistent occipitoposterior (position)
Obstructed labor due to persistent occipitosacral (position)
Obstructed labor due to persistent occipitotransverse (position)

O64.1 Obstructed labor due to breech presentation
Obstructed labor due to buttocks presentation
Obstructed labor due to complete breech presentation
Obstructed labor due to frank breech presentation

O64.2 Obstructed labor due to face presentation
Obstructed labor due to chin presentation

O64.3 Obstructed labor due to brow presentation

O64.4 Obstructed labor due to shoulder presentation
Prolapsed arm
EXCLUDES 1 impacted shoulders (O66.0)
shoulder dystocia (O66.0)

O64.5 Obstructed labor due to compound presentation

O64.8 Obstructed labor due to other malposition and malpresentation
Obstructed labor due to footling presentation
Obstructed labor due to incomplete breech presentation

O64.9 Obstructed labor due to malposition and malpresentation, unspecified

O65 Obstructed labor due to maternal pelvic abnormality

O65.0 Obstructed labor due to deformed pelvis

O65.1 Obstructed labor due to generally contracted pelvis

O65.2 Obstructed labor due to pelvic inlet contraction

O65.3 Obstructed labor due to pelvic outlet and mid-cavity contraction

O65.4 Obstructed labor due to fetopelvic disproportion, unspecified
EXCLUDES 1 dystocia due to abnormality of fetus (O66.2-O66.3)

O65.5 Obstructed labor due to abnormality of maternal pelvic organs
Obstructed labor due to conditions listed in O34.-
Use additional code to identify abnormality of pelvic organs O34.-

O65.8 Obstructed labor due to other maternal pelvic abnormalities

O65.9 Obstructed labor due to maternal pelvic abnormality, unspecified

O66 Other obstructed labor

O66.0 Obstructed labor due to shoulder dystocia
Impacted shoulders
DEF: Obstructed labor due to impacted fetal shoulders. It is an emergency condition that may require cesarean section, forceps delivery, vacuum extraction, or symphysiotomy.

O66.1 Obstructed labor due to locked twins

O66.2 Obstructed labor due to unusually large fetus

O66.3 Obstructed labor due to other abnormalities of fetus
Dystocia due to fetal ascites
Dystocia due to fetal hydrops
Dystocia due to fetal meningomyelocele
Dystocia due to fetal sacral teratoma
Dystocia due to fetal tumor
Dystocia due to hydrocephalic fetus
Use additional code to identify cause of obstruction

O66.4 Failed trial of labor
  O66.40 Failed trial of labor, unspecified
  O66.41 Failed attempted vaginal birth after previous cesarean delivery
    Code first rupture of uterus, if applicable (O71.0-, O71.1)

O66.5 Attempted application of vacuum extractor and forceps
Attempted application of vacuum or forceps, with subsequent delivery by forceps or cesarean delivery

O66.6 Obstructed labor due to other multiple fetuses

O66.8 Other specified obstructed labor
Use additional code to identify cause of obstruction

O66.9 Obstructed labor, unspecified
Dystocia NOS
Fetal dystocia NOS
Maternal dystocia NOS

O67 Labor and delivery complicated by intrapartum hemorrhage, not elsewhere classified
EXCLUDES 1 antepartum hemorrhage NEC (O46.-)
placenta previa (O44.-)
premature separation of placenta [abruptio placentae] (O45.-)
EXCLUDES 2 postpartum hemorrhage (O72.-)

O67.0 Intrapartum hemorrhage with coagulation defect
Intrapartum hemorrhage (excessive) associated with afibrinogenemia
Intrapartum hemorrhage (excessive) associated with disseminated intravascular coagulation
Intrapartum hemorrhage (excessive) associated with hyperfibrinolysis
Intrapartum hemorrhage (excessive) associated with hypofibrinogenemia

O67.8 Other intrapartum hemorrhage
Excessive intrapartum hemorrhage

O67.9 Intrapartum hemorrhage, unspecified

O68 Labor and delivery complicated by abnormality of fetal acid-base balance
Fetal acidemia complicating labor and delivery
Fetal acidosis complicating labor and delivery
Fetal alkalosis complicating labor and delivery
Fetal metabolic acidemia complicating labor and delivery
EXCLUDES 1 fetal stress NOS (O77.9)
labor and delivery complicated by electrocardiographic evidence of fetal stress (O77.8)
labor and delivery complicated by ultrasonic evidence of fetal stress (O77.8)
EXCLUDES 2 abnormality in fetal heart rate or rhythm (O76)
labor and delivery complicated by meconium in amniotic fluid (O77.0)

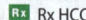

HCC CMS-HCC   Rx Rx HCC   ESR ESRD HCC   COM Commercial HCC   N Newborn: 0   P Pediatric: 0-17   M Maternity: 9-64   A Adult: 15-124

O69 Labor and delivery complicated by umbilical cord complications
AHA: 2016,1Q,5

One of the following 7th characters is to be assigned to each code under category O69. 7th character 0 is for single gestations and multiple gestations where the fetus is unspecified. 7th characters 1 through 9 are for cases of multiple gestations to identify the fetus for which the code applies. The appropriate code from category O30, Multiple gestation, must also be assigned when assigning a code from category O69 that has a 7th character of 1 through 9.
- 0 not applicable or unspecified
- 1 fetus 1
- 2 fetus 2
- 3 fetus 3
- 4 fetus 4
- 5 fetus 5
- 9 other fetus

O69.0 Labor and delivery complicated by prolapse of cord
DEF: Abnormal presentation of the fetus marked by a protruding umbilical cord during labor. It can cause fetal death.

O69.1 Labor and delivery complicated by cord around neck, with compression
EXCLUDES 1 labor and delivery complicated by cord around neck, without compression (O69.81)

O69.2 Labor and delivery complicated by other cord entanglement, with compression
Labor and delivery complicated by compression of cord NOS
Labor and delivery complicated by entanglement of cords of twins in monoamniotic sac
Labor and delivery complicated by knot in cord
EXCLUDES 1 labor and delivery complicated by other cord entanglement, without compression (O69.82)

O69.3 Labor and delivery complicated by short cord

O69.4 Labor and delivery complicated by vasa previa
Labor and delivery complicated by hemorrhage from vasa previa

O69.5 Labor and delivery complicated by vascular lesion of cord
Labor and delivery complicated by cord bruising
Labor and delivery complicated by cord hematoma
Labor and delivery complicated by thrombosis of umbilical vessels

O69.8 Labor and delivery complicated by other cord complications
O69.81 Labor and delivery complicated by cord around neck, without compression
AHA: 2016,1Q,5
O69.82 Labor and delivery complicated by other cord entanglement, without compression
O69.89 Labor and delivery complicated by other cord complications
AHA: 2023,2Q,29

O69.9 Labor and delivery complicated by cord complication, unspecified

O70 Perineal laceration during delivery
INCLUDES episiotomy extended by laceration
EXCLUDES 1 obstetric high vaginal laceration alone (O71.4)
AHA: 2016,2Q,34; 2016,1Q,3-4,5

O70.0 First degree perineal laceration during delivery
Perineal laceration, rupture or tear involving fourchette during delivery
Perineal laceration, rupture or tear involving labia during delivery
Perineal laceration, rupture or tear involving skin during delivery
Perineal laceration, rupture or tear involving vagina during delivery
Perineal laceration, rupture or tear involving vulva during delivery
Slight perineal laceration, rupture or tear during delivery

O70.1 Second degree perineal laceration during delivery
Perineal laceration, rupture or tear during delivery as in O70.0, also involving pelvic floor
Perineal laceration, rupture or tear during delivery as in O70.0, also involving perineal muscles
Perineal laceration, rupture or tear during delivery as in O70.0, also involving vaginal muscles
EXCLUDES 1 perineal laceration involving anal sphincter ▶(O70.2-)◀

O70.2 Third degree perineal laceration during delivery
Perineal laceration, rupture or tear during delivery as in O70.1, also involving anal sphincter
Perineal laceration, rupture or tear during delivery as in O70.1, also involving rectovaginal septum
Perineal laceration, rupture or tear during delivery as in O70.1, also involving sphincter NOS
EXCLUDES 1 anal sphincter tear during delivery without third degree perineal laceration (O70.4)
perineal laceration involving anal or rectal mucosa (O70.3)
AHA: 2016,4Q,53-54

O70.20 Third degree perineal laceration during delivery, unspecified
O70.21 Third degree perineal laceration during delivery, IIIa
Third degree perineal laceration during delivery with less than 50% of external anal sphincter (EAS) thickness torn
O70.22 Third degree perineal laceration during delivery, IIIb
Third degree perineal laceration during delivery with more than 50% external anal sphincter (EAS) thickness torn
O70.23 Third degree perineal laceration during delivery, IIIc
Third degree perineal laceration during delivery with both external anal sphincter (EAS) and internal anal sphincter (IAS) torn

O70.3 Fourth degree perineal laceration during delivery
Perineal laceration, rupture or tear during delivery as in O70.2, also involving anal mucosa
Perineal laceration, rupture or tear during delivery as in O70.2, also involving rectal mucosa

O70.4 Anal sphincter tear complicating delivery, not associated with third degree laceration
EXCLUDES 1 anal sphincter tear with third degree perineal laceration ▶(O70.2-)◀

O70.9 Perineal laceration during delivery, unspecified

O71 Other obstetric trauma
INCLUDES obstetric damage from instruments

O71.0 Rupture of uterus (spontaneous) before onset of labor
EXCLUDES 1 disruption of (current) cesarean delivery wound (O90.0)
laceration of uterus, NEC (O71.81)
O71.00 Rupture of uterus before onset of labor, unspecified trimester
O71.02 Rupture of uterus before onset of labor, second trimester
O71.03 Rupture of uterus before onset of labor, third trimester

O71.1 Rupture of uterus during labor
Rupture of uterus not stated as occurring before onset of labor
EXCLUDES 1 disruption of cesarean delivery wound (O90.0)
laceration of uterus, NEC (O71.81)

O71.2 Postpartum inversion of uterus

O71.3 Obstetric laceration of cervix
Annular detachment of cervix

O71.4 Obstetric high vaginal laceration alone
Laceration of vaginal wall without perineal laceration
EXCLUDES 1 obstetric high vaginal laceration with perineal laceration (O70.-)
AHA: 2016,1Q,5

O71.5 Other obstetric injury to pelvic organs
Obstetric injury to bladder
Obstetric injury to urethra
EXCLUDES 2 obstetric periurethral trauma (O71.82)
AHA: 2014,4Q,18

O71.6 Obstetric damage to pelvic joints and ligaments
Obstetric avulsion of inner symphyseal cartilage
Obstetric damage to coccyx
Obstetric traumatic separation of symphysis (pubis)

O71.7 Obstetric hematoma of pelvis
Obstetric hematoma of perineum
Obstetric hematoma of vagina
Obstetric hematoma of vulva

O71.8 Other specified obstetric trauma

- **O71.81** Laceration of uterus, not elsewhere classified
  - AHA: 2025,1Q,21
- **O71.82** Other specified trauma to perineum and vulva
  - Obstetric periurethral trauma
  - AHA: 2016,1Q,4; 2014,4Q,18
- **O71.89** Other specified obstetric trauma

O71.9 Obstetric trauma, unspecified

O72 Postpartum hemorrhage
INCLUDES: hemorrhage after delivery of fetus or infant

- **O72.0** Third-stage hemorrhage
  - Hemorrhage associated with retained, trapped or adherent placenta
  - Retained placenta NOS
  - Code also type of adherent placenta (O43.2-)
  - AHA: 2019,3Q,11
- **O72.1** Other immediate postpartum hemorrhage
  - Hemorrhage following delivery of placenta
  - Postpartum hemorrhage (atonic) NOS
  - Uterine atony with hemorrhage
  - EXCLUDES 1: uterine atony NOS (O62.2)
    - postpartum atony of uterus without hemorrhage (O75.89)
    - uterine atony without hemorrhage (O62.2)
  - AHA: 2023,2Q,15; 2016,1Q,4
  - DEF: Uterine atony: Failure of the uterine muscles to contract after the fetus and placenta are delivered.
- **O72.2** Delayed and secondary postpartum hemorrhage
  - Hemorrhage associated with retained portions of placenta or membranes after the first 24 hours following delivery of placenta
  - Retained products of conception NOS, following delivery
- **O72.3** Postpartum coagulation defects
  - Postpartum afibrinogenemia
  - Postpartum fibrinolysis

O73 Retained placenta and membranes, without hemorrhage
EXCLUDES 1: placenta accreta (O43.21-)
- placenta increta (O43.22-)
- placenta percreta (O43.23-)

DEF: Postpartum condition resulting from failure to expel placental membrane tissues due to failed contractions of the uterine wall.

- **O73.0** Retained placenta without hemorrhage
  - Adherent placenta, without hemorrhage
  - Trapped placenta without hemorrhage
- **O73.1** Retained portions of placenta and membranes, without hemorrhage
  - Retained products of conception following delivery, without hemorrhage

O74 Complications of anesthesia during labor and delivery
INCLUDES: maternal complications arising from the administration of a general, regional or local anesthetic, analgesic or other sedation during labor and delivery

Use additional code, if applicable, to identify specific complication

- **O74.0** Aspiration pneumonitis due to anesthesia during labor and delivery
  - Inhalation of stomach contents or secretions NOS due to anesthesia during labor and delivery
  - Mendelson's syndrome due to anesthesia during labor and delivery
- **O74.1** Other pulmonary complications of anesthesia during labor and delivery
- **O74.2** Cardiac complications of anesthesia during labor and delivery
- **O74.3** Central nervous system complications of anesthesia during labor and delivery
- **O74.4** Toxic reaction to local anesthesia during labor and delivery
- **O74.5** Spinal and epidural anesthesia-induced headache during labor and delivery
- **O74.6** Other complications of spinal and epidural anesthesia during labor and delivery
- **O74.7** Failed or difficult intubation for anesthesia during labor and delivery
- **O74.8** Other complications of anesthesia during labor and delivery
- **O74.9** Complication of anesthesia during labor and delivery, unspecified

O75 Other complications of labor and delivery, not elsewhere classified
EXCLUDES 2: puerperal (postpartum) infection (O86.-)
- puerperal (postpartum) sepsis (O85)

- **O75.0** Maternal distress during labor and delivery
- **O75.1** Shock during or following labor and delivery
  - Obstetric shock following labor and delivery
- **O75.2** Pyrexia during labor, not elsewhere classified
- **O75.3** Other infection during labor
  - Sepsis during labor
  - Use additional code (B95-B97), to identify infectious agent
  - AHA: 2025,1Q,22
- **O75.4** Other complications of obstetric surgery and procedures
  - Cardiac arrest following obstetric surgery or procedures
  - Cardiac failure following obstetric surgery or procedures
  - Cerebral anoxia following obstetric surgery or procedures
  - Pulmonary edema following obstetric surgery or procedures
  - Use additional code to identify specific complication
  - EXCLUDES 2: complications of anesthesia during labor and delivery (O74.-)
    - disruption of obstetrical (surgical) wound (O90.0-O90.1)
    - hematoma of obstetrical (surgical) wound (O90.2)
    - infection of obstetrical (surgical) wound (O86.0-)
  - AHA: 2025,1Q,21
- **O75.5** Delayed delivery after artificial rupture of membranes
- **O75.8** Other specified complications of labor and delivery
  - **O75.81** Maternal exhaustion complicating labor and delivery
  - **O75.82** Onset (spontaneous) of labor after 37 completed weeks of gestation but before 39 completed weeks gestation, with delivery by (planned) cesarean section
    - Delivery by (planned) cesarean section occurring after 37 completed weeks of gestation but before 39 completed weeks gestation due to (spontaneous) onset of labor
    - Code first to specify reason for planned cesarean section such as:
      - cephalopelvic disproportion (normally formed fetus) (O33.9)
      - previous cesarean delivery (O34.21-)
    - AHA: 2022,2Q,3
  - **O75.89** Other specified complications of labor and delivery
- **O75.9** Complication of labor and delivery, unspecified

O76 Abnormality in fetal heart rate and rhythm complicating labor and delivery
- Depressed fetal heart rate tones complicating labor and delivery
- Fetal bradycardia complicating labor and delivery
- Fetal heart rate abnormal variability complicating labor and delivery
- Fetal heart rate decelerations complicating labor and delivery
- Fetal heart rate irregularity complicating labor and delivery
- Fetal tachycardia complicating labor and delivery
- Non-reassuring fetal heart rate or rhythm complicating labor and delivery
- EXCLUDES 1: fetal stress NOS (O77.9)
  - labor and delivery complicated by electrocardiographic evidence of fetal stress (O77.8)
  - labor and delivery complicated by ultrasonic evidence of fetal stress (O77.8)
- EXCLUDES 2: fetal metabolic acidemia (O68)
  - other fetal stress (O77.0-O77.1)
- AHA: 2013,4Q,118

O77 Other fetal stress complicating labor and delivery
- **O77.0** Labor and delivery complicated by meconium in amniotic fluid
  - AHA: 2022,2Q,16; 2013,4Q,117-118
- **O77.1** Fetal stress in labor or delivery due to drug administration

Chapter 15. Pregnancy, Childbirth and the Puerperium

O77.8 Labor and delivery complicated by other evidence of fetal stress
- Labor and delivery complicated by electrocardiographic evidence of fetal stress
- Labor and delivery complicated by ultrasonic evidence of fetal stress
- EXCLUDES 1: abnormality of fetal acid-base balance (O68)
  - abnormality in fetal heart rate or rhythm (O76)
  - fetal metabolic acidemia (O68)

O77.9 Labor and delivery complicated by fetal stress, unspecified
- EXCLUDES 1: abnormality of fetal acid-base balance (O68)
  - abnormality in fetal heart rate or rhythm (O76)
  - fetal metabolic acidemia (O68)

Encounter for delivery (O80-O82)

O80 Encounter for full-term uncomplicated delivery
- NOTE: Delivery requiring minimal or no assistance, with or without episiotomy, without fetal manipulation [e.g., rotation version] or instrumentation [forceps] of a spontaneous, cephalic, vaginal, full-term, single, live-born infant. This code is for use as a single diagnosis code and is not to be used with any other code from chapter 15.
- Use additional code to indicate outcome of delivery (Z37.0)
- AHA: 2016,4Q,150; 2014,2Q,9

O82 Encounter for cesarean delivery without indication
- Use additional code to indicate outcome of delivery (Z37.0)

Complications predominantly related to the puerperium (O85-O92)

EXCLUDES 2: mental and behavioral disorders associated with the puerperium (F53.-)
- obstetrical tetanus (A34)
- puerperal osteomalacia (M83.0)

O85 Puerperal sepsis
- Postpartum sepsis
- Puerperal peritonitis
- Puerperal pyemia
- Use additional code (B95-B97), to identify infectious agent
- Use additional code (R65.2-) to identify severe sepsis, if applicable
- EXCLUDES 1: fever of unknown origin following delivery (O86.4)
  - obstetric pyemic and septic embolism (O88.3-)
  - puerperal septic thrombophlebitis (O86.81)
- EXCLUDES 2: genital tract infection following delivery (O86.1-)
  - sepsis during labor (O75.3)
  - urinary tract infection following delivery (O86.2-)
- AHA: 2022,2Q,5; 2020,2Q,32; 2019,2Q,39; 2018,4Q,23

O86 Other puerperal infections
- Use additional code (B95-B97), to identify infectious agent
- EXCLUDES 2: infection during labor (O75.3)
  - obstetrical tetanus (A34)

O86.0 Infection of obstetric surgical wound
- Infected cesarean delivery wound following delivery
- Infected perineal repair following delivery
- EXCLUDES 1: complications of procedures, not elsewhere classified (T81.4-)
  - postprocedural fever NOS (R50.82)
  - postprocedural retroperitoneal abscess (K68.11)
- AHA: 2020,2Q,32; 2018,4Q,22-23,62

O86.00 Infection of obstetric surgical wound, unspecified

O86.01 Infection of obstetric surgical wound, superficial incisional site
- Stitch abscess following an obstetrical procedure
- Subcutaneous abscess following an obstetrical procedure

O86.02 Infection of obstetric surgical wound, deep incisional site
- Intramuscular abscess following an obstetrical procedure
- Sub-fascial abscess following an obstetrical procedure
- AHA: 2020,2Q,32

O86.03 Infection of obstetric surgical wound, organ and space site
- Intraabdominal abscess following an obstetrical procedure
- Subphrenic abscess following an obstetrical procedure

O86.04 Sepsis following an obstetrical procedure
- Use additional code to identify the sepsis
- AHA: 2020,2Q,32; 2019,2Q,39

O86.09 Infection of obstetric surgical wound, other surgical site

O86.1 Other infection of genital tract following delivery

O86.11 Cervicitis following delivery

O86.12 Endometritis following delivery

O86.13 Vaginitis following delivery

O86.19 Other infection of genital tract following delivery

O86.2 Urinary tract infection following delivery

O86.20 Urinary tract infection following delivery, unspecified
- Puerperal urinary tract infection NOS
- AHA: 2022,2Q,5

O86.21 Infection of kidney following delivery

O86.22 Infection of bladder following delivery
- Infection of urethra following delivery

O86.29 Other urinary tract infection following delivery

O86.4 Pyrexia of unknown origin following delivery
- Puerperal infection NOS following delivery
- Puerperal pyrexia NOS following delivery
- EXCLUDES 2: pyrexia during labor (O75.2)
- DEF: Fever of unknown origin experienced by the mother after childbirth.

O86.8 Other specified puerperal infections

O86.81 Puerperal septic thrombophlebitis

O86.89 Other specified puerperal infections

O87 Venous complications and hemorrhoids in the puerperium
- INCLUDES: venous complications in labor, delivery and the puerperium
- EXCLUDES 2: obstetric embolism (O88.-)
  - puerperal septic thrombophlebitis (O86.81)
  - venous complications in pregnancy (O22.-)

O87.0 Superficial thrombophlebitis in the puerperium
- Puerperal phlebitis NOS
- Puerperal thrombosis NOS
- Use additional code, if applicable, to identify the superficial vein thrombosis, such as thrombosis of superficial vessels of lower extremities (I80.0-)

O87.1 Deep phlebothrombosis in the puerperium
- Deep vein thrombosis, postpartum
- Pelvic thrombophlebitis, postpartum
- Use additional code to identify the deep vein thrombosis (I82.4-, I82.5-, I82.62-, I82.72-)
- Use additional code, if applicable, for associated long-term (current) use of anticoagulants (Z79.01)

O87.2 Hemorrhoids in the puerperium

O87.3 Cerebral venous thrombosis in the puerperium
- Cerebrovenous sinus thrombosis in the puerperium

O87.4 Varicose veins of lower extremity in the puerperium

O87.8 Other venous complications in the puerperium
- Genital varices in the puerperium

O87.9 Venous complication in the puerperium, unspecified
- Puerperal phlebopathy NOS

O88 Obstetric embolism
- EXCLUDES 1: embolism complicating abortion NOS (O03.2)
  - embolism complicating ectopic or molar pregnancy (O08.2)
  - embolism complicating failed attempted abortion (O07.2)
  - embolism complicating induced abortion (O04.7)
  - embolism complicating spontaneous abortion (O03.2, O03.7)

O88.0 Obstetric air embolism
- DEF: Sudden blocking of the pulmonary artery or right ventricle with air or nitrogen bubbles.

O88.01 Obstetric air embolism in pregnancy

O88.011 Air embolism in pregnancy, first trimester

O88.012 Air embolism in pregnancy, second trimester

O88.013 Air embolism in pregnancy, third trimester

O88.019 Air embolism in pregnancy, unspecified trimester

O88.02 Air embolism in childbirth

Chapter 15. Pregnancy, Childbirth and the Puerperium

- **O88.03** Air embolism in the puerperium
- ✓5th **O88.1** **Amniotic fluid** embolism
  - Anaphylactoid syndrome in pregnancy
  - ✓6th **O88.11** Amniotic fluid embolism in **pregnancy**
    - **O88.111** Amniotic fluid embolism in pregnancy, **first trimester**
    - **O88.112** Amniotic fluid embolism in pregnancy, **second trimester**
    - **O88.113** Amniotic fluid embolism in pregnancy, **third trimester**
    - **O88.119** Amniotic fluid embolism in pregnancy, unspecified trimester
  - **O88.12** Amniotic fluid embolism in **childbirth**
  - **O88.13** Amniotic fluid embolism in the **puerperium**
- ✓5th **O88.2** Obstetric **thromboembolism**
  - ✓6th **O88.21** Thromboembolism in **pregnancy**
    - Obstetric (pulmonary) embolism NOS
    - **O88.211** Thromboembolism in pregnancy, **first trimester**
    - **O88.212** Thromboembolism in pregnancy, **second trimester**
    - **O88.213** Thromboembolism in pregnancy, **third trimester**
    - **O88.219** Thromboembolism in pregnancy, unspecified trimester
  - **O88.22** Thromboembolism in **childbirth**
  - **O88.23** Thromboembolism in the **puerperium**
    - Puerperal (pulmonary) embolism NOS
- ✓5th **O88.3** Obstetric **pyemic and septic embolism**
  - ✓6th **O88.31** Pyemic and septic embolism in **pregnancy**
    - **O88.311** Pyemic and septic embolism in pregnancy, **first trimester**
    - **O88.312** Pyemic and septic embolism in pregnancy, **second trimester**
    - **O88.313** Pyemic and septic embolism in pregnancy, **third trimester**
    - **O88.319** Pyemic and septic embolism in pregnancy, unspecified trimester
  - **O88.32** Pyemic and septic embolism in **childbirth**
  - **O88.33** Pyemic and septic embolism in the **puerperium**
- ✓5th **O88.8** Other obstetric embolism
  - Obstetric fat embolism
  - ✓6th **O88.81** Other embolism in **pregnancy**
    - **O88.811** Other embolism in pregnancy, **first trimester**
    - **O88.812** Other embolism in pregnancy, **second trimester**
    - **O88.813** Other embolism in pregnancy, **third trimester**
    - **O88.819** Other embolism in pregnancy, unspecified trimester
  - **O88.82** Other embolism in **childbirth**
  - **O88.83** Other embolism in the **puerperium**
- ✓4th **O89** Complications of anesthesia during the puerperium
  - INCLUDES maternal complications arising from the administration of a general, regional or local anesthetic, analgesic or other sedation during the puerperium
  - Use additional code, if applicable, to identify specific complication
  - ✓5th **O89.0** **Pulmonary** complications of anesthesia during the puerperium
    - **O89.01** **Aspiration pneumonitis** due to anesthesia during the puerperium
      - Inhalation of stomach contents or secretions NOS due to anesthesia during the puerperium
      - Mendelson's syndrome due to anesthesia during the puerperium
    - **O89.09** Other pulmonary complications of anesthesia during the puerperium
  - **O89.1** **Cardiac** complications of anesthesia during the puerperium
  - **O89.2** **Central nervous system** complications of anesthesia during the puerperium
  - **O89.3** **Toxic reaction** to local anesthesia during the puerperium
  - **O89.4** **Spinal and epidural anesthesia-induced headache** during the puerperium
  - **O89.5** Other complications of **spinal and epidural anesthesia** during the puerperium
  - **O89.6** **Failed or difficult intubation** for anesthesia during the puerperium
  - **O89.8** Other complications of anesthesia during the puerperium
  - **O89.9** Complication of anesthesia during the puerperium, unspecified
- ✓4th **O90** Complications of the puerperium, not elsewhere classified
  - **O90.0** Disruption of cesarean delivery wound
    - Dehiscence of cesarean delivery wound
    - EXCLUDES 1 rupture of uterus (spontaneous) before onset of labor (O71.0-)
    - rupture of uterus during labor (O71.1)
  - **O90.1** Disruption of perineal obstetric wound
    - Disruption of wound of episiotomy
    - Disruption of wound of perineal laceration
    - Secondary perineal tear
  - **O90.2** Hematoma of obstetric wound
  - **O90.3** Peripartum cardiomyopathy
    - Conditions in I42- arising during pregnancy and the puerperium
    - EXCLUDES 1 pre-existing heart disease complicating pregnancy and the puerperium (O99.4-)
    - **AHA:** 2022,3Q,16-17
    - **DEF:** Any structural or functional abnormality of the ventricular myocardium. It is a noninflammatory disease of obscure or unknown etiology with onset during the postpartum period.
  - ✓5th **O90.4** Postpartum acute kidney failure
    - EXCLUDES 1 ▶anuria and oliguria◀ (R34)
    - **AHA:** 2023,4Q,37
    - **O90.41** Hepatorenal syndrome following labor and delivery
    - **O90.49** Other postpartum acute kidney failure
      - Postpartum acute kidney failure
      - Puerperal anuria
      - Puerperal oliguria
  - **O90.5** Postpartum thyroiditis
  - **O90.6** Postpartum mood disturbance
    - Postpartum blues
    - Postpartum dysphoria
    - Postpartum sadness
    - EXCLUDES 1 postpartum depression (F53.0)
    - puerperal psychosis (F53.1)
  - ✓5th **O90.8** Other complications of the puerperium, not elsewhere classified
    - **O90.81** Anemia of the puerperium
      - Postpartum anemia NOS
      - EXCLUDES 1 pre-existing anemia complicating the puerperium (O99.03)
      - **AHA:** 2019,3Q,11
    - **O90.89** Other complications of the puerperium, not elsewhere classified
      - Placental polyp
  - **O90.9** Complication of the puerperium, unspecified
- ✓4th **O91** Infections of breast associated with pregnancy, the puerperium and lactation
  - Use additional code to identify infection
  - ✓5th **O91.0** Infection of nipple associated with pregnancy, the puerperium and lactation
    - ✓6th **O91.01** Infection of nipple associated with **pregnancy**
      - Gestational abscess of nipple
      - **O91.011** Infection of nipple associated with pregnancy, **first trimester**
      - **O91.012** Infection of nipple associated with pregnancy, **second trimester**
      - **O91.013** Infection of nipple associated with pregnancy, **third trimester**
      - **O91.019** Infection of nipple associated with pregnancy, unspecified trimester
    - **O91.02** Infection of nipple associated with the **puerperium**
      - Puerperal abscess of nipple
    - **O91.03** Infection of nipple associated with **lactation**
      - Abscess of nipple associated with lactation

Chapter 15. Pregnancy, Childbirth and the Puerperium

- ✓5th **O91.1** **Abscess of breast associated with pregnancy, the puerperium and lactation**
  - ✓6th **O91.11** Abscess of breast associated with pregnancy
    - Gestational mammary abscess
    - Gestational purulent mastitis
    - Gestational subareolar abscess
    - **O91.111** Abscess of breast associated with pregnancy, first trimester [COM] [M]
    - **O91.112** Abscess of breast associated with pregnancy, second trimester [COM] [M]
    - **O91.113** Abscess of breast associated with pregnancy, third trimester [COM] [M]
    - **O91.119** Abscess of breast associated with pregnancy, unspecified trimester [COM] [M]
  - **O91.12** Abscess of breast associated with the puerperium [M]
    - Puerperal mammary abscess
    - Puerperal purulent mastitis
    - Puerperal subareolar abscess
  - **O91.13** Abscess of breast associated with lactation [M]
    - Mammary abscess associated with lactation
    - Purulent mastitis associated with lactation
    - Subareolar abscess associated with lactation
- ✓5th **O91.2** **Nonpurulent mastitis associated with pregnancy, the puerperium and lactation**
  - ✓6th **O91.21** Nonpurulent mastitis associated with pregnancy
    - Gestational interstitial mastitis
    - Gestational lymphangitis of breast
    - Gestational mastitis NOS
    - Gestational parenchymatous mastitis
    - **O91.211** Nonpurulent mastitis associated with pregnancy, first trimester [COM] [M]
    - **O91.212** Nonpurulent mastitis associated with pregnancy, second trimester [COM] [M]
    - **O91.213** Nonpurulent mastitis associated with pregnancy, third trimester [COM] [M]
    - **O91.219** Nonpurulent mastitis associated with pregnancy, unspecified trimester [COM] [M]
  - **O91.22** Nonpurulent mastitis associated with the puerperium [M]
    - Puerperal interstitial mastitis
    - Puerperal lymphangitis of breast
    - Puerperal mastitis NOS
    - Puerperal parenchymatous mastitis
  - **O91.23** Nonpurulent mastitis associated with lactation [M]
    - Interstitial mastitis associated with lactation
    - Lymphangitis of breast associated with lactation
    - Mastitis NOS associated with lactation
    - Parenchymatous mastitis associated with lactation

- ✓4th **O92** **Other disorders of breast and disorders of lactation associated with pregnancy and the puerperium**
  - ✓5th **O92.0** Retracted nipple associated with pregnancy, the puerperium, and lactation
    - ✓6th **O92.01** Retracted nipple associated with pregnancy
      - **O92.011** Retracted nipple associated with pregnancy, first trimester [COM] [M]
      - **O92.012** Retracted nipple associated with pregnancy, second trimester [COM] [M]
      - **O92.013** Retracted nipple associated with pregnancy, third trimester [COM] [M]
      - **O92.019** Retracted nipple associated with pregnancy, unspecified trimester [COM] [M]
    - **O92.02** Retracted nipple associated with the puerperium [M]
    - **O92.03** Retracted nipple associated with lactation [M]
  - ✓5th **O92.1** Cracked nipple associated with pregnancy, the puerperium, and lactation
    - Fissure of nipple, gestational or puerperal
    - ✓6th **O92.11** Cracked nipple associated with pregnancy
      - **O92.111** Cracked nipple associated with pregnancy, first trimester [COM] [M]
      - **O92.112** Cracked nipple associated with pregnancy, second trimester [COM] [M]
      - **O92.113** Cracked nipple associated with pregnancy, third trimester [COM] [M]
      - **O92.119** Cracked nipple associated with pregnancy, unspecified trimester [COM] [M]
    - **O92.12** Cracked nipple associated with the puerperium [M]
    - **O92.13** Cracked nipple associated with lactation [M]
  - ✓5th **O92.2** Other and unspecified disorders of breast associated with pregnancy and the puerperium
    - **O92.20** Unspecified disorder of breast associated with pregnancy and the puerperium [M]
    - **O92.29** Other disorders of breast associated with pregnancy and the puerperium [M]
  - **O92.3** Agalactia [M]
    - Primary agalactia
    - EXCLUDES 1: elective agalactia (O92.5)
      secondary agalactia (O92.5)
      therapeutic agalactia (O92.5)
    - **DEF:** Absence of milk secretion in a female after delivery.
  - **O92.4** Hypogalactia [M]
  - **O92.5** Suppressed lactation
    - Elective agalactia
    - Secondary agalactia
    - Therapeutic agalactia
    - EXCLUDES 1: primary agalactia (O92.3)
  - **O92.6** Galactorrhea [M]
    - **DEF:** Excessive or persistent milk secretion by the breast that may occur in the absence of nursing.
  - ✓5th **O92.7** Other and unspecified disorders of lactation
    - **O92.70** Unspecified disorders of lactation [M]
    - **O92.79** Other disorders of lactation [M]
      - Puerperal galactocele

Other obstetric conditions, not elsewhere classified (O94-O9A)

- **O94** **Sequelae of complication of pregnancy, childbirth, and the puerperium** [UPD] [M]
  - **NOTE** This category is to be used to indicate conditions in O00-O77.-, O85-O94 and O98-O9A.- as the cause of late effects. The sequelae include conditions specified as such, or as late effects, which may occur at any time after the puerperium
  - Code first condition resulting from (sequela) of complication of pregnancy, childbirth, and the puerperium
  - AHA: 2022,3Q,16-17
- ✓4th **O98** **Maternal infectious and parasitic diseases classifiable elsewhere but complicating pregnancy, childbirth and the puerperium**
  - INCLUDES: the listed conditions when complicating the pregnant state, when aggravated by the pregnancy, or as a reason for obstetric care
  - Use additional code (Chapter 1), to identify specific infectious or parasitic disease
  - EXCLUDES 2: herpes gestationis (O26.4-)
    infectious carrier state (O99.82-, O99.83-)
    obstetrical tetanus (A34)
    puerperal infection (O86.-)
    puerperal sepsis (O85)
    when the reason for maternal care is that the disease is known or suspected to have affected the fetus (O35-O36)
  - ✓5th **O98.0** Tuberculosis complicating pregnancy, childbirth and the puerperium
    - Conditions in A15-A19
    - ✓6th **O98.01** Tuberculosis complicating pregnancy
      - **O98.011** Tuberculosis complicating pregnancy, first trimester [COM] [M]
      - **O98.012** Tuberculosis complicating pregnancy, second trimester [COM] [M]
      - **O98.013** Tuberculosis complicating pregnancy, third trimester [COM] [M]
      - **O98.019** Tuberculosis complicating pregnancy, unspecified trimester [COM] [M]
    - **O98.02** Tuberculosis complicating childbirth [COM] [M]
    - **O98.03** Tuberculosis complicating the puerperium [COM] [M]
  - ✓5th **O98.1** Syphilis complicating pregnancy, childbirth and the puerperium
    - Conditions in A50-A53
    - ✓6th **O98.11** Syphilis complicating pregnancy
      - **O98.111** Syphilis complicating pregnancy, first trimester [COM] [M]
      - **O98.112** Syphilis complicating pregnancy, second trimester [COM] [M]
      - **O98.113** Syphilis complicating pregnancy, third trimester [COM] [M]

	O98.119	Syphilis complicating pregnancy, unspecified trimester
	O98.12	Syphilis complicating childbirth
	O98.13	Syphilis complicating the puerperium

O98.2 Gonorrhea complicating pregnancy, childbirth and the puerperium
Conditions in A54.-

- **O98.21 Gonorrhea complicating pregnancy**
  - O98.211 Gonorrhea complicating pregnancy, first trimester
  - O98.212 Gonorrhea complicating pregnancy, second trimester
  - O98.213 Gonorrhea complicating pregnancy, third trimester
  - O98.219 Gonorrhea complicating pregnancy, unspecified trimester
- O98.22 Gonorrhea complicating childbirth
- O98.23 Gonorrhea complicating the puerperium

O98.3 Other infections with a predominantly sexual mode of transmission complicating pregnancy, childbirth and the puerperium
Conditions in A55-A64
AHA: 2020,1Q,20

- **O98.31 Other infections with a predominantly sexual mode of transmission complicating pregnancy**
  - O98.311 Other infections with a predominantly sexual mode of transmission complicating pregnancy, first trimester
  - O98.312 Other infections with a predominantly sexual mode of transmission complicating pregnancy, second trimester
  - O98.313 Other infections with a predominantly sexual mode of transmission complicating pregnancy, third trimester
  - O98.319 Other infections with a predominantly sexual mode of transmission complicating pregnancy, unspecified trimester
- O98.32 Other infections with a predominantly sexual mode of transmission complicating childbirth
- O98.33 Other infections with a predominantly sexual mode of transmission complicating the puerperium

O98.4 Viral hepatitis complicating pregnancy, childbirth and the puerperium
Conditions in B15-B19

- **O98.41 Viral hepatitis complicating pregnancy**
  - O98.411 Viral hepatitis complicating pregnancy, first trimester
  - O98.412 Viral hepatitis complicating pregnancy, second trimester
  - O98.413 Viral hepatitis complicating pregnancy, third trimester
  - O98.419 Viral hepatitis complicating pregnancy, unspecified trimester
- O98.42 Viral hepatitis complicating childbirth
- O98.43 Viral hepatitis complicating the puerperium

O98.5 Other viral diseases complicating pregnancy, childbirth and the puerperium
Conditions in A80-B09, B25-B34, R87.81-, R87.82-
EXCLUDES 1 human immunodeficiency virus [HIV] disease complicating pregnancy, childbirth and the puerperium (O98.7-)
TIP: Assign a code from this subcategory as the principal or first-listed diagnosis for a patient admitted/presenting during pregnancy, childbirth, or the puerperium because of COVID-19; assign U07.1 and codes for associated manifestations as secondary codes.

- **O98.51 Other viral diseases complicating pregnancy**
  - O98.511 Other viral diseases complicating pregnancy, first trimester
  - O98.512 Other viral diseases complicating pregnancy, second trimester
  - O98.513 Other viral diseases complicating pregnancy, third trimester
  - O98.519 Other viral diseases complicating pregnancy, unspecified trimester
- O98.52 Other viral diseases complicating childbirth
- O98.53 Other viral diseases complicating the puerperium

O98.6 Protozoal diseases complicating pregnancy, childbirth and the puerperium
Conditions in B50-B64

- **O98.61 Protozoal diseases complicating pregnancy**
  - O98.611 Protozoal diseases complicating pregnancy, first trimester
  - O98.612 Protozoal diseases complicating pregnancy, second trimester
  - O98.613 Protozoal diseases complicating pregnancy, third trimester
  - O98.619 Protozoal diseases complicating pregnancy, unspecified trimester
- O98.62 Protozoal diseases complicating childbirth
- O98.63 Protozoal diseases complicating the puerperium

O98.7 Human immunodeficiency virus [HIV] disease complicating pregnancy, childbirth and the puerperium
Use additional code to identify the type of HIV disease:
acquired immune deficiency syndrome (AIDS) (B20)
asymptomatic HIV status (Z21)
HIV positive NOS (Z21)
symptomatic HIV disease (B20)

- **O98.71 Human immunodeficiency virus [HIV] disease complicating pregnancy**
  - O98.711 Human immunodeficiency virus [HIV] disease complicating pregnancy, first trimester
  - O98.712 Human immunodeficiency virus [HIV] disease complicating pregnancy, second trimester
  - O98.713 Human immunodeficiency virus [HIV] disease complicating pregnancy, third trimester
  - O98.719 Human immunodeficiency virus [HIV] disease complicating pregnancy, unspecified trimester
- O98.72 Human immunodeficiency virus [HIV] disease complicating childbirth
- O98.73 Human immunodeficiency virus [HIV] disease complicating the puerperium

O98.8 Other maternal infectious and parasitic diseases complicating pregnancy, childbirth and the puerperium
AHA: 2020,1Q,10

- **O98.81 Other maternal infectious and parasitic diseases complicating pregnancy**
  - O98.811 Other maternal infectious and parasitic diseases complicating pregnancy, first trimester
  - O98.812 Other maternal infectious and parasitic diseases complicating pregnancy, second trimester
  - O98.813 Other maternal infectious and parasitic diseases complicating pregnancy, third trimester
  - O98.819 Other maternal infectious and parasitic diseases complicating pregnancy, unspecified trimester
- O98.82 Other maternal infectious and parasitic diseases complicating childbirth
- O98.83 Other maternal infectious and parasitic diseases complicating the puerperium
  AHA: 2022,2Q,5

O98.9 Unspecified maternal infectious and parasitic disease complicating pregnancy, childbirth and the puerperium

- **O98.91 Unspecified maternal infectious and parasitic disease complicating pregnancy**
  - O98.911 Unspecified maternal infectious and parasitic disease complicating pregnancy, first trimester
  - O98.912 Unspecified maternal infectious and parasitic disease complicating pregnancy, second trimester
  - O98.913 Unspecified maternal infectious and parasitic disease complicating pregnancy, third trimester

O98.919 Unspecified maternal infectious and parasitic disease complicating pregnancy, unspecified trimester COM M

O98.92 Unspecified maternal infectious and parasitic disease complicating childbirth COM M

O98.93 Unspecified maternal infectious and parasitic disease complicating the puerperium COM M

√4ᵗʰ **O99** Other maternal diseases classifiable elsewhere but complicating pregnancy, childbirth and the puerperium
- INCLUDES conditions which complicate the pregnant state, are aggravated by the pregnancy or are a main reason for obstetric care
- Use additional code to identify specific condition
- EXCLUDES 2 when the reason for maternal care is that the condition is known or suspected to have affected the fetus (O35-O36)

√5ᵗʰ **O99.0** Anemia complicating pregnancy, childbirth and the puerperium
- Conditions in D50-D64
- EXCLUDES 1 anemia arising in the puerperium (O90.81)
  postpartum anemia NOS (O90.81)
- AHA: 2019,3Q,11

√6ᵗʰ **O99.01** Anemia complicating pregnancy
- AHA: 2016,1Q,4

O99.011 Anemia complicating pregnancy, first trimester COM M
O99.012 Anemia complicating pregnancy, second trimester COM M
O99.013 Anemia complicating pregnancy, third trimester COM M
O99.019 Anemia complicating pregnancy, unspecified trimester COM M

O99.02 Anemia complicating childbirth COM M
O99.03 Anemia complicating the puerperium COM M
- EXCLUDES 1 postpartum anemia not pre-existing prior to delivery (O90.81)

√5ᵗʰ **O99.1** Other diseases of the blood and blood-forming organs and certain disorders involving the immune mechanism complicating pregnancy, childbirth and the puerperium
- Conditions in D65-D89
- EXCLUDES 1 hemorrhage with coagulation defects (O45.-, O46.0-, O67.0, O72.3)

√6ᵗʰ **O99.11** Other diseases of the blood and blood-forming organs and certain disorders involving the immune mechanism complicating pregnancy

O99.111 Other diseases of the blood and blood-forming organs and certain disorders involving the immune mechanism complicating pregnancy, first trimester COM M
O99.112 Other diseases of the blood and blood-forming organs and certain disorders involving the immune mechanism complicating pregnancy, second trimester COM M
O99.113 Other diseases of the blood and blood-forming organs and certain disorders involving the immune mechanism complicating pregnancy, third trimester COM M
O99.119 Other diseases of the blood and blood-forming organs and certain disorders involving the immune mechanism complicating pregnancy, unspecified trimester COM M

O99.12 Other diseases of the blood and blood-forming organs and certain disorders involving the immune mechanism complicating childbirth COM M
O99.13 Other diseases of the blood and blood-forming organs and certain disorders involving the immune mechanism complicating the puerperium COM M

√5ᵗʰ **O99.2** Endocrine, nutritional and metabolic diseases complicating pregnancy, childbirth and the puerperium
- Conditions in E00-E89
- EXCLUDES 2 diabetes mellitus (O24.-)
  malnutrition (O25.-)
  postpartum thyroiditis (O90.5)

√6ᵗʰ **O99.21** Obesity complicating pregnancy, childbirth, and puerperium
- Use additional code to identify the type of obesity (E66.-)
- AHA: 2021,2Q,10; 2018,4Q,80
- TIP: Do not assign a BMI code (Z68.-) for obese or overweight patients who are pregnant.

O99.210 Obesity complicating pregnancy, unspecified trimester COM M
O99.211 Obesity complicating pregnancy, first trimester COM M
O99.212 Obesity complicating pregnancy, second trimester COM M
O99.213 Obesity complicating pregnancy, third trimester COM M
O99.214 Obesity complicating childbirth COM M
O99.215 Obesity complicating the puerperium COM M

√6ᵗʰ **O99.28** Other endocrine, nutritional and metabolic diseases complicating pregnancy, childbirth and the puerperium
- AHA: 2021,1Q,8

O99.280 Endocrine, nutritional and metabolic diseases complicating pregnancy, unspecified trimester COM M
O99.281 Endocrine, nutritional and metabolic diseases complicating pregnancy, first trimester COM M
O99.282 Endocrine, nutritional and metabolic diseases complicating pregnancy, second trimester COM M
O99.283 Endocrine, nutritional and metabolic diseases complicating pregnancy, third trimester COM M
O99.284 Endocrine, nutritional and metabolic diseases complicating childbirth COM M
O99.285 Endocrine, nutritional and metabolic diseases complicating the puerperium COM M

√5ᵗʰ **O99.3** Mental disorders and diseases of the nervous system complicating pregnancy, childbirth and the puerperium

√6ᵗʰ **O99.31** Alcohol use complicating pregnancy, childbirth, and the puerperium
- Use additional code(s) from F10 to identify manifestations of the alcohol use

O99.310 Alcohol use complicating pregnancy, unspecified trimester COM M
O99.311 Alcohol use complicating pregnancy, first trimester COM M
O99.312 Alcohol use complicating pregnancy, second trimester COM M
O99.313 Alcohol use complicating pregnancy, third trimester COM M
O99.314 Alcohol use complicating childbirth COM M
O99.315 Alcohol use complicating the puerperium COM M

√6ᵗʰ **O99.32** Drug use complicating pregnancy, childbirth, and the puerperium
- Use additional code(s) from F11-F16 and F18-F19 to identify manifestations of the drug use
- AHA: 2018,4Q,69-70; 2018,2Q,10
- TIP: When drug use is documented during pregnancy, assign first a code from this subcategory followed by an additional code from F11-F16 and F18-F19 identifying the specific drug use even if not documented as associated with a physical, mental, or behavioral disorder. According to chapter 15 guidelines, it is the provider's responsibility to state that the condition being treated is *not* affecting the pregnancy.

O99.320 Drug use complicating pregnancy, unspecified trimester COM M
O99.321 Drug use complicating pregnancy, first trimester COM M

- **O99.322** Drug use complicating pregnancy, second trimester
- **O99.323** Drug use complicating pregnancy, third trimester
- **O99.324** Drug use complicating childbirth
- **O99.325** Drug use complicating the puerperium

✓6th **O99.33** **Tobacco use disorder** complicating pregnancy, childbirth, and the puerperium

Smoking complicating pregnancy, childbirth, and the puerperium

Use additional code from category F17 to identify type of tobacco nicotine dependence

- **O99.330** Smoking (tobacco) complicating pregnancy, unspecified trimester
- **O99.331** Smoking (tobacco) complicating pregnancy, first trimester
- **O99.332** Smoking (tobacco) complicating pregnancy, second trimester
- **O99.333** Smoking (tobacco) complicating pregnancy, third trimester
- **O99.334** Smoking (tobacco) complicating childbirth
- **O99.335** Smoking (tobacco) complicating the puerperium

✓6th **O99.34** Other mental disorders complicating pregnancy, childbirth, and the puerperium

Conditions in F01-F09, F20-F52 and F54-F99

EXCLUDES 2: postpartum mood disturbance (O90.6)
postnatal psychosis (F53.1)
puerperal psychosis (F53.1)

- **O99.340** Other mental disorders complicating pregnancy, unspecified trimester
- **O99.341** Other mental disorders complicating pregnancy, first trimester
- **O99.342** Other mental disorders complicating pregnancy, second trimester
- **O99.343** Other mental disorders complicating pregnancy, third trimester
- **O99.344** Other mental disorders complicating childbirth
- **O99.345** Other mental disorders complicating the puerperium

AHA: 2018,4Q,8

✓6th **O99.35** Diseases of the **nervous system** complicating pregnancy, childbirth, and the puerperium

Conditions in G00-G99

EXCLUDES 2: pregnancy related peripheral neuritis (O26.8-)

- **O99.350** Diseases of the nervous system complicating pregnancy, unspecified trimester
- **O99.351** Diseases of the nervous system complicating pregnancy, first trimester
- **O99.352** Diseases of the nervous system complicating pregnancy, second trimester
- **O99.353** Diseases of the nervous system complicating pregnancy, third trimester
- **O99.354** Diseases of the nervous system complicating childbirth
- **O99.355** Diseases of the nervous system complicating the puerperium

✓5th **O99.4** Diseases of the **circulatory system** complicating pregnancy, childbirth and the puerperium

Conditions in I00-I99

EXCLUDES 1: peripartum cardiomyopathy (O90.3)
EXCLUDES 2: hypertensive disorders (O10-O16)
obstetric embolism (O88.-)
venous complications and cerebrovenous sinus thrombosis in labor, childbirth and the puerperium (O87.-)
venous complications and cerebrovenous sinus thrombosis in pregnancy (O22.-)

AHA: 2016,2Q,8

✓6th **O99.41** Diseases of the circulatory system complicating pregnancy

- **O99.411** Diseases of the circulatory system complicating pregnancy, first trimester
- **O99.412** Diseases of the circulatory system complicating pregnancy, second trimester
- **O99.413** Diseases of the circulatory system complicating pregnancy, third trimester
- **O99.419** Diseases of the circulatory system complicating pregnancy, unspecified trimester

- **O99.42** Diseases of the circulatory system complicating childbirth
- **O99.43** Diseases of the circulatory system complicating the puerperium

✓5th **O99.5** Diseases of the **respiratory system** complicating pregnancy, childbirth and the puerperium

Conditions in J00-J99

✓6th **O99.51** Diseases of the respiratory system complicating pregnancy

- **O99.511** Diseases of the respiratory system complicating pregnancy, first trimester
- **O99.512** Diseases of the respiratory system complicating pregnancy, second trimester
- **O99.513** Diseases of the respiratory system complicating pregnancy, third trimester
- **O99.519** Diseases of the respiratory system complicating pregnancy, unspecified trimester

- **O99.52** Diseases of the respiratory system complicating childbirth
- **O99.53** Diseases of the respiratory system complicating the puerperium

✓5th **O99.6** Diseases of the **digestive system** complicating pregnancy, childbirth and the puerperium

Conditions in K00-K93

EXCLUDES 2: hemorrhoids in pregnancy (O22.4-)
liver and biliary tract disorders in pregnancy, childbirth and the puerperium (O26.6-)

✓6th **O99.61** Diseases of the digestive system complicating pregnancy

AHA: 2016,1Q,4

- **O99.611** Diseases of the digestive system complicating pregnancy, first trimester
- **O99.612** Diseases of the digestive system complicating pregnancy, second trimester
- **O99.613** Diseases of the digestive system complicating pregnancy, third trimester
- **O99.619** Diseases of the digestive system complicating pregnancy, unspecified trimester

- **O99.62** Diseases of the digestive system complicating childbirth
- **O99.63** Diseases of the digestive system complicating the puerperium

Chapter 15. Pregnancy, Childbirth and the Puerperium

O99.7 Diseases of the **skin and subcutaneous** tissue complicating pregnancy, childbirth and the puerperium
Conditions in L00-L99
EXCLUDES 2 herpes gestationis (O26.4)
pruritic urticarial papules and plaques of pregnancy (PUPPP) (O26.86)

- **O99.71** Diseases of the skin and subcutaneous tissue complicating **pregnancy**
  - **O99.711** Diseases of the skin and subcutaneous tissue complicating pregnancy, **first trimester** COM M
  - **O99.712** Diseases of the skin and subcutaneous tissue complicating pregnancy, **second trimester** COM M
  - **O99.713** Diseases of the skin and subcutaneous tissue complicating pregnancy, **third trimester** COM M
  - **O99.719** Diseases of the skin and subcutaneous tissue complicating pregnancy, unspecified trimester COM M
- **O99.72** Diseases of the skin and subcutaneous tissue complicating **childbirth**
- **O99.73** Diseases of the skin and subcutaneous tissue complicating the **puerperium** COM M

O99.8 Other specified diseases and conditions complicating pregnancy, childbirth and the puerperium
Conditions in D00-D48, H00-H95, M00-N99, and Q00-Q99
Use additional code to identify condition
EXCLUDES 2 genitourinary infections in pregnancy (O23.-)
infection of genitourinary tract following delivery (O86.1-O86.4)
malignant neoplasm complicating pregnancy, childbirth and the puerperium (O9A.1-)
maternal care for known or suspected abnormality of maternal pelvic organs (O34.-)
postpartum acute kidney failure (O90.49)
traumatic injuries in pregnancy (O9A.2-)

- **O99.81** **Abnormal glucose** complicating pregnancy, childbirth and the puerperium
  EXCLUDES 1 gestational diabetes (O24.4-)
  - **O99.810** Abnormal glucose complicating **pregnancy** COM M
  - **O99.814** Abnormal glucose complicating **childbirth** COM M
  - **O99.815** Abnormal glucose complicating the **puerperium** COM M
- **O99.82** **Streptococcus B carrier state** complicating pregnancy, childbirth and the puerperium
  EXCLUDES 1 carrier of streptococcus group B (GBS) in a nonpregnant woman (Z22.330)
  DEF: *Streptococcus* group B colonization: Bacteria normally found in the vagina or lower intestine of many healthy adult women that may infect the fetus during childbirth, causing mental or physical handicaps or death. Women who test positive for *Streptococcus* group B during pregnancy are considered a "colonized" status and are treated with IV antibiotics at the time of delivery and may also be treated with oral antibiotics during the pregnancy.
  - **O99.820** Streptococcus B carrier state complicating **pregnancy** COM M
  - **O99.824** Streptococcus B carrier state complicating **childbirth** COM M
    AHA: 2019,2Q,8
  - **O99.825** Streptococcus B carrier state complicating the **puerperium** COM M
- **O99.83** Other infection carrier state complicating pregnancy, childbirth and the puerperium
  Use additional code to identify the carrier state (Z22.-)
  - **O99.830** Other infection carrier state complicating **pregnancy** COM M
  - **O99.834** Other infection carrier state complicating **childbirth** COM M
  - **O99.835** Other infection carrier state complicating the **puerperium** COM M
- **O99.84** **Bariatric surgery status** complicating pregnancy, childbirth and the puerperium
  Gastric banding status complicating pregnancy, childbirth and the puerperium
  Gastric bypass status for obesity complicating pregnancy, childbirth and the puerperium
  Obesity surgery status complicating pregnancy, childbirth and the puerperium
  - **O99.840** Bariatric surgery status complicating pregnancy, unspecified trimester COM M
  - **O99.841** Bariatric surgery status complicating pregnancy, **first trimester** COM M
  - **O99.842** Bariatric surgery status complicating pregnancy, **second trimester** COM M
  - **O99.843** Bariatric surgery status complicating pregnancy, **third trimester** COM M
  - **O99.844** Bariatric surgery status complicating **childbirth** COM M
  - **O99.845** Bariatric surgery status complicating the **puerperium** COM M
- **O99.89** Other specified diseases and conditions complicating pregnancy, childbirth and the puerperium
  AHA: 2023,3Q,17; 2020,4Q,36-37
  - **O99.891** Other specified diseases and conditions complicating **pregnancy** COM M
  - **O99.892** Other specified diseases and conditions complicating **childbirth** COM M
  - **O99.893** Other specified diseases and conditions complicating **puerperium** COM M

O9A Maternal malignant neoplasms, traumatic injuries and abuse classifiable elsewhere but complicating pregnancy, childbirth and the puerperium

- **O9A.1** **Malignant neoplasm** complicating pregnancy, childbirth and the puerperium
  Conditions in C00-C96
  Use additional code to identify neoplasm
  EXCLUDES 2 maternal care for benign tumor of corpus uteri (O34.1-)
  maternal care for benign tumor of cervix (O34.4-)
  AHA: 2015,3Q,19
  - **O9A.11** Malignant neoplasm complicating **pregnancy**
    - **O9A.111** Malignant neoplasm complicating pregnancy, **first trimester** COM M
    - **O9A.112** Malignant neoplasm complicating pregnancy, **second trimester** COM M
    - **O9A.113** Malignant neoplasm complicating pregnancy, **third trimester** COM M
    - **O9A.119** Malignant neoplasm complicating pregnancy, unspecified trimester COM M
  - **O9A.12** Malignant neoplasm complicating **childbirth** COM M
  - **O9A.13** Malignant neoplasm complicating the **puerperium** COM M
- **O9A.2** **Injury, poisoning and** certain other consequences of **external causes** complicating pregnancy, childbirth and the puerperium
  Conditions in S00-T88, except T74 and T76
  Use additional code(s) to identify the injury or poisoning
  EXCLUDES 2 physical, sexual and psychological abuse complicating pregnancy, childbirth and the puerperium (O9A.3-, O9A.4-, O9A.5-)
  - **O9A.21** Injury, poisoning and certain other consequences of external causes complicating **pregnancy**
    - **O9A.211** Injury, poisoning and certain other consequences of external causes complicating pregnancy, **first trimester** COM M
    - **O9A.212** Injury, poisoning and certain other consequences of external causes complicating pregnancy, **second trimester** COM M
    - **O9A.213** Injury, poisoning and certain other consequences of external causes complicating pregnancy, **third trimester** COM M
    - **O9A.219** Injury, poisoning and certain other consequences of external causes complicating pregnancy, unspecified trimester
  - **O9A.22** Injury, poisoning and certain other consequences of external causes complicating **childbirth** COM M

O9A.23 Injury, poisoning and certain other consequences of external causes complicating the puerperium

√5th **O9A.3** Physical abuse complicating pregnancy, childbirth and the puerperium
Conditions in T74.11 or T76.11
Use additional code (if applicable):
to identify any associated current injury due to physical abuse
to identify the perpetrator of abuse (Y07.-)
EXCLUDES 2 sexual abuse complicating pregnancy, childbirth and the puerperium (O9A.4)

√6th **O9A.31** Physical abuse complicating pregnancy
  O9A.311 Physical abuse complicating pregnancy, first trimester
  O9A.312 Physical abuse complicating pregnancy, second trimester
  O9A.313 Physical abuse complicating pregnancy, third trimester
  O9A.319 Physical abuse complicating pregnancy, unspecified trimester
O9A.32 Physical abuse complicating childbirth
O9A.33 Physical abuse complicating the puerperium

√5th **O9A.4** Sexual abuse complicating pregnancy, childbirth and the puerperium
Conditions in T74.21 or T76.21
Use additional code (if applicable):
to identify any associated current injury due to sexual abuse
to identify the perpetrator of abuse (Y07.-)

√6th **O9A.41** Sexual abuse complicating pregnancy
  O9A.411 Sexual abuse complicating pregnancy, first trimester
  O9A.412 Sexual abuse complicating pregnancy, second trimester
  O9A.413 Sexual abuse complicating pregnancy, third trimester
  O9A.419 Sexual abuse complicating pregnancy, unspecified trimester
O9A.42 Sexual abuse complicating childbirth
O9A.43 Sexual abuse complicating the puerperium

√5th **O9A.5** Psychological abuse complicating pregnancy, childbirth and the puerperium
Conditions in T74.31 or T76.31
Use additional code to identify the perpetrator of abuse (Y07.-)

√6th **O9A.51** Psychological abuse complicating pregnancy
  O9A.511 Psychological abuse complicating pregnancy, first trimester
  O9A.512 Psychological abuse complicating pregnancy, second trimester
  O9A.513 Psychological abuse complicating pregnancy, third trimester
  O9A.519 Psychological abuse complicating pregnancy, unspecified trimester
O9A.52 Psychological abuse complicating childbirth
O9A.53 Psychological abuse complicating the puerperium

Chapter 16. Certain Conditions Originating in the Perinatal Period (P00–P96)

Chapter-specific Guidelines with Coding Examples

The chapter-specific guidelines from the ICD-10-CM Official Guidelines for Coding and Reporting have been provided below. Along with these guidelines are coding examples, contained in the shaded boxes, that have been developed to help illustrate the coding and/or sequencing guidance found in these guidelines.

For coding and reporting purposes the perinatal period is defined as before birth through the 28th day following birth. The following guidelines are provided for reporting purposes

a. General perinatal rules

1) **Use of Chapter 16 codes**

    Codes in this chapter are never for use on the maternal record. Codes from Chapter 15, the obstetric chapter, are never permitted on the newborn record. Chapter 16 codes may be used throughout the life of the patient if the condition is still present.

2) **Principal diagnosis for birth record**

    When coding the birth episode in a newborn record, assign a code from category Z38, Liveborn infants according to place of birth and type of delivery, as the principal diagnosis. A code from category Z38 is assigned only once, to a newborn at the time of birth. If a newborn is transferred to another institution, a code from category Z38 should not be used at the receiving hospital.

    A code from category Z38 is used only on the newborn record, not on the mother's record.

3) **Use of codes from other chapters with codes from Chapter 16**

    Codes from other chapters may be used with codes from chapter 16 if the codes from the other chapters provide more specific detail. Codes for signs and symptoms may be assigned when a definitive diagnosis has not been established. If the reason for the encounter is a perinatal condition, the code from chapter 16 should be sequenced first.

4) **Use of Chapter 16 codes after the perinatal period**

    Should a condition originate in the perinatal period, and continue throughout the life of the patient, the perinatal code should continue to be used regardless of the patient's age.

    > A 7-year-old patient with history of birth injury that resulted in Erb's palsy is seen for subscapularis release
    >
    > **P14.0**   Erb's paralysis due to birth injury
    >
    > *Explanation:* Although in this instance Erb's palsy is specifically related to a birth injury, it has not resolved and continues to be a health concern. A perinatal code is appropriate even though this patient is beyond the perinatal period.

5) **Birth process or community acquired conditions**

    If a newborn has a condition that may be either due to the birth process or community acquired and the documentation does not indicate which it is, the default is due to the birth process and the code from Chapter 16 should be used. If the condition is community-acquired, a code from Chapter 16 should not be assigned.

    For COVID-19 infection in a newborn, see guideline I.C.16.h.

6) **Code all clinically significant conditions**

    All clinically significant conditions noted on routine newborn examination should be coded. A condition is clinically significant if it requires:

    clinical evaluation; or

    therapeutic treatment; or

    diagnostic procedures; or

    extended length of hospital stay; or

    increased nursing care and/or monitoring; or

    has implications for future health care needs

    Note: The perinatal guidelines listed above are the same as the general coding guidelines for "additional diagnoses", except for the final point regarding implications for future health care needs. Codes should be assigned for conditions that have been specified by the provider as having implications for future health care needs.

b. Observation and evaluation of newborns for suspected conditions not found

1) **Use of Z05 codes**

    Assign a code from category Z05, Observation and evaluation of newborn for suspected diseases and conditions ruled out, to identify those instances when a healthy newborn is evaluated for a suspected condition/disease that is determined after study not to be present. Do not use a code from category Z05 when the patient is documented to have signs or symptoms of a suspected problem; in such cases code the sign or symptom.

2) **Z05 on other than the birth record**

    A code from category Z05 may also be assigned as a principal or first-listed code for readmissions or encounters when the code from category Z38 code no longer applies. Codes from category Z05 are for use only for healthy newborns and infants for which no condition after study is found to be present.

3) **Z05 on a birth record**

    A code from category Z05 is to be used as a secondary code after the code from category Z38, Liveborn infants according to place of birth and type of delivery.

    > Newborn delivered via vaginal delivery; previous ultrasounds showed what appeared to be an abnormality of the right kidney. Kidney function tests were performed and ultrasounds taken and any genitourinary conditions ruled out.
    >
    > **Z38.00**   Single liveborn infant, delivered vaginally
    >
    > **Z05.6**   Observation and evaluation of newborn for suspected genitourinary condition ruled out
    >
    > *Explanation:* The newborn had no signs or symptoms of kidney or other genitourinary condition but was evaluated after delivery due to the abnormal prenatal ultrasound findings. A Z code describing the type and place of birth should be coded first, followed by a Z05 category code for the work performed to rule out a suspected genitourinary condition.

c. Coding additional perinatal diagnoses

1) **Assigning codes for conditions that require treatment**

    Assign codes for conditions that require treatment or further investigation, prolong the length of stay, or require resource utilization.

2) **Codes for conditions specified as having implications for future health care needs**

    Assign codes for conditions that have been specified by the provider as having implications for future health care needs.

    Note: This guideline should not be used for adult patients.

    > An abnormal noise was heard in the left hip of a post-term newborn during a physical examination. The pediatrician would like to follow the patient after discharge as a hip click can be an early sign of hip dysplasia. The newborn was delivered via cesarean at 41 weeks.
    >
    > **Z38.01**   Single liveborn infant, delivered by cesarean
    >
    > **P08.21**   Post-term newborn
    >
    > **R29.4**   Clicking hip
    >
    > *Explanation:* The abnormal hip noise or click is appended as a secondary diagnosis not only because it is an abnormal finding upon examination, but also due to its potential to be part of a bigger health issue. The hip dysplasia has not yet been diagnosed and does not warrant a code at this time.

d. Prematurity and fetal growth retardation

Providers utilize different criteria in determining prematurity. A code for prematurity should not be assigned unless it is documented. Assignment of codes in categories P05, Disorders of newborn related to slow fetal growth and fetal malnutrition, and P07, Disorders of newborn related to short gestation and low birth weight, not elsewhere classified, should be based on the recorded birth weight and estimated gestational age.

When both birth weight and gestational age are available, two codes from category P07 should be assigned, with the code for birth weight sequenced before the code for gestational age.

Chapter 16. Certain Conditions Originating in the Perinatal Period

e. Low birth weight and immaturity status

Codes from category P07, Disorders of newborn related to short gestation and low birth weight, not elsewhere classified, are for use for a child or adult who was premature or had a low birth weight as a newborn and this is affecting the patient's current health status.

See Section I.C.21. Factors influencing health status and contact with health services, Status.

> A 35-year-old patient, who weighed 659 grams at birth, is seen for heart disease documented as being a consequence of the low birth weight
>
> | | |
> |---|---|
> | I51.9 | Heart disease, unspecified |
> | P07.02 | Extremely low birth weight newborn, 500–749 grams |
>
> *Explanation:* A code from subcategories P07.0- and P07.1- is appropriate, regardless of the age of the patient, as long as the documentation provides a clear link between the patient's current illness and the low birth weight.

f. Bacterial sepsis of newborn

Category P36, Bacterial sepsis of newborn, includes congenital sepsis. If a perinate is documented as having sepsis without documentation of congenital or community acquired, the default is congenital and a code from category P36 should be assigned. If the P36 code includes the causal organism, an additional code from category B95, Streptococcus, Staphylococcus, and Enterococcus as the cause of diseases classified elsewhere, or B96, Other bacterial agents as the cause of diseases classified elsewhere, should not be assigned. If the P36 code does not include the causal organism, assign an additional code from category B96. If applicable, use additional codes to identify severe sepsis (R65.2-) and any associated acute organ dysfunction.

> A full-term infant develops severe sepsis 24 hours after discharge from the hospital and is readmitted; cultures identified *E. coli* as the infective agent
>
> | | |
> |---|---|
> | P36.4 | Sepsis of newborn due to Escherichia coli |
> | R65.20 | Severe sepsis without septic shock |
>
> *Explanation:* Even though this newborn was discharged and could have acquired *E. coli* from his/her external environment, due to the lack of documentation specifying specifically how this pathogen was acquired, the default is to code the *E. coli* sepsis as congenital. A code from chapter 1, "Certain Infectious and Parasitic Diseases," is not required because the perinatal sepsis code identifies both the sepsis and the bacteria causing the sepsis.

g. Stillbirth

Code P95, Stillbirth, is only for use in institutions that maintain separate records for stillbirths. No other code should be used with P95. Code P95 should not be used on the mother's record.

h. COVID-19 infection in newborn

For a newborn that tests positive for COVID-19, assign code U07.1, COVID-19, and the appropriate codes for associated manifestation(s) in neonates/newborns in the absence of documentation indicating a specific type of transmission. For a newborn that tests positive for COVID-19 and the provider documents the condition was contracted in utero or during the birth process, assign codes P35.8, Other congenital viral diseases, and U07.1, COVID-19. When coding the birth episode in a newborn record, the appropriate code from category Z38, Liveborn infants according to place of birth and type of delivery, should be assigned as the principal diagnosis.

Chapter 16. Certain Conditions Originating in the Perinatal Period (P00-P96)

NOTE Codes from this chapter are for use on newborn records only, never on maternal records

INCLUDES conditions that have their origin in the fetal or perinatal period (before birth through the first 28 days after birth) even if morbidity occurs later

EXCLUDES 2 congenital malformations, deformations and chromosomal abnormalities (Q00-Q99)
endocrine, nutritional and metabolic diseases (E00-E88)
injury, poisoning and certain other consequences of external causes (S00-T88)
neoplasms (C00-D49)
tetanus neonatorum (A33)

This chapter contains the following blocks:
- P00-P04 Newborn affected by maternal factors and by complications of pregnancy, labor, and delivery
- P05-P08 Disorders of newborn related to length of gestation and fetal growth
- P09 Abnormal findings on neonatal screening
- P10-P15 Birth trauma
- P19-P29 Respiratory and cardiovascular disorders specific to the perinatal period
- P35-P39 Infections specific to the perinatal period
- P50-P61 Hemorrhagic and hematological disorders of newborn
- P70-P74 Transitory endocrine and metabolic disorders specific to newborn
- P76-P78 Digestive system disorders of newborn
- P80-P83 Conditions involving the integument and temperature regulation of newborn
- P84 Other problems with newborn
- P90-P96 Other disorders originating in the perinatal period

Newborn affected by maternal factors and by complications of pregnancy, labor, and delivery (P00-P04)

NOTE These codes are for use when the listed maternal conditions are specified as the cause of confirmed morbidity or potential morbidity which have their origin in the perinatal period (before birth through the first 28 days after birth).

AHA: 2016,4Q,54-55

✓4th P00 Newborn affected by maternal conditions that may be unrelated to present pregnancy

Code first any current condition in newborn

EXCLUDES 2 encounter for observation of newborn for suspected diseases and conditions ruled out (Z05.-)
newborn affected by maternal complications of pregnancy (P01.-)
newborn affected by maternal endocrine and metabolic disorders (P70-P74)
newborn affected by noxious substances transmitted via placenta or breast milk (P04.-)

- **P00.0** Newborn affected by maternal hypertensive disorders
Newborn affected by maternal conditions classifiable to O10-O11, O13-O16

- **P00.1** Newborn affected by maternal renal and urinary tract diseases
Newborn affected by maternal conditions classifiable to N00-N39

- **P00.2** Newborn affected by maternal infectious and parasitic diseases
Newborn affected by maternal infectious disease classifiable to A00-B99, J09 and J10
  - **EXCLUDES 1** maternal genital tract or other localized infections (P00.8)
  - **EXCLUDES 2** infections specific to the perinatal period (P35-P39)
newborn affected by (positive) maternal group B streptococcus (GBS) colonization (P00.82)
  - **AHA:** 2019,2Q,10; 2015,3Q,20

- **P00.3** Newborn affected by other maternal circulatory and respiratory diseases
Newborn affected by maternal conditions classifiable to I00-I99, J00-J99, Q20-Q34 and not included in P00.0, P00.2

- **P00.4** Newborn affected by maternal nutritional disorders
Maternal malnutrition NOS
Newborn affected by maternal disorders classifiable to E40-E64

- **P00.5** Newborn affected by maternal injury
Newborn affected by maternal conditions classifiable to O9A.2-

- **P00.6** Newborn affected by surgical procedure on mother
Newborn affected by amniocentesis
  - **EXCLUDES 1** Cesarean delivery for present delivery (P03.4)
damage to placenta from amniocentesis, Cesarean delivery or surgical induction (P02.1)
previous surgery to uterus or pelvic organs (P03.89)
  - **EXCLUDES 2** newborn affected by complication of (fetal) intrauterine procedure (P96.5)

- **P00.7** Newborn affected by other medical procedures on mother, not elsewhere classified
Newborn affected by radiation to mother
  - **EXCLUDES 1** damage to placenta from amniocentesis, cesarean delivery or surgical induction (P02.1)
newborn affected by other complications of labor and delivery (P03.-)

- ✓5th **P00.8** Newborn affected by other maternal conditions
  - **P00.81** Newborn affected by periodontal disease in mother
  - **P00.82** Newborn affected by (positive) maternal group B streptococcus (GBS) colonization
Contact with positive maternal group B streptococcus
    - **AHA:** 2021,4Q,23
  - **P00.89** Newborn affected by other maternal conditions
Newborn affected by conditions classifiable to T80-T88
Newborn affected by maternal genital tract or other localized infections
Newborn affected by maternal systemic lupus erythematosus
Use additional code to identify infectious agent, if known
    - **EXCLUDES 2** newborn affected by positive maternal group B streptococcus (GBS) colonization (P00.82)
    - **AHA:** 2019,2Q,9

- **P00.9** Newborn affected by unspecified maternal condition

✓4th P01 Newborn affected by maternal complications of pregnancy

Code first any current condition in newborn

EXCLUDES 2 encounter for observation of newborn for suspected diseases and conditions ruled out (Z05.-)

- **P01.0** Newborn affected by incompetent cervix
- **P01.1** Newborn affected by premature rupture of membranes
- **P01.2** Newborn affected by oligohydramnios
  - **EXCLUDES 1** oligohydramnios due to premature rupture of membranes (P01.1)
  - **DEF:** Low amniotic fluid level, resulting in underdeveloped organs in the fetus.
- **P01.3** Newborn affected by polyhydramnios
Newborn affected by hydramnios
  - **DEF:** Excess amniotic fluid surrounding the fetus, typically defined as a total fluid volume of greater than 24 cm.
- **P01.4** Newborn affected by ectopic pregnancy
Newborn affected by abdominal pregnancy
- **P01.5** Newborn affected by multiple pregnancy
Newborn affected by triplet (pregnancy)
Newborn affected by twin (pregnancy)
- **P01.6** Newborn affected by maternal death
- **P01.7** Newborn affected by malpresentation before labor
Newborn affected by breech presentation before labor
Newborn affected by external version before labor
Newborn affected by face presentation before labor
Newborn affected by transverse lie before labor
Newborn affected by unstable lie before labor
  - **AHA:** 2025,1Q,23
- **P01.8** Newborn affected by other maternal complications of pregnancy
- **P01.9** Newborn affected by maternal complication of pregnancy, unspecified

✓4th P02 Newborn affected by complications of placenta, cord and membranes

Code first any current condition in newborn

EXCLUDES 2 encounter for observation of newborn for suspected diseases and conditions ruled out (Z05.-)

- **P02.0** Newborn affected by placenta previa
  - **DEF:** Placenta developed in the lower segment of the uterus that can cause hemorrhaging leading to preterm delivery.
- **P02.1** Newborn affected by other forms of placental separation and hemorrhage
Newborn affected by abruptio placenta
Newborn affected by accidental hemorrhage
Newborn affected by antepartum hemorrhage
Newborn affected by damage to placenta from amniocentesis, cesarean delivery or surgical induction
Newborn affected by maternal blood loss
Newborn affected by premature separation of placenta
- ✓5th **P02.2** Newborn affected by other and unspecified morphological and functional abnormalities of placenta
  - **P02.20** Newborn affected by unspecified morphological and functional abnormalities of placenta

P02.29	**Newborn affected by other morphological and functional abnormalities of placenta**
	Newborn affected by placental dysfunction
	Newborn affected by placental infarction
	Newborn affected by placental insufficiency

P02.3 **Newborn affected by placental transfusion syndromes**
Newborn affected by placental and cord abnormalities resulting in twin-to-twin or other transplacental transfusion

P02.4 **Newborn affected by prolapsed cord**

P02.5 **Newborn affected by other compression of umbilical cord**
Newborn affected by entanglement of umbilical cord
Newborn affected by knot in umbilical cord
Newborn affected by umbilical cord (tightly) around neck
AHA: 2022,1Q,22

✓5th P02.6 **Newborn affected by other and unspecified conditions of umbilical cord**

    P02.60 **Newborn affected by unspecified conditions of umbilical cord**

    P02.69 **Newborn affected by other conditions of umbilical cord**
        Newborn affected by short umbilical cord
        Newborn affected by vasa previa
        EXCLUDES 1   newborn affected by single umbilical artery (Q27.0)

✓5th P02.7 **Newborn affected by chorioamnionitis**
AHA: 2018,4Q,23-24
DEF: Inflammation of the fetal membranes due to maternal infection characterized by fetal tachycardia, respiratory distress, apnea, weak cries, and poor sucking.

    P02.70 **Newborn affected by fetal inflammatory response syndrome** HCC ESR COM
        Newborn affected by FIRS

    P02.78 **Newborn affected by other conditions from chorioamnionitis**
        Newborn affected by amnionitis
        Newborn affected by membranitis
        Newborn affected by placentitis

P02.8 **Newborn affected by other abnormalities of membranes**

P02.9 **Newborn affected by abnormality of membranes, unspecified**

✓4th P03 **Newborn affected by other complications of labor and delivery**
Code first any current condition in newborn
EXCLUDES 2   encounter for observation of newborn for suspected diseases and conditions ruled out (Z05.-)

P03.0 **Newborn affected by breech delivery and extraction**

P03.1 **Newborn affected by other malpresentation, malposition and disproportion during labor and delivery**
Newborn affected by transverse lie
Newborn affected by conditions classifiable to O64-O66
Newborn affected by contracted pelvis
Newborn affected by persistent occipitoposterior

P03.2 **Newborn affected by forceps delivery**

Forceps Assisted Birth

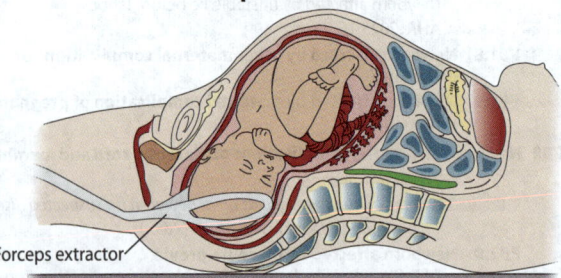

Forceps extractor

P03.3 **Newborn affected by delivery by vacuum extractor [ventouse]**

Vacuum Assisted Birth

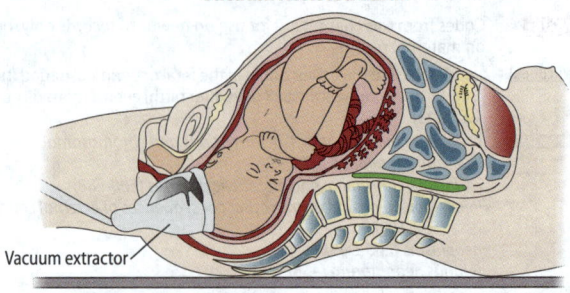

Vacuum extractor

P03.4 **Newborn affected by Cesarean delivery**

P03.5 **Newborn affected by precipitate delivery**
Newborn affected by rapid second stage

P03.6 **Newborn affected by abnormal uterine contractions**
Newborn affected by conditions classifiable to O62.-, except O62.3
Newborn affected by hypertonic labor
Newborn affected by uterine inertia

✓5th P03.8 **Newborn affected by other specified complications of labor and delivery**

    ✓6th P03.81 **Newborn affected by abnormality in fetal (intrauterine) heart rate or rhythm**
        EXCLUDES 1   neonatal cardiac dysrhythmia (P29.1-)

        P03.810 **Newborn affected by abnormality in fetal (intrauterine) heart rate or rhythm before the onset of labor**

        P03.811 **Newborn affected by abnormality in fetal (intrauterine) heart rate or rhythm during labor**

        P03.819 **Newborn affected by abnormality in fetal (intrauterine) heart rate or rhythm, unspecified as to time of onset**

    P03.82 **Meconium passage during delivery**
        EXCLUDES 1   meconium aspiration (P24.00, P24.01)
            meconium staining (P96.83)
        DEF: Fetal intestinal activity that increases in response to a fetomaternal distressed state during delivery. The anal sphincter relaxes and meconium is passed into the amniotic fluid.

    P03.89 **Newborn affected by other specified complications of labor and delivery**
        Newborn affected by abnormality of maternal soft tissues
        Newborn affected by conditions classifiable to O60-O75 and by procedures used in labor and delivery not included in P02.- and P03.0-P03.6
        Newborn affected by induction of labor

P03.9 **Newborn affected by complication of labor and delivery, unspecified**

✓4th P04 **Newborn affected by noxious substances transmitted via placenta or breast milk**
INCLUDES   nonteratogenic effects of substances transmitted via placenta
Code first any current condition in newborn, if applicable
EXCLUDES 2   congenital malformations (Q00-Q99)
    encounter for observation of newborn for suspected diseases and conditions ruled out (Z05.-)
    neonatal jaundice from excessive hemolysis due to drugs or toxins transmitted from mother (P58.4)
    newborn in contact with and (suspected) exposures hazardous to health not transmitted via placenta or breast milk (Z77.-)

    P04.0 **Newborn affected by maternal anesthesia and analgesia in pregnancy, labor and delivery** HCC COM
        Newborn affected by reactions and intoxications from maternal opiates and tranquilizers administered for procedures during pregnancy or labor and delivery
        EXCLUDES 2   newborn affected by other maternal medication (P04.1-)

Chapter 16. Certain Conditions Originating in the Perinatal Period

P04.1 **Newborn affected by other maternal medication**
Code first, if applicable, withdrawal symptoms from maternal use of drugs of addiction (P96.1)
withdrawal symptoms from therapeutic use of drugs in newborn (P96.2)
EXCLUDES 1: dysmorphism due to warfarin (Q86.2)
fetal hydantoin syndrome (Q86.1)
EXCLUDES 2: maternal anesthesia and analgesia in pregnancy, labor and delivery (P04.0)
maternal use of drugs of addiction (P04.4-)
AHA: 2018,4Q,24-25

- **P04.11** Newborn affected by maternal antineoplastic chemotherapy
- **P04.12** Newborn affected by maternal cytotoxic drugs
- **P04.13** Newborn affected by maternal use of anticonvulsants
- **P04.14** Newborn affected by maternal use of opiates
- **P04.15** Newborn affected by maternal use of antidepressants
- **P04.16** Newborn affected by maternal use of amphetamines
- **P04.17** Newborn affected by maternal use of sedative-hypnotics
- **P04.1A** Newborn affected by maternal use of anxiolytics
- **P04.18** Newborn affected by other maternal medication
- **P04.19** Newborn affected by maternal use of unspecified medication

P04.2 **Newborn affected by maternal use of tobacco**
Newborn affected by exposure in utero to tobacco smoke
EXCLUDES 2: newborn exposure to environmental tobacco smoke (P96.81)

P04.3 **Newborn affected by maternal use of alcohol**
EXCLUDES 1: fetal alcohol syndrome (Q86.0)

P04.4 **Newborn affected by maternal use of drugs of addiction**
AHA: 2018,4Q,25

- **P04.40** Newborn affected by maternal use of unspecified drugs of addiction
- **P04.41** Newborn affected by maternal use of cocaine
- **P04.42** Newborn affected by maternal use of hallucinogens
  EXCLUDES 2: newborn affected by other maternal medication (P04.1-)
- **P04.49** Newborn affected by maternal use of other drugs of addiction
  EXCLUDES 2: newborn affected by maternal anesthesia and analgesia (P04.0)
  withdrawal symptoms from maternal use of drugs of addiction (P96.1)

P04.5 **Newborn affected by maternal use of nutritional chemical substances**

P04.6 **Newborn affected by maternal exposure to environmental chemical substances**

P04.8 **Newborn affected by other maternal noxious substances**
AHA: 2018,4Q,25

- **P04.81** Newborn affected by maternal use of cannabis
- **P04.89** Newborn affected by other maternal noxious substances

P04.9 **Newborn affected by maternal noxious substance, unspecified**

Disorders of newborn related to length of gestation and fetal growth (P05-P08)

P05 **Disorders of newborn related to slow fetal growth and fetal malnutrition**
AHA: 2016,4Q,55-56

P05.0 **Newborn light for gestational age**
Newborn light-for-dates
Weight below but length above 10th percentile for gestational age

- **P05.00** Newborn light for gestational age, unspecified weight
- **P05.01** Newborn light for gestational age, less than 500 grams
- **P05.02** Newborn light for gestational age, 500-749 grams
- **P05.03** Newborn light for gestational age, 750-999 grams
- **P05.04** Newborn light for gestational age, 1000-1249 grams
- **P05.05** Newborn light for gestational age, 1250-1499 grams
- **P05.06** Newborn light for gestational age, 1500-1749 grams
- **P05.07** Newborn light for gestational age, 1750-1999 grams
- **P05.08** Newborn light for gestational age, 2000-2499 grams
- **P05.09** Newborn light for gestational age, 2500 grams and over
  Newborn light for gestational age, other

P05.1 **Newborn small for gestational age**
Newborn small-and-light-for-dates
Newborn small-for-dates
Weight and length below 10th percentile for gestational age

- **P05.10** Newborn small for gestational age, unspecified weight
- **P05.11** Newborn small for gestational age, less than 500 grams
- **P05.12** Newborn small for gestational age, 500-749 grams
- **P05.13** Newborn small for gestational age, 750-999 grams
- **P05.14** Newborn small for gestational age, 1000-1249 grams
- **P05.15** Newborn small for gestational age, 1250-1499 grams
- **P05.16** Newborn small for gestational age, 1500-1749 grams
- **P05.17** Newborn small for gestational age, 1750-1999 grams
- **P05.18** Newborn small for gestational age, 2000-2499 grams
- **P05.19** Newborn small for gestational age, other
  Newborn small for gestational age, 2500 grams and over

P05.2 **Newborn affected by fetal (intrauterine) malnutrition not light or small for gestational age**
Infant, not light or small for gestational age, showing signs of fetal malnutrition, such as dry, peeling skin and loss of subcutaneous tissue
EXCLUDES 1: newborn affected by fetal malnutrition with light for gestational age (P05.0-)
newborn affected by fetal malnutrition with small for gestational age (P05.1-)

P05.9 **Newborn affected by slow intrauterine growth, unspecified**
Newborn affected by fetal growth retardation NOS

P07 **Disorders of newborn related to short gestation and low birth weight, not elsewhere classified**
NOTE: When both birth weight and gestational age of the newborn are available, both should be coded with birth weight sequenced before gestational age
INCLUDES: the listed conditions, without further specification, as the cause of morbidity or additional care, in newborn

P07.0 **Extremely low birth weight newborn**
Newborn birth weight 999 g. or less
EXCLUDES 1: low birth weight due to slow fetal growth and fetal malnutrition (P05.-)

- **P07.00** Extremely low birth weight newborn, unspecified weight
- **P07.01** Extremely low birth weight newborn, less than 500 grams
- **P07.02** Extremely low birth weight newborn, 500-749 grams
- **P07.03** Extremely low birth weight newborn, 750-999 grams

Chapter 16. Certain Conditions Originating in the Perinatal Period

P07.1 Other low birth weight newborn
Newborn birth weight 1000-2499 g.
EXCLUDES 1: low birth weight due to slow fetal growth and fetal malnutrition (P05.-)

- **P07.10** Other low birth weight newborn, unspecified weight
- **P07.14** Other low birth weight newborn, 1000-1249 grams
- **P07.15** Other low birth weight newborn, 1250-1499 grams
- **P07.16** Other low birth weight newborn, 1500-1749 grams
- **P07.17** Other low birth weight newborn, 1750-1999 grams
- **P07.18** Other low birth weight newborn, 2000-2499 grams

P07.2 Extreme immaturity of newborn
Less than 28 completed weeks (less than 196 completed days) of gestation.

- **P07.20** Extreme immaturity of newborn, unspecified weeks of gestation
  Gestational age less than 28 completed weeks NOS
- **P07.21** Extreme immaturity of newborn, gestational age less than 23 completed weeks
  Extreme immaturity of newborn, gestational age less than 23 weeks, 0 days
- **P07.22** Extreme immaturity of newborn, gestational age 23 completed weeks
  Extreme immaturity of newborn, gestational age 23 weeks, 0 days through 23 weeks, 6 days
- **P07.23** Extreme immaturity of newborn, gestational age 24 completed weeks
  Extreme immaturity of newborn, gestational age 24 weeks, 0 days through 24 weeks, 6 days
- **P07.24** Extreme immaturity of newborn, gestational age 25 completed weeks
  Extreme immaturity of newborn, gestational age 25 weeks, 0 days through 25 weeks, 6 days
- **P07.25** Extreme immaturity of newborn, gestational age 26 completed weeks
  Extreme immaturity of newborn, gestational age 26 weeks, 0 days through 26 weeks, 6 days
- **P07.26** Extreme immaturity of newborn, gestational age 27 completed weeks
  Extreme immaturity of newborn, gestational age 27 weeks, 0 days through 27 weeks, 6 days

P07.3 Preterm [premature] newborn [other]
28 completed weeks or more but less than 37 completed weeks (196 completed days but less than 259 completed days) of gestation
Prematurity NOS
AHA: 2017,3Q,26

- **P07.30** Preterm newborn, unspecified weeks of gestation
- **P07.31** Preterm newborn, gestational age 28 completed weeks
  Preterm newborn, gestational age 28 weeks, 0 days through 28 weeks, 6 days
- **P07.32** Preterm newborn, gestational age 29 completed weeks
  Preterm newborn, gestational age 29 weeks, 0 days through 29 weeks, 6 days
- **P07.33** Preterm newborn, gestational age 30 completed weeks
  Preterm newborn, gestational age 30 weeks, 0 days through 30 weeks, 6 days
- **P07.34** Preterm newborn, gestational age 31 completed weeks
  Preterm newborn, gestational age 31 weeks, 0 days through 31 weeks, 6 days
- **P07.35** Preterm newborn, gestational age 32 completed weeks
  Preterm newborn, gestational age 32 weeks, 0 days through 32 weeks, 6 days
- **P07.36** Preterm newborn, gestational age 33 completed weeks
  Preterm newborn, gestational age 33 weeks, 0 days through 33 weeks, 6 days
- **P07.37** Preterm newborn, gestational age 34 completed weeks
  Preterm newborn, gestational age 34 weeks, 0 days through 34 weeks, 6 days
- **P07.38** Preterm newborn, gestational age 35 completed weeks
  Preterm newborn, gestational age 35 weeks, 0 days through 35 weeks, 6 days
- **P07.39** Preterm newborn, gestational age 36 completed weeks
  Preterm newborn, gestational age 36 weeks, 0 days through 36 weeks, 6 days

P08 Disorders of newborn related to long gestation and high birth weight
NOTE: When both birth weight and gestational age of the newborn are available, priority of assignment should be given to birth weight
INCLUDES: the listed conditions, without further specification, as causes of morbidity or additional care, in newborn

- **P08.0** Exceptionally large newborn baby
  Usually implies a birth weight of 4500 g. or more
  EXCLUDES 1: syndrome of infant of diabetic mother (P70.1)
  syndrome of infant of mother with gestational diabetes (P70.0)
- **P08.1** Other heavy for gestational age newborn
  Other newborn heavy- or large-for-dates regardless of period of gestation
  Usually implies a birth weight of 4000 g. to 4499 g.
  EXCLUDES 1: newborn with a birth weight of 4500 or more (P08.0)
  syndrome of infant of diabetic mother (P70.1)
  syndrome of infant of mother with gestational diabetes (P70.0)
- **P08.2** Late newborn, not heavy for gestational age
  AHA: 2014,1Q,14
  - **P08.21** Post-term newborn
    Newborn with gestation period over 40 completed weeks to 42 completed weeks
  - **P08.22** Prolonged gestation of newborn
    Newborn with gestation period over 42 completed weeks (294 days or more), not heavy- or large-for-dates.
    Postmaturity NOS

Abnormal findings on neonatal screening (P09)

P09 Abnormal findings on neonatal screening
INCLUDES: abnormal findings on state mandated newborn screens
failed newborn screening
EXCLUDES 2: nonspecific serologic evidence of human immunodeficiency virus [HIV] (R75)
AHA: 2021,4Q,24

- **P09.1** Abnormal findings on neonatal screening for inborn errors of metabolism
- **P09.2** Abnormal findings on neonatal screening for congenital endocrine disease
  Abnormal findings on neonatal screening for congenital adrenal hyperplasia
  Abnormal findings on neonatal screening for hypothyroidism screen
- **P09.3** Abnormal findings on neonatal screening for congenital hematologic disorders
  Abnormal findings for hemoglobinopathy screening
  Abnormal findings on red cell membrane defects screen
  Abnormal findings on sickle cell screen
- **P09.4** Abnormal findings on neonatal screening for cystic fibrosis
- **P09.5** Abnormal findings on neonatal screening for critical congenital heart disease
  Neonatal congenital heart disease screening failure
- **P09.6** Abnormal findings on neonatal hearing screening
  EXCLUDES 2: encounter for hearing examination following failed hearing screening (Z01.110)
- **P09.8** Other abnormal findings on neonatal screening
- **P09.9** Abnormal findings on neonatal screening, unspecified

Birth trauma (P10-P15)

P10 ☑4th **Intracranial laceration and hemorrhage** due to birth injury
  EXCLUDES 1: intracranial hemorrhage of newborn NOS (P52.9)
    intracranial hemorrhage of newborn due to anoxia or hypoxia (P52.-)
    nontraumatic intracranial hemorrhage of newborn (P52.-)

  P10.0 Subdural hemorrhage due to birth injury [HCC] [COM]
    Subdural hematoma (localized) due to birth injury
    EXCLUDES 1: subdural hemorrhage accompanying tentorial tear (P10.4)
  P10.1 Cerebral hemorrhage due to birth injury [HCC] [COM]
  P10.2 Intraventricular hemorrhage due to birth injury [HCC] [COM]
  P10.3 Subarachnoid hemorrhage due to birth injury [HCC] [COM]
  P10.4 Tentorial tear due to birth injury [HCC] [COM]
  P10.8 Other intracranial lacerations and hemorrhages due to birth injury [HCC] [COM]
  P10.9 Unspecified intracranial laceration and hemorrhage due to birth injury [HCC] [COM]

P11 ☑4th **Other birth injuries to central nervous system**
  P11.0 Cerebral edema due to birth injury [HCC] [COM]
  P11.1 Other specified brain damage due to birth injury [HCC] [COM]
  P11.2 Unspecified brain damage due to birth injury [HCC] [COM]
  P11.3 Birth injury to **facial nerve**
    Facial palsy due to birth injury
  P11.4 Birth injury to other cranial nerves
  P11.5 Birth injury to **spine and spinal cord** [HCC] [COM]
    Fracture of spine due to birth injury
  P11.9 Birth injury to central nervous system, unspecified

P12 ☑4th **Birth injury to scalp**

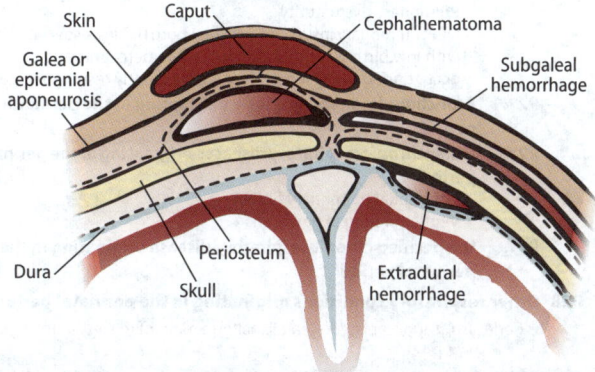
Birth Injuries to Scalp
Skin, Caput, Cephalhematoma, Galea or epicranial aponeurosis, Subgaleal hemorrhage, Periosteum, Dura, Skull, Extradural hemorrhage

  P12.0 Cephalhematoma due to birth injury
    DEF: Condition that occurs in a neonate when blood vessels between the skull and periosteum rupture and blood collects in the subperiosteal space (below the periosteum). It is typically caused by prolonged labor or trauma due to instrument-assisted delivery (e.g., forceps, vacuum extraction), although in rare circumstances, it may indicate a linear skull fracture with intracranial hemorrhage.
  P12.1 Chignon (from vacuum extraction) due to birth injury
    DEF: Artificial swelling of the scalp that occurs when a collection of interstitial fluid and blood forms in the area of the scalp where the suction cup was applied during a vacuum-assisted delivery.
  P12.2 Epicranial subaponeurotic hemorrhage due to birth injury [HCC]
    Subgaleal hemorrhage
  P12.3 Bruising of scalp due to birth injury
  P12.4 Injury of scalp of newborn due to **monitoring equipment**
    Sampling incision of scalp of newborn
    Scalp clip (electrode) injury of newborn
  P12.8 ☑5th Other birth injuries to scalp
    P12.81 Caput succedaneum
      DEF: Swelling of the scalp as a result of pressure being exerted on the head from the vaginal walls, uterus, or instrumentation used in assisting a delivery (e.g., vacuum).
    P12.89 Other birth injuries to scalp
  P12.9 Birth injury to scalp, unspecified

P13 ☑4th **Birth injury to skeleton**
  EXCLUDES 2: birth injury to spine (P11.5)
  P13.0 Fracture of skull due to birth injury
  P13.1 Other birth injuries to skull
    EXCLUDES 1: cephalhematoma (P12.0)
  P13.2 Birth injury to **femur**
  P13.3 Birth injury to other long bones
  P13.4 Fracture of clavicle due to birth injury
  P13.8 Birth injuries to other parts of skeleton
  P13.9 Birth injury to skeleton, unspecified

P14 ☑4th **Birth injury to peripheral nervous system**
  P14.0 Erb's paralysis due to birth injury
    DEF: Erb's paralysis: Most common type of brachial plexus (peripheral nerve) injury in a neonate that involves nerve damage at the level of C5-C6. Synonym(s): Erb's palsy
  P14.1 Klumpke's paralysis due to birth injury
  P14.2 Phrenic nerve paralysis due to birth injury
  P14.3 Other brachial plexus birth injuries
  P14.8 Birth injuries to other parts of peripheral nervous system
  P14.9 Birth injury to peripheral nervous system, unspecified

P15 ☑4th **Other birth injuries**
  P15.0 Birth injury to **liver**
    Rupture of liver due to birth injury
  P15.1 Birth injury to **spleen**
    Rupture of spleen due to birth injury
  P15.2 Sternomastoid injury due to birth injury
  P15.3 Birth injury to **eye**
    Subconjunctival hemorrhage due to birth injury
    Traumatic glaucoma due to birth injury
  P15.4 Birth injury to **face**
    Facial congestion due to birth injury
  P15.5 Birth injury to **external genitalia**
  P15.6 Subcutaneous fat necrosis due to birth injury
  P15.8 Other specified birth injuries
  P15.9 Birth injury, unspecified

Respiratory and cardiovascular disorders specific to the perinatal period (P19-P29)

P19 ☑4th **Metabolic acidemia in newborn**
  INCLUDES: metabolic acidemia in newborn
  P19.0 Metabolic acidemia in newborn first noted **before onset of labor**
  P19.1 Metabolic acidemia in newborn first noted **during labor**
  P19.2 Metabolic acidemia noted **at birth**
  P19.9 Metabolic acidemia in newborn, unspecified

P22 ☑4th **Respiratory distress of newborn**
  AHA: 2019,2Q,29
  P22.0 Respiratory distress syndrome of newborn [HCC] [COM]
    Cardiorespiratory distress syndrome of newborn
    Hyaline membrane disease
    Idiopathic respiratory distress syndrome [IRDS or RDS] of newborn
    Pulmonary hypoperfusion syndrome
    Respiratory distress syndrome, type I
    EXCLUDES 2: respiratory arrest of newborn (P28.81)
      respiratory failure of newborn NOS (P28.5)
    AHA: 2019,2Q,29
    DEF: Severe chest contractions upon air intake and expiratory grunting. The infant appears blue due to oxygen deficiency and has a rapid respiratory rate, formerly called hyaline membrane disease.
  P22.1 Transient tachypnea of newborn
    Idiopathic tachypnea of newborn
    Respiratory distress syndrome, type II
    Wet lung syndrome
    DEF: Rapid, labored breathing of a newborn. It is a short-term problem that begins after birth and lasts about three days.
  P22.8 Other respiratory distress of newborn
    EXCLUDES 1: respiratory arrest of newborn (P28.81)
      respiratory failure of newborn NOS (P28.5)
  P22.9 Respiratory distress of newborn, unspecified
    EXCLUDES 1: respiratory arrest of newborn (P28.81)
      respiratory failure of newborn NOS (P28.5)

P23 Congenital pneumonia
INCLUDES infective pneumonia acquired in utero or during birth
EXCLUDES 1 neonatal pneumonia resulting from aspiration (P24.-)

- **P23.0** Congenital pneumonia due to viral agent
  Use additional code (B97) to identify organism
  EXCLUDES 1 congenital rubella pneumonitis (P35.0)
- **P23.1** Congenital pneumonia due to Chlamydia
- **P23.2** Congenital pneumonia due to staphylococcus
- **P23.3** Congenital pneumonia due to streptococcus, group B
- **P23.4** Congenital pneumonia due to Escherichia coli
- **P23.5** Congenital pneumonia due to Pseudomonas
- **P23.6** Congenital pneumonia due to other bacterial agents
  Congenital pneumonia due to Hemophilus influenzae
  Congenital pneumonia due to Klebsiella pneumoniae
  Congenital pneumonia due to Mycoplasma
  Congenital pneumonia due to Streptococcus, except group B
  Use additional code (B95-B96) to identify organism
- **P23.8** Congenital pneumonia due to other organisms
- **P23.9** Congenital pneumonia, unspecified

P24 Neonatal aspiration
INCLUDES aspiration in utero and during delivery

- **P24.0** Meconium aspiration
  EXCLUDES 1 meconium passage (without aspiration) during delivery (P03.82)
  meconium staining (P96.83)
  DEF: Meconium in the trachea or seen on chest x-ray after birth.
  - **P24.00** Meconium aspiration without respiratory symptoms
    Meconium aspiration NOS
  - **P24.01** Meconium aspiration with respiratory symptoms
    Meconium aspiration pneumonia
    Meconium aspiration pneumonitis
    Meconium aspiration syndrome NOS
    Use additional code to identify any secondary pulmonary hypertension, if applicable (I27.2-)
    DEF: Aspiration of fetal intestinal material during or prior to delivery. It is usually a complication of placental insufficiency, causing pneumonitis and bronchial obstruction (inflammatory reaction of lungs).
- **P24.1** Neonatal aspiration of (clear) amniotic fluid and mucus
  Neonatal aspiration of liquor (amnii)
  - **P24.10** Neonatal aspiration of (clear) amniotic fluid and mucus without respiratory symptoms
    Neonatal aspiration of amniotic fluid and mucus NOS
  - **P24.11** Neonatal aspiration of (clear) amniotic fluid and mucus with respiratory symptoms
    Neonatal aspiration of amniotic fluid and mucus with pneumonia
    Neonatal aspiration of amniotic fluid and mucus with pneumonitis
    Use additional code to identify any secondary pulmonary hypertension, if applicable (I27.2-)
- **P24.2** Neonatal aspiration of blood
  - **P24.20** Neonatal aspiration of blood without respiratory symptoms
    Neonatal aspiration of blood NOS
  - **P24.21** Neonatal aspiration of blood with respiratory symptoms
    Neonatal aspiration of blood with pneumonia
    Neonatal aspiration of blood with pneumonitis
    Use additional code to identify any secondary pulmonary hypertension, if applicable (I27.2-)
- **P24.3** Neonatal aspiration of milk and regurgitated food
  Neonatal aspiration of stomach contents
  - **P24.30** Neonatal aspiration of milk and regurgitated food without respiratory symptoms
    Neonatal aspiration of milk and regurgitated food NOS
  - **P24.31** Neonatal aspiration of milk and regurgitated food with respiratory symptoms
    Neonatal aspiration of milk and regurgitated food with pneumonia
    Neonatal aspiration of milk and regurgitated food with pneumonitis
    Use additional code to identify any secondary pulmonary hypertension, if applicable (I27.2-)
- **P24.8** Other neonatal aspiration
  - **P24.80** Other neonatal aspiration without respiratory symptoms
    Neonatal aspiration NEC
  - **P24.81** Other neonatal aspiration with respiratory symptoms
    Neonatal aspiration pneumonia NEC
    Neonatal aspiration with pneumonia NOS
    Neonatal aspiration with pneumonitis NEC
    Neonatal aspiration with pneumonitis NOS
    Use additional code to identify any secondary pulmonary hypertension, if applicable (I27.2-)
- **P24.9** Neonatal aspiration, unspecified

P25 Interstitial emphysema and related conditions originating in the perinatal period
- **P25.0** Interstitial emphysema originating in the perinatal period
- **P25.1** Pneumothorax originating in the perinatal period
- **P25.2** Pneumomediastinum originating in the perinatal period
- **P25.3** Pneumopericardium originating in the perinatal period
- **P25.8** Other conditions related to interstitial emphysema originating in the perinatal period

P26 Pulmonary hemorrhage originating in the perinatal period
EXCLUDES 1 acute idiopathic hemorrhage in infants over 28 days old (R04.81)

- **P26.0** Tracheobronchial hemorrhage originating in the perinatal period
- **P26.1** Massive pulmonary hemorrhage originating in the perinatal period
- **P26.8** Other pulmonary hemorrhages originating in the perinatal period
- **P26.9** Unspecified pulmonary hemorrhage originating in the perinatal period

P27 Chronic respiratory disease originating in the perinatal period
EXCLUDES 2 respiratory distress of newborn (P22.0-P22.9)

- **P27.0** Wilson-Mikity syndrome
  Pulmonary dysmaturity
  DEF: Pulmonary insufficiency in newborn babies, especially those with low birth weight. Rapid onset of hypercapnia and cyanosis occur during the first month of life frequently resulting in death.
- **P27.1** Bronchopulmonary dysplasia originating in the perinatal period
- **P27.8** Other chronic respiratory diseases originating in the perinatal period
  Congenital pulmonary fibrosis
  Ventilator lung in newborn
- **P27.9** Unspecified chronic respiratory disease originating in the perinatal period

P28 Other respiratory conditions originating in the perinatal period
Code also, if applicable, congenital malformations of the respiratory system (Q30-Q34)

- **P28.0** Primary atelectasis of newborn
  Primary failure to expand terminal respiratory units
  Pulmonary hypoplasia associated with short gestation
  Pulmonary immaturity NOS
- **P28.1** Other and unspecified atelectasis of newborn
  - **P28.10** Unspecified atelectasis of newborn
    Atelectasis of newborn NOS
  - **P28.11** Resorption atelectasis without respiratory distress syndrome
    EXCLUDES 1 resorption atelectasis with respiratory distress syndrome (P22.0)
  - **P28.19** Other atelectasis of newborn
    Partial atelectasis of newborn
    Secondary atelectasis of newborn
- **P28.2** Cyanotic attacks of newborn
  EXCLUDES 1 apnea of newborn (P28.3- - P28.4-)
- **P28.3** Primary sleep apnea of newborn
  Sleep apnea of newborn NOS
  EXCLUDES 2 other apnea of newborn (P28.4-)
  AHA: 2022,4Q,38-39
  DEF: Unexplained cessation of breathing when a neonate makes no respiratory effort for 20 seconds or longer or when a neonate's breathing cessation is accompanied by cyanosis, bradycardia, or hypotonia.
  - **P28.30** Primary sleep apnea of newborn, unspecified
    Transient oxygen desaturation spells of newborn during sleep
  - **P28.31** Primary central sleep apnea of newborn

	P28.32	Primary obstructive sleep apnea of newborn
	P28.33	Primary mixed sleep apnea of newborn
	P28.39	Other primary sleep apnea of newborn

P28.4 Other apnea of newborn
  EXCLUDES 2: primary sleep apnea of newborn (P28.3-)
  AHA: 2022,4Q,38-39
  - **P28.40** Unspecified apnea of newborn
    Apnea of newborn, NOS
    Transient oxygen desaturation spells of newborn
  - **P28.41** Central neonatal apnea of newborn
  - **P28.42** Obstructive apnea of newborn
  - **P28.43** Mixed neonatal apnea of newborn
  - **P28.49** Other apnea of newborn
    Apnea of prematurity

P28.5 Respiratory failure of newborn
  EXCLUDES 2: respiratory arrest of newborn (P28.81)
  respiratory distress of newborn (P22.0)
  AHA: 2019,2Q,29

P28.8 Other specified respiratory conditions of newborn
  - **P28.81** Respiratory arrest of newborn
  - **P28.89** Other specified respiratory conditions of newborn
    Congenital laryngeal stridor
    Sniffles in newborn
    Snuffles in newborn
    EXCLUDES 1: early congenital syphilitic rhinitis (A50.05)

P28.9 Respiratory condition of newborn, unspecified
  Respiratory depression in newborn

P29 Cardiovascular disorders originating in the perinatal period
  EXCLUDES 2: congenital malformations of the circulatory system (Q20-Q28)
  - **P29.0** Neonatal cardiac failure
    Code also associated underlying condition
  - **P29.1** Neonatal cardiac dysrhythmia
    - **P29.11** Neonatal tachycardia
    - **P29.12** Neonatal bradycardia
  - **P29.2** Neonatal hypertension
  - **P29.3** Persistent fetal circulation
    AHA: 2017,4Q,20-21
    - **P29.30** Pulmonary hypertension of newborn
      Persistent pulmonary hypertension of newborn
      DEF: Condition that occurs when pressure within the pulmonary artery is elevated and vascular resistance is observed in the lungs.
    - **P29.38** Other persistent fetal circulation
      Delayed closure of ductus arteriosus
  - **P29.4** Transient myocardial ischemia in newborn
  - **P29.8** Other cardiovascular disorders originating in the perinatal period
    - **P29.81** Cardiac arrest of newborn
    - **P29.89** Other cardiovascular disorders originating in the perinatal period
      AHA: 2014,4Q,23
  - **P29.9** Cardiovascular disorder originating in the perinatal period, unspecified

Infections specific to the perinatal period (P35-P39)

Infections acquired in utero, during birth via the umbilicus, or during the first 28 days after birth
EXCLUDES 2: asymptomatic human immunodeficiency virus [HIV] infection status (Z21)
congenital gonococcal infection (A54.-)
congenital pneumonia (P23.-)
congenital syphilis (A50.-)
human immunodeficiency virus [HIV] disease (B20)
infant botulism (A48.51)
infectious diseases not specific to the perinatal period (A00-B99, J09, J10.-)
intestinal infectious disease (A00-A09)
laboratory evidence of human immunodeficiency virus [HIV] (R75)
tetanus neonatorum (A33)

P35 Congenital viral diseases
  INCLUDES: infections acquired in utero or during birth
  - **P35.0** Congenital rubella syndrome
    Congenital rubella pneumonitis
  - **P35.1** Congenital cytomegalovirus infection
  - **P35.2** Congenital herpesviral [herpes simplex] infection
  - **P35.3** Congenital viral hepatitis
  - **P35.4** Congenital Zika virus disease
    Use additional code to identify manifestations of congenital Zika virus disease
    AHA: 2018,4Q,25-26
  - **P35.8** Other congenital viral diseases
    Congenital varicella [chickenpox]
    AHA: 2020,2Q,13
  - **P35.9** Congenital viral disease, unspecified

P36 Bacterial sepsis of newborn
  INCLUDES: congenital sepsis
  Use additional code(s), if applicable, to identify severe sepsis (R65.2-) and associated acute organ dysfunction(s)
  - **P36.0** Sepsis of newborn due to streptococcus, group B
  - **P36.1** Sepsis of newborn due to other and unspecified streptococci
    - **P36.10** Sepsis of newborn due to unspecified streptococci
    - **P36.19** Sepsis of newborn due to other streptococci
  - **P36.2** Sepsis of newborn due to Staphylococcus aureus
  - **P36.3** Sepsis of newborn due to other and unspecified staphylococci
    - **P36.30** Sepsis of newborn due to unspecified staphylococci
    - **P36.39** Sepsis of newborn due to other staphylococci
  - **P36.4** Sepsis of newborn due to Escherichia coli
  - **P36.5** Sepsis of newborn due to anaerobes
  - **P36.8** Other bacterial sepsis of newborn
    Use additional code from category B96 to identify organism
  - **P36.9** Bacterial sepsis of newborn, unspecified

P37 Other congenital infectious and parasitic diseases
  EXCLUDES 2: congenital syphilis (A50.-)
  infectious neonatal diarrhea (A00-A09)
  necrotizing enterocolitis in newborn (P77.-)
  noninfectious neonatal diarrhea (P78.3)
  ophthalmia neonatorum due to gonococcus (A54.31)
  tetanus neonatorum (A33)
  - **P37.0** Congenital tuberculosis
  - **P37.1** Congenital toxoplasmosis
    Hydrocephalus due to congenital toxoplasmosis
  - **P37.2** Neonatal (disseminated) listeriosis
  - **P37.3** Congenital falciparum malaria
  - **P37.4** Other congenital malaria
  - **P37.5** Neonatal candidiasis
  - **P37.8** Other specified congenital infectious and parasitic diseases
  - **P37.9** Congenital infectious or parasitic disease, unspecified

P38 Omphalitis of newborn
  EXCLUDES 1: omphalitis not of newborn (L08.82)
  tetanus omphalitis (A33)
  umbilical hemorrhage of newborn (P51.-)
  DEF: Omphalitis: Infection and inflammation of the umbilical stump, often due to bacteria that can spread beyond the umbilical stump to the fascia, muscle, or even the umbilical vessels.
  - **P38.1** Omphalitis with mild hemorrhage
  - **P38.9** Omphalitis without hemorrhage
    Omphalitis of newborn NOS

P39 Other infections specific to the perinatal period
  Use additional code to identify organism or specific infection
  - **P39.0** Neonatal infective mastitis
    EXCLUDES 1: breast engorgement of newborn (P83.4)
    noninfective mastitis of newborn (P83.4)
  - **P39.1** Neonatal conjunctivitis and dacryocystitis
    Neonatal chlamydial conjunctivitis
    Ophthalmia neonatorum NOS
    EXCLUDES 1: gonococcal conjunctivitis (A54.31)
  - **P39.2** Intra-amniotic infection affecting newborn, not elsewhere classified
  - **P39.3** Neonatal urinary tract infection
  - **P39.4** Neonatal skin infection
    Neonatal pyoderma
    EXCLUDES 1: pemphigus neonatorum (L00)
    staphylococcal scalded skin syndrome (L00)
  - **P39.8** Other specified infections specific to the perinatal period
  - **P39.9** Infection specific to the perinatal period, unspecified

Hemorrhagic and hematological disorders of newborn (P50-P61)

EXCLUDES 1 congenital stenosis and stricture of bile ducts (Q44.3)
Crigler-Najjar syndrome (E80.5)
Dubin-Johnson syndrome (E80.6)
Gilbert syndrome (E80.4)
hereditary hemolytic anemias (D55-D58)

✓4th P50 Newborn affected by intrauterine (fetal) blood loss
EXCLUDES 1 congenital anemia from intrauterine (fetal) blood loss (P61.3)

- **P50.0** Newborn affected by intrauterine (fetal) blood loss from vasa previa
- **P50.1** Newborn affected by intrauterine (fetal) blood loss from ruptured cord
- **P50.2** Newborn affected by intrauterine (fetal) blood loss from placenta
- **P50.3** Newborn affected by hemorrhage into co-twin
- **P50.4** Newborn affected by hemorrhage into maternal circulation
- **P50.5** Newborn affected by intrauterine (fetal) blood loss from cut end of co-twin's cord
- **P50.8** Newborn affected by other intrauterine (fetal) blood loss
- **P50.9** Newborn affected by intrauterine (fetal) blood loss, unspecified
  Newborn affected by fetal hemorrhage NOS

✓4th P51 Umbilical hemorrhage of newborn
EXCLUDES 1 omphalitis with mild hemorrhage (P38.1)
umbilical hemorrhage from cut end of co-twins cord (P50.5)

- **P51.0** Massive umbilical hemorrhage of newborn
- **P51.8** Other umbilical hemorrhages of newborn
  Slipped umbilical ligature NOS
- **P51.9** Umbilical hemorrhage of newborn, unspecified

✓4th P52 Intracranial nontraumatic hemorrhage of newborn
INCLUDES intracranial hemorrhage due to anoxia or hypoxia
EXCLUDES 1 intracranial hemorrhage due to birth injury (P10.-)
intracranial hemorrhage due to other injury (S06.-)

- **P52.0** Intraventricular (nontraumatic) hemorrhage, grade 1, of newborn HCC COM
  Bleeding into germinal matrix
  Subependymal hemorrhage (without intraventricular extension)
- **P52.1** Intraventricular (nontraumatic) hemorrhage, grade 2, of newborn HCC COM
  Bleeding into ventricle
  Subependymal hemorrhage with intraventricular extension
- ✓5th **P52.2** Intraventricular (nontraumatic) hemorrhage, grade 3 and grade 4, of newborn
  - **P52.21** Intraventricular (nontraumatic) hemorrhage, grade 3, of newborn HCC COM
    Subependymal hemorrhage with intraventricular extension with enlargement of ventricle
  - **P52.22** Intraventricular (nontraumatic) hemorrhage, grade 4, of newborn HCC COM
    Bleeding into cerebral cortex
    Subependymal hemorrhage with intracerebral extension
- **P52.3** Unspecified intraventricular (nontraumatic) hemorrhage of newborn HCC COM
- **P52.4** Intracerebral (nontraumatic) hemorrhage of newborn HCC COM
- **P52.5** Subarachnoid (nontraumatic) hemorrhage of newborn HCC COM
- **P52.6** Cerebellar (nontraumatic) and posterior fossa hemorrhage of newborn HCC COM
- **P52.8** Other intracranial (nontraumatic) hemorrhages of newborn HCC COM
- **P52.9** Intracranial (nontraumatic) hemorrhage of newborn, unspecified HCC COM

P53 Hemorrhagic disease of newborn COM
Vitamin K deficiency of newborn

✓4th P54 Other neonatal hemorrhages
EXCLUDES 1 newborn affected by (intrauterine) blood loss (P50.-)
pulmonary hemorrhage originating in the perinatal period (P26.-)

- **P54.0** Neonatal hematemesis
  EXCLUDES 1 neonatal hematemesis due to swallowed maternal blood (P78.2)
- **P54.1** Neonatal melena
  EXCLUDES 1 neonatal melena due to swallowed maternal blood (P78.2)
- **P54.2** Neonatal rectal hemorrhage
- **P54.3** Other neonatal gastrointestinal hemorrhage
- **P54.4** Neonatal adrenal hemorrhage
- **P54.5** Neonatal cutaneous hemorrhage
  Neonatal bruising
  Neonatal ecchymoses
  Neonatal petechiae
  Neonatal superficial hematomata
  EXCLUDES 2 bruising of scalp due to birth injury (P12.3)
  cephalhematoma due to birth injury (P12.0)
- **P54.6** Neonatal vaginal hemorrhage
  Neonatal pseudomenses
- **P54.8** Other specified neonatal hemorrhages
- **P54.9** Neonatal hemorrhage, unspecified

✓4th P55 Hemolytic disease of newborn

- **P55.0** Rh isoimmunization of newborn HCC COM
  DEF: Incompatible Rh fetal-maternal blood grouping that prematurely destroys red blood cells. Symptoms include jaundice, asphyxia, pulmonary hypertension, edema, respiratory distress, kernicterus, and coagulopathies. It is detected by a Coombs test.
  TIP: A positive Coombs test without documentation of associated Rh isoimmunization should be coded to R79.89 Other specified abnormal findings of blood chemistry.
- **P55.1** ABO isoimmunization of newborn HCC COM
  AHA: 2015,3Q,20
- **P55.8** Other hemolytic diseases of newborn HCC COM
  AHA: 2018,3Q,24
- **P55.9** Hemolytic disease of newborn, unspecified HCC COM

✓4th P56 Hydrops fetalis due to hemolytic disease
EXCLUDES 1 hydrops fetalis NOS (P83.2)

- **P56.0** Hydrops fetalis due to isoimmunization HCC COM
- ✓5th **P56.9** Hydrops fetalis due to other and unspecified hemolytic disease
  - **P56.90** Hydrops fetalis due to unspecified hemolytic disease HCC COM
  - **P56.99** Hydrops fetalis due to other hemolytic disease HCC COM

✓4th P57 Kernicterus

- **P57.0** Kernicterus due to isoimmunization HCC COM
  DEF: Complication of erythroblastosis fetalis associated with severe neural symptoms, high blood bilirubin levels, and nerve cell destruction. It results in bilirubin-pigmented gray matter of the central nervous system.
- **P57.8** Other specified kernicterus HCC COM
  EXCLUDES 1 Crigler-Najjar syndrome (E80.5)
- **P57.9** Kernicterus, unspecified HCC COM

✓4th P58 Neonatal jaundice due to other excessive hemolysis
EXCLUDES 1 jaundice due to isoimmunization (P55-P57)

- **P58.0** Neonatal jaundice due to bruising
- **P58.1** Neonatal jaundice due to bleeding
- **P58.2** Neonatal jaundice due to infection
- **P58.3** Neonatal jaundice due to polycythemia
- ✓5th **P58.4** Neonatal jaundice due to drugs or toxins transmitted from mother or given to newborn
  Code first poisoning due to drug or toxin, if applicable (T36-T65 with fifth or sixth character 1-4)
  Use additional code for adverse effect, if applicable, to identify drug (T36-T50 with fifth or sixth character 5)
  - **P58.41** Neonatal jaundice due to drugs or toxins transmitted from mother
  - **P58.42** Neonatal jaundice due to drugs or toxins given to newborn
- **P58.5** Neonatal jaundice due to swallowed maternal blood
- **P58.8** Neonatal jaundice due to other specified excessive hemolysis
- **P58.9** Neonatal jaundice due to excessive hemolysis, unspecified

✓4th P59 Neonatal jaundice from other and unspecified causes
EXCLUDES 1 jaundice due to inborn errors of metabolism (E70-E88)
kernicterus (P57.-)

- **P59.0** Neonatal jaundice associated with preterm delivery
  Hyperbilirubinemia of prematurity
  Jaundice due to delayed conjugation associated with preterm delivery
  AHA: 2025,1Q,24

Chapter 16. Certain Conditions Originating in the Perinatal Period

P59.1 **Inspissated bile syndrome** [COM]
  DEF: Biliary obstruction in newborn resulting from obstruction of outflow tract.

✓5th **P59.2** **Neonatal jaundice from other and unspecified hepatocellular damage**
  EXCLUDES 1 congenital viral hepatitis (P35.3)
  P59.20 Neonatal jaundice from unspecified hepatocellular damage [COM]
  P59.29 Neonatal jaundice from other hepatocellular damage [COM]
    Neonatal (idiopathic) hepatitis
    Neonatal giant cell hepatitis

P59.3 Neonatal jaundice from breast milk inhibitor
P59.8 Neonatal jaundice from other specified causes
P59.9 Neonatal jaundice, unspecified
  Neonatal physiological jaundice (intense)(prolonged) NOS
  AHA: 2015,3Q,20

P60 Disseminated intravascular coagulation of newborn [COM]
  Defibrination syndrome of newborn

✓4th **P61** **Other perinatal hematological disorders**
  EXCLUDES 1 transient hypogammaglobulinemia of infancy (D80.7)
  P61.0 Transient neonatal thrombocytopenia [COM]
    Neonatal thrombocytopenia due to exchange transfusion
    Neonatal thrombocytopenia due to idiopathic maternal thrombocytopenia
    Neonatal thrombocytopenia due to isoimmunization
    DEF: Temporary decrease in blood platelets of a newborn that is secondary to placental insufficiency.
  P61.1 Polycythemia neonatorum
    DEF: Abnormal increase of total red blood cells of a newborn that results in hyperviscosity, which slows the flow of blood through small blood vessels.
  P61.2 Anemia of prematurity
  P61.3 Congenital anemia from fetal blood loss
  P61.4 Other congenital anemias, not elsewhere classified
    Congenital anemia NOS
  P61.5 Transient neonatal neutropenia [COM]
    EXCLUDES 1 congenital neutropenia (nontransient) (D70.0)
    DEF: Low blood neutrophil counts of newborn that occurs due to maternal hypertension, sepsis, twin-twin transfusion, alloimmunization, and hemolytic disease.
  P61.6 Other transient neonatal disorders of coagulation [COM]
  P61.8 Other specified perinatal hematological disorders
  P61.9 Perinatal hematological disorder, unspecified

Transitory endocrine and metabolic disorders specific to newborn (P70-P74)

INCLUDES transitory endocrine and metabolic disturbances caused by the infant's response to maternal endocrine and metabolic factors, or its adjustment to extrauterine environment

AHA: 2018,2Q,6

✓4th **P70** **Transitory disorders of carbohydrate metabolism specific to newborn**
  P70.0 Syndrome of infant of mother with gestational diabetes
    Newborn (with hypoglycemia) affected by maternal gestational diabetes
    EXCLUDES 1 newborn (with hypoglycemia) affected by maternal (pre-existing) diabetes mellitus (P70.1)
      syndrome of infant of a diabetic mother (P70.1)
  P70.1 Syndrome of infant of a diabetic mother
    Newborn (with hypoglycemia) affected by maternal (pre-existing) diabetes mellitus
    EXCLUDES 1 newborn (with hypoglycemia) affected by maternal gestational diabetes (P70.0)
      syndrome of infant of mother with gestational diabetes (P70.0)
  P70.2 Neonatal diabetes mellitus
  P70.3 Iatrogenic neonatal hypoglycemia
  P70.4 Other neonatal hypoglycemia
    Transitory neonatal hypoglycemia
  P70.8 Other transitory disorders of carbohydrate metabolism of newborn
  P70.9 Transitory disorder of carbohydrate metabolism of newborn, unspecified

✓4th **P71** **Transitory neonatal disorders of calcium and magnesium metabolism**
  P71.0 Cow's milk hypocalcemia in newborn
  P71.1 Other neonatal hypocalcemia
    EXCLUDES 1 neonatal hypoparathyroidism (P71.4)
  P71.2 Neonatal hypomagnesemia

P71.3 Neonatal tetany without calcium or magnesium deficiency
  Neonatal tetany NOS
P71.4 Transitory neonatal hypoparathyroidism
P71.8 Other transitory neonatal disorders of calcium and magnesium metabolism
  AHA: 2016,4Q,54
P71.9 Transitory neonatal disorder of calcium and magnesium metabolism, unspecified

✓4th **P72** **Other transitory neonatal endocrine disorders**
  EXCLUDES 1 congenital hypothyroidism with or without goiter (E03.0-E03.1)
    dyshormogenetic goiter (E07.1)
    dyshormonogenetic goiter (E07.1)
    Pendred's syndrome (E07.1)
  P72.0 Neonatal goiter, not elsewhere classified
    Transitory congenital goiter with normal functioning
  P72.1 Transitory neonatal hyperthyroidism
    Neonatal thyrotoxicosis
  P72.2 Other transitory neonatal disorders of thyroid function, not elsewhere classified
    Transitory neonatal hypothyroidism
  P72.8 Other specified transitory neonatal endocrine disorders
  P72.9 Transitory neonatal endocrine disorder, unspecified

✓4th **P74** **Other transitory neonatal electrolyte and metabolic disturbances**
  AHA: 2018,4Q,26-27
  P74.0 Late metabolic acidosis of newborn
    EXCLUDES 1 (fetal) metabolic acidosis of newborn (P19)
  P74.1 Dehydration of newborn
  ✓5th **P74.2** Disturbances of sodium balance of newborn
    P74.21 Hypernatremia of newborn
    P74.22 Hyponatremia of newborn
  ✓5th **P74.3** Disturbances of potassium balance of newborn
    P74.31 Hyperkalemia of newborn
    P74.32 Hypokalemia of newborn
  ✓5th **P74.4** Other transitory electrolyte disturbances of newborn
    P74.41 Alkalosis of newborn
      Hyperbicarbonatemia
    ✓6th **P74.42** Disturbances of chlorine balance of newborn
      P74.421 Hyperchloremia of newborn
        Hyperchloremic metabolic acidosis
        EXCLUDES 2 late metabolic acidosis of the newborn (P74.0)
      P74.422 Hypochloremia of newborn
    P74.49 Other transitory electrolyte disturbance of newborn
  P74.5 Transitory tyrosinemia of newborn
  P74.6 Transitory hyperammonemia of newborn
  P74.8 Other transitory metabolic disturbances of newborn
    Amino-acid metabolic disorders described as transitory
  P74.9 Transitory metabolic disturbance of newborn, unspecified

Digestive system disorders of newborn (P76-P78)

✓4th **P76** **Other intestinal obstruction of newborn**
  P76.0 Meconium plug syndrome
    Meconium ileus NOS
    EXCLUDES 1 meconium ileus in cystic fibrosis (E84.11)
    DEF: Meconium obstruction of a newborn's intestines, resulting from unusually thick or hard meconium.
  P76.1 Transitory ileus of newborn
    EXCLUDES 1 Hirschsprung's disease (Q43.1)
  P76.2 Intestinal obstruction due to inspissated milk
  P76.8 Other specified intestinal obstruction of newborn
    EXCLUDES 1 intestinal obstruction classifiable to K56.-
  P76.9 Intestinal obstruction of newborn, unspecified

✓4th **P77** **Necrotizing enterocolitis of newborn**
  DEF: Serious intestinal infection and inflammation in preterm infants. Severity is measured by stages and may progress to life-threatening perforation or peritonitis. Resection surgical treatment may be necessary.
  P77.1 Stage 1 necrotizing enterocolitis in newborn [HCC] [COM]
    Necrotizing enterocolitis without pneumatosis, without perforation
    DEF: Broad-spectrum symptoms with nonspecific signs, including feeding intolerance, abdominal distention, bradycardia, and metabolic abnormalities.

☑ Additional Character Required   ✓x7th Placeholder Alert   Manifestation   Unspecified Dx   0 QPP   UPD Unacceptable PDx

P77.2 Stage 2 necrotizing enterocolitis in newborn [HCC] [COM]
Necrotizing enterocolitis with pneumatosis, without perforation
DEF: Radiographic confirmation of necrotizing enterocolitis showing intestinal dilatation, fixed loops of bowels, pneumatosis intestinalis, metabolic acidosis, and thrombocytopenia.

P77.3 Stage 3 necrotizing enterocolitis in newborn [HCC] [COM]
Necrotizing enterocolitis with perforation
Necrotizing enterocolitis with pneumatosis and perforation
DEF: Advanced stage in which an infant demonstrates signs of bowel perforation, septic shock, metabolic acidosis, ascites, disseminated intravascular coagulopathy, and neutropenia.

P77.9 Necrotizing enterocolitis in newborn, unspecified [HCC] [COM]
Necrotizing enterocolitis in newborn, NOS

P78 Other perinatal digestive system disorders
EXCLUDES 1: cystic fibrosis (E84.0-E84.9)
neonatal gastrointestinal hemorrhages (P54.0-P54.3)

P78.0 Perinatal intestinal perforation [HCC] [COM]
Meconium peritonitis

P78.1 Other neonatal peritonitis
Neonatal peritonitis NOS

P78.2 Neonatal hematemesis and melena due to swallowed maternal blood

P78.3 Noninfective neonatal diarrhea
Neonatal diarrhea NOS

P78.8 Other specified perinatal digestive system disorders

- **P78.81 Congenital cirrhosis (of liver)**
- **P78.82 Peptic ulcer of newborn**
- **P78.83 Newborn esophageal reflux**
  Neonatal esophageal reflux
- **P78.84 Gestational alloimmune liver disease** [COM]
  GALD
  Neonatal hemochromatosis
  EXCLUDES 1: hemochromatosis (E83.11-)
  AHA: 2017,4Q,21
  DEF: Severe hepatic injury with onset during fetal development with manifestations beginning during fetal life. It is due to maternal antibodies to fetal hepatic cells (hepatocytes) that cross the placenta into the fetal circulation, causing hepatic cell necrosis.
- **P78.89 Other specified perinatal digestive system disorders**

P78.9 Perinatal digestive system disorder, unspecified

Conditions involving the integument and temperature regulation of newborn (P80-P83)

P80 Hypothermia of newborn
DEF: Decrease in newborn body temperature due to their larger ratio of surface area to body weight, thin skin with blood vessels close to the surface, and a limited amount of subcutaneous fat.

- **P80.0 Cold injury syndrome**
  Severe and usually chronic hypothermia associated with a pink flushed appearance, edema and neurological and biochemical abnormalities.
  EXCLUDES 1: mild hypothermia of newborn (P80.8)
- **P80.8 Other hypothermia of newborn**
  Mild hypothermia of newborn
- **P80.9 Hypothermia of newborn, unspecified**

P81 Other disturbances of temperature regulation of newborn
- **P81.0 Environmental hyperthermia of newborn**
- **P81.8 Other specified disturbances of temperature regulation of newborn**
- **P81.9 Disturbance of temperature regulation of newborn, unspecified**
  Fever of newborn NOS

P83 Other conditions of integument specific to newborn
EXCLUDES 1: congenital malformations of skin and integument (Q80-Q84)
hydrops fetalis due to hemolytic disease (P56.-)
neonatal skin infection (P39.4)
staphylococcal scalded skin syndrome (L00)
EXCLUDES 2: cradle cap (L21.0)
diaper [napkin] dermatitis (L22)

- **P83.0 Sclerema neonatorum**
  DEF: Diffuse, rapidly progressing white, waxy, nonpitting hardening of tissue, usually of legs and feet that is life-threatening. It is found in preterm or debilitated infants. Etiology is unknown.
- **P83.1 Neonatal erythema toxicum**

P83.2 Hydrops fetalis not due to hemolytic disease
Hydrops fetalis NOS
DEF: Severe, life-threatening problem of a newborn characterized by severe edema of the entire body. It is unrelated to immune response.

P83.3 Other and unspecified edema specific to newborn
- **P83.30 Unspecified edema specific to newborn**
- **P83.39 Other edema specific to newborn**

P83.4 Breast engorgement of newborn
Noninfective mastitis of newborn

P83.5 Congenital hydrocele
DEF: Hydrocele: Serous fluid that collects in the tunica vaginalis of the scrotum along the spermatic cord in males.

P83.6 Umbilical polyp of newborn

P83.8 Other specified conditions of integument specific to newborn
AHA: 2017,4Q,21-22
- **P83.81 Umbilical granuloma**
  EXCLUDES 2: granulomatous disorder of the skin and subcutaneous tissue, unspecified (L92.9)
- **P83.88 Other specified conditions of integument specific to newborn**
  Bronze baby syndrome
  Neonatal scleroderma
  Urticaria neonatorum

P83.9 Condition of the integument specific to newborn, unspecified

Other problems with newborn (P84)

P84 Other problems with newborn
Acidemia of newborn
Acidosis of newborn
Anoxia of newborn NOS
Asphyxia of newborn NOS
Hypercapnia of newborn
Hypoxemia of newborn
Hypoxia of newborn NOS
Mixed metabolic and respiratory acidosis of newborn
EXCLUDES 1: intracranial hemorrhage due to anoxia or hypoxia (P52.-)
hypoxic ischemic encephalopathy [HIE] (P91.6-)
late metabolic acidosis of newborn (P74.0)

Other disorders originating in the perinatal period (P90-P96)

P90 Convulsions of newborn [HCC] [COM]
EXCLUDES 1: benign myoclonic epilepsy in infancy (G40.3-)
benign neonatal convulsions (familial) (G40.3-)

P91 Other disturbances of cerebral status of newborn
- **P91.0 Neonatal cerebral ischemia** [HCC] [COM]
  EXCLUDES 1: neonatal cerebral infarction (P91.82-)
- **P91.1 Acquired periventricular cysts of newborn** [HCC] [COM]
- **P91.2 Neonatal cerebral leukomalacia** [HCC] [COM]
  Periventricular leukomalacia
- **P91.3 Neonatal cerebral irritability** [HCC] [COM]
- **P91.4 Neonatal cerebral depression** [HCC] [COM]
- **P91.5 Neonatal coma** [HCC] [COM]
- **P91.6 Hypoxic ischemic encephalopathy [HIE]**
  EXCLUDES 1: neonatal cerebral depression (P91.4)
  neonatal cerebral irritability (P91.3)
  neonatal coma (P91.5)
  AHA: 2017,4Q,22
  - **P91.60 Hypoxic ischemic encephalopathy [HIE], unspecified** [HCC] [COM]
  - **P91.61 Mild hypoxic ischemic encephalopathy [HIE]** [HCC] [COM]
  - **P91.62 Moderate hypoxic ischemic encephalopathy [HIE]** [HCC] [COM]
  - **P91.63 Severe hypoxic ischemic encephalopathy [HIE]** [HCC] [COM]

Chapter 16. Certain Conditions Originating in the Perinatal Period

P91.8 Other specified disturbances of cerebral status of newborn
  AHA: 2017,4Q,22
- **P91.81** Neonatal encephalopathy
  - **P91.811** Neonatal encephalopathy in diseases classified elsewhere [HCC][COM]
    Code first underlying condition, if known, such as:
    congenital cirrhosis (of liver) (P78.81)
    intracranial nontraumatic hemorrhage of newborn (P52.-)
    kernicterus (P57.-)
  - **P91.819** Neonatal encephalopathy, unspecified [HCC][COM]
- **P91.82** Neonatal cerebral infarction
  Neonatal stroke
  Perinatal arterial ischemic stroke
  Perinatal cerebral infarction
  EXCLUDES 1: cerebral infarction (I63.-)
  EXCLUDES 2: intracranial hemorrhage of newborn (P52.-)
  AHA: 2020,4Q,37-38
  - **P91.821** Neonatal cerebral infarction, right side of brain [HCC][ESR][COM]
  - **P91.822** Neonatal cerebral infarction, left side of brain [HCC][ESR][COM]
  - **P91.823** Neonatal cerebral infarction, bilateral [HCC][ESR][COM]
  - **P91.829** Neonatal cerebral infarction, unspecified side [HCC][ESR][COM]
- **P91.88** Other specified disturbances of cerebral status of newborn [HCC][COM]

P91.9 Disturbance of cerebral status of newborn, unspecified [HCC][COM]

P92 Feeding problems of newborn
  EXCLUDES 1: eating disorders (F50.-)
  EXCLUDES 2: feeding problems in child over 28 days old (R63.3-)
  AHA: 2016,3Q,19
- **P92.0** Vomiting of newborn
  EXCLUDES 1: vomiting of child over 28 days old (R11.-)
  - **P92.01** Bilious vomiting of newborn
    EXCLUDES 1: bilious vomiting in child over 28 days old (R11.14)
  - **P92.09** Other vomiting of newborn
    EXCLUDES 1: regurgitation of food in newborn (P92.1)
- **P92.1** Regurgitation and rumination of newborn
- **P92.2** Slow feeding of newborn
- **P92.3** Underfeeding of newborn
- **P92.4** Overfeeding of newborn
- **P92.5** Neonatal difficulty in feeding at breast
  AHA: 2017,1Q,28
- **P92.6** Failure to thrive in newborn
  EXCLUDES 1: failure to thrive in child over 28 days old (R62.51)
- **P92.8** Other feeding problems of newborn
- **P92.9** Feeding problem of newborn, unspecified

P93 Reactions and intoxications due to drugs administered to newborn
  INCLUDES: reactions and intoxications due to drugs administered to fetus affecting newborn
  EXCLUDES 1: jaundice due to drugs or toxins transmitted from mother or given to newborn (P58.4-)
  reactions and intoxications from maternal opiates, tranquilizers and other medication (P04.0-P04.1, P04.4-)
  withdrawal symptoms from maternal use of drugs of addiction (P96.1)
  withdrawal symptoms from therapeutic use of drugs in newborn (P96.2)
- **P93.0** Grey baby syndrome [HCC][COM]
  Grey syndrome from chloramphenicol administration in newborn
- **P93.8** Other reactions and intoxications due to drugs administered to newborn [HCC][COM]
  Use additional code for adverse effect, if applicable, to identify drug (T36-T50 with fifth or sixth character 5)

P94 Disorders of muscle tone of newborn
- **P94.0** Transient neonatal myasthenia gravis
  EXCLUDES 1: myasthenia gravis (G70.0)
- **P94.1** Congenital hypertonia
- **P94.2** Congenital hypotonia
  Floppy baby syndrome, unspecified
- **P94.8** Other disorders of muscle tone of newborn
- **P94.9** Disorder of muscle tone of newborn, unspecified

P95 Stillbirth
  Deadborn fetus NOS
  Fetal death of unspecified cause
  Stillbirth NOS
  EXCLUDES 1: maternal care for intrauterine death (O36.4)
  missed abortion (O02.1)
  outcome of delivery, stillbirth (Z37.1, Z37.3, Z37.4, Z37.7)

P96 Other conditions originating in the perinatal period
- **P96.0** Congenital renal failure
  Uremia of newborn
- **P96.1** Neonatal withdrawal symptoms from maternal use of drugs of addiction [HCC][COM]
  Drug withdrawal syndrome in infant of dependent mother
  Neonatal abstinence syndrome
  EXCLUDES 1: reactions and intoxications from maternal opiates and tranquilizers administered during labor and delivery (P04.0)
  AHA: 2018,4Q,24-25
- **P96.2** Withdrawal symptoms from therapeutic use of drugs in newborn [HCC][COM]
- **P96.3** Wide cranial sutures of newborn
  Neonatal craniotabes
- **P96.5** Complication to newborn due to (fetal) intrauterine procedure
  EXCLUDES 2: newborn affected by amniocentesis (P00.6)
- **P96.8** Other specified conditions originating in the perinatal period
  - **P96.81** Exposure to (parental) (environmental) tobacco smoke in the perinatal period
    EXCLUDES 2: exposure to environmental tobacco smoke after the perinatal period (Z77.22)
    newborn affected by in utero exposure to tobacco (P04.2)
  - **P96.82** Delayed separation of umbilical cord
  - **P96.83** Meconium staining
    EXCLUDES 1: meconium aspiration (P24.00, P24.01)
    meconium passage during delivery (P03.82)
    DEF: Meconium passed in utero causing discoloration on the fetal skin and nails or on the umbilicus. This staining may be incidental or may be an indicator of significant fetal stress that could affect outcomes.
  - **P96.89** Other specified conditions originating in the perinatal period
    Use additional code to specify condition
    AHA: 2023,3Q,3
- **P96.9** Condition originating in the perinatal period, unspecified
  Congenital debility NOS

Chapter 17. Congenital Malformations, Deformations, and Chromosomal Abnormalities (Q00–QA1)

Chapter-specific Guidelines with Coding Examples

The chapter-specific guidelines from the ICD-10-CM Official Guidelines for Coding and Reporting have been provided below. Along with these guidelines are coding examples, contained in the shaded boxes, that have been developed to help illustrate the coding and/or sequencing guidance found in these guidelines.

Assign an appropriate code(s) from categories Q00-**QA1**, Congenital malformations, deformations, and chromosomal abnormalities when a malformation/deformation or chromosomal abnormality is documented. A malformation/deformation/or chromosomal abnormality may be the principal/first-listed diagnosis on a record or a secondary diagnosis.

When a malformation/deformation/or chromosomal abnormality does not have a unique code assignment, assign additional code(s) for any manifestations that may be present.

When the code assignment specifically identifies the malformation/deformation/or chromosomal abnormality, manifestations that are an inherent component of the anomaly should not be coded separately. Additional codes should be assigned for manifestations that are not an inherent component.

> 8-day-old infant with tetralogy of Fallot and pulmonary stenosis
>
> **Q21.3**   **Tetralogy of Fallot**
>
> *Explanation:* Pulmonary stenosis is inherent in the disease process of tetralogy of Fallot. When the code assignment specifically identifies the malformation/deformation/or chromosomal abnormality, manifestations that are inherent components of the anomaly should not be coded separately.

> 7-month-old infant with Down syndrome and common atrioventricular canal
>
> **Q90.9**   **Down syndrome, unspecified**
>
> **Q21.23**   **Complete atrioventricular septal defect**
>
> *Explanation:* While a common atrioventricular canal is often associated with patients with Down syndrome, this manifestation is not an inherent component and may be reported separately. When the code assignment specifically identifies the anomaly, manifestations that are inherent components of the condition should not be coded separately. Additional codes should be assigned for manifestations that are not inherent components.

Codes from Chapter 17 may be used throughout the life of the patient. If a congenital malformation or deformity has been corrected, a personal history code should be used to identify the history of the malformation or deformity. Although present at birth, a malformation/deformation/or chromosomal abnormality may not be identified until later in life. Whenever the condition is diagnosed by the provider, it is appropriate to assign a code from codes Q00-**QA1**. For the birth admission, the appropriate code from category Z38, Liveborn infants, according to place of birth and type of delivery, should be sequenced as the principal diagnosis, followed by any congenital anomaly codes, Q00-**QA1**.

> Three-year-old with history of corrected ventricular septal defect
>
> **Z87.74**   **Personal history of (corrected) congenital malformations of heart and circulatory system**
>
> *Explanation:* If a congenital malformation or deformity has been corrected, a personal history code should be used to identify the history of the malformation or deformity.

> Forty-year-old man with headaches diagnosed with congenital arteriovenous malformation of cerebral vessels by brain scan
>
> **Q28.2**   **Arteriovenous malformation of cerebral vessels**
>
> *Explanation:* Although present at birth, malformations may not be identified until later in life. Whenever a congenital condition is diagnosed by the physician, it is appropriate to assign a code from this chapter.

Chapter 17. Congenital Malformations, Deformations, Chromosomal Abnormalities, and Genetic Disorders (Q00-QA0)

NOTE Codes from this chapter are not for use on maternal records
EXCLUDES 2 inborn errors of metabolism (E70-E88)

This chapter contains the following blocks:
- Q00-Q07 Congenital malformations of the nervous system
- Q10-Q18 Congenital malformations of eye, ear, face and neck
- Q20-Q28 Congenital malformations of the circulatory system
- Q30-Q34 Congenital malformations of the respiratory system
- Q35-Q37 Cleft lip and cleft palate
- Q38-Q45 Other congenital malformations of the digestive system
- Q50-Q56 Congenital malformations of genital organs
- Q60-Q64 Congenital malformations of the urinary system
- Q65-Q79 Congenital malformations and deformations of the musculoskeletal system
- Q80-Q89 Other congenital malformations
- Q90-Q99 Chromosomal abnormalities, not elsewhere classified
- QA0 ▶Genetic disorders, not elsewhere classified◀

Congenital malformations of the nervous system (Q00-Q07)

Q00 Anencephaly and similar malformations

Q00.0 Anencephaly
- Acephaly
- Acrania
- Amyelencephaly
- Hemianencephaly
- Hemicephaly

Q00.1 Craniorachischisis

Q00.2 Iniencephaly

Q01 Encephalocele

INCLUDES
- Arnold-Chiari syndrome, type III
- encephalocystocele
- encephalomyelocele
- hydroencephalocele
- hydromeningocele, cranial
- meningocele, cerebral
- meningoencephalocele

EXCLUDES 1 Meckel-Gruber syndrome (Q61.9)

DEF: Congenital protrusion of brain tissue through a defect in the skull.

- **Q01.0 Frontal encephalocele**
- **Q01.1 Nasofrontal encephalocele**
- **Q01.2 Occipital encephalocele**
- **Q01.8 Encephalocele of other sites**
- **Q01.9 Encephalocele, unspecified**

Q02 Microcephaly

INCLUDES
- hydromicrocephaly
- micrencephalon

Code first, if applicable, congenital Zika virus disease
EXCLUDES 1 Meckel-Gruber syndrome (Q61.9)
AHA: 2018,4Q,26
DEF: Congenital disorder in which the head circumference is more than two standard deviations below the mean for age, sex, race, and gestation and associated with a decreased life expectancy.

Q03 Congenital hydrocephalus

INCLUDES hydrocephalus in newborn
EXCLUDES 1
- acquired hydrocephalus (G91.-)
- Arnold-Chiari syndrome, type II (Q07.0-)
- hydrocephalus due to congenital toxoplasmosis (P37.1)
- hydrocephalus with spina bifida (Q05.0-Q05.4)

DEF: Hydrocephalus: Abnormal buildup of cerebrospinal fluid in the brain causing dilation of the ventricles.

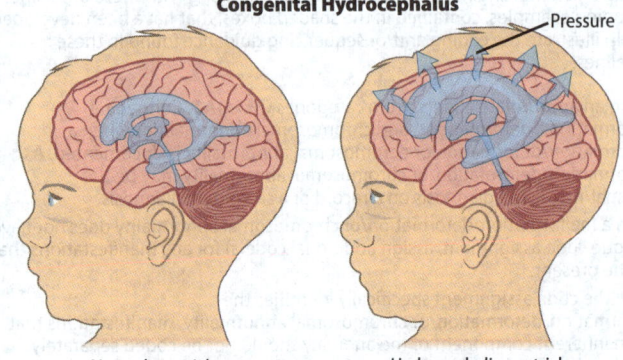

Congenital Hydrocephalus
Normal ventricles — Hydrocephalic ventricles — Pressure

Q03.0 Malformations of aqueduct of Sylvius
- Anomaly of aqueduct of Sylvius
- Obstruction of aqueduct of Sylvius, congenital
- Stenosis of aqueduct of Sylvius

Q03.1 Atresia of foramina of Magendie and Luschka
- Dandy-Walker syndrome

Q03.8 Other congenital hydrocephalus

Q03.9 Congenital hydrocephalus, unspecified

Q04 Other congenital malformations of brain

EXCLUDES 1
- cyclopia (Q87.0)
- macrocephaly (Q75.3)

Q04.0 Congenital malformations of corpus callosum
- Agenesis of corpus callosum

Q04.1 Arhinencephaly

Q04.2 Holoprosencephaly

Q04.3 Other reduction deformities of brain
- Absence of part of brain
- Agenesis of part of brain
- Agyria
- Aplasia of part of brain
- Hydranencephaly
- Hypoplasia of part of brain
- Lissencephaly
- Microgyria
- Pachygyria

EXCLUDES 1 congenital malformations of corpus callosum (Q04.0)

Q04.4 Septo-optic dysplasia of brain

Q04.5 Megalencephaly

Q04.6 Congenital cerebral cysts
- Porencephaly
- Schizencephaly

EXCLUDES 1 acquired porencephalic cyst (G93.0)

Q04.8 Other specified congenital malformations of brain
- Arnold-Chiari syndrome, type IV
- Macrogyria

Q04.9 Congenital malformation of brain, unspecified
- Congenital anomaly NOS of brain
- Congenital deformity NOS of brain
- Congenital disease or lesion NOS of brain
- Multiple anomalies NOS of brain, congenital

Chapter 17. Congenital Malformations, Deformations and Chromosomal Abnormalities

Q05 Spina bifida

INCLUDES
- hydromeningocele (spinal)
- meningocele (spinal)
- meningomyelocele
- myelocele
- myelomeningocele
- rachischisis
- spina bifida (aperta)(cystica)
- syringomyelocele

Use additional code for any associated paraplegia (paraparesis) (G82.2-)

EXCLUDES 1
- Arnold-Chiari syndrome, type II (Q07.0-)
- spina bifida occulta (Q76.0)

DEF: Lack of closure in the vertebral column with protrusion of the spinal cord through the defect, often in the lumbosacral area. This condition can be recognized by the presence of alpha-fetoproteins in the amniotic fluid.

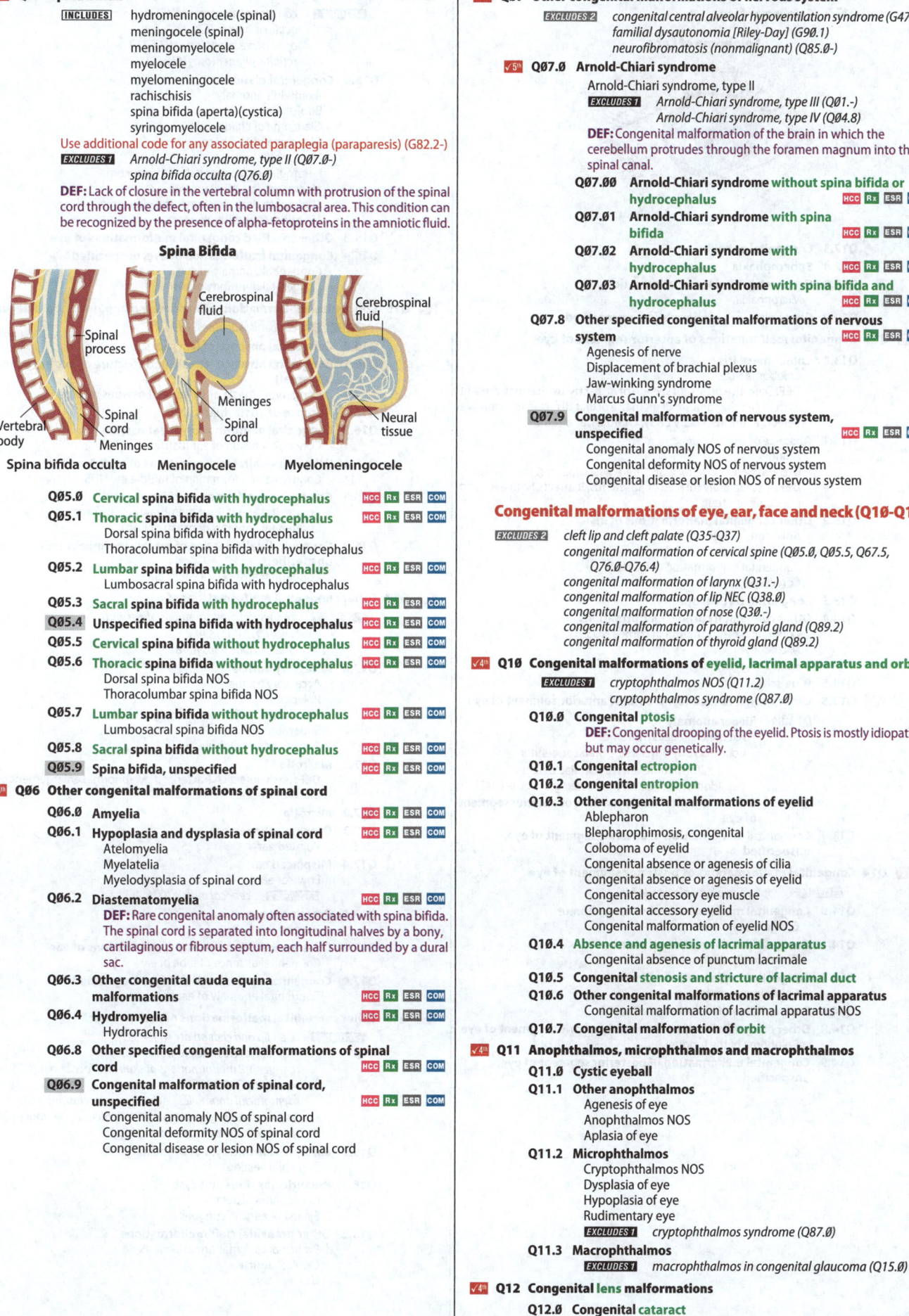

Spina Bifida — Spina bifida occulta, Meningocele, Myelomeningocele

- **Q05.0** Cervical spina bifida with hydrocephalus
- **Q05.1** Thoracic spina bifida with hydrocephalus
  - Dorsal spina bifida with hydrocephalus
  - Thoracolumbar spina bifida with hydrocephalus
- **Q05.2** Lumbar spina bifida with hydrocephalus
  - Lumbosacral spina bifida with hydrocephalus
- **Q05.3** Sacral spina bifida with hydrocephalus
- **Q05.4** Unspecified spina bifida with hydrocephalus
- **Q05.5** Cervical spina bifida without hydrocephalus
- **Q05.6** Thoracic spina bifida without hydrocephalus
  - Dorsal spina bifida NOS
  - Thoracolumbar spina bifida NOS
- **Q05.7** Lumbar spina bifida without hydrocephalus
  - Lumbosacral spina bifida NOS
- **Q05.8** Sacral spina bifida without hydrocephalus
- **Q05.9** Spina bifida, unspecified

Q06 Other congenital malformations of spinal cord

- **Q06.0** Amyelia
- **Q06.1** Hypoplasia and dysplasia of spinal cord
  - Atelomyelia
  - Myelatelia
  - Myelodysplasia of spinal cord
- **Q06.2** Diastematomyelia
  - **DEF:** Rare congenital anomaly often associated with spina bifida. The spinal cord is separated into longitudinal halves by a bony, cartilaginous or fibrous septum, each half surrounded by a dural sac.
- **Q06.3** Other congenital cauda equina malformations
- **Q06.4** Hydromyelia
  - Hydrorachis
- **Q06.8** Other specified congenital malformations of spinal cord
- **Q06.9** Congenital malformation of spinal cord, unspecified
  - Congenital anomaly NOS of spinal cord
  - Congenital deformity NOS of spinal cord
  - Congenital disease or lesion NOS of spinal cord

Q07 Other congenital malformations of nervous system

EXCLUDES 2
- congenital central alveolar hypoventilation syndrome (G47.35)
- familial dysautonomia [Riley-Day] (G90.1)
- neurofibromatosis (nonmalignant) (Q85.0-)

Q07.0 Arnold-Chiari syndrome
Arnold-Chiari syndrome, type II

EXCLUDES 1
- Arnold-Chiari syndrome, type III (Q01.-)
- Arnold-Chiari syndrome, type IV (Q04.8)

DEF: Congenital malformation of the brain in which the cerebellum protrudes through the foramen magnum into the spinal canal.

- **Q07.00** Arnold-Chiari syndrome without spina bifida or hydrocephalus
- **Q07.01** Arnold-Chiari syndrome with spina bifida
- **Q07.02** Arnold-Chiari syndrome with hydrocephalus
- **Q07.03** Arnold-Chiari syndrome with spina bifida and hydrocephalus

- **Q07.8** Other specified congenital malformations of nervous system
  - Agenesis of nerve
  - Displacement of brachial plexus
  - Jaw-winking syndrome
  - Marcus Gunn's syndrome
- **Q07.9** Congenital malformation of nervous system, unspecified
  - Congenital anomaly NOS of nervous system
  - Congenital deformity NOS of nervous system
  - Congenital disease or lesion NOS of nervous system

Congenital malformations of eye, ear, face and neck (Q10-Q18)

EXCLUDES 2
- cleft lip and cleft palate (Q35-Q37)
- congenital malformation of cervical spine (Q05.0, Q05.5, Q67.5, Q76.0-Q76.4)
- congenital malformation of larynx (Q31.-)
- congenital malformation of lip NEC (Q38.0)
- congenital malformation of nose (Q30.-)
- congenital malformation of parathyroid gland (Q89.2)
- congenital malformation of thyroid gland (Q89.2)

Q10 Congenital malformations of eyelid, lacrimal apparatus and orbit

EXCLUDES 1
- cryptophthalmos NOS (Q11.2)
- cryptophthalmos syndrome (Q87.0)

- **Q10.0** Congenital ptosis
  - **DEF:** Congenital drooping of the eyelid. Ptosis is mostly idiopathic, but may occur genetically.
- **Q10.1** Congenital ectropion
- **Q10.2** Congenital entropion
- **Q10.3** Other congenital malformations of eyelid
  - Ablepharon
  - Blepharophimosis, congenital
  - Coloboma of eyelid
  - Congenital absence or agenesis of cilia
  - Congenital absence or agenesis of eyelid
  - Congenital accessory eye muscle
  - Congenital accessory eyelid
  - Congenital malformation of eyelid NOS
- **Q10.4** Absence and agenesis of lacrimal apparatus
  - Congenital absence of punctum lacrimale
- **Q10.5** Congenital stenosis and stricture of lacrimal duct
- **Q10.6** Other congenital malformations of lacrimal apparatus
  - Congenital malformation of lacrimal apparatus NOS
- **Q10.7** Congenital malformation of orbit

Q11 Anophthalmos, microphthalmos and macrophthalmos

- **Q11.0** Cystic eyeball
- **Q11.1** Other anophthalmos
  - Agenesis of eye
  - Anophthalmos NOS
  - Aplasia of eye
- **Q11.2** Microphthalmos
  - Cryptophthalmos NOS
  - Dysplasia of eye
  - Hypoplasia of eye
  - Rudimentary eye
  - **EXCLUDES 1** cryptophthalmos syndrome (Q87.0)
- **Q11.3** Macrophthalmos
  - **EXCLUDES 1** macrophthalmos in congenital glaucoma (Q15.0)

Q12 Congenital lens malformations

- **Q12.0** Congenital cataract

Q12.1 Congenital displaced lens
Q12.2 Coloboma of lens

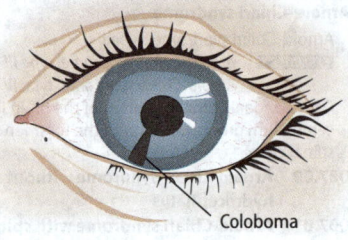
Coloboma of Lens

Q12.3 Congenital aphakia
Q12.4 Spherophakia
Q12.8 Other congenital lens malformations
　　　　Microphakia
Q12.9 Congenital lens malformation, unspecified

✓4th **Q13** Congenital malformations of anterior segment of eye
　Q13.0 Coloboma of iris
　　　Coloboma NOS
　　　DEF: Defective or absent section of ocular tissue that may present as mild cupping or a small pit in the ocular disc due to extensive defects in the iris, ciliary body, choroids, and retina.
　Q13.1 Absence of iris
　　　Aniridia
　　　Use additional code for associated glaucoma (H42)
　　　DEF: Incompletely formed or absent iris. It affects both eyes and is a dominant trait.
　Q13.2 Other congenital malformations of iris
　　　Anisocoria, congenital
　　　Atresia of pupil
　　　Congenital malformation of iris NOS
　　　Corectopia
　Q13.3 Congenital corneal opacity
　Q13.4 Other congenital corneal malformations
　　　Congenital malformation of cornea NOS
　　　Microcornea
　　　Peter's anomaly
　Q13.5 Blue sclera
　✓5th **Q13.8** Other congenital malformations of anterior segment of eye
　　　Q13.81 Rieger anomaly
　　　　　Axenfeld-Rieger syndrome
　　　　　Code also any other associated congenital malformations such as cardiac defects
　　　　　Use additional code for associated glaucoma (H42)
　　　Q13.89 Other congenital malformations of anterior segment of eye
　Q13.9 Congenital malformation of anterior segment of eye, unspecified

✓4th **Q14** Congenital malformations of posterior segment of eye
　EXCLUDES 2　optic nerve hypoplasia (H47.03-)
　Q14.0 Congenital malformation of vitreous humor
　　　Congenital vitreous opacity
　Q14.1 Congenital malformation of retina
　　　Congenital retinal aneurysm
　Q14.2 Congenital malformation of optic disc
　　　Coloboma of optic disc
　Q14.3 Congenital malformation of choroid
　Q14.8 Other congenital malformations of posterior segment of eye
　　　Coloboma of the fundus
　Q14.9 Congenital malformation of posterior segment of eye, unspecified

✓4th **Q15** Other congenital malformations of eye
　EXCLUDES 1　congenital nystagmus (H55.01)
　　　　　ocular albinism (E70.31-)
　　　　　optic nerve hypoplasia (H47.03-)
　　　　　retinitis pigmentosa (H35.52)
　Q15.0 Congenital glaucoma
　　　Axenfeld's anomaly
　　　Buphthalmos
　　　Glaucoma of childhood
　　　Glaucoma of newborn
　　　Hydrophthalmos
　　　Keratoglobus, congenital, with glaucoma
　　　Macrocornea with glaucoma
　　　Macrophthalmos in congenital glaucoma
　　　Megalocornea with glaucoma
　Q15.8 Other specified congenital malformations of eye
　Q15.9 Congenital malformation of eye, unspecified
　　　Congenital anomaly of eye
　　　Congenital deformity of eye

✓4th **Q16** Congenital malformations of ear causing impairment of hearing
　EXCLUDES 1　congenital deafness (H90.-)
　Q16.0 Congenital absence of (ear) auricle
　Q16.1 Congenital absence, atresia and stricture of auditory canal (external)
　　　Congenital atresia or stricture of osseous meatus
　Q16.2 Absence of eustachian tube
　Q16.3 Congenital malformation of ear ossicles
　　　Congenital fusion of ear ossicles
　Q16.4 Other congenital malformations of middle ear
　　　Congenital malformation of middle ear NOS
　Q16.5 Congenital malformation of inner ear
　　　Congenital anomaly of membranous labyrinth
　　　Congenital anomaly of organ of Corti
　Q16.9 Congenital malformation of ear causing impairment of hearing, unspecified
　　　Congenital absence of ear NOS

✓4th **Q17** Other congenital malformations of ear
　EXCLUDES 1　congenital malformations of ear with impairment of hearing (Q16.0-Q16.9)
　　　　　preauricular sinus (Q18.1)
　Q17.0 Accessory auricle
　　　Accessory tragus
　　　Polyotia
　　　Preauricular appendage or tag
　　　Supernumerary ear
　　　Supernumerary lobule
　Q17.1 Macrotia
　　　DEF: Birth defect characterized by abnormal enlargement of the pinna of the ear.
　Q17.2 Microtia
　Q17.3 Other misshapen ear
　　　Pointed ear
　Q17.4 Misplaced ear
　　　Low-set ears
　　　EXCLUDES 1　cervical auricle (Q18.2)
　Q17.5 Prominent ear
　　　Bat ear
　Q17.8 Other specified congenital malformations of ear
　　　Congenital absence of lobe of ear
　Q17.9 Congenital malformation of ear, unspecified
　　　Congenital anomaly of ear NOS

✓4th **Q18** Other congenital malformations of face and neck
　EXCLUDES 1　cleft lip and cleft palate (Q35-Q37)
　　　　　conditions classified to Q67.0-Q67.4
　　　　　congenital malformations of skull and face bones (Q75.-)
　　　　　cyclopia (Q87.0)
　　　　　dentofacial anomalies [including malocclusion] (M26.-)
　　　　　malformation syndromes affecting facial appearance (Q87.0)
　　　　　persistent thyroglossal duct (Q89.2)
　Q18.0 Sinus, fistula and cyst of branchial cleft
　　　Branchial vestige
　Q18.1 Preauricular sinus and cyst
　　　Cervicoaural fistula
　　　Fistula of auricle, congenital
　Q18.2 Other branchial cleft malformations
　　　Branchial cleft malformation NOS
　　　Cervical auricle
　　　Otocephaly

Chapter 17. Congenital Malformations, Deformations and Chromosomal Abnormalities

Q18.3 **Webbing of neck**
Pterygium colli
DEF: Congenital malformation characterized by a thick, triangular skinfold that stretches from the lateral side of the neck across the shoulder. It is associated with genetic conditions such as Turner's and Noonan's syndromes.

Q18.4 **Macrostomia**
DEF: Rare congenital craniofacial bilateral or unilateral anomaly of the mouth due to malformed maxillary and mandibular processes. It results in an abnormally large mouth extending toward the ear.

Q18.5 **Microstomia**

Q18.6 **Macrocheilia**
Hypertrophy of lip, congenital

Q18.7 **Microcheilia**

Q18.8 **Other specified congenital malformations of face and neck**
Medial cyst of face and neck
Medial fistula of face and neck
Medial sinus of face and neck

Q18.9 **Congenital malformation of face and neck, unspecified**
Congenital anomaly NOS of face and neck

Congenital malformations of the circulatory system (Q20-Q28)

Q20 **Congenital malformations of cardiac chambers and connections**
EXCLUDES 1 dextrocardia with situs inversus (Q89.3)
mirror-image atrial arrangement with situs inversus (Q89.3)

Q20.0 **Common arterial trunk**
Persistent truncus arteriosus
EXCLUDES 1 aortic septal defect (Q21.4)

Q20.1 **Double outlet right ventricle**
Taussig-Bing syndrome

Q20.2 **Double outlet left ventricle**

Q20.3 **Discordant ventriculoarterial connection**
Dextrotransposition of aorta
Transposition of great vessels (complete)

Q20.4 **Double inlet ventricle**
Common ventricle
Cor triloculare biatriatum
Single ventricle

Q20.5 **Discordant atrioventricular connection**
Corrected transposition
Levotransposition
Ventricular inversion

Q20.6 **Isomerism of atrial appendages**
Isomerism of atrial appendages with asplenia or polysplenia

Q20.8 **Other congenital malformations of cardiac chambers and connections**
Cor binoculare

Q20.9 **Congenital malformation of cardiac chambers and connections, unspecified**

Q21 **Congenital malformations of cardiac septa**
EXCLUDES 1 acquired cardiac septal defect (I51.0)

Q21.0 **Ventricular septal defect**
Roger's disease

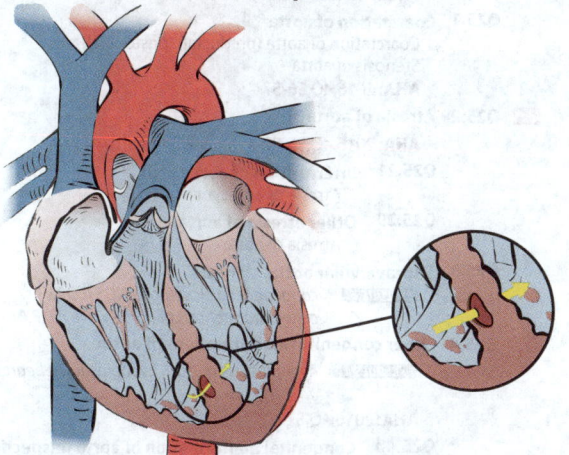
Ventricular Septal Defect

Q21.1 **Atrial septal defect**
EXCLUDES 2 ostium primum atrial septal defect (type I) (Q21.20)
AHA: 2022,4Q,39-40

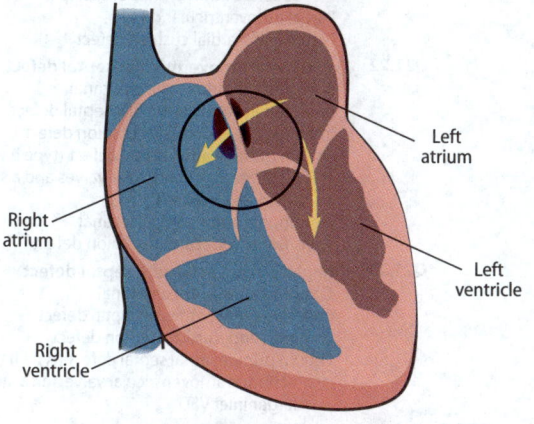
Atrial Septal Defect

Q21.10 Atrial septal defect, unspecified

Q21.11 **Secundum** atrial septal defect
Fenestrated atrial septum
Patent or persistent ostium secundum defect (type II)

Q21.12 **Patent foramen ovale**
Persistent foramen ovale

Q21.13 **Coronary sinus** atrial septal defect
Coronary sinus defect
Unroofed coronary sinus

Q21.14 **Superior sinus venosus** atrial septal defect
Superior vena cava type atrial septal defect

Q21.15 **Inferior sinus venosus** atrial septal defect
Inferior vena cava type atrial septal defect

Q21.16 Sinus venosus atrial septal defect, unspecified
Sinus venosus defect, NOS

Q21.19 Other specified atrial septal defect
Common atrium
Other specified atrial septal abnormality

Q21.2 **Atrioventricular septal defect**
Atrioventricular canal defect
Endocardial cushion defect
Ostium primum atrial septal defect (type I)
AHA: 2022,4Q,39-40

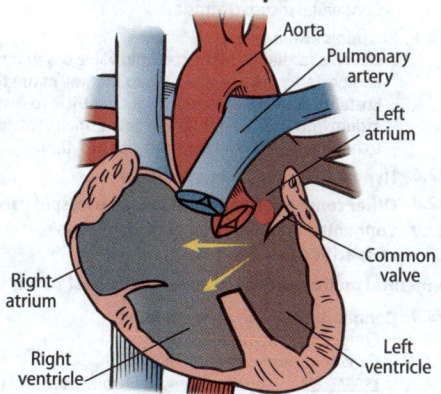
Atrioventricular Septal Defect

Q21.20 **Atrioventricular septal defect, unspecified as to partial or complete**
Atrioventricular canal, NOS
Endocardial cushion defect NOS
Ostium primum atrial septal defect (type I) NOS

Q21.21 Partial atrioventricular septal defect
Incomplete atrioventricular canal
Incomplete atrioventricular septal defect
Incomplete endocardial cushion defect
Ostium primum atrial septal defect (type I) with separate atrioventricular valves
Partial atrioventricular canal
Partial endocardial cushion defect

Q21.22 Transitional atrioventricular septal defect
Intermediate atrioventricular canal
Intermediate atrioventricular septal defect
Intermediate endocardial cushion defect
Ostium primum atrial septal defect (type I) with separate atrioventricular valves and a small or restrictive inlet VSD
Transitional atrioventricular canal
Transitional endocardial cushion defect

Q21.23 Complete atrioventricular septal defect
Common atrioventricular canal
Common atrioventricular septal defect
Common endocardial cushion defect
Ostium primum atrial septal defect (type I) with common atrioventricular valve and a moderate or larger inlet VSD

Q21.3 Tetralogy of Fallot
Ventricular septal defect with pulmonary stenosis or atresia, dextroposition of aorta and hypertrophy of right ventricle.
AHA: 2014,3Q,16

Q21.4 Aortopulmonary septal defect
Aortic septal defect
Aortopulmonary window

Q21.8 Other congenital malformations of cardiac septa
Eisenmenger's defect
Pentalogy of Fallot
Code also, if applicable:
  Eisenmenger's complex (I27.83)
  Eisenmenger's syndrome (I27.83)

Q21.9 Congenital malformation of cardiac septum, unspecified
Septal (heart) defect NOS

Q22 Congenital malformations of pulmonary and tricuspid valves

Q22.0 Pulmonary valve atresia
Q22.1 Congenital pulmonary valve stenosis
Q22.2 Congenital pulmonary valve insufficiency
Congenital pulmonary valve regurgitation
AHA: 2022,4Q,39-40

Q22.3 Other congenital malformations of pulmonary valve
Congenital malformation of pulmonary valve NOS
Supernumerary cusps of pulmonary valve

Q22.4 Congenital tricuspid stenosis
Congenital tricuspid atresia

Q22.5 Ebstein's anomaly
DEF: Malformation of the tricuspid valve characterized by septal and posterior leaflets attaching to the wall of the right ventricle. Ebstein's anomaly causes the right ventricle to fuse with the atrium into a large right atrium and a small ventricle and leads to heart failure and abnormal cardiac rhythm.

Q22.6 Hypoplastic right heart syndrome
Q22.8 Other congenital malformations of tricuspid valve
Q22.9 Congenital malformation of tricuspid valve, unspecified

Q23 Congenital malformations of aortic and mitral valves

Q23.0 Congenital stenosis of aortic valve
Congenital aortic atresia
Congenital aortic stenosis NOS
EXCLUDES 1: congenital stenosis of aortic valve in hypoplastic left heart syndrome (Q23.4)
congenital subaortic stenosis (Q24.4)
supravalvular aortic stenosis (congenital) (Q25.3)

Q23.1 Congenital insufficiency of aortic valve
Congenital aortic insufficiency

Q23.2 Congenital mitral stenosis
Congenital mitral atresia

Q23.3 Congenital mitral insufficiency
Q23.4 Hypoplastic left heart syndrome

Q23.8 Other congenital malformations of aortic and mitral valves
AHA: 2024,4Q,26

Q23.81 Bicuspid aortic valve
Congenital bicuspid aortic valve
Unicuspid (congenital) aortic valve (at birth)
Code also, if applicable, acquired aortic valve disorders, such as:
  aortic (valve) insufficiency (nonrheumatic) (I35.1)
  aortic (valve) stenosis (nonrheumatic) (I35.0)
  aortic (valve) stenosis with insufficiency (nonrheumatic) (I35.2)

Q23.82 Congenital mitral valve cleft leaflet
Cleft mitral valve leaflet at birth

Q23.88 Other congenital malformations of aortic and mitral valves

Q23.9 Congenital malformation of aortic and mitral valves, unspecified

Q24 Other congenital malformations of heart
EXCLUDES 1: endocardial fibroelastosis (I42.4)

Q24.0 Dextrocardia
EXCLUDES 1: dextrocardia with situs inversus (Q89.3)
isomerism of atrial appendages (with asplenia or polysplenia) (Q20.6)
mirror-image atrial arrangement with situs inversus (Q89.3)
DEF: Congenital condition in which the heart is located on the right side of the chest rather than in its normal position on the left.

Q24.1 Levocardia
Q24.2 Cor triatriatum
Q24.3 Pulmonary infundibular stenosis
Subvalvular pulmonic stenosis

Q24.4 Congenital subaortic stenosis
DEF: Congenital heart defect characterized by stenosis of the left ventricular outflow tract due to a fibrous tissue ring or septal hypertrophy below the aortic valve.

Q24.5 Malformation of coronary vessels
Congenital coronary (artery) aneurysm

Q24.6 Congenital heart block
Q24.8 Other specified congenital malformations of heart
Congenital diverticulum of left ventricle
Congenital malformation of myocardium
Congenital malformation of pericardium
Malposition of heart
Uhl's disease

Q24.9 Congenital malformation of heart, unspecified
Congenital anomaly of heart
Congenital disease of heart

Q25 Congenital malformations of great arteries

Q25.0 Patent ductus arteriosus
Patent ductus Botallo
Persistent ductus arteriosus
DEF: Condition in which the normal channel between the pulmonary artery and the aorta fails to close at birth, causing arterial blood to recirculate in the lungs and inhibiting the blood supply to the aorta. **Synonym(s):** PDA.

Q25.1 Coarctation of aorta
Coarctation of aorta (preductal) (postductal)
Stenosis of aorta
AHA: 2016,4Q,56-57

Q25.2 Atresia of aorta
AHA: 2016,4Q,56-57

Q25.21 Interruption of aortic arch
Atresia of aortic arch

Q25.29 Other atresia of aorta
Atresia of aorta

Q25.3 Supravalvular aortic stenosis
EXCLUDES 1: congenital aortic stenosis NOS (Q23.0)
congenital stenosis of aortic valve (Q23.0)

Q25.4 Other congenital malformations of aorta
EXCLUDES 1: hypoplasia of aorta in hypoplastic left heart syndrome (Q23.4)
AHA: 2016,4Q,57

Q25.40 Congenital malformation of aorta unspecified
Q25.41 Absence and aplasia of aorta
Q25.42 Hypoplasia of aorta

Chapter 17. Congenital Malformations, Deformations and Chromosomal Abnormalities

Q25.43 Congenital aneurysm of aorta
  Congenital aneurysm of aortic root
  Congenital aneurysm of aortic sinus
Q25.44 Congenital dilation of aorta
Q25.45 Double aortic arch
  Vascular ring of aorta

Aortic Arch Anomalies

Normal aortic arch — Esophagus, Trachea, Aortic arch

Double aortic arch   Right aortic arch

Q25.46 Tortuous aortic arch
  Persistent convolutions of aortic arch
Q25.47 Right aortic arch
  Persistent right aortic arch
Q25.48 Anomalous origin of subclavian artery
Q25.49 Other congenital malformations of aorta
  Aortic arch
  Bovine arch
Q25.5 Atresia of pulmonary artery
Q25.6 Stenosis of pulmonary artery
  Supravalvular pulmonary stenosis
Q25.7 Other congenital malformations of pulmonary artery
  Q25.71 Coarctation of pulmonary artery
  Q25.72 Congenital pulmonary arteriovenous malformation
    Congenital pulmonary arteriovenous aneurysm
  Q25.79 Other congenital malformations of pulmonary artery
    Aberrant pulmonary artery
    Agenesis of pulmonary artery
    Congenital aneurysm of pulmonary artery
    Congenital anomaly of pulmonary artery
    Hypoplasia of pulmonary artery
Q25.8 Other congenital malformations of other great arteries
Q25.9 Congenital malformation of great arteries, unspecified

Q26 Congenital malformations of great veins
Q26.0 Congenital stenosis of vena cava
  Congenital stenosis of vena cava (inferior)(superior)
Q26.1 Persistent left superior vena cava
Q26.2 Total anomalous pulmonary venous connection
  Total anomalous pulmonary venous return [TAPVR], subdiaphragmatic
  Total anomalous pulmonary venous return [TAPVR], supradiaphragmatic
Q26.3 Partial anomalous pulmonary venous connection
  Partial anomalous pulmonary venous return
Q26.4 Anomalous pulmonary venous connection, unspecified
Q26.5 Anomalous portal venous connection
Q26.6 Portal vein-hepatic artery fistula

Q26.8 Other congenital malformations of great veins
  Absence of vena cava (inferior) (superior)
  Azygos continuation of inferior vena cava
  Persistent left posterior cardinal vein
  Scimitar syndrome
Q26.9 Congenital malformation of great vein, unspecified
  Congenital anomaly of vena cava (inferior) (superior) NOS

Q27 Other congenital malformations of peripheral vascular system
  EXCLUDES 2 anomalies of cerebral and precerebral vessels (Q28.0-Q28.3)
              anomalies of coronary vessels (Q24.5)
              anomalies of pulmonary artery (Q25.5-Q25.7)
              congenital retinal aneurysm (Q14.1)
              hemangioma and lymphangioma (D18.-)
Q27.0 Congenital absence and hypoplasia of umbilical artery
  Single umbilical artery
Q27.1 Congenital renal artery stenosis
Q27.2 Other congenital malformations of renal artery
  Congenital malformation of renal artery NOS
  Multiple renal arteries
Q27.3 Arteriovenous malformation (peripheral)
  Arteriovenous aneurysm
  EXCLUDES 1 acquired arteriovenous aneurysm (I77.0)
  EXCLUDES 2 arteriovenous malformation of cerebral vessels (Q28.2)
              arteriovenous malformation of precerebral vessels (Q28.0)
  DEF: Arteriovenous malformation: Connecting passage between an artery and a vein.
  Q27.30 Arteriovenous malformation, site unspecified
  Q27.31 Arteriovenous malformation of vessel of upper limb
  Q27.32 Arteriovenous malformation of vessel of lower limb
  Q27.33 Arteriovenous malformation of digestive system vessel
    AHA: 2018,3Q,21
  Q27.34 Arteriovenous malformation of renal vessel
  Q27.39 Arteriovenous malformation, other site
Q27.4 Congenital phlebectasia
Q27.8 Other specified congenital malformations of peripheral vascular system
  Absence of peripheral vascular system
  Atresia of peripheral vascular system
  Congenital aneurysm (peripheral)
  Congenital stricture, artery
  Congenital varix
  EXCLUDES 1 arteriovenous malformation (Q27.3-)
Q27.9 Congenital malformation of peripheral vascular system, unspecified
  Anomaly of artery or vein NOS

Q28 Other congenital malformations of circulatory system
  EXCLUDES 1 congenital aneurysm NOS (Q27.8)
              congenital coronary aneurysm (Q24.5)
              ruptured cerebral arteriovenous malformation (I60.8)
              ruptured malformation of precerebral vessels (I72.0)
  EXCLUDES 2 congenital peripheral aneurysm (Q27.8)
              congenital pulmonary aneurysm (Q25.79)
              congenital retinal aneurysm (Q14.1)
Q28.0 Arteriovenous malformation of precerebral vessels
  Congenital arteriovenous precerebral aneurysm (nonruptured)
Q28.1 Other malformations of precerebral vessels
  Congenital malformation of precerebral vessels NOS
  Congenital precerebral aneurysm (nonruptured)
Q28.2 Arteriovenous malformation of cerebral vessels
  Arteriovenous malformation of brain NOS
  Congenital arteriovenous cerebral aneurysm (nonruptured)
Q28.3 Other malformations of cerebral vessels
  Congenital cerebral aneurysm (nonruptured)
  Congenital malformation of cerebral vessels NOS
  Developmental venous anomaly
Q28.8 Other specified congenital malformations of circulatory system
  Congenital aneurysm, specified site NEC
  Spinal vessel anomaly
  EXCLUDES 2 ▶disorders of pyrophosphate metabolism (E83.82-)◀
Q28.9 Congenital malformation of circulatory system, unspecified

Congenital malformations of the respiratory system (Q30-Q34)

✓4ᵗʰ Q30 Congenital malformations of nose
  EXCLUDES 1 congenital deviation of nasal septum (Q67.4)
- Q30.0 Choanal atresia
  - Atresia of nares (anterior) (posterior)
  - Congenital stenosis of nares (anterior) (posterior)
- Q30.1 Agenesis and underdevelopment of nose
  - Congenital absent of nose
- Q30.2 Fissured, notched and cleft nose
- Q30.3 Congenital perforated nasal septum
- Q30.8 Other congenital malformations of nose
  - Accessory nose
  - Congenital anomaly of nasal sinus wall
  - AHA: 2022,2Q,17
- Q30.9 Congenital malformation of nose, unspecified

✓4ᵗʰ Q31 Congenital malformations of larynx
  EXCLUDES 1 congenital laryngeal stridor NOS (P28.89)
- Q31.0 Web of larynx
  - Glottic web of larynx
  - Subglottic web of larynx
  - Web of larynx NOS
  - **DEF:** Congenital malformation of the larynx marked by thin, translucent, or thick fibrotic membrane-like structure between the vocal folds. It is characterized by shortness of breath and stridor.
- Q31.1 Congenital subglottic stenosis
- Q31.2 Laryngeal hypoplasia
- Q31.3 Laryngocele
- Q31.5 Congenital laryngomalacia
- Q31.8 Other congenital malformations of larynx
  - Absence of larynx
  - Agenesis of larynx
  - Atresia of larynx
  - Congenital cleft thyroid cartilage
  - Congenital fissure of epiglottis
  - Congenital stenosis of larynx NEC
  - Posterior cleft of cricoid cartilage
- Q31.9 Congenital malformation of larynx, unspecified

✓4ᵗʰ Q32 Congenital malformations of trachea and bronchus
  EXCLUDES 1 congenital bronchiectasis (Q33.4)
- Q32.0 Congenital tracheomalacia
- Q32.1 Other congenital malformations of trachea
  - Atresia of trachea
  - Congenital anomaly of tracheal cartilage
  - Congenital dilatation of trachea
  - Congenital malformation of trachea
  - Congenital stenosis of trachea
  - Congenital tracheocele
- Q32.2 Congenital bronchomalacia
- Q32.3 Congenital stenosis of bronchus
- Q32.4 Other congenital malformations of bronchus
  - Absence of bronchus
  - Agenesis of bronchus
  - Atresia of bronchus
  - Congenital diverticulum of bronchus
  - Congenital malformation of bronchus NOS

✓4ᵗʰ Q33 Congenital malformations of lung
- Q33.0 Congenital cystic lung
  - Congenital cystic lung disease
  - Congenital honeycomb lung
  - Congenital polycystic lung disease
  - EXCLUDES 1 cystic fibrosis (E84.0)
    cystic lung disease, acquired or unspecified (J98.4)
- Q33.1 Accessory lobe of lung
  - Azygos lobe (fissured), lung
- Q33.2 Sequestration of lung
- Q33.3 Agenesis of lung
  - Congenital absence of lung (lobe)
- Q33.4 Congenital bronchiectasis
- Q33.5 Ectopic tissue in lung
- Q33.6 Congenital hypoplasia and dysplasia of lung
  - EXCLUDES 1 pulmonary hypoplasia associated with short gestation (P28.0)
- Q33.8 Other congenital malformations of lung
- Q33.9 Congenital malformation of lung, unspecified

✓4ᵗʰ Q34 Other congenital malformations of respiratory system
  EXCLUDES 2 congenital central alveolar hypoventilation syndrome (G47.35)
- Q34.0 Anomaly of pleura
- Q34.1 Congenital cyst of mediastinum
- Q34.8 Other specified congenital malformations of respiratory system
  - Atresia of nasopharynx
- Q34.9 Congenital malformation of respiratory system, unspecified
  - Congenital absence of respiratory system
  - Congenital anomaly of respiratory system NOS

Cleft lip and cleft palate (Q35-Q37)

Use additional code to identify associated malformation of the nose (Q30.2)
  EXCLUDES 2 Robin's syndrome (Q87.0)

✓4ᵗʰ Q35 Cleft palate
  INCLUDES fissure of palate
    palatoschisis
  EXCLUDES 1 cleft palate with cleft lip (Q37.-)
  DEF: Congenital fissure or defect of the roof of the mouth opening to the nasal cavity due to failure of embryonic cells to fuse completely.

Cleft Palate

- Q35.1 Cleft hard palate
- Q35.3 Cleft soft palate
- Q35.5 Cleft hard palate with cleft soft palate
- Q35.7 Cleft uvula
- Q35.9 Cleft palate, unspecified
  - Cleft palate NOS

✓4ᵗʰ Q36 Cleft lip
  INCLUDES cheiloschisis
    congenital fissure of lip
    harelip
    labium leporinum
  EXCLUDES 1 cleft lip with cleft palate (Q37.-)
  DEF: Congenital fissure or opening in the upper lip due to failure of embryonic cells to fuse completely.

Cleft Lip

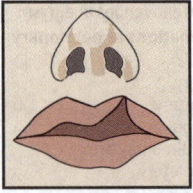
Unilateral incomplete

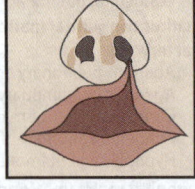
Unilateral complete

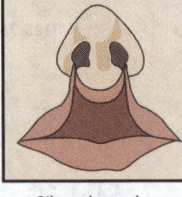
Bilateral complete

- Q36.0 Cleft lip, bilateral
- Q36.1 Cleft lip, median
- Q36.9 Cleft lip, unilateral
  - Cleft lip NOS

✓4ᵗʰ Q37 Cleft palate with cleft lip
  INCLUDES cheilopalatoschisis
- Q37.0 Cleft hard palate with bilateral cleft lip
- Q37.1 Cleft hard palate with unilateral cleft lip
  - Cleft hard palate with cleft lip NOS
- Q37.2 Cleft soft palate with bilateral cleft lip
- Q37.3 Cleft soft palate with unilateral cleft lip
  - Cleft soft palate with cleft lip NOS
- Q37.4 Cleft hard and soft palate with bilateral cleft lip
- Q37.5 Cleft hard and soft palate with unilateral cleft lip
  - Cleft hard and soft palate with cleft lip NOS
- Q37.8 Unspecified cleft palate with bilateral cleft lip

Q37.9 Unspecified cleft palate with unilateral cleft lip [COM]
  Cleft palate with cleft lip NOS

Other congenital malformations of the digestive system (Q38-Q45)

✓4th Q38 Other congenital malformations of tongue, mouth and pharynx
  EXCLUDES 1: dentofacial anomalies (M26.-)
    macrostomia (Q18.4)
    microstomia (Q18.5)

  Q38.0 Congenital malformations of lips, not elsewhere classified
    Congenital fistula of lip
    Congenital malformation of lip NOS
    Van der Woude's syndrome
    EXCLUDES 1: cleft lip (Q36.-)
      cleft lip with cleft palate (Q37.-)
      macrocheilia (Q18.6)
      microcheilia (Q18.7)

  Q38.1 Ankyloglossia
    Tongue tie

  Q38.2 Macroglossia
    Congenital hypertrophy of tongue

  Q38.3 Other congenital malformations of tongue
    Aglossia
    Bifid tongue
    Congenital adhesion of tongue
    Congenital fissure of tongue
    Congenital malformation of tongue NOS
    Double tongue
    Hypoglossia
    Hypoplasia of tongue
    Microglossia

  Q38.4 Congenital malformations of salivary glands and ducts
    Atresia of salivary glands and ducts
    Congenital absence of salivary glands and ducts
    Congenital accessory salivary glands and ducts
    Congenital fistula of salivary gland

  Q38.5 Congenital malformations of palate, not elsewhere classified
    Congenital absence of uvula
    Congenital high arched palate
    Congenital malformation of palate NOS
    EXCLUDES 1: cleft palate (Q35.-)
      cleft palate with cleft lip (Q37.-)

  Q38.6 Other congenital malformations of mouth
    Congenital malformation of mouth NOS

  Q38.7 Congenital pharyngeal pouch
    Congenital diverticulum of pharynx
    EXCLUDES 1: pharyngeal pouch syndrome (D82.1)

  Q38.8 Other congenital malformations of pharynx
    Congenital malformation of pharynx NOS
    Imperforate pharynx

✓4th Q39 Congenital malformations of esophagus

  Q39.0 Atresia of esophagus without fistula [COM]
    Atresia of esophagus NOS

  Q39.1 Atresia of esophagus with tracheo-esophageal fistula [COM]
    Atresia of esophagus with broncho-esophageal fistula

  Q39.2 Congenital tracheo-esophageal fistula without atresia [COM]
    Congenital tracheo-esophageal fistula NOS

  Q39.3 Congenital stenosis and stricture of esophagus [COM]

  Q39.4 Esophageal web [COM]

  Q39.5 Congenital dilatation of esophagus
    Congenital cardiospasm

  Q39.6 Congenital diverticulum of esophagus
    Congenital esophageal pouch

  Q39.8 Other congenital malformations of esophagus
    Congenital absence of esophagus
    Congenital displacement of esophagus
    Congenital duplication of esophagus

  Q39.9 Congenital malformation of esophagus, unspecified

✓4th Q40 Other congenital malformations of upper alimentary tract

  Q40.0 Congenital hypertrophic pyloric stenosis [HCC] [COM]
    Congenital or infantile constriction
    Congenital or infantile hypertrophy
    Congenital or infantile spasm
    Congenital or infantile stenosis
    Congenital or infantile stricture

  Q40.1 Congenital hiatus hernia
    Congenital displacement of cardia through esophageal hiatus
    EXCLUDES 1: congenital diaphragmatic hernia (Q79.0)

  Q40.2 Other specified congenital malformations of stomach
    Congenital displacement of stomach
    Congenital diverticulum of stomach
    Congenital duplication of stomach
    Congenital hourglass stomach
    Megalogastria
    Microgastria

  Q40.3 Congenital malformation of stomach, unspecified

  Q40.8 Other specified congenital malformations of upper alimentary tract

  Q40.9 Congenital malformation of upper alimentary tract, unspecified
    Congenital anomaly of upper alimentary tract
    Congenital deformity of upper alimentary tract

✓4th Q41 Congenital absence, atresia and stenosis of small intestine
  INCLUDES: congenital obstruction, occlusion or stricture of small intestine or intestine NOS
  EXCLUDES 1: cystic fibrosis with intestinal manifestation (E84.11)
    meconium ileus NOS (without cystic fibrosis) (P76.0)

  Q41.0 Congenital absence, atresia and stenosis of duodenum [HCC] [COM]

  Q41.1 Congenital absence, atresia and stenosis of jejunum [HCC] [COM]
    Apple peel syndrome
    Imperforate jejunum

  Q41.2 Congenital absence, atresia and stenosis of ileum [HCC] [COM]

  Q41.8 Congenital absence, atresia and stenosis of other specified parts of small intestine [HCC] [COM]

  Q41.9 Congenital absence, atresia and stenosis of small intestine, part unspecified [HCC] [COM]
    Congenital absence, atresia and stenosis of intestine NOS

✓4th Q42 Congenital absence, atresia and stenosis of large intestine
  INCLUDES: congenital obstruction, occlusion and stricture of large intestine

  Q42.0 Congenital absence, atresia and stenosis of rectum with fistula [HCC] [COM]

  Q42.1 Congenital absence, atresia and stenosis of rectum without fistula [HCC] [COM]
    Imperforate rectum

  Q42.2 Congenital absence, atresia and stenosis of anus with fistula [HCC] [COM]

  Q42.3 Congenital absence, atresia and stenosis of anus without fistula [HCC] [COM]
    Imperforate anus

  Q42.8 Congenital absence, atresia and stenosis of other parts of large intestine [HCC] [COM]

  Q42.9 Congenital absence, atresia and stenosis of large intestine, part unspecified [HCC] [COM]

✓4th Q43 Other congenital malformations of intestine

  Q43.0 Meckel's diverticulum (displaced) (hypertrophic)
    Persistent omphalomesenteric duct
    Persistent vitelline duct
    DEF: Congenital, abnormal remnant of embryonic digestive system development that leaves a sacculation or outpouching from the wall of the small intestine near the terminal part of the ileum made of acid-secreting tissue as in the stomach.

  Q43.1 Hirschsprung's disease [HCC] [COM]
    Aganglionosis
    Congenital (aganglionic) megacolon
    DEF: Congenital enlargement or dilation of the colon, with the absence of nerve cells in a segment of colon distally that causes the inability to defecate.

  Q43.2 Other congenital functional disorders of colon [HCC] [COM]
    Congenital dilatation of colon

  Q43.3 Congenital malformations of intestinal fixation [HCC] [COM]
    Congenital omental, anomalous adhesions [bands]
    Congenital peritoneal adhesions [bands]
    Incomplete rotation of cecum and colon
    Insufficient rotation of cecum and colon
    Jackson's membrane
    Malrotation of colon
    Rotation failure of cecum and colon
    Universal mesentery

  Q43.4 Duplication of intestine

  Q43.5 Ectopic anus

Chapter 17. Congenital Malformations, Deformations and Chromosomal Abnormalities

Q43.6 Congenital fistula of rectum and anus
- EXCLUDES 1: congenital fistula of anus with absence, atresia and stenosis (Q42.2)
  congenital fistula of rectum with absence, atresia and stenosis (Q42.0)
  congenital rectovaginal fistula (Q52.2)
  congenital urethrorectal fistula (Q64.73)
  pilonidal fistula or sinus (L05.-)

Q43.7 Persistent cloaca
- Cloaca NOS

Q43.8 Other specified congenital malformations of intestine
- Congenital blind loop syndrome
- Congenital diverticulitis, colon
- Congenital diverticulum, intestine
- Dolichocolon
- Megaloappendix
- Megaloduodenum
- Microcolon
- Transposition of appendix
- Transposition of colon
- Transposition of intestine
- AHA: 2013,2Q,31

Q43.9 Congenital malformation of intestine, unspecified

✓4th **Q44** Congenital malformations of gallbladder, bile ducts and liver

Q44.0 Agenesis, aplasia and hypoplasia of gallbladder
- Congenital absence of gallbladder

Q44.1 Other congenital malformations of gallbladder
- Congenital malformation of gallbladder NOS
- Intrahepatic gallbladder

Q44.2 Atresia of bile ducts [HCC]

Q44.3 Congenital stenosis and stricture of bile ducts [HCC]

Q44.4 Choledochal cyst

Q44.5 Other congenital malformations of bile ducts
- Accessory hepatic duct
- Biliary duct duplication
- Congenital malformation of bile duct NOS
- Cystic duct duplication

Q44.6 Cystic disease of liver
- Fibrocystic disease of liver

✓5th **Q44.7** Other congenital malformations of liver
- Code also, if applicable, associated malformations affecting other systems
- AHA: 2023,4Q,37-38

  Q44.70 Other congenital malformation of liver, unspecified
  - Congenital malformation of liver, NOS

  Q44.71 Alagille syndrome [HCC]
  - Alagille-Watson syndrome

  Q44.79 Other congenital malformations of liver
  - Accessory liver
  - Congenital absence of liver
  - Congenital hepatomegaly

✓4th **Q45** Other congenital malformations of digestive system
- EXCLUDES 2: congenital diaphragmatic hernia (Q79.0)
  congenital hiatus hernia (Q40.1)

Q45.0 Agenesis, aplasia and hypoplasia of pancreas
- Congenital absence of pancreas

Q45.1 Annular pancreas

Q45.2 Congenital pancreatic cyst

Q45.3 Other congenital malformations of pancreas and pancreatic duct
- Accessory pancreas
- Congenital malformation of pancreas or pancreatic duct NOS
- EXCLUDES 1: congenital diabetes mellitus (E10.-)
  cystic fibrosis (E84.0-E84.9)
  fibrocystic disease of pancreas (E84.-)
  neonatal diabetes mellitus (P70.2)

Q45.8 Other specified congenital malformations of digestive system
- Absence (complete) (partial) of alimentary tract NOS
- Duplication of digestive system
- Malposition, congenital of digestive system

Q45.9 Congenital malformation of digestive system, unspecified
- Congenital anomaly of digestive system
- Congenital deformity of digestive system

Congenital malformations of genital organs (Q50-Q56)

EXCLUDES 1: androgen insensitivity syndrome (E34.5-)
syndromes associated with anomalies in the number and form of chromosomes (Q90-Q99)

✓4th **Q50** Congenital malformations of ovaries, fallopian tubes and broad ligaments

✓5th **Q50.0** Congenital absence of ovary
- EXCLUDES 1: Turner's syndrome (Q96.-)

  Q50.01 Congenital absence of ovary, unilateral
  Q50.02 Congenital absence of ovary, bilateral

Q50.1 Developmental ovarian cyst

Q50.2 Congenital torsion of ovary

✓5th **Q50.3** Other congenital malformations of ovary

  Q50.31 Accessory ovary
  Q50.32 Ovarian streak
  - 46, XX with streak gonads
  Q50.39 Other congenital malformation of ovary
  - Congenital malformation of ovary NOS

Q50.4 Embryonic cyst of fallopian tube
- Fimbrial cyst

Q50.5 Embryonic cyst of broad ligament
- Epoophoron cyst
- Parovarian cyst

Q50.6 Other congenital malformations of fallopian tube and broad ligament
- Absence of fallopian tube and broad ligament
- Accessory fallopian tube and broad ligament
- Atresia of fallopian tube and broad ligament
- Congenital malformation of fallopian tube or broad ligament NOS

✓4th **Q51** Congenital malformations of uterus and cervix

Q51.0 Agenesis and aplasia of uterus
- Congenital absence of uterus

✓5th **Q51.1** Doubling of uterus with doubling of cervix and vagina

  Q51.10 Doubling of uterus with doubling of cervix and vagina without obstruction
  - Doubling of uterus with doubling of cervix and vagina NOS

  Q51.11 Doubling of uterus with doubling of cervix and vagina with obstruction

✓5th **Q51.2** Other doubling of uterus
- Doubling of uterus NOS
- Septate uterus
- AHA: 2018,4Q,27

  Q51.21 Complete doubling of uterus
  - Complete septate uterus
  Q51.22 Partial doubling of uterus
  - Partial septate uterus
  Q51.28 Other and unspecified doubling of uterus
  - Septate uterus NOS

Q51.3 Bicornate uterus
- Bicornate uterus, complete or partial

Q51.4 Unicornate uterus
- Unicornate uterus with or without a separate uterine horn
- Uterus with only one functioning horn

Q51.5 Agenesis and aplasia of cervix
- Congenital absence of cervix

Q51.6 Embryonic cyst of cervix

Q51.7 Congenital fistulae between uterus and digestive and urinary tracts

✓5th **Q51.8** Other congenital malformations of uterus and cervix

  ✓6th **Q51.81** Other congenital malformations of uterus

    Q51.810 Arcuate uterus
    - Arcuatus uterus
    Q51.811 Hypoplasia of uterus
    Q51.818 Other congenital malformations of uterus
    - Mullerian anomaly of uterus NEC

  ✓6th **Q51.82** Other congenital malformations of cervix

    Q51.820 Cervical duplication
    Q51.821 Hypoplasia of cervix
    Q51.828 Other congenital malformations of cervix

Q51.9 Congenital malformation of uterus and cervix, unspecified

✓4th **Q52** Other congenital malformations of female genitalia

Q52.0 Congenital absence of vagina
- Vaginal agenesis, total or partial

[HCC] CMS-HCC   [Rx] Rx HCC   [ESR] ESRD HCC   [COM] Commercial HCC   [N] Newborn: 0   [P] Pediatric: 0-17   [M] Maternity: 9-64   [A] Adult: 15-124

Chapter 17. Congenital Malformations, Deformations and Chromosomal Abnormalities

Q52.1 **Doubling** of vagina
   EXCLUDES 1 doubling of vagina with doubling of uterus and cervix (Q51.1-)
   Q52.10 Doubling of vagina, unspecified
      Septate vagina NOS
   Q52.11 **Transverse** vaginal septum
   Q52.12 **Longitudinal** vaginal septum
      AHA: 2016,4Q,58-59
      Q52.120 Longitudinal vaginal septum, **nonobstructing**
      Q52.121 Longitudinal vaginal septum, **obstructing, right side**
      Q52.122 Longitudinal vaginal septum, **obstructing, left side**
      Q52.123 Longitudinal vaginal septum, **microperforate, right side**
      Q52.124 Longitudinal vaginal septum, **microperforate, left side**
      Q52.129 Other and unspecified longitudinal vaginal septum

Q52.2 Congenital **rectovaginal fistula**
   EXCLUDES 1 cloaca (Q43.7)

Q52.3 **Imperforate hymen**
   DEF: Obstructive anomaly of vagina, characterized by complete closure of the membranous fold around the external opening of the vagina, obstructing the vaginal introitus.

Q52.4 Other congenital malformations of vagina
   Canal of Nuck cyst, congenital
   Congenital malformation of vagina NOS
   Embryonic vaginal cyst
   Gartner's duct cyst
   AHA: 2022,2Q,15

Q52.5 **Fusion of labia**

Q52.6 Congenital malformation of **clitoris**

Q52.7 Other and unspecified congenital malformations of **vulva**
   Q52.70 Unspecified congenital malformations of vulva
      Congenital malformation of vulva NOS
   Q52.71 Congenital **absence** of vulva
   Q52.79 Other congenital malformations of vulva
      Congenital cyst of vulva

Q52.8 Other specified congenital malformations of female genitalia

Q52.9 Congenital malformation of female genitalia, unspecified

Q53 Undescended and ectopic **testicle**
   Q53.0 **Ectopic** testis
      Q53.00 Ectopic testis, unspecified
      Q53.01 Ectopic testis, unilateral
      Q53.02 Ectopic testes, bilateral
   Q53.1 **Undescended** testicle, **unilateral**
      AHA: 2017,4Q,22-23
      Q53.10 Unspecified undescended testicle, unilateral
      Q53.11 Abdominal testis, unilateral
         Q53.111 Unilateral **intraabdominal** testis
         Q53.112 Unilateral **inguinal** testis
      Q53.12 **Ectopic perineal** testis, unilateral
      Q53.13 Unilateral **high scrotal** testis
   Q53.2 **Undescended** testicle, **bilateral**
      AHA: 2017,4Q,22-23
      Q53.20 Undescended testicle, unspecified, bilateral
      Q53.21 Abdominal testis, bilateral
         Q53.211 Bilateral **intraabdominal** testes
         Q53.212 Bilateral **inguinal** testes
      Q53.22 **Ectopic perineal** testis, bilateral
      Q53.23 Bilateral **high scrotal** testes
   Q53.9 Undescended testicle, unspecified
      Cryptorchism NOS

Q54 **Hypospadias**
   EXCLUDES 1 epispadias (Q64.0)
   DEF: Abnormal opening of the urethra on the ventral (underside) surface of the penis.

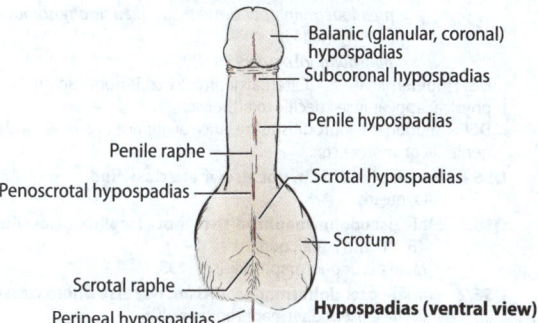

Hypospadias (ventral view)

   Q54.0 Hypospadias, **balanic**
      Hypospadias, coronal
      Hypospadias, glandular
   Q54.1 Hypospadias, **penile**
   Q54.2 Hypospadias, **penoscrotal**
   Q54.3 Hypospadias, **perineal**
   Q54.4 **Congenital chordee**
      Chordee without hypospadias
   Q54.8 Other hypospadias
      Hypospadias with intersex state
   Q54.9 Hypospadias, unspecified

Q55 Other congenital malformations of **male genital organs**
   EXCLUDES 1 congenital hydrocele (P83.5)
      hypospadias (Q54.-)
   Q55.0 Absence and aplasia of testis
      Monorchism
   Q55.1 Hypoplasia of testis and scrotum
      Fusion of testes
   Q55.2 Other and unspecified congenital malformations of **testis and scrotum**
      Q55.20 Unspecified congenital malformations of testis and scrotum
         Congenital malformation of testis or scrotum NOS
      Q55.21 **Polyorchism**
         DEF: Congenital anomaly in which there are more than two testes.
      Q55.22 **Retractile** testis
      Q55.23 Scrotal **transposition**
      Q55.29 Other congenital malformations of testis and scrotum
   Q55.3 Atresia of **vas deferens**
      Code first any associated cystic fibrosis (E84.-)
   Q55.4 Other congenital malformations of vas deferens, epididymis, seminal vesicles and prostate
      Absence or aplasia of prostate
      Absence or aplasia of spermatic cord
      Congenital malformation of vas deferens, epididymis, seminal vesicles or prostate NOS
   Q55.5 Congenital **absence and aplasia of penis**
   Q55.6 Other congenital malformations of **penis**
      Q55.61 **Curvature** of penis (lateral)
      Q55.62 **Hypoplasia** of penis
         Micropenis
      Q55.63 **Congenital torsion** of penis
         EXCLUDES 1 acquired torsion of penis (N48.82)
      Q55.64 **Hidden penis**
         Buried penis
         Concealed penis
         EXCLUDES 1 acquired buried penis (N48.83)
      Q55.69 Other congenital malformation of penis
         Congenital malformation of penis NOS
   Q55.7 Congenital **vasocutaneous fistula**
   Q55.8 Other specified congenital malformations of male genital organs
   Q55.9 Congenital malformation of male genital organ, unspecified
      Congenital anomaly of male genital organ
      Congenital deformity of male genital organ

Q56 Indeterminate sex and pseudohermaphroditism
EXCLUDES 1: 46, XX true hermaphrodite (Q99.1)
androgen insensitivity syndrome (E34.5-)
chimera 46, XX/46, XY true hermaphrodite (Q99.0)
female pseudohermaphroditism with adrenocortical disorder (E25.-)
pseudohermaphroditism with specified chromosomal anomaly (Q96-Q99)
pure gonadal dysgenesis (Q99.1)

DEF: Indeterminate sex: External genitalia that is nondescript, lacking the physical appearance specific to either sex.
DEF: Pseudohermaphroditism: Presence of gonads of one sex and external genitalia of another sex.

- **Q56.0** Hermaphroditism, not elsewhere classified
  Ovotestis
- **Q56.1** Male pseudohermaphroditism, not elsewhere classified
  46, XY with streak gonads
  Male pseudohermaphroditism NOS
- **Q56.2** Female pseudohermaphroditism, not elsewhere classified
  Female pseudohermaphroditism NOS
- **Q56.3** Pseudohermaphroditism, unspecified
- **Q56.4** Indeterminate sex, unspecified
  Ambiguous genitalia

Congenital malformations of the urinary system (Q60-Q64)

Q60 Renal agenesis and other reduction defects of kidney
INCLUDES: congenital absence of kidney
congenital atrophy of kidney
infantile atrophy of kidney

- **Q60.0** Renal agenesis, unilateral
- **Q60.1** Renal agenesis, bilateral
- **Q60.2** Renal agenesis, unspecified
- **Q60.3** Renal hypoplasia, unilateral
- **Q60.4** Renal hypoplasia, bilateral
- **Q60.5** Renal hypoplasia, unspecified
- **Q60.6** Potter's syndrome

Q61 Cystic kidney disease
EXCLUDES 1: acquired cyst of kidney (N28.1)
Potter's syndrome (Q60.6)

- **Q61.0** Congenital renal cyst
  - **Q61.00** Congenital renal cyst, unspecified
    Cyst of kidney NOS (congenital)
  - **Q61.01** Congenital single renal cyst
  - **Q61.02** Congenital multiple renal cysts
- **Q61.1** Polycystic kidney, infantile type
  Polycystic kidney, autosomal recessive
  - **Q61.11** Cystic dilatation of collecting ducts [COM]
  - **Q61.19** Other polycystic kidney, infantile type [COM]
- **Q61.2** Polycystic kidney, adult type
  Polycystic kidney, autosomal dominant
- **Q61.3** Polycystic kidney, unspecified
  AHA: 2016,3Q,22
- **Q61.4** Renal dysplasia
  Multicystic dysplastic kidney
  Multicystic kidney (development)
  Multicystic kidney disease
  Multicystic renal dysplasia
  EXCLUDES 1: polycystic kidney disease (Q61.11-Q61.3)
- **Q61.5** Medullary cystic kidney
  Nephronophthisis
  Sponge kidney NOS
  DEF: Sponge kidney: Dilated collecting tubules that are usually asymptomatic. Calcinosis in tubules may cause renal insufficiency.
- **Q61.8** Other cystic kidney diseases
  Fibrocystic kidney
  Fibrocystic renal degeneration or disease
- **Q61.9** Cystic kidney disease, unspecified
  Meckel-Gruber syndrome

Q62 Congenital obstructive defects of renal pelvis and congenital malformations of ureter
- **Q62.0** Congenital hydronephrosis
- **Q62.1** Congenital occlusion of ureter
  Atresia and stenosis of ureter
  - **Q62.10** Congenital occlusion of ureter, unspecified
  - **Q62.11** Congenital occlusion of ureteropelvic junction
  - **Q62.12** Congenital occlusion of ureterovesical orifice
- **Q62.2** Congenital megaureter
  Congenital dilatation of ureter
- **Q62.3** Other obstructive defects of renal pelvis and ureter
  - **Q62.31** Congenital ureterocele, orthotopic
  - **Q62.32** Cecoureterocele
    Ectopic ureterocele
  - **Q62.39** Other obstructive defects of renal pelvis and ureter
    Ureteropelvic junction obstruction NOS
- **Q62.4** Agenesis of ureter
  Congenital absence ureter
- **Q62.5** Duplication of ureter
  Accessory ureter
  Double ureter
- **Q62.6** Malposition of ureter
  - **Q62.60** Malposition of ureter, unspecified
  - **Q62.61** Deviation of ureter
  - **Q62.62** Displacement of ureter
  - **Q62.63** Anomalous implantation of ureter
    Ectopia of ureter
    Ectopic ureter
  - **Q62.69** Other malposition of ureter
- **Q62.7** Congenital vesico-uretero-renal reflux
- **Q62.8** Other congenital malformations of ureter
  Anomaly of ureter NOS

Q63 Other congenital malformations of kidney
EXCLUDES 1: congenital nephrotic syndrome (N04.-)
- **Q63.0** Accessory kidney
- **Q63.1** Lobulated, fused and horseshoe kidney
- **Q63.2** Ectopic kidney
  Congenital displaced kidney
  Malrotation of kidney
- **Q63.3** Hyperplastic and giant kidney
  Compensatory hypertrophy of kidney
- **Q63.8** Other specified congenital malformations of kidney
  Congenital renal calculi
- **Q63.9** Congenital malformation of kidney, unspecified

Q64 Other congenital malformations of urinary system
- **Q64.0** Epispadias
  EXCLUDES 1: hypospadias (Q54.-)

Epispadias

Normal external urethral orifice
Glans penis
Foreskin (retracted)
Epispadias

Epispadias (dorsal view)

- **Q64.1** Exstrophy of urinary bladder
  - **Q64.10** Exstrophy of urinary bladder, unspecified [COM]
    Ectopia vesicae
  - **Q64.11** Supravesical fissure of urinary bladder [COM]
  - **Q64.12** Cloacal exstrophy of urinary bladder [COM]
  - **Q64.19** Other exstrophy of urinary bladder [COM]
    Extroversion of bladder
- **Q64.2** Congenital posterior urethral valves
- **Q64.3** Other atresia and stenosis of urethra and bladder neck
  - **Q64.31** Congenital bladder neck obstruction
    Congenital obstruction of vesicourethral orifice
  - **Q64.32** Congenital stricture of urethra
  - **Q64.33** Congenital stricture of urinary meatus
  - **Q64.39** Other atresia and stenosis of urethra and bladder neck
    Atresia and stenosis of urethra and bladder neck NOS
- **Q64.4** Malformation of urachus
  Cyst of urachus
  Patent urachus
  Prolapse of urachus
- **Q64.5** Congenital absence of bladder and urethra
- **Q64.6** Congenital diverticulum of bladder

Q64.7 Other and unspecified congenital malformations of bladder and urethra
EXCLUDES 1 congenital prolapse of bladder (mucosa) (Q79.4)
- **Q64.70** Unspecified congenital malformation of bladder and urethra
  - Malformation of bladder or urethra NOS
- **Q64.71** Congenital prolapse of urethra
- **Q64.72** Congenital prolapse of urinary meatus
- **Q64.73** Congenital urethrorectal fistula
- **Q64.74** Double urethra
- **Q64.75** Double urinary meatus
- **Q64.79** Other congenital malformations of bladder and urethra

Q64.8 Other specified congenital malformations of urinary system
Q64.9 Congenital malformation of urinary system, unspecified
Congenital anomaly NOS of urinary system
Congenital deformity NOS of urinary system

Congenital malformations and deformations of the musculoskeletal system (Q65-Q79)

Q65 Congenital deformities of hip
EXCLUDES 1 clicking hip (R29.4)

- **Q65.0** Congenital dislocation of hip, unilateral
  - **Q65.00** Congenital dislocation of unspecified hip, unilateral
  - **Q65.01** Congenital dislocation of right hip, unilateral
  - **Q65.02** Congenital dislocation of left hip, unilateral
- **Q65.1** Congenital dislocation of hip, bilateral
- **Q65.2** Congenital dislocation of hip, unspecified
- **Q65.3** Congenital partial dislocation of hip, unilateral
  - **Q65.30** Congenital partial dislocation of unspecified hip, unilateral
  - **Q65.31** Congenital partial dislocation of right hip, unilateral
  - **Q65.32** Congenital partial dislocation of left hip, unilateral
- **Q65.4** Congenital partial dislocation of hip, bilateral
- **Q65.5** Congenital partial dislocation of hip, unspecified
- **Q65.6** Congenital unstable hip
  - Congenital dislocatable hip
- **Q65.8** Other congenital deformities of hip
  - **Q65.81** Congenital coxa valga
  - **Q65.82** Congenital coxa vara
  - **Q65.89** Other specified congenital deformities of hip
    - Anteversion of femoral neck
    - Congenital acetabular dysplasia
- **Q65.9** Congenital deformity of hip, unspecified

Q66 Congenital deformities of feet
EXCLUDES 1 reduction defects of feet (Q72.-)
valgus deformities (acquired) (M21.0-)
varus deformities (acquired) (M21.1-)
AHA: 2019,4Q,13

- **Q66.0** Congenital talipes equinovarus
  - **Q66.00** Congenital talipes equinovarus, unspecified foot
  - **Q66.01** Congenital talipes equinovarus, right foot
  - **Q66.02** Congenital talipes equinovarus, left foot
- **Q66.1** Congenital talipes calcaneovarus
  - **Q66.10** Congenital talipes calcaneovarus, unspecified foot
  - **Q66.11** Congenital talipes calcaneovarus, right foot
  - **Q66.12** Congenital talipes calcaneovarus, left foot
- **Q66.2** Congenital metatarsus (primus) varus
  AHA: 2016,4Q,59
  - **Q66.21** Congenital metatarsus primus varus
    - **Q66.211** Congenital metatarsus primus varus, right foot
    - **Q66.212** Congenital metatarsus primus varus, left foot
    - **Q66.219** Congenital metatarsus primus varus, unspecified foot
  - **Q66.22** Congenital metatarsus adductus
    - Congenital metatarsus varus
    - **Q66.221** Congenital metatarsus adductus, right foot
    - **Q66.222** Congenital metatarsus adductus, left foot
    - **Q66.229** Congenital metatarsus adductus, unspecified foot
- **Q66.3** Other congenital varus deformities of feet
  - Hallux varus, congenital
  - AHA: 2023,3Q,20
  - **Q66.30** Other congenital varus deformities of feet, unspecified foot
  - **Q66.31** Other congenital varus deformities of feet, right foot
  - **Q66.32** Other congenital varus deformities of feet, left foot
- **Q66.4** Congenital talipes calcaneovalgus
  - **Q66.40** Congenital talipes calcaneovalgus, unspecified foot
  - **Q66.41** Congenital talipes calcaneovalgus, right foot
  - **Q66.42** Congenital talipes calcaneovalgus, left foot
- **Q66.5** Congenital pes planus
  - Congenital flat foot
  - Congenital rigid flat foot
  - Congenital spastic (everted) flat foot
  - EXCLUDES 1 pes planus, acquired (M21.4)
  - **Q66.50** Congenital pes planus, unspecified foot
  - **Q66.51** Congenital pes planus, right foot
  - **Q66.52** Congenital pes planus, left foot
- **Q66.6** Other congenital valgus deformities of feet
  - Congenital metatarsus valgus
- **Q66.7** Congenital pes cavus
  - **Q66.70** Congenital pes cavus, unspecified foot
  - **Q66.71** Congenital pes cavus, right foot
  - **Q66.72** Congenital pes cavus, left foot
- **Q66.8** Other congenital deformities of feet
  - **Q66.80** Congenital vertical talus deformity, unspecified foot
  - **Q66.81** Congenital vertical talus deformity, right foot
  - **Q66.82** Congenital vertical talus deformity, left foot
  - **Q66.89** Other specified congenital deformities of feet
    - Congenital asymmetric talipes
    - Congenital clubfoot NOS
    - Congenital talipes NOS
    - Congenital tarsal coalition
    - Hammer toe, congenital
    - **DEF:** Clubfoot: Congenital anomaly of the foot with the heel elevated and rotated outward and the toes pointing inward.
- **Q66.9** Congenital deformity of feet, unspecified
  - **Q66.90** Congenital deformity of feet, unspecified, unspecified foot
  - **Q66.91** Congenital deformity of feet, unspecified, right foot
  - **Q66.92** Congenital deformity of feet, unspecified, left foot

Q67 Congenital musculoskeletal deformities of head, face, spine and chest
EXCLUDES 1 congenital malformation syndromes classified to Q87.-
Potter's syndrome (Q60.6)

- **Q67.0** Congenital facial asymmetry
- **Q67.1** Congenital compression facies
- **Q67.2** Dolichocephaly
  - EXCLUDES 1 sagittal craniosynostosis (Q75.01)
- **Q67.3** Plagiocephaly
  - EXCLUDES 1 coronal craniosynostosis (Q75.02-)
  - lambdoid craniosynostosis (Q75.04-)
- **Q67.4** Other congenital deformities of skull, face and jaw
  - Congenital depressions in skull
  - Congenital hemifacial atrophy or hypertrophy
  - Deviation of nasal septum, congenital
  - Squashed or bent nose, congenital
  - EXCLUDES 1 dentofacial anomalies [including malocclusion] (M26.-)
  - syphilitic saddle nose (A50.5)
  - **DEF:** Deviated septum: Condition in which the nasal septum, a thin wall composed of cartilage and bone that separates the two nostrils, is crooked or displaced from the midline.
- **Q67.5** Congenital deformity of spine
  - Congenital postural scoliosis
  - Congenital scoliosis NOS
  - EXCLUDES 1 infantile idiopathic scoliosis (M41.0)
  - scoliosis due to congenital bony malformation (Q76.3)
  - AHA: 2014,4Q,26
- **Q67.6** Pectus excavatum
  - Congenital funnel chest
- **Q67.7** Pectus carinatum
  - Congenital pigeon chest
- **Q67.8** Other congenital deformities of chest
  - Congenital deformity of chest wall NOS

Q68 Other congenital musculoskeletal deformities
EXCLUDES 1 reduction defects of limb(s) (Q71-Q73)
EXCLUDES 2 congenital myotonic chondrodystrophy (G71.13)

- **Q68.0** Congenital deformity of sternocleidomastoid muscle
  - Congenital (sternomastoid) torticollis
  - Congenital contracture of sternocleidomastoid (muscle)
  - Sternomastoid tumor (congenital)
- **Q68.1** Congenital deformity of finger(s) and hand
  - Congenital clubfinger
  - Spade-like hand (congenital)
- **Q68.2** Congenital deformity of knee
  - Congenital dislocation of knee
  - Congenital genu recurvatum
- **Q68.3** Congenital bowing of femur
  - **EXCLUDES 1** anteversion of femur (neck) (Q65.89)
- **Q68.4** Congenital bowing of tibia and fibula
- **Q68.5** Congenital bowing of long bones of leg, unspecified
- **Q68.6** Discoid meniscus
- **Q68.8** Other specified congenital musculoskeletal deformities
  - Congenital deformity of clavicle
  - Congenital deformity of elbow
  - Congenital deformity of forearm
  - Congenital deformity of scapula
  - Congenital deformity of wrist
  - Congenital dislocation of elbow
  - Congenital dislocation of shoulder
  - Congenital dislocation of wrist

Q69 Polydactyly
- **Q69.0** Accessory finger(s)
- **Q69.1** Accessory thumb(s)
- **Q69.2** Accessory toe(s)
  - Accessory hallux
- **Q69.9** Polydactyly, unspecified
  - Supernumerary digit(s) NOS

Q70 Syndactyly
- **Q70.0** Fused fingers
  - Complex syndactyly of fingers with synostosis
  - **Q70.00** Fused fingers, unspecified hand
  - **Q70.01** Fused fingers, right hand
  - **Q70.02** Fused fingers, left hand
  - **Q70.03** Fused fingers, bilateral
- **Q70.1** Webbed fingers
  - Simple syndactyly of fingers without synostosis
  - **Q70.10** Webbed fingers, unspecified hand
  - **Q70.11** Webbed fingers, right hand
  - **Q70.12** Webbed fingers, left hand
  - **Q70.13** Webbed fingers, bilateral
- **Q70.2** Fused toes
  - Complex syndactyly of toes with synostosis
  - **Q70.20** Fused toes, unspecified foot
  - **Q70.21** Fused toes, right foot
  - **Q70.22** Fused toes, left foot
  - **Q70.23** Fused toes, bilateral
- **Q70.3** Webbed toes
  - Simple syndactyly of toes without synostosis
  - **Q70.30** Webbed toes, unspecified foot
  - **Q70.31** Webbed toes, right foot
  - **Q70.32** Webbed toes, left foot
  - **Q70.33** Webbed toes, bilateral
- **Q70.4** Polysyndactyly, unspecified
  - **EXCLUDES 1** specified syndactyly of hand and feet - code to specified conditions (Q70.0-Q70.3-)
- **Q70.9** Syndactyly, unspecified
  - Symphalangy NOS

Q71 Reduction defects of upper limb
- **Q71.0** Congenital complete absence of upper limb
  - **Q71.00** Congenital complete absence of unspecified upper limb
  - **Q71.01** Congenital complete absence of right upper limb
  - **Q71.02** Congenital complete absence of left upper limb
  - **Q71.03** Congenital complete absence of upper limb, bilateral
- **Q71.1** Congenital absence of upper arm and forearm with hand present
  - **Q71.10** Congenital absence of unspecified upper arm and forearm with hand present
  - **Q71.11** Congenital absence of right upper arm and forearm with hand present
  - **Q71.12** Congenital absence of left upper arm and forearm with hand present
  - **Q71.13** Congenital absence of upper arm and forearm with hand present, bilateral
- **Q71.2** Congenital absence of both forearm and hand
  - **Q71.20** Congenital absence of both forearm and hand, unspecified upper limb
  - **Q71.21** Congenital absence of both forearm and hand, right upper limb
  - **Q71.22** Congenital absence of both forearm and hand, left upper limb
  - **Q71.23** Congenital absence of both forearm and hand, bilateral
- **Q71.3** Congenital absence of hand and finger
  - **Q71.30** Congenital absence of unspecified hand and finger
  - **Q71.31** Congenital absence of right hand and finger
  - **Q71.32** Congenital absence of left hand and finger
  - **Q71.33** Congenital absence of hand and finger, bilateral
- **Q71.4** Longitudinal reduction defect of radius
  - Clubhand (congenital)
  - Radial clubhand
  - **Q71.40** Longitudinal reduction defect of unspecified radius
  - **Q71.41** Longitudinal reduction defect of right radius
  - **Q71.42** Longitudinal reduction defect of left radius
  - **Q71.43** Longitudinal reduction defect of radius, bilateral
- **Q71.5** Longitudinal reduction defect of ulna
  - **Q71.50** Longitudinal reduction defect of unspecified ulna
  - **Q71.51** Longitudinal reduction defect of right ulna
  - **Q71.52** Longitudinal reduction defect of left ulna
  - **Q71.53** Longitudinal reduction defect of ulna, bilateral
- **Q71.6** Lobster-claw hand
  - **Q71.60** Lobster-claw hand, unspecified hand
  - **Q71.61** Lobster-claw right hand
  - **Q71.62** Lobster-claw left hand
  - **Q71.63** Lobster-claw hand, bilateral
- **Q71.8** Other reduction defects of upper limb
  - **Q71.81** Congenital shortening of upper limb
    - **Q71.811** Congenital shortening of right upper limb
    - **Q71.812** Congenital shortening of left upper limb
    - **Q71.813** Congenital shortening of upper limb, bilateral
    - **Q71.819** Congenital shortening of unspecified upper limb
  - **Q71.89** Other reduction defects of upper limb
    - **Q71.891** Other reduction defects of right upper limb
    - **Q71.892** Other reduction defects of left upper limb
    - **Q71.893** Other reduction defects of upper limb, bilateral
    - **Q71.899** Other reduction defects of unspecified upper limb
- **Q71.9** Unspecified reduction defect of upper limb
  - **Q71.90** Unspecified reduction defect of unspecified upper limb
  - **Q71.91** Unspecified reduction defect of right upper limb
  - **Q71.92** Unspecified reduction defect of left upper limb
  - **Q71.93** Unspecified reduction defect of upper limb, bilateral

Q72 Reduction defects of lower limb
- **Q72.0** Congenital complete absence of lower limb
  - **Q72.00** Congenital complete absence of unspecified lower limb
  - **Q72.01** Congenital complete absence of right lower limb
  - **Q72.02** Congenital complete absence of left lower limb
  - **Q72.03** Congenital complete absence of lower limb, bilateral
- **Q72.1** Congenital absence of thigh and lower leg with foot present
  - **Q72.10** Congenital absence of unspecified thigh and lower leg with foot present
  - **Q72.11** Congenital absence of right thigh and lower leg with foot present
  - **Q72.12** Congenital absence of left thigh and lower leg with foot present
  - **Q72.13** Congenital absence of thigh and lower leg with foot present, bilateral
- **Q72.2** Congenital absence of both lower leg and foot
  - **Q72.20** Congenital absence of both lower leg and foot, unspecified lower limb
  - **Q72.21** Congenital absence of both lower leg and foot, right lower limb

	Q72.22	Congenital absence of both lower leg and foot, **left** lower limb
	Q72.23	Congenital absence of both lower leg and foot, **bilateral**
✓5th **Q72.3**		Congenital **absence of foot and toe(s)**
	Q72.30	Congenital absence of unspecified foot and toe(s)
	Q72.31	Congenital absence of **right** foot and toe(s)
	Q72.32	Congenital absence of **left** foot and toe(s)
	Q72.33	Congenital absence of foot and toe(s), **bilateral**
✓5th **Q72.4**		Longitudinal reduction defect of **femur**
		Proximal femoral focal deficiency
	Q72.40	Longitudinal reduction defect of unspecified femur
	Q72.41	Longitudinal reduction defect of **right** femur
	Q72.42	Longitudinal reduction defect of **left** femur
	Q72.43	Longitudinal reduction defect of femur, **bilateral**
✓5th **Q72.5**		Longitudinal reduction defect of **tibia**
	Q72.50	Longitudinal reduction defect of unspecified tibia
	Q72.51	Longitudinal reduction defect of **right** tibia
	Q72.52	Longitudinal reduction defect of **left** tibia
	Q72.53	Longitudinal reduction defect of tibia, **bilateral**
✓5th **Q72.6**		Longitudinal reduction defect of **fibula**
	Q72.60	Longitudinal reduction defect of unspecified fibula
	Q72.61	Longitudinal reduction defect of **right** fibula
	Q72.62	Longitudinal reduction defect of **left** fibula
	Q72.63	Longitudinal reduction defect of fibula, **bilateral**
✓5th **Q72.7**		**Split foot**
	Q72.70	Split foot, unspecified lower limb
	Q72.71	Split foot, **right** lower limb
	Q72.72	Split foot, **left** lower limb
	Q72.73	Split foot, **bilateral**
✓5th **Q72.8**		Other reduction defects of lower limb
✓6th	Q72.81	Congenital **shortening** of lower limb
	Q72.811	Congenital shortening of **right** lower limb
	Q72.812	Congenital shortening of **left** lower limb
	Q72.813	Congenital shortening of lower limb, **bilateral**
	Q72.819	Congenital shortening of unspecified lower limb
✓6th	Q72.89	Other reduction defects of lower limb
	Q72.891	Other reduction defects of **right** lower limb
	Q72.892	Other reduction defects of **left** lower limb
	Q72.893	Other reduction defects of lower limb, **bilateral**
	Q72.899	Other reduction defects of unspecified lower limb
✓5th **Q72.9**		Unspecified reduction defect of lower limb
	Q72.90	Unspecified reduction defect of unspecified lower limb
	Q72.91	Unspecified reduction defect of **right** lower limb
	Q72.92	Unspecified reduction defect of **left** lower limb
	Q72.93	Unspecified reduction defect of lower limb, **bilateral**
✓4th **Q73**		Reduction defects of unspecified limb
	Q73.0	Congenital **absence** of unspecified limb(s)
		Amelia NOS
	Q73.1	**Phocomelia**, unspecified limb(s)
		Phocomelia NOS
	Q73.8	Other reduction defects of unspecified limb(s)
		Ectromelia of limb NOS
		Hemimelia of limb NOS
		Longitudinal reduction deformity of unspecified limb(s)
		Reduction defect of limb NOS
✓4th **Q74**		Other congenital malformations of limb(s)
	EXCLUDES 1	polydactyly (Q69.-)
		reduction defect of limb (Q71-Q73)
		syndactyly (Q70.-)
	Q74.0	Other congenital malformations of upper limb(s), including shoulder girdle
		Accessory carpal bones
		Cleidocranial dysostosis
		Congenital pseudarthrosis of clavicle
		Macrodactylia (fingers)
		Madelung's deformity
		Radioulnar synostosis
		Sprengel's deformity
		Triphalangeal thumb
	Q74.1	Congenital malformation of knee
		Congenital absence of patella
		Congenital dislocation of patella
		Congenital genu valgum
		Congenital genu varum
		Rudimentary patella
	EXCLUDES 1	congenital dislocation of knee (Q68.2)
		congenital genu recurvatum (Q68.2)
		nail patella syndrome (Q87.2)
	Q74.2	Other congenital malformations of lower limb(s), including pelvic girdle
		Congenital fusion of sacroiliac joint
		Congenital malformation of ankle joint
		Congenital malformation of sacroiliac joint
	EXCLUDES 1	anteversion of femur (neck) (Q65.89)
	Q74.3	Arthrogryposis multiplex congenita
	Q74.8	Other specified congenital malformations of limb(s)
	Q74.9	Unspecified congenital malformation of limb(s)
		Congenital anomaly of limb(s) NOS
✓4th **Q75**		Other congenital malformations of **skull and face bones**
	EXCLUDES 1	congenital malformation of face NOS (Q18.-)
		congenital malformation syndromes classified to Q87.-
		dentofacial anomalies [including malocclusion] (M26.-)
		musculoskeletal deformities of head and face (Q67.0-Q67.4)
		skull defects associated with congenital anomalies of brain such as:
		anencephaly (Q00.0)
		encephalocele (Q01.-)
		hydrocephalus (Q03.-)
		microcephaly (Q02)
✓5th	Q75.0	**Craniosynostosis**
		AHA: 2023,4Q,38-39
		DEF: Congenital condition in which one or more of the cranial sutures fuse prematurely, creating a deformed or aberrant head shape.
▲ ✓6th	Q75.00	**Craniosynostosis, unspecified**
		Craniosynostosis NOS
▲	Q75.001	**Craniosynostosis, unspecified type, unilateral**
▲	Q75.002	**Craniosynostosis, unspecified type, bilateral**
▲	Q75.009	**Craniosynostosis, unspecified**
		Imperfect fusion of skull
	Q75.01	**Sagittal** craniosynostosis
		Non-deformational dolichocephaly
		Non-deformational scaphocephaly
	EXCLUDES 1	plagiocephaly (Q67.3)
✓6th	Q75.02	**Coronal** craniosynostosis
		~~Non-deformational anterior plagiocephaly~~
	EXCLUDES 1	dolichocephaly (Q67.2)
▲	Q75.021	**Coronal craniosynostosis, unilateral**
		Non-deformational anterior plagiocephaly
▲	Q75.022	**Coronal craniosynostosis, bilateral**
		Non-deformational brachycephaly
▲	Q75.029	**Coronal craniosynostosis, unspecified**
	Q75.03	**Metopic** craniosynostosis
		Trigonocephaly
✓6th	Q75.04	**Lambdoid** craniosynostosis
		Non-deformational posterior plagiocephaly
	EXCLUDES 1	dolichocephaly (Q67.2)
	Q75.041	**Lambdoid craniosynostosis, unilateral**
	Q75.042	**Lambdoid craniosynostosis, bilateral**
	Q75.049	**Lambdoid craniosynostosis, unspecified**
✓6th	Q75.05	**Multi-suture** craniosynostosis
	Q75.051	**Cloverleaf skull**
		Kleeblattschaedel skull
	Q75.052	**Pansynostosis**
	Q75.058	**Other multi-suture craniosynostosis**
	EXCLUDES 1	coronal craniosynostosis, bilateral (Q75.022)
		lambdoid craniosynostosis, bilateral (Q75.042)
	Q75.08	Other single-suture craniosynostosis
	Q75.1	**Craniofacial dysostosis**
		Crouzon's disease
	Q75.2	**Hypertelorism**
	Q75.3	**Macrocephaly**

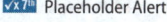
Manifestation

Chapter 17. Congenital Malformations, Deformations and Chromosomal Abnormalities

Q75.4 **Mandibulofacial dysostosis**
Franceschetti syndrome
Treacher Collins syndrome

Q75.5 **Oculomandibular dysostosis**

Q75.8 **Other specified congenital malformations of skull and face bones**
Absence of skull bone, congenital
Congenital deformity of forehead
Platybasia

Q75.9 **Congenital malformation of skull and face bones, unspecified**
Congenital anomaly of face bones NOS
Congenital anomaly of skull NOS

✓4th **Q76** **Congenital malformations of spine and bony thorax**
EXCLUDES 1 congenital musculoskeletal deformities of spine and chest (Q67.5-Q67.8)

Q76.0 **Spina bifida occulta**
EXCLUDES 1 meningocele (spinal) (Q05.-)
spina bifida (aperta) (cystica) (Q05.-)

Q76.1 **Klippel-Feil syndrome**
Cervical fusion syndrome

Q76.2 **Congenital spondylolisthesis**
Congenital spondylolysis
EXCLUDES 1 spondylolisthesis (acquired) (M43.1-)
spondylolysis (acquired) (M43.0-)

Q76.3 **Congenital scoliosis due to congenital bony malformation**
Hemivertebra fusion or failure of segmentation with scoliosis

✓5th **Q76.4** **Other congenital malformations of spine, not associated with scoliosis**

✓6th **Q76.41** **Congenital kyphosis**
Q76.411 Congenital kyphosis, occipito-atlanto-axial region
Q76.412 Congenital kyphosis, cervical region
Q76.413 Congenital kyphosis, cervicothoracic region
Q76.414 Congenital kyphosis, thoracic region
Q76.415 Congenital kyphosis, thoracolumbar region
Q76.419 Congenital kyphosis, unspecified region

✓6th **Q76.42** **Congenital lordosis**
Q76.425 Congenital lordosis, thoracolumbar region
Q76.426 Congenital lordosis, lumbar region
Q76.427 Congenital lordosis, lumbosacral region
Q76.428 Congenital lordosis, sacral and sacrococcygeal region
Q76.429 Congenital lordosis, unspecified region

Q76.49 Other congenital malformations of spine, not associated with scoliosis
Congenital absence of vertebra NOS
Congenital fusion of spine NOS
Congenital malformation of lumbosacral (joint) (region) NOS
Congenital malformation of spine NOS
Hemivertebra NOS
Malformation of spine NOS
Platyspondylisis NOS
Supernumerary vertebra NOS

Q76.5 **Cervical rib**
Supernumerary rib in cervical region

Q76.6 **Other congenital malformations of ribs**
Accessory rib
Congenital absence of rib
Congenital fusion of ribs
Congenital malformation of ribs NOS
EXCLUDES 1 short rib syndrome (Q77.2)

Q76.7 **Congenital malformation of sternum**
Congenital absence of sternum
Sternum bifidum

Q76.8 **Other congenital malformations of bony thorax**

Q76.9 **Congenital malformation of bony thorax, unspecified**

✓4th **Q77** **Osteochondrodysplasia with defects of growth of tubular bones and spine**
EXCLUDES 1 mucopolysaccharidosis (E76.0-E76.3)
EXCLUDES 2 congenital myotonic chondrodystrophy (G71.13)

Q77.0 **Achondrogenesis** COM
Hypochondrogenesis

Q77.1 **Thanatophoric short stature** COM

Q77.2 **Short rib syndrome** COM
Asphyxiating thoracic dysplasia [Jeune]

Q77.3 **Chondrodysplasia punctata** COM
EXCLUDES 1 Rhizomelic chondrodysplasia punctata ▶(E71.540)◀

Q77.4 **Achondroplasia** COM
Hypochondroplasia
Osteosclerosis congenita

Q77.5 **Diastrophic dysplasia** COM

Q77.6 **Chondroectodermal dysplasia** COM
Ellis-van Creveld syndrome

Q77.7 **Spondyloepiphyseal dysplasia** COM

Q77.8 **Other osteochondrodysplasia with defects of growth of tubular bones and spine** COM

Q77.9 **Osteochondrodysplasia with defects of growth of tubular bones and spine, unspecified** COM

✓4th **Q78** **Other osteochondrodysplasias**
EXCLUDES 2 congenital myotonic chondrodystrophy (G71.13)

Q78.0 **Osteogenesis imperfecta** COM
Fragilitas ossium
Osteopsathyrosis

Q78.1 **Polyostotic fibrous dysplasia** COM
Albright(-McCune)(-Sternberg) syndrome

Q78.2 **Osteopetrosis** COM
Albers-Schonberg syndrome
Osteosclerosis NOS
DEF: Rare congenital condition in which the bones are excessively dense, resulting from a discrepancy in the formation and breakdown of bone.

Q78.3 **Progressive diaphyseal dysplasia** COM
Camurati-Engelmann syndrome

Q78.4 **Enchondromatosis** COM
Maffucci's syndrome
Ollier's disease

Q78.5 **Metaphyseal dysplasia** COM
Pyle's syndrome

Q78.6 **Multiple congenital exostoses** COM
Diaphyseal aclasis

Q78.8 **Other specified osteochondrodysplasias** COM
Osteopoikilosis

Q78.9 **Osteochondrodysplasia, unspecified** COM
Chondrodystrophy NOS
Osteodystrophy NOS

✓4th **Q79** **Congenital malformations of musculoskeletal system, not elsewhere classified**
EXCLUDES 2 congenital (sternomastoid) torticollis (Q68.0)

Q79.0 **Congenital diaphragmatic hernia** COM
EXCLUDES 1 congenital hiatus hernia (Q40.1)

Q79.1 **Other congenital malformations of diaphragm** COM
Absence of diaphragm
Congenital malformation of diaphragm NOS
Eventration of diaphragm

Q79.2 **Exomphalos** COM
Omphalocele
EXCLUDES 1 umbilical hernia (K42.-)

Q79.3 **Gastroschisis** COM

Gastroschisis
Herniated small bowel (gastroschisis)
Rectus abdominus m.
Umbilicus
distal
skin
proximal
Defect

Q79.4 **Prune belly syndrome** COM
Congenital prolapse of bladder mucosa
Eagle-Barrett syndrome

✓5th **Q79.5** **Other congenital malformations of abdominal wall**
EXCLUDES 1 umbilical hernia (K42.-)

Q79.51 Congenital hernia of bladder COM
Q79.59 Other congenital malformations of abdominal wall

Q79.6 Ehlers-Danlos syndromes
AHA: 2019,4Q,13-14
DEF: Connective tissue disorder that causes hyperextended skin and joints and results in fragile blood vessels with bleeding, poor wound healing, and subcutaneous pseudotumors.

- Q79.60 Ehlers-Danlos syndrome, unspecified
- Q79.61 Classical Ehlers-Danlos syndrome
  - Classical EDS (cEDS)
- Q79.62 Hypermobile Ehlers-Danlos syndrome
  - Hypermobile EDS (hEDS)
- Q79.63 Vascular Ehlers-Danlos syndrome
  - Vascular EDS (vEDS)
- Q79.69 Other Ehlers-Danlos syndromes

Q79.8 Other congenital malformations of musculoskeletal system
- Absence of muscle
- Absence of tendon
- Accessory muscle
- Amyotrophia congenita
- Congenital constricting bands
- Congenital shortening of tendon
- Poland syndrome

Q79.9 Congenital malformation of musculoskeletal system, unspecified
- Congenital anomaly of musculoskeletal system NOS
- Congenital deformity of musculoskeletal system NOS

Other congenital malformations (Q80-Q89)

Q80 Congenital ichthyosis
EXCLUDES 1: Refsum's disease (G60.1)
DEF: Excessive production of skin cells resulting in red, dry, scaly skin.

- Q80.0 Ichthyosis vulgaris
- Q80.1 X-linked ichthyosis
- Q80.2 Lamellar ichthyosis
  - Collodion baby
- Q80.3 Congenital bullous ichthyosiform erythroderma
- Q80.4 Harlequin fetus
- Q80.8 Other congenital ichthyosis
- Q80.9 Congenital ichthyosis, unspecified

Q81 Epidermolysis bullosa
- Q81.0 Epidermolysis bullosa simplex
  - **EXCLUDES 1:** Cockayne's syndrome (Q87.19)
- Q81.1 Epidermolysis bullosa letalis
  - Herlitz' syndrome
- Q81.2 Epidermolysis bullosa dystrophica
- Q81.8 Other epidermolysis bullosa
- Q81.9 Epidermolysis bullosa, unspecified

Q82 Other congenital malformations of skin
EXCLUDES 1:
- acrodermatitis enteropathica (E83.2)
- congenital erythropoietic porphyria (E80.0)
- pilonidal cyst or sinus (L05.-)
- Sturge-Weber (-Dimitri) syndrome (Q85.89)

- Q82.0 Hereditary lymphedema
- Q82.1 Xeroderma pigmentosum
- Q82.2 Congenital cutaneous mastocytosis
  - Congenital diffuse cutaneous mastocytosis
  - Congenital maculopapular cutaneous mastocytosis
  - Congenital urticaria pigmentosa
  - **EXCLUDES 1:**
    - cutaneous mastocytosis NOS (D47.01)
    - diffuse cutaneous mastocytosis (with onset after newborn period) (D47.01)
    - malignant mastocytosis (C96.2-)
    - systemic mastocytosis (D47.02)
    - urticaria pigmentosa (non-congenital) (with onset after newborn period) (D47.01)
  - **AHA:** 2017,4Q,5
- Q82.3 Incontinentia pigmenti
- Q82.4 Ectodermal dysplasia (anhidrotic)
  - **EXCLUDES 1:** Ellis-van Creveld syndrome (Q77.6)
- Q82.5 Congenital non-neoplastic nevus
  - Birthmark NOS
  - Flammeus Nevus
  - Portwine Nevus
  - Sanguineous Nevus
  - Strawberry Nevus
  - Vascular Nevus NOS
  - Verrucous Nevus
  - **EXCLUDES 2:**
    - araneus nevus (I78.1)
    - Cafe au lait spots (L81.3)
    - lentigo (L81.4)
    - melanocytic nevus (D22.-)
    - nevus NOS (D22.-)
    - pigmented nevus (D22.-)
    - spider nevus (I78.1)
    - stellar nevus (I78.1)
  - **AHA:** 2024,3Q,5
- Q82.6 Congenital sacral dimple
  - Parasacral dimple
  - **EXCLUDES 2:**
    - pilonidal cyst with abscess (L05.01)
    - pilonidal cyst without abscess (L05.91)
  - **AHA:** 2016,4Q,60
- Q82.8 Other specified congenital malformations of skin
  - Abnormal palmar creases
  - Accessory skin tags
  - Benign familial pemphigus [Hailey-Hailey]
  - Congenital poikiloderma
  - Cutis laxa (hyperelastica)
  - Dermatoglyphic anomalies
  - Inherited keratosis palmaris et plantaris
  - Keratosis follicularis [Darier-White]
  - **EXCLUDES 1:** Ehlers-Danlos syndromes (Q79.6-)
  - **EXCLUDES 2:** disorders of pyrophosphate metabolism (E83.82-)
  - **AHA:** 2021,3Q,10; 2016,1Q,17
- Q82.9 Congenital malformation of skin, unspecified

Q83 Congenital malformations of breast
EXCLUDES 2:
- absence of pectoral muscle (Q79.8)
- hypoplasia of breast (N64.82)
- micromastia (N64.82)

- Q83.0 Congenital absence of breast with absent nipple
- Q83.1 Accessory breast
  - Supernumerary breast
- Q83.2 Absent nipple
- Q83.3 Accessory nipple
  - Supernumerary nipple
- Q83.8 Other congenital malformations of breast
- Q83.9 Congenital malformation of breast, unspecified

Q84 Other congenital malformations of integument
- Q84.0 Congenital alopecia
  - Congenital atrichosis
- Q84.1 Congenital morphological disturbances of hair, not elsewhere classified
  - Beaded hair
  - Monilethrix
  - Pili annulati
  - **EXCLUDES 1:** Menkes' kinky hair syndrome (E83.09)
- Q84.2 Other congenital malformations of hair
  - Congenital hypertrichosis
  - Congenital malformation of hair NOS
  - Persistent lanugo
- Q84.3 Anonychia
  - **EXCLUDES 1:** nail patella syndrome (Q87.2)
- Q84.4 Congenital leukonychia
- Q84.5 Enlarged and hypertrophic nails
  - Congenital onychauxis
  - Pachyonychia
- Q84.6 Other congenital malformations of nails
  - Congenital clubnail
  - Congenital koilonychia
  - Congenital malformation of nail NOS
- Q84.8 Other specified congenital malformations of integument
  - Aplasia cutis congenita
- Q84.9 Congenital malformation of integument, unspecified
  - Congenital anomaly of integument NOS
  - Congenital deformity of integument NOS

Q85 Phakomatoses, not elsewhere classified

EXCLUDES 1 *ataxia telangiectasia [Louis-Bar] (G11.3)*
familial dysautonomia [Riley-Day] (G90.1)

Q85.0 Neurofibromatosis (nonmalignant)

Q85.00 Neurofibromatosis, unspecified HCC ESR COM

Q85.01 Neurofibromatosis, type 1 HCC ESR COM
Von Recklinghausen disease

Q85.02 Neurofibromatosis, type 2 HCC ESR COM
Acoustic neurofibromatosis
DEF: Inherited condition with cutaneous lesions, benign tumors of peripheral nerves, and bilateral 8th nerve masses.

Q85.03 Schwannomatosis HCC ESR COM
DEF: Genetic mutation (SMARCB1/INI1) causing multiple benign tumors along the nerve pathways, except on the 8th cranial (vestibular) nerve.

Q85.09 Other neurofibromatosis HCC ESR COM

Q85.1 Tuberous sclerosis HCC Rx ESR COM
Bourneville's disease
Epiloia

Q85.8 Other phakomatoses, not elsewhere classified

EXCLUDES 1 *Meckel-Gruber syndrome (Q61.9)*
AHA: 2022,4Q,40-41; 2021,3Q,12

Q85.81 PTEN hamartoma tumor syndrome HCC Rx ESR COM
PHTS
PTEN related Cowden syndrome
Code also, if applicable, genetic susceptibility to malignant neoplasm (Z15.0-)
AHA: 2022,4Q,41
TIP: PTEN hamartoma tumor syndrome (PHTS) manifests differently in each patient. Separate codes should be assigned in addition to code Q85.81 for any manifestations of PHTS, such as macrocephaly, autism, or learning delays.

Q85.82 Other Cowden syndrome HCC Rx ESR COM

Q85.83 Von Hippel-Lindau syndrome HCC Rx ESR COM
Code also manifestations
AHA: 2023,2Q,16

Q85.89 Other phakomatoses, not elsewhere classified HCC Rx ESR COM
Peutz-Jeghers syndrome
Sturge-Weber(-Dimitri) syndrome

Q85.9 Phakomatosis, unspecified HCC Rx ESR COM
Hamartosis NOS

Q86 Congenital malformation syndromes due to known exogenous causes, not elsewhere classified

EXCLUDES 2 *iodine-deficiency-related hypothyroidism (E00-E02)*
nonteratogenic effects of substances transmitted via placenta or breast milk (P04.-)

Q86.0 Fetal alcohol syndrome (dysmorphic) COM

Q86.1 Fetal hydantoin syndrome COM
Meadow's syndrome

Q86.2 Dysmorphism due to warfarin COM

Q86.8 Other congenital malformation syndromes due to known exogenous causes COM

Q87 Other specified congenital malformation syndromes affecting multiple systems

Use additional code(s) to identify all associated manifestations

Q87.0 Congenital malformation syndromes predominantly affecting facial appearance
Acrocephalopolysyndactyly
Acrocephalosyndactyly [Apert]
Cryptophthalmos syndrome
Cyclopia
Goldenhar syndrome
Moebius syndrome
Oro-facial-digital syndrome
Robin syndrome
Whistling face

Q87.1 Congenital malformation syndromes predominantly associated with short stature

EXCLUDES 1 *Ellis-van Creveld syndrome (Q77.6)*
Smith-Lemli-Opitz syndrome (E78.72)
AHA: 2019,4Q,14-15

Q87.11 Prader-Willi syndrome Rx COM
AHA: 2024,4Q,11

Q87.19 Other congenital malformation syndromes predominantly associated with short stature COM
Aarskog syndrome
Cockayne syndrome
De Lange syndrome
Dubowitz syndrome
Noonan syndrome
Robinow-Silverman-Smith syndrome
Russell-Silver syndrome
Seckel syndrome

Q87.2 Congenital malformation syndromes predominantly involving limbs COM
Holt-Oram syndrome
Klippel-Trenaunay-Weber syndrome
Nail patella syndrome
Rubinstein-Taybi syndrome
Sirenomelia syndrome
Thrombocytopenia with absent radius [TAR] syndrome
VATER syndrome

Q87.3 Congenital malformation syndromes involving early overgrowth COM
Beckwith-Wiedemann syndrome
Sotos syndrome
Weaver syndrome

Q87.4 Marfan syndrome
DEF: Disorder that affects the connective tissue of multiple systems, including disproportionally long or abnormal bone structure and eye and cardiovascular complications.

Q87.40 Marfan syndrome, unspecified Rx COM

Q87.41 Marfan syndrome with cardiovascular manifestations

Q87.410 Marfan syndrome with aortic dilation Rx COM

Q87.418 Marfan syndrome with other cardiovascular manifestations Rx COM

Q87.42 Marfan syndrome with ocular manifestations Rx COM

Q87.43 Marfan syndrome with skeletal manifestation Rx COM

Q87.5 Other congenital malformation syndromes with other skeletal changes COM

Q87.8 Other specified congenital malformation syndromes, not elsewhere classified

EXCLUDES 1 *Zellweger syndrome (E71.510)*
AHA: 2023,4Q,39-40

Q87.81 Alport syndrome COM
Use additional code to identify stage of chronic kidney disease (N18.1-N18.6)

Q87.82 Arterial tortuosity syndrome Rx COM
AHA: 2016,4Q,60-61

Q87.83 Bardet-Biedl syndrome COM

Q87.84 Laurence-Moon syndrome COM

Q87.85 MED13L syndrome COM
Asadollahi-Rauch syndrome
Mediator complex subunit 13L syndrome
Code also, if applicable, any associated manifestations such as:
autism spectrum disorder (F84.0-)
congenital malformations of cardiac septa (Q21.-)
epilepsy and recurrent seizures (G40.-)
intellectual disability (F70-F79)

Q87.86 Kleefstra syndrome Rx COM
AHA: 2024,4Q,27

● **Q87.87 Hao-Fountain Syndrome**
HAFOUS
Use additional code, if applicable, for associated conditions such as:
autism spectrum disorder (F84.0)
developmental speech disorder (F80.-)
epilepsy, by specific type (G40.-)
intellectual disabilities (F70-F79)
pervasive developmental disorders (F84.-)

- **Q87.88** **CTNNB1** syndrome
  Use additional code, if applicable, for associated conditions such as:
  cerebral palsy (G80.-)
  congenital heart malformations (Q20.0-Q24.9)
  developmental disorder of speech and language (F80.-)
  exudative retinopathy (H35.02-)
  intellectual disability (F70-F79)
  microcephaly (Q02)
- **Q87.89** Other specified congenital malformation syndromes, not elsewhere classified   COM

Q89 Other congenital malformations, not elsewhere classified

- **Q89.0** Congenital absence and malformations of **spleen**
  EXCLUDES 1: isomerism of atrial appendages (with asplenia or polysplenia) (Q20.6)
  - **Q89.01** Asplenia (congenital)
    AHA: 2025,1Q,24
  - **Q89.09** Congenital malformations of spleen
    Congenital splenomegaly
- **Q89.1** Congenital malformations of **adrenal gland**
  EXCLUDES 1: adrenogenital disorders (E25.-)
  congenital adrenal hyperplasia (E25.0)
- **Q89.2** Congenital malformations of other endocrine glands
  Congenital malformation of parathyroid or thyroid gland
  Persistent thyroglossal duct
  Thyroglossal cyst
  EXCLUDES 1: congenital goiter (E03.0)
  congenital hypothyroidism (E03.1)
- **Q89.3** Situs inversus   COM
  Dextrocardia with situs inversus
  Mirror-image atrial arrangement with situs inversus
  Situs inversus or transversus abdominalis
  Situs inversus or transversus thoracis
  Transposition of abdominal viscera
  Transposition of thoracic viscera
  EXCLUDES 1: dextrocardia NOS (Q24.0)
  DEF: Congenital anomaly in which the internal thoracic and abdominal organs are transposed laterally and found on the opposite side from the normal position.
- **Q89.4** Conjoined twins   COM
  Craniopagus
  Dicephaly
  Pygopagus
  Thoracopagus
- **Q89.7** Multiple congenital malformations, not elsewhere classified
  Multiple congenital anomalies NOS
  Multiple congenital deformities NOS
  EXCLUDES 1: congenital malformation syndromes affecting multiple systems (Q87.-)
- ▲ **Q89.8** Other specified congenital malformations
  Use additional code(s) to identify all associated manifestations
  AHA: 2021,3Q,12
  - **Q89.81** **Kabuki** syndrome
    Kabuki syndrome, type 1, due to KMT2D mutation
    Kabuki syndrome, type 2, due to KDM6A mutation
    Niikawa-Kuroki syndrome
- • **Q89.89** Other specified congenital malformations
- **Q89.9** Congenital malformation, unspecified
  Congenital anomaly NOS
  Congenital deformity NOS

Chromosomal abnormalities, not elsewhere classified (Q90-Q99)

EXCLUDES 2: mitochondrial metabolic disorders (E88.4-)

Q90 Down syndrome
Code also associated physical condition(s), such as atrioventricular septal defect (Q21.2-)
Use additional code(s) to identify any associated degree of intellectual disabilities (F70-F79)
- **Q90.0** Trisomy 21, **nonmosaicism** (meiotic nondisjunction)   COM
- **Q90.1** Trisomy 21, **mosaicism** (mitotic nondisjunction)   COM
- **Q90.2** Trisomy 21, **translocation**   COM
- **Q90.9** Down syndrome, unspecified   COM
  Trisomy 21 NOS

Q91 Trisomy 18 and Trisomy 13

- **Q91.0** Trisomy **18, nonmosaicism** (meiotic nondisjunction)   Rx COM
- **Q91.1** Trisomy **18, mosaicism** (mitotic nondisjunction)   Rx COM
- **Q91.2** Trisomy **18, translocation**   Rx COM
- **Q91.3** Trisomy 18, unspecified   Rx COM
- **Q91.4** Trisomy **13, nonmosaicism** (meiotic nondisjunction)   Rx COM
- **Q91.5** Trisomy **13, mosaicism** (mitotic nondisjunction)   Rx COM
- **Q91.6** Trisomy **13, translocation**   Rx COM
- **Q91.7** Trisomy 13, unspecified   Rx COM

Q92 Other trisomies and partial trisomies of the autosomes, not elsewhere classified
INCLUDES: unbalanced translocations and insertions
EXCLUDES 1: trisomies of chromosomes 13, 18, 21 (Q90-Q91)

- **Q92.0** **Whole** chromosome trisomy, **nonmosaicism** (meiotic nondisjunction)   Rx COM
- **Q92.1** **Whole** chromosome trisomy, **mosaicism** (mitotic nondisjunction)   Rx COM
- **Q92.2** **Partial** trisomy   Rx COM
  Less than whole arm duplicated
  Whole arm or more duplicated
  EXCLUDES 1: partial trisomy due to unbalanced translocation (Q92.5)
- **Q92.5** **Duplications** with other complex rearrangements   Rx COM
  Partial trisomy due to unbalanced translocations
  Code also any associated deletions due to unbalanced translocations, inversions and insertions (Q93.7)
- **Q92.6** Marker chromosomes
  Individual with marker heterochromatin
  Trisomies due to dicentrics
  Trisomies due to extra rings
  Trisomies due to isochromosomes
  - **Q92.61** Marker chromosomes in **normal** individual   Rx COM
  - **Q92.62** Marker chromosomes in **abnormal** individual   Rx COM
- **Q92.7** Triploidy and polyploidy   Rx COM
- **Q92.8** Other specified trisomies and partial trisomies of autosomes   Rx COM
  Duplications identified by fluorescence in situ hybridization (FISH)
  Duplications identified by in situ hybridization (ISH)
  Duplications seen only at prometaphase
- **Q92.9** Trisomy and partial trisomy of autosomes, unspecified   Rx COM

Q93 Monosomies and deletions from the autosomes, not elsewhere classified

- **Q93.0** **Whole** chromosome monosomy, **nonmosaicism** (meiotic nondisjunction)   Rx COM
- **Q93.1** **Whole** chromosome monosomy, **mosaicism** (mitotic nondisjunction)   Rx COM
- **Q93.2** Chromosome **replaced with ring**, dicentric or isochromosome
- **Q93.3** Deletion of short arm of chromosome 4   Rx COM
  Wolff-Hirschorn syndrome
- **Q93.4** Deletion of short arm of chromosome 5
  Cri-du-chat syndrome
- **Q93.5** Other deletions of **part of a chromosome**
  AHA: 2018,4Q,28
  - **Q93.51** Angelman syndrome   Rx COM
  - **Q93.52** Phelan-McDermid syndrome   Rx COM
    22q13.3 deletion syndrome
    Use additional code(s) to identify any associated conditions, such as:
    autism spectrum disorder (F84.0)
    degree of intellectual disabilities (F70-F79)
    epilepsy and recurrent seizures (G40.-)
    lymphedema (I89.0)
    AHA: 2023,4Q,40-41
  - **Q93.59** Other deletions of part of a chromosome   Rx COM
- **Q93.7** Deletions with other complex rearrangements   Rx COM
  Deletions due to unbalanced translocations, inversions and insertions
  Code also any associated duplications due to unbalanced translocations, inversions and insertions (Q92.5)

Chapter 17. Congenital Malformations, Deformations and Chromosomal Abnormalities

✓5th Q93.8 Other deletions from the autosomes

    Q93.81 Velo-cardio-facial syndrome [Rx] [COM]
        Deletion 22q11.2
        AHA: 2019,3Q,14
        DEF: Microdeletion syndrome affecting multiple organs characterized by a cleft palate, heart defects, an elongated face with almond-shaped eyes, wide nose, small ears, weak immune system, weak musculature, hypothyroidism, short stature, and scoliosis. The deletion occurs at q11.2 on the long arm of the chromosome 22.

    Q93.82 Williams syndrome [Rx] [COM]
        AHA: 2018,4Q,28-29

    Q93.88 Other microdeletions [Rx] [COM]
        Miller-Dieker syndrome
        Smith-Magenis syndrome

    Q93.89 Other deletions from the autosomes [Rx] [COM]
        Deletions identified by fluorescence in situ hybridization (FISH)
        Deletions identified by in situ hybridization (ISH)
        Deletions seen only at prometaphase

    Q93.9 Deletion from autosomes, unspecified [Rx] [COM]

✓4th Q95 Balanced rearrangements and structural markers, not elsewhere classified

    INCLUDES Robertsonian and balanced reciprocal translocations and insertions

    Q95.0 Balanced translocation and insertion in normal individual
    Q95.1 Chromosome inversion in normal individual
    Q95.2 Balanced autosomal rearrangement in abnormal individual [Rx] [COM]
    Q95.3 Balanced sex/autosomal rearrangement in abnormal individual [Rx] [COM]
    Q95.5 Individual with autosomal fragile site
    Q95.8 Other balanced rearrangements and structural markers
    Q95.9 Balanced rearrangement and structural marker, unspecified

✓4th Q96 Turner's syndrome

    EXCLUDES 1 Noonan syndrome (Q87.19)

    Q96.0 Karyotype 45, X [COM]
    Q96.1 Karyotype 46, X iso (Xq) [COM]
        Karyotype 46, isochromosome Xq
    Q96.2 Karyotype 46, X with abnormal sex chromosome, except iso (Xq) [COM]
        Karyotype 46, X with abnormal sex chromosome, except isochromosome Xq
    Q96.3 Mosaicism, 45, X/46, XX or XY [COM]
    Q96.4 Mosaicism, 45, X/other cell line(s) with abnormal sex chromosome [COM]
    Q96.8 Other variants of Turner's syndrome [COM]
    Q96.9 Turner's syndrome, unspecified [COM]

✓4th Q97 Other sex chromosome abnormalities, female phenotype, not elsewhere classified

    EXCLUDES 1 Turner's syndrome (Q96.-)

    Q97.0 Karyotype 47, XXX [COM]
    Q97.1 Female with more than three X chromosomes [COM]
    Q97.2 Mosaicism, lines with various numbers of X chromosomes [COM]
    Q97.3 Female with 46, XY karyotype [COM]
    Q97.8 Other specified sex chromosome abnormalities, female phenotype [COM]
    Q97.9 Sex chromosome abnormality, female phenotype, unspecified [COM]

✓4th Q98 Other sex chromosome abnormalities, male phenotype, not elsewhere classified

    Q98.0 Klinefelter syndrome karyotype 47, XXY [COM]
    Q98.1 Klinefelter syndrome, male with more than two X chromosomes [COM]
    Q98.3 Other male with 46, XX karyotype [COM]
    Q98.4 Klinefelter syndrome, unspecified [COM]
    Q98.5 Karyotype 47, XYY
    Q98.6 Male with structurally abnormal sex chromosome [COM]
    Q98.7 Male with sex chromosome mosaicism [COM]
    Q98.8 Other specified sex chromosome abnormalities, male phenotype
    Q98.9 Sex chromosome abnormality, male phenotype, unspecified [COM]

✓4th Q99 Other chromosome abnormalities, not elsewhere classified

    Q99.0 Chimera 46, XX/46, XY [COM]
        Chimera 46, XX/46, XY true hermaphrodite
    Q99.1 46, XX true hermaphrodite [COM]
        46, XX with streak gonads
        46, XY with streak gonads
        Pure gonadal dysgenesis
    Q99.2 Fragile X chromosome [Rx] [COM]
        Fragile X syndrome
    ✓5th Q99.8 Other specified chromosome abnormalities
        ✓6th Q99.81 Usher syndrome
            Use additional code to identify any auditory and visual manifestations
            Q99.811 Usher syndrome, type 1
            Q99.812 Usher syndrome, type 2
            Q99.813 Usher syndrome, type 3
            Q99.818 Other Usher syndrome
                Usher syndrome, type 4
            Q99.819 Usher syndrome, unspecified
        Q99.89 Other specified chromosome abnormalities
    Q99.9 Chromosomal abnormality, unspecified [COM]

Genetic disorders, not elsewhere classified (QA0)

✓4th QA0 Neurodevelopmental disorders related to specific genetic pathogenic variants

    Code also, if applicable, any associated conditions, such as:
        attention-deficit hyperactivity disorders (F90.-)
        autism spectrum disorder (F84.0)
        developmental and epileptic encephalopathy (G93.45)
        epilepsy, by specific type (G40.-)
        intellectual disabilities (F70-F79)
        pervasive developmental disorders (F84.-)

    ✓5th QA0.0 Neurodevelopmental disorders related to pathogenic variants in specific genes
        ✓6th QA0.01 Neurodevelopmental disorders related to pathogenic variants in certain specific genes
            ✓7th QA0.010 Neurodevelopmental disorders, related to pathogenic variants in ion channel genes
                QA0.0101 SCN2A-related neurodevelopmental disorder
                QA0.0102 CACNA1A-related neurodevelopmental disorder
                QA0.0109 Neurodevelopmental disorder related to pathogenic variant in other ion channel gene
                    SCN8A-related neurodevelopmental disorder
            QA0.011 Neurodevelopmental disorders, related to pathogenic variants in glutamate receptor genes
            QA0.012 Neurodevelopmental disorders, related to pathogenic variants in other receptor genes
            ✓7th QA0.013 Neurodevelopmental disorders, related to pathogenic variants in other transporter and solute carrier genes
                QA0.0131 SLC6A1-related disorder
                    GABA transporter 1 deficiency
                QA0.0139 Neurodevelopmental disorder, related to pathogenic variant in other transporter or solute carrier gene
            ✓7th QA0.014 Neurodevelopmental disorders, related to pathogenic variants in synapse related genes
                QA0.0141 Syntaxin-binding protein 1-related disorder
                    STXBP1-related disorders
                QA0.0142 DLG4-related synaptopathy
                QA0.0149 Neurodevelopmental disorder, related to pathogenic variant in other synapse related gene
                    Other genetic synaptopathy
            ✓7th QA0.015 Neurodevelopmental disorders, related to genes associated with transcription and gene expression

- QA0.0151 **FOXG1 syndrome**
  FOXG1-related disorder
  FOXG1-related encephalopathy
  FOXG1-related neurodevelopmental disorder
- QA0.0159 **Neurodevelopmental disorder, related to other genes associated with transcription and gene expression**
- QA0.8 **Other neurodevelopmental disorders related to pathogenic variants in other specific genes**

Chapter 18. Symptoms, Signs, and Abnormal Clinical and Laboratory Findings, Not Elsewhere Classified (R00–R99)

Chapter-specific Guidelines with Coding Examples

The chapter-specific guidelines from the ICD-10-CM Official Guidelines for Coding and Reporting have been provided below. Along with these guidelines are coding examples, contained in the shaded boxes, that have been developed to help illustrate the coding and/or sequencing guidance found in these guidelines.

Chapter 18 includes symptoms, signs, abnormal results of clinical or other investigative procedures, and ill-defined conditions regarding which no diagnosis classifiable elsewhere is recorded. Signs and symptoms that point to a specific diagnosis have been assigned to a category in other chapters of the classification.

a. Use of symptom codes

Codes that describe symptoms and signs are acceptable for reporting purposes when a related definitive diagnosis has not been established (confirmed) by the provider.

> Tenderness and localized pain in the right upper quadrant; based on presentation, probable gallstones
>
> | R10.11 | Right upper quadrant pain |
> |---|---|
> | R10.811 | Right upper quadrant abdominal tenderness |
>
> *Explanation:* Codes that describe symptoms such as abdominal pain are acceptable for reporting purposes when the provider has not established (confirmed) a definitive diagnosis.

b. Use of a symptom code with a definitive diagnosis code

Codes for signs and symptoms may be reported in addition to a related definitive diagnosis when the sign or symptom is not routinely associated with that diagnosis, such as the various signs and symptoms associated with complex syndromes. The definitive diagnosis code should be sequenced before the symptom code.

Signs or symptoms that are associated routinely with a disease process should not be assigned as additional codes, unless otherwise instructed by the classification.

> Pneumonia with hemoptysis
>
> | J18.9 | Pneumonia, unspecified organism |
> |---|---|
> | R04.2 | Hemoptysis |
>
> *Explanation:* Codes for signs and symptoms may be reported in addition to a related definitive diagnosis when the sign or symptom is not routinely associated with that diagnosis.

> Abdominal pain due to acute appendicitis
>
> | K35.80 | Unspecified acute appendicitis |
> |---|---|
>
> *Explanation:* Codes for signs or symptoms routinely associated with a disease process should not be assigned unless the classification instructs otherwise.

c. Combination codes that include symptoms

ICD-10-CM contains a number of combination codes that identify both the definitive diagnosis and common symptoms of that diagnosis. When using one of these combination codes, an additional code should not be assigned for the symptom.

> IBS with diarrhea
>
> | K58.0 | Irritable bowel syndrome with diarrhea |
> |---|---|
>
> *Explanation:* When a combination code identifies both the definitive diagnosis and the symptom, an additional code should not be assigned for the symptom.

d. Repeated falls

Code R29.6, Repeated falls, is for use for encounters when a patient has recently fallen and the reason for the fall is being investigated.

Code Z91.81, History of falling, is for use when a patient has fallen in the past and is at risk for future falls. When appropriate, both codes R29.6 and Z91.81 may be assigned together.

e. Coma

Code R40.20, Unspecified coma, should be assigned when the underlying cause of the coma is not known, or the cause is a traumatic brain injury and the coma scale is not documented in the medical record.

Do not report codes for unspecified coma, individual or total Glasgow coma scale scores for a patient with a medically induced coma or a sedated patient.

1) Coma scale

The coma scale codes (R40.21- to R40.24-) can be used in conjunction with traumatic brain injury codes. These codes cannot be used with R40.2A, Nontraumatic coma due to underlying condition. They are primarily for use by trauma registries, but they may be used in any setting where this information is collected. The coma scale codes should be sequenced after the diagnosis code(s).

These codes, one from each subcategory, are needed to complete the scale. The 7th character indicates when the scale was recorded. The 7th character should match for all three codes.

At a minimum, report the initial score documented on presentation at your facility. This may be a score from the emergency medicine technician (EMT) or in the emergency department. If desired, a facility may choose to capture multiple coma scale scores.

Assign code R40.24-, Glasgow coma scale, total score, when only the total score is documented in the medical record and not the individual score(s).

If multiple coma scores are captured within the first 24 hours after hospital admission, assign only the code for the score at the time of admission. ICD-10-CM does not classify coma scores that are reported after admission but less than 24 hours later.

See Section I.B.14. for coma scale documentation by clinicians other than patient's provider

> 36-year-old man found down after unknown injury with skull fracture and with concussion and loss of consciousness of unknown duration. Upon hospital admission, the patient was evaluated with the following Glasgow coma scores:
>
> Eye-opening response—3: eyes open to speech
>
> Verbal response—3: random speech with no conversational exchange
>
> Motor response—4: pulls limb away from painful stimulus
>
> | S02.0XXA | Fracture of vault of skull, initial encounter for closed fracture |
> |---|---|
> | S06.0X9A | Concussion with loss of consciousness of unspecified duration, initial encounter |
> | R40.2133 | Coma scale, eyes open, to sound, at hospital admission |
> | R40.2233 | Coma scale, best verbal response, inappropriate words, at hospital admission |
> | R40.2343 | Coma scale, best motor response, flexion withdrawal, at hospital admission |
>
> *Explanation:* When individual scores for the Glasgow coma scale are documented, one code from each category is needed to complete the scale. The seventh character indicates when the scale was recorded and should match for all three codes. Assign a code from subcategory R40.24- Glasgow coma scale, total score, when only the total and not the individual score(s) is documented.

f. Functional quadriplegia

GUIDELINE HAS BEEN DELETED EFFECTIVE OCTOBER 1, 2017

g. SIRS due to non-infectious process

The systemic inflammatory response syndrome (SIRS) can develop as a result of certain non-infectious disease processes, such as trauma, malignant neoplasm, or pancreatitis. When SIRS is documented with a noninfectious condition, and no subsequent infection is documented, the code for the underlying condition, such as an injury, should be assigned, followed by code R65.10, Systemic inflammatory response syndrome (SIRS) of non-infectious origin without acute organ dysfunction, or code R65.11, Systemic inflammatory response syndrome (SIRS) of non-infectious origin with acute organ dysfunction. If an associated acute organ dysfunction is documented, the appropriate code(s) for the specific type of organ dysfunction(s) should be assigned in addition to code R65.11. If acute organ dysfunction is documented, but it cannot be determined if the acute organ dysfunction is associated with SIRS or due to another condition (e.g., directly due to the trauma), the provider should be queried.

> Systemic inflammatory response syndrome (SIRS) due to acute gallstone pancreatitis
>
> **K85.10** Biliary acute pancreatitis without necrosis or infection
>
> **R65.10** Systemic inflammatory response syndrome [SIRS] of non-infectious origin without acute organ dysfunction
>
> *Explanation:* When SIRS is documented with a non-infectious condition without subsequent infection documented, the code for the underlying condition such as pancreatitis should be assigned followed by the appropriate code for SIRS of noninfectious origin, either with or without associated organ dysfunction.

h. **Death NOS**

Code R99, Ill-defined and unknown cause of mortality, is only for use in the very limited circumstance when a patient who has already died is brought into an emergency department or other healthcare facility and is pronounced dead upon arrival. It does not represent the discharge disposition of death.

i. **NIHSS stroke scale**

The NIH stroke scale (NIHSS) codes (R29.7- -) can be used in conjunction with acute stroke codes (I60-I63) to idenICD-10-CM 2026tify the patient's neurological status and the severity of the stroke. The stroke scale codes should be sequenced after the acute stroke diagnosis code(s).

At a minimum, report the initial score documented. If desired, a facility may choose to capture multiple stroke scale scores.

See Section I.B.14. for NIHSS stroke scale documentation by clinicians other than patient's provider

Chapter 18. Symptoms, Signs and Abnormal Clinical and Laboratory Findings, Not Elsewhere Classified (R00-R99)

NOTE This chapter includes symptoms, signs, abnormal results of clinical or other investigative procedures, and ill-defined conditions regarding which no diagnosis classifiable elsewhere is recorded.

Signs and symptoms that point rather definitely to a given diagnosis have been assigned to a category in other chapters of the classification. In general, categories in this chapter include the less well-defined conditions and symptoms that, without the necessary study of the case to establish a final diagnosis, point perhaps equally to two or more diseases or to two or more systems of the body. Practically all categories in the chapter could be designated 'not otherwise specified', 'unknown etiology' or 'transient'. The Alphabetical Index should be consulted to determine which symptoms and signs are to be allocated here and which to other chapters. The residual subcategories, numbered .8, are generally provided for other relevant symptoms that cannot be allocated elsewhere in the classification.

The conditions and signs or symptoms included in categories R00-R94 consist of:

(a) cases for which no more specific diagnosis can be made even after all the facts bearing on the case have been investigated;

(b) signs or symptoms existing at the time of initial encounter that proved to be transient and whose causes could not be determined;

(c) provisional diagnosis in a patient who failed to return for further investigation or care;

(d) cases referred elsewhere for investigation or treatment before the diagnosis was made;

(e) cases in which a more precise diagnosis was not available for any other reason;

(f) certain symptoms, for which supplementary information is provided, that represent important problems in medical care in their own right.

EXCLUDES 2 abnormal findings on antenatal screening of mother (O28.-)
certain conditions originating in the perinatal period (P04-P96)
signs and symptoms classified in the body system chapters
signs and symptoms of breast (N63, N64.5)

AHA: 2017,1Q,6,7

This chapter contains the following blocks:

- R00-R09 Symptoms and signs involving the circulatory and respiratory systems
- R10-R19 Symptoms and signs involving the digestive system and abdomen
- R20-R23 Symptoms and signs involving the skin and subcutaneous tissue
- R25-R29 Symptoms and signs involving the nervous and musculoskeletal systems
- R30-R39 Symptoms and signs involving the genitourinary system
- R40-R46 Symptoms and signs involving cognition, perception, emotional state and behavior
- R47-R49 Symptoms and signs involving speech and voice
- R50-R69 General symptoms and signs
- R70-R79 Abnormal findings on examination of blood, without diagnosis
- R80-R82 Abnormal findings on examination of urine, without diagnosis
- R83-R89 Abnormal findings on examination of other body fluids, substances and tissues, without diagnosis
- R90-R94 Abnormal findings on diagnostic imaging and in function studies, without diagnosis
- R97 Abnormal tumor markers
- R99 Ill-defined and unknown cause of mortality

Symptoms and signs involving the circulatory and respiratory systems (R00-R09)

R00 Abnormalities of heart beat
EXCLUDES 1 abnormalities originating in the perinatal period (P29.1-)
EXCLUDES 2 specified arrhythmias (I47-I49)

R00.0 Tachycardia, unspecified
Rapid heart beat
Sinoauricular tachycardia NOS
Sinus [sinusal] tachycardia NOS
EXCLUDES 1 inappropriate sinus tachycardia, so stated (I47.11)
neonatal tachycardia (P29.11)
paroxysmal tachycardia (I47.-)
AHA: 2022,4Q,46
DEF: Excessively rapid heart rate of more than 100 beats per minute.

R00.1 Bradycardia, unspecified
Sinoatrial bradycardia
Sinus bradycardia
Slow heart beat
Vagal bradycardia
Use additional code for adverse effect, if applicable, to identify drug (T36-T50 with fifth or sixth character 5)
EXCLUDES 1 neonatal bradycardia (P29.12)
AHA: 2020,2Q,23
DEF: Slowed heartbeat, usually defined as a rate fewer than 60 beats per minute. Heart rhythm may be slow as a result of a congenital defect or an acquired problem.

R00.2 Palpitations
Awareness of heart beat

R00.8 Other abnormalities of heart beat

R00.9 Unspecified abnormalities of heart beat

R01 Cardiac murmurs and other cardiac sounds
EXCLUDES 1 cardiac murmurs and sounds originating in the perinatal period (P29.8)

R01.0 Benign and innocent cardiac murmurs
Functional cardiac murmur

R01.1 Cardiac murmur, unspecified
Cardiac bruit NOS
Heart murmur NOS
Systolic murmur NOS

R01.2 Other cardiac sounds
Cardiac dullness, increased or decreased
Precordial friction

R03 Abnormal blood-pressure reading, without diagnosis

R03.0 Elevated blood-pressure reading, without diagnosis of hypertension
NOTE This category is to be used to record an episode of elevated blood pressure in a patient in whom no formal diagnosis of hypertension has been made, or as an isolated incidental finding.

R03.1 Nonspecific low blood-pressure reading
EXCLUDES 1 hypotension (I95.-)
maternal hypotension syndrome (O26.5-)
neurogenic orthostatic hypotension (G90.3)

R04 Hemorrhage from respiratory passages

R04.0 Epistaxis
Hemorrhage from nose
Nosebleed
AHA: 2023,2Q,28

R04.1 Hemorrhage from throat
EXCLUDES 2 hemoptysis (R04.2)

R04.2 Hemoptysis
Blood-stained sputum
Cough with hemorrhage
AHA: 2013,4Q,118

R04.8 Hemorrhage from other sites in respiratory passages

R04.81 Acute idiopathic pulmonary hemorrhage in infants
Acute idiopathic hemorrhage in infants over 28 days old
AIPHI
EXCLUDES 1 perinatal pulmonary hemorrhage (P26.-)
von Willebrand disease (D68.0-)

R04.89 Hemorrhage from other sites in respiratory passages
Pulmonary hemorrhage NOS

R04.9 Hemorrhage from respiratory passages, unspecified

R05 Cough
EXCLUDES 1 paroxysmal cough due to Bordetella pertussis (A37.0-)
smoker's cough (J41.0)
EXCLUDES 2 cough with hemorrhage (R04.2)
AHA: 2021,4Q,24-25; 2016,2Q,33

R05.1 Acute cough

R05.2 Subacute cough

R05.3 Chronic cough
Persistent cough
Refractory cough
Unexplained cough

R05.4 Cough syncope
Code first syncope and collapse (R55)

R05.8 Other specified cough

R05.9 Cough, unspecified

R06 Abnormalities of breathing ✓4th

EXCLUDES 1: acute respiratory distress syndrome (J80)
respiratory arrest (R09.2)
respiratory arrest of newborn (P28.81)
respiratory distress syndrome of newborn (P22.-)
respiratory failure (J96.-)
respiratory failure of newborn (P28.5)

R06.0 Dyspnea ✓5th
EXCLUDES 1: tachypnea NOS (R06.82)
transient tachypnea of newborn (P22.1)

- **R06.00** Dyspnea, unspecified
  AHA: 2017,1Q,26
- **R06.01** Orthopnea
- **R06.02** Shortness of breath
- **R06.03** Acute respiratory distress
  AHA: 2017,4Q,23
- **R06.09** Other forms of dyspnea

R06.1 Stridor
EXCLUDES 1: congenital laryngeal stridor (P28.89)
laryngismus (stridulus) (J38.5)
DEF: Certain type of wheezing described as a loud, constant, musical sound produced when breathing with an obstructed airway, like the inspiratory sound heard when laryngeal or esophageal obstruction is present.

R06.2 Wheezing
EXCLUDES 1: asthma (J45.-)
AHA: 2016,2Q,33
DEF: High-pitched whistling sound during breathing due to stenosis of the respiratory passageway. Wheezing is associated with asthma, sleep apnea, bronchiectasis, bronchiolitis, COPD, and pleural effusion.

R06.3 Periodic breathing
Cheyne-Stokes breathing

R06.4 Hyperventilation
EXCLUDES 1: psychogenic hyperventilation (F45.8)

R06.5 Mouth breathing
EXCLUDES 2: dry mouth NOS (R68.2)

R06.6 Hiccough
EXCLUDES 1: psychogenic hiccough (F45.8)

R06.7 Sneezing

R06.8 Other abnormalities of breathing ✓5th
- **R06.81** Apnea, not elsewhere classified
  Apnea NOS
  EXCLUDES 1: apnea (of) newborn (P28.4-)
  sleep apnea (G47.3-)
  sleep apnea of newborn (primary) (P28.3-)
- **R06.82** Tachypnea, not elsewhere classified
  Tachypnea NOS
  EXCLUDES 1: transitory tachypnea of newborn (P22.1)
- **R06.83** Snoring
- **R06.89** Other abnormalities of breathing
  Breath-holding (spells)
  Sighing

R06.9 Unspecified abnormalities of breathing

R07 Pain in throat and chest ✓4th
EXCLUDES 1: epidemic myalgia (B33.0)
EXCLUDES 2: jaw pain R68.84
pain in breast (N64.4)

R07.0 Pain in throat
EXCLUDES 1: chronic sore throat (J31.2)
sore throat (acute) NOS (J02.9)
EXCLUDES 2: dysphagia (R13.1-)
pain in neck (M54.2)

R07.1 Chest pain on breathing
Painful respiration

R07.2 Precordial pain
DEF: Pain felt in the anterior (front) chest wall over the region of the heart. This type of pain is generally felt slightly to the left of the sternum, but may also extend into the surrounding chest wall region.

R07.8 Other chest pain ✓5th
AHA: 2024,3Q,16
- **R07.81** Pleurodynia
  Pleurodynia NOS
  EXCLUDES 1: epidemic pleurodynia (B33.0)
- **R07.82** Intercostal pain
- **R07.89** Other chest pain
  Anterior chest-wall pain NOS
  AHA: 2021,1Q,42

R07.9 Chest pain, unspecified

R09 Other symptoms and signs involving the circulatory and respiratory system ✓4th
EXCLUDES 1: acute respiratory distress syndrome (J80)
respiratory arrest of newborn (P28.81)
respiratory distress syndrome of newborn (P22.0)
respiratory failure (J96.-)
respiratory failure of newborn (P28.5)

R09.0 Asphyxia and hypoxemia ✓5th
EXCLUDES 1: asphyxia due to carbon monoxide (T58.-)
asphyxia due to foreign body in respiratory tract (T17.-)
birth (intrauterine) asphyxia (P84)
hyperventilation (R06.4)
traumatic asphyxia (T71.-)
EXCLUDES 2: hypercapnia (R06.89)

- **R09.01** Asphyxia
  DEF: Interference of oxygen intake due to obstruction or injury of airways resulting in a lack of oxygen perfusion to the tissues or excessive carbon dioxide in the blood. Can cause unconsciousness or death.
- **R09.02** Hypoxemia
  AHA: 2019,3Q,15
  DEF: Insufficient oxygen in the arterial blood resulting in inadequate delivery of oxygen to the body tissues.

R09.1 Pleurisy
EXCLUDES 1: pleurisy with effusion (J90)

R09.2 Respiratory arrest
Cardiorespiratory failure
EXCLUDES 1: cardiac arrest (I46.-)
respiratory arrest of newborn (P28.81)
respiratory distress of newborn (P22.0)
respiratory failure (J96.-)
respiratory failure of newborn (P28.5)
respiratory insufficiency (R06.89)
respiratory insufficiency of newborn (P28.5)

R09.3 Abnormal sputum
Abnormal amount of sputum
Abnormal color of sputum
Abnormal odor of sputum
Excessive sputum
EXCLUDES 1: blood-stained sputum (R04.2)

R09.8 Other specified symptoms and signs involving the circulatory and respiratory systems ✓5th
- **R09.81** Nasal congestion
- **R09.82** Postnasal drip
- **R09.89** Other specified symptoms and signs involving the circulatory and respiratory systems
  Abnormal chest percussion
  Bruit (arterial)
  Chest tympany
  Choking sensation
  Friction sounds in chest
  Rales
  Weak pulse
  EXCLUDES 2: foreign body in throat (T17.2-)
  wheezing (R06.2)
  AHA: 2021,1Q,42

R09.A Foreign body sensation of the circulatory and respiratory system ✓5th
AHA: 2023,4Q,41-42
- **R09.A0** Foreign body sensation, unspecified
- **R09.A1** Foreign body sensation, nose
- **R09.A2** Foreign body sensation, throat
  Foreign body sensation globus
- **R09.A9** Foreign body sensation, other site

Symptoms and signs involving the digestive system and abdomen (R10-R19)

EXCLUDES 2 congenital or infantile pylorospasm (Q40.0)
gastrointestinal hemorrhage (K92.0-K92.2)
intestinal obstruction (K56.-)
newborn gastrointestinal hemorrhage (P54.0-P54.3)
newborn intestinal obstruction (P76.-)
pylorospasm (K31.3)
signs and symptoms involving the urinary system (R30-R39)
symptoms referable to female genital organs (N94.-)
symptoms referable to male genital organs (N48-N50)

✓4th **R10 Abdominal and pelvic pain**
  EXCLUDES 1 renal colic (N23)
  EXCLUDES 2 ▶costovertebral (angle) tenderness (R39.85)◀
    dorsalgia (M54.-)
    flatulence and related conditions (R14.-)

R10.0 Acute abdomen
  Severe abdominal pain (generalized) (with abdominal rigidity)
  EXCLUDES 1 abdominal rigidity NOS (R19.3)
    generalized abdominal pain NOS (R10.84)
    localized abdominal pain (R10.1-R10.3-)

✓5th **R10.1 Pain localized to upper abdomen**
  EXCLUDES 2 ▶pain localized to flank (R10.A-)◀
    ▶pelvic and perineal pain (R10.2-)◀
  R10.10 Upper abdominal pain, unspecified
  R10.11 Right upper quadrant pain
  R10.12 Left upper quadrant pain
  R10.13 Epigastric pain
    Dyspepsia
    EXCLUDES 1 functional dyspepsia (K30)

Abdominal Pain

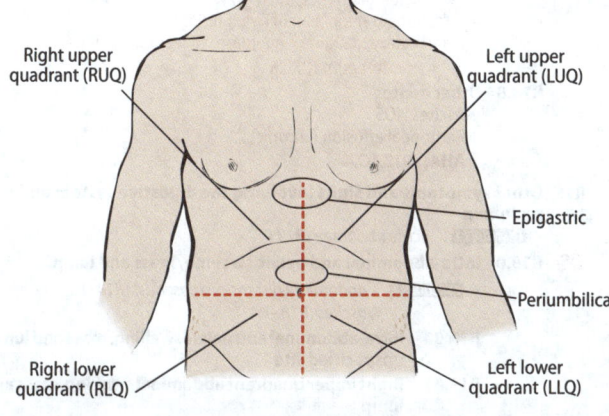

Right upper quadrant (RUQ)
Left upper quadrant (LUQ)
Epigastric
Periumbilical
Right lower quadrant (RLQ)
Left lower quadrant (LLQ)

▲ ✓5th **R10.2 Pelvic and perineal pain**
  EXCLUDES 1 vulvodynia (N94.81)
  EXCLUDES 2 ▶pain localized to other parts of lower abdomen (R10.3-)◀
    ▶pain localized to upper abdomen (R10.1-)◀
•   **R10.20** Pelvic and perineal pain unspecified side
•   **R10.21** Pelvic and perineal pain right side
•   **R10.22** Pelvic and perineal pain left side
•   **R10.23** Pelvic and perineal pain bilateral
  R10.24 Suprapubic pain

✓5th **R10.3 Pain localized to other parts of lower abdomen**
  EXCLUDES 2 ▶pain localized to flank (R10.A-)◀
    ▶pelvic and perineal pain (R10.2-)◀
  R10.30 Lower abdominal pain, unspecified
  R10.31 Right lower quadrant pain
  R10.32 Left lower quadrant pain
  R10.33 Periumbilical pain

✓5th **R10.8 Other abdominal pain**
  ✓6th **R10.81 Abdominal tenderness**
    Abdominal tenderness NOS
    EXCLUDES 2 ▶pain localized to other parts of lower abdomen (R10.3-)◀
      ▶pain localized to upper abdomen (R10.1-)◀
  R10.811 Right upper quadrant abdominal tenderness
  R10.812 Left upper quadrant abdominal tenderness
  R10.813 Right lower quadrant abdominal tenderness
  R10.814 Left lower quadrant abdominal tenderness
  R10.815 Periumbilic abdominal tenderness
  R10.816 Epigastric abdominal tenderness
  R10.817 Generalized abdominal tenderness
  R10.819 Abdominal tenderness, unspecified site

  ✓6th **R10.82 Rebound abdominal tenderness**
    EXCLUDES 2 ▶pain localized to other parts of lower abdomen (R10.3-)◀
      ▶pain localized to upper abdomen (R10.1-)◀
  R10.821 Right upper quadrant rebound tenderness
  R10.822 Left upper quadrant rebound tenderness
  R10.823 Right lower quadrant rebound tenderness
  R10.824 Left lower quadrant rebound tenderness
  R10.825 Periumbilic rebound abdominal tenderness
  R10.826 Epigastric rebound abdominal tenderness
  R10.827 Generalized rebound abdominal tenderness
  R10.829 Rebound abdominal tenderness, unspecified site

  R10.83 Colic
    Colic NOS
    Infantile colic
    EXCLUDES 1 colic in adult and child over 12 months old (R10.84)
    DEF: Inconsolable crying in an otherwise well-fed and healthy infant for more than three hours a day, three days a week, for more than three weeks.

  R10.84 Generalized abdominal pain
    EXCLUDES 1 generalized abdominal pain associated with acute abdomen (R10.0)

•   **R10.85 Abdominal pain of multiple sites**
    EXCLUDES 1 abdominal rigidity NOS (R19.3)
      generalized abdominal pain associated with acute abdomen (R10.0)
      generalized abdominal pain NOS (R10.84)
      localized abdominal pain (R10.1-R10.4-)

•   ✓6th **R10.8A Flank tenderness**
•   **R10.8A1** Right flank tenderness
•   **R10.8A2** Left flank tenderness
•   **R10.8A3** Suprapubic tenderness
•   **R10.8A9** Flank tenderness, unspecified
    Flank tenderness NOS

R10.9 Unspecified abdominal pain

✓5th **R10.A Pain localized to flank**
  Lateral abdomen pain
  Lateral flank pain
  Latus region pain
  EXCLUDES 2 pain localized to other parts of lower abdomen (R10.3-)
    pain localized to upper abdomen (R10.1-)
  R10.A0 Flank pain, unspecified side
  R10.A1 Flank pain, right side
  R10.A2 Flank pain, left side
  R10.A3 Flank pain, bilateral

✓4th **R11 Nausea and vomiting**
  EXCLUDES 1 cyclical vomiting associated with migraine (G43.A-)
    excessive vomiting in pregnancy (O21.-)
    hematemesis (K92.0)
    neonatal hematemesis (P54.0)
    newborn vomiting (P92.0-)
    psychogenic vomiting (F50.89)
    vomiting associated with bulimia nervosa (F50.2-)
    vomiting following gastrointestinal surgery (K91.0)
  AHA: 2017,1Q,28

R11.0 Nausea
  Nausea NOS
  Nausea without vomiting

✓5th **R11.1 Vomiting**
  R11.10 Vomiting, unspecified
    Vomiting NOS
  R11.11 Vomiting without nausea

R11.12 **Projectile** vomiting
R11.13 **Vomiting of fecal matter**
R11.14 **Bilious** vomiting
Bilious emesis
R11.15 **Cyclical** vomiting syndrome unrelated to migraine
Cyclic vomiting syndrome NOS
Persistent vomiting
EXCLUDES 1   cyclical vomiting in migraine (G43.A-)
EXCLUDES 2   bulimia nervosa (F50.20)
diabetes mellitus due to underlying condition (E08.-)
AHA: 2019,4Q,15
• **R11.16** **Cannabis hyperemesis syndrome**
Cannabinoid hyperemesis syndrome
Code also:
cannabis abuse (F12.1-)
cannabis dependence (F12.2-)
cannabis use, unspecified (F12.92-, F12.93, F12.95-, F12.98-, F12.99)
Code also manifestations, such as:
dehydration (E86.0)
electrolyte imbalance (E87.8)
R11.2 **Nausea with vomiting, unspecified**
Persistent nausea with vomiting NOS
AHA: 2020,1Q,8

R12 **Heartburn**
EXCLUDES 1   dyspepsia NOS (R10.13)
functional dyspepsia (K30)

✓4th **R13** **Aphagia and dysphagia**
R13.0 **Aphagia**
Inability to swallow
EXCLUDES 1   psychogenic aphagia (F50.9)
✓5th **R13.1** **Dysphagia**
Code first, if applicable, dysphagia following cerebrovascular disease (I69. with final characters -91)
EXCLUDES 1   psychogenic dysphagia (F45.8)

Swallowing Function

R13.10 **Dysphagia, unspecified**
Difficulty in swallowing NOS
R13.11 Dysphagia, **oral** phase
R13.12 Dysphagia, **oropharyngeal** phase
R13.13 Dysphagia, **pharyngeal** phase
R13.14 Dysphagia, **pharyngoesophageal** phase
R13.19 Other dysphagia
Cervical dysphagia
Neurogenic dysphagia

✓4th **R14** **Flatulence and related conditions**
EXCLUDES 1   psychogenic aerophagy (F45.8)
R14.0 **Abdominal distension (gaseous)**
Bloating
Tympanites (abdominal) (intestinal)
R14.1 Gas pain
R14.2 Eructation
R14.3 Flatulence

✓4th **R15** **Fecal incontinence**
INCLUDES   encopresis NOS
EXCLUDES 1   fecal incontinence of nonorganic origin (F98.1)
R15.0 **Incomplete defecation**
EXCLUDES 1   constipation (K59.0-)
fecal impaction (K56.41)
EXCLUDES 2   ▶constipation (K59.0-)◀
▶fecal impaction (K56.41)◀
R15.1 **Fecal smearing**
Fecal soiling
R15.2 **Fecal urgency**
R15.9 **Full incontinence of feces**
Fecal incontinence NOS

✓4th **R16** **Hepatomegaly and splenomegaly, not elsewhere classified**
R16.0 **Hepatomegaly, not elsewhere classified**
Hepatomegaly NOS
R16.1 **Splenomegaly, not elsewhere classified**
Splenomegaly NOS
R16.2 **Hepatomegaly with splenomegaly, not elsewhere classified**
Hepatosplenomegaly NOS

R17 **Unspecified jaundice**
EXCLUDES 1   neonatal jaundice (P55, P57-P59)

✓4th **R18** **Ascites**
INCLUDES   fluid in peritoneal cavity
EXCLUDES 1   ascites in alcoholic cirrhosis (K70.31)
ascites in alcoholic hepatitis (K70.11)
ascites in toxic liver disease with chronic active hepatitis (K71.51)
DEF: Abnormal accumulation of free fluid in the abdominal cavity, causing distention and tightness in addition to shortness of breath as the fluid accumulates. Ascites is usually an underlying disorder and can be a manifestation of any number of diseases.
R18.0 **Malignant ascites**   HCC UPD
Code first malignancy, such as:
malignant neoplasm of ovary (C56.-)
secondary malignant neoplasm of retroperitoneum and peritoneum (C78.6)
R18.8 **Other ascites**
Ascites NOS
Peritoneal effusion (chronic)
AHA: 2018,1Q,4

✓4th **R19** **Other symptoms and signs involving the digestive system and abdomen**
EXCLUDES 1   acute abdomen (R10.0)
✓5th **R19.0** **Intra-abdominal and pelvic swelling, mass and lump**
EXCLUDES 1   abdominal distension (gaseous) (R14.-)
ascites (R18.-)
R19.00 **Intra-abdominal and pelvic swelling, mass and lump, unspecified site**
R19.01 **Right upper quadrant** abdominal swelling, mass and lump
R19.02 **Left upper quadrant** abdominal swelling, mass and lump
R19.03 **Right lower quadrant** abdominal swelling, mass and lump
R19.04 **Left lower quadrant** abdominal swelling, mass and lump
R19.05 **Periumbilic** swelling, mass or lump
Diffuse or generalized umbilical swelling or mass
R19.06 **Epigastric** swelling, mass or lump
R19.07 **Generalized** intra-abdominal and pelvic swelling, mass and lump
Diffuse or generalized intra-abdominal swelling or mass NOS
Diffuse or generalized pelvic swelling or mass NOS
R19.09 **Other intra-abdominal and pelvic swelling, mass and lump**
✓5th **R19.1** **Abnormal bowel sounds**
R19.11 **Absent** bowel sounds
R19.12 **Hyperactive** bowel sounds
R19.15 **Other abnormal bowel sounds**
Abnormal bowel sounds NOS
R19.2 **Visible peristalsis**
Hyperperistalsis
DEF: Visible movements of muscular attempts to move food through the digestive tract due to pyloric obstruction, stomach obstruction, or intestinal obstruction.

Chapter 18. Symptoms, Signs and Abnormal Clinical and Laboratory Findings

R19.3 Abdominal rigidity
- EXCLUDES 1: abdominal rigidity with severe abdominal pain (R10.0)
- R19.30 Abdominal rigidity, unspecified site
- R19.31 Right upper quadrant abdominal rigidity
- R19.32 Left upper quadrant abdominal rigidity
- R19.33 Right lower quadrant abdominal rigidity
- R19.34 Left lower quadrant abdominal rigidity
- R19.35 Periumbilic abdominal rigidity
- R19.36 Epigastric abdominal rigidity
- R19.37 Generalized abdominal rigidity

R19.4 Change in bowel habit
- EXCLUDES 1: constipation (K59.0-)
- functional diarrhea (K59.1)

R19.5 Other fecal abnormalities
- Abnormal stool color
- Bulky stools
- Mucus in stools
- Occult blood in feces
- Occult blood in stools
- EXCLUDES 1: melena (K92.1)
- neonatal melena (P54.1)
- AHA: 2021,1Q,9; 2019,1Q,32

R19.6 Halitosis

R19.7 Diarrhea, unspecified
- Diarrhea NOS
- EXCLUDES 1: functional diarrhea (K59.1)
- neonatal diarrhea (P78.3)
- psychogenic diarrhea (F45.8)
- AHA: 2021,3Q,3

R19.8 Other specified symptoms and signs involving the digestive system and abdomen

Symptoms and signs involving the skin and subcutaneous tissue (R20-R23)

EXCLUDES 2: symptoms relating to breast (N64.4-N64.5)

R20 Disturbances of skin sensation
- EXCLUDES 1: dissociative anesthesia and sensory loss (F44.6)
- psychogenic disturbances (F45.8)
- R20.0 Anesthesia of skin
- R20.1 Hypoesthesia of skin
- R20.2 Paresthesia of skin
  - Formication
  - Pins and needles
  - Tingling skin
  - EXCLUDES 1: acroparesthesia (I73.8)
- R20.3 Hyperesthesia
- R20.8 Other disturbances of skin sensation
- R20.9 Unspecified disturbances of skin sensation

R21 Rash and other nonspecific skin eruption
- INCLUDES: rash NOS
- EXCLUDES 1: specified type of rash - code to condition
- vesicular eruption (R23.8)

R22 Localized swelling, mass and lump of skin and subcutaneous tissue
- INCLUDES: subcutaneous nodules (localized)(superficial)
- EXCLUDES 1: abnormal findings on diagnostic imaging (R90-R93)
  - edema (R60.-)
  - enlarged lymph nodes (R59.-)
  - localized adiposity (E65)
  - swelling of joint (M25.4-)
- R22.0 Localized swelling, mass and lump, head
- R22.1 Localized swelling, mass and lump, neck
- R22.2 Localized swelling, mass and lump, trunk
  - EXCLUDES 1: intra-abdominal or pelvic mass and lump (R19.0-)
  - intra-abdominal or pelvic swelling (R19.0-)
  - EXCLUDES 2: breast mass and lump (N63)
  - AHA: 2022,3Q,8
- R22.3 Localized swelling, mass and lump, upper limb
  - R22.30 Localized swelling, mass and lump, unspecified upper limb
  - R22.31 Localized swelling, mass and lump, right upper limb
  - R22.32 Localized swelling, mass and lump, left upper limb
  - R22.33 Localized swelling, mass and lump, upper limb, bilateral
- R22.4 Localized swelling, mass and lump, lower limb
  - R22.40 Localized swelling, mass and lump, unspecified lower limb
  - R22.41 Localized swelling, mass and lump, right lower limb
  - R22.42 Localized swelling, mass and lump, left lower limb
  - R22.43 Localized swelling, mass and lump, lower limb, bilateral
- R22.9 Localized swelling, mass and lump, unspecified

R23 Other skin changes
- R23.0 Cyanosis
  - EXCLUDES 1: acrocyanosis (I73.8)
  - cyanotic attacks of newborn (P28.2)
  - DEF: Bluish or purplish discoloration of the skin due to an inadequate oxygen blood level.
- R23.1 Pallor
  - Clammy skin
- R23.2 Flushing
  - Excessive blushing
  - Code first, if applicable, menopausal and female climacteric states (N95.1)
- R23.3 Spontaneous ecchymoses
  - Petechiae
  - EXCLUDES 1: ecchymoses of newborn (P54.5)
  - purpura (D69.-)
- R23.4 Changes in skin texture
  - Desquamation of skin
  - Induration of skin
  - Scaling of skin
  - EXCLUDES 1: epidermal thickening NOS (L85.9)
- R23.8 Other skin changes
- R23.9 Unspecified skin changes

Symptoms and signs involving the nervous and musculoskeletal systems (R25-R29)

R25 Abnormal involuntary movements
- EXCLUDES 1: specific movement disorders (G20-G26)
- stereotyped movement disorders (F98.4)
- tic disorders (F95.-)
- R25.0 Abnormal head movements
- R25.1 Tremor, unspecified
  - EXCLUDES 1: chorea NOS (G25.5)
  - essential tremor (G25.0)
  - hysterical tremor (F44.4)
  - intention tremor (G25.2)
- R25.2 Cramp and spasm
  - EXCLUDES 2: carpopedal spasm (R29.0)
  - charley-horse (M62.831)
  - infantile spasms (G40.4-)
  - muscle spasm of back (M62.830)
  - muscle spasm of calf (M62.831)
- R25.3 Fasciculation
  - Twitching NOS
- R25.8 Other abnormal involuntary movements
- R25.9 Unspecified abnormal involuntary movements

R26 Abnormalities of gait and mobility
- EXCLUDES 1: ataxia NOS (R27.0)
  - hereditary ataxia (G11.-)
  - immobility syndrome (paraplegic) (M62.3)
  - locomotor (syphilitic) ataxia (A52.11)
- R26.0 Ataxic gait
  - Staggering gait
  - AHA: 2022,2Q,12
- R26.1 Paralytic gait
  - Spastic gait
- R26.2 Difficulty in walking, not elsewhere classified
  - EXCLUDES 1: falling (R29.6)
  - unsteadiness on feet (R26.81)
  - AHA: 2016,2Q,7
- R26.8 Other abnormalities of gait and mobility
  - R26.81 Unsteadiness on feet
  - R26.89 Other abnormalities of gait and mobility
    - AHA: 2020,2Q,29
- R26.9 Unspecified abnormalities of gait and mobility

R27 Other lack of coordination
- EXCLUDES 1: ataxic gait (R26.0)
  - hereditary ataxia (G11.-)
  - vertigo NOS (R42)
- R27.0 Ataxia, unspecified
  - EXCLUDES 1: ataxia following cerebrovascular disease (I69. with final characters -93)
- R27.8 Other lack of coordination

Chapter 18. Symptoms, Signs and Abnormal Clinical and Laboratory Findings

R27.9 Unspecified lack of coordination

☑4th **R29** Other symptoms and signs involving the nervous and musculoskeletal systems

R29.0 Tetany
Carpopedal spasm
EXCLUDES 1: hysterical tetany (F44.5)
neonatal tetany (P71.3)
parathyroid tetany (E20.9)
post-thyroidectomy tetany (E89.2)
DEF: Calcium or other mineral imbalance causing voluntary muscles such as hands, feet, or larynx to spasm rhythmically.

R29.1 Meningismus

R29.2 Abnormal reflex
EXCLUDES 2: abnormal pupillary reflex (H57.0)
hyperactive gag reflex (J39.2)
vasovagal reaction or syncope (R55)

R29.3 Abnormal posture

R29.4 Clicking hip
EXCLUDES 1: congenital deformities of hip (Q65.-)

R29.5 Transient paralysis
Code first any associated spinal cord injury (S14.0, S14.1-, S24.0, S24.1-, S34.0-, S34.1-)
EXCLUDES 1: transient ischemic attack (G45.9)

R29.6 Repeated falls
Falling
Tendency to fall
EXCLUDES 2: at risk for falling (Z91.81)
history of falling (Z91.81)
AHA: 2016,2Q,6

☑5th **R29.7** National Institutes of Health Stroke Scale (NIHSS) score
Code first the type of cerebral infarction (I63.-)
AHA: 2016,4Q,61-62
TIP: Codes from this subcategory may be assigned based on medical record documentation from clinicians who are not the patient's provider.

☑6th **R29.70** NIHSS score 0-9
- R29.700 NIHSS score 0
- R29.701 NIHSS score 1
- R29.702 NIHSS score 2
- R29.703 NIHSS score 3
- R29.704 NIHSS score 4
- R29.705 NIHSS score 5
- R29.706 NIHSS score 6
- R29.707 NIHSS score 7
- R29.708 NIHSS score 8
- R29.709 NIHSS score 9

☑6th **R29.71** NIHSS score 10-19
- R29.710 NIHSS score 10
- R29.711 NIHSS score 11
- R29.712 NIHSS score 12
- R29.713 NIHSS score 13
- R29.714 NIHSS score 14
- R29.715 NIHSS score 15
- R29.716 NIHSS score 16
- R29.717 NIHSS score 17
- R29.718 NIHSS score 18
- R29.719 NIHSS score 19

☑6th **R29.72** NIHSS score 20-29
- R29.720 NIHSS score 20
- R29.721 NIHSS score 21
- R29.722 NIHSS score 22
- R29.723 NIHSS score 23
- R29.724 NIHSS score 24
- R29.725 NIHSS score 25
- R29.726 NIHSS score 26
- R29.727 NIHSS score 27
- R29.728 NIHSS score 28
- R29.729 NIHSS score 29

☑6th **R29.73** NIHSS score 30-39
- R29.730 NIHSS score 30
- R29.731 NIHSS score 31
- R29.732 NIHSS score 32
- R29.733 NIHSS score 33
- R29.734 NIHSS score 34
- R29.735 NIHSS score 35
- R29.736 NIHSS score 36
- R29.737 NIHSS score 37
- R29.738 NIHSS score 38
- R29.739 NIHSS score 39

☑6th **R29.74** NIHSS score 40-42
- R29.740 NIHSS score 40
- R29.741 NIHSS score 41
- R29.742 NIHSS score 42

☑5th **R29.8** Other symptoms and signs involving the nervous and musculoskeletal systems

☑6th **R29.81** Other symptoms and signs involving the nervous system

R29.810 Facial weakness
Facial droop
EXCLUDES 1: Bell's palsy (G51.0)
facial weakness following cerebrovascular disease (I69. with final characters -92)

R29.818 Other symptoms and signs involving the nervous system

☑6th **R29.89** Other symptoms and signs involving the musculoskeletal system
EXCLUDES 2: pain in limb (M79.6-)

R29.890 Loss of height
EXCLUDES 1: osteoporosis (M80-M81)

R29.891 Ocular torticollis
EXCLUDES 1: congenital (sternomastoid) torticollis Q68.0
psychogenic torticollis (F45.8)
spasmodic torticollis (G24.3)
torticollis due to birth injury (P15.8)
torticollis NOS M43.6
DEF: Abnormal head posture as a result of a contracted state of cervical muscles to correct a visual disturbance, either double vision or a visual field defect.

R29.898 Other symptoms and signs involving the musculoskeletal system

☑5th **R29.9** Unspecified symptoms and signs involving the nervous and musculoskeletal systems

R29.90 Unspecified symptoms and signs involving the nervous system

R29.91 Unspecified symptoms and signs involving the musculoskeletal system

Symptoms and signs involving the genitourinary system (R30-R39)

☑4th **R30** Pain associated with micturition
EXCLUDES 1: psychogenic pain associated with micturition (F45.8)

R30.0 Dysuria
Strangury

R30.1 Vesical tenesmus
DEF: Feeling of a full bladder even when there is little or no urine in the bladder.

R30.9 Painful micturition, unspecified
Painful urination NOS

☑4th **R31** Hematuria
EXCLUDES 1: hematuria included with underlying conditions, such as:
acute cystitis with hematuria (N30.01)
recurrent and persistent hematuria in glomerular diseases (N02.-)
AHA: 2025,2Q,20-21; 2017,1Q,17

R31.0 Gross hematuria

R31.1 Benign essential microscopic hematuria

☑5th **R31.2** Other microscopic hematuria
AHA: 2016,4Q,62

R31.21 Asymptomatic microscopic hematuria
AMH

R31.29 Other microscopic hematuria

R31.9 Hematuria, unspecified

R32 Unspecified urinary incontinence
Enuresis NOS
- EXCLUDES 1: functional urinary incontinence (R39.81)
nonorganic enuresis (F98.0)
stress incontinence and other specified urinary incontinence (N39.3-N39.4-)
urinary incontinence associated with cognitive impairment (R39.81)

R33 Retention of urine
- EXCLUDES 1: psychogenic retention of urine (F45.8)

R33.0 Drug induced retention of urine
Use additional code for adverse effect, if applicable, to identify drug (T36-T50 with fifth or sixth character 5)

R33.8 Other retention of urine
Code first, if applicable, any causal condition, such as:
enlarged prostate (N40.1)
AHA: 2018,4Q,55

R33.9 Retention of urine, unspecified

R34 Anuria and oliguria
- EXCLUDES 1: anuria and oliguria complicating abortion or ectopic or molar pregnancy (O00-O07, O08.4)
anuria and oliguria complicating pregnancy (O26.83-)
anuria and oliguria complicating the puerperium (O90.49)

R35 Polyuria
Code first, if applicable, any causal condition, such as:
enlarged prostate (N40.1)
- EXCLUDES 1: psychogenic polyuria (F45.8)

R35.0 Frequency of micturition
R35.1 Nocturia
R35.8 Other polyuria
AHA: 2021,4Q,26

R35.81 Nocturnal polyuria
- EXCLUDES 2: nocturnal enuresis (N39.44)

R35.89 Other polyuria
Polyuria NOS

R36 Urethral discharge
R36.0 Urethral discharge without blood
R36.1 Hematospermia
R36.9 Urethral discharge, unspecified
Penile discharge NOS
Urethrorrhea

R37 Sexual dysfunction, unspecified

R39 Other and unspecified symptoms and signs involving the genitourinary system
R39.0 Extravasation of urine
R39.1 Other difficulties with micturition
Code first, if applicable, any causal condition, such as:
enlarged prostate (N40.1)

R39.11 Hesitancy of micturition
R39.12 Poor urinary stream
▶Weak urinary stream◀
R39.13 Splitting of urinary stream
R39.14 Feeling of incomplete bladder emptying
R39.15 Urgency of urination
- EXCLUDES 1: urge incontinence (N39.41, N39.46)
R39.16 Straining to void
R39.19 Other difficulties with micturition
AHA: 2016,4Q,63
R39.191 Need to immediately re-void
R39.192 Position dependent micturition
R39.198 Other difficulties with micturition

R39.2 Extrarenal uremia
Prerenal uremia
- EXCLUDES 1: uremia NOS (N19)

R39.8 Other symptoms and signs involving the genitourinary system
AHA: 2017,4Q,22-23

R39.81 Functional urinary incontinence
Urinary incontinence due to cognitive impairment, or severe physical disability or immobility
- EXCLUDES 1: stress incontinence and other specified urinary incontinence (N39.3-N39.4-)
urinary incontinence NOS (R32)

R39.82 Chronic bladder pain
AHA: 2016,4Q,64

R39.83 Unilateral non-palpable testicle
R39.84 Bilateral non-palpable testicles

R39.85 Costovertebral (angle) tenderness
- EXCLUDES 2: abdominal and pelvic pain (R10.-)
R39.851 Costovertebral (angle) tenderness, right side
R39.852 Costovertebral (angle) tenderness, left side
R39.853 Costovertebral (angle) tenderness, bilateral
R39.859 Costovertebral (angle) tenderness, unspecified side

R39.89 Other symptoms and signs involving the genitourinary system

R39.9 Unspecified symptoms and signs involving the genitourinary system

Symptoms and signs involving cognition, perception, emotional state and behavior (R40-R46)

- EXCLUDES 2: symptoms and signs constituting part of a pattern of mental disorder (F01-F99)

R40 Somnolence, stupor and coma
- EXCLUDES 1: neonatal coma (P91.5)
somnolence, stupor and coma in diabetes (E08-E13)
somnolence, stupor and coma in hepatic failure (K72.-)
somnolence, stupor and coma in hypoglycemia (nondiabetic) (E15)

R40.0 Somnolence
Drowsiness
- EXCLUDES 1: coma (R40.2-)

R40.1 Stupor
Catatonic stupor
Semicoma
- EXCLUDES 1: catatonic schizophrenia (F20.2)
coma (R40.2-)
depressive stupor ▶(F31.-, F32.-, F33.-)◀
dissociative stupor (F44.2)
manic stupor (F30.2)

R40.2 Coma
Code first any associated:
fracture of skull (S02.-)
intracranial injury (S06.-)

NOTE: One code from each subcategory, R40.21-R40.23, is required to complete the coma scale

AHA: 2020,3Q,46; 2019,2Q,12; 2018,4Q,70; 2017,4Q,23-25,95; 2015,2Q,17; 2014,1Q,19

TIP: Codes for individual (R40.21-, R40.22-, R40.23-) or total (R40.24-) coma scale scores may be assigned based on medical record documentation from clinicians who are not the patient's provider.

TIP: It is not appropriate to assign individual (R40.21-, R40.22-, R40.23-) or total (R40.24-) coma scale score codes for patients who are sedated or in medically induced comas, nor in conjunction with code R40.2A.

R40.20 Unspecified coma
Coma NOS
Unconsciousness NOS
AHA: 2021,4Q,112-113; 2021,2Q,5

R40.21 Coma scale, eyes open

The following appropriate 7th character is to be added to subcategory R40.21-, R40.22-, R40.23-, and R40.24-.
0 unspecified time
1 in the field [EMT or ambulance]
2 at arrival to emergency department
3 at hospital admission
4 24 hours or more after hospital admission

R40.211 Coma scale, eyes open, never
Coma scale eye opening score of 1

R40.212 Coma scale, eyes open, to pain
Coma scale eye opening score of 2

R40.213 Coma scale, eyes open, to sound
Coma scale eye opening score of 3

R40.214 Coma scale, eyes open, spontaneous
Coma scale eye opening score of 4

R40.22 Coma scale, best verbal response

R40.221 Coma scale, best verbal response, none
Coma scale verbal score of 1

R40.222 Coma scale, best verbal response, incomprehensible words
Coma scale verbal score of 2
Incomprehensible sounds (2-5 years of age)
Moans/grunts to pain; restless (< 2 years old)

R40.223 Coma scale, best verbal response, inappropriate words
Coma scale verbal score of 3
Inappropriate crying or screaming (< 2 years of age)
Screaming (2-5 years of age)

R40.224 Coma scale, best verbal response, confused conversation
Coma scale verbal score of 4
Inappropriate words (2-5 years of age)
Irritable cries (< 2 years of age)

R40.225 Coma scale, best verbal response, oriented
Coma scale verbal score of 5
Cooing or babbling or crying appropriately (< 2 years of age)
Uses appropriate words (2-5 years of age)

R40.23 Coma scale, best motor response

R40.231 Coma scale, best motor response, none
Coma scale motor score of 1

R40.232 Coma scale, best motor response, extension
Abnormal extensor posturing to pain or noxious stimuli (< 2 years of age)
Coma scale motor score of 2
Extensor posturing to pain or noxious stimuli (2-5 years of age)

R40.233 Coma scale, best motor response, abnormal flexion
Abnormal flexure posturing to pain or noxious stimuli (2-5 years of age)
Coma scale motor score of 3
Flexion/decorticate posturing (< 2 years of age)

R40.234 Coma scale, best motor response, flexion withdrawal
Coma scale motor score of 4
Withdraws from pain or noxious stimuli (2-5 years of age)

R40.235 Coma scale, best motor response, localizes pain
Coma scale motor score of 5
Localizes pain (2-5 years of age)
Withdraws to touch (< 2 years of age)

R40.236 Coma scale, best motor response, obeys commands
Coma scale motor score of 6
Normal or spontaneous movement (< 2 years of age)
Obeys commands (2-5 years of age)

R40.24 Glasgow coma scale, total score
NOTE Assign a code from subcategory R40.24, when only the total coma score is documented
AHA: 2021,2Q,4; 2016,4Q,64-65

R40.241 Glasgow coma scale score 13-15
R40.242 Glasgow coma scale score 9-12
R40.243 Glasgow coma scale score 3-8
R40.244 Other coma, without documented Glasgow coma scale score, or with partial score reported

R40.2A Nontraumatic coma due to underlying condition
Secondary coma
Code first underlying condition
EXCLUDES 1: ▶coma scale, best motor response (R40.24.-)◀
▶coma scale, best verbal response (R40.22.-)◀
▶coma scale, eyes open (R40.21.-)◀
▶Glasgow coma scale, total score (R40.23.-)◀
AHA: 2023,4Q,42

R40.3 Persistent vegetative state
DEF: Persistent wakefulness without consciousness due to a nonfunctioning cerebral cortex.

R40.4 Transient alteration of awareness
AHA: 2020,2Q,24

R41 Other symptoms and signs involving cognitive functions and awareness
EXCLUDES 1: dissociative [conversion] disorders (F44.-)
mild cognitive impairment of uncertain or unknown etiology) (G31.84)

R41.0 Disorientation, unspecified
Confusion NOS
Delirium NOS
EXCLUDES 1: delirium due to known physiological condition (F05)
AHA: 2022,2Q,11; 2019,2Q,34

R41.1 Anterograde amnesia
R41.2 Retrograde amnesia
R41.3 Other amnesia
Amnesia NOS
Memory loss NOS
EXCLUDES 1: amnestic disorder due to known physiologic condition (F04)
amnestic syndrome due to psychoactive substance use (F10-F19 with 5th character .6)
mild memory disturbance due to known physiological condition (F06.8)
transient global amnesia (G45.4)

R41.4 Neurologic neglect syndrome
Asomatognosia
Hemi-akinesia
Hemi-inattention
Hemispatial neglect
Left-sided neglect
Sensory neglect
Visuospatial neglect
EXCLUDES 1: visuospatial deficit (R41.842)

R41.8 Other symptoms and signs involving cognitive functions and awareness

R41.81 Age-related cognitive decline
Senility NOS

R41.82 Altered mental status, unspecified
Change in mental status NOS
EXCLUDES 1: altered level of consciousness (R40.-)
altered mental status due to known condition - code to condition
delirium NOS (R41.0)
AHA: 2012,4Q,97

R41.83 Borderline intellectual functioning
IQ level 71 to 84
EXCLUDES 1: intellectual disabilities (F70-F79)

R41.84 Other specified cognitive deficit
Code first the underlying condition, if known, such as: schizophrenia (F20.-)
EXCLUDES 1: cognitive deficits as sequelae of cerebrovascular disease (I69.01-, I69.11-, I69.21-, I69.31-, I69.81-, I69.91-)

R41.840 Attention and concentration deficit
EXCLUDES 1: attention-deficit hyperactivity disorders (F90.-)

R41.841 Cognitive communication deficit
R41.842 Visuospatial deficit
R41.843 Psychomotor deficit
R41.844 Frontal lobe and executive function deficit

R41.85 Anosognosia
AHA: 2024,4Q,27

R41.89 Other symptoms and signs involving cognitive functions and awareness

Chapter 18. Symptoms, Signs and Abnormal Clinical and Laboratory Findings

R41.9 Unspecified symptoms and signs involving cognitive functions and awareness
Unspecified neurocognitive disorder

R42 Dizziness and giddiness
Light-headedness
Vertigo NOS
EXCLUDES 1: vertiginous syndromes (H81.-)
vertigo from infrasound (T75.23)

√4th R43 Disturbances of smell and taste
- **R43.0** Anosmia
  DEF: Permanent or transient absence of smell that may be congenital or acquired.
- **R43.1** Parosmia
  DEF: Abnormal perception of smell usually triggered by environmental odors.
- **R43.2** Parageusia
  DEF: Abnormal perception of taste.
- **R43.8** Other disturbances of smell and taste
  Mixed disturbance of smell and taste
- **R43.9** Unspecified disturbances of smell and taste

√4th R44 Other symptoms and signs involving general sensations and perceptions
EXCLUDES 1: alcoholic hallucinations (F10.151, F10.251, F10.951)
hallucinations in drug psychosis (F11-F19 with fifth to sixth characters 51)
hallucinations in mood disorders with psychotic symptoms (F30.2, F31.5, F32.3, F33.3)
hallucinations in schizophrenia, schizotypal and delusional disorders (F20-F29)
EXCLUDES 2: disturbances of skin sensation (R20.-)
- **R44.0** Auditory hallucinations
- **R44.1** Visual hallucinations
- **R44.2** Other hallucinations
- **R44.3** Hallucinations, unspecified
  AHA: 2022,2Q,11
- **R44.8** Other symptoms and signs involving general sensations and perceptions
- **R44.9** Unspecified symptoms and signs involving general sensations and perceptions

√4th R45 Symptoms and signs involving emotional state
- **R45.0** Nervousness
  Nervous tension
- **R45.1** Restlessness and agitation
- **R45.2** Unhappiness
- **R45.3** Demoralization and apathy
  EXCLUDES 1: anhedonia (R45.84)
- **R45.4** Irritability and anger
- **R45.5** Hostility
- **R45.6** Violent behavior
- **R45.7** State of emotional shock and stress, unspecified
- **√5th R45.8** Other symptoms and signs involving emotional state
  - **R45.81** Low self-esteem
  - **R45.82** Worries
  - **R45.83** Excessive crying of child, adolescent or adult
    EXCLUDES 1: excessive crying of infant (baby) R68.11
  - **R45.84** Anhedonia
  - **√6th R45.85** Homicidal and suicidal ideations
    EXCLUDES 1: suicide attempt (T14.91)
    - **R45.850** Homicidal ideations
    - **R45.851** Suicidal ideations
      AHA: 2022,1Q,29
      DEF: Thoughts of committing suicide but no actual attempt of suicide has been made.
  - **R45.86** Emotional lability
  - **R45.87** Impulsiveness
  - **R45.88** Nonsuicidal self-harm HCC Rx ESR COM
    Nonsuicidal self-injury
    Nonsuicidal self-mutilation
    Self-inflicted injury without suicidal intent
    Code also injury, if known
    AHA: 2021,4Q,26-27
  - **R45.89** Other symptoms and signs involving emotional state
    Flat affect
    Loneliness

√4th R46 Symptoms and signs involving appearance and behavior
EXCLUDES 1: appearance and behavior in schizophrenia, schizotypal and delusional disorders (F20-F29)
mental and behavioral disorders (F01-F99)
- **R46.0** Very low level of personal hygiene
- **R46.1** Bizarre personal appearance
- **R46.2** Strange and inexplicable behavior
- **R46.3** Overactivity
- **R46.4** Slowness and poor responsiveness
  EXCLUDES 1: stupor (R40.1)
- **R46.5** Suspiciousness and marked evasiveness
- **R46.6** Undue concern and preoccupation with stressful events
- **R46.7** Verbosity and circumstantial detail obscuring reason for contact
- **√5th R46.8** Other symptoms and signs involving appearance and behavior
  - **R46.81** Obsessive-compulsive behavior
    EXCLUDES 1: obsessive-compulsive disorder (F42.-)
  - **R46.89** Other symptoms and signs involving appearance and behavior

Symptoms and signs involving speech and voice (R47-R49)

√4th R47 Speech disturbances, not elsewhere classified
EXCLUDES 1: autism (F84.0)
cluttering (F80.81)
specific developmental disorders of speech and language (F80.-)
stuttering (F80.81)
- **√5th R47.0** Dysphasia and aphasia
  - **R47.01** Aphasia
    EXCLUDES 1: aphasia following cerebrovascular disease (I69. with final characters -20)
    progressive isolated aphasia (G31.01)
  - **R47.02** Dysphasia
    EXCLUDES 1: dysphasia following cerebrovascular disease (I69. with final characters -21)
- **R47.1** Dysarthria and anarthria
  EXCLUDES 1: dysarthria following cerebrovascular disease (I69. with final characters -22)
- **√5th R47.8** Other speech disturbances
  EXCLUDES 1: dysarthria following cerebrovascular disease (I69. with final characters -28)
  - **R47.81** Slurred speech
  - **R47.82** *Fluency disorder in conditions classified elsewhere*
    Stuttering in conditions classified elsewhere
    Code first underlying disease or condition, such as: Parkinson's disease (G20.-)
    EXCLUDES 1: adult onset fluency disorder (F98.5)
    childhood onset fluency disorder (F80.81)
    fluency disorder (stuttering) following cerebrovascular disease (I69. with final characters -23)
  - **R47.89** Other speech disturbances
- **R47.9** Unspecified speech disturbances

√4th R48 Dyslexia and other symbolic dysfunctions, not elsewhere classified
EXCLUDES 1: specific developmental disorders of scholastic skills (F81.-)
- **R48.0** Dyslexia and alexia
- **R48.1** Agnosia
  Astereognosia (astereognosis)
  Autotopagnosia
  EXCLUDES 1: visual object agnosia (R48.3)
  DEF: Inability to recognize common things such as faces, objects, smells, or voices.
- **R48.2** Apraxia
  EXCLUDES 1: apraxia following cerebrovascular disease (I69. with final characters -90)
- **R48.3** Visual agnosia
  Prosopagnosia
  Simultanagnosia (asimultagnosia)
- **R48.8** Other symbolic dysfunctions
  Acalculia
  Agraphia
  AHA: 2017,1Q,27
- **R48.9** Unspecified symbolic dysfunctions

√4th R49 Voice and resonance disorders
EXCLUDES 1: psychogenic voice and resonance disorders (F44.4)
- **R49.0** Dysphonia
  Hoarseness

R49.1 Aphonia
Loss of voice

R49.2 Hypernasality and hyponasality ✓5th
- R49.21 Hypernasality
- R49.22 Hyponasality

R49.8 Other voice and resonance disorders

R49.9 Unspecified voice and resonance disorder
Change in voice NOS
Resonance disorder NOS

General symptoms and signs (R50-R69)

R50 Fever of other and unknown origin ✓4th
  EXCLUDES 1
    chills without fever (R68.83)
    febrile convulsions (R56.0-)
    fever of unknown origin during labor (O75.2)
    fever of unknown origin in newborn (P81.9)
    hypothermia due to illness (R68.0)
    malignant hyperthermia due to anesthesia (T88.3)
    puerperal pyrexia NOS (O86.4)

R50.2 Drug induced fever
Use additional code for adverse effect, if applicable, to identify drug (T36-T50 with fifth or sixth character 5)
  EXCLUDES 1 postvaccination (postimmunization) fever (R50.83)

R50.8 Other specified fever ✓5th

  R50.81 Fever presenting with conditions classified elsewhere
  Code first underlying condition when associated fever is present, such as with:
    leukemia (C91-C95)
    neutropenia (D70.-)
    sickle-cell disease (D57.-)
  AHA: 2020,3Q,22; 2014,4Q,22

  R50.82 Postprocedural fever
    EXCLUDES 1
      postprocedural infection (T81.4-)
      posttransfusion fever (R50.84)
      postvaccination (postimmunization) fever (R50.83)

  R50.83 Postvaccination fever
  Postimmunization fever

  R50.84 Febrile nonhemolytic transfusion reaction
  FNHTR
  Posttransfusion fever

R50.9 Fever, unspecified
Fever NOS
Fever of unknown origin [FUO]
Fever with chills
Fever with rigors
Hyperpyrexia NOS
Persistent fever
Pyrexia NOS

R51 Headache ✓4th
  EXCLUDES 2
    atypical face pain (G50.1)
    migraine and other headache syndromes (G43-G44)
    trigeminal neuralgia (G50.0)
  AHA: 2020,4Q,38-39

  R51.0 Headache with orthostatic component, not elsewhere classified
  Headache with positional component, not elsewhere classified

  R51.9 Headache, unspecified
  Facial pain NOS

R52 Pain, unspecified
Acute pain NOS
Generalized pain NOS
Pain NOS
  EXCLUDES 1
    acute and chronic pain, not elsewhere classified (G89.-)
    localized pain, unspecified type - code to pain by site, such as:
    pain disorders exclusively related to psychological factors (F45.41)
      abdomen pain (R10.-)
      back pain (M54.9)
      breast pain (N64.4)
      chest pain (R07.1-R07.9)
      ear pain (H92.0-)
      eye pain (H57.1)
      headache (R51.9)
      joint pain (M25.5-)
      limb pain (M79.6-)
      lumbar region pain (M54.5-)
      pelvic and perineal pain ▶(R10.2-)◄
      renal colic (N23)
      shoulder pain (M25.51-)
      spine pain (M54.-)
      throat pain (R07.0)
      tongue pain (K14.6)
      tooth pain (K08.8)

R53 Malaise and fatigue ✓4th

  R53.0 Neoplastic (malignant) related fatigue
  Code first associated neoplasm

  R53.1 Weakness
  Asthenia NOS
    EXCLUDES 1
      age-related weakness (R54)
      muscle weakness (generalized) (M62.81)
      sarcopenia (M62.84)
      senile asthenia (R54)
  AHA: 2017,1Q,7; 2015,1Q,25

  R53.2 Functional quadriplegia HCC ESR COM
  Complete immobility due to severe physical disability or frailty
    EXCLUDES 1
      frailty NOS (R54)
      hysterical paralysis (F44.4)
      immobility syndrome (M62.3)
      neurologic quadriplegia (G82.5-)
      quadriplegia (G82.50)
  AHA: 2022,4Q,15; 2016,2Q,6
  DEF: Inability to move due to a nonphysiological condition, such as dementia. The patient has no mental ability to move independently.

  R53.8 Other malaise and fatigue ✓5th
    EXCLUDES 1
      combat exhaustion and fatigue (F43.0)
      congenital debility (P96.9)
      exhaustion and fatigue due to excessive exertion (T73.3)
      exhaustion and fatigue due to exposure (T73.2)
      exhaustion and fatigue due to heat (T67.-)
      exhaustion and fatigue due to pregnancy (O26.8-)
      exhaustion and fatigue due to recurrent depressive episode ▶(F33-)◄
      exhaustion and fatigue due to senile debility (R54)

    R53.81 Other malaise UPD
    Chronic debility
    Debility NOS
    General physical deterioration
    Malaise NOS
    Nervous debility
      EXCLUDES 1 age-related physical debility (R54)
    AHA: 2021,1Q,43

    R53.82 Chronic fatigue, unspecified UPD
      EXCLUDES 1
        chronic fatigue syndrome (G93.32)
        myalgic encephalomyelitis (G93.32)
        other post infection and related fatigue syndromes (G93.39)
        postviral fatigue syndrome (G93.31)

    R53.83 Other fatigue UPD
    Fatigue NOS
    Lack of energy
    Lethargy
    Tiredness
      EXCLUDES 2 exhaustion and fatigue due to depressive episode (F32.-)

Chapter 18. Symptoms, Signs and Abnormal Clinical and Laboratory Findings

R54 Age-related physical debility [UPD] [A]
Frailty
Old age
Senescence
Senile asthenia
Senile debility
- EXCLUDES 1: age-related cognitive decline (R41.81)
  - sarcopenia (M62.84)
  - senile psychosis (F03.-)
  - senility NOS (R41.81)

R55 Syncope and collapse
Blackout
Fainting
Vasovagal attack
- EXCLUDES 1: cardiogenic shock (R57.0)
  - carotid sinus syncope (G90.01)
  - heat syncope (T67.1)
  - neurocirculatory asthenia (F45.8)
  - neurogenic orthostatic hypotension (G90.3)
  - orthostatic hypotension (I95.1)
  - postprocedural shock (T81.1-)
  - psychogenic syncope (F48.8)
  - shock complicating or following abortion or ectopic or molar pregnancy (O00-O07, O08.3)
  - shock complicating or following labor and delivery (O75.1)
  - shock NOS (R57.9)
  - Stokes-Adams attack (I45.9)
  - unconsciousness NOS (R40.2-)

✓4th R56 Convulsions, not elsewhere classified
- EXCLUDES 1: dissociative convulsions and seizures (F44.5)
  - epileptic convulsions and seizures (G40.-)
  - newborn convulsions and seizures (P90)

✓5th R56.0 Febrile convulsions
R56.00 Simple febrile convulsions [HCC] [ESR] [COM]
Febrile convulsion NOS
Febrile seizure NOS
R56.01 Complex febrile convulsions [HCC] [ESR] [COM]
Atypical febrile seizure
Complex febrile seizure
Complicated febrile seizure
- EXCLUDES 1: status epilepticus (G40.901)

R56.1 Post traumatic seizures [HCC] [ESR] [COM]
- EXCLUDES 1: post traumatic epilepsy (G40.-)

R56.9 Unspecified convulsions [HCC] [ESR] [COM]
Convulsion disorder
Fit NOS
Recurrent convulsions
Seizure(s) (convulsive) NOS
AHA: 2022,4Q,46; 2021,1Q,3; 2019,1Q,19

✓4th R57 Shock, not elsewhere classified
- EXCLUDES 1: anaphylactic shock NOS (T78.2)
  - anaphylactic reaction or shock due to adverse food reaction (T78.0-)
  - anaphylactic shock due to adverse effect of correct drug or medicament properly administered (T88.6)
  - anaphylactic shock due to serum (T80.5-)
  - electric shock (T75.4)
  - obstetric shock (O75.1)
  - postprocedural shock (T81.1-)
  - psychic shock (F43.0)
  - shock complicating or following ectopic or molar pregnancy (O00-O07, O08.3)
  - shock due to anesthesia (T88.2)
  - shock due to lightning (T75.01)
  - toxic shock syndrome (A48.3)
  - traumatic shock (T79.4)

R57.0 Cardiogenic shock [HCC] [ESR] [COM]
- EXCLUDES 2: septic shock (R65.21)
AHA: 2020,3Q,26
DEF: Associated with myocardial infarction, cardiac tamponade, and massive pulmonary embolism. Symptoms include mental confusion, reduced blood pressure, tachycardia, pallor, and cold, clammy skin.

R57.1 Hypovolemic shock [HCC] [ESR] [COM]
AHA: 2019,2Q,7

R57.8 Other shock [HCC] [ESR] [COM]
R57.9 Shock, unspecified [HCC] [ESR] [COM]
Failure of peripheral circulation NOS

R58 Hemorrhage, not elsewhere classified
Hemorrhage NOS
- EXCLUDES 1: hemorrhage included with underlying conditions, such as:
  - acute duodenal ulcer with hemorrhage (K26.0)
  - acute gastritis with bleeding (K29.01)
  - ulcerative enterocolitis with rectal bleeding (K51.01)

✓4th R59 Enlarged lymph nodes
- INCLUDES: swollen glands
- EXCLUDES 1: acute lymphadenitis (L04.-)
  - chronic lymphadenitis (I88.1)
  - lymphadenitis NOS (I88.9)
  - mesenteric (acute) (chronic) lymphadenitis (I88.0)

R59.0 Localized enlarged lymph nodes
R59.1 Generalized enlarged lymph nodes
Lymphadenopathy NOS
R59.9 Enlarged lymph nodes, unspecified

✓4th R60 Edema, not elsewhere classified
- EXCLUDES 1: angioneurotic edema (T78.3)
  - ascites (R18.-)
  - cerebral edema (G93.6)
  - cerebral edema due to birth injury (P11.0)
  - edema of larynx (J38.4)
  - edema of nasopharynx (J39.2)
  - edema of pharynx (J39.2)
  - gestational edema (O12.0-)
  - hereditary edema (Q82.0)
  - hydrops fetalis NOS (P83.2)
  - hydrothorax (J94.8)
  - newborn edema (P83.3)
  - pulmonary edema (J81.-)

R60.0 Localized edema
R60.1 Generalized edema
- EXCLUDES 2: nutritional edema (E40-E46)
R60.9 Edema, unspecified
Fluid retention NOS

R61 Generalized hyperhidrosis
Excessive sweating
Night sweats
Secondary hyperhidrosis
Code first, if applicable, menopausal and female climacteric states (N95.1)
- EXCLUDES 1: focal (primary) (secondary) hyperhidrosis (L74.5-)
  - Frey's syndrome (L74.52)
  - localized (primary) (secondary) hyperhidrosis (L74.5-)

✓4th R62 Lack of expected normal physiological development in childhood and adults
- EXCLUDES 1: delayed puberty (E30.0)
  - gonadal dysgenesis (Q99.1)
  - hypopituitarism (E23.0)

R62.0 Delayed milestone in childhood [P]
Delayed attainment of expected physiological developmental stage
Late talker
Late walker

✓5th R62.5 Other and unspecified lack of expected normal physiological development in childhood
- EXCLUDES 1: HIV disease resulting in failure to thrive (B20)
  - physical retardation due to malnutrition (E45)

R62.50 Unspecified lack of expected normal physiological development in childhood
Infantilism NOS

R62.51 Failure to thrive (child) [P]
Failure to gain weight
▶Faltering growth◄
- EXCLUDES 1: failure to thrive in child under 28 days old (P92.6)
AHA: 2018,4Q,82
DEF: Nonorganic failure to thrive (FTT): Symptom of neglect or abuse.
DEF: Organic failure to thrive (FTT): Acute or chronic illness that interferes with nutritional intake, absorption, metabolism excretion, and energy requirements.

R62.52 Short stature (child)
Lack of growth
Physical retardation
Short stature NOS
- EXCLUDES 1: short stature due to endocrine disorder (E34.3-)

R62.59 Other lack of expected normal physiological development in childhood

R62.7 Adult failure to thrive [UPD] [A]

Chapter 18. Symptoms, Signs and Abnormal Clinical and Laboratory Findings

R63 Symptoms and signs concerning food and fluid intake
EXCLUDES 1: bulimia NOS (F50.2-)

R63.0 Anorexia
Loss of appetite
EXCLUDES 1: anorexia nervosa (F50.0-)
loss of appetite of nonorganic origin (F50.89)
AHA: 2018,4Q,82
TIP: Assign an additional code from category Z68 when BMI is documented. BMI can be based on documentation from clinicians who are not the patient's provider.

R63.1 Polydipsia
Excessive thirst

R63.2 Polyphagia
Excessive eating
Hyperalimentation NOS

R63.3 Feeding difficulties
EXCLUDES 2: eating disorders (F50.-)
feeding problems of newborn (P92.-)
infant feeding disorder of nonorganic origin (F98.2-)
AHA: 2021,4Q,27-28; 2017,1Q,28; 2016,3Q,19

- **R63.30** Feeding difficulties, unspecified
- **R63.31** Pediatric feeding disorder, acute
  Pediatric feeding dysfunction, acute
  Code also, if applicable, associated conditions such as:
  aspiration pneumonia (J69.0)
  dysphagia (R13.1-)
  gastro-esophageal reflux disease (K21.-)
  malnutrition (E40-E46)
- **R63.32** Pediatric feeding disorder, chronic
  Pediatric feeding dysfunction, chronic
  Code also, if applicable, associated conditions such as:
  aspiration pneumonia (J69.0)
  dysphagia (R13.1-)
  gastro-esophageal reflux disease (K21.-)
  malnutrition (E40-E46)
- **R63.39** Other feeding difficulties
  Feeding problem (elderly) (infant) NOS
  Picky eater

R63.4 Abnormal weight loss
AHA: 2018,4Q,82
TIP: Assign an additional code from category Z68 when BMI is documented. BMI can be based on documentation from clinicians who are not the patient's provider.

R63.5 Abnormal weight gain
EXCLUDES 1: excessive weight gain in pregnancy (O26.0-)
obesity (E66.-)
AHA: 2018,4Q,82
TIP: Assign an additional code from category Z68 when BMI is documented. BMI can be based on documentation from clinicians who are not the patient's provider.

R63.6 Underweight
Use additional code to identify body mass index (BMI), if known (Z68.-)
EXCLUDES 1: abnormal weight loss (R63.4)
anorexia nervosa (F50.0-)
malnutrition (E40-E46)
AHA: 2018,4Q,82

R63.8 Other symptoms and signs concerning food and fluid intake

R64 Cachexia
EXCLUDES 1: abnormal weight loss (R63.4)
cachexia due to underlying condition (E88.A)
nutritional marasmus (E41)
AHA: 2018,4Q,82; 2017,3Q,24

R65 Symptoms and signs specifically associated with systemic inflammation and infection
AHA: 2019,2Q,38
TIP: When documentation states SIRS with an infection, assign only a code for the infection. ICD-10-CM does not offer a code for SIRS due to infectious process. If sepsis is suspected, query the provider.

R65.1 Systemic inflammatory response syndrome [SIRS] of non-infectious origin
Code first underlying condition, such as:
heatstroke (T67.0-)
injury and trauma (S00-T88)
EXCLUDES 1: sepsis - code to infection
severe sepsis (R65.2)

- **R65.10** Systemic inflammatory response syndrome [SIRS] of non-infectious origin without acute organ dysfunction
  Systemic inflammatory response syndrome (SIRS) NOS
  AHA: 2019,2Q,24
- **R65.11** Systemic inflammatory response syndrome [SIRS] of non-infectious origin with acute organ dysfunction
  Use additional code to identify specific acute organ dysfunction, such as:
  acute kidney failure (N17.-)
  acute respiratory failure (J96.0-)
  critical illness myopathy (G72.81)
  critical illness polyneuropathy (G62.81)
  disseminated intravascular coagulopathy [DIC] (D65)
  encephalopathy (metabolic) (septic) (G93.41)
  hepatic failure (K72.0-)

R65.2 Severe sepsis
Infection with associated acute organ dysfunction
Sepsis with acute organ dysfunction
Sepsis with multiple organ dysfunction
Systemic inflammatory response syndrome due to infectious process with acute organ dysfunction
Code first underlying infection, such as:
infection following a procedure (T81.4-)
infections following infusion, transfusion and therapeutic injection (T80.2-)
puerperal sepsis (O85)
sepsis following (induced) termination of pregnancy (O04.87)
sepsis following complete or unspecified spontaneous abortion (O03.87)
sepsis following ectopic and molar pregnancy (O08.82)
sepsis following incomplete spontaneous abortion (O03.37)
sepsis NOS (A41.9)
Use additional code to identify specific acute organ dysfunction, such as:
acute kidney failure (N17.-)
acute respiratory failure (J96.0-)
critical illness myopathy (G72.81)
critical illness polyneuropathy (G62.81)
disseminated intravascular coagulopathy [DIC] (D65)
encephalopathy (metabolic) (septic) (G93.41)
hepatic failure (K72.0-)
AHA: 2020,2Q,17; 2018,4Q,62-63; 2017,4Q,98-99; 2016,3Q,8

- **R65.20** Severe sepsis without septic shock
  Severe sepsis NOS
  AHA: 2020,2Q,17; 2016,3Q,14; 2013,4Q,119
- **R65.21** Severe sepsis with septic shock
  EXCLUDES 1: ▶postprocedural septic shock (T81.12-)◀
  AHA: 2018,4Q,63

R68 Other general symptoms and signs

R68.0 Hypothermia, not associated with low environmental temperature
EXCLUDES 1: hypothermia NOS (accidental) (T68)
hypothermia due to anesthesia (T88.51)
hypothermia due to low environmental temperature (T68)
newborn hypothermia (P80.-)

R68.1 Nonspecific symptoms peculiar to infancy
EXCLUDES 1: colic, infantile (R10.83)
neonatal cerebral irritability (P91.3)
teething syndrome (K00.7)

- **R68.11** Excessive crying of infant (baby)
  EXCLUDES 1: excessive crying of child, adolescent, or adult (R45.83)

HCC CMS-HCC | Rx Rx HCC | ESR ESRD HCC | COM Commercial HCC | N Newborn: 0 | P Pediatric: 0-17 | M Maternity: 9-64 | A Adult: 15-124

Chapter 18. Symptoms, Signs and Abnormal Clinical and Laboratory Findings

R68.12 **Fussy infant (baby)**
Irritable infant

R68.13 **Apparent life threatening event in infant (ALTE)**
Apparent life threatening event in newborn
Brief resolved unexplained event (BRUE)
Code first confirmed diagnosis, if known
Use additional code(s) for associated signs and symptoms if no confirmed diagnosis established, or if signs and symptoms are not associated routinely with confirmed diagnosis, or provide additional information for cause of ALTE

R68.19 **Other nonspecific symptoms peculiar to infancy**

R68.2 **Dry mouth, unspecified**
EXCLUDES 1: dry mouth due to dehydration (E86.0)
dry mouth due to Sjogren syndrome (M35.0-)
EXCLUDES 2: salivary gland hyposecretion (K11.7)

R68.3 **Clubbing of fingers**
Clubbing of nails
EXCLUDES 1: congenital clubfinger (Q68.1)
DEF: Enlarged soft tissue of the distal fingers that usually occurs in heart and lung diseases.

R68.8 **Other general symptoms and signs**

R68.81 **Early satiety**
DEF: Premature feeling of being full after eating only a small amount of food. The mechanism of satiety is multifactorial.

R68.82 **Decreased libido**
Decreased sexual desire

R68.83 **Chills (without fever)**
Chills NOS
EXCLUDES 1: chills with fever (R50.9)

R68.84 **Jaw pain**
Mandibular pain
Maxilla pain
EXCLUDES 1: temporomandibular joint arthralgia (M26.62-)

R68.89 **Other general symptoms and signs**

R69 **Illness, unspecified**
▶Unknown and unspecified causes of morbidity◀

Abnormal findings on examination of blood, without diagnosis (R70-R79)

EXCLUDES 2: abnormal findings on antenatal screening of mother (O28.-)
abnormalities of lipids (E78.-)
abnormalities of platelets and thrombocytes (D69.-)
abnormalities of white blood cells classified elsewhere (D70-D72)
coagulation hemorrhagic disorders (D65-D68)
diagnostic abnormal findings classified elsewhere - see Alphabetical Index
hemorrhagic and hematological disorders of newborn (P50-P61)

R70 **Elevated erythrocyte sedimentation rate and abnormality of plasma viscosity**

R70.0 **Elevated erythrocyte sedimentation rate**

R70.1 **Abnormal plasma viscosity**

R71 **Abnormality of red blood cells**
EXCLUDES 1: anemias (D50-D64)
anemia of premature infant (P61.2)
benign (familial) polycythemia (D75.0)
congenital anemias (P61.2-P61.4)
newborn anemia due to isoimmunization (P55.-)
polycythemia neonatorum (P61.1)
polycythemia NOS (D75.1)
polycythemia vera (D45)
secondary polycythemia (D75.1)

R71.0 **Precipitous drop in hematocrit**
Drop (precipitous) in hemoglobin
Drop in hematocrit

R71.8 **Other abnormality of red blood cells**
Abnormal red-cell morphology NOS
Abnormal red-cell volume NOS
Anisocytosis
Poikilocytosis

R73 **Elevated blood glucose level**
EXCLUDES 1: diabetes mellitus (E08-E13)
diabetes mellitus in pregnancy, childbirth and the puerperium (O24.-)
neonatal disorders (P70.0-P70.2)
postsurgical hypoinsulinemia (E89.1)

R73.0 **Abnormal glucose**
EXCLUDES 1: abnormal glucose in pregnancy (O99.81-)
diabetes mellitus (E08-E13)
dysmetabolic syndrome X (E88.81-)
gestational diabetes (O24.4-)
glycosuria (R81)
hypoglycemia (E16.2)
type 1 diabetes mellitus, presymptomatic (E10.A-)

R73.01 **Impaired fasting glucose**
Elevated fasting glucose

R73.02 **Impaired glucose tolerance (oral)**
Elevated glucose tolerance

R73.03 **Prediabetes**
Latent diabetes
AHA: 2024,3Q,11; 2016,4Q,65

R73.09 **Other abnormal glucose**
Abnormal glucose NOS
Abnormal non-fasting glucose tolerance

R73.9 **Hyperglycemia, unspecified**

R74 **Abnormal serum enzyme levels**

R74.0 **Nonspecific elevation of levels of transaminase and lactic acid dehydrogenase [LDH]**
AHA: 2020,4Q,39

R74.01 **Elevation of levels of liver transaminase levels**
Elevation of levels of alanine transaminase (ALT)
Elevation of levels of aspartate transaminase (AST)

R74.02 **Elevation of levels of lactic acid dehydrogenase [LDH]**

R74.8 **Abnormal levels of other serum enzymes**
Abnormal level of acid phosphatase
Abnormal level of alkaline phosphatase
Abnormal level of amylase
Abnormal level of lipase [triacylglycerol lipase]
AHA: 2019,2Q,6

R74.9 **Abnormal serum enzyme level, unspecified**

R75 **Inconclusive laboratory evidence of human immunodeficiency virus [HIV]**
Nonconclusive HIV-test finding in infants
EXCLUDES 1: asymptomatic human immunodeficiency virus [HIV] infection status (Z21)
human immunodeficiency virus [HIV] disease (B20)

R76 **Other abnormal immunological findings in serum**

R76.0 **Raised antibody titer**
EXCLUDES 1: isoimmunization in pregnancy (O36.0-O36.1)
isoimmunization affecting newborn (P55.-)
AHA: 2021,1Q,6

R76.1 **Nonspecific reaction to test for tuberculosis**

R76.11 **Nonspecific reaction to tuberculin skin test without active tuberculosis**
Abnormal result of Mantoux test
PPD positive
Tuberculin (skin test) positive
Tuberculin (skin test) reactor
EXCLUDES 1: nonspecific reaction to cell mediated immunity measurement of gamma interferon antigen response without active tuberculosis (R76.12)

R76.12 **Nonspecific reaction to cell mediated immunity measurement of gamma interferon antigen response without active tuberculosis**
Nonspecific reaction to QuantiFERON-TB test (QFT) without active tuberculosis
EXCLUDES 1: nonspecific reaction to tuberculin skin test without active tuberculosis (R76.11)
positive tuberculin skin test (R76.11)

Chapter 18. Symptoms, Signs and Abnormal Clinical and Laboratory Findings

▲ ✓5ᵗʰ **R76.8 Other specified abnormal immunological findings in serum**
Raised level of immunoglobulins NOS
AHA: 2021,1Q,6

● **R76.81 Abnormal rheumatoid factor and anti-citrullinated protein antibody without rheumatoid arthritis**
Abnormal anti-CCP
Abnormal anti-cyclic citrullinated protein antibody and rheumatoid factor
EXCLUDES 1 rheumatoid arthritis with rheumatoid factor (M05.-)

● **R76.89 Other specified abnormal immunological findings in serum**
Raised level of immunoglobulins NOS

R76.9 Abnormal immunological finding in serum, unspecified

✓4ᵗʰ **R77 Other abnormalities of plasma proteins**
EXCLUDES 1 disorders of plasma-protein metabolism (E88.0-)

R77.0 Abnormality of albumin

R77.1 Abnormality of globulin
Hyperglobulinemia NOS

R77.2 Abnormality of alphafetoprotein

R77.8 Other specified abnormalities of plasma proteins

R77.9 Abnormality of plasma protein, unspecified
AHA: 2019,2Q,6

✓4ᵗʰ **R78 Findings of drugs and other substances, not normally found in blood**
Use additional code to identify the any retained foreign body, if applicable (Z18.-)
EXCLUDES 2 mental or behavioral disorders due to psychoactive substance use (F10-F19)

R78.0 Finding of alcohol in blood
Use additional external cause code (Y90.-), for detail regarding alcohol level

R78.1 Finding of opiate drug in blood

R78.2 Finding of cocaine in blood

R78.3 Finding of hallucinogen in blood

R78.4 Finding of other drugs of addictive potential in blood

R78.5 Finding of other psychotropic drug in blood

R78.6 Finding of steroid agent in blood

✓5ᵗʰ **R78.7 Finding of abnormal level of heavy metals in blood**

R78.71 Abnormal lead level in blood
EXCLUDES 1 lead poisoning (T56.0-)

R78.79 Finding of abnormal level of heavy metals in blood

✓5ᵗʰ **R78.8 Finding of other specified substances, not normally found in blood**

R78.81 Bacteremia
EXCLUDES 1 sepsis — code to specified infection
AHA: 2025,1Q,20
DEF: Laboratory finding of bacteria in the blood in the absence of two or more signs of sepsis. Transient in nature, it can progress to septicemia with a severe infectious process.

R78.89 Finding of other specified substances, not normally found in blood
Finding of abnormal level of lithium in blood

R78.9 Finding of unspecified substance, not normally found in blood

✓4ᵗʰ **R79 Other abnormal findings of blood chemistry**
Use additional code to identify any retained foreign body, if applicable (Z18.-)
EXCLUDES 1 asymptomatic hyperuricemia (E79.0)
hyperglycemia NOS (R73.9)
hypoglycemia NOS (E16.2)
neonatal hypoglycemia (P70.3-P70.4)
specific findings indicating disorder of amino-acid metabolism (E70-E72)
specific findings indicating disorder of carbohydrate metabolism (E73-E74)
specific findings indicating disorder of lipid metabolism (E75.-)

R79.0 Abnormal level of blood mineral
Abnormal blood level of cobalt
Abnormal blood level of copper
Abnormal blood level of iron
Abnormal blood level of magnesium
Abnormal blood level of mineral NEC
Abnormal blood level of zinc
EXCLUDES 1 abnormal level of lithium (R78.89)
disorders of mineral metabolism (E83.-)
neonatal hypomagnesemia (P71.2)
nutritional mineral deficiency (E58-E61)

R79.1 Abnormal coagulation profile
Abnormal or prolonged bleeding time
Abnormal or prolonged coagulation time
Abnormal or prolonged partial thromboplastin time [PTT]
Abnormal or prolonged prothrombin time [PT]
Low von Willebrand factor
EXCLUDES 1 coagulation defects (D68.-)
EXCLUDES 2 abnormality of fluid, electrolyte or acid-base balance (E86-E87)

✓5ᵗʰ **R79.8 Other specified abnormal findings of blood chemistry**

R79.81 Abnormal blood-gas level

R79.82 Elevated C-reactive protein [CRP]

R79.83 Abnormal findings of blood amino-acid level
Homocysteinemia
EXCLUDES 1 disorders of amino-acid metabolism (E70-E72)
AHA: 2021,4Q,28

R79.89 Other specified abnormal findings of blood chemistry
AHA: 2019,2Q,6
TIP: Assign for positive Coombs test when not further clarified in the documentation.

R79.9 Abnormal finding of blood chemistry, unspecified

Abnormal findings on examination of urine, without diagnosis (R80-R82)

EXCLUDES 1 abnormal findings on antenatal screening of mother (O28.-)
diagnostic abnormal findings classified elsewhere - see Alphabetical Index
specific findings indicating disorder of amino-acid metabolism (E70-E72)
specific findings indicating disorder of carbohydrate metabolism (E73-E74)

✓4ᵗʰ **R80 Proteinuria**
EXCLUDES 1 gestational proteinuria (O12.1-)

R80.0 Isolated proteinuria
Idiopathic proteinuria
EXCLUDES 1 isolated proteinuria with specific morphological lesion (N06.-)

R80.1 Persistent proteinuria, unspecified

R80.2 Orthostatic proteinuria, unspecified
Postural proteinuria

R80.3 Bence Jones proteinuria

R80.8 Other proteinuria

R80.9 Proteinuria, unspecified
Albuminuria NOS

R81 Glycosuria
EXCLUDES 1 renal glycosuria (E74.818)

✓4ᵗʰ **R82 Other and unspecified abnormal findings in urine**
INCLUDES chromoabnormalities in urine
Use additional code to identify any retained foreign body, if applicable (Z18.-)
EXCLUDES 2 hematuria (R31.-)

R82.0 Chyluria
EXCLUDES 1 filarial chyluria (B74.-)

R82.1 Myoglobinuria

R82.2 Biliuria

R82.3 Hemoglobinuria
EXCLUDES 1 hemoglobinuria due to hemolysis from external causes NEC (D59.6)
hemoglobinuria due to paroxysmal nocturnal [Marchiafava-Micheli] (D59.5)
DEF: Free hemoglobin in blood due to rapid hemolysis of red blood cells. Causes include burns, crushed injury, sickle cell anemia, thalassemia, parasitic infections, or kidney infections.

R82.4 Acetonuria
Ketonuria
DEF: Excessive excretion of acetone in urine that commonly occurs in diabetic acidosis.

R82.5 Elevated urine levels of drugs, medicaments and biological substances
Elevated urine levels of 17-ketosteroids
Elevated urine levels of catecholamines
Elevated urine levels of indoleacetic acid
Elevated urine levels of steroids

R82.6 Abnormal urine levels of substances chiefly nonmedicinal as to source
Abnormal urine level of heavy metals

Chapter 18. Symptoms, Signs and Abnormal Clinical and Laboratory Findings

R82.7 Abnormal findings on microbiological examination of urine
- EXCLUDES 1: colonization status (Z22.-)
- AHA: 2016,4Q,65
  - **R82.71** Bacteriuria
  - **R82.79** Other abnormal findings on microbiological examination of urine
    - Positive culture findings of urine

R82.8 Abnormal findings on cytological and histological examination of urine
- AHA: 2019,4Q,16
  - **R82.81** Pyuria
    - Sterile pyuria
  - **R82.89** Other abnormal findings on cytological and histological examination of urine

R82.9 Other and unspecified abnormal findings in urine
- **R82.90** Unspecified abnormal findings in urine
- **R82.91** Other chromoabnormalities of urine
  - Chromoconversion (dipstick)
  - Idiopathic dipstick converts positive for blood with no cellular forms in sediment
  - EXCLUDES 1: hemoglobinuria (R82.3)
    - myoglobinuria (R82.1)
- **R82.99** Other abnormal findings in urine
  - AHA: 2018,4Q,29-30
  - **R82.991** Hypocitraturia
  - **R82.992** Hyperoxaluria
    - EXCLUDES 1: ▶primary hyperoxaluria (E72.53-)◀
      - ▶secondary hyperoxaluria (E72.54-)◀
  - **R82.993** Hyperuricosuria
  - **R82.994** Hypercalciuria
    - Idiopathic hypercalciuria
  - **R82.998** Other abnormal findings in urine
    - Cells and casts in urine
    - Crystalluria
    - Melanuria

Abnormal findings on examination of other body fluids, substances and tissues, without diagnosis (R83-R89)

- EXCLUDES 1: abnormal findings on antenatal screening of mother (O28.-)
  - diagnostic abnormal findings classified elsewhere - see Alphabetical Index
- EXCLUDES 2: abnormal findings on examination of blood, without diagnosis (R70-R79)
  - abnormal findings on examination of urine, without diagnosis (R80-R82)
  - abnormal tumor markers (R97.-)

R83 Abnormal findings in cerebrospinal fluid
- **R83.0** Abnormal level of enzymes in cerebrospinal fluid
- **R83.1** Abnormal level of hormones in cerebrospinal fluid
- **R83.2** Abnormal level of other drugs, medicaments and biological substances in cerebrospinal fluid
- **R83.3** Abnormal level of substances chiefly nonmedicinal as to source in cerebrospinal fluid
- **R83.4** Abnormal immunological findings in cerebrospinal fluid
- **R83.5** Abnormal microbiological findings in cerebrospinal fluid
  - Positive culture findings in cerebrospinal fluid
  - EXCLUDES 1: colonization status (Z22.-)
- **R83.6** Abnormal cytological findings in cerebrospinal fluid
- **R83.8** Other abnormal findings in cerebrospinal fluid
  - Abnormal chromosomal findings in cerebrospinal fluid
- **R83.9** Unspecified abnormal finding in cerebrospinal fluid

R84 Abnormal findings in specimens from respiratory organs and thorax
- INCLUDES: abnormal findings in bronchial washings
  - abnormal findings in nasal secretions
  - abnormal findings in pleural fluid
  - abnormal findings in sputum
  - abnormal findings in throat scrapings
- EXCLUDES 1: blood-stained sputum (R04.2)
  - **R84.0** Abnormal level of enzymes in specimens from respiratory organs and thorax
  - **R84.1** Abnormal level of hormones in specimens from respiratory organs and thorax
  - **R84.2** Abnormal level of other drugs, medicaments and biological substances in specimens from respiratory organs and thorax
  - **R84.3** Abnormal level of substances chiefly nonmedicinal as to source in specimens from respiratory organs and thorax
  - **R84.4** Abnormal immunological findings in specimens from respiratory organs and thorax
  - **R84.5** Abnormal microbiological findings in specimens from respiratory organs and thorax
    - Positive culture findings in specimens from respiratory organs and thorax
    - EXCLUDES 1: colonization status (Z22.-)
  - **R84.6** Abnormal cytological findings in specimens from respiratory organs and thorax
  - **R84.7** Abnormal histological findings in specimens from respiratory organs and thorax
  - **R84.8** Other abnormal findings in specimens from respiratory organs and thorax
    - Abnormal chromosomal findings in specimens from respiratory organs and thorax
  - **R84.9** Unspecified abnormal finding in specimens from respiratory organs and thorax

R85 Abnormal findings in specimens from digestive organs and abdominal cavity
- INCLUDES: abnormal findings in peritoneal fluid
  - abnormal findings in saliva
- EXCLUDES 1: cloudy peritoneal dialysis effluent (R88.0)
  - fecal abnormalities (R19.5)
  - **R85.0** Abnormal level of enzymes in specimens from digestive organs and abdominal cavity
  - **R85.1** Abnormal level of hormones in specimens from digestive organs and abdominal cavity
  - **R85.2** Abnormal level of other drugs, medicaments and biological substances in specimens from digestive organs and abdominal cavity
  - **R85.3** Abnormal level of substances chiefly nonmedicinal as to source in specimens from digestive organs and abdominal cavity
  - **R85.4** Abnormal immunological findings in specimens from digestive organs and abdominal cavity
  - **R85.5** Abnormal microbiological findings in specimens from digestive organs and abdominal cavity
    - Positive culture findings in specimens from digestive organs and abdominal cavity
    - EXCLUDES 1: colonization status (Z22.-)
  - **R85.6** Abnormal cytological findings in specimens from digestive organs and abdominal cavity
    - **R85.61** Abnormal cytologic smear of anus
      - EXCLUDES 1: abnormal cytological findings in specimens from other digestive organs and abdominal cavity (R85.69)
        - anal intraepithelial neoplasia I [AIN I] (K62.82)
        - anal intraepithelial neoplasia II [AIN II] (K62.82)
        - anal intraepithelial neoplasia III [AIN III] (D01.3)
        - carcinoma in situ of anus (histologically confirmed) (D01.3)
        - dysplasia (mild) (moderate) of anus (histologically confirmed) (K62.82)
        - severe dysplasia of anus (histologically confirmed) (D01.3)
      - EXCLUDES 2: anal high risk human papillomavirus (HPV) DNA test positive (R85.81)
        - anal low risk human papillomavirus (HPV) DNA test positive (R85.82)
      - **R85.610** Atypical squamous cells of undetermined significance on cytologic smear of anus [ASC-US]
      - **R85.611** Atypical squamous cells cannot exclude high grade squamous intraepithelial lesion on cytologic smear of anus [ASC-H]
      - **R85.612** Low grade squamous intraepithelial lesion on cytologic smear of anus [LGSIL]
      - **R85.613** High grade squamous intraepithelial lesion on cytologic smear of anus [HGSIL]
      - **R85.614** Cytologic evidence of malignancy on smear of anus
      - **R85.615** Unsatisfactory cytologic smear of anus
        - Inadequate sample of cytologic smear of anus
      - **R85.616** Satisfactory anal smear but lacking transformation zone
      - **R85.618** Other abnormal cytological findings on specimens from anus

R85.619 Unspecified abnormal cytological findings in specimens from anus
Abnormal anal cytology NOS
Atypical glandular cells of anus NOS

R85.69 Abnormal cytological findings in specimens from other digestive organs and abdominal cavity

R85.7 Abnormal histological findings in specimens from digestive organs and abdominal cavity

R85.8 Other abnormal findings in specimens from digestive organs and abdominal cavity

R85.81 Anal high risk human papillomavirus [HPV] DNA test positive
EXCLUDES 1 — anogenital warts due to human papillomavirus (HPV) (A63.0)
condyloma acuminatum (A63.0)

R85.82 Anal low risk human papillomavirus [HPV] DNA test positive
Use additional code for associated human papillomavirus (B97.7)

R85.89 Other abnormal findings in specimens from digestive organs and abdominal cavity
Abnormal chromosomal findings in specimens from digestive organs and abdominal cavity

R85.9 Unspecified abnormal finding in specimens from digestive organs and abdominal cavity

R86 Abnormal findings in specimens from male genital organs
INCLUDES abnormal findings in prostatic secretions
abnormal findings in semen, seminal fluid
abnormal spermatozoa
EXCLUDES 1 — azoospermia (N46.0-)
oligospermia (N46.1-)

R86.0 Abnormal level of enzymes in specimens from male genital organs

R86.1 Abnormal level of hormones in specimens from male genital organs

R86.2 Abnormal level of other drugs, medicaments and biological substances in specimens from male genital organs

R86.3 Abnormal level of substances chiefly nonmedicinal as to source in specimens from male genital organs

R86.4 Abnormal immunological findings in specimens from male genital organs

R86.5 Abnormal microbiological findings in specimens from male genital organs
Positive culture findings in specimens from male genital organs
EXCLUDES 1 — colonization status (Z22.-)

R86.6 Abnormal cytological findings in specimens from male genital organs

R86.7 Abnormal histological findings in specimens from male genital organs

R86.8 Other abnormal findings in specimens from male genital organs
Abnormal chromosomal findings in specimens from male genital organs

R86.9 Unspecified abnormal finding in specimens from male genital organs

R87 Abnormal findings in specimens from female genital organs
INCLUDES abnormal findings in secretion and smears from cervix uteri
abnormal findings in secretion and smears from vagina
abnormal findings in secretion and smears from vulva

R87.0 Abnormal level of enzymes in specimens from female genital organs

R87.1 Abnormal level of hormones in specimens from female genital organs

R87.2 Abnormal level of other drugs, medicaments and biological substances in specimens from female genital organs

R87.3 Abnormal level of substances chiefly nonmedicinal as to source in specimens from female genital organs

R87.4 Abnormal immunological findings in specimens from female genital organs

R87.5 Abnormal microbiological findings in specimens from female genital organs
Positive culture findings in specimens from female genital organs
EXCLUDES 1 — colonization status (Z22.-)

R87.6 Abnormal cytological findings in specimens from female genital organs

R87.61 Abnormal cytological findings in specimens from cervix uteri
EXCLUDES 1 — abnormal cytological findings in specimens from other female genital organs (R87.69)
abnormal cytological findings in specimens from vagina (R87.62-)
carcinoma in situ of cervix uteri (histologically confirmed) (D06.-)
cervical intraepithelial neoplasia I [CIN I] (N87.0)
cervical intraepithelial neoplasia II [CIN II] (N87.1)
cervical intraepithelial neoplasia III [CIN III] (D06.-)
dysplasia (mild) (moderate) of cervix uteri (histologically confirmed) (N87.-)
severe dysplasia of cervix uteri (histologically confirmed) (D06.-)
EXCLUDES 2 — cervical high risk human papillomavirus (HPV) DNA test positive (R87.810)
cervical low risk human papillomavirus (HPV) DNA test positive (R87.820)

R87.610 Atypical squamous cells of undetermined significance on cytologic smear of cervix [ASC-US]

R87.611 Atypical squamous cells cannot exclude high grade squamous intraepithelial lesion on cytologic smear of cervix [ASC-H]

R87.612 Low grade squamous intraepithelial lesion on cytologic smear of cervix [LGSIL]

R87.613 High grade squamous intraepithelial lesion on cytologic smear of cervix [HGSIL]

R87.614 Cytologic evidence of malignancy on smear of cervix

R87.615 Unsatisfactory cytologic smear of cervix
Inadequate sample of cytologic smear of cervix

R87.616 Satisfactory cervical smear but lacking transformation zone

R87.618 Other abnormal cytological findings on specimens from cervix uteri

R87.619 Unspecified abnormal cytological findings in specimens from cervix uteri
Abnormal cervical cytology NOS
Abnormal Papanicolaou smear of cervix NOS
Abnormal thin preparation smear of cervix NOS
▶Atypical endocervical cells of cervix NOS◀
Atypical endometrial cells of cervix NOS
Atypical glandular cells of cervix NOS

R87.62 Abnormal cytological findings in specimens from vagina
Use additional code to identify acquired absence of uterus and cervix, if applicable (Z90.71-)
EXCLUDES 1 — abnormal cytological findings in specimens from cervix uteri (R87.61-)
abnormal cytological findings in specimens from other female genital organs (R87.69)
carcinoma in situ of vagina (histologically confirmed) (D07.2)
dysplasia (mild) (moderate) of vagina (histologically confirmed) (N89.-)
severe dysplasia of vagina (histologically confirmed) (D07.2)
vaginal intraepithelial neoplasia I [VAIN I] (N89.0)
vaginal intraepithelial neoplasia II [VAIN II] (N89.1)
vaginal intraepithelial neoplasia III [VAIN III] (D07.2)
EXCLUDES 2 — vaginal high risk human papillomavirus (HPV) DNA test positive (R87.811)
vaginal low risk human papillomavirus (HPV) DNA test positive (R87.821)

R87.620 Atypical squamous cells of undetermined significance on cytologic smear of vagina [ASC-US]

Chapter 18. Symptoms, Signs and Abnormal Clinical and Laboratory Findings

R87.621 Atypical squamous cells cannot exclude high grade squamous intraepithelial lesion on cytologic smear of vagina [ASC-H]

R87.622 Low grade squamous intraepithelial lesion on cytologic smear of vagina [LGSIL]

R87.623 High grade squamous intraepithelial lesion on cytologic smear of vagina [HGSIL]

R87.624 Cytologic evidence of malignancy on smear of vagina

R87.625 Unsatisfactory cytologic smear of vagina
Inadequate sample of cytologic smear of vagina

R87.628 Other abnormal cytological findings on specimens from vagina

R87.629 Unspecified abnormal cytological findings in specimens from vagina
Abnormal Papanicolaou smear of vagina NOS
Abnormal thin preparation smear of vagina NOS
Abnormal vaginal cytology NOS
Atypical endocervical cells of vagina NOS
Atypical endometrial cells of vagina NOS
Atypical glandular cells of vagina NOS

R87.69 Abnormal cytological findings in specimens from other female genital organs
Abnormal cytological findings in specimens from female genital organs NOS
EXCLUDES 1 dysplasia of vulva (histologically confirmed) (N90.0-N90.3)

R87.7 Abnormal histological findings in specimens from female genital organs
EXCLUDES 1 carcinoma in situ (histologically confirmed) of female genital organs (D06-D07.3)
cervical intraepithelial neoplasia I [CIN I] (N87.0)
cervical intraepithelial neoplasia II [CIN II] (N87.1)
cervical intraepithelial neoplasia III [CIN III] (D06.-)
dysplasia (mild) (moderate) of cervix uteri (histologically confirmed) (N87.-)
dysplasia (mild) (moderate) of vagina (histologically confirmed) (N89.-)
severe dysplasia of cervix uteri (histologically confirmed) (D06.-)
severe dysplasia of vagina (histologically confirmed) (D07.2)
vaginal intraepithelial neoplasia I [VAIN I] (N89.0)
vaginal intraepithelial neoplasia II [VAIN II] (N89.1)
vaginal intraepithelial neoplasia III [VAIN III] (D07.2)

R87.8 Other abnormal findings in specimens from female genital organs

R87.81 High risk human papillomavirus [HPV] DNA test positive from female genital organs
EXCLUDES 1 anogenital warts due to human papillomavirus (HPV) (A63.0)
condyloma acuminatum (A63.0)

R87.810 Cervical high risk human papillomavirus [HPV] DNA test positive

R87.811 Vaginal high risk human papillomavirus [HPV] DNA test positive

R87.82 Low risk human papillomavirus [HPV] DNA test positive from female genital organs
Use additional code for associated human papillomavirus (B97.7)

R87.820 Cervical low risk human papillomavirus [HPV] DNA test positive

R87.821 Vaginal low risk human papillomavirus [HPV] DNA test positive

R87.89 Other abnormal findings in specimens from female genital organs
Abnormal chromosomal findings in specimens from female genital organs

R87.9 Unspecified abnormal finding in specimens from female genital organs

R88 Abnormal findings in other body fluids and substances

R88.0 Cloudy (hemodialysis) (peritoneal) dialysis effluent

R88.8 Abnormal findings in other body fluids and substances

R89 Abnormal findings in specimens from other organs, systems and tissues
INCLUDES abnormal findings in nipple discharge
abnormal findings in synovial fluid
abnormal findings in wound secretions

R89.0 Abnormal level of enzymes in specimens from other organs, systems and tissues

R89.1 Abnormal level of hormones in specimens from other organs, systems and tissues

R89.2 Abnormal level of other drugs, medicaments and biological substances in specimens from other organs, systems and tissues

R89.3 Abnormal level of substances chiefly nonmedicinal as to source in specimens from other organs, systems and tissues

R89.4 Abnormal immunological findings in specimens from other organs, systems and tissues

R89.5 Abnormal microbiological findings in specimens from other organs, systems and tissues
Positive culture findings in specimens from other organs, systems and tissues
EXCLUDES 1 colonization status (Z22.-)

R89.6 Abnormal cytological findings in specimens from other organs, systems and tissues

R89.7 Abnormal histological findings in specimens from other organs, systems and tissues
AHA: 2025,2Q,5

R89.8 Other abnormal findings in specimens from other organs, systems and tissues
Abnormal chromosomal findings in specimens from other organs, systems and tissues

R89.9 Unspecified abnormal finding in specimens from other organs, systems and tissues

Abnormal findings on diagnostic imaging and in function studies, without diagnosis (R90-R94)

INCLUDES nonspecific abnormal findings on diagnostic imaging by computerized axial tomography [CAT scan]
nonspecific abnormal findings on diagnostic imaging by magnetic resonance imaging [MRI][NMR]
nonspecific abnormal findings on diagnostic imaging by positron emission tomography [PET scan]
nonspecific abnormal findings on diagnostic imaging by thermography
nonspecific abnormal findings on diagnostic imaging by ultrasound [echogram]
nonspecific abnormal findings on diagnostic imaging by X-ray examination
EXCLUDES 1 abnormal findings on antenatal screening of mother (O28.-)
diagnostic abnormal findings classified elsewhere - see Alphabetical Index

R90 Abnormal findings on diagnostic imaging of central nervous system

R90.0 Intracranial space-occupying lesion found on diagnostic imaging of central nervous system

R90.8 Other abnormal findings on diagnostic imaging of central nervous system

R90.81 Abnormal echoencephalogram

R90.82 White matter disease, unspecified

R90.89 Other abnormal findings on diagnostic imaging of central nervous system
Other cerebrovascular abnormality found on diagnostic imaging of central nervous system

R91 Abnormal findings on diagnostic imaging of lung

R91.1 Solitary pulmonary nodule
Coin lesion lung
Solitary pulmonary nodule, subsegmental branch of the bronchial tree

R91.8 Other nonspecific abnormal finding of lung field
Lung mass NOS found on diagnostic imaging of lung
Pulmonary infiltrate NOS
Shadow, lung

R92 Abnormal and inconclusive findings on diagnostic imaging of breast

R92.0 Mammographic microcalcification found on diagnostic imaging of breast
EXCLUDES 2 mammographic calcification (calculus) found on diagnostic imaging of breast (R92.1)
DEF: Calcium and cellular debris deposits in the breast that cannot be felt but can be detected on a mammogram. The deposits can be a sign of cancer, benign conditions, or changes in the breast tissue as a result of inflammation, injury, or an obstructed duct.

Chapter 18. Symptoms, Signs and Abnormal Clinical and Laboratory Findings

- **R92.1** Mammographic calcification found on diagnostic imaging of breast
  - Mammographic calculus found on diagnostic imaging of breast
- **R92.2** Inconclusive mammogram
  - Inconclusive mammogram NEC
  - Inconclusive mammography NEC
  - AHA: 2015,1Q,24
- √5ᵗʰ **R92.3** Mammographic density found on imaging of breast
  - Code also, if applicable, inconclusive mammogram (R92.2)
  - AHA: 2023,4Q,42-44
  - **R92.30** Dense breasts, unspecified
    - Dense breasts NOS
    - Low density
  - √6ᵗʰ **R92.31** Mammographic fatty tissue density of breast
    - Breast Imaging Reporting and Data System (BI-RADS): 1
    - Breast Imaging Reporting and Data System (BI-RADS): A
    - **R92.311** Mammographic fatty tissue density, right breast
    - **R92.312** Mammographic fatty tissue density, left breast
    - **R92.313** Mammographic fatty tissue density, bilateral breasts
  - √6ᵗʰ **R92.32** Mammographic fibroglandular density of breast
    - Breast Imaging Reporting and Data System (BI-RADS): 2
    - Breast Imaging Reporting and Data System (BI-RADS): B
    - **R92.321** Mammographic fibroglandular density, right breast
    - **R92.322** Mammographic fibroglandular density, left breast
    - **R92.323** Mammographic fibroglandular density, bilateral breasts
  - √6ᵗʰ **R92.33** Mammographic heterogeneous density of breast
    - Breast Imaging Reporting and Data System (BI-RADS): 3
    - Breast Imaging Reporting and Data System (BI-RADS): C
    - **R92.331** Mammographic heterogeneous density, right breast
    - **R92.332** Mammographic heterogeneous density, left breast
    - **R92.333** Mammographic heterogeneous density, bilateral breasts
  - √6ᵗʰ **R92.34** Mammographic extreme density of breast
    - Breast Imaging Reporting and Data System (BI-RADS): 4
    - Breast Imaging Reporting and Data System (BI-RADS): D
    - **R92.341** Mammographic extreme density, right breast
    - **R92.342** Mammographic extreme density, left breast
    - **R92.343** Mammographic extreme density, bilateral breasts
- **R92.8** Other abnormal and inconclusive findings on diagnostic imaging of breast

√4ᵗʰ **R93** Abnormal findings on diagnostic imaging of other body structures
- **R93.0** Abnormal findings on diagnostic imaging of skull and head, not elsewhere classified
  - EXCLUDES 1: intracranial space-occupying lesion found on diagnostic imaging (R90.0)
- **R93.1** Abnormal findings on diagnostic imaging of heart and coronary circulation
  - Abnormal echocardiogram NOS
  - Abnormal heart shadow
- **R93.2** Abnormal findings on diagnostic imaging of liver and biliary tract
  - Nonvisualization of gallbladder
- **R93.3** Abnormal findings on diagnostic imaging of other parts of digestive tract
- √5ᵗʰ **R93.4** Abnormal findings on diagnostic imaging of urinary organs
  - EXCLUDES 2: hypertrophy of kidney (N28.81)
  - AHA: 2016,4Q,66
  - **R93.41** Abnormal radiologic findings on diagnostic imaging of renal pelvis, ureter, or bladder
    - Filling defect of bladder found on diagnostic imaging
    - Filling defect of renal pelvis found on diagnostic imaging
    - Filling defect of ureter found on diagnostic imaging
  - √6ᵗʰ **R93.42** Abnormal radiologic findings on diagnostic imaging of kidney
    - **R93.421** Abnormal radiologic findings on diagnostic imaging of right kidney
    - **R93.422** Abnormal radiologic findings on diagnostic imaging of left kidney
    - **R93.429** Abnormal radiologic findings on diagnostic imaging of unspecified kidney
  - **R93.49** Abnormal radiologic findings on diagnostic imaging of other urinary organs
- **R93.5** Abnormal findings on diagnostic imaging of other abdominal regions, including retroperitoneum
- **R93.6** Abnormal findings on diagnostic imaging of limbs
  - EXCLUDES 2: abnormal finding in skin and subcutaneous tissue (R93.8-)
  - AHA: 2020,1Q,14
- **R93.7** Abnormal findings on diagnostic imaging of other parts of musculoskeletal system
  - EXCLUDES 2: abnormal findings on diagnostic imaging of skull (R93.0)
- √5ᵗʰ **R93.8** Abnormal findings on diagnostic imaging of other specified body structures
  - AHA: 2018,4Q,30
  - √6ᵗʰ **R93.81** Abnormal radiologic findings on diagnostic imaging of testis
    - **R93.811** Abnormal radiologic findings on diagnostic imaging of right testicle
    - **R93.812** Abnormal radiologic findings on diagnostic imaging of left testicle
    - **R93.813** Abnormal radiologic findings on diagnostic imaging of testicles, bilateral
    - **R93.819** Abnormal radiologic findings on diagnostic imaging of unspecified testicle
  - **R93.89** Abnormal findings on diagnostic imaging of other specified body structures
    - Abnormal finding by radioisotope localization of placenta
    - Abnormal radiological finding in skin and subcutaneous tissue
    - Mediastinal shift
- **R93.9** Diagnostic imaging inconclusive due to excess body fat of patient

√4ᵗʰ **R94** Abnormal results of function studies
- INCLUDES: abnormal results of radionuclide [radioisotope] uptake studies
  - abnormal results of scintigraphy
- √5ᵗʰ **R94.0** Abnormal results of function studies of central nervous system
  - **R94.01** Abnormal electroencephalogram [EEG]
  - **R94.02** Abnormal brain scan
  - **R94.09** Abnormal results of other function studies of central nervous system
- √5ᵗʰ **R94.1** Abnormal results of function studies of peripheral nervous system and special senses
  - √6ᵗʰ **R94.11** Abnormal results of function studies of eye
    - **R94.110** Abnormal electro-oculogram [EOG]
    - **R94.111** Abnormal electroretinogram [ERG]
      - Abnormal retinal function study
    - **R94.112** Abnormal visually evoked potential [VEP]
    - **R94.113** Abnormal oculomotor study
    - **R94.118** Abnormal results of other function studies of eye
  - √6ᵗʰ **R94.12** Abnormal results of function studies of ear and other special senses
    - AHA: 2016,3Q,17
    - **R94.120** Abnormal auditory function study
    - **R94.121** Abnormal vestibular function study
    - **R94.128** Abnormal results of other function studies of ear and other special senses

Chapter 18. Symptoms, Signs and Abnormal Clinical and Laboratory Findings

- ✓6th **R94.13 Abnormal results of function studies of peripheral nervous system**
  - **R94.130** Abnormal response to nerve stimulation, unspecified
  - **R94.131** Abnormal electromyogram [EMG]
    - EXCLUDES 1 electromyogram of eye (R94.113)
  - **R94.138** Abnormal results of other function studies of peripheral nervous system
- **R94.2 Abnormal results of pulmonary function studies**
  - Reduced ventilatory capacity
  - Reduced vital capacity
- ✓5th **R94.3 Abnormal results of cardiovascular function studies**
  - **R94.30** Abnormal result of cardiovascular function study, unspecified
  - **R94.31** Abnormal electrocardiogram [ECG] [EKG]
    - EXCLUDES 1 long QT syndrome (I45.81)
  - **R94.39** Abnormal result of other cardiovascular function study
    - Abnormal electrophysiological intracardiac studies
    - Abnormal phonocardiogram
    - Abnormal vectorcardiogram
    - **AHA:** 2023,1Q,25
- **R94.4 Abnormal results of kidney function studies**
  - Abnormal renal function test
- **R94.5 Abnormal results of liver function studies**
- **R94.6 Abnormal results of thyroid function studies**
- **R94.7 Abnormal results of other endocrine function studies**
  - EXCLUDES 2 abnormal glucose (R73.0-)
- **R94.8 Abnormal results of function studies of other organs and systems**
  - Abnormal basal metabolic rate [BMR]
  - Abnormal bladder function test
  - Abnormal splenic function test

Abnormal tumor markers (R97)

- ✓4th **R97 Abnormal tumor markers**
  - Elevated tumor associated antigens [TAA]
  - Elevated tumor specific antigens [TSA]
  - **R97.0** Elevated carcinoembryonic antigen [CEA]
  - **R97.1** Elevated cancer antigen 125 [CA 125]
  - ✓5th **R97.2** Elevated prostate specific antigen [PSA]
    - **AHA:** 2016,4Q,66
    - **R97.20** Elevated prostate specific antigen [PSA]
    - **R97.21** Rising PSA following treatment for malignant neoplasm of prostate
      - **AHA:** 2023,2Q,5
  - **R97.8** Other abnormal tumor markers

Ill-defined and unknown cause of mortality (R99)

- **R99 Ill-defined and unknown cause of mortality**
  - Death (unexplained) NOS
  - Unspecified cause of mortality

Chapter 19. Injury, Poisoning, and Certain Other Consequences of External Causes (S00–T88)

Chapter-specific Guidelines with Coding Examples

The chapter-specific guidelines from the ICD-10-CM Official Guidelines for Coding and Reporting have been provided below. Along with these guidelines are coding examples, contained in the shaded boxes, that have been developed to help illustrate the coding and/or sequencing guidance found in these guidelines.

a. Application of 7th characters in Chapter 19

Most categories in chapter 19 have a 7th character requirement for each applicable code. Most categories in this chapter have three 7th character values (with the exception of fractures): A, initial encounter, D, subsequent encounter and S, sequela. Categories for traumatic fractures have additional 7th character values. While the patient may be seen by a new or different provider over the course of treatment for an injury, assignment of the 7th character is based on whether the patient is undergoing active treatment and not whether the provider is seeing the patient for the first time.

For complication codes, active treatment refers to treatment for the condition described by the code, even though it may be related to an earlier precipitating problem. For example, code T84.50XA, Infection and inflammatory reaction due to unspecified internal joint prosthesis, initial encounter, is used when active treatment is provided for the infection, even though the condition relates to the prosthetic device, implant or graft that was placed at a previous encounter.

7th character "A", initial encounter is used for each encounter where the patient is receiving active treatment for the condition.

Patient evaluated after fall from a skateboard onto the sidewalk, x-rays identify a nondisplaced fracture to the distal pole of the right scaphoid bone. The patient is placed in a cast.	
S62.014A	Nondisplaced fracture of distal pole of navicular [scaphoid] bone of right wrist, initial encounter for closed fracture
V00.131A	Fall from skateboard, initial encounter
Y93.51	Activity, roller skating (inline) and skateboarding
Y92.480	Sidewalk as the place of occurrence of the external cause
Y99.8	Other external cause status

Explanation: This fracture would be coded with a seventh character A for initial encounter because the patient received x-rays to identify the site of the fracture and treatment was rendered; this would be considered active treatment.

7th character "D" subsequent encounter is used for encounters after the patient has completed active treatment of the condition and is receiving routine care for the condition during the healing or recovery phase.

Patient seen in follow-up after fall from a skateboard onto the sidewalk resulted in casting of the right arm. X-rays are taken to evaluate how well the nondisplaced fracture to the distal pole of the right scaphoid bone is healing. The physician feels the fracture is healing appropriately; no adjustments to the cast are made.	
S62.014D	Nondisplaced fracture of distal pole of navicular [scaphoid] bone of right wrist, subsequent encounter for fracture with routine healing
V00.131D	Fall from skateboard, subsequent encounter

Explanation: This fracture would be coded with a seventh character D for subsequent encounter, whether the same physician who provided the initial cast application or a different physician is now seeing the patient. Although the patient received x-rays, the intent of the x-rays was to assess how the fracture was healing. There was no active treatment rendered and the visit is therefore considered a subsequent encounter.

The aftercare Z codes should not be used for aftercare for conditions such as injuries or poisonings, where 7th characters are provided to identify subsequent care. For example, for aftercare of an injury, assign the acute injury code with the 7th character "D" (subsequent encounter).

7th character "S", sequela, is for use for complications or conditions that arise as a direct result of a condition, such as scar formation after a burn. The scars are sequelae of the burn. When using 7th character "S", it is necessary to use both the injury code that precipitated the sequela and the code for the sequela itself. The "S" is added only to the injury code, not the sequela code. The 7th character "S" identifies the injury responsible for the sequela. The specific type of sequela (e.g. scar) is sequenced first, followed by the injury code.

See Section I.B.10. Sequelae, (Late Effects)

Patient with a history of a nondisplaced fracture to the distal pole of the right scaphoid bone due to a fall from a skateboard is seen for evaluation of arthritis to the right wrist that has developed as a consequence of the traumatic fracture.	
M12.531	Traumatic arthropathy, right wrist
S62.014S	Nondisplaced fracture of distal pole of navicular [scaphoid] bone of right wrist, sequela
V00.131S	Fall from skateboard, sequela

Explanation: The code identifying the specific sequela condition (traumatic arthritis) should be coded first followed by the injury that instigated the development of the sequela (fracture). The scaphoid fracture injury code is given a 7th character S for sequela to represent its role as the inciting injury. The fracture has healed and is not being managed or treated on this admit and therefore is not applicable as a first listed or principal diagnosis. However, it is directly related to the development of the arthritis and should be appended as a secondary code to signify this cause and effect relationship.

b. Coding of injuries

When coding injuries, assign separate codes for each injury unless a combination code is provided, in which case the combination code is assigned. Codes from category T07, Unspecified multiple injuries should not be assigned in the inpatient setting unless information for a more specific code is not available. Traumatic injury codes (S00-T14.9) are not to be used for normal, healing surgical wounds or to identify complications of surgical wounds.

11-year-old girl fell from her horse, resulting in a laceration to her right forearm with several large pieces of wooden fragments embedded in the wound as well as abrasions to her right ear; in addition, her right shoulder was dislocated.	
S43.004A	Unspecified dislocation of right shoulder joint, initial encounter
S51.821A	Laceration with foreign body of right forearm, initial encounter
S00.411A	Abrasion of right ear, initial encounter
V80.010A	Animal-rider injured by fall from or being thrown from horse in noncollision accident, initial encounter
Y93.52	Activity, horseback riding

Explanation: Each separate injury should be reported. The patient's injury to the forearm is reported with one combination code that captures both the laceration and the foreign body.

The code for the most serious injury, as determined by the provider and the focus of treatment, is sequenced first.

1) **Superficial injuries**

   Superficial injuries such as abrasions or contusions are not coded when associated with more severe injuries of the same site.

2) **Primary injury with damage to nerves/blood vessels**

   When a primary injury results in minor damage to peripheral nerves or blood vessels, the primary injury is sequenced first with additional code(s) for injuries to nerves and spinal cord (such as category S04), and/or injury to blood vessels (such as category S15). When the primary injury is to the blood vessels or nerves, that injury should be sequenced first.

3) **Iatrogenic injuries**

   Injury codes from Chapter 19 should not be assigned for injuries that occur during, or as a result of, a medical intervention. Assign the appropriate complication code(s).

c. Coding of traumatic fractures

The principles of multiple coding of injuries should be followed in coding fractures. Fractures of specified sites are coded individually by site in accordance with both the provisions within categories S02, S12, S22, S32, S42, S49, S52, S59, S62, S72, S79, S82, S89, S92 and the level of detail furnished by medical record content.

A fracture not indicated as open or closed should be coded to closed. A fracture not indicated whether displaced or not displaced should be coded to displaced.

More specific guidelines are as follows:

1) Initial vs. subsequent encounter for fractures

Traumatic fractures are coded using the appropriate 7th character for initial encounter (A, B, C) for each encounter where the patient is receiving active treatment for the fracture. The appropriate 7th character for initial encounter should also be assigned for a patient who delayed seeking treatment for the fracture or nonunion.

Fractures are coded using the appropriate 7th character for subsequent care for encounters after the patient has completed active treatment of the fracture and is receiving routine care for the fracture during the healing or recovery phase.

Care for complications of surgical treatment for fracture repairs during the healing or recovery phase should be coded with the appropriate complication codes.

Care of complications of fractures, such as malunion and nonunion, should be reported with the appropriate 7th character for subsequent care with nonunion (K, M, N,) or subsequent care with malunion (P, Q, R).

Malunion/nonunion: The appropriate 7th character for initial encounter should also be assigned for a patient who delayed seeking treatment for the fracture or nonunion.

> Female patient fell during a forest hiking excursion almost six months ago and until recently did not feel she needed to seek medical attention for her left ankle pain; x-rays show nonunion of lateral malleolus and surgery has been scheduled
>
> **S82.62XA** Displaced fracture of lateral malleolus of left fibula, initial encounter for closed fracture
>
> **W01.0XXA** Fall on same level from slipping, tripping and stumbling without subsequent striking against object, initial encounter
>
> **Y92.821** Forest as place of occurrence of the external cause
>
> **Y93.01** Activity, walking, marching and hiking
>
> **Y99.8** Other external cause status
>
> *Explanation:* A seventh character of A is used for the lateral malleolus nonunion fracture to signify that the fracture is receiving active treatment. The delayed care for the fracture has resulted in a nonunion, but capturing the nonunion in the seventh character is trumped by the provision of active care.

The open fracture designations in the assignment of the 7th character for fractures of the forearm, femur and lower leg, including ankle are based on the Gustilo open fracture classification. When the Gustilo classification type is not specified for an open fracture, the 7th character for open fracture type I or II should be assigned (B, E, H, M, Q).

A code from category M80, not a traumatic fracture code, should be used for any patient with known osteoporosis who suffers a fracture, even if the patient had a minor fall or trauma, if that fall or trauma would not usually break a normal, healthy bone.

See Section I.C.13. Osteoporosis.

The aftercare Z codes should not be used for aftercare for traumatic fractures. For aftercare of a traumatic fracture, assign the acute fracture code with the appropriate 7th character.

2) Multiple fractures sequencing

Multiple fractures are sequenced in accordance with the severity of the fracture.

3) Physeal fractures

For physeal fractures, assign only the code identifying the type of physeal fracture. Do not assign a separate code to identify the specific bone that is fractured.

d. Coding of burns and corrosions

The ICD-10-CM makes a distinction between burns and corrosions. The burn codes are for thermal burns, except sunburns, that come from a heat source, such as a fire or hot appliance. The burn codes are also for burns resulting from electricity and radiation. Corrosions are burns due to chemicals. The guidelines are the same for burns and corrosions.

Current burns (T20-T25) are classified by depth, extent and by agent (X code). Burns are classified by depth as first degree (erythema), second degree (blistering), and third degree (full-thickness involvement). Burns of the eye and internal organs (T26-T28) are classified by site, but not by degree.

1) Sequencing of burn and related condition codes

Sequence first the code that reflects the highest degree of burn when more than one burn is present.

a. When the reason for the admission or encounter is for treatment of external multiple burns, sequence first the code that reflects the burn of the highest degree.

b. When a patient has both internal and external burns, the circumstances of admission govern the selection of the principal diagnosis or first-listed diagnosis.

c. When a patient is admitted for burn injuries and other related conditions such as smoke inhalation and/or respiratory failure, the circumstances of admission govern the selection of the principal or first-listed diagnosis.

> Patient referred for minor first-degree burns to multiple sites of her right and left hands as well as severe smoke inhalation. While she was sleeping at home, a candle on her dresser lit the bedroom curtains on fire.
>
> **T59.811A** Toxic effect of smoke, accidental (unintentional), initial encounter
>
> **J70.5** Respiratory conditions due to smoke inhalation
>
> **T23.191A** Burn of first degree of multiple sites of right wrist and hand, initial encounter
>
> **T23.192A** Burn of first degree of multiple sites of left wrist and hand, initial encounter
>
> **X08.8XXA** Exposure to other specified smoke, fire and flames, initial encounter
>
> **Y99.8** Other external cause status
>
> **Y92.003** Bedroom of unspecified non-institutional (private) residence as the place of occurrence of the external cause
>
> **Y93.84** Activity, sleeping
>
> *Explanation:* Based on the documentation, the inhalation injury is more severe than the first-degree burns and is sequenced first. The burns to the hands are appended as secondary diagnoses.

2) Burns of the same anatomic site

Classify burns of the same anatomic site and on the same side but of different degrees to the subcategory identifying the highest degree recorded in the diagnosis (e.g., for second and third degree burns of right thigh, assign only code T24.311-).

3) Non-healing burns

Non-healing burns are coded as acute burns.

Necrosis of burned skin should be coded as a non-healed burn.

4) Infected burn

For any documented infected burn site, use an additional code for the infection.

5) Assign separate codes for each burn site

When coding burns, assign separate codes for each burn site. Category T30, Burn and corrosion, body region unspecified is extremely vague and should rarely be used.

Codes for burns of "multiple sites" should only be assigned when the medical record documentation does not specify the individual sites.

6) Burns and corrosions classified according to extent of body surface involved

Assign codes from category T31, Burns classified according to extent of body surface involved, or T32, Corrosions classified according to extent of body surface involved, for acute burns or corrosions when the site of the burn or corrosion is not specified or when there is a need for additional data. It is advisable to use category T31 as additional coding when needed to provide data for evaluating burn mortality, such as that needed by burn units. It is also advisable to use category T31 as an additional code for reporting purposes when there is mention of a third-degree burn involving 20 percent or more of the body surface. Codes from categories T31 and T32 should not be used for sequelae of burns or corrosions.

Categories T31 and T32 are based on the classic "rule of nines" in estimating body surface involved: head and neck are assigned nine percent, each arm nine percent, each leg 18 percent, the anterior trunk 18 percent, posterior trunk 18 percent, and genitalia one percent. Providers may change these percentage assignments where necessary to accommodate infants and children who have proportionately larger heads than adults, and patients who have large buttocks, thighs, or abdomen that involve burns.

> Patient seen for dressing change after he accidentally spilled acetic acid on himself two days ago. The second-degree burns to his right thigh, covering about 3 percent of his body surface, are healing appropriately.
>
> | T54.2X1D | Toxic effect of corrosive acids and acid-like substances, accidental (unintentional), subsequent encounter |
> |---|---|
> | T24.611D | Corrosion of second degree of right thigh, subsequent encounter |
> | T32.0 | Corrosions involving less than 10% of body surface |
>
> *Explanation:* Code T32.0 provides additional information as to how much of the patient's body was affected by the corrosive substance.

7) Encounters for treatment of sequela of burns
Encounters for the treatment of the late effects of burns or corrosions (i.e., scars or joint contractures) should be coded with a burn or corrosion code with the 7th character "S" for sequela.

8) Sequelae with a late effect code and current burn
When appropriate, both a code for a current burn or corrosion with 7th character "A" or "D" and a burn or corrosion code with 7th character "S" may be assigned on the same record (when both a current burn and sequelae of an old burn exist). Burns and corrosions do not heal at the same rate and a current healing wound may still exist with sequela of a healed burn or corrosion.

See Section I.B.10. Sequela (Late Effects)

> Female patient seen for second-degree burn to the left ear; she also has significant scarring on her left elbow from a third-degree burn from childhood
>
> | T20.212A | Burn of second degree of left ear [any part, except ear drum], initial encounter |
> |---|---|
> | L90.5 | Scar conditions and fibrosis of skin |
> | T22.322S | Burn of third degree of left elbow, sequela |
>
> *Explanation:* The patient is being seen for management of a current second-degree burn, which is reflected in the code by appending the seventh character of A, indicating active treatment or management of this burn. The elbow scarring is a sequela of a previous third-degree burn. The sequela condition precedes the original burn injury, which is appended with a seventh character of S.

9) Use of an external cause code with burns and corrosions
An external cause code should be used with burns and corrosions to identify the source and intent of the burn, as well as the place where it occurred.

e. Adverse effects, poisoning, underdosing and toxic effects
Codes in categories T36-T65 are combination codes that include the substance that was taken as well as the intent. No additional external cause code is required for poisonings, toxic effects, adverse effects and underdosing codes.

1) Do not code directly from the Table of Drugs
Do not code directly from the Table of Drugs and Chemicals. Always refer back to the Tabular List.

2) Use as many codes as necessary to describe
Use as many codes as necessary to describe completely all drugs, medicinal or biological substances.

3) If the same code would describe the causative agent
If the same code would describe the causative agent for more than one adverse reaction, poisoning, toxic effect or underdosing, assign the code only once.

4) If two or more drugs, medicinal or biological substances
If two or more drugs, medicinal or biological substances are taken, code each individually unless a combination code is listed in the Table of Drugs and Chemicals.

If multiple unspecified drugs, medicinal or biological substances were taken, assign the appropriate code from subcategory T50.91, Poisoning by, adverse effect of and underdosing of multiple unspecified drugs, medicaments and biological substances.

5) The occurrence of drug toxicity is classified in ICD-10-CM as follows:
(a) Adverse effect
When coding an adverse effect of a drug that has been correctly prescribed and properly administered, assign the appropriate code for the nature of the adverse effect followed by the appropriate code for the adverse effect of the drug (T36-T50). The code for the drug should have a 5th or 6th character "5" (for example T36.0X5-) Examples of the nature of an adverse effect are tachycardia, delirium, gastrointestinal hemorrhaging, vomiting, hypokalemia, hepatitis, renal failure, or respiratory failure.

(b) Poisoning
When coding a poisoning or reaction to the improper use of a medication (e.g., overdose, wrong substance given or taken in error, wrong route of administration), first assign the appropriate code from categories T36-T50. The poisoning codes have an associated intent as their 5th or 6th character (accidental, intentional self-harm, assault and undetermined). If the intent of the poisoning is unknown or unspecified, code the intent as accidental intent. The undetermined intent is only for use if the documentation in the record specifies that the intent cannot be determined. Use additional code(s) for all manifestations of poisonings.

If there is also a diagnosis of abuse or dependence of the substance, the abuse or dependence is assigned as an additional code.

Examples of poisoning include:
(i) Error was made in drug prescription
Errors made in drug prescription or in the administration of the drug by provider, nurse, patient, or other person.
(ii) Overdose of a drug intentionally taken
If an overdose of a drug was intentionally taken or administered and resulted in drug toxicity, it would be coded as a poisoning.
(iii) Nonprescribed drug taken with correctly prescribed and properly administered drug
If a nonprescribed drug or medicinal agent was taken in combination with a correctly prescribed and properly administered drug, any drug toxicity or other reaction resulting from the interaction of the two drugs would be classified as a poisoning.
(iv) Interaction of drug(s) and alcohol
When a reaction results from the interaction of a drug(s) and alcohol, this would be classified as poisoning.

See Section I.C.4. if poisoning is the result of insulin pump malfunctions.

For Sequela (Late Effects) see Section I.B.10.

(c) Underdosing
Underdosing refers to taking less of a medication than is prescribed by a provider or a manufacturer's instruction. Discontinuing the use of a prescribed medication on the patient's own initiative (not directed by the patient's provider) is also classified as an underdosing. For underdosing, assign the code from categories T36-T50 (fifth or sixth character "6"). Documentation of a change in the patient's condition is not required in order to assign an underdosing code. Documentation that the patient is taking less of a medication than is prescribed or discontinued the prescribed medication is sufficient for code assignment.

Codes for underdosing should never be assigned as principal or first-listed codes. If a patient has a relapse or exacerbation of the medical condition for which the drug is prescribed because of the reduction in dose, then the medical condition itself should be coded.

Noncompliance (Z91.12-, Z91.13-, Z91.14- and Z91.A4-) or complication of care (Y63.6-Y63.9) codes are to be used with an underdosing code to indicate intent, if known.

> Patient referred for atrial fibrillation with history of chronic atrial fibrillation for which she is prescribed amiodarone. Financial concerns have left the patient unable to pay for her prescriptions and she has been skipping her amiodarone dose every other day to offset the cost.
>
> | I48.20 | Chronic atrial fibrillation, unspecified |
> |---|---|
> | T46.2X6A | Underdosing of other antidysrhythmic drugs, initial encounter |
> | Z91.120 | Patient's intentional underdosing of medication regimen due to financial hardship |
>
> *Explanation:* By skipping her amiodarone pill every other day, the patient's atrial fibrillation returned. The condition for which the drug was being taken is reported first, followed by an underdosing code to show that the patient was not adhering to her prescription regiment. The Z code helps elaborate on the patient's social and/or economic circumstances that led to the patient taking less then what she was prescribed.

(d) Toxic effects

When a harmful substance is ingested or comes in contact with a person, this is classified as a toxic effect. The toxic effect codes are in categories T51–T65. When coding a toxic effect, assign the toxic effect code first, followed by codes for all associated manifestations of the toxic effect.

Toxic effect codes have an associated intent: accidental, intentional self-harm, assault and undetermined.

For Sequela (Late Effects) see Section I.B.10. Sequela

f. Adult and child abuse, neglect and other maltreatment

Sequence first the appropriate code from categories T74, Adult and child abuse, neglect and other maltreatment, confirmed, or T76, Adult and child abuse, neglect and other maltreatment, suspected, for abuse, neglect and other maltreatment, followed by any accompanying mental health or injury code(s).

If the documentation in the medical record states abuse or neglect, it is coded as confirmed (T74.-). It is coded as suspected if it is documented as suspected (T76.-).

For cases of confirmed abuse or neglect an external cause code from the assault section (X92-Y09) should be added to identify the cause of any physical injuries. A perpetrator code (Y07) should be added when the perpetrator of the abuse is known. For suspected cases of abuse or neglect, do not report external cause or perpetrator code.

If a suspected case of abuse, neglect or mistreatment is ruled out during an encounter code Z04.71, Encounter for examination and observation following alleged physical adult abuse, ruled out, or code Z04.72, Encounter for examination and observation following alleged child physical abuse, ruled out, should be used, not a code from T76.

If a suspected case of alleged rape or sexual abuse is ruled out during an encounter code Z04.41, Encounter for examination and observation following alleged adult rape or code Z04.42, Encounter for examination and observation following alleged child rape, should be used, not a code from T76.

If a suspected case of forced sexual exploitation or forced labor exploitation is ruled out during an encounter, code Z04.81, Encounter for examination and observation of victim following forced sexual exploitation, or code Z04.82, Encounter for examination and observation of victim following forced labor exploitation, should be used, not a code from T76.

See Section I.C.15. Abuse in a pregnant patient.

g. Complications of care

1) General guidelines for complications of care
(a) Documentation of complications of care
See Section I.B.16. for information on documentation of complications of care.

2) Pain due to medical devices

Pain associated with devices, implants or grafts left in a surgical site (for example painful hip prosthesis) is assigned to the appropriate code(s) found in Chapter 19, Injury, poisoning, and certain other consequences of external causes. Specific codes for pain due to medical devices are found in the T code section of the ICD-10-CM. Use additional code(s) from category G89 to identify acute or chronic pain due to presence of the device, implant or graft (G89.18 or G89.28).

	Chronic left breast pain secondary to breast implant
T85.848A	Pain due to other internal prosthetic devices, implants and grafts, initial encounter
N64.4	Mastodynia
G89.28	Other chronic postprocedural pain

Explanation: As the pain is a complication related to the breast implant, the complication code is sequenced first. The T code does not describe the site or type of pain, so additional codes may be appended to indicate that the patient is experiencing chronic pain in the breast.

3) Transplant complications
(a) Transplant complications other than kidney

Codes under category T86, Complications of transplanted organs and tissues, are for use for both complications and rejection of transplanted organs. A transplant complication code is only assigned if the complication affects the function of the transplanted organ. Two codes are required to fully describe a transplant complication: the appropriate code from category T86 and a secondary code that identifies the complication.

Pre-existing conditions or conditions that develop after the transplant are not coded as complications unless they affect the function of the transplanted organs.

See I.C.21. for transplant organ removal status
See I.C.2. for malignant neoplasm associated with transplanted organ.
See I.C.1.d.4. for sequencing of sepsis due to infection in transplanted organ

(b) Kidney transplant complications

Patients who have undergone kidney transplant may still have some form of chronic kidney disease (CKD) because the kidney transplant may not fully restore kidney function. Code T86.1- should be assigned for documented complications of a kidney transplant, such as transplant failure or rejection or other transplant complication. Code T86.1- should not be assigned for post kidney transplant patients who have chronic kidney (CKD) unless a transplant complication such as transplant failure or rejection is documented. If the documentation is unclear as to whether the patient has a complication of the transplant, query the provider.

Conditions that affect the function of the transplanted kidney, other than CKD, should be assigned a code from subcategory T86.1, Complications of transplanted organ, Kidney, and a secondary code that identifies the complication.

For patients with CKD following a kidney transplant, but who do not have a complication such as failure or rejection, *see section I.C.14. Chronic kidney disease and kidney transplant status.*

See I.C.1.d.4. for sequencing of sepsis due to infection in transplanted organ

	Patient seen for chronic kidney disease stage 2; history of successful kidney transplant with no complications identified
N18.2	Chronic kidney disease, stage 2 (mild)
Z94.0	Kidney transplant status

Explanation: This patient's stage 2 CKD is not indicated as being due to the transplanted kidney but instead is just the residual disease the patient had prior to the transplant.

4) Complication codes that include the external cause

As with certain other T codes, some of the complications of care codes have the external cause included in the code. The code includes the nature of the complication as well as the type of procedure that caused the complication. No external cause code indicating the type of procedure is necessary for these codes.

5) Complications of care codes within the body system chapters

Intraoperative and postprocedural complication codes are found within the body system chapters with codes specific to the organs and structures of that body system. These codes should be sequenced first, followed by a code(s) for the specific complication, if applicable.

	Postprocedural ischemic infarction of the left middle cerebral artery due to cardiac surgery
I97.820	Postprocedural cerebrovascular infarction following cardiac surgery
I63.512	Cerebral infarction due to unspecified occlusion or stenosis of left middle cerebral artery

Explanation: The infarction was caused by the cardiac procedure and is coded as a postprocedural complication. The postprocedural cerebrovascular infarction is the first-listed diagnosis, followed by the code for the infarction itself.

Complication codes from the body system chapters should be assigned for intraoperative and postprocedural complications (e.g., the appropriate complication code from chapter 9 would be assigned for a vascular intraoperative or postprocedural complication) unless the complication is specifically indexed to a T code in chapter 19.

Muscle/Tendon Table

ICD-10-CM categorizes certain muscles and tendons in the upper and lower extremities by their action (e.g., extension, flexion), their anatomical location (e.g., posterior, anterior), and/or whether they are intrinsic or extrinsic to a certain anatomical area. The Muscle/Tendon Table is provided at the beginning of chapters 13 and 19 as a resource to help users when code selection depends on one or more of these characteristics. A **TIP** has been placed at those categories and/or subcategories that relate to this table. Please note that this table is not all-inclusive, and proper code assignment should be based on the provider's documentation.

Body Region	Muscle	Extensor Tendon	Flexor Tendon	Other Tendon
Shoulder				
	Deltoid	Posterior deltoid	Anterior deltoid	
	Rotator cuff			
	Infraspinatus			Infraspinatus
	Subscapularis			Subscapularis
	Supraspinatus			Supraspinatus
	Teres minor			Teres minor
	Teres major	Teres major		
Upper arm				
	Anterior muscles			
	Biceps brachii — long head		Biceps brachii — long head	
	Biceps brachii — short head		Biceps brachii — short head	
	Brachialis		Brachialis	
	Coracobrachialis		Coracobrachialis	
	Posterior muscles			
	Triceps brachii	Triceps brachii		
Forearm				
	Anterior muscles			
	Flexors			
	Deep			
	Flexor digitorum profundus		Flexor digitorum profundus	
	Flexor pollicis longus		Flexor pollicis longus	
	Intermediate			
	Flexor digitorum superficialis		Flexor digitorum superficialis	
	Superficial			
	Flexor carpi radialis		Flexor carpi radialis	
	Flexor carpi ulnaris		Flexor carpi ulnaris	
	Palmaris longus		Palmaris longus	
	Pronators			
	Pronator quadratus			Pronator quadratus
	Pronator teres			Pronator teres
	Posterior muscles			
	Extensors			
	Deep			
	Abductor pollicis longus			Abductor pollicis longus
	Extensor indicis	Extensor indicis		
	Extensor pollicis brevis	Extensor pollicis brevis		
	Extensor pollicis longus	Extensor pollicis longus		
	Superficial			
	Brachioradialis			Brachioradialis
	Extensor carpi radialis brevis	Extensor carpi radialis brevis		
	Extensor carpi radialis longus	Extensor carpi radialis longus		
	Extensor carpi ulnaris	Extensor carpi ulnaris		
	Extensor digiti minimi	Extensor digiti minimi		
	Extensor digitorum	Extensor digitorum		
	Anconeus	Anconeus		
	Supinator			Supinator

Muscle/Tendon Table

Body Region	Muscle	Extensor Tendon	Flexor Tendon	Other Tendon
Hand				
Extrinsic — attach to a site in the forearm as well as a site in the hand with action related to hand movement at the wrist				
	Extensor carpi radialis brevis	Extensor carpi radialis brevis		
	Extensor carpi radialis longus	Extensor carpi radialis longus		
	Extensor carpi ulnaris	Extensor carpi ulnaris		
	Flexor carpi radialis		Flexor carpi radialis	
	Flexor carpi ulnaris		Flexor carpi ulnaris	
	Flexor digitorum superficialis		Flexor digitorum superficialis	
	Palmaris longus		Palmaris longus	
Extrinsic — attach to a site in the forearm as well as a site in the hand with action in the hand related to finger movement				
	Adductor pollicis longus			Adductor pollicis longus
	Extensor digiti minimi	Extensor digiti minimi		
	Extensor digitorum	Extensor digitorum		
	Extensor indicis	Extensor indicis		
	Flexor digitorum profundus		Flexor digitorum profundus	
	Flexor digitorum superficialis		Flexor digitorum superficialis	
Extrinsic — attach to a site in the forearm as well as a site in the hand with action in the hand related to thumb movement				
	Extensor pollicis brevis	Extensor pollicis brevis		
	Extensor pollicis longus	Extensor pollicis longus		
	Flexor pollicis longus		Flexor pollicis longus	
Intrinsic — found within the hand only				
	Adductor pollicis			Adductor pollicis
	Dorsal interossei	Dorsal interossei	Dorsal interossei	
	Lumbricals	Lumbricals	Lumbricals	
	Palmaris brevis			Palmaris brevis
	Palmar interossei	Palmar interossei	Palmar interossei	
	Hypothenar muscles			
	Abductor digiti minimi			Abductor digiti minimi
	Flexor digiti minimi brevis		Flexor digiti minimi brevis	
	Opponens digiti minimi		Opponens digiti minimi	
	Thenar muscles			
	Abductor pollicis brevis			Abductor pollicis brevis
	Flexor pollicis brevis		Flexor pollicis brevis	
	Opponens pollicis		Opponens pollicis	
Thigh				
	Anterior muscles			
	Iliopsoas		Iliopsoas	
	Pectineus		Pectineus	
	Quadriceps	Quadriceps		
	Rectus femoris	Rectus femoris — Extends knee	Rectus femoris — Flexes hip	
	Vastus intermedius	Vastus intermedius		
	Vastus lateralis	Vastus lateralis		
	Vastus medialis	Vastus medialis		
	Sartorius		Sartorius	
	Medial muscles			
	Adductor brevis			Adductor brevis
	Adductor longus			Adductor longus
	Adductor magnus			Adductor magnus
	Gracilis			Gracilis
	Obturator externus			Obturator externus
	Posterior muscles			
	Hamstring	Hamstring — Extends hip	Hamstring — Flexes knee	
	Biceps femoris	Biceps femoris	Biceps femoris	
	Semimembranosus	Semimembranosus	Semimembranosus	
	Semitendinosus	Semitendinosus	Semitendinosus	

Body Region	Muscle	Extensor Tendon	Flexor Tendon	Other Tendon
Lower leg				
	Anterior muscles			
	Extensor digitorum longus	Extensor digitorum longus		
	Extensor hallucis longus	Extensor hallucis longus		
	Fibularis (peroneus) tertius	Fibularis (peroneus) tertius		
	Tibialis anterior	Tibialis anterior		Tibialis anterior
	Lateral muscles			
	Fibularis (peroneus) brevis		Fibularis (peroneus) brevis	
	Fibularis (peroneus) longus		Fibularis (peroneus) longus	
	Posterior muscles			
	Deep			
	Flexor digitorum longus		Flexor digitorum longus	
	Flexor hallucis longus		Flexor hallucis longus	
	Popliteus		Popliteus	
	Tibialis posterior		Tibialis posterior	
	Superficial			
	Gastrocnemius		Gastrocnemius	
	Plantaris		Plantaris	
	Soleus		Soleus	
				Calcaneal (Achilles)
Ankle/Foot				
Extrinsic — attach to a site in the lower leg as well as a site in the foot with action related to foot movement at the ankle				
	Plantaris		Plantaris	
	Soleus		Soleus	
	Tibialis anterior	Tibialis anterior		
	Tibialis posterior		Tibialis posterior	
Extrinsic — attach to a site in the lower leg as well as a site in the foot with action in the foot related to toe movement				
	Extensor digitorum longus	Extensor digitorum longus		
	Extensor hallucis longus	Extensor hallucis longus		
	Flexor digitorum longus		Flexor digitorum longus	
	Flexor hallucis longus		Flexor hallucis longus	
Intrinsic — found within the ankle/foot only				
	Dorsal muscles			
	Extensor digitorum brevis	Extensor digitorum brevis		
	Extensor hallucis brevis	Extensor hallucis brevis		
	Plantar muscles			
	Abductor digiti minimi		Abductor digiti minimi	
	Abductor hallucis		Abductor hallucis	
	Dorsal interossei	Dorsal interossei	Dorsal interossei	
	Flexor digiti minimi brevis		Flexor digiti minimi brevis	
	Flexor digitorum brevis		Flexor digitorum brevis	
	Flexor hallucis brevis		Flexor hallucis brevis	
	Lumbricals	Lumbricals	Lumbricals	
	Quadratus plantae		Quadratus plantae	
	Plantar interossei	Plantar interossei	Plantar interossei	

Chapter 19. Injury, Poisoning and Certain Other Consequences of External Causes (S00-T88)

NOTE Use secondary code(s) from Chapter 20, External causes of morbidity, to indicate cause of injury. Codes within the T section that include the external cause do not require an additional external cause code.

Use additional code to identify any retained foreign body, if applicable (Z18.-)

EXCLUDES 1 birth trauma (P10-P15)
obstetric trauma (O70-O71)

EXCLUDES 2 ▶birth trauma (P10-P15)◀
▶obstetric trauma (O70-O71)◀

NOTE The chapter uses the S-section for coding different types of injuries related to single body regions and the T-section to cover injuries to unspecified body regions as well as poisoning and certain other consequences of external causes.

AHA: 2016,2Q,3-7; 2015,4Q,35-38; 2015,3Q,37-39,40; 2015,2Q,6; 2015,1Q,3-21
TIP: The specific site of an injury can be determined from the radiology report when authenticated by a radiologist and available at the time of code assignment.

This chapter contains the following blocks:

S00-S09	Injuries to the head
S10-S19	Injuries to the neck
S20-S29	Injuries to the thorax
S30-S39	Injuries to the abdomen, lower back, lumbar spine, pelvis and external genitals
S40-S49	Injuries to the shoulder and upper arm
S50-S59	Injuries to the elbow and forearm
S60-S69	Injuries to the wrist, hand and fingers
S70-S79	Injuries to the hip and thigh
S80-S89	Injuries to the knee and lower leg
S90-S99	Injuries to the ankle and foot
T07	Injuries involving multiple body regions
T14	Injury of unspecified body region
T15-T19	Effects of foreign body entering through natural orifice
T20-T25	Burns and corrosions of external body surface, specified by site
T26-T28	Burns and corrosions confined to eye and internal organs
T30-T32	Burns and corrosions of multiple and unspecified body regions
T33-T34	Frostbite
T36-T50	Poisoning by, adverse effect of and underdosing of drugs, medicaments and biological substances
T51-T65	Toxic effects of substances chiefly nonmedicinal as to source
T66-T78	Other and unspecified effects of external causes
T79	Certain early complications of trauma
T80-T88	Complications of surgical and medical care, not elsewhere classified

Injuries to the head (S00-S09)

INCLUDES
injuries of ear
injuries of eye
injuries of face [any part]
injuries of gum
injuries of jaw
injuries of oral cavity
injuries of palate
injuries of periocular area
injuries of scalp
injuries of temporomandibular joint area
injuries of tongue
injuries of tooth

Code also for any associated infection

EXCLUDES 2 burns and corrosions (T20-T32)
effects of foreign body in ear (T16)
effects of foreign body in larynx (T17.3)
effects of foreign body in mouth NOS (T18.0)
effects of foreign body in nose (T17.0-T17.1)
effects of foreign body in pharynx (T17.2)
effects of foreign body on external eye (T15.-)
frostbite (T33-T34)
insect bite or sting, venomous (T63.4)

S00 **Superficial injury of head**

EXCLUDES 1 diffuse cerebral contusion (S06.2-)
focal cerebral contusion (S06.3-)
injury of eye and orbit (S05.-)
open wound of head (S01.-)

The appropriate 7th character is to be added to each code from category S00.
A initial encounter
D subsequent encounter
S sequela

S00.0 **Superficial injury of scalp**
- S00.00 Unspecified superficial injury of scalp
- S00.01 Abrasion of scalp
- S00.02 Blister (nonthermal) of scalp
- S00.03 Contusion of scalp
  Bruise of scalp
  Hematoma of scalp
- S00.04 External constriction of part of scalp
- S00.05 Superficial foreign body of scalp
  Splinter in the scalp
- S00.06 Insect bite (nonvenomous) of scalp
- S00.07 Other superficial bite of scalp
  EXCLUDES 1 open bite of scalp (S01.05)

S00.1 **Contusion of eyelid and periocular area**
Black eye
EXCLUDES 2 contusion of eyeball and orbital tissues (S05.1-)
- S00.10 Contusion of unspecified eyelid and periocular area
- S00.11 Contusion of right eyelid and periocular area
- S00.12 Contusion of left eyelid and periocular area

S00.2 **Other and unspecified superficial injuries of eyelid and periocular area**
EXCLUDES 2 superficial injury of conjunctiva and cornea (S05.0-)

- S00.20 Unspecified superficial injury of eyelid and periocular area
  - S00.201 Unspecified superficial injury of right eyelid and periocular area
  - S00.202 Unspecified superficial injury of left eyelid and periocular area
  - S00.209 Unspecified superficial injury of unspecified eyelid and periocular area

- S00.21 Abrasion of eyelid and periocular area
  - S00.211 Abrasion of right eyelid and periocular area
  - S00.212 Abrasion of left eyelid and periocular area
  - S00.219 Abrasion of unspecified eyelid and periocular area

- S00.22 Blister (nonthermal) of eyelid and periocular area
  - S00.221 Blister (nonthermal) of right eyelid and periocular area
  - S00.222 Blister (nonthermal) of left eyelid and periocular area
  - S00.229 Blister (nonthermal) of unspecified eyelid and periocular area

- S00.24 External constriction of eyelid and periocular area
  - S00.241 External constriction of right eyelid and periocular area
  - S00.242 External constriction of left eyelid and periocular area
  - S00.249 External constriction of unspecified eyelid and periocular area

- S00.25 Superficial foreign body of eyelid and periocular area
  Splinter of eyelid and periocular area
  EXCLUDES 2 retained foreign body in eyelid (H02.81-)
  - S00.251 Superficial foreign body of right eyelid and periocular area
  - S00.252 Superficial foreign body of left eyelid and periocular area
  - S00.259 Superficial foreign body of unspecified eyelid and periocular area

- S00.26 Insect bite (nonvenomous) of eyelid and periocular area
  - S00.261 Insect bite (nonvenomous) of right eyelid and periocular area
  - S00.262 Insect bite (nonvenomous) of left eyelid and periocular area
  - S00.269 Insect bite (nonvenomous) of unspecified eyelid and periocular area

- S00.27 Other superficial bite of eyelid and periocular area
  EXCLUDES 1 open bite of eyelid and periocular area (S01.15)
  - S00.271 Other superficial bite of right eyelid and periocular area
  - S00.272 Other superficial bite of left eyelid and periocular area
  - S00.279 Other superficial bite of unspecified eyelid and periocular area

S00.3 **Superficial injury of nose**
- S00.30 Unspecified superficial injury of nose
- S00.31 Abrasion of nose
- S00.32 Blister (nonthermal) of nose

Chapter 19. Injury, Poisoning and Certain Other Consequences of External Causes

S00.33 Contusion of nose
- Bruise of nose
- Hematoma of nose

S00.34 External constriction of nose

S00.35 Superficial foreign body of nose
- Splinter in the nose

S00.36 Insect bite (nonvenomous) of nose

S00.37 Other superficial bite of nose
- EXCLUDES 1 open bite of nose (S01.25)

S00.4 Superficial injury of ear
- **S00.40** Unspecified superficial injury of ear
  - S00.401 Unspecified superficial injury of right ear
  - S00.402 Unspecified superficial injury of left ear
  - S00.409 Unspecified superficial injury of unspecified ear
- **S00.41** Abrasion of ear
  - S00.411 Abrasion of right ear
  - S00.412 Abrasion of left ear
  - S00.419 Abrasion of unspecified ear
- **S00.42** Blister (nonthermal) of ear
  - S00.421 Blister (nonthermal) of right ear
  - S00.422 Blister (nonthermal) of left ear
  - S00.429 Blister (nonthermal) of unspecified ear
- **S00.43** Contusion of ear
  - Bruise of ear
  - Hematoma of ear
  - S00.431 Contusion of right ear
  - S00.432 Contusion of left ear
  - S00.439 Contusion of unspecified ear
- **S00.44** External constriction of ear
  - S00.441 External constriction of right ear
  - S00.442 External constriction of left ear
  - S00.449 External constriction of unspecified ear
- **S00.45** Superficial foreign body of ear
  - Splinter in the ear
  - S00.451 Superficial foreign body of right ear
  - S00.452 Superficial foreign body of left ear
  - S00.459 Superficial foreign body of unspecified ear
- **S00.46** Insect bite (nonvenomous) of ear
  - S00.461 Insect bite (nonvenomous) of right ear
  - S00.462 Insect bite (nonvenomous) of left ear
  - S00.469 Insect bite (nonvenomous) of unspecified ear
- **S00.47** Other superficial bite of ear
  - EXCLUDES 1 open bite of ear (S01.35)
  - S00.471 Other superficial bite of right ear
  - S00.472 Other superficial bite of left ear
  - S00.479 Other superficial bite of unspecified ear

S00.5 Superficial injury of lip and oral cavity
- **S00.50** Unspecified superficial injury of lip and oral cavity
  - S00.501 Unspecified superficial injury of lip
  - S00.502 Unspecified superficial injury of oral cavity
- **S00.51** Abrasion of lip and oral cavity
  - S00.511 Abrasion of lip
  - S00.512 Abrasion of oral cavity
- **S00.52** Blister (nonthermal) of lip and oral cavity
  - S00.521 Blister (nonthermal) of lip
  - S00.522 Blister (nonthermal) of oral cavity
- **S00.53** Contusion of lip and oral cavity
  - S00.531 Contusion of lip
    - Bruise of lip
    - Hematoma of lip
  - S00.532 Contusion of oral cavity
    - Bruise of oral cavity
    - Hematoma of oral cavity
- **S00.54** External constriction of lip and oral cavity
  - S00.541 External constriction of lip
  - S00.542 External constriction of oral cavity
- **S00.55** Superficial foreign body of lip and oral cavity
  - S00.551 Superficial foreign body of lip
    - Splinter of lip and oral cavity
  - S00.552 Superficial foreign body of oral cavity
    - Splinter of lip and oral cavity
- **S00.56** Insect bite (nonvenomous) of lip and oral cavity
  - S00.561 Insect bite (nonvenomous) of lip
  - S00.562 Insect bite (nonvenomous) of oral cavity
- **S00.57** Other superficial bite of lip and oral cavity
  - S00.571 Other superficial bite of lip
    - EXCLUDES 1 open bite of lip (S01.551)
  - S00.572 Other superficial bite of oral cavity
    - EXCLUDES 1 open bite of oral cavity (S01.552)

S00.8 Superficial injury of other parts of head
- Superficial injuries of face [any part]
- **S00.80** Unspecified superficial injury of other part of head
- **S00.81** Abrasion of other part of head
- **S00.82** Blister (nonthermal) of other part of head
- **S00.83** Contusion of other part of head
  - Bruise of other part of head
  - Hematoma of other part of head
- **S00.84** External constriction of other part of head
- **S00.85** Superficial foreign body of other part of head
  - Splinter in other part of head
- **S00.86** Insect bite (nonvenomous) of other part of head
- **S00.87** Other superficial bite of other part of head
  - EXCLUDES 1 open bite of other part of head (S01.85)

S00.9 Superficial injury of unspecified part of head
- **S00.90** Unspecified superficial injury of unspecified part of head
- **S00.91** Abrasion of unspecified part of head
- **S00.92** Blister (nonthermal) of unspecified part of head
- **S00.93** Contusion of unspecified part of head
  - Bruise of head
  - Hematoma of head
- **S00.94** External constriction of unspecified part of head
- **S00.95** Superficial foreign body of unspecified part of head
  - Splinter of head
- **S00.96** Insect bite (nonvenomous) of unspecified part of head
- **S00.97** Other superficial bite of unspecified part of head
  - EXCLUDES 1 open bite of head (S01.95)

S01 Open wound of head
- Code also any associated:
  - injury of cranial nerve (S04.-)
  - injury of muscle and tendon of head (S09.1-)
  - intracranial injury (S06.-)
  - wound infection
- EXCLUDES 1 open skull fracture (S02.- with 7th character B)
- EXCLUDES 2 injury of eye and orbit (S05.-)
  - traumatic amputation of part of head (S08.-)

The appropriate 7th character is to be added to each code from category S01.
- A initial encounter
- D subsequent encounter
- S sequela

S01.0 Open wound of scalp
- EXCLUDES 1 avulsion of scalp (S08.0-)
- **S01.00** Unspecified open wound of scalp
- **S01.01** Laceration without foreign body of scalp
- **S01.02** Laceration with foreign body of scalp
- **S01.03** Puncture wound without foreign body of scalp
- **S01.04** Puncture wound with foreign body of scalp
- **S01.05** Open bite of scalp
  - Bite of scalp NOS
  - EXCLUDES 1 superficial bite of scalp (S00.06, S00.07-)

Chapter 19. Injury, Poisoning and Certain Other Consequences of External Causes

- **S01.1** Open wound of **eyelid and periocular area**
  Open wound of eyelid and periocular area with or without involvement of lacrimal passages
  - **S01.10** Unspecified open wound of eyelid and periocular area
    - **S01.101** Unspecified open wound of **right** eyelid and periocular area
    - **S01.102** Unspecified open wound of **left** eyelid and periocular area
    - **S01.109** Unspecified open wound of unspecified eyelid and periocular area
  - **S01.11** **Laceration without foreign body** of eyelid and periocular area
    - **S01.111** Laceration without foreign body of **right** eyelid and periocular area
    - **S01.112** Laceration without foreign body of **left** eyelid and periocular area
    - **S01.119** Laceration without foreign body of unspecified eyelid and periocular area
  - **S01.12** **Laceration with foreign body** of eyelid and periocular area
    - **S01.121** Laceration with foreign body of **right** eyelid and periocular area
    - **S01.122** Laceration with foreign body of **left** eyelid and periocular area
    - **S01.129** Laceration with foreign body of unspecified eyelid and periocular area
  - **S01.13** **Puncture wound without foreign body** of eyelid and periocular area
    - **S01.131** Puncture wound without foreign body of **right** eyelid and periocular area
    - **S01.132** Puncture wound without foreign body of **left** eyelid and periocular area
    - **S01.139** Puncture wound without foreign body of unspecified eyelid and periocular area
  - **S01.14** **Puncture wound with foreign body** of eyelid and periocular area
    - **S01.141** Puncture wound with foreign body of **right** eyelid and periocular area
    - **S01.142** Puncture wound with foreign body of **left** eyelid and periocular area
    - **S01.149** Puncture wound with foreign body of unspecified eyelid and periocular area
  - **S01.15** **Open bite** of eyelid and periocular area
    Bite of eyelid and periocular area NOS
    EXCLUDES 1 superficial bite of eyelid and periocular area (S00.26, S00.27)
    - **S01.151** Open bite of **right** eyelid and periocular area
    - **S01.152** Open bite of **left** eyelid and periocular area
    - **S01.159** Open bite of unspecified eyelid and periocular area
- **S01.2** Open wound of **nose**
  - **S01.20** Unspecified open wound of nose
  - **S01.21** **Laceration without foreign body** of nose
  - **S01.22** **Laceration with foreign body** of nose
  - **S01.23** **Puncture wound without foreign body** of nose
  - **S01.24** **Puncture wound with foreign body** of nose
  - **S01.25** **Open bite** of nose
    Bite of nose NOS
    EXCLUDES 1 superficial bite of nose (S00.36, S00.37)
- **S01.3** Open wound of **ear**
  - **S01.30** Unspecified open wound of ear
    - **S01.301** Unspecified open wound of **right** ear
    - **S01.302** Unspecified open wound of **left** ear
    - **S01.309** Unspecified open wound of unspecified ear
  - **S01.31** **Laceration without foreign body** of ear
    - **S01.311** Laceration without foreign body of **right** ear
    - **S01.312** Laceration without foreign body of **left** ear
    - **S01.319** Laceration without foreign body of unspecified ear
  - **S01.32** **Laceration with foreign body** of ear
    - **S01.321** Laceration with foreign body of **right** ear
    - **S01.322** Laceration with foreign body of **left** ear
    - **S01.329** Laceration with foreign body of unspecified ear
  - **S01.33** **Puncture wound without foreign body** of ear
    - **S01.331** Puncture wound without foreign body of **right** ear
    - **S01.332** Puncture wound without foreign body of **left** ear
    - **S01.339** Puncture wound without foreign body of unspecified ear
  - **S01.34** **Puncture wound with foreign body** of ear
    - **S01.341** Puncture wound with foreign body of **right** ear
    - **S01.342** Puncture wound with foreign body of **left** ear
    - **S01.349** Puncture wound with foreign body of unspecified ear
  - **S01.35** **Open bite** of ear
    Bite of ear NOS
    EXCLUDES 1 superficial bite of ear (S00.46, S00.47)
    - **S01.351** Open bite of **right** ear
    - **S01.352** Open bite of **left** ear
    - **S01.359** Open bite of unspecified ear
- **S01.4** Open wound of **cheek and temporomandibular area**
  - **S01.40** Unspecified open wound of cheek and temporomandibular area
    - **S01.401** Unspecified open wound of **right** cheek and temporomandibular area
    - **S01.402** Unspecified open wound of **left** cheek and temporomandibular area
    - **S01.409** Unspecified open wound of unspecified cheek and temporomandibular area
  - **S01.41** **Laceration without foreign body** of cheek and temporomandibular area
    - **S01.411** Laceration without foreign body of **right** cheek and temporomandibular area
    - **S01.412** Laceration without foreign body of **left** cheek and temporomandibular area
    - **S01.419** Laceration without foreign body of unspecified cheek and temporomandibular area
  - **S01.42** **Laceration with foreign body** of cheek and temporomandibular area
    - **S01.421** Laceration with foreign body of **right** cheek and temporomandibular area
    - **S01.422** Laceration with foreign body of **left** cheek and temporomandibular area
    - **S01.429** Laceration with foreign body of unspecified cheek and temporomandibular area
  - **S01.43** **Puncture wound without foreign body** of cheek and temporomandibular area
    - **S01.431** Puncture wound without foreign body of **right** cheek and temporomandibular area
    - **S01.432** Puncture wound without foreign body of **left** cheek and temporomandibular area
    - **S01.439** Puncture wound without foreign body of unspecified cheek and temporomandibular area
  - **S01.44** **Puncture wound with foreign body** of cheek and temporomandibular area
    - **S01.441** Puncture wound with foreign body of **right** cheek and temporomandibular area
    - **S01.442** Puncture wound with foreign body of **left** cheek and temporomandibular area
    - **S01.449** Puncture wound with foreign body of unspecified cheek and temporomandibular area
  - **S01.45** **Open bite** of cheek and temporomandibular area
    Bite of cheek and temporomandibular area NOS
    EXCLUDES 2 superficial bite of cheek and temporomandibular area (S00.86, S00.87)
    - **S01.451** Open bite of **right** cheek and temporomandibular area
    - **S01.452** Open bite of **left** cheek and temporomandibular area
    - **S01.459** Open bite of unspecified cheek and temporomandibular area

HCC CMS-HCC | **Rx** Rx HCC | **ESR** ESRD HCC | **COM** Commercial HCC | **N** Newborn: 0 | **P** Pediatric: 0-17 | **M** Maternity: 9-64 | **A** Adult: 15-124

Chapter 19. Injury, Poisoning and Certain Other Consequences of External Causes

✓5th S01.5 Open wound of lip and oral cavity
EXCLUDES 2 tooth dislocation (S03.2)
tooth fracture (S02.5)

- ✓6th **S01.50** Unspecified open wound of lip and oral cavity
  - ✓7th **S01.501** Unspecified open wound of lip
  - ✓7th **S01.502** Unspecified open wound of oral cavity
- ✓6th **S01.51** Laceration of lip and oral cavity without foreign body
  - ✓7th **S01.511** Laceration without foreign body of lip
  - ✓7th **S01.512** Laceration without foreign body of oral cavity
- ✓6th **S01.52** Laceration of lip and oral cavity with foreign body
  - ✓7th **S01.521** Laceration with foreign body of lip
  - ✓7th **S01.522** Laceration with foreign body of oral cavity
- ✓6th **S01.53** Puncture wound of lip and oral cavity without foreign body
  - ✓7th **S01.531** Puncture wound without foreign body of lip
  - ✓7th **S01.532** Puncture wound without foreign body of oral cavity
- ✓6th **S01.54** Puncture wound of lip and oral cavity with foreign body
  - ✓7th **S01.541** Puncture wound with foreign body of lip
  - ✓7th **S01.542** Puncture wound with foreign body of oral cavity
- ✓6th **S01.55** Open bite of lip and oral cavity
  - ✓7th **S01.551** Open bite of lip
    - Bite of lip NOS
    - **EXCLUDES 1** superficial bite of lip (S00.571)
  - ✓7th **S01.552** Open bite of oral cavity
    - Bite of oral cavity NOS
    - **EXCLUDES 1** superficial bite of oral cavity (S00.572)

✓5th S01.8 Open wound of other parts of head
- ✓x7th **S01.80** Unspecified open wound of other part of head
- ✓x7th **S01.81** Laceration without foreign body of other part of head
- ✓x7th **S01.82** Laceration with foreign body of other part of head
- ✓x7th **S01.83** Puncture wound without foreign body of other part of head
- ✓x7th **S01.84** Puncture wound with foreign body of other part of head
- ✓x7th **S01.85** Open bite of other part of head
  - Bite of other part of head NOS
  - **EXCLUDES 1** superficial bite of other part of head (S00.87)

✓5th S01.9 Open wound of unspecified part of head
- ✓x7th **S01.90** Unspecified open wound of unspecified part of head
- ✓x7th **S01.91** Laceration without foreign body of unspecified part of head
- ✓x7th **S01.92** Laceration with foreign body of unspecified part of head
- ✓x7th **S01.93** Puncture wound without foreign body of unspecified part of head
- ✓x7th **S01.94** Puncture wound with foreign body of unspecified part of head
- ✓x7th **S01.95** Open bite of unspecified part of head
  - Bite of head NOS
  - **EXCLUDES 1** superficial bite of head NOS (S00.97)

✓4th S02 Fracture of skull and facial bones
NOTE A fracture not indicated as open or closed should be coded to closed.

Code also any associated intracranial injury (S06.-)
AHA: 2021,1Q,6; 2017,1Q,42; 2016,4Q,66-67

The appropriate 7th character is to be added to each code from category S02.
- A initial encounter for closed fracture
- B initial encounter for open fracture
- D subsequent encounter for fracture with routine healing
- G subsequent encounter for fracture with delayed healing
- K subsequent encounter for fracture with nonunion
- S sequela

- ✓x7th **S02.0** Fracture of vault of skull
  - Fracture of frontal bone
  - Fracture of parietal bone

✓5th S02.1 Fracture of base of skull
EXCLUDES 2 lateral orbital wall (S02.84-)
medial orbital wall (S02.83-)
orbital floor (S02.3-)
AHA: 2019,4Q,16-17

- ✓6th **S02.10** Unspecified fracture of base of skull
  - ✓7th **S02.101** Fracture of base of skull, right side
  - ✓7th **S02.102** Fracture of base of skull, left side
  - ✓7th **S02.109** Fracture of base of skull, unspecified side
- ✓6th **S02.11** Fracture of occiput
  - ✓7th **S02.110** Type I occipital condyle fracture, unspecified side
  - ✓7th **S02.111** Type II occipital condyle fracture, unspecified side
  - ✓7th **S02.112** Type III occipital condyle fracture, unspecified side
  - ✓7th **S02.113** Unspecified occipital condyle fracture
  - ✓7th **S02.118** Other fracture of occiput, unspecified side
  - ✓7th **S02.119** Unspecified fracture of occiput
  - ✓7th **S02.11A** Type I occipital condyle fracture, right side
  - ✓7th **S02.11B** Type I occipital condyle fracture, left side
  - ✓7th **S02.11C** Type II occipital condyle fracture, right side
  - ✓7th **S02.11D** Type II occipital condyle fracture, left side
  - ✓7th **S02.11E** Type III occipital condyle fracture, right side
  - ✓7th **S02.11F** Type III occipital condyle fracture, left side
  - ✓7th **S02.11G** Other fracture of occiput, right side
  - ✓7th **S02.11H** Other fracture of occiput, left side
- ✓6th **S02.12** Fracture of orbital roof
  - **AHA:** 2019,4Q,16-17
  - ✓7th **S02.121** Fracture of orbital roof, right side
  - ✓7th **S02.122** Fracture of orbital roof, left side
  - ✓7th **S02.129** Fracture of orbital roof, unspecified side
- ✓x7th **S02.19** Other fracture of base of skull
  - Fracture of anterior fossa of base of skull
  - Fracture of ethmoid sinus
  - Fracture of frontal sinus
  - Fracture of middle fossa of base of skull
  - Fracture of posterior fossa of base of skull
  - Fracture of sphenoid
  - Fracture of temporal bone

- ✓x7th **S02.2** Fracture of nasal bones

✓5th S02.3 Fracture of orbital floor
Fracture of inferior orbital wall
EXCLUDES 1 orbit NOS (S02.85)
EXCLUDES 2 lateral orbital wall (S02.84-)
medial orbital wall (S02.83-)
orbital roof (S02.1-)

- ✓x7th **S02.30** Fracture of orbital floor, unspecified side
- ✓x7th **S02.31** Fracture of orbital floor, right side
- ✓x7th **S02.32** Fracture of orbital floor, left side

✓5th S02.4 Fracture of malar, maxillary and zygoma bones
Fracture of superior maxilla
Fracture of upper jaw (bone)
Fracture of zygomatic process of temporal bone

- ✓6th **S02.40** Fracture of malar, maxillary and zygoma bones, unspecified
  - ✓7th **S02.400** Malar fracture, unspecified side
  - ✓7th **S02.401** Maxillary fracture, unspecified side

✓ Additional Character Required   ✓x7th Placeholder Alert   Manifestation   Unspecified Dx   Q QPP   UPD Unacceptable PDx

	S02.402	Zygomatic fracture, unspecified side	HCC ESR
	S02.40A	Malar fracture, right side	HCC ESR
	S02.40B	Malar fracture, left side	HCC ESR
	S02.40C	Maxillary fracture, right side	HCC ESR
	S02.40D	Maxillary fracture, left side	HCC ESR
	S02.40E	Zygomatic fracture, right side	HCC ESR
	S02.40F	Zygomatic fracture, left side	HCC ESR

√6th S02.41 LeFort fracture

DEF: Named for Rene Le Fort, these fractures describe different combinations of multiple fractures that occur from significant force to the midface. A common denominator in all three types of LeFort fractures is fracture of the pterygoid processes, which are two bony plates resembling wings that extend downward from the sphenoid bone.

LeFort Fracture Types

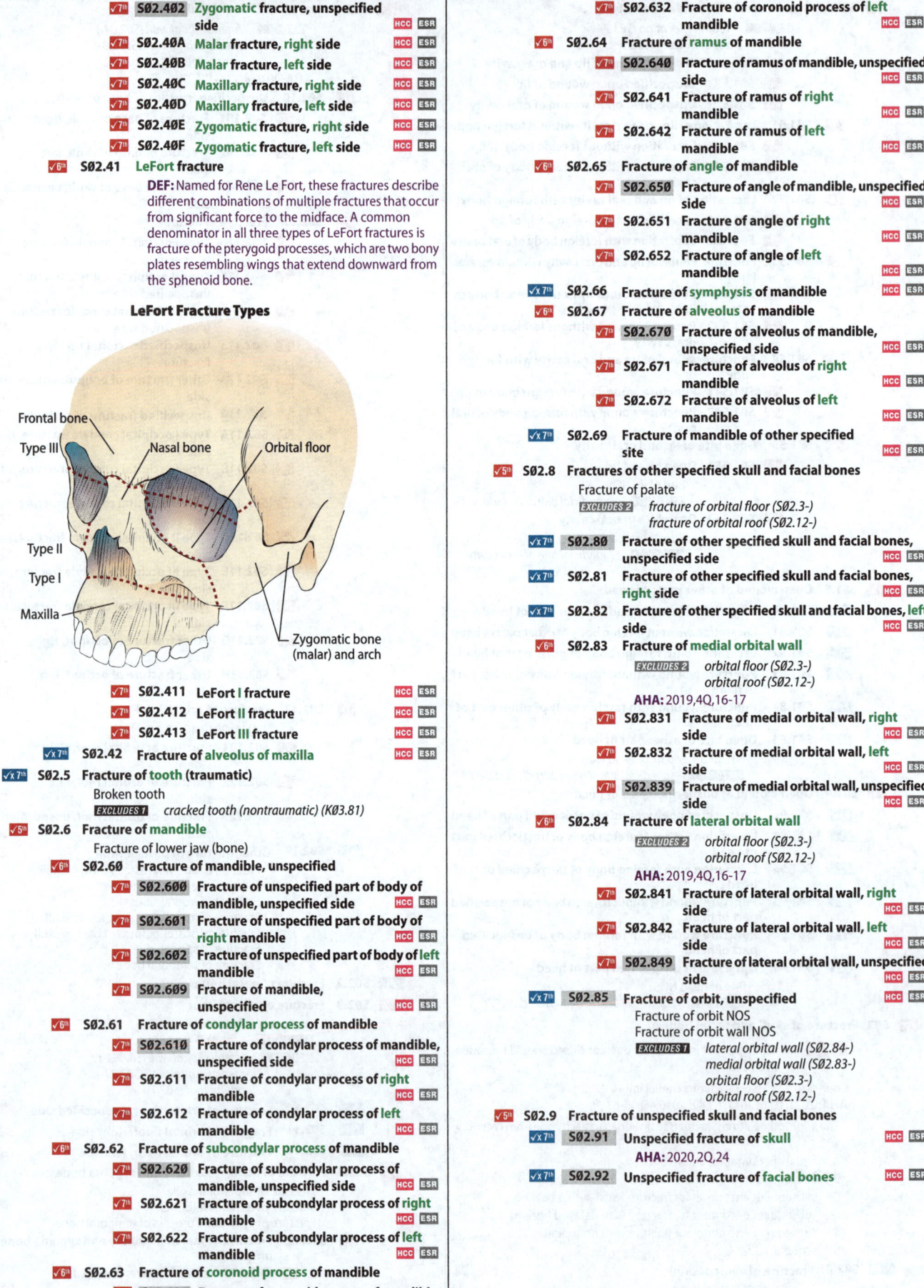

	S02.411	LeFort I fracture	HCC ESR
	S02.412	LeFort II fracture	HCC ESR
	S02.413	LeFort III fracture	HCC ESR

√x 7th S02.42 Fracture of alveolus of maxilla HCC ESR

√x 7th S02.5 Fracture of tooth (traumatic)
Broken tooth
EXCLUDES 1 cracked tooth (nontraumatic) (K03.81)

√5th S02.6 Fracture of mandible
Fracture of lower jaw (bone)

√6th S02.60 Fracture of mandible, unspecified
	S02.600	Fracture of unspecified part of body of mandible, unspecified side	HCC ESR
	S02.601	Fracture of unspecified part of body of right mandible	HCC ESR
	S02.602	Fracture of unspecified part of body of left mandible	HCC ESR
	S02.609	Fracture of mandible, unspecified	

√6th S02.61 Fracture of condylar process of mandible
	S02.610	Fracture of condylar process of mandible, unspecified side	HCC ESR
	S02.611	Fracture of condylar process of right mandible	HCC ESR
	S02.612	Fracture of condylar process of left mandible	HCC ESR

√6th S02.62 Fracture of subcondylar process of mandible
	S02.620	Fracture of subcondylar process of mandible, unspecified side	HCC ESR
	S02.621	Fracture of subcondylar process of right mandible	HCC ESR
	S02.622	Fracture of subcondylar process of left mandible	HCC ESR

√6th S02.63 Fracture of coronoid process of mandible
| | S02.630 | Fracture of coronoid process of mandible, unspecified side | HCC ESR |
| | S02.631 | Fracture of coronoid process of right mandible | HCC ESR |

| | S02.632 | Fracture of coronoid process of left mandible | HCC ESR |

√6th S02.64 Fracture of ramus of mandible
	S02.640	Fracture of ramus of mandible, unspecified side	HCC ESR
	S02.641	Fracture of ramus of right mandible	HCC ESR
	S02.642	Fracture of ramus of left mandible	HCC ESR

√6th S02.65 Fracture of angle of mandible
	S02.650	Fracture of angle of mandible, unspecified side	HCC ESR
	S02.651	Fracture of angle of right mandible	HCC ESR
	S02.652	Fracture of angle of left mandible	HCC ESR

√x 7th S02.66 Fracture of symphysis of mandible HCC ESR

√6th S02.67 Fracture of alveolus of mandible
	S02.670	Fracture of alveolus of mandible, unspecified side	HCC ESR
	S02.671	Fracture of alveolus of right mandible	HCC ESR
	S02.672	Fracture of alveolus of left mandible	HCC ESR

√x 7th S02.69 Fracture of mandible of other specified site HCC ESR

√5th S02.8 Fractures of other specified skull and facial bones
Fracture of palate
EXCLUDES 2 fracture of orbital floor (S02.3-)
fracture of orbital roof (S02.12-)

√x 7th S02.80 Fracture of other specified skull and facial bones, unspecified side HCC ESR
√x 7th S02.81 Fracture of other specified skull and facial bones, right side HCC ESR
√x 7th S02.82 Fracture of other specified skull and facial bones, left side HCC ESR

√6th S02.83 Fracture of medial orbital wall
EXCLUDES 2 orbital floor (S02.3-)
orbital roof (S02.12-)
AHA: 2019,4Q,16-17
	S02.831	Fracture of medial orbital wall, right side	HCC ESR
	S02.832	Fracture of medial orbital wall, left side	HCC ESR
	S02.839	Fracture of medial orbital wall, unspecified side	HCC ESR

√6th S02.84 Fracture of lateral orbital wall
EXCLUDES 2 orbital floor (S02.3-)
orbital roof (S02.12-)
AHA: 2019,4Q,16-17
	S02.841	Fracture of lateral orbital wall, right side	HCC ESR
	S02.842	Fracture of lateral orbital wall, left side	HCC ESR
	S02.849	Fracture of lateral orbital wall, unspecified side	HCC ESR

√x 7th S02.85 Fracture of orbit, unspecified
Fracture of orbit NOS
Fracture of orbit wall NOS
EXCLUDES 1 lateral orbital wall (S02.84-)
medial orbital wall (S02.83-)
orbital floor (S02.3-)
orbital roof (S02.12-)

√5th S02.9 Fracture of unspecified skull and facial bones
√x 7th S02.91 Unspecified fracture of skull HCC ESR
AHA: 2020,2Q,24
√x 7th S02.92 Unspecified fracture of facial bones HCC ESR

S03 Dislocation and sprain of joints and ligaments of head

INCLUDES
avulsion of joint (capsule) or ligament of head
laceration of cartilage, joint (capsule) or ligament of head
sprain of cartilage, joint (capsule) or ligament of head
traumatic hemarthrosis of joint or ligament of head
traumatic rupture of joint or ligament of head
traumatic subluxation of joint or ligament of head
traumatic tear of joint or ligament of head

Code also any associated open wound

EXCLUDES 2 strain of muscle or tendon of head (S09.1)

The appropriate 7th character is to be added to each code from category S03.
- A initial encounter
- D subsequent encounter
- S sequela

S03.0 Dislocation of jaw
Dislocation of jaw (cartilage) (meniscus)
Dislocation of mandible
Dislocation of temporomandibular (joint)
AHA: 2016,4Q,67

- S03.00 Dislocation of jaw, unspecified side
- S03.01 Dislocation of jaw, right side
- S03.02 Dislocation of jaw, left side
- S03.03 Dislocation of jaw, bilateral

S03.1 Dislocation of septal cartilage of nose
S03.2 Dislocation of tooth
S03.4 Sprain of jaw
Sprain of temporomandibular (joint) (ligament)
AHA: 2016,4Q,67

- S03.40 Sprain of jaw, unspecified side
- S03.41 Sprain of jaw, right side
- S03.42 Sprain of jaw, left side
- S03.43 Sprain of jaw, bilateral

S03.8 Sprain of joints and ligaments of other parts of head
S03.9 Sprain of joints and ligaments of unspecified parts of head

S04 Injury of cranial nerve

The selection of side should be based on the side of the body being affected

Code first any associated intracranial injury (S06.-)
Code also any associated:
 open wound of head (S01.-)
 skull fracture (S02.-)

The appropriate 7th character is to be added to each code from category S04.
- A initial encounter
- D subsequent encounter
- S sequela

S04.0 Injury of optic nerve and pathways
Use additional code to identify any visual field defect or blindness (H53.4-, H54.-)

- **S04.01 Injury of optic nerve**
  Injury of 2nd cranial nerve
  - S04.011 Injury of optic nerve, right eye
  - S04.012 Injury of optic nerve, left eye
  - S04.019 Injury of optic nerve, unspecified eye
    Injury of optic nerve NOS
- **S04.02 Injury of optic chiasm**
- **S04.03 Injury of optic tract and pathways**
  Injury of optic radiation
  - S04.031 Injury of optic tract and pathways, right side
  - S04.032 Injury of optic tract and pathways, left side
  - S04.039 Injury of optic tract and pathways, unspecified side
    Injury of optic tract and pathways NOS
- **S04.04 Injury of visual cortex**
  - S04.041 Injury of visual cortex, right side
  - S04.042 Injury of visual cortex, left side
  - S04.049 Injury of visual cortex, unspecified side
    Injury of visual cortex NOS

S04.1 Injury of oculomotor nerve
Injury of 3rd cranial nerve

- S04.10 Injury of oculomotor nerve, unspecified side
- S04.11 Injury of oculomotor nerve, right side
- S04.12 Injury of oculomotor nerve, left side

S04.2 Injury of trochlear nerve
Injury of 4th cranial nerve

- S04.20 Injury of trochlear nerve, unspecified side
- S04.21 Injury of trochlear nerve, right side
- S04.22 Injury of trochlear nerve, left side

S04.3 Injury of trigeminal nerve
Injury of 5th cranial nerve

- S04.30 Injury of trigeminal nerve, unspecified side
- S04.31 Injury of trigeminal nerve, right side
- S04.32 Injury of trigeminal nerve, left side

S04.4 Injury of abducent nerve
Injury of 6th cranial nerve

- S04.40 Injury of abducent nerve, unspecified side
- S04.41 Injury of abducent nerve, right side
- S04.42 Injury of abducent nerve, left side

S04.5 Injury of facial nerve
Injury of 7th cranial nerve

- S04.50 Injury of facial nerve, unspecified side
- S04.51 Injury of facial nerve, right side
- S04.52 Injury of facial nerve, left side

S04.6 Injury of acoustic nerve
Injury of 8th cranial nerve
Injury of auditory nerve

- S04.60 Injury of acoustic nerve, unspecified side
- S04.61 Injury of acoustic nerve, right side
- S04.62 Injury of acoustic nerve, left side

S04.7 Injury of accessory nerve
Injury of 11th cranial nerve

- S04.70 Injury of accessory nerve, unspecified side
- S04.71 Injury of accessory nerve, right side
- S04.72 Injury of accessory nerve, left side

S04.8 Injury of other cranial nerves

- **S04.81 Injury of olfactory [1st] nerve**
  - S04.811 Injury of olfactory [1st] nerve, right side
  - S04.812 Injury of olfactory [1st] nerve, left side
  - S04.819 Injury of olfactory [1st] nerve, unspecified side
- **S04.89 Injury of other cranial nerves**
  Injury of vagus [10th] nerve
  - S04.891 Injury of other cranial nerves, right side
  - S04.892 Injury of other cranial nerves, left side
  - S04.899 Injury of other cranial nerves, unspecified side

S04.9 Injury of unspecified cranial nerve

S05 Injury of eye and orbit

INCLUDES open wound of eye and orbit
EXCLUDES 2
2nd cranial [optic] nerve injury (S04.0-)
3rd cranial [oculomotor] nerve injury (S04.1-)
open wound of eyelid and periocular area (S01.1-)
orbital bone fracture (S02.1-, S02.3-, S02.8-)
superficial injury of eyelid (S00.1-S00.2)

The appropriate 7th character is to be added to each code from category S05.
- A initial encounter
- D subsequent encounter
- S sequela

S05.0 Injury of conjunctiva and corneal abrasion without foreign body
EXCLUDES 1
foreign body in conjunctival sac (T15.1)
foreign body in cornea (T15.0)

- S05.00 Injury of conjunctiva and corneal abrasion without foreign body, unspecified eye
- S05.01 Injury of conjunctiva and corneal abrasion without foreign body, right eye
- S05.02 Injury of conjunctiva and corneal abrasion without foreign body, left eye

S05.1 Contusion of eyeball and orbital tissues
Traumatic hyphema
EXCLUDES 2: black eye NOS (S00.1)
contusion of eyelid and periocular area (S00.1)

- **S05.10** Contusion of eyeball and orbital tissues, unspecified eye
- **S05.11** Contusion of eyeball and orbital tissues, right eye
- **S05.12** Contusion of eyeball and orbital tissues, left eye

S05.2 Ocular laceration and rupture with prolapse or loss of intraocular tissue

- **S05.20** Ocular laceration and rupture with prolapse or loss of intraocular tissue, unspecified eye
- **S05.21** Ocular laceration and rupture with prolapse or loss of intraocular tissue, right eye
- **S05.22** Ocular laceration and rupture with prolapse or loss of intraocular tissue, left eye

S05.3 Ocular laceration without prolapse or loss of intraocular tissue
Laceration of eye NOS
AHA: 2022,1Q,33
DEF: Tear in ocular tissue without displacing structures that is due to blunt trauma. It is characterized by pain, redness, and decreased vision.

- **S05.30** Ocular laceration without prolapse or loss of intraocular tissue, unspecified eye
- **S05.31** Ocular laceration without prolapse or loss of intraocular tissue, right eye
- **S05.32** Ocular laceration without prolapse or loss of intraocular tissue, left eye

S05.4 Penetrating wound of orbit with or without foreign body
EXCLUDES 2: retained (old) foreign body following penetrating wound in orbit (H05.5-)

- **S05.40** Penetrating wound of orbit with or without foreign body, unspecified eye
- **S05.41** Penetrating wound of orbit with or without foreign body, right eye
- **S05.42** Penetrating wound of orbit with or without foreign body, left eye

S05.5 Penetrating wound with foreign body of eyeball
EXCLUDES 2: retained (old) intraocular foreign body (H44.6-, H44.7)

- **S05.50** Penetrating wound with foreign body of unspecified eyeball
- **S05.51** Penetrating wound with foreign body of right eyeball
- **S05.52** Penetrating wound with foreign body of left eyeball

S05.6 Penetrating wound without foreign body of eyeball
Ocular penetration NOS

- **S05.60** Penetrating wound without foreign body of unspecified eyeball
- **S05.61** Penetrating wound without foreign body of right eyeball
- **S05.62** Penetrating wound without foreign body of left eyeball

S05.7 Avulsion of eye
Traumatic enucleation

- **S05.70** Avulsion of unspecified eye
- **S05.71** Avulsion of right eye
- **S05.72** Avulsion of left eye

S05.8 Other injuries of eye and orbit
Lacrimal duct injury

- **S05.8X** Other injuries of eye and orbit
  - **S05.8X1** Other injuries of right eye and orbit
  - **S05.8X2** Other injuries of left eye and orbit
  - **S05.8X9** Other injuries of unspecified eye and orbit

S05.9 Unspecified injury of eye and orbit
Injury of eye NOS

- **S05.90** Unspecified injury of unspecified eye and orbit
- **S05.91** Unspecified injury of right eye and orbit
- **S05.92** Unspecified injury of left eye and orbit

S06 Intracranial injury

NOTE 7th characters D and S do not apply to codes in category S06 with 6th character 7 – death due to brain injury prior to regaining consciousness, or 8 – death due to other cause prior to regaining consciousness.

INCLUDES: traumatic brain injury

Code also any associated:
  open wound of head (S01.-)
  skull fracture (S02.-)
Use additional code, if applicable, to identify mild neurocognitive disorders due to known physiological condition (F06.7-)
EXCLUDES 1: head injury NOS (S09.90)
AHA: 2022,4Q,42-45; 2017,4Q,25; 2017,1Q,42; 2015,3Q,37
TIP: Do not assign Z87.820 Personal history of traumatic brain injury, when residual conditions persist after an intracranial injury. The codes for the residual conditions should be first listed, followed by a code from category S06 using seventh character S to identify sequelae.

▶The appropriate 7th character is to be added to each code from category S06, except as described in the NOTE above.◀
- A initial encounter
- D subsequent encounter
- S sequela

S06.0 Concussion
Commotio cerebri
EXCLUDES 1: concussion with other intracranial injuries classified in subcategories S06.1- to S06.6-, and S06.81- to S06.89-, code to specified intracranial injury
AHA: 2016,4Q,67-68

- **S06.0X** Concussion
  - **S06.0X0** Concussion without loss of consciousness
  - **S06.0X1** Concussion with loss of consciousness of 30 minutes or less
    Concussion with brief loss of consciousness
  - **S06.0XA** Concussion with loss of consciousness status unknown
    Concussion NOS
  - **S06.0X9** Concussion with loss of consciousness of unspecified duration

S06.1 Traumatic cerebral edema
Diffuse traumatic cerebral edema
Focal traumatic cerebral edema
AHA: 2019,3Q,35; 2015,1Q,12-13

- **S06.1X** Traumatic cerebral edema
  - **S06.1X0** Traumatic cerebral edema without loss of consciousness
  - **S06.1X1** Traumatic cerebral edema with loss of consciousness of 30 minutes or less
    Traumatic cerebral edema with brief loss of consciousness
  - **S06.1X2** Traumatic cerebral edema with loss of consciousness of 31 minutes to 59 minutes
  - **S06.1X3** Traumatic cerebral edema with loss of consciousness of 1 hour to 5 hours 59 minutes
  - **S06.1X4** Traumatic cerebral edema with loss of consciousness of 6 hours to 24 hours
  - **S06.1X5** Traumatic cerebral edema with loss of consciousness greater than 24 hours with return to pre-existing conscious level
  - **S06.1X6** Traumatic cerebral edema with loss of consciousness greater than 24 hours without return to pre-existing conscious level with patient surviving
  - **S06.1X7** Traumatic cerebral edema with loss of consciousness of any duration with death due to brain injury prior to regaining consciousness
  - **S06.1X8** Traumatic cerebral edema with loss of consciousness of any duration with death due to other cause prior to regaining consciousness

Chapter 19. Injury, Poisoning and Certain Other Consequences of External Causes

- √7th **S06.1XA** Traumatic cerebral edema with loss of consciousness status unknown [HCC] [ESR]
  Traumatic cerebral edema NOS
- √7th **S06.1X9** Traumatic cerebral edema with loss of consciousness of unspecified duration [HCC] [ESR]

√5th **S06.2** Diffuse traumatic brain injury
  Diffuse axonal brain injury
  Use additional code, if applicable, for traumatic brain compression or herniation (S06.A-)
  EXCLUDES 1 traumatic diffuse cerebral edema (S06.1X-)
  AHA: 2020,3Q,46

√6th **S06.2X** Diffuse traumatic brain injury
  - √7th **S06.2X0** Diffuse traumatic brain injury without loss of consciousness [HCC] [ESR]
  - √7th **S06.2X1** Diffuse traumatic brain injury with loss of consciousness of 30 minutes or less [HCC] [ESR]
    Diffuse traumatic brain injury with brief loss of consciousness
  - √7th **S06.2X2** Diffuse traumatic brain injury with loss of consciousness of 31 minutes to 59 minutes [HCC] [ESR]
  - √7th **S06.2X3** Diffuse traumatic brain injury with loss of consciousness of 1 hour to 5 hours 59 minutes [HCC] [ESR] [COM]
  - √7th **S06.2X4** Diffuse traumatic brain injury with loss of consciousness of 6 hours to 24 hours [HCC] [ESR] [COM]
  - √7th **S06.2X5** Diffuse traumatic brain injury with loss of consciousness greater than 24 hours with return to pre-existing conscious levels [HCC] [ESR] [COM]
  - √7th **S06.2X6** Diffuse traumatic brain injury with loss of consciousness greater than 24 hours without return to pre-existing conscious level with patient surviving [HCC] [ESR] [COM]
  - √7th **S06.2X7** Diffuse traumatic brain injury with loss of consciousness of any duration with death due to brain injury prior to regaining consciousness
  - √7th **S06.2X8** Diffuse traumatic brain injury with loss of consciousness of any duration with death due to other cause prior to regaining consciousness
  - √7th **S06.2XA** Diffuse traumatic brain injury with loss of consciousness status unknown [HCC] [ESR]
    Diffuse traumatic brain injury NOS
  - √7th **S06.2X9** Diffuse traumatic brain injury with loss of consciousness of unspecified duration [HCC] [ESR]

√5th **S06.3** Focal traumatic brain injury
  Use additional code, if applicable, for traumatic brain compression or herniation (S06.A-)
  EXCLUDES 2 any condition classifiable to S06.4-S06.6
  focal cerebral edema (S06.1)
  AHA: 2020,3Q,46; 2019,3Q,35; 2015,1Q,12-13

√6th **S06.30** Unspecified focal traumatic brain injury
  - √7th **S06.300** Unspecified focal traumatic brain injury without loss of consciousness [HCC] [ESR]
  - √7th **S06.301** Unspecified focal traumatic brain injury with loss of consciousness of 30 minutes or less [HCC] [ESR]
    Unspecified focal traumatic brain injury with brief loss of consciousness
  - √7th **S06.302** Unspecified focal traumatic brain injury with loss of consciousness of 31 minutes to 59 minutes [HCC] [ESR]
  - √7th **S06.303** Unspecified focal traumatic brain injury with loss of consciousness of 1 hour to 5 hours 59 minutes [HCC] [ESR] [COM]
  - √7th **S06.304** Unspecified focal traumatic brain injury with loss of consciousness of 6 hours to 24 hours [HCC] [ESR] [COM]
  - √7th **S06.305** Unspecified focal traumatic brain injury with loss of consciousness greater than 24 hours with return to pre-existing conscious level [HCC] [ESR] [COM]
  - √7th **S06.306** Unspecified focal traumatic brain injury with loss of consciousness greater than 24 hours without return to pre-existing conscious level with patient surviving [HCC] [ESR] [COM]
  - √7th **S06.307** Unspecified focal traumatic brain injury with loss of consciousness of any duration with death due to brain injury prior to regaining consciousness
  - √7th **S06.308** Unspecified focal traumatic brain injury with loss of consciousness of any duration with death due to other cause prior to regaining consciousness
  - √7th **S06.30A** Unspecified focal traumatic brain injury with loss of consciousness status unknown [HCC] [ESR]
    Unspecified focal traumatic brain injury NOS
  - √7th **S06.309** Unspecified focal traumatic brain injury with loss of consciousness of unspecified duration [HCC] [ESR]

√6th **S06.31** Contusion and laceration of right cerebrum
  - √7th **S06.310** Contusion and laceration of right cerebrum without loss of consciousness [HCC] [ESR]
  - √7th **S06.311** Contusion and laceration of right cerebrum with loss of consciousness of 30 minutes or less [HCC] [ESR]
    Contusion and laceration of right cerebrum with brief loss of consciousness
  - √7th **S06.312** Contusion and laceration of right cerebrum with loss of consciousness of 31 minutes to 59 minutes [HCC] [ESR]
  - √7th **S06.313** Contusion and laceration of right cerebrum with loss of consciousness of 1 hour to 5 hours 59 minutes [HCC] [ESR] [COM]
  - √7th **S06.314** Contusion and laceration of right cerebrum with loss of consciousness of 6 hours to 24 hours [HCC] [ESR] [COM]
  - √7th **S06.315** Contusion and laceration of right cerebrum with loss of consciousness greater than 24 hours with return to pre-existing conscious level [HCC] [ESR] [COM]
  - √7th **S06.316** Contusion and laceration of right cerebrum with loss of consciousness greater than 24 hours without return to pre-existing conscious level with patient surviving [HCC] [ESR] [COM]
  - √7th **S06.317** Contusion and laceration of right cerebrum with loss of consciousness of any duration with death due to brain injury prior to regaining consciousness
  - √7th **S06.318** Contusion and laceration of right cerebrum with loss of consciousness of any duration with death due to other cause prior to regaining consciousness
  - √7th **S06.31A** Contusion and laceration of right cerebrum with loss of consciousness status unknown [HCC] [ESR]
    Contusion and laceration of right cerebrum NOS
  - √7th **S06.319** Contusion and laceration of right cerebrum with loss of consciousness of unspecified duration [HCC] [ESR]

√6th **S06.32** Contusion and laceration of left cerebrum
  - √7th **S06.320** Contusion and laceration of left cerebrum without loss of consciousness [HCC] [ESR]
  - √7th **S06.321** Contusion and laceration of left cerebrum with loss of consciousness of 30 minutes or less [HCC] [ESR]
    Contusion and laceration of left cerebrum with brief loss of consciousness
  - √7th **S06.322** Contusion and laceration of left cerebrum with loss of consciousness of 31 minutes to 59 minutes [HCC] [ESR]
  - √7th **S06.323** Contusion and laceration of left cerebrum with loss of consciousness of 1 hour to 5 hours 59 minutes [HCC] [ESR] [COM]
  - √7th **S06.324** Contusion and laceration of left cerebrum with loss of consciousness of 6 hours to 24 hours [HCC] [ESR] [COM]
  - √7th **S06.325** Contusion and laceration of left cerebrum with loss of consciousness greater than 24 hours with return to pre-existing conscious level [HCC] [ESR] [COM]

✓ Additional Character Required | √x7th Placeholder Alert | Manifestation | Unspecified Dx | Q QPP | UPD Unacceptable PDx

- **S06.326** Contusion and laceration of left cerebrum with loss of consciousness greater than 24 hours without return to pre-existing conscious level with patient surviving [HCC] [ESR] [COM]
- **S06.327** Contusion and laceration of left cerebrum with loss of consciousness of any duration with death due to brain injury prior to regaining consciousness
- **S06.328** Contusion and laceration of left cerebrum with loss of consciousness of any duration with death due to other cause prior to regaining consciousness
- **S06.32A** Contusion and laceration of left cerebrum with loss of consciousness status unknown [HCC] [ESR]
  - Contusion and laceration of left cerebrum NOS
- **S06.329** Contusion and laceration of left cerebrum with loss of consciousness of unspecified duration [HCC] [ESR]

S06.33 Contusion and laceration of cerebrum, unspecified
- **S06.330** Contusion and laceration of cerebrum, unspecified, without loss of consciousness
- **S06.331** Contusion and laceration of cerebrum, unspecified, with loss of consciousness of 30 minutes or less [HCC] [ESR]
  - Contusion and laceration of cerebrum, unspecified, with brief loss of consciousness
- **S06.332** Contusion and laceration of cerebrum, unspecified, with loss of consciousness of 31 minutes to 59 minutes [HCC] [ESR]
- **S06.333** Contusion and laceration of cerebrum, unspecified, with loss of consciousness of 1 hour to 5 hours 59 minutes [HCC] [ESR] [COM]
- **S06.334** Contusion and laceration of cerebrum, unspecified, with loss of consciousness of 6 hours to 24 hours [HCC] [ESR] [COM]
- **S06.335** Contusion and laceration of cerebrum, unspecified, with loss of consciousness greater than 24 hours with return to pre-existing conscious level [HCC] [ESR] [COM]
- **S06.336** Contusion and laceration of cerebrum, unspecified, with loss of consciousness greater than 24 hours without return to pre-existing conscious level with patient surviving [HCC] [ESR] [COM]
- **S06.337** Contusion and laceration of cerebrum, unspecified, with loss of consciousness of any duration with death due to brain injury prior to regaining consciousness
- **S06.338** Contusion and laceration of cerebrum, unspecified, with loss of consciousness of any duration with death due to other cause prior to regaining consciousness
- **S06.33A** Contusion and laceration of cerebrum, unspecified, with loss of consciousness status unknown [HCC] [ESR]
  - Contusion and laceration of cerebrum NOS
- **S06.339** Contusion and laceration of cerebrum, unspecified, with loss of consciousness of unspecified duration [HCC] [ESR]

S06.34 Traumatic hemorrhage of right cerebrum
  - Traumatic intracerebral hemorrhage and hematoma of right cerebrum
- **S06.340** Traumatic hemorrhage of right cerebrum without loss of consciousness [HCC] [ESR]
- **S06.341** Traumatic hemorrhage of right cerebrum with loss of consciousness of 30 minutes or less
  - Traumatic hemorrhage of right cerebrum with brief loss of consciousness
- **S06.342** Traumatic hemorrhage of right cerebrum with loss of consciousness of 31 minutes to 59 minutes [HCC] [ESR]
- **S06.343** Traumatic hemorrhage of right cerebrum with loss of consciousness of 1 hours to 5 hours 59 minutes [HCC] [ESR] [COM]
- **S06.344** Traumatic hemorrhage of right cerebrum with loss of consciousness of 6 hours to 24 hours [HCC] [ESR] [COM]
- **S06.345** Traumatic hemorrhage of right cerebrum with loss of consciousness greater than 24 hours with return to pre-existing conscious level [HCC] [ESR] [COM]
- **S06.346** Traumatic hemorrhage of right cerebrum with loss of consciousness greater than 24 hours without return to pre-existing conscious level with patient surviving [HCC] [ESR] [COM]
- **S06.347** Traumatic hemorrhage of right cerebrum with loss of consciousness of any duration with death due to brain injury prior to regaining consciousness
- **S06.348** Traumatic hemorrhage of right cerebrum with loss of consciousness of any duration with death due to other cause prior to regaining consciousness
- **S06.34A** Traumatic hemorrhage of right cerebrum with loss of consciousness status unknown [HCC] [ESR]
  - Traumatic hemorrhage of right cerebrum NOS
- **S06.349** Traumatic hemorrhage of right cerebrum with loss of consciousness of unspecified duration [HCC] [ESR]

S06.35 Traumatic hemorrhage of left cerebrum
  - Traumatic intracerebral hemorrhage and hematoma of left cerebrum
- **S06.350** Traumatic hemorrhage of left cerebrum without loss of consciousness [HCC] [ESR]
- **S06.351** Traumatic hemorrhage of left cerebrum with loss of consciousness of 30 minutes or less
  - Traumatic hemorrhage of left cerebrum with brief loss of consciousness
- **S06.352** Traumatic hemorrhage of left cerebrum with loss of consciousness of 31 minutes to 59 minutes
- **S06.353** Traumatic hemorrhage of left cerebrum with loss of consciousness of 1 hours to 5 hours 59 minutes [HCC] [ESR] [COM]
- **S06.354** Traumatic hemorrhage of left cerebrum with loss of consciousness of 6 hours to 24 hours [HCC] [ESR] [COM]
- **S06.355** Traumatic hemorrhage of left cerebrum with loss of consciousness greater than 24 hours with return to pre-existing conscious level [HCC] [ESR] [COM]
- **S06.356** Traumatic hemorrhage of left cerebrum with loss of consciousness greater than 24 hours without return to pre-existing conscious level with patient surviving [HCC] [ESR] [COM]
- **S06.357** Traumatic hemorrhage of left cerebrum with loss of consciousness of any duration with death due to brain injury prior to regaining consciousness
- **S06.358** Traumatic hemorrhage of left cerebrum with loss of consciousness of any duration with death due to other cause prior to regaining consciousness
- **S06.35A** Traumatic hemorrhage of left cerebrum with loss of consciousness status unknown [HCC] [ESR]
  - Traumatic hemorrhage of left cerebrum NOS
- **S06.359** Traumatic hemorrhage of left cerebrum with loss of consciousness of unspecified duration [HCC] [ESR]

S06.36 Traumatic hemorrhage of cerebrum, unspecified
  - Traumatic intracerebral hemorrhage and hematoma, unspecified
- **S06.360** Traumatic hemorrhage of cerebrum, unspecified, without loss of consciousness [HCC] [ESR]

S06.361 Traumatic hemorrhage of cerebrum, unspecified, with loss of consciousness of 30 minutes or less [HCC] [ESR]
  Traumatic hemorrhage of cerebrum, unspecified, with brief loss of consciousness

S06.362 Traumatic hemorrhage of cerebrum, unspecified, with loss of consciousness of 31 minutes to 59 minutes [HCC] [ESR]

S06.363 Traumatic hemorrhage of cerebrum, unspecified, with loss of consciousness of 1 hours to 5 hours 59 minutes [HCC] [ESR] [COM]

S06.364 Traumatic hemorrhage of cerebrum, unspecified, with loss of consciousness of 6 hours to 24 hours [HCC] [ESR] [COM]

S06.365 Traumatic hemorrhage of cerebrum, unspecified, with loss of consciousness greater than 24 hours with return to pre-existing conscious level [HCC] [ESR] [COM]

S06.366 Traumatic hemorrhage of cerebrum, unspecified, with loss of consciousness greater than 24 hours without return to pre-existing conscious level with patient surviving [HCC] [ESR] [COM]

S06.367 Traumatic hemorrhage of cerebrum, unspecified, with loss of consciousness of any duration with death due to brain injury prior to regaining consciousness

S06.368 Traumatic hemorrhage of cerebrum, unspecified, with loss of consciousness of any duration with death due to other cause prior to regaining consciousness

S06.36A Traumatic hemorrhage of cerebrum, unspecified, with loss of consciousness status unknown [HCC] [ESR]
  Traumatic hemorrhage of cerebrum NOS

S06.369 Traumatic hemorrhage of cerebrum, unspecified, with loss of consciousness of unspecified duration [HCC] [ESR]

S06.37 Contusion, laceration, and hemorrhage of cerebellum

S06.370 Contusion, laceration, and hemorrhage of cerebellum without loss of consciousness [HCC] [ESR]

S06.371 Contusion, laceration, and hemorrhage of cerebellum with loss of consciousness of 30 minutes or less [HCC] [ESR]
  Contusion, laceration, and hemorrhage of cerebellum with brief loss of consciousness

S06.372 Contusion, laceration, and hemorrhage of cerebellum with loss of consciousness of 31 minutes to 59 minutes [HCC] [ESR]

S06.373 Contusion, laceration, and hemorrhage of cerebellum with loss of consciousness of 1 hour to 5 hours 59 minutes [HCC] [ESR] [COM]

S06.374 Contusion, laceration, and hemorrhage of cerebellum with loss of consciousness of 6 hours to 24 hours [HCC] [ESR] [COM]

S06.375 Contusion, laceration, and hemorrhage of cerebellum with loss of consciousness greater than 24 hours with return to pre-existing conscious level [HCC] [ESR] [COM]

S06.376 Contusion, laceration, and hemorrhage of cerebellum with loss of consciousness greater than 24 hours without return to pre-existing conscious level with patient surviving [HCC] [ESR] [COM]

S06.377 Contusion, laceration, and hemorrhage of cerebellum with loss of consciousness of any duration with death due to brain injury prior to regaining consciousness

S06.378 Contusion, laceration, and hemorrhage of cerebellum with loss of consciousness of any duration with death due to other cause prior to regaining consciousness

S06.37A Contusion, laceration, and hemorrhage of cerebellum with loss of consciousness status unknown [HCC] [ESR]
  Contusion, laceration, and hemorrhage of cerebellum NOS

S06.379 Contusion, laceration, and hemorrhage of cerebellum with loss of consciousness of unspecified duration [HCC] [ESR]

S06.38 Contusion, laceration, and hemorrhage of brainstem

S06.380 Contusion, laceration, and hemorrhage of brainstem without loss of consciousness [HCC] [ESR]

S06.381 Contusion, laceration, and hemorrhage of brainstem with loss of consciousness of 30 minutes or less [HCC] [ESR]
  Contusion, laceration, and hemorrhage of brainstem with brief loss of consciousness

S06.382 Contusion, laceration, and hemorrhage of brainstem with loss of consciousness of 31 minutes to 59 minutes [HCC] [ESR]

S06.383 Contusion, laceration, and hemorrhage of brainstem with loss of consciousness of 1 hour to 5 hours 59 minutes [HCC] [ESR] [COM]

S06.384 Contusion, laceration, and hemorrhage of brainstem with loss of consciousness of 6 hours to 24 hours [HCC] [ESR] [COM]

S06.385 Contusion, laceration, and hemorrhage of brainstem with loss of consciousness greater than 24 hours with return to pre-existing conscious level [HCC] [ESR] [COM]

S06.386 Contusion, laceration, and hemorrhage of brainstem with loss of consciousness greater than 24 hours without return to pre-existing conscious level with patient surviving [HCC] [ESR] [COM]

S06.387 Contusion, laceration, and hemorrhage of brainstem with loss of consciousness of any duration with death due to brain injury prior to regaining consciousness

S06.388 Contusion, laceration, and hemorrhage of brainstem with loss of consciousness of any duration with death due to other cause prior to regaining consciousness

S06.38A Contusion, laceration, and hemorrhage of brainstem with loss of consciousness status unknown [HCC] [ESR]
  Contusion, laceration, and hemorrhage of brainstem NOS

S06.389 Contusion, laceration, and hemorrhage of brainstem with loss of consciousness of unspecified duration [HCC] [ESR]

S06.4 Epidural hemorrhage
  Extradural hemorrhage (traumatic)
  Extradural hemorrhage NOS
  DEF: Epidural space: Space between the endosteum of the cranium (skull) and the dura mater, the outermost layer of a three-layer membrane that covers the brain.

S06.4X Epidural hemorrhage

S06.4X0 Epidural hemorrhage without loss of consciousness [HCC] [ESR]

S06.4X1 Epidural hemorrhage with loss of consciousness of 30 minutes or less [HCC] [ESR]
  Epidural hemorrhage with brief loss of consciousness

S06.4X2 Epidural hemorrhage with loss of consciousness of 31 minutes to 59 minutes [HCC] [ESR]

S06.4X3 Epidural hemorrhage with loss of consciousness of 1 hour to 5 hours 59 minutes [HCC] [ESR] [COM]

S06.4X4 Epidural hemorrhage with loss of consciousness of 6 hours to 24 hours [HCC] [ESR] [COM]

S06.4X5 Epidural hemorrhage with loss of consciousness greater than 24 hours with return to pre-existing conscious level [HCC] [ESR] [COM]

- **S06.4X6** Epidural hemorrhage with loss of consciousness greater than 24 hours without return to pre-existing conscious level with patient surviving HCC ESR COM
- **S06.4X7** Epidural hemorrhage with loss of consciousness of any duration with death due to brain injury prior to regaining consciousness
- **S06.4X8** Epidural hemorrhage with loss of consciousness of any duration with death due to other causes prior to regaining consciousness
- **S06.4XA** Epidural hemorrhage with loss of consciousness status unknown HCC ESR
  - Epidural hemorrhage NOS
- **S06.4X9** Epidural hemorrhage with loss of consciousness of unspecified duration HCC ESR

S06.5 Traumatic subdural hemorrhage
Use additional code, if applicable, for traumatic brain compression or herniation (S06.A-)
AHA: 2021,2Q,5; 2021,1Q,4
DEF: Subdural: Potential space between the dura mater and arachnoid membrane around the brain.

- **S06.5X** Traumatic subdural hemorrhage
  - **S06.5X0** Traumatic subdural hemorrhage without loss of consciousness HCC ESR
  - **S06.5X1** Traumatic subdural hemorrhage with loss of consciousness of 30 minutes or less HCC ESR
    - Traumatic subdural hemorrhage with brief loss of consciousness
  - **S06.5X2** Traumatic subdural hemorrhage with loss of consciousness of 31 minutes to 59 minutes HCC ESR
  - **S06.5X3** Traumatic subdural hemorrhage with loss of consciousness of 1 hour to 5 hours 59 minutes HCC ESR
  - **S06.5X4** Traumatic subdural hemorrhage with loss of consciousness of 6 hours to 24 hours HCC ESR COM
  - **S06.5X5** Traumatic subdural hemorrhage with loss of consciousness greater than 24 hours with return to pre-existing conscious level HCC ESR COM
  - **S06.5X6** Traumatic subdural hemorrhage with loss of consciousness greater than 24 hours without return to pre-existing conscious level with patient surviving HCC ESR COM
  - **S06.5X7** Traumatic subdural hemorrhage with loss of consciousness of any duration with death due to brain injury before regaining consciousness
  - **S06.5X8** Traumatic subdural hemorrhage with loss of consciousness of any duration with death due to other cause before regaining consciousness
  - **S06.5XA** Traumatic subdural hemorrhage with loss of consciousness status unknown HCC ESR
    - Traumatic subdural hemorrhage NOS
    - **AHA:** 2022,4Q,44
  - **S06.5X9** Traumatic subdural hemorrhage with loss of consciousness of unspecified duration HCC ESR

S06.6 Traumatic subarachnoid hemorrhage
Use additional code, if applicable, for traumatic brain compression or herniation (S06.A-)
AHA: 2021,2Q,5; 2021,1Q,4
DEF: Subarachnoid: Space located between the arachnoid membrane and the pia mater that contains cerebrospinal fluid.

- **S06.6X** Traumatic subarachnoid hemorrhage
  - **S06.6X0** Traumatic subarachnoid hemorrhage without loss of consciousness HCC ESR
  - **S06.6X1** Traumatic subarachnoid hemorrhage with loss of consciousness of 30 minutes or less HCC ESR
    - Traumatic subarachnoid hemorrhage with brief loss of consciousness
  - **S06.6X2** Traumatic subarachnoid hemorrhage with loss of consciousness of 31 minutes to 59 minutes HCC ESR
  - **S06.6X3** Traumatic subarachnoid hemorrhage with loss of consciousness of 1 hour to 5 hours 59 minutes HCC ESR COM
  - **S06.6X4** Traumatic subarachnoid hemorrhage with loss of consciousness of 6 hours to 24 hours HCC ESR COM
  - **S06.6X5** Traumatic subarachnoid hemorrhage with loss of consciousness greater than 24 hours with return to pre-existing conscious level HCC ESR COM
  - **S06.6X6** Traumatic subarachnoid hemorrhage with loss of consciousness greater than 24 hours without return to pre-existing conscious level with patient surviving HCC ESR COM
  - **S06.6X7** Traumatic subarachnoid hemorrhage with loss of consciousness of any duration with death due to brain injury prior to regaining consciousness
  - **S06.6X8** Traumatic subarachnoid hemorrhage with loss of consciousness of any duration with death due to other cause prior to regaining consciousness
  - **S06.6XA** Traumatic subarachnoid hemorrhage with loss of consciousness status unknown HCC ESR
    - Traumatic subarachnoid hemorrhage NOS
    - **AHA:** 2022,4Q,44
  - **S06.6X9** Traumatic subarachnoid hemorrhage with loss of consciousness of unspecified duration HCC ESR

S06.8 Other specified intracranial injuries
- **S06.81** Injury of right internal carotid artery, intracranial portion, not elsewhere classified
  - **S06.810** Injury of right internal carotid artery, intracranial portion, not elsewhere classified without loss of consciousness
  - **S06.811** Injury of right internal carotid artery, intracranial portion, not elsewhere classified with loss of consciousness of 30 minutes or less HCC ESR
    - Injury of right internal carotid artery, intracranial portion, not elsewhere classified with brief loss of consciousness
  - **S06.812** Injury of right internal carotid artery, intracranial portion, not elsewhere classified with loss of consciousness of 31 minutes to 59 minutes HCC ESR
  - **S06.813** Injury of right internal carotid artery, intracranial portion, not elsewhere classified with loss of consciousness of 1 hour to 5 hours 59 minutes HCC ESR COM
  - **S06.814** Injury of right internal carotid artery, intracranial portion, not elsewhere classified with loss of consciousness of 6 hours to 24 hours HCC ESR COM
  - **S06.815** Injury of right internal carotid artery, intracranial portion, not elsewhere classified with loss of consciousness greater than 24 hours with return to pre-existing conscious level HCC ESR
  - **S06.816** Injury of right internal carotid artery, intracranial portion, not elsewhere classified with loss of consciousness greater than 24 hours without return to pre-existing conscious level with patient surviving HCC ESR COM
  - **S06.817** Injury of right internal carotid artery, intracranial portion, not elsewhere classified with loss of consciousness of any duration with death due to brain injury prior to regaining consciousness
  - **S06.818** Injury of right internal carotid artery, intracranial portion, not elsewhere classified with loss of consciousness of any duration with death due to other cause prior to regaining consciousness

S06.81A Injury of right internal carotid artery, intracranial portion, not elsewhere classified with loss of consciousness status unknown
Injury of right internal carotid artery, intracranial portion, not elsewhere classified NOS

S06.819 Injury of right internal carotid artery, intracranial portion, not elsewhere classified with loss of consciousness of unspecified duration

S06.82 Injury of left internal carotid artery, intracranial portion, not elsewhere classified

S06.820 Injury of left internal carotid artery, intracranial portion, not elsewhere classified without loss of consciousness

S06.821 Injury of left internal carotid artery, intracranial portion, not elsewhere classified with loss of consciousness of 30 minutes or less
Injury of left internal carotid artery, intracranial portion, not elsewhere classified with brief loss of consciousness

S06.822 Injury of left internal carotid artery, intracranial portion, not elsewhere classified with loss of consciousness of 31 minutes to 59 minutes

S06.823 Injury of left internal carotid artery, intracranial portion, not elsewhere classified with loss of consciousness of 1 hour to 5 hours 59 minutes

S06.824 Injury of left internal carotid artery, intracranial portion, not elsewhere classified with loss of consciousness of 6 hours to 24 hours

S06.825 Injury of left internal carotid artery, intracranial portion, not elsewhere classified with loss of consciousness greater than 24 hours with return to pre-existing conscious level

S06.826 Injury of left internal carotid artery, intracranial portion, not elsewhere classified with loss of consciousness greater than 24 hours without return to pre-existing conscious level with patient surviving

S06.827 Injury of left internal carotid artery, intracranial portion, not elsewhere classified with loss of consciousness of any duration with death due to brain injury prior to regaining consciousness

S06.828 Injury of left internal carotid artery, intracranial portion, not elsewhere classified with loss of consciousness of any duration with death due to other cause prior to regaining consciousness

S06.82A Injury of left internal carotid artery, intracranial portion, not elsewhere classified with loss of consciousness status unknown
Injury of left internal carotid artery, intracranial portion, not elsewhere classified NOS

S06.829 Injury of left internal carotid artery, intracranial portion, not elsewhere classified with loss of consciousness of unspecified duration

S06.8A Primary blast injury of brain, not elsewhere classified
Code also, if applicable, focal traumatic brain injury (S06.3-)
EXCLUDES 2 traumatic cerebral edema (S06.1)

S06.8A0 Primary blast injury of brain, not elsewhere classified without loss of consciousness

S06.8A1 Primary blast injury of brain, not elsewhere classified with loss of consciousness of 30 minutes or less
Primary blast injury of brain, not elsewhere classified with brief loss of consciousness

S06.8A2 Primary blast injury of brain, not elsewhere classified with loss of consciousness of 31 minutes to 59 minutes

S06.8A3 Primary blast injury of brain, not elsewhere classified with loss of consciousness of 1 hour to 5 hours 59 minutes

S06.8A4 Primary blast injury of brain, not elsewhere classified with loss of consciousness of 6 hours to 24 hours

S06.8A5 Primary blast injury of brain, not elsewhere classified with loss of consciousness greater than 24 hours with return to pre-existing conscious level

S06.8A6 Primary blast injury of brain, not elsewhere classified with loss of consciousness greater than 24 hours without return to pre-existing conscious level with patient surviving

S06.8A7 Primary blast injury of brain, not elsewhere classified with loss of consciousness of any duration with death due to brain injury prior to regaining consciousness

S06.8A8 Primary blast injury of brain, not elsewhere classified with loss of consciousness of any duration with death due to other cause prior to regaining consciousness

S06.8AA Primary blast injury of brain, not elsewhere classified with loss of consciousness status unknown
Primary blast injury of brain NOS

S06.8A9 Primary blast injury of brain, not elsewhere classified with loss of consciousness of unspecified duration

S06.89 Other specified intracranial injury
EXCLUDES 1 concussion (S06.0X-)
AHA: 2024,2Q,15

S06.890 Other specified intracranial injury without loss of consciousness

S06.891 Other specified intracranial injury with loss of consciousness of 30 minutes or less
Other specified intracranial injury with brief loss of consciousness

S06.892 Other specified intracranial injury with loss of consciousness of 31 minutes to 59 minutes

S06.893 Other specified intracranial injury with loss of consciousness of 1 hour to 5 hours 59 minutes

S06.894 Other specified intracranial injury with loss of consciousness of 6 hours to 24 hours

S06.895 Other specified intracranial injury with loss of consciousness greater than 24 hours with return to pre-existing conscious level

S06.896 Other specified intracranial injury with loss of consciousness greater than 24 hours without return to pre-existing conscious level with patient surviving

S06.897 Other specified intracranial injury with loss of consciousness of any duration with death due to brain injury prior to regaining consciousness

S06.898 Other specified intracranial injury with loss of consciousness of any duration with death due to other cause prior to regaining consciousness

S06.89A Other specified intracranial injury with loss of consciousness status unknown

S06.899 Other specified intracranial injury with loss of consciousness of unspecified duration

Chapter 19. Injury, Poisoning and Certain Other Consequences of External Causes

S06.9 Unspecified intracranial injury
Brain injury NOS
Head injury NOS with loss of consciousness
Traumatic brain injury NOS
EXCLUDES 1 conditions classifiable to S06.0- to S06.8- code to specified intracranial injury
head injury NOS (S09.90)
AHA: 2020,3Q,46; 2020,2Q,31

- **S06.9X Unspecified intracranial injury**
  - **S06.9X0** Unspecified intracranial injury without loss of consciousness
  - **S06.9X1** Unspecified intracranial injury with loss of consciousness of 30 minutes or less
    Unspecified intracranial injury with brief loss of consciousness
  - **S06.9X2** Unspecified intracranial injury with loss of consciousness of 31 minutes to 59 minutes
  - **S06.9X3** Unspecified intracranial injury with loss of consciousness of 1 hour to 5 hours 59 minutes
  - **S06.9X4** Unspecified intracranial injury with loss of consciousness of 6 hours to 24 hours
  - **S06.9X5** Unspecified intracranial injury with loss of consciousness greater than 24 hours with return to pre-existing conscious level
  - **S06.9X6** Unspecified intracranial injury with loss of consciousness greater than 24 hours without return to pre-existing conscious level with patient surviving
  - **S06.9X7** Unspecified intracranial injury with loss of consciousness of any duration with death due to brain injury prior to regaining consciousness
  - **S06.9X8** Unspecified intracranial injury with loss of consciousness of any duration with death due to other cause prior to regaining consciousness
  - **S06.9XA** Unspecified intracranial injury with loss of consciousness status unknown
  - **S06.9X9** Unspecified intracranial injury with loss of consciousness of unspecified duration

S06.A Traumatic brain compression and herniation
Traumatic cerebral compression
Code first the underlying traumatic brain injury, such as:
  diffuse traumatic brain injury (S06.2-)
  focal traumatic brain injury (S06.3-)
  traumatic subarachnoid hemorrhage (S06.6-)
  traumatic subdural hemorrhage (S06.5-)
AHA: 2021,4Q,29

- **S06.A0 Traumatic brain compression without herniation**
  Traumatic brain compression NOS
  Traumatic cerebral compression NOS
- **S06.A1 Traumatic brain compression with herniation**
  Traumatic brain herniation
  Traumatic brainstem compression with herniation
  Traumatic cerebellar compression with herniation
  Traumatic cerebral compression with herniation

S07 Crushing injury of head
Use additional code for all associated injuries, such as:
  intracranial injuries (S06.-)
  skull fractures (S02.-)

The appropriate 7th character is to be added to each code from category S07.
- A initial encounter
- D subsequent encounter
- S sequela

- **S07.0** Crushing injury of face
- **S07.1** Crushing injury of skull
- **S07.8** Crushing injury of other parts of head
- **S07.9** Crushing injury of head, part unspecified

S08 Avulsion and traumatic amputation of part of head
An amputation not identified as partial or complete should be coded to complete

The appropriate 7th character is to be added to each code from category S08.
- A initial encounter
- D subsequent encounter
- S sequela

- **S08.0** Avulsion of scalp
- **S08.1 Traumatic amputation of ear**
  - **S08.11 Complete traumatic amputation of ear**
    - **S08.111** Complete traumatic amputation of right ear
    - **S08.112** Complete traumatic amputation of left ear
    - **S08.119** Complete traumatic amputation of unspecified ear
  - **S08.12 Partial traumatic amputation of ear**
    - **S08.121** Partial traumatic amputation of right ear
    - **S08.122** Partial traumatic amputation of left ear
    - **S08.129** Partial traumatic amputation of unspecified ear
- **S08.8 Traumatic amputation of other parts of head**
  - **S08.81 Traumatic amputation of nose**
    - **S08.811** Complete traumatic amputation of nose
    - **S08.812** Partial traumatic amputation of nose
  - **S08.89** Traumatic amputation of other parts of head

S09 Other and unspecified injuries of head

The appropriate 7th character is to be added to each code from category S09.
- A initial encounter
- D subsequent encounter
- S sequela

- **S09.0** Injury of blood vessels of head, not elsewhere classified
  EXCLUDES 1 injury of cerebral blood vessels (S06.-)
  injury of precerebral blood vessels (S15.-)
- **S09.1 Injury of muscle and tendon of head**
  Code also any associated open wound (S01.-)
  EXCLUDES 2 sprain to joints and ligament of head (S03.9)
  - **S09.10** Unspecified injury of muscle and tendon of head
    Injury of muscle and tendon of head NOS
  - **S09.11** Strain of muscle and tendon of head
  - **S09.12** Laceration of muscle and tendon of head
  - **S09.19** Other specified injury of muscle and tendon of head
- **S09.2 Traumatic rupture of ear drum**
  EXCLUDES 1 traumatic rupture of ear drum due to blast injury (S09.31-)
  - **S09.20** Traumatic rupture of unspecified ear drum
  - **S09.21** Traumatic rupture of right ear drum
  - **S09.22** Traumatic rupture of left ear drum
- **S09.3 Other specified and unspecified injury of middle and inner ear**
  EXCLUDES 1 injury to ear NOS (S09.91-)
  EXCLUDES 2 injury to external ear (S00.4-, S01.3-, S08.1-)
  - **S09.30 Unspecified injury of middle and inner ear**
    - **S09.301** Unspecified injury of right middle and inner ear
    - **S09.302** Unspecified injury of left middle and inner ear
    - **S09.309** Unspecified injury of unspecified middle and inner ear
  - **S09.31 Primary blast injury of ear**
    Blast injury of ear NOS
    - **S09.311** Primary blast injury of right ear
    - **S09.312** Primary blast injury of left ear
    - **S09.313** Primary blast injury of ear, bilateral
    - **S09.319** Primary blast injury of unspecified ear
  - **S09.39 Other specified injury of middle and inner ear**
    Secondary blast injury to ear
    - **S09.391** Other specified injury of right middle and inner ear
    - **S09.392** Other specified injury of left middle and inner ear

| HCC CMS-HCC | Rx Rx HCC | ESR ESRD HCC | COM Commercial HCC | N Newborn: 0 | P Pediatric: 0-17 | M Maternity: 9-64 | A Adult: 15-124 |

Chapter 19. Injury, Poisoning and Certain Other Consequences of External Causes

- ✓7th **S09.399** Other specified injury of unspecified middle and inner ear
- ✓x7th **S09.8** Other specified injuries of head
- ✓5th **S09.9** Unspecified injury of face and head
  - ✓x7th **S09.90** Unspecified injury of head
    - Head injury NOS
    - EXCLUDES 1: brain injury NOS (S06.9-)
      head injury NOS with loss of consciousness (S06.9-)
      intracranial injury NOS (S06.9-)
  - ✓x7th **S09.91** Unspecified injury of ear
    - Injury of ear NOS
  - ✓x7th **S09.92** Unspecified injury of nose
    - Injury of nose NOS
  - ✓x7th **S09.93** Unspecified injury of face
    - Injury of face NOS
    - AHA: 2019,2Q,23

Injuries to the neck (S10-S19)

INCLUDES: injuries of nape
injuries of supraclavicular region
injuries of throat

EXCLUDES 2: burns and corrosions (T20-T32)
effects of foreign body in esophagus (T18.1)
effects of foreign body in larynx (T17.3)
effects of foreign body in pharynx (T17.2)
effects of foreign body in trachea (T17.4)
frostbite (T33-T34)
insect bite or sting, venomous (T63.4)

- ✓4th **S10** Superficial injury of neck

  The appropriate 7th character is to be added to each code from category S10.
  - A initial encounter
  - D subsequent encounter
  - S sequela

  - ✓x7th **S10.0** Contusion of throat
    - Contusion of cervical esophagus
    - Contusion of larynx
    - Contusion of pharynx
    - Contusion of trachea
  - ✓5th **S10.1** Other and unspecified superficial injuries of throat
    - ✓x7th **S10.10** Unspecified superficial injuries of throat
    - ✓x7th **S10.11** Abrasion of throat
    - ✓x7th **S10.12** Blister (nonthermal) of throat
    - ✓x7th **S10.14** External constriction of part of throat
    - ✓x7th **S10.15** Superficial foreign body of throat
      - Splinter in the throat
    - ✓x7th **S10.16** Insect bite (nonvenomous) of throat
    - ✓x7th **S10.17** Other superficial bite of throat
      - EXCLUDES 1: open bite of throat (S11.85)
  - ✓5th **S10.8** Superficial injury of other specified parts of neck
    - ✓x7th **S10.80** Unspecified superficial injury of other specified part of neck
    - ✓x7th **S10.81** Abrasion of other specified part of neck
    - ✓x7th **S10.82** Blister (nonthermal) of other specified part of neck
    - ✓x7th **S10.83** Contusion of other specified part of neck
    - ✓x7th **S10.84** External constriction of other specified part of neck
    - ✓x7th **S10.85** Superficial foreign body of other specified part of neck
      - Splinter in other specified part of neck
    - ✓x7th **S10.86** Insect bite of other specified part of neck
    - ✓x7th **S10.87** Other superficial bite of other specified part of neck
      - EXCLUDES 1: open bite of other specified parts of neck (S11.85)
  - ✓5th **S10.9** Superficial injury of unspecified part of neck
    - ✓x7th **S10.90** Unspecified superficial injury of unspecified part of neck
    - ✓x7th **S10.91** Abrasion of unspecified part of neck
    - ✓x7th **S10.92** Blister (nonthermal) of unspecified part of neck
    - ✓x7th **S10.93** Contusion of unspecified part of neck
    - ✓x7th **S10.94** External constriction of unspecified part of neck
    - ✓x7th **S10.95** Superficial foreign body of unspecified part of neck
    - ✓x7th **S10.96** Insect bite of unspecified part of neck
  - ✓x7th **S10.97** Other superficial bite of unspecified part of neck

- ✓4th **S11** Open wound of neck

  Code also any associated:
  spinal cord injury (S14.0, S14.1-)
  wound infection

  EXCLUDES 2: open fracture of vertebra (S12.- with 7th character B)

  The appropriate 7th character is to be added to each code from category S11.
  - A initial encounter
  - D subsequent encounter
  - S sequela

  - ✓5th **S11.0** Open wound of larynx and trachea
    - ✓6th **S11.01** Open wound of larynx
      - EXCLUDES 2: open wound of vocal cord (S11.03)
      - ✓7th **S11.011** Laceration without foreign body of larynx
      - ✓7th **S11.012** Laceration with foreign body of larynx
      - ✓7th **S11.013** Puncture wound without foreign body of larynx
      - ✓7th **S11.014** Puncture wound with foreign body of larynx
      - ✓7th **S11.015** Open bite of larynx
        - Bite of larynx NOS
      - ✓7th **S11.019** Unspecified open wound of larynx
    - ✓6th **S11.02** Open wound of trachea
      - Open wound of cervical trachea
      - Open wound of trachea NOS
      - EXCLUDES 2: open wound of thoracic trachea (S27.5-)
      - ✓7th **S11.021** Laceration without foreign body of trachea
      - ✓7th **S11.022** Laceration with foreign body of trachea
      - ✓7th **S11.023** Puncture wound without foreign body of trachea
      - ✓7th **S11.024** Puncture wound with foreign body of trachea
      - ✓7th **S11.025** Open bite of trachea
        - Bite of trachea NOS
      - ✓7th **S11.029** Unspecified open wound of trachea
    - ✓6th **S11.03** Open wound of vocal cord
      - ✓7th **S11.031** Laceration without foreign body of vocal cord
      - ✓7th **S11.032** Laceration with foreign body of vocal cord
      - ✓7th **S11.033** Puncture wound without foreign body of vocal cord
      - ✓7th **S11.034** Puncture wound with foreign body of vocal cord
      - ✓7th **S11.035** Open bite of vocal cord
        - Bite of vocal cord NOS
      - ✓7th **S11.039** Unspecified open wound of vocal cord
  - ✓5th **S11.1** Open wound of thyroid gland
    - ✓x7th **S11.10** Unspecified open wound of thyroid gland
    - ✓x7th **S11.11** Laceration without foreign body of thyroid gland
    - ✓x7th **S11.12** Laceration with foreign body of thyroid gland
    - ✓x7th **S11.13** Puncture wound without foreign body of thyroid gland
    - ✓x7th **S11.14** Puncture wound with foreign body of thyroid gland
    - ✓x7th **S11.15** Open bite of thyroid gland
      - Bite of thyroid gland NOS
  - ✓5th **S11.2** Open wound of pharynx and cervical esophagus
    - EXCLUDES 1: open wound of esophagus NOS (S27.8-)
    - ✓x7th **S11.20** Unspecified open wound of pharynx and cervical esophagus
    - ✓x7th **S11.21** Laceration without foreign body of pharynx and cervical esophagus
    - ✓x7th **S11.22** Laceration with foreign body of pharynx and cervical esophagus
    - ✓x7th **S11.23** Puncture wound without foreign body of pharynx and cervical esophagus
    - ✓x7th **S11.24** Puncture wound with foreign body of pharynx and cervical esophagus
    - ✓x7th **S11.25** Open bite of pharynx and cervical esophagus
      - Bite of pharynx and cervical esophagus NOS
  - ✓5th **S11.8** Open wound of other specified parts of neck
    - ✓x7th **S11.80** Unspecified open wound of other specified part of neck
    - ✓x7th **S11.81** Laceration without foreign body of other specified part of neck

---

✓ Additional Character Required | ✓x7th Placeholder Alert | Manifestation | Unspecified Dx | Q QPP | UPD Unacceptable PDx

Chapter 19. Injury, Poisoning and Certain Other Consequences of External Causes

- S11.82 **Laceration with foreign body** of other specified part of neck
- S11.83 **Puncture wound without foreign body** of other specified part of neck
- S11.84 **Puncture wound with foreign body** of other specified part of neck
- S11.85 **Open bite** of other specified part of neck
  - Bite of other specified part of neck NOS
  - EXCLUDES 1: superficial bite of other specified part of neck (S10.87)
- S11.89 Other open wound of other specified part of neck
- **S11.9 Open wound of unspecified part of neck**
  - S11.90 Unspecified open wound of unspecified part of neck
  - S11.91 **Laceration without foreign body** of unspecified part of neck
  - S11.92 **Laceration with foreign body** of unspecified part of neck
  - S11.93 **Puncture wound without foreign body** of unspecified part of neck
  - S11.94 **Puncture wound with foreign body** of unspecified part of neck
  - S11.95 **Open bite** of unspecified part of neck
    - Bite of neck NOS
    - EXCLUDES 1: superficial bite of neck (S10.97)

S12 Fracture of cervical vertebra and other parts of neck

NOTE: A fracture not indicated as displaced or nondisplaced should be coded to displaced.

A fracture not indicated as open or closed should be coded to closed.

INCLUDES:
- fracture of cervical neural arch
- fracture of cervical spine
- fracture of cervical spinous process
- fracture of cervical transverse process
- fracture of cervical vertebral arch
- fracture of neck

Code first any associated cervical spinal cord injury (S14.0, S14.1-)
AHA: 2024,2Q,23; 2021,1Q,6; 2018,2Q,12; 2015,3Q,37-39

The appropriate 7th character is to be added to all codes from subcategories S12.0-S12.6.
- A initial encounter for closed fracture
- B initial encounter for open fracture
- D subsequent encounter for fracture with routine healing
- G subsequent encounter for fracture with delayed healing
- K subsequent encounter for fracture with nonunion
- S sequela

- **S12.0 Fracture of first cervical vertebra**
  - Atlas
  - S12.00 Unspecified fracture of first cervical vertebra
    - S12.000 Unspecified **displaced** fracture of first cervical vertebra
    - S12.001 Unspecified **nondisplaced** fracture of first cervical vertebra
  - S12.01 **Stable burst** fracture of first cervical vertebra
  - S12.02 **Unstable burst** fracture of first cervical vertebra
  - S12.03 **Posterior arch** fracture of first cervical vertebra
    - S12.030 **Displaced** posterior arch fracture of first cervical vertebra
    - S12.031 **Nondisplaced** posterior arch fracture of first cervical vertebra
  - S12.04 **Lateral mass** fracture of first cervical vertebra
    - S12.040 **Displaced** lateral mass fracture of first cervical vertebra
    - S12.041 **Nondisplaced** lateral mass fracture of first cervical vertebra
  - S12.09 Other fracture of first cervical vertebra
    - S12.090 Other **displaced** fracture of first cervical vertebra
    - S12.091 Other **nondisplaced** fracture of first cervical vertebra
- **S12.1 Fracture of second cervical vertebra**
  - Axis
  - S12.10 Unspecified fracture of second cervical vertebra
    - S12.100 Unspecified **displaced** fracture of second cervical vertebra
    - S12.101 Unspecified **nondisplaced** fracture of second cervical vertebra
  - S12.11 **Type II dens** fracture
    - S12.110 **Anterior displaced** Type II dens fracture
    - S12.111 **Posterior displaced** Type II dens fracture
    - S12.112 **Nondisplaced** Type II dens fracture
  - S12.12 Other dens fracture
    - S12.120 Other **displaced** dens fracture
    - S12.121 Other **nondisplaced** dens fracture
  - S12.13 Unspecified traumatic **spondylolisthesis** of second cervical vertebra
    - S12.130 Unspecified traumatic **displaced** spondylolisthesis of second cervical vertebra
    - S12.131 Unspecified traumatic **nondisplaced** spondylolisthesis of second cervical vertebra
  - S12.14 **Type III** traumatic **spondylolisthesis** of second cervical vertebra
  - S12.15 Other traumatic **spondylolisthesis** of second cervical vertebra
    - S12.150 Other traumatic **displaced** spondylolisthesis of second cervical vertebra
    - S12.151 Other traumatic **nondisplaced** spondylolisthesis of second cervical vertebra
  - S12.19 Other fracture of second cervical vertebra
    - S12.190 Other **displaced** fracture of second cervical vertebra
    - S12.191 Other **nondisplaced** fracture of second cervical vertebra
- **S12.2 Fracture of third cervical vertebra**
  - S12.20 Unspecified fracture of third cervical vertebra
    - S12.200 Unspecified **displaced** fracture of third cervical vertebra
    - S12.201 Unspecified **nondisplaced** fracture of third cervical vertebra
  - S12.23 Unspecified traumatic **spondylolisthesis** of third cervical vertebra
    - S12.230 Unspecified traumatic **displaced** spondylolisthesis of third cervical vertebra
    - S12.231 Unspecified traumatic **nondisplaced** spondylolisthesis of third cervical vertebra
  - S12.24 **Type III** traumatic **spondylolisthesis** of third cervical vertebra
  - S12.25 Other traumatic spondylolisthesis of third cervical vertebra
    - S12.250 Other traumatic **displaced** spondylolisthesis of third cervical vertebra
    - S12.251 Other traumatic **nondisplaced** spondylolisthesis of third cervical vertebra
  - S12.29 Other fracture of third cervical vertebra
    - S12.290 Other **displaced** fracture of third cervical vertebra
    - S12.291 Other **nondisplaced** fracture of third cervical vertebra
- **S12.3 Fracture of fourth cervical vertebra**
  - S12.30 Unspecified fracture of fourth cervical vertebra
    - S12.300 Unspecified **displaced** fracture of fourth cervical vertebra
    - S12.301 Unspecified **nondisplaced** fracture of fourth cervical vertebra
  - S12.33 Unspecified traumatic **spondylolisthesis** of fourth cervical vertebra
    - S12.330 Unspecified traumatic **displaced** spondylolisthesis of fourth cervical vertebra

Chapter 19. Injury, Poisoning and Certain Other Consequences of External Causes

- ✓7th **S12.331** Unspecified traumatic nondisplaced spondylolisthesis of fourth cervical vertebra `HCC` `ESR` `COM` `Q`
- ✓x 7th **S12.34** Type III traumatic spondylolisthesis of fourth cervical vertebra `HCC` `ESR` `COM` `Q`
- ✓6th **S12.35** Other traumatic spondylolisthesis of fourth cervical vertebra
  - ✓7th **S12.350** Other traumatic displaced spondylolisthesis of fourth cervical vertebra `HCC` `ESR` `COM` `Q`
  - ✓7th **S12.351** Other traumatic nondisplaced spondylolisthesis of fourth cervical vertebra `HCC` `ESR` `COM` `Q`
- ✓6th **S12.39** Other fracture of fourth cervical vertebra
  - ✓7th **S12.390** Other displaced fracture of fourth cervical vertebra `HCC` `ESR` `COM` `Q`
  - ✓7th **S12.391** Other nondisplaced fracture of fourth cervical vertebra `HCC` `ESR` `COM` `Q`
- ✓5th **S12.4** Fracture of fifth cervical vertebra
  - **S12.40** Unspecified fracture of fifth cervical vertebra
    - ✓7th **S12.400** Unspecified displaced fracture of fifth cervical vertebra `HCC` `ESR` `COM` `Q`
    - ✓7th **S12.401** Unspecified nondisplaced fracture of fifth cervical vertebra `HCC` `ESR` `COM` `Q`
  - ✓6th **S12.43** Unspecified traumatic spondylolisthesis of fifth cervical vertebra
    - ✓7th **S12.430** Unspecified traumatic displaced spondylolisthesis of fifth cervical vertebra `HCC` `ESR` `COM` `Q`
    - ✓7th **S12.431** Unspecified traumatic nondisplaced spondylolisthesis of fifth cervical vertebra `HCC` `ESR` `COM` `Q`
  - ✓x 7th **S12.44** Type III traumatic spondylolisthesis of fifth cervical vertebra `HCC` `ESR` `COM` `Q`
  - ✓6th **S12.45** Other traumatic spondylolisthesis of fifth cervical vertebra
    - ✓7th **S12.450** Other traumatic displaced spondylolisthesis of fifth cervical vertebra `HCC` `ESR` `COM` `Q`
    - ✓7th **S12.451** Other traumatic nondisplaced spondylolisthesis of fifth cervical vertebra `HCC` `ESR` `COM` `Q`
  - ✓6th **S12.49** Other fracture of fifth cervical vertebra
    - ✓7th **S12.490** Other displaced fracture of fifth cervical vertebra `HCC` `ESR` `COM` `Q`
    - ✓7th **S12.491** Other nondisplaced fracture of fifth cervical vertebra `HCC` `ESR` `COM` `Q`
- ✓5th **S12.5** Fracture of sixth cervical vertebra
  - ✓6th **S12.50** Unspecified fracture of sixth cervical vertebra
    - ✓7th **S12.500** Unspecified displaced fracture of sixth cervical vertebra `HCC` `ESR` `COM` `Q`
    - ✓7th **S12.501** Unspecified nondisplaced fracture of sixth cervical vertebra `HCC` `ESR` `COM` `Q`
  - ✓6th **S12.53** Unspecified traumatic spondylolisthesis of sixth cervical vertebra
    - ✓7th **S12.530** Unspecified traumatic displaced spondylolisthesis of sixth cervical vertebra `HCC` `ESR` `COM` `Q`
    - ✓7th **S12.531** Unspecified traumatic nondisplaced spondylolisthesis of sixth cervical vertebra `HCC` `ESR` `COM` `Q`
  - ✓x 7th **S12.54** Type III traumatic spondylolisthesis of sixth cervical vertebra `HCC` `ESR` `COM` `Q`
  - ✓6th **S12.55** Other traumatic spondylolisthesis of sixth cervical vertebra
    - ✓7th **S12.550** Other traumatic displaced spondylolisthesis of sixth cervical vertebra `HCC` `ESR` `COM` `Q`
    - ✓7th **S12.551** Other traumatic nondisplaced spondylolisthesis of sixth cervical vertebra `HCC` `ESR` `COM` `Q`
  - ✓6th **S12.59** Other fracture of sixth cervical vertebra
    - ✓7th **S12.590** Other displaced fracture of sixth cervical vertebra `HCC` `ESR` `COM` `Q`
    - ✓7th **S12.591** Other nondisplaced fracture of sixth cervical vertebra `HCC` `ESR` `COM` `Q`
- ✓5th **S12.6** Fracture of seventh cervical vertebra
  - ✓6th **S12.60** Unspecified fracture of seventh cervical vertebra
    - ✓7th **S12.600** Unspecified displaced fracture of seventh cervical vertebra `HCC` `ESR` `COM` `Q`
    - ✓7th **S12.601** Unspecified nondisplaced fracture of seventh cervical vertebra `HCC` `ESR` `COM` `Q`
  - ✓6th **S12.63** Unspecified traumatic spondylolisthesis of seventh cervical vertebra
    - ✓7th **S12.630** Unspecified traumatic displaced spondylolisthesis of seventh cervical vertebra `HCC` `ESR` `COM` `Q`
    - ✓7th **S12.631** Unspecified traumatic nondisplaced spondylolisthesis of seventh cervical vertebra `HCC` `ESR` `COM` `Q`
  - ✓x 7th **S12.64** Type III traumatic spondylolisthesis of seventh cervical vertebra `HCC` `ESR` `COM` `Q`
  - ✓6th **S12.65** Other traumatic spondylolisthesis of seventh cervical vertebra
    - ✓7th **S12.650** Other traumatic displaced spondylolisthesis of seventh cervical vertebra `HCC` `ESR` `COM` `Q`
    - ✓7th **S12.651** Other traumatic nondisplaced spondylolisthesis of seventh cervical vertebra `HCC` `ESR` `COM` `Q`
  - ✓6th **S12.69** Other fracture of seventh cervical vertebra
    - ✓7th **S12.690** Other displaced fracture of seventh cervical vertebra `HCC` `ESR` `COM` `Q`
    - ✓7th **S12.691** Other nondisplaced fracture of seventh cervical vertebra `HCC` `ESR` `COM` `Q`
- ✓x 7th **S12.8** Fracture of other parts of neck
  - ▶Fracture of hyoid bone◀
  - ▶Fracture of larynx◀
  - ▶Fracture of thyroid cartilage◀
  - ▶Fracture of trachea◀

  > The appropriate 7th character is to be added to code S12.8.
  > A   initial encounter
  > D   subsequent encounter
  > S   sequela

- ✓x 7th **S12.9** Fracture of neck, unspecified `HCC` `ESR` `COM` `Q`
  - Fracture of cervical spine NOS
  - Fracture of cervical vertebra NOS
  - Fracture of neck NOS

  > The appropriate 7th character is to be added to code S12.9.
  > A   initial encounter
  > D   subsequent encounter
  > S   sequela

- ✓4th **S13** Dislocation and sprain of joints and ligaments at neck level

  INCLUDES   avulsion of joint or ligament at neck level
  laceration of cartilage, joint or ligament at neck level
  sprain of cartilage, joint or ligament at neck level
  traumatic hemarthrosis of joint or ligament at neck level
  traumatic rupture of joint or ligament at neck level
  traumatic subluxation of joint or ligament at neck level
  traumatic tear of joint or ligament at neck level

  Code also any associated open wound
  EXCLUDES 2   strain of muscle or tendon at neck level (S16.1)

  > The appropriate 7th character is to be added to each code from category S13.
  > A   initial encounter
  > D   subsequent encounter
  > S   sequela

  - ✓x 7th **S13.0** Traumatic rupture of cervical intervertebral disc
    - **EXCLUDES 1**   rupture or displacement (nontraumatic) of cervical intervertebral disc NOS (M50.-)
  - ✓5th **S13.1** Subluxation and dislocation of cervical vertebrae
    - Code also any associated:
      - open wound of neck (S11.-)
      - spinal cord injury (S14.1-)
    - **EXCLUDES 2**   fracture of cervical vertebrae (S12.0-S12.3-)
    - ✓6th **S13.10** Subluxation and dislocation of unspecified cervical vertebrae
      - ✓7th **S13.100** Subluxation of unspecified cervical vertebrae
      - ✓7th **S13.101** Dislocation of unspecified cervical vertebrae

---

✓ Additional Character Required   ✓x 7th Placeholder Alert   Manifestation   Unspecified Dx   Q QPP   UPD Unacceptable PDx

S13.11 Subluxation and dislocation of C0/C1 cervical vertebrae
Subluxation and dislocation of atlantooccipital joint
Subluxation and dislocation of atloidooccipital joint
Subluxation and dislocation of occipitoatloid joint

- S13.110 Subluxation of C0/C1 cervical vertebrae
- S13.111 Dislocation of C0/C1 cervical vertebrae

S13.12 Subluxation and dislocation of C1/C2 cervical vertebrae
Subluxation and dislocation of atlantoaxial joint

- S13.120 Subluxation of C1/C2 cervical vertebrae
- S13.121 Dislocation of C1/C2 cervical vertebrae

S13.13 Subluxation and dislocation of C2/C3 cervical vertebrae
- S13.130 Subluxation of C2/C3 cervical vertebrae
- S13.131 Dislocation of C2/C3 cervical vertebrae

S13.14 Subluxation and dislocation of C3/C4 cervical vertebrae
- S13.140 Subluxation of C3/C4 cervical vertebrae
- S13.141 Dislocation of C3/C4 cervical vertebrae

S13.15 Subluxation and dislocation of C4/C5 cervical vertebrae
- S13.150 Subluxation of C4/C5 cervical vertebrae
- S13.151 Dislocation of C4/C5 cervical vertebrae

S13.16 Subluxation and dislocation of C5/C6 cervical vertebrae
- S13.160 Subluxation of C5/C6 cervical vertebrae
- S13.161 Dislocation of C5/C6 cervical vertebrae

S13.17 Subluxation and dislocation of C6/C7 cervical vertebrae
- S13.170 Subluxation of C6/C7 cervical vertebrae
- S13.171 Dislocation of C6/C7 cervical vertebrae

S13.18 Subluxation and dislocation of C7/T1 cervical vertebrae
- S13.180 Subluxation of C7/T1 cervical vertebrae
- S13.181 Dislocation of C7/T1 cervical vertebrae

S13.2 Dislocation of other and unspecified parts of neck
- S13.20 Dislocation of unspecified parts of neck
- S13.29 Dislocation of other parts of neck

S13.4 Sprain of ligaments of cervical spine
Sprain of anterior longitudinal (ligament), cervical
Sprain of atlanto-axial (joints)
Sprain of atlanto-occipital (joints)
Whiplash injury of cervical spine

S13.5 Sprain of thyroid region
Sprain of cricoarytenoid (joint) (ligament)
Sprain of cricothyroid (joint) (ligament)
Sprain of thyroid cartilage

S13.8 Sprain of joints and ligaments of other parts of neck

S13.9 Sprain of joints and ligaments of unspecified parts of neck

S14 Injury of nerves and spinal cord at neck level

NOTE Code to highest level of cervical cord injury

Code also any associated:
fracture of cervical vertebra (S12.0- — S12.6.-)
open wound of neck (S11.-)
transient paralysis (R29.5)

AHA: 2024,2Q,23

The appropriate 7th character is to be added to each code from category S14.
- A initial encounter
- D subsequent encounter
- S sequela

S14.0 Concussion and edema of cervical spinal cord

S14.1 Other and unspecified injuries of cervical spinal cord

S14.10 Unspecified injury of cervical spinal cord
- S14.101 Unspecified injury at C1 level of cervical spinal cord
- S14.102 Unspecified injury at C2 level of cervical spinal cord
- S14.103 Unspecified injury at C3 level of cervical spinal cord
- S14.104 Unspecified injury at C4 level of cervical spinal cord
- S14.105 Unspecified injury at C5 level of cervical spinal cord
- S14.106 Unspecified injury at C6 level of cervical spinal cord
- S14.107 Unspecified injury at C7 level of cervical spinal cord
- S14.108 Unspecified injury at C8 level of cervical spinal cord
- S14.109 Unspecified injury at unspecified level of cervical spinal cord
  Injury of cervical spinal cord NOS

S14.11 Complete lesion of cervical spinal cord
- S14.111 Complete lesion at C1 level of cervical spinal cord
- S14.112 Complete lesion at C2 level of cervical spinal cord
- S14.113 Complete lesion at C3 level of cervical spinal cord
- S14.114 Complete lesion at C4 level of cervical spinal cord
- S14.115 Complete lesion at C5 level of cervical spinal cord
- S14.116 Complete lesion at C6 level of cervical spinal cord
- S14.117 Complete lesion at C7 level of cervical spinal cord
- S14.118 Complete lesion at C8 level of cervical spinal cord
- S14.119 Complete lesion at unspecified level of cervical spinal cord

S14.12 Central cord syndrome of cervical spinal cord
- S14.121 Central cord syndrome at C1 level of cervical spinal cord
- S14.122 Central cord syndrome at C2 level of cervical spinal cord
- S14.123 Central cord syndrome at C3 level of cervical spinal cord
- S14.124 Central cord syndrome at C4 level of cervical spinal cord
- S14.125 Central cord syndrome at C5 level of cervical spinal cord
- S14.126 Central cord syndrome at C6 level of cervical spinal cord
- S14.127 Central cord syndrome at C7 level of cervical spinal cord
- S14.128 Central cord syndrome at C8 level of cervical spinal cord
- S14.129 Central cord syndrome at unspecified level of cervical spinal cord

S14.13 Anterior cord syndrome of cervical spinal cord
- S14.131 Anterior cord syndrome at C1 level of cervical spinal cord
- S14.132 Anterior cord syndrome at C2 level of cervical spinal cord
- S14.133 Anterior cord syndrome at C3 level of cervical spinal cord
- S14.134 Anterior cord syndrome at C4 level of cervical spinal cord
- S14.135 Anterior cord syndrome at C5 level of cervical spinal cord
- S14.136 Anterior cord syndrome at C6 level of cervical spinal cord
- S14.137 Anterior cord syndrome at C7 level of cervical spinal cord
- S14.138 Anterior cord syndrome at C8 level of cervical spinal cord
- S14.139 Anterior cord syndrome at unspecified level of cervical spinal cord

S14.14 Brown-Sequard syndrome of cervical spinal cord
- S14.141 Brown-Sequard syndrome at C1 level of cervical spinal cord
- S14.142 Brown-Sequard syndrome at C2 level of cervical spinal cord
- S14.143 Brown-Sequard syndrome at C3 level of cervical spinal cord
- S14.144 Brown-Sequard syndrome at C4 level of cervical spinal cord

Chapter 19. Injury, Poisoning and Certain Other Consequences of External Causes

- **S14.145** Brown-Sequard syndrome at C5 level of cervical spinal cord [HCC] [ESR] [COM]
- **S14.146** Brown-Sequard syndrome at C6 level of cervical spinal cord [HCC] [ESR] [COM]
- **S14.147** Brown-Sequard syndrome at C7 level of cervical spinal cord [HCC] [ESR] [COM]
- **S14.148** Brown-Sequard syndrome at C8 level of cervical spinal cord [HCC] [ESR] [COM]
- **S14.149** Brown-Sequard syndrome at unspecified level of cervical spinal cord [HCC] [ESR] [COM]

S14.15 Other incomplete lesions of cervical spinal cord
Incomplete lesion of cervical spinal cord NOS
Posterior cord syndrome of cervical spinal cord

- **S14.151** Other incomplete lesion at C1 level of cervical spinal cord [HCC] [ESR] [COM]
- **S14.152** Other incomplete lesion at C2 level of cervical spinal cord [HCC] [ESR] [COM]
- **S14.153** Other incomplete lesion at C3 level of cervical spinal cord [HCC] [ESR] [COM]
- **S14.154** Other incomplete lesion at C4 level of cervical spinal cord [HCC] [ESR] [COM]
- **S14.155** Other incomplete lesion at C5 level of cervical spinal cord [HCC] [ESR] [COM]
- **S14.156** Other incomplete lesion at C6 level of cervical spinal cord [HCC] [ESR] [COM]
- **S14.157** Other incomplete lesion at C7 level of cervical spinal cord [HCC] [ESR] [COM]
- **S14.158** Other incomplete lesion at C8 level of cervical spinal cord [HCC] [ESR] [COM]
- **S14.159** Other incomplete lesion at unspecified level of cervical spinal cord [HCC] [ESR] [COM]

S14.2 Injury of nerve root of cervical spine
S14.3 Injury of brachial plexus
S14.4 Injury of peripheral nerves of neck
S14.5 Injury of cervical sympathetic nerves
S14.8 Injury of other specified nerves of neck
S14.9 Injury of unspecified nerves of neck

S15 Injury of blood vessels at neck level
Code also any associated open wound (S11.-)

The appropriate 7th character is to be added to each code from category S15.
- A initial encounter
- D subsequent encounter
- S sequela

S15.0 Injury of carotid artery of neck
Injury of carotid artery (common) (external) (internal, extracranial portion)
Injury of carotid artery NOS

EXCLUDES 1 injury of internal carotid artery, intracranial portion (S06.8)

S15.00 Unspecified injury of carotid artery
- **S15.001** Unspecified injury of right carotid artery
- **S15.002** Unspecified injury of left carotid artery
- **S15.009** Unspecified injury of unspecified carotid artery

S15.01 Minor laceration of carotid artery
Incomplete transection of carotid artery
Laceration of carotid artery NOS
Superficial laceration of carotid artery
- **S15.011** Minor laceration of right carotid artery
- **S15.012** Minor laceration of left carotid artery
- **S15.019** Minor laceration of unspecified carotid artery

S15.02 Major laceration of carotid artery
Complete transection of carotid artery
Traumatic rupture of carotid artery
- **S15.021** Major laceration of right carotid artery
- **S15.022** Major laceration of left carotid artery
- **S15.029** Major laceration of unspecified carotid artery

S15.09 Other specified injury of carotid artery
- **S15.091** Other specified injury of right carotid artery
- **S15.092** Other specified injury of left carotid artery
- **S15.099** Other specified injury of unspecified carotid artery

S15.1 Injury of vertebral artery

S15.10 Unspecified injury of vertebral artery
- **S15.101** Unspecified injury of right vertebral artery
- **S15.102** Unspecified injury of left vertebral artery
- **S15.109** Unspecified injury of unspecified vertebral artery

S15.11 Minor laceration of vertebral artery
Incomplete transection of vertebral artery
Laceration of vertebral artery NOS
Superficial laceration of vertebral artery
- **S15.111** Minor laceration of right vertebral artery
- **S15.112** Minor laceration of left vertebral artery
- **S15.119** Minor laceration of unspecified vertebral artery

S15.12 Major laceration of vertebral artery
Complete transection of vertebral artery
Traumatic rupture of vertebral artery
- **S15.121** Major laceration of right vertebral artery
- **S15.122** Major laceration of left vertebral artery
- **S15.129** Major laceration of unspecified vertebral artery

S15.19 Other specified injury of vertebral artery
- **S15.191** Other specified injury of right vertebral artery
- **S15.192** Other specified injury of left vertebral artery
- **S15.199** Other specified injury of unspecified vertebral artery

S15.2 Injury of external jugular vein

S15.20 Unspecified injury of external jugular vein
- **S15.201** Unspecified injury of right external jugular vein
- **S15.202** Unspecified injury of left external jugular vein
- **S15.209** Unspecified injury of unspecified external jugular vein

S15.21 Minor laceration of external jugular vein
Incomplete transection of external jugular vein
Laceration of external jugular vein NOS
Superficial laceration of external jugular vein
- **S15.211** Minor laceration of right external jugular vein
- **S15.212** Minor laceration of left external jugular vein
- **S15.219** Minor laceration of unspecified external jugular vein

S15.22 Major laceration of external jugular vein
Complete transection of external jugular vein
Traumatic rupture of external jugular vein
- **S15.221** Major laceration of right external jugular vein
- **S15.222** Major laceration of left external jugular vein
- **S15.229** Major laceration of unspecified external jugular vein

S15.29 Other specified injury of external jugular vein
- **S15.291** Other specified injury of right external jugular vein
- **S15.292** Other specified injury of left external jugular vein
- **S15.299** Other specified injury of unspecified external jugular vein

S15.3 Injury of internal jugular vein

S15.30 Unspecified injury of internal jugular vein
- **S15.301** Unspecified injury of right internal jugular vein
- **S15.302** Unspecified injury of left internal jugular vein
- **S15.309** Unspecified injury of unspecified internal jugular vein

S15.31 Minor laceration of internal jugular vein
Incomplete transection of internal jugular vein
Laceration of internal jugular vein NOS
Superficial laceration of internal jugular vein
- **S15.311** Minor laceration of right internal jugular vein

- S15.312 Minor laceration of left internal jugular vein
- S15.319 Minor laceration of unspecified internal jugular vein
- S15.32 **Major laceration** of internal jugular vein
  - Complete transection of internal jugular vein
  - Traumatic rupture of internal jugular vein
  - S15.321 Major laceration of right internal jugular vein
  - S15.322 Major laceration of left internal jugular vein
  - S15.329 Major laceration of unspecified internal jugular vein
- S15.39 Other specified injury of internal jugular vein
  - S15.391 Other specified injury of right internal jugular vein
  - S15.392 Other specified injury of left internal jugular vein
  - S15.399 Other specified injury of unspecified internal jugular vein
- S15.8 Injury of other specified blood vessels at neck level
- S15.9 Injury of unspecified blood vessel at neck level

S16 Injury of muscle, fascia and tendon at neck level

Code also any associated open wound (S11.-)

EXCLUDES 2: sprain of joint or ligament at neck level (S13.9)

The appropriate 7th character is to be added to each code from category S16.
- A initial encounter
- D subsequent encounter
- S sequela

- S16.1 Strain of muscle, fascia and tendon at neck level
- S16.2 Laceration of muscle, fascia and tendon at neck level
- S16.8 Other specified injury of muscle, fascia and tendon at neck level
- S16.9 Unspecified injury of muscle, fascia and tendon at neck level

S17 Crushing injury of neck

Use additional code for all associated injuries, such as:
- injury of blood vessels (S15.-)
- open wound of neck (S11.-)
- spinal cord injury (S14.0, S14.1-)
- vertebral fracture (S12.0- — S12.3-)

The appropriate 7th character is to be added to each code from category S17.
- A initial encounter
- D subsequent encounter
- S sequela

- S17.0 Crushing injury of larynx and trachea
- S17.8 Crushing injury of other specified parts of neck
- S17.9 Crushing injury of neck, part unspecified

S19 Other specified and unspecified injuries of neck

The appropriate 7th character is to be added to each code from category S19.
- A initial encounter
- D subsequent encounter
- S sequela

- S19.8 Other specified injuries of neck
  - S19.80 Other specified injuries of unspecified part of neck
  - S19.81 Other specified injuries of larynx
  - S19.82 Other specified injuries of cervical trachea
    - EXCLUDES 2: other specified injury of thoracic trachea (S27.5-)
  - S19.83 Other specified injuries of vocal cord
  - S19.84 Other specified injuries of thyroid gland
  - S19.85 Other specified injuries of pharynx and cervical esophagus
    - AHA: 2022,1Q,27
  - S19.89 Other specified injuries of other specified part of neck
- S19.9 Unspecified injury of neck

Injuries to the thorax (S20-S29)

INCLUDES:
- injuries of breast
- injuries of chest (wall)
- injuries of interscapular area

EXCLUDES 2:
- burns and corrosions (T20-T32)
- effects of foreign body in bronchus (T17.5)
- effects of foreign body in esophagus (T18.1)
- effects of foreign body in lung (T17.8)
- effects of foreign body in trachea (T17.4)
- frostbite (T33-T34)
- injuries of axilla
- injuries of clavicle
- injuries of scapular region
- injuries of shoulder
- insect bite or sting, venomous (T63.4)

S20 Superficial injury of thorax

AHA: 2020,4Q,39

The appropriate 7th character is to be added to each code from category S20.
- A initial encounter
- D subsequent encounter
- S sequela

- S20.0 **Contusion** of breast
  - S20.00 Contusion of breast, unspecified breast
  - S20.01 Contusion of right breast
  - S20.02 Contusion of left breast
- S20.1 Other and unspecified superficial injuries of breast
  - S20.10 Unspecified superficial injuries of breast
    - S20.101 Unspecified superficial injuries of breast, right breast
    - S20.102 Unspecified superficial injuries of breast, left breast
    - S20.109 Unspecified superficial injuries of breast, unspecified breast
  - S20.11 **Abrasion** of breast
    - S20.111 Abrasion of breast, right breast
    - S20.112 Abrasion of breast, left breast
    - S20.119 Abrasion of breast, unspecified breast
  - S20.12 **Blister** (nonthermal) of breast
    - S20.121 Blister (nonthermal) of breast, right breast
    - S20.122 Blister (nonthermal) of breast, left breast
    - S20.129 Blister (nonthermal) of breast, unspecified breast
  - S20.14 **External constriction** of part of breast
    - S20.141 External constriction of part of breast, right breast
    - S20.142 External constriction of part of breast, left breast
    - S20.149 External constriction of part of breast, unspecified breast
  - S20.15 Superficial **foreign body** of breast
    - Splinter in the breast
    - S20.151 Superficial foreign body of breast, right breast
    - S20.152 Superficial foreign body of breast, left breast
    - S20.159 Superficial foreign body of breast, unspecified breast
  - S20.16 **Insect bite** (nonvenomous) of breast
    - S20.161 Insect bite (nonvenomous) of breast, right breast
    - S20.162 Insect bite (nonvenomous) of breast, left breast
    - S20.169 Insect bite (nonvenomous) of breast, unspecified breast
  - S20.17 Other superficial **bite** of breast
    - EXCLUDES 1: open bite of breast (S21.05-)
    - S20.171 Other superficial bite of breast, right breast
    - S20.172 Other superficial bite of breast, left breast
    - S20.179 Other superficial bite of breast, unspecified breast
- S20.2 Contusion of thorax
  - S20.20 Contusion of thorax, unspecified
  - S20.21 Contusion of front wall of thorax
    - S20.211 Contusion of right front wall of thorax

- S20.212 Contusion of left front wall of thorax
- S20.213 Contusion of bilateral front wall of thorax
- S20.214 Contusion of middle front wall of thorax
- S20.219 Contusion of unspecified front wall of thorax
- S20.22 Contusion of back wall of thorax
  - S20.221 Contusion of right back wall of thorax
  - S20.222 Contusion of left back wall of thorax
  - S20.223 Contusion of bilateral back wall of thorax
  - S20.224 Contusion of middle back wall of thorax
  - S20.229 Contusion of unspecified back wall of thorax
- S20.3 Other and unspecified superficial injuries of front wall of thorax
  - S20.30 Unspecified superficial injuries of front wall of thorax
    - S20.301 Unspecified superficial injuries of right front wall of thorax
    - S20.302 Unspecified superficial injuries of left front wall of thorax
    - S20.303 Unspecified superficial injuries of bilateral front wall of thorax
    - S20.304 Unspecified superficial injuries of middle front wall of thorax
    - S20.309 Unspecified superficial injuries of unspecified front wall of thorax
  - S20.31 Abrasion of front wall of thorax
    - S20.311 Abrasion of right front wall of thorax
    - S20.312 Abrasion of left front wall of thorax
    - S20.313 Abrasion of bilateral front wall of thorax
    - S20.314 Abrasion of middle front wall of thorax
    - S20.319 Abrasion of unspecified front wall of thorax
  - S20.32 Blister (nonthermal) of front wall of thorax
    - S20.321 Blister (nonthermal) of right front wall of thorax
    - S20.322 Blister (nonthermal) of left front wall of thorax
    - S20.323 Blister (nonthermal) of bilateral front wall of thorax
    - S20.324 Blister (nonthermal) of middle front wall of thorax
    - S20.329 Blister (nonthermal) of unspecified front wall of thorax
  - S20.34 External constriction of front wall of thorax
    - S20.341 External constriction of right front wall of thorax
    - S20.342 External constriction of left front wall of thorax
    - S20.343 External constriction of bilateral front wall of thorax
    - S20.344 External constriction of middle front wall of thorax
    - S20.349 External constriction of unspecified front wall of thorax
  - S20.35 Superficial foreign body of front wall of thorax
    Splinter in front wall of thorax
    - S20.351 Superficial foreign body of right front wall of thorax
    - S20.352 Superficial foreign body of left front wall of thorax
    - S20.353 Superficial foreign body of bilateral front wall of thorax
    - S20.354 Superficial foreign body of middle front wall of thorax
    - S20.359 Superficial foreign body of unspecified front wall of thorax
  - S20.36 Insect bite (nonvenomous) of front wall of thorax
    - S20.361 Insect bite (nonvenomous) of right front wall of thorax
    - S20.362 Insect bite (nonvenomous) of left front wall of thorax
    - S20.363 Insect bite (nonvenomous) of bilateral front wall of thorax
    - S20.364 Insect bite (nonvenomous) of middle front wall of thorax
    - S20.369 Insect bite (nonvenomous) of unspecified front wall of thorax
  - S20.37 Other superficial bite of front wall of thorax
    EXCLUDES 1 open bite of front wall of thorax (S21.15)
    - S20.371 Other superficial bite of right front wall of thorax
    - S20.372 Other superficial bite of left front wall of thorax
    - S20.373 Other superficial bite of bilateral front wall of thorax
    - S20.374 Other superficial bite of middle front wall of thorax
    - S20.379 Other superficial bite of unspecified front wall of thorax
- S20.4 Other and unspecified superficial injuries of back wall of thorax
  - S20.40 Unspecified superficial injuries of back wall of thorax
    - S20.401 Unspecified superficial injuries of right back wall of thorax
    - S20.402 Unspecified superficial injuries of left back wall of thorax
    - S20.409 Unspecified superficial injuries of unspecified back wall of thorax
  - S20.41 Abrasion of back wall of thorax
    - S20.411 Abrasion of right back wall of thorax
    - S20.412 Abrasion of left back wall of thorax
    - S20.419 Abrasion of unspecified back wall of thorax
  - S20.42 Blister (nonthermal) of back wall of thorax
    - S20.421 Blister (nonthermal) of right back wall of thorax
    - S20.422 Blister (nonthermal) of left back wall of thorax
    - S20.429 Blister (nonthermal) of unspecified back wall of thorax
  - S20.44 External constriction of back wall of thorax
    - S20.441 External constriction of right back wall of thorax
    - S20.442 External constriction of left back wall of thorax
    - S20.449 External constriction of unspecified back wall of thorax
  - S20.45 Superficial foreign body of back wall of thorax
    Splinter of back wall of thorax
    - S20.451 Superficial foreign body of right back wall of thorax
    - S20.452 Superficial foreign body of left back wall of thorax
    - S20.459 Superficial foreign body of unspecified back wall of thorax
  - S20.46 Insect bite (nonvenomous) of back wall of thorax
    - S20.461 Insect bite (nonvenomous) of right back wall of thorax
    - S20.462 Insect bite (nonvenomous) of left back wall of thorax
    - S20.469 Insect bite (nonvenomous) of unspecified back wall of thorax
  - S20.47 Other superficial bite of back wall of thorax
    EXCLUDES 1 open bite of back wall of thorax (S21.25)
    - S20.471 Other superficial bite of right back wall of thorax
    - S20.472 Other superficial bite of left back wall of thorax
    - S20.479 Other superficial bite of unspecified back wall of thorax
- S20.9 Superficial injury of unspecified parts of thorax
  EXCLUDES 1 contusion of thorax NOS (S20.20)
  - S20.90 Unspecified superficial injury of unspecified parts of thorax
    Superficial injury of thoracic wall NOS
  - S20.91 Abrasion of unspecified parts of thorax
  - S20.92 Blister (nonthermal) of unspecified parts of thorax
  - S20.94 External constriction of unspecified parts of thorax
  - S20.95 Superficial foreign body of unspecified parts of thorax
    Splinter in thorax NOS
  - S20.96 Insect bite (nonvenomous) of unspecified parts of thorax
  - S20.97 Other superficial bite of unspecified parts of thorax
    EXCLUDES 1 open bite of thorax NOS (S21.95)

S21 Open wound of thorax

Code also any associated injury, such as:
injury of heart (S26.-)
injury of intrathoracic organs (S27.-)
rib fracture (S22.3-, S22.4-)
spinal cord injury (S24.0-, S24.1-)
traumatic hemopneumothorax (S27.3)
traumatic hemothorax (S27.1)
traumatic pneumothorax (S27.0)
wound infection

EXCLUDES 1 traumatic amputation (partial) of thorax (S28.1)

The appropriate 7th character is to be added to each code from category S21.
- A initial encounter
- D subsequent encounter
- S sequela

S21.0 Open wound of breast

- **S21.00** Unspecified open wound of breast
  - **S21.001** Unspecified open wound of right breast
  - **S21.002** Unspecified open wound of left breast
  - **S21.009** Unspecified open wound of unspecified breast
- **S21.01** Laceration without foreign body of breast
  - **S21.011** Laceration without foreign body of right breast
  - **S21.012** Laceration without foreign body of left breast
  - **S21.019** Laceration without foreign body of unspecified breast
- **S21.02** Laceration with foreign body of breast
  - **S21.021** Laceration with foreign body of right breast
  - **S21.022** Laceration with foreign body of left breast
  - **S21.029** Laceration with foreign body of unspecified breast
- **S21.03** Puncture wound without foreign body of breast
  - **S21.031** Puncture wound without foreign body of right breast
  - **S21.032** Puncture wound without foreign body of left breast
  - **S21.039** Puncture wound without foreign body of unspecified breast
- **S21.04** Puncture wound with foreign body of breast
  - **S21.041** Puncture wound with foreign body of right breast
  - **S21.042** Puncture wound with foreign body of left breast
  - **S21.049** Puncture wound with foreign body of unspecified breast
- **S21.05** Open bite of breast
  Bite of breast NOS
  EXCLUDES 1 superficial bite of breast (S20.17)
  - **S21.051** Open bite of right breast
  - **S21.052** Open bite of left breast
  - **S21.059** Open bite of unspecified breast

S21.1 Open wound of front wall of thorax without penetration into thoracic cavity

Open wound of chest without penetration into thoracic cavity

- **S21.10** Unspecified open wound of front wall of thorax without penetration into thoracic cavity
  - **S21.101** Unspecified open wound of right front wall of thorax without penetration into thoracic cavity
  - **S21.102** Unspecified open wound of left front wall of thorax without penetration into thoracic cavity
  - **S21.109** Unspecified open wound of unspecified front wall of thorax without penetration into thoracic cavity
- **S21.11** Laceration without foreign body of front wall of thorax without penetration into thoracic cavity
  - **S21.111** Laceration without foreign body of right front wall of thorax without penetration into thoracic cavity
  - **S21.112** Laceration without foreign body of left front wall of thorax without penetration into thoracic cavity
  - **S21.119** Laceration without foreign body of unspecified front wall of thorax without penetration into thoracic cavity
- **S21.12** Laceration with foreign body of front wall of thorax without penetration into thoracic cavity
  - **S21.121** Laceration with foreign body of right front wall of thorax without penetration into thoracic cavity
  - **S21.122** Laceration with foreign body of left front wall of thorax without penetration into thoracic cavity
  - **S21.129** Laceration with foreign body of unspecified front wall of thorax without penetration into thoracic cavity
- **S21.13** Puncture wound without foreign body of front wall of thorax without penetration into thoracic cavity
  - **S21.131** Puncture wound without foreign body of right front wall of thorax without penetration into thoracic cavity
  - **S21.132** Puncture wound without foreign body of left front wall of thorax without penetration into thoracic cavity
  - **S21.139** Puncture wound without foreign body of unspecified front wall of thorax without penetration into thoracic cavity
- **S21.14** Puncture wound with foreign body of front wall of thorax without penetration into thoracic cavity
  - **S21.141** Puncture wound with foreign body of right front wall of thorax without penetration into thoracic cavity
  - **S21.142** Puncture wound with foreign body of left front wall of thorax without penetration into thoracic cavity
  - **S21.149** Puncture wound with foreign body of unspecified front wall of thorax without penetration into thoracic cavity
- **S21.15** Open bite of front wall of thorax without penetration into thoracic cavity
  Bite of front wall of thorax NOS
  EXCLUDES 1 superficial bite of front wall of thorax (S20.37)
  - **S21.151** Open bite of right front wall of thorax without penetration into thoracic cavity
  - **S21.152** Open bite of left front wall of thorax without penetration into thoracic cavity
  - **S21.159** Open bite of unspecified front wall of thorax without penetration into thoracic cavity

S21.2 Open wound of back wall of thorax without penetration into thoracic cavity

- **S21.20** Unspecified open wound of back wall of thorax without penetration into thoracic cavity
  - **S21.201** Unspecified open wound of right back wall of thorax without penetration into thoracic cavity
  - **S21.202** Unspecified open wound of left back wall of thorax without penetration into thoracic cavity
  - **S21.209** Unspecified open wound of unspecified back wall of thorax without penetration into thoracic cavity
- **S21.21** Laceration without foreign body of back wall of thorax without penetration into thoracic cavity
  - **S21.211** Laceration without foreign body of right back wall of thorax without penetration into thoracic cavity
  - **S21.212** Laceration without foreign body of left back wall of thorax without penetration into thoracic cavity
  - **S21.219** Laceration without foreign body of unspecified back wall of thorax without penetration into thoracic cavity
- **S21.22** Laceration with foreign body of back wall of thorax without penetration into thoracic cavity
  - **S21.221** Laceration with foreign body of right back wall of thorax without penetration into thoracic cavity
  - **S21.222** Laceration with foreign body of left back wall of thorax without penetration into thoracic cavity
  - **S21.229** Laceration with foreign body of unspecified back wall of thorax without penetration into thoracic cavity

- **S21.23** Puncture wound without foreign body of back wall of thorax without penetration into thoracic cavity
  - **S21.231** Puncture wound without foreign body of right back wall of thorax without penetration into thoracic cavity
  - **S21.232** Puncture wound without foreign body of left back wall of thorax without penetration into thoracic cavity
  - **S21.239** Puncture wound without foreign body of unspecified back wall of thorax without penetration into thoracic cavity
- **S21.24** Puncture wound with foreign body of back wall of thorax without penetration into thoracic cavity
  - **S21.241** Puncture wound with foreign body of right back wall of thorax without penetration into thoracic cavity
  - **S21.242** Puncture wound with foreign body of left back wall of thorax without penetration into thoracic cavity
  - **S21.249** Puncture wound with foreign body of unspecified back wall of thorax without penetration into thoracic cavity
- **S21.25** Open bite of back wall of thorax without penetration into thoracic cavity
  Bite of back wall of thorax NOS
  EXCLUDES 1 superficial bite of back wall of thorax (S20.47)
  - **S21.251** Open bite of right back wall of thorax without penetration into thoracic cavity
  - **S21.252** Open bite of left back wall of thorax without penetration into thoracic cavity
  - **S21.259** Open bite of unspecified back wall of thorax without penetration into thoracic cavity

- **S21.3** Open wound of front wall of thorax with penetration into thoracic cavity
  Open wound of chest with penetration into thoracic cavity
  - **S21.30** Unspecified open wound of front wall of thorax with penetration into thoracic cavity
    - **S21.301** Unspecified open wound of right front wall of thorax with penetration into thoracic cavity
    - **S21.302** Unspecified open wound of left front wall of thorax with penetration into thoracic cavity
    - **S21.309** Unspecified open wound of unspecified front wall of thorax with penetration into thoracic cavity
  - **S21.31** Laceration without foreign body of front wall of thorax with penetration into thoracic cavity
    - **S21.311** Laceration without foreign body of right front wall of thorax with penetration into thoracic cavity
    - **S21.312** Laceration without foreign body of left front wall of thorax with penetration into thoracic cavity
    - **S21.319** Laceration without foreign body of unspecified front wall of thorax with penetration into thoracic cavity
  - **S21.32** Laceration with foreign body of front wall of thorax with penetration into thoracic cavity
    - **S21.321** Laceration with foreign body of right front wall of thorax with penetration into thoracic cavity
    - **S21.322** Laceration with foreign body of left front wall of thorax with penetration into thoracic cavity
    - **S21.329** Laceration with foreign body of unspecified front wall of thorax with penetration into thoracic cavity
  - **S21.33** Puncture wound without foreign body of front wall of thorax with penetration into thoracic cavity
    - **S21.331** Puncture wound without foreign body of right front wall of thorax with penetration into thoracic cavity
    - **S21.332** Puncture wound without foreign body of left front wall of thorax with penetration into thoracic cavity
    - **S21.339** Puncture wound without foreign body of unspecified front wall of thorax with penetration into thoracic cavity
  - **S21.34** Puncture wound with foreign body of front wall of thorax with penetration into thoracic cavity
    - **S21.341** Puncture wound with foreign body of right front wall of thorax with penetration into thoracic cavity
    - **S21.342** Puncture wound with foreign body of left front wall of thorax with penetration into thoracic cavity
    - **S21.349** Puncture wound with foreign body of unspecified front wall of thorax with penetration into thoracic cavity
  - **S21.35** Open bite of front wall of thorax with penetration into thoracic cavity
    EXCLUDES 1 superficial bite of front wall of thorax (S20.37)
    - **S21.351** Open bite of right front wall of thorax with penetration into thoracic cavity
    - **S21.352** Open bite of left front wall of thorax with penetration into thoracic cavity
    - **S21.359** Open bite of unspecified front wall of thorax with penetration into thoracic cavity

- **S21.4** Open wound of back wall of thorax with penetration into thoracic cavity
  - **S21.40** Unspecified open wound of back wall of thorax with penetration into thoracic cavity
    - **S21.401** Unspecified open wound of right back wall of thorax with penetration into thoracic cavity
    - **S21.402** Unspecified open wound of left back wall of thorax with penetration into thoracic cavity
    - **S21.409** Unspecified open wound of unspecified back wall of thorax with penetration into thoracic cavity
  - **S21.41** Laceration without foreign body of back wall of thorax with penetration into thoracic cavity
    - **S21.411** Laceration without foreign body of right back wall of thorax with penetration into thoracic cavity
    - **S21.412** Laceration without foreign body of left back wall of thorax with penetration into thoracic cavity
    - **S21.419** Laceration without foreign body of unspecified back wall of thorax with penetration into thoracic cavity
  - **S21.42** Laceration with foreign body of back wall of thorax with penetration into thoracic cavity
    - **S21.421** Laceration with foreign body of right back wall of thorax with penetration into thoracic cavity
    - **S21.422** Laceration with foreign body of left back wall of thorax with penetration into thoracic cavity
    - **S21.429** Laceration with foreign body of unspecified back wall of thorax with penetration into thoracic cavity
  - **S21.43** Puncture wound without foreign body of back wall of thorax with penetration into thoracic cavity
    - **S21.431** Puncture wound without foreign body of right back wall of thorax with penetration into thoracic cavity
    - **S21.432** Puncture wound without foreign body of left back wall of thorax with penetration into thoracic cavity
    - **S21.439** Puncture wound without foreign body of unspecified back wall of thorax with penetration into thoracic cavity
  - **S21.44** Puncture wound with foreign body of back wall of thorax with penetration into thoracic cavity
    - **S21.441** Puncture wound with foreign body of right back wall of thorax with penetration into thoracic cavity
    - **S21.442** Puncture wound with foreign body of left back wall of thorax with penetration into thoracic cavity
    - **S21.449** Puncture wound with foreign body of unspecified back wall of thorax with penetration into thoracic cavity

Chapter 19. Injury, Poisoning and Certain Other Consequences of External Causes

- ✓6th **S21.45** Open bite of back wall of thorax with penetration into thoracic cavity
  Bite of back wall of thorax NOS
  EXCLUDES 1 superficial bite of back wall of thorax (S20.47)
  - ✓7th **S21.451** Open bite of right back wall of thorax with penetration into thoracic cavity
  - ✓7th **S21.452** Open bite of left back wall of thorax with penetration into thoracic cavity
  - ✓7th **S21.459** Open bite of unspecified back wall of thorax with penetration into thoracic cavity
- ✓5th **S21.9** Open wound of unspecified part of thorax
  Open wound of thoracic wall NOS
  - ✓x7th **S21.90** Unspecified open wound of unspecified part of thorax
  - ✓x7th **S21.91** Laceration without foreign body of unspecified part of thorax
  - ✓x7th **S21.92** Laceration with foreign body of unspecified part of thorax
  - ✓x7th **S21.93** Puncture wound without foreign body of unspecified part of thorax
  - ✓x7th **S21.94** Puncture wound with foreign body of unspecified part of thorax
  - ✓x7th **S21.95** Open bite of unspecified part of thorax
    EXCLUDES 1 superficial bite of thorax (S20.97)

- ✓4th **S22** Fracture of rib(s), sternum and thoracic spine
  NOTE: A fracture not indicated as displaced or nondisplaced should be coded to displaced
  A fracture not indicated as open or closed should be coded to closed
  INCLUDES: fracture of thoracic neural arch
  fracture of thoracic spinous process
  fracture of thoracic transverse process
  fracture of thoracic vertebra
  fracture of thoracic vertebral arch
  Code also, if applicable, any associated condition such as:
  injury of intrathoracic organ (S27.-)
  spinal cord injury (S24.0-, S24.1-)
  traumatic hemopneumothorax (S27.2)
  traumatic hemothorax (S27.1-)
  traumatic pneumothorax (S27.0)
  EXCLUDES 1 transection of thorax (S28.1)
  EXCLUDES 2 fracture of clavicle (S42.0-)
  fracture of scapula (S42.1-)
  AHA: 2021,1Q,6; 2018,2Q,12; 2015,3Q,37-39

  The appropriate 7th character is to be added to each code from category S22.
  - A initial encounter for closed fracture
  - B initial encounter for open fracture
  - D subsequent encounter for fracture with routine healing
  - G subsequent encounter for fracture with delayed healing
  - K subsequent encounter for fracture with nonunion
  - S sequela

  - ✓5th **S22.0** Fracture of thoracic vertebra
    - ✓6th **S22.00** Fracture of unspecified thoracic vertebra
      - ✓7th **S22.000** Wedge compression fracture of unspecified thoracic vertebra HCC ESR COM Q
      - ✓7th **S22.001** Stable burst fracture of unspecified thoracic vertebra HCC ESR COM Q
      - ✓7th **S22.002** Unstable burst fracture of unspecified thoracic vertebra HCC ESR COM Q
      - ✓7th **S22.008** Other fracture of unspecified thoracic vertebra HCC ESR COM Q
      - ✓7th **S22.009** Unspecified fracture of unspecified thoracic vertebra HCC ESR COM Q
    - ✓6th **S22.01** Fracture of first thoracic vertebra
      - ✓7th **S22.010** Wedge compression fracture of first thoracic vertebra HCC ESR COM Q
      - ✓7th **S22.011** Stable burst fracture of first thoracic vertebra HCC ESR COM Q
      - ✓7th **S22.012** Unstable burst fracture of first thoracic vertebra HCC ESR COM Q
      - ✓7th **S22.018** Other fracture of first thoracic vertebra HCC ESR COM Q
      - ✓7th **S22.019** Unspecified fracture of first thoracic vertebra HCC ESR COM Q
    - ✓6th **S22.02** Fracture of second thoracic vertebra
      - ✓7th **S22.020** Wedge compression fracture of second thoracic vertebra HCC ESR COM Q
      - ✓7th **S22.021** Stable burst fracture of second thoracic vertebra HCC ESR COM Q
      - ✓7th **S22.022** Unstable burst fracture of second thoracic vertebra HCC ESR COM Q
      - ✓7th **S22.028** Other fracture of second thoracic vertebra HCC ESR COM Q
      - ✓7th **S22.029** Unspecified fracture of second thoracic vertebra HCC ESR COM Q
    - ✓6th **S22.03** Fracture of third thoracic vertebra
      - ✓7th **S22.030** Wedge compression fracture of third thoracic vertebra HCC ESR COM Q
      - ✓7th **S22.031** Stable burst fracture of third thoracic vertebra HCC ESR COM Q
      - ✓7th **S22.032** Unstable burst fracture of third thoracic vertebra HCC ESR COM Q
      - ✓7th **S22.038** Other fracture of third thoracic vertebra HCC ESR COM Q
      - ✓7th **S22.039** Unspecified fracture of third thoracic vertebra HCC ESR COM Q
    - ✓6th **S22.04** Fracture of fourth thoracic vertebra
      - ✓7th **S22.040** Wedge compression fracture of fourth thoracic vertebra HCC ESR COM Q
      - ✓7th **S22.041** Stable burst fracture of fourth thoracic vertebra HCC ESR COM Q
      - ✓7th **S22.042** Unstable burst fracture of fourth thoracic vertebra HCC ESR COM Q
      - ✓7th **S22.048** Other fracture of fourth thoracic vertebra HCC ESR COM Q
      - ✓7th **S22.049** Unspecified fracture of fourth thoracic vertebra HCC ESR COM Q
    - ✓6th **S22.05** Fracture of T5-T6 vertebra
      - ✓7th **S22.050** Wedge compression fracture of T5-T6 vertebra HCC ESR COM Q
      - ✓7th **S22.051** Stable burst fracture of T5-T6 vertebra HCC ESR COM Q
      - ✓7th **S22.052** Unstable burst fracture of T5-T6 vertebra HCC ESR COM Q
      - ✓7th **S22.058** Other fracture of T5-T6 vertebra HCC ESR COM Q
      - ✓7th **S22.059** Unspecified fracture of T5-T6 vertebra HCC ESR COM Q
    - ✓6th **S22.06** Fracture of T7-T8 vertebra
      - ✓7th **S22.060** Wedge compression fracture of T7-T8 vertebra HCC ESR COM Q
      - ✓7th **S22.061** Stable burst fracture of T7-T8 vertebra HCC ESR COM Q
      - ✓7th **S22.062** Unstable burst fracture of T7-T8 vertebra HCC ESR COM Q
      - ✓7th **S22.068** Other fracture of T7-T8 thoracic vertebra HCC ESR COM Q
      - ✓7th **S22.069** Unspecified fracture of T7-T8 vertebra HCC ESR COM Q
    - ✓6th **S22.07** Fracture of T9-T10 vertebra
      - ✓7th **S22.070** Wedge compression fracture of T9-T10 vertebra HCC ESR COM Q
      - ✓7th **S22.071** Stable burst fracture of T9-T10 vertebra HCC ESR COM Q
      - ✓7th **S22.072** Unstable burst fracture of T9-T10 vertebra HCC ESR COM Q
      - ✓7th **S22.078** Other fracture of T9-T10 vertebra HCC ESR COM Q
      - ✓7th **S22.079** Unspecified fracture of T9-T10 vertebra HCC ESR COM Q
    - ✓6th **S22.08** Fracture of T11-T12 vertebra
      - ✓7th **S22.080** Wedge compression fracture of T11-T12 vertebra HCC ESR COM Q
      - ✓7th **S22.081** Stable burst fracture of T11-T12 vertebra HCC ESR COM Q
      - ✓7th **S22.082** Unstable burst fracture of T11-T12 vertebra HCC ESR COM Q
      - ✓7th **S22.088** Other fracture of T11-T12 vertebra HCC ESR COM Q

HCC CMS-HCC | Rx Rx HCC | ESR ESRD HCC | COM Commercial HCC | N Newborn: 0 | P Pediatric: 0-17 | M Maternity: 9-64 | A Adult: 15-124

Chapter 19. Injury, Poisoning and Certain Other Consequences of External Causes

- ✓7th **S22.089** Unspecified fracture of T11-T12 vertebra HCC ESR COM Q
  - AHA: 2024,4Q,19
- ✓5th **S22.2** Fracture of sternum
  - DEF: Break in flat bone (breast bone) in the anterior thorax caused by blunt trauma to the anterior chest.
  - ✓x7th **S22.20** Unspecified fracture of sternum Q
  - ✓x7th **S22.21** Fracture of manubrium Q
  - ✓x7th **S22.22** Fracture of body of sternum Q
  - ✓x7th **S22.23** Sternal manubrial dissociation Q
  - ✓x7th **S22.24** Fracture of xiphoid process Q
- ✓5th **S22.3** Fracture of one rib
  - AHA: 2021,1Q,5
  - ✓x7th **S22.31** Fracture of one rib, right side Q
  - ✓x7th **S22.32** Fracture of one rib, left side Q
  - ✓x7th **S22.39** Fracture of one rib, unspecified side Q
- ✓5th **S22.4** Multiple fractures of ribs
  - Fractures of two or more ribs
  - EXCLUDES 1: flail chest (S22.5-)
  - AHA: 2021,1Q,5
  - ✓x7th **S22.41** Multiple fractures of ribs, right side Q
  - ✓x7th **S22.42** Multiple fractures of ribs, left side Q
  - ✓x7th **S22.43** Multiple fractures of ribs, bilateral Q
  - ✓x7th **S22.49** Multiple fractures of ribs, unspecified side Q
- ✓x7th **S22.5** Flail chest Q
- ✓x7th **S22.9** Fracture of bony thorax, part unspecified Q

✓4th **S23** Dislocation and sprain of joints and ligaments of thorax
- INCLUDES:
  - avulsion of joint or ligament of thorax
  - laceration of cartilage, joint or ligament of thorax
  - sprain of cartilage, joint or ligament of thorax
  - traumatic hemarthrosis of joint or ligament of thorax
  - traumatic rupture of joint or ligament of thorax
  - traumatic subluxation of joint or ligament of thorax
  - traumatic tear of joint or ligament of thorax
- Code also any associated open wound
- EXCLUDES 2:
  - dislocation, sprain of sternoclavicular joint (S43.2, S43.6)
  - strain of muscle or tendon of thorax (S29.01-)

The appropriate 7th character is to be added to each code from category S23.
- A initial encounter
- D subsequent encounter
- S sequela

- ✓x7th **S23.0** Traumatic rupture of thoracic intervertebral disc
  - EXCLUDES 1: rupture or displacement (nontraumatic) of thoracic intervertebral disc NOS (M51.- with fifth character 4)
- ✓5th **S23.1** Subluxation and dislocation of thoracic vertebra
  - Code also any associated:
    - open wound of thorax (S21.-)
    - spinal cord injury (S24.0-, S24.1-)
  - EXCLUDES 2: fracture of thoracic vertebrae (S22.0-)
  - ✓6th **S23.10** Subluxation and dislocation of unspecified thoracic vertebra
    - ✓7th **S23.100** Subluxation of unspecified thoracic vertebra
    - ✓7th **S23.101** Dislocation of unspecified thoracic vertebra
  - ✓6th **S23.11** Subluxation and dislocation of T1/T2 thoracic vertebra
    - ✓7th **S23.110** Subluxation of T1/T2 thoracic vertebra
    - ✓7th **S23.111** Dislocation of T1/T2 thoracic vertebra
  - ✓6th **S23.12** Subluxation and dislocation of T2/T3-T3/T4 thoracic vertebra
    - ✓7th **S23.120** Subluxation of T2/T3 thoracic vertebra
    - ✓7th **S23.121** Dislocation of T2/T3 thoracic vertebra
    - ✓7th **S23.122** Subluxation of T3/T4 thoracic vertebra
    - ✓7th **S23.123** Dislocation of T3/T4 thoracic vertebra
  - ✓6th **S23.13** Subluxation and dislocation of T4/T5-T5/T6 thoracic vertebra
    - ✓7th **S23.130** Subluxation of T4/T5 thoracic vertebra
    - ✓7th **S23.131** Dislocation of T4/T5 thoracic vertebra
    - ✓7th **S23.132** Subluxation of T5/T6 thoracic vertebra
    - ✓7th **S23.133** Dislocation of T5/T6 thoracic vertebra
  - ✓6th **S23.14** Subluxation and dislocation of T6/T7-T7/T8 thoracic vertebra
    - ✓7th **S23.140** Subluxation of T6/T7 thoracic vertebra
    - ✓7th **S23.141** Dislocation of T6/T7 thoracic vertebra
    - ✓7th **S23.142** Subluxation of T7/T8 thoracic vertebra
    - ✓7th **S23.143** Dislocation of T7/T8 thoracic vertebra
  - ✓6th **S23.15** Subluxation and dislocation of T8/T9-T9/T10 thoracic vertebra
    - ✓7th **S23.150** Subluxation of T8/T9 thoracic vertebra
    - ✓7th **S23.151** Dislocation of T8/T9 thoracic vertebra
    - ✓7th **S23.152** Subluxation of T9/T10 thoracic vertebra
    - ✓7th **S23.153** Dislocation of T9/T10 thoracic vertebra
  - ✓6th **S23.16** Subluxation and dislocation of T10/T11-T11/T12 thoracic vertebra
    - ✓7th **S23.160** Subluxation of T10/T11 thoracic vertebra
    - ✓7th **S23.161** Dislocation of T10/T11 thoracic vertebra
    - ✓7th **S23.162** Subluxation of T11/T12 thoracic vertebra
    - ✓7th **S23.163** Dislocation of T11/T12 thoracic vertebra
  - ✓6th **S23.17** Subluxation and dislocation of T12/L1 thoracic vertebra
    - ✓7th **S23.170** Subluxation of T12/L1 thoracic vertebra
    - ✓7th **S23.171** Dislocation of T12/L1 thoracic vertebra
- ✓5th **S23.2** Dislocation of other and unspecified parts of thorax
  - ✓x7th **S23.20** Dislocation of unspecified part of thorax
  - ✓x7th **S23.29** Dislocation of other parts of thorax
- ✓x7th **S23.3** Sprain of ligaments of thoracic spine
- ✓5th **S23.4** Sprain of ribs and sternum
  - ✓x7th **S23.41** Sprain of ribs
  - ✓6th **S23.42** Sprain of sternum
    - ✓7th **S23.420** Sprain of sternoclavicular (joint) (ligament)
    - ✓7th **S23.421** Sprain of chondrosternal joint
    - ✓7th **S23.428** Other sprain of sternum
    - ✓7th **S23.429** Unspecified sprain of sternum
- ✓x7th **S23.8** Sprain of other specified parts of thorax
- ✓x7th **S23.9** Sprain of unspecified parts of thorax

✓4th **S24** Injury of nerves and spinal cord at thorax level
- NOTE: Code to highest level of thoracic spinal cord injury.
  - Injuries to the spinal cord (S24.0 and S24.1) refer to the cord level and not bone level injury, and can affect nerve roots at and below the level given.
- Code also any associated:
  - fracture of thoracic vertebra (S22.0-)
  - open wound of thorax (S21.-)
  - transient paralysis (R29.5)
- EXCLUDES 2: injury of brachial plexus (S14.3)

The appropriate 7th character is to be added to each code from category S24.
- A initial encounter
- D subsequent encounter
- S sequela

- ✓x7th **S24.0** Concussion and edema of thoracic spinal cord HCC ESR COM
- ✓5th **S24.1** Other and unspecified injuries of thoracic spinal cord
  - ✓6th **S24.10** Unspecified injury of thoracic spinal cord
    - ✓7th **S24.101** Unspecified injury at T1 level of thoracic spinal cord HCC ESR COM
    - ✓7th **S24.102** Unspecified injury at T2-T6 level of thoracic spinal cord HCC ESR COM
    - ✓7th **S24.103** Unspecified injury at T7-T10 level of thoracic spinal cord HCC ESR COM
    - ✓7th **S24.104** Unspecified injury at T11-T12 level of thoracic spinal cord HCC ESR COM
    - ✓7th **S24.109** Unspecified injury at unspecified level of thoracic spinal cord HCC ESR COM
      - Injury of thoracic spinal cord NOS
  - ✓6th **S24.11** Complete lesion of thoracic spinal cord
    - ✓7th **S24.111** Complete lesion at T1 level of thoracic spinal cord
    - ✓7th **S24.112** Complete lesion at T2-T6 level of thoracic spinal cord HCC ESR COM
    - ✓7th **S24.113** Complete lesion at T7-T10 level of thoracic spinal cord HCC ESR COM

- **S24.114** Complete lesion at **T11-T12** level of thoracic spinal cord `HCC` `ESR` `COM`
- **S24.119** Complete lesion at unspecified level of thoracic spinal cord `HCC` `ESR` `COM`
- **S24.13** Anterior cord syndrome of thoracic spinal cord
  - **S24.131** Anterior cord syndrome at **T1** level of thoracic spinal cord
  - **S24.132** Anterior cord syndrome at **T2-T6** level of thoracic spinal cord `HCC` `ESR` `COM`
  - **S24.133** Anterior cord syndrome at **T7-T10** level of thoracic spinal cord `HCC` `ESR` `COM`
  - **S24.134** Anterior cord syndrome at **T11-T12** level of thoracic spinal cord `HCC` `ESR` `COM`
  - **S24.139** Anterior cord syndrome at unspecified level of thoracic spinal cord `HCC` `ESR` `COM`
- **S24.14** Brown-Sequard syndrome of thoracic spinal cord
  - **S24.141** Brown-Sequard syndrome at **T1** level of thoracic spinal cord `HCC` `ESR` `COM`
  - **S24.142** Brown-Sequard syndrome at **T2-T6** level of thoracic spinal cord `HCC` `ESR` `COM`
  - **S24.143** Brown-Sequard syndrome at **T7-T10** level of thoracic spinal cord
  - **S24.144** Brown-Sequard syndrome at **T11-T12** level of thoracic spinal cord
  - **S24.149** Brown-Sequard syndrome at unspecified level of thoracic spinal cord `HCC` `ESR` `COM`
- **S24.15** Other incomplete lesions of thoracic spinal cord
  - Incomplete lesion of thoracic spinal cord NOS
  - Posterior cord syndrome of thoracic spinal cord
  - **S24.151** Other incomplete lesion at **T1** level of thoracic spinal cord `HCC` `ESR` `COM`
  - **S24.152** Other incomplete lesion at **T2-T6** level of thoracic spinal cord `HCC` `ESR` `COM`
  - **S24.153** Other incomplete lesion at **T7-T10** level of thoracic spinal cord `HCC` `ESR` `COM`
  - **S24.154** Other incomplete lesion at **T11-T12** level of thoracic spinal cord
  - **S24.159** Other incomplete lesion at unspecified level of thoracic spinal cord `HCC` `ESR` `COM`
- **S24.2** Injury of nerve root of thoracic spine
- **S24.3** Injury of peripheral nerves of thorax
- **S24.4** Injury of thoracic sympathetic nervous system
  - Injury of cardiac plexus
  - Injury of esophageal plexus
  - Injury of pulmonary plexus
  - Injury of stellate ganglion
  - Injury of thoracic sympathetic ganglion
- **S24.8** Injury of other specified nerves of thorax
- **S24.9** Injury of unspecified nerve of thorax
- **S25** Injury of blood vessels of thorax
  - Code also any associated open wound (S21.-)
  - The appropriate 7th character is to be added to each code from category S25.
    - A   initial encounter
    - D   subsequent encounter
    - S   sequela
  - **S25.0** Injury of thoracic aorta
    - Injury of aorta NOS
    - **S25.00** Unspecified injury of thoracic aorta
    - **S25.01** Minor laceration of thoracic aorta
      - Incomplete transection of thoracic aorta
      - Laceration of thoracic aorta NOS
      - Superficial laceration of thoracic aorta
    - **S25.02** Major laceration of thoracic aorta
      - Complete transection of thoracic aorta
      - Traumatic rupture of thoracic aorta
    - **S25.09** Other specified injury of thoracic aorta
  - **S25.1** Injury of innominate or subclavian artery
    - **S25.10** Unspecified injury of innominate or subclavian artery
      - **S25.101** Unspecified injury of **right** innominate or subclavian artery
      - **S25.102** Unspecified injury of **left** innominate or subclavian artery
      - **S25.109** Unspecified injury of unspecified innominate or subclavian artery
    - **S25.11** Minor laceration of innominate or subclavian artery
      - Incomplete transection of innominate or subclavian artery
      - Laceration of innominate or subclavian artery NOS
      - Superficial laceration of innominate or subclavian artery
      - **S25.111** Minor laceration of **right** innominate or subclavian artery
      - **S25.112** Minor laceration of **left** innominate or subclavian artery
      - **S25.119** Minor laceration of unspecified innominate or subclavian artery
    - **S25.12** Major laceration of innominate or subclavian artery
      - Complete transection of innominate or subclavian artery
      - Traumatic rupture of innominate or subclavian artery
      - **S25.121** Major laceration of **right** innominate or subclavian artery
      - **S25.122** Major laceration of **left** innominate or subclavian artery
      - **S25.129** Major laceration of unspecified innominate or subclavian artery
    - **S25.19** Other specified injury of innominate or subclavian artery
      - **S25.191** Other specified injury of **right** innominate or subclavian artery
      - **S25.192** Other specified injury of **left** innominate or subclavian artery
      - **S25.199** Other specified injury of unspecified innominate or subclavian artery
  - **S25.2** Injury of superior vena cava
    - Injury of vena cava NOS
    - **S25.20** Unspecified injury of superior vena cava
    - **S25.21** Minor laceration of superior vena cava
      - Incomplete transection of superior vena cava
      - Laceration of superior vena cava NOS
      - Superficial laceration of superior vena cava
    - **S25.22** Major laceration of superior vena cava
      - Complete transection of superior vena cava
      - Traumatic rupture of superior vena cava
    - **S25.29** Other specified injury of superior vena cava
  - **S25.3** Injury of innominate or subclavian vein
    - **S25.30** Unspecified injury of innominate or subclavian vein
      - **S25.301** Unspecified injury of **right** innominate or subclavian vein
      - **S25.302** Unspecified injury of **left** innominate or subclavian vein
      - **S25.309** Unspecified injury of unspecified innominate or subclavian vein
    - **S25.31** Minor laceration of innominate or subclavian vein
      - Incomplete transection of innominate or subclavian vein
      - Laceration of innominate or subclavian vein NOS
      - Superficial laceration of innominate or subclavian vein
      - **S25.311** Minor laceration of **right** innominate or subclavian vein
      - **S25.312** Minor laceration of **left** innominate or subclavian vein
      - **S25.319** Minor laceration of unspecified innominate or subclavian vein
    - **S25.32** Major laceration of innominate or subclavian vein
      - Complete transection of innominate or subclavian vein
      - Traumatic rupture of innominate or subclavian vein
      - **S25.321** Major laceration of **right** innominate or subclavian vein
      - **S25.322** Major laceration of **left** innominate or subclavian vein
      - **S25.329** Major laceration of unspecified innominate or subclavian vein
    - **S25.39** Other specified injury of innominate or subclavian vein
      - **S25.391** Other specified injury of **right** innominate or subclavian vein
      - **S25.392** Other specified injury of **left** innominate or subclavian vein
      - **S25.399** Other specified injury of unspecified innominate or subclavian vein
  - **S25.4** Injury of pulmonary blood vessels
    - **S25.40** Unspecified injury of pulmonary blood vessels
      - **S25.401** Unspecified injury of **right** pulmonary blood vessels

---

`HCC` CMS-HCC `Rx` Rx HCC `ESR` ESRD HCC `COM` Commercial HCC **N** Newborn: 0 **P** Pediatric: 0-17 **M** Maternity: 9-64 **A** Adult: 15-124

Chapter 19. Injury, Poisoning and Certain Other Consequences of External Causes

- **S25.402** Unspecified injury of **left** pulmonary blood vessels
- **S25.409** Unspecified injury of unspecified pulmonary blood vessels
- **S25.41** **Minor laceration** of pulmonary blood vessels
  - Incomplete transection of pulmonary blood vessels
  - Laceration of pulmonary blood vessels NOS
  - Superficial laceration of pulmonary blood vessels
  - **S25.411** Minor laceration of **right** pulmonary blood vessels
  - **S25.412** Minor laceration of **left** pulmonary blood vessels
  - **S25.419** Minor laceration of unspecified pulmonary blood vessels
- **S25.42** **Major laceration** of pulmonary blood vessels
  - Complete transection of pulmonary blood vessels
  - Traumatic rupture of pulmonary blood vessels
  - **S25.421** Major laceration of **right** pulmonary blood vessels
  - **S25.422** Major laceration of **left** pulmonary blood vessels
  - **S25.429** Major laceration of unspecified pulmonary blood vessels
- **S25.49** Other specified injury of pulmonary blood vessels
  - **S25.491** Other specified injury of **right** pulmonary blood vessels
  - **S25.492** Other specified injury of **left** pulmonary blood vessels
  - **S25.499** Other specified injury of unspecified pulmonary blood vessels
- **S25.5** Injury of **intercostal blood vessels**
  - **S25.50** Unspecified injury of intercostal blood vessels
    - **S25.501** Unspecified injury of intercostal blood vessels, **right** side
    - **S25.502** Unspecified injury of intercostal blood vessels, **left** side
    - **S25.509** Unspecified injury of intercostal blood vessels, unspecified side
  - **S25.51** **Laceration** of intercostal blood vessels
    - **S25.511** Laceration of intercostal blood vessels, **right** side
    - **S25.512** Laceration of intercostal blood vessels, **left** side
    - **S25.519** Laceration of intercostal blood vessels, unspecified side
  - **S25.59** Other specified injury of intercostal blood vessels
    - **S25.591** Other specified injury of intercostal blood vessels, **right** side
    - **S25.592** Other specified injury of intercostal blood vessels, **left** side
    - **S25.599** Other specified injury of intercostal blood vessels, unspecified side
- **S25.8** Injury of other blood vessels of thorax
  - Injury of azygos vein
  - Injury of mammary artery or vein
  - **S25.80** Unspecified injury of other blood vessels of thorax
    - **S25.801** Unspecified injury of other blood vessels of thorax, **right** side
    - **S25.802** Unspecified injury of other blood vessels of thorax, **left** side
    - **S25.809** Unspecified injury of other blood vessels of thorax, unspecified side
  - **S25.81** **Laceration** of other blood vessels of thorax
    - **S25.811** Laceration of other blood vessels of thorax, **right** side
    - **S25.812** Laceration of other blood vessels of thorax, **left** side
    - **S25.819** Laceration of other blood vessels of thorax, unspecified side
  - **S25.89** Other specified injury of other blood vessels of thorax
    - **S25.891** Other specified injury of other blood vessels of thorax, **right** side
    - **S25.892** Other specified injury of other blood vessels of thorax, **left** side
    - **S25.899** Other specified injury of other blood vessels of thorax, unspecified side
- **S25.9** Injury of unspecified blood vessel of thorax
  - **S25.90** Unspecified injury of unspecified blood vessel of thorax
  - **S25.91** **Laceration** of unspecified blood vessel of thorax
  - **S25.99** Other specified injury of unspecified blood vessel of thorax

S26 Injury of heart

Code also any associated:
- open wound of thorax (S21.-)
- traumatic hemopneumothorax (S27.2)
- traumatic hemothorax (S27.1)
- traumatic pneumothorax (S27.0)

The appropriate 7th character is to be added to each code from category S26.
- A initial encounter
- D subsequent encounter
- S sequela

- **S26.0** Injury of heart **with hemopericardium**
  - **S26.00** Unspecified injury of heart with hemopericardium
  - **S26.01** **Contusion** of heart with hemopericardium
  - **S26.02** **Laceration** of heart with hemopericardium
    - **S26.020** **Mild** laceration of heart with hemopericardium
      - Laceration of heart without penetration of heart chamber
    - **S26.021** **Moderate** laceration of heart with hemopericardium
      - Laceration of heart with penetration of heart chamber
    - **S26.022** **Major** laceration of heart with hemopericardium
      - Laceration of heart with penetration of multiple heart chambers
  - **S26.09** Other injury of heart with hemopericardium
- **S26.1** Injury of heart **without hemopericardium**
  - **S26.10** Unspecified injury of heart without hemopericardium
  - **S26.11** **Contusion** of heart without hemopericardium
  - **S26.12** **Laceration** of heart without hemopericardium
  - **S26.19** Other injury of heart without hemopericardium
- **S26.9** Injury of heart, unspecified with or without hemopericardium
  - **S26.90** Unspecified injury of heart, unspecified with or without hemopericardium
  - **S26.91** **Contusion** of heart, unspecified with or without hemopericardium
    - **DEF:** Bruising within the heart muscle, with no mention of an open wound, usually caused by blunt chest trauma in motor vehicle accidents, falling from great heights, or receiving CPR.
  - **S26.92** **Laceration** of heart, unspecified with or without hemopericardium
    - Laceration of heart NOS
    - **AHA:** 2019,2Q,24
  - **S26.99** Other injury of heart, unspecified with or without hemopericardium

S27 Injury of other and unspecified intrathoracic organs

Code also any associated open wound of thorax (S21.-)

EXCLUDES 2: injury of cervical esophagus (S10-S19)
injury of trachea (cervical) (S10-S19)

The appropriate 7th character is to be added to each code from category S27.
- A initial encounter
- D subsequent encounter
- S sequela

- **S27.0** Traumatic pneumothorax
  - EXCLUDES 1: spontaneous pneumothorax (J93.-)
- **S27.1** Traumatic hemothorax
- **S27.2** Traumatic hemopneumothorax
- **S27.3** Other and unspecified injuries of **lung**
  - **S27.30** Unspecified injury of lung
    - **S27.301** Unspecified injury of lung, **unilateral**
    - **S27.302** Unspecified injury of lung, **bilateral**
    - **S27.309** Unspecified injury of lung, unspecified
  - **S27.31** **Primary blast** injury of lung
    - Blast injury of lung NOS
    - **S27.311** Primary blast injury of lung, **unilateral**
    - **S27.312** Primary blast injury of lung, **bilateral**
    - **S27.319** Primary blast injury of lung, unspecified

Chapter 19. Injury, Poisoning and Certain Other Consequences of External Causes

- **S27.32** Contusion of lung
  - **DEF:** Bruising of the lung without mention of an open wound.
  - **S27.321** Contusion of lung, unilateral
  - **S27.322** Contusion of lung, bilateral
  - **S27.329** Contusion of lung, unspecified
- **S27.33** Laceration of lung
  - **S27.331** Laceration of lung, unilateral
  - **S27.332** Laceration of lung, bilateral
  - **S27.339** Laceration of lung, unspecified
- **S27.39** Other injuries of lung
  - Secondary blast injury of lung
  - **S27.391** Other injuries of lung, unilateral
  - **S27.392** Other injuries of lung, bilateral
  - **S27.399** Other injuries of lung, unspecified
- **S27.4** Injury of bronchus
  - **S27.40** Unspecified injury of bronchus
    - **S27.401** Unspecified injury of bronchus, unilateral
    - **S27.402** Unspecified injury of bronchus, bilateral
    - **S27.409** Unspecified injury of bronchus, unspecified
  - **S27.41** Primary blast injury of bronchus
    - Blast injury of bronchus NOS
    - **S27.411** Primary blast injury of bronchus, unilateral
    - **S27.412** Primary blast injury of bronchus, bilateral
    - **S27.419** Primary blast injury of bronchus, unspecified
  - **S27.42** Contusion of bronchus
    - **S27.421** Contusion of bronchus, unilateral
    - **S27.422** Contusion of bronchus, bilateral
    - **S27.429** Contusion of bronchus, unspecified
  - **S27.43** Laceration of bronchus
    - **S27.431** Laceration of bronchus, unilateral
    - **S27.432** Laceration of bronchus, bilateral
    - **S27.439** Laceration of bronchus, unspecified
  - **S27.49** Other injury of bronchus
    - Secondary blast injury of bronchus
    - **S27.491** Other injury of bronchus, unilateral
    - **S27.492** Other injury of bronchus, bilateral
    - **S27.499** Other injury of bronchus, unspecified
- **S27.5** Injury of thoracic trachea
  - **S27.50** Unspecified injury of thoracic trachea
  - **S27.51** Primary blast injury of thoracic trachea
    - Blast injury of thoracic trachea NOS
  - **S27.52** Contusion of thoracic trachea
  - **S27.53** Laceration of thoracic trachea
  - **S27.59** Other injury of thoracic trachea
    - Secondary blast injury of thoracic trachea
- **S27.6** Injury of pleura
  - **S27.60** Unspecified injury of pleura
  - **S27.63** Laceration of pleura
  - **S27.69** Other injury of pleura
- **S27.8** Injury of other specified intrathoracic organs
  - **S27.80** Injury of diaphragm
    - **S27.802** Contusion of diaphragm
    - **S27.803** Laceration of diaphragm
    - **S27.808** Other injury of diaphragm
    - **S27.809** Unspecified injury of diaphragm
  - **S27.81** Injury of esophagus (thoracic part)
    - **S27.812** Contusion of esophagus (thoracic part)
    - **S27.813** Laceration of esophagus (thoracic part)
    - **S27.818** Other injury of esophagus (thoracic part)
    - **S27.819** Unspecified injury of esophagus (thoracic part)
  - **S27.89** Injury of other specified intrathoracic organs
    - Injury of lymphatic thoracic duct
    - Injury of thymus gland
    - **S27.892** Contusion of other specified intrathoracic organs
    - **S27.893** Laceration of other specified intrathoracic organs
    - **S27.898** Other injury of other specified intrathoracic organs
    - **S27.899** Unspecified injury of other specified intrathoracic organs
- **S27.9** Injury of unspecified intrathoracic organ

- **S28** Crushing injury of thorax, and traumatic amputation of part of thorax

  > The appropriate 7th character is to be added to each code from category S28.
  > A initial encounter
  > D subsequent encounter
  > S sequela

  - **S28.0** Crushed chest
    - Use additional code for all associated injuries
    - **EXCLUDES 1** flail chest (S22.5)
  - **S28.1** Traumatic amputation (partial) of part of thorax, except breast
  - **S28.2** Traumatic amputation of breast
    - **S28.21** Complete traumatic amputation of breast
      - Traumatic amputation of breast NOS
      - **S28.211** Complete traumatic amputation of right breast
      - **S28.212** Complete traumatic amputation of left breast
      - **S28.219** Complete traumatic amputation of unspecified breast
    - **S28.22** Partial traumatic amputation of breast
      - **S28.221** Partial traumatic amputation of right breast
      - **S28.222** Partial traumatic amputation of left breast
      - **S28.229** Partial traumatic amputation of unspecified breast

- **S29** Other and unspecified injuries of thorax
  - Code also any associated open wound (S21.-)

  > The appropriate 7th character is to be added to each code from category S29.
  > A initial encounter
  > D subsequent encounter
  > S sequela

  - **S29.0** Injury of muscle and tendon at thorax level
    - **S29.00** Unspecified injury of muscle and tendon of thorax
      - **S29.001** Unspecified injury of muscle and tendon of front wall of thorax
      - **S29.002** Unspecified injury of muscle and tendon of back wall of thorax
      - **S29.009** Unspecified injury of muscle and tendon of unspecified wall of thorax
    - **S29.01** Strain of muscle and tendon of thorax
      - **S29.011** Strain of muscle and tendon of front wall of thorax
      - **S29.012** Strain of muscle and tendon of back wall of thorax
      - **S29.019** Strain of muscle and tendon of unspecified wall of thorax
    - **S29.02** Laceration of muscle and tendon of thorax
      - **S29.021** Laceration of muscle and tendon of front wall of thorax
      - **S29.022** Laceration of muscle and tendon of back wall of thorax
      - **S29.029** Laceration of muscle and tendon of unspecified wall of thorax
    - **S29.09** Other injury of muscle and tendon of thorax
      - **S29.091** Other injury of muscle and tendon of front wall of thorax
      - **S29.092** Other injury of muscle and tendon of back wall of thorax
      - **S29.099** Other injury of muscle and tendon of unspecified wall of thorax
  - **S29.8** Other specified injuries of thorax
  - **S29.9** Unspecified injury of thorax

Injuries to the abdomen, lower back, lumbar spine, pelvis and external genitals (S30-S39)

INCLUDES
- injuries to the abdominal wall
- injuries to the anus
- injuries to the buttock
- injuries to the external genitalia
- injuries to the flank
- injuries to the groin

EXCLUDES 2
- burns and corrosions (T20-T32)
- effects of foreign body in anus and rectum (T18.5)
- effects of foreign body in genitourinary tract (T19.-)
- effects of foreign body in stomach, small intestine and colon (T18.2-T18.4)
- frostbite (T33-T34)
- insect bite or sting, venomous (T63.4)

S30 Superficial injury of abdomen, lower back, pelvis and external genitals

EXCLUDES 2 superficial injury of hip (S70.-)

The appropriate 7th character is to be added to each code from category S30.
- A initial encounter
- D subsequent encounter
- S sequela

- **S30.0** Contusion of lower back and pelvis
  - Contusion of buttock
- **S30.1** Contusion of abdominal wall
  - ~~Contusion of flank~~
  - ~~Contusion of groin~~
  - **S30.11** Contusion of abdominal wall
  - **S30.12** Contusion of groin
  - **S30.13** Contusion of flank (latus) region
- **S30.2** Contusion of external genital organs
  - **S30.20** Contusion of unspecified external genital organ
    - **S30.201** Contusion of unspecified external genital organ, male
    - **S30.202** Contusion of unspecified external genital organ, female
  - **S30.21** Contusion of penis
  - **S30.22** Contusion of scrotum and testes
  - **S30.23** Contusion of vagina and vulva
- **S30.3** Contusion of anus
- **S30.8** Other superficial injuries of abdomen, lower back, pelvis and external genitals
  - **S30.81** Abrasion of abdomen, lower back, pelvis and external genitals
    - **S30.810** Abrasion of lower back and pelvis
    - **S30.811** Abrasion of abdominal wall
    - **S30.812** Abrasion of penis
    - **S30.813** Abrasion of scrotum and testes
    - **S30.814** Abrasion of vagina and vulva
    - **S30.815** Abrasion of unspecified external genital organs, male
    - **S30.816** Abrasion of unspecified external genital organs, female
    - **S30.817** Abrasion of anus
    - **S30.81A** Abrasion of flank
  - **S30.82** Blister (nonthermal) of abdomen, lower back, pelvis and external genitals
    - **S30.820** Blister (nonthermal) of lower back and pelvis
    - **S30.821** Blister (nonthermal) of abdominal wall
    - **S30.822** Blister (nonthermal) of penis
    - **S30.823** Blister (nonthermal) of scrotum and testes
    - **S30.824** Blister (nonthermal) of vagina and vulva
    - **S30.825** Blister (nonthermal) of unspecified external genital organs, male
    - **S30.826** Blister (nonthermal) of unspecified external genital organs, female
    - **S30.827** Blister (nonthermal) of anus
    - **S30.82A** Blister (nonthermal) of flank
  - **S30.84** External constriction of abdomen, lower back, pelvis and external genitals
    - **S30.840** External constriction of lower back and pelvis
    - **S30.841** External constriction of abdominal wall
    - **S30.842** External constriction of penis
      - Hair tourniquet syndrome of penis
      - Use additional cause code to identify the constricting item (W49.0-)
    - **S30.843** External constriction of scrotum and testes
    - **S30.844** External constriction of vagina and vulva
    - **S30.845** External constriction of unspecified external genital organs, male
    - **S30.846** External constriction of unspecified external genital organs, female
    - **S30.84A** External constriction of flank
  - **S30.85** Superficial foreign body of abdomen, lower back, pelvis and external genitals
    - Splinter in the abdomen, lower back, pelvis and external genitals
    - **S30.850** Superficial foreign body of lower back and pelvis
    - **S30.851** Superficial foreign body of abdominal wall
    - **S30.852** Superficial foreign body of penis
    - **S30.853** Superficial foreign body of scrotum and testes
    - **S30.854** Superficial foreign body of vagina and vulva
    - **S30.855** Superficial foreign body of unspecified external genital organs, male
    - **S30.856** Superficial foreign body of unspecified external genital organs, female
    - **S30.857** Superficial foreign body of anus
    - **S30.85A** Superficial foreign body of flank
  - **S30.86** Insect bite (nonvenomous) of abdomen, lower back, pelvis and external genitals
    - **S30.860** Insect bite (nonvenomous) of lower back and pelvis
    - **S30.861** Insect bite (nonvenomous) of abdominal wall
    - **S30.862** Insect bite (nonvenomous) of penis
    - **S30.863** Insect bite (nonvenomous) of scrotum and testes
    - **S30.864** Insect bite (nonvenomous) of vagina and vulva
    - **S30.865** Insect bite (nonvenomous) of unspecified external genital organs, male
    - **S30.866** Insect bite (nonvenomous) of unspecified external genital organs, female
    - **S30.867** Insect bite (nonvenomous) of anus
    - **S30.86A** Insect bite (nonvenomous) of flank
  - **S30.87** Other superficial bite of abdomen, lower back, pelvis and external genitals
    - **EXCLUDES 1** open bite of abdomen, lower back, pelvis and external genitals (S31.05, S31.15, S31.25, S31.35, S31.45, S31.55)
    - **S30.870** Other superficial bite of lower back and pelvis
    - **S30.871** Other superficial bite of abdominal wall
    - **S30.872** Other superficial bite of penis
    - **S30.873** Other superficial bite of scrotum and testes
    - **S30.874** Other superficial bite of vagina and vulva
    - **S30.875** Other superficial bite of unspecified external genital organs, male
    - **S30.876** Other superficial bite of unspecified external genital organs, female
    - **S30.877** Other superficial bite of anus
    - **S30.87A** Other superficial bite of flank
- **S30.9** Unspecified superficial injury of abdomen, lower back, pelvis and external genitals
  - **S30.91** Unspecified superficial injury of lower back and pelvis
  - **S30.92** Unspecified superficial injury of abdominal wall
  - **S30.93** Unspecified superficial injury of penis
  - **S30.94** Unspecified superficial injury of scrotum and testes
  - **S30.95** Unspecified superficial injury of vagina and vulva
  - **S30.96** Unspecified superficial injury of unspecified external genital organs, male
  - **S30.97** Unspecified superficial injury of unspecified external genital organs, female
  - **S30.98** Unspecified superficial injury of anus
  - **S30.9A** Unspecified superficial injury of flank

S31 Open wound of abdomen, lower back, pelvis and external genitals

Code also any associated:
 spinal cord injury (S24.0-, S24.1-, S34.0-, S34.1-)
 wound infection

EXCLUDES 1 traumatic amputation of part of abdomen, lower back and pelvis (S38.2-, S38.3)

EXCLUDES 2 open fracture of pelvis (S32.1- - S32.9 with 7th character B)
 open wound of hip (S71.00-S71.02)

The appropriate 7th character is to be added to each code from category S31.
- A initial encounter
- D subsequent encounter
- S sequela

S31.0 Open wound of lower back and pelvis

S31.00 Unspecified open wound of lower back and pelvis
- **S31.000** Unspecified open wound of lower back and pelvis without penetration into retroperitoneum
  Unspecified open wound of lower back and pelvis NOS
- **S31.001** Unspecified open wound of lower back and pelvis with penetration into retroperitoneum

S31.01 Laceration without foreign body of lower back and pelvis
- **S31.010** Laceration without foreign body of lower back and pelvis without penetration into retroperitoneum
  Laceration without foreign body of lower back and pelvis NOS
- **S31.011** Laceration without foreign body of lower back and pelvis with penetration into retroperitoneum

S31.02 Laceration with foreign body of lower back and pelvis
- **S31.020** Laceration with foreign body of lower back and pelvis without penetration into retroperitoneum
  Laceration with foreign body of lower back and pelvis NOS
- **S31.021** Laceration with foreign body of lower back and pelvis with penetration into retroperitoneum

S31.03 Puncture wound without foreign body of lower back and pelvis
- **S31.030** Puncture wound without foreign body of lower back and pelvis without penetration into retroperitoneum
  Puncture wound without foreign body of lower back and pelvis NOS
- **S31.031** Puncture wound without foreign body of lower back and pelvis with penetration into retroperitoneum

S31.04 Puncture wound with foreign body of lower back and pelvis
- **S31.040** Puncture wound with foreign body of lower back and pelvis without penetration into retroperitoneum
  Puncture wound with foreign body of lower back and pelvis NOS
- **S31.041** Puncture wound with foreign body of lower back and pelvis with penetration into retroperitoneum

S31.05 Open bite of lower back and pelvis
Bite of lower back and pelvis NOS
EXCLUDES 1 superficial bite of lower back and pelvis (S30.860, S30.870)
- **S31.050** Open bite of lower back and pelvis without penetration into retroperitoneum
  Open bite of lower back and pelvis NOS
- **S31.051** Open bite of lower back and pelvis with penetration into retroperitoneum

S31.1 Open wound of abdominal wall without penetration into peritoneal cavity
Open wound of abdominal wall NOS
EXCLUDES 2 open wound of abdominal wall with penetration into peritoneal cavity (S31.6-)

S31.10 Unspecified open wound of abdominal wall without penetration into peritoneal cavity
- **S31.100** Unspecified open wound of abdominal wall, right upper quadrant without penetration into peritoneal cavity
- **S31.101** Unspecified open wound of abdominal wall, left upper quadrant without penetration into peritoneal cavity
- **S31.102** Unspecified open wound of abdominal wall, epigastric region without penetration into peritoneal cavity
- **S31.103** Unspecified open wound of abdominal wall, right lower quadrant without penetration into peritoneal cavity
- **S31.104** Unspecified open wound of abdominal wall, left lower quadrant without penetration into peritoneal cavity
- **S31.105** Unspecified open wound of abdominal wall, periumbilic region without penetration into peritoneal cavity
- **S31.106** Unspecified open wound of abdominal wall, right flank without penetration into peritoneal cavity
- **S31.107** Unspecified open wound of abdominal wall, left flank without penetration into peritoneal cavity
- **S31.109** Unspecified open wound of abdominal wall, unspecified quadrant without penetration into peritoneal cavity
  Unspecified open wound of abdominal wall NOS
- **S31.10A** Unspecified open wound of abdominal wall, unspecified flank without penetration into peritoneal cavity
  Open wound of abdominal wall of flank NOS without penetration into peritoneal cavity

S31.11 Laceration without foreign body of abdominal wall without penetration into peritoneal cavity
- **S31.110** Laceration without foreign body of abdominal wall, right upper quadrant without penetration into peritoneal cavity
- **S31.111** Laceration without foreign body of abdominal wall, left upper quadrant without penetration into peritoneal cavity
- **S31.112** Laceration without foreign body of abdominal wall, epigastric region without penetration into peritoneal cavity
- **S31.113** Laceration without foreign body of abdominal wall, right lower quadrant without penetration into peritoneal cavity
- **S31.114** Laceration without foreign body of abdominal wall, left lower quadrant without penetration into peritoneal cavity
- **S31.115** Laceration without foreign body of abdominal wall, periumbilic region without penetration into peritoneal cavity
- **S31.116** Laceration without foreign body of abdominal wall, right flank without penetration into peritoneal cavity
- **S31.117** Laceration without foreign body of abdominal wall, left flank without penetration into peritoneal cavity
- **S31.119** Laceration without foreign body of abdominal wall, unspecified quadrant without penetration into peritoneal cavity
- **S31.11A** Laceration without foreign body of abdominal wall, unspecified flank without penetration into peritoneal cavity
  Laceration without foreign body of flank NOS without penetration into peritoneal cavity

S31.12 Laceration with foreign body of abdominal wall without penetration into peritoneal cavity
- **S31.120** Laceration of abdominal wall with foreign body, right upper quadrant without penetration into peritoneal cavity
- **S31.121** Laceration of abdominal wall with foreign body, left upper quadrant without penetration into peritoneal cavity
- **S31.122** Laceration of abdominal wall with foreign body, epigastric region without penetration into peritoneal cavity
- **S31.123** Laceration of abdominal wall with foreign body, right lower quadrant without penetration into peritoneal cavity
- **S31.124** Laceration of abdominal wall with foreign body, left lower quadrant without penetration into peritoneal cavity

- S31.125 Laceration of abdominal wall with foreign body, periumbilic region without penetration into peritoneal cavity
- S31.126 Laceration with foreign body of abdominal wall, right flank without penetration into peritoneal cavity
- S31.127 Laceration with foreign body of abdominal wall, left flank without penetration into peritoneal cavity
- S31.129 Laceration of abdominal wall with foreign body, unspecified quadrant without penetration into peritoneal cavity
- S31.12A Laceration with foreign body of abdominal wall unspecified flank without penetration into peritoneal cavity
  Laceration with foreign body of abdominal wall of flank NOS without penetration into peritoneal cavity

- S31.13 **Puncture wound** of abdominal wall **without foreign body** without penetration into peritoneal cavity
  - S31.130 Puncture wound of abdominal wall without foreign body, **right upper quadrant** without penetration into peritoneal cavity
  - S31.131 Puncture wound of abdominal wall without foreign body, **left upper quadrant** without penetration into peritoneal cavity
  - S31.132 Puncture wound of abdominal wall without foreign body, **epigastric region** without penetration into peritoneal cavity
  - S31.133 Puncture wound of abdominal wall without foreign body, **right lower quadrant** without penetration into peritoneal cavity
  - S31.134 Puncture wound of abdominal wall without foreign body, **left lower quadrant** without penetration into peritoneal cavity
  - S31.135 Puncture wound of abdominal wall without foreign body, **periumbilic region** without penetration into peritoneal cavity
  - S31.136 Puncture wound of abdominal wall without foreign body, **right flank** without penetration into peritoneal cavity
  - S31.137 Puncture wound of abdominal wall without foreign body, **left flank** without penetration into peritoneal cavity
  - S31.139 Puncture wound of abdominal wall without foreign body, unspecified quadrant without penetration into peritoneal cavity
  - S31.13A Puncture wound of abdominal wall without foreign body, unspecified flank without penetration into peritoneal cavity
    Puncture wound of abdominal wall of flank NOS without foreign body

- S31.14 **Puncture wound** of abdominal wall **with foreign body** without penetration into peritoneal cavity
  - S31.140 Puncture wound of abdominal wall with foreign body, **right upper quadrant** without penetration into peritoneal cavity
  - S31.141 Puncture wound of abdominal wall with foreign body, **left upper quadrant** without penetration into peritoneal cavity
  - S31.142 Puncture wound of abdominal wall with foreign body, **epigastric region** without penetration into peritoneal cavity
  - S31.143 Puncture wound of abdominal wall with foreign body, **right lower quadrant** without penetration into peritoneal cavity
  - S31.144 Puncture wound of abdominal wall with foreign body, **left lower quadrant** without penetration into peritoneal cavity
  - S31.145 Puncture wound of abdominal wall with foreign body, **periumbilic region** without penetration into peritoneal cavity
  - S31.146 Puncture wound of abdominal wall with foreign body, **right flank** without penetration into peritoneal cavity
  - S31.147 Puncture wound of abdominal wall with foreign body, **left flank** without penetration into peritoneal cavity
  - S31.149 Puncture wound of abdominal wall with foreign body, unspecified quadrant without penetration into peritoneal cavity
  - S31.14A Puncture wound of abdominal wall with foreign body, unspecified flank without penetration into peritoneal cavity
    Puncture wound of abdominal wall with foreign body of flank NOS without penetration into peritoneal cavity

- S31.15 **Open bite** of abdominal wall without penetration into peritoneal cavity
  Bite of abdominal wall NOS
  EXCLUDES 1 superficial bite of abdominal wall (S30.871)
  - S31.150 Open bite of abdominal wall, **right upper quadrant** without penetration into peritoneal cavity
  - S31.151 Open bite of abdominal wall, **left upper quadrant** without penetration into peritoneal cavity
  - S31.152 Open bite of abdominal wall, **epigastric region** without penetration into peritoneal cavity
  - S31.153 Open bite of abdominal wall, **right lower quadrant** without penetration into peritoneal cavity
  - S31.154 Open bite of abdominal wall, **left lower quadrant** without penetration into peritoneal cavity
  - S31.155 Open bite of abdominal wall, **periumbilic region** without penetration into peritoneal cavity
  - S31.156 Open bite of abdominal wall, **right flank** without penetration into peritoneal cavity
  - S31.157 Open bite of abdominal wall, **left flank** without penetration into peritoneal cavity
  - S31.159 Open bite of abdominal wall, unspecified quadrant without penetration into peritoneal cavity
  - S31.15A Open bite of abdominal wall, unspecified flank without penetration into peritoneal cavity
    Open bite of abdominal wall of flank NOS without penetration into peritoneal cavity

- S31.2 **Open wound of penis**
  - S31.20 Unspecified open wound of penis
  - S31.21 **Laceration without foreign body** of penis
  - S31.22 **Laceration with foreign body** of penis
  - S31.23 **Puncture wound without foreign body** of penis
  - S31.24 **Puncture wound with foreign body** of penis
  - S31.25 **Open bite** of penis
    Bite of penis NOS
    EXCLUDES 1 superficial bite of penis (S30.862, S30.872)

- S31.3 **Open wound of scrotum and testes**
  - S31.30 Unspecified open wound of scrotum and testes
  - S31.31 **Laceration without foreign body** of scrotum and testes
  - S31.32 **Laceration with foreign body** of scrotum and testes
  - S31.33 **Puncture wound without foreign body** of scrotum and testes
  - S31.34 **Puncture wound with foreign body** of scrotum and testes
  - S31.35 **Open bite** of scrotum and testes
    Bite of scrotum and testes NOS
    EXCLUDES 1 superficial bite of scrotum and testes (S30.863, S30.873)

- S31.4 **Open wound of vagina and vulva**
  EXCLUDES 1 injury to vagina and vulva during delivery (O70.-, O71.4)
  - S31.40 Unspecified open wound of vagina and vulva
  - S31.41 **Laceration without foreign body** of vagina and vulva
  - S31.42 **Laceration with foreign body** of vagina and vulva
  - S31.43 **Puncture wound without foreign body** of vagina and vulva
  - S31.44 **Puncture wound with foreign body** of vagina and vulva
  - S31.45 **Open bite** of vagina and vulva
    Bite of vagina and vulva NOS
    EXCLUDES 1 superficial bite of vagina and vulva (S30.864, S30.874)

S31.5 Open wound of unspecified external genital organs

EXCLUDES 1: traumatic amputation of external genital organs (S38.21, S38.22)

- **S31.50** Unspecified open wound of unspecified external genital organs
  - **S31.501** Unspecified open wound of unspecified external genital organs, male
  - **S31.502** Unspecified open wound of unspecified external genital organs, female
- **S31.51** Laceration without foreign body of unspecified external genital organs
  - **S31.511** Laceration without foreign body of unspecified external genital organs, male
  - **S31.512** Laceration without foreign body of unspecified external genital organs, female
- **S31.52** Laceration with foreign body of unspecified external genital organs
  - **S31.521** Laceration with foreign body of unspecified external genital organs, male
  - **S31.522** Laceration with foreign body of unspecified external genital organs, female
- **S31.53** Puncture wound without foreign body of unspecified external genital organs
  - **S31.531** Puncture wound without foreign body of unspecified external genital organs, male
  - **S31.532** Puncture wound without foreign body of unspecified external genital organs, female
- **S31.54** Puncture wound with foreign body of unspecified external genital organs
  - **S31.541** Puncture wound with foreign body of unspecified external genital organs, male
  - **S31.542** Puncture wound with foreign body of unspecified external genital organs, female
- **S31.55** Open bite of unspecified external genital organs

  Bite of unspecified external genital organs NOS

  EXCLUDES 1: superficial bite of unspecified external genital organs (S30.865, S30.866, S30.875, S30.876)
  - **S31.551** Open bite of unspecified external genital organs, male
  - **S31.552** Open bite of unspecified external genital organs, female

S31.6 Open wound of abdominal wall with penetration into peritoneal cavity

AHA: 2023,3Q,8

- **S31.60** Unspecified open wound of abdominal wall with penetration into peritoneal cavity
  - **S31.600** Unspecified open wound of abdominal wall, right upper quadrant with penetration into peritoneal cavity
  - **S31.601** Unspecified open wound of abdominal wall, left upper quadrant with penetration into peritoneal cavity
  - **S31.602** Unspecified open wound of abdominal wall, epigastric region with penetration into peritoneal cavity
  - **S31.603** Unspecified open wound of abdominal wall, right lower quadrant with penetration into peritoneal cavity
  - **S31.604** Unspecified open wound of abdominal wall, left lower quadrant with penetration into peritoneal cavity
  - **S31.605** Unspecified open wound of abdominal wall, periumbilic region with penetration into peritoneal cavity
  - **S31.606** Unspecified open wound of abdominal wall, right flank with penetration into peritoneal cavity
  - **S31.607** Unspecified open wound of abdominal wall, left flank with penetration into peritoneal cavity
  - **S31.609** Unspecified open wound of abdominal wall, unspecified quadrant with penetration into peritoneal cavity
  - **S31.60A** Unspecified open wound of abdominal wall, unspecified flank with penetration into peritoneal cavity

    Unspecified open wound of abdominal wall of flank NOS, with penetration into peritoneal cavity
- **S31.61** Laceration without foreign body of abdominal wall with penetration into peritoneal cavity
  - **S31.610** Laceration without foreign body of abdominal wall, right upper quadrant with penetration into peritoneal cavity
  - **S31.611** Laceration without foreign body of abdominal wall, left upper quadrant with penetration into peritoneal cavity
  - **S31.612** Laceration without foreign body of abdominal wall, epigastric region with penetration into peritoneal cavity
  - **S31.613** Laceration without foreign body of abdominal wall, right lower quadrant with penetration into peritoneal cavity
  - **S31.614** Laceration without foreign body of abdominal wall, left lower quadrant with penetration into peritoneal cavity
  - **S31.615** Laceration without foreign body of abdominal wall, periumbilic region with penetration into peritoneal cavity
  - **S31.616** Laceration without foreign body of abdominal wall, right flank with penetration into peritoneal cavity
  - **S31.617** Laceration without foreign body of abdominal wall, left flank with penetration into peritoneal cavity
  - **S31.619** Laceration without foreign body of abdominal wall, unspecified quadrant with penetration into peritoneal cavity
  - **S31.61A** Laceration without foreign body of abdominal wall, unspecified flank with penetration into peritoneal cavity

    Laceration without foreign body of abdominal wall of flank NOS, with penetration into peritoneal cavity
- **S31.62** Laceration with foreign body of abdominal wall with penetration into peritoneal cavity
  - **S31.620** Laceration with foreign body of abdominal wall, right upper quadrant with penetration into peritoneal cavity
  - **S31.621** Laceration with foreign body of abdominal wall, left upper quadrant with penetration into peritoneal cavity
  - **S31.622** Laceration with foreign body of abdominal wall, epigastric region with penetration into peritoneal cavity
  - **S31.623** Laceration with foreign body of abdominal wall, right lower quadrant with penetration into peritoneal cavity
  - **S31.624** Laceration with foreign body of abdominal wall, left lower quadrant with penetration into peritoneal cavity
  - **S31.625** Laceration with foreign body of abdominal wall, periumbilic region with penetration into peritoneal cavity
  - **S31.626** Laceration with foreign body of abdominal wall, right flank with penetration into peritoneal cavity
  - **S31.627** Laceration with foreign body of abdominal wall, left flank with penetration into peritoneal cavity
  - **S31.629** Laceration with foreign body of abdominal wall, unspecified quadrant with penetration into peritoneal cavity
  - **S31.62A** Laceration with foreign body of abdominal wall, unspecified flank with penetration into peritoneal cavity

    Laceration with foreign body of abdominal wall, flank NOS, with penetration into peritoneal cavity
- **S31.63** Puncture wound without foreign body of abdominal wall with penetration into peritoneal cavity
  - **S31.630** Puncture wound without foreign body of abdominal wall, right upper quadrant with penetration into peritoneal cavity
  - **S31.631** Puncture wound without foreign body of abdominal wall, left upper quadrant with penetration into peritoneal cavity

Chapter 19. Injury, Poisoning and Certain Other Consequences of External Causes

- ✓7th **S31.632** Puncture wound without foreign body of abdominal wall, *epigastric region* with penetration into peritoneal cavity
- ✓7th **S31.633** Puncture wound without foreign body of abdominal wall, *right lower quadrant* with penetration into peritoneal cavity
- ✓7th **S31.634** Puncture wound without foreign body of abdominal wall, *left lower quadrant* with penetration into peritoneal cavity
- ✓7th **S31.635** Puncture wound without foreign body of abdominal wall, *periumbilic region* with penetration into peritoneal cavity
- • ✓7th **S31.636** Puncture wound of abdominal wall without foreign body, *right flank* with penetration into peritoneal cavity
- • ✓7th **S31.637** Puncture wound of abdominal wall without foreign body, *left flank* with penetration into peritoneal cavity
- ✓7th **S31.639** Puncture wound without foreign body of abdominal wall, unspecified quadrant with penetration into peritoneal cavity
- • ✓7th **S31.63A** Puncture wound of abdominal wall without foreign body, unspecified flank with penetration into peritoneal cavity
   - Puncture wound of abdominal wall without foreign body, flank NOS, with penetration into peritoneal cavity

- ✓6th **S31.64** **Puncture wound with foreign body** of abdominal wall with penetration into peritoneal cavity
  - ✓7th **S31.640** Puncture wound with foreign body of abdominal wall, *right upper quadrant* with penetration into peritoneal cavity
  - ✓7th **S31.641** Puncture wound with foreign body of abdominal wall, *left upper quadrant* with penetration into peritoneal cavity
  - ✓7th **S31.642** Puncture wound with foreign body of abdominal wall, *epigastric region* with penetration into peritoneal cavity
  - ✓7th **S31.643** Puncture wound with foreign body of abdominal wall, *right lower quadrant* with penetration into peritoneal cavity
  - ✓7th **S31.644** Puncture wound with foreign body of abdominal wall, *left lower quadrant* with penetration into peritoneal cavity
  - ✓7th **S31.645** Puncture wound with foreign body of abdominal wall, *periumbilic region* with penetration into peritoneal cavity
  - • ✓7th **S31.646** Puncture wound of abdominal wall with foreign body, *right flank* with penetration into peritoneal cavity
  - • ✓7th **S31.647** Puncture wound of abdominal wall with foreign body, *left flank* with penetration into peritoneal cavity
  - ✓7th **S31.649** Puncture wound with foreign body of abdominal wall, unspecified quadrant with penetration into peritoneal cavity
  - • ✓7th **S31.64A** Puncture wound of abdominal wall with foreign body, unspecified flank with penetration into peritoneal cavity
    - Puncture wound of abdominal wall with foreign body, flank NOS, with penetration into peritoneal cavity

- ✓6th **S31.65** **Open bite** of abdominal wall with penetration into peritoneal cavity
   - **EXCLUDES 1** *superficial bite of abdominal wall (S30.861, S30.871)*
  - ✓7th **S31.650** Open bite of abdominal wall, *right upper quadrant* with penetration into peritoneal cavity
  - ✓7th **S31.651** Open bite of abdominal wall, *left upper quadrant* with penetration into peritoneal cavity
  - ✓7th **S31.652** Open bite of abdominal wall, *epigastric region* with penetration into peritoneal cavity
  - ✓7th **S31.653** Open bite of abdominal wall, *right lower quadrant* with penetration into peritoneal cavity
  - ✓7th **S31.654** Open bite of abdominal wall, *left lower quadrant* with penetration into peritoneal cavity
  - ✓7th **S31.655** Open bite of abdominal wall, *periumbilic region* with penetration into peritoneal cavity
  - • ✓7th **S31.656** Open bite of abdominal wall, *right flank* with penetration into peritoneal cavity
  - • ✓7th **S31.657** Open bite of abdominal wall, *left flank* with penetration into peritoneal cavity
  - ✓7th **S31.659** Open bite of abdominal wall, unspecified quadrant with penetration into peritoneal cavity
  - • ✓7th **S31.65A** Open bite of abdominal wall, unspecified flank with penetration into peritoneal cavity
    - Open bite of abdominal wall, flank NOS, with penetration into peritoneal cavity

- ✓5th **S31.8** Open wound of other parts of abdomen, lower back and pelvis
  - ✓6th **S31.80** Open wound of unspecified buttock
    - ✓7th **S31.801** **Laceration without foreign body** of unspecified buttock
    - ✓7th **S31.802** **Laceration with foreign body** of unspecified buttock
    - ✓7th **S31.803** **Puncture wound without foreign body** of unspecified buttock
    - ✓7th **S31.804** **Puncture wound with foreign body** of unspecified buttock
    - ✓7th **S31.805** **Open bite** of unspecified buttock
      - Bite of buttock NOS
      - **EXCLUDES 1** *superficial bite of buttock (S30.870)*
    - ✓7th **S31.809** Unspecified open wound of unspecified buttock
  - ✓6th **S31.81** Open wound of right buttock
    - ✓7th **S31.811** **Laceration without foreign body** of right buttock
    - ✓7th **S31.812** **Laceration with foreign body** of right buttock
    - ✓7th **S31.813** **Puncture wound without foreign body** of right buttock
    - ✓7th **S31.814** **Puncture wound with foreign body** of right buttock
    - ✓7th **S31.815** **Open bite** of right buttock
      - Bite of right buttock NOS
      - **EXCLUDES 1** *superficial bite of buttock (S30.870)*
    - ✓7th **S31.819** Unspecified open wound of right buttock
  - ✓6th **S31.82** Open wound of left buttock
    - ✓7th **S31.821** **Laceration without foreign body** of left buttock
    - ✓7th **S31.822** **Laceration with foreign body** of left buttock
    - ✓7th **S31.823** **Puncture wound without foreign body** of left buttock
    - ✓7th **S31.824** **Puncture wound with foreign body** of left buttock
    - ✓7th **S31.825** **Open bite** of left buttock
      - Bite of left buttock NOS
      - **EXCLUDES 1** *superficial bite of buttock (S30.870)*
    - ✓7th **S31.829** Unspecified open wound of left buttock
  - ✓6th **S31.83** Open wound of anus
    - ✓7th **S31.831** **Laceration without foreign body** of anus
    - ✓7th **S31.832** **Laceration with foreign body** of anus
    - ✓7th **S31.833** **Puncture wound without foreign body** of anus
    - ✓7th **S31.834** **Puncture wound with foreign body** of anus
    - ✓7th **S31.835** **Open bite** of anus
      - Bite of anus NOS
      - **EXCLUDES 1** *superficial bite of anus (S30.877)*
    - ✓7th **S31.839** Unspecified open wound of anus

Chapter 19. Injury, Poisoning and Certain Other Consequences of External Causes

✓4th S32 Fracture of lumbar spine and pelvis

NOTE A fracture not indicated as displaced or nondisplaced should be coded to displaced.

A fracture not indicated as opened or closed should be coded to closed.

INCLUDES
fracture of lumbosacral neural arch
fracture of lumbosacral spinous process
fracture of lumbosacral transverse process
fracture of lumbosacral vertebra
fracture of lumbosacral vertebral arch

Code first any associated spinal cord and spinal nerve injury (S34.-)
EXCLUDES 1 transection of abdomen (S38.3)
EXCLUDES 2 fracture of hip NOS (S72.0-)
AHA: 2021,1Q,6; 2018,2Q,12; 2015,3Q,37-39; 2012,4Q,93

The appropriate 7th character is to be added to each code from category S32.
- A initial encounter for closed fracture
- B initial encounter for open fracture
- D subsequent encounter for fracture with routine healing
- G subsequent encounter for fracture with delayed healing
- K subsequent encounter for fracture with nonunion
- S sequela

✓5th S32.0 Fracture of lumbar vertebra
Fracture of lumbar spine NOS

✓6th S32.00 Fracture of unspecified lumbar vertebra
- ✓7th S32.000 Wedge compression fracture of unspecified lumbar vertebra [HCC] [ESR] [COM] [Q]
- ✓7th S32.001 Stable burst fracture of unspecified lumbar vertebra [HCC] [ESR] [COM] [Q]
- ✓7th S32.002 Unstable burst fracture of unspecified lumbar vertebra [HCC] [ESR] [COM] [Q]
- ✓7th S32.008 Other fracture of unspecified lumbar vertebra
- ✓7th S32.009 Unspecified fracture of unspecified lumbar vertebra

✓6th S32.01 Fracture of first lumbar vertebra
- ✓7th S32.010 Wedge compression fracture of first lumbar vertebra [HCC] [ESR] [COM] [Q]
- ✓7th S32.011 Stable burst fracture of first lumbar vertebra [HCC] [ESR] [COM] [Q]
- ✓7th S32.012 Unstable burst fracture of first lumbar vertebra [HCC] [ESR] [COM] [Q]
- ✓7th S32.018 Other fracture of first lumbar vertebra [HCC] [ESR] [COM] [Q]
- ✓7th S32.019 Unspecified fracture of first lumbar vertebra [HCC] [ESR] [COM] [Q]

✓6th S32.02 Fracture of second lumbar vertebra
- ✓7th S32.020 Wedge compression fracture of second lumbar vertebra [HCC] [ESR] [COM] [Q]
- ✓7th S32.021 Stable burst fracture of second lumbar vertebra [HCC] [ESR] [COM] [Q]
- ✓7th S32.022 Unstable burst fracture of second lumbar vertebra [HCC] [ESR] [COM] [Q]
- ✓7th S32.028 Other fracture of second lumbar vertebra [HCC] [ESR] [COM] [Q]
- ✓7th S32.029 Unspecified fracture of second lumbar vertebra [HCC] [ESR] [COM] [Q]

✓6th S32.03 Fracture of third lumbar vertebra
- ✓7th S32.030 Wedge compression fracture of third lumbar vertebra [HCC] [ESR] [COM] [Q]
- ✓7th S32.031 Stable burst fracture of third lumbar vertebra [HCC] [ESR] [COM] [Q]
- ✓7th S32.032 Unstable burst fracture of third lumbar vertebra [HCC] [ESR] [COM] [Q]
- ✓7th S32.038 Other fracture of third lumbar vertebra [HCC] [ESR] [COM] [Q]
- ✓7th S32.039 Unspecified fracture of third lumbar vertebra [HCC] [ESR] [COM] [Q]

✓6th S32.04 Fracture of fourth lumbar vertebra
- ✓7th S32.040 Wedge compression fracture of fourth lumbar vertebra [HCC] [ESR] [COM] [Q]
- ✓7th S32.041 Stable burst fracture of fourth lumbar vertebra [HCC] [ESR] [COM] [Q]
- ✓7th S32.042 Unstable burst fracture of fourth lumbar vertebra [HCC] [ESR] [COM] [Q]
- ✓7th S32.048 Other fracture of fourth lumbar vertebra [HCC] [ESR] [COM] [Q]
- ✓7th S32.049 Unspecified fracture of fourth lumbar vertebra [HCC] [ESR] [COM] [Q]

✓6th S32.05 Fracture of fifth lumbar vertebra
- ✓7th S32.050 Wedge compression fracture of fifth lumbar vertebra [HCC] [ESR] [COM] [Q]
- ✓7th S32.051 Stable burst fracture of fifth lumbar vertebra [HCC] [ESR] [COM] [Q]
- ✓7th S32.052 Unstable burst fracture of fifth lumbar vertebra [HCC] [ESR] [COM] [Q]
- ✓7th S32.058 Other fracture of fifth lumbar vertebra [HCC] [ESR] [COM] [Q]
- ✓7th S32.059 Unspecified fracture of fifth lumbar vertebra [HCC] [ESR] [COM] [Q]

✓5th S32.1 Fracture of sacrum
NOTE For vertical fractures, code to most medial fracture extension

Use two codes if both a vertical and transverse fracture are present

Code also any associated fracture of pelvic ring (S32.8-)

- ✓x 7th S32.10 Unspecified fracture of sacrum [HCC] [ESR] [COM] [Q]

✓6th S32.11 Zone I fracture of sacrum
Vertical sacral ala fracture of sacrum

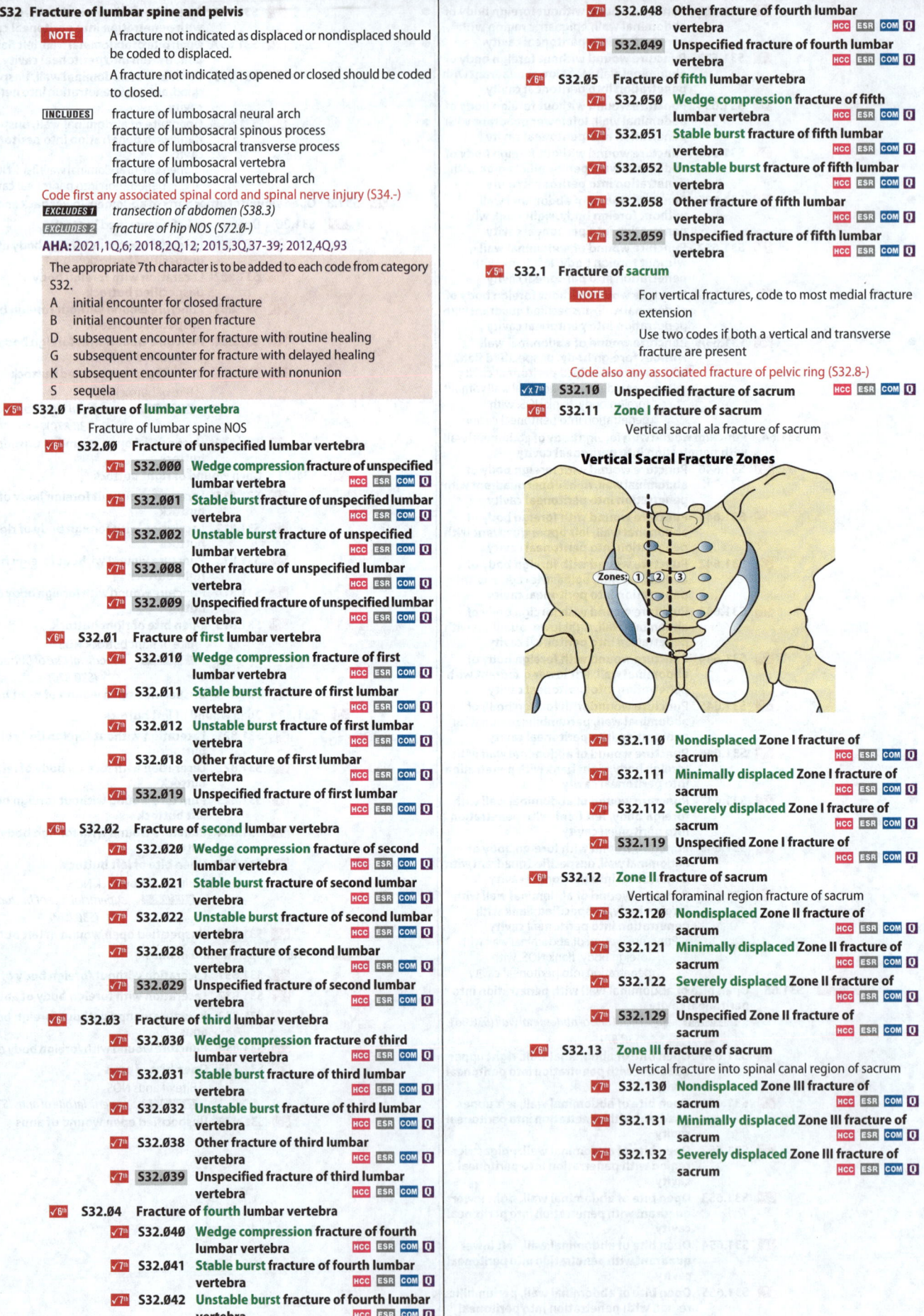

Vertical Sacral Fracture Zones
Zones: ① ② ③

- ✓7th S32.110 Nondisplaced Zone I fracture of sacrum [HCC] [ESR] [COM] [Q]
- ✓7th S32.111 Minimally displaced Zone I fracture of sacrum [HCC] [ESR] [COM] [Q]
- ✓7th S32.112 Severely displaced Zone I fracture of sacrum [HCC] [ESR] [COM] [Q]
- ✓7th S32.119 Unspecified Zone I fracture of sacrum [HCC] [ESR] [COM] [Q]

✓6th S32.12 Zone II fracture of sacrum
Vertical foraminal region fracture of sacrum
- ✓7th S32.120 Nondisplaced Zone II fracture of sacrum [HCC] [ESR] [COM] [Q]
- ✓7th S32.121 Minimally displaced Zone II fracture of sacrum [HCC] [ESR] [COM] [Q]
- ✓7th S32.122 Severely displaced Zone II fracture of sacrum [HCC] [ESR] [COM] [Q]
- ✓7th S32.129 Unspecified Zone II fracture of sacrum [HCC] [ESR] [COM] [Q]

✓6th S32.13 Zone III fracture of sacrum
Vertical fracture into spinal canal region of sacrum
- ✓7th S32.130 Nondisplaced Zone III fracture of sacrum [HCC] [ESR] [COM] [Q]
- ✓7th S32.131 Minimally displaced Zone III fracture of sacrum [HCC] [ESR] [COM] [Q]
- ✓7th S32.132 Severely displaced Zone III fracture of sacrum [HCC] [ESR] [COM] [Q]

[HCC] CMS-HCC   [Rx] Rx HCC   [ESR] ESRD HCC   [COM] Commercial HCC   [N] Newborn: 0   [P] Pediatric: 0-17   [M] Maternity: 9-64   [A] Adult: 15-124

	S32.139	Unspecified Zone III fracture of sacrum

Transverse Sacral Fracture Types

Type 1   Type 2   Type 3   Type 4

	S32.14	**Type 1** fracture of sacrum

Transverse flexion fracture of sacrum without displacement

	S32.15	**Type 2** fracture of sacrum

Transverse flexion fracture of sacrum with posterior displacement

	S32.16	**Type 3** fracture of sacrum

Transverse extension fracture of sacrum with anterior displacement

	S32.17	**Type 4** fracture of sacrum

Transverse segmental comminution of upper sacrum

	S32.19	Other fracture of sacrum
	S32.2	Fracture of **coccyx**
	S32.3	Fracture of **ilium**

EXCLUDES 1: fracture of ilium with associated disruption of pelvic ring (S32.8-)

- S32.30 Unspecified fracture of ilium
  - S32.301 Unspecified fracture of **right** ilium
  - S32.302 Unspecified fracture of **left** ilium
  - S32.309 Unspecified fracture of unspecified ilium
- S32.31 **Avulsion** fracture of ilium
  - S32.311 **Displaced** avulsion fracture of **right** ilium
  - S32.312 **Displaced** avulsion fracture of **left** ilium
  - S32.313 **Displaced** avulsion fracture of unspecified ilium
  - S32.314 **Nondisplaced** avulsion fracture of **right** ilium
  - S32.315 **Nondisplaced** avulsion fracture of **left** ilium
  - S32.316 **Nondisplaced** avulsion fracture of unspecified ilium
- S32.39 Other fracture of ilium
  - S32.391 Other fracture of **right** ilium
  - S32.392 Other fracture of **left** ilium
  - S32.399 Other fracture of unspecified ilium
- S32.4 Fracture of **acetabulum**

Code also any associated fracture of pelvic ring (S32.8-)
AHA: 2016,3Q,16

- S32.40 Unspecified fracture of acetabulum
  - S32.401 Unspecified fracture of **right** acetabulum
  - S32.402 Unspecified fracture of **left** acetabulum
  - S32.409 Unspecified fracture of unspecified acetabulum
- S32.41 Fracture of **anterior wall** of acetabulum
  - S32.411 **Displaced** fracture of anterior wall of **right** acetabulum
  - S32.412 **Displaced** fracture of anterior wall of **left** acetabulum
  - S32.413 **Displaced** fracture of anterior wall of unspecified acetabulum
  - S32.414 **Nondisplaced** fracture of anterior wall of **right** acetabulum
  - S32.415 **Nondisplaced** fracture of anterior wall of **left** acetabulum
  - S32.416 **Nondisplaced** fracture of anterior wall of unspecified acetabulum
- S32.42 Fracture of **posterior wall** of acetabulum
  - S32.421 **Displaced** fracture of posterior wall of **right** acetabulum
  - S32.422 **Displaced** fracture of posterior wall of **left** acetabulum
  - S32.423 **Displaced** fracture of posterior wall of unspecified acetabulum
  - S32.424 **Nondisplaced** fracture of posterior wall of **right** acetabulum
  - S32.425 **Nondisplaced** fracture of posterior wall of **left** acetabulum
  - S32.426 **Nondisplaced** fracture of posterior wall of unspecified acetabulum
- S32.43 Fracture of **anterior column** [iliopubic] of acetabulum
  - S32.431 **Displaced** fracture of anterior column [iliopubic] of **right** acetabulum
  - S32.432 **Displaced** fracture of anterior column [iliopubic] of **left** acetabulum
  - S32.433 **Displaced** fracture of anterior column [iliopubic] of unspecified acetabulum
  - S32.434 **Nondisplaced** fracture of anterior column [iliopubic] of **right** acetabulum
  - S32.435 **Nondisplaced** fracture of anterior column [iliopubic] of **left** acetabulum
  - S32.436 **Nondisplaced** fracture of anterior column [iliopubic] of unspecified acetabulum
- S32.44 Fracture of **posterior column** [ilioischial] of acetabulum
  - S32.441 **Displaced** fracture of posterior column [ilioischial] of **right** acetabulum
  - S32.442 **Displaced** fracture of posterior column [ilioischial] of **left** acetabulum
  - S32.443 **Displaced** fracture of posterior column [ilioischial] of unspecified acetabulum
  - S32.444 **Nondisplaced** fracture of posterior column [ilioischial] of **right** acetabulum
  - S32.445 **Nondisplaced** fracture of posterior column [ilioischial] of **left** acetabulum
  - S32.446 **Nondisplaced** fracture of posterior column [ilioischial] of unspecified acetabulum
- S32.45 **Transverse** fracture of acetabulum
  - S32.451 **Displaced** transverse fracture of **right** acetabulum
  - S32.452 **Displaced** transverse fracture of **left** acetabulum
  - S32.453 **Displaced** transverse fracture of unspecified acetabulum
  - S32.454 **Nondisplaced** transverse fracture of **right** acetabulum
  - S32.455 **Nondisplaced** transverse fracture of **left** acetabulum
  - S32.456 **Nondisplaced** transverse fracture of unspecified acetabulum
- S32.46 **Associated transverse-posterior** fracture of acetabulum
  - S32.461 **Displaced** associated transverse-posterior fracture of **right** acetabulum

S32.462–S32.9 — Chapter 19. Injury, Poisoning and Certain Other Consequences of External Causes

- √7th **S32.462** Displaced associated transverse-posterior fracture of left acetabulum
- √7th **S32.463** Displaced associated transverse-posterior fracture of unspecified acetabulum
- √7th **S32.464** Nondisplaced associated transverse-posterior fracture of right acetabulum
- √7th **S32.465** Nondisplaced associated transverse-posterior fracture of left acetabulum
- √7th **S32.466** Nondisplaced associated transverse-posterior fracture of unspecified acetabulum
- √6th **S32.47** Fracture of medial wall of acetabulum
  - √7th **S32.471** Displaced fracture of medial wall of right acetabulum
  - √7th **S32.472** Displaced fracture of medial wall of left acetabulum
  - √7th **S32.473** Displaced fracture of medial wall of unspecified acetabulum
  - √7th **S32.474** Nondisplaced fracture of medial wall of right acetabulum
  - √7th **S32.475** Nondisplaced fracture of medial wall of left acetabulum
  - √7th **S32.476** Nondisplaced fracture of medial wall of unspecified acetabulum
- √6th **S32.48** Dome fracture of acetabulum
  - √7th **S32.481** Displaced dome fracture of right acetabulum
  - √7th **S32.482** Displaced dome fracture of left acetabulum
  - √7th **S32.483** Displaced dome fracture of unspecified acetabulum
  - √7th **S32.484** Nondisplaced dome fracture of right acetabulum
  - √7th **S32.485** Nondisplaced dome fracture of left acetabulum
  - √7th **S32.486** Nondisplaced dome fracture of unspecified acetabulum
- √6th **S32.49** Other specified fracture of acetabulum
  - √7th **S32.491** Other specified fracture of right acetabulum
  - √7th **S32.492** Other specified fracture of left acetabulum
  - √7th **S32.499** Other specified fracture of unspecified acetabulum
- √5th **S32.5** Fracture of pubis
  - EXCLUDES 1: fracture of pubis with associated disruption of pelvic ring (S32.8-)
  - √6th **S32.50** Unspecified fracture of pubis
    - √7th **S32.501** Unspecified fracture of right pubis
    - √7th **S32.502** Unspecified fracture of left pubis
    - √7th **S32.509** Unspecified fracture of unspecified pubis
  - √6th **S32.51** Fracture of superior rim of pubis
    - √7th **S32.511** Fracture of superior rim of right pubis
    - √7th **S32.512** Fracture of superior rim of left pubis
    - √7th **S32.519** Fracture of superior rim of unspecified pubis
  - √6th **S32.59** Other specified fracture of pubis
    - √7th **S32.591** Other specified fracture of right pubis
    - √7th **S32.592** Other specified fracture of left pubis
    - √7th **S32.599** Other specified fracture of unspecified pubis

- √5th **S32.6** Fracture of ischium
  - EXCLUDES 1: fracture of ischium with associated disruption of pelvic ring (S32.8-)
  - √6th **S32.60** Unspecified fracture of ischium
    - √7th **S32.601** Unspecified fracture of right ischium
    - √7th **S32.602** Unspecified fracture of left ischium
    - √7th **S32.609** Unspecified fracture of unspecified ischium
  - √6th **S32.61** Avulsion fracture of ischium
    - √7th **S32.611** Displaced avulsion fracture of right ischium
    - √7th **S32.612** Displaced avulsion fracture of left ischium
    - √7th **S32.613** Displaced avulsion fracture of unspecified ischium
    - √7th **S32.614** Nondisplaced avulsion fracture of right ischium
    - √7th **S32.615** Nondisplaced avulsion fracture of left ischium
    - √7th **S32.616** Nondisplaced avulsion fracture of unspecified ischium
  - √6th **S32.69** Other specified fracture of ischium
    - √7th **S32.691** Other specified fracture of right ischium
    - √7th **S32.692** Other specified fracture of left ischium
    - √7th **S32.699** Other specified fracture of unspecified ischium
- √5th **S32.8** Fracture of other parts of pelvis
  - Code also any associated:
    fracture of acetabulum (S32.4-)
    sacral fracture (S32.1-)

  Fractures Disrupting Pelvic Circle
  Pelvic circle — Stable
  Unstable (two-place fracture)
  Pelvic Bones: Iliac crest, Anterior superior iliac spine, Ischial spine, Acetabulum, Femur, Ilium, L5, Sacrum, Coccyx, Pubis, Ischium, Pubic symphysis

  - √6th **S32.81** Multiple fractures of pelvis with disruption of pelvic ring
    Multiple pelvic fractures with disruption of pelvic circle
    - √7th **S32.810** Multiple fractures of pelvis with stable disruption of pelvic ring
    - √7th **S32.811** Multiple fractures of pelvis with unstable disruption of pelvic ring
  - √x7th **S32.82** Multiple fractures of pelvis without disruption of pelvic ring
    Multiple pelvic fractures without disruption of pelvic circle
  - √x7th **S32.89** Fracture of other parts of pelvis
- √x7th **S32.9** Fracture of unspecified parts of lumbosacral spine and pelvis
  Fracture of lumbosacral spine NOS
  Fracture of pelvis NOS
  AHA: 2012,4Q,93

S33 Dislocation and sprain of joints and ligaments of lumbar spine and pelvis

INCLUDES
- avulsion of joint or ligament of lumbar spine and pelvis
- laceration of cartilage, joint or ligament of lumbar spine and pelvis
- sprain of cartilage, joint or ligament of lumbar spine and pelvis
- traumatic hemarthrosis of joint or ligament of lumbar spine and pelvis
- traumatic rupture of joint or ligament of lumbar spine and pelvis
- traumatic subluxation of joint or ligament of lumbar spine and pelvis
- traumatic tear of joint or ligament of lumbar spine and pelvis

Code also any associated open wound

EXCLUDES 1
- nontraumatic rupture or displacement of lumbar intervertebral disc NOS (M51.-)
- obstetric damage to pelvic joints and ligaments (O71.6)

EXCLUDES 2
- dislocation and sprain of joints and ligaments of hip (S73.-)
- strain of muscle of lower back and pelvis (S39.01-)

The appropriate 7th character is to be added to each code from category S33.
- A initial encounter
- D subsequent encounter
- S sequela

S33.0 Traumatic rupture of lumbar intervertebral disc

EXCLUDES 1 rupture or displacement (nontraumatic) of lumbar intervertebral disc NOS (M51.- with fifth character 6)

S33.1 Subluxation and dislocation of lumbar vertebra

Code also any associated:
- open wound of abdomen, lower back and pelvis (S31)
- spinal cord injury (S24.0, S24.1-, S34.0-, S34.1-)

EXCLUDES 2 fracture of lumbar vertebrae (S32.0-)

- **S33.10** Subluxation and dislocation of unspecified lumbar vertebra
  - **S33.100** Subluxation of unspecified lumbar vertebra
  - **S33.101** Dislocation of unspecified lumbar vertebra
- **S33.11** Subluxation and dislocation of L1/L2 lumbar vertebra
  - **S33.110** Subluxation of L1/L2 lumbar vertebra
  - **S33.111** Dislocation of L1/L2 lumbar vertebra
- **S33.12** Subluxation and dislocation of L2/L3 lumbar vertebra
  - **S33.120** Subluxation of L2/L3 lumbar vertebra
  - **S33.121** Dislocation of L2/L3 lumbar vertebra
- **S33.13** Subluxation and dislocation of L3/L4 lumbar vertebra
  - **S33.130** Subluxation of L3/L4 lumbar vertebra
  - **S33.131** Dislocation of L3/L4 lumbar vertebra
- **S33.14** Subluxation and dislocation of L4/L5 lumbar vertebra
  - **S33.140** Subluxation of L4/L5 lumbar vertebra
  - **S33.141** Dislocation of L4/L5 lumbar vertebra

S33.2 Dislocation of sacroiliac and sacrococcygeal joint

S33.3 Dislocation of other and unspecified parts of lumbar spine and pelvis
- **S33.30** Dislocation of unspecified parts of lumbar spine and pelvis
- **S33.39** Dislocation of other parts of lumbar spine and pelvis

S33.4 Traumatic rupture of symphysis pubis

S33.5 Sprain of ligaments of lumbar spine

S33.6 Sprain of sacroiliac joint

S33.8 Sprain of other parts of lumbar spine and pelvis

S33.9 Sprain of unspecified parts of lumbar spine and pelvis

S34 Injury of lumbar and sacral spinal cord and nerves at abdomen, lower back and pelvis level

NOTE Code to highest level of lumbar cord injury.

Injuries to the spinal cord (S34.0 and S34.1) refer to the cord level and not bone level injury, and can affect nerve roots at and below the level given.

Code also any associated:
- fracture of vertebra (S22.0-, S32.0-)
- open wound of abdomen, lower back and pelvis (S31.-)
- transient paralysis (R29.5)

The appropriate 7th character is to be added to each code from category S34.
- A initial encounter
- D subsequent encounter
- S sequela

S34.0 Concussion and edema of lumbar and sacral spinal cord
- **S34.01** Concussion and edema of lumbar spinal cord
- **S34.02** Concussion and edema of sacral spinal cord
  - Concussion and edema of conus medullaris

S34.1 Other and unspecified injury of lumbar and sacral spinal cord
- **S34.10** Unspecified injury to lumbar spinal cord
  - **S34.101** Unspecified injury to L1 level of lumbar spinal cord
    - Unspecified injury to lumbar spinal cord level 1
  - **S34.102** Unspecified injury to L2 level of lumbar spinal cord
    - Unspecified injury to lumbar spinal cord level 2
  - **S34.103** Unspecified injury to L3 level of lumbar spinal cord
    - Unspecified injury to lumbar spinal cord level 3
  - **S34.104** Unspecified injury to L4 level of lumbar spinal cord
    - Unspecified injury to lumbar spinal cord level 4
  - **S34.105** Unspecified injury to L5 level of lumbar spinal cord
    - Unspecified injury to lumbar spinal cord level 5
  - **S34.109** Unspecified injury to unspecified level of lumbar spinal cord
- **S34.11** Complete lesion of lumbar spinal cord
  - **S34.111** Complete lesion of L1 level of lumbar spinal cord
    - Complete lesion of lumbar spinal cord level 1
  - **S34.112** Complete lesion of L2 level of lumbar spinal cord
    - Complete lesion of lumbar spinal cord level 2
  - **S34.113** Complete lesion of L3 level of lumbar spinal cord
    - Complete lesion of lumbar spinal cord level 3
  - **S34.114** Complete lesion of L4 level of lumbar spinal cord
    - Complete lesion of lumbar spinal cord level 4
  - **S34.115** Complete lesion of L5 level of lumbar spinal cord
    - Complete lesion of lumbar spinal cord level 5
  - **S34.119** Complete lesion of unspecified level of lumbar spinal cord
- **S34.12** Incomplete lesion of lumbar spinal cord
  - **S34.121** Incomplete lesion of L1 level of lumbar spinal cord
    - Incomplete lesion of lumbar spinal cord level 1
  - **S34.122** Incomplete lesion of L2 level of lumbar spinal cord
    - Incomplete lesion of lumbar spinal cord level 2

Chapter 19. Injury, Poisoning and Certain Other Consequences of External Causes

- ☑7th **S34.123** Incomplete lesion of L3 level of lumbar spinal cord [HCC] [ESR] [COM]
  - Incomplete lesion of lumbar spinal cord level 3
- ☑7th **S34.124** Incomplete lesion of L4 level of lumbar spinal cord [HCC] [ESR] [COM]
  - Incomplete lesion of lumbar spinal cord level 4
- ☑7th **S34.125** Incomplete lesion of L5 level of lumbar spinal cord [HCC] [ESR] [COM]
  - Incomplete lesion of lumbar spinal cord level 5
- ☑7th **S34.129** Incomplete lesion of unspecified level of lumbar spinal cord [HCC] [ESR] [COM]
- ☑6th **S34.13** Other and unspecified injury to sacral spinal cord
  - Other injury to conus medullaris
  - ☑7th **S34.131** Complete lesion of sacral spinal cord [HCC] [ESR] [COM]
    - Complete lesion of conus medullaris
  - ☑7th **S34.132** Incomplete lesion of sacral spinal cord [HCC] [ESR] [COM]
    - Incomplete lesion of conus medullaris
  - ☑7th **S34.139** Unspecified injury to sacral spinal cord [HCC] [ESR] [COM]
    - Unspecified injury of conus medullaris
- ☑5th **S34.2** Injury of nerve root of lumbar and sacral spine
  - ☑x7th **S34.21** Injury of nerve root of lumbar spine
  - ☑x7th **S34.22** Injury of nerve root of sacral spine
- ☑x7th **S34.3** Injury of cauda equina [HCC] [ESR] [COM]
- ☑x7th **S34.4** Injury of lumbosacral plexus
- ☑x7th **S34.5** Injury of lumbar, sacral and pelvic sympathetic nerves
  - Injury of celiac ganglion or plexus
  - Injury of hypogastric plexus
  - Injury of mesenteric plexus (inferior) (superior)
  - Injury of splanchnic nerve
- ☑x7th **S34.6** Injury of peripheral nerve(s) at abdomen, lower back and pelvis level
- ☑x7th **S34.8** Injury of other nerves at abdomen, lower back and pelvis level
- ☑x7th **S34.9** Injury of unspecified nerves at abdomen, lower back and pelvis level
- ☑4th **S35** Injury of blood vessels at abdomen, lower back and pelvis level
  - Code also any associated open wound (S31.-)

  > The appropriate 7th character is to be added to each code from category S35.
  > A initial encounter
  > D subsequent encounter
  > S sequela

  - ☑5th **S35.0** Injury of abdominal aorta
    - EXCLUDES 1 injury of aorta NOS (S25.0)
    - ☑x7th **S35.00** Unspecified injury of abdominal aorta
    - ☑x7th **S35.01** Minor laceration of abdominal aorta
      - Incomplete transection of abdominal aorta
      - Laceration of abdominal aorta NOS
      - Superficial laceration of abdominal aorta
    - ☑x7th **S35.02** Major laceration of abdominal aorta
      - Complete transection of abdominal aorta
      - Traumatic rupture of abdominal aorta
    - ☑x7th **S35.09** Other injury of abdominal aorta
  - ☑5th **S35.1** Injury of inferior vena cava
    - Injury of hepatic vein
    - EXCLUDES 1 injury of vena cava NOS (S25.2)
    - ☑x7th **S35.10** Unspecified injury of inferior vena cava
    - ☑x7th **S35.11** Minor laceration of inferior vena cava
      - Incomplete transection of inferior vena cava
      - Laceration of inferior vena cava NOS
      - Superficial laceration of inferior vena cava
    - ☑x7th **S35.12** Major laceration of inferior vena cava
      - Complete transection of inferior vena cava
      - Traumatic rupture of inferior vena cava
    - ☑x7th **S35.19** Other injury of inferior vena cava
  - ☑5th **S35.2** Injury of celiac or mesenteric artery and branches
    - ☑6th **S35.21** Injury of celiac artery
      - ☑7th **S35.211** Minor laceration of celiac artery
        - Incomplete transection of celiac artery
        - Laceration of celiac artery NOS
        - Superficial laceration of celiac artery
      - ☑7th **S35.212** Major laceration of celiac artery
        - Complete transection of celiac artery
        - Traumatic rupture of celiac artery
      - ☑7th **S35.218** Other injury of celiac artery
      - ☑7th **S35.219** Unspecified injury of celiac artery
    - ☑6th **S35.22** Injury of superior mesenteric artery
      - ☑7th **S35.221** Minor laceration of superior mesenteric artery
        - Incomplete transection of superior mesenteric artery
        - Laceration of superior mesenteric artery NOS
        - Superficial laceration of superior mesenteric artery
      - ☑7th **S35.222** Major laceration of superior mesenteric artery
        - Complete transection of superior mesenteric artery
        - Traumatic rupture of superior mesenteric artery
      - ☑7th **S35.228** Other injury of superior mesenteric artery
      - ☑7th **S35.229** Unspecified injury of superior mesenteric artery
    - ☑6th **S35.23** Injury of inferior mesenteric artery
      - ☑7th **S35.231** Minor laceration of inferior mesenteric artery
        - Incomplete transection of inferior mesenteric artery
        - Laceration of inferior mesenteric artery NOS
        - Superficial laceration of inferior mesenteric artery
      - ☑7th **S35.232** Major laceration of inferior mesenteric artery
        - Complete transection of inferior mesenteric artery
        - Traumatic rupture of inferior mesenteric artery
      - ☑7th **S35.238** Other injury of inferior mesenteric artery
      - ☑7th **S35.239** Unspecified injury of inferior mesenteric artery
    - ☑6th **S35.29** Injury of branches of celiac and mesenteric artery
      - Injury of gastric artery
      - Injury of gastroduodenal artery
      - Injury of hepatic artery
      - Injury of splenic artery
      - ☑7th **S35.291** Minor laceration of branches of celiac and mesenteric artery
        - Incomplete transection of branches of celiac and mesenteric artery
        - Laceration of branches of celiac and mesenteric artery NOS
        - Superficial laceration of branches of celiac and mesenteric artery
      - ☑7th **S35.292** Major laceration of branches of celiac and mesenteric artery
        - Complete transection of branches of celiac and mesenteric artery
        - Traumatic rupture of branches of celiac and mesenteric artery
      - ☑7th **S35.298** Other injury of branches of celiac and mesenteric artery
      - ☑7th **S35.299** Unspecified injury of branches of celiac and mesenteric artery
  - ☑5th **S35.3** Injury of portal or splenic vein and branches
    - ☑6th **S35.31** Injury of portal vein
      - ☑7th **S35.311** Laceration of portal vein
      - ☑7th **S35.318** Other specified injury of portal vein
      - ☑7th **S35.319** Unspecified injury of portal vein
    - ☑6th **S35.32** Injury of splenic vein
      - ☑7th **S35.321** Laceration of splenic vein
      - ☑7th **S35.328** Other specified injury of splenic vein
      - ☑7th **S35.329** Unspecified injury of splenic vein

[HCC] CMS-HCC   [Rx] Rx HCC   [ESR] ESRD HCC   [COM] Commercial HCC   [N] Newborn: 0   [P] Pediatric: 0-17   [M] Maternity: 9-64   [A] Adult: 15-124

- **S35.33** Injury of superior mesenteric vein
  - **S35.331** Laceration of superior mesenteric vein
  - **S35.338** Other specified injury of superior mesenteric vein
  - **S35.339** Unspecified injury of superior mesenteric vein
- **S35.34** Injury of inferior mesenteric vein
  - **S35.341** Laceration of inferior mesenteric vein
  - **S35.348** Other specified injury of inferior mesenteric vein
  - **S35.349** Unspecified injury of inferior mesenteric vein
- **S35.4** Injury of renal blood vessels
  - **S35.40** Unspecified injury of renal blood vessel
    - **S35.401** Unspecified injury of right renal artery
    - **S35.402** Unspecified injury of left renal artery
    - **S35.403** Unspecified injury of unspecified renal artery
    - **S35.404** Unspecified injury of right renal vein
    - **S35.405** Unspecified injury of left renal vein
    - **S35.406** Unspecified injury of unspecified renal vein
  - **S35.41** Laceration of renal blood vessel
    - **S35.411** Laceration of right renal artery
    - **S35.412** Laceration of left renal artery
    - **S35.413** Laceration of unspecified renal artery
    - **S35.414** Laceration of right renal vein
    - **S35.415** Laceration of left renal vein
    - **S35.416** Laceration of unspecified renal vein
  - **S35.49** Other specified injury of renal blood vessel
    - **S35.491** Other specified injury of right renal artery
    - **S35.492** Other specified injury of left renal artery
    - **S35.493** Other specified injury of unspecified renal artery
    - **S35.494** Other specified injury of right renal vein
    - **S35.495** Other specified injury of left renal vein
    - **S35.496** Other specified injury of unspecified renal vein
- **S35.5** Injury of iliac blood vessels
  - **S35.50** Injury of unspecified iliac blood vessel(s)
  - **S35.51** Injury of iliac artery or vein
    - Injury of hypogastric artery or vein
    - **S35.511** Injury of right iliac artery
    - **S35.512** Injury of left iliac artery
    - **S35.513** Injury of unspecified iliac artery
    - **S35.514** Injury of right iliac vein
    - **S35.515** Injury of left iliac vein
    - **S35.516** Injury of unspecified iliac vein
  - **S35.53** Injury of uterine artery or vein
    - **S35.531** Injury of right uterine artery
    - **S35.532** Injury of left uterine artery
    - **S35.533** Injury of unspecified uterine artery
    - **S35.534** Injury of right uterine vein
    - **S35.535** Injury of left uterine vein
    - **S35.536** Injury of unspecified uterine vein
  - **S35.59** Injury of other iliac blood vessels
- **S35.8** Injury of other blood vessels at abdomen, lower back and pelvis level
  - Injury of ovarian artery or vein
  - **S35.8X** Injury of other blood vessels at abdomen, lower back and pelvis level
    - **S35.8X1** Laceration of other blood vessels at abdomen, lower back and pelvis level
    - **S35.8X8** Other specified injury of other blood vessels at abdomen, lower back and pelvis level
    - **S35.8X9** Unspecified injury of other blood vessels at abdomen, lower back and pelvis level
- **S35.9** Injury of unspecified blood vessel at abdomen, lower back and pelvis level
  - **S35.90** Unspecified injury of unspecified blood vessel at abdomen, lower back and pelvis level
  - **S35.91** Laceration of unspecified blood vessel at abdomen, lower back and pelvis level
  - **S35.99** Other specified injury of unspecified blood vessel at abdomen, lower back and pelvis level

- **S36** Injury of intra-abdominal organs
  - Code also any associated open wound (S31.-)
  - The appropriate 7th character is to be added to each code from category S36.
    - A initial encounter
    - D subsequent encounter
    - S sequela
  - **S36.0** Injury of spleen
    - **AHA:** 2015,2Q,36; 2015,1Q,10
    - **S36.00** Unspecified injury of spleen
    - **S36.02** Contusion of spleen
      - **S36.020** Minor contusion of spleen
        - Contusion of spleen less than 2 cm
      - **S36.021** Major contusion of spleen
        - Contusion of spleen greater than 2 cm
      - **S36.029** Unspecified contusion of spleen
    - **S36.03** Laceration of spleen
      - **S36.030** Superficial (capsular) laceration of spleen
        - Laceration of spleen less than 1 cm
        - Minor laceration of spleen
      - **S36.031** Moderate laceration of spleen
        - Laceration of spleen 1 to 3 cm
      - **S36.032** Major laceration of spleen
        - Avulsion of spleen
        - Laceration of spleen greater than 3 cm
        - Massive laceration of spleen
        - Multiple moderate lacerations of spleen
        - Stellate laceration of spleen
      - **S36.039** Unspecified laceration of spleen
    - **S36.09** Other injury of spleen
  - **S36.1** Injury of liver and gallbladder and bile duct
    - **S36.11** Injury of liver
      - **AHA:** 2024,1Q,25
      - **S36.112** Contusion of liver
      - **S36.113** Laceration of liver, unspecified degree
      - **S36.114** Minor laceration of liver
        - Laceration involving capsule only, or, without significant involvement of hepatic parenchyma [i.e., less than 1 cm deep]
      - **S36.115** Moderate laceration of liver
        - Laceration involving parenchyma but without major disruption of parenchyma [i.e., less than 10 cm long and less than 3 cm deep]
      - **S36.116** Major laceration of liver
        - Laceration with significant disruption of hepatic parenchyma [i.e., greater than 10 cm long and 3 cm deep]
        - Multiple moderate lacerations, with or without hematoma
        - Stellate laceration of liver
      - **S36.118** Other injury of liver
      - **S36.119** Unspecified injury of liver
    - **S36.12** Injury of gallbladder
      - **S36.122** Contusion of gallbladder
      - **S36.123** Laceration of gallbladder
      - **S36.128** Other injury of gallbladder
      - **S36.129** Unspecified injury of gallbladder
    - **S36.13** Injury of bile duct
  - **S36.2** Injury of pancreas
    - **S36.20** Unspecified injury of pancreas
      - **S36.200** Unspecified injury of head of pancreas
      - **S36.201** Unspecified injury of body of pancreas
      - **S36.202** Unspecified injury of tail of pancreas
      - **S36.209** Unspecified injury of unspecified part of pancreas
    - **S36.22** Contusion of pancreas
      - **S36.220** Contusion of head of pancreas

S36.221–S36.99 — Chapter 19. Injury, Poisoning and Certain Other Consequences of External Causes

- S36.221 Contusion of body of pancreas
- S36.222 Contusion of tail of pancreas
- S36.229 Contusion of unspecified part of pancreas
- S36.23 Laceration of pancreas, unspecified degree
  - S36.230 Laceration of head of pancreas, unspecified degree
  - S36.231 Laceration of body of pancreas, unspecified degree
  - S36.232 Laceration of tail of pancreas, unspecified degree
  - S36.239 Laceration of unspecified part of pancreas, unspecified degree
- S36.24 Minor laceration of pancreas
  - S36.240 Minor laceration of head of pancreas
  - S36.241 Minor laceration of body of pancreas
  - S36.242 Minor laceration of tail of pancreas
  - S36.249 Minor laceration of unspecified part of pancreas
- S36.25 Moderate laceration of pancreas
  - S36.250 Moderate laceration of head of pancreas
  - S36.251 Moderate laceration of body of pancreas
  - S36.252 Moderate laceration of tail of pancreas
  - S36.259 Moderate laceration of unspecified part of pancreas
- S36.26 Major laceration of pancreas
  - S36.260 Major laceration of head of pancreas
  - S36.261 Major laceration of body of pancreas
  - S36.262 Major laceration of tail of pancreas
  - S36.269 Major laceration of unspecified part of pancreas
- S36.29 Other injury of pancreas
  - S36.290 Other injury of head of pancreas
  - S36.291 Other injury of body of pancreas
  - S36.292 Other injury of tail of pancreas
  - S36.299 Other injury of unspecified part of pancreas
- S36.3 Injury of stomach
  - S36.30 Unspecified injury of stomach
  - S36.32 Contusion of stomach
  - S36.33 Laceration of stomach
  - S36.39 Other injury of stomach
- S36.4 Injury of small intestine
  - S36.40 Unspecified injury of small intestine
    - S36.400 Unspecified injury of duodenum
    - S36.408 Unspecified injury of other part of small intestine
    - S36.409 Unspecified injury of unspecified part of small intestine
  - S36.41 Primary blast injury of small intestine
    Blast injury of small intestine NOS
    - S36.410 Primary blast injury of duodenum
    - S36.418 Primary blast injury of other part of small intestine
    - S36.419 Primary blast injury of unspecified part of small intestine
  - S36.42 Contusion of small intestine
    - S36.420 Contusion of duodenum
    - S36.428 Contusion of other part of small intestine
    - S36.429 Contusion of unspecified part of small intestine
  - S36.43 Laceration of small intestine
    - S36.430 Laceration of duodenum
    - S36.438 Laceration of other part of small intestine
    - S36.439 Laceration of unspecified part of small intestine
  - S36.49 Other injury of small intestine
    - S36.490 Other injury of duodenum
    - S36.498 Other injury of other part of small intestine
      AHA: 2023,3Q,8
    - S36.499 Other injury of unspecified part of small intestine
- S36.5 Injury of colon
  EXCLUDES 2 injury of rectum (S36.6-)
  - S36.50 Unspecified injury of colon
    - S36.500 Unspecified injury of ascending [right] colon
    - S36.501 Unspecified injury of transverse colon
    - S36.502 Unspecified injury of descending [left] colon
    - S36.503 Unspecified injury of sigmoid colon
    - S36.508 Unspecified injury of other part of colon
    - S36.509 Unspecified injury of unspecified part of colon
  - S36.51 Primary blast injury of colon
    Blast injury of colon NOS
    - S36.510 Primary blast injury of ascending [right] colon
    - S36.511 Primary blast injury of transverse colon
    - S36.512 Primary blast injury of descending [left] colon
    - S36.513 Primary blast injury of sigmoid colon
    - S36.518 Primary blast injury of other part of colon
    - S36.519 Primary blast injury of unspecified part of colon
  - S36.52 Contusion of colon
    - S36.520 Contusion of ascending [right] colon
    - S36.521 Contusion of transverse colon
    - S36.522 Contusion of descending [left] colon
    - S36.523 Contusion of sigmoid colon
    - S36.528 Contusion of other part of colon
    - S36.529 Contusion of unspecified part of colon
  - S36.53 Laceration of colon
    - S36.530 Laceration of ascending [right] colon
    - S36.531 Laceration of transverse colon
    - S36.532 Laceration of descending [left] colon
    - S36.533 Laceration of sigmoid colon
    - S36.538 Laceration of other part of colon
    - S36.539 Laceration of unspecified part of colon
  - S36.59 Other injury of colon
    Secondary blast injury of colon
    AHA: 2023,3Q,8
    - S36.590 Other injury of ascending [right] colon
    - S36.591 Other injury of transverse colon
    - S36.592 Other injury of descending [left] colon
    - S36.593 Other injury of sigmoid colon
    - S36.598 Other injury of other part of colon
    - S36.599 Other injury of unspecified part of colon
- S36.6 Injury of rectum
  - S36.60 Unspecified injury of rectum
  - S36.61 Primary blast injury of rectum
    Blast injury of rectum NOS
  - S36.62 Contusion of rectum
  - S36.63 Laceration of rectum
  - S36.69 Other injury of rectum
    Secondary blast injury of rectum
- S36.8 Injury of other intra-abdominal organs
  - S36.81 Injury of peritoneum
  - S36.89 Injury of other intra-abdominal organs
    Injury of retroperitoneum
    - S36.892 Contusion of other intra-abdominal organs
    - S36.893 Laceration of other intra-abdominal organs
    - S36.898 Other injury of other intra-abdominal organs
    - S36.899 Unspecified injury of other intra-abdominal organs
- S36.9 Injury of unspecified intra-abdominal organ
  - S36.90 Unspecified injury of unspecified intra-abdominal organ
  - S36.92 Contusion of unspecified intra-abdominal organ
  - S36.93 Laceration of unspecified intra-abdominal organ
  - S36.99 Other injury of unspecified intra-abdominal organ

S37 Injury of urinary and pelvic organs

Code also any associated open wound (S31.-)

EXCLUDES 1 obstetric trauma to pelvic organs (O71.-)

EXCLUDES 2 injury of peritoneum (S36.81)
injury of retroperitoneum (S36.89-)

The appropriate 7th character is to be added to each code from category S37.
- A initial encounter
- D subsequent encounter
- S sequela

S37.0 Injury of kidney
EXCLUDES 2 acute kidney injury (nontraumatic) (N17.9)

- **S37.00** Unspecified injury of kidney
  - S37.001 Unspecified injury of right kidney
  - S37.002 Unspecified injury of left kidney
  - S37.009 Unspecified injury of unspecified kidney
- **S37.01** Minor contusion of kidney
  - Contusion of kidney less than 2 cm
  - Contusion of kidney NOS
  - S37.011 Minor contusion of right kidney
  - S37.012 Minor contusion of left kidney
  - S37.019 Minor contusion of unspecified kidney
- **S37.02** Major contusion of kidney
  - Contusion of kidney greater than 2 cm
  - S37.021 Major contusion of right kidney
  - S37.022 Major contusion of left kidney
  - S37.029 Major contusion of unspecified kidney
- **S37.03** Laceration of kidney, unspecified degree
  - S37.031 Laceration of right kidney, unspecified degree
  - S37.032 Laceration of left kidney, unspecified degree
  - S37.039 Laceration of unspecified kidney, unspecified degree
- **S37.04** Minor laceration of kidney
  - Laceration of kidney less than 1 cm
  - S37.041 Minor laceration of right kidney
  - S37.042 Minor laceration of left kidney
  - S37.049 Minor laceration of unspecified kidney
- **S37.05** Moderate laceration of kidney
  - Laceration of kidney 1 to 3 cm
  - S37.051 Moderate laceration of right kidney
  - S37.052 Moderate laceration of left kidney
  - S37.059 Moderate laceration of unspecified kidney
- **S37.06** Major laceration of kidney
  - Avulsion of kidney
  - Laceration of kidney greater than 3 cm
  - Massive laceration of kidney
  - Multiple moderate lacerations of kidney
  - Stellate laceration of kidney
  - S37.061 Major laceration of right kidney
  - S37.062 Major laceration of left kidney
  - S37.069 Major laceration of unspecified kidney
- **S37.09** Other injury of kidney
  - S37.091 Other injury of right kidney
  - S37.092 Other injury of left kidney
  - S37.099 Other injury of unspecified kidney

S37.1 Injury of ureter
- S37.10 Unspecified injury of ureter
- S37.12 Contusion of ureter
- S37.13 Laceration of ureter
- S37.19 Other injury of ureter

S37.2 Injury of bladder
- S37.20 Unspecified injury of bladder
- S37.22 Contusion of bladder
- S37.23 Laceration of bladder
- S37.29 Other injury of bladder

S37.3 Injury of urethra
- S37.30 Unspecified injury of urethra
- S37.32 Contusion of urethra
- S37.33 Laceration of urethra
- S37.39 Other injury of urethra

S37.4 Injury of ovary
- **S37.40** Unspecified injury of ovary
  - S37.401 Unspecified injury of ovary, unilateral
  - S37.402 Unspecified injury of ovary, bilateral
  - S37.409 Unspecified injury of ovary, unspecified
- **S37.42** Contusion of ovary
  - S37.421 Contusion of ovary, unilateral
  - S37.422 Contusion of ovary, bilateral
  - S37.429 Contusion of ovary, unspecified
- **S37.43** Laceration of ovary
  - S37.431 Laceration of ovary, unilateral
  - S37.432 Laceration of ovary, bilateral
  - S37.439 Laceration of ovary, unspecified
- **S37.49** Other injury of ovary
  - S37.491 Other injury of ovary, unilateral
  - S37.492 Other injury of ovary, bilateral
  - S37.499 Other injury of ovary, unspecified

S37.5 Injury of fallopian tube
- **S37.50** Unspecified injury of fallopian tube
  - S37.501 Unspecified injury of fallopian tube, unilateral
  - S37.502 Unspecified injury of fallopian tube, bilateral
  - S37.509 Unspecified injury of fallopian tube, unspecified
- **S37.51** Primary blast injury of fallopian tube
  - Blast injury of fallopian tube NOS
  - S37.511 Primary blast injury of fallopian tube, unilateral
  - S37.512 Primary blast injury of fallopian tube, bilateral
  - S37.519 Primary blast injury of fallopian tube, unspecified
- **S37.52** Contusion of fallopian tube
  - S37.521 Contusion of fallopian tube, unilateral
  - S37.522 Contusion of fallopian tube, bilateral
  - S37.529 Contusion of fallopian tube, unspecified
- **S37.53** Laceration of fallopian tube
  - S37.531 Laceration of fallopian tube, unilateral
  - S37.532 Laceration of fallopian tube, bilateral
  - S37.539 Laceration of fallopian tube, unspecified
- **S37.59** Other injury of fallopian tube
  - Secondary blast injury of fallopian tube
  - S37.591 Other injury of fallopian tube, unilateral
  - S37.592 Other injury of fallopian tube, bilateral
  - S37.599 Other injury of fallopian tube, unspecified

S37.6 Injury of uterus
EXCLUDES 1 injury to gravid uterus (O9A.2-)
injury to uterus during delivery (O71.-)

- S37.60 Unspecified injury of uterus
- S37.62 Contusion of uterus
- S37.63 Laceration of uterus
- S37.69 Other injury of uterus

S37.8 Injury of other urinary and pelvic organs
- **S37.81** Injury of adrenal gland
  - S37.812 Contusion of adrenal gland
  - S37.813 Laceration of adrenal gland
  - S37.818 Other injury of adrenal gland
  - S37.819 Unspecified injury of adrenal gland
- **S37.82** Injury of prostate
  - S37.822 Contusion of prostate
  - S37.823 Laceration of prostate
  - S37.828 Other injury of prostate
  - S37.829 Unspecified injury of prostate
- **S37.89** Injury of other urinary and pelvic organ
  - S37.892 Contusion of other urinary and pelvic organ

- **S37.893** Laceration of other urinary and pelvic organ
- **S37.898** Other injury of other urinary and pelvic organ
- **S37.899** Unspecified injury of other urinary and pelvic organ
- **S37.9** Injury of unspecified urinary and pelvic organ
  - **S37.90** Unspecified injury of unspecified urinary and pelvic organ
  - **S37.92** Contusion of unspecified urinary and pelvic organ
  - **S37.93** Laceration of unspecified urinary and pelvic organ
  - **S37.99** Other injury of unspecified urinary and pelvic organ
- **S38** Crushing injury and traumatic amputation of abdomen, lower back, pelvis and external genitals

  NOTE An amputation not identified as partial or complete should be coded to complete

  The appropriate 7th character is to be added to each code from category S38.
  - A initial encounter
  - D subsequent encounter
  - S sequela

  - **S38.0** Crushing injury of external genital organs
    Use additional code for any associated injuries
    - **S38.00** Crushing injury of unspecified external genital organs
      - **S38.001** Crushing injury of unspecified external genital organs, male
      - **S38.002** Crushing injury of unspecified external genital organs, female
    - **S38.01** Crushing injury of penis
    - **S38.02** Crushing injury of scrotum and testis
    - **S38.03** Crushing injury of vulva
  - **S38.1** Crushing injury of abdomen, lower back, and pelvis
    Use additional code for all associated injuries, such as:
    fracture of thoracic or lumbar spine and pelvis (S22.0-, S32.-)
    injury to intra-abdominal organs (S36.-)
    injury to urinary and pelvic organs (S37.-)
    open wound of abdominal wall (S31.-)
    spinal cord injury (S34.0, S34.1-)
    EXCLUDES 2 crushing injury of external genital organs (S38.0-)
  - **S38.2** Traumatic amputation of external genital organs
    - **S38.21** Traumatic amputation of female external genital organs
      Traumatic amputation of clitoris
      Traumatic amputation of labium (majus) (minus)
      Traumatic amputation of vulva
      - **S38.211** Complete traumatic amputation of female external genital organs
      - **S38.212** Partial traumatic amputation of female external genital organs
    - **S38.22** Traumatic amputation of penis
      - **S38.221** Complete traumatic amputation of penis
      - **S38.222** Partial traumatic amputation of penis
    - **S38.23** Traumatic amputation of scrotum and testis
      - **S38.231** Complete traumatic amputation of scrotum and testis
      - **S38.232** Partial traumatic amputation of scrotum and testis
  - **S38.3** Transection (partial) of abdomen
- **S39** Other and unspecified injuries of abdomen, lower back, pelvis and external genitals
  Code also any associated open wound (S31.-)
  EXCLUDES 2 sprain of joints and ligaments of lumbar spine and pelvis (S33.-)

  The appropriate 7th character is to be added to each code from category S39.
  - A initial encounter
  - D subsequent encounter
  - S sequela

  - **S39.0** Injury of muscle, fascia and tendon of abdomen, lower back and pelvis
    - **S39.00** Unspecified injury of muscle, fascia and tendon of abdomen, lower back and pelvis
      - **S39.001** Unspecified injury of muscle, fascia and tendon of abdomen
      - **S39.002** Unspecified injury of muscle, fascia and tendon of lower back
      - **S39.003** Unspecified injury of muscle, fascia and tendon of pelvis
    - **S39.01** Strain of muscle, fascia and tendon of abdomen, lower back and pelvis
      - **S39.011** Strain of muscle, fascia and tendon of abdomen
      - **S39.012** Strain of muscle, fascia and tendon of lower back
      - **S39.013** Strain of muscle, fascia and tendon of pelvis
    - **S39.02** Laceration of muscle, fascia and tendon of abdomen, lower back and pelvis
      - **S39.021** Laceration of muscle, fascia and tendon of abdomen
      - **S39.022** Laceration of muscle, fascia and tendon of lower back
      - **S39.023** Laceration of muscle, fascia and tendon of pelvis
    - **S39.09** Other injury of muscle, fascia and tendon of abdomen, lower back and pelvis
      - **S39.091** Other injury of muscle, fascia and tendon of abdomen
      - **S39.092** Other injury of muscle, fascia and tendon of lower back
      - **S39.093** Other injury of muscle, fascia and tendon of pelvis
  - **S39.8** Other specified injuries of abdomen, lower back, pelvis and external genitals
    - **S39.81** Other specified injuries of abdomen
    - **S39.82** Other specified injuries of lower back
    - **S39.83** Other specified injuries of pelvis
    - **S39.84** Other specified injuries of external genitals
      - **S39.840** Fracture of corpus cavernosum penis
      - **S39.848** Other specified injuries of external genitals
  - **S39.9** Unspecified injury of abdomen, lower back, pelvis and external genitals
    - **S39.91** Unspecified injury of abdomen
    - **S39.92** Unspecified injury of lower back
    - **S39.93** Unspecified injury of pelvis
    - **S39.94** Unspecified injury of external genitals

Injuries to the shoulder and upper arm (S40-S49)

INCLUDES injuries of axilla
injuries of scapular region
EXCLUDES 2 burns and corrosions (T20-T32)
frostbite (T33-T34)
injuries of elbow (S50-S59)
insect bite or sting, venomous (T63.4)

- **S40** Superficial injury of shoulder and upper arm

  The appropriate 7th character is to be added to each code from category S40.
  - A initial encounter
  - D subsequent encounter
  - S sequela

  - **S40.0** Contusion of shoulder and upper arm
    - **S40.01** Contusion of shoulder
      - **S40.011** Contusion of right shoulder
      - **S40.012** Contusion of left shoulder
      - **S40.019** Contusion of unspecified shoulder
    - **S40.02** Contusion of upper arm
      - **S40.021** Contusion of right upper arm
      - **S40.022** Contusion of left upper arm
      - **S40.029** Contusion of unspecified upper arm
  - **S40.2** Other superficial injuries of shoulder
    - **S40.21** Abrasion of shoulder
      - **S40.211** Abrasion of right shoulder
      - **S40.212** Abrasion of left shoulder
      - **S40.219** Abrasion of unspecified shoulder
    - **S40.22** Blister (nonthermal) of shoulder
      - **S40.221** Blister (nonthermal) of right shoulder
      - **S40.222** Blister (nonthermal) of left shoulder
      - **S40.229** Blister (nonthermal) of unspecified shoulder

Chapter 19. Injury, Poisoning and Certain Other Consequences of External Causes

S40.24 External constriction of shoulder
- S40.241 External constriction of right shoulder
- S40.242 External constriction of left shoulder
- S40.249 External constriction of unspecified shoulder

S40.25 Superficial foreign body of shoulder
Splinter in the shoulder
- S40.251 Superficial foreign body of right shoulder
- S40.252 Superficial foreign body of left shoulder
- S40.259 Superficial foreign body of unspecified shoulder

S40.26 Insect bite (nonvenomous) of shoulder
- S40.261 Insect bite (nonvenomous) of right shoulder
- S40.262 Insect bite (nonvenomous) of left shoulder
- S40.269 Insect bite (nonvenomous) of unspecified shoulder

S40.27 Other superficial bite of shoulder
EXCLUDES 1 open bite of shoulder (S41.05)
- S40.271 Other superficial bite of right shoulder
- S40.272 Other superficial bite of left shoulder
- S40.279 Other superficial bite of unspecified shoulder

S40.8 Other superficial injuries of upper arm

S40.81 Abrasion of upper arm
- S40.811 Abrasion of right upper arm
- S40.812 Abrasion of left upper arm
- S40.819 Abrasion of unspecified upper arm

S40.82 Blister (nonthermal) of upper arm
- S40.821 Blister (nonthermal) of right upper arm
- S40.822 Blister (nonthermal) of left upper arm
- S40.829 Blister (nonthermal) of unspecified upper arm

S40.84 External constriction of upper arm
- S40.841 External constriction of right upper arm
- S40.842 External constriction of left upper arm
- S40.849 External constriction of unspecified upper arm

S40.85 Superficial foreign body of upper arm
Splinter in the upper arm
- S40.851 Superficial foreign body of right upper arm
- S40.852 Superficial foreign body of left upper arm
- S40.859 Superficial foreign body of unspecified upper arm

S40.86 Insect bite (nonvenomous) of upper arm
- S40.861 Insect bite (nonvenomous) of right upper arm
- S40.862 Insect bite (nonvenomous) of left upper arm
- S40.869 Insect bite (nonvenomous) of unspecified upper arm

S40.87 Other superficial bite of upper arm
EXCLUDES 1 open bite of upper arm (S41.14)
EXCLUDES 2 other superficial bite of shoulder (S40.27-)
- S40.871 Other superficial bite of right upper arm
- S40.872 Other superficial bite of left upper arm
- S40.879 Other superficial bite of unspecified upper arm

S40.9 Unspecified superficial injury of shoulder and upper arm

S40.91 Unspecified superficial injury of shoulder
- S40.911 Unspecified superficial injury of right shoulder
- S40.912 Unspecified superficial injury of left shoulder
- S40.919 Unspecified superficial injury of unspecified shoulder

S40.92 Unspecified superficial injury of upper arm
- S40.921 Unspecified superficial injury of right upper arm
- S40.922 Unspecified superficial injury of left upper arm
- S40.929 Unspecified superficial injury of unspecified upper arm

S41 Open wound of shoulder and upper arm
Code also any associated wound infection
EXCLUDES 1 traumatic amputation of shoulder and upper arm (S48.-)
EXCLUDES 2 open fracture of shoulder and upper arm (S42.- with 7th character B or C)

The appropriate 7th character is to be added to each code from category S41.
- A initial encounter
- D subsequent encounter
- S sequela

S41.0 Open wound of shoulder

S41.00 Unspecified open wound of shoulder
- S41.001 Unspecified open wound of right shoulder
- S41.002 Unspecified open wound of left shoulder
- S41.009 Unspecified open wound of unspecified shoulder

S41.01 Laceration without foreign body of shoulder
- S41.011 Laceration without foreign body of right shoulder
- S41.012 Laceration without foreign body of left shoulder
- S41.019 Laceration without foreign body of unspecified shoulder

S41.02 Laceration with foreign body of shoulder
- S41.021 Laceration with foreign body of right shoulder
- S41.022 Laceration with foreign body of left shoulder
- S41.029 Laceration with foreign body of unspecified shoulder

S41.03 Puncture wound without foreign body of shoulder
- S41.031 Puncture wound without foreign body of right shoulder
- S41.032 Puncture wound without foreign body of left shoulder
- S41.039 Puncture wound without foreign body of unspecified shoulder

S41.04 Puncture wound with foreign body of shoulder
- S41.041 Puncture wound with foreign body of right shoulder
- S41.042 Puncture wound with foreign body of left shoulder
- S41.049 Puncture wound with foreign body of unspecified shoulder

S41.05 Open bite of shoulder
Bite of shoulder NOS
EXCLUDES 1 superficial bite of shoulder (S40.27)
- S41.051 Open bite of right shoulder
- S41.052 Open bite of left shoulder
- S41.059 Open bite of unspecified shoulder

S41.1 Open wound of upper arm

S41.10 Unspecified open wound of upper arm
AHA: 2016,3Q,24
- S41.101 Unspecified open wound of right upper arm
- S41.102 Unspecified open wound of left upper arm
- S41.109 Unspecified open wound of unspecified upper arm

S41.11 Laceration without foreign body of upper arm
- S41.111 Laceration without foreign body of right upper arm
- S41.112 Laceration without foreign body of left upper arm
- S41.119 Laceration without foreign body of unspecified upper arm

S41.12 Laceration with foreign body of upper arm
- S41.121 Laceration with foreign body of right upper arm
- S41.122 Laceration with foreign body of left upper arm
- S41.129 Laceration with foreign body of unspecified upper arm

S41.13 Puncture wound without foreign body of upper arm
AHA: 2016,3Q,24
- S41.131 Puncture wound without foreign body of right upper arm

	✓7th	S41.132	Puncture wound without foreign body of left upper arm
	✓7th	S41.139	Puncture wound without foreign body of unspecified upper arm

✓6th **S41.14** Puncture wound with foreign body of upper arm
   AHA: 2016,3Q,24
   ✓7th S41.141 Puncture wound with foreign body of right upper arm
   ✓7th S41.142 Puncture wound with foreign body of left upper arm
   ✓7th S41.149 Puncture wound with foreign body of unspecified upper arm

✓6th **S41.15** Open bite of upper arm
   Bite of upper arm NOS
   EXCLUDES 1 superficial bite of upper arm (S40.87)
   ✓7th S41.151 Open bite of right upper arm
   ✓7th S41.152 Open bite of left upper arm
   ✓7th S41.159 Open bite of unspecified upper arm

✓4th **S42** Fracture of shoulder and upper arm

   NOTE A fracture not indicated as displaced or nondisplaced should be coded to displaced
   A fracture not indicated as open or closed should be coded to closed
   EXCLUDES 1 traumatic amputation of shoulder and upper arm (S48.-)
   EXCLUDES 2 periprosthetic fracture around internal prosthetic shoulder joint (M97.3)

   AHA: 2018,2Q,12; 2015,3Q,37-39
   DEF: Diaphysis: Central shaft of a long bone.
   DEF: Epiphysis: Proximal and distal rounded ends of a long bone, communicates with the joint.
   DEF: Metaphysis: Section of a long bone located between the epiphysis and diaphysis at the proximal and distal ends.
   DEF: Physis (growth plate): Narrow zone of cartilaginous tissue between the epiphysis and metaphysis at each end of a long bone. In childhood, proliferation of cells in this zone lengthens the bone. As the bone matures, this area thins, ossification eventually fusing into solid bone and growth stops. **Synonym(s):** Epiphyseal plate.

   The appropriate 7th character is to be added to all codes from category S42 [unless otherwise indicated].
   A initial encounter for closed fracture
   B initial encounter for open fracture
   D subsequent encounter for fracture with routine healing
   G subsequent encounter for fracture with delayed healing
   K subsequent encounter for fracture with nonunion
   P subsequent encounter for fracture with malunion
   S sequela

✓5th **S42.0** Fracture of clavicle
   ✓6th **S42.00** Fracture of unspecified part of clavicle
      ✓7th S42.001 Fracture of unspecified part of right clavicle
      ✓7th S42.002 Fracture of unspecified part of left clavicle
      ✓7th S42.009 Fracture of unspecified part of unspecified clavicle
         AHA: 2012,4Q,93
   ✓6th **S42.01** Fracture of sternal end of clavicle
      ✓7th S42.011 Anterior displaced fracture of sternal end of right clavicle
      ✓7th S42.012 Anterior displaced fracture of sternal end of left clavicle
      ✓7th S42.013 Anterior displaced fracture of sternal end of unspecified clavicle
         Displaced fracture of sternal end of clavicle NOS
      ✓7th S42.014 Posterior displaced fracture of sternal end of right clavicle
      ✓7th S42.015 Posterior displaced fracture of sternal end of left clavicle
      ✓7th S42.016 Posterior displaced fracture of sternal end of unspecified clavicle
      ✓7th S42.017 Nondisplaced fracture of sternal end of right clavicle
      ✓7th S42.018 Nondisplaced fracture of sternal end of left clavicle
      ✓7th S42.019 Nondisplaced fracture of sternal end of unspecified clavicle

   ✓6th **S42.02** Fracture of shaft of clavicle
      ✓7th S42.021 Displaced fracture of shaft of right clavicle
      ✓7th S42.022 Displaced fracture of shaft of left clavicle
      ✓7th S42.023 Displaced fracture of shaft of unspecified clavicle
      ✓7th S42.024 Nondisplaced fracture of shaft of right clavicle
      ✓7th S42.025 Nondisplaced fracture of shaft of left clavicle
      ✓7th S42.026 Nondisplaced fracture of shaft of unspecified clavicle

   ✓6th **S42.03** Fracture of lateral end of clavicle
      Fracture of acromial end of clavicle
      ✓7th S42.031 Displaced fracture of lateral end of right clavicle
      ✓7th S42.032 Displaced fracture of lateral end of left clavicle
      ✓7th S42.033 Displaced fracture of lateral end of unspecified clavicle
      ✓7th S42.034 Nondisplaced fracture of lateral end of right clavicle
      ✓7th S42.035 Nondisplaced fracture of lateral end of left clavicle
      ✓7th S42.036 Nondisplaced fracture of lateral end of unspecified clavicle

✓5th **S42.1** Fracture of scapula
   ✓6th **S42.10** Fracture of unspecified part of scapula
      ✓7th S42.101 Fracture of unspecified part of scapula, right shoulder
      ✓7th S42.102 Fracture of unspecified part of scapula, left shoulder
      ✓7th S42.109 Fracture of unspecified part of scapula, unspecified shoulder
   ✓6th **S42.11** Fracture of body of scapula
      ✓7th S42.111 Displaced fracture of body of scapula, right shoulder
      ✓7th S42.112 Displaced fracture of body of scapula, left shoulder
      ✓7th S42.113 Displaced fracture of body of scapula, unspecified shoulder
      ✓7th S42.114 Nondisplaced fracture of body of scapula, right shoulder
      ✓7th S42.115 Nondisplaced fracture of body of scapula, left shoulder
      ✓7th S42.116 Nondisplaced fracture of body of scapula, unspecified shoulder
   ✓6th **S42.12** Fracture of acromial process
      ✓7th S42.121 Displaced fracture of acromial process, right shoulder
      ✓7th S42.122 Displaced fracture of acromial process, left shoulder
      ✓7th S42.123 Displaced fracture of acromial process, unspecified shoulder
      ✓7th S42.124 Nondisplaced fracture of acromial process, right shoulder
      ✓7th S42.125 Nondisplaced fracture of acromial process, left shoulder
      ✓7th S42.126 Nondisplaced fracture of acromial process, unspecified shoulder
   ✓6th **S42.13** Fracture of coracoid process
      ✓7th S42.131 Displaced fracture of coracoid process, right shoulder
      ✓7th S42.132 Displaced fracture of coracoid process, left shoulder
      ✓7th S42.133 Displaced fracture of coracoid process, unspecified shoulder
      ✓7th S42.134 Nondisplaced fracture of coracoid process, right shoulder
      ✓7th S42.135 Nondisplaced fracture of coracoid process, left shoulder
      ✓7th S42.136 Nondisplaced fracture of coracoid process, unspecified shoulder
   ✓6th **S42.14** Fracture of glenoid cavity of scapula
      ✓7th S42.141 Displaced fracture of glenoid cavity of scapula, right shoulder

Chapter 19. Injury, Poisoning and Certain Other Consequences of External Causes

- ✓7th **S42.142** Displaced fracture of glenoid cavity of scapula, left shoulder Q
- ✓7th **S42.143** Displaced fracture of glenoid cavity of scapula, unspecified shoulder Q
- ✓7th **S42.144** Nondisplaced fracture of glenoid cavity of scapula, right shoulder Q
- ✓7th **S42.145** Nondisplaced fracture of glenoid cavity of scapula, left shoulder Q
- ✓7th **S42.146** Nondisplaced fracture of glenoid cavity of scapula, unspecified shoulder Q

- ✓6th **S42.15** Fracture of neck of scapula
  - ✓7th **S42.151** Displaced fracture of neck of scapula, right shoulder Q
  - ✓7th **S42.152** Displaced fracture of neck of scapula, left shoulder Q
  - ✓7th **S42.153** Displaced fracture of neck of scapula, unspecified shoulder Q
  - ✓7th **S42.154** Nondisplaced fracture of neck of scapula, right shoulder Q
  - ✓7th **S42.155** Nondisplaced fracture of neck of scapula, left shoulder Q
  - ✓7th **S42.156** Nondisplaced fracture of neck of scapula, unspecified shoulder Q

- ✓6th **S42.19** Fracture of other part of scapula
  - ✓7th **S42.191** Fracture of other part of scapula, right shoulder Q
  - ✓7th **S42.192** Fracture of other part of scapula, left shoulder Q
  - ✓7th **S42.199** Fracture of other part of scapula, unspecified shoulder Q

- ✓5th **S42.2** Fracture of upper end of humerus
  Fracture of proximal end of humerus
  EXCLUDES 2 fracture of shaft of humerus (S42.3-)
  physeal fracture of upper end of humerus (S49.0-)

  - ✓6th **S42.20** Unspecified fracture of upper end of humerus
    - ✓7th **S42.201** Unspecified fracture of upper end of right humerus Q
    - ✓7th **S42.202** Unspecified fracture of upper end of left humerus Q
    - ✓7th **S42.209** Unspecified fracture of upper end of unspecified humerus Q

  - ✓6th **S42.21** Unspecified fracture of surgical neck of humerus
    Fracture of neck of humerus NOS
    - ✓7th **S42.211** Unspecified displaced fracture of surgical neck of right humerus Q
    - ✓7th **S42.212** Unspecified displaced fracture of surgical neck of left humerus Q
    - ✓7th **S42.213** Unspecified displaced fracture of surgical neck of unspecified humerus Q
    - ✓7th **S42.214** Unspecified nondisplaced fracture of surgical neck of right humerus Q
    - ✓7th **S42.215** Unspecified nondisplaced fracture of surgical neck of left humerus Q
    - ✓7th **S42.216** Unspecified nondisplaced fracture of surgical neck of unspecified humerus Q

  - ✓6th **S42.22** 2-part fracture of surgical neck of humerus
    - ✓7th **S42.221** 2-part displaced fracture of surgical neck of right humerus Q
    - ✓7th **S42.222** 2-part displaced fracture of surgical neck of left humerus Q
    - ✓7th **S42.223** 2-part displaced fracture of surgical neck of unspecified humerus Q
    - ✓7th **S42.224** 2-part nondisplaced fracture of surgical neck of right humerus Q
    - ✓7th **S42.225** 2-part nondisplaced fracture of surgical neck of left humerus Q
    - ✓7th **S42.226** 2-part nondisplaced fracture of surgical neck of unspecified humerus Q

  - ✓6th **S42.23** 3-part fracture of surgical neck of humerus
    - ✓7th **S42.231** 3-part fracture of surgical neck of right humerus Q
    - ✓7th **S42.232** 3-part fracture of surgical neck of left humerus Q
    - ✓7th **S42.239** 3-part fracture of surgical neck of unspecified humerus Q

  - ✓6th **S42.24** 4-part fracture of surgical neck of humerus
    - ✓7th **S42.241** 4-part fracture of surgical neck of right humerus Q
    - ✓7th **S42.242** 4-part fracture of surgical neck of left humerus Q
    - ✓7th **S42.249** 4-part fracture of surgical neck of unspecified humerus Q

  - ✓6th **S42.25** Fracture of greater tuberosity of humerus
    - ✓7th **S42.251** Displaced fracture of greater tuberosity of right humerus Q
    - ✓7th **S42.252** Displaced fracture of greater tuberosity of left humerus Q
    - ✓7th **S42.253** Displaced fracture of greater tuberosity of unspecified humerus Q
    - ✓7th **S42.254** Nondisplaced fracture of greater tuberosity of right humerus Q
    - ✓7th **S42.255** Nondisplaced fracture of greater tuberosity of left humerus Q
    - ✓7th **S42.256** Nondisplaced fracture of greater tuberosity of unspecified humerus Q

  - ✓6th **S42.26** Fracture of lesser tuberosity of humerus
    - ✓7th **S42.261** Displaced fracture of lesser tuberosity of right humerus Q
    - ✓7th **S42.262** Displaced fracture of lesser tuberosity of left humerus Q
    - ✓7th **S42.263** Displaced fracture of lesser tuberosity of unspecified humerus Q
    - ✓7th **S42.264** Nondisplaced fracture of lesser tuberosity of right humerus Q
    - ✓7th **S42.265** Nondisplaced fracture of lesser tuberosity of left humerus Q
    - ✓7th **S42.266** Nondisplaced fracture of lesser tuberosity of unspecified humerus Q

  - ✓6th **S42.27** Torus fracture of upper end of humerus

    > The appropriate 7th character is to be added to all codes in subcategory S42.27
    > A initial encounter for closed fracture
    > D subsequent encounter for fracture with routine healing
    > G subsequent encounter for fracture with delayed healing
    > K subsequent encounter for fracture with nonunion
    > P subsequent encounter for fracture with malunion
    > S sequela

    - ✓7th **S42.271** Torus fracture of upper end of right humerus Q
    - ✓7th **S42.272** Torus fracture of upper end of left humerus Q
    - ✓7th **S42.279** Torus fracture of upper end of unspecified humerus Q

  - ✓6th **S42.29** Other fracture of upper end of humerus
    Fracture of anatomical neck of humerus
    Fracture of articular head of humerus
    AHA: 2024,2Q,24; 2019,1Q,18
    - ✓7th **S42.291** Other displaced fracture of upper end of right humerus Q
    - ✓7th **S42.292** Other displaced fracture of upper end of left humerus Q
    - ✓7th **S42.293** Other displaced fracture of upper end of unspecified humerus Q
    - ✓7th **S42.294** Other nondisplaced fracture of upper end of right humerus Q
    - ✓7th **S42.295** Other nondisplaced fracture of upper end of left humerus Q
    - ✓7th **S42.296** Other nondisplaced fracture of upper end of unspecified humerus Q

- ✓5th **S42.3** Fracture of shaft of humerus
  Fracture of humerus NOS
  Fracture of upper arm NOS
  EXCLUDES 2 physeal fractures of upper end of humerus (S49.0-)
  physeal fractures of lower end of humerus (S49.1-)

  - ✓6th **S42.30** Unspecified fracture of shaft of humerus
    - ✓7th **S42.301** Unspecified fracture of shaft of humerus, right arm Q
    - ✓7th **S42.302** Unspecified fracture of shaft of humerus, left arm Q
    - ✓7th **S42.309** Unspecified fracture of shaft of humerus, unspecified arm Q

- ✓6th **S42.31 Greenstick** fracture of shaft of humerus

  > The appropriate 7th character is to be added to all codes in subcategory S42.31
  > A initial encounter for closed fracture
  > D subsequent encounter for fracture with routine healing
  > G subsequent encounter for fracture with delayed healing
  > K subsequent encounter for fracture with nonunion
  > P subsequent encounter for fracture with malunion
  > S sequela

  - ✓7th **S42.311** Greenstick fracture of shaft of humerus, **right** arm
  - ✓7th **S42.312** Greenstick fracture of shaft of humerus, **left** arm
  - ✓7th **S42.319** Greenstick fracture of shaft of humerus, unspecified arm

- ✓6th **S42.32 Transverse** fracture of shaft of humerus
  - ✓7th **S42.321** **Displaced** transverse fracture of shaft of humerus, **right** arm
  - ✓7th **S42.322** **Displaced** transverse fracture of shaft of humerus, **left** arm
  - ✓7th **S42.323** **Displaced** transverse fracture of shaft of humerus, unspecified arm
  - ✓7th **S42.324** **Nondisplaced** transverse fracture of shaft of humerus, **right** arm
  - ✓7th **S42.325** **Nondisplaced** transverse fracture of shaft of humerus, **left** arm
  - ✓7th **S42.326** **Nondisplaced** transverse fracture of shaft of humerus, unspecified arm

- ✓6th **S42.33 Oblique** fracture of shaft of humerus
  - ✓7th **S42.331** **Displaced** oblique fracture of shaft of humerus, **right** arm
  - ✓7th **S42.332** **Displaced** oblique fracture of shaft of humerus, **left** arm
  - ✓7th **S42.333** **Displaced** oblique fracture of shaft of humerus, unspecified arm
  - ✓7th **S42.334** **Nondisplaced** oblique fracture of shaft of humerus, **right** arm
  - ✓7th **S42.335** **Nondisplaced** oblique fracture of shaft of humerus, **left** arm
  - ✓7th **S42.336** **Nondisplaced** oblique fracture of shaft of humerus, unspecified arm

- ✓6th **S42.34 Spiral** fracture of shaft of humerus
  - ✓7th **S42.341** **Displaced** spiral fracture of shaft of humerus, **right** arm
  - ✓7th **S42.342** **Displaced** spiral fracture of shaft of humerus, **left** arm
  - ✓7th **S42.343** **Displaced** spiral fracture of shaft of humerus, unspecified arm
  - ✓7th **S42.344** **Nondisplaced** spiral fracture of shaft of humerus, **right** arm
  - ✓7th **S42.345** **Nondisplaced** spiral fracture of shaft of humerus, **left** arm
  - ✓7th **S42.346** **Nondisplaced** spiral fracture of shaft of humerus, unspecified arm

- ✓6th **S42.35 Comminuted** fracture of shaft of humerus
  - ✓7th **S42.351** **Displaced** comminuted fracture of shaft of humerus, **right** arm
  - ✓7th **S42.352** **Displaced** comminuted fracture of shaft of humerus, **left** arm
  - ✓7th **S42.353** **Displaced** comminuted fracture of shaft of humerus, unspecified arm
  - ✓7th **S42.354** **Nondisplaced** comminuted fracture of shaft of humerus, **right** arm
  - ✓7th **S42.355** **Nondisplaced** comminuted fracture of shaft of humerus, **left** arm
  - ✓7th **S42.356** **Nondisplaced** comminuted fracture of shaft of humerus, unspecified arm

- ✓6th **S42.36 Segmental** fracture of shaft of humerus
  - ✓7th **S42.361** **Displaced** segmental fracture of shaft of humerus, **right** arm
  - ✓7th **S42.362** **Displaced** segmental fracture of shaft of humerus, **left** arm
  - ✓7th **S42.363** **Displaced** segmental fracture of shaft of humerus, unspecified arm
  - ✓7th **S42.364** **Nondisplaced** segmental fracture of shaft of humerus, **right** arm
  - ✓7th **S42.365** **Nondisplaced** segmental fracture of shaft of humerus, **left** arm
  - ✓7th **S42.366** **Nondisplaced** segmental fracture of shaft of humerus, unspecified arm

- ✓6th **S42.39 Other** fracture of shaft of humerus
  - ✓7th **S42.391** Other fracture of shaft of **right** humerus
  - ✓7th **S42.392** Other fracture of shaft of **left** humerus
  - ✓7th **S42.399** Other fracture of shaft of unspecified humerus

- ✓5th **S42.4 Fracture of lower end of humerus**
  Fracture of distal end of humerus
  EXCLUDES 2 fracture of shaft of humerus (S42.3-)
  physeal fracture of lower end of humerus (S49.1-)

  - ✓6th **S42.40 Unspecified** fracture of lower end of humerus
    Fracture of elbow NOS
    - ✓7th **S42.401** Unspecified fracture of lower end of **right** humerus
    - ✓7th **S42.402** Unspecified fracture of lower end of **left** humerus
    - ✓7th **S42.409** Unspecified fracture of lower end of unspecified humerus

  - ✓6th **S42.41 Simple supracondylar** fracture **without intercondylar** fracture of humerus
    - ✓7th **S42.411** **Displaced** simple supracondylar fracture without intercondylar fracture of **right** humerus
    - ✓7th **S42.412** **Displaced** simple supracondylar fracture without intercondylar fracture of **left** humerus
    - ✓7th **S42.413** **Displaced** simple supracondylar fracture without intercondylar fracture of unspecified humerus
    - ✓7th **S42.414** **Nondisplaced** simple supracondylar fracture without intercondylar fracture of **right** humerus
    - ✓7th **S42.415** **Nondisplaced** simple supracondylar fracture without intercondylar fracture of **left** humerus
    - ✓7th **S42.416** **Nondisplaced** simple supracondylar fracture without intercondylar fracture of unspecified humerus

  - ✓6th **S42.42 Comminuted supracondylar** fracture **without intercondylar** fracture of humerus
    - ✓7th **S42.421** **Displaced** comminuted supracondylar fracture without intercondylar fracture of **right** humerus
    - ✓7th **S42.422** **Displaced** comminuted supracondylar fracture without intercondylar fracture of **left** humerus
    - ✓7th **S42.423** **Displaced** comminuted supracondylar fracture without intercondylar fracture of unspecified humerus
    - ✓7th **S42.424** **Nondisplaced** comminuted supracondylar fracture without intercondylar fracture of **right** humerus
    - ✓7th **S42.425** **Nondisplaced** comminuted supracondylar fracture without intercondylar fracture of **left** humerus
    - ✓7th **S42.426** **Nondisplaced** comminuted supracondylar fracture without intercondylar fracture of unspecified humerus

  - ✓6th **S42.43 Fracture (avulsion) of lateral epicondyle** of humerus
    - ✓7th **S42.431** **Displaced** fracture (avulsion) of lateral epicondyle of **right** humerus
    - ✓7th **S42.432** **Displaced** fracture (avulsion) of lateral epicondyle of **left** humerus
    - ✓7th **S42.433** **Displaced** fracture (avulsion) of lateral epicondyle of unspecified humerus
    - ✓7th **S42.434** **Nondisplaced** fracture (avulsion) of lateral epicondyle of **right** humerus
    - ✓7th **S42.435** **Nondisplaced** fracture (avulsion) of lateral epicondyle of **left** humerus
    - ✓7th **S42.436** **Nondisplaced** fracture (avulsion) of lateral epicondyle of unspecified humerus

  - ✓6th **S42.44 Fracture (avulsion) of medial epicondyle** of humerus
    - ✓7th **S42.441** **Displaced** fracture (avulsion) of medial epicondyle of **right** humerus

- **S42.442** Displaced fracture (avulsion) of medial epicondyle of left humerus
- **S42.443** Displaced fracture (avulsion) of medial epicondyle of unspecified humerus
- **S42.444** Nondisplaced fracture (avulsion) of medial epicondyle of right humerus
- **S42.445** Nondisplaced fracture (avulsion) of medial epicondyle of left humerus
- **S42.446** Nondisplaced fracture (avulsion) of medial epicondyle of unspecified humerus
- **S42.447** Incarcerated fracture (avulsion) of medial epicondyle of right humerus
- **S42.448** Incarcerated fracture (avulsion) of medial epicondyle of left humerus
- **S42.449** Incarcerated fracture (avulsion) of medial epicondyle of unspecified humerus

S42.45 Fracture of lateral condyle of humerus
Fracture of capitellum of humerus
- **S42.451** Displaced fracture of lateral condyle of right humerus
- **S42.452** Displaced fracture of lateral condyle of left humerus
- **S42.453** Displaced fracture of lateral condyle of unspecified humerus
- **S42.454** Nondisplaced fracture of lateral condyle of right humerus
- **S42.455** Nondisplaced fracture of lateral condyle of left humerus
- **S42.456** Nondisplaced fracture of lateral condyle of unspecified humerus

S42.46 Fracture of medial condyle of humerus
Trochlea fracture of humerus
- **S42.461** Displaced fracture of medial condyle of right humerus
- **S42.462** Displaced fracture of medial condyle of left humerus
- **S42.463** Displaced fracture of medial condyle of unspecified humerus
- **S42.464** Nondisplaced fracture of medial condyle of right humerus
- **S42.465** Nondisplaced fracture of medial condyle of left humerus
- **S42.466** Nondisplaced fracture of medial condyle of unspecified humerus

S42.47 Transcondylar fracture of humerus
- **S42.471** Displaced transcondylar fracture of right humerus
- **S42.472** Displaced transcondylar fracture of left humerus
- **S42.473** Displaced transcondylar fracture of unspecified humerus
- **S42.474** Nondisplaced transcondylar fracture of right humerus
- **S42.475** Nondisplaced transcondylar fracture of left humerus
- **S42.476** Nondisplaced transcondylar fracture of unspecified humerus

S42.48 Torus fracture of lower end of humerus

> The appropriate 7th character is to be added to all codes in subcategory S42.48.
> A initial encounter for closed fracture
> D subsequent encounter for fracture with routine healing
> G subsequent encounter for fracture with delayed healing
> K subsequent encounter for fracture with nonunion
> P subsequent encounter for fracture with malunion
> S sequela

- **S42.481** Torus fracture of lower end of right humerus
- **S42.482** Torus fracture of lower end of left humerus
- **S42.489** Torus fracture of lower end of unspecified humerus

S42.49 Other fracture of lower end of humerus
- **S42.491** Other displaced fracture of lower end of right humerus
- **S42.492** Other displaced fracture of lower end of left humerus
- **S42.493** Other displaced fracture of lower end of unspecified humerus
- **S42.494** Other nondisplaced fracture of lower end of right humerus
- **S42.495** Other nondisplaced fracture of lower end of left humerus
- **S42.496** Other nondisplaced fracture of lower end of unspecified humerus

S42.9 Fracture of shoulder girdle, part unspecified
Fracture of shoulder NOS
- **S42.90** Fracture of unspecified shoulder girdle, part unspecified
- **S42.91** Fracture of right shoulder girdle, part unspecified
- **S42.92** Fracture of left shoulder girdle, part unspecified

S43 Dislocation and sprain of joints and ligaments of shoulder girdle
INCLUDES avulsion of joint or ligament of shoulder girdle
laceration of cartilage, joint or ligament of shoulder girdle
sprain of cartilage, joint or ligament of shoulder girdle
traumatic hemarthrosis of joint or ligament of shoulder girdle
traumatic rupture of joint or ligament of shoulder girdle
traumatic subluxation of joint or ligament of shoulder girdle
traumatic tear of joint or ligament of shoulder girdle
Code also any associated open wound
EXCLUDES 2 strain of muscle, fascia and tendon of shoulder and upper arm (S46.-)

> The appropriate 7th character is to be added to each code from category S43.
> A initial encounter
> D subsequent encounter
> S sequela

S43.0 Subluxation and dislocation of shoulder joint
Dislocation of glenohumeral joint
Subluxation of glenohumeral joint

- **S43.00** Unspecified subluxation and dislocation of shoulder joint
  Dislocation of humerus NOS
  Subluxation of humerus NOS
  - **S43.001** Unspecified subluxation of right shoulder joint
  - **S43.002** Unspecified subluxation of left shoulder joint
  - **S43.003** Unspecified subluxation of unspecified shoulder joint
  - **S43.004** Unspecified dislocation of right shoulder joint
  - **S43.005** Unspecified dislocation of left shoulder joint
  - **S43.006** Unspecified dislocation of unspecified shoulder joint

- **S43.01** Anterior subluxation and dislocation of humerus
  - **S43.011** Anterior subluxation of right humerus
  - **S43.012** Anterior subluxation of left humerus
  - **S43.013** Anterior subluxation of unspecified humerus
  - **S43.014** Anterior dislocation of right humerus
  - **S43.015** Anterior dislocation of left humerus
  - **S43.016** Anterior dislocation of unspecified humerus

- **S43.02** Posterior subluxation and dislocation of humerus
  - **S43.021** Posterior subluxation of right humerus
  - **S43.022** Posterior subluxation of left humerus
  - **S43.023** Posterior subluxation of unspecified humerus
  - **S43.024** Posterior dislocation of right humerus
  - **S43.025** Posterior dislocation of left humerus
  - **S43.026** Posterior dislocation of unspecified humerus

- **S43.03** Inferior subluxation and dislocation of humerus
  - **S43.031** Inferior subluxation of right humerus
  - **S43.032** Inferior subluxation of left humerus
  - **S43.033** Inferior subluxation of unspecified humerus
  - **S43.034** Inferior dislocation of right humerus

- ✓7th **S43.035** Inferior dislocation of left humerus
- ✓7th **S43.036** Inferior dislocation of unspecified humerus
- ✓6th **S43.08** Other subluxation and dislocation of shoulder joint
  - ✓7th **S43.081** Other subluxation of right shoulder joint
  - ✓7th **S43.082** Other subluxation of left shoulder joint
  - ✓7th **S43.083** Other subluxation of unspecified shoulder joint
  - ✓7th **S43.084** Other dislocation of right shoulder joint
  - ✓7th **S43.085** Other dislocation of left shoulder joint
  - ✓7th **S43.086** Other dislocation of unspecified shoulder joint
- ✓5th **S43.1** Subluxation and dislocation of acromioclavicular joint
  - ✓6th **S43.10** Unspecified dislocation of acromioclavicular joint
    - ✓7th **S43.101** Unspecified dislocation of right acromioclavicular joint
    - ✓7th **S43.102** Unspecified dislocation of left acromioclavicular joint
    - ✓7th **S43.109** Unspecified dislocation of unspecified acromioclavicular joint
  - ✓6th **S43.11** Subluxation of acromioclavicular joint
    - ✓7th **S43.111** Subluxation of right acromioclavicular joint
    - ✓7th **S43.112** Subluxation of left acromioclavicular joint
    - ✓7th **S43.119** Subluxation of unspecified acromioclavicular joint
  - ✓6th **S43.12** Dislocation of acromioclavicular joint, 100%-200% displacement
    - ✓7th **S43.121** Dislocation of right acromioclavicular joint, 100%-200% displacement
    - ✓7th **S43.122** Dislocation of left acromioclavicular joint, 100%-200% displacement
    - ✓7th **S43.129** Dislocation of unspecified acromioclavicular joint, 100%-200% displacement
  - ✓6th **S43.13** Dislocation of acromioclavicular joint, greater than 200% displacement
    - ✓7th **S43.131** Dislocation of right acromioclavicular joint, greater than 200% displacement
    - ✓7th **S43.132** Dislocation of left acromioclavicular joint, greater than 200% displacement
    - ✓7th **S43.139** Dislocation of unspecified acromioclavicular joint, greater than 200% displacement
  - ✓6th **S43.14** Inferior dislocation of acromioclavicular joint
    - ✓7th **S43.141** Inferior dislocation of right acromioclavicular joint
    - ✓7th **S43.142** Inferior dislocation of left acromioclavicular joint
    - ✓7th **S43.149** Inferior dislocation of unspecified acromioclavicular joint
  - ✓6th **S43.15** Posterior dislocation of acromioclavicular joint
    - ✓7th **S43.151** Posterior dislocation of right acromioclavicular joint
    - ✓7th **S43.152** Posterior dislocation of left acromioclavicular joint
    - ✓7th **S43.159** Posterior dislocation of unspecified acromioclavicular joint
- ✓5th **S43.2** Subluxation and dislocation of sternoclavicular joint
  - ✓6th **S43.20** Unspecified subluxation and dislocation of sternoclavicular joint
    - ✓7th **S43.201** Unspecified subluxation of right sternoclavicular joint
    - ✓7th **S43.202** Unspecified subluxation of left sternoclavicular joint
    - ✓7th **S43.203** Unspecified subluxation of unspecified sternoclavicular joint
    - ✓7th **S43.204** Unspecified dislocation of right sternoclavicular joint
    - ✓7th **S43.205** Unspecified dislocation of left sternoclavicular joint
    - ✓7th **S43.206** Unspecified dislocation of unspecified sternoclavicular joint
  - ✓6th **S43.21** Anterior subluxation and dislocation of sternoclavicular joint
    - ✓7th **S43.211** Anterior subluxation of right sternoclavicular joint
    - ✓7th **S43.212** Anterior subluxation of left sternoclavicular joint
    - ✓7th **S43.213** Anterior subluxation of unspecified sternoclavicular joint
    - ✓7th **S43.214** Anterior dislocation of right sternoclavicular joint
    - ✓7th **S43.215** Anterior dislocation of left sternoclavicular joint
    - ✓7th **S43.216** Anterior dislocation of unspecified sternoclavicular joint
  - ✓6th **S43.22** Posterior subluxation and dislocation of sternoclavicular joint
    - ✓7th **S43.221** Posterior subluxation of right sternoclavicular joint
    - ✓7th **S43.222** Posterior subluxation of left sternoclavicular joint
    - ✓7th **S43.223** Posterior subluxation of unspecified sternoclavicular joint
    - ✓7th **S43.224** Posterior dislocation of right sternoclavicular joint
    - ✓7th **S43.225** Posterior dislocation of left sternoclavicular joint
    - ✓7th **S43.226** Posterior dislocation of unspecified sternoclavicular joint
- ✓5th **S43.3** Subluxation and dislocation of other and unspecified parts of shoulder girdle
  - ✓6th **S43.30** Subluxation and dislocation of unspecified parts of shoulder girdle
    - Dislocation of shoulder girdle NOS
    - Subluxation of shoulder girdle NOS
    - ✓7th **S43.301** Subluxation of unspecified parts of right shoulder girdle
    - ✓7th **S43.302** Subluxation of unspecified parts of left shoulder girdle
    - ✓7th **S43.303** Subluxation of unspecified parts of unspecified shoulder girdle
    - ✓7th **S43.304** Dislocation of unspecified parts of right shoulder girdle
    - ✓7th **S43.305** Dislocation of unspecified parts of left shoulder girdle
    - ✓7th **S43.306** Dislocation of unspecified parts of unspecified shoulder girdle
  - ✓6th **S43.31** Subluxation and dislocation of scapula
    - ✓7th **S43.311** Subluxation of right scapula
    - ✓7th **S43.312** Subluxation of left scapula
    - ✓7th **S43.313** Subluxation of unspecified scapula
    - ✓7th **S43.314** Dislocation of right scapula
    - ✓7th **S43.315** Dislocation of left scapula
    - ✓7th **S43.316** Dislocation of unspecified scapula
  - ✓6th **S43.39** Subluxation and dislocation of other parts of shoulder girdle
    - ✓7th **S43.391** Subluxation of other parts of right shoulder girdle
    - ✓7th **S43.392** Subluxation of other parts of left shoulder girdle
    - ✓7th **S43.393** Subluxation of other parts of unspecified shoulder girdle
    - ✓7th **S43.394** Dislocation of other parts of right shoulder girdle
    - ✓7th **S43.395** Dislocation of other parts of left shoulder girdle
    - ✓7th **S43.396** Dislocation of other parts of unspecified shoulder girdle
- ✓5th **S43.4** Sprain of shoulder joint
  - ✓6th **S43.40** Unspecified sprain of shoulder joint
    - ✓7th **S43.401** Unspecified sprain of right shoulder joint
    - ✓7th **S43.402** Unspecified sprain of left shoulder joint
    - ✓7th **S43.409** Unspecified sprain of unspecified shoulder joint
  - ✓6th **S43.41** Sprain of coracohumeral (ligament)
    - ✓7th **S43.411** Sprain of right coracohumeral (ligament)
    - ✓7th **S43.412** Sprain of left coracohumeral (ligament)
    - ✓7th **S43.419** Sprain of unspecified coracohumeral (ligament)
  - ✓6th **S43.42** Sprain of rotator cuff capsule
    - EXCLUDES 1 rotator cuff syndrome (complete) (incomplete), not specified as traumatic (M75.1-)
    - EXCLUDES 2 injury of tendon of rotator cuff (S46.0-)
    - ✓7th **S43.421** Sprain of right rotator cuff capsule
    - ✓7th **S43.422** Sprain of left rotator cuff capsule
    - ✓7th **S43.429** Sprain of unspecified rotator cuff capsule

Chapter 19. Injury, Poisoning and Certain Other Consequences of External Causes

- ✓6th **S43.43** **Superior glenoid labrum** lesion
  SLAP lesion
  AHA: 2024,2Q,24; 2019,2Q,26
  DEF: Detachment injury of the superior aspect of the glenoid labrum, which is the ring of fibrocartilage attached to the rim of the glenoid cavity of the scapula.
  - ✓7th **S43.431** Superior glenoid labrum lesion of **right** shoulder
  - ✓7th **S43.432** Superior glenoid labrum lesion of **left** shoulder
  - ✓7th **S43.439** Superior glenoid labrum lesion of **unspecified** shoulder
- ✓6th **S43.49** Other sprain of shoulder joint
  - ✓7th **S43.491** Other sprain of **right** shoulder joint
  - ✓7th **S43.492** Other sprain of **left** shoulder joint
  - ✓7th **S43.499** Other sprain of unspecified shoulder joint
- ✓5th **S43.5** Sprain of **acromioclavicular** joint
  Sprain of acromioclavicular ligament
  - ✓x 7th **S43.50** Sprain of unspecified acromioclavicular joint
  - ✓x 7th **S43.51** Sprain of **right** acromioclavicular joint
  - ✓x 7th **S43.52** Sprain of **left** acromioclavicular joint
- ✓5th **S43.6** Sprain of **sternoclavicular** joint
  - ✓x 7th **S43.60** Sprain of unspecified sternoclavicular joint
  - ✓x 7th **S43.61** Sprain of **right** sternoclavicular joint
  - ✓x 7th **S43.62** Sprain of **left** sternoclavicular joint
- ✓5th **S43.8** Sprain of other specified parts of shoulder girdle
  - ✓x 7th **S43.80** Sprain of other specified parts of unspecified shoulder girdle
  - ✓x 7th **S43.81** Sprain of other specified parts of **right** shoulder girdle
  - ✓x 7th **S43.82** Sprain of other specified parts of **left** shoulder girdle
- ✓5th **S43.9** Sprain of unspecified parts of shoulder girdle
  - ✓x 7th **S43.90** Sprain of unspecified parts of unspecified shoulder girdle
    Sprain of shoulder girdle NOS
  - ✓x 7th **S43.91** Sprain of unspecified parts of **right** shoulder girdle
  - ✓x 7th **S43.92** Sprain of unspecified parts of **left** shoulder girdle

✓4th S44 Injury of nerves at shoulder and upper arm level

Code also any associated open wound (S41.-)
EXCLUDES 2 injury of brachial plexus (S14.3-)

The appropriate 7th character is to be added to each code from category S44.
- A initial encounter
- D subsequent encounter
- S sequela

- ✓5th **S44.0** Injury of **ulnar nerve** at upper arm level
  EXCLUDES 1 ulnar nerve NOS (S54.0)
  - ✓x 7th **S44.00** Injury of ulnar nerve at upper arm level, unspecified arm
  - ✓x 7th **S44.01** Injury of ulnar nerve at upper arm level, **right** arm
  - ✓x 7th **S44.02** Injury of ulnar nerve at upper arm level, **left** arm
- ✓5th **S44.1** Injury of **median nerve** at upper arm level
  EXCLUDES 1 median nerve NOS (S54.1)
  - ✓x 7th **S44.10** Injury of median nerve at upper arm level, unspecified arm
  - ✓x 7th **S44.11** Injury of median nerve at upper arm level, **right** arm
  - ✓x 7th **S44.12** Injury of median nerve at upper arm level, **left** arm
- ✓5th **S44.2** Injury of **radial nerve** at upper arm level
  EXCLUDES 1 radial nerve NOS (S54.2)
  - ✓x 7th **S44.20** Injury of radial nerve at upper arm level, unspecified arm
  - ✓x 7th **S44.21** Injury of radial nerve at upper arm level, **right** arm
  - ✓x 7th **S44.22** Injury of radial nerve at upper arm level, **left** arm
- ✓5th **S44.3** Injury of **axillary nerve**
  - ✓x 7th **S44.30** Injury of axillary nerve, unspecified arm
  - ✓x 7th **S44.31** Injury of axillary nerve, **right** arm
  - ✓x 7th **S44.32** Injury of axillary nerve, **left** arm
- ✓5th **S44.4** Injury of **musculocutaneous nerve**
  - ✓x 7th **S44.40** Injury of musculocutaneous nerve, unspecified arm
  - ✓x 7th **S44.41** Injury of musculocutaneous nerve, **right** arm
  - ✓x 7th **S44.42** Injury of musculocutaneous nerve, **left** arm
- ✓5th **S44.5** Injury of **cutaneous sensory nerve** at shoulder and upper arm level
  - ✓x 7th **S44.50** Injury of cutaneous sensory nerve at shoulder and upper arm level, unspecified arm
  - ✓x 7th **S44.51** Injury of cutaneous sensory nerve at shoulder and upper arm level, **right** arm
  - ✓x 7th **S44.52** Injury of cutaneous sensory nerve at shoulder and upper arm level, **left** arm
- ✓5th **S44.8** Injury of other nerves at shoulder and upper arm level
  - ✓6th **S44.8X** Injury of other nerves at shoulder and upper arm level
    - ✓7th **S44.8X1** Injury of other nerves at shoulder and upper arm level, **right** arm
    - ✓7th **S44.8X2** Injury of other nerves at shoulder and upper arm level, **left** arm
    - ✓7th **S44.8X9** Injury of other nerves at shoulder and upper arm level, unspecified arm
- ✓5th **S44.9** Injury of unspecified nerve at shoulder and upper arm level
  - ✓x 7th **S44.90** Injury of unspecified nerve at shoulder and upper arm level, unspecified arm
  - ✓x 7th **S44.91** Injury of unspecified nerve at shoulder and upper arm level, **right** arm
  - ✓x 7th **S44.92** Injury of unspecified nerve at shoulder and upper arm level, **left** arm

✓4th S45 Injury of blood vessels at shoulder and upper arm level

Code also any associated open wound (S41.-)
EXCLUDES 2 injury of subclavian artery (S25.1)
injury of subclavian vein (S25.3)

The appropriate 7th character is to be added to each code from category S45.
- A initial encounter
- D subsequent encounter
- S sequela

- ✓5th **S45.0** Injury of **axillary artery**
  - ✓6th **S45.00** Unspecified injury of axillary artery
    - ✓7th **S45.001** Unspecified injury of axillary artery, **right** side
    - ✓7th **S45.002** Unspecified injury of axillary artery, **left** side
    - ✓7th **S45.009** Unspecified injury of axillary artery, unspecified side
  - ✓6th **S45.01** **Laceration** of axillary artery
    - ✓7th **S45.011** Laceration of axillary artery, **right** side
    - ✓7th **S45.012** Laceration of axillary artery, **left** side
    - ✓7th **S45.019** Laceration of axillary artery, unspecified side
  - ✓6th **S45.09** Other specified injury of axillary artery
    - ✓7th **S45.091** Other specified injury of axillary artery, **right** side
    - ✓7th **S45.092** Other specified injury of axillary artery, **left** side
    - ✓7th **S45.099** Other specified injury of axillary artery, unspecified side
- ✓5th **S45.1** Injury of **brachial artery**
  - ✓6th **S45.10** Unspecified injury of brachial artery
    - ✓7th **S45.101** Unspecified injury of brachial artery, **right** side
    - ✓7th **S45.102** Unspecified injury of brachial artery, **left** side
    - ✓7th **S45.109** Unspecified injury of brachial artery, unspecified side
  - ✓6th **S45.11** **Laceration** of brachial artery
    - ✓7th **S45.111** Laceration of brachial artery, **right** side
    - ✓7th **S45.112** Laceration of brachial artery, **left** side
    - ✓7th **S45.119** Laceration of brachial artery, unspecified side
  - ✓6th **S45.19** Other specified injury of brachial artery
    - ✓7th **S45.191** Other specified injury of brachial artery, **right** side
    - ✓7th **S45.192** Other specified injury of brachial artery, **left** side
    - ✓7th **S45.199** Other specified injury of brachial artery, unspecified side
- ✓5th **S45.2** Injury of **axillary or brachial vein**
  - ✓6th **S45.20** Unspecified injury of axillary or brachial vein
    - ✓7th **S45.201** Unspecified injury of axillary or brachial vein, **right** side

- ✓7th **S45.202** Unspecified injury of axillary or brachial vein, **left** side
- ✓7th **S45.209** Unspecified injury of axillary or brachial vein, unspecified side
- ✓6th **S45.21** **Laceration** of axillary or brachial vein
  - ✓7th **S45.211** Laceration of axillary or brachial vein, **right** side
  - ✓7th **S45.212** Laceration of axillary or brachial vein, **left** side
  - ✓7th **S45.219** Laceration of axillary or brachial vein, unspecified side
- ✓6th **S45.29** Other specified injury of axillary or brachial vein
  - ✓7th **S45.291** Other specified injury of axillary or brachial vein, **right** side
  - ✓7th **S45.292** Other specified injury of axillary or brachial vein, **left** side
  - ✓7th **S45.299** Other specified injury of axillary or brachial vein, unspecified side
- ✓5th **S45.3** Injury of **superficial vein** at shoulder and upper arm level
  - ✓6th **S45.30** Unspecified injury of superficial vein at shoulder and upper arm level
    - ✓7th **S45.301** Unspecified injury of superficial vein at shoulder and upper arm level, **right** arm
    - ✓7th **S45.302** Unspecified injury of superficial vein at shoulder and upper arm level, **left** arm
    - ✓7th **S45.309** Unspecified injury of superficial vein at shoulder and upper arm level, unspecified arm
  - ✓6th **S45.31** **Laceration** of superficial vein at shoulder and upper arm level
    - ✓7th **S45.311** Laceration of superficial vein at shoulder and upper arm level, **right** arm
    - ✓7th **S45.312** Laceration of superficial vein at shoulder and upper arm level, **left** arm
    - ✓7th **S45.319** Laceration of superficial vein at shoulder and upper arm level, unspecified arm
  - ✓6th **S45.39** Other specified injury of superficial vein at shoulder and upper arm level
    - ✓7th **S45.391** Other specified injury of superficial vein at shoulder and upper arm level, **right** arm
    - ✓7th **S45.392** Other specified injury of superficial vein at shoulder and upper arm level, **left** arm
    - ✓7th **S45.399** Other specified injury of superficial vein at shoulder and upper arm level, unspecified arm
- ✓5th **S45.8** Injury of other specified blood vessels at shoulder and upper arm level
  - ✓6th **S45.80** Unspecified injury of other specified blood vessels at shoulder and upper arm level
    - ✓7th **S45.801** Unspecified injury of other specified blood vessels at shoulder and upper arm level, **right** arm
    - ✓7th **S45.802** Unspecified injury of other specified blood vessels at shoulder and upper arm level, **left** arm
    - ✓7th **S45.809** Unspecified injury of other specified blood vessels at shoulder and upper arm level, unspecified arm
  - ✓6th **S45.81** **Laceration** of other specified blood vessels at shoulder and upper arm level
    - ✓7th **S45.811** Laceration of other specified blood vessels at shoulder and upper arm level, **right** arm
    - ✓7th **S45.812** Laceration of other specified blood vessels at shoulder and upper arm level, **left** arm
    - ✓7th **S45.819** Laceration of other specified blood vessels at shoulder and upper arm level, unspecified arm
  - ✓6th **S45.89** Other specified injury of other specified blood vessels at shoulder and upper arm level
    - ✓7th **S45.891** Other specified injury of other specified blood vessels at shoulder and upper arm level, **right** arm
    - ✓7th **S45.892** Other specified injury of other specified blood vessels at shoulder and upper arm level, **left** arm
    - ✓7th **S45.899** Other specified injury of other specified blood vessels at shoulder and upper arm level, unspecified arm
- ✓5th **S45.9** Injury of unspecified blood vessel at shoulder and upper arm level
  - ✓6th **S45.90** Unspecified injury of unspecified blood vessel at shoulder and upper arm level
    - ✓7th **S45.901** Unspecified injury of unspecified blood vessel at shoulder and upper arm level, **right** arm
    - ✓7th **S45.902** Unspecified injury of unspecified blood vessel at shoulder and upper arm level, **left** arm
    - ✓7th **S45.909** Unspecified injury of unspecified blood vessel at shoulder and upper arm level, unspecified arm
  - ✓6th **S45.91** **Laceration** of unspecified blood vessel at shoulder and upper arm level
    - ✓7th **S45.911** Laceration of unspecified blood vessel at shoulder and upper arm level, **right** arm
    - ✓7th **S45.912** Laceration of unspecified blood vessel at shoulder and upper arm level, **left** arm
    - ✓7th **S45.919** Laceration of unspecified blood vessel at shoulder and upper arm level, unspecified arm
  - ✓6th **S45.99** Other specified injury of unspecified blood vessel at shoulder and upper arm level
    - ✓7th **S45.991** Other specified injury of unspecified blood vessel at shoulder and upper arm level, **right** arm
    - ✓7th **S45.992** Other specified injury of unspecified blood vessel at shoulder and upper arm level, **left** arm
    - ✓7th **S45.999** Other specified injury of unspecified blood vessel at shoulder and upper arm level, unspecified arm

- ✓4th **S46** **Injury of muscle, fascia and tendon at shoulder and upper arm level**

  Code also any associated open wound (S41.-)

  EXCLUDES 2 injury of muscle, fascia and tendon at elbow (S56.-)
  sprain of joints and ligaments of shoulder girdle (S43.9)

  TIP: Refer to the Muscle/Tendon table at the beginning of this chapter.

  The appropriate 7th character is to be added to each code from category S46.
  A   initial encounter
  D   subsequent encounter
  S   sequela

  - ✓5th **S46.0** Injury of muscle(s) and tendon(s) of the **rotator cuff** of shoulder
    - ✓6th **S46.00** Unspecified injury of muscle(s) and tendon(s) of the rotator cuff of shoulder
      - ✓7th **S46.001** Unspecified injury of muscle(s) and tendon(s) of the rotator cuff of **right** shoulder
      - ✓7th **S46.002** Unspecified injury of muscle(s) and tendon(s) of the rotator cuff of **left** shoulder
      - ✓7th **S46.009** Unspecified injury of muscle(s) and tendon(s) of the rotator cuff of unspecified shoulder
    - ✓6th **S46.01** **Strain** of muscle(s) and tendon(s) of the rotator cuff of shoulder
      - ✓7th **S46.011** Strain of muscle(s) and tendon(s) of the rotator cuff of **right** shoulder
      - ✓7th **S46.012** Strain of muscle(s) and tendon(s) of the rotator cuff of **left** shoulder
      - ✓7th **S46.019** Strain of muscle(s) and tendon(s) of the rotator cuff of unspecified shoulder
    - ✓6th **S46.02** **Laceration** of muscle(s) and tendon(s) of the rotator cuff of shoulder
      - ✓7th **S46.021** Laceration of muscle(s) and tendon(s) of the rotator cuff of **right** shoulder
      - ✓7th **S46.022** Laceration of muscle(s) and tendon(s) of the rotator cuff of **left** shoulder
      - ✓7th **S46.029** Laceration of muscle(s) and tendon(s) of the rotator cuff of unspecified shoulder
    - ✓6th **S46.09** Other injury of muscle(s) and tendon(s) of the rotator cuff of shoulder
      - ✓7th **S46.091** Other injury of muscle(s) and tendon(s) of the rotator cuff of **right** shoulder
      - ✓7th **S46.092** Other injury of muscle(s) and tendon(s) of the rotator cuff of **left** shoulder
      - ✓7th **S46.099** Other injury of muscle(s) and tendon(s) of the rotator cuff of unspecified shoulder

S46.1 Injury of muscle, fascia and tendon of long head of biceps

- **S46.10** Unspecified injury of muscle, fascia and tendon of long head of biceps
  - S46.101 Unspecified injury of muscle, fascia and tendon of long head of biceps, **right** arm
  - S46.102 Unspecified injury of muscle, fascia and tendon of long head of biceps, **left** arm
  - S46.109 Unspecified injury of muscle, fascia and tendon of long head of biceps, unspecified arm
- **S46.11 Strain** of muscle, fascia and tendon of long head of biceps
  - AHA: 2020,1Q,38; 2019,2Q,27
  - S46.111 Strain of muscle, fascia and tendon of long head of biceps, **right** arm
  - S46.112 Strain of muscle, fascia and tendon of long head of biceps, **left** arm
  - S46.119 Strain of muscle, fascia and tendon of long head of biceps, unspecified arm
- **S46.12 Laceration** of muscle, fascia and tendon of long head of biceps
  - S46.121 Laceration of muscle, fascia and tendon of long head of biceps, **right** arm
  - S46.122 Laceration of muscle, fascia and tendon of long head of biceps, **left** arm
  - S46.129 Laceration of muscle, fascia and tendon of long head of biceps, unspecified arm
- **S46.19** Other injury of muscle, fascia and tendon of long head of biceps
  - S46.191 Other injury of muscle, fascia and tendon of long head of biceps, **right** arm
  - S46.192 Other injury of muscle, fascia and tendon of long head of biceps, **left** arm
  - S46.199 Other injury of muscle, fascia and tendon of long head of biceps, unspecified arm

S46.2 Injury of muscle, fascia and tendon of other parts of biceps

- **S46.20** Unspecified injury of muscle, fascia and tendon of other parts of biceps
  - S46.201 Unspecified injury of muscle, fascia and tendon of other parts of biceps, **right** arm
  - S46.202 Unspecified injury of muscle, fascia and tendon of other parts of biceps, **left** arm
  - S46.209 Unspecified injury of muscle, fascia and tendon of other parts of biceps, unspecified arm
- **S46.21 Strain** of muscle, fascia and tendon of other parts of biceps
  - S46.211 Strain of muscle, fascia and tendon of other parts of biceps, **right** arm
  - S46.212 Strain of muscle, fascia and tendon of other parts of biceps, **left** arm
  - S46.219 Strain of muscle, fascia and tendon of other parts of biceps, unspecified arm
- **S46.22 Laceration** of muscle, fascia and tendon of other parts of biceps
  - S46.221 Laceration of muscle, fascia and tendon of other parts of biceps, **right** arm
  - S46.222 Laceration of muscle, fascia and tendon of other parts of biceps, **left** arm
  - S46.229 Laceration of muscle, fascia and tendon of other parts of biceps, unspecified arm
- **S46.29** Other injury of muscle, fascia and tendon of other parts of biceps
  - S46.291 Other injury of muscle, fascia and tendon of other parts of biceps, **right** arm
  - S46.292 Other injury of muscle, fascia and tendon of other parts of biceps, **left** arm
  - S46.299 Other injury of muscle, fascia and tendon of other parts of biceps, unspecified arm

S46.3 Injury of muscle, fascia and tendon of triceps

- **S46.30** Unspecified injury of muscle, fascia and tendon of triceps
  - S46.301 Unspecified injury of muscle, fascia and tendon of triceps, **right** arm
  - S46.302 Unspecified injury of muscle, fascia and tendon of triceps, **left** arm
  - S46.309 Unspecified injury of muscle, fascia and tendon of triceps, unspecified arm
- **S46.31 Strain** of muscle, fascia and tendon of triceps
  - S46.311 Strain of muscle, fascia and tendon of triceps, **right** arm
  - S46.312 Strain of muscle, fascia and tendon of triceps, **left** arm
  - S46.319 Strain of muscle, fascia and tendon of triceps, unspecified arm
- **S46.32 Laceration** of muscle, fascia and tendon of triceps
  - S46.321 Laceration of muscle, fascia and tendon of triceps, **right** arm
  - S46.322 Laceration of muscle, fascia and tendon of triceps, **left** arm
  - S46.329 Laceration of muscle, fascia and tendon of triceps, unspecified arm
- **S46.39** Other injury of muscle, fascia and tendon of triceps
  - S46.391 Other injury of muscle, fascia and tendon of triceps, **right** arm
  - S46.392 Other injury of muscle, fascia and tendon of triceps, **left** arm
  - S46.399 Other injury of muscle, fascia and tendon of triceps, unspecified arm

S46.8 Injury of other muscles, fascia and tendons at shoulder and upper arm level

- **S46.80** Unspecified injury of other muscles, fascia and tendons at shoulder and upper arm level
  - S46.801 Unspecified injury of other muscles, fascia and tendons at shoulder and upper arm level, **right** arm
  - S46.802 Unspecified injury of other muscles, fascia and tendons at shoulder and upper arm level, **left** arm
  - S46.809 Unspecified injury of other muscles, fascia and tendons at shoulder and upper arm level, unspecified arm
- **S46.81 Strain** of other muscles, fascia and tendons at shoulder and upper arm level
  - S46.811 Strain of other muscles, fascia and tendons at shoulder and upper arm level, **right** arm
  - S46.812 Strain of other muscles, fascia and tendons at shoulder and upper arm level, **left** arm
  - S46.819 Strain of other muscles, fascia and tendons at shoulder and upper arm level, unspecified arm
- **S46.82 Laceration** of other muscles, fascia and tendons at shoulder and upper arm level
  - S46.821 Laceration of other muscles, fascia and tendons at shoulder and upper arm level, **right** arm
  - S46.822 Laceration of other muscles, fascia and tendons at shoulder and upper arm level, **left** arm
  - S46.829 Laceration of other muscles, fascia and tendons at shoulder and upper arm level, unspecified arm
- **S46.89** Other injury of other muscles, fascia and tendons at shoulder and upper arm level
  - S46.891 Other injury of other muscles, fascia and tendons at shoulder and upper arm level, **right** arm
  - S46.892 Other injury of other muscles, fascia and tendons at shoulder and upper arm level, **left** arm
  - S46.899 Other injury of other muscles, fascia and tendons at shoulder and upper arm level, unspecified arm

S46.9 Injury of unspecified muscle, fascia and tendon at shoulder and upper arm level

- **S46.90** Unspecified injury of unspecified muscle, fascia and tendon at shoulder and upper arm level
  - S46.901 Unspecified injury of unspecified muscle, fascia and tendon at shoulder and upper arm level, **right** arm
  - S46.902 Unspecified injury of unspecified muscle, fascia and tendon at shoulder and upper arm level, **left** arm
  - S46.909 Unspecified injury of unspecified muscle, fascia and tendon at shoulder and upper arm level, unspecified arm
- **S46.91 Strain** of unspecified muscle, fascia and tendon at shoulder and upper arm level
  - S46.911 Strain of unspecified muscle, fascia and tendon at shoulder and upper arm level, **right** arm
  - S46.912 Strain of unspecified muscle, fascia and tendon at shoulder and upper arm level, **left** arm

S46.919 Strain of unspecified muscle, fascia and tendon at shoulder and upper arm level, unspecified arm

S46.92 Laceration of unspecified muscle, fascia and tendon at shoulder and upper arm level
- **S46.921** Laceration of unspecified muscle, fascia and tendon at shoulder and upper arm level, right arm
- **S46.922** Laceration of unspecified muscle, fascia and tendon at shoulder and upper arm level, left arm
- **S46.929** Laceration of unspecified muscle, fascia and tendon at shoulder and upper arm level, unspecified arm

S46.99 Other injury of unspecified muscle, fascia and tendon at shoulder and upper arm level
- **S46.991** Other injury of unspecified muscle, fascia and tendon at shoulder and upper arm level, right arm
- **S46.992** Other injury of unspecified muscle, fascia and tendon at shoulder and upper arm level, left arm
- **S46.999** Other injury of unspecified muscle, fascia and tendon at shoulder and upper arm level, unspecified arm

S47 Crushing injury of shoulder and upper arm
Use additional code for all associated injuries
EXCLUDES 2: crushing injury of elbow (S57.0-)

The appropriate 7th character is to be added to each code from category S47.
- A initial encounter
- D subsequent encounter
- S sequela

S47.1 Crushing injury of right shoulder and upper arm
S47.2 Crushing injury of left shoulder and upper arm
S47.9 Crushing injury of shoulder and upper arm, unspecified arm

S48 Traumatic amputation of shoulder and upper arm
An amputation not identified as partial or complete should be coded to complete
EXCLUDES 1: traumatic amputation at elbow level (S58.0)

The appropriate 7th character is to be added to each code from category S48.
- A initial encounter
- D subsequent encounter
- S sequela

S48.0 Traumatic amputation at shoulder joint
- **S48.01** Complete traumatic amputation at shoulder joint
  - **S48.011** Complete traumatic amputation at right shoulder joint
  - **S48.012** Complete traumatic amputation at left shoulder joint
  - **S48.019** Complete traumatic amputation at unspecified shoulder joint
- **S48.02** Partial traumatic amputation at shoulder joint
  - **S48.021** Partial traumatic amputation at right shoulder joint
  - **S48.022** Partial traumatic amputation at left shoulder joint
  - **S48.029** Partial traumatic amputation at unspecified shoulder joint

S48.1 Traumatic amputation at level between shoulder and elbow
- **S48.11** Complete traumatic amputation at level between shoulder and elbow
  - **S48.111** Complete traumatic amputation at level between right shoulder and elbow
  - **S48.112** Complete traumatic amputation at level between left shoulder and elbow
  - **S48.119** Complete traumatic amputation at level between unspecified shoulder and elbow
- **S48.12** Partial traumatic amputation at level between shoulder and elbow
  - **S48.121** Partial traumatic amputation at level between right shoulder and elbow
  - **S48.122** Partial traumatic amputation at level between left shoulder and elbow
  - **S48.129** Partial traumatic amputation at level between unspecified shoulder and elbow

S48.9 Traumatic amputation of shoulder and upper arm, level unspecified
- **S48.91** Complete traumatic amputation of shoulder and upper arm, level unspecified
  - **S48.911** Complete traumatic amputation of right shoulder and upper arm, level unspecified
  - **S48.912** Complete traumatic amputation of left shoulder and upper arm, level unspecified
  - **S48.919** Complete traumatic amputation of unspecified shoulder and upper arm, level unspecified
- **S48.92** Partial traumatic amputation of shoulder and upper arm, level unspecified
  - **S48.921** Partial traumatic amputation of right shoulder and upper arm, level unspecified
  - **S48.922** Partial traumatic amputation of left shoulder and upper arm, level unspecified
  - **S48.929** Partial traumatic amputation of unspecified shoulder and upper arm, level unspecified

S49 Other and unspecified injuries of shoulder and upper arm
AHA: 2018,2Q,12; 2018,1Q,3

The appropriate 7th character is to be added to each code from subcategories S49.0 and S49.1.
- A initial encounter for closed fracture
- D subsequent encounter for fracture with routine healing
- G subsequent encounter for fracture with delayed healing
- K subsequent encounter for fracture with nonunion
- P subsequent encounter for fracture with malunion
- S sequela

S49.0 Physeal fracture of upper end of humerus
AHA: 2019,4Q,56
- **S49.00** Unspecified physeal fracture of upper end of humerus
  - **S49.001** Unspecified physeal fracture of upper end of humerus, right arm
  - **S49.002** Unspecified physeal fracture of upper end of humerus, left arm
  - **S49.009** Unspecified physeal fracture of upper end of humerus, unspecified arm
- **S49.01** Salter-Harris Type I physeal fracture of upper end of humerus
  - **S49.011** Salter-Harris Type I physeal fracture of upper end of humerus, right arm
  - **S49.012** Salter-Harris Type I physeal fracture of upper end of humerus, left arm
  - **S49.019** Salter-Harris Type I physeal fracture of upper end of humerus, unspecified arm
- **S49.02** Salter-Harris Type II physeal fracture of upper end of humerus
  - **S49.021** Salter-Harris Type II physeal fracture of upper end of humerus, right arm
  - **S49.022** Salter-Harris Type II physeal fracture of upper end of humerus, left arm
  - **S49.029** Salter-Harris Type II physeal fracture of upper end of humerus, unspecified arm
- **S49.03** Salter-Harris Type III physeal fracture of upper end of humerus
  - **S49.031** Salter-Harris Type III physeal fracture of upper end of humerus, right arm
  - **S49.032** Salter-Harris Type III physeal fracture of upper end of humerus, left arm
  - **S49.039** Salter-Harris Type III physeal fracture of upper end of humerus, unspecified arm
- **S49.04** Salter-Harris Type IV physeal fracture of upper end of humerus
  - **S49.041** Salter-Harris Type IV physeal fracture of upper end of humerus, right arm

- **S49.042** Salter-Harris Type IV physeal fracture of upper end of humerus, left arm
- **S49.049** Salter-Harris Type IV physeal fracture of upper end of humerus, unspecified

S49.09 Other physeal fracture of upper end of humerus
- **S49.091** Other physeal fracture of upper end of humerus, right arm
- **S49.092** Other physeal fracture of upper end of humerus, left arm
- **S49.099** Other physeal fracture of upper end of humerus, unspecified arm

S49.1 Physeal fracture of lower end of humerus
AHA: 2019,4Q,56

S49.10 Unspecified physeal fracture of lower end of humerus
- **S49.101** Unspecified physeal fracture of lower end of humerus, right arm
- **S49.102** Unspecified physeal fracture of lower end of humerus, left arm
- **S49.109** Unspecified physeal fracture of lower end of humerus, unspecified arm

S49.11 Salter-Harris Type I physeal fracture of lower end of humerus
- **S49.111** Salter-Harris Type I physeal fracture of lower end of humerus, right arm
- **S49.112** Salter-Harris Type I physeal fracture of lower end of humerus, left arm
- **S49.119** Salter-Harris Type I physeal fracture of lower end of humerus, unspecified arm

S49.12 Salter-Harris Type II physeal fracture of lower end of humerus
- **S49.121** Salter-Harris Type II physeal fracture of lower end of humerus, right arm
- **S49.122** Salter-Harris Type II physeal fracture of lower end of humerus, left arm
- **S49.129** Salter-Harris Type II physeal fracture of lower end of humerus, unspecified arm

S49.13 Salter-Harris Type III physeal fracture of lower end of humerus
- **S49.131** Salter-Harris Type III physeal fracture of lower end of humerus, right arm
- **S49.132** Salter-Harris Type III physeal fracture of lower end of humerus, left arm
- **S49.139** Salter-Harris Type III physeal fracture of lower end of humerus, unspecified arm

S49.14 Salter-Harris Type IV physeal fracture of lower end of humerus
- **S49.141** Salter-Harris Type IV physeal fracture of lower end of humerus, right arm
- **S49.142** Salter-Harris Type IV physeal fracture of lower end of humerus, left arm
- **S49.149** Salter-Harris Type IV physeal fracture of lower end of humerus, unspecified arm

S49.19 Other physeal fracture of lower end of humerus
- **S49.191** Other physeal fracture of lower end of humerus, right arm
- **S49.192** Other physeal fracture of lower end of humerus, left arm
- **S49.199** Other physeal fracture of lower end of humerus, unspecified arm

S49.8 Other specified injuries of shoulder and upper arm

The appropriate 7th character is to be added to each code in subcategory S49.8.
- A initial encounter
- D subsequent encounter
- S sequela

- **S49.80** Other specified injuries of shoulder and upper arm, unspecified arm
- **S49.81** Other specified injuries of right shoulder and upper arm
- **S49.82** Other specified injuries of left shoulder and upper arm

S49.9 Unspecified injury of shoulder and upper arm

The appropriate 7th character is to be added to each code in subcategory S49.9.
- A initial encounter
- D subsequent encounter
- S sequela

- **S49.90** Unspecified injury of shoulder and upper arm, unspecified
- **S49.91** Unspecified injury of right shoulder and upper arm
- **S49.92** Unspecified injury of left shoulder and upper arm

Injuries to the elbow and forearm (S50-S59)

EXCLUDES 2: burns and corrosions (T20-T32)
frostbite (T33-T34)
injuries of wrist and hand (S60-S69)
insect bite or sting, venomous (T63.4)

S50 Superficial injury of elbow and forearm
EXCLUDES 2: superficial injury of wrist and hand (S60.-)

The appropriate 7th character is to be added to each code from category S50.
- A initial encounter
- D subsequent encounter
- S sequela

S50.0 Contusion of elbow
- **S50.00** Contusion of unspecified elbow
- **S50.01** Contusion of right elbow
- **S50.02** Contusion of left elbow

S50.1 Contusion of forearm
- **S50.10** Contusion of unspecified forearm
- **S50.11** Contusion of right forearm
- **S50.12** Contusion of left forearm

S50.3 Other superficial injuries of elbow
- **S50.31** Abrasion of elbow
  - **S50.311** Abrasion of right elbow
  - **S50.312** Abrasion of left elbow
  - **S50.319** Abrasion of unspecified elbow
- **S50.32** Blister (nonthermal) of elbow
  - **S50.321** Blister (nonthermal) of right elbow
  - **S50.322** Blister (nonthermal) of left elbow
  - **S50.329** Blister (nonthermal) of unspecified elbow
- **S50.34** External constriction of elbow
  - **S50.341** External constriction of right elbow
  - **S50.342** External constriction of left elbow
  - **S50.349** External constriction of unspecified elbow
- **S50.35** Superficial foreign body of elbow
  Splinter in the elbow
  - **S50.351** Superficial foreign body of right elbow
  - **S50.352** Superficial foreign body of left elbow
  - **S50.359** Superficial foreign body of unspecified elbow
- **S50.36** Insect bite (nonvenomous) of elbow
  - **S50.361** Insect bite (nonvenomous) of right elbow
  - **S50.362** Insect bite (nonvenomous) of left elbow
  - **S50.369** Insect bite (nonvenomous) of unspecified elbow
- **S50.37** Other superficial bite of elbow
  EXCLUDES 1: open bite of elbow (S51.05)
  - **S50.371** Other superficial bite of right elbow
  - **S50.372** Other superficial bite of left elbow
  - **S50.379** Other superficial bite of unspecified elbow

S50.8 Other superficial injuries of forearm
- **S50.81** Abrasion of forearm
  - **S50.811** Abrasion of right forearm
  - **S50.812** Abrasion of left forearm
  - **S50.819** Abrasion of unspecified forearm
- **S50.82** Blister (nonthermal) of forearm
  - **S50.821** Blister (nonthermal) of right forearm
  - **S50.822** Blister (nonthermal) of left forearm

Chapter 19. Injury, Poisoning and Certain Other Consequences of External Causes

- ✓7th **S50.829** Blister (nonthermal) of unspecified forearm
- ✓6th **S50.84** **External constriction** of forearm
  - ✓7th **S50.841** External constriction of **right** forearm
  - ✓7th **S50.842** External constriction of **left** forearm
  - ✓7th **S50.849** External constriction of unspecified forearm
- ✓6th **S50.85** Superficial **foreign body** of forearm
  Splinter in the forearm
  - ✓7th **S50.851** Superficial foreign body of **right** forearm
  - ✓7th **S50.852** Superficial foreign body of **left** forearm
  - ✓7th **S50.859** Superficial foreign body of unspecified forearm
- ✓6th **S50.86** **Insect bite** (nonvenomous) of forearm
  - ✓7th **S50.861** Insect bite (nonvenomous) of **right** forearm
  - ✓7th **S50.862** Insect bite (nonvenomous) of **left** forearm
  - ✓7th **S50.869** Insect bite (nonvenomous) of unspecified forearm
- ✓6th **S50.87** Other superficial **bite** of forearm
  EXCLUDES 1 open bite of forearm (S51.85)
  - ✓7th **S50.871** Other superficial bite of **right** forearm
  - ✓7th **S50.872** Other superficial bite of **left** forearm
  - ✓7th **S50.879** Other superficial bite of unspecified forearm
- ✓5th **S50.9** Unspecified superficial injury of elbow and forearm
  - ✓6th **S50.90** Unspecified superficial injury of **elbow**
    - ✓7th **S50.901** Unspecified superficial injury of **right** elbow
    - ✓7th **S50.902** Unspecified superficial injury of **left** elbow
    - ✓7th **S50.909** Unspecified superficial injury of unspecified elbow
  - ✓6th **S50.91** Unspecified superficial injury of **forearm**
    - ✓7th **S50.911** Unspecified superficial injury of **right** forearm
    - ✓7th **S50.912** Unspecified superficial injury of **left** forearm
    - ✓7th **S50.919** Unspecified superficial injury of unspecified forearm

- ✓4th **S51** **Open wound of elbow and forearm**
  Code also any associated wound infection
  EXCLUDES 1 open fracture of elbow and forearm (S52.- with open fracture 7th character)
  traumatic amputation of elbow and forearm (S58.-)
  EXCLUDES 2 open wound of wrist and hand (S61.-)

  The appropriate 7th character is to be added to each code from category S51.
  A   initial encounter
  D   subsequent encounter
  S   sequela

  - ✓5th **S51.0** Open wound of **elbow**
    - ✓6th **S51.00** Unspecified open wound of elbow
      - ✓7th **S51.001** Unspecified open wound of **right** elbow
        AHA: 2012,4Q,108
      - ✓7th **S51.002** Unspecified open wound of **left** elbow
      - ✓7th **S51.009** Unspecified open wound of unspecified elbow
        Open wound of elbow NOS
    - ✓6th **S51.01** **Laceration without foreign body** of elbow
      - ✓7th **S51.011** Laceration without foreign body of **right** elbow
      - ✓7th **S51.012** Laceration without foreign body of **left** elbow
      - ✓7th **S51.019** Laceration without foreign body of unspecified elbow
    - ✓6th **S51.02** **Laceration with foreign body** of elbow
      - ✓7th **S51.021** Laceration with foreign body of **right** elbow
      - ✓7th **S51.022** Laceration with foreign body of **left** elbow
      - ✓7th **S51.029** Laceration with foreign body of unspecified elbow
    - ✓6th **S51.03** **Puncture wound without foreign body** of elbow
      - ✓7th **S51.031** Puncture wound without foreign body of **right** elbow
      - ✓7th **S51.032** Puncture wound without foreign body of **left** elbow
      - ✓7th **S51.039** Puncture wound without foreign body of unspecified elbow
    - ✓6th **S51.04** **Puncture wound with foreign body** of elbow
      - ✓7th **S51.041** Puncture wound with foreign body of **right** elbow
      - ✓7th **S51.042** Puncture wound with foreign body of **left** elbow
      - ✓7th **S51.049** Puncture wound with foreign body of unspecified elbow
    - ✓6th **S51.05** **Open bite** of elbow
      Bite of elbow NOS
      EXCLUDES 1 superficial bite of elbow (S50.36, S50.37)
      - ✓7th **S51.051** Open bite, **right** elbow
      - ✓7th **S51.052** Open bite, **left** elbow
      - ✓7th **S51.059** Open bite, unspecified elbow
  - ✓5th **S51.8** Open wound of **forearm**
    EXCLUDES 2 open wound of elbow (S51.0-)
    - ✓6th **S51.80** Unspecified open wound of forearm
      AHA: 2016,3Q,24
      - ✓7th **S51.801** Unspecified open wound of **right** forearm
      - ✓7th **S51.802** Unspecified open wound of **left** forearm
      - ✓7th **S51.809** Unspecified open wound of unspecified forearm
        Open wound of forearm NOS
    - ✓6th **S51.81** **Laceration without foreign body** of forearm
      - ✓7th **S51.811** Laceration without foreign body of **right** forearm
      - ✓7th **S51.812** Laceration without foreign body of **left** forearm
      - ✓7th **S51.819** Laceration without foreign body of unspecified forearm
    - ✓6th **S51.82** **Laceration with foreign body** of forearm
      - ✓7th **S51.821** Laceration with foreign body of **right** forearm
      - ✓7th **S51.822** Laceration with foreign body of **left** forearm
      - ✓7th **S51.829** Laceration with foreign body of unspecified forearm
    - ✓6th **S51.83** **Puncture wound without foreign body** of forearm
      AHA: 2016,3Q,24
      - ✓7th **S51.831** Puncture wound without foreign body of **right** forearm
      - ✓7th **S51.832** Puncture wound without foreign body of **left** forearm
      - ✓7th **S51.839** Puncture wound without foreign body of unspecified forearm
    - ✓6th **S51.84** **Puncture wound with foreign body** of forearm
      AHA: 2016,3Q,24
      - ✓7th **S51.841** Puncture wound with foreign body of **right** forearm
      - ✓7th **S51.842** Puncture wound with foreign body of **left** forearm
      - ✓7th **S51.849** Puncture wound with foreign body of unspecified forearm
    - ✓6th **S51.85** **Open bite** of forearm
      Bite of forearm NOS
      EXCLUDES 1 superficial bite of forearm (S50.86, S50.87)
      - ✓7th **S51.851** Open bite of **right** forearm
      - ✓7th **S51.852** Open bite of **left** forearm
      - ✓7th **S51.859** Open bite of unspecified forearm

| HCC | CMS-HCC | Rx | Rx HCC | ESR | ESRD HCC | COM | Commercial HCC | N | Newborn: 0 | P | Pediatric: 0-17 | M | Maternity: 9-64 | A | Adult: 15-124 |

S52 Fracture of forearm

NOTE A fracture not indicated as displaced or nondisplaced should be coded to displaced.

A fracture not indicated as open or closed should be coded to closed.

The open fracture designations are based on the Gustilo open fracture classification.

EXCLUDES 1 traumatic amputation of forearm (S58.-)
EXCLUDES 2 fracture at wrist and hand level (S62.-)
periprosthetic fracture around internal prosthetic elbow joint (M97.4)

AHA: 2018,2Q,12; 2016,1Q,33; 2015,3Q,37-39
DEF: Diaphysis: Central shaft of a long bone.
DEF: Epiphysis: Proximal and distal rounded ends of a long bone, communicates with the joint.
DEF: Metaphysis: Section of a long bone located between the epiphysis and diaphysis at the proximal and distal ends.
DEF: Physis (growth plate): Narrow zone of cartilaginous tissue between the epiphysis and metaphysis at each end of a long bone. In childhood, proliferation of cells in this zone lengthens the bone. As the bone matures, this area thins, ossification eventually fusing into solid bone and growth stops. **Synonym(s):** Epiphyseal plate.

The appropriate 7th character is to be added to all codes from category S52 [unless otherwise indicated].
- initial encounter for open fracture NOS
- A initial encounter for closed fracture
- B initial encounter for open fracture type I or II
- C initial encounter for open fracture type IIIA, IIIB, or IIIC
- D subsequent encounter for closed fracture with routine healing
- E subsequent encounter for open fracture type I or II with routine healing
- F subsequent encounter for open fracture type IIIA, IIIB, or IIIC with routine healing
- G subsequent encounter for closed fracture with delayed healing
- H subsequent encounter for open fracture type I or II with delayed healing
- J subsequent encounter for open fracture type IIIA, IIIB, or IIIC with delayed healing
- K subsequent encounter for closed fracture with nonunion
- M subsequent encounter for open fracture type I or II with nonunion
- N subsequent encounter for open fracture type IIIA, IIIB, or IIIC with nonunion
- P subsequent encounter for closed fracture with malunion
- Q subsequent encounter for open fracture type I or II with malunion
- R subsequent encounter for open fracture type IIIA, IIIB, or IIIC with malunion
- S sequela

S52.0 Fracture of upper end of ulna
Fracture of proximal end of ulna
EXCLUDES 2 fracture of elbow NOS (S42.40-)
fractures of shaft of ulna (S52.2-)

S52.00 Unspecified fracture of upper end of ulna
- **S52.001** Unspecified fracture of upper end of right ulna
- **S52.002** Unspecified fracture of upper end of left ulna
- **S52.009** Unspecified fracture of upper end of unspecified ulna

S52.01 Torus fracture of upper end of ulna

The appropriate 7th character is to be added to all codes in subcategory S52.01
- A initial encounter for closed fracture
- D subsequent encounter for fracture with routine healing
- G subsequent encounter for fracture with delayed healing
- K subsequent encounter for fracture with nonunion
- P subsequent encounter for fracture with malunion
- S sequela

- **S52.011** Torus fracture of upper end of right ulna
- **S52.012** Torus fracture of upper end of left ulna
- **S52.019** Torus fracture of upper end of unspecified ulna

S52.02 Fracture of olecranon process without intraarticular extension of ulna
- **S52.021** Displaced fracture of olecranon process without intraarticular extension of right ulna
- **S52.022** Displaced fracture of olecranon process without intraarticular extension of left ulna
- **S52.023** Displaced fracture of olecranon process without intraarticular extension of unspecified ulna
- **S52.024** Nondisplaced fracture of olecranon process without intraarticular extension of right ulna
- **S52.025** Nondisplaced fracture of olecranon process without intraarticular extension of left ulna
- **S52.026** Nondisplaced fracture of olecranon process without intraarticular extension of unspecified ulna

S52.03 Fracture of olecranon process with intraarticular extension of ulna
- **S52.031** Displaced fracture of olecranon process with intraarticular extension of right ulna
- **S52.032** Displaced fracture of olecranon process with intraarticular extension of left ulna
- **S52.033** Displaced fracture of olecranon process with intraarticular extension of unspecified ulna
- **S52.034** Nondisplaced fracture of olecranon process with intraarticular extension of right ulna
- **S52.035** Nondisplaced fracture of olecranon process with intraarticular extension of left ulna
- **S52.036** Nondisplaced fracture of olecranon process with intraarticular extension of unspecified ulna

S52.04 Fracture of coronoid process of ulna
- **S52.041** Displaced fracture of coronoid process of right ulna
- **S52.042** Displaced fracture of coronoid process of left ulna
- **S52.043** Displaced fracture of coronoid process of unspecified ulna
- **S52.044** Nondisplaced fracture of coronoid process of right ulna
- **S52.045** Nondisplaced fracture of coronoid process of left ulna
- **S52.046** Nondisplaced fracture of coronoid process of unspecified ulna

S52.09 Other fracture of upper end of ulna
- **S52.091** Other fracture of upper end of right ulna
- **S52.092** Other fracture of upper end of left ulna
- **S52.099** Other fracture of upper end of unspecified ulna

S52.1 Fracture of upper end of radius
Fracture of proximal end of radius
EXCLUDES 2 fracture of shaft of radius (S52.3-)
physeal fractures of upper end of radius (S59.2-)

S52.10 Unspecified fracture of upper end of radius
- **S52.101** Unspecified fracture of upper end of right radius
- **S52.102** Unspecified fracture of upper end of left radius
- **S52.109** Unspecified fracture of upper end of unspecified radius

S52.11 Torus fracture of upper end of radius

The appropriate 7th character is to be added to all codes in subcategory S52.11
- A initial encounter for closed fracture
- D subsequent encounter for fracture with routine healing
- G subsequent encounter for fracture with delayed healing
- K subsequent encounter for fracture with nonunion
- P subsequent encounter for fracture with malunion
- S sequela

- S52.111 Torus fracture of upper end of right radius
- S52.112 Torus fracture of upper end of left radius
- S52.119 Torus fracture of upper end of unspecified radius

S52.12 Fracture of head of radius
- S52.121 Displaced fracture of head of right radius
- S52.122 Displaced fracture of head of left radius
- S52.123 Displaced fracture of head of unspecified radius
- S52.124 Nondisplaced fracture of head of right radius
- S52.125 Nondisplaced fracture of head of left radius
- S52.126 Nondisplaced fracture of head of unspecified radius

S52.13 Fracture of neck of radius
- S52.131 Displaced fracture of neck of right radius
- S52.132 Displaced fracture of neck of left radius
- S52.133 Displaced fracture of neck of unspecified radius
- S52.134 Nondisplaced fracture of neck of right radius
- S52.135 Nondisplaced fracture of neck of left radius
- S52.136 Nondisplaced fracture of neck of unspecified radius

S52.18 Other fracture of upper end of radius
- S52.181 Other fracture of upper end of right radius
- S52.182 Other fracture of upper end of left radius
- S52.189 Other fracture of upper end of unspecified radius

S52.2 Fracture of shaft of ulna

S52.20 Unspecified fracture of shaft of ulna
Fracture of ulna NOS
- S52.201 Unspecified fracture of shaft of right ulna
- S52.202 Unspecified fracture of shaft of left ulna
- S52.209 Unspecified fracture of shaft of unspecified ulna

S52.21 Greenstick fracture of shaft of ulna

The appropriate 7th character is to be added to all codes in subcategory S52.21
- A initial encounter for closed fracture
- D subsequent encounter for fracture with routine healing
- G subsequent encounter for fracture with delayed healing
- K subsequent encounter for fracture with nonunion
- P subsequent encounter for fracture with malunion
- S sequela

- S52.211 Greenstick fracture of shaft of right ulna
- S52.212 Greenstick fracture of shaft of left ulna
- S52.219 Greenstick fracture of shaft of unspecified ulna

S52.22 Transverse fracture of shaft of ulna
- S52.221 Displaced transverse fracture of shaft of right ulna
- S52.222 Displaced transverse fracture of shaft of left ulna
- S52.223 Displaced transverse fracture of shaft of unspecified ulna
- S52.224 Nondisplaced transverse fracture of shaft of right ulna
- S52.225 Nondisplaced transverse fracture of shaft of left ulna
- S52.226 Nondisplaced transverse fracture of shaft of unspecified ulna

S52.23 Oblique fracture of shaft of ulna
- S52.231 Displaced oblique fracture of shaft of right ulna
- S52.232 Displaced oblique fracture of shaft of left ulna
- S52.233 Displaced oblique fracture of shaft of unspecified ulna
- S52.234 Nondisplaced oblique fracture of shaft of right ulna
- S52.235 Nondisplaced oblique fracture of shaft of left ulna
- S52.236 Nondisplaced oblique fracture of shaft of unspecified ulna

S52.24 Spiral fracture of shaft of ulna
- S52.241 Displaced spiral fracture of shaft of ulna, right arm
- S52.242 Displaced spiral fracture of shaft of ulna, left arm
- S52.243 Displaced spiral fracture of shaft of ulna, unspecified arm
- S52.244 Nondisplaced spiral fracture of shaft of ulna, right arm
- S52.245 Nondisplaced spiral fracture of shaft of ulna, left arm
- S52.246 Nondisplaced spiral fracture of shaft of ulna, unspecified arm

S52.25 Comminuted fracture of shaft of ulna
- S52.251 Displaced comminuted fracture of shaft of ulna, right arm
- S52.252 Displaced comminuted fracture of shaft of ulna, left arm
- S52.253 Displaced comminuted fracture of shaft of ulna, unspecified arm
- S52.254 Nondisplaced comminuted fracture of shaft of ulna, right arm
- S52.255 Nondisplaced comminuted fracture of shaft of ulna, left arm
- S52.256 Nondisplaced comminuted fracture of shaft of ulna, unspecified arm

S52.26 Segmental fracture of shaft of ulna
- S52.261 Displaced segmental fracture of shaft of ulna, right arm
- S52.262 Displaced segmental fracture of shaft of ulna, left arm
- S52.263 Displaced segmental fracture of shaft of ulna, unspecified arm
- S52.264 Nondisplaced segmental fracture of shaft of ulna, right arm
- S52.265 Nondisplaced segmental fracture of shaft of ulna, left arm
- S52.266 Nondisplaced segmental fracture of shaft of ulna, unspecified arm

S52.27 Monteggia's fracture of ulna
Fracture of upper shaft of ulna with dislocation of radial head
- S52.271 Monteggia's fracture of right ulna
- S52.272 Monteggia's fracture of left ulna
- S52.279 Monteggia's fracture of unspecified ulna

S52.28 Bent bone of ulna
- S52.281 Bent bone of right ulna
- S52.282 Bent bone of left ulna
- S52.283 Bent bone of unspecified ulna

- ✓6th **S52.29** Other fracture of shaft of ulna
  - ✓7th **S52.291** Other fracture of shaft of right ulna
  - ✓7th **S52.292** Other fracture of shaft of left ulna
  - ✓7th **S52.299** Other fracture of shaft of unspecified ulna
- ✓5th **S52.3** Fracture of shaft of radius
  - ✓6th **S52.30** Unspecified fracture of shaft of radius
    - ✓7th **S52.301** Unspecified fracture of shaft of right radius
    - ✓7th **S52.302** Unspecified fracture of shaft of left radius
    - ✓7th **S52.309** Unspecified fracture of shaft of unspecified radius
  - ✓6th **S52.31** Greenstick fracture of shaft of radius

    The appropriate 7th character is to be added to all codes in subcategory S52.31.
    - A initial encounter for closed fracture
    - D subsequent encounter for fracture with routine healing
    - G subsequent encounter for fracture with delayed healing
    - K subsequent encounter for fracture with nonunion
    - P subsequent encounter for fracture with malunion
    - S sequela

    - ✓7th **S52.311** Greenstick fracture of shaft of radius, right arm
    - ✓7th **S52.312** Greenstick fracture of shaft of radius, left arm
    - ✓7th **S52.319** Greenstick fracture of shaft of radius, unspecified arm
  - ✓6th **S52.32** Transverse fracture of shaft of radius
    - ✓7th **S52.321** Displaced transverse fracture of shaft of right radius
    - ✓7th **S52.322** Displaced transverse fracture of shaft of left radius
    - ✓7th **S52.323** Displaced transverse fracture of shaft of unspecified radius
    - ✓7th **S52.324** Nondisplaced transverse fracture of shaft of right radius
    - ✓7th **S52.325** Nondisplaced transverse fracture of shaft of left radius
    - ✓7th **S52.326** Nondisplaced transverse fracture of shaft of unspecified radius
  - ✓6th **S52.33** Oblique fracture of shaft of radius
    - ✓7th **S52.331** Displaced oblique fracture of shaft of right radius
    - ✓7th **S52.332** Displaced oblique fracture of shaft of left radius
    - ✓7th **S52.333** Displaced oblique fracture of shaft of unspecified radius
    - ✓7th **S52.334** Nondisplaced oblique fracture of shaft of right radius
    - ✓7th **S52.335** Nondisplaced oblique fracture of shaft of left radius
    - ✓7th **S52.336** Nondisplaced oblique fracture of shaft of unspecified radius
  - ✓6th **S52.34** Spiral fracture of shaft of radius
    - ✓7th **S52.341** Displaced spiral fracture of shaft of radius, right arm
    - ✓7th **S52.342** Displaced spiral fracture of shaft of radius, left arm
    - ✓7th **S52.343** Displaced spiral fracture of shaft of radius, unspecified arm
    - ✓7th **S52.344** Nondisplaced spiral fracture of shaft of radius, right arm
    - ✓7th **S52.345** Nondisplaced spiral fracture of shaft of radius, left arm
    - ✓7th **S52.346** Nondisplaced spiral fracture of shaft of radius, unspecified arm
  - ✓6th **S52.35** Comminuted fracture of shaft of radius
    - ✓7th **S52.351** Displaced comminuted fracture of shaft of radius, right arm
    - ✓7th **S52.352** Displaced comminuted fracture of shaft of radius, left arm
    - ✓7th **S52.353** Displaced comminuted fracture of shaft of radius, unspecified arm
    - ✓7th **S52.354** Nondisplaced comminuted fracture of shaft of radius, right arm
    - ✓7th **S52.355** Nondisplaced comminuted fracture of shaft of radius, left arm
    - ✓7th **S52.356** Nondisplaced comminuted fracture of shaft of radius, unspecified arm
  - ✓6th **S52.36** Segmental fracture of shaft of radius
    - ✓7th **S52.361** Displaced segmental fracture of shaft of radius, right arm
    - ✓7th **S52.362** Displaced segmental fracture of shaft of radius, left arm
    - ✓7th **S52.363** Displaced segmental fracture of shaft of radius, unspecified arm
    - ✓7th **S52.364** Nondisplaced segmental fracture of shaft of radius, right arm
    - ✓7th **S52.365** Nondisplaced segmental fracture of shaft of radius, left arm
    - ✓7th **S52.366** Nondisplaced segmental fracture of shaft of radius, unspecified arm
  - ✓6th **S52.37** Galeazzi's fracture

    Fracture of lower shaft of radius with radioulnar joint dislocation
    - ✓7th **S52.371** Galeazzi's fracture of right radius
    - ✓7th **S52.372** Galeazzi's fracture of left radius
    - ✓7th **S52.379** Galeazzi's fracture of unspecified radius
  - ✓6th **S52.38** Bent bone of radius
    - ✓7th **S52.381** Bent bone of right radius
    - ✓7th **S52.382** Bent bone of left radius
    - ✓7th **S52.389** Bent bone of unspecified radius
  - ✓6th **S52.39** Other fracture of shaft of radius
    - ✓7th **S52.391** Other fracture of shaft of radius, right arm
    - ✓7th **S52.392** Other fracture of shaft of radius, left arm
    - ✓7th **S52.399** Other fracture of shaft of radius, unspecified arm
- ✓5th **S52.5** Fracture of lower end of radius

  Fracture of distal end of radius

  EXCLUDES 2 physeal fractures of lower end of radius (S59.2-)

  DEF: Fracture of the distal end of the radius above the wrist, most commonly caused by a fall onto an outstretched hand.
  - ✓6th **S52.50** Unspecified fracture of the lower end of radius
    - ✓7th **S52.501** Unspecified fracture of the lower end of right radius
    - ✓7th **S52.502** Unspecified fracture of the lower end of left radius
    - ✓7th **S52.509** Unspecified fracture of the lower end of unspecified radius
  - ✓6th **S52.51** Fracture of radial styloid process
    - ✓7th **S52.511** Displaced fracture of right radial styloid process
    - ✓7th **S52.512** Displaced fracture of left radial styloid process
    - ✓7th **S52.513** Displaced fracture of unspecified radial styloid process
    - ✓7th **S52.514** Nondisplaced fracture of right radial styloid process
    - ✓7th **S52.515** Nondisplaced fracture of left radial styloid process
    - ✓7th **S52.516** Nondisplaced fracture of unspecified radial styloid process
  - ✓6th **S52.52** Torus fracture of lower end of radius

    The appropriate 7th character is to be added to all codes in subcategory S52.52.
    - A initial encounter for closed fracture
    - D subsequent encounter for fracture with routine healing
    - G subsequent encounter for fracture with delayed healing
    - K subsequent encounter for fracture with nonunion
    - P subsequent encounter for fracture with malunion
    - S sequela

    - ✓7th **S52.521** Torus fracture of lower end of right radius
    - ✓7th **S52.522** Torus fracture of lower end of left radius

- **S52.529** Torus fracture of lower end of unspecified radius
- **S52.53** **Colles'** fracture
  - AHA: 2016,2Q,4
  - DEF: Fracture of the radius at the wrist in which the distal fragment is pushed posteriorly. The dorsal angulation of the fragment results in the wrist cocking up.
  - **S52.531** Colles' fracture of right radius
  - **S52.532** Colles' fracture of left radius
  - **S52.539** Colles' fracture of unspecified radius
- **S52.54** **Smith's** fracture
  - **S52.541** Smith's fracture of right radius
  - **S52.542** Smith's fracture of left radius
  - **S52.549** Smith's fracture of unspecified radius
- **S52.55** Other **extraarticular** fracture of lower end of radius
  - **S52.551** Other extraarticular fracture of lower end of right radius
  - **S52.552** Other extraarticular fracture of lower end of left radius
  - **S52.559** Other extraarticular fracture of lower end of unspecified radius
- **S52.56** **Barton's** fracture
  - **S52.561** Barton's fracture of right radius
  - **S52.562** Barton's fracture of left radius
  - **S52.569** Barton's fracture of unspecified radius
- **S52.57** Other **intraarticular** fracture of lower end of radius
  - **S52.571** Other intraarticular fracture of lower end of right radius
  - **S52.572** Other intraarticular fracture of lower end of left radius
  - **S52.579** Other intraarticular fracture of lower end of unspecified radius
- **S52.59** Other fractures of lower end of radius
  - AHA: 2019,3Q,9
  - **S52.591** Other fractures of lower end of right radius
  - **S52.592** Other fractures of lower end of left radius
  - **S52.599** Other fractures of lower end of unspecified radius
- **S52.6** Fracture of **lower end of ulna**
  - **S52.60** Unspecified fracture of lower end of ulna
    - **S52.601** Unspecified fracture of lower end of right ulna
    - **S52.602** Unspecified fracture of lower end of left ulna
    - **S52.609** Unspecified fracture of lower end of unspecified ulna
  - **S52.61** Fracture of ulna **styloid process**
    - **S52.611** Displaced fracture of right ulna styloid process
    - **S52.612** Displaced fracture of left ulna styloid process
    - **S52.613** Displaced fracture of unspecified ulna styloid process
    - **S52.614** Nondisplaced fracture of right ulna styloid process
    - **S52.615** Nondisplaced fracture of left ulna styloid process
    - **S52.616** Nondisplaced fracture of unspecified ulna styloid process
- **S52.62** **Torus** fracture of lower end of ulna
  - The appropriate 7th character is to be added to all codes in subcategory S52.62.
    - A initial encounter for closed fracture
    - D subsequent encounter for fracture with routine healing
    - G subsequent encounter for fracture with delayed healing
    - K subsequent encounter for fracture with nonunion
    - P subsequent encounter for fracture with malunion
    - S sequela
  - **S52.621** Torus fracture of lower end of right ulna
  - **S52.622** Torus fracture of lower end of left ulna
  - **S52.629** Torus fracture of lower end of unspecified ulna
- **S52.69** Other fracture of lower end of ulna
  - AHA: 2019,3Q,9
  - **S52.691** Other fracture of lower end of right ulna
  - **S52.692** Other fracture of lower end of left ulna
  - **S52.699** Other fracture of lower end of unspecified ulna
- **S52.9** Unspecified fracture of **forearm**
  - **S52.90** Unspecified fracture of unspecified forearm
  - **S52.91** Unspecified fracture of right forearm
  - **S52.92** Unspecified fracture of left forearm

S53 Dislocation and sprain of joints and ligaments of elbow

INCLUDES
- avulsion of joint or ligament of elbow
- laceration of cartilage, joint or ligament of elbow
- sprain of cartilage, joint or ligament of elbow
- traumatic hemarthrosis of joint or ligament of elbow
- traumatic rupture of joint or ligament of elbow
- traumatic subluxation of joint or ligament of elbow
- traumatic tear of joint or ligament of elbow

Code also any associated open wound

EXCLUDES 2: strain of muscle, fascia and tendon at forearm level (S56.-)

The appropriate 7th character is to be added to each code from category S53.
- A initial encounter
- D subsequent encounter
- S sequela

- **S53.0** Subluxation and dislocation of **radial head**
  - Dislocation of radiohumeral joint
  - Subluxation of radiohumeral joint
  - EXCLUDES 1: Monteggia's fracture-dislocation (S52.27-)
  - **S53.00** Unspecified subluxation and dislocation of radial head
    - **S53.001** Unspecified subluxation of right radial head
    - **S53.002** Unspecified subluxation of left radial head
    - **S53.003** Unspecified subluxation of unspecified radial head
    - **S53.004** Unspecified dislocation of right radial head
    - **S53.005** Unspecified dislocation of left radial head
    - **S53.006** Unspecified dislocation of unspecified radial head
  - **S53.01** Anterior subluxation and dislocation of radial head
    - Anteriomedial subluxation and dislocation of radial head
    - **S53.011** Anterior subluxation of right radial head
    - **S53.012** Anterior subluxation of left radial head
    - **S53.013** Anterior subluxation of unspecified radial head
    - **S53.014** Anterior dislocation of right radial head
    - **S53.015** Anterior dislocation of left radial head
    - **S53.016** Anterior dislocation of unspecified radial head
  - **S53.02** Posterior subluxation and dislocation of radial head
    - Posteriolateral subluxation and dislocation of radial head
    - **S53.021** Posterior subluxation of right radial head
    - **S53.022** Posterior subluxation of left radial head

- S53.023 Posterior subluxation of unspecified radial head
- S53.024 Posterior dislocation of right radial head
- S53.025 Posterior dislocation of left radial head
- S53.026 Posterior dislocation of unspecified radial head
- S53.03 Nursemaid's elbow
  - S53.031 Nursemaid's elbow, right elbow
  - S53.032 Nursemaid's elbow, left elbow
  - S53.033 Nursemaid's elbow, unspecified elbow
- S53.09 Other subluxation and dislocation of radial head
  - S53.091 Other subluxation of right radial head
  - S53.092 Other subluxation of left radial head
  - S53.093 Other subluxation of unspecified radial head
  - S53.094 Other dislocation of right radial head
  - S53.095 Other dislocation of left radial head
  - S53.096 Other dislocation of unspecified radial head
- S53.1 Subluxation and dislocation of ulnohumeral joint
  - Subluxation and dislocation of elbow NOS
  - EXCLUDES 1 dislocation of radial head alone (S53.0-)
- S53.10 Unspecified subluxation and dislocation of ulnohumeral joint
  - S53.101 Unspecified subluxation of right ulnohumeral joint
  - S53.102 Unspecified subluxation of left ulnohumeral joint
  - S53.103 Unspecified subluxation of unspecified ulnohumeral joint
  - S53.104 Unspecified dislocation of right ulnohumeral joint
  - S53.105 Unspecified dislocation of left ulnohumeral joint
  - S53.106 Unspecified dislocation of unspecified ulnohumeral joint
- S53.11 Anterior subluxation and dislocation of ulnohumeral joint
  - S53.111 Anterior subluxation of right ulnohumeral joint
  - S53.112 Anterior subluxation of left ulnohumeral joint
  - S53.113 Anterior subluxation of unspecified ulnohumeral joint
  - S53.114 Anterior dislocation of right ulnohumeral joint
    - AHA: 2012,4Q,108
  - S53.115 Anterior dislocation of left ulnohumeral joint
  - S53.116 Anterior dislocation of unspecified ulnohumeral joint
- S53.12 Posterior subluxation and dislocation of ulnohumeral joint
  - S53.121 Posterior subluxation of right ulnohumeral joint
  - S53.122 Posterior subluxation of left ulnohumeral joint
  - S53.123 Posterior subluxation of unspecified ulnohumeral joint
  - S53.124 Posterior dislocation of right ulnohumeral joint
  - S53.125 Posterior dislocation of left ulnohumeral joint
  - S53.126 Posterior dislocation of unspecified ulnohumeral joint
- S53.13 Medial subluxation and dislocation of ulnohumeral joint
  - S53.131 Medial subluxation of right ulnohumeral joint
  - S53.132 Medial subluxation of left ulnohumeral joint
  - S53.133 Medial subluxation of unspecified ulnohumeral joint
  - S53.134 Medial dislocation of right ulnohumeral joint
  - S53.135 Medial dislocation of left ulnohumeral joint
  - S53.136 Medial dislocation of unspecified ulnohumeral joint
- S53.14 Lateral subluxation and dislocation of ulnohumeral joint
  - S53.141 Lateral subluxation of right ulnohumeral joint
  - S53.142 Lateral subluxation of left ulnohumeral joint
  - S53.143 Lateral subluxation of unspecified ulnohumeral joint
  - S53.144 Lateral dislocation of right ulnohumeral joint
  - S53.145 Lateral dislocation of left ulnohumeral joint
  - S53.146 Lateral dislocation of unspecified ulnohumeral joint
- S53.19 Other subluxation and dislocation of ulnohumeral joint
  - S53.191 Other subluxation of right ulnohumeral joint
  - S53.192 Other subluxation of left ulnohumeral joint
  - S53.193 Other subluxation of unspecified ulnohumeral joint
  - S53.194 Other dislocation of right ulnohumeral joint
  - S53.195 Other dislocation of left ulnohumeral joint
  - S53.196 Other dislocation of unspecified ulnohumeral joint
- S53.2 Traumatic rupture of radial collateral ligament
  - EXCLUDES 1 sprain of radial collateral ligament NOS (S53.43-)
  - S53.20 Traumatic rupture of unspecified radial collateral ligament
  - S53.21 Traumatic rupture of right radial collateral ligament
  - S53.22 Traumatic rupture of left radial collateral ligament
- S53.3 Traumatic rupture of ulnar collateral ligament
  - EXCLUDES 1 sprain of ulnar collateral ligament (S53.44-)
  - S53.30 Traumatic rupture of unspecified ulnar collateral ligament
  - S53.31 Traumatic rupture of right ulnar collateral ligament
  - S53.32 Traumatic rupture of left ulnar collateral ligament
- S53.4 Sprain of elbow
  - EXCLUDES 2 traumatic rupture of radial collateral ligament (S53.2-)
  - traumatic rupture of ulnar collateral ligament (S53.3-)
  - S53.40 Unspecified sprain of elbow
    - S53.401 Unspecified sprain of right elbow
    - S53.402 Unspecified sprain of left elbow
    - S53.409 Unspecified sprain of unspecified elbow
      - Sprain of elbow NOS
  - S53.41 Radiohumeral (joint) sprain
    - S53.411 Radiohumeral (joint) sprain of right elbow
    - S53.412 Radiohumeral (joint) sprain of left elbow
    - S53.419 Radiohumeral (joint) sprain of unspecified elbow
  - S53.42 Ulnohumeral (joint) sprain
    - S53.421 Ulnohumeral (joint) sprain of right elbow
    - S53.422 Ulnohumeral (joint) sprain of left elbow
    - S53.429 Ulnohumeral (joint) sprain of unspecified elbow
  - S53.43 Radial collateral ligament sprain
    - S53.431 Radial collateral ligament sprain of right elbow
    - S53.432 Radial collateral ligament sprain of left elbow
    - S53.439 Radial collateral ligament sprain of unspecified elbow
  - S53.44 Ulnar collateral ligament sprain
    - S53.441 Ulnar collateral ligament sprain of right elbow
    - S53.442 Ulnar collateral ligament sprain of left elbow
    - S53.449 Ulnar collateral ligament sprain of unspecified elbow
  - S53.49 Other sprain of elbow
    - S53.491 Other sprain of right elbow
    - S53.492 Other sprain of left elbow
    - S53.499 Other sprain of unspecified elbow

S54 Injury of nerves at forearm level

Code also any associated open wound (S51.-)

EXCLUDES 2 injury of nerves at wrist and hand level (S64.-)

The appropriate 7th character is to be added to each code from category S54.
- A initial encounter
- D subsequent encounter
- S sequela

S54.0 Injury of ulnar nerve at forearm level
Injury of ulnar nerve NOS
- S54.00 Injury of ulnar nerve at forearm level, unspecified arm
- S54.01 Injury of ulnar nerve at forearm level, right arm
- S54.02 Injury of ulnar nerve at forearm level, left arm

S54.1 Injury of median nerve at forearm level
Injury of median nerve NOS
- S54.10 Injury of median nerve at forearm level, unspecified arm
- S54.11 Injury of median nerve at forearm level, right arm
- S54.12 Injury of median nerve at forearm level, left arm

S54.2 Injury of radial nerve at forearm level
Injury of radial nerve NOS
- S54.20 Injury of radial nerve at forearm level, unspecified arm
- S54.21 Injury of radial nerve at forearm level, right arm
- S54.22 Injury of radial nerve at forearm level, left arm

S54.3 Injury of cutaneous sensory nerve at forearm level
- S54.30 Injury of cutaneous sensory nerve at forearm level, unspecified arm
- S54.31 Injury of cutaneous sensory nerve at forearm level, right arm
- S54.32 Injury of cutaneous sensory nerve at forearm level, left arm

S54.8 Injury of other nerves at forearm level
- S54.8X Injury of other nerves at forearm level
  - S54.8X1 Injury of other nerves at forearm level, right arm
  - S54.8X2 Injury of other nerves at forearm level, left arm
  - S54.8X9 Injury of other nerves at forearm level, unspecified arm

S54.9 Injury of unspecified nerve at forearm level
- S54.90 Injury of unspecified nerve at forearm level, unspecified arm
- S54.91 Injury of unspecified nerve at forearm level, right arm
- S54.92 Injury of unspecified nerve at forearm level, left arm

S55 Injury of blood vessels at forearm level

Code also any associated open wound (S51.-)

EXCLUDES 2 injury of blood vessels at wrist and hand level (S65.-)
injury of brachial vessels (S45.1-S45.2)

The appropriate 7th character is to be added to each code from category S55.
- A initial encounter
- D subsequent encounter
- S sequela

S55.0 Injury of ulnar artery at forearm level
- S55.00 Unspecified injury of ulnar artery at forearm level
  - S55.001 Unspecified injury of ulnar artery at forearm level, right arm
  - S55.002 Unspecified injury of ulnar artery at forearm level, left arm
  - S55.009 Unspecified injury of ulnar artery at forearm level, unspecified arm
- S55.01 Laceration of ulnar artery at forearm level
  - S55.011 Laceration of ulnar artery at forearm level, right arm
  - S55.012 Laceration of ulnar artery at forearm level, left arm
  - S55.019 Laceration of ulnar artery at forearm level, unspecified arm
- S55.09 Other specified injury of ulnar artery at forearm level
  - S55.091 Other specified injury of ulnar artery at forearm level, right arm
  - S55.092 Other specified injury of ulnar artery at forearm level, left arm
  - S55.099 Other specified injury of ulnar artery at forearm level, unspecified arm

S55.1 Injury of radial artery at forearm level
- S55.10 Unspecified injury of radial artery at forearm level
  - S55.101 Unspecified injury of radial artery at forearm level, right arm
  - S55.102 Unspecified injury of radial artery at forearm level, left arm
  - S55.109 Unspecified injury of radial artery at forearm level, unspecified arm
- S55.11 Laceration of radial artery at forearm level
  - S55.111 Laceration of radial artery at forearm level, right arm
  - S55.112 Laceration of radial artery at forearm level, left arm
  - S55.119 Laceration of radial artery at forearm level, unspecified arm
- S55.19 Other specified injury of radial artery at forearm level
  - S55.191 Other specified injury of radial artery at forearm level, right arm
  - S55.192 Other specified injury of radial artery at forearm level, left arm
  - S55.199 Other specified injury of radial artery at forearm level, unspecified arm

S55.2 Injury of vein at forearm level
- S55.20 Unspecified injury of vein at forearm level
  - S55.201 Unspecified injury of vein at forearm level, right arm
  - S55.202 Unspecified injury of vein at forearm level, left arm
  - S55.209 Unspecified injury of vein at forearm level, unspecified arm
- S55.21 Laceration of vein at forearm level
  - S55.211 Laceration of vein at forearm level, right arm
  - S55.212 Laceration of vein at forearm level, left arm
  - S55.219 Laceration of vein at forearm level, unspecified arm
- S55.29 Other specified injury of vein at forearm level
  - S55.291 Other specified injury of vein at forearm level, right arm
  - S55.292 Other specified injury of vein at forearm level, left arm
  - S55.299 Other specified injury of vein at forearm level, unspecified arm

S55.8 Injury of other blood vessels at forearm level
- S55.80 Unspecified injury of other blood vessels at forearm level
  - S55.801 Unspecified injury of other blood vessels at forearm level, right arm
  - S55.802 Unspecified injury of other blood vessels at forearm level, left arm
  - S55.809 Unspecified injury of other blood vessels at forearm level, unspecified arm
- S55.81 Laceration of other blood vessels at forearm level
  - S55.811 Laceration of other blood vessels at forearm level, right arm
  - S55.812 Laceration of other blood vessels at forearm level, left arm
  - S55.819 Laceration of other blood vessels at forearm level, unspecified arm
- S55.89 Other specified injury of other blood vessels at forearm level
  - S55.891 Other specified injury of other blood vessels at forearm level, right arm
  - S55.892 Other specified injury of other blood vessels at forearm level, left arm
  - S55.899 Other specified injury of other blood vessels at forearm level, unspecified arm

S55.9 Injury of unspecified blood vessel at forearm level
- S55.90 Unspecified injury of unspecified blood vessel at forearm level
  - S55.901 Unspecified injury of unspecified blood vessel at forearm level, right arm
  - S55.902 Unspecified injury of unspecified blood vessel at forearm level, left arm
  - S55.909 Unspecified injury of unspecified blood vessel at forearm level, unspecified arm

- ✓6th **S55.91** Laceration of unspecified blood vessel at forearm level
  - ✓7th **S55.911** Laceration of unspecified blood vessel at forearm level, right arm
  - ✓7th **S55.912** Laceration of unspecified blood vessel at forearm level, left arm
  - ✓7th **S55.919** Laceration of unspecified blood vessel at forearm level, unspecified arm
- ✓6th **S55.99** Other specified injury of unspecified blood vessel at forearm level
  - ✓7th **S55.991** Other specified injury of unspecified blood vessel at forearm level, right arm
  - ✓7th **S55.992** Other specified injury of unspecified blood vessel at forearm level, left arm
  - ✓7th **S55.999** Other specified injury of unspecified blood vessel at forearm level, unspecified arm

- ✓4th **S56** Injury of muscle, fascia and tendon at forearm level
  Code also any associated open wound (S51.-)
  EXCLUDES 2: injury of muscle, fascia and tendon at or below wrist (S66.-)
  sprain of joints and ligaments of elbow (S53.4-)
  TIP: Refer to the Muscle/Tendon table at the beginning of this chapter

  The appropriate 7th character is to be added to each code from category S56.
  A initial encounter
  D subsequent encounter
  S sequela

  - ✓5th **S56.0** Injury of flexor muscle, fascia and tendon of thumb at forearm level
    - ✓6th **S56.00** Unspecified injury of flexor muscle, fascia and tendon of thumb at forearm level
      - ✓7th **S56.001** Unspecified injury of flexor muscle, fascia and tendon of right thumb at forearm level
      - ✓7th **S56.002** Unspecified injury of flexor muscle, fascia and tendon of left thumb at forearm level
      - ✓7th **S56.009** Unspecified injury of flexor muscle, fascia and tendon of unspecified thumb at forearm level
    - ✓6th **S56.01** Strain of flexor muscle, fascia and tendon of thumb at forearm level
      - ✓7th **S56.011** Strain of flexor muscle, fascia and tendon of right thumb at forearm level
      - ✓7th **S56.012** Strain of flexor muscle, fascia and tendon of left thumb at forearm level
      - ✓7th **S56.019** Strain of flexor muscle, fascia and tendon of unspecified thumb at forearm level
    - ✓6th **S56.02** Laceration of flexor muscle, fascia and tendon of thumb at forearm level
      - ✓7th **S56.021** Laceration of flexor muscle, fascia and tendon of right thumb at forearm level
      - ✓7th **S56.022** Laceration of flexor muscle, fascia and tendon of left thumb at forearm level
      - ✓7th **S56.029** Laceration of flexor muscle, fascia and tendon of unspecified thumb at forearm level
    - ✓6th **S56.09** Other injury of flexor muscle, fascia and tendon of thumb at forearm level
      - ✓7th **S56.091** Other injury of flexor muscle, fascia and tendon of right thumb at forearm level
      - ✓7th **S56.092** Other injury of flexor muscle, fascia and tendon of left thumb at forearm level
      - ✓7th **S56.099** Other injury of flexor muscle, fascia and tendon of unspecified thumb at forearm level
  - ✓5th **S56.1** Injury of flexor muscle, fascia and tendon of other and unspecified finger at forearm level
    - ✓6th **S56.10** Unspecified injury of flexor muscle, fascia and tendon of other and unspecified finger at forearm level
      - ✓7th **S56.101** Unspecified injury of flexor muscle, fascia and tendon of right index finger at forearm level
      - ✓7th **S56.102** Unspecified injury of flexor muscle, fascia and tendon of left index finger at forearm level
      - ✓7th **S56.103** Unspecified injury of flexor muscle, fascia and tendon of right middle finger at forearm level
      - ✓7th **S56.104** Unspecified injury of flexor muscle, fascia and tendon of left middle finger at forearm level
      - ✓7th **S56.105** Unspecified injury of flexor muscle, fascia and tendon of right ring finger at forearm level
      - ✓7th **S56.106** Unspecified injury of flexor muscle, fascia and tendon of left ring finger at forearm level
      - ✓7th **S56.107** Unspecified injury of flexor muscle, fascia and tendon of right little finger at forearm level
      - ✓7th **S56.108** Unspecified injury of flexor muscle, fascia and tendon of left little finger at forearm level
      - ✓7th **S56.109** Unspecified injury of flexor muscle, fascia and tendon of unspecified finger at forearm level
    - ✓6th **S56.11** Strain of flexor muscle, fascia and tendon of other and unspecified finger at forearm level
      - ✓7th **S56.111** Strain of flexor muscle, fascia and tendon of right index finger at forearm level
      - ✓7th **S56.112** Strain of flexor muscle, fascia and tendon of left index finger at forearm level
      - ✓7th **S56.113** Strain of flexor muscle, fascia and tendon of right middle finger at forearm level
      - ✓7th **S56.114** Strain of flexor muscle, fascia and tendon of left middle finger at forearm level
      - ✓7th **S56.115** Strain of flexor muscle, fascia and tendon of right ring finger at forearm level
      - ✓7th **S56.116** Strain of flexor muscle, fascia and tendon of left ring finger at forearm level
      - ✓7th **S56.117** Strain of flexor muscle, fascia and tendon of right little finger at forearm level
      - ✓7th **S56.118** Strain of flexor muscle, fascia and tendon of left little finger at forearm level
      - ✓7th **S56.119** Strain of flexor muscle, fascia and tendon of finger of unspecified finger at forearm level
    - ✓6th **S56.12** Laceration of flexor muscle, fascia and tendon of other and unspecified finger at forearm level
      - ✓7th **S56.121** Laceration of flexor muscle, fascia and tendon of right index finger at forearm level
      - ✓7th **S56.122** Laceration of flexor muscle, fascia and tendon of left index finger at forearm level
      - ✓7th **S56.123** Laceration of flexor muscle, fascia and tendon of right middle finger at forearm level
      - ✓7th **S56.124** Laceration of flexor muscle, fascia and tendon of left middle finger at forearm level
      - ✓7th **S56.125** Laceration of flexor muscle, fascia and tendon of right ring finger at forearm level
      - ✓7th **S56.126** Laceration of flexor muscle, fascia and tendon of left ring finger at forearm level
      - ✓7th **S56.127** Laceration of flexor muscle, fascia and tendon of right little finger at forearm level
      - ✓7th **S56.128** Laceration of flexor muscle, fascia and tendon of left little finger at forearm level
      - ✓7th **S56.129** Laceration of flexor muscle, fascia and tendon of unspecified finger at forearm level
    - ✓6th **S56.19** Other injury of flexor muscle, fascia and tendon of other and unspecified finger at forearm level
      - ✓7th **S56.191** Other injury of flexor muscle, fascia and tendon of right index finger at forearm level
      - ✓7th **S56.192** Other injury of flexor muscle, fascia and tendon of left index finger at forearm level
      - ✓7th **S56.193** Other injury of flexor muscle, fascia and tendon of right middle finger at forearm level
      - ✓7th **S56.194** Other injury of flexor muscle, fascia and tendon of left middle finger at forearm level
      - ✓7th **S56.195** Other injury of flexor muscle, fascia and tendon of right ring finger at forearm level
      - ✓7th **S56.196** Other injury of flexor muscle, fascia and tendon of left ring finger at forearm level
      - ✓7th **S56.197** Other injury of flexor muscle, fascia and tendon of right little finger at forearm level
      - ✓7th **S56.198** Other injury of flexor muscle, fascia and tendon of left little finger at forearm level
      - ✓7th **S56.199** Other injury of flexor muscle, fascia and tendon of unspecified finger at forearm level

✓ Additional Character Required ✓x7th Placeholder Alert Manifestation Unspecified Dx Q QPP UPD Unacceptable PDx

- **S56.2** Injury of other flexor muscle, fascia and tendon at forearm level
  - **S56.20** Unspecified injury of other flexor muscle, fascia and tendon at forearm level
    - S56.201 Unspecified injury of other flexor muscle, fascia and tendon at forearm level, right arm
    - S56.202 Unspecified injury of other flexor muscle, fascia and tendon at forearm level, left arm
    - S56.209 Unspecified injury of other flexor muscle, fascia and tendon at forearm level, unspecified arm
  - **S56.21** Strain of other flexor muscle, fascia and tendon at forearm level
    - S56.211 Strain of other flexor muscle, fascia and tendon at forearm level, right arm
    - S56.212 Strain of other flexor muscle, fascia and tendon at forearm level, left arm
    - S56.219 Strain of other flexor muscle, fascia and tendon at forearm level, unspecified arm
  - **S56.22** Laceration of other flexor muscle, fascia and tendon at forearm level
    - S56.221 Laceration of other flexor muscle, fascia and tendon at forearm level, right arm
    - S56.222 Laceration of other flexor muscle, fascia and tendon at forearm level, left arm
    - S56.229 Laceration of other flexor muscle, fascia and tendon at forearm level, unspecified arm
  - **S56.29** Other injury of other flexor muscle, fascia and tendon at forearm level
    - S56.291 Other injury of other flexor muscle, fascia and tendon at forearm level, right arm
    - S56.292 Other injury of other flexor muscle, fascia and tendon at forearm level, left arm
    - S56.299 Other injury of other flexor muscle, fascia and tendon at forearm level, unspecified arm
- **S56.3** Injury of extensor or abductor muscles, fascia and tendons of thumb at forearm level
  - **S56.30** Unspecified injury of extensor or abductor muscles, fascia and tendons of thumb at forearm level
    - S56.301 Unspecified injury of extensor or abductor muscles, fascia and tendons of right thumb at forearm level
    - S56.302 Unspecified injury of extensor or abductor muscles, fascia and tendons of left thumb at forearm level
    - S56.309 Unspecified injury of extensor or abductor muscles, fascia and tendons of unspecified thumb at forearm level
  - **S56.31** Strain of extensor or abductor muscles, fascia and tendons of thumb at forearm level
    - S56.311 Strain of extensor or abductor muscles, fascia and tendons of right thumb at forearm level
    - S56.312 Strain of extensor or abductor muscles, fascia and tendons of left thumb at forearm level
    - S56.319 Strain of extensor or abductor muscles, fascia and tendons of unspecified thumb at forearm level
  - **S56.32** Laceration of extensor or abductor muscles, fascia and tendons of thumb at forearm level
    - S56.321 Laceration of extensor or abductor muscles, fascia and tendons of right thumb at forearm level
    - S56.322 Laceration of extensor or abductor muscles, fascia and tendons of left thumb at forearm level
    - S56.329 Laceration of extensor or abductor muscles, fascia and tendons of unspecified thumb at forearm level
  - **S56.39** Other injury of extensor or abductor muscles, fascia and tendons of thumb at forearm level
    - S56.391 Other injury of extensor or abductor muscles, fascia and tendons of right thumb at forearm level
    - S56.392 Other injury of extensor or abductor muscles, fascia and tendons of left thumb at forearm level
    - S56.399 Other injury of extensor or abductor muscles, fascia and tendons of unspecified thumb at forearm level
- **S56.4** Injury of extensor muscle, fascia and tendon of other and unspecified finger at forearm level
  - **S56.40** Unspecified injury of extensor muscle, fascia and tendon of other and unspecified finger at forearm level
    - S56.401 Unspecified injury of extensor muscle, fascia and tendon of right index finger at forearm level
    - S56.402 Unspecified injury of extensor muscle, fascia and tendon of left index finger at forearm level
    - S56.403 Unspecified injury of extensor muscle, fascia and tendon of right middle finger at forearm level
    - S56.404 Unspecified injury of extensor muscle, fascia and tendon of left middle finger at forearm level
    - S56.405 Unspecified injury of extensor muscle, fascia and tendon of right ring finger at forearm level
    - S56.406 Unspecified injury of extensor muscle, fascia and tendon of left ring finger at forearm level
    - S56.407 Unspecified injury of extensor muscle, fascia and tendon of right little finger at forearm level
    - S56.408 Unspecified injury of extensor muscle, fascia and tendon of left little finger at forearm level
    - S56.409 Unspecified injury of extensor muscle, fascia and tendon of unspecified finger at forearm level
  - **S56.41** Strain of extensor muscle, fascia and tendon of other and unspecified finger at forearm level
    - S56.411 Strain of extensor muscle, fascia and tendon of right index finger at forearm level
    - S56.412 Strain of extensor muscle, fascia and tendon of left index finger at forearm level
    - S56.413 Strain of extensor muscle, fascia and tendon of right middle finger at forearm level
    - S56.414 Strain of extensor muscle, fascia and tendon of left middle finger at forearm level
    - S56.415 Strain of extensor muscle, fascia and tendon of right ring finger at forearm level
    - S56.416 Strain of extensor muscle, fascia and tendon of left ring finger at forearm level
    - S56.417 Strain of extensor muscle, fascia and tendon of right little finger at forearm level
    - S56.418 Strain of extensor muscle, fascia and tendon of left little finger at forearm level
    - S56.419 Strain of extensor muscle, fascia and tendon of finger, unspecified finger at forearm level
  - **S56.42** Laceration of extensor muscle, fascia and tendon of other and unspecified finger at forearm level
    - S56.421 Laceration of extensor muscle, fascia and tendon of right index finger at forearm level
    - S56.422 Laceration of extensor muscle, fascia and tendon of left index finger at forearm level
    - S56.423 Laceration of extensor muscle, fascia and tendon of right middle finger at forearm level
    - S56.424 Laceration of extensor muscle, fascia and tendon of left middle finger at forearm level
    - S56.425 Laceration of extensor muscle, fascia and tendon of right ring finger at forearm level
    - S56.426 Laceration of extensor muscle, fascia and tendon of left ring finger at forearm level
    - S56.427 Laceration of extensor muscle, fascia and tendon of right little finger at forearm level
    - S56.428 Laceration of extensor muscle, fascia and tendon of left little finger at forearm level
    - S56.429 Laceration of extensor muscle, fascia and tendon of unspecified finger at forearm level
  - **S56.49** Other injury of extensor muscle, fascia and tendon of other and unspecified finger at forearm level
    - S56.491 Other injury of extensor muscle, fascia and tendon of right index finger at forearm level

Chapter 19. Injury, Poisoning and Certain Other Consequences of External Causes

S56.492–S58.011

- S56.492 Other injury of extensor muscle, fascia and tendon of left index finger at forearm level
- S56.493 Other injury of extensor muscle, fascia and tendon of right middle finger at forearm level
- S56.494 Other injury of extensor muscle, fascia and tendon of left middle finger at forearm level
- S56.495 Other injury of extensor muscle, fascia and tendon of right ring finger at forearm level
- S56.496 Other injury of extensor muscle, fascia and tendon of left ring finger at forearm level
- S56.497 Other injury of extensor muscle, fascia and tendon of right little finger at forearm level
- S56.498 Other injury of extensor muscle, fascia and tendon of left little finger at forearm level
- S56.499 Other injury of extensor muscle, fascia and tendon of unspecified finger at forearm level

- S56.5 Injury of other extensor muscle, fascia and tendon at forearm level
  - S56.50 Unspecified injury of other extensor muscle, fascia and tendon at forearm level
    - S56.501 Unspecified injury of other extensor muscle, fascia and tendon at forearm level, right arm
    - S56.502 Unspecified injury of other extensor muscle, fascia and tendon at forearm level, left arm
    - S56.509 Unspecified injury of other extensor muscle, fascia and tendon at forearm level, unspecified arm
  - S56.51 Strain of other extensor muscle, fascia and tendon at forearm level
    - S56.511 Strain of other extensor muscle, fascia and tendon at forearm level, right arm
    - S56.512 Strain of other extensor muscle, fascia and tendon at forearm level, left arm
    - S56.519 Strain of other extensor muscle, fascia and tendon at forearm level, unspecified arm
  - S56.52 Laceration of other extensor muscle, fascia and tendon at forearm level
    - S56.521 Laceration of other extensor muscle, fascia and tendon at forearm level, right arm
    - S56.522 Laceration of other extensor muscle, fascia and tendon at forearm level, left arm
    - S56.529 Laceration of other extensor muscle, fascia and tendon at forearm level, unspecified arm
  - S56.59 Other injury of other extensor muscle, fascia and tendon at forearm level
    - S56.591 Other injury of other extensor muscle, fascia and tendon at forearm level, right arm
    - S56.592 Other injury of other extensor muscle, fascia and tendon at forearm level, left arm
    - S56.599 Other injury of other extensor muscle, fascia and tendon at forearm level, unspecified arm

- S56.8 Injury of other muscles, fascia and tendons at forearm level
  - S56.80 Unspecified injury of other muscles, fascia and tendons at forearm level
    - S56.801 Unspecified injury of other muscles, fascia and tendons at forearm level, right arm
    - S56.802 Unspecified injury of other muscles, fascia and tendons at forearm level, left arm
    - S56.809 Unspecified injury of other muscles, fascia and tendons at forearm level, unspecified arm
  - S56.81 Strain of other muscles, fascia and tendons at forearm level
    - S56.811 Strain of other muscles, fascia and tendons at forearm level, right arm
    - S56.812 Strain of other muscles, fascia and tendons at forearm level, left arm
    - S56.819 Strain of other muscles, fascia and tendons at forearm level, unspecified arm
  - S56.82 Laceration of other muscles, fascia and tendons at forearm level
    - S56.821 Laceration of other muscles, fascia and tendons at forearm level, right arm
    - S56.822 Laceration of other muscles, fascia and tendons at forearm level, left arm
    - S56.829 Laceration of other muscles, fascia and tendons at forearm level, unspecified arm
  - S56.89 Other injury of other muscles, fascia and tendons at forearm level
    - S56.891 Other injury of other muscles, fascia and tendons at forearm level, right arm
    - S56.892 Other injury of other muscles, fascia and tendons at forearm level, left arm
    - S56.899 Other injury of other muscles, fascia and tendons at forearm level, unspecified arm

- S56.9 Injury of unspecified muscles, fascia and tendons at forearm level
  - S56.90 Unspecified injury of unspecified muscles, fascia and tendons at forearm level
    - S56.901 Unspecified injury of unspecified muscles, fascia and tendons at forearm level, right arm
    - S56.902 Unspecified injury of unspecified muscles, fascia and tendons at forearm level, left arm
    - S56.909 Unspecified injury of unspecified muscles, fascia and tendons at forearm level, unspecified arm
  - S56.91 Strain of unspecified muscles, fascia and tendons at forearm level
    - S56.911 Strain of unspecified muscles, fascia and tendons at forearm level, right arm
    - S56.912 Strain of unspecified muscles, fascia and tendons at forearm level, left arm
    - S56.919 Strain of unspecified muscles, fascia and tendons at forearm level, unspecified arm
  - S56.92 Laceration of unspecified muscles, fascia and tendons at forearm level
    - S56.921 Laceration of unspecified muscles, fascia and tendons at forearm level, right arm
    - S56.922 Laceration of unspecified muscles, fascia and tendons at forearm level, left arm
    - S56.929 Laceration of unspecified muscles, fascia and tendons at forearm level, unspecified arm
  - S56.99 Other injury of unspecified muscles, fascia and tendons at forearm level
    - S56.991 Other injury of unspecified muscles, fascia and tendons at forearm level, right arm
    - S56.992 Other injury of unspecified muscles, fascia and tendons at forearm level, left arm
    - S56.999 Other injury of unspecified muscles, fascia and tendons at forearm level, unspecified arm

S57 Crushing injury of elbow and forearm

Use additional code(s) for all associated injuries

EXCLUDES 2 crushing injury of wrist and hand (S67.-)

The appropriate 7th character is to be added to each code from category S57.
- A initial encounter
- D subsequent encounter
- S sequela

- S57.0 Crushing injury of elbow
  - S57.00 Crushing injury of unspecified elbow
  - S57.01 Crushing injury of right elbow
  - S57.02 Crushing injury of left elbow
- S57.8 Crushing injury of forearm
  - S57.80 Crushing injury of unspecified forearm
  - S57.81 Crushing injury of right forearm
  - S57.82 Crushing injury of left forearm

S58 Traumatic amputation of elbow and forearm

An amputation not identified as partial or complete should be coded to complete

EXCLUDES 1 traumatic amputation of wrist and hand (S68.-)

The appropriate 7th character is to be added to each code from category S58.
- A initial encounter
- D subsequent encounter
- S sequela

- S58.0 Traumatic amputation at elbow level
  - S58.01 Complete traumatic amputation at elbow level
    - S58.011 Complete traumatic amputation at elbow level, right arm

- S58.012 Complete traumatic amputation at elbow level, left arm [HCC] [ESR] [COM]
- S58.019 Complete traumatic amputation at elbow level, unspecified arm [HCC] [ESR] [COM]
- S58.02 Partial traumatic amputation at elbow level
  - S58.021 Partial traumatic amputation at elbow level, right arm [HCC] [ESR] [COM]
  - S58.022 Partial traumatic amputation at elbow level, left arm [HCC] [ESR] [COM]
  - S58.029 Partial traumatic amputation at elbow level, unspecified arm [HCC] [ESR] [COM]
- S58.1 Traumatic amputation at level between elbow and wrist
  - S58.11 Complete traumatic amputation at level between elbow and wrist
    - S58.111 Complete traumatic amputation at level between elbow and wrist, right arm [HCC] [ESR] [COM]
    - S58.112 Complete traumatic amputation at level between elbow and wrist, left arm [HCC] [ESR] [COM]
    - S58.119 Complete traumatic amputation at level between elbow and wrist, unspecified arm [HCC] [ESR] [COM]
  - S58.12 Partial traumatic amputation at level between elbow and wrist
    - S58.121 Partial traumatic amputation at level between elbow and wrist, right arm [HCC] [ESR] [COM]
    - S58.122 Partial traumatic amputation at level between elbow and wrist, left arm [HCC] [ESR] [COM]
    - S58.129 Partial traumatic amputation at level between elbow and wrist, unspecified arm [HCC] [ESR] [COM]
- S58.9 Traumatic amputation of forearm, level unspecified
  - EXCLUDES 1: traumatic amputation of wrist (S68.-)
  - S58.91 Complete traumatic amputation of forearm, level unspecified
    - S58.911 Complete traumatic amputation of right forearm, level unspecified [HCC] [ESR] [COM]
    - S58.912 Complete traumatic amputation of left forearm, level unspecified [HCC] [ESR] [COM]
    - S58.919 Complete traumatic amputation of unspecified forearm, level unspecified [HCC] [ESR] [COM]
  - S58.92 Partial traumatic amputation of forearm, level unspecified
    - S58.921 Partial traumatic amputation of right forearm, level unspecified [HCC] [ESR] [COM]
    - S58.922 Partial traumatic amputation of left forearm, level unspecified [HCC] [ESR] [COM]
    - S58.929 Partial traumatic amputation of unspecified forearm, level unspecified [HCC] [ESR] [COM]

S59 Other and unspecified injuries of elbow and forearm

EXCLUDES 2: other and unspecified injuries of wrist and hand (S69.-)
AHA: 2018,2Q,12; 2018,1Q,3; 2015,3Q,37-39

The appropriate 7th character is to be added to each code from subcategories S59.0, S59.1, and S59.2.
- A initial encounter for closed fracture
- D subsequent encounter for fracture with routine healing
- G subsequent encounter for fracture with delayed healing
- K subsequent encounter for fracture with nonunion
- P subsequent encounter for fracture with malunion
- S sequela

- S59.0 Physeal fracture of lower end of ulna
  - AHA: 2019,4Q,56
  - S59.00 Unspecified physeal fracture of lower end of ulna
    - S59.001 Unspecified physeal fracture of lower end of ulna, right arm [Q]
    - S59.002 Unspecified physeal fracture of lower end of ulna, left arm [Q]
    - S59.009 Unspecified physeal fracture of lower end of ulna, unspecified arm [Q]
  - S59.01 Salter-Harris Type I physeal fracture of lower end of ulna
    - S59.011 Salter-Harris Type I physeal fracture of lower end of ulna, right arm [Q]
    - S59.012 Salter-Harris Type I physeal fracture of lower end of ulna, left arm [Q]
    - S59.019 Salter-Harris Type I physeal fracture of lower end of ulna, unspecified arm [Q]
  - S59.02 Salter-Harris Type II physeal fracture of lower end of ulna
    - S59.021 Salter-Harris Type II physeal fracture of lower end of ulna, right arm [Q]
    - S59.022 Salter-Harris Type II physeal fracture of lower end of ulna, left arm [Q]
    - S59.029 Salter-Harris Type II physeal fracture of lower end of ulna, unspecified arm [Q]
  - S59.03 Salter-Harris Type III physeal fracture of lower end of ulna
    - S59.031 Salter-Harris Type III physeal fracture of lower end of ulna, right arm [Q]
    - S59.032 Salter-Harris Type III physeal fracture of lower end of ulna, left arm [Q]
    - S59.039 Salter-Harris Type III physeal fracture of lower end of ulna, unspecified arm [Q]
  - S59.04 Salter-Harris Type IV physeal fracture of lower end of ulna
    - S59.041 Salter-Harris Type IV physeal fracture of lower end of ulna, right arm [Q]
    - S59.042 Salter-Harris Type IV physeal fracture of lower end of ulna, left arm [Q]
    - S59.049 Salter-Harris Type IV physeal fracture of lower end of ulna, unspecified arm [Q]
  - S59.09 Other physeal fracture of lower end of ulna
    - S59.091 Other physeal fracture of lower end of ulna, right arm [Q]
    - S59.092 Other physeal fracture of lower end of ulna, left arm [Q]
    - S59.099 Other physeal fracture of lower end of ulna, unspecified arm [Q]
- S59.1 Physeal fracture of upper end of radius
  - AHA: 2019,4Q,56
  - S59.10 Unspecified physeal fracture of upper end of radius
    - S59.101 Unspecified physeal fracture of upper end of radius, right arm [Q]
    - S59.102 Unspecified physeal fracture of upper end of radius, left arm [Q]
    - S59.109 Unspecified physeal fracture of upper end of radius, unspecified arm [Q]
  - S59.11 Salter-Harris Type I physeal fracture of upper end of radius
    - S59.111 Salter-Harris Type I physeal fracture of upper end of radius, right arm [Q]
    - S59.112 Salter-Harris Type I physeal fracture of upper end of radius, left arm [Q]
    - S59.119 Salter-Harris Type I physeal fracture of upper end of radius, unspecified arm [Q]
  - S59.12 Salter-Harris Type II physeal fracture of upper end of radius
    - S59.121 Salter-Harris Type II physeal fracture of upper end of radius, right arm [Q]
    - S59.122 Salter-Harris Type II physeal fracture of upper end of radius, left arm [Q]
    - S59.129 Salter-Harris Type II physeal fracture of upper end of radius, unspecified arm [Q]
  - S59.13 Salter-Harris Type III physeal fracture of upper end of radius
    - S59.131 Salter-Harris Type III physeal fracture of upper end of radius, right arm [Q]
    - S59.132 Salter-Harris Type III physeal fracture of upper end of radius, left arm [Q]
    - S59.139 Salter-Harris Type III physeal fracture of upper end of radius, unspecified arm [Q]
  - S59.14 Salter-Harris Type IV physeal fracture of upper end of radius
    - S59.141 Salter-Harris Type IV physeal fracture of upper end of radius, right arm [Q]
    - S59.142 Salter-Harris Type IV physeal fracture of upper end of radius, left arm [Q]
    - S59.149 Salter-Harris Type IV physeal fracture of upper end of radius, unspecified arm [Q]
  - S59.19 Other physeal fracture of upper end of radius
    - S59.191 Other physeal fracture of upper end of radius, right arm [Q]

[HCC] CMS-HCC [Rx] Rx HCC [ESR] ESRD HCC [COM] Commercial HCC [N] Newborn: 0 [P] Pediatric: 0-17 [M] Maternity: 9-64 [A] Adult: 15-124

Chapter 19. Injury, Poisoning and Certain Other Consequences of External Causes

- **S59.192** Other physeal fracture of upper end of radius, left arm
- **S59.199** Other physeal fracture of upper end of radius, unspecified arm
- **S59.2** Physeal fracture of lower end of radius
  - AHA: 2019,4Q,56
  - **S59.20** Unspecified physeal fracture of lower end of radius
    - **S59.201** Unspecified physeal fracture of lower end of radius, right arm
    - **S59.202** Unspecified physeal fracture of lower end of radius, left arm
    - **S59.209** Unspecified physeal fracture of lower end of radius, unspecified arm
  - **S59.21** Salter-Harris Type I physeal fracture of lower end of radius
    - **S59.211** Salter-Harris Type I physeal fracture of lower end of radius, right arm
    - **S59.212** Salter-Harris Type I physeal fracture of lower end of radius, left arm
    - **S59.219** Salter-Harris Type I physeal fracture of lower end of radius, unspecified arm
  - **S59.22** Salter-Harris Type II physeal fracture of lower end of radius
    - **S59.221** Salter-Harris Type II physeal fracture of lower end of radius, right arm
    - **S59.222** Salter-Harris Type II physeal fracture of lower end of radius, left arm
    - **S59.229** Salter-Harris Type II physeal fracture of lower end of radius, unspecified arm
  - **S59.23** Salter-Harris Type III physeal fracture of lower end of radius
    - **S59.231** Salter-Harris Type III physeal fracture of lower end of radius, right arm
    - **S59.232** Salter-Harris Type III physeal fracture of lower end of radius, left arm
    - **S59.239** Salter-Harris Type III physeal fracture of lower end of radius, unspecified arm
  - **S59.24** Salter-Harris Type IV physeal fracture of lower end of radius
    - **S59.241** Salter-Harris Type IV physeal fracture of lower end of radius, right arm
    - **S59.242** Salter-Harris Type IV physeal fracture of lower end of radius, left arm
    - **S59.249** Salter-Harris Type IV physeal fracture of lower end of radius, unspecified arm
  - **S59.29** Other physeal fracture of lower end of radius
    - **S59.291** Other physeal fracture of lower end of radius, right arm
    - **S59.292** Other physeal fracture of lower end of radius, left arm
    - **S59.299** Other physeal fracture of lower end of radius, unspecified arm
- **S59.8** Other specified injuries of elbow and forearm

  The appropriate 7th character is to be added to each code in subcategory S59.8.
  - A initial encounter
  - D subsequent encounter
  - S sequela

  - **S59.80** Other specified injuries of elbow
    - **S59.801** Other specified injuries of right elbow
    - **S59.802** Other specified injuries of left elbow
    - **S59.809** Other specified injuries of unspecified elbow
  - **S59.81** Other specified injuries of forearm
    - **S59.811** Other specified injuries right forearm
    - **S59.812** Other specified injuries left forearm
    - **S59.819** Other specified injuries unspecified forearm
- **S59.9** Unspecified injury of elbow and forearm

  The appropriate 7th character is to be added to each code in subcategory S59.9.
  - A initial encounter
  - D subsequent encounter
  - S sequela

  - **S59.90** Unspecified injury of elbow
    - **S59.901** Unspecified injury of right elbow
    - **S59.902** Unspecified injury of left elbow
    - **S59.909** Unspecified injury of unspecified elbow
  - **S59.91** Unspecified injury of forearm
    - **S59.911** Unspecified injury of right forearm
    - **S59.912** Unspecified injury of left forearm
    - **S59.919** Unspecified injury of unspecified forearm

Injuries to the wrist, hand and fingers (S60-S69)

EXCLUDES 2: burns and corrosions (T20-T32)
frostbite (T33-T34)
insect bite or sting, venomous (T63.4)

- **S60** Superficial injury of wrist, hand and fingers

  The appropriate 7th character is to be added to each code from category S60.
  - A initial encounter
  - D subsequent encounter
  - S sequela

  - **S60.0** Contusion of finger without damage to nail
    - EXCLUDES 1: contusion involving nail (matrix) (S60.1)
    - **S60.00** Contusion of unspecified finger without damage to nail
      - Contusion of finger(s) NOS
    - **S60.01** Contusion of thumb without damage to nail
      - **S60.011** Contusion of right thumb without damage to nail
      - **S60.012** Contusion of left thumb without damage to nail
      - **S60.019** Contusion of unspecified thumb without damage to nail
    - **S60.02** Contusion of index finger without damage to nail
      - **S60.021** Contusion of right index finger without damage to nail
      - **S60.022** Contusion of left index finger without damage to nail
      - **S60.029** Contusion of unspecified index finger without damage to nail
    - **S60.03** Contusion of middle finger without damage to nail
      - **S60.031** Contusion of right middle finger without damage to nail
      - **S60.032** Contusion of left middle finger without damage to nail
      - **S60.039** Contusion of unspecified middle finger without damage to nail
    - **S60.04** Contusion of ring finger without damage to nail
      - **S60.041** Contusion of right ring finger without damage to nail
      - **S60.042** Contusion of left ring finger without damage to nail
      - **S60.049** Contusion of unspecified ring finger without damage to nail
    - **S60.05** Contusion of little finger without damage to nail
      - **S60.051** Contusion of right little finger without damage to nail
      - **S60.052** Contusion of left little finger without damage to nail
      - **S60.059** Contusion of unspecified little finger without damage to nail
  - **S60.1** Contusion of finger with damage to nail
    - **S60.10** Contusion of unspecified finger with damage to nail
    - **S60.11** Contusion of thumb with damage to nail
      - **S60.111** Contusion of right thumb with damage to nail
      - **S60.112** Contusion of left thumb with damage to nail
      - **S60.119** Contusion of unspecified thumb with damage to nail
    - **S60.12** Contusion of index finger with damage to nail
      - **S60.121** Contusion of right index finger with damage to nail
      - **S60.122** Contusion of left index finger with damage to nail
      - **S60.129** Contusion of unspecified index finger with damage to nail
    - **S60.13** Contusion of middle finger with damage to nail
      - **S60.131** Contusion of right middle finger with damage to nail

- **S60.132** Contusion of left middle finger with damage to nail
- **S60.139** Contusion of unspecified middle finger with damage to nail
- **S60.14** Contusion of ring finger with damage to nail
  - **S60.141** Contusion of right ring finger with damage to nail
  - **S60.142** Contusion of left ring finger with damage to nail
  - **S60.149** Contusion of unspecified ring finger with damage to nail
- **S60.15** Contusion of little finger with damage to nail
  - **S60.151** Contusion of right little finger with damage to nail
  - **S60.152** Contusion of left little finger with damage to nail
  - **S60.159** Contusion of unspecified little finger with damage to nail
- **S60.2** Contusion of wrist and hand
  - *EXCLUDES 2* contusion of fingers (S60.0-, S60.1-)
  - **S60.21** Contusion of wrist
    - **S60.211** Contusion of right wrist
    - **S60.212** Contusion of left wrist
    - **S60.219** Contusion of unspecified wrist
  - **S60.22** Contusion of hand
    - **S60.221** Contusion of right hand
    - **S60.222** Contusion of left hand
    - **S60.229** Contusion of unspecified hand
- **S60.3** Other superficial injuries of thumb
  - **S60.31** Abrasion of thumb
    - **S60.311** Abrasion of right thumb
    - **S60.312** Abrasion of left thumb
    - **S60.319** Abrasion of unspecified thumb
  - **S60.32** Blister (nonthermal) of thumb
    - **S60.321** Blister (nonthermal) of right thumb
    - **S60.322** Blister (nonthermal) of left thumb
    - **S60.329** Blister (nonthermal) of unspecified thumb
  - **S60.34** External constriction of thumb
    - Hair tourniquet syndrome of thumb
    - Use additional cause code to identify the constricting item (W49.0-)
    - **S60.341** External constriction of right thumb
    - **S60.342** External constriction of left thumb
    - **S60.349** External constriction of unspecified thumb
  - **S60.35** Superficial foreign body of thumb
    - Splinter in the thumb
    - **S60.351** Superficial foreign body of right thumb
    - **S60.352** Superficial foreign body of left thumb
    - **S60.359** Superficial foreign body of unspecified thumb
  - **S60.36** Insect bite (nonvenomous) of thumb
    - **S60.361** Insect bite (nonvenomous) of right thumb
    - **S60.362** Insect bite (nonvenomous) of left thumb
    - **S60.369** Insect bite (nonvenomous) of unspecified thumb
  - **S60.37** Other superficial bite of thumb
    - *EXCLUDES 1* open bite of thumb (S61.05-, S61.15-)
    - **S60.371** Other superficial bite of right thumb
    - **S60.372** Other superficial bite of left thumb
    - **S60.379** Other superficial bite of unspecified thumb
  - **S60.39** Other superficial injuries of thumb
    - **S60.391** Other superficial injuries of right thumb
    - **S60.392** Other superficial injuries of left thumb
    - **S60.399** Other superficial injuries of unspecified thumb
- **S60.4** Other superficial injuries of other fingers
  - **S60.41** Abrasion of fingers
    - **S60.410** Abrasion of right index finger
    - **S60.411** Abrasion of left index finger
    - **S60.412** Abrasion of right middle finger
    - **S60.413** Abrasion of left middle finger
    - **S60.414** Abrasion of right ring finger
    - **S60.415** Abrasion of left ring finger
    - **S60.416** Abrasion of right little finger
    - **S60.417** Abrasion of left little finger
    - **S60.418** Abrasion of other finger
      - Abrasion of specified finger with unspecified laterality
    - **S60.419** Abrasion of unspecified finger
  - **S60.42** Blister (nonthermal) of fingers
    - **S60.420** Blister (nonthermal) of right index finger
    - **S60.421** Blister (nonthermal) of left index finger
    - **S60.422** Blister (nonthermal) of right middle finger
    - **S60.423** Blister (nonthermal) of left middle finger
    - **S60.424** Blister (nonthermal) of right ring finger
    - **S60.425** Blister (nonthermal) of left ring finger
    - **S60.426** Blister (nonthermal) of right little finger
    - **S60.427** Blister (nonthermal) of left little finger
    - **S60.428** Blister (nonthermal) of other finger
      - Blister (nonthermal) of specified finger with unspecified laterality
    - **S60.429** Blister (nonthermal) of unspecified finger
  - **S60.44** External constriction of fingers
    - Hair tourniquet syndrome of finger
    - Use additional cause code to identify the constricting item (W49.0-)
    - **S60.440** External constriction of right index finger
    - **S60.441** External constriction of left index finger
    - **S60.442** External constriction of right middle finger
    - **S60.443** External constriction of left middle finger
    - **S60.444** External constriction of right ring finger
    - **S60.445** External constriction of left ring finger
    - **S60.446** External constriction of right little finger
    - **S60.447** External constriction of left little finger
    - **S60.448** External constriction of other finger
      - External constriction of specified finger with unspecified laterality
    - **S60.449** External constriction of unspecified finger
  - **S60.45** Superficial foreign body of fingers
    - Splinter in the finger(s)
    - **S60.450** Superficial foreign body of right index finger
    - **S60.451** Superficial foreign body of left index finger
    - **S60.452** Superficial foreign body of right middle finger
    - **S60.453** Superficial foreign body of left middle finger
    - **S60.454** Superficial foreign body of right ring finger
    - **S60.455** Superficial foreign body of left ring finger
    - **S60.456** Superficial foreign body of right little finger
    - **S60.457** Superficial foreign body of left little finger
    - **S60.458** Superficial foreign body of other finger
      - Superficial foreign body of specified finger with unspecified laterality
    - **S60.459** Superficial foreign body of unspecified finger
  - **S60.46** Insect bite (nonvenomous) of fingers
    - **S60.460** Insect bite (nonvenomous) of right index finger
    - **S60.461** Insect bite (nonvenomous) of left index finger
    - **S60.462** Insect bite (nonvenomous) of right middle finger
    - **S60.463** Insect bite (nonvenomous) of left middle finger
    - **S60.464** Insect bite (nonvenomous) of right ring finger
    - **S60.465** Insect bite (nonvenomous) of left ring finger
    - **S60.466** Insect bite (nonvenomous) of right little finger
    - **S60.467** Insect bite (nonvenomous) of left little finger

- ✓7th **S60.468** Insect bite (nonvenomous) of other finger
  - Insect bite (nonvenomous) of specified finger with unspecified laterality
- ✓7th **S60.469** Insect bite (nonvenomous) of unspecified finger

✓6th **S60.47** Other superficial bite of fingers
  - EXCLUDES 1 — open bite of fingers (S61.25-, S61.35-)
  - ✓7th **S60.470** Other superficial bite of right index finger
  - ✓7th **S60.471** Other superficial bite of left index finger
  - ✓7th **S60.472** Other superficial bite of right middle finger
  - ✓7th **S60.473** Other superficial bite of left middle finger
  - ✓7th **S60.474** Other superficial bite of right ring finger
  - ✓7th **S60.475** Other superficial bite of left ring finger
  - ✓7th **S60.476** Other superficial bite of right little finger
  - ✓7th **S60.477** Other superficial bite of left little finger
  - ✓7th **S60.478** Other superficial bite of other finger
    - Other superficial bite of specified finger with unspecified laterality
  - ✓7th **S60.479** Other superficial bite of unspecified finger

✓5th **S60.5** Other superficial injuries of hand
  - EXCLUDES 2 — superficial injuries of fingers (S60.3-, S60.4-)

  ✓6th **S60.51** Abrasion of hand
  - ✓7th **S60.511** Abrasion of right hand
  - ✓7th **S60.512** Abrasion of left hand
  - ✓7th **S60.519** Abrasion of unspecified hand

  ✓6th **S60.52** Blister (nonthermal) of hand
  - ✓7th **S60.521** Blister (nonthermal) of right hand
  - ✓7th **S60.522** Blister (nonthermal) of left hand
  - ✓7th **S60.529** Blister (nonthermal) of unspecified hand

  ✓6th **S60.54** External constriction of hand
  - ✓7th **S60.541** External constriction of right hand
  - ✓7th **S60.542** External constriction of left hand
  - ✓7th **S60.549** External constriction of unspecified hand

  ✓6th **S60.55** Superficial foreign body of hand
  - Splinter in the hand
  - ✓7th **S60.551** Superficial foreign body of right hand
  - ✓7th **S60.552** Superficial foreign body of left hand
  - ✓7th **S60.559** Superficial foreign body of unspecified hand

  ✓6th **S60.56** Insect bite (nonvenomous) of hand
  - ✓7th **S60.561** Insect bite (nonvenomous) of right hand
  - ✓7th **S60.562** Insect bite (nonvenomous) of left hand
  - ✓7th **S60.569** Insect bite (nonvenomous) of unspecified hand

  ✓6th **S60.57** Other superficial bite of hand
  - EXCLUDES 1 — open bite of hand (S61.45-)
  - ✓7th **S60.571** Other superficial bite of hand of right hand
  - ✓7th **S60.572** Other superficial bite of hand of left hand
  - ✓7th **S60.579** Other superficial bite of hand of unspecified hand

✓5th **S60.8** Other superficial injuries of wrist

  ✓6th **S60.81** Abrasion of wrist
  - ✓7th **S60.811** Abrasion of right wrist
  - ✓7th **S60.812** Abrasion of left wrist
  - ✓7th **S60.819** Abrasion of unspecified wrist

  ✓6th **S60.82** Blister (nonthermal) of wrist
  - ✓7th **S60.821** Blister (nonthermal) of right wrist
  - ✓7th **S60.822** Blister (nonthermal) of left wrist
  - ✓7th **S60.829** Blister (nonthermal) of unspecified wrist

  ✓6th **S60.84** External constriction of wrist
  - ✓7th **S60.841** External constriction of right wrist
  - ✓7th **S60.842** External constriction of left wrist
  - ✓7th **S60.849** External constriction of unspecified wrist

  ✓6th **S60.85** Superficial foreign body of wrist
  - Splinter in the wrist
  - ✓7th **S60.851** Superficial foreign body of right wrist
  - ✓7th **S60.852** Superficial foreign body of left wrist
  - ✓7th **S60.859** Superficial foreign body of unspecified wrist

  ✓6th **S60.86** Insect bite (nonvenomous) of wrist
  - ✓7th **S60.861** Insect bite (nonvenomous) of right wrist
  - ✓7th **S60.862** Insect bite (nonvenomous) of left wrist
  - ✓7th **S60.869** Insect bite (nonvenomous) of unspecified wrist

  ✓6th **S60.87** Other superficial bite of wrist
  - EXCLUDES 1 — open bite of wrist (S61.55)
  - ✓7th **S60.871** Other superficial bite of right wrist
  - ✓7th **S60.872** Other superficial bite of left wrist
  - ✓7th **S60.879** Other superficial bite of unspecified wrist

✓5th **S60.9** Unspecified superficial injury of wrist, hand and fingers

  ✓6th **S60.91** Unspecified superficial injury of wrist
  - ✓7th **S60.911** Unspecified superficial injury of right wrist
  - ✓7th **S60.912** Unspecified superficial injury of left wrist
  - ✓7th **S60.919** Unspecified superficial injury of unspecified wrist

  S60.92 Unspecified superficial injury of hand
  - ✓7th **S60.921** Unspecified superficial injury of right hand
  - ✓7th **S60.922** Unspecified superficial injury of left hand
  - ✓7th **S60.929** Unspecified superficial injury of unspecified hand

  ✓6th **S60.93** Unspecified superficial injury of thumb
  - ✓7th **S60.931** Unspecified superficial injury of right thumb
  - ✓7th **S60.932** Unspecified superficial injury of left thumb
  - ✓7th **S60.939** Unspecified superficial injury of unspecified thumb

  ✓6th **S60.94** Unspecified superficial injury of other fingers
  - ✓7th **S60.940** Unspecified superficial injury of right index finger
  - ✓7th **S60.941** Unspecified superficial injury of left index finger
  - ✓7th **S60.942** Unspecified superficial injury of right middle finger
  - ✓7th **S60.943** Unspecified superficial injury of left middle finger
  - ✓7th **S60.944** Unspecified superficial injury of right ring finger
  - ✓7th **S60.945** Unspecified superficial injury of left ring finger
  - ✓7th **S60.946** Unspecified superficial injury of right little finger
  - ✓7th **S60.947** Unspecified superficial injury of left little finger
  - ✓7th **S60.948** Unspecified superficial injury of other finger
    - Unspecified superficial injury of specified finger with unspecified laterality
  - ✓7th **S60.949** Unspecified superficial injury of unspecified finger

✓4th **S61** Open wound of wrist, hand and fingers
  - Code also any associated wound infection
  - EXCLUDES 1 — open fracture of wrist, hand and finger (S62.- with 7th character B)
  - traumatic amputation of wrist and hand (S68.-)

  The appropriate 7th character is to be added to each code from category S61.
  - A initial encounter
  - D subsequent encounter
  - S sequela

✓5th **S61.0** Open wound of thumb without damage to nail
  - EXCLUDES 1 — open wound of thumb with damage to nail (S61.1-)

  ✓6th **S61.00** Unspecified open wound of thumb without damage to nail
  - ✓7th **S61.001** Unspecified open wound of right thumb without damage to nail
  - ✓7th **S61.002** Unspecified open wound of left thumb without damage to nail
  - ✓7th **S61.009** Unspecified open wound of unspecified thumb without damage to nail

  ✓6th **S61.01** Laceration without foreign body of thumb without damage to nail
  - ✓7th **S61.011** Laceration without foreign body of right thumb without damage to nail
  - ✓7th **S61.012** Laceration without foreign body of left thumb without damage to nail

☑ Additional Character Required   ✓x7th Placeholder Alert   Manifestation   Unspecified Dx   Q QPP   UPD Unacceptable PDx

Chapter 19. Injury, Poisoning and Certain Other Consequences of External Causes

- ✓7th **S61.019** Laceration without foreign body of unspecified thumb without damage to nail
- ✓6th **S61.02** Laceration with foreign body of thumb without damage to nail
  - ✓7th **S61.021** Laceration with foreign body of right thumb without damage to nail
  - ✓7th **S61.022** Laceration with foreign body of left thumb without damage to nail
  - ✓7th **S61.029** Laceration with foreign body of unspecified thumb without damage to nail
- ✓6th **S61.03** Puncture wound without foreign body of thumb without damage to nail
  - ✓7th **S61.031** Puncture wound without foreign body of right thumb without damage to nail
  - ✓7th **S61.032** Puncture wound without foreign body of left thumb without damage to nail
  - ✓7th **S61.039** Puncture wound without foreign body of unspecified thumb without damage to nail
- ✓6th **S61.04** Puncture wound with foreign body of thumb without damage to nail
  - ✓7th **S61.041** Puncture wound with foreign body of right thumb without damage to nail
  - ✓7th **S61.042** Puncture wound with foreign body of left thumb without damage to nail
  - ✓7th **S61.049** Puncture wound with foreign body of unspecified thumb without damage to nail
- ✓6th **S61.05** Open bite of thumb without damage to nail
  Bite of thumb NOS
  EXCLUDES 1 superficial bite of thumb (S60.36-, S60.37-)
  - ✓7th **S61.051** Open bite of right thumb without damage to nail
  - ✓7th **S61.052** Open bite of left thumb without damage to nail
  - ✓7th **S61.059** Open bite of unspecified thumb without damage to nail
- ✓5th **S61.1** Open wound of thumb with damage to nail
  - ✓6th **S61.10** Unspecified open wound of thumb with damage to nail
    - ✓7th **S61.101** Unspecified open wound of right thumb with damage to nail
    - ✓7th **S61.102** Unspecified open wound of left thumb with damage to nail
    - ✓7th **S61.109** Unspecified open wound of unspecified thumb with damage to nail
  - ✓6th **S61.11** Laceration without foreign body of thumb with damage to nail
    - ✓7th **S61.111** Laceration without foreign body of right thumb with damage to nail
    - ✓7th **S61.112** Laceration without foreign body of left thumb with damage to nail
    - ✓7th **S61.119** Laceration without foreign body of unspecified thumb with damage to nail
  - ✓6th **S61.12** Laceration with foreign body of thumb with damage to nail
    - ✓7th **S61.121** Laceration with foreign body of right thumb with damage to nail
    - ✓7th **S61.122** Laceration with foreign body of left thumb with damage to nail
    - ✓7th **S61.129** Laceration with foreign body of unspecified thumb with damage to nail
  - ✓6th **S61.13** Puncture wound without foreign body of thumb with damage to nail
    - ✓7th **S61.131** Puncture wound without foreign body of right thumb with damage to nail
    - ✓7th **S61.132** Puncture wound without foreign body of left thumb with damage to nail
    - ✓7th **S61.139** Puncture wound without foreign body of unspecified thumb with damage to nail
  - ✓6th **S61.14** Puncture wound with foreign body of thumb with damage to nail
    - ✓7th **S61.141** Puncture wound with foreign body of right thumb with damage to nail
    - ✓7th **S61.142** Puncture wound with foreign body of left thumb with damage to nail
    - ✓7th **S61.149** Puncture wound with foreign body of unspecified thumb with damage to nail
  - ✓6th **S61.15** Open bite of thumb with damage to nail
    Bite of thumb with damage to nail NOS
    EXCLUDES 1 superficial bite of thumb (S60.36-, S60.37-)
    - ✓7th **S61.151** Open bite of right thumb with damage to nail
    - ✓7th **S61.152** Open bite of left thumb with damage to nail
    - ✓7th **S61.159** Open bite of unspecified thumb with damage to nail
- ✓5th **S61.2** Open wound of other finger without damage to nail
  EXCLUDES 1 open wound of finger involving nail (matrix) (S61.3-)
  EXCLUDES 2 open wound of thumb without damage to nail (S61.0-)
  - ✓6th **S61.20** Unspecified open wound of other finger without damage to nail
    - ✓7th **S61.200** Unspecified open wound of right index finger without damage to nail
    - ✓7th **S61.201** Unspecified open wound of left index finger without damage to nail
    - ✓7th **S61.202** Unspecified open wound of right middle finger without damage to nail
    - ✓7th **S61.203** Unspecified open wound of left middle finger without damage to nail
    - ✓7th **S61.204** Unspecified open wound of right ring finger without damage to nail
    - ✓7th **S61.205** Unspecified open wound of left ring finger without damage to nail
    - ✓7th **S61.206** Unspecified open wound of right little finger without damage to nail
    - ✓7th **S61.207** Unspecified open wound of left little finger without damage to nail
    - ✓7th **S61.208** Unspecified open wound of other finger without damage to nail
      Unspecified open wound of specified finger with unspecified laterality without damage to nail
    - ✓7th **S61.209** Unspecified open wound of unspecified finger without damage to nail
  - ✓6th **S61.21** Laceration without foreign body of finger without damage to nail
    - ✓7th **S61.210** Laceration without foreign body of right index finger without damage to nail
    - ✓7th **S61.211** Laceration without foreign body of left index finger without damage to nail
    - ✓7th **S61.212** Laceration without foreign body of right middle finger without damage to nail
    - ✓7th **S61.213** Laceration without foreign body of left middle finger without damage to nail
    - ✓7th **S61.214** Laceration without foreign body of right ring finger without damage to nail
    - ✓7th **S61.215** Laceration without foreign body of left ring finger without damage to nail
    - ✓7th **S61.216** Laceration without foreign body of right little finger without damage to nail
    - ✓7th **S61.217** Laceration without foreign body of left little finger without damage to nail
    - ✓7th **S61.218** Laceration without foreign body of other finger without damage to nail
      Laceration without foreign body of specified finger with unspecified laterality without damage to nail
    - ✓7th **S61.219** Laceration without foreign body of unspecified finger without damage to nail
  - ✓6th **S61.22** Laceration with foreign body of finger without damage to nail
    - ✓7th **S61.220** Laceration with foreign body of right index finger without damage to nail
    - ✓7th **S61.221** Laceration with foreign body of left index finger without damage to nail
    - ✓7th **S61.222** Laceration with foreign body of right middle finger without damage to nail
    - ✓7th **S61.223** Laceration with foreign body of left middle finger without damage to nail
    - ✓7th **S61.224** Laceration with foreign body of right ring finger without damage to nail
    - ✓7th **S61.225** Laceration with foreign body of left ring finger without damage to nail
    - ✓7th **S61.226** Laceration with foreign body of right little finger without damage to nail
    - ✓7th **S61.227** Laceration with foreign body of left little finger without damage to nail
    - ✓7th **S61.228** Laceration with foreign body of other finger without damage to nail
      Laceration with foreign body of specified finger with unspecified laterality without damage to nail
    - ✓7th **S61.229** Laceration with foreign body of unspecified finger without damage to nail

Chapter 19. Injury, Poisoning and Certain Other Consequences of External Causes S61.23–S61.335

- **S61.23** Puncture wound without foreign body of finger without damage to nail
  - **S61.230** Puncture wound without foreign body of right index finger without damage to nail
  - **S61.231** Puncture wound without foreign body of left index finger without damage to nail
  - **S61.232** Puncture wound without foreign body of right middle finger without damage to nail
  - **S61.233** Puncture wound without foreign body of left middle finger without damage to nail
  - **S61.234** Puncture wound without foreign body of right ring finger without damage to nail
  - **S61.235** Puncture wound without foreign body of left ring finger without damage to nail
  - **S61.236** Puncture wound without foreign body of right little finger without damage to nail
  - **S61.237** Puncture wound without foreign body of left little finger without damage to nail
  - **S61.238** Puncture wound without foreign body of other finger without damage to nail
    Puncture wound without foreign body of specified finger with unspecified laterality without damage to nail
  - **S61.239** Puncture wound without foreign body of unspecified finger without damage to nail
- **S61.24** Puncture wound with foreign body of finger without damage to nail
  - **S61.240** Puncture wound with foreign body of right index finger without damage to nail
  - **S61.241** Puncture wound with foreign body of left index finger without damage to nail
  - **S61.242** Puncture wound with foreign body of right middle finger without damage to nail
  - **S61.243** Puncture wound with foreign body of left middle finger without damage to nail
  - **S61.244** Puncture wound with foreign body of right ring finger without damage to nail
  - **S61.245** Puncture wound with foreign body of left ring finger without damage to nail
  - **S61.246** Puncture wound with foreign body of right little finger without damage to nail
  - **S61.247** Puncture wound with foreign body of left little finger without damage to nail
  - **S61.248** Puncture wound with foreign body of other finger without damage to nail
    Puncture wound with foreign body of specified finger with unspecified laterality without damage to nail
  - **S61.249** Puncture wound with foreign body of unspecified finger without damage to nail
- **S61.25** Open bite of finger without damage to nail
  Bite of finger without damage to nail NOS
  EXCLUDES 1 superficial bite of finger (S60.46-, S60.47-)
  - **S61.250** Open bite of right index finger without damage to nail
  - **S61.251** Open bite of left index finger without damage to nail
  - **S61.252** Open bite of right middle finger without damage to nail
  - **S61.253** Open bite of left middle finger without damage to nail
  - **S61.254** Open bite of right ring finger without damage to nail
  - **S61.255** Open bite of left ring finger without damage to nail
  - **S61.256** Open bite of right little finger without damage to nail
  - **S61.257** Open bite of left little finger without damage to nail
  - **S61.258** Open bite of other finger without damage to nail
    Open bite of specified finger with unspecified laterality without damage to nail
  - **S61.259** Open bite of unspecified finger without damage to nail
- **S61.3** Open wound of other finger with damage to nail
  - **S61.30** Unspecified open wound of finger with damage to nail
    - **S61.300** Unspecified open wound of right index finger with damage to nail
    - **S61.301** Unspecified open wound of left index finger with damage to nail
    - **S61.302** Unspecified open wound of right middle finger with damage to nail
    - **S61.303** Unspecified open wound of left middle finger with damage to nail
    - **S61.304** Unspecified open wound of right ring finger with damage to nail
    - **S61.305** Unspecified open wound of left ring finger with damage to nail
    - **S61.306** Unspecified open wound of right little finger with damage to nail
    - **S61.307** Unspecified open wound of left little finger with damage to nail
    - **S61.308** Unspecified open wound of other finger with damage to nail
      Unspecified open wound of specified finger with unspecified laterality with damage to nail
    - **S61.309** Unspecified open wound of unspecified finger with damage to nail
  - **S61.31** Laceration without foreign body of finger with damage to nail
    - **S61.310** Laceration without foreign body of right index finger with damage to nail
    - **S61.311** Laceration without foreign body of left index finger with damage to nail
    - **S61.312** Laceration without foreign body of right middle finger with damage to nail
    - **S61.313** Laceration without foreign body of left middle finger with damage to nail
    - **S61.314** Laceration without foreign body of right ring finger with damage to nail
    - **S61.315** Laceration without foreign body of left ring finger with damage to nail
    - **S61.316** Laceration without foreign body of right little finger with damage to nail
    - **S61.317** Laceration without foreign body of left little finger with damage to nail
    - **S61.318** Laceration without foreign body of other finger with damage to nail
      Laceration without foreign body of specified finger with unspecified laterality with damage to nail
    - **S61.319** Laceration without foreign body of unspecified finger with damage to nail
  - **S61.32** Laceration with foreign body of finger with damage to nail
    - **S61.320** Laceration with foreign body of right index finger with damage to nail
    - **S61.321** Laceration with foreign body of left index finger with damage to nail
    - **S61.322** Laceration with foreign body of right middle finger with damage to nail
    - **S61.323** Laceration with foreign body of left middle finger with damage to nail
    - **S61.324** Laceration with foreign body of right ring finger with damage to nail
    - **S61.325** Laceration with foreign body of left ring finger with damage to nail
    - **S61.326** Laceration with foreign body of right little finger with damage to nail
    - **S61.327** Laceration with foreign body of left little finger with damage to nail
    - **S61.328** Laceration with foreign body of other finger with damage to nail
      Laceration with foreign body of specified finger with unspecified laterality with damage to nail
    - **S61.329** Laceration with foreign body of unspecified finger with damage to nail
  - **S61.33** Puncture wound without foreign body of finger with damage to nail
    - **S61.330** Puncture wound without foreign body of right index finger with damage to nail
    - **S61.331** Puncture wound without foreign body of left index finger with damage to nail
    - **S61.332** Puncture wound without foreign body of right middle finger with damage to nail
    - **S61.333** Puncture wound without foreign body of left middle finger with damage to nail
    - **S61.334** Puncture wound without foreign body of right ring finger with damage to nail
    - **S61.335** Puncture wound without foreign body of left ring finger with damage to nail

Additional Character Required · Placeholder Alert · Manifestation · Unspecified Dx · QPP · Unacceptable PDx

- √7ᵗʰ **S61.336** Puncture wound without foreign body of right little finger with damage to nail
- √7ᵗʰ **S61.337** Puncture wound without foreign body of left little finger with damage to nail
- √7ᵗʰ **S61.338** Puncture wound without foreign body of other finger with damage to nail
  - Puncture wound without foreign body of specified finger with unspecified laterality with damage to nail
- √7ᵗʰ **S61.339** Puncture wound without foreign body of unspecified finger with damage to nail

√6ᵗʰ **S61.34** Puncture wound with foreign body of finger with damage to nail
- √7ᵗʰ **S61.340** Puncture wound with foreign body of right index finger with damage to nail
- √7ᵗʰ **S61.341** Puncture wound with foreign body of left index finger with damage to nail
- √7ᵗʰ **S61.342** Puncture wound with foreign body of right middle finger with damage to nail
- √7ᵗʰ **S61.343** Puncture wound with foreign body of left middle finger with damage to nail
- √7ᵗʰ **S61.344** Puncture wound with foreign body of right ring finger with damage to nail
- √7ᵗʰ **S61.345** Puncture wound with foreign body of left ring finger with damage to nail
- √7ᵗʰ **S61.346** Puncture wound with foreign body of right little finger with damage to nail
- √7ᵗʰ **S61.347** Puncture wound with foreign body of left little finger with damage to nail
- √7ᵗʰ **S61.348** Puncture wound with foreign body of other finger with damage to nail
  - Puncture wound with foreign body of specified finger with unspecified laterality with damage to nail
- √7ᵗʰ **S61.349** Puncture wound with foreign body of unspecified finger with damage to nail

√6ᵗʰ **S61.35** Open bite of finger with damage to nail
- Bite of finger with damage to nail NOS
- **EXCLUDES 1** superficial bite of finger (S60.46-, S60.47-)
- √7ᵗʰ **S61.350** Open bite of right index finger with damage to nail
- √7ᵗʰ **S61.351** Open bite of left index finger with damage to nail
- √7ᵗʰ **S61.352** Open bite of right middle finger with damage to nail
- √7ᵗʰ **S61.353** Open bite of left middle finger with damage to nail
- √7ᵗʰ **S61.354** Open bite of right ring finger with damage to nail
- √7ᵗʰ **S61.355** Open bite of left ring finger with damage to nail
- √7ᵗʰ **S61.356** Open bite of right little finger with damage to nail
- √7ᵗʰ **S61.357** Open bite of left little finger with damage to nail
- √7ᵗʰ **S61.358** Open bite of other finger with damage to nail
  - Open bite of specified finger with unspecified laterality with damage to nail
- √7ᵗʰ **S61.359** Open bite of unspecified finger with damage to nail

√5ᵗʰ **S61.4** Open wound of hand
√6ᵗʰ **S61.40** Unspecified open wound of hand
- √7ᵗʰ **S61.401** Unspecified open wound of right hand
- √7ᵗʰ **S61.402** Unspecified open wound of left hand
- √7ᵗʰ **S61.409** Unspecified open wound of unspecified hand

√6ᵗʰ **S61.41** Laceration without foreign body of hand
- √7ᵗʰ **S61.411** Laceration without foreign body of right hand
- √7ᵗʰ **S61.412** Laceration without foreign body of left hand
- √7ᵗʰ **S61.419** Laceration without foreign body of unspecified hand

√6ᵗʰ **S61.42** Laceration with foreign body of hand
- √7ᵗʰ **S61.421** Laceration with foreign body of right hand
- √7ᵗʰ **S61.422** Laceration with foreign body of left hand
- √7ᵗʰ **S61.429** Laceration with foreign body of unspecified hand

√6ᵗʰ **S61.43** Puncture wound without foreign body of hand
- √7ᵗʰ **S61.431** Puncture wound without foreign body of right hand
- √7ᵗʰ **S61.432** Puncture wound without foreign body of left hand
- √7ᵗʰ **S61.439** Puncture wound without foreign body of unspecified hand

√6ᵗʰ **S61.44** Puncture wound with foreign body of hand
- √7ᵗʰ **S61.441** Puncture wound with foreign body of right hand
- √7ᵗʰ **S61.442** Puncture wound with foreign body of left hand
- √7ᵗʰ **S61.449** Puncture wound with foreign body of unspecified hand

√6ᵗʰ **S61.45** Open bite of hand
- Bite of hand NOS
- **EXCLUDES 1** superficial bite of hand (S60.56-, S60.57-)
- √7ᵗʰ **S61.451** Open bite of right hand
- √7ᵗʰ **S61.452** Open bite of left hand
- √7ᵗʰ **S61.459** Open bite of unspecified hand

√5ᵗʰ **S61.5** Open wound of wrist
√6ᵗʰ **S61.50** Unspecified open wound of wrist
- √7ᵗʰ **S61.501** Unspecified open wound of right wrist
- √7ᵗʰ **S61.502** Unspecified open wound of left wrist
- √7ᵗʰ **S61.509** Unspecified open wound of unspecified wrist

√6ᵗʰ **S61.51** Laceration without foreign body of wrist
- √7ᵗʰ **S61.511** Laceration without foreign body of right wrist
- √7ᵗʰ **S61.512** Laceration without foreign body of left wrist
- √7ᵗʰ **S61.519** Laceration without foreign body of unspecified wrist

√6ᵗʰ **S61.52** Laceration with foreign body of wrist
- √7ᵗʰ **S61.521** Laceration with foreign body of right wrist
- √7ᵗʰ **S61.522** Laceration with foreign body of left wrist
- √7ᵗʰ **S61.529** Laceration with foreign body of unspecified wrist

√6ᵗʰ **S61.53** Puncture wound without foreign body of wrist
- √7ᵗʰ **S61.531** Puncture wound without foreign body of right wrist
- √7ᵗʰ **S61.532** Puncture wound without foreign body of left wrist
- √7ᵗʰ **S61.539** Puncture wound without foreign body of unspecified wrist

√6ᵗʰ **S61.54** Puncture wound with foreign body of wrist
- √7ᵗʰ **S61.541** Puncture wound with foreign body of right wrist
- √7ᵗʰ **S61.542** Puncture wound with foreign body of left wrist
- √7ᵗʰ **S61.549** Puncture wound with foreign body of unspecified wrist

√6ᵗʰ **S61.55** Open bite of wrist
- Bite of wrist NOS
- **EXCLUDES 1** superficial bite of wrist (S60.86-, S60.87-)
- √7ᵗʰ **S61.551** Open bite of right wrist
- √7ᵗʰ **S61.552** Open bite of left wrist
- √7ᵗʰ **S61.559** Open bite of unspecified wrist

S62 Fracture at wrist and hand level

NOTE A fracture not indicated as displaced or nondisplaced should be coded to displaced

A fracture not indicated as open or closed should be coded to closed

EXCLUDES 1 traumatic amputation of wrist and hand (S68.-)
EXCLUDES 2 fracture of distal parts of ulna and radius (S52.-)
AHA: 2018,2Q,12; 2015,3Q,37-39

The appropriate 7th character is to be added to each code from category S62.
- A initial encounter for closed fracture
- B initial encounter for open fracture
- D subsequent encounter for fracture with routine healing
- G subsequent encounter for fracture with delayed healing
- K subsequent encounter for fracture with nonunion
- P subsequent encounter for fracture with malunion
- S sequela

S62.0 Fracture of navicular [scaphoid] bone of wrist

- **S62.00** Unspecified fracture of navicular [scaphoid] bone of wrist
  - S62.001 Unspecified fracture of navicular [scaphoid] bone of right wrist
  - S62.002 Unspecified fracture of navicular [scaphoid] bone of left wrist
    - **AHA:** 2012,4Q,106
  - S62.009 Unspecified fracture of navicular [scaphoid] bone of unspecified wrist
- **S62.01** Fracture of distal pole of navicular [scaphoid] bone of wrist
  Fracture of volar tuberosity of navicular [scaphoid] bone of wrist
  - S62.011 Displaced fracture of distal pole of navicular [scaphoid] bone of right wrist
  - S62.012 Displaced fracture of distal pole of navicular [scaphoid] bone of left wrist
  - S62.013 Displaced fracture of distal pole of navicular [scaphoid] bone of unspecified wrist
  - S62.014 Nondisplaced fracture of distal pole of navicular [scaphoid] bone of right wrist
  - S62.015 Nondisplaced fracture of distal pole of navicular [scaphoid] bone of left wrist
  - S62.016 Nondisplaced fracture of distal pole of navicular [scaphoid] bone of unspecified wrist
- **S62.02** Fracture of middle third of navicular [scaphoid] bone of wrist
  - S62.021 Displaced fracture of middle third of navicular [scaphoid] bone of right wrist
  - S62.022 Displaced fracture of middle third of navicular [scaphoid] bone of left wrist
  - S62.023 Displaced fracture of middle third of navicular [scaphoid] bone of unspecified wrist
  - S62.024 Nondisplaced fracture of middle third of navicular [scaphoid] bone of right wrist
  - S62.025 Nondisplaced fracture of middle third of navicular [scaphoid] bone of left wrist
  - S62.026 Nondisplaced fracture of middle third of navicular [scaphoid] bone of unspecified wrist
- **S62.03** Fracture of proximal third of navicular [scaphoid] bone of wrist
  - S62.031 Displaced fracture of proximal third of navicular [scaphoid] bone of right wrist
  - S62.032 Displaced fracture of proximal third of navicular [scaphoid] bone of left wrist
  - S62.033 Displaced fracture of proximal third of navicular [scaphoid] bone of unspecified wrist
  - S62.034 Nondisplaced fracture of proximal third of navicular [scaphoid] bone of right wrist
  - S62.035 Nondisplaced fracture of proximal third of navicular [scaphoid] bone of left wrist
  - S62.036 Nondisplaced fracture of proximal third of navicular [scaphoid] bone of unspecified wrist

S62.1 Fracture of other and unspecified carpal bone(s)

EXCLUDES 2 fracture of scaphoid of wrist (S62.0-)

- **S62.10** Fracture of unspecified carpal bone
  Fracture of wrist NOS
  - S62.101 Fracture of unspecified carpal bone, right wrist
  - S62.102 Fracture of unspecified carpal bone, left wrist
    - **AHA:** 2012,4Q,95
  - S62.109 Fracture of unspecified carpal bone, unspecified wrist
- **S62.11** Fracture of triquetrum [cuneiform] bone of wrist
  - S62.111 Displaced fracture of triquetrum [cuneiform] bone, right wrist
  - S62.112 Displaced fracture of triquetrum [cuneiform] bone, left wrist
  - S62.113 Displaced fracture of triquetrum [cuneiform] bone, unspecified wrist
  - S62.114 Nondisplaced fracture of triquetrum [cuneiform] bone, right wrist
  - S62.115 Nondisplaced fracture of triquetrum [cuneiform] bone, left wrist
  - S62.116 Nondisplaced fracture of triquetrum [cuneiform] bone, unspecified wrist
- **S62.12** Fracture of lunate [semilunar]
  - S62.121 Displaced fracture of lunate [semilunar], right wrist
  - S62.122 Displaced fracture of lunate [semilunar], left wrist
  - S62.123 Displaced fracture of lunate [semilunar], unspecified wrist
  - S62.124 Nondisplaced fracture of lunate [semilunar], right wrist
  - S62.125 Nondisplaced fracture of lunate [semilunar], left wrist
  - S62.126 Nondisplaced fracture of lunate [semilunar], unspecified wrist
- **S62.13** Fracture of capitate [os magnum] bone
  - S62.131 Displaced fracture of capitate [os magnum] bone, right wrist
  - S62.132 Displaced fracture of capitate [os magnum] bone, left wrist
  - S62.133 Displaced fracture of capitate [os magnum] bone, unspecified wrist
  - S62.134 Nondisplaced fracture of capitate [os magnum] bone, right wrist
  - S62.135 Nondisplaced fracture of capitate [os magnum] bone, left wrist
  - S62.136 Nondisplaced fracture of capitate [os magnum] bone, unspecified wrist
- **S62.14** Fracture of body of hamate [unciform] bone
  Fracture of hamate [unciform] bone NOS
  - S62.141 Displaced fracture of body of hamate [unciform] bone, right wrist
  - S62.142 Displaced fracture of body of hamate [unciform] bone, left wrist
  - S62.143 Displaced fracture of body of hamate [unciform] bone, unspecified wrist
  - S62.144 Nondisplaced fracture of body of hamate [unciform] bone, right wrist
  - S62.145 Nondisplaced fracture of body of hamate [unciform] bone, left wrist
  - S62.146 Nondisplaced fracture of body of hamate [unciform] bone, unspecified wrist
- **S62.15** Fracture of hook process of hamate [unciform] bone
  Fracture of unciform process of hamate [unciform] bone
  - S62.151 Displaced fracture of hook process of hamate [unciform] bone, right wrist
  - S62.152 Displaced fracture of hook process of hamate [unciform] bone, left wrist

- **S62.153** Displaced fracture of hook process of hamate [unciform] bone, unspecified wrist
- **S62.154** Nondisplaced fracture of hook process of hamate [unciform] bone, right wrist
- **S62.155** Nondisplaced fracture of hook process of hamate [unciform] bone, left wrist
- **S62.156** Nondisplaced fracture of hook process of hamate [unciform] bone, unspecified wrist

S62.16 Fracture of pisiform
- **S62.161** Displaced fracture of pisiform, right wrist
- **S62.162** Displaced fracture of pisiform, left wrist
- **S62.163** Displaced fracture of pisiform, unspecified wrist
- **S62.164** Nondisplaced fracture of pisiform, right wrist
- **S62.165** Nondisplaced fracture of pisiform, left wrist
- **S62.166** Nondisplaced fracture of pisiform, unspecified wrist

S62.17 Fracture of trapezium [larger multangular]
- **S62.171** Displaced fracture of trapezium [larger multangular], right wrist
- **S62.172** Displaced fracture of trapezium [larger multangular], left wrist
- **S62.173** Displaced fracture of trapezium [larger multangular], unspecified wrist
- **S62.174** Nondisplaced fracture of trapezium [larger multangular], right wrist
- **S62.175** Nondisplaced fracture of trapezium [larger multangular], left wrist
- **S62.176** Nondisplaced fracture of trapezium [larger multangular], unspecified wrist

S62.18 Fracture of trapezoid [smaller multangular]
- **S62.181** Displaced fracture of trapezoid [smaller multangular], right wrist
- **S62.182** Displaced fracture of trapezoid [smaller multangular], left wrist
- **S62.183** Displaced fracture of trapezoid [smaller multangular], unspecified wrist
- **S62.184** Nondisplaced fracture of trapezoid [smaller multangular], right wrist
- **S62.185** Nondisplaced fracture of trapezoid [smaller multangular], left wrist
- **S62.186** Nondisplaced fracture of trapezoid [smaller multangular], unspecified wrist

S62.2 Fracture of first metacarpal bone

S62.20 Unspecified fracture of first metacarpal bone
- **S62.201** Unspecified fracture of first metacarpal bone, right hand
- **S62.202** Unspecified fracture of first metacarpal bone, left hand
- **S62.209** Unspecified fracture of first metacarpal bone, unspecified hand

S62.21 Bennett's fracture
DEF: Intra-articular, two-part fracture at the base of the first metacarpal bone (thumb) on the ulnar side at the carpometacarpal (CMC) joint.
- **S62.211** Bennett's fracture, right hand
- **S62.212** Bennett's fracture, left hand
- **S62.213** Bennett's fracture, unspecified hand

S62.22 Rolando's fracture
DEF: Comminuted, three part intra-articular fracture at the base of the thumb metacarpal.
- **S62.221** Displaced Rolando's fracture, right hand
- **S62.222** Displaced Rolando's fracture, left hand
- **S62.223** Displaced Rolando's fracture, unspecified hand
- **S62.224** Nondisplaced Rolando's fracture, right hand
- **S62.225** Nondisplaced Rolando's fracture, left hand
- **S62.226** Nondisplaced Rolando's fracture, unspecified hand

S62.23 Other fracture of base of first metacarpal bone
- **S62.231** Other displaced fracture of base of first metacarpal bone, right hand
- **S62.232** Other displaced fracture of base of first metacarpal bone, left hand
- **S62.233** Other displaced fracture of base of first metacarpal bone, unspecified hand
- **S62.234** Other nondisplaced fracture of base of first metacarpal bone, right hand
- **S62.235** Other nondisplaced fracture of base of first metacarpal bone, left hand
- **S62.236** Other nondisplaced fracture of base of first metacarpal bone, unspecified hand

S62.24 Fracture of shaft of first metacarpal bone
- **S62.241** Displaced fracture of shaft of first metacarpal bone, right hand
- **S62.242** Displaced fracture of shaft of first metacarpal bone, left hand
- **S62.243** Displaced fracture of shaft of first metacarpal bone, unspecified hand
- **S62.244** Nondisplaced fracture of shaft of first metacarpal bone, right hand
- **S62.245** Nondisplaced fracture of shaft of first metacarpal bone, left hand
- **S62.246** Nondisplaced fracture of shaft of first metacarpal bone, unspecified hand

S62.25 Fracture of neck of first metacarpal bone
- **S62.251** Displaced fracture of neck of first metacarpal bone, right hand
- **S62.252** Displaced fracture of neck of first metacarpal bone, left hand
- **S62.253** Displaced fracture of neck of first metacarpal bone, unspecified hand
- **S62.254** Nondisplaced fracture of neck of first metacarpal bone, right hand
- **S62.255** Nondisplaced fracture of neck of first metacarpal bone, left hand
- **S62.256** Nondisplaced fracture of neck of first metacarpal bone, unspecified hand

S62.29 Other fracture of first metacarpal bone
- **S62.291** Other fracture of first metacarpal bone, right hand
- **S62.292** Other fracture of first metacarpal bone, left hand
- **S62.299** Other fracture of first metacarpal bone, unspecified hand

S62.3 Fracture of other and unspecified metacarpal bone
EXCLUDES 2 fracture of first metacarpal bone (S62.2-)

S62.30 Unspecified fracture of other metacarpal bone
- **S62.300** Unspecified fracture of second metacarpal bone, right hand
- **S62.301** Unspecified fracture of second metacarpal bone, left hand
- **S62.302** Unspecified fracture of third metacarpal bone, right hand
- **S62.303** Unspecified fracture of third metacarpal bone, left hand
- **S62.304** Unspecified fracture of fourth metacarpal bone, right hand
- **S62.305** Unspecified fracture of fourth metacarpal bone, left hand
- **S62.306** Unspecified fracture of fifth metacarpal bone, right hand
- **S62.307** Unspecified fracture of fifth metacarpal bone, left hand
- **S62.308** Unspecified fracture of other metacarpal bone
  Unspecified fracture of specified metacarpal bone with unspecified laterality
- **S62.309** Unspecified fracture of unspecified metacarpal bone

S62.31 Displaced fracture of base of other metacarpal bone
- **S62.310** Displaced fracture of base of second metacarpal bone, right hand
- **S62.311** Displaced fracture of base of second metacarpal bone, left hand

- S62.312 Displaced fracture of base of third metacarpal bone, right hand
- S62.313 Displaced fracture of base of third metacarpal bone, left hand
- S62.314 Displaced fracture of base of fourth metacarpal bone, right hand
- S62.315 Displaced fracture of base of fourth metacarpal bone, left hand
- S62.316 Displaced fracture of base of fifth metacarpal bone, right hand
- S62.317 Displaced fracture of base of fifth metacarpal bone, left hand
- S62.318 Displaced fracture of base of other metacarpal bone
  - Displaced fracture of base of specified metacarpal bone with unspecified laterality
- S62.319 Displaced fracture of base of unspecified metacarpal bone

S62.32 Displaced fracture of shaft of other metacarpal bone
- S62.320 Displaced fracture of shaft of second metacarpal bone, right hand
- S62.321 Displaced fracture of shaft of second metacarpal bone, left hand
- S62.322 Displaced fracture of shaft of third metacarpal bone, right hand
- S62.323 Displaced fracture of shaft of third metacarpal bone, left hand
- S62.324 Displaced fracture of shaft of fourth metacarpal bone, right hand
- S62.325 Displaced fracture of shaft of fourth metacarpal bone, left hand
- S62.326 Displaced fracture of shaft of fifth metacarpal bone, right hand
- S62.327 Displaced fracture of shaft of fifth metacarpal bone, left hand
- S62.328 Displaced fracture of shaft of other metacarpal bone
  - Displaced fracture of shaft of specified metacarpal bone with unspecified laterality
- S62.329 Displaced fracture of shaft of unspecified metacarpal bone

S62.33 Displaced fracture of neck of other metacarpal bone
- S62.330 Displaced fracture of neck of second metacarpal bone, right hand
- S62.331 Displaced fracture of neck of second metacarpal bone, left hand
- S62.332 Displaced fracture of neck of third metacarpal bone, right hand
- S62.333 Displaced fracture of neck of third metacarpal bone, left hand
- S62.334 Displaced fracture of neck of fourth metacarpal bone, right hand
- S62.335 Displaced fracture of neck of fourth metacarpal bone, left hand
- S62.336 Displaced fracture of neck of fifth metacarpal bone, right hand
- S62.337 Displaced fracture of neck of fifth metacarpal bone, left hand
- S62.338 Displaced fracture of neck of other metacarpal bone
  - Displaced fracture of neck of specified metacarpal bone with unspecified laterality
- S62.339 Displaced fracture of neck of unspecified metacarpal bone

S62.34 Nondisplaced fracture of base of other metacarpal bone
- S62.340 Nondisplaced fracture of base of second metacarpal bone, right hand
- S62.341 Nondisplaced fracture of base of second metacarpal bone, left hand
- S62.342 Nondisplaced fracture of base of third metacarpal bone, right hand
- S62.343 Nondisplaced fracture of base of third metacarpal bone, left hand
- S62.344 Nondisplaced fracture of base of fourth metacarpal bone, right hand
- S62.345 Nondisplaced fracture of base of fourth metacarpal bone, left hand
- S62.346 Nondisplaced fracture of base of fifth metacarpal bone, right hand
- S62.347 Nondisplaced fracture of base of fifth metacarpal bone, left hand
- S62.348 Nondisplaced fracture of base of other metacarpal bone
  - Nondisplaced fracture of base of specified metacarpal bone with unspecified laterality
- S62.349 Nondisplaced fracture of base of unspecified metacarpal bone

S62.35 Nondisplaced fracture of shaft of other metacarpal bone
- S62.350 Nondisplaced fracture of shaft of second metacarpal bone, right hand
- S62.351 Nondisplaced fracture of shaft of second metacarpal bone, left hand
- S62.352 Nondisplaced fracture of shaft of third metacarpal bone, right hand
- S62.353 Nondisplaced fracture of shaft of third metacarpal bone, left hand
- S62.354 Nondisplaced fracture of shaft of fourth metacarpal bone, right hand
- S62.355 Nondisplaced fracture of shaft of fourth metacarpal bone, left hand
- S62.356 Nondisplaced fracture of shaft of fifth metacarpal bone, right hand
- S62.357 Nondisplaced fracture of shaft of fifth metacarpal bone, left hand
- S62.358 Nondisplaced fracture of shaft of other metacarpal bone
  - Nondisplaced fracture of shaft of specified metacarpal bone with unspecified laterality
- S62.359 Nondisplaced fracture of shaft of unspecified metacarpal bone

S62.36 Nondisplaced fracture of neck of other metacarpal bone
- S62.360 Nondisplaced fracture of neck of second metacarpal bone, right hand
- S62.361 Nondisplaced fracture of neck of second metacarpal bone, left hand
- S62.362 Nondisplaced fracture of neck of third metacarpal bone, right hand
- S62.363 Nondisplaced fracture of neck of third metacarpal bone, left hand
- S62.364 Nondisplaced fracture of neck of fourth metacarpal bone, right hand
- S62.365 Nondisplaced fracture of neck of fourth metacarpal bone, left hand
- S62.366 Nondisplaced fracture of neck of fifth metacarpal bone, right hand
- S62.367 Nondisplaced fracture of neck of fifth metacarpal bone, left hand
- S62.368 Nondisplaced fracture of neck of other metacarpal bone
  - Nondisplaced fracture of neck of specified metacarpal bone with unspecified laterality
- S62.369 Nondisplaced fracture of neck of unspecified metacarpal bone

S62.39 Other fracture of other metacarpal bone
- S62.390 Other fracture of second metacarpal bone, right hand
- S62.391 Other fracture of second metacarpal bone, left hand
- S62.392 Other fracture of third metacarpal bone, right hand
- S62.393 Other fracture of third metacarpal bone, left hand
- S62.394 Other fracture of fourth metacarpal bone, right hand
- S62.395 Other fracture of fourth metacarpal bone, left hand
- S62.396 Other fracture of fifth metacarpal bone, right hand
- S62.397 Other fracture of fifth metacarpal bone, left hand

- **S62.398** Other fracture of other metacarpal bone
  Other fracture of specified metacarpal bone with unspecified laterality
- **S62.399** Other fracture of unspecified metacarpal bone

S62.5 Fracture of thumb

- **S62.50** Fracture of unspecified phalanx of thumb
  - **S62.501** Fracture of unspecified phalanx of right thumb
  - **S62.502** Fracture of unspecified phalanx of left thumb
  - **S62.509** Fracture of unspecified phalanx of unspecified thumb
- **S62.51** Fracture of proximal phalanx of thumb
  - **S62.511** Displaced fracture of proximal phalanx of right thumb
  - **S62.512** Displaced fracture of proximal phalanx of left thumb
  - **S62.513** Displaced fracture of proximal phalanx of unspecified thumb
  - **S62.514** Nondisplaced fracture of proximal phalanx of right thumb
  - **S62.515** Nondisplaced fracture of proximal phalanx of left thumb
  - **S62.516** Nondisplaced fracture of proximal phalanx of unspecified thumb
- **S62.52** Fracture of distal phalanx of thumb
  - **S62.521** Displaced fracture of distal phalanx of right thumb
  - **S62.522** Displaced fracture of distal phalanx of left thumb
  - **S62.523** Displaced fracture of distal phalanx of unspecified thumb
  - **S62.524** Nondisplaced fracture of distal phalanx of right thumb
  - **S62.525** Nondisplaced fracture of distal phalanx of left thumb
  - **S62.526** Nondisplaced fracture of distal phalanx of unspecified thumb

S62.6 Fracture of other and unspecified finger(s)

EXCLUDES 2   fracture of thumb (S62.5-)

- **S62.60** Fracture of unspecified phalanx of finger
  - **S62.600** Fracture of unspecified phalanx of right index finger
  - **S62.601** Fracture of unspecified phalanx of left index finger
  - **S62.602** Fracture of unspecified phalanx of right middle finger
  - **S62.603** Fracture of unspecified phalanx of left middle finger
  - **S62.604** Fracture of unspecified phalanx of right ring finger
  - **S62.605** Fracture of unspecified phalanx of left ring finger
  - **S62.606** Fracture of unspecified phalanx of right little finger
  - **S62.607** Fracture of unspecified phalanx of left little finger
  - **S62.608** Fracture of unspecified phalanx of other finger
    Fracture of unspecified phalanx of specified finger with unspecified laterality
  - **S62.609** Fracture of unspecified phalanx of unspecified finger
- **S62.61** Displaced fracture of proximal phalanx of finger
  - **S62.610** Displaced fracture of proximal phalanx of right index finger
  - **S62.611** Displaced fracture of proximal phalanx of left index finger
  - **S62.612** Displaced fracture of proximal phalanx of right middle finger
  - **S62.613** Displaced fracture of proximal phalanx of left middle finger
  - **S62.614** Displaced fracture of proximal phalanx of right ring finger
  - **S62.615** Displaced fracture of proximal phalanx of left ring finger
  - **S62.616** Displaced fracture of proximal phalanx of right little finger
  - **S62.617** Displaced fracture of proximal phalanx of left little finger
  - **S62.618** Displaced fracture of proximal phalanx of other finger
    Displaced fracture of proximal phalanx of specified finger with unspecified laterality
  - **S62.619** Displaced fracture of proximal phalanx of unspecified finger
- **S62.62** Displaced fracture of middle phalanx of finger
  - **S62.620** Displaced fracture of middle phalanx of right index finger
  - **S62.621** Displaced fracture of middle phalanx of left index finger
  - **S62.622** Displaced fracture of middle phalanx of right middle finger
  - **S62.623** Displaced fracture of middle phalanx of left middle finger
  - **S62.624** Displaced fracture of middle phalanx of right ring finger
  - **S62.625** Displaced fracture of middle phalanx of left ring finger
  - **S62.626** Displaced fracture of middle phalanx of right little finger
  - **S62.627** Displaced fracture of middle phalanx of left little finger
  - **S62.628** Displaced fracture of middle phalanx of other finger
    Displaced fracture of middle phalanx of specified finger with unspecified laterality
  - **S62.629** Displaced fracture of middle phalanx of unspecified finger
- **S62.63** Displaced fracture of distal phalanx of finger
  - **S62.630** Displaced fracture of distal phalanx of right index finger
  - **S62.631** Displaced fracture of distal phalanx of left index finger
  - **S62.632** Displaced fracture of distal phalanx of right middle finger
  - **S62.633** Displaced fracture of distal phalanx of left middle finger
  - **S62.634** Displaced fracture of distal phalanx of right ring finger
  - **S62.635** Displaced fracture of distal phalanx of left ring finger
  - **S62.636** Displaced fracture of distal phalanx of right little finger
  - **S62.637** Displaced fracture of distal phalanx of left little finger
  - **S62.638** Displaced fracture of distal phalanx of other finger
    Displaced fracture of distal phalanx of specified finger with unspecified laterality
  - **S62.639** Displaced fracture of distal phalanx of unspecified finger
- **S62.64** Nondisplaced fracture of proximal phalanx of finger
  - **S62.640** Nondisplaced fracture of proximal phalanx of right index finger
  - **S62.641** Nondisplaced fracture of proximal phalanx of left index finger
  - **S62.642** Nondisplaced fracture of proximal phalanx of right middle finger
  - **S62.643** Nondisplaced fracture of proximal phalanx of left middle finger
  - **S62.644** Nondisplaced fracture of proximal phalanx of right ring finger
  - **S62.645** Nondisplaced fracture of proximal phalanx of left ring finger
  - **S62.646** Nondisplaced fracture of proximal phalanx of right little finger
  - **S62.647** Nondisplaced fracture of proximal phalanx of left little finger
  - **S62.648** Nondisplaced fracture of proximal phalanx of other finger
    Nondisplaced fracture of proximal phalanx of specified finger with unspecified laterality
  - **S62.649** Nondisplaced fracture of proximal phalanx of unspecified finger

- **S62.65** Nondisplaced fracture of middle phalanx of finger
  - S62.650 Nondisplaced fracture of middle phalanx of right index finger
  - S62.651 Nondisplaced fracture of middle phalanx of left index finger
  - S62.652 Nondisplaced fracture of middle phalanx of right middle finger
  - S62.653 Nondisplaced fracture of middle phalanx of left middle finger
  - S62.654 Nondisplaced fracture of middle phalanx of right ring finger
  - S62.655 Nondisplaced fracture of middle phalanx of left ring finger
  - S62.656 Nondisplaced fracture of middle phalanx of right little finger
  - S62.657 Nondisplaced fracture of middle phalanx of left little finger
  - S62.658 Nondisplaced fracture of middle phalanx of other finger
    Nondisplaced fracture of middle phalanx of specified finger with unspecified laterality
  - S62.659 Nondisplaced fracture of middle phalanx of unspecified finger
- **S62.66** Nondisplaced fracture of distal phalanx of finger
  - S62.660 Nondisplaced fracture of distal phalanx of right index finger
  - S62.661 Nondisplaced fracture of distal phalanx of left index finger
  - S62.662 Nondisplaced fracture of distal phalanx of right middle finger
  - S62.663 Nondisplaced fracture of distal phalanx of left middle finger
  - S62.664 Nondisplaced fracture of distal phalanx of right ring finger
  - S62.665 Nondisplaced fracture of distal phalanx of left ring finger
  - S62.666 Nondisplaced fracture of distal phalanx of right little finger
  - S62.667 Nondisplaced fracture of distal phalanx of left little finger
  - S62.668 Nondisplaced fracture of distal phalanx of other finger
    Nondisplaced fracture of distal phalanx of specified finger with unspecified laterality
  - S62.669 Nondisplaced fracture of distal phalanx of unspecified finger
- ▲ **S62.9** Unspecified fracture of hand
  - ▲ S62.90 Unspecified fracture of unspecified hand
  - ▲ S62.91 Unspecified fracture of right hand
  - ▲ S62.92 Unspecified fracture of left hand

S63 Dislocation and sprain of joints and ligaments at wrist and hand level

INCLUDES
- avulsion of joint or ligament at wrist and hand level
- laceration of cartilage, joint or ligament at wrist and hand level
- sprain of cartilage, joint or ligament at wrist and hand level
- traumatic hemarthrosis of joint or ligament at wrist and hand level
- traumatic rupture of joint or ligament at wrist and hand level
- traumatic subluxation of joint or ligament at wrist and hand level
- traumatic tear of joint or ligament at wrist and hand level

Code also any associated open wound

EXCLUDES 2 strain of muscle, fascia and tendon of wrist and hand (S66.-)

The appropriate 7th character is to be added to each code from category S63.
A initial encounter
D subsequent encounter
S sequela

- **S63.0** Subluxation and dislocation of wrist and hand joints
  - **S63.00** Unspecified subluxation and dislocation of wrist and hand
    Dislocation of carpal bone NOS
    Dislocation of distal end of radius NOS
    Subluxation of carpal bone NOS
    Subluxation of distal end of radius NOS
    - S63.001 Unspecified subluxation of right wrist and hand
    - S63.002 Unspecified subluxation of left wrist and hand
    - S63.003 Unspecified subluxation of unspecified wrist and hand
    - S63.004 Unspecified dislocation of right wrist and hand
    - S63.005 Unspecified dislocation of left wrist and hand
    - S63.006 Unspecified dislocation of unspecified wrist and hand
  - **S63.01** Subluxation and dislocation of distal radioulnar joint
    - S63.011 Subluxation of distal radioulnar joint of right wrist
    - S63.012 Subluxation of distal radioulnar joint of left wrist
    - S63.013 Subluxation of distal radioulnar joint of unspecified wrist
    - S63.014 Dislocation of distal radioulnar joint of right wrist
    - S63.015 Dislocation of distal radioulnar joint of left wrist
    - S63.016 Dislocation of distal radioulnar joint of unspecified wrist
  - **S63.02** Subluxation and dislocation of radiocarpal joint
    - S63.021 Subluxation of radiocarpal joint of right wrist
    - S63.022 Subluxation of radiocarpal joint of left wrist
    - S63.023 Subluxation of radiocarpal joint of unspecified wrist
    - S63.024 Dislocation of radiocarpal joint of right wrist
    - S63.025 Dislocation of radiocarpal joint of left wrist
    - S63.026 Dislocation of radiocarpal joint of unspecified wrist
  - **S63.03** Subluxation and dislocation of midcarpal joint
    - S63.031 Subluxation of midcarpal joint of right wrist
    - S63.032 Subluxation of midcarpal joint of left wrist
    - S63.033 Subluxation of midcarpal joint of unspecified wrist
    - S63.034 Dislocation of midcarpal joint of right wrist
    - S63.035 Dislocation of midcarpal joint of left wrist
    - S63.036 Dislocation of midcarpal joint of unspecified wrist
  - **S63.04** Subluxation and dislocation of carpometacarpal joint of thumb
    EXCLUDES 2 interphalangeal subluxation and dislocation of thumb (S63.1-)
    - S63.041 Subluxation of carpometacarpal joint of right thumb
    - S63.042 Subluxation of carpometacarpal joint of left thumb
    - S63.043 Subluxation of carpometacarpal joint of unspecified thumb
    - S63.044 Dislocation of carpometacarpal joint of right thumb
    - S63.045 Dislocation of carpometacarpal joint of left thumb
    - S63.046 Dislocation of carpometacarpal joint of unspecified thumb
  - **S63.05** Subluxation and dislocation of other carpometacarpal joint
    EXCLUDES 2 subluxation and dislocation of carpometacarpal joint of thumb (S63.04-)
    - S63.051 Subluxation of other carpometacarpal joint of right hand
    - S63.052 Subluxation of other carpometacarpal joint of left hand
    - S63.053 Subluxation of other carpometacarpal joint of unspecified hand
    - S63.054 Dislocation of other carpometacarpal joint of right hand
    - S63.055 Dislocation of other carpometacarpal joint of left hand
    - S63.056 Dislocation of other carpometacarpal joint of unspecified hand

- **S63.06** Subluxation and dislocation of metacarpal (bone), proximal end
  - S63.061 Subluxation of metacarpal (bone), proximal end of right hand
  - S63.062 Subluxation of metacarpal (bone), proximal end of left hand
  - S63.063 Subluxation of metacarpal (bone), proximal end of unspecified hand
  - S63.064 Dislocation of metacarpal (bone), proximal end of right hand
  - S63.065 Dislocation of metacarpal (bone), proximal end of left hand
  - S63.066 Dislocation of metacarpal (bone), proximal end of unspecified hand
- **S63.07** Subluxation and dislocation of distal end of ulna
  - S63.071 Subluxation of distal end of right ulna
  - S63.072 Subluxation of distal end of left ulna
  - S63.073 Subluxation of distal end of unspecified ulna
  - S63.074 Dislocation of distal end of right ulna
  - S63.075 Dislocation of distal end of left ulna
  - S63.076 Dislocation of distal end of unspecified ulna
- **S63.09** Other subluxation and dislocation of wrist and hand
  - S63.091 Other subluxation of right wrist and hand
  - S63.092 Other subluxation of left wrist and hand
  - S63.093 Other subluxation of unspecified wrist and hand
  - S63.094 Other dislocation of right wrist and hand
  - S63.095 Other dislocation of left wrist and hand
  - S63.096 Other dislocation of unspecified wrist and hand
- **S63.1** Subluxation and dislocation of thumb
  - **S63.10** Unspecified subluxation and dislocation of thumb
    - S63.101 Unspecified subluxation of right thumb
    - S63.102 Unspecified subluxation of left thumb
    - S63.103 Unspecified subluxation of unspecified thumb
    - S63.104 Unspecified dislocation of right thumb
    - S63.105 Unspecified dislocation of left thumb
    - S63.106 Unspecified dislocation of unspecified thumb
  - **S63.11** Subluxation and dislocation of metacarpophalangeal joint of thumb
    - S63.111 Subluxation of metacarpophalangeal joint of right thumb
    - S63.112 Subluxation of metacarpophalangeal joint of left thumb
    - S63.113 Subluxation of metacarpophalangeal joint of unspecified thumb
    - S63.114 Dislocation of metacarpophalangeal joint of right thumb
    - S63.115 Dislocation of metacarpophalangeal joint of left thumb
    - S63.116 Dislocation of metacarpophalangeal joint of unspecified thumb
  - **S63.12** Subluxation and dislocation of interphalangeal joint of thumb
    - S63.121 Subluxation of interphalangeal joint of right thumb
    - S63.122 Subluxation of interphalangeal joint of left thumb
    - S63.123 Subluxation of interphalangeal joint of unspecified thumb
    - S63.124 Dislocation of interphalangeal joint of right thumb
    - S63.125 Dislocation of interphalangeal joint of left thumb
    - S63.126 Dislocation of interphalangeal joint of unspecified thumb
- **S63.2** Subluxation and dislocation of other finger(s)
  - EXCLUDES 2 subluxation and dislocation of thumb (S63.1-)
  - **S63.20** Unspecified subluxation of other finger
    - S63.200 Unspecified subluxation of right index finger
    - S63.201 Unspecified subluxation of left index finger
    - S63.202 Unspecified subluxation of right middle finger
    - S63.203 Unspecified subluxation of left middle finger
    - S63.204 Unspecified subluxation of right ring finger
    - S63.205 Unspecified subluxation of left ring finger
    - S63.206 Unspecified subluxation of right little finger
    - S63.207 Unspecified subluxation of left little finger
    - S63.208 Unspecified subluxation of other finger
      Unspecified subluxation of specified finger with unspecified laterality
    - S63.209 Unspecified subluxation of unspecified finger
  - **S63.21** Subluxation of metacarpophalangeal joint of finger
    - S63.210 Subluxation of metacarpophalangeal joint of right index finger
    - S63.211 Subluxation of metacarpophalangeal joint of left index finger
    - S63.212 Subluxation of metacarpophalangeal joint of right middle finger
    - S63.213 Subluxation of metacarpophalangeal joint of left middle finger
    - S63.214 Subluxation of metacarpophalangeal joint of right ring finger
    - S63.215 Subluxation of metacarpophalangeal joint of left ring finger
    - S63.216 Subluxation of metacarpophalangeal joint of right little finger
    - S63.217 Subluxation of metacarpophalangeal joint of left little finger
    - S63.218 Subluxation of metacarpophalangeal joint of other finger
      Subluxation of metacarpophalangeal joint of specified finger with unspecified laterality
    - S63.219 Subluxation of metacarpophalangeal joint of unspecified finger
  - **S63.22** Subluxation of unspecified interphalangeal joint of finger
    - S63.220 Subluxation of unspecified interphalangeal joint of right index finger
    - S63.221 Subluxation of unspecified interphalangeal joint of left index finger
    - S63.222 Subluxation of unspecified interphalangeal joint of right middle finger
    - S63.223 Subluxation of unspecified interphalangeal joint of left middle finger
    - S63.224 Subluxation of unspecified interphalangeal joint of right ring finger
    - S63.225 Subluxation of unspecified interphalangeal joint of left ring finger
    - S63.226 Subluxation of unspecified interphalangeal joint of right little finger
    - S63.227 Subluxation of unspecified interphalangeal joint of left little finger
    - S63.228 Subluxation of unspecified interphalangeal joint of other finger
      Subluxation of unspecified interphalangeal joint of specified finger with unspecified laterality
    - S63.229 Subluxation of unspecified interphalangeal joint of unspecified finger
  - **S63.23** Subluxation of proximal interphalangeal joint of finger
    - S63.230 Subluxation of proximal interphalangeal joint of right index finger
    - S63.231 Subluxation of proximal interphalangeal joint of left index finger
    - S63.232 Subluxation of proximal interphalangeal joint of right middle finger
    - S63.233 Subluxation of proximal interphalangeal joint of left middle finger
    - S63.234 Subluxation of proximal interphalangeal joint of right ring finger
    - S63.235 Subluxation of proximal interphalangeal joint of left ring finger
    - S63.236 Subluxation of proximal interphalangeal joint of right little finger
    - S63.237 Subluxation of proximal interphalangeal joint of left little finger

- S63.238 **Subluxation of proximal interphalangeal joint of other finger**
  Subluxation of proximal interphalangeal joint of specified finger with unspecified laterality
- S63.239 **Subluxation of proximal interphalangeal joint of unspecified finger**

S63.24 Subluxation of distal interphalangeal joint of finger
- S63.240 **Subluxation of distal interphalangeal joint of right index finger**
- S63.241 **Subluxation of distal interphalangeal joint of left index finger**
- S63.242 **Subluxation of distal interphalangeal joint of right middle finger**
- S63.243 **Subluxation of distal interphalangeal joint of left middle finger**
- S63.244 **Subluxation of distal interphalangeal joint of right ring finger**
- S63.245 **Subluxation of distal interphalangeal joint of left ring finger**
- S63.246 **Subluxation of distal interphalangeal joint of right little finger**
- S63.247 **Subluxation of distal interphalangeal joint of left little finger**
- S63.248 **Subluxation of distal interphalangeal joint of other finger**
  Subluxation of distal interphalangeal joint of specified finger with unspecified laterality
- S63.249 **Subluxation of distal interphalangeal joint of unspecified finger**

S63.25 Unspecified dislocation of other finger
- S63.250 **Unspecified dislocation of right index finger**
- S63.251 **Unspecified dislocation of left index finger**
- S63.252 **Unspecified dislocation of right middle finger**
- S63.253 **Unspecified dislocation of left middle finger**
- S63.254 **Unspecified dislocation of right ring finger**
- S63.255 **Unspecified dislocation of left ring finger**
- S63.256 **Unspecified dislocation of right little finger**
- S63.257 **Unspecified dislocation of left little finger**
- S63.258 **Unspecified dislocation of other finger**
  Unspecified dislocation of specified finger with unspecified laterality
- S63.259 **Unspecified dislocation of unspecified finger**
  Unspecified dislocation of unspecified finger with unspecified laterality

S63.26 Dislocation of metacarpophalangeal joint of finger
- S63.260 **Dislocation of metacarpophalangeal joint of right index finger**
- S63.261 **Dislocation of metacarpophalangeal joint of left index finger**
- S63.262 **Dislocation of metacarpophalangeal joint of right middle finger**
- S63.263 **Dislocation of metacarpophalangeal joint of left middle finger**
- S63.264 **Dislocation of metacarpophalangeal joint of right ring finger**
- S63.265 **Dislocation of metacarpophalangeal joint of left ring finger**
- S63.266 **Dislocation of metacarpophalangeal joint of right little finger**
- S63.267 **Dislocation of metacarpophalangeal joint of left little finger**
- S63.268 **Dislocation of metacarpophalangeal joint of other finger**
  Dislocation of metacarpophalangeal joint of specified finger with unspecified laterality
- S63.269 **Dislocation of metacarpophalangeal joint of unspecified finger**

S63.27 Dislocation of unspecified interphalangeal joint of finger
- S63.270 **Dislocation of unspecified interphalangeal joint of right index finger**
- S63.271 **Dislocation of unspecified interphalangeal joint of left index finger**
- S63.272 **Dislocation of unspecified interphalangeal joint of right middle finger**
- S63.273 **Dislocation of unspecified interphalangeal joint of left middle finger**
- S63.274 **Dislocation of unspecified interphalangeal joint of right ring finger**
- S63.275 **Dislocation of unspecified interphalangeal joint of left ring finger**
- S63.276 **Dislocation of unspecified interphalangeal joint of right little finger**
- S63.277 **Dislocation of unspecified interphalangeal joint of left little finger**
- S63.278 **Dislocation of unspecified interphalangeal joint of other finger**
  Dislocation of unspecified interphalangeal joint of specified finger with unspecified laterality
- S63.279 **Dislocation of unspecified interphalangeal joint of unspecified finger**
  Dislocation of unspecified interphalangeal joint of unspecified finger without specified laterality

S63.28 Dislocation of proximal interphalangeal joint of finger
- S63.280 **Dislocation of proximal interphalangeal joint of right index finger**
- S63.281 **Dislocation of proximal interphalangeal joint of left index finger**
- S63.282 **Dislocation of proximal interphalangeal joint of right middle finger**
- S63.283 **Dislocation of proximal interphalangeal joint of left middle finger**
- S63.284 **Dislocation of proximal interphalangeal joint of right ring finger**
- S63.285 **Dislocation of proximal interphalangeal joint of left ring finger**
- S63.286 **Dislocation of proximal interphalangeal joint of right little finger**
- S63.287 **Dislocation of proximal interphalangeal joint of left little finger**
- S63.288 **Dislocation of proximal interphalangeal joint of other finger**
  Dislocation of proximal interphalangeal joint of specified finger with unspecified laterality
- S63.289 **Dislocation of proximal interphalangeal joint of unspecified finger**

S63.29 Dislocation of distal interphalangeal joint of finger
- S63.290 **Dislocation of distal interphalangeal joint of right index finger**
- S63.291 **Dislocation of distal interphalangeal joint of left index finger**
- S63.292 **Dislocation of distal interphalangeal joint of right middle finger**
- S63.293 **Dislocation of distal interphalangeal joint of left middle finger**
- S63.294 **Dislocation of distal interphalangeal joint of right ring finger**
- S63.295 **Dislocation of distal interphalangeal joint of left ring finger**
- S63.296 **Dislocation of distal interphalangeal joint of right little finger**
- S63.297 **Dislocation of distal interphalangeal joint of left little finger**
- S63.298 **Dislocation of distal interphalangeal joint of other finger**
  Dislocation of distal interphalangeal joint of specified finger with unspecified laterality
- S63.299 **Dislocation of distal interphalangeal joint of unspecified finger**

S63.3 Traumatic rupture of ligament of wrist

S63.30 Traumatic rupture of unspecified ligament of wrist
- S63.301 **Traumatic rupture of unspecified ligament of right wrist**
- S63.302 **Traumatic rupture of unspecified ligament of left wrist**
- S63.309 **Traumatic rupture of unspecified ligament of unspecified wrist**

S63.31 Traumatic rupture of collateral ligament of wrist
- S63.311 **Traumatic rupture of collateral ligament of right wrist**

- **S63.312** Traumatic rupture of collateral ligament of left wrist [7th]
- **S63.319** Traumatic rupture of collateral ligament of unspecified wrist [7th]
- **S63.32** Traumatic rupture of radiocarpal ligament [6th]
  - **S63.321** Traumatic rupture of right radiocarpal ligament [7th]
  - **S63.322** Traumatic rupture of left radiocarpal ligament [7th]
  - **S63.329** Traumatic rupture of unspecified radiocarpal ligament [7th]
- **S63.33** Traumatic rupture of ulnocarpal (palmar) ligament [6th]
  - **S63.331** Traumatic rupture of right ulnocarpal (palmar) ligament [7th]
  - **S63.332** Traumatic rupture of left ulnocarpal (palmar) ligament [7th]
  - **S63.339** Traumatic rupture of unspecified ulnocarpal (palmar) ligament [7th]
- **S63.39** Traumatic rupture of other ligament of wrist [6th]
  - **S63.391** Traumatic rupture of other ligament of right wrist [7th]
  - **S63.392** Traumatic rupture of other ligament of left wrist [7th]
  - **S63.399** Traumatic rupture of other ligament of unspecified wrist [7th]
- **S63.4** Traumatic rupture of ligament of finger at metacarpophalangeal and interphalangeal joint(s) [5th]
  - **S63.40** Traumatic rupture of unspecified ligament of finger at metacarpophalangeal and interphalangeal joint [6th]
    - **S63.400** Traumatic rupture of unspecified ligament of right index finger at metacarpophalangeal and interphalangeal joint [7th]
    - **S63.401** Traumatic rupture of unspecified ligament of left index finger at metacarpophalangeal and interphalangeal joint [7th]
    - **S63.402** Traumatic rupture of unspecified ligament of right middle finger at metacarpophalangeal and interphalangeal joint [7th]
    - **S63.403** Traumatic rupture of unspecified ligament of left middle finger at metacarpophalangeal and interphalangeal joint [7th]
    - **S63.404** Traumatic rupture of unspecified ligament of right ring finger at metacarpophalangeal and interphalangeal joint [7th]
    - **S63.405** Traumatic rupture of unspecified ligament of left ring finger at metacarpophalangeal and interphalangeal joint [7th]
    - **S63.406** Traumatic rupture of unspecified ligament of right little finger at metacarpophalangeal and interphalangeal joint [7th]
    - **S63.407** Traumatic rupture of unspecified ligament of left little finger at metacarpophalangeal and interphalangeal joint [7th]
    - **S63.408** Traumatic rupture of unspecified ligament of other finger at metacarpophalangeal and interphalangeal joint [7th]
      Traumatic rupture of unspecified ligament of specified finger with unspecified laterality at metacarpophalangeal and interphalangeal joint
    - **S63.409** Traumatic rupture of unspecified ligament of unspecified finger at metacarpophalangeal and interphalangeal joint [7th]
  - **S63.41** Traumatic rupture of collateral ligament of finger at metacarpophalangeal and interphalangeal joint [6th]
    - **S63.410** Traumatic rupture of collateral ligament of right index finger at metacarpophalangeal and interphalangeal joint [7th]
    - **S63.411** Traumatic rupture of collateral ligament of left index finger at metacarpophalangeal and interphalangeal joint [7th]
    - **S63.412** Traumatic rupture of collateral ligament of right middle finger at metacarpophalangeal and interphalangeal joint [7th]
    - **S63.413** Traumatic rupture of collateral ligament of left middle finger at metacarpophalangeal and interphalangeal joint [7th]
    - **S63.414** Traumatic rupture of collateral ligament of right ring finger at metacarpophalangeal and interphalangeal joint [7th]
    - **S63.415** Traumatic rupture of collateral ligament of left ring finger at metacarpophalangeal and interphalangeal joint [7th]
    - **S63.416** Traumatic rupture of collateral ligament of right little finger at metacarpophalangeal and interphalangeal joint [7th]
    - **S63.417** Traumatic rupture of collateral ligament of left little finger at metacarpophalangeal and interphalangeal joint [7th]
    - **S63.418** Traumatic rupture of collateral ligament of other finger at metacarpophalangeal and interphalangeal joint [7th]
      Traumatic rupture of collateral ligament of specified finger with unspecified laterality at metacarpophalangeal and interphalangeal joint
    - **S63.419** Traumatic rupture of collateral ligament of unspecified finger at metacarpophalangeal and interphalangeal joint [7th]
  - **S63.42** Traumatic rupture of palmar ligament of finger at metacarpophalangeal and interphalangeal joint [6th]
    - **S63.420** Traumatic rupture of palmar ligament of right index finger at metacarpophalangeal and interphalangeal joint [7th]
    - **S63.421** Traumatic rupture of palmar ligament of left index finger at metacarpophalangeal and interphalangeal joint [7th]
    - **S63.422** Traumatic rupture of palmar ligament of right middle finger at metacarpophalangeal and interphalangeal joint [7th]
    - **S63.423** Traumatic rupture of palmar ligament of left middle finger at metacarpophalangeal and interphalangeal joint [7th]
    - **S63.424** Traumatic rupture of palmar ligament of right ring finger at metacarpophalangeal and interphalangeal joint [7th]
    - **S63.425** Traumatic rupture of palmar ligament of left ring finger at metacarpophalangeal and interphalangeal joint [7th]
    - **S63.426** Traumatic rupture of palmar ligament of right little finger at metacarpophalangeal and interphalangeal joint [7th]
    - **S63.427** Traumatic rupture of palmar ligament of left little finger at metacarpophalangeal and interphalangeal joint [7th]
    - **S63.428** Traumatic rupture of palmar ligament of other finger at metacarpophalangeal and interphalangeal joint [7th]
      Traumatic rupture of palmar ligament of specified finger with unspecified laterality at metacarpophalangeal and interphalangeal joint
    - **S63.429** Traumatic rupture of palmar ligament of unspecified finger at metacarpophalangeal and interphalangeal joint [7th]
  - **S63.43** Traumatic rupture of volar plate of finger at metacarpophalangeal and interphalangeal joint [6th]
    - **S63.430** Traumatic rupture of volar plate of right index finger at metacarpophalangeal and interphalangeal joint [7th]
    - **S63.431** Traumatic rupture of volar plate of left index finger at metacarpophalangeal and interphalangeal joint [7th]
    - **S63.432** Traumatic rupture of volar plate of right middle finger at metacarpophalangeal and interphalangeal joint [7th]
    - **S63.433** Traumatic rupture of volar plate of left middle finger at metacarpophalangeal and interphalangeal joint [7th]
    - **S63.434** Traumatic rupture of volar plate of right ring finger at metacarpophalangeal and interphalangeal joint [7th]

- S63.435 [7th] Traumatic rupture of volar plate of left ring finger at metacarpophalangeal and interphalangeal joint
- S63.436 [7th] Traumatic rupture of volar plate of right little finger at metacarpophalangeal and interphalangeal joint
- S63.437 [7th] Traumatic rupture of volar plate of left little finger at metacarpophalangeal and interphalangeal joint
- S63.438 [7th] Traumatic rupture of volar plate of other finger at metacarpophalangeal and interphalangeal joint
  - Traumatic rupture of volar plate of specified finger with unspecified laterality at metacarpophalangeal and interphalangeal joint
- S63.439 [7th] Traumatic rupture of volar plate of unspecified finger at metacarpophalangeal and interphalangeal joint

S63.49 [6th] Traumatic rupture of other ligament of finger at metacarpophalangeal and interphalangeal joint
- S63.490 [7th] Traumatic rupture of other ligament of right index finger at metacarpophalangeal and interphalangeal joint
- S63.491 [7th] Traumatic rupture of other ligament of left index finger at metacarpophalangeal and interphalangeal joint
- S63.492 [7th] Traumatic rupture of other ligament of right middle finger at metacarpophalangeal and interphalangeal joint
- S63.493 [7th] Traumatic rupture of other ligament of left middle finger at metacarpophalangeal and interphalangeal joint
- S63.494 [7th] Traumatic rupture of other ligament of right ring finger at metacarpophalangeal and interphalangeal joint
- S63.495 [7th] Traumatic rupture of other ligament of left ring finger at metacarpophalangeal and interphalangeal joint
- S63.496 [7th] Traumatic rupture of other ligament of right little finger at metacarpophalangeal and interphalangeal joint
- S63.497 [7th] Traumatic rupture of other ligament of left little finger at metacarpophalangeal and interphalangeal joint
- S63.498 [7th] Traumatic rupture of other ligament of other finger at metacarpophalangeal and interphalangeal joint
  - Traumatic rupture of ligament of specified finger with unspecified laterality at metacarpophalangeal and interphalangeal joint
- S63.499 [7th] Traumatic rupture of other ligament of unspecified finger at metacarpophalangeal and interphalangeal joint

S63.5 [5th] Other and unspecified sprain of wrist

S63.50 [6th] Unspecified sprain of wrist
- S63.501 [7th] Unspecified sprain of right wrist
- S63.502 [7th] Unspecified sprain of left wrist
- S63.509 [7th] Unspecified sprain of unspecified wrist

S63.51 [6th] Sprain of carpal (joint)
- S63.511 [7th] Sprain of carpal joint of right wrist
- S63.512 [7th] Sprain of carpal joint of left wrist
- S63.519 [7th] Sprain of carpal joint of unspecified wrist

S63.52 [6th] Sprain of radiocarpal joint
  - EXCLUDES 1: traumatic rupture of radiocarpal ligament (S63.32-)
- S63.521 [7th] Sprain of radiocarpal joint of right wrist
- S63.522 [7th] Sprain of radiocarpal joint of left wrist
- S63.529 [7th] Sprain of radiocarpal joint of unspecified wrist

S63.59 [6th] Other specified sprain of wrist
- S63.591 [7th] Other specified sprain of right wrist
- S63.592 [7th] Other specified sprain of left wrist
- S63.599 [7th] Other specified sprain of unspecified wrist

S63.6 [5th] Other and unspecified sprain of finger(s)

EXCLUDES 1: traumatic rupture of ligament of finger at metacarpophalangeal and interphalangeal joint(s) (S63.4-)

S63.60 [6th] Unspecified sprain of thumb
- S63.601 [7th] Unspecified sprain of right thumb
- S63.602 [7th] Unspecified sprain of left thumb
- S63.609 [7th] Unspecified sprain of unspecified thumb

S63.61 [6th] Unspecified sprain of other and unspecified finger(s)
- S63.610 [7th] Unspecified sprain of right index finger
- S63.611 [7th] Unspecified sprain of left index finger
- S63.612 [7th] Unspecified sprain of right middle finger
- S63.613 [7th] Unspecified sprain of left middle finger
- S63.614 [7th] Unspecified sprain of right ring finger
- S63.615 [7th] Unspecified sprain of left ring finger
- S63.616 [7th] Unspecified sprain of right little finger
- S63.617 [7th] Unspecified sprain of left little finger
- S63.618 [7th] Unspecified sprain of other finger
  - Unspecified sprain of specified finger with unspecified laterality
- S63.619 [7th] Unspecified sprain of unspecified finger

S63.62 [6th] Sprain of interphalangeal joint of thumb
- S63.621 [7th] Sprain of interphalangeal joint of right thumb
- S63.622 [7th] Sprain of interphalangeal joint of left thumb
- S63.629 [7th] Sprain of interphalangeal joint of unspecified thumb

S63.63 [6th] Sprain of interphalangeal joint of other and unspecified finger(s)
- S63.630 [7th] Sprain of interphalangeal joint of right index finger
- S63.631 [7th] Sprain of interphalangeal joint of left index finger
- S63.632 [7th] Sprain of interphalangeal joint of right middle finger
- S63.633 [7th] Sprain of interphalangeal joint of left middle finger
- S63.634 [7th] Sprain of interphalangeal joint of right ring finger
- S63.635 [7th] Sprain of interphalangeal joint of left ring finger
- S63.636 [7th] Sprain of interphalangeal joint of right little finger
- S63.637 [7th] Sprain of interphalangeal joint of left little finger
- S63.638 [7th] Sprain of interphalangeal joint of other finger
- S63.639 [7th] Sprain of interphalangeal joint of unspecified finger

S63.64 [6th] Sprain of metacarpophalangeal joint of thumb
- S63.641 [7th] Sprain of metacarpophalangeal joint of right thumb
- S63.642 [7th] Sprain of metacarpophalangeal joint of left thumb
- S63.649 [7th] Sprain of metacarpophalangeal joint of unspecified thumb

S63.65 [6th] Sprain of metacarpophalangeal joint of other and unspecified finger(s)
- S63.650 [7th] Sprain of metacarpophalangeal joint of right index finger
- S63.651 [7th] Sprain of metacarpophalangeal joint of left index finger
- S63.652 [7th] Sprain of metacarpophalangeal joint of right middle finger
- S63.653 [7th] Sprain of metacarpophalangeal joint of left middle finger
- S63.654 [7th] Sprain of metacarpophalangeal joint of right ring finger
- S63.655 [7th] Sprain of metacarpophalangeal joint of left ring finger
- S63.656 [7th] Sprain of metacarpophalangeal joint of right little finger
- S63.657 [7th] Sprain of metacarpophalangeal joint of left little finger

Chapter 19. Injury, Poisoning and Certain Other Consequences of External Causes

- **S63.658** Sprain of metacarpophalangeal joint of other finger
  - Sprain of metacarpophalangeal joint of specified finger with unspecified laterality
- **S63.659** Sprain of metacarpophalangeal joint of unspecified finger
- **S63.68** Other sprain of thumb
  - **S63.681** Other sprain of right thumb
  - **S63.682** Other sprain of left thumb
  - **S63.689** Other sprain of unspecified thumb
- **S63.69** Other sprain of other and unspecified finger(s)
  - **S63.690** Other sprain of right index finger
  - **S63.691** Other sprain of left index finger
  - **S63.692** Other sprain of right middle finger
  - **S63.693** Other sprain of left middle finger
  - **S63.694** Other sprain of right ring finger
  - **S63.695** Other sprain of left ring finger
  - **S63.696** Other sprain of right little finger
  - **S63.697** Other sprain of left little finger
  - **S63.698** Other sprain of other finger
    - Other sprain of specified finger with unspecified laterality
  - **S63.699** Other sprain of unspecified finger
- **S63.8** Sprain of other part of wrist and hand
  - **S63.8X** Sprain of other part of wrist and hand
    - **S63.8X1** Sprain of other part of right wrist and hand
    - **S63.8X2** Sprain of other part of left wrist and hand
    - **S63.8X9** Sprain of other part of unspecified wrist and hand
- **S63.9** Sprain of unspecified part of wrist and hand
  - **S63.90** Sprain of unspecified part of unspecified wrist and hand
  - **S63.91** Sprain of unspecified part of right wrist and hand
  - **S63.92** Sprain of unspecified part of left wrist and hand

S64 Injury of nerves at wrist and hand level

Code also any associated open wound (S61.-)

The appropriate 7th character is to be added to each code from category S64.
- A initial encounter
- D subsequent encounter
- S sequela

- **S64.0** Injury of ulnar nerve at wrist and hand level
  - **S64.00** Injury of ulnar nerve at wrist and hand level of unspecified arm
  - **S64.01** Injury of ulnar nerve at wrist and hand level of right arm
  - **S64.02** Injury of ulnar nerve at wrist and hand level of left arm
- **S64.1** Injury of median nerve at wrist and hand level
  - **S64.10** Injury of median nerve at wrist and hand level of unspecified arm
  - **S64.11** Injury of median nerve at wrist and hand level of right arm
  - **S64.12** Injury of median nerve at wrist and hand level of left arm
- **S64.2** Injury of radial nerve at wrist and hand level
  - **S64.20** Injury of radial nerve at wrist and hand level of unspecified arm
  - **S64.21** Injury of radial nerve at wrist and hand level of right arm
  - **S64.22** Injury of radial nerve at wrist and hand level of left arm
- **S64.3** Injury of digital nerve of thumb
  - **S64.30** Injury of digital nerve of unspecified thumb
  - **S64.31** Injury of digital nerve of right thumb
  - **S64.32** Injury of digital nerve of left thumb
- **S64.4** Injury of digital nerve of other and unspecified finger
  - **S64.40** Injury of digital nerve of unspecified finger
  - **S64.49** Injury of digital nerve of other finger
    - **S64.490** Injury of digital nerve of right index finger
    - **S64.491** Injury of digital nerve of left index finger
    - **S64.492** Injury of digital nerve of right middle finger
    - **S64.493** Injury of digital nerve of left middle finger
    - **S64.494** Injury of digital nerve of right ring finger
    - **S64.495** Injury of digital nerve of left ring finger
    - **S64.496** Injury of digital nerve of right little finger
    - **S64.497** Injury of digital nerve of left little finger
    - **S64.498** Injury of digital nerve of other finger
      - Injury of digital nerve of specified finger with unspecified laterality
- **S64.8** Injury of other nerves at wrist and hand level
  - **S64.8X** Injury of other nerves at wrist and hand level
    - **S64.8X1** Injury of other nerves at wrist and hand level of right arm
    - **S64.8X2** Injury of other nerves at wrist and hand level of left arm
    - **S64.8X9** Injury of other nerves at wrist and hand level of unspecified arm
- **S64.9** Injury of unspecified nerve at wrist and hand level
  - **S64.90** Injury of unspecified nerve at wrist and hand level of unspecified arm
  - **S64.91** Injury of unspecified nerve at wrist and hand level of right arm
  - **S64.92** Injury of unspecified nerve at wrist and hand level of left arm

S65 Injury of blood vessels at wrist and hand level

Code also any associated open wound (S61.-)

The appropriate 7th character is to be added to each code from category S65.
- A initial encounter
- D subsequent encounter
- S sequela

- **S65.0** Injury of ulnar artery at wrist and hand level
  - **S65.00** Unspecified injury of ulnar artery at wrist and hand level
    - **S65.001** Unspecified injury of ulnar artery at wrist and hand level of right arm
    - **S65.002** Unspecified injury of ulnar artery at wrist and hand level of left arm
    - **S65.009** Unspecified injury of ulnar artery at wrist and hand level of unspecified arm
  - **S65.01** Laceration of ulnar artery at wrist and hand level
    - **S65.011** Laceration of ulnar artery at wrist and hand level of right arm
    - **S65.012** Laceration of ulnar artery at wrist and hand level of left arm
    - **S65.019** Laceration of ulnar artery at wrist and hand level of unspecified arm
  - **S65.09** Other specified injury of ulnar artery at wrist and hand level
    - **S65.091** Other specified injury of ulnar artery at wrist and hand level of right arm
    - **S65.092** Other specified injury of ulnar artery at wrist and hand level of left arm
    - **S65.099** Other specified injury of ulnar artery at wrist and hand level of unspecified arm
- **S65.1** Injury of radial artery at wrist and hand level
  - **S65.10** Unspecified injury of radial artery at wrist and hand level
    - **S65.101** Unspecified injury of radial artery at wrist and hand level of right arm
    - **S65.102** Unspecified injury of radial artery at wrist and hand level of left arm
    - **S65.109** Unspecified injury of radial artery at wrist and hand level of unspecified arm
  - **S65.11** Laceration of radial artery at wrist and hand level
    - **S65.111** Laceration of radial artery at wrist and hand level of right arm
    - **S65.112** Laceration of radial artery at wrist and hand level of left arm
    - **S65.119** Laceration of radial artery at wrist and hand level of unspecified arm
  - **S65.19** Other specified injury of radial artery at wrist and hand level
    - **S65.191** Other specified injury of radial artery at wrist and hand level of right arm
    - **S65.192** Other specified injury of radial artery at wrist and hand level of left arm

- **S65.199** Other specified injury of radial artery at wrist and hand level of unspecified arm

S65.2 Injury of superficial palmar arch

- **S65.20** Unspecified injury of superficial palmar arch
  - **S65.201** Unspecified injury of superficial palmar arch of right hand
  - **S65.202** Unspecified injury of superficial palmar arch of left hand
  - **S65.209** Unspecified injury of superficial palmar arch of unspecified hand
- **S65.21** Laceration of superficial palmar arch
  - **S65.211** Laceration of superficial palmar arch of right hand
  - **S65.212** Laceration of superficial palmar arch of left hand
  - **S65.219** Laceration of superficial palmar arch of unspecified hand
- **S65.29** Other specified injury of superficial palmar arch
  - **S65.291** Other specified injury of superficial palmar arch of right hand
  - **S65.292** Other specified injury of superficial palmar arch of left hand
  - **S65.299** Other specified injury of superficial palmar arch of unspecified hand

S65.3 Injury of deep palmar arch

- **S65.30** Unspecified injury of deep palmar arch
  - **S65.301** Unspecified injury of deep palmar arch of right hand
  - **S65.302** Unspecified injury of deep palmar arch of left hand
  - **S65.309** Unspecified injury of deep palmar arch of unspecified hand
- **S65.31** Laceration of deep palmar arch
  - **S65.311** Laceration of deep palmar arch of right hand
  - **S65.312** Laceration of deep palmar arch of left hand
  - **S65.319** Laceration of deep palmar arch of unspecified hand
- **S65.39** Other specified injury of deep palmar arch
  - **S65.391** Other specified injury of deep palmar arch of right hand
  - **S65.392** Other specified injury of deep palmar arch of left hand
  - **S65.399** Other specified injury of deep palmar arch of unspecified hand

S65.4 Injury of blood vessel of thumb

- **S65.40** Unspecified injury of blood vessel of thumb
  - **S65.401** Unspecified injury of blood vessel of right thumb
  - **S65.402** Unspecified injury of blood vessel of left thumb
  - **S65.409** Unspecified injury of blood vessel of unspecified thumb
- **S65.41** Laceration of blood vessel of thumb
  - **S65.411** Laceration of blood vessel of right thumb
  - **S65.412** Laceration of blood vessel of left thumb
  - **S65.419** Laceration of blood vessel of unspecified thumb
- **S65.49** Other specified injury of blood vessel of thumb
  - **S65.491** Other specified injury of blood vessel of right thumb
  - **S65.492** Other specified injury of blood vessel of left thumb
  - **S65.499** Other specified injury of blood vessel of unspecified thumb

S65.5 Injury of blood vessel of other and unspecified finger

- **S65.50** Unspecified injury of blood vessel of other and unspecified finger
  - **S65.500** Unspecified injury of blood vessel of right index finger
  - **S65.501** Unspecified injury of blood vessel of left index finger
  - **S65.502** Unspecified injury of blood vessel of right middle finger
  - **S65.503** Unspecified injury of blood vessel of left middle finger
  - **S65.504** Unspecified injury of blood vessel of right ring finger
  - **S65.505** Unspecified injury of blood vessel of left ring finger
  - **S65.506** Unspecified injury of blood vessel of right little finger
  - **S65.507** Unspecified injury of blood vessel of left little finger
  - **S65.508** Unspecified injury of blood vessel of other finger
    Unspecified injury of blood vessel of specified finger with unspecified laterality
  - **S65.509** Unspecified injury of blood vessel of unspecified finger
- **S65.51** Laceration of blood vessel of other and unspecified finger
  - **S65.510** Laceration of blood vessel of right index finger
  - **S65.511** Laceration of blood vessel of left index finger
  - **S65.512** Laceration of blood vessel of right middle finger
  - **S65.513** Laceration of blood vessel of left middle finger
  - **S65.514** Laceration of blood vessel of right ring finger
  - **S65.515** Laceration of blood vessel of left ring finger
  - **S65.516** Laceration of blood vessel of right little finger
  - **S65.517** Laceration of blood vessel of left little finger
  - **S65.518** Laceration of blood vessel of other finger
    Laceration of blood vessel of specified finger with unspecified laterality
  - **S65.519** Laceration of blood vessel of unspecified finger
- **S65.59** Other specified injury of blood vessel of other and unspecified finger
  - **S65.590** Other specified injury of blood vessel of right index finger
  - **S65.591** Other specified injury of blood vessel of left index finger
  - **S65.592** Other specified injury of blood vessel of right middle finger
  - **S65.593** Other specified injury of blood vessel of left middle finger
  - **S65.594** Other specified injury of blood vessel of right ring finger
  - **S65.595** Other specified injury of blood vessel of left ring finger
  - **S65.596** Other specified injury of blood vessel of right little finger
  - **S65.597** Other specified injury of blood vessel of left little finger
  - **S65.598** Other specified injury of blood vessel of other finger
    Other specified injury of blood vessel of specified finger with unspecified laterality
  - **S65.599** Other specified injury of blood vessel of unspecified finger

S65.8 Injury of other blood vessels at wrist and hand level

- **S65.80** Unspecified injury of other blood vessels at wrist and hand level
  - **S65.801** Unspecified injury of other blood vessels at wrist and hand level of right arm
  - **S65.802** Unspecified injury of other blood vessels at wrist and hand level of left arm
  - **S65.809** Unspecified injury of other blood vessels at wrist and hand level of unspecified arm
- **S65.81** Laceration of other blood vessels at wrist and hand level
  - **S65.811** Laceration of other blood vessels at wrist and hand level of right arm
  - **S65.812** Laceration of other blood vessels at wrist and hand level of left arm
  - **S65.819** Laceration of other blood vessels at wrist and hand level of unspecified arm
- **S65.89** Other specified injury of other blood vessels at wrist and hand level
  - **S65.891** Other specified injury of other blood vessels at wrist and hand level of right arm

- **S65.892** Other specified injury of other blood vessels at wrist and hand level of *left* arm
- **S65.899** Other specified injury of other blood vessels at wrist and hand level of unspecified arm

- **S65.9** Injury of unspecified blood vessel at *wrist and hand level*
  - **S65.90** Unspecified injury of unspecified blood vessel at wrist and hand level
    - **S65.901** Unspecified injury of unspecified blood vessel at wrist and hand level of *right* arm
    - **S65.902** Unspecified injury of unspecified blood vessel at wrist and hand level of *left* arm
    - **S65.909** Unspecified injury of unspecified blood vessel at wrist and hand level of unspecified arm
  - **S65.91** *Laceration* of unspecified blood vessel at wrist and hand level
    - **S65.911** Laceration of unspecified blood vessel at wrist and hand level of *right* arm
    - **S65.912** Laceration of unspecified blood vessel at wrist and hand level of *left* arm
    - **S65.919** Laceration of unspecified blood vessel at wrist and hand level of unspecified arm
  - **S65.99** Other specified injury of unspecified blood vessel at wrist and hand level
    - **S65.991** Other specified injury of unspecified blood vessel at wrist and hand of *right* arm
    - **S65.992** Other specified injury of unspecified blood vessel at wrist and hand of *left* arm
    - **S65.999** Other specified injury of unspecified blood vessel at wrist and hand of unspecified arm

- **S66 Injury of muscle, fascia and tendon at wrist and hand level**

  Code also any associated open wound (S61.-)

  EXCLUDES 2 *sprain of joints and ligaments of wrist and hand (S63.-)*

  TIP: Refer to the Muscle/Tendon table at the beginning of this chapter.

  The appropriate 7th character is to be added to each code from category S66.
  - A initial encounter
  - D subsequent encounter
  - S sequela

  - **S66.0** Injury of *long flexor* muscle, fascia and tendon of *thumb* at wrist and hand level
    - **S66.00** Unspecified injury of long flexor muscle, fascia and tendon of thumb at wrist and hand level
      - **S66.001** Unspecified injury of long flexor muscle, fascia and tendon of *right* thumb at wrist and hand level
      - **S66.002** Unspecified injury of long flexor muscle, fascia and tendon of *left* thumb at wrist and hand level
      - **S66.009** Unspecified injury of long flexor muscle, fascia and tendon of unspecified thumb at wrist and hand level
    - **S66.01** *Strain* of long flexor muscle, fascia and tendon of thumb at wrist and hand level
      - **S66.011** Strain of long flexor muscle, fascia and tendon of *right* thumb at wrist and hand level
      - **S66.012** Strain of long flexor muscle, fascia and tendon of *left* thumb at wrist and hand level
      - **S66.019** Strain of long flexor muscle, fascia and tendon of unspecified thumb at wrist and hand level
    - **S66.02** *Laceration* of long flexor muscle, fascia and tendon of thumb at wrist and hand level
      - **S66.021** Laceration of long flexor muscle, fascia and tendon of *right* thumb at wrist and hand level
      - **S66.022** Laceration of long flexor muscle, fascia and tendon of *left* thumb at wrist and hand level
      - **S66.029** Laceration of long flexor muscle, fascia and tendon of unspecified thumb at wrist and hand level
    - **S66.09** Other specified injury of long flexor muscle, fascia and tendon of thumb at wrist and hand level
      - **S66.091** Other specified injury of long flexor muscle, fascia and tendon of *right* thumb at wrist and hand level
      - **S66.092** Other specified injury of long flexor muscle, fascia and tendon of *left* thumb at wrist and hand level
      - **S66.099** Other specified injury of long flexor muscle, fascia and tendon of unspecified thumb at wrist and hand level

  - **S66.1** Injury of *flexor* muscle, fascia and tendon of other and unspecified *finger* at wrist and hand level

    EXCLUDES 2 *injury of long flexor muscle, fascia and tendon of thumb at wrist and hand level (S66.0-)*

    - **S66.10** Unspecified injury of flexor muscle, fascia and tendon of other and unspecified finger at wrist and hand level
      - **S66.100** Unspecified injury of flexor muscle, fascia and tendon of *right index* finger at wrist and hand level
      - **S66.101** Unspecified injury of flexor muscle, fascia and tendon of *left index* finger at wrist and hand level
      - **S66.102** Unspecified injury of flexor muscle, fascia and tendon of *right middle* finger at wrist and hand level
      - **S66.103** Unspecified injury of flexor muscle, fascia and tendon of *left middle* finger at wrist and hand level
      - **S66.104** Unspecified injury of flexor muscle, fascia and tendon of *right ring* finger at wrist and hand level
      - **S66.105** Unspecified injury of flexor muscle, fascia and tendon of *left ring* finger at wrist and hand level
      - **S66.106** Unspecified injury of flexor muscle, fascia and tendon of *right little* finger at wrist and hand level
      - **S66.107** Unspecified injury of flexor muscle, fascia and tendon of *left little* finger at wrist and hand level
      - **S66.108** Unspecified injury of flexor muscle, fascia and tendon of other finger at wrist and hand level

        Unspecified injury of flexor muscle, fascia and tendon of specified finger with unspecified laterality at wrist and hand level
      - **S66.109** Unspecified injury of flexor muscle, fascia and tendon of unspecified finger at wrist and hand level
    - **S66.11** *Strain* of flexor muscle, fascia and tendon of other and unspecified finger at wrist and hand level
      - **S66.110** Strain of flexor muscle, fascia and tendon of *right index* finger at wrist and hand level
      - **S66.111** Strain of flexor muscle, fascia and tendon of *left index* finger at wrist and hand level
      - **S66.112** Strain of flexor muscle, fascia and tendon of *right middle* finger at wrist and hand level
      - **S66.113** Strain of flexor muscle, fascia and tendon of *left middle* finger at wrist and hand level
      - **S66.114** Strain of flexor muscle, fascia and tendon of *right ring* finger at wrist and hand level
      - **S66.115** Strain of flexor muscle, fascia and tendon of *left ring* finger at wrist and hand level
      - **S66.116** Strain of flexor muscle, fascia and tendon of *right little* finger at wrist and hand level
      - **S66.117** Strain of flexor muscle, fascia and tendon of *left little* finger at wrist and hand level
      - **S66.118** Strain of flexor muscle, fascia and tendon of other finger at wrist and hand level

        Strain of flexor muscle, fascia and tendon of specified finger with unspecified laterality at wrist and hand level
      - **S66.119** Strain of flexor muscle, fascia and tendon of unspecified finger at wrist and hand level
    - **S66.12** *Laceration* of flexor muscle, fascia and tendon of other and unspecified finger at wrist and hand level
      - **S66.120** Laceration of flexor muscle, fascia and tendon of *right index* finger at wrist and hand level
      - **S66.121** Laceration of flexor muscle, fascia and tendon of *left index* finger at wrist and hand level
      - **S66.122** Laceration of flexor muscle, fascia and tendon of *right middle* finger at wrist and hand level

- S66.123 Laceration of flexor muscle, fascia and tendon of left middle finger at wrist and hand level
- S66.124 Laceration of flexor muscle, fascia and tendon of right ring finger at wrist and hand level
- S66.125 Laceration of flexor muscle, fascia and tendon of left ring finger at wrist and hand level
- S66.126 Laceration of flexor muscle, fascia and tendon of right little finger at wrist and hand level
- S66.127 Laceration of flexor muscle, fascia and tendon of left little finger at wrist and hand level
- S66.128 Laceration of flexor muscle, fascia and tendon of other finger at wrist and hand level

  Laceration of flexor muscle, fascia and tendon of specified finger with unspecified laterality at wrist and hand level

- S66.129 Laceration of flexor muscle, fascia and tendon of unspecified finger at wrist and hand level

- S66.19 Other injury of flexor muscle, fascia and tendon of other and unspecified finger at wrist and hand level
  - S66.190 Other injury of flexor muscle, fascia and tendon of right index finger at wrist and hand level
  - S66.191 Other injury of flexor muscle, fascia and tendon of left index finger at wrist and hand level
  - S66.192 Other injury of flexor muscle, fascia and tendon of right middle finger at wrist and hand level
  - S66.193 Other injury of flexor muscle, fascia and tendon of left middle finger at wrist and hand level
  - S66.194 Other injury of flexor muscle, fascia and tendon of right ring finger at wrist and hand level
  - S66.195 Other injury of flexor muscle, fascia and tendon of left ring finger at wrist and hand level
  - S66.196 Other injury of flexor muscle, fascia and tendon of right little finger at wrist and hand level
  - S66.197 Other injury of flexor muscle, fascia and tendon of left little finger at wrist and hand level
  - S66.198 Other injury of flexor muscle, fascia and tendon of other finger at wrist and hand level

    Other injury of flexor muscle, fascia and tendon of specified finger with unspecified laterality at wrist and hand level

  - S66.199 Other injury of flexor muscle, fascia and tendon of unspecified finger at wrist and hand level

- S66.2 Injury of extensor muscle, fascia and tendon of thumb at wrist and hand level
  - S66.20 Unspecified injury of extensor muscle, fascia and tendon of thumb at wrist and hand level
    - S66.201 Unspecified injury of extensor muscle, fascia and tendon of right thumb at wrist and hand level
    - S66.202 Unspecified injury of extensor muscle, fascia and tendon of left thumb at wrist and hand level
    - S66.209 Unspecified injury of extensor muscle, fascia and tendon of unspecified thumb at wrist and hand level
  - S66.21 Strain of extensor muscle, fascia and tendon of thumb at wrist and hand level
    - S66.211 Strain of extensor muscle, fascia and tendon of right thumb at wrist and hand level
    - S66.212 Strain of extensor muscle, fascia and tendon of left thumb at wrist and hand level
    - S66.219 Strain of extensor muscle, fascia and tendon of unspecified thumb at wrist and hand level
  - S66.22 Laceration of extensor muscle, fascia and tendon of thumb at wrist and hand level
    - S66.221 Laceration of extensor muscle, fascia and tendon of right thumb at wrist and hand level
    - S66.222 Laceration of extensor muscle, fascia and tendon of left thumb at wrist and hand level
    - S66.229 Laceration of extensor muscle, fascia and tendon of unspecified thumb at wrist and hand level
  - S66.29 Other specified injury of extensor muscle, fascia and tendon of thumb at wrist and hand level
    - S66.291 Other specified injury of extensor muscle, fascia and tendon of right thumb at wrist and hand level
    - S66.292 Other specified injury of extensor muscle, fascia and tendon of left thumb at wrist and hand level
    - S66.299 Other specified injury of extensor muscle, fascia and tendon of unspecified thumb at wrist and hand level

- S66.3 Injury of extensor muscle, fascia and tendon of other and unspecified finger at wrist and hand level

  EXCLUDES 2 injury of extensor muscle, fascia and tendon of thumb at wrist and hand level (S66.2-)

  - S66.30 Unspecified injury of extensor muscle, fascia and tendon of other and unspecified finger at wrist and hand level
    - S66.300 Unspecified injury of extensor muscle, fascia and tendon of right index finger at wrist and hand level
    - S66.301 Unspecified injury of extensor muscle, fascia and tendon of left index finger at wrist and hand level
    - S66.302 Unspecified injury of extensor muscle, fascia and tendon of right middle finger at wrist and hand level
    - S66.303 Unspecified injury of extensor muscle, fascia and tendon of left middle finger at wrist and hand level
    - S66.304 Unspecified injury of extensor muscle, fascia and tendon of right ring finger at wrist and hand level
    - S66.305 Unspecified injury of extensor muscle, fascia and tendon of left ring finger at wrist and hand level
    - S66.306 Unspecified injury of extensor muscle, fascia and tendon of right little finger at wrist and hand level
    - S66.307 Unspecified injury of extensor muscle, fascia and tendon of left little finger at wrist and hand level
    - S66.308 Unspecified injury of extensor muscle, fascia and tendon of other finger at wrist and hand level

      Unspecified injury of extensor muscle, fascia and tendon of specified finger with unspecified laterality at wrist and hand level

    - S66.309 Unspecified injury of extensor muscle, fascia and tendon of unspecified finger at wrist and hand level
  - S66.31 Strain of extensor muscle, fascia and tendon of other and unspecified finger at wrist and hand level
    - S66.310 Strain of extensor muscle, fascia and tendon of right index finger at wrist and hand level
    - S66.311 Strain of extensor muscle, fascia and tendon of left index finger at wrist and hand level
    - S66.312 Strain of extensor muscle, fascia and tendon of right middle finger at wrist and hand level
    - S66.313 Strain of extensor muscle, fascia and tendon of left middle finger at wrist and hand level
    - S66.314 Strain of extensor muscle, fascia and tendon of right ring finger at wrist and hand level
    - S66.315 Strain of extensor muscle, fascia and tendon of left ring finger at wrist and hand level

- **S66.316** Strain of extensor muscle, fascia and tendon of right little finger at wrist and hand level
- **S66.317** Strain of extensor muscle, fascia and tendon of left little finger at wrist and hand level
- **S66.318** Strain of extensor muscle, fascia and tendon of other finger at wrist and hand level
  - Strain of extensor muscle, fascia and tendon of specified finger with unspecified laterality at wrist and hand level
- **S66.319** Strain of extensor muscle, fascia and tendon of unspecified finger at wrist and hand level
- **S66.32** Laceration of extensor muscle, fascia and tendon of other and unspecified finger at wrist and hand level
  - **S66.320** Laceration of extensor muscle, fascia and tendon of right index finger at wrist and hand level
  - **S66.321** Laceration of extensor muscle, fascia and tendon of left index finger at wrist and hand level
  - **S66.322** Laceration of extensor muscle, fascia and tendon of right middle finger at wrist and hand level
  - **S66.323** Laceration of extensor muscle, fascia and tendon of left middle finger at wrist and hand level
  - **S66.324** Laceration of extensor muscle, fascia and tendon of right ring finger at wrist and hand level
  - **S66.325** Laceration of extensor muscle, fascia and tendon of left ring finger at wrist and hand level
  - **S66.326** Laceration of extensor muscle, fascia and tendon of right little finger at wrist and hand level
  - **S66.327** Laceration of extensor muscle, fascia and tendon of left little finger at wrist and hand level
  - **S66.328** Laceration of extensor muscle, fascia and tendon of other finger at wrist and hand level
    - Laceration of extensor muscle, fascia and tendon of specified finger with unspecified laterality at wrist and hand level
  - **S66.329** Laceration of extensor muscle, fascia and tendon of unspecified finger at wrist and hand level
- **S66.39** Other injury of extensor muscle, fascia and tendon of other and unspecified finger at wrist and hand level
  - **S66.390** Other injury of extensor muscle, fascia and tendon of right index finger at wrist and hand level
  - **S66.391** Other injury of extensor muscle, fascia and tendon of left index finger at wrist and hand level
  - **S66.392** Other injury of extensor muscle, fascia and tendon of right middle finger at wrist and hand level
  - **S66.393** Other injury of extensor muscle, fascia and tendon of left middle finger at wrist and hand level
  - **S66.394** Other injury of extensor muscle, fascia and tendon of right ring finger at wrist and hand level
  - **S66.395** Other injury of extensor muscle, fascia and tendon of left ring finger at wrist and hand level
  - **S66.396** Other injury of extensor muscle, fascia and tendon of right little finger at wrist and hand level
  - **S66.397** Other injury of extensor muscle, fascia and tendon of left little finger at wrist and hand level
  - **S66.398** Other injury of extensor muscle, fascia and tendon of other finger at wrist and hand level
    - Other injury of extensor muscle, fascia and tendon of specified finger with unspecified laterality at wrist and hand level
  - **S66.399** Other injury of extensor muscle, fascia and tendon of unspecified finger at wrist and hand level
- **S66.4** Injury of intrinsic muscle, fascia and tendon of thumb at wrist and hand level
  - **S66.40** Unspecified injury of intrinsic muscle, fascia and tendon of thumb at wrist and hand level
    - **S66.401** Unspecified injury of intrinsic muscle, fascia and tendon of right thumb at wrist and hand level
    - **S66.402** Unspecified injury of intrinsic muscle, fascia and tendon of left thumb at wrist and hand level
    - **S66.409** Unspecified injury of intrinsic muscle, fascia and tendon of unspecified thumb at wrist and hand level
  - **S66.41** Strain of intrinsic muscle, fascia and tendon of thumb at wrist and hand level
    - **S66.411** Strain of intrinsic muscle, fascia and tendon of right thumb at wrist and hand level
    - **S66.412** Strain of intrinsic muscle, fascia and tendon of left thumb at wrist and hand level
    - **S66.419** Strain of intrinsic muscle, fascia and tendon of unspecified thumb at wrist and hand level
  - **S66.42** Laceration of intrinsic muscle, fascia and tendon of thumb at wrist and hand level
    - **S66.421** Laceration of intrinsic muscle, fascia and tendon of right thumb at wrist and hand level
    - **S66.422** Laceration of intrinsic muscle, fascia and tendon of left thumb at wrist and hand level
    - **S66.429** Laceration of intrinsic muscle, fascia and tendon of unspecified thumb at wrist and hand level
  - **S66.49** Other specified injury of intrinsic muscle, fascia and tendon of thumb at wrist and hand level
    - **S66.491** Other specified injury of intrinsic muscle, fascia and tendon of right thumb at wrist and hand level
    - **S66.492** Other specified injury of intrinsic muscle, fascia and tendon of left thumb at wrist and hand level
    - **S66.499** Other specified injury of intrinsic muscle, fascia and tendon of unspecified thumb at wrist and hand level
- **S66.5** Injury of intrinsic muscle, fascia and tendon of other and unspecified finger at wrist and hand level
  - EXCLUDES 2: injury of intrinsic muscle, fascia and tendon of thumb at wrist and hand level (S66.4-)
  - **S66.50** Unspecified injury of intrinsic muscle, fascia and tendon of other and unspecified finger at wrist and hand level
    - **S66.500** Unspecified injury of intrinsic muscle, fascia and tendon of right index finger at wrist and hand level
    - **S66.501** Unspecified injury of intrinsic muscle, fascia and tendon of left index finger at wrist and hand level
    - **S66.502** Unspecified injury of intrinsic muscle, fascia and tendon of right middle finger at wrist and hand level
    - **S66.503** Unspecified injury of intrinsic muscle, fascia and tendon of left middle finger at wrist and hand level
    - **S66.504** Unspecified injury of intrinsic muscle, fascia and tendon of right ring finger at wrist and hand level
    - **S66.505** Unspecified injury of intrinsic muscle, fascia and tendon of left ring finger at wrist and hand level
    - **S66.506** Unspecified injury of intrinsic muscle, fascia and tendon of right little finger at wrist and hand level

- S66.507 Unspecified injury of intrinsic muscle, fascia and tendon of left little finger at wrist and hand level
- S66.508 Unspecified injury of intrinsic muscle, fascia and tendon of other finger at wrist and hand level
  - Unspecified injury of intrinsic muscle, fascia and tendon of specified finger with unspecified laterality at wrist and hand level
- S66.509 Unspecified injury of intrinsic muscle, fascia and tendon of unspecified finger at wrist and hand level

- S66.51 Strain of intrinsic muscle, fascia and tendon of other and unspecified finger at wrist and hand level
  - S66.510 Strain of intrinsic muscle, fascia and tendon of right index finger at wrist and hand level
  - S66.511 Strain of intrinsic muscle, fascia and tendon of left index finger at wrist and hand level
  - S66.512 Strain of intrinsic muscle, fascia and tendon of right middle finger at wrist and hand level
  - S66.513 Strain of intrinsic muscle, fascia and tendon of left middle finger at wrist and hand level
  - S66.514 Strain of intrinsic muscle, fascia and tendon of right ring finger at wrist and hand level
  - S66.515 Strain of intrinsic muscle, fascia and tendon of left ring finger at wrist and hand level
  - S66.516 Strain of intrinsic muscle, fascia and tendon of right little finger at wrist and hand level
  - S66.517 Strain of intrinsic muscle, fascia and tendon of left little finger at wrist and hand level
  - S66.518 Strain of intrinsic muscle, fascia and tendon of other finger at wrist and hand level
    - Strain of intrinsic muscle, fascia and tendon of specified finger with unspecified laterality at wrist and hand level
  - S66.519 Strain of intrinsic muscle, fascia and tendon of unspecified finger at wrist and hand level

- S66.52 Laceration of intrinsic muscle, fascia and tendon of other and unspecified finger at wrist and hand level
  - S66.520 Laceration of intrinsic muscle, fascia and tendon of right index finger at wrist and hand level
  - S66.521 Laceration of intrinsic muscle, fascia and tendon of left index finger at wrist and hand level
  - S66.522 Laceration of intrinsic muscle, fascia and tendon of right middle finger at wrist and hand level
  - S66.523 Laceration of intrinsic muscle, fascia and tendon of left middle finger at wrist and hand level
  - S66.524 Laceration of intrinsic muscle, fascia and tendon of right ring finger at wrist and hand level
  - S66.525 Laceration of intrinsic muscle, fascia and tendon of left ring finger at wrist and hand level
  - S66.526 Laceration of intrinsic muscle, fascia and tendon of right little finger at wrist and hand level
  - S66.527 Laceration of intrinsic muscle, fascia and tendon of left little finger at wrist and hand level
  - S66.528 Laceration of intrinsic muscle, fascia and tendon of other finger at wrist and hand level
    - Laceration of intrinsic muscle, fascia and tendon of specified finger with unspecified laterality at wrist and hand level
  - S66.529 Laceration of intrinsic muscle, fascia and tendon of unspecified finger at wrist and hand level

- S66.59 Other injury of intrinsic muscle, fascia and tendon of other and unspecified finger at wrist and hand level
  - S66.590 Other injury of intrinsic muscle, fascia and tendon of right index finger at wrist and hand level
  - S66.591 Other injury of intrinsic muscle, fascia and tendon of left index finger at wrist and hand level
  - S66.592 Other injury of intrinsic muscle, fascia and tendon of right middle finger at wrist and hand level
  - S66.593 Other injury of intrinsic muscle, fascia and tendon of left middle finger at wrist and hand level
  - S66.594 Other injury of intrinsic muscle, fascia and tendon of right ring finger at wrist and hand level
  - S66.595 Other injury of intrinsic muscle, fascia and tendon of left ring finger at wrist and hand level
  - S66.596 Other injury of intrinsic muscle, fascia and tendon of right little finger at wrist and hand level
  - S66.597 Other injury of intrinsic muscle, fascia and tendon of left little finger at wrist and hand level
  - S66.598 Other injury of intrinsic muscle, fascia and tendon of other finger at wrist and hand level
    - Other injury of intrinsic muscle, fascia and tendon of specified finger with unspecified laterality at wrist and hand level
  - S66.599 Other injury of intrinsic muscle, fascia and tendon of unspecified finger at wrist and hand level

- S66.8 Injury of other specified muscles, fascia and tendons at wrist and hand level
  - S66.80 Unspecified injury of other specified muscles, fascia and tendons at wrist and hand level
    - S66.801 Unspecified injury of other specified muscles, fascia and tendons at wrist and hand level, right hand
    - S66.802 Unspecified injury of other specified muscles, fascia and tendons at wrist and hand level, left hand
    - S66.809 Unspecified injury of other specified muscles, fascia and tendons at wrist and hand level, unspecified hand
  - S66.81 Strain of other specified muscles, fascia and tendons at wrist and hand level
    - S66.811 Strain of other specified muscles, fascia and tendons at wrist and hand level, right hand
    - S66.812 Strain of other specified muscles, fascia and tendons at wrist and hand level, left hand
    - S66.819 Strain of other specified muscles, fascia and tendons at wrist and hand level, unspecified hand
  - S66.82 Laceration of other specified muscles, fascia and tendons at wrist and hand level
    - S66.821 Laceration of other specified muscles, fascia and tendons at wrist and hand level, right hand
    - S66.822 Laceration of other specified muscles, fascia and tendons at wrist and hand level, left hand
    - S66.829 Laceration of other specified muscles, fascia and tendons at wrist and hand level, unspecified hand
  - S66.89 Other injury of other specified muscles, fascia and tendons at wrist and hand level
    - S66.891 Other injury of other specified muscles, fascia and tendons at wrist and hand level, right hand
    - S66.892 Other injury of other specified muscles, fascia and tendons at wrist and hand level, left hand
    - S66.899 Other injury of other specified muscles, fascia and tendons at wrist and hand level, unspecified hand

S66.9 Injury of unspecified muscle, fascia and tendon at wrist and hand level

S66.90 Unspecified injury of unspecified muscle, fascia and tendon at wrist and hand level
- **S66.901** Unspecified injury of unspecified muscle, fascia and tendon at wrist and hand level, right hand
- **S66.902** Unspecified injury of unspecified muscle, fascia and tendon at wrist and hand level, left hand
- **S66.909** Unspecified injury of unspecified muscle, fascia and tendon at wrist and hand level, unspecified hand

S66.91 Strain of unspecified muscle, fascia and tendon at wrist and hand level
- **S66.911** Strain of unspecified muscle, fascia and tendon at wrist and hand level, right hand
- **S66.912** Strain of unspecified muscle, fascia and tendon at wrist and hand level, left hand
- **S66.919** Strain of unspecified muscle, fascia and tendon at wrist and hand level, unspecified hand

S66.92 Laceration of unspecified muscle, fascia and tendon at wrist and hand level
- **S66.921** Laceration of unspecified muscle, fascia and tendon at wrist and hand level, right hand
- **S66.922** Laceration of unspecified muscle, fascia and tendon at wrist and hand level, left hand
- **S66.929** Laceration of unspecified muscle, fascia and tendon at wrist and hand level, unspecified hand

S66.99 Other injury of unspecified muscle, fascia and tendon at wrist and hand level
- **S66.991** Other injury of unspecified muscle, fascia and tendon at wrist and hand level, right hand
- **S66.992** Other injury of unspecified muscle, fascia and tendon at wrist and hand level, left hand
- **S66.999** Other injury of unspecified muscle, fascia and tendon at wrist and hand level, unspecified hand

S67 Crushing injury of wrist, hand and fingers

Use additional code for all associated injuries, such as:
- fracture of wrist and hand (S62.-)
- open wound of wrist and hand (S61.-)

The appropriate 7th character is to be added to each code from category S67.
- A initial encounter
- D subsequent encounter
- S sequela

S67.0 Crushing injury of thumb
- **S67.00** Crushing injury of unspecified thumb
- **S67.01** Crushing injury of right thumb
- **S67.02** Crushing injury of left thumb

S67.1 Crushing injury of other and unspecified finger(s)
EXCLUDES 2 crushing injury of thumb (S67.0-)
- **S67.10** Crushing injury of unspecified finger(s)
- **S67.19** Crushing injury of other finger(s)
  - **S67.190** Crushing injury of right index finger
  - **S67.191** Crushing injury of left index finger
  - **S67.192** Crushing injury of right middle finger
  - **S67.193** Crushing injury of left middle finger
  - **S67.194** Crushing injury of right ring finger
  - **S67.195** Crushing injury of left ring finger
  - **S67.196** Crushing injury of right little finger
  - **S67.197** Crushing injury of left little finger
  - **S67.198** Crushing injury of other finger
    Crushing injury of specified finger with unspecified laterality

S67.2 Crushing injury of hand
EXCLUDES 2 crushing injury of fingers (S67.1-)
crushing injury of thumb (S67.0-)
- **S67.20** Crushing injury of unspecified hand
- **S67.21** Crushing injury of right hand
- **S67.22** Crushing injury of left hand

S67.3 Crushing injury of wrist
- **S67.30** Crushing injury of unspecified wrist
- **S67.31** Crushing injury of right wrist
- **S67.32** Crushing injury of left wrist

S67.4 Crushing injury of wrist and hand
EXCLUDES 1 crushing injury of hand alone (S67.2-)
crushing injury of wrist alone (S67.3-)
EXCLUDES 2 crushing injury of fingers (S67.1-)
crushing injury of thumb (S67.0-)
- **S67.40** Crushing injury of unspecified wrist and hand
- **S67.41** Crushing injury of right wrist and hand
- **S67.42** Crushing injury of left wrist and hand

S67.9 Crushing injury of unspecified part(s) of wrist, hand and fingers
- **S67.90** Crushing injury of unspecified part(s) of unspecified wrist, hand and fingers
- **S67.91** Crushing injury of unspecified part(s) of right wrist, hand and fingers
- **S67.92** Crushing injury of unspecified part(s) of left wrist, hand and fingers

S68 Traumatic amputation of wrist, hand and fingers

An amputation not identified as partial or complete should be coded to complete.

The appropriate 7th character is to be added to each code from category S68.
- A initial encounter
- D subsequent encounter
- S sequela

S68.0 Traumatic metacarpophalangeal amputation of thumb
Traumatic amputation of thumb NOS

S68.01 Complete traumatic metacarpophalangeal amputation of thumb
- **S68.011** Complete traumatic metacarpophalangeal amputation of right thumb
- **S68.012** Complete traumatic metacarpophalangeal amputation of left thumb
- **S68.019** Complete traumatic metacarpophalangeal amputation of unspecified thumb

S68.02 Partial traumatic metacarpophalangeal amputation of thumb
- **S68.021** Partial traumatic metacarpophalangeal amputation of right thumb
- **S68.022** Partial traumatic metacarpophalangeal amputation of left thumb
- **S68.029** Partial traumatic metacarpophalangeal amputation of unspecified thumb

S68.1 Traumatic metacarpophalangeal amputation of other and unspecified finger
Traumatic amputation of finger NOS
EXCLUDES 2 traumatic metacarpophalangeal amputation of thumb (S68.0-)

S68.11 Complete traumatic metacarpophalangeal amputation of other and unspecified finger
- **S68.110** Complete traumatic metacarpophalangeal amputation of right index finger
- **S68.111** Complete traumatic metacarpophalangeal amputation of left index finger
- **S68.112** Complete traumatic metacarpophalangeal amputation of right middle finger
- **S68.113** Complete traumatic metacarpophalangeal amputation of left middle finger
- **S68.114** Complete traumatic metacarpophalangeal amputation of right ring finger
- **S68.115** Complete traumatic metacarpophalangeal amputation of left ring finger
- **S68.116** Complete traumatic metacarpophalangeal amputation of right little finger
- **S68.117** Complete traumatic metacarpophalangeal amputation of left little finger
- **S68.118** Complete traumatic metacarpophalangeal amputation of other finger
  Complete traumatic metacarpophalangeal amputation of specified finger with unspecified laterality
- **S68.119** Complete traumatic metacarpophalangeal amputation of unspecified finger

- **S68.12** Partial traumatic metacarpophalangeal amputation of other and unspecified finger
  - **S68.120** Partial traumatic metacarpophalangeal amputation of right index finger
  - **S68.121** Partial traumatic metacarpophalangeal amputation of left index finger
  - **S68.122** Partial traumatic metacarpophalangeal amputation of right middle finger
  - **S68.123** Partial traumatic metacarpophalangeal amputation of left middle finger
  - **S68.124** Partial traumatic metacarpophalangeal amputation of right ring finger
  - **S68.125** Partial traumatic metacarpophalangeal amputation of left ring finger
  - **S68.126** Partial traumatic metacarpophalangeal amputation of right little finger
  - **S68.127** Partial traumatic metacarpophalangeal amputation of left little finger
  - **S68.128** Partial traumatic metacarpophalangeal amputation of other finger
    - Partial traumatic metacarpophalangeal amputation of specified finger with unspecified laterality
  - **S68.129** Partial traumatic metacarpophalangeal amputation of unspecified finger

- **S68.4** Traumatic amputation of hand at wrist level
  - Traumatic amputation of hand NOS
  - Traumatic amputation of wrist
  - **S68.41** Complete traumatic amputation of hand at wrist level
    - **S68.411** Complete traumatic amputation of right hand at wrist level
    - **S68.412** Complete traumatic amputation of left hand at wrist level
    - **S68.419** Complete traumatic amputation of unspecified hand at wrist level
  - **S68.42** Partial traumatic amputation of hand at wrist level
    - **S68.421** Partial traumatic amputation of right hand at wrist level
    - **S68.422** Partial traumatic amputation of left hand at wrist level
    - **S68.429** Partial traumatic amputation of unspecified hand at wrist level

- **S68.5** Traumatic transphalangeal amputation of thumb
  - Traumatic interphalangeal joint amputation of thumb
  - **S68.51** Complete traumatic transphalangeal amputation of thumb
    - **S68.511** Complete traumatic transphalangeal amputation of right thumb
    - **S68.512** Complete traumatic transphalangeal amputation of left thumb
    - **S68.519** Complete traumatic transphalangeal amputation of unspecified thumb
  - **S68.52** Partial traumatic transphalangeal amputation of thumb
    - **S68.521** Partial traumatic transphalangeal amputation of right thumb
    - **S68.522** Partial traumatic transphalangeal amputation of left thumb
    - **S68.529** Partial traumatic transphalangeal amputation of unspecified thumb

- **S68.6** Traumatic transphalangeal amputation of other and unspecified finger
  - **S68.61** Complete traumatic transphalangeal amputation of other and unspecified finger(s)
    - **S68.610** Complete traumatic transphalangeal amputation of right index finger
    - **S68.611** Complete traumatic transphalangeal amputation of left index finger
    - **S68.612** Complete traumatic transphalangeal amputation of right middle finger
    - **S68.613** Complete traumatic transphalangeal amputation of left middle finger
    - **S68.614** Complete traumatic transphalangeal amputation of right ring finger
    - **S68.615** Complete traumatic transphalangeal amputation of left ring finger
    - **S68.616** Complete traumatic transphalangeal amputation of right little finger
    - **S68.617** Complete traumatic transphalangeal amputation of left little finger
    - **S68.618** Complete traumatic transphalangeal amputation of other finger
      - Complete traumatic transphalangeal amputation of specified finger with unspecified laterality
    - **S68.619** Complete traumatic transphalangeal amputation of unspecified finger
  - **S68.62** Partial traumatic transphalangeal amputation of other and unspecified finger
    - **S68.620** Partial traumatic transphalangeal amputation of right index finger
    - **S68.621** Partial traumatic transphalangeal amputation of left index finger
    - **S68.622** Partial traumatic transphalangeal amputation of right middle finger
    - **S68.623** Partial traumatic transphalangeal amputation of left middle finger
    - **S68.624** Partial traumatic transphalangeal amputation of right ring finger
    - **S68.625** Partial traumatic transphalangeal amputation of left ring finger
    - **S68.626** Partial traumatic transphalangeal amputation of right little finger
    - **S68.627** Partial traumatic transphalangeal amputation of left little finger
    - **S68.628** Partial traumatic transphalangeal amputation of other finger
      - Partial traumatic transphalangeal amputation of specified finger with unspecified laterality
    - **S68.629** Partial traumatic transphalangeal amputation of unspecified finger

- **S68.7** Traumatic transmetacarpal amputation of hand
  - **S68.71** Complete traumatic transmetacarpal amputation of hand
    - **S68.711** Complete traumatic transmetacarpal amputation of right hand
    - **S68.712** Complete traumatic transmetacarpal amputation of left hand
    - **S68.719** Complete traumatic transmetacarpal amputation of unspecified hand
  - **S68.72** Partial traumatic transmetacarpal amputation of hand
    - **S68.721** Partial traumatic transmetacarpal amputation of right hand
    - **S68.722** Partial traumatic transmetacarpal amputation of left hand
    - **S68.729** Partial traumatic transmetacarpal amputation of unspecified hand

- **S69** Other and unspecified injuries of wrist, hand and finger(s)

  > The appropriate 7th character is to be added to each code from category S69.
  > A initial encounter
  > D subsequent encounter
  > S sequela

  - **S69.8** Other specified injuries of wrist, hand and finger(s)
    - **S69.80** Other specified injuries of unspecified wrist, hand and finger(s)
    - **S69.81** Other specified injuries of right wrist, hand and finger(s)
    - **S69.82** Other specified injuries of left wrist, hand and finger(s)
  - **S69.9** Unspecified injury of wrist, hand and finger(s)
    - **S69.90** Unspecified injury of unspecified wrist, hand and finger(s)
    - **S69.91** Unspecified injury of right wrist, hand and finger(s)
    - **S69.92** Unspecified injury of left wrist, hand and finger(s)

Injuries to the hip and thigh (S70-S79)

EXCLUDES 2: burns and corrosions (T20-T32)
frostbite (T33-T34)
snake bite (T63.0-)
venomous insect bite or sting (T63.4-)

✓4th S70 Superficial injury of hip and thigh

The appropriate 7th character is to be added to each code from category S70.
- A initial encounter
- D subsequent encounter
- S sequela

✓5th S70.0 Contusion of hip
- ✓x7th S70.00 Contusion of unspecified hip
- ✓x7th S70.01 Contusion of right hip
- ✓x7th S70.02 Contusion of left hip

✓5th S70.1 Contusion of thigh
- ✓x7th S70.10 Contusion of unspecified thigh
- ✓x7th S70.11 Contusion of right thigh
- ✓x7th S70.12 Contusion of left thigh

✓5th S70.2 Other superficial injuries of hip
- ✓6th S70.21 Abrasion of hip
  - ✓7th S70.211 Abrasion, right hip
  - ✓7th S70.212 Abrasion, left hip
  - ✓7th S70.219 Abrasion, unspecified hip
- ✓6th S70.22 Blister (nonthermal) of hip
  - ✓7th S70.221 Blister (nonthermal), right hip
  - ✓7th S70.222 Blister (nonthermal), left hip
  - ✓7th S70.229 Blister (nonthermal), unspecified hip
- ✓6th S70.24 External constriction of hip
  - ✓7th S70.241 External constriction, right hip
  - ✓7th S70.242 External constriction, left hip
  - ✓7th S70.249 External constriction, unspecified hip
- ✓6th S70.25 Superficial foreign body of hip
  - Splinter in the hip
  - ✓7th S70.251 Superficial foreign body, right hip
  - ✓7th S70.252 Superficial foreign body, left hip
  - ✓7th S70.259 Superficial foreign body, unspecified hip
- ✓6th S70.26 Insect bite (nonvenomous) of hip
  - ✓7th S70.261 Insect bite (nonvenomous), right hip
  - ✓7th S70.262 Insect bite (nonvenomous), left hip
  - ✓7th S70.269 Insect bite (nonvenomous), unspecified hip
- ✓6th S70.27 Other superficial bite of hip
  - **EXCLUDES 1:** open bite of hip (S71.05-)
  - ✓7th S70.271 Other superficial bite of hip, right hip
  - ✓7th S70.272 Other superficial bite of hip, left hip
  - ✓7th S70.279 Other superficial bite of hip, unspecified hip

✓5th S70.3 Other superficial injuries of thigh
- ✓6th S70.31 Abrasion of thigh
  - ✓7th S70.311 Abrasion, right thigh
  - ✓7th S70.312 Abrasion, left thigh
  - ✓7th S70.319 Abrasion, unspecified thigh
- ✓6th S70.32 Blister (nonthermal) of thigh
  - ✓7th S70.321 Blister (nonthermal), right thigh
  - ✓7th S70.322 Blister (nonthermal), left thigh
  - ✓7th S70.329 Blister (nonthermal), unspecified thigh
- ✓6th S70.34 External constriction of thigh
  - ✓7th S70.341 External constriction, right thigh
  - ✓7th S70.342 External constriction, left thigh
  - ✓7th S70.349 External constriction, unspecified thigh
- ✓6th S70.35 Superficial foreign body of thigh
  - Splinter in the thigh
  - ✓7th S70.351 Superficial foreign body, right thigh
  - ✓7th S70.352 Superficial foreign body, left thigh
  - ✓7th S70.359 Superficial foreign body, unspecified thigh
- ✓6th S70.36 Insect bite (nonvenomous) of thigh
  - ✓7th S70.361 Insect bite (nonvenomous), right thigh
  - ✓7th S70.362 Insect bite (nonvenomous), left thigh
  - ✓7th S70.369 Insect bite (nonvenomous), unspecified thigh
- ✓6th S70.37 Other superficial bite of thigh
  - **EXCLUDES 1:** open bite of thigh (S71.15)
  - ✓7th S70.371 Other superficial bite of right thigh
  - ✓7th S70.372 Other superficial bite of left thigh
  - ✓7th S70.379 Other superficial bite of unspecified thigh

✓5th S70.9 Unspecified superficial injury of hip and thigh
- ✓6th S70.91 Unspecified superficial injury of hip
  - ✓7th S70.911 Unspecified superficial injury of right hip
  - ✓7th S70.912 Unspecified superficial injury of left hip
  - ✓7th S70.919 Unspecified superficial injury of unspecified hip
- ✓6th S70.92 Unspecified superficial injury of thigh
  - ✓7th S70.921 Unspecified superficial injury of right thigh
  - ✓7th S70.922 Unspecified superficial injury of left thigh
  - ✓7th S70.929 Unspecified superficial injury of unspecified thigh

✓4th S71 Open wound of hip and thigh

Code also any associated wound infection
EXCLUDES 1: open fracture of hip and thigh (S72.-)
traumatic amputation of hip and thigh (S78.-)
EXCLUDES 2: bite of venomous animal (T63.-)
open wound of ankle, foot and toes (S91.-)
open wound of knee and lower leg (S81.-)

The appropriate 7th character is to be added to each code from category S71.
- A initial encounter
- D subsequent encounter
- S sequela

✓5th S71.0 Open wound of hip
- ✓6th S71.00 Unspecified open wound of hip
  - ✓7th S71.001 Unspecified open wound, right hip
  - ✓7th S71.002 Unspecified open wound, left hip
  - ✓7th S71.009 Unspecified open wound, unspecified hip
- ✓6th S71.01 Laceration without foreign body of hip
  - ✓7th S71.011 Laceration without foreign body, right hip
  - ✓7th S71.012 Laceration without foreign body, left hip
  - ✓7th S71.019 Laceration without foreign body, unspecified hip
- ✓6th S71.02 Laceration with foreign body of hip
  - ✓7th S71.021 Laceration with foreign body, right hip
  - ✓7th S71.022 Laceration with foreign body, left hip
  - ✓7th S71.029 Laceration with foreign body, unspecified hip
- ✓6th S71.03 Puncture wound without foreign body of hip
  - ✓7th S71.031 Puncture wound without foreign body, right hip
  - ✓7th S71.032 Puncture wound without foreign body, left hip
  - ✓7th S71.039 Puncture wound without foreign body, unspecified hip
- ✓6th S71.04 Puncture wound with foreign body of hip
  - ✓7th S71.041 Puncture wound with foreign body, right hip
  - ✓7th S71.042 Puncture wound with foreign body, left hip
  - ✓7th S71.049 Puncture wound with foreign body, unspecified hip
- ✓6th S71.05 Open bite of hip
  - Bite of hip NOS
  - **EXCLUDES 1:** superficial bite of hip (S70.26, S70.27)
  - ✓7th S71.051 Open bite, right hip
  - ✓7th S71.052 Open bite, left hip
  - ✓7th S71.059 Open bite, unspecified hip

✓5th S71.1 Open wound of thigh
- ✓6th S71.10 Unspecified open wound of thigh
  - **AHA:** 2016,3Q,24
  - ✓7th S71.101 Unspecified open wound, right thigh

HCC CMS-HCC | Rx Rx HCC | ESR ESRD HCC | COM Commercial HCC | N Newborn: 0 | P Pediatric: 0-17 | M Maternity: 9-64 | A Adult: 15-124

- **S71.102** Unspecified open wound, left thigh
- **S71.109** Unspecified open wound, unspecified thigh
- **S71.11** **Laceration without foreign body** of thigh
  - **S71.111** Laceration without foreign body, right thigh
  - **S71.112** Laceration without foreign body, left thigh
  - **S71.119** Laceration without foreign body, unspecified thigh
- **S71.12** **Laceration with foreign body** of thigh
  - **S71.121** Laceration with foreign body, right thigh
  - **S71.122** Laceration with foreign body, left thigh
  - **S71.129** Laceration with foreign body, unspecified thigh
- **S71.13** **Puncture wound without foreign body** of thigh
  - AHA: 2023,3Q,12; 2016,3Q,24
  - **S71.131** Puncture wound without foreign body, right thigh
  - **S71.132** Puncture wound without foreign body, left thigh
  - **S71.139** Puncture wound without foreign body, unspecified thigh
- **S71.14** **Puncture wound with foreign body** of thigh
  - AHA: 2016,3Q,24
  - **S71.141** Puncture wound with foreign body, right thigh
  - **S71.142** Puncture wound with foreign body, left thigh
  - **S71.149** Puncture wound with foreign body, unspecified thigh
- **S71.15** **Open bite** of thigh
  - Bite of thigh NOS
  - EXCLUDES 1: superficial bite of thigh (S70.37-)
  - **S71.151** Open bite, right thigh
  - **S71.152** Open bite, left thigh
  - **S71.159** Open bite, unspecified thigh

S72 **Fracture of femur**

NOTE A fracture not indicated as displaced or nondisplaced should be coded to displaced.

A fracture not indicated as open or closed should be coded to closed.

The open fracture designations are based on the Gustilo open fracture classification.

EXCLUDES 1: traumatic amputation of hip and thigh (S78.-)
EXCLUDES 2: fracture of foot (S92.-)
fracture of lower leg and ankle (S82.-)
periprosthetic fracture of prosthetic implant of hip (M97.0-)

AHA: 2023,3Q,12; 2018,2Q,12; 2016,1Q,33; 2015,3Q,37-39; 2015,1Q,17; 2013,4Q,128

DEF: Diaphysis: Central shaft of a long bone.
DEF: Epiphysis: Proximal and distal rounded ends of a long bone communicates with the joint.
DEF: Metaphysis: Section of a long bone located between the epiphysis and diaphysis at the proximal and distal ends.
DEF: Physis (growth plate): Narrow zone of cartilaginous tissue between the epiphysis and metaphysis at each end of a long bone. In childhood, proliferation of cells in this zone lengthens the bone. As the bone matures, this area thins, ossification eventually fusing into solid bone and growth stops. *Synonym(s):* Epiphyseal plate.

The appropriate 7th character is to be added to all codes from category S72 [unless otherwise indicated].

-   initial encounter for open fracture NOS
- A initial encounter for closed fracture
- B initial encounter for open fracture type I or II
- C initial encounter for open fracture type IIIA, IIIB, or IIIC
- D subsequent encounter for closed fracture with routine healing
- E subsequent encounter for open fracture type I or II with routine healing
- F subsequent encounter for open fracture type IIIA, IIIB, or IIIC with routine healing
- G subsequent encounter for closed fracture with delayed healing
- H subsequent encounter for open fracture type I or II with delayed healing
- J subsequent encounter for open fracture type IIIA, IIIB, or IIIC with delayed healing
- K subsequent encounter for closed fracture with nonunion
- M subsequent encounter for open fracture type I or II with nonunion
- N subsequent encounter for open fracture type IIIA, IIIB, or IIIC with nonunion
- P subsequent encounter for closed fracture with malunion
- Q subsequent encounter for open fracture type I or II with malunion
- R subsequent encounter for open fracture type IIIA, IIIB, or IIIC with malunion
- S sequela

- **S72.0** **Fracture of head and neck** of femur
  - EXCLUDES 2: physeal fracture of lower end of femur (S79.1-)
  - physeal fracture of upper end of femur (S79.0-)
  - AHA: 2016,3Q,16
  - **S72.00** Fracture of unspecified part of neck of femur
    - Fracture of hip NOS
    - Fracture of neck of femur NOS
    - **S72.001** Fracture of unspecified part of neck of right femur
    - **S72.002** Fracture of unspecified part of neck of left femur
    - **S72.009** Fracture of unspecified part of neck of unspecified femur
  - **S72.01** Unspecified **intracapsular** fracture of femur
    - Subcapital fracture of femur
    - **S72.011** Unspecified intracapsular fracture of right femur
    - **S72.012** Unspecified intracapsular fracture of left femur
    - **S72.019** Unspecified intracapsular fracture of unspecified femur

S72.02 Fracture of epiphysis (separation) (upper) of femur
Transepiphyseal fracture of femur
EXCLUDES 1 capital femoral epiphyseal fracture (pediatric) of femur (S79.01-)
Salter-Harris Type I physeal fracture of upper end of femur (S79.01-)

- S72.021 Displaced fracture of epiphysis (separation) (upper) of right femur
- S72.022 Displaced fracture of epiphysis (separation) (upper) of left femur
- S72.023 Displaced fracture of epiphysis (separation) (upper) of unspecified femur
- S72.024 Nondisplaced fracture of epiphysis (separation) (upper) of right femur
- S72.025 Nondisplaced fracture of epiphysis (separation) (upper) of left femur
- S72.026 Nondisplaced fracture of epiphysis (separation) (upper) of unspecified femur

S72.03 Midcervical fracture of femur
Transcervical fracture of femur NOS

- S72.031 Displaced midcervical fracture of right femur
- S72.032 Displaced midcervical fracture of left femur
- S72.033 Displaced midcervical fracture of unspecified femur
- S72.034 Nondisplaced midcervical fracture of right femur
- S72.035 Nondisplaced midcervical fracture of left femur
- S72.036 Nondisplaced midcervical fracture of unspecified femur

S72.04 Fracture of base of neck of femur
Cervicotrochanteric fracture of femur

- S72.041 Displaced fracture of base of neck of right femur
- S72.042 Displaced fracture of base of neck of left femur
- S72.043 Displaced fracture of base of neck of unspecified femur
- S72.044 Nondisplaced fracture of base of neck of right femur
- S72.045 Nondisplaced fracture of base of neck of left femur
- S72.046 Nondisplaced fracture of base of neck of unspecified femur

S72.05 Unspecified fracture of head of femur
Fracture of head of femur NOS

- S72.051 Unspecified fracture of head of right femur
- S72.052 Unspecified fracture of head of left femur
- S72.059 Unspecified fracture of head of unspecified femur

S72.06 Articular fracture of head of femur

- S72.061 Displaced articular fracture of head of right femur
- S72.062 Displaced articular fracture of head of left femur
- S72.063 Displaced articular fracture of head of unspecified femur
- S72.064 Nondisplaced articular fracture of head of right femur
- S72.065 Nondisplaced articular fracture of head of left femur
- S72.066 Nondisplaced articular fracture of head of unspecified femur

S72.09 Other fracture of head and neck of femur

- S72.091 Other fracture of head and neck of right femur
- S72.092 Other fracture of head and neck of left femur
- S72.099 Other fracture of head and neck of unspecified femur

S72.1 Pertrochanteric fracture
AHA: 2016,3Q,16

S72.10 Unspecified trochanteric fracture of femur
Fracture of trochanter NOS

- S72.101 Unspecified trochanteric fracture of right femur
- S72.102 Unspecified trochanteric fracture of left femur
- S72.109 Unspecified trochanteric fracture of unspecified femur

S72.11 Fracture of greater trochanter of femur

- S72.111 Displaced fracture of greater trochanter of right femur
- S72.112 Displaced fracture of greater trochanter of left femur
- S72.113 Displaced fracture of greater trochanter of unspecified femur
- S72.114 Nondisplaced fracture of greater trochanter of right femur
- S72.115 Nondisplaced fracture of greater trochanter of left femur
- S72.116 Nondisplaced fracture of greater trochanter of unspecified femur

S72.12 Fracture of lesser trochanter of femur

- S72.121 Displaced fracture of lesser trochanter of right femur
- S72.122 Displaced fracture of lesser trochanter of left femur
- S72.123 Displaced fracture of lesser trochanter of unspecified femur
- S72.124 Nondisplaced fracture of lesser trochanter of right femur
- S72.125 Nondisplaced fracture of lesser trochanter of left femur
- S72.126 Nondisplaced fracture of lesser trochanter of unspecified femur

S72.13 Apophyseal fracture of femur
EXCLUDES 1 chronic (nontraumatic) slipped upper femoral epiphysis (M93.0-)

- S72.131 Displaced apophyseal fracture of right femur
- S72.132 Displaced apophyseal fracture of left femur
- S72.133 Displaced apophyseal fracture of unspecified femur
- S72.134 Nondisplaced apophyseal fracture of right femur
- S72.135 Nondisplaced apophyseal fracture of left femur
- S72.136 Nondisplaced apophyseal fracture of unspecified femur

S72.14 Intertrochanteric fracture of femur

- S72.141 Displaced intertrochanteric fracture of right femur
- S72.142 Displaced intertrochanteric fracture of left femur
- S72.143 Displaced intertrochanteric fracture of unspecified femur
- S72.144 Nondisplaced intertrochanteric fracture of right femur
- S72.145 Nondisplaced intertrochanteric fracture of left femur
- S72.146 Nondisplaced intertrochanteric fracture of unspecified femur

S72.2 Subtrochanteric fracture of femur

- S72.21 Displaced subtrochanteric fracture of right femur
- S72.22 Displaced subtrochanteric fracture of left femur
- S72.23 Displaced subtrochanteric fracture of unspecified femur
- S72.24 Nondisplaced subtrochanteric fracture of right femur

- **S72.25** Nondisplaced subtrochanteric fracture of left femur
- **S72.26** Nondisplaced subtrochanteric fracture of unspecified femur
- **S72.3** Fracture of shaft of femur
  - **S72.30** Unspecified fracture of shaft of femur
    - **S72.301** Unspecified fracture of shaft of right femur
    - **S72.302** Unspecified fracture of shaft of left femur
    - **S72.309** Unspecified fracture of shaft of unspecified femur
  - **S72.32** Transverse fracture of shaft of femur
    - **S72.321** Displaced transverse fracture of shaft of right femur
    - **S72.322** Displaced transverse fracture of shaft of left femur
    - **S72.323** Displaced transverse fracture of shaft of unspecified femur
    - **S72.324** Nondisplaced transverse fracture of shaft of right femur
    - **S72.325** Nondisplaced transverse fracture of shaft of left femur
    - **S72.326** Nondisplaced transverse fracture of shaft of unspecified femur
  - **S72.33** Oblique fracture of shaft of femur
    - **S72.331** Displaced oblique fracture of shaft of right femur
    - **S72.332** Displaced oblique fracture of shaft of left femur
    - **S72.333** Displaced oblique fracture of shaft of unspecified femur
    - **S72.334** Nondisplaced oblique fracture of shaft of right femur
    - **S72.335** Nondisplaced oblique fracture of shaft of left femur
    - **S72.336** Nondisplaced oblique fracture of shaft of unspecified femur
  - **S72.34** Spiral fracture of shaft of femur
    - **S72.341** Displaced spiral fracture of shaft of right femur
    - **S72.342** Displaced spiral fracture of shaft of left femur
    - **S72.343** Displaced spiral fracture of shaft of unspecified femur
    - **S72.344** Nondisplaced spiral fracture of shaft of right femur
    - **S72.345** Nondisplaced spiral fracture of shaft of left femur
    - **S72.346** Nondisplaced spiral fracture of shaft of unspecified femur
  - **S72.35** Comminuted fracture of shaft of femur
    - **S72.351** Displaced comminuted fracture of shaft of right femur
    - **S72.352** Displaced comminuted fracture of shaft of left femur
    - **S72.353** Displaced comminuted fracture of shaft of unspecified femur
    - **S72.354** Nondisplaced comminuted fracture of shaft of right femur
    - **S72.355** Nondisplaced comminuted fracture of shaft of left femur
    - **S72.356** Nondisplaced comminuted fracture of shaft of unspecified femur
  - **S72.36** Segmental fracture of shaft of femur
    - **S72.361** Displaced segmental fracture of shaft of right femur
    - **S72.362** Displaced segmental fracture of shaft of left femur
    - **S72.363** Displaced segmental fracture of shaft of unspecified femur
    - **S72.364** Nondisplaced segmental fracture of shaft of right femur
    - **S72.365** Nondisplaced segmental fracture of shaft of left femur
    - **S72.366** Nondisplaced segmental fracture of shaft of unspecified femur
  - **S72.39** Other fracture of shaft of femur
    - **S72.391** Other fracture of shaft of right femur
    - **S72.392** Other fracture of shaft of left femur
    - **S72.399** Other fracture of shaft of unspecified femur
- **S72.4** Fracture of lower end of femur
  - Fracture of distal end of femur
  - **EXCLUDES 2** fracture of shaft of femur (S72.3-)
    - physeal fracture of lower end of femur (S79.1-)
  - **AHA:** 2016,4Q,42
  - **S72.40** Unspecified fracture of lower end of femur
    - **AHA:** 2018,1Q,21; 2016,4Q,42
    - **S72.401** Unspecified fracture of lower end of right femur
    - **S72.402** Unspecified fracture of lower end of left femur
    - **S72.409** Unspecified fracture of lower end of unspecified femur
  - **S72.41** Unspecified condyle fracture of lower end of femur
    - Condyle fracture of femur NOS
    - **S72.411** Displaced unspecified condyle fracture of lower end of right femur
    - **S72.412** Displaced unspecified condyle fracture of lower end of left femur
    - **S72.413** Displaced unspecified condyle fracture of lower end of unspecified femur
    - **S72.414** Nondisplaced unspecified condyle fracture of lower end of right femur
    - **S72.415** Nondisplaced unspecified condyle fracture of lower end of left femur
    - **S72.416** Nondisplaced unspecified condyle fracture of lower end of unspecified femur
  - **S72.42** Fracture of lateral condyle of femur
    - **S72.421** Displaced fracture of lateral condyle of right femur
    - **S72.422** Displaced fracture of lateral condyle of left femur
    - **S72.423** Displaced fracture of lateral condyle of unspecified femur
    - **S72.424** Nondisplaced fracture of lateral condyle of right femur
    - **S72.425** Nondisplaced fracture of lateral condyle of left femur
    - **S72.426** Nondisplaced fracture of lateral condyle of unspecified femur
  - **S72.43** Fracture of medial condyle of femur
    - **S72.431** Displaced fracture of medial condyle of right femur
    - **S72.432** Displaced fracture of medial condyle of left femur
    - **S72.433** Displaced fracture of medial condyle of unspecified femur
    - **S72.434** Nondisplaced fracture of medial condyle of right femur
    - **S72.435** Nondisplaced fracture of medial condyle of left femur
    - **S72.436** Nondisplaced fracture of medial condyle of unspecified femur
  - **S72.44** Fracture of lower epiphysis (separation) of femur
    - **EXCLUDES 1** Salter-Harris Type I physeal fracture of lower end of femur (S79.11-)
    - **S72.441** Displaced fracture of lower epiphysis (separation) of right femur
    - **S72.442** Displaced fracture of lower epiphysis (separation) of left femur
    - **S72.443** Displaced fracture of lower epiphysis (separation) of unspecified femur
    - **S72.444** Nondisplaced fracture of lower epiphysis (separation) of right femur
    - **S72.445** Nondisplaced fracture of lower epiphysis (separation) of left femur

- ✓ S72.446 **Nondisplaced** fracture of lower epiphysis (separation) of unspecified femur [HCC] [ESR] [Q]
- ✓6th S72.45 **Supracondylar** fracture **without intracondylar extension** of lower end of femur
  - Supracondylar fracture of lower end of femur NOS
  - EXCLUDES 1: supracondylar fracture with intracondylar extension of lower end of femur (S72.46-)
  - ✓7th S72.451 **Displaced** supracondylar fracture without intracondylar extension of lower end of **right** femur [HCC] [ESR] [Q]
  - ✓7th S72.452 **Displaced** supracondylar fracture without intracondylar extension of lower end of **left** femur [HCC] [ESR] [Q]
  - ✓7th S72.453 **Displaced** supracondylar fracture without intracondylar extension of lower end of **unspecified** femur [HCC] [ESR] [Q]
  - ✓7th S72.454 **Nondisplaced** supracondylar fracture without intracondylar extension of lower end of **right** femur [HCC] [ESR] [Q]
  - ✓7th S72.455 **Nondisplaced** supracondylar fracture without intracondylar extension of lower end of **left** femur [HCC] [ESR] [Q]
  - ✓7th S72.456 **Nondisplaced** supracondylar fracture without intracondylar extension of lower end of **unspecified** femur [HCC] [ESR] [Q]
- ✓6th S72.46 **Supracondylar** fracture **with intracondylar extension** of lower end of femur
  - EXCLUDES 1: supracondylar fracture without intracondylar extension of lower end of femur (S72.45-)
  - ✓7th S72.461 **Displaced** supracondylar fracture with intracondylar extension of lower end of **right** femur [HCC] [ESR] [Q]
  - ✓7th S72.462 **Displaced** supracondylar fracture with intracondylar extension of lower end of **left** femur [HCC] [ESR] [Q]
  - ✓7th S72.463 **Displaced** supracondylar fracture with intracondylar extension of lower end of **unspecified** femur [HCC] [ESR] [Q]
  - ✓7th S72.464 **Nondisplaced** supracondylar fracture with intracondylar extension of lower end of **right** femur [HCC] [ESR] [Q]
  - ✓7th S72.465 **Nondisplaced** supracondylar fracture with intracondylar extension of lower end of **left** femur [HCC] [ESR] [Q]
  - ✓7th S72.466 **Nondisplaced** supracondylar fracture with intracondylar extension of lower end of **unspecified** femur [HCC] [ESR] [Q]
- ✓6th S72.47 **Torus** fracture of lower end of femur

  > The appropriate 7th character is to be added to all codes in subcategory S72.47.
  > A initial encounter for closed fracture
  > D subsequent encounter for fracture with routine healing
  > G subsequent encounter for fracture with delayed healing
  > K subsequent encounter for fracture with nonunion
  > P subsequent encounter for fracture with malunion
  > S sequela

  - ✓7th S72.471 Torus fracture of lower end of **right** femur [HCC] [ESR] [Q]
  - ✓7th S72.472 Torus fracture of lower end of **left** femur [HCC] [ESR] [Q]
  - ✓7th S72.479 Torus fracture of lower end of unspecified femur [HCC] [ESR] [Q]
- ✓6th S72.49 Other fracture of lower end of femur
  - ✓7th S72.491 Other fracture of lower end of **right** femur [HCC] [ESR] [Q]
  - ✓7th S72.492 Other fracture of lower end of **left** femur [HCC] [ESR] [Q]
  - ✓7th S72.499 Other fracture of lower end of unspecified femur [HCC] [ESR] [Q]
- ✓5th S72.8 **Other** fracture of femur
  - ✓6th S72.8X **Other** fracture of femur
    - ✓7th S72.8X1 Other fracture of **right** femur [HCC] [ESR] [Q]
    - ✓7th S72.8X2 Other fracture of **left** femur [HCC] [ESR] [Q]
    - ✓7th S72.8X9 Other fracture of unspecified femur [HCC] [ESR] [Q]
- ✓5th S72.9 **Unspecified** fracture of femur
  - Fracture of thigh NOS
  - Fracture of upper leg NOS
  - EXCLUDES 1: fracture of hip NOS (S72.00-, S72.01-)
  - ✓x7th S72.90 **Unspecified** fracture of unspecified femur [HCC] [ESR] [Q]
    - AHA: 2012,4Q,93
  - ✓x7th S72.91 **Unspecified** fracture of **right** femur [HCC] [ESR] [Q]
  - ✓x7th S72.92 **Unspecified** fracture of **left** femur [HCC] [ESR] [Q]
- ✓4th **S73** **Dislocation and sprain of joint and ligaments of hip**
  - INCLUDES:
    - avulsion of joint or ligament of hip
    - laceration of cartilage, joint or ligament of hip
    - sprain of cartilage, joint or ligament of hip
    - traumatic hemarthrosis of joint or ligament of hip
    - traumatic rupture of joint or ligament of hip
    - traumatic subluxation of joint or ligament of hip
    - traumatic tear of joint or ligament of hip
  - Code also any associated open wound
  - EXCLUDES 2: strain of muscle, fascia and tendon of hip and thigh (S76.-)

  > The appropriate 7th character is to be added to each code from category S73.
  > A initial encounter
  > D subsequent encounter
  > S sequela

  - ✓5th S73.0 **Subluxation and dislocation of hip**
    - EXCLUDES 2: dislocation and subluxation of hip prosthesis (T84.020, T84.021)
    - ✓6th S73.00 Unspecified subluxation and dislocation of hip
      - Dislocation of hip NOS
      - Subluxation of hip NOS
      - ✓7th S73.001 **Unspecified subluxation** of **right** hip [HCC] [ESR]
      - ✓7th S73.002 **Unspecified subluxation** of **left** hip [HCC] [ESR]
      - ✓7th S73.003 **Unspecified subluxation** of unspecified hip [HCC] [ESR]
      - ✓7th S73.004 **Unspecified dislocation** of **right** hip [HCC] [ESR]
      - ✓7th S73.005 **Unspecified dislocation** of **left** hip [HCC] [ESR]
      - ✓7th S73.006 **Unspecified dislocation** of unspecified hip [HCC] [ESR]
    - ✓6th S73.01 **Posterior** subluxation and dislocation of hip
      - ✓7th S73.011 **Posterior subluxation** of **right** hip [HCC] [ESR]
      - ✓7th S73.012 **Posterior subluxation** of **left** hip [HCC] [ESR]
      - ✓7th S73.013 **Posterior subluxation** of unspecified hip [HCC] [ESR]
      - ✓7th S73.014 **Posterior dislocation** of **right** hip [HCC] [ESR]
      - ✓7th S73.015 **Posterior dislocation** of **left** hip [HCC] [ESR]
      - ✓7th S73.016 **Posterior dislocation** of unspecified hip [HCC] [ESR]
    - ✓6th S73.02 **Obturator** subluxation and dislocation of hip
      - ✓7th S73.021 **Obturator subluxation** of **right** hip [HCC] [ESR]
      - ✓7th S73.022 **Obturator subluxation** of **left** hip [HCC] [ESR]
      - ✓7th S73.023 **Obturator subluxation** of unspecified hip [HCC] [ESR]
      - ✓7th S73.024 **Obturator dislocation** of **right** hip [HCC] [ESR]
      - ✓7th S73.025 **Obturator dislocation** of **left** hip [HCC] [ESR]
      - ✓7th S73.026 **Obturator dislocation** of unspecified hip [HCC] [ESR]
    - ✓6th S73.03 **Other anterior** subluxation and dislocation of hip
      - ✓7th S73.031 Other anterior **subluxation** of **right** hip [HCC] [ESR]
      - ✓7th S73.032 Other anterior **subluxation** of **left** hip [HCC] [ESR]
      - ✓7th S73.033 Other anterior **subluxation** of unspecified hip [HCC] [ESR]

- **S73.034** Other anterior dislocation of right hip [7th] HCC ESR
- **S73.035** Other anterior dislocation of left hip [7th] HCC ESR
- **S73.036** Other anterior dislocation of unspecified hip [7th] HCC ESR
- **S73.04** Central subluxation and dislocation of hip [6th]
  - **S73.041** Central subluxation of right hip [7th] HCC ESR
  - **S73.042** Central subluxation of left hip [7th] HCC ESR
  - **S73.043** Central subluxation of unspecified hip [7th] HCC ESR
  - **S73.044** Central dislocation of right hip [7th] HCC ESR
  - **S73.045** Central dislocation of left hip [7th] HCC ESR
  - **S73.046** Central dislocation of unspecified hip [7th] HCC ESR
- **S73.1** Sprain of hip [5th]
  - AHA: 2014,4Q,25
  - **S73.10** Unspecified sprain of hip [6th]
    - **S73.101** Unspecified sprain of right hip [7th]
    - **S73.102** Unspecified sprain of left hip [7th]
    - **S73.109** Unspecified sprain of unspecified hip [7th]
  - **S73.11** Iliofemoral ligament sprain of hip [6th]
    - **S73.111** Iliofemoral ligament sprain of right hip [7th]
    - **S73.112** Iliofemoral ligament sprain of left hip [7th]
    - **S73.119** Iliofemoral ligament sprain of unspecified hip [7th]
  - **S73.12** Ischiocapsular (ligament) sprain of hip [6th]
    - **S73.121** Ischiocapsular ligament sprain of right hip [7th]
    - **S73.122** Ischiocapsular ligament sprain of left hip [7th]
    - **S73.129** Ischiocapsular ligament sprain of unspecified hip [7th]
  - **S73.19** Other sprain of hip [6th]
    - **S73.191** Other sprain of right hip [7th]
    - **S73.192** Other sprain of left hip [7th]
    - **S73.199** Other sprain of unspecified hip [7th]
- **S74** Injury of nerves at hip and thigh level [4th]
  - Code also any associated open wound (S71.-)
  - EXCLUDES 2: injury of nerves at ankle and foot level (S94.-)
  - injury of nerves at lower leg level (S84.-)

  The appropriate 7th character is to be added to each code from category S74.
  - A initial encounter
  - D subsequent encounter
  - S sequela

  - **S74.0** Injury of sciatic nerve at hip and thigh level [5th]
    - **S74.00** Injury of sciatic nerve at hip and thigh level, unspecified leg [7th]
    - **S74.01** Injury of sciatic nerve at hip and thigh level, right leg [7th]
    - **S74.02** Injury of sciatic nerve at hip and thigh level, left leg [7th]
  - **S74.1** Injury of femoral nerve at hip and thigh level [5th]
    - **S74.10** Injury of femoral nerve at hip and thigh level, unspecified leg [7th]
    - **S74.11** Injury of femoral nerve at hip and thigh level, right leg [7th]
    - **S74.12** Injury of femoral nerve at hip and thigh level, left leg [7th]
  - **S74.2** Injury of cutaneous sensory nerve at hip and thigh level [5th]
    - **S74.20** Injury of cutaneous sensory nerve at hip and thigh level, unspecified leg [7th]
    - **S74.21** Injury of cutaneous sensory nerve at hip and thigh level, right leg [7th]
    - **S74.22** Injury of cutaneous sensory nerve at hip and thigh level, left leg [7th]
  - **S74.8** Injury of other nerves at hip and thigh level [5th]
    - **S74.8X** Injury of other nerves at hip and thigh level [6th]
      - **S74.8X1** Injury of other nerves at hip and thigh level, right leg [7th]
      - **S74.8X2** Injury of other nerves at hip and thigh level, left leg [7th]
      - **S74.8X9** Injury of other nerves at hip and thigh level, unspecified leg [7th]
  - **S74.9** Injury of unspecified nerve at hip and thigh level [5th]
    - **S74.90** Injury of unspecified nerve at hip and thigh level, unspecified leg [7th]
    - **S74.91** Injury of unspecified nerve at hip and thigh level, right leg [7th]
    - **S74.92** Injury of unspecified nerve at hip and thigh level, left leg [7th]
- **S75** Injury of blood vessels at hip and thigh level [4th]
  - Code also any associated open wound (S71.-)
  - EXCLUDES 2: injury of blood vessels at lower leg level (S85.-)
  - injury of popliteal artery (S85.0)

  The appropriate 7th character is to be added to each code from category S75.
  - A initial encounter
  - D subsequent encounter
  - S sequela

  - **S75.0** Injury of femoral artery [5th]
    - **S75.00** Unspecified injury of femoral artery [6th]
      - **S75.001** Unspecified injury of femoral artery, right leg [7th]
      - **S75.002** Unspecified injury of femoral artery, left leg [7th]
      - **S75.009** Unspecified injury of femoral artery, unspecified leg [7th]
    - **S75.01** Minor laceration of femoral artery [6th]
      - Incomplete transection of femoral artery
      - Laceration of femoral artery NOS
      - Superficial laceration of femoral artery
      - **S75.011** Minor laceration of femoral artery, right leg [7th]
      - **S75.012** Minor laceration of femoral artery, left leg [7th]
      - **S75.019** Minor laceration of femoral artery, unspecified leg [7th]
    - **S75.02** Major laceration of femoral artery [6th]
      - Complete transection of femoral artery
      - Traumatic rupture of femoral artery
      - AHA: 2023,3Q,12
      - **S75.021** Major laceration of femoral artery, right leg [7th]
      - **S75.022** Major laceration of femoral artery, left leg [7th]
      - **S75.029** Major laceration of femoral artery, unspecified leg [7th]
    - **S75.09** Other specified injury of femoral artery [6th]
      - **S75.091** Other specified injury of femoral artery, right leg [7th]
      - **S75.092** Other specified injury of femoral artery, left leg [7th]
      - **S75.099** Other specified injury of femoral artery, unspecified leg [7th]
  - **S75.1** Injury of femoral vein at hip and thigh level [5th]
    - **S75.10** Unspecified injury of femoral vein at hip and thigh level [6th]
      - **S75.101** Unspecified injury of femoral vein at hip and thigh level, right leg [7th]
      - **S75.102** Unspecified injury of femoral vein at hip and thigh level, left leg [7th]
      - **S75.109** Unspecified injury of femoral vein at hip and thigh level, unspecified leg [7th]
    - **S75.11** Minor laceration of femoral vein at hip and thigh level [6th]
      - Incomplete transection of femoral vein at hip and thigh level
      - Laceration of femoral vein at hip and thigh level NOS
      - Superficial laceration of femoral vein at hip and thigh level
      - **S75.111** Minor laceration of femoral vein at hip and thigh level, right leg [7th]
      - **S75.112** Minor laceration of femoral vein at hip and thigh level, left leg [7th]
      - **S75.119** Minor laceration of femoral vein at hip and thigh level, unspecified leg [7th]
    - **S75.12** Major laceration of femoral vein at hip and thigh level [6th]
      - Complete transection of femoral vein at hip and thigh level
      - Traumatic rupture of femoral vein at hip and thigh level
      - AHA: 2023,3Q,12
      - **S75.121** Major laceration of femoral vein at hip and thigh level, right leg [7th]
      - **S75.122** Major laceration of femoral vein at hip and thigh level, left leg [7th]
      - **S75.129** Major laceration of femoral vein at hip and thigh level, unspecified leg [7th]

S75.19 Other specified injury of femoral vein at hip and thigh level
- **S75.191** Other specified injury of femoral vein at hip and thigh level, **right** leg
- **S75.192** Other specified injury of femoral vein at hip and thigh level, **left** leg
- **S75.199** Other specified injury of femoral vein at hip and thigh level, unspecified leg

S75.2 Injury of greater saphenous vein at hip and thigh level
  EXCLUDES 1 greater saphenous vein NOS (S85.3)

- **S75.20** Unspecified injury of greater saphenous vein at hip and thigh level
  - **S75.201** Unspecified injury of greater saphenous vein at hip and thigh level, **right** leg
  - **S75.202** Unspecified injury of greater saphenous vein at hip and thigh level, **left** leg
  - **S75.209** Unspecified injury of greater saphenous vein at hip and thigh level, unspecified leg

- **S75.21** Minor laceration of greater saphenous vein at hip and thigh level
  Incomplete transection of greater saphenous vein at hip and thigh level
  Laceration of greater saphenous vein at hip and thigh level NOS
  Superficial laceration of greater saphenous vein at hip and thigh level
  - **S75.211** Minor laceration of greater saphenous vein at hip and thigh level, **right** leg
  - **S75.212** Minor laceration of greater saphenous vein at hip and thigh level, **left** leg
  - **S75.219** Minor laceration of greater saphenous vein at hip and thigh level, unspecified leg

- **S75.22** Major laceration of greater saphenous vein at hip and thigh level
  Complete transection of greater saphenous vein at hip and thigh level
  Traumatic rupture of greater saphenous vein at hip and thigh level
  - **S75.221** Major laceration of greater saphenous vein at hip and thigh level, **right** leg
  - **S75.222** Major laceration of greater saphenous vein at hip and thigh level, **left** leg
  - **S75.229** Major laceration of greater saphenous vein at hip and thigh level, unspecified leg

- **S75.29** Other specified injury of greater saphenous vein at hip and thigh level
  - **S75.291** Other specified injury of greater saphenous vein at hip and thigh level, **right** leg
  - **S75.292** Other specified injury of greater saphenous vein at hip and thigh level, **left** leg
  - **S75.299** Other specified injury of greater saphenous vein at hip and thigh level, unspecified leg

S75.8 Injury of other blood vessels at hip and thigh level

- **S75.80** Unspecified injury of other blood vessels at hip and thigh level
  - **S75.801** Unspecified injury of other blood vessels at hip and thigh level, **right** leg
  - **S75.802** Unspecified injury of other blood vessels at hip and thigh level, **left** leg
  - **S75.809** Unspecified injury of other blood vessels at hip and thigh level, unspecified leg

- **S75.81** Laceration of other blood vessels at hip and thigh level
  - **S75.811** Laceration of other blood vessels at hip and thigh level, **right** leg
  - **S75.812** Laceration of other blood vessels at hip and thigh level, **left** leg
  - **S75.819** Laceration of other blood vessels at hip and thigh level, unspecified leg

- **S75.89** Other specified injury of other blood vessels at hip and thigh level
  - **S75.891** Other specified injury of other blood vessels at hip and thigh level, **right** leg
  - **S75.892** Other specified injury of other blood vessels at hip and thigh level, **left** leg
  - **S75.899** Other specified injury of other blood vessels at hip and thigh level, unspecified leg

S75.9 Injury of unspecified blood vessel at hip and thigh level

- **S75.90** Unspecified injury of unspecified blood vessel at hip and thigh level
  - **S75.901** Unspecified injury of unspecified blood vessel at hip and thigh level, **right** leg
  - **S75.902** Unspecified injury of unspecified blood vessel at hip and thigh level, **left** leg
  - **S75.909** Unspecified injury of unspecified blood vessel at hip and thigh level, unspecified leg

- **S75.91** Laceration of unspecified blood vessel at hip and thigh level
  - **S75.911** Laceration of unspecified blood vessel at hip and thigh level, **right** leg
  - **S75.912** Laceration of unspecified blood vessel at hip and thigh level, **left** leg
  - **S75.919** Laceration of unspecified blood vessel at hip and thigh level, unspecified leg

- **S75.99** Other specified injury of unspecified blood vessel at hip and thigh level
  - **S75.991** Other specified injury of unspecified blood vessel at hip and thigh level, **right** leg
  - **S75.992** Other specified injury of unspecified blood vessel at hip and thigh level, **left** leg
  - **S75.999** Other specified injury of unspecified blood vessel at hip and thigh level, unspecified leg

S76 Injury of muscle, fascia and tendon at hip and thigh level
  Code also any associated open wound (S71.-)
  EXCLUDES 2 injury of muscle, fascia and tendon at lower leg level (S86)
  sprain of joint and ligament of hip (S73.1)
  TIP: Refer to the Muscle/Tendon table at the beginning of this chapter.

> The appropriate 7th character is to be added to each code from category S76.
> A initial encounter
> D subsequent encounter
> S sequela

S76.0 Injury of muscle, fascia and tendon of hip

- **S76.00** Unspecified injury of muscle, fascia and tendon of hip
  - **S76.001** Unspecified injury of muscle, fascia and tendon of **right** hip
  - **S76.002** Unspecified injury of muscle, fascia and tendon of **left** hip
  - **S76.009** Unspecified injury of muscle, fascia and tendon of unspecified hip

- **S76.01** Strain of muscle, fascia and tendon of hip
  - **S76.011** Strain of muscle, fascia and tendon of **right** hip
  - **S76.012** Strain of muscle, fascia and tendon of **left** hip
  - **S76.019** Strain of muscle, fascia and tendon of unspecified hip

- **S76.02** Laceration of muscle, fascia and tendon of hip
  - **S76.021** Laceration of muscle, fascia and tendon of **right** hip
  - **S76.022** Laceration of muscle, fascia and tendon of **left** hip
  - **S76.029** Laceration of muscle, fascia and tendon of unspecified hip

- **S76.09** Other specified injury of muscle, fascia and tendon of hip
  - **S76.091** Other specified injury of muscle, fascia and tendon of **right** hip
  - **S76.092** Other specified injury of muscle, fascia and tendon of **left** hip
  - **S76.099** Other specified injury of muscle, fascia and tendon of unspecified hip

S76.1 Injury of quadriceps muscle, fascia and tendon
  Injury of patellar ligament (tendon)

- **S76.10** Unspecified injury of quadriceps muscle, fascia and tendon
  - **S76.101** Unspecified injury of **right** quadriceps muscle, fascia and tendon
  - **S76.102** Unspecified injury of **left** quadriceps muscle, fascia and tendon
  - **S76.109** Unspecified injury of unspecified quadriceps muscle, fascia and tendon

- ✓6th **S76.11** Strain of quadriceps muscle, fascia and tendon
  - ✓7th S76.111 Strain of right quadriceps muscle, fascia and tendon
  - ✓7th S76.112 Strain of left quadriceps muscle, fascia and tendon
  - ✓7th S76.119 Strain of unspecified quadriceps muscle, fascia and tendon
- ✓6th **S76.12** Laceration of quadriceps muscle, fascia and tendon
  - ✓7th S76.121 Laceration of right quadriceps muscle, fascia and tendon
  - ✓7th S76.122 Laceration of left quadriceps muscle, fascia and tendon
  - ✓7th S76.129 Laceration of unspecified quadriceps muscle, fascia and tendon
- ✓6th **S76.19** Other specified injury of quadriceps muscle, fascia and tendon
  - ✓7th S76.191 Other specified injury of right quadriceps muscle, fascia and tendon
  - ✓7th S76.192 Other specified injury of left quadriceps muscle, fascia and tendon
  - ✓7th S76.199 Other specified injury of unspecified quadriceps muscle, fascia and tendon
- ✓5th **S76.2** Injury of adductor muscle, fascia and tendon of thigh
  - ✓6th **S76.20** Unspecified injury of adductor muscle, fascia and tendon of thigh
    - ✓7th S76.201 Unspecified injury of adductor muscle, fascia and tendon of right thigh
    - ✓7th S76.202 Unspecified injury of adductor muscle, fascia and tendon of left thigh
    - ✓7th S76.209 Unspecified injury of adductor muscle, fascia and tendon of unspecified thigh
  - ✓6th **S76.21** Strain of adductor muscle, fascia and tendon of thigh
    - ✓7th S76.211 Strain of adductor muscle, fascia and tendon of right thigh
    - ✓7th S76.212 Strain of adductor muscle, fascia and tendon of left thigh
    - ✓7th S76.219 Strain of adductor muscle, fascia and tendon of unspecified thigh
  - ✓6th **S76.22** Laceration of adductor muscle, fascia and tendon of thigh
    - ✓7th S76.221 Laceration of adductor muscle, fascia and tendon of right thigh
    - ✓7th S76.222 Laceration of adductor muscle, fascia and tendon of left thigh
    - ✓7th S76.229 Laceration of adductor muscle, fascia and tendon of unspecified thigh
  - ✓6th **S76.29** Other injury of adductor muscle, fascia and tendon of thigh
    - ✓7th S76.291 Other injury of adductor muscle, fascia and tendon of right thigh
    - ✓7th S76.292 Other injury of adductor muscle, fascia and tendon of left thigh
    - ✓7th S76.299 Other injury of adductor muscle, fascia and tendon of unspecified thigh
- ✓5th **S76.3** Injury of muscle, fascia and tendon of the posterior muscle group at thigh level
  - ✓6th **S76.30** Unspecified injury of muscle, fascia and tendon of the posterior muscle group at thigh level
    - ✓7th S76.301 Unspecified injury of muscle, fascia and tendon of the posterior muscle group at thigh level, right thigh
    - ✓7th S76.302 Unspecified injury of muscle, fascia and tendon of the posterior muscle group at thigh level, left thigh
    - ✓7th S76.309 Unspecified injury of muscle, fascia and tendon of the posterior muscle group at thigh level, unspecified thigh
  - ✓6th **S76.31** Strain of muscle, fascia and tendon of the posterior muscle group at thigh level
    - ✓7th S76.311 Strain of muscle, fascia and tendon of the posterior muscle group at thigh level, right thigh
    - ✓7th S76.312 Strain of muscle, fascia and tendon of the posterior muscle group at thigh level, left thigh
    - ✓7th S76.319 Strain of muscle, fascia and tendon of the posterior muscle group at thigh level, unspecified thigh
  - ✓6th **S76.32** Laceration of muscle, fascia and tendon of the posterior muscle group at thigh level
    - ✓7th S76.321 Laceration of muscle, fascia and tendon of the posterior muscle group at thigh level, right thigh
    - ✓7th S76.322 Laceration of muscle, fascia and tendon of the posterior muscle group at thigh level, left thigh
    - ✓7th S76.329 Laceration of muscle, fascia and tendon of the posterior muscle group at thigh level, unspecified thigh
  - ✓6th **S76.39** Other specified injury of muscle, fascia and tendon of the posterior muscle group at thigh level
    - ✓7th S76.391 Other specified injury of muscle, fascia and tendon of the posterior muscle group at thigh level, right thigh
    - ✓7th S76.392 Other specified injury of muscle, fascia and tendon of the posterior muscle group at thigh level, left thigh
    - ✓7th S76.399 Other specified injury of muscle, fascia and tendon of the posterior muscle group at thigh level, unspecified thigh
- ✓5th **S76.8** Injury of other specified muscles, fascia and tendons at thigh level
  - ✓6th **S76.80** Unspecified injury of other specified muscles, fascia and tendons at thigh level
    - ✓7th S76.801 Unspecified injury of other specified muscles, fascia and tendons at thigh level, right thigh
    - ✓7th S76.802 Unspecified injury of other specified muscles, fascia and tendons at thigh level, left thigh
    - ✓7th S76.809 Unspecified injury of other specified muscles, fascia and tendons at thigh level, unspecified thigh
  - ✓6th **S76.81** Strain of other specified muscles, fascia and tendons at thigh level
    - ✓7th S76.811 Strain of other specified muscles, fascia and tendons at thigh level, right thigh
    - ✓7th S76.812 Strain of other specified muscles, fascia and tendons at thigh level, left thigh
    - ✓7th S76.819 Strain of other specified muscles, fascia and tendons at thigh level, unspecified thigh
  - ✓6th **S76.82** Laceration of other specified muscles, fascia and tendons at thigh level
    - ✓7th S76.821 Laceration of other specified muscles, fascia and tendons at thigh level, right thigh
    - ✓7th S76.822 Laceration of other specified muscles, fascia and tendons at thigh level, left thigh
    - ✓7th S76.829 Laceration of other specified muscles, fascia and tendons at thigh level, unspecified thigh
  - ✓6th **S76.89** Other injury of other specified muscles, fascia and tendons at thigh level
    - ✓7th S76.891 Other injury of other specified muscles, fascia and tendons at thigh level, right thigh
    - ✓7th S76.892 Other injury of other specified muscles, fascia and tendons at thigh level, left thigh
    - ✓7th S76.899 Other injury of other specified muscles, fascia and tendons at thigh level, unspecified thigh
- ✓5th **S76.9** Injury of unspecified muscles, fascia and tendons at thigh level
  - ✓6th **S76.90** Unspecified injury of unspecified muscles, fascia and tendons at thigh level
    - ✓7th S76.901 Unspecified injury of unspecified muscles, fascia and tendons at thigh level, right thigh
    - ✓7th S76.902 Unspecified injury of unspecified muscles, fascia and tendons at thigh level, left thigh
    - ✓7th S76.909 Unspecified injury of unspecified muscles, fascia and tendons at thigh level, unspecified thigh
  - ✓6th **S76.91** Strain of unspecified muscles, fascia and tendons at thigh level
    - ✓7th S76.911 Strain of unspecified muscles, fascia and tendons at thigh level, right thigh
    - ✓7th S76.912 Strain of unspecified muscles, fascia and tendons at thigh level, left thigh
    - ✓7th S76.919 Strain of unspecified muscles, fascia and tendons at thigh level, unspecified thigh
  - ✓6th **S76.92** Laceration of unspecified muscles, fascia and tendons at thigh level
    - ✓7th S76.921 Laceration of unspecified muscles, fascia and tendons at thigh level, right thigh
    - ✓7th S76.922 Laceration of unspecified muscles, fascia and tendons at thigh level, left thigh

Chapter 19. Injury, Poisoning and Certain Other Consequences of External Causes

- ✓7th **S76.929** Laceration of unspecified muscles, fascia and tendons at thigh level, unspecified thigh
- ✓6th **S76.99** Other specified injury of unspecified muscles, fascia and tendons at thigh level
  - ✓7th **S76.991** Other specified injury of unspecified muscles, fascia and tendons at thigh level, right thigh
  - ✓7th **S76.992** Other specified injury of unspecified muscles, fascia and tendons at thigh level, left thigh
  - ✓7th **S76.999** Other specified injury of unspecified muscles, fascia and tendons at thigh level, unspecified thigh

✓4th **S77** **Crushing injury** of hip and thigh

Use additional code(s) for all associated injuries

EXCLUDES 2: crushing injury of ankle and foot (S97.-)
crushing injury of lower leg (S87.-)

The appropriate 7th character is to be added to each code from category S77.
- A initial encounter
- D subsequent encounter
- S sequela

- ✓5th **S77.0** Crushing injury of hip
  - ✓x7th **S77.00** Crushing injury of unspecified hip
  - ✓x7th **S77.01** Crushing injury of right hip
  - ✓x7th **S77.02** Crushing injury of left hip
- ✓5th **S77.1** Crushing injury of thigh
  - ✓x7th **S77.10** Crushing injury of unspecified thigh
  - ✓x7th **S77.11** Crushing injury of right thigh
  - ✓x7th **S77.12** Crushing injury of left thigh
- ✓5th **S77.2** Crushing injury of hip with thigh
  - ✓x7th **S77.20** Crushing injury of unspecified hip with thigh
  - ✓x7th **S77.21** Crushing injury of right hip with thigh
  - ✓x7th **S77.22** Crushing injury of left hip with thigh

✓4th **S78** **Traumatic amputation** of hip and thigh

An amputation not identified as partial or complete should be coded to complete

EXCLUDES 1: traumatic amputation of knee (S88.0-)

The appropriate 7th character is to be added to each code from category S78.
- A initial encounter
- D subsequent encounter
- S sequela

- ✓5th **S78.0** Traumatic amputation at hip joint
  - ✓6th **S78.01** Complete traumatic amputation at hip joint
    - ✓7th **S78.011** Complete traumatic amputation at right hip joint [HCC ESR COM]
    - ✓7th **S78.012** Complete traumatic amputation at left hip joint [HCC ESR COM]
    - ✓7th **S78.019** Complete traumatic amputation at unspecified hip joint [HCC ESR COM]
  - ✓6th **S78.02** Partial traumatic amputation at hip joint
    - ✓7th **S78.021** Partial traumatic amputation at right hip joint [HCC ESR COM]
    - ✓7th **S78.022** Partial traumatic amputation at left hip joint [HCC ESR COM]
    - ✓7th **S78.029** Partial traumatic amputation at unspecified hip joint [HCC ESR COM]
- ✓5th **S78.1** Traumatic amputation at level between hip and knee

  EXCLUDES 1: traumatic amputation of knee (S88.0-)

  - ✓6th **S78.11** Complete traumatic amputation at level between hip and knee
    - ✓7th **S78.111** Complete traumatic amputation at level between right hip and knee [HCC ESR COM]
    - ✓7th **S78.112** Complete traumatic amputation at level between left hip and knee [HCC ESR COM]
    - ✓7th **S78.119** Complete traumatic amputation at level between unspecified hip and knee
  - ✓6th **S78.12** Partial traumatic amputation at level between hip and knee
    - ✓7th **S78.121** Partial traumatic amputation at level between right hip and knee [HCC ESR COM]
    - ✓7th **S78.122** Partial traumatic amputation at level between left hip and knee [HCC ESR COM]
    - ✓7th **S78.129** Partial traumatic amputation at level between unspecified hip and knee [HCC ESR COM]
- ✓5th **S78.9** Traumatic amputation of hip and thigh, level unspecified
  - ✓6th **S78.91** Complete traumatic amputation of hip and thigh, level unspecified
    - ✓7th **S78.911** Complete traumatic amputation of right hip and thigh, level unspecified [HCC ESR COM]
    - ✓7th **S78.912** Complete traumatic amputation of left hip and thigh, level unspecified [HCC ESR COM]
    - ✓7th **S78.919** Complete traumatic amputation of unspecified hip and thigh, level unspecified [HCC ESR COM]
  - ✓6th **S78.92** Partial traumatic amputation of hip and thigh, level unspecified
    - ✓7th **S78.921** Partial traumatic amputation of right hip and thigh, level unspecified [HCC ESR COM]
    - ✓7th **S78.922** Partial traumatic amputation of left hip and thigh, level unspecified [HCC ESR COM]
    - ✓7th **S78.929** Partial traumatic amputation of unspecified hip and thigh, level unspecified [HCC ESR COM]

✓4th **S79** Other and unspecified injuries of hip and thigh

NOTE: A fracture not indicated as open or closed should be coded to closed

AHA: 2018,2Q,12; 2018,1Q,3; 2015,3Q,37-39

The appropriate 7th character is to be added to each code from subcategories S79.0 and S79.1.
- A initial encounter for closed fracture
- D subsequent encounter for fracture with routine healing
- G subsequent encounter for fracture with delayed healing
- K subsequent encounter for fracture with nonunion
- P subsequent encounter for fracture with malunion
- S sequela

- ✓5th **S79.0** **Physeal fracture** of upper end of femur

  EXCLUDES 1: apophyseal fracture of upper end of femur (S72.13-)
  nontraumatic slipped upper femoral epiphysis (M93.0-)

  AHA: 2019,4Q,56

  - ✓6th **S79.00** Unspecified physeal fracture of upper end of femur
    - ✓7th **S79.001** Unspecified physeal fracture of upper end of right femur [HCC ESR COM Q]
    - ✓7th **S79.002** Unspecified physeal fracture of upper end of left femur [HCC ESR COM Q]
    - ✓7th **S79.009** Unspecified physeal fracture of upper end of unspecified femur [HCC ESR COM Q]
  - ✓6th **S79.01** **Salter-Harris Type I** physeal fracture of upper end of femur

    Acute on chronic slipped capital femoral epiphysis (traumatic)
    Acute slipped capital femoral epiphysis (traumatic)
    Capital femoral epiphyseal fracture

    EXCLUDES 1: chronic slipped upper femoral epiphysis (nontraumatic) (M93.02-)

    - ✓7th **S79.011** Salter-Harris Type I physeal fracture of upper end of right femur [HCC ESR COM Q]
    - ✓7th **S79.012** Salter-Harris Type I physeal fracture of upper end of left femur [HCC ESR COM Q]
    - ✓7th **S79.019** Salter-Harris Type I physeal fracture of upper end of unspecified femur [HCC ESR COM Q]
  - ✓6th **S79.09** Other physeal fracture of upper end of femur
    - ✓7th **S79.091** Other physeal fracture of upper end of right femur [HCC ESR COM Q]
    - ✓7th **S79.092** Other physeal fracture of upper end of left femur [HCC ESR COM Q]
    - ✓7th **S79.099** Other physeal fracture of upper end of unspecified femur [HCC ESR COM Q]

[HCC] CMS-HCC [Rx] Rx HCC [ESR] ESRD HCC [COM] Commercial HCC [N] Newborn: 0 [P] Pediatric: 0-17 [M] Maternity: 9-64 [A] Adult: 15-124

S79.1 Physeal fracture of lower end of femur
AHA: 2019,4Q,56

- **S79.10** Unspecified physeal fracture of lower end of femur
  - S79.101 Unspecified physeal fracture of lower end of right femur
  - S79.102 Unspecified physeal fracture of lower end of left femur
  - S79.109 Unspecified physeal fracture of lower end of unspecified femur
- **S79.11** Salter-Harris Type I physeal fracture of lower end of femur
  - S79.111 Salter-Harris Type I physeal fracture of lower end of right femur
  - S79.112 Salter-Harris Type I physeal fracture of lower end of left femur
  - S79.119 Salter-Harris Type I physeal fracture of lower end of unspecified femur
- **S79.12** Salter-Harris Type II physeal fracture of lower end of femur
  - S79.121 Salter-Harris Type II physeal fracture of lower end of right femur
  - S79.122 Salter-Harris Type II physeal fracture of lower end of left femur
  - S79.129 Salter-Harris Type II physeal fracture of lower end of unspecified femur
- **S79.13** Salter-Harris Type III physeal fracture of lower end of femur
  - S79.131 Salter-Harris Type III physeal fracture of lower end of right femur
  - S79.132 Salter-Harris Type III physeal fracture of lower end of left femur
  - S79.139 Salter-Harris Type III physeal fracture of lower end of unspecified femur
- **S79.14** Salter-Harris Type IV physeal fracture of lower end of femur
  - S79.141 Salter-Harris Type IV physeal fracture of lower end of right femur
  - S79.142 Salter-Harris Type IV physeal fracture of lower end of left femur
  - S79.149 Salter-Harris Type IV physeal fracture of lower end of unspecified femur
- **S79.19** Other physeal fracture of lower end of femur
  - S79.191 Other physeal fracture of lower end of right femur
  - S79.192 Other physeal fracture of lower end of left femur
  - S79.199 Other physeal fracture of lower end of unspecified femur

S79.8 Other specified injuries of hip and thigh

The appropriate 7th character is to be added to each code in subcategory S79.8.
- A initial encounter
- D subsequent encounter
- S sequela

- **S79.81** Other specified injuries of hip
  - S79.811 Other specified injuries of right hip
  - S79.812 Other specified injuries of left hip
  - S79.819 Other specified injuries of unspecified hip
- **S79.82** Other specified injuries of thigh
  - S79.821 Other specified injuries of right thigh
  - S79.822 Other specified injuries of left thigh
  - S79.829 Other specified injuries of unspecified thigh

S79.9 Unspecified injury of hip and thigh

The appropriate 7th character is to be added to each code in subcategory S79.9.
- A initial encounter
- D subsequent encounter
- S sequela

- **S79.91** Unspecified injury of hip
  - S79.911 Unspecified injury of right hip
  - S79.912 Unspecified injury of left hip
  - S79.919 Unspecified injury of unspecified hip
- **S79.92** Unspecified injury of thigh
  - S79.921 Unspecified injury of right thigh
  - S79.922 Unspecified injury of left thigh
  - S79.929 Unspecified injury of unspecified thigh

Injuries to the knee and lower leg (S80-S89)

EXCLUDES 2: burns and corrosions (T20-T32)
frostbite (T33-T34)
injuries of ankle and foot, except fracture of ankle and malleolus (S90-S99)
insect bite or sting, venomous (T63.4)

S80 Superficial injury of knee and lower leg

EXCLUDES 2: superficial injury of ankle and foot (S90.-)

The appropriate 7th character is to be added to each code from category S80.
- A initial encounter
- D subsequent encounter
- S sequela

S80.0 Contusion of knee
- S80.00 Contusion of unspecified knee
- S80.01 Contusion of right knee
- S80.02 Contusion of left knee

S80.1 Contusion of lower leg
- S80.10 Contusion of unspecified lower leg
- S80.11 Contusion of right lower leg
- S80.12 Contusion of left lower leg

S80.2 Other superficial injuries of knee
- **S80.21** Abrasion of knee
  - S80.211 Abrasion, right knee
  - S80.212 Abrasion, left knee
  - S80.219 Abrasion, unspecified knee
- **S80.22** Blister (nonthermal) of knee
  - S80.221 Blister (nonthermal), right knee
  - S80.222 Blister (nonthermal), left knee
  - S80.229 Blister (nonthermal), unspecified knee
- **S80.24** External constriction of knee
  - S80.241 External constriction, right knee
  - S80.242 External constriction, left knee
  - S80.249 External constriction, unspecified knee
- **S80.25** Superficial foreign body of knee
  Splinter in the knee
  - S80.251 Superficial foreign body, right knee
  - S80.252 Superficial foreign body, left knee
  - S80.259 Superficial foreign body, unspecified knee
- **S80.26** Insect bite (nonvenomous) of knee
  - S80.261 Insect bite (nonvenomous), right knee
  - S80.262 Insect bite (nonvenomous), left knee
  - S80.269 Insect bite (nonvenomous), unspecified knee
- **S80.27** Other superficial bite of knee
  EXCLUDES 1: open bite of knee (S81.05-)
  - S80.271 Other superficial bite of right knee
  - S80.272 Other superficial bite of left knee
  - S80.279 Other superficial bite of unspecified knee

S80.8 Other superficial injuries of lower leg
- **S80.81** Abrasion of lower leg
  - S80.811 Abrasion, right lower leg
  - S80.812 Abrasion, left lower leg
  - S80.819 Abrasion, unspecified lower leg
- **S80.82** Blister (nonthermal) of lower leg
  - S80.821 Blister (nonthermal), right lower leg
  - S80.822 Blister (nonthermal), left lower leg
  - S80.829 Blister (nonthermal), unspecified lower leg
- **S80.84** External constriction of lower leg
  - S80.841 External constriction, right lower leg
  - S80.842 External constriction, left lower leg
  - S80.849 External constriction, unspecified lower leg

- ✓6th **S80.85** Superficial foreign body of lower leg
  Splinter in the lower leg
  - ✓7th **S80.851** Superficial foreign body, right lower leg
  - ✓7th **S80.852** Superficial foreign body, left lower leg
  - ✓7th **S80.859** Superficial foreign body, unspecified lower leg
- ✓6th **S80.86** Insect bite (nonvenomous) of lower leg
  - ✓7th **S80.861** Insect bite (nonvenomous), right lower leg
  - ✓7th **S80.862** Insect bite (nonvenomous), left lower leg
  - ✓7th **S80.869** Insect bite (nonvenomous), unspecified lower leg
- ✓6th **S80.87** Other superficial bite of lower leg
  - EXCLUDES 1 open bite of lower leg (S81.85-)
  - ✓7th **S80.871** Other superficial bite, right lower leg
  - ✓7th **S80.872** Other superficial bite, left lower leg
  - ✓7th **S80.879** Other superficial bite, unspecified lower leg
- ✓5th **S80.9** Unspecified superficial injury of knee and lower leg
  - ✓6th **S80.91** Unspecified superficial injury of knee
    - ✓7th **S80.911** Unspecified superficial injury of right knee
    - ✓7th **S80.912** Unspecified superficial injury of left knee
    - ✓7th **S80.919** Unspecified superficial injury of unspecified knee
  - ✓6th **S80.92** Unspecified superficial injury of lower leg
    - ✓7th **S80.921** Unspecified superficial injury of right lower leg
    - ✓7th **S80.922** Unspecified superficial injury of left lower leg
    - ✓7th **S80.929** Unspecified superficial injury of unspecified lower leg

- ✓4th **S81** Open wound of knee and lower leg
  Code also any associated wound infection
  EXCLUDES 1 open fracture of knee and lower leg (S82.-)
  traumatic amputation of lower leg (S88.-)
  EXCLUDES 2 open wound of ankle and foot (S91.-)

  The appropriate 7th character is to be added to each code from category S81.
  A initial encounter
  D subsequent encounter
  S sequela

  - ✓5th **S81.0** Open wound of knee
    - ✓6th **S81.00** Unspecified open wound of knee
      - ✓7th **S81.001** Unspecified open wound, right knee
      - ✓7th **S81.002** Unspecified open wound, left knee
      - ✓7th **S81.009** Unspecified open wound, unspecified knee
    - ✓6th **S81.01** Laceration without foreign body of knee
      - ✓7th **S81.011** Laceration without foreign body, right knee
      - ✓7th **S81.012** Laceration without foreign body, left knee
      - ✓7th **S81.019** Laceration without foreign body, unspecified knee
    - ✓6th **S81.02** Laceration with foreign body of knee
      - ✓7th **S81.021** Laceration with foreign body, right knee
      - ✓7th **S81.022** Laceration with foreign body, left knee
      - ✓7th **S81.029** Laceration with foreign body, unspecified knee
    - ✓6th **S81.03** Puncture wound without foreign body of knee
      AHA: 2025,1Q,31
      - ✓7th **S81.031** Puncture wound without foreign body, right knee
      - ✓7th **S81.032** Puncture wound without foreign body, left knee
      - ✓7th **S81.039** Puncture wound without foreign body, unspecified knee
    - ✓6th **S81.04** Puncture wound with foreign body of knee
      - ✓7th **S81.041** Puncture wound with foreign body, right knee
      - ✓7th **S81.042** Puncture wound with foreign body, left knee
      - ✓7th **S81.049** Puncture wound with foreign body, unspecified knee
  - ✓6th **S81.05** Open bite of knee
    Bite of knee NOS
    EXCLUDES 1 superficial bite of knee (S80.27-)
    - ✓7th **S81.051** Open bite, right knee
    - ✓7th **S81.052** Open bite, left knee
    - ✓7th **S81.059** Open bite, unspecified knee
  - ✓5th **S81.8** Open wound of lower leg
    - ✓6th **S81.80** Unspecified open wound of lower leg
      AHA: 2016,3Q,24
      - ✓7th **S81.801** Unspecified open wound, right lower leg
      - ✓7th **S81.802** Unspecified open wound, left lower leg
      - ✓7th **S81.809** Unspecified open wound, unspecified lower leg
    - ✓6th **S81.81** Laceration without foreign body of lower leg
      - ✓7th **S81.811** Laceration without foreign body, right lower leg
      - ✓7th **S81.812** Laceration without foreign body, left lower leg
      - ✓7th **S81.819** Laceration without foreign body, unspecified lower leg
    - ✓6th **S81.82** Laceration with foreign body of lower leg
      - ✓7th **S81.821** Laceration with foreign body, right lower leg
      - ✓7th **S81.822** Laceration with foreign body, left lower leg
      - ✓7th **S81.829** Laceration with foreign body, unspecified lower leg
    - ✓6th **S81.83** Puncture wound without foreign body of lower leg
      AHA: 2016,3Q,24
      - ✓7th **S81.831** Puncture wound without foreign body, right lower leg
      - ✓7th **S81.832** Puncture wound without foreign body, left lower leg
      - ✓7th **S81.839** Puncture wound without foreign body, unspecified lower leg
    - ✓6th **S81.84** Puncture wound with foreign body of lower leg
      AHA: 2016,3Q,24
      - ✓7th **S81.841** Puncture wound with foreign body, right lower leg
      - ✓7th **S81.842** Puncture wound with foreign body, left lower leg
      - ✓7th **S81.849** Puncture wound with foreign body, unspecified lower leg
    - ✓6th **S81.85** Open bite of lower leg
      Bite of lower leg NOS
      EXCLUDES 1 superficial bite of lower leg (S80.86-, S80.87-)
      - ✓7th **S81.851** Open bite, right lower leg
      - ✓7th **S81.852** Open bite, left lower leg
      - ✓7th **S81.859** Open bite, unspecified lower leg

Chapter 19. Injury, Poisoning and Certain Other Consequences of External Causes

S82 Fracture of lower leg, including ankle

NOTE
A fracture not indicated as displaced or nondisplaced should be coded to displaced

A fracture not indicated as open or closed should be coded to closed

The open fracture designations are based on the Gustilo open fracture classification.

INCLUDES fracture of malleolus
EXCLUDES 1 traumatic amputation of lower leg (S88.-)
EXCLUDES 2 fracture of foot, except ankle (S92.-)
periprosthetic fracture around internal prosthetic ankle joint (M97.2)
periprosthetic fracture around internal prosthetic implant of knee joint (M97.1-)

AHA: 2018,2Q,12; 2016,1Q,33; 2015,3Q,37-39
DEF: Diaphysis: Central shaft of a long bone.
DEF: Epiphysis: Proximal and distal rounded ends of a long bone, communicates with the joint.
DEF: Metaphysis: Section of a long bone located between the epiphysis and diaphysis at the proximal and distal ends.
DEF: Physis (growth plate): Narrow zone of cartilaginous tissue between the epiphysis and metaphysis at each end of a long bone. In childhood, proliferation of cells in this zone lengthens the bone. As the bone matures, this area thins, ossification eventually fusing into solid bone and growth stops. **Synonym(s):** Epiphyseal plate.

The appropriate 7th character is to be added to all codes from category S82 [unless otherwise indicated].
- initial encounter for open fracture NOS
- A initial encounter for closed fracture
- B initial encounter for open fracture type I or II
- C initial encounter for open fracture type IIIA, IIIB, or IIIC
- D subsequent encounter for closed fracture with routine healing
- E subsequent encounter for open fracture type I or II with routine healing
- F subsequent encounter for open fracture type IIIA, IIIB, or IIIC with routine healing
- G subsequent encounter for closed fracture with delayed healing
- H subsequent encounter for open fracture type I or II with delayed healing
- J subsequent encounter for open fracture type IIIA, IIIB, or IIIC with delayed healing
- K subsequent encounter for closed fracture with nonunion
- M subsequent encounter for open fracture type I or II with nonunion
- N subsequent encounter for open fracture type IIIA, IIIB, or IIIC with nonunion
- P subsequent encounter for closed fracture with malunion
- Q subsequent encounter for open fracture type I or II with malunion
- R subsequent encounter for open fracture type IIIA, IIIB, or IIIC with malunion
- S sequela

S82.0 Fracture of patella
Knee cap

S82.00 Unspecified fracture of patella
- S82.001 Unspecified fracture of right patella
- S82.002 Unspecified fracture of left patella
- S82.009 Unspecified fracture of unspecified patella

S82.01 Osteochondral fracture of patella
- S82.011 Displaced osteochondral fracture of right patella
- S82.012 Displaced osteochondral fracture of left patella
- S82.013 Displaced osteochondral fracture of unspecified patella
- S82.014 Nondisplaced osteochondral fracture of right patella
- S82.015 Nondisplaced osteochondral fracture of left patella
- S82.016 Nondisplaced osteochondral fracture of unspecified patella

S82.02 Longitudinal fracture of patella
- S82.021 Displaced longitudinal fracture of right patella
- S82.022 Displaced longitudinal fracture of left patella
- S82.023 Displaced longitudinal fracture of unspecified patella
- S82.024 Nondisplaced longitudinal fracture of right patella
- S82.025 Nondisplaced longitudinal fracture of left patella
- S82.026 Nondisplaced longitudinal fracture of unspecified patella

S82.03 Transverse fracture of patella
- S82.031 Displaced transverse fracture of right patella
- S82.032 Displaced transverse fracture of left patella
- S82.033 Displaced transverse fracture of unspecified patella
- S82.034 Nondisplaced transverse fracture of right patella
- S82.035 Nondisplaced transverse fracture of left patella
- S82.036 Nondisplaced transverse fracture of unspecified patella

S82.04 Comminuted fracture of patella
- S82.041 Displaced comminuted fracture of right patella
- S82.042 Displaced comminuted fracture of left patella
- S82.043 Displaced comminuted fracture of unspecified patella
- S82.044 Nondisplaced comminuted fracture of right patella
- S82.045 Nondisplaced comminuted fracture of left patella
- S82.046 Nondisplaced comminuted fracture of unspecified patella

S82.09 Other fracture of patella
- S82.091 Other fracture of right patella
- S82.092 Other fracture of left patella
- S82.099 Other fracture of unspecified patella

S82.1 Fracture of upper end of tibia
Fracture of proximal end of tibia
EXCLUDES 2 fracture of shaft of tibia (S82.2-)
physeal fracture of upper end of tibia (S89.0-)

S82.10 Unspecified fracture of upper end of tibia
- S82.101 Unspecified fracture of upper end of right tibia
- S82.102 Unspecified fracture of upper end of left tibia
- S82.109 Unspecified fracture of upper end of unspecified tibia

S82.11 Fracture of tibial spine
- S82.111 Displaced fracture of right tibial spine
- S82.112 Displaced fracture of left tibial spine
- S82.113 Displaced fracture of unspecified tibial spine
- S82.114 Nondisplaced fracture of right tibial spine
- S82.115 Nondisplaced fracture of left tibial spine
- S82.116 Nondisplaced fracture of unspecified tibial spine

S82.12 Fracture of lateral condyle of tibia
- S82.121 Displaced fracture of lateral condyle of right tibia
- S82.122 Displaced fracture of lateral condyle of left tibia
- S82.123 Displaced fracture of lateral condyle of unspecified tibia
- S82.124 Nondisplaced fracture of lateral condyle of right tibia
- S82.125 Nondisplaced fracture of lateral condyle of left tibia
- S82.126 Nondisplaced fracture of lateral condyle of unspecified tibia

S82.13 Fracture of medial condyle of tibia
- S82.131 Displaced fracture of medial condyle of right tibia

- √7th S82.132 **Displaced** fracture of medial condyle of **left** tibia ♀
- √7th S82.133 **Displaced** fracture of medial condyle of unspecified tibia ♀
- √7th S82.134 **Nondisplaced** fracture of medial condyle of **right** tibia ♀
- √7th S82.135 **Nondisplaced** fracture of medial condyle of **left** tibia ♀
- √7th S82.136 **Nondisplaced** fracture of medial condyle of unspecified tibia ♀
- √6th S82.14 **Bicondylar** fracture of tibia
    - Fracture of tibial plateau NOS
    - √7th S82.141 **Displaced** bicondylar fracture of **right** tibia ♀
    - √7th S82.142 **Displaced** bicondylar fracture of **left** tibia ♀
    - √7th S82.143 **Displaced** bicondylar fracture of unspecified tibia ♀
    - √7th S82.144 **Nondisplaced** bicondylar fracture of **right** tibia ♀
    - √7th S82.145 **Nondisplaced** bicondylar fracture of **left** tibia ♀
    - √7th S82.146 **Nondisplaced** bicondylar fracture of unspecified tibia ♀
- √6th S82.15 **Fracture of tibial tuberosity**
    - √7th S82.151 **Displaced** fracture of **right** tibial tuberosity ♀
    - √7th S82.152 **Displaced** fracture of **left** tibial tuberosity ♀
    - √7th S82.153 **Displaced** fracture of unspecified tibial tuberosity ♀
    - √7th S82.154 **Nondisplaced** fracture of **right** tibial tuberosity ♀
    - √7th S82.155 **Nondisplaced** fracture of **left** tibial tuberosity ♀
    - √7th S82.156 **Nondisplaced** fracture of unspecified tibial tuberosity ♀
- √6th S82.16 **Torus** fracture of upper end of tibia

    > The appropriate 7th character is to be added to all codes in subcategory S82.16.
    > A initial encounter for closed fracture
    > D subsequent encounter for fracture with routine healing
    > G subsequent encounter for fracture with delayed healing
    > K subsequent encounter for fracture with nonunion
    > P subsequent encounter for fracture with malunion
    > S sequela

    - √7th S82.161 Torus fracture of upper end of **right** tibia ♀
    - √7th S82.162 Torus fracture of upper end of **left** tibia ♀
    - √7th S82.169 Torus fracture of upper end of unspecified tibia ♀
- √6th S82.19 **Other** fracture of upper end of tibia
    - √7th S82.191 Other fracture of upper end of **right** tibia ♀
    - √7th S82.192 Other fracture of upper end of **left** tibia ♀
    - √7th S82.199 Other fracture of upper end of unspecified tibia ♀
- √5th S82.2 **Fracture of shaft of tibia**
    - √6th S82.20 **Unspecified** fracture of shaft of tibia
        - Fracture of tibia NOS
        - √7th S82.201 **Unspecified** fracture of shaft of **right** tibia ♀
        - √7th S82.202 **Unspecified** fracture of shaft of **left** tibia ♀
        - √7th S82.209 **Unspecified** fracture of shaft of unspecified tibia ♀
    - √6th S82.22 **Transverse** fracture of shaft of tibia
        - √7th S82.221 **Displaced** transverse fracture of shaft of **right** tibia ♀
        - √7th S82.222 **Displaced** transverse fracture of shaft of **left** tibia ♀
        - √7th S82.223 **Displaced** transverse fracture of shaft of unspecified tibia ♀
        - √7th S82.224 **Nondisplaced** transverse fracture of shaft of **right** tibia ♀
        - √7th S82.225 **Nondisplaced** transverse fracture of shaft of **left** tibia ♀
        - √7th S82.226 **Nondisplaced** transverse fracture of shaft of unspecified tibia ♀
    - √6th S82.23 **Oblique** fracture of shaft of tibia
        - √7th S82.231 **Displaced** oblique fracture of shaft of **right** tibia ♀
        - √7th S82.232 **Displaced** oblique fracture of shaft of **left** tibia ♀
        - √7th S82.233 **Displaced** oblique fracture of shaft of unspecified tibia ♀
        - √7th S82.234 **Nondisplaced** oblique fracture of shaft of **right** tibia ♀
        - √7th S82.235 **Nondisplaced** oblique fracture of shaft of **left** tibia ♀
        - √7th S82.236 **Nondisplaced** oblique fracture of shaft of unspecified tibia ♀
    - √6th S82.24 **Spiral** fracture of shaft of tibia
        - Toddler fracture
        - √7th S82.241 **Displaced** spiral fracture of shaft of **right** tibia ♀
        - √7th S82.242 **Displaced** spiral fracture of shaft of **left** tibia ♀
        - √7th S82.243 **Displaced** spiral fracture of shaft of unspecified tibia ♀
        - √7th S82.244 **Nondisplaced** spiral fracture of shaft of **right** tibia ♀
        - √7th S82.245 **Nondisplaced** spiral fracture of shaft of **left** tibia ♀
        - √7th S82.246 **Nondisplaced** spiral fracture of shaft of unspecified tibia ♀
    - √6th S82.25 **Comminuted** fracture of shaft of tibia
        - √7th S82.251 **Displaced** comminuted fracture of shaft of **right** tibia ♀
        - √7th S82.252 **Displaced** comminuted fracture of shaft of **left** tibia ♀
        - √7th S82.253 **Displaced** comminuted fracture of shaft of unspecified tibia ♀
        - √7th S82.254 **Nondisplaced** comminuted fracture of shaft of **right** tibia ♀
        - √7th S82.255 **Nondisplaced** comminuted fracture of shaft of **left** tibia ♀
        - √7th S82.256 **Nondisplaced** comminuted fracture of shaft of unspecified tibia ♀
    - √6th S82.26 **Segmental** fracture of shaft of tibia
        - √7th S82.261 **Displaced** segmental fracture of shaft of **right** tibia ♀
        - √7th S82.262 **Displaced** segmental fracture of shaft of **left** tibia ♀
        - √7th S82.263 **Displaced** segmental fracture of shaft of unspecified tibia ♀
        - √7th S82.264 **Nondisplaced** segmental fracture of shaft of **right** tibia ♀
        - √7th S82.265 **Nondisplaced** segmental fracture of shaft of **left** tibia ♀
        - √7th S82.266 **Nondisplaced** segmental fracture of shaft of unspecified tibia ♀
    - √6th S82.29 **Other** fracture of shaft of tibia
        - √7th S82.291 Other fracture of shaft of **right** tibia ♀
        - √7th S82.292 Other fracture of shaft of **left** tibia ♀
        - √7th S82.299 Other fracture of shaft of unspecified tibia ♀
- √5th S82.3 **Fracture of lower end of tibia**
    - *EXCLUDES 1* bimalleolar fracture of lower leg (S82.84-)
      fracture of medial malleolus alone (S82.5-)
      Maisonneuve's fracture (S82.86-)
      pilon fracture of distal tibia (S82.87-)
      trimalleolar fractures of lower leg (S82.85-)
    - √6th S82.30 **Unspecified** fracture of lower end of tibia
        - √7th S82.301 Unspecified fracture of lower end of **right** tibia ♀
        - √7th S82.302 Unspecified fracture of lower end of **left** tibia ♀
        - √7th S82.309 Unspecified fracture of lower end of unspecified tibia ♀

S82.31 Torus fracture of lower end of tibia

The appropriate 7th character is to be added to all codes in subcategory S82.31.
- A initial encounter for closed fracture
- D subsequent encounter for fracture with routine healing
- G subsequent encounter for fracture with delayed healing
- K subsequent encounter for fracture with nonunion
- P subsequent encounter for fracture with malunion
- S sequela

- S82.311 Torus fracture of lower end of right tibia
- S82.312 Torus fracture of lower end of left tibia
- S82.319 Torus fracture of lower end of unspecified tibia

S82.39 Other fracture of lower end of tibia
AHA: 2015,1Q,25
- S82.391 Other fracture of lower end of right tibia
- S82.392 Other fracture of lower end of left tibia
- S82.399 Other fracture of lower end of unspecified tibia

S82.4 Fracture of shaft of fibula
EXCLUDES 2: fracture of lateral malleolus alone (S82.6-)

S82.40 Unspecified fracture of shaft of fibula
- S82.401 Unspecified fracture of shaft of right fibula
- S82.402 Unspecified fracture of shaft of left fibula
- S82.409 Unspecified fracture of shaft of unspecified fibula

S82.42 Transverse fracture of shaft of fibula
- S82.421 Displaced transverse fracture of shaft of right fibula
- S82.422 Displaced transverse fracture of shaft of left fibula
- S82.423 Displaced transverse fracture of shaft of unspecified fibula
- S82.424 Nondisplaced transverse fracture of shaft of right fibula
- S82.425 Nondisplaced transverse fracture of shaft of left fibula
- S82.426 Nondisplaced transverse fracture of shaft of unspecified fibula

S82.43 Oblique fracture of shaft of fibula
- S82.431 Displaced oblique fracture of shaft of right fibula
- S82.432 Displaced oblique fracture of shaft of left fibula
- S82.433 Displaced oblique fracture of shaft of unspecified fibula
- S82.434 Nondisplaced oblique fracture of shaft of right fibula
- S82.435 Nondisplaced oblique fracture of shaft of left fibula
- S82.436 Nondisplaced oblique fracture of shaft of unspecified fibula

S82.44 Spiral fracture of shaft of fibula
- S82.441 Displaced spiral fracture of shaft of right fibula
- S82.442 Displaced spiral fracture of shaft of left fibula
- S82.443 Displaced spiral fracture of shaft of unspecified fibula
- S82.444 Nondisplaced spiral fracture of shaft of right fibula
- S82.445 Nondisplaced spiral fracture of shaft of left fibula
- S82.446 Nondisplaced spiral fracture of shaft of unspecified fibula

S82.45 Comminuted fracture of shaft of fibula
- S82.451 Displaced comminuted fracture of shaft of right fibula
- S82.452 Displaced comminuted fracture of shaft of left fibula
- S82.453 Displaced comminuted fracture of shaft of unspecified fibula
- S82.454 Nondisplaced comminuted fracture of shaft of right fibula
- S82.455 Nondisplaced comminuted fracture of shaft of left fibula
- S82.456 Nondisplaced comminuted fracture of shaft of unspecified fibula

S82.46 Segmental fracture of shaft of fibula
- S82.461 Displaced segmental fracture of shaft of right fibula
- S82.462 Displaced segmental fracture of shaft of left fibula
- S82.463 Displaced segmental fracture of shaft of unspecified fibula
- S82.464 Nondisplaced segmental fracture of shaft of right fibula
- S82.465 Nondisplaced segmental fracture of shaft of left fibula
- S82.466 Nondisplaced segmental fracture of shaft of unspecified fibula

S82.49 Other fracture of shaft of fibula
- S82.491 Other fracture of shaft of right fibula
- S82.492 Other fracture of shaft of left fibula
- S82.499 Other fracture of shaft of unspecified fibula

S82.5 Fracture of medial malleolus
EXCLUDES 1: pilon fracture of distal tibia (S82.87-)
Salter-Harris type III of lower end of tibia (S89.13-)
Salter-Harris type IV of lower end of tibia (S89.14-)

- S82.51 Displaced fracture of medial malleolus of right tibia
- S82.52 Displaced fracture of medial malleolus of left tibia
- S82.53 Displaced fracture of medial malleolus of unspecified tibia
- S82.54 Nondisplaced fracture of medial malleolus of right tibia
- S82.55 Nondisplaced fracture of medial malleolus of left tibia
- S82.56 Nondisplaced fracture of medial malleolus of unspecified tibia

S82.6 Fracture of lateral malleolus
EXCLUDES 1: pilon fracture of distal tibia (S82.87-)

- S82.61 Displaced fracture of lateral malleolus of right fibula
- S82.62 Displaced fracture of lateral malleolus of left fibula
- S82.63 Displaced fracture of lateral malleolus of unspecified fibula
- S82.64 Nondisplaced fracture of lateral malleolus of right fibula
- S82.65 Nondisplaced fracture of lateral malleolus of left fibula
- S82.66 Nondisplaced fracture of lateral malleolus of unspecified fibula

S82.8 Other fractures of lower leg

S82.81 Torus fracture of upper end of fibula

The appropriate 7th character is to be added to all codes in subcategory S82.81
- A initial encounter for closed fracture
- D subsequent encounter for fracture with routine healing
- G subsequent encounter for fracture with delayed healing
- K subsequent encounter for fracture with nonunion
- P subsequent encounter for fracture with malunion
- S sequela

- S82.811 Torus fracture of upper end of right fibula
- S82.812 Torus fracture of upper end of left fibula
- S82.819 Torus fracture of upper end of unspecified fibula

S82.82 Torus fracture of lower end of fibula

The appropriate 7th character is to be added to all codes in subcategory S82.82.
- A initial encounter for closed fracture
- D subsequent encounter for fracture with routine healing
- G subsequent encounter for fracture with delayed healing
- K subsequent encounter for fracture with nonunion
- P subsequent encounter for fracture with malunion
- S sequela

- S82.821 Torus fracture of lower end of right fibula
- S82.822 Torus fracture of lower end of left fibula
- S82.829 Torus fracture of lower end of unspecified fibula

S82.83 Other fracture of upper and lower end of fibula
AHA: 2015,1Q,25
- S82.831 Other fracture of upper and lower end of right fibula
- S82.832 Other fracture of upper and lower end of left fibula
- S82.839 Other fracture of upper and lower end of unspecified fibula

S82.84 Bimalleolar fracture of lower leg

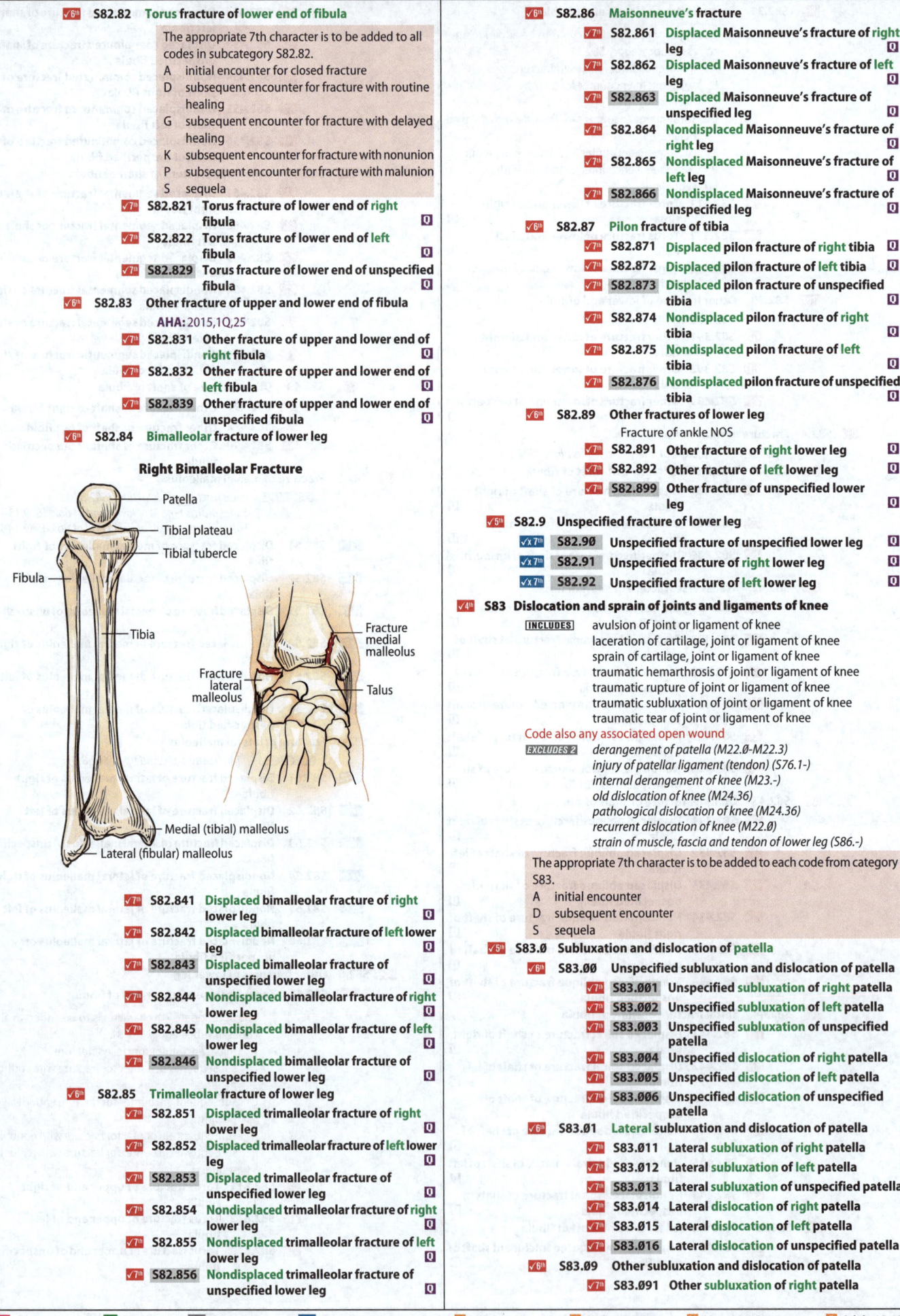

Right Bimalleolar Fracture

- S82.841 Displaced bimalleolar fracture of right lower leg
- S82.842 Displaced bimalleolar fracture of left lower leg
- S82.843 Displaced bimalleolar fracture of unspecified lower leg
- S82.844 Nondisplaced bimalleolar fracture of right lower leg
- S82.845 Nondisplaced bimalleolar fracture of left lower leg
- S82.846 Nondisplaced bimalleolar fracture of unspecified lower leg

S82.85 Trimalleolar fracture of lower leg
- S82.851 Displaced trimalleolar fracture of right lower leg
- S82.852 Displaced trimalleolar fracture of left lower leg
- S82.853 Displaced trimalleolar fracture of unspecified lower leg
- S82.854 Nondisplaced trimalleolar fracture of right lower leg
- S82.855 Nondisplaced trimalleolar fracture of left lower leg
- S82.856 Nondisplaced trimalleolar fracture of unspecified lower leg

S82.86 Maisonneuve's fracture
- S82.861 Displaced Maisonneuve's fracture of right leg
- S82.862 Displaced Maisonneuve's fracture of left leg
- S82.863 Displaced Maisonneuve's fracture of unspecified leg
- S82.864 Nondisplaced Maisonneuve's fracture of right leg
- S82.865 Nondisplaced Maisonneuve's fracture of left leg
- S82.866 Nondisplaced Maisonneuve's fracture of unspecified leg

S82.87 Pilon fracture of tibia
- S82.871 Displaced pilon fracture of right tibia
- S82.872 Displaced pilon fracture of left tibia
- S82.873 Displaced pilon fracture of unspecified tibia
- S82.874 Nondisplaced pilon fracture of right tibia
- S82.875 Nondisplaced pilon fracture of left tibia
- S82.876 Nondisplaced pilon fracture of unspecified tibia

S82.89 Other fractures of lower leg
Fracture of ankle NOS
- S82.891 Other fracture of right lower leg
- S82.892 Other fracture of left lower leg
- S82.899 Other fracture of unspecified lower leg

S82.9 Unspecified fracture of lower leg
- S82.90 Unspecified fracture of unspecified lower leg
- S82.91 Unspecified fracture of right lower leg
- S82.92 Unspecified fracture of left lower leg

S83 Dislocation and sprain of joints and ligaments of knee

INCLUDES
- avulsion of joint or ligament of knee
- laceration of cartilage, joint or ligament of knee
- sprain of cartilage, joint or ligament of knee
- traumatic hemarthrosis of joint or ligament of knee
- traumatic rupture of joint or ligament of knee
- traumatic subluxation of joint or ligament of knee
- traumatic tear of joint or ligament of knee

Code also any associated open wound

EXCLUDES 2
- derangement of patella (M22.0-M22.3)
- injury of patellar ligament (tendon) (S76.1-)
- internal derangement of knee (M23.-)
- old dislocation of knee (M24.36)
- pathological dislocation of knee (M24.36)
- recurrent dislocation of knee (M22.0)
- strain of muscle, fascia and tendon of lower leg (S86.-)

The appropriate 7th character is to be added to each code from category S83.
- A initial encounter
- D subsequent encounter
- S sequela

S83.0 Subluxation and dislocation of patella
S83.00 Unspecified subluxation and dislocation of patella
- S83.001 Unspecified subluxation of right patella
- S83.002 Unspecified subluxation of left patella
- S83.003 Unspecified subluxation of unspecified patella
- S83.004 Unspecified dislocation of right patella
- S83.005 Unspecified dislocation of left patella
- S83.006 Unspecified dislocation of unspecified patella

S83.01 Lateral subluxation and dislocation of patella
- S83.011 Lateral subluxation of right patella
- S83.012 Lateral subluxation of left patella
- S83.013 Lateral subluxation of unspecified patella
- S83.014 Lateral dislocation of right patella
- S83.015 Lateral dislocation of left patella
- S83.016 Lateral dislocation of unspecified patella

S83.09 Other subluxation and dislocation of patella
- S83.091 Other subluxation of right patella

- S83.092 Other subluxation of left patella
- S83.093 Other subluxation of unspecified patella
- S83.094 Other dislocation of right patella
- S83.095 Other dislocation of left patella
- S83.096 Other dislocation of unspecified patella

S83.1 Subluxation and dislocation of knee

EXCLUDES 2: instability of knee prosthesis (T84.022, T84.023)

- S83.10 Unspecified subluxation and dislocation of knee
  - S83.101 Unspecified subluxation of right knee
  - S83.102 Unspecified subluxation of left knee
  - S83.103 Unspecified subluxation of unspecified knee
  - S83.104 Unspecified dislocation of right knee
  - S83.105 Unspecified dislocation of left knee
  - S83.106 Unspecified dislocation of unspecified knee
- S83.11 Anterior subluxation and dislocation of proximal end of tibia
  Posterior subluxation and dislocation of distal end of femur
  - S83.111 Anterior subluxation of proximal end of tibia, right knee
  - S83.112 Anterior subluxation of proximal end of tibia, left knee
  - S83.113 Anterior subluxation of proximal end of tibia, unspecified knee
  - S83.114 Anterior dislocation of proximal end of tibia, right knee
  - S83.115 Anterior dislocation of proximal end of tibia, left knee
  - S83.116 Anterior dislocation of proximal end of tibia, unspecified knee
- S83.12 Posterior subluxation and dislocation of proximal end of tibia
  Anterior dislocation of distal end of femur
  - S83.121 Posterior subluxation of proximal end of tibia, right knee
  - S83.122 Posterior subluxation of proximal end of tibia, left knee
  - S83.123 Posterior subluxation of proximal end of tibia, unspecified knee
  - S83.124 Posterior dislocation of proximal end of tibia, right knee
  - S83.125 Posterior dislocation of proximal end of tibia, left knee
  - S83.126 Posterior dislocation of proximal end of tibia, unspecified knee
- S83.13 Medial subluxation and dislocation of proximal end of tibia
  - S83.131 Medial subluxation of proximal end of tibia, right knee
  - S83.132 Medial subluxation of proximal end of tibia, left knee
  - S83.133 Medial subluxation of proximal end of tibia, unspecified knee
  - S83.134 Medial dislocation of proximal end of tibia, right knee
  - S83.135 Medial dislocation of proximal end of tibia, left knee
  - S83.136 Medial dislocation of proximal end of tibia, unspecified knee
- S83.14 Lateral subluxation and dislocation of proximal end of tibia
  - S83.141 Lateral subluxation of proximal end of tibia, right knee
  - S83.142 Lateral subluxation of proximal end of tibia, left knee
  - S83.143 Lateral subluxation of proximal end of tibia, unspecified knee
  - S83.144 Lateral dislocation of proximal end of tibia, right knee
  - S83.145 Lateral dislocation of proximal end of tibia, left knee
  - S83.146 Lateral dislocation of proximal end of tibia, unspecified knee
- S83.19 Other subluxation and dislocation of knee
  - S83.191 Other subluxation of right knee
  - S83.192 Other subluxation of left knee
  - S83.193 Other subluxation of unspecified knee
  - S83.194 Other dislocation of right knee
  - S83.195 Other dislocation of left knee
  - S83.196 Other dislocation of unspecified knee

S83.2 Tear of meniscus, current injury

EXCLUDES 1: old bucket-handle tear (M23.2)
AHA: 2019,2Q,26

- S83.20 Tear of unspecified meniscus, current injury
  Tear of meniscus of knee NOS
  - S83.200 Bucket-handle tear of unspecified meniscus, current injury, right knee
  - S83.201 Bucket-handle tear of unspecified meniscus, current injury, left knee
  - S83.202 Bucket-handle tear of unspecified meniscus, current injury, unspecified knee
  - S83.203 Other tear of unspecified meniscus, current injury, right knee
  - S83.204 Other tear of unspecified meniscus, current injury, left knee
  - S83.205 Other tear of unspecified meniscus, current injury, unspecified knee
  - S83.206 Unspecified tear of unspecified meniscus, current injury, right knee
  - S83.207 Unspecified tear of unspecified meniscus, current injury, left knee
  - S83.209 Unspecified tear of unspecified meniscus, current injury, unspecified knee
- S83.21 Bucket-handle tear of medial meniscus, current injury
  - S83.211 Bucket-handle tear of medial meniscus, current injury, right knee
  - S83.212 Bucket-handle tear of medial meniscus, current injury, left knee
  - S83.219 Bucket-handle tear of medial meniscus, current injury, unspecified knee
- S83.22 Peripheral tear of medial meniscus, current injury
  - S83.221 Peripheral tear of medial meniscus, current injury, right knee
  - S83.222 Peripheral tear of medial meniscus, current injury, left knee
  - S83.229 Peripheral tear of medial meniscus, current injury, unspecified knee
- S83.23 Complex tear of medial meniscus, current injury
  - S83.231 Complex tear of medial meniscus, current injury, right knee
  - S83.232 Complex tear of medial meniscus, current injury, left knee
  - S83.239 Complex tear of medial meniscus, current injury, unspecified knee
- S83.24 Other tear of medial meniscus, current injury
  - S83.241 Other tear of medial meniscus, current injury, right knee
  - S83.242 Other tear of medial meniscus, current injury, left knee
  - S83.249 Other tear of medial meniscus, current injury, unspecified knee
- S83.25 Bucket-handle tear of lateral meniscus, current injury
  - S83.251 Bucket-handle tear of lateral meniscus, current injury, right knee
  - S83.252 Bucket-handle tear of lateral meniscus, current injury, left knee
  - S83.259 Bucket-handle tear of lateral meniscus, current injury, unspecified knee
- S83.26 Peripheral tear of lateral meniscus, current injury
  - S83.261 Peripheral tear of lateral meniscus, current injury, right knee
  - S83.262 Peripheral tear of lateral meniscus, current injury, left knee
  - S83.269 Peripheral tear of lateral meniscus, current injury, unspecified knee
- S83.27 Complex tear of lateral meniscus, current injury
  - S83.271 Complex tear of lateral meniscus, current injury, right knee
  - S83.272 Complex tear of lateral meniscus, current injury, left knee
  - S83.279 Complex tear of lateral meniscus, current injury, unspecified knee
- S83.28 Other tear of lateral meniscus, current injury
  - S83.281 Other tear of lateral meniscus, current injury, right knee
  - S83.282 Other tear of lateral meniscus, current injury, left knee

- **S83.289** Other tear of lateral meniscus, current injury, unspecified knee
- **S83.3** Tear of articular cartilage of knee, current
  - **S83.30** Tear of articular cartilage of unspecified knee, current
  - **S83.31** Tear of articular cartilage of right knee, current
  - **S83.32** Tear of articular cartilage of left knee, current
- **S83.4** Sprain of collateral ligament of knee
  - **S83.40** Sprain of unspecified collateral ligament of knee
    - **S83.401** Sprain of unspecified collateral ligament of right knee
    - **S83.402** Sprain of unspecified collateral ligament of left knee
    - **S83.409** Sprain of unspecified collateral ligament of unspecified knee
  - **S83.41** Sprain of medial collateral ligament of knee
    Sprain of tibial collateral ligament
    - **S83.411** Sprain of medial collateral ligament of right knee
    - **S83.412** Sprain of medial collateral ligament of left knee
    - **S83.419** Sprain of medial collateral ligament of unspecified knee
  - **S83.42** Sprain of lateral collateral ligament of knee
    Sprain of fibular collateral ligament
    - **S83.421** Sprain of lateral collateral ligament of right knee
    - **S83.422** Sprain of lateral collateral ligament of left knee
    - **S83.429** Sprain of lateral collateral ligament of unspecified knee
- **S83.5** Sprain of cruciate ligament of knee
  AHA: 2016,2Q,3
  - **S83.50** Sprain of unspecified cruciate ligament of knee
    - **S83.501** Sprain of unspecified cruciate ligament of right knee
    - **S83.502** Sprain of unspecified cruciate ligament of left knee
    - **S83.509** Sprain of unspecified cruciate ligament of unspecified knee
  - **S83.51** Sprain of anterior cruciate ligament of knee
    - **S83.511** Sprain of anterior cruciate ligament of right knee
    - **S83.512** Sprain of anterior cruciate ligament of left knee
    - **S83.519** Sprain of anterior cruciate ligament of unspecified knee
  - **S83.52** Sprain of posterior cruciate ligament of knee
    - **S83.521** Sprain of posterior cruciate ligament of right knee
    - **S83.522** Sprain of posterior cruciate ligament of left knee
    - **S83.529** Sprain of posterior cruciate ligament of unspecified knee
- **S83.6** Sprain of the superior tibiofibular joint and ligament
  - **S83.60** Sprain of the superior tibiofibular joint and ligament, unspecified knee
  - **S83.61** Sprain of the superior tibiofibular joint and ligament, right knee
  - **S83.62** Sprain of the superior tibiofibular joint and ligament, left knee
- **S83.8** Sprain of other specified parts of knee
  - **S83.8X** Sprain of other specified parts of knee
    - **S83.8X1** Sprain of other specified parts of right knee
    - **S83.8X2** Sprain of other specified parts of left knee
    - **S83.8X9** Sprain of other specified parts of unspecified knee
- **S83.9** Sprain of unspecified site of knee
  - **S83.90** Sprain of unspecified site of unspecified knee
  - **S83.91** Sprain of unspecified site of right knee
  - **S83.92** Sprain of unspecified site of left knee

- **S84** Injury of nerves at lower leg level
  Code also any associated open wound (S81.-)
  EXCLUDES 2 injury of nerves at ankle and foot level (S94.-)

  The appropriate 7th character is to be added to each code from category S84.
  A initial encounter
  D subsequent encounter
  S sequela
  - **S84.0** Injury of tibial nerve at lower leg level
    - **S84.00** Injury of tibial nerve at lower leg level, unspecified leg
    - **S84.01** Injury of tibial nerve at lower leg level, right leg
    - **S84.02** Injury of tibial nerve at lower leg level, left leg
  - **S84.1** Injury of peroneal nerve at lower leg level
    - **S84.10** Injury of peroneal nerve at lower leg level, unspecified leg
    - **S84.11** Injury of peroneal nerve at lower leg level, right leg
    - **S84.12** Injury of peroneal nerve at lower leg level, left leg
  - **S84.2** Injury of cutaneous sensory nerve at lower leg level
    - **S84.20** Injury of cutaneous sensory nerve at lower leg level, unspecified leg
    - **S84.21** Injury of cutaneous sensory nerve at lower leg level, right leg
    - **S84.22** Injury of cutaneous sensory nerve at lower leg level, left leg
  - **S84.8** Injury of other nerves at lower leg level
    - **S84.80** Injury of other nerves at lower leg level
      - **S84.801** Injury of other nerves at lower leg level, right leg
      - **S84.802** Injury of other nerves at lower leg level, left leg
      - **S84.809** Injury of other nerves at lower leg level, unspecified leg
  - **S84.9** Injury of unspecified nerve at lower leg level
    - **S84.90** Injury of unspecified nerve at lower leg level, unspecified leg
    - **S84.91** Injury of unspecified nerve at lower leg level, right leg
    - **S84.92** Injury of unspecified nerve at lower leg level, left leg

- **S85** Injury of blood vessels at lower leg level
  Code also any associated open wound (S81.-)
  EXCLUDES 2 injury of blood vessels at ankle and foot level (S95.-)

  The appropriate 7th character is to be added to each code from category S85.
  A initial encounter
  D subsequent encounter
  S sequela
  - **S85.0** Injury of popliteal artery
    - **S85.00** Unspecified injury of popliteal artery
      - **S85.001** Unspecified injury of popliteal artery, right leg
      - **S85.002** Unspecified injury of popliteal artery, left leg
      - **S85.009** Unspecified injury of popliteal artery, unspecified leg
    - **S85.01** Laceration of popliteal artery
      - **S85.011** Laceration of popliteal artery, right leg
      - **S85.012** Laceration of popliteal artery, left leg
      - **S85.019** Laceration of popliteal artery, unspecified leg
    - **S85.09** Other specified injury of popliteal artery
      - **S85.091** Other specified injury of popliteal artery, right leg
      - **S85.092** Other specified injury of popliteal artery, left leg
      - **S85.099** Other specified injury of popliteal artery, unspecified leg
  - **S85.1** Injury of tibial artery
    - **S85.10** Unspecified injury of unspecified tibial artery
      Injury of tibial artery NOS
      - **S85.101** Unspecified injury of unspecified tibial artery, right leg
      - **S85.102** Unspecified injury of unspecified tibial artery, left leg

- S85.109 Unspecified injury of unspecified tibial artery, unspecified leg
- S85.11 Laceration of unspecified tibial artery
  - S85.111 Laceration of unspecified tibial artery, right leg
  - S85.112 Laceration of unspecified tibial artery, left leg
  - S85.119 Laceration of unspecified tibial artery, unspecified leg
- S85.12 Other specified injury of unspecified tibial artery
  - S85.121 Other specified injury of unspecified tibial artery, right leg
  - S85.122 Other specified injury of unspecified tibial artery, left leg
  - S85.129 Other specified injury of unspecified tibial artery, unspecified leg
- S85.13 Unspecified injury of anterior tibial artery
  - S85.131 Unspecified injury of anterior tibial artery, right leg
  - S85.132 Unspecified injury of anterior tibial artery, left leg
  - S85.139 Unspecified injury of anterior tibial artery, unspecified leg
- S85.14 Laceration of anterior tibial artery
  - S85.141 Laceration of anterior tibial artery, right leg
  - S85.142 Laceration of anterior tibial artery, left leg
  - S85.149 Laceration of anterior tibial artery, unspecified leg
- S85.15 Other specified injury of anterior tibial artery
  - S85.151 Other specified injury of anterior tibial artery, right leg
  - S85.152 Other specified injury of anterior tibial artery, left leg
  - S85.159 Other specified injury of anterior tibial artery, unspecified leg
- S85.16 Unspecified injury of posterior tibial artery
  - S85.161 Unspecified injury of posterior tibial artery, right leg
  - S85.162 Unspecified injury of posterior tibial artery, left leg
  - S85.169 Unspecified injury of posterior tibial artery, unspecified leg
- S85.17 Laceration of posterior tibial artery
  - S85.171 Laceration of posterior tibial artery, right leg
  - S85.172 Laceration of posterior tibial artery, left leg
  - S85.179 Laceration of posterior tibial artery, unspecified leg
- S85.18 Other specified injury of posterior tibial artery
  - S85.181 Other specified injury of posterior tibial artery, right leg
  - S85.182 Other specified injury of posterior tibial artery, left leg
  - S85.189 Other specified injury of posterior tibial artery, unspecified leg
- S85.2 Injury of peroneal artery
  - S85.20 Unspecified injury of peroneal artery
    - S85.201 Unspecified injury of peroneal artery, right leg
    - S85.202 Unspecified injury of peroneal artery, left leg
    - S85.209 Unspecified injury of peroneal artery, unspecified leg
  - S85.21 Laceration of peroneal artery
    - S85.211 Laceration of peroneal artery, right leg
    - S85.212 Laceration of peroneal artery, left leg
    - S85.219 Laceration of peroneal artery, unspecified leg
  - S85.29 Other specified injury of peroneal artery
    - S85.291 Other specified injury of peroneal artery, right leg
    - S85.292 Other specified injury of peroneal artery, left leg
    - S85.299 Other specified injury of peroneal artery, unspecified leg

- S85.3 Injury of greater saphenous vein at lower leg level
  Injury of greater saphenous vein NOS
  Injury of saphenous vein NOS
  - S85.30 Unspecified injury of greater saphenous vein at lower leg level
    - S85.301 Unspecified injury of greater saphenous vein at lower leg level, right leg
    - S85.302 Unspecified injury of greater saphenous vein at lower leg level, left leg
    - S85.309 Unspecified injury of greater saphenous vein at lower leg level, unspecified leg
  - S85.31 Laceration of greater saphenous vein at lower leg level
    - S85.311 Laceration of greater saphenous vein at lower leg level, right leg
    - S85.312 Laceration of greater saphenous vein at lower leg level, left leg
    - S85.319 Laceration of greater saphenous vein at lower leg level, unspecified leg
  - S85.39 Other specified injury of greater saphenous vein at lower leg level
    - S85.391 Other specified injury of greater saphenous vein at lower leg level, right leg
    - S85.392 Other specified injury of greater saphenous vein at lower leg level, left leg
    - S85.399 Other specified injury of greater saphenous vein at lower leg level, unspecified leg
- S85.4 Injury of lesser saphenous vein at lower leg level
  - S85.40 Unspecified injury of lesser saphenous vein at lower leg level
    - S85.401 Unspecified injury of lesser saphenous vein at lower leg level, right leg
    - S85.402 Unspecified injury of lesser saphenous vein at lower leg level, left leg
    - S85.409 Unspecified injury of lesser saphenous vein at lower leg level, unspecified leg
  - S85.41 Laceration of lesser saphenous vein at lower leg level
    - S85.411 Laceration of lesser saphenous vein at lower leg level, right leg
    - S85.412 Laceration of lesser saphenous vein at lower leg level, left leg
    - S85.419 Laceration of lesser saphenous vein at lower leg level, unspecified leg
  - S85.49 Other specified injury of lesser saphenous vein at lower leg level
    - S85.491 Other specified injury of lesser saphenous vein at lower leg level, right leg
    - S85.492 Other specified injury of lesser saphenous vein at lower leg level, left leg
    - S85.499 Other specified injury of lesser saphenous vein at lower leg level, unspecified leg
- S85.5 Injury of popliteal vein
  - S85.50 Unspecified injury of popliteal vein
    - S85.501 Unspecified injury of popliteal vein, right leg
    - S85.502 Unspecified injury of popliteal vein, left leg
    - S85.509 Unspecified injury of popliteal vein, unspecified leg
  - S85.51 Laceration of popliteal vein
    - S85.511 Laceration of popliteal vein, right leg
    - S85.512 Laceration of popliteal vein, left leg
    - S85.519 Laceration of popliteal vein, unspecified leg
  - S85.59 Other specified injury of popliteal vein
    - S85.591 Other specified injury of popliteal vein, right leg
    - S85.592 Other specified injury of popliteal vein, left leg
    - S85.599 Other specified injury of popliteal vein, unspecified leg
- S85.8 Injury of other blood vessels at lower leg level
  - S85.80 Unspecified injury of other blood vessels at lower leg level
    - S85.801 Unspecified injury of other blood vessels at lower leg level, right leg
    - S85.802 Unspecified injury of other blood vessels at lower leg level, left leg
    - S85.809 Unspecified injury of other blood vessels at lower leg level, unspecified leg

- **S85.81** 6th **Laceration** of other blood vessels at lower leg level
  - **S85.811** 7th Laceration of other blood vessels at lower leg level, **right** leg
  - **S85.812** 7th Laceration of other blood vessels at lower leg level, **left** leg
  - **S85.819** 7th Laceration of other blood vessels at lower leg level, unspecified leg
- **S85.89** 6th Other specified injury of other blood vessels at lower leg level
  - **S85.891** 7th Other specified injury of other blood vessels at lower leg level, **right** leg
  - **S85.892** 7th Other specified injury of other blood vessels at lower leg level, **left** leg
  - **S85.899** 7th Other specified injury of other blood vessels at lower leg level, unspecified leg
- **S85.9** 5th Injury of unspecified blood vessel at lower leg level
  - **S85.90** 6th Unspecified injury of unspecified blood vessel at lower leg level
    - **S85.901** 7th Unspecified injury of unspecified blood vessel at lower leg level, **right** leg
    - **S85.902** 7th Unspecified injury of unspecified blood vessel at lower leg level, **left** leg
    - **S85.909** 7th Unspecified injury of unspecified blood vessel at lower leg level, unspecified leg
  - **S85.91** 6th **Laceration** of unspecified blood vessel at lower leg level
    - **S85.911** 7th Laceration of unspecified blood vessel at lower leg level, **right** leg
    - **S85.912** 7th Laceration of unspecified blood vessel at lower leg level, **left** leg
    - **S85.919** 7th Laceration of unspecified blood vessel at lower leg level, unspecified leg
  - **S85.99** 6th Other specified injury of unspecified blood vessel at lower leg level
    - **S85.991** 7th Other specified injury of unspecified blood vessel at lower leg level, **right** leg
    - **S85.992** 7th Other specified injury of unspecified blood vessel at lower leg level, **left** leg
    - **S85.999** 7th Other specified injury of unspecified blood vessel at lower leg level, unspecified leg
- **S86** 4th **Injury of muscle, fascia and tendon at lower leg level**

  Code also any associated open wound (S81.-)

  EXCLUDES 2 injury of muscle, fascia and tendon at ankle (S96.-)
  injury of patellar ligament (tendon) (S76.1-)
  sprain of joints and ligaments of knee (S83.-)

  TIP: Refer to the Muscle/Tendon table at the beginning of this chapter.

  The appropriate 7th character is to be added to each code from category S86.
  - A initial encounter
  - D subsequent encounter
  - S sequela
  - **S86.0** 5th **Injury of Achilles tendon**
    - **S86.00** 6th Unspecified injury of Achilles tendon
      - **S86.001** 7th Unspecified injury of **right** Achilles tendon
      - **S86.002** 7th Unspecified injury of **left** Achilles tendon
      - **S86.009** 7th Unspecified injury of unspecified Achilles tendon
    - **S86.01** 6th **Strain** of Achilles tendon
      - **S86.011** 7th Strain of **right** Achilles tendon
      - **S86.012** 7th Strain of **left** Achilles tendon
      - **S86.019** 7th Strain of unspecified Achilles tendon
    - **S86.02** 6th **Laceration** of Achilles tendon
      - **S86.021** 7th Laceration of **right** Achilles tendon
      - **S86.022** 7th Laceration of **left** Achilles tendon
      - **S86.029** 7th Laceration of unspecified Achilles tendon
    - **S86.09** 6th Other specified injury of Achilles tendon
      - **S86.091** 7th Other specified injury of **right** Achilles tendon
      - **S86.092** 7th Other specified injury of **left** Achilles tendon
      - **S86.099** 7th Other specified injury of unspecified Achilles tendon
  - **S86.1** 5th Injury of other muscle(s) and tendon(s) of **posterior muscle group** at lower leg level
    - **S86.10** 6th Unspecified injury of other muscle(s) and tendon(s) of posterior muscle group at lower leg level
      - **S86.101** 7th Unspecified injury of other muscle(s) and tendon(s) of posterior muscle group at lower leg level, **right** leg
      - **S86.102** 7th Unspecified injury of other muscle(s) and tendon(s) of posterior muscle group at lower leg level, **left** leg
      - **S86.109** 7th Unspecified injury of other muscle(s) and tendon(s) of posterior muscle group at lower leg level, unspecified leg
    - **S86.11** 6th **Strain** of other muscle(s) and tendon(s) of posterior muscle group at lower leg level
      - **S86.111** 7th Strain of other muscle(s) and tendon(s) of posterior muscle group at lower leg level, **right** leg
      - **S86.112** 7th Strain of other muscle(s) and tendon(s) of posterior muscle group at lower leg level, **left** leg
      - **S86.119** 7th Strain of other muscle(s) and tendon(s) of posterior muscle group at lower leg level, unspecified
    - **S86.12** 6th **Laceration** of other muscle(s) and tendon(s) of posterior muscle group at lower leg level
      - **S86.121** 7th Laceration of other muscle(s) and tendon(s) of posterior muscle group at lower leg level, **right** leg
      - **S86.122** 7th Laceration of other muscle(s) and tendon(s) of posterior muscle group at lower leg level, **left** leg
      - **S86.129** 7th Laceration of other muscle(s) and tendon(s) of posterior muscle group at lower leg level, unspecified
    - **S86.19** 6th Other injury of other muscle(s) and tendon(s) of posterior muscle group at lower leg level
      - **S86.191** 7th Other injury of other muscle(s) and tendon(s) of posterior muscle group at lower leg level, **right** leg
      - **S86.192** 7th Other injury of other muscle(s) and tendon(s) of posterior muscle group at lower leg level, **left** leg
      - **S86.199** 7th Other injury of other muscle(s) and tendon(s) of posterior muscle group at lower leg level, unspecified leg
  - **S86.2** 5th Injury of muscle(s) and tendon(s) of **anterior muscle group** at lower leg level
    - **S86.20** 6th Unspecified injury of muscle(s) and tendon(s) of anterior muscle group at lower leg level
      - **S86.201** 7th Unspecified injury of muscle(s) and tendon(s) of anterior muscle group at lower leg level, **right** leg
      - **S86.202** 7th Unspecified injury of muscle(s) and tendon(s) of anterior muscle group at lower leg level, **left** leg
      - **S86.209** 7th Unspecified injury of muscle(s) and tendon(s) of anterior muscle group at lower leg level, unspecified leg
    - **S86.21** 6th **Strain** of muscle(s) and tendon(s) of anterior muscle group at lower leg level
      - **S86.211** 7th Strain of muscle(s) and tendon(s) of anterior muscle group at lower leg level, **right** leg
      - **S86.212** 7th Strain of muscle(s) and tendon(s) of anterior muscle group at lower leg level, **left** leg
      - **S86.219** 7th Strain of muscle(s) and tendon(s) of anterior muscle group at lower leg level, unspecified leg
    - **S86.22** 6th **Laceration** of muscle(s) and tendon(s) of anterior muscle group at lower leg level
      - **S86.221** 7th Laceration of muscle(s) and tendon(s) of anterior muscle group at lower leg level, **right** leg
      - **S86.222** 7th Laceration of muscle(s) and tendon(s) of anterior muscle group at lower leg level, **left** leg
      - **S86.229** 7th Laceration of muscle(s) and tendon(s) of anterior muscle group at lower leg level, unspecified leg

- **S86.29** Other injury of muscle(s) and tendon(s) of anterior muscle group at lower leg level
  - **S86.291** Other injury of muscle(s) and tendon(s) of anterior muscle group at lower leg level, right leg
  - **S86.292** Other injury of muscle(s) and tendon(s) of anterior muscle group at lower leg level, left leg
  - **S86.299** Other injury of muscle(s) and tendon(s) of anterior muscle group at lower leg level, unspecified leg
- **S86.3** Injury of muscle(s) and tendon(s) of peroneal muscle group at lower leg level
  - **S86.30** Unspecified injury of muscle(s) and tendon(s) of peroneal muscle group at lower leg level
    - **S86.301** Unspecified injury of muscle(s) and tendon(s) of peroneal muscle group at lower leg level, right leg
    - **S86.302** Unspecified injury of muscle(s) and tendon(s) of peroneal muscle group at lower leg level, left leg
    - **S86.309** Unspecified injury of muscle(s) and tendon(s) of peroneal muscle group at lower leg level, unspecified leg
  - **S86.31** Strain of muscle(s) and tendon(s) of peroneal muscle group at lower leg level
    - **S86.311** Strain of muscle(s) and tendon(s) of peroneal muscle group at lower leg level, right leg
    - **S86.312** Strain of muscle(s) and tendon(s) of peroneal muscle group at lower leg level, left leg
    - **S86.319** Strain of muscle(s) and tendon(s) of peroneal muscle group at lower leg level, unspecified leg
  - **S86.32** Laceration of muscle(s) and tendon(s) of peroneal muscle group at lower leg level
    - **S86.321** Laceration of muscle(s) and tendon(s) of peroneal muscle group at lower leg level, right leg
    - **S86.322** Laceration of muscle(s) and tendon(s) of peroneal muscle group at lower leg level, left leg
    - **S86.329** Laceration of muscle(s) and tendon(s) of peroneal muscle group at lower leg level, unspecified leg
  - **S86.39** Other injury of muscle(s) and tendon(s) of peroneal muscle group at lower leg level
    - **S86.391** Other injury of muscle(s) and tendon(s) of peroneal muscle group at lower leg level, right leg
    - **S86.392** Other injury of muscle(s) and tendon(s) of peroneal muscle group at lower leg level, left leg
    - **S86.399** Other injury of muscle(s) and tendon(s) of peroneal muscle group at lower leg level, unspecified leg
- **S86.8** Injury of other muscles and tendons at lower leg level
  - **S86.80** Unspecified injury of other muscles and tendons at lower leg level
    - **S86.801** Unspecified injury of other muscle(s) and tendon(s) at lower leg level, right leg
    - **S86.802** Unspecified injury of other muscle(s) and tendon(s) at lower leg level, left leg
    - **S86.809** Unspecified injury of other muscle(s) and tendon(s) at lower leg level, unspecified leg
  - **S86.81** Strain of other muscles and tendons at lower leg level
    - **S86.811** Strain of other muscle(s) and tendon(s) at lower leg level, right leg
    - **S86.812** Strain of other muscle(s) and tendon(s) at lower leg level, left leg
    - **S86.819** Strain of other muscle(s) and tendon(s) at lower leg level, unspecified leg
  - **S86.82** Laceration of other muscles and tendons at lower leg level
    - **S86.821** Laceration of other muscle(s) and tendon(s) at lower leg level, right leg
    - **S86.822** Laceration of other muscle(s) and tendon(s) at lower leg level, left leg
    - **S86.829** Laceration of other muscle(s) and tendon(s) at lower leg level, unspecified leg
  - **S86.89** Other injury of other muscles and tendons at lower leg level
    - **S86.891** Other injury of other muscle(s) and tendon(s) at lower leg level, right leg
    - **S86.892** Other injury of other muscle(s) and tendon(s) at lower leg level, left leg
    - **S86.899** Other injury of other muscle(s) and tendon(s) at lower leg level, unspecified leg
- **S86.9** Injury of unspecified muscle and tendon at lower leg level
  - **S86.90** Unspecified injury of unspecified muscle and tendon at lower leg level
    - **S86.901** Unspecified injury of unspecified muscle(s) and tendon(s) at lower leg level, right leg
    - **S86.902** Unspecified injury of unspecified muscle(s) and tendon(s) at lower leg level, left leg
    - **S86.909** Unspecified injury of unspecified muscle(s) and tendon(s) at lower leg level, unspecified leg
  - **S86.91** Strain of unspecified muscle and tendon at lower leg level
    - **S86.911** Strain of unspecified muscle(s) and tendon(s) at lower leg level, right leg
    - **S86.912** Strain of unspecified muscle(s) and tendon(s) at lower leg level, left leg
    - **S86.919** Strain of unspecified muscle(s) and tendon(s) at lower leg level, unspecified leg
  - **S86.92** Laceration of unspecified muscle and tendon at lower leg level
    - **S86.921** Laceration of unspecified muscle(s) and tendon(s) at lower leg level, right leg
    - **S86.922** Laceration of unspecified muscle(s) and tendon(s) at lower leg level, left leg
    - **S86.929** Laceration of unspecified muscle(s) and tendon(s) at lower leg level, unspecified leg
  - **S86.99** Other injury of unspecified muscle and tendon at lower leg level
    - **S86.991** Other injury of unspecified muscle(s) and tendon(s) at lower leg level, right leg
    - **S86.992** Other injury of unspecified muscle(s) and tendon(s) at lower leg level, left leg
    - **S86.999** Other injury of unspecified muscle(s) and tendon(s) at lower leg level, unspecified leg

S87 Crushing injury of lower leg

Use additional code(s) for all associated injuries

EXCLUDES 2 crushing injury of ankle and foot (S97.-)

The appropriate 7th character is to be added to each code from category S87.
- A initial encounter
- D subsequent encounter
- S sequela

- **S87.0** Crushing injury of knee
  - **S87.00** Crushing injury of unspecified knee
  - **S87.01** Crushing injury of right knee
  - **S87.02** Crushing injury of left knee
- **S87.8** Crushing injury of lower leg
  - **S87.80** Crushing injury of unspecified lower leg
  - **S87.81** Crushing injury of right lower leg
  - **S87.82** Crushing injury of left lower leg

S88 Traumatic amputation of lower leg

An amputation not identified as partial or complete should be coded to complete

EXCLUDES 1 traumatic amputation of ankle and foot (S98.-)

The appropriate 7th character is to be added to each code from category S88.
- A initial encounter
- D subsequent encounter
- S sequela

- **S88.0** Traumatic amputation at knee level
  - **S88.01** Complete traumatic amputation at knee level
    - AHA: 2023,1Q,27,29
    - **S88.011** Complete traumatic amputation at knee level, right lower leg

Chapter 19. Injury, Poisoning and Certain Other Consequences of External Causes

- **S88.012** Complete traumatic amputation at knee level, left lower leg [HCC] [ESR] [COM]
- **S88.019** Complete traumatic amputation at knee level, unspecified lower leg [HCC] [ESR] [COM]
- **S88.02** Partial traumatic amputation at knee level
  - **S88.021** Partial traumatic amputation at knee level, right lower leg [HCC] [ESR] [COM]
  - **S88.022** Partial traumatic amputation at knee level, left lower leg [HCC] [ESR] [COM]
  - **S88.029** Partial traumatic amputation at knee level, unspecified lower leg [HCC] [ESR] [COM]
- **S88.1** Traumatic amputation at level between knee and ankle
  - **S88.11** Complete traumatic amputation at level between knee and ankle
    - **S88.111** Complete traumatic amputation at level between knee and ankle, right lower leg [HCC] [ESR] [COM]
    - **S88.112** Complete traumatic amputation at level between knee and ankle, left lower leg [HCC] [ESR] [COM]
    - **S88.119** Complete traumatic amputation at level between knee and ankle, unspecified lower leg [HCC] [ESR] [COM]
  - **S88.12** Partial traumatic amputation at level between knee and ankle
    - **S88.121** Partial traumatic amputation at level between knee and ankle, right lower leg [HCC] [ESR] [COM]
    - **S88.122** Partial traumatic amputation at level between knee and ankle, left lower leg [HCC] [ESR] [COM]
    - **S88.129** Partial traumatic amputation at level between knee and ankle, unspecified lower leg [HCC] [ESR] [COM]
- **S88.9** Traumatic amputation of lower leg, level unspecified
  - **S88.91** Complete traumatic amputation of lower leg, level unspecified
    - **S88.911** Complete traumatic amputation of right lower leg, level unspecified [HCC] [ESR] [COM]
    - **S88.912** Complete traumatic amputation of left lower leg, level unspecified [HCC] [ESR] [COM]
    - **S88.919** Complete traumatic amputation of unspecified lower leg, level unspecified [HCC] [ESR] [COM]
  - **S88.92** Partial traumatic amputation of lower leg, level unspecified
    - **S88.921** Partial traumatic amputation of right lower leg, level unspecified [HCC] [ESR] [COM]
    - **S88.922** Partial traumatic amputation of left lower leg, level unspecified [HCC] [ESR] [COM]
    - **S88.929** Partial traumatic amputation of unspecified lower leg, level unspecified [HCC] [ESR] [COM]

S89 Other and unspecified injuries of lower leg

NOTE A fracture not indicated as open or closed should be coded to closed.

EXCLUDES 2 other and unspecified injuries of ankle and foot (S99.-)

AHA: 2018,2Q,12; 2018,1Q,3; 2015,3Q,37-39

The appropriate 7th character is to be added to each code from subcategories S89.0, S89.1, S89.2, and S89.3.
- A initial encounter for closed fracture
- D subsequent encounter for fracture with routine healing
- G subsequent encounter for fracture with delayed healing
- K subsequent encounter for fracture with nonunion
- P subsequent encounter for fracture with malunion
- S sequela

- **S89.0** Physeal fracture of upper end of tibia
  - **AHA:** 2019,4Q,56
  - **S89.00** Unspecified physeal fracture of upper end of tibia
    - **S89.001** Unspecified physeal fracture of upper end of right tibia Q
    - **S89.002** Unspecified physeal fracture of upper end of left tibia Q
    - **S89.009** Unspecified physeal fracture of upper end of unspecified tibia Q
  - **S89.01** Salter-Harris Type I physeal fracture of upper end of tibia
    - **S89.011** Salter-Harris Type I physeal fracture of upper end of right tibia Q
    - **S89.012** Salter-Harris Type I physeal fracture of upper end of left tibia Q
    - **S89.019** Salter-Harris Type I physeal fracture of upper end of unspecified tibia Q
  - **S89.02** Salter-Harris Type II physeal fracture of upper end of tibia
    - **S89.021** Salter-Harris Type II physeal fracture of upper end of right tibia Q
    - **S89.022** Salter-Harris Type II physeal fracture of upper end of left tibia Q
    - **S89.029** Salter-Harris Type II physeal fracture of upper end of unspecified tibia Q
  - **S89.03** Salter-Harris Type III physeal fracture of upper end of tibia
    - **S89.031** Salter-Harris Type III physeal fracture of upper end of right tibia Q
    - **S89.032** Salter-Harris Type III physeal fracture of upper end of left tibia Q
    - **S89.039** Salter-Harris Type III physeal fracture of upper end of unspecified tibia Q
  - **S89.04** Salter-Harris Type IV physeal fracture of upper end of tibia
    - **S89.041** Salter-Harris Type IV physeal fracture of upper end of right tibia Q
    - **S89.042** Salter-Harris Type IV physeal fracture of upper end of left tibia Q
    - **S89.049** Salter-Harris Type IV physeal fracture of upper end of unspecified tibia Q
  - **S89.09** Other physeal fracture of upper end of tibia
    - **S89.091** Other physeal fracture of upper end of right tibia Q
    - **S89.092** Other physeal fracture of upper end of left tibia Q
    - **S89.099** Other physeal fracture of upper end of unspecified tibia Q
- **S89.1** Physeal fracture of lower end of tibia
  - **AHA:** 2019,4Q,56
  - **S89.10** Unspecified physeal fracture of lower end of tibia
    - **S89.101** Unspecified physeal fracture of lower end of right tibia Q
    - **S89.102** Unspecified physeal fracture of lower end of left tibia Q
    - **S89.109** Unspecified physeal fracture of lower end of unspecified tibia Q
  - **S89.11** Salter-Harris Type I physeal fracture of lower end of tibia
    - **S89.111** Salter-Harris Type I physeal fracture of lower end of right tibia Q
    - **S89.112** Salter-Harris Type I physeal fracture of lower end of left tibia Q
    - **S89.119** Salter-Harris Type I physeal fracture of lower end of unspecified tibia Q
  - **S89.12** Salter-Harris Type II physeal fracture of lower end of tibia
    - **S89.121** Salter-Harris Type II physeal fracture of lower end of right tibia Q
    - **S89.122** Salter-Harris Type II physeal fracture of lower end of left tibia Q
    - **S89.129** Salter-Harris Type II physeal fracture of lower end of unspecified tibia Q
  - **S89.13** Salter-Harris Type III physeal fracture of lower end of tibia
    - **EXCLUDES 1** fracture of medial malleolus (adult) (S82.5-)
    - **S89.131** Salter-Harris Type III physeal fracture of lower end of right tibia Q
    - **S89.132** Salter-Harris Type III physeal fracture of lower end of left tibia Q
    - **S89.139** Salter-Harris Type III physeal fracture of lower end of unspecified tibia Q
  - **S89.14** Salter-Harris Type IV physeal fracture of lower end of tibia
    - **EXCLUDES 1** fracture of medial malleolus (adult) (S82.5-)
    - **S89.141** Salter-Harris Type IV physeal fracture of lower end of right tibia Q
    - **S89.142** Salter-Harris Type IV physeal fracture of lower end of left tibia Q

[HCC] CMS-HCC [Rx] Rx HCC [ESR] ESRD HCC [COM] Commercial HCC [N] Newborn: 0 [P] Pediatric: 0-17 [M] Maternity: 9-64 [A] Adult: 15-124

Chapter 19. Injury, Poisoning and Certain Other Consequences of External Causes

- ☑7ᵗʰ **S89.149** Salter-Harris Type IV physeal fracture of lower end of unspecified tibia 🅠
- ☑6ᵗʰ **S89.19** Other physeal fracture of lower end of tibia
  - ☑7ᵗʰ **S89.191** Other physeal fracture of lower end of right tibia 🅠
  - ☑7ᵗʰ **S89.192** Other physeal fracture of lower end of left tibia 🅠
  - ☑7ᵗʰ **S89.199** Other physeal fracture of lower end of unspecified tibia 🅠
- ☑5ᵗʰ **S89.2** Physeal fracture of upper end of fibula
  - **AHA:** 2019,4Q,56
  - ☑6ᵗʰ **S89.20** Unspecified physeal fracture of upper end of fibula
    - ☑7ᵗʰ **S89.201** Unspecified physeal fracture of upper end of right fibula 🅠
    - ☑7ᵗʰ **S89.202** Unspecified physeal fracture of upper end of left fibula 🅠
    - ☑7ᵗʰ **S89.209** Unspecified physeal fracture of upper end of unspecified fibula 🅠
  - ☑6ᵗʰ **S89.21** Salter-Harris Type I physeal fracture of upper end of fibula
    - ☑7ᵗʰ **S89.211** Salter-Harris Type I physeal fracture of upper end of right fibula 🅠
    - ☑7ᵗʰ **S89.212** Salter-Harris Type I physeal fracture of upper end of left fibula 🅠
    - ☑7ᵗʰ **S89.219** Salter-Harris Type I physeal fracture of upper end of unspecified fibula 🅠
  - ☑6ᵗʰ **S89.22** Salter-Harris Type II physeal fracture of upper end of fibula
    - ☑7ᵗʰ **S89.221** Salter-Harris Type II physeal fracture of upper end of right fibula 🅠
    - ☑7ᵗʰ **S89.222** Salter-Harris Type II physeal fracture of upper end of left fibula 🅠
    - ☑7ᵗʰ **S89.229** Salter-Harris Type II physeal fracture of upper end of unspecified fibula 🅠
  - ☑6ᵗʰ **S89.29** Other physeal fracture of upper end of fibula
    - ☑7ᵗʰ **S89.291** Other physeal fracture of upper end of right fibula 🅠
    - ☑7ᵗʰ **S89.292** Other physeal fracture of upper end of left fibula 🅠
    - ☑7ᵗʰ **S89.299** Other physeal fracture of upper end of unspecified fibula 🅠
- ☑5ᵗʰ **S89.3** Physeal fracture of lower end of fibula
  - **AHA:** 2019,4Q,56
  - ☑6ᵗʰ **S89.30** Unspecified physeal fracture of lower end of fibula
    - ☑7ᵗʰ **S89.301** Unspecified physeal fracture of lower end of right fibula 🅠
    - ☑7ᵗʰ **S89.302** Unspecified physeal fracture of lower end of left fibula 🅠
    - ☑7ᵗʰ **S89.309** Unspecified physeal fracture of lower end of unspecified fibula 🅠
  - ☑6ᵗʰ **S89.31** Salter-Harris Type I physeal fracture of lower end of fibula
    - ☑7ᵗʰ **S89.311** Salter-Harris Type I physeal fracture of lower end of right fibula 🅠
    - ☑7ᵗʰ **S89.312** Salter-Harris Type I physeal fracture of lower end of left fibula 🅠
    - ☑7ᵗʰ **S89.319** Salter-Harris Type I physeal fracture of lower end of unspecified fibula 🅠
  - ☑6ᵗʰ **S89.32** Salter-Harris Type II physeal fracture of lower end of fibula
    - ☑7ᵗʰ **S89.321** Salter-Harris Type II physeal fracture of lower end of right fibula 🅠
    - ☑7ᵗʰ **S89.322** Salter-Harris Type II physeal fracture of lower end of left fibula 🅠
    - ☑7ᵗʰ **S89.329** Salter-Harris Type II physeal fracture of lower end of unspecified fibula 🅠
  - ☑6ᵗʰ **S89.39** Other physeal fracture of lower end of fibula
    - ☑7ᵗʰ **S89.391** Other physeal fracture of lower end of right fibula 🅠
    - ☑7ᵗʰ **S89.392** Other physeal fracture of lower end of left fibula 🅠
    - ☑7ᵗʰ **S89.399** Other physeal fracture of lower end of unspecified fibula 🅠

- ☑5ᵗʰ **S89.8** Other specified injuries of lower leg

  The appropriate 7th character is to be added to each code in subcategory S89.8.
  - A initial encounter
  - D subsequent encounter
  - S sequela

  - ☑x7ᵗʰ **S89.80** Other specified injuries of unspecified lower leg
  - ☑x7ᵗʰ **S89.81** Other specified injuries of right lower leg
  - ☑x7ᵗʰ **S89.82** Other specified injuries of left lower leg

- ☑5ᵗʰ **S89.9** Unspecified injury of lower leg

  The appropriate 7th character is to be added to each code in subcategory S89.9.
  - A initial encounter
  - D subsequent encounter
  - S sequela

  - ☑x7ᵗʰ **S89.90** Unspecified injury of unspecified lower leg
  - ☑x7ᵗʰ **S89.91** Unspecified injury of right lower leg
  - ☑x7ᵗʰ **S89.92** Unspecified injury of left lower leg

Injuries to the ankle and foot (S90-S99)

EXCLUDES 2 burns and corrosions (T20-T32)
fracture of ankle and malleolus (S82.-)
frostbite (T33-T34)
insect bite or sting, venomous (T63.4)

- ☑4ᵗʰ **S90** Superficial injury of ankle, foot and toes

  The appropriate 7th character is to be added to each code from category S90.
  - A initial encounter
  - D subsequent encounter
  - S sequela

  - ☑5ᵗʰ **S90.0** Contusion of ankle
    - ☑x7ᵗʰ **S90.00** Contusion of unspecified ankle
    - ☑x7ᵗʰ **S90.01** Contusion of right ankle
    - ☑x7ᵗʰ **S90.02** Contusion of left ankle
  - ☑5ᵗʰ **S90.1** Contusion of toe without damage to nail
    - ☑6ᵗʰ **S90.11** Contusion of great toe without damage to nail
      - ☑7ᵗʰ **S90.111** Contusion of right great toe without damage to nail
      - ☑7ᵗʰ **S90.112** Contusion of left great toe without damage to nail
      - ☑7ᵗʰ **S90.119** Contusion of unspecified great toe without damage to nail
    - ☑6ᵗʰ **S90.12** Contusion of lesser toe without damage to nail
      - ☑7ᵗʰ **S90.121** Contusion of right lesser toe(s) without damage to nail
      - ☑7ᵗʰ **S90.122** Contusion of left lesser toe(s) without damage to nail
      - ☑7ᵗʰ **S90.129** Contusion of unspecified lesser toe(s) without damage to nail
        Contusion of toe NOS
  - ☑5ᵗʰ **S90.2** Contusion of toe with damage to nail
    - ☑6ᵗʰ **S90.21** Contusion of great toe with damage to nail
      - ☑7ᵗʰ **S90.211** Contusion of right great toe with damage to nail
      - ☑7ᵗʰ **S90.212** Contusion of left great toe with damage to nail
      - ☑7ᵗʰ **S90.219** Contusion of unspecified great toe with damage to nail
    - ☑6ᵗʰ **S90.22** Contusion of lesser toe with damage to nail
      - ☑7ᵗʰ **S90.221** Contusion of right lesser toe(s) with damage to nail
      - ☑7ᵗʰ **S90.222** Contusion of left lesser toe(s) with damage to nail
      - ☑7ᵗʰ **S90.229** Contusion of unspecified lesser toe(s) with damage to nail
  - ☑5ᵗʰ **S90.3** Contusion of foot
    - **EXCLUDES 2** contusion of toes (S90.1-, S90.2-)
    - ☑x7ᵗʰ **S90.30** Contusion of unspecified foot
      Contusion of foot NOS
    - ☑x7ᵗʰ **S90.31** Contusion of right foot
    - ☑x7ᵗʰ **S90.32** Contusion of left foot

☑ Additional Character Required   ☑x7ᵗʰ Placeholder Alert   Manifestation   Unspecified Dx   🅠 QPP   UPD Unacceptable PDx

- **S90.4** Other superficial injuries of toe
  - **S90.41** Abrasion of toe
    - S90.411 Abrasion, right great toe
    - S90.412 Abrasion, left great toe
    - S90.413 Abrasion, unspecified great toe
    - S90.414 Abrasion, right lesser toe(s)
    - S90.415 Abrasion, left lesser toe(s)
    - S90.416 Abrasion, unspecified lesser toe(s)
  - **S90.42** Blister (nonthermal) of toe
    - S90.421 Blister (nonthermal), right great toe
    - S90.422 Blister (nonthermal), left great toe
    - S90.423 Blister (nonthermal), unspecified great toe
    - S90.424 Blister (nonthermal), right lesser toe(s)
    - S90.425 Blister (nonthermal), left lesser toe(s)
    - S90.426 Blister (nonthermal), unspecified lesser toe(s)
  - **S90.44** External constriction of toe
    - Hair tourniquet syndrome of toe
    - S90.441 External constriction, right great toe
    - S90.442 External constriction, left great toe
    - S90.443 External constriction, unspecified great toe
    - S90.444 External constriction, right lesser toe(s)
    - S90.445 External constriction, left lesser toe(s)
    - S90.446 External constriction, unspecified lesser toe(s)
  - **S90.45** Superficial foreign body of toe
    - Splinter in the toe
    - S90.451 Superficial foreign body, right great toe
    - S90.452 Superficial foreign body, left great toe
    - S90.453 Superficial foreign body, unspecified great toe
    - S90.454 Superficial foreign body, right lesser toe(s)
    - S90.455 Superficial foreign body, left lesser toe(s)
    - S90.456 Superficial foreign body, unspecified lesser toe(s)
  - **S90.46** Insect bite (nonvenomous) of toe
    - S90.461 Insect bite (nonvenomous), right great toe
    - S90.462 Insect bite (nonvenomous), left great toe
    - S90.463 Insect bite (nonvenomous), unspecified great toe
    - S90.464 Insect bite (nonvenomous), right lesser toe(s)
    - S90.465 Insect bite (nonvenomous), left lesser toe(s)
    - S90.466 Insect bite (nonvenomous), unspecified lesser toe(s)
  - **S90.47** Other superficial bite of toe
    - EXCLUDES 1 open bite of toe (S91.15-, S91.25-)
    - S90.471 Other superficial bite of right great toe
    - S90.472 Other superficial bite of left great toe
    - S90.473 Other superficial bite of unspecified great toe
    - S90.474 Other superficial bite of right lesser toe(s)
    - S90.475 Other superficial bite of left lesser toe(s)
    - S90.476 Other superficial bite of unspecified lesser toe(s)
- **S90.5** Other superficial injuries of ankle
  - **S90.51** Abrasion of ankle
    - S90.511 Abrasion, right ankle
    - S90.512 Abrasion, left ankle
    - S90.519 Abrasion, unspecified ankle
  - **S90.52** Blister (nonthermal) of ankle
    - S90.521 Blister (nonthermal), right ankle
    - S90.522 Blister (nonthermal), left ankle
    - S90.529 Blister (nonthermal), unspecified ankle
  - **S90.54** External constriction of ankle
    - S90.541 External constriction, right ankle
    - S90.542 External constriction, left ankle
    - S90.549 External constriction, unspecified ankle
  - **S90.55** Superficial foreign body of ankle
    - Splinter in the ankle
    - S90.551 Superficial foreign body, right ankle
    - S90.552 Superficial foreign body, left ankle
    - S90.559 Superficial foreign body, unspecified ankle
  - **S90.56** Insect bite (nonvenomous) of ankle
    - S90.561 Insect bite (nonvenomous), right ankle
    - S90.562 Insect bite (nonvenomous), left ankle
    - S90.569 Insect bite (nonvenomous), unspecified ankle
  - **S90.57** Other superficial bite of ankle
    - EXCLUDES 1 open bite of ankle (S91.05-)
    - S90.571 Other superficial bite of ankle, right ankle
    - S90.572 Other superficial bite of ankle, left ankle
    - S90.579 Other superficial bite of ankle, unspecified ankle
- **S90.8** Other superficial injuries of foot
  - **S90.81** Abrasion of foot
    - S90.811 Abrasion, right foot
    - S90.812 Abrasion, left foot
    - S90.819 Abrasion, unspecified foot
  - **S90.82** Blister (nonthermal) of foot
    - S90.821 Blister (nonthermal), right foot
    - S90.822 Blister (nonthermal), left foot
    - S90.829 Blister (nonthermal), unspecified foot
  - **S90.84** External constriction of foot
    - S90.841 External constriction, right foot
    - S90.842 External constriction, left foot
    - S90.849 External constriction, unspecified foot
  - **S90.85** Superficial foreign body of foot
    - Splinter in the foot
    - S90.851 Superficial foreign body, right foot
    - S90.852 Superficial foreign body, left foot
    - S90.859 Superficial foreign body, unspecified foot
  - **S90.86** Insect bite (nonvenomous) of foot
    - S90.861 Insect bite (nonvenomous), right foot
    - S90.862 Insect bite (nonvenomous), left foot
    - S90.869 Insect bite (nonvenomous), unspecified foot
  - **S90.87** Other superficial bite of foot
    - EXCLUDES 1 open bite of foot (S91.35-)
    - S90.871 Other superficial bite of right foot
    - S90.872 Other superficial bite of left foot
    - S90.879 Other superficial bite of unspecified foot
- **S90.9** Unspecified superficial injury of ankle, foot and toe
  - **S90.91** Unspecified superficial injury of ankle
    - S90.911 Unspecified superficial injury of right ankle
    - S90.912 Unspecified superficial injury of left ankle
    - S90.919 Unspecified superficial injury of unspecified ankle
  - **S90.92** Unspecified superficial injury of foot
    - S90.921 Unspecified superficial injury of right foot
    - S90.922 Unspecified superficial injury of left foot
    - S90.929 Unspecified superficial injury of unspecified foot
  - **S90.93** Unspecified superficial injury of toes
    - S90.931 Unspecified superficial injury of right great toe
    - S90.932 Unspecified superficial injury of left great toe
    - S90.933 Unspecified superficial injury of unspecified great toe
    - S90.934 Unspecified superficial injury of right lesser toe(s)
    - S90.935 Unspecified superficial injury of left lesser toe(s)
    - S90.936 Unspecified superficial injury of unspecified lesser toe(s)

S91 Open wound of ankle, foot and toes

Code also any associated wound infection

EXCLUDES 1 open fracture of ankle, foot and toes (S92.- with 7th character B)
traumatic amputation of ankle and foot (S98.-)

AHA: 2021,1Q,7

The appropriate 7th character is to be added to each code from category S91.
- A initial encounter
- D subsequent encounter
- S sequela

S91.0 Open wound of ankle

- **S91.00** Unspecified open wound of ankle
  - S91.001 Unspecified open wound, right ankle
  - S91.002 Unspecified open wound, left ankle
  - S91.009 Unspecified open wound, unspecified ankle
- **S91.01** Laceration without foreign body of ankle
  - S91.011 Laceration without foreign body, right ankle
  - S91.012 Laceration without foreign body, left ankle
  - S91.019 Laceration without foreign body, unspecified ankle
- **S91.02** Laceration with foreign body of ankle
  - S91.021 Laceration with foreign body, right ankle
  - S91.022 Laceration with foreign body, left ankle
  - S91.029 Laceration with foreign body, unspecified ankle
- **S91.03** Puncture wound without foreign body of ankle
  - S91.031 Puncture wound without foreign body, right ankle
  - S91.032 Puncture wound without foreign body, left ankle
  - S91.039 Puncture wound without foreign body, unspecified ankle
- **S91.04** Puncture wound with foreign body of ankle
  - S91.041 Puncture wound with foreign body, right ankle
  - S91.042 Puncture wound with foreign body, left ankle
  - S91.049 Puncture wound with foreign body, unspecified ankle
- **S91.05** Open bite of ankle
  - **EXCLUDES 1** superficial bite of ankle (S90.56-, S90.57-)
  - S91.051 Open bite, right ankle
  - S91.052 Open bite, left ankle
  - S91.059 Open bite, unspecified ankle

S91.1 Open wound of toe without damage to nail

- **S91.10** Unspecified open wound of toe without damage to nail
  - S91.101 Unspecified open wound of right great toe without damage to nail
  - S91.102 Unspecified open wound of left great toe without damage to nail
  - S91.103 Unspecified open wound of unspecified great toe without damage to nail
  - S91.104 Unspecified open wound of right lesser toe(s) without damage to nail
  - S91.105 Unspecified open wound of left lesser toe(s) without damage to nail
  - S91.106 Unspecified open wound of unspecified lesser toe(s) without damage to nail
  - S91.109 Unspecified open wound of unspecified toe(s) without damage to nail
- **S91.11** Laceration without foreign body of toe without damage to nail
  - S91.111 Laceration without foreign body of right great toe without damage to nail
  - S91.112 Laceration without foreign body of left great toe without damage to nail
  - S91.113 Laceration without foreign body of unspecified great toe without damage to nail
  - S91.114 Laceration without foreign body of right lesser toe(s) without damage to nail
  - S91.115 Laceration without foreign body of left lesser toe(s) without damage to nail
  - S91.116 Laceration without foreign body of unspecified lesser toe(s) without damage to nail
  - S91.119 Laceration without foreign body of unspecified toe without damage to nail
- **S91.12** Laceration with foreign body of toe without damage to nail
  - S91.121 Laceration with foreign body of right great toe without damage to nail
  - S91.122 Laceration with foreign body of left great toe without damage to nail
  - S91.123 Laceration with foreign body of unspecified great toe without damage to nail
  - S91.124 Laceration with foreign body of right lesser toe(s) without damage to nail
  - S91.125 Laceration with foreign body of left lesser toe(s) without damage to nail
  - S91.126 Laceration with foreign body of unspecified lesser toe(s) without damage to nail
  - S91.129 Laceration with foreign body of unspecified toe(s) without damage to nail
- **S91.13** Puncture wound without foreign body of toe without damage to nail
  - S91.131 Puncture wound without foreign body of right great toe without damage to nail
  - S91.132 Puncture wound without foreign body of left great toe without damage to nail
  - S91.133 Puncture wound without foreign body of unspecified great toe without damage to nail
  - S91.134 Puncture wound without foreign body of right lesser toe(s) without damage to nail
  - S91.135 Puncture wound without foreign body of left lesser toe(s) without damage to nail
  - S91.136 Puncture wound without foreign body of unspecified lesser toe(s) without damage to nail
  - S91.139 Puncture wound without foreign body of unspecified toe(s) without damage to nail
- **S91.14** Puncture wound with foreign body of toe without damage to nail
  - S91.141 Puncture wound with foreign body of right great toe without damage to nail
  - S91.142 Puncture wound with foreign body of left great toe without damage to nail
  - S91.143 Puncture wound with foreign body of unspecified great toe without damage to nail
  - S91.144 Puncture wound with foreign body of right lesser toe(s) without damage to nail
  - S91.145 Puncture wound with foreign body of left lesser toe(s) without damage to nail
  - S91.146 Puncture wound with foreign body of unspecified lesser toe(s) without damage to nail
  - S91.149 Puncture wound with foreign body of unspecified toe(s) without damage to nail
- **S91.15** Open bite of toe without damage to nail
  - Bite of toe NOS
  - **EXCLUDES 1** superficial bite of toe (S90.46-, S90.47-)
  - S91.151 Open bite of right great toe without damage to nail
  - S91.152 Open bite of left great toe without damage to nail
  - S91.153 Open bite of unspecified great toe without damage to nail
  - S91.154 Open bite of right lesser toe(s) without damage to nail
  - S91.155 Open bite of left lesser toe(s) without damage to nail
  - S91.156 Open bite of unspecified lesser toe(s) without damage to nail
  - S91.159 Open bite of unspecified toe(s) without damage to nail

S91.2 Open wound of toe with damage to nail

- **S91.20** Unspecified open wound of toe with damage to nail
  - S91.201 Unspecified open wound of right great toe with damage to nail
  - S91.202 Unspecified open wound of left great toe with damage to nail

- √7th **S91.203** Unspecified open wound of unspecified great toe with damage to nail
- √7th **S91.204** Unspecified open wound of right lesser toe(s) with damage to nail
- √7th **S91.205** Unspecified open wound of left lesser toe(s) with damage to nail
- √7th **S91.206** Unspecified open wound of unspecified lesser toe(s) with damage to nail
- √7th **S91.209** Unspecified open wound of unspecified toe(s) with damage to nail

√6th **S91.21 Laceration without foreign body** of toe with damage to nail
- √7th **S91.211** Laceration without foreign body of right great toe with damage to nail
- √7th **S91.212** Laceration without foreign body of left great toe with damage to nail
- √7th **S91.213** Laceration without foreign body of unspecified great toe with damage to nail
- √7th **S91.214** Laceration without foreign body of right lesser toe(s) with damage to nail
- √7th **S91.215** Laceration without foreign body of left lesser toe(s) with damage to nail
- √7th **S91.216** Laceration without foreign body of unspecified lesser toe(s) with damage to nail
- √7th **S91.219** Laceration without foreign body of unspecified toe(s) with damage to nail

√6th **S91.22 Laceration with foreign body** of toe with damage to nail
- √7th **S91.221** Laceration with foreign body of right great toe with damage to nail
- √7th **S91.222** Laceration with foreign body of left great toe with damage to nail
- √7th **S91.223** Laceration with foreign body of unspecified great toe with damage to nail
- √7th **S91.224** Laceration with foreign body of right lesser toe(s) with damage to nail
- √7th **S91.225** Laceration with foreign body of left lesser toe(s) with damage to nail
- √7th **S91.226** Laceration with foreign body of unspecified lesser toe(s) with damage to nail
- √7th **S91.229** Laceration with foreign body of unspecified toe(s) with damage to nail

√6th **S91.23 Puncture wound without foreign body** of toe with damage to nail
- √7th **S91.231** Puncture wound without foreign body of right great toe with damage to nail
- √7th **S91.232** Puncture wound without foreign body of left great toe with damage to nail
- √7th **S91.233** Puncture wound without foreign body of unspecified great toe with damage to nail
- √7th **S91.234** Puncture wound without foreign body of right lesser toe(s) with damage to nail
- √7th **S91.235** Puncture wound without foreign body of left lesser toe(s) with damage to nail
- √7th **S91.236** Puncture wound without foreign body of unspecified lesser toe(s) with damage to nail
- √7th **S91.239** Puncture wound without foreign body of unspecified toe(s) with damage to nail

√6th **S91.24 Puncture wound with foreign body** of toe with damage to nail
- √7th **S91.241** Puncture wound with foreign body of right great toe with damage to nail
- √7th **S91.242** Puncture wound with foreign body of left great toe with damage to nail
- √7th **S91.243** Puncture wound with foreign body of unspecified great toe with damage to nail
- √7th **S91.244** Puncture wound with foreign body of right lesser toe(s) with damage to nail
- √7th **S91.245** Puncture wound with foreign body of left lesser toe(s) with damage to nail
- √7th **S91.246** Puncture wound with foreign body of unspecified lesser toe(s) with damage to nail
- √7th **S91.249** Puncture wound with foreign body of unspecified toe(s) with damage to nail

√6th **S91.25 Open bite** of toe with damage to nail
  Bite of toe with damage to nail NOS
  EXCLUDES 1   superficial bite of toe (S90.46-, S90.47-)
- √7th **S91.251** Open bite of right great toe with damage to nail
- √7th **S91.252** Open bite of left great toe with damage to nail
- √7th **S91.253** Open bite of unspecified great toe with damage to nail
- √7th **S91.254** Open bite of right lesser toe(s) with damage to nail
- √7th **S91.255** Open bite of left lesser toe(s) with damage to nail
- √7th **S91.256** Open bite of unspecified lesser toe(s) with damage to nail
- √7th **S91.259** Open bite of unspecified toe(s) with damage to nail

√5th **S91.3 Open wound** of foot
  √6th **S91.30** Unspecified open wound of foot
  - √7th **S91.301** Unspecified open wound, right foot
  - √7th **S91.302** Unspecified open wound, left foot
  - √7th **S91.309** Unspecified open wound, unspecified foot

  √6th **S91.31 Laceration without foreign body** of foot
  - √7th **S91.311** Laceration without foreign body, right foot
  - √7th **S91.312** Laceration without foreign body, left foot
  - √7th **S91.319** Laceration without foreign body, unspecified foot

  √6th **S91.32 Laceration with foreign body** of foot
  - √7th **S91.321** Laceration with foreign body, right foot
  - √7th **S91.322** Laceration with foreign body, left foot
  - √7th **S91.329** Laceration with foreign body, unspecified foot

  √6th **S91.33 Puncture wound without foreign body** of foot
  - √7th **S91.331** Puncture wound without foreign body, right foot
  - √7th **S91.332** Puncture wound without foreign body, left foot
  - √7th **S91.339** Puncture wound without foreign body, unspecified foot

  √6th **S91.34 Puncture wound with foreign body** of foot
  - √7th **S91.341** Puncture wound with foreign body, right foot
  - √7th **S91.342** Puncture wound with foreign body, left foot
  - √7th **S91.349** Puncture wound with foreign body, unspecified foot

  √6th **S91.35 Open bite** of foot
    EXCLUDES 1   superficial bite of foot (S90.86-, S90.87-)
  - √7th **S91.351** Open bite, right foot
  - √7th **S91.352** Open bite, left foot
  - √7th **S91.359** Open bite, unspecified foot

√4th **S92 Fracture of foot and toe, except ankle**

NOTE A fracture not indicated as displaced or nondisplaced should be coded to displaced

A fracture not indicated as open or closed should be coded to closed.

EXCLUDES 2   fracture of ankle (S82.-)
fracture of malleolus (S82.-)
traumatic amputation of ankle and foot (S98.-)

AHA: 2018,2Q,12; 2015,3Q,37-39

The appropriate 7th character is to be added to each code from category S92.
A initial encounter for closed fracture
B initial encounter for open fracture
D subsequent encounter for fracture with routine healing
G subsequent encounter for fracture with delayed healing
K subsequent encounter for fracture with nonunion
P subsequent encounter for fracture with malunion
S sequela

√5th **S92.0 Fracture of calcaneus**
  Heel bone
  Os calcis
  EXCLUDES 2   physeal fracture of calcaneus (S99.0-)

  √6th **S92.00** Unspecified fracture of calcaneus
  - √7th **S92.001** Unspecified fracture of right calcaneus Q
  - √7th **S92.002** Unspecified fracture of left calcaneus Q
  - √7th **S92.009** Unspecified fracture of unspecified calcaneus Q

S92.01 Fracture of body of calcaneus
- **S92.011** Displaced fracture of body of right calcaneus
- **S92.012** Displaced fracture of body of left calcaneus
- **S92.013** Displaced fracture of body of unspecified calcaneus
- **S92.014** Nondisplaced fracture of body of right calcaneus
- **S92.015** Nondisplaced fracture of body of left calcaneus
- **S92.016** Nondisplaced fracture of body of unspecified calcaneus

S92.02 Fracture of anterior process of calcaneus
- **S92.021** Displaced fracture of anterior process of right calcaneus
- **S92.022** Displaced fracture of anterior process of left calcaneus
- **S92.023** Displaced fracture of anterior process of unspecified calcaneus
- **S92.024** Nondisplaced fracture of anterior process of right calcaneus
- **S92.025** Nondisplaced fracture of anterior process of left calcaneus
- **S92.026** Nondisplaced fracture of anterior process of unspecified calcaneus

S92.03 Avulsion fracture of tuberosity of calcaneus
- **S92.031** Displaced avulsion fracture of tuberosity of right calcaneus
- **S92.032** Displaced avulsion fracture of tuberosity of left calcaneus
- **S92.033** Displaced avulsion fracture of tuberosity of unspecified calcaneus
- **S92.034** Nondisplaced avulsion fracture of tuberosity of right calcaneus
- **S92.035** Nondisplaced avulsion fracture of tuberosity of left calcaneus
- **S92.036** Nondisplaced avulsion fracture of tuberosity of unspecified calcaneus

S92.04 Other fracture of tuberosity of calcaneus
- **S92.041** Displaced other fracture of tuberosity of right calcaneus
- **S92.042** Displaced other fracture of tuberosity of left calcaneus
- **S92.043** Displaced other fracture of tuberosity of unspecified calcaneus
- **S92.044** Nondisplaced other fracture of tuberosity of right calcaneus
- **S92.045** Nondisplaced other fracture of tuberosity of left calcaneus
- **S92.046** Nondisplaced other fracture of tuberosity of unspecified calcaneus

S92.05 Other extraarticular fracture of calcaneus
- **S92.051** Displaced other extraarticular fracture of right calcaneus
- **S92.052** Displaced other extraarticular fracture of left calcaneus
- **S92.053** Displaced other extraarticular fracture of unspecified calcaneus
- **S92.054** Nondisplaced other extraarticular fracture of right calcaneus
- **S92.055** Nondisplaced other extraarticular fracture of left calcaneus
- **S92.056** Nondisplaced other extraarticular fracture of unspecified calcaneus

S92.06 Intraarticular fracture of calcaneus
- **S92.061** Displaced intraarticular fracture of right calcaneus
- **S92.062** Displaced intraarticular fracture of left calcaneus
- **S92.063** Displaced intraarticular fracture of unspecified calcaneus
- **S92.064** Nondisplaced intraarticular fracture of right calcaneus
- **S92.065** Nondisplaced intraarticular fracture of left calcaneus
- **S92.066** Nondisplaced intraarticular fracture of unspecified calcaneus

S92.1 Fracture of talus
Astragalus

S92.10 Unspecified fracture of talus
- **S92.101** Unspecified fracture of right talus
- **S92.102** Unspecified fracture of left talus
- **S92.109** Unspecified fracture of unspecified talus

S92.11 Fracture of neck of talus
- **S92.111** Displaced fracture of neck of right talus
- **S92.112** Displaced fracture of neck of left talus
- **S92.113** Displaced fracture of neck of unspecified talus
- **S92.114** Nondisplaced fracture of neck of right talus
- **S92.115** Nondisplaced fracture of neck of left talus
- **S92.116** Nondisplaced fracture of neck of unspecified talus

S92.12 Fracture of body of talus
- **S92.121** Displaced fracture of body of right talus
- **S92.122** Displaced fracture of body of left talus
- **S92.123** Displaced fracture of body of unspecified talus
- **S92.124** Nondisplaced fracture of body of right talus
- **S92.125** Nondisplaced fracture of body of left talus
- **S92.126** Nondisplaced fracture of body of unspecified talus

S92.13 Fracture of posterior process of talus
- **S92.131** Displaced fracture of posterior process of right talus
- **S92.132** Displaced fracture of posterior process of left talus
- **S92.133** Displaced fracture of posterior process of unspecified talus
- **S92.134** Nondisplaced fracture of posterior process of right talus
- **S92.135** Nondisplaced fracture of posterior process of left talus
- **S92.136** Nondisplaced fracture of posterior process of unspecified talus

S92.14 Dome fracture of talus
EXCLUDES 1 osteochondritis dissecans (M93.2)
- **S92.141** Displaced dome fracture of right talus
- **S92.142** Displaced dome fracture of left talus
- **S92.143** Displaced dome fracture of unspecified talus
- **S92.144** Nondisplaced dome fracture of right talus
- **S92.145** Nondisplaced dome fracture of left talus
- **S92.146** Nondisplaced dome fracture of unspecified talus

S92.15 Avulsion fracture (chip fracture) of talus
- **S92.151** Displaced avulsion fracture (chip fracture) of right talus
- **S92.152** Displaced avulsion fracture (chip fracture) of left talus
- **S92.153** Displaced avulsion fracture (chip fracture) of unspecified talus
- **S92.154** Nondisplaced avulsion fracture (chip fracture) of right talus
- **S92.155** Nondisplaced avulsion fracture (chip fracture) of left talus
- **S92.156** Nondisplaced avulsion fracture (chip fracture) of unspecified talus

S92.19 Other fracture of talus
- **S92.191** Other fracture of right talus
- **S92.192** Other fracture of left talus
- **S92.199** Other fracture of unspecified talus

S92.2 Fracture of other and unspecified tarsal bone(s)

- **S92.20** Fracture of unspecified tarsal bone(s)
  - S92.201 Fracture of unspecified tarsal bone(s) of right foot
  - S92.202 Fracture of unspecified tarsal bone(s) of left foot
  - S92.209 Fracture of unspecified tarsal bone(s) of unspecified foot
- **S92.21** Fracture of cuboid bone
  - S92.211 Displaced fracture of cuboid bone of right foot
  - S92.212 Displaced fracture of cuboid bone of left foot
  - S92.213 Displaced fracture of cuboid bone of unspecified foot
  - S92.214 Nondisplaced fracture of cuboid bone of right foot
  - S92.215 Nondisplaced fracture of cuboid bone of left foot
  - S92.216 Nondisplaced fracture of cuboid bone of unspecified foot
- **S92.22** Fracture of lateral cuneiform
  - S92.221 Displaced fracture of lateral cuneiform of right foot
  - S92.222 Displaced fracture of lateral cuneiform of left foot
  - S92.223 Displaced fracture of lateral cuneiform of unspecified foot
  - S92.224 Nondisplaced fracture of lateral cuneiform of right foot
  - S92.225 Nondisplaced fracture of lateral cuneiform of left foot
  - S92.226 Nondisplaced fracture of lateral cuneiform of unspecified foot
- **S92.23** Fracture of intermediate cuneiform
  - S92.231 Displaced fracture of intermediate cuneiform of right foot
  - S92.232 Displaced fracture of intermediate cuneiform of left foot
  - S92.233 Displaced fracture of intermediate cuneiform of unspecified foot
  - S92.234 Nondisplaced fracture of intermediate cuneiform of right foot
  - S92.235 Nondisplaced fracture of intermediate cuneiform of left foot
  - S92.236 Nondisplaced fracture of intermediate cuneiform of unspecified foot
- **S92.24** Fracture of medial cuneiform
  - S92.241 Displaced fracture of medial cuneiform of right foot
  - S92.242 Displaced fracture of medial cuneiform of left foot
  - S92.243 Displaced fracture of medial cuneiform of unspecified foot
  - S92.244 Nondisplaced fracture of medial cuneiform of right foot
  - S92.245 Nondisplaced fracture of medial cuneiform of left foot
  - S92.246 Nondisplaced fracture of medial cuneiform of unspecified foot
- **S92.25** Fracture of navicular [scaphoid] of foot
  - S92.251 Displaced fracture of navicular [scaphoid] of right foot
  - S92.252 Displaced fracture of navicular [scaphoid] of left foot
  - S92.253 Displaced fracture of navicular [scaphoid] of unspecified foot
  - S92.254 Nondisplaced fracture of navicular [scaphoid] of right foot
  - S92.255 Nondisplaced fracture of navicular [scaphoid] of left foot
  - S92.256 Nondisplaced fracture of navicular [scaphoid] of unspecified foot

S92.3 Fracture of metatarsal bone(s)

EXCLUDES 2: physeal fracture of metatarsal (S99.1-)
AHA: 2018, 1Q, 3

- **S92.30** Fracture of unspecified metatarsal bone(s)
  - S92.301 Fracture of unspecified metatarsal bone(s), right foot
  - S92.302 Fracture of unspecified metatarsal bone(s), left foot
  - S92.309 Fracture of unspecified metatarsal bone(s), unspecified foot
- **S92.31** Fracture of first metatarsal bone
  - S92.311 Displaced fracture of first metatarsal bone, right foot
  - S92.312 Displaced fracture of first metatarsal bone, left foot
  - S92.313 Displaced fracture of first metatarsal bone, unspecified foot
  - S92.314 Nondisplaced fracture of first metatarsal bone, right foot
  - S92.315 Nondisplaced fracture of first metatarsal bone, left foot
  - S92.316 Nondisplaced fracture of first metatarsal bone, unspecified foot
- **S92.32** Fracture of second metatarsal bone
  - S92.321 Displaced fracture of second metatarsal bone, right foot
  - S92.322 Displaced fracture of second metatarsal bone, left foot
  - S92.323 Displaced fracture of second metatarsal bone, unspecified foot
  - S92.324 Nondisplaced fracture of second metatarsal bone, right foot
  - S92.325 Nondisplaced fracture of second metatarsal bone, left foot
  - S92.326 Nondisplaced fracture of second metatarsal bone, unspecified foot
- **S92.33** Fracture of third metatarsal bone
  - S92.331 Displaced fracture of third metatarsal bone, right foot
  - S92.332 Displaced fracture of third metatarsal bone, left foot
  - S92.333 Displaced fracture of third metatarsal bone, unspecified foot
  - S92.334 Nondisplaced fracture of third metatarsal bone, right foot
  - S92.335 Nondisplaced fracture of third metatarsal bone, left foot
  - S92.336 Nondisplaced fracture of third metatarsal bone, unspecified foot
- **S92.34** Fracture of fourth metatarsal bone
  - S92.341 Displaced fracture of fourth metatarsal bone, right foot
  - S92.342 Displaced fracture of fourth metatarsal bone, left foot
  - S92.343 Displaced fracture of fourth metatarsal bone, unspecified foot
  - S92.344 Nondisplaced fracture of fourth metatarsal bone, right foot
  - S92.345 Nondisplaced fracture of fourth metatarsal bone, left foot
  - S92.346 Nondisplaced fracture of fourth metatarsal bone, unspecified foot
- **S92.35** Fracture of fifth metatarsal bone
  - S92.351 Displaced fracture of fifth metatarsal bone, right foot
  - S92.352 Displaced fracture of fifth metatarsal bone, left foot
  - S92.353 Displaced fracture of fifth metatarsal bone, unspecified foot
  - S92.354 Nondisplaced fracture of fifth metatarsal bone, right foot
  - S92.355 Nondisplaced fracture of fifth metatarsal bone, left foot
  - S92.356 Nondisplaced fracture of fifth metatarsal bone, unspecified foot

S92.4 Fracture of great toe
EXCLUDES 2: physeal fracture of phalanx of toe (S99.2-)

- **S92.40** Unspecified fracture of great toe
  - S92.401 Displaced unspecified fracture of right great toe
  - S92.402 Displaced unspecified fracture of left great toe
  - S92.403 Displaced unspecified fracture of unspecified great toe
  - S92.404 Nondisplaced unspecified fracture of right great toe
  - S92.405 Nondisplaced unspecified fracture of left great toe
  - S92.406 Nondisplaced unspecified fracture of unspecified great toe
- **S92.41** Fracture of proximal phalanx of great toe
  - S92.411 Displaced fracture of proximal phalanx of right great toe
  - S92.412 Displaced fracture of proximal phalanx of left great toe
  - S92.413 Displaced fracture of proximal phalanx of unspecified great toe
  - S92.414 Nondisplaced fracture of proximal phalanx of right great toe
  - S92.415 Nondisplaced fracture of proximal phalanx of left great toe
  - S92.416 Nondisplaced fracture of proximal phalanx of unspecified great toe
- **S92.42** Fracture of distal phalanx of great toe
  - S92.421 Displaced fracture of distal phalanx of right great toe
  - S92.422 Displaced fracture of distal phalanx of left great toe
  - S92.423 Displaced fracture of distal phalanx of unspecified great toe
  - S92.424 Nondisplaced fracture of distal phalanx of right great toe
  - S92.425 Nondisplaced fracture of distal phalanx of left great toe
  - S92.426 Nondisplaced fracture of distal phalanx of unspecified great toe
- **S92.49** Other fracture of great toe
  - S92.491 Other fracture of right great toe
  - S92.492 Other fracture of left great toe
  - S92.499 Other fracture of unspecified great toe

S92.5 Fracture of lesser toe(s)
EXCLUDES 2: physeal fracture of phalanx of toe (S99.2-)

- **S92.50** Unspecified fracture of lesser toe(s)
  - S92.501 Displaced unspecified fracture of right lesser toe(s)
  - S92.502 Displaced unspecified fracture of left lesser toe(s)
  - S92.503 Displaced unspecified fracture of unspecified lesser toe(s)
  - S92.504 Nondisplaced unspecified fracture of right lesser toe(s)
  - S92.505 Nondisplaced unspecified fracture of left lesser toe(s)
  - S92.506 Nondisplaced unspecified fracture of unspecified lesser toe(s)
- **S92.51** Fracture of proximal phalanx of lesser toe(s)
  - S92.511 Displaced fracture of proximal phalanx of right lesser toe(s)
  - S92.512 Displaced fracture of proximal phalanx of left lesser toe(s)
  - S92.513 Displaced fracture of proximal phalanx of unspecified lesser toe(s)
  - S92.514 Nondisplaced fracture of proximal phalanx of right lesser toe(s)
  - S92.515 Nondisplaced fracture of proximal phalanx of left lesser toe(s)
  - S92.516 Nondisplaced fracture of proximal phalanx of unspecified lesser toe(s)
- **S92.52** Fracture of middle phalanx of lesser toe(s)
  - S92.521 Displaced fracture of middle phalanx of right lesser toe(s)
  - S92.522 Displaced fracture of middle phalanx of left lesser toe(s)
  - S92.523 Displaced fracture of middle phalanx of unspecified lesser toe(s)
  - S92.524 Nondisplaced fracture of middle phalanx of right lesser toe(s)
  - S92.525 Nondisplaced fracture of middle phalanx of left lesser toe(s)
  - S92.526 Nondisplaced fracture of middle phalanx of unspecified lesser toe(s)
- **S92.53** Fracture of distal phalanx of lesser toe(s)
  - S92.531 Displaced fracture of distal phalanx of right lesser toe(s)
  - S92.532 Displaced fracture of distal phalanx of left lesser toe(s)
  - S92.533 Displaced fracture of distal phalanx of unspecified lesser toe(s)
  - S92.534 Nondisplaced fracture of distal phalanx of right lesser toe(s)
  - S92.535 Nondisplaced fracture of distal phalanx of left lesser toe(s)
  - S92.536 Nondisplaced fracture of distal phalanx of unspecified lesser toe(s)
- **S92.59** Other fracture of lesser toe(s)
  - S92.591 Other fracture of right lesser toe(s)
  - S92.592 Other fracture of left lesser toe(s)
  - S92.599 Other fracture of unspecified lesser toe(s)

S92.8 Other fracture of foot, except ankle
- **S92.81** Other fracture of foot
  - Sesamoid fracture of foot
  - **AHA:** 2016, 4Q, 68
  - S92.811 Other fracture of right foot
  - S92.812 Other fracture of left foot
  - S92.819 Other fracture of unspecified foot

S92.9 Unspecified fracture of foot and toe
- **S92.90** Unspecified fracture of foot
  - S92.901 Unspecified fracture of right foot
  - S92.902 Unspecified fracture of left foot
  - S92.909 Unspecified fracture of unspecified foot
- **S92.91** Unspecified fracture of toe
  - S92.911 Unspecified fracture of right toe(s)
  - S92.912 Unspecified fracture of left toe(s)
  - S92.919 Unspecified fracture of unspecified toe(s)

S93 Dislocation and sprain of joints and ligaments at ankle, foot and toe level
INCLUDES
- avulsion of joint or ligament of ankle, foot and toe
- laceration of cartilage, joint or ligament of ankle, foot and toe
- sprain of cartilage, joint or ligament of ankle, foot and toe
- traumatic hemarthrosis of joint or ligament of ankle, foot and toe
- traumatic rupture of joint or ligament of ankle, foot and toe
- traumatic subluxation of joint or ligament of ankle, foot and toe
- traumatic tear of joint or ligament of ankle, foot and toe

Code also any associated open wound
EXCLUDES 2: strain of muscle and tendon of ankle and foot (S96.-)

The appropriate 7th character is to be added to each code from category S93.
- A initial encounter
- D subsequent encounter
- S sequela

S93.0 Subluxation and dislocation of ankle joint
Subluxation and dislocation of astragalus
Subluxation and dislocation of fibula, lower end
Subluxation and dislocation of talus
Subluxation and dislocation of tibia, lower end

- S93.01 Subluxation of right ankle joint
- S93.02 Subluxation of left ankle joint
- S93.03 Subluxation of unspecified ankle joint
- S93.04 Dislocation of right ankle joint
- S93.05 Dislocation of left ankle joint
- S93.06 Dislocation of unspecified ankle joint

- **S93.1** Subluxation and dislocation of toe
  - **S93.10** Unspecified subluxation and dislocation of toe
    Dislocation of toe NOS
    Subluxation of toe NOS
    - **S93.101** Unspecified subluxation of right toe(s)
    - **S93.102** Unspecified subluxation of left toe(s)
    - **S93.103** Unspecified subluxation of unspecified toe(s)
    - **S93.104** Unspecified dislocation of right toe(s)
    - **S93.105** Unspecified dislocation of left toe(s)
    - **S93.106** Unspecified dislocation of unspecified toe(s)
  - **S93.11** Dislocation of interphalangeal joint
    - **S93.111** Dislocation of interphalangeal joint of right great toe
    - **S93.112** Dislocation of interphalangeal joint of left great toe
    - **S93.113** Dislocation of interphalangeal joint of unspecified great toe
    - **S93.114** Dislocation of interphalangeal joint of right lesser toe(s)
    - **S93.115** Dislocation of interphalangeal joint of left lesser toe(s)
    - **S93.116** Dislocation of interphalangeal joint of unspecified lesser toe(s)
    - **S93.119** Dislocation of interphalangeal joint of unspecified toe(s)
  - **S93.12** Dislocation of metatarsophalangeal joint
    - **S93.121** Dislocation of metatarsophalangeal joint of right great toe
    - **S93.122** Dislocation of metatarsophalangeal joint of left great toe
    - **S93.123** Dislocation of metatarsophalangeal joint of unspecified great toe
    - **S93.124** Dislocation of metatarsophalangeal joint of right lesser toe(s)
    - **S93.125** Dislocation of metatarsophalangeal joint of left lesser toe(s)
    - **S93.126** Dislocation of metatarsophalangeal joint of unspecified lesser toe(s)
    - **S93.129** Dislocation of metatarsophalangeal joint of unspecified toe(s)
  - **S93.13** Subluxation of interphalangeal joint
    - **S93.131** Subluxation of interphalangeal joint of right great toe
    - **S93.132** Subluxation of interphalangeal joint of left great toe
    - **S93.133** Subluxation of interphalangeal joint of unspecified great toe
    - **S93.134** Subluxation of interphalangeal joint of right lesser toe(s)
    - **S93.135** Subluxation of interphalangeal joint of left lesser toe(s)
    - **S93.136** Subluxation of interphalangeal joint of unspecified lesser toe(s)
    - **S93.139** Subluxation of interphalangeal joint of unspecified toe(s)
  - **S93.14** Subluxation of metatarsophalangeal joint
    - **S93.141** Subluxation of metatarsophalangeal joint of right great toe
    - **S93.142** Subluxation of metatarsophalangeal joint of left great toe
    - **S93.143** Subluxation of metatarsophalangeal joint of unspecified great toe
    - **S93.144** Subluxation of metatarsophalangeal joint of right lesser toe(s)
    - **S93.145** Subluxation of metatarsophalangeal joint of left lesser toe(s)
    - **S93.146** Subluxation of metatarsophalangeal joint of unspecified lesser toe(s)
    - **S93.149** Subluxation of metatarsophalangeal joint of unspecified toe(s)
- **S93.3** Subluxation and dislocation of foot
  EXCLUDES 2 dislocation of toe (S93.1-)
  - **S93.30** Unspecified subluxation and dislocation of foot
    Dislocation of foot NOS
    Subluxation of foot NOS
    - **S93.301** Unspecified subluxation of right foot
    - **S93.302** Unspecified subluxation of left foot
    - **S93.303** Unspecified subluxation of unspecified foot
    - **S93.304** Unspecified dislocation of right foot
    - **S93.305** Unspecified dislocation of left foot
    - **S93.306** Unspecified dislocation of unspecified foot
  - **S93.31** Subluxation and dislocation of tarsal joint
    - **S93.311** Subluxation of tarsal joint of right foot
    - **S93.312** Subluxation of tarsal joint of left foot
    - **S93.313** Subluxation of tarsal joint of unspecified foot
    - **S93.314** Dislocation of tarsal joint of right foot
    - **S93.315** Dislocation of tarsal joint of left foot
    - **S93.316** Dislocation of tarsal joint of unspecified foot
  - **S93.32** Subluxation and dislocation of tarsometatarsal joint
    - **S93.321** Subluxation of tarsometatarsal joint of right foot
    - **S93.322** Subluxation of tarsometatarsal joint of left foot
    - **S93.323** Subluxation of tarsometatarsal joint of unspecified foot
    - **S93.324** Dislocation of tarsometatarsal joint of right foot
    - **S93.325** Dislocation of tarsometatarsal joint of left foot
    - **S93.326** Dislocation of tarsometatarsal joint of unspecified foot
  - **S93.33** Other subluxation and dislocation of foot
    - **S93.331** Other subluxation of right foot
    - **S93.332** Other subluxation of left foot
    - **S93.333** Other subluxation of unspecified foot
    - **S93.334** Other dislocation of right foot
    - **S93.335** Other dislocation of left foot
    - **S93.336** Other dislocation of unspecified foot
- **S93.4** Sprain of ankle
  EXCLUDES 2 injury of Achilles tendon (S86.0-)
  - **S93.40** Sprain of unspecified ligament of ankle
    Sprain of ankle NOS
    Sprained ankle NOS
    - **S93.401** Sprain of unspecified ligament of right ankle
    - **S93.402** Sprain of unspecified ligament of left ankle
    - **S93.409** Sprain of unspecified ligament of unspecified ankle
  - **S93.41** Sprain of calcaneofibular ligament
    - **S93.411** Sprain of calcaneofibular ligament of right ankle
    - **S93.412** Sprain of calcaneofibular ligament of left ankle
    - **S93.419** Sprain of calcaneofibular ligament of unspecified ankle
  - **S93.42** Sprain of deltoid ligament
    - **S93.421** Sprain of deltoid ligament of right ankle
    - **S93.422** Sprain of deltoid ligament of left ankle
    - **S93.429** Sprain of deltoid ligament of unspecified ankle
  - **S93.43** Sprain of tibiofibular ligament
    - **S93.431** Sprain of tibiofibular ligament of right ankle
    - **S93.432** Sprain of tibiofibular ligament of left ankle
    - **S93.439** Sprain of tibiofibular ligament of unspecified ankle
  - **S93.49** Sprain of other ligament of ankle
    Sprain of internal collateral ligament
    Sprain of talofibular ligament
    - **S93.491** Sprain of other ligament of right ankle
    - **S93.492** Sprain of other ligament of left ankle
    - **S93.499** Sprain of other ligament of unspecified ankle
- **S93.5** Sprain of toe
  - **S93.50** Unspecified sprain of toe
    - **S93.501** Unspecified sprain of right great toe
    - **S93.502** Unspecified sprain of left great toe
    - **S93.503** Unspecified sprain of unspecified great toe

- S93.504 Unspecified sprain of right lesser toe(s)
- S93.505 Unspecified sprain of left lesser toe(s)
- S93.506 Unspecified sprain of unspecified lesser toe(s)
- S93.509 Unspecified sprain of unspecified toe(s)
- S93.51 Sprain of interphalangeal joint of toe
  - S93.511 Sprain of interphalangeal joint of right great toe
  - S93.512 Sprain of interphalangeal joint of left great toe
  - S93.513 Sprain of interphalangeal joint of unspecified great toe
  - S93.514 Sprain of interphalangeal joint of right lesser toe(s)
  - S93.515 Sprain of interphalangeal joint of left lesser toe(s)
  - S93.516 Sprain of interphalangeal joint of unspecified lesser toe(s)
  - S93.519 Sprain of interphalangeal joint of unspecified toe(s)
- S93.52 Sprain of metatarsophalangeal joint of toe
  - S93.521 Sprain of metatarsophalangeal joint of right great toe
  - S93.522 Sprain of metatarsophalangeal joint of left great toe
  - S93.523 Sprain of metatarsophalangeal joint of unspecified great toe
  - S93.524 Sprain of metatarsophalangeal joint of right lesser toe(s)
  - S93.525 Sprain of metatarsophalangeal joint of left lesser toe(s)
  - S93.526 Sprain of metatarsophalangeal joint of unspecified lesser toe(s)
  - S93.529 Sprain of metatarsophalangeal joint of unspecified toe(s)
- S93.6 Sprain of foot
  - EXCLUDES 2: sprain of metatarsophalangeal joint of toe (S93.52-) sprain of toe (S93.5-)
  - S93.60 Unspecified sprain of foot
    - S93.601 Unspecified sprain of right foot
    - S93.602 Unspecified sprain of left foot
    - S93.609 Unspecified sprain of unspecified foot
  - S93.61 Sprain of tarsal ligament of foot
    - S93.611 Sprain of tarsal ligament of right foot
    - S93.612 Sprain of tarsal ligament of left foot
    - S93.619 Sprain of tarsal ligament of unspecified foot
  - S93.62 Sprain of tarsometatarsal ligament of foot
    - S93.621 Sprain of tarsometatarsal ligament of right foot
    - S93.622 Sprain of tarsometatarsal ligament of left foot
    - S93.629 Sprain of tarsometatarsal ligament of unspecified foot
  - S93.69 Other sprain of foot
    - S93.691 Other sprain of right foot
    - S93.692 Other sprain of left foot
    - S93.699 Other sprain of unspecified foot
- S94 Injury of nerves at ankle and foot level
  - Code also any associated open wound (S91.-)
  - The appropriate 7th character is to be added to each code from category S94.
    - A initial encounter
    - D subsequent encounter
    - S sequela
  - S94.0 Injury of lateral plantar nerve
    - S94.00 Injury of lateral plantar nerve, unspecified leg
    - S94.01 Injury of lateral plantar nerve, right leg
    - S94.02 Injury of lateral plantar nerve, left leg
  - S94.1 Injury of medial plantar nerve
    - S94.10 Injury of medial plantar nerve, unspecified leg
    - S94.11 Injury of medial plantar nerve, right leg
    - S94.12 Injury of medial plantar nerve, left leg
  - S94.2 Injury of deep peroneal nerve at ankle and foot level
    - Injury of terminal, lateral branch of deep peroneal nerve
    - S94.20 Injury of deep peroneal nerve at ankle and foot level, unspecified leg
    - S94.21 Injury of deep peroneal nerve at ankle and foot level, right leg
    - S94.22 Injury of deep peroneal nerve at ankle and foot level, left leg
  - S94.3 Injury of cutaneous sensory nerve at ankle and foot level
    - S94.30 Injury of cutaneous sensory nerve at ankle and foot level, unspecified leg
    - S94.31 Injury of cutaneous sensory nerve at ankle and foot level, right leg
    - S94.32 Injury of cutaneous sensory nerve at ankle and foot level, left leg
  - S94.8 Injury of other nerves at ankle and foot level
    - S94.8X Injury of other nerves at ankle and foot level
      - S94.8X1 Injury of other nerves at ankle and foot level, right leg
      - S94.8X2 Injury of other nerves at ankle and foot level, left leg
      - S94.8X9 Injury of other nerves at ankle and foot level, unspecified leg
  - S94.9 Injury of unspecified nerve at ankle and foot level
    - S94.90 Injury of unspecified nerve at ankle and foot level, unspecified leg
    - S94.91 Injury of unspecified nerve at ankle and foot level, right leg
    - S94.92 Injury of unspecified nerve at ankle and foot level, left leg
- S95 Injury of blood vessels at ankle and foot level
  - Code also any associated open wound (S91.-)
  - EXCLUDES 2: injury of posterior tibial artery and vein (S85.1-, S85.8-)
  - The appropriate 7th character is to be added to each code from category S95.
    - A initial encounter
    - D subsequent encounter
    - S sequela
  - S95.0 Injury of dorsal artery of foot
    - S95.00 Unspecified injury of dorsal artery of foot
      - S95.001 Unspecified injury of dorsal artery of right foot
      - S95.002 Unspecified injury of dorsal artery of left foot
      - S95.009 Unspecified injury of dorsal artery of unspecified foot
    - S95.01 Laceration of dorsal artery of foot
      - S95.011 Laceration of dorsal artery of right foot
      - S95.012 Laceration of dorsal artery of left foot
      - S95.019 Laceration of dorsal artery of unspecified foot
    - S95.09 Other specified injury of dorsal artery of foot
      - S95.091 Other specified injury of dorsal artery of right foot
      - S95.092 Other specified injury of dorsal artery of left foot
      - S95.099 Other specified injury of dorsal artery of unspecified foot
  - S95.1 Injury of plantar artery of foot
    - S95.10 Unspecified injury of plantar artery of foot
      - S95.101 Unspecified injury of plantar artery of right foot
      - S95.102 Unspecified injury of plantar artery of left foot
      - S95.109 Unspecified injury of plantar artery of unspecified foot
    - S95.11 Laceration of plantar artery of foot
      - S95.111 Laceration of plantar artery of right foot
      - S95.112 Laceration of plantar artery of left foot
      - S95.119 Laceration of plantar artery of unspecified foot
    - S95.19 Other specified injury of plantar artery of foot
      - S95.191 Other specified injury of plantar artery of right foot
      - S95.192 Other specified injury of plantar artery of left foot

- **S95.199** Other specified injury of plantar artery of unspecified foot
- **S95.2** Injury of *dorsal vein* of foot
  - **S95.20** Unspecified injury of dorsal vein of foot
    - **S95.201** Unspecified injury of dorsal vein of *right* foot
    - **S95.202** Unspecified injury of dorsal vein of *left* foot
    - **S95.209** Unspecified injury of dorsal vein of unspecified foot
  - **S95.21** *Laceration* of dorsal vein of foot
    - **S95.211** Laceration of dorsal vein of *right* foot
    - **S95.212** Laceration of dorsal vein of *left* foot
    - **S95.219** Laceration of dorsal vein of unspecified foot
  - **S95.29** Other specified injury of dorsal vein of foot
    - **S95.291** Other specified injury of dorsal vein of *right* foot
    - **S95.292** Other specified injury of dorsal vein of *left* foot
    - **S95.299** Other specified injury of dorsal vein of unspecified foot
- **S95.8** Injury of other blood vessels at ankle and foot level
  - **S95.80** Unspecified injury of other blood vessels at ankle and foot level
    - **S95.801** Unspecified injury of other blood vessels at ankle and foot level, *right* leg
    - **S95.802** Unspecified injury of other blood vessels at ankle and foot level, *left* leg
    - **S95.809** Unspecified injury of other blood vessels at ankle and foot level, unspecified leg
  - **S95.81** *Laceration* of other blood vessels at ankle and foot level
    - **S95.811** Laceration of other blood vessels at ankle and foot level, *right* leg
    - **S95.812** Laceration of other blood vessels at ankle and foot level, *left* leg
    - **S95.819** Laceration of other blood vessels at ankle and foot level, unspecified leg
  - **S95.89** Other specified injury of other blood vessels at ankle and foot level
    - **S95.891** Other specified injury of other blood vessels at ankle and foot level, *right* leg
    - **S95.892** Other specified injury of other blood vessels at ankle and foot level, *left* leg
    - **S95.899** Other specified injury of other blood vessels at ankle and foot level, unspecified leg
- **S95.9** Injury of unspecified blood vessel at ankle and foot level
  - **S95.90** Unspecified injury of unspecified blood vessel at ankle and foot level
    - **S95.901** Unspecified injury of unspecified blood vessel at ankle and foot level, *right* leg
    - **S95.902** Unspecified injury of unspecified blood vessel at ankle and foot level, *left* leg
    - **S95.909** Unspecified injury of unspecified blood vessel at ankle and foot level, unspecified leg
  - **S95.91** *Laceration* of unspecified blood vessel at ankle and foot level
    - **S95.911** Laceration of unspecified blood vessel at ankle and foot level, *right* leg
    - **S95.912** Laceration of unspecified blood vessel at ankle and foot level, *left* leg
    - **S95.919** Laceration of unspecified blood vessel at ankle and foot level, unspecified leg
  - **S95.99** Other specified injury of unspecified blood vessel at ankle and foot level
    - **S95.991** Other specified injury of unspecified blood vessel at ankle and foot level, *right* leg
    - **S95.992** Other specified injury of unspecified blood vessel at ankle and foot level, *left* leg
    - **S95.999** Other specified injury of unspecified blood vessel at ankle and foot level, unspecified leg

- **S96** Injury of muscle and tendon at ankle and foot level
  Code also any associated open wound (S91.-)
  EXCLUDES 2 injury of Achilles tendon (S86.0-)
  sprain of joints and ligaments of ankle and foot (S93.-)
  TIP: Refer to the Muscle/Tendon table at the beginning of this chapter.

  The appropriate 7th character is to be added to each code from category S96.
  A initial encounter
  D subsequent encounter
  S sequela

  - **S96.0** Injury of muscle and tendon of *long flexor muscle of toe* at ankle and foot level
    - **S96.00** Unspecified injury of muscle and tendon of long flexor muscle of toe at ankle and foot level
      - **S96.001** Unspecified injury of muscle and tendon of long flexor muscle of toe at ankle and foot level, *right* foot
      - **S96.002** Unspecified injury of muscle and tendon of long flexor muscle of toe at ankle and foot level, *left* foot
      - **S96.009** Unspecified injury of muscle and tendon of long flexor muscle of toe at ankle and foot level, unspecified foot
    - **S96.01** *Strain* of muscle and tendon of long flexor muscle of toe at ankle and foot level
      - **S96.011** Strain of muscle and tendon of long flexor muscle of toe at ankle and foot level, *right* foot
      - **S96.012** Strain of muscle and tendon of long flexor muscle of toe at ankle and foot level, *left* foot
      - **S96.019** Strain of muscle and tendon of long flexor muscle of toe at ankle and foot level, unspecified foot
    - **S96.02** *Laceration* of muscle and tendon of long flexor muscle of toe at ankle and foot level
      - **S96.021** Laceration of muscle and tendon of long flexor muscle of toe at ankle and foot level, *right* foot
      - **S96.022** Laceration of muscle and tendon of long flexor muscle of toe at ankle and foot level, *left* foot
      - **S96.029** Laceration of muscle and tendon of long flexor muscle of toe at ankle and foot level, unspecified foot
    - **S96.09** Other injury of muscle and tendon of long flexor muscle of toe at ankle and foot level
      - **S96.091** Other injury of muscle and tendon of long flexor muscle of toe at ankle and foot level, *right* foot
      - **S96.092** Other injury of muscle and tendon of long flexor muscle of toe at ankle and foot level, *left* foot
      - **S96.099** Other injury of muscle and tendon of long flexor muscle of toe at ankle and foot level, unspecified foot
  - **S96.1** Injury of muscle and tendon of *long extensor muscle of toe* at ankle and foot level
    - **S96.10** Unspecified injury of muscle and tendon of long extensor muscle of toe at ankle and foot level
      - **S96.101** Unspecified injury of muscle and tendon of long extensor muscle of toe at ankle and foot level, *right* foot
      - **S96.102** Unspecified injury of muscle and tendon of long extensor muscle of toe at ankle and foot level, *left* foot
      - **S96.109** Unspecified injury of muscle and tendon of long extensor muscle of toe at ankle and foot level, unspecified foot
    - **S96.11** *Strain* of muscle and tendon of long extensor muscle of toe at ankle and foot level
      - **S96.111** Strain of muscle and tendon of long extensor muscle of toe at ankle and foot level, *right* foot
      - **S96.112** Strain of muscle and tendon of long extensor muscle of toe at ankle and foot level, *left* foot
      - **S96.119** Strain of muscle and tendon of long extensor muscle of toe at ankle and foot level, unspecified foot

- **S96.12** Laceration of muscle and tendon of long extensor muscle of toe at ankle and foot level
  - S96.121 Laceration of muscle and tendon of long extensor muscle of toe at ankle and foot level, right foot
  - S96.122 Laceration of muscle and tendon of long extensor muscle of toe at ankle and foot level, left foot
  - S96.129 Laceration of muscle and tendon of long extensor muscle of toe at ankle and foot level, unspecified foot
- **S96.19** Other specified injury of muscle and tendon of long extensor muscle of toe at ankle and foot level
  - S96.191 Other specified injury of muscle and tendon of long extensor muscle of toe at ankle and foot level, right foot
  - S96.192 Other specified injury of muscle and tendon of long extensor muscle of toe at ankle and foot level, left foot
  - S96.199 Other specified injury of muscle and tendon of long extensor muscle of toe at ankle and foot level, unspecified foot

S96.2 Injury of intrinsic muscle and tendon at ankle and foot level
- **S96.20** Unspecified injury of intrinsic muscle and tendon at ankle and foot level
  - S96.201 Unspecified injury of intrinsic muscle and tendon at ankle and foot level, right foot
  - S96.202 Unspecified injury of intrinsic muscle and tendon at ankle and foot level, left foot
  - S96.209 Unspecified injury of intrinsic muscle and tendon at ankle and foot level, unspecified foot
- **S96.21** Strain of intrinsic muscle and tendon at ankle and foot level
  - S96.211 Strain of intrinsic muscle and tendon at ankle and foot level, right foot
  - S96.212 Strain of intrinsic muscle and tendon at ankle and foot level, left foot
  - S96.219 Strain of intrinsic muscle and tendon at ankle and foot level, unspecified foot
- **S96.22** Laceration of intrinsic muscle and tendon at ankle and foot level
  - S96.221 Laceration of intrinsic muscle and tendon at ankle and foot level, right foot
  - S96.222 Laceration of intrinsic muscle and tendon at ankle and foot level, left foot
  - S96.229 Laceration of intrinsic muscle and tendon at ankle and foot level, unspecified foot
- **S96.29** Other specified injury of intrinsic muscle and tendon at ankle and foot level
  - S96.291 Other specified injury of intrinsic muscle and tendon at ankle and foot level, right foot
  - S96.292 Other specified injury of intrinsic muscle and tendon at ankle and foot level, left foot
  - S96.299 Other specified injury of intrinsic muscle and tendon at ankle and foot level, unspecified foot

S96.8 Injury of other specified muscles and tendons at ankle and foot level
- **S96.80** Unspecified injury of other specified muscles and tendons at ankle and foot level
  - S96.801 Unspecified injury of other specified muscles and tendons at ankle and foot level, right foot
  - S96.802 Unspecified injury of other specified muscles and tendons at ankle and foot level, left foot
  - S96.809 Unspecified injury of other specified muscles and tendons at ankle and foot level, unspecified foot
- **S96.81** Strain of other specified muscles and tendons at ankle and foot level
  - S96.811 Strain of other specified muscles and tendons at ankle and foot level, right foot
  - S96.812 Strain of other specified muscles and tendons at ankle and foot level, left foot
  - S96.819 Strain of other specified muscles and tendons at ankle and foot level, unspecified foot
- **S96.82** Laceration of other specified muscles and tendons at ankle and foot level
  - S96.821 Laceration of other specified muscles and tendons at ankle and foot level, right foot
  - S96.822 Laceration of other specified muscles and tendons at ankle and foot level, left foot
  - S96.829 Laceration of other specified muscles and tendons at ankle and foot level, unspecified foot
- **S96.89** Other specified injury of other specified muscles and tendons at ankle and foot level
  - S96.891 Other specified injury of other specified muscles and tendons at ankle and foot level, right foot
  - S96.892 Other specified injury of other specified muscles and tendons at ankle and foot level, left foot
  - S96.899 Other specified injury of other specified muscles and tendons at ankle and foot level, unspecified foot

S96.9 Injury of unspecified muscle and tendon at ankle and foot level
- **S96.90** Unspecified injury of unspecified muscle and tendon at ankle and foot level
  - S96.901 Unspecified injury of unspecified muscle and tendon at ankle and foot level, right foot
  - S96.902 Unspecified injury of unspecified muscle and tendon at ankle and foot level, left foot
  - S96.909 Unspecified injury of unspecified muscle and tendon at ankle and foot level, unspecified foot
- **S96.91** Strain of unspecified muscle and tendon at ankle and foot level
  - S96.911 Strain of unspecified muscle and tendon at ankle and foot level, right foot
  - S96.912 Strain of unspecified muscle and tendon at ankle and foot level, left foot
  - S96.919 Strain of unspecified muscle and tendon at ankle and foot level, unspecified foot
- **S96.92** Laceration of unspecified muscle and tendon at ankle and foot level
  - S96.921 Laceration of unspecified muscle and tendon at ankle and foot level, right foot
  - S96.922 Laceration of unspecified muscle and tendon at ankle and foot level, left foot
  - S96.929 Laceration of unspecified muscle and tendon at ankle and foot level, unspecified foot
- **S96.99** Other specified injury of unspecified muscle and tendon at ankle and foot level
  - S96.991 Other specified injury of unspecified muscle and tendon at ankle and foot level, right foot
  - S96.992 Other specified injury of unspecified muscle and tendon at ankle and foot level, left foot
  - S96.999 Other specified injury of unspecified muscle and tendon at ankle and foot level, unspecified foot

S97 Crushing injury of ankle and foot
Use additional code(s) for all associated injuries

The appropriate 7th character is to be added to each code from category S97.
- A initial encounter
- D subsequent encounter
- S sequela

S97.0 Crushing injury of ankle
- S97.00 Crushing injury of unspecified ankle
- S97.01 Crushing injury of right ankle
- S97.02 Crushing injury of left ankle

S97.1 Crushing injury of toe
- **S97.10** Crushing injury of unspecified toe(s)
  - S97.101 Crushing injury of unspecified right toe(s)
  - S97.102 Crushing injury of unspecified left toe(s)
  - S97.109 Crushing injury of unspecified toe(s)
    Crushing injury of toe NOS
- **S97.11** Crushing injury of great toe
  - S97.111 Crushing injury of right great toe

Chapter 19. Injury, Poisoning and Certain Other Consequences of External Causes

- S97.112 Crushing injury of left great toe
- S97.119 Crushing injury of unspecified great toe
- **S97.12 Crushing injury of lesser toe(s)**
  - S97.121 Crushing injury of right lesser toe(s)
  - S97.122 Crushing injury of left lesser toe(s)
  - S97.129 Crushing injury of unspecified lesser toe(s)
- **S97.8 Crushing injury of foot**
  - S97.80 Crushing injury of unspecified foot
    Crushing injury of foot NOS
  - S97.81 Crushing injury of right foot
  - S97.82 Crushing injury of left foot

S98 Traumatic amputation of ankle and foot
An amputation not identified as partial or complete should be coded to complete

The appropriate 7th character is to be added to each code from category S98.
- A initial encounter
- D subsequent encounter
- S sequela

- **S98.0 Traumatic amputation of foot at ankle level**
  - **S98.01 Complete traumatic amputation of foot at ankle level**
    - S98.011 Complete traumatic amputation of right foot at ankle level
    - S98.012 Complete traumatic amputation of left foot at ankle level
    - S98.019 Complete traumatic amputation of unspecified foot at ankle level
  - **S98.02 Partial traumatic amputation of foot at ankle level**
    - S98.021 Partial traumatic amputation of right foot at ankle level
    - S98.022 Partial traumatic amputation of left foot at ankle level
    - S98.029 Partial traumatic amputation of unspecified foot at ankle level
- **S98.1 Traumatic amputation of one toe**
  - **S98.11 Complete traumatic amputation of great toe**
    - S98.111 Complete traumatic amputation of right great toe
    - S98.112 Complete traumatic amputation of left great toe
    - S98.119 Complete traumatic amputation of unspecified great toe
  - **S98.12 Partial traumatic amputation of great toe**
    - S98.121 Partial traumatic amputation of right great toe
    - S98.122 Partial traumatic amputation of left great toe
    - S98.129 Partial traumatic amputation of unspecified great toe
  - **S98.13 Complete traumatic amputation of one lesser toe**
    Traumatic amputation of toe NOS
    - S98.131 Complete traumatic amputation of one right lesser toe
    - S98.132 Complete traumatic amputation of one left lesser toe
    - S98.139 Complete traumatic amputation of one unspecified lesser toe
  - **S98.14 Partial traumatic amputation of one lesser toe**
    - S98.141 Partial traumatic amputation of one right lesser toe
    - S98.142 Partial traumatic amputation of one left lesser toe
    - S98.149 Partial traumatic amputation of one unspecified lesser toe
- **S98.2 Traumatic amputation of two or more lesser toes**
  - **S98.21 Complete traumatic amputation of two or more lesser toes**
    - S98.211 Complete traumatic amputation of two or more right lesser toes
    - S98.212 Complete traumatic amputation of two or more left lesser toes
    - S98.219 Complete traumatic amputation of two or more unspecified lesser toes
  - **S98.22 Partial traumatic amputation of two or more lesser toes**
    - S98.221 Partial traumatic amputation of two or more right lesser toes
    - S98.222 Partial traumatic amputation of two or more left lesser toes
    - S98.229 Partial traumatic amputation of two or more unspecified lesser toes
- **S98.3 Traumatic amputation of midfoot**
  - **S98.31 Complete traumatic amputation of midfoot**
    - S98.311 Complete traumatic amputation of right midfoot
    - S98.312 Complete traumatic amputation of left midfoot
    - S98.319 Complete traumatic amputation of unspecified midfoot
  - **S98.32 Partial traumatic amputation of midfoot**
    - S98.321 Partial traumatic amputation of right midfoot
    - S98.322 Partial traumatic amputation of left midfoot
    - S98.329 Partial traumatic amputation of unspecified midfoot
- **S98.9 Traumatic amputation of foot, level unspecified**
  - **S98.91 Complete traumatic amputation of foot, level unspecified**
    - S98.911 Complete traumatic amputation of right foot, level unspecified
    - S98.912 Complete traumatic amputation of left foot, level unspecified
    - S98.919 Complete traumatic amputation of unspecified foot, level unspecified
  - **S98.92 Partial traumatic amputation of foot, level unspecified**
    - S98.921 Partial traumatic amputation of right foot, level unspecified
    - S98.922 Partial traumatic amputation of left foot, level unspecified
    - S98.929 Partial traumatic amputation of unspecified foot, level unspecified

S99 Other and unspecified injuries of ankle and foot
AHA: 2018,2Q,12; 2018,1Q,3; 2016,4Q,68-69

- **S99.0 Physeal fracture of calcaneus**
  AHA: 2019,4Q,56

  The appropriate 7th character is to be added to each code from subcategory S99.0.
  - A initial encounter for closed fracture
  - B initial encounter for open fracture
  - D subsequent encounter for fracture with routine healing
  - G subsequent encounter for fracture with delayed healing
  - K subsequent encounter for fracture with nonunion
  - P subsequent encounter for fracture with malunion
  - S sequela

  - **S99.00 Unspecified physeal fracture of calcaneus**
    - S99.001 Unspecified physeal fracture of right calcaneus
    - S99.002 Unspecified physeal fracture of left calcaneus
    - S99.009 Unspecified physeal fracture of unspecified calcaneus
  - **S99.01 Salter-Harris Type I physeal fracture of calcaneus**
    - S99.011 Salter-Harris Type I physeal fracture of right calcaneus
    - S99.012 Salter-Harris Type I physeal fracture of left calcaneus
    - S99.019 Salter-Harris Type I physeal fracture of unspecified calcaneus
  - **S99.02 Salter-Harris Type II physeal fracture of calcaneus**
    - S99.021 Salter-Harris Type II physeal fracture of right calcaneus
    - S99.022 Salter-Harris Type II physeal fracture of left calcaneus

- S99.029 Salter-Harris Type II physeal fracture of unspecified calcaneus
- √6th S99.03 Salter-Harris Type III physeal fracture of calcaneus
  - S99.031 Salter-Harris Type III physeal fracture of right calcaneus
  - S99.032 Salter-Harris Type III physeal fracture of left calcaneus
  - S99.039 Salter-Harris Type III physeal fracture of unspecified calcaneus
- √6th S99.04 Salter-Harris Type IV physeal fracture of calcaneus
  - S99.041 Salter-Harris Type IV physeal fracture of right calcaneus
  - S99.042 Salter-Harris Type IV physeal fracture of left calcaneus
  - S99.049 Salter-Harris Type IV physeal fracture of unspecified calcaneus
- √6th S99.09 Other physeal fracture of calcaneus
  - S99.091 Other physeal fracture of right calcaneus
  - S99.092 Other physeal fracture of left calcaneus
  - S99.099 Other physeal fracture of unspecified calcaneus
- √5th S99.1 Physeal fracture of metatarsal
  - AHA: 2019,4Q,56

  The appropriate 7th character is to be added to each code from subcategory S99.1.
  - A initial encounter for closed fracture
  - B initial encounter for open fracture
  - D subsequent encounter for fracture with routine healing
  - G subsequent encounter for fracture with delayed healing
  - K subsequent encounter for fracture with nonunion
  - P subsequent encounter for fracture with malunion
  - S sequela

  - √6th S99.10 Unspecified physeal fracture of metatarsal
    - S99.101 Unspecified physeal fracture of right metatarsal
    - S99.102 Unspecified physeal fracture of left metatarsal
    - S99.109 Unspecified physeal fracture of unspecified metatarsal
  - √6th S99.11 Salter-Harris Type I physeal fracture of metatarsal
    - S99.111 Salter-Harris Type I physeal fracture of right metatarsal
    - S99.112 Salter-Harris Type I physeal fracture of left metatarsal
    - S99.119 Salter-Harris Type I physeal fracture of unspecified metatarsal
  - √6th S99.12 Salter-Harris Type II physeal fracture of metatarsal
    - S99.121 Salter-Harris Type II physeal fracture of right metatarsal
    - S99.122 Salter-Harris Type II physeal fracture of left metatarsal
    - S99.129 Salter-Harris Type II physeal fracture of unspecified metatarsal
  - √6th S99.13 Salter-Harris Type III physeal fracture of metatarsal
    - S99.131 Salter-Harris Type III physeal fracture of right metatarsal
    - S99.132 Salter-Harris Type III physeal fracture of left metatarsal
    - S99.139 Salter-Harris Type III physeal fracture of unspecified metatarsal
  - √6th S99.14 Salter-Harris Type IV physeal fracture of metatarsal
    - S99.141 Salter-Harris Type IV physeal fracture of right metatarsal
    - S99.142 Salter-Harris Type IV physeal fracture of left metatarsal
    - S99.149 Salter-Harris Type IV physeal fracture of unspecified metatarsal
  - √6th S99.19 Other physeal fracture of metatarsal
    - S99.191 Other physeal fracture of right metatarsal
    - S99.192 Other physeal fracture of left metatarsal
    - S99.199 Other physeal fracture of unspecified metatarsal

- √5th S99.2 Physeal fracture of phalanx of toe
  - AHA: 2019,4Q,56

  The appropriate 7th character is to be added to each code from subcategories S99.2.
  - A initial encounter for closed fracture
  - B initial encounter for open fracture
  - D subsequent encounter for fracture with routine healing
  - G subsequent encounter for fracture with delayed healing
  - K subsequent encounter for fracture with nonunion
  - P subsequent encounter for fracture with malunion
  - S sequela

  - √6th S99.20 Unspecified physeal fracture of phalanx of toe
    - S99.201 Unspecified physeal fracture of right toe
    - S99.202 Unspecified physeal fracture of left toe
    - S99.209 Unspecified physeal fracture of unspecified toe
  - √6th S99.21 Salter-Harris Type I physeal fracture of phalanx of toe
    - S99.211 Salter-Harris Type I physeal fracture of phalanx of right toe
    - S99.212 Salter-Harris Type I physeal fracture of phalanx of left toe
    - S99.219 Salter-Harris Type I physeal fracture of phalanx of unspecified toe
  - √6th S99.22 Salter-Harris Type II physeal fracture of phalanx of toe
    - S99.221 Salter-Harris Type II physeal fracture of phalanx of right toe
    - S99.222 Salter-Harris Type II physeal fracture of phalanx of left toe
    - S99.229 Salter-Harris Type II physeal fracture of phalanx of unspecified toe
  - √6th S99.23 Salter-Harris Type III physeal fracture of phalanx of toe
    - S99.231 Salter-Harris Type III physeal fracture of phalanx of right toe
    - S99.232 Salter-Harris Type III physeal fracture of phalanx of left toe
    - S99.239 Salter-Harris Type III physeal fracture of phalanx of unspecified toe
  - √6th S99.24 Salter-Harris Type IV physeal fracture of phalanx of toe
    - S99.241 Salter-Harris Type IV physeal fracture of phalanx of right toe
    - S99.242 Salter-Harris Type IV physeal fracture of phalanx of left toe
    - S99.249 Salter-Harris Type IV physeal fracture of phalanx of unspecified toe
  - √6th S99.29 Other physeal fracture of phalanx of toe
    - S99.291 Other physeal fracture of phalanx of right toe
    - S99.292 Other physeal fracture of phalanx of left toe
    - S99.299 Other physeal fracture of phalanx of unspecified toe

- √5th S99.8 Other specified injuries of ankle and foot

  The appropriate 7th character is to be added to each code from subcategory S99.8.
  - A initial encounter
  - D subsequent encounter
  - S sequela

  - √6th S99.81 Other specified injuries of ankle
    - S99.811 Other specified injuries of right ankle
    - S99.812 Other specified injuries of left ankle
    - S99.819 Other specified injuries of unspecified ankle
  - √6th S99.82 Other specified injuries of foot
    - S99.821 Other specified injuries of right foot
    - S99.822 Other specified injuries of left foot
    - S99.829 Other specified injuries of unspecified foot

S99.9 Unspecified injury of ankle and foot

The appropriate 7th character is to be added to each code from subcategory S99.9.
- A initial encounter
- D subsequent encounter
- S sequela

S99.91 Unspecified injury of ankle
- S99.911 Unspecified injury of right ankle
- S99.912 Unspecified injury of left ankle
- S99.919 Unspecified injury of unspecified ankle

S99.92 Unspecified injury of foot
- S99.921 Unspecified injury of right foot
- S99.922 Unspecified injury of left foot
- S99.929 Unspecified injury of unspecified foot

INJURY, POISONING AND CERTAIN OTHER CONSEQUENCES OF EXTERNAL CAUSES (T07-T88)

Injuries involving multiple body regions (T07)

EXCLUDES 1: burns and corrosions (T20-T32)
frostbite (T33-T34)
insect bite or sting, venomous (T63.4)
sunburn (L55.-)

T07 Unspecified multiple injuries
EXCLUDES 1: injury NOS (T14.90)
AHA: 2017,4Q,26

The appropriate 7th character is to be added to code T07.
- A initial encounter
- D subsequent encounter
- S sequela

Injury of unspecified body region (T14)

T14 Injury of unspecified body region
EXCLUDES 1: multiple unspecified injuries (T07)
AHA: 2017,4Q,26

The appropriate 7th character is to be added to each code from category T14.
- A initial encounter
- D subsequent encounter
- S sequela

T14.8 Other injury of unspecified body region
Abrasion NOS
Contusion NOS
Crush injury NOS
Fracture NOS
Skin injury NOS
Vascular injury NOS
Wound NOS

T14.9 Unspecified injury
- T14.90 Injury, unspecified
  Injury NOS
- T14.91 Suicide attempt HCC Rx ESR COM
  Attempted suicide NOS

Effects of foreign body entering through natural orifice (T15-T19)

Use additional code, if known, for foreign body entering into or through a natural orifice (W44.-)

EXCLUDES 2: foreign body accidentally left in operation wound (T81.5-)
foreign body in penetrating wound - see open wound by body region
residual foreign body in soft tissue (M79.5)
splinter, without open wound - see superficial injury by body region

T15 Foreign body on external eye
EXCLUDES 2: foreign body in penetrating wound of orbit and eye ball (S05.4-, S05.5-)
open wound of eyelid and periocular area (S01.1-)
retained (old) foreign body in penetrating wound of orbit and eye ball (H05.5-, H44.6-, H44.7-)
retained foreign body in eyelid (H02.8-)
superficial foreign body of eyelid and periocular area (S00.25-)

The appropriate 7th character is to be added to each code from category T15.
- A initial encounter
- D subsequent encounter
- S sequela

T15.0 Foreign body in cornea
- T15.00 Foreign body in cornea, unspecified eye
- T15.01 Foreign body in cornea, right eye
- T15.02 Foreign body in cornea, left eye

T15.1 Foreign body in conjunctival sac
- T15.10 Foreign body in conjunctival sac, unspecified eye
- T15.11 Foreign body in conjunctival sac, right eye
- T15.12 Foreign body in conjunctival sac, left eye

T15.8 Foreign body in other and multiple parts of external eye
Foreign body in lacrimal punctum
- T15.80 Foreign body in other and multiple parts of external eye, unspecified eye
- T15.81 Foreign body in other and multiple parts of external eye, right eye
- T15.82 Foreign body in other and multiple parts of external eye, left eye

T15.9 Foreign body on external eye, part unspecified
- T15.90 Foreign body on external eye, part unspecified, unspecified eye
- T15.91 Foreign body on external eye, part unspecified, right eye
- T15.92 Foreign body on external eye, part unspecified, left eye

T16 Foreign body in ear
INCLUDES: foreign body in auditory canal

The appropriate 7th character is to be added to each code from category T16.
- A initial encounter
- D subsequent encounter
- S sequela

- T16.1 Foreign body in right ear
- T16.2 Foreign body in left ear
- T16.9 Foreign body in ear, unspecified ear

T17 Foreign body in respiratory tract
The appropriate 7th character is to be added to each code from category T17.
- A initial encounter
- D subsequent encounter
- S sequela

- T17.0 Foreign body in nasal sinus
- T17.1 Foreign body in nostril
  Foreign body in nose NOS
- T17.2 Foreign body in pharynx
  Foreign body in nasopharynx
  Foreign body in throat NOS
  - T17.20 Unspecified foreign body in pharynx
    - T17.200 Unspecified foreign body in pharynx causing asphyxiation
    - T17.208 Unspecified foreign body in pharynx causing other injury

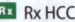

- ✓6th **T17.21** Gastric contents in pharynx
  Aspiration of gastric contents into pharynx
  Vomitus in pharynx
  - ✓7th **T17.210** Gastric contents in pharynx causing asphyxiation
  - ✓7th **T17.218** Gastric contents in pharynx causing other injury
- ✓6th **T17.22** Food in pharynx
  Bones in pharynx
  Seeds in pharynx
  - ✓7th **T17.220** Food in pharynx causing asphyxiation
  - ✓7th **T17.228** Food in pharynx causing other injury
- ✓6th **T17.29** Other foreign object in pharynx
  - ✓7th **T17.290** Other foreign object in pharynx causing asphyxiation
  - ✓7th **T17.298** Other foreign object in pharynx causing other injury
- ✓5th **T17.3** Foreign body in larynx
  - ✓6th **T17.30** Unspecified foreign body in larynx
    - ✓7th **T17.300** Unspecified foreign body in larynx causing asphyxiation
    - ✓7th **T17.308** Unspecified foreign body in larynx causing other injury
  - ✓6th **T17.31** Gastric contents in larynx
    Aspiration of gastric contents into larynx
    Vomitus in larynx
    - ✓7th **T17.310** Gastric contents in larynx causing asphyxiation
    - ✓7th **T17.318** Gastric contents in larynx causing other injury
  - ✓6th **T17.32** Food in larynx
    Bones in larynx
    Seeds in larynx
    - ✓7th **T17.320** Food in larynx causing asphyxiation
    - ✓7th **T17.328** Food in larynx causing other injury
  - ✓6th **T17.39** Other foreign object in larynx
    - ✓7th **T17.390** Other foreign object in larynx causing asphyxiation
    - ✓7th **T17.398** Other foreign object in larynx causing other injury
- ✓5th **T17.4** Foreign body in trachea
  - ✓6th **T17.40** Unspecified foreign body in trachea
    - ✓7th **T17.400** Unspecified foreign body in trachea causing asphyxiation
    - ✓7th **T17.408** Unspecified foreign body in trachea causing other injury
  - ✓6th **T17.41** Gastric contents in trachea
    Aspiration of gastric contents into trachea
    Vomitus in trachea
    - ✓7th **T17.410** Gastric contents in trachea causing asphyxiation
    - ✓7th **T17.418** Gastric contents in trachea causing other injury
  - ✓6th **T17.42** Food in trachea
    Bones in trachea
    Seeds in trachea
    - ✓7th **T17.420** Food in trachea causing asphyxiation
    - ✓7th **T17.428** Food in trachea causing other injury
  - ✓6th **T17.49** Other foreign object in trachea
    - ✓7th **T17.490** Other foreign object in trachea causing asphyxiation
    - ✓7th **T17.498** Other foreign object in trachea causing other injury
- ✓5th **T17.5** Foreign body in bronchus
  - ✓6th **T17.50** Unspecified foreign body in bronchus
    - ✓7th **T17.500** Unspecified foreign body in bronchus causing asphyxiation
    - ✓7th **T17.508** Unspecified foreign body in bronchus causing other injury
  - ✓6th **T17.51** Gastric contents in bronchus
    Aspiration of gastric contents into bronchus
    Vomitus in bronchus
    - ✓7th **T17.510** Gastric contents in bronchus causing asphyxiation
    - ✓7th **T17.518** Gastric contents in bronchus causing other injury
  - ✓6th **T17.52** Food in bronchus
    Bones in bronchus
    Seeds in bronchus
    - ✓7th **T17.520** Food in bronchus causing asphyxiation
    - ✓7th **T17.528** Food in bronchus causing other injury
  - ✓6th **T17.59** Other foreign object in bronchus
    - ✓7th **T17.590** Other foreign object in bronchus causing asphyxiation
    - ✓7th **T17.598** Other foreign object in bronchus causing other injury
- ✓5th **T17.8** Foreign body in other parts of respiratory tract
  Foreign body in bronchioles
  Foreign body in lung
  - ✓6th **T17.80** Unspecified foreign body in other parts of respiratory tract
    - ✓7th **T17.800** Unspecified foreign body in other parts of respiratory tract causing asphyxiation
    - ✓7th **T17.808** Unspecified foreign body in other parts of respiratory tract causing other injury
  - ✓6th **T17.81** Gastric contents in other parts of respiratory tract
    Aspiration of gastric contents into other parts of respiratory tract
    Vomitus in other parts of respiratory tract
    - ✓7th **T17.810** Gastric contents in other parts of respiratory tract causing asphyxiation
    - ✓7th **T17.818** Gastric contents in other parts of respiratory tract causing other injury
  - ✓6th **T17.82** Food in other parts of respiratory tract
    Bones in other parts of respiratory tract
    Seeds in other parts of respiratory tract
    - ✓7th **T17.820** Food in other parts of respiratory tract causing asphyxiation
    - ✓7th **T17.828** Food in other parts of respiratory tract causing other injury
  - ✓6th **T17.89** Other foreign object in other parts of respiratory tract
    - ✓7th **T17.890** Other foreign object in other parts of respiratory tract causing asphyxiation
    - ✓7th **T17.898** Other foreign object in other parts of respiratory tract causing other injury
- ✓5th **T17.9** Foreign body in respiratory tract, part unspecified
  - ✓6th **T17.90** Unspecified foreign body in respiratory tract, part unspecified
    - ✓7th **T17.900** Unspecified foreign body in respiratory tract, part unspecified causing asphyxiation
    - ✓7th **T17.908** Unspecified foreign body in respiratory tract, part unspecified causing other injury
  - ✓6th **T17.91** Gastric contents in respiratory tract, part unspecified
    Aspiration of gastric contents into respiratory tract, part unspecified
    Vomitus in trachea respiratory tract, part unspecified
    - ✓7th **T17.910** Gastric contents in respiratory tract, part unspecified causing asphyxiation
    - ✓7th **T17.918** Gastric contents in respiratory tract, part unspecified causing other injury
  - ✓6th **T17.92** Food in respiratory tract, part unspecified
    Bones in respiratory tract, part unspecified
    Seeds in respiratory tract, part unspecified
    - ✓7th **T17.920** Food in respiratory tract, part unspecified causing asphyxiation
    - ✓7th **T17.928** Food in respiratory tract, part unspecified causing other injury
  - ✓6th **T17.99** Other foreign object in respiratory tract, part unspecified
    - ✓7th **T17.990** Other foreign object in respiratory tract, part unspecified in causing asphyxiation
      AHA: 2019,3Q,15
    - ✓7th **T17.998** Other foreign object in respiratory tract, part unspecified causing other injury

✓4th **T18** Foreign body in alimentary tract

EXCLUDES 2 foreign body in pharynx (T17.2-)

The appropriate 7th character is to be added to each code from category T18.
  A   initial encounter
  D   subsequent encounter
  S   sequela

✓x 7th **T18.0** Foreign body in mouth

Chapter 19. Injury, Poisoning and Certain Other Consequences of External Causes

T18.1 Foreign body in **esophagus**
  EXCLUDES 2: *foreign body in respiratory tract (T17.-)*

  T18.10 Unspecified foreign body in esophagus
  - **T18.100** Unspecified foreign body in esophagus **causing compression of trachea**
    - Unspecified foreign body in esophagus causing obstruction of respiration
  - **T18.108** Unspecified foreign body in esophagus **causing other injury**

  T18.11 **Gastric contents** in esophagus
  - Vomitus in esophagus
  - **T18.110** Gastric contents in esophagus **causing compression of trachea**
    - Gastric contents in esophagus causing obstruction of respiration
  - **T18.118** Gastric contents in esophagus **causing other injury**

  T18.12 **Food** in esophagus
  - Bones in esophagus
  - Seeds in esophagus
  - **T18.120** Food in esophagus **causing compression of trachea**
    - Food in esophagus causing obstruction of respiration
  - **T18.128** Food in esophagus **causing other injury**

  T18.19 Other foreign object in esophagus
  - AHA: 2022,1Q,27; 2015,1Q,23
  - **T18.190** Other foreign object in esophagus **causing compression of trachea**
    - Other foreign body in esophagus causing obstruction of respiration
    - **TIP:** Any foreign object lodged in the esophagus requires immediate treatment and is considered an injury. Assign this code when there is respiratory compromise or compression. If no respiratory compromise or compression is documented, assign code T18.198-.
  - **T18.198** Other foreign object in esophagus **causing other injury**
    - **TIP:** Any foreign object lodged in the esophagus requires immediate treatment and is considered an injury. Assign this code when there is no respiratory compromise or compression. If respiratory compromise or compression is documented, assign code T18.190-.

T18.2 Foreign body in **stomach**
T18.3 Foreign body in **small intestine**
T18.4 Foreign body in **colon**
T18.5 Foreign body in **anus and rectum**
  - Foreign body in rectosigmoid (junction)
T18.8 Foreign body in other parts of alimentary tract
T18.9 Foreign body of alimentary tract, part unspecified
  - Foreign body in digestive system NOS
  - Swallowed foreign body NOS

T19 Foreign body in genitourinary tract
  EXCLUDES 2: *complications due to implanted mesh (T83.7-)*
  mechanical complications of contraceptive device (intrauterine) (vaginal) (T83.3-)
  presence of contraceptive device (intrauterine) (vaginal) (Z97.5)

  The appropriate 7th character is to be added to each code from category T19.
  - A initial encounter
  - D subsequent encounter
  - S sequela

T19.0 Foreign body in **urethra**
T19.1 Foreign body in **bladder**
T19.2 Foreign body in **vulva and vagina**
T19.3 Foreign body in **uterus**
T19.4 Foreign body in **penis**
T19.8 Foreign body in other parts of genitourinary tract
T19.9 Foreign body in genitourinary tract, part unspecified

BURNS AND CORROSIONS (T20-T32)

INCLUDES:
- burns (thermal) from electrical heating appliances
- burns (thermal) from electricity
- burns (thermal) from flame
- burns (thermal) from friction
- burns (thermal) from hot air and hot gases
- burns (thermal) from hot objects
- burns (thermal) from lightning
- burns (thermal) from radiation
- chemical burn [corrosion] (external) (internal)
- scalds

EXCLUDES 2: *erythema [dermatitis] ab igne (L59.0)*
radiation-related disorders of the skin and subcutaneous tissue (L55-L59)
sunburn (L55.-)

AHA: 2016,2Q,4

Burns and corrosions of external body surface, specified by site (T20-T25)

INCLUDES:
- burns and corrosions of first degree [erythema]
- burns and corrosions of second degree [blisters] [epidermal loss]
- burns and corrosions of third degree [deep necrosis of underlying tissue] [full-thickness skin loss]

Use additional code from category T31 or T32 to identify extent of body surface involved

T20 Burn and corrosion of head, face, and neck
  EXCLUDES 2: *burn and corrosion of ear drum (T28.41, T28.91)*
  burn and corrosion of eye and adnexa (T26.-)
  burn and corrosion of mouth and pharynx (T28.0)

  AHA: 2015,1Q,18-19

  The appropriate 7th character is to be added to each code from category T20.
  - A initial encounter
  - D subsequent encounter
  - S sequela

T20.0 Burn of unspecified degree of head, face, and neck
  Use additional external cause code to identify the source, place and intent of the burn (X00-X19, X75-X77, X96-X98, Y92)

  T20.00 Burn of unspecified degree of head, face, and neck, unspecified site
  T20.01 Burn of unspecified degree of **ear** [any part, except ear drum]
    EXCLUDES 2: *burn of ear drum (T28.41-)*
    - **T20.011** Burn of unspecified degree of **right** ear [any part, except ear drum]
    - **T20.012** Burn of unspecified degree of **left** ear [any part, except ear drum]
    - **T20.019** Burn of unspecified degree of unspecified ear [any part, except ear drum]
  T20.02 Burn of unspecified degree of **lip(s)**
  T20.03 Burn of unspecified degree of **chin**
  T20.04 Burn of unspecified degree of **nose** (septum)
  T20.05 Burn of unspecified degree of **scalp** [any part]
  T20.06 Burn of unspecified degree of **forehead and cheek**
  T20.07 Burn of unspecified degree of **neck**
  T20.09 Burn of unspecified degree of **multiple sites** of head, face, and neck

T20.1 Burn of **first degree** of head, face, and neck
  Use additional external cause code to identify the source, place and intent of the burn (X00-X19, X75-X77, X96-X98, Y92)

  T20.10 Burn of first degree of head, face, and neck, unspecified site
  T20.11 Burn of first degree of **ear** [any part, except ear drum]
    EXCLUDES 2: *burn of ear drum (T28.41-)*
    - **T20.111** Burn of first degree of **right** ear [any part, except ear drum]
    - **T20.112** Burn of first degree of **left** ear [any part, except ear drum]
    - **T20.119** Burn of first degree of unspecified ear [any part, except ear drum]
  T20.12 Burn of first degree of **lip(s)**
  T20.13 Burn of first degree of **chin**
  T20.14 Burn of first degree of **nose** (septum)
  T20.15 Burn of first degree of **scalp** [any part]
  T20.16 Burn of first degree of **forehead and cheek**
  T20.17 Burn of first degree of **neck**

Chapter 19. Injury, Poisoning and Certain Other Consequences of External Causes

T20.19 Burn of first degree of multiple sites of head, face, and neck

Degree of Burns

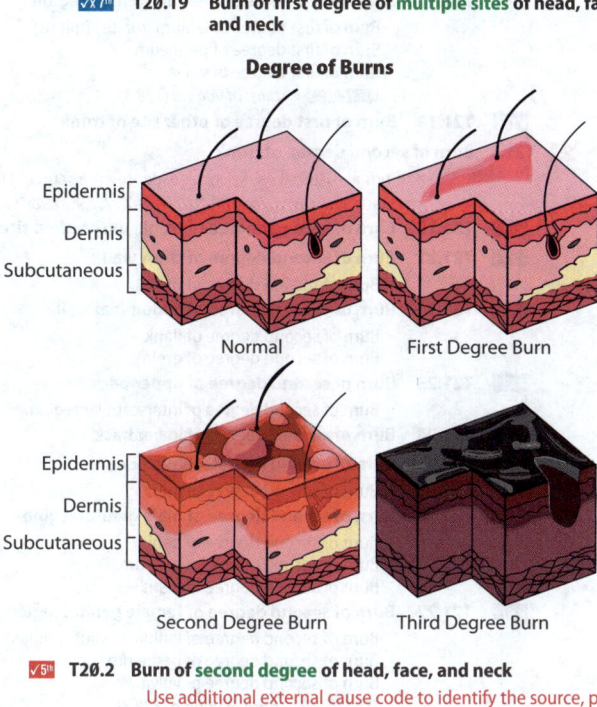

Normal / First Degree Burn / Second Degree Burn / Third Degree Burn

- **T20.2** Burn of second degree of head, face, and neck
  Use additional external cause code to identify the source, place and intent of the burn (X00-X19, X75-X77, X96-X98, Y92)
  - T20.20 Burn of second degree of head, face, and neck, unspecified site
  - T20.21 Burn of second degree of ear [any part, except ear drum]
    EXCLUDES 2 burn of ear drum (T28.41-)
    - T20.211 Burn of second degree of right ear [any part, except ear drum]
    - T20.212 Burn of second degree of left ear [any part, except ear drum]
    - T20.219 Burn of second degree of unspecified ear [any part, except ear drum]
  - T20.22 Burn of second degree of lip(s)
  - T20.23 Burn of second degree of chin
  - T20.24 Burn of second degree of nose (septum)
  - T20.25 Burn of second degree of scalp [any part]
  - T20.26 Burn of second degree of forehead and cheek
  - T20.27 Burn of second degree of neck
  - T20.29 Burn of second degree of multiple sites of head, face, and neck

- **T20.3** Burn of third degree of head, face, and neck
  Use additional external cause code to identify the source, place and intent of the burn (X00-X19, X75-X77, X96-X98, Y92)
  - T20.30 Burn of third degree of head, face, and neck, unspecified site
  - T20.31 Burn of third degree of ear [any part, except ear drum]
    EXCLUDES 2 burn of ear drum (T28.41-)
    AHA: 2015,1Q,18
    - T20.311 Burn of third degree of right ear [any part, except ear drum]
    - T20.312 Burn of third degree of left ear [any part, except ear drum]
    - T20.319 Burn of third degree of unspecified ear [any part, except ear drum]
  - T20.32 Burn of third degree of lip(s)
  - T20.33 Burn of third degree of chin
  - T20.34 Burn of third degree of nose (septum)
  - T20.35 Burn of third degree of scalp [any part]
  - T20.36 Burn of third degree of forehead and cheek
  - T20.37 Burn of third degree of neck
  - T20.39 Burn of third degree of multiple sites of head, face, and neck

- **T20.4** Corrosion of unspecified degree of head, face, and neck
  Code first (T51-T65) to identify chemical and intent
  Use additional external cause code to identify place (Y92)
  - T20.40 Corrosion of unspecified degree of head, face, and neck, unspecified site
  - T20.41 Corrosion of unspecified degree of ear [any part, except ear drum]
    EXCLUDES 2 corrosion of ear drum (T28.91-)
    - T20.411 Corrosion of unspecified degree of right ear [any part, except ear drum]
    - T20.412 Corrosion of unspecified degree of left ear [any part, except ear drum]
    - T20.419 Corrosion of unspecified degree of unspecified ear [any part, except ear drum]
  - T20.42 Corrosion of unspecified degree of lip(s)
  - T20.43 Corrosion of unspecified degree of chin
  - T20.44 Corrosion of unspecified degree of nose (septum)
  - T20.45 Corrosion of unspecified degree of scalp [any part]
  - T20.46 Corrosion of unspecified degree of forehead and cheek
  - T20.47 Corrosion of unspecified degree of neck
  - T20.49 Corrosion of unspecified degree of multiple sites of head, face, and neck

- **T20.5** Corrosion of first degree of head, face, and neck
  Code first (T51-T65) to identify chemical and intent
  Use additional external cause code to identify place (Y92)
  - T20.50 Corrosion of first degree of head, face, and neck, unspecified site
  - T20.51 Corrosion of first degree of ear [any part, except ear drum]
    EXCLUDES 2 corrosion of ear drum (T28.91-)
    - T20.511 Corrosion of first degree of right ear [any part, except ear drum]
    - T20.512 Corrosion of first degree of left ear [any part, except ear drum]
    - T20.519 Corrosion of first degree of unspecified ear [any part, except ear drum]
  - T20.52 Corrosion of first degree of lip(s)
  - T20.53 Corrosion of first degree of chin
  - T20.54 Corrosion of first degree of nose (septum)
  - T20.55 Corrosion of first degree of scalp [any part]
  - T20.56 Corrosion of first degree of forehead and cheek
  - T20.57 Corrosion of first degree of neck
  - T20.59 Corrosion of first degree of multiple sites of head, face, and neck

- **T20.6** Corrosion of second degree of head, face, and neck
  Code first (T51-T65) to identify chemical and intent
  Use additional external cause code to identify place (Y92)
  - T20.60 Corrosion of second degree of head, face, and neck, unspecified site
  - T20.61 Corrosion of second degree of ear [any part, except ear drum]
    EXCLUDES 2 corrosion of ear drum (T28.91-)
    - T20.611 Corrosion of second degree of right ear [any part, except ear drum]
    - T20.612 Corrosion of second degree of left ear [any part, except ear drum]
    - T20.619 Corrosion of second degree of unspecified ear [any part, except ear drum]
  - T20.62 Corrosion of second degree of lip(s)
  - T20.63 Corrosion of second degree of chin
  - T20.64 Corrosion of second degree of nose (septum)
  - T20.65 Corrosion of second degree of scalp [any part]
  - T20.66 Corrosion of second degree of forehead and cheek
  - T20.67 Corrosion of second degree of neck
  - T20.69 Corrosion of second degree of multiple sites of head, face, and neck

- **T20.7** Corrosion of third degree of head, face, and neck
  Code first (T51-T65) to identify chemical and intent
  Use additional external cause code to identify place (Y92)
  - T20.70 Corrosion of third degree of head, face, and neck, unspecified site

Chapter 19. Injury, Poisoning and Certain Other Consequences of External Causes

T20.71 ✓6ᵗʰ Corrosion of third degree of ear [any part, except ear drum]
    EXCLUDES 2: corrosion of ear drum (T28.91-)
    ✓7ᵗʰ **T20.711** Corrosion of third degree of right ear [any part, except ear drum] COM
    ✓7ᵗʰ **T20.712** Corrosion of third degree of left ear [any part, except ear drum] COM
    ✓7ᵗʰ **T20.719** Corrosion of third degree of unspecified ear [any part, except ear drum] COM

✓x7ᵗʰ **T20.72** Corrosion of third degree of lip(s) COM
✓x7ᵗʰ **T20.73** Corrosion of third degree of chin COM
✓x7ᵗʰ **T20.74** Corrosion of third degree of nose (septum) COM
✓x7ᵗʰ **T20.75** Corrosion of third degree of scalp [any part] COM
✓x7ᵗʰ **T20.76** Corrosion of third degree of forehead and cheek COM
✓x7ᵗʰ **T20.77** Corrosion of third degree of neck COM
✓x7ᵗʰ **T20.79** Corrosion of third degree of multiple sites of head, face, and neck COM

✓4ᵗʰ T21 Burn and corrosion of trunk
INCLUDES: burns and corrosion of hip region
EXCLUDES 2: burns and corrosion of axilla (T22.- with fifth character 4)
burns and corrosion of scapular region (T22.- with fifth character 6)
burns and corrosion of shoulder (T22.- with fifth character 5)

The appropriate 7th character is to be added to each code from category T21.
A initial encounter
D subsequent encounter
S sequela

✓5ᵗʰ **T21.0** Burn of unspecified degree of trunk
Use additional external cause code to identify the source, place and intent of the burn (X00-X19, X75-X77, X96-X98, Y92)

  ✓x7ᵗʰ **T21.00** Burn of unspecified degree of trunk, unspecified site
  ✓x7ᵗʰ **T21.01** Burn of unspecified degree of chest wall
    Burn of unspecified degree of breast
  ✓x7ᵗʰ **T21.02** Burn of unspecified degree of abdominal wall
    Burn of unspecified degree of flank
    Burn of unspecified degree of groin
  ✓x7ᵗʰ **T21.03** Burn of unspecified degree of upper back
    Burn of unspecified degree of interscapular region
  ✓x7ᵗʰ **T21.04** Burn of unspecified degree of lower back
  ✓x7ᵗʰ **T21.05** Burn of unspecified degree of buttock
    Burn of unspecified degree of anus
  ✓x7ᵗʰ **T21.06** Burn of unspecified degree of male genital region
    Burn of unspecified degree of penis
    Burn of unspecified degree of scrotum
    Burn of unspecified degree of testis
  ✓x7ᵗʰ **T21.07** Burn of unspecified degree of female genital region
    Burn of unspecified degree of labium (majus) (minus)
    Burn of unspecified degree of perineum
    Burn of unspecified degree of vulva
    EXCLUDES 2: burn of vagina (T28.3)
  ✓x7ᵗʰ **T21.09** Burn of unspecified degree of other site of trunk

✓5ᵗʰ **T21.1** Burn of first degree of trunk
Use additional external cause code to identify the source, place and intent of the burn (X00-X19, X75-X77, X96-X98, Y92)

  ✓x7ᵗʰ **T21.10** Burn of first degree of trunk, unspecified site
  ✓x7ᵗʰ **T21.11** Burn of first degree of chest wall
    Burn of first degree of breast
  ✓x7ᵗʰ **T21.12** Burn of first degree of abdominal wall
    Burn of first degree of flank
    Burn of first degree of groin
  ✓x7ᵗʰ **T21.13** Burn of first degree of upper back
    Burn of first degree of interscapular region
  ✓x7ᵗʰ **T21.14** Burn of first degree of lower back
  ✓x7ᵗʰ **T21.15** Burn of first degree of buttock
    Burn of first degree of anus
  ✓x7ᵗʰ **T21.16** Burn of first degree of male genital region
    Burn of first degree of penis
    Burn of first degree of scrotum
    Burn of first degree of testis
  ✓x7ᵗʰ **T21.17** Burn of first degree of female genital region
    Burn of first degree of labium (majus) (minus)
    Burn of first degree of perineum
    Burn of first degree of vulva
    EXCLUDES 2: burn of vagina (T28.3)
  ✓x7ᵗʰ **T21.19** Burn of first degree of other site of trunk

✓5ᵗʰ **T21.2** Burn of second degree of trunk
Use additional external cause code to identify the source, place and intent of the burn (X00-X19, X75-X77, X96-X98, Y92)

  ✓x7ᵗʰ **T21.20** Burn of second degree of trunk, unspecified site
  ✓x7ᵗʰ **T21.21** Burn of second degree of chest wall
    Burn of second degree of breast
  ✓x7ᵗʰ **T21.22** Burn of second degree of abdominal wall
    Burn of second degree of flank
    Burn of second degree of groin
  ✓x7ᵗʰ **T21.23** Burn of second degree of upper back
    Burn of second degree of interscapular region
  ✓x7ᵗʰ **T21.24** Burn of second degree of lower back
  ✓x7ᵗʰ **T21.25** Burn of second degree of buttock
    Burn of second degree of anus
  ✓x7ᵗʰ **T21.26** Burn of second degree of male genital region
    Burn of second degree of penis
    Burn of second degree of scrotum
    Burn of second degree of testis
  ✓x7ᵗʰ **T21.27** Burn of second degree of female genital region
    Burn of second degree of labium (majus) (minus)
    Burn of second degree of perineum
    Burn of second degree of vulva
    EXCLUDES 2: burn of vagina (T28.3)
  ✓x7ᵗʰ **T21.29** Burn of second degree of other site of trunk

✓5ᵗʰ **T21.3** Burn of third degree of trunk
Use additional external cause code to identify the source, place and intent of the burn (X00-X19, X75-X77, X96-X98, Y92)

  ✓x7ᵗʰ **T21.30** Burn of third degree of trunk, unspecified site COM
  ✓x7ᵗʰ **T21.31** Burn of third degree of chest wall COM
    Burn of third degree of breast
    AHA: 2016,2Q,5
  ✓x7ᵗʰ **T21.32** Burn of third degree of abdominal wall COM
    Burn of third degree of flank
    Burn of third degree of groin
  ✓x7ᵗʰ **T21.33** Burn of third degree of upper back COM
    Burn of third degree of interscapular region
  ✓x7ᵗʰ **T21.34** Burn of third degree of lower back COM
  ✓x7ᵗʰ **T21.35** Burn of third degree of buttock COM
    Burn of third degree of anus
  ✓x7ᵗʰ **T21.36** Burn of third degree of male genital region COM
    Burn of third degree of penis
    Burn of third degree of scrotum
    Burn of third degree of testis
  ✓x7ᵗʰ **T21.37** Burn of third degree of female genital region COM
    Burn of third degree of labium (majus) (minus)
    Burn of third degree of perineum
    Burn of third degree of vulva
    EXCLUDES 2: burn of vagina (T28.3)
  ✓x7ᵗʰ **T21.39** Burn of third degree of other site of trunk COM

✓5ᵗʰ **T21.4** Corrosion of unspecified degree of trunk
Code first (T51-T65) to identify chemical and intent
Use additional external cause code to identify place (Y92)

  ✓x7ᵗʰ **T21.40** Corrosion of unspecified degree of trunk, unspecified site
  ✓x7ᵗʰ **T21.41** Corrosion of unspecified degree of chest wall
    Corrosion of unspecified degree of breast
  ✓x7ᵗʰ **T21.42** Corrosion of unspecified degree of abdominal wall
    Corrosion of unspecified degree of flank
    Corrosion of unspecified degree of groin
  ✓x7ᵗʰ **T21.43** Corrosion of unspecified degree of upper back
    Corrosion of unspecified degree of interscapular region
  ✓x7ᵗʰ **T21.44** Corrosion of unspecified degree of lower back
  ✓x7ᵗʰ **T21.45** Corrosion of unspecified degree of buttock
    Corrosion of unspecified degree of anus

- **T21.46** Corrosion of unspecified degree of male genital region
  - Corrosion of unspecified degree of penis
  - Corrosion of unspecified degree of scrotum
  - Corrosion of unspecified degree of testis
- **T21.47** Corrosion of unspecified degree of female genital region
  - Corrosion of unspecified degree of labium (majus) (minus)
  - Corrosion of unspecified degree of perineum
  - Corrosion of unspecified degree of vulva
  - EXCLUDES 2: corrosion of vagina (T28.8)
- **T21.49** Corrosion of unspecified degree of other site of trunk

T21.5 Corrosion of first degree of trunk
Code first (T51-T65) to identify chemical and intent
Use additional external cause code to identify place (Y92)

- **T21.50** Corrosion of first degree of trunk, unspecified site
- **T21.51** Corrosion of first degree of chest wall
  - Corrosion of first degree of breast
- **T21.52** Corrosion of first degree of abdominal wall
  - Corrosion of first degree of flank
  - Corrosion of first degree of groin
- **T21.53** Corrosion of first degree of upper back
  - Corrosion of first degree of interscapular region
- **T21.54** Corrosion of first degree of lower back
- **T21.55** Corrosion of first degree of buttock
  - Corrosion of first degree of anus
- **T21.56** Corrosion of first degree of male genital region
  - Corrosion of first degree of penis
  - Corrosion of first degree of scrotum
  - Corrosion of first degree of testis
- **T21.57** Corrosion of first degree of female genital region
  - Corrosion of first degree of labium (majus) (minus)
  - Corrosion of first degree of perineum
  - Corrosion of first degree of vulva
  - EXCLUDES 2: corrosion of vagina (T28.8)
- **T21.59** Corrosion of first degree of other site of trunk

T21.6 Corrosion of second degree of trunk
Code first (T51-T65) to identify chemical and intent
Use additional external cause code to identify place (Y92)

- **T21.60** Corrosion of second degree of trunk, unspecified site
- **T21.61** Corrosion of second degree of chest wall
  - Corrosion of second degree of breast
- **T21.62** Corrosion of second degree of abdominal wall
  - Corrosion of second degree of flank
  - Corrosion of second degree of groin
- **T21.63** Corrosion of second degree of upper back
  - Corrosion of second degree of interscapular region
- **T21.64** Corrosion of second degree of lower back
- **T21.65** Corrosion of second degree of buttock
  - Corrosion of second degree of anus
- **T21.66** Corrosion of second degree of male genital region
  - Corrosion of second degree of penis
  - Corrosion of second degree of scrotum
  - Corrosion of second degree of testis
- **T21.67** Corrosion of second degree of female genital region
  - Corrosion of second degree of labium (majus) (minus)
  - Corrosion of second degree of perineum
  - Corrosion of second degree of vulva
  - EXCLUDES 2: corrosion of vagina (T28.8)
- **T21.69** Corrosion of second degree of other site of trunk

T21.7 Corrosion of third degree of trunk
Code first (T51-T65) to identify chemical and intent
Use additional external cause code to identify place (Y92)

- **T21.70** Corrosion of third degree of trunk, unspecified site
- **T21.71** Corrosion of third degree of chest wall
  - Corrosion of third degree of breast
- **T21.72** Corrosion of third degree of abdominal wall
  - Corrosion of third degree of flank
  - Corrosion of third degree of groin
- **T21.73** Corrosion of third degree of upper back
  - Corrosion of third degree of interscapular region
- **T21.74** Corrosion of third degree of lower back
- **T21.75** Corrosion of third degree of buttock
  - Corrosion of third degree of anus
- **T21.76** Corrosion of third degree of male genital region
  - Corrosion of third degree of penis
  - Corrosion of third degree of scrotum
  - Corrosion of third degree of testis
- **T21.77** Corrosion of third degree of female genital region
  - Corrosion of third degree of labium (majus) (minus)
  - Corrosion of third degree of perineum
  - Corrosion of third degree of vulva
  - EXCLUDES 2: corrosion of vagina (T28.8)
- **T21.79** Corrosion of third degree of other site of trunk

T22 Burn and corrosion of shoulder and upper limb, except wrist and hand
EXCLUDES 2: burn and corrosion of interscapular region (T21.-)
burn and corrosion of wrist and hand (T23.-)

The appropriate 7th character is to be added to each code from category T22.
- A initial encounter
- D subsequent encounter
- S sequela

T22.0 Burn of unspecified degree of shoulder and upper limb, except wrist and hand
Use additional external cause code to identify the source, place and intent of the burn (X00-X19, X75-X77, X96-X98, Y92)

- **T22.00** Burn of unspecified degree of shoulder and upper limb, except wrist and hand, unspecified site
- **T22.01** Burn of unspecified degree of forearm
  - **T22.011** Burn of unspecified degree of right forearm
  - **T22.012** Burn of unspecified degree of left forearm
  - **T22.019** Burn of unspecified degree of unspecified forearm
- **T22.02** Burn of unspecified degree of elbow
  - **T22.021** Burn of unspecified degree of right elbow
  - **T22.022** Burn of unspecified degree of left elbow
  - **T22.029** Burn of unspecified degree of unspecified elbow
- **T22.03** Burn of unspecified degree of upper arm
  - **T22.031** Burn of unspecified degree of right upper arm
  - **T22.032** Burn of unspecified degree of left upper arm
  - **T22.039** Burn of unspecified degree of unspecified upper arm
- **T22.04** Burn of unspecified degree of axilla
  - **T22.041** Burn of unspecified degree of right axilla
  - **T22.042** Burn of unspecified degree of left axilla
  - **T22.049** Burn of unspecified degree of unspecified axilla
- **T22.05** Burn of unspecified degree of shoulder
  - **T22.051** Burn of unspecified degree of right shoulder
  - **T22.052** Burn of unspecified degree of left shoulder
  - **T22.059** Burn of unspecified degree of unspecified shoulder
- **T22.06** Burn of unspecified degree of scapular region
  - **T22.061** Burn of unspecified degree of right scapular region
  - **T22.062** Burn of unspecified degree of left scapular region
  - **T22.069** Burn of unspecified degree of unspecified scapular region
- **T22.09** Burn of unspecified degree of multiple sites of shoulder and upper limb, except wrist and hand
  - **T22.091** Burn of unspecified degree of multiple sites of right shoulder and upper limb, except wrist and hand
  - **T22.092** Burn of unspecified degree of multiple sites of left shoulder and upper limb, except wrist and hand
  - **T22.099** Burn of unspecified degree of multiple sites of unspecified shoulder and upper limb, except wrist and hand

T22.1 Burn of first degree of shoulder and upper limb, except wrist and hand

Use additional external cause code to identify the source, place and intent of the burn (X00-X19, X75-X77, X96-X98, Y92)

- **T22.10** Burn of first degree of shoulder and upper limb, except wrist and hand, unspecified site
- **T22.11** Burn of first degree of forearm
  - T22.111 Burn of first degree of right forearm
  - T22.112 Burn of first degree of left forearm
  - T22.119 Burn of first degree of unspecified forearm
- **T22.12** Burn of first degree of elbow
  - T22.121 Burn of first degree of right elbow
  - T22.122 Burn of first degree of left elbow
  - T22.129 Burn of first degree of unspecified elbow
- **T22.13** Burn of first degree of upper arm
  - T22.131 Burn of first degree of right upper arm
  - T22.132 Burn of first degree of left upper arm
  - T22.139 Burn of first degree of unspecified upper arm
- **T22.14** Burn of first degree of axilla
  - T22.141 Burn of first degree of right axilla
  - T22.142 Burn of first degree of left axilla
  - T22.149 Burn of first degree of unspecified axilla
- **T22.15** Burn of first degree of shoulder
  - T22.151 Burn of first degree of right shoulder
  - T22.152 Burn of first degree of left shoulder
  - T22.159 Burn of first degree of unspecified shoulder
- **T22.16** Burn of first degree of scapular region
  - T22.161 Burn of first degree of right scapular region
  - T22.162 Burn of first degree of left scapular region
  - T22.169 Burn of first degree of unspecified scapular region
- **T22.19** Burn of first degree of multiple sites of shoulder and upper limb, except wrist and hand
  - T22.191 Burn of first degree of multiple sites of right shoulder and upper limb, except wrist and hand
  - T22.192 Burn of first degree of multiple sites of left shoulder and upper limb, except wrist and hand
  - T22.199 Burn of first degree of multiple sites of unspecified shoulder and upper limb, except wrist and hand

T22.2 Burn of second degree of shoulder and upper limb, except wrist and hand

Use additional external cause code to identify the source, place and intent of the burn (X00-X19, X75-X77, X96-X98, Y92)

- **T22.20** Burn of second degree of shoulder and upper limb, except wrist and hand, unspecified site
- **T22.21** Burn of second degree of forearm
  - T22.211 Burn of second degree of right forearm
  - T22.212 Burn of second degree of left forearm
  - T22.219 Burn of second degree of unspecified forearm
- **T22.22** Burn of second degree of elbow
  - T22.221 Burn of second degree of right elbow
  - T22.222 Burn of second degree of left elbow
  - T22.229 Burn of second degree of unspecified elbow
- **T22.23** Burn of second degree of upper arm
  - T22.231 Burn of second degree of right upper arm
  - T22.232 Burn of second degree of left upper arm
  - T22.239 Burn of second degree of unspecified upper arm
- **T22.24** Burn of second degree of axilla
  - T22.241 Burn of second degree of right axilla
  - T22.242 Burn of second degree of left axilla
  - T22.249 Burn of second degree of unspecified axilla
- **T22.25** Burn of second degree of shoulder
  - T22.251 Burn of second degree of right shoulder
  - T22.252 Burn of second degree of left shoulder
  - T22.259 Burn of second degree of unspecified shoulder
- **T22.26** Burn of second degree of scapular region
  - T22.261 Burn of second degree of right scapular region
  - T22.262 Burn of second degree of left scapular region
  - T22.269 Burn of second degree of unspecified scapular region
- **T22.29** Burn of second degree of multiple sites of shoulder and upper limb, except wrist and hand
  - T22.291 Burn of second degree of multiple sites of right shoulder and upper limb, except wrist and hand
  - T22.292 Burn of second degree of multiple sites of left shoulder and upper limb, except wrist and hand
  - T22.299 Burn of second degree of multiple sites of unspecified shoulder and upper limb, except wrist and hand

T22.3 Burn of third degree of shoulder and upper limb, except wrist and hand

Use additional external cause code to identify the source, place and intent of the burn (X00-X19, X75-X77, X96-X98, Y92)

- **T22.30** Burn of third degree of shoulder and upper limb, except wrist and hand, unspecified site
- **T22.31** Burn of third degree of forearm
  - T22.311 Burn of third degree of right forearm
  - T22.312 Burn of third degree of left forearm
  - T22.319 Burn of third degree of unspecified forearm
- **T22.32** Burn of third degree of elbow
  - T22.321 Burn of third degree of right elbow
  - T22.322 Burn of third degree of left elbow
  - T22.329 Burn of third degree of unspecified elbow
- **T22.33** Burn of third degree of upper arm
  - T22.331 Burn of third degree of right upper arm
  - T22.332 Burn of third degree of left upper arm
  - T22.339 Burn of third degree of unspecified upper arm
- **T22.34** Burn of third degree of axilla
  - T22.341 Burn of third degree of right axilla
  - T22.342 Burn of third degree of left axilla
  - T22.349 Burn of third degree of unspecified axilla
- **T22.35** Burn of third degree of shoulder
  - T22.351 Burn of third degree of right shoulder
  - T22.352 Burn of third degree of left shoulder
  - T22.359 Burn of third degree of unspecified shoulder
- **T22.36** Burn of third degree of scapular region
  - T22.361 Burn of third degree of right scapular region
  - T22.362 Burn of third degree of left scapular region
  - T22.369 Burn of third degree of unspecified scapular region
- **T22.39** Burn of third degree of multiple sites of shoulder and upper limb, except wrist and hand
  - T22.391 Burn of third degree of multiple sites of right shoulder and upper limb, except wrist and hand
  - T22.392 Burn of third degree of multiple sites of left shoulder and upper limb, except wrist and hand
  - T22.399 Burn of third degree of multiple sites of unspecified shoulder and upper limb, except wrist and hand

T22.4 Corrosion of unspecified degree of shoulder and upper limb, except wrist and hand

Code first (T51-T65) to identify chemical and intent
Use additional external cause code to identify place (Y92)

- **T22.40** Corrosion of unspecified degree of shoulder and upper limb, except wrist and hand, unspecified site
- **T22.41** Corrosion of unspecified degree of forearm
  - **T22.411** Corrosion of unspecified degree of right forearm
  - **T22.412** Corrosion of unspecified degree of left forearm
  - **T22.419** Corrosion of unspecified degree of unspecified forearm
- **T22.42** Corrosion of unspecified degree of elbow
  - **T22.421** Corrosion of unspecified degree of right elbow
  - **T22.422** Corrosion of unspecified degree of left elbow
  - **T22.429** Corrosion of unspecified degree of unspecified elbow
- **T22.43** Corrosion of unspecified degree of upper arm
  - **T22.431** Corrosion of unspecified degree of right upper arm
  - **T22.432** Corrosion of unspecified degree of left upper arm
  - **T22.439** Corrosion of unspecified degree of unspecified upper arm
- **T22.44** Corrosion of unspecified degree of axilla
  - **T22.441** Corrosion of unspecified degree of right axilla
  - **T22.442** Corrosion of unspecified degree of left axilla
  - **T22.449** Corrosion of unspecified degree of unspecified axilla
- **T22.45** Corrosion of unspecified degree of shoulder
  - **T22.451** Corrosion of unspecified degree of right shoulder
  - **T22.452** Corrosion of unspecified degree of left shoulder
  - **T22.459** Corrosion of unspecified degree of unspecified shoulder
- **T22.46** Corrosion of unspecified degree of scapular region
  - **T22.461** Corrosion of unspecified degree of right scapular region
  - **T22.462** Corrosion of unspecified degree of left scapular region
  - **T22.469** Corrosion of unspecified degree of unspecified scapular region
- **T22.49** Corrosion of unspecified degree of multiple sites of shoulder and upper limb, except wrist and hand
  - **T22.491** Corrosion of unspecified degree of multiple sites of right shoulder and upper limb, except wrist and hand
  - **T22.492** Corrosion of unspecified degree of multiple sites of left shoulder and upper limb, except wrist and hand
  - **T22.499** Corrosion of unspecified degree of multiple sites of unspecified shoulder and upper limb, except wrist and hand

T22.5 Corrosion of first degree of shoulder and upper limb, except wrist and hand

Code first (T51-T65) to identify chemical and intent
Use additional external cause code to identify place (Y92)

- **T22.50** Corrosion of first degree of shoulder and upper limb, except wrist and hand unspecified site
- **T22.51** Corrosion of first degree of forearm
  - **T22.511** Corrosion of first degree of right forearm
  - **T22.512** Corrosion of first degree of left forearm
  - **T22.519** Corrosion of first degree of unspecified forearm
- **T22.52** Corrosion of first degree of elbow
  - **T22.521** Corrosion of first degree of right elbow
  - **T22.522** Corrosion of first degree of left elbow
  - **T22.529** Corrosion of first degree of unspecified elbow
- **T22.53** Corrosion of first degree of upper arm
  - **T22.531** Corrosion of first degree of right upper arm
  - **T22.532** Corrosion of first degree of left upper arm
  - **T22.539** Corrosion of first degree of unspecified upper arm
- **T22.54** Corrosion of first degree of axilla
  - **T22.541** Corrosion of first degree of right axilla
  - **T22.542** Corrosion of first degree of left axilla
  - **T22.549** Corrosion of first degree of unspecified axilla
- **T22.55** Corrosion of first degree of shoulder
  - **T22.551** Corrosion of first degree of right shoulder
  - **T22.552** Corrosion of first degree of left shoulder
  - **T22.559** Corrosion of first degree of unspecified shoulder
- **T22.56** Corrosion of first degree of scapular region
  - **T22.561** Corrosion of first degree of right scapular region
  - **T22.562** Corrosion of first degree of left scapular region
  - **T22.569** Corrosion of first degree of unspecified scapular region
- **T22.59** Corrosion of first degree of multiple sites of shoulder and upper limb, except wrist and hand
  - **T22.591** Corrosion of first degree of multiple sites of right shoulder and upper limb, except wrist and hand
  - **T22.592** Corrosion of first degree of multiple sites of left shoulder and upper limb, except wrist and hand
  - **T22.599** Corrosion of first degree of multiple sites of unspecified shoulder and upper limb, except wrist and hand

T22.6 Corrosion of second degree of shoulder and upper limb, except wrist and hand

Code first (T51-T65) to identify chemical and intent
Use additional external cause code to identify place (Y92)

- **T22.60** Corrosion of second degree of shoulder and upper limb, except wrist and hand, unspecified site
- **T22.61** Corrosion of second degree of forearm
  - **T22.611** Corrosion of second degree of right forearm
  - **T22.612** Corrosion of second degree of left forearm
  - **T22.619** Corrosion of second degree of unspecified forearm
- **T22.62** Corrosion of second degree of elbow
  - **T22.621** Corrosion of second degree of right elbow
  - **T22.622** Corrosion of second degree of left elbow
  - **T22.629** Corrosion of second degree of unspecified elbow
- **T22.63** Corrosion of second degree of upper arm
  - **T22.631** Corrosion of second degree of right upper arm
  - **T22.632** Corrosion of second degree of left upper arm
  - **T22.639** Corrosion of second degree of unspecified upper arm
- **T22.64** Corrosion of second degree of axilla
  - **T22.641** Corrosion of second degree of right axilla
  - **T22.642** Corrosion of second degree of left axilla
  - **T22.649** Corrosion of second degree of unspecified axilla
- **T22.65** Corrosion of second degree of shoulder
  - **T22.651** Corrosion of second degree of right shoulder
  - **T22.652** Corrosion of second degree of left shoulder
  - **T22.659** Corrosion of second degree of unspecified shoulder
- **T22.66** Corrosion of second degree of scapular region
  - **T22.661** Corrosion of second degree of right scapular region
  - **T22.662** Corrosion of second degree of left scapular region
  - **T22.669** Corrosion of second degree of unspecified scapular region
- **T22.69** Corrosion of second degree of multiple sites of shoulder and upper limb, except wrist and hand
  - **T22.691** Corrosion of second degree of multiple sites of right shoulder and upper limb, except wrist and hand

- ✓7th **T22.692** Corrosion of second degree of multiple sites of **left** shoulder and upper limb, except wrist and hand
- ✓7th **T22.699** Corrosion of second degree of multiple sites of unspecified shoulder and upper limb, except wrist and hand

✓5th **T22.7** Corrosion of **third degree** of shoulder and upper limb, except wrist and hand
Code first (T51-T65) to identify chemical and intent
Use additional external cause code to identify place (Y92)

- ✓x 7th **T22.70** Corrosion of third degree of shoulder and upper limb, except wrist and hand, unspecified site COM
- ✓6th **T22.71** Corrosion of third degree of **forearm**
  - ✓7th **T22.711** Corrosion of third degree of **right** forearm COM
  - ✓7th **T22.712** Corrosion of third degree of **left** forearm COM
  - ✓7th **T22.719** Corrosion of third degree of unspecified forearm COM
- ✓6th **T22.72** Corrosion of third degree of **elbow**
  - ✓7th **T22.721** Corrosion of third degree of **right** elbow COM
  - ✓7th **T22.722** Corrosion of third degree of **left** elbow COM
  - ✓7th **T22.729** Corrosion of third degree of unspecified elbow COM
- ✓6th **T22.73** Corrosion of third degree of **upper arm**
  - ✓7th **T22.731** Corrosion of third degree of **right** upper arm COM
  - ✓7th **T22.732** Corrosion of third degree of **left** upper arm COM
  - ✓7th **T22.739** Corrosion of third degree of unspecified upper arm COM
- ✓6th **T22.74** Corrosion of third degree of **axilla**
  - ✓7th **T22.741** Corrosion of third degree of **right** axilla COM
  - ✓7th **T22.742** Corrosion of third degree of **left** axilla COM
  - ✓7th **T22.749** Corrosion of third degree of unspecified axilla COM
- ✓6th **T22.75** Corrosion of third degree of **shoulder**
  - ✓7th **T22.751** Corrosion of third degree of **right** shoulder COM
  - ✓7th **T22.752** Corrosion of third degree of **left** shoulder COM
  - ✓7th **T22.759** Corrosion of third degree of unspecified shoulder COM
- ✓6th **T22.76** Corrosion of third degree of **scapular region**
  - ✓7th **T22.761** Corrosion of third degree of **right** scapular region COM
  - ✓7th **T22.762** Corrosion of third degree of **left** scapular region COM
  - ✓7th **T22.769** Corrosion of third degree of unspecified scapular region COM
- ✓6th **T22.79** Corrosion of third degree of **multiple sites** of shoulder and upper limb, except wrist and hand
  - ✓7th **T22.791** Corrosion of third degree of multiple sites of **right** shoulder and upper limb, except wrist and hand COM
  - ✓7th **T22.792** Corrosion of third degree of multiple sites of **left** shoulder and upper limb, except wrist and hand COM
  - ✓7th **T22.799** Corrosion of third degree of multiple sites of unspecified shoulder and upper limb, except wrist and hand COM

✓4th **T23** Burn and corrosion of wrist and hand
AHA: 2015,1Q,19

The appropriate 7th character is to be added to each code from category T23.
- A initial encounter
- D subsequent encounter
- S sequela

✓5th **T23.0** Burn of unspecified degree of wrist and hand
Use additional external cause code to identify the source, place and intent of the burn (X00-X19, X75-X77, X96-X98, Y92)

- ✓6th **T23.00** Burn of unspecified degree of hand, unspecified site
  - ✓7th **T23.001** Burn of unspecified degree of **right** hand, unspecified site
  - ✓7th **T23.002** Burn of unspecified degree of **left** hand, unspecified site
  - ✓7th **T23.009** Burn of unspecified degree of unspecified hand, unspecified site
- ✓6th **T23.01** Burn of unspecified degree of **thumb** (nail)
  - ✓7th **T23.011** Burn of unspecified degree of **right** thumb (nail)
  - ✓7th **T23.012** Burn of unspecified degree of **left** thumb (nail)
  - ✓7th **T23.019** Burn of unspecified degree of unspecified thumb (nail)
- ✓6th **T23.02** Burn of unspecified degree of **single finger** (nail) except thumb
  - ✓7th **T23.021** Burn of unspecified degree of single **right** finger (nail) except thumb
  - ✓7th **T23.022** Burn of unspecified degree of single **left** finger (nail) except thumb
  - ✓7th **T23.029** Burn of unspecified degree of unspecified single finger (nail) except thumb
- ✓6th **T23.03** Burn of unspecified degree of **multiple fingers** (nail), **not including thumb**
  - ✓7th **T23.031** Burn of unspecified degree of multiple **right** fingers (nail), not including thumb
  - ✓7th **T23.032** Burn of unspecified degree of multiple **left** fingers (nail), not including thumb
  - ✓7th **T23.039** Burn of unspecified degree of unspecified multiple fingers (nail), not including thumb
- ✓6th **T23.04** Burn of unspecified degree of **multiple fingers** (nail), **including thumb**
  - ✓7th **T23.041** Burn of unspecified degree of multiple **right** fingers (nail), including thumb
  - ✓7th **T23.042** Burn of unspecified degree of multiple **left** fingers (nail), including thumb
  - ✓7th **T23.049** Burn of unspecified degree of unspecified multiple fingers (nail), including thumb
- ✓6th **T23.05** Burn of unspecified degree of **palm**
  - ✓7th **T23.051** Burn of unspecified degree of **right** palm
  - ✓7th **T23.052** Burn of unspecified degree of **left** palm
  - ✓7th **T23.059** Burn of unspecified degree of unspecified palm
- ✓6th **T23.06** Burn of unspecified degree of **back of hand**
  - ✓7th **T23.061** Burn of unspecified degree of back of **right** hand
  - ✓7th **T23.062** Burn of unspecified degree of back of **left** hand
  - ✓7th **T23.069** Burn of unspecified degree of back of unspecified hand
- ✓6th **T23.07** Burn of unspecified degree of **wrist**
  - ✓7th **T23.071** Burn of unspecified degree of **right** wrist
  - ✓7th **T23.072** Burn of unspecified degree of **left** wrist
  - ✓7th **T23.079** Burn of unspecified degree of unspecified wrist
- ✓6th **T23.09** Burn of unspecified degree of **multiple sites** of wrist and hand
  - ✓7th **T23.091** Burn of unspecified degree of multiple sites of **right** wrist and hand
  - ✓7th **T23.092** Burn of unspecified degree of multiple sites of **left** wrist and hand
  - ✓7th **T23.099** Burn of unspecified degree of multiple sites of unspecified wrist and hand

✓5th **T23.1** Burn of **first degree** of wrist and hand
Use additional external cause code to identify the source, place and intent of the burn (X00-X19, X75-X77, X96-X98, Y92)

- ✓6th **T23.10** Burn of first degree of hand, unspecified site
  - ✓7th **T23.101** Burn of first degree of **right** hand, unspecified site

	T23.102	Burn of first degree of left hand, unspecified site
	T23.109	Burn of first degree of unspecified hand, unspecified site
T23.11		Burn of first degree of thumb (nail)
	T23.111	Burn of first degree of right thumb (nail)
	T23.112	Burn of first degree of left thumb (nail)
	T23.119	Burn of first degree of unspecified thumb (nail)
T23.12		Burn of first degree of single finger (nail) except thumb
	T23.121	Burn of first degree of single right finger (nail) except thumb
	T23.122	Burn of first degree of single left finger (nail) except thumb
	T23.129	Burn of first degree of unspecified single finger (nail) except thumb
T23.13		Burn of first degree of multiple fingers (nail), not including thumb
	T23.131	Burn of first degree of multiple right fingers (nail), not including thumb
	T23.132	Burn of first degree of multiple left fingers (nail), not including thumb
	T23.139	Burn of first degree of unspecified multiple fingers (nail), not including thumb
T23.14		Burn of first degree of multiple fingers (nail), including thumb
	T23.141	Burn of first degree of multiple right fingers (nail), including thumb
	T23.142	Burn of first degree of multiple left fingers (nail), including thumb
	T23.149	Burn of first degree of unspecified multiple fingers (nail), including thumb
T23.15		Burn of first degree of palm
	T23.151	Burn of first degree of right palm
	T23.152	Burn of first degree of left palm
	T23.159	Burn of first degree of unspecified palm
T23.16		Burn of first degree of back of hand
	T23.161	Burn of first degree of back of right hand
	T23.162	Burn of first degree of back of left hand
	T23.169	Burn of first degree of back of unspecified hand
T23.17		Burn of first degree of wrist
	T23.171	Burn of first degree of right wrist
	T23.172	Burn of first degree of left wrist
	T23.179	Burn of first degree of unspecified wrist
T23.19		Burn of first degree of multiple sites of wrist and hand
	T23.191	Burn of first degree of multiple sites of right wrist and hand
	T23.192	Burn of first degree of multiple sites of left wrist and hand
	T23.199	Burn of first degree of multiple sites of unspecified wrist and hand

T23.2 Burn of second degree of wrist and hand

Use additional external cause code to identify the source, place and intent of the burn (X00-X19, X75-X77, X96-X98, Y92)

	T23.20	Burn of second degree of hand, unspecified site
	T23.201	Burn of second degree of right hand, unspecified site
	T23.202	Burn of second degree of left hand, unspecified site
	T23.209	Burn of second degree of unspecified hand, unspecified site
T23.21		Burn of second degree of thumb (nail)
	T23.211	Burn of second degree of right thumb (nail)
	T23.212	Burn of second degree of left thumb (nail)
	T23.219	Burn of second degree of unspecified thumb (nail)
T23.22		Burn of second degree of single finger (nail) except thumb
	T23.221	Burn of second degree of single right finger (nail) except thumb
	T23.222	Burn of second degree of single left finger (nail) except thumb
	T23.229	Burn of second degree of unspecified single finger (nail) except thumb
T23.23		Burn of second degree of multiple fingers (nail), not including thumb
	T23.231	Burn of second degree of multiple right fingers (nail), not including thumb
	T23.232	Burn of second degree of multiple left fingers (nail), not including thumb
	T23.239	Burn of second degree of unspecified multiple fingers (nail), not including thumb
T23.24		Burn of second degree of multiple fingers (nail), including thumb
	T23.241	Burn of second degree of multiple right fingers (nail), including thumb
	T23.242	Burn of second degree of multiple left fingers (nail), including thumb
	T23.249	Burn of second degree of unspecified multiple fingers (nail), including thumb
T23.25		Burn of second degree of palm
	T23.251	Burn of second degree of right palm
	T23.252	Burn of second degree of left palm
	T23.259	Burn of second degree of unspecified palm
T23.26		Burn of second degree of back of hand
	T23.261	Burn of second degree of back of right hand
	T23.262	Burn of second degree of back of left hand
	T23.269	Burn of second degree of back of unspecified hand
T23.27		Burn of second degree of wrist
	T23.271	Burn of second degree of right wrist
	T23.272	Burn of second degree of left wrist
	T23.279	Burn of second degree of unspecified wrist
T23.29		Burn of second degree of multiple sites of wrist and hand
	T23.291	Burn of second degree of multiple sites of right wrist and hand
	T23.292	Burn of second degree of multiple sites of left wrist and hand
	T23.299	Burn of second degree of multiple sites of unspecified wrist and hand

T23.3 Burn of third degree of wrist and hand

Use additional external cause code to identify the source, place and intent of the burn (X00-X19, X75-X77, X96-X98, Y92)

| | T23.30 | Burn of third degree of hand, unspecified site |

AHA: 2016,2Q,5

	T23.301	Burn of third degree of right hand, unspecified site
	T23.302	Burn of third degree of left hand, unspecified site
	T23.309	Burn of third degree of unspecified hand, unspecified site
T23.31		Burn of third degree of thumb (nail)
	T23.311	Burn of third degree of right thumb (nail)
	T23.312	Burn of third degree of left thumb (nail)
	T23.319	Burn of third degree of unspecified thumb (nail)
T23.32		Burn of third degree of single finger (nail) except thumb
	T23.321	Burn of third degree of single right finger (nail) except thumb
	T23.322	Burn of third degree of single left finger (nail) except thumb
	T23.329	Burn of third degree of unspecified single finger (nail) except thumb
T23.33		Burn of third degree of multiple fingers (nail), not including thumb
	T23.331	Burn of third degree of multiple right fingers (nail), not including thumb
	T23.332	Burn of third degree of multiple left fingers (nail), not including thumb
	T23.339	Burn of third degree of unspecified multiple fingers (nail), not including thumb
T23.34		Burn of third degree of multiple fingers (nail), including thumb
	T23.341	Burn of third degree of multiple right fingers (nail), including thumb

- **T23.342** Burn of third degree of multiple left fingers (nail), including thumb
- **T23.349** Burn of third degree of unspecified multiple fingers (nail), including thumb
- **T23.35** Burn of third degree of palm
  - **T23.351** Burn of third degree of right palm
  - **T23.352** Burn of third degree of left palm
  - **T23.359** Burn of third degree of unspecified palm
- **T23.36** Burn of third degree of back of hand
  - **T23.361** Burn of third degree of back of right hand
  - **T23.362** Burn of third degree of back of left hand
  - **T23.369** Burn of third degree of back of unspecified hand
- **T23.37** Burn of third degree of wrist
  - **T23.371** Burn of third degree of right wrist
  - **T23.372** Burn of third degree of left wrist
  - **T23.379** Burn of third degree of unspecified wrist
- **T23.39** Burn of third degree of multiple sites of wrist and hand
  - **T23.391** Burn of third degree of multiple sites of right wrist and hand
  - **T23.392** Burn of third degree of multiple sites of left wrist and hand
  - **T23.399** Burn of third degree of multiple sites of unspecified wrist and hand

T23.4 Corrosion of unspecified degree of wrist and hand

Code first (T51-T65) to identify chemical and intent
Use additional external cause code to identify place (Y92)

- **T23.40** Corrosion of unspecified degree of hand, unspecified site
  - **T23.401** Corrosion of unspecified degree of right hand, unspecified site
  - **T23.402** Corrosion of unspecified degree of left hand, unspecified site
  - **T23.409** Corrosion of unspecified degree of unspecified hand, unspecified site
- **T23.41** Corrosion of unspecified degree of thumb (nail)
  - **T23.411** Corrosion of unspecified degree of right thumb (nail)
  - **T23.412** Corrosion of unspecified degree of left thumb (nail)
  - **T23.419** Corrosion of unspecified degree of unspecified thumb (nail)
- **T23.42** Corrosion of unspecified degree of single finger (nail) except thumb
  - **T23.421** Corrosion of unspecified degree of single right finger (nail) except thumb
  - **T23.422** Corrosion of unspecified degree of single left finger (nail) except thumb
  - **T23.429** Corrosion of unspecified degree of unspecified single finger (nail) except thumb
- **T23.43** Corrosion of unspecified degree of multiple fingers (nail), not including thumb
  - **T23.431** Corrosion of unspecified degree of multiple right fingers (nail), not including thumb
  - **T23.432** Corrosion of unspecified degree of multiple left fingers (nail), not including thumb
  - **T23.439** Corrosion of unspecified degree of unspecified multiple fingers (nail), not including thumb
- **T23.44** Corrosion of unspecified degree of multiple fingers (nail), including thumb
  - **T23.441** Corrosion of unspecified degree of multiple right fingers (nail), including thumb
  - **T23.442** Corrosion of unspecified degree of multiple left fingers (nail), including thumb
  - **T23.449** Corrosion of unspecified degree of unspecified multiple fingers (nail), including thumb
- **T23.45** Corrosion of unspecified degree of palm
  - **T23.451** Corrosion of unspecified degree of right palm
  - **T23.452** Corrosion of unspecified degree of left palm
  - **T23.459** Corrosion of unspecified degree of unspecified palm
- **T23.46** Corrosion of unspecified degree of back of hand
  - **T23.461** Corrosion of unspecified degree of back of right hand
  - **T23.462** Corrosion of unspecified degree of back of left hand
  - **T23.469** Corrosion of unspecified degree of back of unspecified hand
- **T23.47** Corrosion of unspecified degree of wrist
  - **T23.471** Corrosion of unspecified degree of right wrist
  - **T23.472** Corrosion of unspecified degree of left wrist
  - **T23.479** Corrosion of unspecified degree of unspecified wrist
- **T23.49** Corrosion of unspecified degree of multiple sites of wrist and hand
  - **T23.491** Corrosion of unspecified degree of multiple sites of right wrist and hand
  - **T23.492** Corrosion of unspecified degree of multiple sites of left wrist and hand
  - **T23.499** Corrosion of unspecified degree of multiple sites of unspecified wrist and hand

T23.5 Corrosion of first degree of wrist and hand

Code first (T51-T65) to identify chemical and intent
Use additional external cause code to identify place (Y92)

- **T23.50** Corrosion of first degree of hand, unspecified site
  - **T23.501** Corrosion of first degree of right hand, unspecified site
  - **T23.502** Corrosion of first degree of left hand, unspecified site
  - **T23.509** Corrosion of first degree of unspecified hand, unspecified site
- **T23.51** Corrosion of first degree of thumb (nail)
  - **T23.511** Corrosion of first degree of right thumb (nail)
  - **T23.512** Corrosion of first degree of left thumb (nail)
  - **T23.519** Corrosion of first degree of unspecified thumb (nail)
- **T23.52** Corrosion of first degree of single finger (nail) except thumb
  - **T23.521** Corrosion of first degree of single right finger (nail) except thumb
  - **T23.522** Corrosion of first degree of single left finger (nail) except thumb
  - **T23.529** Corrosion of first degree of unspecified single finger (nail) except thumb
- **T23.53** Corrosion of first degree of multiple fingers (nail), not including thumb
  - **T23.531** Corrosion of first degree of multiple right fingers (nail), not including thumb
  - **T23.532** Corrosion of first degree of multiple left fingers (nail), not including thumb
  - **T23.539** Corrosion of first degree of unspecified multiple fingers (nail), not including thumb
- **T23.54** Corrosion of first degree of multiple fingers (nail), including thumb
  - **T23.541** Corrosion of first degree of multiple right fingers (nail), including thumb
  - **T23.542** Corrosion of first degree of multiple left fingers (nail), including thumb
  - **T23.549** Corrosion of first degree of unspecified multiple fingers (nail), including thumb
- **T23.55** Corrosion of first degree of palm
  - **T23.551** Corrosion of first degree of right palm
  - **T23.552** Corrosion of first degree of left palm
  - **T23.559** Corrosion of first degree of unspecified palm
- **T23.56** Corrosion of first degree of back of hand
  - **T23.561** Corrosion of first degree of back of right hand
  - **T23.562** Corrosion of first degree of back of left hand

- ✓7th T23.569 Corrosion of first degree of back of unspecified hand
- ✓6th **T23.57** Corrosion of first degree of wrist
  - ✓7th T23.571 Corrosion of first degree of right wrist
  - ✓7th T23.572 Corrosion of first degree of left wrist
  - ✓7th T23.579 Corrosion of first degree of unspecified wrist
- ✓6th **T23.59** Corrosion of first degree of multiple sites of wrist and hand
  - ✓7th T23.591 Corrosion of first degree of multiple sites of right wrist and hand
  - ✓7th T23.592 Corrosion of first degree of multiple sites of left wrist and hand
  - ✓7th T23.599 Corrosion of first degree of multiple sites of unspecified wrist and hand
- ✓5th **T23.6** Corrosion of second degree of wrist and hand
  - Code first (T51-T65) to identify chemical and intent
  - Use additional external cause code to identify place (Y92)
  - ✓6th **T23.60** Corrosion of second degree of hand, unspecified site
    - ✓7th T23.601 Corrosion of second degree of right hand, unspecified site
    - ✓7th T23.602 Corrosion of second degree of left hand, unspecified site
    - ✓7th T23.609 Corrosion of second degree of unspecified hand, unspecified site
  - ✓6th **T23.61** Corrosion of second degree of thumb (nail)
    - ✓7th T23.611 Corrosion of second degree of right thumb (nail)
    - ✓7th T23.612 Corrosion of second degree of left thumb (nail)
    - ✓7th T23.619 Corrosion of second degree of unspecified thumb (nail)
  - ✓6th **T23.62** Corrosion of second degree of single finger (nail) except thumb
    - ✓7th T23.621 Corrosion of second degree of single right finger (nail) except thumb
    - ✓7th T23.622 Corrosion of second degree of single left finger (nail) except thumb
    - ✓7th T23.629 Corrosion of second degree of unspecified single finger (nail) except thumb
  - ✓6th **T23.63** Corrosion of second degree of multiple fingers (nail), not including thumb
    - ✓7th T23.631 Corrosion of second degree of multiple right fingers (nail), not including thumb
    - ✓7th T23.632 Corrosion of second degree of multiple left fingers (nail), not including thumb
    - ✓7th T23.639 Corrosion of second degree of unspecified multiple fingers (nail), not including thumb
  - ✓6th **T23.64** Corrosion of second degree of multiple fingers (nail), including thumb
    - ✓7th T23.641 Corrosion of second degree of multiple right fingers (nail), including thumb
    - ✓7th T23.642 Corrosion of second degree of multiple left fingers (nail), including thumb
    - ✓7th T23.649 Corrosion of second degree of unspecified multiple fingers (nail), including thumb
  - ✓6th **T23.65** Corrosion of second degree of palm
    - ✓7th T23.651 Corrosion of second degree of right palm
    - ✓7th T23.652 Corrosion of second degree of left palm
    - ✓7th T23.659 Corrosion of second degree of unspecified palm
  - ✓6th **T23.66** Corrosion of second degree of back of hand
    - ✓7th T23.661 Corrosion of second degree back of right hand
    - ✓7th T23.662 Corrosion of second degree back of left hand
    - ✓7th T23.669 Corrosion of second degree back of unspecified hand
  - ✓6th **T23.67** Corrosion of second degree of wrist
    - ✓7th T23.671 Corrosion of second degree of right wrist
    - ✓7th T23.672 Corrosion of second degree of left wrist
    - ✓7th T23.679 Corrosion of second degree of unspecified wrist
  - ✓6th **T23.69** Corrosion of second degree of multiple sites of wrist and hand
    - ✓7th T23.691 Corrosion of second degree of multiple sites of right wrist and hand
    - ✓7th T23.692 Corrosion of second degree of multiple sites of left wrist and hand
    - ✓7th T23.699 Corrosion of second degree of multiple sites of unspecified wrist and hand
- ✓5th **T23.7** Corrosion of third degree of wrist and hand
  - Code first (T51-T65) to identify chemical and intent
  - Use additional external cause code to identify place (Y92)
  - ✓6th **T23.70** Corrosion of third degree of hand, unspecified site
    - ✓7th T23.701 Corrosion of third degree of right hand, unspecified site [COM]
    - ✓7th T23.702 Corrosion of third degree of left hand, unspecified site [COM]
    - ✓7th T23.709 Corrosion of third degree of unspecified hand, unspecified site [COM]
  - ✓6th **T23.71** Corrosion of third degree of thumb (nail)
    - ✓7th T23.711 Corrosion of third degree of right thumb (nail) [COM]
    - ✓7th T23.712 Corrosion of third degree of left thumb (nail) [COM]
    - ✓7th T23.719 Corrosion of third degree of unspecified thumb (nail) [COM]
  - ✓6th **T23.72** Corrosion of third degree of single finger (nail) except thumb
    - ✓7th T23.721 Corrosion of third degree of single right finger (nail) except thumb [COM]
    - ✓7th T23.722 Corrosion of third degree of single left finger (nail) except thumb [COM]
    - ✓7th T23.729 Corrosion of third degree of unspecified single finger (nail) except thumb [COM]
  - ✓6th **T23.73** Corrosion of third degree of multiple fingers (nail), not including thumb
    - ✓7th T23.731 Corrosion of third degree of multiple right fingers (nail), not including thumb [COM]
    - ✓7th T23.732 Corrosion of third degree of multiple left fingers (nail), not including thumb [COM]
    - ✓7th T23.739 Corrosion of third degree of unspecified multiple fingers (nail), not including thumb [COM]
  - ✓6th **T23.74** Corrosion of third degree of multiple fingers (nail), including thumb
    - ✓7th T23.741 Corrosion of third degree of multiple right fingers (nail), including thumb [COM]
    - ✓7th T23.742 Corrosion of third degree of multiple left fingers (nail), including thumb [COM]
    - ✓7th T23.749 Corrosion of third degree of unspecified multiple fingers (nail), including thumb [COM]
  - ✓6th **T23.75** Corrosion of third degree of palm
    - ✓7th T23.751 Corrosion of third degree of right palm [COM]
    - ✓7th T23.752 Corrosion of third degree of left palm [COM]
    - ✓7th T23.759 Corrosion of third degree of unspecified palm [COM]
  - ✓6th **T23.76** Corrosion of third degree of back of hand
    - ✓7th T23.761 Corrosion of third degree of back of right hand [COM]
    - ✓7th T23.762 Corrosion of third degree of back of left hand [COM]
    - ✓7th T23.769 Corrosion of third degree back of unspecified hand [COM]
  - ✓6th **T23.77** Corrosion of third degree of wrist
    - ✓7th T23.771 Corrosion of third degree of right wrist [COM]
    - ✓7th T23.772 Corrosion of third degree of left wrist [COM]
    - ✓7th T23.779 Corrosion of third degree of unspecified wrist [COM]
  - ✓6th **T23.79** Corrosion of third degree of multiple sites of wrist and hand
    - ✓7th T23.791 Corrosion of third degree of multiple sites of right wrist and hand [COM]
    - ✓7th T23.792 Corrosion of third degree of multiple sites of left wrist and hand [COM]
    - ✓7th T23.799 Corrosion of third degree of multiple sites of unspecified wrist and hand [COM]

T24 Burn and corrosion of lower limb, except ankle and foot

EXCLUDES 2 burn and corrosion of ankle and foot (T25.-)
burn and corrosion of hip region (T21.-)

The appropriate 7th character is to be added to each code from category T24.
- A initial encounter
- D subsequent encounter
- S sequela

T24.0 Burn of unspecified degree of lower limb, except ankle and foot
Use additional external cause code to identify the source, place and intent of the burn (X00-X19, X75-X77, X96-X98, Y92)

- **T24.00** Burn of unspecified degree of unspecified site of lower limb, except ankle and foot
  - T24.001 Burn of unspecified degree of unspecified site of right lower limb, except ankle and foot
  - T24.002 Burn of unspecified degree of unspecified site of left lower limb, except ankle and foot
  - T24.009 Burn of unspecified degree of unspecified site of unspecified lower limb, except ankle and foot
- **T24.01** Burn of unspecified degree of thigh
  - T24.011 Burn of unspecified degree of right thigh
  - T24.012 Burn of unspecified degree of left thigh
  - T24.019 Burn of unspecified degree of unspecified thigh
- **T24.02** Burn of unspecified degree of knee
  - T24.021 Burn of unspecified degree of right knee
  - T24.022 Burn of unspecified degree of left knee
  - T24.029 Burn of unspecified degree of unspecified knee
- **T24.03** Burn of unspecified degree of lower leg
  - T24.031 Burn of unspecified degree of right lower leg
  - T24.032 Burn of unspecified degree of left lower leg
  - T24.039 Burn of unspecified degree of unspecified lower leg
- **T24.09** Burn of unspecified degree of multiple sites of lower limb, except ankle and foot
  - T24.091 Burn of unspecified degree of multiple sites of right lower limb, except ankle and foot
  - T24.092 Burn of unspecified degree of multiple sites of left lower limb, except ankle and foot
  - T24.099 Burn of unspecified degree of multiple sites of unspecified lower limb, except ankle and foot

T24.1 Burn of first degree of lower limb, except ankle and foot
Use additional external cause code to identify the source, place and intent of the burn (X00-X19, X75-X77, X96-X98, Y92)

- **T24.10** Burn of first degree of unspecified site of lower limb, except ankle and foot
  - T24.101 Burn of first degree of unspecified site of right lower limb, except ankle and foot
  - T24.102 Burn of first degree of unspecified site of left lower limb, except ankle and foot
  - T24.109 Burn of first degree of unspecified site of unspecified lower limb, except ankle and foot
- **T24.11** Burn of first degree of thigh
  - T24.111 Burn of first degree of right thigh
  - T24.112 Burn of first degree of left thigh
  - T24.119 Burn of first degree of unspecified thigh
- **T24.12** Burn of first degree of knee
  - T24.121 Burn of first degree of right knee
  - T24.122 Burn of first degree of left knee
  - T24.129 Burn of first degree of unspecified knee
- **T24.13** Burn of first degree of lower leg
  - T24.131 Burn of first degree of right lower leg
  - T24.132 Burn of first degree of left lower leg
  - T24.139 Burn of first degree of unspecified lower leg
- **T24.19** Burn of first degree of multiple sites of lower limb, except ankle and foot
  - T24.191 Burn of first degree of multiple sites of right lower limb, except ankle and foot
  - T24.192 Burn of first degree of multiple sites of left lower limb, except ankle and foot
  - T24.199 Burn of first degree of multiple sites of unspecified lower limb, except ankle and foot

T24.2 Burn of second degree of lower limb, except ankle and foot
Use additional external cause code to identify the source, place and intent of the burn (X00-X19, X75-X77, X96-X98, Y92)

- **T24.20** Burn of second degree of unspecified site of lower limb, except ankle and foot
  - T24.201 Burn of second degree of unspecified site of right lower limb, except ankle and foot
  - T24.202 Burn of second degree of unspecified site of left lower limb, except ankle and foot
  - T24.209 Burn of second degree of unspecified site of unspecified lower limb, except ankle and foot
- **T24.21** Burn of second degree of thigh
  - T24.211 Burn of second degree of right thigh
  - T24.212 Burn of second degree of left thigh
  - T24.219 Burn of second degree of unspecified thigh
- **T24.22** Burn of second degree of knee
  - T24.221 Burn of second degree of right knee
  - T24.222 Burn of second degree of left knee
  - T24.229 Burn of second degree of unspecified knee
- **T24.23** Burn of second degree of lower leg
  - T24.231 Burn of second degree of right lower leg
  - T24.232 Burn of second degree of left lower leg
  - T24.239 Burn of second degree of unspecified lower leg
- **T24.29** Burn of second degree of multiple sites of lower limb, except ankle and foot
  - T24.291 Burn of second degree of multiple sites of right lower limb, except ankle and foot
  - T24.292 Burn of second degree of multiple sites of left lower limb, except ankle and foot
  - T24.299 Burn of second degree of multiple sites of unspecified lower limb, except ankle and foot

T24.3 Burn of third degree of lower limb, except ankle and foot
Use additional external cause code to identify the source, place and intent of the burn (X00-X19, X75-X77, X96-X98, Y92)

- **T24.30** Burn of third degree of unspecified site of lower limb, except ankle and foot
  - T24.301 Burn of third degree of unspecified site of right lower limb, except ankle and foot **COM**
  - T24.302 Burn of third degree of unspecified site of left lower limb, except ankle and foot **COM**
  - T24.309 Burn of third degree of unspecified site of unspecified lower limb, except ankle and foot
- **T24.31** Burn of third degree of thigh
  - T24.311 Burn of third degree of right thigh **COM**
  - T24.312 Burn of third degree of left thigh **COM**
  - T24.319 Burn of third degree of unspecified thigh **COM**
- **T24.32** Burn of third degree of knee
  - T24.321 Burn of third degree of right knee **COM**
  - T24.322 Burn of third degree of left knee **COM**
  - T24.329 Burn of third degree of unspecified knee **COM**
- **T24.33** Burn of third degree of lower leg
  - T24.331 Burn of third degree of right lower leg **COM**
  - T24.332 Burn of third degree of left lower leg **COM**
  - T24.339 Burn of third degree of unspecified lower leg **COM**

Chapter 19. Injury, Poisoning and Certain Other Consequences of External Causes

- **T25.42** Corrosion of unspecified degree of foot
  - EXCLUDES 2: corrosion of unspecified degree of toe(s) (nail) (T25.43-)
  - **T25.421** Corrosion of unspecified degree of right foot
  - **T25.422** Corrosion of unspecified degree of left foot
  - **T25.429** Corrosion of unspecified degree of unspecified foot
- **T25.43** Corrosion of unspecified degree of toe(s) (nail)
  - **T25.431** Corrosion of unspecified degree of right toe(s) (nail)
  - **T25.432** Corrosion of unspecified degree of left toe(s) (nail)
  - **T25.439** Corrosion of unspecified degree of unspecified toe(s) (nail)
- **T25.49** Corrosion of unspecified degree of multiple sites of ankle and foot
  - **T25.491** Corrosion of unspecified degree of multiple sites of right ankle and foot
  - **T25.492** Corrosion of unspecified degree of multiple sites of left ankle and foot
  - **T25.499** Corrosion of unspecified degree of multiple sites of unspecified ankle and foot

T25.5 Corrosion of first degree of ankle and foot
Code first (T51-T65) to identify chemical and intent
Use additional external cause code to identify place (Y92)

- **T25.51** Corrosion of first degree of ankle
  - **T25.511** Corrosion of first degree of right ankle
  - **T25.512** Corrosion of first degree of left ankle
  - **T25.519** Corrosion of first degree of unspecified ankle
- **T25.52** Corrosion of first degree of foot
  - EXCLUDES 2: corrosion of first degree of toe(s) (nail) (T25.53-)
  - **T25.521** Corrosion of first degree of right foot
  - **T25.522** Corrosion of first degree of left foot
  - **T25.529** Corrosion of first degree of unspecified foot
- **T25.53** Corrosion of first degree of toe(s) (nail)
  - **T25.531** Corrosion of first degree of right toe(s) (nail)
  - **T25.532** Corrosion of first degree of left toe(s) (nail)
  - **T25.539** Corrosion of first degree of unspecified toe(s) (nail)
- **T25.59** Corrosion of first degree of multiple sites of ankle and foot
  - **T25.591** Corrosion of first degree of multiple sites of right ankle and foot
  - **T25.592** Corrosion of first degree of multiple sites of left ankle and foot
  - **T25.599** Corrosion of first degree of multiple sites of unspecified ankle and foot

T25.6 Corrosion of second degree of ankle and foot
Code first (T51-T65) to identify chemical and intent
Use additional external cause code to identify place (Y92)

- **T25.61** Corrosion of second degree of ankle
  - **T25.611** Corrosion of second degree of right ankle
  - **T25.612** Corrosion of second degree of left ankle
  - **T25.619** Corrosion of second degree of unspecified ankle
- **T25.62** Corrosion of second degree of foot
  - EXCLUDES 2: corrosion of second degree of toe(s) (nail) (T25.63-)
  - **T25.621** Corrosion of second degree of right foot
  - **T25.622** Corrosion of second degree of left foot
  - **T25.629** Corrosion of second degree of unspecified foot
- **T25.63** Corrosion of second degree of toe(s) (nail)
  - **T25.631** Corrosion of second degree of right toe(s) (nail)
  - **T25.632** Corrosion of second degree of left toe(s) (nail)
  - **T25.639** Corrosion of second degree of unspecified toe(s) (nail)
- **T25.69** Corrosion of second degree of multiple sites of ankle and foot
  - **T25.691** Corrosion of second degree of right ankle and foot
  - **T25.692** Corrosion of second degree of left ankle and foot
  - **T25.699** Corrosion of second degree of unspecified ankle and foot

T25.7 Corrosion of third degree of ankle and foot
Code first (T51-T65) to identify chemical and intent
Use additional external cause code to identify place (Y92)

- **T25.71** Corrosion of third degree of ankle
  - **T25.711** Corrosion of third degree of right ankle
  - **T25.712** Corrosion of third degree of left ankle
  - **T25.719** Corrosion of third degree of unspecified ankle
- **T25.72** Corrosion of third degree of foot
  - EXCLUDES 2: corrosion of third degree of toe(s) (nail) (T25.73-)
  - **T25.721** Corrosion of third degree of right foot
  - **T25.722** Corrosion of third degree of left foot
  - **T25.729** Corrosion of third degree of unspecified foot
- **T25.73** Corrosion of third degree of toe(s) (nail)
  - **T25.731** Corrosion of third degree of right toe(s) (nail)
  - **T25.732** Corrosion of third degree of left toe(s) (nail)
  - **T25.739** Corrosion of third degree of unspecified toe(s) (nail)
- **T25.79** Corrosion of third degree of multiple sites of ankle and foot
  - **T25.791** Corrosion of third degree of multiple sites of right ankle and foot
  - **T25.792** Corrosion of third degree of multiple sites of left ankle and foot
  - **T25.799** Corrosion of third degree of multiple sites of unspecified ankle and foot

Burns and corrosions confined to eye and internal organs (T26-T28)

T26 Burn and corrosion confined to eye and adnexa

The appropriate 7th character is to be added to each code from category T26.
- A initial encounter
- D subsequent encounter
- S sequela

T26.0 Burn of eyelid and periocular area
Use additional external cause code to identify the source, place and intent of the burn (X00-X19, X75-X77, X96-X98, Y92)
- **T26.00** Burn of unspecified eyelid and periocular area
- **T26.01** Burn of right eyelid and periocular area
- **T26.02** Burn of left eyelid and periocular area

T26.1 Burn of cornea and conjunctival sac
Use additional external cause code to identify the source, place and intent of the burn (X00-X19, X75-X77, X96-X98, Y92)
- **T26.10** Burn of cornea and conjunctival sac, unspecified eye
- **T26.11** Burn of cornea and conjunctival sac, right eye
- **T26.12** Burn of cornea and conjunctival sac, left eye

T26.2 Burn with resulting rupture and destruction of eyeball
Use additional external cause code to identify the source, place and intent of the burn (X00-X19, X75-X77, X96-X98, Y92)
- **T26.20** Burn with resulting rupture and destruction of unspecified eyeball
- **T26.21** Burn with resulting rupture and destruction of right eyeball
- **T26.22** Burn with resulting rupture and destruction of left eyeball

T26.3 Burns of other specified parts of eye and adnexa
Use additional external cause code to identify the source, place and intent of the burn (X00-X19, X75-X77, X96-X98, Y92)
- T26.30 Burns of other specified parts of unspecified eye and adnexa
- T26.31 Burns of other specified parts of right eye and adnexa
- T26.32 Burns of other specified parts of left eye and adnexa

T26.4 Burn of eye and adnexa, part unspecified
Use additional external cause code to identify the source, place and intent of the burn (X00-X19, X75-X77, X96-X98, Y92)
- T26.40 Burn of unspecified eye and adnexa, part unspecified
- T26.41 Burn of right eye and adnexa, part unspecified
- T26.42 Burn of left eye and adnexa, part unspecified

T26.5 Corrosion of eyelid and periocular area
Code first (T51-T65) to identify chemical and intent
Use additional external cause code to identify place (Y92)
- T26.50 Corrosion of unspecified eyelid and periocular area
- T26.51 Corrosion of right eyelid and periocular area
- T26.52 Corrosion of left eyelid and periocular area

T26.6 Corrosion of cornea and conjunctival sac
Code first (T51-T65) to identify chemical and intent
Use additional external cause code to identify place (Y92)
- T26.60 Corrosion of cornea and conjunctival sac, unspecified eye
- T26.61 Corrosion of cornea and conjunctival sac, right eye
- T26.62 Corrosion of cornea and conjunctival sac, left eye

T26.7 Corrosion with resulting rupture and destruction of eyeball
Code first (T51-T65) to identify chemical and intent
Use additional external cause code to identify place (Y92)
- T26.70 Corrosion with resulting rupture and destruction of unspecified eyeball
- T26.71 Corrosion with resulting rupture and destruction of right eyeball
- T26.72 Corrosion with resulting rupture and destruction of left eyeball

T26.8 Corrosions of other specified parts of eye and adnexa
Code first (T51-T65) to identify chemical and intent
Use additional external cause code to identify place (Y92)
- T26.80 Corrosions of other specified parts of unspecified eye and adnexa
- T26.81 Corrosions of other specified parts of right eye and adnexa
- T26.82 Corrosions of other specified parts of left eye and adnexa

T26.9 Corrosion of eye and adnexa, part unspecified
Code first (T51-T65) to identify chemical and intent
Use additional external cause code to identify place (Y92)
- T26.90 Corrosion of unspecified eye and adnexa, part unspecified
- T26.91 Corrosion of right eye and adnexa, part unspecified
- T26.92 Corrosion of left eye and adnexa, part unspecified

T27 Burn and corrosion of respiratory tract
Use additional external cause code to identify place (Y92)
Use additional external cause code to identify the source and intent of the burn (X00-X19, X75-X77, X96-X98)

The appropriate 7th character is to be added to each code from category T27.
- A initial encounter
- D subsequent encounter
- S sequela

- T27.0 Burn of larynx and trachea
- T27.1 Burn involving larynx and trachea with lung
- T27.2 Burn of other parts of respiratory tract
  - Burn of thoracic cavity
- T27.3 Burn of respiratory tract, part unspecified
- T27.4 Corrosion of larynx and trachea
  - Code first (T51-T65) to identify chemical and intent
- T27.5 Corrosion involving larynx and trachea with lung
  - Code first (T51-T65) to identify chemical and intent
- T27.6 Corrosion of other parts of respiratory tract
  - Code first (T51-T65) to identify chemical and intent
- T27.7 Corrosion of respiratory tract, part unspecified
  - Code first (T51-T65) to identify chemical and intent

T28 Burn and corrosion of other internal organs
Use additional external cause code to identify place (Y92)
Use additional external cause code to identify the source and intent of the burn (X00-X19, X75-X77, X96-X98)

The appropriate 7th character is to be added to each code from category T28.
- A initial encounter
- D subsequent encounter
- S sequela

- T28.0 Burn of mouth and pharynx
- T28.1 Burn of esophagus
- T28.2 Burn of other parts of alimentary tract
- T28.3 Burn of internal genitourinary organs
- T28.4 Burns of other and unspecified internal organs
  - T28.40 Burn of unspecified internal organ
  - T28.41 Burn of ear drum
    - T28.411 Burn of right ear drum
    - T28.412 Burn of left ear drum
    - T28.419 Burn of unspecified ear drum
  - T28.49 Burn of other internal organ
- T28.5 Corrosion of mouth and pharynx
  - Code first (T51-T65) to identify chemical and intent
- T28.6 Corrosion of esophagus
  - Code first (T51-T65) to identify chemical and intent
- T28.7 Corrosion of other parts of alimentary tract
  - Code first (T51-T65) to identify chemical and intent
- T28.8 Corrosion of internal genitourinary organs
  - Code first (T51-T65) to identify chemical and intent
- T28.9 Corrosions of other and unspecified internal organs
  - Code first (T51-T65) to identify chemical and intent
  - T28.90 Corrosions of unspecified internal organs
  - T28.91 Corrosions of ear drum
    - T28.911 Corrosions of right ear drum
    - T28.912 Corrosions of left ear drum
    - T28.919 Corrosions of unspecified ear drum
  - T28.99 Corrosions of other internal organs

Burns and corrosions of multiple and unspecified body regions (T30-T32)

T30 Burn and corrosion, body region unspecified
- T30.0 Burn of unspecified body region, unspecified degree
  - Burn NOS
  - Multiple burns NOS
  - This code is not for inpatient use. Code to specified site and degree of burns
- T30.4 Corrosion of unspecified body region, unspecified degree
  - Corrosion NOS
  - Multiple corrosion NOS
  - This code is not for inpatient use. Code to specified site and degree of corrosion

T31 Burns classified according to extent of body surface involved
NOTE This category is to be used as the primary code only when the site of the burn is unspecified. It should be used as a supplementary code with categories T20-T25 when the site is specified.

- T31.0 Burns involving less than 10% of body surface
- T31.1 Burns involving 10-19% of body surface
  - T31.10 Burns involving 10-19% of body surface with 0% to 9% third degree burns
    - Burns involving 10-19% of body surface NOS
  - T31.11 Burns involving 10-19% of body surface with 10-19% third degree burns
- T31.2 Burns involving 20-29% of body surface
  - T31.20 Burns involving 20-29% of body surface with 0% to 9% third degree burns
    - Burns involving 20-29% of body surface NOS
  - T31.21 Burns involving 20-29% of body surface with 10-19% third degree burns
  - T31.22 Burns involving 20-29% of body surface with 20-29% third degree burns

Chapter 19. Injury, Poisoning and Certain Other Consequences of External Causes

✓5th T31.3   Burns involving 30-39% of body surface
- T31.30 Burns involving 30-39% of body surface with 0% to 9% third degree burns COM
  - Burns involving 30-39% of body surface NOS
- T31.31 Burns involving 30-39% of body surface with 10-19% third degree burns HCC ESR COM
- T31.32 Burns involving 30-39% of body surface with 20-29% third degree burns HCC ESR COM
- T31.33 Burns involving 30-39% of body surface with 30-39% third degree burns HCC ESR COM

✓5th T31.4   Burns involving 40-49% of body surface
- T31.40 Burns involving 40-49% of body surface with 0% to 9% third degree burns COM
  - Burns involving 40-49% of body surface NOS
- T31.41 Burns involving 40-49% of body surface with 10-19% third degree burns HCC ESR COM
- T31.42 Burns involving 40-49% of body surface with 20-29% third degree burns HCC ESR COM
- T31.43 Burns involving 40-49% of body surface with 30-39% third degree burns HCC ESR COM
- T31.44 Burns involving 40-49% of body surface with 40-49% third degree burns HCC ESR COM

✓5th T31.5   Burns involving 50-59% of body surface
- T31.50 Burns involving 50-59% of body surface with 0% to 9% third degree burns COM
  - Burns involving 50-59% of body surface NOS
- T31.51 Burns involving 50-59% of body surface with 10-19% third degree burns HCC ESR COM
- T31.52 Burns involving 50-59% of body surface with 20-29% third degree burns HCC ESR COM
- T31.53 Burns involving 50-59% of body surface with 30-39% third degree burns HCC ESR COM
- T31.54 Burns involving 50-59% of body surface with 40-49% third degree burns HCC ESR COM
- T31.55 Burns involving 50-59% of body surface with 50-59% third degree burns HCC ESR COM

✓5th T31.6   Burns involving 60-69% of body surface
- T31.60 Burns involving 60-69% of body surface with 0% to 9% third degree burns COM
  - Burns involving 60-69% of body surface NOS
- T31.61 Burns involving 60-69% of body surface with 10-19% third degree burns HCC ESR COM
- T31.62 Burns involving 60-69% of body surface with 20-29% third degree burns HCC ESR COM
- T31.63 Burns involving 60-69% of body surface with 30-39% third degree burns HCC ESR COM
- T31.64 Burns involving 60-69% of body surface with 40-49% third degree burns HCC ESR COM
- T31.65 Burns involving 60-69% of body surface with 50-59% third degree burns HCC ESR COM
- T31.66 Burns involving 60-69% of body surface with 60-69% third degree burns HCC ESR COM

✓5th T31.7   Burns involving 70-79% of body surface
- T31.70 Burns involving 70-79% of body surface with 0% to 9% third degree burns COM
  - Burns involving 70-79% of body surface NOS
- T31.71 Burns involving 70-79% of body surface with 10-19% third degree burns HCC ESR COM
- T31.72 Burns involving 70-79% of body surface with 20-29% third degree burns HCC ESR COM
- T31.73 Burns involving 70-79% of body surface with 30-39% third degree burns HCC ESR COM
- T31.74 Burns involving 70-79% of body surface with 40-49% third degree burns HCC ESR COM
- T31.75 Burns involving 70-79% of body surface with 50-59% third degree burns HCC ESR COM
- T31.76 Burns involving 70-79% of body surface with 60-69% third degree burns HCC ESR COM
- T31.77 Burns involving 70-79% of body surface with 70-79% third degree burns HCC ESR COM

✓5th T31.8   Burns involving 80-89% of body surface
- T31.80 Burns involving 80-89% of body surface with 0% to 9% third degree burns COM
  - Burns involving 80-89% of body surface NOS
- T31.81 Burns involving 80-89% of body surface with 10-19% third degree burns HCC ESR COM
- T31.82 Burns involving 80-89% of body surface with 20-29% third degree burns HCC ESR COM
- T31.83 Burns involving 80-89% of body surface with 30-39% third degree burns HCC ESR COM
- T31.84 Burns involving 80-89% of body surface with 40-49% third degree burns HCC ESR COM
- T31.85 Burns involving 80-89% of body surface with 50-59% third degree burns HCC ESR COM
- T31.86 Burns involving 80-89% of body surface with 60-69% third degree burns HCC ESR COM
- T31.87 Burns involving 80-89% of body surface with 70-79% third degree burns HCC ESR COM
- T31.88 Burns involving 80-89% of body surface with 80-89% third degree burns HCC ESR COM

✓5th T31.9   Burns involving 90% or more of body surface
- T31.90 Burns involving 90% or more of body surface with 0% to 9% third degree burns COM
  - Burns involving 90% or more of body surface NOS
- T31.91 Burns involving 90% or more of body surface with 10-19% third degree burns HCC ESR COM
- T31.92 Burns involving 90% or more of body surface with 20-29% third degree burns HCC ESR COM
- T31.93 Burns involving 90% or more of body surface with 30-39% third degree burns HCC ESR COM
- T31.94 Burns involving 90% or more of body surface with 40-49% third degree burns HCC ESR COM
- T31.95 Burns involving 90% or more of body surface with 50-59% third degree burns HCC ESR COM
- T31.96 Burns involving 90% or more of body surface with 60-69% third degree burns HCC ESR COM
- T31.97 Burns involving 90% or more of body surface with 70-79% third degree burns HCC ESR COM
- T31.98 Burns involving 90% or more of body surface with 80-89% third degree burns HCC ESR COM
- T31.99 Burns involving 90% or more of body surface with 90% or more third degree burns HCC ESR COM

Rule of Nines Estimation of Total Body Surface Burned

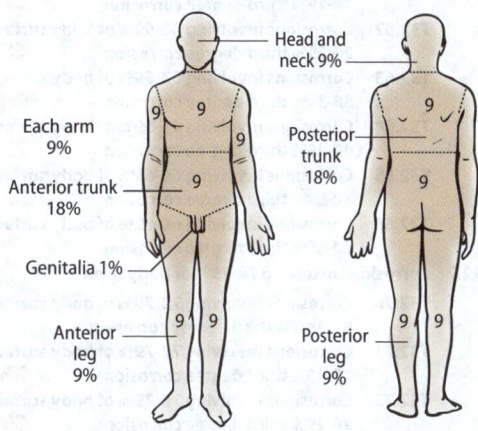

Head and neck 9%; Each arm 9%; Anterior trunk 18%; Posterior trunk 18%; Genitalia 1%; Anterior leg 9%; Posterior leg 9%

✓4th T32   Corrosions classified according to extent of body surface involved

NOTE: This category is to be used as the primary code only when the site of the corrosion is unspecified. It may be used as a supplementary code with categories T20-T25 when the site is specified.

- T32.0 Corrosions involving less than 10% of body surface
- **✓5th T32.1   Corrosions involving 10-19% of body surface**
  - T32.10 Corrosions involving 10-19% of body surface with 0% to 9% third degree corrosion COM
    - Corrosions involving 10-19% of body surface NOS
  - T32.11 Corrosions involving 10-19% of body surface with 10-19% third degree corrosion HCC ESR COM
- **✓5th T32.2   Corrosions involving 20-29% of body surface**
  - T32.20 Corrosions involving 20-29% of body surface with 0% to 9% third degree corrosion COM
  - T32.21 Corrosions involving 20-29% of body surface with 10-19% third degree corrosion HCC ESR COM
  - T32.22 Corrosions involving 20-29% of body surface with 20-29% third degree corrosion HCC ESR COM

Chapter 19. Injury, Poisoning and Certain Other Consequences of External Causes

T32.3 Corrosions involving 30-39% of body surface
- **T32.30** Corrosions involving 30-39% of body surface with 0% to 9% third degree corrosion
- **T32.31** Corrosions involving 30-39% of body surface with 10-19% third degree corrosion
- **T32.32** Corrosions involving 30-39% of body surface with 20-29% third degree corrosion
- **T32.33** Corrosions involving 30-39% of body surface with 30-39% third degree corrosion

T32.4 Corrosions involving 40-49% of body surface
- **T32.40** Corrosions involving 40-49% of body surface with 0% to 9% third degree corrosion
- **T32.41** Corrosions involving 40-49% of body surface with 10-19% third degree corrosion
- **T32.42** Corrosions involving 40-49% of body surface with 20-29% third degree corrosion
- **T32.43** Corrosions involving 40-49% of body surface with 30-39% third degree corrosion
- **T32.44** Corrosions involving 40-49% of body surface with 40-49% third degree corrosion

T32.5 Corrosions involving 50-59% of body surface
- **T32.50** Corrosions involving 50-59% of body surface with 0% to 9% third degree corrosion
- **T32.51** Corrosions involving 50-59% of body surface with 10-19% third degree corrosion
- **T32.52** Corrosions involving 50-59% of body surface with 20-29% third degree corrosion
- **T32.53** Corrosions involving 50-59% of body surface with 30-39% third degree corrosion
- **T32.54** Corrosions involving 50-59% of body surface with 40-49% third degree corrosion
- **T32.55** Corrosions involving 50-59% of body surface with 50-59% third degree corrosion

T32.6 Corrosions involving 60-69% of body surface
- **T32.60** Corrosions involving 60-69% of body surface with 0% to 9% third degree corrosion
- **T32.61** Corrosions involving 60-69% of body surface with 10-19% third degree corrosion
- **T32.62** Corrosions involving 60-69% of body surface with 20-29% third degree corrosion
- **T32.63** Corrosions involving 60-69% of body surface with 30-39% third degree corrosion
- **T32.64** Corrosions involving 60-69% of body surface with 40-49% third degree corrosion
- **T32.65** Corrosions involving 60-69% of body surface with 50-59% third degree corrosion
- **T32.66** Corrosions involving 60-69% of body surface with 60-69% third degree corrosion

T32.7 Corrosions involving 70-79% of body surface
- **T32.70** Corrosions involving 70-79% of body surface with 0% to 9% third degree corrosion
- **T32.71** Corrosions involving 70-79% of body surface with 10-19% third degree corrosion
- **T32.72** Corrosions involving 70-79% of body surface with 20-29% third degree corrosion
- **T32.73** Corrosions involving 70-79% of body surface with 30-39% third degree corrosion
- **T32.74** Corrosions involving 70-79% of body surface with 40-49% third degree corrosion
- **T32.75** Corrosions involving 70-79% of body surface with 50-59% third degree corrosion
- **T32.76** Corrosions involving 70-79% of body surface with 60-69% third degree corrosion
- **T32.77** Corrosions involving 70-79% of body surface with 70-79% third degree corrosion

T32.8 Corrosions involving 80-89% of body surface
- **T32.80** Corrosions involving 80-89% of body surface with 0% to 9% third degree corrosion
- **T32.81** Corrosions involving 80-89% of body surface with 10-19% third degree corrosion
- **T32.82** Corrosions involving 80-89% of body surface with 20-29% third degree corrosion
- **T32.83** Corrosions involving 80-89% of body surface with 30-39% third degree corrosion
- **T32.84** Corrosions involving 80-89% of body surface with 40-49% third degree corrosion
- **T32.85** Corrosions involving 80-89% of body surface with 50-59% third degree corrosion
- **T32.86** Corrosions involving 80-89% of body surface with 60-69% third degree corrosion
- **T32.87** Corrosions involving 80-89% of body surface with 70-79% third degree corrosion
- **T32.88** Corrosions involving 80-89% of body surface with 80-89% third degree corrosion

T32.9 Corrosions involving 90% or more of body surface
- **T32.90** Corrosions involving 90% or more of body surface with 0% to 9% third degree corrosion
- **T32.91** Corrosions involving 90% or more of body surface with 10-19% third degree corrosion
- **T32.92** Corrosions involving 90% or more of body surface with 20-29% third degree corrosion
- **T32.93** Corrosions involving 90% or more of body surface with 30-39% third degree corrosion
- **T32.94** Corrosions involving 90% or more of body surface with 40-49% third degree corrosion
- **T32.95** Corrosions involving 90% or more of body surface with 50-59% third degree corrosion
- **T32.96** Corrosions involving 90% or more of body surface with 60-69% third degree corrosion
- **T32.97** Corrosions involving 90% or more of body surface with 70-79% third degree corrosion
- **T32.98** Corrosions involving 90% or more of body surface with 80-89% third degree corrosion
- **T32.99** Corrosions involving 90% or more of body surface with 90% or more third degree corrosion

Frostbite (T33-T34)

EXCLUDES 2: hypothermia and other effects of reduced temperature (T68, T69.-)

T33 Superficial frostbite

INCLUDES: frostbite with partial thickness skin loss

The appropriate 7th character is to be added to each code from category T33.
- A initial encounter
- D subsequent encounter
- S sequela

T33.0 Superficial frostbite of head
- **T33.01** Superficial frostbite of ear
  - **T33.011** Superficial frostbite of right ear
  - **T33.012** Superficial frostbite of left ear
  - **T33.019** Superficial frostbite of unspecified ear
- **T33.02** Superficial frostbite of nose
- **T33.09** Superficial frostbite of other part of head

T33.1 Superficial frostbite of neck
T33.2 Superficial frostbite of thorax
T33.3 Superficial frostbite of abdominal wall, lower back and pelvis
T33.4 Superficial frostbite of arm

EXCLUDES 2: superficial frostbite of wrist and hand (T33.5-)

- **T33.40** Superficial frostbite of unspecified arm
- **T33.41** Superficial frostbite of right arm
- **T33.42** Superficial frostbite of left arm

T33.5 Superficial frostbite of wrist, hand, and fingers
- **T33.51** Superficial frostbite of wrist
  - **T33.511** Superficial frostbite of right wrist
  - **T33.512** Superficial frostbite of left wrist
  - **T33.519** Superficial frostbite of unspecified wrist
- **T33.52** Superficial frostbite of hand

  EXCLUDES 2: superficial frostbite of fingers (T33.53-)
  - **T33.521** Superficial frostbite of right hand
  - **T33.522** Superficial frostbite of left hand
  - **T33.529** Superficial frostbite of unspecified hand
- **T33.53** Superficial frostbite of finger(s)
  - **T33.531** Superficial frostbite of right finger(s)
  - **T33.532** Superficial frostbite of left finger(s)
  - **T33.539** Superficial frostbite of unspecified finger(s)

- **T33.6** Superficial frostbite of hip and thigh
  - **T33.60** Superficial frostbite of unspecified hip and thigh
  - **T33.61** Superficial frostbite of right hip and thigh
  - **T33.62** Superficial frostbite of left hip and thigh
- **T33.7** Superficial frostbite of knee and lower leg
  - EXCLUDES 2: superficial frostbite of ankle and foot (T33.8-)
  - **T33.70** Superficial frostbite of unspecified knee and lower leg
  - **T33.71** Superficial frostbite of right knee and lower leg
  - **T33.72** Superficial frostbite of left knee and lower leg
- **T33.8** Superficial frostbite of ankle, foot, and toe(s)
  - **T33.81** Superficial frostbite of ankle
    - **T33.811** Superficial frostbite of right ankle
    - **T33.812** Superficial frostbite of left ankle
    - **T33.819** Superficial frostbite of unspecified ankle
  - **T33.82** Superficial frostbite of foot
    - **T33.821** Superficial frostbite of right foot
    - **T33.822** Superficial frostbite of left foot
    - **T33.829** Superficial frostbite of unspecified foot
  - **T33.83** Superficial frostbite of toe(s)
    - **T33.831** Superficial frostbite of right toe(s)
    - **T33.832** Superficial frostbite of left toe(s)
    - **T33.839** Superficial frostbite of unspecified toe(s)
- **T33.9** Superficial frostbite of other and unspecified sites
  - **T33.90** Superficial frostbite of unspecified sites
    - Superficial frostbite NOS
  - **T33.99** Superficial frostbite of other sites
    - Superficial frostbite of leg NOS
    - Superficial frostbite of trunk NOS

- **T34** Frostbite with tissue necrosis

  The appropriate 7th character is to be added to each code from category T34.
  - A initial encounter
  - D subsequent encounter
  - S sequela

- **T34.0** Frostbite with tissue necrosis of head
  - **T34.01** Frostbite with tissue necrosis of ear
    - **T34.011** Frostbite with tissue necrosis of right ear
    - **T34.012** Frostbite with tissue necrosis of left ear
    - **T34.019** Frostbite with tissue necrosis of unspecified ear
  - **T34.02** Frostbite with tissue necrosis of nose
  - **T34.09** Frostbite with tissue necrosis of other part of head
- **T34.1** Frostbite with tissue necrosis of neck
- **T34.2** Frostbite with tissue necrosis of thorax
- **T34.3** Frostbite with tissue necrosis of abdominal wall, lower back and pelvis
- **T34.4** Frostbite with tissue necrosis of arm
  - EXCLUDES 2: frostbite with tissue necrosis of wrist and hand (T34.5-)
  - **T34.40** Frostbite with tissue necrosis of unspecified arm
  - **T34.41** Frostbite with tissue necrosis of right arm
  - **T34.42** Frostbite with tissue necrosis of left arm
- **T34.5** Frostbite with tissue necrosis of wrist, hand, and finger(s)
  - **T34.51** Frostbite with tissue necrosis of wrist
    - **T34.511** Frostbite with tissue necrosis of right wrist
    - **T34.512** Frostbite with tissue necrosis of left wrist
    - **T34.519** Frostbite with tissue necrosis of unspecified wrist
  - **T34.52** Frostbite with tissue necrosis of hand
    - EXCLUDES 2: frostbite with tissue necrosis of finger(s) (T34.53-)
    - **T34.521** Frostbite with tissue necrosis of right hand
    - **T34.522** Frostbite with tissue necrosis of left hand
    - **T34.529** Frostbite with tissue necrosis of unspecified hand
  - **T34.53** Frostbite with tissue necrosis of finger(s)
    - **T34.531** Frostbite with tissue necrosis of right finger(s)
    - **T34.532** Frostbite with tissue necrosis of left finger(s)
    - **T34.539** Frostbite with tissue necrosis of unspecified finger(s)
- **T34.6** Frostbite with tissue necrosis of hip and thigh
  - **T34.60** Frostbite with tissue necrosis of unspecified hip and thigh
  - **T34.61** Frostbite with tissue necrosis of right hip and thigh
  - **T34.62** Frostbite with tissue necrosis of left hip and thigh
- **T34.7** Frostbite with tissue necrosis of knee and lower leg
  - EXCLUDES 2: frostbite with tissue necrosis of ankle and foot (T34.8-)
  - **T34.70** Frostbite with tissue necrosis of unspecified knee and lower leg
  - **T34.71** Frostbite with tissue necrosis of right knee and lower leg
  - **T34.72** Frostbite with tissue necrosis of left knee and lower leg
- **T34.8** Frostbite with tissue necrosis of ankle, foot, and toe(s)
  - **T34.81** Frostbite with tissue necrosis of ankle
    - **T34.811** Frostbite with tissue necrosis of right ankle
    - **T34.812** Frostbite with tissue necrosis of left ankle
    - **T34.819** Frostbite with tissue necrosis of unspecified ankle
  - **T34.82** Frostbite with tissue necrosis of foot
    - **T34.821** Frostbite with tissue necrosis of right foot
    - **T34.822** Frostbite with tissue necrosis of left foot
    - **T34.829** Frostbite with tissue necrosis of unspecified foot
  - **T34.83** Frostbite with tissue necrosis of toe(s)
    - **T34.831** Frostbite with tissue necrosis of right toe(s)
    - **T34.832** Frostbite with tissue necrosis of left toe(s)
    - **T34.839** Frostbite with tissue necrosis of unspecified toe(s)
- **T34.9** Frostbite with tissue necrosis of other and unspecified sites
  - **T34.90** Frostbite with tissue necrosis of unspecified sites
    - Frostbite with tissue necrosis NOS
  - **T34.99** Frostbite with tissue necrosis of other sites
    - Frostbite with tissue necrosis of leg NOS
    - Frostbite with tissue necrosis of trunk NOS

Poisoning by, adverse effects of and underdosing of drugs, medicaments and biological substances (T36-T50)

INCLUDES adverse effect of correct substance properly administered
poisoning by overdose of substance
poisoning by wrong substance given or taken in error
underdosing by (inadvertently) (deliberately) taking less substance than prescribed or instructed

Code first, for adverse effects, the nature of the adverse effect, such as:
 adverse effect NOS (T88.7)
 aspirin gastritis (K29.-)
 blood disorders (D56-D76)
 contact dermatitis (L23-L25)
 dermatitis due to substances taken internally (L27.-)
 nephropathy (N14.0-N14.2)

NOTE The drug giving rise to the adverse effect should be identified by use of codes from categories T36-T50 with fifth or sixth character 5.

Use additional code(s) to specify:
 manifestations of poisoning
 underdosing or failure in dosage during medical and surgical care (Y63.6, Y63.8-Y63.9)
 underdosing of medication regimen (Z91.12-, Z91.13-)

EXCLUDES 1 toxic reaction to local anesthesia in pregnancy (O29.3-)
EXCLUDES 2 abuse and dependence of psychoactive substances (F10-F19)
 abuse of non-dependence-producing substances (F55.-)
 drug reaction and poisoning affecting newborn (P00-P96)
 immunodeficiency due to drugs (D84.821)
 pathological drug intoxication (inebriation) (F10-F19)

AHA: 2018,4Q,71; 2016,2Q,8; 2015,3Q,22

✓4th T36 Poisoning by, adverse effect of and underdosing of systemic antibiotics

EXCLUDES 1 antineoplastic antibiotics (T45.1-)
 locally applied antibiotic NEC (T49.0)
 topically used antibiotic for ear, nose and throat (T49.6)
 topically used antibiotic for eye (T49.5)

The appropriate 7th character is to be added to each code from category T36.
 A initial encounter
 D subsequent encounter
 S sequela

- ✓5th **T36.0** Poisoning by, adverse effect of and underdosing of penicillins
  - ✓6th **T36.0X** Poisoning by, adverse effect of and underdosing of penicillins
    - ✓7th **T36.0X1** Poisoning by penicillins, accidental (unintentional)
      Poisoning by penicillins NOS
    - ✓7th **T36.0X2** Poisoning by penicillins, intentional self-harm HCC Rx ESR COM
    - ✓7th **T36.0X3** Poisoning by penicillins, assault
    - ✓7th **T36.0X4** Poisoning by penicillins, undetermined
    - ✓7th **T36.0X5** Adverse effect of penicillins UPD
    - ✓7th **T36.0X6** Underdosing of penicillins UPD
- ✓5th **T36.1** Poisoning by, adverse effect of and underdosing of cephalosporins and other beta-lactam antibiotics
  - ✓6th **T36.1X** Poisoning by, adverse effect of and underdosing of cephalosporins and other beta-lactam antibiotics
    - ✓7th **T36.1X1** Poisoning by cephalosporins and other beta-lactam antibiotics, accidental (unintentional)
      Poisoning by cephalosporins and other beta-lactam antibiotics NOS
    - ✓7th **T36.1X2** Poisoning by cephalosporins and other beta-lactam antibiotics, intentional self-harm HCC Rx ESR COM
    - ✓7th **T36.1X3** Poisoning by cephalosporins and other beta-lactam antibiotics, assault
    - ✓7th **T36.1X4** Poisoning by cephalosporins and other beta-lactam antibiotics, undetermined
    - ✓7th **T36.1X5** Adverse effect of cephalosporins and other beta-lactam antibiotics UPD
    - ✓7th **T36.1X6** Underdosing of cephalosporins and other beta-lactam antibiotics UPD
- ✓5th **T36.2** Poisoning by, adverse effect of and underdosing of chloramphenicol group
  - ✓6th **T36.2X** Poisoning by, adverse effect of and underdosing of chloramphenicol group
    - ✓7th **T36.2X1** Poisoning by chloramphenicol group, accidental (unintentional)
      Poisoning by chloramphenicol group NOS
    - ✓7th **T36.2X2** Poisoning by chloramphenicol group, intentional self-harm HCC Rx ESR COM
    - ✓7th **T36.2X3** Poisoning by chloramphenicol group, assault
    - ✓7th **T36.2X4** Poisoning by chloramphenicol group, undetermined
    - ✓7th **T36.2X5** Adverse effect of chloramphenicol group UPD
    - ✓7th **T36.2X6** Underdosing of chloramphenicol group UPD
- ✓5th **T36.3** Poisoning by, adverse effect of and underdosing of macrolides
  - ✓6th **T36.3X** Poisoning by, adverse effect of and underdosing of macrolides
    - ✓7th **T36.3X1** Poisoning by macrolides, accidental (unintentional)
      Poisoning by macrolides NOS
    - ✓7th **T36.3X2** Poisoning by macrolides, intentional self-harm HCC Rx ESR COM
    - ✓7th **T36.3X3** Poisoning by macrolides, assault
    - ✓7th **T36.3X4** Poisoning by macrolides, undetermined
    - ✓7th **T36.3X5** Adverse effect of macrolides UPD
    - ✓7th **T36.3X6** Underdosing of macrolides UPD
- ✓5th **T36.4** Poisoning by, adverse effect of and underdosing of tetracyclines
  - ✓6th **T36.4X** Poisoning by, adverse effect of and underdosing of tetracyclines
    - ✓7th **T36.4X1** Poisoning by tetracyclines, accidental (unintentional)
      Poisoning by tetracyclines NOS
    - ✓7th **T36.4X2** Poisoning by tetracyclines, intentional self-harm HCC Rx ESR COM
    - ✓7th **T36.4X3** Poisoning by tetracyclines, assault
    - ✓7th **T36.4X4** Poisoning by tetracyclines, undetermined
    - ✓7th **T36.4X5** Adverse effect of tetracyclines UPD
    - ✓7th **T36.4X6** Underdosing of tetracyclines UPD
- ✓5th **T36.5** Poisoning by, adverse effect of and underdosing of aminoglycosides
  Poisoning by, adverse effect of and underdosing of streptomycin
  - ✓6th **T36.5X** Poisoning by, adverse effect of and underdosing of aminoglycosides
    - ✓7th **T36.5X1** Poisoning by aminoglycosides, accidental (unintentional)
      Poisoning by aminoglycosides NOS
    - ✓7th **T36.5X2** Poisoning by aminoglycosides, intentional self-harm HCC Rx ESR COM
    - ✓7th **T36.5X3** Poisoning by aminoglycosides, assault
    - ✓7th **T36.5X4** Poisoning by aminoglycosides, undetermined
    - ✓7th **T36.5X5** Adverse effect of aminoglycosides UPD
    - ✓7th **T36.5X6** Underdosing of aminoglycosides UPD
- ✓5th **T36.6** Poisoning by, adverse effect of and underdosing of rifampicins
  - ✓6th **T36.6X** Poisoning by, adverse effect of and underdosing of rifampicins
    - ✓7th **T36.6X1** Poisoning by rifampicins, accidental (unintentional)
      Poisoning by rifampicins NOS
    - ✓7th **T36.6X2** Poisoning by rifampicins, intentional self-harm HCC Rx ESR COM
    - ✓7th **T36.6X3** Poisoning by rifampicins, assault
    - ✓7th **T36.6X4** Poisoning by rifampicins, undetermined
    - ✓7th **T36.6X5** Adverse effect of rifampicins UPD
    - ✓7th **T36.6X6** Underdosing of rifampicins UPD
- ✓5th **T36.7** Poisoning by, adverse effect of and underdosing of antifungal antibiotics, systemically used
  - ✓6th **T36.7X** Poisoning by, adverse effect of and underdosing of antifungal antibiotics, systemically used
    - ✓7th **T36.7X1** Poisoning by antifungal antibiotics, systemically used, accidental (unintentional)
      Poisoning by antifungal antibiotics, systemically used NOS
    - ✓7th **T36.7X2** Poisoning by antifungal antibiotics, systemically used, intentional self-harm HCC Rx ESR COM
    - ✓7th **T36.7X3** Poisoning by antifungal antibiotics, systemically used, assault
    - ✓7th **T36.7X4** Poisoning by antifungal antibiotics, systemically used, undetermined
    - ✓7th **T36.7X5** Adverse effect of antifungal antibiotics, systemically used UPD

HCC CMS-HCC   Rx Rx HCC   ESR ESRD HCC   COM Commercial HCC   N Newborn: 0   P Pediatric: 0-17   M Maternity: 9-64   A Adult: 15-124

- **T36.7X6** **Underdosing** of antifungal antibiotics, systemically used [UPD]
- **T36.8** Poisoning by, adverse effect of and underdosing of other systemic antibiotics
  - **T36.8X** Poisoning by, adverse effect of and underdosing of other systemic antibiotics
    AHA: 2017,1Q,39
    - **T36.8X1** Poisoning by other systemic antibiotics, **accidental (unintentional)**
      Poisoning by other systemic antibiotics NOS
    - **T36.8X2** Poisoning by other systemic antibiotics, **intentional self-harm** [HCC][Rx][ESR][COM]
    - **T36.8X3** Poisoning by other systemic antibiotics, **assault**
    - **T36.8X4** Poisoning by other systemic antibiotics, **undetermined**
    - **T36.8X5** **Adverse effect** of other systemic antibiotics [UPD]
    - **T36.8X6** **Underdosing** of other systemic antibiotics [UPD]
- **T36.9** Poisoning by, adverse effect of and underdosing of unspecified systemic antibiotic
  - **T36.91** Poisoning by unspecified systemic antibiotic, **accidental (unintentional)**
    Poisoning by systemic antibiotic NOS
  - **T36.92** Poisoning by unspecified systemic antibiotic, **intentional self-harm** [HCC][Rx][ESR][COM]
  - **T36.93** Poisoning by unspecified systemic antibiotic, **assault**
  - **T36.94** Poisoning by unspecified systemic antibiotic, **undetermined**
  - **T36.95** **Adverse effect** of unspecified systemic antibiotic [UPD]
  - **T36.96** **Underdosing** of unspecified systemic antibiotic [UPD]
- **T36.A** Poisoning by, adverse effect of and underdosing of fluoroquinolone antibiotics
  - **T36.AX** Poisoning by, adverse effect of and underdosing of **fluoroquinolone antibiotics**
    - **T36.AX1** Poisoning by fluoroquinolone antibiotics, **accidental (unintentional)**
      Poisoning by fluoroquinolone antibiotics NOS
    - **T36.AX2** Poisoning by fluoroquinolone antibiotics, **intentional self-harm**
    - **T36.AX3** Poisoning by fluoroquinolone antibiotics, **assault**
    - **T36.AX4** Poisoning by fluoroquinolone antibiotics, **undetermined**
    - **T36.AX5** **Adverse effect** of fluoroquinolone antibiotics
    - **T36.AX6** **Underdosing** of fluoroquinolone antibiotics

- **T37** Poisoning by, adverse effect of and underdosing of other systemic anti-infectives and antiparasitics
  EXCLUDES 1: anti-infectives topically used for ear, nose and throat (T49.6-)
  anti-infectives topically used for eye (T49.5-)
  locally applied anti-infectives NEC (T49.0-)

  > The appropriate 7th character is to be added to each code from category T37.
  > A initial encounter
  > D subsequent encounter
  > S sequela

  - **T37.0** Poisoning by, adverse effect of and underdosing of sulfonamides
    - **T37.0X** Poisoning by, adverse effect of and underdosing of sulfonamides
      - **T37.0X1** Poisoning by sulfonamides, **accidental (unintentional)**
        Poisoning by sulfonamides NOS
      - **T37.0X2** Poisoning by sulfonamides, **intentional self-harm** [HCC][Rx][ESR][COM]
      - **T37.0X3** Poisoning by sulfonamides, **assault**
      - **T37.0X4** Poisoning by sulfonamides, **undetermined**
      - **T37.0X5** **Adverse effect** of sulfonamides [UPD]
      - **T37.0X6** **Underdosing** of sulfonamides [UPD]
  - **T37.1** Poisoning by, adverse effect of and underdosing of antimycobacterial drugs
    EXCLUDES 1: rifampicins (T36.6-)
    streptomycin (T36.5-)
    - **T37.1X** Poisoning by, adverse effect of and underdosing of **antimycobacterial drugs**
      - **T37.1X1** Poisoning by antimycobacterial drugs, **accidental (unintentional)**
        Poisoning by antimycobacterial drugs NOS
      - **T37.1X2** Poisoning by antimycobacterial drugs, **intentional self-harm** [HCC][Rx][ESR][COM]
      - **T37.1X3** Poisoning by antimycobacterial drugs, **assault**
      - **T37.1X4** Poisoning by antimycobacterial drugs, **undetermined**
      - **T37.1X5** **Adverse effect** of antimycobacterial drugs [UPD]
      - **T37.1X6** **Underdosing** of antimycobacterial drugs [UPD]
  - **T37.2** Poisoning by, adverse effect of and underdosing of antimalarials and drugs acting on other blood protozoa
    EXCLUDES 1: hydroxyquinoline derivatives (T37.8-)
    - **T37.2X** Poisoning by, adverse effect of and underdosing of **antimalarials and drugs acting on other blood protozoa**
      - **T37.2X1** Poisoning by antimalarials and drugs acting on other blood protozoa, **accidental (unintentional)**
        Poisoning by antimalarials and drugs acting on other blood protozoa NOS
      - **T37.2X2** Poisoning by antimalarials and drugs acting on other blood protozoa, **intentional self-harm** [HCC][Rx][ESR][COM]
      - **T37.2X3** Poisoning by antimalarials and drugs acting on other blood protozoa, **assault**
      - **T37.2X4** Poisoning by antimalarials and drugs acting on other blood protozoa, **undetermined**
      - **T37.2X5** **Adverse effect** of antimalarials and drugs acting on other blood protozoa [UPD]
      - **T37.2X6** **Underdosing** of antimalarials and drugs acting on other blood protozoa [UPD]
  - **T37.3** Poisoning by, adverse effect of and underdosing of other antiprotozoal drugs
    - **T37.3X** Poisoning by, adverse effect of and underdosing of **other antiprotozoal drugs**
      - **T37.3X1** Poisoning by other antiprotozoal drugs, **accidental (unintentional)**
        Poisoning by other antiprotozoal drugs NOS
      - **T37.3X2** Poisoning by other antiprotozoal drugs, **intentional self-harm** [HCC][Rx][ESR][COM]
      - **T37.3X3** Poisoning by other antiprotozoal drugs, **assault**
      - **T37.3X4** Poisoning by other antiprotozoal drugs, **undetermined**
      - **T37.3X5** **Adverse effect** of other antiprotozoal drugs [UPD]
      - **T37.3X6** **Underdosing** of other antiprotozoal drugs [UPD]
  - **T37.4** Poisoning by, adverse effect of and underdosing of anthelminthics
    - **T37.4X** Poisoning by, adverse effect of and underdosing of **anthelminthics**
      - **T37.4X1** Poisoning by anthelminthics, **accidental (unintentional)**
        Poisoning by anthelminthics NOS
      - **T37.4X2** Poisoning by anthelminthics, **intentional self-harm** [HCC][Rx][ESR][COM]
      - **T37.4X3** Poisoning by anthelminthics, **assault**
      - **T37.4X4** Poisoning by anthelminthics, **undetermined**
      - **T37.4X5** **Adverse effect** of anthelminthics [UPD]
      - **T37.4X6** **Underdosing** of anthelminthics [UPD]

T37.5 Poisoning by, adverse effect of and underdosing of antiviral drugs

EXCLUDES 1: amantadine (T42.8-)
cytarabine (T45.1-)

- **T37.5X** Poisoning by, adverse effect of and underdosing of antiviral drugs
  - **T37.5X1** Poisoning by antiviral drugs, accidental (unintentional)
    Poisoning by antiviral drugs NOS
  - **T37.5X2** Poisoning by antiviral drugs, intentional self-harm [HCC Rx ESR COM]
  - **T37.5X3** Poisoning by antiviral drugs, assault
  - **T37.5X4** Poisoning by antiviral drugs, undetermined
  - **T37.5X5** Adverse effect of antiviral drugs [UPD]
  - **T37.5X6** Underdosing of antiviral drugs [UPD]

T37.8 Poisoning by, adverse effect of and underdosing of other specified systemic anti-infectives and antiparasitics

Poisoning by, adverse effect of and underdosing of hydroxyquinoline derivatives

EXCLUDES 1: antimalarial drugs (T37.2-)

- **T37.8X** Poisoning by, adverse effect of and underdosing of other specified systemic anti-infectives and antiparasitics
  - **T37.8X1** Poisoning by other specified systemic anti-infectives and antiparasitics, accidental (unintentional)
    Poisoning by other specified systemic anti-infectives and antiparasitics NOS
  - **T37.8X2** Poisoning by other specified systemic anti-infectives and antiparasitics, intentional self-harm [HCC Rx ESR COM]
  - **T37.8X3** Poisoning by other specified systemic anti-infectives and antiparasitics, assault
  - **T37.8X4** Poisoning by other specified systemic anti-infectives and antiparasitics, undetermined
  - **T37.8X5** Adverse effect of other specified systemic anti-infectives and antiparasitics [UPD]
  - **T37.8X6** Underdosing of other specified systemic anti-infectives and antiparasitics [UPD]

T37.9 Poisoning by, adverse effect of and underdosing of unspecified systemic anti-infective and antiparasitics

- **T37.91** Poisoning by unspecified systemic anti-infective and antiparasitics, accidental (unintentional)
  Poisoning by, adverse effect of and underdosing of systemic anti-infective and antiparasitics NOS
- **T37.92** Poisoning by unspecified systemic anti-infective and antiparasitics, intentional self-harm [HCC Rx ESR COM]
- **T37.93** Poisoning by unspecified systemic anti-infective and antiparasitics, assault
- **T37.94** Poisoning by unspecified systemic anti-infective and antiparasitics, undetermined
- **T37.95** Adverse effect of unspecified systemic anti-infective and antiparasitic [UPD]
- **T37.96** Underdosing of unspecified systemic anti-infectives and antiparasitics [UPD]

T38 Poisoning by, adverse effect of and underdosing of hormones and their synthetic substitutes and antagonists, not elsewhere classified

EXCLUDES 1: mineralocorticoids and their antagonists (T50.0-)
oxytocic hormones (T48.0-)
parathyroid hormones and derivatives (T50.9-)

The appropriate 7th character is to be added to each code from category T38.
- A initial encounter
- D subsequent encounter
- S sequela

T38.0 Poisoning by, adverse effect of and underdosing of glucocorticoids and synthetic analogues

EXCLUDES 1: glucocorticoids, topically used (T49.-)

- **T38.0X** Poisoning by, adverse effect of and underdosing of glucocorticoids and synthetic analogues
  - **T38.0X1** Poisoning by glucocorticoids and synthetic analogues, accidental (unintentional)
    Poisoning by glucocorticoids and synthetic analogues NOS
  - **T38.0X2** Poisoning by glucocorticoids and synthetic analogues, intentional self-harm [HCC Rx ESR COM]
  - **T38.0X3** Poisoning by glucocorticoids and synthetic analogues, assault
  - **T38.0X4** Poisoning by glucocorticoids and synthetic analogues, undetermined
  - **T38.0X5** Adverse effect of glucocorticoids and synthetic analogues [UPD]
  - **T38.0X6** Underdosing of glucocorticoids and synthetic analogues [UPD]

T38.1 Poisoning by, adverse effect of and underdosing of thyroid hormones and substitutes

- **T38.1X** Poisoning by, adverse effect of and underdosing of thyroid hormones and substitutes
  - **T38.1X1** Poisoning by thyroid hormones and substitutes, accidental (unintentional)
    Poisoning by thyroid hormones and substitutes NOS
  - **T38.1X2** Poisoning by thyroid hormones and substitutes, intentional self-harm [HCC Rx ESR COM]
  - **T38.1X3** Poisoning by thyroid hormones and substitutes, assault
  - **T38.1X4** Poisoning by thyroid hormones and substitutes, undetermined
  - **T38.1X5** Adverse effect of thyroid hormones and substitutes [UPD]
  - **T38.1X6** Underdosing of thyroid hormones and substitutes [UPD]

T38.2 Poisoning by, adverse effect of and underdosing of antithyroid drugs

- **T38.2X** Poisoning by, adverse effect of and underdosing of antithyroid drugs
  - **T38.2X1** Poisoning by antithyroid drugs, accidental (unintentional)
    Poisoning by antithyroid drugs NOS
  - **T38.2X2** Poisoning by antithyroid drugs, intentional self-harm [HCC Rx ESR COM]
  - **T38.2X3** Poisoning by antithyroid drugs, assault
  - **T38.2X4** Poisoning by antithyroid drugs, undetermined
  - **T38.2X5** Adverse effect of antithyroid drugs [UPD]
  - **T38.2X6** Underdosing of antithyroid drugs [UPD]

T38.3 Poisoning by, adverse effect of and underdosing of insulin and oral hypoglycemic [antidiabetic] drugs

- **T38.3X** Poisoning by, adverse effect of and underdosing of insulin and oral hypoglycemic [antidiabetic] drugs
  - **T38.3X1** Poisoning by insulin and oral hypoglycemic [antidiabetic] drugs, accidental (unintentional)
    Poisoning by insulin and oral hypoglycemic [antidiabetic] drugs NOS
  - **T38.3X2** Poisoning by insulin and oral hypoglycemic [antidiabetic] drugs, intentional self-harm [HCC Rx ESR COM]
  - **T38.3X3** Poisoning by insulin and oral hypoglycemic [antidiabetic] drugs, assault
  - **T38.3X4** Poisoning by insulin and oral hypoglycemic [antidiabetic] drugs, undetermined
  - **T38.3X5** Adverse effect of insulin and oral hypoglycemic [antidiabetic] drugs [UPD]
  - **T38.3X6** Underdosing of insulin and oral hypoglycemic [antidiabetic] drugs [UPD]

T38.4 Poisoning by, adverse effect of and underdosing of oral contraceptives

Poisoning by, adverse effect of and underdosing of multiple- and single-ingredient oral contraceptive preparations

- **T38.4X** Poisoning by, adverse effect of and underdosing of oral contraceptives
  - **T38.4X1** Poisoning by oral contraceptives, accidental (unintentional)
    Poisoning by oral contraceptives NOS
  - **T38.4X2** Poisoning by oral contraceptives, intentional self-harm [HCC Rx ESR COM]
  - **T38.4X3** Poisoning by oral contraceptives, assault
  - **T38.4X4** Poisoning by oral contraceptives, undetermined
  - **T38.4X5** Adverse effect of oral contraceptives [UPD]
  - **T38.4X6** Underdosing of oral contraceptives [UPD]

HCC CMS-HCC | Rx Rx HCC | ESR ESRD HCC | COM Commercial HCC | N Newborn: 0 | P Pediatric: 0-17 | M Maternity: 9-64 | A Adult: 15-124

T38.5 Poisoning by, adverse effect of and underdosing of other estrogens and progestogens

Poisoning by, adverse effect of and underdosing of estrogens and progestogens mixtures and substitutes

- **T38.5X** Poisoning by, adverse effect of and underdosing of other estrogens and progestogens
  - **T38.5X1** Poisoning by other estrogens and progestogens, accidental (unintentional)
    - Poisoning by other estrogens and progestogens NOS
  - **T38.5X2** Poisoning by other estrogens and progestogens, intentional self-harm
  - **T38.5X3** Poisoning by other estrogens and progestogens, assault
  - **T38.5X4** Poisoning by other estrogens and progestogens, undetermined
  - **T38.5X5** Adverse effect of other estrogens and progestogens
  - **T38.5X6** Underdosing of other estrogens and progestogens

T38.6 Poisoning by, adverse effect of and underdosing of antigonadotrophins, antiestrogens, antiandrogens, not elsewhere classified

Poisoning by, adverse effect of and underdosing of tamoxifen

- **T38.6X** Poisoning by, adverse effect of and underdosing of antigonadotrophins, antiestrogens, antiandrogens, not elsewhere classified
  - **T38.6X1** Poisoning by antigonadotrophins, antiestrogens, antiandrogens, not elsewhere classified, accidental (unintentional)
    - Poisoning by antigonadotrophins, antiestrogens, antiandrogens, not elsewhere classified NOS
  - **T38.6X2** Poisoning by antigonadotrophins, antiestrogens, antiandrogens, not elsewhere classified, intentional self-harm
  - **T38.6X3** Poisoning by antigonadotrophins, antiestrogens, antiandrogens, not elsewhere classified, assault
  - **T38.6X4** Poisoning by antigonadotrophins, antiestrogens, antiandrogens, not elsewhere classified, undetermined
  - **T38.6X5** Adverse effect of antigonadotrophins, antiestrogens, antiandrogens, not elsewhere classified
  - **T38.6X6** Underdosing of antigonadotrophins, antiestrogens, antiandrogens, not elsewhere classified

T38.7 Poisoning by, adverse effect of and underdosing of androgens and anabolic congeners

- **T38.7X** Poisoning by, adverse effect of and underdosing of androgens and anabolic congeners
  - **T38.7X1** Poisoning by androgens and anabolic congeners, accidental (unintentional)
    - Poisoning by androgens and anabolic congeners NOS
  - **T38.7X2** Poisoning by androgens and anabolic congeners, intentional self-harm
  - **T38.7X3** Poisoning by androgens and anabolic congeners, assault
  - **T38.7X4** Poisoning by androgens and anabolic congeners, undetermined
  - **T38.7X5** Adverse effect of androgens and anabolic congeners
  - **T38.7X6** Underdosing of androgens and anabolic congeners

T38.8 Poisoning by, adverse effect of and underdosing of other and unspecified hormones and synthetic substitutes

- **T38.80** Poisoning by, adverse effect of and underdosing of unspecified hormones and synthetic substitutes
  - **T38.801** Poisoning by unspecified hormones and synthetic substitutes, accidental (unintentional)
    - Poisoning by unspecified hormones and synthetic substitutes NOS
  - **T38.802** Poisoning by unspecified hormones and synthetic substitutes, intentional self-harm
  - **T38.803** Poisoning by unspecified hormones and synthetic substitutes, assault
  - **T38.804** Poisoning by unspecified hormones and synthetic substitutes, undetermined
  - **T38.805** Adverse effect of unspecified hormones and synthetic substitutes
  - **T38.806** Underdosing of unspecified hormones and synthetic substitutes

- **T38.81** Poisoning by, adverse effect of and underdosing of anterior pituitary [adenohypophyseal] hormones
  - **T38.811** Poisoning by anterior pituitary [adenohypophyseal] hormones, accidental (unintentional)
    - Poisoning by anterior pituitary [adenohypophyseal] hormones NOS
  - **T38.812** Poisoning by anterior pituitary [adenohypophyseal] hormones, intentional self-harm
  - **T38.813** Poisoning by anterior pituitary [adenohypophyseal] hormones, assault
  - **T38.814** Poisoning by anterior pituitary [adenohypophyseal] hormones, undetermined
  - **T38.815** Adverse effect of anterior pituitary [adenohypophyseal] hormones
  - **T38.816** Underdosing of anterior pituitary [adenohypophyseal] hormones

- **T38.89** Poisoning by, adverse effect of and underdosing of other hormones and synthetic substitutes
  - **T38.891** Poisoning by other hormones and synthetic substitutes, accidental (unintentional)
    - Poisoning by other hormones and synthetic substitutes NOS
  - **T38.892** Poisoning by other hormones and synthetic substitutes, intentional self-harm
  - **T38.893** Poisoning by other hormones and synthetic substitutes, assault
  - **T38.894** Poisoning by other hormones and synthetic substitutes, undetermined
  - **T38.895** Adverse effect of other hormones and synthetic substitutes
  - **T38.896** Underdosing of other hormones and synthetic substitutes

T38.9 Poisoning by, adverse effect of and underdosing of other and unspecified hormone antagonists

- **T38.90** Poisoning by, adverse effect of and underdosing of unspecified hormone antagonists
  - **T38.901** Poisoning by unspecified hormone antagonists, accidental (unintentional)
    - Poisoning by unspecified hormone antagonists NOS
  - **T38.902** Poisoning by unspecified hormone antagonists, intentional self-harm
  - **T38.903** Poisoning by unspecified hormone antagonists, assault
  - **T38.904** Poisoning by unspecified hormone antagonists, undetermined
  - **T38.905** Adverse effect of unspecified hormone antagonists
  - **T38.906** Underdosing of unspecified hormone antagonists

- **T38.99** Poisoning by, adverse effect of and underdosing of other hormone antagonists
  - **T38.991** Poisoning by other hormone antagonists, accidental (unintentional)
    - Poisoning by other hormone antagonists NOS
  - **T38.992** Poisoning by other hormone antagonists, intentional self-harm
  - **T38.993** Poisoning by other hormone antagonists, assault
  - **T38.994** Poisoning by other hormone antagonists, undetermined
  - **T38.995** Adverse effect of other hormone antagonists
  - **T38.996** Underdosing of other hormone antagonists

T39 Poisoning by, adverse effect of and underdosing of nonopioid analgesics, antipyretics and antirheumatics

> The appropriate 7th character is to be added to each code from category T39.
> A initial encounter
> D subsequent encounter
> S sequela

T39.0 Poisoning by, adverse effect of and underdosing of salicylates

T39.01 Poisoning by, adverse effect of and underdosing of aspirin
Poisoning by, adverse effect of and underdosing of acetylsalicylic acid

- **T39.011** Poisoning by aspirin, accidental (unintentional)
- **T39.012** Poisoning by aspirin, intentional self-harm [HCC] [Rx] [ESR] [COM]
- **T39.013** Poisoning by aspirin, assault
- **T39.014** Poisoning by aspirin, undetermined
- **T39.015** Adverse effect of aspirin [UPD]
  AHA: 2016,1Q,15
- **T39.016** Underdosing of aspirin [UPD]

T39.09 Poisoning by, adverse effect of and underdosing of other salicylates

- **T39.091** Poisoning by salicylates, accidental (unintentional)
  Poisoning by salicylates NOS
- **T39.092** Poisoning by salicylates, intentional self-harm [HCC] [Rx] [ESR] [COM]
- **T39.093** Poisoning by salicylates, assault
- **T39.094** Poisoning by salicylates, undetermined
- **T39.095** Adverse effect of salicylates [UPD]
- **T39.096** Underdosing of salicylates [UPD]

T39.1 Poisoning by, adverse effect of and underdosing of 4-Aminophenol derivatives

T39.1X Poisoning by, adverse effect of and underdosing of 4-Aminophenol derivatives

- **T39.1X1** Poisoning by 4-Aminophenol derivatives, accidental (unintentional)
  Poisoning by 4-Aminophenol derivatives NOS
- **T39.1X2** Poisoning by 4-Aminophenol derivatives, intentional self-harm [HCC] [Rx] [ESR] [COM]
- **T39.1X3** Poisoning by 4-Aminophenol derivatives, assault
- **T39.1X4** Poisoning by 4-Aminophenol derivatives, undetermined
- **T39.1X5** Adverse effect of 4-Aminophenol derivatives [UPD]
- **T39.1X6** Underdosing of 4-Aminophenol derivatives [UPD]

T39.2 Poisoning by, adverse effect of and underdosing of pyrazolone derivatives

T39.2X Poisoning by, adverse effect of and underdosing of pyrazolone derivatives

- **T39.2X1** Poisoning by pyrazolone derivatives, accidental (unintentional)
  Poisoning by pyrazolone derivatives NOS
- **T39.2X2** Poisoning by pyrazolone derivatives, intentional self-harm [HCC] [Rx] [ESR] [COM]
- **T39.2X3** Poisoning by pyrazolone derivatives, assault
- **T39.2X4** Poisoning by pyrazolone derivatives, undetermined
- **T39.2X5** Adverse effect of pyrazolone derivatives [UPD]
- **T39.2X6** Underdosing of pyrazolone derivatives [UPD]

T39.3 Poisoning by, adverse effect of and underdosing of other nonsteroidal anti-inflammatory drugs [NSAID]

T39.31 Poisoning by, adverse effect of and underdosing of propionic acid derivatives
Poisoning by, adverse effect of and underdosing of fenoprofen
Poisoning by, adverse effect of and underdosing of flurbiprofen
Poisoning by, adverse effect of and underdosing of ibuprofen
Poisoning by, adverse effect of and underdosing of ketoprofen
Poisoning by, adverse effect of and underdosing of naproxen
Poisoning by, adverse effect of and underdosing of oxaprozin

- **T39.311** Poisoning by propionic acid derivatives, accidental (unintentional)
- **T39.312** Poisoning by propionic acid derivatives, intentional self-harm [HCC] [Rx] [ESR] [COM]
- **T39.313** Poisoning by propionic acid derivatives, assault
- **T39.314** Poisoning by propionic acid derivatives, undetermined
- **T39.315** Adverse effect of propionic acid derivatives [UPD]
- **T39.316** Underdosing of propionic acid derivatives [UPD]

T39.39 Poisoning by, adverse effect of and underdosing of other nonsteroidal anti-inflammatory drugs [NSAID]

- **T39.391** Poisoning by other nonsteroidal anti-inflammatory drugs [NSAID], accidental (unintentional)
  Poisoning by other nonsteroidal anti-inflammatory drugs NOS
- **T39.392** Poisoning by other nonsteroidal anti-inflammatory drugs [NSAID], intentional self-harm [HCC] [Rx] [ESR] [COM]
- **T39.393** Poisoning by other nonsteroidal anti-inflammatory drugs [NSAID], assault
- **T39.394** Poisoning by other nonsteroidal anti-inflammatory drugs [NSAID], undetermined
- **T39.395** Adverse effect of other nonsteroidal anti-inflammatory drugs [NSAID] [UPD]
- **T39.396** Underdosing of other nonsteroidal anti-inflammatory drugs [NSAID] [UPD]

T39.4 Poisoning by, adverse effect of and underdosing of antirheumatics, not elsewhere classified

EXCLUDES 1 poisoning by, adverse effect of and underdosing of glucocorticoids (T38.0-)
poisoning by, adverse effect of and underdosing of salicylates (T39.0-)

T39.4X Poisoning by, adverse effect of and underdosing of antirheumatics, not elsewhere classified

- **T39.4X1** Poisoning by antirheumatics, not elsewhere classified, accidental (unintentional)
  Poisoning by antirheumatics, not elsewhere classified NOS
- **T39.4X2** Poisoning by antirheumatics, not elsewhere classified, intentional self-harm [HCC] [Rx] [ESR] [COM]
- **T39.4X3** Poisoning by antirheumatics, not elsewhere classified, assault
- **T39.4X4** Poisoning by antirheumatics, not elsewhere classified, undetermined
- **T39.4X5** Adverse effect of antirheumatics, not elsewhere classified [UPD]
- **T39.4X6** Underdosing of antirheumatics, not elsewhere classified [UPD]

T39.8 Poisoning by, adverse effect of and underdosing of other nonopioid analgesics and antipyretics, not elsewhere classified

T39.8X Poisoning by, adverse effect of and underdosing of other nonopioid analgesics and antipyretics, not elsewhere classified

- **T39.8X1** Poisoning by other nonopioid analgesics and antipyretics, not elsewhere classified, accidental (unintentional)
  Poisoning by other nonopioid analgesics and antipyretics, not elsewhere classified NOS

[HCC] CMS-HCC [Rx] Rx HCC [ESR] ESRD HCC [COM] Commercial HCC [N] Newborn: 0 [P] Pediatric: 0-17 [M] Maternity: 9-64 [A] Adult: 15-124

Chapter 19. Injury, Poisoning and Certain Other Consequences of External Causes

- **T39.8X2** Poisoning by other nonopioid analgesics and antipyretics, not elsewhere classified, intentional self-harm [HCC Rx ESR COM]
- **T39.8X3** Poisoning by other nonopioid analgesics and antipyretics, not elsewhere classified, assault
- **T39.8X4** Poisoning by other nonopioid analgesics and antipyretics, not elsewhere classified, undetermined
- **T39.8X5** Adverse effect of other nonopioid analgesics and antipyretics, not elsewhere classified [UPD]
- **T39.8X6** Underdosing of other nonopioid analgesics and antipyretics, not elsewhere classified [UPD]

T39.9 Poisoning by, adverse effect of and underdosing of unspecified nonopioid analgesic, antipyretic and antirheumatic
- **T39.91** Poisoning by unspecified nonopioid analgesic, antipyretic and antirheumatic, accidental (unintentional)
  Poisoning by nonopioid analgesic, antipyretic and antirheumatic NOS
- **T39.92** Poisoning by unspecified nonopioid analgesic, antipyretic and antirheumatic, intentional self-harm [HCC Rx ESR COM]
- **T39.93** Poisoning by unspecified nonopioid analgesic, antipyretic and antirheumatic, assault
- **T39.94** Poisoning by unspecified nonopioid analgesic, antipyretic and antirheumatic, undetermined
- **T39.95** Adverse effect of unspecified nonopioid analgesic, antipyretic and antirheumatic [UPD]
- **T39.96** Underdosing of unspecified nonopioid analgesic, antipyretic and antirheumatic

T40 Poisoning by, adverse effect of and underdosing of narcotics and psychodysleptics [hallucinogens]

EXCLUDES 2 drug dependence and related mental and behavioral disorders due to psychoactive substance use (F10.-F19.-)

The appropriate 7th character is to be added to each code from category T40.
- A initial encounter
- D subsequent encounter
- S sequela

T40.0 Poisoning by, adverse effect of and underdosing of opium
- **T40.0X** Poisoning by, adverse effect of and underdosing of opium
  - **T40.0X1** Poisoning by opium, accidental (unintentional) [HCC ESR COM]
    Poisoning by opium NOS
  - **T40.0X2** Poisoning by opium, intentional self-harm [HCC Rx ESR COM]
  - **T40.0X3** Poisoning by opium, assault
  - **T40.0X4** Poisoning by opium, undetermined [HCC ESR COM]
  - **T40.0X5** Adverse effect of opium [UPD]
  - **T40.0X6** Underdosing of opium [UPD]

T40.1 Poisoning by and adverse effect of heroin
- **T40.1X** Poisoning by and adverse effect of heroin
  - **T40.1X1** Poisoning by heroin, accidental (unintentional) [HCC ESR COM]
    Poisoning by heroin NOS
  - **T40.1X2** Poisoning by heroin, intentional self-harm [HCC Rx ESR COM]
  - **T40.1X3** Poisoning by heroin, assault
  - **T40.1X4** Poisoning by heroin, undetermined [HCC ESR COM]

T40.2 Poisoning by, adverse effect of and underdosing of other opioids
- **T40.2X** Poisoning by, adverse effect of and underdosing of other opioids
  - **T40.2X1** Poisoning by other opioids, accidental (unintentional) [HCC ESR COM]
    Poisoning by other opioids NOS
  - **T40.2X2** Poisoning by other opioids, intentional self-harm [HCC Rx ESR COM]
  - **T40.2X3** Poisoning by other opioids, assault
  - **T40.2X4** Poisoning by other opioids, undetermined [HCC ESR COM]
  - **T40.2X5** Adverse effect of other opioids [UPD]
    AHA: 2020,2Q,24
  - **T40.2X6** Underdosing of other opioids [UPD]

T40.3 Poisoning by, adverse effect of and underdosing of methadone
- **T40.3X** Poisoning by, adverse effect of and underdosing of methadone
  - **T40.3X1** Poisoning by methadone, accidental (unintentional) [HCC ESR COM]
    Poisoning by methadone NOS
  - **T40.3X2** Poisoning by methadone, intentional self-harm [HCC Rx ESR COM]
  - **T40.3X3** Poisoning by methadone, assault
  - **T40.3X4** Poisoning by methadone, undetermined [HCC ESR COM]
  - **T40.3X5** Adverse effect of methadone [UPD]
  - **T40.3X6** Underdosing of methadone [UPD]

T40.4 Poisoning by, adverse effect of and underdosing of other synthetic narcotics
AHA: 2020,4Q,40
- **T40.41** Poisoning by, adverse effect of and underdosing of fentanyl or fentanyl analogs
  - **T40.411** Poisoning by fentanyl or fentanyl analogs, accidental (unintentional) [HCC ESR COM]
  - **T40.412** Poisoning by fentanyl or fentanyl analogs, intentional self-harm [HCC Rx ESR COM]
  - **T40.413** Poisoning by fentanyl or fentanyl analogs, assault
  - **T40.414** Poisoning by fentanyl or fentanyl analogs, undetermined [HCC ESR COM]
  - **T40.415** Adverse effect of fentanyl or fentanyl analogs [UPD]
  - **T40.416** Underdosing of fentanyl or fentanyl analogs [UPD]
- **T40.42** Poisoning by, adverse effect of and underdosing of tramadol
  - **T40.421** Poisoning by tramadol, accidental (unintentional) [HCC ESR COM]
  - **T40.422** Poisoning by tramadol, intentional self-harm [HCC Rx ESR COM]
  - **T40.423** Poisoning by tramadol, assault
  - **T40.424** Poisoning by tramadol, undetermined [HCC ESR COM]
  - **T40.425** Adverse effect of tramadol [UPD]
  - **T40.426** Underdosing of tramadol [UPD]
- **T40.49** Poisoning by, adverse effect of and underdosing of other synthetic narcotics
  - **T40.491** Poisoning by other synthetic narcotics, accidental (unintentional) [HCC ESR COM]
  - **T40.492** Poisoning by other synthetic narcotics, intentional self-harm [HCC Rx ESR COM]
  - **T40.493** Poisoning by other synthetic narcotics, assault
  - **T40.494** Poisoning by other synthetic narcotics, undetermined [HCC ESR COM]
  - **T40.495** Adverse effect of other synthetic narcotics [UPD]
  - **T40.496** Underdosing of other synthetic narcotics [UPD]

T40.5 Poisoning by, adverse effect of and underdosing of cocaine
- **T40.5X** Poisoning by, adverse effect of and underdosing of cocaine
  - **T40.5X1** Poisoning by cocaine, accidental (unintentional) [HCC ESR COM]
    Poisoning by cocaine NOS
    AHA: 2016,2Q,8
  - **T40.5X2** Poisoning by cocaine, intentional self-harm [HCC Rx ESR COM]
  - **T40.5X3** Poisoning by cocaine, assault
  - **T40.5X4** Poisoning by cocaine, undetermined [HCC ESR COM]
  - **T40.5X5** Adverse effect of cocaine [UPD]
  - **T40.5X6** Underdosing of cocaine [UPD]

T40.6 Poisoning by, adverse effect of and underdosing of other and unspecified narcotics

- **T40.60** Poisoning by, adverse effect of and underdosing of unspecified narcotics
  - **T40.601** Poisoning by unspecified narcotics, accidental (unintentional)
    - Poisoning by narcotics NOS
  - **T40.602** Poisoning by unspecified narcotics, intentional self-harm
  - **T40.603** Poisoning by unspecified narcotics, assault
  - **T40.604** Poisoning by unspecified narcotics, undetermined
  - **T40.605** Adverse effect of unspecified narcotics
  - **T40.606** Underdosing of unspecified narcotics
- **T40.69** Poisoning by, adverse effect of and underdosing of other narcotics
  - **T40.691** Poisoning by other narcotics, accidental (unintentional)
    - Poisoning by other narcotics NOS
  - **T40.692** Poisoning by other narcotics, intentional self-harm
  - **T40.693** Poisoning by other narcotics, assault
  - **T40.694** Poisoning by other narcotics, undetermined
  - **T40.695** Adverse effect of other narcotics
  - **T40.696** Underdosing of other narcotics

T40.7 Poisoning by, adverse effect of and underdosing of cannabis (derivatives)

- **T40.71** Poisoning by, adverse effect of and underdosing of cannabis (derivatives)
  - AHA: 2021,4Q,30
  - **T40.711** Poisoning by cannabis, accidental (unintentional)
  - **T40.712** Poisoning by cannabis, intentional self-harm
  - **T40.713** Poisoning by cannabis, assault
  - **T40.714** Poisoning by cannabis, undetermined
  - **T40.715** Adverse effect of cannabis
  - **T40.716** Underdosing of cannabis
- **T40.72** Poisoning by, adverse effect of and underdosing of synthetic cannabinoids
  - AHA: 2021,4Q,30
  - **T40.721** Poisoning by synthetic cannabinoids, accidental (unintentional)
  - **T40.722** Poisoning by synthetic cannabinoids, intentional self-harm
  - **T40.723** Poisoning by synthetic cannabinoids, assault
  - **T40.724** Poisoning by synthetic cannabinoids, undetermined
  - **T40.725** Adverse effect of synthetic cannabinoids
  - **T40.726** Underdosing of synthetic cannabinoids

T40.8 Poisoning by and adverse effect of lysergide [LSD]

- **T40.8X** Poisoning by and adverse effect of lysergide [LSD]
  - **T40.8X1** Poisoning by lysergide [LSD], accidental (unintentional)
    - Poisoning by lysergide [LSD] NOS
  - **T40.8X2** Poisoning by lysergide [LSD], intentional self-harm
  - **T40.8X3** Poisoning by lysergide [LSD], assault
  - **T40.8X4** Poisoning by lysergide [LSD], undetermined

T40.9 Poisoning by, adverse effect of and underdosing of other and unspecified psychodysleptics [hallucinogens]

- **T40.90** Poisoning by, adverse effect of and underdosing of unspecified psychodysleptics [hallucinogens]
  - **T40.901** Poisoning by unspecified psychodysleptics [hallucinogens], accidental (unintentional)
  - **T40.902** Poisoning by unspecified psychodysleptics [hallucinogens], intentional self-harm
  - **T40.903** Poisoning by unspecified psychodysleptics [hallucinogens], assault
  - **T40.904** Poisoning by unspecified psychodysleptics [hallucinogens], undetermined
  - **T40.905** Adverse effect of unspecified psychodysleptics [hallucinogens]
  - **T40.906** Underdosing of unspecified psychodysleptics [hallucinogens]
- **T40.99** Poisoning by, adverse effect of and underdosing of other psychodysleptics [hallucinogens]
  - **T40.991** Poisoning by other psychodysleptics [hallucinogens], accidental (unintentional)
    - Poisoning by other psychodysleptics [hallucinogens] NOS
  - **T40.992** Poisoning by other psychodysleptics [hallucinogens], intentional self-harm
  - **T40.993** Poisoning by other psychodysleptics [hallucinogens], assault
  - **T40.994** Poisoning by other psychodysleptics [hallucinogens], undetermined
  - **T40.995** Adverse effect of other psychodysleptics [hallucinogens]
  - **T40.996** Underdosing of other psychodysleptics [hallucinogens]

T41 Poisoning by, adverse effect of and underdosing of anesthetics and therapeutic gases

EXCLUDES 1: benzodiazepines (T42.4-)
cocaine (T40.5-)
complications of anesthesia during labor and delivery (O74.-)
complications of anesthesia during pregnancy (O29.-)
complications of anesthesia during the puerperium (O89.-)
opioids (T40.0-T40.2-)

The appropriate 7th character is to be added to each code from category T41.
- A initial encounter
- D subsequent encounter
- S sequela

T41.0 Poisoning by, adverse effect of and underdosing of inhaled anesthetics

EXCLUDES 1: oxygen (T41.5-)

- **T41.0X** Poisoning by, adverse effect of and underdosing of inhaled anesthetics
  - **T41.0X1** Poisoning by inhaled anesthetics, accidental (unintentional)
    - Poisoning by inhaled anesthetics NOS
  - **T41.0X2** Poisoning by inhaled anesthetics, intentional self-harm
  - **T41.0X3** Poisoning by inhaled anesthetics, assault
  - **T41.0X4** Poisoning by inhaled anesthetics, undetermined
  - **T41.0X5** Adverse effect of inhaled anesthetics
  - **T41.0X6** Underdosing of inhaled anesthetics

T41.1 Poisoning by, adverse effect of and underdosing of intravenous anesthetics

Poisoning by, adverse effect of and underdosing of thiobarbiturates

- **T41.1X** Poisoning by, adverse effect of and underdosing of intravenous anesthetics
  - **T41.1X1** Poisoning by intravenous anesthetics, accidental (unintentional)
    - Poisoning by intravenous anesthetics NOS
  - **T41.1X2** Poisoning by intravenous anesthetics, intentional self-harm
  - **T41.1X3** Poisoning by intravenous anesthetics, assault
  - **T41.1X4** Poisoning by intravenous anesthetics, undetermined
  - **T41.1X5** Adverse effect of intravenous anesthetics
  - **T41.1X6** Underdosing of intravenous anesthetics

Chapter 19. Injury, Poisoning and Certain Other Consequences of External Causes

T41.2 Poisoning by, adverse effect of and underdosing of other and unspecified general anesthetics

- **T41.20** Poisoning by, adverse effect of and underdosing of unspecified general anesthetics
  - **T41.201** Poisoning by unspecified general anesthetics, accidental (unintentional)
    Poisoning by general anesthetics NOS
  - **T41.202** Poisoning by unspecified general anesthetics, intentional self-harm [HCC Rx ESR COM]
  - **T41.203** Poisoning by unspecified general anesthetics, assault
  - **T41.204** Poisoning by unspecified general anesthetics, undetermined
  - **T41.205** Adverse effect of unspecified general anesthetics [UPD]
    AHA: 2016,4Q,73
  - **T41.206** Underdosing of unspecified general anesthetics [UPD]
- **T41.29** Poisoning by, adverse effect of and underdosing of other general anesthetics
  - **T41.291** Poisoning by other general anesthetics, accidental (unintentional)
    Poisoning by other general anesthetics NOS
  - **T41.292** Poisoning by other general anesthetics, intentional self-harm [HCC Rx ESR COM]
  - **T41.293** Poisoning by other general anesthetics, assault
  - **T41.294** Poisoning by other general anesthetics, undetermined
  - **T41.295** Adverse effect of other general anesthetics [UPD]
  - **T41.296** Underdosing of other general anesthetics [UPD]

T41.3 Poisoning by, adverse effect of and underdosing of local anesthetics
  Cocaine (topical)
  EXCLUDES 2: poisoning by cocaine used as a central nervous system stimulant (T40.5X1-T40.5X4)

- **T41.3X** Poisoning by, adverse effect of and underdosing of local anesthetics
  - **T41.3X1** Poisoning by local anesthetics, accidental (unintentional)
    Poisoning by local anesthetics NOS
  - **T41.3X2** Poisoning by local anesthetics, intentional self-harm [HCC Rx ESR COM]
  - **T41.3X3** Poisoning by local anesthetics, assault
  - **T41.3X4** Poisoning by local anesthetics, undetermined
  - **T41.3X5** Adverse effect of local anesthetics [UPD]
  - **T41.3X6** Underdosing of local anesthetics [UPD]

T41.4 Poisoning by, adverse effect of and underdosing of unspecified anesthetic
- **T41.41** Poisoning by unspecified anesthetic, accidental (unintentional)
  Poisoning by anesthetic NOS
- **T41.42** Poisoning by unspecified anesthetic, intentional self-harm [HCC Rx ESR COM]
- **T41.43** Poisoning by unspecified anesthetic, assault
- **T41.44** Poisoning by unspecified anesthetic, undetermined
- **T41.45** Adverse effect of unspecified anesthetic [UPD]
- **T41.46** Underdosing of unspecified anesthetics [UPD]

T41.5 Poisoning by, adverse effect of and underdosing of therapeutic gases
- **T41.5X** Poisoning by, adverse effect of and underdosing of therapeutic gases
  - **T41.5X1** Poisoning by therapeutic gases, accidental (unintentional)
    Poisoning by therapeutic gases NOS
  - **T41.5X2** Poisoning by therapeutic gases, intentional self-harm [HCC Rx ESR COM]
  - **T41.5X3** Poisoning by therapeutic gases, assault
  - **T41.5X4** Poisoning by therapeutic gases, undetermined
  - **T41.5X5** Adverse effect of therapeutic gases [UPD]
  - **T41.5X6** Underdosing of therapeutic gases [UPD]

T42 Poisoning by, adverse effect of and underdosing of antiepileptic, sedative- hypnotic and antiparkinsonism drugs
  EXCLUDES 2: drug dependence and related mental and behavioral disorders due to psychoactive substance use (F10.-- F19.-)

> The appropriate 7th character is to be added to each code from category T42.
> A initial encounter
> D subsequent encounter
> S sequela

T42.0 Poisoning by, adverse effect of and underdosing of hydantoin derivatives
- **T42.0X** Poisoning by, adverse effect of and underdosing of hydantoin derivatives
  - **T42.0X1** Poisoning by hydantoin derivatives, accidental (unintentional)
    Poisoning by hydantoin derivatives NOS
  - **T42.0X2** Poisoning by hydantoin derivatives, intentional self-harm [HCC Rx ESR COM]
  - **T42.0X3** Poisoning by hydantoin derivatives, assault
  - **T42.0X4** Poisoning by hydantoin derivatives, undetermined
  - **T42.0X5** Adverse effect of hydantoin derivatives [UPD]
  - **T42.0X6** Underdosing of hydantoin derivatives [UPD]

T42.1 Poisoning by, adverse effect of and underdosing of iminostilbenes
  Poisoning by, adverse effect of and underdosing of carbamazepine
- **T42.1X** Poisoning by, adverse effect of and underdosing of iminostilbenes
  - **T42.1X1** Poisoning by iminostilbenes, accidental (unintentional)
    Poisoning by iminostilbenes NOS
  - **T42.1X2** Poisoning by iminostilbenes, intentional self-harm [HCC Rx ESR COM]
  - **T42.1X3** Poisoning by iminostilbenes, assault
  - **T42.1X4** Poisoning by iminostilbenes, undetermined
  - **T42.1X5** Adverse effect of iminostilbenes [UPD]
  - **T42.1X6** Underdosing of iminostilbenes [UPD]

T42.2 Poisoning by, adverse effect of and underdosing of succinimides and oxazolidinediones
- **T42.2X** Poisoning by, adverse effect of and underdosing of succinimides and oxazolidinediones
  - **T42.2X1** Poisoning by succinimides and oxazolidinediones, accidental (unintentional)
    Poisoning by succinimides and oxazolidinediones NOS
  - **T42.2X2** Poisoning by succinimides and oxazolidinediones, intentional self-harm [HCC Rx ESR COM]
  - **T42.2X3** Poisoning by succinimides and oxazolidinediones, assault
  - **T42.2X4** Poisoning by succinimides and oxazolidinediones, undetermined
  - **T42.2X5** Adverse effect of succinimides and oxazolidinediones [UPD]
  - **T42.2X6** Underdosing of succinimides and oxazolidinediones [UPD]

T42.3 Poisoning by, adverse effect of and underdosing of barbiturates
  EXCLUDES 1: poisoning by, adverse effect of and underdosing of thiobarbiturates (T41.1-)
- **T42.3X** Poisoning by, adverse effect of and underdosing of barbiturates
  - **T42.3X1** Poisoning by barbiturates, accidental (unintentional)
    Poisoning by barbiturates NOS
  - **T42.3X2** Poisoning by barbiturates, intentional self-harm [HCC Rx ESR COM]
  - **T42.3X3** Poisoning by barbiturates, assault
  - **T42.3X4** Poisoning by barbiturates, undetermined
  - **T42.3X5** Adverse effect of barbiturates [UPD]
  - **T42.3X6** Underdosing of barbiturates [UPD]

T42.4 Poisoning by, adverse effect of and underdosing of benzodiazepines

- **T42.4X** Poisoning by, adverse effect of and underdosing of benzodiazepines
  - **T42.4X1** Poisoning by benzodiazepines, accidental (unintentional)
    Poisoning by benzodiazepines NOS
  - **T42.4X2** Poisoning by benzodiazepines, intentional self-harm [HCC Rx ESR COM]
  - **T42.4X3** Poisoning by benzodiazepines, assault
  - **T42.4X4** Poisoning by benzodiazepines, undetermined
  - **T42.4X5** Adverse effect of benzodiazepines [UPD]
  - **T42.4X6** Underdosing of benzodiazepines [UPD]

T42.5 Poisoning by, adverse effect of and underdosing of mixed antiepileptics

- **T42.5X** Poisoning by, adverse effect of and underdosing of antiepileptics
  - **T42.5X1** Poisoning by mixed antiepileptics, accidental (unintentional)
    Poisoning by mixed antiepileptics NOS
  - **T42.5X2** Poisoning by mixed antiepileptics, intentional self-harm [HCC Rx ESR COM]
  - **T42.5X3** Poisoning by mixed antiepileptics, assault
  - **T42.5X4** Poisoning by mixed antiepileptics, undetermined
  - **T42.5X5** Adverse effect of mixed antiepileptics [UPD]
  - **T42.5X6** Underdosing of mixed antiepileptics [UPD]

T42.6 Poisoning by, adverse effect of and underdosing of other antiepileptic and sedative-hypnotic drugs

Poisoning by, adverse effect of and underdosing of methaqualone
Poisoning by, adverse effect of and underdosing of valproic acid

EXCLUDES 1 poisoning by, adverse effect of and underdosing of carbamazepine (T42.1-)

- **T42.6X** Poisoning by, adverse effect of and underdosing of other antiepileptic and sedative-hypnotic drugs
  - **T42.6X1** Poisoning by other antiepileptic and sedative-hypnotic drugs, accidental (unintentional)
    Poisoning by other antiepileptic and sedative-hypnotic drugs NOS
  - **T42.6X2** Poisoning by other antiepileptic and sedative-hypnotic drugs, intentional self-harm [HCC Rx ESR COM]
  - **T42.6X3** Poisoning by other antiepileptic and sedative-hypnotic drugs, assault
  - **T42.6X4** Poisoning by other antiepileptic and sedative-hypnotic drugs, undetermined
  - **T42.6X5** Adverse effect of other antiepileptic and sedative-hypnotic drugs [UPD]
  - **T42.6X6** Underdosing of other antiepileptic and sedative-hypnotic drugs [UPD]

T42.7 Poisoning by, adverse effect of and underdosing of unspecified antiepileptic and sedative-hypnotic drugs

- **T42.71** Poisoning by unspecified antiepileptic and sedative-hypnotic drugs, accidental (unintentional)
  Poisoning by antiepileptic and sedative-hypnotic drugs NOS
- **T42.72** Poisoning by unspecified antiepileptic and sedative-hypnotic drugs, intentional self-harm [HCC Rx ESR COM]
- **T42.73** Poisoning by unspecified antiepileptic and sedative-hypnotic drugs, assault
- **T42.74** Poisoning by unspecified antiepileptic and sedative-hypnotic drugs, undetermined
- **T42.75** Adverse effect of unspecified antiepileptic and sedative-hypnotic drugs [UPD]
- **T42.76** Underdosing of unspecified antiepileptic and sedative-hypnotic drugs [UPD]

T42.8 Poisoning by, adverse effect of and underdosing of antiparkinsonism drugs and other central muscle-tone depressants

Poisoning by, adverse effect of and underdosing of amantadine

- **T42.8X** Poisoning by, adverse effect of and underdosing of antiparkinsonism drugs and other central muscle-tone depressants
  - **T42.8X1** Poisoning by antiparkinsonism drugs and other central muscle-tone depressants, accidental (unintentional)
    Poisoning by antiparkinsonism drugs and other central muscle-tone depressants NOS
  - **T42.8X2** Poisoning by antiparkinsonism drugs and other central muscle-tone depressants, intentional self-harm [HCC Rx ESR COM]
  - **T42.8X3** Poisoning by antiparkinsonism drugs and other central muscle-tone depressants, assault
  - **T42.8X4** Poisoning by antiparkinsonism drugs and other central muscle-tone depressants, undetermined
  - **T42.8X5** Adverse effect of antiparkinsonism drugs and other central muscle-tone depressants [UPD]
  - **T42.8X6** Underdosing of antiparkinsonism drugs and other central muscle-tone depressants [UPD]

T43 Poisoning by, adverse effect of and underdosing of psychotropic drugs, not elsewhere classified

EXCLUDES 1
- appetite depressants (T50.5-)
- barbiturates (T42.3-)
- benzodiazepines (T42.4-)
- methaqualone (T42.6-)
- psychodysleptics [hallucinogens] (T40.7-T40.9-)

EXCLUDES 2 drug dependence and related mental and behavioral disorders due to psychoactive substance use (F10.- – F19.-)

> The appropriate 7th character is to be added to each code from category T43.
> A initial encounter
> D subsequent encounter
> S sequela

T43.0 Poisoning by, adverse effect of and underdosing of tricyclic and tetracyclic antidepressants

- **T43.01** Poisoning by, adverse effect of and underdosing of tricyclic antidepressants
  - **T43.011** Poisoning by tricyclic antidepressants, accidental (unintentional)
    Poisoning by tricyclic antidepressants NOS
  - **T43.012** Poisoning by tricyclic antidepressants, intentional self-harm [HCC Rx ESR COM]
  - **T43.013** Poisoning by tricyclic antidepressants, assault
  - **T43.014** Poisoning by tricyclic antidepressants, undetermined
  - **T43.015** Adverse effect of tricyclic antidepressants [UPD]
  - **T43.016** Underdosing of tricyclic antidepressants [UPD]
- **T43.02** Poisoning by, adverse effect of and underdosing of tetracyclic antidepressants
  - **T43.021** Poisoning by tetracyclic antidepressants, accidental (unintentional)
    Poisoning by tetracyclic antidepressants NOS
  - **T43.022** Poisoning by tetracyclic antidepressants, intentional self-harm [HCC Rx ESR COM]
  - **T43.023** Poisoning by tetracyclic antidepressants, assault
  - **T43.024** Poisoning by tetracyclic antidepressants, undetermined
  - **T43.025** Adverse effect of tetracyclic antidepressants [UPD]
  - **T43.026** Underdosing of tetracyclic antidepressants [UPD]

Chapter 19. Injury, Poisoning and Certain Other Consequences of External Causes

- ✓5th **T43.1** Poisoning by, adverse effect of and underdosing of monoamine-oxidase-inhibitor antidepressants
  - ✓6th **T43.1X** Poisoning by, adverse effect of and underdosing of monoamine-oxidase-inhibitor antidepressants
    - ✓7th **T43.1X1** Poisoning by monoamine-oxidase-inhibitor antidepressants, accidental (unintentional)
      Poisoning by monoamine-oxidase-inhibitor antidepressants NOS
    - ✓7th **T43.1X2** Poisoning by monoamine-oxidase-inhibitor antidepressants, intentional self-harm [HCC] [Rx] [ESR] [COM]
    - ✓7th **T43.1X3** Poisoning by monoamine-oxidase-inhibitor antidepressants, assault
    - ✓7th **T43.1X4** Poisoning by monoamine-oxidase-inhibitor antidepressants, undetermined
    - ✓7th **T43.1X5** Adverse effect of monoamine-oxidase-inhibitor antidepressants [UPD]
    - ✓7th **T43.1X6** Underdosing of monoamine-oxidase-inhibitor antidepressants [UPD]
- ✓5th **T43.2** Poisoning by, adverse effect of and underdosing of other and unspecified antidepressants
  - ✓6th **T43.20** Poisoning by, adverse effect of and underdosing of unspecified antidepressants
    - ✓7th **T43.201** Poisoning by unspecified antidepressants, accidental (unintentional)
      Poisoning by antidepressants NOS
    - ✓7th **T43.202** Poisoning by unspecified antidepressants, intentional self-harm [HCC] [Rx] [ESR] [COM]
    - ✓7th **T43.203** Poisoning by unspecified antidepressants, assault
    - ✓7th **T43.204** Poisoning by unspecified antidepressants, undetermined
    - ✓7th **T43.205** Adverse effect of unspecified antidepressants [UPD]
      Antidepressant discontinuation syndrome
    - ✓7th **T43.206** Underdosing of unspecified antidepressants [UPD]
  - ✓6th **T43.21** Poisoning by, adverse effect of and underdosing of selective serotonin and norepinephrine reuptake inhibitors
    Poisoning by, adverse effect of and underdosing of SSNRI antidepressants
    - ✓7th **T43.211** Poisoning by selective serotonin and norepinephrine reuptake inhibitors, accidental (unintentional)
    - ✓7th **T43.212** Poisoning by selective serotonin and norepinephrine reuptake inhibitors, intentional self-harm [HCC] [Rx] [ESR] [COM]
    - ✓7th **T43.213** Poisoning by selective serotonin and norepinephrine reuptake inhibitors, assault
    - ✓7th **T43.214** Poisoning by selective serotonin and norepinephrine reuptake inhibitors, undetermined
    - ✓7th **T43.215** Adverse effect of selective serotonin and norepinephrine reuptake inhibitors [UPD]
    - ✓7th **T43.216** Underdosing of selective serotonin and norepinephrine reuptake inhibitors [UPD]
  - ✓6th **T43.22** Poisoning by, adverse effect of and underdosing of selective serotonin reuptake inhibitors
    Poisoning by, adverse effect of and underdosing of SSRI antidepressants
    - ✓7th **T43.221** Poisoning by selective serotonin reuptake inhibitors, accidental (unintentional)
    - ✓7th **T43.222** Poisoning by selective serotonin reuptake inhibitors, intentional self-harm [HCC] [Rx] [ESR] [COM]
    - ✓7th **T43.223** Poisoning by selective serotonin reuptake inhibitors, assault
    - ✓7th **T43.224** Poisoning by selective serotonin reuptake inhibitors, undetermined
    - ✓7th **T43.225** Adverse effect of selective serotonin reuptake inhibitors [UPD]
      AHA: 2024,4Q,16; 2022,2Q,11
    - ✓7th **T43.226** Underdosing of selective serotonin reuptake inhibitors [UPD]
  - ✓6th **T43.29** Poisoning by, adverse effect of and underdosing of other antidepressants
    - ✓7th **T43.291** Poisoning by other antidepressants, accidental (unintentional)
      Poisoning by other antidepressants NOS
    - ✓7th **T43.292** Poisoning by other antidepressants, intentional self-harm [HCC] [Rx] [ESR] [COM]
    - ✓7th **T43.293** Poisoning by other antidepressants, assault
    - ✓7th **T43.294** Poisoning by other antidepressants, undetermined
    - ✓7th **T43.295** Adverse effect of other antidepressants [UPD]
    - ✓7th **T43.296** Underdosing of other antidepressants [UPD]
- ✓5th **T43.3** Poisoning by, adverse effect of and underdosing of phenothiazine antipsychotics and neuroleptics
  - ✓6th **T43.3X** Poisoning by, adverse effect of and underdosing of phenothiazine antipsychotics and neuroleptics
    - ✓7th **T43.3X1** Poisoning by phenothiazine antipsychotics and neuroleptics, accidental (unintentional)
      Poisoning by phenothiazine antipsychotics and neuroleptics NOS
    - ✓7th **T43.3X2** Poisoning by phenothiazine antipsychotics and neuroleptics, intentional self-harm [HCC] [Rx] [ESR] [COM]
    - ✓7th **T43.3X3** Poisoning by phenothiazine antipsychotics and neuroleptics, assault
    - ✓7th **T43.3X4** Poisoning by phenothiazine antipsychotics and neuroleptics, undetermined
    - ✓7th **T43.3X5** Adverse effect of phenothiazine antipsychotics and neuroleptics [UPD]
    - ✓7th **T43.3X6** Underdosing of phenothiazine antipsychotics and neuroleptics [UPD]
- ✓5th **T43.4** Poisoning by, adverse effect of and underdosing of butyrophenone and thiothixene neuroleptics
  - ✓6th **T43.4X** Poisoning by, adverse effect of and underdosing of butyrophenone and thiothixene neuroleptics
    - ✓7th **T43.4X1** Poisoning by butyrophenone and thiothixene neuroleptics, accidental (unintentional)
      Poisoning by butyrophenone and thiothixene neuroleptics NOS
    - ✓7th **T43.4X2** Poisoning by butyrophenone and thiothixene neuroleptics, intentional self-harm [HCC] [Rx] [ESR] [COM]
    - ✓7th **T43.4X3** Poisoning by butyrophenone and thiothixene neuroleptics, assault
    - ✓7th **T43.4X4** Poisoning by butyrophenone and thiothixene neuroleptics, undetermined
    - ✓7th **T43.4X5** Adverse effect of butyrophenone and thiothixene neuroleptics [UPD]
    - ✓7th **T43.4X6** Underdosing of butyrophenone and thiothixene neuroleptics [UPD]
- ✓5th **T43.5** Poisoning by, adverse effect of and underdosing of other and unspecified antipsychotics and neuroleptics
  - EXCLUDES 1 poisoning by, adverse effect of and underdosing of rauwolfia (T46.5-)
  - ✓6th **T43.50** Poisoning by, adverse effect of and underdosing of unspecified antipsychotics and neuroleptics
    - ✓7th **T43.501** Poisoning by unspecified antipsychotics and neuroleptics, accidental (unintentional)
      Poisoning by antipsychotics and neuroleptics NOS
    - ✓7th **T43.502** Poisoning by unspecified antipsychotics and neuroleptics, intentional self-harm [HCC] [Rx] [ESR] [COM]
    - ✓7th **T43.503** Poisoning by unspecified antipsychotics and neuroleptics, assault
    - ✓7th **T43.504** Poisoning by unspecified antipsychotics and neuroleptics, undetermined
    - ✓7th **T43.505** Adverse effect of unspecified antipsychotics and neuroleptics [UPD]
      AHA: 2022,4Q,24
    - ✓7th **T43.506** Underdosing of unspecified antipsychotics and neuroleptics [UPD]

T43.59 Poisoning by, adverse effect of and underdosing of other antipsychotics and neuroleptics
AHA: 2017,1Q,40

- **T43.591** Poisoning by other antipsychotics and neuroleptics, accidental (unintentional)
  Poisoning by other antipsychotics and neuroleptics NOS
- **T43.592** Poisoning by other antipsychotics and neuroleptics, intentional self-harm [HCC][Rx][ESR][COM]
- **T43.593** Poisoning by other antipsychotics and neuroleptics, assault
- **T43.594** Poisoning by other antipsychotics and neuroleptics, undetermined
- **T43.595** Adverse effect of other antipsychotics and neuroleptics [UPD]
  AHA: 2022,2Q,11
- **T43.596** Underdosing of other antipsychotics and neuroleptics [UPD]

T43.6 Poisoning by, adverse effect of and underdosing of psychostimulants
EXCLUDES 1 poisoning by, adverse effect of and underdosing of cocaine (T40.5-)

T43.60 Poisoning by, adverse effect of and underdosing of unspecified psychostimulant
- **T43.601** Poisoning by unspecified psychostimulants, accidental (unintentional) [HCC][ESR][COM]
  Poisoning by psychostimulants NOS
- **T43.602** Poisoning by unspecified psychostimulants, intentional self-harm [HCC][Rx][ESR][COM]
- **T43.603** Poisoning by unspecified psychostimulants, assault
- **T43.604** Poisoning by unspecified psychostimulants, undetermined [HCC][ESR][COM]
- **T43.605** Adverse effect of unspecified psychostimulants [UPD]
- **T43.606** Underdosing of unspecified psychostimulants [UPD]

T43.61 Poisoning by, adverse effect of and underdosing of caffeine
- **T43.611** Poisoning by caffeine, accidental (unintentional) [HCC][ESR][COM]
  Poisoning by caffeine NOS
- **T43.612** Poisoning by caffeine, intentional self-harm [HCC][Rx][ESR][COM]
- **T43.613** Poisoning by caffeine, assault
- **T43.614** Poisoning by caffeine, undetermined [HCC][ESR][COM]
- **T43.615** Adverse effect of caffeine [UPD]
- **T43.616** Underdosing of caffeine [UPD]

T43.62 Poisoning by, adverse effect of and underdosing of amphetamines
- **T43.621** Poisoning by amphetamines, accidental (unintentional) [HCC][ESR][COM]
  Poisoning by amphetamines NOS
  AHA: 2021,3Q,8
- **T43.622** Poisoning by amphetamines, intentional self-harm [HCC][Rx][ESR][COM]
- **T43.623** Poisoning by amphetamines, assault
- **T43.624** Poisoning by amphetamines, undetermined [HCC][ESR][COM]
- **T43.625** Adverse effect of amphetamines [UPD]
- **T43.626** Underdosing of amphetamines [UPD]

T43.63 Poisoning by, adverse effect of and underdosing of methylphenidate
- **T43.631** Poisoning by methylphenidate, accidental (unintentional) [HCC][ESR][COM]
  Poisoning by methylphenidate NOS
- **T43.632** Poisoning by methylphenidate, intentional self-harm [HCC][Rx][ESR][COM]
- **T43.633** Poisoning by methylphenidate, assault
- **T43.634** Poisoning by methylphenidate, undetermined [HCC][ESR][COM]
- **T43.635** Adverse effect of methylphenidate [UPD]
- **T43.636** Underdosing of methylphenidate [UPD]

T43.64 Poisoning by ecstasy
Poisoning by 3,4-methylenedioxymethamphetamine
Poisoning by MDMA
AHA: 2018,4Q,30-31

- **T43.641** Poisoning by ecstasy, accidental (unintentional) [HCC][ESR][COM]
  Poisoning by ecstasy NOS
- **T43.642** Poisoning by ecstasy, intentional self-harm [HCC][Rx][ESR][COM]
- **T43.643** Poisoning by ecstasy, assault
- **T43.644** Poisoning by ecstasy, undetermined [HCC][ESR][COM]

T43.65 Poisoning by, adverse effect of and underdosing of methamphetamines
AHA: 2022,4Q,45-47

- **T43.651** Poisoning by methamphetamines, accidental (unintentional) [HCC][ESR][COM]
  Poisoning by methamphetamines NOS
  AHA: 2022,4Q,46
- **T43.652** Poisoning by methamphetamines, intentional self-harm [HCC][Rx][ESR][COM]
- **T43.653** Poisoning by methamphetamines, assault
- **T43.654** Poisoning by methamphetamines, undetermined [HCC][ESR][COM]
- **T43.655** Adverse effect of methamphetamines [UPD]
  AHA: 2022,4Q,46
- **T43.656** Underdosing of methamphetamines [UPD]

T43.69 Poisoning by, adverse effect of and underdosing of other psychostimulants
- **T43.691** Poisoning by other psychostimulants, accidental (unintentional) [HCC][ESR][COM]
  Poisoning by other psychostimulants NOS
- **T43.692** Poisoning by other psychostimulants, intentional self-harm [HCC][Rx][ESR][COM]
- **T43.693** Poisoning by other psychostimulants, assault
- **T43.694** Poisoning by other psychostimulants, undetermined [HCC][ESR][COM]
- **T43.695** Adverse effect of other psychostimulants [UPD]
- **T43.696** Underdosing of other psychostimulants [UPD]

T43.8 Poisoning by, adverse effect of and underdosing of other psychotropic drugs

T43.8X Poisoning by, adverse effect of and underdosing of other psychotropic drugs
- **T43.8X1** Poisoning by other psychotropic drugs, accidental (unintentional)
  Poisoning by other psychotropic drugs NOS
- **T43.8X2** Poisoning by other psychotropic drugs, intentional self-harm [HCC][Rx][ESR][COM]
- **T43.8X3** Poisoning by other psychotropic drugs, assault
- **T43.8X4** Poisoning by other psychotropic drugs, undetermined
- **T43.8X5** Adverse effect of other psychotropic drugs [UPD]
- **T43.8X6** Underdosing of other psychotropic drugs [UPD]

T43.9 Poisoning by, adverse effect of and underdosing of unspecified psychotropic drug
- **T43.91** Poisoning by unspecified psychotropic drug, accidental (unintentional)
  Poisoning by psychotropic drug NOS
- **T43.92** Poisoning by unspecified psychotropic drug, intentional self-harm [HCC][Rx][ESR][COM]
- **T43.93** Poisoning by unspecified psychotropic drug, assault
- **T43.94** Poisoning by unspecified psychotropic drug, undetermined
- **T43.95** Adverse effect of unspecified psychotropic drug [UPD]
- **T43.96** Underdosing of unspecified psychotropic drug [UPD]

[HCC] CMS-HCC [Rx] Rx HCC [ESR] ESRD HCC [COM] Commercial HCC N Newborn: 0 P Pediatric: 0-17 M Maternity: 9-64 A Adult: 15-124

T44 Poisoning by, adverse effect of and underdosing of drugs primarily affecting the autonomic nervous system

> The appropriate 7th character is to be added to each code from category T44.
> A initial encounter
> D subsequent encounter
> S sequela

T44.0 Poisoning by, adverse effect of and underdosing of anticholinesterase agents

T44.0X Poisoning by, adverse effect of and underdosing of anticholinesterase agents

- **T44.0X1** Poisoning by anticholinesterase agents, accidental (unintentional)
  Poisoning by anticholinesterase agents NOS
- **T44.0X2** Poisoning by anticholinesterase agents, intentional self-harm
- **T44.0X3** Poisoning by anticholinesterase agents, assault
- **T44.0X4** Poisoning by anticholinesterase agents, undetermined
- **T44.0X5** Adverse effect of anticholinesterase agents
- **T44.0X6** Underdosing of anticholinesterase agents

T44.1 Poisoning by, adverse effect of and underdosing of other parasympathomimetics [cholinergics]

T44.1X Poisoning by, adverse effect of and underdosing of other parasympathomimetics [cholinergics]

- **T44.1X1** Poisoning by other parasympathomimetics [cholinergics], accidental (unintentional)
  Poisoning by other parasympathomimetics [cholinergics] NOS
- **T44.1X2** Poisoning by other parasympathomimetics [cholinergics], intentional self-harm
- **T44.1X3** Poisoning by other parasympathomimetics [cholinergics], assault
- **T44.1X4** Poisoning by other parasympathomimetics [cholinergics], undetermined
- **T44.1X5** Adverse effect of other parasympathomimetics [cholinergics]
- **T44.1X6** Underdosing of other parasympathomimetics [cholinergics]

T44.2 Poisoning by, adverse effect of and underdosing of ganglionic blocking drugs

T44.2X Poisoning by, adverse effect of and underdosing of ganglionic blocking drugs

- **T44.2X1** Poisoning by ganglionic blocking drugs, accidental (unintentional)
  Poisoning by ganglionic blocking drugs NOS
- **T44.2X2** Poisoning by ganglionic blocking drugs, intentional self-harm
- **T44.2X3** Poisoning by ganglionic blocking drugs, assault
- **T44.2X4** Poisoning by ganglionic blocking drugs, undetermined
- **T44.2X5** Adverse effect of ganglionic blocking drugs
- **T44.2X6** Underdosing of ganglionic blocking drugs

T44.3 Poisoning by, adverse effect of and underdosing of other parasympatholytics [anticholinergics and antimuscarinics] and spasmolytics

Poisoning by, adverse effect of and underdosing of papaverine

T44.3X Poisoning by, adverse effect of and underdosing of other parasympatholytics [anticholinergics and antimuscarinics] and spasmolytics

- **T44.3X1** Poisoning by other parasympatholytics [anticholinergics and antimuscarinics] and spasmolytics, accidental (unintentional)
  Poisoning by other parasympatholytics [anticholinergics and antimuscarinics] and spasmolytics NOS
- **T44.3X2** Poisoning by other parasympatholytics [anticholinergics and antimuscarinics] and spasmolytics, intentional self-harm
- **T44.3X3** Poisoning by other parasympatholytics [anticholinergics and antimuscarinics] and spasmolytics, assault
- **T44.3X4** Poisoning by other parasympatholytics [anticholinergics and antimuscarinics] and spasmolytics, undetermined
- **T44.3X5** Adverse effect of other parasympatholytics [anticholinergics and antimuscarinics] and spasmolytics
- **T44.3X6** Underdosing of other parasympatholytics [anticholinergics and antimuscarinics] and spasmolytics

T44.4 Poisoning by, adverse effect of and underdosing of predominantly alpha-adrenoreceptor agonists

Poisoning by, adverse effect of and underdosing of metaraminol

T44.4X Poisoning by, adverse effect of and underdosing of predominantly alpha-adrenoreceptor agonists

- **T44.4X1** Poisoning by predominantly alpha-adrenoreceptor agonists, accidental (unintentional)
  Poisoning by predominantly alpha-adrenoreceptor agonists NOS
- **T44.4X2** Poisoning by predominantly alpha-adrenoreceptor agonists, intentional self-harm
- **T44.4X3** Poisoning by predominantly alpha-adrenoreceptor agonists, assault
- **T44.4X4** Poisoning by predominantly alpha-adrenoreceptor agonists, undetermined
- **T44.4X5** Adverse effect of predominantly alpha-adrenoreceptor agonists
- **T44.4X6** Underdosing of predominantly alpha-adrenoreceptor agonists

T44.5 Poisoning by, adverse effect of and underdosing of predominantly beta-adrenoreceptor agonists

EXCLUDES 1 poisoning by, adverse effect of and underdosing of beta-adrenoreceptor agonists used in asthma therapy (T48.6-)

T44.5X Poisoning by, adverse effect of and underdosing of predominantly beta-adrenoreceptor agonists

- **T44.5X1** Poisoning by predominantly beta-adrenoreceptor agonists, accidental (unintentional)
  Poisoning by predominantly beta-adrenoreceptor agonists NOS
- **T44.5X2** Poisoning by predominantly beta-adrenoreceptor agonists, intentional self-harm
- **T44.5X3** Poisoning by predominantly beta-adrenoreceptor agonists, assault
- **T44.5X4** Poisoning by predominantly beta-adrenoreceptor agonists, undetermined
- **T44.5X5** Adverse effect of predominantly beta-adrenoreceptor agonists
- **T44.5X6** Underdosing of predominantly beta-adrenoreceptor agonists

T44.6 Poisoning by, adverse effect of and underdosing of alpha-adrenoreceptor antagonists

EXCLUDES 1 poisoning by, adverse effect of and underdosing of ergot alkaloids (T48.0)

T44.6X Poisoning by, adverse effect of and underdosing of alpha-adrenoreceptor antagonists

- **T44.6X1** Poisoning by alpha-adrenoreceptor antagonists, accidental (unintentional)
  Poisoning by alpha-adrenoreceptor antagonists NOS
- **T44.6X2** Poisoning by alpha-adrenoreceptor antagonists, intentional self-harm
- **T44.6X3** Poisoning by alpha-adrenoreceptor antagonists, assault
- **T44.6X4** Poisoning by alpha-adrenoreceptor antagonists, undetermined
- **T44.6X5** Adverse effect of alpha-adrenoreceptor antagonists
- **T44.6X6** Underdosing of alpha-adrenoreceptor antagonists

Chapter 19. Injury, Poisoning and Certain Other Consequences of External Causes

- ✓5th **T44.7** Poisoning by, adverse effect of and underdosing of beta-adrenoreceptor antagonists
  - ✓6th **T44.7X** Poisoning by, adverse effect of and underdosing of beta-adrenoreceptor antagonists
    - ✓7th **T44.7X1** Poisoning by beta-adrenoreceptor antagonists, accidental (unintentional)
      Poisoning by beta-adrenoreceptor antagonists NOS
    - ✓7th **T44.7X2** Poisoning by beta-adrenoreceptor antagonists, intentional self-harm HCC Rx ESR COM
    - ✓7th **T44.7X3** Poisoning by beta-adrenoreceptor antagonists, assault
    - ✓7th **T44.7X4** Poisoning by beta-adrenoreceptor antagonists, undetermined
    - ✓7th **T44.7X5** Adverse effect of beta-adrenoreceptor antagonists UPD
    - ✓7th **T44.7X6** Underdosing of beta-adrenoreceptor antagonists UPD
- ✓5th **T44.8** Poisoning by, adverse effect of and underdosing of centrally-acting and adrenergic-neuron- blocking agents
  - EXCLUDES 2: poisoning by, adverse effect of and underdosing of clonidine (T46.5)
    poisoning by, adverse effect of and underdosing of guanethidine (T46.5)
  - ✓6th **T44.8X** Poisoning by, adverse effect of and underdosing of centrally-acting and adrenergic- neuron-blocking agents
    - ✓7th **T44.8X1** Poisoning by centrally-acting and adrenergic-neuron-blocking agents, accidental (unintentional)
      Poisoning by centrally-acting and adrenergic-neuron-blocking agents NOS
    - ✓7th **T44.8X2** Poisoning by centrally-acting and adrenergic-neuron-blocking agents, intentional self-harm HCC Rx ESR COM
    - ✓7th **T44.8X3** Poisoning by centrally-acting and adrenergic-neuron-blocking agents, assault
    - ✓7th **T44.8X4** Poisoning by centrally-acting and adrenergic-neuron-blocking agents, undetermined
    - ✓7th **T44.8X5** Adverse effect of centrally-acting and adrenergic-neuron-blocking agents UPD
    - ✓7th **T44.8X6** Underdosing of centrally-acting and adrenergic-neuron-blocking agents UPD
- ✓5th **T44.9** Poisoning by, adverse effect of and underdosing of other and unspecified drugs primarily affecting the autonomic nervous system
  Poisoning by, adverse effect of and underdosing of drug stimulating both alpha and beta-adrenoreceptors
  - ✓6th **T44.90** Poisoning by, adverse effect of and underdosing of unspecified drugs primarily affecting the autonomic nervous system
    - ✓7th **T44.901** Poisoning by unspecified drugs primarily affecting the autonomic nervous system, accidental (unintentional)
      Poisoning by unspecified drugs primarily affecting the autonomic nervous system NOS
    - ✓7th **T44.902** Poisoning by unspecified drugs primarily affecting the autonomic nervous system, intentional self-harm HCC Rx ESR COM
    - ✓7th **T44.903** Poisoning by unspecified drugs primarily affecting the autonomic nervous system, assault
    - ✓7th **T44.904** Poisoning by unspecified drugs primarily affecting the autonomic nervous system, undetermined
    - ✓7th **T44.905** Adverse effect of unspecified drugs primarily affecting the autonomic nervous system UPD
    - ✓7th **T44.906** Underdosing of unspecified drugs primarily affecting the autonomic nervous system UPD
  - ✓6th **T44.99** Poisoning by, adverse effect of and underdosing of other drugs primarily affecting the autonomic nervous system
    - ✓7th **T44.991** Poisoning by other drug primarily affecting the autonomic nervous system, accidental (unintentional)
      Poisoning by other drugs primarily affecting the autonomic nervous system NOS
    - ✓7th **T44.992** Poisoning by other drugs primarily affecting the autonomic nervous system, intentional self-harm HCC Rx ESR COM
    - ✓7th **T44.993** Poisoning by other drugs primarily affecting the autonomic nervous system, assault
    - ✓7th **T44.994** Poisoning by other drugs primarily affecting the autonomic nervous system, undetermined
    - ✓7th **T44.995** Adverse effect of other drug primarily affecting the autonomic nervous system UPD
    - ✓7th **T44.996** Underdosing of other drug primarily affecting the autonomic nervous system UPD
- ✓4th **T45** Poisoning by, adverse effect of and underdosing of primarily systemic and hematological agents, not elsewhere classified

  > The appropriate 7th character is to be added to each code from category T45.
  > A initial encounter
  > D subsequent encounter
  > S sequela

  - ✓5th **T45.0** Poisoning by, adverse effect of and underdosing of antiallergic and antiemetic drugs
    - EXCLUDES 1: poisoning by, adverse effect of and underdosing of phenothiazine-based neuroleptics (T43.3)
    - ✓6th **T45.0X** Poisoning by, adverse effect of and underdosing of antiallergic and antiemetic drugs
      - ✓7th **T45.0X1** Poisoning by antiallergic and antiemetic drugs, accidental (unintentional)
        Poisoning by antiallergic and antiemetic drugs NOS
      - ✓7th **T45.0X2** Poisoning by antiallergic and antiemetic drugs, intentional self-harm HCC Rx ESR COM
      - ✓7th **T45.0X3** Poisoning by antiallergic and antiemetic drugs, assault
      - ✓7th **T45.0X4** Poisoning by antiallergic and antiemetic drugs, undetermined
      - ✓7th **T45.0X5** Adverse effect of antiallergic and antiemetic drugs UPD
      - ✓7th **T45.0X6** Underdosing of antiallergic and antiemetic drugs UPD
  - ✓5th **T45.1** Poisoning by, adverse effect of and underdosing of antineoplastic and immunosuppressive drugs
    - EXCLUDES 1: poisoning by, adverse effect of and underdosing of immune checkpoint inhibitors and immunostimulant drugs (T45.A)
      poisoning by, adverse effect of and underdosing of tamoxifen (T38.6)
    - AHA: 2019,1Q,17,20; 2014,4Q,22
    - ✓6th **T45.1X** Poisoning by, adverse effect of and underdosing of antineoplastic and immunosuppressive drugs
      - ✓7th **T45.1X1** Poisoning by antineoplastic and immunosuppressive drugs, accidental (unintentional)
        Poisoning by antineoplastic and immunosuppressive drugs NOS
      - ✓7th **T45.1X2** Poisoning by antineoplastic and immunosuppressive drugs, intentional self-harm HCC Rx ESR COM
      - ✓7th **T45.1X3** Poisoning by antineoplastic and immunosuppressive drugs, assault
      - ✓7th **T45.1X4** Poisoning by antineoplastic and immunosuppressive drugs, undetermined
      - ✓7th **T45.1X5** Adverse effect of antineoplastic and immunosuppressive drugs UPD
        AHA: 2024,1Q,25; 2023,2Q,10; 2021,3Q,4; 2020,4Q,11; 2020,3Q,22; 2019,2Q,24,28
      - ✓7th **T45.1X6** Underdosing of antineoplastic and immunosuppressive drugs UPD

Chapter 19. Injury, Poisoning and Certain Other Consequences of External Causes

T45.2 Poisoning by, adverse effect of and underdosing of vitamins
EXCLUDES 2: poisoning by, adverse effect of and underdosing of iron (T45.4)
poisoning by, adverse effect of and underdosing of nicotinic acid (derivatives) (T46.7)
poisoning by, adverse effect of and underdosing of vitamin K (T45.7)

- **T45.2X** Poisoning by, adverse effect of and underdosing of vitamins
  - **T45.2X1** Poisoning by vitamins, accidental (unintentional)
    - Poisoning by vitamins NOS
  - **T45.2X2** Poisoning by vitamins, intentional self-harm [HCC Rx ESR COM]
  - **T45.2X3** Poisoning by vitamins, assault
  - **T45.2X4** Poisoning by vitamins, undetermined
  - **T45.2X5** Adverse effect of vitamins [UPD]
  - **T45.2X6** Underdosing of vitamins [UPD]
    - EXCLUDES 1: vitamin deficiencies (E50-E56)

T45.3 Poisoning by, adverse effect of and underdosing of enzymes
- **T45.3X** Poisoning by, adverse effect of and underdosing of enzymes
  - **T45.3X1** Poisoning by enzymes, accidental (unintentional)
    - Poisoning by enzymes NOS
  - **T45.3X2** Poisoning by enzymes, intentional self-harm [HCC Rx ESR COM]
  - **T45.3X3** Poisoning by enzymes, assault
  - **T45.3X4** Poisoning by enzymes, undetermined
  - **T45.3X5** Adverse effect of enzymes [UPD]
  - **T45.3X6** Underdosing of enzymes [UPD]

T45.4 Poisoning by, adverse effect of and underdosing of iron and its compounds
- **T45.4X** Poisoning by, adverse effect of and underdosing of iron and its compounds
  - **T45.4X1** Poisoning by iron and its compounds, accidental (unintentional)
    - Poisoning by iron and its compounds NOS
  - **T45.4X2** Poisoning by iron and its compounds, intentional self-harm [HCC Rx ESR COM]
  - **T45.4X3** Poisoning by iron and its compounds, assault
  - **T45.4X4** Poisoning by iron and its compounds, undetermined
  - **T45.4X5** Adverse effect of iron and its compounds [UPD]
  - **T45.4X6** Underdosing of iron and its compounds [UPD]
    - EXCLUDES 1: iron deficiency (E61.1)

T45.5 Poisoning by, adverse effect of and underdosing of anticoagulants and antithrombotic drugs
- **T45.51** Poisoning by, adverse effect of and underdosing of anticoagulants
  - **T45.511** Poisoning by anticoagulants, accidental (unintentional)
    - Poisoning by anticoagulants NOS
  - **T45.512** Poisoning by anticoagulants, intentional self-harm [HCC Rx ESR COM]
  - **T45.513** Poisoning by anticoagulants, assault
  - **T45.514** Poisoning by anticoagulants, undetermined
  - **T45.515** Adverse effect of anticoagulants [UPD]
    - AHA: 2021,1Q,4; 2016,1Q,14; 2013,2Q,34
  - **T45.516** Underdosing of anticoagulants [UPD]
- **T45.52** Poisoning by, adverse effect of and underdosing of antithrombotic drugs
  - Poisoning by, adverse effect of and underdosing of antiplatelet drugs
  - EXCLUDES 2: poisoning by, adverse effect of and underdosing of acetylsalicylic acid (T39.01-)
  - poisoning by, adverse effect of and underdosing of aspirin (T39.01-)
  - **T45.521** Poisoning by antithrombotic drugs, accidental (unintentional)
    - Poisoning by antithrombotic drug NOS
  - **T45.522** Poisoning by antithrombotic drugs, intentional self-harm [HCC Rx ESR COM]
  - **T45.523** Poisoning by antithrombotic drugs, assault
  - **T45.524** Poisoning by antithrombotic drugs, undetermined
  - **T45.525** Adverse effect of antithrombotic drugs [UPD]
    - AHA: 2016,1Q,15
  - **T45.526** Underdosing of antithrombotic drugs [UPD]

T45.6 Poisoning by, adverse effect of and underdosing of fibrinolysis-affecting drugs
- **T45.60** Poisoning by, adverse effect of and underdosing of unspecified fibrinolysis-affecting drugs
  - **T45.601** Poisoning by unspecified fibrinolysis-affecting drugs, accidental (unintentional)
    - Poisoning by fibrinolysis-affecting drug NOS
  - **T45.602** Poisoning by unspecified fibrinolysis-affecting drugs, intentional self-harm [HCC Rx ESR COM]
  - **T45.603** Poisoning by unspecified fibrinolysis-affecting drugs, assault
  - **T45.604** Poisoning by unspecified fibrinolysis-affecting drugs, undetermined
  - **T45.605** Adverse effect of unspecified fibrinolysis-affecting drugs [UPD]
  - **T45.606** Underdosing of unspecified fibrinolysis-affecting drugs [UPD]
- **T45.61** Poisoning by, adverse effect of and underdosing of thrombolytic drugs
  - **T45.611** Poisoning by thrombolytic drug, accidental (unintentional)
    - Poisoning by thrombolytic drug NOS
  - **T45.612** Poisoning by thrombolytic drug, intentional self-harm [HCC Rx ESR COM]
  - **T45.613** Poisoning by thrombolytic drug, assault
  - **T45.614** Poisoning by thrombolytic drug, undetermined
  - **T45.615** Adverse effect of thrombolytic drugs [UPD]
    - AHA: 2017,2Q,9
  - **T45.616** Underdosing of thrombolytic drugs [UPD]
- **T45.62** Poisoning by, adverse effect of and underdosing of hemostatic drugs
  - **T45.621** Poisoning by hemostatic drug, accidental (unintentional)
    - Poisoning by hemostatic drug NOS
  - **T45.622** Poisoning by hemostatic drug, intentional self-harm [HCC Rx ESR COM]
  - **T45.623** Poisoning by hemostatic drug, assault
  - **T45.624** Poisoning by hemostatic drug, undetermined
  - **T45.625** Adverse effect of hemostatic drug [UPD]
  - **T45.626** Underdosing of hemostatic drugs [UPD]
- **T45.69** Poisoning by, adverse effect of and underdosing of other fibrinolysis-affecting drugs
  - **T45.691** Poisoning by other fibrinolysis-affecting drugs, accidental (unintentional)
    - Poisoning by other fibrinolysis-affecting drug NOS
  - **T45.692** Poisoning by other fibrinolysis-affecting drugs, intentional self-harm [HCC Rx ESR COM]
  - **T45.693** Poisoning by other fibrinolysis-affecting drugs, assault
  - **T45.694** Poisoning by other fibrinolysis-affecting drugs, undetermined
  - **T45.695** Adverse effect of other fibrinolysis-affecting drugs [UPD]
  - **T45.696** Underdosing of other fibrinolysis-affecting drugs [UPD]

T45.7 Poisoning by, adverse effect of and underdosing of anticoagulant antagonists, vitamin K and other coagulants
- **T45.7X** Poisoning by, adverse effect of and underdosing of anticoagulant antagonists, vitamin K and other coagulants
  - **T45.7X1** Poisoning by anticoagulant antagonists, vitamin K and other coagulants, accidental (unintentional)
    - Poisoning by anticoagulant antagonists, vitamin K and other coagulants NOS

☑ Additional Character Required ✓x7th Placeholder Alert Manifestation Unspecified Dx Q QPP UPD Unacceptable PDx

- T45.7X2 Poisoning by anticoagulant antagonists, vitamin K and other coagulants, intentional self-harm [HCC] [Rx] [ESR] [COM]
- T45.7X3 Poisoning by anticoagulant antagonists, vitamin K and other coagulants, assault
- T45.7X4 Poisoning by anticoagulant antagonists, vitamin K and other coagulants, undetermined
- T45.7X5 Adverse effect of anticoagulant antagonists, vitamin K and other coagulants [UPD]
- T45.7X6 Underdosing of anticoagulant antagonist, vitamin K and other coagulants [UPD]
  - EXCLUDES 1: vitamin K deficiency (E56.1)

T45.8 Poisoning by, adverse effect of and underdosing of other primarily systemic and hematological agents
Poisoning by, adverse effect of and underdosing of liver preparations and other antianemic agents
Poisoning by, adverse effect of and underdosing of natural blood and blood products
Poisoning by, adverse effect of and underdosing of plasma substitute

EXCLUDES 2:
- poisoning by, adverse effect of and underdosing of immunoglobulin (T50.Z1)
- poisoning by, adverse effect of and underdosing of iron (T45.4)
- transfusion reactions (T80.-)

- T45.8X Poisoning by, adverse effect of and underdosing of other primarily systemic and hematological agents
  - T45.8X1 Poisoning by other primarily systemic and hematological agents, accidental (unintentional)
    Poisoning by other primarily systemic and hematological agents NOS
  - T45.8X2 Poisoning by other primarily systemic and hematological agents, intentional self-harm [HCC] [Rx] [ESR] [COM]
  - T45.8X3 Poisoning by other primarily systemic and hematological agents, assault
  - T45.8X4 Poisoning by other primarily systemic and hematological agents, undetermined
  - T45.8X5 Adverse effect of other primarily systemic and hematological agents [UPD]
    AHA: 2016,4Q,42
  - T45.8X6 Underdosing of other primarily systemic and hematological agents [UPD]

T45.9 Poisoning by, adverse effect of and underdosing of unspecified primarily systemic and hematological agent
- T45.91 Poisoning by unspecified primarily systemic and hematological agent, accidental (unintentional)
  Poisoning by primarily systemic and hematological agent NOS
- T45.92 Poisoning by unspecified primarily systemic and hematological agent, intentional self-harm [HCC] [Rx] [ESR] [COM]
- T45.93 Poisoning by unspecified primarily systemic and hematological agent, assault
- T45.94 Poisoning by unspecified primarily systemic and hematological agent, undetermined
- T45.95 Adverse effect of unspecified primarily systemic and hematological agent [UPD]
- T45.96 Underdosing of unspecified primarily systemic and hematological agent [UPD]

T45.A Poisoning by, adverse effect of and underdosing of immune checkpoint inhibitors and immunostimulant drugs
EXCLUDES 1: poisoning by, adverse effect of and underdosing of antineoplastic and immunosuppressive drug (T45.1)
AHA: 2024,4Q,28

- T45.AX Poisoning by, adverse effect of and underdosing of immune checkpoint inhibitors and immunostimulant drugs
  - T45.AX1 Poisoning by immune checkpoint inhibitors and immunostimulant drugs, accidental (unintentional)
    Poisoning by immune checkpoint inhibitors and immunosuppressive drugs NOS
  - T45.AX2 Poisoning by immune checkpoint inhibitors and immunostimulant drugs, intentional self-harm [HCC] [Rx] [ESR] [COM]
  - T45.AX3 Poisoning by immune checkpoint inhibitors and immunostimulant drugs, assault
  - T45.AX4 Poisoning by immune checkpoint inhibitors and immunostimulant drugs, undetermined
  - T45.AX5 Adverse effect of immune checkpoint inhibitors and immunostimulant drugs
  - T45.AX6 Underdosing of immune checkpoint inhibitors and immunostimulant drugs

T46 Poisoning by, adverse effect of and underdosing of agents primarily affecting the cardiovascular system
EXCLUDES 1: poisoning by, adverse effect of and underdosing of metaraminol (T44.4)

The appropriate 7th character is to be added to each code from category T46.
- A initial encounter
- D subsequent encounter
- S sequela

T46.0 Poisoning by, adverse effect of and underdosing of cardiac-stimulant glycosides and drugs of similar action
- T46.0X Poisoning by, adverse effect of and underdosing of cardiac-stimulant glycosides and drugs of similar action
  - T46.0X1 Poisoning by cardiac-stimulant glycosides and drugs of similar action, accidental (unintentional)
    Poisoning by cardiac-stimulant glycosides and drugs of similar action NOS
  - T46.0X2 Poisoning by cardiac-stimulant glycosides and drugs of similar action, intentional self-harm [HCC] [Rx] [ESR] [COM]
  - T46.0X3 Poisoning by cardiac-stimulant glycosides and drugs of similar action, assault
  - T46.0X4 Poisoning by cardiac-stimulant glycosides and drugs of similar action, undetermined
  - T46.0X5 Adverse effect of cardiac-stimulant glycosides and drugs of similar action [UPD]
  - T46.0X6 Underdosing of cardiac-stimulant glycosides and drugs of similar action [UPD]

T46.1 Poisoning by, adverse effect of and underdosing of calcium-channel blockers
- T46.1X Poisoning by, adverse effect of and underdosing of calcium-channel blockers
  - T46.1X1 Poisoning by calcium-channel blockers, accidental (unintentional)
    Poisoning by calcium-channel blockers NOS
  - T46.1X2 Poisoning by calcium-channel blockers, intentional self-harm [HCC] [Rx] [ESR] [COM]
  - T46.1X3 Poisoning by calcium-channel blockers, assault
  - T46.1X4 Poisoning by calcium-channel blockers, undetermined
  - T46.1X5 Adverse effect of calcium-channel blockers [UPD]
  - T46.1X6 Underdosing of calcium-channel blockers [UPD]
    AHA: 2023,1Q,39

T46.2 Poisoning by, adverse effect of and underdosing of other antidysrhythmic drugs, not elsewhere classified
EXCLUDES 1: poisoning by, adverse effect of and underdosing of beta-adrenoreceptor antagonists (T44.7-)

- T46.2X Poisoning by, adverse effect of and underdosing of other antidysrhythmic drugs
  - T46.2X1 Poisoning by other antidysrhythmic drugs, accidental (unintentional)
    Poisoning by other antidysrhythmic drugs NOS
  - T46.2X2 Poisoning by other antidysrhythmic drugs, intentional self-harm [HCC] [Rx] [ESR] [COM]
  - T46.2X3 Poisoning by other antidysrhythmic drugs, assault
  - T46.2X4 Poisoning by other antidysrhythmic drugs, undetermined
  - T46.2X5 Adverse effect of other antidysrhythmic drugs [UPD]
  - T46.2X6 Underdosing of other antidysrhythmic drugs [UPD]

Chapter 19. Injury, Poisoning and Certain Other Consequences of External Causes

- **T46.3** Poisoning by, adverse effect of and underdosing of coronary vasodilators
  Poisoning by, adverse effect of and underdosing of dipyridamole
  EXCLUDES 1 poisoning by, adverse effect of and underdosing of calcium-channel blockers (T46.1)
  - **T46.3X** Poisoning by, adverse effect of and underdosing of coronary vasodilators
    - **T46.3X1** Poisoning by coronary vasodilators, accidental (unintentional)
      Poisoning by coronary vasodilators NOS
    - **T46.3X2** Poisoning by coronary vasodilators, intentional self-harm
    - **T46.3X3** Poisoning by coronary vasodilators, assault
    - **T46.3X4** Poisoning by coronary vasodilators, undetermined
    - **T46.3X5** Adverse effect of coronary vasodilators
    - **T46.3X6** Underdosing of coronary vasodilators

- **T46.4** Poisoning by, adverse effect of and underdosing of angiotensin-converting-enzyme inhibitors
  - **T46.4X** Poisoning by, adverse effect of and underdosing of angiotensin-converting-enzyme inhibitors
    - **T46.4X1** Poisoning by angiotensin-converting-enzyme inhibitors, accidental (unintentional)
      Poisoning by angiotensin-converting-enzyme inhibitors NOS
    - **T46.4X2** Poisoning by angiotensin-converting-enzyme inhibitors, intentional self-harm
    - **T46.4X3** Poisoning by angiotensin-converting-enzyme inhibitors, assault
    - **T46.4X4** Poisoning by angiotensin-converting-enzyme inhibitors, undetermined
    - **T46.4X5** Adverse effect of angiotensin-converting-enzyme inhibitors
    - **T46.4X6** Underdosing of angiotensin-converting-enzyme inhibitors

- **T46.5** Poisoning by, adverse effect of and underdosing of other antihypertensive drugs
  EXCLUDES 2 poisoning by, adverse effect of and underdosing of beta-adrenoreceptor antagonists (T44.7)
  poisoning by, adverse effect of and underdosing of calcium-channel blockers (T46.1)
  poisoning by, adverse effect of and underdosing of diuretics (T50.0-T50.2)
  - **T46.5X** Poisoning by, adverse effect of and underdosing of other antihypertensive drugs
    - **T46.5X1** Poisoning by other antihypertensive drugs, accidental (unintentional)
      Poisoning by other antihypertensive drugs NOS
    - **T46.5X2** Poisoning by other antihypertensive drugs, intentional self-harm
    - **T46.5X3** Poisoning by other antihypertensive drugs, assault
    - **T46.5X4** Poisoning by other antihypertensive drugs, undetermined
    - **T46.5X5** Adverse effect of other antihypertensive drugs
    - **T46.5X6** Underdosing of other antihypertensive drugs
      AHA: 2023,1Q,39; 2022,1Q,36

- **T46.6** Poisoning by, adverse effect of and underdosing of antihyperlipidemic and antiarteriosclerotic drugs
  - **T46.6X** Poisoning by, adverse effect of and underdosing of antihyperlipidemic and antiarteriosclerotic drugs
    - **T46.6X1** Poisoning by antihyperlipidemic and antiarteriosclerotic drugs, accidental (unintentional)
      Poisoning by antihyperlipidemic and antiarteriosclerotic drugs NOS
    - **T46.6X2** Poisoning by antihyperlipidemic and antiarteriosclerotic drugs, intentional self-harm
    - **T46.6X3** Poisoning by antihyperlipidemic and antiarteriosclerotic drugs, assault
    - **T46.6X4** Poisoning by antihyperlipidemic and antiarteriosclerotic drugs, undetermined
    - **T46.6X5** Adverse effect of antihyperlipidemic and antiarteriosclerotic drugs
    - **T46.6X6** Underdosing of antihyperlipidemic and antiarteriosclerotic drugs

- **T46.7** Poisoning by, adverse effect of and underdosing of peripheral vasodilators
  Poisoning by, adverse effect of and underdosing of nicotinic acid (derivatives)
  EXCLUDES 1 poisoning by, adverse effect of and underdosing of papaverine (T44.3)
  - **T46.7X** Poisoning by, adverse effect of and underdosing of peripheral vasodilators
    - **T46.7X1** Poisoning by peripheral vasodilators, accidental (unintentional)
      Poisoning by peripheral vasodilators NOS
    - **T46.7X2** Poisoning by peripheral vasodilators, intentional self-harm
    - **T46.7X3** Poisoning by peripheral vasodilators, assault
    - **T46.7X4** Poisoning by peripheral vasodilators, undetermined
    - **T46.7X5** Adverse effect of peripheral vasodilators
    - **T46.7X6** Underdosing of peripheral vasodilators

- **T46.8** Poisoning by, adverse effect of and underdosing of antivaricose drugs, including sclerosing agents
  - **T46.8X** Poisoning by, adverse effect of and underdosing of antivaricose drugs, including sclerosing agents
    - **T46.8X1** Poisoning by antivaricose drugs, including sclerosing agents, accidental (unintentional)
      Poisoning by antivaricose drugs, including sclerosing agents NOS
    - **T46.8X2** Poisoning by antivaricose drugs, including sclerosing agents, intentional self-harm
    - **T46.8X3** Poisoning by antivaricose drugs, including sclerosing agents, assault
    - **T46.8X4** Poisoning by antivaricose drugs, including sclerosing agents, undetermined
    - **T46.8X5** Adverse effect of antivaricose drugs, including sclerosing agents
    - **T46.8X6** Underdosing of antivaricose drugs, including sclerosing agents

- **T46.9** Poisoning by, adverse effect of and underdosing of other and unspecified agents primarily affecting the cardiovascular system
  - **T46.90** Poisoning by, adverse effect of and underdosing of unspecified agents primarily affecting the cardiovascular system
    - **T46.901** Poisoning by unspecified agents primarily affecting the cardiovascular system, accidental (unintentional)
    - **T46.902** Poisoning by unspecified agents primarily affecting the cardiovascular system, intentional self-harm
    - **T46.903** Poisoning by unspecified agents primarily affecting the cardiovascular system, assault
    - **T46.904** Poisoning by unspecified agents primarily affecting the cardiovascular system, undetermined
    - **T46.905** Adverse effect of unspecified agents primarily affecting the cardiovascular system
    - **T46.906** Underdosing of unspecified agents primarily affecting the cardiovascular system
  - **T46.99** Poisoning by, adverse effect of and underdosing of other agents primarily affecting the cardiovascular system
    - **T46.991** Poisoning by other agents primarily affecting the cardiovascular system, accidental (unintentional)
    - **T46.992** Poisoning by other agents primarily affecting the cardiovascular system, intentional self-harm

Chapter 19. Injury, Poisoning and Certain Other Consequences of External Causes

- T46.993 Poisoning by other agents primarily affecting the cardiovascular system, assault
- T46.994 Poisoning by other agents primarily affecting the cardiovascular system, undetermined
- T46.995 Adverse effect of other agents primarily affecting the cardiovascular system
- T46.996 Underdosing of other agents primarily affecting the cardiovascular system

T47 Poisoning by, adverse effect of and underdosing of agents primarily affecting the gastrointestinal system

> The appropriate 7th character is to be added to each code from category T47.
> A initial encounter
> D subsequent encounter
> S sequela

- T47.0 Poisoning by, adverse effect of and underdosing of histamine H2-receptor blockers
  - T47.0X Poisoning by, adverse effect of and underdosing of histamine H2-receptor blockers
    - T47.0X1 Poisoning by histamine H2-receptor blockers, accidental (unintentional)
      Poisoning by histamine H2-receptor blockers NOS
    - T47.0X2 Poisoning by histamine H2-receptor blockers, intentional self-harm
    - T47.0X3 Poisoning by histamine H2-receptor blockers, assault
    - T47.0X4 Poisoning by histamine H2-receptor blockers, undetermined
    - T47.0X5 Adverse effect of histamine H2-receptor blockers
    - T47.0X6 Underdosing of histamine H2-receptor blockers

- T47.1 Poisoning by, adverse effect of and underdosing of other antacids and anti-gastric-secretion drugs
  - T47.1X Poisoning by, adverse effect of and underdosing of other antacids and anti-gastric-secretion drugs
    - T47.1X1 Poisoning by other antacids and anti-gastric-secretion drugs, accidental (unintentional)
      Poisoning by other antacids and anti-gastric-secretion drugs NOS
    - T47.1X2 Poisoning by other antacids and anti-gastric-secretion drugs, intentional self-harm
    - T47.1X3 Poisoning by other antacids and anti-gastric-secretion drugs, assault
    - T47.1X4 Poisoning by other antacids and anti-gastric-secretion drugs, undetermined
    - T47.1X5 Adverse effect of other antacids and anti-gastric-secretion drugs
    - T47.1X6 Underdosing of other antacids and anti-gastric-secretion drugs

- T47.2 Poisoning by, adverse effect of and underdosing of stimulant laxatives
  - T47.2X Poisoning by, adverse effect of and underdosing of stimulant laxatives
    - T47.2X1 Poisoning by stimulant laxatives, accidental (unintentional)
      Poisoning by stimulant laxatives NOS
    - T47.2X2 Poisoning by stimulant laxatives, intentional self-harm
    - T47.2X3 Poisoning by stimulant laxatives, assault
    - T47.2X4 Poisoning by stimulant laxatives, undetermined
    - T47.2X5 Adverse effect of stimulant laxatives
    - T47.2X6 Underdosing of stimulant laxatives

- T47.3 Poisoning by, adverse effect of and underdosing of saline and osmotic laxatives
  - T47.3X Poisoning by and adverse effect of saline and osmotic laxatives
    - T47.3X1 Poisoning by saline and osmotic laxatives, accidental (unintentional)
      Poisoning by saline and osmotic laxatives NOS
    - T47.3X2 Poisoning by saline and osmotic laxatives, intentional self-harm
    - T47.3X3 Poisoning by saline and osmotic laxatives, assault
    - T47.3X4 Poisoning by saline and osmotic laxatives, undetermined
    - T47.3X5 Adverse effect of saline and osmotic laxatives
    - T47.3X6 Underdosing of saline and osmotic laxatives

- T47.4 Poisoning by, adverse effect of and underdosing of other laxatives
  - T47.4X Poisoning by, adverse effect of and underdosing of other laxatives
    - T47.4X1 Poisoning by other laxatives, accidental (unintentional)
      Poisoning by other laxatives NOS
    - T47.4X2 Poisoning by other laxatives, intentional self-harm
    - T47.4X3 Poisoning by other laxatives, assault
    - T47.4X4 Poisoning by other laxatives, undetermined
    - T47.4X5 Adverse effect of other laxatives
    - T47.4X6 Underdosing of other laxatives

- T47.5 Poisoning by, adverse effect of and underdosing of digestants
  - T47.5X Poisoning by, adverse effect of and underdosing of digestants
    - T47.5X1 Poisoning by digestants, accidental (unintentional)
      Poisoning by digestants NOS
    - T47.5X2 Poisoning by digestants, intentional self-harm
    - T47.5X3 Poisoning by digestants, assault
    - T47.5X4 Poisoning by digestants, undetermined
    - T47.5X5 Adverse effect of digestants
    - T47.5X6 Underdosing of digestants

- T47.6 Poisoning by, adverse effect of and underdosing of antidiarrheal drugs
  > EXCLUDES 2 poisoning by, adverse effect of and underdosing of systemic antibiotics and other anti-infectives (T36-T37)
  - T47.6X Poisoning by, adverse effect of and underdosing of antidiarrheal drugs
    - T47.6X1 Poisoning by antidiarrheal drugs, accidental (unintentional)
      Poisoning by antidiarrheal drugs NOS
    - T47.6X2 Poisoning by antidiarrheal drugs, intentional self-harm
    - T47.6X3 Poisoning by antidiarrheal drugs, assault
    - T47.6X4 Poisoning by antidiarrheal drugs, undetermined
    - T47.6X5 Adverse effect of antidiarrheal drugs
    - T47.6X6 Underdosing of antidiarrheal drugs

- T47.7 Poisoning by, adverse effect of and underdosing of emetics
  - T47.7X Poisoning by, adverse effect of and underdosing of emetics
    - T47.7X1 Poisoning by emetics, accidental (unintentional)
      Poisoning by emetics NOS
    - T47.7X2 Poisoning by emetics, intentional self-harm
    - T47.7X3 Poisoning by emetics, assault
    - T47.7X4 Poisoning by emetics, undetermined
    - T47.7X5 Adverse effect of emetics
    - T47.7X6 Underdosing of emetics

- T47.8 Poisoning by, adverse effect of and underdosing of other agents primarily affecting gastrointestinal system
  - T47.8X Poisoning by, adverse effect of and underdosing of other agents primarily affecting gastrointestinal system
    - T47.8X1 Poisoning by other agents primarily affecting gastrointestinal system, accidental (unintentional)
      Poisoning by other agents primarily affecting gastrointestinal system NOS
    - T47.8X2 Poisoning by other agents primarily affecting gastrointestinal system, intentional self-harm

Chapter 19. Injury, Poisoning and Certain Other Consequences of External Causes

- ✓7th **T47.8X3** Poisoning by other agents primarily affecting gastrointestinal system, **assault**
- ✓7th **T47.8X4** Poisoning by other agents primarily affecting gastrointestinal system, **undetermined**
- ✓7th **T47.8X5** **Adverse effect** of other agents primarily affecting gastrointestinal system [UPD]
- ✓7th **T47.8X6** **Underdosing** of other agents primarily affecting gastrointestinal system [UPD]

✓5th **T47.9** Poisoning by, adverse effect of and underdosing of unspecified agents primarily affecting the gastrointestinal system
- ✓x7th **T47.91** Poisoning by unspecified agents primarily affecting the gastrointestinal system, **accidental (unintentional)**
  - Poisoning by agents primarily affecting the gastrointestinal system NOS
- ✓x7th **T47.92** Poisoning by unspecified agents primarily affecting the gastrointestinal system, **intentional self-harm** [HCC] [Rx] [ESR] [COM]
- ✓x7th **T47.93** Poisoning by unspecified agents primarily affecting the gastrointestinal system, **assault**
- ✓x7th **T47.94** Poisoning by unspecified agents primarily affecting the gastrointestinal system, **undetermined**
- ✓x7th **T47.95** **Adverse effect** of unspecified agents primarily affecting the gastrointestinal system [UPD]
- ✓x7th **T47.96** **Underdosing** of unspecified agents primarily affecting the gastrointestinal system [UPD]

✓4th **T48** Poisoning by, adverse effect of and underdosing of agents primarily acting on smooth and skeletal muscles and the respiratory system

> The appropriate 7th character is to be added to each code from category T48.
> A   initial encounter
> D   subsequent encounter
> S   sequela

✓5th **T48.0** Poisoning by, adverse effect of and underdosing of oxytocic drugs
  EXCLUDES 1 poisoning by, adverse effect of and underdosing of estrogens, progestogens and antagonists (T38.4-T38.6)
- ✓6th **T48.0X** Poisoning by, adverse effect of and underdosing of **oxytocic drugs**
  - ✓7th **T48.0X1** Poisoning by oxytocic drugs, **accidental (unintentional)**
    - Poisoning by oxytocic drugs NOS
  - ✓7th **T48.0X2** Poisoning by oxytocic drugs, **intentional self-harm** [HCC] [Rx] [ESR] [COM]
  - ✓7th **T48.0X3** Poisoning by oxytocic drugs, **assault**
  - ✓7th **T48.0X4** Poisoning by oxytocic drugs, **undetermined**
  - ✓7th **T48.0X5** **Adverse effect** of oxytocic drugs [UPD]
  - ✓7th **T48.0X6** **Underdosing** of oxytocic drugs [UPD]

✓5th **T48.1** Poisoning by, adverse effect of and underdosing of skeletal muscle relaxants [neuromuscular blocking agents]
- ✓6th **T48.1X** Poisoning by, adverse effect of and underdosing of **skeletal muscle relaxants** [neuromuscular blocking agents]
  - ✓7th **T48.1X1** Poisoning by skeletal muscle relaxants [neuromuscular blocking agents], **accidental (unintentional)**
    - Poisoning by skeletal muscle relaxants [neuromuscular blocking agents] NOS
  - ✓7th **T48.1X2** Poisoning by skeletal muscle relaxants [neuromuscular blocking agents], **intentional self-harm** [HCC] [Rx] [ESR] [COM]
  - ✓7th **T48.1X3** Poisoning by skeletal muscle relaxants [neuromuscular blocking agents], **assault**
  - ✓7th **T48.1X4** Poisoning by skeletal muscle relaxants [neuromuscular blocking agents], **undetermined**
  - ✓7th **T48.1X5** **Adverse effect** of skeletal muscle relaxants [neuromuscular blocking agents] [UPD]
  - ✓7th **T48.1X6** **Underdosing** of skeletal muscle relaxants [neuromuscular blocking agents] [UPD]

✓5th **T48.2** Poisoning by, adverse effect of and underdosing of other and unspecified drugs acting on muscles
- ✓6th **T48.20** Poisoning by, adverse effect of and underdosing of unspecified drugs acting on muscles
  - ✓7th **T48.201** Poisoning by unspecified drugs acting on muscles, **accidental (unintentional)**
    - Poisoning by unspecified drugs acting on muscles NOS
  - ✓7th **T48.202** Poisoning by unspecified drugs acting on muscles, **intentional self-harm** [HCC] [Rx] [ESR] [COM]
  - ✓7th **T48.203** Poisoning by unspecified drugs acting on muscles, **assault**
  - ✓7th **T48.204** Poisoning by unspecified drugs acting on muscles, **undetermined**
  - ✓7th **T48.205** **Adverse effect** of unspecified drugs acting on muscles [UPD]
  - ✓7th **T48.206** **Underdosing** of unspecified drugs acting on muscles [UPD]
- ✓6th **T48.29** Poisoning by, adverse effect of and underdosing of other drugs acting on muscles
  - ✓7th **T48.291** Poisoning by other drugs acting on muscles, **accidental (unintentional)**
    - Poisoning by other drugs acting on muscles NOS
  - ✓7th **T48.292** Poisoning by other drugs acting on muscles, **intentional self-harm** [HCC] [Rx] [ESR] [COM]
  - ✓7th **T48.293** Poisoning by other drugs acting on muscles, **assault**
  - ✓7th **T48.294** Poisoning by other drugs acting on muscles, **undetermined**
  - ✓7th **T48.295** **Adverse effect** of other drugs acting on muscles [UPD]
  - ✓7th **T48.296** **Underdosing** of other drugs acting on muscles [UPD]

✓5th **T48.3** Poisoning by, adverse effect of and underdosing of antitussives
- ✓6th **T48.3X** Poisoning by, adverse effect of and underdosing of **antitussives**
  - ✓7th **T48.3X1** Poisoning by antitussives, **accidental (unintentional)**
    - Poisoning by antitussives NOS
  - ✓7th **T48.3X2** Poisoning by antitussives, **intentional self-harm** [HCC] [Rx] [ESR] [COM]
  - ✓7th **T48.3X3** Poisoning by antitussives, **assault**
  - ✓7th **T48.3X4** Poisoning by antitussives, **undetermined**
  - ✓7th **T48.3X5** **Adverse effect** of antitussives [UPD]
  - ✓7th **T48.3X6** **Underdosing** of antitussives [UPD]

✓5th **T48.4** Poisoning by, adverse effect of and underdosing of expectorants
- ✓6th **T48.4X** Poisoning by, adverse effect of and underdosing of **expectorants**
  - ✓7th **T48.4X1** Poisoning by expectorants, **accidental (unintentional)**
    - Poisoning by expectorants NOS
  - ✓7th **T48.4X2** Poisoning by expectorants, **intentional self-harm** [HCC] [Rx] [ESR] [COM]
  - ✓7th **T48.4X3** Poisoning by expectorants, **assault**
  - ✓7th **T48.4X4** Poisoning by expectorants, **undetermined**
  - ✓7th **T48.4X5** **Adverse effect** of expectorants [UPD]
  - ✓7th **T48.4X6** **Underdosing** of expectorants [UPD]

✓5th **T48.5** Poisoning by, adverse effect of and underdosing of other anti-common-cold drugs
  Poisoning by, adverse effect of and underdosing of decongestants
  EXCLUDES 2 poisoning by, adverse effect of and underdosing of antipyretics, NEC (T39.9-)
  poisoning by, adverse effect of and underdosing of non-steroidal antiinflammatory drugs (T39.3-)
  poisoning by, adverse effect of and underdosing of salicylates (T39.0-)
- ✓6th **T48.5X** Poisoning by, adverse effect of and underdosing of other anti-common-cold drugs
  - ✓7th **T48.5X1** Poisoning by other anti-common-cold drugs, **accidental (unintentional)**
    - Poisoning by other anti-common-cold drugs NOS
  - ✓7th **T48.5X2** Poisoning by other anti-common-cold drugs, **intentional self-harm** [HCC] [Rx] [ESR] [COM]

■ Additional Character Required   ✓x7th Placeholder Alert   Manifestation   Unspecified Dx   Q QPP   UPD Unacceptable PDx

Chapter 19. Injury, Poisoning and Certain Other Consequences of External Causes

- 7th **T48.5X3** Poisoning by other anti-common-cold drugs, assault
- 7th **T48.5X4** Poisoning by other anti-common-cold drugs, undetermined
- 7th **T48.5X5** Adverse effect of other anti-common-cold drugs [UPD]
- 7th **T48.5X6** Underdosing of other anti-common-cold drugs [UPD]

5th **T48.6** Poisoning by, adverse effect of and underdosing of antiasthmatics, not elsewhere classified
Poisoning by, adverse effect of and underdosing of beta-adrenoreceptor agonists used in asthma therapy
EXCLUDES 1 poisoning by, adverse effect of and underdosing of anterior pituitary [adenohypophyseal] hormones (T38.8)
poisoning by, adverse effect of and underdosing of beta-adrenoreceptor agonists not used in asthma therapy (T44.5)

6th **T48.6X** Poisoning by, adverse effect of and underdosing of antiasthmatics
- 7th **T48.6X1** Poisoning by antiasthmatics, accidental (unintentional)
  Poisoning by antiasthmatics NOS
- 7th **T48.6X2** Poisoning by antiasthmatics, intentional self-harm [HCC][Rx][ESR][COM]
- 7th **T48.6X3** Poisoning by antiasthmatics, assault
- 7th **T48.6X4** Poisoning by antiasthmatics, undetermined
- 7th **T48.6X5** Adverse effect of antiasthmatics [UPD]
- 7th **T48.6X6** Underdosing of antiasthmatics [UPD]
  AHA: 2024,1Q,23

5th **T48.9** Poisoning by, adverse effect of and underdosing of other and unspecified agents primarily acting on the respiratory system

6th **T48.90** Poisoning by, adverse effect of and underdosing of unspecified agents primarily acting on the respiratory system
- 7th **T48.901** Poisoning by unspecified agents primarily acting on the respiratory system, accidental (unintentional)
- 7th **T48.902** Poisoning by unspecified agents primarily acting on the respiratory system, intentional self-harm [HCC][Rx][ESR][COM]
- 7th **T48.903** Poisoning by unspecified agents primarily acting on the respiratory system, assault
- 7th **T48.904** Poisoning by unspecified agents primarily acting on the respiratory system, undetermined
- 7th **T48.905** Adverse effect of unspecified agents primarily acting on the respiratory system [UPD]
- 7th **T48.906** Underdosing of unspecified agents primarily acting on the respiratory system [UPD]

6th **T48.99** Poisoning by, adverse effect of and underdosing of other agents primarily acting on the respiratory system
- 7th **T48.991** Poisoning by other agents primarily acting on the respiratory system, accidental (unintentional)
- 7th **T48.992** Poisoning by other agents primarily acting on the respiratory system, intentional self-harm [HCC][Rx][ESR][COM]
- 7th **T48.993** Poisoning by other agents primarily acting on the respiratory system, assault
- 7th **T48.994** Poisoning by other agents primarily acting on the respiratory system, undetermined
- 7th **T48.995** Adverse effect of other agents primarily acting on the respiratory system [UPD]
- 7th **T48.996** Underdosing of other agents primarily acting on the respiratory system [UPD]

4th **T49** Poisoning by, adverse effect of and underdosing of topical agents primarily affecting skin and mucous membrane and by ophthalmological, otorhinolaryngological and dental drugs
INCLUDES poisoning by, adverse effect of and underdosing of glucocorticoids, topically used

The appropriate 7th character is to be added to each code from category T49.
- A initial encounter
- D subsequent encounter
- S sequela

5th **T49.0** Poisoning by, adverse effect of and underdosing of local antifungal, anti-infective and anti-inflammatory drugs

6th **T49.0X** Poisoning by, adverse effect of and underdosing of local antifungal, anti-infective and anti-inflammatory drugs
- 7th **T49.0X1** Poisoning by local antifungal, anti-infective and anti-inflammatory drugs, accidental (unintentional)
  Poisoning by local antifungal, anti-infective and anti-inflammatory drugs NOS
- 7th **T49.0X2** Poisoning by local antifungal, anti-infective and anti-inflammatory drugs, intentional self-harm [HCC][Rx][ESR][COM]
- 7th **T49.0X3** Poisoning by local antifungal, anti-infective and anti-inflammatory drugs, assault
- 7th **T49.0X4** Poisoning by local antifungal, anti-infective and anti-inflammatory drugs, undetermined
- 7th **T49.0X5** Adverse effect of local antifungal, anti-infective and anti-inflammatory drugs [UPD]
- 7th **T49.0X6** Underdosing of local antifungal, anti-infective and anti-inflammatory drugs [UPD]

5th **T49.1** Poisoning by, adverse effect of and underdosing of antipruritics

6th **T49.1X** Poisoning by, adverse effect of and underdosing of antipruritics
- 7th **T49.1X1** Poisoning by antipruritics, accidental (unintentional)
  Poisoning by antipruritics NOS
- 7th **T49.1X2** Poisoning by antipruritics, intentional self-harm [HCC][Rx][ESR][COM]
- 7th **T49.1X3** Poisoning by antipruritics, assault
- 7th **T49.1X4** Poisoning by antipruritics, undetermined
- 7th **T49.1X5** Adverse effect of antipruritics [UPD]
- 7th **T49.1X6** Underdosing of antipruritics [UPD]

5th **T49.2** Poisoning by, adverse effect of and underdosing of local astringents and local detergents

6th **T49.2X** Poisoning by, adverse effect of and underdosing of local astringents and local detergents
- 7th **T49.2X1** Poisoning by local astringents and local detergents, accidental (unintentional)
  Poisoning by local astringents and local detergents NOS
- 7th **T49.2X2** Poisoning by local astringents and local detergents, intentional self-harm [HCC][Rx][ESR][COM]
- 7th **T49.2X3** Poisoning by local astringents and local detergents, assault
- 7th **T49.2X4** Poisoning by local astringents and local detergents, undetermined
- 7th **T49.2X5** Adverse effect of local astringents and local detergents [UPD]
- 7th **T49.2X6** Underdosing of local astringents and local detergents [UPD]

5th **T49.3** Poisoning by, adverse effect of and underdosing of emollients, demulcents and protectants

6th **T49.3X** Poisoning by, adverse effect of and underdosing of emollients, demulcents and protectants
- 7th **T49.3X1** Poisoning by emollients, demulcents and protectants, accidental (unintentional)
  Poisoning by emollients, demulcents and protectants NOS
- 7th **T49.3X2** Poisoning by emollients, demulcents and protectants, intentional self-harm [HCC][Rx][ESR][COM]
- 7th **T49.3X3** Poisoning by emollients, demulcents and protectants, assault

---

[HCC] CMS-HCC [Rx] Rx HCC [ESR] ESRD HCC [COM] Commercial HCC [N] Newborn: 0 [P] Pediatric: 0-17 [M] Maternity: 9-64 [A] Adult: 15-124

Chapter 19. Injury, Poisoning and Certain Other Consequences of External Causes

- T49.3X4 Poisoning by emollients, demulcents and protectants, **undetermined**
- T49.3X5 **Adverse effect** of emollients, demulcents and protectants
- T49.3X6 **Underdosing** of emollients, demulcents and protectants

- T49.4 Poisoning by, adverse effect of and underdosing of keratolytics, keratoplastics, and other hair treatment drugs and preparations
  - T49.4X Poisoning by, adverse effect of and underdosing of **keratolytics, keratoplastics, and other hair treatment drugs and preparations**
    - T49.4X1 Poisoning by keratolytics, keratoplastics, and other hair treatment drugs and preparations, **accidental** (unintentional)
      Poisoning by keratolytics, keratoplastics, and other hair treatment drugs and preparations NOS
    - T49.4X2 Poisoning by keratolytics, keratoplastics, and other hair treatment drugs and preparations, **intentional self-harm**
    - T49.4X3 Poisoning by keratolytics, keratoplastics, and other hair treatment drugs and preparations, **assault**
    - T49.4X4 Poisoning by keratolytics, keratoplastics, and other hair treatment drugs and preparations, **undetermined**
    - T49.4X5 **Adverse effect** of keratolytics, keratoplastics, and other hair treatment drugs and preparations
    - T49.4X6 **Underdosing** of keratolytics, keratoplastics, and other hair treatment drugs and preparations

- T49.5 Poisoning by, adverse effect of and underdosing of ophthalmological drugs and preparations
  - T49.5X Poisoning by, adverse effect of and underdosing of **ophthalmological drugs and preparations**
    - T49.5X1 Poisoning by ophthalmological drugs and preparations, **accidental** (unintentional)
      Poisoning by ophthalmological drugs and preparations NOS
    - T49.5X2 Poisoning by ophthalmological drugs and preparations, **intentional self-harm**
    - T49.5X3 Poisoning by ophthalmological drugs and preparations, **assault**
    - T49.5X4 Poisoning by ophthalmological drugs and preparations, **undetermined**
    - T49.5X5 **Adverse effect** of ophthalmological drugs and preparations
    - T49.5X6 **Underdosing** of ophthalmological drugs and preparations

- T49.6 Poisoning by, adverse effect of and underdosing of otorhinolaryngological drugs and preparations
  - T49.6X Poisoning by, adverse effect of and underdosing of **otorhinolaryngological drugs and preparations**
    - T49.6X1 Poisoning by otorhinolaryngological drugs and preparations, **accidental** (unintentional)
      Poisoning by otorhinolaryngological drugs and preparations NOS
    - T49.6X2 Poisoning by otorhinolaryngological drugs and preparations, **intentional self-harm**
    - T49.6X3 Poisoning by otorhinolaryngological drugs and preparations, **assault**
    - T49.6X4 Poisoning by otorhinolaryngological drugs and preparations, **undetermined**
    - T49.6X5 **Adverse effect** of otorhinolaryngological drugs and preparations
    - T49.6X6 **Underdosing** of otorhinolaryngological drugs and preparations

- T49.7 Poisoning by, adverse effect of and underdosing of dental drugs, topically applied
  - T49.7X Poisoning by, adverse effect of and underdosing of **dental drugs, topically applied**
    - T49.7X1 Poisoning by dental drugs, topically applied, **accidental** (unintentional)
      Poisoning by dental drugs, topically applied NOS
    - T49.7X2 Poisoning by dental drugs, topically applied, **intentional self-harm**
    - T49.7X3 Poisoning by dental drugs, topically applied, **assault**
    - T49.7X4 Poisoning by dental drugs, topically applied, **undetermined**
    - T49.7X5 **Adverse effect** of dental drugs, topically applied
    - T49.7X6 **Underdosing** of dental drugs, topically applied

- T49.8 Poisoning by, adverse effect of and underdosing of other topical agents
  Poisoning by, adverse effect of and underdosing of spermicides
  - T49.8X Poisoning by, adverse effect of and underdosing of **other topical agents**
    - T49.8X1 Poisoning by other topical agents, **accidental** (unintentional)
      Poisoning by other topical agents NOS
    - T49.8X2 Poisoning by other topical agents, **intentional self-harm**
    - T49.8X3 Poisoning by other topical agents, **assault**
    - T49.8X4 Poisoning by other topical agents, **undetermined**
    - T49.8X5 **Adverse effect** of other topical agents
    - T49.8X6 **Underdosing** of other topical agents

- T49.9 Poisoning by, adverse effect of and underdosing of unspecified topical agent
  - T49.91 Poisoning by unspecified topical agent, **accidental** (unintentional)
  - T49.92 Poisoning by unspecified topical agent, **intentional self-harm**
  - T49.93 Poisoning by unspecified topical agent, **assault**
  - T49.94 Poisoning by unspecified topical agent, **undetermined**
  - T49.95 **Adverse effect** of unspecified topical agent
  - T49.96 **Underdosing** of unspecified topical agent

- T50 Poisoning by, adverse effect of and underdosing of diuretics and other and unspecified drugs, medicaments and biological substances

  The appropriate 7th character is to be added to each code from category T50.
  - A initial encounter
  - D subsequent encounter
  - S sequela

  - T50.0 Poisoning by, adverse effect of and underdosing of mineralocorticoids and their antagonists
    - T50.0X Poisoning by, adverse effect of and underdosing of **mineralocorticoids** and their antagonists
      - T50.0X1 Poisoning by mineralocorticoids and their antagonists, **accidental** (unintentional)
        Poisoning by mineralocorticoids and their antagonists NOS
      - T50.0X2 Poisoning by mineralocorticoids and their antagonists, **intentional self-harm**
      - T50.0X3 Poisoning by mineralocorticoids and their antagonists, **assault**
      - T50.0X4 Poisoning by mineralocorticoids and their antagonists, **undetermined**
      - T50.0X5 **Adverse effect** of mineralocorticoids and their antagonists
      - T50.0X6 **Underdosing** of mineralocorticoids and their antagonists

  - T50.1 Poisoning by, adverse effect of and underdosing of loop [high-ceiling] diuretics
    - T50.1X Poisoning by, adverse effect of and underdosing of **loop [high-ceiling] diuretics**
      - T50.1X1 Poisoning by loop [high-ceiling] diuretics, **accidental** (unintentional)
        Poisoning by loop [high-ceiling] diuretics NOS
      - T50.1X2 Poisoning by loop [high-ceiling] diuretics, **intentional self-harm**
      - T50.1X3 Poisoning by loop [high-ceiling] diuretics, **assault**
      - T50.1X4 Poisoning by loop [high-ceiling] diuretics, **undetermined**

Additional Character Required | Placeholder Alert | Manifestation | Unspecified Dx | QPP | UPD Unacceptable PDx

- ✓7th **T50.1X5** Adverse effect of loop [high-ceiling] diuretics [UPD]
- ✓7th **T50.1X6** Underdosing of loop [high-ceiling] diuretics [UPD]
- ✓5th **T50.2** Poisoning by, adverse effect of and underdosing of carbonic-anhydrase inhibitors, benzothiadiazides and other diuretics
  - Poisoning by, adverse effect of and underdosing of acetazolamide
  - ✓6th **T50.2X** Poisoning by, adverse effect of and underdosing of carbonic-anhydrase inhibitors, benzothiadiazides and other diuretics
    - ✓7th **T50.2X1** Poisoning by carbonic-anhydrase inhibitors, benzothiadiazides and other diuretics, accidental (unintentional)
      - Poisoning by carbonic-anhydrase inhibitors, benzothiadiazides and other diuretics NOS
    - ✓7th **T50.2X2** Poisoning by carbonic-anhydrase inhibitors, benzothiadiazides and other diuretics, intentional self-harm [HCC] [Rx] [ESR] [COM]
    - ✓7th **T50.2X3** Poisoning by carbonic-anhydrase inhibitors, benzothiadiazides and other diuretics, assault
    - ✓7th **T50.2X4** Poisoning by carbonic-anhydrase inhibitors, benzothiadiazides and other diuretics, undetermined
    - ✓7th **T50.2X5** Adverse effect of carbonic-anhydrase inhibitors, benzothiadiazides and other diuretics [UPD]
    - ✓7th **T50.2X6** Underdosing of carbonic-anhydrase inhibitors, benzothiadiazides and other diuretics [UPD]
- ✓5th **T50.3** Poisoning by, adverse effect of and underdosing of electrolytic, caloric and water-balance agents
  - Poisoning by, adverse effect of and underdosing of oral rehydration salts
  - ✓6th **T50.3X** Poisoning by, adverse effect of and underdosing of electrolytic, caloric and water-balance agents
    - ✓7th **T50.3X1** Poisoning by electrolytic, caloric and water-balance agents, accidental (unintentional)
      - Poisoning by electrolytic, caloric and water-balance agents NOS
    - ✓7th **T50.3X2** Poisoning by electrolytic, caloric and water-balance agents, intentional self-harm [HCC] [Rx] [ESR] [COM]
    - ✓7th **T50.3X3** Poisoning by electrolytic, caloric and water-balance agents, assault
    - ✓7th **T50.3X4** Poisoning by electrolytic, caloric and water-balance agents, undetermined
    - ✓7th **T50.3X5** Adverse effect of electrolytic, caloric and water-balance agents [UPD]
      - AHA: 2022,2Q,10
    - ✓7th **T50.3X6** Underdosing of electrolytic, caloric and water-balance agents [UPD]
- ✓5th **T50.4** Poisoning by, adverse effect of and underdosing of drugs affecting uric acid metabolism
  - ✓6th **T50.4X** Poisoning by, adverse effect of and underdosing of drugs affecting uric acid metabolism
    - ✓7th **T50.4X1** Poisoning by drugs affecting uric acid metabolism, accidental (unintentional)
      - Poisoning by drugs affecting uric acid metabolism NOS
    - ✓7th **T50.4X2** Poisoning by drugs affecting uric acid metabolism, intentional self-harm [HCC] [Rx] [ESR] [COM]
    - ✓7th **T50.4X3** Poisoning by drugs affecting uric acid metabolism, assault
    - ✓7th **T50.4X4** Poisoning by drugs affecting uric acid metabolism, undetermined
    - ✓7th **T50.4X5** Adverse effect of drugs affecting uric acid metabolism [UPD]
    - ✓7th **T50.4X6** Underdosing of drugs affecting uric acid metabolism [UPD]
- ✓5th **T50.5** Poisoning by, adverse effect of and underdosing of appetite depressants
  - ✓6th **T50.5X** Poisoning by, adverse effect of and underdosing of appetite depressants
    - ✓7th **T50.5X1** Poisoning by appetite depressants, accidental (unintentional)
      - Poisoning by appetite depressants NOS
    - ✓7th **T50.5X2** Poisoning by appetite depressants, intentional self-harm [HCC] [Rx] [ESR] [COM]
    - ✓7th **T50.5X3** Poisoning by appetite depressants, assault
    - ✓7th **T50.5X4** Poisoning by appetite depressants, undetermined
    - ✓7th **T50.5X5** Adverse effect of appetite depressants [UPD]
    - ✓7th **T50.5X6** Underdosing of appetite depressants [UPD]
- ✓5th **T50.6** Poisoning by, adverse effect of and underdosing of antidotes and chelating agents
  - Poisoning by, adverse effect of and underdosing of alcohol deterrents
  - ✓6th **T50.6X** Poisoning by, adverse effect of and underdosing of antidotes and chelating agents
    - ✓7th **T50.6X1** Poisoning by antidotes and chelating agents, accidental (unintentional)
      - Poisoning by antidotes and chelating agents NOS
    - ✓7th **T50.6X2** Poisoning by antidotes and chelating agents, intentional self-harm [HCC] [Rx] [ESR] [COM]
    - ✓7th **T50.6X3** Poisoning by antidotes and chelating agents, assault
    - ✓7th **T50.6X4** Poisoning by antidotes and chelating agents, undetermined
    - ✓7th **T50.6X5** Adverse effect of antidotes and chelating agents [UPD]
    - ✓7th **T50.6X6** Underdosing of antidotes and chelating agents [UPD]
- ✓5th **T50.7** Poisoning by, adverse effect of and underdosing of analeptics and opioid receptor antagonists
  - ✓6th **T50.7X** Poisoning by, adverse effect of and underdosing of analeptics and opioid receptor antagonists
    - ✓7th **T50.7X1** Poisoning by analeptics and opioid receptor antagonists, accidental (unintentional)
      - Poisoning by analeptics and opioid receptor antagonists NOS
    - ✓7th **T50.7X2** Poisoning by analeptics and opioid receptor antagonists, intentional self-harm [HCC] [Rx] [ESR] [COM]
    - ✓7th **T50.7X3** Poisoning by analeptics and opioid receptor antagonists, assault
    - ✓7th **T50.7X4** Poisoning by analeptics and opioid receptor antagonists, undetermined
    - ✓7th **T50.7X5** Adverse effect of analeptics and opioid receptor antagonists [UPD]
    - ✓7th **T50.7X6** Underdosing of analeptics and opioid receptor antagonists [UPD]
- ✓5th **T50.8** Poisoning by, adverse effect of and underdosing of diagnostic agents
  - ✓6th **T50.8X** Poisoning by, adverse effect of and underdosing of diagnostic agents
    - ✓7th **T50.8X1** Poisoning by diagnostic agents, accidental (unintentional)
      - Poisoning by diagnostic agents NOS
    - ✓7th **T50.8X2** Poisoning by diagnostic agents, intentional self-harm [HCC] [Rx] [ESR] [COM]
    - ✓7th **T50.8X3** Poisoning by diagnostic agents, assault
    - ✓7th **T50.8X4** Poisoning by diagnostic agents, undetermined
    - ✓7th **T50.8X5** Adverse effect of diagnostic agents [UPD]
      - AHA: 2023,3Q,4; 2022,4Q,33; 2021,3Q,9-10
    - ✓7th **T50.8X6** Underdosing of diagnostic agents [UPD]
- ✓5th **T50.A** Poisoning by, adverse effect of and underdosing of bacterial vaccines
  - ✓6th **T50.A1** Poisoning by, adverse effect of and underdosing of pertussis vaccine, including combinations with a pertussis component
    - ✓7th **T50.A11** Poisoning by pertussis vaccine, including combinations with a pertussis component, accidental (unintentional)
    - ✓7th **T50.A12** Poisoning by pertussis vaccine, including combinations with a pertussis component, intentional self-harm [HCC] [Rx] [ESR] [COM]
    - ✓7th **T50.A13** Poisoning by pertussis vaccine, including combinations with a pertussis component, assault
    - ✓7th **T50.A14** Poisoning by pertussis vaccine, including combinations with a pertussis component, undetermined

- ✓7th **T50.A15** Adverse effect of pertussis vaccine, including combinations with a pertussis component [UPD]
- ✓7th **T50.A16** Underdosing of pertussis vaccine, including combinations with a pertussis component [UPD]
- ✓6th **T50.A2** Poisoning by, adverse effect of and underdosing of mixed bacterial vaccines without a pertussis component
  - ✓7th **T50.A21** Poisoning by mixed bacterial vaccines without a pertussis component, accidental (unintentional)
  - ✓7th **T50.A22** Poisoning by mixed bacterial vaccines without a pertussis component, intentional self-harm [HCC] [Rx] [ESR] [COM]
  - ✓7th **T50.A23** Poisoning by mixed bacterial vaccines without a pertussis component, assault
  - ✓7th **T50.A24** Poisoning by mixed bacterial vaccines without a pertussis component, undetermined
  - ✓7th **T50.A25** Adverse effect of mixed bacterial vaccines without a pertussis component [UPD]
  - ✓7th **T50.A26** Underdosing of mixed bacterial vaccines without a pertussis component [UPD]
- ✓6th **T50.A9** Poisoning by, adverse effect of and underdosing of other bacterial vaccines
  - ✓7th **T50.A91** Poisoning by other bacterial vaccines, accidental (unintentional)
  - ✓7th **T50.A92** Poisoning by other bacterial vaccines, intentional self-harm [HCC] [Rx] [ESR] [COM]
  - ✓7th **T50.A93** Poisoning by other bacterial vaccines, assault
  - ✓7th **T50.A94** Poisoning by other bacterial vaccines, undetermined
  - ✓7th **T50.A95** Adverse effect of other bacterial vaccines [UPD]
  - ✓7th **T50.A96** Underdosing of other bacterial vaccines [UPD]
- ✓5th **T50.B** Poisoning by, adverse effect of and underdosing of viral vaccines
  - ✓6th **T50.B1** Poisoning by, adverse effect of and underdosing of smallpox vaccines
    - ✓7th **T50.B11** Poisoning by smallpox vaccines, accidental (unintentional)
    - ✓7th **T50.B12** Poisoning by smallpox vaccines, intentional self-harm [HCC] [Rx] [ESR] [COM]
    - ✓7th **T50.B13** Poisoning by smallpox vaccines, assault
    - ✓7th **T50.B14** Poisoning by smallpox vaccines, undetermined
    - ✓7th **T50.B15** Adverse effect of smallpox vaccines [UPD]
    - ✓7th **T50.B16** Underdosing of smallpox vaccines [UPD]
  - ✓6th **T50.B9** Poisoning by, adverse effect of and underdosing of other viral vaccines
    - ✓7th **T50.B91** Poisoning by other viral vaccines, accidental (unintentional)
    - ✓7th **T50.B92** Poisoning by other viral vaccines, intentional self-harm [HCC] [Rx] [ESR] [COM]
    - ✓7th **T50.B93** Poisoning by other viral vaccines, assault
    - ✓7th **T50.B94** Poisoning by other viral vaccines, undetermined
    - ✓7th **T50.B95** Adverse effect of other viral vaccines [UPD]
      - AHA: 2021,1Q,43
    - ✓7th **T50.B96** Underdosing of other viral vaccines [UPD]
- ✓5th **T50.Z** Poisoning by, adverse effect of and underdosing of other vaccines and biological substances
  - ✓6th **T50.Z1** Poisoning by, adverse effect of and underdosing of immunoglobulin
    - ✓7th **T50.Z11** Poisoning by immunoglobulin, accidental (unintentional)
    - ✓7th **T50.Z12** Poisoning by immunoglobulin, intentional self-harm [HCC] [Rx] [ESR] [COM]
    - ✓7th **T50.Z13** Poisoning by immunoglobulin, assault
    - ✓7th **T50.Z14** Poisoning by immunoglobulin, undetermined
    - ✓7th **T50.Z15** Adverse effect of immunoglobulin [UPD]
    - ✓7th **T50.Z16** Underdosing of immunoglobulin [UPD]
  - ✓6th **T50.Z9** Poisoning by, adverse effect of and underdosing of other vaccines and biological substances
    - ✓7th **T50.Z91** Poisoning by other vaccines and biological substances, accidental (unintentional)
    - ✓7th **T50.Z92** Poisoning by other vaccines and biological substances, intentional self-harm [HCC] [Rx] [ESR] [COM]
    - ✓7th **T50.Z93** Poisoning by other vaccines and biological substances, assault
    - ✓7th **T50.Z94** Poisoning by other vaccines and biological substances, undetermined
    - ✓7th **T50.Z95** Adverse effect of other vaccines and biological substances [UPD]
      - AHA: 2020,1Q,18
    - ✓7th **T50.Z96** Underdosing of other vaccines and biological substances [UPD]
- ✓5th **T50.9** Poisoning by, adverse effect of and underdosing of other and unspecified drugs, medicaments and biological substances
  - ✓6th **T50.90** Poisoning by, adverse effect of and underdosing of unspecified drugs, medicaments and biological substances
    - ✓7th **T50.901** Poisoning by unspecified drugs, medicaments and biological substances, accidental (unintentional)
    - ✓7th **T50.902** Poisoning by unspecified drugs, medicaments and biological substances, intentional self-harm [HCC] [Rx] [ESR] [COM]
    - ✓7th **T50.903** Poisoning by unspecified drugs, medicaments and biological substances, assault
    - ✓7th **T50.904** Poisoning by unspecified drugs, medicaments and biological substances, undetermined
    - ✓7th **T50.905** Adverse effect of unspecified drugs, medicaments and biological substances
    - ✓7th **T50.906** Underdosing of unspecified drugs, medicaments and biological substances
  - ✓6th **T50.91** Poisoning by, adverse effect of and underdosing of multiple unspecified drugs, medicaments and biological substances
    - Multiple drug ingestion NOS
    - Code also any specific drugs, medicaments and biological substances
    - ✓7th **T50.911** Poisoning by multiple unspecified drugs, medicaments and biological substances, accidental (unintentional)
    - ✓7th **T50.912** Poisoning by multiple unspecified drugs, medicaments and biological substances, intentional self-harm [HCC] [Rx] [ESR] [COM]
    - ✓7th **T50.913** Poisoning by multiple unspecified drugs, medicaments and biological substances, assault
    - ✓7th **T50.914** Poisoning by multiple unspecified drugs, medicaments and biological substances, undetermined
    - ✓7th **T50.915** Adverse effect of multiple unspecified drugs, medicaments and biological substances [UPD]
    - ✓7th **T50.916** Underdosing of multiple unspecified drugs, medicaments and biological substances [UPD]
  - ✓6th **T50.99** Poisoning by, adverse effect of and underdosing of other drugs, medicaments and biological substances
    - ✓7th **T50.991** Poisoning by other drugs, medicaments and biological substances, accidental (unintentional)
    - ✓7th **T50.992** Poisoning by other drugs, medicaments and biological substances, intentional self-harm [HCC] [Rx] [ESR] [COM]
    - ✓7th **T50.993** Poisoning by other drugs, medicaments and biological substances, assault
    - ✓7th **T50.994** Poisoning by other drugs, medicaments and biological substances, undetermined
    - ✓7th **T50.995** Adverse effect of other drugs, medicaments and biological substances
      - AHA: 2023,3Q,4
    - ✓7th **T50.996** Underdosing of other drugs, medicaments and biological substances

Toxic effects of substances chiefly nonmedicinal as to source (T51-T65)

NOTE When no intent is indicated code to accidental. Undetermined intent is only for use when there is specific documentation in the record that the intent of the toxic effect cannot be determined.

Use additional code(s) for all associated manifestations of toxic effect, such as:
 personal history of foreign body fully removed (Z87.821)
 respiratory conditions due to external agents (J60-J70)
 to identify any retained foreign body, if applicable (Z18.-)

EXCLUDES 1 contact with and (suspected) exposure to toxic substances (Z77.-)

AHA: 2017,1Q,39-40

T51 Toxic effect of alcohol

The appropriate 7th character is to be added to each code from category T51.
- A initial encounter
- D subsequent encounter
- S sequela

T51.0 Toxic effect of ethanol
Toxic effect of ethyl alcohol

EXCLUDES 2 acute alcohol intoxication or "hangover" effects (F10.129, F10.229, F10.929)
 drunkenness (F10.129, F10.229, F10.929)
 pathological alcohol intoxication (F10.129, F10.229, F10.929)

T51.0X Toxic effect of ethanol
- T51.0X1 Toxic effect of ethanol, accidental (unintentional)
  Toxic effect of ethanol NOS
- T51.0X2 Toxic effect of ethanol, intentional self-harm
- T51.0X3 Toxic effect of ethanol, assault
- T51.0X4 Toxic effect of ethanol, undetermined

T51.1 Toxic effect of methanol
Toxic effect of methyl alcohol

T51.1X Toxic effect of methanol
- T51.1X1 Toxic effect of methanol, accidental (unintentional)
  Toxic effect of methanol NOS
- T51.1X2 Toxic effect of methanol, intentional self-harm
- T51.1X3 Toxic effect of methanol, assault
- T51.1X4 Toxic effect of methanol, undetermined

T51.2 Toxic effect of 2-Propanol
Toxic effect of isopropyl alcohol

T51.2X Toxic effect of 2-Propanol
- T51.2X1 Toxic effect of 2-Propanol, accidental (unintentional)
  Toxic effect of 2-Propanol NOS
- T51.2X2 Toxic effect of 2-Propanol, intentional self-harm
- T51.2X3 Toxic effect of 2-Propanol, assault
- T51.2X4 Toxic effect of 2-Propanol, undetermined

T51.3 Toxic effect of fusel oil
Toxic effect of amyl alcohol
Toxic effect of butyl [1-butanol] alcohol
Toxic effect of propyl [1-propanol] alcohol

T51.3X Toxic effect of fusel oil
- T51.3X1 Toxic effect of fusel oil, accidental (unintentional)
  Toxic effect of fusel oil NOS
- T51.3X2 Toxic effect of fusel oil, intentional self-harm
- T51.3X3 Toxic effect of fusel oil, assault
- T51.3X4 Toxic effect of fusel oil, undetermined

T51.8 Toxic effect of other alcohols

T51.8X Toxic effect of other alcohols
- T51.8X1 Toxic effect of other alcohols, accidental (unintentional)
  Toxic effect of other alcohols NOS
- T51.8X2 Toxic effect of other alcohols, intentional self-harm
- T51.8X3 Toxic effect of other alcohols, assault
- T51.8X4 Toxic effect of other alcohols, undetermined

T51.9 Toxic effect of unspecified alcohol
- T51.91 Toxic effect of unspecified alcohol, accidental (unintentional)
- T51.92 Toxic effect of unspecified alcohol, intentional self-harm
- T51.93 Toxic effect of unspecified alcohol, assault
- T51.94 Toxic effect of unspecified alcohol, undetermined

T52 Toxic effect of organic solvents

EXCLUDES 1 halogen derivatives of aliphatic and aromatic hydrocarbons (T53.-)

The appropriate 7th character is to be added to each code from category T52.
- A initial encounter
- D subsequent encounter
- S sequela

T52.0 Toxic effects of petroleum products
Toxic effects of ether petroleum
Toxic effects of gasoline [petrol]
Toxic effects of kerosene [paraffin oil]
Toxic effects of naphtha petroleum
Toxic effects of paraffin wax
Toxic effects of spirit petroleum

T52.0X Toxic effects of petroleum products
- T52.0X1 Toxic effect of petroleum products, accidental (unintentional)
  Toxic effects of petroleum products NOS
- T52.0X2 Toxic effect of petroleum products, intentional self-harm
- T52.0X3 Toxic effect of petroleum products, assault
- T52.0X4 Toxic effect of petroleum products, undetermined

T52.1 Toxic effects of benzene

EXCLUDES 1 homologues of benzene (T52.2)
 nitroderivatives and aminoderivatives of benzene and its homologues (T65.3)

T52.1X Toxic effects of benzene
- T52.1X1 Toxic effect of benzene, accidental (unintentional)
  Toxic effects of benzene NOS
- T52.1X2 Toxic effect of benzene, intentional self-harm
- T52.1X3 Toxic effect of benzene, assault
- T52.1X4 Toxic effect of benzene, undetermined

T52.2 Toxic effects of homologues of benzene
Toxic effects of toluene [methylbenzene]
Toxic effects of xylene [dimethylbenzene]

T52.2X Toxic effects of homologues of benzene
- T52.2X1 Toxic effect of homologues of benzene, accidental (unintentional)
  Toxic effects of homologues of benzene NOS
- T52.2X2 Toxic effect of homologues of benzene, intentional self-harm
- T52.2X3 Toxic effect of homologues of benzene, assault
- T52.2X4 Toxic effect of homologues of benzene, undetermined

T52.3 Toxic effects of glycols

T52.3X Toxic effects of glycols
- T52.3X1 Toxic effect of glycols, accidental (unintentional)
  Toxic effects of glycols NOS
- T52.3X2 Toxic effect of glycols, intentional self-harm
- T52.3X3 Toxic effect of glycols, assault
- T52.3X4 Toxic effect of glycols, undetermined

T52.4 Toxic effects of ketones

T52.4X Toxic effects of ketones
- T52.4X1 Toxic effect of ketones, accidental (unintentional)
  Toxic effects of ketones NOS
- T52.4X2 Toxic effect of ketones, intentional self-harm
- T52.4X3 Toxic effect of ketones, assault
- T52.4X4 Toxic effect of ketones, undetermined

T52.8 Toxic effects of other organic solvents

T52.8X Toxic effects of other organic solvents
- T52.8X1 Toxic effect of other organic solvents, accidental (unintentional)
  Toxic effects of other organic solvents NOS
- T52.8X2 Toxic effect of other organic solvents, intentional self-harm [HCC] [Rx] [ESR] [COM]
- T52.8X3 Toxic effect of other organic solvents, assault
- T52.8X4 Toxic effect of other organic solvents, undetermined

T52.9 Toxic effects of unspecified organic solvent
- T52.91 Toxic effect of unspecified organic solvent, accidental (unintentional)
- T52.92 Toxic effect of unspecified organic solvent, intentional self-harm [HCC] [Rx] [ESR] [COM]
- T52.93 Toxic effect of unspecified organic solvent, assault
- T52.94 Toxic effect of unspecified organic solvent, undetermined

T53 Toxic effect of halogen derivatives of aliphatic and aromatic hydrocarbons

The appropriate 7th character is to be added to each code from category T53.
- A initial encounter
- D subsequent encounter
- S sequela

T53.0 Toxic effects of carbon tetrachloride
Toxic effects of tetrachloromethane

T53.0X Toxic effects of carbon tetrachloride
- T53.0X1 Toxic effect of carbon tetrachloride, accidental (unintentional)
  Toxic effects of carbon tetrachloride NOS
- T53.0X2 Toxic effect of carbon tetrachloride, intentional self-harm [HCC] [Rx] [ESR] [COM]
- T53.0X3 Toxic effect of carbon tetrachloride, assault
- T53.0X4 Toxic effect of carbon tetrachloride, undetermined

T53.1 Toxic effects of chloroform
Toxic effects of trichloromethane

T53.1X Toxic effects of chloroform
- T53.1X1 Toxic effect of chloroform, accidental (unintentional)
  Toxic effects of chloroform NOS
- T53.1X2 Toxic effect of chloroform, intentional self-harm [HCC] [Rx] [ESR] [COM]
- T53.1X3 Toxic effect of chloroform, assault
- T53.1X4 Toxic effect of chloroform, undetermined

T53.2 Toxic effects of trichloroethylene
Toxic effects of trichloroethene

T53.2X Toxic effects of trichloroethylene
- T53.2X1 Toxic effect of trichloroethylene, accidental (unintentional)
  Toxic effects of trichloroethylene NOS
- T53.2X2 Toxic effect of trichloroethylene, intentional self-harm [HCC] [Rx] [ESR] [COM]
- T53.2X3 Toxic effect of trichloroethylene, assault
- T53.2X4 Toxic effect of trichloroethylene, undetermined

T53.3 Toxic effects of tetrachloroethylene
Toxic effect of tetrachloroethene
Toxic effects of perchloroethylene

T53.3X Toxic effects of tetrachloroethylene
- T53.3X1 Toxic effect of tetrachloroethylene, accidental (unintentional)
  Toxic effects of tetrachloroethylene NOS
- T53.3X2 Toxic effect of tetrachloroethylene, intentional self-harm [HCC] [Rx] [ESR] [COM]
- T53.3X3 Toxic effect of tetrachloroethylene, assault
- T53.3X4 Toxic effect of tetrachloroethylene, undetermined

T53.4 Toxic effects of dichloromethane
Toxic effects of methylene chloride

T53.4X Toxic effects of dichloromethane
- T53.4X1 Toxic effect of dichloromethane, accidental (unintentional)
  Toxic effects of dichloromethane NOS
- T53.4X2 Toxic effect of dichloromethane, intentional self-harm [HCC] [Rx] [ESR] [COM]
- T53.4X3 Toxic effect of dichloromethane, assault
- T53.4X4 Toxic effect of dichloromethane, undetermined

T53.5 Toxic effects of chlorofluorocarbons

T53.5X Toxic effects of chlorofluorocarbons
- T53.5X1 Toxic effect of chlorofluorocarbons, accidental (unintentional)
  Toxic effects of chlorofluorocarbons NOS
- T53.5X2 Toxic effect of chlorofluorocarbons, intentional self-harm [HCC] [Rx] [ESR] [COM]
- T53.5X3 Toxic effect of chlorofluorocarbons, assault
- T53.5X4 Toxic effect of chlorofluorocarbons, undetermined

T53.6 Toxic effects of other halogen derivatives of aliphatic hydrocarbons

T53.6X Toxic effects of other halogen derivatives of aliphatic hydrocarbons
- T53.6X1 Toxic effect of other halogen derivatives of aliphatic hydrocarbons, accidental (unintentional)
  Toxic effects of other halogen derivatives of aliphatic hydrocarbons NOS
- T53.6X2 Toxic effect of other halogen derivatives of aliphatic hydrocarbons, intentional self-harm [HCC] [Rx] [ESR] [COM]
- T53.6X3 Toxic effect of other halogen derivatives of aliphatic hydrocarbons, assault
- T53.6X4 Toxic effect of other halogen derivatives of aliphatic hydrocarbons, undetermined

T53.7 Toxic effects of other halogen derivatives of aromatic hydrocarbons

T53.7X Toxic effects of other halogen derivatives of aromatic hydrocarbons
- T53.7X1 Toxic effect of other halogen derivatives of aromatic hydrocarbons, accidental (unintentional)
  Toxic effects of other halogen derivatives of aromatic hydrocarbons NOS
- T53.7X2 Toxic effect of other halogen derivatives of aromatic hydrocarbons, intentional self-harm [HCC] [Rx] [ESR] [COM]
- T53.7X3 Toxic effect of other halogen derivatives of aromatic hydrocarbons, assault
- T53.7X4 Toxic effect of other halogen derivatives of aromatic hydrocarbons, undetermined

T53.9 Toxic effects of unspecified halogen derivatives of aliphatic and aromatic hydrocarbons
- T53.91 Toxic effect of unspecified halogen derivatives of aliphatic and aromatic hydrocarbons, accidental (unintentional)
- T53.92 Toxic effect of unspecified halogen derivatives of aliphatic and aromatic hydrocarbons, intentional self-harm [HCC] [Rx] [ESR] [COM]
- T53.93 Toxic effect of unspecified halogen derivatives of aliphatic and aromatic hydrocarbons, assault
- T53.94 Toxic effect of unspecified halogen derivatives of aliphatic and aromatic hydrocarbons, undetermined

T54 Toxic effect of corrosive substances

The appropriate 7th character is to be added to each code from category T54.
- A initial encounter
- D subsequent encounter
- S sequela

T54.0 Toxic effects of phenol and phenol homologues

T54.0X Toxic effects of phenol and phenol homologues
- T54.0X1 Toxic effect of phenol and phenol homologues, accidental (unintentional)
  Toxic effects of phenol and phenol homologues NOS
- T54.0X2 Toxic effect of phenol and phenol homologues, intentional self-harm [HCC] [Rx] [ESR] [COM]

✓7th T54.0X3 Toxic effect of phenol and phenol homologues, assault
✓7th T54.0X4 Toxic effect of phenol and phenol homologues, undetermined

✓5th **T54.1 Toxic effects of other corrosive organic compounds**
  ✓6th T54.1X Toxic effects of other corrosive organic compounds
    ✓7th T54.1X1 Toxic effect of other corrosive organic compounds, accidental (unintentional)
        Toxic effects of other corrosive organic compounds NOS
    ✓7th T54.1X2 Toxic effect of other corrosive organic compounds, intentional self-harm [HCC] [Rx] [ESR] [COM]
    ✓7th T54.1X3 Toxic effect of other corrosive organic compounds, assault
    ✓7th T54.1X4 Toxic effect of other corrosive organic compounds, undetermined

✓5th **T54.2 Toxic effects of corrosive acids and acid-like substances**
    Toxic effects of hydrochloric acid
    Toxic effects of sulfuric acid
  ✓6th T54.2X Toxic effects of corrosive acids and acid-like substances
    ✓7th T54.2X1 Toxic effect of corrosive acids and acid-like substances, accidental (unintentional)
        Toxic effects of corrosive acids and acid-like substances NOS
    ✓7th T54.2X2 Toxic effect of corrosive acids and acid-like substances, intentional self-harm [HCC] [Rx] [ESR] [COM]
    ✓7th T54.2X3 Toxic effect of corrosive acids and acid-like substances, assault
    ✓7th T54.2X4 Toxic effect of corrosive acids and acid-like substances, undetermined

✓5th **T54.3 Toxic effects of corrosive alkalis and alkali-like substances**
    Toxic effects of potassium hydroxide
    Toxic effects of sodium hydroxide
  ✓6th T54.3X Toxic effects of corrosive alkalis and alkali-like substances
    ✓7th T54.3X1 Toxic effect of corrosive alkalis and alkali-like substances, accidental (unintentional)
        Toxic effects of corrosive alkalis and alkali-like substances NOS
    ✓7th T54.3X2 Toxic effect of corrosive alkalis and alkali-like substances, intentional self-harm [HCC] [Rx] [ESR] [COM]
    ✓7th T54.3X3 Toxic effect of corrosive alkalis and alkali-like substances, assault
    ✓7th T54.3X4 Toxic effect of corrosive alkalis and alkali-like substances, undetermined

✓5th **T54.9 Toxic effects of unspecified corrosive substance**
  ✓x7th T54.91 Toxic effect of unspecified corrosive substance, accidental (unintentional)
  ✓x7th T54.92 Toxic effect of unspecified corrosive substance, intentional self-harm [HCC] [Rx] [ESR] [COM]
  ✓x7th T54.93 Toxic effect of unspecified corrosive substance, assault
  ✓x7th T54.94 Toxic effect of unspecified corrosive substance, undetermined

✓4th **T55 Toxic effect of soaps and detergents**

> The appropriate 7th character is to be added to each code from category T55.
> A initial encounter
> D subsequent encounter
> S sequela

✓5th **T55.0 Toxic effect of soaps**
  ✓6th T55.0X Toxic effect of soaps
    ✓7th T55.0X1 Toxic effect of soaps, accidental (unintentional)
        Toxic effect of soaps NOS
    ✓7th T55.0X2 Toxic effect of soaps, intentional self-harm [HCC] [Rx] [ESR] [COM]
    ✓7th T55.0X3 Toxic effect of soaps, assault
    ✓7th T55.0X4 Toxic effect of soaps, undetermined

✓5th **T55.1 Toxic effect of detergents**
  ✓6th T55.1X Toxic effect of detergents
    ✓7th T55.1X1 Toxic effect of detergents, accidental (unintentional)
        Toxic effect of detergents NOS
    ✓7th T55.1X2 Toxic effect of detergents, intentional self-harm [HCC] [Rx] [ESR] [COM]
    ✓7th T55.1X3 Toxic effect of detergents, assault
    ✓7th T55.1X4 Toxic effect of detergents, undetermined

✓4th **T56 Toxic effect of metals**
  INCLUDES toxic effects of fumes and vapors of metals
            toxic effects of metals from all sources, except medicinal substances
  Use additional code to identify any retained metal foreign body, if applicable (Z18.0-, T18.1-)
  EXCLUDES 1 arsenic and its compounds (T57.0)
              manganese and its compounds (T57.2)

> The appropriate 7th character is to be added to each code from category T56.
> A initial encounter
> D subsequent encounter
> S sequela

✓5th **T56.0 Toxic effects of lead and its compounds**
  ✓6th T56.0X Toxic effects of lead and its compounds
    ✓7th T56.0X1 Toxic effect of lead and its compounds, accidental (unintentional)
        Toxic effects of lead and its compounds NOS
    ✓7th T56.0X2 Toxic effect of lead and its compounds, intentional self-harm [HCC] [Rx] [ESR] [COM]
    ✓7th T56.0X3 Toxic effect of lead and its compounds, assault
    ✓7th T56.0X4 Toxic effect of lead and its compounds, undetermined

✓5th **T56.1 Toxic effects of mercury and its compounds**
  ✓6th T56.1X Toxic effects of mercury and its compounds
    ✓7th T56.1X1 Toxic effect of mercury and its compounds, accidental (unintentional)
        Toxic effects of mercury and its compounds NOS
    ✓7th T56.1X2 Toxic effect of mercury and its compounds, intentional self-harm [HCC] [Rx] [ESR] [COM]
    ✓7th T56.1X3 Toxic effect of mercury and its compounds, assault
    ✓7th T56.1X4 Toxic effect of mercury and its compounds, undetermined

✓5th **T56.2 Toxic effects of chromium and its compounds**
  ✓6th T56.2X Toxic effects of chromium and its compounds
    ✓7th T56.2X1 Toxic effect of chromium and its compounds, accidental (unintentional)
        Toxic effects of chromium and its compounds NOS
    ✓7th T56.2X2 Toxic effect of chromium and its compounds, intentional self-harm [HCC] [Rx] [ESR] [COM]
    ✓7th T56.2X3 Toxic effect of chromium and its compounds, assault
    ✓7th T56.2X4 Toxic effect of chromium and its compounds, undetermined

✓5th **T56.3 Toxic effects of cadmium and its compounds**
  ✓6th T56.3X Toxic effects of cadmium and its compounds
    ✓7th T56.3X1 Toxic effect of cadmium and its compounds, accidental (unintentional)
        Toxic effects of cadmium and its compounds NOS
    ✓7th T56.3X2 Toxic effect of cadmium and its compounds, intentional self-harm [HCC] [Rx] [ESR] [COM]
    ✓7th T56.3X3 Toxic effect of cadmium and its compounds, assault
    ✓7th T56.3X4 Toxic effect of cadmium and its compounds, undetermined

- **T56.4** Toxic effects of copper and its compounds
  - **T56.4X** Toxic effects of copper and its compounds
    - **T56.4X1** Toxic effect of copper and its compounds, accidental (unintentional)
      Toxic effects of copper and its compounds NOS
    - **T56.4X2** Toxic effect of copper and its compounds, intentional self-harm
    - **T56.4X3** Toxic effect of copper and its compounds, assault
    - **T56.4X4** Toxic effect of copper and its compounds, undetermined
- **T56.5** Toxic effects of zinc and its compounds
  - **T56.5X** Toxic effects of zinc and its compounds
    - **T56.5X1** Toxic effect of zinc and its compounds, accidental (unintentional)
      Toxic effects of zinc and its compounds NOS
    - **T56.5X2** Toxic effect of zinc and its compounds, intentional self-harm
    - **T56.5X3** Toxic effect of zinc and its compounds, assault
    - **T56.5X4** Toxic effect of zinc and its compounds, undetermined
- **T56.6** Toxic effects of tin and its compounds
  - **T56.6X** Toxic effects of tin and its compounds
    - **T56.6X1** Toxic effect of tin and its compounds, accidental (unintentional)
      Toxic effects of tin and its compounds NOS
    - **T56.6X2** Toxic effect of tin and its compounds, intentional self-harm
    - **T56.6X3** Toxic effect of tin and its compounds, assault
    - **T56.6X4** Toxic effect of tin and its compounds, undetermined
- **T56.7** Toxic effects of beryllium and its compounds
  - **T56.7X** Toxic effects of beryllium and its compounds
    - **T56.7X1** Toxic effect of beryllium and its compounds, accidental (unintentional)
      Toxic effects of beryllium and its compounds NOS
    - **T56.7X2** Toxic effect of beryllium and its compounds, intentional self-harm
    - **T56.7X3** Toxic effect of beryllium and its compounds, assault
    - **T56.7X4** Toxic effect of beryllium and its compounds, undetermined
- **T56.8** Toxic effects of other metals
  - **T56.81** Toxic effect of thallium
    - **T56.811** Toxic effect of thallium, accidental (unintentional)
      Toxic effect of thallium NOS
    - **T56.812** Toxic effect of thallium, intentional self-harm
    - **T56.813** Toxic effect of thallium, assault
    - **T56.814** Toxic effect of thallium, undetermined
  - **T56.82** Toxic effect of gadolinium
    EXCLUDES 1 adverse effect of diagnostic agents (T50.8X5-)
    AHA: 2023,4Q,44-45
    - **T56.821** Toxic effect of gadolinium, accidental (unintentional)
      Toxic effect of gadolinium NOS
    - **T56.822** Toxic effect of gadolinium, intentional self-harm
    - **T56.823** Toxic effect of gadolinium, assault
    - **T56.824** Toxic effect of gadolinium, undetermined
  - **T56.89** Toxic effects of other metals
    - **T56.891** Toxic effect of other metals, accidental (unintentional)
      Toxic effects of other metals NOS
    - **T56.892** Toxic effect of other metals, intentional self-harm
    - **T56.893** Toxic effect of other metals, assault
    - **T56.894** Toxic effect of other metals, undetermined
- **T56.9** Toxic effects of unspecified metal
  - **T56.91** Toxic effect of unspecified metal, accidental (unintentional)
  - **T56.92** Toxic effect of unspecified metal, intentional self-harm
  - **T56.93** Toxic effect of unspecified metal, assault
  - **T56.94** Toxic effect of unspecified metal, undetermined
- **T57** Toxic effect of other inorganic substances

  The appropriate 7th character is to be added to each code from category T57.
  - A initial encounter
  - D subsequent encounter
  - S sequela

  - **T57.0** Toxic effect of arsenic and its compounds
    - **T57.0X** Toxic effect of arsenic and its compounds
      - **T57.0X1** Toxic effect of arsenic and its compounds, accidental (unintentional)
        Toxic effect of arsenic and its compounds NOS
      - **T57.0X2** Toxic effect of arsenic and its compounds, intentional self-harm
      - **T57.0X3** Toxic effect of arsenic and its compounds, assault
      - **T57.0X4** Toxic effect of arsenic and its compounds, undetermined
  - **T57.1** Toxic effect of phosphorus and its compounds
    EXCLUDES 1 organophosphate insecticides (T60.0)
    - **T57.1X** Toxic effect of phosphorus and its compounds
      - **T57.1X1** Toxic effect of phosphorus and its compounds, accidental (unintentional)
        Toxic effect of phosphorus and its compounds NOS
      - **T57.1X2** Toxic effect of phosphorus and its compounds, intentional self-harm
      - **T57.1X3** Toxic effect of phosphorus and its compounds, assault
      - **T57.1X4** Toxic effect of phosphorus and its compounds, undetermined
  - **T57.2** Toxic effect of manganese and its compounds
    - **T57.2X** Toxic effect of manganese and its compounds
      - **T57.2X1** Toxic effect of manganese and its compounds, accidental (unintentional)
        Toxic effect of manganese and its compounds NOS
      - **T57.2X2** Toxic effect of manganese and its compounds, intentional self-harm
      - **T57.2X3** Toxic effect of manganese and its compounds, assault
      - **T57.2X4** Toxic effect of manganese and its compounds, undetermined
  - **T57.3** Toxic effect of hydrogen cyanide
    - **T57.3X** Toxic effect of hydrogen cyanide
      - **T57.3X1** Toxic effect of hydrogen cyanide, accidental (unintentional)
        Toxic effect of hydrogen cyanide NOS
      - **T57.3X2** Toxic effect of hydrogen cyanide, intentional self-harm
      - **T57.3X3** Toxic effect of hydrogen cyanide, assault
      - **T57.3X4** Toxic effect of hydrogen cyanide, undetermined
  - **T57.8** Toxic effect of other specified inorganic substances
    - **T57.8X** Toxic effect of other specified inorganic substances
      - **T57.8X1** Toxic effect of other specified inorganic substances, accidental (unintentional)
        Toxic effect of other specified inorganic substances NOS
      - **T57.8X2** Toxic effect of other specified inorganic substances, intentional self-harm
      - **T57.8X3** Toxic effect of other specified inorganic substances, assault
      - **T57.8X4** Toxic effect of other specified inorganic substances, undetermined

T57.9 Toxic effect of unspecified inorganic substance
- T57.91 Toxic effect of unspecified inorganic substance, accidental (unintentional)
- T57.92 Toxic effect of unspecified inorganic substance, intentional self-harm
- T57.93 Toxic effect of unspecified inorganic substance, assault
- T57.94 Toxic effect of unspecified inorganic substance, undetermined

T58 Toxic effect of carbon monoxide
INCLUDES: asphyxiation from carbon monoxide
toxic effect of carbon monoxide from all sources

The appropriate 7th character is to be added to each code from category T58.
- A initial encounter
- D subsequent encounter
- S sequela

T58.0 Toxic effect of carbon monoxide from motor vehicle exhaust
Toxic effect of exhaust gas from gas engine
Toxic effect of exhaust gas from motor pump
- T58.01 Toxic effect of carbon monoxide from motor vehicle exhaust, accidental (unintentional)
- T58.02 Toxic effect of carbon monoxide from motor vehicle exhaust, intentional self-harm
- T58.03 Toxic effect of carbon monoxide from motor vehicle exhaust, assault
- T58.04 Toxic effect of carbon monoxide from motor vehicle exhaust, undetermined

T58.1 Toxic effect of carbon monoxide from utility gas
Toxic effect of acetylene
Toxic effect of gas NOS used for lighting, heating, cooking
Toxic effect of water gas
- T58.11 Toxic effect of carbon monoxide from utility gas, accidental (unintentional)
- T58.12 Toxic effect of carbon monoxide from utility gas, intentional self-harm
- T58.13 Toxic effect of carbon monoxide from utility gas, assault
- T58.14 Toxic effect of carbon monoxide from utility gas, undetermined

T58.2 Toxic effect of carbon monoxide from incomplete combustion of other domestic fuels
Toxic effect of carbon monoxide from incomplete combustion of coal, coke, kerosene, wood
- T58.2X Toxic effect of carbon monoxide from incomplete combustion of other domestic fuels
  - T58.2X1 Toxic effect of carbon monoxide from incomplete combustion of other domestic fuels, accidental (unintentional)
  - T58.2X2 Toxic effect of carbon monoxide from incomplete combustion of other domestic fuels, intentional self-harm
  - T58.2X3 Toxic effect of carbon monoxide from incomplete combustion of other domestic fuels, assault
  - T58.2X4 Toxic effect of carbon monoxide from incomplete combustion of other domestic fuels, undetermined

T58.8 Toxic effect of carbon monoxide from other source
Toxic effect of carbon monoxide from blast furnace gas
Toxic effect of carbon monoxide from fuels in industrial use
Toxic effect of carbon monoxide from kiln vapor
- T58.8X Toxic effect of carbon monoxide from other source
  - T58.8X1 Toxic effect of carbon monoxide from other source, accidental (unintentional)
  - T58.8X2 Toxic effect of carbon monoxide from other source, intentional self-harm
  - T58.8X3 Toxic effect of carbon monoxide from other source, assault
  - T58.8X4 Toxic effect of carbon monoxide from other source, undetermined

T58.9 Toxic effect of carbon monoxide from unspecified source
- T58.91 Toxic effect of carbon monoxide from unspecified source, accidental (unintentional)
- T58.92 Toxic effect of carbon monoxide from unspecified source, intentional self-harm
- T58.93 Toxic effect of carbon monoxide from unspecified source, assault
- T58.94 Toxic effect of carbon monoxide from unspecified source, undetermined

T59 Toxic effect of other gases, fumes and vapors
INCLUDES: aerosol propellants
EXCLUDES 1: chlorofluorocarbons (T53.5)

The appropriate 7th character is to be added to each code from category T59.
- A initial encounter
- D subsequent encounter
- S sequela

T59.0 Toxic effect of nitrogen oxides
- T59.0X Toxic effect of nitrogen oxides
  - T59.0X1 Toxic effect of nitrogen oxides, accidental (unintentional)
    Toxic effect of nitrogen oxides NOS
  - T59.0X2 Toxic effect of nitrogen oxides, intentional self-harm
  - T59.0X3 Toxic effect of nitrogen oxides, assault
  - T59.0X4 Toxic effect of nitrogen oxides, undetermined

T59.1 Toxic effect of sulfur dioxide
- T59.1X Toxic effect of sulfur dioxide
  - T59.1X1 Toxic effect of sulfur dioxide, accidental (unintentional)
    Toxic effect of sulfur dioxide NOS
  - T59.1X2 Toxic effect of sulfur dioxide, intentional self-harm
  - T59.1X3 Toxic effect of sulfur dioxide, assault
  - T59.1X4 Toxic effect of sulfur dioxide, undetermined

T59.2 Toxic effect of formaldehyde
- T59.2X Toxic effect of formaldehyde
  - T59.2X1 Toxic effect of formaldehyde, accidental (unintentional)
    Toxic effect of formaldehyde NOS
  - T59.2X2 Toxic effect of formaldehyde, intentional self-harm
  - T59.2X3 Toxic effect of formaldehyde, assault
  - T59.2X4 Toxic effect of formaldehyde, undetermined

T59.3 Toxic effect of lacrimogenic gas
Toxic effect of tear gas
- T59.3X Toxic effect of lacrimogenic gas
  - T59.3X1 Toxic effect of lacrimogenic gas, accidental (unintentional)
    Toxic effect of lacrimogenic gas NOS
  - T59.3X2 Toxic effect of lacrimogenic gas, intentional self-harm
  - T59.3X3 Toxic effect of lacrimogenic gas, assault
  - T59.3X4 Toxic effect of lacrimogenic gas, undetermined

T59.4 Toxic effect of chlorine gas
- T59.4X Toxic effect of chlorine gas
  - T59.4X1 Toxic effect of chlorine gas, accidental (unintentional)
    Toxic effect of chlorine gas NOS
  - T59.4X2 Toxic effect of chlorine gas, intentional self-harm
  - T59.4X3 Toxic effect of chlorine gas, assault
  - T59.4X4 Toxic effect of chlorine gas, undetermined

T59.5 Toxic effect of fluorine gas and hydrogen fluoride
- T59.5X Toxic effect of fluorine gas and hydrogen fluoride
  - T59.5X1 Toxic effect of fluorine gas and hydrogen fluoride, accidental (unintentional)
    Toxic effect of fluorine gas and hydrogen fluoride NOS
  - T59.5X2 Toxic effect of fluorine gas and hydrogen fluoride, intentional self-harm
  - T59.5X3 Toxic effect of fluorine gas and hydrogen fluoride, assault
  - T59.5X4 Toxic effect of fluorine gas and hydrogen fluoride, undetermined

Chapter 19. Injury, Poisoning and Certain Other Consequences of External Causes

T59.6 Toxic effect of hydrogen sulfide
- **T59.6X** Toxic effect of hydrogen sulfide
  - **T59.6X1** Toxic effect of hydrogen sulfide, accidental (unintentional)
    Toxic effect of hydrogen sulfide NOS
  - **T59.6X2** Toxic effect of hydrogen sulfide, intentional self-harm [HCC Rx ESR COM]
  - **T59.6X3** Toxic effect of hydrogen sulfide, assault
  - **T59.6X4** Toxic effect of hydrogen sulfide, undetermined

T59.7 Toxic effect of carbon dioxide
- **T59.7X** Toxic effect of carbon dioxide
  - **T59.7X1** Toxic effect of carbon dioxide, accidental (unintentional)
    Toxic effect of carbon dioxide NOS
  - **T59.7X2** Toxic effect of carbon dioxide, intentional self-harm [HCC Rx ESR COM]
  - **T59.7X3** Toxic effect of carbon dioxide, assault
  - **T59.7X4** Toxic effect of carbon dioxide, undetermined

T59.8 Toxic effect of other specified gases, fumes and vapors
- **T59.81** Toxic effect of smoke
  Smoke inhalation
  EXCLUDES 2 toxic effect of cigarette (tobacco) smoke (T65.22-)
  - **T59.811** Toxic effect of smoke, accidental (unintentional)
    Toxic effect of smoke NOS
    AHA: 2013,4Q,121
  - **T59.812** Toxic effect of smoke, intentional self-harm [HCC Rx ESR COM]
  - **T59.813** Toxic effect of smoke, assault
  - **T59.814** Toxic effect of smoke, undetermined
- **T59.89** Toxic effect of other specified gases, fumes and vapors
  - **T59.891** Toxic effect of other specified gases, fumes and vapors, accidental (unintentional)
  - **T59.892** Toxic effect of other specified gases, fumes and vapors, intentional self-harm [HCC Rx ESR COM]
  - **T59.893** Toxic effect of other specified gases, fumes and vapors, assault
  - **T59.894** Toxic effect of other specified gases, fumes and vapors, undetermined

T59.9 Toxic effect of unspecified gases, fumes and vapors
- **T59.91** Toxic effect of unspecified gases, fumes and vapors, accidental (unintentional)
- **T59.92** Toxic effect of unspecified gases, fumes and vapors, intentional self-harm [HCC Rx ESR COM]
- **T59.93** Toxic effect of unspecified gases, fumes and vapors, assault
- **T59.94** Toxic effect of unspecified gases, fumes and vapors, undetermined

T60 Toxic effect of pesticides
INCLUDES toxic effect of wood preservatives

The appropriate 7th character is to be added to each code from category T60.
- A initial encounter
- D subsequent encounter
- S sequela

T60.0 Toxic effect of organophosphate and carbamate insecticides
- **T60.0X** Toxic effect of organophosphate and carbamate insecticides
  - **T60.0X1** Toxic effect of organophosphate and carbamate insecticides, accidental (unintentional)
    Toxic effect of organophosphate and carbamate insecticides NOS
  - **T60.0X2** Toxic effect of organophosphate and carbamate insecticides, intentional self-harm [HCC Rx ESR COM]
  - **T60.0X3** Toxic effect of organophosphate and carbamate insecticides, assault
  - **T60.0X4** Toxic effect of organophosphate and carbamate insecticides, undetermined

T60.1 Toxic effect of halogenated insecticides
EXCLUDES 1 chlorinated hydrocarbon (T53.-)
- **T60.1X** Toxic effect of halogenated insecticides
  - **T60.1X1** Toxic effect of halogenated insecticides, accidental (unintentional)
    Toxic effect of halogenated insecticides NOS
  - **T60.1X2** Toxic effect of halogenated insecticides, intentional self-harm [HCC Rx ESR COM]
  - **T60.1X3** Toxic effect of halogenated insecticides, assault
  - **T60.1X4** Toxic effect of halogenated insecticides, undetermined

T60.2 Toxic effect of other insecticides
- **T60.2X** Toxic effect of other insecticides
  - **T60.2X1** Toxic effect of other insecticides, accidental (unintentional)
    Toxic effect of other insecticides NOS
  - **T60.2X2** Toxic effect of other insecticides, intentional self-harm [HCC Rx ESR COM]
  - **T60.2X3** Toxic effect of other insecticides, assault
  - **T60.2X4** Toxic effect of other insecticides, undetermined

T60.3 Toxic effect of herbicides and fungicides
- **T60.3X** Toxic effect of herbicides and fungicides
  - **T60.3X1** Toxic effect of herbicides and fungicides, accidental (unintentional)
    Toxic effect of herbicides and fungicides NOS
  - **T60.3X2** Toxic effect of herbicides and fungicides, intentional self-harm [HCC Rx ESR COM]
  - **T60.3X3** Toxic effect of herbicides and fungicides, assault
  - **T60.3X4** Toxic effect of herbicides and fungicides, undetermined

T60.4 Toxic effect of rodenticides
EXCLUDES 1 strychnine and its salts (T65.1)
thallium (T56.81-)
- **T60.4X** Toxic effect of rodenticides
  - **T60.4X1** Toxic effect of rodenticides, accidental (unintentional)
    Toxic effect of rodenticides NOS
  - **T60.4X2** Toxic effect of rodenticides, intentional self-harm [HCC Rx ESR COM]
  - **T60.4X3** Toxic effect of rodenticides, assault
  - **T60.4X4** Toxic effect of rodenticides, undetermined

T60.8 Toxic effect of other pesticides
- **T60.8X** Toxic effect of other pesticides
  - **T60.8X1** Toxic effect of other pesticides, accidental (unintentional)
    Toxic effect of other pesticides NOS
  - **T60.8X2** Toxic effect of other pesticides, intentional self-harm [HCC Rx ESR COM]
  - **T60.8X3** Toxic effect of other pesticides, assault
  - **T60.8X4** Toxic effect of other pesticides, undetermined

T60.9 Toxic effect of unspecified pesticide
- **T60.91** Toxic effect of unspecified pesticide, accidental (unintentional)
- **T60.92** Toxic effect of unspecified pesticide, intentional self-harm [HCC Rx ESR COM]
- **T60.93** Toxic effect of unspecified pesticide, assault
- **T60.94** Toxic effect of unspecified pesticide, undetermined

Chapter 19. Injury, Poisoning and Certain Other Consequences of External Causes

T61 Toxic effect of noxious substances eaten as seafood

EXCLUDES 1
allergic reaction to food, such as:
toxic effect of aflatoxin and other mycotoxins (T64)
toxic effect of cyanides (T65.0-)
toxic effect of harmful algae bloom (T65.82-)
toxic effect of hydrogen cyanide (T57.3-)
toxic effect of mercury (T56.1-)
toxic effect of red tide (T65.82-)
anaphylactic reaction or shock due to adverse food reaction (T78.0-)
bacterial foodborne intoxications (A05.-)
dermatitis (L23.6, L25.4, L27.2)
food protein-induced enterocolitis syndrome (K52.21)
food protein-induced enteropathy (K52.22)
gastroenteritis (noninfective) (K52.29)

The appropriate 7th character is to be added to each code from category T61.
- A initial encounter
- D subsequent encounter
- S sequela

- **T61.0** Ciguatera fish poisoning
  - T61.01 Ciguatera fish poisoning, accidental (unintentional)
  - T61.02 Ciguatera fish poisoning, intentional self-harm
  - T61.03 Ciguatera fish poisoning, assault
  - T61.04 Ciguatera fish poisoning, undetermined
- **T61.1** Scombroid fish poisoning
  Histamine-like syndrome
  - T61.11 Scombroid fish poisoning, accidental (unintentional)
  - T61.12 Scombroid fish poisoning, intentional self-harm
  - T61.13 Scombroid fish poisoning, assault
  - T61.14 Scombroid fish poisoning, undetermined
- **T61.7** Other fish and shellfish poisoning
  - **T61.77** Other fish poisoning
    - T61.771 Other fish poisoning, accidental (unintentional)
    - T61.772 Other fish poisoning, intentional self-harm
    - T61.773 Other fish poisoning, assault
    - T61.774 Other fish poisoning, undetermined
  - **T61.78** Other shellfish poisoning
    - T61.781 Other shellfish poisoning, accidental (unintentional)
    - T61.782 Other shellfish poisoning, intentional self-harm
    - T61.783 Other shellfish poisoning, assault
    - T61.784 Other shellfish poisoning, undetermined
- **T61.8** Toxic effect of other seafood
  - **T61.8X** Toxic effect of other seafood
    - T61.8X1 Toxic effect of other seafood, accidental (unintentional)
    - T61.8X2 Toxic effect of other seafood, intentional self-harm
    - T61.8X3 Toxic effect of other seafood, assault
    - T61.8X4 Toxic effect of other seafood, undetermined
- **T61.9** Toxic effect of unspecified seafood
  - T61.91 Toxic effect of unspecified seafood, accidental (unintentional)
  - T61.92 Toxic effect of unspecified seafood, intentional self-harm
  - T61.93 Toxic effect of unspecified seafood, assault
  - T61.94 Toxic effect of unspecified seafood, undetermined

T62 Toxic effect of other noxious substances eaten as food

EXCLUDES 1
allergic reaction to food, such as:
toxic effect of aflatoxin and other mycotoxins (T64)
toxic effect of cyanides (T65.0-)
toxic effect of hydrogen cyanide (T57.3-)
toxic effect of mercury (T56.1-)
anaphylactic shock (reaction) due to adverse food reaction (T78.0-)
bacterial food borne intoxications (A05.-)
dermatitis (L23.6, L25.4, L27.2)
food protein-induced enterocolitis syndrome (K52.21)
food protein-induced enteropathy (K52.22)
gastroenteritis (noninfective) (K52.29)

The appropriate 7th character is to be added to each code from category T62.
- A initial encounter
- D subsequent encounter
- S sequela

- **T62.0** Toxic effect of ingested mushrooms
  - **T62.0X** Toxic effect of ingested mushrooms
    - T62.0X1 Toxic effect of ingested mushrooms, accidental (unintentional)
      Toxic effect of ingested mushrooms NOS
    - T62.0X2 Toxic effect of ingested mushrooms, intentional self-harm
    - T62.0X3 Toxic effect of ingested mushrooms, assault
    - T62.0X4 Toxic effect of ingested mushrooms, undetermined
- **T62.1** Toxic effect of ingested berries
  - **T62.1X** Toxic effect of ingested berries
    - T62.1X1 Toxic effect of ingested berries, accidental (unintentional)
      Toxic effect of ingested berries NOS
    - T62.1X2 Toxic effect of ingested berries, intentional self-harm
    - T62.1X3 Toxic effect of ingested berries, assault
    - T62.1X4 Toxic effect of ingested berries, undetermined
- **T62.2** Toxic effect of other ingested (parts of) plant(s)
  - **T62.2X** Toxic effect of other ingested (parts of) plant(s)
    - T62.2X1 Toxic effect of other ingested (parts of) plant(s), accidental (unintentional)
      Toxic effect of other ingested (parts of) plant(s) NOS
    - T62.2X2 Toxic effect of other ingested (parts of) plant(s), intentional self-harm
    - T62.2X3 Toxic effect of other ingested (parts of) plant(s), assault
    - T62.2X4 Toxic effect of other ingested (parts of) plant(s), undetermined
- **T62.8** Toxic effect of other specified noxious substances eaten as food
  - **T62.8X** Toxic effect of other specified noxious substances eaten as food
    - T62.8X1 Toxic effect of other specified noxious substances eaten as food, accidental (unintentional)
      Toxic effect of other specified noxious substances eaten as food NOS
    - T62.8X2 Toxic effect of other specified noxious substances eaten as food, intentional self-harm
    - T62.8X3 Toxic effect of other specified noxious substances eaten as food, assault
    - T62.8X4 Toxic effect of other specified noxious substances eaten as food, undetermined
- **T62.9** Toxic effect of unspecified noxious substance eaten as food
  - T62.91 Toxic effect of unspecified noxious substance eaten as food, accidental (unintentional)
    Toxic effect of unspecified noxious substance eaten as food NOS
  - T62.92 Toxic effect of unspecified noxious substance eaten as food, intentional self-harm
  - T62.93 Toxic effect of unspecified noxious substance eaten as food, assault
  - T62.94 Toxic effect of unspecified noxious substance eaten as food, undetermined

T63 Toxic effect of contact with venomous animals and plants

INCLUDES: bite or touch of venomous animal
pricked or stuck by thorn or leaf

EXCLUDES 2: *ingestion of toxic animal or plant (T61.-, T62.-)*

The appropriate 7th character is to be added to each code from category T63.
- A initial encounter
- D subsequent encounter
- S sequela

T63.0 Toxic effect of snake venom

T63.00 Toxic effect of unspecified snake venom
- T63.001 Toxic effect of unspecified snake venom, accidental (unintentional)
  - Toxic effect of unspecified snake venom NOS
- T63.002 Toxic effect of unspecified snake venom, intentional self-harm
- T63.003 Toxic effect of unspecified snake venom, assault
- T63.004 Toxic effect of unspecified snake venom, undetermined

T63.01 Toxic effect of rattlesnake venom
- T63.011 Toxic effect of rattlesnake venom, accidental (unintentional)
  - Toxic effect of rattlesnake venom NOS
- T63.012 Toxic effect of rattlesnake venom, intentional self-harm
- T63.013 Toxic effect of rattlesnake venom, assault
- T63.014 Toxic effect of rattlesnake venom, undetermined

T63.02 Toxic effect of coral snake venom
- T63.021 Toxic effect of coral snake venom, accidental (unintentional)
  - Toxic effect of coral snake venom NOS
- T63.022 Toxic effect of coral snake venom, intentional self-harm
- T63.023 Toxic effect of coral snake venom, assault
- T63.024 Toxic effect of coral snake venom, undetermined

T63.03 Toxic effect of taipan venom
- T63.031 Toxic effect of taipan venom, accidental (unintentional)
  - Toxic effect of taipan venom NOS
- T63.032 Toxic effect of taipan venom, intentional self-harm
- T63.033 Toxic effect of taipan venom, assault
- T63.034 Toxic effect of taipan venom, undetermined

T63.04 Toxic effect of cobra venom
- T63.041 Toxic effect of cobra venom, accidental (unintentional)
  - Toxic effect of cobra venom NOS
- T63.042 Toxic effect of cobra venom, intentional self-harm
- T63.043 Toxic effect of cobra venom, assault
- T63.044 Toxic effect of cobra venom, undetermined

T63.06 Toxic effect of venom of other North and South American snake
- T63.061 Toxic effect of venom of other North and South American snake, accidental (unintentional)
  - Toxic effect of venom of other North and South American snake NOS
- T63.062 Toxic effect of venom of other North and South American snake, intentional self-harm
- T63.063 Toxic effect of venom of other North and South American snake, assault
- T63.064 Toxic effect of venom of other North and South American snake, undetermined

T63.07 Toxic effect of venom of other Australian snake
- T63.071 Toxic effect of venom of other Australian snake, accidental (unintentional)
  - Toxic effect of venom of other Australian snake NOS
- T63.072 Toxic effect of venom of other Australian snake, intentional self-harm
- T63.073 Toxic effect of venom of other Australian snake, assault
- T63.074 Toxic effect of venom of other Australian snake, undetermined

T63.08 Toxic effect of venom of other African and Asian snake
- T63.081 Toxic effect of venom of other African and Asian snake, accidental (unintentional)
  - Toxic effect of venom of other African and Asian snake NOS
- T63.082 Toxic effect of venom of other African and Asian snake, intentional self-harm
- T63.083 Toxic effect of venom of other African and Asian snake, assault
- T63.084 Toxic effect of venom of other African and Asian snake, undetermined

T63.09 Toxic effect of venom of other snake
- T63.091 Toxic effect of venom of other snake, accidental (unintentional)
  - Toxic effect of venom of other snake NOS
- T63.092 Toxic effect of venom of other snake, intentional self-harm
- T63.093 Toxic effect of venom of other snake, assault
- T63.094 Toxic effect of venom of other snake, undetermined

T63.1 Toxic effect of venom of other reptiles

T63.11 Toxic effect of venom of gila monster
- T63.111 Toxic effect of venom of gila monster, accidental (unintentional)
  - Toxic effect of venom of gila monster NOS
- T63.112 Toxic effect of venom of gila monster, intentional self-harm
- T63.113 Toxic effect of venom of gila monster, assault
- T63.114 Toxic effect of venom of gila monster, undetermined

T63.12 Toxic effect of venom of other venomous lizard
- T63.121 Toxic effect of venom of other venomous lizard, accidental (unintentional)
  - Toxic effect of venom of other venomous lizard NOS
- T63.122 Toxic effect of venom of other venomous lizard, intentional self-harm
- T63.123 Toxic effect of venom of other venomous lizard, assault
- T63.124 Toxic effect of venom of other venomous lizard, undetermined

T63.19 Toxic effect of venom of other reptiles
- T63.191 Toxic effect of venom of other reptiles, accidental (unintentional)
  - Toxic effect of venom of other reptiles NOS
- T63.192 Toxic effect of venom of other reptiles, intentional self-harm
- T63.193 Toxic effect of venom of other reptiles, assault
- T63.194 Toxic effect of venom of other reptiles, undetermined

T63.2 Toxic effect of venom of scorpion

T63.2X Toxic effect of venom of scorpion
- T63.2X1 Toxic effect of venom of scorpion, accidental (unintentional)
  - Toxic effect of venom of scorpion NOS
- T63.2X2 Toxic effect of venom of scorpion, intentional self-harm
- T63.2X3 Toxic effect of venom of scorpion, assault
- T63.2X4 Toxic effect of venom of scorpion, undetermined

T63.3 Toxic effect of venom of spider

T63.30 Toxic effect of unspecified spider venom
- T63.301 Toxic effect of unspecified spider venom, accidental (unintentional)
- T63.302 Toxic effect of unspecified spider venom, intentional self-harm
- T63.303 Toxic effect of unspecified spider venom, assault
- T63.304 Toxic effect of unspecified spider venom, undetermined

- ✓6th **T63.31** Toxic effect of venom of black widow spider
  - ✓7th **T63.311** Toxic effect of venom of black widow spider, accidental (unintentional)
  - ✓7th **T63.312** Toxic effect of venom of black widow spider, intentional self-harm [HCC] [Rx] [ESR] [COM]
  - ✓7th **T63.313** Toxic effect of venom of black widow spider, assault
  - ✓7th **T63.314** Toxic effect of venom of black widow spider, undetermined
- ✓6th **T63.32** Toxic effect of venom of tarantula
  - ✓7th **T63.321** Toxic effect of venom of tarantula, accidental (unintentional)
  - ✓7th **T63.322** Toxic effect of venom of tarantula, intentional self-harm [HCC] [Rx] [ESR] [COM]
  - ✓7th **T63.323** Toxic effect of venom of tarantula, assault
  - ✓7th **T63.324** Toxic effect of venom of tarantula, undetermined
- ✓6th **T63.33** Toxic effect of venom of brown recluse spider
  - ✓7th **T63.331** Toxic effect of venom of brown recluse spider, accidental (unintentional)
  - ✓7th **T63.332** Toxic effect of venom of brown recluse spider, intentional self-harm [HCC] [Rx] [ESR] [COM]
  - ✓7th **T63.333** Toxic effect of venom of brown recluse spider, assault
  - ✓7th **T63.334** Toxic effect of venom of brown recluse spider, undetermined
- ✓6th **T63.39** Toxic effect of venom of other spider
  - ✓7th **T63.391** Toxic effect of venom of other spider, accidental (unintentional)
  - ✓7th **T63.392** Toxic effect of venom of other spider, intentional self-harm [HCC] [Rx] [ESR] [COM]
  - ✓7th **T63.393** Toxic effect of venom of other spider, assault
  - ✓7th **T63.394** Toxic effect of venom of other spider, undetermined
- ✓5th **T63.4** Toxic effect of venom of other arthropods
  - Use additional code, if applicable, for anaphylactic shock (T78.2)
  - ✓6th **T63.41** Toxic effect of venom of centipedes and venomous millipedes
    - ✓7th **T63.411** Toxic effect of venom of centipedes and venomous millipedes, accidental (unintentional)
    - ✓7th **T63.412** Toxic effect of venom of centipedes and venomous millipedes, intentional self-harm [HCC] [Rx] [ESR] [COM]
    - ✓7th **T63.413** Toxic effect of venom of centipedes and venomous millipedes, assault
    - ✓7th **T63.414** Toxic effect of venom of centipedes and venomous millipedes, undetermined
  - ✓6th **T63.42** Toxic effect of venom of ants
    - ✓7th **T63.421** Toxic effect of venom of ants, accidental (unintentional)
    - ✓7th **T63.422** Toxic effect of venom of ants, intentional self-harm [HCC] [Rx] [ESR] [COM]
    - ✓7th **T63.423** Toxic effect of venom of ants, assault
    - ✓7th **T63.424** Toxic effect of venom of ants, undetermined
  - ✓6th **T63.43** Toxic effect of venom of caterpillars
    - ✓7th **T63.431** Toxic effect of venom of caterpillars, accidental (unintentional)
    - ✓7th **T63.432** Toxic effect of venom of caterpillars, intentional self-harm [HCC] [Rx] [ESR] [COM]
    - ✓7th **T63.433** Toxic effect of venom of caterpillars, assault
    - ✓7th **T63.434** Toxic effect of venom of caterpillars, undetermined
  - ✓6th **T63.44** Toxic effect of venom of bees
    - ✓7th **T63.441** Toxic effect of venom of bees, accidental (unintentional)
    - ✓7th **T63.442** Toxic effect of venom of bees, intentional self-harm [HCC] [Rx] [ESR] [COM]
    - ✓7th **T63.443** Toxic effect of venom of bees, assault
    - ✓7th **T63.444** Toxic effect of venom of bees, undetermined
  - ✓6th **T63.45** Toxic effect of venom of hornets
    - ✓7th **T63.451** Toxic effect of venom of hornets, accidental (unintentional)
    - ✓7th **T63.452** Toxic effect of venom of hornets, intentional self-harm [HCC] [Rx] [ESR] [COM]
    - ✓7th **T63.453** Toxic effect of venom of hornets, assault
    - ✓7th **T63.454** Toxic effect of venom of hornets, undetermined
  - ✓6th **T63.46** Toxic effect of venom of wasps
    - Toxic effect of yellow jacket
    - ✓7th **T63.461** Toxic effect of venom of wasps, accidental (unintentional)
    - ✓7th **T63.462** Toxic effect of venom of wasps, intentional self-harm [HCC] [Rx] [ESR] [COM]
    - ✓7th **T63.463** Toxic effect of venom of wasps, assault
    - ✓7th **T63.464** Toxic effect of venom of wasps, undetermined
  - ✓6th **T63.48** Toxic effect of venom of other arthropod
    - ✓7th **T63.481** Toxic effect of venom of other arthropod, accidental (unintentional)
    - ✓7th **T63.482** Toxic effect of venom of other arthropod, intentional self-harm [HCC] [Rx] [ESR] [COM]
    - ✓7th **T63.483** Toxic effect of venom of other arthropod, assault
    - ✓7th **T63.484** Toxic effect of venom of other arthropod, undetermined
- ✓5th **T63.5** Toxic effect of contact with venomous fish
  - EXCLUDES 2 — poisoning by ingestion of fish (T61.-)
  - ✓6th **T63.51** Toxic effect of contact with stingray
    - ✓7th **T63.511** Toxic effect of contact with stingray, accidental (unintentional)
    - ✓7th **T63.512** Toxic effect of contact with stingray, intentional self-harm [HCC] [Rx] [ESR] [COM]
    - ✓7th **T63.513** Toxic effect of contact with stingray, assault
    - ✓7th **T63.514** Toxic effect of contact with stingray, undetermined
  - ✓6th **T63.59** Toxic effect of contact with other venomous fish
    - ✓7th **T63.591** Toxic effect of contact with other venomous fish, accidental (unintentional)
    - ✓7th **T63.592** Toxic effect of contact with other venomous fish, intentional self-harm [HCC] [Rx] [ESR] [COM]
    - ✓7th **T63.593** Toxic effect of contact with other venomous fish, assault
    - ✓7th **T63.594** Toxic effect of contact with other venomous fish, undetermined
- ✓5th **T63.6** Toxic effect of contact with other venomous marine animals
  - EXCLUDES 1 — sea-snake venom (T63.09)
  - EXCLUDES 2 — poisoning by ingestion of shellfish (T61.78-)
  - ✓6th **T63.61** Toxic effect of contact with Portuguese Man-o-war
    - Toxic effect of contact with bluebottle
    - ✓7th **T63.611** Toxic effect of contact with Portuguese Man-o-war, accidental (unintentional)
    - ✓7th **T63.612** Toxic effect of contact with Portuguese Man-o-war, intentional self-harm [HCC] [Rx] [ESR] [COM]
    - ✓7th **T63.613** Toxic effect of contact with Portuguese Man-o-war, assault
    - ✓7th **T63.614** Toxic effect of contact with Portuguese Man-o-war, undetermined
  - ✓6th **T63.62** Toxic effect of contact with other jellyfish
    - ✓7th **T63.621** Toxic effect of contact with other jellyfish, accidental (unintentional)
    - ✓7th **T63.622** Toxic effect of contact with other jellyfish, intentional self-harm [HCC] [Rx] [ESR] [COM]
    - ✓7th **T63.623** Toxic effect of contact with other jellyfish, assault
    - ✓7th **T63.624** Toxic effect of contact with other jellyfish, undetermined
  - ✓6th **T63.63** Toxic effect of contact with sea anemone
    - ✓7th **T63.631** Toxic effect of contact with sea anemone, accidental (unintentional)
    - ✓7th **T63.632** Toxic effect of contact with sea anemone, intentional self-harm [HCC] [Rx] [ESR] [COM]
    - ✓7th **T63.633** Toxic effect of contact with sea anemone, assault
    - ✓7th **T63.634** Toxic effect of contact with sea anemone, undetermined

Chapter 19. Injury, Poisoning and Certain Other Consequences of External Causes

- **T63.69** Toxic effect of contact with other venomous marine animals
  - **T63.691** Toxic effect of contact with other venomous marine animals, accidental (unintentional)
  - **T63.692** Toxic effect of contact with other venomous marine animals, intentional self-harm
  - **T63.693** Toxic effect of contact with other venomous marine animals, assault
  - **T63.694** Toxic effect of contact with other venomous marine animals, undetermined
- **T63.7** Toxic effect of contact with venomous plant
  - **T63.71** Toxic effect of contact with venomous marine plant
    - **T63.711** Toxic effect of contact with venomous marine plant, accidental (unintentional)
    - **T63.712** Toxic effect of contact with venomous marine plant, intentional self-harm
    - **T63.713** Toxic effect of contact with venomous marine plant, assault
    - **T63.714** Toxic effect of contact with venomous marine plant, undetermined
  - **T63.79** Toxic effect of contact with other venomous plant
    - **T63.791** Toxic effect of contact with other venomous plant, accidental (unintentional)
    - **T63.792** Toxic effect of contact with other venomous plant, intentional self-harm
    - **T63.793** Toxic effect of contact with other venomous plant, assault
    - **T63.794** Toxic effect of contact with other venomous plant, undetermined
- **T63.8** Toxic effect of contact with other venomous animals
  - **T63.81** Toxic effect of contact with venomous frog
    - EXCLUDES 1 contact with nonvenomous frog (W62.0)
    - **T63.811** Toxic effect of contact with venomous frog, accidental (unintentional)
    - **T63.812** Toxic effect of contact with venomous frog, intentional self-harm
    - **T63.813** Toxic effect of contact with venomous frog, assault
    - **T63.814** Toxic effect of contact with venomous frog, undetermined
  - **T63.82** Toxic effect of contact with venomous toad
    - EXCLUDES 1 contact with nonvenomous toad (W62.1)
    - **T63.821** Toxic effect of contact with venomous toad, accidental (unintentional)
    - **T63.822** Toxic effect of contact with venomous toad, intentional self-harm
    - **T63.823** Toxic effect of contact with venomous toad, assault
    - **T63.824** Toxic effect of contact with venomous toad, undetermined
  - **T63.83** Toxic effect of contact with other venomous amphibian
    - EXCLUDES 1 contact with nonvenomous amphibian (W62.9)
    - **T63.831** Toxic effect of contact with other venomous amphibian, accidental (unintentional)
    - **T63.832** Toxic effect of contact with other venomous amphibian, intentional self-harm
    - **T63.833** Toxic effect of contact with other venomous amphibian, assault
    - **T63.834** Toxic effect of contact with other venomous amphibian, undetermined
  - **T63.89** Toxic effect of contact with other venomous animals
    - **T63.891** Toxic effect of contact with other venomous animals, accidental (unintentional)
    - **T63.892** Toxic effect of contact with other venomous animals, intentional self-harm
    - **T63.893** Toxic effect of contact with other venomous animals, assault
    - **T63.894** Toxic effect of contact with other venomous animals, undetermined
- **T63.9** Toxic effect of contact with unspecified venomous animal
  - **T63.91** Toxic effect of contact with unspecified venomous animal, accidental (unintentional)
  - **T63.92** Toxic effect of contact with unspecified venomous animal, intentional self-harm
  - **T63.93** Toxic effect of contact with unspecified venomous animal, assault
  - **T63.94** Toxic effect of contact with unspecified venomous animal, undetermined

T64 Toxic effect of aflatoxin and other mycotoxin food contaminants

The appropriate 7th character is to be added to each code from category T64.
- A initial encounter
- D subsequent encounter
- S sequela

- **T64.0** Toxic effect of aflatoxin
  - **T64.01** Toxic effect of aflatoxin, accidental (unintentional)
  - **T64.02** Toxic effect of aflatoxin, intentional self-harm
  - **T64.03** Toxic effect of aflatoxin, assault
  - **T64.04** Toxic effect of aflatoxin, undetermined
- **T64.8** Toxic effect of other mycotoxin food contaminants
  - **T64.81** Toxic effect of other mycotoxin food contaminants, accidental (unintentional)
  - **T64.82** Toxic effect of other mycotoxin food contaminants, intentional self-harm
  - **T64.83** Toxic effect of other mycotoxin food contaminants, assault
  - **T64.84** Toxic effect of other mycotoxin food contaminants, undetermined

T65 Toxic effect of other and unspecified substances

The appropriate 7th character is to be added to each code from category T65.
- A initial encounter
- D subsequent encounter
- S sequela

- **T65.0** Toxic effect of cyanides
  - EXCLUDES 1 hydrogen cyanide (T57.3-)
  - **T65.0X** Toxic effect of cyanides
    - **T65.0X1** Toxic effect of cyanides, accidental (unintentional)
      Toxic effect of cyanides NOS
    - **T65.0X2** Toxic effect of cyanides, intentional self-harm
    - **T65.0X3** Toxic effect of cyanides, assault
    - **T65.0X4** Toxic effect of cyanides, undetermined
- **T65.1** Toxic effect of strychnine and its salts
  - **T65.1X** Toxic effect of strychnine and its salts
    - **T65.1X1** Toxic effect of strychnine and its salts, accidental (unintentional)
      Toxic effect of strychnine and its salts NOS
    - **T65.1X2** Toxic effect of strychnine and its salts, intentional self-harm
    - **T65.1X3** Toxic effect of strychnine and its salts, assault
    - **T65.1X4** Toxic effect of strychnine and its salts, undetermined
- **T65.2** Toxic effect of tobacco and nicotine
  - EXCLUDES 2 nicotine dependence (F17.-)
  - **T65.21** Toxic effect of chewing tobacco
    - **T65.211** Toxic effect of chewing tobacco, accidental (unintentional)
      Toxic effect of chewing tobacco NOS
    - **T65.212** Toxic effect of chewing tobacco, intentional self-harm
    - **T65.213** Toxic effect of chewing tobacco, assault
    - **T65.214** Toxic effect of chewing tobacco, undetermined

T65.22 Toxic effect of tobacco cigarettes
Toxic effect of tobacco smoke
Use additional code for exposure to second hand tobacco smoke (Z57.31, Z77.22)

- √7th **T65.221** Toxic effect of tobacco cigarettes, accidental (unintentional)
  Toxic effect of tobacco cigarettes NOS
- √7th **T65.222** Toxic effect of tobacco cigarettes, intentional self-harm HCC Rx ESR COM
- √7th **T65.223** Toxic effect of tobacco cigarettes, assault
- √7th **T65.224** Toxic effect of tobacco cigarettes, undetermined

√6th T65.29 Toxic effect of other tobacco and nicotine
- √7th **T65.291** Toxic effect of other tobacco and nicotine, accidental (unintentional)
  Toxic effect of other tobacco and nicotine NOS
- √7th **T65.292** Toxic effect of other tobacco and nicotine, intentional self-harm HCC Rx ESR COM
- √7th **T65.293** Toxic effect of other tobacco and nicotine, assault
- √7th **T65.294** Toxic effect of other tobacco and nicotine, undetermined

√5th T65.3 Toxic effect of nitroderivatives and aminoderivatives of benzene and its homologues
Toxic effect of aniline [benzenamine]
Toxic effect of nitrobenzene
Toxic effect of trinitrotoluene

√6th T65.3X Toxic effect of nitroderivatives and aminoderivatives of benzene and its homologues
- √7th **T65.3X1** Toxic effect of nitroderivatives and aminoderivatives of benzene and its homologues, accidental (unintentional)
  Toxic effect of nitroderivatives and aminoderivatives of benzene and its homologues NOS
- √7th **T65.3X2** Toxic effect of nitroderivatives and aminoderivatives of benzene and its homologues, intentional self-harm HCC Rx ESR COM
- √7th **T65.3X3** Toxic effect of nitroderivatives and aminoderivatives of benzene and its homologues, assault
- √7th **T65.3X4** Toxic effect of nitroderivatives and aminoderivatives of benzene and its homologues, undetermined

√5th T65.4 Toxic effect of carbon disulfide
√6th T65.4X Toxic effect of carbon disulfide
- √7th **T65.4X1** Toxic effect of carbon disulfide, accidental (unintentional)
  Toxic effect of carbon disulfide NOS
- √7th **T65.4X2** Toxic effect of carbon disulfide, intentional self-harm HCC Rx ESR COM
- √7th **T65.4X3** Toxic effect of carbon disulfide, assault
- √7th **T65.4X4** Toxic effect of carbon disulfide, undetermined

√5th T65.5 Toxic effect of nitroglycerin and other nitric acids and esters
Toxic effect of 1,2,3-Propanetriol trinitrate

√6th T65.5X Toxic effect of nitroglycerin and other nitric acids and esters
- √7th **T65.5X1** Toxic effect of nitroglycerin and other nitric acids and esters, accidental (unintentional)
  Toxic effect of nitroglycerin and other nitric acids and esters NOS
- √7th **T65.5X2** Toxic effect of nitroglycerin and other nitric acids and esters, intentional self-harm HCC Rx ESR COM
- √7th **T65.5X3** Toxic effect of nitroglycerin and other nitric acids and esters, assault
- √7th **T65.5X4** Toxic effect of nitroglycerin and other nitric acids and esters, undetermined

√5th T65.6 Toxic effect of paints and dyes, not elsewhere classified
√6th T65.6X Toxic effect of paints and dyes, not elsewhere classified
- √7th **T65.6X1** Toxic effect of paints and dyes, not elsewhere classified, accidental (unintentional)
  Toxic effect of paints and dyes NOS
- √7th **T65.6X2** Toxic effect of paints and dyes, not elsewhere classified, intentional self-harm HCC Rx ESR COM
- √7th **T65.6X3** Toxic effect of paints and dyes, not elsewhere classified, assault
- √7th **T65.6X4** Toxic effect of paints and dyes, not elsewhere classified, undetermined

√5th T65.8 Toxic effect of other specified substances
√6th T65.81 Toxic effect of latex
- √7th **T65.811** Toxic effect of latex, accidental (unintentional)
  Toxic effect of latex NOS
- √7th **T65.812** Toxic effect of latex, intentional self-harm HCC Rx ESR COM
- √7th **T65.813** Toxic effect of latex, assault
- √7th **T65.814** Toxic effect of latex, undetermined

√6th T65.82 Toxic effect of harmful algae and algae toxins
Toxic effect of blue-green algae bloom
Toxic effect of (harmful) algae bloom NOS
Toxic effect of brown tide
Toxic effect of cyanobacteria bloom
Toxic effect of Florida red tide
Toxic effect of pfiesteria piscicida
Toxic effect of red tide

- √7th **T65.821** Toxic effect of harmful algae and algae toxins, accidental (unintentional)
  Toxic effect of harmful algae and algae toxins NOS
- √7th **T65.822** Toxic effect of harmful algae and algae toxins, intentional self-harm HCC Rx ESR COM
- √7th **T65.823** Toxic effect of harmful algae and algae toxins, assault
- √7th **T65.824** Toxic effect of harmful algae and algae toxins, undetermined

√6th T65.83 Toxic effect of fiberglass
- √7th **T65.831** Toxic effect of fiberglass, accidental (unintentional)
  Toxic effect of fiberglass NOS
- √7th **T65.832** Toxic effect of fiberglass, intentional self-harm HCC Rx ESR COM
- √7th **T65.833** Toxic effect of fiberglass, assault
- √7th **T65.834** Toxic effect of fiberglass, undetermined

√6th T65.84 Toxic effect of xylazine
Use additional code(s) for all associated manifestations, such as:
cellulitis and acute lymphangitis (L03.-)
cutaneous abscess, furuncle and carbuncle (L02.-)
non-pressure chronic ulcer of lower limb, not elsewhere classified (L97.-)
non-pressure chronic ulcer of skin, not elsewhere classified (L98.4-)

- √7th **T65.841** Toxic effect of xylazine, accidental (unintentional)
  Toxic effect of xylazine NOS
- √7th **T65.842** Toxic effect of xylazine, intentional self-harm
- √7th **T65.843** Toxic effect of xylazine, assault
- √7th **T65.844** Toxic effect of xylazine, undetermined

√6th T65.89 Toxic effect of other specified substances
- √7th **T65.891** Toxic effect of other specified substances, accidental (unintentional)
  Toxic effect of other specified substances NOS
  AHA: 2018,1Q,5
- √7th **T65.892** Toxic effect of other specified substances, intentional self-harm HCC Rx ESR COM
- √7th **T65.893** Toxic effect of other specified substances, assault
- √7th **T65.894** Toxic effect of other specified substances, undetermined

√5th T65.9 Toxic effect of unspecified substance
- √x7th **T65.91** Toxic effect of unspecified substance, accidental (unintentional)
  Poisoning NOS
- √x7th **T65.92** Toxic effect of unspecified substance, intentional self-harm HCC Rx ESR COM
- √x7th **T65.93** Toxic effect of unspecified substance, assault
- √x7th **T65.94** Toxic effect of unspecified substance, undetermined

---

HCC CMS-HCC Rx Rx HCC ESR ESRD HCC COM Commercial HCC N Newborn: 0 P Pediatric: 0-17 M Maternity: 9-64 A Adult: 15-124

Other and unspecified effects of external causes (T66-T78)

T66 Radiation sickness, unspecified
> EXCLUDES 1: specified adverse effects of radiation, such as:
> radiation gastroenteritis and colitis (K52.0)
> radiation pneumonitis (J70.0)
> radiation related disorders of the skin and subcutaneous tissue (L55-L59)
> radiation sunburn (L55.-)
> burns (T20-T31)
> leukemia (C91-C95)

The appropriate 7th character is to be added to code T66.
- A initial encounter
- D subsequent encounter
- S sequela

T67 Effects of heat and light
> EXCLUDES 1: erythema [dermatitis] ab igne (L59.0)
> malignant hyperpyrexia due to anesthesia (T88.3)
> radiation-related disorders of the skin and subcutaneous tissue (L55-L59)
>
> EXCLUDES 2: burns (T20-T31)
> sunburn (L55.-)
> sweat disorder due to heat (L74-L75)

The appropriate 7th character is to be added to each code from category T67.
- A initial encounter
- D subsequent encounter
- S sequela

T67.0 Heatstroke and sunstroke
> Use additional code(s) to identify any associated complications of heatstroke, such as:
> coma and stupor (R40.-)
> rhabdomyolysis (M62.82)
> systemic inflammatory response syndrome (R65.1-)
> AHA: 2019,4Q,17-18
> DEF: Headache, vertigo, cramps, and elevated body temperature due to prolonged exposure to high environmental temperatures that requires emergency intervention.

- **T67.01** Heatstroke and sunstroke
  - Heat apoplexy
  - Heat pyrexia
  - Siriasis
  - Thermoplegia
- **T67.02** Exertional heatstroke
- **T67.09** Other heatstroke and sunstroke

T67.1 Heat syncope
- Heat collapse

T67.2 Heat cramp

T67.3 Heat exhaustion, anhydrotic
- Heat prostration due to water depletion
> EXCLUDES 1: heat exhaustion due to salt depletion (T67.4)

T67.4 Heat exhaustion due to salt depletion
- Heat prostration due to salt (and water) depletion

T67.5 Heat exhaustion, unspecified
- Heat prostration NOS

T67.6 Heat fatigue, transient

T67.7 Heat edema

T67.8 Other effects of heat and light

T67.9 Effect of heat and light, unspecified

T68 Hypothermia
- Accidental hypothermia
- Hypothermia NOS
> Use additional code to identify source of exposure:
> exposure to excessive cold of man-made origin (W93)
> exposure to excessive cold of natural origin (X31)
>
> EXCLUDES 1: hypothermia following anesthesia (T88.51)
> hypothermia of newborn (P80.-)
> hypothermia not associated with low environmental temperature (R68.0)
>
> EXCLUDES 2: frostbite (T33-T34)

The appropriate 7th character is to be added to code T68.
- A initial encounter
- D subsequent encounter
- S sequela

T69 Other effects of reduced temperature
> Use additional code to identify source of exposure:
> exposure to excessive cold of man-made origin (W93)
> exposure to excessive cold of natural origin (X31)
>
> EXCLUDES 2: frostbite (T33-T34)

The appropriate 7th character is to be added to each code from category T69.
- A initial encounter
- D subsequent encounter
- S sequela

T69.0 Immersion hand and foot
- **T69.01** Immersion hand
  - **T69.011** Immersion hand, right hand
  - **T69.012** Immersion hand, left hand
  - **T69.019** Immersion hand, unspecified hand
- **T69.02** Immersion foot
  - Trench foot
  - **T69.021** Immersion foot, right foot
  - **T69.022** Immersion foot, left foot
  - **T69.029** Immersion foot, unspecified foot

T69.1 Chilblains
> DEF: Red, swollen, itchy skin primarily affecting the fingers and toes, nose and ears, and legs. Chilblains follows damp-cold exposure, and can also be associated with pruritus and a burning feeling.

T69.8 Other specified effects of reduced temperature

T69.9 Effect of reduced temperature, unspecified

T70 Effects of air pressure and water pressure

The appropriate 7th character is to be added to each code from category T70.
- A initial encounter
- D subsequent encounter
- S sequela

T70.0 Otitic barotrauma
- Aero-otitis media
- Effects of change in ambient atmospheric pressure or water pressure on ears

T70.1 Sinus barotrauma
- Aerosinusitis
- Effects of change in ambient atmospheric pressure on sinuses

T70.2 Other and unspecified effects of high altitude
> EXCLUDES 2: polycythemia due to high altitude (D75.1)

- **T70.20** Unspecified effects of high altitude
- **T70.29** Other effects of high altitude
  - Alpine sickness
  - Anoxia due to high altitude
  - Barotrauma NOS
  - Hypobaropathy
  - Mountain sickness

T70.3 Caisson disease [decompression sickness]
- Compressed-air disease
- Diver's palsy or paralysis
> DEF: Rapid reduction in air pressure while breathing compressed air. Symptoms include skin lesions, joint pains, and respiratory and neurological problems.

T70.4 Effects of high-pressure fluids
- Hydraulic jet injection (industrial)
- Pneumatic jet injection (industrial)
- Traumatic jet injection (industrial)

T70.8 Other effects of air pressure and water pressure

T70.9 Effect of air pressure and water pressure, unspecified

T71 Asphyxiation

Mechanical suffocation
Traumatic suffocation

EXCLUDES 1
acute respiratory distress (syndrome) (J80)
anoxia due to high altitude (T70.2)
asphyxia from carbon monoxide (T58.-)
asphyxia from inhalation of food or foreign body (T17.-)
asphyxia from other gases, fumes and vapors (T59.-)
asphyxia NOS (R09.01)
respiratory distress (syndrome) in newborn (P22.-)

The appropriate 7th character is to be added to each code from category T71.
- A initial encounter
- D subsequent encounter
- S sequela

T71.1 Asphyxiation due to mechanical threat to breathing
Suffocation due to mechanical threat to breathing

T71.11 Asphyxiation due to smothering under pillow
- T71.111 Asphyxiation due to smothering under pillow, accidental
  Asphyxiation due to smothering under pillow NOS
- T71.112 Asphyxiation due to smothering under pillow, intentional self-harm HCC Rx ESR COM
- T71.113 Asphyxiation due to smothering under pillow, assault
- T71.114 Asphyxiation due to smothering under pillow, undetermined

T71.12 Asphyxiation due to plastic bag
- T71.121 Asphyxiation due to plastic bag, accidental
  Asphyxiation due to plastic bag NOS
- T71.122 Asphyxiation due to plastic bag, intentional self-harm HCC Rx ESR COM
- T71.123 Asphyxiation due to plastic bag, assault
- T71.124 Asphyxiation due to plastic bag, undetermined

T71.13 Asphyxiation due to being trapped in bed linens
- T71.131 Asphyxiation due to being trapped in bed linens, accidental
  Asphyxiation due to being trapped in bed linens NOS
- T71.132 Asphyxiation due to being trapped in bed linens, intentional self-harm HCC Rx ESR COM
- T71.133 Asphyxiation due to being trapped in bed linens, assault
- T71.134 Asphyxiation due to being trapped in bed linens, undetermined

T71.14 Asphyxiation due to smothering under another person's body (in bed)
- T71.141 Asphyxiation due to smothering under another person's body (in bed), accidental
  Asphyxiation due to smothering under another person's body (in bed) NOS
- T71.143 Asphyxiation due to smothering under another person's body (in bed), assault
- T71.144 Asphyxiation due to smothering under another person's body (in bed), undetermined

T71.15 Asphyxiation due to smothering in furniture
- T71.151 Asphyxiation due to smothering in furniture, accidental
  Asphyxiation due to smothering in furniture NOS
- T71.152 Asphyxiation due to smothering in furniture, intentional self-harm HCC Rx ESR COM
- T71.153 Asphyxiation due to smothering in furniture, assault
- T71.154 Asphyxiation due to smothering in furniture, undetermined

T71.16 Asphyxiation due to hanging
Hanging by window shade cord

Use additional code for any associated injuries, such as:
crushing injury of neck (S17.-)
fracture of cervical vertebrae (S12.0-S12.2-)
open wound of neck (S11.-)

- T71.161 Asphyxiation due to hanging, accidental
  Asphyxiation due to hanging NOS
  Hanging NOS
- T71.162 Asphyxiation due to hanging, intentional self-harm HCC Rx ESR COM
- T71.163 Asphyxiation due to hanging, assault
- T71.164 Asphyxiation due to hanging, undetermined

T71.19 Asphyxiation due to mechanical threat to breathing due to other causes
- T71.191 Asphyxiation due to mechanical threat to breathing due to other causes, accidental
  Asphyxiation due to other causes NOS
- T71.192 Asphyxiation due to mechanical threat to breathing due to other causes, intentional self-harm HCC Rx ESR COM
- T71.193 Asphyxiation due to mechanical threat to breathing due to other causes, assault
- T71.194 Asphyxiation due to mechanical threat to breathing due to other causes, undetermined

T71.2 Asphyxiation due to systemic oxygen deficiency due to low oxygen content in ambient air
Suffocation due to systemic oxygen deficiency due to low oxygen content in ambient air

- T71.20 Asphyxiation due to systemic oxygen deficiency due to low oxygen content in ambient air due to unspecified cause
- T71.21 Asphyxiation due to cave-in or falling earth
  Use additional code for any associated cataclysm (X34-X38)

T71.22 Asphyxiation due to being trapped in a car trunk
- T71.221 Asphyxiation due to being trapped in a car trunk, accidental
- T71.222 Asphyxiation due to being trapped in a car trunk, intentional self-harm HCC Rx ESR COM
- T71.223 Asphyxiation due to being trapped in a car trunk, assault
- T71.224 Asphyxiation due to being trapped in a car trunk, undetermined

T71.23 Asphyxiation due to being trapped in a (discarded) refrigerator
- T71.231 Asphyxiation due to being trapped in a (discarded) refrigerator, accidental
- T71.232 Asphyxiation due to being trapped in a (discarded) refrigerator, intentional self-harm HCC Rx ESR COM
- T71.233 Asphyxiation due to being trapped in a (discarded) refrigerator, assault
- T71.234 Asphyxiation due to being trapped in a (discarded) refrigerator, undetermined

- T71.29 Asphyxiation due to being trapped in other low oxygen environment

T71.9 Asphyxiation due to unspecified cause
Suffocation (by strangulation) due to unspecified cause
Suffocation NOS
Systemic oxygen deficiency due to low oxygen content in ambient air due to unspecified cause
Systemic oxygen deficiency due to mechanical threat to breathing due to unspecified cause
Traumatic asphyxia NOS

T73 Effects of other deprivation

The appropriate 7th character is to be added to each code from category T73.
- A initial encounter
- D subsequent encounter
- S sequela

T73.0 Starvation
Deprivation of food

T73.1 Deprivation of water

T73.2 Exhaustion due to exposure

Chapter 19. Injury, Poisoning and Certain Other Consequences of External Causes

- ✓x7ᵗʰ **T73.3** Exhaustion due to excessive exertion
  Exhaustion due to overexertion
- ✓x7ᵗʰ **T73.8** Other effects of deprivation
- ✓x7ᵗʰ **T73.9** Effect of deprivation, unspecified

✓4ᵗʰ **T74** Adult and child abuse, neglect and other maltreatment, confirmed
  Use additional code, if applicable, to identify any associated current injury
  Use additional external cause code to identify perpetrator, if known (Y07.-)
  EXCLUDES 1 abuse and maltreatment in pregnancy (O9A.3-, O9A.4-, O9A.5-)
  adult and child maltreatment, suspected (T76.-)

  The appropriate 7th character is to be added to each code from category T74.
  A initial encounter
  D subsequent encounter
  S sequela

- ✓5ᵗʰ **T74.0** Neglect or abandonment, confirmed
  - ✓x7ᵗʰ **T74.01** Adult neglect or abandonment, confirmed A
  - ✓x7ᵗʰ **T74.02** Child neglect or abandonment, confirmed P
- ✓5ᵗʰ **T74.1** Physical abuse, confirmed
  EXCLUDES 2 sexual abuse (T74.2-)
  - ✓x7ᵗʰ **T74.11** Adult physical abuse, confirmed A
  - ✓x7ᵗʰ **T74.12** Child physical abuse, confirmed P
    EXCLUDES 2 shaken infant syndrome (T74.4)
- ✓5ᵗʰ **T74.2** Sexual abuse, confirmed
  Rape, confirmed
  Sexual assault, confirmed
  - ✓x7ᵗʰ **T74.21** Adult sexual abuse, confirmed A
  - ✓x7ᵗʰ **T74.22** Child sexual abuse, confirmed P
- ✓5ᵗʰ **T74.3** Psychological abuse, confirmed
  Bullying and intimidation, confirmed
  Intimidation through social media, confirmed
  Target of threatened harm, confirmed
  Target of threatened physical violence, confirmed
  Target of threatened sexual abuse, confirmed
  - ✓x7ᵗʰ **T74.31** Adult psychological abuse, confirmed A
  - ✓x7ᵗʰ **T74.32** Child psychological abuse, confirmed P
- ✓x7ᵗʰ **T74.4** Shaken infant syndrome P
- ✓5ᵗʰ **T74.5** Forced sexual exploitation, confirmed
  AHA: 2018,4Q,32-33,65
  - ✓x7ᵗʰ **T74.51** Adult forced sexual exploitation, confirmed A
  - ✓x7ᵗʰ **T74.52** Child sexual exploitation, confirmed P
- ✓5ᵗʰ **T74.6** Forced labor exploitation, confirmed
  AHA: 2018,4Q,32-33,65
  - ✓x7ᵗʰ **T74.61** Adult forced labor exploitation, confirmed A
  - ✓x7ᵗʰ **T74.62** Child forced labor exploitation, confirmed P
- ✓5ᵗʰ **T74.9** Unspecified maltreatment, confirmed
  - ✓x7ᵗʰ **T74.91** Unspecified adult maltreatment, confirmed A
  - ✓x7ᵗʰ **T74.92** Unspecified child maltreatment, confirmed P
- ✓5ᵗʰ **T74.A** Financial abuse, confirmed
  AHA: 2023,1Q,4
  - ✓x7ᵗʰ **T74.A1** Adult financial abuse, confirmed A
  - ✓x7ᵗʰ **T74.A2** Child financial abuse, confirmed P

✓4ᵗʰ **T75** Other and unspecified effects of other external causes
  EXCLUDES 1 adverse effects NEC (T78.-)
  EXCLUDES 2 burns (electric) (T20-T31)

  The appropriate 7th character is to be added to each code from category T75.
  A initial encounter
  D subsequent encounter
  S sequela

- ✓5ᵗʰ **T75.0** Effects of lightning
  Struck by lightning
  - ✓x7ᵗʰ **T75.00** Unspecified effects of lightning
    Struck by lightning NOS
  - ✓x7ᵗʰ **T75.01** Shock due to being struck by lightning
  - ✓x7ᵗʰ **T75.09** Other effects of lightning
    Use additional code for other effects of lightning

- ✓x7ᵗʰ **T75.1** Unspecified effects of drowning and nonfatal submersion
  Immersion
  EXCLUDES 1 specified effects of drowning - code to effects
  AHA: 2023,1Q,25
- ✓5ᵗʰ **T75.2** Effects of vibration
  - ✓x7ᵗʰ **T75.20** Unspecified effects of vibration
  - ✓x7ᵗʰ **T75.21** Pneumatic hammer syndrome
  - ✓x7ᵗʰ **T75.22** Traumatic vasospastic syndrome
  - ✓x7ᵗʰ **T75.23** Vertigo from infrasound
    EXCLUDES 1 vertigo NOS (R42)
  - ✓x7ᵗʰ **T75.29** Other effects of vibration
- ✓x7ᵗʰ **T75.3** Motion sickness
  Airsickness
  Seasickness
  Travel sickness
  Use additional external cause code to identify vehicle or type of motion (Y92.81-)
- ✓x7ᵗʰ **T75.4** Electrocution
  Shock from electric current
  Shock from electroshock gun (taser)
- ✓5ᵗʰ **T75.8** Other specified effects of external causes
  - ✓x7ᵗʰ **T75.81** Effects of abnormal gravitation [G] forces
  - ✓x7ᵗʰ **T75.82** Effects of weightlessness
  - ●✓6ᵗʰ **T75.83** Effects of war theater
    Use additional code to identify associated manifestations
    - ●✓7ᵗʰ **T75.830** Gulf war illness
      Gulf war syndrome
    - ●✓7ᵗʰ **T75.838** Effects of other war theater
  - ✓x7ᵗʰ **T75.89** Other specified effects of external causes

✓4ᵗʰ **T76** Adult and child abuse, neglect and other maltreatment, suspected
  Use additional code, if applicable, to identify any associated current injury
  EXCLUDES 1 adult and child maltreatment, confirmed (T74.-)
  suspected abuse and maltreatment in pregnancy (O9A.3-, O9A.4-, O9A.5-)
  suspected adult physical abuse, ruled out (Z04.71)
  suspected adult sexual abuse, ruled out (Z04.41)
  suspected child physical abuse, ruled out (Z04.72)
  suspected child sexual abuse, ruled out (Z04.42)
  AHA: 2018,4Q,72

  The appropriate 7th character is to be added to each code from category T76.
  A initial encounter
  D subsequent encounter
  S sequela

- ✓5ᵗʰ **T76.0** Neglect or abandonment, suspected
  - ✓x7ᵗʰ **T76.01** Adult neglect or abandonment, suspected A
  - ✓x7ᵗʰ **T76.02** Child neglect or abandonment, suspected P
- ✓5ᵗʰ **T76.1** Physical abuse, suspected
  - ✓x7ᵗʰ **T76.11** Adult physical abuse, suspected A
  - ✓x7ᵗʰ **T76.12** Child physical abuse, suspected P
    AHA: 2019,2Q,12
- ✓5ᵗʰ **T76.2** Sexual abuse, suspected
  Rape, suspected
  EXCLUDES 1 alleged abuse, ruled out (Z04.7)
  - ✓x7ᵗʰ **T76.21** Adult sexual abuse, suspected A
  - ✓x7ᵗʰ **T76.22** Child sexual abuse, suspected P
- ✓5ᵗʰ **T76.3** Psychological abuse, suspected
  Bullying and intimidation, suspected
  Intimidation through social media, suspected
  Target of threatened harm, suspected
  Target of threatened physical violence, suspected
  Target of threatened sexual abuse, suspected
  - ✓x7ᵗʰ **T76.31** Adult psychological abuse, suspected A
  - ✓x7ᵗʰ **T76.32** Child psychological abuse, suspected P
- ✓5ᵗʰ **T76.5** Forced sexual exploitation, suspected
  AHA: 2018,4Q,32-33,65
  - ✓x7ᵗʰ **T76.51** Adult forced sexual exploitation, suspected A
  - ✓x7ᵗʰ **T76.52** Child sexual exploitation, suspected P
- ✓5ᵗʰ **T76.6** Forced labor exploitation, suspected
  AHA: 2018,4Q,32-33,65
  - ✓x7ᵗʰ **T76.61** Adult forced labor exploitation, suspected A

- **T76.62** Child forced labor exploitation, suspected
- **T76.9** Unspecified maltreatment, suspected
  - **T76.91** Unspecified adult maltreatment, suspected
  - **T76.92** Unspecified child maltreatment, suspected
- **T76.A** Financial abuse, suspected
  - AHA: 2023,1Q,4
  - **T76.A1** Adult financial abuse, suspected
  - **T76.A2** Child financial abuse, suspected

T78 Adverse effects, not elsewhere classified

EXCLUDES 2 complications of surgical and medical care NEC (T80-T88)

The appropriate 7th character is to be added to each code from category T78.
- A initial encounter
- D subsequent encounter
- S sequela

- **T78.0** Anaphylactic reaction due to food
  - Anaphylactic reaction due to adverse food reaction
  - Anaphylactic shock or reaction due to nonpoisonous foods
  - Anaphylactoid reaction due to food
  - **T78.00** Anaphylactic reaction due to unspecified food
  - **T78.01** Anaphylactic reaction due to peanuts
  - **T78.02** Anaphylactic reaction due to shellfish (crustaceans)
  - **T78.03** Anaphylactic reaction due to other fish
  - **T78.04** Anaphylactic reaction due to fruits and vegetables
  - **T78.05** Anaphylactic reaction due to tree nuts and seeds
    - EXCLUDES 2 anaphylactic reaction due to peanuts (T78.01)
  - **T78.06** Anaphylactic reaction due to food additives
  - **T78.07** Anaphylactic reaction due to milk and dairy products
    - **T78.070** Anaphylactic reaction due to milk and dairy products with tolerance to baked milk
      - EXCLUDES 1 Anaphylactic reaction due to milk and dairy products with reactivity to baked milk (T78.071)
    - **T78.071** Anaphylactic reaction due to milk and dairy products with reactivity to baked milk
      - EXCLUDES 1 Anaphylactic reaction due to milk and dairy products with tolerance to baked milk (T78.070)
    - **T78.079** Anaphylactic reaction due to milk and dairy products, unspecified
  - **T78.08** Anaphylactic reaction due to eggs
    - **T78.080** Anaphylactic reaction due to egg with tolerance to baked egg
      - EXCLUDES 1 Anaphylactic reaction due to egg with reactivity to baked egg (T78.081)
    - **T78.081** Anaphylactic reaction due to egg with reactivity to baked egg
      - EXCLUDES 1 Anaphylactic reaction due to egg with tolerance to baked egg (T78.080)
    - **T78.089** Anaphylactic reaction due to eggs, unspecified
  - **T78.09** Anaphylactic reaction due to other food products

- **T78.1** Other adverse food reactions, not elsewhere classified
  - Use additional code to identify the type of reaction, if applicable
  - EXCLUDES 1 anaphylactic reaction or shock due to adverse food reaction (T78.0-)
  - anaphylactic reaction due to food (T78.0-)
  - bacterial food borne intoxications (A05.-)
  - EXCLUDES 2 allergic and dietetic gastroenteritis and colitis (K52.29)
  - allergic rhinitis due to food (J30.5)
  - dermatitis due to food in contact with skin (L23.6, L24.6, L25.4)
  - dermatitis due to ingested food (L27.2)
  - food protein-induced enterocolitis syndrome (K52.21)
  - food protein-induced enteropathy (K52.22)
  - **T78.11** Other adverse food reactions due to milk and dairy products
    - **T78.110** Other adverse food reactions due to milk and dairy products with tolerance to baked milk
      - EXCLUDES 1 Other adverse food reaction due to milk and dairy products with reactivity to baked milk (T78.111)
    - **T78.111** Other adverse food reaction due to milk and dairy products with reactivity to baked milk
      - EXCLUDES 1 Other adverse food reaction due to milk and dairy products with tolerance to baked milk (T78.110)
    - **T78.119** Other adverse food reaction due to milk and dairy products with baked milk tolerance/reactivity, unspecified
  - **T78.12** Other adverse food reaction due to eggs
    - **T78.120** Other adverse food reaction due to egg with tolerance to baked egg
      - EXCLUDES 1 Other adverse food reaction due to egg with reactivity to baked egg (T78.121)
    - **T78.121** Other adverse food reaction due to egg with reactivity to baked egg
      - EXCLUDES 1 Other adverse food reaction due to egg with tolerance to baked egg (T78.120)
    - **T78.129** Other adverse food reaction due to egg with baked egg tolerance/reactivity, unspecified
  - **T78.19** Other adverse food reactions, not elsewhere classified

- **T78.2** Anaphylactic shock, unspecified
  - Allergic shock
  - Anaphylactic reaction
  - Anaphylaxis
  - EXCLUDES 1 anaphylactic reaction or shock due to adverse effect of correct medicinal substance properly administered (T88.6)
  - anaphylactic reaction or shock due to adverse food reaction (T78.0-)
  - anaphylactic reaction or shock due to serum (T80.5-)

- **T78.3** Angioneurotic edema
  - Allergic angioedema
  - Giant urticaria
  - Quincke's edema
  - EXCLUDES 1 serum urticaria (T80.6-)
  - urticaria (L50.-)

- **T78.4** Other and unspecified allergy
  - EXCLUDES 1 specified types of allergic reaction such as:
    - allergic diarrhea (K52.29)
    - allergic gastroenteritis and colitis (K52.29)
    - dermatitis (L23-L25, L27.-)
    - food protein-induced enterocolitis syndrome (K52.21)
    - food protein-induced enteropathy (K52.22)
    - hay fever (J30.1)
  - **T78.40** Allergy, unspecified
    - Allergic reaction NOS
    - Hypersensitivity NOS
  - **T78.41** Arthus phenomenon
    - Arthus reaction

Chapter 19. Injury, Poisoning and Certain Other Consequences of External Causes

T78.49 Other allergy
AHA: 2021,1Q,42

T78.8 Other adverse effects, not elsewhere classified

Certain early complications of trauma (T79)

T79 Certain early complications of trauma, not elsewhere classified
EXCLUDES 2: acute respiratory distress syndrome (J80)
complications occurring during or following medical procedures (T80-T88)
complications of surgical and medical care NEC (T80-T88)
newborn respiratory distress syndrome (P22.0)

The appropriate 7th character is to be added to each code from category T79.
A initial encounter
D subsequent encounter
S sequela

T79.0 Air embolism (traumatic)
EXCLUDES 1: air embolism complicating abortion or ectopic or molar pregnancy (O00-O07, O08.2)
air embolism complicating pregnancy, childbirth and the puerperium (O88.0)
air embolism following infusion, transfusion, and therapeutic injection (T80.0)
air embolism following procedure NEC (T81.7-)
DEF: Arterial or venous obstruction due to the introduction of air bubbles into the blood vessels following surgery or trauma.

T79.1 Fat embolism (traumatic)
EXCLUDES 1: fat embolism complicating:
abortion or ectopic or molar pregnancy (O00-O07, O08.2)
pregnancy, childbirth and the puerperium (O88.8)
DEF: Arterial blockage due to the entrance of fat into the circulatory system after a fracture of the large bones or administration of corticosteroids.

T79.2 Traumatic secondary and recurrent hemorrhage and seroma

T79.4 Traumatic shock
Shock (immediate) (delayed) following injury
EXCLUDES 1: anaphylactic shock due to adverse food reaction (T78.0-)
anaphylactic shock due to correct medicinal substance properly administered (T88.6)
anaphylactic shock due to serum (T80.5-)
anaphylactic shock NOS (T78.2)
electric shock (T75.4)
nontraumatic shock NEC (R57.-)
obstetric shock (O75.1)
postprocedural shock (T81.1-)
septic shock (R65.21)
shock complicating abortion or ectopic or molar pregnancy (O00-O07, O08.3)
shock due to anesthesia (T88.2)
shock due to lightning (T75.01)
shock NOS (R57.9)

T79.5 Traumatic anuria
Crush syndrome
Renal failure following crushing

T79.6 Traumatic ischemia of muscle
Traumatic rhabdomyolysis
Volkmann's ischemic contracture
EXCLUDES 2: anterior tibial syndrome (M76.8)
compartment syndrome (traumatic) (T79.A-)
nontraumatic ischemia of muscle (M62.2-)
AHA: 2019,2Q,12

T79.7 Traumatic subcutaneous emphysema
EXCLUDES 2: emphysema NOS (J43)
emphysema (subcutaneous) resulting from a procedure (T81.82)

T79.A Traumatic compartment syndrome
EXCLUDES 1: fibromyalgia (M79.7)
nontraumatic compartment syndrome (M79.A-)
EXCLUDES 2: traumatic ischemic infarction of muscle (T79.6)
DEF: Compression of nerves and blood vessels within an enclosed muscle space due to previous trauma, which leads to impaired blood flow and muscle and nerve damage.

T79.A0 Compartment syndrome, unspecified
Compartment syndrome NOS

T79.A1 Traumatic compartment syndrome of upper extremity
Traumatic compartment syndrome of shoulder, arm, forearm, wrist, hand, and fingers

T79.A11 Traumatic compartment syndrome of right upper extremity

T79.A12 Traumatic compartment syndrome of left upper extremity

T79.A19 Traumatic compartment syndrome of unspecified upper extremity

T79.A2 Traumatic compartment syndrome of lower extremity
Traumatic compartment syndrome of hip, buttock, thigh, leg, foot, and toes

T79.A21 Traumatic compartment syndrome of right lower extremity

T79.A22 Traumatic compartment syndrome of left lower extremity

T79.A29 Traumatic compartment syndrome of unspecified lower extremity

T79.A3 Traumatic compartment syndrome of abdomen

T79.A9 Traumatic compartment syndrome of other sites

T79.8 Other early complications of trauma

T79.9 Unspecified early complication of trauma

Complications of surgical and medical care, not elsewhere classified (T80-T88)

Use additional code for adverse effect, if applicable, to identify drug (T36-T50 with fifth or sixth character 5)
Use additional code(s) to identify the specified condition resulting from the complication
Use additional code to identify devices involved and details of circumstances (Y62-Y82)

EXCLUDES 2 any encounters with medical care for postprocedural conditions in which no complications are present, such as:
artificial opening status (Z93.-)
closure of external stoma (Z43.-)
fitting and adjustment of external prosthetic device (Z44.-)
burns and corrosions from local applications and irradiation (T20-T32)
complications of surgical procedures during pregnancy, childbirth and the puerperium (O00-O9A)
mechanical complication of respirator [ventilator] (J95.850)
poisoning and toxic effects of drugs and chemicals (T36-T65 with fifth or sixth character 1-4 or 6)
postprocedural fever (R50.82)
specified complications classified elsewhere, such as:
cerebrospinal fluid leak from spinal puncture (G97.0)
colostomy malfunction (K94.0-)
disorders of fluid and electrolyte imbalance (E86-E87)
functional disturbances following cardiac surgery (I97.0-I97.1)
intraoperative and postprocedural complications of specified body systems (D78.-, E36.-, E89.-, G97.3-, G97.4, H59.3-, H59.-, H95.2-, H95.3, I97.4-, I97.5, J95.6-, J95.7, K91.6-, L76.-, M96.-, N99.-)
ostomy complications (J95.0-, K94.-, N99.5-)
postgastric surgery syndromes (K91.1)
postlaminectomy syndrome NEC (M96.1)
postmastectomy lymphedema syndrome (I97.2)
postsurgical blind-loop syndrome (K91.2)
ventilator associated pneumonia (J95.851)

AHA: 2015,1Q,15

✓4th T80 Complications following infusion, transfusion and therapeutic injection

INCLUDES complications following perfusion
EXCLUDES 2 bone marrow transplant rejection (T86.01)
febrile nonhemolytic transfusion reaction (R50.84)
fluid overload due to transfusion (E87.71)
posttransfusion purpura (D69.51)
transfusion (red blood cell) associated hemochromatosis (E83.111)
transfusion associated circulatory overload (TACO) (E87.71)
transfusion related acute lung injury (TRALI) (J95.84)

The appropriate 7th character is to be added to each code from category T80.
A initial encounter
D subsequent encounter
S sequela

✓x 7th T80.0 Air embolism following infusion, transfusion and therapeutic injection

✓x 7th T80.1 Vascular complications following infusion, transfusion and therapeutic injection
Use additional code to identify the vascular complication
EXCLUDES 2 extravasation of vesicant agent (T80.81-)
infiltration of vesicant agent (T80.81-)
postprocedural vascular complications (T81.7-)
vascular complications specified as due to prosthetic devices, implants and grafts (T82.8-, T83.8-, T84.8-, T85.8-)

✓5th T80.2 Infections following infusion, transfusion and therapeutic injection
Use additional code (R65.2-) to identify severe sepsis, if applicable
Use additional code to identify the specific infection, such as: sepsis (A41.9)
EXCLUDES 2 infections specified as due to prosthetic devices, implants and grafts (T82.6-T82.7, T83.5-T83.6, T84.5-T84.7, T85.7)
postprocedural infections (T81.4-)

AHA: 2018,4Q,62

✓6th T80.21 Infection due to central venous catheter
Infection due to pulmonary artery catheter (Swan-Ganz catheter)
AHA: 2019,1Q,13-14
DEF: Central venous catheter: Catheter positioned in the superior vena cava or right atrium and introduced through a large vein, such as the jugular or subclavian, and used to measure venous pressure or administer fluids or medication.
TIP: Code assignment is based on the location of the catheter and not how the catheter is being used; for example, for hemodialysis. Infections resulting from catheters that are not central lines should be coded to T82.7-.

✓7th T80.211 Bloodstream infection due to central venous catheter
Bloodstream infection due to Hickman catheter
Bloodstream infection due to peripherally inserted central catheter (PICC)
Bloodstream infection due to portacath (port-a-cath)
Bloodstream infection due to pulmonary artery catheter
Bloodstream infection due to triple lumen catheter
Bloodstream infection due to umbilical venous catheter
Catheter-related bloodstream infection (CRBSI) NOS
Central line-associated bloodstream infection (CLABSI)
AHA: 2019,1Q,13,14; 2018,4Q,89

✓7th T80.212 Local infection due to central venous catheter
Exit or insertion site infection
Local infection due to Hickman catheter
Local infection due to peripherally inserted central catheter (PICC)
Local infection due to portacath (port-a-cath)
Local infection due to pulmonary artery catheter
Local infection due to triple lumen catheter
Local infection due to umbilical venous catheter
Port or reservoir infection
Tunnel infection

✓7th T80.218 Other infection due to central venous catheter
Other central line-associated infection
Other infection due to Hickman catheter
Other infection due to peripherally inserted central catheter (PICC)
Other infection due to portacath (port-a-cath)
Other infection due to pulmonary artery catheter
Other infection due to triple lumen catheter
Other infection due to umbilical venous catheter

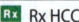

             T80.219 Unspecified infection due to central venous catheter
                        Central line-associated infection NOS
                        Unspecified infection due to Hickman catheter
                        Unspecified infection due to peripherally inserted central catheter (PICC)
                        Unspecified infection due to portacath (port-a-cath)
                        Unspecified infection due to pulmonary artery catheter
                        Unspecified infection due to triple lumen catheter
                        Unspecified infection due to umbilical venous catheter
      T80.22 Acute infection following transfusion, infusion, or injection of blood and blood products
      T80.29 Infection following other infusion, transfusion and therapeutic injection
   T80.3 ABO incompatibility reaction due to transfusion of blood or blood products
          EXCLUDES 1   minor blood group antigens reactions (Duffy) (E) (K) (Kell) (Kidd) (Lewis) (M) (N) (P) (S) (T80.A-)
      T80.30 ABO incompatibility reaction due to transfusion of blood or blood products, unspecified
                  ABO incompatibility blood transfusion NOS
                  Reaction to ABO incompatibility from transfusion NOS
      T80.31 ABO incompatibility with hemolytic transfusion reaction
             T80.310 ABO incompatibility with acute hemolytic transfusion reaction
                        ABO incompatibility with hemolytic transfusion reaction less than 24 hours after transfusion
                        Acute hemolytic transfusion reaction (AHTR) due to ABO incompatibility
             T80.311 ABO incompatibility with delayed hemolytic transfusion reaction
                        ABO incompatibility with hemolytic transfusion reaction 24 hours or more after transfusion
                        Delayed hemolytic transfusion reaction (DHTR) due to ABO incompatibility
             T80.319 ABO incompatibility with hemolytic transfusion reaction, unspecified
                        ABO incompatibility with hemolytic transfusion reaction at unspecified time after transfusion
                        Hemolytic transfusion reaction (HTR) due to ABO incompatibility NOS
      T80.39 Other ABO incompatibility reaction due to transfusion of blood or blood products
                  Delayed serologic transfusion reaction (DSTR) from ABO incompatibility
                  Other ABO incompatible blood transfusion
                  Other reaction to ABO incompatible blood transfusion
   T80.4 Rh incompatibility reaction due to transfusion of blood or blood products
          Reaction due to incompatibility of Rh antigens (C) (c) (D) (E) (e)
      T80.40 Rh incompatibility reaction due to transfusion of blood or blood products, unspecified
                  Reaction due to Rh factor in transfusion NOS
                  Rh incompatible blood transfusion NOS
      T80.41 Rh incompatibility with hemolytic transfusion reaction
             T80.410 Rh incompatibility with acute hemolytic transfusion reaction
                        Acute hemolytic transfusion reaction (AHTR) due to Rh incompatibility
                        Rh incompatibility with hemolytic transfusion reaction less than 24 hours after transfusion
             T80.411 Rh incompatibility with delayed hemolytic transfusion reaction
                        Delayed hemolytic transfusion reaction (DHTR) due to Rh incompatibility
                        Rh incompatibility with hemolytic transfusion reaction 24 hours or more after transfusion
             T80.419 Rh incompatibility with hemolytic transfusion reaction, unspecified
                        Hemolytic transfusion reaction (HTR) due to Rh incompatibility NOS
                        Rh incompatibility with hemolytic transfusion reaction at unspecified time after transfusion
      T80.49 Other Rh incompatibility reaction due to transfusion of blood or blood products
                  Delayed serologic transfusion reaction (DSTR) from Rh incompatibility
                  Other reaction to Rh incompatible blood transfusion
   T80.A Non-ABO incompatibility reaction due to transfusion of blood or blood products
          Reaction due to incompatibility of minor antigens (Duffy) (Kell) (Kidd) (Lewis) (M) (N) (P) (S)
      T80.A0 Non-ABO incompatibility reaction due to transfusion of blood or blood products, unspecified
                  Non-ABO antigen incompatibility reaction from transfusion NOS
      T80.A1 Non-ABO incompatibility with hemolytic transfusion reaction
             T80.A10 Non-ABO incompatibility with acute hemolytic transfusion reaction
                        Acute hemolytic transfusion reaction (AHTR) due to non-ABO incompatibility
                        Non-ABO incompatibility with hemolytic transfusion reaction less than 24 hours after transfusion
             T80.A11 Non-ABO incompatibility with delayed hemolytic transfusion reaction
                        Delayed hemolytic transfusion reaction (DHTR) due to non-ABO incompatibility
                        Non-ABO incompatibility with hemolytic transfusion reaction 24 or more hours after transfusion
             T80.A19 Non-ABO incompatibility with hemolytic transfusion reaction, unspecified
                        Hemolytic transfusion reaction (HTR) due to non-ABO incompatibility NOS
                        Non-ABO incompatibility with hemolytic transfusion reaction at unspecified time after transfusion
      T80.A9 Other non-ABO incompatibility reaction due to transfusion of blood or blood products
                  Delayed serologic transfusion reaction (DSTR) from non-ABO incompatibility
                  Other reaction to non-ABO incompatible blood transfusion
   T80.5 Anaphylactic reaction due to serum
          Allergic shock due to serum
          Anaphylactic shock due to serum
          Anaphylactoid reaction due to serum
          Anaphylaxis due to serum
          EXCLUDES 1   ABO incompatibility reaction due to transfusion of blood or blood products (T80.3-)
                      allergic reaction or shock NOS (T78.2)
                      anaphylactic reaction or shock due to adverse effect of correct medicinal substance properly administered (T88.6)
                      anaphylactic reaction or shock NOS (T78.2)
                      other serum reaction (T80.6-)
          DEF: Life-threatening hypersensitivity to a foreign serum causing respiratory distress, vascular collapse, and shock.
      T80.51 Anaphylactic reaction due to administration of blood and blood products
      T80.52 Anaphylactic reaction due to vaccination
              AHA: 2021,1Q,43
      T80.59 Anaphylactic reaction due to other serum
   T80.6 Other serum reactions
          Intoxication by serum
          Protein sickness
          Serum rash
          Serum sickness
          Serum urticaria
          EXCLUDES 2   serum hepatitis (B16-B19)
          DEF: Serum sickness: Hypersensitivity to a foreign serum that causes fever, hives, swelling, and lymphadenopathy.
      T80.61 Other serum reaction due to administration of blood and blood products

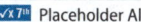

T80.62 – T81.30
Chapter 19. Injury, Poisoning and Certain Other Consequences of External Causes

- ✓x 7th **T80.62** Other serum reaction **due to vaccination**
  AHA: 2021,1Q,42
- ✓x 7th **T80.69** Other serum reaction due to other serum
  Code also, if applicable, arthropathy in hypersensitivity reactions classified elsewhere (M36.4)
- ✓5th **T80.8** Other complications following infusion, transfusion and therapeutic injection
  - ✓6th **T80.81** Extravasation of vesicant agent
    Infiltration of vesicant agent
    - ✓7th **T80.810** Extravasation of vesicant antineoplastic chemotherapy
      Infiltration of vesicant antineoplastic chemotherapy
    - ✓7th **T80.818** Extravasation of other vesicant agent
      Infiltration of other vesicant agent
  - ✓x 7th **T80.82** Complication of immune effector cellular therapy
    Complication of chimeric antigen receptor (CAR-T) cell therapy
    Complication of IEC therapy
    Use additional code to identify the specific complication, such as:
    cytokine release syndrome (D89.83-)
    immune effector cell-associated neurotoxicity syndrome (G92.0-)
    EXCLUDES 2: adverse effect of immune checkpoint inhibitors and immunostimulant drugs (T45.AX5)
    complication of bone marrow transplant (T86.0)
    complication of stem cell transplant (T86.5)
    AHA: 2021,4Q,31
  - ✓x 7th **T80.89** Other complications following infusion, transfusion and therapeutic injection
    Delayed serologic transfusion reaction (DSTR), unspecified incompatibility
    Use additional code to identify graft-versus-host reaction, if applicable, (D89.81-)
    AHA: 2020,4Q,14
- ✓5th **T80.9** Unspecified complication following infusion, transfusion and therapeutic injection
  - ✓x 7th **T80.90** Unspecified complication **following infusion and therapeutic injection**
  - ✓6th **T80.91** **Hemolytic transfusion reaction,** unspecified incompatibility
    EXCLUDES 1: ABO incompatibility with hemolytic transfusion reaction (T80.31-)
    non-ABO incompatibility with hemolytic transfusion reaction (T80.A1-)
    Rh incompatibility with hemolytic transfusion reaction (T80.41-)
    - ✓7th **T80.910** **Acute** hemolytic transfusion reaction, unspecified incompatibility
    - ✓7th **T80.911** **Delayed** hemolytic transfusion reaction, unspecified incompatibility
    - ✓7th **T80.919** Hemolytic transfusion reaction, unspecified incompatibility, unspecified as acute or delayed
      Hemolytic transfusion reaction NOS
  - ✓x 7th **T80.92** Unspecified transfusion reaction
    Transfusion reaction NOS

- ✓4th **T81** Complications of procedures, not elsewhere classified
  Use additional code for adverse effect, if applicable, to identify drug (T36-T50 with fifth or sixth character 5)
  EXCLUDES 2: complications following immunization (T88.0-T88.1)
  complications following infusion, transfusion and therapeutic injection (T80.-)
  complications of transplanted organs and tissue (T86.-)
  specified complications classified elsewhere, such as:
  complication of prosthetic devices, implants and grafts (T82-T85)
  dermatitis due to drugs and medicaments (L23.3, L24.4, L25.1, L27.0-L27.1)
  endosseous dental implant failure (M27.6-)
  floppy iris syndrome (IFIS) (intraoperative) (H21.81)
  intraoperative and postprocedural complications of specific body system (D78.-, E36.-, E89.-, G97.3-, G97.4, H59.3-, H59.-, H95.2-, H95.3, I97.4-, I97.5, J95, K91.-, L76.-, M96.-, N99.-)
  ostomy complications (J95.0-, K94.-, N99.5-)
  plateau iris syndrome (post-iridectomy) (postprocedural) H21.82
  poisoning and toxic effects of drugs and chemicals (T36-T65 with fifth or sixth character 1-4)
  AHA: 2019,2Q,21

  The appropriate 7th character is to be added to each code from category T81.
  A initial encounter
  D subsequent encounter
  S sequela

  - ✓5th **T81.1** Postprocedural shock
    Shock during or resulting from a procedure, not elsewhere classified
    EXCLUDES 1: anaphylactic shock NOS (T78.2)
    anaphylactic shock due to correct substance properly administered (T88.6)
    anaphylactic shock due to serum (T80.5-)
    electric shock (T75.4)
    obstetric shock (O75.1)
    shock due to anesthesia (T88.2)
    shock following abortion or ectopic or molar pregnancy (O00-O07, O08.3)
    traumatic shock (T79.4)
    AHA: 2021,1Q,13
    - ✓x 7th **T81.10** Postprocedural shock unspecified
      Collapse NOS during or resulting from a procedure, not elsewhere classified
      Postprocedural failure of peripheral circulation
      Postprocedural shock NOS
    - ✓x 7th **T81.11** Postprocedural **cardiogenic** shock ESR
    - ✓x 7th **T81.12** Postprocedural **septic** shock ESR UPD
      Postprocedural endotoxic shock resulting from a procedure, not elsewhere classified
      Postprocedural gram-negative shock resulting from a procedure, not elsewhere classified
      Code first underlying infection
      Use additional code, to identify any associated acute organ dysfunction, if applicable
      AHA: 2018,4Q,63
    - ✓x 7th **T81.19** Other postprocedural shock
      Postprocedural hypovolemic shock
  - ✓5th **T81.3** Disruption of wound, not elsewhere classified
    Disruption of any suture materials or other closure methods
    EXCLUDES 1: breakdown (mechanical) of permanent sutures (T85.612)
    displacement of permanent sutures (T85.622)
    disruption of cesarean delivery wound (O90.0)
    disruption of perineal obstetric wound (O90.1)
    mechanical complication of permanent sutures NEC (T85.692)
    AHA: 2014,1Q,23
    - ✓x 7th **T81.30** Disruption of wound, unspecified
      Disruption of wound NOS

Chapter 19. Injury, Poisoning and Certain Other Consequences of External Causes

T81.31 Disruption of external operation (surgical) wound, not elsewhere classified
Dehiscence of operation wound NOS
Disruption of operation wound NOS
Disruption or dehiscence of closure of cornea
Disruption or dehiscence of closure of mucosa
Disruption or dehiscence of closure of skin and subcutaneous tissue
Full-thickness skin disruption or dehiscence
Superficial disruption or dehiscence of operation wound

EXCLUDES 1 dehiscence of amputation stump (T87.81)

T81.32 Disruption of internal operation (surgical) wound, not elsewhere classified
AHA: 2024,4Q,29-30; 2020,2Q,22; 2017,3Q,4

- **T81.320** Disruption or dehiscence of gastrointestinal tract anastomosis, repair, or closure
- **T81.321** Disruption or dehiscence of closure of internal operation (surgical) wound of abdominal wall muscle or fascia
- **T81.328** Disruption or dehiscence of closure of other specified internal operation (surgical) wound
  Disruption or dehiscence of closure of muscle or muscle flap (other than abdominal wall muscle)
  Disruption or dehiscence of closure of ribs or rib cage
  Disruption or dehiscence of closure of skull or craniotomy
  Disruption or dehiscence of closure of sternum or sternotomy
  Disruption or dehiscence of closure of superficial or muscular fascia (other than abdominal wall fascia)
  Disruption or dehiscence of closure of tendon or ligament
- **T81.329** Deep disruption or dehiscence of operation wound, unspecified
  Deep disruption or dehiscence of operation wound NOS

T81.33 Disruption of traumatic injury wound repair
Disruption or dehiscence of closure of traumatic laceration (external) (internal)

T81.4 Infection following a procedure
Wound abscess following a procedure
Code also, if applicable, disruption of internal operation (surgical) wound (T81.32-)
Use additional code (R65.2-) to identify severe sepsis, if applicable
Use additional code to identify infection

EXCLUDES 2 bleb associated endophthalmitis (H59.4-)
infection due to infusion, transfusion and therapeutic injection (T80.2-)
infection due to prosthetic devices, implants and grafts (T82.6-T82.7, T83.5-T83.6, T84.5-T84.7, T85.7)
obstetric surgical wound infection (O86.0-)
postprocedural fever NOS (R50.82)
postprocedural retroperitoneal abscess (K68.11)

AHA: 2024,1Q,19; 2018,4Q,33-34,62; 2014,1Q,23

- **T81.40** Infection following a procedure, unspecified
- **T81.41** Infection following a procedure, superficial incisional surgical site
  Stitch abscess following a procedure
  Subcutaneous abscess following a procedure
- **T81.42** Infection following a procedure, deep incisional surgical site
  Intra-muscular abscess following a procedure
- **T81.43** Infection following a procedure, organ and space surgical site
  Intra-abdominal abscess following a procedure
  Subphrenic abscess following a procedure
- **T81.44** Sepsis following a procedure
  Use additional code to identify the sepsis
- **T81.49** Infection following a procedure, other surgical site

T81.5 Complications of foreign body accidentally left in body following procedure
AHA: 2014,4Q,24

- **T81.50** Unspecified complication of foreign body accidentally left in body following procedure
  - **T81.500** Unspecified complication of foreign body accidentally left in body following surgical operation
  - **T81.501** Unspecified complication of foreign body accidentally left in body following infusion or transfusion
  - **T81.502** Unspecified complication of foreign body accidentally left in body following kidney dialysis
  - **T81.503** Unspecified complication of foreign body accidentally left in body following injection or immunization
  - **T81.504** Unspecified complication of foreign body accidentally left in body following endoscopic examination
  - **T81.505** Unspecified complication of foreign body accidentally left in body following heart catheterization
  - **T81.506** Unspecified complication of foreign body accidentally left in body following aspiration, puncture or other catheterization
  - **T81.507** Unspecified complication of foreign body accidentally left in body following removal of catheter or packing
  - **T81.508** Unspecified complication of foreign body accidentally left in body following other procedure
  - **T81.509** Unspecified complication of foreign body accidentally left in body following unspecified procedure

- **T81.51** Adhesions due to foreign body accidentally left in body following procedure
  - **T81.510** Adhesions due to foreign body accidentally left in body following surgical operation
  - **T81.511** Adhesions due to foreign body accidentally left in body following infusion or transfusion
  - **T81.512** Adhesions due to foreign body accidentally left in body following kidney dialysis
  - **T81.513** Adhesions due to foreign body accidentally left in body following injection or immunization
  - **T81.514** Adhesions due to foreign body accidentally left in body following endoscopic examination
  - **T81.515** Adhesions due to foreign body accidentally left in body following heart catheterization
  - **T81.516** Adhesions due to foreign body accidentally left in body following aspiration, puncture or other catheterization
  - **T81.517** Adhesions due to foreign body accidentally left in body following removal of catheter or packing
  - **T81.518** Adhesions due to foreign body accidentally left in body following other procedure
  - **T81.519** Adhesions due to foreign body accidentally left in body following unspecified procedure

- **T81.52** Obstruction due to foreign body accidentally left in body following procedure
  - **T81.520** Obstruction due to foreign body accidentally left in body following surgical operation
  - **T81.521** Obstruction due to foreign body accidentally left in body following infusion or transfusion
  - **T81.522** Obstruction due to foreign body accidentally left in body following kidney dialysis
  - **T81.523** Obstruction due to foreign body accidentally left in body following injection or immunization
  - **T81.524** Obstruction due to foreign body accidentally left in body following endoscopic examination
  - **T81.525** Obstruction due to foreign body accidentally left in body following heart catheterization
  - **T81.526** Obstruction due to foreign body accidentally left in body following aspiration, puncture or other catheterization
  - **T81.527** Obstruction due to foreign body accidentally left in body following removal of catheter or packing

T81.528 Obstruction due to foreign body accidentally left in body following other procedure

T81.529 Obstruction due to foreign body accidentally left in body following unspecified procedure

T81.53 Perforation due to foreign body accidentally left in body following procedure

- **T81.530** Perforation due to foreign body accidentally left in body following surgical operation
- **T81.531** Perforation due to foreign body accidentally left in body following infusion or transfusion
- **T81.532** Perforation due to foreign body accidentally left in body following kidney dialysis
- **T81.533** Perforation due to foreign body accidentally left in body following injection or immunization
- **T81.534** Perforation due to foreign body accidentally left in body following endoscopic examination
- **T81.535** Perforation due to foreign body accidentally left in body following heart catheterization
- **T81.536** Perforation due to foreign body accidentally left in body following aspiration, puncture or other catheterization
- **T81.537** Perforation due to foreign body accidentally left in body following removal of catheter or packing
- **T81.538** Perforation due to foreign body accidentally left in body following other procedure
- **T81.539** Perforation due to foreign body accidentally left in body following unspecified procedure

T81.59 Other complications of foreign body accidentally left in body following procedure

EXCLUDES 2: obstruction or perforation due to prosthetic devices and implants intentionally left in body (T82.0-T82.5, T83.0-T83.4, T83.7, T84.0-T84.4, T85.0-T85.6)

- **T81.590** Other complications of foreign body accidentally left in body following surgical operation
  AHA: 2025,2Q,10
- **T81.591** Other complications of foreign body accidentally left in body following infusion or transfusion
- **T81.592** Other complications of foreign body accidentally left in body following kidney dialysis
- **T81.593** Other complications of foreign body accidentally left in body following injection or immunization
- **T81.594** Other complications of foreign body accidentally left in body following endoscopic examination
- **T81.595** Other complications of foreign body accidentally left in body following heart catheterization
- **T81.596** Other complications of foreign body accidentally left in body following aspiration, puncture or other catheterization
- **T81.597** Other complications of foreign body accidentally left in body following removal of catheter or packing
- **T81.598** Other complications of foreign body accidentally left in body following other procedure
- **T81.599** Other complications of foreign body accidentally left in body following unspecified procedure

T81.6 Acute reaction to foreign substance accidentally left during a procedure

EXCLUDES 2: complications of foreign body accidentally left in body cavity or operation wound following procedure (T81.5-)

T81.60 Unspecified acute reaction to foreign substance accidentally left during a procedure

T81.61 Aseptic peritonitis due to foreign substance accidentally left during a procedure
Chemical peritonitis

T81.69 Other acute reaction to foreign substance accidentally left during a procedure

T81.7 Vascular complications following a procedure, not elsewhere classified
Air embolism following procedure NEC
Phlebitis or thrombophlebitis resulting from a procedure

EXCLUDES 1: embolism complicating abortion or ectopic or molar pregnancy (O00-O07, O08.2)
embolism complicating pregnancy, childbirth and the puerperium (O88.-)
traumatic embolism (T79.0)

EXCLUDES 2: embolism due to prosthetic devices, implants and grafts (T82.8-, T83.81, T84.8-, T85.81-)
embolism following infusion, transfusion and therapeutic injection (T80.0)

AHA: 2019,2Q,22

T81.71 Complication of artery following a procedure, not elsewhere classified

- **T81.710** Complication of mesenteric artery following a procedure, not elsewhere classified
- **T81.711** Complication of renal artery following a procedure, not elsewhere classified
- **T81.718** Complication of other artery following a procedure, not elsewhere classified
  AHA: 2024,4Q,19; 2019,2Q,21-22
- **T81.719** Complication of unspecified artery following a procedure, not elsewhere classified

T81.72 Complication of vein following a procedure, not elsewhere classified

T81.8 Other complications of procedures, not elsewhere classified

EXCLUDES 2: hypothermia following anesthesia (T88.51)
malignant hyperpyrexia due to anesthesia (T88.3)

T81.81 Complication of inhalation therapy

T81.82 Emphysema (subcutaneous) resulting from a procedure

T81.83 Persistent postprocedural fistula
Code also, if applicable, disruption of internal operation (surgical) wound (T81.32-)
Use additional code, if known, for site of fistula such as:
 anal fistula (K60.3-)
 anorectal fistula (K60.5-)
 bladder fistula (N32.2)
 other female intestinal-genital tract fistulae (N82.4)
AHA: 2024,3Q,4; 2023,1Q,30; 2017,3Q,3-4

T81.89 Other complications of procedures, not elsewhere classified
Use additional code to specify complication, such as:
 postprocedural delirium (F05)
AHA: 2014,1Q,23

T81.9 Unspecified complication of procedure

T82 Complications of cardiac and vascular prosthetic devices, implants and grafts

EXCLUDES 2: failure and rejection of transplanted organs and tissue (T86.-)
AHA: 2020,3Q,36-37

The appropriate 7th character is to be added to each code from category T82.
 A initial encounter
 D subsequent encounter
 S sequela

T82.0 Mechanical complication of heart valve prosthesis
Mechanical complication of artificial heart valve

EXCLUDES 1: mechanical complication of biological heart valve graft (T82.22-)

T82.01 Breakdown (mechanical) of heart valve prosthesis

T82.02 Displacement of heart valve prosthesis
Malposition of heart valve prosthesis

T82.03 Leakage of heart valve prosthesis

T82.09 Other mechanical complication of heart valve prosthesis
Obstruction (mechanical) of heart valve prosthesis
Perforation of heart valve prosthesis
Protrusion of heart valve prosthesis

Chapter 19. Injury, Poisoning and Certain Other Consequences of External Causes

T82.1 Mechanical complication of cardiac electronic device
- **T82.11** Breakdown (mechanical) of cardiac electronic device
  - T82.110 Breakdown (mechanical) of cardiac electrode
  - T82.111 Breakdown (mechanical) of cardiac pulse generator (battery)
  - T82.118 Breakdown (mechanical) of other cardiac electronic device
  - T82.119 Breakdown (mechanical) of unspecified cardiac electronic device
- **T82.12** Displacement of cardiac electronic device
  - Malposition of cardiac electronic device
  - T82.120 Displacement of cardiac electrode
  - T82.121 Displacement of cardiac pulse generator (battery)
  - T82.128 Displacement of other cardiac electronic device
  - T82.129 Displacement of unspecified cardiac electronic device
- **T82.19** Other mechanical complication of cardiac electronic device
  - Leakage of cardiac electronic device
  - Obstruction of cardiac electronic device
  - Perforation of cardiac electronic device
  - Protrusion of cardiac electronic device
  - T82.190 Other mechanical complication of cardiac electrode
  - T82.191 Other mechanical complication of cardiac pulse generator (battery)
  - T82.198 Other mechanical complication of other cardiac electronic device
  - T82.199 Other mechanical complication of unspecified cardiac device

T82.2 Mechanical complication of coronary artery bypass graft and biological heart valve graft
EXCLUDES 1: mechanical complication of artificial heart valve prosthesis (T82.0-)
- **T82.21** Mechanical complication of coronary artery bypass graft
  - T82.211 Breakdown (mechanical) of coronary artery bypass graft
  - T82.212 Displacement of coronary artery bypass graft
    - Malposition of coronary artery bypass graft
  - T82.213 Leakage of coronary artery bypass graft
  - T82.218 Other mechanical complication of coronary artery bypass graft
    - Obstruction, mechanical of coronary artery bypass graft
    - Perforation of coronary artery bypass graft
    - Protrusion of coronary artery bypass graft
- **T82.22** Mechanical complication of biological heart valve graft
  - T82.221 Breakdown (mechanical) of biological heart valve graft
  - T82.222 Displacement of biological heart valve graft
    - Malposition of biological heart valve graft
  - T82.223 Leakage of biological heart valve graft
  - T82.228 Other mechanical complication of biological heart valve graft
    - Obstruction of biological heart valve graft
    - Perforation of biological heart valve graft
    - Protrusion of biological heart valve graft

T82.3 Mechanical complication of other vascular grafts
- **T82.31** Breakdown (mechanical) of other vascular grafts
  - T82.310 Breakdown (mechanical) of aortic (bifurcation) graft (replacement)
    - AHA: 2020,3Q,3-8
  - T82.311 Breakdown (mechanical) of carotid arterial graft (bypass)
  - T82.312 Breakdown (mechanical) of femoral arterial graft (bypass)
  - T82.318 Breakdown (mechanical) of other vascular grafts
  - T82.319 Breakdown (mechanical) of unspecified vascular grafts
- **T82.32** Displacement of other vascular grafts
  - Malposition of other vascular grafts
  - T82.320 Displacement of aortic (bifurcation) graft (replacement)
  - T82.321 Displacement of carotid arterial graft (bypass)
  - T82.322 Displacement of femoral arterial graft (bypass)
  - T82.328 Displacement of other vascular grafts
  - T82.329 Displacement of unspecified vascular grafts
- **T82.33** Leakage of other vascular grafts
  - T82.330 Leakage of aortic (bifurcation) graft (replacement)
    - AHA: 2020,3Q,3-8
  - T82.331 Leakage of carotid arterial graft (bypass)
  - T82.332 Leakage of femoral arterial graft (bypass)
  - T82.338 Leakage of other vascular grafts
  - T82.339 Leakage of unspecified vascular graft
- **T82.39** Other mechanical complication of other vascular grafts
  - Obstruction (mechanical) of other vascular grafts
  - Perforation of other vascular grafts
  - Protrusion of other vascular grafts
  - T82.390 Other mechanical complication of aortic (bifurcation) graft (replacement)
    - AHA: 2020,3Q,3-5
  - T82.391 Other mechanical complication of carotid arterial graft (bypass)
  - T82.392 Other mechanical complication of femoral arterial graft (bypass)
  - T82.398 Other mechanical complication of other vascular grafts
  - T82.399 Other mechanical complication of unspecified vascular grafts

T82.4 Mechanical complication of vascular dialysis catheter
Mechanical complication of hemodialysis catheter
EXCLUDES 1: mechanical complication of intraperitoneal dialysis catheter (T85.62)
- **T82.41** Breakdown (mechanical) of vascular dialysis catheter
- **T82.42** Displacement of vascular dialysis catheter
  - Malposition of vascular dialysis catheter
- **T82.43** Leakage of vascular dialysis catheter
- **T82.49** Other complication of vascular dialysis catheter
  - Obstruction (mechanical) of vascular dialysis catheter
  - Perforation of vascular dialysis catheter
  - Protrusion of vascular dialysis catheter

T82.5 Mechanical complication of other cardiac and vascular devices and implants
EXCLUDES 2: mechanical complication of epidural and subdural infusion catheter (T85.61)
- **T82.51** Breakdown (mechanical) of other cardiac and vascular devices and implants
  - T82.510 Breakdown (mechanical) of surgically created arteriovenous fistula
    - AHA: 2020,3Q,36
  - T82.511 Breakdown (mechanical) of surgically created arteriovenous shunt
    - AHA: 2020,3Q,37
  - T82.512 Breakdown (mechanical) of artificial heart
  - T82.513 Breakdown (mechanical) of balloon (counterpulsation) device
  - T82.514 Breakdown (mechanical) of infusion catheter
  - T82.515 Breakdown (mechanical) of umbrella device
  - T82.518 Breakdown (mechanical) of other cardiac and vascular devices and implants
  - T82.519 Breakdown (mechanical) of unspecified cardiac and vascular devices and implants

- **T82.52** Displacement of other cardiac and vascular devices and implants
  - Malposition of other cardiac and vascular devices and implants
  - **T82.520** Displacement of surgically created arteriovenous fistula
    - AHA: 2020,3Q,36
  - **T82.521** Displacement of surgically created arteriovenous shunt
  - **T82.522** Displacement of artificial heart
  - **T82.523** Displacement of balloon (counterpulsation) device
  - **T82.524** Displacement of infusion catheter
    - AHA: 2020,2Q,21; 2019,3Q,15
  - **T82.525** Displacement of umbrella device
  - **T82.528** Displacement of other cardiac and vascular devices and implants
  - **T82.529** Displacement of unspecified cardiac and vascular devices and implants
- **T82.53** Leakage of other cardiac and vascular devices and implants
  - **T82.530** Leakage of surgically created arteriovenous fistula
    - AHA: 2020,3Q,36
  - **T82.531** Leakage of surgically created arteriovenous shunt
  - **T82.532** Leakage of artificial heart
  - **T82.533** Leakage of balloon (counterpulsation) device
  - **T82.534** Leakage of infusion catheter
  - **T82.535** Leakage of umbrella device
  - **T82.538** Leakage of other cardiac and vascular devices and implants
  - **T82.539** Leakage of unspecified cardiac and vascular devices and implants
- **T82.59** Other mechanical complication of other cardiac and vascular devices and implants
  - Obstruction (mechanical) of other cardiac and vascular devices and implants
  - Perforation of other cardiac and vascular devices and implants
  - Protrusion of other cardiac and vascular devices and implants
  - **T82.590** Other mechanical complication of surgically created arteriovenous fistula
    - AHA: 2020,3Q,36
  - **T82.591** Other mechanical complication of surgically created arteriovenous shunt
  - **T82.592** Other mechanical complication of artificial heart
  - **T82.593** Other mechanical complication of balloon (counterpulsation) device
  - **T82.594** Other mechanical complication of infusion catheter
  - **T82.595** Other mechanical complication of umbrella device
  - **T82.598** Other mechanical complication of other cardiac and vascular devices and implants
  - **T82.599** Other mechanical complication of unspecified cardiac and vascular devices and implants
- **T82.6** Infection and inflammatory reaction due to cardiac valve prosthesis
  - Use additional code to identify infection
  - AHA: 2025,1Q,19,20
- **T82.7** Infection and inflammatory reaction due to other cardiac and vascular devices, implants and grafts
  - Use additional code to identify infection
  - AHA: 2019,1Q,13-14
  - **DEF:** Midline catheter: Long peripheral catheter introduced via the cephalic, basilic, brachial, or median cubital veins in the upper arm and positioned so that the tip is level or near the level of the axilla and distal to the shoulder. Midline catheters are typically used for IV access, fluid replacement, and medication administration.
  - **TIP:** Assign this code for infections and/or cellulitis resulting from catheters that are not centrally placed (e.g., midline catheters).
- **T82.8** Other specified complications of cardiac and vascular prosthetic devices, implants and grafts
  - AHA: 2016,4Q,70
  - **T82.81** Embolism due to cardiac and vascular prosthetic devices, implants and grafts
    - **T82.817** Embolism due to cardiac prosthetic devices, implants and grafts
    - **T82.818** Embolism due to vascular prosthetic devices, implants and grafts
  - **T82.82** Fibrosis due to cardiac and vascular prosthetic devices, implants and grafts
    - **T82.827** Fibrosis due to cardiac prosthetic devices, implants and grafts
    - **T82.828** Fibrosis due to vascular prosthetic devices, implants and grafts
  - **T82.83** Hemorrhage due to cardiac and vascular prosthetic devices, implants and grafts
    - **T82.837** Hemorrhage due to cardiac prosthetic devices, implants and grafts
    - **T82.838** Hemorrhage due to vascular prosthetic devices, implants and grafts
      - AHA: 2020,3Q,36-37
  - **T82.84** Pain due to cardiac and vascular prosthetic devices, implants and grafts
    - **T82.847** Pain due to cardiac prosthetic devices, implants and grafts
    - **T82.848** Pain due to vascular prosthetic devices, implants and grafts
  - **T82.85** Stenosis due to cardiac and vascular prosthetic devices, implants and grafts
    - **T82.855** Stenosis of coronary artery stent
      - In-stent stenosis (restenosis) of coronary artery stent
      - Restenosis of coronary artery stent
      - AHA: 2025,2Q,26; 2025,1Q,20; 2021,3Q,6-7
    - **T82.856** Stenosis of peripheral vascular stent
      - In-stent stenosis (restenosis) of peripheral vascular stent
      - Restenosis of peripheral vascular stent
    - **T82.857** Stenosis of other cardiac prosthetic devices, implants and grafts
      - AHA: 2025,1Q,19
    - **T82.858** Stenosis of other vascular prosthetic devices, implants and grafts
  - **T82.86** Thrombosis of cardiac and vascular prosthetic devices, implants and grafts
    - AHA: 2023,2Q,7
    - **T82.867** Thrombosis due to cardiac prosthetic devices, implants and grafts
    - **T82.868** Thrombosis due to vascular prosthetic devices, implants and grafts
  - **T82.89** Other specified complication of cardiac and vascular prosthetic devices, implants and grafts
    - **T82.897** Other specified complication of cardiac prosthetic devices, implants and grafts
      - AHA: 2019,2Q,33
    - **T82.898** Other specified complication of vascular prosthetic devices, implants and grafts
      - AHA: 2020,3Q,3-5
- **T82.9** Unspecified complication of cardiac and vascular prosthetic device, implant and graft

Chapter 19. Injury, Poisoning and Certain Other Consequences of External Causes

T83 Complications of genitourinary prosthetic devices, implants and grafts

EXCLUDES 2: failure and rejection of transplanted organs and tissue (T86.-)

AHA: 2016,4Q,70-71

The appropriate 7th character is to be added to each code from category T83.
- A initial encounter
- D subsequent encounter
- S sequela

T83.0 Mechanical complication of urinary catheter

EXCLUDES 2: complications of stoma of urinary tract (N99.5-)

- **T83.01 Breakdown (mechanical) of urinary catheter**
  - T83.010 Breakdown (mechanical) of cystostomy catheter
  - T83.011 Breakdown (mechanical) of indwelling urethral catheter
  - T83.012 Breakdown (mechanical) of nephrostomy catheter
  - T83.018 Breakdown (mechanical) of other urinary catheter
    - Breakdown (mechanical) of Hopkins catheter
    - Breakdown (mechanical) of ileostomy catheter
    - Breakdown (mechanical) urostomy catheter

- **T83.02 Displacement of urinary catheter**
  - Malposition of urinary catheter
  - T83.020 Displacement of cystostomy catheter
  - T83.021 Displacement of indwelling urethral catheter
  - T83.022 Displacement of nephrostomy catheter
  - T83.028 Displacement of other urinary catheter
    - Displacement of Hopkins catheter
    - Displacement of ileostomy catheter
    - Displacement of urostomy catheter

- **T83.03 Leakage of urinary catheter**
  - T83.030 Leakage of cystostomy catheter
    - AHA: 2021,4Q,18
  - T83.031 Leakage of indwelling urethral catheter
  - T83.032 Leakage of nephrostomy catheter
  - T83.038 Leakage of other urinary catheter
    - Leakage of Hopkins catheter
    - Leakage of ileostomy catheter
    - Leakage of urostomy catheter

- **T83.09 Other mechanical complication of urinary catheter**
  - Obstruction (mechanical) of urinary catheter
  - Perforation of urinary catheter
  - Protrusion of urinary catheter
  - T83.090 Other mechanical complication of cystostomy catheter
  - T83.091 Other mechanical complication of indwelling urethral catheter
  - T83.092 Other mechanical complication of nephrostomy catheter
  - T83.098 Other mechanical complication of other urinary catheter
    - Other mechanical complication of Hopkins catheter
    - Other mechanical complication of ileostomy catheter
    - Other mechanical complication of urostomy catheter

T83.1 Mechanical complication of other urinary devices and implants

- **T83.11 Breakdown (mechanical) of other urinary devices and implants**
  - T83.110 Breakdown (mechanical) of urinary electronic stimulator device
    - EXCLUDES 2: breakdown (mechanical) of electrode (lead) for sacral nerve neurostimulator (T85.111)
    - breakdown (mechanical) of implanted electronic sacral neurostimulator, pulse generator or receiver (T85.113)
  - T83.111 Breakdown (mechanical) of implanted urinary sphincter
  - T83.112 Breakdown (mechanical) of indwelling ureteral stent
  - T83.113 Breakdown (mechanical) of other urinary stents
    - Breakdown (mechanical) of ileal conduit stent
    - Breakdown (mechanical) of nephroureteral stent
  - T83.118 Breakdown (mechanical) of other urinary devices and implants

- **T83.12 Displacement of other urinary devices and implants**
  - Malposition of other urinary devices and implants
  - T83.120 Displacement of urinary electronic stimulator device
    - EXCLUDES 2: displacement of electrode (lead) for sacral nerve neurostimulator (T85.121)
    - displacement of implanted electronic sacral neurostimulator, pulse generator or receiver (T85.123)
  - T83.121 Displacement of implanted urinary sphincter
  - T83.122 Displacement of indwelling ureteral stent
  - T83.123 Displacement of other urinary stents
    - Displacement of ileal conduit stent
    - Displacement of nephroureteral stent
  - T83.128 Displacement of other urinary devices and implants

- **T83.19 Other mechanical complication of other urinary devices and implants**
  - Leakage of other urinary devices and implants
  - Obstruction (mechanical) of other urinary devices and implants
  - Perforation of other urinary devices and implants
  - Protrusion of other urinary devices and implants
  - T83.190 Other mechanical complication of urinary electronic stimulator device
    - EXCLUDES 2: other mechanical complication of electrode (lead) for sacral nerve neurostimulator (T85.191)
    - other mechanical complication of implanted electronic sacral neurostimulator, pulse generator or receiver (T85.193)
  - T83.191 Other mechanical complication of implanted urinary sphincter
  - T83.192 Other mechanical complication of indwelling ureteral stent
  - T83.193 Other mechanical complication of other urinary stent
    - Other mechanical complication of ileal conduit stent
    - Other mechanical complication of nephroureteral stent
  - T83.198 Other mechanical complication of other urinary devices and implants

T83.2 Mechanical complication of graft of urinary organ

- **T83.21** Breakdown (mechanical) of graft of urinary organ
- **T83.22** Displacement of graft of urinary organ
  - Malposition of graft of urinary organ
- **T83.23** Leakage of graft of urinary organ
- **T83.24** Erosion of graft of urinary organ
- **T83.25** Exposure of graft of urinary organ
- **T83.29** Other mechanical complication of graft of urinary organ
  - Obstruction (mechanical) of graft of urinary organ
  - Perforation of graft of urinary organ
  - Protrusion of graft of urinary organ

T83.3 Mechanical complication of intrauterine contraceptive device

- **T83.31** Breakdown (mechanical) of intrauterine contraceptive device
- **T83.32** Displacement of intrauterine contraceptive device
  - Malposition of intrauterine contraceptive device
  - Missing string of intrauterine contraceptive device
  - AHA: 2018,1Q,5
- **T83.39** Other mechanical complication of intrauterine contraceptive device
  - Leakage of intrauterine contraceptive device
  - Obstruction (mechanical) of intrauterine contraceptive device
  - Perforation of intrauterine contraceptive device
  - Protrusion of intrauterine contraceptive device

T83.4 Mechanical complication of other prosthetic devices, implants and grafts of genital tract

- **T83.41** Breakdown (mechanical) of other prosthetic devices, implants and grafts of genital tract
  - **T83.410** Breakdown (mechanical) of implanted penile prosthesis
    - Breakdown (mechanical) of penile prosthesis cylinder
    - Breakdown (mechanical) of penile prosthesis pump
    - Breakdown (mechanical) of penile prosthesis reservoir
  - **T83.411** Breakdown (mechanical) of implanted testicular prosthesis
  - **T83.418** Breakdown (mechanical) of other prosthetic devices, implants and grafts of genital tract
- **T83.42** Displacement of other prosthetic devices, implants and grafts of genital tract
  - Malposition of other prosthetic devices, implants and grafts of genital tract
  - **T83.420** Displacement of implanted penile prosthesis
    - Displacement of penile prosthesis cylinder
    - Displacement of penile prosthesis pump
    - Displacement of penile prosthesis reservoir
  - **T83.421** Displacement of implanted testicular prosthesis
  - **T83.428** Displacement of other prosthetic devices, implants and grafts of genital tract
    - AHA: 2018,1Q,5
- **T83.49** Other mechanical complication of other prosthetic devices, implants and grafts of genital tract
  - Leakage of other prosthetic devices, implants and grafts of genital tract
  - Obstruction, mechanical of other prosthetic devices, implants and grafts of genital tract
  - Perforation of other prosthetic devices, implants and grafts of genital tract
  - Protrusion of other prosthetic devices, implants and grafts of genital tract
  - **T83.490** Other mechanical complication of implanted penile prosthesis
    - Other mechanical complication of penile prosthesis cylinder
    - Other mechanical complication of penile prosthesis pump
    - Other mechanical complication of penile prosthesis reservoir
  - **T83.491** Other mechanical complication of implanted testicular prosthesis
  - **T83.498** Other mechanical complication of other prosthetic devices, implants and grafts of genital tract

T83.5 Infection and inflammatory reaction due to prosthetic device, implant and graft in urinary system

Use additional code to identify infection

- **T83.51** Infection and inflammatory reaction due to urinary catheter
  - EXCLUDES 2: complications of stoma of urinary tract (N99.5-)
  - AHA: 2019,3Q,17
  - **T83.510** Infection and inflammatory reaction due to cystostomy catheter
  - **T83.511** Infection and inflammatory reaction due to indwelling urethral catheter
    - AHA: 2022,2Q,7
  - **T83.512** Infection and inflammatory reaction due to nephrostomy catheter
  - **T83.518** Infection and inflammatory reaction due to other urinary catheter
    - Infection and inflammatory reaction due to Hopkins catheter
    - Infection and inflammatory reaction due to ileostomy catheter
    - Infection and inflammatory reaction due to urostomy catheter
- **T83.59** Infection and inflammatory reaction due to prosthetic device, implant and graft in urinary system
  - **T83.590** Infection and inflammatory reaction due to implanted urinary neurostimulation device
    - EXCLUDES 2: infection and inflammatory reaction due to electrode lead of sacral nerve neurostimulator (T85.732)
    - infection and inflammatory reaction due to pulse generator or receiver of sacral nerve neurostimulator (T85.734)
  - **T83.591** Infection and inflammatory reaction due to implanted urinary sphincter
  - **T83.592** Infection and inflammatory reaction due to indwelling ureteral stent
  - **T83.593** Infection and inflammatory reaction due to other urinary stents
    - Infection and inflammatory reaction due to ileal conduit stents
    - Infection and inflammatory reaction due to nephroureteral stent
  - **T83.598** Infection and inflammatory reaction due to other prosthetic device, implant and graft in urinary system
    - AHA: 2020,3Q,25

T83.6 Infection and inflammatory reaction due to prosthetic device, implant and graft in genital tract

Use additional code to identify infection

- **T83.61** Infection and inflammatory reaction due to implanted penile prosthesis
  - Infection and inflammatory reaction due to penile prosthesis cylinder
  - Infection and inflammatory reaction due to penile prosthesis pump
  - Infection and inflammatory reaction due to penile prosthesis reservoir
- **T83.62** Infection and inflammatory reaction due to implanted testicular prosthesis
- **T83.69** Infection and inflammatory reaction due to other prosthetic device, implant and graft in genital tract

T83.7 Complications due to implanted mesh and other prosthetic materials

- **T83.71** Erosion of implanted mesh and other prosthetic materials
  - **T83.711** Erosion of implanted vaginal mesh to surrounding organ or tissue
    - Erosion of implanted vaginal mesh into pelvic floor muscles

Chapter 19. Injury, Poisoning and Certain Other Consequences of External Causes

- ✓7th **T83.712** Erosion of implanted urethral mesh to surrounding organ or tissue ESR
  - Erosion of implanted female urethral sling
  - Erosion of implanted male urethral sling
  - Erosion of implanted urethral mesh into pelvic floor muscles
- ✓7th **T83.713** Erosion of implanted urethral bulking agent to surrounding organ or tissue ESR
- ✓7th **T83.714** Erosion of implanted ureteral bulking agent to surrounding organ or tissue ESR
- ✓7th **T83.718** Erosion of other implanted mesh to organ or tissue ESR
- ✓7th **T83.719** Erosion of other prosthetic materials to surrounding organ or tissue ESR

✓6th **T83.72** Exposure of implanted mesh and other prosthetic materials into surrounding organ or tissue
  - Extrusion of implanted mesh
- ✓7th **T83.721** Exposure of implanted vaginal mesh into vagina
  - Exposure of implanted vaginal mesh through vaginal wall
- ✓7th **T83.722** Exposure of implanted urethral mesh into urethra ESR
  - Exposure of implanted female urethral sling
  - Exposure of implanted male urethral sling
  - Exposure of implanted urethral mesh through urethral wall
- ✓7th **T83.723** Exposure of implanted urethral bulking agent into urethra ESR
- ✓7th **T83.724** Exposure of implanted ureteral bulking agent into ureter ESR
- ✓7th **T83.728** Exposure of other implanted mesh into organ or tissue ESR
- ✓7th **T83.729** Exposure of other prosthetic materials into organ or tissue ESR

✓x 7th **T83.79** Other specified complications due to other genitourinary prosthetic materials ESR

✓5th **T83.8** Other specified complications of genitourinary prosthetic devices, implants and grafts
- ✓x 7th **T83.81** Embolism due to genitourinary prosthetic devices, implants and grafts ESR
- ✓x 7th **T83.82** Fibrosis due to genitourinary prosthetic devices, implants and grafts ESR
- ✓x 7th **T83.83** Hemorrhage due to genitourinary prosthetic devices, implants and grafts ESR
  - AHA: 2025,2Q,21
- ✓x 7th **T83.84** Pain due to genitourinary prosthetic devices, implants and grafts ESR
- ✓x 7th **T83.85** Stenosis due to genitourinary prosthetic devices, implants and grafts ESR
- ✓x 7th **T83.86** Thrombosis due to genitourinary prosthetic devices, implants and grafts ESR
  - AHA: 2024,3Q,6
- ✓x 7th **T83.89** Other specified complication of genitourinary prosthetic devices, implants and grafts ESR
  - AHA: 2022,3Q,13; 2016,1Q,19

✓x 7th **T83.9** Unspecified complication of genitourinary prosthetic device, implant and graft ESR

✓4th **T84** Complications of internal orthopedic prosthetic devices, implants and grafts
  EXCLUDES 2: failure and rejection of transplanted organs and tissues (T86.-)
  fracture of bone following insertion of orthopedic implant, joint prosthesis or bone plate (M96.6)

The appropriate 7th character is to be added to each code from category T84.
  A initial encounter
  D subsequent encounter
  S sequela

✓5th **T84.0** Mechanical complication of internal joint prosthesis
- ✓6th **T84.01** Broken internal joint prosthesis
  - Breakage (fracture) of prosthetic joint
  - Broken prosthetic joint implant
  - EXCLUDES 1: periprosthetic joint implant fracture (M97.-)
  - AHA: 2016,4Q,42
  - ✓7th **T84.010** Broken internal right hip prosthesis ESR
  - ✓7th **T84.011** Broken internal left hip prosthesis ESR
  - ✓7th **T84.012** Broken internal right knee prosthesis ESR
  - ✓7th **T84.013** Broken internal left knee prosthesis ESR
  - ✓7th **T84.018** Broken internal joint prosthesis, other site
    - Use additional code to identify the joint (Z96.6-)
  - ✓7th **T84.019** Broken internal joint prosthesis, unspecified site ESR
- ✓6th **T84.02** Dislocation of internal joint prosthesis
  - Instability of internal joint prosthesis
  - Subluxation of internal joint prosthesis
  - AHA: 2019,2Q,27
  - ✓7th **T84.020** Dislocation of internal right hip prosthesis ESR
  - ✓7th **T84.021** Dislocation of internal left hip prosthesis ESR
  - ✓7th **T84.022** Instability of internal right knee prosthesis ESR
  - ✓7th **T84.023** Instability of internal left knee prosthesis ESR
  - ✓7th **T84.028** Dislocation of other internal joint prosthesis
    - Use additional code to identify the joint (Z96.6-)
  - ✓7th **T84.029** Dislocation of unspecified internal joint prosthesis ESR
- ✓6th **T84.03** Mechanical loosening of internal prosthetic joint
  - Aseptic loosening of prosthetic joint
  - ✓7th **T84.030** Mechanical loosening of internal right hip prosthetic joint ESR
  - ✓7th **T84.031** Mechanical loosening of internal left hip prosthetic joint ESR
  - ✓7th **T84.032** Mechanical loosening of internal right knee prosthetic joint ESR
  - ✓7th **T84.033** Mechanical loosening of internal left knee prosthetic joint ESR
  - ✓7th **T84.038** Mechanical loosening of other internal prosthetic joint
    - Use additional code to identify the joint (Z96.6-)
  - ✓7th **T84.039** Mechanical loosening of unspecified internal prosthetic joint ESR
- ✓6th **T84.05** Periprosthetic osteolysis of internal prosthetic joint
  - Use additional code to identify major osseous defect, if applicable (M89.7-)
  - ✓7th **T84.050** Periprosthetic osteolysis of internal prosthetic right hip joint ESR
  - ✓7th **T84.051** Periprosthetic osteolysis of internal prosthetic left hip joint ESR
  - ✓7th **T84.052** Periprosthetic osteolysis of internal prosthetic right knee joint ESR
  - ✓7th **T84.053** Periprosthetic osteolysis of internal prosthetic left knee joint ESR
  - ✓7th **T84.058** Periprosthetic osteolysis of other internal prosthetic joint
    - Use additional code to identify the joint (Z96.6-)
  - ✓7th **T84.059** Periprosthetic osteolysis of unspecified internal prosthetic joint ESR
- ✓6th **T84.06** Wear of articular bearing surface of internal prosthetic joint
  - ✓7th **T84.060** Wear of articular bearing surface of internal prosthetic right hip joint ESR
  - ✓7th **T84.061** Wear of articular bearing surface of internal prosthetic left hip joint ESR
  - ✓7th **T84.062** Wear of articular bearing surface of internal prosthetic right knee joint ESR
  - ✓7th **T84.063** Wear of articular bearing surface of internal prosthetic left knee joint ESR
  - ✓7th **T84.068** Wear of articular bearing surface of other internal prosthetic joint ESR
    - Use additional code to identify the joint (Z96.6-)
  - ✓7th **T84.069** Wear of articular bearing surface of unspecified internal prosthetic joint ESR

T84.09 Other mechanical complication of internal joint prosthesis
Prosthetic joint implant failure NOS
AHA: 2019,1Q,20

- **T84.090** Other mechanical complication of internal right hip prosthesis
- **T84.091** Other mechanical complication of internal left hip prosthesis
- **T84.092** Other mechanical complication of internal right knee prosthesis
- **T84.093** Other mechanical complication of internal left knee prosthesis
- **T84.098** Other mechanical complication of other internal joint prosthesis
  Use additional code to identify the joint (Z96.6-)
- **T84.099** Other mechanical complication of unspecified internal joint prosthesis

T84.1 Mechanical complication of internal fixation device of bones of limb
EXCLUDES 2: mechanical complication of internal fixation device of bones of feet (T84.2-)
mechanical complication of internal fixation device of bones of fingers (T84.2-)
mechanical complication of internal fixation device of bones of hands (T84.2-)
mechanical complication of internal fixation device of bones of toes (T84.2-)

T84.11 Breakdown (mechanical) of internal fixation device of bones of limb
- **T84.110** Breakdown (mechanical) of internal fixation device of right humerus
- **T84.111** Breakdown (mechanical) of internal fixation device of left humerus
- **T84.112** Breakdown (mechanical) of internal fixation device of bone of right forearm
- **T84.113** Breakdown (mechanical) of internal fixation device of bone of left forearm
- **T84.114** Breakdown (mechanical) of internal fixation device of right femur
- **T84.115** Breakdown (mechanical) of internal fixation device of left femur
- **T84.116** Breakdown (mechanical) of internal fixation device of bone of right lower leg
- **T84.117** Breakdown (mechanical) of internal fixation device of bone of left lower leg
- **T84.119** Breakdown (mechanical) of internal fixation device of unspecified bone of limb

T84.12 Displacement of internal fixation device of bones of limb
Malposition of internal fixation device of bones of limb
- **T84.120** Displacement of internal fixation device of right humerus
- **T84.121** Displacement of internal fixation device of left humerus
- **T84.122** Displacement of internal fixation device of bone of right forearm
- **T84.123** Displacement of internal fixation device of bone of left forearm
- **T84.124** Displacement of internal fixation device of right femur
- **T84.125** Displacement of internal fixation device of left femur
- **T84.126** Displacement of internal fixation device of bone of right lower leg
- **T84.127** Displacement of internal fixation device of bone of left lower leg
- **T84.129** Displacement of internal fixation device of unspecified bone of limb

T84.19 Other mechanical complication of internal fixation device of bones of limb
Obstruction (mechanical) of internal fixation device of bones of limb
Perforation of internal fixation device of bones of limb
Protrusion of internal fixation device of bones of limb
- **T84.190** Other mechanical complication of internal fixation device of right humerus
- **T84.191** Other mechanical complication of internal fixation device of left humerus
- **T84.192** Other mechanical complication of internal fixation device of bone of right forearm
- **T84.193** Other mechanical complication of internal fixation device of bone of left forearm
- **T84.194** Other mechanical complication of internal fixation device of right femur
- **T84.195** Other mechanical complication of internal fixation device of left femur
- **T84.196** Other mechanical complication of internal fixation device of bone of right lower leg
- **T84.197** Other mechanical complication of internal fixation device of bone of left lower leg
- **T84.199** Other mechanical complication of internal fixation device of unspecified bone of limb

T84.2 Mechanical complication of internal fixation device of other bones

T84.21 Breakdown (mechanical) of internal fixation device of other bones
- **T84.210** Breakdown (mechanical) of internal fixation device of bones of hand and fingers
- **T84.213** Breakdown (mechanical) of internal fixation device of bones of foot and toes
- **T84.216** Breakdown (mechanical) of internal fixation device of vertebrae
- **T84.218** Breakdown (mechanical) of internal fixation device of other bones

T84.22 Displacement of internal fixation device of other bones
Malposition of internal fixation device of other bones
- **T84.220** Displacement of internal fixation device of bones of hand and fingers
- **T84.223** Displacement of internal fixation device of bones of foot and toes
- **T84.226** Displacement of internal fixation device of vertebrae
- **T84.228** Displacement of internal fixation device of other bones

T84.29 Other mechanical complication of internal fixation device of other bones
Obstruction (mechanical) of internal fixation device of other bones
Perforation of internal fixation device of other bones
Protrusion of internal fixation device of other bones
- **T84.290** Other mechanical complication of internal fixation device of bones of hand and fingers
- **T84.293** Other mechanical complication of internal fixation device of bones of foot and toes
- **T84.296** Other mechanical complication of internal fixation device of vertebrae
  AHA: 2024,2Q,12
- **T84.298** Other mechanical complication of internal fixation device of other bones

T84.3 Mechanical complication of other bone devices, implants and grafts
EXCLUDES 2: other complications of bone graft (T86.83-)

T84.31 Breakdown (mechanical) of other bone devices, implants and grafts
- **T84.310** Breakdown (mechanical) of electronic bone stimulator
- **T84.318** Breakdown (mechanical) of other bone devices, implants and grafts

Chapter 19. Injury, Poisoning and Certain Other Consequences of External Causes

- ✓6th **T84.32** Displacement of other bone devices, implants and grafts
  - Malposition of other bone devices, implants and grafts
  - ✓7th **T84.320** Displacement of electronic bone stimulator [ESR]
  - ✓7th **T84.328** Displacement of other bone devices, implants and grafts [ESR]
    - AHA: 2014,4Q,28
- ✓6th **T84.39** Other mechanical complication of other bone devices, implants and grafts
  - Obstruction (mechanical) of other bone devices, implants and grafts
  - Perforation of other bone devices, implants and grafts
  - Protrusion of other bone devices, implants and grafts
  - ✓7th **T84.390** Other mechanical complication of electronic bone stimulator [ESR]
  - ✓7th **T84.398** Other mechanical complication of other bone devices, implants and grafts [ESR]
- ✓5th **T84.4** Mechanical complication of other internal orthopedic devices, implants and grafts
  - ✓6th **T84.41** Breakdown (mechanical) of other internal orthopedic devices, implants and grafts
    - ✓7th **T84.410** Breakdown (mechanical) of muscle and tendon graft [ESR]
    - ✓7th **T84.418** Breakdown (mechanical) of other internal orthopedic devices, implants and grafts [ESR]
  - ✓6th **T84.42** Displacement of other internal orthopedic devices, implants and grafts
    - Malposition of other internal orthopedic devices, implants and grafts
    - ✓7th **T84.420** Displacement of muscle and tendon graft [ESR]
    - ✓7th **T84.428** Displacement of other internal orthopedic devices, implants and grafts [ESR]
  - ✓6th **T84.49** Other mechanical complication of other internal orthopedic devices, implants and grafts
    - Mechanical complication of other internal orthopedic devices, implants and grafts NOS
    - Obstruction (mechanical) of other internal orthopedic devices, implants and grafts
    - Perforation of other internal orthopedic devices, implants and grafts
    - Protrusion of other internal orthopedic devices, implants and grafts
    - ✓7th **T84.490** Other mechanical complication of muscle and tendon graft [ESR]
    - ✓7th **T84.498** Other mechanical complication of other internal orthopedic devices, implants and grafts [ESR]
- ✓5th **T84.5** Infection and inflammatory reaction due to internal joint prosthesis
  - Use additional code to identify infection
  - AHA: 2019,3Q,16; 2015,1Q,16
  - ✓x7th **T84.50** Infection and inflammatory reaction due to unspecified internal joint prosthesis [ESR]
  - ✓x7th **T84.51** Infection and inflammatory reaction due to internal right hip prosthesis [ESR]
  - ✓x7th **T84.52** Infection and inflammatory reaction due to internal left hip prosthesis [ESR]
  - ✓x7th **T84.53** Infection and inflammatory reaction due to internal right knee prosthesis [ESR]
  - ✓x7th **T84.54** Infection and inflammatory reaction due to internal left knee prosthesis [ESR]
  - ✓x7th **T84.59** Infection and inflammatory reaction due to other internal joint prosthesis [ESR]
- ✓5th **T84.6** Infection and inflammatory reaction due to internal fixation device
  - Use additional code to identify infection
  - ✓x7th **T84.60** Infection and inflammatory reaction due to internal fixation device of unspecified site [ESR]
  - ✓6th **T84.61** Infection and inflammatory reaction due to internal fixation device of arm
    - ✓7th **T84.610** Infection and inflammatory reaction due to internal fixation device of right humerus [ESR]
    - ✓7th **T84.611** Infection and inflammatory reaction due to internal fixation device of left humerus [ESR]
    - ✓7th **T84.612** Infection and inflammatory reaction due to internal fixation device of right radius [ESR]
    - ✓7th **T84.613** Infection and inflammatory reaction due to internal fixation device of left radius [ESR]
    - ✓7th **T84.614** Infection and inflammatory reaction due to internal fixation device of right ulna [ESR]
    - ✓7th **T84.615** Infection and inflammatory reaction due to internal fixation device of left ulna [ESR]
    - ✓7th **T84.619** Infection and inflammatory reaction due to internal fixation device of unspecified bone of arm [ESR]
  - ✓6th **T84.62** Infection and inflammatory reaction due to internal fixation device of leg
    - ✓7th **T84.620** Infection and inflammatory reaction due to internal fixation device of right femur [ESR]
    - ✓7th **T84.621** Infection and inflammatory reaction due to internal fixation device of left femur [ESR]
    - ✓7th **T84.622** Infection and inflammatory reaction due to internal fixation device of right tibia [ESR]
    - ✓7th **T84.623** Infection and inflammatory reaction due to internal fixation device of left tibia [ESR]
    - ✓7th **T84.624** Infection and inflammatory reaction due to internal fixation device of right fibula [ESR]
    - ✓7th **T84.625** Infection and inflammatory reaction due to internal fixation device of left fibula [ESR]
    - ✓7th **T84.629** Infection and inflammatory reaction due to internal fixation device of unspecified bone of leg [ESR]
  - ✓x7th **T84.63** Infection and inflammatory reaction due to internal fixation device of spine [ESR]
  - ✓x7th **T84.69** Infection and inflammatory reaction due to internal fixation device of other site [ESR]
- ✓x7th **T84.7** Infection and inflammatory reaction due to other internal orthopedic prosthetic devices, implants and grafts [ESR]
  - Use additional code to identify infection
- ✓5th **T84.8** Other specified complications of internal orthopedic prosthetic devices, implants and grafts
  - ✓x7th **T84.81** Embolism due to internal orthopedic prosthetic devices, implants and grafts [ESR]
  - ✓x7th **T84.82** Fibrosis due to internal orthopedic prosthetic devices, implants and grafts [ESR]
    - AHA: 2025,1Q,25
  - ✓x7th **T84.83** Hemorrhage due to internal orthopedic prosthetic devices, implants and grafts [ESR]
  - ✓x7th **T84.84** Pain due to internal orthopedic prosthetic devices, implants and grafts [ESR]
    - AHA: 2024,2Q,12
  - ✓x7th **T84.85** Stenosis due to internal orthopedic prosthetic devices, implants and grafts [ESR]
  - ✓x7th **T84.86** Thrombosis due to internal orthopedic prosthetic devices, implants and grafts [ESR]
  - ✓x7th **T84.89** Other specified complication of internal orthopedic prosthetic devices, implants and grafts [ESR]
- ✓x7th **T84.9** Unspecified complication of internal orthopedic prosthetic device, implant and graft [ESR]

- ✓4th **T85** Complications of other internal prosthetic devices, implants and grafts
  - EXCLUDES 2: failure and rejection of transplanted organs and tissue (T86.-)
  - AHA: 2023,2Q,7; 2016,4Q,71-72

  The appropriate 7th character is to be added to each code from category T85.
  - A initial encounter
  - D subsequent encounter
  - S sequela

  - ✓5th **T85.0** Mechanical complication of ventricular intracranial (communicating) shunt
    - ✓x7th **T85.01** Breakdown (mechanical) of ventricular intracranial (communicating) shunt [ESR]

Additional Character Required | ✓x7th Placeholder Alert | Manifestation | Unspecified Dx | Q QPP | UPD Unacceptable PDx

T85.02 Displacement of ventricular intracranial (communicating) shunt
Malposition of ventricular intracranial (communicating) shunt

T85.03 Leakage of ventricular intracranial (communicating) shunt

T85.09 Other mechanical complication of ventricular intracranial (communicating) shunt
Obstruction (mechanical) of ventricular intracranial (communicating) shunt
Perforation of ventricular intracranial (communicating) shunt
Protrusion of ventricular intracranial (communicating) shunt

T85.1 Mechanical complication of implanted electronic stimulator of nervous system

T85.11 Breakdown (mechanical) of implanted electronic stimulator of nervous system

T85.110 Breakdown (mechanical) of implanted electronic neurostimulator of brain electrode (lead)

T85.111 Breakdown (mechanical) of implanted electronic neurostimulator of peripheral nerve electrode (lead)
Breakdown of electrode (lead) for cranial nerve neurostimulators
Breakdown of electrode (lead) for gastric neurostimulator
Breakdown of electrode (lead) for sacral nerve neurostimulator
Breakdown of electrode (lead) for vagal nerve neurostimulators

T85.112 Breakdown (mechanical) of implanted electronic neurostimulator of spinal cord electrode (lead)

T85.113 Breakdown (mechanical) of implanted electronic neurostimulator, generator
Breakdown (mechanical) of implanted electronic neurostimulator generator, brain, peripheral, gastric, spinal
Breakdown (mechanical) of implanted electronic sacral neurostimulator, pulse generator or receiver

T85.118 Breakdown (mechanical) of other implanted electronic stimulator of nervous system

T85.12 Displacement of implanted electronic stimulator of nervous system
Malposition of implanted electronic stimulator of nervous system

T85.120 Displacement of implanted electronic neurostimulator of brain electrode (lead)

T85.121 Displacement of implanted electronic neurostimulator of peripheral nerve electrode (lead)
Displacement of electrode (lead) for cranial nerve neurostimulators
Displacement of electrode (lead) for gastric neurostimulator
Displacement of electrode (lead) for sacral nerve neurostimulator
Displacement of electrode (lead) for vagal nerve neurostimulators

T85.122 Displacement of implanted electronic neurostimulator of spinal cord electrode (lead)

T85.123 Displacement of implanted electronic neurostimulator, generator
Displacement of implanted electronic neurostimulator generator, brain, peripheral, gastric, spinal
Displacement of implanted electronic sacral neurostimulator, pulse generator or receiver

T85.128 Displacement of other implanted electronic stimulator of nervous system

T85.19 Other mechanical complication of implanted electronic stimulator of nervous system
Leakage of implanted electronic stimulator of nervous system
Obstruction (mechanical) of implanted electronic stimulator of nervous system
Perforation of implanted electronic stimulator of nervous system
Protrusion of implanted electronic stimulator of nervous system

T85.190 Other mechanical complication of implanted electronic neurostimulator of brain electrode (lead)

T85.191 Other mechanical complication of implanted electronic neurostimulator of peripheral nerve electrode (lead)
Other mechanical complication of electrode (lead) for cranial nerve neurostimulators
Other mechanical complication of electrode (lead) for gastric neurostimulator
Other mechanical complication of electrode (lead) for sacral nerve neurostimulator
Other mechanical complication of electrode (lead) for vagal nerve neurostimulators

T85.192 Other mechanical complication of implanted electronic neurostimulator of spinal cord electrode (lead)

T85.193 Other mechanical complication of implanted electronic neurostimulator, generator
Other mechanical complication of implanted electronic neurostimulator generator, brain, peripheral, gastric, spinal
Other mechanical complication of implanted electronic sacral neurostimulator, pulse generator or receiver

T85.199 Other mechanical complication of other implanted electronic stimulator of nervous system

T85.2 Mechanical complication of intraocular lens

T85.21 Breakdown (mechanical) of intraocular lens

T85.22 Displacement of intraocular lens
Malposition of intraocular lens

T85.29 Other mechanical complication of intraocular lens
Obstruction (mechanical) of intraocular lens
Perforation of intraocular lens
Protrusion of intraocular lens

T85.3 Mechanical complication of other ocular prosthetic devices, implants and grafts
EXCLUDES 2 other complications of corneal graft (T86.84-)

T85.31 Breakdown (mechanical) of other ocular prosthetic devices, implants and grafts

T85.310 Breakdown (mechanical) of prosthetic orbit of right eye

T85.311 Breakdown (mechanical) of prosthetic orbit of left eye

T85.318 Breakdown (mechanical) of other ocular prosthetic devices, implants and grafts

T85.32 Displacement of other ocular prosthetic devices, implants and grafts
Malposition of other ocular prosthetic devices, implants and grafts

T85.320 Displacement of prosthetic orbit of right eye

T85.321 Displacement of prosthetic orbit of left eye

T85.328 Displacement of other ocular prosthetic devices, implants and grafts

T85.39 Other mechanical complication of other ocular prosthetic devices, implants and grafts
Obstruction (mechanical) of other ocular prosthetic devices, implants and grafts
Perforation of other ocular prosthetic devices, implants and grafts
Protrusion of other ocular prosthetic devices, implants and grafts

T85.390 Other mechanical complication of prosthetic orbit of right eye

T85.391 Other mechanical complication of prosthetic orbit of left eye

- **T85.398** Other mechanical complication of other ocular prosthetic devices, implants and grafts
- **T85.4** Mechanical complication of breast prosthesis and implant
  - **T85.41** Breakdown (mechanical) of breast prosthesis and implant
  - **T85.42** Displacement of breast prosthesis and implant
    - Malposition of breast prosthesis and implant
  - **T85.43** Leakage of breast prosthesis and implant
  - **T85.44** Capsular contracture of breast implant
  - **T85.49** Other mechanical complication of breast prosthesis and implant
    - Obstruction (mechanical) of breast prosthesis and implant
    - Perforation of breast prosthesis and implant
    - Protrusion of breast prosthesis and implant
- **T85.5** Mechanical complication of gastrointestinal prosthetic devices, implants and grafts
  - **T85.51** Breakdown (mechanical) of gastrointestinal prosthetic devices, implants and grafts
    - **T85.510** Breakdown (mechanical) of bile duct prosthesis
    - **T85.511** Breakdown (mechanical) of esophageal anti-reflux device
    - **T85.518** Breakdown (mechanical) of other gastrointestinal prosthetic devices, implants and grafts
  - **T85.52** Displacement of gastrointestinal prosthetic devices, implants and grafts
    - Malposition of gastrointestinal prosthetic devices, implants and grafts
    - **T85.520** Displacement of bile duct prosthesis
    - **T85.521** Displacement of esophageal anti-reflux device
    - **T85.528** Displacement of other gastrointestinal prosthetic devices, implants and grafts
  - **T85.59** Other mechanical complication of gastrointestinal prosthetic devices, implants and
    - Obstruction, mechanical of gastrointestinal prosthetic devices, implants and grafts
    - Perforation of gastrointestinal prosthetic devices, implants and grafts
    - Protrusion of gastrointestinal prosthetic devices, implants and grafts
    - **T85.590** Other mechanical complication of bile duct prosthesis
    - **T85.591** Other mechanical complication of esophageal anti-reflux device
    - **T85.598** Other mechanical complication of other gastrointestinal prosthetic devices, implants and grafts
- **T85.6** Mechanical complication of other specified internal and external prosthetic devices, implants and grafts
  - **T85.61** Breakdown (mechanical) of other specified internal prosthetic devices, implants and grafts
    - **T85.610** Breakdown (mechanical) of cranial or spinal infusion catheter
      - Breakdown (mechanical) of epidural infusion catheter
      - Breakdown (mechanical) of intrathecal infusion catheter
      - Breakdown (mechanical) of subarachnoid infusion catheter
      - Breakdown (mechanical) of subdural infusion catheter
    - **T85.611** Breakdown (mechanical) of intraperitoneal dialysis catheter
      - EXCLUDES 1: mechanical complication of vascular dialysis catheter (T82.4-)
    - **T85.612** Breakdown (mechanical) of permanent sutures
      - EXCLUDES 1: mechanical complication of permanent (wire) suture used in bone repair (T84.1-T84.2)
    - **T85.613** Breakdown (mechanical) of artificial skin graft and decellularized allodermis
      - Failure of artificial skin graft and decellularized allodermis
      - Non-adherence of artificial skin graft and decellularized allodermis
      - Poor incorporation of artificial skin graft and decellularized allodermis
      - Shearing of artificial skin graft and decellularized allodermis
    - **T85.614** Breakdown (mechanical) of insulin pump
    - **T85.615** Breakdown (mechanical) of other nervous system device, implant or graft
      - Breakdown (mechanical) of intrathecal infusion pump
    - **T85.618** Breakdown (mechanical) of other specified internal prosthetic devices, implants and grafts
  - **T85.62** Displacement of other specified internal prosthetic devices, implants and grafts
    - Malposition of other specified internal prosthetic devices, implants and grafts
    - **T85.620** Displacement of cranial or spinal infusion catheter
      - Displacement of epidural infusion catheter
      - Displacement of intrathecal infusion catheter
      - Displacement of subarachnoid infusion catheter
      - Displacement of subdural infusion catheter
    - **T85.621** Displacement of intraperitoneal dialysis catheter
      - EXCLUDES 1: mechanical complication of vascular dialysis catheter (T82.4-)
    - **T85.622** Displacement of permanent sutures
      - EXCLUDES 1: mechanical complication of permanent (wire) suture used in bone repair (T84.1-T84.2)
    - **T85.623** Displacement of artificial skin graft and decellularized allodermis
      - Dislodgement of artificial skin graft and decellularized allodermis
    - **T85.624** Displacement of insulin pump
    - **T85.625** Displacement of other nervous system device, implant or graft
      - Displacement of intrathecal infusion pump
    - **T85.628** Displacement of other specified internal prosthetic devices, implants and grafts
  - **T85.63** Leakage of other specified internal prosthetic devices, implants and grafts
    - **T85.630** Leakage of cranial or spinal infusion catheter
      - Leakage of epidural infusion catheter
      - Leakage of intrathecal infusion catheter
      - Leakage of subarachnoid infusion catheter
      - Leakage of subdural infusion catheter
      - AHA: 2022,3Q,24
    - **T85.631** Leakage of intraperitoneal dialysis catheter
      - EXCLUDES 1: mechanical complication of vascular dialysis catheter (T82.4)
    - **T85.633** Leakage of insulin pump
    - **T85.635** Leakage of other nervous system device, implant or graft
      - Leakage of intrathecal infusion pump
    - **T85.638** Leakage of other specified internal prosthetic devices, implants and grafts

- **T85.69** Other mechanical complication of other specified internal prosthetic devices, implants and grafts
  - Obstruction, mechanical of other specified internal prosthetic devices, implants and grafts
  - Perforation of other specified internal prosthetic devices, implants and grafts
  - Protrusion of other specified internal prosthetic devices, implants and grafts
  - **T85.690** Other mechanical complication of cranial or spinal infusion catheter
    - Other mechanical complication of epidural infusion catheter
    - Other mechanical complication of intrathecal infusion catheter
    - Other mechanical complication of subarachnoid infusion catheter
    - Other mechanical complication of subdural infusion catheter
  - **T85.691** Other mechanical complication of intraperitoneal dialysis catheter
    - EXCLUDES 1: mechanical complication of vascular dialysis catheter (T82.4)
  - **T85.692** Other mechanical complication of permanent sutures
    - EXCLUDES 1: mechanical complication of permanent (wire) suture used in bone repair (T84.1-T84.2)
  - **T85.693** Other mechanical complication of artificial skin graft and decellularized allodermis
  - **T85.694** Other mechanical complication of insulin pump
  - **T85.695** Other mechanical complication of other nervous system device, implant or graft
    - Other mechanical complication of intrathecal infusion pump
  - **T85.698** Other mechanical complication of other specified internal prosthetic devices, implants and grafts
    - Mechanical complication of nonabsorbable surgical material NOS
- **T85.7** Infection and inflammatory reaction due to other internal prosthetic devices, implants and grafts
  - Use additional code to identify infection
  - **T85.71** Infection and inflammatory reaction due to peritoneal dialysis catheter
  - **T85.72** Infection and inflammatory reaction due to insulin pump
  - **T85.73** Infection and inflammatory reaction due to nervous system devices, implants and graft
    - **T85.730** Infection and inflammatory reaction due to ventricular intracranial (communicating) shunt
    - **T85.731** Infection and inflammatory reaction due to implanted electronic neurostimulator of brain, electrode (lead)
    - **T85.732** Infection and inflammatory reaction due to implanted electronic neurostimulator of peripheral nerve, electrode (lead)
      - Infection and inflammatory reaction due to electrode (lead) for cranial nerve neurostimulators
      - Infection and inflammatory reaction due to electrode (lead) for gastric neurostimulator
      - Infection and inflammatory reaction due to electrode (lead) for sacral nerve neurostimulator
      - Infection and inflammatory reaction due to electrode (lead) for vagal nerve neurostimulators
    - **T85.733** Infection and inflammatory reaction due to implanted electronic neurostimulator of spinal cord, electrode (lead)
    - **T85.734** Infection and inflammatory reaction due to implanted electronic neurostimulator, generator
      - Generator pocket infection
    - **T85.735** Infection and inflammatory reaction due to cranial or spinal infusion catheter
      - Infection and inflammatory reaction due to epidural catheter
      - Infection and inflammatory reaction due to intrathecal infusion catheter
      - Infection and inflammatory reaction due to subarachnoid catheter
      - Infection and inflammatory reaction due to subdural catheter
    - **T85.738** Infection and inflammatory reaction due to other nervous system device, implant or graft
      - Infection and inflammatory reaction due to intrathecal infusion pump
  - **T85.79** Infection and inflammatory reaction due to other internal prosthetic devices, implants and grafts
    - **AHA:** 2023,2Q,27; 2022,2Q,7
- **T85.8** Other specified complications of internal prosthetic devices, implants and grafts, not elsewhere classified
  - **T85.81** Embolism due to internal prosthetic devices, implants and grafts, not elsewhere classified
    - **T85.810** Embolism due to nervous system prosthetic devices, implants and grafts
    - **T85.818** Embolism due to other internal prosthetic devices, implants and grafts
  - **T85.82** Fibrosis due to internal prosthetic devices, implants and grafts, not elsewhere classified
    - **T85.820** Fibrosis due to nervous system prosthetic devices, implants and grafts
    - **T85.828** Fibrosis due to other internal prosthetic devices, implants and grafts
  - **T85.83** Hemorrhage due to internal prosthetic devices, implants and grafts, not elsewhere classified
    - **T85.830** Hemorrhage due to nervous system prosthetic devices, implants and grafts
    - **T85.838** Hemorrhage due to other internal prosthetic devices, implants and grafts
  - **T85.84** Pain due to internal prosthetic devices, implants and grafts, not elsewhere classified
    - **T85.840** Pain due to nervous system prosthetic devices, implants and grafts
    - **T85.848** Pain due to other internal prosthetic devices, implants and grafts
  - **T85.85** Stenosis due to internal prosthetic devices, implants and grafts, not elsewhere classified
    - **T85.850** Stenosis due to nervous system prosthetic devices, implants and grafts
    - **T85.858** Stenosis due to other internal prosthetic devices, implants and grafts
  - **T85.86** Thrombosis due to internal prosthetic devices, implants and grafts, not elsewhere classified
    - **AHA:** 2024,2Q,7
    - **T85.860** Thrombosis due to nervous system prosthetic devices, implants and grafts
    - **T85.868** Thrombosis due to other internal prosthetic devices, implants and grafts
  - **T85.89** Other specified complication of internal prosthetic devices, implants and grafts, not elsewhere classified
    - Erosion or breakdown of subcutaneous device pocket
    - **AHA:** 2024,2Q,8
    - **T85.890** Other specified complication of nervous system prosthetic devices, implants and grafts
    - **T85.898** Other specified complication of other internal prosthetic devices, implants and grafts
- **T85.9** Unspecified complication of internal prosthetic device, implant and graft
  - Complication of internal prosthetic device, implant and graft NOS

HCC CMS-HCC | Rx Rx HCC | ESR ESRD HCC | COM Commercial HCC | N Newborn: 0 | P Pediatric: 0-17 | M Maternity: 9-64 | A Adult: 15-124

Chapter 19. Injury, Poisoning and Certain Other Consequences of External Causes

T86 Complications of transplanted organs and tissue
  Use additional code to identify other transplant complications, such as:
    graft-versus-host disease (D89.81-)
    malignancy associated with organ transplant (C80.2)
    post-transplant lymphoproliferative disorders (PTLD) (D47.Z1)
  AHA: 2020,1Q,18

- **T86.0** Complications of bone marrow transplant
  - **T86.00** Unspecified complication of bone marrow transplant
  - **T86.01** Bone marrow transplant rejection
  - **T86.02** Bone marrow transplant failure
  - **T86.03** Bone marrow transplant infection
  - **T86.09** Other complications of bone marrow transplant
    AHA: 2023,3Q,19

- **T86.1** Complications of kidney transplant
  - **T86.10** Unspecified complication of kidney transplant
  - **T86.11** Kidney transplant rejection
  - **T86.12** Kidney transplant failure
    AHA: 2013,1Q,24
  - **T86.13** Kidney transplant infection
    Use additional code to specify infection
  - **T86.19** Other complication of kidney transplant
    AHA: 2019,2Q,7

- **T86.2** Complications of heart transplant
  EXCLUDES 1: complication of:
    artificial heart device (T82.5-)
    heart-lung transplant (T86.3-)
  - **T86.20** Unspecified complication of heart transplant
  - **T86.21** Heart transplant rejection
  - **T86.22** Heart transplant failure
  - **T86.23** Heart transplant infection
    Use additional code to specify infection
  - **T86.29** Other complications of heart transplant
    - **T86.290** Cardiac allograft vasculopathy
      EXCLUDES 1: atherosclerosis of coronary arteries (I25.75-, I25.76-, I25.81-)
    - **T86.298** Other complications of heart transplant

- **T86.3** Complications of heart-lung transplant
  - **T86.30** Unspecified complication of heart-lung transplant
  - **T86.31** Heart-lung transplant rejection
  - **T86.32** Heart-lung transplant failure
  - **T86.33** Heart-lung transplant infection
    Use additional code to specify infection
  - **T86.39** Other complications of heart-lung transplant

- **T86.4** Complications of liver transplant
  - **T86.40** Unspecified complication of liver transplant
  - **T86.41** Liver transplant rejection
  - **T86.42** Liver transplant failure
  - **T86.43** Liver transplant infection
    Use additional code to identify infection, such as:
      cytomegalovirus (CMV) infection (B25.-)
  - **T86.49** Other complications of liver transplant

- **T86.5** Complications of stem cell transplant
  Complications from stem cells from peripheral blood
  Complications from stem cells from umbilical cord
  AHA: 2020,4Q,14

- **T86.8** Complications of other transplanted organs and tissues
  - **T86.81** Complications of lung transplant
    EXCLUDES 1: complication of heart-lung transplant (T86.3-)
    - **T86.810** Lung transplant rejection
    - **T86.811** Lung transplant failure
    - **T86.812** Lung transplant infection
      Use additional code to specify infection
    - **T86.818** Other complications of lung transplant
      AHA: 2019,2Q,6
    - **T86.819** Unspecified complication of lung transplant
  - **T86.82** Complications of skin graft (allograft) (autograft)
    EXCLUDES 2: complication of artificial skin graft (T85.693)
    - **T86.820** Skin graft (allograft) rejection
    - **T86.821** Skin graft (allograft) (autograft) failure
    - **T86.822** Skin graft (allograft) (autograft) infection
      Use additional code to specify infection
    - **T86.828** Other complications of skin graft (allograft) (autograft)
    - **T86.829** Unspecified complication of skin graft (allograft) (autograft)
  - **T86.83** Complications of bone graft
    EXCLUDES 2: mechanical complications of bone graft (T84.3-)
    - **T86.830** Bone graft rejection
    - **T86.831** Bone graft failure
    - **T86.832** Bone graft infection
      Use additional code to specify infection
    - **T86.838** Other complications of bone graft
      AHA: 2023,1Q,30
    - **T86.839** Unspecified complication of bone graft
  - **T86.84** Complications of corneal transplant
    EXCLUDES 2: mechanical complications of corneal graft (T85.3-)
    AHA: 2020,4Q,40
    - **T86.840** Corneal transplant rejection
      - **T86.8401** Corneal transplant rejection, right eye
      - **T86.8402** Corneal transplant rejection, left eye
      - **T86.8403** Corneal transplant rejection, bilateral
      - **T86.8409** Corneal transplant rejection, unspecified eye
    - **T86.841** Corneal transplant failure
      - **T86.8411** Corneal transplant failure, right eye
      - **T86.8412** Corneal transplant failure, left eye
      - **T86.8413** Corneal transplant failure, bilateral
      - **T86.8419** Corneal transplant failure, unspecified eye
    - **T86.842** Corneal transplant infection
      Use additional code to specify infection
      - **T86.8421** Corneal transplant infection, right eye
      - **T86.8422** Corneal transplant infection, left eye
      - **T86.8423** Corneal transplant infection, bilateral
      - **T86.8429** Corneal transplant infection, unspecified eye
    - **T86.848** Other complications of corneal transplant
      - **T86.8481** Other complications of corneal transplant, right eye
      - **T86.8482** Other complications of corneal transplant, left eye
      - **T86.8483** Other complications of corneal transplant, bilateral
      - **T86.8489** Other complications of corneal transplant, unspecified eye
    - **T86.849** Unspecified complication of corneal transplant
      - **T86.8491** Unspecified complication of corneal transplant, right eye
      - **T86.8492** Unspecified complication of corneal transplant, left eye
      - **T86.8493** Unspecified complication of corneal transplant, bilateral
      - **T86.8499** Unspecified complication of corneal transplant, unspecified eye

Chapter 19. Injury, Poisoning and Certain Other Consequences of External Causes

- **T86.85** Complication of intestine transplant
  - **T86.850** Intestine transplant rejection
  - **T86.851** Intestine transplant failure
  - **T86.852** Intestine transplant infection
    Use additional code to specify infection
  - **T86.858** Other complications of intestine transplant
  - **T86.859** Unspecified complication of intestine transplant
- **T86.89** Complications of other transplanted tissue
  Transplant failure or rejection of pancreas
  AHA: 2020,1Q,18
  - **T86.890** Other transplanted tissue rejection
  - **T86.891** Other transplanted tissue failure
  - **T86.892** Other transplanted tissue infection
    Use additional code to specify infection
  - **T86.898** Other complications of other transplanted tissue
  - **T86.899** Unspecified complication of other transplanted tissue
- **T86.9** Complication of unspecified transplanted organ and tissue
  - **T86.90** Unspecified complication of unspecified transplanted organ and tissue
  - **T86.91** Unspecified transplanted organ and tissue rejection
  - **T86.92** Unspecified transplanted organ and tissue failure
  - **T86.93** Unspecified transplanted organ and tissue infection
    Use additional code to specify infection
  - **T86.99** Other complications of unspecified transplanted organ and tissue

T87 Complications peculiar to reattachment and amputation

- **T87.0** Complications of reattached (part of) upper extremity
  - **T87.0X** Complications of reattached (part of) upper extremity
    - **T87.0X1** Complications of reattached (part of) right upper extremity
    - **T87.0X2** Complications of reattached (part of) left upper extremity
    - **T87.0X9** Complications of reattached (part of) unspecified upper extremity
- **T87.1** Complications of reattached (part of) lower extremity
  - **T87.1X** Complications of reattached (part of) lower extremity
    - **T87.1X1** Complications of reattached (part of) right lower extremity
    - **T87.1X2** Complications of reattached (part of) left lower extremity
    - **T87.1X9** Complications of reattached (part of) unspecified lower extremity
- **T87.2** Complications of other reattached body part
- **T87.3** Neuroma of amputation stump
  DEF: Non-neoplastic tumor generated at the proximal end of severed, partially transected, or injured nerve following amputation.
  - **T87.30** Neuroma of amputation stump, unspecified extremity
  - **T87.31** Neuroma of amputation stump, right upper extremity
  - **T87.32** Neuroma of amputation stump, left upper extremity
  - **T87.33** Neuroma of amputation stump, right lower extremity
  - **T87.34** Neuroma of amputation stump, left lower extremity
- **T87.4** Infection of amputation stump
  - **T87.40** Infection of amputation stump, unspecified extremity
  - **T87.41** Infection of amputation stump, right upper extremity
  - **T87.42** Infection of amputation stump, left upper extremity
  - **T87.43** Infection of amputation stump, right lower extremity
  - **T87.44** Infection of amputation stump, left lower extremity
- **T87.5** Necrosis of amputation stump
  - **T87.50** Necrosis of amputation stump, unspecified extremity
  - **T87.51** Necrosis of amputation stump, right upper extremity
  - **T87.52** Necrosis of amputation stump, left upper extremity
  - **T87.53** Necrosis of amputation stump, right lower extremity
  - **T87.54** Necrosis of amputation stump, left lower extremity
- **T87.8** Other complications of amputation stump
  - **T87.81** Dehiscence of amputation stump
  - **T87.89** Other complications of amputation stump
    Amputation stump contracture
    Amputation stump contracture of next proximal joint
    Amputation stump edema
    Amputation stump flexion
    Amputation stump hematoma
    EXCLUDES 2 phantom limb syndrome (G54.6-G54.7)
    AHA: 2022,3Q,11
- **T87.9** Unspecified complications of amputation stump

T88 Other complications of surgical and medical care, not elsewhere classified

EXCLUDES 2 complication following infusion, transfusion and therapeutic injection (T80.-)
complication following procedure NEC (T81.-)
complications of anesthesia in labor and delivery (O74.-)
complications of anesthesia in pregnancy (O29.-)
complications of anesthesia in puerperium (O89.-)
complications of devices, implants and grafts (T82-T85)
complications of obstetric surgery and procedure (O75.4)
dermatitis due to drugs and medicaments (L23.3, L24.4, L25.1, L27.0-L27.1)
poisoning and toxic effects of drugs and chemicals (T36-T65 with fifth or sixth character 1-4)
specified complications classified elsewhere

The appropriate 7th character is to be added to each code from category T88.
- A   initial encounter
- D   subsequent encounter
- S   sequela

- **T88.0** Infection following immunization
  Sepsis following immunization
  AHA: 2018,4Q,62-63
- **T88.1** Other complications following immunization, not elsewhere classified
  Generalized vaccinia
  Rash following immunization
  EXCLUDES 1 vaccinia not from vaccine (B08.011)
  EXCLUDES 2 anaphylactic shock due to serum (T80.5-)
  other serum reactions (T80.6-)
  postimmunization arthropathy (M02.2)
  postimmunization encephalitis (G04.02)
  postimmunization fever (R50.83)
- **T88.2** Shock due to anesthesia
  Use additional code for adverse effect, if applicable, to identify drug (T41.- with fifth or sixth character 5)
  EXCLUDES 1 complications of anesthesia (in):
  labor and delivery (O74.-)
  postprocedural shock NOS (T81.1-)
  pregnancy (O29.-)
  puerperium (O89.-)
- **T88.3** Malignant hyperthermia due to anesthesia
  Use additional code for adverse effect, if applicable, to identify drug (T41.- with fifth or sixth character 5)
- **T88.4** Failed or difficult intubation
- **T88.5** Other complications of anesthesia
  Use additional code for adverse effect, if applicable, to identify drug (T41.- with fifth or sixth character 5)
  - **T88.51** Hypothermia following anesthesia

T88.52 Failed moderate sedation during procedure
Failed conscious sedation during procedure
EXCLUDES 2 personal history of failed moderate sedation (Z92.83)

T88.53 Unintended awareness under general anesthesia during procedure
EXCLUDES 2 personal history of unintended awareness under general anesthesia (Z92.84)
AHA: 2016,4Q,72-73

T88.59 Other complications of anesthesia

T88.6 Anaphylactic reaction due to adverse effect of correct drug or medicament properly administered
Anaphylactic shock due to adverse effect of correct drug or medicament properly administered
Anaphylactoid reaction NOS
Use additional code for adverse effect, if applicable, to identify drug (T36-T50 with fifth or sixth character 5)
EXCLUDES 1 anaphylactic reaction due to serum (T80.5-)
anaphylactic shock or reaction due to adverse food reaction (T78.0-)
AHA: 2020,1Q,18

T88.7 Unspecified adverse effect of drug or medicament
Drug hypersensitivity NOS
Drug reaction NOS
Use additional code for adverse effect, if applicable, to identify drug (T36-T50 with fifth or sixth character 5)
EXCLUDES 1 specified adverse effects of drugs and medicaments (A00-R94 and T80-T88.6, T88.8)

T88.8 Other specified complications of surgical and medical care, not elsewhere classified
Use additional code to identify the complication
AHA: 2022,2Q,7

T88.9 Complication of surgical and medical care, unspecified

Chapter 20. External Causes of Morbidity (V00–Y99)

Chapter-specific Guidelines with Coding Examples

The chapter-specific guidelines from the ICD-10-CM Official Guidelines for Coding and Reporting have been provided below. Along with these guidelines are coding examples, contained in the shaded boxes, that have been developed to help illustrate the coding and/or sequencing guidance found in these guidelines.

The external causes of morbidity codes should never be sequenced as the first-listed or principal diagnosis.

External cause codes are intended to provide data for injury research and evaluation of injury prevention strategies. These codes capture how the injury or health condition happened (cause), the intent (unintentional or accidental; or intentional, such as suicide or assault), the place where the event occurred the activity of the patient at the time of the event, and the person's status (e.g., civilian, military).

There is no national requirement for mandatory ICD-10-CM external cause code reporting. Unless a provider is subject to a state-based external cause code reporting mandate or these codes are required by a particular payer, reporting of ICD-10-CM codes in Chapter 20, External Causes of Morbidity, is not required. In the absence of a mandatory reporting requirement, providers are encouraged to voluntarily report external cause codes, as they provide valuable data for injury research and evaluation of injury prevention strategies.

a. General external cause coding guidelines

1) Used with any code in the range of A00.0–T88.9, Z00–Z99

An external cause code may be used with any code in the range of A00.0-T88.9, Z00-Z99, classification that represents a health condition due to an external cause. Though they are most applicable to injuries, they are also valid for use with such things as infections or diseases due to an external source, and other health conditions, such as a heart attack that occurs during strenuous physical activity.

> Actinic reticuloid due to tanning bed use
>
> **L57.1** Actinic reticuloid
>
> **W89.1XXA** Exposure to tanning bed, initial encounter
>
> *Explanation:* An external cause code may be used with any code in the range of A00.0–T88.9, Z00–Z99, classifications that describe health conditions due to an external cause. Code W89.1 Exposure to tanning bed requires a seventh character of A to report this initial encounter, with a placeholder X for the fifth and sixth characters.

2) External cause code used for length of treatment

Assign the external cause code, with the appropriate 7th character (initial encounter, subsequent encounter or sequela) for each encounter for which the injury or condition is being treated.

Most categories in chapter 20 have a 7th character requirement for each applicable code. Most categories in this chapter have three 7th character values: A, initial encounter, D, subsequent encounter and S, sequela. While the patient may be seen by a new or different provider over the course of treatment for an injury or condition, assignment of the 7th character for external cause should match the 7th character of the code assigned for the associated injury or condition for the encounter.

3) Use the full range of external cause codes

Use the full range of external cause codes to completely describe the cause, the intent, the place of occurrence, and if applicable, the activity of the patient at the time of the event, and the patient's status, for all injuries, and other health conditions due to an external cause.

4) Assign as many external cause codes as necessary

Assign as many external cause codes as necessary to fully explain each cause. If only one external code can be recorded, assign the code most related to the principal diagnosis.

5) The selection of the appropriate external cause code

The selection of the appropriate external cause code is guided by the Alphabetic Index of External Causes and by Inclusion and Exclusion notes in the Tabular List.

6) External cause code can never be a principal diagnosis

An external cause code can never be a principal (first-listed) diagnosis.

7) Combination external cause codes

Certain of the external cause codes are combination codes that identify sequential events that result in an injury, such as a fall which results in striking against an object. The injury may be due to either event or both.

The combination external cause code used should correspond to the sequence of events regardless of which caused the most serious injury.

> Toddler tripped and fell while walking and struck his head on an end table, sustaining a scalp contusion
>
> **S00.03XA** Contusion of scalp, initial encounter
>
> **W01.190A** Fall on same level from slipping, tripping and stumbling with subsequent striking against furniture, initial encounter
>
> *Explanation:* Combination external cause codes identify sequential events that result in an injury, such as a fall resulting in striking against an object. The injury may be due to either or both events.

8) No external cause code needed in certain circumstances

No external cause code from Chapter 20 is needed if the external cause and intent are included in a code from another chapter (e.g., T36.0X1-, Poisoning by penicillins, accidental (unintentional)).

b. Place of occurrence guideline

Codes from category Y92, Place of occurrence of the external cause, are secondary codes for use after other external cause codes to identify the location of the patient at the time of injury or other condition.

Generally, a place of occurrence code is assigned only once, at the initial encounter for treatment. However, in the rare instance that a new injury occurs during hospitalization, an additional place of occurrence code may be assigned. No 7th characters are used for Y92.

Do not use place of occurrence code Y92.9 if the place is not stated or is not applicable.

> A farmer was working in his barn and sustained a foot contusion when the horse stepped on his left foot
>
> **S90.32XA** Contusion of left foot, initial encounter
>
> **W55.19XA** Other contact with horse, initial encounter
>
> **Y92.71** Barn as the place of occurrence of the external cause
>
> *Explanation:* A place-of-occurrence code from category Y92 is assigned at the initial encounter to identify the location of the patient at the time the injury occurred.

c. Activity code

Assign a code from category Y93, Activity code, to describe the activity of the patient at the time the injury or other health condition occurred.

An activity code is used only once, at the initial encounter for treatment. Only one code from Y93 should be recorded on a medical record.

The activity codes are not applicable to poisonings, adverse effects, misadventures or sequela.

Do not assign Y93.9, Unspecified activity, if the activity is not stated.

A code from category Y93 is appropriate for use with external cause and intent codes if identifying the activity provides additional information about the event.

> Ranch hand who was grooming a horse sustained a foot contusion when the horse stepped on his left foot
>
> **S90.32XA** Contusion of left foot, initial encounter
>
> **W55.19XA** Other contact with horse, initial encounter
>
> **Y93.K3** Activity, grooming and shearing an animal
>
> *Explanation:* One activity code from category Y93 is assigned at the initial encounter only to describe the activity of the patient at the time the injury occurred.

d. Place of occurrence, activity, and status codes used with other external cause code

When applicable, place of occurrence, activity, and external cause status codes are sequenced after the main external cause code(s). Regardless of the number of external cause codes assigned, generally there should be only one place of occurrence code, one activity code, and one external cause status code assigned to an encounter. However, in the rare instance that a new injury occurs during hospitalization, an additional place of occurrence code may be assigned.

e. **If the reporting format limits the number of external cause codes**

If the reporting format limits the number of external cause codes that can be used in reporting clinical data, report the code for the cause/intent most related to the principal diagnosis. If the format permits capture of additional external cause codes, the cause/intent, including medical misadventures, of the additional events should be reported rather than the codes for place, activity, or external status.

f. **Multiple external cause coding guidelines**

More than one external cause code is required to fully describe the external cause of an illness or injury. The assignment of external cause codes should be sequenced in the following priority:

If two or more events cause separate injuries, an external cause code should be assigned for each cause. The first-listed external cause code will be selected in the following order:

External codes for child and adult abuse take priority over all other external cause codes.

See Section I.C.19., Child and Adult abuse guidelines.

External cause codes for terrorism events take priority over all other external cause codes except child and adult abuse.

External cause codes for cataclysmic events take priority over all other external cause codes except child and adult abuse and terrorism.

External cause codes for transport accidents take priority over all other external cause codes except cataclysmic events, child and adult abuse and terrorism.

Activity and external cause status codes are assigned following all causal (intent) external cause codes.

The first-listed external cause code should correspond to the cause of the most serious diagnosis due to an assault, accident, or self-harm, following the order of hierarchy listed above..

> 30-year-old man accidentally discharged his hunting rifle, sustaining an open gunshot wound, with no retained bullet fragments, to the right thigh, which caused him to fall down the stairs, resulting in closed displaced comminuted fracture of his left radial shaft
>
> | | |
> |---|---|
> | S71.131A | Puncture wound without foreign body, right thigh, initial encounter |
> | W33.02XA | Accidental discharge of hunting rifle, initial encounter |
> | S52.352A | Displaced comminuted fracture of shaft of radius, left arm, initial encounter for closed fracture |
> | W10.9XXA | Fall (on) (from) unspecified stairs and steps, initial encounter |
>
> *Explanation:* If two or more events cause separate injuries, an external cause code should be assigned for each cause.

g. **Child and adult abuse guideline**

Adult and child abuse, neglect and maltreatment are classified as assault. Any of the assault codes may be used to indicate the external cause of any injury resulting from the confirmed abuse.

For confirmed cases of abuse, neglect and maltreatment, when the perpetrator is known, a code from Y07, Perpetrator of maltreatment and neglect, should accompany any other assault codes.

See Section I.C.19. Adult and child abuse, neglect and other maltreatment

h. **Unknown or undetermined intent guideline**

If the intent (accident, self-harm, assault) of the cause of an injury or other condition is unknown or unspecified, code the intent as accidental intent. All transport accident categories assume accidental intent.

1) **Use of undetermined intent**

External cause codes for events of undetermined intent are only for use if the documentation in the record specifies that the intent cannot be determined.

i. **Sequelae (late effects) of external cause guidelines**

1) **Sequelae external cause codes**

Sequela are reported using the external cause code with the 7th character "S" for sequela. These codes should be used with any report of a late effect or sequela resulting from a previous injury.

See Section I.B.10. Sequela (Late Effects)

2) **Sequela external cause code with a related current injury**

A sequela external cause code should never be used with a related current nature of injury code.

3) **Use of sequela external cause codes for subsequent visits**

Use a late effect external cause code for subsequent visits when a late effect of the initial injury is being treated. Do not use a late effect external cause code for subsequent visits for follow-up care (e.g., to assess healing, to receive rehabilitative therapy) of the injury when no late effect of the injury has been documented.

j. **Terrorism guidelines**

1) **Cause of injury identified by the Federal Government (FBI) as terrorism**

When the cause of an injury is identified by the Federal Government (FBI) as terrorism, the first-listed external cause code should be a code from category Y38, Terrorism. The definition of terrorism employed by the FBI is found at the inclusion note at the beginning of category Y38. Use additional code for place of occurrence (Y92.-). More than one Y38 code may be assigned if the injury is the result of more than one mechanism of terrorism.

2) **Cause of an injury is suspected to be the result of terrorism**

When the cause of an injury is suspected to be the result of terrorism a code from category Y38 should not be assigned. Suspected cases should be classified as assault.

3) **Code Y38.9, Terrorism, secondary effects**

Assign code Y38.9, Terrorism, secondary effects, for conditions occurring subsequent to the terrorist event. This code should not be assigned for conditions that are due to the initial terrorist act.

It is acceptable to assign code Y38.9 with another code from Y38 if there is an injury due to the initial terrorist event and an injury that is a subsequent result of the terrorist event.

k. **External cause status**

A code from category Y99, External cause status, should be assigned whenever any other external cause code is assigned for an encounter, including an Activity code, except for the events noted below. Assign a code from category Y99, External cause status, to indicate the work status of the person at the time the event occurred. The status code indicates whether the event occurred during military activity, whether a non-military person was at work, whether an individual including a student or volunteer was involved in a non-work activity at the time of the causal event.

A code from Y99, External cause status, should be assigned, when applicable, with other external cause codes, such as transport accidents and falls. The external cause status codes are not applicable to poisonings, adverse effects, misadventures or late effects.

Do not assign a code from category Y99 if no other external cause codes (cause, activity) are applicable for the encounter.

An external cause status code is used only once, at the initial encounter for treatment. Only one code from Y99 should be recorded on a medical record.

Do not assign code Y99.9, Unspecified external cause status, if the status is not stated.

Chapter 20. External Causes of Morbidity (V00-Y99)

NOTE This chapter permits the classification of environmental events and circumstances as the cause of injury, and other adverse effects. Where a code from this section is applicable, it is intended that it shall be used secondary to a code from another chapter of the Classification indicating the nature of the condition. Most often, the condition will be classifiable to Chapter 19, Injury, poisoning and certain other consequences of external causes (S00-T88). Other conditions that may be stated to be due to external causes are classified in Chapters I to XVIII. For these conditions, codes from Chapter 20 should be used to provide additional information as to the cause of the condition.

AHA: 2018,4Q,58-60

This chapter contains the following blocks:

V00-V09	Pedestrian injured in transport accident
V00-V99	Transport accidents
V00-X58	Accidents
V10-V19	Pedal cycle rider injured in transport accident
V20-V29	Motorcycle rider injured in transport accident
V30-V39	Occupant of three-wheeled motor vehicle injured in transport accident
V40-V49	Car occupant injured in transport accident
V50-V59	Occupant of pick-up truck or van injured in transport accident
V60-V69	Occupant of heavy transport vehicle injured in transport accident
V70-V79	Bus occupant injured in transport accident
V80-V89	Other land transport accidents
V90-V94	Water transport accidents
V95-V97	Air and space transport accidents
V98-V99	Other and unspecified transport accidents
W00-W19	Slipping, tripping, stumbling and falls
W00-X58	Other external causes of accidental injury
W20-W49	Exposure to inanimate mechanical forces
W50-W64	Exposure to animate mechanical forces
W65-W74	Accidental non-transport drowning and submersion
W85-W99	Exposure to electric current, radiation and extreme ambient air temperature and pressure
X00-X08	Exposure to smoke, fire and flames
X10-X19	Contact with heat and hot substances
X30-X39	Exposure to forces of nature
X50	Overexertion and strenuous or repetitive movements
X52-X58	Accidental exposure to other specified factors
X71-X83	Intentional self-harm
X92-Y08	Assault
Y21-Y33	Event of undetermined intent
Y35-Y38	Legal intervention, operations of war, military operations, and terrorism
Y62-Y69	Misadventures to patients during surgical and medical care
Y62-Y84	Complications of medical and surgical care
Y70-Y82	Medical devices associated with adverse incidents in diagnostic and therapeutic use
Y83-Y84	Surgical and other medical procedures as the cause of abnormal reaction of the patient, or of later complication, without mention of misadventure at the time of the procedure
Y90-Y99	Supplementary factors related to causes of morbidity classified elsewhere

ACCIDENTS (V00-X58)

AHA: 2018,2Q,7-8

Transport accidents (V00-V99)

NOTE This section is structured in 12 groups. Those relating to land transport accidents (V00-V89) reflect the victim's mode of transport and are subdivided to identify the victim's 'counterpart' or the type of event. The vehicle of which the injured person is an occupant is identified in the first two characters since it is seen as the most important factor to identify for prevention purposes. A transport accident is one in which the vehicle involved must be moving or running or in use for transport purposes at the time of the accident.

Use additional code to identify:
 airbag injury (W22.1)
 type of street or road (Y92.4-)
 use of cellular telephone and other electronic equipment at the time of the transport accident (Y93.C-)

EXCLUDES 1 agricultural vehicles in stationary use or maintenance (W31.-)
 assault by crashing of motor vehicle (Y03.-)
 automobile or motor cycle in stationary use or maintenance - code to type of accident
 crashing of motor vehicle, undetermined intent (Y32)
 intentional self-harm by crashing of motor vehicle (X82)

EXCLUDES 2 transport accidents due to cataclysm (X34-X38)

NOTE Definitions related to transport accidents:

(a) A transport accident (V00-V99) is any accident involving a device designed primarily for, or used at the time primarily for, conveying persons or good from one place to another.

(b) A public highway [trafficway] or street is the entire width between property lines (or other boundary lines) of land open to the public as a matter of right or custom for purposes of moving persons or property from one place to another. A roadway is that part of the public highway designed, improved and customarily used for vehicular traffic.

(c) A traffic accident is any vehicle accident occurring on the public highway [i.e. originating on, terminating on, or involving a vehicle partially on the highway]. A vehicle accident is assumed to have occurred on the public highway unless another place is specified, except in the case of accidents involving only off-road motor vehicles, which are classified as nontraffic accidents unless the contrary is stated.

(d) A nontraffic accident is any vehicle accident that occurs entirely in any place other than a public highway.

(e) A pedestrian is any person involved in an accident who was not at the time of the accident riding in or on a motor vehicle, railway train, streetcar or animal-drawn or other vehicle, or on a pedal cycle or animal. This includes, a person changing a tire, working on a parked car, or a person on foot. It also includes the user of a pedestrian conveyance such as a baby stroller, ice-skates, skis, sled, roller skates, a skateboard, nonmotorized or motorized wheelchair, motorized mobility scooter, or nonmotorized scooter.

(f) A driver is an occupant of a transport vehicle who is operating or intending to operate it.

(g) A passenger is any occupant of a transport vehicle other than the driver, except a person traveling on the outside of the vehicle.

(h) A person on the outside of a vehicle is any person being transported by a vehicle but not occupying the space normally reserved for the driver or passengers, or the space intended for the transport of property. This includes a person travelling on the bodywork, bumper, fender, roof, running board or step of a vehicle, as well as, hanging on the outside of the vehicle.

(i) A pedal cycle is any land transport vehicle operated solely by nonmotorized pedals including a bicycle or tricycle.

(j) A pedal cyclist is any person riding a pedal cycle or in a sidecar or trailer attached to a pedal cycle.

(k) A motorcycle is a two-wheeled motor vehicle with one or two riding saddles and sometimes with a third wheel for the support of a sidecar. The sidecar is considered part of the motorcycle. This includes a moped, motor scooter, or motorized bicycle.

(l) A motorcycle rider is any person riding a motorcycle or in a sidecar or trailer attached to the motorcycle.

(m) A three-wheeled motor vehicle is a motorized tricycle designed primarily for on-road use. This includes a motor-driven tricycle, a motorized rickshaw, or a three-wheeled motor car.

(n) A car [automobile] is a four-wheeled motor vehicle designed primarily for carrying up to 7 persons. A trailer being towed by the car is considered part of the car. It does not include a van or minivan — see definition (o).

(o) A pick-up truck or van is a four or six-wheeled motor vehicle designed for carrying passengers as well as property or cargo weighing less than the local limit for classification as a heavy goods vehicle, and not requiring a special driver's license. This includes a minivan and a sport-utility vehicle (SUV).

(p) A heavy transport vehicle is a motor vehicle designed primarily for carrying property, meeting local criteria for classification as a heavy goods vehicle in terms of weight and requiring a special driver's license.

(q) A bus (coach) is a motor vehicle designed or adapted primarily for carrying more than 10 passengers, and requiring a special driver's license.

(r) A railway train or railway vehicle is any device, with or without freight or passenger cars couple to it, designed for traffic on a railway track. This includes subterranean (subways) or elevated trains.

(s) A streetcar, is a device designed and used primarily for transporting passengers within a municipality, running on rails, usually subject to normal traffic control signals, and operated principally on a right-of-way that forms part of the roadway. This includes a tram or trolley that runs on rails. A trailer being towed by a streetcar is considered part of the streetcar.

(t) A special vehicle mainly used on industrial premises is a motor vehicle designed primarily for use within the buildings and premises of industrial or commercial establishments. This includes battery-powered airport passenger vehicles or baggage/mail trucks, forklifts, coal-cars in a coal mine, logging cars and trucks used in mines or quarries.

(u) A special vehicle mainly used in agriculture is a motor vehicle designed specifically for use in farming and agriculture (horticulture), to work the land, tend and harvest crops and transport materials on the farm. This includes harvesters, farm machinery and tractor and trailers.

(v) A special construction vehicle is a motor vehicle designed specifically for use on construction and demolition sites. This includes bulldozers, diggers, earth levellers, dump trucks, backhoes, front-end loaders, pavers, and mechanical shovels.

(w) A special all-terrain vehicle is a motor vehicle of special design to enable it to negotiate over rough or soft terrain, snow or sand. Examples of special design are high construction, special wheels and tires, tracks, and support on a cushion of air. This includes snow mobiles, All-terrain vehicles (ATV), and dune buggies. It does not include passenger vehicle designated as Sport Utility Vehicles. (SUV)

(x) A watercraft is any device designed for transporting passengers or goods on water. This includes motor or sailboats, ships, and hovercraft.

(y) An aircraft is any device for transporting passengers or goods in the air. This includes hot-air balloons, gliders, helicopters and airplanes.

(z) A military vehicle is any motorized vehicle operating on a public roadway owned by the military and being operated by a member of the military.

Pedestrian injured in transport accident (V00-V09)

INCLUDES person changing tire on transport vehicle
person examining engine of vehicle broken down in (on side of) road

EXCLUDES 1 fall due to non-transport collision with other person (W03)
pedestrian on foot falling (slipping) on ice and snow (W00.-)
struck or bumped by another person (W51)

The appropriate 7th character is to be added to each code from categories V00-V09.
- A initial encounter
- D subsequent encounter
- S sequela

V00 Pedestrian conveyance accident

Use additional place of occurrence and activity external cause codes, if known (Y92.-, Y93.-)

EXCLUDES 1 collision with another person without fall (W51)
fall due to person on foot colliding with another person on foot (W03)
fall from non-moving wheelchair, nonmotorized scooter and motorized mobility scooter without collision (W05.-)
pedestrian (conveyance) collision with other land transport vehicle (V01-V09)
pedestrian on foot falling (slipping) on ice and snow (W00.-)

- **V00.0 Pedestrian on foot injured in collision with pedestrian conveyance**
  - **V00.01 Pedestrian on foot injured in collision with roller-skater**
  - **V00.02 Pedestrian on foot injured in collision with skateboarder**
  - **V00.03 Pedestrian on foot injured in collision with standing micro-mobility pedestrian conveyance**
    - **V00.031 Pedestrian on foot injured in collision with rider of standing electric scooter**
    - **V00.038 Pedestrian on foot injured in collision with rider of other standing micro-mobility pedestrian conveyance**
      Pedestrian on foot injured in collision with rider of hoverboard
      Pedestrian on foot injured in collision with rider of segway
  - **V00.09 Pedestrian on foot injured in collision with other pedestrian conveyance**

- **V00.1 Rolling-type pedestrian conveyance accident**
  EXCLUDES 1 accident with baby stroller (V00.82-)
  accident with motorized mobility scooter (V00.83-)
  accident with wheelchair (powered) (V00.81-)
  - **V00.11 In-line roller-skate accident**
    - **V00.111 Fall from in-line roller-skates**
    - **V00.112 In-line roller-skater colliding with stationary object**
    - **V00.118 Other in-line roller-skate accident**
      EXCLUDES 1 roller-skater collision with other land transport vehicle (V01-V09 with 5th character 1)
  - **V00.12 Non-in-line roller-skate accident**
    - **V00.121 Fall from non-in-line roller-skates**
    - **V00.122 Non-in-line roller-skater colliding with stationary object**
    - **V00.128 Other non-in-line roller-skating accident**
      EXCLUDES 1 roller-skater collision with other land transport vehicle (V01-V09 with 5th character 1)
  - **V00.13 Skateboard accident**
    - **V00.131 Fall from skateboard**
    - **V00.132 Skateboarder colliding with stationary object**
    - **V00.138 Other skateboard accident**
      EXCLUDES 1 skateboarder collision with other land transport vehicle (V01-V09 with 5th character 2)
  - **V00.14 Scooter (nonmotorized) accident**
    EXCLUDES 1 motor scooter accident (V20-V29)
    - **V00.141 Fall from scooter (nonmotorized)**
    - **V00.142 Scooter (nonmotorized) colliding with stationary object**
    - **V00.148 Other scooter (nonmotorized) accident**
      EXCLUDES 1 scooter (nonmotorized) collision with other land transport vehicle (V01-V09 with fifth character 9)
  - **V00.15 Heelies accident**
    Rolling shoe
    Wheeled shoe
    Wheelies accident
    - **V00.151 Fall from heelies**
    - **V00.152 Heelies colliding with stationary object**
    - **V00.158 Other heelies accident**
  - **V00.18 Accident on other rolling-type pedestrian conveyance**
    - **V00.181 Fall from other rolling-type pedestrian conveyance**
    - **V00.182 Pedestrian on other rolling-type pedestrian conveyance colliding with stationary object**
    - **V00.188 Other accident on other rolling-type pedestrian conveyance**

- **V00.2 Gliding-type pedestrian conveyance accident**
  - **V00.21 Ice-skates accident**
    - **V00.211 Fall from ice-skates**
    - **V00.212 Ice-skater colliding with stationary object**
    - **V00.218 Other ice-skates accident**
      EXCLUDES 1 ice-skater collision with other land transport vehicle (V01-V09 with 5th character 9)
  - **V00.22 Sled accident**
    - **V00.221 Fall from sled**
    - **V00.222 Sledder colliding with stationary object**
    - **V00.228 Other sled accident**
      EXCLUDES 1 sled collision with other land transport vehicle (V01-V09 with 5th character 9)
  - **V00.28 Other gliding-type pedestrian conveyance accident**
    - **V00.281 Fall from other gliding-type pedestrian conveyance**
    - **V00.282 Pedestrian on other gliding-type pedestrian conveyance colliding with stationary object**
    - **V00.288 Other accident on other gliding-type pedestrian conveyance**
      EXCLUDES 1 gliding-type pedestrian conveyance collision with other land transport vehicle (V01-V09 with 5th character 9)

- **V00.3 Flat-bottomed pedestrian conveyance accident**
  - **V00.31 Snowboard accident**
    - **V00.311 Fall from snowboard**
    - **V00.312 Snowboarder colliding with stationary object**

- **V00.318** Other snowboard accident
  - EXCLUDES 1: snowboarder collision with other land transport vehicle (V01-V09 with 5th character 9)
- **V00.32** Snow-ski accident
  - **V00.321** Fall from snow-skis
  - **V00.322** Snow-skier colliding with stationary object
  - **V00.328** Other snow-ski accident
    - EXCLUDES 1: snow-skier collision with other land transport vehicle (V01-V09 with 5th character 9)
- **V00.38** Other flat-bottomed pedestrian conveyance accident
  - **V00.381** Fall from other flat-bottomed pedestrian conveyance
  - **V00.382** Pedestrian on other flat-bottomed pedestrian conveyance colliding with stationary object
  - **V00.388** Other accident on other flat-bottomed pedestrian conveyance

V00.8 Accident on other pedestrian conveyance

- **V00.81** Accident with wheelchair (powered)
  - **V00.811** Fall from moving wheelchair (powered)
    - EXCLUDES 1: fall from non-moving wheelchair (W05.0)
  - **V00.812** Wheelchair (powered) colliding with stationary object
  - **V00.818** Other accident with wheelchair (powered)
- **V00.82** Accident with baby stroller
  - **V00.821** Fall from baby stroller
  - **V00.822** Baby stroller colliding with stationary object
  - **V00.828** Other accident with baby stroller
- **V00.83** Accident with motorized mobility scooter
  - **V00.831** Fall from motorized mobility scooter
    - EXCLUDES 1: fall from non-moving motorized mobility scooter (W05.2)
  - **V00.832** Motorized mobility scooter colliding with stationary object
  - **V00.838** Other accident with motorized mobility scooter
- **V00.84** Accident with standing micro-mobility pedestrian conveyance
  - **V00.841** Fall from standing electric scooter
  - **V00.842** Pedestrian on standing electric scooter colliding with stationary object
  - **V00.848** Other accident with standing micro-mobility pedestrian conveyance
    - Accident with hoverboard
    - Accident with segway
- **V00.89** Accident on other pedestrian conveyance
  - **V00.891** Fall from other pedestrian conveyance
  - **V00.892** Pedestrian on other pedestrian conveyance colliding with stationary object
  - **V00.898** Other accident on other pedestrian conveyance
    - EXCLUDES 1: other pedestrian (conveyance) collision with other land transport vehicle (V01-V09 with 5th character 9)

V01 Pedestrian injured in collision with pedal cycle

V01.0 Pedestrian injured in collision with pedal cycle in nontraffic accident

- **V01.00** Pedestrian on foot injured in collision with pedal cycle in nontraffic accident
  - Pedestrian NOS injured in collision with pedal cycle in nontraffic accident
- **V01.01** Pedestrian on roller-skates injured in collision with pedal cycle in nontraffic accident
- **V01.02** Pedestrian on skateboard injured in collision with pedal cycle in nontraffic accident
- **V01.03** Pedestrian on standing micro-mobility pedestrian conveyance injured in collision with pedal cycle in nontraffic accident
  - **V01.031** Pedestrian on standing electric scooter injured in collision with pedal cycle in nontraffic accident
  - **V01.038** Pedestrian on other standing micro-mobility pedestrian conveyance injured in collision with pedal cycle in nontraffic accident
    - Pedestrian on hoverboard injured in collision with pedal cycle in nontraffic accident
    - Pedestrian on segway injured in collision with pedal cycle in nontraffic accident
- **V01.09** Pedestrian with other conveyance injured in collision with pedal cycle in nontraffic accident
  - Pedestrian in motorized mobility scooter injured in collision with pedal cycle in nontraffic accident
  - Pedestrian in wheelchair (powered) injured in collision with pedal cycle in nontraffic accident
  - Pedestrian on ice-skates injured in collision with pedal cycle in nontraffic accident
  - Pedestrian on nonmotorized scooter injured in collision with pedal cycle in nontraffic accident
  - Pedestrian on sled injured in collision with pedal cycle in nontraffic accident
  - Pedestrian on snowboard injured in collision with pedal cycle in nontraffic accident
  - Pedestrian on snow-skis injured in collision with pedal cycle in nontraffic accident
  - Pedestrian with baby stroller injured in collision with pedal cycle in nontraffic accident

V01.1 Pedestrian injured in collision with pedal cycle in traffic accident

- **V01.10** Pedestrian on foot injured in collision with pedal cycle in traffic accident
  - Pedestrian NOS injured in collision with pedal cycle in traffic accident
- **V01.11** Pedestrian on roller-skates injured in collision with pedal cycle in traffic accident
- **V01.12** Pedestrian on skateboard injured in collision with pedal cycle in traffic accident
- **V01.13** Pedestrian on standing micro-mobility pedestrian conveyance injured in collision with pedal cycle in traffic accident
  - **V01.131** Pedestrian on standing electric scooter injured in collision with pedal cycle in traffic accident
  - **V01.138** Pedestrian on other standing micro-mobility pedestrian conveyance injured in collision with pedal cycle in traffic accident
    - Pedestrian on hoverboard injured in collision with pedal cycle in traffic accident
    - Pedestrian on segway injured in collision with pedal cycle in traffic accident
- **V01.19** Pedestrian with other conveyance injured in collision with pedal cycle in traffic accident
  - Pedestrian in motorized mobility scooter injured in collision with pedal cycle in traffic accident
  - Pedestrian in wheelchair (powered) injured in collision with pedal cycle in traffic accident
  - Pedestrian on ice-skates injured in collision with pedal cycle in traffic accident
  - Pedestrian on nonmotorized scooter injured in collision with pedal cycle in traffic accident
  - Pedestrian on sled injured in collision with pedal cycle in traffic accident
  - Pedestrian on snowboard injured in collision with pedal cycle in traffic accident
  - Pedestrian on snow-skis injured in collision with pedal cycle in traffic accident
  - Pedestrian with baby stroller injured in collision with pedal cycle in traffic accident

V01.9 Pedestrian injured in collision with pedal cycle, unspecified whether traffic or nontraffic accident

- **V01.90** Pedestrian on foot injured in collision with pedal cycle, unspecified whether traffic or nontraffic accident
  - Pedestrian NOS injured in collision with pedal cycle, unspecified whether traffic or nontraffic accident

---

| Additional Character Required | Placeholder Alert | Manifestation | Unspecified Dx | QPP | Unacceptable PDx |

Chapter 20. External Causes of Morbidity

- **V01.91** Pedestrian on roller-skates injured in collision with pedal cycle, unspecified whether traffic or nontraffic accident
- **V01.92** Pedestrian on skateboard injured in collision with pedal cycle, unspecified whether traffic or nontraffic accident
- **V01.93** Pedestrian on standing micro-mobility pedestrian conveyance injured in collision with pedal cycle, unspecified whether traffic or nontraffic accident
  - **V01.931** Pedestrian on standing electric scooter injured in collision with pedal cycle, unspecified whether traffic or nontraffic accident
  - **V01.938** Pedestrian on other standing micro-mobility pedestrian conveyance injured in collision with pedal cycle, unspecified whether traffic or nontraffic accident
    - Pedestrian on hoverboard injured in collision with pedal cycle, unspecified whether traffic or nontraffic accident
    - Pedestrian on segway injured in collision with pedal cycle, unspecified whether traffic or nontraffic accident
- **V01.99** Pedestrian with other conveyance injured in collision with pedal cycle, unspecified whether traffic or nontraffic accident
  - Pedestrian in motorized mobility scooter injured in collision with pedal cycle, unspecified whether traffic or nontraffic accident
  - Pedestrian in wheelchair (powered) injured in collision with pedal cycle, unspecified whether traffic or nontraffic accident
  - Pedestrian on ice-skates injured in collision with pedal cycle unspecified, whether traffic or nontraffic accident
  - Pedestrian on nonmotorized scooter injured in collision with pedal cycle, unspecified whether traffic or nontraffic accident
  - Pedestrian on sled injured in collision with pedal cycle unspecified, whether traffic or nontraffic accident
  - Pedestrian on snowboard injured in collision with pedal cycle, unspecified whether traffic or nontraffic accident
  - Pedestrian on snow-skis injured in collision with pedal cycle, unspecified whether traffic or nontraffic accident
  - Pedestrian with baby stroller injured in collision with pedal cycle, unspecified whether traffic or nontraffic accident

- **V02** Pedestrian injured in collision with two- or three-wheeled motor vehicle
  - **V02.0** Pedestrian injured in collision with two- or three-wheeled motor vehicle in nontraffic accident
    - **V02.00** Pedestrian on foot injured in collision with two- or three-wheeled motor vehicle in nontraffic accident
      - Pedestrian NOS injured in collision with two- or three-wheeled motor vehicle in nontraffic accident
    - **V02.01** Pedestrian on roller-skates injured in collision with two- or three-wheeled motor vehicle in nontraffic accident
    - **V02.02** Pedestrian on skateboard injured in collision with two- or three-wheeled motor vehicle in nontraffic accident
    - **V02.03** Pedestrian on standing micro-mobility pedestrian conveyance injured in collision with two- or three-wheeled motor vehicle in nontraffic accident
      - **V02.031** Pedestrian on standing electric scooter injured in collision with two- or three-wheeled motor vehicle in nontraffic accident
      - **V02.038** Pedestrian on other standing micro-mobility pedestrian conveyance injured in collision with two- or three-wheeled motor vehicle in nontraffic accident
        - Pedestrian on hoverboard injured in collision with two-or three wheeled motor vehicle in nontraffic accident
        - Pedestrian on segway injured in collision with two- or three-wheeled motor vehicle in nontraffic accident
    - **V02.09** Pedestrian with other conveyance injured in collision with two- or three-wheeled motor vehicle in nontraffic accident
      - Pedestrian in motorized mobility scooter injured in collision with two- or three-wheeled motor vehicle in nontraffic accident
      - Pedestrian in wheelchair (powered) injured in collision with two- or three-wheeled motor vehicle in nontraffic accident
      - Pedestrian on ice-skates injured in collision with two- or three-wheeled motor vehicle in nontraffic accident
      - Pedestrian on nonmotorized scooter injured in collision with two- or three-wheeled motor vehicle in nontraffic accident
      - Pedestrian on sled injured in collision with two- or three-wheeled motor vehicle in nontraffic accident
      - Pedestrian on snowboard injured in collision with two- or three-wheeled motor vehicle in nontraffic accident
      - Pedestrian on snow-skis injured in collision with two- or three-wheeled motor vehicle in nontraffic accident
      - Pedestrian with baby stroller injured in collision with two- or three-wheeled motor vehicle in nontraffic accident
  - **V02.1** Pedestrian injured in collision with two- or three-wheeled motor vehicle in traffic accident
    - **V02.10** Pedestrian on foot injured in collision with two- or three-wheeled motor vehicle in traffic accident
      - Pedestrian NOS injured in collision with two- or three-wheeled motor vehicle in traffic accident
    - **V02.11** Pedestrian on roller-skates injured in collision with two- or three-wheeled motor vehicle in traffic accident
    - **V02.12** Pedestrian on skateboard injured in collision with two- or three-wheeled motor vehicle in traffic accident
    - **V02.13** Pedestrian on standing micro-mobility pedestrian conveyance injured in collision with two- or three-wheeled motor vehicle in traffic accident
      - **V02.131** Pedestrian on standing electric scooter injured in collision with two- or three-wheeled motor vehicle in traffic accident
      - **V02.138** Pedestrian on other standing micro-mobility pedestrian conveyance injured in collision with two- or three-wheeled motor vehicle in traffic accident
        - Pedestrian on hoverboard injured in collision with two-or three wheeled motor vehicle in traffic accident
        - Pedestrian on segway injured in collision with two- or three-wheeled motor vehicle in traffic accident
    - **V02.19** Pedestrian with other conveyance injured in collision with two- or three-wheeled motor vehicle in traffic accident
      - Pedestrian in motorized mobility scooter injured in collision with two- or three-wheeled motor vehicle in traffic accident
      - Pedestrian in wheelchair (powered) injured in collision with two- or three-wheeled motor vehicle in traffic accident
      - Pedestrian on ice-skates injured in collision with two- or three-wheeled motor vehicle in traffic accident
      - Pedestrian on nonmotorized scooter injured in collision with two- or three-wheeled motor vehicle in traffic accident
      - Pedestrian on sled injured in collision with two- or three-wheeled motor vehicle in traffic accident
      - Pedestrian on snowboard injured in collision with two- or three-wheeled motor vehicle in traffic accident
      - Pedestrian on snow-skis injured in collision with two- or three-wheeled motor vehicle in traffic accident
      - Pedestrian with baby stroller injured in collision with two- or three-wheeled motor vehicle in traffic accident

CMS-HCC | Rx HCC | ESRD HCC | Commercial HCC | Newborn: 0 | Pediatric: 0-17 | Maternity: 9-64 | Adult: 15-124

Chapter 20. External Causes of Morbidity

V02.9 Pedestrian injured in collision with two- or three-wheeled motor vehicle, unspecified whether traffic or nontraffic accident

    V02.90 Pedestrian on foot injured in collision with two- or three-wheeled motor vehicle, unspecified whether traffic or nontraffic accident
        Pedestrian NOS injured in collision with two- or three-wheeled motor vehicle, unspecified whether traffic or nontraffic accident

    V02.91 Pedestrian on roller-skates injured in collision with two- or three-wheeled motor vehicle, unspecified whether traffic or nontraffic accident

    V02.92 Pedestrian on skateboard injured in collision with two- or three-wheeled motor vehicle, unspecified whether traffic or nontraffic accident

    V02.93 Pedestrian on standing micro-mobility pedestrian conveyance injured in collision with two- or three-wheeled motor vehicle, unspecified whether traffic or nontraffic accident

        V02.931 Pedestrian on standing electric scooter injured in collision with two- or three wheeled motor vehicle, unspecified whether traffic or nontraffic accident

        V02.938 Pedestrian on other standing micro-mobility pedestrian conveyance injured in collision with two- or three wheeled motor vehicle, unspecified whether traffic or nontraffic accident
            Pedestrian on hoverboard injured in collision with two-three-wheeled motor vehicle, unspecified whether traffic or nontraffic accident
            Pedestrian on segway injured in collision with two- or three wheeled motor vehicle, unspecified whether traffic or nontraffic accident

    V02.99 Pedestrian with other conveyance injured in collision with two- or three-wheeled motor vehicle, unspecified whether traffic or nontraffic accident
        Pedestrian in motorized mobility scooter injured in collision with two- or three wheeled motor vehicle, unspecified whether traffic or nontraffic accident
        Pedestrian in wheelchair (powered) injured in collision with two- or three-wheeled motor vehicle, unspecified whether traffic or nontraffic accident
        Pedestrian on ice-skates injured in collision with two- or three-wheeled motor vehicle, unspecified whether traffic or nontraffic accident
        Pedestrian on nonmotorized scooter injured in collision with two- or three-wheeled motor vehicle, unspecified whether traffic or nontraffic accident
        Pedestrian on sled injured in collision with two- or three-wheeled motor vehicle, unspecified whether traffic or nontraffic accident
        Pedestrian on snowboard injured in collision with two- or three-wheeled motor vehicle, unspecified whether traffic or nontraffic accident
        Pedestrian on snow-skis injured in collision with two- or three-wheeled motor vehicle, unspecified whether traffic or nontraffic accident
        Pedestrian with baby stroller injured in collision with two- or three-wheeled motor vehicle, unspecified whether traffic or nontraffic accident

V03 Pedestrian injured in collision with car, pick-up truck or van

  V03.0 Pedestrian injured in collision with car, pick-up truck or van in nontraffic accident

    V03.00 Pedestrian on foot injured in collision with car, pick-up truck or van in nontraffic accident
        Pedestrian NOS injured in collision with car, pick-up truck or van in nontraffic accident

    V03.01 Pedestrian on roller-skates injured in collision with car, pick-up truck or van in nontraffic accident

    V03.02 Pedestrian on skateboard injured in collision with car, pick-up truck or van in nontraffic accident

    V03.03 Pedestrian on standing micro-mobility pedestrian conveyance injured in collision with car, pick-up or van in nontraffic accident

        V03.031 Pedestrian on standing electric scooter injured in collision with car, pick-up or van in nontraffic accident

        V03.038 Pedestrian on other standing micro-mobility pedestrian conveyance injured in collision with car, pick-up or van in nontraffic accident
            Pedestrian on hoverboard injured in collision with car, pick-up or van in nontraffic accident
            Pedestrian on segway injured in collision with car, pick-up or van in nontraffic accident

    V03.09 Pedestrian with other conveyance injured in collision with car, pick-up truck or van in nontraffic accident
        Pedestrian in motorized mobility scooter injured in collision with car, pick-up truck or van in nontraffic accident
        Pedestrian in wheelchair (powered) injured in collision with car, pick-up truck or van in nontraffic accident
        Pedestrian on ice-skates injured in collision with car, pick-up truck or van in nontraffic accident
        Pedestrian on nonmotorized scooter injured in collision with car, pick-up truck or van in nontraffic accident
        Pedestrian on sled injured in collision with car, pick-up truck or van in nontraffic accident
        Pedestrian on snowboard injured in collision with car, pick-up truck or van in nontraffic accident
        Pedestrian on snow-skis injured in collision with car, pick-up truck or van in nontraffic accident
        Pedestrian with baby stroller injured in collision with car, pick-up truck or van in nontraffic accident

  V03.1 Pedestrian injured in collision with car, pick-up truck or van in traffic accident

    V03.10 Pedestrian on foot injured in collision with car, pick-up truck or van in traffic accident
        Pedestrian NOS injured in collision with car, pick-up truck or van in traffic accident

    V03.11 Pedestrian on roller-skates injured in collision with car, pick-up truck or van in traffic accident

    V03.12 Pedestrian on skateboard injured in collision with car, pick-up truck or van in traffic accident

    V03.13 Pedestrian on standing micro-mobility pedestrian conveyance injured in collision with car, pick-up or van in traffic accident

        V03.131 Pedestrian on standing electric scooter injured in collision with car, pick-up or van in traffic accident

        V03.138 Pedestrian on other standing micro-mobility pedestrian conveyance injured in collision with car, pick-up or van in traffic accident
            Pedestrian on hoverboard injured in collision with car, pick-up or van in traffic accident
            Pedestrian on segway injured in collision with car, pick-up or van in traffic accident

    V03.19 Pedestrian with other conveyance injured in collision with car, pick-up truck or van in traffic accident
        Pedestrian in motorized mobility scooter injured in collision with car, pick-up truck or van in nontraffic accident
        Pedestrian in wheelchair (powered) injured in collision with car, pick-up truck or van in traffic accident
        Pedestrian on ice-skates injured in collision with car, pick-up truck or van in traffic accident
        Pedestrian on nonmotorized scooter injured in collision with car, pick-up truck or van in nontraffic accident
        Pedestrian on sled injured in collision with car, pick-up truck or van in traffic accident
        Pedestrian on snowboard injured in collision with car, pick-up truck or van in traffic accident
        Pedestrian on snow-skis injured in collision with car, pick-up truck or van in traffic accident
        Pedestrian with baby stroller injured in collision with car, pick-up truck or van in traffic accident

  V03.9 Pedestrian injured in collision with car, pick-up truck or van, unspecified whether traffic or nontraffic accident

    V03.90 Pedestrian on foot injured in collision with car, pick-up truck or van, unspecified whether traffic or nontraffic accident
        Pedestrian NOS injured in collision with car, pick-up truck or van, unspecified whether traffic or nontraffic accident

    V03.91 Pedestrian on roller-skates injured in collision with car, pick-up truck or van, unspecified whether traffic or nontraffic accident

√x 7th **V03.92** Pedestrian **on skateboard** injured in collision with car, pick-up truck or van, unspecified whether traffic or nontraffic accident

√6th **V03.93** Pedestrian on standing micro-mobility pedestrian conveyance injured in collision with car, pick-up or van, unspecified whether traffic or nontraffic accident

√7th **V03.931** Pedestrian **on standing electric scooter** injured in collision with car, pick-up or van, unspecified whether traffic or nontraffic accident

√7th **V03.938** Pedestrian on other standing micro-mobility pedestrian conveyance injured in collision with car, pick-up or van, unspecified whether traffic or nontraffic accident

Pedestrian on hoverboard injured in collision with car, pick-up or van, unspecified whether traffic or nontraffic accident

Pedestrian on segway injured in collision with car, pick-up or van, unspecified whether traffic or nontraffic accident

√x 7th **V03.99** Pedestrian with other conveyance injured in collision with car, pick-up truck or van, unspecified whether traffic or nontraffic accident

Pedestrian in motorized mobility scooter injured in collision with car, pick-up truck or van, unspecified whether traffic or nontraffic accident

Pedestrian in wheelchair (powered) injured in collision with car, pick-up truck or van, unspecified whether traffic or nontraffic accident

Pedestrian on ice-skates injured in collision with car, pick-up truck or van, unspecified whether traffic or nontraffic accident

Pedestrian on nonmotorized scooter injured in collision with car, pick-up truck or van, unspecified whether traffic or nontraffic accident

Pedestrian on sled injured in collision with car, pick-up truck or van in nontraffic accident

Pedestrian on snowboard injured in collision with car, pick-up truck or van, unspecified whether traffic or nontraffic accident

Pedestrian on snow-skis injured in collision with car, pick-up truck or van, unspecified whether traffic or nontraffic accident

Pedestrian with baby stroller injured in collision with car, pick-up truck or van, unspecified whether traffic or nontraffic accident

√4th **V04** Pedestrian injured in collision with heavy transport vehicle or bus

EXCLUDES 1 pedestrian injured in collision with military vehicle (V09.01, V09.21)

√5th **V04.0** Pedestrian injured in collision with heavy transport vehicle or bus **in nontraffic accident**

√x 7th **V04.00** Pedestrian **on foot** injured in collision with heavy transport vehicle or bus in nontraffic accident

Pedestrian NOS injured in collision with heavy transport vehicle or bus in nontraffic accident

√x 7th **V04.01** Pedestrian **on roller-skates** injured in collision with heavy transport vehicle or bus in nontraffic accident

√x 7th **V04.02** Pedestrian **on skateboard** injured in collision with heavy transport vehicle or bus in nontraffic accident

√6th **V04.03** Pedestrian on standing micro-mobility pedestrian conveyance injured in collision with heavy transport vehicle or bus in nontraffic accident

√7th **V04.031** Pedestrian **on standing electric scooter** injured in collision with heavy transport vehicle or bus in nontraffic accident

√7th **V04.038** Pedestrian on other standing micro-mobility pedestrian conveyance injured in collision with heavy transport vehicle or bus in nontraffic accident

Pedestrian on hoverboard injured in collision with heavy transport vehicle or bus in nontraffic accident

Pedestrian on segway injured in collision with heavy transport vehicle or bus in nontraffic accident

√x 7th **V04.09** Pedestrian with other conveyance injured in collision with heavy transport vehicle or bus in nontraffic accident

Pedestrian in motorized mobility scooter injured in collision with heavy transport vehicle or bus in nontraffic accident

Pedestrian in wheelchair (powered) injured in collision with heavy transport vehicle or bus in nontraffic accident

Pedestrian on ice-skates injured in collision with heavy transport vehicle or bus in nontraffic accident

Pedestrian on nonmotorized scooter injured in collision with heavy transport vehicle or bus in nontraffic accident

Pedestrian on sled injured in collision with heavy transport vehicle or bus in nontraffic accident

Pedestrian on snowboard injured in collision with heavy transport vehicle or bus in nontraffic accident

Pedestrian on snow-skis injured in collision with heavy transport vehicle or bus in nontraffic accident

Pedestrian with baby stroller injured in collision with heavy transport vehicle or bus in nontraffic accident

√5th **V04.1** Pedestrian injured in collision with heavy transport vehicle or bus **in traffic accident**

√x 7th **V04.10** Pedestrian **on foot** injured in collision with heavy transport vehicle or bus in traffic accident

Pedestrian NOS injured in collision with heavy transport vehicle or bus in traffic accident

√x 7th **V04.11** Pedestrian **on roller-skates** injured in collision with heavy transport vehicle or bus in traffic accident

√x 7th **V04.12** Pedestrian **on skateboard** injured in collision with heavy transport vehicle or bus in traffic accident

√6th **V04.13** Pedestrian on standing micro-mobility pedestrian conveyance injured in collision with heavy transport vehicle or bus in traffic accident

√7th **V04.131** Pedestrian **on standing electric scooter** injured in collision with heavy transport vehicle or bus in traffic accident

√7th **V04.138** Pedestrian on other standing micro-mobility pedestrian conveyance injured in collision with heavy transport vehicle or bus in traffic accident

Pedestrian on hoverboard injured in collision with heavy transport vehicle or bus in traffic accident

Pedestrian on segway injured in collision with heavy transport vehicle or bus in traffic accident

√x 7th **V04.19** Pedestrian with other conveyance injured in collision with heavy transport vehicle or bus in traffic accident

Pedestrian in motorized mobility scooter injured in collision with heavy transport vehicle or bus in traffic accident

Pedestrian in wheelchair (powered) injured in collision with heavy transport vehicle or bus in traffic accident

Pedestrian on ice-skates injured in collision with heavy transport vehicle or bus in traffic accident

Pedestrian on nonmotorized scooter injured in collision with heavy transport vehicle or bus in traffic accident

Pedestrian on sled injured in collision with heavy transport vehicle or bus in traffic accident

Pedestrian on snowboard injured in collision with heavy transport vehicle or bus in traffic accident

Pedestrian on snow-skis injured in collision with heavy transport vehicle or bus in traffic accident

Pedestrian with baby stroller injured in collision with heavy transport vehicle or bus in traffic accident

√5th **V04.9** Pedestrian injured in collision with heavy transport vehicle or bus, unspecified whether traffic or nontraffic accident

√x 7th **V04.90** Pedestrian **on foot** injured in collision with heavy transport vehicle or bus, unspecified whether traffic or nontraffic accident

Pedestrian NOS injured in collision with heavy transport vehicle or bus, unspecified whether traffic or nontraffic accident

√x 7th **V04.91** Pedestrian **on roller-skates** injured in collision with heavy transport vehicle or bus, unspecified whether traffic or nontraffic accident

√x 7th **V04.92** Pedestrian **on skateboard** injured in collision with heavy transport vehicle or bus, unspecified whether traffic or nontraffic accident

 CMS-HCC   Rx HCC   ESRD HCC   COM Commercial HCC   N Newborn: 0   P Pediatric: 0-17   M Maternity: 9-64   A Adult: 15-124

- V04.93 **Pedestrian on standing micro-mobility pedestrian conveyance injured in collision with heavy transport vehicle or bus, unspecified whether traffic or nontraffic accident**
  - V04.931 **Pedestrian on standing electric scooter injured in collision with heavy transport vehicle or bus, unspecified whether traffic or nontraffic accident**
  - V04.938 **Pedestrian on other standing micro-mobility pedestrian conveyance injured in collision with heavy transport vehicle or bus, unspecified whether traffic or nontraffic accident**
    - Pedestrian on hoverboard injured in collision with heavy transport vehicle or bus, unspecified whether traffic or nontraffic accident
    - Pedestrian on segway injured in collision with heavy transport vehicle or bus, unspecified whether traffic or nontraffic accident
- V04.99 **Pedestrian with other conveyance injured in collision with heavy transport vehicle or bus, unspecified whether traffic or nontraffic accident**
  - Pedestrian in motorized mobility scooter injured in collision with heavy transport vehicle or bus, unspecified whether traffic or nontraffic accident
  - Pedestrian in wheelchair (powered) injured in collision with heavy transport vehicle or bus, unspecified whether traffic or nontraffic accident
  - Pedestrian on ice-skates injured in collision with heavy transport vehicle or bus, unspecified whether traffic or nontraffic accident
  - Pedestrian on nonmotorized scooter injured in collision with heavy transport vehicle or bus, unspecified whether traffic or nontraffic accident
  - Pedestrian on sled injured in collision with heavy transport vehicle or bus, unspecified whether traffic or nontraffic accident
  - Pedestrian on snowboard injured in collision with heavy transport vehicle or bus, unspecified whether traffic or nontraffic accident
  - Pedestrian on snow-skis injured in collision with heavy transport vehicle or bus, unspecified whether traffic or nontraffic accident
  - Pedestrian with baby stroller injured in collision with heavy transport vehicle or bus, unspecified whether traffic or nontraffic accident

V05 Pedestrian injured in collision with railway train or railway vehicle

- V05.0 **Pedestrian injured in collision with railway train or railway vehicle in nontraffic accident**
  - V05.00 **Pedestrian on foot injured in collision with railway train or railway vehicle in nontraffic accident**
    - Pedestrian NOS injured in collision with railway train or railway vehicle in nontraffic accident
  - V05.01 **Pedestrian on roller-skates injured in collision with railway train or railway vehicle in nontraffic accident**
  - V05.02 **Pedestrian on skateboard injured in collision with railway train or railway vehicle in nontraffic accident**
  - V05.03 **Pedestrian on standing micro-mobility pedestrian conveyance injured in collision with railway train or railway vehicle in nontraffic accident**
    - V05.031 **Pedestrian on standing electric scooter injured in collision with railway train or railway vehicle in nontraffic accident**
    - V05.038 **Pedestrian on other standing micro-mobility pedestrian conveyance injured in collision with railway train or railway vehicle in nontraffic accident**
      - Pedestrian on hoverboard injured in collision with railway train or railway vehicle in nontraffic accident
      - Pedestrian on segway injured in collision with railway train or railway vehicle in nontraffic accident
  - V05.09 **Pedestrian with other conveyance injured in collision with railway train or railway vehicle in nontraffic accident**
    - Pedestrian in motorized mobility scooter injured in collision with railway train or railway vehicle in nontraffic accident
    - Pedestrian in wheelchair (powered) injured in collision with railway train or railway vehicle in nontraffic accident
    - Pedestrian on ice-skates injured in collision with railway train or railway vehicle in nontraffic accident
    - Pedestrian on nonmotorized scooter injured in collision with railway train or railway vehicle in nontraffic accident
    - Pedestrian on sled injured in collision with railway train or railway vehicle in nontraffic accident
    - Pedestrian on snowboard injured in collision with railway train or railway vehicle in nontraffic accident
    - Pedestrian on snow-skis injured in collision with railway train or railway vehicle in nontraffic accident
    - Pedestrian with baby stroller injured in collision with railway train or railway vehicle in nontraffic accident
- V05.1 **Pedestrian injured in collision with railway train or railway vehicle in traffic accident**
  - V05.10 **Pedestrian on foot injured in collision with railway train or railway vehicle in traffic accident**
    - Pedestrian NOS injured in collision with railway train or railway vehicle in traffic accident
  - V05.11 **Pedestrian on roller-skates injured in collision with railway train or railway vehicle in traffic accident**
  - V05.12 **Pedestrian on skateboard injured in collision with railway train or railway vehicle in traffic accident**
  - V05.13 **Pedestrian on standing micro-mobility pedestrian conveyance injured in collision with railway train or railway vehicle in traffic accident**
    - V05.131 **Pedestrian on standing electric scooter injured in collision with railway train or railway vehicle in traffic accident**
    - V05.138 **Pedestrian on other standing micro-mobility pedestrian conveyance injured in collision with railway train or railway vehicle in traffic accident**
      - Pedestrian on hoverboard injured in collision with railway train or railway vehicle in traffic accident
      - Pedestrian on segway injured in collision with railway train or railway vehicle in traffic accident
  - V05.19 **Pedestrian with other conveyance injured in collision with railway train or railway vehicle in traffic accident**
    - Pedestrian in motorized mobility scooter injured in collision with railway train or railway vehicle in traffic accident
    - Pedestrian in wheelchair (powered) injured in collision with railway train or railway vehicle in traffic accident
    - Pedestrian on ice-skates injured in collision with railway train or railway vehicle in traffic accident
    - Pedestrian on nonmotorized scooter injured in collision with railway train or railway vehicle in traffic accident
    - Pedestrian on sled injured in collision with railway train or railway vehicle in traffic accident
    - Pedestrian on snowboard injured in collision with railway train or railway vehicle in traffic accident
    - Pedestrian on snow-skis injured in collision with railway train or railway vehicle in traffic accident
    - Pedestrian with baby stroller injured in collision with railway train or railway vehicle in traffic accident
- V05.9 **Pedestrian injured in collision with railway train or railway vehicle, unspecified whether traffic or nontraffic accident**
  - V05.90 **Pedestrian on foot injured in collision with railway train or railway vehicle, unspecified whether traffic or nontraffic accident**
    - Pedestrian NOS injured in collision with railway train or railway vehicle, unspecified whether traffic or nontraffic accident
  - V05.91 **Pedestrian on roller-skates injured in collision with railway train or railway vehicle, unspecified whether traffic or nontraffic accident**
  - V05.92 **Pedestrian on skateboard injured in collision with railway train or railway vehicle, unspecified whether traffic or nontraffic accident**

Chapter 20. External Causes of Morbidity

- ✓6th **V05.93** Pedestrian on standing micro-mobility pedestrian conveyance injured in collision with railway train or railway vehicle, unspecified whether traffic or nontraffic accident
  - ✓7th **V05.931** Pedestrian on standing electric scooter injured in collision with railway train or railway vehicle, unspecified whether traffic or nontraffic accident
  - ✓7th **V05.938** Pedestrian on other standing micro-mobility pedestrian conveyance injured in collision with railway train or railway vehicle, unspecified whether traffic or nontraffic accident
    - Pedestrian on hoverboard injured in collision with railway train or railway vehicle, unspecified whether traffic or nontraffic accident
    - Pedestrian on segway injured in collision with railway train or railway vehicle, unspecified whether traffic or nontraffic accident
- ✓x7th **V05.99** Pedestrian with other conveyance injured in collision with railway train or railway vehicle, unspecified whether traffic or nontraffic accident
  - Pedestrian in motorized mobility scooter injured in collision with railway train or railway vehicle, unspecified whether traffic or nontraffic
  - Pedestrian in wheelchair (powered) injured in collision with railway train or railway vehicle, unspecified whether traffic or nontraffic
  - Pedestrian on ice-skates injured in collision with railway train or railway vehicle, unspecified whether traffic or nontraffic
  - Pedestrian on nonmotorized scooter injured in collision with railway train or railway vehicle, unspecified whether traffic or nontraffic
  - Pedestrian on sled injured in collision with railway train or railway vehicle, unspecified whether traffic or nontraffic
  - Pedestrian on snowboard injured in collision with railway train or railway vehicle, unspecified whether traffic or nontraffic
  - Pedestrian on snow-skis injured in collision with railway train or railway vehicle, unspecified whether traffic or nontraffic
  - Pedestrian with baby stroller injured in collision with railway train or railway vehicle, unspecified whether traffic or nontraffic

- ✓4th **V06** Pedestrian injured in collision with other nonmotor vehicle
  - INCLUDES: collision with animal-drawn vehicle, animal being ridden, nonpowered streetcar
  - EXCLUDES 1: pedestrian injured in collision with pedestrian conveyance (V00.0-)
  - ✓5th **V06.0** Pedestrian injured in collision with other nonmotor vehicle in nontraffic accident
    - ✓x7th **V06.00** Pedestrian on foot injured in collision with other nonmotor vehicle in nontraffic accident
      - Pedestrian NOS injured in collision with other nonmotor vehicle in nontraffic accident
    - ✓x7th **V06.01** Pedestrian on roller-skates injured in collision with other nonmotor vehicle in nontraffic accident
    - ✓x7th **V06.02** Pedestrian on skateboard injured in collision with other nonmotor vehicle in nontraffic accident
    - ✓6th **V06.03** Pedestrian on standing micro-mobility pedestrian conveyance injured in collision with other nonmotor vehicle in nontraffic accident
      - ✓7th **V06.031** Pedestrian on standing electric scooter injured in collision with other nonmotor vehicle in nontraffic accident
      - ✓7th **V06.038** Pedestrian on other standing micro-mobility pedestrian conveyance injured in collision with other nonmotor vehicle in nontraffic accident
        - Pedestrian on hoverboard injured in collision with other nonmotor vehicle in nontraffic accident
        - Pedestrian on segway injured in collision with other nonmotor vehicle in nontraffic accident
    - ✓x7th **V06.09** Pedestrian with other conveyance injured in collision with other nonmotor vehicle in nontraffic accident
      - Pedestrian in motorized mobility scooter injured in collision with other nonmotor vehicle in nontraffic accident
      - Pedestrian in wheelchair (powered) injured in collision with other nonmotor vehicle in nontraffic accident
      - Pedestrian on ice-skates injured in collision with other nonmotor vehicle in nontraffic accident
      - Pedestrian on nonmotorized scooter injured in collision with other nonmotor vehicle in nontraffic accident
      - Pedestrian on sled injured in collision with other nonmotor vehicle in nontraffic accident
      - Pedestrian on snowboard injured in collision with other nonmotor vehicle in nontraffic accident
      - Pedestrian on snow-skis injured in collision with other nonmotor vehicle in nontraffic accident
      - Pedestrian with baby stroller injured in collision with other nonmotor vehicle in nontraffic accident
  - ✓5th **V06.1** Pedestrian injured in collision with other nonmotor vehicle in traffic accident
    - ✓x7th **V06.10** Pedestrian on foot injured in collision with other nonmotor vehicle in traffic accident
      - Pedestrian NOS injured in collision with other nonmotor vehicle in traffic accident
    - ✓x7th **V06.11** Pedestrian on roller-skates injured in collision with other nonmotor vehicle in traffic accident
    - ✓x7th **V06.12** Pedestrian on skateboard injured in collision with other nonmotor vehicle in traffic accident
    - ✓6th **V06.13** Pedestrian on standing micro-mobility pedestrian conveyance injured in collision with other nonmotor vehicle in traffic accident
      - ✓7th **V06.131** Pedestrian on standing electric scooter injured in collision with other nonmotor vehicle in traffic accident
      - ✓7th **V06.138** Pedestrian on other standing micro-mobility pedestrian conveyance injured in collision with other nonmotor vehicle in traffic accident
        - Pedestrian on hoverboard injured in collision with other nonmotor vehicle in traffic accident
        - Pedestrian on segway injured in collision with other nonmotor vehicle in traffic accident
    - ✓x7th **V06.19** Pedestrian with other conveyance injured in collision with other nonmotor vehicle in traffic accident
      - Pedestrian in motorized mobility scooter injured in collision with other nonmotor vehicle in traffic accident
      - Pedestrian in wheelchair (powered) injured in collision with other nonmotor vehicle in traffic accident
      - Pedestrian on ice-skates injured in collision with other nonmotor vehicle in traffic accident
      - Pedestrian on nonmotorized scooter injured in collision with other nonmotor vehicle in traffic accident
      - Pedestrian on sled injured in collision with other nonmotor vehicle in traffic accident
      - Pedestrian on snowboard injured in collision with other nonmotor vehicle in traffic accident
      - Pedestrian on snow-skis injured in collision with other nonmotor vehicle in traffic accident
      - Pedestrian with baby stroller injured in collision with other nonmotor vehicle in traffic accident
  - ✓5th **V06.9** Pedestrian injured in collision with other nonmotor vehicle, unspecified whether traffic or nontraffic accident
    - ✓x7th **V06.90** Pedestrian on foot injured in collision with other nonmotor vehicle, unspecified whether traffic or nontraffic accident
      - Pedestrian NOS injured in collision with other nonmotor vehicle, unspecified whether traffic or nontraffic accident
    - ✓x7th **V06.91** Pedestrian on roller-skates injured in collision with other nonmotor vehicle, unspecified whether traffic or nontraffic accident
    - ✓x7th **V06.92** Pedestrian on skateboard injured in collision with other nonmotor vehicle, unspecified whether traffic or nontraffic accident

- **V06.93** Pedestrian on standing micro-mobility pedestrian conveyance injured in collision with other nonmotor vehicle, unspecified whether traffic or nontraffic accident
  - **V06.931** Pedestrian on standing electric scooter injured in collision with other nonmotor vehicle, unspecified whether traffic or nontraffic accident
  - **V06.938** Pedestrian on other standing micro-mobility pedestrian conveyance injured in collision with other nonmotor vehicle, unspecified whether traffic or nontraffic accident
    - ▶Pedestrian on hoverboard injured in collision with other nonmotor vehicle, unspecified whether traffic or nontraffic accident◀
    - Pedestrian on segway injured in collision with other nonmotor vehicle, unspecified whether traffic or nontraffic accident
- **V06.99** Pedestrian with other conveyance injured in collision with other nonmotor vehicle, unspecified whether traffic or nontraffic accident
  - Pedestrian in motorized mobility scooter injured in collision with other nonmotorized vehicle, unspecified whether traffic or nontraffic accident
  - Pedestrian in wheelchair (powered) injured in collision with other nonmotor vehicle, unspecified whether traffic or nontraffic accident
  - Pedestrian on ice-skates injured in collision with other nonmotor vehicle, unspecified whether traffic or nontraffic accident
  - Pedestrian on nonmotorized scooter injured in collision with other nonmotor vehicle, unspecified whether traffic or nontraffic accident
  - Pedestrian on sled injured in collision with other nonmotor vehicle, unspecified whether traffic or nontraffic accident
  - Pedestrian on snowboard injured in collision with other nonmotor vehicle, unspecified whether traffic or nontraffic accident
  - Pedestrian on snow-skis injured in collision with other nonmotor vehicle, unspecified whether traffic or nontraffic accident
  - Pedestrian with baby stroller injured in collision with other nonmotor vehicle, unspecified whether traffic or nontraffic accident

V09 Pedestrian injured in other and unspecified transport accidents

- **V09.0** Pedestrian injured in nontraffic accident involving other and unspecified motor vehicles
  - **V09.00** Pedestrian injured in nontraffic accident involving unspecified motor vehicles
  - **V09.01** Pedestrian injured in nontraffic accident involving military vehicle
  - **V09.09** Pedestrian injured in nontraffic accident involving other motor vehicles
    - Pedestrian injured in nontraffic accident by special vehicle
- **V09.1** Pedestrian injured in unspecified nontraffic accident
- **V09.2** Pedestrian injured in traffic accident involving other and unspecified motor vehicles
  - **V09.20** Pedestrian injured in traffic accident involving unspecified motor vehicles
  - **V09.21** Pedestrian injured in traffic accident involving military vehicle
  - **V09.29** Pedestrian injured in traffic accident involving other motor vehicles
- **V09.3** Pedestrian injured in unspecified traffic accident
- **V09.9** Pedestrian injured in unspecified transport accident

Pedal cycle rider injured in transport accident (V10-V19)

INCLUDES any non-motorized vehicle, excluding an animal-drawn vehicle, or a sidecar or trailer attached to the pedal cycle

EXCLUDES 2 rupture of pedal cycle tire (W37.0)

The appropriate 7th character is to be added to each code from categories V10-V19.
- A initial encounter
- D subsequent encounter
- S sequela

V10 Pedal cycle rider injured in collision with pedestrian or animal

EXCLUDES 1 pedal cycle rider collision with animal-drawn vehicle or animal being ridden (V16.-)

- **V10.0** Pedal cycle driver injured in collision with pedestrian or animal in nontraffic accident
- **V10.1** Pedal cycle passenger injured in collision with pedestrian or animal in nontraffic accident
- **V10.2** Unspecified pedal cyclist injured in collision with pedestrian or animal in nontraffic accident
- **V10.3** Person boarding or alighting a pedal cycle injured in collision with pedestrian or animal
- **V10.4** Pedal cycle driver injured in collision with pedestrian or animal in traffic accident
- **V10.5** Pedal cycle passenger injured in collision with pedestrian or animal in traffic accident
- **V10.9** Unspecified pedal cyclist injured in collision with pedestrian or animal in traffic accident

V11 Pedal cycle rider injured in collision with other pedal cycle

- **V11.0** Pedal cycle driver injured in collision with other pedal cycle in nontraffic accident
- **V11.1** Pedal cycle passenger injured in collision with other pedal cycle in nontraffic accident
- **V11.2** Unspecified pedal cyclist injured in collision with other pedal cycle in nontraffic accident
- **V11.3** Person boarding or alighting a pedal cycle injured in collision with other pedal cycle
- **V11.4** Pedal cycle driver injured in collision with other pedal cycle in traffic accident
- **V11.5** Pedal cycle passenger injured in collision with other pedal cycle in traffic accident
- **V11.9** Unspecified pedal cyclist injured in collision with other pedal cycle in traffic accident

V12 Pedal cycle rider injured in collision with two- or three-wheeled motor vehicle

- **V12.0** Pedal cycle driver injured in collision with two- or three-wheeled motor vehicle in nontraffic accident
- **V12.1** Pedal cycle passenger injured in collision with two- or three-wheeled motor vehicle in nontraffic accident
- **V12.2** Unspecified pedal cyclist injured in collision with two- or three-wheeled motor vehicle in nontraffic accident
- **V12.3** Person boarding or alighting a pedal cycle injured in collision with two- or three-wheeled motor vehicle
- **V12.4** Pedal cycle driver injured in collision with two- or three-wheeled motor vehicle in traffic accident
- **V12.5** Pedal cycle passenger injured in collision with two- or three-wheeled motor vehicle in traffic accident
- **V12.9** Unspecified pedal cyclist injured in collision with two- or three-wheeled motor vehicle in traffic accident

V13 Pedal cycle rider injured in collision with car, pick-up truck or van

- **V13.0** Pedal cycle driver injured in collision with car, pick-up truck or van in nontraffic accident
- **V13.1** Pedal cycle passenger injured in collision with car, pick-up truck or van in nontraffic accident
- **V13.2** Unspecified pedal cyclist injured in collision with car, pick-up truck or van in nontraffic accident
- **V13.3** Person boarding or alighting a pedal cycle injured in collision with car, pick-up truck or van
- **V13.4** Pedal cycle driver injured in collision with car, pick-up truck or van in traffic accident
- **V13.5** Pedal cycle passenger injured in collision with car, pick-up truck or van in traffic accident
- **V13.9** Unspecified pedal cyclist injured in collision with car, pick-up truck or van in traffic accident

V14 Pedal cycle rider injured in collision with heavy transport vehicle or bus

EXCLUDES 1 pedal cycle rider injured in collision with military vehicle (V19.81)

- **V14.0** Pedal cycle driver injured in collision with heavy transport vehicle or bus in nontraffic accident

Chapter 20. External Causes of Morbidity

- **V14.1** Pedal cycle passenger injured in collision with heavy transport vehicle or bus in nontraffic accident
- **V14.2** Unspecified pedal cyclist injured in collision with heavy transport vehicle or bus in nontraffic accident
- **V14.3** Person boarding or alighting a pedal cycle injured in collision with heavy transport vehicle or bus
- **V14.4** Pedal cycle driver injured in collision with heavy transport vehicle or bus in traffic accident
- **V14.5** Pedal cycle passenger injured in collision with heavy transport vehicle or bus in traffic accident
- **V14.9** Unspecified pedal cyclist injured in collision with heavy transport vehicle or bus in traffic accident

V15 Pedal cycle rider injured in collision with railway train or railway vehicle
- **V15.0** Pedal cycle driver injured in collision with railway train or railway vehicle in nontraffic accident
- **V15.1** Pedal cycle passenger injured in collision with railway train or railway vehicle in nontraffic accident
- **V15.2** Unspecified pedal cyclist injured in collision with railway train or railway vehicle in nontraffic accident
- **V15.3** Person boarding or alighting a pedal cycle injured in collision with railway train or railway vehicle
- **V15.4** Pedal cycle driver injured in collision with railway train or railway vehicle in traffic accident
- **V15.5** Pedal cycle passenger injured in collision with railway train or railway vehicle in traffic accident
- **V15.9** Unspecified pedal cyclist injured in collision with railway train or railway vehicle in traffic accident

V16 Pedal cycle rider injured in collision with other nonmotor vehicle
> INCLUDES collision with animal-drawn vehicle, animal being ridden, streetcar
- **V16.0** Pedal cycle driver injured in collision with other nonmotor vehicle in nontraffic accident
- **V16.1** Pedal cycle passenger injured in collision with other nonmotor vehicle in nontraffic accident
- **V16.2** Unspecified pedal cyclist injured in collision with other nonmotor vehicle in nontraffic accident
- **V16.3** Person boarding or alighting a pedal cycle injured in collision with other nonmotor vehicle in nontraffic accident
- **V16.4** Pedal cycle driver injured in collision with other nonmotor vehicle in traffic accident
- **V16.5** Pedal cycle passenger injured in collision with other nonmotor vehicle in traffic accident
- **V16.9** Unspecified pedal cyclist injured in collision with other nonmotor vehicle in traffic accident

V17 Pedal cycle rider injured in collision with fixed or stationary object
- **V17.0** Pedal cycle driver injured in collision with fixed or stationary object in nontraffic accident
- **V17.1** Pedal cycle passenger injured in collision with fixed or stationary object in nontraffic accident
- **V17.2** Unspecified pedal cyclist injured in collision with fixed or stationary object in nontraffic accident
- **V17.3** Person boarding or alighting a pedal cycle injured in collision with fixed or stationary object
- **V17.4** Pedal cycle driver injured in collision with fixed or stationary object in traffic accident
- **V17.5** Pedal cycle passenger injured in collision with fixed or stationary object in traffic accident
- **V17.9** Unspecified pedal cyclist injured in collision with fixed or stationary object in traffic accident

V18 Pedal cycle rider injured in noncollision transport accident
> INCLUDES fall or thrown from pedal cycle (without antecedent collision)
> overturning pedal cycle NOS
> overturning pedal cycle without collision
- **V18.0** Pedal cycle driver injured in noncollision transport accident in nontraffic accident
- **V18.1** Pedal cycle passenger injured in noncollision transport accident in nontraffic accident
- **V18.2** Unspecified pedal cyclist injured in noncollision transport accident in nontraffic accident
- **V18.3** Person boarding or alighting a pedal cycle injured in noncollision transport accident
- **V18.4** Pedal cycle driver injured in noncollision transport accident in traffic accident
- **V18.5** Pedal cycle passenger injured in noncollision transport accident in traffic accident
- **V18.9** Unspecified pedal cyclist injured in noncollision transport accident in traffic accident

V19 Pedal cycle rider injured in other and unspecified transport accidents
- **V19.0** Pedal cycle driver injured in collision with other and unspecified motor vehicles in nontraffic accident
  - **V19.00** Pedal cycle driver injured in collision with unspecified motor vehicles in nontraffic accident
  - **V19.09** Pedal cycle driver injured in collision with other motor vehicles in nontraffic accident
- **V19.1** Pedal cycle passenger injured in collision with other and unspecified motor vehicles in nontraffic accident
  - **V19.10** Pedal cycle passenger injured in collision with unspecified motor vehicles in nontraffic accident
  - **V19.19** Pedal cycle passenger injured in collision with other motor vehicles in nontraffic accident
- **V19.2** Unspecified pedal cyclist injured in collision with other and unspecified motor vehicles in nontraffic accident
  - **V19.20** Unspecified pedal cyclist injured in collision with unspecified motor vehicles in nontraffic accident
    Pedal cycle collision NOS, nontraffic
  - **V19.29** Unspecified pedal cyclist injured in collision with other motor vehicles in nontraffic accident
- **V19.3** Pedal cyclist (driver) (passenger) injured in unspecified nontraffic accident
  Pedal cycle accident NOS, nontraffic
  Pedal cyclist injured in nontraffic accident NOS
- **V19.4** Pedal cycle driver injured in collision with other and unspecified motor vehicles in traffic accident
  - **V19.40** Pedal cycle driver injured in collision with unspecified motor vehicles in traffic accident
  - **V19.49** Pedal cycle driver injured in collision with other motor vehicles in traffic accident
- **V19.5** Pedal cycle passenger injured in collision with other and unspecified motor vehicles in traffic accident
  - **V19.50** Pedal cycle passenger injured in collision with unspecified motor vehicles in traffic accident
  - **V19.59** Pedal cycle passenger injured in collision with other motor vehicles in traffic accident
- **V19.6** Unspecified pedal cyclist injured in collision with other and unspecified motor vehicles in traffic accident
  - **V19.60** Unspecified pedal cyclist injured in collision with unspecified motor vehicles in traffic accident
    Pedal cycle collision NOS (traffic)
  - **V19.69** Unspecified pedal cyclist injured in collision with other motor vehicles in traffic accident
- **V19.8** Pedal cyclist (driver) (passenger) injured in other specified transport accidents
  - **V19.81** Pedal cyclist (driver) (passenger) injured in transport accident with military vehicle
  - **V19.88** Pedal cyclist (driver) (passenger) injured in other specified transport accidents
- **V19.9** Pedal cyclist (driver) (passenger) injured in unspecified traffic accident
  Pedal cycle accident NOS

Motorcycle rider injured in transport accident (V20-V29)

> INCLUDES electric bicycle
> e-bike
> e-bicycle
> moped
> motorcycle with sidecar
> motorized bicycle
> motor scooter
>
> EXCLUDES 1 three-wheeled motor vehicle (V30-V39)
>
> AHA: 2022,4Q,47

The appropriate 7th character is to be added to each code from categories V20-V29.
A   initial encounter
D   subsequent encounter
S   sequela

V20 Motorcycle rider injured in collision with pedestrian or animal
> EXCLUDES 1 motorcycle rider collision with animal-drawn vehicle or animal being ridden (V26.-)
- **V20.0** Motorcycle driver injured in collision with pedestrian or animal in nontraffic accident
  - **V20.01** Electric (assisted) bicycle driver injured in collision with pedestrian or animal in nontraffic accident
  - **V20.09** Other motorcycle driver injured in collision with pedestrian or animal in nontraffic accident
- **V20.1** Motorcycle passenger injured in collision with pedestrian or animal in nontraffic accident
  - **V20.11** Electric (assisted) bicycle passenger injured in collision with pedestrian or animal in nontraffic accident

Chapter 20. External Causes of Morbidity

- V20.19 Other motorcycle passenger injured in collision with pedestrian or animal in nontraffic accident
- **V20.2** Unspecified motorcycle rider injured in collision with pedestrian or animal in nontraffic accident
  - V20.21 Unspecified electric (assisted) bicycle rider injured in collision with pedestrian or animal in nontraffic accident
  - V20.29 Unspecified rider of other motorcycle injured in collision with pedestrian or animal in nontraffic accident
- **V20.3** Person boarding or alighting a motorcycle injured in collision with pedestrian or animal
  - V20.31 Person boarding or alighting an electric (assisted) bicycle injured in collision with pedestrian or animal
  - V20.39 Person boarding or alighting other motorcycle injured in collision with pedestrian or animal
- **V20.4** Motorcycle driver injured in collision with pedestrian or animal in traffic accident
  - V20.41 Electric (assisted) bicycle driver injured in collision with pedestrian or animal in traffic accident
  - V20.49 Other motorcycle driver injured in collision with pedestrian or animal in traffic accident
- **V20.5** Motorcycle passenger injured in collision with pedestrian or animal in traffic accident
  - V20.51 Electric (assisted) bicycle passenger injured in collision with pedestrian or animal in traffic accident
  - V20.59 Other motorcycle passenger injured in collision with pedestrian or animal in traffic accident
- **V20.9** Unspecified motorcycle rider injured in collision with pedestrian or animal in traffic accident
  - V20.91 Unspecified electric (assisted) bicycle rider injured in collision with pedestrian or animal in traffic accident
  - V20.99 Unspecified rider of other motorcycle injured in collision with pedestrian or animal in traffic accident

V21 Motorcycle rider injured in collision with pedal cycle

- **V21.0** Motorcycle driver injured in collision with pedal cycle in nontraffic accident
  - V21.01 Electric (assisted) bicycle driver injured in collision with pedal cycle in nontraffic accident
  - V21.09 Other motorcycle driver injured in collision with pedal cycle in nontraffic accident
- **V21.1** Motorcycle passenger injured in collision with pedal cycle in nontraffic accident
  - V21.11 Electric (assisted) bicycle passenger injured in collision with pedal cycle in nontraffic accident
  - V21.19 Other motorcycle passenger injured in collision with pedal cycle in nontraffic accident
- **V21.2** Unspecified motorcycle rider injured in collision with pedal cycle in nontraffic accident
  - V21.21 Unspecified electric (assisted) bicycle rider injured in collision with pedal cycle in nontraffic accident
  - V21.29 Unspecified rider of other motorcycle injured in collision with pedal cycle in nontraffic accident
- **V21.3** Person boarding or alighting a motorcycle injured in collision with pedal cycle
  - V21.31 Person boarding or alighting an electric (assisted) bicycle injured in collision with pedal cycle
  - V21.39 Person boarding or alighting other motorcycle injured in collision with pedal cycle
- **V21.4** Motorcycle driver injured in collision with pedal cycle in traffic accident
  - V21.41 Electric (assisted) bicycle driver injured in collision with pedal cycle in traffic accident
  - V21.49 Other motorcycle driver injured in collision with pedal cycle in traffic accident
- **V21.5** Motorcycle passenger injured in collision with pedal cycle in traffic accident
  - V21.51 Electric (assisted) bicycle passenger injured in collision with pedal cycle in traffic accident
  - V21.59 Other motorcycle passenger injured in collision with pedal cycle in traffic accident
- **V21.9** Unspecified motorcycle rider injured in collision with pedal cycle in traffic accident
  - V21.91 Unspecified electric (assisted) bicycle rider injured in collision with pedal cycle in traffic accident
  - V21.99 Unspecified rider of other motorcycle injured in collision with pedal cycle in traffic accident

V22 Motorcycle rider injured in collision with two- or three-wheeled motor vehicle

- **V22.0** Motorcycle driver injured in collision with two- or three-wheeled motor vehicle in nontraffic accident
  - V22.01 Electric (assisted) bicycle driver injured in collision with two- or three-wheeled motor vehicle in nontraffic accident
  - V22.09 Other motorcycle driver injured in collision with two- or three-wheeled motor vehicle in nontraffic accident
- **V22.1** Motorcycle passenger injured in collision with two- or three-wheeled motor vehicle in nontraffic accident
  - V22.11 Electric (assisted) bicycle passenger injured in collision with two- or three-wheeled motor vehicle in nontraffic accident
  - V22.19 Other motorcycle passenger injured in collision with two- or three-wheeled motor vehicle in nontraffic accident
- **V22.2** Unspecified motorcycle rider injured in collision with two- or three-wheeled motor vehicle in nontraffic accident
  - V22.21 Unspecified electric (assisted) bicycle rider injured in collision with two- or three-wheeled motor vehicle in nontraffic accident
  - V22.29 Unspecified rider of other motorcycle injured in collision with two- or three-wheeled motor vehicle in nontraffic accident
- **V22.3** Person boarding or alighting a motorcycle injured in collision with two- or three-wheeled motor vehicle
  - V22.31 Person boarding or alighting an electric (assisted) bicycle injured in collision with two- or three-wheeled motor vehicle
  - V22.39 Person boarding or alighting other motorcycle injured in collision with two- or three-wheeled motor vehicle
- **V22.4** Motorcycle driver injured in collision with two- or three-wheeled motor vehicle in traffic accident
  - V22.41 Electric (assisted) bicycle driver injured in collision with two- or three-wheeled motor vehicle in traffic accident
  - V22.49 Other motorcycle driver injured in collision with two- or three-wheeled motor vehicle in traffic accident
- **V22.5** Motorcycle passenger injured in collision with two- or three-wheeled motor vehicle in traffic accident
  - V22.51 Electric (assisted) bicycle passenger injured in collision with two- or three-wheeled motor vehicle in traffic accident
  - V22.59 Other motorcycle passenger injured in collision with two- or three-wheeled motor vehicle in traffic accident
- **V22.9** Unspecified motorcycle rider injured in collision with two- or three-wheeled motor vehicle in traffic accident
  - V22.91 Unspecified electric (assisted) bicycle rider injured in collision with two- or three-wheeled motor vehicle in traffic accident
  - V22.99 Unspecified rider of other motorcycle injured in collision with two- or three-wheeled motor vehicle in traffic accident

V23 Motorcycle rider injured in collision with car, pick-up truck or van

- **V23.0** Motorcycle driver injured in collision with car, pick-up truck or van in nontraffic accident
  - V23.01 Electric (assisted) bicycle driver injured in collision with car, pick-up truck or van in nontraffic accident
  - V23.09 Other motorcycle driver injured in collision with car, pick-up truck or van in nontraffic accident
- **V23.1** Motorcycle passenger injured in collision with car, pick-up truck or van in nontraffic accident
  - V23.11 Electric (assisted) bicycle passenger injured in collision with car, pick-up truck or van in nontraffic accident
  - V23.19 Other motorcycle passenger injured in collision with car, pick-up truck or van in nontraffic accident
- **V23.2** Unspecified motorcycle rider injured in collision with car, pick-up truck or van in nontraffic accident
  - V23.21 Unspecified electric (assisted) bicycle rider injured in collision with car, pick-up truck or van in nontraffic accident
  - V23.29 Unspecified rider of other motorcycle injured in collision with car, pick-up truck or van in nontraffic accident
- **V23.3** Person boarding or alighting a motorcycle injured in collision with car, pick-up truck or van
  - V23.31 Person boarding or alighting an electric (assisted) bicycle injured in collision with car, pick-up truck or van

- **V23.39** Person boarding or alighting other motorcycle injured in collision with car, pick-up truck or van
- **V23.4** Motorcycle driver injured in collision with car, pick-up truck or van in traffic accident
  - **V23.41** Electric (assisted) bicycle driver injured in collision with car, pick-up truck or van in traffic accident
  - **V23.49** Other motorcycle driver injured in collision with car, pick-up truck or van in traffic accident
- **V23.5** Motorcycle passenger injured in collision with car, pick-up truck or van in traffic accident
  - **V23.51** Electric (assisted) bicycle passenger injured in collision with car, pick-up truck or van in traffic accident
  - **V23.59** Other motorcycle passenger injured in collision with car, pick-up truck or van in traffic accident
- **V23.9** Unspecified motorcycle rider injured in collision with car, pick-up truck or van in traffic accident
  - **V23.91** Unspecified electric (assisted) bicycle rider injured in collision with car, pick-up truck or van in traffic accident
  - **V23.99** Unspecified rider of other motorcycle injured in collision with car, pick-up truck or van in traffic accident

V24 Motorcycle rider injured in collision with heavy transport vehicle or bus

EXCLUDES 1 motorcycle rider injured in collision with military vehicle (V29.818)

- **V24.0** Motorcycle driver injured in collision with heavy transport vehicle or bus in nontraffic accident
  - **V24.01** Electric (assisted) bicycle driver injured in collision with heavy transport vehicle or bus in nontraffic accident
  - **V24.09** Other motorcycle driver injured in collision with heavy transport vehicle or bus in nontraffic accident
- **V24.1** Motorcycle passenger injured in collision with heavy transport vehicle or bus in nontraffic accident
  - **V24.11** Electric (assisted) bicycle passenger injured in collision with heavy transport vehicle or bus in nontraffic accident
  - **V24.19** Other motorcycle passenger injured in collision with heavy transport vehicle or bus in nontraffic accident
- **V24.2** Unspecified motorcycle rider injured in collision with heavy transport vehicle or bus in nontraffic accident
  - **V24.21** Unspecified electric (assisted) bicycle rider injured in collision with heavy transport vehicle or bus in nontraffic accident
  - **V24.29** Unspecified rider of other motorcycle injured in collision with heavy transport vehicle or bus in nontraffic accident
- **V24.3** Person boarding or alighting a motorcycle injured in collision with heavy transport vehicle or bus
  - **V24.31** Person boarding or alighting an electric (assisted) bicycle injured in collision with heavy transport vehicle or bus
  - **V24.39** Person boarding or alighting other motorcycle injured in collision with heavy transport vehicle or bus
- **V24.4** Motorcycle driver injured in collision with heavy transport vehicle or bus in traffic accident
  - **V24.41** Electric (assisted) bicycle driver injured in collision with heavy transport vehicle or bus in traffic accident
  - **V24.49** Other motorcycle driver injured in collision with heavy transport vehicle or bus in traffic accident
- **V24.5** Motorcycle passenger injured in collision with heavy transport vehicle or bus in traffic accident
  - **V24.51** Electric (assisted) bicycle passenger injured in collision with heavy transport vehicle or bus in traffic accident
  - **V24.59** Other motorcycle passenger injured in collision with heavy transport vehicle or bus in traffic accident
- **V24.9** Unspecified motorcycle rider injured in collision with heavy transport vehicle or bus in traffic accident
  - **V24.91** Unspecified electric (assisted) bicycle rider injured in collision with heavy transport vehicle or bus in traffic accident
  - **V24.99** Unspecified rider of other motorcycle injured in collision with heavy transport vehicle or bus in traffic accident

V25 Motorcycle rider injured in collision with railway train or railway vehicle

- **V25.0** Motorcycle driver injured in collision with railway train or railway vehicle in nontraffic accident
  - **V25.01** Electric (assisted) bicycle driver injured in collision with railway train or railway vehicle in nontraffic accident
  - **V25.09** Other motorcycle driver injured in collision with railway train or railway vehicle in nontraffic accident
- **V25.1** Motorcycle passenger injured in collision with railway train or railway vehicle in nontraffic accident
  - **V25.11** Electric (assisted) bicycle passenger injured in collision with railway train or railway vehicle in nontraffic accident
  - **V25.19** Other motorcycle passenger injured in collision with railway train or railway vehicle in nontraffic accident
- **V25.2** Unspecified motorcycle rider injured in collision with railway train or railway vehicle in nontraffic accident
  - **V25.21** Unspecified electric (assisted) bicycle rider injured in collision with railway train or railway vehicle in nontraffic accident
  - **V25.29** Unspecified rider of other motorcycle injured in collision with railway train or railway vehicle in nontraffic accident
- **V25.3** Person boarding or alighting a motorcycle injured in collision with railway train or railway vehicle
  - **V25.31** Person boarding or alighting an electric (assisted) bicycle injured in collision with railway train or railway vehicle
  - **V25.39** Person boarding or alighting other motorcycle injured in collision with railway train or railway vehicle
- **V25.4** Motorcycle driver injured in collision with railway train or railway vehicle in traffic accident
  - **V25.41** Electric (assisted) bicycle driver injured in collision with railway train or railway vehicle in traffic accident
  - **V25.49** Other motorcycle driver injured in collision with railway train or railway vehicle in traffic accident
- **V25.5** Motorcycle passenger injured in collision with railway train or railway vehicle in traffic accident
  - **V25.51** Electric (assisted) bicycle passenger injured in collision with railway train or railway vehicle in traffic accident
  - **V25.59** Other motorcycle passenger injured in collision with railway train or railway vehicle in traffic accident
- **V25.9** Unspecified motorcycle rider injured in collision with railway train or railway vehicle in traffic accident
  - **V25.91** Unspecified electric (assisted) bicycle rider injured in collision with railway train or railway vehicle in traffic accident
  - **V25.99** Unspecified rider of other motorcycle injured in collision with railway train or railway vehicle in traffic accident

V26 Motorcycle rider injured in collision with other nonmotor vehicle

INCLUDES collision with animal-drawn vehicle, animal being ridden, streetcar

- **V26.0** Motorcycle driver injured in collision with other nonmotor vehicle in nontraffic accident
  - **V26.01** Electric (assisted) bicycle driver injured in collision with other nonmotor vehicle in nontraffic accident
  - **V26.09** Other motorcycle driver injured in collision with other nonmotor vehicle in nontraffic accident
- **V26.1** Motorcycle passenger injured in collision with other nonmotor vehicle in nontraffic accident
  - **V26.11** Electric (assisted) bicycle passenger injured in collision with other nonmotor vehicle in nontraffic accident
  - **V26.19** Other motorcycle passenger injured in collision with other nonmotor vehicle in nontraffic accident
- **V26.2** Unspecified motorcycle rider injured in collision with other nonmotor vehicle in nontraffic accident
  - **V26.21** Unspecified electric (assisted) bicycle rider injured in collision with other nonmotor vehicle in nontraffic accident
  - **V26.29** Unspecified rider of other motorcycle injured in collision with other nonmotor vehicle in nontraffic accident
- **V26.3** Person boarding or alighting a motorcycle injured in collision with other nonmotor vehicle
  - **V26.31** Person boarding or alighting an electric (assisted) bicycle injured in collision with other nonmotor vehicle

- ✓x7th **V26.39** Person boarding or alighting other motorcycle injured in collision with other nonmotor vehicle
- ✓5th **V26.4** Motorcycle driver injured in collision with other nonmotor vehicle in traffic accident
  - ✓x7th **V26.41** Electric (assisted) bicycle driver injured in collision with other nonmotor vehicle in traffic accident
  - ✓x7th **V26.49** Other motorcycle driver injured in collision with other nonmotor vehicle in traffic accident
- ✓5th **V26.5** Motorcycle passenger injured in collision with other nonmotor vehicle in traffic accident
  - ✓x7th **V26.51** Electric (assisted) bicycle passenger injured in collision with other nonmotor vehicle in traffic accident
  - ✓x7th **V26.59** Other motorcycle passenger injured in collision with other nonmotor vehicle in traffic accident
- ✓5th **V26.9** Unspecified motorcycle rider injured in collision with other nonmotor vehicle in traffic accident
  - ✓x7th **V26.91** Unspecified electric (assisted) bicycle rider injured in collision with other nonmotor vehicle in traffic accident
  - ✓x7th **V26.99** Unspecified rider of other motorcycle injured in collision with other nonmotor vehicle in traffic accident

✓4th **V27** Motorcycle rider injured in collision with fixed or stationary object
- ✓5th **V27.0** Motorcycle driver injured in collision with fixed or stationary object in nontraffic accident
  - ✓x7th **V27.01** Electric (assisted) bicycle driver injured in collision with fixed or stationary object in nontraffic accident
  - ✓x7th **V27.09** Other motorcycle driver injured in collision with fixed or stationary object in nontraffic accident
- ✓5th **V27.1** Motorcycle passenger injured in collision with fixed or stationary object in nontraffic accident
  - ✓x7th **V27.11** Electric (assisted) bicycle passenger injured in collision with fixed or stationary object in nontraffic accident
  - ✓x7th **V27.19** Other motorcycle passenger injured in collision with fixed or stationary object in nontraffic accident
- ✓5th **V27.2** Unspecified motorcycle rider injured in collision with fixed or stationary object in nontraffic accident
  - ✓x7th **V27.21** Unspecified electric (assisted) bicycle rider injured in collision with fixed or stationary object in nontraffic accident
  - ✓x7th **V27.29** Unspecified rider of other motorcycle injured in collision with fixed or stationary object in nontraffic accident
- ✓5th **V27.3** Person boarding or alighting a motorcycle injured in collision with fixed or stationary object
  - ✓x7th **V27.31** Person boarding or alighting an electric (assisted) bicycle injured in collision with fixed or stationary object
  - ✓x7th **V27.39** Person boarding or alighting other motorcycle injured in collision with fixed or stationary object
- ✓5th **V27.4** Motorcycle driver injured in collision with fixed or stationary object in traffic accident
  - ✓x7th **V27.41** Electric (assisted) bicycle driver injured in collision with fixed or stationary object in traffic accident
  - ✓x7th **V27.49** Other motorcycle driver injured in collision with fixed or stationary object in traffic accident
- ✓5th **V27.5** Motorcycle passenger injured in collision with fixed or stationary object in traffic accident
  - ✓x7th **V27.51** Electric (assisted) bicycle passenger injured in collision with fixed or stationary object in traffic accident
  - ✓x7th **V27.59** Other motorcycle passenger injured in collision with fixed or stationary object in traffic accident
- ✓5th **V27.9** Unspecified motorcycle rider injured in collision with fixed or stationary object in traffic accident
  - ✓x7th **V27.91** Unspecified electric (assisted) bicycle rider injured in collision with fixed or stationary object in traffic accident
  - ✓x7th **V27.99** Unspecified rider of other motorcycle injured in collision with fixed or stationary object in traffic accident

✓4th **V28** Motorcycle rider injured in noncollision transport accident
- INCLUDES: fall or thrown from motorcycle (without antecedent collision)
  - overturning motorcycle NOS
  - overturning motorcycle without collision
- ✓5th **V28.0** Motorcycle driver injured in noncollision transport accident in nontraffic accident
  - ✓x7th **V28.01** Electric (assisted) bicycle driver injured in noncollision transport accident in nontraffic accident
  - ✓x7th **V28.09** Other motorcycle driver injured in noncollision transport accident in nontraffic accident
- ✓5th **V28.1** Motorcycle passenger injured in noncollision transport accident in nontraffic accident
  - ✓x7th **V28.11** Electric (assisted) bicycle passenger injured in noncollision transport accident in nontraffic accident
  - ✓x7th **V28.19** Other motorcycle passenger injured in noncollision transport accident in nontraffic accident
- ✓5th **V28.2** Unspecified motorcycle rider injured in noncollision transport accident in nontraffic accident
  - ✓x7th **V28.21** Unspecified electric (assisted) bicycle rider injured in noncollision transport accident in nontraffic accident
  - ✓x7th **V28.29** Unspecified rider of other motorcycle injured in noncollision transport accident in nontraffic accident
- ✓5th **V28.3** Person boarding or alighting a motorcycle injured in noncollision transport accident
  - ✓x7th **V28.31** Person boarding or alighting an electric (assisted) bicycle injured in noncollision transport accident
  - ✓x7th **V28.39** Person boarding or alighting other motorcycle injured in noncollision transport accident
- ✓5th **V28.4** Motorcycle driver injured in noncollision transport accident in traffic accident
  - ✓x7th **V28.41** Electric (assisted) bicycle driver injured in noncollision transport accident in traffic accident
  - ✓x7th **V28.49** Other motorcycle driver injured in noncollision transport accident in traffic accident
- ✓5th **V28.5** Motorcycle passenger injured in noncollision transport accident in traffic accident
  - ✓x7th **V28.51** Electric (assisted) bicycle passenger injured in noncollision transport accident in traffic accident
  - ✓x7th **V28.59** Other motorcycle passenger injured in noncollision transport accident in traffic accident
- ✓5th **V28.9** Unspecified motorcycle rider injured in noncollision transport accident in traffic accident
  - ✓x7th **V28.91** Unspecified electric (assisted) bicycle rider injured in noncollision transport accident in traffic accident
  - ✓x7th **V28.99** Unspecified rider of other motorcycle injured in noncollision transport accident in traffic accident

✓4th **V29** Motorcycle rider injured in other and unspecified transport accidents
- ✓5th **V29.0** Motorcycle driver injured in collision with other and unspecified motor vehicles in nontraffic accident
  - ✓6th **V29.00** Motorcycle driver injured in collision with unspecified motor vehicles in nontraffic accident
    - ✓7th **V29.001** Electric (assisted) bicycle driver injured in collision with unspecified motor vehicles in nontraffic accident
    - ✓7th **V29.008** Other motorcycle driver injured in collision with unspecified motor vehicles in nontraffic accident
  - ✓6th **V29.09** Motorcycle driver injured in collision with other motor vehicles in nontraffic accident
    - ✓7th **V29.091** Electric (assisted) bicycle driver injured in collision with other motor vehicles in nontraffic accident
    - ✓7th **V29.098** Other motorcycle driver injured in collision with other motor vehicles in nontraffic accident
- ✓5th **V29.1** Motorcycle passenger injured in collision with other and unspecified motor vehicles in nontraffic accident
  - ✓6th **V29.10** Motorcycle passenger injured in collision with unspecified motor vehicles in nontraffic accident
    - ✓7th **V29.101** Electric (assisted) bicycle passenger injured in collision with unspecified motor vehicles in nontraffic accident
    - ✓7th **V29.108** Other motorcycle passenger injured in collision with unspecified motor vehicles in nontraffic accident
  - ✓6th **V29.19** Motorcycle passenger injured in collision with other motor vehicles in nontraffic accident
    - ✓7th **V29.191** Electric (assisted) bicycle passenger injured in collision with other motor vehicles in nontraffic accident
    - ✓7th **V29.198** Other motorcycle passenger injured in collision with other motor vehicles in nontraffic accident
- ✓5th **V29.2** Unspecified motorcycle rider injured in collision with other and unspecified motor vehicles in nontraffic accident
  - ✓6th **V29.20** Unspecified motorcycle rider injured in collision with unspecified motor vehicles in nontraffic accident
    - ✓7th **V29.201** Unspecified electric (assisted) bicycle rider injured in collision with unspecified motor vehicles in nontraffic accident

---

■ Additional Character Required   ✓x7th Placeholder Alert   Manifestation   Unspecified Dx   ℚ QPP   UPD Unacceptable PDx

Chapter 20. External Causes of Morbidity

- ☑7th **V29.208** Unspecified rider of other motorcycle injured in collision with unspecified motor vehicles in nontraffic accident
  - *Motorcycle collision NOS, nontraffic*
- ☑6th **V29.29** Unspecified motorcycle rider injured in collision with other motor vehicles in nontraffic accident
  - ☑7th **V29.291** Unspecified electric (assisted) bicycle rider injured in collision with other motor vehicles in nontraffic accident
  - ☑7th **V29.298** Unspecified rider of other motorcycle injured in collision with other motor vehicles in nontraffic accident
- ☑5th **V29.3** Motorcycle rider (driver) (passenger) injured in unspecified nontraffic accident
  - ☑x7th **V29.31** Electric (assisted) bicycle (driver) (passenger) injured in unspecified nontraffic accident
  - ☑x7th **V29.39** Other motorcycle (driver) (passenger) injured in unspecified nontraffic accident
    - *Motorcycle accident NOS, nontraffic*
    - *Motorcycle rider injured in nontraffic accident NOS*
- ☑5th **V29.4** Motorcycle driver injured in collision with other and unspecified motor vehicles in traffic accident
  - ☑6th **V29.40** Motorcycle driver injured in collision with unspecified motor vehicles in traffic accident
    - ☑7th **V29.401** Electric (assisted) bicycle driver injured in collision with unspecified motor vehicles in traffic accident
    - ☑7th **V29.408** Other motorcycle driver injured in collision with unspecified motor vehicles in traffic accident
  - ☑6th **V29.49** Motorcycle driver injured in collision with other motor vehicles in traffic accident
    - ☑7th **V29.491** Electric (assisted) bicycle driver injured in collision with other motor vehicles in traffic accident
    - ☑7th **V29.498** Other motorcycle driver injured in collision with other motor vehicles in traffic accident
- ☑5th **V29.5** Motorcycle passenger injured in collision with other and unspecified motor vehicles in traffic accident
  - ☑6th **V29.50** Motorcycle passenger injured in collision with unspecified motor vehicles in traffic accident
    - ☑7th **V29.501** Electric (assisted) bicycle passenger injured in collision with unspecified motor vehicles in traffic accident
    - ☑7th **V29.508** Other motorcycle passenger injured in collision with unspecified motor vehicles in traffic accident
  - ☑6th **V29.59** Motorcycle passenger injured in collision with other motor vehicles in traffic accident
    - ☑7th **V29.591** Electric (assisted) bicycle passenger injured in collision with other motor vehicles in traffic accident
    - ☑7th **V29.598** Other motorcycle passenger injured in collision with other motor vehicles in traffic accident
- ☑5th **V29.6** Unspecified motorcycle rider injured in collision with other and unspecified motor vehicles in traffic accident
  - ☑6th **V29.60** Unspecified motorcycle rider injured in collision with unspecified motor vehicles in traffic accident
    - ☑7th **V29.601** Unspecified electric (assisted) bicycle rider injured in collision with unspecified motor vehicles in traffic accident
    - ☑7th **V29.608** Unspecified rider of other motorcycle injured in collision with unspecified motor vehicles in traffic accident
      - *Motorcycle collision NOS (traffic)*
  - ☑6th **V29.69** Unspecified motorcycle rider injured in collision with other motor vehicles in traffic accident
    - ☑7th **V29.691** Unspecified electric (assisted) bicycle rider injured in collision with other motor vehicles in traffic accident
    - ☑7th **V29.698** Unspecified rider of other motorcycle injured in collision with other motor vehicles in traffic accident
- ☑5th **V29.8** Motorcycle rider (driver) (passenger) injured in other specified transport accidents
  - ☑6th **V29.81** Motorcycle rider (driver) (passenger) injured in transport accident with military vehicle
    - ☑7th **V29.811** Electric (assisted) bicycle rider (driver) (passenger) injured in transport accident with military vehicle
    - ☑7th **V29.818** Rider (driver) (passenger) of other motorcycle injured in transport accident with military vehicle
  - ☑6th **V29.88** Motorcycle rider (driver) (passenger) injured in other specified transport accidents
    - ☑7th **V29.881** Electric (assisted) bicycle rider (driver) (passenger) injured in other specified transport accidents
    - ☑7th **V29.888** Rider (driver) (passenger) of other motorcycle injured in other specified transport accidents
- ☑5th **V29.9** Motorcycle rider (driver) (passenger) injured in unspecified traffic accident
  - ☑x7th **V29.91** Electric (assisted) bicycle rider (driver) (passenger) injured in unspecified traffic accident
  - ☑x7th **V29.99** Rider (driver) (passenger) of other motorcycle injured in unspecified traffic accident
    - *Motorcycle accident NOS*

Occupant of three-wheeled motor vehicle injured in transport accident (V30-V39)

INCLUDES motorized tricycle
motorized rickshaw
three-wheeled motor car

EXCLUDES 1 all-terrain vehicles (V86.-)
motorcycle with sidecar (V20-V29)
vehicle designed primarily for off-road use (V86.-)

The appropriate 7th character is to be added to each code from categories V30-V39.
- A initial encounter
- D subsequent encounter
- S sequela

- ☑4th **V30** Occupant of three-wheeled motor vehicle injured in collision with pedestrian or animal
  - **EXCLUDES 1** *three-wheeled motor vehicle collision with animal-drawn vehicle or animal being ridden (V36.-)*
  - ☑x7th **V30.0** Driver of three-wheeled motor vehicle injured in collision with pedestrian or animal in nontraffic accident
  - ☑x7th **V30.1** Passenger in three-wheeled motor vehicle injured in collision with pedestrian or animal in nontraffic accident
  - ☑x7th **V30.2** Person on outside of three-wheeled motor vehicle injured in collision with pedestrian or animal in nontraffic accident
  - ☑x7th **V30.3** Unspecified occupant of three-wheeled motor vehicle injured in collision with pedestrian or animal in nontraffic accident
  - ☑x7th **V30.4** Person boarding or alighting a three-wheeled motor vehicle injured in collision with pedestrian or animal
  - ☑x7th **V30.5** Driver of three-wheeled motor vehicle injured in collision with pedestrian or animal in traffic accident
  - ☑x7th **V30.6** Passenger in three-wheeled motor vehicle injured in collision with pedestrian or animal in traffic accident
  - ☑x7th **V30.7** Person on outside of three-wheeled motor vehicle injured in collision with pedestrian or animal in traffic accident
  - ☑x7th **V30.9** Unspecified occupant of three-wheeled motor vehicle injured in collision with pedestrian or animal in traffic accident
- ☑4th **V31** Occupant of three-wheeled motor vehicle injured in collision with pedal cycle
  - ☑x7th **V31.0** Driver of three-wheeled motor vehicle injured in collision with pedal cycle in nontraffic accident
  - ☑x7th **V31.1** Passenger in three-wheeled motor vehicle injured in collision with pedal cycle in nontraffic accident
  - ☑x7th **V31.2** Person on outside of three-wheeled motor vehicle injured in collision with pedal cycle in nontraffic accident
  - ☑x7th **V31.3** Unspecified occupant of three-wheeled motor vehicle injured in collision with pedal cycle in nontraffic accident
  - ☑x7th **V31.4** Person boarding or alighting a three-wheeled motor vehicle injured in collision with pedal cycle
  - ☑x7th **V31.5** Driver of three-wheeled motor vehicle injured in collision with pedal cycle in traffic accident
  - ☑x7th **V31.6** Passenger in three-wheeled motor vehicle injured in collision with pedal cycle in traffic accident
  - ☑x7th **V31.7** Person on outside of three-wheeled motor vehicle injured in collision with pedal cycle in traffic accident
  - ☑x7th **V31.9** Unspecified occupant of three-wheeled motor vehicle injured in collision with pedal cycle in traffic accident
- ☑4th **V32** Occupant of three-wheeled motor vehicle injured in collision with two- or three-wheeled motor vehicle
  - ☑x7th **V32.0** Driver of three-wheeled motor vehicle injured in collision with two- or three-wheeled motor vehicle in nontraffic accident
  - ☑x7th **V32.1** Passenger in three-wheeled motor vehicle injured in collision with two- or three-wheeled motor vehicle in nontraffic accident

- **V32.2** Person on outside of three-wheeled motor vehicle injured in collision with two- or three-wheeled motor vehicle in nontraffic accident
- **V32.3** Unspecified occupant of three-wheeled motor vehicle injured in collision with two- or three-wheeled motor vehicle in nontraffic accident
- **V32.4** Person boarding or alighting a three-wheeled motor vehicle injured in collision with two- or three-wheeled motor vehicle
- **V32.5** Driver of three-wheeled motor vehicle injured in collision with two- or three-wheeled motor vehicle in traffic accident
- **V32.6** Passenger in three-wheeled motor vehicle injured in collision with two- or three-wheeled motor vehicle in traffic accident
- **V32.7** Person on outside of three-wheeled motor vehicle injured in collision with two- or three-wheeled motor vehicle in traffic accident
- **V32.9** Unspecified occupant of three-wheeled motor vehicle injured in collision with two- or three-wheeled motor vehicle in traffic accident

V33 Occupant of three-wheeled motor vehicle injured in collision with car, pick-up truck or van
- **V33.0** Driver of three-wheeled motor vehicle injured in collision with car, pick-up truck or van in nontraffic accident
- **V33.1** Passenger in three-wheeled motor vehicle injured in collision with car, pick-up truck or van in nontraffic accident
- **V33.2** Person on outside of three-wheeled motor vehicle injured in collision with car, pick-up truck or van in nontraffic accident
- **V33.3** Unspecified occupant of three-wheeled motor vehicle injured in collision with car, pick-up truck or van in nontraffic accident
- **V33.4** Person boarding or alighting a three-wheeled motor vehicle injured in collision with car, pick-up truck or van
- **V33.5** Driver of three-wheeled motor vehicle injured in collision with car, pick-up truck or van in traffic accident
- **V33.6** Passenger in three-wheeled motor vehicle injured in collision with car, pick-up truck or van in traffic accident
- **V33.7** Person on outside of three-wheeled motor vehicle injured in collision with car, pick-up truck or van in traffic accident
- **V33.9** Unspecified occupant of three-wheeled motor vehicle injured in collision with car, pick-up truck or van in traffic accident

V34 Occupant of three-wheeled motor vehicle injured in collision with heavy transport vehicle or bus
> **EXCLUDES 1** occupant of three-wheeled motor vehicle injured in collision with military vehicle (V39.81)

- **V34.0** Driver of three-wheeled motor vehicle injured in collision with heavy transport vehicle or bus in nontraffic accident
- **V34.1** Passenger in three-wheeled motor vehicle injured in collision with heavy transport vehicle or bus in nontraffic accident
- **V34.2** Person on outside of three-wheeled motor vehicle injured in collision with heavy transport vehicle or bus in nontraffic accident
- **V34.3** Unspecified occupant of three-wheeled motor vehicle injured in collision with heavy transport vehicle or bus in nontraffic accident
- **V34.4** Person boarding or alighting a three-wheeled motor vehicle injured in collision with heavy transport vehicle or bus
- **V34.5** Driver of three-wheeled motor vehicle injured in collision with heavy transport vehicle or bus in traffic accident
- **V34.6** Passenger in three-wheeled motor vehicle injured in collision with heavy transport vehicle or bus in traffic accident
- **V34.7** Person on outside of three-wheeled motor vehicle injured in collision with heavy transport vehicle or bus in traffic accident
- **V34.9** Unspecified occupant of three-wheeled motor vehicle injured in collision with heavy transport vehicle or bus in traffic accident

V35 Occupant of three-wheeled motor vehicle injured in collision with railway train or railway vehicle
- **V35.0** Driver of three-wheeled motor vehicle injured in collision with railway train or railway vehicle in nontraffic accident
- **V35.1** Passenger in three-wheeled motor vehicle injured in collision with railway train or railway vehicle in nontraffic accident
- **V35.2** Person on outside of three-wheeled motor vehicle injured in collision with railway train or railway vehicle in nontraffic accident
- **V35.3** Unspecified occupant of three-wheeled motor vehicle injured in collision with railway train or railway vehicle in nontraffic accident
- **V35.4** Person boarding or alighting a three-wheeled motor vehicle injured in collision with railway train or railway vehicle
- **V35.5** Driver of three-wheeled motor vehicle injured in collision with railway train or railway vehicle in traffic accident
- **V35.6** Passenger in three-wheeled motor vehicle injured in collision with railway train or railway vehicle in traffic accident
- **V35.7** Person on outside of three-wheeled motor vehicle injured in collision with railway train or railway vehicle in traffic accident
- **V35.9** Unspecified occupant of three-wheeled motor vehicle injured in collision with railway train or railway vehicle in traffic accident

V36 Occupant of three-wheeled motor vehicle injured in collision with other nonmotor vehicle
> **INCLUDES** collision with animal-drawn vehicle, animal being ridden, streetcar

- **V36.0** Driver of three-wheeled motor vehicle injured in collision with other nonmotor vehicle in nontraffic accident
- **V36.1** Passenger in three-wheeled motor vehicle injured in collision with other nonmotor vehicle in nontraffic accident
- **V36.2** Person on outside of three-wheeled motor vehicle injured in collision with other nonmotor vehicle in nontraffic accident
- **V36.3** Unspecified occupant of three-wheeled motor vehicle injured in collision with other nonmotor vehicle in nontraffic accident
- **V36.4** Person boarding or alighting a three-wheeled motor vehicle injured in collision with other nonmotor vehicle
- **V36.5** Driver of three-wheeled motor vehicle injured in collision with other nonmotor vehicle in traffic accident
- **V36.6** Passenger in three-wheeled motor vehicle injured in collision with other nonmotor vehicle in traffic accident
- **V36.7** Person on outside of three-wheeled motor vehicle injured in collision with other nonmotor vehicle in traffic accident
- **V36.9** Unspecified occupant of three-wheeled motor vehicle injured in collision with other nonmotor vehicle in traffic accident

V37 Occupant of three-wheeled motor vehicle injured in collision with fixed or stationary object
- **V37.0** Driver of three-wheeled motor vehicle injured in collision with fixed or stationary object in nontraffic accident
- **V37.1** Passenger in three-wheeled motor vehicle injured in collision with fixed or stationary object in nontraffic accident
- **V37.2** Person on outside of three-wheeled motor vehicle injured in collision with fixed or stationary object in nontraffic accident
- **V37.3** Unspecified occupant of three-wheeled motor vehicle injured in collision with fixed or stationary object in nontraffic accident
- **V37.4** Person boarding or alighting a three-wheeled motor vehicle injured in collision with fixed or stationary object
- **V37.5** Driver of three-wheeled motor vehicle injured in collision with fixed or stationary object in traffic accident
- **V37.6** Passenger in three-wheeled motor vehicle injured in collision with fixed or stationary object in traffic accident
- **V37.7** Person on outside of three-wheeled motor vehicle injured in collision with fixed or stationary object in traffic accident
- **V37.9** Unspecified occupant of three-wheeled motor vehicle injured in collision with fixed or stationary object in traffic accident

V38 Occupant of three-wheeled motor vehicle injured in noncollision transport accident
> **INCLUDES** fall or thrown from three-wheeled motor vehicle
> overturning of three-wheeled motor vehicle NOS
> overturning of three-wheeled motor vehicle without collision

- **V38.0** Driver of three-wheeled motor vehicle injured in noncollision transport accident in nontraffic accident
- **V38.1** Passenger in three-wheeled motor vehicle injured in noncollision transport accident in nontraffic accident
- **V38.2** Person on outside of three-wheeled motor vehicle injured in noncollision transport accident in nontraffic accident
- **V38.3** Unspecified occupant of three-wheeled motor vehicle injured in noncollision transport accident in nontraffic accident
- **V38.4** Person boarding or alighting a three-wheeled motor vehicle injured in noncollision transport accident
- **V38.5** Driver of three-wheeled motor vehicle injured in noncollision transport accident in traffic accident
- **V38.6** Passenger in three-wheeled motor vehicle injured in noncollision transport accident in traffic accident
- **V38.7** Person on outside of three-wheeled motor vehicle injured in noncollision transport accident in traffic accident
- **V38.9** Unspecified occupant of three-wheeled motor vehicle injured in noncollision transport accident in traffic accident

V39 Occupant of three-wheeled motor vehicle injured in other and unspecified transport accidents
- **V39.0** Driver of three-wheeled motor vehicle injured in collision with other and unspecified motor vehicles in nontraffic accident
  - **V39.00** Driver of three-wheeled motor vehicle injured in collision with unspecified motor vehicles in nontraffic accident
  - **V39.09** Driver of three-wheeled motor vehicle injured in collision with other motor vehicles in nontraffic accident

Chapter 20. External Causes of Morbidity

- **V39.1** Passenger in three-wheeled motor vehicle injured in collision with other and unspecified motor vehicles in nontraffic accident
  - **V39.10** Passenger in three-wheeled motor vehicle injured in collision with unspecified motor vehicles in nontraffic accident
  - **V39.19** Passenger in three-wheeled motor vehicle injured in collision with other motor vehicles in nontraffic accident
- **V39.2** Unspecified occupant of three-wheeled motor vehicle injured in collision with other and unspecified motor vehicles in nontraffic accident
  - **V39.20** Unspecified occupant of three-wheeled motor vehicle injured in collision with unspecified motor vehicles in nontraffic accident
    Collision NOS involving three-wheeled motor vehicle, nontraffic
  - **V39.29** Unspecified occupant of three-wheeled motor vehicle injured in collision with other motor vehicles in nontraffic accident
- **V39.3** Occupant (driver) (passenger) of three-wheeled motor vehicle injured in unspecified nontraffic accident
    Accident NOS involving three-wheeled motor vehicle, nontraffic
    Occupant of three-wheeled motor vehicle injured in nontraffic accident NOS
- **V39.4** Driver of three-wheeled motor vehicle injured in collision with other and unspecified motor vehicles in traffic accident
  - **V39.40** Driver of three-wheeled motor vehicle injured in collision with unspecified motor vehicles in traffic accident
  - **V39.49** Driver of three-wheeled motor vehicle injured in collision with other motor vehicles in traffic accident
- **V39.5** Passenger in three-wheeled motor vehicle injured in collision with other and unspecified motor vehicles in traffic accident
  - **V39.50** Passenger in three-wheeled motor vehicle injured in collision with unspecified motor vehicles in traffic accident
  - **V39.59** Passenger in three-wheeled motor vehicle injured in collision with other motor vehicles in traffic accident
- **V39.6** Unspecified occupant of three-wheeled motor vehicle injured in collision with other and unspecified motor vehicles in traffic accident
  - **V39.60** Unspecified occupant of three-wheeled motor vehicle injured in collision with unspecified motor vehicles in traffic accident
    Collision NOS involving three-wheeled motor vehicle (traffic)
  - **V39.69** Unspecified occupant of three-wheeled motor vehicle injured in collision with other motor vehicles in traffic accident
- **V39.8** Occupant (driver) (passenger) of three-wheeled motor vehicle injured in other specified transport accidents
  - **V39.81** Occupant (driver) (passenger) of three-wheeled motor vehicle injured in transport accident with military vehicle
  - **V39.89** Occupant (driver) (passenger) of three-wheeled motor vehicle injured in other specified transport accidents
- **V39.9** Occupant (driver) (passenger) of three-wheeled motor vehicle injured in unspecified traffic accident
    Accident NOS involving three-wheeled motor vehicle

Car occupant injured in transport accident (V40-V49)

INCLUDES a four-wheeled motor vehicle designed primarily for carrying passengers
automobile (pulling a trailer or camper)

EXCLUDES 1 bus (V50-V59)
minibus (V50-V59)
minivan (V50-V59)
motorcoach (V70-V79)
pick-up truck (V50-V59)
sport utility vehicle (SUV) (V50-V59)

> The appropriate 7th character is to be added to each code from categories V40-V49.
> A   initial encounter
> D   subsequent encounter
> S   sequela

- **V40** Car occupant injured in collision with pedestrian or animal
  EXCLUDES 1 car collision with animal-drawn vehicle or animal being ridden (V46.-)
  - **V40.0** Car driver injured in collision with pedestrian or animal in nontraffic accident
  - **V40.1** Car passenger injured in collision with pedestrian or animal in nontraffic accident
  - **V40.2** Person on outside of car injured in collision with pedestrian or animal in nontraffic accident
  - **V40.3** Unspecified car occupant injured in collision with pedestrian or animal in nontraffic accident
  - **V40.4** Person boarding or alighting a car injured in collision with pedestrian or animal
  - **V40.5** Car driver injured in collision with pedestrian or animal in traffic accident
  - **V40.6** Car passenger injured in collision with pedestrian or animal in traffic accident
  - **V40.7** Person on outside of car injured in collision with pedestrian or animal in traffic accident
  - **V40.9** Unspecified car occupant injured in collision with pedestrian or animal in traffic accident
- **V41** Car occupant injured in collision with pedal cycle
  - **V41.0** Car driver injured in collision with pedal cycle in nontraffic accident
  - **V41.1** Car passenger injured in collision with pedal cycle in nontraffic accident
  - **V41.2** Person on outside of car injured in collision with pedal cycle in nontraffic accident
  - **V41.3** Unspecified car occupant injured in collision with pedal cycle in nontraffic accident
  - **V41.4** Person boarding or alighting a car injured in collision with pedal cycle
  - **V41.5** Car driver injured in collision with pedal cycle in traffic accident
  - **V41.6** Car passenger injured in collision with pedal cycle in traffic accident
  - **V41.7** Person on outside of car injured in collision with pedal cycle in traffic accident
  - **V41.9** Unspecified car occupant injured in collision with pedal cycle in traffic accident
- **V42** Car occupant injured in collision with two- or three-wheeled motor vehicle
  - **V42.0** Car driver injured in collision with two- or three-wheeled motor vehicle in nontraffic accident
  - **V42.1** Car passenger injured in collision with two- or three-wheeled motor vehicle in nontraffic accident
  - **V42.2** Person on outside of car injured in collision with two- or three-wheeled motor vehicle in nontraffic accident
  - **V42.3** Unspecified car occupant injured in collision with two- or three-wheeled motor vehicle in nontraffic accident
  - **V42.4** Person boarding or alighting a car injured in collision with two- or three-wheeled motor vehicle
  - **V42.5** Car driver injured in collision with two- or three-wheeled motor vehicle in traffic accident
  - **V42.6** Car passenger injured in collision with two- or three-wheeled motor vehicle in traffic accident
  - **V42.7** Person on outside of car injured in collision with two- or three-wheeled motor vehicle in traffic accident
  - **V42.9** Unspecified car occupant injured in collision with two- or three-wheeled motor vehicle in traffic accident
- **V43** Car occupant injured in collision with car, pick-up truck or van
  - **V43.0** Car driver injured in collision with car, pick-up truck or van in nontraffic accident
    - **V43.01** Car driver injured in collision with sport utility vehicle in nontraffic accident
    - **V43.02** Car driver injured in collision with other type car in nontraffic accident
    - **V43.03** Car driver injured in collision with pick-up truck in nontraffic accident
    - **V43.04** Car driver injured in collision with van in nontraffic accident
  - **V43.1** Car passenger injured in collision with car, pick-up truck or van in nontraffic accident
    - **V43.11** Car passenger injured in collision with sport utility vehicle in nontraffic accident
    - **V43.12** Car passenger injured in collision with other type car in nontraffic accident
    - **V43.13** Car passenger injured in collision with pick-up truck in nontraffic accident
    - **V43.14** Car passenger injured in collision with van in nontraffic accident
  - **V43.2** Person on outside of car injured in collision with car, pick-up truck or van in nontraffic accident
    - **V43.21** Person on outside of car injured in collision with sport utility vehicle in nontraffic accident

- V43.22 Person on outside of car injured in collision with other type car in nontraffic accident
- V43.23 Person on outside of car injured in collision with pick-up truck in nontraffic accident
- V43.24 Person on outside of car injured in collision with van in nontraffic accident
- V43.3 Unspecified car occupant injured in collision with car, pick-up truck or van in nontraffic accident
  - V43.31 Unspecified car occupant injured in collision with sport utility vehicle in nontraffic accident
  - V43.32 Unspecified car occupant injured in collision with other type car in nontraffic accident
  - V43.33 Unspecified car occupant injured in collision with pick-up truck in nontraffic accident
  - V43.34 Unspecified car occupant injured in collision with van in nontraffic accident
- V43.4 Person boarding or alighting a car injured in collision with car, pick-up truck or van
  - V43.41 Person boarding or alighting a car injured in collision with sport utility vehicle
  - V43.42 Person boarding or alighting a car injured in collision with other type car
  - V43.43 Person boarding or alighting a car injured in collision with pick-up truck
  - V43.44 Person boarding or alighting a car injured in collision with van
- V43.5 Car driver injured in collision with car, pick-up truck or van in traffic accident
  - V43.51 Car driver injured in collision with sport utility vehicle in traffic accident
  - V43.52 Car driver injured in collision with other type car in traffic accident
  - V43.53 Car driver injured in collision with pick-up truck in traffic accident
  - V43.54 Car driver injured in collision with van in traffic accident
- V43.6 Car passenger injured in collision with car, pick-up truck or van in traffic accident
  - V43.61 Car passenger injured in collision with sport utility vehicle in traffic accident
  - V43.62 Car passenger injured in collision with other type car in traffic accident
  - V43.63 Car passenger injured in collision with pick-up truck in traffic accident
  - V43.64 Car passenger injured in collision with van in traffic accident
- V43.7 Person on outside of car injured in collision with car, pick-up truck or van in traffic accident
  - V43.71 Person on outside of car injured in collision with sport utility vehicle in traffic accident
  - V43.72 Person on outside of car injured in collision with other type car in traffic accident
  - V43.73 Person on outside of car injured in collision with pick-up truck in traffic accident
  - V43.74 Person on outside of car injured in collision with van in traffic accident
- V43.9 Unspecified car occupant injured in collision with car, pick-up truck or van in traffic accident
  - V43.91 Unspecified car occupant injured in collision with sport utility vehicle in traffic accident
  - V43.92 Unspecified car occupant injured in collision with other type car in traffic accident
  - V43.93 Unspecified car occupant injured in collision with pick-up truck in traffic accident
  - V43.94 Unspecified car occupant injured in collision with van in traffic accident
- V44 Car occupant injured in collision with heavy transport vehicle or bus
  - EXCLUDES 1: car occupant injured in collision with military vehicle (V49.81)
  - V44.0 Car driver injured in collision with heavy transport vehicle or bus in nontraffic accident
  - V44.1 Car passenger injured in collision with heavy transport vehicle or bus in nontraffic accident
  - V44.2 Person on outside of car injured in collision with heavy transport vehicle or bus in nontraffic accident
  - V44.3 Unspecified car occupant injured in collision with heavy transport vehicle or bus in nontraffic accident
  - V44.4 Person boarding or alighting a car injured in collision with heavy transport vehicle or bus
  - V44.5 Car driver injured in collision with heavy transport vehicle or bus in traffic accident
  - V44.6 Car passenger injured in collision with heavy transport vehicle or bus in traffic accident
  - V44.7 Person on outside of car injured in collision with heavy transport vehicle or bus in traffic accident
  - V44.9 Unspecified car occupant injured in collision with heavy transport vehicle or bus in traffic accident
- V45 Car occupant injured in collision with railway train or railway vehicle
  - V45.0 Car driver injured in collision with railway train or railway vehicle in nontraffic accident
  - V45.1 Car passenger injured in collision with railway train or railway vehicle in nontraffic accident
  - V45.2 Person on outside of car injured in collision with railway train or railway vehicle in nontraffic accident
  - V45.3 Unspecified car occupant injured in collision with railway train or railway vehicle in nontraffic accident
  - V45.4 Person boarding or alighting a car injured in collision with railway train or railway vehicle
  - V45.5 Car driver injured in collision with railway train or railway vehicle in traffic accident
  - V45.6 Car passenger injured in collision with railway train or railway vehicle in traffic accident
  - V45.7 Person on outside of car injured in collision with railway train or railway vehicle in traffic accident
  - V45.9 Unspecified car occupant injured in collision with railway train or railway vehicle in traffic accident
- V46 Car occupant injured in collision with other nonmotor vehicle
  - INCLUDES: collision with animal-drawn vehicle, animal being ridden, streetcar
  - V46.0 Car driver injured in collision with other nonmotor vehicle in nontraffic accident
  - V46.1 Car passenger injured in collision with other nonmotor vehicle in nontraffic accident
  - V46.2 Person on outside of car injured in collision with other nonmotor vehicle in nontraffic accident
  - V46.3 Unspecified car occupant injured in collision with other nonmotor vehicle in nontraffic accident
  - V46.4 Person boarding or alighting a car injured in collision with other nonmotor vehicle
  - V46.5 Car driver injured in collision with other nonmotor vehicle in traffic accident
  - V46.6 Car passenger injured in collision with other nonmotor vehicle in traffic accident
  - V46.7 Person on outside of car injured in collision with other nonmotor vehicle in traffic accident
  - V46.9 Unspecified car occupant injured in collision with other nonmotor vehicle in traffic accident
- V47 Car occupant injured in collision with fixed or stationary object
  - AHA: 2016,4Q,73
  - V47.0 Car driver injured in collision with fixed or stationary object in nontraffic accident
  - V47.1 Car passenger injured in collision with fixed or stationary object in nontraffic accident
  - V47.2 Person on outside of car injured in collision with fixed or stationary object in nontraffic accident
  - V47.3 Unspecified car occupant injured in collision with fixed or stationary object in nontraffic accident
  - V47.4 Person boarding or alighting a car injured in collision with fixed or stationary object
  - V47.5 Car driver injured in collision with fixed or stationary object in traffic accident
  - V47.6 Car passenger injured in collision with fixed or stationary object in traffic accident
  - V47.7 Person on outside of car injured in collision with fixed or stationary object in traffic accident
  - V47.9 Unspecified car occupant injured in collision with fixed or stationary object in traffic accident
- V48 Car occupant injured in noncollision transport accident
  - INCLUDES: overturning car NOS
  - overturning car without collision
  - V48.0 Car driver injured in noncollision transport accident in nontraffic accident
  - V48.1 Car passenger injured in noncollision transport accident in nontraffic accident
  - V48.2 Person on outside of car injured in noncollision transport accident in nontraffic accident
  - V48.3 Unspecified car occupant injured in noncollision transport accident in nontraffic accident
  - V48.4 Person boarding or alighting a car injured in noncollision transport accident

- ✓x7ᵗʰ **V48.5** Car driver injured in noncollision transport accident *in traffic accident*
- ✓x7ᵗʰ **V48.6** Car passenger injured in noncollision transport accident *in traffic accident*
- ✓x7ᵗʰ **V48.7** Person on outside of car injured in noncollision transport accident *in traffic accident*
- ✓x7ᵗʰ **V48.9** Unspecified car occupant injured in noncollision transport accident *in traffic accident*

✓4ᵗʰ **V49** Car occupant injured in other and unspecified transport accidents

- ✓5ᵗʰ **V49.0** Driver injured in collision with other and unspecified motor vehicles *in nontraffic accident*
  - ✓x7ᵗʰ **V49.00** Driver injured in collision with unspecified motor vehicles in nontraffic accident
  - ✓x7ᵗʰ **V49.09** Driver injured in collision with other motor vehicles in nontraffic accident
- ✓5ᵗʰ **V49.1** Passenger injured in collision with other and unspecified motor vehicles *in nontraffic accident*
  - ✓x7ᵗʰ **V49.10** Passenger injured in collision with unspecified motor vehicles in nontraffic accident
  - ✓x7ᵗʰ **V49.19** Passenger injured in collision with other motor vehicles in nontraffic accident
- ✓5ᵗʰ **V49.2** Unspecified car occupant injured in collision with other and unspecified motor vehicles *in nontraffic accident*
  - ✓x7ᵗʰ **V49.20** Unspecified car occupant injured in collision with unspecified motor vehicles in nontraffic accident
    Car collision NOS, nontraffic
  - ✓x7ᵗʰ **V49.29** Unspecified car occupant injured in collision with other motor vehicles in nontraffic accident
- ✓x7ᵗʰ **V49.3** Car occupant (driver) (passenger) injured in unspecified nontraffic accident
    Car accident NOS, nontraffic
    Car occupant injured in nontraffic accident NOS
- ✓5ᵗʰ **V49.4** Driver injured in collision with other and unspecified motor vehicles *in traffic accident*
  - ✓x7ᵗʰ **V49.40** Driver injured in collision with unspecified motor vehicles in traffic accident
  - ✓x7ᵗʰ **V49.49** Driver injured in collision with other motor vehicles in traffic accident
- ✓5ᵗʰ **V49.5** Passenger injured in collision with other and unspecified motor vehicles *in traffic accident*
  - ✓x7ᵗʰ **V49.50** Passenger injured in collision with unspecified motor vehicles in traffic accident
  - ✓x7ᵗʰ **V49.59** Passenger injured in collision with other motor vehicles in traffic accident
- ✓5ᵗʰ **V49.6** Unspecified car occupant injured in collision with other and unspecified motor vehicles *in traffic accident*
  - ✓x7ᵗʰ **V49.60** Unspecified car occupant injured in collision with unspecified motor vehicles in traffic accident
    Car collision NOS (traffic)
  - ✓x7ᵗʰ **V49.69** Unspecified car occupant injured in collision with other motor vehicles in traffic accident
- ✓5ᵗʰ **V49.8** Car occupant (driver) (passenger) injured in other specified transport accidents
  - ✓x7ᵗʰ **V49.81** Car occupant (driver) (passenger) injured in transport accident with *military vehicle*
  - ✓x7ᵗʰ **V49.88** Car occupant (driver) (passenger) injured in other specified transport accidents
- ✓x7ᵗʰ **V49.9** Car occupant (driver) (passenger) injured in unspecified traffic accident
    Car accident NOS

Occupant of pick-up truck or van injured in transport accident (V50-V59)

> **INCLUDES** a four or six wheel motor vehicle designed primarily for carrying passengers and property but weighing less than the local limit for classification as a heavy goods vehicle
> minibus
> minivan
> sport utility vehicle (SUV)
> truck
> van
>
> **EXCLUDES 1** heavy transport vehicle (V60-V69)

The appropriate 7th character is to be added to each code from categories V50-V59.
- A initial encounter
- D subsequent encounter
- S sequela

✓4ᵗʰ **V50** Occupant of pick-up truck or van injured in collision with pedestrian or animal
> **EXCLUDES 1** pick-up truck or van collision with animal-drawn vehicle or animal being ridden (V56.-)

- ✓x7ᵗʰ **V50.0** Driver of pick-up truck or van injured in collision with pedestrian or animal *in nontraffic accident*
- ✓x7ᵗʰ **V50.1** Passenger in pick-up truck or van injured in collision with pedestrian or animal *in nontraffic accident*
- ✓x7ᵗʰ **V50.2** Person on outside of pick-up truck or van injured in collision with pedestrian or animal *in nontraffic accident*
- ✓x7ᵗʰ **V50.3** Unspecified occupant of pick-up truck or van injured in collision with pedestrian or animal *in nontraffic accident*
- ✓x7ᵗʰ **V50.4** Person boarding or alighting a pick-up truck or van injured in collision with pedestrian or animal
- ✓x7ᵗʰ **V50.5** Driver of pick-up truck or van injured in collision with pedestrian or animal *in traffic accident*
- ✓x7ᵗʰ **V50.6** Passenger in pick-up truck or van injured in collision with pedestrian or animal *in traffic accident*
- ✓x7ᵗʰ **V50.7** Person on outside of pick-up truck or van injured in collision with pedestrian or animal *in traffic accident*
- ✓x7ᵗʰ **V50.9** Unspecified occupant of pick-up truck or van injured in collision with pedestrian or animal *in traffic accident*

✓4ᵗʰ **V51** Occupant of pick-up truck or van injured in collision with pedal cycle
- ✓x7ᵗʰ **V51.0** Driver of pick-up truck or van injured in collision with pedal cycle *in nontraffic accident*
- ✓x7ᵗʰ **V51.1** Passenger in pick-up truck or van injured in collision with pedal cycle *in nontraffic accident*
- ✓x7ᵗʰ **V51.2** Person on outside of pick-up truck or van injured in collision with pedal cycle *in nontraffic accident*
- ✓x7ᵗʰ **V51.3** Unspecified occupant of pick-up truck or van injured in collision with pedal cycle *in nontraffic accident*
- ✓x7ᵗʰ **V51.4** Person boarding or alighting a pick-up truck or van injured in collision with pedal cycle
- ✓x7ᵗʰ **V51.5** Driver of pick-up truck or van injured in collision with pedal cycle *in traffic accident*
- ✓x7ᵗʰ **V51.6** Passenger in pick-up truck or van injured in collision with pedal cycle *in traffic accident*
- ✓x7ᵗʰ **V51.7** Person on outside of pick-up truck or van injured in collision with pedal cycle *in traffic accident*
- ✓x7ᵗʰ **V51.9** Unspecified occupant of pick-up truck or van injured in collision with pedal cycle *in traffic accident*

✓4ᵗʰ **V52** Occupant of pick-up truck or van injured in collision with two- or three-wheeled motor vehicle
- ✓x7ᵗʰ **V52.0** Driver of pick-up truck or van injured in collision with two- or three-wheeled motor vehicle *in nontraffic accident*
- ✓x7ᵗʰ **V52.1** Passenger in pick-up truck or van injured in collision with two- or three-wheeled motor vehicle *in nontraffic accident*
- ✓x7ᵗʰ **V52.2** Person on outside of pick-up truck or van injured in collision with two- or three-wheeled motor vehicle *in nontraffic accident*
- ✓x7ᵗʰ **V52.3** Unspecified occupant of pick-up truck or van injured in collision with two- or three-wheeled motor vehicle *in nontraffic accident*
- ✓x7ᵗʰ **V52.4** Person boarding or alighting a pick-up truck or van injured in collision with two- or three-wheeled motor vehicle
- ✓x7ᵗʰ **V52.5** Driver of pick-up truck or van injured in collision with two- or three-wheeled motor vehicle *in traffic accident*
- ✓x7ᵗʰ **V52.6** Passenger in pick-up truck or van injured in collision with two- or three-wheeled motor vehicle *in traffic accident*
- ✓x7ᵗʰ **V52.7** Person on outside of pick-up truck or van injured in collision with two- or three-wheeled motor vehicle *in traffic accident*
- ✓x7ᵗʰ **V52.9** Unspecified occupant of pick-up truck or van injured in collision with two- or three-wheeled motor vehicle *in traffic accident*

Chapter 20. External Causes of Morbidity

- ☑4ᵗʰ **V53** Occupant of pick-up truck or van injured in collision with car, pick-up truck or van
  - ✓x7ᵗʰ **V53.0** Driver of pick-up truck or van injured in collision with car, pick-up truck or van in nontraffic accident
  - ✓x7ᵗʰ **V53.1** Passenger in pick-up truck or van injured in collision with car, pick-up truck or van in nontraffic accident
  - ✓x7ᵗʰ **V53.2** Person on outside of pick-up truck or van injured in collision with car, pick-up truck or van in nontraffic accident
  - ✓x7ᵗʰ **V53.3** Unspecified occupant of pick-up truck or van injured in collision with car, pick-up truck or van in nontraffic accident
  - ✓x7ᵗʰ **V53.4** Person boarding or alighting a pick-up truck or van injured in collision with car, pick-up truck or van
  - ✓x7ᵗʰ **V53.5** Driver of pick-up truck or van injured in collision with car, pick-up truck or van in traffic accident
  - ✓x7ᵗʰ **V53.6** Passenger in pick-up truck or van injured in collision with car, pick-up truck or van in traffic accident
  - ✓x7ᵗʰ **V53.7** Person on outside of pick-up truck or van injured in collision with car, pick-up truck or van in traffic accident
  - ✓x7ᵗʰ **V53.9** Unspecified occupant of pick-up truck or van injured in collision with car, pick-up truck or van in traffic accident

- ☑4ᵗʰ **V54** Occupant of pick-up truck or van injured in collision with heavy transport vehicle or bus
  - **EXCLUDES 1** occupant of pick-up truck or van injured in collision with military vehicle (V59.81)
  - ✓x7ᵗʰ **V54.0** Driver of pick-up truck or van injured in collision with heavy transport vehicle or bus in nontraffic accident
  - ✓x7ᵗʰ **V54.1** Passenger in pick-up truck or van injured in collision with heavy transport vehicle or bus in nontraffic accident
  - ✓x7ᵗʰ **V54.2** Person on outside of pick-up truck or van injured in collision with heavy transport vehicle or bus in nontraffic accident
  - ✓x7ᵗʰ **V54.3** Unspecified occupant of pick-up truck or van injured in collision with heavy transport vehicle or bus in nontraffic accident
  - ✓x7ᵗʰ **V54.4** Person boarding or alighting a pick-up truck or van injured in collision with heavy transport vehicle or bus
  - ✓x7ᵗʰ **V54.5** Driver of pick-up truck or van injured in collision with heavy transport vehicle or bus in traffic accident
  - ✓x7ᵗʰ **V54.6** Passenger in pick-up truck or van injured in collision with heavy transport vehicle or bus in traffic accident
  - ✓x7ᵗʰ **V54.7** Person on outside of pick-up truck or van injured in collision with heavy transport vehicle or bus in traffic accident
  - ✓x7ᵗʰ **V54.9** Unspecified occupant of pick-up truck or van injured in collision with heavy transport vehicle or bus in traffic accident

- ☑4ᵗʰ **V55** Occupant of pick-up truck or van injured in collision with railway train or railway vehicle
  - ✓x7ᵗʰ **V55.0** Driver of pick-up truck or van injured in collision with railway train or railway vehicle in nontraffic accident
  - ✓x7ᵗʰ **V55.1** Passenger in pick-up truck or van injured in collision with railway train or railway vehicle in nontraffic accident
  - ✓x7ᵗʰ **V55.2** Person on outside of pick-up truck or van injured in collision with railway train or railway vehicle in nontraffic accident
  - ✓x7ᵗʰ **V55.3** Unspecified occupant of pick-up truck or van injured in collision with railway train or railway vehicle in nontraffic accident
  - ✓x7ᵗʰ **V55.4** Person boarding or alighting a pick-up truck or van injured in collision with railway train or railway vehicle
  - ✓x7ᵗʰ **V55.5** Driver of pick-up truck or van injured in collision with railway train or railway vehicle in traffic accident
  - ✓x7ᵗʰ **V55.6** Passenger in pick-up truck or van injured in collision with railway train or railway vehicle in traffic accident
  - ✓x7ᵗʰ **V55.7** Person on outside of pick-up truck or van injured in collision with railway train or railway vehicle in traffic accident
  - ✓x7ᵗʰ **V55.9** Unspecified occupant of pick-up truck or van injured in collision with railway train or railway vehicle in traffic accident

- ☑4ᵗʰ **V56** Occupant of pick-up truck or van injured in collision with other nonmotor vehicle
  - **INCLUDES** collision with animal-drawn vehicle, animal being ridden, streetcar
  - ✓x7ᵗʰ **V56.0** Driver of pick-up truck or van injured in collision with other nonmotor vehicle in nontraffic accident
  - ✓x7ᵗʰ **V56.1** Passenger in pick-up truck or van injured in collision with other nonmotor vehicle in nontraffic accident
  - ✓x7ᵗʰ **V56.2** Person on outside of pick-up truck or van injured in collision with other nonmotor vehicle in nontraffic accident
  - ✓x7ᵗʰ **V56.3** Unspecified occupant of pick-up truck or van injured in collision with other nonmotor vehicle in nontraffic accident
  - ✓x7ᵗʰ **V56.4** Person boarding or alighting a pick-up truck or van injured in collision with other nonmotor vehicle
  - ✓x7ᵗʰ **V56.5** Driver of pick-up truck or van injured in collision with other nonmotor vehicle in traffic accident
  - ✓x7ᵗʰ **V56.6** Passenger in pick-up truck or van injured in collision with other nonmotor vehicle in traffic accident
  - ✓x7ᵗʰ **V56.7** Person on outside of pick-up truck or van injured in collision with other nonmotor vehicle in traffic accident
  - ✓x7ᵗʰ **V56.9** Unspecified occupant of pick-up truck or van injured in collision with other nonmotor vehicle in traffic accident

- ☑4ᵗʰ **V57** Occupant of pick-up truck or van injured in collision with fixed or stationary object
  - ✓x7ᵗʰ **V57.0** Driver of pick-up truck or van injured in collision with fixed or stationary object in nontraffic accident
  - ✓x7ᵗʰ **V57.1** Passenger in pick-up truck or van injured in collision with fixed or stationary object in nontraffic accident
  - ✓x7ᵗʰ **V57.2** Person on outside of pick-up truck or van injured in collision with fixed or stationary object in nontraffic accident
  - ✓x7ᵗʰ **V57.3** Unspecified occupant of pick-up truck or van injured in collision with fixed or stationary object in nontraffic accident
  - ✓x7ᵗʰ **V57.4** Person boarding or alighting a pick-up truck or van injured in collision with fixed or stationary object
  - ✓x7ᵗʰ **V57.5** Driver of pick-up truck or van injured in collision with fixed or stationary object in traffic accident
  - ✓x7ᵗʰ **V57.6** Passenger in pick-up truck or van injured in collision with fixed or stationary object in traffic accident
  - ✓x7ᵗʰ **V57.7** Person on outside of pick-up truck or van injured in collision with fixed or stationary object in traffic accident
  - ✓x7ᵗʰ **V57.9** Unspecified occupant of pick-up truck or van injured in collision with fixed or stationary object in traffic accident

- ☑4ᵗʰ **V58** Occupant of pick-up truck or van injured in noncollision transport accident
  - **INCLUDES** overturning pick-up truck or van NOS
    overturning pick-up truck or van without collision
  - ✓x7ᵗʰ **V58.0** Driver of pick-up truck or van injured in noncollision transport accident in nontraffic accident
  - ✓x7ᵗʰ **V58.1** Passenger in pick-up truck or van injured in noncollision transport accident in nontraffic accident
  - ✓x7ᵗʰ **V58.2** Person on outside of pick-up truck or van injured in noncollision transport accident in nontraffic accident
  - ✓x7ᵗʰ **V58.3** Unspecified occupant of pick-up truck or van injured in noncollision transport accident in nontraffic accident
  - ✓x7ᵗʰ **V58.4** Person boarding or alighting a pick-up truck or van injured in noncollision transport accident
  - ✓x7ᵗʰ **V58.5** Driver of pick-up truck or van injured in noncollision transport accident in traffic accident
  - ✓x7ᵗʰ **V58.6** Passenger in pick-up truck or van injured in noncollision transport accident in traffic accident
  - ✓x7ᵗʰ **V58.7** Person on outside of pick-up truck or van injured in noncollision transport accident in traffic accident
  - ✓x7ᵗʰ **V58.9** Unspecified occupant of pick-up truck or van injured in noncollision transport accident in traffic accident

- ☑4ᵗʰ **V59** Occupant of pick-up truck or van injured in other and unspecified transport accidents
  - ☑5ᵗʰ **V59.0** Driver of pick-up truck or van injured in collision with other and unspecified motor vehicles in nontraffic accident
    - ✓x7ᵗʰ **V59.00** Driver of pick-up truck or van injured in collision with unspecified motor vehicles in nontraffic accident
    - ✓x7ᵗʰ **V59.09** Driver of pick-up truck or van injured in collision with other motor vehicles in nontraffic accident
  - ☑5ᵗʰ **V59.1** Passenger in pick-up truck or van injured in collision with other and unspecified motor vehicles in nontraffic accident
    - ✓x7ᵗʰ **V59.10** Passenger in pick-up truck or van injured in collision with unspecified motor vehicles in nontraffic accident
    - ✓x7ᵗʰ **V59.19** Passenger in pick-up truck or van injured in collision with other motor vehicles in nontraffic accident
  - ☑5ᵗʰ **V59.2** Unspecified occupant of pick-up truck or van injured in collision with other and unspecified motor vehicles in nontraffic accident
    - ✓x7ᵗʰ **V59.20** Unspecified occupant of pick-up truck or van injured in collision with unspecified motor vehicles in nontraffic accident
      Collision NOS involving pick-up truck or van, nontraffic
    - ✓x7ᵗʰ **V59.29** Unspecified occupant of pick-up truck or van injured in collision with other motor vehicles in nontraffic accident
  - ✓x7ᵗʰ **V59.3** Occupant (driver) (passenger) of pick-up truck or van injured in unspecified nontraffic accident
    Accident NOS involving pick-up truck or van, nontraffic
    Occupant of pick-up truck or van injured in nontraffic accident NOS
  - ☑5ᵗʰ **V59.4** Driver of pick-up truck or van injured in collision with other and unspecified motor vehicles in traffic accident
    - ✓x7ᵗʰ **V59.40** Driver of pick-up truck or van injured in collision with unspecified motor vehicles in traffic accident
    - ✓x7ᵗʰ **V59.49** Driver of pick-up truck or van injured in collision with other motor vehicles in traffic accident

---

✓ Additional Character Required ✓x7ᵗʰ Placeholder Alert Manifestation Unspecified Dx Q QPP UPD Unacceptable PDx

- ✓5th **V59.5** Passenger in pick-up truck or van injured in collision with other and unspecified motor vehicles in traffic accident
  - ✓x7th **V59.50** Passenger in pick-up truck or van injured in collision with unspecified motor vehicles in traffic accident
  - ✓x7th **V59.59** Passenger in pick-up truck or van injured in collision with other motor vehicles in traffic accident
- ✓5th **V59.6** Unspecified occupant of pick-up truck or van injured in collision with other and unspecified motor vehicles in traffic accident
  - ✓x7th **V59.60** Unspecified occupant of pick-up truck or van injured in collision with unspecified motor vehicles in traffic accident
    Collision NOS involving pick-up truck or van (traffic)
  - ✓x7th **V59.69** Unspecified occupant of pick-up truck or van injured in collision with other motor vehicles in traffic accident
- ✓5th **V59.8** Occupant (driver) (passenger) of pick-up truck or van injured in other specified transport accidents
  - ✓x7th **V59.81** Occupant (driver) (passenger) of pick-up truck or van injured in transport accident with military vehicle
  - ✓x7th **V59.88** Occupant (driver) (passenger) of pick-up truck or van injured in other specified transport accidents
- ✓x7th **V59.9** Occupant (driver) (passenger) of pick-up truck or van injured in unspecified traffic accident
  Accident NOS involving pick-up truck or van

Occupant of heavy transport vehicle injured in transport accident (V60-V69)

INCLUDES 18 wheeler
armored car
panel truck

EXCLUDES 1 bus
motorcoach

The appropriate 7th character is to be added to each code from categories V60-V69.
- A initial encounter
- D subsequent encounter
- S sequela

- ✓4th **V60** Occupant of heavy transport vehicle injured in collision with pedestrian or animal
  EXCLUDES 1 heavy transport vehicle collision with animal-drawn vehicle or animal being ridden (V66.-)
  - ✓x7th **V60.0** Driver of heavy transport vehicle injured in collision with pedestrian or animal in nontraffic accident
  - ✓x7th **V60.1** Passenger in heavy transport vehicle injured in collision with pedestrian or animal in nontraffic accident
  - ✓x7th **V60.2** Person on outside of heavy transport vehicle injured in collision with pedestrian or animal in nontraffic accident
  - ✓x7th **V60.3** Unspecified occupant of heavy transport vehicle injured in collision with pedestrian or animal in nontraffic accident
  - ✓x7th **V60.4** Person boarding or alighting a heavy transport vehicle injured in collision with pedestrian or animal
  - ✓x7th **V60.5** Driver of heavy transport vehicle injured in collision with pedestrian or animal in traffic accident
  - ✓x7th **V60.6** Passenger in heavy transport vehicle injured in collision with pedestrian or animal in traffic accident
  - ✓x7th **V60.7** Person on outside of heavy transport vehicle injured in collision with pedestrian or animal in traffic accident
  - ✓x7th **V60.9** Unspecified occupant of heavy transport vehicle injured in collision with pedestrian or animal in traffic accident
- ✓4th **V61** Occupant of heavy transport vehicle injured in collision with pedal cycle
  - ✓x7th **V61.0** Driver of heavy transport vehicle injured in collision with pedal cycle in nontraffic accident
  - ✓x7th **V61.1** Passenger in heavy transport vehicle injured in collision with pedal cycle in nontraffic accident
  - ✓x7th **V61.2** Person on outside of heavy transport vehicle injured in collision with pedal cycle in nontraffic accident
  - ✓x7th **V61.3** Unspecified occupant of heavy transport vehicle injured in collision with pedal cycle in nontraffic accident
  - ✓x7th **V61.4** Person boarding or alighting a heavy transport vehicle injured in collision with pedal cycle while boarding or alighting
  - ✓x7th **V61.5** Driver of heavy transport vehicle injured in collision with pedal cycle in traffic accident
  - ✓x7th **V61.6** Passenger in heavy transport vehicle injured in collision with pedal cycle in traffic accident
  - ✓x7th **V61.7** Person on outside of heavy transport vehicle injured in collision with pedal cycle in traffic accident
  - ✓x7th **V61.9** Unspecified occupant of heavy transport vehicle injured in collision with pedal cycle in traffic accident

- ✓4th **V62** Occupant of heavy transport vehicle injured in collision with two- or three-wheeled motor vehicle
  - ✓x7th **V62.0** Driver of heavy transport vehicle injured in collision with two- or three-wheeled motor vehicle in nontraffic accident
  - ✓x7th **V62.1** Passenger in heavy transport vehicle injured in collision with two- or three-wheeled motor vehicle in nontraffic accident
  - ✓x7th **V62.2** Person on outside of heavy transport vehicle injured in collision with two- or three-wheeled motor vehicle in nontraffic accident
  - ✓x7th **V62.3** Unspecified occupant of heavy transport vehicle injured in collision with two- or three-wheeled motor vehicle in nontraffic accident
  - ✓x7th **V62.4** Person boarding or alighting a heavy transport vehicle injured in collision with two- or three-wheeled motor vehicle
  - ✓x7th **V62.5** Driver of heavy transport vehicle injured in collision with two- or three-wheeled motor vehicle in traffic accident
  - ✓x7th **V62.6** Passenger in heavy transport vehicle injured in collision with two- or three-wheeled motor vehicle in traffic accident
  - ✓x7th **V62.7** Person on outside of heavy transport vehicle injured in collision with two- or three-wheeled motor vehicle in traffic accident
  - ✓x7th **V62.9** Unspecified occupant of heavy transport vehicle injured in collision with two- or three-wheeled motor vehicle in traffic accident
- ✓4th **V63** Occupant of heavy transport vehicle injured in collision with car, pick-up truck or van
  - ✓x7th **V63.0** Driver of heavy transport vehicle injured in collision with car, pick-up truck or van in nontraffic accident
  - ✓x7th **V63.1** Passenger in heavy transport vehicle injured in collision with car, pick-up truck or van in nontraffic accident
  - ✓x7th **V63.2** Person on outside of heavy transport vehicle injured in collision with car, pick-up truck or van in nontraffic accident
  - ✓x7th **V63.3** Unspecified occupant of heavy transport vehicle injured in collision with car, pick-up truck or van in nontraffic accident
  - ✓x7th **V63.4** Person boarding or alighting a heavy transport vehicle injured in collision with car, pick-up truck or van
  - ✓x7th **V63.5** Driver of heavy transport vehicle injured in collision with car, pick-up truck or van in traffic accident
  - ✓x7th **V63.6** Passenger in heavy transport vehicle injured in collision with car, pick-up truck or van in traffic accident
  - ✓x7th **V63.7** Person on outside of heavy transport vehicle injured in collision with car, pick-up truck or van in traffic accident
  - ✓x7th **V63.9** Unspecified occupant of heavy transport vehicle injured in collision with car, pick-up truck or van in traffic accident
- ✓4th **V64** Occupant of heavy transport vehicle injured in collision with heavy transport vehicle or bus
  EXCLUDES 1 occupant of heavy transport vehicle injured in collision with military vehicle (V69.81)
  - ✓x7th **V64.0** Driver of heavy transport vehicle injured in collision with heavy transport vehicle or bus in nontraffic accident
  - ✓x7th **V64.1** Passenger in heavy transport vehicle injured in collision with heavy transport vehicle or bus in nontraffic accident
  - ✓x7th **V64.2** Person on outside of heavy transport vehicle injured in collision with heavy transport vehicle or bus in nontraffic accident
  - ✓x7th **V64.3** Unspecified occupant of heavy transport vehicle injured in collision with heavy transport vehicle or bus in nontraffic accident
  - ✓x7th **V64.4** Person boarding or alighting a heavy transport vehicle injured in collision with heavy transport vehicle or bus while boarding or alighting
  - ✓x7th **V64.5** Driver of heavy transport vehicle injured in collision with heavy transport vehicle or bus in traffic accident
  - ✓x7th **V64.6** Passenger in heavy transport vehicle injured in collision with heavy transport vehicle or bus in traffic accident
  - ✓x7th **V64.7** Person on outside of heavy transport vehicle injured in collision with heavy transport vehicle or bus in traffic accident
  - ✓x7th **V64.9** Unspecified occupant of heavy transport vehicle injured in collision with heavy transport vehicle or bus in traffic accident
- ✓4th **V65** Occupant of heavy transport vehicle injured in collision with railway train or railway vehicle
  - ✓x7th **V65.0** Driver of heavy transport vehicle injured in collision with railway train or railway vehicle in nontraffic accident
  - ✓x7th **V65.1** Passenger in heavy transport vehicle injured in collision with railway train or railway vehicle in nontraffic accident
  - ✓x7th **V65.2** Person on outside of heavy transport vehicle injured in collision with railway train or railway vehicle in nontraffic accident
  - ✓x7th **V65.3** Unspecified occupant of heavy transport vehicle injured in collision with railway train or railway vehicle in nontraffic accident
  - ✓x7th **V65.4** Person boarding or alighting a heavy transport vehicle injured in collision with railway train or railway vehicle
  - ✓x7th **V65.5** Driver of heavy transport vehicle injured in collision with railway train or railway vehicle in traffic accident

- ✓x7th **V65.6** Passenger in heavy transport vehicle injured in collision with railway train or railway vehicle in traffic accident
- ✓x7th **V65.7** Person on outside of heavy transport vehicle injured in collision with railway train or railway vehicle in traffic accident
- ✓x7th **V65.9** Unspecified occupant of heavy transport vehicle injured in collision with railway train or railway vehicle in traffic accident

✓4th **V66** Occupant of heavy transport vehicle injured in collision with other nonmotor vehicle
  - INCLUDES: collision with animal-drawn vehicle, animal being ridden, streetcar
- ✓x7th **V66.0** Driver of heavy transport vehicle injured in collision with other nonmotor vehicle in nontraffic accident
- ✓x7th **V66.1** Passenger in heavy transport vehicle injured in collision with other nonmotor vehicle in nontraffic accident
- ✓x7th **V66.2** Person on outside of heavy transport vehicle injured in collision with other nonmotor vehicle in nontraffic accident
- ✓x7th **V66.3** Unspecified occupant of heavy transport vehicle injured in collision with other nonmotor vehicle in nontraffic accident
- ✓x7th **V66.4** Person boarding or alighting a heavy transport vehicle injured in collision with other nonmotor vehicle
- ✓x7th **V66.5** Driver of heavy transport vehicle injured in collision with other nonmotor vehicle in traffic accident
- ✓x7th **V66.6** Passenger in heavy transport vehicle injured in collision with other nonmotor vehicle in traffic accident
- ✓x7th **V66.7** Person on outside of heavy transport vehicle injured in collision with other nonmotor vehicle in traffic accident
- ✓x7th **V66.9** Unspecified occupant of heavy transport vehicle injured in collision with other nonmotor vehicle in traffic accident

✓4th **V67** Occupant of heavy transport vehicle injured in collision with fixed or stationary object
- ✓x7th **V67.0** Driver of heavy transport vehicle injured in collision with fixed or stationary object in nontraffic accident
- ✓x7th **V67.1** Passenger in heavy transport vehicle injured in collision with fixed or stationary object in nontraffic accident
- ✓x7th **V67.2** Person on outside of heavy transport vehicle injured in collision with fixed or stationary object in nontraffic accident
- ✓x7th **V67.3** Unspecified occupant of heavy transport vehicle injured in collision with fixed or stationary object in nontraffic accident
- ✓x7th **V67.4** Person boarding or alighting a heavy transport vehicle injured in collision with fixed or stationary object
- ✓x7th **V67.5** Driver of heavy transport vehicle injured in collision with fixed or stationary object in traffic accident
- ✓x7th **V67.6** Passenger in heavy transport vehicle injured in collision with fixed or stationary object in traffic accident
- ✓x7th **V67.7** Person on outside of heavy transport vehicle injured in collision with fixed or stationary object in traffic accident
- ✓x7th **V67.9** Unspecified occupant of heavy transport vehicle injured in collision with fixed or stationary object in traffic accident

✓4th **V68** Occupant of heavy transport vehicle injured in noncollision transport accident
  - INCLUDES: overturning heavy transport vehicle NOS
    overturning heavy transport vehicle without collision
- ✓x7th **V68.0** Driver of heavy transport vehicle injured in noncollision transport accident in nontraffic accident
- ✓x7th **V68.1** Passenger in heavy transport vehicle injured in noncollision transport accident in nontraffic accident
- ✓x7th **V68.2** Person on outside of heavy transport vehicle injured in noncollision transport accident in nontraffic accident
- ✓x7th **V68.3** Unspecified occupant of heavy transport vehicle injured in noncollision transport accident in nontraffic accident
- ✓x7th **V68.4** Person boarding or alighting a heavy transport vehicle injured in noncollision transport accident
- ✓x7th **V68.5** Driver of heavy transport vehicle injured in noncollision transport accident in traffic accident
- ✓x7th **V68.6** Passenger in heavy transport vehicle injured in noncollision transport accident in traffic accident
- ✓x7th **V68.7** Person on outside of heavy transport vehicle injured in noncollision transport accident in traffic accident
- ✓x7th **V68.9** Unspecified occupant of heavy transport vehicle injured in noncollision transport accident in traffic accident

✓4th **V69** Occupant of heavy transport vehicle injured in other and unspecified transport accidents
  - ✓5th **V69.0** Driver of heavy transport vehicle injured in collision with other and unspecified motor vehicles in nontraffic accident
    - ✓x7th **V69.00** Driver of heavy transport vehicle injured in collision with unspecified motor vehicles in nontraffic accident
    - ✓x7th **V69.09** Driver of heavy transport vehicle injured in collision with other motor vehicles in nontraffic accident
  - ✓5th **V69.1** Passenger in heavy transport vehicle injured in collision with other and unspecified motor vehicles in nontraffic accident
    - ✓x7th **V69.10** Passenger in heavy transport vehicle injured in collision with unspecified motor vehicles in nontraffic accident
    - ✓x7th **V69.19** Passenger in heavy transport vehicle injured in collision with other motor vehicles in nontraffic accident
  - ✓5th **V69.2** Unspecified occupant of heavy transport vehicle injured in collision with other and unspecified motor vehicles in nontraffic accident
    - ✓x7th **V69.20** Unspecified occupant of heavy transport vehicle injured in collision with unspecified motor vehicles in nontraffic accident
      - Collision NOS involving heavy transport vehicle, nontraffic
    - ✓x7th **V69.29** Unspecified occupant of heavy transport vehicle injured in collision with other motor vehicles in nontraffic accident
  - ✓x7th **V69.3** Occupant (driver) (passenger) of heavy transport vehicle injured in unspecified nontraffic accident
    - Accident NOS involving heavy transport vehicle, nontraffic
    - Occupant of heavy transport vehicle injured in nontraffic accident NOS
  - ✓5th **V69.4** Driver of heavy transport vehicle injured in collision with other and unspecified motor vehicles in traffic accident
    - ✓x7th **V69.40** Driver of heavy transport vehicle injured in collision with unspecified motor vehicles in traffic accident
    - ✓x7th **V69.49** Driver of heavy transport vehicle injured in collision with other motor vehicles in traffic accident
  - ✓5th **V69.5** Passenger in heavy transport vehicle injured in collision with other and unspecified motor vehicles in traffic accident
    - ✓x7th **V69.50** Passenger in heavy transport vehicle injured in collision with unspecified motor vehicles in traffic accident
    - ✓x7th **V69.59** Passenger in heavy transport vehicle injured in collision with other motor vehicles in traffic accident
  - ✓5th **V69.6** Unspecified occupant of heavy transport vehicle injured in collision with other and unspecified motor vehicles in traffic accident
    - ✓x7th **V69.60** Unspecified occupant of heavy transport vehicle injured in collision with unspecified motor vehicles in traffic accident
      - Collision NOS involving heavy transport vehicle (traffic)
    - ✓x7th **V69.69** Unspecified occupant of heavy transport vehicle injured in collision with other motor vehicles in traffic accident
  - ✓5th **V69.8** Occupant (driver) (passenger) of heavy transport vehicle injured in other specified transport accidents
    - ✓x7th **V69.81** Occupant (driver) (passenger) of heavy transport vehicle injured in transport accidents with military vehicle
    - ✓x7th **V69.88** Occupant (driver) (passenger) of heavy transport vehicle injured in other specified transport accidents
  - ✓x7th **V69.9** Occupant (driver) (passenger) of heavy transport vehicle injured in unspecified traffic accident
    - Accident NOS involving heavy transport vehicle

Bus occupant injured in transport accident (V70-V79)

INCLUDES: motorcoach
EXCLUDES 1: minibus (V50-V59)

The appropriate 7th character is to be added to each code from categories V70-V79.
- A initial encounter
- D subsequent encounter
- S sequela

✓4th **V70** Bus occupant injured in collision with pedestrian or animal
  - EXCLUDES 1: bus collision with animal-drawn vehicle or animal being ridden (V76.-)
- ✓x7th **V70.0** Driver of bus injured in collision with pedestrian or animal in nontraffic accident
- ✓x7th **V70.1** Passenger on bus injured in collision with pedestrian or animal in nontraffic accident
- ✓x7th **V70.2** Person on outside of bus injured in collision with pedestrian or animal in nontraffic accident
- ✓x7th **V70.3** Unspecified occupant of bus injured in collision with pedestrian or animal in nontraffic accident
- ✓x7th **V70.4** Person boarding or alighting from bus injured in collision with pedestrian or animal
- ✓x7th **V70.5** Driver of bus injured in collision with pedestrian or animal in traffic accident

Chapter 20. External Causes of Morbidity

- √x7th **V70.6** Passenger on bus injured in collision with pedestrian or animal in traffic accident
- √x7th **V70.7** Person on outside of bus injured in collision with pedestrian or animal in traffic accident
- √x7th **V70.9** Unspecified occupant of bus injured in collision with pedestrian or animal in traffic accident

√4th **V71** Bus occupant injured in collision with pedal cycle
- √x7th **V71.0** Driver of bus injured in collision with pedal cycle in nontraffic accident
- √x7th **V71.1** Passenger on bus injured in collision with pedal cycle in nontraffic accident
- √x7th **V71.2** Person on outside of bus injured in collision with pedal cycle in nontraffic accident
- √x7th **V71.3** Unspecified occupant of bus injured in collision with pedal cycle in nontraffic accident
- √x7th **V71.4** Person boarding or alighting from bus injured in collision with pedal cycle
- √x7th **V71.5** Driver of bus injured in collision with pedal cycle in traffic accident
- √x7th **V71.6** Passenger on bus injured in collision with pedal cycle in traffic accident
- √x7th **V71.7** Person on outside of bus injured in collision with pedal cycle in traffic accident
- √x7th **V71.9** Unspecified occupant of bus injured in collision with pedal cycle in traffic accident

√4th **V72** Bus occupant injured in collision with two- or three-wheeled motor vehicle
- √x7th **V72.0** Driver of bus injured in collision with two- or three-wheeled motor vehicle in nontraffic accident
- √x7th **V72.1** Passenger on bus injured in collision with two- or three-wheeled motor vehicle in nontraffic accident
- √x7th **V72.2** Person on outside of bus injured in collision with two- or three-wheeled motor vehicle in nontraffic accident
- √x7th **V72.3** Unspecified occupant of bus injured in collision with two- or three-wheeled motor vehicle in nontraffic accident
- √x7th **V72.4** Person boarding or alighting from bus injured in collision with two- or three-wheeled motor vehicle
- √x7th **V72.5** Driver of bus injured in collision with two- or three-wheeled motor vehicle in traffic accident
- √x7th **V72.6** Passenger on bus injured in collision with two- or three-wheeled motor vehicle in traffic accident
- √x7th **V72.7** Person on outside of bus injured in collision with two- or three-wheeled motor vehicle in traffic accident
- √x7th **V72.9** Unspecified occupant of bus injured in collision with two- or three-wheeled motor vehicle in traffic accident

√4th **V73** Bus occupant injured in collision with car, pick-up truck or van
- √x7th **V73.0** Driver of bus injured in collision with car, pick-up truck or van in nontraffic accident
- √x7th **V73.1** Passenger on bus injured in collision with car, pick-up truck or van in nontraffic accident
- √x7th **V73.2** Person on outside of bus injured in collision with car, pick-up truck or van in nontraffic accident
- √x7th **V73.3** Unspecified occupant of bus injured in collision with car, pick-up truck or van in nontraffic accident
- √x7th **V73.4** Person boarding or alighting from bus injured in collision with car, pick-up truck or van
- √x7th **V73.5** Driver of bus injured in collision with car, pick-up truck or van in traffic accident
- √x7th **V73.6** Passenger on bus injured in collision with car, pick-up truck or van in traffic accident
- √x7th **V73.7** Person on outside of bus injured in collision with car, pick-up truck or van in traffic accident
- √x7th **V73.9** Unspecified occupant of bus injured in collision with car, pick-up truck or van in traffic accident

√4th **V74** Bus occupant injured in collision with heavy transport vehicle or bus
  - EXCLUDES 1 bus occupant injured in collision with military vehicle (V79.81)
- √x7th **V74.0** Driver of bus injured in collision with heavy transport vehicle or bus in nontraffic accident
- √x7th **V74.1** Passenger on bus injured in collision with heavy transport vehicle or bus in nontraffic accident
- √x7th **V74.2** Person on outside of bus injured in collision with heavy transport vehicle or bus in nontraffic accident
- √x7th **V74.3** Unspecified occupant of bus injured in collision with heavy transport vehicle or bus in nontraffic accident
- √x7th **V74.4** Person boarding or alighting from bus injured in collision with heavy transport vehicle or bus
- √x7th **V74.5** Driver of bus injured in collision with heavy transport vehicle or bus in traffic accident
- √x7th **V74.6** Passenger on bus injured in collision with heavy transport vehicle or bus in traffic accident
- √x7th **V74.7** Person on outside of bus injured in collision with heavy transport vehicle or bus in traffic accident
- √x7th **V74.9** Unspecified occupant of bus injured in collision with heavy transport vehicle or bus in traffic accident

√4th **V75** Bus occupant injured in collision with railway train or railway vehicle
- √x7th **V75.0** Driver of bus injured in collision with railway train or railway vehicle in nontraffic accident
- √x7th **V75.1** Passenger on bus injured in collision with railway train or railway vehicle in nontraffic accident
- √x7th **V75.2** Person on outside of bus injured in collision with railway train or railway vehicle in nontraffic accident
- √x7th **V75.3** Unspecified occupant of bus injured in collision with railway train or railway vehicle in nontraffic accident
- √x7th **V75.4** Person boarding or alighting from bus injured in collision with railway train or railway vehicle
- √x7th **V75.5** Driver of bus injured in collision with railway train or railway vehicle in traffic accident
- √x7th **V75.6** Passenger on bus injured in collision with railway train or railway vehicle in traffic accident
- √x7th **V75.7** Person on outside of bus injured in collision with railway train or railway vehicle in traffic accident
- √x7th **V75.9** Unspecified occupant of bus injured in collision with railway train or railway vehicle in traffic accident

√4th **V76** Bus occupant injured in collision with other nonmotor vehicle
  - INCLUDES collision with animal-drawn vehicle, animal being ridden, streetcar
- √x7th **V76.0** Driver of bus injured in collision with other nonmotor vehicle in nontraffic accident
- √x7th **V76.1** Passenger on bus injured in collision with other nonmotor vehicle in nontraffic accident
- √x7th **V76.2** Person on outside of bus injured in collision with other nonmotor vehicle in nontraffic accident
- √x7th **V76.3** Unspecified occupant of bus injured in collision with other nonmotor vehicle in nontraffic accident
- √x7th **V76.4** Person boarding or alighting from bus injured in collision with other nonmotor vehicle
- √x7th **V76.5** Driver of bus injured in collision with other nonmotor vehicle in traffic accident
- √x7th **V76.6** Passenger on bus injured in collision with other nonmotor vehicle in traffic accident
- √x7th **V76.7** Person on outside of bus injured in collision with other nonmotor vehicle in traffic accident
- √x7th **V76.9** Unspecified occupant of bus injured in collision with other nonmotor vehicle in traffic accident

√4th **V77** Bus occupant injured in collision with fixed or stationary object
- √x7th **V77.0** Driver of bus injured in collision with fixed or stationary object in nontraffic accident
- √x7th **V77.1** Passenger on bus injured in collision with fixed or stationary object in nontraffic accident
- √x7th **V77.2** Person on outside of bus injured in collision with fixed or stationary object in nontraffic accident
- √x7th **V77.3** Unspecified occupant of bus injured in collision with fixed or stationary object in nontraffic accident
- √x7th **V77.4** Person boarding or alighting from bus injured in collision with fixed or stationary object
- √x7th **V77.5** Driver of bus injured in collision with fixed or stationary object in traffic accident
- √x7th **V77.6** Passenger on bus injured in collision with fixed or stationary object in traffic accident
- √x7th **V77.7** Person on outside of bus injured in collision with fixed or stationary object in traffic accident
- √x7th **V77.9** Unspecified occupant of bus injured in collision with fixed or stationary object in traffic accident

√4th **V78** Bus occupant injured in noncollision transport accident
  - INCLUDES overturning bus NOS
             overturning bus without collision
- √x7th **V78.0** Driver of bus injured in noncollision transport accident in nontraffic accident
- √x7th **V78.1** Passenger on bus injured in noncollision transport accident in nontraffic accident
- √x7th **V78.2** Person on outside of bus injured in noncollision transport accident in nontraffic accident
- √x7th **V78.3** Unspecified occupant of bus injured in noncollision transport accident in nontraffic accident
- √x7th **V78.4** Person boarding or alighting from bus injured in noncollision transport accident

Chapter 20. External Causes of Morbidity

- ✓x7th **V78.5** Driver of bus injured in noncollision transport accident in traffic accident
- ✓x7th **V78.6** Passenger on bus injured in noncollision transport accident in traffic accident
- ✓x7th **V78.7** Person on outside of bus injured in noncollision transport accident in traffic accident
- ✓x7th **V78.9** Unspecified occupant of bus injured in noncollision transport accident in traffic accident

- ✓4th **V79** Bus occupant injured in other and unspecified transport accidents
  - ✓5th **V79.0** Driver of bus injured in collision with other and unspecified motor vehicles in nontraffic accident
    - ✓x7th **V79.00** Driver of bus injured in collision with unspecified motor vehicles in nontraffic accident
    - ✓x7th **V79.09** Driver of bus injured in collision with other motor vehicles in nontraffic accident
  - ✓5th **V79.1** Passenger on bus injured in collision with other and unspecified motor vehicles in nontraffic accident
    - ✓x7th **V79.10** Passenger on bus injured in collision with unspecified motor vehicles in nontraffic accident
    - ✓x7th **V79.19** Passenger on bus injured in collision with other motor vehicles in nontraffic accident
  - ✓5th **V79.2** Unspecified bus occupant injured in collision with other and unspecified motor vehicles in nontraffic accident
    - ✓x7th **V79.20** Unspecified bus occupant injured in collision with unspecified motor vehicles in nontraffic accident
      - Bus collision NOS, nontraffic
    - ✓x7th **V79.29** Unspecified bus occupant injured in collision with other motor vehicles in nontraffic accident
  - ✓x7th **V79.3** Bus occupant (driver) (passenger) injured in unspecified nontraffic accident
    - Bus accident NOS, nontraffic
    - Bus occupant injured in nontraffic accident NOS
  - ✓5th **V79.4** Driver of bus injured in collision with other and unspecified motor vehicles in traffic accident
    - ✓x7th **V79.40** Driver of bus injured in collision with unspecified motor vehicles in traffic accident
    - ✓x7th **V79.49** Driver of bus injured in collision with other motor vehicles in traffic accident
  - ✓5th **V79.5** Passenger on bus injured in collision with other and unspecified motor vehicles in traffic accident
    - ✓x7th **V79.50** Passenger on bus injured in collision with unspecified motor vehicles in traffic accident
    - ✓x7th **V79.59** Passenger on bus injured in collision with other motor vehicles in traffic accident
  - ✓5th **V79.6** Unspecified bus occupant injured in collision with other and unspecified motor vehicles in traffic accident
    - ✓x7th **V79.60** Unspecified bus occupant injured in collision with unspecified motor vehicles in traffic accident
      - Bus collision NOS (traffic)
    - ✓x7th **V79.69** Unspecified bus occupant injured in collision with other motor vehicles in traffic accident
  - ✓5th **V79.8** Bus occupant (driver) (passenger) injured in other specified transport accidents
    - ✓x7th **V79.81** Bus occupant (driver) (passenger) injured in transport accidents with military vehicle
    - ✓x7th **V79.88** Bus occupant (driver) (passenger) injured in other specified transport accidents
  - ✓x7th **V79.9** Bus occupant (driver) (passenger) injured in unspecified traffic accident
    - Bus accident NOS

Other land transport accidents (V80-V89)

The appropriate 7th character is to be added to each code from categories V80-V89.
- A   initial encounter
- D   subsequent encounter
- S   sequela

- ✓4th **V80** Animal-rider or occupant of animal-drawn vehicle injured in transport accident
  - ✓5th **V80.0** Animal-rider or occupant of animal drawn vehicle injured by fall from or being thrown from animal or animal-drawn vehicle in noncollision accident
    - ✓6th **V80.01** Animal-rider injured by fall from or being thrown from animal in noncollision accident
      - ✓7th **V80.010** Animal-rider injured by fall from or being thrown from horse in noncollision accident
      - ✓7th **V80.018** Animal-rider injured by fall from or being thrown from other animal in noncollision accident
    - ✓x7th **V80.02** Occupant of animal-drawn vehicle injured by fall from or being thrown from animal-drawn vehicle in noncollision accident
      - Overturning animal-drawn vehicle NOS
      - Overturning animal-drawn vehicle without collision
  - ✓5th **V80.1** Animal-rider or occupant of animal-drawn vehicle injured in collision with pedestrian or animal
    - EXCLUDES 1 animal-rider or animal-drawn vehicle collision with animal-drawn vehicle or animal being ridden (V80.7)
    - ✓x7th **V80.11** Animal-rider injured in collision with pedestrian or animal
    - ✓x7th **V80.12** Occupant of animal-drawn vehicle injured in collision with pedestrian or animal
  - ✓5th **V80.2** Animal-rider or occupant of animal-drawn vehicle injured in collision with pedal cycle
    - ✓x7th **V80.21** Animal-rider injured in collision with pedal cycle
    - ✓x7th **V80.22** Occupant of animal-drawn vehicle injured in collision with pedal cycle
  - ✓5th **V80.3** Animal-rider or occupant of animal-drawn vehicle injured in collision with two- or three-wheeled motor vehicle
    - ✓x7th **V80.31** Animal-rider injured in collision with two- or three-wheeled motor vehicle
    - ✓x7th **V80.32** Occupant of animal-drawn vehicle injured in collision with two- or three-wheeled motor vehicle
  - ✓5th **V80.4** Animal-rider or occupant of animal-drawn vehicle injured in collision with car, pick-up truck, van, heavy transport vehicle or bus
    - EXCLUDES 1 animal-rider injured in collision with military vehicle (V80.910)
      - occupant of animal-drawn vehicle injured in collision with military vehicle (V80.920)
    - ✓x7th **V80.41** Animal-rider injured in collision with car, pick-up truck, van, heavy transport vehicle or bus
    - ✓x7th **V80.42** Occupant of animal-drawn vehicle injured in collision with car, pick-up truck, van, heavy transport vehicle or bus
  - ✓5th **V80.5** Animal-rider or occupant of animal-drawn vehicle injured in collision with other specified motor vehicle
    - ✓x7th **V80.51** Animal-rider injured in collision with other specified motor vehicle
    - ✓x7th **V80.52** Occupant of animal-drawn vehicle injured in collision with other specified motor vehicle
  - ✓5th **V80.6** Animal-rider or occupant of animal-drawn vehicle injured in collision with railway train or railway vehicle
    - ✓x7th **V80.61** Animal-rider injured in collision with railway train or railway vehicle
    - ✓x7th **V80.62** Occupant of animal-drawn vehicle injured in collision with railway train or railway vehicle
  - ✓5th **V80.7** Animal-rider or occupant of animal-drawn vehicle injured in collision with other nonmotor vehicles
    - ✓6th **V80.71** Animal-rider or occupant of animal-drawn vehicle injured in collision with animal being ridden
      - ✓7th **V80.710** Animal-rider injured in collision with other animal being ridden
      - ✓7th **V80.711** Occupant of animal-drawn vehicle injured in collision with animal being ridden
    - ✓6th **V80.72** Animal-rider or occupant of animal-drawn vehicle injured in collision with other animal-drawn vehicle
      - ✓7th **V80.720** Animal-rider injured in collision with animal-drawn vehicle
      - ✓7th **V80.721** Occupant of animal-drawn vehicle injured in collision with other animal-drawn vehicle
    - ✓6th **V80.73** Animal-rider or occupant of animal-drawn vehicle injured in collision with streetcar
      - ✓7th **V80.730** Animal-rider injured in collision with streetcar
      - ✓7th **V80.731** Occupant of animal-drawn vehicle injured in collision with streetcar
    - ✓6th **V80.79** Animal-rider or occupant of animal-drawn vehicle injured in collision with other nonmotor vehicles
      - ✓7th **V80.790** Animal-rider injured in collision with other nonmotor vehicles
      - ✓7th **V80.791** Occupant of animal-drawn vehicle injured in collision with other nonmotor vehicles
  - ✓5th **V80.8** Animal-rider or occupant of animal-drawn vehicle injured in collision with fixed or stationary object
    - ✓x7th **V80.81** Animal-rider injured in collision with fixed or stationary object
    - ✓x7th **V80.82** Occupant of animal-drawn vehicle injured in collision with fixed or stationary object

Additional Character Required | ✓x7th Placeholder Alert | Manifestation | Unspecified Dx | QPP | UPD Unacceptable PDx

Chapter 20. External Causes of Morbidity

V80.9 Animal-rider or occupant of animal-drawn vehicle injured in other and unspecified transport accidents

 V80.91 Animal-rider injured in other and unspecified transport accidents

  V80.910 Animal-rider injured in transport accident with military vehicle

  V80.918 Animal-rider injured in other transport accident

  V80.919 Animal-rider injured in unspecified transport accident
   Animal rider accident NOS

 V80.92 Occupant of animal-drawn vehicle injured in other and unspecified transport accidents

  V80.920 Occupant of animal-drawn vehicle injured in transport accident with military vehicle

  V80.928 Occupant of animal-drawn vehicle injured in other transport accident

  V80.929 Occupant of animal-drawn vehicle injured in unspecified transport accident
   Animal-drawn vehicle accident NOS

V81 Occupant of railway train or railway vehicle injured in transport accident
 INCLUDES derailment of railway train or railway vehicle
   person on outside of train
 EXCLUDES 1 streetcar (V82.-)

 V81.0 Occupant of railway train or railway vehicle injured in collision with motor vehicle in nontraffic accident
  EXCLUDES 1 occupant of railway train or railway vehicle injured due to collision with military vehicle (V81.83)

 V81.1 Occupant of railway train or railway vehicle injured in collision with motor vehicle in traffic accident
  EXCLUDES 1 occupant of railway train or railway vehicle injured due to collision with military vehicle (V81.83)

 V81.2 Occupant of railway train or railway vehicle injured in collision with or hit by rolling stock

 V81.3 Occupant of railway train or railway vehicle injured in collision with other object
  Railway collision NOS

 V81.4 Person injured while boarding or alighting from railway train or railway vehicle

 V81.5 Occupant of railway train or railway vehicle injured by fall in railway train or railway vehicle

 V81.6 Occupant of railway train or railway vehicle injured by fall from railway train or railway vehicle

 V81.7 Occupant of railway train or railway vehicle injured in derailment without antecedent collision

 V81.8 Occupant of railway train or railway vehicle injured in other specified railway accidents

  V81.81 Occupant of railway train or railway vehicle injured due to explosion or fire on train

  V81.82 Occupant of railway train or railway vehicle injured due to object falling onto train
   Occupant of railway train or railway vehicle injured due to falling earth onto train
   Occupant of railway train or railway vehicle injured due to falling rocks onto train
   Occupant of railway train or railway vehicle injured due to falling snow onto train
   Occupant of railway train or railway vehicle injured due to falling trees onto train

  V81.83 Occupant of railway train or railway vehicle injured due to collision with military vehicle

  V81.89 Occupant of railway train or railway vehicle injured due to other specified railway accident

 V81.9 Occupant of railway train or railway vehicle injured in unspecified railway accident
  Railway accident NOS

V82 Occupant of powered streetcar injured in transport accident
 INCLUDES interurban electric car
   person on outside of streetcar
   tram (car)
   trolley (car)
 EXCLUDES 1 bus (V70-V79)
   motorcoach (V70-V79)
   nonpowered streetcar (V76.-)
   train (V81.-)

 V82.0 Occupant of streetcar injured in collision with motor vehicle in nontraffic accident

 V82.1 Occupant of streetcar injured in collision with motor vehicle in traffic accident

 V82.2 Occupant of streetcar injured in collision with or hit by rolling stock

 V82.3 Occupant of streetcar injured in collision with other object
  EXCLUDES 1 collision with animal-drawn vehicle or animal being ridden (V82.8)

 V82.4 Person injured while boarding or alighting from streetcar

 V82.5 Occupant of streetcar injured by fall in streetcar
  EXCLUDES 1 fall in streetcar:
   while boarding or alighting (V82.4)
   with antecedent collision (V82.0-V82.3)

 V82.6 Occupant of streetcar injured by fall from streetcar
  EXCLUDES 1 fall from streetcar:
   while boarding or alighting (V82.4)
   with antecedent collision (V82.0-V82.3)

 V82.7 Occupant of streetcar injured in derailment without antecedent collision
  EXCLUDES 1 occupant of streetcar injured in derailment with antecedent collision (V82.0-V82.3)

 V82.8 Occupant of streetcar injured in other specified transport accidents
  Streetcar collision with military vehicle
  Streetcar collision with train or nonmotor vehicles

 V82.9 Occupant of streetcar injured in unspecified traffic accident
  Streetcar accident NOS

V83 Occupant of special vehicle mainly used on industrial premises injured in transport accident
 INCLUDES battery-powered airport passenger vehicle
   battery-powered truck (baggage) (mail)
   coal-car in mine
   forklift (truck)
   logging car
   self-propelled industrial truck
   station baggage truck (powered)
   tram, truck, or tub (powered) in mine or quarry
 EXCLUDES 1 special construction vehicles (V85.-)
   special industrial vehicle in stationary use or maintenance (W31.-)

 V83.0 Driver of special industrial vehicle injured in traffic accident

 V83.1 Passenger of special industrial vehicle injured in traffic accident

 V83.2 Person on outside of special industrial vehicle injured in traffic accident

 V83.3 Unspecified occupant of special industrial vehicle injured in traffic accident

 V83.4 Person injured while boarding or alighting from special industrial vehicle

 V83.5 Driver of special industrial vehicle injured in nontraffic accident

 V83.6 Passenger of special industrial vehicle injured in nontraffic accident

 V83.7 Person on outside of special industrial vehicle injured in nontraffic accident

 V83.9 Unspecified occupant of special industrial vehicle injured in nontraffic accident
  Special-industrial-vehicle accident NOS

V84 Occupant of special vehicle mainly used in agriculture injured in transport accident
 INCLUDES self-propelled farm machinery
   tractor (and trailer)
 EXCLUDES 1 animal-powered farm machinery accident (W30.8-)
   contact with combine harvester (W30.0)
   special agricultural vehicle in stationary use or maintenance (W30.-)

 V84.0 Driver of special agricultural vehicle injured in traffic accident

 V84.1 Passenger of special agricultural vehicle injured in traffic accident

 V84.2 Person on outside of special agricultural vehicle injured in traffic accident

 V84.3 Unspecified occupant of special agricultural vehicle injured in traffic accident

 V84.4 Person injured while boarding or alighting from special agricultural vehicle

 V84.5 Driver of special agricultural vehicle injured in nontraffic accident

 V84.6 Passenger of special agricultural vehicle injured in nontraffic accident

 V84.7 Person on outside of special agricultural vehicle injured in nontraffic accident

 V84.9 Unspecified occupant of special agricultural vehicle injured in nontraffic accident
  Special-agricultural-vehicle accident NOS

Chapter 20. External Causes of Morbidity

- ☑4th **V85** Occupant of special construction vehicle injured in transport accident
  - INCLUDES:
    - bulldozer
    - digger
    - dump truck
    - earth-leveller
    - mechanical shovel
    - road-roller
  - EXCLUDES 1: special construction vehicle in stationary use or maintenance (W31.-)
    - special industrial vehicle (V83.-)

  - ✓x 7th **V85.0** Driver of special construction vehicle injured in traffic accident
  - ✓x 7th **V85.1** Passenger of special construction vehicle injured in traffic accident
  - ✓x 7th **V85.2** Person on outside of special construction vehicle injured in traffic accident
  - ✓x 7th **V85.3** Unspecified occupant of special construction vehicle injured in traffic accident
  - ✓x 7th **V85.4** Person injured while boarding or alighting from special construction vehicle
  - ✓x 7th **V85.5** Driver of special construction vehicle injured in nontraffic accident
  - ✓x 7th **V85.6** Passenger of special construction vehicle injured in nontraffic accident
  - ✓x 7th **V85.7** Person on outside of special construction vehicle injured in nontraffic accident
  - ✓x 7th **V85.9** Unspecified occupant of special construction vehicle injured in nontraffic accident
    - Special-construction-vehicle accident NOS

- ☑4th **V86** Occupant of special all-terrain or other off-road motor vehicle, injured in transport accident
  - EXCLUDES 1: special all-terrain vehicle in stationary use or maintenance (W31.-)
    - sport-utility vehicle (V50-V59)
    - three-wheeled motor vehicle designed for on-road use (V30-V39)
  - AHA: 2017,4Q,26

  - ☑5th **V86.0** Driver of special all-terrain or other off-road motor vehicle injured in traffic accident
    - ✓x 7th **V86.01** Driver of ambulance or fire engine injured in traffic accident
    - ✓x 7th **V86.02** Driver of snowmobile injured in traffic accident
    - ✓x 7th **V86.03** Driver of dune buggy injured in traffic accident
    - ✓x 7th **V86.04** Driver of military vehicle injured in traffic accident
    - ✓x 7th **V86.05** Driver of 3- or 4- wheeled all-terrain vehicle (ATV) injured in traffic accident
    - ✓x 7th **V86.06** Driver of dirt bike or motor/cross bike injured in traffic accident
    - ✓x 7th **V86.09** Driver of other special all-terrain or other off-road motor vehicle injured in traffic accident
      - Driver of go cart injured in traffic accident
      - Driver of golf cart injured in traffic accident

  - ☑5th **V86.1** Passenger of special all-terrain or other off-road motor vehicle injured in traffic accident
    - ✓x 7th **V86.11** Passenger of ambulance or fire engine injured in traffic accident
    - ✓x 7th **V86.12** Passenger of snowmobile injured in traffic accident
    - ✓x 7th **V86.13** Passenger of dune buggy injured in traffic accident
    - ✓x 7th **V86.14** Passenger of military vehicle injured in traffic accident
    - ✓x 7th **V86.15** Passenger of 3- or 4- wheeled all-terrain vehicle (ATV) injured in traffic accident
    - ✓x 7th **V86.16** Passenger of dirt bike or motor/cross bike injured in traffic accident
    - ✓x 7th **V86.19** Passenger of other special all-terrain or other off-road motor vehicle injured in traffic accident
      - Passenger of go cart injured in traffic accident
      - Passenger of golf cart injured in traffic accident

  - ☑5th **V86.2** Person on outside of special all-terrain or other off-road motor vehicle injured in traffic accident
    - ✓x 7th **V86.21** Person on outside of ambulance or fire engine injured in traffic accident
    - ✓x 7th **V86.22** Person on outside of snowmobile injured in traffic accident
    - ✓x 7th **V86.23** Person on outside of dune buggy injured in traffic accident
    - ✓x 7th **V86.24** Person on outside of military vehicle injured in traffic accident
    - ✓x 7th **V86.25** Person on outside of 3- or 4- wheeled all-terrain vehicle (ATV) injured in traffic accident
    - ✓x 7th **V86.26** Person on outside of dirt bike or motor/cross bike injured in traffic accident
    - ✓x 7th **V86.29** Person on outside of other special all-terrain or other off-road motor vehicle injured in traffic accident
      - Person on outside of go cart in traffic accident
      - Person on outside of golf cart injured in traffic accident

  - ☑5th **V86.3** Unspecified occupant of special all-terrain or other off-road motor vehicle injured in traffic accident
    - ✓x 7th **V86.31** Unspecified occupant of ambulance or fire engine injured in traffic accident
    - ✓x 7th **V86.32** Unspecified occupant of snowmobile injured in traffic accident
    - ✓x 7th **V86.33** Unspecified occupant of dune buggy injured in traffic accident
    - ✓x 7th **V86.34** Unspecified occupant of military vehicle injured in traffic accident
    - ✓x 7th **V86.35** Unspecified occupant of 3- or 4- wheeled all-terrain vehicle (ATV) injured in traffic accident
    - ✓x 7th **V86.36** Unspecified occupant of dirt bike or motor/cross bike injured in traffic accident
    - ✓x 7th **V86.39** Unspecified occupant of other special all-terrain or other off-road motor vehicle injured in traffic accident
      - Unspecified occupant of go cart injured in traffic accident
      - Unspecified occupant of golf cart injured in traffic accident

  - ☑5th **V86.4** Person injured while boarding or alighting from special all-terrain or other off-road motor vehicle
    - ✓x 7th **V86.41** Person injured while boarding or alighting from ambulance or fire engine
    - ✓x 7th **V86.42** Person injured while boarding or alighting from snowmobile
    - ✓x 7th **V86.43** Person injured while boarding or alighting from dune buggy
    - ✓x 7th **V86.44** Person injured while boarding or alighting from military vehicle
    - ✓x 7th **V86.45** Person injured while boarding or alighting from a 3- or 4- wheeled all-terrain vehicle (ATV)
    - ✓x 7th **V86.46** Person injured while boarding or alighting from a dirt bike or motor/cross bike
    - ✓x 7th **V86.49** Person injured while boarding or alighting from other special all-terrain or other off-road motor vehicle
      - Person injured while boarding or alighting from go cart
      - Person injured while boarding or alighting from golf cart

  - ☑5th **V86.5** Driver of special all-terrain or other off-road motor vehicle injured in nontraffic accident
    - ✓x 7th **V86.51** Driver of ambulance or fire engine injured in nontraffic accident
    - ✓x 7th **V86.52** Driver of snowmobile injured in nontraffic accident
    - ✓x 7th **V86.53** Driver of dune buggy injured in nontraffic accident
    - ✓x 7th **V86.54** Driver of military vehicle injured in nontraffic accident
    - ✓x 7th **V86.55** Driver of 3- or 4- wheeled all-terrain vehicle (ATV) injured in nontraffic accident
    - ✓x 7th **V86.56** Driver of dirt bike or motor/cross bike injured in nontraffic accident
    - ✓x 7th **V86.59** Driver of other special all-terrain or other off-road motor vehicle injured in nontraffic accident
      - Driver of go cart injured in nontraffic accident
      - Driver of golf cart injured in nontraffic accident

  - ☑5th **V86.6** Passenger of special all-terrain or other off-road motor vehicle injured in nontraffic accident
    - ✓x 7th **V86.61** Passenger of ambulance or fire engine injured in nontraffic accident
    - ✓x 7th **V86.62** Passenger of snowmobile injured in nontraffic accident
    - ✓x 7th **V86.63** Passenger of dune buggy injured in nontraffic accident
    - ✓x 7th **V86.64** Passenger of military vehicle injured in nontraffic accident
    - ✓x 7th **V86.65** Passenger of 3- or 4- wheeled all-terrain vehicle (ATV) injured in nontraffic accident
    - ✓x 7th **V86.66** Passenger of dirt bike or motor/cross bike injured in nontraffic accident
    - ✓x 7th **V86.69** Passenger of other special all-terrain or other off-road motor vehicle injured in nontraffic accident
      - Passenger of go cart injured in nontraffic accident
      - Passenger of golf cart injured in nontraffic accident

  - ☑5th **V86.7** Person on outside of special all-terrain or other off-road motor vehicle injured in nontraffic accident
    - ✓x 7th **V86.71** Person on outside of ambulance or fire engine injured in nontraffic accident

Chapter 20. External Causes of Morbidity

- ✓x7th **V86.72** Person on outside of snowmobile injured in nontraffic accident
- ✓x7th **V86.73** Person on outside of dune buggy injured in nontraffic accident
- ✓x7th **V86.74** Person on outside of military vehicle injured in nontraffic accident
- ✓x7th **V86.75** Person on outside of 3- or 4- wheeled all-terrain vehicle (ATV) injured in nontraffic accident
- ✓x7th **V86.76** Person on outside of dirt bike or motor/cross bike injured in nontraffic accident
- ✓x7th **V86.79** Person on outside of other special all-terrain or other off-road motor vehicles injured in nontraffic accident
    - Person on outside of go cart injured in nontraffic accident
    - Person on outside of golf cart injured in nontraffic accident
- ✓5th **V86.9** Unspecified occupant of special all-terrain or other off-road motor vehicle injured in nontraffic accident
  - ✓x7th **V86.91** Unspecified occupant of ambulance or fire engine injured in nontraffic accident
  - ✓x7th **V86.92** Unspecified occupant of snowmobile injured in nontraffic accident
  - ✓x7th **V86.93** Unspecified occupant of dune buggy injured in nontraffic accident
  - ✓x7th **V86.94** Unspecified occupant of military vehicle injured in nontraffic accident
  - ✓x7th **V86.95** Unspecified occupant of 3- or 4- wheeled all-terrain vehicle (ATV) injured in nontraffic accident
  - ✓x7th **V86.96** Unspecified occupant of dirt bike or motor/cross bike injured in nontraffic accident
  - ✓x7th **V86.99** Unspecified occupant of other special all-terrain or other off-road motor vehicle injured in nontraffic accident
    - Off-road motor-vehicle accident NOS
    - Other motor-vehicle accident NOS
    - Unspecified occupant of go cart injured in nontraffic accident
    - Unspecified occupant of golf cart injured in nontraffic accident

- ✓4th **V87** Traffic accident of specified type but victim's mode of transport unknown
  - EXCLUDES 1 *collision involving:*
    - *pedal cycle (V10-V19)*
    - *pedestrian (V01-V09)*
  - ✓x7th **V87.0** Person injured in collision between car and two- or three-wheeled powered vehicle (traffic)
  - ✓x7th **V87.1** Person injured in collision between other motor vehicle and two- or three-wheeled motor vehicle (traffic)
  - ✓x7th **V87.2** Person injured in collision between car and pick-up truck or van (traffic)
  - ✓x7th **V87.3** Person injured in collision between car and bus (traffic)
  - ✓x7th **V87.4** Person injured in collision between car and heavy transport vehicle (traffic)
  - ✓x7th **V87.5** Person injured in collision between heavy transport vehicle and bus (traffic)
  - ✓x7th **V87.6** Person injured in collision between railway train or railway vehicle and car (traffic)
  - ✓x7th **V87.7** Person injured in collision between other specified motor vehicles (traffic)
  - ✓x7th **V87.8** Person injured in other specified noncollision transport accidents involving motor vehicle (traffic)
  - ✓x7th **V87.9** Person injured in other specified (collision)(noncollision) transport accidents involving nonmotor vehicle (traffic)

- ✓4th **V88** Nontraffic accident of specified type but victim's mode of transport unknown
  - EXCLUDES 1 *collision involving:*
    - *pedal cycle (V10-V19)*
    - *pedestrian (V01-V09)*
  - ✓x7th **V88.0** Person injured in collision between car and two- or three-wheeled motor vehicle, nontraffic
  - ✓x7th **V88.1** Person injured in collision between other motor vehicle and two- or three-wheeled motor vehicle, nontraffic
  - ✓x7th **V88.2** Person injured in collision between car and pick-up truck or van, nontraffic
  - ✓x7th **V88.3** Person injured in collision between car and bus, nontraffic
  - ✓x7th **V88.4** Person injured in collision between car and heavy transport vehicle, nontraffic
  - ✓x7th **V88.5** Person injured in collision between heavy transport vehicle and bus, nontraffic
  - ✓x7th **V88.6** Person injured in collision between railway train or railway vehicle and car, nontraffic
- ✓x7th **V88.7** Person injured in collision between other specified motor vehicle, nontraffic
- ✓x7th **V88.8** Person injured in other specified noncollision transport accidents involving motor vehicle, nontraffic
- ✓x7th **V88.9** Person injured in other specified (collision)(noncollision) transport accidents involving nonmotor vehicle, nontraffic

- ✓4th **V89** Motor- or nonmotor-vehicle accident, type of vehicle unspecified
  - ✓x7th **V89.0** Person injured in unspecified motor-vehicle accident, nontraffic
    - Motor-vehicle accident NOS, nontraffic
  - ✓x7th **V89.1** Person injured in unspecified nonmotor-vehicle accident, nontraffic
    - Nonmotor-vehicle accident NOS (nontraffic)
  - ✓x7th **V89.2** Person injured in unspecified motor-vehicle accident, traffic
    - Motor-vehicle accident [MVA] NOS
    - Road (traffic) accident [RTA] NOS
  - ✓x7th **V89.3** Person injured in unspecified nonmotor-vehicle accident, traffic
    - Nonmotor-vehicle traffic accident NOS
  - ✓x7th **V89.9** Person injured in unspecified vehicle accident
    - Collision NOS

Water transport accidents (V90-V94)

The appropriate 7th character is to be added to each code from categories V90-V94.
- A initial encounter
- D subsequent encounter
- S sequela

- ✓4th **V90** Drowning and submersion due to accident to watercraft
  - EXCLUDES 1 *civilian water transport accident involving military watercraft (V94.81-)*
    - *fall into water not from watercraft (W16.-)*
    - *military watercraft accident in military or war operations (Y36.0-, Y37.0-)*
    - *water-transport-related drowning or submersion without accident to watercraft (V92.-)*
  - ✓5th **V90.0** Drowning and submersion due to watercraft overturning
    - ✓x7th **V90.00** Drowning and submersion due to merchant ship overturning
    - ✓x7th **V90.01** Drowning and submersion due to passenger ship overturning
      - Drowning and submersion due to Ferry-boat overturning
      - Drowning and submersion due to Liner overturning
    - ✓x7th **V90.02** Drowning and submersion due to fishing boat overturning
    - ✓x7th **V90.03** Drowning and submersion due to other powered watercraft overturning
      - Drowning and submersion due to Hovercraft (on open water) overturning
      - Drowning and submersion due to Jet ski overturning
    - ✓x7th **V90.04** Drowning and submersion due to sailboat overturning
    - ✓x7th **V90.05** Drowning and submersion due to canoe or kayak overturning
    - ✓x7th **V90.06** Drowning and submersion due to (nonpowered) inflatable craft overturning
    - ✓x7th **V90.08** Drowning and submersion due to other unpowered watercraft overturning
      - Drowning and submersion due to windsurfer overturning
    - ✓x7th **V90.09** Drowning and submersion due to unspecified watercraft overturning
      - Drowning and submersion due to boat NOS overturning
      - Drowning and submersion due to ship NOS overturning
      - Drowning and submersion due to watercraft NOS overturning
  - ✓5th **V90.1** Drowning and submersion due to watercraft sinking
    - ✓x7th **V90.10** Drowning and submersion due to merchant ship sinking
    - ✓x7th **V90.11** Drowning and submersion due to passenger ship sinking
      - Drowning and submersion due to Ferry-boat sinking
      - Drowning and submersion due to Liner sinking
    - ✓x7th **V90.12** Drowning and submersion due to fishing boat sinking

	V90.13	Drowning and submersion due to other powered watercraft sinking
		Drowning and submersion due to Hovercraft (on open water) sinking
		Drowning and submersion due to Jet ski sinking
✓x 7th	**V90.14**	Drowning and submersion due to sailboat sinking
✓x 7th	**V90.15**	Drowning and submersion due to canoe or kayak sinking
✓x 7th	**V90.16**	Drowning and submersion due to (nonpowered) inflatable craft sinking
✓x 7th	**V90.18**	Drowning and submersion due to other unpowered watercraft sinking
✓x 7th	**V90.19**	Drowning and submersion due to unspecified watercraft sinking
		Drowning and submersion due to boat NOS sinking
		Drowning and submersion due to ship NOS sinking
		Drowning and submersion due to watercraft NOS sinking

✓5th **V90.2** Drowning and submersion due to falling or jumping from burning watercraft

✓x 7th	**V90.20**	Drowning and submersion due to falling or jumping from burning merchant ship
✓x 7th	**V90.21**	Drowning and submersion due to falling or jumping from burning passenger ship
		Drowning and submersion due to falling or jumping from burning Ferry-boat
		Drowning and submersion due to falling or jumping from burning Liner
✓x 7th	**V90.22**	Drowning and submersion due to falling or jumping from burning fishing boat
✓x 7th	**V90.23**	Drowning and submersion due to falling or jumping from other burning powered watercraft
		Drowning and submersion due to falling and jumping from burning Hovercraft (on open water)
		Drowning and submersion due to falling and jumping from burning Jet ski
✓x 7th	**V90.24**	Drowning and submersion due to falling or jumping from burning sailboat
✓x 7th	**V90.25**	Drowning and submersion due to falling or jumping from burning canoe or kayak
✓x 7th	**V90.26**	Drowning and submersion due to falling or jumping from burning (nonpowered) inflatable craft
✓x 7th	**V90.27**	Drowning and submersion due to falling or jumping from burning water-skis
✓x 7th	**V90.28**	Drowning and submersion due to falling or jumping from other burning unpowered watercraft
		Drowning and submersion due to falling and jumping from burning surf-board
		Drowning and submersion due to falling and jumping from burning windsurfer
✓x 7th	**V90.29**	Drowning and submersion due to falling or jumping from unspecified burning watercraft
		Drowning and submersion due to falling or jumping from burning boat NOS
		Drowning and submersion due to falling or jumping from burning ship NOS
		Drowning and submersion due to falling or jumping from burning watercraft NOS

✓5th **V90.3** Drowning and submersion due to falling or jumping from crushed watercraft

✓x 7th	**V90.30**	Drowning and submersion due to falling or jumping from crushed merchant ship
✓x 7th	**V90.31**	Drowning and submersion due to falling or jumping from crushed passenger ship
		Drowning and submersion due to falling and jumping from crushed Ferry boat
		Drowning and submersion due to falling and jumping from crushed Liner
✓x 7th	**V90.32**	Drowning and submersion due to falling or jumping from crushed fishing boat
✓x 7th	**V90.33**	Drowning and submersion due to falling or jumping from other crushed powered watercraft
		Drowning and submersion due to falling and jumping from crushed Hovercraft
		Drowning and submersion due to falling and jumping from crushed Jet ski
✓x 7th	**V90.34**	Drowning and submersion due to falling or jumping from crushed sailboat
✓x 7th	**V90.35**	Drowning and submersion due to falling or jumping from crushed canoe or kayak
✓x 7th	**V90.36**	Drowning and submersion due to falling or jumping from crushed (nonpowered) inflatable craft
✓x 7th	**V90.37**	Drowning and submersion due to falling or jumping from crushed water-skis
✓x 7th	**V90.38**	Drowning and submersion due to falling or jumping from other crushed unpowered watercraft
		Drowning and submersion due to falling and jumping from crushed surf-board
		Drowning and submersion due to falling and jumping from crushed windsurfer
✓x 7th	**V90.39**	Drowning and submersion due to falling or jumping from crushed unspecified watercraft
		Drowning and submersion due to falling and jumping from crushed boat NOS
		Drowning and submersion due to falling and jumping from crushed ship NOS
		Drowning and submersion due to falling and jumping from crushed watercraft NOS

✓5th **V90.8** Drowning and submersion due to other accident to watercraft

✓x 7th	**V90.80**	Drowning and submersion due to other accident to merchant ship
✓x 7th	**V90.81**	Drowning and submersion due to other accident to passenger ship
		Drowning and submersion due to other accident to Ferry-boat
		Drowning and submersion due to other accident to Liner
✓x 7th	**V90.82**	Drowning and submersion due to other accident to fishing boat
✓x 7th	**V90.83**	Drowning and submersion due to other accident to other powered watercraft
		Drowning and submersion due to other accident to Hovercraft (on open water)
		Drowning and submersion due to other accident to Jet ski
✓x 7th	**V90.84**	Drowning and submersion due to other accident to sailboat
✓x 7th	**V90.85**	Drowning and submersion due to other accident to canoe or kayak
✓x 7th	**V90.86**	Drowning and submersion due to other accident to (nonpowered) inflatable craft
✓x 7th	**V90.87**	Drowning and submersion due to other accident to water-skis
✓x 7th	**V90.88**	Drowning and submersion due to other accident to other unpowered watercraft
		Drowning and submersion due to other accident to surf-board
		Drowning and submersion due to other accident to windsurfer
✓x 7th	**V90.89**	Drowning and submersion due to other accident to unspecified watercraft
		Drowning and submersion due to other accident to boat NOS
		Drowning and submersion due to other accident to ship NOS
		Drowning and submersion due to other accident to watercraft NOS

✓4th **V91** Other injury due to accident to watercraft

INCLUDES any injury except drowning and submersion as a result of an accident to watercraft

EXCLUDES 1 civilian water transport accident involving military watercraft (V94.81-)

military watercraft accident in military or war operations (Y36, Y37.-)

EXCLUDES 2 drowning and submersion due to accident to watercraft (V90.-)

✓5th **V91.0** Burn due to watercraft on fire

EXCLUDES 1 burn from localized fire or explosion on board ship without accident to watercraft (V93.-)

✓x 7th	**V91.00**	Burn due to merchant ship on fire
✓x 7th	**V91.01**	Burn due to passenger ship on fire
		Burn due to Ferry-boat on fire
		Burn due to Liner on fire
✓x 7th	**V91.02**	Burn due to fishing boat on fire
✓x 7th	**V91.03**	Burn due to other powered watercraft on fire
		Burn due to Hovercraft (on open water) on fire
		Burn due to Jet ski on fire
✓x 7th	**V91.04**	Burn due to sailboat on fire
✓x 7th	**V91.05**	Burn due to canoe or kayak on fire
✓x 7th	**V91.06**	Burn due to (nonpowered) inflatable craft on fire
✓x 7th	**V91.07**	Burn due to water-skis on fire
✓x 7th	**V91.08**	Burn due to other unpowered watercraft on fire

V91.09 Burn due to unspecified watercraft on fire
  Burn due to boat NOS on fire
  Burn due to ship NOS on fire
  Burn due to watercraft NOS on fire

V91.1 Crushed between watercraft and other watercraft or other object due to collision
  Crushed by lifeboat after abandoning ship in a collision
  NOTE: Select the specified type of watercraft that the victim was on at the time of the collision

V91.10 Crushed between merchant ship and other watercraft or other object due to collision

V91.11 Crushed between passenger ship and other watercraft or other object due to collision
  Crushed between Ferry-boat and other watercraft or other object due to collision
  Crushed between Liner and other watercraft or other object due to collision

V91.12 Crushed between fishing boat and other watercraft or other object due to collision

V91.13 Crushed between other powered watercraft and other watercraft or other object due to collision
  Crushed between Hovercraft (on open water) and other watercraft or other object due to collision
  Crushed between Jet ski and other watercraft or other object due to collision

V91.14 Crushed between sailboat and other watercraft or other object due to collision

V91.15 Crushed between canoe or kayak and other watercraft or other object due to collision

V91.16 Crushed between (nonpowered) inflatable craft and other watercraft or other object due to collision

V91.18 Crushed between other unpowered watercraft and other watercraft or other object due to collision
  Crushed between surfboard and other watercraft or other object due to collision
  Crushed between windsurfer and other watercraft or other object due to collision

V91.19 Crushed between unspecified watercraft and other watercraft or other object due to collision
  Crushed between boat NOS and other watercraft or other object due to collision
  Crushed between ship NOS and other watercraft or other object due to collision
  Crushed between watercraft NOS and other watercraft or other object due to collision

V91.2 Fall due to collision between watercraft and other watercraft or other object
  Fall while remaining on watercraft after collision
  NOTE: Select the specified type of watercraft that the victim was on at the time of the collision
  EXCLUDES 1: crushed between watercraft and other watercraft and other object due to collision (V91.1-)
  drowning and submersion due to falling from crushed watercraft (V90.3-)

V91.20 Fall due to collision between merchant ship and other watercraft or other object

V91.21 Fall due to collision between passenger ship and other watercraft or other object
  Fall due to collision between Ferry-boat and other watercraft or other object
  Fall due to collision between Liner and other watercraft or other object

V91.22 Fall due to collision between fishing boat and other watercraft or other object

V91.23 Fall due to collision between other powered watercraft and other watercraft or other object
  Fall due to collision between Hovercraft (on open water) and other watercraft or other object
  Fall due to collision between Jet ski and other watercraft or other object

V91.24 Fall due to collision between sailboat and other watercraft or other object

V91.25 Fall due to collision between canoe or kayak and other watercraft or other object

V91.26 Fall due to collision between (nonpowered) inflatable craft and other watercraft or other object

V91.29 Fall due to collision between unspecified watercraft and other watercraft or other object
  Fall due to collision between boat NOS and other watercraft or other object
  Fall due to collision between ship NOS and other watercraft or other object
  Fall due to collision between watercraft NOS and other watercraft or other object

V91.3 Hit or struck by falling object due to accident to watercraft
  Hit or struck by falling object (part of damaged watercraft or other object) after falling or jumping from damaged watercraft
  EXCLUDES 2: drowning or submersion due to fall or jumping from damaged watercraft (V90.2-, V90.3-)

V91.30 Hit or struck by falling object due to accident to merchant ship

V91.31 Hit or struck by falling object due to accident to passenger ship
  Hit or struck by falling object due to accident to Ferry-boat
  Hit or struck by falling object due to accident to Liner

V91.32 Hit or struck by falling object due to accident to fishing boat

V91.33 Hit or struck by falling object due to accident to other powered watercraft
  Hit or struck by falling object due to accident to Hovercraft (on open water)
  Hit or struck by falling object due to accident to Jet ski

V91.34 Hit or struck by falling object due to accident to sailboat

V91.35 Hit or struck by falling object due to accident to canoe or kayak

V91.36 Hit or struck by falling object due to accident to (nonpowered) inflatable craft

V91.37 Hit or struck by falling object due to accident to water-skis
  Hit by water-skis after jumping off of waterskis

V91.38 Hit or struck by falling object due to accident to other unpowered watercraft
  Hit or struck by object after falling off damaged windsurfer
  Hit or struck by surf-board after falling off damaged surf-board

V91.39 Hit or struck by falling object due to accident to unspecified watercraft
  Hit or struck by falling object due to accident to boat NOS
  Hit or struck by falling object due to accident to ship NOS
  Hit or struck by falling object due to accident to watercraft NOS

V91.8 Other injury due to other accident to watercraft

V91.80 Other injury due to other accident to merchant ship

V91.81 Other injury due to other accident to passenger ship
  Other injury due to other accident to Ferry-boat
  Other injury due to other accident to Liner

V91.82 Other injury due to other accident to fishing boat

V91.83 Other injury due to other accident to other powered watercraft
  Other injury due to other accident to Hovercraft (on open water)
  Other injury due to other accident to Jet ski

V91.84 Other injury due to other accident to sailboat

V91.85 Other injury due to other accident to canoe or kayak

V91.86 Other injury due to other accident to (nonpowered) inflatable craft

V91.87 Other injury due to other accident to water-skis

V91.88 Other injury due to other accident to other unpowered watercraft
  Other injury due to other accident to surf-board
  Other injury due to other accident to windsurfer

V91.89 Other injury due to other accident to unspecified watercraft
  Other injury due to other accident to boat NOS
  Other injury due to other accident to ship NOS
  Other injury due to other accident to watercraft NOS

V92 Drowning and submersion due to accident on board watercraft, without accident to watercraft

EXCLUDES 1
- civilian water transport accident involving military watercraft (V94.81-)
- drowning or submersion of diver who voluntarily jumps from boat not involved in an accident (W16.711, W16.721)
- drowning or submersion due to accident to watercraft (V90-V91)
- fall into water without watercraft (W16.-)
- military watercraft accident in military or war operations (Y36, Y37)

V92.0 Drowning and submersion due to fall off watercraft
Drowning and submersion due to fall from gangplank of watercraft
Drowning and submersion due to fall overboard watercraft

EXCLUDES 2 hitting head on object or bottom of body of water due to fall from watercraft (V94.0-)

- **V92.00** Drowning and submersion due to fall off merchant ship
- **V92.01** Drowning and submersion due to fall off passenger ship
  - Drowning and submersion due to fall off Ferry-boat
  - Drowning and submersion due to fall off Liner
- **V92.02** Drowning and submersion due to fall off fishing boat
- **V92.03** Drowning and submersion due to fall off other powered watercraft
  - Drowning and submersion due to fall off Hovercraft (on open water)
  - Drowning and submersion due to fall off Jet ski
- **V92.04** Drowning and submersion due to fall off sailboat
- **V92.05** Drowning and submersion due to fall off canoe or kayak
- **V92.06** Drowning and submersion due to fall off (nonpowered) inflatable craft
- **V92.07** Drowning and submersion due to fall off water-skis
  - **EXCLUDES 1**
    - drowning and submersion due to falling off burning water-skis (V90.27)
    - drowning and submersion due to falling off crushed water-skis (V90.37)
    - hit by boat while water-skiing NOS (V94.-)
- **V92.08** Drowning and submersion due to fall off other unpowered watercraft
  - Drowning and submersion due to fall off surf-board
  - Drowning and submersion due to fall off windsurfer
  - **EXCLUDES 1**
    - drowning and submersion due to fall off burning unpowered watercraft (V90.28)
    - drowning and submersion due to fall off crushed unpowered watercraft (V90.38)
    - drowning and submersion due to fall off damaged unpowered watercraft (V90.88)
    - drowning and submersion due to rider of nonpowered watercraft being hit by other watercraft (V94.-)
    - other injury due to rider of nonpowered watercraft being hit by other watercraft (V94.-)
- **V92.09** Drowning and submersion due to fall off unspecified watercraft
  - Drowning and submersion due to fall off boat NOS
  - Drowning and submersion due to fall off ship
  - Drowning and submersion due to fall off watercraft NOS

V92.1 Drowning and submersion due to being thrown overboard by motion of watercraft

EXCLUDES 1
- drowning and submersion due to fall off surf-board (V92.08)
- drowning and submersion due to fall off water-skis (V92.07)
- drowning and submersion due to fall off windsurfer (V92.08)

- **V92.10** Drowning and submersion due to being thrown overboard by motion of merchant ship
- **V92.11** Drowning and submersion due to being thrown overboard by motion of passenger ship
  - Drowning and submersion due to being thrown overboard by motion of Ferry-boat
  - Drowning and submersion due to being thrown overboard by motion of Liner
- **V92.12** Drowning and submersion due to being thrown overboard by motion of fishing boat
- **V92.13** Drowning and submersion due to being thrown overboard by motion of other powered watercraft
  - Drowning and submersion due to being thrown overboard by motion of Hovercraft
- **V92.14** Drowning and submersion due to being thrown overboard by motion of sailboat
- **V92.15** Drowning and submersion due to being thrown overboard by motion of canoe or kayak
- **V92.16** Drowning and submersion due to being thrown overboard by motion of (nonpowered) inflatable craft
- **V92.19** Drowning and submersion due to being thrown overboard by motion of unspecified watercraft
  - Drowning and submersion due to being thrown overboard by motion of boat NOS
  - Drowning and submersion due to being thrown overboard by motion of ship NOS
  - Drowning and submersion due to being thrown overboard by motion of watercraft NOS

V92.2 Drowning and submersion due to being washed overboard from watercraft
Code first any associated cataclysm (X37.0-)

- **V92.20** Drowning and submersion due to being washed overboard from merchant ship
- **V92.21** Drowning and submersion due to being washed overboard from passenger ship
  - Drowning and submersion due to being washed overboard from Ferry-boat
  - Drowning and submersion due to being washed overboard from Liner
- **V92.22** Drowning and submersion due to being washed overboard from fishing boat
- **V92.23** Drowning and submersion due to being washed overboard from other powered watercraft
  - Drowning and submersion due to being washed overboard from Hovercraft (on open water)
  - Drowning and submersion due to being washed overboard from Jet ski
- **V92.24** Drowning and submersion due to being washed overboard from sailboat
- **V92.25** Drowning and submersion due to being washed overboard from canoe or kayak
- **V92.26** Drowning and submersion due to being washed overboard from (nonpowered) inflatable craft
- **V92.27** Drowning and submersion due to being washed overboard from water-skis
  - **EXCLUDES 1** drowning and submersion due to fall off water-skis (V92.07)
- **V92.28** Drowning and submersion due to being washed overboard from other unpowered watercraft
  - Drowning and submersion due to being washed overboard from surf-board
  - Drowning and submersion due to being washed overboard from windsurfer
- **V92.29** Drowning and submersion due to being washed overboard from unspecified watercraft
  - Drowning and submersion due to being washed overboard from boat NOS
  - Drowning and submersion due to being washed overboard from ship NOS
  - Drowning and submersion due to being washed overboard from watercraft NOS

V93 Other injury due to accident on board watercraft, without accident to watercraft

EXCLUDES 1
- civilian water transport accident involving military watercraft (V94.81-)
- military watercraft accident in military or war operations (Y36, Y37.-)
- other injury due to accident to watercraft (V91.-)

EXCLUDES 2 drowning and submersion due to accident on board watercraft, without accident to watercraft (V92.-)

V93.0 Burn due to localized fire on board watercraft
EXCLUDES 1 burn due to watercraft on fire (V91.0-)

- **V93.00** Burn due to localized fire on board merchant vessel
- **V93.01** Burn due to localized fire on board passenger vessel
  - Burn due to localized fire on board Ferry-boat
  - Burn due to localized fire on board Liner
- **V93.02** Burn due to localized fire on board fishing boat

Chapter 20. External Causes of Morbidity

- ✓x7th **V93.03** Burn due to localized fire on board other powered watercraft
  - Burn due to localized fire on board Hovercraft
  - Burn due to localized fire on board Jet ski
- ✓x7th **V93.04** Burn due to localized fire on board sailboat
- ✓x7th **V93.09** Burn due to localized fire on board unspecified watercraft
  - Burn due to localized fire on board boat NOS
  - Burn due to localized fire on board ship NOS
  - Burn due to localized fire on board watercraft NOS

✓5th **V93.1** Other burn on board watercraft
  - Burn due to source other than fire on board watercraft
  - EXCLUDES 1   burn due to watercraft on fire (V91.0-)
- ✓x7th **V93.10** Other burn on board merchant vessel
- ✓x7th **V93.11** Other burn on board passenger vessel
  - Other burn on board Ferry-boat
  - Other burn on board Liner
- ✓x7th **V93.12** Other burn on board fishing boat
- ✓x7th **V93.13** Other burn on board other powered watercraft
  - Other burn on board Hovercraft
  - Other burn on board Jet ski
- ✓x7th **V93.14** Other burn on board sailboat
- ✓x7th **V93.19** Other burn on board unspecified watercraft
  - Other burn on board boat NOS
  - Other burn on board ship NOS
  - Other burn on board watercraft NOS

✓5th **V93.2** Heat exposure on board watercraft
  - EXCLUDES 1   exposure to man-made heat not aboard watercraft (W92)
  - exposure to natural heat while on board watercraft (X30)
  - exposure to sunlight while on board watercraft (X32)
  - EXCLUDES 2   burn due to fire on board watercraft (V93.0-)
- ✓x7th **V93.20** Heat exposure on board merchant ship
- ✓x7th **V93.21** Heat exposure on board passenger ship
  - Heat exposure on board Ferry-boat
  - Heat exposure on board Liner
- ✓x7th **V93.22** Heat exposure on board fishing boat
- ✓x7th **V93.23** Heat exposure on board other powered watercraft
  - Heat exposure on board hovercraft
- ✓x7th **V93.24** Heat exposure on board sailboat
- ✓x7th **V93.29** Heat exposure on board unspecified watercraft
  - Heat exposure on board boat NOS
  - Heat exposure on board ship NOS
  - Heat exposure on board watercraft NOS

✓5th **V93.3** Fall on board watercraft
  - EXCLUDES 1   fall due to collision of watercraft (V91.2-)
- ✓x7th **V93.30** Fall on board merchant ship
- ✓x7th **V93.31** Fall on board passenger ship
  - Fall on board Ferry-boat
  - Fall on board Liner
- ✓x7th **V93.32** Fall on board fishing boat
- ✓x7th **V93.33** Fall on board other powered watercraft
  - Fall on board Hovercraft (on open water)
  - Fall on board Jet ski
- ✓x7th **V93.34** Fall on board sailboat
- ✓x7th **V93.35** Fall on board canoe or kayak
- ✓x7th **V93.36** Fall on board (nonpowered) inflatable craft
- ✓x7th **V93.38** Fall on board other unpowered watercraft
- ✓x7th **V93.39** Fall on board unspecified watercraft
  - Fall on board boat NOS
  - Fall on board ship NOS
  - Fall on board watercraft NOS

✓5th **V93.4** Struck by falling object on board watercraft
  - Hit by falling object on board watercraft
  - EXCLUDES 1   struck by falling object due to accident to watercraft (V91.3)
- ✓x7th **V93.40** Struck by falling object on merchant ship
- ✓x7th **V93.41** Struck by falling object on passenger ship
  - Struck by falling object on Ferry-boat
  - Struck by falling object on Liner
- ✓x7th **V93.42** Struck by falling object on fishing boat
- ✓x7th **V93.43** Struck by falling object on other powered watercraft
  - Struck by falling object on Hovercraft
- ✓x7th **V93.44** Struck by falling object on sailboat
- ✓x7th **V93.48** Struck by falling object on other unpowered watercraft
- ✓x7th **V93.49** Struck by falling object on unspecified watercraft

✓5th **V93.5** Explosion on board watercraft
  - Boiler explosion on steamship
  - EXCLUDES 2   fire on board watercraft (V93.0-)
- ✓x7th **V93.50** Explosion on board merchant ship
- ✓x7th **V93.51** Explosion on board passenger ship
  - Explosion on board Ferry-boat
  - Explosion on board Liner
- ✓x7th **V93.52** Explosion on board fishing boat
- ✓x7th **V93.53** Explosion on board other powered watercraft
  - Explosion on board Hovercraft
  - Explosion on board Jet ski
- ✓x7th **V93.54** Explosion on board sailboat
- ✓x7th **V93.59** Explosion on board unspecified watercraft
  - Explosion on board boat NOS
  - Explosion on board ship NOS
  - Explosion on board watercraft NOS

✓5th **V93.6** Machinery accident on board watercraft
  - EXCLUDES 1   machinery explosion on board watercraft (V93.4-)
  - machinery fire on board watercraft (V93.0-)
- ✓x7th **V93.60** Machinery accident on board merchant ship
- ✓x7th **V93.61** Machinery accident on board passenger ship
  - Machinery accident on board Ferry-boat
  - Machinery accident on board Liner
- ✓x7th **V93.62** Machinery accident on board fishing boat
- ✓x7th **V93.63** Machinery accident on board other powered watercraft
  - Machinery accident on board Hovercraft
- ✓x7th **V93.64** Machinery accident on board sailboat
- ✓x7th **V93.69** Machinery accident on board unspecified watercraft
  - Machinery accident on board boat NOS
  - Machinery accident on board ship NOS
  - Machinery accident on board watercraft NOS

✓5th **V93.8** Other injury due to other accident on board watercraft
  - Accidental poisoning by gases or fumes on watercraft
- ✓x7th **V93.80** Other injury due to other accident on board merchant ship
- ✓x7th **V93.81** Other injury due to other accident on board passenger ship
  - Other injury due to other accident on board Ferry-boat
  - Other injury due to other accident on board Liner
- ✓x7th **V93.82** Other injury due to other accident on board fishing boat
- ✓x7th **V93.83** Other injury due to other accident on board other powered watercraft
  - Other injury due to other accident on board Hovercraft
  - Other injury due to other accident on board Jet ski
- ✓x7th **V93.84** Other injury due to other accident on board sailboat
- ✓x7th **V93.85** Other injury due to other accident on board canoe or kayak
- ✓x7th **V93.86** Other injury due to other accident on board (nonpowered) inflatable craft
- ✓x7th **V93.87** Other injury due to other accident on board water-skis
  - Hit or struck by object while waterskiing
- ✓x7th **V93.88** Other injury due to other accident on board other unpowered watercraft
  - Hit or struck by object while on board windsurfer
  - Hit or struck by object while surfing
- ✓x7th **V93.89** Other injury due to other accident on board unspecified watercraft
  - Other injury due to other accident on board boat NOS
  - Other injury due to other accident on board ship NOS
  - Other injury due to other accident on board watercraft NOS

✓4th **V94** Other and unspecified water transport accidents
  - EXCLUDES 1   military watercraft accidents in military or war operations (Y36, Y37)
- ✓x7th **V94.0** Hitting object or bottom of body of water due to fall from watercraft
  - EXCLUDES 2   drowning and submersion due to fall from watercraft (V92.0-)

V94.1 Bather struck by watercraft
Swimmer hit by watercraft
- **V94.11** Bather struck by powered watercraft
- **V94.12** Bather struck by nonpowered watercraft

V94.2 Rider of nonpowered watercraft struck by other watercraft
- **V94.21** Rider of nonpowered watercraft struck by other nonpowered watercraft
  - Canoer hit by other nonpowered watercraft
  - Surfer hit by other nonpowered watercraft
  - Windsurfer hit by other nonpowered watercraft
- **V94.22** Rider of nonpowered watercraft struck by powered watercraft
  - Canoer hit by motorboat
  - Surfer hit by motorboat
  - Windsurfer hit by motorboat

V94.3 Injury to rider of (inflatable) watercraft being pulled behind other watercraft
- **V94.31** Injury to rider of (inflatable) recreational watercraft being pulled behind other watercraft
  - Injury to rider of inner-tube pulled behind motor boat
- **V94.32** Injury to rider of non-recreational watercraft being pulled behind other watercraft
  - Injury to occupant of dingy being pulled behind boat or ship
  - Injury to occupant of life-raft being pulled behind boat or ship

V94.4 Injury to barefoot water-skier
Injury to person being pulled behind boat or ship

V94.8 Other water transport accident
- **V94.81** Water transport accident involving military watercraft
  - **V94.810** Civilian watercraft involved in water transport accident with military watercraft
    - Passenger on civilian watercraft injured due to accident with military watercraft
  - **V94.811** Civilian in water injured by military watercraft
  - **V94.818** Other water transport accident involving military watercraft
- **V94.89** Other water transport accident

V94.9 Unspecified water transport accident
Water transport accident NOS

Air and space transport accidents (V95-V97)

EXCLUDES 1 *military aircraft accidents in military or war operations (Y36, Y37)*

The appropriate 7th character is to be added to each code from categories V95-V97.
- A initial encounter
- D subsequent encounter
- S sequela

V95 Accident to powered aircraft causing injury to occupant

V95.0 Helicopter accident injuring occupant
- **V95.00** Unspecified helicopter accident injuring occupant
- **V95.01** Helicopter crash injuring occupant
- **V95.02** Forced landing of helicopter injuring occupant
- **V95.03** Helicopter collision injuring occupant
  - Helicopter collision with any object, fixed, movable or moving
- **V95.04** Helicopter fire injuring occupant
- **V95.05** Helicopter explosion injuring occupant
- **V95.09** Other helicopter accident injuring occupant

V95.1 Ultralight, microlight or powered-glider accident injuring occupant
- **V95.10** Unspecified ultralight, microlight or powered-glider accident injuring occupant
- **V95.11** Ultralight, microlight or powered-glider crash injuring occupant
- **V95.12** Forced landing of ultralight, microlight or powered-glider injuring occupant
- **V95.13** Ultralight, microlight or powered-glider collision injuring occupant
  - Ultralight, microlight or powered-glider collision with any object, fixed, movable or moving
- **V95.14** Ultralight, microlight or powered-glider fire injuring occupant
- **V95.15** Ultralight, microlight or powered-glider explosion injuring occupant
- **V95.19** Other ultralight, microlight or powered-glider accident injuring occupant

V95.2 Other private fixed-wing aircraft accident injuring occupant
- **V95.20** Unspecified accident to other private fixed-wing aircraft, injuring occupant
- **V95.21** Other private fixed-wing aircraft crash injuring occupant
- **V95.22** Forced landing of other private fixed-wing aircraft injuring occupant
- **V95.23** Other private fixed-wing aircraft collision injuring occupant
  - Other private fixed-wing aircraft collision with any object, fixed, movable or moving
- **V95.24** Other private fixed-wing aircraft fire injuring occupant
- **V95.25** Other private fixed-wing aircraft explosion injuring occupant
- **V95.29** Other accident to other private fixed-wing aircraft injuring occupant

V95.3 Commercial fixed-wing aircraft accident injuring occupant
- **V95.30** Unspecified accident to commercial fixed-wing aircraft injuring occupant
- **V95.31** Commercial fixed-wing aircraft crash injuring occupant
- **V95.32** Forced landing of commercial fixed-wing aircraft injuring occupant
- **V95.33** Commercial fixed-wing aircraft collision injuring occupant
  - Commercial fixed-wing aircraft collision with any object, fixed, movable or moving
- **V95.34** Commercial fixed-wing aircraft fire injuring occupant
- **V95.35** Commercial fixed-wing aircraft explosion injuring occupant
- **V95.39** Other accident to commercial fixed-wing aircraft injuring occupant

V95.4 Spacecraft accident injuring occupant
- **V95.40** Unspecified spacecraft accident injuring occupant
- **V95.41** Spacecraft crash injuring occupant
- **V95.42** Forced landing of spacecraft injuring occupant
- **V95.43** Spacecraft collision injuring occupant
  - Spacecraft collision with any object, fixed, moveable or moving
- **V95.44** Spacecraft fire injuring occupant
- **V95.45** Spacecraft explosion injuring occupant
- **V95.49** Other spacecraft accident injuring occupant

V95.8 Other powered aircraft accidents injuring occupant

V95.9 Unspecified aircraft accident injuring occupant
Air transport accident NOS
Aircraft accident NOS

V96 Accident to nonpowered aircraft causing injury to occupant

V96.0 Balloon accident injuring occupant
- **V96.00** Unspecified balloon accident injuring occupant
- **V96.01** Balloon crash injuring occupant
- **V96.02** Forced landing of balloon injuring occupant
- **V96.03** Balloon collision injuring occupant
  - Balloon collision with any object, fixed, moveable or moving
- **V96.04** Balloon fire injuring occupant
- **V96.05** Balloon explosion injuring occupant
- **V96.09** Other balloon accident injuring occupant

V96.1 Hang-glider accident injuring occupant
- **V96.10** Unspecified hang-glider accident injuring occupant
- **V96.11** Hang-glider crash injuring occupant
- **V96.12** Forced landing of hang-glider injuring occupant
- **V96.13** Hang-glider collision injuring occupant
  - Hang-glider collision with any object, fixed, moveable or moving
- **V96.14** Hang-glider fire injuring occupant
- **V96.15** Hang-glider explosion injuring occupant
- **V96.19** Other hang-glider accident injuring occupant

V96.2 Glider (nonpowered) accident injuring occupant
- **V96.20** Unspecified glider (nonpowered) accident injuring occupant

Chapter 20. External Causes of Morbidity

V96.21–W03

- ✓x7th **V96.21** Glider (nonpowered) crash injuring occupant
- ✓x7th **V96.22** Forced landing of glider (nonpowered) injuring occupant
- ✓x7th **V96.23** Glider (nonpowered) collision injuring occupant
  - Glider (nonpowered) collision with any object, fixed, moveable or moving
- ✓x7th **V96.24** Glider (nonpowered) fire injuring occupant
- ✓x7th **V96.25** Glider (nonpowered) explosion injuring occupant
- ✓x7th **V96.29** Other glider (nonpowered) accident injuring occupant

- ✓x7th **V96.8** Other nonpowered-aircraft accidents injuring occupant
  - Kite carrying a person accident injuring occupant
- ✓x7th **V96.9** Unspecified nonpowered-aircraft accident injuring occupant
  - Nonpowered-aircraft accident NOS

✓4th **V97** Other specified air transport accidents

- ✓x7th **V97.0** Occupant of aircraft injured in other specified air transport accidents
  - Fall in, on or from aircraft in air transport accident
  - EXCLUDES 1: accident while boarding or alighting aircraft (V97.1)
- ✓x7th **V97.1** Person injured while boarding or alighting from aircraft
- ✓5th **V97.2** Parachutist accident
  - ✓x7th **V97.21** Parachutist entangled in object
    - Parachutist landing in tree
  - ✓x7th **V97.22** Parachutist injured on landing
  - ✓x7th **V97.29** Other parachutist accident
- ✓5th **V97.3** Person on ground injured in air transport accident
  - ✓x7th **V97.31** Hit by object falling from aircraft
    - Hit by crashing aircraft
    - Injured by aircraft hitting car
    - Injured by aircraft hitting house
  - ✓x7th **V97.32** Injured by rotating propeller
  - ✓x7th **V97.33** Sucked into jet engine
  - ✓x7th **V97.39** Other injury to person on ground due to air transport accident
- ✓5th **V97.8** Other air transport accidents, not elsewhere classified
  - EXCLUDES 1: aircraft accident NOS (V95.9)
  - exposure to changes in air pressure during ascent or descent (W94.-)
  - ✓6th **V97.81** Air transport accident involving military aircraft
    - ✓7th **V97.810** Civilian aircraft involved in air transport accident with military aircraft
      - Passenger in civilian aircraft injured due to accident with military aircraft
    - ✓7th **V97.811** Civilian injured by military aircraft
    - ✓7th **V97.818** Other air transport accident involving military aircraft
  - ✓x7th **V97.89** Other air transport accidents, not elsewhere classified
    - Injury from machinery on aircraft

Other and unspecified transport accidents (V98-V99)

EXCLUDES 1: vehicle accident, type of vehicle unspecified (V89.-)

The appropriate 7th character is to be added to each code from categories V98-V99.
- A initial encounter
- D subsequent encounter
- S sequela

✓4th **V98** Other specified transport accidents

- ✓x7th **V98.0** Accident to, on or involving cable-car, not on rails
  - Caught or dragged by cable-car, not on rails
  - Fall or jump from cable-car, not on rails
  - Object thrown from or in cable-car, not on rails
- ✓x7th **V98.1** Accident to, on or involving land-yacht
- ✓x7th **V98.2** Accident to, on or involving ice yacht
- ✓x7th **V98.3** Accident to, on or involving ski lift
  - Accident to, on or involving ski chair-lift
  - Accident to, on or involving ski-lift with gondola
- ✓x7th **V98.8** Other specified transport accidents

✓x7th **V99** Unspecified transport accident

OTHER EXTERNAL CAUSES OF ACCIDENTAL INJURY (W00-X58)

Slipping, tripping, stumbling and falls (W00-W19)

EXCLUDES 1:
- assault involving a fall (Y01-Y02)
- fall from animal (V80.-)
- fall (in) (from) machinery (in operation) (W28-W31)
- fall (in) (from) transport vehicle (V01-V99)
- intentional self-harm involving a fall (X80-X81)

EXCLUDES 2:
- at risk for fall (history of fall) Z91.81
- fall (in) (from) burning building (X00.-)
- fall into fire (X00-X04, X08)

The appropriate 7th character is to be added to each code from categories W00-W19.
- A initial encounter
- D subsequent encounter
- S sequela

✓4th **W00** Fall due to ice and snow

INCLUDES: pedestrian on foot falling (slipping) on ice and snow

EXCLUDES 1:
- fall on (from) ice and snow involving pedestrian conveyance (V00.-)
- fall from stairs and steps not due to ice and snow (W10.-)

AHA: 2016,2Q,4

- ✓x7th **W00.0** Fall on same level due to ice and snow
- ✓x7th **W00.1** Fall from stairs and steps due to ice and snow
- ✓x7th **W00.2** Other fall from one level to another due to ice and snow
- ✓x7th **W00.9** Unspecified fall due to ice and snow

✓4th **W01** Fall on same level from slipping, tripping and stumbling

INCLUDES: fall on moving sidewalk

EXCLUDES 1:
- fall due to bumping (striking) against object (W18.0-)
- fall in shower or bathtub (W18.2-)
- fall off or from toilet (W18.1-)
- fall on same level from slipping, tripping and stumbling due to ice or snow (W00.0)
- fall on same level NOS (W18.30)
- slipping, tripping and stumbling NOS (W18.40)
- slipping, tripping and stumbling without falling (W18.4-)

- ✓x7th **W01.0** Fall on same level from slipping, tripping and stumbling without subsequent striking against object
  - Falling over animal
- ✓5th **W01.1** Fall on same level from slipping, tripping and stumbling with subsequent striking against object
  - ✓x7th **W01.10** Fall on same level from slipping, tripping and stumbling with subsequent striking against unspecified object
  - ✓6th **W01.11** Fall on same level from slipping, tripping and stumbling with subsequent striking against sharp object
    - ✓7th **W01.110** Fall on same level from slipping, tripping and stumbling with subsequent striking against sharp glass
    - ✓7th **W01.111** Fall on same level from slipping, tripping and stumbling with subsequent striking against power tool or machine
    - ✓7th **W01.118** Fall on same level from slipping, tripping and stumbling with subsequent striking against other sharp object
    - ✓7th **W01.119** Fall on same level from slipping, tripping and stumbling with subsequent striking against unspecified sharp object
  - ✓6th **W01.19** Fall on same level from slipping, tripping and stumbling with subsequent striking against other object
    - ✓7th **W01.190** Fall on same level from slipping, tripping and stumbling with subsequent striking against furniture
    - ✓7th **W01.198** Fall on same level from slipping, tripping and stumbling with subsequent striking against other object

✓x7th **W03** Other fall on same level due to collision with another person
- Fall due to non-transport collision with other person
- EXCLUDES 1:
  - collision with another person without fall (W51)
  - crushed or pushed by a crowd or human stampede (W52)
  - fall due to ice or snow (W00)
  - fall involving pedestrian conveyance (V00-V09)
  - fall on same level NOS (W18.30)

AHA: 2012,4Q,108

Chapter 20. External Causes of Morbidity

- ✓x 7th **W04** Fall while being carried or supported by other persons
  - Accidentally dropped while being carried
- ✓4th **W05** Fall from non-moving wheelchair, nonmotorized scooter and motorized mobility scooter
  - EXCLUDES 1: fall from moving motorized mobility scooter (V00.831)
    - fall from moving wheelchair (powered) (V00.811)
    - fall from nonmotorized scooter (V00.141)
  - ✓x 7th **W05.0** Fall from non-moving wheelchair
    - AHA: 2019,2Q,27
  - ✓x 7th **W05.1** Fall from non-moving nonmotorized scooter
  - ✓x 7th **W05.2** Fall from non-moving motorized mobility scooter
- ✓x 7th **W06** Fall from bed
- ✓x 7th **W07** Fall from chair
- ✓x 7th **W08** Fall from other furniture
  - Fall from stool
- ✓4th **W09** Fall on and from playground equipment
  - EXCLUDES 1: fall involving recreational machinery (W31)
  - ✓x 7th **W09.0** Fall on or from playground slide
  - ✓x 7th **W09.1** Fall from playground swing
  - ✓x 7th **W09.2** Fall on or from jungle gym
  - ✓x 7th **W09.8** Fall on or from other playground equipment
- ✓4th **W10** Fall on and from stairs and steps
  - EXCLUDES 1: Fall from stairs and steps due to ice and snow (W00.1)
  - ✓x 7th **W10.0** Fall (on)(from) escalator
  - ✓x 7th **W10.1** Fall (on)(from) sidewalk curb
  - ✓x 7th **W10.2** Fall (on)(from) incline
    - Fall (on) (from) ramp
  - ✓x 7th **W10.8** Fall (on) (from) other stairs and steps
  - ✓x 7th **W10.9** Fall (on) (from) unspecified stairs and steps
- ✓x 7th **W11** Fall on and from ladder
- ✓x 7th **W12** Fall on and from scaffolding
- ✓4th **W13** Fall from, out of or through building or structure
  - ✓x 7th **W13.0** Fall from, out of or through balcony
    - Fall from, out of or through railing
  - ✓x 7th **W13.1** Fall from, out of or through bridge
  - ✓x 7th **W13.2** Fall from, out of or through roof
  - ✓x 7th **W13.3** Fall through floor
  - ✓x 7th **W13.4** Fall from, out of or through window
    - EXCLUDES 2: fall with subsequent striking against sharp glass (W01.110-)
  - ✓x 7th **W13.8** Fall from, out of or through other building or structure
    - Fall from, out of or through flag-pole
    - Fall from, out of or through viaduct
    - Fall from, out of or through wall
  - ✓x 7th **W13.9** Fall from, out of or through building, not otherwise specified
    - EXCLUDES 1: collapse of a building or structure (W20.-)
      - fall or jump from burning building or structure (X00.-)
- ✓x 7th **W14** Fall from tree
- ✓x 7th **W15** Fall from cliff
- ✓4th **W16** Fall, jump or diving into water
  - EXCLUDES 1: accidental non-watercraft drowning and submersion not involving fall (W65-W74)
    - effects of air pressure from diving (W94.-)
    - fall into water from watercraft (V90-V94)
    - hitting an object or against bottom when falling from watercraft (V94.0)
  - EXCLUDES 2: striking or hitting diving board (W21.4)
  - ✓5th **W16.0** Fall into swimming pool
    - Fall into swimming pool NOS
    - EXCLUDES 1: fall into empty swimming pool (W17.3)
    - ✓6th **W16.01** Fall into swimming pool striking water surface
      - ✓7th **W16.011** Fall into swimming pool striking water surface causing drowning and submersion
        - EXCLUDES 1: drowning and submersion while in swimming pool without fall (W67)
      - ✓7th **W16.012** Fall into swimming pool striking water surface causing other injury
    - ✓6th **W16.02** Fall into swimming pool striking bottom
      - ✓7th **W16.021** Fall into swimming pool striking bottom causing drowning and submersion
        - EXCLUDES 1: drowning and submersion while in swimming pool without fall (W67)
      - ✓7th **W16.022** Fall into swimming pool striking bottom causing other injury
    - ✓6th **W16.03** Fall into swimming pool striking wall
      - ✓7th **W16.031** Fall into swimming pool striking wall causing drowning and submersion
        - EXCLUDES 1: drowning and submersion while in swimming pool without fall (W67)
      - ✓7th **W16.032** Fall into swimming pool striking wall causing other injury
  - ✓5th **W16.1** Fall into natural body of water
    - Fall into lake
    - Fall into open sea
    - Fall into river
    - Fall into stream
    - ✓6th **W16.11** Fall into natural body of water striking water surface
      - ✓7th **W16.111** Fall into natural body of water striking water surface causing drowning and submersion
        - EXCLUDES 1: drowning and submersion while in natural body of water without fall (W69)
      - ✓7th **W16.112** Fall into natural body of water striking water surface causing other injury
    - ✓6th **W16.12** Fall into natural body of water striking bottom
      - ✓7th **W16.121** Fall into natural body of water striking bottom causing drowning and submersion
        - EXCLUDES 1: drowning and submersion while in natural body of water without fall (W69)
      - ✓7th **W16.122** Fall into natural body of water striking bottom causing other injury
    - ✓6th **W16.13** Fall into natural body of water striking side
      - ✓7th **W16.131** Fall into natural body of water striking side causing drowning and submersion
        - EXCLUDES 1: drowning and submersion while in natural body of water without fall (W69)
      - ✓7th **W16.132** Fall into natural body of water striking side causing other injury
  - ✓5th **W16.2** Fall in (into) filled bathtub or bucket of water
    - ✓6th **W16.21** Fall in (into) filled bathtub
      - EXCLUDES 1: fall into empty bathtub (W18.2)
      - ✓7th **W16.211** Fall in (into) filled bathtub causing drowning and submersion
        - EXCLUDES 1: drowning and submersion while in filled bathtub without fall (W65)
      - ✓7th **W16.212** Fall in (into) filled bathtub causing other injury
    - ✓6th **W16.22** Fall in (into) bucket of water
      - ✓7th **W16.221** Fall in (into) bucket of water causing drowning and submersion
      - ✓7th **W16.222** Fall in (into) bucket of water causing other injury
  - ✓5th **W16.3** Fall into other water
    - Fall into fountain
    - Fall into reservoir
    - ✓6th **W16.31** Fall into other water striking water surface
      - ✓7th **W16.311** Fall into other water striking water surface causing drowning and submersion
        - EXCLUDES 1: drowning and submersion while in other water without fall (W73)
      - ✓7th **W16.312** Fall into other water striking water surface causing other injury
    - ✓6th **W16.32** Fall into other water striking bottom
      - ✓7th **W16.321** Fall into other water striking bottom causing drowning and submersion
        - EXCLUDES 1: drowning and submersion while in other water without fall (W73)

- **W16.322** Fall into other water striking bottom causing other injury
- **W16.33** Fall into other water striking wall
  - **W16.331** Fall into other water striking wall causing drowning and submersion
    - EXCLUDES 1: drowning and submersion while in other water without fall (W73)
  - **W16.332** Fall into other water striking wall causing other injury
- **W16.4** Fall into unspecified water
  - **W16.41** Fall into unspecified water causing drowning and submersion
  - **W16.42** Fall into unspecified water causing other injury
- **W16.5** Jumping or diving into swimming pool
  - **W16.51** Jumping or diving into swimming pool striking water surface
    - **W16.511** Jumping or diving into swimming pool striking water surface causing drowning and submersion
      - EXCLUDES 1: drowning and submersion while in swimming pool without jumping or diving (W67)
    - **W16.512** Jumping or diving into swimming pool striking water surface causing other injury
  - **W16.52** Jumping or diving into swimming pool striking bottom
    - **W16.521** Jumping or diving into swimming pool striking bottom causing drowning and submersion
      - EXCLUDES 1: drowning and submersion while in swimming pool without jumping or diving (W67)
    - **W16.522** Jumping or diving into swimming pool striking bottom causing other injury
  - **W16.53** Jumping or diving into swimming pool striking wall
    - **W16.531** Jumping or diving into swimming pool striking wall causing drowning and submersion
      - EXCLUDES 1: drowning and submersion while in swimming pool without jumping or diving (W67)
    - **W16.532** Jumping or diving into swimming pool striking wall causing other injury
- **W16.6** Jumping or diving into natural body of water
  - Jumping or diving into lake
  - Jumping or diving into open sea
  - Jumping or diving into river
  - Jumping or diving into stream
  - **W16.61** Jumping or diving into natural body of water striking water surface
    - **W16.611** Jumping or diving into natural body of water striking water surface causing drowning and submersion
      - EXCLUDES 1: drowning and submersion while in natural body of water without jumping or diving (W69)
    - **W16.612** Jumping or diving into natural body of water striking water surface causing other injury
  - **W16.62** Jumping or diving into natural body of water striking bottom
    - **W16.621** Jumping or diving into natural body of water striking bottom causing drowning and submersion
      - EXCLUDES 1: drowning and submersion while in natural body of water without jumping or diving (W69)
    - **W16.622** Jumping or diving into natural body of water striking bottom causing other injury
- **W16.7** Jumping or diving from boat
  - EXCLUDES 1: fall from boat into water - see watercraft accident (V90-V94)
  - **W16.71** Jumping or diving from boat striking water surface
    - **W16.711** Jumping or diving from boat striking water surface causing drowning and submersion
    - **W16.712** Jumping or diving from boat striking water surface causing other injury
  - **W16.72** Jumping or diving from boat striking bottom
    - **W16.721** Jumping or diving from boat striking bottom causing drowning and submersion
    - **W16.722** Jumping or diving from boat striking bottom causing other injury
- **W16.8** Jumping or diving into other water
  - Jumping or diving into fountain
  - Jumping or diving into reservoir
  - **W16.81** Jumping or diving into other water striking water surface
    - **W16.811** Jumping or diving into other water striking water surface causing drowning and submersion
      - EXCLUDES 1: drowning and submersion while in other water without jumping or diving (W73)
    - **W16.812** Jumping or diving into other water striking water surface causing other injury
  - **W16.82** Jumping or diving into other water striking bottom
    - **W16.821** Jumping or diving into other water striking bottom causing drowning and submersion
      - EXCLUDES 1: drowning and submersion while in other water without jumping or diving (W73)
    - **W16.822** Jumping or diving into other water striking bottom causing other injury
  - **W16.83** Jumping or diving into other water striking wall
    - **W16.831** Jumping or diving into other water striking wall causing drowning and submersion
      - EXCLUDES 1: drowning and submersion while in other water without jumping or diving (W73)
    - **W16.832** Jumping or diving into other water striking wall causing other injury
- **W16.9** Jumping or diving into unspecified water
  - **W16.91** Jumping or diving into unspecified water causing drowning and submersion
  - **W16.92** Jumping or diving into unspecified water causing other injury

W17 Other fall from one level to another

- **W17.0** Fall into well
- **W17.1** Fall into storm drain or manhole
- **W17.2** Fall into hole
  - Fall into pit
- **W17.3** Fall into empty swimming pool
  - EXCLUDES 1: fall into filled swimming pool (W16.0-)
- **W17.4** Fall from dock
- **W17.8** Other fall from one level to another
  - **W17.81** Fall down embankment (hill)
  - **W17.82** Fall from (out of) grocery cart
    - Fall due to grocery cart tipping over
  - **W17.89** Other fall from one level to another
    - Fall from cherry picker
    - Fall from lifting device
    - Fall from mobile elevated work platform [MEWP]
    - Fall from sky lift
    - **AHA:** 2015, 2Q, 6

W18 Other slipping, tripping and stumbling and falls

- **W18.0** Fall due to bumping against object
  - Striking against object with subsequent fall
  - EXCLUDES 1: fall on same level due to slipping, tripping, or stumbling with subsequent striking against object (W01.1-)
  - **W18.00** Striking against unspecified object with subsequent fall
  - **W18.01** Striking against sports equipment with subsequent fall
  - **W18.02** Striking against glass with subsequent fall
  - **W18.09** Striking against other object with subsequent fall
- **W18.1** Fall from or off toilet
  - **W18.11** Fall from or off toilet without subsequent striking against object
    - Fall from (off) toilet NOS
  - **W18.12** Fall from or off toilet with subsequent striking against object

Chapter 20. External Causes of Morbidity

- **W18.2** Fall in (into) shower or empty bathtub
  - EXCLUDES 1: fall in full bathtub causing drowning or submersion (W16.21-)
- **W18.3** Other and unspecified fall on same level
  - **W18.30** Fall on same level, unspecified
  - **W18.31** Fall on same level due to stepping on an object
    - Fall on same level due to stepping on an animal
    - EXCLUDES 1: slipping, tripping and stumbling without fall due to stepping on animal (W18.41)
  - **W18.39** Other fall on same level
- **W18.4** Slipping, tripping and stumbling without falling
  - EXCLUDES 1: collision with another person without fall (W51)
  - **W18.40** Slipping, tripping and stumbling without falling, unspecified
  - **W18.41** Slipping, tripping and stumbling without falling due to stepping on object
    - Slipping, tripping and stumbling without falling due to stepping on animal
    - EXCLUDES 1: slipping, tripping and stumbling with fall due to stepping on animal (W18.31)
  - **W18.42** Slipping, tripping and stumbling without falling due to stepping into hole or opening
  - **W18.43** Slipping, tripping and stumbling without falling due to stepping from one level to another
  - **W18.49** Other slipping, tripping and stumbling without falling
- **W19** Unspecified fall
  - Accidental fall NOS
  - AHA: 2012,4Q,95

Exposure to inanimate mechanical forces (W20-W49)

EXCLUDES 1: assault (X92-Y09)
contact or collision with animals or persons (W50-W64)
exposure to inanimate mechanical forces involving military or war operations (Y36.-, Y37.-)
intentional self-harm (X71-X83)

The appropriate 7th character is to be added to each code from categories W20-W49.
- A initial encounter
- D subsequent encounter
- S sequela

- **W20** Struck by thrown, projected or falling object
  - Code first any associated:
    - cataclysm (X34-X39)
    - lightning strike (T75.00)
  - EXCLUDES 1: falling object in machinery accident (W24, W28-W31)
    falling object in transport accident (V01-V99)
    object set in motion by explosion (W35-W40)
    object set in motion by firearm (W32-W34)
    struck by thrown sports equipment (W21.-)
  - **W20.0** Struck by falling object in cave-in
    - EXCLUDES 2: asphyxiation due to cave-in (T71.21)
  - **W20.1** Struck by object due to collapse of building
    - EXCLUDES 1: struck by object due to collapse of burning building (X00.2, X02.2)
  - **W20.8** Other cause of strike by thrown, projected or falling object
    - EXCLUDES 1: struck by thrown sports equipment (W21.-)
- **W21** Striking against or struck by sports equipment
  - EXCLUDES 1: assault with sports equipment (Y08.0-)
    striking against or struck by sports equipment with subsequent fall (W18.01)
  - **W21.0** Struck by hit or thrown ball
    - **W21.00** Struck by hit or thrown ball, unspecified type
    - **W21.01** Struck by football
    - **W21.02** Struck by soccer ball
    - **W21.03** Struck by baseball
    - **W21.04** Struck by golf ball
    - **W21.05** Struck by basketball
    - **W21.06** Struck by volleyball
    - **W21.07** Struck by softball
    - **W21.09** Struck by other hit or thrown ball
  - **W21.1** Struck by bat, racquet or club
    - **W21.11** Struck by baseball bat
    - **W21.12** Struck by tennis racquet
    - **W21.13** Struck by golf club
    - **W21.19** Struck by other bat, racquet or club
  - **W21.2** Struck by hockey stick or puck
    - **W21.21** Struck by hockey stick
      - **W21.210** Struck by ice hockey stick
      - **W21.211** Struck by field hockey stick
    - **W21.22** Struck by hockey puck
      - **W21.220** Struck by ice hockey puck
      - **W21.221** Struck by field hockey puck
  - **W21.3** Struck by sports foot wear
    - **W21.31** Struck by shoe cleats
      - Stepped on by shoe cleats
    - **W21.32** Struck by skate blades
      - Skated over by skate blades
    - **W21.39** Struck by other sports foot wear
  - **W21.4** Striking against diving board
    - Use additional code for subsequent falling into water, if applicable (W16.-)
  - **W21.8** Striking against or struck by other sports equipment
    - **W21.81** Striking against or struck by football helmet
    - **W21.89** Striking against or struck by other sports equipment
  - **W21.9** Striking against or struck by unspecified sports equipment
- **W22** Striking against or struck by other objects
  - EXCLUDES 1: striking against or struck by object with subsequent fall (W18.09)
  - **W22.0** Striking against stationary object
    - EXCLUDES 1: striking against stationary sports equipment (W21.8)
    - **W22.01** Walked into wall
    - **W22.02** Walked into lamppost
    - **W22.03** Walked into furniture
    - **W22.04** Striking against wall of swimming pool
      - **W22.041** Striking against wall of swimming pool causing drowning and submersion
        - EXCLUDES 1: drowning and submersion while swimming without striking against wall (W67)
      - **W22.042** Striking against wall of swimming pool causing other injury
    - **W22.09** Striking against other stationary object
  - **W22.1** Striking against or struck by automobile airbag
    - **W22.10** Striking against or struck by unspecified automobile airbag
    - **W22.11** Striking against or struck by driver side automobile airbag
    - **W22.12** Striking against or struck by front passenger side automobile airbag
    - **W22.19** Striking against or struck by other automobile airbag
  - **W22.8** Striking against or struck by other objects
    - Striking against or struck by object NOS
    - EXCLUDES 1: struck by thrown, projected or falling object (W20.-)
- **W23** Caught, crushed, jammed or pinched in or between objects
  - EXCLUDES 1: injury caused by cutting or piercing instruments (W25-W27)
    injury caused by firearms malfunction (W32.1, W33.1-, W34.1-)
    injury caused by lifting and transmission devices (W24.-)
    injury caused by machinery (W28-W31)
    injury caused by nonpowered hand tools (W27.-)
    injury caused by struck by thrown, projected or falling object (W20.-)
    injury caused by transport vehicle being used as a means of transportation (V01-V99)
  - **W23.0** Caught, crushed, jammed, or pinched between moving objects
  - **W23.1** Caught, crushed, jammed, or pinched between stationary objects
  - **W23.2** Caught, crushed, jammed or pinched between a moving and stationary object
    - AHA: 2022,4Q,48

W24 Contact with lifting and transmission devices, not elsewhere classified
EXCLUDES 1 *transport accidents (V01-V99)*

W24.0 Contact with lifting devices, not elsewhere classified
Contact with chain hoist
Contact with drive belt
Contact with pulley (block)

W24.1 Contact with transmission devices, not elsewhere classified
Contact with transmission belt or cable

W25 Contact with sharp glass
Code first any associated:
  injury due to flying glass from explosion or firearm discharge (W32-W40)
  transport accident (V00-V99)
EXCLUDES 1 *fall on same level due to slipping, tripping and stumbling with subsequent striking against sharp glass (W01.110-)*
  striking against sharp glass with subsequent fall (W18.02-)
EXCLUDES 2 *glass embedded in skin (W45.-)*

W26 Contact with other sharp objects
EXCLUDES 2 *sharp object(s) embedded in skin (W45.-)*
AHA: 2016,4Q,73

W26.0 Contact with knife
EXCLUDES 1 *contact with electric knife (W29.1)*

W26.1 Contact with sword or dagger

W26.2 Contact with edge of stiff paper
Paper cut

W26.8 Contact with other sharp object(s), not elsewhere classified
Contact with tin can lid

W26.9 Contact with unspecified sharp object(s)

W27 Contact with nonpowered hand tool

W27.0 Contact with workbench tool
Contact with auger
Contact with axe
Contact with chisel
Contact with handsaw
Contact with screwdriver

W27.1 Contact with garden tool
Contact with hoe
Contact with nonpowered lawn mower
Contact with pitchfork
Contact with rake

W27.2 Contact with scissors

W27.3 Contact with needle (sewing)
EXCLUDES 1 *contact with hypodermic needle (W46.-)*

W27.4 Contact with kitchen utensil
Contact with can-opener NOS
Contact with fork
Contact with ice-pick

W27.5 Contact with paper-cutter

W27.8 Contact with other nonpowered hand tool
Contact with nonpowered sewing machine
Contact with shovel

W28 Contact with powered lawn mower
Powered lawn mower (commercial) (residential)
EXCLUDES 1 *contact with nonpowered lawn mower (W27.1)*
EXCLUDES 2 *exposure to electric current (W86.-)*

W29 Contact with other powered hand tools and household machinery
EXCLUDES 1 *contact with commercial machinery (W31.82)*
  contact with hot household appliance (X15)
  contact with nonpowered hand tool (W27.-)
  exposure to electric current (W86)

W29.0 Contact with powered kitchen appliance
Contact with blender
Contact with can-opener
Contact with garbage disposal
Contact with mixer

W29.1 Contact with electric knife

W29.2 Contact with other powered household machinery
Contact with electric fan
Contact with powered dryer (clothes) (powered) (spin)
Contact with sewing machine
Contact with washing-machine

W29.3 Contact with powered garden and outdoor hand tools and machinery
Contact with chainsaw
Contact with edger
Contact with garden cultivator (tiller)
Contact with hedge trimmer
Contact with other powered garden tool
EXCLUDES 1 *contact with powered lawn mower (W28)*

W29.4 Contact with nail gun

W29.8 Contact with other powered hand tools and household machinery
Contact with do-it-yourself tool NOS

W30 Contact with agricultural machinery
INCLUDES animal-powered farm machine
EXCLUDES 1 *agricultural transport vehicle accident (V01-V99)*
  explosion of grain store (W40.8)
  exposure to electric current (W86.-)

W30.0 Contact with combine harvester
Contact with reaper
Contact with thresher

W30.1 Contact with power take-off devices (PTO)

W30.2 Contact with hay derrick

W30.3 Contact with grain storage elevator
EXCLUDES 1 *explosion of grain store (W40.8)*

W30.8 Contact with other specified agricultural machinery

W30.81 Contact with agricultural transport vehicle in stationary use
Contact with agricultural transport vehicle under repair, not on public roadway
EXCLUDES 1 *agricultural transport vehicle accident (V01-V99)*

W30.89 Contact with other specified agricultural machinery

W30.9 Contact with unspecified agricultural machinery
Contact with farm machinery NOS

W31 Contact with other and unspecified machinery
EXCLUDES 1 *contact with agricultural machinery (W30.-)*
  contact with machinery in transport under own power or being towed by a vehicle (V01-V99)
  exposure to electric current (W86)

W31.0 Contact with mining and earth-drilling machinery
Contact with bore or drill (land) (seabed)
Contact with shaft hoist
Contact with shaft lift
Contact with undercutter

W31.1 Contact with metalworking machines
Contact with abrasive wheel
Contact with forging machine
Contact with lathe
Contact with mechanical shears
Contact with metal drilling machine
Contact with metal sawing machine
Contact with milling machine
Contact with power press
Contact with rolling-mill

W31.2 Contact with powered woodworking and forming machines
Contact with band saw
Contact with bench saw
Contact with circular saw
Contact with molding machine
Contact with overhead plane
Contact with powered saw
Contact with radial saw
Contact with sander
EXCLUDES 1 *nonpowered woodworking tools (W27.0)*

W31.3 Contact with prime movers
Contact with gas turbine
Contact with internal combustion engine
Contact with steam engine
Contact with water driven turbine

W31.8 Contact with other specified machinery

W31.81 Contact with recreational machinery
Contact with roller coaster

W31.82 Contact with other commercial machinery
Contact with commercial electric fan
Contact with commercial kitchen appliances
Contact with commercial powered dryer (clothes) (powered) (spin)
Contact with commercial sewing machine
Contact with commercial washing-machine

EXCLUDES 1 contact with household machinery (W29.-)
contact with powered lawn mower (W28)

W31.83 Contact with special construction vehicle in stationary use
Contact with special construction vehicle under repair, not on public roadway

EXCLUDES 1 special construction vehicle accident (V01-V99)

W31.89 Contact with other specified machinery

W31.9 Contact with unspecified machinery
Contact with machinery NOS

W32 Accidental handgun discharge and malfunction
INCLUDES accidental discharge and malfunction of gun for single hand use
accidental discharge and malfunction of pistol
accidental discharge and malfunction of revolver
handgun discharge and malfunction NOS

EXCLUDES 1 accidental airgun discharge and malfunction (W34.010, W34.110)
accidental BB gun discharge and malfunction (W34.010, W34.110)
accidental pellet gun discharge and malfunction (W34.010, W34.110)
accidental shotgun discharge and malfunction (W33.01, W33.11)
assault by handgun discharge (X93)
handgun discharge involving legal intervention (Y35.0-)
handgun discharge involving military or war operations (Y36.4-)
intentional self-harm by handgun discharge (X72)
Very pistol discharge and malfunction (W34.09, W34.19)

W32.0 Accidental handgun discharge

W32.1 Accidental handgun malfunction
Injury due to explosion of handgun (parts)
Injury due to malfunction of mechanism or component of handgun
Injury due to recoil of handgun
Powder burn from handgun

W33 Accidental rifle, shotgun and larger firearm discharge and malfunction
INCLUDES rifle, shotgun and larger firearm discharge and malfunction NOS

EXCLUDES 1 accidental airgun discharge and malfunction (W34.010, W34.110)
accidental BB gun discharge and malfunction (W34.010, W34.110)
accidental handgun discharge and malfunction (W32.-)
accidental pellet gun discharge and malfunction (W34.010, W34.110)
assault by rifle, shotgun and larger firearm discharge (X94)
firearm discharge involving legal intervention (Y35.0-)
firearm discharge involving military or war operations (Y36.4-)
intentional self-harm by rifle, shotgun and larger firearm discharge (X73)

W33.0 Accidental rifle, shotgun and larger firearm discharge

W33.00 Accidental discharge of unspecified larger firearm
Discharge of unspecified larger firearm NOS

W33.01 Accidental discharge of shotgun
Discharge of shotgun NOS

W33.02 Accidental discharge of hunting rifle
Discharge of hunting rifle NOS

W33.03 Accidental discharge of machine gun
Discharge of machine gun NOS

W33.09 Accidental discharge of other larger firearm
Discharge of other larger firearm NOS

W33.1 Accidental rifle, shotgun and larger firearm malfunction
Injury due to explosion of rifle, shotgun and larger firearm (parts)
Injury due to malfunction of mechanism or component of rifle, shotgun and larger firearm
Injury due to piercing, cutting, crushing or pinching due to (by) slide trigger mechanism, scope or other gun part
Injury due to recoil of rifle, shotgun and larger firearm
Powder burn from rifle, shotgun and larger firearm

W33.10 Accidental malfunction of unspecified larger firearm
Malfunction of unspecified larger firearm NOS

W33.11 Accidental malfunction of shotgun
Malfunction of shotgun NOS

W33.12 Accidental malfunction of hunting rifle
Malfunction of hunting rifle NOS

W33.13 Accidental malfunction of machine gun
Malfunction of machine gun NOS

W33.19 Accidental malfunction of other larger firearm
Malfunction of other larger firearm NOS

W34 Accidental discharge and malfunction from other and unspecified firearms and guns

W34.0 Accidental discharge from other and unspecified firearms and guns

W34.00 Accidental discharge from unspecified firearms or gun
Discharge from firearm NOS
Gunshot wound NOS
Shot NOS

W34.01 Accidental discharge of gas, air or spring-operated guns

W34.010 Accidental discharge of airgun
Accidental discharge of BB gun
Accidental discharge of pellet gun

W34.011 Accidental discharge of paintball gun
Accidental injury due to paintball discharge

W34.018 Accidental discharge of other gas, air or spring-operated gun

W34.09 Accidental discharge from other specified firearms
Accidental discharge from Very pistol [flare]

W34.1 Accidental malfunction from other and unspecified firearms and guns

W34.10 Accidental malfunction from unspecified firearms or gun
Firearm malfunction NOS

W34.11 Accidental malfunction of gas, air or spring-operated guns

W34.110 Accidental malfunction of airgun
Accidental malfunction of BB gun
Accidental malfunction of pellet gun

W34.111 Accidental malfunction of paintball gun
Accidental injury due to paintball gun malfunction

W34.118 Accidental malfunction of other gas, air or spring-operated gun

W34.19 Accidental malfunction from other specified firearms
Accidental malfunction from Very pistol [flare]

W35 Explosion and rupture of boiler
EXCLUDES 1 explosion and rupture of boiler on watercraft (V93.4)

W36 Explosion and rupture of gas cylinder

W36.1 Explosion and rupture of aerosol can
W36.2 Explosion and rupture of air tank
W36.3 Explosion and rupture of pressurized-gas tank
W36.8 Explosion and rupture of other gas cylinder
W36.9 Explosion and rupture of unspecified gas cylinder

W37 Explosion and rupture of pressurized tire, pipe or hose

W37.0 Explosion of bicycle tire
W37.8 Explosion and rupture of other pressurized tire, pipe or hose

W38 Explosion and rupture of other specified pressurized devices

W39 Discharge of firework

Chapter 20. External Causes of Morbidity

W40 **Explosion of other materials**
  EXCLUDES 1: assault by explosive material (X96)
  explosion involving legal intervention (Y35.1-)
  explosion involving military or war operations (Y36.0-, Y36.2-)
  intentional self-harm by explosive material (X75)

- **W40.0** Explosion of blasting material
  Explosion of blasting cap
  Explosion of detonator
  Explosion of dynamite
  Explosion of explosive (any) used in blasting operations

- **W40.1** Explosion of explosive gases
  Explosion of acetylene
  Explosion of butane
  Explosion of coal gas
  Explosion of explosive gas
  Explosion of fire damp
  Explosion of gasoline fumes
  Explosion in mine NOS
  Explosion of methane
  Explosion of propane

- **W40.8** Explosion of other specified explosive materials
  Explosion in dump NOS
  Explosion in factory NOS
  Explosion in grain store
  Explosion in munitions
  EXCLUDES 1: explosion involving legal intervention (Y35.1-)
  explosion involving military or war operations (Y36.0-, Y36.2-)

- **W40.9** Explosion of unspecified explosive materials
  Explosion NOS

W42 **Exposure to noise**

- **W42.0** Exposure to supersonic waves
- **W42.9** Exposure to other noise
  Exposure to sound waves NOS

W44 **Foreign body entering into or through a natural orifice**
  EXCLUDES 2: contact with other sharp objects (W26)
  contact with sharp glass (W25)
  foreign body or object entering through skin (W45)
  AHA: 2023,4Q,45-46

- **W44.A** Battery entering into or through a natural orifice
  - **W44.A0** Battery unspecified, entering into or through a natural orifice
  - **W44.A1** Button battery entering into or through a natural orifice
  - **W44.A9** Other batteries entering into or through a natural orifice
    ▶Cylindrical battery entering into or through a natural orifice◀

- **W44.B** Plastic entering into or through a natural orifice
  - **W44.B0** Plastic object unspecified, entering into or through a natural orifice
  - **W44.B1** Plastic bead entering into or through a natural orifice
    EXCLUDES 2: plastic jewelry entering into or through a natural orifice (W44.B4)
  - **W44.B2** Plastic coin entering into or through a natural orifice
  - **W44.B3** Plastic toy and toy part entering into or through a natural orifice
  - **W44.B4** Plastic jewelry entering into or through a natural orifice
    EXCLUDES 2: plastic bead entering into or through a natural orifice (W44.B1)
  - **W44.B5** Plastic bottle entering into or through a natural orifice
  - **W44.B9** Other plastic object entering into or through a natural orifice

- **W44.C** Glass entering into or through a natural orifice
  - **W44.C0** Glass unspecified, entering into or through a natural orifice
  - **W44.C1** Sharp glass entering into or through a natural orifice
    Glass shard entering into or through a natural orifice
  - **W44.C2** Intact glass entering into or through a natural orifice
    Intact glass bottle entering into or through a natural orifice

- **W44.D** Magnetic metal entering into or through a natural orifice
  - **W44.D0** Magnetic metal object unspecified, entering into or through a natural orifice
  - **W44.D1** Magnetic metal bead entering into or through a natural orifice
  - **W44.D2** Magnetic metal coin entering into or through a natural orifice
  - **W44.D3** Magnetic metal toy entering into or through a natural orifice
  - **W44.D4** Magnetic metal jewelry entering into or through a natural orifice
  - **W44.D9** Other magnetic metal objects entering into or through a natural orifice

- **W44.E** Non-magnetic metal entering into or through a natural orifice
  - **W44.E0** Non-magnetic metal object unspecified, entering into or through a natural orifice
  - **W44.E1** Non-magnetic metal bead entering into or through a natural orifice
  - **W44.E2** Non-magnetic metal coin entering into or through a natural orifice
  - **W44.E3** Non-magnetic metal toy entering into or through a natural orifice
  - **W44.E4** Non-magnetic metal jewelry entering into or through a natural orifice
  - **W44.E9** Other non-magnetic metal objects entering into or through a natural orifice
    Bottle cap entering into or through a natural orifice
    Can lid entering into or through a natural orifice
    Pull tab entering into or through a natural orifice

- **W44.F** Objects of natural or organic material entering into or through a natural orifice
  - **W44.F0** Objects of natural or organic material unspecified, entering into or through a natural orifice
  - **W44.F1** Bezoar entering into or through a natural orifice
  - **W44.F2** Rubber band entering into or through a natural orifice
  - **W44.F3** Food entering into or through a natural orifice
  - **W44.F4** Insect entering into or through a natural orifice
  - **W44.F9** Other object of natural or organic material, entering into or through a natural orifice

- **W44.G** Other non-organic objects entering into or through a natural orifice
  - **W44.G0** Other non-organic objects unspecified, entering into or through a natural orifice
  - **W44.G1** Audio device entering into or through a natural orifice
    Ear buds
    Hearing aids
  - **W44.G2** Combination metal and plastic toy and toy part entering into or through natural orifice
  - **W44.G3** Combination metal and plastic jewelry entering into or through a natural orifice
  - **W44.G9** Other non-organic objects entering into or through a natural orifice

- **W44.H** Other sharp object entering into or through a natural orifice
  - **W44.H0** Other sharp object unspecified, entering into or through a natural orifice
  - **W44.H1** Needle entering into or through a natural orifice
    Dart entering into or through a natural orifice
    Hypodermic needle entering into or through a natural orifice
    Safety pin entering into or through a natural orifice
    Sewing needle entering into or through a natural orifice
  - **W44.H2** Knife, sword or dagger entering into or through a natural orifice
  - **W44.H9** Other sharp object entering into or through a natural orifice
    Shard pottery entering into or through a natural orifice

- **W44.8** Other foreign body entering into or through a natural orifice
- **W44.9** Unspecified foreign body entering into or through a natural orifice
  Foreign body NOS entering into or through a natural orifice

W45 **Foreign body or object entering through skin**
  INCLUDES: foreign body or object embedded in skin
  nail embedded in skin
  EXCLUDES 2: contact with hand tools (nonpowered) (powered) (W27-W29)
  contact with other sharp objects (W26.-)
  contact with sharp glass (W25.-)
  struck by objects (W20-W22)

- **W45.0** Nail entering through skin
- **W45.3** Fishing hook entering through skin

Chapter 20. External Causes of Morbidity

- **W45.8** Other foreign body or object entering through skin
  - Splinter in skin NOS
- **W46** Contact with hypodermic needle
  - **W46.0** Contact with hypodermic needle
    - Hypodermic needle stick NOS
  - **W46.1** Contact with contaminated hypodermic needle
- **W49** Exposure to other inanimate mechanical forces
  - INCLUDES: exposure to abnormal gravitational [G] forces
    - exposure to inanimate mechanical forces NEC
  - EXCLUDES 1: exposure to inanimate mechanical forces involving military or war operations (Y36.-, Y37.-)
  - **W49.0** Item causing external constriction
    - **W49.01** Hair causing external constriction
    - **W49.02** String or thread causing external constriction
    - **W49.03** Rubber band causing external constriction
    - **W49.04** Ring or other jewelry causing external constriction
    - **W49.09** Other specified item causing external constriction
  - **W49.9** Exposure to other inanimate mechanical forces

Exposure to animate mechanical forces (W50-W64)

EXCLUDES 1: toxic effect of contact with venomous animals and plants (T63.-)

The appropriate 7th character is to be added to each code from categories W50-W64.
- A initial encounter
- D subsequent encounter
- S sequela

- **W50** Accidental hit, strike, kick, twist, bite or scratch by another person
  - INCLUDES: hit, strike, kick, twist, bite, or scratch by another person NOS
  - EXCLUDES 1: assault by bodily force (Y04)
    - struck by objects (W20-W22)
  - **W50.0** Accidental hit or strike by another person
    - Hit or strike by another person NOS
  - **W50.1** Accidental kick by another person
    - Kick by another person NOS
  - **W50.2** Accidental twist by another person
    - Twist by another person NOS
  - **W50.3** Accidental bite by another person
    - Bite by another person NOS
    - Human bite
  - **W50.4** Accidental scratch by another person
    - Scratch by another person NOS
- **W51** Accidental striking against or bumped into by another person
  - EXCLUDES 1: assault by striking against or bumping into by another person (Y04.2)
    - fall due to collision with another person (W03)
- **W52** Crushed, pushed or stepped on by crowd or human stampede
  - Crushed, pushed or stepped on by crowd or human stampede with or without fall
- **W53** Contact with rodent
  - INCLUDES: contact with saliva, feces or urine of rodent
  - **W53.0** Contact with mouse
    - **W53.01** Bitten by mouse
    - **W53.09** Other contact with mouse
  - **W53.1** Contact with rat
    - **W53.11** Bitten by rat
    - **W53.19** Other contact with rat
  - **W53.2** Contact with squirrel
    - **W53.21** Bitten by squirrel
    - **W53.29** Other contact with squirrel
  - **W53.8** Contact with other rodent
    - **W53.81** Bitten by other rodent
    - **W53.89** Other contact with other rodent
- **W54** Contact with dog
  - INCLUDES: contact with saliva, feces or urine of dog
  - **W54.0** Bitten by dog
  - **W54.1** Struck by dog
    - Knocked over by dog
  - **W54.8** Other contact with dog

- **W55** Contact with other mammals
  - INCLUDES: contact with saliva, feces or urine of mammal
  - EXCLUDES 1: animal being ridden - see transport accidents
    - bitten or struck by dog (W54)
    - bitten or struck by rodent (W53.-)
    - contact with marine mammals (W56.-)
  - **W55.0** Contact with cat
    - **W55.01** Bitten by cat
    - **W55.03** Scratched by cat
    - **W55.09** Other contact with cat
  - **W55.1** Contact with horse
    - **W55.11** Bitten by horse
    - **W55.12** Struck by horse
    - **W55.19** Other contact with horse
  - **W55.2** Contact with cow
    - Contact with bull
    - **W55.21** Bitten by cow
    - **W55.22** Struck by cow
      - Gored by bull
    - **W55.29** Other contact with cow
  - **W55.3** Contact with other hoof stock
    - Contact with goats
    - Contact with sheep
    - **W55.31** Bitten by other hoof stock
    - **W55.32** Struck by other hoof stock
      - Gored by goat
      - Gored by ram
    - **W55.39** Other contact with other hoof stock
  - **W55.4** Contact with pig
    - **W55.41** Bitten by pig
    - **W55.42** Struck by pig
    - **W55.49** Other contact with pig
  - **W55.5** Contact with raccoon
    - **W55.51** Bitten by raccoon
    - **W55.52** Struck by raccoon
    - **W55.59** Other contact with raccoon
  - **W55.8** Contact with other mammals
    - **W55.81** Bitten by other mammals
    - **W55.82** Struck by other mammals
    - **W55.89** Other contact with other mammals
- **W56** Contact with nonvenomous marine animal
  - EXCLUDES 1: contact with venomous marine animal (T63.-)
  - **W56.0** Contact with dolphin
    - **W56.01** Bitten by dolphin
    - **W56.02** Struck by dolphin
    - **W56.09** Other contact with dolphin
  - **W56.1** Contact with sea lion
    - **W56.11** Bitten by sea lion
    - **W56.12** Struck by sea lion
    - **W56.19** Other contact with sea lion
  - **W56.2** Contact with orca
    - Contact with killer whale
    - **W56.21** Bitten by orca
    - **W56.22** Struck by orca
    - **W56.29** Other contact with orca
  - **W56.3** Contact with other marine mammals
    - **W56.31** Bitten by other marine mammals
    - **W56.32** Struck by other marine mammals
    - **W56.39** Other contact with other marine mammals
  - **W56.4** Contact with shark
    - **W56.41** Bitten by shark
    - **W56.42** Struck by shark
    - **W56.49** Other contact with shark
  - **W56.5** Contact with other fish
    - **W56.51** Bitten by other fish
    - **W56.52** Struck by other fish
    - **W56.59** Other contact with other fish

Additional Character Required | Placeholder Alert | 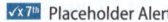 Manifestation | Unspecified Dx | QPP | Unacceptable PDx

Chapter 20. External Causes of Morbidity

- ✓5th **W56.8** Contact with other nonvenomous marine animals
  - ✓x7th **W56.81** Bitten by other nonvenomous marine animals
  - ✓x7th **W56.82** Struck by other nonvenomous marine animals
  - ✓x7th **W56.89** Other contact with other nonvenomous marine animals
- ✓x7th **W57** Bitten or stung by nonvenomous insect and other nonvenomous arthropods
  - EXCLUDES 1 contact with venomous insects and arthropods (T63.2-, T63.3-, T63.4-)
- ✓4th **W58** Contact with crocodile or alligator
  - ✓5th **W58.0** Contact with alligator
    - ✓x7th **W58.01** Bitten by alligator
    - ✓x7th **W58.02** Struck by alligator
    - ✓x7th **W58.03** Crushed by alligator
    - ✓x7th **W58.09** Other contact with alligator
  - ✓5th **W58.1** Contact with crocodile
    - ✓x7th **W58.11** Bitten by crocodile
    - ✓x7th **W58.12** Struck by crocodile
    - ✓x7th **W58.13** Crushed by crocodile
    - ✓x7th **W58.19** Other contact with crocodile
- ✓4th **W59** Contact with other nonvenomous reptiles
  - EXCLUDES 1 contact with venomous reptile (T63.0-, T63.1-)
  - ✓5th **W59.0** Contact with nonvenomous lizards
    - ✓x7th **W59.01** Bitten by nonvenomous lizards
    - ✓x7th **W59.02** Struck by nonvenomous lizards
    - ✓x7th **W59.09** Other contact with nonvenomous lizards
      Exposure to nonvenomous lizards
  - ✓5th **W59.1** Contact with nonvenomous snakes
    - ✓x7th **W59.11** Bitten by nonvenomous snake
    - ✓x7th **W59.12** Struck by nonvenomous snake
    - ✓x7th **W59.13** Crushed by nonvenomous snake
    - ✓x7th **W59.19** Other contact with nonvenomous snake
  - ✓5th **W59.2** Contact with turtles
    - EXCLUDES 1 contact with tortoises (W59.8-)
    - ✓x7th **W59.21** Bitten by turtle
    - ✓x7th **W59.22** Struck by turtle
    - ✓x7th **W59.29** Other contact with turtle
      Exposure to turtles
  - ✓5th **W59.8** Contact with other nonvenomous reptiles
    - ✓x7th **W59.81** Bitten by other nonvenomous reptiles
    - ✓x7th **W59.82** Struck by other nonvenomous reptiles
    - ✓x7th **W59.83** Crushed by other nonvenomous reptiles
    - ✓x7th **W59.89** Other contact with other nonvenomous reptiles
- ✓x7th **W60** Contact with nonvenomous plant thorns and spines and sharp leaves
  - EXCLUDES 1 contact with venomous plants (T63.7-)
- ✓4th **W61** Contact with birds (domestic) (wild)
  - INCLUDES contact with excreta of birds
  - ✓5th **W61.0** Contact with parrot
    - ✓x7th **W61.01** Bitten by parrot
    - ✓x7th **W61.02** Struck by parrot
    - ✓x7th **W61.09** Other contact with parrot
      Exposure to parrots
  - ✓5th **W61.1** Contact with macaw
    - ✓x7th **W61.11** Bitten by macaw
    - ✓x7th **W61.12** Struck by macaw
    - ✓x7th **W61.19** Other contact with macaw
      Exposure to macaws
  - ✓5th **W61.2** Contact with other psittacines
    - ✓x7th **W61.21** Bitten by other psittacines
    - ✓x7th **W61.22** Struck by other psittacines
    - ✓x7th **W61.29** Other contact with other psittacines
      Exposure to other psittacines
  - ✓5th **W61.3** Contact with chicken
    - ✓x7th **W61.32** Struck by chicken
    - ✓x7th **W61.33** Pecked by chicken
    - ✓x7th **W61.39** Other contact with chicken
      Exposure to chickens
  - ✓5th **W61.4** Contact with turkey
    - ✓x7th **W61.42** Struck by turkey
    - ✓x7th **W61.43** Pecked by turkey
    - ✓x7th **W61.49** Other contact with turkey
  - ✓5th **W61.5** Contact with goose
    - ✓x7th **W61.51** Bitten by goose
    - ✓x7th **W61.52** Struck by goose
    - ✓x7th **W61.59** Other contact with goose
  - ✓5th **W61.6** Contact with duck
    - ✓x7th **W61.61** Bitten by duck
    - ✓x7th **W61.62** Struck by duck
    - ✓x7th **W61.69** Other contact with duck
  - ✓5th **W61.9** Contact with other birds
    - ✓x7th **W61.91** Bitten by other birds
    - ✓x7th **W61.92** Struck by other birds
    - ✓x7th **W61.99** Other contact with other birds
      Contact with bird NOS
- ✓4th **W62** Contact with nonvenomous amphibians
  - EXCLUDES 1 contact with venomous amphibians (T63.81-T63.83)
  - ✓x7th **W62.0** Contact with nonvenomous frogs
  - ✓x7th **W62.1** Contact with nonvenomous toads
  - ✓x7th **W62.9** Contact with other nonvenomous amphibians
- ✓x7th **W64** Exposure to other animate mechanical forces
  - INCLUDES exposure to nonvenomous animal NOS
  - EXCLUDES 1 contact with venomous animal (T63.-)

Accidental non-transport drowning and submersion (W65-W74)

EXCLUDES 1 accidental drowning and submersion due to fall into water (W16.-)
accidental drowning and submersion due to water transport accident (V90.-, V92.-)
EXCLUDES 2 accidental drowning and submersion due to cataclysm (X34-X39)

The appropriate 7th character is to be added to each code from categories W65-W74.
- A initial encounter
- D subsequent encounter
- S sequela

- ✓x7th **W65** Accidental drowning and submersion while in bath-tub
  - EXCLUDES 1 accidental drowning and submersion due to fall in (into) bathtub (W16.211)
- ✓x7th **W67** Accidental drowning and submersion while in swimming-pool
  - EXCLUDES 1 accidental drowning and submersion due to fall into swimming pool (W16.011, W16.021, W16.031)
  accidental drowning and submersion due to striking into wall of swimming pool (W22.041)
  - **AHA:** 2023,1Q,25
- ✓x7th **W69** Accidental drowning and submersion while in natural water
  Accidental drowning and submersion while in lake
  Accidental drowning and submersion while in open sea
  Accidental drowning and submersion while in river
  Accidental drowning and submersion while in stream
  - EXCLUDES 1 accidental drowning and submersion due to fall into natural body of water (W16.111, W16.121, W16.131)
- ✓x7th **W73** Other specified cause of accidental non-transport drowning and submersion
  Accidental drowning and submersion while in quenching tank
  Accidental drowning and submersion while in reservoir
  - EXCLUDES 1 accidental drowning and submersion due to fall into other water (W16.311, W16.321, W16.331)
- ✓x7th **W74** Unspecified cause of accidental drowning and submersion
  Drowning NOS

Exposure to electric current, radiation and extreme ambient air temperature and pressure (W85-W99)

EXCLUDES 1 exposure to:
  failure in dosage of radiation or temperature during surgical and medical care (Y63.2-Y63.5)
  lightning (T75.0-)
  natural cold (X31)
  natural heat (X30)
  natural radiation NOS (X39)
  radiological procedure and radiotherapy (Y84.2)
  sunlight (X32)

AHA: 2018,2Q,7-8

The appropriate 7th character is to be added to each code from categories W85-W99.
  A initial encounter
  D subsequent encounter
  S sequela

W85 Exposure to electric transmission lines
  Broken power line

W86 Exposure to other specified electric current
  W86.0 Exposure to domestic wiring and appliances
  W86.1 Exposure to industrial wiring, appliances and electrical machinery
    Exposure to conductors
    Exposure to control apparatus
    Exposure to electrical equipment and machinery
    Exposure to transformers
  W86.8 Exposure to other electric current
    Exposure to wiring and appliances in or on farm (not farmhouse)
    Exposure to wiring and appliances in or on public building
    Exposure to wiring and appliances in or on residential institutions
    Exposure to wiring and appliances in or on schools
    Exposure to wiring and appliances outdoors

W88 Exposure to ionizing radiation
  EXCLUDES 1 exposure to sunlight (X32)
  W88.0 Exposure to X-rays
  W88.1 Exposure to radioactive isotopes
  W88.8 Exposure to other ionizing radiation

W89 Exposure to man-made visible and ultraviolet light
  INCLUDES exposure to welding light (arc)
  EXCLUDES 2 exposure to sunlight (X32)
  W89.0 Exposure to welding light (arc)
  W89.1 Exposure to tanning bed
  W89.8 Exposure to other man-made visible and ultraviolet light
  W89.9 Exposure to unspecified man-made visible and ultraviolet light

W90 Exposure to other nonionizing radiation
  EXCLUDES 2 exposure to sunlight (X32)
  AHA: 2019,1Q,21
  W90.0 Exposure to radiofrequency
  W90.1 Exposure to infrared radiation
  W90.2 Exposure to laser radiation
  W90.8 Exposure to other nonionizing radiation

W92 Exposure to excessive heat of man-made origin

W93 Exposure to excessive cold of man-made origin
  W93.0 Contact with or inhalation of dry ice
    W93.01 Contact with dry ice
    W93.02 Inhalation of dry ice
  W93.1 Contact with or inhalation of liquid air
    W93.11 Contact with liquid air
      Contact with liquid hydrogen
      Contact with liquid nitrogen
    W93.12 Inhalation of liquid air
      Inhalation of liquid hydrogen
      Inhalation of liquid nitrogen
  W93.2 Prolonged exposure in deep freeze unit or refrigerator
  W93.8 Exposure to other excessive cold of man-made origin

W94 Exposure to high and low air pressure and changes in air pressure
  W94.0 Exposure to prolonged high air pressure
  W94.1 Exposure to prolonged low air pressure
    W94.11 Exposure to residence or prolonged visit at high altitude
    W94.12 Exposure to other prolonged low air pressure
  W94.2 Exposure to rapid changes in air pressure during ascent
    W94.21 Exposure to reduction in atmospheric pressure while surfacing from deep-water diving
    W94.22 Exposure to reduction in atmospheric pressure while surfacing from underground
    W94.23 Exposure to sudden change in air pressure in aircraft during ascent
    W94.29 Exposure to other rapid changes in air pressure during ascent
  W94.3 Exposure to rapid changes in air pressure during descent
    W94.31 Exposure to sudden change in air pressure in aircraft during descent
    W94.32 Exposure to high air pressure from rapid descent in water
    W94.39 Exposure to other rapid changes in air pressure during descent

W99 Exposure to other man-made environmental factors

Exposure to smoke, fire and flames (X00-X08)

EXCLUDES 1 arson (X97)
EXCLUDES 2 explosions (W35-W40)
  lightning (T75.0-)
  transport accident (V01-V99)

AHA: 2018,2Q,7-8

The appropriate 7th character is to be added to each code from categories X00-X08.
  A initial encounter
  D subsequent encounter
  S sequela

X00 Exposure to uncontrolled fire in building or structure
  INCLUDES conflagration in building or structure
  Code first any associated cataclysm
  EXCLUDES 2 exposure to ignition or melting of nightwear (X05)
    exposure to ignition or melting of other clothing and apparel (X06.-)
    exposure to other specified smoke, fire and flames (X08.-)
  AHA: 2016,2Q,5
  X00.0 Exposure to flames in uncontrolled fire in building or structure
  X00.1 Exposure to smoke in uncontrolled fire in building or structure
  X00.2 Injury due to collapse of burning building or structure in uncontrolled fire
    EXCLUDES 1 injury due to collapse of building not on fire (W20.1)
  X00.3 Fall from burning building or structure in uncontrolled fire
  X00.4 Hit by object from burning building or structure in uncontrolled fire
    AHA: 2016,2Q,4
  X00.5 Jump from burning building or structure in uncontrolled fire
  X00.8 Other exposure to uncontrolled fire in building or structure

X01 Exposure to uncontrolled fire, not in building or structure
  INCLUDES exposure to forest fire
  X01.0 Exposure to flames in uncontrolled fire, not in building or structure
  X01.1 Exposure to smoke in uncontrolled fire, not in building or structure
  X01.3 Fall due to uncontrolled fire, not in building or structure
  X01.4 Hit by object due to uncontrolled fire, not in building or structure
  X01.8 Other exposure to uncontrolled fire, not in building or structure

X02 Exposure to controlled fire in building or structure
  INCLUDES exposure to fire in fireplace
    exposure to fire in stove
  X02.0 Exposure to flames in controlled fire in building or structure
  X02.1 Exposure to smoke in controlled fire in building or structure
  X02.2 Injury due to collapse of burning building or structure in controlled fire
    EXCLUDES 1 injury due to collapse of building not on fire (W20.1)
  X02.3 Fall from burning building or structure in controlled fire
  X02.4 Hit by object from burning building or structure in controlled fire
  X02.5 Jump from burning building or structure in controlled fire
  X02.8 Other exposure to controlled fire in building or structure

X03 Exposure to controlled fire, not in building or structure
INCLUDES exposure to bon fire
exposure to camp-fire
exposure to trash fire

- X03.0 Exposure to flames in controlled fire, not in building or structure
- X03.1 Exposure to smoke in controlled fire, not in building or structure
- X03.3 Fall due to controlled fire, not in building or structure
- X03.4 Hit by object due to controlled fire, not in building or structure
- X03.8 Other exposure to controlled fire, not in building or structure

X04 Exposure to ignition of highly flammable material
Exposure to ignition of gasoline
Exposure to ignition of kerosene
Exposure to ignition of petrol

EXCLUDES 2 exposure to ignition or melting of nightwear (X05)
exposure to ignition or melting of other clothing and apparel (X06)

AHA: 2016,2Q,4

X05 Exposure to ignition or melting of nightwear
EXCLUDES 2 exposure to uncontrolled fire in building or structure (X00.-)
exposure to controlled fire in building or structure (X02.-)
exposure to controlled fire, not in building or structure (X03.-)
exposure to ignition of highly flammable materials (X04.-)
exposure to uncontrolled fire, not in building or structure (X01.-)

X06 Exposure to ignition or melting of other clothing and apparel
EXCLUDES 2 exposure to uncontrolled fire in building or structure (X00.-)
exposure to controlled fire in building or structure (X02.-)
exposure to controlled fire, not in building or structure (X03.-)
exposure to ignition of highly flammable materials (X04.-)
exposure to uncontrolled fire, not in building or structure (X01.-)

- X06.0 Exposure to ignition of plastic jewelry
- X06.1 Exposure to melting of plastic jewelry
- X06.2 Exposure to ignition of other clothing and apparel
- X06.3 Exposure to melting of other clothing and apparel

X08 Exposure to other specified smoke, fire and flames
- X08.0 Exposure to bed fire
  Exposure to mattress fire
  - X08.00 Exposure to bed fire due to unspecified burning material
  - X08.01 Exposure to bed fire due to burning cigarette
  - X08.09 Exposure to bed fire due to other burning material
- X08.1 Exposure to sofa fire
  - X08.10 Exposure to sofa fire due to unspecified burning material
  - X08.11 Exposure to sofa fire due to burning cigarette
  - X08.19 Exposure to sofa fire due to other burning material
- X08.2 Exposure to other furniture fire
  - X08.20 Exposure to other furniture fire due to unspecified burning material
  - X08.21 Exposure to other furniture fire due to burning cigarette
  - X08.29 Exposure to other furniture fire due to other burning material
- X08.8 Exposure to other specified smoke, fire and flames

Contact with heat and hot substances (X10-X19)
EXCLUDES 1 exposure to excessive natural heat (X30)
exposure to fire and flames (X00-X08)

AHA: 2018,2Q,7-8

The appropriate 7th character is to be added to each code from categories X10-X19.
- A initial encounter
- D subsequent encounter
- S sequela

X10 Contact with hot drinks, food, fats and cooking oils
- X10.0 Contact with hot drinks
- X10.1 Contact with hot food
- X10.2 Contact with fats and cooking oils

X11 Contact with hot tap-water
INCLUDES contact with boiling tap-water
contact with boiling water NOS
EXCLUDES 1 contact with water heated on stove (X12)

- X11.0 Contact with hot water in bath or tub
  EXCLUDES 1 contact with running hot water in bath or tub (X11.1)
- X11.1 Contact with running hot water
  Contact with hot water running out of hose
  Contact with hot water running out of tap
- X11.8 Contact with other hot tap-water
  Contact with hot tap-water NOS
  Contact with hot water in bucket

X12 Contact with other hot fluids
Contact with water heated on stove
EXCLUDES 1 hot (liquid) metals (X18)

X13 Contact with steam and other hot vapors
- X13.0 Inhalation of steam and other hot vapors
- X13.1 Other contact with steam and other hot vapors

X14 Contact with hot air and other hot gases
- X14.0 Inhalation of hot air and gases
- X14.1 Other contact with hot air and other hot gases

X15 Contact with hot household appliances
EXCLUDES 1 contact with heating appliances (X16)
contact with powered household appliances (W29.-)
exposure to controlled fire in building or structure due to household appliance (X02.8)
exposure to household appliances electrical current (W86.0)

- X15.0 Contact with hot stove (kitchen)
- X15.1 Contact with hot toaster
- X15.2 Contact with hotplate
- X15.3 Contact with hot saucepan or skillet
  Contact with hot cooking pan
  Contact with hot cooking pot
- X15.8 Contact with other hot household appliances
  Contact with cooker
  Contact with kettle
  Contact with light bulbs

X16 Contact with hot heating appliances, radiators and pipes
EXCLUDES 1 contact with powered appliances (W29.-)
exposure to controlled fire in building or structure due to appliance (X02.8)
exposure to industrial appliances electrical current (W86.1)

X17 Contact with hot engines, machinery and tools
EXCLUDES 1 contact with hot heating appliances, radiators and pipes (X16)
contact with hot household appliances (X15)

X18 Contact with other hot metals
Contact with liquid metal

X19 Contact with other heat and hot substances
EXCLUDES 1 objects that are not normally hot, e.g., an object made hot by a house fire (X00-X08)

Exposure to forces of nature (X30-X39)
AHA: 2018,2Q,7-8

The appropriate 7th character is to be added to each code from categories X30-X39.
- A initial encounter
- D subsequent encounter
- S sequela

X30 Exposure to excessive natural heat
Exposure to excessive heat as the cause of sunstroke
Exposure to heat NOS
EXCLUDES 1 excessive heat of man-made origin (W92)
exposure to man-made radiation (W89)
exposure to sunlight (X32)
exposure to tanning bed (W89)

Chapter 20. External Causes of Morbidity

X31 Exposure to excessive natural cold
Excessive cold as the cause of chilblains NOS
Excessive cold as the cause of immersion foot or hand
Exposure to cold NOS
Exposure to weather conditions
EXCLUDES 1 cold of man-made origin (W93.-)
contact with or inhalation of dry ice (W93.-)
contact with or inhalation of liquefied gas (W93.-)

X32 Exposure to sunlight
EXCLUDES 1 man-made radiation (tanning bed) (W89)
EXCLUDES 2 radiation-related disorders of the skin and subcutaneous tissue (L55-L59)

X34 Earthquake
EXCLUDES 2 tidal wave (tsunami) due to earthquake (X37.41)

X35 Volcanic eruption
EXCLUDES 2 tidal wave (tsunami) due to volcanic eruption (X37.41)

X36 Avalanche, landslide and other earth movements
INCLUDES victim of mudslide of cataclysmic nature
EXCLUDES 1 earthquake (X34)
EXCLUDES 2 transport accident involving collision with avalanche or landslide not in motion (V01-V99)

   X36.0 Collapse of dam or man-made structure causing earth movement

   X36.1 Avalanche, landslide, or mudslide

X37 Cataclysmic storm
   X37.0 Hurricane
Storm surge
Typhoon
   X37.1 Tornado
Cyclone
Twister
   X37.2 Blizzard (snow)(ice)
   X37.3 Dust storm
   X37.4 Tidalwave
      X37.41 Tidal wave due to earthquake or volcanic eruption
Tidal wave NOS
Tsunami
      X37.42 Tidal wave due to storm
      X37.43 Tidal wave due to landslide
   X37.8 Other cataclysmic storms
Cloudburst
Torrential rain
EXCLUDES 2 flood (X38)
   X37.9 Unspecified cataclysmic storm
Storm NOS
EXCLUDES 1 collapse of dam or man-made structure causing earth movement (X36.0)

X38 Flood
Flood arising from remote storm
Flood of cataclysmic nature arising from melting snow
Flood resulting directly from storm
EXCLUDES 1 collapse of dam or man-made structure causing earth movement (X36.0)
tidal wave caused by storm (X37.42)
tidal wave NOS (X37.41)

X39 Exposure to other forces of nature
   X39.0 Exposure to natural radiation
EXCLUDES 1 contact with and (suspected) exposure to radon and other naturally occurring radiation (Z77.123)
exposure to man-made radiation (W88-W90)
exposure to sunlight (X32)
      X39.01 Exposure to radon
      X39.08 Exposure to other natural radiation
   X39.8 Other exposure to forces of nature

Overexertion and strenuous or repetitive movements (X50)

X50 Overexertion and strenuous or repetitive movements
AHA: 2018,2Q,7-8; 2016,4Q,73-74

The appropriate 7th character is to be added to each code from category X50.
A initial encounter
D subsequent encounter
S sequela

   X50.0 Overexertion from strenuous movement or load
Lifting heavy objects
Lifting weights
   X50.1 Overexertion from prolonged static or awkward postures
Prolonged bending
Prolonged kneeling
Prolonged reaching
Prolonged sitting
Prolonged standing
Prolonged twisting
Static bending
Static kneeling
Static reaching
Static sitting
Static standing
Static twisting
   X50.3 Overexertion from repetitive movements
Use of hand as hammer
EXCLUDES 2 overuse from prolonged static or awkward postures (X50.1)
   X50.9 Other and unspecified overexertion or strenuous movements or postures
Contact pressure
Contact stress

Accidental exposure to other specified factors (X52-X58)

AHA: 2018,2Q,7-8

The appropriate 7th character is to be added to each code from categories X52-X58.
A initial encounter
D subsequent encounter
S sequela

X52 Prolonged stay in weightless environment
Weightlessness in spacecraft (simulator)

X58 Exposure to other specified factors
Accident NOS
Exposure NOS

Intentional self-harm (X71-X83)

Purposely self-inflicted injury
Suicide (attempted)

The appropriate 7th character is to be added to each code from categories X71-X83.
A initial encounter
D subsequent encounter
S sequela

X71 Intentional self-harm by drowning and submersion
   X71.0 Intentional self-harm by drowning and submersion while in bathtub
   X71.1 Intentional self-harm by drowning and submersion while in swimming pool
   X71.2 Intentional self-harm by drowning and submersion after jump into swimming pool
   X71.3 Intentional self-harm by drowning and submersion in natural water
   X71.8 Other intentional self-harm by drowning and submersion
   X71.9 Intentional self-harm by drowning and submersion, unspecified

X72 Intentional self-harm by handgun discharge
Intentional self-harm by gun for single hand use
Intentional self-harm by pistol
Intentional self-harm by revolver
EXCLUDES 1 Very pistol (X74.8)

X73 Intentional self-harm by rifle, shotgun and larger firearm discharge
EXCLUDES 1 airgun (X74.01)
   X73.0 Intentional self-harm by shotgun discharge

	X73.1	Intentional self-harm by hunting rifle discharge
	X73.2	Intentional self-harm by machine gun discharge
	X73.8	Intentional self-harm by other larger firearm discharge
	X73.9	Intentional self-harm by unspecified larger firearm discharge

- **X74** Intentional self-harm by other and unspecified firearm and gun discharge
  - **X74.0** Intentional self-harm by gas, air or spring-operated guns
    - X74.01 Intentional self-harm by airgun
      - Intentional self-harm by BB gun discharge
      - Intentional self-harm by pellet gun discharge
    - X74.02 Intentional self-harm by paintball gun
    - X74.09 Intentional self-harm by other gas, air or spring-operated gun
  - X74.8 Intentional self-harm by other firearm discharge
    - Intentional self-harm by Very pistol [flare] discharge
  - X74.9 Intentional self-harm by unspecified firearm discharge
- X75 Intentional self-harm by explosive material
- X76 Intentional self-harm by smoke, fire and flames
- **X77** Intentional self-harm by steam, hot vapors and hot objects
  - X77.0 Intentional self-harm by steam or hot vapors
  - X77.1 Intentional self-harm by hot tap water
  - X77.2 Intentional self-harm by other hot fluids
  - X77.3 Intentional self-harm by hot household appliances
  - X77.8 Intentional self-harm by other hot objects
  - X77.9 Intentional self-harm by unspecified hot objects
- **X78** Intentional self-harm by sharp object
  - X78.0 Intentional self-harm by sharp glass
  - X78.1 Intentional self-harm by knife
  - X78.2 Intentional self-harm by sword or dagger
  - X78.8 Intentional self-harm by other sharp object
    - **AHA:** 2022,1Q,27
  - X78.9 Intentional self-harm by unspecified sharp object
- X79 Intentional self-harm by blunt object
- X80 Intentional self-harm by jumping from a high place
  - Intentional fall from one level to another
- **X81** Intentional self-harm by jumping or lying in front of moving object
  - X81.0 Intentional self-harm by jumping or lying in front of motor vehicle
  - X81.1 Intentional self-harm by jumping or lying in front of (subway) train
  - X81.8 Intentional self-harm by jumping or lying in front of other moving object
- **X82** Intentional self-harm by crashing of motor vehicle
  - X82.0 Intentional collision of motor vehicle with other motor vehicle
  - X82.1 Intentional collision of motor vehicle with train
  - X82.2 Intentional collision of motor vehicle with tree
  - X82.8 Other intentional self-harm by crashing of motor vehicle
- **X83** Intentional self-harm by other specified means
  - *EXCLUDES 1* intentional self-harm by poisoning or contact with toxic substance - see Table of Drugs and Chemicals
  - X83.0 Intentional self-harm by crashing of aircraft
  - X83.1 Intentional self-harm by electrocution
  - X83.2 Intentional self-harm by exposure to extremes of cold
  - X83.8 Intentional self-harm by other specified means

Assault (X92-Y09)

INCLUDES homicide
injuries inflicted by another person with intent to injure or kill, by any means

EXCLUDES 1 injuries due to legal intervention (Y35.-)
injuries due to operations of war (Y36.-)
injuries due to terrorism (Y38.-)

The appropriate 7th character is to be added to each code from categories X92-Y04 and Y08.
- A initial encounter
- D subsequent encounter
- S sequela

- **X92** Assault by drowning and submersion
  - X92.0 Assault by drowning and submersion while in bathtub
  - X92.1 Assault by drowning and submersion while in swimming pool
  - X92.2 Assault by drowning and submersion after push into swimming pool
  - X92.3 Assault by drowning and submersion in natural water
  - X92.8 Other assault by drowning and submersion
  - X92.9 Assault by drowning and submersion, unspecified
- X93 Assault by handgun discharge
  - Assault by discharge of gun for single hand use
  - Assault by discharge of pistol
  - Assault by discharge of revolver
  - *EXCLUDES 1* Very pistol (X95.8)
- **X94** Assault by rifle, shotgun and larger firearm discharge
  - *EXCLUDES 1* airgun (X95.01)
  - X94.0 Assault by shotgun
  - X94.1 Assault by hunting rifle
  - X94.2 Assault by machine gun
  - X94.8 Assault by other larger firearm discharge
  - X94.9 Assault by unspecified larger firearm discharge
- **X95** Assault by other and unspecified firearm and gun discharge
  - **X95.0** Assault by gas, air or spring-operated guns
    - X95.01 Assault by airgun discharge
      - Assault by BB gun discharge
      - Assault by pellet gun discharge
    - X95.02 Assault by paintball gun discharge
    - X95.09 Assault by other gas, air or spring-operated gun
  - X95.8 Assault by other firearm discharge
    - Assault by Very pistol [flare] discharge
  - X95.9 Assault by unspecified firearm discharge
    - **AHA:** 2025,1Q,31; 2023,3Q,8,12
- **X96** Assault by explosive material
  - *EXCLUDES 1* incendiary device (X97)
    terrorism involving explosive material (Y38.2-)
  - X96.0 Assault by antipersonnel bomb
    - *EXCLUDES 1* antipersonnel bomb use in military or war (Y36.2-)
  - X96.1 Assault by gasoline bomb
  - X96.2 Assault by letter bomb
  - X96.3 Assault by fertilizer bomb
  - X96.4 Assault by pipe bomb
  - X96.8 Assault by other specified explosive
  - X96.9 Assault by unspecified explosive
- X97 Assault by smoke, fire and flames
  - Assault by arson
  - Assault by cigarettes
  - Assault by incendiary device
- **X98** Assault by steam, hot vapors and hot objects
  - X98.0 Assault by steam or hot vapors
  - X98.1 Assault by hot tap water
  - X98.2 Assault by hot fluids
  - X98.3 Assault by hot household appliances
  - X98.8 Assault by other hot objects
  - X98.9 Assault by unspecified hot objects
- **X99** Assault by sharp object
  - *EXCLUDES 1* assault by strike by sports equipment (Y08.0-)
  - X99.0 Assault by sharp glass

X99.1 Assault by knife
X99.2 Assault by sword or dagger
X99.8 Assault by other sharp object
X99.9 Assault by unspecified sharp object
 Assault by stabbing NOS

Y00 Assault by blunt object
 EXCLUDES 1 assault by strike by sports equipment (Y08.0-)

Y01 Assault by pushing from high place

Y02 Assault by pushing or placing victim in front of moving object
 Y02.0 Assault by pushing or placing victim in front of motor vehicle
 Y02.1 Assault by pushing or placing victim in front of (subway) train
 Y02.8 Assault by pushing or placing victim in front of other moving object

Y03 Assault by crashing of motor vehicle
 Y03.0 Assault by being hit or run over by motor vehicle
 Y03.8 Other assault by crashing of motor vehicle

Y04 Assault by bodily force
 EXCLUDES 1 assault by:
  submersion (X92.-)
  use of weapon (X93-X95, X99, Y00)
 Y04.0 Assault by unarmed brawl or fight
 Y04.1 Assault by human bite
 Y04.2 Assault by strike against or bumped into by another person
 Y04.8 Assault by other bodily force
  Assault by bodily force NOS

Y07 Perpetrator of assault, maltreatment and neglect
 NOTE Codes from this category are for use only in cases of confirmed abuse (T74.-)
 Selection of the correct perpetrator code is based on the relationship between the perpetrator and the victim
 INCLUDES perpetrator of abandonment
  perpetrator of emotional neglect
  perpetrator of mental cruelty
  perpetrator of physical abuse
  perpetrator of physical neglect
  perpetrator of sexual abuse
  perpetrator of torture
  perpetrator of verbal abuse
 Y07.0 Spouse or partner, perpetrator of maltreatment and neglect
  Spouse or partner, perpetrator of maltreatment and neglect against spouse or partner
  AHA: 2023,1Q,5
  Y07.01 Husband, perpetrator of maltreatment and neglect
   Y07.010 Husband, current, perpetrator of maltreatment and neglect
   Y07.011 Husband, former, perpetrator of maltreatment and neglect
  Y07.02 Wife, perpetrator of maltreatment and neglect
   Y07.020 Wife, current, perpetrator of maltreatment and neglect
   Y07.021 Wife, former, perpetrator of maltreatment and neglect
  Y07.03 Male partner, perpetrator of maltreatment and neglect
   Male intimate or dating partner, perpetrator of maltreatment and neglect
   Y07.030 Male partner, current, perpetrator of maltreatment and neglect
   Y07.031 Male partner, former, perpetrator of maltreatment and neglect
  Y07.04 Female partner, perpetrator of maltreatment and neglect
   Female intimate or dating partner, perpetrator of maltreatment and neglect
   Y07.040 Female partner, current, perpetrator of maltreatment and neglect
   Y07.041 Female partner, former, perpetrator of maltreatment and neglect
  Y07.05 Non-binary partner, perpetrator of maltreatment and neglect
   Gender non-conforming partner, perpetrator of maltreatment and neglect
   Y07.050 Non-binary partner, current, perpetrator of maltreatment and neglect
   Y07.051 Non-binary partner, former, perpetrator of maltreatment and neglect
 Y07.1 Parent (adoptive) (biological), perpetrator of maltreatment and neglect
  Y07.11 Biological father, perpetrator of maltreatment and neglect
  Y07.12 Biological mother, perpetrator of maltreatment and neglect
  Y07.13 Adoptive father, perpetrator of maltreatment and neglect
  Y07.14 Adoptive mother, perpetrator of maltreatment and neglect
 Y07.4 Other family member, perpetrator of maltreatment and neglect
  AHA: 2023,1Q,5
  Y07.41 Sibling, perpetrator of maltreatment and neglect
   EXCLUDES 1 stepsibling, perpetrator of maltreatment and neglect (Y07.435, Y07.436)
   Y07.410 Brother, perpetrator of maltreatment and neglect
   Y07.411 Sister, perpetrator of maltreatment and neglect
  Y07.42 Foster parent, perpetrator of maltreatment and neglect
   Y07.420 Foster father, perpetrator of maltreatment and neglect
   Y07.421 Foster mother, perpetrator of maltreatment and neglect
  Y07.43 Stepparent or stepsibling, perpetrator of maltreatment and neglect
   Y07.430 Stepfather, perpetrator of maltreatment and neglect
   Y07.432 Male friend of parent (co-residing in household), perpetrator of maltreatment and neglect
   Y07.433 Stepmother, perpetrator of maltreatment and neglect
   Y07.434 Female friend of parent (co-residing in household), perpetrator of maltreatment and neglect
   Y07.435 Stepbrother, perpetrator of maltreatment and neglect
   Y07.436 Stepsister, perpetrator of maltreatment and neglect
  Y07.44 Child, perpetrator of maltreatment and neglect
   Adopted child, perpetrator of maltreatment and neglect
   Biological child, perpetrator of maltreatment and neglect
   Daughter, perpetrator of maltreatment and neglect
   Foster child, perpetrator of maltreatment and neglect
   In-law child, perpetrator of maltreatment and neglect
   Non-binary child, perpetrator of maltreatment and neglect
   Son, perpetrator of maltreatment and neglect
   Stepchild, perpetrator of maltreatment and neglect
  Y07.45 Grandchild, perpetrator of maltreatment and neglect
   Adopted grandchild, perpetrator of maltreatment and neglect
   Biological grandchild, perpetrator of maltreatment and neglect
   Foster grandchild, perpetrator of maltreatment and neglect
   Granddaughter, perpetrator of maltreatment and neglect
   Grandson, perpetrator of maltreatment and neglect
   In-law grandchild, perpetrator of maltreatment and neglect
   Non-binary grandchild, perpetrator of maltreatment and neglect
   Step grandchild, perpetrator of maltreatment and neglect
  Y07.46 Grandparent, perpetrator of maltreatment and neglect
   Grandfather, perpetrator of maltreatment and neglect
   Grandmother, perpetrator of maltreatment and neglect
   Non-binary grandparent, perpetrator of maltreatment and neglect
  Y07.47 Parental sibling, perpetrator of maltreatment and neglect
   Aunt, perpetrator of maltreatment and neglect
   Non-binary parental sibling, perpetrator of maltreatment and neglect
   Uncle, perpetrator of maltreatment and neglect

- ✓6th **Y07.49** Other family member, perpetrator of maltreatment and neglect
  - **Y07.490** Male cousin, perpetrator of maltreatment and neglect
  - **Y07.491** Female cousin, perpetrator of maltreatment and neglect
  - **Y07.499** Other family member, perpetrator of maltreatment and neglect
- ✓5th **Y07.5** Non-family member, perpetrator of maltreatment and neglect
  - AHA: 2023,1Q,5
  - **Y07.50** Unspecified non-family member, perpetrator of maltreatment and neglect
  - ✓6th **Y07.51** Daycare provider, perpetrator of maltreatment and neglect
    - **Y07.510** At-home childcare provider, perpetrator of maltreatment and neglect
    - **Y07.511** Daycare center childcare provider, perpetrator of maltreatment and neglect
    - **Y07.512** At-home adultcare provider, perpetrator of maltreatment and neglect
    - **Y07.513** Adultcare center provider, perpetrator of maltreatment and neglect
    - **Y07.519** Unspecified daycare provider, perpetrator of maltreatment and neglect
  - ✓6th **Y07.52** Healthcare provider, perpetrator of maltreatment and neglect
    - **Y07.521** Mental health provider, perpetrator of maltreatment and neglect
    - **Y07.528** Other therapist or healthcare provider, perpetrator of maltreatment and neglect
      - Nurse perpetrator of maltreatment and neglect
      - Occupational therapist perpetrator of maltreatment and neglect
      - Physical therapist perpetrator of maltreatment and neglect
      - Speech therapist perpetrator of maltreatment and neglect
    - **Y07.529** Unspecified healthcare provider, perpetrator of maltreatment and neglect
  - **Y07.53** Teacher or instructor, perpetrator of maltreatment and neglect
    - Coach, perpetrator of maltreatment and neglect
  - **Y07.54** Acquaintance or friend, perpetrator of maltreatment and neglect
  - **Y07.59** Other non-family member, perpetrator of maltreatment and neglect
- **Y07.6** Multiple perpetrators of maltreatment and neglect
  - AHA: 2018,4Q,32
- **Y07.9** Unspecified perpetrator of maltreatment and neglect
- ✓4th **Y08** Assault by other specified means
  - ✓5th **Y08.0** Assault by strike by sport equipment
    - ✓x7th **Y08.01** Assault by strike by hockey stick
    - ✓x7th **Y08.02** Assault by strike by baseball bat
    - ✓x7th **Y08.09** Assault by strike by other specified type of sport equipment
  - ✓5th **Y08.8** Assault by other specified means
    - ✓x7th **Y08.81** Assault by crashing of aircraft
    - ✓x7th **Y08.89** Assault by other specified means
- **Y09** Assault by unspecified means
  - Assassination (attempted) NOS
  - Homicide (attempted) NOS
  - Manslaughter (attempted) NOS
  - Murder (attempted) NOS

Event of undetermined intent (Y21-Y33)

Undetermined intent is only for use when there is specific documentation in the record that the intent of the injury cannot be determined. If no such documentation is present, code to accidental (unintentional).

The appropriate 7th character is to be added to each code from categories Y21-Y33.
- A initial encounter
- D subsequent encounter
- S sequela

- ✓4th **Y21** Drowning and submersion, undetermined intent
  - ✓x7th **Y21.0** Drowning and submersion while in bathtub, undetermined intent
  - ✓x7th **Y21.1** Drowning and submersion after fall into bathtub, undetermined intent
  - ✓x7th **Y21.2** Drowning and submersion while in swimming pool, undetermined intent
  - ✓x7th **Y21.3** Drowning and submersion after fall into swimming pool, undetermined intent
  - ✓x7th **Y21.4** Drowning and submersion in natural water, undetermined intent
  - ✓x7th **Y21.8** Other drowning and submersion, undetermined intent
  - ✓x7th **Y21.9** Unspecified drowning and submersion, undetermined intent
- ✓x7th **Y22** Handgun discharge, undetermined intent
  - Discharge of gun for single hand use, undetermined intent
  - Discharge of pistol, undetermined intent
  - Discharge of revolver, undetermined intent
  - EXCLUDES 2 Very pistol (Y24.8)
- ✓4th **Y23** Rifle, shotgun and larger firearm discharge, undetermined intent
  - EXCLUDES 2 airgun (Y24.0)
  - ✓x7th **Y23.0** Shotgun discharge, undetermined intent
  - ✓x7th **Y23.1** Hunting rifle discharge, undetermined intent
  - ✓x7th **Y23.2** Military firearm discharge, undetermined intent
  - ✓x7th **Y23.3** Machine gun discharge, undetermined intent
  - ✓x7th **Y23.8** Other larger firearm discharge, undetermined intent
  - ✓x7th **Y23.9** Unspecified larger firearm discharge, undetermined intent
- ✓4th **Y24** Other and unspecified firearm discharge, undetermined intent
  - ✓x7th **Y24.0** Airgun discharge, undetermined intent
    - BB gun discharge, undetermined intent
    - Pellet gun discharge, undetermined intent
  - ✓x7th **Y24.8** Other firearm discharge, undetermined intent
    - Paintball gun discharge, undetermined intent
    - Very pistol [flare] discharge, undetermined intent
  - ✓x7th **Y24.9** Unspecified firearm discharge, undetermined intent
- ✓x7th **Y25** Contact with explosive material, undetermined intent
- ✓x7th **Y26** Exposure to smoke, fire and flames, undetermined intent
- ✓4th **Y27** Contact with steam, hot vapors and hot objects, undetermined intent
  - ✓x7th **Y27.0** Contact with steam and hot vapors, undetermined intent
  - ✓x7th **Y27.1** Contact with hot tap water, undetermined intent
  - ✓x7th **Y27.2** Contact with hot fluids, undetermined intent
  - ✓x7th **Y27.3** Contact with hot household appliance, undetermined intent
  - ✓x7th **Y27.8** Contact with other hot objects, undetermined intent
  - ✓x7th **Y27.9** Contact with unspecified hot objects, undetermined intent
- ✓4th **Y28** Contact with sharp object, undetermined intent
  - ✓x7th **Y28.0** Contact with sharp glass, undetermined intent
  - ✓x7th **Y28.1** Contact with knife, undetermined intent
  - ✓x7th **Y28.2** Contact with sword or dagger, undetermined intent
  - ✓x7th **Y28.8** Contact with other sharp object, undetermined intent
  - ✓x7th **Y28.9** Contact with unspecified sharp object, undetermined intent
- ✓x7th **Y29** Contact with blunt object, undetermined intent
- ✓x7th **Y30** Falling, jumping or pushed from a high place, undetermined intent
  - Victim falling from one level to another, undetermined intent
- ✓x7th **Y31** Falling, lying or running before or into moving object, undetermined intent
- ✓x7th **Y32** Crashing of motor vehicle, undetermined intent
- ✓x7th **Y33** Other specified events, undetermined intent

Chapter 20. External Causes of Morbidity

Legal intervention, operations of war, military operations, and terrorism (Y35-Y38)

The appropriate 7th character is to be added to each code from categories Y35-Y38.
- A initial encounter
- D subsequent encounter
- S sequela

Y35 Legal intervention

INCLUDES any injury sustained as a result of an encounter with any law enforcement official, serving in any capacity at the time of the encounter, whether on-duty or off-duty. Includes injury to law enforcement official, suspect and bystander

AHA: 2019,4Q,18-19

Y35.0 Legal intervention involving firearm discharge

Y35.00 Legal intervention involving unspecified firearm discharge
Legal intervention involving gunshot wound
Legal intervention involving shot NOS

- **Y35.001** Legal intervention involving unspecified firearm discharge, law enforcement official injured
- **Y35.002** Legal intervention involving unspecified firearm discharge, bystander injured
- **Y35.003** Legal intervention involving unspecified firearm discharge, suspect injured
- **Y35.009** Legal intervention involving unspecified firearm discharge, unspecified person injured

Y35.01 Legal intervention involving injury by machine gun
- **Y35.011** Legal intervention involving injury by machine gun, law enforcement official injured
- **Y35.012** Legal intervention involving injury by machine gun, bystander injured
- **Y35.013** Legal intervention involving injury by machine gun, suspect injured
- **Y35.019** Legal intervention involving injury by machine gun, unspecified person injured

Y35.02 Legal intervention involving injury by handgun
- **Y35.021** Legal intervention involving injury by handgun, law enforcement official injured
- **Y35.022** Legal intervention involving injury by handgun, bystander injured
- **Y35.023** Legal intervention involving injury by handgun, suspect injured
- **Y35.029** Legal intervention involving injury by handgun, unspecified person injured

Y35.03 Legal intervention involving injury by rifle pellet
- **Y35.031** Legal intervention involving injury by rifle pellet, law enforcement official injured
- **Y35.032** Legal intervention involving injury by rifle pellet, bystander injured
- **Y35.033** Legal intervention involving injury by rifle pellet, suspect injured
- **Y35.039** Legal intervention involving injury by rifle pellet, unspecified person injured

Y35.04 Legal intervention involving injury by rubber bullet
- **Y35.041** Legal intervention involving injury by rubber bullet, law enforcement official injured
- **Y35.042** Legal intervention involving injury by rubber bullet, bystander injured
- **Y35.043** Legal intervention involving injury by rubber bullet, suspect injured
- **Y35.049** Legal intervention involving injury by rubber bullet, unspecified person injured

Y35.09 Legal intervention involving other firearm discharge
- **Y35.091** Legal intervention involving other firearm discharge, law enforcement official injured
- **Y35.092** Legal intervention involving other firearm discharge, bystander injured
- **Y35.093** Legal intervention involving other firearm discharge, suspect injured
- **Y35.099** Legal intervention involving other firearm discharge, unspecified person injured

Y35.1 Legal intervention involving explosives

Y35.10 Legal intervention involving unspecified explosives
- **Y35.101** Legal intervention involving unspecified explosives, law enforcement official injured
- **Y35.102** Legal intervention involving unspecified explosives, bystander injured
- **Y35.103** Legal intervention involving unspecified explosives, suspect injured
- **Y35.109** Legal intervention involving unspecified explosives, unspecified person injured

Y35.11 Legal intervention involving injury by dynamite
- **Y35.111** Legal intervention involving injury by dynamite, law enforcement official injured
- **Y35.112** Legal intervention involving injury by dynamite, bystander injured
- **Y35.113** Legal intervention involving injury by dynamite, suspect injured
- **Y35.119** Legal intervention involving injury by dynamite, unspecified person injured

Y35.12 Legal intervention involving injury by explosive shell
- **Y35.121** Legal intervention involving injury by explosive shell, law enforcement official injured
- **Y35.122** Legal intervention involving injury by explosive shell, bystander injured
- **Y35.123** Legal intervention involving injury by explosive shell, suspect injured
- **Y35.129** Legal intervention involving injury by explosive shell, unspecified person injured

Y35.19 Legal intervention involving other explosives
Legal intervention involving injury by grenade
Legal intervention involving injury by mortar bomb

- **Y35.191** Legal intervention involving other explosives, law enforcement official injured
- **Y35.192** Legal intervention involving other explosives, bystander injured
- **Y35.193** Legal intervention involving other explosives, suspect injured
- **Y35.199** Legal intervention involving other explosives, unspecified person injured

Y35.2 Legal intervention involving gas
Legal intervention involving asphyxiation by gas
Legal intervention involving poisoning by gas

Y35.20 Legal intervention involving unspecified gas
- **Y35.201** Legal intervention involving unspecified gas, law enforcement official injured
- **Y35.202** Legal intervention involving unspecified gas, bystander injured
- **Y35.203** Legal intervention involving unspecified gas, suspect injured
- **Y35.209** Legal intervention involving unspecified gas, unspecified person injured

Y35.21 Legal intervention involving injury by tear gas
- **Y35.211** Legal intervention involving injury by tear gas, law enforcement official injured
- **Y35.212** Legal intervention involving injury by tear gas, bystander injured
- **Y35.213** Legal intervention involving injury by tear gas, suspect injured
- **Y35.219** Legal intervention involving injury by tear gas, unspecified person injured

Y35.29 Legal intervention involving other gas
- **Y35.291** Legal intervention involving other gas, law enforcement official injured
- **Y35.292** Legal intervention involving other gas, bystander injured
- **Y35.293** Legal intervention involving other gas, suspect injured
- **Y35.299** Legal intervention involving other gas, unspecified person injured

Y35.3 Legal intervention involving blunt objects
Legal intervention involving being hit or struck by blunt object

Y35.30 Legal intervention involving unspecified blunt objects
- **Y35.301** Legal intervention involving unspecified blunt objects, law enforcement official injured
- **Y35.302** Legal intervention involving unspecified blunt objects, bystander injured

- **Y35.303** Legal intervention involving unspecified blunt objects, suspect injured
- **Y35.309** Legal intervention involving unspecified blunt objects, unspecified person injured
- **Y35.31** Legal intervention involving baton
  - **Y35.311** Legal intervention involving baton, law enforcement official injured
  - **Y35.312** Legal intervention involving baton, bystander injured
  - **Y35.313** Legal intervention involving baton, suspect injured
  - **Y35.319** Legal intervention involving baton, unspecified person injured
- **Y35.39** Legal intervention involving other blunt objects
  - **Y35.391** Legal intervention involving other blunt objects, law enforcement official injured
  - **Y35.392** Legal intervention involving other blunt objects, bystander injured
  - **Y35.393** Legal intervention involving other blunt objects, suspect injured
  - **Y35.399** Legal intervention involving other blunt objects, unspecified person injured
- **Y35.4** Legal intervention involving sharp objects
  - Legal intervention involving being cut by sharp objects
  - Legal intervention involving being stabbed by sharp objects
  - **Y35.40** Legal intervention involving unspecified sharp objects
    - **Y35.401** Legal intervention involving unspecified sharp objects, law enforcement official injured
    - **Y35.402** Legal intervention involving unspecified sharp objects, bystander injured
    - **Y35.403** Legal intervention involving unspecified sharp objects, suspect injured
    - **Y35.409** Legal intervention involving unspecified sharp objects, unspecified person injured
  - **Y35.41** Legal intervention involving bayonet
    - **Y35.411** Legal intervention involving bayonet, law enforcement official injured
    - **Y35.412** Legal intervention involving bayonet, bystander injured
    - **Y35.413** Legal intervention involving bayonet, suspect injured
    - **Y35.419** Legal intervention involving bayonet, unspecified person injured
  - **Y35.49** Legal intervention involving other sharp objects
    - **Y35.491** Legal intervention involving other sharp objects, law enforcement official injured
    - **Y35.492** Legal intervention involving other sharp objects, bystander injured
    - **Y35.493** Legal intervention involving other sharp objects, suspect injured
    - **Y35.499** Legal intervention involving other sharp objects, unspecified person injured
- **Y35.8** Legal intervention involving other specified means
  - AHA: 2019,4Q,19
  - **Y35.81** Legal intervention involving manhandling
    - **Y35.811** Legal intervention involving manhandling, law enforcement official injured
    - **Y35.812** Legal intervention involving manhandling, bystander injured
    - **Y35.813** Legal intervention involving manhandling, suspect injured
    - **Y35.819** Legal intervention involving manhandling, unspecified person injured
  - **Y35.83** Legal intervention involving a conducted energy device
    - Electroshock device (taser)
    - Stun gun
    - **Y35.831** Legal intervention involving a conducted energy device, law enforcement official injured
    - **Y35.832** Legal intervention involving a conducted energy device, bystander injured
    - **Y35.833** Legal intervention involving a conducted energy device, suspect injured
    - **Y35.839** Legal intervention involving a conducted energy device, unspecified person injured
  - **Y35.89** Legal intervention involving other specified means
    - **Y35.891** Legal intervention involving other specified means, law enforcement official injured
    - **Y35.892** Legal intervention involving other specified means, bystander injured
    - **Y35.893** Legal intervention involving other specified means, suspect injured
      - AHA: 2018,1Q,5
    - **Y35.899** Legal intervention involving other specified means, unspecified person injured
- **Y35.9** Legal intervention, means unspecified
  - **Y35.91** Legal intervention, means unspecified, law enforcement official injured
  - **Y35.92** Legal intervention, means unspecified, bystander injured
  - **Y35.93** Legal intervention, means unspecified, suspect injured
  - **Y35.99** Legal intervention, means unspecified, unspecified person injured

Y36 Operations of war

INCLUDES injuries to military personnel and civilians caused by war, civil insurrection, and peacekeeping missions

EXCLUDES 1 injury to military personnel occurring during peacetime military operations (Y37.-)
military vehicles involved in transport accidents with non-military vehicle during peacetime (V09.01, V09.21, V19.81, V29.818, V39.81, V49.81, V59.81, V69.81, V79.81)

AHA: 2014,3Q,4

- **Y36.0** War operations involving explosion of marine weapons
  - **Y36.00** War operations involving explosion of unspecified marine weapon
    - War operations involving underwater blast NOS
    - **Y36.000** War operations involving explosion of unspecified marine weapon, military personnel
    - **Y36.001** War operations involving explosion of unspecified marine weapon, civilian
  - **Y36.01** War operations involving explosion of depth-charge
    - **Y36.010** War operations involving explosion of depth-charge, military personnel
    - **Y36.011** War operations involving explosion of depth-charge, civilian
  - **Y36.02** War operations involving explosion of marine mine
    - War operations involving explosion of marine mine, at sea or in harbor
    - **Y36.020** War operations involving explosion of marine mine, military personnel
    - **Y36.021** War operations involving explosion of marine mine, civilian
  - **Y36.03** War operations involving explosion of sea-based artillery shell
    - **Y36.030** War operations involving explosion of sea-based artillery shell, military personnel
    - **Y36.031** War operations involving explosion of sea-based artillery shell, civilian
  - **Y36.04** War operations involving explosion of torpedo
    - **Y36.040** War operations involving explosion of torpedo, military personnel
    - **Y36.041** War operations involving explosion of torpedo, civilian
  - **Y36.05** War operations involving accidental detonation of onboard marine weapons
    - **Y36.050** War operations involving accidental detonation of onboard marine weapons, military personnel
    - **Y36.051** War operations involving accidental detonation of onboard marine weapons, civilian
  - **Y36.09** War operations involving explosion of other marine weapons
    - **Y36.090** War operations involving explosion of other marine weapons, military personnel
    - **Y36.091** War operations involving explosion of other marine weapons, civilian

Y36.1 War operations involving destruction of aircraft

- **Y36.10** War operations involving unspecified destruction of aircraft
  - **Y36.100** War operations involving unspecified destruction of aircraft, military personnel
  - **Y36.101** War operations involving unspecified destruction of aircraft, civilian
- **Y36.11** War operations involving destruction of aircraft due to enemy fire or explosives
  - War operations involving destruction of aircraft due to air to air missile
  - War operations involving destruction of aircraft due to explosive placed on aircraft
  - War operations involving destruction of aircraft due to rocket propelled grenade [RPG]
  - War operations involving destruction of aircraft due to small arms fire
  - War operations involving destruction of aircraft due to surface to air missile
  - **Y36.110** War operations involving destruction of aircraft due to enemy fire or explosives, military personnel
  - **Y36.111** War operations involving destruction of aircraft due to enemy fire or explosives, civilian
- **Y36.12** War operations involving destruction of aircraft due to collision with other aircraft
  - **Y36.120** War operations involving destruction of aircraft due to collision with other aircraft, military personnel
  - **Y36.121** War operations involving destruction of aircraft due to collision with other aircraft, civilian
- **Y36.13** War operations involving destruction of aircraft due to onboard fire
  - **Y36.130** War operations involving destruction of aircraft due to onboard fire, military personnel
  - **Y36.131** War operations involving destruction of aircraft due to onboard fire, civilian
- **Y36.14** War operations involving destruction of aircraft due to accidental detonation of onboard munitions and explosives
  - **Y36.140** War operations involving destruction of aircraft due to accidental detonation of onboard munitions and explosives, military personnel
  - **Y36.141** War operations involving destruction of aircraft due to accidental detonation of onboard munitions and explosives, civilian
- **Y36.19** War operations involving other destruction of aircraft
  - **Y36.190** War operations involving other destruction of aircraft, military personnel
  - **Y36.191** War operations involving other destruction of aircraft, civilian

Y36.2 War operations involving other explosions and fragments

EXCLUDES 1
- war operations involving explosion of aircraft (Y36.1-)
- war operations involving explosion of marine weapons (Y36.0-)
- war operations involving explosion of nuclear weapons (Y36.5-)
- war operations involving explosion occurring after cessation of hostilities (Y36.8-)

- **Y36.20** War operations involving unspecified explosion and fragments
  - War operations involving air blast NOS
  - War operations involving blast fragments NOS
  - War operations involving blast NOS
  - War operations involving blast wave NOS
  - War operations involving blast wind NOS
  - War operations involving explosion of bomb NOS
  - War operations involving explosion NOS
  - **Y36.200** War operations involving unspecified explosion and fragments, military personnel
  - **Y36.201** War operations involving unspecified explosion and fragments, civilian
- **Y36.21** War operations involving explosion of aerial bomb
  - **Y36.210** War operations involving explosion of aerial bomb, military personnel
  - **Y36.211** War operations involving explosion of aerial bomb, civilian
- **Y36.22** War operations involving explosion of guided missile
  - **Y36.220** War operations involving explosion of guided missile, military personnel
  - **Y36.221** War operations involving explosion of guided missile, civilian
- **Y36.23** War operations involving explosion of improvised explosive device [IED]
  - War operations involving explosion of person-borne improvised explosive device [IED]
  - War operations involving explosion of roadside improvised explosive device [IED]
  - War operations involving explosion of vehicle-borne improvised explosive device [IED]
  - **Y36.230** War operations involving explosion of improvised explosive device [IED], military personnel
  - **Y36.231** War operations involving explosion of improvised explosive device [IED], civilian
- **Y36.24** War operations involving explosion due to accidental detonation and discharge of own munitions or munitions launch device
  - **Y36.240** War operations involving explosion due to accidental detonation and discharge of own munitions or munitions launch device, military personnel
  - **Y36.241** War operations involving explosion due to accidental detonation and discharge of own munitions or munitions launch device, civilian
- **Y36.25** War operations involving fragments from munitions
  - **Y36.250** War operations involving fragments from munitions, military personnel
  - **Y36.251** War operations involving fragments from munitions, civilian
- **Y36.26** War operations involving fragments of improvised explosive device [IED]
  - War operations involving fragments of person-borne improvised explosive device [IED]
  - War operations involving fragments of roadside improvised explosive device [IED]
  - War operations involving fragments of vehicle-borne improvised explosive device [IED]
  - **Y36.260** War operations involving fragments of improvised explosive device [IED], military personnel
  - **Y36.261** War operations involving fragments of improvised explosive device [IED], civilian
- **Y36.27** War operations involving fragments from weapons
  - **Y36.270** War operations involving fragments from weapons, military personnel
  - **Y36.271** War operations involving fragments from weapons, civilian
- **Y36.29** War operations involving other explosions and fragments
  - War operations involving explosion of grenade
  - War operations involving explosions of land mine
  - War operations involving shrapnel NOS
  - **Y36.290** War operations involving other explosions and fragments, military personnel
  - **Y36.291** War operations involving other explosions and fragments, civilian

Y36.3 War operations involving fires, conflagrations and hot substances

War operations involving smoke, fumes, and heat from fires, conflagrations and hot substances

EXCLUDES 1
- war operations involving fires and conflagrations aboard military aircraft (Y36.1-)
- war operations involving fires and conflagrations aboard military watercraft (Y36.0-)
- war operations involving fires and conflagrations caused indirectly by conventional weapons (Y36.2-)
- war operations involving fires and thermal effects of nuclear weapons (Y36.53-)

- **Y36.30** War operations involving unspecified fire, conflagration and hot substance
  - **Y36.300** War operations involving unspecified fire, conflagration and hot substance, military personnel
  - **Y36.301** War operations involving unspecified fire, conflagration and hot substance, civilian

- **Y36.31** War operations involving gasoline bomb
  War operations involving incendiary bomb
  War operations involving petrol bomb
  - **Y36.310** War operations involving gasoline bomb, military personnel
  - **Y36.311** War operations involving gasoline bomb, civilian
- **Y36.32** War operations involving incendiary bullet
  - **Y36.320** War operations involving incendiary bullet, military personnel
  - **Y36.321** War operations involving incendiary bullet, civilian
- **Y36.33** War operations involving flamethrower
  - **Y36.330** War operations involving flamethrower, military personnel
  - **Y36.331** War operations involving flamethrower, civilian
- **Y36.39** War operations involving other fires, conflagrations and hot substances
  - **Y36.390** War operations involving other fires, conflagrations and hot substances, military personnel
  - **Y36.391** War operations involving other fires, conflagrations and hot substances, civilian

Y36.4 War operations involving firearm discharge and other forms of conventional warfare

- **Y36.41** War operations involving rubber bullets
  - **Y36.410** War operations involving rubber bullets, military personnel
  - **Y36.411** War operations involving rubber bullets, civilian
- **Y36.42** War operations involving firearms pellets
  - **Y36.420** War operations involving firearms pellets, military personnel
  - **Y36.421** War operations involving firearms pellets, civilian
- **Y36.43** War operations involving other firearms discharge
  War operations involving bullets NOS
  EXCLUDES 1: war operations involving munitions fragments (Y36.25-)
  war operations involving incendiary bullets (Y36.32-)
  - **Y36.430** War operations involving other firearms discharge, military personnel
  - **Y36.431** War operations involving other firearms discharge, civilian
- **Y36.44** War operations involving unarmed hand to hand combat
  EXCLUDES 1: war operations involving combat using blunt or piercing object (Y36.45-)
  war operations involving intentional restriction of air and airway (Y36.46-)
  war operations involving unintentional restriction of air and airway (Y36.47-)
  - **Y36.440** War operations involving unarmed hand to hand combat, military personnel
  - **Y36.441** War operations involving unarmed hand to hand combat, civilian
- **Y36.45** War operations involving combat using blunt or piercing object
  - **Y36.450** War operations involving combat using blunt or piercing object, military personnel
  - **Y36.451** War operations involving combat using blunt or piercing object, civilian
- **Y36.46** War operations involving intentional restriction of air and airway
  - **Y36.460** War operations involving intentional restriction of air and airway, military personnel
  - **Y36.461** War operations involving intentional restriction of air and airway, civilian
- **Y36.47** War operations involving unintentional restriction of air and airway
  - **Y36.470** War operations involving unintentional restriction of air and airway, military personnel
  - **Y36.471** War operations involving unintentional restriction of air and airway, civilian
- **Y36.49** War operations involving other forms of conventional warfare
  - **Y36.490** War operations involving other forms of conventional warfare, military personnel
  - **Y36.491** War operations involving other forms of conventional warfare, civilian

Y36.5 War operations involving nuclear weapons
War operations involving dirty bomb NOS

- **Y36.50** War operations involving unspecified effect of nuclear weapon
  - **Y36.500** War operations involving unspecified effect of nuclear weapon, military personnel
  - **Y36.501** War operations involving unspecified effect of nuclear weapon, civilian
- **Y36.51** War operations involving direct blast effect of nuclear weapon
  War operations involving blast pressure of nuclear weapon
  - **Y36.510** War operations involving direct blast effect of nuclear weapon, military personnel
  - **Y36.511** War operations involving direct blast effect of nuclear weapon, civilian
- **Y36.52** War operations involving indirect blast effect of nuclear weapon
  War operations involving being struck or crushed by blast debris of nuclear weapon
  War operations involving being thrown by blast of nuclear weapon
  - **Y36.520** War operations involving indirect blast effect of nuclear weapon, military personnel
  - **Y36.521** War operations involving indirect blast effect of nuclear weapon, civilian
- **Y36.53** War operations involving thermal radiation effect of nuclear weapon
  War operation involving fireball effects from nuclear weapon
  War operations involving direct heat from nuclear weapon
  - **Y36.530** War operations involving thermal radiation effect of nuclear weapon, military personnel
  - **Y36.531** War operations involving thermal radiation effect of nuclear weapon, civilian
- **Y36.54** War operation involving nuclear radiation effects of nuclear weapon
  War operation involving acute radiation exposure from nuclear weapon
  War operation involving exposure to immediate ionizing radiation from nuclear weapon
  War operation involving fallout exposure from nuclear weapon
  War operation involving secondary effects of nuclear weapons
  - **Y36.540** War operation involving nuclear radiation effects of nuclear weapon, military personnel
  - **Y36.541** War operation involving nuclear radiation effects of nuclear weapon, civilian
- **Y36.59** War operation involving other effects of nuclear weapons
  - **Y36.590** War operation involving other effects of nuclear weapons, military personnel
  - **Y36.591** War operation involving other effects of nuclear weapons, civilian

Y36.6 War operations involving biological weapons

- **Y36.6X** War operations involving biological weapons
  - **Y36.6X0** War operations involving biological weapons, military personnel
  - **Y36.6X1** War operations involving biological weapons, civilian

Y36.7 War operations involving chemical weapons and other forms of unconventional warfare
EXCLUDES 1: war operations involving incendiary devices (Y36.3-, Y36.5-)

- **Y36.7X** War operations involving chemical weapons and other forms of unconventional warfare
  - **Y36.7X0** War operations involving chemical weapons and other forms of unconventional warfare, military personnel

- **Y36.7X1** War operations involving chemical weapons and other forms of unconventional warfare, *civilian*

- **Y36.8** War operations occurring *after cessation of hostilities*
  War operations classifiable to categories Y36.0-Y36.8 but occurring after cessation of hostilities
  - **Y36.81** Explosion of *mine* placed during war operations but exploding after cessation of hostilities
    - **Y36.810** Explosion of mine placed during war operations but exploding after cessation of hostilities, *military personnel*
    - **Y36.811** Explosion of mine placed during war operations but exploding after cessation of hostilities, *civilian*
  - **Y36.82** Explosion of *bomb* placed during war operations but exploding after cessation of hostilities
    - **Y36.820** Explosion of bomb placed during war operations but exploding after cessation of hostilities, *military personnel*
    - **Y36.821** Explosion of bomb placed during war operations but exploding after cessation of hostilities, *civilian*
  - **Y36.88** Other war operations occurring after cessation of hostilities
    - **Y36.880** Other war operations occurring after cessation of hostilities, *military personnel*
    - **Y36.881** Other war operations occurring after cessation of hostilities, *civilian*
  - **Y36.89** Unspecified war operations occurring after cessation of hostilities
    - **Y36.890** Unspecified war operations occurring after cessation of hostilities, *military personnel*
    - **Y36.891** Unspecified war operations occurring after cessation of hostilities, *civilian*

- **Y36.9** Other and unspecified war operations
  - **Y36.90** War operations, unspecified
  - **Y36.91** War operations involving unspecified *weapon of mass destruction* [WMD]
  - **Y36.92** War operations involving *friendly fire*

- **Y36.A** Blast overpressure in war operations
  Code also type of explosive, if known
  accidental detonation of onboard munitions (Y36.140)
  explosion of grenade (Y36.290)
  explosion of torpedo (Y36.040)
  improvised explosive device (Y36.230)
  - **Y36.A1** *Low level* blast overpressure in war operations
    LLB overpressure in war operations
    Low level blast overpressure due to explosion in war operations
  - **Y36.A2** *High level* blast overpressure in war operations
    High level blast overpressure due to explosion in war operations
    HLB overpressure in war operations

- **Y37** Military operations
  INCLUDES injuries to military personnel and civilians occurring during peacetime on military property and during routine military exercises and operations
  EXCLUDES 1 military aircraft involved in aircraft accident with civilian aircraft (V97.81-)
  military vehicles involved in transport accident with civilian vehicle (V09.01, V09.21, V19.81, V29.818, V39.81, V49.81, V59.81, V69.81, V79.81)
  military watercraft involved in water transport accident with civilian watercraft (V94.81-)
  war operations (Y36.-)

  - **Y37.0** Military operations involving *explosion of marine weapons*
    - **Y37.00** Military operations involving explosion of unspecified marine weapon
      Military operations involving underwater blast NOS
      - **Y37.000** Military operations involving explosion of unspecified marine weapon, *military personnel*
      - **Y37.001** Military operations involving explosion of unspecified marine weapon, *civilian*
    - **Y37.01** Military operations involving explosion of *depth-charge*
      - **Y37.010** Military operations involving explosion of depth-charge, *military personnel*
      - **Y37.011** Military operations involving explosion of depth-charge, *civilian*
    - **Y37.02** Military operations involving explosion of *marine mine*
      Military operations involving explosion of marine mine, at sea or in harbor
      - **Y37.020** Military operations involving explosion of marine mine, *military personnel*
      - **Y37.021** Military operations involving explosion of marine mine, *civilian*
    - **Y37.03** Military operations involving explosion of *sea-based artillery shell*
      - **Y37.030** Military operations involving explosion of sea-based artillery shell, *military personnel*
      - **Y37.031** Military operations involving explosion of sea-based artillery shell, *civilian*
    - **Y37.04** Military operations involving explosion of *torpedo*
      - **Y37.040** Military operations involving explosion of torpedo, *military personnel*
      - **Y37.041** Military operations involving explosion of torpedo, *civilian*
    - **Y37.05** Military operations involving accidental detonation of *onboard marine weapons*
      - **Y37.050** Military operations involving accidental detonation of onboard marine weapons, *military personnel*
      - **Y37.051** Military operations involving accidental detonation of onboard marine weapons, *civilian*
    - **Y37.09** Military operations involving explosion of other marine weapons
      - **Y37.090** Military operations involving explosion of other marine weapons, *military personnel*
      - **Y37.091** Military operations involving explosion of other marine weapons, *civilian*

  - **Y37.1** Military operations involving *destruction of aircraft*
    - **Y37.10** Military operations involving unspecified destruction of aircraft
      - **Y37.100** Military operations involving unspecified destruction of aircraft, *military personnel*
      - **Y37.101** Military operations involving unspecified destruction of aircraft, *civilian*
    - **Y37.11** Military operations involving destruction of aircraft *due to enemy fire or explosives*
      Military operations involving destruction of aircraft due to air to air missile
      Military operations involving destruction of aircraft due to explosive placed on aircraft
      Military operations involving destruction of aircraft due to rocket propelled grenade [RPG]
      Military operations involving destruction of aircraft due to small arms fire
      Military operations involving destruction of aircraft due to surface to air missile
      - **Y37.110** Military operations involving destruction of aircraft due to enemy fire or explosives, *military personnel*
      - **Y37.111** Military operations involving destruction of aircraft due to enemy fire or explosives, *civilian*
    - **Y37.12** Military operations involving destruction of aircraft *due to collision with other aircraft*
      - **Y37.120** Military operations involving destruction of aircraft due to collision with other aircraft, *military personnel*
      - **Y37.121** Military operations involving destruction of aircraft due to collision with other aircraft, *civilian*
    - **Y37.13** Military operations involving destruction of aircraft *due to onboard fire*
      - **Y37.130** Military operations involving destruction of aircraft due to onboard fire, *military personnel*
      - **Y37.131** Military operations involving destruction of aircraft due to onboard fire, *civilian*
    - **Y37.14** Military operations involving destruction of aircraft due to *accidental detonation of onboard munitions and explosives*
      - **Y37.140** Military operations involving destruction of aircraft due to accidental detonation of onboard munitions and explosives, *military personnel*
      - **Y37.141** Military operations involving destruction of aircraft due to accidental detonation of onboard munitions and explosives, *civilian*

- **Y37.19** Military operations involving other destruction of aircraft
  - **Y37.190** Military operations involving other destruction of aircraft, military personnel
  - **Y37.191** Military operations involving other destruction of aircraft, civilian
- **Y37.2** Military operations involving other explosions and fragments
  - EXCLUDES 1: military operations involving explosion of aircraft (Y37.1-)
  - military operations involving explosion of marine weapons (Y37.0-)
  - military operations involving explosion of nuclear weapons (Y37.5-)
  - **Y37.20** Military operations involving unspecified explosion and fragments
    - Military operations involving air blast NOS
    - Military operations involving blast fragments NOS
    - Military operations involving blast NOS
    - Military operations involving blast wave NOS
    - Military operations involving blast wind NOS
    - Military operations involving explosion of bomb NOS
    - Military operations involving explosion NOS
    - **Y37.200** Military operations involving unspecified explosion and fragments, military personnel
    - **Y37.201** Military operations involving unspecified explosion and fragments, civilian
  - **Y37.21** Military operations involving explosion of aerial bomb
    - **Y37.210** Military operations involving explosion of aerial bomb, military personnel
    - **Y37.211** Military operations involving explosion of aerial bomb, civilian
  - **Y37.22** Military operations involving explosion of guided missile
    - **Y37.220** Military operations involving explosion of guided missile, military personnel
    - **Y37.221** Military operations involving explosion of guided missile, civilian
  - **Y37.23** Military operations involving explosion of improvised explosive device [IED]
    - Military operations involving explosion of person-borne improvised explosive device [IED]
    - Military operations involving explosion of roadside improvised explosive device [IED]
    - Military operations involving explosion of vehicle-borne improvised explosive device [IED]
    - **Y37.230** Military operations involving explosion of improvised explosive device [IED], military personnel
    - **Y37.231** Military operations involving explosion of improvised explosive device [IED], civilian
  - **Y37.24** Military operations involving explosion due to accidental detonation and discharge of own munitions or munitions launch device
    - **Y37.240** Military operations involving explosion due to accidental detonation and discharge of own munitions or munitions launch device, military personnel
    - **Y37.241** Military operations involving explosion due to accidental detonation and discharge of own munitions or munitions launch device, civilian
  - **Y37.25** Military operations involving fragments from munitions
    - **Y37.250** Military operations involving fragments from munitions, military personnel
    - **Y37.251** Military operations involving fragments from munitions, civilian
  - **Y37.26** Military operations involving fragments of improvised explosive device [IED]
    - Military operations involving fragments of person-borne improvised explosive device [IED]
    - Military operations involving fragments of roadside improvised explosive device [IED]
    - Military operations involving fragments of vehicle-borne improvised explosive device [IED]
    - **Y37.260** Military operations involving fragments of improvised explosive device [IED], military personnel
    - **Y37.261** Military operations involving fragments of improvised explosive device [IED], civilian
  - **Y37.27** Military operations involving fragments from weapons
    - **Y37.270** Military operations involving fragments from weapons, military personnel
    - **Y37.271** Military operations involving fragments from weapons, civilian
  - **Y37.29** Military operations involving other explosions and fragments
    - Military operations involving explosion of grenade
    - Military operations involving explosions of land mine
    - Military operations involving shrapnel NOS
    - **Y37.290** Military operations involving other explosions and fragments, military personnel
    - **Y37.291** Military operations involving other explosions and fragments, civilian
- **Y37.3** Military operations involving fires, conflagrations and hot substances
  - Military operations involving smoke, fumes, and heat from fires, conflagrations and hot substances
  - EXCLUDES 1: military operations involving fires and conflagrations aboard military aircraft (Y37.1-)
  - military operations involving fires and conflagrations aboard military watercraft (Y37.0-)
  - military operations involving fires and conflagrations caused indirectly by conventional weapons (Y37.2-)
  - military operations involving fires and thermal effects of nuclear weapons (Y36.53-)
  - **Y37.30** Military operations involving unspecified fire, conflagration and hot substance
    - **Y37.300** Military operations involving unspecified fire, conflagration and hot substance, military personnel
    - **Y37.301** Military operations involving unspecified fire, conflagration and hot substance, civilian
  - **Y37.31** Military operations involving gasoline bomb
    - Military operations involving incendiary bomb
    - Military operations involving petrol bomb
    - **Y37.310** Military operations involving gasoline bomb, military personnel
    - **Y37.311** Military operations involving gasoline bomb, civilian
  - **Y37.32** Military operations involving incendiary bullet
    - **Y37.320** Military operations involving incendiary bullet, military personnel
    - **Y37.321** Military operations involving incendiary bullet, civilian
  - **Y37.33** Military operations involving flamethrower
    - **Y37.330** Military operations involving flamethrower, military personnel
    - **Y37.331** Military operations involving flamethrower, civilian
  - **Y37.39** Military operations involving other fires, conflagrations and hot substances
    - **Y37.390** Military operations involving other fires, conflagrations and hot substances, military personnel
    - **Y37.391** Military operations involving other fires, conflagrations and hot substances, civilian
- **Y37.4** Military operations involving firearm discharge and other forms of conventional warfare
  - **Y37.41** Military operations involving rubber bullets
    - **Y37.410** Military operations involving rubber bullets, military personnel
    - **Y37.411** Military operations involving rubber bullets, civilian
  - **Y37.42** Military operations involving firearms pellets
    - **Y37.420** Military operations involving firearms pellets, military personnel
    - **Y37.421** Military operations involving firearms pellets, civilian
  - **Y37.43** Military operations involving other firearms discharge
    - Military operations involving bullets NOS
    - EXCLUDES 1: military operations involving munitions fragments (Y37.25-)
    - military operations involving incendiary bullets (Y37.32-)
    - **Y37.430** Military operations involving other firearms discharge, military personnel

Chapter 20. External Causes of Morbidity

- ✓6th **Y37.431** Military operations involving other firearms discharge, civilian
- ✓6th **Y37.44** Military operations involving unarmed hand to hand combat
  - EXCLUDES 1: military operations involving combat using blunt or piercing object (Y37.45-)
  - military operations involving intentional restriction of air and airway (Y37.46-)
  - military operations involving unintentional restriction of air and airway (Y37.47-)
  - ✓7th **Y37.440** Military operations involving unarmed hand to hand combat, military personnel
  - ✓7th **Y37.441** Military operations involving unarmed hand to hand combat, civilian
- ✓6th **Y37.45** Military operations involving combat using blunt or piercing object
  - ✓7th **Y37.450** Military operations involving combat using blunt or piercing object, military personnel
  - ✓7th **Y37.451** Military operations involving combat using blunt or piercing object, civilian
- ✓6th **Y37.46** Military operations involving intentional restriction of air and airway
  - ✓7th **Y37.460** Military operations involving intentional restriction of air and airway, military personnel
  - ✓7th **Y37.461** Military operations involving intentional restriction of air and airway, civilian
- ✓6th **Y37.47** Military operations involving unintentional restriction of air and airway
  - ✓7th **Y37.470** Military operations involving unintentional restriction of air and airway, military personnel
  - ✓7th **Y37.471** Military operations involving unintentional restriction of air and airway, civilian
- ✓6th **Y37.49** Military operations involving other forms of conventional warfare
  - ✓7th **Y37.490** Military operations involving other forms of conventional warfare, military personnel
  - ✓7th **Y37.491** Military operations involving other forms of conventional warfare, civilian
- ✓5th **Y37.5** Military operations involving nuclear weapons
  - Military operation involving dirty bomb NOS
  - ✓6th **Y37.50** Military operations involving unspecified effect of nuclear weapon
    - ✓7th **Y37.500** Military operations involving unspecified effect of nuclear weapon, military personnel
    - ✓7th **Y37.501** Military operations involving unspecified effect of nuclear weapon, civilian
  - ✓6th **Y37.51** Military operations involving direct blast effect of nuclear weapon
    - Military operations involving blast pressure of nuclear weapon
    - ✓7th **Y37.510** Military operations involving direct blast effect of nuclear weapon, military personnel
    - ✓7th **Y37.511** Military operations involving direct blast effect of nuclear weapon, civilian
  - ✓6th **Y37.52** Military operations involving indirect blast effect of nuclear weapon
    - Military operations involving being struck or crushed by blast debris of nuclear weapon
    - Military operations involving being thrown by blast of nuclear weapon
    - ✓7th **Y37.520** Military operations involving indirect blast effect of nuclear weapon, military personnel
    - ✓7th **Y37.521** Military operations involving indirect blast effect of nuclear weapon, civilian
  - ✓6th **Y37.53** Military operations involving thermal radiation effect of nuclear weapon
    - Military operation involving fireball effects from nuclear weapon
    - Military operations involving direct heat from nuclear weapon
    - ✓7th **Y37.530** Military operations involving thermal radiation effect of nuclear weapon, military personnel
    - ✓7th **Y37.531** Military operations involving thermal radiation effect of nuclear weapon, civilian
  - ✓6th **Y37.54** Military operation involving nuclear radiation effects of nuclear weapon
    - Military operation involving acute radiation exposure from nuclear weapon
    - Military operation involving exposure to immediate ionizing radiation from nuclear weapon
    - Military operation involving fallout exposure from nuclear weapon
    - Military operation involving secondary effects of nuclear weapons
    - ✓7th **Y37.540** Military operation involving nuclear radiation effects of nuclear weapon, military personnel
    - ✓7th **Y37.541** Military operation involving nuclear radiation effects of nuclear weapon, civilian
  - ✓6th **Y37.59** Military operation involving other effects of nuclear weapons
    - ✓7th **Y37.590** Military operation involving other effects of nuclear weapons, military personnel
    - ✓7th **Y37.591** Military operation involving other effects of nuclear weapons, civilian
- ✓5th **Y37.6** Military operations involving biological weapons
  - ✓6th **Y37.6X** Military operations involving biological weapons
    - ✓7th **Y37.6X0** Military operations involving biological weapons, military personnel
    - ✓7th **Y37.6X1** Military operations involving biological weapons, civilian
- ✓5th **Y37.7** Military operations involving chemical weapons and other forms of unconventional warfare
  - EXCLUDES 1: military operations involving incendiary devices (Y36.3-, Y36.5-)
  - ✓6th **Y37.7X** Military operations involving chemical weapons and other forms of unconventional warfare
    - ✓7th **Y37.7X0** Military operations involving chemical weapons and other forms of unconventional warfare, military personnel
    - ✓7th **Y37.7X1** Military operations involving chemical weapons and other forms of unconventional warfare, civilian
- ✓5th **Y37.9** Other and unspecified military operations
  - ✓x7th **Y37.90** Military operations, unspecified
  - ✓x7th **Y37.91** Military operations involving unspecified weapon of mass destruction [WMD]
  - ✓x7th **Y37.92** Military operations involving friendly fire
- ● ✓5th **Y37.A** Blast overpressure in military operations
  - Code also type of explosive, if known
    - accidental detonation of onboard munitions (Y37.140)
    - explosion of grenade (Y37.290)
    - explosion of torpedo (Y37.040)
    - improvised explosive device (Y37.230)
- ● ✓x7th **Y37.A1** Low level blast overpressure in military operations
  - LLB overpressure in military operations
  - Low level blast overpressure due to explosion in military operations
- ● ✓x7th **Y37.A2** High level blast overpressure in military operations
  - High level blast overpressure due to explosion in military operations
  - HLB overpressure in military operations
- ✓4th **Y38** Terrorism
  - NOTE: These codes are for use to identify injuries resulting from the unlawful use of force or violence against persons or property to intimidate or coerce a Government, the civilian population, or any segment thereof, in furtherance of political or social objective
  - Use additional code for place of occurrence (Y92.-)
  - ✓5th **Y38.0** Terrorism involving explosion of marine weapons
    - Terrorism involving depth-charge
    - Terrorism involving marine mine
    - Terrorism involving mine NOS, at sea or in harbor
    - Terrorism involving sea-based artillery shell
    - Terrorism involving torpedo
    - Terrorism involving underwater blast
    - ✓6th **Y38.0X** Terrorism involving explosion of marine weapons
      - ✓7th **Y38.0X1** Terrorism involving explosion of marine weapons, public safety official injured
      - ✓7th **Y38.0X2** Terrorism involving explosion of marine weapons, civilian injured

Chapter 20. External Causes of Morbidity

- ☑7th **Y38.0X3** Terrorism involving explosion of marine weapons, terrorist injured
- ☑5th **Y38.1** Terrorism involving destruction of aircraft
    - Terrorism involving aircraft being shot down
    - Terrorism involving aircraft burned
    - Terrorism involving aircraft exploded
    - Terrorism involving aircraft used as a weapon
    - ☑6th **Y38.1X** Terrorism involving destruction of aircraft
        - ☑7th **Y38.1X1** Terrorism involving destruction of aircraft, public safety official injured
        - ☑7th **Y38.1X2** Terrorism involving destruction of aircraft, civilian injured
        - ☑7th **Y38.1X3** Terrorism involving destruction of aircraft, terrorist injured
- ☑5th **Y38.2** Terrorism involving other explosions and fragments
    - Terrorism involving antipersonnel (fragments) bomb
    - Terrorism involving blast NOS
    - Terrorism involving explosion (fragments) of artillery shell
    - Terrorism involving explosion (fragments) of bomb
    - Terrorism involving explosion (fragments) of grenade
    - Terrorism involving explosion (fragments) of guided missile
    - Terrorism involving explosion (fragments) of land mine
    - Terrorism involving explosion (fragments) of rocket
    - Terrorism involving explosion (fragments) of shell
    - Terrorism involving explosion of breech block
    - Terrorism involving explosion of cannon block
    - Terrorism involving explosion of mortar bomb
    - Terrorism involving explosion of munitions
    - Terrorism involving explosion NOS
    - Terrorism involving mine NOS, on land
    - Terrorism involving shrapnel
    - **EXCLUDES 1** *terrorism involving explosion of nuclear weapon (Y38.5)*
    - *terrorism involving suicide bomber (Y38.81)*
    - ☑6th **Y38.2X** Terrorism involving other explosions and fragments
        - ☑7th **Y38.2X1** Terrorism involving other explosions and fragments, public safety official injured
        - ☑7th **Y38.2X2** Terrorism involving other explosions and fragments, civilian injured
        - ☑7th **Y38.2X3** Terrorism involving other explosions and fragments, terrorist injured
- ☑5th **Y38.3** Terrorism involving fires, conflagration and hot substances
    - Terrorism involving conflagration NOS
    - Terrorism involving fire NOS
    - Terrorism involving petrol bomb
    - **EXCLUDES 1** *terrorism involving fire or heat of nuclear weapon (Y38.5)*
    - ☑6th **Y38.3X** Terrorism involving fires, conflagration and hot substances
        - ☑7th **Y38.3X1** Terrorism involving fires, conflagration and hot substances, public safety official injured
        - ☑7th **Y38.3X2** Terrorism involving fires, conflagration and hot substances, civilian injured
        - ☑7th **Y38.3X3** Terrorism involving fires, conflagration and hot substances, terrorist injured
- ☑5th **Y38.4** Terrorism involving firearms
    - Terrorism involving carbine bullet
    - Terrorism involving machine gun bullet
    - Terrorism involving pellets (shotgun)
    - Terrorism involving pistol bullet
    - Terrorism involving rifle bullet
    - Terrorism involving rubber (rifle) bullet
    - ☑6th **Y38.4X** Terrorism involving firearms
        - ☑7th **Y38.4X1** Terrorism involving firearms, public safety official injured
        - ☑7th **Y38.4X2** Terrorism involving firearms, civilian injured
        - ☑7th **Y38.4X3** Terrorism involving firearms, terrorist injured
- ☑5th **Y38.5** Terrorism involving nuclear weapons
    - Terrorism involving blast effects of nuclear weapon
    - Terrorism involving exposure to ionizing radiation from nuclear weapon
    - Terrorism involving fireball effect of nuclear weapon
    - Terrorism involving heat from nuclear weapon
    - ☑6th **Y38.5X** Terrorism involving nuclear weapons
        - ☑7th **Y38.5X1** Terrorism involving nuclear weapons, public safety official injured
        - ☑7th **Y38.5X2** Terrorism involving nuclear weapons, civilian injured
        - ☑7th **Y38.5X3** Terrorism involving nuclear weapons, terrorist injured
- ☑5th **Y38.6** Terrorism involving biological weapons
    - Terrorism involving anthrax
    - Terrorism involving cholera
    - Terrorism involving smallpox
    - ☑6th **Y38.6X** Terrorism involving biological weapons
        - ☑7th **Y38.6X1** Terrorism involving biological weapons, public safety official injured
        - ☑7th **Y38.6X2** Terrorism involving biological weapons, civilian injured
        - ☑7th **Y38.6X3** Terrorism involving biological weapons, terrorist injured
- ☑5th **Y38.7** Terrorism involving chemical weapons
    - Terrorism involving gases, fumes, chemicals
    - Terrorism involving hydrogen cyanide
    - Terrorism involving phosgene
    - Terrorism involving sarin
    - ☑6th **Y38.7X** Terrorism involving chemical weapons
        - ☑7th **Y38.7X1** Terrorism involving chemical weapons, public safety official injured
        - ☑7th **Y38.7X2** Terrorism involving chemical weapons, civilian injured
        - ☑7th **Y38.7X3** Terrorism involving chemical weapons, terrorist injured
- ☑5th **Y38.8** Terrorism involving other and unspecified means
    - ☑x7th **Y38.80** Terrorism involving unspecified means
        - Terrorism NOS
    - ☑6th **Y38.81** Terrorism involving suicide bomber
        - ☑7th **Y38.811** Terrorism involving suicide bomber, public safety official injured
        - ☑7th **Y38.812** Terrorism involving suicide bomber, civilian injured
    - ☑6th **Y38.89** Terrorism involving other means
        - Terrorism involving drowning and submersion
        - Terrorism involving lasers
        - Terrorism involving piercing or stabbing instruments
        - ☑7th **Y38.891** Terrorism involving other means, public safety official injured
        - ☑7th **Y38.892** Terrorism involving other means, civilian injured
        - ☑7th **Y38.893** Terrorism involving other means, terrorist injured
- ☑5th **Y38.9** Terrorism, secondary effects
    - **NOTE** This code is for use to identify conditions occurring subsequent to a terrorist attack not those that are due to the initial terrorist attack
    - ☑6th **Y38.9X** Terrorism, secondary effects
        - ☑7th **Y38.9X1** Terrorism, secondary effects, public safety official injured
        - ☑7th **Y38.9X2** Terrorism, secondary effects, civilian injured

COMPLICATIONS OF MEDICAL AND SURGICAL CARE (Y62-Y84)

INCLUDES complications of medical devices
surgical and medical procedures as the cause of abnormal reaction of the patient, or of later complication, without mention of misadventure at the time of the procedure

Misadventures to patients during surgical and medical care (Y62-Y69)

EXCLUDES 1 *surgical and medical procedures as the cause of abnormal reaction of the patient, without mention of misadventure at the time of the procedure (Y83-Y84)*
EXCLUDES 2 *breakdown or malfunctioning of medical device (during procedure) (after implantation) (ongoing use) (Y70-Y82)*

- ☑4th **Y62** Failure of sterile precautions during surgical and medical care
    - **Y62.0** Failure of sterile precautions during surgical operation
    - **Y62.1** Failure of sterile precautions during infusion or transfusion
    - **Y62.2** Failure of sterile precautions during kidney dialysis and other perfusion **Rx** **ESR**
    - **Y62.3** Failure of sterile precautions during injection or immunization
    - **Y62.4** Failure of sterile precautions during endoscopic examination
    - **Y62.5** Failure of sterile precautions during heart catheterization
    - **Y62.6** Failure of sterile precautions during aspiration, puncture and other catheterization
    - **Y62.8** Failure of sterile precautions during other surgical and medical care

	Y62.9	Failure of sterile precautions during unspecified surgical and medical care
✓4th	**Y63**	**Failure in dosage during surgical and medical care**
		EXCLUDES 2: accidental overdose of drug or wrong drug given in error (T36-T50)
	Y63.0	Excessive amount of blood or other fluid given during transfusion or infusion
	Y63.1	Incorrect dilution of fluid used during infusion
	Y63.2	Overdose of radiation given during therapy
	Y63.3	Inadvertent exposure of patient to radiation during medical care
	Y63.4	Failure in dosage in electroshock or insulin-shock therapy
	Y63.5	Inappropriate temperature in local application and packing
	Y63.6	Underdosing and nonadministration of necessary drug, medicament or biological substance
		AHA: 2018,4Q,72
	Y63.8	Failure in dosage during other surgical and medical care
		AHA: 2018,4Q,72
	Y63.9	Failure in dosage during unspecified surgical and medical care
		AHA: 2018,4Q,72
✓4th	**Y64**	**Contaminated medical or biological substances**
	Y64.0	Contaminated medical or biological substance, transfused or infused
	Y64.1	Contaminated medical or biological substance, injected or used for immunization
	Y64.8	Contaminated medical or biological substance administered by other means
	Y64.9	Contaminated medical or biological substance administered by unspecified means
		Administered contaminated medical or biological substance NOS
✓4th	**Y65**	**Other misadventures during surgical and medical care**
	Y65.0	Mismatched blood in transfusion
	Y65.1	Wrong fluid used in infusion
	Y65.2	Failure in suture or ligature during surgical operation
	Y65.3	Endotracheal tube wrongly placed during anesthetic procedure
	Y65.4	Failure to introduce or to remove other tube or instrument
		AHA: 2025,2Q,10
	✓5th Y65.5	Performance of wrong procedure (operation)
		Y65.51 Performance of wrong procedure (operation) on correct patient
		Wrong device implanted into correct surgical site
		EXCLUDES 1: performance of correct procedure (operation) on wrong side or body part (Y65.53)
		Y65.52 Performance of procedure (operation) on patient not scheduled for surgery
		Performance of procedure (operation) intended for another patient
		Performance of procedure (operation) on wrong patient
		Y65.53 Performance of correct procedure (operation) on wrong side or body part
		Performance of correct procedure (operation) on wrong side
		Performance of correct procedure (operation) on wrong site
	Y65.8	Other specified misadventures during surgical and medical care
		AHA: 2022,1Q,22; 2019,2Q,23-24
	Y66	**Nonadministration of surgical and medical care**
		Premature cessation of surgical and medical care
		EXCLUDES 1: DNR status (Z66)
		palliative care (Z51.5)
	Y69	**Unspecified misadventure during surgical and medical care**

Medical devices associated with adverse incidents in diagnostic and therapeutic use (Y70-Y82)

INCLUDES: breakdown or malfunction of medical devices (during use) (after implantation) (ongoing use)

EXCLUDES 2: later complications following use of medical devices without breakdown or malfunctioning of device (Y83-Y84)
misadventure to patients during surgical and medical care, classifiable to (Y62-Y69)
surgical and other medical procedures as the cause of abnormal reaction of the patient, or of later complication, without mention of misadventure at the time of the procedure (Y83-Y84)

✓4th	**Y70**	**Anesthesiology devices associated with adverse incidents**
	Y70.0	Diagnostic and monitoring anesthesiology devices associated with adverse incidents
	Y70.1	Therapeutic (nonsurgical) and rehabilitative anesthesiology devices associated with adverse incidents
	Y70.2	Prosthetic and other implants, materials and accessory anesthesiology devices associated with adverse incidents
	Y70.3	Surgical instruments, materials and anesthesiology devices (including sutures) associated with adverse incidents
	Y70.8	Miscellaneous anesthesiology devices associated with adverse incidents, not elsewhere classified
✓4th	**Y71**	**Cardiovascular devices associated with adverse incidents**
	Y71.0	Diagnostic and monitoring cardiovascular devices associated with adverse incidents
	Y71.1	Therapeutic (nonsurgical) and rehabilitative cardiovascular devices associated with adverse incidents
	Y71.2	Prosthetic and other implants, materials and accessory cardiovascular devices associated with adverse incidents
	Y71.3	Surgical instruments, materials and cardiovascular devices (including sutures) associated with adverse incidents
	Y71.8	Miscellaneous cardiovascular devices associated with adverse incidents, not elsewhere classified
✓4th	**Y72**	**Otorhinolaryngological devices associated with adverse incidents**
	Y72.0	Diagnostic and monitoring otorhinolaryngological devices associated with adverse incidents
	Y72.1	Therapeutic (nonsurgical) and rehabilitative otorhinolaryngological devices associated with adverse incidents
	Y72.2	Prosthetic and other implants, materials and accessory otorhinolaryngological devices associated with adverse incidents
	Y72.3	Surgical instruments, materials and otorhinolaryngological devices (including sutures) associated with adverse incidents
	Y72.8	Miscellaneous otorhinolaryngological devices associated with adverse incidents, not elsewhere classified
✓4th	**Y73**	**Gastroenterology and urology devices associated with adverse incidents**
	Y73.0	Diagnostic and monitoring gastroenterology and urology devices associated with adverse incidents
	Y73.1	Therapeutic (nonsurgical) and rehabilitative gastroenterology and urology devices associated with adverse incidents
	Y73.2	Prosthetic and other implants, materials and accessory gastroenterology and urology devices associated with adverse incidents
	Y73.3	Surgical instruments, materials and gastroenterology and urology devices (including sutures) associated with adverse incidents
	Y73.8	Miscellaneous gastroenterology and urology devices associated with adverse incidents, not elsewhere classified
✓4th	**Y74**	**General hospital and personal-use devices associated with adverse incidents**
	Y74.0	Diagnostic and monitoring general hospital and personal-use devices associated with adverse incidents
	Y74.1	Therapeutic (nonsurgical) and rehabilitative general hospital and personal-use devices associated with adverse incidents
	Y74.2	Prosthetic and other implants, materials and accessory general hospital and personal-use devices associated with adverse incidents
	Y74.3	Surgical instruments, materials and general hospital and personal-use devices (including sutures) associated with adverse incidents
	Y74.8	Miscellaneous general hospital and personal-use devices associated with adverse incidents, not elsewhere classified
✓4th	**Y75**	**Neurological devices associated with adverse incidents**
	Y75.0	Diagnostic and monitoring neurological devices associated with adverse incidents
	Y75.1	Therapeutic (nonsurgical) and rehabilitative neurological devices associated with adverse incidents
	Y75.2	Prosthetic and other implants, materials and neurological devices associated with adverse incidents
	Y75.3	Surgical instruments, materials and neurological devices (including sutures) associated with adverse incidents
	Y75.8	Miscellaneous neurological devices associated with adverse incidents, not elsewhere classified
✓4th	**Y76**	**Obstetric and gynecological devices associated with adverse incidents**
	Y76.0	Diagnostic and monitoring obstetric and gynecological devices associated with adverse incidents
	Y76.1	Therapeutic (nonsurgical) and rehabilitative obstetric and gynecological devices associated with adverse incidents
	Y76.2	Prosthetic and other implants, materials and accessory obstetric and gynecological devices associated with adverse incidents

- **Y76.3** Surgical instruments, materials and obstetric and gynecological devices (including sutures) associated with adverse incidents
- **Y76.8** Miscellaneous obstetric and gynecological devices associated with adverse incidents, not elsewhere classified

✓4th **Y77** Ophthalmic devices associated with adverse incidents
- **Y77.0** Diagnostic and monitoring ophthalmic devices associated with adverse incidents
- ✓5th **Y77.1** Therapeutic (nonsurgical) and rehabilitative ophthalmic devices associated with adverse incidents
  AHA: 2020,4Q,41
  - **Y77.11** Contact lens associated with adverse incidents
    Rigid gas permeable contact lens associated with adverse incidents
    Soft (hydrophilic) contact lens associated with adverse incidents
  - **Y77.19** Other therapeutic (nonsurgical) and rehabilitative ophthalmic devices associated with adverse incidents
- **Y77.2** Prosthetic and other implants, materials and accessory ophthalmic devices associated with adverse incidents
- **Y77.3** Surgical instruments, materials and ophthalmic devices (including sutures) associated with adverse incidents
- **Y77.8** Miscellaneous ophthalmic devices associated with adverse incidents, not elsewhere classified

✓4th **Y78** Radiological devices associated with adverse incidents
- **Y78.0** Diagnostic and monitoring radiological devices associated with adverse incidents
- **Y78.1** Therapeutic (nonsurgical) and rehabilitative radiological devices associated with adverse incidents
- **Y78.2** Prosthetic and other implants, materials and accessory radiological devices associated with adverse incidents
- **Y78.3** Surgical instruments, materials and radiological devices (including sutures) associated with adverse incidents
- **Y78.8** Miscellaneous radiological devices associated with adverse incidents, not elsewhere classified

✓4th **Y79** Orthopedic devices associated with adverse incidents
- **Y79.0** Diagnostic and monitoring orthopedic devices associated with adverse incidents
- **Y79.1** Therapeutic (nonsurgical) and rehabilitative orthopedic devices associated with adverse incidents
- **Y79.2** Prosthetic and other implants, materials and accessory orthopedic devices associated with adverse incidents
- **Y79.3** Surgical instruments, materials and orthopedic devices (including sutures) associated with adverse incidents
- **Y79.8** Miscellaneous orthopedic devices associated with adverse incidents, not elsewhere classified

✓4th **Y80** Physical medicine devices associated with adverse incidents
- **Y80.0** Diagnostic and monitoring physical medicine devices associated with adverse incidents
- **Y80.1** Therapeutic (nonsurgical) and rehabilitative physical medicine devices associated with adverse incidents
- **Y80.2** Prosthetic and other implants, materials and accessory physical medicine devices associated with adverse incidents
- **Y80.3** Surgical instruments, materials and physical medicine devices (including sutures) associated with adverse incidents
- **Y80.8** Miscellaneous physical medicine devices associated with adverse incidents, not elsewhere classified

✓4th **Y81** General- and plastic-surgery devices associated with adverse incidents
- **Y81.0** Diagnostic and monitoring general- and plastic-surgery devices associated with adverse incidents
- **Y81.1** Therapeutic (nonsurgical) and rehabilitative general- and plastic-surgery devices associated with adverse incidents
- **Y81.2** Prosthetic and other implants, materials and accessory general- and plastic-surgery devices associated with adverse incidents
- **Y81.3** Surgical instruments, materials and general- and plastic-surgery devices (including sutures) associated with adverse incidents
- **Y81.8** Miscellaneous general- and plastic-surgery devices associated with adverse incidents, not elsewhere classified

✓4th **Y82** Other and unspecified medical devices associated with adverse incidents
- **Y82.8** Other medical devices associated with adverse incidents
- **Y82.9** Unspecified medical devices associated with adverse incidents

Surgical and other medical procedures as the cause of abnormal reaction of the patient, or of later complication, without mention of misadventure at the time of the procedure (Y83-Y84)

EXCLUDES 1 misadventures to patients during surgical and medical care, classifiable to (Y62-Y69)
EXCLUDES 2 breakdown or malfunctioning of medical device (during procedure) (after implantation) (ongoing use) (Y70-Y82)

✓4th **Y83** Surgical operation and other surgical procedures as the cause of abnormal reaction of the patient, or of later complication, without mention of misadventure at the time of the procedure
- **Y83.0** Surgical operation with transplant of whole organ as the cause of abnormal reaction of the patient, or of later complication, without mention of misadventure at the time of the procedure
- **Y83.1** Surgical operation with implant of artificial internal device as the cause of abnormal reaction of the patient, or of later complication, without mention of misadventure at the time of the procedure
- **Y83.2** Surgical operation with anastomosis, bypass or graft as the cause of abnormal reaction of the patient, or of later complication, without mention of misadventure at the time of the procedure
- **Y83.3** Surgical operation with formation of external stoma as the cause of abnormal reaction of the patient, or of later complication, without mention of misadventure at the time of the procedure
- **Y83.4** Other reconstructive surgery as the cause of abnormal reaction of the patient, or of later complication, without mention of misadventure at the time of the procedure
- **Y83.5** Amputation of limb(s) as the cause of abnormal reaction of the patient, or of later complication, without mention of misadventure at the time of the procedure
- **Y83.6** Removal of other organ (partial) (total) as the cause of abnormal reaction of the patient, or of later complication, without mention of misadventure at the time of the procedure
- **Y83.8** Other surgical procedures as the cause of abnormal reaction of the patient, or of later complication, without mention of misadventure at the time of the procedure
  AHA: 2023,2Q,14
- **Y83.9** Surgical procedure, unspecified as the cause of abnormal reaction of the patient, or of later complication, without mention of misadventure at the time of the procedure

✓4th **Y84** Other medical procedures as the cause of abnormal reaction of the patient, or of later complication, without mention of misadventure at the time of the procedure
- **Y84.0** Cardiac catheterization as the cause of abnormal reaction of the patient, or of later complication, without mention of misadventure at the time of the procedure
- **Y84.1** Kidney dialysis as the cause of abnormal reaction of the patient, or of later complication, without mention of misadventure at the time of the procedure
- **Y84.2** Radiological procedure and radiotherapy as the cause of abnormal reaction of the patient, or of later complication, without mention of misadventure at the time of the procedure
  AHA: 2019,1Q,21; 2017,1Q,33
- **Y84.3** Shock therapy as the cause of abnormal reaction of the patient, or of later complication, without mention of misadventure at the time of the procedure
- **Y84.4** Aspiration of fluid as the cause of abnormal reaction of the patient, or of later complication, without mention of misadventure at the time of the procedure
- **Y84.5** Insertion of gastric or duodenal sound as the cause of abnormal reaction of the patient, or of later complication, without mention of misadventure at the time of the procedure
- **Y84.6** Urinary catheterization as the cause of abnormal reaction of the patient, or of later complication, without mention of misadventure at the time of the procedure
  AHA: 2025,2Q,20
- **Y84.7** Blood-sampling as the cause of abnormal reaction of the patient, or of later complication, without mention of misadventure at the time of the procedure
- **Y84.8** Other medical procedures as the cause of abnormal reaction of the patient, or of later complication, without mention of misadventure at the time of the procedure
  AHA: 2024,1Q,26; 2023,2Q,28; 2021,1Q,5; 2014,4Q,24
- **Y84.9** Medical procedure, unspecified as the cause of abnormal reaction of the patient, or of later complication, without mention of misadventure at the time of the procedure

Supplementary factors related to causes of morbidity classified elsewhere (Y90-Y99)

NOTE These categories may be used to provide supplementary information concerning causes of morbidity. They are not to be used for single-condition coding.

Y90 Evidence of alcohol involvement determined by blood alcohol level
Code first any associated alcohol related disorders (F10)
- Y90.0 Blood alcohol level of less than 20 mg/100 ml
- Y90.1 Blood alcohol level of 20-39 mg/100 ml
- Y90.2 Blood alcohol level of 40-59 mg/100 ml
- Y90.3 Blood alcohol level of 60-79 mg/100 ml
- Y90.4 Blood alcohol level of 80-99 mg/100 ml
- Y90.5 Blood alcohol level of 100-119 mg/100 ml
- Y90.6 Blood alcohol level of 120-199 mg/100 ml
- Y90.7 Blood alcohol level of 200-239 mg/100 ml
- Y90.8 Blood alcohol level of 240 mg/100 ml or more
- Y90.9 Presence of alcohol in blood, level not specified

Y92 Place of occurrence of the external cause
Place of occurrence should be recorded only at the initial encounter for treatment
The following category is for use, when relevant, to identify the place of occurrence of the external cause. Use in conjunction with an activity code.

- **Y92.0** Non-institutional (private) residence as the place of occurrence of the external cause
  - EXCLUDES 1: abandoned or derelict house (Y92.89)
    home under construction but not yet occupied (Y92.6-)
    institutional place of residence (Y92.1-)

  - **Y92.00** Unspecified non-institutional (private) residence as the place of occurrence of the external cause
    - Y92.000 Kitchen of unspecified non-institutional (private) residence as the place of occurrence of the external cause
    - Y92.001 Dining room of unspecified non-institutional (private) residence as the place of occurrence of the external cause
    - Y92.002 Bathroom of unspecified non-institutional (private) residence as the place of occurrence of the external cause
    - Y92.003 Bedroom of unspecified non-institutional (private) residence as the place of occurrence of the external cause
    - Y92.007 Garden or yard of unspecified non-institutional (private) residence as the place of occurrence of the external cause
    - Y92.008 Other place in unspecified non-institutional (private) residence as the place of occurrence of the external cause
    - Y92.009 Unspecified place in unspecified non-institutional (private) residence as the place of occurrence of the external cause
      Home (NOS) as the place of occurrence of the external cause

  - **Y92.01** Single-family non-institutional (private) house as the place of occurrence of the external cause
    Farmhouse as the place of occurrence of the external cause
    - EXCLUDES 1: barn (Y92.71)
      chicken coop or hen house (Y92.72)
      farm field (Y92.73)
      orchard (Y92.74)
      single family mobile home or trailer (Y92.02-)
      slaughter house (Y92.86)
    - Y92.010 Kitchen of single-family (private) house as the place of occurrence of the external cause
    - Y92.011 Dining room of single-family (private) house as the place of occurrence of the external cause
    - Y92.012 Bathroom of single-family (private) house as the place of occurrence of the external cause
    - Y92.013 Bedroom of single-family (private) house as the place of occurrence of the external cause
    - Y92.014 Private driveway to single-family (private) house as the place of occurrence of the external cause
    - Y92.015 Private garage of single-family (private) house as the place of occurrence of the external cause
    - Y92.016 Swimming-pool in single-family (private) house or garden as the place of occurrence of the external cause
      AHA: 2023, 1Q, 25
    - Y92.017 Garden or yard in single-family (private) house as the place of occurrence of the external cause
    - Y92.018 Other place in single-family (private) house as the place of occurrence of the external cause
    - Y92.019 Unspecified place in single-family (private) house as the place of occurrence of the external cause

  - **Y92.02** Mobile home as the place of occurrence of the external cause
    - Y92.020 Kitchen in mobile home as the place of occurrence of the external cause
    - Y92.021 Dining room in mobile home as the place of occurrence of the external cause
    - Y92.022 Bathroom in mobile home as the place of occurrence of the external cause
    - Y92.023 Bedroom in mobile home as the place of occurrence of the external cause
    - Y92.024 Driveway of mobile home as the place of occurrence of the external cause
    - Y92.025 Garage of mobile home as the place of occurrence of the external cause
    - Y92.026 Swimming-pool of mobile home as the place of occurrence of the external cause
    - Y92.027 Garden or yard of mobile home as the place of occurrence of the external cause
    - Y92.028 Other place in mobile home as the place of occurrence of the external cause
    - Y92.029 Unspecified place in mobile home as the place of occurrence of the external cause

  - **Y92.03** Apartment as the place of occurrence of the external cause
    Condominium as the place of occurrence of the external cause
    Co-op apartment as the place of occurrence of the external cause
    - Y92.030 Kitchen in apartment as the place of occurrence of the external cause
    - Y92.031 Bathroom in apartment as the place of occurrence of the external cause
    - Y92.032 Bedroom in apartment as the place of occurrence of the external cause
    - Y92.038 Other place in apartment as the place of occurrence of the external cause
    - Y92.039 Unspecified place in apartment as the place of occurrence of the external cause

  - **Y92.04** Boarding-house as the place of occurrence of the external cause
    - Y92.040 Kitchen in boarding-house as the place of occurrence of the external cause
    - Y92.041 Bathroom in boarding-house as the place of occurrence of the external cause
    - Y92.042 Bedroom in boarding-house as the place of occurrence of the external cause
    - Y92.043 Driveway of boarding-house as the place of occurrence of the external cause
    - Y92.044 Garage of boarding-house as the place of occurrence of the external cause
    - Y92.045 Swimming-pool of boarding-house as the place of occurrence of the external cause
    - Y92.046 Garden or yard of boarding-house as the place of occurrence of the external cause
    - Y92.048 Other place in boarding-house as the place of occurrence of the external cause
    - Y92.049 Unspecified place in boarding-house as the place of occurrence of the external cause

  - **Y92.09** Other non-institutional residence as the place of occurrence of the external cause
    AHA: 2017, 2Q, 10
    - Y92.090 Kitchen in other non-institutional residence as the place of occurrence of the external cause
    - Y92.091 Bathroom in other non-institutional residence as the place of occurrence of the external cause

- **Y92.092** Bedroom in other non-institutional residence as the place of occurrence of the external cause
- **Y92.093** Driveway of other non-institutional residence as the place of occurrence of the external cause
- **Y92.094** Garage of other non-institutional residence as the place of occurrence of the external cause
- **Y92.095** Swimming-pool of other non-institutional residence as the place of occurrence of the external cause
- **Y92.096** Garden or yard of other non-institutional residence as the place of occurrence of the external cause
- **Y92.098** Other place in other non-institutional residence as the place of occurrence of the external cause
- **Y92.099** Unspecified place in other non-institutional residence as the place of occurrence of the external cause

✓5th **Y92.1** Institutional (nonprivate) residence as the place of occurrence of the external cause
- **Y92.10** Unspecified residential institution as the place of occurrence of the external cause
- ✓6th **Y92.11** Children's home and orphanage as the place of occurrence of the external cause
  - **Y92.110** Kitchen in children's home and orphanage as the place of occurrence of the external cause
  - **Y92.111** Bathroom in children's home and orphanage as the place of occurrence of the external cause
  - **Y92.112** Bedroom in children's home and orphanage as the place of occurrence of the external cause
  - **Y92.113** Driveway of children's home and orphanage as the place of occurrence of the external cause
  - **Y92.114** Garage of children's home and orphanage as the place of occurrence of the external cause
  - **Y92.115** Swimming-pool of children's home and orphanage as the place of occurrence of the external cause
  - **Y92.116** Garden or yard of children's home and orphanage as the place of occurrence of the external cause
  - **Y92.118** Other place in children's home and orphanage as the place of occurrence of the external cause
  - **Y92.119** Unspecified place in children's home and orphanage as the place of occurrence of the external cause
- ✓6th **Y92.12** Nursing home as the place of occurrence of the external cause
  - Home for the sick as the place of occurrence of the external cause
  - Hospice as the place of occurrence of the external cause
  - AHA: 2017,2Q,10
  - **Y92.120** Kitchen in nursing home as the place of occurrence of the external cause
  - **Y92.121** Bathroom in nursing home as the place of occurrence of the external cause
  - **Y92.122** Bedroom in nursing home as the place of occurrence of the external cause
  - **Y92.123** Driveway of nursing home as the place of occurrence of the external cause
  - **Y92.124** Garage of nursing home as the place of occurrence of the external cause
  - **Y92.125** Swimming-pool of nursing home as the place of occurrence of the external cause
  - **Y92.126** Garden or yard of nursing home as the place of occurrence of the external cause
  - **Y92.128** Other place in nursing home as the place of occurrence of the external cause
  - **Y92.129** Unspecified place in nursing home as the place of occurrence of the external cause
- ✓6th **Y92.13** Military base as the place of occurrence of the external cause
  - EXCLUDES 1 military training grounds (Y92.84)
  - **Y92.130** Kitchen on military base as the place of occurrence of the external cause
  - **Y92.131** Mess hall on military base as the place of occurrence of the external cause
  - **Y92.133** Barracks on military base as the place of occurrence of the external cause
  - **Y92.135** Garage on military base as the place of occurrence of the external cause
  - **Y92.136** Swimming-pool on military base as the place of occurrence of the external cause
  - **Y92.137** Garden or yard on military base as the place of occurrence of the external cause
  - **Y92.138** Other place on military base as the place of occurrence of the external cause
  - **Y92.139** Unspecified place military base as the place of occurrence of the external cause
- ✓6th **Y92.14** Prison as the place of occurrence of the external cause
  - **Y92.140** Kitchen in prison as the place of occurrence of the external cause
  - **Y92.141** Dining room in prison as the place of occurrence of the external cause
  - **Y92.142** Bathroom in prison as the place of occurrence of the external cause
  - **Y92.143** Cell of prison as the place of occurrence of the external cause
  - **Y92.146** Swimming-pool of prison as the place of occurrence of the external cause
  - **Y92.147** Courtyard of prison as the place of occurrence of the external cause
  - **Y92.148** Other place in prison as the place of occurrence of the external cause
  - **Y92.149** Unspecified place in prison as the place of occurrence of the external cause
- ✓6th **Y92.15** Reform school as the place of occurrence of the external cause
  - **Y92.150** Kitchen in reform school as the place of occurrence of the external cause
  - **Y92.151** Dining room in reform school as the place of occurrence of the external cause
  - **Y92.152** Bathroom in reform school as the place of occurrence of the external cause
  - **Y92.153** Bedroom in reform school as the place of occurrence of the external cause
  - **Y92.154** Driveway of reform school as the place of occurrence of the external cause
  - **Y92.155** Garage of reform school as the place of occurrence of the external cause
  - **Y92.156** Swimming-pool of reform school as the place of occurrence of the external cause
  - **Y92.157** Garden or yard of reform school as the place of occurrence of the external cause
  - **Y92.158** Other place in reform school as the place of occurrence of the external cause
  - **Y92.159** Unspecified place in reform school as the place of occurrence of the external cause
- ✓6th **Y92.16** School dormitory as the place of occurrence of the external cause
  - EXCLUDES 1 reform school as the place of occurrence of the external cause (Y92.15-)
  - school buildings and grounds as the place of occurrence of the external cause (Y92.2-)
  - school sports and athletic areas as the place of occurrence of the external cause (Y92.3-)
  - **Y92.160** Kitchen in school dormitory as the place of occurrence of the external cause
  - **Y92.161** Dining room in school dormitory as the place of occurrence of the external cause
  - **Y92.162** Bathroom in school dormitory as the place of occurrence of the external cause
  - **Y92.163** Bedroom in school dormitory as the place of occurrence of the external cause
  - **Y92.168** Other place in school dormitory as the place of occurrence of the external cause
  - **Y92.169** Unspecified place in school dormitory as the place of occurrence of the external cause
- ✓6th **Y92.19** Other specified residential institution as the place of occurrence of the external cause
  - AHA: 2017,2Q,10
  - **Y92.190** Kitchen in other specified residential institution as the place of occurrence of the external cause

Y92.191 Dining room in other specified residential institution as the place of occurrence of the external cause
Y92.192 Bathroom in other specified residential institution as the place of occurrence of the external cause
Y92.193 Bedroom in other specified residential institution as the place of occurrence of the external cause
Y92.194 Driveway of other specified residential institution as the place of occurrence of the external cause
Y92.195 Garage of other specified residential institution as the place of occurrence of the external cause
Y92.196 Pool of other specified residential institution as the place of occurrence of the external cause
Y92.197 Garden or yard of other specified residential institution as the place of occurrence of the external cause
Y92.198 Other place in other specified residential institution as the place of occurrence of the external cause
Y92.199 Unspecified place in other specified residential institution as the place of occurrence of the external cause

Y92.2 School, other institution and public administrative area as the place of occurrence of the external cause
Building and adjacent grounds used by the general public or by a particular group of the public

EXCLUDES 1: building under construction as the place of occurrence of the external cause (Y92.6)
residential institution as the place of occurrence of the external cause (Y92.1)
school dormitory as the place of occurrence of the external cause (Y92.16-)
sports and athletics area of schools as the place of occurrence of the external cause (Y92.3-)

Y92.21 School (private) (public) (state) as the place of occurrence of the external cause
  Y92.210 Daycare center as the place of occurrence of the external cause
  Y92.211 Elementary school as the place of occurrence of the external cause
    Kindergarten as the place of occurrence of the external cause
  Y92.212 Middle school as the place of occurrence of the external cause
  Y92.213 High school as the place of occurrence of the external cause
    AHA: 2012,4Q,108
  Y92.214 College as the place of occurrence of the external cause
    University as the place of occurrence of the external cause
  Y92.215 Trade school as the place of occurrence of the external cause
  Y92.218 Other school as the place of occurrence of the external cause
  Y92.219 Unspecified school as the place of occurrence of the external cause

Y92.22 Religious institution as the place of occurrence of the external cause
  Church as the place of occurrence of the external cause
  Mosque as the place of occurrence of the external cause
  Synagogue as the place of occurrence of the external cause

Y92.23 Hospital as the place of occurrence of the external cause
  EXCLUDES 1: ambulatory (outpatient) health services establishments (Y92.53-)
  home for the sick as the place of occurrence of the external cause (Y92.12-)
  hospice as the place of occurrence of the external cause (Y92.12-)
  nursing home as the place of occurrence of the external cause (Y92.12-)

  Y92.230 Patient room in hospital as the place of occurrence of the external cause
  Y92.231 Patient bathroom in hospital as the place of occurrence of the external cause
  Y92.232 Corridor of hospital as the place of occurrence of the external cause
  Y92.233 Cafeteria of hospital as the place of occurrence of the external cause
  Y92.234 Operating room of hospital as the place of occurrence of the external cause
  Y92.238 Other place in hospital as the place of occurrence of the external cause
  Y92.239 Unspecified place in hospital as the place of occurrence of the external cause

Y92.24 Public administrative building as the place of occurrence of the external cause
  Y92.240 Courthouse as the place of occurrence of the external cause
  Y92.241 Library as the place of occurrence of the external cause
  Y92.242 Post office as the place of occurrence of the external cause
  Y92.243 City hall as the place of occurrence of the external cause
  Y92.248 Other public administrative building as the place of occurrence of the external cause

Y92.25 Cultural building as the place of occurrence of the external cause
  Y92.250 Art Gallery as the place of occurrence of the external cause
  Y92.251 Museum as the place of occurrence of the external cause
  Y92.252 Music hall as the place of occurrence of the external cause
  Y92.253 Opera house as the place of occurrence of the external cause
  Y92.254 Theater (live) as the place of occurrence of the external cause
  Y92.258 Other cultural public building as the place of occurrence of the external cause

Y92.26 Movie house or cinema as the place of occurrence of the external cause

Y92.29 Other specified public building as the place of occurrence of the external cause
  Assembly hall as the place of occurrence of the external cause
  Clubhouse as the place of occurrence of the external cause

Y92.3 Sports and athletics area as the place of occurrence of the external cause

Y92.31 Athletic court as the place of occurrence of the external cause
  EXCLUDES 1: tennis court in private home or garden (Y92.09)
  Y92.310 Basketball court as the place of occurrence of the external cause
  Y92.311 Squash court as the place of occurrence of the external cause
  Y92.312 Tennis court as the place of occurrence of the external cause
  Y92.318 Other athletic court as the place of occurrence of the external cause

Y92.32 Athletic field as the place of occurrence of the external cause
  Y92.320 Baseball field as the place of occurrence of the external cause
  Y92.321 Football field as the place of occurrence of the external cause
  Y92.322 Soccer field as the place of occurrence of the external cause
  Y92.328 Other athletic field as the place of occurrence of the external cause
    Cricket field as the place of occurrence of the external cause
    Hockey field as the place of occurrence of the external cause

Y92.33 Skating rink as the place of occurrence of the external cause
  Y92.330 Ice skating rink (indoor) (outdoor) as the place of occurrence of the external cause
  Y92.331 Roller skating rink as the place of occurrence of the external cause

Y92.34 Swimming pool (public) as the place of occurrence of the external cause
  EXCLUDES 1: swimming pool in private home or garden (Y92.016)

Y92.39 Other specified sports and athletic area as the place of occurrence of the external cause
  Golf-course as the place of occurrence of the external cause
  Gymnasium as the place of occurrence of the external cause
  Riding-school as the place of occurrence of the external cause
  Stadium as the place of occurrence of the external cause

Y92.4 **Street, highway and other paved roadways** as the place of occurrence of the external cause
  EXCLUDES 1 private driveway of residence (Y92.014, Y92.024, Y92.043, Y92.093, Y92.113, Y92.123, Y92.154, Y92.194)

  Y92.41 **Street and highway** as the place of occurrence of the external cause
    Y92.410 **Unspecified street and highway** as the place of occurrence of the external cause
      Road NOS as the place of occurrence of the external cause
    Y92.411 **Interstate** highway as the place of occurrence of the external cause
      Freeway as the place of occurrence of the external cause
      Motorway as the place of occurrence of the external cause
    Y92.412 **Parkway** as the place of occurrence of the external cause
    Y92.413 **State road** as the place of occurrence of the external cause
    Y92.414 **Local residential or business street** as the place of occurrence of the external cause
    Y92.415 **Exit ramp or entrance ramp** of street or highway as the place of occurrence of the external cause

  Y92.48 Other paved roadways as the place of occurrence of the external cause
    Y92.480 **Sidewalk** as the place of occurrence of the external cause
    Y92.481 **Parking lot** as the place of occurrence of the external cause
    Y92.482 **Bike path** as the place of occurrence of the external cause
    Y92.488 Other paved roadways as the place of occurrence of the external cause

Y92.5 **Trade and service area** as the place of occurrence of the external cause
  EXCLUDES 1 garage in private home (Y92.015)
    schools and other public administration buildings (Y92.2-)

  Y92.51 **Private commercial establishments** as the place of occurrence of the external cause
    Y92.510 **Bank** as the place of occurrence of the external cause
    Y92.511 **Restaurant or cafe** as the place of occurrence of the external cause
    Y92.512 **Supermarket, store or market** as the place of occurrence of the external cause
    Y92.513 **Shop** (commercial) as the place of occurrence of the external cause

  Y92.52 **Service areas** as the place of occurrence of the external cause
    Y92.520 **Airport** as the place of occurrence of the external cause
    Y92.521 **Bus station** as the place of occurrence of the external cause
    Y92.522 **Railway station** as the place of occurrence of the external cause
    Y92.523 **Highway rest stop** as the place of occurrence of the external cause
    Y92.524 **Gas station** as the place of occurrence of the external cause
      Petroleum station as the place of occurrence of the external cause
      Service station as the place of occurrence of the external cause

  Y92.53 **Ambulatory health services establishments** as the place of occurrence of the external cause
    Y92.530 **Ambulatory surgery center** as the place of occurrence of the external cause
      Outpatient surgery center, including that connected with a hospital as the place of occurrence of the external cause
      Same day surgery center, including that connected with a hospital as the place of occurrence of the external cause
    Y92.531 **Health care provider office** as the place of occurrence of the external cause
      Physician office as the place of occurrence of the external cause
    Y92.532 **Urgent care center** as the place of occurrence of the external cause
    Y92.538 **Other ambulatory health services establishments** as the place of occurrence of the external cause
      AHA: 2019,1Q,21

  Y92.59 Other trade areas as the place of occurrence of the external cause
    Casino as the place of occurrence of the external cause
    Garage (commercial) as the place of occurrence of the external cause
    Hotel as the place of occurrence of the external cause
    Office building as the place of occurrence of the external cause
    Radio or television station as the place of occurrence of the external cause
    Shopping mall as the place of occurrence of the external cause
    Warehouse as the place of occurrence of the external cause

Y92.6 **Industrial and construction area** as the place of occurrence of the external cause
  Y92.61 **Building** [any] **under construction** as the place of occurrence of the external cause
  Y92.62 **Dock or shipyard** as the place of occurrence of the external cause
    Dockyard as the place of occurrence of the external cause
    Dry dock as the place of occurrence of the external cause
    Shipyard as the place of occurrence of the external cause
  Y92.63 **Factory** as the place of occurrence of the external cause
    Factory building as the place of occurrence of the external cause
    Factory premises as the place of occurrence of the external cause
    Industrial yard as the place of occurrence of the external cause
  Y92.64 **Mine or pit** as the place of occurrence of the external cause
    Mine as the place of occurrence of the external cause
  Y92.65 **Oil rig** as the place of occurrence of the external cause
    Pit (coal) (gravel) (sand) as the place of occurrence of the external cause
  Y92.69 Other specified industrial and construction area as the place of occurrence of the external cause
    Gasworks as the place of occurrence of the external cause
    Power-station (coal) (nuclear) (oil) as the place of occurrence of the external cause
    Tunnel under construction as the place of occurrence of the external cause
    Workshop as the place of occurrence of the external cause

Y92.7 **Farm** as the place of occurrence of the external cause
  Ranch as the place of occurrence of the external cause
  EXCLUDES 1 farmhouse and home premises of farm (Y92.01-)

  Y92.71 **Barn** as the place of occurrence of the external cause
  Y92.72 **Chicken coop** as the place of occurrence of the external cause
    Hen house as the place of occurrence of the external cause
  Y92.73 **Farm field** as the place of occurrence of the external cause
  Y92.74 **Orchard** as the place of occurrence of the external cause
  Y92.79 Other farm location as the place of occurrence of the external cause

Y92.8 Other places as the place of occurrence of the external cause

Y92.81 Transport vehicle as the place of occurrence of the external cause
EXCLUDES 1 transport accidents (V00-V99)
- **Y92.810** Car as the place of occurrence of the external cause
- **Y92.811** Bus as the place of occurrence of the external cause
- **Y92.812** Truck as the place of occurrence of the external cause
- **Y92.813** Airplane as the place of occurrence of the external cause
- **Y92.814** Boat as the place of occurrence of the external cause
- **Y92.815** Train as the place of occurrence of the external cause
- **Y92.816** Subway car as the place of occurrence of the external cause
- **Y92.818** Other transport vehicle as the place of occurrence of the external cause

Y92.82 Wilderness area
- **Y92.820** Desert as the place of occurrence of the external cause
- **Y92.821** Forest as the place of occurrence of the external cause
- **Y92.828** Other wilderness area as the place of occurrence of the external cause
    - Marsh as the place of occurrence of the external cause
    - Mountain as the place of occurrence of the external cause
    - Prairie as the place of occurrence of the external cause
    - Swamp as the place of occurrence of the external cause

Y92.83 Recreation area as the place of occurrence of the external cause
- **Y92.830** Public park as the place of occurrence of the external cause
- **Y92.831** Amusement park as the place of occurrence of the external cause
- **Y92.832** Beach as the place of occurrence of the external cause
    - Seashore as the place of occurrence of the external cause
- **Y92.833** Campsite as the place of occurrence of the external cause
- **Y92.834** Zoological garden (Zoo) as the place of occurrence of the external cause
- **Y92.838** Other recreation area as the place of occurrence of the external cause

Y92.84 Military training ground as the place of occurrence of the external cause
Y92.85 Railroad track as the place of occurrence of the external cause
Y92.86 Slaughter house as the place of occurrence of the external cause
Y92.89 Other specified places as the place of occurrence of the external cause
- Derelict house as the place of occurrence of the external cause

Y92.9 Unspecified place or not applicable

Y93 Activity codes

NOTE Category Y93 is provided for use to indicate the activity of the person seeking healthcare for an injury or health condition, such as a heart attack while shoveling snow, which resulted from, or was contributed to, by the activity. These codes are appropriate for use for both acute injuries, such as those from chapter 19, and conditions that are due to the long-term, cumulative effects of an activity, such as those from chapter 13. They are also appropriate for use with external cause codes for cause and intent if identifying the activity provides additional information on the event. These codes should be used in conjunction with codes for external cause status (Y99) and place of occurrence (Y92).

This section contains the following broad activity categories:

- Y93.0 Activities involving walking and running
- Y93.1 Activities involving water and water craft
- Y93.2 Activities involving ice and snow
- Y93.3 Activities involving climbing, rappelling, and jumping off
- Y93.4 Activities involving dancing and other rhythmic movement
- Y93.5 Activities involving other sports and athletics played individually
- Y93.6 Activities involving other sports and athletics played as a team or group
- Y93.7 Activities involving other specified sports and athletics
- Y93.A Activities involving other cardiorespiratory exercise
- Y93.B Activities involving other muscle strengthening exercises
- Y93.C Activities involving computer technology and electronic devices
- Y93.D Activities involving arts and handcrafts
- Y93.E Activities involving personal hygiene and interior property and clothing maintenance
- Y93.F Activities involving caregiving
- Y93.G Activities involving food preparation, cooking and grilling
- Y93.H Activities involving exterior property and land maintenance, building and construction
- Y93.I Activities involving roller coasters and other types of external motion
- Y93.J Activities involving playing musical instrument
- Y93.K Activities involving animal care
- Y93.L ▶Other outdoor activity◀
- Y93.8 Activities, other specified
- Y93.9 Activity, unspecified

Y93.0 Activities involving walking and running
EXCLUDES 1 activity, walking an animal (Y93.K1)
activity, walking or running on a treadmill (Y93.A1)
- **Y93.01** Activity, walking, marching and hiking
    - Activity, walking, marching and hiking on level or elevated terrain
    - EXCLUDES 1 activity, mountain climbing (Y93.31)
- **Y93.02** Activity, running

Y93.1 Activities involving water and water craft
EXCLUDES 1 activities involving ice (Y93.2-)
- **Y93.11** Activity, swimming
- **Y93.12** Activity, springboard and platform diving
- **Y93.13** Activity, water polo
- **Y93.14** Activity, water aerobics and water exercise
- **Y93.15** Activity, underwater diving and snorkeling
    - Activity, SCUBA diving
- **Y93.16** Activity, rowing, canoeing, kayaking, rafting and tubing
    - Activity, canoeing, kayaking, rafting and tubing in calm and turbulent water
- **Y93.17** Activity, water skiing and wake boarding
- **Y93.18** Activity, surfing, windsurfing and boogie boarding
    - Activity, water sliding
- **Y93.19** Activity, other involving water and watercraft
    - Activity involving water NOS
    - Activity, parasailing
    - Activity, water survival training and testing

Y93.2 Activities involving ice and snow
EXCLUDES 1 activity, shoveling ice and snow (Y93.H1)
- **Y93.21** Activity, ice skating
    - Activity, figure skating (singles) (pairs)
    - Activity, ice dancing
    - EXCLUDES 1 activity, ice hockey (Y93.22)
- **Y93.22** Activity, ice hockey

Y93.23	**Activity,** snow **(alpine) (downhill)** skiing, snowboarding, sledding, tobogganing and snow tubing	
	EXCLUDES 1 *activity, cross country skiing (Y93.24)*	
Y93.24	**Activity,** cross country skiing	
	Activity, nordic skiing	
Y93.29	**Activity, other involving ice and snow**	
	Activity involving ice and snow NOS	
✓5th Y93.3	**Activities involving climbing, rappelling and jumping off**	
	EXCLUDES 1 *activity, hiking on level or elevated terrain (Y93.01)*	
	activity, jumping rope (Y93.56)	
	activity, trampoline jumping (Y93.44)	
Y93.31	**Activity,** mountain climbing, rock climbing and wall climbing	
Y93.32	**Activity,** rappelling	
Y93.33	**Activity,** BASE jumping	
	Activity, Building, Antenna, Span, Earth jumping	
Y93.34	**Activity,** bungee jumping	
Y93.35	**Activity,** hang gliding	
Y93.39	**Activity, other involving climbing, rappelling and jumping off**	
✓5th Y93.4	**Activities involving dancing and other rhythmic movement**	
	EXCLUDES 1 *activity, martial arts (Y93.75)*	
Y93.41	**Activity,** dancing	
	AHA: 2012,4Q,108	
Y93.42	**Activity,** yoga	
Y93.43	**Activity,** gymnastics	
	Activity, rhythmic gymnastics	
	EXCLUDES 1 *activity, trampolining (Y93.44)*	
Y93.44	**Activity,** trampolining	
Y93.45	**Activity,** cheerleading	
Y93.49	**Activity, other involving dancing and other rhythmic movements**	
✓5th Y93.5	**Activities involving other sports and athletics played individually**	
	EXCLUDES 1 *activity, dancing (Y93.41)*	
	activity, gymnastic (Y93.43)	
	activity, trampolining (Y93.44)	
	activity, yoga (Y93.42)	
Y93.51	**Activity,** roller skating **(inline)** and skateboarding	
Y93.52	**Activity,** horseback riding	
Y93.53	**Activity,** golf	
Y93.54	**Activity,** bowling	
Y93.55	**Activity,** bike riding	
Y93.56	**Activity,** jumping rope	
Y93.57	**Activity,** non-running track and field events	
	EXCLUDES 1 *activity, running (any form) (Y93.02)*	
Y93.59	**Activity, other involving other sports and athletics played individually**	
	EXCLUDES 1 *activities involving climbing, rappelling, and jumping (Y93.3-)*	
	activities involving ice and snow (Y93.2-)	
	activities involving walking and running (Y93.0-)	
	activities involving water and watercraft (Y93.1-)	
✓5th Y93.6	**Activities involving other sports and athletics played as a team or group**	
	EXCLUDES 1 *activity, ice hockey (Y93.22)*	
	activity, water polo (Y93.13)	
Y93.61	**Activity,** American tackle football	
	Activity, football NOS	
Y93.62	**Activity,** American flag or touch football	
Y93.63	**Activity,** rugby	
Y93.64	**Activity,** baseball	
	Activity, softball	
Y93.65	**Activity,** lacrosse and field hockey	
Y93.66	**Activity,** soccer	
Y93.67	**Activity,** basketball	
Y93.68	**Activity,** volleyball **(beach) (court)**	
Y93.6A	**Activity, physical games generally associated with** school recess, summer camp and children	
	Activity, capture the flag	
	Activity, dodge ball	
	Activity, four square	
	Activity, kickball	
Y93.69	**Activity, other involving other sports and athletics played as a team or group**	
	Activity, cricket	

✓5th Y93.7	**Activities involving other specified sports and athletics**	
Y93.71	**Activity,** boxing	
Y93.72	**Activity,** wrestling	
Y93.73	**Activity,** racquet and hand **sports**	
	Activity, handball	
	Activity, racquetball	
	Activity, squash	
	Activity, tennis	
Y93.74	**Activity,** frisbee	
	Activity, ultimate frisbee	
Y93.75	**Activity,** martial arts	
	Activity, combatives	
Y93.79	**Activity, other specified sports and athletics**	
	EXCLUDES 1 *sports and athletics activities specified in categories Y93.0-Y93.6*	
✓5th Y93.A	**Activities involving other cardiorespiratory exercise**	
	Activities involving physical training	
Y93.A1	**Activity,** exercise machines **primarily for cardiorespiratory conditioning**	
	Activity, elliptical and stepper machines	
	Activity, stationary bike	
	Activity, treadmill	
Y93.A2	**Activity,** calisthenics	
	Activity, jumping jacks	
	Activity, warm up and cool down	
Y93.A3	**Activity,** aerobic and step exercise	
Y93.A4	**Activity,** circuit training	
Y93.A5	**Activity,** obstacle course	
	Activity, challenge course	
	Activity, confidence course	
Y93.A6	**Activity,** grass drills	
	Activity, guerilla drills	
Y93.A9	**Activity, other involving cardiorespiratory exercise**	
	EXCLUDES 1 *activities involving cardiorespiratory exercise specified in categories Y93.0-Y93.7*	
✓5th Y93.B	**Activities involving other muscle strengthening exercises**	
Y93.B1	**Activity,** exercise machines **primarily for muscle strengthening**	
Y93.B2	**Activity,** push-ups, pull-ups, sit-ups	
Y93.B3	**Activity,** free weights	
	Activity, barbells	
	Activity, dumbbells	
Y93.B4	**Activity,** pilates	
Y93.B9	**Activity, other involving muscle strengthening exercises**	
	EXCLUDES 1 *activities involving muscle strengthening specified in categories Y93.0-Y93.A*	
✓5th Y93.C	**Activities involving computer technology and electronic devices**	
	EXCLUDES 1 *activity, electronic musical keyboard or instruments (Y93.J-)*	
Y93.C1	**Activity,** computer keyboarding	
	Activity, electronic game playing using keyboard or other stationary device	
Y93.C2	**Activity,** hand held interactive electronic device	
	Activity, cellular telephone and communication device	
	Activity, electronic game playing using interactive device	
	EXCLUDES 1 *activity, electronic game playing using keyboard or other stationary device (Y93.C1)*	
Y93.C9	**Activity, other involving computer technology and electronic devices**	
✓5th Y93.D	**Activities involving arts and handcrafts**	
	EXCLUDES 1 *activities involving playing musical instrument (Y93.J-)*	
Y93.D1	**Activity,** knitting and crocheting	
Y93.D2	**Activity,** sewing	
Y93.D3	**Activity,** furniture building and finishing	
	Activity, furniture repair	
Y93.D9	**Activity, other involving arts and handcrafts**	

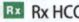

Y93.E Activities involving personal hygiene and interior property and clothing maintenance

EXCLUDES 1: activities involving cooking and grilling (Y93.G-)
activities involving caregiving (Y93.F-)
activities involving exterior property and land maintenance, building and construction (Y93.H-)
activity, dishwashing (Y93.G1)
activity, food preparation (Y93.G1)
activity, gardening (Y93.H2)

- **Y93.E1** Activity, personal bathing and showering
- **Y93.E2** Activity, laundry
- **Y93.E3** Activity, vacuuming
- **Y93.E4** Activity, ironing
- **Y93.E5** Activity, floor mopping and cleaning
- **Y93.E6** Activity, residential relocation
  Activity, packing up and unpacking involved in moving to a new residence
- **Y93.E8** Activity, other personal hygiene
- **Y93.E9** Activity, other interior property and clothing maintenance

Y93.F Activities involving caregiving
Activity involving the provider of caregiving
- **Y93.F1** Activity, caregiving, bathing
- **Y93.F2** Activity, caregiving, lifting
- **Y93.F9** Activity, other caregiving

Y93.G Activities involving food preparation, cooking and grilling
- **Y93.G1** Activity, food preparation and clean up
  Activity, dishwashing
- **Y93.G2** Activity, grilling and smoking food
- **Y93.G3** Activity, cooking and baking
  Activity, use of stove, oven and microwave oven
- **Y93.G9** Activity, other involving cooking and grilling

Y93.H Activities involving exterior property and land maintenance, building and construction
- **Y93.H1** Activity, digging, shoveling and raking
  Activity, dirt digging
  Activity, raking leaves
  Activity, snow shoveling
- **Y93.H2** Activity, gardening and landscaping
  Activity, pruning, trimming shrubs, weeding
- **Y93.H3** Activity, building and construction
- **Y93.H9** Activity, other involving exterior property and land maintenance, building and construction

Y93.I Activities involving roller coasters and other types of external motion
- **Y93.I1** Activity, rollercoaster riding
- **Y93.I9** Activity, other involving external motion

Y93.J Activities involving playing musical instrument
Activity involving playing electric musical instrument
- **Y93.J1** Activity, piano playing
  Activity, musical keyboard (electronic) playing
- **Y93.J2** Activity, drum and other percussion instrument playing
- **Y93.J3** Activity, string instrument playing
- **Y93.J4** Activity, winds and brass instrument playing

Y93.K Activities involving animal care
EXCLUDES 1: activity, horseback riding (Y93.52)
- **Y93.K1** Activity, walking an animal
- **Y93.K2** Activity, milking an animal
- **Y93.K3** Activity, grooming and shearing an animal
- **Y93.K9** Activity, other involving animal care

Y93.L Other outdoor activity
- **Y93.L1** Activity, splitting wood
- **Y93.L9** Activity, other outdoor activity

Y93.8 Activities, other specified
- **Y93.81** Activity, refereeing a sports activity
- **Y93.82** Activity, spectator at an event
- **Y93.83** Activity, rough housing and horseplay
- **Y93.84** Activity, sleeping
- **Y93.85** Activity, choking game
  Activity, blackout game
  Activity, fainting game
  Activity, pass out game
  AHA: 2016,4Q,74-76
- **Y93.89** Activity, other specified

Y93.9 Activity, unspecified

Y95 Nosocomial condition
AHA: 2013,4Q,119

Y99 External cause status
NOTE A single code from category Y99 should be used in conjunction with the external cause code(s) assigned to a record to indicate the status of the person at the time the event occurred.

- **Y99.0** Civilian activity done for income or pay
  Civilian activity done for financial or other compensation
  EXCLUDES 1: military activity (Y99.1)
  volunteer activity (Y99.2)
- **Y99.1** Military activity
  EXCLUDES 1: activity of off duty military personnel (Y99.8)
- **Y99.2** Volunteer activity
  EXCLUDES 1: activity of child or other family member assisting in compensated work of other family member (Y99.8)
- **Y99.8** Other external cause status
  Activity of child or other family member assisting in compensated work of other family member
  Activity NEC
  Hobby not done for income
  Leisure activity
  Off-duty activity of military personnel
  Recreation or sport not for income or while a student
  Student activity
  EXCLUDES 1: civilian activity done for income or compensation (Y99.0)
  military activity (Y99.1)
  AHA: 2012,4Q,108
- **Y99.9** Unspecified external cause status

Chapter 21. Factors Influencing Health Status and Contact with Health Services (Z00–Z99)

Chapter-specific Guidelines with Coding Examples

The chapter-specific guidelines from the d Official Guidelines for Coding and Reporting have been provided below. Along with these guidelines are coding examples, contained in the shaded boxes, that have been developed to help illustrate the coding and/or sequencing guidance found in these guidelines.

Note: The chapter-specific guidelines provide additional information about the use of Z codes for specified encounters.

a. Use of Z Codes in any healthcare setting

Z codes are for use in any healthcare setting. Z codes may be used as either a first-listed (principal diagnosis code in the inpatient setting) or secondary code, depending on the circumstances of the encounter. Certain Z codes may only be used as first-listed or principal diagnosis.

> Patient with middle lobe lung cancer presents for initiation of chemotherapy
>
> Z51.11   Encounter for antineoplastic chemotherapy
> C34.2   Malignant neoplasm of middle lobe, bronchus or lung
>
> *Explanation:* A Z code can be used as first-listed in this situation based on guidelines in this chapter as well as chapter 2, "Neoplasms."

> Patient has chronic lymphocytic leukemia for which the patient had previous chemotherapy and is now in remission
>
> C91.11   Chronic lymphocytic leukemia of B-cell type in remission
> Z92.21   Personal history of antineoplastic chemotherapy
>
> *Explanation:* The personal history Z code is used to describe a secondary (supplementary) diagnosis to identify that this patient has had chemotherapy in the past.

b. Z Codes indicate a reason for an encounter or provide additional information about a patient encounter

Z codes are not procedure codes. A corresponding procedure code must accompany a Z code to describe any procedure performed.

c. Categories of Z Codes

1) Contact/exposure

Category Z20 indicates contact with, and suspected exposure to, communicable diseases. These codes are for patients who are suspected to have been exposed to a disease by close personal contact with an infected individual or are in an area where a disease is epidemic.

Category Z77, Other contact with and (suspected) exposures hazardous to health, indicates contact with and suspected exposures hazardous to health.

Contact/exposure codes may be used as a first-listed code to explain an encounter for testing, or, more commonly, as a secondary code to identify a potential risk.

2) Inoculations and vaccinations

Code Z23 is for encounters for inoculations and vaccinations. It indicates that a patient is being seen to receive a prophylactic inoculation against a disease. Procedure codes are required to identify the actual administration of the injection and the type(s) of immunizations given. Code Z23 may be used as a secondary code if the inoculation is given as a routine part of preventive health care, such as a well-baby visit.

3) Status

Status codes indicate that a patient is either a carrier of a disease or has the sequelae or residual of a past disease or condition. This includes such things as the presence of prosthetic or mechanical devices resulting from past treatment. A status code is informative, because the status may affect the course of treatment and its outcome. A status code is distinct from a history code. The history code indicates that the patient no longer has the condition.

A status code should not be used with a diagnosis code from one of the body system chapters, if the diagnosis code includes the information provided by the status code. For example, code Z94.1, Heart transplant status, should not be used with a code from subcategory T86.2, Complications of heart transplant. The status code does not provide additional information. The complication code indicates that the patient is a heart transplant patient.

For encounters for weaning from a mechanical ventilator, assign a code from subcategory J96.1, Chronic respiratory failure, followed by code Z99.11, Dependence on respirator [ventilator] status.

The status Z codes/categories are:

Z14   Genetic carrier
       Genetic carrier status indicates that a person carries a gene, associated with a particular disease, which may be passed to offspring who may develop that disease. The person does not have the disease and is not at risk of developing the disease.

Z15   Genetic susceptibility to disease
       Genetic susceptibility indicates that a person has a gene that increases the risk of that person developing the disease.
       Codes from category Z15 should **generally** not be used as principal or first-listed codes. If the patient has the condition to which he/she is susceptible, and that condition is the reason for the encounter, the code for the current condition should be sequenced first. If the patient is being seen for follow-up after completed treatment for this condition, and the condition no longer exists, a follow-up code should be sequenced first, followed by the appropriate personal history and genetic susceptibility codes. If the purpose of the encounter is genetic counseling associated with procreative management, code Z31.5, Encounter for genetic counseling, should be assigned as the first-listed code, followed by a code from category Z15. Additional codes should be assigned for any applicable family or personal history.

Z16   Resistance to antimicrobial drugs
       This **category** indicates that a patient has a condition that is resistant to antimicrobial drug treatment. Sequence the infection code first.

Z17   Estrogen, and other hormones and factors receptor status
Z18   Retained foreign body fragments
Z19   Hormone sensitivity malignancy status
Z21   Asymptomatic HIV infection status
       This code indicates that a patient has tested positive for HIV but has manifested no signs or symptoms of the disease.

Z22   Carrier of infectious disease
       Carrier status indicates that a person harbors the specific organisms of a disease without manifest symptoms and is capable of transmitting the infection.

Z28.3 Underimmunization status
       See Section I.B.14. for underimmunization documentation by clinicians other than the patient's provider.

Z33.1 Pregnant state, incidental
       This code is a secondary code only for use when the pregnancy is in no way complicating the reason for visit. Otherwise, a code from the obstetric chapter is required.

Z66   Do not resuscitate
       This code may be used when it is documented by the provider that a patient is on do not resuscitate status at any time during the stay.

Z67   Blood type
Z68   Body mass index (BMI)
       BMI codes should only be assigned when there is an associated, reportable diagnosis (such as obesity or anorexia) documented by the patient's provider.
       Do not assign BMI codes during pregnancy. When the documentation reflects fluctuating BMI values during the current encounter for an associated reportable condition, assign a code for the most severe value.
       See Section I.B.14. for BMI documentation by clinicians other than the patient's provider.

Z74.01 Bed confinement status
Z76.82 Awaiting organ transplant status
Z78   Other specified health status
       Code Z78.1, Physical restraint status, may be used when it is documented by the provider that a patient has been put in restraints during the current encounter. Please note that this code should not be reported when it is documented by the provider that a patient is temporarily restrained during a procedure.

Z79 Long-term (current) drug therapy
Codes from this category indicate a patient's continuous use of a prescribed drug (including such things as aspirin therapy) for the long-term treatment of a condition or for prophylactic use. It is not for use for patients who have addictions to drugs. This subcategory is not for use of medications for detoxification or maintenance programs to prevent withdrawal symptoms (e.g., methadone maintenance for opiate dependence). Assign the appropriate code for the drug use, abuse, or dependence instead.

Assign a code from Z79 if the patient is receiving a medication for an extended period as a prophylactic measure (such as for the prevention of deep vein thrombosis) or as treatment of a chronic condition (such as arthritis) or a disease requiring a lengthy course of treatment (such as cancer). Do not assign a code from category Z79 for medication being administered for a brief period of time to treat an acute illness or injury (such as a course of antibiotics to treat acute bronchitis).

Z88 Allergy status to drugs, medicaments and biological substances
Except: Z88.9, Allergy status to unspecified drugs, medicaments and biological substances status

Z89 Acquired absence of limb
Z90 Acquired absence of organs, not elsewhere classified
Z91.0- Allergy status, other than to drugs and biological substances
Z92.82 Status post administration of tPA (rtPA) in a different facility within the last 24 hours prior to admission to a current facility

Assign code Z92.82, Status post administration of tPA (rtPA) in a different facility within the last 24 hours prior to admission to current facility, as a secondary diagnosis when a patient is received by transfer into a facility and documentation indicates they were administered tissue plasminogen activator (tPA) within the last 24 hours prior to admission to the current facility.

This guideline applies even if the patient is still receiving the tPA at the time they are received into the current facility.

The appropriate code for the condition for which the tPA was administered (such as cerebrovascular disease or myocardial infarction) should be assigned first.

Code Z92.82 is only applicable to the receiving facility record and not to the transferring facility record.

Z93 Artificial opening status
Z94 Transplanted organ and tissue status
Z95 Presence of cardiac and vascular implants and grafts
Z96 Presence of other functional implants
Z97 Presence of other devices
Z98 Other postprocedural states
Assign code Z98.85, Transplanted organ removal status, to indicate that a transplanted organ has been previously removed. This code should not be assigned for the encounter in which the transplanted organ is removed. The complication necessitating removal of the transplant organ should be assigned for that encounter.
See section I.C.19. for information on the coding of organ transplant complications.

Z99 Dependence on enabling machines and devices, not elsewhere classified
Note: Categories Z89-Z90 and Z93-Z99 are for use only if there are no complications or malfunctions of the organ or tissue replaced, the amputation site or the equipment on which the patient is dependent.

4) History (of)

There are two types of history Z codes, personal and family. Personal history codes explain a patient's past medical condition that no longer exists and is not receiving any treatment, but that has the potential for recurrence, and therefore may require continued monitoring.

Family history codes are for use when a patient has a family member(s) who has had a particular disease that causes the patient to be at higher risk of also contracting the disease.

Personal history codes may be used in conjunction with follow-up codes and family history codes may be used in conjunction with screening codes to explain the need for a test or procedure. History codes are also acceptable on any medical record regardless of the reason for visit. A history of an illness, even if no longer present, is important information that may alter the type of treatment ordered.

The reason for the encounter (for example, screening or counseling) should be sequenced first and the appropriate personal and/or family history code(s) should be assigned as additional diagnos(es).

The history Z code categories are:
Z80 Family history of primary malignant neoplasm
Z81 Family history of mental and behavioral disorders
Z82 Family history of certain disabilities and chronic diseases (leading to disablement)
Z83 Family history of other specific disorders
Z84 Family history of other conditions
Z85 Personal history of malignant neoplasm
Z86 Personal history of certain other diseases
Z87 Personal history of other diseases and conditions
Z91.4- Personal history of psychological trauma, not elsewhere classified
Z91.5- Personal history of self-harm
Z91.81 History of falling
Z91.82 Personal history of military deployment
Z91.85 Personal history of military service
Z92 Personal history of medical treatment
Except: Z92.0, Personal history of contraception
Except: Z92.82, Status post administration of tPA (rtPA) in a different facility within the last 24 hours prior to admission to a current facility

5) Screening

Screening is the testing for disease or disease precursors in seemingly well individuals so that early detection and treatment can be provided for those who test positive for the disease (e.g., screening mammogram).

The testing of a person to rule out or confirm a suspected diagnosis because the patient has some sign or symptom is a diagnostic examination, not a screening. In these cases, the sign or symptom is used to explain the reason for the test.

A screening code may be a first-listed code if the reason for the visit is specifically the screening exam. It may also be used as an additional code if the screening is done during an office visit for other health problems. A screening code is not necessary if the screening is inherent to a routine examination, such as a pap smear done during a routine pelvic examination.

Should a condition be discovered during the screening then the code for the condition may be assigned as an additional diagnosis.

> Prostate screening of healthy 50-year-old male patient; PSA noted to be elevated but normal digital rectal exam
>
> **Z12.5**   **Encounter for screening for malignant neoplasm of prostate**
>
> **R97.20**   **Elevated prostate specific antigen [PSA]**
>
> *Explanation:* The patient had no signs or symptoms of any prostate-related illness prior to coming in for the screening. The screening code is appropriately used as the first-listed code to signify that this was for routine screening. The elevated PSA is reported as a secondary diagnosis to reflect that an abnormal lab value was found as a result of the screening procedure(s).

The Z code indicates that a screening exam is planned. A procedure code is required to confirm that the screening was performed.

The screening Z codes/categories:
Z11 Encounter for screening for infectious and parasitic diseases
Z12 Encounter for screening for malignant neoplasms
Z13 Encounter for screening for other diseases and disorders
Except: Z13.9, Encounter for screening, unspecified
Z36 Encounter for antenatal screening for mother

6) Observation

There are three observation Z code categories. They are for use in very limited circumstances when a person is being observed for a suspected condition that is ruled out. The observation codes are not for use if an injury or illness or any signs or symptoms related to the suspected condition are present. In such cases the diagnosis/symptom code is used with the corresponding external cause code.

The observation codes are primarily to be used as a principal/first-listed diagnosis. An observation code may be assigned as a secondary diagnosis code when the patient is being observed for a condition that is ruled out and is unrelated to the principal/first-listed diagnosis. Also, when the principal diagnosis is required to be a code from category Z38, Liveborn infants according to place of birth and type of delivery. Then a code from category Z05, Encounter for observation and evaluation of newborn for suspected diseases and conditions ruled out, is sequenced after the Z38 code. Additional codes may be used in addition to the observation code but only if they are unrelated to the suspected condition being observed.

Codes from subcategory Z03.7, Encounter for suspected maternal and fetal conditions ruled out, may either be used as a first-listed or as an additional code assignment depending on the case. They are for use in very limited circumstances on a maternal record when an encounter is for a suspected maternal or fetal condition that is ruled out during that encounter (for example, a maternal or fetal condition may be suspected due to an abnormal test result). These codes should not be used when the condition is confirmed. In those cases, the confirmed condition should be coded. In addition, these codes are not for use if an illness or any signs or symptoms related to the suspected condition or problem are present. In such cases the diagnosis/symptom code is used.

Additional codes may be used in addition to the code from subcategory Z03.7, but only if they are unrelated to the suspected condition being evaluated.

Codes from subcategory Z03.7 may not be used for encounters for antenatal screening of mother. *See Section I.C.21. Screening.*

For encounters for suspected fetal condition that are inconclusive following testing and evaluation, assign the appropriate code from category O35, O36, O40 or O41.

The observation Z code categories:

- Z03 Encounter for medical observation for suspected diseases and conditions ruled out
- Z04 Encounter for examination and observation for other reasons
  Except: Z04.9, Encounter for examination and observation for unspecified reason
- Z05 Encounter for observation and evaluation of newborn for suspected diseases and conditions ruled out

7) **Aftercare**

Aftercare visit codes cover situations when the initial treatment of a disease has been performed and the patient requires continued care during the healing or recovery phase, or for the long-term consequences of the disease. The aftercare Z code should not be used if treatment is directed at a current, acute disease. The diagnosis code is to be used in these cases.

The aftercare Z codes should also not be used for aftercare for injuries. For aftercare of an injury, assign the acute injury code with the appropriate 7th character (for subsequent encounter).

The aftercare codes are generally first listed to explain the specific reason for the encounter. An aftercare code may be reported as an additional code when a specific type of aftercare is provided in addition to the reason for the encounter. An example of this would be the closure of a colostomy during an encounter for treatment of another condition.

Aftercare codes should be used in conjunction with other aftercare codes or diagnosis codes to provide better detail on the specifics of an aftercare encounter visit, unless otherwise directed by the classification. The sequencing of multiple aftercare codes depends on the circumstances of the encounter.

> Patient presents for third round of gemcitabine and first dose of antineoplastic radiation therapy for advanced pancreatic carcinoma
>
> **Z51.11 Encounter for antineoplastic chemotherapy**
> **Z51.0 Encounter for antineoplastic radiation therapy**
> **C25.9 Malignant neoplasm of pancreas, unspecified**
>
> *Explanation:* Gemcitabine is an antineoplastic chemotherapy. Since the encounter was solely to administer antineoplastic treatment, both forms of treatment are reported and either code can be the first-listed diagnosis, followed by the neoplastic condition code. Aftercare codes are typically not assigned for current treatment of disease; however, Z51.0 and subcategory Z51.1 are an exception to this standard.

Certain aftercare Z code categories need a secondary diagnosis code to describe the resolving condition or sequelae. For others, the condition is included in the code title.

Additional Z code aftercare category terms include fitting and adjustment, and attention to artificial openings.

Status Z codes may be used with aftercare Z codes to indicate the nature of the aftercare. For example code Z95.1, Presence of aortocoronary bypass graft, may be used with code Z48.812, Encounter for surgical aftercare following surgery on the circulatory system, to indicate the surgery for which the aftercare is being performed. A status code should not be used when the aftercare code indicates the type of status, such as using Z43.0, Encounter for attention to tracheostomy, with Z93.0, Tracheostomy status.

The aftercare codes are generally found in the following categories:

- Z42 Encounter for plastic and reconstructive surgery following medical procedure or healed injury
- Z43 Encounter for attention to artificial openings
- Z44 Encounter for fitting and adjustment of external prosthetic device
- Z45 Encounter for adjustment and management of implanted device
- Z46 Encounter for fitting and adjustment of other devices
- Z47 Orthopedic aftercare
- Z48 Encounter for other postprocedural aftercare
- Z49 Encounter for care involving renal dialysis
- Z51 Encounter for other aftercare and medical care

8) **Follow-up**

The follow-up codes are used to explain continuing surveillance following completed treatment of a disease, condition, or injury. They imply that the condition has been fully treated and no longer exists. They should not be confused with aftercare codes, or injury codes with a 7th character for subsequent encounter, that explain ongoing care of a healing condition or its sequelae. Follow-up codes may be used in conjunction with history codes to provide the full picture of the healed condition and its treatment. The follow-up code is sequenced first, followed by the history code.

A follow-up code may be used to explain multiple visits. Should a condition be found to have recurred on the follow-up visit, then the diagnosis code for the condition should be assigned in place of the follow-up code.

The follow-up Z codes/categories:

- Z08 Encounter for follow-up examination after completed treatment for malignant neoplasm
- Z09 Encounter for follow-up examination after completed treatment for conditions other than malignant neoplasm

Codes Z08, Encounter for follow-up examination after completed treatment for malignant neoplasm, and Z09, Encounter for follow up examination after completed treatment for conditions other than malignant neoplasm, may be assigned following any type of completed treatment modality (including both medical and surgical treatments).

- Z39 Encounter for maternal postpartum care and examination

> Follow-up for patient several months after completing a regime of IV antibiotics for recurrent pneumonia; lungs are clear and pneumonia is resolved
>
> **Z09 Encounter for follow-up examination after completed treatment for conditions other than malignant neoplasm**
> **Z87.01 Personal history of pneumonia (recurrent)**
>
> *Explanation:* Code Z09 identifies the follow-up visit as being unrelated to a malignant neoplasm, and code Z87 describes the condition that has now resolved.

> Follow-up for patient several months after completing a regime of IV antibiotics for recurrent pneumonia; pneumonia has recurred, and a new antibiotic regimen has been prescribed
>
> **J18.9 Pneumonia, unspecified organism**
>
> *Explanation:* Since the follow-up exam for pneumonia determined that the pneumonia was not resolved or recurred, code Z09 Encounter for follow-up examination after completed treatment for conditions other than malignant neoplasm, no longer applies. Instead the first-listed code describes the pneumonia.

9) **Donor**

Codes in category Z52, Donors of organs and tissues, are used for living individuals who are donating blood or other body tissue. These codes are for individuals donating for others, as well as for self-donations. They are not used to identify cadaveric donations.

10) **Counseling**

Counseling Z codes are used when a patient or family member receives assistance in the aftermath of an illness or injury, or when support is required in coping with family or social problems.

The counseling Z codes/categories:

- Z30.0- Encounter for general counseling and advice on contraception
- Z31.5 Encounter for procreative genetic counseling
- Z31.6- Encounter for general counseling and advice on procreation
- Z32.2 Encounter for childbirth instruction
- Z32.3 Encounter for childcare instruction
- Z69 Encounter for mental health services for victim and perpetrator of abuse
- Z70 Counseling related to sexual attitude, behavior and orientation
- Z71 Persons encountering health services for other counseling and medical advice, not elsewhere classified
  Note: Code Z71.84, Encounter for health counseling related to travel, is to be used for health risk and safety counseling for future travel purposes.

Code Z71.85, Encounter for immunization safety counseling, is to be used for counseling of the patient or caregiver regarding the safety of a vaccine. This code should not be used for the provision of general information regarding risks and potential side effects during routine encounters for the administration of vaccines.

Code Z71.87, Encounter for pediatric-to-adult transition counseling, should be assigned when pediatric-to-adult transition counseling is the sole reason for the encounter or when this counseling is provided in addition to other services, such as treatment of a chronic condition. If both transition counseling and treatment of a medical condition are provided during the same encounter, the code(s) for the medical condition(s) treated and code Z71.87 should be assigned, with sequencing depending on the circumstances of the encounter.

Z76.81   Expectant mother prebirth pediatrician visit

11) Encounters for obstetrical and reproductive services

See Section I.C.15. Pregnancy, Childbirth, and the Puerperium, for further instruction on the use of these codes.

Z codes for pregnancy are for use in those circumstances when none of the problems or complications included in the codes from the Obstetrics chapter exist (a routine prenatal visit or postpartum care). Codes in category Z34, Encounter for supervision of normal pregnancy, are always first-listed and are not to be used with any other code from the OB chapter.

Codes in category Z3A, Weeks of gestation, may be assigned to provide additional information about the pregnancy. Category Z3A codes should not be assigned for pregnancies with abortive outcomes (categories O00-O08), elective termination of pregnancy (code Z33.2), nor for postpartum conditions, as category Z3A is not applicable to these conditions. The date of the admission should be used to determine weeks of gestation for inpatient admissions that encompass more than one gestational week.

The outcome of delivery, category Z37, should be included on all maternal delivery records. It is always a secondary code.

Codes in category Z37 should not be used on the newborn record.

Z codes for family planning (contraceptive) or procreative management and counseling should be included on an obstetric record either during the pregnancy or the postpartum stage, if applicable.

Z codes/categories for obstetrical and reproductive services:

Z30	Encounter for contraceptive management
Z31	Encounter for procreative management
Z32.2	Encounter for childbirth instruction
Z32.3	Encounter for childcare instruction
Z33	Pregnant state
Z34	Encounter for supervision of normal pregnancy
Z36	Encounter for antenatal screening of mother
Z3A	Weeks of gestation
Z37	Outcome of delivery
Z39	Encounter for maternal postpartum care and examination
Z76.81	Expectant mother prebirth pediatrician visit

12) Routine and administrative examinations

The Z codes allow for the description of encounters for routine examinations, such as, a general check-up, or, examinations for administrative purposes, such as, a pre-employment physical. The codes are not to be used if the examination is for diagnosis of a suspected condition or for treatment purposes. In such cases the diagnosis code is used. During a routine exam, should a diagnosis or condition be discovered, it should be coded as an additional code. Pre-existing and chronic conditions and history codes may also be included as additional codes as long as the examination is for administrative purposes and not focused on any particular condition.

Some of the codes for routine health examinations distinguish between "with" and "without" abnormal findings. Code assignment depends on the information that is known at the time the encounter is being coded. For example, if no abnormal findings were found during the examination, but the encounter is being coded before test results are back, it is acceptable to assign the code for "without abnormal findings." When assigning a code for "with abnormal findings," additional code(s) should be assigned to identify the specific abnormal finding(s).

> 12-month-old boy presented for well-child visit; pediatrician notices some eczema on the child's scalp and back of the knees
>
> **Z00.121**   **Encounter for routine child health examination with abnormal findings**
>
> **L30.9**   **Dermatitis, unspecified**
>
> *Explanation:* The Z code identifying that this is a routine well-child visit is reported first. Because an abnormal finding (eczema) was documented, a code for this condition may also be appended.

Pre-operative examination and pre-procedural laboratory examination Z codes are for use only in those situations when a patient is being cleared for a procedure or surgery and no treatment is given.

The Z codes/categories for routine and administrative examinations:

Z00	Encounter for general examination without complaint, suspected or reported diagnosis
Z01	Encounter for other special examination without complaint, suspected or reported diagnosis
Z02	Encounter for administrative examination
	Except: Z02.9, Encounter for administrative examinations, unspecified
Z32.0-	Encounter for pregnancy test

13) Miscellaneous Z codes

The miscellaneous Z codes capture a number of other health care encounters that do not fall into one of the other categories. Some of these codes identify the reason for the encounter; others are for use as additional codes that provide useful information on circumstances that may affect a patient's care and treatment.

Prophylactic organ removal

For encounters specifically for prophylactic removal of an organ (such as prophylactic removal of breasts due to a genetic susceptibility to cancer or a family history of cancer), the principal or first-listed code should be a code from subcategory Z40.0, Encounter for prophylactic surgery for risk factors related to malignant neoplasms, or subcategory Z40.8, Encounter for other prophylactic surgery. If applicable, assign additional code(s) to identify any associated risk factor (such as genetic susceptibility or family history).

If the patient has a malignancy of one site and is having prophylactic removal at another site to prevent either a new primary malignancy or metastatic disease, a code for the malignancy should also be assigned in addition to a code from subcategory Z40.0, Encounter for prophylactic surgery for risk factors related to malignant neoplasms. A Z40.0 code should not be assigned if the patient is having organ removal for treatment of a malignancy, such as the removal of the testes for the treatment of prostate cancer.

Miscellaneous Z codes/subcategories/categories:

Z28	Immunization not carried out
	Except: Z28.3-, Underimmunization status
Z29	Encounter for other prophylactic measures
Z40	Encounter for prophylactic surgery
Z41	Encounter for procedures for purposes other than remedying health state
	Except: Z41.9, Encounter for procedure for purposes other than remedying health state, unspecified
Z53	Persons encountering health services for specific procedures and treatment, not carried out
Z72	Problems related to lifestyle
	Note: These codes should be assigned only when the documentation specifies that the patient has an associated problem
Z73	Problems related to life management difficulty
	Note: These codes should be assigned only when the documentation specifies that the patient has an associated problem.
Z74	Problems related to care provider dependency
	Except: Z74.01, Bed confinement status
Z75	Problems related to medical facilities and other health care
Z76.0	Encounter for issue of repeat prescription
Z76.3	Healthy person accompanying sick person
Z76.4	Other boarder to healthcare facility
Z76.5	Malingerer [conscious simulation]
Z91.1-	Patient's noncompliance with medical treatment and regimen
Z91.A-	Caregiver's noncompliance with patient's medical treatment and regimen

Z91.B	**Personal risk factor of exposure to diethylstilbestrol**	
Z91.83	Wandering in diseases classified elsewhere	
Z91.84-	Oral health risk factors	
Z91.89	Other specified personal risk factors, not elsewhere classified	

See Section I.B.14. for Z55-Z65 Persons with potential health hazards related to socioeconomic and psychosocial circumstances, documentation by clinicians other than the patient's provider

14) Nonspecific Z codes

Certain Z codes are so non-specific, or potentially redundant with other codes in the classification, that there can be little justification for their use in the inpatient setting. Their use in the outpatient setting should be limited to those instances when there is no further documentation to permit more precise coding. Otherwise, any sign or symptom or any other reason for visit that is captured in another code should be used.

Nonspecific Z codes/categories:

Z02.9	Encounter for administrative examinations, unspecified
Z04.9	Encounter for examination and observation for unspecified reason
Z13.9	Encounter for screening, unspecified
Z41.9	Encounter for procedure for purposes other than remedying health state, unspecified
Z52.9	Donor of unspecified organ or tissue
Z86.59	Personal history of other mental and behavioral disorders
Z88.9	Allergy status to unspecified drugs, medicaments and biological substances status
Z92.0	Personal history of contraception

15) Z codes that may only be principal/first-listed diagnosis

The following Z codes/**subcategories**/categories may only be reported as the principal/first-listed diagnosis, except when there are multiple encounters on the same day and the medical records for the encounters are combined:

Z00	Encounter for general examination without complaint, suspected or reported diagnosis
	Except: Z00.6
Z01	Encounter for other special examination without complaint, suspected or reported diagnosis
Z02	Encounter for administrative examination
Z04	Encounter for examination and observation for other reasons
Z33.2	Encounter for elective termination of pregnancy
Z31.81	Encounter for male factor infertility in female patient
Z31.83	Encounter for assisted reproductive fertility procedure cycle
Z31.84	Encounter for fertility preservation procedure
Z34	Encounter for supervision of normal pregnancy
Z39	Encounter for maternal postpartum care and examination
Z38	Liveborn infants according to place of birth and type of delivery
Z40	Encounter for prophylactic surgery
Z42	Encounter for plastic and reconstructive surgery following medical procedure or healed injury
Z51.0	Encounter for antineoplastic radiation therapy
Z51.1-	Encounter for antineoplastic chemotherapy and immunotherapy
Z52	Donors of organs and tissues
	Except: Z52.9, Donor of unspecified organ or tissue
Z76.1	Encounter for health supervision and care of foundling
Z76.2	Encounter for health supervision and care of other healthy infant and child
Z99.12	Encounter for respirator [ventilator] dependence during power failure

---

Female patient seen at 32 weeks' gestation to check the progress of her first pregnancy

Z34.03	**Encounter for supervision of normal first pregnancy, third trimester**
Z3A.32	**32 weeks gestation of pregnancy**

Explanation: Category Z34 is appropriate as a first-listed diagnosis. Category Z3A helps to clarify at which point in the pregnancy the patient was provided supervision.

16) Newborns and infants

See Section I.C.16. Newborn (Perinatal) Guidelines, for further instruction on the use of these codes.

Newborn Z codes/subcategories/categories:

Z76.1	Encounter for health supervision and care of foundling
Z00.1-	Encounter for routine child health examination
Z38	Liveborn infants according to place of birth and type of delivery

17) Social determinants of health

Social determinants of health (SDOH) codes describing social problems, conditions, or risk factors that influence a patient's health should be assigned when this information is documented in the patient's medical record. Assign as many SDOH codes as are necessary to describe all of the social problems, conditions, or risk factors documented during the current episode of care. For example, a patient who lives alone may suffer an acute injury temporarily impacting their ability to perform routine activities of daily living. When documented as such, this would support assignment of code Z60.2, Problems related to living alone. However, merely living alone, without documentation of a risk or unmet need for assistance at home, would not support assignment of code Z60.2. Documentation by a clinician (or patient-reported information that is signed off by a clinician) that the patient expressed concerns with access and availability of food would support assignment of code Z59.41, Food insecurity. **Similarly, medical record documentation indicating the patient is experiencing homelessness would support assignment of a code from subcategory Z59.0, Homelessness.**

For social determinants of health classified to chapter 21, such as information found in categories Z55-Z65, Persons with potential health hazards related to socioeconomic and psychosocial circumstances, code assignment may be based on medical record documentation from clinicians involved in the care of the patient who are not the patient's provider since this information represents social information, rather than medical diagnoses. For example, coding professionals may utilize documentation of social information from social workers, community health workers, case managers, or nurses, if their documentation is included in the official medical record.

Patient self-reported documentation may be used to assign codes for social determinants of health, as long as the patient self-reported information is signed-off by and incorporated into the medical record by either a clinician or provider.

Social determinants of health codes are located primarily in these Z code categories:

Z55	Problems related to education and literacy
Z56	Problems related to employment and unemployment
Z57	Occupational exposure to risk factors
Z58	Problems related to physical environment
Z59	Problems related to housing and economic circumstances
Z60	Problems related to social environment
Z62	Problems related to upbringing
Z63	Other problems related to primary support group, including family circumstances
Z64	Problems related to certain psychosocial circumstances
Z65	Problems related to other psychosocial circumstances

See Section I.B.14. Documentation by Clinicians Other than the Patient's Provider.

Chapter 21. Factors Influencing Health Status and Contact With Health Services (Z00-Z99)

NOTE Z codes represent reasons for encounters. A corresponding procedure code must accompany a Z code if a procedure is performed. Categories Z00-Z99 are provided for occasions when circumstances other than a disease, injury or external cause classifiable to categories A00-Y89 are recorded as "diagnoses" or "problems." This can arise in two main ways:

(a) When a person who may or may not be sick encounters the health services for some specific purpose, such as to receive limited care or service for a current condition, to donate an organ or tissue, to receive prophylactic vaccination (immunization), or to discuss a problem which is in itself not a disease or injury.

(b) When some circumstance or problem is present which influences the person's health status but is not in itself a current illness or injury.

AHA: 2018,4Q,60-61

This chapter contains the following blocks:

Z00-Z13	Persons encountering health services for examinations
Z14-Z15	Genetic carrier and genetic susceptibility to disease
Z16	Resistance to antimicrobial drugs
Z17	estrogen, and other hormones and factors receptor status
Z18	Retained foreign body fragments
Z19	Hormone sensitivity malignancy status
Z20-Z29	Persons with potential health hazards related to communicable diseases
Z30-Z39	Persons encountering health services in circumstances related to reproduction
Z40-Z53	Encounters for other specific health care
Z55-Z65	Persons with potential health hazards related to socioeconomic and psychosocial circumstances
Z66	Do not resuscitate status
Z67	Blood type
Z68	Body mass index (BMI)
Z69-Z76	Persons encountering health services in other circumstances
Z77-Z99	Persons with potential health hazards related to family and personal history and certain conditions influencing health status

Persons encountering health services for examinations (Z00-Z13)

NOTE Nonspecific abnormal findings disclosed at the time of these examinations are classified to categories R70-R94.

EXCLUDES 1 examinations related to pregnancy and reproduction (Z30-Z36, Z39.-)
EXCLUDES 2 ▶examinations related to pregnancy and reproduction (Z30-Z36, Z39.-)◀

Z00 Encounter for general examination without complaint, suspected or reported diagnosis
  EXCLUDES 1 encounter for examination for administrative purposes (Z02.-)
  EXCLUDES 2 encounter for pre-procedural examinations (Z01.81-)
  special screening examinations (Z11-Z13)
  AHA: 2017,4Q,95

  Z00.0 Encounter for general adult medical examination
  Encounter for adult periodic examination (annual) (physical) and any associated laboratory and radiologic examinations
    EXCLUDES 1 encounter for examination of sign or symptom - code to sign or symptom
    general health check-up of infant or child (Z00.12.-)

    Z00.00 Encounter for general adult medical examination without abnormal findings
    Encounter for adult health check-up NOS
    AHA: 2016,1Q,36

    Z00.01 Encounter for general adult medical examination with abnormal findings
    Use additional code to identify abnormal findings
    AHA: 2016,1Q,35-36

  Z00.1 Encounter for newborn, infant and child health examinations

    Z00.11 Newborn health examination
    Health check for child under 29 days old
    Use additional code to identify any abnormal findings
    EXCLUDES 1 health check for child over 28 days old (Z00.12.-)

      Z00.110 Health examination for newborn under 8 days old
      Health check for newborn under 8 days old

      Z00.111 Health examination for newborn 8 to 28 days old
      Health check for newborn 8 to 28 days old
      Newborn weight check

    Z00.12 Encounter for routine child health examination
    Health check (routine) for child over 28 days old
    Immunizations appropriate for age
    Routine developmental screening of infant or child
    Routine vison and hearing testing
    EXCLUDES 1 health check for child under 29 days old (Z00.11.-)
    health supervision of foundling or other healthy infant or child (Z76.1-Z76.2)
    newborn health examination (Z00.11.-)
    AHA: 2018,4Q,36

      Z00.121 Encounter for routine child health examination with abnormal findings
      Use additional code to identify abnormal findings
      AHA: 2024,4Q,6; 2016,1Q,34-35

      Z00.129 Encounter for routine child health examination without abnormal findings
      Encounter for routine child health examination NOS
      AHA: 2016,1Q,34

  Z00.2 Encounter for examination for period of rapid growth in childhood

  Z00.3 Encounter for examination for adolescent development state
  Encounter for puberty development state

  Z00.5 Encounter for examination of potential donor of organ and tissue

  Z00.6 Encounter for examination for normal comparison and control in clinical research program
  Examination of participant or control in clinical research program

  Z00.7 Encounter for examination for period of delayed growth in childhood

    Z00.70 Encounter for examination for period of delayed growth in childhood without abnormal findings

    Z00.71 Encounter for examination for period of delayed growth in childhood with abnormal findings
    Use additional code to identify abnormal findings

  Z00.8 Encounter for other general examination
  Encounter for health examination in population surveys

Z01 Encounter for other special examination without complaint, suspected or reported diagnosis
  INCLUDES routine examination of specific system
  NOTE Codes from category Z01 represent the reason for the encounter. A separate procedure code is required to identify any examinations or procedures performed
  EXCLUDES 1 encounter for examination for administrative purposes (Z02.-)
  encounter for examination for suspected conditions, proven not to exist (Z03.-)
  ~~encounter for laboratory and radiologic examinations as a component of general medical examinations (Z00.0-)~~
  encounter for laboratory, radiologic and imaging examinations for sign(s) and symptom(s) - code to the sign(s) or symptom(s)
  EXCLUDES 2 ▶encounter for laboratory and radiologic examinations as a component of general medical examinations (Z00.0-)◀
  screening examinations (Z11-Z13)

  Z01.0 Encounter for examination of eyes and vision
    EXCLUDES 1 examination for driving license (Z02.4)

    Z01.00 Encounter for examination of eyes and vision without abnormal findings
    Encounter for examination of eyes and vision NOS

    Z01.01 Encounter for examination of eyes and vision with abnormal findings
    Use additional code to identify abnormal findings
    AHA: 2016,4Q,21

Chapter 21. Factors Influencing Health Status and Contact With Health Services

Z01.02 **Encounter for examination of eyes and vision following failed vision screening**
- EXCLUDES 1: encounter for examination of eyes and vision with abnormal findings (Z01.01)
- encounter for examination of eyes and vision without abnormal findings (Z01.00)
- AHA: 2019,4Q,20

Z01.020 Encounter for examination of eyes and vision following failed vision screening without abnormal findings `PDx`

Z01.021 Encounter for examination of eyes and vision following failed vision screening with abnormal findings `PDx`
- Use additional code to identify abnormal findings

Z01.1 **Encounter for examination of ears and hearing**

Z01.10 Encounter for examination of ears and hearing without abnormal findings `PDx`
- Encounter for examination of ears and hearing NOS
- AHA: 2016,4Q,24

Z01.11 **Encounter for examination of ears and hearing with abnormal findings**
- AHA: 2016,3Q,17-18

Z01.110 Encounter for hearing examination following failed hearing screening `PDx`

Z01.118 Encounter for examination of ears and hearing with other abnormal findings `PDx`
- Use additional code to identify abnormal findings

Z01.12 Encounter for hearing conservation and treatment `PDx`

Z01.2 **Encounter for dental examination and cleaning**

Z01.20 Encounter for dental examination and cleaning without abnormal findings `PDx`
- Encounter for dental examination and cleaning NOS

Z01.21 Encounter for dental examination and cleaning with abnormal findings `PDx`
- Use additional code to identify abnormal findings

Z01.3 **Encounter for examination of blood pressure**

Z01.30 Encounter for examination of blood pressure without abnormal findings `PDx`
- Encounter for examination of blood pressure NOS

Z01.31 Encounter for examination of blood pressure with abnormal findings `PDx`
- Use additional code to identify abnormal findings

Z01.4 **Encounter for gynecological examination**
- EXCLUDES 2: pregnancy examination or test (Z32.0-)
- routine examination for contraceptive maintenance (Z30.4-)

Z01.41 **Encounter for routine gynecological examination**
- Encounter for general gynecological examination with or without cervical smear
- Encounter for gynecological examination (general) (routine) NOS
- Encounter for pelvic examination (annual) (periodic)
- Use additional code:
  - for screening for human papillomavirus, if applicable, (Z11.51)
  - for screening vaginal pap smear, if applicable (Z12.72)
  - to identify acquired absence of uterus, if applicable (Z90.71-)
- EXCLUDES 1: gynecologic examination status-post hysterectomy for malignant condition (Z08)
- screening cervical pap smear not a part of a routine gynecological examination (Z12.4)

Z01.411 Encounter for gynecological examination (general) (routine) with abnormal findings `PDx`
- Use additional code to identify abnormal findings

Z01.419 Encounter for gynecological examination (general) (routine) without abnormal findings `PDx`

Z01.42 Encounter for cervical smear to confirm findings of recent normal smear following initial abnormal smear `PDx`

Z01.8 **Encounter for other specified special examinations**

Z01.81 **Encounter for preprocedural examinations**
- Encounter for preoperative examinations
- Encounter for radiological and imaging examinations as part of preprocedural examination
- TIP: Assign a code for the condition necessitating surgery and any findings as additional diagnoses.

Z01.810 Encounter for preprocedural cardiovascular examination `PDx`

Z01.811 Encounter for preprocedural respiratory examination `PDx`

Z01.812 Encounter for preprocedural laboratory examination `PDx`
- Blood and urine tests prior to treatment or procedure
- AHA: 2023,2Q,3; 2020,3Q,14

Z01.818 Encounter for other preprocedural examination `PDx`
- Encounter for examinations prior to antineoplastic chemotherapy
- Encounter for preprocedural examination NOS

Z01.82 Encounter for allergy testing `PDx`
- EXCLUDES 1: encounter for antibody response examination (Z01.84)

Z01.83 Encounter for blood typing
- Encounter for Rh typing

Z01.84 Encounter for antibody response examination
- Encounter for immunity status testing
- EXCLUDES 1: encounter for allergy testing (Z01.82)
- AHA: 2020,2Q,11

Z01.89 Encounter for other specified special examinations `PDx`

Z02 **Encounter for administrative examination**

Z02.0 Encounter for examination for admission to educational institution
- Encounter for examination for admission to preschool (education)
- Encounter for examination for re-admission to school following illness or medical treatment

Z02.1 Encounter for pre-employment examination `PDx`

Z02.2 Encounter for examination for admission to residential institution
- EXCLUDES 1: examination for admission to prison (Z02.89)

Z02.3 Encounter for examination for recruitment to armed forces `PDx`

Z02.4 Encounter for examination for driving license `PDx`

Z02.5 Encounter for examination for participation in sport `PDx`
- EXCLUDES 1: blood-alcohol and blood-drug test (Z02.83)

Z02.6 Encounter for examination for insurance purposes `PDx`

Z02.7 **Encounter for issue of medical certificate**
- EXCLUDES 1: encounter for general medical examination (Z00-Z01, Z02.0-Z02.6, Z02.8-Z02.9)

Z02.71 Encounter for disability determination `PDx`
- Encounter for issue of medical certificate of incapacity
- Encounter for issue of medical certificate of invalidity

Z02.79 Encounter for issue of other medical certificate `PDx`

Z02.8 **Encounter for other administrative examinations**

Z02.81 Encounter for paternity testing `PDx`

Z02.82 Encounter for adoption services `PDx`

Z02.83 Encounter for blood-alcohol and blood-drug test `PDx`
- Use additional code for findings of alcohol or drugs in blood (R78.-)

Z02.84 Encounter for child welfare exam
- Encounter for child welfare screening exam
- EXCLUDES 2: encounter for examination and observation for alleged child physical abuse (Z04.72)
- encounter for examination and observation for alleged child rape (Z04.42)
- AHA: 2023,4Q,49

Z02.89 Encounter for other administrative examinations [PDx]
- Encounter for examination for admission to prison
- Encounter for examination for admission to summer camp
- Encounter for immigration examination
- Encounter for naturalization examination
- Encounter for premarital examination
  - EXCLUDES 1: health supervision of foundling or other healthy infant or child (Z76.1-Z76.2)

Z02.9 Encounter for administrative examinations, unspecified [PDx]

✓4th Z03 Encounter for **medical observation** for suspected diseases and conditions ruled out

This category is to be used when a person without a diagnosis is suspected of having an abnormal condition, without signs or symptoms, which requires study, but after examination and observation, is ruled out. This category is also for use for administrative and legal observation status.

- EXCLUDES 1:
  - contact with and (suspected) exposures hazardous to health (Z77.-)
  - encounter for observation and evaluation of newborn for suspected diseases and conditions ruled out (Z05.-)
  - person with feared complaint in whom no diagnosis is made (Z71.1)
  - signs or symptoms under study - code to signs or symptoms

AHA: 2020,2Q,8; 2018,2Q,7-8; 2017,4Q,27

Z03.6 Encounter for observation for suspected **toxic effect from ingested substance** ruled out
- Encounter for observation for suspected adverse effect from drug
- Encounter for observation for suspected poisoning

✓5th Z03.7 Encounter for suspected **maternal and fetal conditions** ruled out
- Encounter for suspected maternal and fetal conditions not found
  - EXCLUDES 1: known or suspected fetal anomalies affecting management of mother, not ruled out (O26.-, O35.-, O36.-, O40.-, O41.-)

Z03.71 Encounter for suspected problem with **amniotic cavity and membrane** ruled out [M]
- Encounter for suspected oligohydramnios ruled out
- Encounter for suspected polyhydramnios ruled out

Z03.72 Encounter for suspected **placental problem** ruled out [M]

Z03.73 Encounter for suspected **fetal anomaly** ruled out [M]

Z03.74 Encounter for suspected **problem with fetal growth** ruled out [M]

Z03.75 Encounter for suspected **cervical shortening** ruled out [M]

Z03.79 Encounter for other suspected maternal and fetal conditions ruled out [M]

✓5th Z03.8 Encounter for **observation** for other suspected diseases and conditions ruled out

✓6th Z03.81 Encounter for observation for suspected **exposure to biological agents** ruled out

Z03.810 Encounter for observation for suspected exposure to **anthrax** ruled out

Z03.818 Encounter for observation for suspected exposure to other biological agents ruled out

AHA: 2020,2Q,8; 2020,1Q,34-36

TIP: Possible or actual exposure to COVID-19 should be coded using Z20.822 Contact with and (suspected) exposure to COVID-19, even when the COVID-19 infection has been ruled out.

✓6th Z03.82 Encounter for observation for suspected **foreign body** ruled out
- EXCLUDES 1:
  - retained foreign body (Z18.-)
  - residual foreign body in soft tissue (M79.5)
  - retained foreign body in eyelid (H02.81)
- EXCLUDES 2: confirmed foreign body ingestion or aspiration including:
  - foreign body in alimentary tract (T18)
  - foreign body in ear (T16)
  - foreign body in respiratory tract (T17)
  - foreign body on external eye (T15)

AHA: 2020,4Q,42

Z03.821 Encounter for observation for suspected **ingested** foreign body ruled out

Z03.822 Encounter for observation for suspected **aspirated (inhaled)** foreign body ruled out

Z03.823 Encounter for observation for suspected **inserted (injected)** foreign body ruled out
- Encounter for observation for suspected inserted (injected) foreign body in eye ruled out
- Encounter for observation for suspected inserted (injected) foreign body in orifice ruled out
- Encounter for observation for suspected inserted (injected) foreign body in skin ruled out

Z03.83 Encounter for observation for suspected conditions related to **home physiologic monitoring device** ruled out
- Encounter for observation for apnea alarm without findings
- Encounter for observation for bradycardia alarm without findings
- Encounter for observation for malfunction of home cardiorespiratory monitor
- Encounter for observation for non-specific findings home physiologic monitoring device
- Encounter for observation for pulse oximeter alarm without findings
  - EXCLUDES 1:
    - apnea NOS (R06.81)
    - neonatal bradycardia (P29.12)
    - newborn apnea (P28.4-)
    - primary sleep apnea of newborn (P28.3-)
    - sleep apnea (G47.3-)

AHA: 2022,4Q,51

Z03.89 Encounter for observation for other suspected diseases and conditions ruled out

✓4th Z04 Encounter for examination and observation for other reasons

This category is to be used when a person without a diagnosis is suspected of having an abnormal condition, without signs or symptoms, which requires study, but after examination and observation, is ruled-out. This category is also for use for administrative and legal observation status.

- INCLUDES: encounter for examination for medicolegal reasons

AHA: 2018,2Q,7-8

Z04.1 Encounter for examination and observation following **transport accident** [PDx]
- EXCLUDES 1: encounter for examination and observation following work accident (Z04.2)

AHA: 2019,2Q,11; 2018,2Q,8

Z04.2 Encounter for examination and observation following **work accident** [PDx]

Z04.3 Encounter for examination and observation following other accident [PDx]

✓5th Z04.4 Encounter for examination and observation following **alleged rape**
- Encounter for examination and observation of victim following alleged rape
- Encounter for examination and observation of victim following alleged sexual abuse

Z04.41 Encounter for examination and observation following alleged **adult** rape [PDx][A]
- Suspected adult rape, ruled out
- Suspected adult sexual abuse, ruled out

Z04.42 Encounter for examination and observation following alleged **child** rape [PDx][P]
- Suspected child rape, ruled out
- Suspected child sexual abuse, ruled out

Z04.6 Encounter for **general psychiatric examination, requested by authority** [PDx]

✓5th Z04.7 Encounter for examination and observation following alleged **physical abuse**

Z04.71 Encounter for examination and observation following alleged **adult** physical abuse [PDx][A]
- Suspected adult physical abuse, ruled out
  - EXCLUDES 1:
    - confirmed case of adult physical abuse (T74.-)
    - encounter for examination and observation following alleged adult sexual abuse (Z04.41)
    - suspected case of adult physical abuse, not ruled out (T76.-)

HCC CMS-HCC | Rx Rx HCC | ESR ESRD HCC | COM Commercial HCC | PDx Primary Dx Only | N Newborn: 0 | P Pediatric: 0-17 | M Maternity: 9-64 | A Adult: 15-124

Z04.72 Encounter for examination and observation following alleged child physical abuse [PDx] [P]
Suspected child physical abuse, ruled out
EXCLUDES 1 confirmed case of child physical abuse (T74.-)
encounter for examination and observation following alleged child sexual abuse (Z04.42)
suspected case of child physical abuse, not ruled out (T76.-)

✓5th **Z04.8** Encounter for examination and observation for other specified reasons
Encounter for examination and observation for request for expert evidence
AHA: 2018,4Q,32,35,72

Z04.81 Encounter for examination and observation of victim following forced sexual exploitation [PDx]

Z04.82 Encounter for examination and observation of victim following forced labor exploitation [PDx]

Z04.89 Encounter for examination and observation for other specified reasons [PDx]

Z04.9 Encounter for examination and observation for unspecified reason [PDx]
Encounter for observation NOS

✓4th **Z05** Encounter for observation and evaluation of newborn for suspected diseases and conditions ruled out
This category is to be used for newborns, within the neonatal period (the first 28 days of life), who are suspected of having an abnormal condition, but without signs or symptoms, and which, after examination and observation, is ruled out.
AHA: 2022,1Q,17-18; 2017,4Q,27; 2016,4Q,77

Z05.0 Observation and evaluation of newborn for suspected cardiac condition ruled out [N]

Z05.1 Observation and evaluation of newborn for suspected infectious condition ruled out [N]
AHA: 2019,2Q,10

Z05.2 Observation and evaluation of newborn for suspected neurological condition ruled out [N]

Z05.3 Observation and evaluation of newborn for suspected respiratory condition ruled out [N]

✓5th **Z05.4** Observation and evaluation of newborn for suspected genetic, metabolic or immunologic condition ruled out

Z05.41 Observation and evaluation of newborn for suspected genetic condition ruled out [N]
AHA: 2016,4Q,55

Z05.42 Observation and evaluation of newborn for suspected metabolic condition ruled out [N]

Z05.43 Observation and evaluation of newborn for suspected immunologic condition ruled out [N]

Z05.5 Observation and evaluation of newborn for suspected gastrointestinal condition ruled out [N]

Z05.6 Observation and evaluation of newborn for suspected genitourinary condition ruled out [N]

✓5th **Z05.7** Observation and evaluation of newborn for suspected skin, subcutaneous, musculoskeletal and connective tissue condition ruled out

Z05.71 Observation and evaluation of newborn for suspected skin and subcutaneous tissue condition ruled out [N]

Z05.72 Observation and evaluation of newborn for suspected musculoskeletal condition ruled out [N]

Z05.73 Observation and evaluation of newborn for suspected connective tissue condition ruled out [N]

✓5th **Z05.8** Observation and evaluation of newborn for other specified suspected condition ruled out
AHA: 2023,4Q,48; 2022,1Q,17-18

Z05.81 Observation and evaluation of newborn for suspected condition related to home physiologic monitoring device ruled out [N]
Encounter for observation of newborn for apnea alarm without findings
Encounter for observation of newborn for bradycardia alarm without findings
Encounter for observation of newborn for malfunction of home cardiorespiratory monitor
Encounter for observation of newborn for non-specific findings home physiologic monitoring device
Encounter for observation of newborn for pulse oximeter alarm without findings
EXCLUDES 1 encounter for observation for suspected conditions related to home physiologic monitoring device ruled out (Z03.83)
neonatal bradycardia (P29.12)
other newborn apnea (P28.4-)
primary sleep apnea of newborn (P28.3-)

Z05.89 Observation and evaluation of newborn for other specified suspected condition ruled out [N]

Z05.9 Observation and evaluation of newborn for unspecified suspected condition ruled out [N]

Z08 Encounter for follow-up examination after completed treatment for malignant neoplasm
Medical surveillance following completed treatment
Use additional code to identify any acquired absence of organs (Z90.-)
Use additional code to identify the personal history of malignant neoplasm (Z85.-)
EXCLUDES 1 aftercare following medical care (Z43-Z49, Z51)
AHA: 2020,3Q,30

Z09 Encounter for follow-up examination after completed treatment for conditions other than malignant neoplasm
Medical surveillance following completed treatment
Use additional code to identify any applicable history of disease code (Z86.-, Z87.-)
EXCLUDES 1 aftercare following medical care (Z43-Z49, Z51)
surveillance of contraception (Z30.4-)
surveillance of prosthetic and other medical devices (Z44-Z46)
AHA: 2022,3Q,4; 2021,1Q,33; 2020,2Q,10; 2017,1Q,9; 2015,1Q,8

✓4th **Z11** Encounter for screening for infectious and parasitic diseases
Screening is the testing for disease or disease precursors in asymptomatic individuals so that early detection and treatment can be provided for those who test positive for the disease.
EXCLUDES 1 encounter for diagnostic examination - code to sign or symptom

Z11.0 Encounter for screening for intestinal infectious diseases

Z11.1 Encounter for screening for respiratory tuberculosis
Encounter for screening for active tuberculosis disease

Z11.2 Encounter for screening for other bacterial diseases

Z11.3 Encounter for screening for infections with a predominantly sexual mode of transmission
EXCLUDES 2 encounter for screening for human immunodeficiency virus [HIV] (Z11.4)
encounter for screening for human papillomavirus (Z11.51)

Z11.4 Encounter for screening for human immunodeficiency virus [HIV]

✓5th **Z11.5** Encounter for screening for other viral diseases
EXCLUDES 2 encounter for screening for viral intestinal disease (Z11.0)

Z11.51 Encounter for screening for human papillomavirus (HPV)

Z11.52 Encounter for screening for COVID-19
AHA: 2023,2Q,3; 2021,1Q,27,37,41

Z11.59 Encounter for screening for other viral diseases
AHA: 2020,3Q,14

Z11.6 Encounter for screening for other protozoal diseases and helminthiases
EXCLUDES 2 encounter for screening for protozoal intestinal disease (Z11.0)

Z11.7 Encounter for testing for latent tuberculosis infection
AHA: 2019,4Q,20

Chapter 21. Factors Influencing Health Status and Contact With Health Services

- **Z11.8** Encounter for screening for other infectious and parasitic diseases
  - Encounter for screening for chlamydia
  - Encounter for screening for mycoses
  - Encounter for screening for rickettsial
  - Encounter for screening for spirochetal
- **Z11.9** Encounter for screening for infectious and parasitic diseases, unspecified

- ✓4th **Z12** Encounter for screening for malignant neoplasms
  - Screening is the testing for disease or disease precursors in asymptomatic individuals so that early detection and treatment can be provided for those who test positive for the disease.
  - Use additional code to identify any family history of malignant neoplasm (Z80.-)
  - EXCLUDES 1: encounter for diagnostic examination - code to sign or symptom
  - **Z12.0** Encounter for screening for malignant neoplasm of stomach
  - ✓5th **Z12.1** Encounter for screening for malignant neoplasm of intestinal tract
    - AHA: 2017,1Q,8,9
    - **Z12.10** Encounter for screening for malignant neoplasm of intestinal tract, unspecified
    - **Z12.11** Encounter for screening for malignant neoplasm of colon
      - Encounter for screening colonoscopy NOS
      - AHA: 2019,1Q,32-33; 2018,1Q,6
      - TIP: Surveillance colonoscopies are a type of screening exam used to screen for malignancies in those patients with history of polyps and/or cancer (previously removed). If polyps or cancer are removed during the colonoscopy, code the appropriate neoplasm code instead of Z12.11.
    - **Z12.12** Encounter for screening for malignant neoplasm of rectum
      - AHA: 2018,1Q,6
    - **Z12.13** Encounter for screening for malignant neoplasm of small intestine
  - **Z12.2** Encounter for screening for malignant neoplasm of respiratory organs
  - ✓5th **Z12.3** Encounter for screening for malignant neoplasm of breast
    - **Z12.31** Encounter for screening mammogram for malignant neoplasm of breast
      - EXCLUDES 1: inconclusive mammogram (R92.2)
      - AHA: 2023,4Q,44; 2015,1Q,24
    - **Z12.39** Encounter for other screening for malignant neoplasm of breast
  - **Z12.4** Encounter for screening for malignant neoplasm of cervix
    - Encounter for screening pap smear for malignant neoplasm of cervix
    - EXCLUDES 1: when screening is part of general gynecological examination (Z01.4-)
    - EXCLUDES 2: encounter for screening for human papillomavirus (Z11.51)
  - **Z12.5** Encounter for screening for malignant neoplasm of prostate
  - **Z12.6** Encounter for screening for malignant neoplasm of bladder
  - ✓5th **Z12.7** Encounter for screening for malignant neoplasm of other genitourinary organs
    - **Z12.71** Encounter for screening for malignant neoplasm of testis
    - **Z12.72** Encounter for screening for malignant neoplasm of vagina
      - Vaginal pap smear status-post hysterectomy for non-malignant condition
      - Use additional code to identify acquired absence of uterus (Z90.71-)
      - EXCLUDES 1: vaginal pap smear status-post hysterectomy for malignant conditions (Z08)
    - **Z12.73** Encounter for screening for malignant neoplasm of ovary
    - **Z12.79** Encounter for screening for malignant neoplasm of other genitourinary organs
  - ✓5th **Z12.8** Encounter for screening for malignant neoplasm of other sites
    - **Z12.81** Encounter for screening for malignant neoplasm of oral cavity
    - **Z12.82** Encounter for screening for malignant neoplasm of nervous system
    - **Z12.83** Encounter for screening for malignant neoplasm of skin
    - **Z12.89** Encounter for screening for malignant neoplasm of other sites
      - AHA: 2021,1Q,14
  - **Z12.9** Encounter for screening for malignant neoplasm, site unspecified

- ✓4th **Z13** Encounter for screening for other diseases and disorders
  - Screening is the testing for disease or disease precursors in asymptomatic individuals so that early detection and treatment can be provided for those who test positive for the disease.
  - EXCLUDES 1: encounter for diagnostic examination - code to sign or symptom
  - **Z13.0** Encounter for screening for diseases of the blood and blood-forming organs and certain disorders involving the immune mechanism
  - **Z13.1** Encounter for screening for diabetes mellitus
  - ✓5th **Z13.2** Encounter for screening for nutritional, metabolic and other endocrine disorders
    - **Z13.21** Encounter for screening for nutritional disorder
    - ✓6th **Z13.22** Encounter for screening for metabolic disorder
      - **Z13.220** Encounter for screening for lipoid disorders
        - Encounter for screening for cholesterol level
        - Encounter for screening for hypercholesterolemia
        - Encounter for screening for hyperlipidemia
      - **Z13.228** Encounter for screening for other metabolic disorders
    - **Z13.29** Encounter for screening for other suspected endocrine disorder
      - EXCLUDES 2: encounter for screening for diabetes mellitus (Z13.1)
  - ✓5th **Z13.3** Encounter for screening examination for mental health and behavioral disorders
    - AHA: 2018,4Q,35-36
    - **Z13.30** Encounter for screening examination for mental health and behavioral disorders, unspecified
    - **Z13.31** Encounter for screening for depression
      - Encounter for screening for depression for child or adolescent
      - Encounter for screening for depression, adult
    - **Z13.32** Encounter for screening for maternal depression
      - Encounter for screening for perinatal depression
    - **Z13.39** Encounter for screening examination for other mental health and behavioral disorders
      - Encounter for screening for alcoholism
      - Encounter for screening for intellectual disabilities
  - ✓5th **Z13.4** Encounter for screening for certain developmental disorders in childhood
    - Encounter for development testing of infant or child
    - Encounter for screening for developmental handicaps in early childhood
    - EXCLUDES 2: encounter for routine child health examination (Z00.12-)
    - AHA: 2018,4Q,36
    - **Z13.40** Encounter for screening for unspecified developmental delays
    - **Z13.41** Encounter for autism screening
    - **Z13.42** Encounter for screening for global developmental delays (milestones)
      - Encounter for screening for developmental handicaps in early childhood
    - **Z13.49** Encounter for screening for other developmental delays
  - **Z13.5** Encounter for screening for eye and ear disorders
    - EXCLUDES 2: encounter for general hearing examination (Z01.1-)
    - encounter for general vision examination (Z01.0-)
    - AHA: 2016,3Q,17
  - **Z13.6** Encounter for screening for cardiovascular disorders
  - ✓5th **Z13.7** Encounter for screening for genetic and chromosomal anomalies
    - EXCLUDES 1: genetic testing for procreative management (Z31.4-)
    - **Z13.71** Encounter for nonprocreative screening for genetic disease carrier status
    - **Z13.79** Encounter for other screening for genetic and chromosomal anomalies
  - ✓5th **Z13.8** Encounter for screening for other specified diseases and disorders
    - EXCLUDES 2: screening for malignant neoplasms (Z12.-)
    - ✓6th **Z13.81** Encounter for screening for digestive system disorders
      - **Z13.810** Encounter for screening for upper gastrointestinal disorder

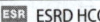

	Z13.811	Encounter for screening for lower gastrointestinal disorder
		EXCLUDES 1 encounter for screening for intestinal infectious disease (Z11.0)
	Z13.818	Encounter for screening for other digestive system disorders
✓6th	Z13.82	Encounter for screening for musculoskeletal disorder
	Z13.820	Encounter for screening for osteoporosis
	Z13.828	Encounter for screening for other musculoskeletal disorder
	Z13.83	Encounter for screening for respiratory disorder NEC
		EXCLUDES 1 encounter for screening for respiratory tuberculosis (Z11.1)
	Z13.84	Encounter for screening for dental disorders
✓6th	Z13.85	Encounter for screening for nervous system disorders
	Z13.850	Encounter for screening for traumatic brain injury
	Z13.858	Encounter for screening for other nervous system disorders
	Z13.88	Encounter for screening for disorder due to exposure to contaminants
		EXCLUDES 1 those exposed to contaminants without suspected disorders (Z57.-, Z77.-)
	Z13.89	Encounter for screening for other disorder
		Encounter for screening for genitourinary disorders
Z13.9		Encounter for screening, unspecified

Genetic carrier and genetic susceptibility to disease (Z14-Z15)

✓4th **Z14 Genetic carrier**
DEF: Individuals carrying a gene mutation associated with a certain disease that typically do not develop the disease but are able to pass the mutated genes to offspring.

✓5th Z14.0 **Hemophilia A** carrier
    Z14.01 **Asymptomatic** hemophilia A carrier
    Z14.02 **Symptomatic** hemophilia A carrier
Z14.1 **Cystic fibrosis** carrier
Z14.8 Genetic carrier of other disease

✓4th **Z15 Genetic susceptibility to disease**
    INCLUDES confirmed abnormal gene
Use additional code, if applicable, for any associated family history of the disease (Z80-Z84)
EXCLUDES 1 chromosomal anomalies (Q90-Q99)

✓5th Z15.0 Genetic susceptibility to **malignant neoplasm**
Code first, if applicable, any current malignant neoplasm (C00-C75, C81-C96)
Use additional code, if applicable, for any personal history of malignant neoplasm (Z85.-)

    Z15.01 Genetic susceptibility to malignant neoplasm of breast
    Z15.02 Genetic susceptibility to malignant neoplasm of ovary
    Z15.03 Genetic susceptibility to malignant neoplasm of prostate
    Z15.04 Genetic susceptibility to malignant neoplasm of endometrium
•   Z15.05 Genetic susceptibility to malignant neoplasm of fallopian tube(s)
• ✓6th Z15.06 Genetic susceptibility to malignant neoplasm of digestive system
•   Z15.060 Genetic susceptibility to colorectal cancer
        Z15.068 Genetic susceptibility to other malignant neoplasm of digestive system
            Genetic susceptibility to biliary tract cancer
            Genetic susceptibility to gastric cancer
            Genetic susceptibility to pancreatic cancer
            Genetic susceptibility to small bowel cancer
•   Z15.07 Genetic susceptibility to malignant neoplasm of urinary tract
    Z15.09 Genetic susceptibility to other malignant neoplasm
        AHA: 2021,1Q,14

Z15.1 Genetic susceptibility to **epilepsy and neurodevelopmental disorders**
Code also, if applicable, related disorders such as:
  developmental and epileptic encephalopathy (G93.45)
  developmental disorder of speech and language (F80.-)
  developmental disorders of scholastic skills (F81.-)
  epilepsy, by specific type (G40.-)
  intellectual disabilities (F70-F79)
  other neurodevelopmental disorder (F88)
  pervasive developmental disorders (F84.-)
AHA: 2024,4Q,31

Z15.2 Genetic susceptibility to **obesity**
Code also, if applicable, any associated manifestations, such as:
  other obesity (E66.8-)
  polyphagia (R63.2)
Use additional code to identify body mass index (BMI), if known (Z68.-)
AHA: 2024,4Q,31

• Z15.3 Genetic susceptibility to **kidney disease**
Code also, if applicable, hypertension (I10-I1A)

✓5th Z15.8 Genetic susceptibility to other disease
    Z15.81 Genetic susceptibility to **multiple endocrine neoplasia [MEN]**
        EXCLUDES 1 multiple endocrine neoplasia [MEN] syndromes (E31.2-)
    DEF: Group of conditions in which several endocrine glands grow excessively (such as in adenomatous hyperplasia) and/or develop benign or malignant tumors. Tumors and hyperplasia associated with MEN often produce excess hormones, which impede normal physiology. There is no comprehensive cure known for MEN syndrome. Treatment is directed at the hyperplasia or tumors in each individual gland. Tumors are usually surgically removed and oral medications or hormonal injections are used to correct hormone imbalances.
    Z15.89 Genetic susceptibility to other disease

Resistance to antimicrobial drugs (Z16)

✓4th **Z16 Resistance to antimicrobial drugs**
NOTE The codes in this category are provided for use as additional codes to identify the resistance and non-responsiveness of a condition to antimicrobial drugs.
Code first the infection
EXCLUDES 1 Methicillin resistant Staphylococcus aureus infection (A49.02)
  Methicillin resistant Staphylococcus aureus pneumonia (J15.212)
  sepsis due to Methicillin resistant Staphylococcus aureus (A41.02)

✓5th Z16.1 Resistance to **beta lactam** antibiotics
    Z16.10 Resistance to unspecified beta lactam antibiotics UPD
    Z16.11 Resistance to **penicillins** UPD
        Resistance to amoxicillin
        Resistance to ampicillin
    Z16.12 **Extended spectrum beta lactamase** (ESBL) resistance UPD
        EXCLUDES 2 Methicillin resistant Staphylococcus aureus infection in diseases classified elsewhere (B95.62)
    Z16.13 Resistance to **carbapenem** UPD
        AHA: 2023,4Q,47
    Z16.19 Resistance to other specified beta lactam antibiotics UPD
        Resistance to cephalosporins

✓5th Z16.2 Resistance to other antibiotics
    Z16.20 Resistance to unspecified antibiotic UPD
        Resistance to antibiotics NOS
    Z16.21 Resistance to **vancomycin** UPD
    Z16.22 Resistance to **vancomycin related** antibiotics UPD
    Z16.23 Resistance to **quinolones and fluoroquinolones** UPD
    Z16.24 Resistance to **multiple** antibiotics UPD
    Z16.29 Resistance to other single specified antibiotic UPD
        Resistance to aminoglycosides
        Resistance to macrolides
        Resistance to sulfonamides
        Resistance to tetracyclines

Z16.3 Resistance to other antimicrobial drugs
EXCLUDES 1: resistance to antibiotics (Z16.1-, Z16.2-)

- **Z16.30** Resistance to unspecified antimicrobial drugs
  - Drug resistance NOS
- **Z16.31** Resistance to antiparasitic drug(s)
  - Resistance to quinine and related compounds
- **Z16.32** Resistance to antifungal drug(s)
- **Z16.33** Resistance to antiviral drug(s)
- **Z16.34** Resistance to antimycobacterial drug(s)
  - Resistance to tuberculostatics
  - **Z16.341** Resistance to single antimycobacterial drug
    - Resistance to antimycobacterial drug NOS
  - **Z16.342** Resistance to multiple antimycobacterial drugs
- **Z16.35** Resistance to multiple antimicrobial drugs
  - EXCLUDES 1: resistance to multiple antibiotics only (Z16.24)
- **Z16.39** Resistance to other specified antimicrobial drug

Estrogen, and other hormones and factors receptor status (Z17)

Z17 Estrogen, and other hormones and factors receptor status
NOTE: Use one code, as available, for each receptor: Z17.0, Z17.1, Z17.2-, Z17.3-

Code first malignant neoplasm, such as:
  malignant neoplasm of breast (C50.-)
  malignant neoplasm of ovary (C56.-)
AHA: 2022,3Q,14
DEF: Receptor status of breast cancer cells for the hormone estrogen that is used to help determine treatment and evaluate prognosis. ER+ breast cancer responds to hormone therapies while ER- breast cancer does not.

- **Z17.0** Estrogen receptor positive status [ER+]
- **Z17.1** Estrogen receptor negative status [ER-]
- **Z17.2** Progesterone receptor status
  - AHA: 2024,4Q,31
  - **Z17.21** Progesterone receptor positive status
    - PR+
  - **Z17.22** Progesterone receptor negative status
    - PR-
- **Z17.3** Human epidermal growth factor 2 receptor
  - AHA: 2024,4Q,31
  - **Z17.31** Human epidermal growth factor receptor 2 positive status
    - HER2+
  - **Z17.32** Human epidermal growth factor receptor 2 negative status
    - HER2-
- **Z17.4** Combined receptor status
  - NOTE: Assign a code from subcategory Z17.4- when only a combined receptor status is documented
  - AHA: 2024,4Q,31
  - **Z17.41** Hormone receptor positive
    - HR+
    - **Z17.410** Hormone receptor positive with human epidermal growth factor receptor 2 positive status
      - HR+ with HER2+
    - **Z17.411** Hormone receptor positive with human epidermal growth factor receptor 2 negative status
      - HR+ with HER2-
  - **Z17.42** Hormone receptor negative
    - HR-
    - **Z17.420** Hormone receptor negative with human epidermal growth factor receptor 2 positive status
      - HR- with HER2+
    - **Z17.421** Hormone receptor negative with human epidermal growth factor receptor 2 negative status
      - HR- with HER2-
      - TNBC
      - Triple negative breast cancer

Retained foreign body fragments (Z18)

Z18 Retained foreign body fragments
INCLUDES:
  embedded fragment (status)
  embedded splinter (status)
  retained foreign body status
EXCLUDES 1:
  artificial joint prosthesis status (Z96.6-)
  foreign body accidentally left during a procedure (T81.5-)
  foreign body entering through orifice (T15-T19)
  in situ cardiac device (Z95.-)
  organ or tissue replaced by means other than transplant (Z96.-, Z97.-)
  organ or tissue replaced by transplant (Z94.-)
  personal history of retained foreign body fully removed Z87.821
  superficial foreign body (non-embedded splinter) - code to superficial foreign body, by site
AHA: 2023,2Q,27
DEF: Embedded or retained fragment, splinter, or foreign body, natural or synthetic that can cause infection.

- **Z18.0** Retained radioactive fragments
  - **Z18.01** Retained depleted uranium fragments
  - **Z18.09** Other retained radioactive fragments
    - Other retained depleted isotope fragments
    - Retained nontherapeutic radioactive fragments
- **Z18.1** Retained metal fragments
  - EXCLUDES 1: retained radioactive metal fragments (Z18.01-Z18.09)
  - **Z18.10** Retained metal fragments, unspecified
    - Retained metal fragment NOS
  - **Z18.11** Retained magnetic metal fragments
  - **Z18.12** Retained nonmagnetic metal fragments
- **Z18.2** Retained plastic fragments
  - Acrylics fragments
  - Diethylhexyl phthalates fragments
  - Isocyanate fragments
- **Z18.3** Retained organic fragments
  - **Z18.31** Retained animal quills or spines
  - **Z18.32** Retained tooth
  - **Z18.33** Retained wood fragments
  - **Z18.39** Other retained organic fragments
- **Z18.8** Other specified retained foreign body
  - **Z18.81** Retained glass fragments
  - **Z18.83** Retained stone or crystalline fragments
    - Retained concrete or cement fragments
  - **Z18.89** Other specified retained foreign body fragments
- **Z18.9** Retained foreign body fragments, unspecified material

Hormone sensitivity malignancy status (Z19)

Z19 Hormone sensitivity malignancy status
Code first malignant neoplasm — see Table of Neoplasms, by site, malignant
AHA: 2016,4Q,76

- **Z19.1** Hormone sensitive malignancy status
- **Z19.2** Hormone resistant malignancy status
  - Castrate resistant prostate malignancy status

Persons with potential health hazards related to communicable diseases (Z20-Z29)

Z20 Contact with and (suspected) exposure to communicable diseases
EXCLUDES 1:
  carrier of infectious disease (Z22.-)
  diagnosed current infectious or parasitic disease - see Alphabetic Index
EXCLUDES 2:
  personal history of infectious and parasitic diseases (Z86.1-)

- **Z20.0** Contact with and (suspected) exposure to intestinal infectious diseases
  - **Z20.01** Contact with and (suspected) exposure to intestinal infectious diseases due to Escherichia coli (E. coli)
  - **Z20.09** Contact with and (suspected) exposure to other intestinal infectious diseases
- **Z20.1** Contact with and (suspected) exposure to tuberculosis
- **Z20.2** Contact with and (suspected) exposure to infections with a predominantly sexual mode of transmission
- **Z20.3** Contact with and (suspected) exposure to rabies
- **Z20.4** Contact with and (suspected) exposure to rubella
- **Z20.5** Contact with and (suspected) exposure to viral hepatitis

Chapter 21. Factors Influencing Health Status and Contact With Health Services

Z20.6 Contact with and (suspected) exposure to human immunodeficiency virus [HIV]
- EXCLUDES 1: asymptomatic human immunodeficiency virus [HIV] HIV infection status (Z21)

Z20.7 Contact with and (suspected) exposure to pediculosis, acariasis and other infestations

Z20.8 Contact with and (suspected) exposure to other communicable diseases

- **Z20.81** Contact with and (suspected) exposure to other bacterial communicable diseases
  - **Z20.810** Contact with and (suspected) exposure to anthrax
  - **Z20.811** Contact with and (suspected) exposure to meningococcus
  - **Z20.818** Contact with and (suspected) exposure to other bacterial communicable diseases
    - AHA: 2019,2Q,10

- **Z20.82** Contact with and (suspected) exposure to other viral communicable diseases
  - **Z20.820** Contact with and (suspected) exposure to varicella
  - **Z20.821** Contact with and (suspected) exposure to Zika virus
    - AHA: 2018,4Q,35,64
  - **Z20.822** Contact with and (suspected) exposure to COVID-19
    - Contact with and (suspected) exposure to SARS-CoV-2
    - AHA: 2023,2Q,3; 2022,2Q,28-29; 2021,4Q,109; 2021,1Q,27-29,37-38,41
  - **Z20.828** Contact with and (suspected) exposure to other viral communicable diseases
    - AHA: 2022,3Q,4; 2021,1Q,37-38; 2020,4Q,99; 2020,3Q,14-15; 2020,2Q,4,8; 2020,1Q,34-36

- **Z20.89** Contact with and (suspected) exposure to other communicable diseases

Z20.9 Contact with and (suspected) exposure to unspecified communicable disease

Z21 Asymptomatic human immunodeficiency virus [HIV] infection status
- HIV positive NOS
- Code first human immunodeficiency virus [HIV] disease complicating pregnancy, childbirth and the puerperium, if applicable (O98.7-)
- EXCLUDES 1:
  - acquired immunodeficiency syndrome (B20)
  - contact with human immunodeficiency virus [HIV] (Z20.6)
  - exposure to human immunodeficiency virus [HIV] (Z20.6)
  - human immunodeficiency virus [HIV] disease (B20)
  - inconclusive laboratory evidence of human immunodeficiency virus [HIV] (R75)
- AHA: 2022,1Q,36; 2019,1Q,8-11
- DEF: Phase of human immunodeficiency virus (HIV) infection with no clinical symptoms. This phase may last for 10 years or more.

Z22 Carrier of infectious disease
- INCLUDES:
  - colonization status
  - suspected carrier
- EXCLUDES 2: carrier of viral hepatitis (B18.-)

- **Z22.0** Carrier of typhoid
- **Z22.1** Carrier of other intestinal infectious diseases
- **Z22.2** Carrier of diphtheria
- **Z22.3** Carrier of other specified bacterial diseases
  - **Z22.31** Carrier of bacterial disease due to meningococci
  - **Z22.32** Carrier of bacterial disease due to staphylococci
    - **Z22.321** Carrier or suspected carrier of Methicillin susceptible Staphylococcus aureus
      - MSSA colonization
    - **Z22.322** Carrier or suspected carrier of Methicillin resistant Staphylococcus aureus
      - MRSA colonization
      - DEF: Carriers (colonization) of methicillin resistant *Staphylococcus aureus* (MRSA) have MRSA on their skin or in their body but do not exhibit signs of infection. These individuals are able to pass MRSA on to others who may develop an infection.

  - **Z22.33** Carrier of bacterial disease due to streptococci
    - **Z22.330** Carrier of Group B streptococcus
      - EXCLUDES 1: carrier of streptococcus group B (GBS) complicating pregnancy, childbirth and the puerperium (O99.82-)
    - **Z22.338** Carrier of other streptococcus
  - **Z22.34** Carrier of Acinetobacter baumannii
    - AHA: 2023,4Q,47
    - **Z22.340** Carrier of carbapenem-resistant Acinetobacter baumannii
    - **Z22.341** Carrier of carbapenem-sensitive Acinetobacter baumannii
    - **Z22.349** Carrier of Acinetobacter baumannii, unspecified
  - **Z22.35** Carrier of Enterobacterales
    - Carrier of E. coli
    - Carrier of K. pneumoniae
    - AHA: 2023,4Q,47
    - **Z22.350** Carrier of carbapenem-resistant Enterobacterales
    - **Z22.358** Carrier of other Enterobacterales
      - Carrier of carbapenem-sensitive Enterobacterales
      - Carrier of ESBL-producing Enterobacterales
      - Carrier of extended-spectrum beta-lactamase producing Enterobacterales
    - **Z22.359** Carrier of Enterobacterales, unspecified
  - **Z22.39** Carrier of other specified bacterial diseases

- **Z22.4** Carrier of infections with a predominantly sexual mode of transmission
- **Z22.6** Carrier of human T-lymphotropic virus type-1 [HTLV-1] infection
- **Z22.7** Latent tuberculosis
  - Latent tuberculosis infection (LTBI)
  - EXCLUDES 1:
    - nonspecific reaction to cell mediated immunity measurement of gamma interferon antigen response without active tuberculosis (R76.12)
    - nonspecific reaction to tuberculin skin test without active tuberculosis (R76.11)
  - AHA: 2019,4Q,19
- **Z22.8** Carrier of other infectious diseases
- **Z22.9** Carrier of infectious disease, unspecified

Z23 Encounter for immunization
- NOTE: Procedure codes are required to identify the types of immunizations given
- Code first any routine childhood examination
- Code also, if applicable, encounter for immunization safety counseling (Z71.85)

Z28 Immunization not carried out and underimmunization status
- INCLUDES: vaccination not carried out
- Code also, if applicable, encounter for immunization safety counseling (Z71.85)

- **Z28.0** Immunization not carried out because of contraindication
  - DEF: Contraindication: Situation where a drug, surgery, or other procedure may negatively affect or cause harm to a patient.
  - **Z28.01** Immunization not carried out because of acute illness of patient
  - **Z28.02** Immunization not carried out because of chronic illness or condition of patient
  - **Z28.03** Immunization not carried out because of immune compromised state of patient
  - **Z28.04** Immunization not carried out because of patient allergy to vaccine or component
  - **Z28.09** Immunization not carried out because of other contraindication

- **Z28.1** Immunization not carried out because of patient decision for reasons of belief or group pressure
  - Immunization not carried out because of religious belief
- **Z28.2** Immunization not carried out because of patient decision for other and unspecified reason
  - **Z28.20** Immunization not carried out because of patient decision for unspecified reason
  - **Z28.21** Immunization not carried out because of patient refusal
  - **Z28.29** Immunization not carried out because of patient decision for other reason

Z28.3 Underimmunization status

Use additional code, if applicable, to identify:
immunization not carried out because of contraindication (Z28.0-)
immunization not carried out because of patient decision for other and unspecified reason (Z28.2-)
immunization not carried out because of patient decision for reasons of belief or group pressure (Z28.1)
immunization not carried out for other reason (Z28.8-)

AHA: 2022,1Q,4-5

Z28.31 Underimmunization for COVID-19 status

NOTE: These codes should not be used for individuals who are not eligible for the COVID-19 vaccines, as determined by the healthcare provider.

- Z28.310 Unvaccinated for COVID-19
- Z28.311 Partially vaccinated for COVID-19

Z28.39 Other underimmunization status
Delinquent immunization status
Lapsed immunization schedule status

Z28.8 Immunization not carried out for other reason

Z28.81 Immunization not carried out due to patient having had the disease

Z28.82 Immunization not carried out because of caregiver refusal
Immunization not carried out because of guardian refusal
Immunization not carried out because of parent refusal

EXCLUDES 1 immunization not carried out because of caregiver refusal because of religious belief (Z28.1)

Z28.83 Immunization not carried out due to unavailability of vaccine
Delay in delivery of vaccine
Lack of availability of vaccine
Manufacturer delay of vaccine

AHA: 2018,4Q,36

Z28.89 Immunization not carried out for other reason

Z28.9 Immunization not carried out for unspecified reason

Z29 Encounter for other prophylactic measures

EXCLUDES 1 desensitization to allergens (Z51.6)
prophylactic surgery (Z40.-)

AHA: 2016,4Q,78-79

Z29.1 Encounter for prophylactic immunotherapy
Encounter for administration of immunoglobulin

- Z29.11 Encounter for prophylactic immunotherapy for respiratory syncytial virus (RSV)
- Z29.12 Encounter for prophylactic antivenin
- Z29.13 Encounter for prophylactic Rho(D) immune globulin
  AHA: 2019,3Q,5
- Z29.14 Encounter for prophylactic rabies immune globin

Z29.3 Encounter for prophylactic fluoride administration

Z29.8 Encounter for other specified prophylactic measures

AHA: 2023,4Q,49; 2022,2Q,27

- Z29.81 Encounter for HIV pre-exposure prophylaxis
  Code also, if applicable, risk factors for HIV, such as:
  contact with and (suspected) exposure to human immunodeficiency virus [HIV] (Z20.6)
  high risk sexual behavior (Z72.5-)
- Z29.89 Encounter for other specified prophylactic measures

Z29.9 Encounter for prophylactic measures, unspecified

Persons encountering health services in circumstances related to reproduction (Z30-Z39)

Z30 Encounter for contraceptive management

AHA: 2016,4Q,78

DEF: Contraceptive management to prevent pregnancy. Methods include oral medications, intrauterine devices, and surgical procedures for males and females (sterilization).

Z30.0 Encounter for general counseling and advice on contraception

Z30.01 Encounter for initial prescription of contraceptives

EXCLUDES 1 encounter for surveillance of contraceptives (Z30.4-)

- Z30.011 Encounter for initial prescription of contraceptive pills
- Z30.012 Encounter for prescription of emergency contraception
  Encounter for postcoital contraception
- Z30.013 Encounter for initial prescription of injectable contraceptive
- Z30.014 Encounter for initial prescription of intrauterine contraceptive device
  EXCLUDES 1 encounter for insertion of intrauterine contraceptive device (Z30.430, Z30.432)
- Z30.015 Encounter for initial prescription of vaginal ring hormonal contraceptive
- Z30.016 Encounter for initial prescription of transdermal patch hormonal contraceptive device
- Z30.017 Encounter for initial prescription of implantable subdermal contraceptive
- Z30.018 Encounter for initial prescription of other contraceptives
  Encounter for initial prescription of barrier contraception
  Encounter for initial prescription of diaphragm
- Z30.019 Encounter for initial prescription of contraceptives, unspecified

Z30.02 Counseling and instruction in natural family planning to avoid pregnancy

Z30.09 Encounter for other general counseling and advice on contraception
Encounter for family planning advice NOS

Z30.2 Encounter for sterilization
AHA: 2021,3Q,13

Z30.4 Encounter for surveillance of contraceptives

Z30.40 Encounter for surveillance of contraceptives, unspecified

Z30.41 Encounter for surveillance of contraceptive pills
Encounter for repeat prescription for contraceptive pill

Z30.42 Encounter for surveillance of injectable contraceptive

Z30.43 Encounter for surveillance of intrauterine contraceptive device

- Z30.430 Encounter for insertion of intrauterine contraceptive device
- Z30.431 Encounter for routine checking of intrauterine contraceptive device
- Z30.432 Encounter for removal of intrauterine contraceptive device
- Z30.433 Encounter for removal and reinsertion of intrauterine contraceptive device
  Encounter for replacement of intrauterine contraceptive device

Z30.44 Encounter for surveillance of vaginal ring hormonal contraceptive device

Z30.45 Encounter for surveillance of transdermal patch hormonal contraceptive device

Z30.46 Encounter for surveillance of implantable subdermal contraceptive
Encounter for checking, reinsertion or removal of implantable subdermal contraceptive

Z30.49 Encounter for surveillance of other contraceptives
Encounter for surveillance of barrier contraception
Encounter for surveillance of diaphragm

Z30.8 Encounter for other contraceptive management
Encounter for postvasectomy sperm count
Encounter for routine examination for contraceptive maintenance

EXCLUDES 1 sperm count following sterilization reversal (Z31.42)
sperm count for fertility testing (Z31.41)

Z30.9 Encounter for contraceptive management, unspecified

Z31 Encounter for procreative management

EXCLUDES 2 complications associated with artificial fertilization (N98.-)
female infertility (N97.-)
male infertility (N46.-)

Z31.0 Encounter for reversal of previous sterilization

Z31.4 Encounter for procreative investigation and testing
EXCLUDES 1 postvasectomy sperm count (Z30.8)

Z31.41 Encounter for fertility testing
Encounter for fallopian tube patency testing
Encounter for sperm count for fertility testing

Z31.42 Aftercare following sterilization reversal
Sperm count following sterilization reversal

Chapter 21. Factors Influencing Health Status and Contact With Health Services

Z31.43 Encounter for genetic testing of female for procreative management
Use additional code for recurrent pregnancy loss, if applicable (N96, O26.2-)
EXCLUDES 1: nonprocreative genetic testing (Z13.7-)

- **Z31.430** Encounter of female for testing for genetic disease carrier status for procreative management
- **Z31.438** Encounter for other genetic testing of female for procreative management

Z31.44 Encounter for genetic testing of male for procreative management
EXCLUDES 1: nonprocreative genetic testing (Z13.7-)

- **Z31.440** Encounter of male for testing for genetic disease carrier status for procreative management
- **Z31.441** Encounter for testing of male partner of patient with recurrent pregnancy loss
- **Z31.448** Encounter for other genetic testing of male for procreative management

Z31.49 Encounter for other procreative investigation and testing

Z31.5 Encounter for procreative genetic counseling
AHA: 2017,4Q,27

Z31.6 Encounter for general counseling and advice on procreation
- **Z31.61** Procreative counseling and advice using natural family planning
- **Z31.62** Encounter for fertility preservation counseling
  - Encounter for fertility preservation counseling prior to cancer therapy
  - Encounter for fertility preservation counseling prior to surgical removal of gonads
- **Z31.69** Encounter for other general counseling and advice on procreation

Z31.7 Encounter for procreative management and counseling for gestational carrier
EXCLUDES 1: pregnant state, gestational carrier (Z33.3)
AHA: 2016,4Q,78

Z31.8 Encounter for other procreative management
- **Z31.81** Encounter for male factor infertility in female patient
- **Z31.82** Encounter for Rh incompatibility status
  AHA: 2015,3Q,40; 2014,4Q,17
- **Z31.83** Encounter for assisted reproductive fertility procedure cycle
  Patient undergoing in vitro fertilization cycle
  Use additional code to identify the type of infertility
  EXCLUDES 1: pre-cycle diagnosis and testing - code to reason for encounter
  AHA: 2022,2Q,15-16
- **Z31.84** Encounter for fertility preservation procedure
  Encounter for fertility preservation procedure prior to cancer therapy
  Encounter for fertility preservation procedure prior to surgical removal of gonads
- **Z31.89** Encounter for other procreative management

Z31.9 Encounter for procreative management, unspecified

Z32 Encounter for pregnancy test and childbirth and childcare instruction

Z32.0 Encounter for pregnancy test
- **Z32.00** Encounter for pregnancy test, result unknown
  Encounter for pregnancy test NOS
- **Z32.01** Encounter for pregnancy test, result positive
- **Z32.02** Encounter for pregnancy test, result negative

Z32.2 Encounter for childbirth instruction

Z32.3 Encounter for childcare instruction
Encounter for prenatal or postpartum childcare instruction

Z33 Pregnant state

Z33.1 Pregnant state, incidental
Pregnancy NOS
Pregnant state NOS
EXCLUDES 1: complications of pregnancy (O00-O9A)
pregnant state, gestational carrier (Z33.3)

Z33.2 Encounter for elective termination of pregnancy
EXCLUDES 1: early fetal death with retention of dead fetus (O02.1)
late fetal death (O36.4)
spontaneous abortion (O03)
AHA: 2024,3Q,9; 2023,2Q,15; 2022,1Q,20
TIP: Do not assign a code from category Z3A with this code.

Z33.3 Pregnant state, gestational carrier
EXCLUDES 1: encounter for procreative management and counseling for gestational carrier (Z31.7)
AHA: 2016,4Q,78

Z34 Encounter for supervision of normal pregnancy
EXCLUDES 1: any complication of pregnancy (O00-O9A)
encounter for pregnancy test (Z32.0-)
encounter for supervision of high risk pregnancy (O09.-)
AHA: 2019,3Q,5; 2014,4Q,17

Z34.0 Encounter for supervision of normal first pregnancy
- **Z34.00** Encounter for supervision of normal first pregnancy, unspecified trimester
- **Z34.01** Encounter for supervision of normal first pregnancy, first trimester
- **Z34.02** Encounter for supervision of normal first pregnancy, second trimester
- **Z34.03** Encounter for supervision of normal first pregnancy, third trimester

Z34.8 Encounter for supervision of other normal pregnancy
- **Z34.80** Encounter for supervision of other normal pregnancy, unspecified trimester
- **Z34.81** Encounter for supervision of other normal pregnancy, first trimester
- **Z34.82** Encounter for supervision of other normal pregnancy, second trimester
- **Z34.83** Encounter for supervision of other normal pregnancy, third trimester

Z34.9 Encounter for supervision of normal pregnancy, unspecified
- **Z34.90** Encounter for supervision of normal pregnancy, unspecified, unspecified trimester
- **Z34.91** Encounter for supervision of normal pregnancy, unspecified, first trimester
- **Z34.92** Encounter for supervision of normal pregnancy, unspecified, second trimester
- **Z34.93** Encounter for supervision of normal pregnancy, unspecified, third trimester

Z36 Encounter for antenatal screening of mother
INCLUDES: encounter for placental sample (taken vaginally)
screening is the testing for disease or disease precursors in asymptomatic individuals so that early detection and treatment can be provided for those who test positive for the disease.
EXCLUDES 1: diagnostic examination - code to sign or symptom
encounter for suspected maternal and fetal conditions ruled out (Z03.7-)
suspected fetal condition affecting management of pregnancy - code to condition in Chapter 15
EXCLUDES 2: abnormal findings on antenatal screening of mother (O28.-)
genetic counseling and testing (Z31.43-, Z31.5)
routine prenatal care (Z34)
AHA: 2017,4Q,28

- **Z36.0** Encounter for antenatal screening for chromosomal anomalies
- **Z36.1** Encounter for antenatal screening for raised alphafetoprotein level
  Encounter for antenatal screening for elevated maternal serum alphafetoprotein level
  DEF: High levels of alpha-fetoprotein (AFP) that may indicate a possibility of spina bifida and other neural tube defects, anencephaly, or omphalocele in the fetus.
- **Z36.2** Encounter for other antenatal screening follow-up
  Non-visualized anatomy on a previous scan
- **Z36.3** Encounter for antenatal screening for malformations
  Screening for a suspected anomaly
- **Z36.4** Encounter for antenatal screening for fetal growth retardation
  Intrauterine growth restriction (IUGR)/small-for-dates
- **Z36.5** Encounter for antenatal screening for isoimmunization

Chapter 21. Factors Influencing Health Status and Contact With Health Services

Z36.8 Encounter for other antenatal screening
- **Z36.81** Encounter for antenatal screening for **hydrops fetalis**
  - **DEF:** Hydrops fetalis: Abnormal accumulation of fluid in two or more parts of the fetus, such as ascites, effusion of the pleural or pericardial tissues, or edema.
- **Z36.82** Encounter for antenatal screening for **nuchal translucency**
- **Z36.83** Encounter for fetal screening for **congenital cardiac abnormalities**
- **Z36.84** Encounter for antenatal screening for **fetal lung maturity**
- **Z36.85** Encounter for antenatal screening for **Streptococcus B**
- **Z36.86** Encounter for antenatal screening for **cervical length**
  - Screening for risk of pre-term labor
- **Z36.87** Encounter for antenatal screening for **uncertain dates**
- **Z36.88** Encounter for antenatal screening for **fetal macrosomia**
  - Screening for large-for-dates
- **Z36.89** Encounter for other specified antenatal screening
- **Z36.8A** Encounter for antenatal screening for other genetic defects

Z36.9 Encounter for antenatal screening, unspecified

Z3A Weeks of gestation

NOTE Codes from category Z3A are for use, only on the maternal record, to indicate the weeks of gestation of the pregnancy, if known.

Code first obstetric condition or encounter for delivery ▶(O09-O60, O80-O82, O94-O9A)◀

AHA: 2022,2Q,3; 2019,2Q,11; 2016,2Q,34; 2014,3Q,17; 2014,2Q,9; 2013,2Q,33

TIP: Do not assign a code from this category with codes from categories O00-O08 or code Z33.2.

- **Z3A.0** Weeks of gestation of pregnancy, unspecified or less than 10 weeks
  - **Z3A.00** Weeks of gestation of pregnancy not specified
  - **Z3A.01** Less than 8 weeks gestation of pregnancy
  - **Z3A.08** 8 weeks gestation of pregnancy
  - **Z3A.09** 9 weeks gestation of pregnancy
- **Z3A.1** Weeks of gestation of pregnancy, weeks 10-19
  - **Z3A.10** 10 weeks gestation of pregnancy
  - **Z3A.11** 11 weeks gestation of pregnancy
  - **Z3A.12** 12 weeks gestation of pregnancy
  - **Z3A.13** 13 weeks gestation of pregnancy
  - **Z3A.14** 14 weeks gestation of pregnancy
  - **Z3A.15** 15 weeks gestation of pregnancy
  - **Z3A.16** 16 weeks gestation of pregnancy
  - **Z3A.17** 17 weeks gestation of pregnancy
  - **Z3A.18** 18 weeks gestation of pregnancy
  - **Z3A.19** 19 weeks gestation of pregnancy
- **Z3A.2** Weeks of gestation of pregnancy, weeks 20-29
  - **Z3A.20** 20 weeks gestation of pregnancy
  - **Z3A.21** 21 weeks gestation of pregnancy
  - **Z3A.22** 22 weeks gestation of pregnancy
  - **Z3A.23** 23 weeks gestation of pregnancy
  - **Z3A.24** 24 weeks gestation of pregnancy
  - **Z3A.25** 25 weeks gestation of pregnancy
  - **Z3A.26** 26 weeks gestation of pregnancy
  - **Z3A.27** 27 weeks gestation of pregnancy
  - **Z3A.28** 28 weeks gestation of pregnancy
  - **Z3A.29** 29 weeks gestation of pregnancy
- **Z3A.3** Weeks of gestation of pregnancy, weeks 30-39
  - **Z3A.30** 30 weeks gestation of pregnancy
  - **Z3A.31** 31 weeks gestation of pregnancy
  - **Z3A.32** 32 weeks gestation of pregnancy
  - **Z3A.33** 33 weeks gestation of pregnancy
  - **Z3A.34** 34 weeks gestation of pregnancy
  - **Z3A.35** 35 weeks gestation of pregnancy
  - **Z3A.36** 36 weeks gestation of pregnancy
  - **Z3A.37** 37 weeks gestation of pregnancy
  - **Z3A.38** 38 weeks gestation of pregnancy
  - **Z3A.39** 39 weeks gestation of pregnancy
- **Z3A.4** Weeks of gestation of pregnancy, weeks 40 or greater
  - **AHA:** 2014,4Q,23
  - **Z3A.40** 40 weeks gestation of pregnancy
  - **Z3A.41** 41 weeks gestation of pregnancy
  - **Z3A.42** 42 weeks gestation of pregnancy
  - **Z3A.49** Greater than 42 weeks gestation of pregnancy

Z37 Outcome of delivery

This category is intended for use as an additional code to identify the outcome of delivery on the mother's record. It is not for use on the newborn record.

EXCLUDES 1 stillbirth (P95)

- **Z37.0** Single live birth
  - **AHA:** 2024,3Q,9; 2016,2Q,34; 2014,2Q,9
- **Z37.1** Single stillbirth
- **Z37.2** Twins, both liveborn
- **Z37.3** Twins, one liveborn and one stillborn
- **Z37.4** Twins, both stillborn
- **Z37.5** Other multiple births, all liveborn
  - **Z37.50** Multiple births, unspecified, all liveborn
  - **Z37.51** Triplets, all liveborn
  - **Z37.52** Quadruplets, all liveborn
  - **Z37.53** Quintuplets, all liveborn
  - **Z37.54** Sextuplets, all liveborn
  - **Z37.59** Other multiple births, all liveborn
- **Z37.6** Other multiple births, some liveborn
  - **Z37.60** Multiple births, unspecified, some liveborn
  - **Z37.61** Triplets, some liveborn
  - **Z37.62** Quadruplets, some liveborn
  - **Z37.63** Quintuplets, some liveborn
  - **Z37.64** Sextuplets, some liveborn
  - **Z37.69** Other multiple births, some liveborn
- **Z37.7** Other multiple births, all stillborn
- **Z37.9** Outcome of delivery, unspecified
  - Multiple birth NOS
  - Single birth NOS

Z38 Liveborn infants according to place of birth and type of delivery

This category is for use as the principal code on the initial record of a newborn baby. It is to be used for the initial birth record only. It is not to be used on the mother's record.

AHA: 2020,2Q,13; 2017,2Q,5-7; 2016,3Q,18; 2015,2Q,15

TIP: For attending physician services, a code from this category can be reported as first listed every time the physician visits the newborn during the birth admission.

- **Z38.0** Single liveborn infant, born in hospital
  - Single liveborn infant, born in birthing center or other health care facility
  - **Z38.00** Single liveborn infant, delivered vaginally
  - **Z38.01** Single liveborn infant, delivered by cesarean
- **Z38.1** Single liveborn infant, born outside hospital
- **Z38.2** Single liveborn infant, unspecified as to place of birth
  - Single liveborn infant NOS
- **Z38.3** Twin liveborn infant, born in hospital
  - **Z38.30** Twin liveborn infant, delivered vaginally
  - **Z38.31** Twin liveborn infant, delivered by cesarean
- **Z38.4** Twin liveborn infant, born outside hospital
- **Z38.5** Twin liveborn infant, unspecified as to place of birth
- **Z38.6** Other multiple liveborn infant, born in hospital
  - **Z38.61** Triplet liveborn infant, delivered vaginally

- **Z38.62** Triplet liveborn infant, delivered by cesarean
- **Z38.63** Quadruplet liveborn infant, delivered vaginally
- **Z38.64** Quadruplet liveborn infant, delivered by cesarean
- **Z38.65** Quintuplet liveborn infant, delivered vaginally
- **Z38.66** Quintuplet liveborn infant, delivered by cesarean
- **Z38.68** Other multiple liveborn infant, delivered vaginally
- **Z38.69** Other multiple liveborn infant, delivered by cesarean
- **Z38.7** Other multiple liveborn infant, born outside hospital
- **Z38.8** Other multiple liveborn infant, unspecified as to place of birth

Z39 Encounter for maternal postpartum care and examination

- **Z39.0** Encounter for care and examination of mother immediately after delivery
  - Care and observation in uncomplicated cases when the delivery occurs outside a healthcare facility
  - EXCLUDES 1: care for postpartum complication - see Alphabetic Index
  - AHA: 2021,3Q,13
- **Z39.1** Encounter for care and examination of lactating mother
  - Encounter for supervision of lactation
  - EXCLUDES 1: disorders of lactation (O92.-)
- **Z39.2** Encounter for routine postpartum follow-up

Encounters for other specific health care (Z40-Z53)

Categories Z40-Z53 are intended for use to indicate a reason for care. They may be used for patients who have already been treated for a disease or injury, but who are receiving aftercare or prophylactic care, or care to consolidate the treatment, or to deal with a residual state.

EXCLUDES 2: follow-up examination for medical surveillance after treatment (Z08-Z09)

Z40 Encounter for prophylactic surgery

EXCLUDES 1: organ donations (Z52.-)
therapeutic organ removal - code to condition

DEF: Treatment measure intended to prevent or ward off a disease or condition.

- **Z40.0** Encounter for prophylactic surgery for risk factors related to malignant neoplasms
  - Admission for prophylactic organ removal
  - ▶Use additional code to identify risk factor, such as genetic susceptibility to malignant neoplasm (Z15.-)◀
  - AHA: 2017,4Q,28-29
  - **Z40.00** Encounter for prophylactic removal of unspecified organ
  - **Z40.01** Encounter for prophylactic removal of breast
  - **Z40.02** Encounter for prophylactic removal of ovary(s)
    - ~~Encounter for prophylactic removal of ovary(s) and fallopian tube(s)~~
  - **Z40.03** Encounter for prophylactic removal of fallopian tube(s)
  - **Z40.09** Encounter for prophylactic removal of other organ
- **Z40.8** Encounter for other prophylactic surgery
  - **Z40.81** Encounter for prophylactic surgery for removal of ovary(s) for persons without known genetic/familial risk factors
    - Encounter for prophylactic oophorectomy for persons without known genetic/familial risk factors
  - **Z40.82** Encounter for prophylactic surgery for removal of fallopian tube(s) for persons without known genetic/familial risk factors
    - Encounter for prophylactic salpingectomy for persons without known genetic/familial risk factors
    - Opportunistic salpingectomy
  - **Z40.89** Encounter for other prophylactic surgery
- **Z40.9** Encounter for prophylactic surgery, unspecified

Z41 Encounter for procedures for purposes other than remedying health state

- **Z41.1** Encounter for cosmetic surgery
  - Encounter for cosmetic breast implant
  - Encounter for cosmetic procedure
  - EXCLUDES 1: encounter for plastic and reconstructive surgery following medical procedure or healed injury (Z42.-)
  - encounter for post-mastectomy breast implantation (Z42.1)
- **Z41.2** Encounter for routine and ritual male circumcision
  - AHA: 2018,3Q,15
  - **TIP:** This code should only be reported when the circumcision is elective (unrelated to a specific diagnosis) and was not performed during the birth admission.
- **Z41.3** Encounter for ear piercing
- **Z41.8** Encounter for other procedures for purposes other than remedying health state
- **Z41.9** Encounter for procedure for purposes other than remedying health state, unspecified

Z42 Encounter for plastic and reconstructive surgery following medical procedure or healed injury

EXCLUDES 1: encounter for cosmetic plastic surgery (Z41.1)
encounter for plastic surgery for treatment of current injury - code to relevent injury

- **Z42.1** Encounter for breast reconstruction following mastectomy
  - EXCLUDES 1: deformity and disproportion of reconstructed breast (N65.1-)
- **Z42.8** Encounter for other plastic and reconstructive surgery following medical procedure or healed injury
  - AHA: 2017,1Q,42

Z43 Encounter for attention to artificial openings

INCLUDES: closure of artificial openings
passage of sounds or bougies through artificial openings
reforming artificial openings
removal of catheter from artificial openings
toilet or cleansing of artificial openings

EXCLUDES 1: complications of external stoma (J95.0-, K94.-, N99.5-)
EXCLUDES 2: fitting and adjustment of prosthetic and other devices (Z44-Z46)

AHA: 2019,2Q,33

- **Z43.0** Encounter for attention to tracheostomy
- **Z43.1** Encounter for attention to gastrostomy
  - EXCLUDES 2: artificial opening status only, without need for care (Z93.-)
- **Z43.2** Encounter for attention to ileostomy
- **Z43.3** Encounter for attention to colostomy
- **Z43.4** Encounter for attention to other artificial openings of digestive tract
- **Z43.5** Encounter for attention to cystostomy
- **Z43.6** Encounter for attention to other artificial openings of urinary tract
  - Encounter for attention to nephrostomy
  - Encounter for attention to ureterostomy
  - Encounter for attention to urethrostomy
- **Z43.7** Encounter for attention to artificial vagina
- **Z43.8** Encounter for attention to other artificial openings
- **Z43.9** Encounter for attention to unspecified artificial opening

Z44 Encounter for fitting and adjustment of external prosthetic device

INCLUDES: removal or replacement of external prosthetic device
EXCLUDES 1: malfunction or other complications of device - see Alphabetical Index
presence of prosthetic device (Z97.-)

- **Z44.0** Encounter for fitting and adjustment of artificial arm
  - **Z44.00** Encounter for fitting and adjustment of unspecified artificial arm
    - **Z44.001** Encounter for fitting and adjustment of unspecified right artificial arm
    - **Z44.002** Encounter for fitting and adjustment of unspecified left artificial arm
    - **Z44.009** Encounter for fitting and adjustment of unspecified artificial arm, unspecified arm

Z44.01 Encounter for fitting and adjustment of complete artificial arm
- **Z44.011** Encounter for fitting and adjustment of complete right artificial arm
- **Z44.012** Encounter for fitting and adjustment of complete left artificial arm
- **Z44.019** Encounter for fitting and adjustment of complete artificial arm, unspecified arm

Z44.02 Encounter for fitting and adjustment of partial artificial arm
- **Z44.021** Encounter for fitting and adjustment of partial artificial right arm
- **Z44.022** Encounter for fitting and adjustment of partial artificial left arm
- **Z44.029** Encounter for fitting and adjustment of partial artificial arm, unspecified arm

Z44.1 Encounter for fitting and adjustment of artificial leg
- **Z44.10** Encounter for fitting and adjustment of unspecified artificial leg
  - **Z44.101** Encounter for fitting and adjustment of unspecified right artificial leg
  - **Z44.102** Encounter for fitting and adjustment of unspecified left artificial leg
  - **Z44.109** Encounter for fitting and adjustment of unspecified artificial leg, unspecified leg
- **Z44.11** Encounter for fitting and adjustment of complete artificial leg
  - **Z44.111** Encounter for fitting and adjustment of complete right artificial leg
  - **Z44.112** Encounter for fitting and adjustment of complete left artificial leg
  - **Z44.119** Encounter for fitting and adjustment of complete artificial leg, unspecified leg
- **Z44.12** Encounter for fitting and adjustment of partial artificial leg
  - **Z44.121** Encounter for fitting and adjustment of partial artificial right leg
  - **Z44.122** Encounter for fitting and adjustment of partial artificial left leg
  - **Z44.129** Encounter for fitting and adjustment of partial artificial leg, unspecified leg

Z44.2 Encounter for fitting and adjustment of artificial eye
- EXCLUDES 1: mechanical complication of ocular prosthesis (T85.3)
- **Z44.20** Encounter for fitting and adjustment of artificial eye, unspecified
- **Z44.21** Encounter for fitting and adjustment of artificial right eye
- **Z44.22** Encounter for fitting and adjustment of artificial left eye

Z44.3 Encounter for fitting and adjustment of external breast prosthesis
- EXCLUDES 1: complications of breast implant (T85.4-)
  encounter for adjustment or removal of breast implant (Z45.81-)
  encounter for breast reconstruction following mastectomy (Z42.1)
  encounter for initial breast implant insertion for cosmetic breast augmentation (Z41.1)
- **Z44.30** Encounter for fitting and adjustment of external breast prosthesis, unspecified breast
- **Z44.31** Encounter for fitting and adjustment of external right breast prosthesis
- **Z44.32** Encounter for fitting and adjustment of external left breast prosthesis

Z44.8 Encounter for fitting and adjustment of other external prosthetic devices

Z44.9 Encounter for fitting and adjustment of unspecified external prosthetic device

Z45 Encounter for adjustment and management of implanted device
- INCLUDES: removal or replacement of implanted device
- EXCLUDES 1: malfunction or other complications of device - see Alphabetical Index
- EXCLUDES 2: encounter for fitting and adjustment of non-implanted device (Z46.-)

Z45.0 Encounter for adjustment and management of cardiac device
- **TIP:** Assign an additional code for the associated condition if that condition requires constant intervention from the device, as in cases of sick sinus syndrome. For conditions that do not require constant intervention from the device, as in cases of ventricular fibrillation, an additional code for the associated condition should be assigned only if the patient is experiencing the condition and the device is firing during the current admission.
- **Z45.01** Encounter for adjustment and management of cardiac pacemaker
  Encounter for adjustment and management of cardiac resynchronization therapy pacemaker (CRT-P)
  - EXCLUDES 1: encounter for adjustment and management of automatic implantable cardiac defibrillator with synchronous cardiac pacemaker (Z45.02)
  - **Z45.010** Encounter for checking and testing of cardiac pacemaker pulse generator [battery]
    Encounter for replacing cardiac pacemaker pulse generator [battery]
  - **Z45.018** Encounter for adjustment and management of other part of cardiac pacemaker
    - EXCLUDES 1: presence of other part of cardiac pacemaker (Z95.0)
    - EXCLUDES 2: presence of prosthetic and other devices (Z95.1-Z95.5, Z95.811-Z97)
- **Z45.02** Encounter for adjustment and management of automatic implantable cardiac defibrillator
  Encounter for adjustment and management of automatic implantable cardiac defibrillator with synchronous cardiac pacemaker
  Encounter for adjustment and management of cardiac resynchronization therapy defibrillator (CRT-D)
  - **AHA:** 2024,1Q,21-22
- **Z45.09** Encounter for adjustment and management of other cardiac device

Z45.1 Encounter for adjustment and management of infusion pump

Z45.2 Encounter for adjustment and management of vascular access device
  Encounter for adjustment and management of vascular catheters
  - EXCLUDES 1: encounter for adjustment and management of renal dialysis catheter (Z49.01)
  - **AHA:** 2020,2Q,21; 2018,3Q,20

Z45.3 Encounter for adjustment and management of implanted devices of the special senses
- **Z45.31** Encounter for adjustment and management of implanted visual substitution device
- **Z45.32** Encounter for adjustment and management of implanted hearing device
  - EXCLUDES 1: encounter for fitting and adjustment of hearing aid (Z46.1)
  - **Z45.320** Encounter for adjustment and management of bone conduction device
  - **Z45.321** Encounter for adjustment and management of cochlear device
  - **Z45.328** Encounter for adjustment and management of other implanted hearing device

Z45.4 Encounter for adjustment and management of implanted nervous system device
- **Z45.41** Encounter for adjustment and management of cerebrospinal fluid drainage device
  Encounter for adjustment and management of cerebral ventricular (communicating) shunt

Z45.42 **Encounter for adjustment and management of neurostimulator**
Encounter for adjustment and management of brain neurostimulator
Encounter for adjustment and management of gastric neurostimulator
Encounter for adjustment and management of peripheral nerve neurostimulator
Encounter for adjustment and management of sacral nerve neurostimulator
Encounter for adjustment and management of spinal cord neurostimulator
Encounter for adjustment and management of vagus nerve neurostimulator

Z45.49 **Encounter for adjustment and management of other implanted nervous system device**
AHA: 2014,3Q,19

✓5th **Z45.8** **Encounter for adjustment and management of other implanted devices**

✓6th **Z45.81** **Encounter for adjustment or removal of breast implant**
Encounter for elective implant exchange (different material) (different size)
Encounter for removal of tissue expander with or without synchronous insertion of permanent implant
EXCLUDES 1 complications of breast implant (T85.4-)
encounter for breast reconstruction following mastectomy (Z42.1)
encounter for initial breast implant insertion for cosmetic breast augmentation (Z41.1)

Z45.811 **Encounter for adjustment or removal of right breast implant**
Z45.812 **Encounter for adjustment or removal of left breast implant**
Z45.819 **Encounter for adjustment or removal of unspecified breast implant**

Z45.82 **Encounter for adjustment or removal of myringotomy device (stent) (tube)**

Z45.89 **Encounter for adjustment and management of other implanted devices**
AHA: 2014,4Q,26-28

Z45.9 **Encounter for adjustment and management of unspecified implanted device**

✓4th **Z46** **Encounter for fitting and adjustment of other devices**
INCLUDES removal or replacement of other device
EXCLUDES 1 malfunction or other complications of device - see Alphabetical Index
EXCLUDES 2 encounter for fitting and management of implanted devices (Z45.-)
issue of repeat prescription only (Z76.0)
presence of prosthetic and other devices (Z95-Z97)

Z46.0 **Encounter for fitting and adjustment of spectacles and contact lenses**

Z46.1 **Encounter for fitting and adjustment of hearing aid**
EXCLUDES 1 encounter for adjustment and management of implanted hearing device (Z45.32-)

Z46.2 **Encounter for fitting and adjustment of other devices related to nervous system and special senses**
EXCLUDES 2 encounter for adjustment and management of implanted nervous system device (Z45.4-)
encounter for adjustment and management of implanted visual substitution device (Z45.31)

Z46.3 **Encounter for fitting and adjustment of dental prosthetic device**
Encounter for fitting and adjustment of dentures

Z46.4 **Encounter for fitting and adjustment of orthodontic device**

✓5th **Z46.5** **Encounter for fitting and adjustment of other gastrointestinal appliance and device**
EXCLUDES 1 encounter for attention to artificial openings of digestive tract (Z43.1-Z43.4)

Z46.51 **Encounter for fitting and adjustment of gastric lap band**
Z46.59 **Encounter for fitting and adjustment of other gastrointestinal appliance and device**

Z46.6 **Encounter for fitting and adjustment of urinary device**
EXCLUDES 2 attention to artificial openings of urinary tract (Z43.5, Z43.6)

✓5th **Z46.8** **Encounter for fitting and adjustment of other specified devices**

Z46.81 **Encounter for fitting and adjustment of insulin pump**
Encounter for insulin pump instruction and training
Encounter for insulin pump titration

Z46.82 **Encounter for fitting and adjustment of non-vascular catheter**

Z46.89 **Encounter for fitting and adjustment of other specified devices**
Encounter for fitting and adjustment of wheelchair

Z46.9 **Encounter for fitting and adjustment of unspecified device**

✓4th **Z47** **Orthopedic aftercare**
EXCLUDES 1 aftercare for healing fracture - code to fracture with 7th character D

Z47.1 **Aftercare following joint replacement surgery**
Use additional code to identify the joint (Z96.6-)
AHA: 2020,1Q,23

Z47.2 **Encounter for removal of internal fixation device**
EXCLUDES 1 encounter for adjustment of internal fixation device for fracture treatment - code to fracture with appropriate 7th character
encounter for removal of external fixation device - code to fracture with 7th character D
infection or inflammatory reaction to internal fixation device (T84.6-)
mechanical complication of internal fixation device (T84.1-)

✓5th **Z47.3** **Aftercare following explantation of joint prosthesis**
Aftercare following explantation of joint prosthesis, staged procedure
Encounter for joint prosthesis insertion following prior explantation of joint prosthesis
AHA: 2020,1Q,23; 2015,1Q,16
TIP: For staged removal of elbow joint prosthesis, assign code Z47.1.

Z47.31 **Aftercare following explantation of shoulder joint prosthesis**
EXCLUDES 1 acquired absence of shoulder joint following prior explantation of shoulder joint prosthesis (Z89.23-)
shoulder joint prosthesis explantation status (Z89.23-)

Z47.32 **Aftercare following explantation of hip joint prosthesis**
EXCLUDES 1 acquired absence of hip joint following prior explantation of hip joint prosthesis (Z89.62-)
hip joint prosthesis explantation status (Z89.62-)

Z47.33 **Aftercare following explantation of knee joint prosthesis**
EXCLUDES 1 acquired absence of knee joint following prior explantation of knee prosthesis (Z89.52-)
knee joint prosthesis explantation status (Z89.52-)

✓5th **Z47.8** **Encounter for other orthopedic aftercare**

Z47.81 **Encounter for orthopedic aftercare following surgical amputation**
Use additional code to identify the limb amputated (Z89.-)

Z47.82 **Encounter for orthopedic aftercare following scoliosis surgery**

Z47.89 **Encounter for other orthopedic aftercare**
AHA: 2015,1Q,8

Chapter 21. Factors Influencing Health Status and Contact With Health Services

✓4th Z48 Encounter for other postprocedural aftercare
- EXCLUDES 1: encounter for aftercare following injury - code to Injury, by site, with appropriate 7th character for subsequent encounter
  encounter for follow-up examination after completed treatment (Z08-Z09)
- EXCLUDES 2: encounter for attention to artificial openings (Z43.-)
  encounter for fitting and adjustment of prosthetic and other devices (Z44-Z46)
- AHA: 2015,4Q,38; 2015,1Q,6-7

✓5th Z48.0 Encounter for attention to dressings, sutures and drains
- EXCLUDES 1: encounter for planned postprocedural wound closure (Z48.1)

- **Z48.00 Encounter for change or removal of nonsurgical wound dressing**
  - Encounter for change or removal of wound dressing NOS
- **Z48.01 Encounter for change or removal of surgical wound dressing**
  - AHA: 2019,2Q,33
- **Z48.02 Encounter for removal of sutures**
  - Encounter for removal of staples
- **Z48.03 Encounter for change or removal of drains**
  - AHA: 2019,2Q,33

Z48.1 Encounter for planned postprocedural wound closure
- EXCLUDES 1: encounter for attention to dressings and sutures (Z48.0-)

✓5th Z48.2 Encounter for aftercare following organ transplant
- **Z48.21 Encounter for aftercare following heart transplant** [HCC] [Rx] [ESR] [COM]
- **Z48.22 Encounter for aftercare following kidney transplant** [Rx] [COM]
- **Z48.23 Encounter for aftercare following liver transplant** [HCC] [Rx] [ESR] [COM]
- **Z48.24 Encounter for aftercare following lung transplant** [HCC] [Rx] [ESR] [COM]
- **✓6th Z48.28 Encounter for aftercare following multiple organ transplant**
  - **Z48.280 Encounter for aftercare following heart-lung transplant** [HCC] [Rx] [ESR] [COM]
  - **Z48.288 Encounter for aftercare following multiple organ transplant**
- **✓6th Z48.29 Encounter for aftercare following other organ transplant**
  - **Z48.290 Encounter for aftercare following bone marrow transplant** [HCC] [Rx] [ESR] [COM]
  - **Z48.298 Encounter for aftercare following other organ transplant**

Z48.3 Aftercare following surgery for neoplasm
- Use additional code to identify the neoplasm

✓5th Z48.8 Encounter for other specified postprocedural aftercare
- **✓6th Z48.81 Encounter for surgical aftercare following surgery on specified body systems**
  - These codes identify the body system requiring aftercare. They are for use in conjunction with other aftercare codes to fully explain the aftercare encounter. The condition treated should also be coded if still present.
  - EXCLUDES 1: aftercare for injury - code the injury with 7th character D
    aftercare following surgery for neoplasm (Z48.3)
  - EXCLUDES 2: aftercare following organ transplant (Z48.2-)
    orthopedic aftercare (Z47.-)
  - AHA: 2015,4Q,38
  - **Z48.810 Encounter for surgical aftercare following surgery on the sense organs**
  - **Z48.811 Encounter for surgical aftercare following surgery on the nervous system**
    - EXCLUDES 2: encounter for surgical aftercare following surgery on the sense organs (Z48.810)
  - **Z48.812 Encounter for surgical aftercare following surgery on the circulatory system**
    - AHA: 2012,4Q,96
  - **Z48.813 Encounter for surgical aftercare following surgery on the respiratory system**
    - AHA: 2019,2Q,33
  - **Z48.814 Encounter for surgical aftercare following surgery on the teeth or oral cavity**
  - **Z48.815 Encounter for surgical aftercare following surgery on the digestive system**
  - **Z48.816 Encounter for surgical aftercare following surgery on the genitourinary system**
    - EXCLUDES 1: encounter for aftercare following sterilization reversal (Z31.42)
  - **Z48.817 Encounter for surgical aftercare following surgery on the skin and subcutaneous tissue**
- **Z48.89 Encounter for other specified surgical aftercare**

✓4th Z49 Encounter for care involving renal dialysis
- Code also associated end stage renal disease (N18.6)

✓5th Z49.0 Preparatory care for renal dialysis
- Encounter for dialysis instruction and training
- **Z49.01 Encounter for fitting and adjustment of extracorporeal dialysis catheter** [Rx] [ESR]
  - Removal or replacement of renal dialysis catheter
  - Toilet or cleansing of renal dialysis catheter
- **Z49.02 Encounter for fitting and adjustment of peritoneal dialysis catheter** [Rx] [ESR]

✓5th Z49.3 Encounter for adequacy testing for dialysis
- **Z49.31 Encounter for adequacy testing for hemodialysis** [Rx] [ESR]
- **Z49.32 Encounter for adequacy testing for peritoneal dialysis** [Rx] [ESR]
  - Encounter for peritoneal equilibration test

✓4th Z51 Encounter for other aftercare and medical care
- Code also condition requiring care
- EXCLUDES 1: follow-up examination after treatment (Z08-Z09)

- **Z51.0 Encounter for antineoplastic radiation therapy** [PDx]
  - AHA: 2017,4Q,103
  - TIP: Do not assign when admission is for insertion/implantation of radioactive elements. Assign a code for the malignancy instead. Any complications related to the radioactive elements should be assigned as secondary diagnoses.

- **✓5th Z51.1 Encounter for antineoplastic chemotherapy and immunotherapy**
  - EXCLUDES 2: encounter for chemotherapy and immunotherapy for nonneoplastic condition - code to condition
  - **Z51.11 Encounter for antineoplastic chemotherapy** [PDx]
    - AHA: 2025,2Q,16; 2022,1Q,16; 2015,3Q,19
  - **Z51.12 Encounter for antineoplastic immunotherapy** [PDx]
    - AHA: 2024,1Q,24

- **Z51.5 Encounter for palliative care**
  - AHA: 2022,1Q,18; 2020,4Q,98; 2017,1Q,48

- **Z51.6 Encounter for desensitization to allergens**
  - AHA: 2025,2Q,16; 2016,4Q,77

- **✓5th Z51.8 Encounter for other specified aftercare**
  - EXCLUDES 1: holiday relief care (Z75.5)
  - **Z51.81 Encounter for therapeutic drug level monitoring**
    - Code also any long-term (current) drug therapy (Z79.-)
    - EXCLUDES 1: encounter for blood-drug test for administrative or medicolegal reasons (Z02.83)
    - DEF: Drug monitoring: Measurement of the level of a specific drug in the body or measurement of a specific function to assess effectiveness of a drug.
  - **Z51.89 Encounter for other specified aftercare**
    - AHA: 2012,4Q,95-97

- **Z51.A Encounter for sepsis aftercare**
  - AHA: 2024,4Q,34

✓4th Z52 Donors of organs and tissues
- INCLUDES: autologous and other living donors
- EXCLUDES 1: cadaveric donor - omit code
  examination of potential donor (Z00.5)
- AHA: 2012,4Q,99

✓5th Z52.0 Blood donor
- **✓6th Z52.00 Unspecified blood donor**
  - **Z52.000 Unspecified donor, whole blood** [PDx]
  - **Z52.001 Unspecified donor, stem cells** [PDx]
  - **Z52.008 Unspecified donor, other blood** [PDx]
- **✓6th Z52.01 Autologous blood donor**
  - **Z52.010 Autologous donor, whole blood** [PDx]
  - **Z52.011 Autologous donor, stem cells** [PDx]
  - **Z52.018 Autologous donor, other blood** [PDx]

Chapter 21. Factors Influencing Health Status and Contact With Health Services

Z52.09 Other blood donor
  Volunteer donor
  - **Z52.090** Other blood donor, whole blood [PDx]
  - **Z52.091** Other blood donor, stem cells [PDx]
  - **Z52.098** Other blood donor, other blood [PDx]

Z52.1 Skin donor
  - **Z52.10** Skin donor, unspecified [PDx]
  - **Z52.11** Skin donor, autologous [PDx]
  - **Z52.19** Skin donor, other [PDx]

Z52.2 Bone donor
  - **Z52.20** Bone donor, unspecified [PDx]
  - **Z52.21** Bone donor, autologous [PDx]
  - **Z52.29** Bone donor, other [PDx]

Z52.3 Bone marrow donor [PDx]

Z52.4 Kidney donor [PDx]

Z52.5 Cornea donor [PDx]

Z52.6 Liver donor [PDx]

Z52.8 Donor of other specified organs or tissues
  - **Z52.81** Egg (Oocyte) donor
    - **Z52.810** Egg (Oocyte) donor under age 35, anonymous recipient [PDx]
      Egg donor under age 35 NOS
    - **Z52.811** Egg (Oocyte) donor under age 35, designated recipient [PDx]
    - **Z52.812** Egg (Oocyte) donor age 35 and over, anonymous recipient [PDx]
      Egg donor age 35 and over NOS
    - **Z52.813** Egg (Oocyte) donor age 35 and over, designated recipient [PDx]
    - **Z52.819** Egg (Oocyte) donor, unspecified [PDx]
  - **Z52.89** Donor of other specified organs or tissues [PDx]

Z52.9 Donor of unspecified organ or tissue
  Donor NOS

Z53 Persons encountering health services for specific procedures and treatment, not carried out

Z53.0 Procedure and treatment not carried out because of contraindication
  - **Z53.01** Procedure and treatment not carried out due to patient smoking
  - **Z53.09** Procedure and treatment not carried out because of other contraindication

Z53.1 Procedure and treatment not carried out because of patient's decision for reasons of belief and group pressure

Z53.2 Procedure and treatment not carried out because of patient's decision for other and unspecified reasons
  - **Z53.20** Procedure and treatment not carried out because of patient's decision for unspecified reasons
  - **Z53.21** Procedure and treatment not carried out due to patient leaving prior to being seen by health care provider
  - **Z53.29** Procedure and treatment not carried out because of patient's decision for other reasons

Z53.3 Procedure converted to open procedure
  AHA: 2016,4Q,79
  - **Z53.31** Laparoscopic surgical procedure converted to open procedure [UPD]
  - **Z53.32** Thoracoscopic surgical procedure converted to open procedure [UPD]
  - **Z53.33** Arthroscopic surgical procedure converted to open procedure [UPD]
  - **Z53.39** Other specified procedure converted to open procedure [UPD]

Z53.8 Procedure and treatment not carried out for other reasons

Z53.9 Procedure and treatment not carried out, unspecified reason

Persons with potential health hazards related to socioeconomic and psychosocial circumstances (Z55-Z65)

AHA: 2021,4Q,34-37; 2019,4Q,66; 2018,4Q,58,73; 2018,1Q,18
DEF: Social determinants of health: Socioeconomic factors that can affect a person's health, including both environmental and societal conditions such as education and literacy, employment, health behaviors, housing, lack of adequate food or water, occupational exposure to risk factors, social support, transportation, and violence. Tracking social needs that impact patients allows providers to identify population health trends and to promote the personalized care that addresses the medical and social needs of individual patients. **Synonym(s):** SDOH.
TIP: Because codes in these categories represent social information rather than medical diagnoses, they can be assigned based on documentation by nonphysician clinicians involved in the care of these patients as well as self-reported documentation from the patient, as long as the information is approved and incorporated into the medical record by a clinician or provider.

Z55 Problems related to education and literacy
  EXCLUDES 1 disorders of psychological development (F80-F89)

Z55.0 Illiteracy and low-level literacy

Z55.1 Schooling unavailable and unattainable

Z55.2 Failed school examinations

Z55.3 Underachievement in school

Z55.4 Educational maladjustment and discord with teachers and classmates

Z55.5 Less than a high school diploma [UPD]
  No general equivalence degree (GED)

Z55.6 Problems related to health literacy [UPD]
  Difficulty understanding health related information
  Difficulty understanding medication instructions
  Problem completing medical forms
  AHA: 2023,1Q,6

Z55.8 Other problems related to education and literacy
  Problems related to inadequate teaching

Z55.9 Problems related to education and literacy, unspecified
  Academic problems NOS

Z56 Problems related to employment and unemployment
  EXCLUDES 2 occupational exposure to risk factors (Z57.-)
  problems related to housing and economic circumstances (Z59.-)

Z56.0 Unemployment, unspecified

Z56.1 Change of job

Z56.2 Threat of job loss

Z56.3 Stressful work schedule

Z56.4 Discord with boss and workmates

Z56.5 Uncongenial work environment
  Difficult conditions at work

Z56.6 Other physical and mental strain related to work
  ▶Workplace stress◀

Z56.8 Other problems related to employment
  - **Z56.81** Sexual harassment on the job
  - **Z56.82** Military deployment status
    Individual (civilian or military) currently deployed in theater or in support of military war, peacekeeping and humanitarian operations
  - **Z56.89** Other problems related to employment
    ▶Furloughed◀
    ▶Underemployed◀

Z56.9 Unspecified problems related to employment
  Occupational problems NOS

Z57 Occupational exposure to risk factors

Z57.0 Occupational exposure to noise

Z57.1 Occupational exposure to radiation

Z57.2 Occupational exposure to dust

Z57.3 Occupational exposure to other air contaminants
  - **Z57.31** Occupational exposure to environmental tobacco smoke
    EXCLUDES 2 exposure to environmental tobacco smoke (Z77.22)
  - **Z57.39** Occupational exposure to other air contaminants

Z57.4 Occupational exposure to toxic agents in agriculture
  Occupational exposure to solids, liquids, gases or vapors in agriculture

Z57.5 Occupational exposure to toxic agents in other industries
  Occupational exposure to solids, liquids, gases or vapors in other industries

Z57.6 Occupational exposure to extreme temperature

Z57.7 Occupational exposure to vibration

Z57.8 Occupational exposure to other risk factors
Z57.9 Occupational exposure to unspecified risk factor

Z58 Problems related to physical environment
EXCLUDES 2 occupational exposure (Z57.-)

Z58.6 Inadequate drinking-water supply
Lack of safe drinking water
EXCLUDES 2 deprivation of water (T73.1)

Z58.8 Other problems related to physical environment
AHA: 2023,1Q,6

- **Z58.81** Basic services unavailable in physical environment
  - Unable to obtain internet service, due to unavailability in geographic area
  - Unable to obtain telephone service, due to unavailability in geographic area
  - Unable to obtain utilities, due to inadequate physical environment
- **Z58.89** Other problems related to physical environment

Z59 Problems related to housing and economic circumstances
EXCLUDES 2 problems related to upbringing (Z62.-)

Z59.0 Homelessness
- **Z59.00** Homelessness unspecified
- **Z59.01** Sheltered homelessness
  - Doubled up
  - Living in a shelter such as: motel, scattered site housing, temporary or transitional living situation
- **Z59.02** Unsheltered homelessness
  - ▶Lives in a homeless encampment◀
  - Residing in place not meant for human habitation such as: abandoned buildings, cars, parks, sidewalk
  - Residing on the street

Z59.1 Inadequate housing
EXCLUDES 2 problems related to the natural and physical environment (Z77.1-)
AHA: 2023,1Q,6

- **Z59.10** Inadequate housing, unspecified
  - Inadequate housing NOS
- **Z59.11** Inadequate housing environmental temperature
  - Lack of air conditioning
  - Lack of heating
- **Z59.12** Inadequate housing utilities
  - Lack of electricity services
  - Lack of gas services
  - Lack of oil services
  - Lack of water services
  - **EXCLUDES 2**
    - basic services unavailable in physical environment (Z58.81)
    - ▶financial insecurity, difficulty paying for utilities (Z59.861)◀
    - lack of adequate food (Z59.4-)
    - other problems related to housing and economic circumstances (Z59.8-)
- **Z59.19** Other inadequate housing
  - Pest infestation
  - ▶Poor housing weatherization◀
  - Restriction of space
  - Technical defects in home preventing adequate care
  - Unsatisfactory surroundings

Z59.2 Discord with neighbors, lodgers and landlord
Z59.3 Problems related to living in residential institution
Boarding-school resident
EXCLUDES 1 institutional upbringing (Z62.22)

Z59.4 Lack of adequate food
EXCLUDES 2
- deprivation of food (T73.0)
- effects of hunger (T73.0)
- inappropriate diet or eating habits (Z72.4)
- malnutrition (E40-E46)

- **Z59.41** Food insecurity
- **Z59.48** Other specified lack of adequate food
  - Inadequate food
  - Lack of food

Z59.5 Extreme poverty
Z59.6 Low income

Z59.7 Insufficient social insurance and welfare support
Insufficient social and welfare insurance
AHA: 2024,4Q,34

- **Z59.71** Insufficient health insurance coverage
  - Inadequate social insurance
  - Insufficient social insurance
  - No health insurance coverage
- **Z59.72** Insufficient welfare support
  - Inadequate welfare support

Z59.8 Other problems related to housing and economic circumstances
AHA: 2022,4Q,52

- **Z59.81** Housing instability, housed
  - Foreclosure on home loan
  - Past due on rent or mortgage
  - Unwanted multiple moves in the last 12 months
  - **Z59.811** Housing instability, housed, with risk of homelessness
    - Imminent risk of homelessness
  - **Z59.812** Housing instability, housed, homelessness in past 12 months
  - **Z59.819** Housing instability, housed unspecified
    - **EXCLUDES 2**
      - extreme poverty (Z59.5)
      - financial insecurity ▶(Z59.86-)◀
      - low income (Z59.6)
      - material hardship due to limited financial resources, not elsewhere classified (Z59.87)

- **Z59.82** Transportation insecurity
  - Excessive transportation time
  - Inaccessible transportation
  - Inadequate transportation
  - Lack of transportation
  - Unaffordable transportation
  - Unreliable transportation
  - Unsafe transportation
  - **EXCLUDES 2** unavailability and inaccessibility of healthcare facilities (Z75.3)

- **Z59.86** Financial insecurity
  - ~~Bankruptcy~~
  - Burdensome debt
  - Economic strain
  - Financial strain
  - Money problems
  - Running out of money
  - Unable to make ends meet
  - **EXCLUDES 2**
    - extreme poverty (Z59.5)
    - low income (Z59.6)
    - material hardship, not elsewhere classified (Z59.87)
  - **Z59.861** Financial insecurity, difficulty paying for utilities
    - Difficulty paying for electricity
    - Difficulty paying for heat
    - Difficulty paying for oil
    - Difficulty paying water bill
    - Utility disconnect notice due to inability to pay
    - **EXCLUDES 2** inadequate housing utilities (Z59.12)
  - **Z59.868** Other specified financial insecurity
    - Bankruptcy
  - **Z59.869** Financial insecurity, unspecified

- **Z59.87** Material hardship due to limited financial resources, not elsewhere classified
  - ~~Unable to obtain adequate utilities due to limited financial resources~~
  - Material deprivation due to limited financial resources
  - Unable to obtain adequate childcare due to limited financial resources
  - Unable to obtain adequate clothing due to limited financial resources
  - Unable to obtain basic needs due to limited financial resources
  - **EXCLUDES 2**
    - extreme poverty (Z59.5)
    - financial insecurity, not elsewhere classified ▶(Z59.86-)◀
    - low income (Z59.6)

	Z59.89	**Other problems related to housing and economic circumstances** UPD
		Foreclosure on loan
		Isolated dwelling
		Problems with creditors
	Z59.9	**Problem related to housing and economic circumstances, unspecified**

✓4th **Z60 Problems related to social environment**

- **Z60.0 Problems of adjustment to life-cycle transitions**
  - Empty nest syndrome
  - Phase of life problem
  - Problem with adjustment to retirement [pension]
- **Z60.2 Problems related to living alone**
- **Z60.3 Acculturation difficulty**
  - Problem with migration
  - Problem with social transplantation
  - **DEF:** Problem adapting to a different culture or environment not based on any coexisting mental disorder.
- **Z60.4 Social exclusion and rejection**
  - Exclusion and rejection on the basis of personal characteristics, such as unusual physical appearance, illness or behavior.
  - Social isolation
  - EXCLUDES 1 target of adverse discrimination such as for racial or religious reasons (Z60.5)
- **Z60.5 Target of (perceived) adverse discrimination and persecution**
  - EXCLUDES 1 social exclusion and rejection (Z60.4)
- **Z60.8 Other problems related to social environment**
  - Inadequate social support
  - Lack of emotional support
- **Z60.9 Problem related to social environment, unspecified**

✓4th **Z62 Problems related to upbringing**

INCLUDES current and past negative life events in childhood
current and past problems of a child related to upbringing

EXCLUDES 2 maltreatment syndrome (T74.-)
problems related to housing and economic circumstances (Z59.-)

- **Z62.0 Inadequate parental supervision and control**
- **Z62.1 Parental overprotection**
- ✓5th **Z62.2 Upbringing away from parents**
  - EXCLUDES 1 problems with boarding school (Z59.3)
  - AHA: 2023,4Q,49
  - **Z62.21 Child in welfare custody** P
    - Child in foster care
    - Child in welfare guardianship
  - **Z62.22 Institutional upbringing**
    - Child living in group home
    - Child living in orphanage
    - Code also, if applicable, child in welfare custody (Z62.21)
  - **Z62.23 Child in custody of non-parental relative** UPD P
    - Child in care of non-parental family member
    - Child in custody of grandparent
    - Child in kinship care
    - Guardianship by non-parental relative
    - Code also, if applicable, child in welfare custody (Z62.21)
  - **Z62.24 Child in custody of non-relative guardian** UPD P
    - Code also, if applicable, child in welfare custody (Z62.21)
  - **Z62.29 Other upbringing away from parents**
- **Z62.3 Hostility towards and scapegoating of child** P
- **Z62.6 Inappropriate (excessive) parental pressure**

✓5th **Z62.8 Other specified problems related to upbringing**

Code also, if applicable:
- absence of family member (Z63.3-)
- disappearance and death of family member (Z63.4)
- disruption of family by separation and divorce (Z63.5)
- other specified problems related to primary support group (Z63.8)
- other stressful life events affecting family and household (Z63.7-)

- ✓6th **Z62.81 Personal history of abuse in childhood**
  - Personal history of abuse in adolescence
  - AHA: 2023,1Q,6
  - **Z62.810 Personal history of physical and sexual abuse in childhood**
    - EXCLUDES 1 current child physical abuse (T74.12, T76.12)
    - current child sexual abuse (T74.22, T76.22)
  - **Z62.811 Personal history of psychological abuse in childhood**
    - EXCLUDES 1 current child psychological abuse (T74.32, T76.32)
  - **Z62.812 Personal history of neglect in childhood**
    - EXCLUDES 1 current child neglect (T74.02, T76.02)
  - **Z62.813 Personal history of forced labor or sexual exploitation in childhood**
    - AHA: 2018,4Q,32,35
  - **Z62.814 Personal history of child financial abuse** UPD
    - EXCLUDES 1 current child financial abuse (T74.A2)
  - **Z62.815 Personal history of intimate partner abuse in childhood** UPD
    - EXCLUDES 2 adult and child abuse, neglect and other maltreatment, confirmed (T74.-)
  - **Z62.819 Personal history of unspecified abuse in childhood**
    - EXCLUDES 1 current child abuse NOS (T74.92, T76.92)
- ✓6th **Z62.82 Parent-child conflict**
  - AHA: 2023,4Q,49
  - **Z62.820 Parent-biological child conflict**
    - Parent-child problem NOS
  - **Z62.821 Parent-adopted child conflict**
  - **Z62.822 Parent-foster child conflict**
  - **Z62.823 Parent-step child conflict** UPD
- ✓6th **Z62.83 Non-parental relative or guardian-child conflict**
  - AHA: 2023,4Q,50
  - **Z62.831 Non-parental relative-child conflict** UPD
    - Grandparent-child conflict
    - Kinship-care child conflict
    - Non-parental relative legal guardian-child conflict
    - Other relative-child conflict
    - EXCLUDES 1 group home staff-child conflict (Z62.833)
  - **Z62.832 Non-relative guardian-child conflict** UPD
    - EXCLUDES 1 group home staff-child conflict (Z62.833)
  - **Z62.833 Group home staff-child conflict** UPD
- ✓6th **Z62.89 Other specified problems related to upbringing**
  - **Z62.890 Parent-child estrangement NEC**
  - **Z62.891 Sibling rivalry**
  - **Z62.892 Runaway [from current living environment]** UPD
    - Child leaving living situation without permission
    - AHA: 2023,4Q,50
  - **Z62.898 Other specified problems related to upbringing**
- **Z62.9 Problem related to upbringing, unspecified**

Z63 Other problems related to primary support group, including family circumstances

EXCLUDES 2: maltreatment syndrome (T74.-, T76)
parent-child problems (Z62.-)
problems related to negative life events in childhood (Z62.-)
problems related to upbringing (Z62.-)

- **Z63.0** Problems in relationship with **spouse or partner**
  Relationship distress with spouse or intimate partner
  EXCLUDES 1: counseling for spousal or partner abuse problems (Z69.1)
  counseling related to sexual attitude, behavior, and orientation (Z70.-)
- **Z63.1** Problems in relationship with **in-laws**
- **Z63.3** Absence of family member
  EXCLUDES 1: absence of family member due to disappearance and death (Z63.4)
  absence of family member due to separation and divorce (Z63.5)
  - **Z63.31** Absence of family member due to military deployment
    Individual or family affected by other family member being on military deployment
    EXCLUDES 1: family disruption due to return of family member from military deployment (Z63.71)
  - **Z63.32** Other absence of family member
- **Z63.4** Disappearance and death of family member
  Assumed death of family member
  Bereavement
  AHA: 2014,1Q,25
- **Z63.5** Disruption of family by separation and divorce
  Marital estrangement
- **Z63.6** Dependent relative needing care at home
- **Z63.7** Other stressful life events affecting family and household
  - **Z63.71** Stress on family due to return of family member from military deployment
    Individual or family affected by family member having returned from military deployment (current or past conflict)
  - **Z63.72** Alcoholism and drug addiction in family
  - **Z63.79** Other stressful life events affecting family and household
    Anxiety (normal) about sick person in family
    Health problems within family
    Ill or disturbed family member
    Isolated family
- **Z63.8** Other specified problems related to primary support group
  Family discord NOS
  Family estrangement NOS
  High expressed emotional level within family
  Inadequate family support NOS
  Inadequate or distorted communication within family
- **Z63.9** Problem related to primary support group, unspecified
  Relationship disorder NOS

Z64 Problems related to certain psychosocial circumstances

- **Z64.0** Problems related to unwanted pregnancy
- **Z64.1** Problems related to multiparity
- **Z64.4** Discord with counselors
  Discord with probation officer
  Discord with social worker

Z65 Problems related to other psychosocial circumstances

- **Z65.0** Conviction in civil and criminal proceedings without imprisonment
- **Z65.1** Imprisonment and other incarceration
- **Z65.2** Problems related to release from prison
- **Z65.3** Problems related to other legal circumstances
  Arrest
  Child custody or support proceedings
  Litigation
  Prosecution
- **Z65.4** Victim of crime and terrorism
  Victim of torture
- **Z65.5** Exposure to disaster, war and other hostilities
  EXCLUDES 1: target of perceived discrimination or persecution (Z60.5)
- **Z65.8** Other specified problems related to psychosocial circumstances
  At risk for feeling loneliness
  Religious or spiritual problem
- **Z65.9** Problem related to unspecified psychosocial circumstances

Do not resuscitate status (Z66)

- **Z66** Do not resuscitate
  DNR status
  DEF: Medical order written by a physician that instructs others not to perform cardiopulmonary resuscitation (CPR), intubation, or advanced cardiac life support (ACLS). It prevents unnecessary invasive treatment to prolong life should breathing stop or cardiac arrest occur.

Blood type (Z67)

- **Z67** Blood type
  AHA: 2015,3Q,40
  - **Z67.1** Type A blood
    - **Z67.10** Type A blood, Rh positive
    - **Z67.11** Type A blood, Rh negative
  - **Z67.2** Type B blood
    - **Z67.20** Type B blood, Rh positive
    - **Z67.21** Type B blood, Rh negative
  - **Z67.3** Type AB blood
    - **Z67.30** Type AB blood, Rh positive
    - **Z67.31** Type AB blood, Rh negative
  - **Z67.4** Type O blood
    - **Z67.40** Type O blood, Rh positive
    - **Z67.41** Type O blood, Rh negative
  - **Z67.9** Unspecified blood type
    - **Z67.90** Unspecified blood type, Rh positive
    - **Z67.91** Unspecified blood type, Rh negative
  - **Z67.A** Duffy phenotype
    AHA: 2024,4Q,32
    - **Z67.A1** Duffy null
      Duffy phenotype Fy(a-b-)
    - **Z67.A2** Duffy a positive
      Duffy phenotype Fy(a+b-)
    - **Z67.A3** Duffy b positive
      Duffy phenotype Fy(a-b+)
    - **Z67.A4** Duffy a and b positive
      Duffy phenotype Fy(a+b+)

Body mass index [BMI] (Z68)

- **Z68** Body mass index [BMI]
  Kilograms per meters squared
  NOTE: BMI adult codes are for use for persons 20 years of age or older
  BMI pediatric codes are for use for persons 2-19 years of age. These percentiles are based on the growth charts published by the Centers for Disease Control and Prevention (CDC)
  AHA: 2022,3Q,6; 2019,4Q,19,57; 2018,4Q,73,77-83; 2017,1Q,39
  DEF: Index used to help determine whether an individual is underweight, a healthy weight, overweight, or obese.
  TIP: A BMI code may be assigned based on medical record documentation from clinicians who are not the patient's provider. However, the BMI must be associated with a condition that meets the definition of a reportable diagnosis, per the ICD-10-CM Official Guidelines for Coding and Reporting, and that condition can only be reported when documented by the patient's provider.
  - **Z68.1** Body mass index [BMI] 19.9 or less, adult
    AHA: 2024,4Q,13
  - **Z68.2** Body mass index [BMI] 20-29, adult
    - **Z68.20** Body mass index [BMI] 20.0-20.9, adult
    - **Z68.21** Body mass index [BMI] 21.0-21.9, adult
    - **Z68.22** Body mass index [BMI] 22.0-22.9, adult
    - **Z68.23** Body mass index [BMI] 23.0-23.9, adult
    - **Z68.24** Body mass index [BMI] 24.0-24.9, adult
    - **Z68.25** Body mass index [BMI] 25.0-25.9, adult
    - **Z68.26** Body mass index [BMI] 26.0-26.9, adult
    - **Z68.27** Body mass index [BMI] 27.0-27.9, adult
    - **Z68.28** Body mass index [BMI] 28.0-28.9, adult
    - **Z68.29** Body mass index [BMI] 29.0-29.9, adult
  - **Z68.3** Body mass index [BMI] 30-39, adult
    - **Z68.30** Body mass index [BMI] 30.0-30.9, adult
    - **Z68.31** Body mass index [BMI] 31.0-31.9, adult
    - **Z68.32** Body mass index [BMI] 32.0-32.9, adult
    - **Z68.33** Body mass index [BMI] 33.0-33.9, adult

Chapter 21. Factors Influencing Health Status and Contact With Health Services

- **Z68.34** Body mass index [BMI] 34.0-34.9, adult [UPD] [A]
- **Z68.35** Body mass index [BMI] 35.0-35.9, adult [UPD] [A]
- **Z68.36** Body mass index [BMI] 36.0-36.9, adult [UPD] [A]
- **Z68.37** Body mass index [BMI] 37.0-37.9, adult [UPD] [A]
- **Z68.38** Body mass index [BMI] 38.0-38.9, adult [UPD] [A]
- **Z68.39** Body mass index [BMI] 39.0-39.9, adult [UPD] [A]

√5th **Z68.4** Body mass index [BMI] 40 or greater, adult
- **Z68.41** Body mass index [BMI] 40.0-44.9, adult [HCC] [ESR] [UPD] [A]
- **Z68.42** Body mass index [BMI] 45.0-49.9, adult [HCC] [ESR] [UPD] [A]
- **Z68.43** Body mass index [BMI] 50.0-59.9, adult [HCC] [ESR] [UPD] [A]
- **Z68.44** Body mass index [BMI] 60.0-69.9, adult [HCC] [ESR] [UPD] [A]
- **Z68.45** Body mass index [BMI] 70 or greater, adult [HCC] [ESR] [UPD] [A]

√5th **Z68.5** Body mass index [BMI] pediatric
  AHA: 2024,4Q,33; 2018,4Q,81-82
- **Z68.51** Body mass index [BMI] pediatric, less than 5th percentile for age [UPD]
- **Z68.52** Body mass index [BMI] pediatric, 5th percentile to less than 85th percentile for age [UPD]
- **Z68.53** Body mass index [BMI] pediatric, 85th percentile to less than 95th percentile for age [UPD]
- **Z68.54** Body mass index [BMI] pediatric, 95th percentile for age to less than 120% of the 95th percentile for age [UPD]
- **Z68.55** Body mass index [BMI] pediatric, 120% of the 95th percentile for age to less than 140% of the 95th percentile for age [UPD]
- **Z68.56** Body mass index [BMI] pediatric, greater than or equal to 140% of the 95th percentile for age [HCC] [ESR] [UPD]

Persons encountering health services in other circumstances (Z69-Z76)

√4th **Z69** Encounter for mental health services for victim and perpetrator of abuse
  INCLUDES counseling for victims and perpetrators of abuse

√5th **Z69.0** Encounter for mental health services for child abuse problems
  √6th **Z69.01** Encounter for mental health services for parental child abuse
    Z69.010 Encounter for mental health services for victim of parental child abuse [P]
      Encounter for mental health services for victim of child abuse by parent
      Encounter for mental health services for victim of child neglect by parent
      Encounter for mental health services for victim of child psychological abuse by parent
      Encounter for mental health services for victim of child sexual abuse by parent
    Z69.011 Encounter for mental health services for perpetrator of parental child abuse
      Encounter for mental health services for perpetrator of parental child neglect
      Encounter for mental health services for perpetrator of parental child psychological abuse
      Encounter for mental health services for perpetrator of parental child sexual abuse
      EXCLUDES 1 encounter for mental health services for non-parental child abuse (Z69.02-)

  √6th **Z69.02** Encounter for mental health services for non-parental child abuse
    Z69.020 Encounter for mental health services for victim of non-parental child abuse [P]
      Encounter for mental health services for victim of non-parental child neglect
      Encounter for mental health services for victim of non-parental child psychological abuse
      Encounter for mental health services for victim of non-parental child sexual abuse
    Z69.021 Encounter for mental health services for perpetrator of non-parental child abuse
      Encounter for mental health services for perpetrator of non-parental child neglect
      Encounter for mental health services for perpetrator of non-parental child psychological abuse
      Encounter for mental health services for perpetrator of non-parental child sexual abuse

√5th **Z69.1** Encounter for mental health services for spousal or partner abuse problems
  Z69.11 Encounter for mental health services for victim of spousal or partner abuse
    Encounter for mental health services for victim of spouse or partner neglect
    Encounter for mental health services for victim of spouse or partner psychological abuse
    Encounter for mental health services for victim of spouse or partner violence, physical
  Z69.12 Encounter for mental health services for perpetrator of spousal or partner abuse
    Encounter for mental health services for perpetrator of spouse or partner neglect
    Encounter for mental health services for perpetrator of spouse or partner psychological abuse
    Encounter for mental health services for perpetrator of spouse or partner violence, physical
    Encounter for mental health services for perpetrator of spouse or partner violence, sexual

√5th **Z69.8** Encounter for mental health services for victim or perpetrator of other abuse
  Z69.81 Encounter for mental health services for victim of other abuse
    Encounter for mental health services for victim of non-spousal adult abuse
    Encounter for mental health services for victim of spouse or partner violence, sexual
    Encounter for rape victim counseling
  Z69.82 Encounter for mental health services for perpetrator of other abuse
    Encounter for mental health services for perpetrator of non-spousal adult abuse

√4th **Z70** Counseling related to sexual attitude, behavior and orientation
  INCLUDES encounter for mental health services for sexual attitude, behavior and orientation
  EXCLUDES 2 contraceptive or procreative counseling (Z30-Z31)

- **Z70.0** Counseling related to sexual attitude
- **Z70.1** Counseling related to patient's sexual behavior and orientation
    Patient concerned regarding impotence
    Patient concerned regarding non-responsiveness
    Patient concerned regarding promiscuity
    Patient concerned regarding sexual orientation
- **Z70.2** Counseling related to sexual behavior and orientation of third party
    Advice sought regarding sexual behavior and orientation of child
    Advice sought regarding sexual behavior and orientation of partner
    Advice sought regarding sexual behavior and orientation of spouse
- **Z70.3** Counseling related to combined concerns regarding sexual attitude, behavior and orientation
- **Z70.8** Other sex counseling
    Encounter for sex education
- **Z70.9** Sex counseling, unspecified

Chapter 21. Factors Influencing Health Status and Contact With Health Services

✓4th Z71 Persons encountering health services for other counseling and medical advice, not elsewhere classified
EXCLUDES 2: contraceptive or procreation counseling (Z30-Z31)
sex counseling (Z70.-)

Z71.0 Person encountering health services to consult on behalf of another person
Person encountering health services to seek advice or treatment for non-attending third party
EXCLUDES 2: anxiety (normal) about sick person in family (Z63.7)
expectant (adoptive) parent(s) pre-birth pediatrician visit (Z76.81)

Z71.1 Person with feared health complaint in whom no diagnosis is made
"Worried well"
Person encountering health services in which problem was normal state
Person encountering health services with feared condition which was not demonstrated
EXCLUDES 1: medical observation for suspected diseases and conditions proven not to exist (Z03.-)

Z71.2 Person consulting for explanation of examination or test findings

Z71.3 Dietary counseling and surveillance
Use additional code for any associated underlying medical condition
Use additional code to identify body mass index (BMI), if known (Z68.-)

✓5th Z71.4 Alcohol abuse counseling and surveillance
Use additional code for alcohol abuse or dependence (F10.-)

Z71.41 Alcohol abuse counseling and surveillance of alcoholic

Z71.42 Counseling for family member of alcoholic
Counseling for significant other, partner, or friend of alcoholic

✓5th Z71.5 Drug abuse counseling and surveillance
Use additional code for drug abuse or dependence (F11-F16, F18-F19)

Z71.51 Drug abuse counseling and surveillance of drug abuser

Z71.52 Counseling for family member of drug abuser
Counseling for significant other, partner, or friend of drug abuser

Z71.6 Tobacco abuse counseling
Use additional code for nicotine dependence (F17.-)

Z71.7 Human immunodeficiency virus [HIV] counseling

✓5th Z71.8 Other specified counseling
EXCLUDES 2: counseling for contraception (Z30.0-)
AHA: 2017,4Q,27

Z71.81 Spiritual or religious counseling

Z71.82 Exercise counseling

Z71.83 Encounter for nonprocreative genetic counseling
EXCLUDES 1: counseling for procreative genetics (Z31.5)
counseling for procreative management (Z31.6)

Z71.84 Encounter for health counseling related to travel
Encounter for health risk and safety counseling for (international) travel
Code also, if applicable, encounter for immunization (Z23)
EXCLUDES 2: encounter for administrative examination (Z02.-)
encounter for other special examination without complaint, suspected or reported diagnosis (Z01.-)
AHA: 2019,4Q,20,57

Z71.85 Encounter for immunization safety counseling
Encounter for vaccine product safety counseling
Code also, if applicable, encounter for immunization (Z23)
Code also, if applicable, immunization not carried out (Z28.-)
EXCLUDES 1: encounter for health counseling related to travel (Z71.84)
AHA: 2021,4Q,34

Z71.87 Encounter for pediatric-to-adult transition counseling
Code also chronic condition, if applicable, such as:
autism spectrum disorder (F84.0)
congenital malformations of the circulatory system (Q20-Q28)
cystic fibrosis (E84-)
sickle-cell disorder (D57-)
AHA: 2022,4Q,51

Z71.88 Encounter for counseling for socioeconomic factors
AHA: 2022,4Q,51

Z71.89 Other specified counseling

Z71.9 Counseling, unspecified
Encounter for medical advice NOS

✓4th Z72 Problems related to lifestyle
EXCLUDES 2: problems related to life-management difficulty (Z73.-)
problems related to socioeconomic and psychosocial circumstances (Z55-Z65)

Z72.0 Tobacco use
Tobacco use NOS
EXCLUDES 1: history of tobacco dependence (Z87.891)
nicotine dependence (F17.2-)
tobacco dependence (F17.2-)
tobacco use during pregnancy (O99.33-)

Z72.3 Lack of physical exercise

Z72.4 Inappropriate diet and eating habits
EXCLUDES 1: behavioral eating disorders of infancy or childhood (F98.2-F98.3)
eating disorders (F50.-)
lack of adequate food (Z59.48)
malnutrition and other nutritional deficiencies (E40-E64)

✓5th Z72.5 High risk sexual behavior
Promiscuity
EXCLUDES 1: paraphilias (F65)

Z72.51 High risk heterosexual behavior

Z72.52 High risk homosexual behavior

Z72.53 High risk bisexual behavior

Z72.6 Gambling and betting
EXCLUDES 1: compulsive or pathological gambling (F63.0)

✓5th Z72.8 Other problems related to lifestyle

✓6th Z72.81 Antisocial behavior
EXCLUDES 1: conduct disorders (F91.-)

Z72.810 Child and adolescent antisocial behavior
Antisocial behavior (child) (adolescent) without manifest psychiatric disorder
Delinquency NOS
Group delinquency
Offenses in the context of gang membership
Stealing in company with others
Truancy from school

Z72.811 Adult antisocial behavior
Adult antisocial behavior without manifest psychiatric disorder

✓6th Z72.82 Problems related to sleep

Z72.820 Sleep deprivation
Lack of adequate sleep
EXCLUDES 1: insomnia (G47.0-)

Z72.821 Inadequate sleep hygiene
Bad sleep habits
Irregular sleep habits
Unhealthy sleep wake schedule
EXCLUDES 1: insomnia (F51.0-, G47.0-)

Z72.823 Risk of suffocation (smothering) under another while sleeping
Child-caregiver co-sleeping
Infant bed-sharing
AHA: 2022,4Q,51

Z72.89 Other problems related to lifestyle
Self-damaging behavior

Z72.9 Problem related to lifestyle, unspecified

✓4th Z73 Problems related to life management difficulty
EXCLUDES 2: problems related to socioeconomic and psychosocial circumstances (Z55-Z65)
DEF: State of emotional, mental, and physical exhaustion causing difficulties in managing personal, school, or work circumstances. It is usually due to prolonged stress or poor interpersonal relationship skills or parenting skills.

Z73.0 Burn-out

Chapter 21. Factors Influencing Health Status and Contact With Health Services

- **Z73.1** Type A behavior pattern
- **Z73.2** Lack of relaxation and leisure
- **Z73.3** Stress, not elsewhere classified
  - Physical and mental strain NOS
  - EXCLUDES 1: stress related to employment or unemployment (Z56.-)
- **Z73.4** Inadequate social skills, not elsewhere classified
- **Z73.5** Social role conflict, not elsewhere classified
- **Z73.6** Limitation of activities due to disability
  - EXCLUDES 1: care-provider dependency (Z74.-)
- **Z73.8** Other problems related to life management difficulty
  - **Z73.81** Behavioral insomnia of childhood
    - DEF: Behaviors on the part of the child or caregivers that cause negative compliance with a child's sleep schedule resulting in lack of adequate sleep.
    - **Z73.810** Behavioral insomnia of childhood, sleep-onset association type
    - **Z73.811** Behavioral insomnia of childhood, limit setting type
    - **Z73.812** Behavioral insomnia of childhood, combined type
    - **Z73.819** Behavioral insomnia of childhood, unspecified type
  - **Z73.82** Dual sensory impairment
  - **Z73.89** Other problems related to life management difficulty
- **Z73.9** Problem related to life management difficulty, unspecified
- **Z74** Problems related to care provider dependency
  - EXCLUDES 2: dependence on enabling machines or devices NEC (Z99.-)
  - **Z74.0** Reduced mobility
    - **Z74.01** Bed confinement status
      - Bedridden
    - **Z74.09** Other reduced mobility
      - Chair ridden
      - Reduced mobility NOS
      - EXCLUDES 2: wheelchair dependence (Z99.3)
  - **Z74.1** Need for assistance with personal care
  - **Z74.2** Need for assistance at home and no other household member able to render care
  - **Z74.3** Need for continuous supervision
  - **Z74.8** Other problems related to care provider dependency
  - **Z74.9** Problem related to care provider dependency, unspecified
- **Z75** Problems related to medical facilities and other health care
  - **Z75.0** Medical services not available in home
    - EXCLUDES 1: no other household member able to render care (Z74.2)
  - **Z75.1** Person awaiting admission to adequate facility elsewhere
  - **Z75.2** Other waiting period for investigation and treatment
  - **Z75.3** Unavailability and inaccessibility of health-care facilities
    - EXCLUDES 1: bed unavailable (Z75.1)
  - **Z75.4** Unavailability and inaccessibility of other helping agencies
  - **Z75.5** Holiday relief care
  - **Z75.8** Other problems related to medical facilities and other health care
  - **Z75.9** Unspecified problem related to medical facilities and other health care
- **Z76** Persons encountering health services in other circumstances
  - **Z76.0** Encounter for issue of repeat prescription
    - Encounter for issue of repeat prescription for appliance
    - Encounter for issue of repeat prescription for medicaments
    - Encounter for issue of repeat prescription for spectacles
    - EXCLUDES 2: issue of medical certificate (Z02.7)
    - repeat prescription for contraceptive (Z30.4-)
  - **Z76.1** Encounter for health supervision and care of foundling
  - **Z76.2** Encounter for health supervision and care of other healthy infant and child
    - Encounter for medical or nursing care or supervision of healthy infant under circumstances such as adverse socioeconomic conditions at home
    - Encounter for medical or nursing care or supervision of healthy infant under circumstances such as awaiting foster or adoptive placement
    - Encounter for medical or nursing care or supervision of healthy infant under circumstances such as maternal illness
    - Encounter for medical or nursing care or supervision of healthy infant under circumstances such as number of children at home preventing or interfering with normal care
  - **Z76.3** Healthy person accompanying sick person
  - **Z76.4** Other boarder to healthcare facility
    - EXCLUDES 1: homelessness (Z59.0-)
  - **Z76.5** Malingerer [conscious simulation]
    - Person feigning illness (with obvious motivation)
    - EXCLUDES 1: factitious disorder (F68.1-, F68.A)
    - peregrinating patient (F68.1-)
    - DEF: Act of intentionally exaggerating an illness or disability in order to receive personal gain or to avoid punishment or responsibility.
  - **Z76.8** Persons encountering health services in other specified circumstances
    - **Z76.81** Expectant parent(s) prebirth pediatrician visit
      - Pre-adoption pediatrician visit for adoptive parent(s)
    - **Z76.82** Awaiting organ transplant status
      - Patient waiting for organ availability
    - **Z76.89** Persons encountering health services in other specified circumstances
      - Persons encountering health services NOS
      - AHA: 2014,2Q,10

Persons with potential health hazards related to family and personal history and certain conditions influencing health status (Z77-Z99)

Code also any follow-up examination (Z08-Z09)

- **Z77** Other contact with and (suspected) exposures hazardous to health
  - INCLUDES: contact with and (suspected) exposures to potential hazards to health
  - EXCLUDES 2: contact with and (suspected) exposure to communicable diseases (Z20.-)
    - exposure to (parental) (environmental) tobacco smoke in the perinatal period (P96.81)
    - newborn affected by noxious substances transmitted via placenta or breast milk (P04.-)
    - occupational exposure to risk factors (Z57.-)
    - retained foreign body (Z18.-)
    - retained foreign body fully removed (Z87.821)
    - toxic effects of substances chiefly nonmedicinal as to source (T51-T65)
  - **Z77.0** Contact with and (suspected) exposure to hazardous, chiefly nonmedicinal, chemicals
    - **Z77.01** Contact with and (suspected) exposure to hazardous metals
      - **Z77.010** Contact with and (suspected) exposure to arsenic
      - **Z77.011** Contact with and (suspected) exposure to lead
      - **Z77.012** Contact with and (suspected) exposure to uranium
        - EXCLUDES 1: retained depleted uranium fragments (Z18.01)
      - **Z77.018** Contact with and (suspected) exposure to other hazardous metals
        - Contact with and (suspected) exposure to chromium compounds
        - Contact with and (suspected) exposure to nickel dust
    - **Z77.02** Contact with and (suspected) exposure to hazardous aromatic compounds
      - **Z77.020** Contact with and (suspected) exposure to aromatic amines
      - **Z77.021** Contact with and (suspected) exposure to benzene
      - **Z77.028** Contact with and (suspected) exposure to other hazardous aromatic compounds
        - Aromatic dyes NOS
        - Polycyclic aromatic hydrocarbons
    - **Z77.09** Contact with and (suspected) exposure to other hazardous, chiefly nonmedicinal, chemicals
      - **Z77.090** Contact with and (suspected) exposure to asbestos
      - **Z77.098** Contact with and (suspected) exposure to other hazardous, chiefly nonmedicinal, chemicals
        - Dyes NOS
  - **Z77.1** Contact with and (suspected) exposure to environmental pollution and hazards in the physical environment
    - **Z77.11** Contact with and (suspected) exposure to environmental pollution
      - **Z77.110** Contact with and (suspected) exposure to air pollution
      - **Z77.111** Contact with and (suspected) exposure to water pollution

Chapter 21. Factors Influencing Health Status and Contact With Health Services

- **Z77.112** Contact with and (suspected) exposure to **soil** pollution
- **Z77.118** Contact with and (suspected) exposure to other environmental pollution
- ✓6th **Z77.12** Contact with and (suspected) exposure to **hazards in the physical environment**
  - **Z77.120** Contact with and (suspected) exposure to **mold** (toxic)
  - **Z77.121** Contact with and (suspected) exposure to **harmful algae and algae toxins**
    - Contact with and (suspected) exposure to (harmful) algae bloom NOS
    - Contact with and (suspected) exposure to blue-green algae bloom
    - Contact with and (suspected) exposure to brown tide
    - Contact with and (suspected) exposure to cyanobacteria bloom
    - Contact with and (suspected) exposure to Florida red tide
    - Contact with and (suspected) exposure to pfiesteria piscicida
    - Contact with and (suspected) exposure to red tide
  - **Z77.122** Contact with and (suspected) exposure to **noise**
  - **Z77.123** Contact with and (suspected) exposure to **radon and other naturally occurring radiation**
    - EXCLUDES 2: radiation exposure as the cause of a confirmed condition (W88-W90, X39.0-)
    - radiation sickness NOS (T66)
  - **Z77.128** Contact with and (suspected) exposure to other hazards in the physical environment
- ✓5th **Z77.2** Contact with and (suspected) exposure to other hazardous substances
  - **Z77.21** Contact with and (suspected) exposure to potentially hazardous **body fluids**
  - **Z77.22** Contact with and (suspected) exposure to **environmental tobacco smoke** (acute) (chronic)
    - Exposure to second hand tobacco smoke (acute) (chronic)
    - Passive smoking (acute) (chronic)
    - EXCLUDES 1: nicotine dependence (F17.-)
    - tobacco use (Z72.0)
    - EXCLUDES 2: occupational exposure to environmental tobacco smoke (Z57.31)
  - **Z77.29** Contact with and (suspected) exposure to other hazardous substances
    - AHA: 2016,2Q,33
- ● ✓5th **Z77.3** Contact with and (suspected) exposure to **war theater**
  - ● **Z77.31** Contact with and (suspected) exposure to **Gulf War theater**
    - Contact with and (suspected) exposure to Persian Gulf War theater
  - ● **Z77.39** Contact with and (suspected) exposure to other war theater
    - Agent Orange exposure
- **Z77.9** Other contact with and (suspected) exposures hazardous to health
- ✓4th **Z78** Other specified health status
  - EXCLUDES 2: asymptomatic human immunodeficiency virus [HIV] infection status (Z21)
  - postprocedural status (Z93-Z99)
  - sex reassignment status (Z87.890)
  - **Z78.0** Asymptomatic menopausal state [A]
    - Menopausal state NOS
    - Postmenopausal status NOS
    - EXCLUDES 2: symptomatic menopausal state (N95.1)
  - **Z78.1** Physical restraint status
    - EXCLUDES 1: physical restraint due to a procedure - omit code
    - DEF: Application of mechanical restraining devices or manual restraints to limit physical mobility of a patient.
  - **Z78.9** Other specified health status

- ✓4th **Z79** Long term (current) drug therapy
  - INCLUDES: long term (current) drug use for prophylactic purposes
  - Code also any therapeutic drug level monitoring (Z51.81)
  - EXCLUDES 2: drug abuse and dependence (F11-F19)
    - drug use complicating pregnancy, childbirth, and the puerperium (O99.32-)
  - AHA: 2024,2Q,26; 2021,1Q,12
- ✓5th **Z79.0** Long term (current) use of anticoagulants and antithrombotics/antiplatelets
  - EXCLUDES 2: long term (current) use of aspirin (Z79.82)
  - **Z79.01** Long term (current) use of **anticoagulants**
    - AHA: 2023,2Q,28; 2022,2Q,17; 2021,1Q,4; 2020,2Q,20
  - **Z79.02** Long term (current) use of **antithrombotics/antiplatelets** UPD
- **Z79.1** Long term (current) use of **non-steroidal anti-inflammatories (NSAID)** UPD
  - EXCLUDES 2: long term (current) use of aspirin (Z79.82)
- **Z79.2** Long term (current) use of **antibiotics** UPD
- **Z79.3** Long term (current) use of **hormonal contraceptives**
  - Long term (current) use of birth control pill or patch
- **Z79.4** Long term (current) use of **insulin** HCC Rx ESR COM
  - EXCLUDES 2: long-term (current) use of injectable non-insulin antidiabetic drugs (Z79.85)
    - long term (current) use of oral antidiabetic drugs (Z79.84)
    - long term (current) use of oral hypoglycemic drugs (Z79.84)
  - AHA: 2020,3Q,31
- ✓5th **Z79.5** Long term (current) use of steroids
  - **Z79.51** Long term (current) use of **inhaled steroids** UPD
  - **Z79.52** Long term (current) use of **systemic steroids** UPD
    - AHA: 2024,3Q,14
- ✓5th **Z79.6** Long term (current) use of **immunomodulators and immunosuppressants**
  - EXCLUDES 2: long term (current) use of steroids (Z79.5-)
    - long term (current) use of agents affecting estrogen receptors and estrogen levels (Z79.81-)
  - AHA: 2022,4Q,50
  - **Z79.60** Long term (current) use of unspecified immunomodulators and immunosuppressants UPD
  - **Z79.61** Long term (current) use of **immunomodulator** UPD
    - Long term (current) use of apremilast
    - Long term (current) use of immunomodulatory imide drug
    - Long term (current) use of lenalidomide
    - Long term (current) use of pomalidomide
  - ✓6th **Z79.62** Long term (current) use of **immunosuppressant**
    - **Z79.620** Long term (current) use of **immunosuppressive biologic** UPD
      - Long term (current) use of adalimumab
      - Long term (current) use of etanercept
      - Long term (current) use of infliximab
      - Long term (current) use of monoclonal antibodies
    - **Z79.621** Long term (current) use of **calcineurin inhibitor** UPD
      - Long term (current) use of cyclosporine
      - Long term (current) use of tacrolimus
    - **Z79.622** Long term (current) use of **Janus kinase inhibitor** UPD
      - Long term (current) use of tofacitinib
    - **Z79.623** Long term (current) use of **mammalian target of rapamycin (mTOR) inhibitor** UPD
      - Long term (current) use of sirolimus
    - **Z79.624** Long term (current) use of **inhibitors of nucleotide synthesis** UPD
      - Long term (current) use of azathioprine
      - Long term (current) use of mycophenolate
      - Long term (current) use of purine synthesis (IMDH) inhibitors

HCC CMS-HCC | Rx Rx HCC | ESR ESRD HCC | COM Commercial HCC | PDx Primary Dx Only | N Newborn: 0 | P Pediatric: 0-17 | M Maternity: 9-64 | A Adult: 15-124

Chapter 21. Factors Influencing Health Status and Contact With Health Services

Z79.63 **Long term (current) use of chemotherapeutic agent**
- **Z79.630** **Long term (current) use of alkylating agent** `UPD`
  - Long term (current) use of chlorambucil
  - Long term (current) use of cisplatin
  - Long term (current) use of cyclophosphamide
- **Z79.631** **Long term (current) use of antimetabolite agent** `UPD`
  - Long term (current) use of 5-fluorouracil
  - Long term (current) use of 6-mercaptopurine
  - Long term (current) use of cytarabine
  - Long term (current) use of methotrexate
- **Z79.632** **Long term (current) use of antitumor antibiotic** `UPD`
  - Long term (current) use of bleomycin
  - Long term (current) use of doxorubicin
  - Long term (current) use of mitomycin C
- **Z79.633** **Long term (current) use of mitotic inhibitor** `UPD`
  - Long term (current) use of paclitaxel
  - Long term (current) use of plant alkaloids
  - Long term (current) use of vinblastine
  - Long term (current) use of vincristine
- **Z79.634** **Long term (current) use of topoisomerase inhibitor** `UPD`
  - Long term (current) use of etoposide
  - Long term (current) use of irinotecan
  - Long term (current) use of topotecan

Z79.64 **Long term (current) use of myelosuppressive agent** `UPD`
- Long term (current) use of hydroxyurea

Z79.69 **Long term (current) use of other immunomodulators and immunosuppressants** `UPD`

Z79.8 **Other long term (current) drug therapy**
- **Z79.81** **Long term (current) use of agents affecting estrogen receptors and estrogen levels**
  - Code first, if applicable:
    - malignant neoplasm of breast (C50.-)
    - malignant neoplasm of prostate (C61)
  - Use additional code, if applicable, to identify:
    - estrogen receptor positive status (Z17.0)
    - family history of breast cancer (Z80.3)
    - genetic susceptibility to malignant neoplasm (cancer) (Z15.0-)
    - personal history of breast cancer (Z85.3)
    - personal history of prostate cancer (Z85.46)
    - postmenopausal status (Z78.0)
  - EXCLUDES 1: hormone replacement therapy (Z79.890)
  - **AHA:** 2022,3Q,14
  - **Z79.810** **Long term (current) use of selective estrogen receptor modulators (SERMs)** `UPD`
    - Long term (current) use of toremifene (Fareston)
    - Long term (current) use of raloxifene (Evista)
    - Long term (current) use of tamoxifen (Nolvadex)
  - **Z79.811** **Long term (current) use of aromatase inhibitors** `UPD`
    - Long term (current) use of anastrozole (Arimidex)
    - Long term (current) use of exemestane (Aromasin)
    - Long term (current) use of letrozole (Femara)
  - **Z79.818** **Long term (current) use of other agents affecting estrogen receptors and estrogen levels** `UPD`
    - Long term (current) use of estrogen receptor downregulators
    - Long term (current) use of fulvestrant (Faslodex)
    - Long term (current) use of gonadotropin-releasing hormone (GnRH) agonist
    - Long term (current) use of goserelin acetate (Zoladex)
    - Long term (current) use of leuprolide acetate (leuprorelin) (Lupron)
    - Long term (current) use of megestrol acetate (Megace)

- **Z79.82** **Long term (current) use of aspirin**
- **Z79.83** **Long term (current) use of bisphosphonates** `UPD`
  - **AHA:** 2016,4Q,42
- **Z79.84** **Long term (current) use of oral hypoglycemic drugs** `UPD`
  - Long term (current) use of oral antidiabetic drugs
  - EXCLUDES 2: long-term (current) use of injectable non-insulin antidiabetic drugs (Z79.85)
  - long term (current) use of insulin (Z79.4)
  - **AHA:** 2020,3Q,31; 2016,4Q,76
- **Z79.85** **Long-term (current) use of injectable non-insulin antidiabetic drugs** `UPD`
  - EXCLUDES 2: long term (current) use of insulin (Z79.4)
  - long term (current) use of oral hypoglycemic drugs (Z79.84)
  - **AHA:** 2022,4Q,50
- **Z79.89** **Other long term (current) drug therapy**
  - **Z79.890** **Hormone replacement therapy** `UPD`
  - **Z79.891** **Long term (current) use of opiate analgesic**
    - Long term (current) use of methadone for pain management
    - EXCLUDES 1: methadone use NOS (F11.9-)
    - use of methadone for treatment of heroin addiction (F11.2-)
  - **Z79.899** **Other long term (current) drug therapy**
    - **AHA:** 2023,3Q,17-18; 2020,4Q,11; 2020,3Q,31; 2020,2Q,14; 2015,4Q,34; 2015,3Q,21

Z80 **Family history of primary malignant neoplasm**
- **Z80.0** **Family history of malignant neoplasm of digestive organs** `UPD`
  - Conditions classifiable to C15-C26
  - **AHA:** 2018,1Q,6
- **Z80.1** **Family history of malignant neoplasm of trachea, bronchus and lung** `UPD`
  - Conditions classifiable to C33-C34
- **Z80.2** **Family history of malignant neoplasm of other respiratory and intrathoracic organs** `UPD`
  - Conditions classifiable to C30-C32, C37-C39
- **Z80.3** **Family history of malignant neoplasm of breast** `UPD`
  - Conditions classifiable to C50.-
- **Z80.4** **Family history of malignant neoplasm of genital organs**
  - Conditions classifiable to C51-C63
  - **Z80.41** **Family history of malignant neoplasm of ovary** `UPD`
  - **Z80.42** **Family history of malignant neoplasm of prostate** `UPD`
  - **Z80.43** **Family history of malignant neoplasm of testis** `UPD`
  - **Z80.44** **Family history of malignant neoplasm of fallopian tube(s)**
  - **Z80.49** **Family history of malignant neoplasm of other genital organs** `UPD`
- **Z80.5** **Family history of malignant neoplasm of urinary tract**
  - Conditions classifiable to C64-C68
  - **Z80.51** **Family history of malignant neoplasm of kidney** `UPD`
  - **Z80.52** **Family history of malignant neoplasm of bladder** `UPD`
  - **Z80.59** **Family history of malignant neoplasm of other urinary tract organ** `UPD`

- **Z80.6** Family history of leukemia
  Conditions classifiable to C91-C95
- **Z80.7** Family history of other malignant neoplasms of lymphoid, hematopoietic and related tissues
  Conditions classifiable to C81-C90, C96.-
- **Z80.8** Family history of malignant neoplasm of other organs or systems
  Conditions classifiable to C00-C14, C40-C49, C69-C79
- **Z80.9** Family history of malignant neoplasm, unspecified
  Conditions classifiable to C80.1

Z81 Family history of mental and behavioral disorders

- **Z81.0** Family history of intellectual disabilities
  Conditions classifiable to F70-F79
- **Z81.1** Family history of alcohol abuse and dependence
  Conditions classifiable to F10.-
- **Z81.2** Family history of tobacco abuse and dependence
  Conditions classifiable to F17.-
- **Z81.3** Family history of other psychoactive substance abuse and dependence
  Conditions classifiable to F11-F16, F18-F19
- **Z81.4** Family history of other substance abuse and dependence
  Conditions classifiable to F55
- **Z81.8** Family history of other mental and behavioral disorders
  Conditions classifiable elsewhere in F01-F99

Z82 Family history of certain disabilities and chronic diseases (leading to disablement)

- **Z82.0** Family history of epilepsy and other diseases of the nervous system
  Conditions classifiable to G00-G99
- **Z82.1** Family history of blindness and visual loss
  Conditions classifiable to H54.-
- **Z82.2** Family history of deafness and hearing loss
  Conditions classifiable to H90-H91
- **Z82.3** Family history of stroke
  Conditions classifiable to I60-I64
- **Z82.4** Family history of ischemic heart disease and other diseases of the circulatory system
  Conditions classifiable to I00-I5A, I65-I99
  - **Z82.41** Family history of sudden cardiac death
  - **Z82.49** Family history of ischemic heart disease and other diseases of the circulatory system
- **Z82.5** Family history of asthma and other chronic lower respiratory diseases
  Conditions classifiable to J40-J47
  EXCLUDES 2 family history of other diseases of the respiratory system (Z83.6)
- **Z82.6** Family history of arthritis and other diseases of the musculoskeletal system and connective tissue
  Conditions classifiable to M00-M99
  - **Z82.61** Family history of arthritis
  - **Z82.62** Family history of osteoporosis
  - **Z82.69** Family history of other diseases of the musculoskeletal system and connective tissue
- **Z82.7** Family history of congenital malformations, deformations and chromosomal abnormalities
  Conditions classifiable to Q00-Q99
  - **Z82.71** Family history of polycystic kidney
  - **Z82.79** Family history of other congenital malformations, deformations and chromosomal abnormalities
- **Z82.8** Family history of other disabilities and chronic diseases leading to disablement, not elsewhere classified

Z83 Family history of other specific disorders

EXCLUDES 2 contact with and (suspected) exposure to communicable disease in the family (Z20.-)

- **Z83.0** Family history of human immunodeficiency virus [HIV] disease
  Conditions classifiable to B20
- **Z83.1** Family history of other infectious and parasitic diseases
  Conditions classifiable to A00-B19, B25-B94, B99
- **Z83.2** Family history of diseases of the blood and blood-forming organs and certain disorders involving the immune mechanism
  Conditions classifiable to D50-D89
- **Z83.3** Family history of diabetes mellitus
  Conditions classifiable to E08-E13
- **Z83.4** Family history of other endocrine, nutritional and metabolic diseases
  Conditions classifiable to E00-E07, E15-E88
  - **Z83.41** Family history of multiple endocrine neoplasia [MEN] syndrome
  - **Z83.42** Family history of familial hypercholesterolemia
    AHA: 2016,4Q,77
  - **Z83.43** Family history of other disorder of lipoprotein metabolism and other lipidemias
    AHA: 2018,4Q,6,35
    - **Z83.430** Family history of elevated lipoprotein(a)
      Family history of elevated Lp(a)
    - **Z83.438** Family history of other disorder of lipoprotein metabolism and other lipidemia
      Family history of familial combined hyperlipidemia
  - **Z83.49** Family history of other endocrine, nutritional and metabolic diseases
- **Z83.5** Family history of eye and ear disorders
  - **Z83.51** Family history of eye disorders
    Conditions classifiable to H00-H53, H55-H59
    EXCLUDES 2 family history of blindness and visual loss (Z82.1)
    - **Z83.511** Family history of glaucoma
    - **Z83.518** Family history of other specified eye disorder
  - **Z83.52** Family history of ear disorders
    Conditions classifiable to H60-H83, H92-H95
    EXCLUDES 2 family history of deafness and hearing loss (Z82.2)
- **Z83.6** Family history of other diseases of the respiratory system
  Conditions classifiable to J00-J39, J60-J99
  EXCLUDES 2 family history of asthma and other chronic lower respiratory diseases (Z82.5)
- **Z83.7** Family history of diseases of the digestive system
  Conditions classifiable to D12, K00-K93
  - **Z83.71** Family history of colonic polyps
    EXCLUDES 2 family history of malignant neoplasm of digestive organs (Z80.0)
    AHA: 2023,4Q,47-48; 2021,1Q,14
    - **Z83.710** Family history of adenomatous and serrated polyps
      Conditions classifiable to D12.-
      Family history of tubular adenoma polyps
      Family history of tubulovillous adenoma polyps
      Family history of villous adenoma polyps
    - **Z83.711** Family history of hyperplastic colon polyps
    - **Z83.718** Family history of other colon polyps
      Family history of inflammatory colon polyps
    - **Z83.719** Family history of colon polyps, unspecified
      Family history of colon polyps NOS
  - **Z83.72** Family history of familial adenomatous polyposis
    AHA: 2024,4Q,33
  - **Z83.79** Family history of other diseases of the digestive system

Z84 Family history of other conditions

- **Z84.0** Family history of diseases of the skin and subcutaneous tissue
  Conditions classifiable to L00-L99
- **Z84.1** Family history of disorders of kidney and ureter
  Conditions classifiable to N00-N29
  - **Z84.11** Family history of APOL1-mediated kidney disease [AMKD]
  - **Z84.19** Family history of other disorders of kidney and ureter
- **Z84.2** Family history of other diseases of the genitourinary system
  Conditions classifiable to N30-N99
- **Z84.3** Family history of consanguinity

Chapter 21. Factors Influencing Health Status and Contact With Health Services

√5th **Z84.8 Family history of other specified conditions**
- **Z84.81 Family history of carrier of genetic disease** UPD
  - AHA: 2021,1Q,14
- **Z84.82 Family history of sudden infant death syndrome** UPD
  - Family history of SIDS
  - AHA: 2016,4Q,77
- **Z84.89 Family history of other specified conditions** UPD
- **Z84.A Family history of exposure to diethylstilbestrol**
  - DES granddaughter or grandson
  - Family history of DES exposure
  - Third generation DES exposure

√4th **Z85 Personal history of malignant neoplasm**
  Code first any follow-up examination after treatment of malignant neoplasm (Z08)
  Use additional code to identify:
    alcohol use and dependence (F10.-)
    exposure to environmental tobacco smoke (Z77.22)
    history of tobacco dependence (Z87.891)
    occupational exposure to environmental tobacco smoke (Z57.31)
    tobacco dependence (F17.-)
    tobacco use (Z72.0)
  EXCLUDES 2 personal history of benign neoplasm (Z86.01-)
              personal history of carcinoma-in-situ (Z86.00-)
  AHA: 2022,3Q,28; 2020,3Q,30; 2018,4Q,64

√5th **Z85.0 Personal history of malignant neoplasm of digestive organs**
  AHA: 2017,1Q,9
  - **Z85.00 Personal history of malignant neoplasm of unspecified digestive organ**
  - **Z85.01 Personal history of malignant neoplasm of esophagus**
    Conditions classifiable to C15
  - √6th **Z85.02 Personal history of malignant neoplasm of stomach**
    - **Z85.020 Personal history of malignant carcinoid tumor of stomach**
      Conditions classifiable to C7A.092
    - **Z85.028 Personal history of other malignant neoplasm of stomach**
      Conditions classifiable to C16
  - √6th **Z85.03 Personal history of malignant neoplasm of large intestine**
    - **Z85.030 Personal history of malignant carcinoid tumor of large intestine**
      Conditions classifiable to C7A.022-C7A.025, C7A.029
    - **Z85.038 Personal history of other malignant neoplasm of large intestine**
      Conditions classifiable to C18
  - √6th **Z85.04 Personal history of malignant neoplasm of rectum, rectosigmoid junction, and anus**
    - **Z85.040 Personal history of malignant carcinoid tumor of rectum**
      Conditions classifiable to C7A.026
    - **Z85.048 Personal history of other malignant neoplasm of rectum, rectosigmoid junction, and anus**
      Conditions classifiable to C19-C21
  - **Z85.05 Personal history of malignant neoplasm of liver**
    Conditions classifiable to C22
  - √6th **Z85.06 Personal history of malignant neoplasm of small intestine**
    - **Z85.060 Personal history of malignant carcinoid tumor of small intestine**
      Conditions classifiable to C7A.01-
    - **Z85.068 Personal history of other malignant neoplasm of small intestine**
      Conditions classifiable to C17
  - **Z85.07 Personal history of malignant neoplasm of pancreas**
    Conditions classifiable to C25
  - **Z85.09 Personal history of malignant neoplasm of other digestive organs**

√5th **Z85.1 Personal history of malignant neoplasm of trachea, bronchus and lung**
  - √6th **Z85.11 Personal history of malignant neoplasm of bronchus and lung**
    - **Z85.110 Personal history of malignant carcinoid tumor of bronchus and lung**
      Conditions classifiable to C7A.090
    - **Z85.118 Personal history of other malignant neoplasm of bronchus and lung**
      Conditions classifiable to C34
  - **Z85.12 Personal history of malignant neoplasm of trachea**
    Conditions classifiable to C33

√5th **Z85.2 Personal history of malignant neoplasm of other respiratory and intrathoracic organs**
  - **Z85.20 Personal history of malignant neoplasm of unspecified respiratory organ**
  - **Z85.21 Personal history of malignant neoplasm of larynx**
    Conditions classifiable to C32
  - **Z85.22 Personal history of malignant neoplasm of nasal cavities, middle ear, and accessory sinuses**
    Conditions classifiable to C30-C31
  - √6th **Z85.23 Personal history of malignant neoplasm of thymus**
    - **Z85.230 Personal history of malignant carcinoid tumor of thymus**
      Conditions classifiable to C7A.091
    - **Z85.238 Personal history of other malignant neoplasm of thymus**
      Conditions classifiable to C37
  - **Z85.29 Personal history of malignant neoplasm of other respiratory and intrathoracic organs**

Z85.3 Personal history of malignant neoplasm of breast
  Conditions classifiable to C50.-

√5th **Z85.4 Personal history of malignant neoplasm of genital organs**
  Conditions classifiable to C51-C63
  - **Z85.40 Personal history of malignant neoplasm of unspecified female genital organ**
  - **Z85.41 Personal history of malignant neoplasm of cervix uteri**
  - **Z85.42 Personal history of malignant neoplasm of other parts of uterus**
  - **Z85.43 Personal history of malignant neoplasm of ovary**
  - **Z85.44 Personal history of malignant neoplasm of other female genital organs**
    AHA: 2024,2Q,11
  - **Z85.45 Personal history of malignant neoplasm of unspecified male genital organ**
  - **Z85.46 Personal history of malignant neoplasm of prostate**
    AHA: 2023,2Q,5
  - **Z85.47 Personal history of malignant neoplasm of testis**
  - **Z85.48 Personal history of malignant neoplasm of epididymis**
  - **Z85.49 Personal history of malignant neoplasm of other male genital organs**
  - **Z85.4A Personal history of malignant neoplasm of fallopian tube(s)**

√5th **Z85.5 Personal history of malignant neoplasm of urinary tract**
  Conditions classifiable to C64-C68
  - **Z85.50 Personal history of malignant neoplasm of unspecified urinary tract organ**
  - **Z85.51 Personal history of malignant neoplasm of bladder**
  - √6th **Z85.52 Personal history of malignant neoplasm of kidney**
    EXCLUDES 1 personal history of malignant neoplasm of renal pelvis (Z85.53)
    - **Z85.520 Personal history of malignant carcinoid tumor of kidney**
      Conditions classifiable to C7A.093
    - **Z85.528 Personal history of other malignant neoplasm of kidney**
      Conditions classifiable to C64
  - **Z85.53 Personal history of malignant neoplasm of renal pelvis**
  - **Z85.54 Personal history of malignant neoplasm of ureter**
  - **Z85.59 Personal history of malignant neoplasm of other urinary tract organ**

Z85.6 Personal history of leukemia
  Conditions classifiable to C91-C95
  EXCLUDES 1 leukemia in remission C91.0-C95.9 with 5th character 1

√5th **Z85.7 Personal history of other malignant neoplasms of lymphoid, hematopoietic and related tissues**
  - **Z85.71 Personal history of Hodgkin lymphoma**
    Conditions classifiable to C81
  - **Z85.72 Personal history of non-Hodgkin lymphomas**
    Conditions classifiable to C82-C85
    AHA: 2022,3Q,28

Chapter 21. Factors Influencing Health Status and Contact With Health Services

Z85.79 **Personal history of other malignant neoplasms of lymphoid, hematopoietic and related tissues**
Conditions classifiable to C88-C90, C96
EXCLUDES 1: multiple myeloma in remission (C90.01)
plasma cell leukemia in remission (C90.11)
plasmacytoma in remission (C90.21)

Z85.8 **Personal history of malignant neoplasms of other organs and systems**
Conditions classifiable to C00-C14, C40-C49, C69-C75, C7A.098, C76-C79

Z85.81 **Personal history of malignant neoplasm of lip, oral cavity, and pharynx**
Conditions classifiable to C00-C14

- **Z85.810** Personal history of malignant neoplasm of tongue
- **Z85.818** Personal history of malignant neoplasm of other sites of lip, oral cavity, and pharynx
- **Z85.819** Personal history of malignant neoplasm of unspecified site of lip, oral cavity, and pharynx

Z85.82 **Personal history of malignant neoplasm of skin**

- **Z85.820** Personal history of malignant melanoma of skin
  Conditions classifiable to C43
  AHA: 2022,3Q,9
- **Z85.821** Personal history of Merkel cell carcinoma
  Conditions classifiable to C4A
- **Z85.828** Personal history of other malignant neoplasm of skin
  Conditions classifiable to C44

Z85.83 **Personal history of malignant neoplasm of bone and soft tissue**
Conditions classifiable to C40-C41; C45-C49

- **Z85.830** Personal history of malignant neoplasm of bone
- **Z85.831** Personal history of malignant neoplasm of soft tissue
  EXCLUDES 2: personal history of malignant neoplasm of skin (Z85.82-)

Z85.84 **Personal history of malignant neoplasm of eye and nervous tissue**
Conditions classifiable to C69-C72

- **Z85.840** Personal history of malignant neoplasm of eye
- **Z85.841** Personal history of malignant neoplasm of brain
- **Z85.848** Personal history of malignant neoplasm of other parts of nervous tissue

Z85.85 **Personal history of malignant neoplasm of endocrine glands**
Conditions classifiable to C73-C75

- **Z85.850** Personal history of malignant neoplasm of thyroid
- **Z85.858** Personal history of malignant neoplasm of other endocrine glands
  AHA: 2024,2Q,10

Z85.89 **Personal history of malignant neoplasm of other organs and systems**
Conditions classifiable to C7A.098, C76, C77-C79

Z85.9 **Personal history of malignant neoplasm, unspecified**
Conditions classifiable to C7A.00, C80.1

Z86 **Personal history of certain other diseases**
Code first any follow-up examination after treatment (Z09)

Z86.0 **Personal history of in-situ and benign neoplasms and neoplasms of uncertain behavior**
EXCLUDES 2: personal history of malignant neoplasms (Z85.-)
AHA: 2017,1Q,9

Z86.00 **Personal history of in-situ neoplasm**
Conditions classifiable to D00-D09
AHA: 2019,4Q,20

- **Z86.000** Personal history of in-situ neoplasm of breast
  Conditions classifiable to D05
- **Z86.001** Personal history of in-situ neoplasm of cervix uteri
  Conditions classifiable to D06
  Personal history of cervical intraepithelial neoplasia III [CIN III]
- **Z86.002** Personal history of in-situ neoplasm of other and unspecified genital organs
  Conditions classifiable to D07
  Personal history of high-grade prostatic intraepithelial neoplasia III [HGPIN III]
  Personal history of vaginal intraepithelial neoplasia III [VAIN III]
  Personal history of vulvar intraepithelial neoplasia III [VIN III]
- **Z86.003** Personal history of in-situ neoplasm of oral cavity, esophagus and stomach
  Conditions classifiable to D00
- **Z86.004** Personal history of in-situ neoplasm of other and unspecified digestive organs
  Conditions classifiable to D01
  Personal history of anal intraepithelial neoplasia (AIN III)
- **Z86.005** Personal history of in-situ neoplasm of middle ear and respiratory system
  Conditions classifiable to D02
- **Z86.006** Personal history of melanoma in-situ
  Conditions classifiable to D03
  EXCLUDES 2: sites other than skin - code to personal history of in-situ neoplasm of the site
- **Z86.007** Personal history of in-situ neoplasm of skin
  Conditions classifiable to D04
  Personal history of carcinoma in situ of skin
- **Z86.008** Personal history of in-situ neoplasm of other site
  Conditions classifiable to D09
- **Z86.00A** Personal history of in-situ neoplasm of the fallopian tube(s)

Z86.01 **Personal history of benign neoplasm**

Z86.010 **Personal history of colon polyps**
Personal history of colorectal polyps
Personal history of rectal polyps
AHA: 2024,4Q,33; 2021,1Q,14; 2017,1Q,14

- **Z86.0100** Personal history of colon polyps, unspecified
  Personal history of colon polyps NOS
- **Z86.0101** Personal history of adenomatous and serrated colon polyps
  Personal history of sessile adenomatous colon polyp
  Personal history of sessile serrated colon polyp
  Personal history of traditional serrated adenoma polyps
  Personal history of tubular adenoma polyps
  Personal history of tubulovillous adenoma polyps
  Personal history of villous adenoma polyps
- **Z86.0102** Personal history of hyperplastic colon polyps
- **Z86.0109** Personal history of other colon polyps

Z86.011 Personal history of benign neoplasm of the brain
Z86.012 Personal history of benign carcinoid tumor
Z86.018 Personal history of other benign neoplasm
AHA: 2017,1Q,14

Z86.03 Personal history of neoplasm of uncertain behavior

Z86.1 **Personal history of infectious and parasitic diseases**
Conditions classifiable to A00-B89, B99
EXCLUDES 1: personal history of infectious diseases specific to a body system
sequelae of infectious and parasitic diseases (B90-B94)

- **Z86.11** Personal history of tuberculosis
- **Z86.12** Personal history of poliomyelitis
- **Z86.13** Personal history of malaria
- **Z86.14** Personal history of Methicillin resistant Staphylococcus aureus infection
  Personal history of MRSA infection
- **Z86.15** Personal history of latent tuberculosis infection

Z86.16 Personal history of COVID-19
EXCLUDES 1: post COVID-19 condition (U09.9)
AHA: 2021,4Q,107-108; 2021,1Q,28-29,33-35,40-41,44-45

Z86.19 Personal history of other infectious and parasitic diseases
AHA: 2022,3Q,4; 2021,1Q,33-34,40; 2020,3Q,13; 2020,2Q,10,12

Z86.2 Personal history of diseases of the blood and blood-forming organs and certain disorders involving the immune mechanism
Conditions classifiable to D50-D89

Z86.3 Personal history of endocrine, nutritional and metabolic diseases
Conditions classifiable to E00-E88

Z86.31 Personal history of diabetic foot ulcer
EXCLUDES 2: current diabetic foot ulcer (E08.621, E09.621, E10.621, E11.621, E13.621)

Z86.32 Personal history of gestational diabetes
Personal history of conditions classifiable to O24.4-
EXCLUDES 1: gestational diabetes mellitus in current pregnancy (O24.4-)

Z86.39 Personal history of other endocrine, nutritional and metabolic disease
AHA: 2020,1Q,12

Z86.5 Personal history of mental and behavioral disorders
Conditions classifiable to F40-F59

Z86.51 Personal history of combat and operational stress reaction

Z86.59 Personal history of other mental and behavioral disorders

Z86.6 Personal history of diseases of the nervous system and sense organs
Conditions classifiable to G00-G99, H00-H95

Z86.61 Personal history of infections of the central nervous system
Personal history of encephalitis
Personal history of meningitis

Z86.69 Personal history of other diseases of the nervous system and sense organs
AHA: 2016,4Q,24

Z86.7 Personal history of diseases of the circulatory system
Conditions classifiable to I00-I99
EXCLUDES 2: old myocardial infarction (I25.2)
personal history of anaphylactic shock (Z87.892)
postmyocardial infarction syndrome (I24.1)

Z86.71 Personal history of venous thrombosis and embolism
- Z86.711 Personal history of pulmonary embolism
- Z86.718 Personal history of other venous thrombosis and embolism
  AHA: 2020,2Q,20

Z86.72 Personal history of thrombophlebitis

Z86.73 Personal history of transient ischemic attack (TIA), and cerebral infarction without residual deficits
Personal history of prolonged reversible ischemic neurological deficit (PRIND)
Personal history of stroke NOS without residual deficits
EXCLUDES 1: personal history of traumatic brain injury (Z87.820)
sequelae of cerebrovascular disease (I69.-)
AHA: 2023,1Q,37; 2012,4Q,92

Z86.74 Personal history of sudden cardiac arrest
Personal history of sudden cardiac death successfully resuscitated
AHA: 2024,1Q,27

Z86.79 Personal history of other diseases of the circulatory system
AHA: 2022,2Q,14; 2020,1Q,12

Z87 Personal history of other diseases and conditions
Code first any follow-up examination after treatment (Z09)
AHA: 2022,4Q,50-51

Z87.0 Personal history of diseases of the respiratory system
Conditions classifiable to J00-J99

Z87.01 Personal history of pneumonia (recurrent)

Z87.09 Personal history of other diseases of the respiratory system

Z87.1 Personal history of diseases of the digestive system
Conditions classifiable to K00-K93

Z87.11 Personal history of peptic ulcer disease

Z87.19 Personal history of other diseases of the digestive system
AHA: 2017,1Q,14

Z87.2 Personal history of diseases of the skin and subcutaneous tissue
Conditions classifiable to L00-L99
EXCLUDES 2: personal history of diabetic foot ulcer (Z86.31)

Z87.3 Personal history of diseases of the musculoskeletal system and connective tissue
Conditions classifiable to M00-M99
EXCLUDES 2: personal history of (healed) traumatic fracture (Z87.81)

Z87.31 Personal history of (healed) nontraumatic fracture

Z87.310 Personal history of (healed) osteoporosis fracture
Personal history of (healed) collapsed vertebra due to osteoporosis
Personal history of (healed) fragility fracture
TIP: Assign for history of osteoporosis fractures that have resolved, even when a code from category M80 indicating current osteoporosis fracture is also reported.

Z87.311 Personal history of (healed) other pathological fracture
Personal history of (healed) collapsed vertebra NOS
EXCLUDES 2: personal history of osteoporosis fracture (Z87.310)

Z87.312 Personal history of (healed) stress fracture
Personal history of (healed) fatigue fracture

Z87.39 Personal history of other diseases of the musculoskeletal system and connective tissue

Z87.4 Personal history of diseases of the genitourinary system
Conditions classifiable to N00-N99

Z87.41 Personal history of dysplasia of the female genital tract
EXCLUDES 1: personal history of intraepithelial neoplasia III of female genital tract ▶(Z86.001, Z86.008, Z86.00A)◀
personal history of malignant neoplasm of female genital tract ▶(Z85.40-Z85.44, Z85.4A)◀

- Z87.410 Personal history of cervical dysplasia
- Z87.411 Personal history of vaginal dysplasia
- Z87.412 Personal history of vulvar dysplasia

Z87.42 Personal history of other diseases of the female genital tract

Z87.43 Personal history of diseases of the male genital organs

Z87.430 Personal history of prostatic dysplasia
EXCLUDES 1: personal history of malignant neoplasm of prostate (Z85.46)

Z87.438 Personal history of other diseases of male genital organs

Z87.44 Personal history of diseases of the urinary system
EXCLUDES 1: personal history of malignant neoplasm of cervix uteri (Z85.41)

- Z87.440 Personal history of urinary (tract) infections
- Z87.441 Personal history of nephrotic syndrome
- Z87.442 Personal history of urinary calculi
  Personal history of kidney stones
- Z87.448 Personal history of other diseases of urinary system

Z87.5 Personal history of complications of pregnancy, childbirth and the puerperium
Conditions classifiable to O00-O9A
EXCLUDES 2: recurrent pregnancy loss (N96)

Z87.51 Personal history of pre-term labor
EXCLUDES 1: current pregnancy with history of pre-term labor (O09.21-)

Z87.59 Personal history of other complications of pregnancy, childbirth and the puerperium
Personal history of trophoblastic disease

Z87.6 Personal history of certain (corrected) conditions arising in the perinatal period
Conditions classifiable to P00-P96
EXCLUDES 1: personal history of (corrected) congenital malformations (Z87.7-)

Z87.61 Personal history of (corrected) necrotizing enterocolitis of newborn

Z87.68 Personal history of other (corrected) conditions arising in the perinatal period [UPD]

√5th **Z87.7** Personal history of (corrected) congenital malformations
Conditions classifiable to Q00-Q89 that have been repaired or corrected
EXCLUDES 2 congenital malformations that have been partially corrected or repaired but which still require medical treatment - code to condition
other postprocedural states (Z98.-)
personal history of medical treatment (Z92.-)
presence of cardiac and vascular implants and grafts (Z95.-)
presence of other devices (Z97.-)
presence of other functional implants (Z96.-)
transplanted organ and tissue status (Z94.-)

√6th **Z87.71** Personal history of (corrected) congenital malformations of genitourinary system
 Z87.710 Personal history of (corrected) hypospadias
 Z87.718 Personal history of other specified (corrected) congenital malformations of genitourinary system

√6th **Z87.72** Personal history of (corrected) congenital malformations of nervous system and sense organs
 Z87.720 Personal history of (corrected) congenital malformations of eye
 Z87.721 Personal history of (corrected) congenital malformations of ear
 Z87.728 Personal history of other specified (corrected) congenital malformations of nervous system and sense organs

√6th **Z87.73** Personal history of (corrected) congenital malformations of digestive system
 Z87.730 Personal history of (corrected) cleft lip and palate
 Z87.731 Personal history of (corrected) tracheoesophageal fistula or atresia [UPD]
 Z87.732 Personal history of (corrected) persistent cloaca or cloacal malformations [UPD]
 Z87.738 Personal history of other specified (corrected) congenital malformations of digestive system

 Z87.74 Personal history of (corrected) congenital malformations of heart and circulatory system
 Z87.75 Personal history of (corrected) congenital malformations of respiratory system

√6th **Z87.76** Personal history of (corrected) congenital malformations of integument, limbs and musculoskeletal system
 Z87.760 Personal history of (corrected) congenital diaphragmatic hernia or other congenital diaphragm malformations [UPD]
 Z87.761 Personal history of (corrected) gastroschisis [UPD]
 Z87.762 Personal history of (corrected) prune belly malformation [UPD]
 Z87.763 Personal history of other (corrected) congenital abdominal wall malformations [UPD]
 Z87.768 Personal history of other specified (corrected) congenital malformations of integument, limbs and musculoskeletal system [UPD]

√6th **Z87.79** Personal history of other (corrected) congenital malformations
 Z87.790 Personal history of (corrected) congenital malformations of face and neck
 Z87.798 Personal history of other (corrected) congenital malformations

√5th **Z87.8** Personal history of other specified conditions
EXCLUDES 2 personal history of self harm (Z91.5-)
 Z87.81 Personal history of (healed) traumatic fracture
 EXCLUDES 2 personal history of (healed) nontraumatic fracture (Z87.31-)

√6th **Z87.82** Personal history of other (healed) physical injury and trauma
Conditions classifiable to S00-T88, except traumatic fractures
 Z87.820 Personal history of traumatic brain injury
 EXCLUDES 1 personal history of transient ischemic attack (TIA), and cerebral infarction without residual deficits (Z86.73)
 Z87.821 Personal history of retained foreign body fully removed
 Z87.828 Personal history of other (healed) physical injury and trauma

√6th **Z87.89** Personal history of other specified conditions
 Z87.890 Personal history of sex reassignment
 Z87.891 Personal history of nicotine dependence
 EXCLUDES 1 current nicotine dependence (F17.2-)
 AHA: 2017,2Q,27
 Z87.892 Personal history of anaphylaxis
 Code also allergy status such as:
 allergy status to drugs, medicaments and biological substances (Z88.-)
 allergy status, other than to drugs and biological substances (Z91.0-)
 AHA: 2025,2Q,16
 Z87.898 Personal history of other specified conditions
 AHA: 2013,1Q,21

√4th **Z88** Allergy status to drugs, medicaments and biological substances
EXCLUDES 2 allergy status, other than to drugs and biological substances (Z91.0-)
AHA: 2025,2Q,16; 2015,3Q,23
 Z88.0 Allergy status to penicillin
 Z88.1 Allergy status to other antibiotic agents
 Z88.2 Allergy status to sulfonamides
 Z88.3 Allergy status to other anti-infective agents
 Z88.4 Allergy status to anesthetic agent
 Z88.5 Allergy status to narcotic agent
 Z88.6 Allergy status to analgesic agent
 Z88.7 Allergy status to serum and vaccine
 Z88.8 Allergy status to other drugs, medicaments and biological substances
 Z88.9 Allergy status to unspecified drugs, medicaments and biological substances

√4th **Z89** Acquired absence of limb
INCLUDES amputation status
postprocedural loss of limb
post-traumatic loss of limb
EXCLUDES 1 acquired deformities of limbs (M20-M21)
congenital absence of limbs (Q71-Q73)

√5th **Z89.0** Acquired absence of thumb and other finger(s)
 √6th **Z89.01** Acquired absence of thumb
  Z89.011 Acquired absence of right thumb
  Z89.012 Acquired absence of left thumb
  Z89.019 Acquired absence of unspecified thumb
 √6th **Z89.02** Acquired absence of other finger(s)
  EXCLUDES 2 acquired absence of thumb (Z89.01-)
  Z89.021 Acquired absence of right finger(s)
  Z89.022 Acquired absence of left finger(s)
  Z89.029 Acquired absence of unspecified finger(s)

√5th **Z89.1** Acquired absence of hand and wrist
 √6th **Z89.11** Acquired absence of hand
  Z89.111 Acquired absence of right hand [COM]
  Z89.112 Acquired absence of left hand [COM]
  Z89.119 Acquired absence of unspecified hand [COM]
 √6th **Z89.12** Acquired absence of wrist
  Disarticulation at wrist
  Z89.121 Acquired absence of right wrist [COM]
  Z89.122 Acquired absence of left wrist [COM]
  Z89.129 Acquired absence of unspecified wrist [COM]

Chapter 21. Factors Influencing Health Status and Contact With Health Services

Z89.2 Acquired absence of upper limb above wrist
- **Z89.20** Acquired absence of upper limb, unspecified level
  - **Z89.201** Acquired absence of right upper limb, unspecified level
  - **Z89.202** Acquired absence of left upper limb, unspecified level
  - **Z89.209** Acquired absence of unspecified upper limb, unspecified level
    Acquired absence of arm NOS
- **Z89.21** Acquired absence of upper limb below elbow
  - **Z89.211** Acquired absence of right upper limb below elbow
  - **Z89.212** Acquired absence of left upper limb below elbow
  - **Z89.219** Acquired absence of unspecified upper limb below elbow
- **Z89.22** Acquired absence of upper limb above elbow
  Disarticulation at elbow
  - **Z89.221** Acquired absence of right upper limb above elbow
  - **Z89.222** Acquired absence of left upper limb above elbow
  - **Z89.229** Acquired absence of unspecified upper limb above elbow
- **Z89.23** Acquired absence of shoulder
  Acquired absence of shoulder joint following explantation of shoulder joint prosthesis, with or without presence of antibiotic-impregnated cement spacer
  - **Z89.231** Acquired absence of right shoulder
  - **Z89.232** Acquired absence of left shoulder
  - **Z89.239** Acquired absence of unspecified shoulder

Z89.4 Acquired absence of toe(s), foot, and ankle
- **Z89.41** Acquired absence of great toe
  - **Z89.411** Acquired absence of right great toe
  - **Z89.412** Acquired absence of left great toe
  - **Z89.419** Acquired absence of unspecified great toe
- **Z89.42** Acquired absence of other toe(s)
  EXCLUDES 2: acquired absence of great toe (Z89.41-)
  - **Z89.421** Acquired absence of other right toe(s)
  - **Z89.422** Acquired absence of other left toe(s)
  - **Z89.429** Acquired absence of other toe(s), unspecified side
- **Z89.43** Acquired absence of foot
  - **Z89.431** Acquired absence of right foot
  - **Z89.432** Acquired absence of left foot
  - **Z89.439** Acquired absence of unspecified foot
- **Z89.44** Acquired absence of ankle
  Disarticulation of ankle
  - **Z89.441** Acquired absence of right ankle
  - **Z89.442** Acquired absence of left ankle
  - **Z89.449** Acquired absence of unspecified ankle

Z89.5 Acquired absence of leg below knee
- **Z89.51** Acquired absence of leg below knee
  - **Z89.511** Acquired absence of right leg below knee
  - **Z89.512** Acquired absence of left leg below knee
  - **Z89.519** Acquired absence of unspecified leg below knee
- **Z89.52** Acquired absence of knee
  Acquired absence of knee joint following explantation of knee joint prosthesis, with or without presence of antibiotic-impregnated cement spacer
  - **Z89.521** Acquired absence of right knee
  - **Z89.522** Acquired absence of left knee
  - **Z89.529** Acquired absence of unspecified knee

Z89.6 Acquired absence of leg above knee
- **Z89.61** Acquired absence of leg above knee
  Acquired absence of leg NOS
  Disarticulation at knee
  - **Z89.611** Acquired absence of right leg above knee
  - **Z89.612** Acquired absence of left leg above knee
  - **Z89.619** Acquired absence of unspecified leg above knee
- **Z89.62** Acquired absence of hip
  Acquired absence of hip joint following explantation of hip joint prosthesis, with or without presence of antibiotic-impregnated cement spacer
  Disarticulation at hip
  - **Z89.621** Acquired absence of right hip joint
  - **Z89.622** Acquired absence of left hip joint
  - **Z89.629** Acquired absence of unspecified hip joint

Z89.9 Acquired absence of limb, unspecified

Z90 Acquired absence of organs, not elsewhere classified
  INCLUDES: postprocedural or post-traumatic loss of body part NEC
  EXCLUDES 1: congenital absence - see Alphabetical Index
  EXCLUDES 2: postprocedural absence of endocrine glands (E89.-)

- **Z90.0** Acquired absence of part of head and neck
  - **Z90.01** Acquired absence of eye
  - **Z90.02** Acquired absence of larynx
  - **Z90.09** Acquired absence of other part of head and neck
    Acquired absence of nose
    EXCLUDES 2: teeth (K08.1)
- **Z90.1** Acquired absence of breast and nipple
  AHA: 2022,3Q,8
  - **Z90.10** Acquired absence of unspecified breast and nipple
  - **Z90.11** Acquired absence of right breast and nipple
  - **Z90.12** Acquired absence of left breast and nipple
  - **Z90.13** Acquired absence of bilateral breasts and nipples
- **Z90.2** Acquired absence of lung [part of]
- **Z90.3** Acquired absence of stomach [part of]
- **Z90.4** Acquired absence of other specified parts of digestive tract
  - **Z90.41** Acquired absence of pancreas
    Code also exocrine pancreatic insufficiency (K86.81)
    Use additional code to identify any associated:
      diabetes mellitus, postpancreatectomy (E13.-)
      insulin use (Z79.4)
    AHA: 2024,2Q,10
    - **Z90.410** Acquired total absence of pancreas
      Acquired absence of pancreas NOS
    - **Z90.411** Acquired partial absence of pancreas
  - **Z90.49** Acquired absence of other specified parts of digestive tract
- **Z90.5** Acquired absence of kidney
- **Z90.6** Acquired absence of other parts of urinary tract
  Acquired absence of bladder
- **Z90.7** Acquired absence of genital organ(s)
  EXCLUDES 1: personal history of sex reassignment (Z87.890)
  EXCLUDES 2: female genital mutilation status (N90.81-)
  - **Z90.71** Acquired absence of cervix and uterus
    - **Z90.710** Acquired absence of both cervix and uterus
      Acquired absence of uterus NOS
      Status post total hysterectomy
    - **Z90.711** Acquired absence of uterus with remaining cervical stump
      Status post partial hysterectomy with remaining cervical stump
    - **Z90.712** Acquired absence of cervix with remaining uterus
  - **Z90.72** Acquired absence of ovaries
    - **Z90.721** Acquired absence of ovaries, unilateral
    - **Z90.722** Acquired absence of ovaries, bilateral
  - **Z90.79** Acquired absence of other genital organ(s)
    AHA: 2023,2Q,5
- **Z90.8** Acquired absence of other organs
  - **Z90.81** Acquired absence of spleen
  - **Z90.89** Acquired absence of other organs
    AHA: 2023,3Q,13

Chapter 21. Factors Influencing Health Status and Contact With Health Services

- ✓4th **Z91** **Personal risk factors, not elsewhere classified**
  - EXCLUDES 2: contact with and (suspected) exposures hazardous to health (Z77.-)
    - exposure to pollution and other problems related to physical environment (Z77.1-)
    - female genital mutilation status (N90.81-)
    - occupational exposure to risk factors (Z57.-)
    - personal history of physical injury and trauma (Z87.81, Z87.82-)
  - ✓5th **Z91.0** **Allergy status, other than to drugs and biological substances**
    - EXCLUDES 2: allergy status to drugs, medicaments, and biological substances (Z88.-)
    - ✓6th **Z91.01** **Food allergy status**
      - EXCLUDES 2: food additives allergy status (Z91.02)
      - **Z91.010** Allergy to peanuts
      - ▲ ✓7th **Z91.011** Allergy to milk products
        - EXCLUDES 1: lactose intolerance (E73.-)
        - **Z91.0110** Allergy to milk products, unspecified
        - **Z91.0111** Allergy to milk products with tolerance to baked milk
          - EXCLUDES 1: allergy to milk products with reactivity to baked milk (Z91.0112)
        - **Z91.0112** Allergy to milk products with reactivity to baked milk
          - EXCLUDES 1: allergy to milk products with tolerance to baked milk (Z91.0111)
      - ▲ ✓7th **Z91.012** Allergy to eggs
        - **Z91.0120** Allergy to eggs, unspecified
        - **Z91.0121** Allergy to eggs with tolerance to baked egg
          - EXCLUDES 1: allergy to eggs with reactivity to baked egg (Z91.0122)
        - **Z91.0122** Allergy to eggs with reactivity to baked egg
          - EXCLUDES 1: allergy to egg with tolerance to baked egg (Z91.0121)
      - **Z91.013** Allergy to seafood
        - Allergy to octopus or squid ink
        - Allergy to shellfish
      - **Z91.014** Allergy to mammalian meats
        - Allergy to beef
        - Allergy to lamb
        - Allergy to pork
        - Allergy to red meats
        - AHA: 2021,4Q,33
      - **Z91.018** Allergy to other foods
        - Allergy to nuts other than peanuts
    - **Z91.02** Food additives allergy status
    - ✓6th **Z91.03** **Insect allergy status**
      - **Z91.030** Bee allergy status
      - **Z91.038** Other insect allergy status
    - ✓6th **Z91.04** **Nonmedicinal substance allergy status**
      - **Z91.040** Latex allergy status
        - Latex sensitivity status
      - **Z91.041** Radiographic dye allergy status
        - Allergy status to contrast media used for diagnostic X-ray procedure
      - **Z91.048** Other nonmedicinal substance allergy status
    - **Z91.09** Other allergy status, other than to drugs and biological substances

  - ✓5th **Z91.1** **Patient's noncompliance with medical treatment and regimen**
    - Code also, if applicable, to identify underdosing of specific drug (T36-T50 with final character 6)
    - EXCLUDES 2: caregiver noncompliance with patient's medical treatment and regimen (Z91.A-)
    - AHA: 2022,4Q,49
    - ✓6th **Z91.11** **Patient's noncompliance with dietary regimen**
      - Code also, if applicable, food insecurity (Z59.4-)
      - **Z91.110** Patient's noncompliance with dietary regimen due to financial hardship [UPD]
      - **Z91.118** Patient's noncompliance with dietary regimen for other reason [UPD]
        - Inability to comply with dietary regimen
      - **Z91.119** Patient's noncompliance with dietary regimen due to unspecified reason [UPD]
    - ✓6th **Z91.12** **Patient's intentional underdosing of medication regimen**
      - Code first underdosing of medication (T36-T50) with fifth or sixth character 6
      - AHA: 2018,4Q,72
      - **Z91.120** Patient's intentional underdosing of medication regimen due to financial hardship
      - **Z91.128** Patient's intentional underdosing of medication regimen for other reason
    - ✓6th **Z91.13** **Patient's unintentional underdosing of medication regimen**
      - Code first underdosing of medication (T36-T50) with fifth or sixth character 6
      - AHA: 2018,4Q,72
      - **Z91.130** Patient's unintentional underdosing of medication regimen due to age-related debility
      - **Z91.138** Patient's unintentional underdosing of medication regimen for other reason
    - ✓6th **Z91.14** **Patient's other noncompliance with medication regimen**
      - Patient's underdosing of medication NOS
      - Code first, if applicable, adverse effect of underdosing (T36-T50)
      - AHA: 2023,1Q,7; 2022,1Q,36; 2018,4Q,72
      - **Z91.141** Patient's other noncompliance with medication regimen due to financial hardship [UPD]
      - **Z91.148** Patient's other noncompliance with medication regimen for other reason [UPD]
    - ✓6th **Z91.15** **Patient's noncompliance with renal dialysis**
      - AHA: 2023,1Q,7
      - **Z91.151** Patient's noncompliance with renal dialysis due to financial hardship [Rx] [ESR] [UPD]
      - **Z91.158** Patient's noncompliance with renal dialysis for other reason [Rx] [ESR] [UPD]
    - ✓6th **Z91.19** **Patient's noncompliance with other medical treatment and regimen**
      - Patient's nonadherence to medical treatment
      - **Z91.190** Patient's noncompliance with other medical treatment and regimen due to financial hardship [UPD]
      - **Z91.198** Patient's noncompliance with other medical treatment and regimen for other reason [UPD]
        - AHA: 2024,1Q,23
      - **Z91.199** Patient's noncompliance with other medical treatment and regimen due to unspecified reason [UPD]
  - ✓5th **Z91.A** **Caregiver's noncompliance with patient's medical treatment and regimen**
    - AHA: 2023,4Q,48; 2022,4Q,49
    - ✓6th **Z91.A1** **Caregiver's noncompliance with patient's dietary regimen**
      - Caregiver's inability to comply with patient's dietary regimen
      - Code also, if applicable, food insecurity (Z59.4-)
      - **Z91.A10** Caregiver's noncompliance with patient's dietary regimen due to financial hardship [UPD]
      - **Z91.A18** Caregiver's noncompliance with patient's dietary regimen for other reason [UPD]

Z91.A2 Caregiver's intentional underdosing of patient's medication regimen
Code first underdosing of medication (T36-T50) with fifth or sixth character 6

- **Z91.A20** Caregiver's intentional underdosing of patient's medication regimen due to financial hardship [UPD]
- **Z91.A28** Caregiver's intentional underdosing of medication regimen for other reason [UPD]

Z91.A3 Caregiver's unintentional underdosing of patient's medication regimen [UPD]
Code first underdosing of medication (T36-T50) with fifth or sixth character 6

Z91.A4 Caregiver's other noncompliance with patient's medication regimen
Caregiver's underdosing of patient's medication NOS
Caregiver's underdosing with patient's medication NOS

- **Z91.A41** Caregiver's other noncompliance with patient's medication regimen due to financial hardship [UPD]
- **Z91.A48** Caregiver's other noncompliance with patient's medication regimen for other reason [UPD]

Z91.A5 Caregiver's noncompliance with patient's renal dialysis
- **Z91.A51** Caregiver's noncompliance with patient's renal dialysis due to financial hardship [Rx] [ESR] [UPD]
- **Z91.A58** Caregiver's noncompliance with patient's renal dialysis for other reason [Rx] [ESR]

Z91.A9 Caregiver's noncompliance with patient's other medical treatment and regimen
Caregiver's nonadherence to patient's medical treatment

- **Z91.A91** Caregiver's noncompliance with patient's other medical treatment and regimen due to financial hardship [UPD]
- **Z91.A98** Caregiver's noncompliance with patient's other medical treatment and regimen for other reason [UPD]

Z91.4 Personal history of psychological trauma, not elsewhere classified
AHA: 2023,1Q,7

Z91.41 Personal history of adult abuse
EXCLUDES 2 personal history of abuse in childhood (Z62.81-)

- **Z91.410** Personal history of adult physical and sexual abuse [A]
  - *EXCLUDES 1* current adult physical abuse (T74.11, T76.11)
  - current adult sexual abuse (T74.21, T76.11)
- **Z91.411** Personal history of adult psychological abuse [A]
- **Z91.412** Personal history of adult neglect
  - *EXCLUDES 1* current adult neglect (T74.01, T76.01)
- **Z91.413** Personal history of adult financial abuse [UPD]
- **Z91.414** Personal history of adult intimate partner abuse [UPD]
- **Z91.419** Personal history of unspecified adult abuse [A]

Z91.42 Personal history of forced labor or sexual exploitation
AHA: 2018,4Q,32,35

Z91.49 Other personal history of psychological trauma, not elsewhere classified

Z91.5 Personal history of self-harm
Code also mental health disorder, if known
AHA: 2021,4Q,33

Z91.51 Personal history of suicidal behavior [UPD]
Personal history of parasuicide
Personal history of self-poisoning
Personal history of suicide attempt

Z91.52 Personal history of nonsuicidal self-harm [UPD]
Personal history of nonsuicidal self-injury
Personal history of self-inflicted injury without suicidal intent
Personal history of self-mutilation

Z91.8 Other specified personal risk factors, not elsewhere classified

Z91.81 History of falling
At risk for falling

Z91.82 Personal history of military deployment [A]
Individual (civilian or military) with past history of military war, peacekeeping and humanitarian deployment (current or past conflict)
Returned from military deployment
EXCLUDES 2 personal history of military service (Z91.85)

Z91.83 Wandering in diseases classified elsewhere
Code first underlying disorder such as:
Alzheimer's disease (G30.-)
autism or pervasive developmental disorder (F84.-)
intellectual disabilities (F70-F79)
unspecified dementia with behavioral disturbance (F03.9-, F03.A-, F03.B-, F03.C-)

Z91.84 Oral health risk factors
AHA: 2017,4Q,29

- **Z91.841** Risk for dental caries, low
- **Z91.842** Risk for dental caries, moderate
- **Z91.843** Risk for dental caries, high
- **Z91.849** Unspecified risk for dental caries

Z91.85 Personal history of military service [UPD]
Personal history of serving in the armed forces
Personal history of veteran
EXCLUDES 2 personal history of military deployment (Z91.82)
AHA: 2023,4Q,48

Z91.89 Other specified personal risk factors, not elsewhere classified
Increased risk for social isolation
AHA: 2017,1Q,45

Z91.B Personal risk factor of exposure to diethylstilbestrol
DES daughter or son
Personal risk factor of exposure to DES
Personal risk factor of exposure to DES in utero
Second generation DES exposure
Code also, associated conditions, such as:
conditions classifiable to C50.-
osteoporosis (M80.-)
premature menopause (E28.31-)

Z92 Personal history of medical treatment
EXCLUDES 2 postprocedural states (Z98.-)

Z92.0 Personal history of contraception
EXCLUDES 1 counseling or management of current contraceptive practices (Z30.-)
long term (current) use of contraception (Z79.3)
presence of (intrauterine) contraceptive device (Z97.5)

Z92.2 Personal history of drug therapy
EXCLUDES 2 long term (current) drug therapy (Z79.-)

Z92.21 Personal history of antineoplastic chemotherapy
Z92.22 Personal history of monoclonal drug therapy
EXCLUDES 2 personal history of immune checkpoint inhibitor therapy (Z92.26)
Z92.23 Personal history of estrogen therapy
Z92.24 Personal history of steroid therapy
- **Z92.240** Personal history of inhaled steroid therapy
- **Z92.241** Personal history of systemic steroid therapy
  Personal history of steroid therapy NOS
Z92.25 Personal history of immunosuppression therapy
EXCLUDES 2 personal history of steroid therapy (Z92.24)
Z92.26 Personal history of immune checkpoint inhibitor therapy
Personal history of ICI drug therapy
AHA: 2024,4Q,34
Z92.29 Personal history of other drug therapy

Z92.3 Personal history of irradiation
Personal history of exposure to therapeutic radiation
EXCLUDES 1 exposure to radiation in the physical environment (Z77.12)
occupational exposure to radiation (Z57.1)

Chapter 21. Factors Influencing Health Status and Contact With Health Services

Z92.8 ✓5ᵗʰ **Personal history of other medical treatment**
- **Z92.81** Personal history of **extracorporeal membrane oxygenation** (ECMO)
- **Z92.82** Status post administration of tPA (rtPA) in a different facility within the last 24 hours prior to admission to current facility [UPD]
  - Code first condition requiring tPA administration, such as:
    - acute cerebral infarction (I63.-)
    - acute myocardial infarction (I21.-, I22.-)
  - AHA: 2013,4Q,124
- **Z92.83** Personal history of **failed moderate sedation**
  - Personal history of failed conscious sedation
  - EXCLUDES 2: failed moderate sedation during procedure (T88.52)
- **Z92.84** Personal history of **unintended awareness under general anesthesia**
  - EXCLUDES 2: unintended awareness under general anesthesia during procedure (T88.53)
  - AHA: 2016,4Q,72-73,77
- ✓6ᵗʰ **Z92.85** Personal history of cellular therapy
  - EXCLUDES 2: personal history of immune checkpoint inhibitor therapy (Z92.26)
  - AHA: 2021,4Q,33-34
  - **Z92.850** Personal history of **Chimeric Antigen Receptor T-cell therapy** [UPD]
    - Personal history of CAR T-cell therapy
  - **Z92.858** Personal history of other cellular therapy [UPD]
  - **Z92.859** Personal history of cellular therapy, unspecified [UPD]
- **Z92.86** Personal history of **gene therapy** [UPD]
  - AHA: 2021,4Q,33-34
- **Z92.89** Personal history of other medical treatment
  - AHA: 2020,1Q,18

✓4ᵗʰ **Z93 Artificial opening status**
- EXCLUDES 1: artificial openings requiring attention or management (Z43.-)
  - complications of external stoma (J95.0-, K94.-, N99.5-)
- **Z93.0** **Tracheostomy** status [HCC] [ESR] [COM]
  - AHA: 2013,4Q,129
- **Z93.1** **Gastrostomy** status [HCC] [ESR] [COM]
- **Z93.2** **Ileostomy** status [HCC] [ESR] [COM]
  - Ileal pouch status
  - Kock pouch status
- **Z93.3** **Colostomy** status [HCC] [ESR] [COM]
- **Z93.4** Other artificial openings of gastrointestinal tract status [HCC] [ESR] [COM]
- ✓5ᵗʰ **Z93.5** **Cystostomy** status
  - **Z93.50** Unspecified cystostomy status [HCC] [ESR] [COM]
  - **Z93.51** **Cutaneous-vesicostomy** status [HCC] [ESR] [COM]
  - **Z93.52** **Appendico-vesicostomy** status [HCC] [ESR] [COM]
  - **Z93.59** Other cystostomy status [HCC] [ESR] [COM]
- **Z93.6** Other artificial openings of **urinary tract** status [HCC] [ESR] [COM]
  - Nephrostomy status
  - Ureterostomy status
  - Urethrostomy status
- **Z93.8** Other artificial opening status [HCC] [ESR] [COM]
- **Z93.9** Artificial opening status, unspecified [HCC] [ESR] [COM]

✓4ᵗʰ **Z94 Transplanted organ and tissue status**
- INCLUDES: organ or tissue replaced by heterogenous or homogenous transplant
- EXCLUDES 1: complications of transplanted organ or tissue - see Alphabetical Index
- EXCLUDES 2: presence of vascular grafts (Z95.-)
- **Z94.0** **Kidney** transplant status [Rx] [COM]
- **Z94.1** **Heart** transplant status [HCC] [Rx] [COM]
  - EXCLUDES 1: artificial heart status (Z95.812)
    - heart-valve replacement status (Z95.2-Z95.4)
- **Z94.2** **Lung** transplant status [HCC] [Rx] [ESR] [COM]
- **Z94.3** **Heart and lungs** transplant status [HCC] [Rx] [ESR] [COM]
- **Z94.4** **Liver** transplant status [HCC] [Rx] [ESR] [COM]
- **Z94.5** **Skin** transplant status
  - Autogenous skin transplant status
- **Z94.6** **Bone** transplant status
- **Z94.7** **Corneal** transplant status

✓5ᵗʰ **Z94.8** Other transplanted organ and tissue status
- **Z94.81** **Bone marrow** transplant status [HCC] [Rx] [ESR] [COM]
- **Z94.82** **Intestine** transplant status [HCC] [Rx] [ESR] [COM]
- **Z94.83** **Pancreas** transplant status [HCC] [Rx] [ESR] [COM]
- **Z94.84** **Stem cells** transplant status [HCC] [Rx] [ESR] [COM]
- **Z94.89** Other transplanted organ and tissue status
- **Z94.9** Transplanted organ and tissue status, unspecified

✓4ᵗʰ **Z95 Presence of cardiac and vascular implants and grafts**
- EXCLUDES 2: complications of cardiac and vascular devices, implants and grafts (T82.-)
- **Z95.0** Presence of **cardiac pacemaker**
  - Presence of cardiac resynchronization therapy (CRT-P) pacemaker
  - EXCLUDES 1: adjustment or management of cardiac device (Z45.0-)
    - adjustment or management of cardiac pacemaker (Z45.0)
    - presence of automatic (implantable) cardiac defibrillator with synchronous cardiac pacemaker (Z95.810)
  - AHA: 2022,2Q,14; 2019,1Q,33
  - **TIP:** Assign an additional code for the associated condition if that condition requires constant intervention from the device, as in cases of sick sinus syndrome. For conditions that do not require constant intervention from the device, as in cases of ventricular fibrillation, an additional code for the associated condition should be assigned only if the patient is experiencing the condition and the device is firing during the current admission.
- **Z95.1** Presence of **aortocoronary bypass graft**
  - Presence of coronary artery bypass graft
- **Z95.2** Presence of **prosthetic heart valve**
  - Presence of heart valve NOS
- **Z95.3** Presence of **xenogenic heart valve**
- **Z95.4** Presence of other heart-valve replacement
- **Z95.5** Presence of **coronary angioplasty** implant and graft
  - EXCLUDES 1: coronary angioplasty status without implant and graft (Z98.61)
- ✓5ᵗʰ **Z95.8** Presence of other cardiac and vascular implants and grafts
  - ✓6ᵗʰ **Z95.81** Presence of other cardiac implants and grafts
    - **Z95.810** Presence of **automatic (implantable) cardiac defibrillator**
      - Presence of automatic (implantable) cardiac defibrillator with synchronous cardiac pacemaker
      - Presence of cardiac resynchronization therapy defibrillator (CRT-D)
      - Presence of cardioverter-defibrillator (ICD)
      - AHA: 2022,2Q,14; 2019,1Q,33
      - **TIP:** Assign an additional code for the associated condition if that condition requires constant intervention from the device, as in cases of sick sinus syndrome. For conditions that do not require constant intervention from the device, as in cases of ventricular fibrillation, an additional code for the associated condition should be assigned only if the patient is experiencing the condition and the device is firing during the current admission.
    - **Z95.811** Presence of **heart assist device** [HCC] [ESR] [COM]
    - **Z95.812** Presence of **fully implantable artificial heart** [HCC] [ESR] [COM]
    - **Z95.818** Presence of other cardiac implants and grafts
  - ✓6ᵗʰ **Z95.82** Presence of other vascular implants and grafts
    - **Z95.820** Peripheral **vascular angioplasty status** with implants and grafts
      - EXCLUDES 1: peripheral vascular angioplasty without implant and graft (Z98.62)
    - **Z95.828** Presence of other vascular implants and grafts
      - Presence of intravascular prosthesis NEC
- **Z95.9** Presence of cardiac and vascular implant and graft, unspecified

✓4ᵗʰ **Z96 Presence of other functional implants**
- EXCLUDES 2: complications of internal prosthetic devices, implants and grafts (T82-T85)
  - fitting and adjustment of prosthetic and other devices (Z44-Z46)
- **Z96.0** Presence of **urogenital** implants

	Z96.1	Presence of intraocular lens
		Presence of pseudophakia
✓5th	Z96.2	Presence of otological and audiological implants
	Z96.20	Presence of otological and audiological implant, unspecified
	Z96.21	Cochlear implant status
	Z96.22	Myringotomy tube(s) status
	Z96.29	Presence of other otological and audiological implants
		Presence of bone-conduction hearing device
		Presence of eustachian tube stent
		Stapes replacement
	Z96.3	Presence of artificial larynx
✓5th	Z96.4	Presence of endocrine implants
	Z96.41	Presence of insulin pump (external) (internal)
	Z96.49	Presence of other endocrine implants
	Z96.5	Presence of tooth-root and mandibular implants
✓5th	Z96.6	Presence of orthopedic joint implants
		AHA: 2019,3Q,16
	Z96.60	Presence of unspecified orthopedic joint implant
✓6th	Z96.61	Presence of artificial shoulder joint
	Z96.611	Presence of right artificial shoulder joint
	Z96.612	Presence of left artificial shoulder joint
	Z96.619	Presence of unspecified artificial shoulder joint
✓6th	Z96.62	Presence of artificial elbow joint
	Z96.621	Presence of right artificial elbow joint
	Z96.622	Presence of left artificial elbow joint
	Z96.629	Presence of unspecified artificial elbow joint
✓6th	Z96.63	Presence of artificial wrist joint
	Z96.631	Presence of right artificial wrist joint
	Z96.632	Presence of left artificial wrist joint
	Z96.639	Presence of unspecified artificial wrist joint
✓6th	Z96.64	Presence of artificial hip joint
		Hip-joint replacement (partial) (total)
	Z96.641	Presence of right artificial hip joint
	Z96.642	Presence of left artificial hip joint
	Z96.643	Presence of artificial hip joint, bilateral
	Z96.649	Presence of unspecified artificial hip joint
✓6th	Z96.65	Presence of artificial knee joint
	Z96.651	Presence of right artificial knee joint
	Z96.652	Presence of left artificial knee joint
	Z96.653	Presence of artificial knee joint, bilateral
	Z96.659	Presence of unspecified artificial knee joint
✓6th	Z96.66	Presence of artificial ankle joint
	Z96.661	Presence of right artificial ankle joint
	Z96.662	Presence of left artificial ankle joint
	Z96.669	Presence of unspecified artificial ankle joint
✓6th	Z96.69	Presence of other orthopedic joint implants
	Z96.691	Finger-joint replacement of right hand
	Z96.692	Finger-joint replacement of left hand
	Z96.693	Finger-joint replacement, bilateral
	Z96.698	Presence of other orthopedic joint implants
	Z96.7	Presence of other bone and tendon implants
		Presence of skull plate
✓5th	Z96.8	Presence of other specified functional implants
	Z96.81	Presence of artificial skin
	Z96.82	Presence of neurostimulator
		Presence of brain neurostimulator
		Presence of gastric neurostimulator
		Presence of peripheral nerve neurostimulator
		Presence of sacral nerve neurostimulator
		Presence of spinal cord neurostimulator
		Presence of vagus nerve neurostimulator
		AHA: 2019,4Q,19
	Z96.89	Presence of other specified functional implants
	Z96.9	Presence of functional implant, unspecified
✓4th	Z97	Presence of other devices
	EXCLUDES 1	complications of internal prosthetic devices, implants and grafts (T82-T85)
	EXCLUDES 2	fitting and adjustment of prosthetic and other devices (Z44-Z46)
		presence of cerebrospinal fluid drainage device (Z98.2)
	Z97.0	Presence of artificial eye
✓5th	Z97.1	Presence of artificial limb (complete) (partial)
	Z97.10	Presence of artificial limb (complete) (partial), unspecified
	Z97.11	Presence of artificial right arm (complete) (partial)
	Z97.12	Presence of artificial left arm (complete) (partial)
	Z97.13	Presence of artificial right leg (complete) (partial)
	Z97.14	Presence of artificial left leg (complete) (partial)
	Z97.15	Presence of artificial arms, bilateral (complete) (partial)
	Z97.16	Presence of artificial legs, bilateral (complete) (partial)
	Z97.2	Presence of dental prosthetic device (complete) (partial)
		Presence of dentures (complete) (partial)
	Z97.3	Presence of spectacles and contact lenses
	Z97.4	Presence of external hearing-aid
	Z97.5	Presence of (intrauterine) contraceptive device
	EXCLUDES 1	checking, reinsertion or removal of implantable subdermal contraceptive (Z30.46)
		checking, reinsertion or removal of intrauterine contraceptive device (Z30.43-)
	Z97.8	Presence of other specified devices
✓4th	Z98	Other postprocedural states
	EXCLUDES 2	aftercare (Z43-Z49, Z51)
		follow-up medical care (Z08-Z09)
		▶Fontan related circulation (I27.84-)◀
		postprocedural complication - see Alphabetical Index
	Z98.0	Intestinal bypass and anastomosis status
	EXCLUDES 2	bariatric surgery status (Z98.84)
		gastric bypass status (Z98.84)
		obesity surgery status (Z98.84)
	Z98.1	Arthrodesis status
		AHA: 2024,1Q,23
	Z98.2	Presence of cerebrospinal fluid drainage device
		Presence of CSF shunt
	Z98.3	Post therapeutic collapse of lung status
		Code first underlying disease
✓5th	Z98.4	Cataract extraction status
		Use additional code to identify intraocular lens implant status (Z96.1)
	EXCLUDES 1	aphakia (H27.0)
	Z98.41	Cataract extraction status, right eye
	Z98.42	Cataract extraction status, left eye
	Z98.49	Cataract extraction status, unspecified eye
✓5th	Z98.5	Sterilization status
	EXCLUDES 1	female infertility (N97.-)
		male infertility (N46.-)
	Z98.51	Tubal ligation status
	Z98.52	Vasectomy status
✓5th	Z98.6	Angioplasty status
	Z98.61	Coronary angioplasty status
	EXCLUDES 1	coronary angioplasty status with implant and graft (Z95.5)
	Z98.62	Peripheral vascular angioplasty status
	EXCLUDES 1	peripheral vascular angioplasty status with implant and graft (Z95.820)
✓5th	Z98.8	Other specified postprocedural states
✓6th	Z98.81	Dental procedure status
	Z98.810	Dental sealant status
	Z98.811	Dental restoration status
		Dental crown status
		Dental fillings status
	Z98.818	Other dental procedure status
	Z98.82	Breast implant status
	EXCLUDES 1	breast implant removal status (Z98.86)
		AHA: 2022,3Q,8
	Z98.83	Filtering (vitreous) bleb after glaucoma surgery status
	EXCLUDES 1	inflammation (infection) of postprocedural bleb (H59.4-)
		AHA: 2020,3Q,29

Chapter 21. Factors Influencing Health Status and Contact With Health Services

Z98.84 **Bariatric surgery status**
Gastric banding status
Gastric bypass status for obesity
Obesity surgery status
EXCLUDES 1 bariatric surgery status complicating pregnancy, childbirth, or the puerperium (O99.84)
EXCLUDES 2 intestinal bypass and anastomosis status (Z98.0)
AHA: 2020,1Q,12

Z98.85 **Transplanted organ removal status**
Transplanted organ previously removed due to complication, failure, rejection or infection
EXCLUDES 1 encounter for removal of transplanted organ - code to complication of transplanted organ (T86.-)

Z98.86 **Personal history of breast implant removal**

✓6th **Z98.87** **Personal history of in utero procedure**

Z98.870 **Personal history of in utero procedure during pregnancy**
EXCLUDES 2 complications from in utero procedure for current pregnancy (O35.7)
supervision of current pregnancy with history of in utero procedure during previous pregnancy (O09.82-)

Z98.871 **Personal history of in utero procedure while a fetus**

✓6th **Z98.89** **Other specified postprocedural states**

Z98.890 **Other specified postprocedural states**
Personal history of surgery, not elsewhere classified
AHA: 2023,3Q,13

Z98.891 **History of uterine scar from previous surgery**
EXCLUDES 1 maternal care due to uterine scar from previous surgery (O34.2-)
AHA: 2016,4Q,51-52,76

✓4th **Z99** **Dependence on enabling machines and devices, not elsewhere classified**
AHA: 2020,1Q,11

Z99.0 **Dependence on aspirator**

✓5th **Z99.1** **Dependence on respirator**
Dependence on ventilator

Z99.11 **Dependence on respirator [ventilator] status** `HCC` `ESR` `COM`
▶Ventilator status◀
AHA: 2015,1Q,21

Z99.12 **Encounter for respirator [ventilator] dependence during power failure** `HCC` `ESR` `COM` `PDx`
EXCLUDES 1 mechanical complication of respirator [ventilator] (J95.850)

Z99.2 **Dependence on renal dialysis** `Rx` `ESR`
Hemodialysis status
Peritoneal dialysis status
Presence of arteriovenous shunt for dialysis
Renal dialysis status NOS
EXCLUDES 1 encounter for fitting and adjustment of dialysis catheter (Z49.0-)
EXCLUDES 2 noncompliance with renal dialysis (Z91.15-)
AHA: 2022,3Q,15; 2016,1Q,12; 2013,4Q,125

Z99.3 **Dependence on wheelchair**
Wheelchair confinement status
Code first cause of dependence, such as:
muscular dystrophy (G71.0-)
obesity (E66.-)

✓5th **Z99.8** **Dependence on other enabling machines and devices**

Z99.81 **Dependence on supplemental oxygen**
Dependence on long-term oxygen
AHA: 2013,4Q,129

Z99.89 **Dependence on other enabling machines and devices**
Dependence on machine or device NOS
AHA: 2020,1Q,11

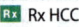 CMS-HCC   Rx HCC   ESRD HCC 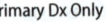 Commercial HCC   Primary Dx Only 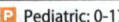 Newborn: 0 **P** Pediatric: 0-17 **M** Maternity: 9-64 **A** Adult: 15-124

Chapter 22. Codes for Special Purposes (U00–U85)

Chapter-specific Guidelines

- U07.0 Vaping-related disorder (see Section I.C.10.e., Vaping-related disorders)
- U07.1 COVID-19 (see Section I.C.1.g.1., COVID-19 infection)
- U09.9 Post COVID-19 condition, unspecified (see Section I.C.1.g.1.m.)

Chapter 22. Codes for Special Purposes (U00-U85)

This chapter contains the following blocks:

U00-U85 Provisional assignment of new diseases of uncertain etiology or emergency use

Provisional assignment of new diseases of uncertain etiology or emergency use (U00-U49)

✓4th U07 Emergency use of U07

U07.0 Vaping-related disorder
Dabbing related lung damage
Dabbing related lung injury
E-cigarette, or vaping, product use associated lung injury [EVALI]
Electronic cigarette related lung damage
Electronic cigarette related lung injury

Use additional code, to identify manifestations, such as:
  abdominal pain (R10.84)
  acute respiratory distress syndrome (J80)
  diarrhea (R19.7)
  drug-induced interstitial lung disorder (J70.4)
  lipoid pneumonia (J69.1)
  weight loss (R63.4)

DEF: Respiratory illness or injury caused by harmful aerosolized substances and chemicals produced by electronic cigarettes, vapes, e-pipes, and other battery-powered vaping devices. Symptoms may include shortness of breath and fever, while some patients experience severe, sometimes fatal, lung damage. *Synonym(s):* e-cigarette and vaping product use-associated lung injury, EVALI.

U07.1 COVID-19
Use additional code to identify pneumonia or other manifestations, such as:
Use additional code, if applicable, for associated conditions such as:
  COVID-19 associated coagulopathy (D68.8)
  disseminated intravascular coagulation (D65)
  hypercoagulable states (D68.69)
  pneumonia due to COVID-19 (J12.82)
  thrombophilia (D68.69)

EXCLUDES 2 coronavirus as the cause of diseases classified elsewhere (B97.2-)
pneumonia due to SARS-associated coronavirus (J12.81)

AHA: 2025,1Q,3,34; 2022,2Q,28; 2021,4Q,101,107-108; 2021,1Q,25-30,31-49; 2020,4Q,14,99; 2020,3Q,9-16; 2020,2Q,3-13

DEF: First diagnosed in December 2019 in China, coronavirus disease 2019 (COVID-19) is a respiratory infection caused by a newly identified (novel) virus not previously seen in humans, known as severe acute respiratory syndrome coronavirus 2 (SARS-CoV-2). Symptoms of this lower respiratory illness include fever, dry cough, and tiredness that may progress to include difficulty breathing. Older patients and those with high blood pressure, heart problems, and diabetes are more likely to develop serious symptoms of the illness. *Synonym(s):* SARS-CoV-2, coronavirus disease 2019.

TIP: Code U07.1 should not be assigned based solely on a positive COVID-19 blood test. A confirmed diagnosis of COVID-19 must be documented by the provider. If the diagnosis is unclear, a query should be submitted to the provider for clarification.

✓4th U09 Post COVID-19 condition

U09.9 Post COVID-19 condition, unspecified

NOTE This code enables establishment of a link with COVID-19.

This code is not to be used in cases that are still presenting with active COVID-19. However, an exception is made in cases of re-infection with COVID-19, occurring with a condition related to prior COVID-19.

Post-acute sequela of COVID-19
Code first the specific condition related to COVID-19 if known, such as:
  chronic respiratory failure (J96.1-)
  loss of smell (R43.8)
  loss of taste (R43.8)
  multisystem inflammatory syndrome (M35.81)
  pulmonary embolism (I26.-)
  pulmonary fibrosis (J84.10)

AHA: 2021,4Q,31-32,102-106

Appendixes

Appendix A: Valid 3-character ICD-10-CM Codes

A09	Infectious gastroenteritis and colitis, unspecified
A33	Tetanus neonatorum
A34	Obstetrical tetanus
A35	Other tetanus
A46	Erysipelas
A55	Chlamydial lymphogranuloma (venereum)
A57	Chancroid
A58	Granuloma inguinale
A64	Unspecified sexually transmitted disease
A65	Nonvenereal syphilis
A70	Chlamydia psittaci infections
A78	Q fever
A86	Unspecified viral encephalitis
A89	Unspecified viral infection of central nervous system
A90	Dengue fever [classical dengue]
A91	Dengue hemorrhagic fever
A94	Unspecified arthropod-borne viral fever
A99	Unspecified viral hemorrhagic fever
B03	Smallpox
B04	Monkeypox
B09	Unspecified viral infection characterized by skin and mucous membrane lesions
B20	Human immunodeficiency virus [HIV] disease
B49	Unspecified mycosis
B54	Unspecified malaria
B59	Pneumocystosis
B64	Unspecified protozoal disease
B72	Dracunculiasis
B75	Trichinellosis
B79	Trichuriasis
B80	Enterobiasis
B86	Scabies
B89	Unspecified parasitic disease
B91	Sequelae of poliomyelitis
B92	Sequelae of leprosy
C01	Malignant neoplasm of base of tongue
C07	Malignant neoplasm of parotid gland
C12	Malignant neoplasm of pyriform sinus
C19	Malignant neoplasm of rectosigmoid junction
C20	Malignant neoplasm of rectum
C23	Malignant neoplasm of gallbladder
C33	Malignant neoplasm of trachea
C37	Malignant neoplasm of thymus
C52	Malignant neoplasm of vagina
C55	Malignant neoplasm of uterus, part unspecified
C58	Malignant neoplasm of placenta
C61	Malignant neoplasm of prostate
C73	Malignant neoplasm of thyroid gland
D34	Benign neoplasm of thyroid gland
D45	Polycythemia vera
D62	Acute posthemorrhagic anemia
D65	Disseminated intravascular coagulation [defibrination syndrome]
D66	Hereditary factor VIII deficiency
D67	Hereditary factor IX deficiency
D77	Other disorders of blood and blood-forming organs in diseases classified elsewhere
E02	Subclinical iodine-deficiency hypothyroidism
E15	Nondiabetic hypoglycemic coma
E35	Disorders of endocrine glands in diseases classified elsewhere
E40	Kwashiorkor
E41	Nutritional marasmus
E42	Marasmic kwashiorkor
E43	Unspecified severe protein-calorie malnutrition
E45	Retarded development following protein-calorie malnutrition
E46	Unspecified protein-calorie malnutrition
E52	Niacin deficiency [pellagra]
E54	Ascorbic acid deficiency
E58	Dietary calcium deficiency
E59	Dietary selenium deficiency
E60	Dietary zinc deficiency
E65	Localized adiposity
E68	Sequelae of hyperalimentation
F04	Amnestic disorder due to known physiological condition
F05	Delirium due to known physiological condition
F09	Unspecified mental disorder due to known physiological condition
F21	Schizotypal disorder
F22	Delusional disorders
F23	Brief psychotic disorder
F24	Shared psychotic disorder
F28	Other psychotic disorder not due to a substance or known physiological condition
F29	Unspecified psychosis not due to a substance or known physiological condition
F39	Unspecified mood [affective] disorder
F42	Obsessive-compulsive disorder
F54	Psychological and behavioral factors associated with disorders or diseases classified elsewhere
F59	Unspecified behavioral syndromes associated with physiological disturbances and physical factors
F66	Other sexual disorders
F69	Unspecified disorder of adult personality and behavior
F70	Mild intellectual disabilities
F71	Moderate intellectual disabilities
F72	Severe intellectual disabilities
F73	Profound intellectual disabilities
F79	Unspecified intellectual disabilities
F82	Specific developmental disorder of motor function
F88	Other disorders of psychological development
F89	Unspecified disorder of psychological development
F99	Mental disorder, not otherwise specified
G01	Meningitis in bacterial diseases classified elsewhere
G02	Meningitis in other infectious and parasitic diseases classified elsewhere
G07	Intracranial and intraspinal abscess and granuloma in diseases classified elsewhere
G08	Intracranial and intraspinal phlebitis and thrombophlebitis
G09	Sequelae of inflammatory diseases of central nervous system
G10	Huntington's disease
G14	Postpolio syndrome
G26	Extrapyramidal and movement disorders in diseases classified elsewhere
G53	Cranial nerve disorders in diseases classified elsewhere
G55	Nerve root and plexus compressions in diseases classified elsewhere
G59	Mononeuropathy in diseases classified elsewhere
G63	Polyneuropathy in diseases classified elsewhere
G64	Other disorders of peripheral nervous system
G94	Other disorders of brain in diseases classified elsewhere
H22	Disorders of iris and ciliary body in diseases classified elsewhere
H28	Cataract in diseases classified elsewhere
H32	Chorioretinal disorders in diseases classified elsewhere
H42	Glaucoma in diseases classified elsewhere
I00	Rheumatic fever without heart involvement
I10	Essential (primary) hypertension
I32	Pericarditis in diseases classified elsewhere
I38	Endocarditis, valve unspecified
I39	Endocarditis and heart valve disorders in diseases classified elsewhere
I41	Myocarditis in diseases classified elsewhere
I43	Cardiomyopathy in diseases classified elsewhere
I52	Other heart disorders in diseases classified elsewhere
I5A	Non-ischemic myocardial injury (non-traumatic)
I76	Septic arterial embolism
I81	Portal vein thrombosis
I96	Gangrene, not elsewhere classified
J00	Acute nasopharyngitis (common cold)
J13	Pneumonia due to Streptococcus pneumoniae
J14	Pneumonia due to Hemophilus influenzae

Appendix A: Valid 3-character ICD-10-CM Codes

J17	Pneumonia in diseases classified elsewhere
J22	Unspecified acute lower respiratory infection
J36	Peritonsillar abscess
J40	Bronchitis, not specified as acute or chronic
J42	Unspecified chronic bronchitis
J60	Coalworker's pneumoconiosis
J61	Pneumoconiosis due to asbestos and other mineral fibers
J64	Unspecified pneumoconiosis
J65	Pneumoconiosis associated with tuberculosis
J80	Acute respiratory distress syndrome
J90	Pleural effusion, not elsewhere classified
J99	Respiratory disorders in diseases classified elsewhere
K23	Disorders of esophagus in diseases classified elsewhere
K30	Functional dyspepsia
K36	Other appendicitis
K37	Unspecified appendicitis
K67	Disorders of peritoneum in infectious diseases classified elsewhere
K77	Liver disorders in diseases classified elsewhere
K87	Disorders of gallbladder, biliary tract and pancreas in diseases classified elsewhere
L00	Staphylococcal scalded skin syndrome
L14	Bullous disorders in diseases classified elsewhere
L22	Diaper dermatitis
L26	Exfoliative dermatitis
L42	Pityriasis rosea
L45	Papulosquamous disorders in diseases classified elsewhere
L52	Erythema nodosum
L54	Erythema in diseases classified elsewhere
L62	Nail disorders in diseases classified elsewhere
L80	Vitiligo
L83	Acanthosis nigricans
L84	Corns and callosities
L86	Keratoderma in diseases classified elsewhere
L88	Pyoderma gangrenosum
L99	Other disorders of skin and subcutaneous tissue in diseases classified elsewhere
N08	Glomerular disorders in diseases classified elsewhere
N10	Acute tubulo-interstitial nephritis
N12	Tubulo-interstitial nephritis, not specified as acute or chronic
N16	Renal tubulo-interstitial disorders in diseases classified elsewhere
N19	Unspecified kidney failure
N22	Calculus of urinary tract in diseases classified elsewhere
N23	Unspecified renal colic
N29	Other disorders of kidney and ureter in diseases classified elsewhere
N33	Bladder disorders in diseases classified elsewhere
N37	Urethral disorders in diseases classified elsewhere
N51	Disorders of male genital organs in diseases classified elsewhere
N61	Inflammatory disorders of breast
N62	Hypertrophy of breast
N72	Inflammatory disease of cervix uteri
N74	Female pelvic inflammatory disorders in diseases classified elsewhere
N86	Erosion and ectropion of cervix uteri
N96	Recurrent pregnancy loss
O68	Labor and delivery complicated by abnormality of fetal acid-base balance
O76	Abnormality in fetal heart rate and rhythm complicating labor and delivery
O80	Encounter for full-term uncomplicated delivery
O82	Encounter for cesarean delivery without indication
O85	Puerperal sepsis
O94	Sequelae of complication of pregnancy, childbirth, and the puerperium
P53	Hemorrhagic disease of newborn
P60	Disseminated intravascular coagulation of newborn
P84	Other problems with newborn
P90	Convulsions of newborn
P95	Stillbirth
Q02	Microcephaly
R12	Heartburn
R17	Unspecified jaundice
R21	Rash and other nonspecific skin eruption
R32	Unspecified urinary incontinence
R34	Anuria and oliguria
R37	Sexual dysfunction, unspecified
R42	Dizziness and giddiness
R52	Pain, unspecified
R54	Age-related physical debility
R55	Syncope and collapse
R58	Hemorrhage, not elsewhere classified
R61	Generalized hyperhidrosis
R64	Cachexia
R69	Illness, unspecified
R75	Inconclusive laboratory evidence of human immunodeficiency virus [HIV]
R81	Glycosuria
R99	Ill-defined and unknown cause of mortality
Y09	Assault by unspecified means
Y66	Nonadministration of surgical and medical care
Y69	Unspecified misadventure during surgical and medical care
Y95	Nosocomial condition
Z08	Encounter for follow-up examination after completed treatment for malignant neoplasm
Z09	Encounter for follow-up examination after completed treatment for conditions other than malignant neoplasm
Z21	Asymptomatic human immunodeficiency virus [HIV] infection status
Z23	Encounter for immunization
Z66	Do not resuscitate

Appendix B: Pharmacology List 2026

This section enables the coder to quickly review drugs, drug actions, and indications that are often associated with overlooked or undocumented diagnoses. The coder should review the patient's medication record and know what condition the physician is treating with the prescribed medication based on documentation in the medical record. When documentation is lacking, the coder can reference this section to locate the drug, determine the drug action, confirm drug indications, and when necessary query the physician. When applicable, some of the drugs provided in this resource have also been mapped to their appropriate Z code for long-term drug use.

Drug	Z Code	Drug Action/Classification	Indications
5-fluorouracil (5-FU) [fluorouracil]	Z79.631	Antimetabolite agent	Skin, colorectal, breast, stomach, and pancreas cancer
6-mercaptopurine (6-MP) [mercaptopurine]	Z79.631	Antimetabolite agent	Acute lymphoblastic leukemia
Abilify [aripiprazole]		Antipsychotic	Depression; bipolar I disorder; schizophrenia; autism symptoms
Acarbose [acarbose]	Z79.84	Oral hypoglycemic	Diabetes mellitus
Acetaminophen with codeine [acetaminophen/codeine phosphate]	Z79.891	Analgesic, narcotic	Moderate to severe pain
Aclasta [zoledronic acid]	Z79.83	Bisphosphonate	Osteoporosis in postmenopausal women; Paget's disease
Actemra [tocilizumab]	Z79.620	Immunosuppressive biologic/monoclonal antibody	Rheumatoid arthritis; systemic sclerosis-associated interstitial lung disease; giant cell arteritis; polyarticular or systemic juvenile idiopathic arthritis; cytokine release syndrome; COVID-19 for certain pediatric and adult populations
Actimmune [interferon gamma-1b]	Z79.69	Other immunosuppressant/immunomodulator	Chronic granulomatous disease; malignant osteopetrosis
Activella [estradiol/norethindrone acetate]	Z79.890	Estrogen therapy	Menopause symptoms; vaginal and vulvar atrophy; osteoporosis prevention
Actonel [risedronate sodium]	Z79.83	Bisphosphonate	Osteoporosis; Paget's disease
Actoplus Met [metformin hydrochloride/pioglitazone hydrochloride]	Z79.84	Oral hypoglycemic	Diabetes mellitus
Actos [pioglitazone hydrochloride]	Z79.84	Oral hypoglycemic	Diabetes mellitus
Aczone [dapsone]		Acne agent, topical	Acne vulgaris
Adderall XR [amphetamine aspartate and sulfate/dextroamphetamine saccharate and sulfate]		CNS stimulant	Attention deficit hyperactivity disorder (ADHD)
Adlarity [donepezil hydrochloride]		Acetylcholinesterase/cholinesterase inhibitors	Dementia due to Alzheimer's
Admelog [insulin lispro]	Z79.4	Insulin	Diabetes mellitus
Advair [fluticasone propionate/salmeterol xinafoate]	Z79.51	Corticosteroid – inhaled/antiasthmatic	Prophylaxis and treatment of asthma and COPD
Advil [ibuprofen]	Z79.1	Nonsteroidal anti-inflammatory drug (NSAID)	Pain or fever relief
Afrezza [human insulin recombinant]		Insulin – inhaled	Diabetes mellitus
Agamree [vamorolone]	Z79.52	Corticosteroid	Duchenne muscular dystrophy
Aggrastat [tirofiban hydrochloride]	Z79.02	Antiplatelet	Unstable angina; heart attacks
Aimovig [erenumab-aooe]	Z79.620	Immunosuppressive biologic/monoclonal antibody	Migraine headache prevention
AirDuo RespiClick [fluticasone propionate/salmeterol xinafoate]	Z79.51	Corticosteroid – inhaled/antiasthmatic	Asthma
Aklief [trifarotene]		Acne agent, topical	Acne vulgaris
Aldactone [spironolactone]		Cardiovascular agent; antihypertensive agent; diuretic; electrolytic and renal agent	Severe heart failure; ascites associated with cirrhosis; hypokalemia; hypertension; fluid retention in heart failure, cirrhosis, and nephrotic syndrome
Aleve [naproxen sodium]	Z79.1	Nonsteroidal anti-inflammatory drug (NSAID)	Reduction of temporary aches and pains
Allegra allergy [fexofenadine hydrochloride]		Antihistamine	Seasonal allergic rhinitis
Allopurinol [allopurinol]		Antigout	Gouty arthritis; renal calculus; hyperuricemia; hyperuricemia secondary to leukemia; hyperuricemia secondary to lymphoma
Alora [estradiol]	Z79.890	Estrogen therapy	Menopause symptoms
Alphagan P [brimonidine tartrate]		Antiglaucoma agent (ophthalmic); antihypertensive, ocular	Open angle glaucoma or another condition in which pressure in the eye is too high (ocular hypertension)
Alprazolam [alprazolam]		Antianxiety; sedative/hypnotic	Anxiety and panic disorders
Altabax [retapamulin]	Z79.2	Antibiotic, topical	Skin infections
Altace [ramipril]		ACE inhibitor	Congestive heart failure; hypertension
Alvesco [ciclesonide]	Z79.51	Corticosteroid – inhaled; antiasthmatic	Prophylaxis and treatment of asthma
Amaryl [glimepiride]	Z79.84	Oral hypoglycemic	Diabetes mellitus
Ambien [zolpidem tartrate]		CNS depressant; anxiolytic/sedative/hypnotic	Insomnia
Amikacin [amikacin sulfate]	Z79.2	Antibiotic	Gram-negative bacterial infections such as Pseudomonas, Escherichia coli (E. coli), Proteus, Klebsiella-Enterobacter-Serratia

Drug	Z Code	Drug Action/Classification	Indications
Amitriptyline HCl [amitriptyline hydrochloride]		Antidepressant	Depression
Amoxicillin [amoxicillin]	Z79.2	Antibiotic	Treatment of infections with a broad spectrum of bactericidal activity against many gram-positive and gram-negative microorganisms; otitis media, gonorrhea, skin, respiratory, gastrointestinal, and genitourinary infections
Ampicillin [ampicillin sodium]	Z79.2	Antibiotic	Bacterial infections
Ampyra [dalfampridine]		Potassium channel blocker	Improvement in walking in patients with multiple sclerosis
Amrix [cyclobenzaprine hydrochloride]			Adjunct to rest and physical therapy for muscle spasms
Anaprox DS [naproxen sodium]	Z79.1	Nonsteroidal anti-inflammatory drug (NSAID)	Pain, inflammation or fever relief
Anastrozole [anastrozole]	Z79.811	Aromatase inhibitor	Postmenopausal breast cancer
Androderm [testosterone]	Z79.890	Testosterone therapy – topical	Primary hypogonadism; hypogonadotropic hypogonadism
AndroGel [testosterone]	Z79.890	Testosterone therapy – topical	Primary hypogonadism; hypogonadotropic hypogonadism
Angeliq [drospirenone/estradiol]	Z79.890	Estrogen therapy	Menopause symptoms
Angiomax [bivalirudin]	Z79.02	Antithrombotic	Prevention of blood clots
Antineoplastic/chemotherapy		Antineoplastic	Cancer
Aphexda [motixafortide]		Immunostimulant	Multiple myeloma
Apidra [insulin glulisine recombinant]	Z79.4	Insulin	Diabetes mellitus
Aranelle [ethinyl estradiol/norethindrone]	Z79.3	Contraceptive	Prevention of pregnancy; acne
Aranesp [darbepoetin alfa]		Erythropoiesis-stimulating agent (ESA)	Treatment of anemia in disorders such as CKD and neoplasms
Aredia [pamidronate disodium]	Z79.83	Bisphosphonate	Osteoporosis
Argatroban [argatroban]	Z79.02	Antithrombotic	Prophylaxis and treatment of venous thrombosis in thrombocytopenia patients
Aricept [donepezil hydrochloride]		Acetylcholinesterase/cholinesterase inhibitors	Dementia due to Alzheimer's
Arimidex [anastrozole]	Z79.811	Aromatase inhibitor; antineoplastic	Postmenopausal breast cancer
Arixtra [fondaparinux sodium]	Z79.01	Anticoagulant	Venous thrombosis and pulmonary embolism
Arnuity Ellipta [fluticasone furoate]	Z79.51	Corticosteroid – inhaled; antiasthmatic	Prophylaxis and treatment of asthma
Aromasin [exemestane]	Z79.811	Aromatase inhibitor	Postmenopausal breast cancer
Arthrotec [diclofenac sodium/misoprostol]	Z79.1	Nonsteroidal anti-inflammatory drug (NSAID)-prostaglandin combo	Treatment of patients with osteoarthritis or rheumatoid arthritis who may develop stomach ulcers from taking nonsteroidal anti-inflammatory drugs (NSAIDs) alone
Asmanex [mometasone furoate]	Z79.51	Corticosteroid – inhaled; antiasthmatic	Prophylaxis and treatment of asthma
Astagraf XL [tacrolimus]	Z79.621	Calcineurin inhibitor; immunosuppressant	Prophylaxis of organ transplant rejection
Atelvia [risedronate sodium]	Z79.83	Bisphosphonate	Osteoporosis
Atenolol [atenolol]		Beta blocker	Angina pectoris; hypertension; acute myocardial infarction
Ativan [lorazepam]		Antianxiety; sedative/hypnotic	Anxiety disorder associated with depressive symptoms; controls tension, agitation, irritability, and insomnia
Atripla [efavirenz/emtricitabine/tenofovir disoproxil fumarate]		Antiretroviral	HIV
Atrovent HFA [ipratropium bromide]		Antiasthmatic/bronchodilator	Chronic bronchitis, emphysema; bronchial asthma
Augmentin [amoxicillin/clavulanate potassium]	Z79.2	Antibiotic	Bacterial infections of the middle ear, lower respiratory, sinus, skin and skin structures; urinary tract infections
Augtyro [repotrectinib]		Kinase inhibitor	ROS1-Positive non-small cell lung cancer
Avapro [irbesartan]		Antihypertensive	Hypertension
Avelox [moxifloxacin hydrochloride]	Z79.2	Antibiotic	Bacterial infections of the skin, sinuses, lungs, or stomach; plague
Aviane-28 [ethinyl estradiol/levonorgestrel]	Z79.3	Contraceptive	Prevention of pregnancy
Avonex [interferon beta-1a]	Z79.69	Other immunosuppressant/immunomodulator	Treatment of relapsing multiple sclerosis
Axid AR [nizatidine]		Histamine H2-receptor antagonist	Acid/peptic disorder; gastroesophageal reflux; duodenal, gastric, and peptic ulcers
Ayvakit [avapritinib]		Multikinase inhibitor	Unresectable or metastatic gastrointestinal stromal tumor (GIST); advanced systemic mastocytosis
Azactam [aztreonam]	Z79.2	Antibiotic	Severe bacterial infections
Azithromycin [azithromycin]	Z79.2	Antibiotic	Bacterial infections
Azstarys [serdexmethylphenidate and dexmethylphenidate]		CNS stimulant	Attention deficit hyperactivity disorder (ADHD)
Bactrim [sulfamethoxazole/trimethoprim]	Z79.2	Antibiotic	Urinary tract infections; acute otitis media; acute exacerbation of chronic bronchitis; shigellosis; Pneumocystis carinii infections
Basaglar [insulin glargine]	Z79.4	Insulin	Diabetes mellitus

Drug	Z Code	Drug Action/Classification	Indications
Bayer [acetylsalicylic acid]	Z79.82	Aspirin	Prophylaxis and treatment of heart attacks, angina or strokes; reduction of fever, pain, and inflammation
Benztropine mesylate [benztropine mesylate]		Anticholinergic antiparkinson agent	Parkinson's disease
Betaseron [interferon beta-1b]	Z79.69	Other immunosuppressant/ immunomodulator	Treatment of relapsing multiple sclerosis
Betoptic [betaxolol hydrochloride]		Beta blocker; ophthalmic glaucoma agent	Lowering of intraocular pressure; also used for treatment of ocular hypertension and chronic open-angle glaucoma
Beyaz [drospirenone/ethinyl estradiol/ levomefolate calcium]	Z79.3	Contraceptive	Prevention of pregnancy; acne vulgaris
Beyfortus [nirsevimab-alip]	Z79.620	Immunostimulant; monoclonal antibody	Lower respiratory tract disease (LRTD) caused by RSV
Biaxin XL [clarithromycin]	Z79.2	Antibiotic	Acid/peptic disorder or ulcer; acute exacerbation chronic bronchitis; human immunodeficiency virus; lower and upper respiratory tract infection; sinus infection; prophylaxis mycobacterium avium complex; pharyngitis; pneumonia; tonsillitis
Bijuva [estradiol/progesterone]	Z79.890	Estrogen/progesterone therapy	Menopausal symptoms
Biktarvy [bictegravir sodium/emtricitabine/ tenofovir alafenamide fumarate]		Antiretroviral	HIV
Biltricide [praziquantel]		Antiparasitic	Infections from Schistosoma species and liver flukes
Bimzelx [bimekizumab]	Z79.69	Other immunosuppressant/ immunomodulator	Plaque psoriasis
Binosto [alendronate sodium]	Z79.83	Bisphosphonate	Osteoporosis
Bleomycin [bleomycin]	Z79.632	Antitumor antibiotic	Squamous cell carcinoma; Hodgkin's disease; non-Hodgkin's lymphoma; malignant pleural effusion; testicular cancer
Brenzavvy [bexagliflozin]	Z79.84	Oral hypoglycemic	Diabetes mellitus
Breo Ellipta [fluticasone furoate/vilanterol trifenatate]	Z79.51	Corticosteroid – inhaled; antiasthmatic	Asthma and COPD
Brexafemme [ibrexafungerp]		Antifungal	Vulvovaginal candidiasis
Briellyn [ethinyl estradiol/norethindrone]	Z79.3	Contraceptive	Prevention of pregnancy
Brilinta [ticagrelor]	Z79.02	Antiplatelet	Unstable angina; heart attacks; prevention of blood clots
Brisdelle [paroxetine mesylate]		Selective serotonin reuptake inhibitor (SSRI)	Vasomotor symptoms related to menopause
Briumvi [ublituximab-xiiy]	Z79.620	Immunosuppressive biologic; monoclonal antibody	Multiple sclerosis
Bufferin [aspirin]	Z79.82	Aspirin	Pain, reduce fever or inflammation; prophylaxis and treatment of heart attack, stroke, angina
Buprenorphine HCl and Naloxone HCl [buprenorphine hydrochloride/naloxone hydrochloride]	Z79.891	Analgesic, narcotic	Opioid addiction
Buspirone HCl [buspirone hydrochloride]		Antianxiety	Generalized anxiety disorder
Busulfex [busulfan]	Z79.630	Chemotherapeutic alkylating agent	Chronic myelogenous leukemia
Butrans [buprenorphine]	Z79.891	Analgesic, narcotic	Chronic pain
Bydureon bcise [exenatide]	Z79.85	Antidiabetic – non-insulin injectable	Diabetes mellitus
Byetta [exenatide]	Z79.85	Antidiabetic – non-insulin injectable	Diabetes mellitus
Caldolor [ibuprofen]	Z79.1	Nonsteroidal anti-inflammatory drug (NSAID)	Pain or fever relief
Cambia [diclofenac potassium]	Z79.1	Nonsteroidal anti-inflammatory drug (NSAID)	Migraine headache
Camila [norethindrone]	Z79.3	Contraceptive	Prevention of pregnancy; menstrual disorders
Camptosar [irinotecan]	Z79.634	Topoisomerase inhibitor	Metastatic colon or rectal cancer
Camzyos [mavacamten]		Cardiovascular agent	Symptomatic obstructive hypertrophic cardiomyopathy (HCM)
Caplyta [lumateperone]		Antipsychotic	Schizophrenia
Cardizem CD [diltiazem hydrochloride]		Calcium channel blocker	Chronic stable angina; angina due to coronary artery spasm; hypertension
Cardura [doxazosin mesylate]		Antiadrenergic; antihypertensive	Benign prostatic hyperplasia; hypertension
Carmustine [carmustine]	Z79.630	Chemotherapeutic alkylating agent	Brain tumors; Hodgkin's disease; multiple myeloma; non-Hodgkin's lymphoma
Cefazolin sodium [cefazolin sodium]	Z79.2	Antibiotic	Bacterial infections
Cefepime hydrochloride [cefepime hydrochloride]	Z79.2	Antibiotic	Bacterial infections
Cefprozil [cefprozil]	Z79.2	Antibiotic	Bacterial infections
Ceftriaxone [ceftriaxone sodium]	Z79.2	Antibiotic	Bacterial infections
Cefuroxime sodium [cefuroxime sodium]	Z79.2	Antibiotic	Bacterial infections

Drug	Z Code	Drug Action/Classification	Indications
Celebrex [celecoxib]	Z79.1	Nonsteroidal anti-inflammatory drug (NSAID)	Osteoarthritis; rheumatoid arthritis; juvenile rheumatoid arthritis; ankylosing spondylitis; acute pain; primary dysmenorrhea
Celestone Soluspan [betamethasone acetate/betamethasone sodium phosphate]	Z79.52	Corticosteroid; antiasthmatic	Asthma; severe inflammation
Celexa [citalopram hydrobromide]		Antidepressant	Depression
CellCept [mycophenolate mofetil]	Z79.624	Inhibitors of nucleotide synthesis; immunosuppressant	Prophylaxis of organ transplant rejection
Centany [mupirocin]	Z79.2	Antibiotic, topical	Bacterial skin infections
Cephalexin [cephalexin]	Z79.2	Antibiotic	Bacterial infections
Cerubidine [daunorubicin hydrochloride]	Z79.632	Antitumor antibiotic	Leukemia
Chlorambucil [chlorambucil]	Z79.630	Chemotherapeutic alkylating agent	Chronic lymphocytic leukemia; malignant lymphoma
Cibinqo [abrocitinib]	Z79.622	Janus kinase (JAK) inhibitor	Atopic dermatitis
Cimduo [lamivudine/tenofovir disoproxil fumarate]		Antiretroviral	HIV
Cipro [ciprofloxacin hydrochloride]	Z79.2	Antibiotic	Cystitis; infectious diarrhea; gonorrhea; bone and joint infection; gastrointestinal tract infection; lower and upper respiratory tract infection; sinus infection; urinary tract infection; nosocomial pneumonia; chronic prostatitis
Ciprofloxacin [ciprofloxacin]	Z79.2	Antibiotic	Bacterial infections
Cisplatin [cisplatin]	Z79.630	Chemotherapeutic alkylating agent	Cancer
Clarithromycin [clarithromycin]	Z79.2	Antibiotic	Skin and respiratory bacterial infections; stomach ulcers caused by Helicobacter pylori
Claritin [loratadine]		Antihistamine	Seasonal allergic rhinitis; chronic idiopathic urticaria
Cleocin [clindamycin phosphate]	Z79.2	Antibiotic	Bacterial infections
Climara [estradiol]	Z79.890	Estrogen therapy	Osteoporosis; menopausal symptoms; vaginal and vulvar atrophy; hypoestrogenism; ovarian failure
Clindamycin [clindamycin phosphate]	Z79.2	Antibiotic	Bacterial infections
Clonazepam [clonazepam]		Anticonvulsant	Absence, akinetic, and myoclonic epilepsy; Lennox-Gastaut syndrome; panic disorders
Clonidine HCl [clonidine hydrochloride]		Antihypertensive	Hypertension
Clopidogrel bisulfate [clopidogrel bisulfate]	Z79.02	Antiplatelet	Unstable angina; heart attacks; prevention of blood clots
Codeine [codeine sulfate]	Z79.891	Analgesic, narcotic	Mild to moderate pain
Colace [docusate sodium]		Gastrointestinal agent; laxative, stool softener	Constipation
Colazal [balsalazide]		Anti-inflammatory	Ulcerative colitis
Colocort [hydrocortisone]	Z79.52	Corticosteroid	Inflammation of the colon
Columvi [glofitamab-gxbm]	Z79.620	Monoclonal antibody	Large B-cell lymphoma
CombiPatch [ethinyl estradiol/norethindrone acetate]	Z79.890	Estrogen therapy	Menopause symptoms; vaginal and vulvar atrophy; osteoporosis prevention
Combivent Respimat [ipratropium bromide/albuterol sulfate]		Antiasthmatic/bronchodilator	Chronic bronchitis, emphysema; bronchial asthma
Compro [prochlorperazine]		Antiemetic; antipsychotic	Nausea and vomiting; manic phase of bipolar syndrome or schizophrenia
Copaxone [glatiramer acetate]	Z79.69	Other immunosuppressant/immunomodulator	Multiple sclerosis
Coreg [carvedilol]		Beta blocker	Hypertension; chronic heart failure; left ventricular dysfunction following myocardial infarction
Coreg CR [carvedilol phosphate]		Beta blocker	Hypertension; chronic heart failure; left ventricular dysfunction following myocardial infarction
Cortef [hydrocortisone]	Z79.52	Corticosteroid	Severe inflammation
Cortenema [hydrocortisone]	Z79.52	Corticosteroid	Inflammation of the colon
Cortifoam [hydrocortisone acetate]	Z79.52	Corticosteroid	Colon and rectum inflammation
Cosentyx [secukinumab]	Z79.620	Immunosuppressive biologic; monoclonal antibody	Plaque psoriasis; psoriatic arthritis; ankylosing spondylitis
Cozaar [losartan potassium]		Antihypertensive	Hypertension
Crestor [rosuvastatin calcium]		HMG-CoA reductase inhibitor (statin)	Hypercholesterolemia; hyperlipidemia; hyperproteinemia
Cyclosporine [cyclosporine]	Z79.621	Calcineurin inhibitor	Prophylaxis of organ transplant rejection
Cyltezo [adalimumab-adbm]	Z79.620	Immunosuppressive biologic; monoclonal antibody	Rheumatoid arthritis; juvenile idiopathic arthritis; psoriatic arthritis; Crohn's disease; ulcerative colitis; plaque psoriasis
Cymbalta [duloxetine hydrochloride]		Antidepressant, serotonin and norepinephrine reuptake inhibitor (SNRI)	Major depressive disorder; general anxiety disorder; fibromyalgia; diabetic peripheral neuropathy; chronic musculoskeletal pain

Drug	Z Code	Drug Action/Classification	Indications
Cytarabine [cytarabine]	Z79.631	Antimetabolite agent	Leukemia
Cytomel [liothyronine sodium]		Thyroid hormone	Hypothyroidism or prevention of euthyroid goiters
Cytoxan [cyclophosphamide]	Z79.630	Chemotherapeutic alkylating agent	Cancer
Daptomycin [daptomycin]	Z79.2	Antibiotic	Bacterial infections of the skin, underlying tissues, and bloodstream
Daybue [trofinetide]		CNS agent	Rett syndrome
Daypro [oxaprozin]	Z79.1	Nonsteroidal anti-inflammatory drug (NSAID)	Osteoarthritis; rheumatoid arthritis; juvenile rheumatoid arthritis
Daysee [ethinyl estradiol/levonorgestrel]	Z79.3	Contraceptive	Prevention of pregnancy
Defencath [taurolidine, heparin]	Z79.01	Antimicrobial; anticoagulant	Catheter-related bloodstream infections
Delestrogen [estradiol valerate]	Z79.890	Estrogen therapy	Menopause symptoms
Demerol [meperidine hydrochloride]	Z79.891	Analgesic, narcotic	Moderate to severe pain
Depakote [divalproex sodium]		Anticonvulsant	Bipolar affective disorder; complex absence, complex partial and mixed pattern epilepsy; migraine headache
Depo-Medrol [methylprednisolone acetate]	Z79.52	Corticosteroid	Arthritis; joint disorders
Depo-Provera [medroxyprogesterone acetate]	Z79.3	Contraceptive	Prevention of pregnancy
Depo-SubQ Provera [medroxyprogesterone acetate]	Z79.3	Contraceptive	Prevention of pregnancy; menstrual disorder pain
Descovy [emtricitabine/tenofovir alafenamide]		Antiretroviral	HIV
Desogestrel/ethinyl estradiol [desogestrel/ethinyl estradiol]	Z79.3	Contraceptive	Prevention of pregnancy
Detrol [tolterodine tartrate]		Muscarinic receptor antagonist	Overactive bladders in patients with urinary frequency, urgency, or urge incontinence
Dexamethasone Intensol [dexamethasone]	Z79.52	Corticosteroid	Arthritis; allergic disorders; breathing disorders; inflammation; lupus
Dexilant [dexlansoprazole]		Proton pump inhibitor	Erosive esophagitis; heartburn; nonerosive gastroesophageal reflux disease
DiaBeta [glyburide]	Z79.84	Oral hypoglycemic	Diabetes mellitus
Diclegis [doxylamine succinate/pyridoxine hydrochloride]		Antiemetic	Nausea/vomiting in pregnancy
Dificid [fidaxomicin]	Z79.2	Antibiotic	Clostridium difficile
Diflucan [fluconazole]		Antifungal	Oropharyngeal and esophageal candidiasis; cryptococcal meningitis in AIDS patients; vaginal candidiasis
Digoxin [digoxin]		Antiarrhythmic; inotropic agent	Heart failure; atrial flutter; atrial fibrillation; supraventricular tachycardia
Dilantin [phenytoin sodium]		Anticonvulsant	Grand mal and psychomotor seizures
Dilaudid [hydromorphone hydrochloride]	Z79.891	Analgesic, narcotic	Moderate to severe pain
Diovan [valsartan]		Antihypertensive	Hypertension; heart failure; post-myocardial infarction
Diskets [methadone hydrochloride]		Opioid agonist	Treatment of opioid addiction
Disulfiram [disulfiram]		Alcohol treatment	Alcoholism
Divigel [estradiol]	Z79.890	Estrogen therapy – topical	Menopause symptoms
Dovato [dolutegravir sodium/lamivudine]		Antiretroviral	HIV
Doxorubicin [doxorubicin]	Z79.632	Antitumor antibiotic	Hodgkin lymphoma; non-Hodgkin lymphoma; specific types of cancers and leukemias
Doxycycline [doxycycline]	Z79.2	Antibiotic	Bacterial infections; acne
Duavee [bazedoxifene acetate/conjugated estrogens]	Z79.890	Estrogen therapy	Menopause symptoms; osteoporosis
Duetact [glimepiride/pioglitazone hydrochloride]	Z79.84	Oral hypoglycemic	Diabetes mellitus
Duexis [famotidine/ibuprofen]	Z79.1	Nonsteroidal anti-inflammatory drug (NSAID)	Osteoarthritis and rheumatoid arthritis; reduce risk of upper gastrointestinal ulcers
Dulera [formoterol fumarate/mometasone furoate]	Z79.51	Corticosteroid – inhaled; antiasthmatic	Asthma
Dupixent [dupilumab]	Z79.620	Immunosuppressive biologic; monoclonal antibody	Atopic dermatitis; asthma; chronic rhinosinusitis with nasal polyps; eosinophilic esophagitis; prurigo nodularis
Duramorph PF [morphine sulfate]	Z79.891	Analgesic, narcotic	Moderate to severe pain
Durlaza [aspirin]	Z79.82	Aspirin	Pain; inflammation; prevention of heart attack, stroke, angina
Dymista [azelastine/fluticasone]		Corticosteroid – intranasal	Seasonal allergies
E.E.S. [erythromycin ethylsuccinate]	Z79.2	Antibiotic	Bacterial infections
Efavirenz (efavirenz)		Antiretroviral	HIV

Drug	Z Code	Drug Action/Classification	Indications
Effexor XR [venlafaxine hydrochloride]		Antidepressant, serotonin and norepinephrine reuptake inhibitors (SNRIs)	Major depressive disorder; social anxiety disorder; panic disorder
Effient [prasugrel hydrochloride]	Z79.02	Antiplatelet	Reduce risk of heart attack or stroke
Elestrin [estradiol]	Z79.890	Estrogen therapy	Menopause symptoms
Elfabrio [pegunigalsidase alfa-iwxj]		Enzyme replacement therapy	Fabry disease
Eligard [leuprolide acetate]	Z79.818	Agents affecting estrogen receptors and estrogen levels	Palliative treatment of prostate cancer symptoms
Eliquis [apixaban]	Z79.01	Anticoagulant	Venous thrombosis
Elrexfio [elranatamab-bcmm]	Z79.620	Monoclonal antibody	Multiple myeloma
Enbrel [etanercept]	Z79.620	Immunosuppressive biologic; antirheumatic	Rheumatoid arthritis; polyarticular juvenile idiopathic arthritis; psoriatic arthritis; ankylosing spondylitis; plaque psoriasis
Enjaymo [sutimlimab-jome]	Z79.69	Other immunosuppressant/immunomodulator	Decreases need for red blood cell transfusion due to breakdown of red blood cells (hemolysis) in adults with cold agglutinin disease (CAD)
Enpresse-28 [ethinyl estradiol/levonorgestrel]	Z79.3	Contraceptive	Prevention of pregnancy
Entocort EC [budesonide]	Z79.52	Corticosteroid	Crohn's disease; ulcerative colitis
Entresto [sacubitril/valsartan]		Angiotensin II receptor blocker; neprilysin inhibitor	Chronic heart failure
Entyvio [vedolizumab]	Z79.620	Immunosuppressive biologic; monoclonal antibody	Crohn's disease; ulcerative colitis
Envarsus XR [tacrolimus]	Z79.621	Calcineurin inhibitor	Prophylaxis of organ transplant rejection
Epinephrine [epinephrine]		Bronchodilator, cardiotonic	Hypotension associated with septic shock; anaphylaxis
Epivir, Epivir-HBV [lamivudine]		Antiretroviral	HIV; chronic hepatitis B
Epkinly [epcoritamab-bysp]	Z79.620	Monoclonal antibody	Large B-cell lymphoma; high-grade B-cell lymphoma
Eptifibatide [eptifibatide]	Z79.02	Antiplatelet	Unstable angina; heart attacks; prevention of blood clots
Erelzi [etanercept-szzs]	Z79.620	Immunosuppressive biologic	Rheumatoid arthritis; polyarticular juvenile idiopathic arthritis; psoriatic arthritis; ankylosing spondylitis
Ertapenem [ertapenem sodium]	Z79.2	Antibiotic	Bacterial infections of the stomach, urinary tract, pelvis, skin, and lung
ERYC [erythromycin]	Z79.2	Antibiotic	Respiratory tract infections
Erygel [erythromycin]	Z79.2	Antibiotic, topical	Bacterial skin infections
EryPed [erythromycin ethylsuccinate]	Z79.2	Antibiotic	Bacterial infections; rheumatic fever attacks
Ery-Tab [erythromycin]	Z79.2	Antibiotic	Bacterial infections
Erythrocin [erythromycin lactobionate]	Z79.2	Antibiotic	Bacterial infections
Erythromycin [erythromycin]	Z79.2	Antibiotic	Respiratory tract infections
Estrace [estradiol]	Z79.890	Estrogen therapy	Vaginal cream for treatment of vaginal and vulvar atrophy
EstroGel [estradiol]	Z79.890	Estrogen therapy – topical	Menopause symptoms
Etoposide [etoposide]	Z79.634	Topoisomerase inhibitor	Small cell lung cancer
Evista [raloxifene hydrochloride]	Z79.810	Selective estrogen receptor modulator (SERM)	Osteoporosis in postmenopausal women
Exemestane [exemestane]	Z79.811	Aromatase inhibitor	Postmenopausal breast cancer
Exxua [gepirone]		Antidepressant	Major depressive disorder
Fareston [toremifene citrate]	Z79.810	Selective estrogen receptor modulator (SERM)	Postmenopausal breast cancer
Farxiga [dapagliflozin propanediol]	Z79.84	Oral hypoglycemic	Diabetes mellitus
Faslodex [fulvestrant]	Z79.818	Agents affecting estrogen receptors and estrogen levels	Hormone-related breast cancer; metastatic breast cancer
Feldene [piroxicam]	Z79.1	Nonsteroidal anti-inflammatory drug (NSAID)	Treatment of pain and inflammation due to arthritis
Femara [letrozole]	Z79.811	Aromatase inhibitor	Postmenopausal breast cancer
Femhrt [ethinyl estradiol/norethindrone acetate]	Z79.3, Z79.890	Contraceptive; estrogen therapy	Prevention of pregnancy; menopause symptoms; osteoporosis prevention
Femring [estradiol acetate]	Z79.890	Estrogen therapy	Osteoporosis prevention; menopausal symptoms; hypoestrogenism; ovarian failure
Fentanyl citrate [fentanyl citrate]	Z79.891	Analgesic, narcotic	Postprocedural or chronic pain
Fentora [fentanyl citrate]	Z79.891	Analgesic, narcotic	Breakthrough cancer pain
Fetroja [cefiderocol]	Z79.2	Antibiotic	Complicated urinary tract infections; hospital-acquired bacterial pneumonia; ventilator-associated bacterial pneumonia
Fiasp [insulin aspart]	Z79.4	Insulin	Diabetes mellitus
Filspari [sparsentan]		Endothelin and angiotensin II receptor antagonist	Primary immunoglobulin A nephropathy (IgAN)

Drug	Z Code	Drug Action/Classification	Indications
Fioricet with codeine [acetaminophen/butalbital/caffeine/codeine phosphate]	Z79.891	Analgesic, narcotic	Tension headaches
Firmagon [degarelix]	Z79.890	Hormone therapy	Prostate cancer
Flagyl [metronidazole]	Z79.2	Antibiotic	Bacterial infections
Flavoxate HCl [flavoxate hydrochloride]		Urinary antispasmodic	Relief of dysuria, urgency, nocturia, suprapubic pain, frequency, and incontinence associated with cystitis, prostatitis, urethritis, and urethrocystitis/urethrotrigonitis
Flomax [tamsulosin hydrochloride]		Antiadrenergic	Benign prostatic hyperplasia
Flonase allergy relief [fluticasone propionate]		Corticosteroid – intranasal	Perennial and seasonal allergic rhinitis
Flovent HFA [fluticasone propionate]	Z79.51	Corticosteroid – inhaled; antiasthmatic	Asthma
Fosamax [alendronate sodium]	Z79.83	Bisphosphonate	Osteoporosis; Paget's disease
Fosinopril sodium [fosinopril sodium]		ACE inhibitor	Hypertension; heart failure
Fosrenol [lanthanum carbonate]		Phosphate binder	End-stage renal disease (ESRD)
Fragmin [dalteparin sodium]	Z79.01	Anticoagulant	Venous thrombosis
Fruzaqla [fruquintinib]		Kinase inhibitor	Colorectal cancer
Gengraf [cyclosporine]	Z79.621	Calcineurin inhibitor	Prophylaxis of organ transplant rejection
Gentamicin sulfate [gentamicin sulfate]	Z79.2	Antibiotic	Severe bacterial infections
Gildagia [ethinyl estradiol/norethindrone]	Z79.3	Contraceptive	Prevention of pregnancy
Gildess 24 FE [ethinyl estradiol/norethindrone acetate]	Z79.3	Contraceptive	Prevention of pregnancy
Glimepiride [glimepiride]	Z79.84	Oral hypoglycemic	Diabetes mellitus
Glucotrol XL [glipizide]	Z79.84	Oral hypoglycemic	Diabetes mellitus
Glumetza [metformin hydrochloride]	Z79.84	Oral hypoglycemic	Diabetes mellitus
Glyburide (micronized) [glyburide]	Z79.84	Oral hypoglycemic	Diabetes mellitus
Glynase [glyburide]	Z79.84	Oral hypoglycemic	Diabetes mellitus
Glyset [miglitol]	Z79.84	Oral hypoglycemic	Diabetes mellitus
Harvoni [ledipasvir/sofosbuvir]		Antiviral	Chronic hepatitis C
Heparin sodium [heparin sodium]	Z79.01	Anticoagulant	Prophylaxis and treatment of venous thrombosis, pulmonary embolism; prevention of cerebral thrombosis; treatment of consumptive coagulopathies
Hiprex [methenamine]	Z79.2	Antibiotic	Recurring bladder infection
Humalog [insulin lispro recombinant]	Z79.4	Insulin	Diabetes mellitus
Humira [adalimumab]	Z79.620	Immunosuppressive biologic; monoclonal antibody	Rheumatoid arthritis; juvenile idiopathic arthritis; psoriatic arthritis; Crohn's disease; ulcerative colitis; plaque psoriasis; hidradenitis suppurativa; uveitis
Humulin R [insulin recombinant]	Z79.4	Insulin	Diabetes mellitus
Hycamtin [topotecan hydrochloride]	Z79.634	Topoisomerase inhibitor	Ovarian cancer; small cell lung cancer; cervical cancer
Hydrocodone [acetaminophen/hydrocodone bitartrate]	Z79.891	Analgesic, narcotic	Moderate to severe pain
Hydrocodone bitartrate and acetaminophen [acetaminophen/ hydrocodone bitartrate]	Z79.891	Analgesic, narcotic	Moderate to severe pain
Hydrocortisone [hydrocortisone]	Z79.52	Corticosteroid	Addison's disease; arthritis; immune disorders; allergies; breathing problems
Hydromorphone HCl [hydromorphone hydrochloride]	Z79.891	Analgesic, narcotic	Moderate to severe pain
Hydroxyurea [hydroxyurea]	Z79.64	Myelosuppressive agent	Pain related to sickle cell disease; chronic myeloid leukemia; ovarian cancer; skin cancer
Hyrimoz [adalimumab-adaz]	Z79.620	Immunosuppressive biologic; monoclonal antibody	Rheumatoid arthritis; juvenile idiopathic arthritis; psoriatic arthritis; Crohn's disease; ulcerative colitis; plaque psoriasis; ankylosing spondylitis
Hyzaar [hydrochlorothiazide/ losartan potassium]		Antihypertensive	Hypertension
Ibsrela [tenapanor hydrochloride]		NHE-3 inhibitor	Irritable bowel syndrome with constipation (IBS-C)
Ibuprofen [ibuprofen]	Z79.1	Nonsteroidal anti-inflammatory drug (NSAID)	Pain or fever relief
Imitrex [sumatriptan succinate]		Antimigraine	Migraine headache
Imjudo [tremelimumab]	Z79.620	Immunosuppressive biologic; monoclonal antibody	Unresectable hepatocellular carcinoma
Imuran [azathioprine]	Z79.624	Inhibitors of nucleotide synthesis; antirheumatic; immunosuppressant	Rheumatoid arthritis; prophylaxis of organ transplant rejection
Indocin [indomethacin]	Z79.1	Nonsteroidal anti-inflammatory drug (NSAID)	Treatment of pain and inflammation
Inpefa [sotagliflozin]		Cardiovascular agent	Heart failure

Drug	Z Code	Drug Action/Classification	Indications
Intron A [interferon alfa 2-b]	Z79.69	Other immunosuppressant/immunomodulator	Cancer; hepatitis
Invanz [ertapenem sodium]	Z79.2	Antibiotic	Bacterial infections of the stomach, urinary tract, pelvis, skin, and lung
Invokamet [canagliflozin/metformin hydrochloride]	Z79.84	Oral hypoglycemic	Diabetes mellitus
Invokana [canagliflozin]	Z79.84	Oral hypoglycemic	Diabetes mellitus
Isoniazid [isoniazid]	Z79.2	Antibiotic	Tuberculosis
Isoproterenol hydrochloride [isoproterenol hydrochloride]		Adrenergic agent/catecholamine	Shock; cardiac arrest; heart failure; bronchospasm
Isopto Carpine [pilocarpine hydrochloride]		Cholinergic parasympathomimetic agent	Reduction of intraocular pressure in open-angle glaucoma or ocular hypertension; management of acute angle-closure glaucoma
Isordil Titradose [isosorbide dinitrate]		Smooth muscle relaxant	Acute anginal attacks
Isturisa [osilodrostat]		Cortisol synthesis inhibitor	Cushing's disease in adults
Ixempra [ixabepilone]	Z79.633	Mitotic inhibitor	Advanced breast cancer
Izervay [avacincaptad pegol]		Anti-angiogenic ophthalmic agent	Geographic atrophy due to age-related macular degeneration
Jantoven [warfarin sodium]	Z79.01	Anticoagulant	Venous thrombosis, pulmonary embolism; prevention of cerebral thrombosis; treatment of consumptive coagulopathies
Janumet [metformin hydrochloride/sitagliptin phosphate]	Z79.84	Oral hypoglycemic	Diabetes mellitus
Januvia [sitagliptin phosphate]	Z79.84	Oral hypoglycemic	Diabetes mellitus
Jaypirca [pirtobrutinib]		Kinase inhibitor	Mantle cell lymphoma
Jentadueto [linagliptin/metformin hydrochloride]]	Z79.84	Oral hypoglycemic	Diabetes mellitus
Jesduvroq [daprodustat]		Erythropoiesis-stimulating agent (ESA)	Treatment of anemia in CKD patients on dialysis
Junel [ethinyl estradiol/norethindrone acetate]	Z79.3	Contraceptive	Prevention of pregnancy
Katerzia [amlodipine benzoate]		Antihypertensive	Hypertension; coronary artery disease (CAD); chronic stable angina; prinzmetal's angina; variant angina
Kazano [alogliptin benzoate/metformin hydrochloride]	Z79.84	Oral hypoglycemic	Diabetes mellitus
Kenalog-10; Kenalog-40 [triamcinolone acetonide]	Z79.52	Corticosteroid	Gouty arthritis; bursitis; tenosynovitis; epicondylitis; rheumatoid arthritis; synovitis; osteoarthritis
Keytruda [pembrolizumab]	Z79.620	Immunosuppressive biologic; monoclonal antibody	Unresectable or metastatic melanoma
Kimmtrak [tebentafusp-tebn]		Antineoplastic	Uveal melanoma
Klaron [sulfacetamide sodium]	Z79.2	Antibiotic, topical	Acne vulgaris
Klonopin [clonazepam]		Anticonvulsant; CNS depressant	Epilepsy; seizures; panic disorder
Klor-Con [potassium chloride]		Mineral; electrolyte	Hypokalemia
Kombiglyze [metformin hydrochloride/saxagliptin hydrochloride]	Z79.84	Oral hypoglycemic	Diabetes mellitus
K-Tab [potassium chloride]		Mineral; electrolyte	Hypokalemia
Lamisil [terbinafine hydrochloride]		Antifungal	Tinea cruris (jock itch); T. pedis (athlete's foot); T. corporis (ringworm)
Lanoxin [digoxin]		Antiarrhythmic; inotropic agent	Congestive heart failure; chronic atrial fibrillation
Lantus [insulin glargine recombinant]	Z79.4	Insulin	Diabetes mellitus
Lasix [furosemide]		Antihypertensive; diuretic	Hypertension; edema associated with heart failure and renal disease
Leqembi [lecanemab-irmb]		Amyloid beta-directed antibody	Dementia due to Alzheimer's
Lescol XL [fluvastatin sodium]		HMG-CoA reductase inhibitor (statin)	Hypercholesterolemia; hyperlipidemia; hyperlipoproteinemia
Letrozole [letrozole]	Z79.811	Aromatase inhibitor; antineoplastic	Postmenopausal breast cancer
Leukeran [chlorambucil]	Z79.630	Chemotherapeutic alkylating agent	Cancer
Levemir [insulin detemir recombinant]	Z79.4	Insulin	Diabetes mellitus
Levonest [levonorgestrel/ethinyl estradiol]	Z79.3	Contraceptive	Prevention of pregnancy; menstrual disorders; acne
Levoxyl [levothyroxine sodium]	Z79.890	Thyroid hormone	Hypothyroidism; pituitary thyrotropin suppression
Lexapro [escitalopram oxalate]		Antidepressant, selective serotonin reuptake inhibitor (SSRI)	Depression; anxiety
Lialda [mesalamine]		Anti-inflammatory	Ulcerative colitis
Lidocaine HCl [lidocaine hydrochloride]		Antiarrhythmic	Management of ventricular arrhythmias or during cardiac manipulation, such as cardiac surgery
Liletta [levonorgestrel]	Z79.3	Contraceptive	Intrauterine device to prevent pregnancy

Drug	Z Code	Drug Action/Classification	Indications
Lincocin [lincocin hydrochloride]	Z79.2	Antibiotic	Severe bacterial infections
Lipitor [atorvastatin calcium]		HMG-CoA reductase inhibitor (statin)	Hypercholesterolemia; hyperlipidemia; hyperproteinemia
Lisinopril [lisinopril]		ACE inhibitor	Congestive heart failure; hypertension
Litfulo [ritlecitinib]		Multikinase inhibitor	Alopecia areata
Lithium carbonate [lithium carbonate]		Antimanic	Control of manic episodes in bipolar disorders
Livtencity [maribavir]		Antiviral	Post-transplant CMV infection/disease
Lo Loestrin Fe [ethinyl estradiol/norethindrone acetate]	Z79.3	Contraceptive	Prevention of pregnancy
Locoid [hydrocortisone butyrate]	Z79.52	Corticosteroid – topical	Atopic dermatitis; other dermatoses
Lomotil [diphenoxylate hydrochloride/atropine sulfate]		Antidiarrheal	Symptoms of chronic and functional diarrhea
Lopid [gemfibrozil]		Lipid regulating agent	Hypercholesterolemia; hyperlipidemia; hyperlipoproteinemia; hypertriglyceridemia
Lopressor [metoprolol tartrate]		Beta blocker	Angina pectoris; hypertension; acute myocardial infarction
Loqtorzi [toripalimab-tpzi]	Z79.620	Monoclonal antibody	Nasopharyngeal carcinoma
Lorazepam [lorazepam]		Antianxiety; sedative/hypnotic; anticonvulsant; antiemetic	Anxiety disorder associated with depressive symptoms; controls tension, agitation, irritability, and insomnia
Loryna [drospirenone/ethinyl estradiol]	Z79.3	Contraceptive	Prevention of pregnancy
LoSeasonique [ethinyl estradiol/levonorgestrel]	Z79.3	Contraceptive	Prevention of pregnancy
Lotensin [benazepril hydrochloride]		ACE inhibitor	Hypertension
Lotrel [amlodipine besylate/benazepril hydrochloride]		Antihypertensive	Hypertension
Lovastatin [lovastatin]		HMG-CoA reductase inhibitor (statin)	Hypercholesterolemia; hyperlipidemia; hyperlipoproteinemia
Lovenox [enoxaparin sodium]	Z79.01	Anticoagulant	Venous thrombosis and pulmonary embolism
Low-Ogestrel-28 [norgestrel/ethinyl estradiol]	Z79.3	Contraceptive	Prevention of pregnancy
Lupkynis [voclosporin]	Z79.621	Calcineurin inhibitor; immunosuppressant	Lupus nephritis
Lupron Depot [leuprolide acetate]	Z79.818	Agents affecting estrogen receptors and estrogen levels; antineoplastic	Endometriosis symptoms; uterine fibroids; symptoms of prostate cancer
Macrobid [nitrofurantoin]	Z79.2	Antibiotic	Urinary tract infections
Macrodantin [nitrofurantoin]	Z79.2	Antibiotic	Urinary tract infections
Meclizine hydrochloride [meclizine hydrochloride]		Antihistamine; antiemetic	Nausea, vomiting, and dizziness associated with motion sickness; symptoms of vertigo
Medrol [methylprednisolone]	Z79.52	Corticosteroid	Allergic and edematous states; collagen disorders
Megace ES [megestrol acetate]	Z79.818	Agents affecting estrogen receptors and estrogen levels; progestin; antineoplastic	Endometrial or advanced breast cancers; weight loss due to AIDS
Menest [esterified estrogens]	Z79.890	Estrogen therapy	Menopause symptoms; ovarian failure
Menostar [estradiol]	Z79.890	Estrogen therapy	Menopause symptoms; osteoporosis prevention
Mepron [atovaquone]	Z79.2	Antibiotic	Pneumonia due to Pneumocystis jirovecii
Merrem [meropenem]	Z79.2	Antibiotic	Bacterial infections of skin or stomach; bacterial meningitis
Mesalamine [mesalamine]		Anti-inflammatory	Ulcerative colitis
Metformin [metformin hydrochloride]	Z79.84	Oral hypoglycemic	Diabetes mellitus
Methadone HCl [methadone hydrochloride]	Z79.891	Analgesic, narcotic; opioid agonist	Pain; treatment of opioid addiction
Methadose [methadone hydrochloride]	Z79.891	Analgesic, narcotic; opioid agonist	Acute and chronic pain
Methergine [methylergonovine maleate]		Oxytocic agent	Routine management of postpartum hemorrhage after delivery of placenta
Methotrexate sodium [methotrexate sodium]	Z79.631	Antimetabolite agent	Cancer
Methylprednisolone [methylprednisolone]	Z79.52	Corticosteroid	Inflammatory disorders
Metronidazole [metronidazole]	Z79.2	Antibiotic	Bacterial infections
Miacalcin [calcitonin salmon]		Calcitonin	Hypercalcemia; osteoporosis; Paget's disease
Miebo [perfluorhexyloctane]		Ophthalmic anti-inflammatory agent	Dry eye disease
Minivelle [estradiol]	Z79.890	Estrogen therapy	Menopause symptoms; osteoporosis prevention
Minocin [minocycline hydrochloride]	Z79.2	Antibiotic	Bacterial infections; acne
Mirena [levonorgestrel]	Z79.3	Contraceptive	Intrauterine device for prevention of pregnancy; menstrual disorders
Mitomycin [mitomycin]	Z79.632	Antitumor antibiotic; antineoplastic	Stomach and pancreas cancer
Mobic [meloxicam]	Z79.1	Nonsteroidal anti-inflammatory drug (NSAID)	Treatment of pain and inflammation due to osteoarthritis and rheumatoid arthritis

Drug	Z Code	Drug Action/Classification	Indications
Monoclonal antibodies	Z79.620	Immunosuppressive biologic	Cancer; prophylaxis of organ transplant rejection
Monodox [doxycycline]	Z79.2	Antibiotic	Bacterial infections; acne
Mono-Linyah [norgestimate/ethinyl estradiol]	Z79.3	Contraceptive	Prevention of pregnancy; menstrual disorders; acne
Monurol [fosfomycin trometamine]	Z79.2	Antibiotic	Bacterial bladder infections
Morphine sulfate [morphine sulfate]	Z79.891	Analgesic, narcotic	Moderate to severe pain
Motrin IB [ibuprofen]	Z79.1	Nonsteroidal anti-inflammatory drug (NSAID)	Pain or fever relief
Mounjaro [tirzepatide]	Z79.85	Antidiabetic – non-insulin injectable	Diabetes mellitus
MS Contin [morphine sulfate]	Z79.891	Analgesic, narcotic	Moderate to severe pain
Multaq [dronedarone hydrochloride]		Antiarrhythmic	Atrial fibrillation; atrial flutter
Mycobutin [rifabutin]	Z79.2	Antibiotic	Mycobacterium avium complex (MAC) prophylactic in HIV patients
Mytesi [crofelemer]		Antidiarrheal	Diarrhea occurring in HIV/AIDs patient's on anti-retroviral therapy
Nabumetone [nabumetone]	Z79.1	Nonsteroidal anti-inflammatory drug (NSAID)	Osteoarthritis and rheumatoid arthritis
Nalfon [fenoprofen calcium]	Z79.1	Nonsteroidal anti-inflammatory drug (NSAID)	Pain or inflammation relief; osteoarthritis; rheumatoid arthritis
Namzaric [memantine/donepezil hydrochlorides]		Acetylcholinesterase/cholinesterase inhibitors	Dementia due to Alzheimer's
Naprelan [naproxen sodium]	Z79.1	Nonsteroidal anti-inflammatory drug (NSAID)	Pain or inflammation relief
Naprosyn [naproxen]	Z79.1	Nonsteroidal anti-inflammatory drug (NSAID)	Rheumatoid, gouty arthritis and osteoarthritis; ankylosing spondylitis; bursitis; dysmenorrhea; pain, mild to moderate; tendonitis
Natazia [estradiol valerate/dienogest]	Z79.3	Contraceptive	Prevention of pregnancy; menstrual disorders
Nebupent [pentamidine isethionate]	Z79.2	Antibiotic; antifungal	Fungal infections; Pneumocystis jirovecii (carinii) pneumonia in HIV patients
Nefazodone HCl [nefazodone hydrochloride]		Antidepressant	Depression
Nembutal sodium [pentobarbital sodium]		Sedative/hypnotic	Insomnia; adjunct medication in diagnostic procedures or for emergency use with convulsive disorders
NeoProfen [ibuprofen lysine]	Z79.1	Nonsteroidal anti-inflammatory drug (NSAID)	Pain or fever relief in premature infants
Neoral [cyclosporine]	Z79.621	Calcineurin inhibitor	Prophylaxis of organ transplant rejection; rheumatoid arthritis; psoriasis
Neosporin [bacitracin, neomycin]	Z79.2	Antibiotic, topical	Bacterial skin infections
Neurontin [gabapentin]		Anticonvulsant	Postherpetic neuralgia; partial onset seizures
Nexium [esomeprazole magnesium]		Proton pump inhibitor	Gastroesophageal reflux disease (GERD); erosive esophagitis
Nexletol [bempedoic acid]		Antihyperlipidemic	Heterozygous familial hypercholesterolemia; established atherosclerotic cardiovascular disease requiring additional lowering of LDL-C
Nexplanon [etonogestrel]	Z79.3	Contraceptive	Implantable device used for prevention of pregnancy
Ngenla [somatrogon-ghla]		Growth hormone	Growth failure
Nitrofurantoin [nitrofurantoin]	Z79.2	Antibiotic	Bacterial urinary tract infections
Nitrostat [nitroglycerin]		Muscle relaxant; antianginal; antihypertensive; coronary vasodilator	Angina pectoris; heart failure associated with myocardial infarction; hypertension, perioperative; surgery, adjunct
Norpace [disopyramide phosphate]		Antiarrhythmic	Coronary artery disease; prevention, recurrence, and control of unifocal, multifocal, and paired PVCs
Norvasc [amlodipine besylate]		Antihypertensive	Hypertension; coronary artery disease (CAD); chronic stable angina; prinzmetal's angina; variant angina
Novolin [insulin recombinant]	Z79.4	Insulin	Diabetes mellitus
Novolog [insulin aspart recombinant]	Z79.4	Insulin	Diabetes mellitus
Nucynta [tapentadol hydrochloride]	Z79.891	Analgesic, narcotic	Moderate to severe pain
NuvaRing [etonogestrel/ethinyl estradiol]	Z79.3	Contraceptive	Vaginal ring to prevent pregnancy
Ogsiveo [nirogacestat]		Antineoplastic	Desmoid tumors
Ojjaara [momelotinib]	Z79.622	Janus kinase (JAK) inhibitor	Myelofibrosis
Olumiant [baricitinib]	Z79.622	Janus kinase (JAK) inhibitor	Rheumatoid arthritis
Omvoh [mirikizumab-mrkz]	Z79.620	Monoclonal antibody	Ulcerative colitis
Opdualag [nivolumab and relatlimab-rmbw]		Antineoplastic combination	Unresectable or metastatic melanoma
Oracea [doxycycline]	Z79.2	Antibiotic	Rosacea
Orapred ODT [prednisolone sodium phosphate]	Z79.52	Corticosteroid	Inflammatory disorders
Orbactiv [oritavancin diphosphate]	Z79.2	Antibiotic	Bacterial skin infections

Drug	Z Code	Drug Action/Classification	Indications
Orencia [abatacept]	Z79.69	Other immunosuppressant/ immunomodulator	Rheumatoid arthritis; polyarticular juvenile idiopathic arthritis; psoriatic arthritis; prophylaxis of acute graft versus host disease (aGVHD)
Orilissa [elagolix]	Z79.890	Hormone therapy	Pain associated with endometriosis
Orphenadrine citrate [orphenadrine citrate]		Muscle relaxant	Acute spasms, tension, and post-trauma cases
Orserdu [elacestrant]	Z79.818	Agents affecting estrogen receptors and estrogen levels	Advanced or metastatic breast cancer
Oseni [alogliptin benzoate/pioglitazone hydrochloride]	Z79.84	Oral hypoglycemic	Diabetes mellitus
Osphena [ospemifene]	Z79.810	Selective estrogen receptor modulator (SERM)	Postmenopausal dyspareunia due to vaginal atrophy; osteoporosis; menopausal symptoms
Otezla [apremilast]	Z79.61	Immunomodulator; antirheumatic	Psoriatic arthritis; plaque psoriasis; oral ulcers associated with Behcet's disease
Oxazepam [oxazepam]		Antianxiety	Anxiety, tension, and withdrawal from alcohol
Oxbryta [voxelotor]		Hemoglobin S polymerization inhibitor	Sickle cell disease
Oxycodone HCl [oxycodone hydrochloride]	Z79.891	Analgesic, narcotic	Moderate to severe pain
OxyContin [oxycodone hydrochloride]	Z79.891	Analgesic, narcotic	Moderate to severe pain
Ozempic [semaglutide]	Z79.85	Antidiabetic – non-insulin injectable	Diabetes mellitus
Paclitaxel [paclitaxel]	Z79.633	Mitotic inhibitor	Cancer of the breast, ovaries, and lung; AIDS-related Kaposi's sarcoma
Paxil [paroxetine hydrochloride]		Antidepressant; selective serotonin reuptake inhibitor (SSRI)	Obsessive-compulsive disorder; major depressive disorder; panic disorder; social anxiety disorder; generalized anxiety disorder; posttraumatic stress disorder
Paxlovid [nirmatrelvir, ritonavir]		Antiviral	COVID-19
PediaPred [prednisolone sodium phosphate]	Z79.52	Corticosteroid	Inflammatory disorders
PegIntron [peginterferon alfa-2b]	Z79.69	Other immunosuppressant/ immunomodulator; antiviral	Hepatitis C
Penicillin-VK [penicillin V potassium]	Z79.2	Antibiotic	Chorea, prevention; endocarditis, prevention, secondary to tooth extraction; erysipelas; infections of the skin, skin structures, and upper respiratory tract; rheumatic fever, prophylaxis; scarlet fever; Vincent's gingivitis; Vincent's pharyngitis
Pentam [pentamidine isethionate]	Z79.2	Antibiotic; antifungal	Severe bacterial lung infections; fungal infections; Pneumocystis jirovecii (carinii) pneumonia
Pentasa [mesalamine]		Anti-inflammatory	Crohn's disease; ulcerative colitis
Pepcid AC [famotidine]		Histamine H2-receptor inhibitor	Acid/peptic disorder; adenoma, secretory; gastroesophageal reflux; duodenal and gastric ulcer; Zollinger-Ellison syndrome
Percocet [oxycodone hydrochloride/acetaminophen]	Z79.891	Analgesic, narcotic	Moderate to severe pain
Persantine [dipyridamole]	Z79.02	Antiplatelet	Prevention of blood clots after heart valve surgery
Pfizerpen [penicillin g potassium]	Z79.2	Antibiotic	Severe bacterial infections
Phenobarbital [phenobarbital sodium]		Anticonvulsant	Grand mal epilepsy; sedative
Piqray [alpelisib]		Kinase inhibitor	Postmenopausal advanced or metastatic breast cancer
Pitocin [oxytocin]		Uterotonic	Induction or stimulation of labor at term; control of bleeding after childbirth
Plan B One-Step [levonorgestrel]	Z79.3	Contraceptive	Prevention of pregnancy
Plavix [clopidogrel bisulfate]	Z79.02	Antiplatelet	Lessening of the chance of heart attack or stroke
Pluvicto [lutetium Lu 177 vipivotide tetraxetan]		Radioligand therapeutic agent	Metastatic castration-resistant prostate cancer (mCRPC)
Pomalyst [pomalidomide]	Z79.61	Immunomodulator; antineoplastic	Multiple myeloma; Kaposi sarcoma
Pombiliti [cipaglucosidase alfa-atga]		Lysosomal enzyme	Pompe disease
Ponstel [mefenamic acid]	Z79.1	Nonsteroidal anti-inflammatory drug (NSAID)	Mild to moderate pain; primary dysmenorrhea
Ponvory [ponesimod]	Z79.69	Other immunosuppressant/ immunomodulator	Relapsing forms of multiple sclerosis (MS)
Pradaxa [dabigatran etexilate mesylate]	Z79.01	Anticoagulant	Prophylaxis and treatment of blood clots in patients with atrial fibrillation
Prasugrel [prasugrel hydrochloride]	Z79.02	Antiplatelet	Lessening the chance of heart attack or stroke
Pravastatin sodium [pravastatin sodium]		HMG-CoA reductase inhibitor (statin)	Hypercholesterolemia; hyperlipidemia; hyperlipoproteinemia
Prednisolone [prednisolone]	Z79.52	Corticosteroid	Inflammatory disorders
Prednisone [prednisone]	Z79.52	Corticosteroid	Immunosuppressant effects; relief of inflammation; used in arthritis, polymyositis and other systemic diseases
Pregnyl [chorionic gonadotropin]		Gonadotropic hormone	Prepubertal cryptorchidism; hypogonadism; corpus luteum insufficiency and infertility

Drug	Z Code	Drug Action/Classification	Indications
Prempro [conjugated estrogens/medroxyprogesterone acetate]	Z79.890	Estrogen/progesterone therapy	Menopause symptoms; osteoporosis; atrophic vaginitis
Prevacid [lansoprazole]		Proton pump inhibitor	Acid/peptic disorder; erosive esophagitis; duodenal ulcer; Zollinger-Ellison syndrome
Prezcobix [darunavir/cobicistat]		Antiretroviral	HIV
Prezista [darunavir]		Antiretroviral	HIV
Priftin [rifapentine]	Z79.2	Antibiotic	Tuberculosis
Prilosec [omeprazole magnesium]		Proton pump inhibitor	Acid/peptic disorder; endocrine adenoma; erosive esophagitis; systemic mastocytosis; gastroesophageal reflux; duodenal, peptic and gastric ulcer; Zollinger-Ellison syndrome
Primaxin [cilastatin sodium/imipenem]	Z79.2	Antibiotic	Bacterial septicemia; endocarditis; bacterial infections of the skin, lower respiratory tract, intra-abdomen, bones, and joints
Pristiq [desvenlafaxine]		Antidepressant; serotonin and norepinephrine reuptake inhibitor (SNRI)	Major depressive disorder
Procardia [nifedipine]		Calcium channel blocker	Vasospastic angina; chronic stable angina; hypertension
Prograf [tacrolimus]	Z79.621	Calcineurin inhibitor	Prophylaxis of organ transplant rejection
Prolia [denosumab]	Z79.620	Immunosuppressive biologic; monoclonal antibody	Osteoporosis
Promethazine hydrochloride [promethazine hydrochloride]		Anesthesia, adjunct to; antiemetic; antihistamine; antitussive/expectorant; sedative/hypnotic; vertigo/motion sickness; vomiting	Anesthesia; adjunct; angioedema; conjunctivitis; dermographism; hypersensitivity, motion sickness; pain; perennial, seasonal, and allergic rhinitis; sedation, obstetrical; urticaria
Propranolol hydrochloride [propranolol hydrochloride]		Beta blocker	Angina pectoris; hypertension; cardiac arrhythmias
Protonix [pantoprazole sodium]		Proton pump inhibitor	Short-term treatment and maintenance therapy of erosive esophagitis associated with gastroesophageal reflux disease (GERD)
Protopic [tacrolimus]	Z79.621	Calcineurin inhibitor	Atomic dermatitis (eczema)
Proventil-HFA [albuterol sulfate]		Antiasthmatic/bronchodilator	Asthma
Provera [medroxyprogesterone acetate]	Z79.3, Z79.890	Contraceptive; progestin; antineoplastic	Prevention of pregnancy; amenorrhea; carcinoma, endometrium, adjunct; carcinoma, renal; hemorrhage
Prozac [fluoxetine hydrochloride]		Selective serotonin reuptake inhibitor (SSRI)	Bulimia nervosa; depression; obsessive-compulsive disorder
Pulmicort [budesonide]	Z79.51	Corticosteroid – inhaled; antiasthmatic	Prophylaxis and treatment of asthma
Qalsody [tofersen]		CNS agent	Amyotrophic lateral sclerosis
Qelbree [viloxazine hydrochloride]		Selective norepinephrine reuptake inhibitor	Attention deficit hyperactivity disorder (ADHD)
Qnasl [beclomethasone dipropionate]		Corticosteroid – intranasal	Perennial and seasonal allergies; vasomotor rhinitis
Qtern [dapagliflozin/saxagliptin]	Z79.84	Oral hypoglycemic	Diabetes mellitus
Quinapril hydrochloride [quinapril hydrochloride]		ACE inhibitor	Hypertension; heart failure
Qulipta [atogepant]		Calcitonin gene-related peptide inhibitor	Migraine headache prevention
Quviviq [daridorexant hydrochloride]		CNS depressant	Insomnia
Qvar Redihaler [beclomethasone dipropionate]	Z79.51	Corticosteroid – inhaled; antiasthmatic	Prophylaxis and treatment of asthma
Raloxifene HCl [raloxifene hydrochloride]	Z79.810	Selective estrogen receptor modulator (SERM)	Osteoporosis in postmenopausal women
Rapaflo [silodosin]		Antiadrenergic	Benign prostatic hyperplasia
Rapamune [sirolimus]	Z79.623	Mammalian target of rapamycin (mTOR) inhibitor	Prophylaxis of organ transplant rejection
Rayos [prednisone]	Z79.52	Corticosteroid; antiasthmatic	Arthritis; blood disorders; allergies; asthma
Rebif [interferon beta-1a]	Z79.69	Other immunosuppressant/immunomodulator	Treatment of relapsing multiple sclerosis
Reclast [zoledronic acid]	Z79.83	Bisphosphonate	Osteoporosis; Paget's disease; bone cancer
Relenza [zanamivir]		Antiviral	Treat and prevent influenza A and B
Relyvrio [sodium phenylbutyrate/taurursodiol]		Central nervous system agent	Amyotrophic lateral sclerosis (ALS)
Remicade [infliximab]	Z79.620	Immunosuppressive biologic; monoclonal antibody	Ankylosing spondylitis; psoriatic arthritis; rheumatoid arthritis; Crohn's disease; ulcerative colitis
Renvela [sevelamer carbonate]		Phosphate binder	Chronic kidney disease (CKD) on dialysis
Repaglinide [repaglinide]	Z79.84	Oral hypoglycemic	Diabetes mellitus
Restasis [cyclosporine ophthalmic emulsion]	Z79.621	Calcineurin inhibitor	Ocular inflammation due to keratoconjunctivitis sicca
Restoril [temazepam]		Sedative/hypnotic	Insomnia
Retrovir [zidovudine]		Antiretroviral	HIV

Drug	Z Code	Drug Action/Classification	Indications
Revlimid [lenalidomide]	Z79.61	Immunomodulator; antineoplastic	Multiple myeloma following autologous stem cell transplant; myelodysplastic syndromes; mantle cell lymphoma
Reyvow [lasmiditan]		Antimigraine	Migraine headache
Rezzayo [rezafungin]		Antifungal	Candidemia; invasive candidiasis
Rifadin [rifampin]	Z79.2	Antibiotic	Tuberculosis
Rimactane [rifampin]	Z79.2	Antibiotic	Tuberculosis
Rinvoq [upadacitinib]	Z79.622	Janus kinase (JAK) inhibitor	Rheumatoid arthritis; psoriatic arthritis; ankylosing spondylitis; ulcerative colitis
Risperdal [risperidone]		Antipsychotic/antimanic	Schizophrenia; bipolar I disorder
Ritalin [methylphenidate hydrochloride]		CNS stimulant	Attention deficit hyperactivity disorder (ADHD); narcolepsy
Rituxan [rituximab]	Z79.620	Immunosuppressive biologic; monoclonal antibody	Non-Hodgkin's lymphoma; chronic lymphocytic leukemia; rheumatoid arthritis; granulomatosis with polyangiitis; pemphigus vulgaris
Roxicodone [oxycodone hydrochloride]	Z79.891	Analgesic, narcotic	Pain relief
Rukobia [fostemsavir tromethamine]		Antiretroviral	HIV
Rybelsus [semaglutide]	Z79.84	Oral hypoglycemic	Diabetes mellitus
Rystiggo [rozanolixizumab-noli]		Antineoplastic	Myasthenia gravis
Ryzneuta [efbemalenograstim alfa-vuxw]		Immunostimulant	Neutropenia
Sabril [vigabatrin]		Anticonvulsant	Refractory complex partial seizures
Sandimmune [cyclosporine]	Z79.621	Calcineurin inhibitor	Prophylaxis of organ transplant rejection
Savaysa [edoxaban tosylate]	Z79.01	Anticoagulant	Prophylaxis and treatment of venous thrombosis, pulmonary embolism; prevention of blood clots due to atrial fibrillation
Scemblix [asciminib hydrochloride]		Kinase inhibitor	Philadelphia chromosome-positive chronic myeloid leukemia
Seasonale [levonorgestrel/ethinyl estradiol]	Z79.3	Contraceptive	Prevention of pregnancy
Seasonique [ethinyl estradiol/levonorgestrel]	Z79.3	Contraceptive	Prevention of pregnancy
Septra [sulfamethoxazole trimethoprim]	Z79.2	Antibiotic	Urinary tract infections; acute otitis media; acute exacerbations of chronic bronchitis; shigellosis
Serevent [salmeterol xinafoate]		Bronchodilator	Asthma
Seromycin [cycloserine]	Z79.2	Antibiotic	Tuberculosis; urinary tract infections
Seroquel XR [quetiapine fumarate]		Antipsychotic	Schizophrenia; bipolar disorder; major depressive disorder
Silvadene [silver sulfadiazine]	Z79.2	Antibiotic, topical	Wound sepsis due to second/third degree burns
Simulect [basiliximab]	Z79.620	Immunosuppressive biologic; monoclonal antibody	Prophylaxis of organ transplant rejection
Sinemet [carbidopa/levodopa]		Antiparkinsonism	Parkinson's disease
Singulair [montelukast sodium]		Antiasthmatic	Asthma; exercise-induced bronchoconstriction; perennial and seasonal allergic rhinitis
Sirolimus [sirolimus]	Z79.623	Mammalian target of rapamycin (mTOR) inhibitor	Prophylaxis of organ transplant rejection
Sitagliptin [sitagliptin/metformin hydrochloride]	Z79.84	Oral hypoglycemic	Diabetes mellitus
Sivextro [tedizolid phosphate]	Z79.2	Antibiotic	Skin infections including MRSA
Skyclarys [omaveloxolone]		CNS stimulant	Friedrich's ataxia
Skyla [levonorgestrel]	Z79.3	Contraceptive	Intrauterine device to prevent pregnancy
Skyrizi [risankizumab]	Z79.620	Immunosuppressive biologic; monoclonal antibody	Plaque psoriasis
Sodium nitroprusside [sodium nitroprusside]		Vasodilator	Hypertensive crisis; control surgical bleeding; acute congestive heart failure
Soliqua [insulin glargine/lixisenatide]	Z79.4	Insulin	Diabetes mellitus
Solodyn [minocycline hydrochloride]	Z79.2	Antibiotic	Bacterial infections
Solosec [secnidazole]	Z79.2	Antibiotic	Bacterial vaginal inflammation; trichomoniasis
Soltamox [tamoxifen citrate]	Z79.810	Selective estrogen receptor modulator (SERM)	Breast cancer
Solu-Cortef [hydrocortisone sodium succinate]	Z79.52	Corticosteroid; antiasthmatic	Asthma; severe inflammation; allergic reactions
Solu-Medrol [methylprednisolone sodium succinate]	Z79.52	Corticosteroid	Anti-inflammatory and antiallergenic for shock and ulcerative colitis
Sotyktu [deucravacitinib]		Multikinase inhibitor	Plaque psoriasis
Spiriva [tiotropium bromide]		Antiasthmatic/bronchodilator	Chronic obstructive pulmonary disease (COPD); asthma
Sprintec [norgestimate/ethinyl estradiol]	Z79.3	Contraceptive	Prevention of pregnancy
Stelara [ustekinumab]	Z79.620	Immunosuppressive biologic; monoclonal antibody	Plaque psoriasis; psoriatic arthritis; Crohn's disease; ulcerative colitis

Appendix B: Pharmacology List 2026

Drug	Z Code	Drug Action/Classification	Indications
Strattera [atomoxetine hydrochloride]		CNS stimulant	Attention deficit hyperactivity disorder (ADHD)
Streptomycin sulfate [streptomycin sulfate]	Z79.2	Antibiotic	Severe bacterial infections
Suboxone [buprenorphine/naloxone]		Opioid agonist	Treatment of opioid addiction
Sunlenca [lenacapavir]		Antiretroviral	HIV
Supprelin LA [histrelin acetate]	Z79.818	Agents affecting estrogen receptors and estrogen levels	Precocious puberty
Suprax [cefixime]	Z79.2	Antibiotic	Bacterial infections
Sylatron [peginterferon alfa-2b]	Z79.69	Other immunosuppressant/immunomodulator	Prevention of recurrent malignant melanoma
Symbicort [budesonide/formoterol fumarate dihydrate]	Z79.51	Corticosteroid – inhaled; antiasthmatic	Prophylaxis and treatment of asthma and COPD
Symbyax [olanzapine/fluoxetine]		Antidepressant	Acute depressive episodes associated with bipolar I disorder; treatment-resistant depression
Symlin [pramlintide]	Z79.85	Antidiabetic – non-insulin injectable	Diabetes mellitus
Symtuza [darunavir/cobicistat/emtricitabine/tenofovir alafenamide]		Antiretroviral	HIV
Synarel [nafarelin acetate]	Z79.818	Agents affecting estrogen receptors and estrogen levels	Endometriosis symptoms; precocious puberty
Synercid [dalfopristin/quinupristin]	Z79.2	Antibiotic	Severe blood infections
Synjardy [empagliflozin/metformin hydrochloride]	Z79.84	Oral hypoglycemic	Diabetes mellitus
Synthroid [levothyroxine sodium]	Z79.890	Thyroid hormone	Hypothyroidism
Tacrolimus [tacrolimus]	Z79.621	Calcineurin inhibitor	Prophylaxis of organ transplant rejection
Talicia [omeprazole magnesium/ amoxicillin/ rifabutin]	Z79.2	Combination antibiotic	Helicobacter pylori
Taltz [ixekizumab]	Z79.620	Immunosuppressive biologic; monoclonal antibody	Plaque psoriasis; psoriatic arthritis; ankylosing spondylitis; axial spondyloarthritis
Talvey [talquetamab-tgvs]		Antineoplastic	Multiple myeloma
Tamiflu [oseltamivir phosphate]		Antiviral	Treatment and prevention of influenza A and B
Tamoxifen citrate [tamoxifen citrate]	Z79.810	Selective estrogen receptor modulator (SERM)	Metastatic breast cancer in postmenopausal women
Tavneos [avacopan]	Z79.69	Other immunosuppressant/immunomodulator	ANCA-associated vasculitis
Taxotere [docetaxel]	Z79.633	Mitotic inhibitor	Cancer
Tazicef [ceftazidime]	Z79.2	Antibiotic	Confirmed or suspected bacterial infections
Teflaro [ceftaroline fosamil]	Z79.2	Antibiotic	Bacterial skin infections; pneumonia
Tegretol [carbamazepine]		Anticonvulsant; analgesic	Epilepsy, especially with complex symptomatology; specific analgesic for trigeminal neuralgia
Temozolomide [temozolomide]	Z79.630	Chemotherapeutic alkylating agent	Chronic myelogenous leukemia
Tenormin [atenolol]		Beta blocker	Angina pectoris; hypertension; acute myocardial infarction
Terazosin HCl [terazosin hydrochloride]		Antiadrenergic	Benign prostatic hypertrophy; hypertension
Terlivaz [terlipressin]		Antidiuretic hormone	Kidney function in hepatorenal syndrome
Testim [testosterone]	Z79.890	Testosterone therapy – topical	Primary hypogonadism
Tetracycline [tetracycline]	Z79.2	Antibiotic	Bacterial infections
Thalomid [thalidomide]	Z79.61	Immunomodulator	Multiple myeloma; erythema nodosum leprosum
Tiazac [diltiazem hydrochloride]		Calcium channel blocker	Chronic stable angina; atrial fibrillation; atrial flutter; hypertension; paroxysmal supraventricular tachycardia
Tobradex [tobramycin/dexamethasone]		Aminoglycoside ocular anti-infective; anti-inflammatory	Infectious conjunctivitis; dermatosis, corticosteroid-responsive with secondary infection; foreign body in eye; corneal inflammation; uveitis
Tobramycin [dexamethasone/tobramycin]	Z79.2	Antibiotic	Bacterial eye infections
Topamax [topiramate]		Anticonvulsant	Epilepsy; primary generalized tonic-clonic seizures; seizures associated with Lennox-Gastaut syndrome; migraine headache
Toprol-XL [metoprolol succinate]		Beta blocker	Angina pectoris; hypertension
Toremifene citrate [toremifene citrate]	Z79.810	Selective estrogen receptor modulator (SERM)	Metastatic breast cancer in postmenopausal women
Torisel [temsirolimus]	Z79.623	Mammalian target of rapamycin (mTOR) inhibitor	Renal cell carcinoma
Toujeo Solostar [insulin glargine recombinant]	Z79.4	Insulin	Diabetes mellitus
Tradjenta [linagliptin]	Z79.84	Oral hypoglycemic	Diabetes mellitus
Trazodone HCl [trazodone hydrochloride]		Antidepressant	Depression

Drug	Z Code	Drug Action/Classification	Indications
Trelegy Ellipta [fluticasone furoate/ umeclidinium bromide/vilanterol trifenatate]	Z79.51	Corticosteroid – inhaled; antiasthmatic	COPD
Trelstar [triptorelin pamoate]	Z79.818	Agents affecting estrogen receptors and estrogen levels	Palliative treatment of prostate cancer symptoms
Tremfya [guselkumab]	Z79.620	Immunosuppressive biologic; monoclonal antibody	Plaque psoriasis
Tresiba [insulin degludec]	Z79.4	Insulin	Diabetes mellitus
Triamterene and hydrochlorothiazide [triamterene/ hydrochlorothiazide]		Antihypertensive; diuretic	Edema; hypertension
Trijardy XR [empagliflozin/linagliptin/ metformin hydrochloride]	Z79.84	Oral hypoglycemic	Diabetes mellitus
Tri-Lo-Estarylla [ethinyl estradiol/ norgestimate]	Z79.3	Contraceptive	Prevention of pregnancy
Tri-Lo-Sprintec [ethinyl estradiol/ norgestimate]	Z79.3	Contraceptive	Prevention of pregnancy
Trimethoprim [trimethoprim]	Z79.2	Antibiotic	Acute exacerbation chronic bronchitis; travelers' diarrhea; infections of the middle, lower respiratory tract, and urinary tract; pneumonia, pneumocystis; shigellosis
Triptodur [triptorelin]	Z79.818	Agents affecting estrogen receptors and estrogen levels	Precocious puberty
Tri-Sprintec [ethinyl estradiol/norgestimate]	Z79.3	Contraceptive	Prevention of pregnancy; acne
Trokendi XR [topiramate]		Anticonvulsant	Epilepsy; primary generalized tonic-clonic seizures; seizures associated with Lennox-Gastaut syndrome; migraine headache
Trulicity [dulaglutide]	Z79.85	Antidiabetic – non-insulin injectable	Diabetes mellitus
Truqap [capivasertib]		Antineoplastic; kinase inhibitor	Breast cancer
Truvada [emtricitabine/tenofovir disoproxil fumarate]		Antiretroviral	HIV
Turalio [pexidartinib]		Kinase inhibitor	Symptomatic tenosynovial giant cell tumor
Tygacil [tigecycline]	Z79.2	Antibiotic	Bacterial skin or digestive system infections; pneumonia
Tzield [teplizumab-mzwv]	Z79.85	Antidiabetic – non-insulin injectable	Delay onset of stage 3 type 1 diabetes
Ubrelvy [ubrogepant]		Calcitonin gene-related peptide inhibitor	Migraine headache
Unasyn [ampicillin sodium/sulbactam sodium]	Z79.2	Antibiotic	Bacterial infections
Vabomere [meropenem; vaborbactam]	Z79.2	Antibiotic	Complicated urinary tract infections; pyelonephritis
Vabysmo [faricimab-svoa]		Anti-angiogenic ophthalmic agent	Neovascular age-related macular degeneration; diabetic macular edema
Vagifem [estradiol]	Z79.890	Estrogen therapy	Menopause symptoms
Valium [diazepam]		Antianxiety; muscle relaxant; anticonvulsant	Anxiety, tension, withdrawal from alcohol; muscle spasms and anticonvulsant therapy; epilepsy, generalized tonic-clonic; status epilepticus; stiff-person syndrome; tetanus
Vancocin HCl [vancomycin hydrochloride]	Z79.2	Antibiotic	Severe bacterial infections
Vancomycin HCl [vancomycin hydrochloride]	Z79.2	Antibiotic	Severe bacterial infections
Vanflyta [quizartinib]		Kinase inhibitor	Acute myeloid leukemia
Varenicline tartrate [varenicline tartrate]		Smoking cessation aid	Nicotine addiction; smoking
Vasotec [enalaprilat maleate]		ACE inhibitor	Congestive heart failure; hypertension
Velivet [desogestrel/ethinyl estradiol]	Z79.3	Contraceptive	Prevention of pregnancy
Velsipity [etrasimod]		Anti-inflammatory	Ulcerative colitis
Venlafaxine HCl [venlafaxine hydrochloride]		Antidepressant, serotonin and norepinephrine reuptake inhibitor (SNRI)	Major depressive disorder; social anxiety disorder; panic disorder
Ventolin HFA [albuterol sulfate]		Antiasthmatic/bronchodilator	Asthma
Veozah [fezolinetant]		CNS agent	Menopause symptoms
Verapamil HCL [verapamil hydrochloride]		Calcium channel blocker	Angina pectoris; chronic stable angina; atrial fibrillation; atrial flutter; paroxysmal supraventricular tachycardia; ventricular arrhythmia; hypertension
Viagra [sildenafil citrate]		Phosphodiesterase-5 (PDE5) inhibitor	Erectile dysfunction
Vibativ [telavancin hydrochloride]	Z79.2	Antibiotic	Pneumonia; severe bacterial skin infections
Vibramycin [doxycycline calcium]	Z79.2	Antibiotic	Bacterial infections
Victoza [liraglutide]	Z79.85	Antidiabetic – non-insulin injectable	Diabetes mellitus
Vinblastine sulfate [vinblastine sulfate]	Z79.633	Mitotic inhibitor	Cancer
Vincristine sulfate PFS [vincristine sulfate]	Z79.633	Mitotic inhibitor	Cancer
Virazole [ribavirin]		Antiviral	Respiratory syncytial virus (RSV)
Viread [tenofovir disoproxil fumarate]		Antiretroviral	HIV; chronic hepatitis B

Appendix B: Pharmacology List 2026

Drug	Z Code	Drug Action/Classification	Indications
Voltaren Arthritis Pain [diclofenac sodium]	Z79.1	Nonsteroidal anti-inflammatory drug (NSAID)	Treatment of pain, inflammation, and joint stiffness due to arthritis
Vonjo [pacritinib]		Multikinase inhibitor	Treats intermediate or high-risk primary or secondary myelofibrosis in adults with low platelets
Voquezna [vonoprazan, amoxicillin, and clarithromycin]	Z79.2	Antibiotic, antimicrobial; potassium-competitive acid blocker	Helicobacter pylori
Vtama [tapinarof]		Topical antipsoriatic	Plaque psoriasis
Vumerity [diroximel fumarate]	Z79.69	Other immunosuppressant/immunomodulator	Relapsing forms of multiple sclerosis (MS)
Vytorin [ezetimibe/simvastatin]		HMG-CoA reductase inhibitor (statin); cholesterol absorption inhibitor	Hyperlipidemia; hypercholesterolemia
Wakix [pitolisant hydrochloride]		CNS stimulant	Narcolepsy
Warfarin sodium [warfarin sodium]	Z79.01	Anticoagulant	Prophylaxis and treatment of venous thrombosis; treatment of atrial fibrillation with embolization (pulmonary embolism), arrhythmias, myocardial infarction, and stroke prevention
Wellbutrin SR, Wellbutrin XL [bupropion hydrochloride]		Antidepressant	Depression
Xacduro [sulbactam, durlobactam]	Z79.2	Antibiotic	Hospital-acquired bacterial pneumonia and ventilator-associated bacterial pneumonia caused by Acinetobacter baumannii-calcoaceticus complex
Xalatan [latanoprost]		Prostaglandin F2? analogue	Glaucoma, open-angle; ocular hypertension
Xanax, Xanax XR [alprazolam]		Antianxiety; sedative/hypnotic	Anxiety disorders with panic disorder and depression
Xarelto [rivaroxaban]	Z79.01	Anticoagulant	Prophylaxis and treatment of venous thrombosis, pulmonary embolism; prevention of blood clots due to atrial fibrillation
Xdemvy [lotilaner]		Antiparasitic	Demodex blepharitis
Xeljanz, Xeljanz XR [tofacitinib citrate]	Z79.622	Janus kinase (JAK) inhibitor	Rheumatoid arthritis; psoriatic arthritis
Xeloda [capecitabine]	Z79.631	Antimetabolite agent	Cancer of the breast, colon, colorectal
Xelstrym [dextroamphetamine]		CNS stimulant	Attention deficit hyperactivity disorder (ADHD)
Xenleta [lefamulin acetate]	Z79.2	Antibiotic	Community-acquired bacterial pneumonia
Xgeva [denosumab]	Z79.620	Immunosuppressive biologic; monoclonal antibody	Treatment and prevention of bone resorption and prevention of bone fracture
Xifaxan [rifaximin]	Z79.2	Antibiotic	E. coli diarrhea
Xigduo XR [dapagliflozin/metformin hydrochloride]	Z79.84	Oral hypoglycemic	Diabetes mellitus
Xpovio [selinexor]		Antineoplastic	Multiple myeloma in adults
Xulane [ethinyl estradiol/norelgestromin]	Z79.3	Contraceptive	Prevention of pregnancy
Xultophy 100/3.6 [insulin degludec/liraglutide]	Z79.4	Insulin	Diabetes mellitus
Xyrem [sodium oxybate]		CNS depressant; anxiolytic/sedative/hypnotic	Cataplexy and/or excessive daytime sleepiness in narcolepsy
Xyzal Allergy 24Hr [levocetirizine dihydrochloride]		Antihistamine	Perennial allergic rhinitis; chronic idiopathic urticaria
Yasmin [drospirenone/ethinyl estradiol]	Z79.3	Contraceptive	Prevention of pregnancy
Yaz [drospirenone/ethinyl estradiol]	Z79.3	Contraceptive	Prevention of pregnancy; menstrual disorders
Zavzpret [zavegepant]		Calcitonin gene-related peptide inhibitor	Migraine headache
Zerbaxa [ceftolozane sulfate/tazobactam sodium]	Z79.2	Antibiotic	Complicated urinary tract and intra-abdominal infections
Zestoretic [lisinopril/hydrochlorothiazide]		ACE inhibitor	Congestive heart failure; hypertension
Zestril [lisinopril]		ACE inhibitor	Congestive heart failure; hypertension
Zetia [ezetimibe]		Antihyperlipidemic	Hypercholesterolemia; sitosterolemia
Ziac [bisoprolol fumarate/hydrochlorothiazide]		Antihypertensive	Hypertension
Zilbrysq [zilucoplan]	Z79.69	Other immunosuppressant/immunomodulator	Myasthenia gravis
Zipsor [diclofenac potassium]	Z79.1	Nonsteroidal anti-inflammatory drug (NSAID)	Pain and inflammation relief
Zithromax [azithromycin]	Z79.2	Antibiotic	Infections of the cervix, lower respiratory tract, skin and skin structures, urethra, nongonococcal; mycobacterium avium complex; pharyngitis, streptococcal pneumonia; tonsillitis
Zocor [simvastatin]		HMG-CoA reductase inhibitor (statin)	Hypercholesterolemia; hyperlipidemia; hyperlipoproteinemia; hypertriglyceridemia
Zoladex [goserelin acetate]	Z79.818	Agents affecting estrogen receptors and estrogen levels	Palliative treatment of prostate cancer and breast cancer symptoms; endometriosis
Zoloft [sertraline hydrochloride]		Antidepressant	Anxiety with panic disorder and depression; obsessive-compulsive disorder

Drug	Z Code	Drug Action/Classification	Indications
Zometa [zoledronic acid]	Z79.83	Bisphosphonate	Multiple myeloma; Paget's disease
Zortress [everolimus]	Z79.623	Mammalian target of rapamycin (mTOR) inhibitor	Prophylaxis of organ transplant rejection
Zovia 1/50E-28 [ethinyl estradiol/ethynodiol diacetate]	Z79.3	Contraceptive	Prevention of pregnancy
Zovirax [acyclovir]		Antiviral	Genital herpes and herpes zoster infections
Zubsolv [buprenorphine/naloxone]		Opioid agonist	Treatment of opioid addiction
Zurzuvae [zuranolone]		CNS agent	Postpartum depression
Zyloprim [allopurinol]		Antigout	Gouty arthritis; renal calculus; hyperuricemia; hyperuricemia secondary to leukemia; hyperuricemia secondary to lymphoma
Zynyz [retifanlimab-dlwr]	Z79.60	Immune checkpoint inhibitor; immunosuppressant	Merkel cell carcinoma
Zyprexa [olanzapine]		Antipsychotic/antimanic	Psychotic disorders; schizophrenia
Zyrtec allergy [cetirizine hydrochloride]		Antihistamine	Perennial and seasonal allergic rhinitis; chronic urticaria
Zyvox [linezolid]	Z79.2	Antibiotic	Severe bacterial infections

Appendix C: Z Codes for Long-Term Drug Use with Associated Drugs

This resource correlates the Z codes that are used to identify current long-term drug use with a list of drugs that are typically categorized to that class of drug. These lists are not all-inclusive, providing only the more commonly used drugs.

Z79.01 Long term (current) use of anticoagulants
- Arixtra
- Defencath
- Eliquis
- Fragmin
- Heparin
- Jantoven
- Lovenox
- Pradaxa
- Savaysa
- Warfarin
- Xarelto

Z79.02 Long term (current) use of antithrombotics/ antiplatelets
- Aggrastat
- Angiomax
- Argatroban
- Brilinta
- Clopidogrel bisulfate
- Effient
- Eptifibatide
- Persantine
- Plavix
- Prasugrel

Z79.1 Long term (current) use of non-steroidal anti-inflammatories (NSAID)
- Advil
- Aleve
- Anaprox DS
- Arthrotec
- Caldolor
- Cambia
- Celebrex
- Daypro
- Duexis
- Feldene
- Ibuprofen
- Indocin
- Mobic
- Motrin IB
- Nabumetone
- Nalfon
- Naprelan
- Naprosyn
- NeoProfen
- Ponstel
- Voltaren Arthritis Pain
- Zipsor

Z79.2 Long term (current) use of antibiotics
- Altabax
- Amikacin
- Amoxicillin
- Ampicillin
- Augmentin
- Avelox
- Azactam
- Azithromycin
- Bactrim
- Biaxin XL
- Cefazolin sodium
- Cefepime hydrochloride
- Cefprozil
- Ceftriaxone
- Cefuroxime sodium
- Centany
- Cephalexin
- Cipro
- Ciprofloxacin
- Clarithromycin
- Cleocin
- Clindamycin
- Daptomycin
- Dificid
- Doxycycline
- E.E.S.
- Ertapenem
- ERYC
- Erygel
- EryPed
- Ery-Tab
- Erythrocin
- Erythromycin
- Fetroja
- Flagyl
- Gentamicin sulfate
- Hiprex
- Invanz
- Isoniazid
- Klaron
- Lincocin
- Macrobid
- Macrodantin
- Mepron
- Merrem
- Metronidazole
- Minocin
- Monodox
- Monurol
- Mycobutin
- Nebupent
- Neosporin
- Nitrofurantoin
- Oracea
- Orbactiv
- Penicillin-VK
- Pentam
- Pfizerpen
- Priftin
- Primaxin
- Rifadin
- Rimactane
- Septra
- Seromycin
- Silvadene
- Sivextro
- Solodyn
- Solosec
- Streptomycin sulfate
- Suprax
- Synercid
- Talicia
- Tazicef
- Teflaro
- Tetracycline
- Tobramycin
- Trimethoprim
- Tygacil
- Unasyn
- Vabomere
- Vancocin HCl
- Vancomycin HCl
- Vibativ
- Vibramycin
- Voquezna
- Xacduro
- Xenleta
- Xifaxan
- Zerbaxa
- Zithromax
- Zyvox

Z79.3 Long term (current) use of hormonal contraceptives
- Aranelle
- Aviane-28
- Beyaz
- Briellyn
- Camila
- Daysee
- Depo-Provera
- Depo-SubQ Provera
- Desogestrel/ethinyl estradiol
- Enpresse-28
- Femhrt
- Gildagia
- Gildess 24 FE
- Junel
- Levonest
- Liletta
- Lo Loestrin Fe
- Loryna
- LoSeasonique
- Low-Ogestrel-28
- Mirena
- Mono-Linyah
- Natazia
- Nexplanon
- NuvaRing
- Plan B One-Step
- Provera
- Seasonale
- Seasonique
- Skyla
- Sprintec
- Tri-Lo-Estarylla
- Tri-Lo-Sprintec
- Tri-Sprintec
- Velivet
- Xulane
- Yasmin
- Yaz
- Zovia 1/50E-28

Z79.4 Long term (current) use of insulin
- Admelog
- Apidra
- Basaglar
- Fiasp
- Humalog
- Humulin R
- Lantus
- Levemir
- Novolin
- Novolog
- Soliqua
- Toujeo Solostar
- Tresiba
- Xultophy 100/3.6

Z79.51 Long term (current) use of inhaled steroids
- Advair
- AirDuo RespiClick
- Alvesco
- Arnuity Ellipta
- Asmanex
- Breo Ellipta
- Dulera
- Flovent HFA
- Pulmicort
- Qvar Redihaler
- Symbicort
- Trelegy Ellipta

Z79.52 Long term (current) use of systemic steroids
- Agamree
- Celestone Soluspan
- Colocort
- Cortef
- Cortenema
- Cortifoam
- Depo-Medrol
- Dexamethasone Intensol
- Entocort EC
- Hydrocortisone
- Kenalog-10
- Kenalog-40
- Locoid
- Medrol
- Methylprednisolone
- Orapred ODT
- PediaPred
- Prednisolone
- Prednisone
- Rayos
- Solu-Cortef
- Solu-Medrol

Z79.61 Long term (current) use of immunomodulator
- Otezla
- Pomalyst
- Revlimid
- Thalomid

Z79.620 Long term (current) use of immunosuppressive biologic
- Actemra
- Aimovig
- Beyfortus
- Briumvi
- Columvi
- Cosentyx
- Cyltezo
- Dupixent
- Elrexfio
- Enbrel
- Entyvio
- Epkinly
- Humira
- Hyrimoz
- Imjudo
- Keytruda
- Loqtorzi
- Monoclonal antibodies
- Omvoh
- Prolia
- Remicade
- Rituxan
- Simulect
- Skyrizi
- Stelara
- Taltz
- Tremfya
- Xgeva

Z79.621 Long term (current) use of calcineurin inhibitor
- Astagraf XL
- Cyclosporine
- Envarsus XR
- Gengraf
- Lupkynis
- Neoral
- Prograf
- Protopic
- Restasis
- Sandimmune
- Tacrolimus

Appendix C: Z Codes for Long-Term Drug Use with Associated Drugs

Z79.622 **Long term (current) use of Janus kinase inhibitor**
- Cibinqo
- Ojjaara
- Olumiant
- Rinvoq
- Xeljanz
- Xeljanz XR

Z79.623 **Long term (current) use of mammalian target of rapamycin (mTOR) inhibitor**
- Rapamune
- Sirolimus
- Torisel
- Zortress

Z79.624 **Long term (current) use of inhibitors of nucleotide synthesis**
- CellCept
- Imuran

Z79.630 **Long term (current) use of alkylating agent**
- Busulfex
- Carmustine
- Chlorambucil
- Cisplatin
- Cytoxan
- Leukeran
- Temozolomide

Z79.631 **Long term (current) use of antimetabolite agent**
- 5-fluorouracil (5-FU)
- 6-mercaptopurine (6-MP)
- Cytarabine
- Methotrexate sodium
- Xeloda

Z79.632 **Long term (current) use of antitumor antibiotic**
- Bleomycin
- Cerubidine
- Doxorubicin
- Mitomycin

Z79.633 **Long term (current) use of mitotic inhibitor**
- Ixempra
- Paclitaxel
- Taxotere
- Vinblastine sulfate
- Vincristine sulfate PFS

Z79.634 **Long term (current) use of topoisomerase inhibitor**
- Camptosar
- Etoposide
- Hycamtin

Z79.64 **Long term (current) use of myelosuppressive agent**
- Hydroxyurea

Z79.69 **Long term (current) use of other immunomodulators and immunosuppressants**
- Actimmune
- Avonex
- Betaseron
- Bimzelx-bkzx
- Copaxone
- Enjaymo
- Intron A
- Orencia
- PegIntron
- Ponvory
- Rebif
- Sylatron
- Tavneos
- Vumerity
- Zilbrysq
- Zynyz

Z79.810 **Long term (current) use of selective estrogen receptor modulators (SERMs)**
- Evista
- Fareston
- Osphena
- Raloxifene HCl
- Soltamox
- Tamoxifen citrate
- Toremifene citrate

Z79.811 **Long term (current) use of aromatase inhibitors**
- Anastrozole
- Arimidex
- Aromasin
- Exemestane
- Femara
- Letrozole

Z79.818 **Long term (current) use of other agents affecting estrogen receptors and estrogen levels**
- Eligard
- Faslodex
- Lupron Depot
- Megace ES
- Orserdu
- Supprelin LA
- Synarel
- Trelstar
- Triptodur
- Zoladex

Z79.82 **Long term (current) use of aspirin**
- Bayer
- Bufferin
- Durlaza

Z79.83 **Long term (current) use of bisphosphonates**
- Aclasta
- Actonel
- Aredia
- Atelvia
- Binosto
- Fosamax
- Reclast
- Zometa

Z79.84 **Long term (current) use of oral hypoglycemic drugs**
- Acarbose
- Actoplus Met
- Actos
- Amaryl
- Brenzavvy
- DiaBeta
- Duetact
- Farxiga
- Glimepiride
- Glucotrol XL
- Glumetza
- Glyburide
- Glynase
- Glyset
- Invokamet
- Invokana
- Janumet
- Januvia
- Jentadueto
- Kazano
- Kombiglyze
- Metformin
- Oseni
- Qtern
- Repaglinide
- Rybelsus
- Sitagliptin
- Synjardy
- Tradjenta
- Trijardy XR
- Xigduo XR

Z79.85 **Long-term (current) use of injectable non-insulin antidiabetic drugs**
- Bydureon bcise
- Byetta
- Mounjaro
- Ozempic
- Symlin
- Trulicity
- Tzield
- Victoza

Z79.890 **Hormone replacement therapy**
- Activella
- Alora
- Androderm
- AndroGel
- Angeliq
- Bijuva
- Climara
- CombiPatch
- Delestrogen
- Divigel
- Duavee
- Elestrin
- Estrace
- EstroGel
- Femhrt
- Femring
- Firmagon
- Levoxyl
- Menest
- Menostar
- Minivelle
- Orilissa
- Prempro
- Provera
- Synthroid
- Testim
- Vagifem

Z79.891 **Long term (current) use of opiate analgesic**
- Acetaminophen with codeine
- Buprenorphine HCl and Naloxone HCl
- Butrans
- Codeine
- Demerol
- Dilaudid
- Duramorph PF
- Fentanyl citrate
- Fentora
- Fioricet with codeine
- Hydrocodone
- Hydrocodone bitartrate and acetaminophen
- Hydromorphone HCl
- Methadone HCl
- Methadose
- Morphine sulfate
- MS Contin
- Nucynta
- Oxycodone HCl
- OxyContin
- Percocet
- Roxicodone

Appendix D: Z Codes Only as Principal/First-Listed Diagnosis

Z00.00	Z01.12	Z02.3	Z04.72	Z34.92	Z38.8	Z52.010	Z52.813
Z00.01	Z01.20	Z02.4	Z04.81	Z34.93	Z39.0	Z52.011	Z52.819
Z00.110	Z01.21	Z02.5	Z04.82	Z38.00	Z39.1	Z52.018	Z52.89
Z00.111	Z01.30	Z02.6	Z04.89	Z38.01	Z39.2	Z52.090	Z76.1
Z00.121	Z01.31	Z02.71	Z04.9	Z38.1	Z40.00	Z52.091	Z76.2
Z00.129	Z01.411	Z02.79	Z31.81	Z38.2	Z40.01	Z52.098	Z99.12
Z00.2	Z01.419	Z02.81	Z31.83	Z38.30	Z40.02	Z52.10	
Z00.3	Z01.42	Z02.82	Z31.84	Z38.31	Z40.03	Z52.11	
Z00.5	Z01.810	Z02.83	Z33.2	Z38.4	Z40.09	Z52.19	
Z00.70	Z01.811	Z02.84	Z34.00	Z38.5	Z40.8	Z52.20	
Z00.71	Z01.812	Z02.89	Z34.01	Z38.61	Z40.9	Z52.21	
Z00.8	Z01.818	Z02.9	Z34.02	Z38.62	Z42.1	Z52.29	
Z01.00	Z01.82	Z04.1	Z34.03	Z38.63	Z42.8	Z52.3	
Z01.01	Z01.83	Z04.2	Z34.80	Z38.64	Z51.0	Z52.4	
Z01.020	Z01.84	Z04.3	Z34.81	Z38.65	Z51.11	Z52.5	
Z01.021	Z01.89	Z04.41	Z34.82	Z38.66	Z51.12	Z52.6	
Z01.10	Z02.0	Z04.42	Z34.83	Z38.68	Z52.000	Z52.810	
Z01.110	Z02.1	Z04.6	Z34.90	Z38.69	Z52.001	Z52.811	
Z01.118	Z02.2	Z04.71	Z34.91	Z38.7	Z52.008	Z52.812	

Appendix E: Centers for Medicare & Medicaid Services Hierarchical Condition Categories (CMS-HCC)

In the 1970s, Medicare began demonstration projects that contracted with health maintenance organizations (HMOs) to provide care for Medicare beneficiaries in exchange for prospective payments. In 1985, this project changed from demonstration status to a regular part of the Medicare program, Medicare Part C. The Balanced Budget Act (BBA) of 1997 named Medicare's Part C managed care program Medicare+Choice, and the Medicare Modernization Act (MMA) of 2003 again renamed it to Medicare Advantage (MA).

Medicare is one of the world's largest health insurance programs, and about one-third of the beneficiaries on Medicare are enrolled in an MA private health care plan. Due to the great variance in the health status of Medicare beneficiaries, risk adjustment provides a means of adequately compensating those plans with large numbers of seriously ill patients while not overburdening other plans that have healthier individuals. Medicare Advantage (MA) plans have been using the Hierarchical Condition Category (HCC) risk adjustment model since 2004.

The Risk Adjustment Model

The primary purpose of a risk adjustment model is to predict (on average) the future health care costs for specific consortiums enrolled in Medicare Advantage (MA) health plans. CMS is then able to provide capitation payments to these private health plans. Capitation payments are an incentive for health plans to enroll not only healthier individuals but those with chronic conditions or who are more seriously ill by removing some of the financial burden.

The MA risk adjustment model uses HCCs to assess the disease burden of its enrollees. HCC diagnostic groupings were created after examining claims data so that enrollees with similar disease processes, and consequently similar health care expenditures, could be pooled into a larger data set in which an average expenditure rate could be determined. The medical conditions included in HCC categories are those that were determined to most predictably affect the health status and health care costs of any individual. Several important principles to the risk adjustment model and the development of the HCC categories include but are not limited to:

1. The HCC diagnostic categories should be clinically meaningful.
   - Diagnostic categories are well-defined.
   - Clinically specific diseases or medical conditions are grouped to each category.
2. The HCC diagnostic categories should predict medical expenditures.
   - The diagnoses grouped to a specific category should have as close to the same cost burden not only in the current year but also in the future.
3. The HCC diagnostic categories should have adequate sample sizes and discretionary categories excluded to be as accurate and stable in their estimate of costs as possible.
   - A diagnostic category that groups extremely rare diseases or conditions would not be reliably effective in determining current or future costs.
   - Codes that are not credible as cost predictors or may be subject to coding variation should be excluded, when possible.
4. The HCC diagnostic categories should be both hierarchical and additive.
   - Hierarchical measurement is used within a specific disease process.
   - Disease processes that are unrelated to each other are measured additively.
5. The diagnostic classification should encourage specificity and should not reward coding proliferation.
   - More diagnosis codes and vague diagnosis codes do not equal greater disease burden.

Beginning in CY 2024, CMS finalized implementing a revised version of the CMS-HCC risk-adjustment model. This model will be phased-in with proposed completion in CY2026 and has the same structure as the 2020 CMS-HCC risk-adjustment model currently used for payment in that it incorporates all of the following:

- Updated data years used for model calibration
- Updated denominator year used in determining the average per capita predicted expenditures to create relative factors in the model
- A clinical reclassification of the hierarchical condition categories (HCCs) using ICD-10-CM codes

The model will use more recent data and denominator year and reflect a reclassification by which CMS rebuilt the condition categories to reflect diagnosis coding under the ICD-10-CM diagnosis classification system. CMS assessed conditions that are coded more frequently for Medicare Advantage, and as a result the proposed model includes additional constraints and the removal of several HCCs in order to reduce the impact on risk scores of MA coding variation. The 2024 CMS-HCC V28 model has 115 payment HCCs, up from 86 in the current model. This increase in HCCs is due to newly created HCCs added to the model and the splitting of several existing HCCs resulting from changes in the structure and clinical specificity of codes from ICD-9 to ICD-10, as well as changes in clinical concepts for some conditions. The model results in more appropriate relative weights because they reflect more recent utilization, coding, and expenditure patterns. Beneficiary risk scores or plan average risk scores may change depending on each individual beneficiary's combination of diagnoses or the clinical profile of a plan's enrollee population.

To guide the reclassification process, CMS applied its longstanding 10 Principles of Risk Adjustment that were used to create the original CMS-HCC diagnosis classification system. Both the panel of clinicians and analyses of cost data informed CMS's creation of the revised condition categories. The new categories reflect more clinical specificity and validity available through ICD-10 coding and better reflects recent cost and utilization patterns. The new categories and updated HCCs also reflect possible changes to physician coding patterns that have developed as a result of the transition to ICD-10 that the current model does not. Changes to the condition categories are based on each category's ability to predict costs for Medicare Parts A and B benefits. Condition categories that do not predict costs well or do not have well-specified diagnosis coding are not included in the model.

Risk Adjustment Factors

The CMS-HCC risk adjustment model uses "risk adjustment factors" to calculate a risk score for each member. This score summarizes that particular patient's expected cost of care relative to other members'. Each member's risk score is based on demographic and health status information and is calculated as the sum of these demographic and health factors weighted by their estimated marginal contributions to total risk. The model also takes into account where the patient resides (community or institutional), Medicaid eligibility (full or partial benefits), the patient's Medicare enrollment status (new or established), age, disability status, whether the patient is frail or has end-stage renal disease (ESRD), and even prescription drug use.

No procedure codes, ICD-10-PCS or CPT, are included in the MA risk adjustment model. The model relies solely on diagnostic and demographic data. Not all ICD-10-CM diagnoses map to an HCC, and there is no specific code sequencing involved. The CMS-HCC model is additive as well as hierarchical. The additive functionality allows a patient to have more than one HCC category assigned, providing a more complete clinical picture and prediction of resource consumption. The hierarchical aspect of the model provides a means of ranking diagnoses that are similar in disease process, by severity. The hierarchy of the condition categories ensures the patient's conditions are classified to the most severe condition within the related group. Less severe conditions within a particular hierarchy are superseded by more severe diagnoses within the same group. The hierarchy and additive relationship permits this model to characterize the person's illness level within each disease process, while still allowing the effects of unrelated disease processes to be counted in the patient's overall score.

Certain combinations of coexisting diagnoses for an individual can increase medical costs. The CMS-HCC model adjusts for these higher costs by the addition of "disease interaction" factors. For each patient, multiple HCCs assigned, along with demographic and disease interaction factors, are used to calculate a single, combined risk adjustment factor (RAF). The RAF score for an individual member represents all of the HCCs that have been submitted from all sources for that member to CMS during the course of an entire calendar year.

There are separate CMS-HCC models for new enrollees and continuing enrollees. The new enrollee model uses demographic factors only, such as age, sex, and disability status, and is used when the enrollee has less than 12 months of medical history. The community model accounts for age, sex, original reason for Medicare entitlement (age or disability), Medicaid eligibility, and clinical conditions as measured by HCCs. In the second step, expected costs are adjusted for outliers based on the member's risk score and whether the patient has ESRD.

Demographic data (age, sex, eligibility) as well as health status (diagnoses codes submitted on claims to CMS) of an MA population are used to determine the reimbursement to the health plan to care for their members.

CMS considers a RAF score of 1.0 as the benchmark to indicate the score of the average healthy patient with the same demographic and diagnostic factors. These patients are expected to use average or lower-than-average resources. When the RAF score is higher than 1.0, CMS considers the patient to be sicker than the average patient with the same criteria and expects greater-than-average resource utilization. Beginning in PY2026 100% of the RAF score will be based on the 2024 CMS-HCC model.

Appendix E: Centers for Medicare & Medicaid Services Hierarchical Condition Categories (CMS-HCC)

A low RAF score may accurately indicate a healthier patient, but it may also falsely indicate a healthier patient due to incomplete or inaccurate coding, incomplete or insufficient record documentation, or patients who fail to complete an annual assessment.

A high RAF score may accurately indicate a sicker patient, or it may be falsely inflated from overcoding due to diagnoses that are reported but not documented, or from copying and pasting from previous encounters or problem lists of resolved conditions.

Documentation Requirements

Payment is made per HCC category (not per diagnosis code). No matter how many times in the year the diagnosis codes are reported, a single payment is made to the MA plan each year. Each year the list of HCCs and the RAF for each patient is "reset." This means the annual health assessment is extremely important, and adequate documentation is critical. Accurate risk adjustment payment relies on complete medical record documentation and diagnosis coding. CMS requires that all applicable diagnosis codes be reported and that all diagnoses be reported to the highest level of specificity and that these be substantiated by the medical record.

> **CMS's Guiding Principle:**
> The risk adjustment diagnosis must be based on clinical medical record documentation from a face-to-face encounter, coded according to the *ICD-10-CM Guidelines for Coding and Reporting*; assigned based on dates of service within the data collection period, submitted to the MA organization from an appropriate risk adjustment provider type and an appropriate risk adjustment physician data source.

A "face-to-face" health service encounter between a patient and healthcare provider describes an encounter between the patient and the provider (MD, DO), including qualified nonphysician practitioners (NPP) (e.g., nurse practitioner or physician's assistant), which is face-to-face with the patient. CMS provides a current listing of acceptable physician specialty types for risk adjustment data submission within the 2012 Regional Technical Assistance Participant Guide. The only exception to the face-to-face encounter requirement is pathology services (professional component only). Due to the 2019 Coronavirus Disease (COVID-19) pandemic, CMS is allowing MA organizations to submit diagnoses from telehealth services that meet the risk adjustment face-to-face requirement when the services are provided using interactive audio and video telecommunications systems that permit real-time interactive communication. Currently, CMS does not provide a listing of all services that are considered face-to-face visits for risk adjustment data, but does provide guidance on what types of services are not acceptable for risk adjustment in the Participant Guide. For example, diagnostic radiology does not qualify because diagnostic radiologists typically do not document confirmed diagnoses. Other examples of services that are not acceptable include diagnostic reports that have not been interpreted, such as laboratory reports.

It is essential that the medical record documentation show evidence by provider authentication that the direct face-to-face service was personally furnished by the physician or qualified NPP. Examples of these services include office visits, hospital visits, preoperative anesthesia assessment, and surgical and invasive procedures.

Risk adjustment relies on annual health information. Each enrollee is assigned an individual risk score based on the health status information obtained from the diagnosis codes on the claims. The CMS-HCC model relies on ICD-10-CM coding specificity for accurate risk adjustment by using the most specific code available that is substantiated by the documentation in the medical record. Providers should fully document and accurately code the evaluation and management of all severe and chronic conditions to ensure a full, complete, and accurate clinical record of the patient's condition and reflect the work involved in caring for the patient, particularly those with complex and challenging health issues. All conditions affecting the treatment or management of the patient's health should be documented at least once a year, as applicable to care provided, to accurately describe the true complexity and severity of the patient's health. If the diagnosis coding on the claim is not accurate or complete, the claim may indicate that the provider did much less medical decision-making, evaluation, and management than was actually performed.

Documentation to support or validate risk adjustment conditions may be found anywhere in the note for the face-to-face encounter. It is important to ensure that the note accurately reflects all chronic conditions that affect the health and care of the patient. Each encounter must be unique and reflect only that visit as it occurred. Insufficient documentation influences the assignment of diagnosis codes and directly affects the patient's risk score.

Documentation should properly validate all reported conditions. Each page of progress notes should be properly authenticated and include the patient's name and the date.

Providers should document each clinical diagnosis to the highest degree of specificity per encounter, including all complications and/or manifestations, including clear links to causal conditions. Only confirmed conditions should be documented—no rule-out conditions or abnormal findings without clinical significance. All known conditions, including chronic conditions, that affect the care and treatment of the patient at least once per year should be noted.

Providers should specifically document the condition and clinical significance, and any pertinent changes, using terminology such as decreased, increased, worsening, improving, or unchanged, or abnormal findings.

Documentation Tips

- Document all cause-and-effect relationships.
- Report the most specific diagnosis code available that is supported by the documentation.
- Include all current diagnoses as part of the current medical decision-making, and document for every visit.
- Identify diagnoses that are current or chronic problems rather than a past medical history or previous resolved condition.
- Document history of heart attack, status codes, etc., that affect the patient's care as "history of" or "PMH" when they no longer exist or are not current conditions.
- Ensure each progress note has the date, signature, and credentials/specialty.
- Document the thought processes used to assess each condition.
- Know high revenue HCCs that are often undiagnosed or undercoded.
- Avoid "unspecified" codes.
- Ensure the codes reported are accurate.
- Ensure each encounter is billed.
- Review rejection reports, and audit reports to assess risks.

Audits

Because reimbursement is by patient, rather than based on an average of the entire population, and is based upon documentation, there is the potential for upcoding. Audits are conducted by the MA plan and CMS recovery auditors.

Initial Validation Audit (IVA)

CMS requires that the MA plan validate HCCs. This is usually performed by an independent auditor working with the plan or a contracted vendor to validate the MA plan's data submitted to CMS.

The MA plan submits the one best medical record that supports each HCC identified for the beneficiary.

Risk Adjustment Data Validation Audit

Risk adjustment data validation (RADV) audits were introduced in 2011 and updated for 2015. They are performed by CMS to validate the integrity and accuracy of risk-adjusted payments by verifying that the diagnosis codes the MA plans submit are supported by the medical record documentation for a member. On March 30, 2020, CMS suspended all RADV activities due to the 2019 coronavirus public health emergency (PHE). On June 12, 2025, CMS resumed audit activities and initiated the first round of PY 2019 RADV audits.

MA plans can be selected by CMS for RADV audits annually and if chosen are required to submit their members' medical records to CMS. Providers are required to assist the MA plan by providing the medical record documentation included in the audit. Even though each diagnosis needs to be reported only once in a calendar year, during a RADV audit up to five dates of service may be submitted to support any one HCC.

To be validated, medical record documentation must meet certain criteria and standards. Even if the diagnosis is documented and coded correctly, any deficiency in the documentation can make the encounter and the HCC invalid. Diagnoses that cannot be validated are considered payment errors. The results of the audit are communicated to the MA plan, which then communicates these results to the provider. Under- and overpayments are subject to payment adjustment. The results of RADV audits can be extrapolated over the MA plan population to calculate potential payment errors and overpayments/recoupments. Regulations include a RADV appeal process, a document dispute process, and a procedure for obtaining physician-signature attestations.

The following items are reviewed during the validation process:

- The record is for the correct enrollee.
- The record is from the correct calendar year for the payment year being audited.
- The record is legible.
- The date of service is present on the records and is for a face-to-face visit.
- The record is from a valid provider type.
- Valid credentials and/or a valid physician specialty are documented on the record.
- The record contains a signature from an acceptable type of physician.
- There is a diagnosis on the record.
- The diagnosis supports an HCC.
- The diagnosis supports the submitted HCC.

Mitigate audit risk by coding each reportable diagnosis each time it meets reporting guidelines. Audit regularly to assess areas of risk and in need of improvement and to capture conditions documented but not coded. Check for additional qualifying HCCs. Ensure claims are submitted and that corrected claims are submitted when indicated. There are three claims submission deadlines: January, March, and September. CMS adjusts each member's risk score twice a year, with the final reconciliation in August of the year after the plan year.

If providers emphasize correct coding and documentation and perform internal audits to determine where the risks are and prepare for audits, incorrect payment is less likely.

For additional information on risk adjustment coding, see Optum's *Risk Adjustment Coding and HCC Guide*.

Appendix F: Centers for Medicare & Medicaid Services Quality Payment Program

In 2015, in an effort to repeal the faulty Medicare sustainable growth rate (SGR), focus on quality of patient outcomes, and control Medicare spending, Congress passed the Medicare Access and CHIP Reauthorization Act (MACRA), which included sweeping changes for practitioners who provide services reimbursed under the Medicare physician fee schedule (MPFS). MACRA repealed the Medicare SGR methodology used for updating the MPFS and replaced it with the Quality Payment Program (QPP).

Under the QPP, providers who demonstrate success at controlling costs while providing high-quality care to their patients are eligible to earn increased payments. Clinicians who successfully report on determined criteria receive a larger payment. Beginning with the 2022 payment year and beyond, the maximum negative payment adjustment for those who do not participate or do not fulfill the defined requirements during each performance year will be up to 9 percent of Medicare Part B reimbursements. Payment adjustments (positive, neutral, or negative) received for the 2027 payment year will be based on the MIPS final score for the 2025 performance year.

Passage of the Medicare Access and CHIP Reauthorization Act of 2015

The final rule for implementing MACRA was published November 4, 2016. The final rule primarily provided details on how the QPP was to be implemented, including requiring the secretary of Health and Human Services (HHS) to sunset the value-based (VM) modifier incentive program, the Medicare electronic health record (EHR) incentive program, and the Physician Quality Reporting System (PQRS), and incorporated these incentive programs into the QPP.

Replacement of the Sustainable Growth Rate

Under the SGR, if overall physician costs were higher than a targeted Medicare expenditure, payments were reduced across the board. With the SGR method, payments to clinicians would have resulted in substantial cuts.

Because the QPP replaces the SGR methodology, the following revisions were detailed in MACRA:

- Established conversion factor updates:
  - a Medicare physician fee schedule conversion factor adjustment of 0.5 percent in 2016–2019 and a conversion factor adjustment of 0.00 percent for 2020–2026
  - the qualifying participant (QP) alternative payment models (APM) conversion factor of 0.75 percent and a nonqualifying provider APM conversion factor of 0.25 percent for 2026 and each subsequent year

Under the QPP, the Centers for Medicare and Medicaid Services (CMS) aims to:

- Support quality of patient care improvement by focusing on better outcomes for patients, decreasing provider burden, and preserving the independent clinical practice
- Promote the adoption of APMs, which align incentives across healthcare stakeholders
- Advance existing efforts of delivery system reform, including ensuring a smooth transition to a new system that promotes high-quality, efficient care through unification of CMS legacy programs such as the EHR incentive program

Quality Payment Program Established

The MACRA final rule established the Quality Payment Program (QPP) effective January 1, 2017. Within the QPP there are two interrelated pathways: Advanced Alternative Payment Models (APM) and the Merit-based Incentive Payment System (MIPS).

Eligible clinicians (EC) select the track/pathway—MIPS or advanced APMs—they wish to participate in based on the practice size, specialty, location, and patient population. Unlike previous quality initiatives, a provider does not have to enroll in the QPP. However, groups wishing to participate in the MIPS program via the Consumer Assessment of Healthcare Providers and Systems (CAHPS) for MIPS survey measures or CMS Web Interface (WI) must register by June 30 each year. Note that beginning with the 2022 performance period, the CMS WI will no longer be available as a submission or collection type. The CAHPS for MIPS survey is an optional quality measure that groups participating in MIPS can elect to administer.

In the 2020 Physician Fee Schedule Final Rule, CMS finalized a new participation framework to begin in 2021 known as MIPS Value Pathways (MVPs). The MVPs allow for a more cohesive participation experience by connecting activities and measures that are relevant to a specialty, medical condition, or a particular population. Due to the 2019 Coronavirus public health emergency (PHE), CMS postponed the implementation of MVPs as a reporting option for MIPS measures and activities until 2023. CMS finalized proposed updates for the criteria, process, and MVP implementation and finalized 12 MVPs for the 2023 performance year. Beginning with 2025 performance year there are 22 finalized MVPs. For additional and updated information on MVPs, see https://qpp.cms.gov/mips/mips-value-pathways.

Merit-based Incentive Payment System

MIPS is the track for clinicians who opt to participate in traditional Medicare as opposed to participating through an advanced APM. In doing so, clinicians may earn a payment adjustment related to evidence-based and practice-specific quality data. As a result, depending on the degree and success of performance in all four categories, clinicians receive one of the following:

- Positive payment adjustment in which additional compensation is received
- Neutral payment adjustment that neither increases nor reduces Medicare payments
- Negative payment adjustment of up to 9 percent of Medicare payment furnished in calendar year (CY) 2026

Participation in the MIPS track is determined based on the amount billed to Medicare and the number of beneficiaries seen per year. The following provider types are eligible for participation if they meet or exceed at least one of the following criteria:

- Medicare billings are greater than $90,000.
- More than 200 covered services are provided to Medicare Part B patients.
- Care is provided to more than 200 Medicare patients each year.

The following clinician types are considered ECs:

- Physicians (MD, DO, DDS, DMD, DPM, OD)
- Physician assistants (PA)
- Nurse practitioners (NP)
- Clinical nurse specialists (CNS)
- Certified registered nurse anesthetists (CRNA)
- Physical therapists (PT)
- Occupational therapists (OT)
- Qualified speech-language pathologists
- Qualified audiologists
- Clinical psychologists
- Osteopathic practitioners
- Chiropractor
- Registered dieticians or nutrition professionals
- Clinical social workers
- Certified nurse midwives

Anatomy of MIPS

A measurement-based regime creates a single reporting framework for physicians that comprise four performance categories:

- Quality
- Improvement Activities (IA)
- Promoting Interoperability
- Cost

MIPS eligible clinicians may participate in the program as an individual clinician, group, virtual group, or APM entity. Each of the four performance categories has been weighted, with greatest emphasis placed on the Quality category. Performance category weights for individuals, groups, and virtual groups placed the Quality category at 30 percent, Promoting Interoperability is second at 25 percent, IA at 15 percent, and Cost at 30 percent. Performance category weights for APM entities reporting traditional MIPS are weighted differently than these participation levels. The emphasis is still on the Quality category at 50 percent, Promoting Interoperability is second at 30 percent, Improvement Activities is third at 20 percent, and Cost is at 0 percent. Beginning with the 2022 performance period regardless of participation level (e.g., individual, group, etc.) the quality and cost performance categories will be equally weighted at 30%.

The 2023 MIPS performance threshold equates to 75 points out of a possible 100 points. Simply put, eligible clinicians are required to score 75 points to avoid up to a negative 9 percent payment adjustment.

Appendix F: Centers for Medicare & Medicaid Services Quality Payment Program

Quality Performance
Under the MIPS Quality performance category, ECs and groups must select six measures from a listing of almost 200 measures, with at least one of the six measures being an outcome measure, high-priority measure (in absences of outcome measure), or complete specialty measure set. Patient outcomes such as mortality, whether a patient is readmitted to the hospital, and the patient's experience are areas that CMS and the healthcare industry seek to improve. An outcome measure is the way CMS can quantify changes in the health of an individual, groups of individuals, and even certain populations that they can attribute back to a specific intervention or series of interventions.

Quality measures are tools for quantifying, or measuring, healthcare processes and patient outcomes and perceptions, as well as organizational structure and/or systems linked to the ability to provide high-quality healthcare. These measures play an important role under the MIPS. Reporting should be done on a minimum of half of the EC's or group practice's Medicare Part B patients. Performance data is reported for 75 percent of the patients who qualify for each measure.

Improvement Activities
The IA category assesses to what degree a clinician participates in activities designed to improve clinical practices. ECs are required to attest that they have participated in two high-weighted activities, one high-weighted activity and two medium-weighted activities, or four medium-weighted activities. The activities may be selected from an expanded inventory of more than 100 activities across eight subcategories for 90 consecutive days. These eight subcategories include:

- Expanded practice access
- Population management
- Care coordination
- Beneficiary engagement
- Patient safety and practice assessment
- Achieving health equity
- Integrating behavioral and mental health
- Emergency preparedness and response

This category was created with some inherent flexibility; for example, for groups with 15 or fewer participants, nonpatient-facing clinicians (e.g., pathologists), or those ECs in a rural or health professional shortage area (HPSA) receive two times the points when they report activities for at least 90 consecutive days.

Promoting Interoperability
CMS wants to encourage and promote the use of certified EHR technology (CEHRT) among providers and, in particular, the use of interoperability and sharing of information among clinicians and between providers and patients. In response to the 21st Century Cures Act Final Rule, CMS updated the CEHRT requirements to include technology certified to the 2015 Edition Cures Update certification criteria, the current 2015 Edition certification criteria, or a combination of both criteria to collect and report PI data.

Successful reporting of measures in this category require the EC to report measures from the four objectives and measures based exclusively on the 2015 edition of CEHRT and, as applicable, claim an exclusion. Exclusions are reported by submitting a "0" in addition to the exclusion type that applies to the EC because some measures may be associated with more than one exclusion.

The PI performance category contains four objectives:

- E-Prescribing
- Health Information Exchange
- Provider to Patient Exchange
- Public Health and Clinical Data Exchange

Data collected for each of the four objectives must be submitted for the same minimum continuous 90 days (unless an exclusion is applicable).

Cost
In this performance category, CMS determines an EC or group practice's cost score by calculating data from two measures previously included in the value-based payment modifier that involves the total cost of care for attributed beneficiaries and what Medicare spends per beneficiary. This amount is the total of both Medicare Part A and B payments from three days before through 30 days after a beneficiary has had an inpatient hospitalization episode. CMS then determines which ECs and practices have an adequate number of beneficiaries and hospitalizations associated with them. This number is compared with national benchmarks established for the performance period.

There are a total of 35 cost measures:

- Episode-based cost measures based on a range of procedures, acute inpatient medical conditions, and chronic conditions
- Population-based cost measures focused more broadly on primary and inpatient care.

For procedure episodes, the case minimum established is 10 with credit for the episodes going to the clinician who performs the procedure. For acute inpatient medical condition episodes, the case minimum is set at 20, and credit is assigned to each clinician who bills the inpatient evaluation and management (E/M) claim lines during a triggered inpatient hospitalization under a TIN that furnishes at least 30 percent of the inpatient E/M claim lines during that particular hospitalization.

Clinicians have no additional submission responsibilities associated with this category as the score is determined from Medicare administrative claims data.

The category also has separate benchmarks. The Cost score is determined and compared with those benchmarks with points assigned based on the decile system in a similar manner to the Quality performance category with some differences such as:

- Benchmarks for performance are for the *same* year versus prior year performance.
- Scores are determined once case minimum requirements for each of the two measures in this category have been met.

MIPS Scoring
CMS uses scoring to determine an EC's successful participation in the QPP and thereby determine if the clinician's reimbursement will be negative, neutral, or positive.

The scoring methodology is a unified approach across all performance categories, allowing eligible clinicians to understand what is expected so they can perform successfully in the MIPS. For more information and details on QPP, see https:/qpp.cms.gov.

Notes

Notes

Illustrations

Chapter 3. Diseases of the Blood and Blood-forming Organs and Certain Disorders Involving the Immune Mechanism (D50–D89)

Red Blood Cells

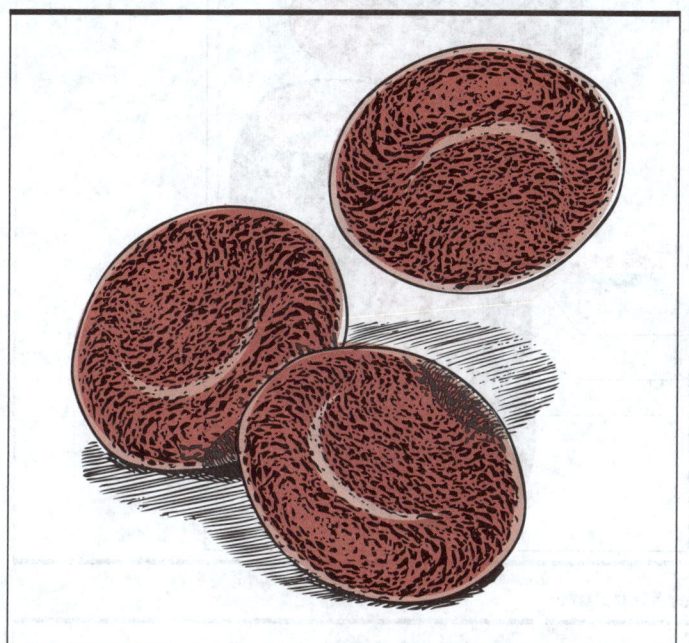

White Blood Cell

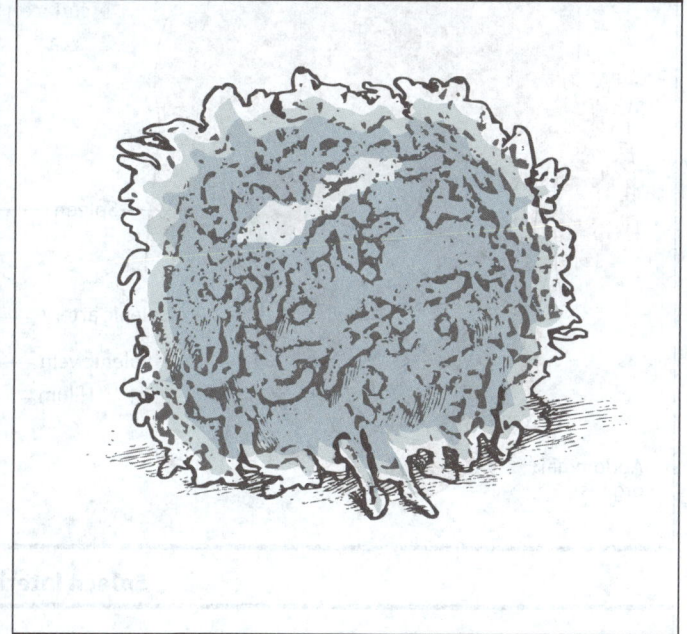

Platelet

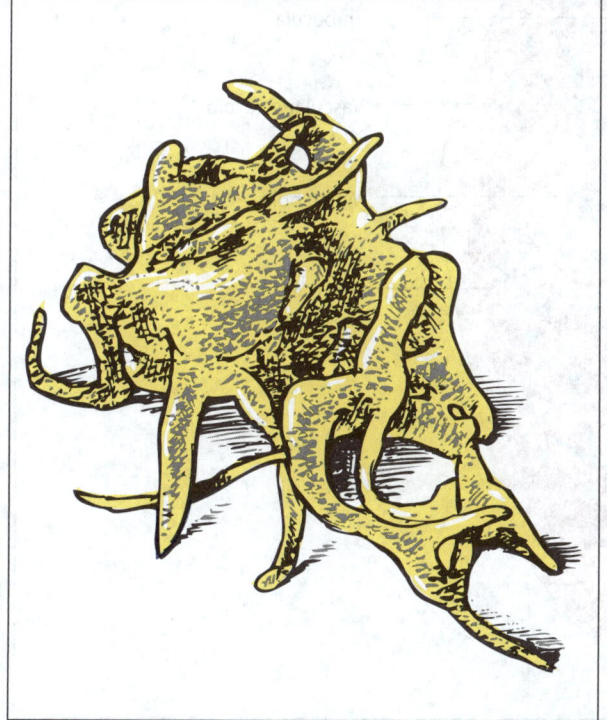

Coagulation

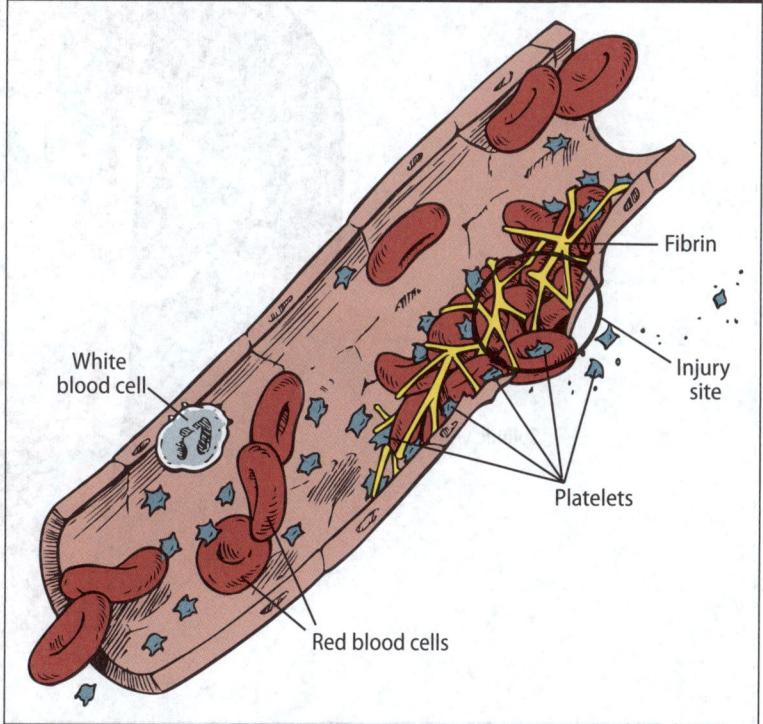

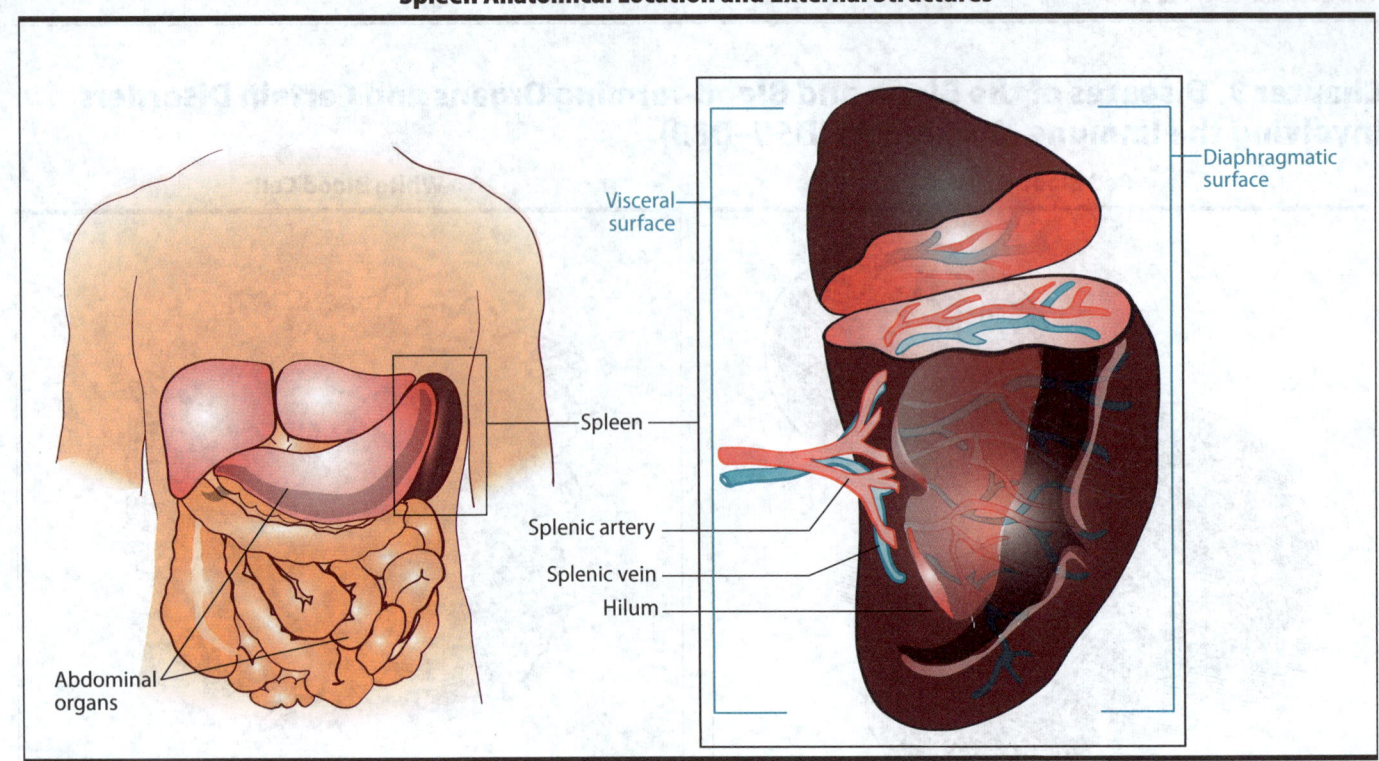

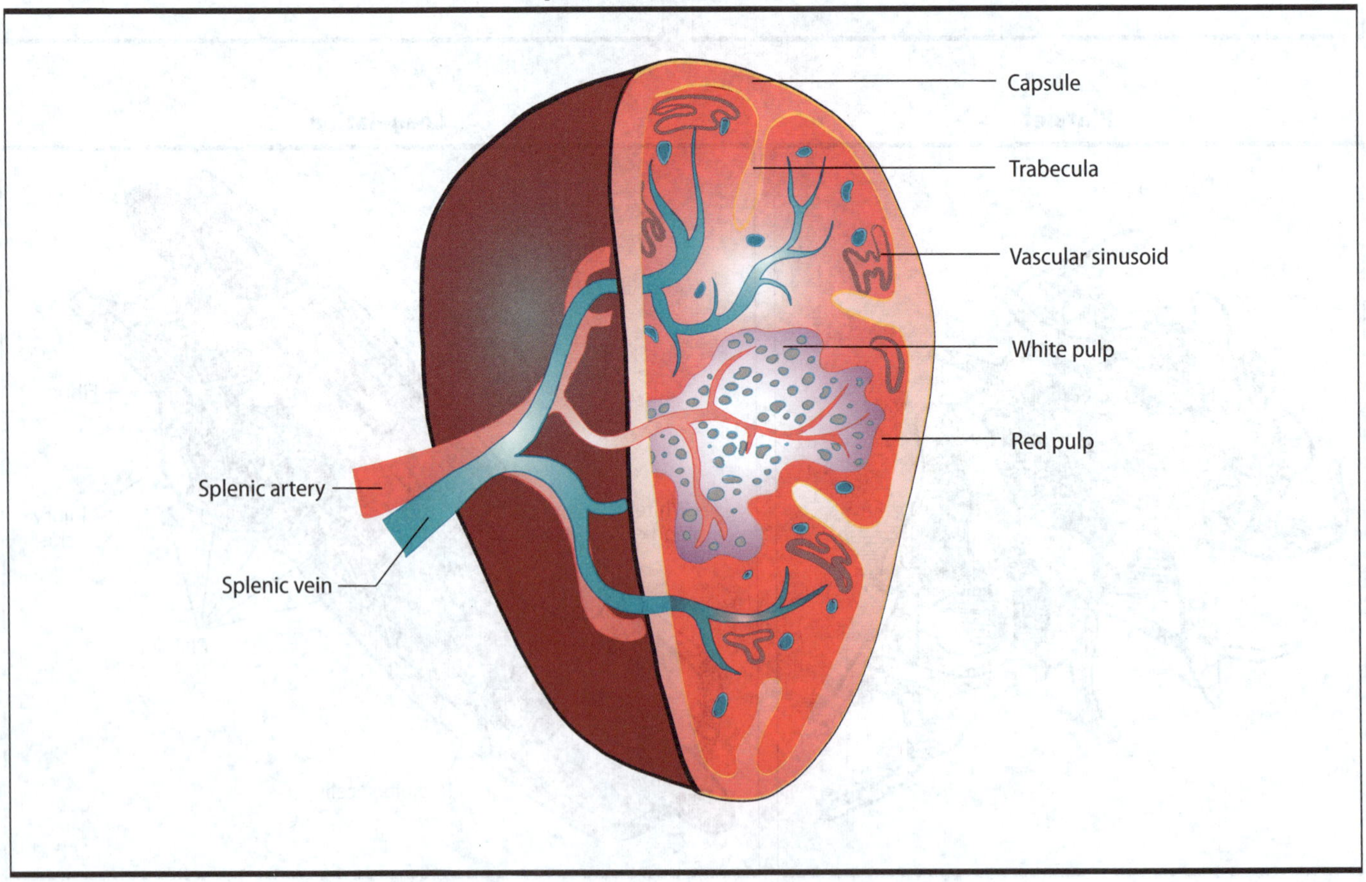

Chapter 4. Endocrine, Nutritional and Metabolic Diseases (E00–E89)

Endocrine System

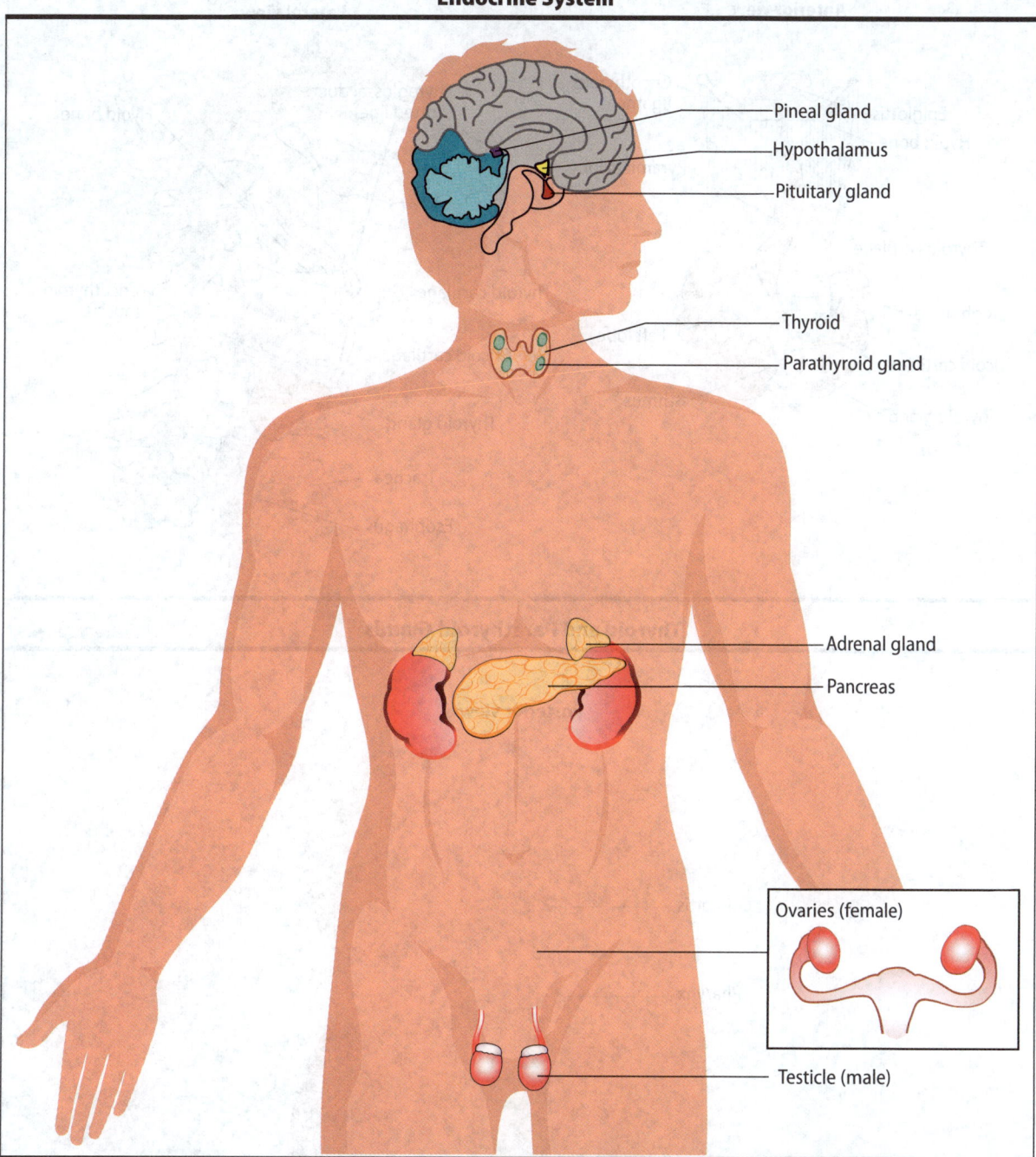

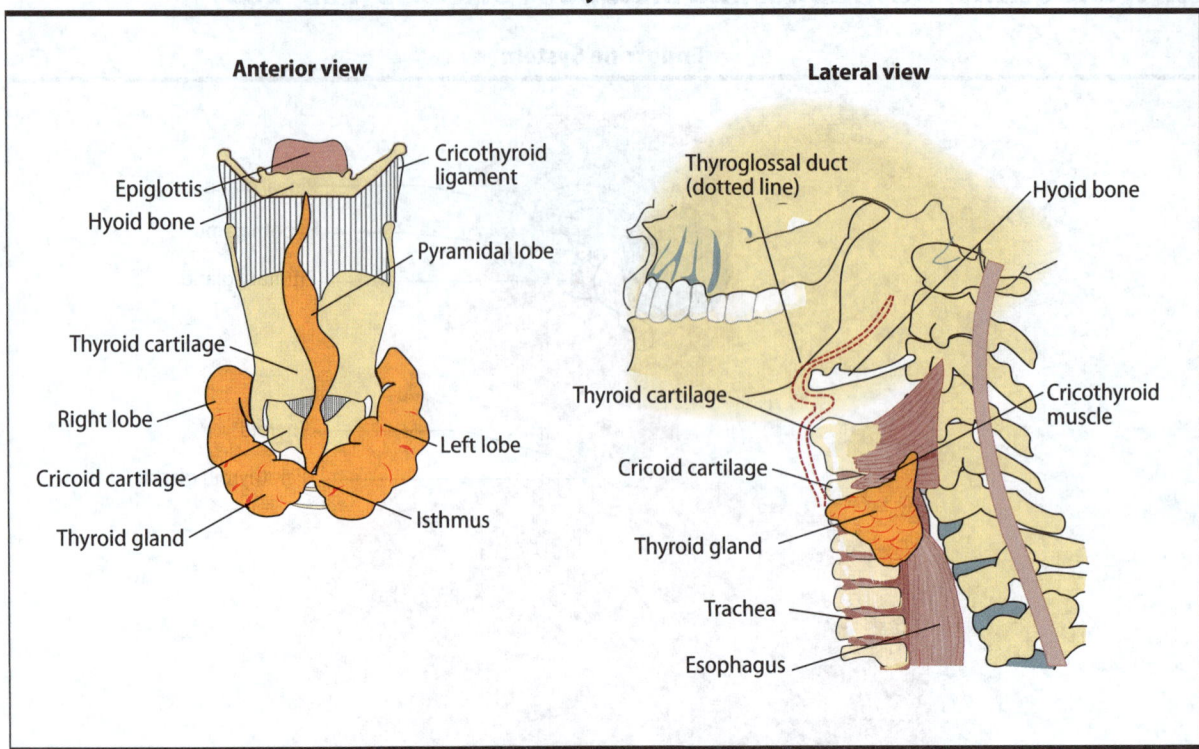

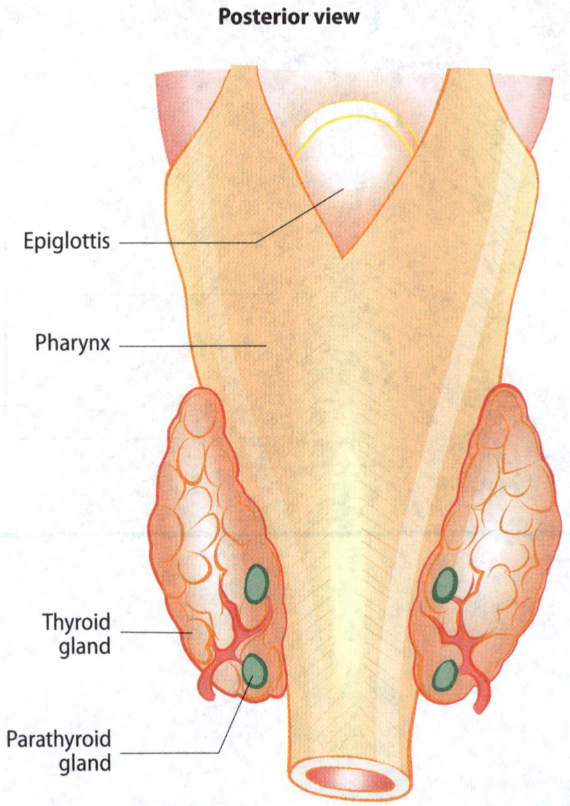

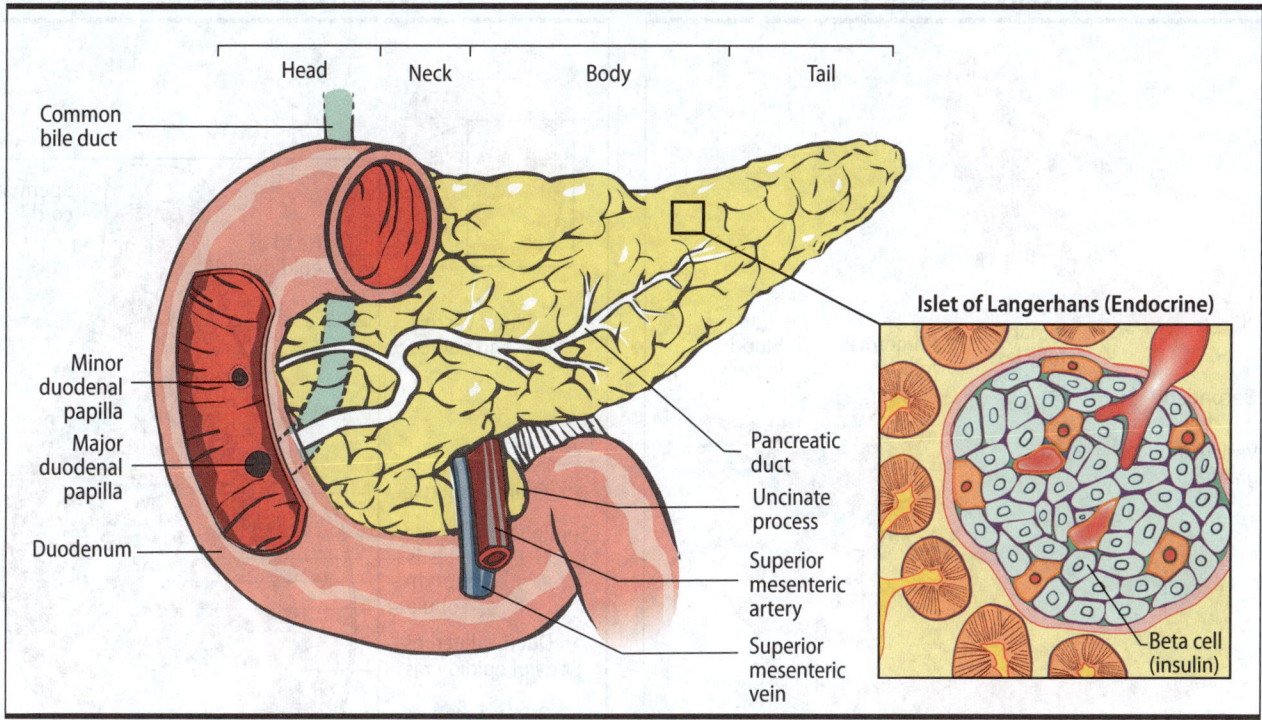

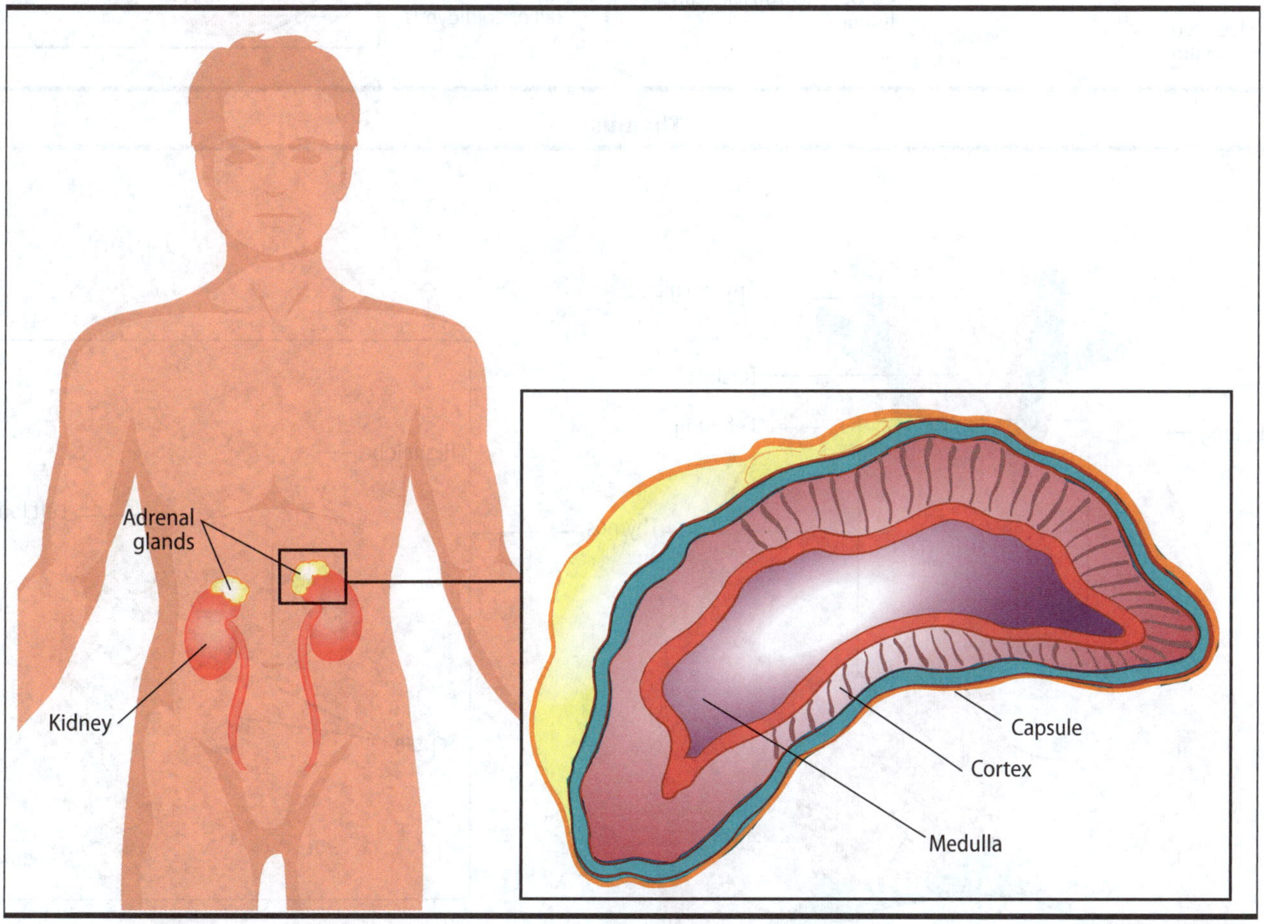

Structure of an Ovary

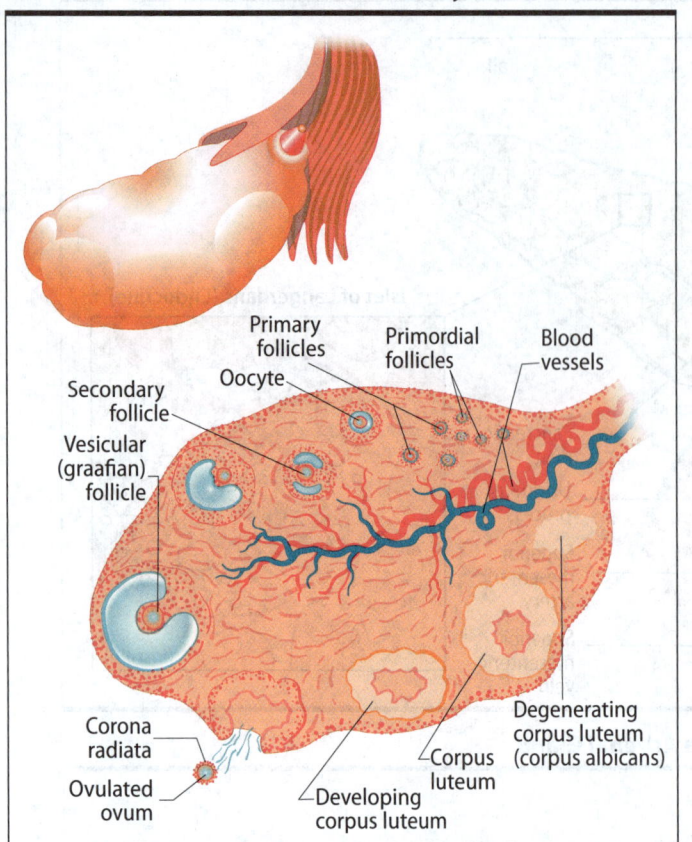

Testis and Associated Structures

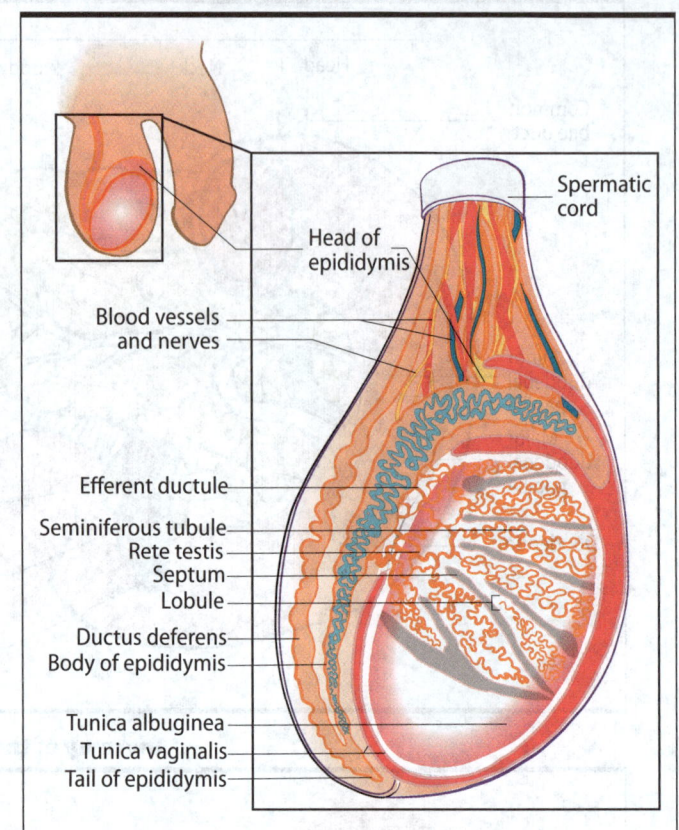

Thymus

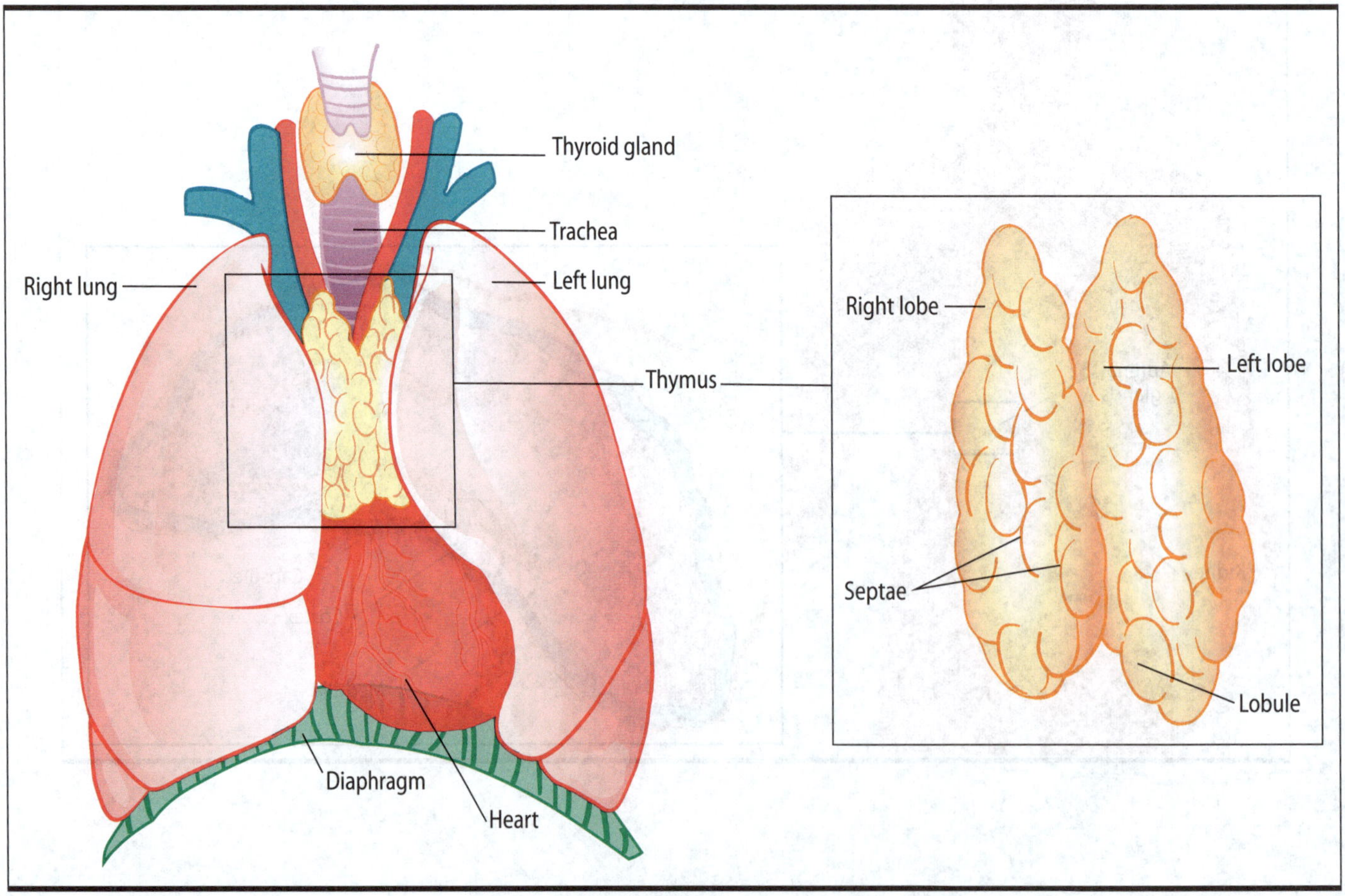

Chapter 6. Diseases of the Nervous System (GØØ–G99)

Brain

Cranial Nerves

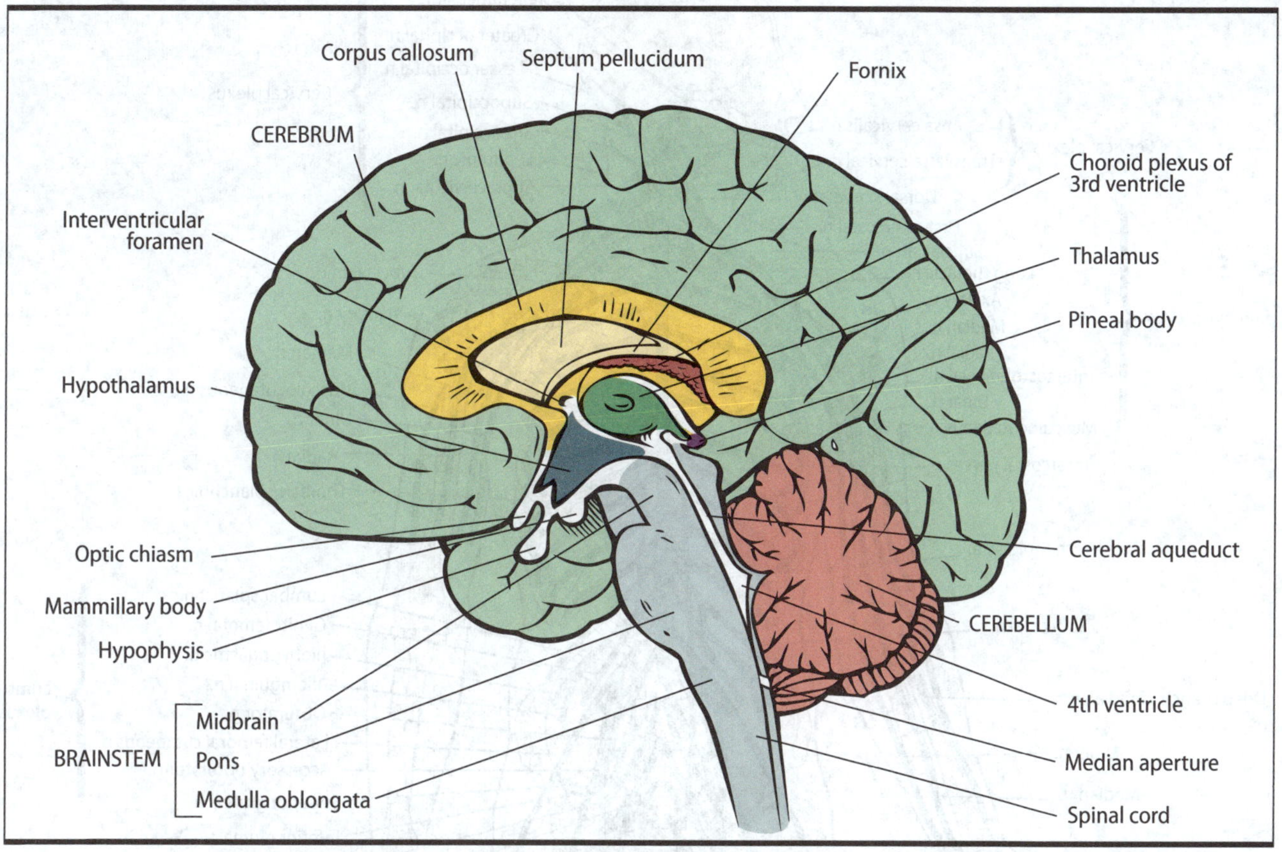

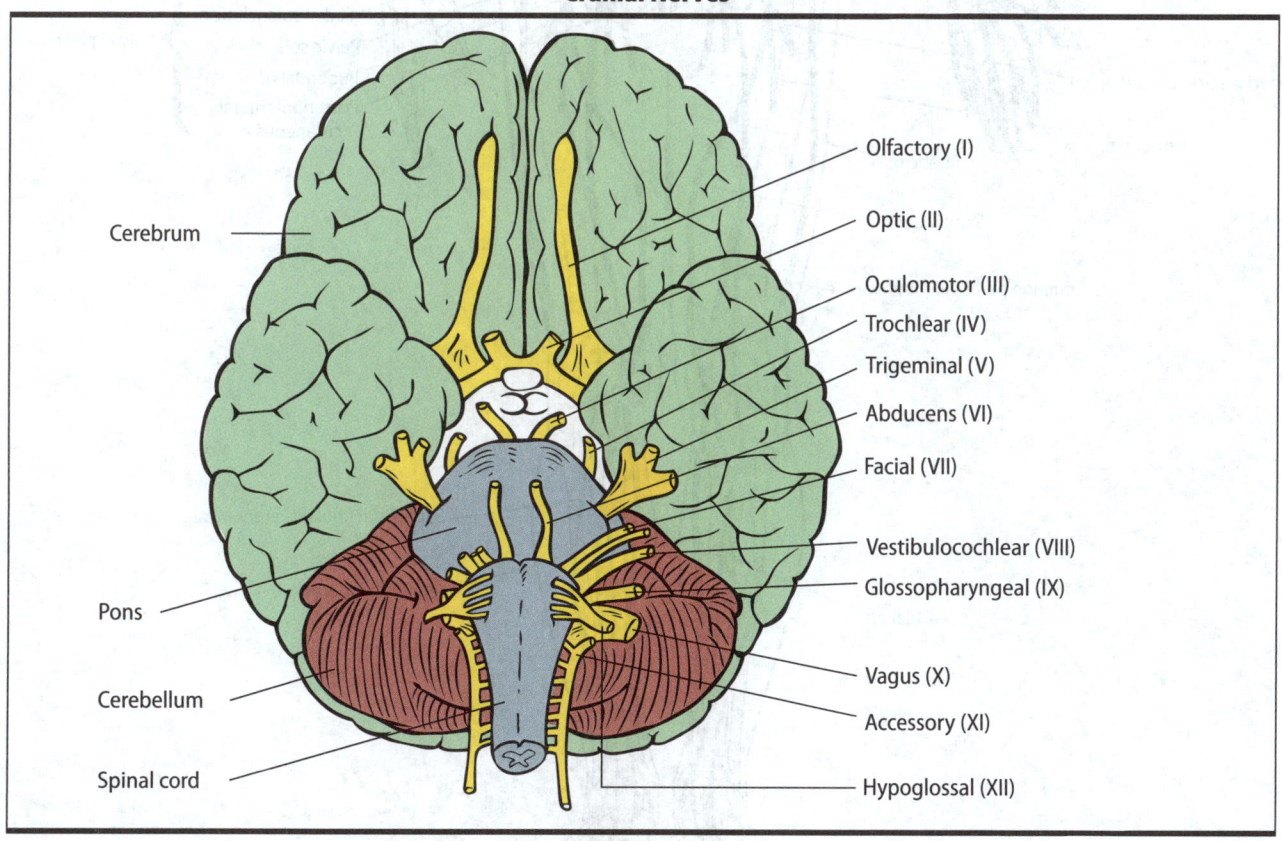

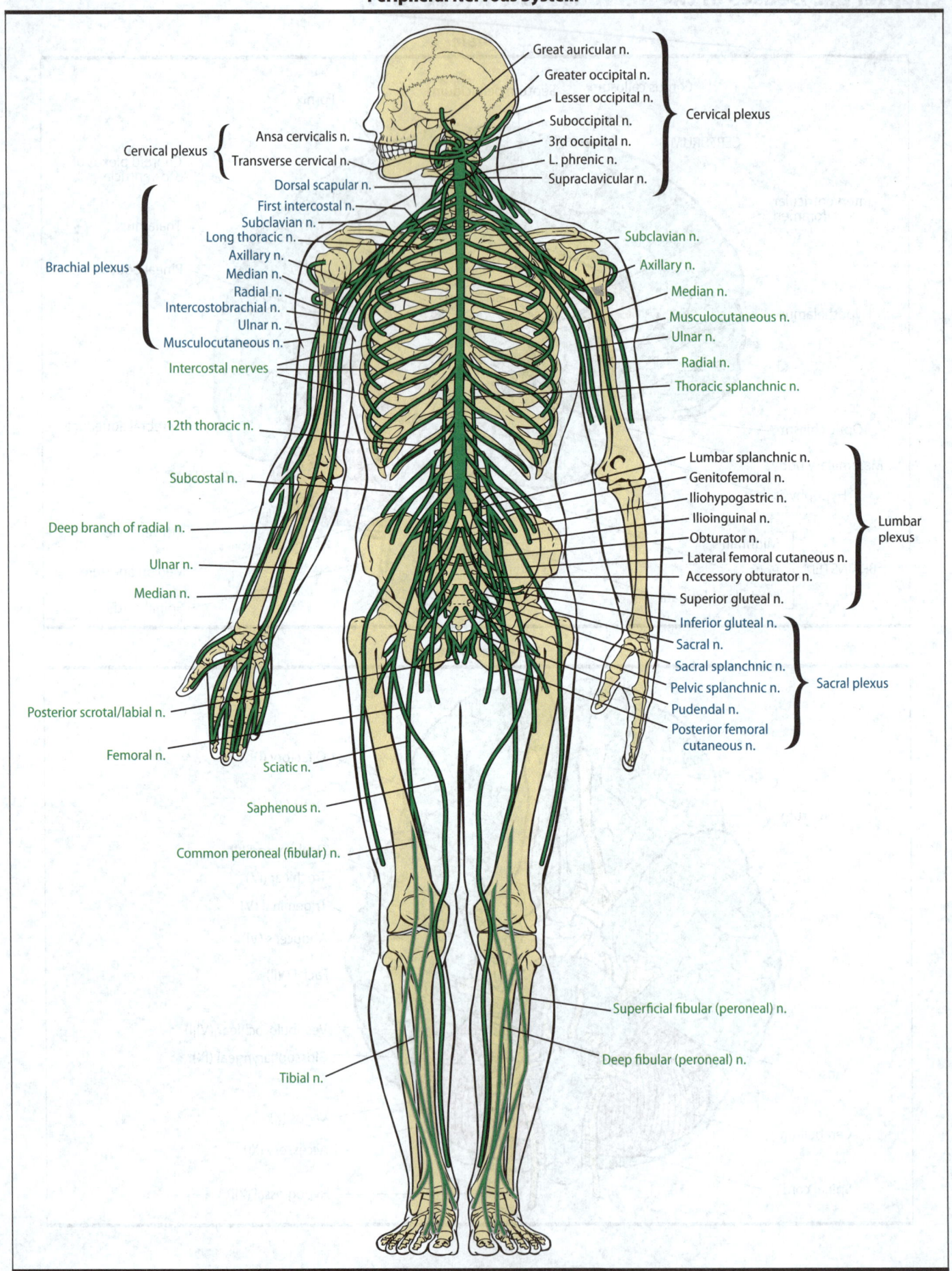

Spinal Cord and Spinal Nerves

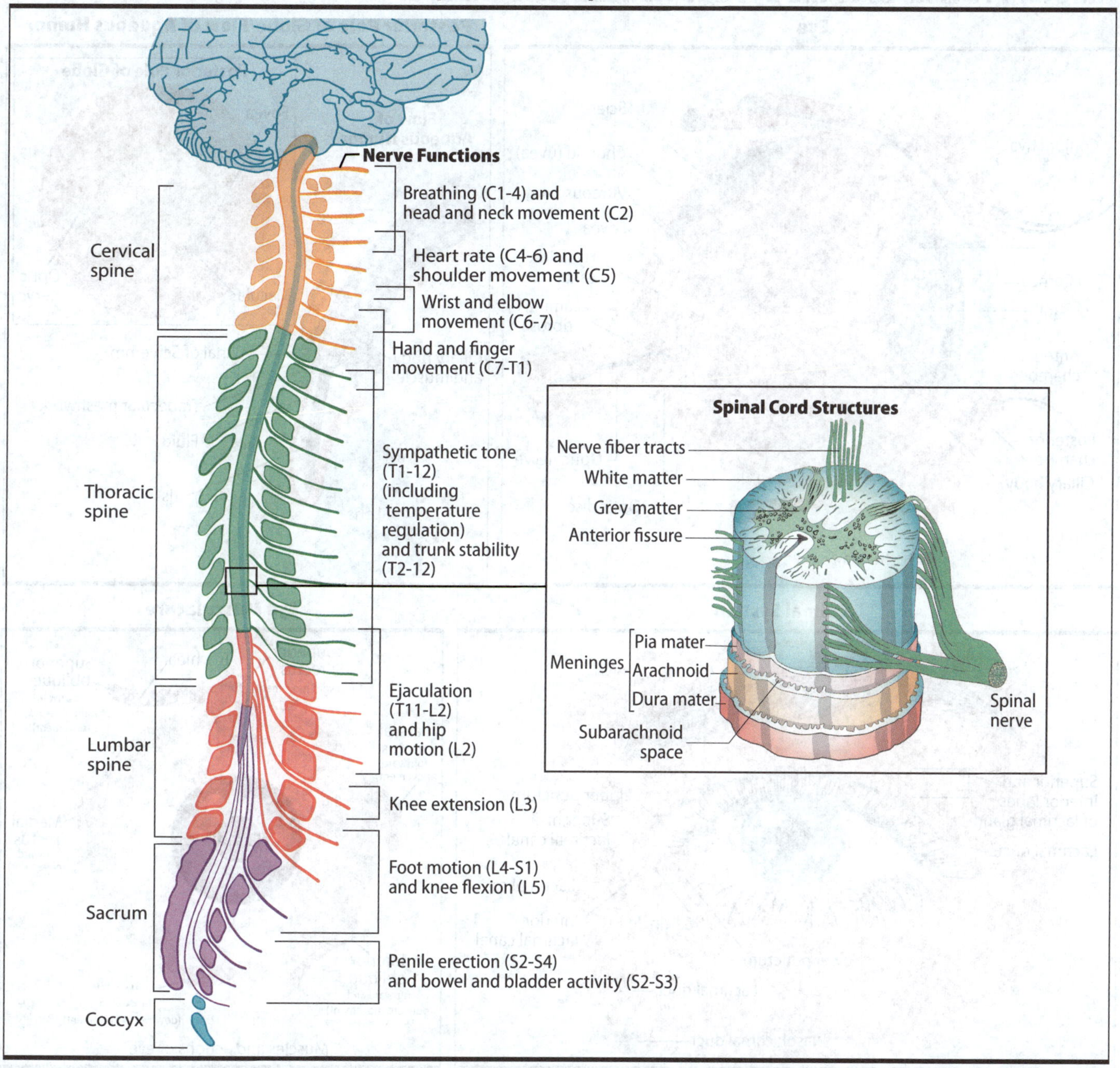

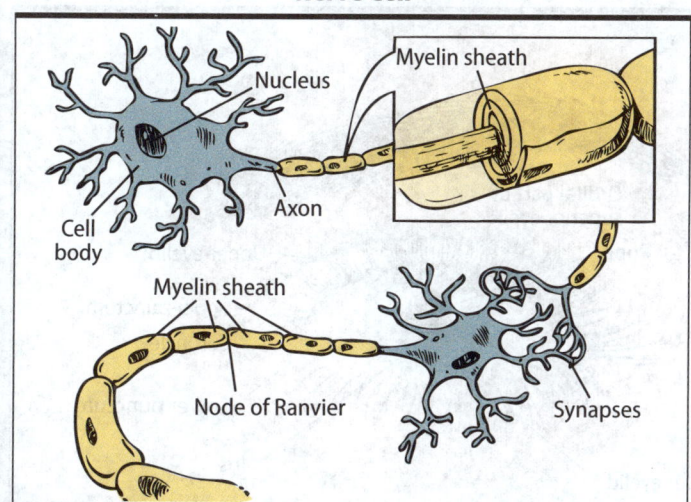
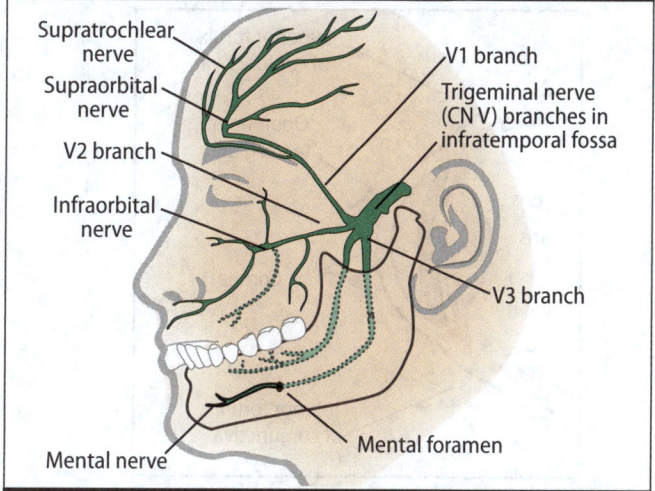

Chapter 7. Diseases of the Eye and Adnexa (H00–H59)

Eye
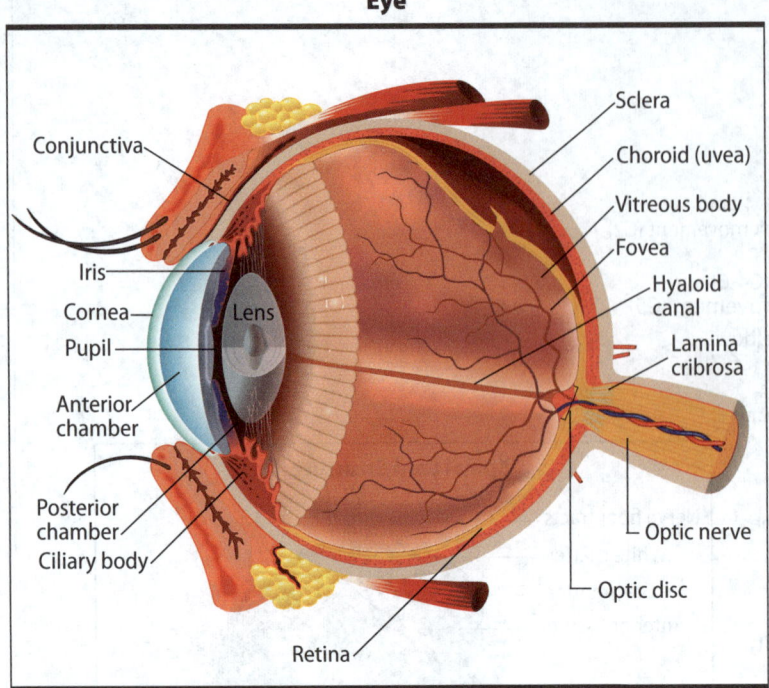

Posterior Pole of Globe/Flow of Aqueous Humor
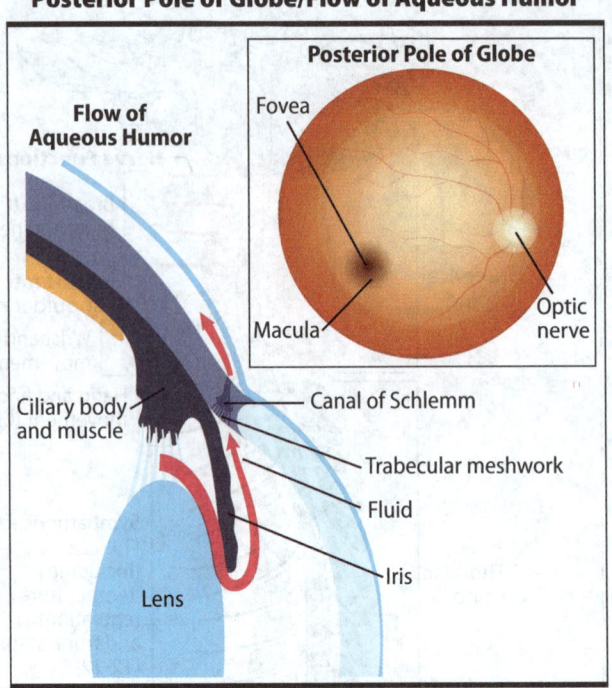

Lacrimal System
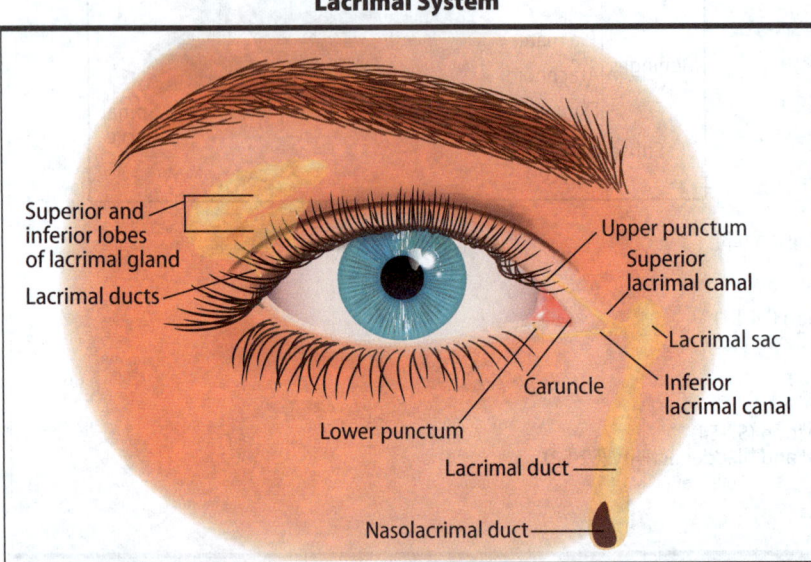

Eye Musculature
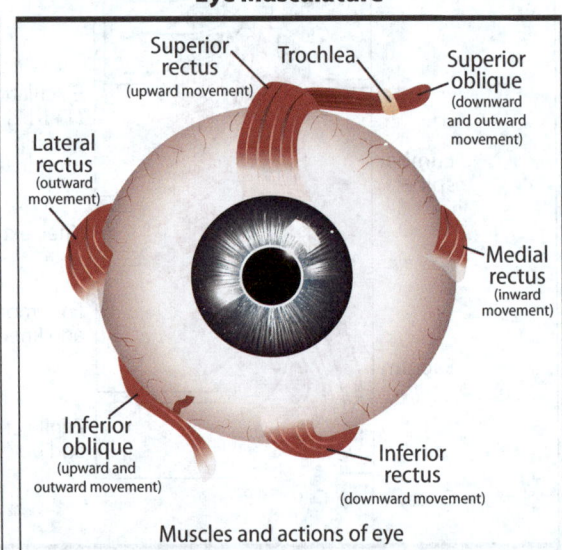

Eyelid Structures
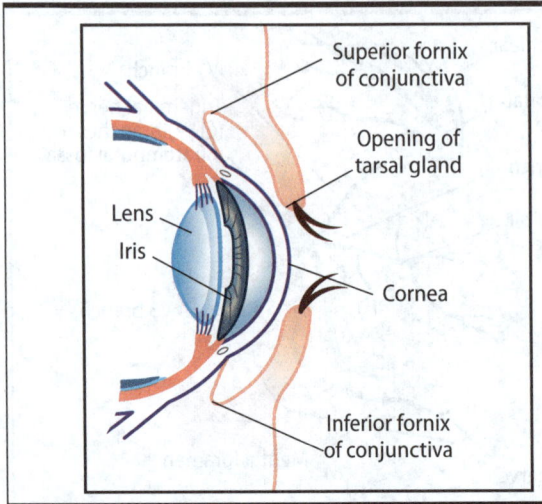
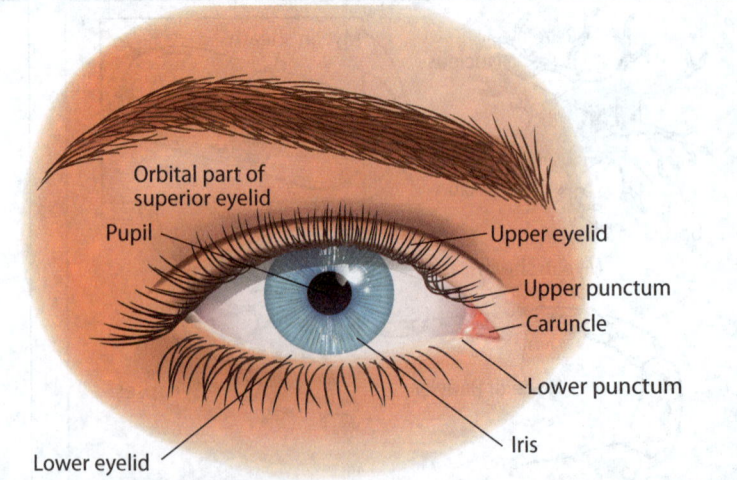

Chapter 8. Diseases of the Ear and Mastoid Process (H60–H95)

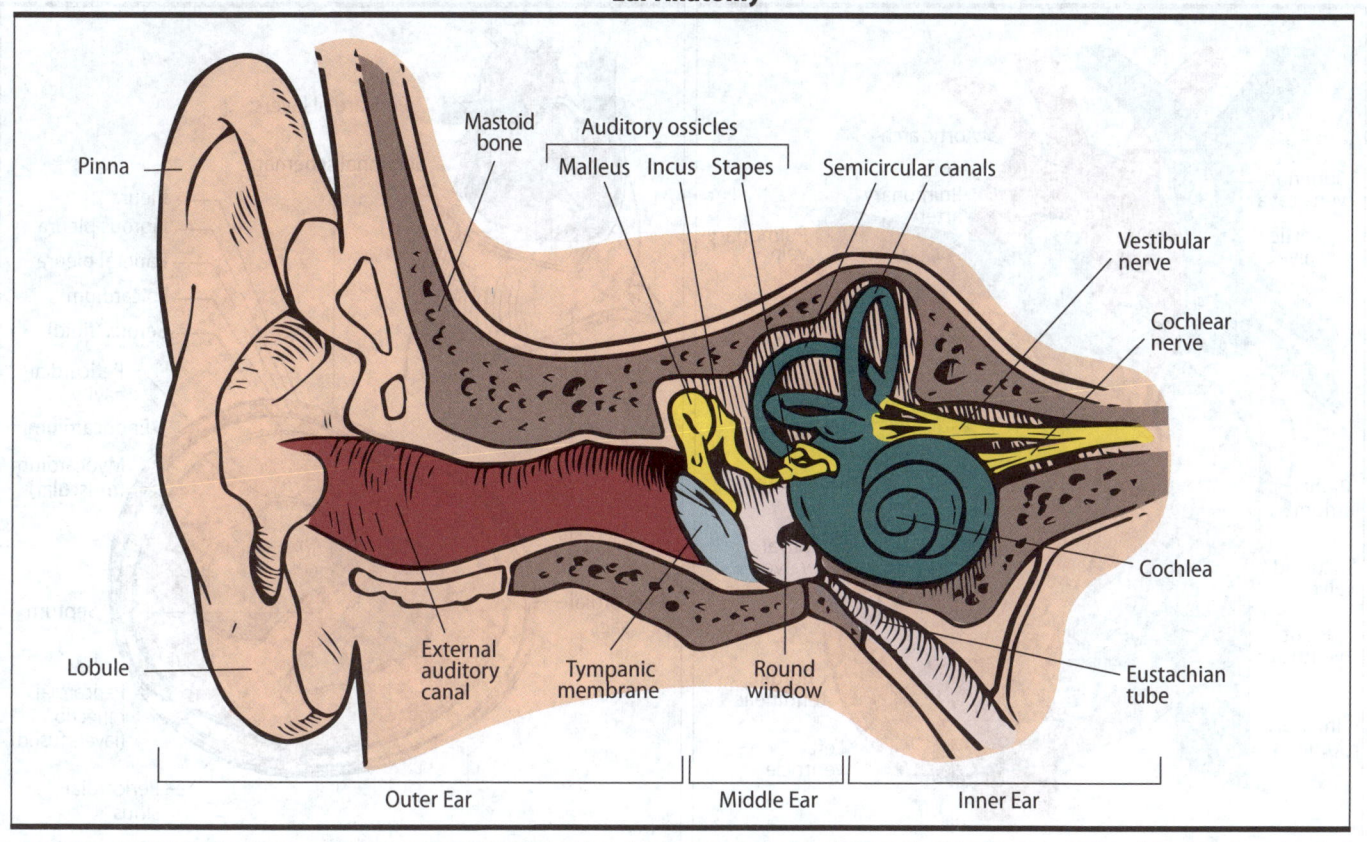

Ear Anatomy

Chapter 9. Diseases of the Circulatory System (I00–I99)

Anatomy of the Heart

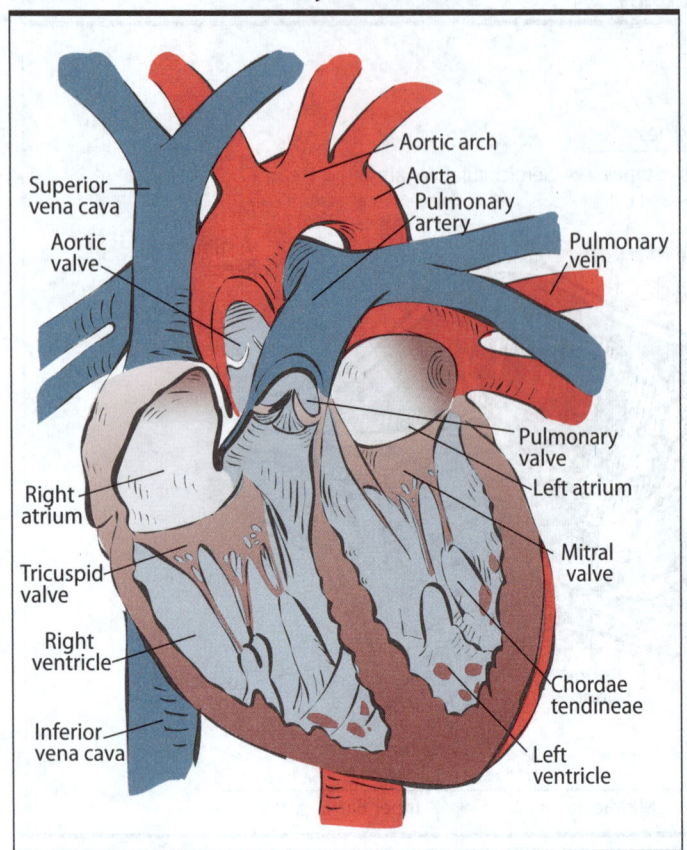

Heart Cross Section

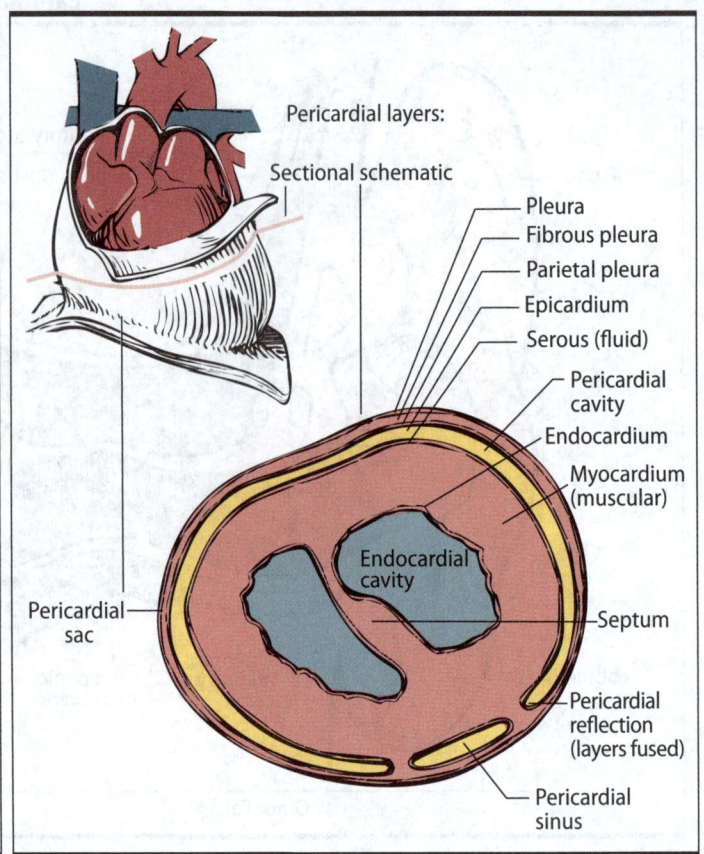

Heart Valves

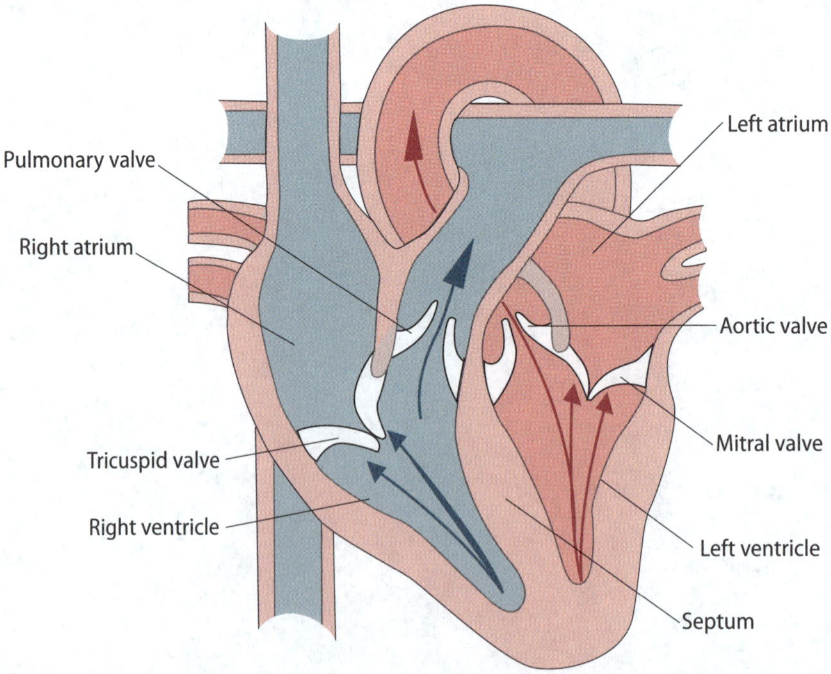

Schematic shows valves of the heart as blood is pumped out. The septum is the wall dividing the left and right ventricles. The papillary muscles and chordae tendineae (above right) function to open and close the atrioventricular valves

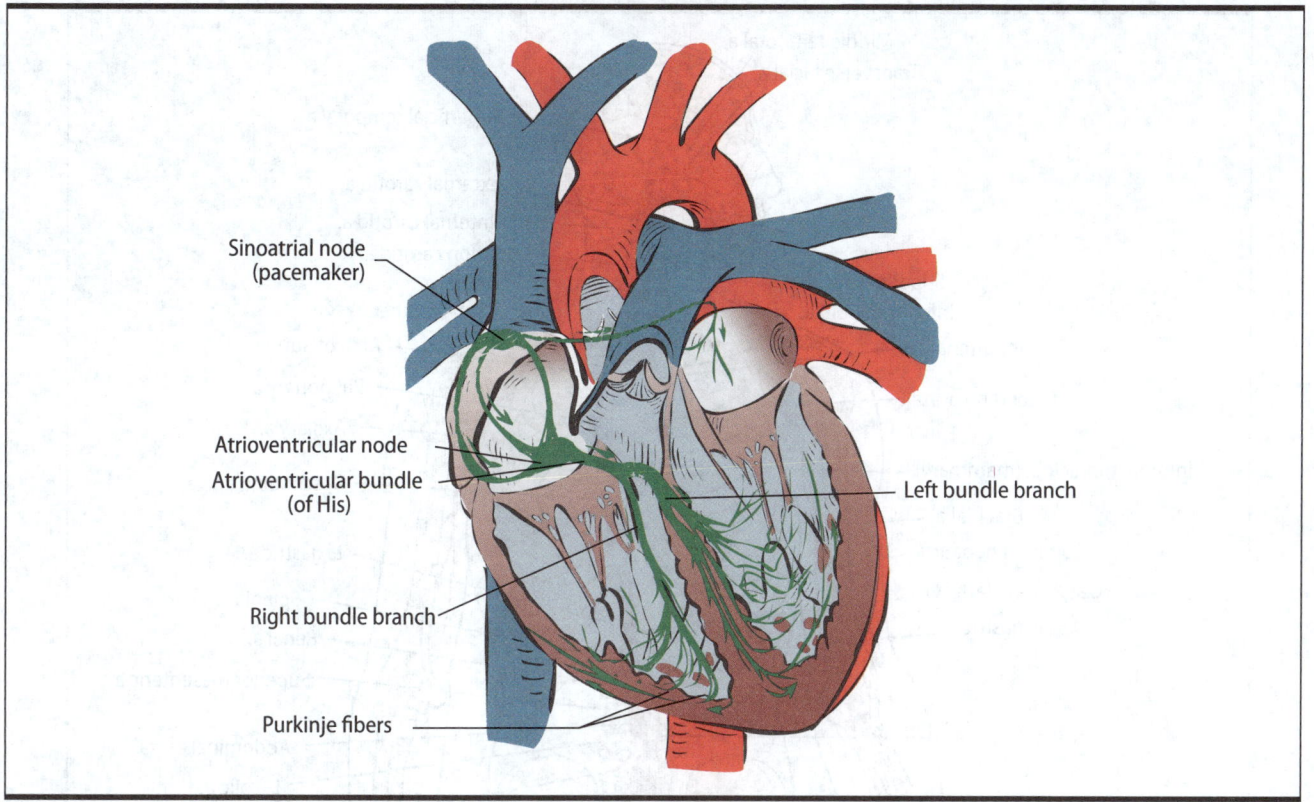

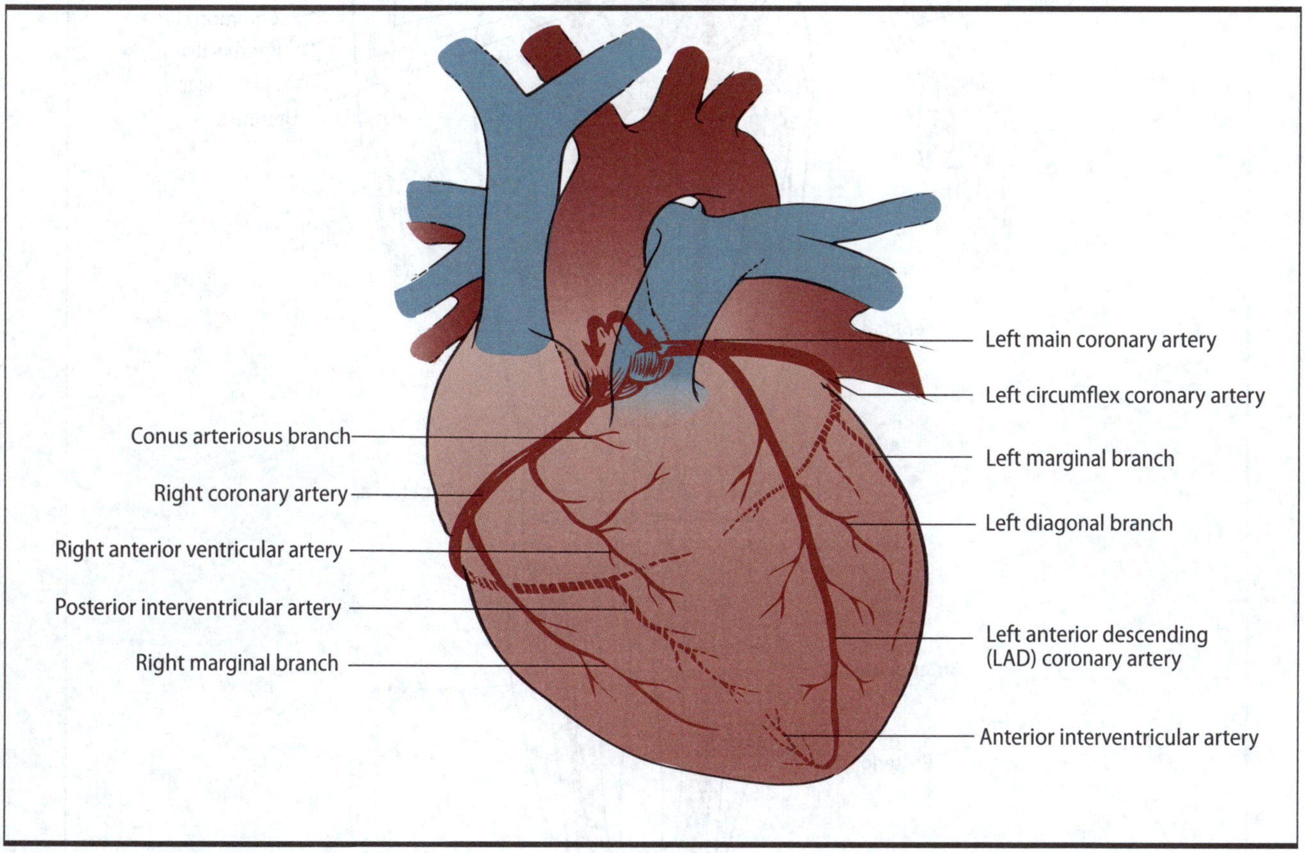

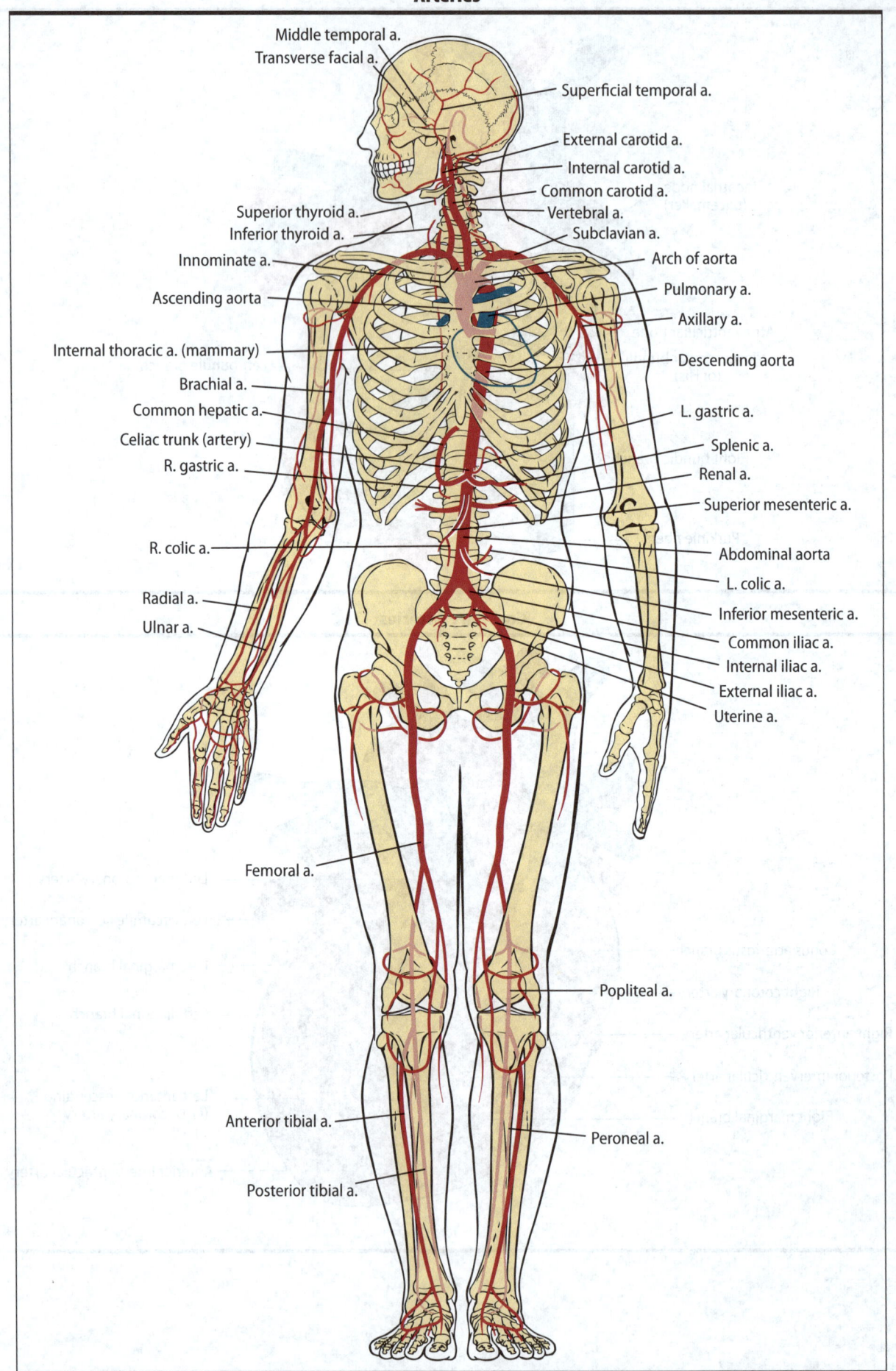

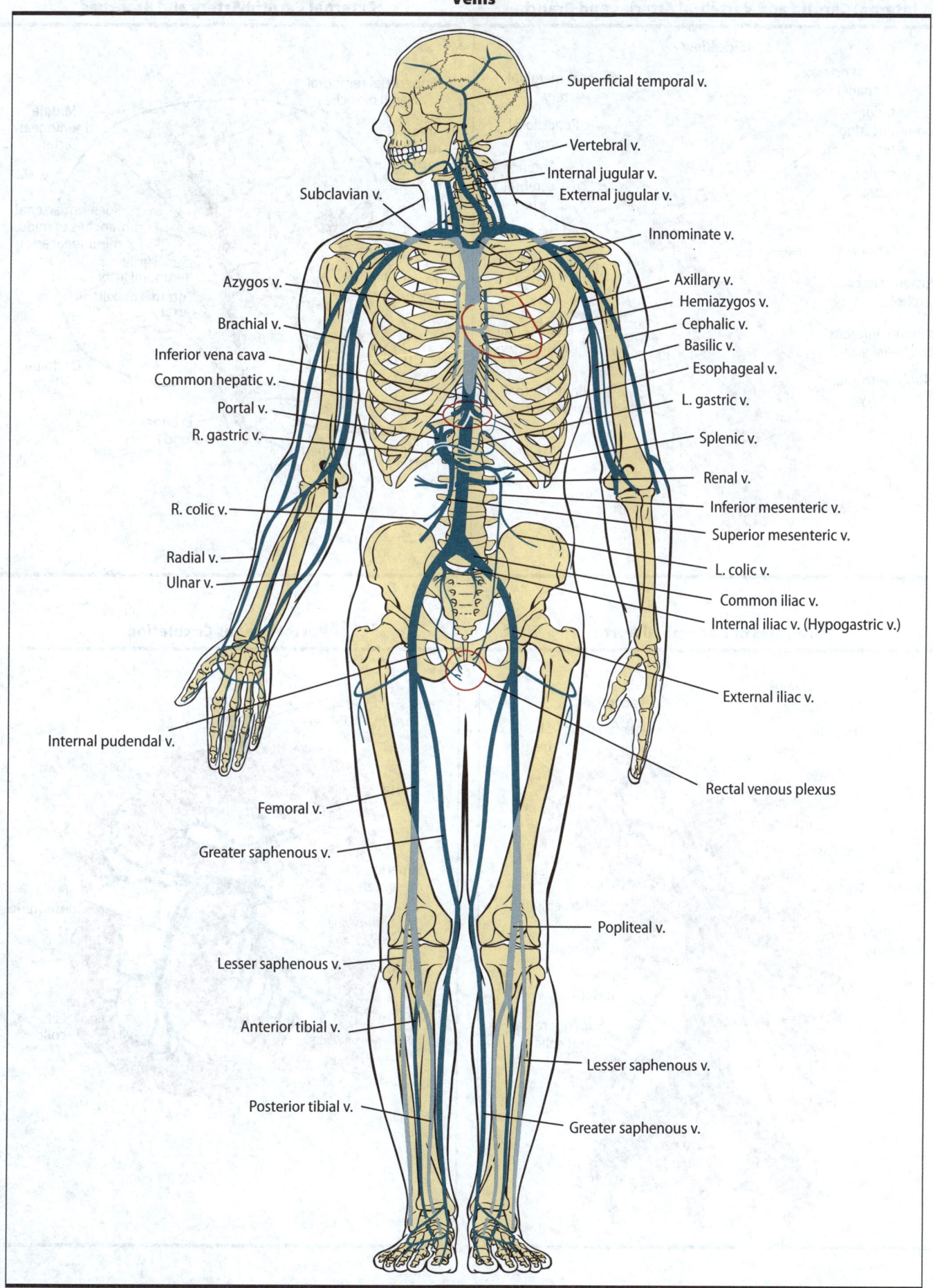

Internal Carotid and Vertebral Arteries and Branches

External Carotid Artery and Branches

Branches of Abdominal Aorta

Portal Venous Circulation

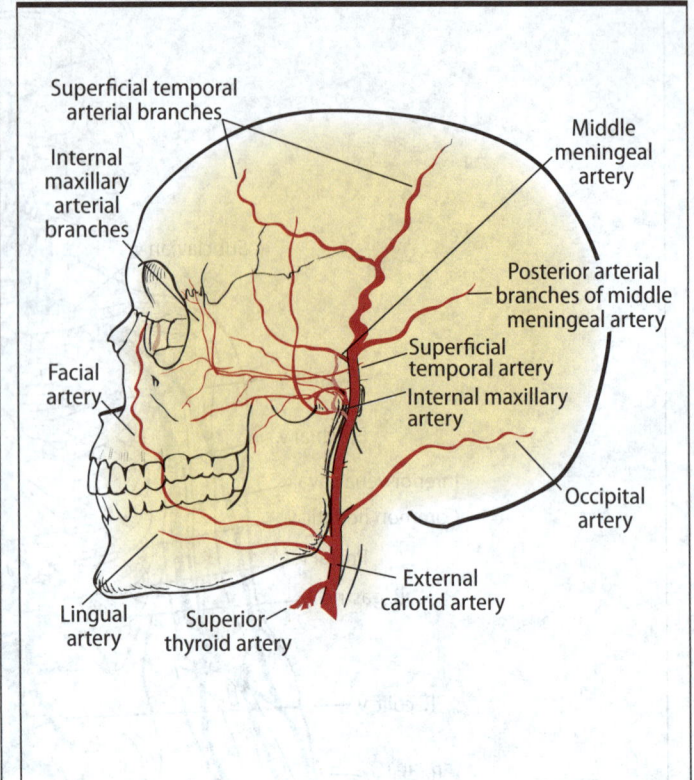
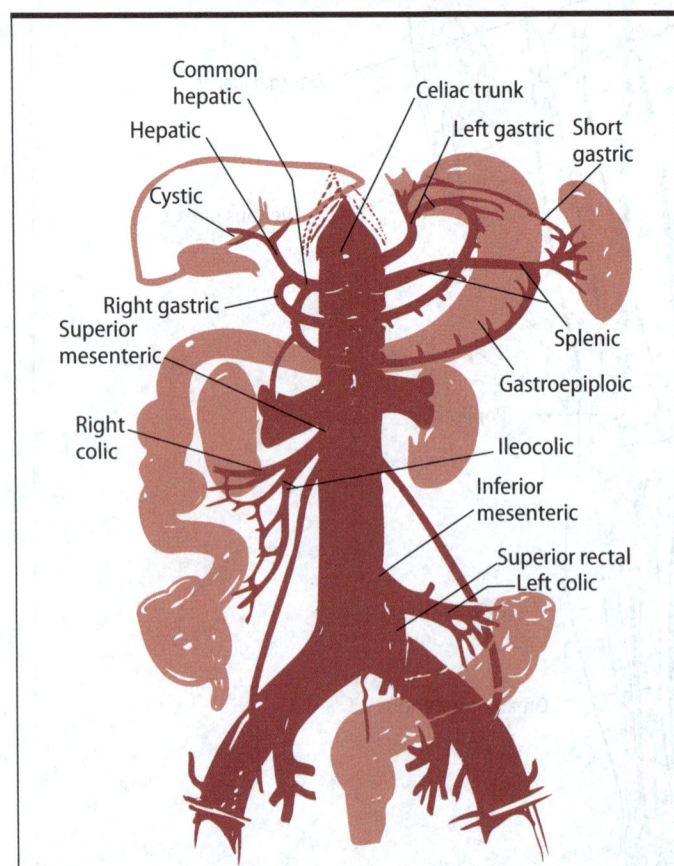
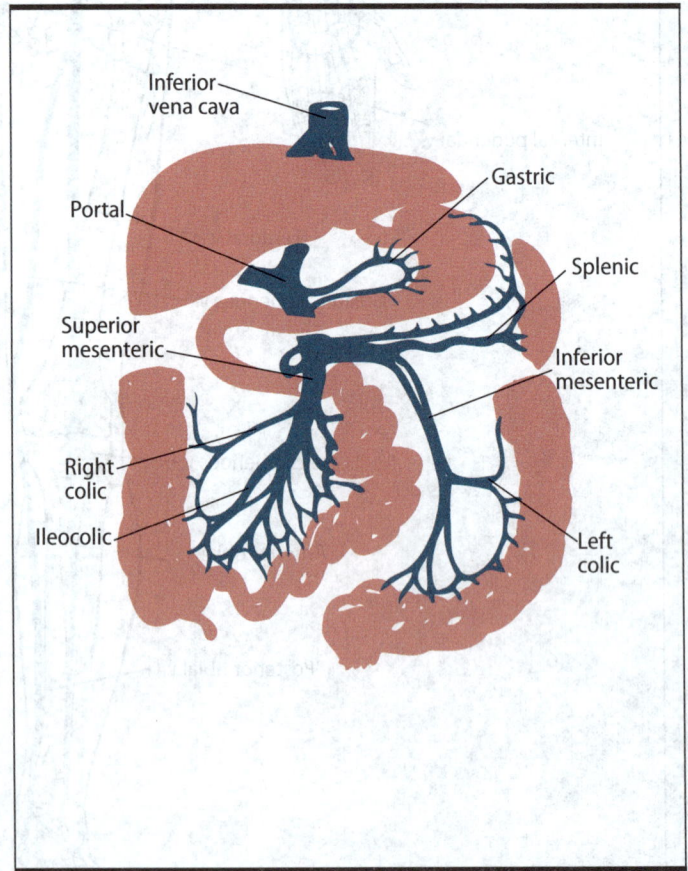

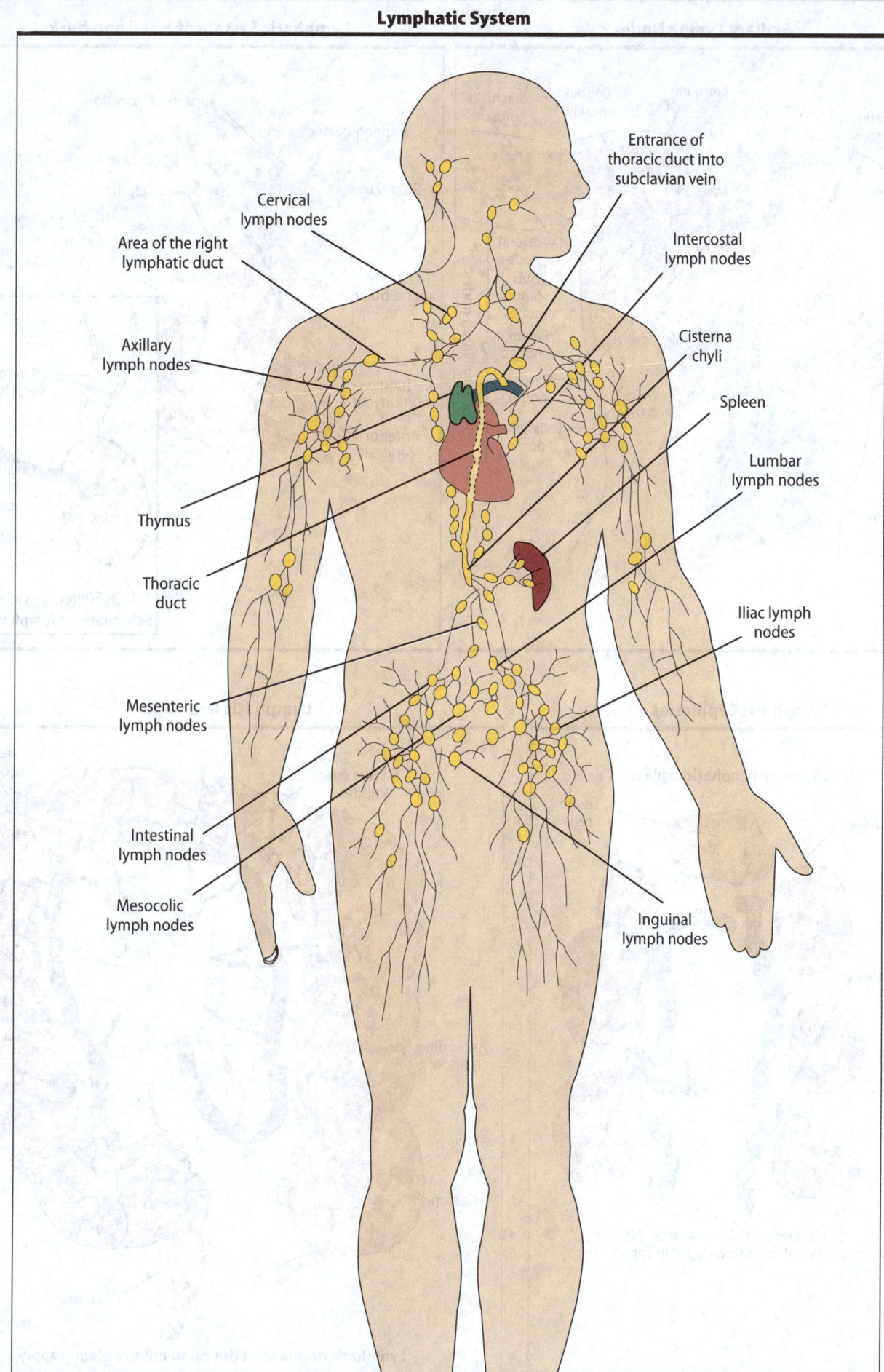

Axillary Lymph Nodes

Lymphatic System of Head and Neck

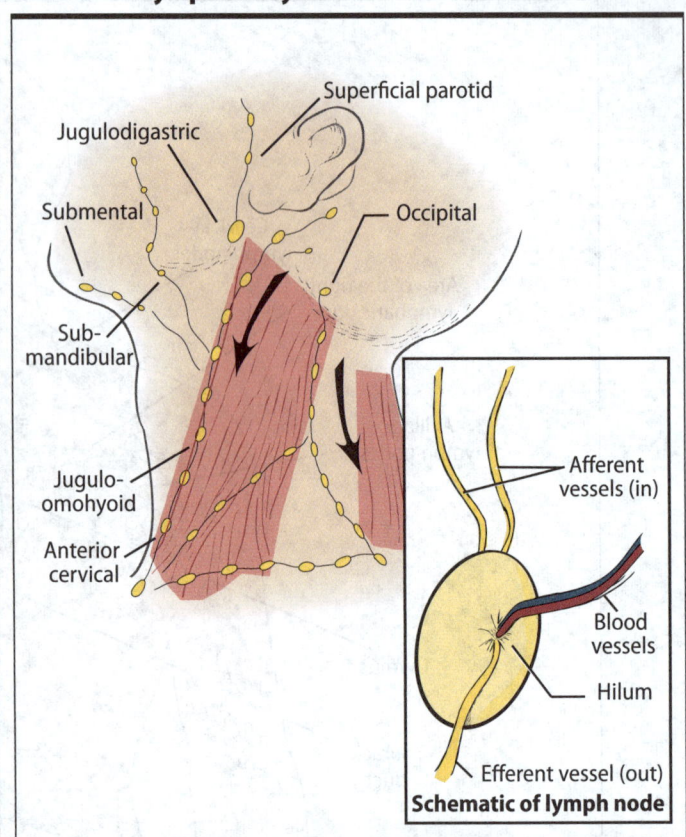

Lymphatic Capillaries

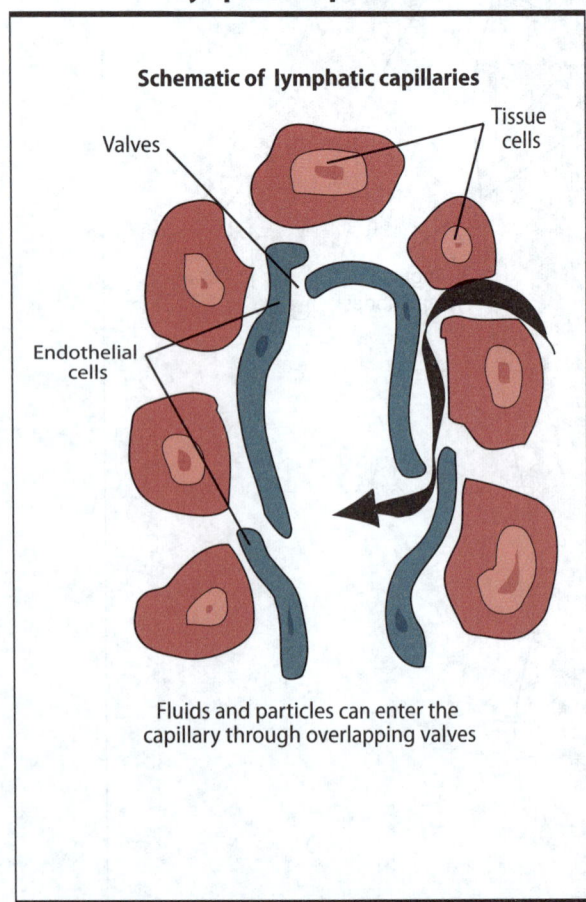

Lymphatic Drainage

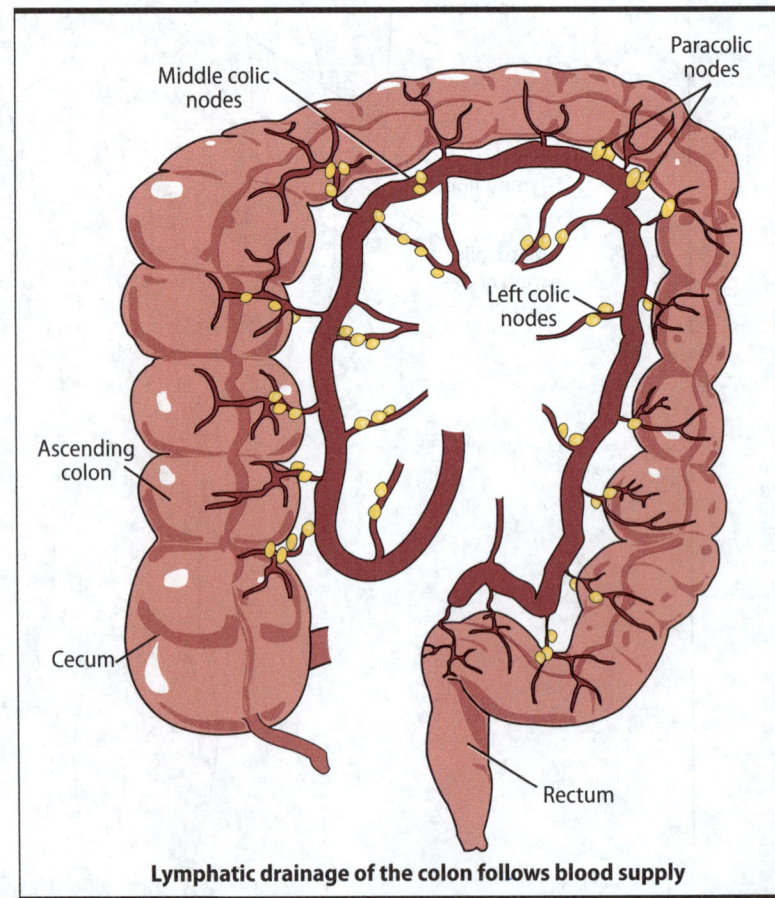

Lymphatic drainage of the colon follows blood supply

Chapter 10. Diseases of the Respiratory System (JØØ-J99, UØ7.Ø)

Respiratory System

Upper Respiratory System

Nasal Cavity

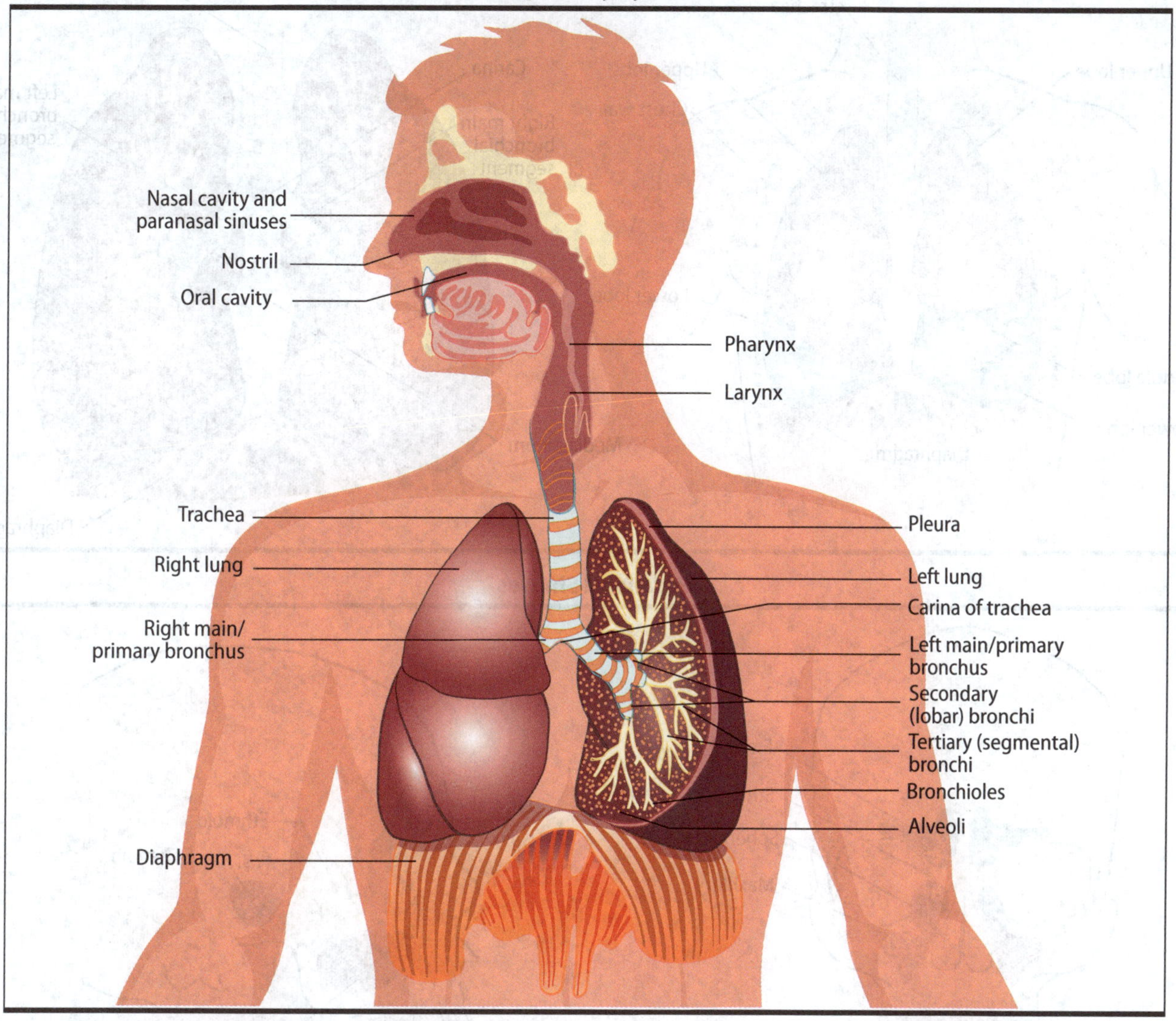

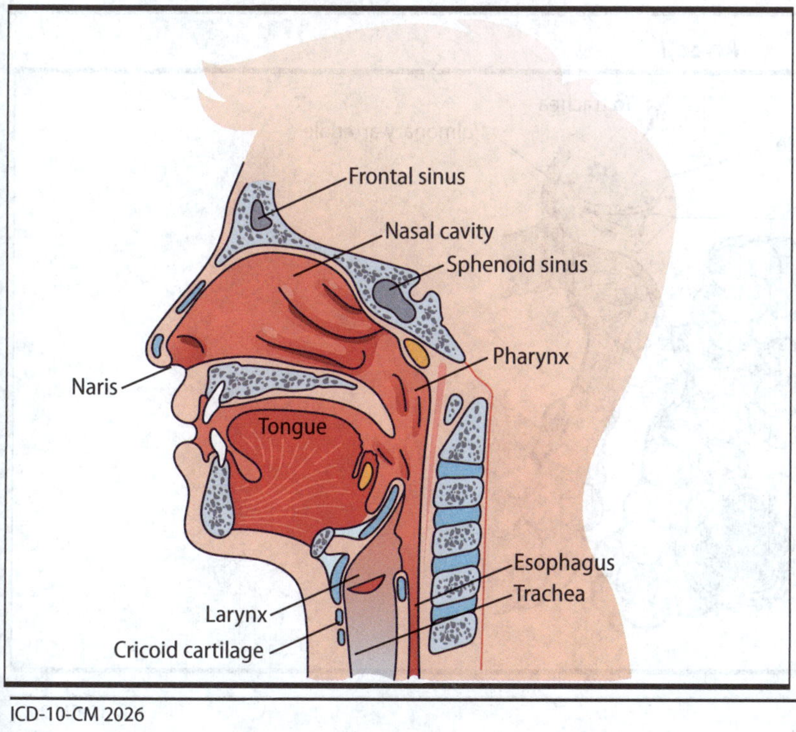

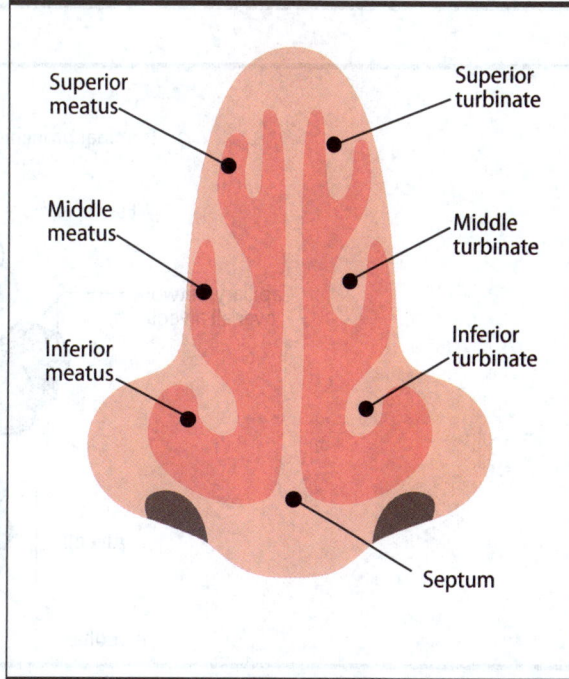

Lower Respiratory System

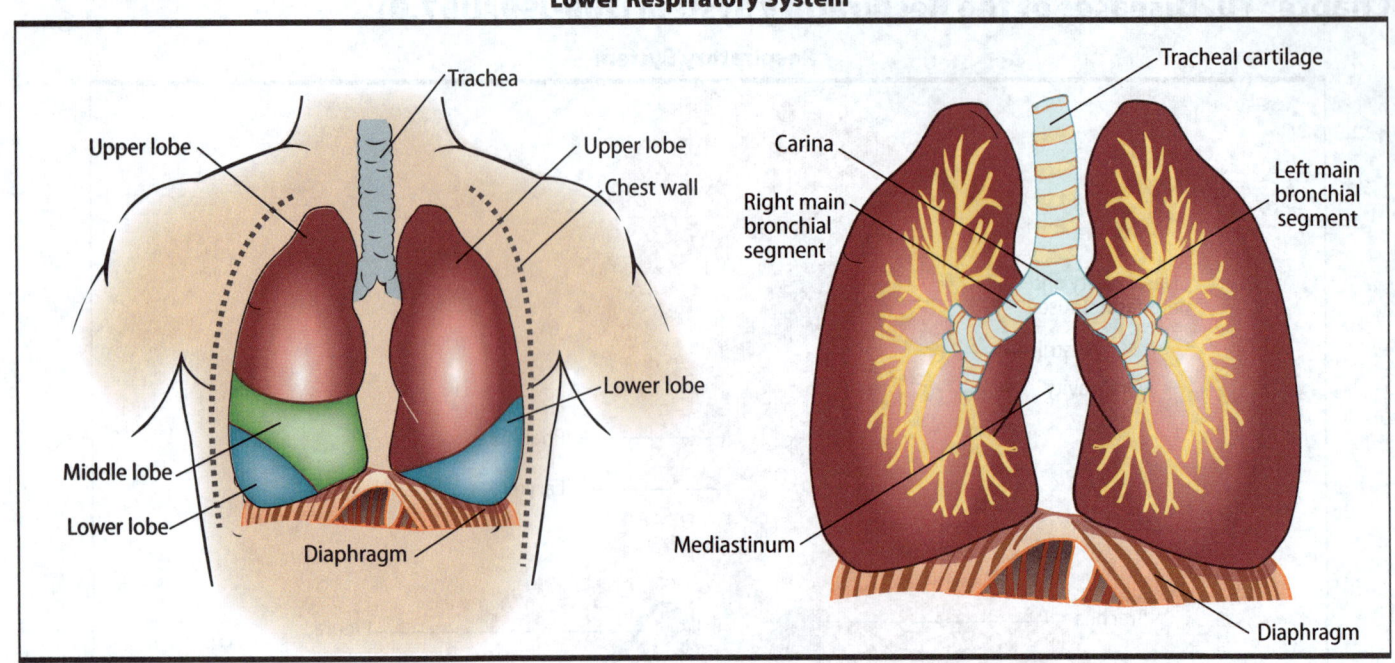

Paranasal Sinuses

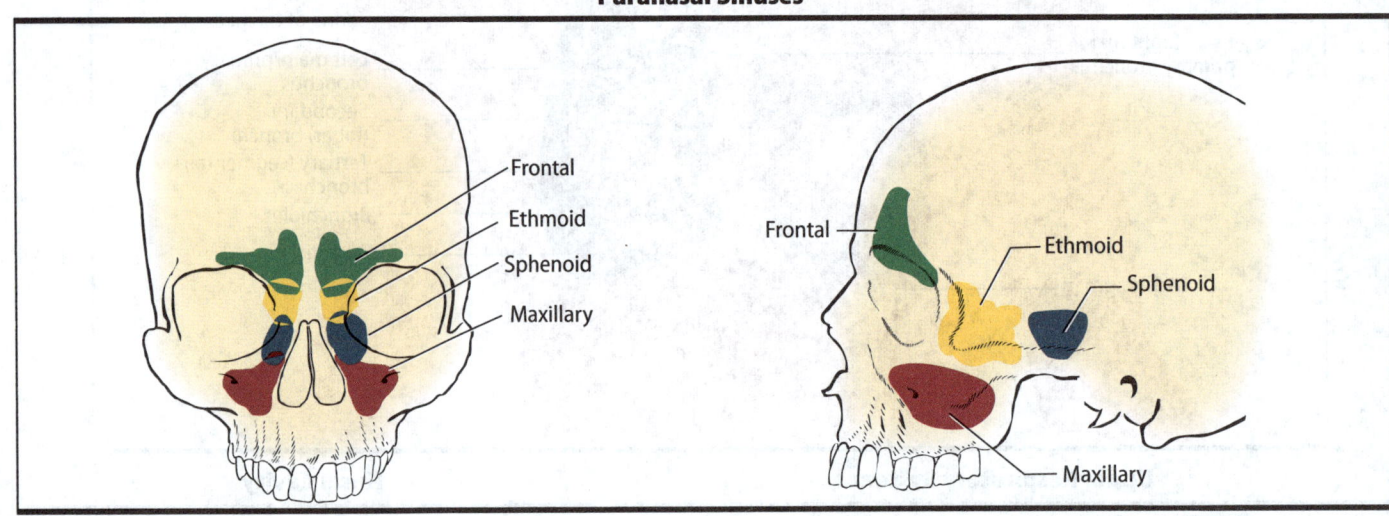

Alveoli

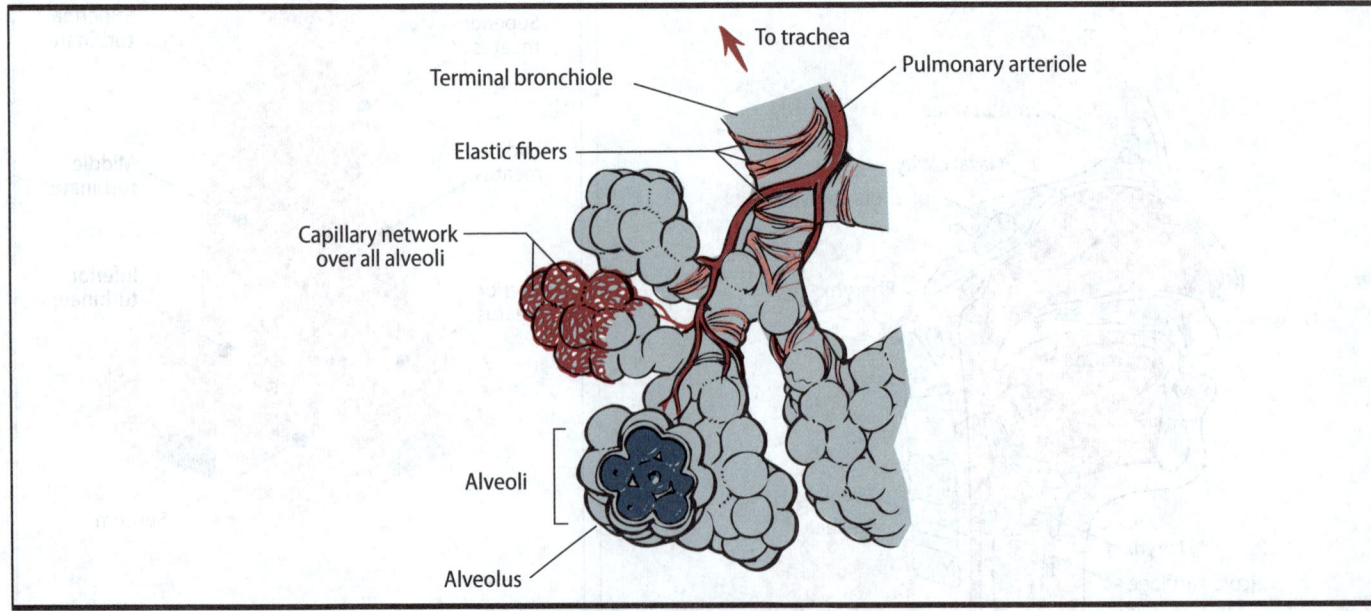

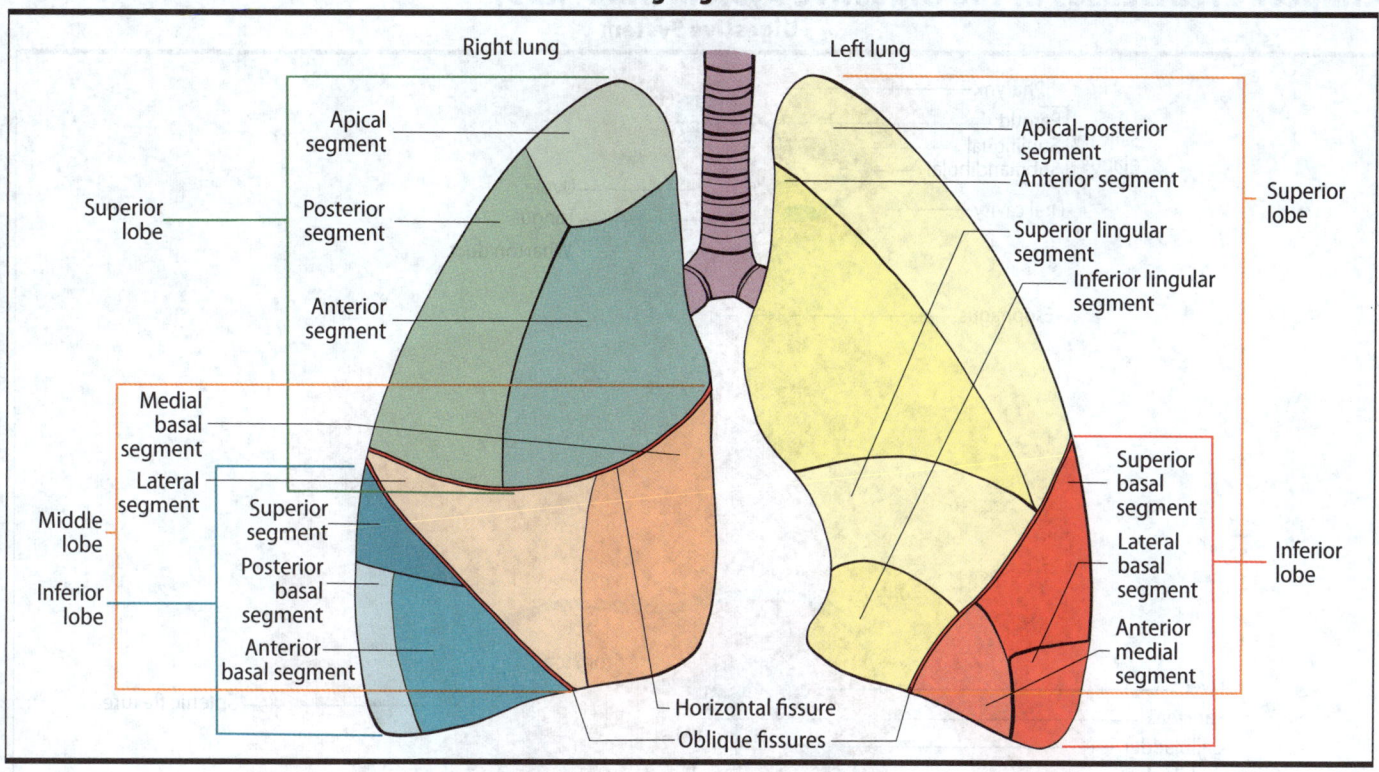

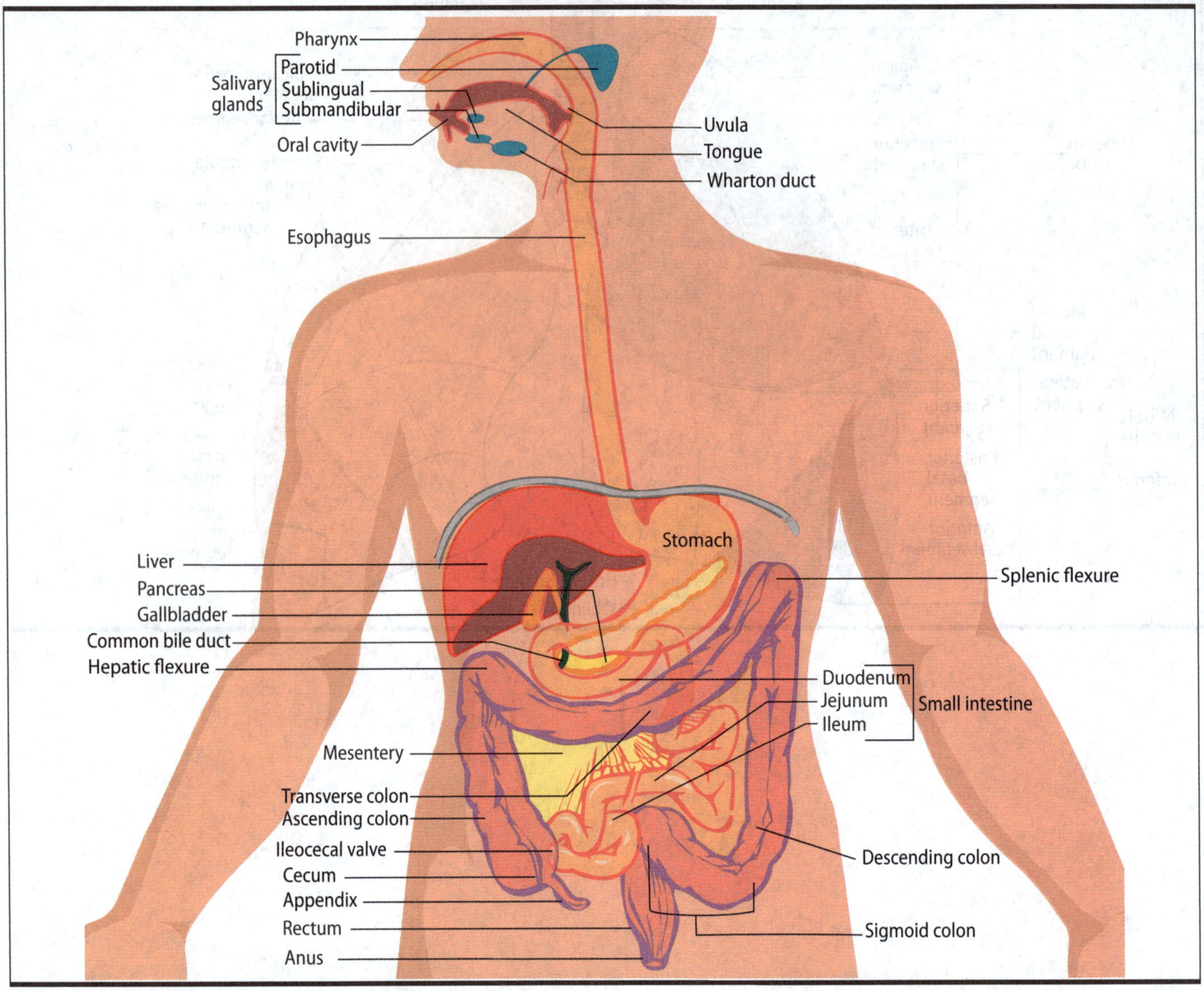

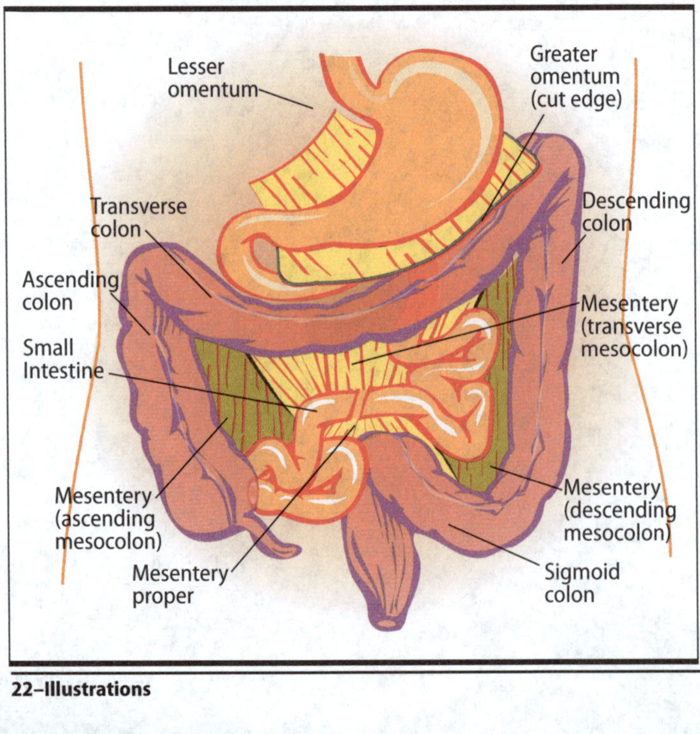

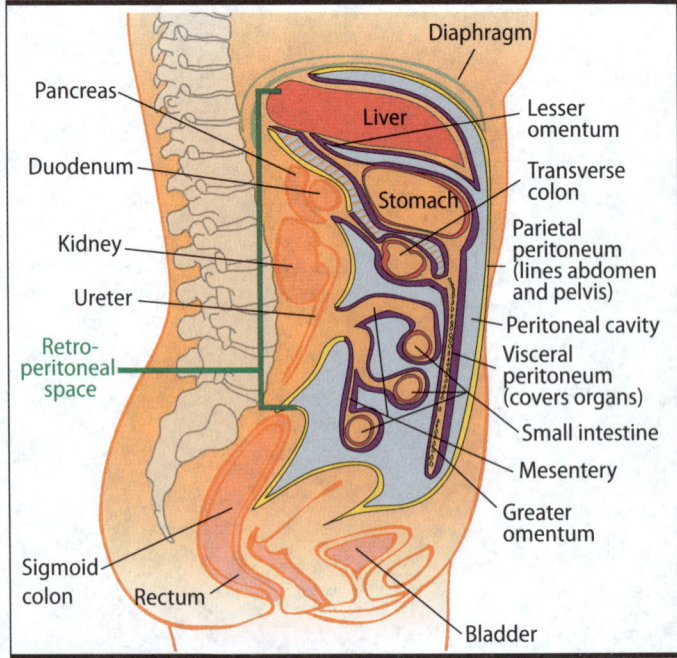

Chapter 12. Diseases of the Skin and Subcutaneous Tissue (L00–L99)

Nail Anatomy

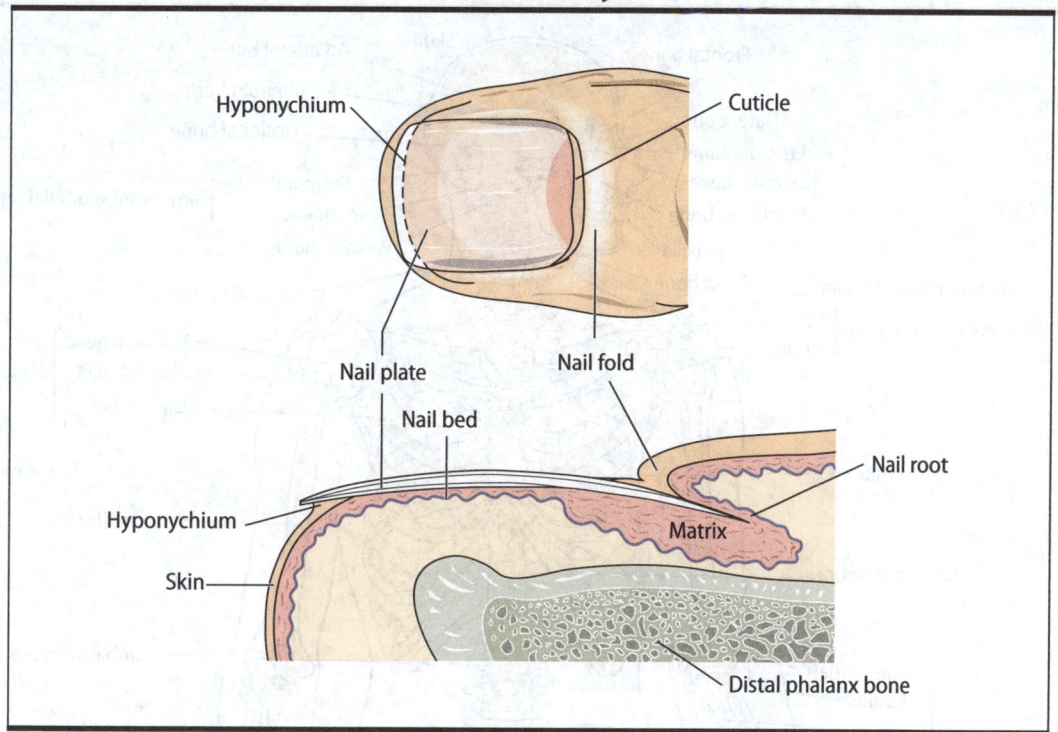

Skin and Subcutaneous Tissue

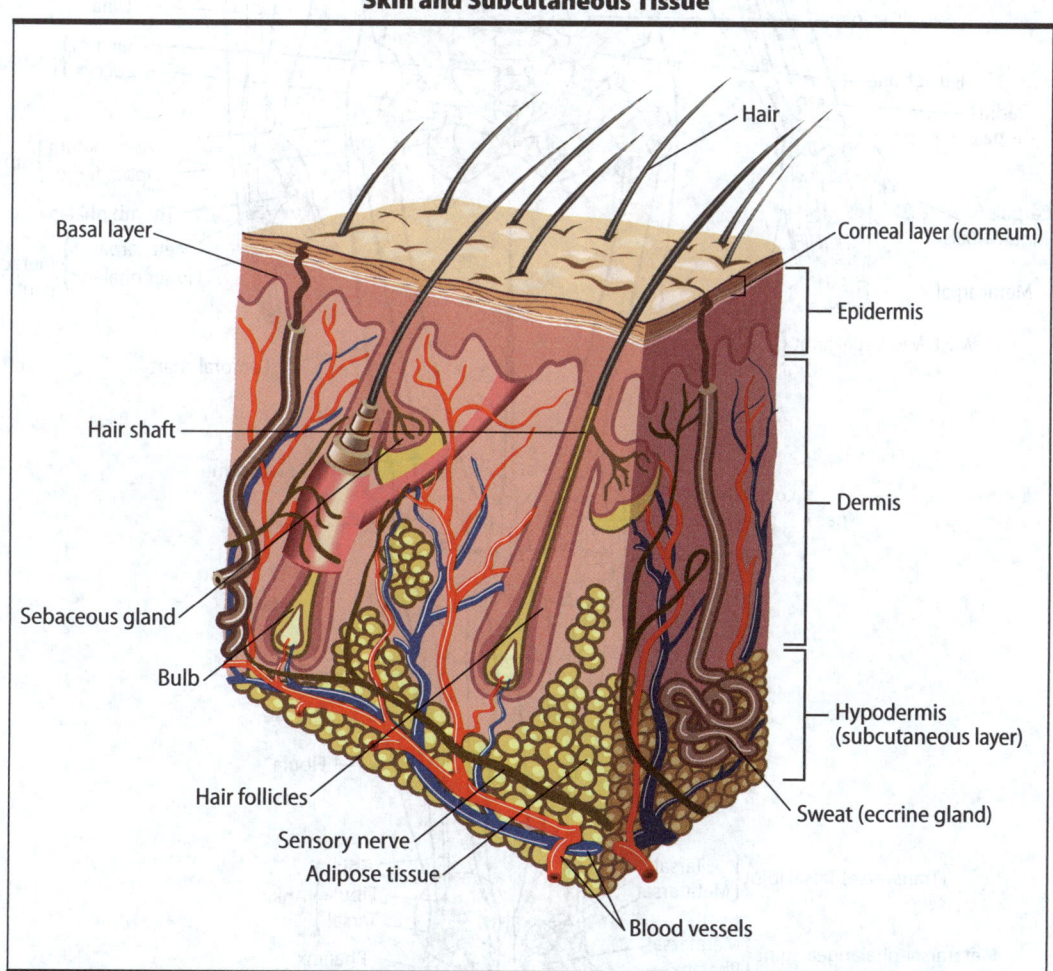

Chapter 13. Diseases of the Musculoskeletal System and Connective Tissue (M00–M99)

Bones and Joints

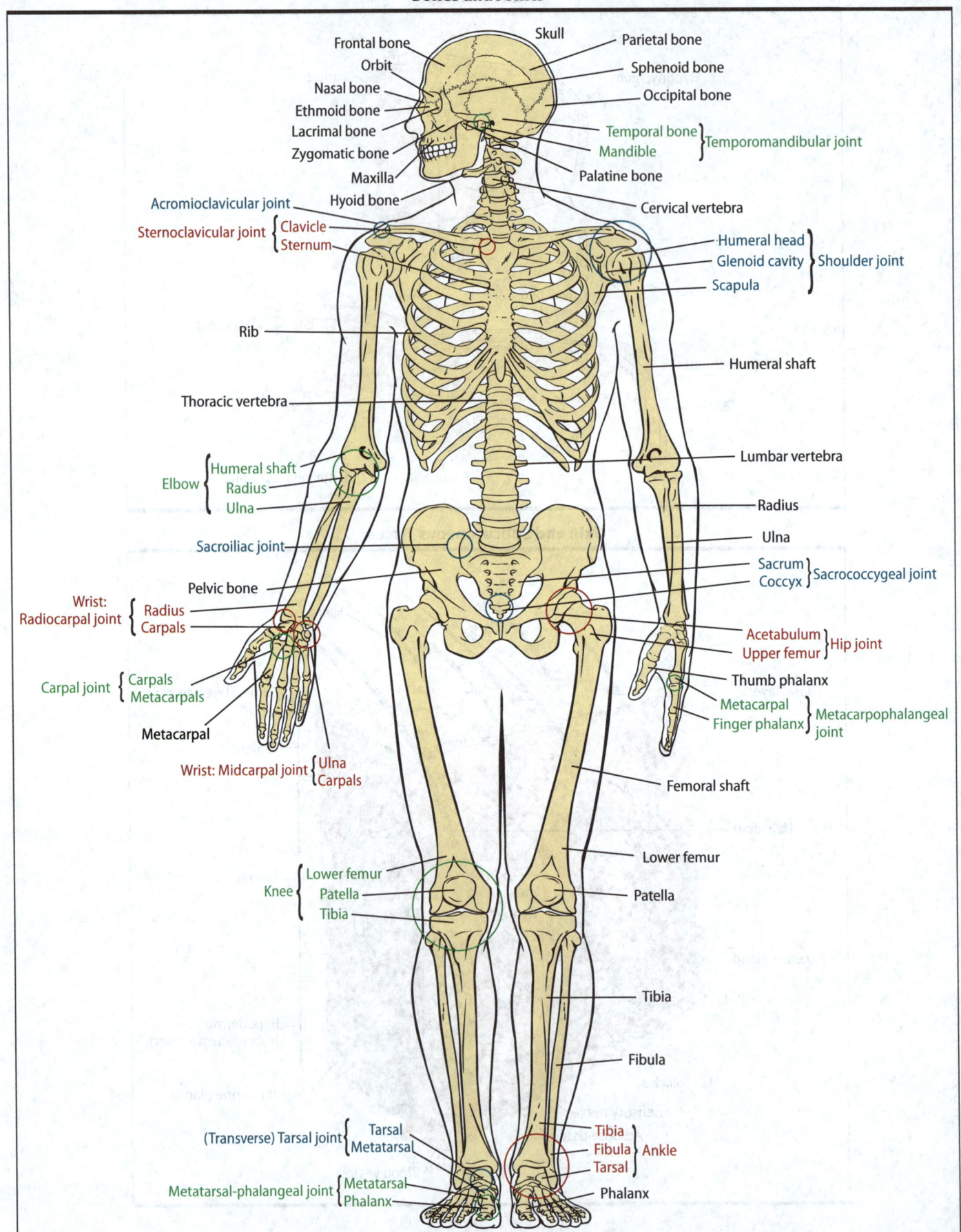

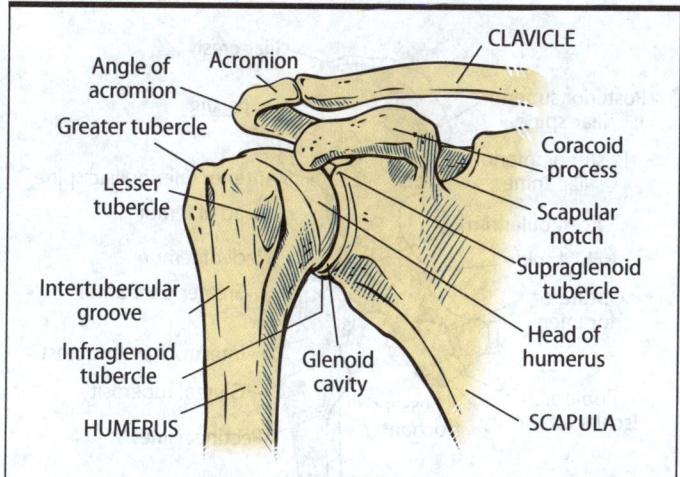
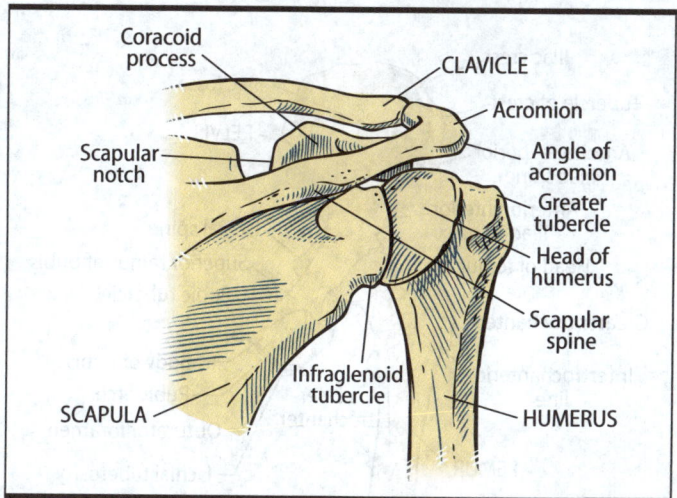
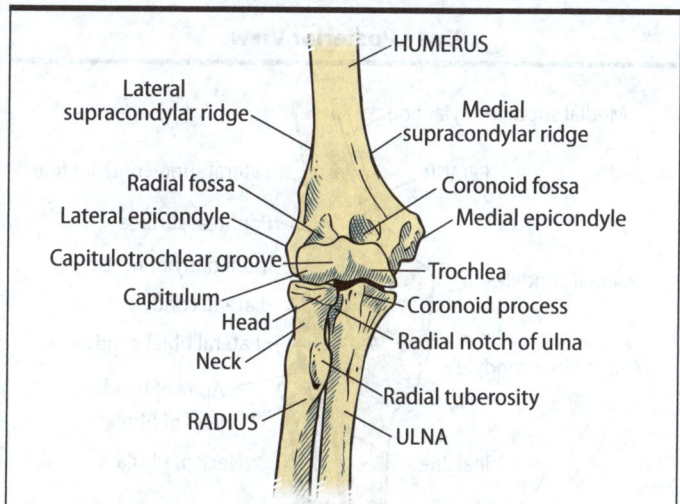
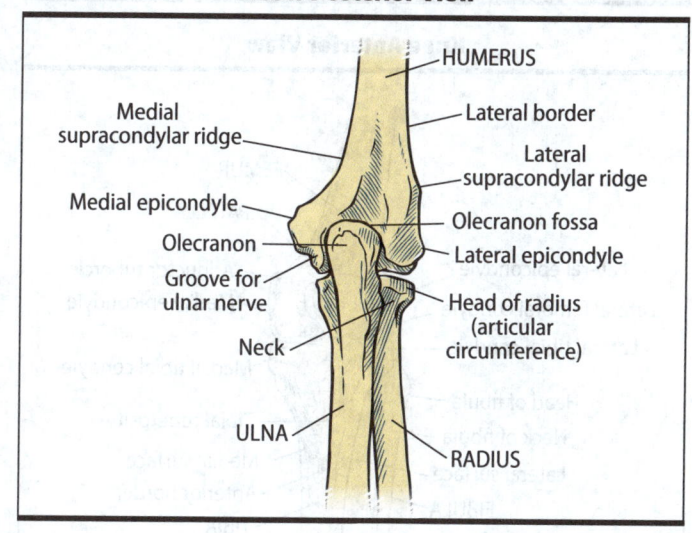
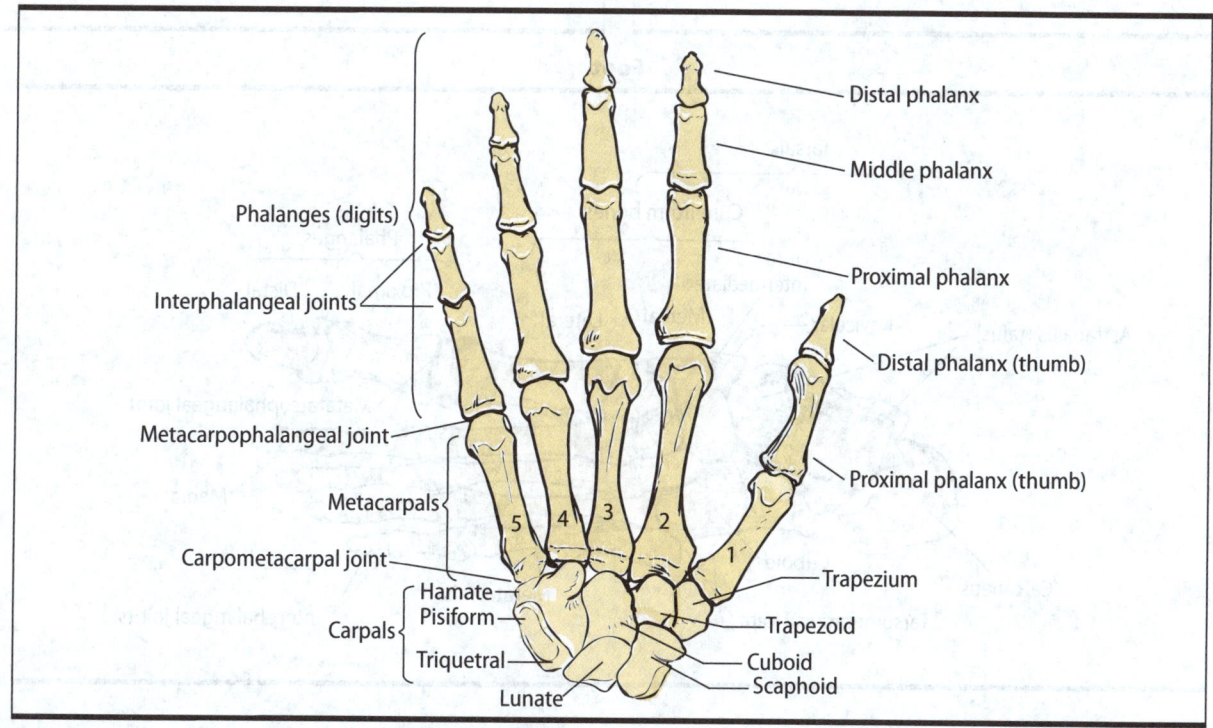

Hip Anterior View

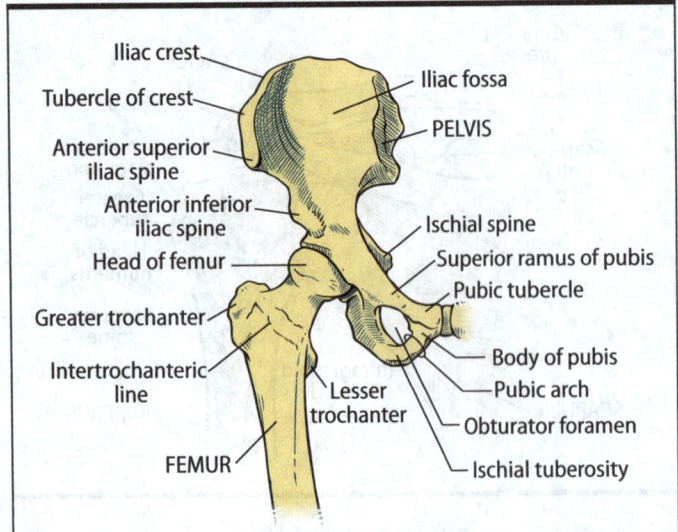

Hip Posterior View

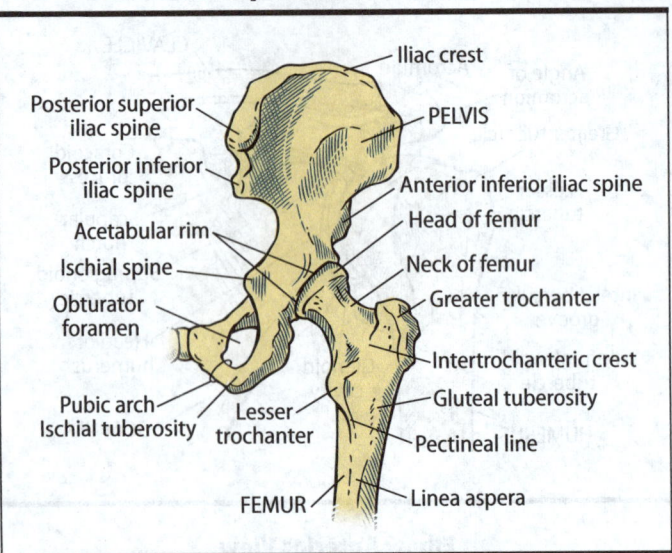

Knee Anterior View

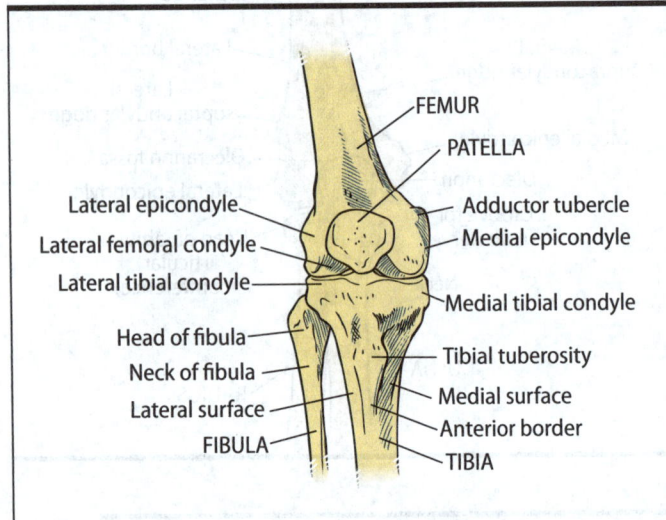

Knee Posterior View

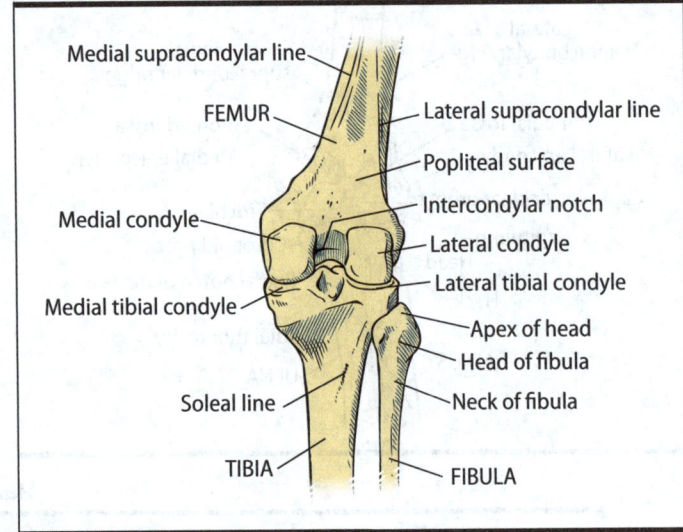

Foot

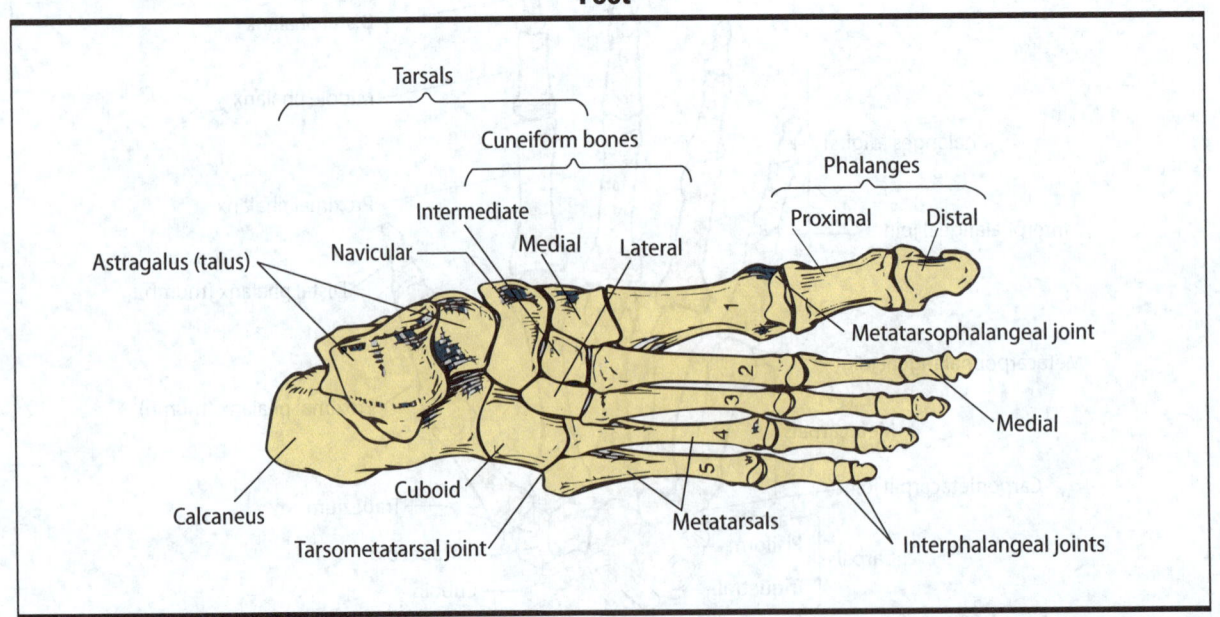

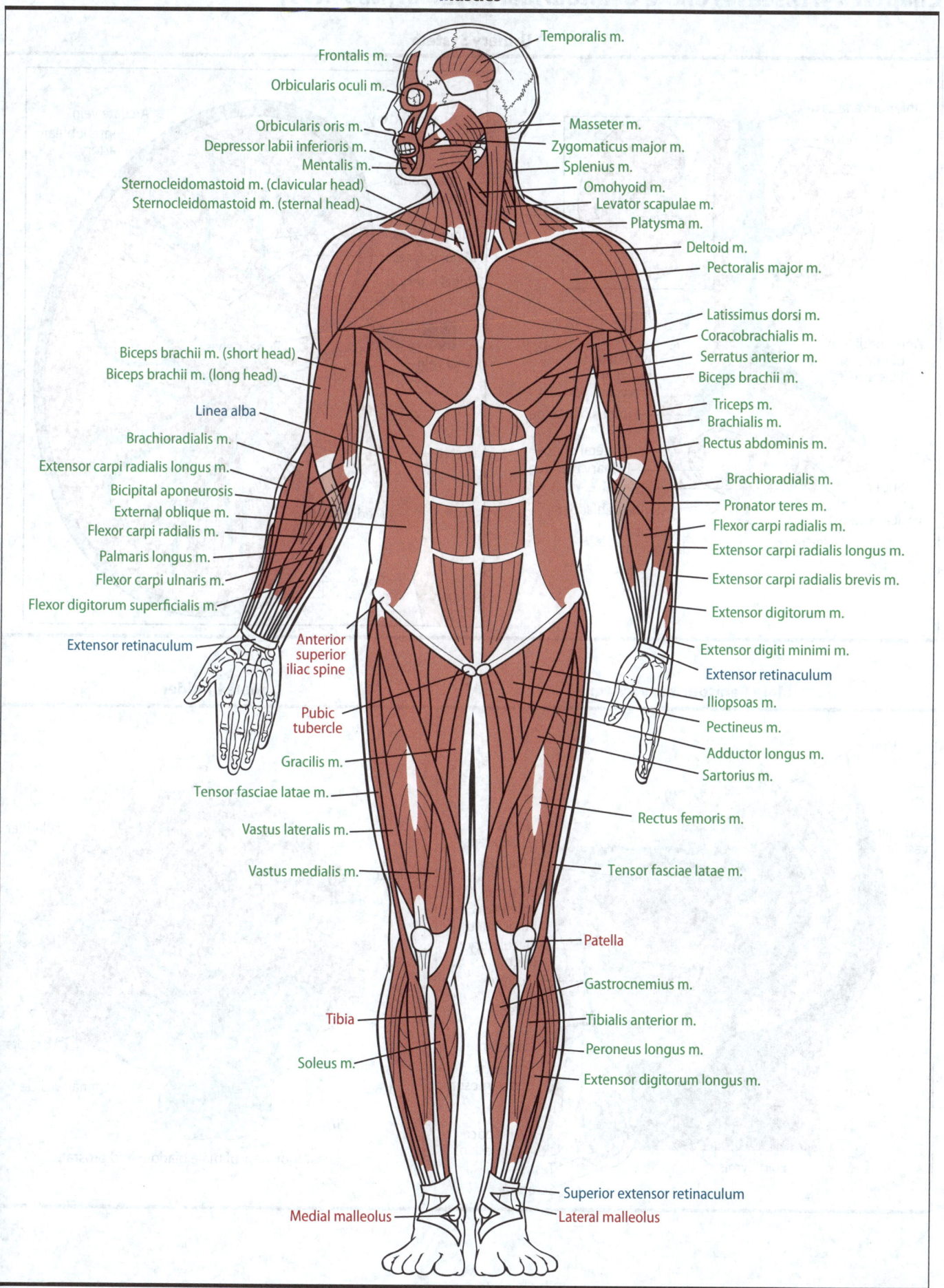

Chapter 14. Diseases of the Genitourinary System (NØØ–N99)

Urinary System

Male Genitourinary System

Male Bladder

Posterior view of male bladder and prostate

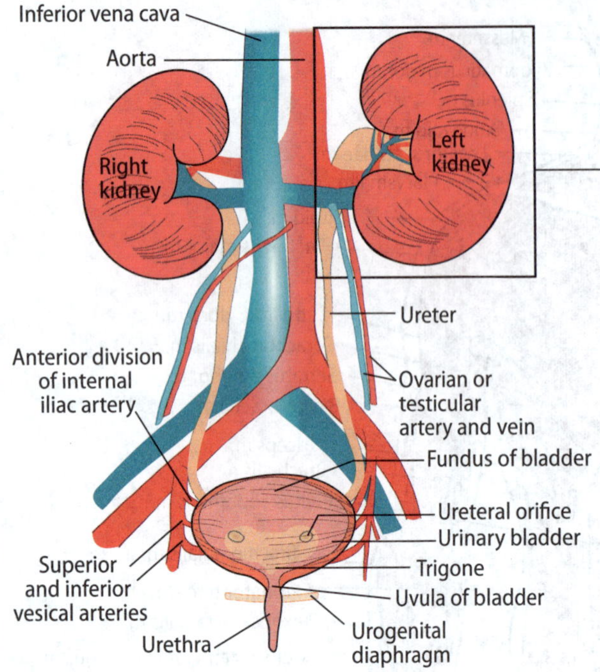

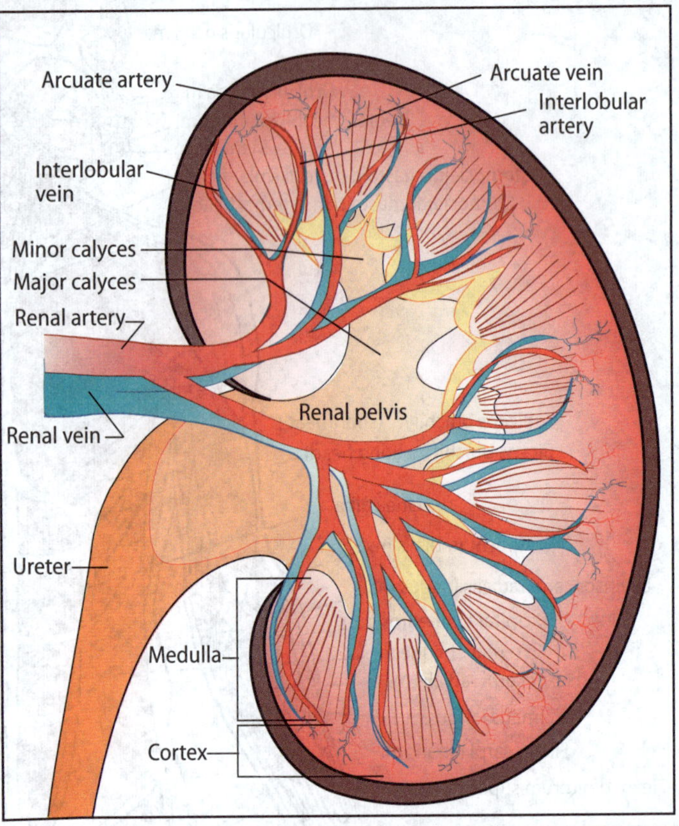

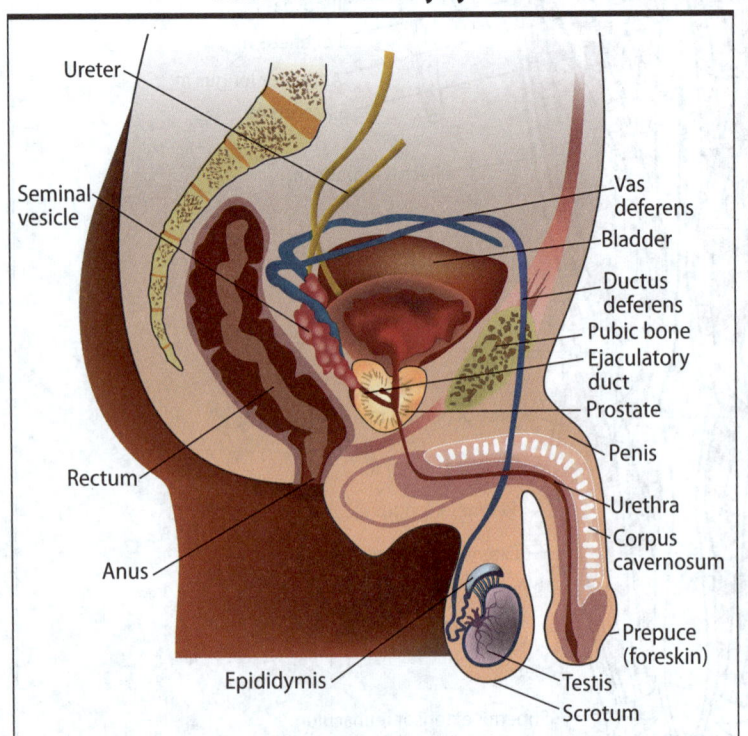

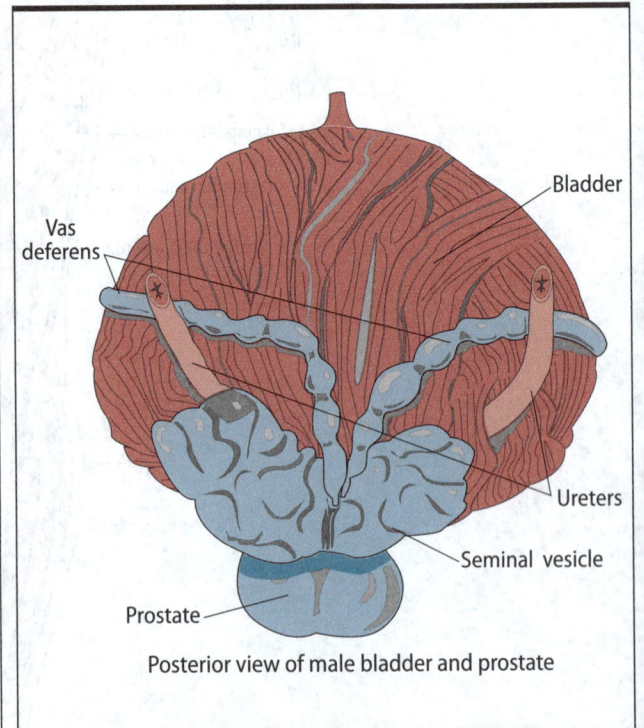

Female Genitourinary System

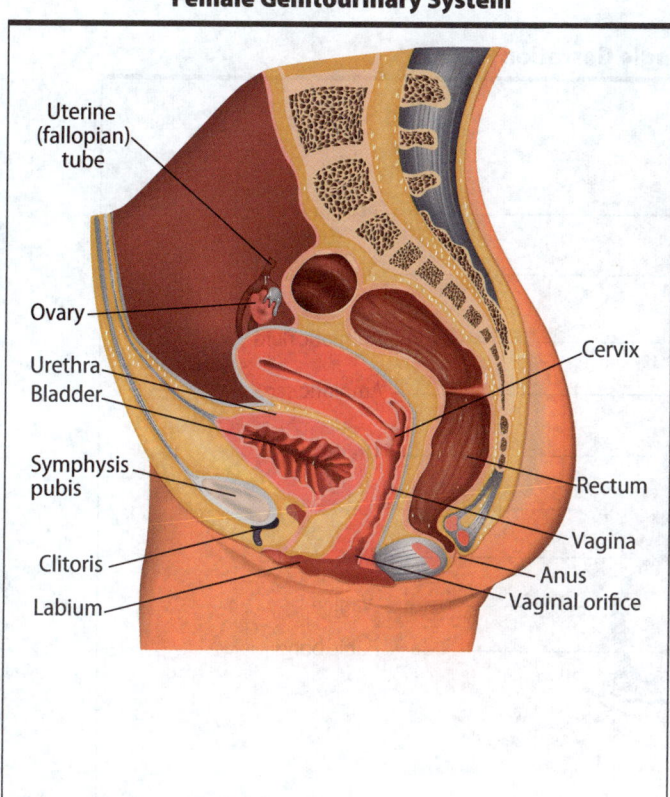

Female Bladder

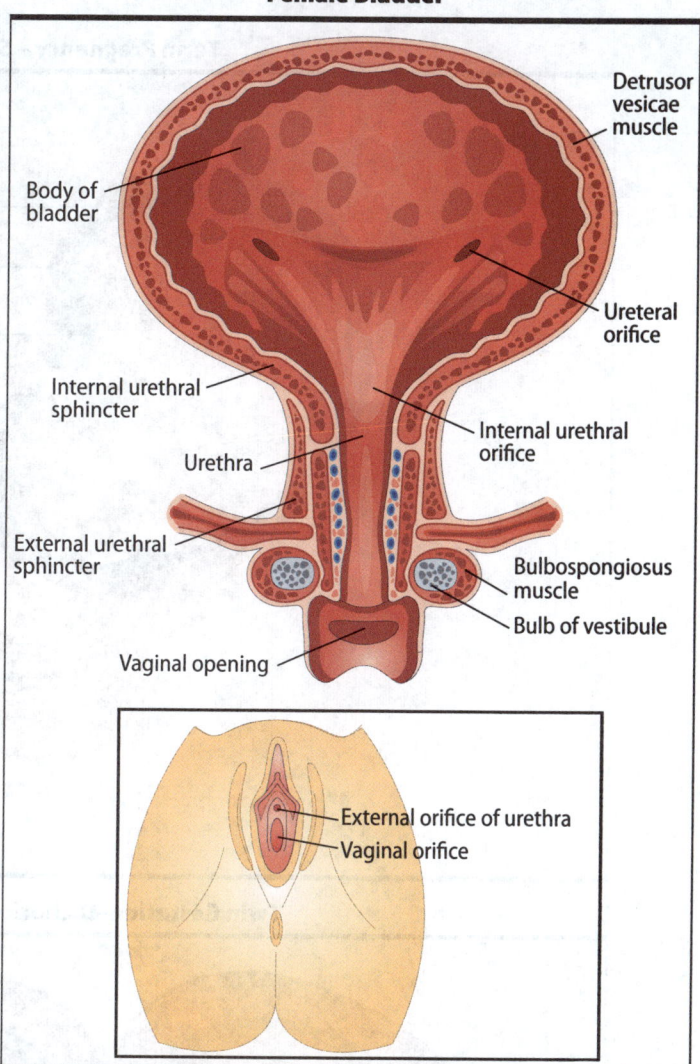

Female Internal Genitalia

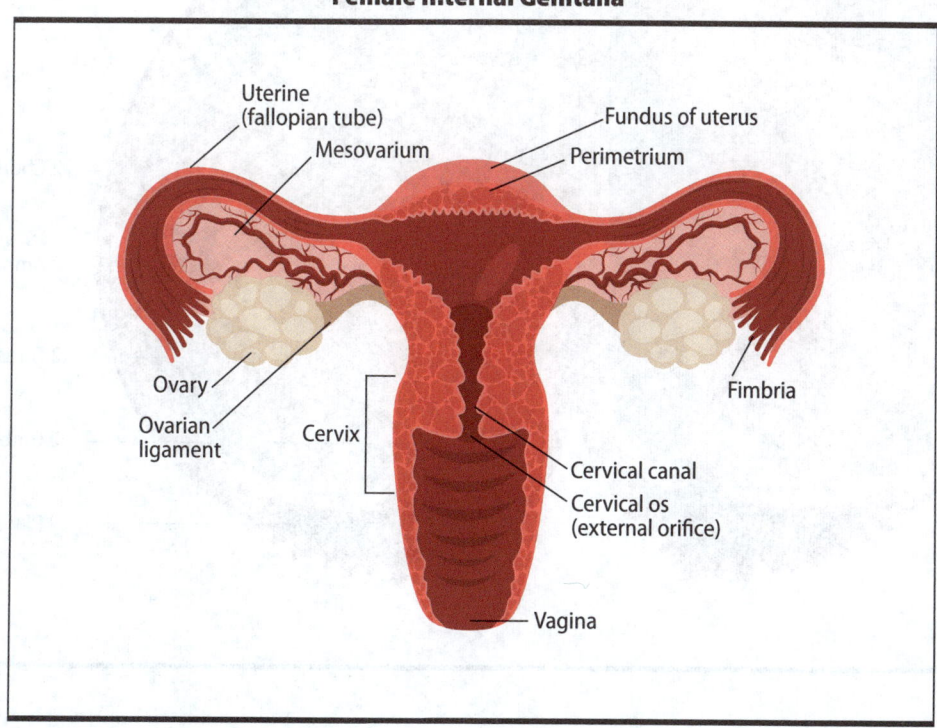

Chapter 15. Pregnancy, Childbirth and the Puerperium (O00–O9A)

Term Pregnancy – Single Gestation

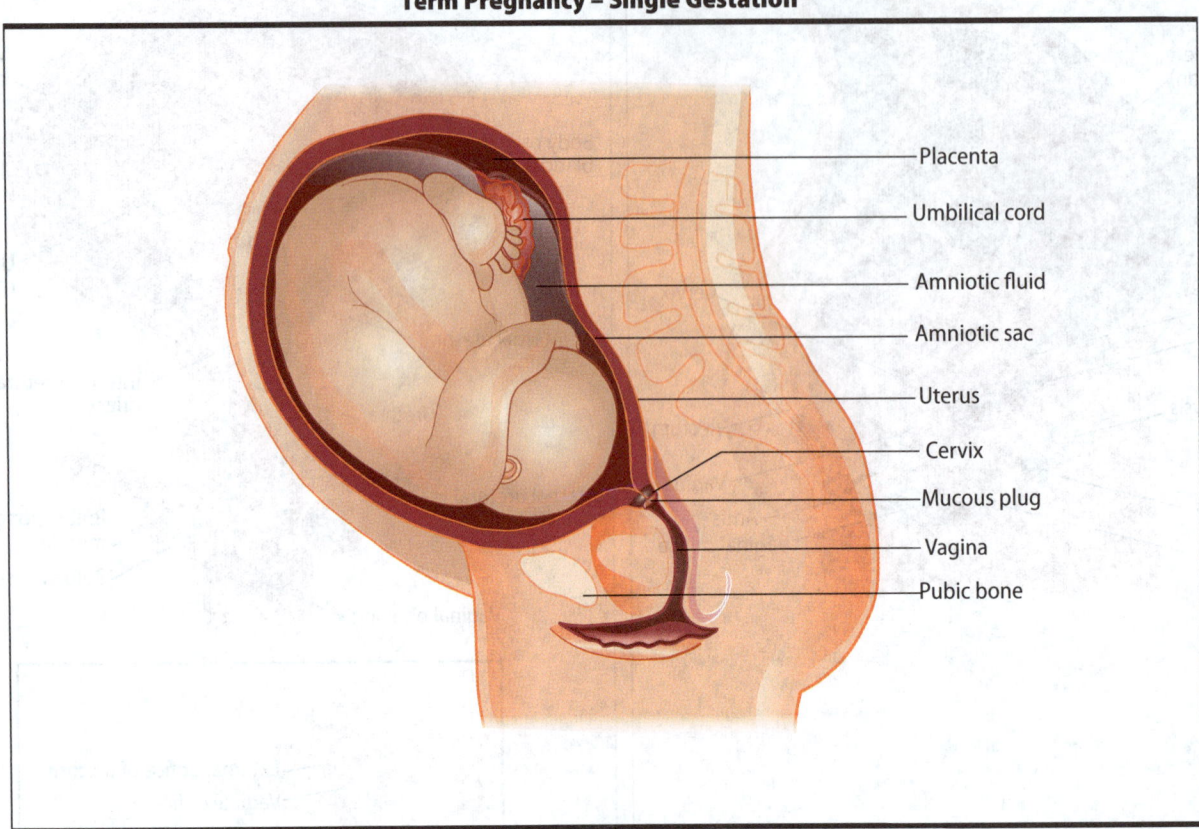

Twin Gestation–Dichorionic–Diamniotic (DI-DI)

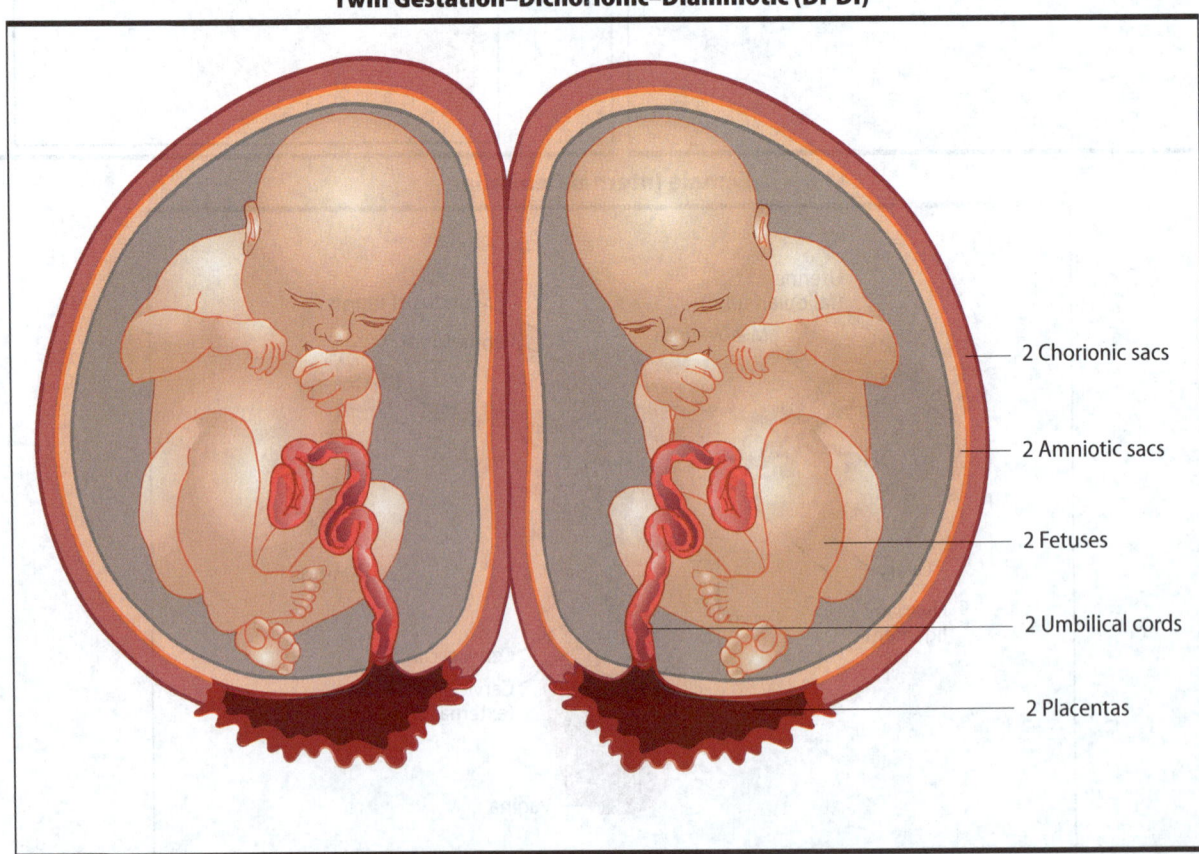

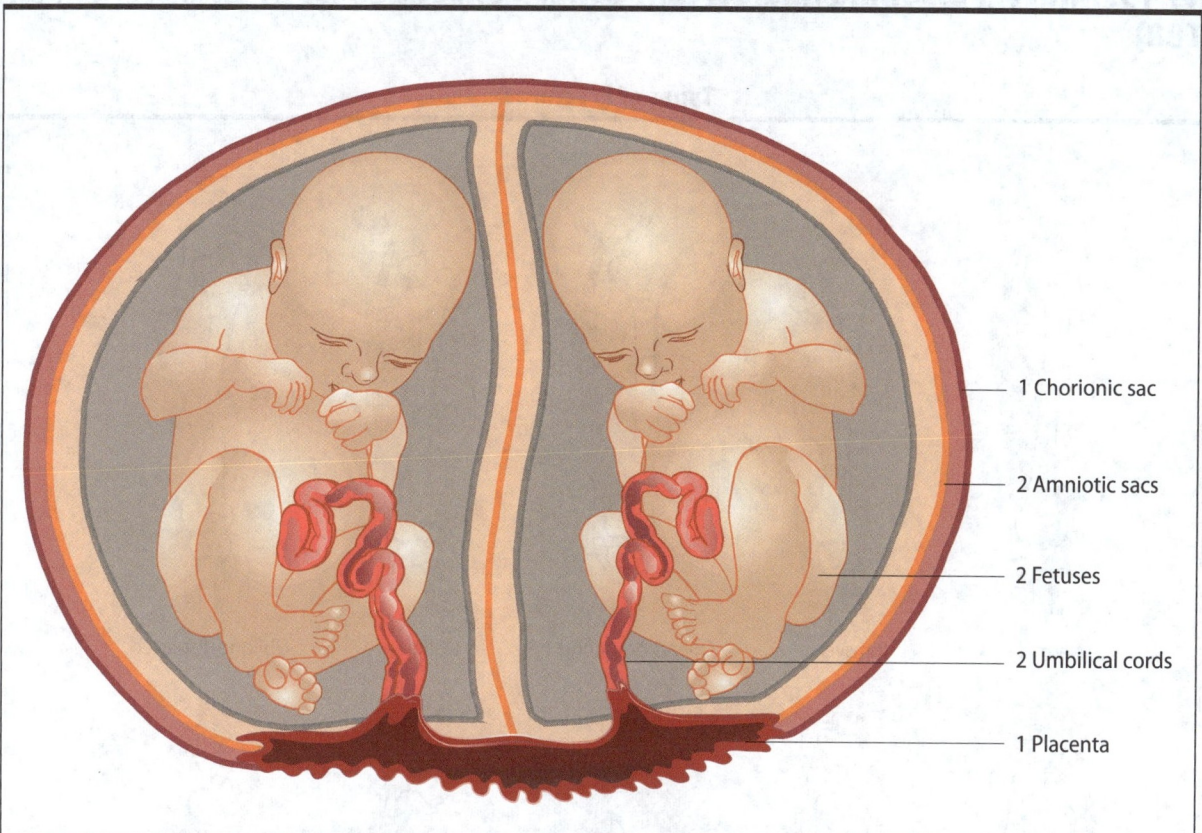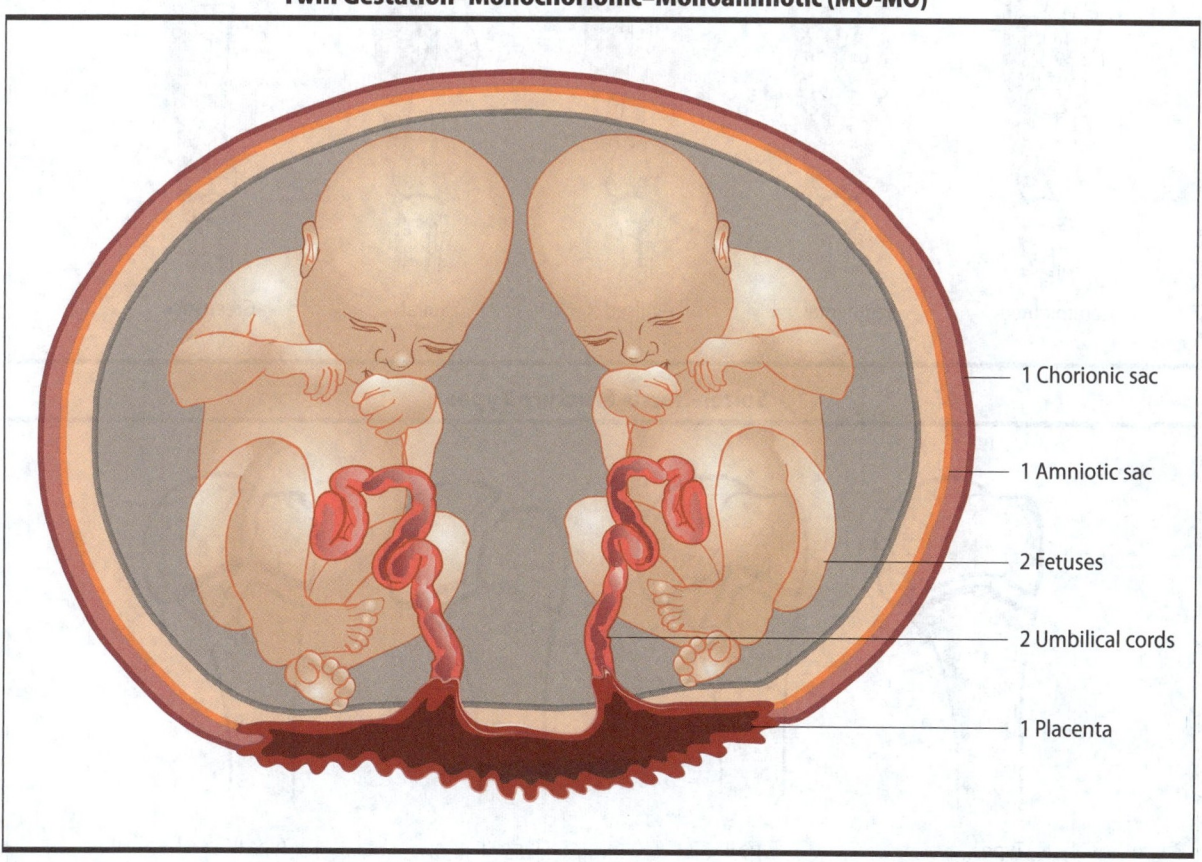

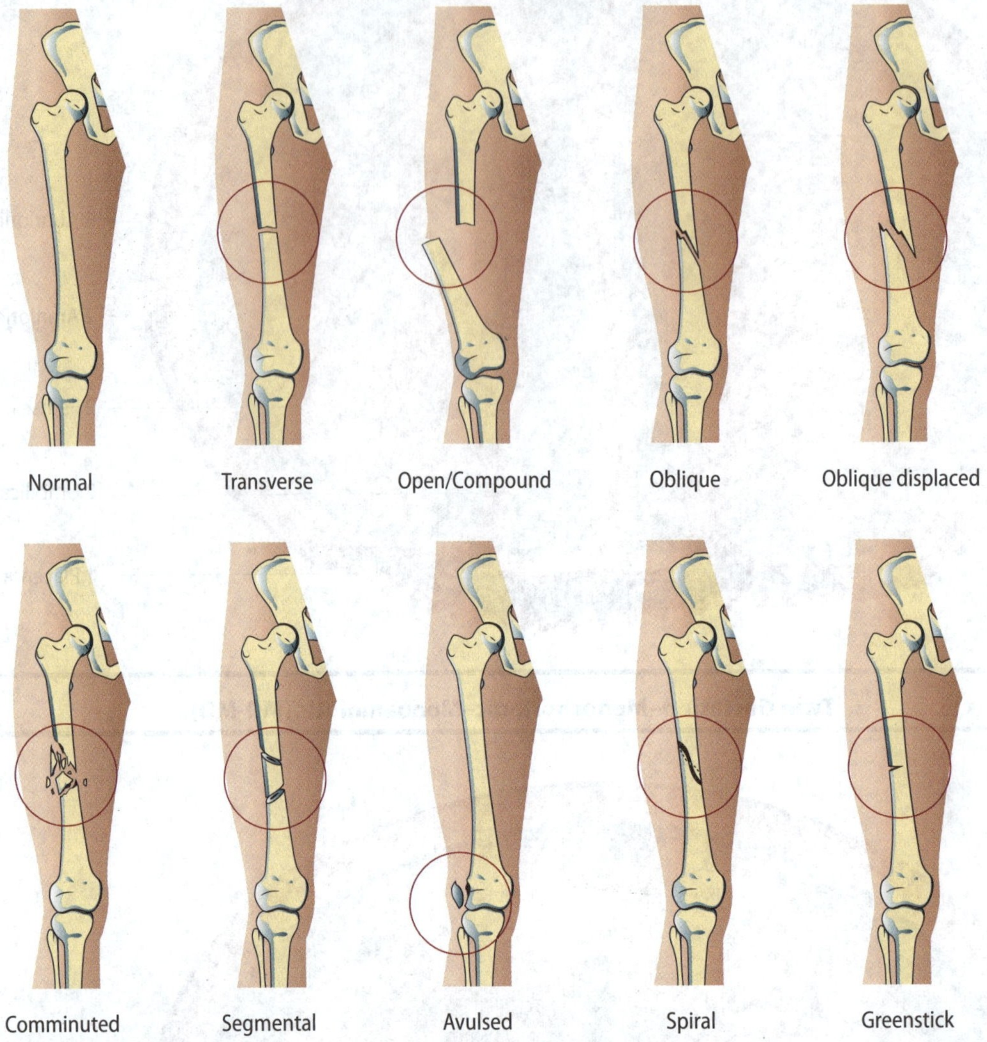

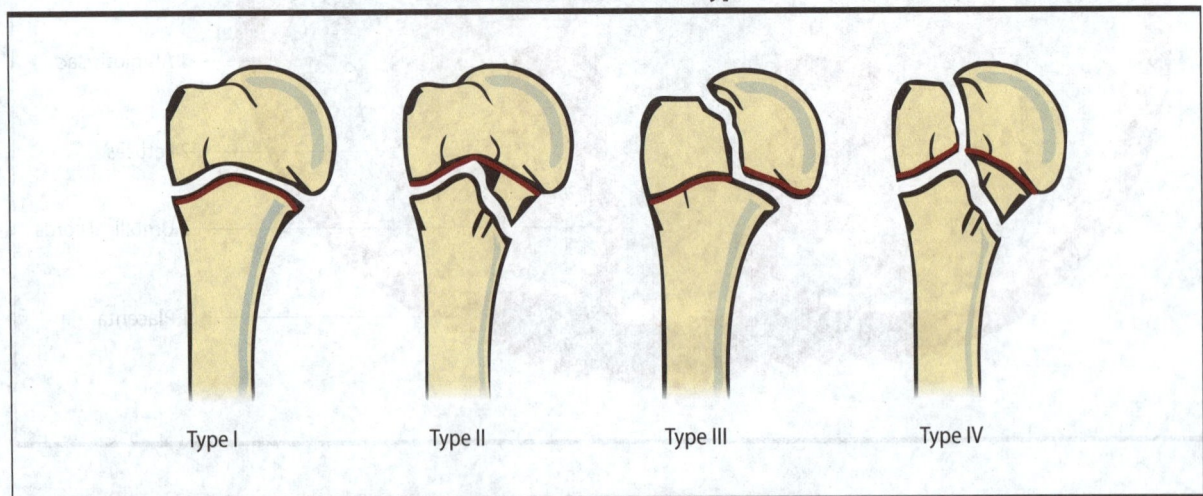